INCLUDES NETTER'S ANATOMY ART

D0807554

2 0 1 4
ICD-10-CM
D R A F T

Carol J. Buck
MS, CPC, CPC-H, CCS-P

Former Program Director
Medical Secretary Programs
Northwest Technical College
East Grand Forks, Minnesota

ELSEVIER
SAUNDERS

3251 Riverport Lane
St. Louis, Missouri 63043

2014 ICD-10-CM DRAFT

ISBN: 978-1-4557-2290-7

Notices

Knowledge and best practice in this field are constantly changing. As new research and experience broaden our understanding, changes in research methods, professional practices, or medical treatment may become necessary.

Practitioners and researchers must always rely on their own experience and knowledge in evaluating and using any information, methods, compounds, or experiments described herein. In using such information or methods they should be mindful of their own safety and the safety of others, including parties for whom they have a professional responsibility.

With respect to any drug or pharmaceutical products identified, readers are advised to check the most current information provided (i) on procedures featured or (ii) by the manufacturer of each product to be administered, to verify the recommended dose or formula, the method and duration of administration, and contraindications. It is the responsibility of practitioners, relying on their own experience and knowledge of their patients, to make diagnoses, to determine dosages and the best treatment for each individual patient, and to take all appropriate safety precautions.

To the fullest extent of the law, neither the Publisher nor the authors, contributors, or editors, assume any liability for any injury and/or damage to persons or property as a matter of products liability, negligence or otherwise, or from any use or operation of any methods, products, instructions, or ideas contained in the material herein.

Library of Congress Cataloging-in-Publication Data

Buck, Carol J., author.
  2014 ICD-10-CM draft / Carol J. Buck. -- 2014.
    p. ; cm.
  Includes index.
  Preceded by: 2013 ICD-10-CM draft / Carol J. Buck. c2013.
  ISBN 978-1-4557-2290-7 (pbk. : alk. paper)
  I. Buck, Carol J. 2013 ICD-10-CM draft. Preceded by (work): II. Title.
  [DNLM: 1. International statistical classification of diseases and related health problems.
10th revision. Clinical modification. 2. Disease--classification. 3. Forms and Records Control--methods.
4. International Classification of Diseases. 5. Medical Records. WB 15]
  RB115
  616.001'2--dc23

2013019280

Content Strategy Director: Jeanne R. Olson
Senior Content Development Specialist: Jenna Price
Publishing Services Manager: Pat Joiner
Senior Designer: Amy Buxton

Printed in the United States of America

Last digit is the print number: 9 8 7 6 5 4 3

CONTENTS

ICD-10-CM

SYMBOLS AND CONVENTIONS

Illustrations and Items

The ICD-10-CM Tabular List contains illustrations, pictures, and items to assist you in understanding difficult terminology, diseases/conditions, or coding in a specific category. Items are always printed in ████████ ink so that the added material is not mistaken for official notations or instructions. ████████ ink is used for other annotations in the text. Your ideas on what other descriptions or illustrations should be in future editions of this text are always appreciated.

Annotated

Throughout the manual, revisions, additions, and deleted codes or words are indicated by the following symbols:

- ◄▦ **Revised:** Revisions within the line or code from the previous edition are indicated by the arrow.
- ◄ **New:** Additions to the previous edition are indicated by the triangle.
- ~~deleted~~ **Deleted:** Deletions from the previous edition are struck through.

ICD-10-CM Tabular List Symbols

Throughout this text revisions and additions are indicated by the following symbols:

- ● **Use Additional Character(s):** The red stop sign cautions that the code requires additional character(s) to ensure the greatest specificity.
- X For codes less than 6 characters that require a 7th character a placeholder X should be assigned for all characters less than 6. The 7th character must always be the 7th character of a code.
- ● **Unacceptable Principal Diagnosis:** These codes have a blue dot before them and give additional information or describe the circumstances affecting the health care encounter but are unacceptable as principal diagnosis in the *Definitions of Medicare Code Edits,* Version 30 (MCE) for inpatient admission.
- OGCR The *Official Guidelines for Coding and Reporting* symbol includes the placement of a portion of a guideline as that guideline pertains to the code by which it is located. The complete OGCR are located in Part I.
- ▦ **Unspecified:** The highlight indicates that although the code is valid as a principal (first-listed) diagnosis, it is not as specific as other codes without the highlight.
- ▦ **Includes:** This note appears immediately under a three-character code title to further define or give examples of the content of the category and is highlighted in ▦ for easier reference.

Excludes Notes

The ICD-10-CM has two types of excludes notes. Each note has a different definition for use, but they are both similar in that they indicate that codes excluded from each other are independent of each other.

Excludes1

A type 1 Excludes note is a pure excludes. It means "NOT CODED HERE!" An Excludes1 note indicates that the code excluded should never be used at the same time as the code above the Excludes1 note. An Excludes1 is for use when two conditions cannot occur together, such as a congenital form versus an acquired form of the same condition.

Excludes2

A type 2 Excludes note represents "NOT INCLUDED HERE." An Excludes2 note indicates that the condition excluded is not part of the condition it is excluded from but a patient may have both conditions at the same time. When an Excludes2 note appears under a code, it is acceptable to use both the code and the excluded code together.

- ▦ **Code first:** The words indicate an instructional note that directs the coder to sequence the underlying condition before the manifestation. "Code first" is highlighted in ▦ for easier reference.
- ▦ **Use additional:** The words indicate an instructional note that another code may be needed and are highlighted in ▦ for easier reference.

Certain conditions have both an underlying etiology and multiple body system manifestations due to the underlying etiology. For such conditions the ICD-10-CM has a coding convention that requires the underlying condition be sequenced first, followed by the manifestation. Wherever such a combination exists, there is a "use additional code" note at the etiology code and a "code first" note at the manifestation code. These instructional notes indicate the proper sequencing order of the codes, etiology followed by manifestation.

In most cases the manifestation codes will have in the code title, "in diseases classified elsewhere." Codes with this title are a component of the etiology/manifestation convention. The code title indicates that it is a manifestation code. "In diseases classified elsewhere" codes are never permitted to be used as first-listed or principal diagnosis codes. They must be used in conjunction with an underlying condition code, and they must be listed following the underlying condition.

- ▦ **Code also:** A "code also" note instructs that two codes may be required to fully describe a condition, but the sequencing of the two codes is discretionary, depending on the severity of the conditions and the reason for the encounter.
- ✎✎ Indicates **complications and comorbidities and major complications and comorbidities** according to the *Medicare Severity Diagnosis Related Groups (MS-DRGs), Definitions Manual,* Version 30.

HAC is a **Hospital-Acquired Condition** that, when present as a secondary diagnosis in an inpatient setting, is a higher cost, higher volume, or both, and results in a higher MS-DRG assignment according to the *Medicare Severity Diagnosis Related Groups (MS-DRGs), Definitions Manual*, Version 30.

Present on Admission: These code categories represent circumstances regarding the health care encounter or factors influencing health status that do not represent a current disease or injury or are always present on admission according to the *Medicare Severity Diagnosis Related Groups (MS-DRGs), Definitions Manual*, Version 30.

Age conflict: The *Definitions of Medicare Code Edits* (MCE) detects inconsistencies between a patient's age and diagnosis. For example, a 5-year-old patient with benign prostatic hypertrophy or a 78-year-old pregnant female.

The diagnosis is clinically and virtually impossible in a patient of the stated age. Therefore, either the diagnosis or the age is presumed to be incorrect. There are four age categories for diagnoses in the *Definitions of Medicare Code Edits*, Version 30 (MCE):

N
- Newborn. Age of 0 years; a subset of diagnoses intended only for newborns and neonates (e.g., fetal distress, perinatal jaundice).

P
- Pediatric. Age range is 0-17 years inclusive (e.g., Reye's syndrome, routine child health exam).

M
- Maternity. Age range is 12-55 years inclusive (e.g., diabetes in pregnancy, antepartum pulmonary complication).

A
- Adult. Age range is 15-124 years inclusive (e.g., senile delirium, mature cataract).

♀♂ **Sex conflict:** *Definitions of Medicare Code Edits*, Version 30 (MCE) detects inconsistencies between a patient's sex and any diagnosis or procedure on the patient's record. For example, a male patient with cervical cancer (diagnosis) or a female patient with a prostatectomy (procedure). In both instances, the indicated diagnosis or the procedure conflicts with the stated sex of the patient. Therefore, either the patient's diagnosis, procedure, or sex is presumed to be incorrect.

Manifestation Code: Describes the manifestation of an underlying disease, not the disease itself, and therefore, should not be assigned as a principal diagnosis, according to the *Definitions of Medicare Code Edits*, Version 30 (MCE).

ICD-10-CM Tabular

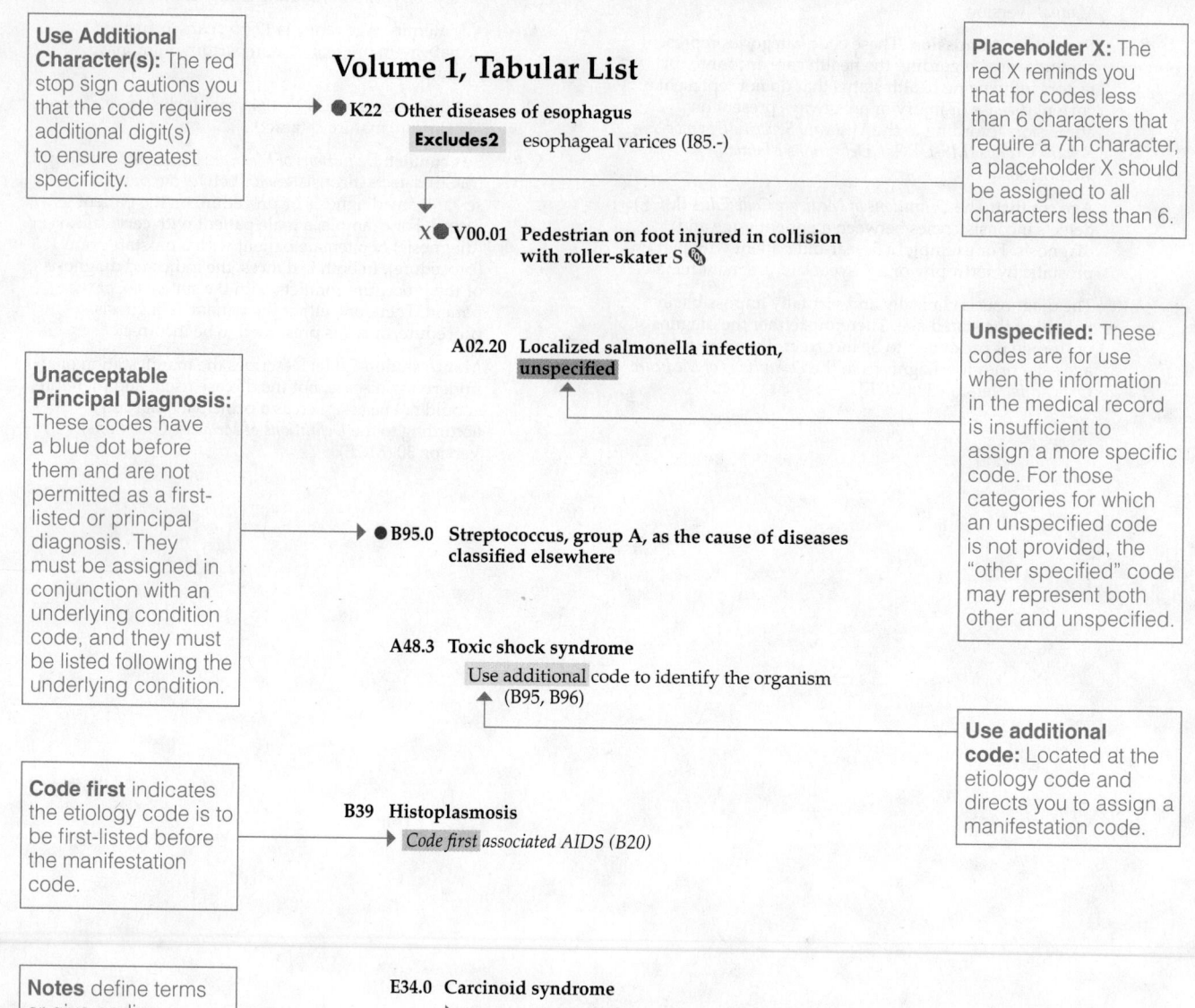

Use Additional Character(s): The red stop sign cautions you that the code requires additional digit(s) to ensure greatest specificity.

Volume 1, Tabular List

● **K22 Other diseases of esophagus**

    Excludes2   esophageal varices (I85.-)

X ● **V00.01 Pedestrian on foot injured in collision with roller-skater S** 🔄

Placeholder X: The red X reminds you that for codes less than 6 characters that require a 7th character, a placeholder X should be assigned to all characters less than 6.

A02.20 Localized salmonella infection, unspecified

Unacceptable Principal Diagnosis: These codes have a blue dot before them and are not permitted as a first-listed or principal diagnosis. They must be assigned in conjunction with an underlying condition code, and they must be listed following the underlying condition.

● **B95.0 Streptococcus, group A, as the cause of diseases classified elsewhere**

Unspecified: These codes are for use when the information in the medical record is insufficient to assign a more specific code. For those categories for which an unspecified code is not provided, the "other specified" code may represent both other and unspecified.

A48.3 Toxic shock syndrome

    Use additional code to identify the organism (B95, B96)

Use additional code: Located at the etiology code and directs you to assign a manifestation code.

Code first indicates the etiology code is to be first-listed before the manifestation code.

B39 Histoplasmosis

    Code first associated AIDS (B20)

Notes define terms or give coding instructions.

E34.0 Carcinoid syndrome

    Note: May be used as an additional code to identify functional activity associated with a carcinoid tumor.

Codes or index entries are for purposes of illustration only and may not be current.

OGCR Section I.C.6.B.5. ◄────────────────────

Neoplasm Related Pain Code G89.3 is assigned to pain documented as being related, associated or due to cancer, primary or secondary malignancy, or tumor. This code is assigned regardless of whether the pain is acute or chronic.

> **OGCR:** The *Official Guidelines for Coding and Reporting* are placed near the codes to which they refer and are highlighted.

I70.2 **Atherosclerosis of native arteries of the extremities**
Mönckeberg's (medial) sclerosis

Use additional code, if applicable, to identify chronic total occlusion of artery of extremity (I70.92)

> **code, if applicable,** directs the coder to other conditions that may be appropriate to report.

> The word "and" should be interpreted to mean either "and" or "or" when it appears in a statement.

I74 **Arterial embolism and thrombosis**
Includes embolic infarction
embolic occlusion
thrombotic infarction
thrombotic occlusion

Codes or index entries are for purposes of illustration only and may not be current.

Bold typeface is used on all codes and titles.

I83.001 **Varicose veins of unspecified lower extremity with ulcer of thigh**

"with" should be interpreted to mean "associated with" or "due to."

K73.2 **Chronic active hepatitis, not elsewhere classified**

"not elsewhere classified" or NEC identifies a code that is assigned only when the information at hand specifies a condition for which no more specific code is available.

"not otherwise specified" or NOS is equivalent to unspecified.

W13.9 **Fall from, out of or through building, not otherwise specified**

Excludes1 means "NOT CODED HERE!" An Excludes1 note indicates that the code excluded should never be assigned at the same time as the code above the Excludes1 note.

M19 **Other and unspecified osteoarthritis**
Excludes1   polyarthritis (M15.-)
Excludes2   arthrosis of spine (M47.-)
              hallux rigidus (M20.2)
              osteoarthritis of spine (M47.-)

Excludes2 represents "NOT INCLUDED HERE." An Excludes2 note indicates that the condition excluded is not part of the condition represented by the code, but a patient may have both conditions at the same time and it is acceptable to use both the code and the excluded code together, when appropriate.

Includes: This note appears immediately under a three-character code title to further define, or give examples of, the content.

A06 **Amebiasis**
Includes   infection due to Entamoeba histolytica

E26.01 **Conn's syndrome**
Code also adrenal adenoma (D35.0)

Code also instructs that two codes may be required to fully describe a condition, but this note does not provide sequencing direction.

Codes titled "other" or "other specified" are for use when the information in the medical record provides detail for which a specific code does not exist.

E25.8 **Other adrenogenital disorders**

Codes or index entries are for purposes of illustration only and may not be current.

O00.2 Ovarian pregnancy **M** ◄─ **Maternity DX** (Diagnosis) for ages 12-55 according to the *Definitions of Medicare Code Edits* (MCE)

P02.20 Newborn (suspected to be) affected by unspecified morphological and functional abnormalities of placenta **N**

Newborn, Age 0, according to the *Definitions of Medicare Code Edits* (MCE)

L21.0 Seborrhea capitis
    Cradle cap **P**

Pediatric Age, 0-17, according to the *Definitions of Medicare Code Edits* (MCE)

G30.1 Alzheimer's disease with late onset **A** ◄─ **Adult Age,** 15-124, according to the *Definitions of Medicare Code Edits* (MCE)

Females Only according to the *Definitions of Medicare Code Edits* (MCE)

B37.3 Candidiasis of vulva and vagina ♀

C60.1 Malignant neoplasm of glans penis ♂ ◄─ **Males Only** according to the *Definitions of Medicare Code Edits* (MCE)

Unacceptable PDX according to the *Definitions of Medicare Code Edits* (MCE)

● H16.8 Other keratitis

▸ H22 *Disorders of iris and ciliary body in diseases classified elsewhere*
    Code first *underlying disease, such as:*
      gout (M1A-, M10.-)

Manifestation according to the *Definitions of Medicare Code Edits* (MCE)

G14 Postpolio syndrome 🔗 ◄─ **Present On Admission** (POA) according to the *Medicare Severity Diagnosis Related Groups* (MS-DRGs)
  Includes Postpolio myelitic syndrome
  Excludes1 sequelae of poliomyelitis (B91)

T81.512 Adhesions due to foreign body accidentally left in body following kidney dialysis 🔗 ◄─ **Hospital-Acquired Condition** according to the *Medicare Severity Diagnosis Related Groups* (MS-DRGs)

R57.1 Hypovolemic shock 🔗

Major Complication/ Comorbidity (MCC) according to the *Medicare Severity Diagnosis Related Groups* (MS-DRGs)

B25.1 Cytomegaloviral hepatitis 🔗 ◄─ **Complication/ Comorbidity** (CC) according to the *Medicare Severity Diagnosis Related Groups* (MS-DRGs)

Codes or index entries are for purposes of illustration only and may not be current.

Alphabetic Index

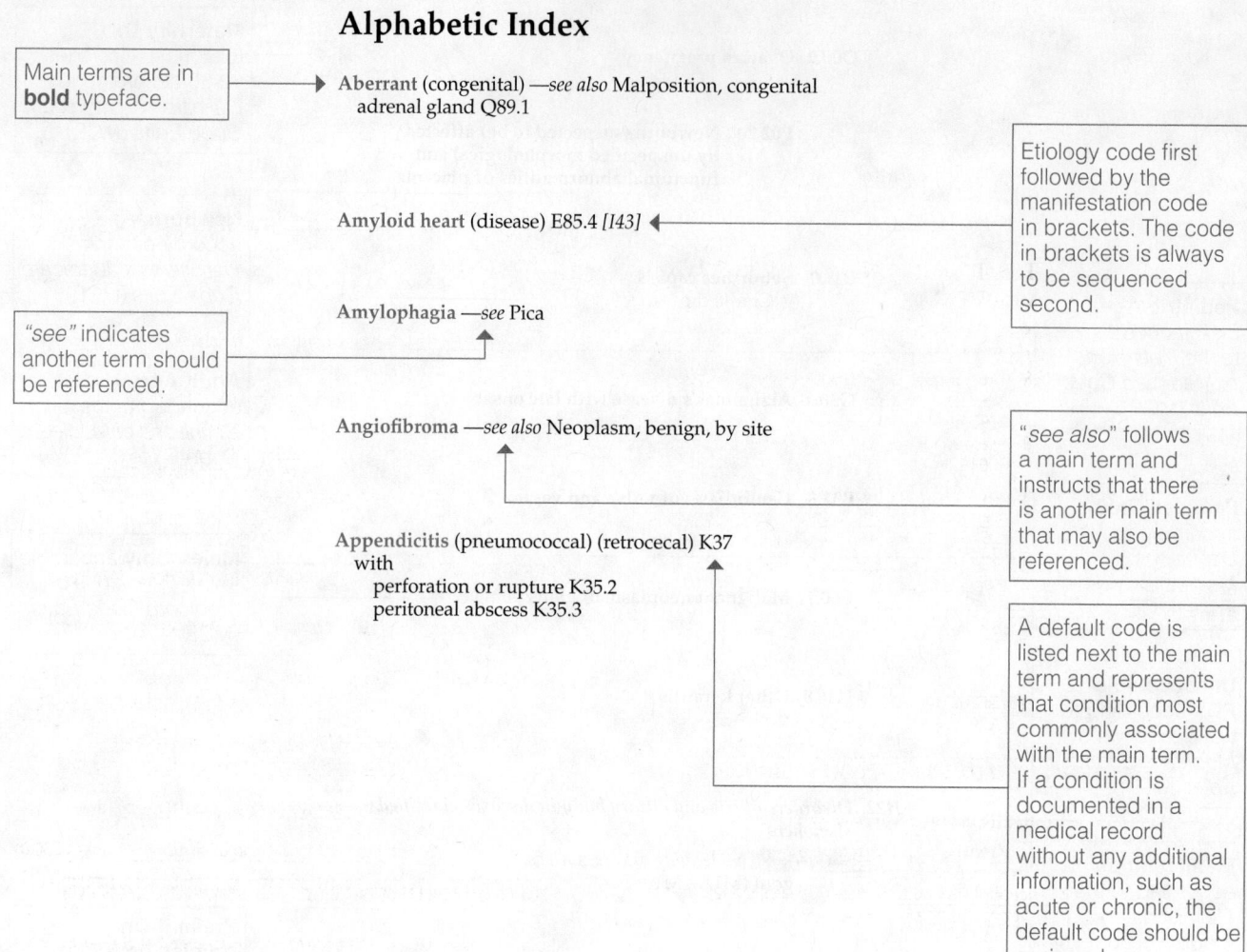

Main terms are in **bold** typeface.

Aberrant (congenital) —*see also* Malposition, congenital
adrenal gland Q89.1

Etiology code first followed by the manifestation code in brackets. The code in brackets is always to be sequenced second.

Amyloid heart (disease) E85.4 *[I43]*

"see" indicates another term should be referenced.

Amylophagia —*see* Pica

Angiofibroma —*see also* Neoplasm, benign, by site

"see also" follows a main term and instructs that there is another main term that may also be referenced.

Appendicitis (pneumococcal) (retrocecal) K37
with
perforation or rupture K35.2
peritoneal abscess K35.3

A default code is listed next to the main term and represents that condition most commonly associated with the main term. If a condition is documented in a medical record without any additional information, such as acute or chronic, the default code should be assigned.

Codes or index entries are for purposes of illustration only and may not be current.

CHAPTER 1

CERTAIN INFECTIOUS AND PARASITIC DISEASES (A00-B99)

Use additional code to identify resistance to antimicrobial drugs (Z16.-)

Excludes1 ~~infectious and parasitic diseases complicating pregnancy, childbirth and the puerperium (O98.-)~~

~~influenza and other acute respiratory infections (J00-J22)~~

Excludes2 infectious and parasitic diseases complicating pregnancy, childbirth and the puerperium (O98.-)

influenza and other acute respiratory infections (J00-J22)

RICKETTSIOSES (A75-A79)

A75 Typhus fever

Excludes1 rickettsiosis due to Ehrlichia sennetsu (A79.<u>281</u>)

VIRAL AND PRION INFECTIONS OF THE CENTRAL NERVOUS SYSTEM (A80-A89)

A85 Other viral encephalitis, not elsewhere classified

Excludes1 encephalitis due to: <u>cytomegalovirus (B25.8)</u> ~~cytomegalovirus (B25.8)~~

encephalitis due to herpesvirus NEC (B10.0-)

encephalitis due to herpesvirus [herpes simplex] (B00.4)

encephalitis due to measles virus (B05.0)

encephalitis due to mumps virus (B26.2)

encephalitis due to poliomyelitis virus (A80.-)

encephalitis due to zoster (B02.0)

OTHER HUMAN HERPESVIRUSES (B10)

B10 Other human herpesviruses

Excludes2 human herpesvirus 3 (B01.-, B02.-)

PEDICULOSIS, ACARIASIS AND OTHER INFESTATIONS (B85-B89)

B85 Pediculosis and phthiriasis

B85.4 Mixed pediculosis and phthiriasis
  Infestation classifiable to more than one of the categories B85.0-~~B85.3~~

CHAPTER 2

NEOPLASMS (C00-D49)

MALIGNANT NEOPLASMS OF LIP, ORAL CAVITY AND PHARYNX (C00-C14)

C13 Malignant neoplasm of hypopharynx

C13.1 Malignant neoplasm of aryepiglottic fold, hypopharyngeal aspect

Malignant neoplasm of aryepiglottic fold, marginal zone

Malignant neoplasm of interarytenoid fold, marginal zone

~~Malignant neoplasm of aryepiglottic fold marginal zone~~

~~Malignant neoplasm of interarytenoid fold marginal zone~~

MALIGNANT NEOPLASMS OF RESPIRATORY AND INTRATHORACIC ORGANS (C30-C39)

C32 Malignant neoplasm of larynx

C32.1 Malignant neoplasm of supraglottis

Excludes2 malignant neoplasm of aryepiglottic fold or interarytenoid fold:<u>,</u> hypopharyngeal aspect (C13.1)

~~NOS~~malignant neoplasm of aryepiglottic fold or interarytenoid fold, marginal zone (C13.1)

~~hypopharyngeal aspect (C13.1)~~

~~marginal zone~~malignant neoplasm of aryepiglottic fold or interarytenoid fold NOS (C13.1)

MALIGNANT NEOPLASMS OF BONE AND ARTICULAR CARTILAGE (C40-C41)

C41 Malignant neoplasm of bone and articular cartilage of other and unspecified sites

Excludes1 malignant neoplasm of cartilage of: <u>ear (C49.0)</u> ~~ear~~malignant neoplasm of cartilage of eyelid (C49.0)

~~eyelid (C49.0)~~

malignant neoplasm of cartilage of larynx (C32.3)

malignant neoplasm of cartilage of limbs (C40.-)

malignant neoplasm of cartilage of nose (C30.0)

MALIGNANT NEOPLASMS OF MESOTHELIAL AND SOFT TISSUE (C45-C49)

C49 Malignant neoplasm of other connective and soft tissue

Excludes1 malignant neoplasm of connective tissue of breast (C50.-)

MALIGNANT NEOPLASMS OF THYROID AND OTHER ENDOCRINE GLANDS (C73-C75)

C75 Malignant neoplasm of other endocrine glands and related structures

Excludes1 malignant neoplasm of ovary (C56.-)

MALIGNANT NEOPLASMS OF LYMPHOID, HEMATOPOIETIC AND RELATED TISSUE (C81-C96)

C88 Malignant immunoproliferative diseases and certain other B-cell lymphomas

Excludes1 B-cell lymphoma, unspecified ~~C85.1~~<u>(C85.1-)</u>

NEOPLASMS OF UNCERTAIN BEHAVIOR, POLYCYTHEMIA VERA AND MYELODYSPLASTIC SYNDROMES (D37-D48)

Excludes1 neoplasms of unspecified behavior (D49.-)

D48 Neoplasm of uncertain behavior of other and unspecified sites

D48.5 Neoplasm of uncertain behavior of skin

Excludes1 neoplasm of uncertain behavior of skin of genital organs (D39.8, D40.<u>78</u>)

NEOPLASMS OF UNSPECIFIED BEHAVIOR (D49)

D49   Neoplasms of unspecified behavior

D49.2   Neoplasm of unspecified behavior of bone, soft tissue, and skin

Excludes1   neoplasm of unspecified behavior of bone marrow (D49.89)

CHAPTER 3

DISEASES OF THE BLOOD AND BLOOD-FORMING ORGANS AND CERTAIN DISORDERS INVOLVING THE IMMUNE MECHANISM (D50-D89)

COAGULATION DEFECTS, PURPURA AND OTHER HEMORRHAGIC CONDITIONS (D65-D69)

D68   Other coagulation defects

Excludes1   coagulation defects complicating: abortion or ectopic or molar pregnancy (O00-O07, O08.1)

~~abortion or ectopic or molar pregnancy (O00-O07, O08.1)~~

coagulation defects complicating pregnancy, childbirth and the puerperium (O45.0, O46.0, O67.0, O72.3)

OTHER DISORDERS OF BLOOD AND BLOOD-FORMING ORGANS (D70-D77)

D77   *Other disorders of blood and blood-forming organs in diseases classified elsewhere*

Code first underlying disease, such as:
amyloidosis (E85.-)

Excludes1   splenitis, splenomegaly in: late syphilis (A52.79)

~~late syphilis (A52.79)~~

splenitis, splenomegaly in tuberculosis (A18.85)

CHAPTER 4

ENDOCRINE, NUTRITIONAL AND METABOLIC DISEASES (E00-E89)

DIABETES MELLITUS (E08-E13)

E08   Diabetes mellitus due to underlying condition

E08.2   Diabetes mellitus due to underlying condition with kidney complications

E08.22   Diabetes mellitus due to underlying condition with diabetic chronic kidney disease

~~Diabetes mellitus due to underlying condition with chronic kidney disease due to conditions classified to .21 and .22~~

E08.3   Diabetes mellitus due to underlying condition with ophthalmic complications

E08.39   Diabetes mellitus due to underlying condition with other diabetic ophthalmic complication

Use additional code to identify manifestation, such as: diabetic glaucoma (H40-H42)

E09   Drug or chemical induced diabetes mellitus

E09.2   Drug or chemical induced diabetes mellitus with kidney complications

E09.22   Drug or chemical induced diabetes mellitus with diabetic chronic kidney disease

~~Drug or chemical induced diabetes mellitus with chronic kidney disease due to conditions classified to .21 and .22~~

E09.3   Drug or chemical induced diabetes mellitus with ophthalmic complications

E09.39   Drug or chemical induced diabetes mellitus with other diabetic ophthalmic complication

Use additional code to identify manifestation, such as: diabetic glaucoma (H40-H42)

E10   Type 1 diabetes mellitus

E10.2   Type 1 diabetes mellitus with kidney complications

E10.22   Type 1 diabetes mellitus with diabetic chronic kidney disease

~~Type 1 diabetes mellitus with chronic kidney disease due to conditions classified to .21 and .22~~

E10.3   Type 1 diabetes mellitus with ophthalmic complications

E10.39   Type 1 diabetes mellitus with other diabetic ophthalmic complication

Use additional code to identify manifestation, such as: diabetic glaucoma (H40-H42)

E11   Type 2 diabetes mellitus

E11.2   Type 2 diabetes mellitus with kidney complications

E11.22   Type 2 diabetes mellitus with diabetic chronic kidney disease

~~Type 2 diabetes mellitus with chronic kidney disease due to conditions classified to .21 and .22~~

E11.3   Type 2 diabetes mellitus with ophthalmic complications

E11.39   Type 2 diabetes mellitus with other diabetic ophthalmic complication

Use additional code to identify manifestation, such as: diabetic glaucoma (H40-H42)

E13   Other specified diabetes mellitus

E13.2   Other specified diabetes mellitus with kidney complications

E13.22   Other specified diabetes mellitus with diabetic chronic kidney disease

~~Other specified diabetes mellitus with chronic kidney disease due to conditions classified to .21 and .22~~

E13.3   Other specified diabetes mellitus with ophthalmic complications

E13.39   Other specified diabetes mellitus with other diabetic ophthalmic complication

Use additional code to identify manifestation, such as: diabetic glaucoma (H40-H42)

DISORDERS OF OTHER ENDOCRINE GLANDS (E20-E35)

E27   Other disorders of adrenal gland

E27.1   Primary adrenocortical insufficiency

Excludes1   amyloidosis (E85.-)

E35   *Disorders of endocrine glands in diseases classified elsewhere*

Code first underlying disease, such as:
~~tuberculous calcification of adrenal gland (B90.8)~~

Use additional code , if applicable, to identify:
sequelae of tuberculosis of other organs (B90.8)

OTHER NUTRITIONAL DEFICIENCIES (E50-E64)

E55   Vitamin D deficiency

Excludes1   osteoporosis (M80.-)

E55.0   Rickets, active

Infantile ~~O~~osteomalacia

Juvenile ~~O~~osteomalacia

METABOLIC DISORDERS (E70-E88)

E71   Disorders of branched-chain amino-acid metabolism and fatty-acid metabolism

E71.4   Disorders of carnitine metabolism

E71.43   Iatrogenic carnitine deficiency

Carnitine deficiency due to: hemodialysis ~~hemodialysis~~

Carnitine deficiency due to Valproic acid therapy

E72   Other disorders of amino-acid metabolism

Excludes1   disorders of:
gout (~~M1A~~M1A.-, M10.-)

E79   Disorders of purine and pyrimidine metabolism

Excludes1   gout (~~M1A~~M1A.-M10.-)

E83   Disorders of mineral metabolism

E83.3   Disorders of phosphorus metabolism and phosphatases

Excludes1   osteoporosis (M80.-)

E86   Volume depletion

Excludes1   postprocedural hypovolemic shock (T81.1~~1~~9)

E87   Other disorders of fluid, electrolyte and acid-base balance

E87.2   Acidosis

Excludes1   diabetic acidosis - see categories E08-E10, E13 with ketoacidosis

CHAPTER 5

MENTAL, BEHAVIORAL AND NEURODEVELOPMENTAL DISORDERS (F01-F99)

MENTAL AND BEHAVIORAL DISORDERS DUE TO PSYCHOACTIVE SUBSTANCE USE (F10-F19)

F15   Other stimulant related disorders

Includes   ~~C~~caffeine

MOOD [AFFECTIVE] DISORDERS (F30-F39)

F32   Major depressive disorder, single episode

Excludes1   bipolar disorder (F31.-)
manic episode (F30.-)

ANXIETY, DISSOCIATIVE, STRESS-RELATED, SOMATOFORM AND OTHER NONPSYCHOTIC MENTAL DISORDERS (F40-F48)

F42   Obsessive-compulsive disorder

Excludes2   obsessive-compulsive symptoms occurring in:
depression (F32-F33)
~~depression (F32-F33)~~
obsessive-compulsive symptoms occurring in schizophrenia (F20.-)

BEHAVIORAL SYNDROMES ASSOCIATED WITH PHYSIOLOGICAL DISTURBANCES AND PHYSICAL FACTORS (F50-F59)

F51   Sleep disorders not due to a substance or known physiological condition

F51.0   Insomnia not due to a substance or known physiological condition

Excludes2   drug-related insomnia (F11.182, F11.282, F11.982, F13.182, F13.282, F13.982, F14.182, F14.282, F14.982, F15.182, F15.282, F15.982, F19.182, F19.282, F19.982)

F51.1   Hypersomnia not due to a substance or known physiological condition

Excludes2   drug-related hypersomnia (F11.182, F11.282, F11.982, F13.182, F13.282, F13.982, F14.182, F14.282, F14.982, F15.182, F15.282, F15.982, F19.182, F19.282, F19.982)

BEHAVIORAL AND EMOTIONAL DISORDERS WITH ONSET USUALLY OCCURRING IN CHILDHOOD AND ADOLESCENCE (F90-F98)

F94   Disorders of social functioning with onset specific to childhood and adolescence

F94.2   Disinhibited attachment disorder of childhood

Excludes1   reactive attachment disorder of childhood (F94.~~1~~1)

F98   Other behavioral and emotional disorders with onset usually occurring in childhood and adolescence

F98.1   Encopresis not due to a substance or known physiological condition

Excludes1   encopresis NOS (R15.-)

CHAPTER 6

DISEASES OF THE NERVOUS SYSTEM (G00-G99)

INFLAMMATORY DISEASES OF THE CENTRAL NERVOUS SYSTEM (G00-G09)

G07   *Intracranial and intraspinal abscess and granuloma in diseases classified elsewhere*

Code first ~~—~~underlying disease, such as:

G08   Intracranial and intraspinal phlebitis and thrombophlebitis

Excludes1   intracranial phlebitis and thrombophlebitis complicating:
~~nonpyogenic intraspinal phlebitis and thrombophlebitis (G95.1)~~

Excludes2   intracranial phlebitis and thrombophlebitis complicating nonpyogenic intraspinal phlebitis and thrombophlebitis (G95.1)

OTHER DEGENERATIVE DISEASES OF THE NERVOUS SYSTEM (G30-G32)

G32 Other degenerative disorders of nervous system in diseases classified elsewhere

   G32.0 *Subacute combined degeneration of spinal cord in diseases classified elsewhere*

   G32.8 Other specified degenerative disorders of nervous system in diseases classified elsewhere

      Code first underlying disease, such as:
         amyloidosis cerebral degeneration (E85.-)

      G32.81 *Cerebellar ataxia in diseases classified elsewhere*

         Code first underlying disease, such as:
            celiac disease (with gluten ataxia) (K90.0)
            non-celiac gluten ataxia (M35.9)

EPISODIC AND PAROXYSMAL DISORDERS (G40-G47)

G43 Migraine

   Excludes1 headache NOS (R51)

   Excludes2 headache syndromes (G44.-)

G47 Sleep disorders

   G47.0 Insomnia

      Excludes2 drug related insomnia F11.182, F11.282, F11.982, F13.182, F13.282, F13.982, F14.182, F14.282, F14.982, F15.182, F15.282, F15.982, F19.182, F19.282, F19.982
         drug-related insomnia (F11.182, F11.282, F11.982, F13.182, F13.282, F13.982, F14.182, F14.282, F14.982, F15.182, F15.282, F15.982, F19.182, F19.282, F19.982)

   G47.1 Hypersomnia

      Excludes2 drug-related hypersomnia F11.182, F11.282, F11.982, F13.182, F13.282, F13.982, F14.182, F14.282, F14.982, F15.182, F15.282, F15.982, F19.182, F19.282, F19.982
         drug-related hypersomnia (F11.182, F11.282, F11.982, F13.182, F13.282, F13.982, F14.182, F14.282, F14.982, F15.182, F15.282, F15.982, F19.182, F19.282, F19.982)

   G47.3 Sleep apnea

      Excludes1 apnea NOS R06.81(R06.81)

   G47.4 Narcolepsy and cataplexy

      G47.42 Narcolepsy in conditions classified elsewhere
         Code first underlying condition

NERVE, NERVE ROOT AND PLEXUS DISORDERS (G50-G59)

G54 Nerve root and plexus disorders

   Excludes1 neuritis or radiculitis: brachial NOS (M54.13) brachial NOS (M54.13)
      neuritis or radiculitis lumbar NOS (M54.16)
      neuritis or radiculitis lumbosacral NOS (M54.17)
      neuritis or radiculitis thoracic NOS (M54.14)

G55 *Nerve root and plexus compressions in diseases classified elsewhere*

   Excludes1 nerve root compression (due to) (in) spondylosis (M47.0-M47.2.-)

G59 *Mononeuropathy in diseases classified elsewhere*

   Excludes1 diabetic mononeuropathy (E09-E148-E13 with .41)

POLYNEUROPATHIES AND OTHER DISORDERS OF THE PERIPHERAL NERVOUS SYSTEM (G60-G65)

G63 *Polyneuropathy in diseases classified elsewhere*

   Code first underlying disease, such as:
      amyloidosis (E85.-)

OTHER DISORDERS OF THE NERVOUS SYSTEM (G89-G99)

G99 Other disorders of nervous system in diseases classified elsewhere

   G99.0 *Autonomic neuropathy in diseases classified elsewhere*

      Code first underlying disease, such as:
         amyloidosis (E85.-)
         gout (M1AM1A.-, M10.-)

      Excludes1 diabetic autonomic neuropathy (E09-148-E13 with .43)

   G99.8 *Other specified disorders of nervous system in diseases classified elsewhere*

      Code first underlying disorder, such as:
         amyloidosis (E85.-)

CHAPTER 7

DISEASES OF THE EYE AND ADNEXA (H00-H59)

DISORDERS OF SCLERA, CORNEA, IRIS AND CILIARY BODY (H15-H22)

H22 *Disorders of iris and ciliary body in diseases classified elsewhere*

   Code first underlying disease, such as:
      gout (M1AM1A.-, M10.-)
      leprosy (A30.-)
      parasitic disease (B89)

DISORDERS OF LENS (H25-H28)

H28 *Cataract in diseases classified elsewhere*

   Excludes1 cataract in diabetes mellitus (E08.33, E09.33, E10.33, E11.33, E13.33E08.36, E09.36, E10.36, E11.36, E13.36)

DISORDERS OF CHOROID AND RETINA (H30-H36)

H35 Other retinal disorders

   Excludes2 diabetic retinal disorders (E08.311-E08.359, E09.311- E09.359, E10.311- E10.359, E11.311-E11.359, E13.311-E08.359, E09.311-E09.359, E10.311-E10.359, E11.311-E11.359, E13.311-E13.359)

   H35.0 Background retinopathy and retinal vascular changes
      Code also any associated hypertension (I10.-)

GLAUCOMA (H40-H42)

H42 *Glaucoma in diseases classified elsewhere*

   Code first underlying condition, such as:
      amyloidosis (E85.-)

VISUAL DISTURBANCES AND BLINDNESS (H53-H54)

H53 Visual disturbances

   H53.4 Visual field defects

      H53.46 Homonymous bilateral field defects
         Homonymous hemianop(s)ia
         Quadrant anop(s)ia
         Homonymous hemianopsia
         Quadrant anopia
         Quadrant anopsia

CHAPTER 8

DISEASES OF THE EAR AND MASTOID PROCESS (H60-H95)

DISEASES OF EXTERNAL EAR (H60-H62)

H61 Other disorders of external ear

H61.1 Noninfective disorders of pinna

Excludes2 gouty tophi of ear (~~M1A-, M10~~M1A.-)

H62 Disorders of external ear in diseases classified elsewhere

H62.8 Other disorders of external ear in diseases classified elsewhere

Code first underlying disease, such as:
gout (~~M1A~~M1A.-, M10.-)

DISEASES OF MIDDLE EAR AND MASTOID (H65-H75)

H66 Suppurative and unspecified otitis media

~~Use additional code for any associated perforated tympanic membrane (H72.-)~~

H66.1 Chronic tubotympanic suppurative otitis media

Use additional code for any associated perforated tympanic membrane (H72.-)

H66.2 Chronic atticoantral suppurative otitis media

Use additional code for any associated perforated tympanic membrane (H72.-)

H66.3 Other chronic suppurative otitis media

Use additional code for any associated perforated tympanic membrane (H72.-)

H66.4 Suppurative otitis media, unspecified

Use additional code for any associated perforated tympanic membrane (H72.-)

H66.9 Otitis media, unspecified

Use additional code for any associated perforated tympanic membrane (H72.-)

CHAPTER 9

DISEASES OF THE CIRCULATORY SYSTEM (I00-I99)

ACUTE RHEUMATIC FEVER (I00-I02)

I00 Rheumatic fever without heart involvement

Excludes1 rheumatic fever with heart involvement (I01.0 -I01.9)

ISCHEMIC HEART DISEASES (I20-I25)

I23 Certain current complications following ST elevation (STEMI) and non-ST elevation (NSTEMI) myocardial infarction (within the 28 day period)

~~**Note:** A code from category I23 must be used in conjunction with a code from category I21 or category I22. The I23 code should be sequenced first, if it is the reason for encounter, or, it should be sequenced after the I21 or I22 code if the complication of the MI occurs during the encounter for the MI.~~

I25 Chronic ischemic heart disease

I25.7 Atherosclerosis of coronary artery bypass graft(s) and coronary artery of transplanted heart with angina pectoris

I25.71 Atherosclerosis of autologous vein coronary artery bypass graft(s) with angina pectoris

I25.718 Atherosclerosis of autologous vein coronary artery bypass graft(s) with other forms of angina pectoris

Excludes1 other forms of angina pectoris without atherosclerosis of autologous vein coronary artery bypass graft(s) (I20.8)

I25.79 Atherosclerosis of other coronary artery bypass graft(s) with angina pectoris

I25.798 Atherosclerosis of other coronary artery bypass graft(s) with other forms of angina pectoris

Excludes1 other forms of angina pectoris without atherosclerosis of other coronary artery bypass graft(s) (I20.8)

PULMONARY HEART DISEASE AND DISEASES OF PULMONARY CIRCULATION (I26-I28)

I26 Pulmonary embolism

Excludes2 pulmonary embolism complicating abortion, ectopic or molar pregnancy (O00-O07, O08.2)
pulmonary embolism complicating pregnancy, childbirth and the puerperium (O88.-)
~~pulmonary embolism complicating: abortion, ectopic or molar pregnancy (O00-O07, O08.2) pregnancy, childbirth and the puerperium (O88.-)~~

OTHER FORMS OF HEART DISEASE (I30-I52)

I42 Cardiomyopathy

Code first pre-existing cardiomyopathy complicating pregnancy and puerperium (O99.4)

I43 *Cardiomyopathy in diseases classified elsewhere*

Code first underlying disease, such as:
amyloidosis (E85.-)

I47 Paroxysmal tachycardia

Excludes1 tachycardia: NOS (R00.0)
sinoauricular tachycardia NOS (R00.0)
~~sinoauricularus [sinusal] tachycardia NOS (R00.0)~~
~~sinus [sinusal] NOS (R00.0)~~

I49 Other cardiac arrhythmias

Excludes1 bradycardia: NOS (R00.1)
~~NOS (R00.1)~~
~~sinoatrial (R00.1)~~
~~sinus (R00.1)~~
~~vagal (R00.1)~~
sinoatrial bradycardia (R00.1)
sinus bradycardia (R00.1)
vagal bradycardia (R00.1)

I50 Heart failure

CEREBROVASCULAR DISEASES (I60-I69)

I68   Cerebrovascular disorders in diseases classified elsewhere

   I68.0   Cerebral amyloid angiopathy

      Code first underlying amyloidosis (E85.-)

DISEASES OF ARTERIES, ARTERIOLES AND CAPILLARIES (I70-I79)

I70   Atherosclerosis

   I70.2   Atherosclerosis of native arteries of the extremities

      I70.23   **Atherosclerosis of native arteries of right leg with ulceration**

         Use additional code to identify severity of ulcer (L97.- with fifth character 1)

      I70.24   **Atherosclerosis of native arteries of left leg with ulceration**

         Use additional code to identify severity of ulcer (L97.- with fifth character 2)

      I70.26   **Atherosclerosis of native arteries of extremities with gangrene**

         Use additional code to identify the severity of any ulcer (L97.-, L98.49-), if applicable

   I70.3   Atherosclerosis of unspecified type of bypass graft(s) of the extremities

      I70.33   **Atherosclerosis of unspecified type of bypass graft(s) of the right leg with ulceration**

         Use additional code to identify severity of ulcer (L97.- with fifth character 1)

      I70.34   **Atherosclerosis of unspecified type of bypass graft(s) of the left leg with ulceration**

         Use additional code to identify severity of ulcer (L97.- with fifth character 2)

      I70.36   **Atherosclerosis of unspecified type of bypass graft(s) of the extremities with gangrene**

         Use additional code to identify the severity of any ulcer (L97.-, L98.49-), if applicable

   I70.4   Atherosclerosis of autologous vein bypass graft(s) of the extremities

      I70.43   **Atherosclerosis of autologous vein bypass graft(s) of the right leg with ulceration**

         Use additional code to identify severity of ulcer (L97.- with fifth character 1)

      I70.44   **Atherosclerosis of autologous vein bypass graft(s) of the left leg with ulceration**

         Use additional code to identify severity of ulcer (L97.- with fifth character 2)

      I70.46   **Atherosclerosis of autologous vein bypass graft(s) of the extremities with gangrene**

         Use additional code to identify the severity of any ulcer (L97.-, L98.49-), if applicable

   I70.5   Atherosclerosis of nonautologous biological bypass graft(s) of the extremities

      I70.53   **Atherosclerosis of nonautologous biological bypass graft(s) of the right leg with ulceration**

         Use additional code to identify severity of ulcer (L97.- with fifth character 1)

      I70.54   **Atherosclerosis of nonautologous biological bypass graft(s) of the left leg with ulceration**

         Use additional code to identify severity of ulcer (L97.- with fifth character 2)

      I70.56   **Atherosclerosis of nonautologous biological bypass graft(s) of the extremities with gangrene**

         Use additional code to identify the severity of any ulcer (L97.-, L98.49-), if applicable

   I70.6   Atherosclerosis of nonbiological bypass graft(s) of the extremities

      I70.63   **Atherosclerosis of nonbiological bypass graft(s) of the right leg with ulceration**

         Use additional code to identify severity of ulcer (L97.- with fifth character 1)

      I70.64   **Atherosclerosis of nonbiological bypass graft(s) of the left leg with ulceration**

         Use additional code to identify severity of ulcer (L97.- with fifth character 2)

      I70.66   **Atherosclerosis of nonbiological bypass graft(s) of the extremities with gangrene**

         Use additional code to identify the severity of any ulcer (L97.-, L98.49-), if applicable

   I70.7   Atherosclerosis of other type of bypass graft(s) of the extremities

      I70.73   **Atherosclerosis of other type of bypass graft(s) of the right leg with ulceration**

         Use additional code to identify severity of ulcer (L97.- with fifth character 1)

      I70.74   **Atherosclerosis of other type of bypass graft(s) of the left leg with ulceration**

         Use additional code to identify severity of ulcer (L97.- with fifth character 2)

      I70.76   **Atherosclerosis of other type of bypass graft(s) of the extremities with gangrene**

         Use additional code to identify the severity of any ulcer (L97.-, L98.49-), if applicable

   I70.9   **Other and unspecified atherosclerosis**

      I70.92   **Chronic total occlusion of artery of the extremities**

         Excludes1   acute occlusion of artery of the extremity (I70.2-, I70.3-, I70.4-)

I73   Other peripheral vascular diseases

   Excludes2   frostbite (T33–T34)

I79   Disorders of arteries, arterioles and capillaries in diseases classified elsewhere

   I79.8   Other disorders of arteries, arterioles and capillaries in diseases classified elsewhere

      Code first underlying disease, such as: amyloidosis (E85.-)

      Excludes1   endarteritis: syphilitic endarteritis (A52.09) tuberculous endarteritis (A18.89)

DISEASES OF VEINS, LYMPHATIC VESSELS AND LYMPH NODES, NOT ELSEWHERE CLASSIFIED (I80-I89)

I82 Other venous embolism and thrombosis

I82.4 Acute embolism and thrombosis of deep veins of lower extremity

I82.40 Acute embolism and thrombosis of unspecified deep veins of lower extremity

Excludes1 acute embolism and thrombosis of unspecified deep veins of distal lower extremity (I82.4bZ-) acute embolism and thrombosis of unspecified deep veins of proximal lower extremity (I82.4aY-)

I82.5 Chronic embolism and thrombosis of deep veins of lower extremity

I82.50 Chronic embolism and thrombosis of unspecified deep veins of lower extremity

Excludes1 chronic embolism and thrombosis of unspecified deep veins of distal lower extremity (I82.5bZ-) chronic embolism and thrombosis of unspecified deep veins of proximal lower extremity (I82.5aY-)

CHAPTER 10

DISEASES OF THE RESPIRATORY SYSTEM (J00-J99)

INFLUENZA AND PNEUMONIA (J09-J18)

Excludes2 pneumonia due to solids and liquids (J69.-)

J10 Influenza due to other identified influenza virus

~~Use additional code to identify the virus (B97.-)~~

J13 Pneumonia due to Streptococcus pneumoniae

Code first associated influenza, if applicable (J09.X1, J10.0-, -J11.0-)

J14 Pneumonia due to Hemophilus influenzae

Code first associated influenza, if applicable (J09.X1, J10.0-, -J11.0-)

J15 Bacterial pneumonia, not elsewhere classified

Code first associated influenza, if applicable (J09.X1, J10.0-, -J11.0-)

J16 Pneumonia due to other infectious organisms, not elsewhere classified

Code first associated influenza, if applicable (J09.X1, J10.0-, -J11.0-)

J18 Pneumonia, unspecified organism

Code first associated influenza, if applicable (J09.X1, J10.0-, -J11.0-)

OTHER ACUTE LOWER RESPIRATORY INFECTIONS (J20-J22)

J20 Acute bronchitis

Excludes1 bronchitis NOS (J40) tracheobronchitis NOS (J40)

Excludes2 ~~bronchitis NOS (J40)~~ ~~tracheobronchitis NOS (J40)~~

OTHER DISEASES OF UPPER RESPIRATORY TRACT (J30-J39)

J34 Other and unspecified disorders of nose and nasal sinuses

J34.8 Other specified disorders of nose and nasal sinuses

J34.81 Nasal mucositis (ulcerative)

Code also type of associated therapy, such as: antineoplastic and immunosuppressive drugs (T45.1xX-)

CHRONIC LOWER RESPIRATORY DISEASES (J40-J47)

J40 Bronchitis, not specified as acute or chronic

Excludes1 acute bronchitis (J20.-)

J44 Other chronic obstructive pulmonary disease

Code also type of asthma, if applicable (J45.-):

OTHER RESPIRATORY DISEASES PRINCIPALLY AFFECTING THE INTERSTITIUM (J80-J84)

J84 Other interstitial pulmonary diseases

J84.8 Other specified interstitial pulmonary diseases

J84.89 Other specified interstitial pulmonary diseases

Excludes1 idiopathic non-specific interstitial pneumonitis (J84.84113)

INTRAOPERATIVE AND POSTPROCEDURAL COMPLICATIONS AND DISORDERS OF RESPIRATORY SYSTEM, NOT ELSEWHERE CLASSIFIED (J95)

J95 Intraoperative and postprocedural complications and disorders of respiratory system, not elsewhere classified

Excludes2 pulmonary manifestations due to radiation (J70.0-J70.1)

J95.7 Accidental puncture and laceration of a respiratory system organ or structure during a procedure

Excludes2 postprocedural pneumothorax (J95.811)

OTHER DISEASES OF THE RESPIRATORY SYSTEM (J96-J99)

J99 *Respiratory disorders in diseases classified elsewhere*

Code first underlying disease, such as: amyloidosis (E85.-)

CHAPTER 11

DISEASES OF THE DIGESTIVE SYSTEM (K00-K95)

DISEASES OF ORAL CAVITY AND SALIVARY GLANDS (K00-K14)

K09 Cysts of oral region, not elsewhere classified

K09.0 Developmental odontogenic cysts

Excludes2 keratocysts ~~D16.4, D16.5~~(D16.4, D16.5) odontogenic keratocystic tumors ~~D16.4, D16.5~~(D16.4, D16.5)

K12 Stomatitis and related lesions

K12.3 Oral mucositis (ulcerative)

K12.31 Oral mucositis (ulcerative) due to antineoplastic therapy

Use additional code for adverse effect, if applicable, to identify antineoplastic and immunosuppressive drugs (T45.1xX5)

DISEASES OF APPENDIX (K35-K38)

K35   Acute appendicitis

K35.2   **Acute appendicitis with generalized peritonitis**
~~Appendicitis with peritonitis NOS~~

K35.3   **Acute appendicitis with localized peritonitis**
Acute appendicitis with ~~localized peritonitis with or without rupture or perforation of appendix~~or without perforation or rupture NOS
Acute appendicitis with or without perforation or rupture with localized peritonitis

OTHER DISEASES OF INTESTINES (K55-K64)

K62   Other diseases of anus and rectum

Excludes2   fecal incontinence (R15.-)

K62.8   **Other specified diseases of anus and rectum**

K62.81   **Anal sphincter tear (healed) (nontraumatic) (old)**
Use additional code for any associated fecal incontinence (R15.-)

K62.89   **Other specified diseases of anus and rectum**
Use additional code for any associated fecal incontinence (R15.-)

K63   Other diseases of intestine

K63.0   **Abscess of intestine**

Excludes1   abscess of intestine with ulcerative colitis (K51.014, K51.~~114, K51.~~214, K51.314, K51.414, K51.514, K51.814, K51.914)

K63.2   **Fistula of intestine**

Excludes1   fistula of intestine with ulcerative colitis (K51.013, K51.~~113, K51.~~213, K51.313, K51.413, K51.513, K51.813, K51.913)

DISEASES OF PERITONEUM AND RETROPERITONEUM (K65-K68)

K65   Peritonitis

K65.2   **Spontaneous bacterial peritonitis**

Excludes1   bacterial peritonitis NOS ~~K65.9~~(K65.9)

K67   *Disorders of peritoneum in infectious diseases classified elsewhere*

Code first underlying disease, such as:
helminthiasis (B65.0 --B83.9)

DISEASES OF LIVER (K70-K77)

K72   Hepatic failure, not elsewhere classified

Excludes1   ~~hepatic failure complicating abortion or ectopic or molar pregnancy (O00-O07, O08.8) hepatic failure complicating pregnancy, childbirth and the puerperium (O26.6-)~~

Excludes2   hepatic failure complicating abortion or ectopic or molar pregnancy (O00-O07, O08.8) hepatic failure complicating pregnancy, childbirth and the puerperium (O26.6-)

K76   Other diseases of liver

Excludes2   amyloid degeneration of liver (E85.-)

K77   *Liver disorders in diseases classified elsewhere*

Code first underlying disease, such as:
amyloidosis (E85.-)

DISORDERS OF GALLBLADDER, BILIARY TRACT AND PANCREAS (K80–K87)

K85   Acute pancreatitis

K85.3   **Drug induced acute pancreatitis**
Use additional code to identify drug abuse and dependence (F11.--F17.-)

OTHER DISEASES OF THE DIGESTIVE SYSTEM (K90-K95)

K90   Intestinal malabsorption

K90.0   **Celiac disease**
Use additional code for associated disorders including:
dermatitis herpetiformis (L13.0)
gluten ataxia (G32.81)

K92   Other diseases of digestive system

K92.8   **Other specified diseases of the digestive system**

K92.81   **Gastrointestinal mucositis (ulcerative)**
Code also type of associated therapy, such as:
antineoplastic and immunosuppressive drugs (T45.1xX-)

K95   Complications of bariatric procedures

K95.0   **Complications of gastric band procedure**

K95.01   **Infection due to gastric band procedure**
Use additional code to specify type of infection or organism, such as:
bacterial and viral infectious agents ~~(B95-, B96~~(B95.-, B96.-)

K95.8   **Complications of other bariatric procedure**

K95.81   **Infection due to other bariatric procedure**
Use additional code to specify type of infection or organism, such as:
bacterial and viral infectious agents ~~(B95-, B96~~(B95.-, B96.-)

CHAPTER 12

DISEASES OF THE SKIN AND SUBCUTANEOUS TISSUE (L00-L99)

INFECTIONS OF THE SKIN AND SUBCUTANEOUS TISSUE (L00-L08)

L00   Staphylococcal scalded skin syndrome
Use additional code to identify percentage of skin exfoliation (L49.-)

L03   Cellulitis and acute lymphangitis

L03.1   **Cellulitis and acute lymphangitis of other parts of limb**

L03.12   **Acute lymphangitis of other parts of limb**
Excludes2   acute lymphangitis of toes (L03.04-)

URTICARIA AND ERYTHEMA (L49-L54)

L51   Erythema multiforme
Use additional code to identify percentage of skin exfoliation (L49.-)

OTHER DISORDERS OF THE SKIN AND SUBCUTANEOUS TISSUE (L80-L99)

L99   *Other disorders of skin and subcutaneous tissue in diseases classified elsewhere*

Code first underlying disease, such as:
amyloidosis (E85.-)

CHAPTER 13

DISEASES OF THE MUSCULOSKELETAL SYSTEM AND CONNECTIVE TISSUE (M00-M99)

INFECTIOUS ARTHROPATHIES (M00-M02)

M01 Direct infections of joint in infectious and parasitic diseases classified elsewhere

> **Excludes1** ~~arthritis, arthropathy (in):~~
> ~~gonococcal (A54.42)~~
> arthropathy in Lyme disease (A69.23)
> ~~meningococcal (A39.83)~~
> ~~postmeningococcal (A39.84)~~
> ~~mumps (B26.85)~~
> ~~postinfective (M02.-)~~
> ~~reactive (M04.0-)~~
> ~~rubella (B06.82)~~
> ~~sarcoidosis (D86.86)~~
> ~~typhoid fever (A01.04)~~
> ~~tuberculosis (A18.02)~~
> ~~spine (A18.01)~~
> gonococcal arthritis (A54.42)
> meningococcal arthritis (A39.83)
> mumps arthritis (B26.85)
> postinfective arthropathy (M02.-)
> postmeningococcal arthritis (A39.84)
> reactive arthritis (M02.3)
> rubella arthritis (B06.82)
> sarcoidosis arthritis (D86.86)
> typhoid fever arthritis (A01.04)
> tuberculosis arthritis (A18.01-A18.02)

M02 Postinfective and reactive arthropathies

> **Excludes1** ~~postinfectious arthritis (in):~~
> ~~meningococcal~~postmeningococcal arthritis (A39.84)
> mumps arthritis (B26.85)
> rubella arthritis (B06.82)
> syphilis arthritis (late) (A52.77)

INFLAMMATORY POLYARTHROPATHIES (M05-M14)

M08 Juvenile arthritis

  M08.8 Other juvenile arthritis

    M08.88 Other juvenile arthritis, ~~vertebrae~~ other specified site
    Other juvenile arthritis, vertebrae

M1A Chronic gout

> **Excludes1** acute gout (M10.-)

M10 Gout

> **Excludes1** chronic gout (M1A.-)

M12 Other and unspecified arthropathy

  M12.0 Chronic postrheumatic arthropathy [Jaccoud]

    M12.08 Chronic postrheumatic arthropathy [Jaccoud], ~~vertebrae~~other specified site
    Chronic postrheumatic arthropathy [Jaccoud], vertebrae

  M12.2 Villonodular synovitis (pigmented)

    M12.28 Villonodular synovitis (pigmented), ~~vertebrae~~other specified site
    Villonodular synovitis (pigmented), vertebrae

  M12.3 Palindromic rheumatism

    M12.38 Palindromic rheumatism, ~~vertebrae~~other specified site
    Palindromic rheumatism, vertebrae

M12.5 Traumatic arthropathy

> **Excludes1** post-traumatic osteoarthritis ~~(of):~~of first carpometacarpal joint (M18.2-M18.3)
> ~~NOS (M19.1-)~~
> ~~first carpometacarpal joint (M18.2-M18.3)~~
> post-traumatic osteoarthritis of hip (M16.4-M16.5)
> post-traumatic osteoarthritis of knee (M17.2-M17.3)
> ~~other single joints~~post-traumatic osteoarthritis NOS (M19.1-)
> post-traumatic osteoarthritis of other single joints (M19.1-)

  M12.58 Traumatic arthropathy, ~~vertebrae~~other specified site
  Traumatic arthropathy, vertebrae

M12.8 Other specific arthropathies, not elsewhere classified

  M12.88 Other specific arthropathies, not elsewhere classified, ~~vertebrae~~other specified site
  Other specific arthropathies, not elsewhere classified, vertebrae

M14 Arthropathies in other diseases classified elsewhere

> **Excludes1** arthropathy in:
> diabetes mellitus (E08-E13 with ~~4th character 61.~~61.-)

M14.6 Charcôt's joint

> **Excludes1** ~~Charcôt's joint in diabetes mellitus (E08-E13 with final characters~~ ôt's joint in diabetes mellitus (E08-E13 with .610)

M14.8 Arthropathies in other specified diseases classified elsewhere

  Code first underlying disease, such as:
  amyloidosis (E85.-)

OTHER JOINT DISORDERS (M20-M25)

M21 Other acquired deformities of limbs

  M21.6 Other acquired deformities of foot

> **Excludes2** deformities of toe (acquired) (M20.1-~~(~~M20.6)

M25 Other joint disorder, not elsewhere classified

  M25.0 Hemarthrosis

    M25.08 Hemarthrosis, ~~vertebrae~~other specified site
    Hemarthrosis, vertebrae

  M25.1 Fistula of joint

    M25.18 Fistula, ~~vertebrae~~other specified site
    Fistula, vertebrae

DEFORMING DORSOPATHIES (M40-M43)

M43 Other deforming dorsopathies

> **Excludes1** spinal curvature in osteoporosis (M80.-)

SPONDYLOPATHIES (M45-M49)

M47 Spondylosis

  M47.1 Other spondylosis with myelopathy

    ~~M47.17 Other spondylosis with myelopathy, lumbosacral region~~

    ~~M47.18 Other spondylosis with myelopathy, sacral and sacrococcygeal region~~

M49 Spondylopathies in diseases classified elsewhere

> **Excludes1** ~~neuropathic spondylopathy (in):~~
> ~~nonsyphilitic NEC (G98.0)~~
> ~~syringomyelia (G95.0)~~
> ~~tabes dorsalis (A52.11)~~
> ~~spondylitis (in):~~
> gonococcal spondylitis (A54.41)
> ~~syphilis (acquired) (A52.77)~~
> neuropathic [tabes dorsalis] spondylitis
> (A52.11)
> ~~tuberculosis (A18.01)~~
> ~~typhoid fever (A01.05)~~
> neuropathic spondylopathy in syringomyelia
> (G95.0)
> neuropathic spondylopathy in tabes dorsalis
> (A52.11)
> nonsyphilitic neuropathic spondylopathy NEC
> (G98.0)
> spondylitis in syphilis (acquired) (A52.77)
> tuberculous spondylitis (A18.01)
> typhoid fever spondylitis (A01.05)

OTHER DORSOPATHIES (M50-M54)

M50 Cervical disc disorders

M50.0 Cervical disc disorder with myelopathy

M50.01 Cervical disc disorder with myelopathy,
~~occipito-atlanto-axi~~high cervical region
C2-C3 disc disorder with myelopathy
C3-C4 disc disorder with myelopathy

M50.02 Cervical disc disorder with myelopathy, mid-cervical region
C4-C5 disc disorder with myelopathy
C5-C6 disc disorder with myelopathy
C6-C7 disc disorder with myelopathy

M50.03 Cervical disc disorder with myelopathy, cervicothoracic region
C7-T1 disc disorder with myelopathy

M50.1 Cervical disc disorder with radiculopathy

M50.11 Cervical disc disorder with radiculopathy,
~~occipito-atlanto-axi~~high cervical region
C2-C3 disc disorder with radiculopathy
C3 radiculopathy due to disc disorder
C3-C4 disc disorder with radiculopathy
C4 radiculopathy due to disc disorder

M50.12 Cervical disc disorder with radiculopathy, mid-cervical region
C4-C5 disc disorder with radiculopathy
C5 radiculopathy due to disc disorder
C5-C6 disc disorder with radiculopathy
C6 radiculopathy due to disc disorder
C6-C7 disc disorder with radiculopathy
C7 radiculopathy due to disc disorder

M50.13 Cervical disc disorder with radiculopathy, cervicothoracic region
C7-T1 disc disorder with radiculopathy
C8 radiculopathy due to disc disorder

M50.2 Other cervical disc displacement

M50.21 Other cervical disc displacement,
~~occipito-atlanto-axi~~high cervical region
Other C2-C3 cervical disc displacement
Other C3-C4 cervical disc displacement

M50.22 Other cervical disc displacement, mid-cervical region
Other C4-C5 cervical disc displacement
Other C5-C6 cervical disc displacement
Other C6-C7 cervical disc displacement

M50.23 Other cervical disc displacement, cervicothoracic region
Other C7-T1 cervical disc displacement

M50.3 Other cervical disc degeneration

M50.31 Other cervical disc degeneration,
~~occipito-atlanto-axi~~high cervical region
Other C2-C3 cervical disc degeneration
Other C3-C4 cervical disc degeneration

M50.32 Other cervical disc degeneration, mid-cervical region
Other C4-C5 cervical disc degeneration
Other C5-C6 cervical disc degeneration
Other C6-C7 cervical disc degeneration

M50.33 Other cervical disc degeneration, cervicothoracic region
Other C7-T1 cervical disc degeneration

M50.8 Other cervical disc disorders

M50.81 Other cervical disc disorders,
~~occipito-atlanto-axi~~high cervical region
Other C2-C3 cervical disc disorders
Other C3-C4 cervical disc disorders

M50.82 Other cervical disc disorders, mid-cervical region
Other C4-C5 cervical disc disorders
Other C5-C6 cervical disc disorders
Other C6-C7 cervical disc disorders

M50.83 Other cervical disc disorders, cervicothoracic region
Other C7-T1 cervical disc disorders

M50.9 Cervical disc disorder, unspecified

M50.91 Cervical disc disorder, unspecified,
~~occipito-atlanto-axi~~high cervical region
C2-C3 cervical disc disorder, unspecified
C3-C4 cervical disc disorder, unspecified

M50.92 Cervical disc disorder, unspecified, mid-cervical region
C4-C5 cervical disc disorder, unspecified
C5-C6 cervical disc disorder, unspecified
C6-C7 cervical disc disorder, unspecified

M50.93 Cervical disc disorder, unspecified, cervicothoracic region
C7-T1 cervical disc disorder, unspecified

M51 Thoracic, thoracolumbar, and lumbosacral intervertebral disc disorders

M51.0 Thoracic, thoracolumbar and lumbosacral intervertebral disc disorders with myelopathy

~~M51.07   Intervertebral disc disorders with myelopathy, lumbosacral region~~

M54 Dorsalgia

M54.5 Low back pain

> **Excludes1**   low back strain ~~S39.012~~(S39.012)

DISORDERS OF MUSCLES (M60-M63)

> **Excludes1**   myopathy in: amyloidosis (E85.-)
> ~~amyloidosis (E85.-)~~
> myopathy in polyarteritis nodosa (M30.0)
> myopathy in rheumatoid arthritis (M05.32)
> myopathy in scleroderma (M34.-)
> myopathy in Sjögren's syndrome (M35.03)
> myopathy in systemic lupus erythematosus
> (M32.-)

DISORDERS OF BONE DENSITY AND STRUCTURE (M80-M85)

M84 Disorder of continuity of bone

M84.5 Pathological fracture in neoplastic disease

M84.58 Pathological fracture in neoplastic disease,
~~vertebrae~~other specified site
Pathological fracture in neoplastic disease,
vertebrae

OTHER OSTEOPATHIES (M86-M90)

M90 Osteopathies in diseases classified elsewhere

>   **Excludes1**   osteochondritis, osteomyelitis, and osteopathy (in):
>   diabetes mellitus (E08-E13 with ~~4th character~~ .61-)

CHONDROPATHIES (M91-M94)

M91 Juvenile osteochondrosis of hip and pelvis

>   **M91.0** Juvenile osteochondrosis of pelvis
>   Osteochondrosis (juvenile) of: acetabulum
>   ~~acetabulum~~
>   Osteochondrosis (juvenile) of iliac crest [Buchanan]
>   Osteochondrosis (juvenile) of ischiopubic synchondrosis [van Neck]
>   Osteochondrosis (juvenile) of symphysis pubis [Pierson]

INTRAOPERATIVE AND POSTPROCEDURAL COMPLICATIONS AND DISORDERS OF MUSCULOSKELETAL SYSTEM, NOT ELSEWHERE CLASSIFIED (M96)

M96 Intraoperative and postprocedural complications and disorders of musculoskeletal system, not elsewhere classified

>   **M96.8** Other intraoperative and postprocedural complications and disorders of musculoskeletal system, not elsewhere classified
>
>>   **M96.81** Intraoperative hemorrhage and hematoma of a musculoskeletal structure complicating a procedure
>>
>>>   **Excludes1**   intraoperative hemorrhage and hematoma of a musculoskeletal structure due to accidental puncture and laceration during a procedure (M96.82-)

CHAPTER 14

DISEASES OF THE GENITOURINARY SYSTEM (N00-N99)

GLOMERULAR DISEASES (N00-N08)

N02 Recurrent and persistent hematuria

>   **Excludes1**   ~~acute prostatitis with hematuria (N41.01)~~
>   ~~chronic prostatitis with hematuria (N41.11)~~

N07 Hereditary nephropathy, not elsewhere classified

>   **Excludes2**   hereditary amyloid nephropathy (E85.-)
>   non-neuropathic heredofamilial amyloidosis (E85.-)

N08 Glomerular disorders in diseases classified elsewhere

>   *Code first* underlying disease, such as:
>   amyloidosis (E85.-)
>   gout (~~M1A~~M1A.-, M10.-)

ACUTE KIDNEY FAILURE AND CHRONIC KIDNEY DISEASE (N17-N19)

>   **Excludes2**   renal failure: complicating abortion or ectopic or molar pregnancy (O00-O07, O08.4)
>   ~~complicating abortion or ectopic or molar pregnancy (O00-O07, O08.4)~~
>   renal failure following labor and delivery (O90.4)
>   renal failure postprocedural (N99.0)

N18 Chronic kidney disease (CKD)

>   **N18.9** Chronic kidney disease, unspecified
>   ~~Renal disease NOS~~

UROLITHIASIS (N20-N23)

N22 Calculus of urinary tract in diseases classified elsewhere

>   *Code first* underlying disease, such as:
>   gout (~~M1A~~M1A.-, M10.-)

OTHER DISORDERS OF KIDNEY AND URETER (N25-N29)

N28 Other disorders of kidney and ureter, not elsewhere classified

>   **N28.9** Disorder of kidney and ureter, unspecified
>
>>   **Excludes1**   unspecified nephritic syndrome (N05.-)

N29 Other disorders of kidney and ureter in diseases classified elsewhere

>   *Code first* underlying disease, such as:
>   amyloidosis (E85.-)

OTHER DISEASES OF THE URINARY SYSTEM (N30-N39)

N33 Bladder disorders in diseases classified elsewhere

>   **Excludes1**   bladder disorder in: syphilis (A52.76)
>   ~~syphilis (A52.76)~~
>   bladder disorder in tuberculosis (A18.12)
>   ~~cystitis (in):~~
>   candidal ~~infection~~cystitis (B37.41)
>   chlamydial cystitis(A56.01)
>   ~~diphtheritic (A36.85)~~
>   cystitis in gonorrhea (A54.01)
>   ~~syphilitic (A52.76)~~
>   ~~trichomonal infection (A59.03)~~
>   cystitis in neurogenic bladder (N31.-)
>   diphtheritic cystitis (A36.85)
>   syphilitic cystitis (A52.76)
>   trichomonal cystitis (A59.03)

N39 Other disorders of urinary system

>   **Excludes2**   hematuria NOS (R31.-)

INFLAMMATORY DISEASES OF FEMALE PELVIC ORGANS (N70-N77)

N71 Inflammatory disease of uterus, except cervix

>   **Excludes1**   infection of uterus following delivery (O85, O86.-)

N74 *Female pelvic inflammatory disorders in diseases classified elsewhere*

>   **Excludes1**   ~~cervicitis:~~
>   chlamydial cervicitis (A56.02)
>   ~~gonococcal (A54.03)~~
>   ~~herpesviral [herpes simplex] (A60.03)~~
>   ~~syphilitic (A52.76)~~
>   ~~trichomonal (A59.09)~~
>   ~~tuberculous (A18.16)~~
>   ~~pelvic inflammatory disease:~~
>   chlamydial pelvic inflammatory disease (A56.11)
>   gonococcal (~~A54.24~~cervicitis (A54.03)
>   ~~herpesviral [herpes simplex] (A60.09)~~
>   ~~syphilitic (A52.76)~~
>   ~~tuberculous (A18.17)~~
>   gonococcal pelvic inflammatory disease (A54.24)
>   herpesviral [herpes simplex] cervicitis (A60.03)
>   herpesviral [herpes simplex] pelvic inflammatory disease (A60.09)
>   syphilitic cervicitis (A52.76)
>   syphilitic pelvic inflammatory disease (A52.76)
>   trichomonal cervicitis (A59.09)
>   tuberculous cervicitis (A18.16)
>   tuberculous pelvic inflammatory disease (A18.17)

N76   Other inflammation of vagina and vulva

    N76.8   Other specified inflammation of vagina and vulva

        N76.81   Mucositis (ulcerative) of vagina and vulva

            Code also type of associated therapy,
              such as:
              antineoplastic and immunosuppressive
              drugs (T45.1xX-)

N77   Vulvovaginal ulceration and inflammation in diseases classified elsewhere

    N77.1   Vaginitis, vulvitis and vulvovaginitis in diseases classified elsewhere

        Excludes1   vaginitis, vulvitis and ~~vulvovaginitis (in):~~
            candidi~~asal~~ vulvovaginitis (B37.3)
            chlamydial vulvovaginitis (A56.02)
            gonococcal ~~infection~~vulvovaginitis
              (A54.02)
            herpesviral [herpes simplex]
              ~~infection~~vulvovaginitis (A60.04)
            ~~syphilitic, early (A51.0)~~
            ~~syphilitic, late (A52.76)~~
            trichomonal vulvovaginitis (A59.01)
            tuberculous vulvovaginitis (A18.18)
            vulvovaginitis in early syphilis (A51.0)
            vulvovaginitis in late syphilis (A52.76)

NONINFLAMMATORY DISORDERS OF FEMALE GENITAL TRACT (N80-N98)

N81   Female genital prolapse

    N81.6   Rectocele

        Use additional code for any associated fecal
        incontinence, if applicable (R15.-)

        Excludes2   perineocele ~~N81.81~~(N81.81)

INTRAOPERATIVE AND POSTPROCEDURAL COMPLICATIONS AND DISORDERS OF GENITOURINARY SYSTEM, NOT ELSEWHERE CLASSIFIED (N99)

N99   Intraoperative and postprocedural complications and disorders of genitourinary system, not elsewhere classified

    Excludes2   postoophorectomy osteoporosis without
           current pathological fracture (-M81.8)

CHAPTER 15

PREGNANCY, CHILDBIRTH AND THE PUERPERIUM (O00-O9A)

MATERNAL CARE RELATED TO THE FETUS AND AMNIOTIC CAVITY AND POSSIBLE DELIVERY PROBLEMS (O30-O48)

O31   Complications specific to multiple gestation

    Excludes2   malpresentation of one fetus or more (O32.59)

O33   Maternal care for disproportion

    Excludes1   disproportion with obstructed labor (O65-O66)

COMPLICATIONS OF LABOR AND DELIVERY (O60-O77)

O75   Other complications of labor and delivery, not elsewhere classified

    O75.8   Other specified complications of labor and delivery

        O75.82   Onset (spontaneous) of labor after
            37 completed weeks of gestation but before
            39 completed weeks gestation, with delivery
            by (planned) cesarean section

            ~~Use additional code to specify reason for
planned cesarean section such as:
cephalopelvic disproportion (normally
formed fetus) (O33.9)
previous cesarean delivery (O34.21)~~

            *Code first to specify reason for planned cesarean
section such as:*
cephalopelvic disproportion (normally
formed fetus) (O33.9)
previous cesarean delivery (O34.21)

ENCOUNTER FOR DELIVERY (O80-O82)

O80   Encounter for full-term uncomplicated delivery
    Delivery requiring minimal or no assistance, with or without
    episiotomy, without fetal manipulation [e.g., rotation
    version] or instrumentation [forceps] of a spontaneous,
    cephalic, vaginal, full-term, single, live-born infant.
    This code is for use as a single diagnosis code and is not
    to be used with any other code from chapter 15. ~~This
code must be accompanied by a delivery code from the
appropriate procedure classification.~~

O82   Encounter for cesarean delivery without indication
    ~~This code must be accompanied by a delivery code from the
appropriate procedure classification.~~

COMPLICATIONS PREDOMINANTLY RELATED TO THE PUERPERIUM (O85-O92)

O88   Obstetric embolism

    Excludes1   embolism complicating failed attempted
           abortion (O07.2, ~~O07.7~~)

OTHER OBSTETRIC CONDITIONS, NOT ELSEWHERE CLASSIFIED (O94-O9A)

O99   Other maternal diseases classifiable elsewhere but complicating pregnancy, childbirth and the puerperium

    O99.0   Anemia complicating pregnancy, childbirth and the puerperium

        O99.03   Anemia complicating the puerperium

            Excludes1   postpartum anemia not
                pre-existing prior to
                delivery (O90-.81)

CHAPTER 16

CERTAIN CONDITIONS ORIGINATING IN THE PERINATAL PERIOD (P00-P96)

RESPIRATORY AND CARDIOVASCULAR DISORDERS SPECIFIC TO THE PERINATAL PERIOD (P19-P29)

P28   Other respiratory conditions originating in the perinatal period

    P28.8   Other specified respiratory conditions of newborn

        P28.89   Other specified respiratory conditions of newborn

            Excludes1   early congenital syphilitic
                rhinitis (A50.05)

OTHER DISORDERS ORIGINATING IN THE PERINATAL PERIOD (P90-P96)

P92   Feeding problems of newborn

    P92.0   Vomiting of newborn

        P92.01   Bilious vomiting of newborn

            Excludes1   bilious vomiting in child over 28 days old (R11.1~~4~~3)

CHAPTER 17

CONGENITAL MALFORMATIONS, DEFORMATIONS AND CHROMOSOMAL ABNORMALITIES (Q00-Q99)

CONGENITAL MALFORMATIONS OF EYE, EAR, FACE AND NECK (Q10-Q18)

    Excludes2   congenital malformation of: cervical spine (Q05.0, Q05.5, Q67.5, Q76.0-Q76.4)

~~cervical spine (Q05.0, Q05.5, Q67.5, Q76.0-Q76.4)~~

congenital malformation of larynx (Q31.-)

congenital malformation of lip NEC (Q38.0)

congenital malformation of nose (Q30.-)

congenital malformation of parathyroid gland (Q89.2)

congenital malformation of thyroid gland (Q89.2)

OTHER CONGENITAL MALFORMATIONS OF THE DIGESTIVE SYSTEM (Q38-Q45)

Q43   Other congenital malformations of intestine

    Q43.6   Congenital fistula of rectum and anus

        Excludes1   congenital urethrorectal fistula (Q64.7<u>3</u>)

CONGENITAL MALFORMATIONS AND DEFORMATIONS OF THE MUSCULOSKELETAL SYSTEM (Q65-Q79)

Q67   Congenital musculoskeletal deformities of head, face, spine and chest

    Q67.4   Other congenital deformities of skull, face and jaw

        Excludes1   dentofacial anomalies [including malocclusion] (M26<u>.</u>-)

Q70   Syndactyly

    Q70.4   Polysyndactyly, unspecified

        Excludes1   specified syndactyly of hand and feet - code to specified conditions (Q70.0- -Q70.3-)

CHAPTER 18

SYMPTOMS, SIGNS AND ABNORMAL CLINICAL AND LABORATORY FINDINGS, NOT ELSEWHERE CLASSIFIED (R00-R99)

Note: (a) cases for which no more specific diagnosis can be made even after all the facts bearing on the case have been investigated~~:~~<u>;</u>

SYMPTOMS AND SIGNS INVOLVING THE CIRCULATORY AND RESPIRATORY SYSTEMS (R00-R09)

R09   Other symptoms and signs involving the circulatory and respiratory system

    R09.0   Asphyxia and hypoxemia

        Excludes1   traumatic asphyxia (T71<u>.</u>-)

SYMPTOMS AND SIGNS INVOLVING THE GENITOURINARY SYSTEM (R30-R39)

R31   Hematuria

    Excludes1   hematuria included with underlying conditions, such as:

~~acute prostatitis with hematuria (N41.01)~~

SYMPTOMS AND SIGNS INVOLVING COGNITION, PERCEPTION, EMOTIONAL STATE AND BEHAVIOR (R40-R46)

R40   Somnolence, stupor and coma

    R40.2   Coma

        Code first any associated:

~~coma in~~ fracture of skull (S02.-)

~~coma in~~ intracranial injury (S06.-)

~~The appropriate 7th character is to be added to each code from subcategory R40.21-, R40.22-, R40.23-:~~

~~0~~	~~unspecified time~~
~~1~~	~~in the field [EMT or ambulance]~~
~~2~~	~~at arrival to emergency department~~
~~3~~	~~at hospital admission~~
~~4~~	~~24 hours or more after hospital admission~~

Note: ~~A code from each subcategory~~<u>One code from subcategories R40.21-R40-23</u> is required to complete the coma scale

        R40.21   Coma scale, eyes open

The following appropriate 7th character is to be added to subcategory R40.21-:

0	unspecified time
1	in the field [EMT or ambulance]
2	at arrival to emergency department
3	at hospital admission
4	24 hours or more after hospital admission

        R40.22   Coma scale, best verbal response

The following appropriate 7th character is to be added to subcategory R40.22-:

0	unspecified time
1	in the field [EMT or ambulance]
2	at arrival to emergency department
3	at hospital admission
4	24 hours or more after hospital admission

        R40.23   Coma scale, best motor response

The following appropriate 7th character is to be added to subcategory R40.23-:

0	unspecified time
1	in the field [EMT or ambulance]
2	at arrival to emergency department
3	at hospital admission
4	24 hours or more after hospital admission

GENERAL SYMPTOMS AND SIGNS (R50-R69)

R53   Malaise and fatigue

    R53.8   Other malaise and fatigue

        Excludes1   exhaustion and fatigue due to:
              depressive episode (F32.-)
              ~~depressive episode (F32.-)~~
              exhaustion and fatigue due to excessive exertion (T73.3)
              exhaustion and fatigue due to exposure (T73.2)
              exhaustion and fatigue due to heat (T67.-)
              exhaustion and fatigue due to pregnancy (O26.8-)
              exhaustion and fatigue due to recurrent depressive episode (F33)
              exhaustion and fatigue due to senile debility (R54)

R65   Symptoms and signs specifically associated with systemic inflammation and infection

    R65.2   Severe sepsis

        Code first underlying infection, such as:
        sepsis NOS ~~A41.9~~(A41.9)

ABNORMAL FINDINGS ON EXAMINATION OF BLOOD, WITHOUT DIAGNOSIS (R70-R79)

R79   Other abnormal findings of blood chemistry

    Excludes1   specific findings indicating disorder of: amino-acid metabolism (E70-E72)
        ~~amino-acid metabolism (E70-E72)~~
        specific findings indicating disorder of carbohydrate metabolism (E73-E74)
        specific findings indicating disorder of lipid metabolism (E75.-)

ABNORMAL FINDINGS ON EXAMINATION OF URINE, WITHOUT DIAGNOSIS (R80-R82)

    Excludes1   specific findings indicating disorder of: amino-acid metabolism (E70-E72)
        ~~amino-acid metabolism (E70-E72)~~
        specific findings indicating disorder of carbohydrate metabolism (E73-E74)

CHAPTER 19

INJURY, POISONING AND CERTAIN OTHER CONSEQUENCES OF EXTERNAL CAUSES (S00-T88)

INJURIES TO THE HEAD (S00-S09)

S06   Intracranial injury

    S06.2   Diffuse traumatic brain injury

        Excludes1   traumatic diffuse cerebral edema (S06.1xX-)

S07   Crushing injury of head

    Use additional code for all associated injuries, such as:
    intracranial injuries (S06.-)

INJURIES TO THE NECK (S10-S19)

S12   Fracture of cervical vertebra and other parts of neck

    ~~Code also any associated cervical spinal cord injury (S14.0, S14.1-)~~

    Code first any associated cervical spinal cord injury (S14.0, S14.1-)

    S12.8   Fracture of other parts of neck
        Hyoid bone
        Larynx
        Thyroid cartilage
        Trachea
        ~~Hyoid bone~~
        ~~Larynx~~
        ~~Thyroid cartilage~~
        ~~Trachea~~

    S12.9   Fracture of neck, unspecified
        Fracture of neck NOS
        Fracture of cervical spine NOS
        Fracture of cervical vertebra NOS
        ~~Fracture of neck NOS~~
        ~~Fracture of cervical spine NOS~~
        ~~Fracture of cervical vertebra NOS~~

S14   Injury of nerves and spinal cord at neck level

    Code also any associated:
    open wound of neck (S11.-)

INJURIES TO THE THORAX (S20-S29)

S21   Open wound of thorax

    Code also any associated injury ~~(to) (such as)~~, such as:
    injury of heart (S26.-)
    injury of intrathoracic organs (S27.-)

S24   Injury of nerves and spinal cord at thorax level

    Note: Injuries to the spinal cord (S24.0 and S24.1) refer to the cord level and not bone level injury, and can affect nerve roots at and below the level given.

INJURIES TO THE ABDOMEN, LOWER BACK, LUMBAR SPINE, PELVIS AND EXTERNAL GENITALS (S30-S39)

S32   Fracture of lumbar spine and pelvis

    Code first any associated spinal cord and spinal nerve injury (S34.-)

S34   Injury of lumbar and sacral spinal cord and nerves at abdomen, lower back and pelvis level

    Note: Injuries to the spinal cord (S34.0 and S34.1) refer to the cord level and not bone level injury, and can affect nerve roots at and below the level given.

S37   Injury of urinary and pelvic organs

    Excludes1   obstetric trauma to pelvic organs (O71.-)

S38   Crushing injury and traumatic amputation of abdomen, lower back, pelvis and external genitals

    S38.1   Crushing injury of abdomen, lower back, and pelvis

        Use additional code for all associated injuries, such as:
        open wound of abdominal wall (S31.-)

        Excludes2   crushing injury of external genital organs (S38.20-)

INJURIES TO THE ELBOW AND FOREARM (S50-S59)

S54 Injury of nerves at forearm level

S54.8 Injury of other nerves at forearm level

S54.8X ~~Unspecified i~~Injury of other nerves at forearm level

BURNS AND CORROSIONS OF EXTERNAL BODY SURFACE, SPECIFIED BY SITE (T20-T25)

T20 Burn and corrosion of head, face, and neck

T20.5 Corrosion of first degree of head, face, and neck

T20.56 Corrosion of first degree of forehead and cheek

BURNS AND CORROSIONS CONFINED TO EYE AND INTERNAL ORGANS (T26-T28)

T27 Burn and corrosion of respiratory tract

Use additional external cause code to identify the source and intent of the burn (X00-X19, X75-X77, X96-X98)

T28 Burn and corrosion of other internal organs

Use additional external cause code to identify the source and intent of the burn (X00-X19, X75-X77, X96-X98)

BURNS AND CORROSIONS OF MULTIPLE AND UNSPECIFIED BODY REGIONS (T30-T32)

T31 Burns classified according to extent of body surface involved

~~This category is to be used as the primary code only when the site of the burn is unspecified. It should be used as a supplementary code with categories T20-T25 when the site is specified.~~

Note: This category is to be used as the primary code only when the site of the burn is unspecified. It should be used as a supplementary code with categories T20-T25 when the site is specified.

POISONING BY, ADVERSE EFFECTS OF AND UNDERDOSING OF DRUGS, MEDICAMENTS AND BIOLOGICAL SUBSTANCES (T36-T50)

T40 Poisoning by, adverse effect of and underdosing of narcotics and psychodysleptics [hallucinogens]

T40.1 Poisoning by and adverse effect of heroin

T40.1X Poisoning by and adverse effect of heroin

~~T40.1X5 Adverse effect of heroin~~

T40.8 Poisoning by and adverse effect of lysergide [LSD]

T40.8X Poisoning by and adverse effect of lysergide [LSD]

~~T40.8X5 Adverse effect of lysergide [LSD]~~

T41 Poisoning by, adverse effect of and underdosing of anesthetics and therapeutic gases

T41.3 Poisoning by, adverse effect of and underdosing of local anesthetics

Excludes2 poisoning by cocaine used as a central nervous system stimulant (T40.5~~x1-T40.5x~~X1-T40.5X4)

TOXIC EFFECTS OF SUBSTANCES CHIEFLY NONMEDICINAL AS TO SOURCE (T51-T65)

Note: When no intent is indicated code to accidental. Undetermined intent is only for use when there is specific documentation in the record that the intent of the toxic effect cannot be determined.

T61 Toxic effect of noxious substances eaten as seafood

Excludes1 allergic reaction to food, such as: ~~anaphylactic shock (T78.02, T78.05)~~ toxic effect of ~~food contaminants, such as:~~aflatoxin and other mycotoxins (T64) ~~aflatoxin and other mycotoxins (T64)~~ toxic effect of cyanides (T65.0-) toxic effect of harmful algae bloom (T65.82-) toxic effect of hydrogen cyanide (T57.3-) toxic effect of mercury (T56.1-) toxic effect of red tide (T65.82-)

T62 Toxic effect of other noxious substances eaten as food

Excludes1 toxic effect of ~~food contaminants, such as:~~aflatoxin and other mycotoxins (T64) ~~aflatoxin and other mycotoxins (T64)~~ toxic effect of cyanides (T65.0-) toxic effect of hydrogen cyanide (T57.3-) toxic effect of mercury (T56.1-)

T63 Toxic effect of contact with venomous animals and plants

T63.5 Toxic effect of contact with venomous fish

Excludes2 poisoning by ingestion of fish (T61.-)

CERTAIN EARLY COMPLICATIONS OF TRAUMA (T79)

T79 Certain early complications of trauma, not elsewhere classified

T79.0 Air embolism (traumatic)

Excludes1 air embolism complicating: abortion or ectopic or molar pregnancy (O00-O07, O08.2) ~~abortion or ectopic or molar pregnancy (O00-O07, O08.2)~~ air embolism complicating pregnancy, childbirth and the puerperium (O88.0) air embolism following: infusion, transfusion, and therapeutic injection (T80.0) ~~infusion, transfusion, and therapeutic injection (T80.0)~~ air embolism following procedure NEC (T81.7-)

COMPLICATIONS OF SURGICAL AND MEDICAL CARE, NOT ELSEWHERE CLASSIFIED (T80-T88)

Excludes2 specified complications classified elsewhere, such as: disorders of fluid and electrolyte imbalance (E86-E87) ostomy complications (J95.0-, K94.-, N99.5-)

T81 Complications of procedures, not elsewhere classified

Excludes2 specified complications classified elsewhere, such as: intraoperative and postprocedural complications of specific body system (D78.-, E36.-, E89.-, G97.3-, G97.4, H59.3-, H59.-, H95.2-, H95.3, I97.4-, I97.5, J95, K91.-, L76.-, M96.-, N99.-)

T86   Complications of transplanted organs and tissue

T86.8   Complications of other transplanted organs and tissues

T86.82   Complications of skin graft (allograft) (autograft)

Excludes2   complication of artificial skin graft (T85.64~~93~~)

CHAPTER 20

EXTERNAL CAUSES OF MORBIDITY (V00-Y99)

TRANSPORT ACCIDENTS (V00-V99)

Note: ~~This section is structured in 12 groups. Those relating to land transport accidents (V01- V89) reflect the victim's mode of transport and are subdivided to identify the victim's 'counterpart' or the type of event. The vehicle of which the injured person is an occupant is identified in the first two characters since it is seen as the most important factor to identify for prevention purposes. A transport accident is one in which the vehicle involved must be moving or running or in use for transport purposes at the time of the accident.~~

Note: ~~Definitions of transport vehicles:~~

(a) ~~A transport accident is any accident involving a device designed primarily for, or used at the time primarily for, conveying persons or good from one place to another.~~

(b) ~~A public highway [trafficway] or street is the entire width between property lines (or other boundary lines) of land open to the public as a matter of right or custom for purposes of moving persons or property from one place to another. A roadway is that part of the public highway designed, improved and customarily used for vehicular traffic.~~

(c) ~~A traffic accident is any vehicle accident occurring on the public highway [i.e., originating on, terminating on, or involving a vehicle partially on the highway]. A vehicle accident is assumed to have occurred on the public highway unless another place is specified, except in the case of accidents involving only off-road motor vehicles, which are classified as nontraffic accidents unless the contrary is stated.~~

(d) ~~A nontraffic accident is any vehicle accident that occurs entirely in any place other than a public highway.~~

(e) ~~A pedestrian is any person involved in an accident who was not at the time of the accident riding in or on a motor vehicle, railway train, streetcar or animal-drawn or other vehicle, or on a pedal cycle or animal. This includes, a person changing a tire or working on a parked car. It also includes the use of a pedestrian conveyance such as a baby carriage, ice-skates, roller skates, a skateboard, nonmotorized or motorized wheelchair, motorized mobility scooter, or nonmotorized scooter.~~

(f) ~~A driver is an occupant of a transport vehicle who is operating or intending to operate it.~~

(g) ~~A passenger is any occupant of a transport vehicle other than the driver, except a person traveling on the outside of the vehicle.~~

(h) ~~A person on the outside of a vehicle is any person being transported by a vehicle but not occupying the space normally reserved for the driver or passengers, or the space intended for the transport of property. This includes the body, bumper, fender, roof, running board or step of a vehicle.~~

(i) ~~A pedal cycle is any land transport vehicle operated solely by nonmotorized pedals including a bicycle or tricycle.~~

(j) ~~A pedal cyclist is any person riding a pedal cycle or in a sidecar or trailer attached to a pedal cycle.~~

(k) ~~A motorcycle is a two-wheeled motor vehicle with one or two riding saddles and sometimes with a third wheel for the support of a sidecar. The sidecar is considered part of the motorcycle.~~

(l) ~~A motorcycle rider is any person riding a motorcycle or in a sidecar or trailer attached to the motorcycle.~~

(m) ~~A three-wheeled motor vehicle is a motorized tricycle designed primarily for on-road use. This includes a motor-driven tricycle, a motorized rickshaw, or a three-wheeled motor car.~~

(n) ~~A car [automobile] is a four-wheeled motor vehicle designed primarily for carrying up to 7 persons. A trailer being towed by the car is considered part of the car.~~

(o) ~~A pick-up truck or van is a four or six-wheeled motor vehicle designed for carrying passengers as well as property or cargo weighing less than the local limit for classification as a heavy goods vehicle, and not requiring a special driver's license. This includes a minivan and a sport-utility vehicle (SUV).~~

(p) ~~A heavy transport vehicle is a motor vehicle designed primarily for carrying property, meeting local criteria for classification as a heavy goods vehicle in terms of weight and requiring a special driver's license.~~

(q) ~~A bus (coach) is a motor vehicle designed or adapted primarily for carrying more than 10 passengers, and requiring a special driver's license.~~

(r) ~~A railway train or railway vehicle is any device, with or without freight or passenger cars coupled to it, designed for traffic on a railway track. This includes subterranean (subways) or elevated trains.~~

(s) ~~A streetcar is a device designed and used primarily for transporting passengers within a municipality, running on rails, usually subject to normal traffic control signals, and operated principally on a right-of-way that forms part of the roadway. This includes a tram or trolley that runs on rails. A trailer being towed by a streetcar is considered part of the streetcar.~~

(t) ~~A special vehicle mainly used on industrial premises is a motor vehicle designed primarily for use within the buildings and premises of industrial or commercial establishments. This includes battery-powered trucks, forklifts, coal-cars in a coal mine, logging cars and trucks used in mines or quarries.~~

(u) ~~A special vehicle mainly used in agriculture is a motor vehicle designed specifically for use in farming and agriculture (horticulture), to work the land, tend and harvest crops and transport materials on the farm. This includes harvesters, farm machinery and tractor and trailers.~~

(v) ~~A special construction vehicle is a motor vehicle designed specifically for use on construction and demolition sites. This includes bulldozers, diggers, earth levellers, dump trucks, backhoes, front-end loaders, pavers, and mechanical shovels.~~

(w) ~~A special all-terrain vehicle is a motor vehicle of special design to enable it to negotiate over rough or soft terrain, snow or sand. This includes snow mobiles, all-terrain vehicles (ATV), and dune buggies. It does not include passenger vehicle designated as sport utility vehicles (SUV).~~

(x) ~~A watercraft is any device designed for transporting passengers or goods on water. This includes motor or sail boats, ships, and hovercraft.~~

(y) ~~An aircraft is any device for transporting passengers or goods in the air. This includes hot-air balloons, gliders, helicopters and airplanes.~~

(z) ~~A military vehicle is any motorized vehicle operating on a public roadway owned by the military and being operated by a member of the military.~~

This section is structured in 12 groups. Those relating to land transport accidents (V01-V89) reflect the victim's mode of transport and are subdivided to identify the victim's 'counterpart' or the type of event. The vehicle of which the injured person is an occupant is identified in the first two characters since it is seen as the most important factor to identify for prevention purposes. A transport accident is one in which the vehicle involved must be moving or running or in use for transport purposes at the time of the accident.

PEDAL CYCLE RIDER INJURED IN TRANSPORT ACCIDENT (V10-V19)

V10 Pedal cycle rider injured in collision with pedestrian or animal

> **Excludes1**   pedal cycle rider collision with animal-drawn vehicle or animal being ridden (V16.-)

OCCUPANT OF HEAVY TRANSPORT VEHICLE INJURED IN TRANSPORT ACCIDENT (V60-V69)

V69 Occupant of heavy transport vehicle injured in other and unspecified transport accidents

> V69.3 Occupant (driver) (passenger) of heavy transport vehicle injured in unspecified nontraffic accident
> Occupant of heavy transport vehicle injured in nontraffic accident <u>NOS</u>
> ~~NOS~~

WATER TRANSPORT ACCIDENTS (V90-V94)

V91 Other injury due to accident to watercraft

> **Excludes1**   military watercraft accident in military or war operations (Y36, Y37.-)

V92 Drowning and submersion due to accident on board watercraft, without accident to watercraft

> V92.0 Drowning and submersion due to fall off watercraft
>
> > V92.07 Drowning and submersion due to fall off water-skis
> >
> > > **Excludes1**   hit by boat while water-skiing NOS (V94.<u>x</u>X)
> >
> > V92.08 Drowning and submersion due to fall off other unpowered watercraft
> >
> > > **Excludes1**   drowning and submersion due to rider of nonpowered watercraft being hit by other watercraft (V94.<u>-</u>-)
> > > other injury due to rider of nonpowered watercraft being hit by other watercraft (V94.<u>-</u>-)

V93 Other injury due to accident on board watercraft, without accident to watercraft

> **Excludes1**   military watercraft accident in military or war operations (~~Y36, Y37~~<u>Y36, Y37</u>.-)

AIR AND SPACE TRANSPORT ACCIDENTS (V95-V97)

> **Excludes1**   military aircraft accidents in military or war operations (-Y36, Y37)

SLIPPING, TRIPPING, STUMBLING AND FALLS (W00-W19)

> **Excludes1**   fall ~~(in) (from):~~<u>from</u> animal (V80.-)
> ~~animal (V80.-)~~
> <u>fall (in) (from)</u> machinery (in operation) (W28-W31)
> <u>fall (in) (from)</u> transport vehicle (V01-V99)
>
> **Excludes2**   fall (in) (from)<u>:</u> burning building (X00.-)
> ~~burning building (X00.-)~~
> <u>fall</u> into fire (X00-X04, X08-X09)

W16 Fall, jump or diving into water

> **Excludes2**   striking or hitting diving board (W21.3<u>4</u>)

EXPOSURE TO INANIMATE MECHANICAL FORCES (W20-W49)

W20 Struck by thrown, projected or falling object

> **Excludes1**   falling object in: <u>machinery accident (W24, W28-W31)</u>
> ~~machinery accident (W24, W28-W31)~~
> <u>falling object in</u> transport accident (V01-V99)
> object set in motion by<u>:</u> explosion (W35-W40)
> ~~explosion (W35-W40)~~
> object set in motion by firearm (W32-W34)

W33 Accidental rifle, shotgun and larger firearm discharge and malfunction

> **Excludes1**   accidental handgun discharge and malfunction (W32.-)

EXPOSURE TO ANIMATE MECHANICAL FORCES (W50-W64)

W55 Contact with other mammals

> **Excludes1**   contact with marine mammals (W56.<u>x</u>-)

W60 Contact with nonvenomous plant thorns and spines and sharp leaves

> **Excludes1**   contact with venomous plants (T63.<u>x</u><u>7</u>-)

EXPOSURE TO ELECTRIC CURRENT, RADIATION AND EXTREME AMBIENT AIR TEMPERATURE AND PRESSURE (W85-W99)

W94 Exposure to high and low air pressure and changes in air pressure

> W94.3 Exposure to rapid changes in air pressure during descent
>
> > W94.31 Exposure to sudden change in air pressure in aircraft during ~~ascent or~~ descent

EXPOSURE TO SMOKE, FIRE AND FLAMES (X00-X08)

X00 Exposure to uncontrolled fire in building or structure

> **Excludes2**   exposure to ignition or melting of other clothing and apparel (<u>X06.-)</u>

EXPOSURE TO FORCES OF NATURE (X30-X39)

X31 Exposure to excessive natural cold

> **Excludes1**   contact with or inhalation of<u>: dry ice (W93.-)</u>
> ~~dry ice~~<u>contact with or inhalation of liquefied gas (W93.-)</u>
> ~~liquefied gas (W93.-)~~

LEGAL INTERVENTION, OPERATIONS OF WAR, MILITARY OPERATIONS, AND TERRORISM (Y35-Y38)

Y35 Legal intervention

> **Includes**   any injury sustained as a result of an encounter with any law enforcement official, serving in any capacity at the time of the encounter, whether on-duty or off-duty. Includes: injury to law enforcement official, suspect and bystander

SUPPLEMENTARY FACTORS RELATED TO CAUSES OF MORBIDITY CLASSIFIED ELSEWHERE (Y90-Y99)

Y92   Place of occurrence of the external cause

Y92.0   Non-institutional (private) residence as the place of occurrence of the external cause

Y92.00   Unspecified non-institutional (private) residence as the place of occurrence of the external cause

Y92.002   Bathroom of unspecified non-institutional (private) residence single-family (private) house as the place of occurrence of the external cause

Y92.4   Street, highway and other paved roadways as the place of occurrence of the external cause

Excludes1   private driveway of residence (Y92.0x4, ~~Y92.1x3~~14, Y92.024, Y92.043, Y92.093, Y92.113, Y92.123, Y92.154, Y92.194)

Y99   External cause status

Y99.1   Military activity

Excludes2   ~~activity of off duty military personnel (Y99.8)~~

Excludes1   activity of off duty military personnel (Y99.8)

CHAPTER 21

FACTORS INFLUENCING HEALTH STATUS AND CONTACT WITH HEALTH SERVICES (Z00-Z99)

PERSONS ENCOUNTERING HEALTH SERVICES FOR EXAMINATIONS (Z00-Z13)

Z00   Encounter for general examination without complaint, suspected or reported diagnosis

Z00.1   Encounter for newborn, infant and child health examinations

Z00.12   Encounter for routine child health examination

Excludes1   health check for child under 29 days old (Z00.11-)

ENCOUNTERS FOR OTHER SPECIFIC HEALTH CARE (Z40-Z53)

Z46   Encounter for fitting and adjustment of other devices

Z46.8   Encounter for fitting and adjustment of other specified devices

Z46.81   Encounter for fitting and adjustment of insulin pump

PERSONS ENCOUNTERING HEALTH SERVICES IN OTHER CIRCUMSTANCES (Z69-Z76)

Z72   Problems related to lifestyle

Z72.4   Inappropriate diet and eating habits

Excludes1   behavioral eating disorders of infancy or childhood (F98.2.--F98.3)

PERSONS WITH POTENTIAL HEALTH HAZARDS RELATED TO FAMILY AND PERSONAL HISTORY AND CERTAIN CONDITIONS INFLUENCING HEALTH STATUS (Z77-Z99)

Z78   Other specified health status

Excludes2   postprocedural status (Z93--Z99)

Z91   Personal risk factors, not elsewhere classified

Z91.4   Personal history of psychological trauma, not elsewhere classified

Z91.41   Personal history of adult abuse

Z91.410   Personal history of adult physical and sexual abuse

Excludes1   current adult sexual abuse (T74.-21, T76.11)

Z91.8   Other specified personal risk factors, not elsewhere classified

Z91.83   *Wandering in diseases classified elsewhere*

Code first *underlying disorder such as:*
Alzheimer's disease (G30.-)
autism or pervasive developmental disorder (F84.-)

Z94   Transplanted organ and tissue status

Z94.1   Heart transplant status

Excludes1   artificial heart status (Z95.81~~1~~2)

Z95   Presence of cardiac and vascular implants and grafts

Z95.0   Presence of cardiac pacemaker

Excludes1   presence of automatic (implantable) cardiac defibrillator with synchronous cardiac pacemaker ~~Z95.810~~(Z95.810)

PART I

ICD-10-CM Official Guidelines for Coding and Reporting 2014
Narrative changes appear in bold text
Items underlined have been moved within the guidelines since the 2013 version
Italics **are used to indicate revisions to heading changes**

The Centers for Medicare and Medicaid Services (CMS) and the National Center for Health Statistics (NCHS), two departments within the U.S. Federal Government's Department of Health and Human Services (DHHS) provide the following guidelines for coding and reporting using the International Classification of Diseases, 10th Revision, Clinical Modification (ICD-10-CM). These guidelines should be used as a companion document to the official version of the ICD-10-CM as published on the NCHS website. The ICD-10-CM is a morbidity classification published by the United States for classifying diagnoses and reason for visits in all health care settings. The ICD-10-CM is based on the ICD-10, the statistical classification of disease published by the World Health Organization (WHO).

These guidelines have been approved by the four organizations that make up the Cooperating Parties for the ICD-10-CM: the American Hospital Association (AHA), the American Health Information Management Association (AHIMA), CMS, and NCHS.

These guidelines are a set of rules that have been developed to accompany and complement the official conventions and instructions provided within the ICD-10-CM itself. The instructions and conventions of the classification take precedence over guidelines. These guidelines are based on the coding and sequencing instructions in the Tabular List and Alphabetic Index of ICD-10-CM, but provide additional instruction. Adherence to these guidelines when assigning ICD-10-CM diagnosis codes is required under the Health Insurance Portability and Accountability Act (HIPAA). The diagnosis codes (Tabular List and Alphabetic Index) have been adopted under HIPAA for all healthcare settings. A joint effort between the healthcare provider and the coder is essential to achieve complete and accurate documentation, code assignment, and reporting of diagnoses and procedures. These guidelines have been developed to assist both the healthcare provider and the coder in identifying those diagnoses that are to be reported. The importance of consistent, complete documentation in the medical record cannot be overemphasized. Without such documentation accurate coding cannot be achieved. The entire record should be reviewed to determine the specific reason for the encounter and the conditions treated.

The term encounter is used for all settings, including hospital admissions. In the context of these guidelines, the term provider is used throughout the guidelines to mean physician or any qualified health care practitioner who is legally accountable for establishing the patient's diagnosis. Only this set of guidelines, approved by the Cooperating Parties, is official.

The guidelines are organized into sections. Section I includes the structure and conventions of the classification and general guidelines that apply to the entire classification, and chapter-specific guidelines that correspond to the chapters as they are arranged in the classification. Section II includes guidelines for selection of principal diagnosis for non-outpatient settings. Section III includes guidelines for reporting additional diagnoses in non-outpatient settings. Section IV is for outpatient coding and reporting. It is necessary to review all sections of the guidelines to fully understand all of the rules and instructions needed to code properly.

ICD-10-CM Official Guidelines for Coding and Reporting

Section I. Conventions, general coding guidelines and chapter specific guidelines

A. Conventions for the ICD-10-CM
   1. The Alphabetic Index and Tabular List
   2. Format and Structure:
   3. Use of codes for reporting purposes
   4. Placeholder character
   5. 7th Characters
   6. Abbreviations
       a. Alphabetic Index abbreviations
       b. Tabular List abbreviations
   7. Punctuation
   8. Use of "and"
   9. Other and Unspecified codes
       a. "Other" codes
       b. "Unspecified" codes
   10. Includes Notes
   11. Inclusion terms
   12. Excludes Notes
       a. Excludes1
       b. Excludes2
   13. Etiology/manifestation convention ("code first", "use additional code" and "in diseases classified elsewhere" notes)
   14. "And"
   15. "With"
   16. "See" and "See Also"
   17. "Code also note"
   18. Default codes
B. General Coding Guidelines
   1. Locating a code in the ICD-10-CM
   2. Level of Detail in Coding
   3. Code or codes from A00.0 through T88.9, Z00-Z99.8
   4. Signs and symptoms
   5. Conditions that are an integral part of a disease process
   6. Conditions that are not an integral part of a disease process
   7. Multiple coding for a single condition
   8. Acute and Chronic Conditions
   9. Combination Code
   10. Sequela (Late Effects)
   11. Impending or Threatened Condition
   12. Reporting Same Diagnosis Code More than Once
   13. Laterality
   14. Documentation for BMI, *Non-pressure ulcers* and Pressure Ulcer Stages
   15. Syndromes
   16. Documentation of Complications of Care
   17. Borderline Diagnosis
   18. Use of Sign/Symptom/Unspecified Codes
C. Chapter-Specific Coding Guidelines
   1. Chapter 1: Certain Infectious and Parasitic Diseases (A00-B99)
       a. Human Immunodeficiency Virus (HIV) Infections
       b. Infectious agents as the cause of diseases classified to other chapters
       c. Infections resistant to antibiotics
       d. Sepsis, Severe Sepsis, and Septic Shock
       e. Methicillin Resistant *Staphylococcus aureus* (MRSA) Conditions
   2. Chapter 2: Neoplasms (C00-D49)
       a. Treatment directed at the malignancy
       b. Treatment of secondary site
       c. Coding and sequencing of complications
       d. Primary malignancy previously excised
       e. Admissions/Encounters involving chemotherapy, immunotherapy and radiation therapy
       f. Admission/encounter to determine extent of malignancy
       g. Symptoms, signs, and abnormal findings listed in Chapter 18 associated with neoplasms
       h. Admission/encounter for pain control/ management
       i. Malignancy in two or more noncontiguous sites
       j. Disseminated malignant neoplasm, unspecified
       k. Malignant neoplasm without specification of site
       l. Sequencing of neoplasm codes
       m. Current malignancy versus personal history of malignancy
       n. Leukemia, Multiple Myeloma, and Malignant Plasma Cell Neoplasms in remission versus personal history
       o. Aftercare following surgery for neoplasm
       p. Follow-up care for completed treatment of a malignancy
       q. Prophylactic organ removal for prevention of malignancy
       r. Malignant neoplasm associated with transplanted organ
   3. Chapter 3: Disease of the blood and blood-forming organs and certain disorders involving the immune mechanism (D50-D89)
   4. Chapter 4: Endocrine, Nutritional, and Metabolic Diseases (E00-E89)
       a. Diabetes mellitus
   5. Chapter 5: Mental, Behavioral and Neurodevelopmental disorders (F01 – F99)
       a. Pain disorders related to psychological factors
       b. Mental and behavioral disorders due to psychoactive substance use
   6. Chapter 6: Diseases of the Nervous System (G00-G99)
       a. Dominant/nondominant side
       b. Pain - Category G89
   7. Chapter 7: Diseases of the Eye and Adnexa (H00-H59)
       a. Glaucoma
   8. Chapter 8: Diseases of the Ear and Mastoid Process (H60-H95)
   9. Chapter 9: Diseases of the Circulatory System (I00-I99)
       a. Hypertension
       b. Atherosclerotic Coronary Artery Disease and Angina
       c. Intraoperative and Postprocedural Cerebrovascular Accident
       d. Sequelae of Cerebrovascular Disease
       e. Acute myocardial infarction (AMI)

10. Chapter 10: Diseases of the Respiratory System (J00-J99)
    a. Chronic Obstructive Pulmonary Disease [COPD] and Asthma
    b. Acute Respiratory Failure
    c. Influenza due to certain identified influenza viruses
    d. Ventilator associated Pneumonia
11. Chapter 11: Diseases of the Digestive System (K00-K95)
12. Chapter 12: Diseases of the Skin and Subcutaneous Tissue (L00-L99)
    a. Pressure ulcer stage codes
13. Chapter 13: Diseases of the Musculoskeletal System and Connective Tissue (M00-M99)
    a. Site and laterality
    b. Acute traumatic versus chronic or recurrent musculoskeletal conditions
    c. Coding of Pathologic Fractures
    d. Osteoporosis
14. Chapter 14: Diseases of Genitourinary System (N00-N99)
    a. Chronic kidney disease
15. Chapter 15: Pregnancy, Childbirth, and the Puerperium (O00-O9A)
    a. General Rules for Obstetric Cases
    b. Selection of OB Principal or First-listed Diagnosis
    c. Pre-existing conditions versus conditions due to the pregnancy
    d. Pre-existing hypertension in pregnancy
    e. Fetal Conditions Affecting the Management of the Mother
    f. HIV Infection in Pregnancy, Childbirth and the Puerperium
    g. Diabetes mellitus in pregnancy
    h. Long term use of insulin
    i. Gestational (pregnancy induced) diabetes
    j. Sepsis and septic shock complicating abortion, pregnancy, childbirth and the puerperium
    k. Puerperal sepsis
    l. Alcohol and tobacco use during pregnancy, childbirth and the puerperium
    m. Poisoning, toxic effects, adverse effects and underdosing in a pregnant patient
    n. Normal Delivery, Code O80
    o. The Peripartum and Postpartum Periods
    p. Code O94, Sequelae of complication of pregnancy, childbirth, and the puerperium
    q. *Termination of Pregnancy and Spontaneous abortions*
    r. Abuse in a pregnant patient
16. Chapter 16: Certain Conditions Originating in the Perinatal Period (P00-P96)
    a. General Perinatal Rules
    b. Observation and Evaluation of Newborns for Suspected Conditions not Found
    c. Coding Additional Perinatal Diagnoses
    d. Prematurity and Fetal Growth Retardation
    e. Low birth weight and immaturity status
    f. Bacterial Sepsis of Newborn
    g. Stillbirth

17. Chapter 17: Congenital malformations, deformations, and chromosomal abnormalities (Q00-Q99)
18. Chapter 18: Symptoms, signs, and abnormal clinical and laboratory findings, not elsewhere classified (R00-R99)
    a. Use of symptom codes
    b. Use of a symptom code with a definitive diagnosis code
    c. Combination codes that include symptoms
    d. Repeated falls
    e. Coma scale
    f. Functional quadriplegia
    g. SIRS due to Non-Infectious Process
    h. Death NOS
19. Chapter 19: Injury, poisoning, and certain other consequences of external causes (S00-T88)
    a. Application of 7th Characters in Chapter 19
    b. Coding of Injuries
    c. Coding of Traumatic Fractures
    d. Coding of Burns and Corrosions
    e. Adverse Effects, Poisoning, Underdosing and Toxic Effects
    f. Adult and child abuse, neglect and other maltreatment
    g. Complications of care
20. Chapter 20: External Causes of Morbidity (V00-Y99)
    a. General External Cause Coding Guidelines
    b. Place of Occurrence Guideline
    c. Activity Code
    d. Place of Occurrence, Activity, and Status Codes Used with other External Cause Code
    e. If the Reporting Format Limits the Number of External Cause Codes
    f. Multiple External Cause Coding Guidelines
    g. Child and Adult Abuse Guideline
    h. Unknown or Undetermined Intent Guideline
    i. Sequelae (Late Effects) of External Cause Guidelines
    j. Terrorism Guidelines
    k. External cause status
21. Chapter 21: Factors influencing health status and contact with health services (Z00-Z99)
    a. Use of Z codes in any healthcare setting
    b. Z Codes indicate a reason for an encounter
    c. Categories of Z Codes

Section II. Selection of Principal Diagnosis

A. Codes for symptoms, signs, and ill-defined conditions
B. Two or more interrelated conditions, each potentially meeting the definition for principal diagnosis
C. Two or more diagnoses that equally meet the definition for principal diagnosis
D. Two or more comparative or contrasting conditions
E. A symptom(s) followed by contrasting/comparative diagnoses
F. Original treatment plan not carried out
G. Complications of surgery and other medical care
H. Uncertain Diagnosis

I. Admission from Observation Unit
1. Admission Following Medical Observation
2. Admission Following Post-Operative Observation
J. Admission from Outpatient Surgery
K. Admissions/Encounters for Rehabilitation

Section III. Reporting Additional Diagnoses

A. Previous conditions
B. Abnormal findings
C. Uncertain Diagnosis

Section IV. Diagnostic Coding and Reporting Guidelines for Outpatient Services

A. Selection of first-listed condition
1. Outpatient Surgery
2. Observation Stay
B. Codes from A00.0 through T88.9, Z00-Z99
C. Accurate reporting of ICD-10-CM diagnosis codes
D. Codes that describe symptoms and signs
E. Encounters for circumstances other than a disease or injury
F. Level of Detail in Coding
1. ICD-10-CM codes with 3, 4, 5, 6, or 7 characters
2. Use of full number of *characters* required for a code
G. ICD-10-CM code for the diagnosis, condition, problem, or other reason for encounter/visit
H. Uncertain diagnosis
I. Chronic diseases
J. Code all documented conditions that coexist
K. Patients receiving diagnostic services only
L. Patients receiving therapeutic services only
M. Patients receiving preoperative evaluations only
N. Ambulatory surgery
O. Routine outpatient prenatal visits
P. Encounters for general medical examinations with abnormal findings
Q. Encounters for routine health screenings

Appendix I: Present on Admission Reporting Guidelines

Section I. Conventions, general coding guidelines and chapter specific guidelines

The conventions, general guidelines and chapter-specific guidelines are applicable to all health care settings unless otherwise indicated. The conventions and instructions of the classification take precedence over guidelines.

A. **Conventions for the ICD-10-CM**
The conventions for the ICD-10-CM are the general rules for use of the classification independent of the guidelines. These conventions are incorporated within the Alphabetic Index and Tabular List of the ICD-10-CM as instructional notes.

1. **The Alphabetic Index and Tabular List**
The ICD-10-CM is divided into the Alphabetic Index, an alphabetical list of terms and their corresponding code, and the Tabular List, a **structured** list of codes divided into chapters based on body system or condition. The Alphabetic Index consists of the following parts: the Index of Diseases and Injury, the Index of External Causes of Injury, the Table of Neoplasms and the Table of Drugs and Chemicals.
See Section I.C2. General guidelines
See Section I.C.19. Adverse effects, poisoning, underdosing and toxic effects

2. **Format and Structure:**
The ICD-10-CM Tabular List contains categories, subcategories and codes. Characters for categories, subcategories and codes may be either a letter or a number. All categories are 3 characters. A three-character category that has no further subdivision is equivalent to a code. Subcategories are either 4 or 5 characters. Codes may be 3, 4, 5, 6 or 7 characters. That is, each level of subdivision after a category is a subcategory. The final level of subdivision is a code. Codes that have applicable 7th characters are still referred to as codes, not subcategories. A code that has an applicable 7th character is considered invalid without the 7th character.
The ICD-10-CM uses an indented format for ease in reference

3. **Use of codes for reporting purposes**
For reporting purposes only codes are permissible, not categories or subcategories, and any applicable 7th character is required.

4. **Placeholder character**
The ICD-10-CM utilizes a placeholder character "X". The "X" is used as a placeholder at certain codes to allow for future expansion. An example of this is at the poisoning, adverse effect and underdosing codes, categories T36-T50. Where a placeholder exists, the X must be used in order for the code to be considered a valid code.

5. **7th Characters**
Certain ICD-10-CM categories have applicable 7th characters. The applicable 7th character is required for all codes within the category, or as the notes in the Tabular List instruct. The 7th character must always be the 7th character in the data field. If a code that requires a 7th character is not 6 characters, a placeholder X must be used to fill in the empty characters.

6. **Abbreviations**
   a. **Alphabetic Index abbreviations**
   NEC "Not elsewhere classifiable"
   This abbreviation in the Alphabetic Index represents "other specified". When a specific code is not available for a condition the Alphabetic Index directs the coder to the "other specified" code in the Tabular List.
   NOS "Not otherwise specified"
   This abbreviation is the equivalent of unspecified.

b. **Tabular List abbreviations**
   NEC "Not elsewhere classifiable"
   This abbreviation in the Tabular List represents "other specified". When a specific code is not available for a condition the Tabular List includes an NEC entry under a code to identify the code as the "other specified" code.
   NOS "Not otherwise specified"
   This abbreviation is the equivalent of unspecified.

7. **Punctuation**
   [ ] Brackets are used in the Tabular List to enclose synonyms, alternative wording or explanatory phrases. Brackets are used in the Alphabetic Index to identify manifestation codes.
   ( ) Parentheses are used in both the Alphabetic Index and Tabular List to enclose supplementary words that may be present or absent in the statement of a disease or procedure without affecting the code number to which it is assigned. The terms within the parentheses are referred to as nonessential modifiers. **The nonessential modifiers in the Alphabetic Index to Diseases apply to subterms following a main term except when a nonessential modifier and a subentry are mutually exclusive, the subentry takes precedence. For example, in the ICD-10-CM Alphabetic Index under the main term Enteritis, "acute" is a nonessential modifier and "chronic" is a subentry. In this case, the nonessential modifier "acute" does not apply to the subentry "chronic".**
   : Colons are used in the Tabular List after an incomplete term which needs one or more of the modifiers following the colon to make it assignable to a given category.

8. **Use of "and".**
   See Section I.A.14. Use of the term "And"

9. **Other and Unspecified codes**
   a. **"Other" codes**
   Codes titled "other" or "other specified" are for use when the information in the medical record provides detail for which a specific code does not exist. Alphabetic Index entries with NEC in the line designate "other" codes in the Tabular List. These Alphabetic Index entries represent specific disease entities for which no specific code exists so the term is included within an "other" code.

   b. **"Unspecified" codes**
   Codes titled "unspecified" are for use when the information in the medical record is insufficient to assign a more specific code. For those categories for which an unspecified code is not provided, the "other specified" code may represent both other and unspecified.
   See Section I.B.18 Use of Signs/Symptom/ Unspecified Codes

10. **Includes Notes**
    This note appears immediately under a three-character code title to further define, or give examples of, the content of the category.

11. **Inclusion terms**
    List of terms is included under some codes. These terms are the conditions for which that code is to be used. The terms may be synonyms of the code title, or, in the case of "other specified" codes, the terms are a list of the various conditions assigned to that code. The inclusion terms are not necessarily exhaustive. Additional terms found only in the Alphabetic Index may also be assigned to a code.

12. **Excludes Notes**
    The ICD-10-CM has two types of excludes notes. Each type of note has a different definition for use but they are all similar in that they indicate that codes excluded from each other are independent of each other.

    a. **Excludes1**
    A type 1 Excludes note is a pure excludes note. It means "NOT CODED HERE!" An Excludes1 note indicates that the code excluded should never be used at the same time as the code above the Excludes1 note. An Excludes1 is used when two conditions cannot occur together, such as a congenital form versus an acquired form of the same condition.

    b. **Excludes2**
    A Type 2 Excludes note represents "Not included here". An excludes2 note indicates that the condition excluded is not part of the condition represented by the code, but a patient may have both conditions at the same time. When an Excludes2 note appears under a code, it is acceptable to use both the code and the excluded code together, when appropriate.

13. **Etiology/manifestation convention ("code first", "use additional code" and "in diseases classified elsewhere" notes)**
    Certain conditions have both an underlying etiology and multiple body system manifestations due to the underlying etiology. For such conditions, the ICD-10-CM has a coding convention that requires the underlying condition be sequenced first followed by the manifestation. Wherever such a combination exists, there is a "use additional code" note at the etiology code, and a "code first" note at the manifestation code. These instructional notes indicate the proper sequencing order of the codes, etiology followed by manifestation.

    In most cases the manifestation codes will have in the code title, "in diseases classified elsewhere." Codes with this title are a component of the etiology/ manifestation convention. The code title indicates that it is a manifestation code. "In diseases classified elsewhere" codes are never permitted to be used as first-listed or principal diagnosis codes. They must be used in conjunction with an underlying condition code and they must be listed following the underlying condition. See category F02, Dementia in other diseases classified elsewhere, for an example of this convention.

There are manifestation codes that do not have "in diseases classified elsewhere" in the title. For such codes, **there is a "use additional code" note at the etiology code and a "code first" note at the manifestation code and the rules for sequencing apply.**

In addition to the notes in the Tabular List, these conditions also have a specific Alphabetic Index entry structure. In the Alphabetic Index both conditions are listed together with the etiology code first followed by the manifestation codes in brackets. The code in brackets is always to be sequenced second.

An example of the etiology/manifestation convention is dementia in Parkinson's disease. In the Alphabetic Index, code G20 is listed first, followed by code F02.80 or F02.81 in brackets. Code G20 represents the underlying etiology, Parkinson's disease, and must be sequenced first, whereas codes F02.80 and F02.81 represent the manifestation of dementia in diseases classified elsewhere, with or without behavioral disturbance.

"Code first" and "Use additional code" notes are also used as sequencing rules in the classification for certain codes that are not part of an etiology/ manifestation combination.

See Section I.B.7. Multiple coding for a single condition.

14. **"And"**

The word "and" should be interpreted to mean either "and" or "or" when it appears in a title.

For example, cases of "tuberculosis of bones", "tuberculosis of joints" and "tuberculosis of bones and joints" are classified to subcategory A18.0, Tuberculosis of bones and joints.

15. **"With"**

The word "with" should be interpreted to mean "associated with" or "due to" when it appears in a code title, the Alphabetic Index, or an instructional note in the Tabular List.

The word "with" in the Alphabetic Index is sequenced immediately following the main term, not in alphabetical order.

16. **"See" and "See Also"**

The "see" instruction following a main term in the Alphabetic Index indicates that another term should be referenced. It is necessary to go to the main term referenced with the "see" note to locate the correct code.

A "see also" instruction following a main term in the Alphabetic Index instructs that there is another main term that may also be referenced that may provide additional Alphabetic Index entries that may be useful. It is not necessary to follow the "see also" note when the original main term provides the necessary code.

17. **"Code also note"**

A "code also" note instructs that two codes may be required to fully describe a condition, but this note does not provide sequencing direction.

18. **Default codes**

A code listed next to a main term in the ICD-10-CM Alphabetic Index is referred to as a default code. The default code represents that condition that is most commonly associated with the main term, or is the unspecified code for the condition. If a condition is documented in a medical record (for example, appendicitis) without any additional information, such as acute or chronic, the default code should be assigned.

B. **General Coding Guidelines**

1. **Locating a code in the ICD-10-CM**

To select a code in the classification that corresponds to a diagnosis or reason for visit documented in a medical record, first locate the term in the Alphabetic Index, and then verify the code in the Tabular List. Read and be guided by instructional notations that appear in both the Alphabetic Index and the Tabular List.

It is essential to use both the Alphabetic Index and Tabular List when locating and assigning a code. The Alphabetic Index does not always provide the full code. Selection of the full code, including laterality and any applicable 7th character can only be done in the Tabular List. A dash (-) at the end of an Alphabetic Index entry indicates that additional characters are required. Even if a dash is not included at the Alphabetic Index entry, it is necessary to refer to the Tabular List to verify that no 7th character is required.

2. **Level of Detail in Coding**

Diagnosis codes are to be used and reported at their highest number of characters available.

ICD-10-CM diagnosis codes are composed of codes with 3, 4, 5, 6 or 7 characters. Codes with three characters are included in ICD-10-CM as the heading of a category of codes that may be further subdivided by the use of fourth and/or fifth characters and/or sixth characters, which provide greater detail.

A three-character code is to be used only if it is not further subdivided. A code is invalid if it has not been coded to the full number of characters required for that code, including the 7th character, if applicable.

3. **Code or codes from A00.0 through T88.9, Z00-Z99.8**

The appropriate code or codes from A00.0 through T88.9, Z00-Z99.8 must be used to identify diagnoses, symptoms, conditions, problems, complaints or other reason(s) for the encounter/visit.

4. **Signs and symptoms**

Codes that describe symptoms and signs, as opposed to diagnoses, are acceptable for reporting purposes when a related definitive diagnosis has not been established (confirmed) by the provider.

Chapter 18 of ICD-10-CM, Symptoms, Signs, and Abnormal Clinical and Laboratory Findings, Not Elsewhere Classified (codes R00.0 - R99) contains many, but not all codes for symptoms.

See Section I.B.18 Use of Signs/Symptom/ Unspecified Codes

5. Conditions that are an integral part of a disease process

Signs and symptoms that are associated routinely with a disease process should not be assigned as additional codes, unless otherwise instructed by the classification.

6. Conditions that are not an integral part of a disease process

Additional signs and symptoms that may not be associated routinely with a disease process should be coded when present.

7. Multiple coding for a single condition

In addition to the etiology/manifestation convention that requires two codes to fully describe a single condition that affects multiple body systems, there are other single conditions that also require more than one code. "Use additional code" notes are found in the Tabular List at codes that are not part of an etiology/manifestation pair where a secondary code is useful to fully describe a condition. The sequencing rule is the same as the etiology/manifestation pair, "use additional code" indicates that a secondary code should be added.

For example, for bacterial infections that are not included in chapter 1, a secondary code from category B95, Streptococcus, Staphylococcus, and Enterococcus, as the cause of diseases classified elsewhere, or B96, Other bacterial agents as the cause of diseases classified elsewhere, may be required to identify the bacterial organism causing the infection. A "use additional code" note will normally be found at the infectious disease code, indicating a need for the organism code to be added as a secondary code.

"Code first" notes are also under certain codes that are not specifically manifestation codes but may be due to an underlying cause. When there is a "code first" note and an underlying condition is present, the underlying condition should be sequenced first.

"Code, if applicable, any causal condition first", notes indicate that this code may be assigned as a principal diagnosis when the causal condition is unknown or not applicable. If a causal condition is known, then the code for that condition should be sequenced as the principal or first-listed diagnosis.

Multiple codes may be needed for sequela, complication codes and obstetric codes to more fully describe a condition. See the specific guidelines for these conditions for further instruction.

8. Acute and Chronic Conditions

If the same condition is described as both acute (subacute) and chronic, and separate subentries exist in the Alphabetic Index at the same indentation level, code both and sequence the acute (subacute) code first.

9. Combination Code

A combination code is a single code used to classify:

Two diagnoses, or

A diagnosis with an associated secondary process (manifestation)

A diagnosis with an associated complication

Combination codes are identified by referring to subterm entries in the Alphabetic Index and by reading the inclusion and exclusion notes in the Tabular List.

Assign only the combination code when that code fully identifies the diagnostic conditions involved or when the Alphabetic Index so directs. Multiple coding should not be used when the classification provides a combination code that clearly identifies all of the elements documented in the diagnosis. When the combination code lacks necessary specificity in describing the manifestation or complication, an additional code should be used as a secondary code.

10. Sequela (Late Effects)

A sequela is the residual effect (condition produced) after the acute phase of an illness or injury has terminated. There is no time limit on when a sequela code can be used. The residual may be apparent early, such as in cerebral infarction, or it may occur months or years later, such as that due to a previous injury. Coding of sequela generally requires two codes sequenced in the following order: The condition or nature of the sequela is sequenced first. The sequela code is sequenced second.

An exception to the above guidelines are those instances where the code for the sequela is followed by a manifestation code identified in the Tabular List and title, or the sequela code has been expanded (at the fourth, fifth or sixth character levels) to include the manifestation(s). The code for the acute phase of an illness or injury that led to the sequela is never used with a code for the late effect.

See Section I.C.9. Sequelae of cerebrovascular disease

See Section I.C.15. Sequelae of complication of pregnancy, childbirth and the puerperium

See Section I.C.19. Application of 7th characters for Chapter 19

11. Impending or Threatened Condition

Code any condition described at the time of discharge as "impending" or "threatened" as follows:

If it did occur, code as confirmed diagnosis.

If it did not occur, reference the Alphabetic Index to determine if the condition has a subentry term for "impending" or "threatened" and also reference main term entries for "Impending" and for "Threatened."

If the subterms are listed, assign the given code.

If the subterms are not listed, code the existing underlying condition(s) and not the condition described as impending or threatened.

12. Reporting Same Diagnosis Code More than Once
Each unique ICD-10-CM diagnosis code may be reported only once for an encounter. This applies to bilateral conditions when there are no distinct codes identifying laterality or two different conditions classified to the same ICD-10-CM diagnosis code.

13. Laterality
Some ICD-10-CM codes indicate laterality, **specifying whether the condition occurs on the left, right or is bilateral.** If no bilateral code is provided and the condition is bilateral, assign separate codes for both the left and right side. **If the side is not identified in the medical record, assign the code for the unspecified side.**

14. Documentation for BMI, *Non-pressure ulcers* **and Pressure Ulcer Stages**
For the Body Mass Index (BMI), **depth of non-pressure chronic ulcers** and pressure ulcer stage codes, code assignment may be based on medical record documentation from clinicians who are not the patient's provider (i.e., physician or other qualified healthcare practitioner legally accountable for establishing the patient's diagnosis), since this information is typically documented by other clinicians involved in the care of the patient (e.g., a dietitian often documents the BMI and nurses often documents the pressure ulcer stages). However, the associated diagnosis (such as overweight, obesity, or pressure ulcer) must be documented by the patient's provider. If there is conflicting medical record documentation, either from the same clinician or different clinicians, the patient's attending provider should be queried for clarification.

The BMI codes should only be reported as secondary diagnoses. As with all other secondary diagnosis codes, the BMI codes should only be assigned when they meet the definition of a reportable additional diagnosis (see Section III, Reporting Additional Diagnoses).

15. Syndromes
Follow the Alphabetic Index guidance when coding syndromes. In the absence of Alphabetic Index guidance, assign codes for the documented manifestations of the syndrome. **Additional codes for manifestations that are not an integral part of the disease process may also be assigned when the condition does not have a unique code.**

16. Documentation of Complications of Care
Code assignment is based on the provider's documentation of the relationship between the condition and the care or procedure. The guideline extends to any complications of care, regardless of the chapter the code is located in. It is important to note that not all conditions that occur during or following medical care or surgery are classified as complications. There must be a cause-and-effect relationship between the care provided and the condition, and an indication in the documentation that it is a complication. Query the provider for clarification, if the complication is not clearly documented.

17. Borderline Diagnosis
If the provider documents a "borderline" diagnosis at the time of discharge, the diagnosis is coded as confirmed, unless the classification provides a specific entry (e.g., borderline diabetes). If a borderline condition has a specific index entry in ICD-10-CM, it should be coded as such. Since borderline conditions are not uncertain diagnoses, no distinction is made between the care setting (inpatient versus outpatient). Whenever the documentation is unclear regarding a borderline condition, coders are encouraged to query for clarification.

18. Use of Sign/Symptom/Unspecified Codes
Sign/symptom and "unspecified" codes have **acceptable, even necessary, uses. While specific diagnosis codes should be reported when they are supported by the available medical record documentation and clinical knowledge of the patient's health condition, there are instances when signs/symptoms or unspecified codes are the best choices for accurately reflecting the healthcare encounter. Each healthcare encounter should be coded to the level of certainty known for that encounter.**

If a definitive diagnosis has not been established by the end of the encounter, it is appropriate to report codes for sign(s) and/or symptom(s) in lieu of a definitive diagnosis. When sufficient clinical information isn't known or available about a particular health condition to assign a more specific code, it is acceptable to report the appropriate "unspecified" code (e.g., a diagnosis of pneumonia has been determined, but not the specific type). Unspecified codes should be reported when they are the codes that most accurately reflects what is known about the patient's condition at the time of that particular encounter. It would be inappropriate to select a specific code that is not supported by the medical record documentation or conduct medically unnecessary diagnostic testing in order to determine a more specific code.

C. Chapter-Specific Coding Guidelines
In addition to general coding guidelines, there are guidelines for specific diagnoses and/or conditions in the classification. Unless otherwise indicated, these guidelines apply to all health care settings. Please refer to Section II for guidelines on the selection of principal diagnosis.

1. Chapter 1: Certain Infectious and Parasitic Diseases (A00-B99)

a. Human Immunodeficiency Virus (HIV) Infections

1) Code only confirmed cases
Code only confirmed cases of HIV infection/illness. This is an exception to the hospital inpatient guideline Section II, H.

In this context, "confirmation" does not require documentation of positive serology or culture for HIV; the provider's diagnostic statement that the patient is HIV positive, or has an HIV-related illness is sufficient.

2) Selection and sequencing of HIV codes

(a) Patient admitted for HIV-related condition

If a patient is admitted for an HIV-related condition, the principal diagnosis should be B20, Human immunodeficiency virus [HIV] disease followed by additional diagnosis codes for all reported HIV-related conditions.

(b) Patient with HIV disease admitted for unrelated condition

If a patient with HIV disease is admitted for an unrelated condition (such as a traumatic injury), the code for the unrelated condition (e.g., the nature of injury code) should be the principal diagnosis. Other diagnoses would be B20 followed by additional diagnosis codes for all reported HIV-related conditions.

(c) Whether the patient is newly diagnosed

Whether the patient is newly diagnosed or has had previous admissions/encounters for HIV conditions is irrelevant to the sequencing decision.

(d) Asymptomatic human immunodeficiency virus

Z21, Asymptomatic human immunodeficiency virus [HIV] infection status, is to be applied when the patient without any documentation of symptoms is listed as being "HIV positive," "known HIV," "HIV test positive," or similar terminology. Do not use this code if the term "AIDS" is used or if the patient is treated for any HIV-related illness or is described as having any condition(s) resulting from his/her HIV positive status; use B20 in these cases.

(e) Patients with inconclusive HIV serology

Patients with inconclusive HIV serology, but no definitive diagnosis or manifestations of the illness, may be assigned code R75, Inconclusive laboratory evidence of human immunodeficiency virus [HIV].

(f) Previously diagnosed HIV-related illness

Patients with any known prior diagnosis of an HIV-related illness should be coded to B20. Once a patient has developed an HIV-related illness, the patient should always be assigned code B20 on every subsequent admission/encounter. Patients previously diagnosed with any HIV illness (B20) should never be assigned to R75 or Z21, Asymptomatic human immunodeficiency virus [HIV] infection status.

(g) HIV Infection in Pregnancy, Childbirth and the Puerperium

During pregnancy, childbirth or the puerperium, a patient admitted (or presenting for a health care encounter) because of an HIV-related illness should receive a principal diagnosis code of O98.7-, Human immunodeficiency [HIV] disease complicating pregnancy, childbirth and the puerperium, followed by B20 and the code(s) for the HIV-related illness(es). Codes from Chapter 15 always take sequencing priority.

Patients with asymptomatic HIV infection status admitted (or presenting for a health care encounter) during pregnancy, childbirth, or the puerperium should receive codes of O98.7- and Z21.

(h) Encounters for testing for HIV

If a patient is being seen to determine his/her HIV status, use code Z11.4, Encounter for screening for human immunodeficiency virus [HIV]. Use additional codes for any associated high risk behavior.

If a patient with signs or symptoms is being seen for HIV testing, code the signs and symptoms. An additional counseling code Z71.7, Human immunodeficiency virus [HIV] counseling, may be used if counseling is provided during the encounter for the test.

When a patient returns to be informed of his/her HIV test results and the test result is negative, use code Z71.7, Human immunodeficiency virus [HIV] counseling.

If the results are positive, see previous guidelines and assign codes as appropriate.

b. Infectious agents as the cause of diseases classified to other chapters

Certain infections are classified in chapters other than Chapter 1 and no organism is identified as part of the infection code. In these instances, it is necessary to use an additional code from Chapter 1 to identify the organism. A code from category B95, Streptococcus, Staphylococcus, and Enterococcus as the cause of diseases classified to other chapters, B96, Other bacterial agents as the cause of diseases classified to other chapters, or B97, Viral agents as the cause of diseases classified to other chapters, is to be used as an additional code to identify the organism. An instructional note will be found at the infection code advising that an additional organism code is required.

c. Infections resistant to antibiotics

Many bacterial infections are resistant to current antibiotics. It is necessary to identify all infections documented as antibiotic resistant. Assign a code from category Z16, Resistance to antimicrobial drugs, following the infection code only if the infection code does not identify drug resistance.

d. Sepsis, Severe Sepsis, and Septic Shock

1) Coding of Sepsis and Severe Sepsis

(a) Sepsis

For a diagnosis of sepsis, assign the appropriate code for the underlying systemic infection. If the type of infection or causal organism is not further specified, assign code A41.9, Sepsis, unspecified organism.

A code from subcategory R65.2, Severe sepsis, should not be assigned unless severe sepsis or an associated acute organ dysfunction is documented.

(i) Negative or inconclusive blood cultures and sepsis
Negative or inconclusive blood cultures do not preclude a diagnosis of sepsis in patients with clinical evidence of the condition, however, the provider should be queried.

(ii) Urosepsis
The term urosepsis is a nonspecific term. It is not to be considered synonymous with sepsis. It has no default code in the Alphabetic Index. Should a provider use this term, he/she must be queried for clarification.

(iii) Sepsis with organ dysfunction
If a patient has sepsis and associated acute organ dysfunction or multiple organ dysfunction (MOD), follow the instructions for coding severe sepsis.

(iv) Acute organ dysfunction that is not clearly associated with the sepsis
If a patient has sepsis and an acute organ dysfunction, but the medical record documentation indicates that the acute organ dysfunction is related to a medical condition other than the sepsis, do not assign a code from subcategory R65.2, Severe sepsis. An acute organ dysfunction must be associated with the sepsis in order to assign the severe sepsis code. If the documentation is not clear as to whether an acute organ dysfunction is related to the sepsis or another medical condition, query the provider.

(b) Severe sepsis
The coding of severe sepsis requires a minimum of 2 codes: first a code for the underlying systemic infection, followed by a code from subcategory R65.2, Severe sepsis. If the causal organism is not documented, assign code A41.9, Sepsis, unspecified organism, for the infection. Additional code(s) for the associated acute organ dysfunction are also required.

Due to the complex nature of severe sepsis, some cases may require querying the provider prior to assignment of the codes.

2) Septic shock

(a) Septic shock generally refers to circulatory failure associated with severe sepsis, and therefore, it represents a type of acute organ dysfunction.

For all cases of septic shock, the code for the systemic infection should be sequenced first, followed by code R65.21, Severe sepsis with septic shock or code T81.12, Postprocedural septic shock. Any additional codes for the other acute organ dysfunctions should also be assigned. As noted in the sequencing instructions in the Tabular List, the code for septic shock cannot be assigned as a principal diagnosis.

3) Sequencing of severe sepsis
If severe sepsis is present on admission, and meets the definition of principal diagnosis, the underlying systemic infection should be assigned as principal diagnosis followed by the appropriate code from subcategory R65.2 as required by the sequencing rules in the Tabular List. A code from subcategory R65.2 can never be assigned as a principal diagnosis.

When severe sepsis develops during an encounter (it was not present on admission) the underlying systemic infection and the appropriate code from subcategory R65.2 should be assigned as secondary diagnoses.

Severe sepsis may be present on admission but the diagnosis may not be confirmed until sometime after admission. If the documentation is not clear whether severe sepsis was present on admission, the provider should be queried.

4) Sepsis and severe sepsis with a localized infection
If the reason for admission is both sepsis or severe sepsis and a localized infection, such as pneumonia or cellulitis, a code(s) for the underlying systemic infection should be assigned first and the code for the localized infection should be assigned as a secondary diagnosis. If the patient has severe sepsis, a code from subcategory R65.2 should also be assigned as a secondary diagnosis. If the patient is admitted with a localized infection, such as pneumonia, and sepsis/severe sepsis doesn't develop until after admission, the localized infection should be assigned first, followed by the appropriate sepsis/severe sepsis codes.

5) Sepsis due to a postprocedural infection

(a) Documentation of causal relationship
As with all postprocedural complications, code assignment is based on the provider's documentation of the relationship between the infection and the procedure.

(b) Sepsis due to a postprocedural infection
For such cases, the postprocedural infection code, such as, T80.2, Infections following infusion, transfusion, and therapeutic injection, T81.4, Infection following a procedure, T88.0, Infection following immunization, or O86.0, Infection of obstetric surgical wound, should be coded first, followed by the code for the specific infection. If the patient has severe sepsis the appropriate code from subcategory R65.2 should also be assigned with the additional code(s) for any acute organ dysfunction.

(c) Postprocedural infection and postprocedural septic shock

In cases where a postprocedural infection has occurred and has resulted in severe sepsis and postprocedural septic shock, the code for the precipitating complication such as code T81.4, Infection following a procedure, or O86.0, Infection of obstetrical surgical wound should be coded first followed by code R65.21, Severe sepsis with septic shock and a code for the systemic infection.

6) Sepsis and severe sepsis associated with a noninfectious process (condition)

In some cases a noninfectious process (condition), such as trauma, may lead to an infection which can result in sepsis or severe sepsis. If sepsis or severe sepsis is documented as associated with a noninfectious condition, such as a burn or serious injury, and this condition meets the definition for principal diagnosis, the code for the noninfectious condition should be sequenced first, followed by the code for the resulting infection. If severe sepsis, is present a code from subcategory R65.2 should also be assigned with any associated organ dysfunction(s) codes. It is not necessary to assign a code from subcategory R65.1, Systemic inflammatory response syndrome (SIRS) of non-infectious origin, for these cases.

If the infection meets the definition of principal diagnosis it should be sequenced before the non-infectious condition. When both the associated non-infectious condition and the infection meet the definition of principal diagnosis either may be assigned as principal diagnosis.

Only one code from category R65, Symptoms and signs specifically associated with systemic inflammation and infection, should be assigned. Therefore, when a non-infectious condition leads to an infection resulting in severe sepsis, assign the appropriate code from subcategory R65.2, Severe sepsis. Do not additionally assign a code from subcategory R65.1, Systemic inflammatory response syndrome (SIRS) of non-infectious origin.

See Section I.C.18. SIRS due to non-infectious process

7) Sepsis and septic shock complicating abortion, pregnancy, childbirth, and the puerperium

See Section I.C.15. Sepsis and septic shock complicating abortion, pregnancy, childbirth and the puerperium

8) Newborn sepsis

See Section I.C.16. f. Bacterial sepsis of Newborn

e. Methicillin Resistant *Staphylococcus aureus* (MRSA) Conditions

1) Selection and sequencing of MRSA codes

(a) Combination codes for MRSA infection

When a patient is diagnosed with an infection that is due to methicillin resistant *Staphylococcus aureus* (MRSA), and that infection has a combination code that includes the causal organism (e.g., sepsis, pneumonia) assign the appropriate combination code for the condition (e.g., code A41.02, Sepsis due to Methicillin resistant Staphylococcus aureus

or code J15.212, Pneumonia due to Methicillin resistant Staphylococcus aureus). Do not assign code B95.62, Methicillin resistant Staphylococcus aureus infection as the cause of diseases classified elsewhere, as an additional code because the combination code includes the type of infection and the MRSA organism. Do not assign a code from subcategory Z16.11, Resistance to penicillins, as an additional diagnosis.

See Section C.1. for instructions on coding and sequencing of sepsis and severe sepsis.

(b) Other codes for MRSA infection

When there is documentation of a current infection (e.g., wound infection, stitch abscess, urinary tract infection) due to MRSA, and that infection does not have a combination code that includes the causal organism, assign the appropriate code to identify the condition along with code B95.62, Methicillin resistant Staphylococcus aureus infection as the cause of diseases classified elsewhere for the MRSA infection. Do not assign a code from subcategory Z16.11, Resistance to penicillins.

(c) Methicillin susceptible Staphylococcus aureus (MSSA) and MRSA colonization

The condition or state of being colonized or carrying MSSA or MRSA is called colonization or carriage, while an individual person is described as being colonized or being a carrier. Colonization means that MSSA or MSRA is present on or in the body without necessarily causing illness. A positive MRSA colonization test might be documented by the provider as "MRSA screen positive" or "MRSA nasal swab positive".

Assign code Z22.322, Carrier or suspected carrier of Methicillin resistant Staphylococcus aureus, for patients documented as having MRSA colonization. Assign code Z22.321, Carrier or suspected carrier of Methicillin susceptible Staphylococcus aureus, for patient documented as having MSSA colonization. Colonization is not necessarily indicative of a disease process or as the cause of a specific condition the patient may have unless documented as such by the provider.

(d) MRSA colonization and infection

If a patient is documented as having both MRSA colonization and infection during a hospital admission, code Z22.322, Carrier or suspected carrier of Methicillin resistant Staphylococcus aureus, and a code for the MRSA infection may both be assigned.

2. Chapter 2: Neoplasms (C00-D49)
General guidelines

Chapter 2 of the ICD-10-CM contains the codes for most benign and all malignant neoplasms. Certain benign neoplasms, such as prostatic adenomas, may be found in the specific body system chapters. To properly code a neoplasm it is necessary to determine from the record if the neoplasm is benign, in-situ, malignant, or of uncertain histologic behavior. If malignant, any secondary (metastatic) sites should also be determined.

Primary malignant neoplasms overlapping site boundaries

A primary malignant neoplasm that overlaps two or more contiguous (next to each other) sites should be classified to the subcategory/ code .8 ('overlapping lesion'), unless the combination is specifically indexed elsewhere. For multiple neoplasms of the same site that are not contiguous such as tumors in different quadrants of the same breast, codes for each site should be assigned.

Malignant neoplasm of ectopic tissue

Malignant neoplasms of ectopic tissue are to be coded to the site **of origin** mentioned, e.g., ectopic pancreatic malignant neoplasms **involving the stomach** are coded to pancreas, unspecified (C25.9).

The neoplasm table in the Alphabetic Index should be referenced first. However, if the histological term is documented, that term should be referenced first, rather than going immediately to the Neoplasm Table, in order to determine which column in the Neoplasm Table is appropriate. For example, if the documentation indicates "adenoma," refer to the term in the Alphabetic Index to review the entries under this term and the instructional note to "see also neoplasm, by site, benign." The table provides the proper code based on the type of neoplasm and the site. It is important to select the proper column in the table that corresponds to the type of neoplasm. The Tabular List should then be referenced to verify that the correct code has been selected from the table and that a more specific site code does not exist.

See Section I.C.21. Factors influencing health status and contact with health services, Status, for information regarding Z15.0, codes for genetic susceptibility to cancer.

a. Treatment directed at the malignancy

If the treatment is directed at the malignancy, designate the malignancy as the principal diagnosis.

The only exception to this guideline is if a patient admission/encounter is solely for the administration of chemotherapy, immunotherapy or radiation therapy, assign the appropriate Z51.— code as the first-listed or principal diagnosis, and the diagnosis or problem for which the service is being performed as a secondary diagnosis.

b. Treatment of secondary site

When a patient is admitted because of a primary neoplasm with metastasis and treatment is directed toward the secondary site only, the secondary neoplasm is designated as the principal diagnosis even though the primary malignancy is still present.

c. Coding and sequencing of complications

Coding and sequencing of complications associated with the malignancies or with the therapy thereof are subject to the following guidelines:

1) Anemia associated with malignancy

When admission/encounter is for management of an anemia associated with the malignancy, and the treatment is only for anemia, the appropriate code for the malignancy is sequenced as the principal or first-listed diagnosis followed by the appropriate code for the anemia (such as code D63.0, Anemia in neoplastic disease).

2) Anemia associated with chemotherapy, immunotherapy and radiation therapy

When the admission/encounter is for management of an anemia associated with an adverse effect of the administration of chemotherapy or immunotherapy and the only treatment is for the anemia, the anemia code is sequenced first followed by the appropriate codes for the neoplasm and the adverse effect (T45.1X5, Adverse effect of antineoplastic and immunosuppressive drugs).

When the admission/encounter is for management of an anemia associated with an adverse effect of radiotherapy, the anemia code should be sequenced first, followed by the appropriate neoplasm code and code Y84.2, Radiological procedure and radiotherapy as the cause of abnormal reaction of the patient, or of later complication, without mention of misadventure at the time of the procedure.

3) Management of dehydration due to the malignancy

When the admission/encounter is for management of dehydration due to the malignancy and only the dehydration is being treated (intravenous rehydration), the dehydration is sequenced first, followed by the code(s) for the malignancy.

4) Treatment of a complication resulting from a surgical procedure

When the admission/encounter is for treatment of a complication resulting from a surgical procedure, designate the complication as the principal or first-listed diagnosis if treatment is directed at resolving the complication.

d. Primary malignancy previously excised

When a primary malignancy has been previously excised or eradicated from its site and there is no further treatment directed to that site and there is no evidence of any existing primary malignancy, a code from category Z85, Personal history of malignant neoplasm, should be used to indicate the former site of the malignancy. Any mention of extension, invasion, or metastasis to another site is coded as a secondary malignant neoplasm to that site. The secondary site may be the principal or first-listed with the Z85 code used as a secondary code.

e. Admissions/Encounters involving chemotherapy, immunotherapy and radiation therapy

1) Episode of care involves surgical removal of neoplasm

When an episode of care involves the surgical removal of a neoplasm, primary or secondary site, followed by adjunct chemotherapy or radiation treatment during the same episode of care, the code for the neoplasm should be assigned as principal or first-listed diagnosis.

2) Patient admission/encounter solely for administration of chemotherapy, immunotherapy and radiation therapy

If a patient admission/encounter is solely for the administration of chemotherapy, immunotherapy or radiation therapy assign code Z51.0, Encounter for antineoplastic radiation therapy, or Z51.11, Encounter for antineoplastic chemotherapy, or Z51.12, Encounter for antineoplastic immunotherapy as the first-listed or principal diagnosis. If a patient receives more than one of these therapies during the same admission more than one of these codes may be assigned, in any sequence.

The malignancy for which the therapy is being administered should be assigned as a secondary diagnosis.

3) Patient admitted for radiation therapy, chemotherapy or immunotherapy and develops complications

When a patient is admitted for the purpose of radiotherapy, immunotherapy or chemotherapy and develops complications such as uncontrolled nausea and vomiting or dehydration, the principal or first-listed diagnosis is Z51.0, Encounter for antineoplastic radiation therapy, or Z51.11, Encounter for antineoplastic chemotherapy, or Z51.12, Encounter for antineoplastic immunotherapy followed by any codes for the complications.

f. Admission/encounter to determine extent of malignancy

When the reason for admission/encounter is to determine the extent of the malignancy, or for a procedure such as paracentesis or thoracentesis, the primary malignancy or appropriate metastatic site is designated as the principal or first-listed diagnosis, even though chemotherapy or radiotherapy is administered.

g. Symptoms, signs, and abnormal findings listed in Chapter 18 associated with neoplasms

Symptoms, signs, and ill-defined conditions listed in Chapter 18 characteristic of, or associated with, an existing primary or secondary site malignancy cannot be used to replace the malignancy as principal or first-listed diagnosis, regardless of the number of admissions or encounters for treatment and care of the neoplasm.

See section I.C.21. Factors influencing health status and contact with health services, Encounter for prophylactic organ removal.

h. Admission/encounter for pain control/ management

See Section I.C.6. for information on coding admission/ encounter for pain control/management.

i. Malignancy in two or more noncontiguous sites

A patient may have more than one malignant tumor in the same organ. These tumors may

represent different primaries or metastatic disease, depending on the site. Should the documentation be unclear, the provider should be queried as to the status of each tumor so that the correct codes can be assigned.

j. Disseminated malignant neoplasm, unspecified

Code C80.0, Disseminated malignant neoplasm, unspecified, is for use only in those cases where the patient has advanced metastatic disease and no known primary or secondary sites are specified. It should not be used in place of assigning codes for the primary site and all known secondary sites.

k. Malignant neoplasm without specification of site

Code C80.1, Malignant (primary) neoplasm, unspecified, equates to Cancer, unspecified. This code should only be used when no determination can be made as to the primary site of a malignancy. This code should rarely be used in the inpatient setting.

l. Sequencing of neoplasm codes

1) Encounter for treatment of primary malignancy

If the reason for the encounter is for treatment of a primary malignancy, assign the malignancy as the principal/first-listed diagnosis. The primary site is to be sequenced first, followed by any metastatic sites.

2) Encounter for treatment of secondary malignancy

When an encounter is for a primary malignancy with metastasis and treatment is directed toward the metastatic (secondary) site(s) only, the metastatic site(s) is designated as the principal/ first-listed diagnosis. The primary malignancy is coded as an additional code.

3) Malignant neoplasm in a pregnant patient

When a pregnant woman has a malignant neoplasm, a code from subcategory O9A.1-, Malignant neoplasm complicating pregnancy, childbirth, and the puerperium, should be sequenced first, followed by the appropriate code from Chapter 2 to indicate the type of neoplasm.

4) Encounter for complication associated with a neoplasm

When an encounter is for management of a complication associated with a neoplasm, such as dehydration, and the treatment is only for the complication, the complication is coded first, followed by the appropriate code(s) for the neoplasm.

The exception to this guideline is anemia. When the admission/encounter is for management of an anemia associated with the malignancy, and the treatment is only for anemia, the appropriate code for the malignancy is sequenced as the principal or first-listed diagnosis followed by code D63.0, Anemia in neoplastic disease.

5) Complication from surgical procedure for treatment of a neoplasm

When an encounter is for treatment of a complication resulting from a surgical procedure performed for the treatment of the neoplasm, designate the complication as the principal/first-listed diagnosis. See guideline regarding the coding of a current malignancy versus personal history to determine if the code for the neoplasm should also be assigned.

6) Pathologic fracture due to a neoplasm

When an encounter is for a pathological fracture due to a neoplasm, and the focus of treatment is the fracture, a code from subcategory M84.5, Pathological fracture in neoplastic disease, should be sequenced first, followed by the code for the neoplasm.

If the focus of treatment is the neoplasm with an associated pathological fracture, the neoplasm code should be sequenced first, followed by a code from M84.5 for the pathological fracture.

m. Current malignancy versus personal history of malignancy

When a primary malignancy has been excised but further treatment, such as an additional surgery for the malignancy, radiation therapy or chemotherapy is directed to that site, the primary malignancy code should be used until treatment is completed.

When a primary malignancy has been previously excised or eradicated from its site, there is no further treatment (of the malignancy) directed to that site, and there is no evidence of any existing primary malignancy, a code from category Z85, Personal history of malignant neoplasm, should be used to indicate the former site of the malignancy.

See Section I.C.21. Factors influencing health status and contact with health services, History (of)

n. Leukemia, Multiple Myeloma, and Malignant Plasma Cell Neoplasms in remission versus personal history

The categories for leukemia, and category C90, Multiple myeloma and malignant plasma cell neoplasms, have codes indicating whether or not the leukemia has achieved remission. There are also codes Z85.6, Personal history of leukemia, and Z85.79, Personal history of other malignant neoplasms of lymphoid, hematopoietic and related tissues. If the documentation is unclear, as to whether the leukemia has achieved remission, the provider should be queried.

See Section I.C.21. Factors influencing health status and contact with health services, History (of)

o. Aftercare following surgery for neoplasm

See Section I.C.21. Factors influencing health status and contact with health services, Aftercare

p. Follow-up care for completed treatment of a malignancy

See Section I.C.21. Factors influencing health status and contact with health services, Follow-up

q. Prophylactic organ removal for prevention of malignancy

See Section I.C. 21, Factors influencing health status and contact with health services, Prophylactic organ removal

r. Malignant neoplasm associated with transplanted organ

A malignant neoplasm of a transplanted organ should be coded as a transplant complication. Assign first the appropriate code from category T86.-, Complications of transplanted organs and tissue, followed by code C80.2, Malignant neoplasm associated with transplanted organ. Use an additional code for the specific malignancy.

3. Chapter 3: Disease of the blood and blood-forming organs and certain disorders involving the immune mechanism (D50-D89)

Reserved for future guideline expansion

4. Chapter 4: Endocrine, Nutritional, and Metabolic Diseases (E00-E89)

a. Diabetes mellitus

The diabetes mellitus codes are combination codes that include the type of diabetes mellitus, the body system affected, and the complications affecting that body system. As many codes within a particular category as are necessary to describe all of the complications of the disease may be used. They should be sequenced based on the reason for a particular encounter. Assign as many codes from categories E08 – E13 as needed to identify all of the associated conditions that the patient has.

1) Type of diabetes

The age of a patient is not the sole determining factor, though most type 1 diabetics develop the condition before reaching puberty. For this reason type 1 diabetes mellitus is also referred to as juvenile diabetes.

2) Type of diabetes mellitus not documented

If the type of diabetes mellitus is not documented in the medical record the default is E11.-, Type 2 diabetes mellitus.

3) Diabetes mellitus and the use of insulin

If the documentation in a medical record does not indicate the type of diabetes but does indicate that the patient uses insulin, code E11, Type 2 diabetes mellitus, should be assigned. Code Z79.4, Long-term (current) use of insulin, should also be assigned to indicate that the patient uses insulin. Code Z79.4 should not be assigned if insulin is given temporarily to bring a type 2 patient's blood sugar under control during an encounter.

4) Diabetes mellitus in pregnancy and gestational diabetes

See Section I.C.15. Diabetes mellitus in pregnancy.
See Section I.C.15. Gestational (pregnancy induced) diabetes

5) Complications due to insulin pump malfunction

(a) Underdose of insulin due to insulin pump failure

An underdose of insulin due to an insulin pump failure should be assigned to a code from subcategory T85.6, Mechanical complication of other specified internal and external prosthetic devices, implants and grafts, that specifies the type of pump malfunction, as the principal or first-listed code, followed by code T38.3x6-, Underdosing of insulin and oral hypoglycemic [antidiabetic] drugs. Additional codes for the type of diabetes mellitus and any associated complications due to the underdosing should also be assigned.

(b) Overdose of insulin due to insulin pump failure

The principal or first-listed code for an encounter due to an insulin pump malfunction resulting in an overdose of insulin, should also be T85.6-, Mechanical complication of other specified internal and external prosthetic devices, implants and grafts, followed by code T38.3x1-, Poisoning by insulin and oral hypoglycemic [antidiabetic] drugs, accidental (unintentional).

6) Secondary diabetes mellitus

Codes under categories E08, Diabetes mellitus due to underlying condition, E09, Drug or chemical induced diabetes mellitus **and E13, Other specified diabetes mellitus,** identify complications/manifestations associated with secondary diabetes mellitus. Secondary diabetes is always caused by another condition or event (e.g., cystic fibrosis, malignant neoplasm of pancreas, pancreatectomy, adverse effect of drug, or poisoning).

(a) Secondary diabetes mellitus and the use of insulin

For patients who routinely use insulin, code Z79.4, Long-term (current) use of insulin, should also be assigned. Code Z79.4 should not be assigned if insulin is given temporarily to bring a patient's blood sugar under control during an encounter.

(b) Assigning and sequencing secondary diabetes codes and its causes

The sequencing of the secondary diabetes codes in relationship to codes for the cause of the diabetes is based on the Tabular List instructions for categories E08, E09 **and E13.**

(i) Secondary diabetes mellitus due to pancreatectomy For postpancreatectomy diabetes mellitus (lack of insulin due to the surgical removal of all or part of the pancreas), assign code E89.1, Postprocedural hypoinsulinemia. Assign a code from category E13 and a code from subcategory Z90.41-, Acquired absence of pancreas, as additional codes.

(ii) Secondary diabetes due to drugs

Secondary diabetes may be caused by an adverse effect of correctly administered medications, poisoning or sequela of poisoning.

See section I.C.19.e for coding of adverse effects and poisoning, and section I.C.20 for external cause code reporting.

5. **Chapter 5: Mental, Behavioral and *Neurodevelopmental* disorders (F01 – F99)**

a. Pain disorders related to psychological factors

Assign code F45.41, for pain that is exclusively related to psychological disorders. As indicated by the Excludes 1 note under category G89, a code from category G89 should not be assigned with code F45.41

Code F45.42, Pain disorders with related psychological factors, should be used with a code from category G89, Pain, not elsewhere classified, if there is documentation of a psychological component for a patient with acute or chronic pain.

See Section I.C.6. Pain

c. Mental and behavioral disorders due to psychoactive substance use

1) In Remission

Selection of codes for "in remission" for categories F10-F19, Mental and behavioral disorders due to psychoactive substance use (categories F10-F19 with -.21) requires the provider's clinical judgment. The appropriate codes for "in remission" are assigned only on the basis of provider documentation (as defined in the Official Guidelines for Coding and Reporting).

2) Psychoactive Substance Use, Abuse And Dependence

When the provider documentation refers to use, abuse and dependence of the same substance (e.g. alcohol, opioid, cannabis, etc.), only one code should be assigned to identify the pattern of use based on the following hierarchy:

- If both use and abuse are documented, assign only the code for abuse
- If both abuse and dependence are documented, assign only the code for dependence
- If use, abuse and dependence are all documented, assign only the code for dependence
- If both use and dependence are documented, assign only the code for dependence.

3) Psychoactive Substance Use

As with all other diagnoses, the codes for psychoactive substance use (F10.9-, F11.9-, F12.9-, F13.9-, F14.9-, F15.9-, F16.9-) should only be assigned based on provider documentation and when they meet the definition of a reportable diagnosis (see Section III, Reporting Additional Diagnoses). The codes are to be used only when the psychoactive substance use is associated with a mental or behavioral disorder, and such a relationship is documented by the provider.

6. **Chapter 6: Diseases of the Nervous System (G00-G99)**

   a. **Dominant/nondominant side**

   Codes from category G81, Hemiplegia and hemiparesis, and subcategories, G83.1, Monoplegia of lower limb, G83.2, Monoplegia of upper limb, and G83.3, Monoplegia, unspecified, identify whether the dominant or nondominant side is affected. Should the affected side be documented, but not specified as dominant or nondominant, and the classification system does not indicate a default, code selection is as follows:

   - For ambidextrous patients, the default should be dominant.
   - If the left side is affected, the default is non-dominant.
   - If the right side is affected, the default is dominant.

   b. **Pain - Category G89**

   1) **General coding information**

   Codes in category G89, Pain, not elsewhere classified, may be used in conjunction with codes from other categories and chapters to provide more detail about acute or chronic pain and neoplasm-related pain, unless otherwise indicated below.

   If the pain is not specified as acute or chronic, post-thoracotomy, postprocedural, or neoplasm-related, do not assign codes from category G89.

   A code from category G89 should not be assigned if the underlying (definitive) diagnosis is known, unless the reason for the encounter is pain control/management and not management of the underlying condition.

   When an admission or encounter is for a procedure aimed at treating the underlying condition (e.g., spinal fusion, kyphoplasty), a code for the underlying condition (e.g., vertebral fracture, spinal stenosis) should be assigned as the principal diagnosis. No code from category G89 should be assigned.

   (a) **Category G89 Codes as Principal or First-Listed Diagnosis**

   Category G89 codes are acceptable as principal diagnosis or the first-listed code:

   - When pain control or pain management is the reason for the admission/encounter (e.g., a patient with displaced intervertebral disc, nerve impingement and severe back pain presents for injection of steroid into the spinal canal). The underlying cause of the pain should be reported as an additional diagnosis, if known.
   - When a patient is admitted for the insertion of a neurostimulator for pain control, assign the appropriate pain code as the principal or first-listed diagnosis. When an admission or encounter is for a procedure aimed at treating the underlying condition and a

neurostimulator is inserted for pain control during the same admission/encounter, a code for the underlying condition should be assigned as the principal diagnosis and the appropriate pain code should be assigned as a secondary diagnosis.

   (b) **Use of Category G89 Codes in Conjunction with Site Specific Pain Codes**

   (i) **Assigning Category G89 and Site-Specific Pain Codes**

   Codes from category G89 may be used in conjunction with codes that identify the site of pain (including codes from chapter 18) if the category G89 code provides additional information. For example, if the code describes the site of the pain, but does not fully describe whether the pain is acute or chronic, then both codes should be assigned.

   (ii) **Sequencing of Category G89 Codes with Site-Specific Pain Codes**

   The sequencing of category G89 codes with site-specific pain codes (including chapter 18 codes), is dependent on the circumstances of the encounter/admission as follows:

   - If the encounter is for pain control or pain management, assign the code from category G89 followed by the code identifying the specific site of pain (e.g., encounter for pain management for acute neck pain from trauma is assigned code G89.11, Acute pain due to trauma, followed by code M54.2, Cervicalgia, to identify the site of pain).
   - If the encounter is for any other reason except pain control or pain management, and a related definitive diagnosis has not been established (confirmed) by the provider, assign the code for the specific site of pain first, followed by the appropriate code from category G89.

   2) **Pain due to devices, implants and grafts**
   See Section I.C.19. Pain due to medical devices

   3) **Postoperative Pain**
   The provider's documentation should be used to guide the coding of postoperative pain, as well as *Section III. Reporting Additional Diagnoses* and *Section IV. Diagnostic Coding and Reporting in the Outpatient Setting.*

   The default for post-thoracotomy and other postoperative pain not specified as acute or chronic is the code for the acute form.

   Routine or expected postoperative pain immediately after surgery should not be coded.

   (a) **Postoperative pain not associated with specific postoperative complication**
   Postoperative pain not associated with a specific postoperative complication is assigned to the appropriate postoperative pain code in category G89.

(b) Postoperative pain associated with specific postoperative complication

Postoperative pain associated with a specific postoperative complication (such as painful wire sutures) is assigned to the appropriate code(s) found in Chapter 19, Injury, poisoning, and certain other consequences of external causes. If appropriate, use additional code(s) from category G89 to identify acute or chronic pain (G89.18 or G89.28).

4) Chronic pain

Chronic pain is classified to subcategory G89.2. There is no time frame defining when pain becomes chronic pain. The provider's documentation should be used to guide use of these codes.

5) Neoplasm Related Pain

Code G89.3 is assigned to pain documented as being related, associated or due to cancer, primary or secondary malignancy, or tumor. This code is assigned regardless of whether the pain is acute or chronic.

This code may be assigned as the principal or first-listed code when the stated reason for the admission/encounter is documented as pain control/pain management. The underlying neoplasm should be reported as an additional diagnosis.

When the reason for the admission/encounter is management of the neoplasm and the pain associated with the neoplasm is also documented, code G89.3 may be assigned as an additional diagnosis. It is not necessary to assign an additional code for the site of the pain.

See Section I.C.2 for instructions on the sequencing of neoplasms for all other stated reasons for the admission/encounter (except for pain control/pain management).

6) Chronic pain syndrome

Central pain syndrome (G89.0) and chronic pain syndrome (G89.4) are different than the term "chronic pain," and therefore codes should only be used when the provider has specifically documented this condition.

See Section I.C.5. Pain disorders related to psychological factors

7. Chapter 7: Diseases of the Eye and Adnexa (H00-H59)

a. Glaucoma

1) Assigning Glaucoma Codes

Assign as many codes from category H40, Glaucoma, as needed to identify the type of glaucoma, the affected eye, and the glaucoma stage.

2) Bilateral glaucoma with same type and stage

When a patient has bilateral glaucoma and both eyes are documented as being the same type and stage, and there is a code for bilateral glaucoma, report only the code for the type of glaucoma, bilateral, with the seventh character for the stage.

When a patient has bilateral glaucoma and both eyes are documented as being the same type and stage, and the classification does not provide a code for bilateral glaucoma (i.e. subcategories H40.10, H40.11 and H40.20) report only one code for the type of glaucoma with the appropriate seventh character for the stage.

3) Bilateral glaucoma stage with different types or stages

When a patient has bilateral glaucoma and each eye is documented as having a different type or stage, and the classification distinguishes laterality, assign the appropriate code for each eye rather than the code for bilateral glaucoma.

When a patient has bilateral glaucoma and each eye is documented as having a different type, and the classification does not distinguish laterality (i.e. subcategories H40.10, H40.11 and H40.20), assign one code for each type of glaucoma with the appropriate seventh character for the stage.

When a patient has bilateral glaucoma and each eye is documented as having the same type, but different stage, and the classification does not distinguish laterality (i.e. subcategories H40.10, H40.11 and H40.20), assign a code for the type of glaucoma for each eye with the seventh character for the specific glaucoma stage documented for each eye.

4) Patient admitted with glaucoma and stage evolves during the admission

If a patient is admitted with glaucoma and the stage progresses during the admission, assign the code for highest stage documented.

5) Indeterminate stage glaucoma

Assignment of the seventh character "4" for "indeterminate stage" should be based on the clinical documentation. The seventh character "4" is used for glaucomas whose stage cannot be clinically determined. This seventh character should not be confused with the seventh character "0", unspecified, which should be assigned when there is no documentation regarding the stage of the glaucoma.

8. Chapter 8: Diseases of the Ear and Mastoid Process (H60-H95)

Reserved for future guideline expansion

9. Chapter 9: Diseases of the Circulatory System (I00-I99)

a. Hypertension

1) Hypertension with Heart Disease

Heart conditions classified to I50.- or I51.4-I51.9, are assigned to, a code from category I11, Hypertensive heart disease, when a causal relationship is stated (due to hypertension) or implied (hypertensive). Use an additional code from category I50, Heart failure, to identify the type of heart failure in those patients with heart failure.

The same heart conditions (I50.-, I51.4-I51.9) with hypertension, but without a stated causal relationship, are coded separately. Sequence according to the circumstances of the admission/encounter.

2) Hypertensive Chronic Kidney Disease

Assign codes from category I12, Hypertensive chronic kidney disease, when both hypertension and a condition classifiable to category N18, Chronic kidney disease (CKD), are present. Unlike hypertension with heart disease, ICD-10-CM presumes a cause-and-effect relationship and classifies chronic kidney disease with hypertension as hypertensive chronic kidney disease.

The appropriate code from category N18 should be used as a secondary code with a code from category I12 to identify the stage of chronic kidney disease.

See Section I.C.14. Chronic kidney disease.

If a patient has hypertensive chronic kidney disease and acute renal failure, an additional code for the acute renal failure is required.

3) Hypertensive Heart and Chronic Kidney Disease

Assign codes from combination category I13, Hypertensive heart and chronic kidney disease, when both hypertensive kidney disease and hypertensive heart disease are stated in the diagnosis. Assume a relationship between the hypertension and the chronic kidney disease, whether or not the condition is so designated. If heart failure is present, assign an additional code from category I50 to identify the type of heart failure.

The appropriate code from category N18, Chronic kidney disease, should be used as a secondary code with a code from category I13 to identify the stage of chronic kidney disease.

See Section I.C.14. Chronic kidney disease.

The codes in category I13, Hypertensive heart and chronic kidney disease, are combination codes that include hypertension, heart disease and chronic kidney disease. The Includes note at I13 specifies that the conditions included at I11 and I12 are included together in I13. If a patient has hypertension, heart disease and chronic kidney disease then a code from I13 should be used, not individual codes for hypertension, heart disease and chronic kidney disease, or codes from I11 or I12.

For patients with both acute renal failure and chronic kidney disease an additional code for acute renal failure is required.

4) Hypertensive Cerebrovascular Disease

For hypertensive cerebrovascular disease, first assign the appropriate code from categories I60–I69, followed by the appropriate hypertension code.

5) Hypertensive Retinopathy

Subcategory H35.0, Background retinopathy and retinal vascular changes, should be used with a code from category I10 – I15, Hypertensive disease to include the systemic hypertension. The sequencing is based on the reason for the encounter.

6) Hypertension, Secondary

Secondary hypertension is due to an underlying condition. Two codes are required: one to identify the underlying etiology and one from category I15 to identify the hypertension. Sequencing of codes is determined by the reason for admission/encounter.

7) Hypertension, Transient

Assign code R03.0, Elevated blood pressure reading without diagnosis of hypertension, unless patient has an established diagnosis of hypertension. Assign code O13.-, Gestational [pregnancy-induced] hypertension without significant proteinuria, or O14.-, Pre-eclampsia, for transient hypertension of pregnancy.

8) Hypertension, Controlled

This diagnostic statement usually refers to an existing state of hypertension under control by therapy. Assign the appropriate code from categories I10-I15, Hypertensive diseases.

9) Hypertension, Uncontrolled

Uncontrolled hypertension may refer to untreated hypertension or hypertension not responding to current therapeutic regimen. In either case, assign the appropriate code from categories I10-I15, Hypertensive diseases.

b. Atherosclerotic Coronary Artery Disease and Angina

ICD-10-CM has combination codes for atherosclerotic heart disease with angina pectoris. The subcategories for these codes are I25.11, Atherosclerotic heart disease of native coronary artery with angina pectoris and I25.7, Atherosclerosis of coronary artery bypass graft(s) and coronary artery of transplanted heart with angina pectoris.

When using one of these combination codes it is not necessary to use an additional code for angina pectoris. A causal relationship can be assumed in a patient with both atherosclerosis and angina pectoris, unless the documentation indicates the angina is due to something other than the atherosclerosis.

If a patient with coronary artery disease is admitted due to an acute myocardial infarction (AMI), the AMI should be sequenced before the coronary artery disease.

See Section I.C.9. Acute myocardial infarction (AMI)

c. Intraoperative and Postprocedural Cerebrovascular Accident

Medical record documentation should clearly specify the cause-and-effect relationship between the medical intervention and the cerebrovascular accident in order to assign a code for intraoperative or postprocedural cerebrovascular accident.

Proper code assignment depends on whether it was an infarction or hemorrhage and whether it occurred intraoperatively or postoperatively. If it was a cerebral hemorrhage, code assignment depends on the type of procedure performed.

d. **Sequelae of Cerebrovascular Disease**
   1) **Category I69, Sequelae of Cerebrovascular disease**

Category I69 is used to indicate conditions classifiable to categories I60-I67 as the causes of sequela (neurologic deficits), themselves classified elsewhere. These "late effects" include neurologic deficits that persist after initial onset of conditions classifiable to categories I60-I67. The neurologic deficits caused by cerebrovascular disease may be present from the onset or may arise at any time after the onset of the condition classifiable to categories I60-I67.

Codes from category I69, Sequelae of cerebrovascular disease, that specify hemiplegia, hemiparesis and monoplegia identify whether the dominant or nondominant side is affected. Should the affected side be documented, but not specified as dominant or nondominant, and the classification system does not indicate a default, code selection is as follows:
- **For ambidextrous patients, the default should be dominant.**
- **If the left side is affected, the default is non-dominant.**
- **If the right side is affected, the default is dominant.**

   2) **Codes from category I69 with codes from I60-I67**

Codes from category I69 may be assigned on a health care record with codes from I60-I67, if the patient has a current cerebrovascular disease and deficits from an old cerebrovascular disease.

   3) **Codes from category I69** *and Personal history of transient ischemic attack (TIA) and cerebral infarction (Z86.73)*

Codes from category I69 should not be assigned if the patient does not have neurologic deficits.
   See Section I.C.21. 4. History (of) for use of personal history codes

e. **Acute myocardial infarction (AMI)**
   1) **ST elevation myocardial infarction (STEMI) and non ST elevation myocardial infarction (NSTEMI)**

The ICD-10-CM codes for acute myocardial infarction (AMI) identify the site, such as anterolateral wall or true posterior wall. Subcategories I21.0-I21.2 and code I21.3 are used for ST elevation myocardial infarction (STEMI). Code I21.4, Non-ST elevation (NSTEMI) myocardial infarction, is used for non ST elevation myocardial infarction (NSTEMI) and nontransmural MIs.

If NSTEMI evolves to STEMI, assign the STEMI code. If STEMI converts to NSTEMI due to thrombolytic therapy, it is still coded as STEMI.

For encounters occurring while the myocardial infarction is equal to, or less than, four weeks old, including transfers to another acute setting or a postacute setting, and the patient requires continued care for the myocardial infarction, codes from category I21 may continue to be reported. For encounters after the 4 week time frame and the patient is still receiving care related to the myocardial infarction, the appropriate aftercare code should be assigned, rather than a code from category I21. For old or healed myocardial infarctions not requiring further care, code I25.2, Old myocardial infarction, may be assigned.

   2) **Acute myocardial infarction, unspecified**

Code I21.3, ST elevation (STEMI) myocardial infarction of unspecified site, is the default for unspecified acute myocardial infarction. If only STEMI or transmural MI without the site is documented, assign code I21.3.

   3) **AMI documented as nontransmural or subendocardial but site provided**

If an AMI is documented as nontransmural or subendocardial, but the site is provided, it is still coded as a subendocardial AMI.
   See Section I.C.21.3 for information on coding status post administration of tPA in a different facility within the last 24 hours.

   4) **Subsequent acute myocardial infarction**

A code from category I22, Subsequent ST elevation (STEMI) and non ST elevation (NSTEMI) myocardial infarction, is to be used when a patient who has suffered an AMI has a new AMI within the 4 week time frame of the initial AMI. A code from category I22 must be used in conjunction with a code from category I21. The sequencing of the I22 and I21 codes depends on the circumstances of the encounter.

10. **Chapter 10: Diseases of the Respiratory System (J00-J99)**
   a. **Chronic Obstructive Pulmonary Disease [COPD] and Asthma**
      1) **Acute exacerbation of chronic obstructive bronchitis and asthma**

The codes in categories J44 and J45 distinguish between uncomplicated cases and those in acute exacerbation. An acute exacerbation is a worsening or a decompensation of a chronic condition. An acute exacerbation is not equivalent to an infection superimposed on a chronic condition, though an exacerbation may be triggered by an infection.

   b. **Acute Respiratory Failure**
      1) **Acute respiratory failure as principal diagnosis**

A code from subcategory J96.0, Acute respiratory failure, or subcategory J96.2, Acute and chronic respiratory failure, may be assigned as a principal diagnosis when it is the condition established after study to be chiefly responsible for occasioning the admission to the hospital, and the selection is supported by the Alphabetic Index and Tabular List. However, chapter-specific coding guidelines (such as obstetrics, poisoning, HIV, newborn) that provide sequencing direction take precedence.

      2) **Acute respiratory failure as secondary diagnosis**

Respiratory failure may be listed as a secondary diagnosis if it occurs after admission, or if it is

GUIDELINES (ICD-10-CM)

present on admission, but does not meet the definition of principal diagnosis.

3) Sequencing of acute respiratory failure and another acute condition

When a patient is admitted with respiratory failure and another acute condition, (e.g., myocardial infarction, cerebrovascular accident, aspiration pneumonia), the principal diagnosis will not be the same in every situation. This applies whether the other acute condition is a respiratory or nonrespiratory condition. Selection of the principal diagnosis will be dependent on the circumstances of admission. If both the respiratory failure and the other acute condition are equally responsible for occasioning the admission to the hospital, and there are no chapter-specific sequencing rules, the guideline regarding two or more diagnoses that equally meet the definition for principal diagnosis *(Section II, C.)* may be applied in these situations.

If the documentation is not clear as to whether acute respiratory failure and another condition are equally responsible for occasioning the admission, query the provider for clarification.

c. Influenza due to certain identified influenza viruses

Code only confirmed cases of influenza due to certain identified influenza viruses (category J09), **and due to other identified influenza virus (category J10)**. This is an exception to the hospital inpatient guideline Section II, H. (Uncertain Diagnosis).

In this context, "confirmation" does not require documentation of positive laboratory testing specific for avian or other novel influenza A **or other identified influenza virus**. However, coding should be based on the provider's diagnostic statement that the patient has avian influenza, or other novel influenza A, **for category J09, or has another particular identified strain of influenza, such as H1N1 or H3N2, but not identified as novel or variant, for category J10**.

If the provider records "suspected" or "possible" or "probable" avian influenza, **or novel influenza, or other identified influenza, then** the appropriate influenza code from category J11, Influenza due to unidentified influenza virus, should be assigned. A code from category J09, Influenza due to certain identified influenza viruses, should not be assigned **nor should a code from category J10, Influenza due to other identified influenza virus**.

d. Ventilator associated Pneumonia

1) Documentation of Ventilator associated Pneumonia

As with all procedural or postprocedural complications, code assignment is based on the provider's documentation of the relationship between the condition and the procedure.

Code J95.851, Ventilator associated pneumonia, should be assigned only when the provider has documented ventilator associated pneumonia

(VAP). An additional code to identify the organism (e.g., Pseudomonas aeruginosa, code B96.5) should also be assigned. Do not assign an additional code from categories J12-J18 to identify the type of pneumonia.

Code J95.851 should not be assigned for cases where the patient has pneumonia and is on a mechanical ventilator and the provider has not specifically stated that the pneumonia is ventilator-associated pneumonia. If the documentation is unclear as to whether the patient has a pneumonia that is a complication attributable to the mechanical ventilator, query the provider.

2) Ventilator associated Pneumonia Develops after Admission

A patient may be admitted with one type of pneumonia (e.g., code J13, Pneumonia due to Streptococcus pneumonia) and subsequently develop VAP. In this instance, the principal diagnosis would be the appropriate code from categories J12-J18 for the pneumonia diagnosed at the time of admission. Code J95.851, Ventilator associated pneumonia, would be assigned as an additional diagnosis when the provider has also documented the presence of ventilator associated pneumonia.

11. Chapter 11: Diseases of the Digestive System (K00-K95)

Reserved for future guideline expansion

12. Chapter 12: Diseases of the Skin and Subcutaneous Tissue (L00-L99)

a. Pressure ulcer stage codes

1) Pressure ulcer stages

Codes from category L89, Pressure ulcer, are combination codes that identify the site of the pressure ulcer as well as the stage of the ulcer.

The ICD-10-CM classifies pressure ulcer stages based on severity, which is designated by stages 1-4, unspecified stage and unstageable.

Assign as many codes from category L89 as needed to identify all the pressure ulcers the patient has, if applicable.

2) Unstageable pressure ulcers

Assignment of the code for unstageable pressure ulcer (L89.--0) should be based on the clinical documentation. These codes are used for pressure ulcers whose stage cannot be clinically determined (e.g., the ulcer is covered by eschar or has been treated with a skin or muscle graft) and pressure ulcers that are documented as deep tissue injury but not documented as due to trauma. This code should not be confused with the codes for unspecified stage (L89.--9). When there is no documentation regarding the stage of the pressure ulcer, assign the appropriate code for unspecified stage (L89.--9).

3) Documented pressure ulcer stage

Assignment of the pressure ulcer stage code should be guided by clinical documentation of the stage or documentation of the terms found in the Alphabetic Index. For clinical terms describing the stage that are not found in the Alphabetic Index, and there is no documentation of the stage, the provider should be queried.

4) Patients admitted with pressure ulcers documented as healed

No code is assigned if the documentation states that the pressure ulcer is completely healed.

5) Patients admitted with pressure ulcers documented as healing

Pressure ulcers described as healing should be assigned the appropriate pressure ulcer stage code based on the documentation in the medical record. If the documentation does not provide information about the stage of the healing pressure ulcer, assign the appropriate code for unspecified stage.

If the documentation is unclear as to whether the patient has a current (new) pressure ulcer or if the patient is being treated for a healing pressure ulcer, query the provider.

6) Patient admitted with pressure ulcer evolving into another stage during the admission

If a patient is admitted with a pressure ulcer at one stage and it progresses to a higher stage, assign the code for the highest stage reported for that site.

13. Chapter 13: Diseases of the Musculoskeletal System and Connective Tissue (M00-M99)

a. Site and laterality

Most of the codes within Chapter 13 have site and laterality designations. The site represents the bone, joint or the muscle involved. For some conditions where more than one bone, joint or muscle is usually involved, such as osteoarthritis, there is a "multiple sites" code available. For categories where no multiple site code is provided and more than one bone, joint or muscle is involved, multiple codes should be used to indicate the different sites involved.

1) Bone versus joint

For certain conditions, the bone may be affected at the upper or lower end, (e.g., avascular necrosis of bone, M87, Osteoporosis, M80, M81). Though the portion of the bone affected may be at the joint, the site designation will be the bone, not the joint.

b. Acute traumatic versus chronic or recurrent musculoskeletal conditions

Many musculoskeletal conditions are a result of previous injury or trauma to a site, or are recurrent conditions. Bone, joint or muscle conditions that are the result of a healed injury are usually found in chapter 13. Recurrent bone, joint or muscle conditions are also usually found in chapter 13. Any current, acute injury should be coded to the appropriate injury code from chapter 19. Chronic or recurrent conditions should generally be coded with a code from chapter 13. If it is difficult to determine from the documentation in the record which code is best to describe a condition, query the provider.

c. Coding of Pathologic Fractures

7th character A is for use as long as the patient is receiving active treatment for the fracture. Examples of active treatment are: surgical treatment, emergency department encounter, evaluation and treatment by a new physician. 7th character, D is to be used for encounters after the patient has completed active treatment. The other 7th characters, listed under each subcategory in the Tabular List, are to be used for subsequent encounters for treatment of problems associated with the healing, such as malunions, nonunions, and sequelae.

Care for complications of surgical treatment for fracture repairs during the healing or recovery phase should be coded with the appropriate complication codes.

See Section I.C.19. Coding of traumatic fractures.

d. Osteoporosis

Osteoporosis is a systemic condition, meaning that all bones of the musculoskeletal system are affected. Therefore, site is not a component of the codes under category M81, Osteoporosis without current pathological fracture. The site codes under category M80, Osteoporosis with current pathological fracture, identify the site of the fracture, not the osteoporosis.

1) Osteoporosis without pathological fracture

Category M81, Osteoporosis without current pathological fracture, is for use for patients with osteoporosis who do not currently have a pathologic fracture due to the osteoporosis, even if they have had a fracture in the past. For patients with a history of osteoporosis fractures, status code Z87.310, Personal history of (healed) osteoporosis fracture, should follow the code from M81.

2) Osteoporosis with current pathological fracture

Category M80, Osteoporosis with current pathological fracture, is for patients who have a current pathologic fracture at the time of an encounter. The codes under M80 identify the site of the fracture. A code from category M80, not a traumatic fracture code, should be used for any patient with known osteoporosis who suffers a fracture, even if the patient had a minor fall or trauma, if that fall or trauma would not usually break a normal, healthy bone.

14. Chapter 14: Diseases of Genitourinary System (N00-N99)

a. Chronic kidney disease

1) Stages of chronic kidney disease (CKD)

The ICD-10-CM classifies CKD based on severity. The severity of CKD is designated by stages 1-5. Stage 2, code N18.2, equates to mild CKD; stage 3, code N18.3, equates to moderate CKD; and stage 4, code N18.4, equates to severe CKD. Code N18.6, End stage renal disease (ESRD), is assigned when the provider has documented end-stage-renal disease (ESRD).

If both a stage of CKD and ESRD are documented, assign code N18.6 only.

2) Chronic kidney disease and kidney transplant status

Patients who have undergone kidney transplant may still have some form of chronic kidney disease CKD because the kidney transplant may not fully restore kidney function. Therefore, the presence of CKD alone does not constitute a transplant complication. Assign the appropriate N18 code for the patient's stage of CKD and code Z94.0, Kidney transplant status. If a transplant complication such as failure or rejection or other transplant complication is documented, see section I.C.19.g for information on coding complications of a kidney transplant. If the documentation is unclear as to whether the patient has a complication of the transplant, query the provider.

3) Chronic kidney disease with other conditions

Patients with CKD may also suffer from other serious conditions, most commonly diabetes mellitus and hypertension. The sequencing of the CKD code in relationship to codes for other contributing conditions is based on the conventions in the Tabular List.

See I.C.9. Hypertensive chronic kidney disease.
See I.C.19. Chronic kidney disease and kidney transplant complications.

15. Chapter 15: Pregnancy, Childbirth, and the Puerperium (O00-O9A)

a. General Rules for Obstetric Cases

1) Codes from chapter 15 and sequencing priority

Obstetric cases require codes from chapter 15, codes in the range O00-O9A, Pregnancy, Childbirth, and the Puerperium. Chapter 15 codes have sequencing priority over codes from other chapters. Additional codes from other chapters may be used in conjunction with chapter 15 codes to further specify conditions. Should the provider document that the pregnancy is incidental to the encounter, then code Z33.1, Pregnant state, incidental, should be used in place of any chapter 15 codes. It is the provider's responsibility to state that the condition being treated is not affecting the pregnancy.

2) Chapter 15 codes used only on the maternal record

Chapter 15 codes are to be used only on the maternal record, never on the record of the newborn.

3) Final character for trimester

The majority of codes in Chapter 15 have a final character indicating the trimester of pregnancy. The timeframes for the trimesters are indicated at the beginning of the chapter. If trimester is not a component of a code it is because the condition always occurs in a specific trimester, or the concept of trimester of pregnancy is not applicable. Certain codes have characters for only certain trimesters because the condition does not occur in all trimesters, but it may occur in more than just one.

Assignment of the final character for trimester should be based on the provider's documentation of the trimester (or number of weeks) for the current admission/encounter. This applies to the assignment of trimester for pre-existing conditions as well as those that develop during or are due to the pregnancy. The provider's documentation of the number of weeks may be used to assign the appropriate code identifying the trimester.

Whenever delivery occurs during the current admission, and there is an "in childbirth" option for the obstetric complication being coded, the "in childbirth" code should be assigned.

4) Selection of trimester for inpatient admissions that encompass more than one trimester

In instances when a patient is admitted to a hospital for complications of pregnancy during one trimester and remains in the hospital into a subsequent trimester, the trimester character for the antepartum complication code should be assigned on the basis of the trimester when the complication developed, not the trimester of the discharge. If the condition developed prior to the current admission/encounter or represents a pre-existing condition, the trimester character for the trimester at the time of the admission/encounter should be assigned.

5) Unspecified trimester

Each category that includes codes for trimester has a code for "unspecified trimester." The "unspecified trimester" code should rarely be used, such as when the documentation in the record is insufficient to determine the trimester and it is not possible to obtain clarification.

6) 7th character for Fetus Identification

Where applicable, a 7th character is to be assigned for certain categories (O31, O32, O33.3 - O33.6, O35, O36, O40, O41, O60.1, O60.2, O64, and O69) to identify the fetus for which the complication code applies.

Assign 7th character "0":
- For single gestations
- When the documentation in the record is insufficient to determine the fetus affected and it is not possible to obtain clarification.
- When it is not possible to clinically determine which fetus is affected.

b. Selection of OB Principal or First-listed Diagnosis

1) Routine outpatient prenatal visits

For routine outpatient prenatal visits when no complications are present, a code from category Z34, Encounter for supervision of normal pregnancy, should be used as the first-listed diagnosis. These codes should not be used in conjunction with chapter 15 codes.

2) Prenatal outpatient visits for high-risk patients

For routine prenatal outpatient visits for patients with high-risk pregnancies, a code from category O09, Supervision of high-risk pregnancy, should be used as the first-listed diagnosis. Secondary chapter 15 codes may be used in conjunction with these codes if appropriate.

3) Episodes when no delivery occurs
In episodes when no delivery occurs, the principal diagnosis should correspond to the principal complication of the pregnancy which necessitated the encounter. Should more than one complication exist, all of which are treated or monitored, any of the complications codes may be sequenced first.

4) When a delivery occurs
When a delivery occurs, the principal diagnosis should correspond to the main circumstances or complication of the delivery. In cases of cesarean delivery, the selection of the principal diagnosis should be the condition established after study that was responsible for the patient's admission. If the patient was admitted with a condition that resulted in the performance of a cesarean procedure, that condition should be selected as the principal diagnosis. If the reason for the admission/encounter was unrelated to the condition resulting in the cesarean delivery, the condition related to the reason for the admission/encounter should be selected as the principal diagnosis.

5) Outcome of delivery
A code from category Z37, Outcome of delivery, should be included on every maternal record when a delivery has occurred. These codes are not to be used on subsequent records or on the newborn record.

c. Pre-existing conditions versus conditions due to the pregnancy
Certain categories in Chapter 15 distinguish between conditions of the mother that existed prior to pregnancy (pre-existing) and those that are a direct result of pregnancy. When assigning codes from Chapter 15, it is important to assess if a condition was pre-existing prior to pregnancy or developed during or due to the pregnancy in order to assign the correct code.

Categories that do not distinguish between pre-existing and pregnancy-related conditions may be used for either. It is acceptable to use codes specifically for the puerperium with codes complicating pregnancy and childbirth if a condition arises postpartum during the delivery encounter.

d. Pre-existing hypertension in pregnancy
Category O10, Pre-existing hypertension complicating pregnancy, childbirth and the puerperium, includes codes for hypertensive heart and hypertensive chronic kidney disease. When assigning one of the O10 codes that includes hypertensive heart disease or hypertensive chronic kidney disease, it is necessary to add a secondary code from the appropriate hypertension category to specify the type of heart failure or chronic kidney disease.

See Section I.C.9. Hypertension.

e. Fetal Conditions Affecting the Management of the Mother

1) Codes from categories O35 and O36
Codes from categories O35, Maternal care for known or suspected fetal abnormality and damage, and O36, Maternal care for other fetal problems, are assigned only when the fetal condition is actually responsible for modifying the management of the mother, i.e., by requiring diagnostic studies, additional observation, special care, or termination of pregnancy. The fact that the fetal condition exists does not justify assigning a code from this series to the mother's record.

2) In utero surgery
In cases when surgery is performed on the fetus, a diagnosis code from category O35, Maternal care for known or suspected fetal abnormality and damage, should be assigned identifying the fetal condition. Assign the appropriate procedure code for the procedure performed.

No code from Chapter 16, the perinatal codes, should be used on the mother's record to identify fetal conditions. Surgery performed in utero on a fetus is still to be coded as an obstetric encounter.

f. HIV Infection in Pregnancy, Childbirth and the Puerperium
During pregnancy, childbirth or the puerperium, a patient admitted because of an HIV-related illness should receive a principal diagnosis from subcategory O98.7-, Human immunodeficiency [HIV] disease complicating pregnancy, childbirth and the puerperium, followed by the code(s) for the HIV-related illness(es).

Patients with asymptomatic HIV infection status admitted during pregnancy, childbirth, or the puerperium should receive codes of O98.7- and Z21, Asymptomatic human immunodeficiency virus [HIV] infection status.

g. Diabetes mellitus in pregnancy
Diabetes mellitus is a significant complicating factor in pregnancy. Pregnant women who are diabetic should be assigned a code from category O24, Diabetes mellitus in pregnancy, childbirth, and the puerperium, first, followed by the appropriate diabetes code(s) (E08-E13) from Chapter 4.

h. Long term use of insulin
Code Z79.4, Long-term (current) use of insulin, should also be assigned if the diabetes mellitus is being treated with insulin.

i. Gestational (pregnancy induced) diabetes
Gestational (pregnancy induced) diabetes can occur during the second and third trimester of pregnancy in women who were not diabetic prior to pregnancy. Gestational diabetes can cause complications in the pregnancy similar to those of pre-existing diabetes mellitus. It also puts the woman at greater risk of developing diabetes after the pregnancy. Codes for gestational diabetes are in subcategory O24.4, Gestational

diabetes mellitus. No other code from category O24, Diabetes mellitus in pregnancy, childbirth, and the puerperium, should be used with a code from O24.4.

The codes under subcategory O24.4 include diet controlled and insulin controlled. If a patient with gestational diabetes is treated with both diet and insulin, only the code for insulin-controlled is required.

Code Z79.4, Long-term (current) use of insulin, should not be assigned with codes from subcategory O24.4.

An abnormal glucose tolerance in pregnancy is assigned a code from subcategory O99.81, Abnormal glucose complicating pregnancy, childbirth, and the puerperium.

j. Sepsis and septic shock complicating abortion, pregnancy, childbirth and the puerperium

When assigning a chapter 15 code for sepsis complicating abortion, pregnancy, childbirth, and the puerperium, a code for the specific type of infection should be assigned as an additional diagnosis. If severe sepsis is present, a code from subcategory R65.2, Severe sepsis, and code(s) for associated organ dysfunction(s) should also be assigned as additional diagnoses.

k. Puerperal sepsis

Code O85, Puerperal sepsis, should be assigned with a secondary code to identify the causal organism (e.g., for a bacterial infection, assign a code from category B95-B96, Bacterial infections in conditions classified elsewhere). A code from category A40, Streptococcal sepsis, or A41, Other sepsis, should not be used for puerperal sepsis. If applicable, use additional codes to identify severe sepsis (R65.2-) and any associated acute organ dysfunction.

l. Alcohol and tobacco use during pregnancy, childbirth and the puerperium

1) Alcohol use during pregnancy, childbirth and the puerperium

Codes under subcategory O99.31, Alcohol use complicating pregnancy, childbirth, and the puerperium, should be assigned for any pregnancy case when a mother uses alcohol during the pregnancy or postpartum. A secondary code from category F10, Alcohol related disorders, should also be assigned to identify manifestations of the alcohol use.

2) Tobacco use during pregnancy, childbirth and the puerperium

Codes under subcategory O99.33, Smoking (tobacco) complicating pregnancy, childbirth, and the puerperium, should be assigned for any pregnancy case when a mother uses any type of tobacco product during the pregnancy or postpartum. A secondary code from category F17, Nicotine dependence, should also be assigned to identify the type of nicotine dependence.

m. Poisoning, toxic effects, adverse effects and underdosing in a pregnant patient

A code from subcategory O9A.2, Injury, poisoning and certain other consequences of external causes complicating pregnancy, childbirth, and the puerperium, should be sequenced first, followed by the appropriate injury, poisoning, toxic effect, adverse effect or underdosing code, and then the additional code(s) that specifies the condition caused by the poisoning, toxic effect, adverse effect or underdosing.

See Section I.C.19. Adverse effects, poisoning, underdosing and toxic effects.

n. Normal Delivery, Code O80

1) Encounter for full term uncomplicated delivery

Code O80 should be assigned when a woman is admitted for a full-term normal delivery and delivers a single, healthy infant without any complications antepartum, during the delivery, or postpartum during the delivery episode. Code O80 is always a principal diagnosis. It is not to be used if any other code from chapter 15 is needed to describe a current complication of the antenatal, delivery, or perinatal period. Additional codes from other chapters may be used with code O80 if they are not related to or are in any way complicating the pregnancy.

2) Uncomplicated delivery with resolved antepartum complication

Code O80 may be used if the patient had a complication at some point during the pregnancy, but the complication is not present at the time of the admission for delivery.

3) Outcome of delivery for O80

Z37.0, Single live birth, is the only outcome of delivery code appropriate for use with O80.

o. The Peripartum and Postpartum Periods

1) Peripartum and Postpartum periods

The postpartum period begins immediately after delivery and continues for six weeks following delivery. The peripartum period is defined as the last month of pregnancy to five months postpartum.

2) Peripartum and postpartum complication

A postpartum complication is any complication occurring within the six-week period.

3) Pregnancy-related complications after 6 week period

Chapter 15 codes may also be used to describe pregnancy-related complications after the peripartum or postpartum period if the provider documents that a condition is pregnancy related.

4) Admission for routine postpartum care following delivery outside hospital

When the mother delivers outside the hospital prior to admission and is admitted for routine postpartum care and no complications are noted, code Z39.0, Encounter for care and examination of mother immediately after delivery, should be assigned as the principal diagnosis.

5) Pregnancy associated cardiomyopathy
Pregnancy associated cardiomyopathy, code O90.3, is unique in that it may be diagnosed in the third trimester of pregnancy but may continue to progress months after delivery. For this reason, it is referred to as peripartum cardiomyopathy. Code O90.3 is only for use when the cardiomyopathy develops as a result of pregnancy in a woman who did not have pre-existing heart disease.

p. Code O94, Sequelae of complication of pregnancy, childbirth, and the puerperium
1) Code O94
Code O94, Sequelae of complication of pregnancy, childbirth, and the puerperium, is for use in those cases when an initial complication of a pregnancy develops a sequelae requiring care or treatment at a future date.

2) After the initial postpartum period
This code may be used at any time after the initial postpartum period.

3) Sequencing of Code O94
This code, like all sequela codes, is to be sequenced following the code describing the sequelae of the complication.

q. *Termination of Pregnancy and Spontaneous abortions*
1) Abortion with Liveborn Fetus
When an attempted termination of pregnancy results in a liveborn fetus assign code **Z33.2, Encounter for elective termination of pregnancy** and a code from category Z37, Outcome of Delivery.

2) Retained Products of Conception following an abortion
Subsequent encounters for retained products of conception following a spontaneous abortion or elective termination of pregnancy are assigned the appropriate code from category O03, Spontaneous abortion, or codes O07.4, Failed attempted termination of pregnancy without complication and Z33.2, Encounter for elective termination of pregnancy. This advice is appropriate even when the patient was discharged previously with a discharge diagnosis of complete abortion.

3) *Complications leading to abortion*
Codes from Chapter 15 may be used as additional codes to identify any documented complications of the pregnancy in conjunction with codes in categories in O07 and O08.

r. Abuse in a pregnant patient
For suspected or confirmed cases of abuse of a pregnant patient, a code(s) from subcategories O9A.3, Physical abuse complicating pregnancy, childbirth, and the puerperium, O9A.4, Sexual abuse complicating pregnancy, childbirth, and the puerperium, and O9A.5, Psychological abuse complicating pregnancy, childbirth, and the puerperium, should be sequenced first, followed by the appropriate codes (if applicable) to identify any associated current injury due to physical abuse, sexual abuse, and the perpetrator of abuse.

See Section I.C.19. Adult and child abuse, neglect and other maltreatment.

16. Chapter 16: Certain Conditions Originating in the Perinatal Period (P00-P96)
For coding and reporting purposes the perinatal period is defined as before birth through the 28th day following birth. The following guidelines are provided for reporting purposes

a. General Perinatal Rules
1) Use of Chapter 16 Codes
Codes in this chapter are <u>never</u> for use on the maternal record. Codes from Chapter 15, the obstetric chapter, are never permitted on the newborn record. Chapter 16 codes may be used throughout the life of the patient if the condition is still present.

2) Principal Diagnosis for Birth Record
When coding the birth episode in a newborn record, assign a code from category Z38, Liveborn infants according to place of birth and type of delivery, as the principal diagnosis. A code from category Z38 is assigned only once, to a newborn at the time of birth. If a newborn is transferred to another institution, a code from category Z38 should not be used at the receiving hospital.

A code from category Z38 is used only on the newborn record, not on the mother's record.

3) Use of Codes from other Chapters with Codes from Chapter 16
Codes from other chapters may be used with codes from chapter 16 if the codes from the other chapters provide more specific detail. Codes for signs and symptoms may be assigned when a definitive diagnosis has not been established. If the reason for the encounter is a perinatal condition, the code from chapter 16 should be sequenced first.

4) Use of Chapter 16 Codes after the Perinatal Period
Should a condition originate in the perinatal period, and continue throughout the life of the patient, the perinatal code should continue to be used regardless of the patient's age.

5) Birth process or community acquired conditions
If a newborn has a condition that may be either due to the birth process or community acquired and the documentation does not indicate which it is, the default is due to the birth process and the code from Chapter 16 should be used. If the condition is community-acquired, a code from Chapter 16 should not be assigned.

6) Code all clinically significant conditions
All clinically significant conditions noted on routine newborn examination should be coded. A condition is clinically significant if it requires:
- clinical evaluation; or
- therapeutic treatment; or
- diagnostic procedures; or

• extended length of hospital stay; or

• increased nursing care and/or monitoring; or

• has implications for future health care needs

Note: The perinatal guidelines listed above are the same as the general coding guidelines for "additional diagnoses", except for the final point regarding implications for future health care needs. Codes should be assigned for conditions that have been specified by the provider as having implications for future health care needs.

b. Observation and Evaluation of Newborns for Suspected Conditions not Found

Reserved for future expansion

c. Coding Additional Perinatal Diagnoses

1) Assigning codes for conditions that require treatment

Assign codes for conditions that require treatment or further investigation, prolong the length of stay, or require resource utilization.

2) Codes for conditions specified as having implications for future health care needs

Assign codes for conditions that have been specified by the provider as having implications for future health care needs.

Note: This guideline should not be used for adult patients.

d. Prematurity and Fetal Growth Retardation

Providers utilize different criteria in determining prematurity. A code for prematurity should not be assigned unless it is documented. Assignment of codes in categories P05, Disorders of newborn related to slow fetal growth and fetal malnutrition, and P07, Disorders of newborn related to short gestation and low birth weight, not elsewhere classified, should be based on the recorded birth weight and estimated gestational age. Codes from category P05 should not be assigned with codes from category P07.

When both birth weight and gestational age are available, two codes from category P07 should be assigned, with the code for birth weight sequenced before the code for gestational age.

e. Low birth weight and immaturity status

Codes from category P07, Disorders of newborn related to short gestation and low birth weight, not elsewhere classified, are for use for a child or adult who was premature or had a low birth weight as a newborn and this is affecting the patient's current health status.

See Section I.C.21. Factors influencing health status and contact with health services, Status.

f. Bacterial Sepsis of Newborn

Category P36, Bacterial sepsis of newborn, includes congenital sepsis. If a perinate is documented as having sepsis without documentation of congenital or community acquired, the default is congenital and a code from category P36 should be assigned. If the P36 code includes the causal organism, an additional code from category B95, Streptococcus, Staphylococcus, and Enterococcus as the cause of diseases classified elsewhere, or

B96, Other bacterial agents as the cause of diseases classified elsewhere, should not be assigned. If the P36 code does not include the causal organism, assign an additional code from category B96. If applicable, use additional codes to identify severe sepsis (R65.2-) and any associated acute organ dysfunction.

g. Stillbirth

Code P95, Stillbirth, is only for use in institutions that maintain separate records for stillbirths. No other code should be used with P95. Code P95 should not be used on the mother's record.

17. **Chapter 17: Congenital malformations, deformations, and chromosomal abnormalities (Q00-Q99)**

Assign an appropriate code(s) from categories Q00-Q99, Congenital malformations, deformations, and chromosomal abnormalities when a malformation/deformation or chromosomal abnormality is documented. A malformation/deformation/or chromosomal abnormality may be the principal/first-listed diagnosis on a record or a secondary diagnosis.

When a malformation/deformation/or chromosomal abnormality does not have a unique code assignment, assign additional code(s) for any manifestations that may be present.

When the code assignment specifically identifies the malformation/deformation/or chromosomal abnormality, manifestations that are an inherent component of the anomaly should not be coded separately. Additional codes should be assigned for manifestations that are not an inherent component.

Codes from Chapter 17 may be used throughout the life of the patient. If a congenital malformation or deformity has been corrected, a personal history code should be used to identify the history of the malformation or deformity. Although present at birth, malformation/deformation/or chromosomal abnormality may not be identified until later in life. Whenever the condition is diagnosed by the physician, it is appropriate to assign a code from codes Q00-Q99.

For the birth admission, the appropriate code from category Z38, Liveborn infants, according to place of birth and type of delivery, should be sequenced as the principal diagnosis, followed by any congenital anomaly codes, Q00-Q99.

18. **Chapter 18: Symptoms, signs, and abnormal clinical and laboratory findings, not elsewhere classified (R00-R99)**

Chapter 18 includes symptoms, signs, abnormal results of clinical or other investigative procedures, and ill-defined conditions regarding which no diagnosis classifiable elsewhere is recorded. Signs and symptoms that point to a specific diagnosis have been assigned to a category in other chapters of the classification.

a. Use of symptom codes

Codes that describe symptoms and signs are acceptable for reporting purposes when a related definitive diagnosis has not been established (confirmed) by the provider.

b. Use of a symptom code with a definitive diagnosis code

Codes for signs and symptoms may be reported in addition to a related definitive diagnosis when the sign or symptom is not routinely associated with that diagnosis, such as the various signs and symptoms associated with complex syndromes. The definitive diagnosis code should be sequenced before the symptom code.

Signs or symptoms that are associated routinely with a disease process should not be assigned as additional codes, unless otherwise instructed by the classification.

c. Combination codes that include symptoms

ICD-10-CM contains a number of combination codes that identify both the definitive diagnosis and common symptoms of that diagnosis. When using one of these combination codes, an additional code should not be assigned for the symptom.

d. Repeated falls

Code R29.6, Repeated falls, is for use for encounters when a patient has recently fallen and the reason for the fall is being investigated.

Code Z91.81, History of falling, is for use when a patient has fallen in the past and is at risk for future falls. When appropriate, both codes R29.6 and Z91.81 may be assigned together.

e. Coma scale

The coma scale codes (R40.2-) can be used in conjunction with traumatic brain injury codes, acute cerebrovascular disease or sequelae of cerebrovascular disease codes. These codes are primarily for use by trauma registries, but they may be used in any setting where this information is collected. The coma scale codes should be sequenced after the diagnosis code(s).

These codes, one from each subcategory, are needed to complete the scale. The 7th character indicates when the scale was recorded. The 7th character should match for all three codes.

At a minimum, report the initial score documented on presentation at your facility. This may be a score from the emergency medicine technician (EMT) or in the emergency department. If desired, a facility may choose to capture multiple coma scale scores.

Assign code R40.24, Glasgow coma scale, total score, when only the total score is documented in the medical record and not the individual score(s).

f. Functional quadriplegia

Functional quadriplegia (code R53.2) is the lack of ability to use one's limbs or to ambulate due to extreme debility. It is not associated with neurologic deficit or injury, and code R53.2 should not be used for cases of neurologic quadriplegia. It should only be assigned if functional quadriplegia is specifically documented in the medical record.

g. SIRS due to Non-Infectious Process

The systemic inflammatory response syndrome (SIRS) can develop as a result of certain non-infectious disease processes, such as trauma, malignant neoplasm, or pancreatitis. When SIRS is documented with a noninfectious condition, and no subsequent infection is documented, the code for the underlying condition, such as an injury, should be assigned, followed by code R65.10, Systemic inflammatory response syndrome (SIRS) of non-infectious origin without acute organ dysfunction, or code R65.11, Systemic inflammatory response syndrome (SIRS) of non-infectious origin with acute organ dysfunction. If an associated acute organ dysfunction is documented, the appropriate code(s) for the specific type of organ dysfunction(s) should be assigned in addition to code R65.11. If acute organ dysfunction is documented, but it cannot be determined if the acute organ dysfunction is associated with SIRS or due to another condition (e.g., directly due to the trauma), the provider should be queried.

h. Death NOS

Code R99, Ill-defined and unknown cause of mortality, is only for use in the very limited circumstance when a patient who has already died is brought into an emergency department or other healthcare facility and is pronounced dead upon arrival. It does not represent the discharge disposition of death.

19. Chapter 19: Injury, poisoning, and certain other consequences of external causes (S00-T88)

a. Application of 7th Characters in Chapter 19

Most categories in chapter 19 have a 7th character requirement for each applicable code. Most categories in this chapter have three 7th character values (with the exception of fractures): A, initial encounter, D, subsequent encounter and S, sequela. Categories for traumatic fractures have additional 7th character values.

7th character "A", initial encounter is used while the patient is receiving active treatment for the condition. Examples of active treatment are: surgical treatment, emergency department encounter, and evaluation and treatment by a new physician.

7th character "D" subsequent encounter is used for encounters after the patient has received active treatment of the condition and is receiving routine care for the condition during the healing or recovery phase. Examples of subsequent care are: cast change or removal, removal of external or internal fixation device, medication adjustment, other aftercare and follow up visits following treatment of the injury or condition.

The aftercare Z codes should not be used for aftercare for conditions such as injuries or poisonings, where 7th characters are provided to identify subsequent care. For example, for aftercare of an injury, assign the acute injury code with the 7th character "D" (subsequent encounter).

7th character "S", sequela, is for use for complications or conditions that arise as a direct result of a condition, such as scar formation after a burn. The scars are sequelae of the burn. When using 7th character "S", it is necessary to use both the injury code that precipitated the sequela and the code for the sequela itself. The "S" is added only to the injury code, not the sequela code. The 7th character "S" identifies the injury responsible for the sequela. The specific type of sequela (e.g. scar) is sequenced first, followed by the injury code.

b. Coding of Injuries

When coding injuries, assign separate codes for each injury unless a combination code is provided, in which case the combination code is assigned. Code T07, Unspecified multiple injuries should not be assigned in the inpatient setting unless information for a more specific code is not available. Traumatic injury codes (S00-T14.9) are not to be used for normal, healing surgical wounds or to identify complications of surgical wounds.

The code for the most serious injury, as determined by the provider and the focus of treatment, is sequenced first.

1) Superficial injuries

Superficial injuries such as abrasions or contusions are not coded when associated with more severe injuries of the same site.

2) Primary injury with damage to nerves/ blood vessels

When a primary injury results in minor damage to peripheral nerves or blood vessels, the primary injury is sequenced first with additional code(s) for injuries to nerves and spinal cord (such as category S04), and/or injury to blood vessels (such as category S15). When the primary injury is to the blood vessels or nerves, that injury should be sequenced first.

c. Coding of Traumatic Fractures

The principles of multiple coding of injuries should be followed in coding fractures. Fractures of specified sites are coded individually by site in accordance with both the provisions within categories S02, S12, S22, S32, S42, S49, S52, S59, S62, S72, S79, S82, S89, S92 and the level of detail furnished by medical record content.

A fracture not indicated as open or closed should be coded to closed. A fracture not indicated whether displaced or not displaced should be coded to displaced.

More specific guidelines are as follows:

1) Initial vs. Subsequent Encounter for Fractures

Traumatic fractures are coded using the appropriate 7th character for initial encounter (A, B, C) while the patient is receiving active treatment for the fracture. Examples of active treatment are: surgical treatment, emergency department encounter, and evaluation and treatment by a new physician. The appropriate 7th character for initial encounter should also be assigned for a patient who delayed seeking treatment for the fracture or nonunion.

Fractures are coded using the appropriate 7th character for subsequent care for encounters after the patient has completed active treatment of the fracture and is receiving routine care for the fracture during the healing or recovery phase. Examples of fracture aftercare are: cast change or removal, removal of external or internal fixation device, medication adjustment, and follow-up visits following fracture treatment.

Care for complications of surgical treatment for fracture repairs during the healing or recovery phase should be coded with the appropriate complication codes.

Care of complications of fractures, such as malunion and nonunion, should be reported with the appropriate 7th character for subsequent care with nonunion (K, M, N,) or subsequent care with malunion (P, Q, R).

A code from category M80, not a traumatic fracture code, should be used for any patient with known osteoporosis who suffers a fracture, even if the patient had a minor fall or trauma, if that fall or trauma would not usually break a normal, healthy bone.

See Section I.C.13. Osteoporosis.

The aftercare Z codes should not be used for aftercare for traumatic fractures. For aftercare of a traumatic fracture, assign the acute fracture code with the appropriate 7th character.

2) Multiple fractures sequencing

Multiple fractures are sequenced in accordance with the severity of the fracture.

d. Coding of Burns and Corrosions

The ICD-10-CM makes a distinction between burns and corrosions. The burn codes are for thermal burns, except sunburns, that come from a heat source, such as a fire or hot appliance. The burn codes are also for burns resulting from electricity and radiation. Corrosions are burns due to chemicals. The guidelines are the same for burns and corrosions.

Current burns (T20-T25) are classified by depth, extent and by agent (X code). Burns are classified by depth as first degree (erythema), second degree (blistering), and third degree (full-thickness involvement). Burns of the eye and internal organs (T26-T28) are classified by site, but not by degree.

1) Sequencing of burn and related condition codes

Sequence first the code that reflects the highest degree of burn when more than one burn is present.

    a. When the reason for the admission or encounter is for treatment of external multiple burns, sequence first the code that reflects the burn of the highest degree.

b. When a patient has both internal and external burns, the circumstances of admission govern the selection of the principal diagnosis or first-listed diagnosis.

c. When a patient is admitted for burn injuries and other related conditions such as smoke inhalation and/or respiratory failure, the circumstances of admission govern the selection of the principal or first-listed diagnosis.

2) Burns of the same local site

Classify burns of the same local site (three-character category level, T20-T28) but of different degrees to the subcategory identifying the highest degree recorded in the diagnosis.

3) Non-healing burns

Non-healing burns are coded as acute burns.
Necrosis of burned skin should be coded as a non-healed burn.

4) Infected Burn

For any documented infected burn site, use an additional code for the infection.

5) Assign separate codes for each burn site

When coding burns, assign separate codes for each burn site. Category T30, Burn and corrosion, body region unspecified is extremely vague and should rarely be used.

6) Burns and Corrosions Classified According to Extent of Body Surface Involved

Assign codes from category T31, Burns classified according to extent of body surface involved, or T32, Corrosions classified according to extent of body surface involved, when the site of the burn is not specified or when there is a need for additional data. It is advisable to use category T31 as additional coding when needed to provide data for evaluating burn mortality, such as that needed by burn units. It is also advisable to use category T31 as an additional code for reporting purposes when there is mention of a third-degree burn involving 20 percent or more of the body surface.

Categories T31 and T32 are based on the classic "rule of nines" in estimating body surface involved: head and neck are assigned nine percent, each arm nine percent, each leg 18 percent, the anterior trunk 18 percent, posterior trunk 18 percent, and genitalia one percent. Providers may change these percentage assignments where necessary to accommodate infants and children who have proportionately larger heads than adults, and patients who have large buttocks, thighs, or abdomen that involve burns.

7) Encounters for treatment of sequela of burns

Encounters for the treatment of the late effects of burns or corrosions (i.e., scars or joint contractures) should be coded with a burn or corrosion code with the 7th character "S" for sequela.

8) Sequelae with a late effect code and current burn

When appropriate, both a code for a current burn or corrosion with 7th character "A" or "D" and a burn or corrosion code with 7th character "S" may be assigned on the same record (when both a current burn and sequelae of an old burn exist). Burns and corrosions do not heal at the same rate and a current healing wound may still exist with sequela of a healed burn or corrosion.

9) Use of an external cause code with burns and corrosions

An external cause code should be used with burns and corrosions to identify the source and intent of the burn, as well as the place where it occurred.

e. Adverse Effects, Poisoning , Underdosing and Toxic Effects

Codes in categories T36-T65 are combination codes that include the substance that was taken as well as the intent. No additional external cause code is required for poisonings, toxic effects, adverse effects and underdosing codes.

1) Do not code directly from the Table of Drugs

Do not code directly from the Table of Drugs and Chemicals. Always refer back to the Tabular List.

2) Use as many codes as necessary to describe

Use as many codes as necessary to describe completely all drugs, medicinal or biological substances.

3) If the same code would describe the causative agent

If the same code would describe the causative agent for more than one adverse reaction, poisoning, toxic effect or underdosing, assign the code only once.

4) If two or more drugs, medicinal or biological substances

If two or more drugs, medicinal or biological substances are reported, code each individually unless a combination code is listed in the Table of Drugs and Chemicals.

5) The occurrence of drug toxicity is classified in ICD-10-CM as follows:

(a) Adverse Effect

When coding an adverse effect of a drug that has been correctly prescribed and properly administered, assign the appropriate code for the nature of the adverse effect followed by the appropriate code for the adverse effect of the drug (T36-T50). The code for the drug should have a 5th or 6th character "5" (for example T36.0X5-) Examples of the nature of an adverse effect are tachycardia, delirium, gastrointestinal hemorrhaging, vomiting, hypokalemia, hepatitis, renal failure, or respiratory failure.

(b) Poisoning

When coding a poisoning or reaction to the improper use of a medication (e.g., overdose, wrong substance given or taken in error, wrong route of administration), first assign the appropriate code from categories T36-T50. The poisoning codes have an associated intent as their 5th or 6th character (accidental, intentional self-harm, assault and undetermined. Use additional code(s) for all manifestations of poisonings.

If there is also a diagnosis of abuse or dependence of the substance, the abuse or dependence is assigned as an additional code.

Examples of poisoning include:

 (i) Error was made in drug prescription Errors made in drug prescription or in the administration of the drug by provider, nurse, patient, or other person.

 (ii) Overdose of a drug intentionally taken If an overdose of a drug was intentionally taken or administered and resulted in drug toxicity, it would be coded as a poisoning.

 (iii) Nonprescribed drug taken with correctly prescribed and properly administered drug.
If a nonprescribed drug or medicinal agent was taken in combination with a correctly prescribed and properly administered drug, any drug toxicity or other reaction resulting from the interaction of the two drugs would be classified as a poisoning.

 (iv) Interaction of drug(s) and alcohol. When a reaction results from the interaction of a drug(s) and alcohol, this would be classified as poisoning.

See Section I.C.4. if poisoning is the result of insulin pump malfunctions.

(c) Underdosing
Underdosing refers to taking less of a medication than is prescribed by a provider or a manufacturer's instruction. For underdosing, assign the code from categories T36-T50 (fifth or sixth character "6").

Codes for underdosing should never be assigned as principal or first-listed codes. If a patient has a relapse or exacerbation of the medical condition for which the drug is prescribed because of the reduction in dose, then the medical condition itself should be coded.

Noncompliance (Z91.12-, Z91.13-) or complication of care (Y63.6-Y63.9) codes are to be used with an underdosing code to indicate intent, if known.

(d) Toxic Effects
When a harmful substance is ingested or comes in contact with a person, this is classified as a toxic effect. The toxic effect codes are in categories T51-T65.

Toxic effect codes have an associated intent: accidental, intentional self-harm, assault and undetermined.

f. Adult and child abuse, neglect and other maltreatment
Sequence first the appropriate code from categories T74.- (Adult and child abuse, neglect and other maltreatment, confirmed) or T76.- (Adult and child abuse, neglect and other maltreatment, suspected) for abuse, neglect and other maltreatment, followed by any accompanying mental health or injury code(s).

If the documentation in the medical record states abuse or neglect it is coded as confirmed (T74.-). It is coded as suspected if it is documented as suspected (T76.-).

For cases of confirmed abuse or neglect an external cause code from the assault section (X92-Y08) should be added to identify the cause of any physical injuries. A perpetrator code (Y07) should be added when the perpetrator of the abuse is known. For suspected cases of abuse or neglect, do not report external cause or perpetrator code.

If a suspected case of abuse, neglect or mistreatment is ruled out during an encounter code Z04.71, Encounter for examination and observation following alleged physical adult abuse, ruled out, or code Z04.72, Encounter for examination and observation following alleged child physical abuse, ruled out, should be used, not a code from T76.

If a suspected case of alleged rape or sexual abuse is ruled out during an encounter code Z04.41, Encounter for examination and observation following alleged physical adult abuse, ruled out, or code Z04.42, Encounter for examination and observation following alleged rape or sexual abuse, ruled out, should be used, not a code from T76.

See Section I.C.15. Abuse in a pregnant patient.

g. Complications of care
1) General guidelines for complications of care
(a) Documentation of complications of care
See Section I.B.16. for information on documentation of complications of care.

2) Pain due to medical devices
Pain associated with devices, implants or grafts left in a surgical site (for example painful hip prosthesis) is assigned to the appropriate code(s) found in Chapter 19, Injury, poisoning, and certain other consequences of external causes. Specific codes for pain due to medical devices are found in the T code section of the ICD-10-CM. Use additional code(s) from category G89 to identify acute or chronic pain due to presence of the device, implant or graft (G89.18 or G89.28).

3) Transplant complications

(a) Transplant complications other than kidney

Codes under category T86, Complications of transplanted organs and tissues, are for use for both complications and rejection of transplanted organs. A transplant complication code is only assigned if the complication affects the function of the transplanted organ. Two codes are required to fully describe a transplant complication: the appropriate code from category T86 and a secondary code that identifies the complication.

Pre-existing conditions or conditions that develop after the transplant are not coded as complications unless they affect the function of the transplanted organs.

See I.C.21. for transplant organ removal status
See I.C.2. for malignant neoplasm associated with transplanted organ.

(b) Kidney transplant complications

Patients who have undergone kidney transplant may still have some form of chronic kidney disease (CKD) because the kidney transplant may not fully restore kidney function. Code T86.1- should be assigned for documented complications of a kidney transplant, such as transplant failure or rejection or other transplant complication. Code T86.1- should not be assigned for post kidney transplant patients who have chronic kidney (CKD) unless a transplant complication such as transplant failure or rejection is documented. If the documentation is unclear as to whether the patient has a complication of the transplant, query the provider.

Conditions that affect the function of the transplanted kidney, other than CKD, should be assigned a code from subcategory T86.1, Complications of transplanted organ, Kidney, and a secondary code that identifies the complication.

For patients with CKD following a kidney transplant, but who do not have a complication such as failure or rejection, *see section I.C.14. Chronic kidney disease and kidney transplant status.*

4) Complication codes that include the external cause

As with certain other T codes, some of the complications of care codes have the external cause included in the code. The code includes the nature of the complication as well as the type of procedure that caused the complication. No external cause code indicating the type of procedure is necessary for these codes.

5) Complications of care codes within the body system chapters

Intraoperative and postprocedural complication codes are found within the body system chapters with codes specific to the organs and structures of that body system. These codes should be sequenced first, followed by a code(s) for the specific complication, if applicable.

20. Chapter 20: External Causes of Morbidity (V00-Y99)

The external causes of morbidity codes should never be sequenced as the first-listed or principal diagnosis.

External cause codes are intended to provide data for injury research and evaluation of injury prevention strategies. These codes capture how the injury or health condition happened (cause), the intent (unintentional or accidental; or intentional, such as suicide or assault), the place where the event occurred the activity of the patient at the time of the event, and the person's status (e.g., civilian, military).

There is no national requirement for mandatory ICD-10-CM external cause code reporting. Unless a provider is subject to a state-based external cause code reporting mandate or these codes are required by a particular payer, reporting of ICD-10-CM codes in Chapter 20, External Causes of Morbidity, is not required. In the absence of a mandatory reporting requirement, providers are encouraged to voluntarily report external cause codes, as they provide valuable data for injury research and evaluation of injury prevention strategies.

a. General External Cause Coding Guidelines

1) Used with any code in the range of A00.0-T88.9, Z00-Z99

An external cause code may be used with any code in the range of A00.0-T88.9, Z00-Z99, classification that is a health condition due to an external cause. Though they are most applicable to injuries, they are also valid for use with such things as infections or diseases due to an external source, and other health conditions, such as a heart attack that occurs during strenuous physical activity.

2) External cause code used for length of treatment

Assign the external cause code, with the appropriate 7th character (initial encounter, subsequent encounter or sequela) for each encounter for which the injury or condition is being treated.

3) Use the full range of external cause codes

Use the full range of external cause codes to completely describe the cause, the intent, the place of occurrence and if applicable, the activity of the patient at the time of the event, and the patient's status, for all injuries, and other health conditions due to an external cause.

4) Assign as many external cause codes as necessary

Assign as many external cause codes as necessary to fully explain each cause. If only one external code can be recorded, assign the code most related to the principal diagnosis.

5) The selection of the appropriate external cause code

The selection of the appropriate external cause code is guided by the Alphabetic Index of External Causes and by Inclusion and Exclusion notes in the Tabular List.

6) External cause code can never be a principal diagnosis

An external cause code can never be a principal (first-listed) diagnosis.

7) Combination external cause codes

Certain of the external cause codes are combination codes that identify sequential events that result in an injury, such as a fall which results in striking against an object. The injury may be due to either event or both. The combination external cause code used should correspond to the sequence of events regardless of which caused the most serious injury.

8) No external cause code needed in certain circumstances

No external cause code from Chapter 20 is needed if the external cause and intent are included in a code from another chapter (e.g. T36.0X1- Poisoning by penicillins, accidental (unintentional)).

b. Place of Occurrence Guideline

Codes from category Y92, Place of occurrence of the external cause, are secondary codes for use after other external cause codes to identify the location of the patient at the time of injury or other condition.

A place of occurrence code is used only once, at the initial encounter for treatment. No 7th characters are used for Y92. Only one code from Y92 should be recorded on a medical record.

Do not use place of occurrence code Y92.9 if the place is not stated or is not applicable.

c. Activity Code

Assign a code from category Y93, Activity code, to describe the activity of the patient at the time the injury or other health condition occurred.

An activity code is used only once, at the initial encounter for treatment. Only one code from Y93 should be recorded on a medical record.

The activity codes are not applicable to poisonings, adverse effects, misadventures or sequela.

Do not assign Y93.9, Unspecified activity, if the activity is not stated.

A code from category Y93 is appropriate for use with external cause and intent codes if identifying the activity provides additional information about the event.

d. Place of Occurrence, Activity, and Status Codes Used with other External Cause Code

When applicable, place of occurrence, activity, and external cause status codes are sequenced after the main external cause code(s). Regardless of the number of external cause codes assigned, there should be only one place of occurrence code, one activity code, and one external cause status code assigned to an encounter.

e. If the Reporting Format Limits the Number of External Cause Codes

If the reporting format limits the number of external cause codes that can be used in reporting clinical data, report the code for the cause/intent most related to the principal diagnosis. If the format permits capture of additional external cause codes, the cause/intent, including medical misadventures, of the additional events should be reported rather than the codes for place, activity, or external status.

f. Multiple External Cause Coding Guidelines

More than one external cause code is required to fully describe the external cause of an illness or injury. The assignment of external cause codes should be sequenced in the following priority:

If two or more events cause separate injuries, an external cause code should be assigned for each cause. The first-listed external cause code will be selected in the following order:

External codes for child and adult abuse take priority over all other external cause codes.

See Section I.C.19., Child and Adult abuse guidelines.

External codes for terrorism events take priority over all other external cause codes except child and adult abuse.

External cause codes for cataclysmic events take priority over all other external cause codes except child and adult abuse and terrorism.

External cause codes for transport accidents take priority over all other external cause codes except cataclysmic events, child and adult abuse and terrorism.

Activity and external cause status codes are assigned following all causal (intent) external cause codes.

The first-listed external cause code should correspond to the cause of the most serious diagnosis due to an assault, accident, or self-harm, following the order of hierarchy listed above.

g. Child and Adult Abuse Guideline

Adult and child abuse, neglect and maltreatment are classified as assault. Any of the assault codes may be used to indicate the external cause of any injury resulting from the confirmed abuse.

For confirmed cases of abuse, neglect and maltreatment, when the perpetrator is known, a code from Y07, Perpetrator of maltreatment and neglect, should accompany any other assault codes.

See Section I.C.19. Adult and child abuse, neglect and other maltreatment

h. Unknown or Undetermined Intent Guideline

If the intent (accident, self-harm, assault) of the cause of an injury or other condition is unknown or unspecified, code the intent as accidental intent. All transport accident categories assume accidental intent.

1) Use of undetermined intent

External cause codes for events of undetermined intent are only for use if the documentation in the record specifies that the intent cannot be determined.

i. Sequelae (Late Effects) of External Cause Guidelines

1) Sequelae external cause codes

Sequela are reported using the external cause code with the 7th character "S" for sequela. These codes should be used with any report of a late effect or sequela resulting from a previous injury.

2) Sequela external cause code with a related current injury

A sequela external cause code should never be used with a related current nature of injury code.

3) Use of sequela external cause codes for subsequent visits

Use a late effect external cause code for subsequent visits when a late effect of the initial injury is being treated. Do not use a late effect external cause code for subsequent visits for follow-up care (e.g., to assess healing, to receive rehabilitative therapy) of the injury when no late effect of the injury has been documented.

j. Terrorism Guidelines

1) Cause of injury identified by the Federal Government (FBI) as terrorism

When the cause of an injury is identified by the Federal Government (FBI) as terrorism, the first-listed external cause code should be a code from category Y38, Terrorism. The definition of terrorism employed by the FBI is found at the inclusion note at the beginning of category Y38. Use additional code for place of occurrence (Y92.-). More than one Y38 code may be assigned if the injury is the result of more than one mechanism of terrorism.

2) Cause of an injury is suspected to be the result of terrorism

When the cause of an injury is suspected to be the result of terrorism a code from category Y38 should not be assigned. Suspected cases should be classified as assault.

3) Code Y38.9, Terrorism, secondary effects

Assign code Y38.9, Terrorism, secondary effects, for conditions occurring subsequent to the terrorist event. This code should not be assigned for conditions that are due to the initial terrorist act.

It is acceptable to assign code Y38.9 with another code from Y38 if there is an injury due to the initial terrorist event and an injury that is a subsequent result of the terrorist event.

k. External cause status

A code from category Y99, External cause status, should be assigned whenever any other external cause code is assigned for an encounter, including an Activity code, except for the events noted below. Assign a code from category Y99, External cause status, to indicate the work status of the person at the time the event occurred. The status code indicates whether the event occurred during military activity, whether a non-military person was at work, whether an individual including a student or volunteer was involved in a non-work activity at the time of the causal event.

A code from Y99, External cause status, should be assigned, when applicable, with other external cause codes, such as transport accidents and falls. The external cause status codes are not applicable to poisonings, adverse effects, misadventures or late effects.

Do not assign a code from category Y99 if no other external cause codes (cause, activity) are applicable for the encounter.

An external cause status code is used only once, at the initial encounter for treatment. Only one code from Y99 should be recorded on a medical record.

Do not assign code Y99.9, Unspecified external cause status, if the status is not stated.

21. Chapter 21: Factors influencing health status and contact with health services (Z00-Z99)

Note: The chapter specific guidelines provide additional information about the use of Z codes for specified encounters.

a. Use of Z codes in any healthcare setting

Z codes are for use in any healthcare setting. Z codes may be used as either a first-listed (principal diagnosis code in the inpatient setting) or secondary code, depending on the circumstances of the encounter. Certain Z codes may only be used as first-listed or principal diagnosis.

b. Z Codes indicate a reason for an encounter

Z codes are not procedure codes. A corresponding procedure code must accompany a Z code to describe any procedure performed.

c. Categories of Z Codes

1) Contact/Exposure

Category Z20 indicates contact with, and suspected exposure to, communicable diseases. These codes are for patients who do not show any sign or symptom of a disease but are suspected to have been exposed to it by close personal contact with an infected individual or are in an area where a disease is epidemic.

Category Z77, indicates contact with and suspected exposures hazardous to health.

Contact/exposure codes may be used as a first-listed code to explain an encounter for testing, or, more commonly, as a secondary code to identify a potential risk.

2) Inoculations and vaccinations

Code Z23 is for encounters for inoculations and vaccinations. It indicates that a patient is being seen to receive a prophylactic inoculation against a disease. Procedure codes are required to identify the actual administration of the injection and the type(s) of immunizations given. Code Z23 may be used as a secondary code if the inoculation is given as a routine part of preventive health care, such as a well-baby visit.

3) Status

Status codes indicate that a patient is either a carrier of a disease or has the sequelae or residual of a past disease or condition. This includes such things as the presence of prosthetic or mechanical devices resulting from past treatment. A status code is informative, because the status may affect the course of treatment and its outcome. A status code is distinct from a history code. The history code indicates that the patient no longer has the condition.

A status code should not be used with a diagnosis code from one of the body system chapters, if the diagnosis code includes the information provided by the status code. For example, code Z94.1, Heart transplant status, should not be used with a code from subcategory T86.2, Complications of heart transplant. The status code does not provide additional information. The complication code indicates that the patient is a heart transplant patient.

For encounters for weaning from a mechanical ventilator, assign a code from subcategory J96.1, Chronic respiratory failure, followed by code Z99.11, Dependence on respirator [ventilator] status.

The status Z codes/categories are:

Z14   Genetic carrier
       Genetic carrier status indicates that a person carries a gene, associated with a particular disease, which may be passed to offspring who may develop that disease. The person does not have the disease and is not at risk of developing the disease.

Z15   Genetic susceptibility to disease Genetic susceptibility indicates that a person has a gene that increases the risk of that person developing the disease.

Codes from category Z15 should not be used as principal or first-listed codes. If the patient has the condition to which he/she is susceptible, and that condition is the reason for the encounter, the code for the current condition should be sequenced first. If the patient is being seen for follow-up after completed treatment for this condition, and the condition no longer exists, a follow-up code should be sequenced first, followed by the appropriate personal history and genetic susceptibility codes. If the purpose of the encounter is genetic counseling associated with procreative management, code Z31.5, Encounter for genetic counseling, should be assigned as the first-listed code, followed by a code from category Z15. Additional codes should be assigned for any applicable family or personal history.

Z16   Resistance to antimicrobial drugs
       This code indicates that a patient has a condition that is resistant to antimicrobial drug treatment. Sequence the infection code first.

Z17   Estrogen receptor status

Z18   Retained foreign body fragments

Z21   Asymptomatic HIV infection status This code indicates that a patient has tested positive for HIV but has manifested no signs or symptoms of the disease.

Z22   Carrier of infectious disease Carrier status indicates that a person harbors the specific organisms of a disease without manifest symptoms and is capable of transmitting the infection.

Z28.3 Underimmunization status

Z33.1 Pregnant state, incidental This code is a secondary code only for use when the pregnancy is in no way complicating the reason for visit. Otherwise, a code from the obstetric chapter is required.

Z66   Do not resuscitate
This code may be used when it is documented by the provider that a patient is on do not resuscitate status at any time during the stay.

Z67   Blood type

Z68   Body mass index (BMI)

Z74.01 Bed confinement status

Z76.82 Awaiting organ transplant status

Z78   Other specified health status
Code Z78.1, Physical restraint status, may be used when it is documented by the provider that a patient has been put in restraints during the current encounter. Please note that this code should not be reported when it is documented by the provider that a patient is temporarily restrained during a procedure.

Z79   Long-term (current) drug therapy
Codes from this category indicate a patient's continuous use of a prescribed drug (including such things as aspirin therapy) for the long-term treatment of a condition or for prophylactic use. It is not for use for patients who have addictions to drugs. This subcategory is not for use of medications for detoxification or maintenance programs to prevent withdrawal symptoms in patients with drug dependence (e.g., methadone maintenance for opiate dependence). Assign the appropriate code for the drug dependence instead.

Assign a code from Z79 if the patient is receiving a medication for an extended period as a prophylactic measure (such as for the prevention of deep vein thrombosis) or as treatment of a chronic condition (such as arthritis) or a disease requiring a lengthy course of treatment (such as cancer). Do not assign a code from category Z79 for medication being administered for a brief period of time to treat an acute illness or injury (such as a course of antibiotics to treat acute bronchitis).

Z88   Allergy status to drugs, medicaments and biological substances Except: Z88.9, Allergy status to unspecified drugs, medicaments and biological substances status

Z89   Acquired absence of limb

Z90   Acquired absence of organs, not elsewhere classified

Z91.0- Allergy status, other than to drugs and biological substances

Z92.82 Status post administration of tPA (rtPA) in a different facility within the last 24 hours prior to admission to a current facility Assign code Z92.82, Status post administration of tPA (rtPA) in a different facility within the last 24 hours prior to admission to current facility, as a secondary diagnosis when a patient is received by transfer into a facility and documentation indicates they were administered tissue plasminogen activator (tPA) within the last 24 hours prior to admission to the current facility. This guideline applies even if the patient is still receiving the tPA at the time they are received into the current facility. The appropriate code for the condition for which the tPA was administered (such as cerebrovascular disease or myocardial infarction) should be assigned first. Code Z92.82 is only applicable to the receiving facility record and not to the transferring facility record.

Z93 Artificial opening status
Z94 Transplanted organ and tissue status
Z95 Presence of cardiac and vascular implants and grafts
Z96 Presence of other functional implants
Z97 Presence of other devices
Z98 Other postprocedural states

Assign code Z98.85, Transplanted organ removal status, to indicate that a transplanted organ has been previously removed. This code should not be assigned for the encounter in which the transplanted organ is removed. The complication necessitating removal of the transplant organ should be assigned for that encounter.

See section I.C.19. for information on the coding of organ transplant complications.

Z99 Dependence on enabling machines and devices, not elsewhere classified

Note: Categories Z89-Z90 and Z93-Z99 are for use only if there are no complications or malfunctions of the organ or tissue replaced, the amputation site or the equipment on which the patient is dependent.

4) History (of)

There are two types of history Z codes, personal and family. Personal history codes explain a patient's past medical condition that no longer exists and is not receiving any treatment, but that has the potential for recurrence, and therefore may require continued monitoring.

Family history codes are for use when a patient has a family member(s) who has had a particular disease that causes the patient to be at higher risk of also contracting the disease.

Personal history codes may be used in conjunction with follow-up codes and family history codes may be used in conjunction with screening codes to explain the need for a test or procedure. History codes are also acceptable on any medical record regardless of the reason for visit. A history of an illness, even if no longer present, is important information that may alter the type of treatment ordered.

The history Z code categories are:

Z80 Family history of primary malignant neoplasm
Z81 Family history of mental and behavioral disorders
Z82 Family history of certain disabilities and chronic diseases (leading to disablement)
Z83 Family history of other specific disorders
Z84 Family history of other conditions
Z85 Personal history of malignant neoplasm
Z86 Personal history of certain other diseases
Z87 Personal history of other diseases and conditions
Z91.4- Personal history of psychological trauma, not elsewhere classified
Z91.5 Personal history of self-harm
Z91.8- Other specified personal risk factors, not elsewhere classified
Exception:
Z91.83, Wandering in diseases classified elsewhere
Z92 Personal history of medical treatment Except: Z92.0, Personal history of contraception Except: Z92.82, Status post administration of tPA (rtPA) in a different facility within the last 24 hours prior to admission to a current facility

5) Screening

Screening is the testing for disease or disease precursors in seemingly well individuals so that early detection and treatment can be provided for those who test positive for the disease (e.g., screening mammogram).

The testing of a person to rule out or confirm a suspected diagnosis because the patient has some sign or symptom is a diagnostic examination, not a screening. In these cases, the sign or symptom is used to explain the reason for the test.

A screening code may be a first-listed code if the reason for the visit is specifically the screening exam. It may also be used as an additional code if the screening is done during an office visit for other health problems. A screening code is not necessary if the screening is inherent to a routine examination, such as a pap smear done during a routine pelvic examination.

Should a condition be discovered during the screening then the code for the condition may be assigned as an additional diagnosis.

The Z code indicates that a screening exam is planned. A procedure code is required to confirm that the screening was performed.

The screening Z codes/categories:

Z11   Encounter for screening for infectious and parasitic diseases

Z12   Encounter for screening for malignant neoplasms

Z13   Encounter for screening for other diseases and disorders Except: Z13.9, Encounter for screening, unspecified

Z36   Encounter for antenatal screening for mother

6) Observation

There are two observation Z code categories. They are for use in very limited circumstances when a person is being observed for a suspected condition that is ruled out. The observation codes are not for use if an injury or illness or any signs or symptoms related to the suspected condition are present. In such cases the diagnosis/symptom code is used with the corresponding external cause code.

The observation codes are to be used as principal diagnosis only. Additional codes may be used in addition to the observation code but only if they are unrelated to the suspected condition being observed.

Codes from subcategory Z03.7 Encounter for suspected maternal and fetal conditions ruled out, may either be used as a first-listed or as an additional code assignment depending on the case. They are for use in very limited circumstances on a maternal record when an encounter is for a suspected maternal or fetal condition that is ruled out during that encounter (for example, a maternal or fetal condition may be suspected due to an abnormal test result). These codes should not be used when the condition is confirmed. In those cases, the confirmed condition should be coded. In addition, these codes are not for use if an illness or any signs or symptoms related to the suspected condition or problem are present. In such cases the diagnosis/symptom code is used.

Additional codes may be used in addition to the code from subcategory Z03.7, but only if they are unrelated to the suspected condition being evaluated.

Codes from subcategory Z03.7 may not be used for encounters for antenatal screening of mother. *See Section I.C.21. Screening.*

For encounters for suspected fetal condition that are inconclusive following testing and evaluation, assign the appropriate code from category O35, O36, O40 or O41.

The observation Z code categories:

Z03   Encounter for medical observation for suspected diseases and conditions ruled out

Z04   Encounter for examination and observation for other reasons Except: Z04.9, Encounter for examination and observation for unspecified reason

7) Aftercare

Aftercare visit codes cover situations when the initial treatment of a disease has been performed and the patient requires continued care during the healing or recovery phase, or for the long-term consequences of the disease. The aftercare Z code should not be used if treatment is directed at a current, acute disease. The diagnosis code is to be used in these cases.

Exceptions to this rule are codes Z51.0, Encounter for antineoplastic radiation therapy, and codes from subcategory Z51.1, Encounter for antineoplastic chemotherapy and immunotherapy. These codes are to be first-listed, followed by the diagnosis code when a patient's encounter is solely to receive radiation therapy, chemotherapy, or immunotherapy for the treatment of a neoplasm. If the reason for the encounter is more than one type of antineoplastic therapy, code Z51.0 and a code from subcategory Z51.1 may be assigned together, in which case one of these codes would be reported as a secondary diagnosis.

The aftercare Z codes should also not be used for aftercare for injuries. For aftercare of an injury, assign the acute injury code with the appropriate 7th character (for subsequent encounter).

The aftercare codes are generally first-listed to explain the specific reason for the encounter. An aftercare code may be used as an additional code when some type of aftercare is provided in addition to the reason for admission and no diagnosis code is applicable. An example of this would be the closure of a colostomy during an encounter for treatment of another condition.

Aftercare codes should be used in conjunction with other aftercare codes or diagnosis codes to provide better detail on the specifics of an aftercare encounter visit, unless otherwise directed by the classification. Should a patient receive multiple types of antineoplastic therapy during the same encounter, code Z51.0, Encounter for antineoplastic radiation therapy, and codes from subcategory Z51.1, Encounter for antineoplastic chemotherapy and immunotherapy, may be used together on a record. The sequencing of multiple aftercare codes depends on the circumstances of the encounter.

Certain aftercare Z code categories need a secondary diagnosis code to describe the resolving condition or sequelae. For others, the condition is included in the code title.

Additional Z code aftercare category terms include fitting and adjustment, and attention to artificial openings.

Status Z codes may be used with aftercare Z codes to indicate the nature of the aftercare. For example code Z95.1, Presence of aortocoronary bypass graft, may be used with code Z48.812, Encounter for surgical aftercare following surgery on the circulatory system, to indicate the surgery for which the aftercare is being performed. A status code should not be used when the aftercare code indicates the type of status, such as using Z43.0,

Encounter for attention to tracheostomy, with Z93.0, Tracheostomy status.

The aftercare Z category/codes:

Z42	Encounter for plastic and reconstructive surgery following medical procedure or healed injury
Z43	Encounter for attention to artificial openings
Z44	Encounter for fitting and adjustment of external prosthetic device
Z45	Encounter for adjustment and management of implanted device
Z46	Encounter for fitting and adjustment of other devices
Z47	Orthopedic aftercare
Z48	Encounter for other postprocedural aftercare
Z49	Encounter for care involving renal dialysis
Z51	Encounter for other aftercare

8) Follow-up

The follow-up codes are used to explain continuing surveillance following completed treatment of a disease, condition, or injury. They imply that the condition has been fully treated and no longer exists. They should not be confused with aftercare codes, or injury codes with a 7th character for subsequent encounter, that explain ongoing care of a healing condition or its sequelae. Follow-up codes may be used in conjunction with history codes to provide the full picture of the healed condition and its treatment. The follow-up code is sequenced first, followed by the history code.

A follow-up code may be used to explain multiple visits. Should a condition be found to have recurred on the follow-up visit, then the diagnosis code for the condition should be assigned in place of the follow-up code.

The follow-up Z code categories:

Z08	Encounter for follow-up examination after completed treatment for malignant neoplasm
Z09	Encounter for follow-up examination after completed treatment for conditions other than malignant neoplasm
Z39	Encounter for maternal postpartum care and examination

9) Donor

Codes in category Z52, Donors of organs and tissues, are used for living individuals who are donating blood or other body tissue. These codes are only for individuals donating for others, not for self-donations. They are not used to identify cadaveric donations.

10) Counseling

Counseling Z codes are used when a patient or family member receives assistance in the aftermath of an illness or injury, or when support is required in coping with family or social problems. They are not used in conjunction with a diagnosis code when the counseling component of care is considered integral to standard treatment.

The counseling Z codes/categories:

Z30.0-	Encounter for general counseling and advice on contraception
Z31.5	Encounter for genetic counseling
Z31.6-	Encounter for general counseling and advice on procreation
Z32.2	Encounter for childbirth instruction
Z32.3	Encounter for childcare instruction
Z69	Encounter for mental health services for victim and perpetrator of abuse
Z70	Counseling related to sexual attitude, behavior and orientation
Z71	Persons encountering health services for other counseling and medical advice, not elsewhere classified
Z76.81	Expectant mother prebirth pediatrician visit

11) Encounters for Obstetrical and Reproductive Services

See Section I.C.15. Pregnancy, Childbirth, and the Puerperium, for further instruction on the use of these codes.

Z codes for pregnancy are for use in those circumstances when none of the problems or complications included in the codes from the Obstetrics chapter exist (a routine prenatal visit or postpartum care). Codes in category Z34, Encounter for supervision of normal pregnancy, are always first listed and are not to be used with any other code from the OB chapter.

Codes in category Z3A, Weeks of gestation, may be assigned to provide additional information about the pregnancy.

The date of the admission should be used to determine weeks of gestation for inpatient admissions that encompass more than one gestational week.

The outcome of delivery, category Z37, should be included on all maternal delivery records. It is always a secondary code. Codes in category Z37 should not be used on the newborn record.

Z codes for family planning (contraceptive) or procreative management and counseling should be included on an obstetric record either during the pregnancy or the postpartum stage, if applicable.

Z codes/categories for obstetrical and reproductive services:

Z30	Encounter for contraceptive management
Z31	Encounter for procreative management
Z32.2	Encounter for childbirth instruction
Z32.3	Encounter for childcare instruction
Z33	Pregnant state
Z34	Encounter for supervision of normal pregnancy
Z36	Encounter for antenatal screening of mother
Z3A	Weeks of gestation
Z37	Outcome of delivery
Z39	Encounter for maternal postpartum care and examination

GUIDELINES (ICD-10-CM)

Z76.81   Expectant mother prebirth pediatrician visit

12)   Newborns and Infants

See Section I.C.16. Newborn (Perinatal) Guidelines, for further instruction on the use of these codes.

Newborn Z codes/categories:

Z76.1   Encounter for health supervision and care of foundling

Z00.1-   Encounter for routine child health examination

Z38   Liveborn infants according to place of birth and type of delivery

13)   Routine and administrative examinations

The Z codes allow for the description of encounters for routine examinations, such as, a general check-up, or, examinations for administrative purposes, such as, a pre-employment physical. The codes are not to be used if the examination is for diagnosis of a suspected condition or for treatment purposes. In such cases the diagnosis code is used. During a routine exam, should a diagnosis or condition be discovered, it should be coded as an additional code. Pre-existing and chronic conditions and history codes may also be included as additional codes as long as the examination is for administrative purposes and not focused on any particular condition.

Some of the codes for routine health examinations distinguish between "with" and "without" abnormal findings. Code assignment depends on the information that is known at the time the encounter is being coded. For example, if no abnormal findings were found during the examination, but the encounter is being coded before test results are back, it is acceptable to assign the code for "without abnormal findings." When assigning a code for "with abnormal findings," additional code(s) should be assigned to identify the specific abnormal finding(s).

Pre-operative examination and pre-procedural laboratory examination Z codes are for use only in those situations when a patient is being cleared for a procedure or surgery and no treatment is given.

The Z codes/categories for routine and administrative examinations:

Z00   Encounter for general examination without complaint, suspected or reported diagnosis

Z01   Encounter for other special examination without complaint, suspected or reported diagnosis

Z02   Encounter for administrative examination
Except: Z02.9, Encounter for administrative examinations, unspecified

Z32.0-   Encounter for pregnancy test

14)   Miscellaneous Z codes

The miscellaneous Z codes capture a number of other health care encounters that do not fall into one of the other categories. Certain of these codes

identify the reason for the encounter; others are for use as additional codes that provide useful information on circumstances that may affect a patient's care and treatment.

Prophylactic Organ Removal

For encounters specifically for prophylactic removal of an organ (such as prophylactic removal of breasts due to a genetic susceptibility to cancer or a family history of cancer), the principal or first-listed code should be a code from category Z40, Encounter for prophylactic surgery, followed by the appropriate codes to identify the associated risk factor (such as genetic susceptibility or family history).

If the patient has a malignancy of one site and is having prophylactic removal at another site to prevent either a new primary malignancy or metastatic disease, a code for the malignancy should also be assigned in addition to a code from subcategory Z40.0, Encounter for prophylactic surgery for risk factors related to malignant neoplasms. A Z40.0 code should not be assigned if the patient is having organ removal for treatment of a malignancy, such as the removal of the testes for the treatment of prostate cancer.

Miscellaneous Z codes/categories:

Z28   Immunization not carried out
Except: Z28.3, Underimmunization status

Z40   Encounter for prophylactic surgery

Z41   Encounter for procedures for purposes other than remedying health state
Except: Z41.9, Encounter for procedure for purposes other than remedying health state, unspecified

Z53   Persons encountering health services for specific procedures and treatment, not carried out

Z55   Problems related to education and literacy

Z56   Problems related to employment and unemployment

Z57   Occupational exposure to risk factors

Z58   Problems related to physical environment

Z59   Problems related to housing and economic circumstances

Z60   Problems related to social environment

Z62   Problems related to upbringing

Z63   Other problems related to primary support group, including family circumstances

Z64   Problems related to certain psychosocial circumstances

Z65   Problems related to other psychosocial circumstances

Z72   Problems related to lifestyle

Z73   Problems related to life management difficulty

Z74   Problems related to care provider dependency Except: Z74.01, Bed confinement status

Z75 Problems related to medical facilities and other health care

Z76.0 Encounter for issue of repeat prescription

Z76.3 Healthy person accompanying sick person

Z76.4 Other boarder to healthcare facility

Z76.5 Malingerer [conscious simulation]

Z91.1- Patient's noncompliance with medical treatment and regimen

Z91.83 Wandering in diseases classified elsewhere

Z91.89 Other specified personal risk factors, not elsewhere classified

15) Nonspecific Z codes

Certain Z codes are so non-specific, or potentially redundant with other codes in the classification, that there can be little justification for their use in the inpatient setting. Their use in the outpatient setting should be limited to those instances when there is no further documentation to permit more precise coding. Otherwise, any sign or symptom or any other reason for visit that is captured in another code should be used.

Nonspecific Z codes/categories:

Z02.9 Encounter for administrative examinations, unspecified

Z04.9 Encounter for examination and observation for unspecified reason

Z13.9 Encounter for screening, unspecified

Z41.9 Encounter for procedure for purposes other than remedying health state, unspecified

Z52.9 Donor of unspecified organ or tissue

Z86.59 Personal history of other mental and behavioral disorders

Z88.9 Allergy status to unspecified drugs, medicaments and biological substances status

Z92.0 Personal history of contraception

16) Z Codes That May Only be Principal/First-Listed Diagnosis

The following Z codes/categories may only be reported as the principal/first-listed diagnosis, except when there are multiple encounters on the same day and the medical records for the encounters are combined:

Z00 Encounter for general examination without complaint, suspected or reported diagnosis

Z01 Encounter for other special examination without complaint, suspected or reported diagnosis

Z02 Encounter for administrative examination

Z03 Encounter for medical observation for suspected diseases and conditions ruled out

Z04 Encounter for examination and observation for other reasons

Z33.2 Encounter for elective termination of pregnancy

Z31.81 Encounter for male factor infertility in female patient

Z31.82 Encounter for Rh incompatibility status

Z31.83 Encounter for assisted reproductive fertility procedure cycle

Z31.84 Encounter for fertility preservation procedure

Z34 Encounter for supervision of normal pregnancy

Z39 Encounter for maternal postpartum care and examination

Z38 Liveborn infants according to place of birth and type of delivery

Z42 Encounter for plastic and reconstructive surgery following medical procedure or healed injury

Z51.0 Encounter for antineoplastic radiation therapy

Z51.1- Encounter for antineoplastic chemotherapy and immunotherapy

Z52 Donors of organs and tissues Except: Z52.9, Donor of unspecified organ or tissue

Z76.1 Encounter for health supervision and care of foundling

Z76.2 Encounter for health supervision and care of other healthy infant and child

Z99.12 Encounter for respirator [ventilator] dependence during power failure

Section II. Selection of Principal Diagnosis

The circumstances of inpatient admission always govern the selection of principal diagnosis. The principal diagnosis is defined in the Uniform Hospital Discharge Data Set (UHDDS) as "that condition established after study to be chiefly responsible for occasioning the admission of the patient to the hospital for care."

The UHDDS definitions are used by hospitals to report inpatient data elements in a standardized manner. These data elements and their definitions can be found in the July 31, 1985, Federal Register (Vol. 50, No, 147), pp. 31038-40.

Since that time the application of the UHDDS definitions has been expanded to include all nonoutpatient settings (acute care, short term, long term care and psychiatric hospitals; home health agencies; rehab facilities; nursing homes, etc).

In determining principal diagnosis, coding conventions in the ICD-10-CM, the Tabular List and Alphabetic Index take precedence over these official coding guidelines. (See Section I.A., Conventions for the ICD-10-CM)

The importance of consistent, complete documentation in the medical record cannot be overemphasized. Without such documentation the application of all coding guidelines is a difficult, if not impossible, task.

A. Codes for symptoms, signs, and ill-defined conditions

Codes for symptoms, signs, and ill-defined conditions from Chapter 18 are not to be used as principal diagnosis when a related definitive diagnosis has been established.

B. Two or more interrelated conditions, each potentially meeting the definition for principal diagnosis.

When there are two or more interrelated conditions (such as diseases in the same ICD-10-CM chapter or manifestations characteristically associated with a certain disease) potentially meeting the definition of principal diagnosis, either condition may be sequenced first, unless the circumstances of the admission, the therapy provided, the Tabular List, or the Alphabetic Index indicate otherwise.

C. Two or more diagnoses that equally meet the definition for principal diagnosis

In the unusual instance when two or more diagnoses equally meet the criteria for principal diagnosis as determined by the circumstances of admission, diagnostic workup and/or therapy provided, and the Alphabetic Index, Tabular List, or another coding guidelines does not provide sequencing direction, any one of the diagnoses may be sequenced first.

D. Two or more comparative or contrasting conditions.

In those rare instances when two or more contrasting or comparative diagnoses are documented as "either/or" (or similar terminology), they are coded as if the diagnoses were confirmed and the diagnoses are sequenced according to the circumstances of the admission. If no further determination can be made as to which diagnosis should be principal, either diagnosis may be sequenced first.

E. A symptom(s) followed by contrasting/ comparative diagnoses

When a symptom(s) is followed by contrasting/ comparative diagnoses, the symptom code is sequenced first. **However, if the symptom code is integral to the conditions listed, no code for the symptom is reported.** All the contrasting/ comparative diagnoses should be coded as additional diagnoses.

F. Original treatment plan not carried out

Sequence as the principal diagnosis the condition, which after study occasioned the admission to the hospital, even though treatment may not have been carried out due to unforeseen circumstances.

G. Complications of surgery and other medical care

When the admission is for treatment of a complication resulting from surgery or other medical care, the complication code is sequenced as the principal diagnosis. If the complication is classified to the T80-T88 series and the code lacks the necessary specificity in describing the complication, an additional code for the specific complication should be assigned.

H. Uncertain Diagnosis

If the diagnosis documented at the time of discharge is qualified as "probable", "suspected", "likely", "questionable", "possible", or "still to be ruled out", or other similar terms indicating uncertainty, code the condition as if it existed or was established. The bases for these guidelines are the diagnostic workup, arrangements for further workup or observation, and initial therapeutic approach that correspond most closely with the established diagnosis.

Note: This guideline is applicable only to inpatient admissions to short-term, acute, long-term care and psychiatric hospitals.

I. Admission from Observation Unit

1. Admission Following Medical Observation

When a patient is admitted to an observation unit for a medical condition, which either worsens or does not improve, and is subsequently admitted as an inpatient of the same hospital for this same medical condition, the principal diagnosis would be the medical condition which led to the hospital admission.

2. Admission Following Post-Operative Observation

When a patient is admitted to an observation unit to monitor a condition (or complication) that develops following outpatient surgery, and then is subsequently admitted as an inpatient of the same hospital, hospitals should apply the Uniform Hospital Discharge Data Set (UHDDS) definition of principal diagnosis as "that condition established after study to be chiefly responsible for occasioning the admission of the patient to the hospital for care."

J. Admission from Outpatient Surgery

When a patient receives surgery in the hospital's outpatient surgery department and is subsequently admitted for continuing inpatient care at the same hospital, the following guidelines should be followed in selecting the principal diagnosis for the inpatient admission:

- If the reason for the inpatient admission is a complication, assign the complication as the principal diagnosis.
- If no complication, or other condition, is documented as the reason for the inpatient admission, assign the reason for the outpatient surgery as the principal diagnosis.
- If the reason for the inpatient admission is another condition unrelated to the surgery, assign the unrelated condition as the principal diagnosis.

K. *Admissions/Encounters for Rehabilitation*

When the purpose for the admission/encounter is rehabilitation, sequence first the code for the condition for which the service is being performed. For example, for an admission/ encounter for rehabilitation for right-sided dominant hemiplegia following a cerebrovascular infarction, report code I69.351, Hemiplegia and hemiparesis following cerebral infarction affecting right dominant side, as the first-listed or principal diagnosis.

If the condition for which the rehabilitation service is no longer present, report the appropriate aftercare code as the first-listed or principal diagnosis. For example, if a patient with severe degenerative osteoarthritis of the hip, underwent hip replacement and the current encounter/admission is for rehabilitation, report code Z47.1, Aftercare following joint replacement surgery, as the first-listed or principal diagnosis.

See Section I.C.21.c.7, Factors influencing health states and contact with health services, Aftercare.

Section III. Reporting Additional Diagnoses

GENERAL RULES FOR OTHER (ADDITIONAL) DIAGNOSES

For reporting purposes the definition for "other diagnoses" is interpreted as additional conditions that affect patient care in terms of requiring:

clinical evaluation; or
therapeutic treatment; or
diagnostic procedures; or
extended length of hospital stay; or
increased nursing care and/or monitoring.

The UHDDS item #11-b defines Other Diagnoses as "all conditions that coexist at the time of admission, that develop subsequently, or that affect the treatment received and/or the length of stay. Diagnoses that relate to an earlier episode which have no bearing on the current hospital stay are to be excluded." UHDDS definitions apply to inpatients in acute care, short-term, long term care and psychiatric hospital setting. The UHDDS definitions are used by acute care short-term hospitals to report inpatient data elements in a standardized manner. These data elements and their definitions can be found in the July 31, 1985, Federal Register (Vol. 50, No, 147), pp. 31038-40.

Since that time the application of the UHDDS definitions has been expanded to include all nonoutpatient settings (acute care, short term, long term care and psychiatric hospitals; home health agencies; rehab facilities; nursing homes, etc). The following guidelines are to be applied in designating "other diagnoses" when neither the Alphabetic Index nor the Tabular List in ICD-10-CM provide direction. The listing of the diagnoses in the patient record is the responsibility of the attending provider.

A. Previous conditions

If the provider has included a diagnosis in the final diagnostic statement, such as the discharge summary or the face sheet, it should ordinarily be coded. Some providers include in the diagnostic statement resolved conditions or diagnoses and status-post procedures from previous admission that have no bearing on the current stay. Such conditions are not to be reported and are coded only if required by hospital policy.

However, history codes (categories Z80-Z87) may be used as secondary codes if the historical condition or family history has an impact on current care or influences treatment.

B. Abnormal findings

Abnormal findings (laboratory, x-ray, pathologic, and other diagnostic results) are not coded and reported unless the provider indicates their clinical significance. If the findings are outside the normal range and the attending provider has ordered other tests to evaluate the condition or prescribed treatment, it is appropriate to ask the provider whether the abnormal finding should be added.

Please note: This differs from the coding practices in the outpatient setting for coding encounters for diagnostic tests that have been interpreted by a provider.

C. Uncertain Diagnosis

If the diagnosis documented at the time of discharge is qualified as "probable", "suspected", "likely", "questionable", "possible", or "still to be ruled out" or other similar terms indicating uncertainty, code the condition as if it existed or was established. The bases for these guidelines are the diagnostic workup, arrangements for further workup or observation, and initial therapeutic approach that correspond most closely with the established diagnosis.

Note: This guideline is applicable only to inpatient admissions to short-term, acute, long-term care and psychiatric hospitals.

Section IV. Diagnostic Coding and Reporting Guidelines for Outpatient Services

These coding guidelines for outpatient diagnoses have been approved for use by hospitals/ providers in coding and reporting hospital-based outpatient services and provider-based office visits.

Information about the use of certain abbreviations, punctuation, symbols, and other conventions used in the ICD-10-CM Tabular List (code numbers and titles), can be found in Section IA of these guidelines, under "Conventions Used in the Tabular List." **Section I.B. contains general guidelines that apply to the entire classification. Section I.C. contains chapter-specific guidelines that correspond to the chapters as they are arranged in the classification.** Information about the correct sequence to use in finding a code is also described in Section I.

The terms encounter and visit are often used interchangeably in describing outpatient service contacts and, therefore, appear together in these guidelines without distinguishing one from the other.

Though the conventions and general guidelines apply to all settings, coding guidelines for outpatient and provider reporting of diagnoses will vary in a number of instances from those for inpatient diagnoses, recognizing that:

The Uniform Hospital Discharge Data Set (UHDDS) definition of principal diagnosis applies only to inpatients in acute, short-term, long-term care and psychiatric hospitals.

Coding guidelines for inconclusive diagnoses (probable, suspected, rule out, etc.) were developed for inpatient reporting and do not apply to outpatients.

A. Selection of first-listed condition

In the outpatient setting, the term first-listed diagnosis is used in lieu of principal diagnosis.

In determining the first-listed diagnosis the coding conventions of ICD-10-CM, as well as the general and disease specific guidelines take precedence over the outpatient guidelines.

Diagnoses often are not established at the time of the initial encounter/visit. It may take two or more visits before the diagnosis is confirmed.

The most critical rule involves beginning the search for the correct code assignment through the Alphabetic Index. Never begin searching initially in the Tabular List as this will lead to coding errors.

1. Outpatient Surgery

When a patient presents for outpatient surgery (same day surgery), code the reason for the surgery as the first-listed diagnosis (reason for the encounter), even if the surgery is not performed due to a contraindication.

2. Observation Stay

When a patient is admitted for observation for a medical condition, assign a code for the medical condition as the first-listed diagnosis.

When a patient presents for outpatient surgery and develops complications requiring admission to observation, code the reason for the surgery as the first reported diagnosis (reason for the encounter), followed by codes for the complications as secondary diagnoses.

B. Codes from A00.0 through T88.9, Z00-Z99

The appropriate code(s) from A00.0 through T88.9, Z00-Z99 must be used to identify diagnoses, symptoms, conditions, problems, complaints, or other reason(s) for the encounter/visit.

C. Accurate reporting of ICD-10-CM diagnosis codes

For accurate reporting of ICD-10-CM diagnosis codes, the documentation should describe the patient's condition, using terminology which includes specific diagnoses as well as symptoms, problems, or reasons for the encounter. There are ICD-10-CM codes to describe all of these.

D. Codes that describe symptoms and signs

Codes that describe symptoms and signs, as opposed to diagnoses, are acceptable for reporting purposes when a diagnosis has not been established (confirmed) by the provider. Chapter 18 of ICD-10-CM, Symptoms, Signs, and Abnormal Clinical and Laboratory Findings Not Elsewhere Classified (codes R00-R99) contain many, but not all codes for symptoms.

E. Encounters for circumstances other than a disease or injury

ICD-10-CM provides codes to deal with encounters for circumstances other than a disease or injury. The Factors Influencing Health Status and Contact with Health Services codes (Z00-Z99) are provided to deal with occasions when circumstances other than a disease or injury are recorded as diagnosis or problems.

See Section I.C.21. Factors influencing health status and contact with health services.

F. Level of Detail in Coding

1. ICD-10-CM codes with 3, 4, 5, 6 or 7 characters

ICD-10-CM is composed of codes with 3, 4, 5, 6 or 7 characters. Codes with three characters are included in ICD-10-CM as the heading of a category of codes that may be further subdivided by the use of fourth, fifth, sixth or seventh characters to provide greater specificity.

2. Use of full number of *characters* required for a code

A three-character code is to be used only if it is not further subdivided. A code is invalid if it has not been coded to the full number of characters required for that code, including the 7th character, if applicable.

G. ICD-10-CM code for the diagnosis, condition, problem, or other reason for encounter/visit

List first the ICD-10-CM code for the diagnosis, condition, problem, or other reason for encounter/visit shown in the medical record to be chiefly responsible for the services provided. List additional codes that describe any coexisting conditions. In some cases the first-listed diagnosis may be a symptom when a diagnosis has not been established (confirmed) by the physician.

H. Uncertain diagnosis

Do not code diagnoses documented as "probable", "suspected," "questionable," "rule out," or "working diagnosis" or other similar terms indicating uncertainty. Rather, code the condition(s) to the highest degree of certainty for that encounter/visit, such as symptoms, signs, abnormal test results, or other reason for the visit.

Please note: This differs from the coding practices used by short-term, acute care, long-term care and psychiatric hospitals.

I. Chronic diseases

Chronic diseases treated on an ongoing basis may be coded and reported as many times as the patient receives treatment and care for the condition(s)

J. Code all documented conditions that coexist

Code all documented conditions that coexist at the time of the encounter/visit, and require or affect patient care treatment or management. Do not code conditions that were previously treated and no longer exist. However, history codes (categories Z80-Z87) may be used as secondary codes if the historical condition or family history has an impact on current care or influences treatment.

K. Patients receiving diagnostic services only

For patients receiving diagnostic services only during an encounter/visit, sequence first the diagnosis, condition, problem, or other reason for encounter/visit shown in the medical record to be chiefly responsible for the outpatient services provided during the encounter/visit. Codes for other diagnoses (e.g., chronic conditions) may be sequenced as additional diagnoses.

For encounters for routine laboratory/radiology testing in the absence of any signs, symptoms, or associated diagnosis, assign Z01.89, Encounter for other specified special examinations. If routine testing is performed during the same encounter as a test to evaluate a sign, symptom, or diagnosis, it is appropriate to assign both the Z code and the code describing the reason for the non-routine test.

For outpatient encounters for diagnostic tests that have been interpreted by a physician, and the final report is available at the time of coding, code any confirmed or definitive diagnosis(es) documented in the interpretation. Do not code related signs and symptoms as additional diagnoses.

Please note: This differs from the coding practice in the hospital inpatient setting regarding abnormal findings on test results.

L. **Patients receiving therapeutic services only**

For patients receiving therapeutic services only during an encounter/visit, sequence first the diagnosis, condition, problem, or other reason for encounter/visit shown in the medical record to be chiefly responsible for the outpatient services provided during the encounter/visit. Codes for other diagnoses (e.g., chronic conditions) may be sequenced as additional diagnoses.

The only exception to this rule is that when the primary reason for the admission/encounter is chemotherapy or radiation therapy, the appropriate Z code for the service is listed first, and the diagnosis or problem for which the service is being performed listed second.

M. **Patients receiving preoperative evaluations only**

For patients receiving preoperative evaluations only, sequence first a code from subcategory Z01.81, Encounter for pre-procedural examinations, to describe the pre-op consultations. Assign a code for the condition to describe the reason for the surgery as an additional diagnosis. Code also any findings related to the pre-op evaluation.

N. **Ambulatory surgery**

For ambulatory surgery, code the diagnosis for which the surgery was performed. If the postoperative diagnosis is known to be different from the preoperative diagnosis at the time the diagnosis is confirmed, select the postoperative diagnosis for coding, since it is the most definitive.

O. **Routine outpatient prenatal visits**

See Section I.C.15. Routine outpatient prenatal visits.

P. **Encounters for general medical examinations with abnormal findings**

The subcategories for encounters for general medical examinations, Z00.0-, provide codes for with and without abnormal findings. Should a general medical examination result in an abnormal finding, the code for general medical examination with abnormal finding should be assigned as the first-listed diagnosis. A secondary code for the abnormal finding should also be coded.

Q. **Encounters for routine health screenings**

See Section I.C.21. Factors influencing health status and contact with health services, Screening

Appendix I
Present on Admission Reporting Guidelines

Introduction

These guidelines are to be used as a supplement to the *ICD-10-CM Official Guidelines for Coding and Reporting* to facilitate the assignment of the Present on Admission (POA) indicator for each diagnosis and external cause of injury code reported on claim forms (UB-04 and 837 Institutional).

These guidelines are not intended to replace any guidelines in the main body of the *ICD-10-CM Official Guidelines for Coding and Reporting*. The POA guidelines are not intended to provide guidance on when a condition should be coded, but rather, how to apply the POA indicator to the final set of diagnosis codes that have been assigned in accordance with Sections I, II, and III of the official coding guidelines. Subsequent to the assignment of the ICD-10-CM codes, the POA indicator should then be assigned to those conditions that have been coded.

As stated in the Introduction to the ICD-10-CM Official Guidelines for Coding and Reporting, a joint effort between the healthcare provider and the coder is essential to achieve complete and accurate documentation, code assignment, and reporting of diagnoses and procedures. The importance of consistent, complete documentation in the medical record cannot be overemphasized. Medical record documentation from any provider involved in the care and treatment of the patient may be used to support the determination of whether a condition was present on admission or not. In the context of the official coding guidelines, the term "provider" means a physician or any qualified healthcare practitioner who is legally accountable for establishing the patient's diagnosis.

These guidelines are not a substitute for the provider's clinical judgment as to the determination of whether a condition was/was not present on admission. The provider should be queried regarding issues related to the linking of signs/symptoms, timing of test results, and the timing of findings.

General Reporting Requirements

All claims involving inpatient admissions to general acute care hospitals or other facilities that are subject to a law or regulation mandating collection of present on admission information.

Present on admission is defined as present at the time the order for inpatient admission occurs -- conditions that develop during an outpatient encounter, including emergency department, observation, or outpatient surgery, are considered as present on admission.

POA indicator is assigned to principal and secondary diagnoses (as defined in Section II of the Official Guidelines for Coding and Reporting) and the external cause of injury codes.

Issues related to inconsistent, missing, conflicting or unclear documentation must still be resolved by the provider.

If a condition would not be coded and reported based on UHDDS definitions and current official coding guidelines, then the POA indicator would not be reported.

Reporting Options

Y - Yes

N - No

U - Unknown

W - Clinically undetermined

Unreported/Not used - (Exempt from POA reporting)

Reporting Definitions

Y = present at the time of inpatient admission

N = not present at the time of inpatient admission

U = documentation is insufficient to determine if condition is present on admission

W = provider is unable to clinically determine whether condition was present on admission or not

Timeframe for POA Identification and Documentation

There is no required timeframe as to when a provider (per the definition of "provider" used in these guidelines) must identify or document a condition to be present on admission. In some clinical situations, it may not be possible for a provider to make a definitive diagnosis (or a condition may not be recognized or reported by the patient) for a period of time after admission. In some cases it may be several days before the provider arrives at a definitive diagnosis. This does not mean that the condition was not present on admission. Determination of whether the condition was present on admission or not will be based on the applicable POA guideline as identified in this document, or on the provider's best clinical judgment.

If at the time of code assignment the documentation is unclear as to whether a condition was present on admission or not, it is appropriate to query the provider for clarification.

Assigning the POA Indicator

Condition is on the "Exempt from Reporting" list

Leave the "present on admission" field blank if the condition is on the list of ICD-10-CM codes for which this field is not applicable. This is the only circumstance in which the field may be left blank.

POA Explicitly Documented

Assign Y for any condition the provider explicitly documents as being present on admission.

Assign N for any condition the provider explicitly documents as not present at the time of admission.

Conditions diagnosed prior to inpatient admission

Assign "Y" for conditions that were diagnosed prior to admission (example: hypertension, diabetes mellitus, asthma)

Conditions diagnosed during the admission but clearly present before admission

Assign "Y" for conditions diagnosed during the admission that were clearly present but not diagnosed until after admission occurred.

Diagnoses subsequently confirmed after admission are considered present on admission if at the time of admission they are documented as suspected, possible, rule out, differential diagnosis, or constitute an underlying cause of a symptom that is present at the time of admission.

Condition develops during outpatient encounter prior to inpatient admission

Assign Y for any condition that develops during an outpatient encounter prior to a written order for inpatient admission.

Documentation does not indicate whether condition was present on admission

Assign "U" when the medical record documentation is unclear as to whether the condition was present on admission. "U" should not be routinely assigned and used only in very limited circumstances. Coders are encouraged to query the providers when the documentation is unclear.

Documentation states that it cannot be determined whether the condition was or was not present on admission

Assign "W" when the medical record documentation indicates that it cannot be clinically determined whether or not the condition was present on admission.

Chronic condition with acute exacerbation during the admission

If a single code identifies both the chronic condition and the acute exacerbation, see POA guidelines pertaining to combination codes.

If a single code only identifies the chronic condition and not the acute exacerbation (e.g., acute exacerbation of chronic leukemia), assign "Y."

Conditions documented as possible, probable, suspected, or rule out at the time of discharge

If the final diagnosis contains a possible, probable, suspected, or rule out diagnosis, and this diagnosis was based on signs, symptoms or clinical findings suspected at the time of inpatient admission, assign "Y."

If the final diagnosis contains a possible, probable, suspected, or rule out diagnosis, and this diagnosis was based on signs, symptoms or clinical findings that were not present on admission, assign "N".

Conditions documented as impending or threatened at the time of discharge

If the final diagnosis contains an impending or threatened diagnosis, and this diagnosis is based on symptoms or clinical findings that were present on admission, assign "Y".

If the final diagnosis contains an impending or threatened diagnosis, and this diagnosis is based on symptoms or clinical findings that were not present on admission, assign "N".

Acute and Chronic Conditions

Assign "Y" for acute conditions that are present at time of admission and N for acute conditions that are not present at time of admission.

Assign "Y" for chronic conditions, even though the condition may not be diagnosed until after admission.

If a single code identifies both an acute and chronic condition, see the POA guidelines for combination codes.

Combination Codes

Assign "N" if any part of the combination code was not present on admission (e.g., COPD with acute exacerbation and the exacerbation was not present on admission; gastric ulcer that does not start bleeding until after admission; asthma patient develops status asthmaticus after admission)

Assign "Y" if all parts of the combination code were present on admission (e.g., patient with acute prostatitis admitted with hematuria)

If the final diagnosis includes comparative or contrasting diagnoses, and both were present, or suspected, at the time of admission, assign "Y".

For infection codes that include the causal organism, assign "Y" if the infection (or signs of the infection) was present on admission, even though the culture results may not be known until after admission (e.g., patient is admitted with pneumonia and the provider documents pseudomonas as the causal organism a few days later).

Same Diagnosis Code for Two or More Conditions

When the same ICD-10-CM diagnosis code applies to two or more conditions during the same encounter (e.g. two separate conditions classified to the same ICD-10-CM diagnosis code):

Assign "Y" if all conditions represented by the single ICD-10-CM code were present on admission (e.g. bilateral unspecified age-related cataracts).

Assign "N" if any of the conditions represented by the single ICD-10-CM code was not present on admission (e.g. traumatic secondary and recurrent hemorrhage and seroma is assigned to a single code T79.2, but only one of the conditions was present on admission).

Obstetrical conditions

Whether or not the patient delivers during the current hospitalization does not affect assignment of the POA indicator. The determining factor for POA assignment is whether the pregnancy complication or obstetrical condition described by the code was present at the time of admission or not.

If the pregnancy complication or obstetrical condition was present on admission (e.g., patient admitted in preterm labor), assign "Y".

If the pregnancy complication or obstetrical condition was not present on admission (e.g., 2nd degree laceration during delivery, postpartum hemorrhage that occurred during current hospitalization, fetal distress develops after admission), assign "N".

If the obstetrical code includes more than one diagnosis and any of the diagnoses identified by the code were not present on admission assign "N".

(e.g., Category O11, Pre-existing hypertension with pre-eclampsia)

Perinatal conditions

Newborns are not considered to be admitted until after birth. Therefore, any condition present at birth or that developed in utero is considered present at admission and should be assigned "Y". This includes conditions that occur during delivery (e.g., injury during delivery, meconium aspiration, exposure to streptococcus B in the vaginal canal).

Congenital conditions and anomalies

Assign "Y" for congenital conditions and anomalies except for categories Q00-Q99, Congenital anomalies, which are on the exempt list. Congenital conditions are always considered present on admission.

External cause of injury codes

Assign "Y" for any external cause code representing an external cause of morbidity that occurred prior to inpatient admission (e.g., patient fell out of bed at home, patient fell out of bed in emergency room prior to admission)

Assign "N" for any external cause code representing an external cause of morbidity that occurred during inpatient hospitalization (e.g., patient fell out of hospital bed during hospital stay, patient experienced an adverse reaction to a medication administered after inpatient admission)

Categories and Codes
Exempt from Diagnosis Present on Admission Requirement

Note: "Diagnosis present on admission" for these code categories are exempt because they represent circumstances regarding the healthcare encounter or factors influencing health status that do not represent a current disease or injury or are always present on admission

B90-B94, Sequelae of infectious and parasitic diseases

E64, Sequelae of malnutrition and other nutritional deficiencies

I25.2, Old myocardial infarction

I69, Sequelae of cerebrovascular disease

O09, Supervision of high risk pregnancy

O66.5, Attempted application of vacuum extractor and forceps

O80, Encounter for full-term uncomplicated delivery

O94, Sequelae of complication of pregnancy, childbirth, and the puerperium

P00, Newborn (suspected to be) affected by maternal conditions that may be unrelated to present pregnancy

Q00 - Q99, Congenital malformations, deformations and chromosomal abnormalities

S00-T88.9, Injury, poisoning and certain other consequences of external causes with 7th character representing subsequent encounter or sequela

V00-V09, Pedestrian injured in transport accident

Except V00.81-, Accident with wheelchair (powered)

V00.83-, Accident with motorized mobility scooter

V10-V19, Pedal cycle rider injured in transport accident

V20-V29, Motorcycle rider injured in transport accident

V30-V39, Occupant of three-wheeled motor vehicle injured in transport accident

V40-V49, Car occupant injured in transport accident

V50-V59, Occupant of pick-up truck or van injured in transport accident

V60-V69, Occupant of heavy transport vehicle injured in transport accident

V70-V79, Bus occupant injured in transport accident

V80-V89, Other land transport accidents

V90-V94, Water transport accidents

V95-V97, Air and space transport accidents

V98-V99, Other and unspecified transport accidents

W09, Fall on and from playground equipment

W14, Fall from tree

W15, Fall from cliff

W17.0, Fall into well

W17.1, Fall into storm drain or manhole

W18.01 Striking against sports equipment with subsequent fall

W21, Striking against or struck by sports equipment

W30, Contact with agricultural machinery

W31, Contact with other and unspecified machinery

W32-W34, Accidental handgun discharge and malfunction

W35- W40, Exposure to inanimate mechanical forces

W52, Crushed, pushed or stepped on by crowd or human stampede

W56, Contact with nonvenomous marine animal

W58, Contact with crocodile or alligator

W61, Contact with birds (domestic) (wild)

W62, Contact with nonvenomous amphibians

W89, Exposure to man-made visible and ultraviolet light

X02, Exposure to controlled fire in building or structure

X03, Exposure to controlled fire, not in building or structure

X04, Exposure to ignition of highly flammable material

X52, Prolonged stay in weightless environment

X71, Intentional self-harm by drowning and submersion

Except X71.0-, Intentional self-harm by drowning and submersion while in bath tub

X72, Intentional self-harm by handgun discharge

X73, Intentional self-harm by rifle, shotgun and larger firearm discharge

X74, Intentional self-harm by other and unspecified firearm and gun discharge

X75, Intentional self-harm by explosive material

X76, Intentional self-harm by smoke, fire and flames

X77, Intentional self-harm by steam, hot vapors and hot objects

X81, Intentional self-harm by jumping or lying in front of moving object

X82, Intentional self-harm by crashing of motor vehicle

X83, Intentional self-harm by other specified means

Y03, Assault by crashing of motor vehicle

Y07, Perpetrator of assault, maltreatment and neglect

Y08.8, Assault by strike by sports equipment

Y21, Drowning and submersion, undetermined intent

Y22, Handgun discharge, undetermined intent

Y23, Rifle, shotgun and larger firearm discharge, undetermined intent

Y24, Other and unspecified firearm discharge, undetermined intent

Y30, Falling, jumping or pushed from a high place, undetermined intent

Y32, Assault by crashing of motor vehicle, undetermined intent

Y37, Military operations

Y36, Operations of war

Y92, Place of occurrence of the external cause

Y93, Activity code

Y99, External cause status

Z00, Encounter for general examination without complaint, suspected or reported diagnosis

Z01, Encounter for other special examination without complaint, suspected or reported diagnosis

Z02, Encounter for administrative examination

Z03, Encounter for medical observation for suspected diseases and conditions ruled out

Z08, Encounter for follow-up examination following completed treatment for malignant neoplasm

Z09, Encounter for follow-up examination after completed treatment for conditions other than malignant neoplasm

Z11, Encounter for screening for infectious and parasitic diseases

Z11.8, Encounter for screening for other infectious and parasitic diseases

Z12, Encounter for screening for malignant neoplasms

Z13, Encounter for screening for other diseases and disorders

Z13.4, Encounter for screening for certain developmental disorders in childhood

Z13.5, Encounter for screening for eye and ear disorders

Z13.6, Encounter for screening for cardiovascular disorders

Z13.83, Encounter for screening for respiratory disorder NEC

Z13.89, Encounter for screening for other disorder

Z13.89, Encounter for screening for other disorder

Z14, Genetic carrier

Z15, Genetic susceptibility to disease

Z17, Estrogen receptor status

Z18, Retained foreign body fragments

Z22, Carrier of infectious disease

Z23, Encounter for immunization

Z28, Immunization not carried out and underimmunization status

Z28.3, Underimmunization status

Z30, Encounter for contraceptive management

Z31, Encounter for procreative management

Z34, Encounter for supervision of normal pregnancy

Z36, Encounter for antenatal screening of mother

Z37, Outcome of delivery

Z38, Liveborn infants according to place of birth and type of delivery

Z39, Encounter for maternal postpartum care and examination

Z41, Encounter for procedures for purposes other than remedying health state

Z42, Encounter for plastic and reconstructive surgery following medical procedure or healed injury

Z43, Encounter for attention to artificial openings

Z44, Encounter for fitting and adjustment of external prosthetic device

Z45, Encounter for adjustment and management of implanted device

Z46, Encounter for fitting and adjustment of other devices

Z47.8, Encounter for other orthopedic aftercare

Z49, Encounter for care involving renal dialysis

Z51, Encounter for other aftercare

Z51.5, Encounter for palliative care

Z51.8, Encounter for other specified aftercare

Z52, Donors of organs and tissues

Z59, Problems related to housing and economic circumstances

Z63, Other problems related to primary support group, including family circumstances

Z65, Problems related to other psychosocial circumstances

Z65.8 Other specified problems related to psychosocial circumstances

Z67.1 - Z67.9 Blood type

Z68, Body mass index (BMI)

Z72, Problems related to lifestyle

Z74.01, Bed confinement status

Z76, Persons encountering health services in other circumstances

Z77.110- Z77.128, Environmental pollution and hazards in the physical environment

Z78, Other specified health status

Z79, Long term (current) drug therapy

Z80, Family history of primary malignant neoplasm

Z81, Family history of mental and behavioral disorders

Z82, Family history of certain disabilities and chronic diseases (leading to disablement)

Z83, Family history of other specific disorders

Z84, Family history of other conditions

Z85, Personal history of primary malignant neoplasm

Z86, Personal history of certain other diseases

Z87, Personal history of other diseases and conditions

Z87.828, Personal history of other (healed) physical injury and trauma

Z87.891, Personal history of nicotine dependence

Z88, Allergy status to drugs, medicaments and biological substances

Z89, Acquired absence of limb

Z90.710, Acquired absence of both cervix and uterus

Z91.0, Allergy status, other than to drugs and biological substances

Z91.4, Personal history of psychological trauma, not elsewhere classified

Z91.5, Personal history of self-harm

Z91.8, Other specified risk factors, not elsewhere classified

Z92, Personal history of medical treatment

Z93, Artificial opening status

Z94, Transplanted organ and tissue status

Z95, Presence of cardiac and vascular implants and grafts

Z97, Presence of other devices

Z98, Other postprocedural states

Z99, Dependence on enabling machines and devices, not elsewhere classified

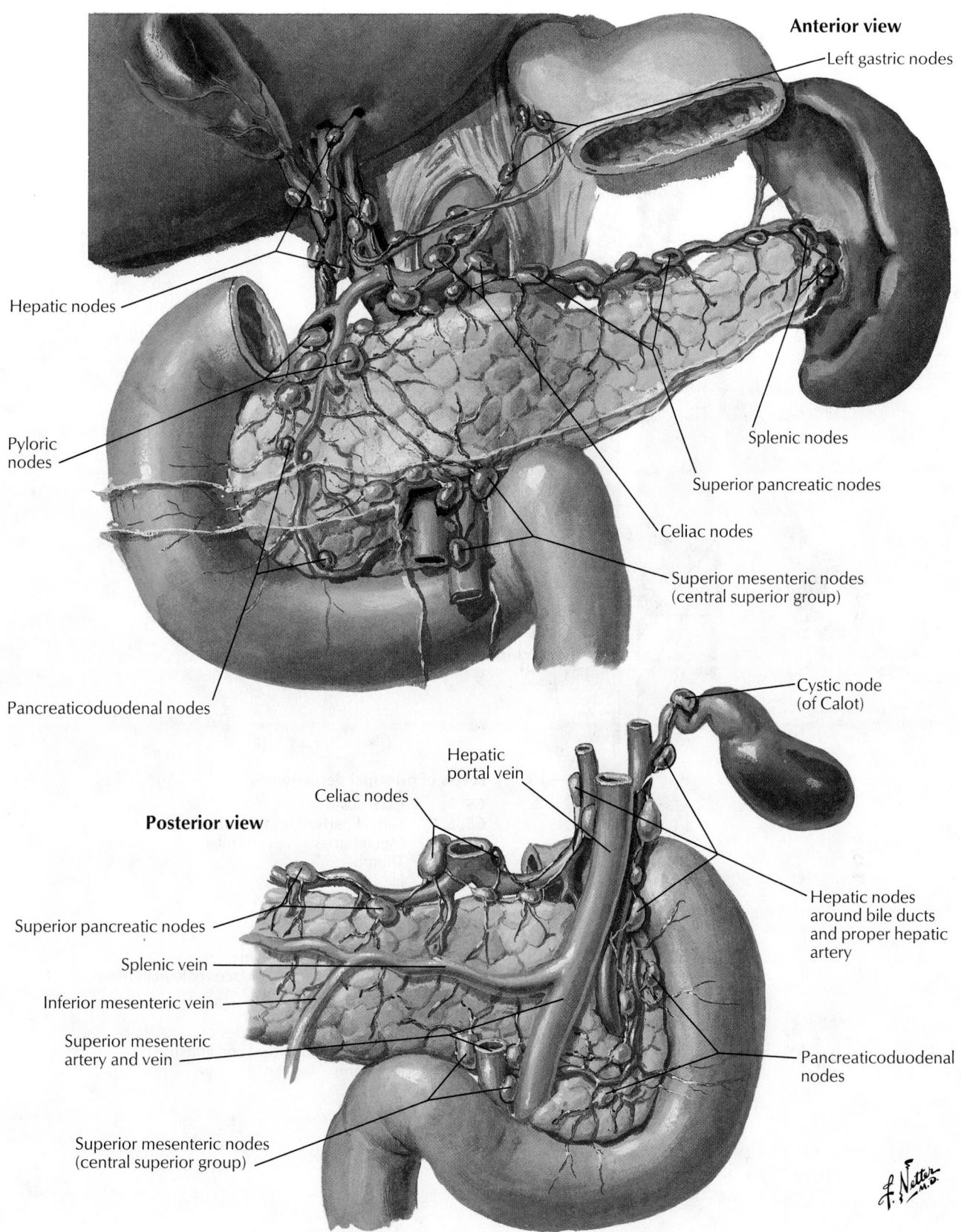

Anterior view

Left gastric nodes

Hepatic nodes

Pyloric nodes

Splenic nodes

Superior pancreatic nodes

Celiac nodes

Superior mesenteric nodes
(central superior group)

Pancreaticoduodenal nodes

Cystic node
(of Calot)

Hepatic
portal vein

Celiac nodes

Posterior view

Hepatic nodes
around bile ducts
and proper hepatic
artery

Superior pancreatic nodes

Splenic vein

Inferior mesenteric vein

Superior mesenteric
artery and vein

Pancreaticoduodenal
nodes

Superior mesenteric nodes
(central superior group)

Plate 315   Lymph Vessels and Nodes of Pancreas. (Netter: Atlas of Human Anatomy, 4 ed, 2006, Saunders.)

Dermatome pattern

Levels of principal dermatomes

C5	Clavicles
C5, 6, 7	Lateral parts of upper limbs
C8; T1	Medial sides of upper limbs
C6	Thumb
C6, 7, 8	Hand
C8	Ring and little fingers
T4	Level of nipples
T10	Level of umbilicus
T12	Inguinal or groin regions
L1, 2, 3, 4	Anterior and inner surfaces of lower limbs
L4, 5; S1	Foot
L4	Medial side of great toe
L5; S1, 2	Outer and posterior sides of lower limbs
S1	Lateral margin of foot and little toe
S2, 3, 4	Perineum

Plate 164 Dermatomes. (Netter: Atlas of Human Anatomy, 4 ed, 2006, Saunders.)

Female: frontal section

Peritoneum
Body of bladder
Fundus of bladder
Interureteric crest
Left ureteric orifice
Trigone of bladder
Neck of bladder
Paravesical endopelvic fascia and vesical venous plexus
Vesical fascia
Tendinous arch of levator ani muscle
Obturator internus muscle
Levator ani muscle
Tendinous arch of pelvic fascia
Urethra
Sphincter urethrae muscle
Perineal membrane
Inferior pubic ramus
Crus of clitoris and ischiocavernosus muscle
Bulb of vestibule and bulbospongiosus muscle
Deep perineal (investing or Gallaudet's) fascia
Superficial perineal (Colles') fascia

Round ligament of uterus
Vagina

Male: frontal section

Body of bladder
Fundus of bladder
Ductus (vas) deferens
Interureteric crest
Right ureteric orifice
Trigone of bladder
Neck of bladder
Paravesical endopelvic fascia and vesical venous plexus
Tendinous arch of levator ani muscle
Uvula of bladder
Obturator internus muscle
Levator ani muscle
Capsule of prostate
Prostate and prostatic urethra
Seminal colliculus
Bulbourethral (Cowper's) gland
Perineal membrane and sphincter urethrae muscle
Bulbous portion of spongy urethra
Corpus spongiosum and bulbospongiosus muscle
Deep perineal (investing or Gallaudet's) fascia

Peritoneum
Internal urethral sphincter
Tendinous arch of pelvic fascia
Anterior recess of ischioanal fossa
Inferior pubic ramus
Crus of penis and ischiocavernosus muscle
Superficial perineal (Colles') fascia

Plate 366   Urinary Bladder: Female and Male. (Netter: Atlas of Human Anatomy, 4 ed, 2006, Saunders.)

Sites of ectopic implantation

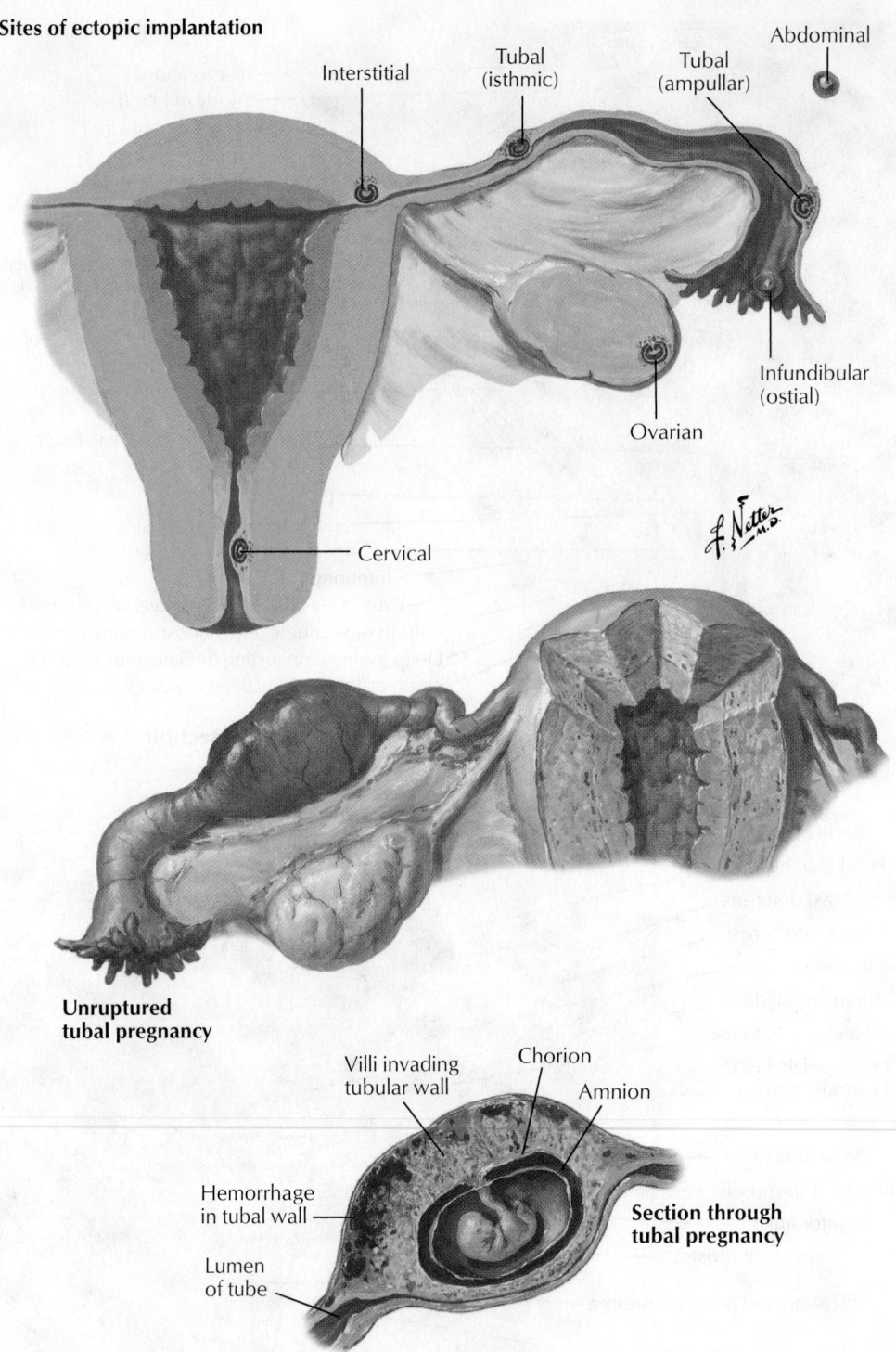

Interstitial

Tubal (isthmic)

Tubal (ampullar)

Abdominal

Infundibular (ostial)

Ovarian

Cervical

Unruptured tubal pregnancy

Villi invading tubular wall

Chorion

Amnion

Hemorrhage in tubal wall

Lumen of tube

Section through tubal pregnancy

Plate 375   Ectopic Pregnancy. (Netter: Atlas of Human Anatomy, 4 ed, 2006, Saunders.)

Skin of penis

Superficial fascia of penis (Colles' fascia)

Deep (Buck's) fascia of penis

Testicular artery

Ductus deferens

Artery to ductus deferens

Genital branch of genitofemoral nerve

Pampiniform (venous) plexus

Epididymis

Appendix of epididymis

Appendix of testis

Testis (covered by visceral layer of tunica vaginalis)

Parietal layer of tunica vaginalis

Superficial inguinal ring

External spermatic fascia

Cremaster muscle and fascia

Septum of scrotum (formed by dartos fascia)

Superficial (dartos) fascia of scrotum

Skin of scrotum

Superficial (dartos) fascia of scrotum

External spermatic fascia

Cremaster muscle and fascia

Internal spermatic fascia

Parietal layer of tunica vaginalis

Epididymis

Testis (covered by visceral layer of tunica vaginalis)

Skin of scrotum

Plate 387   Scrotum and Contents. (Netter: Atlas of Human Anatomy, 4 ed, 2006, Saunders.)

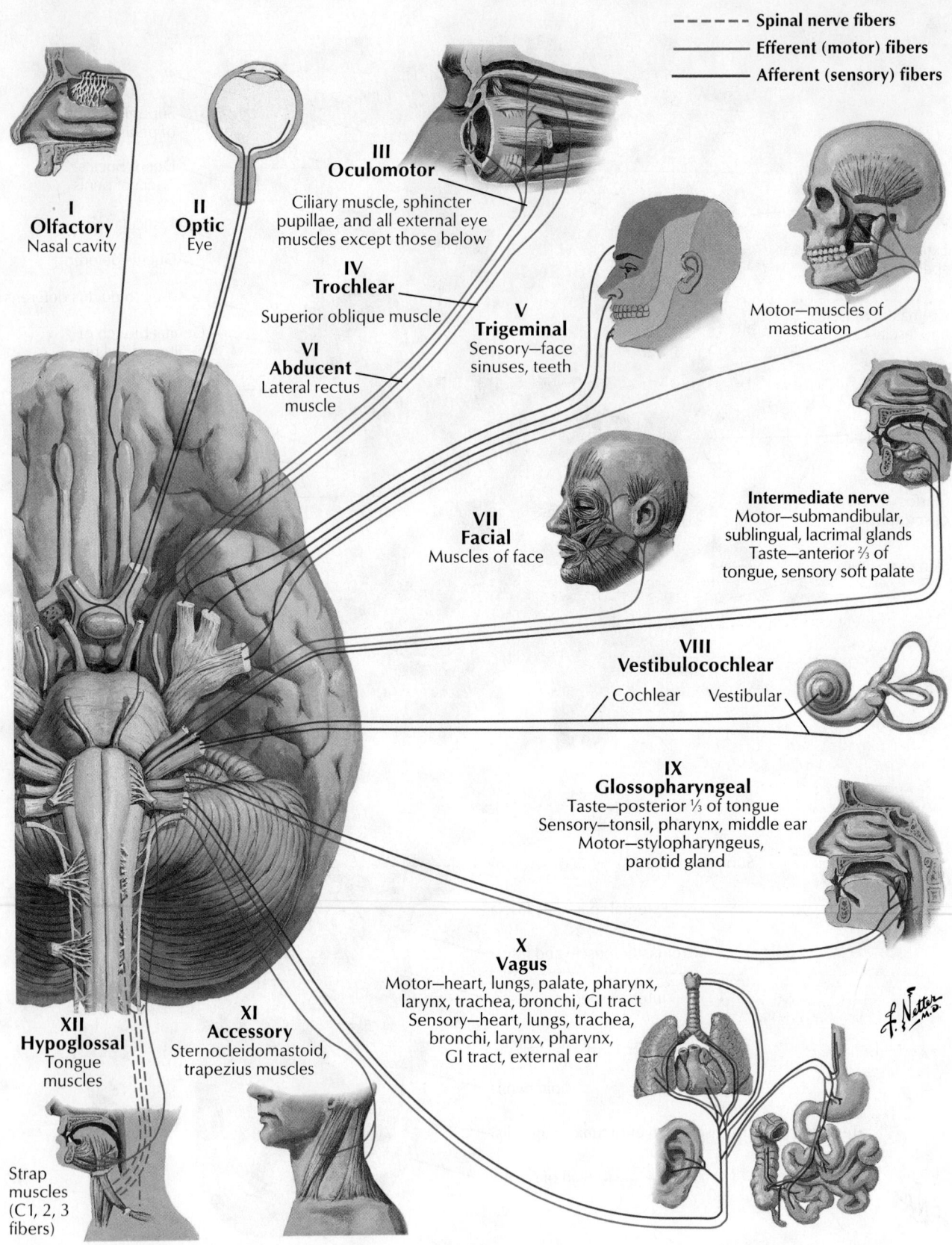

- - - - - - **Spinal nerve fibers**
————— **Efferent (motor) fibers**
————— **Afferent (sensory) fibers**

I
Olfactory
Nasal cavity

II
Optic
Eye

III
Oculomotor
Ciliary muscle, sphincter pupillae, and all external eye muscles except those below

IV
Trochlear
Superior oblique muscle

VI
Abducent
Lateral rectus muscle

V
Trigeminal
Sensory—face sinuses, teeth

Motor—muscles of mastication

VII
Facial
Muscles of face

Intermediate nerve
Motor—submandibular, sublingual, lacrimal glands
Taste—anterior ⅔ of tongue, sensory soft palate

VIII
Vestibulocochlear
Cochlear   Vestibular

IX
Glossopharyngeal
Taste—posterior ⅓ of tongue
Sensory—tonsil, pharynx, middle ear
Motor—stylopharyngeus, parotid gland

X
Vagus
Motor—heart, lungs, palate, pharynx, larynx, trachea, bronchi, GI tract
Sensory—heart, lungs, trachea, bronchi, larynx, pharynx, GI tract, external ear

XII
Hypoglossal
Tongue muscles

XI
Accessory
Sternocleidomastoid, trapezius muscles

Strap muscles (C1, 2, 3 fibers)

Plate 118   Cranial Nerves (Motor and Sensory Distribution): Schema. (Netter: Atlas of Human Anatomy, 4 ed, 2006, Saunders.)

Superior view

Supratrochlear nerve

Medial rectus muscle

Superior oblique muscle

Infratrochlear nerve

Nasociliary nerve

Trochlear nerve (IV)

Common tendinous ring

Ophthalmic nerve (V₁)

Optic nerve (II)

Internal carotid artery and nerve plexus

Oculomotor nerve (III)

Trochlear nerve (IV)

Abducent nerve (VI)

Tentorium cerebelli

Medial branch } Supraorbital nerve
Lateral branch }

Levator palpebrae superioris muscle

Superior rectus muscle

Lacrimal gland

Lacrimal nerve

Lateral rectus muscle

Frontal nerve

Maxillary nerve (V₂)

Meningeal branch of maxillary nerve

Mandibular nerve (V₃)

Lesser petrosal nerve

Meningeal branch of mandibular nerve

Greater petrosal nerve

Trigeminal (semilunar) ganglion

Tentorial (meningeal) branch of ophthalmic nerve

Superior view:
levator palpebrae superioris, superior rectus, and superior oblique muscles partially cut away

Supratrochlear nerve (cut)

Supraorbital nerve branches (cut)

Infratrochlear nerve

Anterior ethmoidal nerve

Optic nerve (II)

Posterior ethmoidal nerve

Superior branch of oculomotor nerve (III) (cut)

Nasociliary nerve

Internal carotid plexus

Trochlear nerve (IV) (cut)

Oculomotor nerve (III)

Abducent nerve (VI)

Long ciliary nerves

Short ciliary nerves

Lacrimal nerve

Ciliary ganglion

Parasympathetic root of ciliary ganglion (from inferior branch of oculomotor nerve)

Sympathetic root of ciliary ganglion (from internal carotid plexus)

Sensory root of ciliary ganglion (from nasociliary nerve)

Branches to inferior and medial rectus muscles

Abducent nerve (VI)

Inferior branch of oculomotor nerve (III)

Lacrimal nerve

Frontal nerve (cut)

Ophthalmic nerve (V₁)

Plate 86 Nerves of Orbit. (Netter: Atlas of Human Anatomy, 4 ed, 2006, Saunders.)

Anterior (palmar) view

Musculocutaneous nerve { Lateral antebrachial cutaneous nerve

Medial antebrachial cutaneous nerve

Radial nerve { Superficial branch

Palmar branch

Ulnar nerve

Palmar digital branches

Median nerve { Palmar branch / Palmar digital branches

Posterior (dorsal) view

Lateral antebrachial cutaneous nerve — **Musculocutaneous nerve**

Medial antebrachial cutaneous nerve

Posterior antebrachial cutaneous nerve

Division between ulnar and radial nerve innervation on dorsum of hand is variable.

Radial nerve

Dorsal branch and dorsal digital branches

Superficial branch and dorsal digital branches

Ulnar nerve

Proper palmar digital branches

Proper palmar digital branches — **Median nerve**

Plate 472   Cutaneous Innervation of Wrist and Hand. (Netter: Atlas of Human Anatomy, 4 ed, 2006, Saunders.)

Anterior view

Deltoid muscle

Coracobrachialis muscle

Biceps brachii muscle { Short head (*cut*)
Long head (*cut*)

Musculocutaneous nerve

Brachialis muscle

Biceps brachii muscle (*cut*) and tendon

Lateral antebrachial cutaneous nerve
(from musculocutaneous nerve)

Radial nerve { Deep branch
Superficial branch

Supinator muscle

Brachioradialis muscle

Radial artery

Pronator teres muscle (*partially cut*)

Median nerve

Flexor pollicis longus muscle

Flexor carpi radialis
tendon (*cut*)

Flexor retinaculum
(transverse carpal
ligament)

Superficial branch
of radial nerve

Recurrent (motor)
branch of
median nerve to
thenar muscles

Common palmar
digital branches
of median nerve

Proper palmar
digital branches
of median nerve

Intercostobrachial nerve

Medial brachial
cutaneous nerve

Radial nerve

Ulnar nerve

Medial antebrachial
cutaneous nerve

Median nerve

Brachial artery

Bicipital aponeurosis

Humeral head (*cut*)
Ulnar head } Pronator teres muscle

Flexor carpi radialis muscle (*cut*)

Humeroulnar head
Radial head } Flexor digitorum
superficialis muscle (*cut*)

Flexor digitorum profundus muscle

Flexor carpi ulnaris muscle

Ulnar artery and nerve

Dorsal branch of ulnar nerve

Flexor digitorum superficialis tendons (*cut*)

Deep palmar branch of ulnar artery and deep branch of ulnar nerve

Superficial branch of ulnar nerve

Superficial palmar arch (*cut*)

Common palmar digital branch of ulnar nerve

Communicating branch of median nerve with ulnar nerve

Proper palmar digital branches of ulnar nerve

Plate 473 Arteries and Nerves of Upper Limb. (Netter: Atlas of Human Anatomy, 4 ed, 2006, Saunders.)

Lateral cutaneous branch of subcostal nerve

Inguinal ligament (Poupart's)

Superficial circumflex iliac vein

Femoral branches of genitofemoral nerve

Lateral femoral cutaneous nerve

Saphenous opening (fossa ovalis)

Fascia lata

Anterior cutaneous branches of femoral nerve

Patellar nerve plexus

Branches of lateral sural cutaneous nerve (from common fibular [peroneal] nerve)

Deep fascia of leg (crural fascia)

Superficial fibular (peroneal) nerve Medial dorsal cutaneous branch

Intermediate dorsal cutaneous branch

Small saphenous vein and lateral dorsal cutaneous nerve (from sural nerve)

Lateral dorsal digital nerve and vein of 5th toe

Dorsal metatarsal veins

Dorsal digital nerves and veins

Superficial epigastric vein

Ilioinguinal nerve (scrotal branch) (usually passes through superficial inguinal ring)

Genital branch of genitofemoral nerve

Femoral vein

Superficial external pudendal vein

Accessory saphenous vein

Great saphenous vein

Cutaneous branches of obturator nerve

Infrapatellar branch of saphenous nerve

Saphenous nerve (terminal branch of femoral nerve)

Great saphenous vein

Dorsal digital nerves

Dorsal venous arch

Dorsal digital nerve and vein of medial side of great toe

Dorsal digital branch of deep fibular (peroneal) nerve

Plate 544 Superficial Nerves and Veins of Lower Limb: Anterior View. (Netter: Atlas of Human Anatomy, 4 ed, 2006, Saunders.)

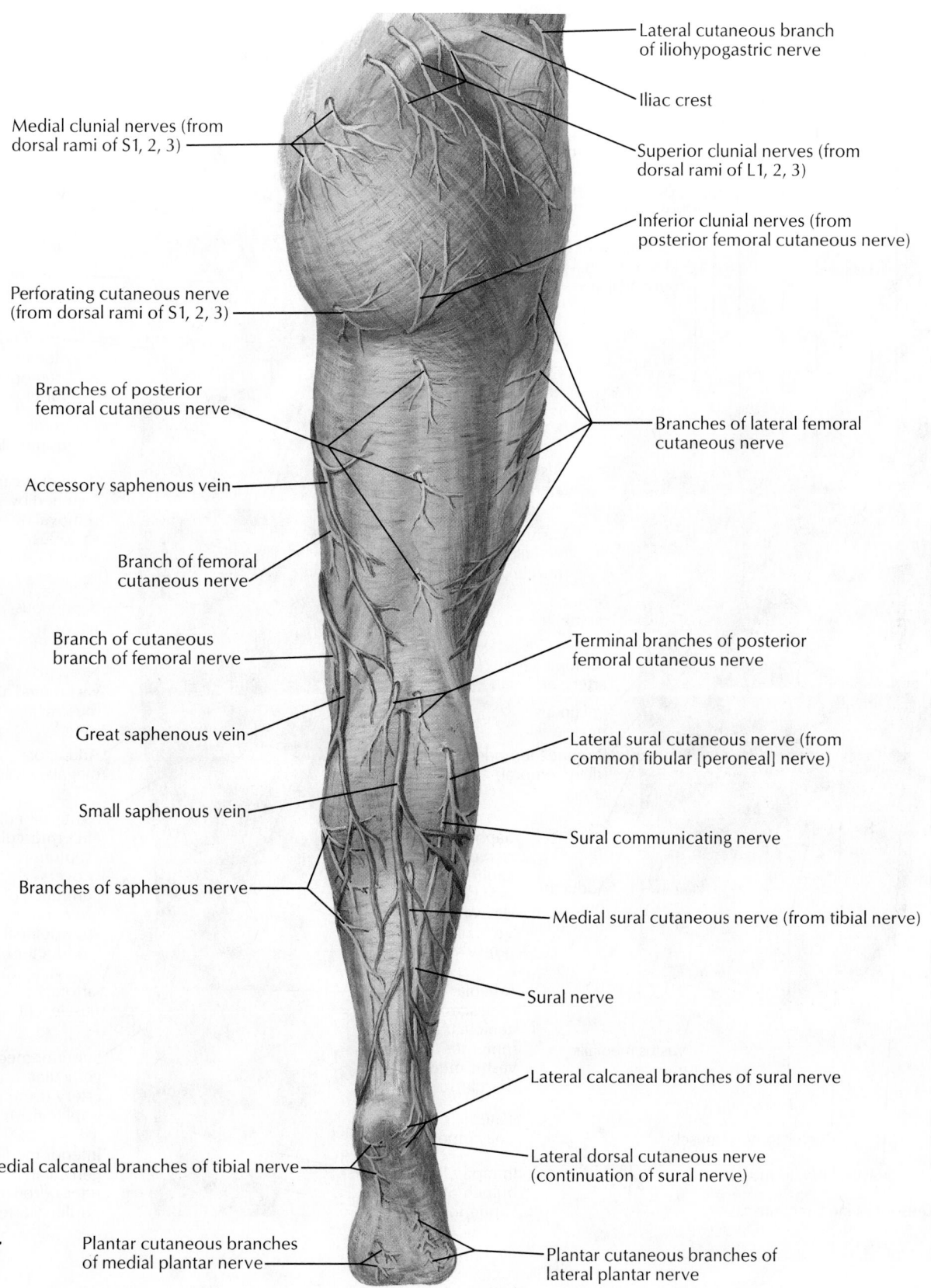

Lateral cutaneous branch of iliohypogastric nerve

Iliac crest

Medial clunial nerves (from dorsal rami of S1, 2, 3)

Superior clunial nerves (from dorsal rami of L1, 2, 3)

Inferior clunial nerves (from posterior femoral cutaneous nerve)

Perforating cutaneous nerve (from dorsal rami of S1, 2, 3)

Branches of posterior femoral cutaneous nerve

Branches of lateral femoral cutaneous nerve

Accessory saphenous vein

Branch of femoral cutaneous nerve

Branch of cutaneous branch of femoral nerve

Terminal branches of posterior femoral cutaneous nerve

Great saphenous vein

Lateral sural cutaneous nerve (from common fibular [peroneal] nerve)

Small saphenous vein

Sural communicating nerve

Branches of saphenous nerve

Medial sural cutaneous nerve (from tibial nerve)

Sural nerve

Lateral calcaneal branches of sural nerve

Medial calcaneal branches of tibial nerve

Lateral dorsal cutaneous nerve (continuation of sural nerve)

Plantar cutaneous branches of medial plantar nerve

Plantar cutaneous branches of lateral plantar nerve

Plate 545   Superficial Nerves and Veins of Lower Limb: Posterior View. (Netter: Atlas of Human Anatomy, 4 ed, 2006, Saunders.)

Superficial dissections

Anterior superior iliac spine

Lateral femoral cutaneous nerve

Inguinal ligament

Iliopsoas muscle

Superficial circumflex iliac vessels

Superficial epigastric vessels

Superficial and Deep external pudendal vessels

Tensor fasciae latae muscle (*retracted*)

Gluteus minimus and medius muscles

Lateral circumflex femoral artery

Rectus femoris muscle

Vastus lateralis muscle

Vastus medialis muscle

Femoral sheath

Femoral nerve, artery, and vein

Pectineus muscle

Profunda femoris (deep femoral) artery

Gracilis muscle

Adductor longus muscle

Saphenous nerve and saphenous branch of descending genicular artery

Sartorius muscle

Vastus medialis muscle

Articular branch of descending genicular artery (emerges from vastus medialis muscle)

Fascia lata (*cut*)

Patellar anastomosis

Rectus femoris muscle

Infrapatellar branch of Saphenous nerve

Vastus lateralis muscle

Tensor fasciae latae muscle

Lateral femoral cutaneous nerve (*cut*)

Sartorius muscle (*cut*)

Iliopsoas muscle

Femoral nerve, artery, and vein

Pectineus muscle

Profunda femoris (deep femoral) artery

Adductor longus muscle

Adductor canal (opened by removal of sartorius muscle)

Saphenous nerve

Nerve to vastus medialis muscle

Adductor magnus muscle

Anteromedial intermuscular septum covers entrance of femoral vessels to popliteal fossa (adductor hiatus)

Sartorius muscle (*cut*)

Superior medial genicular artery (from popliteal artery)

Inferior medial genicular artery (from popliteal artery)

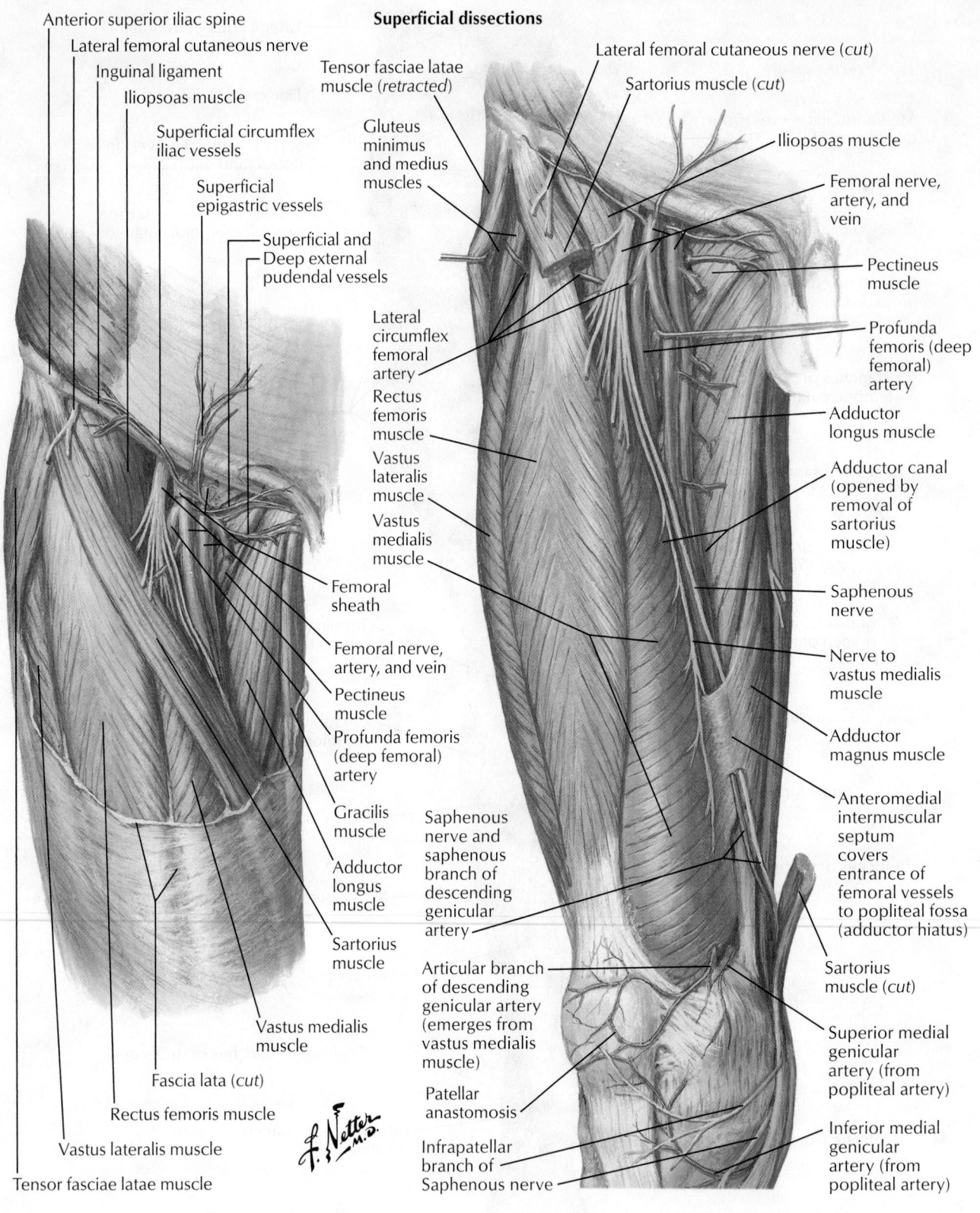

F. Netter M.D.

Plate 500 Arteries and Nerves of Thigh: Anterior Views. (Netter: Atlas of Human Anatomy, 4 ed, 2006, Saunders.)

Deep dissection

Deep circumflex iliac artery

Lateral femoral cutaneous nerve

Sartorius muscle (*cut*)

Iliopsoas muscle

Tensor fasciae latae muscle (*retracted*)

Gluteus medius and minimus muscles

Femoral nerve

Rectus femoris muscle (*cut*)

Ascending, transverse and descending branches of Lateral circumflex femoral artery

Medial circumflex femoral artery

Pectineus muscle (*cut*)

Profunda femoris (deep femoral) artery

Perforating branches

Adductor longus muscle (*cut*)

Vastus lateralis muscle

Vastus intermedius muscle

Rectus femoris muscle (*cut*)

Saphenous nerve

Anteromedial intermuscular septum (*opened*)

Vastus medialis muscle

Quadriceps femoris tendon

Patella and patellar anastomosis

Medial patellar retinaculum

Patellar ligament

External iliac artery and vein

Inguinal ligament (Poupart's)

Femoral artery and vein (*cut*)

Pectineus muscle (*cut*)

Obturator canal

Obturator externus muscle

Adductor longus muscle (*cut*)

Anterior branch and Posterior branch of obturator nerve

Quadratus femoris muscle

Adductor brevis muscle

Branches of posterior branch of obturator nerve

Adductor magnus muscle

Gracilis muscle

Cutaneous branch of obturator nerve

Femoral artery and vein (*cut*)

Descending genicular artery
Articular branch
Saphenous branch

Adductor hiatus

Sartorius muscle (*cut*)

Adductor magnus tendon

Adductor tubercle on medial epicondyle of femur

Superior medial genicular artery (from popliteal artery)

Infrapatellar branch of Saphenous nerve

Inferior medial genicular artery (from popliteal artery)

Plate 501 Arteries and Nerves of Thigh: Posterior View. (Netter: Atlas of Human Anatomy, 4 ed, 2006, Saunders.)

61

Deep dissection

Superior clunial nerves

Gluteus maximus muscle (*cut*)

Medial clunial nerves

Inferior gluteal artery and nerve

Pudendal nerve

Nerve to obturator internus (and superior gemellus)

Posterior femoral cutaneous nerve

Sacrotuberous ligament

Ischial tuberosity

Inferior clunial nerves (*cut*)

Adductor magnus muscle

Gracilis muscle

Sciatic nerve

Muscular branches of sciatic nerve

Semitendinosus muscle (*retracted*)

Semimembranosus muscle

Sciatic nerve

Articular branch

Adductor hiatus

Popliteal vein and artery

Superior medial genicular artery

Medial epicondyle of femur

Tibial nerve

Gastrocnemius muscle (medial head)

Medial sural cutaneous nerve

Small saphenous vein

Iliac crest

Gluteal aponeurosis and gluteus medius muscle (*cut*)

Superior gluteal artery and nerve

Gluteus minimus muscle

Tensor fasciae latae muscle

Piriformis muscle

Gluteus medius muscle (*cut*)

Superior gemellus muscle

Greater trochanter of femur

Obturator internus muscle

Inferior gemellus muscle

Gluteus maximus muscle (*cut*)

Quadratus femoris muscle

Medial circumflex femoral artery

Vastus lateralis muscle and iliotibial tract

Adductor minimus part of adductor magnus muscle

1st perforating artery (from profunda femoris artery)

Adductor magnus muscle

2nd and 3rd perforating arteries (from profunda femoris artery)

4th perforating artery (from profunda femoris artery)

Long head (*retracted*) ⎱ Biceps femoris
Short head ⎰ muscle

Superior lateral genicular artery

Common fibular (peroneal) nerve

Plantaris muscle

Gastrocnemius muscle (lateral head)

Lateral sural cutaneous nerve

Plate 502   Arteries and Nerves of Thigh: Posterior View. (Netter: Atlas of Human Anatomy, 4 ed, 2006, Saunders.)

Horizontal section

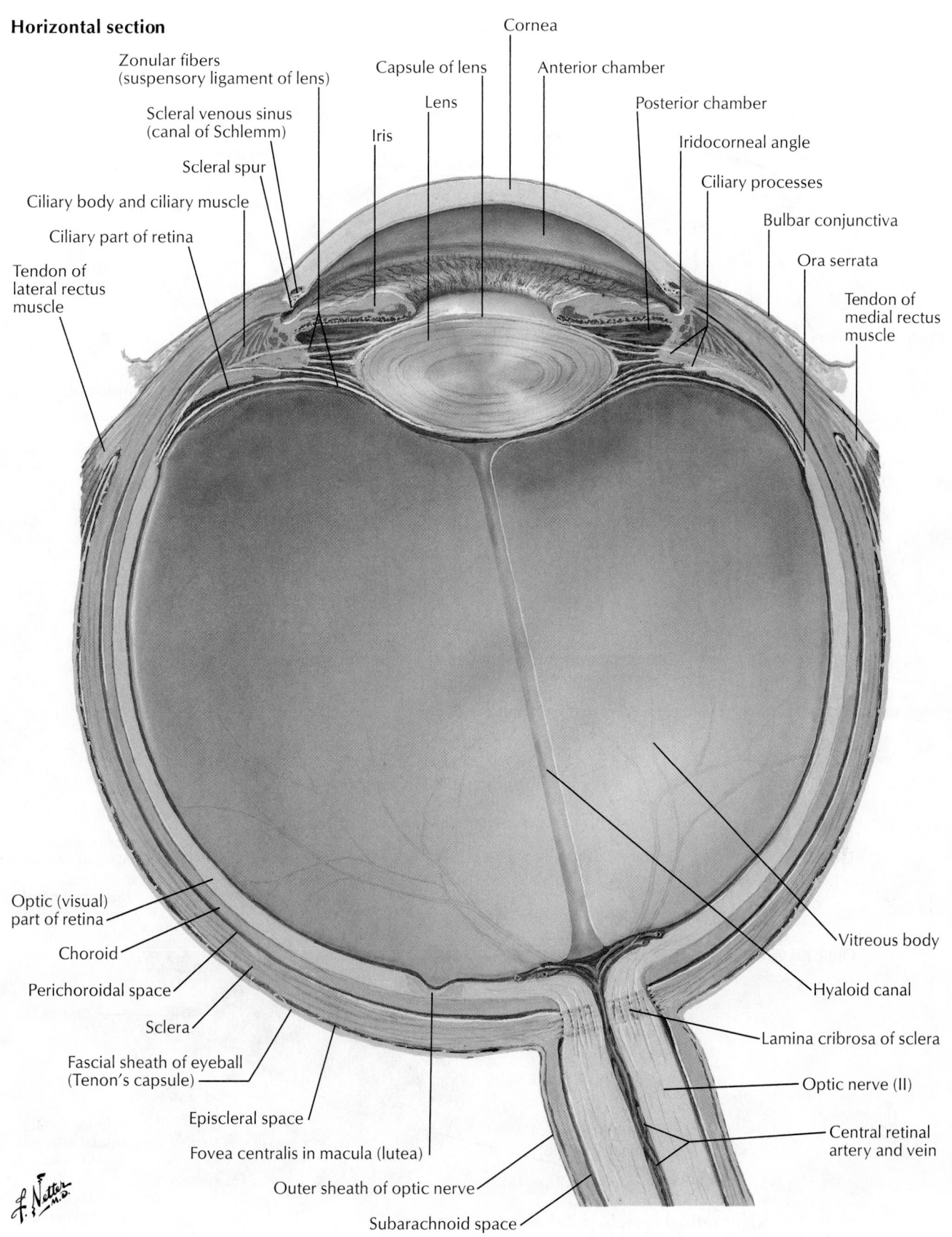

Zonular fibers
(suspensory ligament of lens)

Scleral venous sinus
(canal of Schlemm)

Scleral spur

Ciliary body and ciliary muscle

Ciliary part of retina

Tendon of
lateral rectus
muscle

Capsule of lens

Iris

Lens

Cornea

Anterior chamber

Posterior chamber

Iridocorneal angle

Ciliary processes

Bulbar conjunctiva

Ora serrata

Tendon of
medial rectus
muscle

Optic (visual)
part of retina

Choroid

Perichoroidal space

Sclera

Fascial sheath of eyeball
(Tenon's capsule)

Episcleral space

Fovea centralis in macula (lutea)

Outer sheath of optic nerve

Subarachnoid space

Vitreous body

Hyaloid canal

Lamina cribrosa of sclera

Optic nerve (II)

Central retinal
artery and vein

Plate 87 Eyeball. (Netter: Atlas of Human Anatomy, 4 ed, 2006, Saunders.)

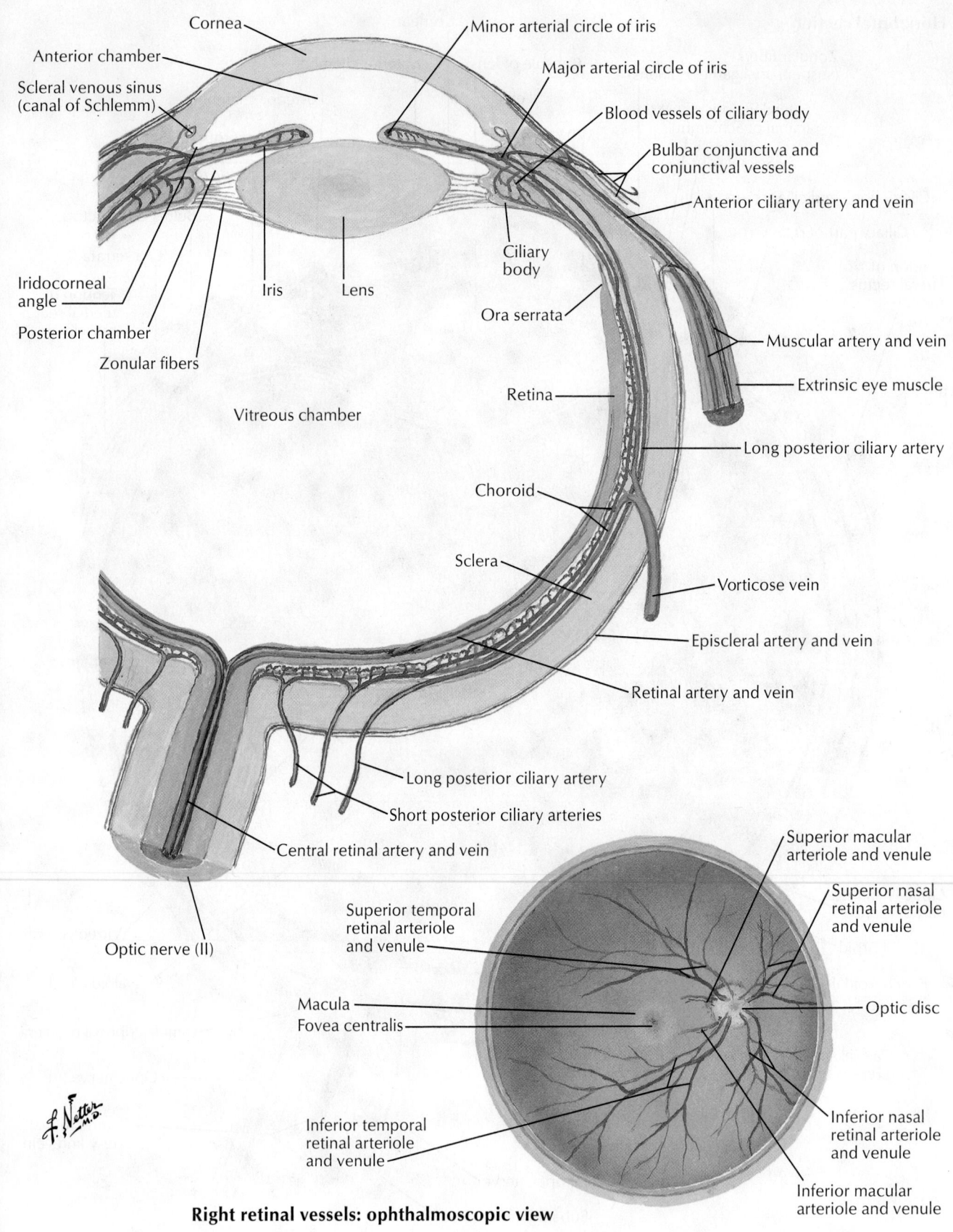

Cornea

Anterior chamber

Scleral venous sinus
(canal of Schlemm)

Minor arterial circle of iris

Major arterial circle of iris

Blood vessels of ciliary body

Bulbar conjunctiva and
conjunctival vessels

Anterior ciliary artery and vein

Iridocorneal
angle

Iris

Lens

Ciliary
body

Posterior chamber

Zonular fibers

Ora serrata

Muscular artery and vein

Extrinsic eye muscle

Vitreous chamber

Retina

Long posterior ciliary artery

Choroid

Sclera

Vorticose vein

Episcleral artery and vein

Retinal artery and vein

Long posterior ciliary artery

Short posterior ciliary arteries

Central retinal artery and vein

Optic nerve (II)

Superior macular
arteriole and venule

Superior nasal
retinal arteriole
and venule

Superior temporal
retinal arteriole
and venule

Macula

Fovea centralis

Optic disc

Inferior nasal
retinal arteriole
and venule

Inferior temporal
retinal arteriole
and venule

Inferior macular
arteriole and venule

Right retinal vessels: ophthalmoscopic view

Plate 90 Intrinsic Arteries and Veins of Eye. (Netter: Atlas of Human Anatomy, 4 ed, 2006, Saunders.)

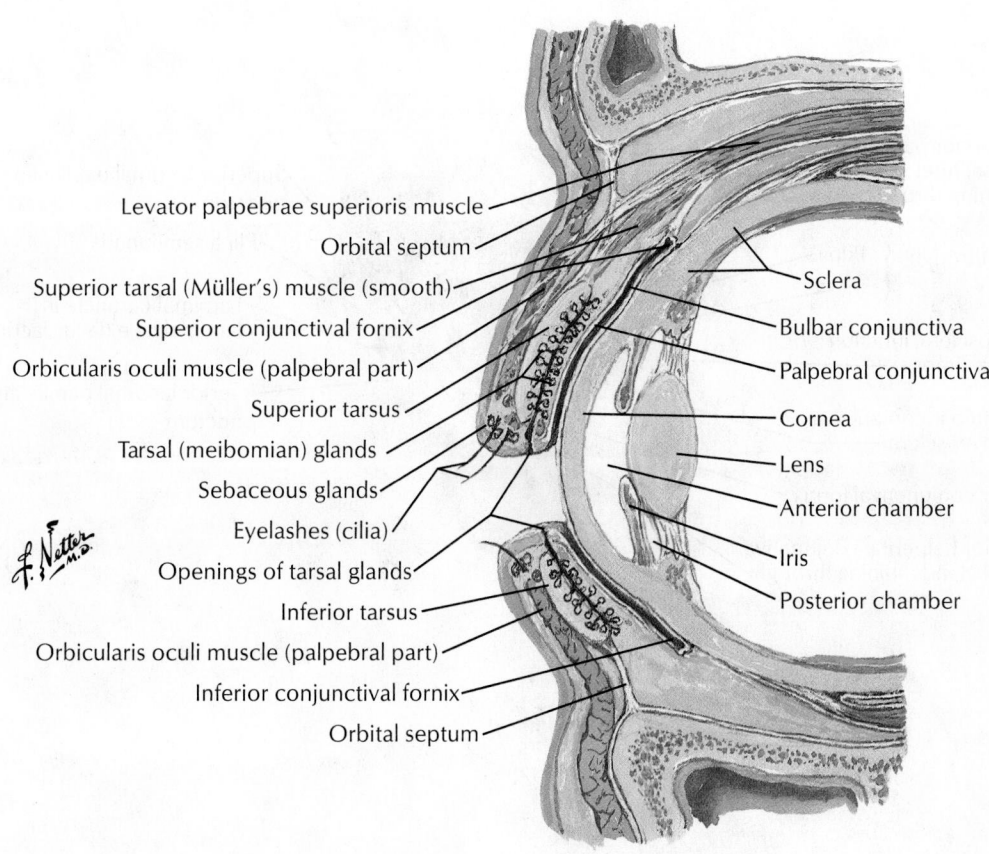

Levator palpebrae superioris muscle

Orbital septum

Superior tarsal (Müller's) muscle (smooth)

Superior conjunctival fornix

Orbicularis oculi muscle (palpebral part)

Superior tarsus

Tarsal (meibomian) glands

Sebaceous glands

Eyelashes (cilia)

Openings of tarsal glands

Inferior tarsus

Orbicularis oculi muscle (palpebral part)

Inferior conjunctival fornix

Orbital septum

Sclera

Bulbar conjunctiva

Palpebral conjunctiva

Cornea

Lens

Anterior chamber

Iris

Posterior chamber

Plate 81, Middle Eyelids. (Netter: Atlas of Human Anatomy, 4 ed, 2006, Saunders.)

Superior palpebral conjunctiva: tarsal (meibomian) glands shining through

Seen through cornea { Pupil Iris }

Corneoscleral junction (corneal limbus)

Bulbar conjunctiva over sclera

Inferior conjunctival fornix

Inferior palpebral conjunctiva: tarsal glands shining through

Superior lacrimal papilla and punctum

Plica semilunaris

Lacrimal caruncle in lacrimal lake (lacus lacrimalis)

Inferior lacrimal papilla and punctum

Plate 81, Upper   Eyelid. (Netter: Atlas of Human Anatomy, 4 ed, 2006, Saunders.)

Orbital part of lacrimal gland

Palpebral part of lacrimal gland

Excretory ducts of lacrimal gland

Plica semilunaris

Lacrimal caruncle

Inferior lacrimal papilla and punctum

Superior lacrimal papilla and punctum

Lacrimal canaliculi

Lacrimal sac

Nasolacrimal duct

Opening of nasolacrimal duct

Frontal bone (cut away)

Orbital part of lacrimal gland

Palpebral part of lacrimal gland

Excretory ducts of lacrimal gland

Plica semilunaris and lacrimal lake

Lacrimal caruncle

Inferior lacrimal papilla and punctum

Opening of nasolacrimal duct

Superior lacrimal papilla and punctum

Lacrimal canaliculi

Lacrimal sac

Nasolacrimal duct

Middle nasal concha

Nasal cavity

Inferior nasal concha (cut)

Inferior nasal meatus

Plate 82 Lacrimal Apparatus. (Netter: Atlas of Human Anatomy, 4 ed, 2006, Saunders.)

Frontal section

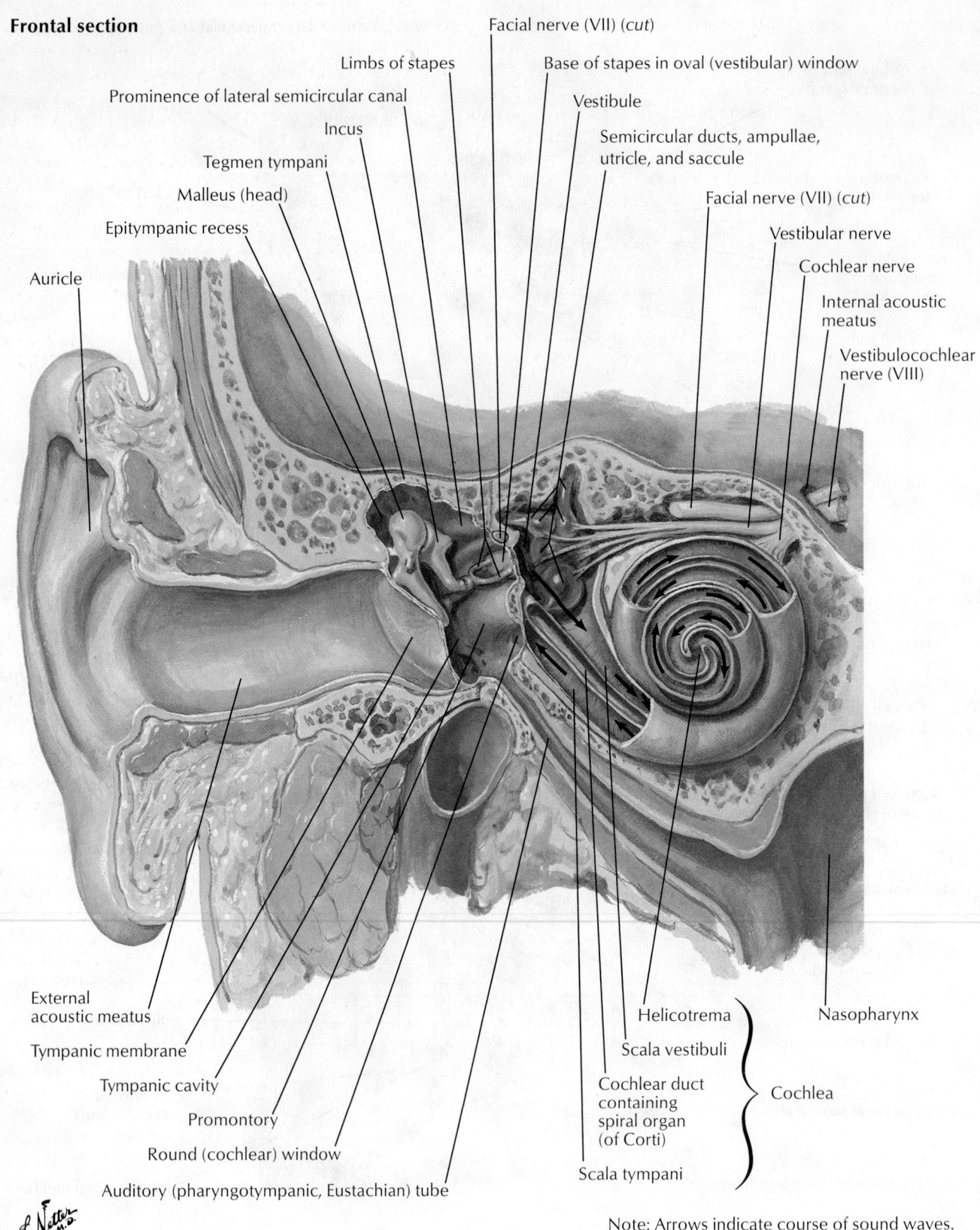

Limbs of stapes

Prominence of lateral semicircular canal

Incus

Tegmen tympani

Malleus (head)

Epitympanic recess

Auricle

Facial nerve (VII) (*cut*)

Base of stapes in oval (vestibular) window

Vestibule

Semicircular ducts, ampullae, utricle, and saccule

Facial nerve (VII) (*cut*)

Vestibular nerve

Cochlear nerve

Internal acoustic meatus

Vestibulocochlear nerve (VIII)

External acoustic meatus

Tympanic membrane

Tympanic cavity

Promontory

Round (cochlear) window

Auditory (pharyngotympanic, Eustachian) tube

Helicotrema

Scala vestibuli

Cochlear duct containing spiral organ (of Corti)

Scala tympani

Nasopharynx

Cochlea

Note: Arrows indicate course of sound waves.

Plate 92   Pathway of Sound Reception. (Netter: Atlas of Human Anatomy, 4 ed, 2006, Saunders.)

68

Medial wall of tympanic cavity: lateral view

Mastoid antrum

Prominence of lateral semicircular canal

Prominence of facial canal

Geniculum (geniculate ganglion) of facial nerve

Greater petrosal nerve

Base of stapes in fossa of oval (vestibular) window

Limbs of stapes

Pyramidal eminence

Chorda tympani nerve (*cut*)

Mastoid cells

Tendon of stapedius muscle

Fossa of round (cochlear) window

Facial nerve (VII) in stylomastoid foramen

Jugular fossa

Tympanic cells

Internal carotid artery

Promontory with tympanic nerve (of Jacobson) and plexus under mucosa

Levator veli palatini muscle

Auditory (pharyngotympanic, Eustachian) tube

Tensor tympani muscle (*tendon cut*)

Plate 94 Tympanic Cavity. (Netter: Atlas of Human Anatomy, 4 ed, 2006, Saunders.)

Dissected right bony labyrinth (otic capsule): membranous labyrinth removed

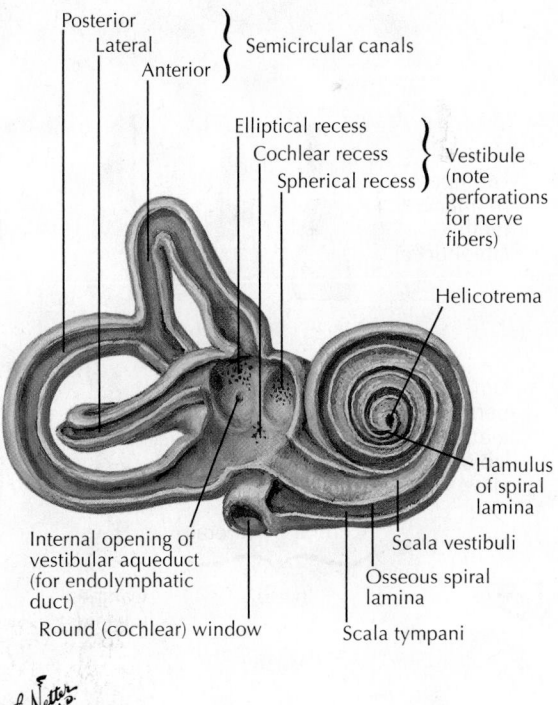

Posterior

Lateral

Anterior

} Semicircular canals

Elliptical recess

Cochlear recess

Spherical recess

} Vestibule (note perforations for nerve fibers)

Helicotrema

Hamulus of spiral lamina

Scala vestibuli

Osseous spiral lamina

Scala tympani

Internal opening of vestibular aqueduct (for endolymphatic duct)

Round (cochlear) window

Otoscopic view of right tympanic membrane

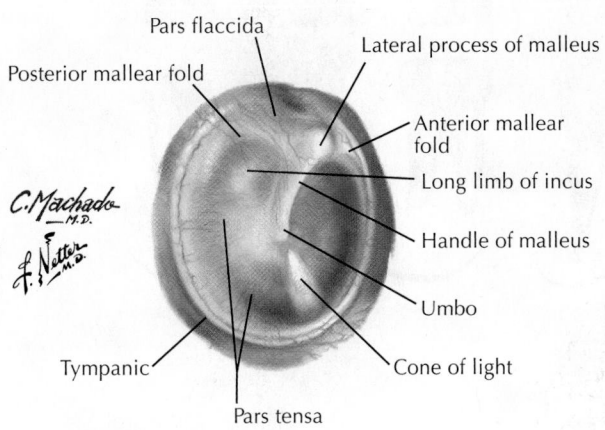

Pars flaccida

Posterior mallear fold

Lateral process of malleus

Anterior mallear fold

Long limb of incus

Handle of malleus

Umbo

Cone of light

Pars tensa

Tympanic

C. Machado M.D.

Plate 93 Tympanic Cavity. (Netter: Atlas of Human Anatomy, 4 ed, 2006, Saunders.)

Plate 95 Bony Membranous Labyrinth. (Netter: Atlas of Human Anatomy, 4 ed, 2006, Saunders.)

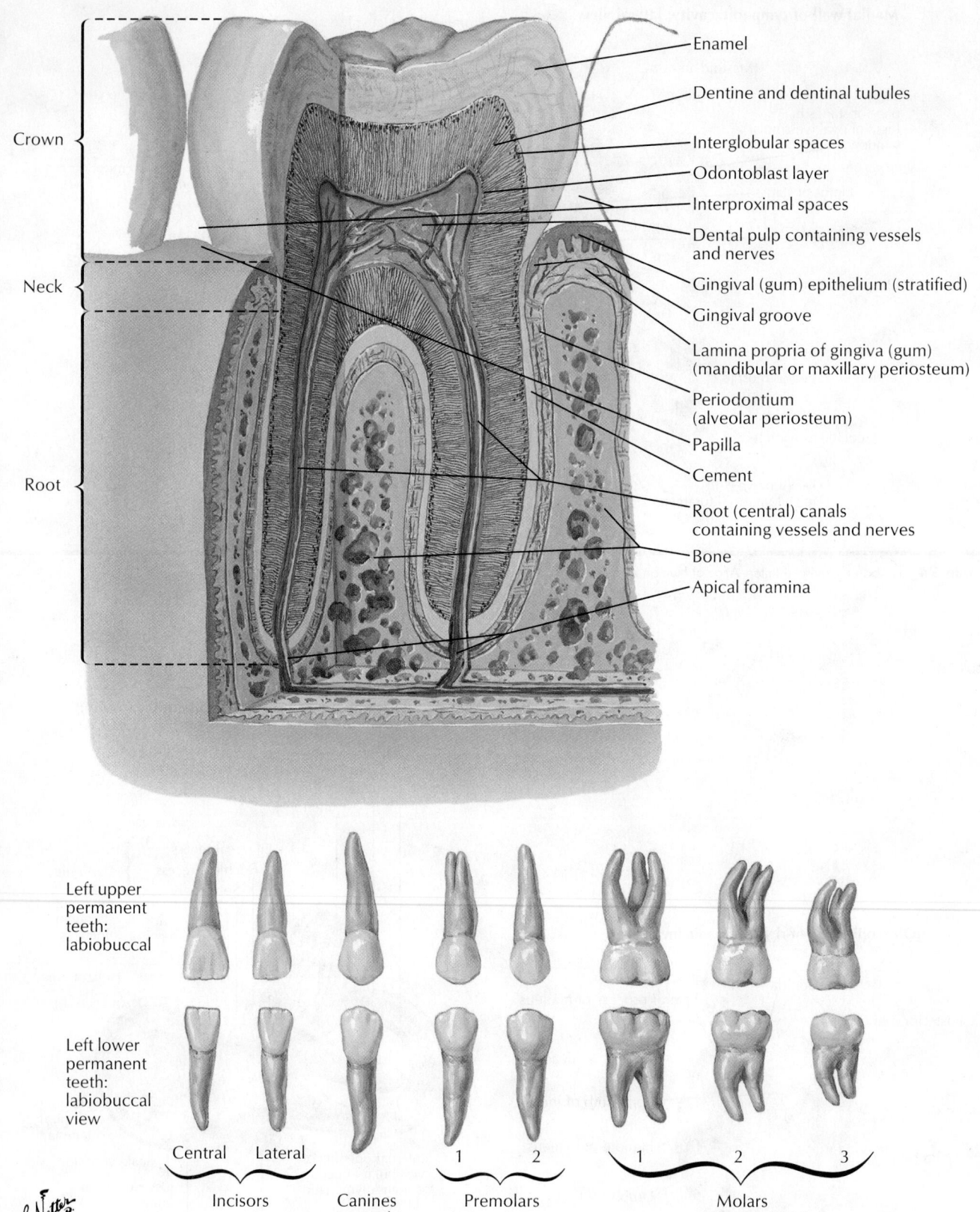

Crown

Neck

Root

Enamel

Dentine and dentinal tubules

Interglobular spaces

Odontoblast layer

Interproximal spaces

Dental pulp containing vessels and nerves

Gingival (gum) epithelium (stratified)

Gingival groove

Lamina propria of gingiva (gum) (mandibular or maxillary periosteum)

Periodontium (alveolar periosteum)

Papilla

Cement

Root (central) canals containing vessels and nerves

Bone

Apical foramina

Left upper permanent teeth: labiobuccal

Left lower permanent teeth: labiobuccal view

Central   Lateral

Incisors

Canines (cuspids)

1   2

Premolars

1   2   3

Molars

Plate 57 Teeth. (Netter: Atlas of Human Anatomy, 4 ed, 2006, Saunders.)

Tongue

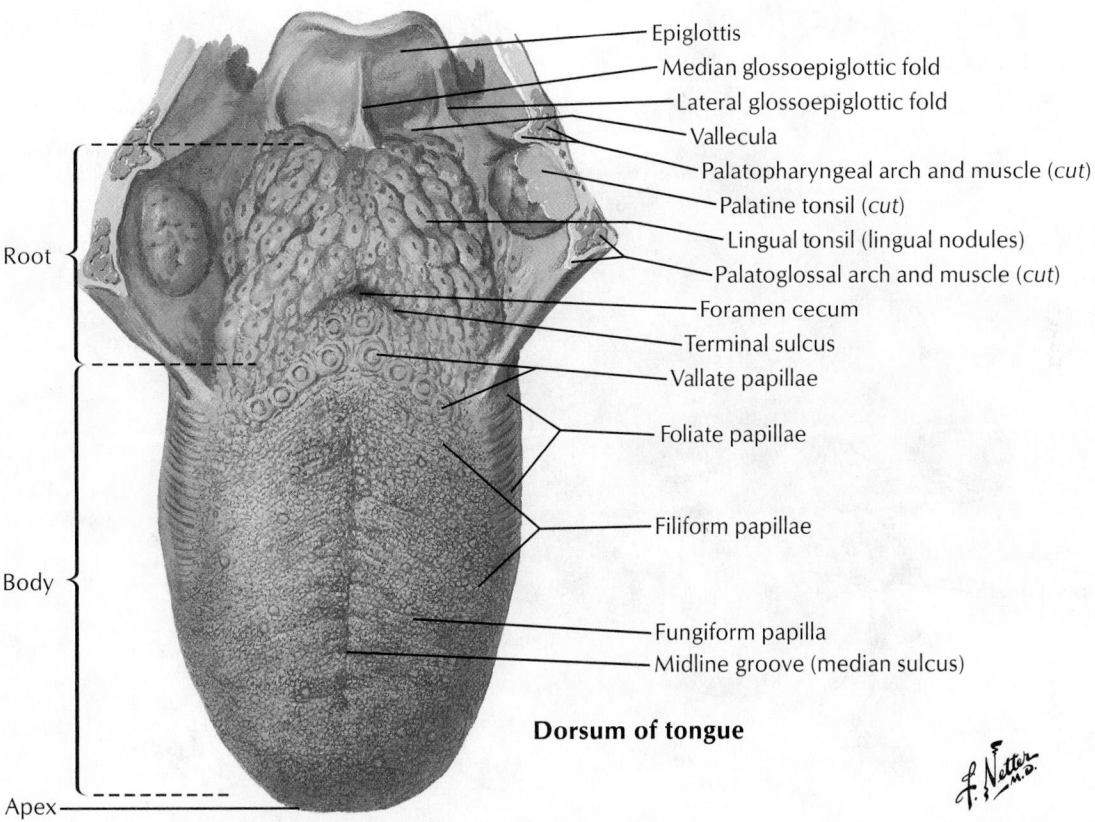

Epiglottis
Median glossoepiglottic fold
Lateral glossoepiglottic fold
Vallecula
Palatopharyngeal arch and muscle (*cut*)
Palatine tonsil (*cut*)
Lingual tonsil (lingual nodules)
Palatoglossal arch and muscle (*cut*)
Foramen cecum
Terminal sulcus
Vallate papillae
Foliate papillae
Filiform papillae
Fungiform papilla
Midline groove (median sulcus)

Root

Body

Apex

Dorsum of tongue

Plate 58   Tongue. (Netter: Atlas of Human Anatomy, 4 ed, 2006, Saunders.)

Frontal sinus

Opening into middle nasal meatus

Orbit

Pterygopalatine fossa

Maxillary sinus

Lateral dissection

Roots of teeth

Plate 49 Paranasal Sinuses. (Netter: Atlas of Human Anatomy, 4 ed, 2006, Saunders.)

Superficial temporal artery and vein and auriculotemporal nerve

Branches of facial nerve

Transverse facial artery

Accessory parotid gland

Parotid duct

Buccinator muscle (cut)

Masseter muscle

Lingual nerve

Submandibular ganglion

Tongue

Frenulum of tongue

Sublingual fold with openings of sublingual ducts

Sublingual caruncle with opening of submandibular duct

Sublingual gland

Submandibular duct

Sublingual artery and vein

Mylohyoid muscle (cut)

Digastric muscle (anterior belly)

Submandibular gland

Facial artery and vein

Hyoid bone

Parotid gland

Retromandibular vein (anterior and posterior branches)

Digastric muscle (posterior belly)

Stylohyoid muscle

External jugular vein

Sternocleidomastoid muscle

Common trunk receiving facial, anterior branch of retromandibular, and lingual veins (common facial vein)

Internal jugular vein

External carotid artery

Parotid gland: totally serous

Submandibular gland: mostly serous, partially mucous

Sublingual gland: almost completely mucous

Plate 61 Salivary Glands. (Netter: Atlas of Human Anatomy, 4 ed, 2006, Saunders.)

Coronary Arteries: Arteriographic Views

Right coronary artery: left anterior oblique view

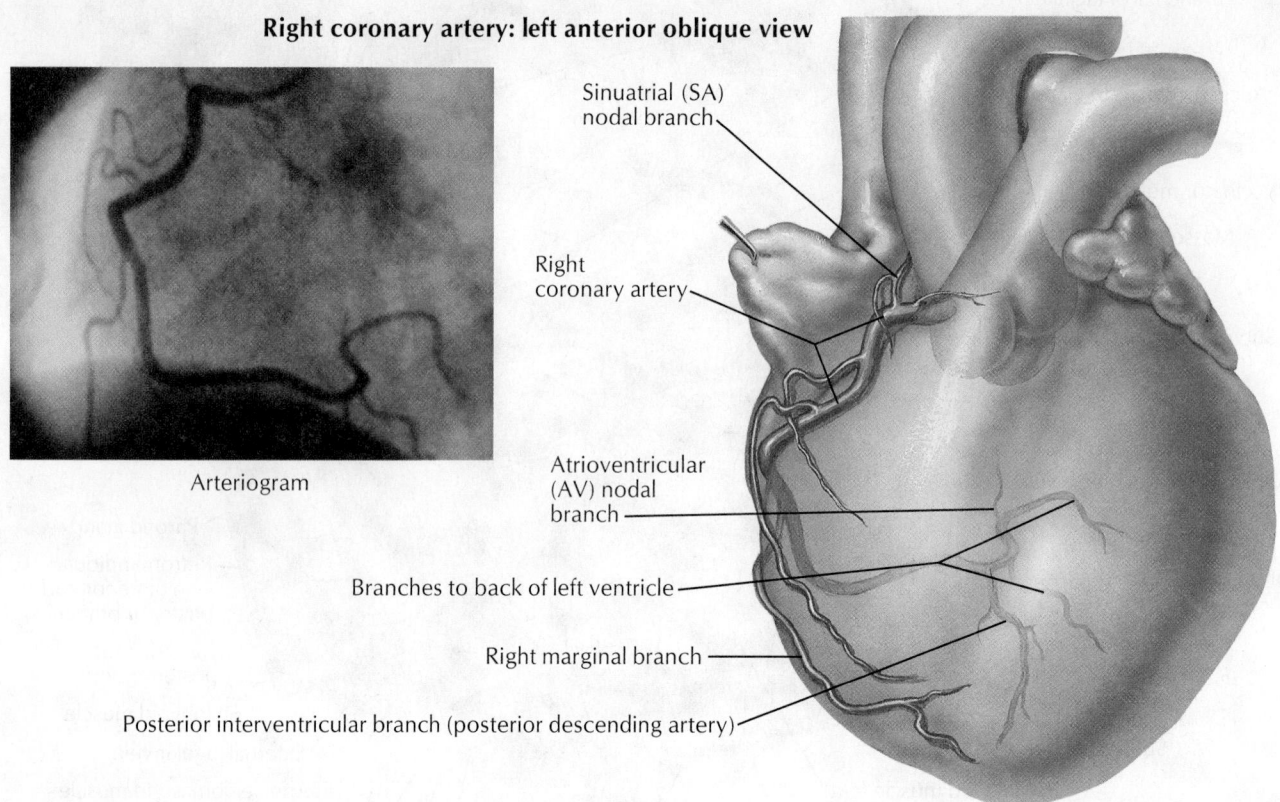

Arteriogram

Sinuatrial (SA) nodal branch

Right coronary artery

Atrioventricular (AV) nodal branch

Branches to back of left ventricle

Right marginal branch

Posterior interventricular branch (posterior descending artery)

Right coronary artery: right anterior oblique view

Sinuatrial (SA) nodal branch

Conus (arteriosus) branch

Right coronary artery

Right marginal branch

Arteriogram

Atrioventricular (AV) nodal branch

Right posterolateral branches (to back of left ventricle)

Posterior interventricular branch (posterior descending artery)

Plate 218 Coronary Arteries: Arteriographic Views. (Netter: Atlas of Human Anatomy, 4 ed, 2006, Saunders.)

74

Left coronary artery: left anterior oblique view

Left coronary artery

Circumflex branch

Arteriogram

Anterior interventricular branch (left anterior descending)

Diagonal branches of anterior interventricular branch

Atrioventricular branch of circumflex branch

Left (obtuse) marginal branch

Posterolateral branches

(Perforating) interventricular septal branches

Left coronary artery: right anterior oblique view

Left coronary artery

Anterior interventricular branch (left anterior descending)

Circumflex branch

(Perforating) interventricular septal branches

Arteriogram

Left (obtuse) marginal branch

Posterolateral branches

Diagonal branch of Anterior interventricular branch

Atrioventricular branch of circumflex branch

Plate 219 Coronary Arteries: Arteriographic Views. (Netter: Atlas of Human Anatomy, 4 ed, 2006, Saunders.)

Corpus callosum

Anterolateral central (lenticulostriate) arteries

Lateral frontobasal (orbitofrontal) artery

Prefrontal artery

Precentral (pre-Rolandic) and central (Rolandic) sulcal arteries

Anterior parietal (postcentral sulcal) artery

Posterior parietal artery

Branch to angular gyrus

Temporal branches (anterior, middle, and posterior)

Middle cerebral artery and branches (deep in lateral cerebral [Sylvian] sulcus)

Anterior communicating artery

Posterior communicating artery

Anterior inferior cerebellar artery (AICA)

Posterior spinal artery

Paracentral artery

Medial frontal branches

Pericallosal artery

Callosomarginal artery

Polar frontal artery

Anterior cerebral arteries

Medial frontobasal (orbitofrontal) artery

Distal medial striate artery (recurrent artery of Heubner)

Internal carotid artery

Anterior choroidal artery

Posterior cerebral artery

Superior cerebellar artery

Basilar and pontine arteries

Labyrinthine (internal acoustic) artery

Vertebral artery

Posterior inferior cerebellar artery (PICA)

Anterior spinal artery

Corpus striatum (caudate and lentiform nuclei)

Anterolateral central (lenticulostriate) arteries

Insula (island of Reil)

Limen of insula

Precentral (pre-Rolandic), central (Rolandic) sulcal, and parietal arteries

Lateral cerebral (Sylvian) sulcus

Temporal branches of middle cerebral artery

Temporal lobe

Middle cerebral artery

Internal carotid artery

Falx cerebri

Callosomarginal arteries and Pericallosal arteries (branches of anterior cerebral arteries)

Trunk of corpus callosum

Internal capsule

Septum pellucidum

Rostrum of corpus callosum

Anterior cerebral arteries

Distal medial striate artery (recurrent artery of Heubner)

Anterior communicating artery

Optic chiasm

Plate 141 Arteries of Brain: Frontal View and Section. (Netter: Atlas of Human Anatomy, 4 ed, 2006, Saunders.)

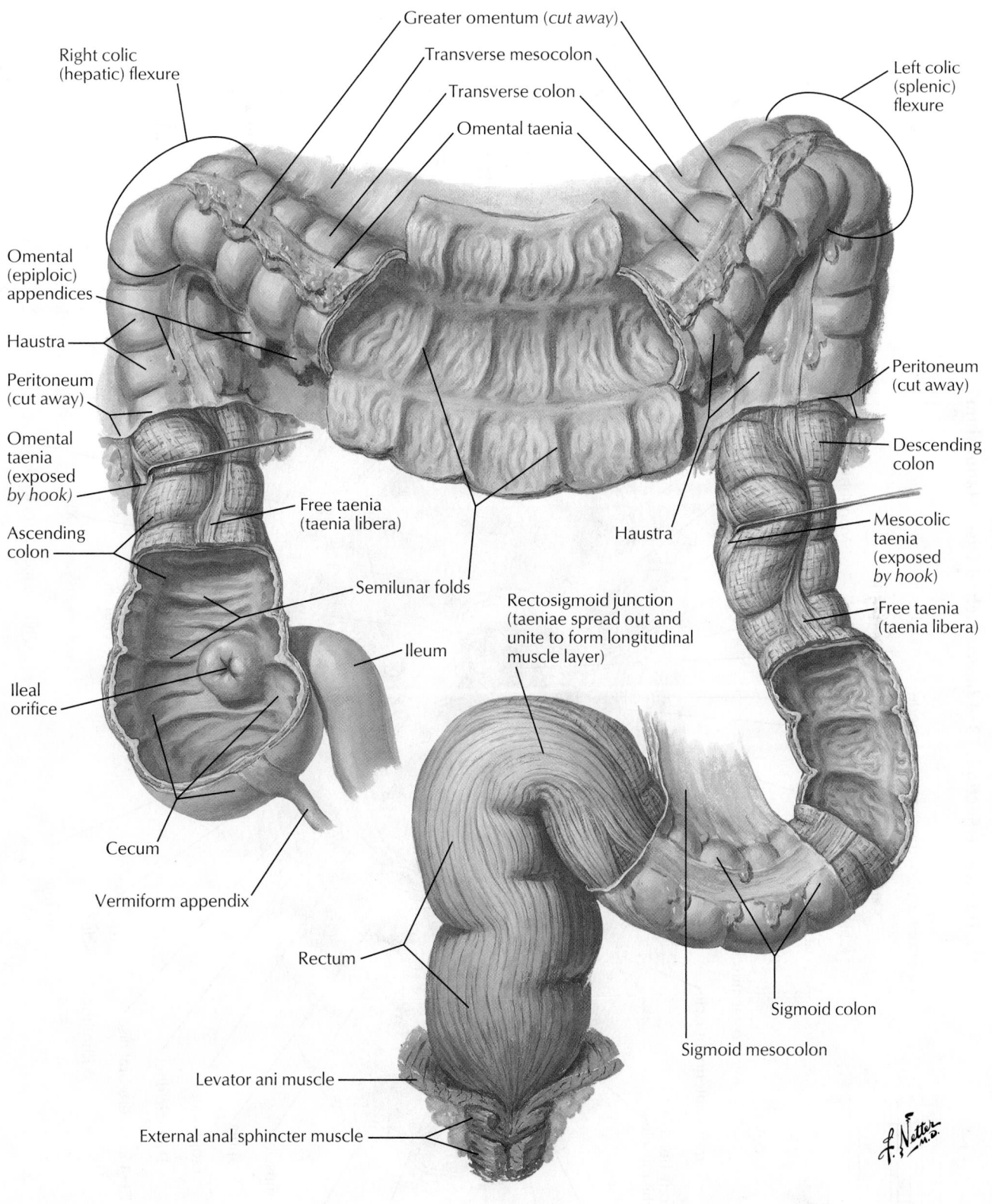

Right colic (hepatic) flexure

Greater omentum (*cut away*)

Transverse mesocolon

Transverse colon

Omental taenia

Left colic (splenic) flexure

Omental (epiploic) appendices

Haustra

Peritoneum (cut away)

Omental taenia (exposed *by hook*)

Ascending colon

Ileal orifice

Cecum

Vermiform appendix

Rectum

Free taenia (taenia libera)

Semilunar folds

Ileum

Rectosigmoid junction (taeniae spread out and unite to form longitudinal muscle layer)

Haustra

Peritoneum (cut away)

Descending colon

Mesocolic taenia (exposed *by hook*)

Free taenia (taenia libera)

Sigmoid colon

Sigmoid mesocolon

Levator ani muscle

External anal sphincter muscle

Plate 284   Mucosa and Musculature of Large Intestine. (Netter: Atlas of Human Anatomy, 4 ed, 2006, Saunders.)

Transverse Section: T3–4 Intervertebral Disc, Manubrium

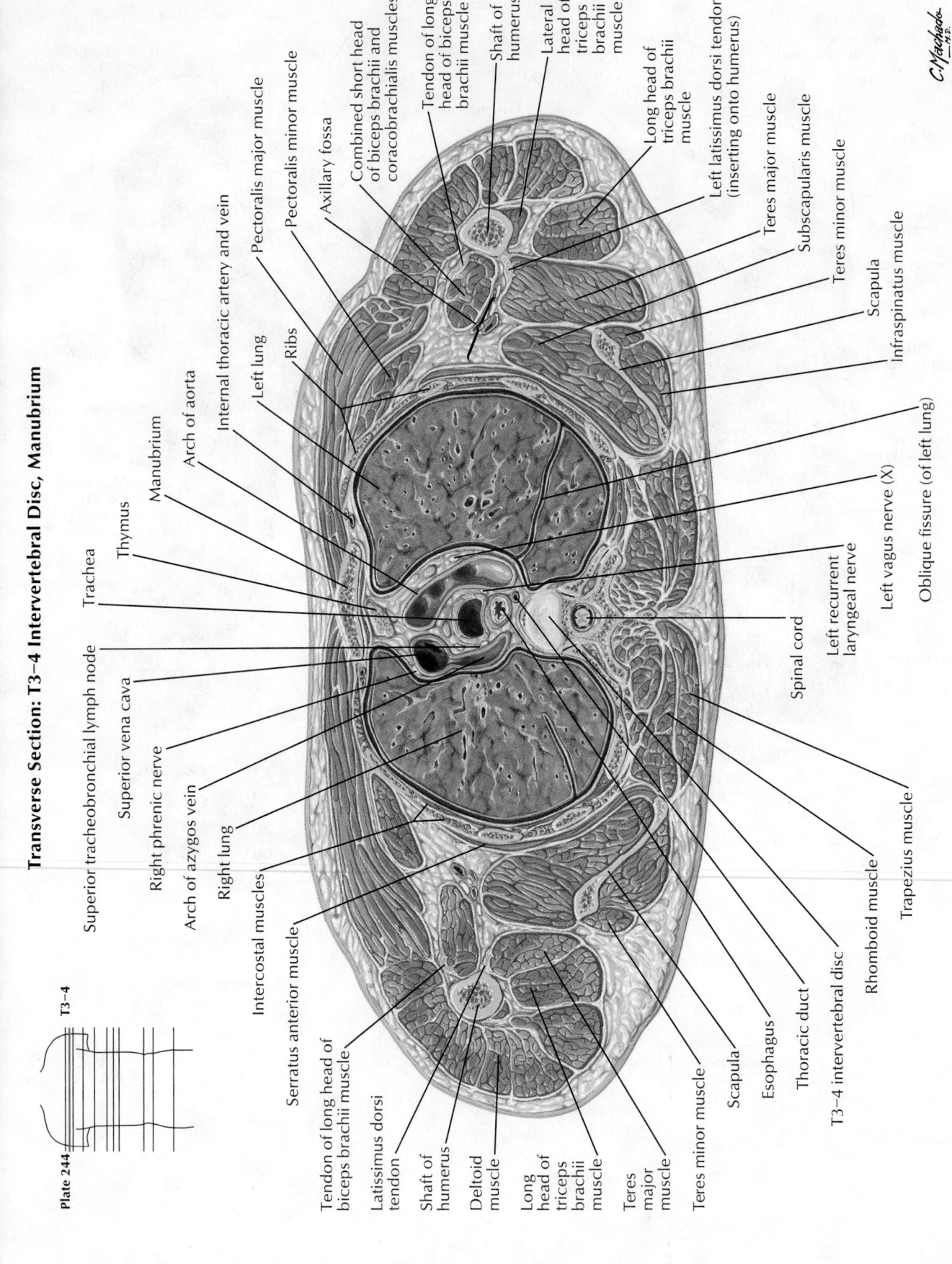

C. Machado _M.D.

Plate 244

T3–4

Plate 244 Cross Section of Thorax at T3-4 Disc Level. (Netter: Atlas of Human Anatomy, 4 ed, 2006, Saunders.)

Right knee in extension: posterior view

Posterior cruciate ligament

Anterior cruciate ligament

Posterior meniscofemoral ligament

Lateral condyle of femur (articular surface)

Popliteus tendon

Fibular collateral ligament

Lateral meniscus

Head of fibula

Adductor tubercle on medial epicondyle of femur

Medial condyle of femur (articular surface)

Medial meniscus

Tibial collateral ligament

Medial condyle of tibia

Plate 509   Knee: Cruciate and Collateral Ligaments. (Netter: Atlas of Human Anatomy, 4 ed, 2006, Saunders.)

Paramedian (sagittal) dissection

Ureter
Uterine (fallopian) tube
Ovary
Ligament of ovary
Round ligament of uterus
Broad ligament (*cut*)
Superior pubic ramus (*cut*)
Inferior pubic ramus (*cut*)
Ischiocavernosus muscle
Body of clitoris
Labia minora
Labium majus

Rectouterine pouch (of Douglas)
Peritoneum (*cut edge*)
Vesicouterine pouch
Rectum
Ureter
Urinary bladder
Vagina
Pelvic diaphragm (levator ani muscle)
Deep transverse perineal muscle (*cut*)
External anal sphincter muscle

Median (sagittal) section

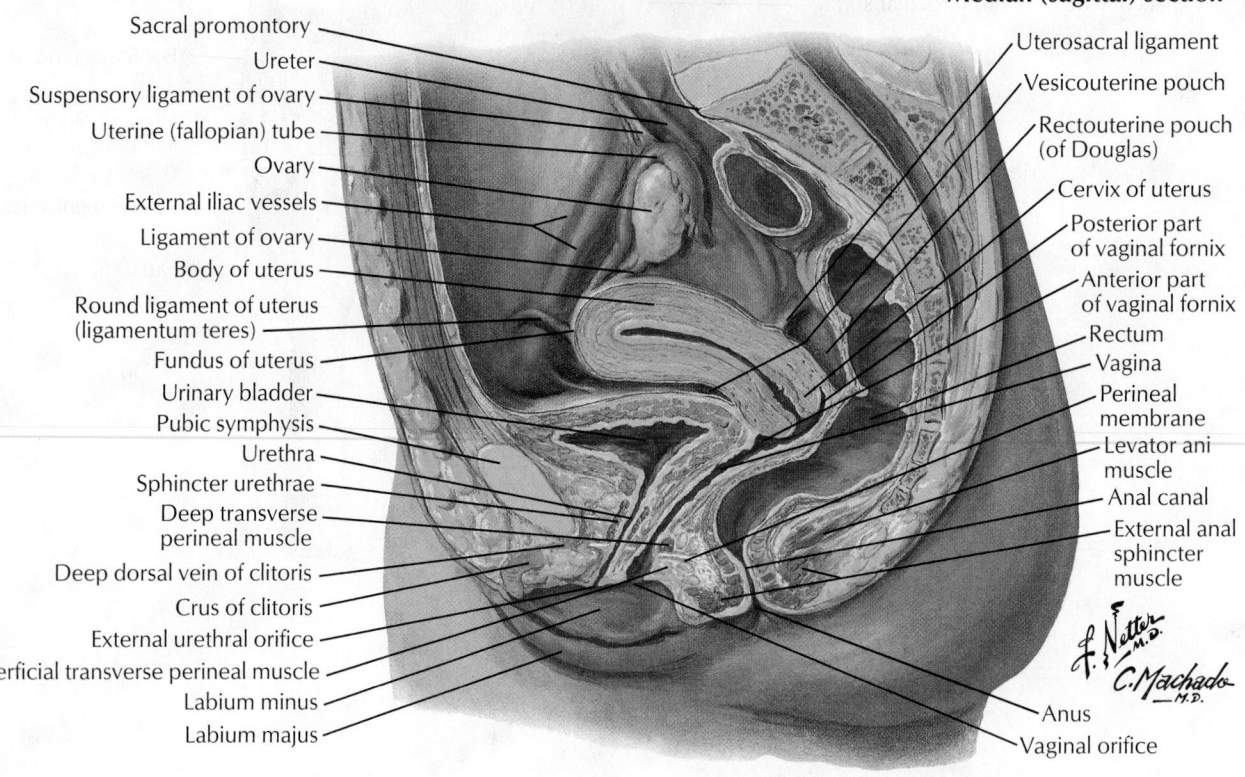

Sacral promontory
Ureter
Suspensory ligament of ovary
Uterine (fallopian) tube
Ovary
External iliac vessels
Ligament of ovary
Body of uterus
Round ligament of uterus (ligamentum teres)
Fundus of uterus
Urinary bladder
Pubic symphysis
Urethra
Sphincter urethrae
Deep transverse perineal muscle
Deep dorsal vein of clitoris
Crus of clitoris
External urethral orifice
Superficial transverse perineal muscle
Labium minus
Labium majus

Uterosacral ligament
Vesicouterine pouch
Rectouterine pouch (of Douglas)
Cervix of uterus
Posterior part of vaginal fornix
Anterior part of vaginal fornix
Rectum
Vagina
Perineal membrane
Levator ani muscle
Anal canal
External anal sphincter muscle
Anus
Vaginal orifice

Plate 360   Pelvic Viscera and Perineum: Female. (Netter: Atlas of Human Anatomy, 4 ed, 2006, Saunders.)

PART II

II

A

Aarskog's syndrome Q87.1

Abandonment —*see* Maltreatment

Abasia (-astasia) (hysterical) F44.4

Abderhalden-Kaufmann-Lignac syndrome
(cystinosis) E72.04

Abdomen, abdominal —*see also* condition
- acute R10.0
- angina K55.1
- muscle deficiency syndrome Q79.4

Abdominalgia —*see* Pain, abdominal

Abduction contracture, hip or other joint —*see*
Contraction, joint

Aberrant (congenital) —*see also* Malposition,
congenital
- adrenal gland Q89.1
- artery (peripheral) Q27.8
  - basilar NEC Q28.1
  - cerebral Q28.3
  - coronary Q24.5
  - digestive system Q27.8
  - eye Q15.8
  - lower limb Q27.8
  - precerebral Q28.1
  - pulmonary Q25.79
  - renal Q27.2
  - retina Q14.1
  - specified site NEC Q27.8
  - subclavian Q27.8
  - upper limb Q27.8
  - vertebral Q28.1
- breast Q83.8
- endocrine gland NEC Q89.2
- hepatic duct Q44.5
- pancreas Q45.3
- parathyroid gland Q89.2
- pituitary gland Q89.2
- sebaceous glands, mucous membrane,
  mouth, congenital Q38.6
- spleen Q89.09
- subclavian artery Q27.8
- thymus (gland) Q89.2
- thyroid gland Q89.2
- vein (peripheral) NEC Q27.8
  - cerebral Q28.3
  - digestive system Q27.8
  - lower limb Q27.8
  - precerebral Q28.1
  - specified site NEC Q27.8
  - upper limb Q27.8

Aberration
- distantial —*see* Disturbance, visual
- mental F99

Abetalipoproteinemia E78.6

Abiotrophy R68.89

Ablatio, ablation
- retinae —*see* Detachment, retina

Ablepharia, ablepharon Q10.3

Abnormal, abnormality, abnormalities —*see
also* Anomaly
- acid-base balance (mixed) E87.4
- albumin R77.0
- alphafetoprotein R77.2
- alveolar ridge K08.9
- anatomical relationship Q89.9
- apertures, congenital, diaphragm
  Q79.1
- auditory perception H93.29-
  - diplacusis —*see* Diplacusis
  - hyperacusis —*see* Hyperacusis
  - recruitment —*see* Recruitment, auditory
  - threshold shift —*see* Shift, auditory
    threshold
- autosomes Q99.9
  - fragile site Q95.5
- basal metabolic rate R94.8
- biosynthesis, testicular androgen
  E29.1
- bleeding time R79.1

Abnormal, abnormality, abnormalities —
(Continued)
- blood level (of)
  - cobalt R79.0
  - copper R79.0
  - iron R79.0
  - lithium R78.89
  - magnesium R79.0
  - mineral NEC R79.0
  - zinc R79.0
- blood pressure
  - elevated R03.0
  - low reading (nonspecific) R03.1
- blood sugar R73.09
- blood-gas level R79.81
- bowel sounds R19.15
  - absent R19.11
  - hyperactive R19.12
- brain scan R94.02
- breathing R06.9
- caloric test R94.138
- cerebrospinal fluid R83.9
  - cytology R83.6
  - drug level R83.2
  - enzyme level R83.0
  - hormones R83.1
  - immunology R83.4
  - microbiology R83.5
  - nonmedicinal level R83.3
  - specified type NEC R83.8
- chemistry, blood R79.9
  - C-reactive protein R79.82
  - drugs —*see* Findings, abnormal, in
    blood
  - gas level R79.81
  - minerals R79.0
  - pancytopenia D61.818
  - PTT R79.1
  - specified NEC R79.89
  - toxins —*see* Findings, abnormal, in
    blood
- chest sounds (friction) (rales) R09.89
- chromosome, chromosomal Q99.9
  - with more than three X chromosomes,
    female Q97.1
  - analysis result R89.8
    - bronchial washings R84.8
    - cerebrospinal fluid R83.8
    - cervix uteri NEC R87.89
    - nasal secretions R84.8
    - nipple discharge R89.8
    - peritoneal fluid R85.89
    - pleural fluid R84.8
    - prostatic secretions R86.8
    - saliva R85.89
    - seminal fluid R86.8
    - sputum R84.8
    - synovial fluid R89.8
    - throat scrapings R84.8
    - vagina R87.89
    - vulva R87.89
    - wound secretions R89.8
  - dicentric replacement Q93.2
  - ring replacement Q93.2
  - sex Q99.8
    - female phenotype Q97.9
      - specified NEC Q97.8
    - male phenotype Q98.9
      - specified NEC Q98.8
    - structural male Q98.6
  - specified NEC Q99.8
- clinical findings NEC R68.89
- coagulation D68.9
  - newborn, transient P61.6
  - profile R79.1
  - time R79.1
- communication —*see* Fistula
- conjunctiva, vascular H11.41-
- coronary artery Q24.5
- cortisol-binding globulin E27.8

Abnormal, abnormality, abnormalities —
(Continued)
- course, eustachian tube Q17.8
- creatinine clearance R94.4
- cytology
  - anus R85.619
    - atypical squamous cells cannot
      exclude high grade squamous
      intraepithelial lesion (ASC-H)
      R85.611
    - atypical squamous cells of
      undetermined significance
      (ASC-US) R85.610
    - cytologic evidence of malignancy
      R85.614
    - high grade squamous intraepithelial
      lesion (HGSIL) R85.613
    - human papillomavirus (HPV) DNA
      test
      - high risk positive R85.81
      - low risk postive R85.82
    - inadequate smear R85.615
    - low grade squamous intraepithelial
      lesion (LGSIL) R85.612
    - satisfactory anal smear but lacking
      transformation zone R85.616
    - specified NEC R85.618
    - unsatisfactory smear R85.615
  - female genital organs —*see* Abnormal,
    Papanicolaou (smear)
- dark adaptation curve H53.61
- dentofacial NEC —*see* Anomaly, dentofacial
- development, developmental Q89.9
  - central nervous system Q07.9
- diagnostic imaging
  - abdomen, abdominal region NEC
    R93.5
  - biliary tract R93.2
  - breast R92.8
  - central nervous system NEC R90.89
  - cerebrovascular NEC R90.89
  - coronary circulation R93.1
  - digestive tract NEC R93.3
  - gastrointestinal (tract) R93.3
  - genitourinary organs R93.8
  - head R93.0
  - heart R93.1
  - intrathoracic organ NEC R93.8
  - limbs R93.6
  - liver R93.2
  - lung (field) R91.8
  - musculoskeletal system NEC R93.7
  - retroperitoneum R93.5
  - site specified NEC R93.8
  - skin and subcutaneous tissue R93.8
  - skull R93.0
  - urinary organs R93.4
- direction, teeth, fully erupted M26.30
- ear ossicles, acquired NEC H74.39-
  - ankylosis —*see* Ankylosis, ear ossicles
  - discontinuity —*see* Discontinuity, ossicles,
    ear
  - partial loss —*see* Loss, ossicles, ear
    (partial)
- Ebstein Q22.5
- echocardiogram R93.1
- echoencephalogram R90.81
- echogram —*see* Abnormal, diagnostic
  imaging
- electrocardiogram [ECG] [EKG] R94.31
- electroencephalogram [EEG] R94.01
- electrolyte —*see* Imbalance, electrolyte
- electromyogram [EMG] R94.131
- electro-oculogram [EOG] R94.110
- electrophysiological intracardiac studies
  R94.39
- electroretinogram [ERG] R94.111
- erythrocytes
  - congenital, with perinatal jaundice D58.9
- feces (color) (contents) (mucus) R19.5

Abnormal, abnormality, abnormalities —
  (Continued)
  finding —*see* Findings, abnormal, without
    diagnosis
  fluid
    amniotic —*see* Abnormal, specimen,
      specified
    cerebrospinal —*see* Abnormal,
      cerebrospinal fluid
    peritoneal —*see* Abnormal, specimen,
      digestive organs
    pleural —*see* Abnormal, specimen,
      respiratory organs
    synovial —*see* Abnormal, specimen,
      specified
    thorax (bronchial washings) (pleural
      fluid) —*see* Abnormal, specimen,
      respiratory organs
    vaginal —*see* Abnormal, specimen, female
      genital organs
  form
    teeth K00.2
    uterus —*see* Anomaly, uterus
  function studies
    auditory R94.120
    bladder R94.8
    brain R94.09
    cardiovascular R94.30
    ear R94.128
    endocrine NEC R94.7
    eye NEC R94.118
    kidney R94.4
    liver R94.5
    nervous system
      central NEC R94.09
      peripheral NEC R94.138
    pancreas R94.8
    placenta R94.8
    pulmonary R94.2
    special senses NEC R94.128
    spleen R94.8
    thyroid R94.6
    vestibular R94.121
  gait —*see* Gait
    hysterical F44.4
  gastrin secretion E16.4
  globulin R77.1
    cortisol-binding E27.8
    thyroid-binding E07.89
  glomerular, minor (*see also* N00-N07 with
    fourth character .0) N05.0
  glucagon secretion E16.3
  glucose tolerance (test) (non-fasting)
    R73.09
  gravitational (G) forces or states (effect of)
    T75.81
  hair (color) (shaft) L67.9
    specified NEC L67.8
  hard tissue formation in pulp (dental)
    K04.3
  head movement R25.0
  heart
    rate R00.9
      specified NEC R00.8
    shadow R93.1
    sounds NEC R01.2
  hemoglobin (disease) (*see also* Disease,
    hemoglobin) D58.2
    trait —*see* Trait, hemoglobin, abnormal
  histology NEC R89.7
  immunological findings R89.4
    in serum R76.9
      specified NEC R76.8
  increase in appetite R63.2
  involuntary movement —*see* Abnormal,
    movement, involuntary
  jaw closure M26.51
  karyotype R89.8
  kidney function test R94.4
  knee jerk R29.2
  leukocyte (cell) (differential) NEC D72.9

Abnormal, abnormality, abnormalities —
  (Continued)
  liver
  loss of
    height R29.890
    weight R63.4
  mammogram NEC R92.8
    calcification (calculus) R92.1
    microcalcification R92.0
  Mantoux test R76.11
  movement (disorder) —*see also* Disorder,
    movement
    head R25.0
    involuntary R25.9
      fasciculation R25.3
      of head R25.0
      spasm R25.2
      specified type NEC R25.8
      tremor R25.1
  myoglobin (Aberdeen) (Annapolis) R89.7
  neonatal screening P09
  oculomotor study R94.113
  palmar creases Q82.8
  Papanicolaou (smear)
    anus R85.619
      atypical squamous cells cannot
        exclude high grade squamous
        intraepithelial lesion (ASC-H)
        R85.611
      atypical squamous cells of undetermined
        significance (ASC-US) R85.610
      cytologic evidence of malignancy
        R85.614
      high grade squamous intraepithelial
        lesion (HGSIL) R85.613
      human papillomavirus (HPV)
        DNA test
        high risk positive R85.81
        low risk postive R85.82
      inadequate smear R85.615
      low grade squamous intraepithelial
        lesion (LGSIL) R85.612
      satisfactory anal smear but lacking
        transformation zone R85.616
      specified NEC R85.618
      unsatisfactory smear R85.615
    bronchial washings R84.6
    cerebrospinal fluid R83.6
    cervix R87.619
      atypical squamous cells cannot
        exclude high grade squamous
        intraepithelial lesion (ASC-H)
        R87.611
      atypical squamous cells of undetermined
        significance (ASC-US) R87.610
      cytologic evidence of malignancy
        R87.614
      high grade squamous intraepithelial
        lesion (HGSIL) R87.613
      inadequate smear R87.615
      low grade squamous intraepithelial
        lesion (LGSIL) R87.612
      non-atypical endometrial cells
        R87.618
      satisfactory cervical smear but
        lacking transformation zone
        R87.616
      specified NEC R87.618
      thin preparaton R87.619
      unsatisfactory smear R87.615
    nasal secretions R84.6
    nipple discharge R89.6
    peritoneal fluid R85.69
    pleural fluid R84.6
    prostatic secretions R86.6
    saliva R85.69
    seminal fluid R86.6
    sites NEC R89.6
    sputum R84.6
    synovial fluid R89.6
    throat scrapings R84.6

Abnormal, abnormality, abnormalities —
  (Continued)
  Papanicolaou (smear) *(Continued)*
    vagina R87.629
      atypical squamous cells cannot
        exclude high grade squamous
        intraepithelial lesion (ASC-H)
        R87.621
      atypical squamous cells of
        undetermined significance
        (ASC-US) R87.620
      cytologic evidence of malignancy
        R87.624
      high grade squamous intraepithelial
        lesion (HGSIL) R87.623
      inadequate smear R87.625
      low grade squamous intraepithelial
        lesion (LGSIL) R87.622
      specified NEC R87.628
      thin preparation R87.629
      unsatisfactory smear R87.625
    vulva R87.69
    wound secretions R89.6
  partial thromboplastin time (PTT) R79.1
  pelvis (bony) —*see* Deformity, pelvis
  percussion, chest (tympany) R09.89
  periods (grossly) —*see* Menstruation
  phonocardiogram R94.39
  plantar reflex R29.2
  plasma
    protein R77.9
      specified NEC R77.8
    viscosity R70.1
  pleural (folds) Q34.0
  posture R29.3
  product of conception O02.9
    specified type NEC O02.89
  prothrombin time (PT) R79.1
  pulmonary
    artery, congenital Q25.79
    function, newborn P28.89
    test results R94.2
  pulsations in neck R00.2
  pupillary H21.56-
    function (reaction) (reflex) —*see* Anomaly,
      pupil, function
  radiological examination —*see* Abnormal,
    diagnostic imaging
  red blood cell (s) (morphology) (volume)
    R71.8
  reflex —*see* Reflex
  renal function test R94.4
  response to nerve stimulation R94.130
  retinal correspondence H53.31
  retinal function study R94.111
  rhythm, heart —*see also* Arrhythmia
  saliva —*see* Abnormal, specimen, digestive
    organs
  scan
    kidney R94.4
    liver R93.2
    thyroid R94.6
  secretion
    gastrin E16.4
    glucagon E16.3
  semen, seminal fluid —*see* Abnormal,
    specimen, male genital organs
  serum level (of)
    acid phosphatase R74.8
    alkaline phosphatase R74.8
    amylase R74.8
    enzymes R74.9
      specified NEC R74.8
    lipase R74.8
    triacylglycerol lipase R74.8
  shape
    gravid uterus —*see* Anomaly, uterus
  sinus venosus Q21.1
  size, tooth, teeth K00.2
  spacing, tooth, teeth, fully erupted
    M26.30

◀ New   ◀▥▥ Revised   ~~deleted~~ Deleted

Abnormal, abnormality, abnormalities — (Continued)
 specimen
  digestive organs (peritoneal fluid) (saliva) R85.9
   cytology R85.69
   drug level R85.2
   enzyme level R85.0
   histology R85.7
   hormones R85.1
   immunology R85.4
   microbiology R85.5
   nonmedicinal level R85.3
   specified type NEC R85.89
  female genital organs (secretions) (smears) R87.9
   cytology R87.69
    cervix R87.619
     human papillomavirus (HPV) DNA test
      high risk positive R87.810
      low risk positive R87.820
     inadequate (unsatisfactory) smear R87.615
     non-atypical endometrial cells R87.618
     specified NEC R87.618 ◀▥
    vagina R87.629
     human papillomavirus (HPV) DNA test
      high risk positive R87.811
      low risk positive R87.821
     inadequate (unsatisfactory) smear R87.625
    vulva R87.69
   drug level R87.2
   enzyme level R87.0
   histological R87.7
   hormones R87.1
   immunology R87.4
   microbiology R87.5
   nonmedicinal level R87.3
   specified type NEC R87.89
  male genital organs (prostatic secretions) (semen) R86.9
   cytology R86.6
   drug level R86.2
   enzyme level R86.0
   histological R86.7
   hormones R86.1
   immunology R86.4
   microbiology R86.5
   nonmedicinal level R86.3
   specified type NEC R86.8
  nipple discharge —see Abnormal, specimen, specified
  respiratory organs (bronchial washings) (nasal secretions) (pleural fluid) (sputum) R84.9
   cytology R84.6
   drug level R84.2
   enzyme level R84.0
   histology R84.7
   hormones R84.1
   immunology R84.4
   microbiology R84.5
   nonmedicinal level R84.3
   specified type NEC R84.8
  specified organ, system and tissue NOS R89.9
   cytology R89.6
   drug level R89.2
   enzyme level R89.0
   histology R89.7
   hormones R89.1
   immunology R89.4
   microbiology R89.5
   nonmedicinal level R89.3
   specified type NEC R89.8
  synovial fluid —see Abnormal, specimen, specified

Abnormal, abnormality, abnormalities — (Continued)
 specimen (Continued)
  thorax (bronchial washings) (pleural fluids) —see Abnormal, specimen, respiratory organs
  vagina (secretion) (smear) R87.629
  vulva (secretion) (smear) R87.69
  wound secretion —see Abnormal, specimen, specified
  spermatozoa —see Abnormal, specimen, male genital organs
 sputum (amount) (color) (odor) R09.3
 stool (color) (contents) (mucus) R19.5
  bloody K92.1
  guaiac positive R19.5
 synchondrosis Q78.8
 thermography (see also Abnormal, diagnostic imaging) R93.8
 thyroid-binding globulin E07.89
 tooth, teeth (form) (size) K00.2
 toxicology (findings) R78.9
 transport protein E88.09
 tumor marker NEC R97.8
 ultrasound results —see Abnormal, diagnostic imaging
 umbilical cord complicating delivery O69.9
 urination NEC R39.19
 urine (constituents) R82.90
  bile R82.2
  cytological examination R82.8
  drugs R82.5
  fat R82.0
  glucose R81
  heavy metals R82.6
  hemoglobin R82.3
  histological examination R82.8
  ketones R82.4
  microbiological examination (culture) R82.7
  myoglobin R82.1
  positive culture R82.7
  protein —see Proteinuria
  specified substance NEC R82.99
   chromoabnormality NEC R82.91
  substances nonmedical R82.6
 uterine hemorrhage —see Hemorrhage, uterus
 vectorcardiogram R94.39
 visually evoked potential (VEP) R94.112
 white blood cells D72.9
  specified NEC D72.89
 X-ray examination —see Abnormal, diagnostic imaging
Abnormity (any organ or part) —see Anomaly
Abocclusion M26.29
 hemolytic disease (newborn) P55.1
 incompatibility reaction ABO —see Complication (s), transfusion, incompatibility reaction, ABO
Abolition, language R48.8
Aborter, habitual or recurrent —see Loss (of), pregnancy, recurrent
Abortion (complete) (spontaneous) O03.9
 with retained products of conception —see Abortion, incomplete
 with ◀
  retained products of conception - see Abortion, incomplete ◀
 attempted (elective) (failed) O07.4
  complicated by O07.30
   afibrinogenemia O07.1
   cardiac arrest O07.36
   chemical damage of pelvic organ (s) O07.34
   circulatory collapse O07.31
   cystitis O07.38
   defibrination syndrome O07.1
   electrolyte imbalance O07.33
   embolism (air) (amniotic fluid) (blood clot) (fat) (pulmonary) (septic) (soap) O07.2
   endometritis O07.0

Abortion (Continued)
 attempted (Continued)
  complicated by (Continued)
   genital tract and pelvic infection O07.0
   hemolysis O07.1
   hemorrhage (delayed) (excessive) O07.1
   infection
    genital tract or pelvic O07.0
    urinary tract tract O07.38
   intravascular coagulation O07.1
   laceration of pelvic organ (s) O07.34
   metabolic disorder O07.33
   oliguria O07.32
   oophoritis O07.0
   parametritis O07.0
   pelvic peritonitis O07.0
   perforation of pelvic organ (s) O07.34
   renal failure or shutdown O07.32
   salpingitis or salpingo-oophoritis O07.0
   sepsis O07.37
   shock O07.31
   specified condition NEC O07.39
   tubular necrosis (renal) O07.32
   uremia O07.32
   urinary tract infection O07.38
   venous complication NEC O07.35
    embolism (air) (amniotic fluid) (blood clot) (fat) (pulmonary) (septic) (soap) O07.2
 complicated (by) (following) O03.80
  afibrinogenemia O03.6
  cardiac arrest O03.86
  chemical damage of pelvic organ (s) O03.84
  circulatory collapse O03.81
  cystitis O03.88
  defibrination syndrome O03.6
  electrolyte imbalance O03.83
  embolism (air) (amniotic fluid) (blood clot) (fat) (pulmonary) (septic) (soap) O03.7
  endometritis O03.5
  genital tract and pelvic infection O03.5
  hemolysis O03.6
  hemorrhage (delayed) (excessive) O03.6
  infection
   genital tract or pelvic O03.5
   urinary tract O03.88
  intravascular coagulation O03.6
  laceration of pelvic organ (s) O03.84
  metabolic disorder O03.83
  oliguria O03.82
  oophoritis O03.5
  parametritis O03.5
  pelvic peritonitis O03.5
  perforation of pelvic organ (s) O03.84
  renal failure or shutdown O03.82
  salpingitis or salpingo-oophoritis O03.5
  sepsis O03.87
  shock O03.81
  specified condition NEC O03.89
  tubular necrosis (renal) O03.82
  uremia O03.82
  urinary tract infection O03.88
  venous complication NEC O03.85
   embolism (air) (amniotic fluid) (blood clot) (fat) (pulmonary) (septic) (soap) O03.7
 failed —see Abortion, attempted
 habitual or recurrent N96
  with current abortion —see categories O03-O06
  without current pregnancy N96
  care in current pregnancy O26.2-
 incomplete (spontaneous) O03.4
  complicated (by) (following) O03.30
   afibrinogenemia O03.1
   cardiac arrest O03.36
   chemical damage of pelvic organ (s) O03.34
   circulatory collapse O03.31
   cystitis O03.38

◀ New   ◀▥ Revised   ~~deleted~~ Deleted

Abortion *(Continued)*
  incomplete *(Continued)*
    complicated *(Continued)*
      defibrination syndrome O03.1
      electrolyte imbalance O03.33
      embolism (air) (amniotic fluid) (blood
          clot) (fat) (pulmonary) (septic)
          (soap) O03.2
      endometritis O03.0
      genital tract and pelvic infection O03.0
      hemolysis O03.1
      hemorrhage (delayed) (excessive)
          O03.1
      infection
        genital tract or pelvic O03.0
        urinary tract O03.38
      intravascular coagulation O03.1
      laceration of pelvic organ (s) O03.34
      metabolic disorder O03.33
      oliguria O03.32
      oophoritis O03.0
      parametritis O03.0
      pelvic peritonitis O03.0
      perforation of pelvic organ (s) O03.34
      renal failure or shutdown O03.32
      salpingitis or salpingo-oophoritis O03.0
      sepsis O03.37
      shock O03.31
      specified condition NEC O03.39
      tubular necrosis (renal) O03.32
      uremia O03.32
      urinary infection O03.38
      venous complication NEC O03.35
        embolism (air) (amniotic fluid) (blood
            clot) (fat) (pulmonary) (septic)
            (soap) O03.2
  induced (encounter for) Z33.2
    complicated by O04.80
      afibrinogenemia O04.6
      cardiac arrest O04.86
      chemical damage of pelvic organ (s)
          O04.84
      circulatory collapse O04.81
      cystitis O04.88
      defibrination syndrome O04.6
      electrolyte imbalance O04.83
      embolism (air) (amniotic fluid) (blood
          clot) (fat) (pulmonary) (septic)
          (soap) O04.7
      endometritis O04.5
      genital tract and pelvic infection O04.5
      hemolysis O04.6
      hemorrhage (delayed) (excessive)
          O04.6
      infection
        genital tract or pelvic O04.5
        urinary tract O04.88
      intravascular coagulation O04.6
      laceration of pelvic organ (s) O04.84
      metabolic disorder O04.83
      oliguria O04.82
      oophoritis O04.5
      parametritis O04.5
      pelvic peritonitis O04.5
      perforation of pelvic organ (s) O04.84
      renal failure or shutdown O04.82
      salpingitis or salpingo-oophoritis O04.5
      sepsis O04.87
      shock O04.81
      specified condition NEC O04.89
      tubular necrosis (renal) O04.82
      uremia O04.82
      urinary tract infection O04.88
      venous complication NEC O04.85
        embolism (air) (amniotic fluid) (blood
            clot) (fat) (pulmonary) (septic)
            (soap) O04.7
  missed O02.1
  spontaneous —*see* Abortion (complete)
      (spontaneous)
    threatened O20.0

Abortion *(Continued)*
  threatened (spontaneous) O20.0
  tubal O00.1
Abortus fever A23.1
Aboulomania F60.7
Abrami's disease D59.8
Abramov-Fiedler myocarditis (acute isolated
    myocarditis) I40.1
Abrasion T14.8
  abdomen, abdominal (wall) S30.811
  alveolar process S00.512
  ankle S90.51-
  antecubital space —*see* Abrasion, elbow
  anus S30.817
  arm (upper) S40.81-
  auditory canal —*see* Abrasion, ear
  auricle —*see* Abrasion, ear
  axilla —*see* Abrasion, arm
  back, lower S30.810
  breast S20.11-
  brow S00.81
  buttock S30.810
  calf —*see* Abrasion, leg
  canthus —*see* Abrasion, eyelid
  cheek S00.81
    internal S00.512
  chest wall —*see* Abrasion, thorax
  chin S00.81
  clitoris S30.814
  cornea S05.0-
  costal region —*see* Abrasion, thorax
  dental K03.1
  digit (s)
    foot —*see* Abrasion, toe
    hand —*see* Abrasion, finger
  ear S00.41-
  elbow S50.31-
  epididymis S30.813
  epigastric region S30.811
  epiglottis S10.11
  esophagus (thoracic) S27.818
    cervical S10.11
  eyebrow —*see* Abrasion, eyelid
  eyelid S00.21-
  face S00.81
  finger (s) S60.41-
    index S60.41-
    little S60.41-
    middle S60.41-
    ring S60.41-
  flank S30.811
  foot (except toe (s) alone) S90.81-
    toe —*see* Abrasion, toe
  forearm S50.81-
    elbow only —*see* Abrasion, elbow
  forehead S00.81
  genital organs, external
    female S30.816
    male S30.815
  groin S30.811
  gum S00.512
  hand S60.51-
  head S00.91
    ear —*see* Abrasion, ear
    eyelid —*see* Abrasion, eyelid
    lip S00.511
    nose S00.31
    oral cavity S00.512
    scalp S00.01
    specified site NEC S00.81
  heel —*see* Abrasion, foot
  hip S70.21-
  inguinal region S30.811
  interscapular region S20.419
  jaw S00.81
  knee S80.21-
  labium (majus) (minus) S30.814
  larynx S10.11
  leg (lower) S80.81-
    knee —*see* Abrasion, knee
    upper —*see* Abrasion, thigh

Abrasion *(Continued)*
  lip S00.511
  lower back S30.810
  lumbar region S30.810
  malar region S00.81
  mammary —*see* Abrasion, breast
  mastoid region S00.81
  mouth S00.512
  nail
    finger —*see* Abrasion, finger
    toe —*see* Abrasion, toe
  nape S10.81
  nasal S00.31
  neck S10.91
    specified site NEC S10.81
    throat S10.11
  nose S00.31
  occipital region S00.01
  oral cavity S00.512
  orbital region —*see* Abrasion, eyelid
  palate S00.512
  palm —*see* Abrasion, hand
  parietal region S00.01
  pelvis S30.810
  penis S30.812
  perineum
    female S30.814
    male S30.810
  periocular area —*see* Abrasion, eyelid
  phalanges
    finger —*see* Abrasion, finger
    toe —*see* Abrasion, toe
  pharynx S10.11
  pinna —*see* Abrasion, ear
  popliteal space —*see* Abrasion, knee
  prepuce S30.812
  pubic region S30.810
  pudendum
    female S30.816
    male S30.815
  sacral region S30.810
  scalp S00.01
  scapular region —*see* Abrasion, shoulder
  scrotum S30.813
  shin —*see* Abrasion, leg
  shoulder S40.21-
  skin NEC T14.8
  sternal region S20.319
  submaxillary region S00.81
  submental region S00.81
  subungual
    finger (s) —*see* Abrasion, finger
    toe (s) —*see* Abrasion, toe
  supraclavicular fossa S10.81
  supraorbital S00.81
  temple S00.81
  temporal region S00.81
  testis S30.813
  thigh S70.31-
  thorax, thoracic (wall) S20.91
    back S20.41-
    front S20.31-
  throat S10.11
  thumb S60.31-
  toe (s) (lesser) S90.416
    great S90.41-
  tongue S00.512
  tooth, teeth (dentifrice) (habitual) (hard
      tissues) (occupational) (ritual)
      (traditional) K03.1
  trachea S10.11
  tunica vaginalis S30.813
  tympanum, tympanic membrane —*see*
      Abrasion, ear
  uvula S00.512
  vagina S30.814
  vocal cords S10.11
  vulva S30.814
  wrist S60.81-
Abrism —*see* Poisoning, food, noxious,
    plant

◄ New   ◄▦ Revised   ~~deleted~~ Deleted

Abruptio placentae O45.9-
  with
    afibrinogenemia O45.01-
    coagulation defect O45.00-
      specified NEC O45.09-
    disseminated intravascular coagulation
      O45.02-
    hypofibrinogenemia O45.01-
  specified NEC O45.8-
Abruption, placenta —see Abruptio placentae
Abscess (connective tissue) (embolic) (fistulous)
    (infective) (metastatic) (multiple)
    (pernicious) (pyogenic) (septic) L02.91
  with
    diverticular disease (intestine) K57.80
      with bleeding K57.81
      large intestine K57.20
        with
          bleeding K57.21
          small intestine K57.40
            with bleeding K57.41
      small intestine K57.00
        with
          bleeding K57.01
          large intestine K57.40
            with bleeding K57.41
    lymphangitis - code by site under
      Abscess
  abdomen, abdominal
    cavity K65.1
    wall L02.211
  abdominopelvic K65.1
  accessory sinus —see Sinusitis
  adrenal (capsule) (gland) E27.8
  alveolar K04.7
    with sinus K04.6
  amebic A06.4
    brain (and liver or lung abscess) A06.6
    genitourinary tract A06.82
    liver (without mention of brain or lung
      abscess) A06.4
    lung (and liver) (without mention of brain
      abscess) A06.5
    specified site NEC A06.89
    spleen A06.89
  anerobic A48.0
  ankle —see Abscess, lower limb
  anorectal K61.2
  antecubital space —see Abscess, upper limb
  antrum (chronic) (Highmore) —see Sinusitis,
    maxillary
  anus K61.0
  apical (tooth) K04.7
    with sinus (alveolar) K04.6
  appendix K35.3
  areola (acute) (chronic) (nonpuerperal) N61
    puerperal, postpartum or gestational —see
      Infection, nipple
  arm (any part) —see Abscess, upper limb
  artery (wall) I77.89
  atheromatous I77.2
  auricle, ear —see Abscess, ear, external
  axilla (region) L02.41-
    lymph gland or node L04.2
  back (any part, except buttock) L02.212
  Bartholin's gland N75.1
    with
      abortion —see Abortion, by type
        complicated by, sepsis
      ectopic or molar pregnancy O08.0
      following ectopic or molar pregnancy
        O08.0
  Bezold's —see Mastoiditis, acute
  bilharziasis B65.1
  bladder (wall) —see Cystitis, specified type
    NEC
  bone (subperiosteal) —see also Osteomyelitis,
    specified type NEC
    accessory sinus (chronic) —see Sinusitis
    chronic or old —see Osteomyelitis, chronic
    jaw (lower) (upper) M27.2

Abscess (Continued)
  bone (Continued)
    mastoid —see Mastoiditis, acute,
      subperiosteal
    petrous —see Petrositis
    spinal (tuberculous) A18.01
      nontuberculous —see Osteomyelitis,
        vertebra
  bowel K63.0
  brain (any part) (cystic) (otogenic) G06.0
    amebic (with abscess of any other site)
      A06.6
    gonococcal A54.82
    pheomycotic (chromomycotic) B43.1
    tuberculous A17.81
  breast (acute) (chronic) (nonpuerperal) N61
    newborn P39.0
    puerperal, postpartum, gestational —see
      Mastitis, obstetric, purulent
  broad ligament N73.2
    acute N73.0
    chronic N73.1
  Brodie's (localized) (chronic) M86.8X-
  bronchi J98.09
  buccal cavity K12.2
  bulbourethral gland N34.0
  bursa M71.00
    ankle M71.07-
    elbow M71.02-
    foot M71.07-
    hand M71.04-
    hip M71.05-
    knee M71.06-
    multiple sites M71.09
    pharyngeal J39.1
    shoulder M71.01-
    specified site NEC M71.08
    wrist M71.03-
  buttock L02.31
  canthus —see Blepharoconjunctivitis
  cartilage —see Disorder, cartilage, specified
    type NEC
  cecum K35.3
  cerebellum, cerebellar G06.0
    sequelae G09
  cerebral (embolic) G06.0
    sequelae G09
  cervical (meaning neck) L02.11
    lymph gland or node L04.0
  cervix (stump) (uteri) —see Cervicitis
  cheek (external) L02.01
    inner K12.2
  chest J86.9
    with fistula J86.0
    wall L02.213
  chin L02.01
  choroid —see Inflammation, chorioretinal
  circumtonsillar J36
  cold (lung) (tuberculous) —see also
      Tuberculosis, abscess, lung
    articular —see Tuberculosis, joint
  colon (wall) K63.0
  colostomy K94.02
  conjunctiva —see Conjunctivitis, acute
  cornea H16.31-
  corpus
    cavernosum N48.21
    luteum —see Oophoritis
  Cowper's gland N34.0
  cranium G06.0
  cul-de-sac (Douglas') (posterior) —see
    Peritonitis, pelvic, female
  cutaneous —see Abscess, by site
  dental K04.7
    with sinus (alveolar) K04.6
  dentoalveolar K04.7
    with sinus K04.6
  diaphragm, diaphragmatic K65.1
  Douglas' cul-de-sac or pouch —see
    Peritonitis, pelvic, female
  Dubois A50.59

Abscess (Continued)
  ear (middle) —see also Otitis, media,
      suppurative
    acute —see Otitis, media, suppurative,
      acute
    external H60.0-
  entamebic —see Abscess, amebic
  enterostomy K94.12
  epididymis N45.4
  epidural G06.2
    brain G06.0
    spinal cord G06.1
  epiglottis J38.7
  epiploon, epiploic K65.1
  erysipelatous —see Erysipelas
  esophagus K20.8
  ethmoid (bone) (chronic) (sinus) J32.2
  external auditory canal —see Abscess, ear,
    external
  extradural G06.2
    brain G06.0
      sequelae G09
    spinal cord G06.1
  extraperitoneal K68.19
  eye —see Endophthalmitis, purulent
  eyelid H00.03-
  face (any part, except ear, eye and nose)
    L02.01
  fallopian tube —see Salpingitis
  fascia M72.8
  fauces J39.1
  fecal K63.0
  femoral (region) —see Abscess, lower
    limb
  filaria, filarial —see Infestation, filarial
  finger (any) —see also Abscess, hand
    nail —see Cellulitis, finger
  foot L02.61-
  forehead L02.01
  frontal sinus (chronic) J32.1
  gallbladder K81.0
  genital organ or tract
    female (external) N76.4
    male N49.9
      multiple sites N49.8
      specified NEC N49.8
  gestational mammary O91.11-
  gestational subareolar O91.11-
  gingival K05.21
  gland, glandular (lymph) (acute) —see
    Lymphadenitis, acute
  gluteal (region) L02.31
  gonorrheal —see Gonococcus
  groin L02.214
  gum K05.21
  hand L02.51-
  head NEC L02.811
    face (any part, except ear, eye and nose)
      L02.01
  heart —see Carditis
  heel —see Abscess, foot
  helminthic —see Infestation, helminth
  hepatic (cholangitic) (hematogenic)
      (lymphogenic) (pylephlebitic) K75.0
    amebic A06.4
  hip (region) —see Abscess, lower limb
  ileocecal K35.3
  ileostomy (bud) K94.12
  iliac (region) L02.214
    fossa K35.3
  infraclavicular (fossa) —see Abscess, upper
    limb
  inguinal (region) L02.214
    lymph gland or node L04.1
  intestine, intestinal NEC K63.0
    rectal K61.1
  intra-abdominal (see also Abscess,
      peritoneum) K65.1
    postoperative T81.4
    retroperitoneal K68.11
  intracranial G06.0

◀ New ◀ Revised ~~deleted~~ Deleted

Abscess *(Continued)*
  intramammary —*see* Abscess, breast
  intraorbital —*see* Abscess, orbit
  intraperitoneal K65.1
  intrasphincteric (anus) K61.4
  intraspinal G06.1
  intratonsillar J36
  ischiorectal (fossa) K61.3
  jaw (bone) (lower) (upper) M27.2
  joint —*see* Arthritis, pyogenic or pyemic
    spine (tuberculous) A18.01
      nontuberculous —*see* Spondylopathy,
        infective
  kidney N15.1
    with calculus N20.0
      with hydronephrosis N13.6
    puerperal (postpartum) O86.21
  knee —*see also* Abscess, lower limb
    joint M00.9
  labium (majus) (minus) N76.4
  lacrimal
    caruncle —*see* Inflammation, lacrimal,
      passages, acute
    gland —*see* Dacryoadenitis
    passages (duct) (sac) —*see* Inflammation,
      lacrimal, passages, acute
  lacunar N34.0
  larynx J38.7
  lateral (alveolar) K04.7
    with sinus K04.6
  leg (any part) —*see* Abscess, lower limb
  lens H27.8
  lingual K14.0
    tonsil J36
  lip K13.0
  Littre's gland N34.0
  liver (cholangitic) (hematogenic)
    (lymphogenic) (pylephlebitic)
    (pyogenic) K75.0
    amebic (due to Entamoeba histolytica)
      (dysenteric) (tropical) A06.4
      with
        brain abscess (and liver or lung
          abscess) A06.6
        lung abscess A06.5
  loin (region) L02.211
  lower limb L02.41-
  lumbar (tuberculous) A18.01
    nontuberculous L02.212
  lung (miliary) (putrid) J85.2
    with pneumonia J85.1
      due to specified organism *(see*
        Pneumonia, in (due to))
    amebic (with liver abscess) A06.5
      with
        brain abscess A06.6
        pneumonia A06.5
  lymph, lymphatic, gland or node (acute) —*see*
    also Lymphadenitis, acute
    mesentery I88.0
  malar M27.2
  mammary gland —*see* Abscess, breast
  marginal, anus K61.0
  mastoid —*see* Mastoiditis, acute
  maxilla, maxillary M27.2
    molar (tooth) K04.7
      with sinus K04.6
    premolar K04.7
    sinus (chronic) J32.0
  mediastinum J85.3
  meibomian gland —*see* Hordeolum
  meninges G06.2
  mesentery, mesenteric K65.1
  mesosalpinx —*see* Salpingitis
  mons pubis L02.215
  mouth (floor) K12.2
  muscle —*see* Myositis, infective
  myocardium I40.0
  nabothian (follicle) —*see* Cervicitis
  nasal J32.9
  nasopharyngeal J39.1

Abscess *(Continued)*
  navel L02.216
    newborn P38.9
      with mild hemorrhage P38.1
      without hemorrhage P38.9
  neck (region) L02.11
    lymph gland or node L04.0
  nephritic —*see* Abscess, kidney
  nipple N61
    associated with
      lactation —*see* Pregnancy, complicated
        by,
      pregnancy —*see* Pregnancy, complicated
        by
  nose (external) (fossa) (septum) J34.0
    sinus (chronic) —*see* Sinusitis
  omentum K65.1
  operative wound T81.4
  orbit, orbital —*see* Cellulitis, orbit
  otogenic G06.0
  ovary, ovarian (corpus luteum) —*see*
    Oophoritis
  oviduct —*see* Oophoritis
  palate (soft) K12.2
    hard M27.2
  palmar (space) —*see* Abscess, hand
  pancreas (duct) —*see* Pancreatitis, acute
  parafrenal N48.21
  parametric, parametrium N73.2
    acute N73.0
    chronic N73.1
  paranephric N15.1
  parapancreatic —*see* Pancreatitis, acute
  parapharyngeal J39.0
  pararectal K61.1
  parasinus —*see* Sinusitis
  parauterine *(see also* Disease, pelvis,
    inflammatory) N73.2
  paravaginal —*see* Vaginitis
  parietal region (scalp) L02.811
  parodontal K05.21
  parotid (duct) (gland) K11.3
    region K12.2
  pectoral (region) L02.213
  pelvis, pelvic
    female —*see* Disease, pelvis, inflammatory
    male, peritoneal K65.1
  penis N48.21
    gonococcal (accessory gland) (periurethral)
      A54.1
  perianal K61.0
  periapical K04.7
    with sinus (alveolar) K04.6
  periappendicular K35.3
  pericardial I30.1
  pericecal K35.3
  pericemental K05.21
  pericholecystic —*see* Cholecystitis, acute
  pericoronal K05.21
  peridental K05.21
  perimetric *(see also* Disease, pelvis,
    inflammatory) N73.2
  perinephric, perinephritic —*see* Abscess,
    kidney
  perineum, perineal (superficial) L02.215
    urethra N34.0
  periodontal (parietal) K05.21
    apical K04.7
  periosteum, periosteal —*see also*
    Osteomyelitis, specified type NEC
    with osteomyelitis —*see also* Osteomyelitis,
      specified type NEC
    acute —*see* Osteomyelitis, acute
    chronic —*see* Osteomyelitis, chronic
  peripharyngeal J39.0
  peripleuritic J86.9
    with fistula J86.0
  periprostatic N41.2
  perirectal K61.1
  perirenal (tissue) —*see* Abscess, kidney
  perisinuous (nose) —*see* Sinusitis

Abscess *(Continued)*
  peritoneum, peritoneal (perforated)
    (ruptured) K65.1
    with appendicitis K35.3
    pelvic
      female —*see* Peritonitis, pelvic, female
      male K65.1
    postoperative T81.4
    puerperal, postpartum, childbirth O85
    tuberculous A18.31
  peritonsillar J36
  perityphlic K35.3
  periureteral N28.89
  periurethral N34.0
    gonococcal (accessory gland) (periurethral)
      A54.1
  periuterine *(see also* Disease, pelvis,
    inflammatory) N73.2
  perivesical —*see* Cystitis, specified type NEC
  petrous bone —*see* Petrositis
  phagedenic NOS L02.91
    chancroid A57
  pharynx, pharyngeal (lateral) J39.1
  pilonidal L05.01
  pituitary (gland) E23.6
  pleura J86.9
    with fistula J86.0
  popliteal —*see* Abscess, lower limb
  postcecal K35.3
  postlaryngeal J38.7
  postnasal J34.0
  postoperative (any site) T81.4
    retroperitoneal K68.11
  postpharyngeal J39.0
  posttonsillar J36
  post-typhoid A01.09
  pouch of Douglas —*see* Peritonitis, pelvic,
    female
  premammary —*see* Abscess, breast
  prepatellar —*see* Abscess, lower limb
  prostate N41.2
    gonococcal (acute) (chronic) A54.22
  psoas muscle K68.12
  puerperal - code by site under Puerperal,
    abscess
  pulmonary —*see* Abscess, lung
  pulp, pulpal (dental) K04.0
  rectovaginal septum K63.0
  rectovesical —*see* Cystitis, specified type NEC
  rectum K61.1
  renal —*see* Abscess, kidney
  retina —*see* Inflammation, chorioretinal
  retrobulbar —*see* Abscess, orbit
  retrocecal K65.1
  retrolaryngeal J38.7
  retromammary —*see* Abscess, breast
  retroperitoneal NEC K68.19
    postprocedural K68.11
  retropharyngeal J39.0
  retrouterine —*see* Peritonitis, pelvic, female
  retrovesical —*see* Cystitis, specified type NEC
  root, tooth K04.7
    with sinus (alveolar) K04.6
  round ligament *(see also* Disease, pelvis,
    inflammatory) N73.2
  rupture (spontaneous) NOS L02.91
  sacrum (tuberculous) A18.01
    nontuberculous M46.28
  salivary (duct) (gland) K11.3
  scalp (any part) L02.811
  scapular —*see* Osteomyelitis, specified type
    NEC
  sclera —*see* Scleritis
  scrofulous (tuberculous) A18.2
  scrotum N49.2
  seminal vesicle N49.0
  septal, dental K04.7
    with sinus (alveolar) K04.6
  serous —*see* Periostitis
  shoulder (region) —*see* Abscess, upper limb
  sigmoid K63.0

Abscess *(Continued)*

sinus (accessory) (chronic) (nasal) —*see also* Sinusitis
   intracranial venous (any) G06.0
Skene's duct or gland N34.0
skin —*see* Abscess, by site
specified site NEC L02.818
spermatic cord N49.1
sphenoidal (sinus) (chronic) J32.3
spinal cord (any part) (staphylococcal) G06.1
   tuberculous A17.81
spine (column) (tuberculous) A18.01
   epidural G06.1
   nontuberculous —*see* Osteomyelitis, vertebra
spleen D73.3
   amebic A06.89
stitch T81.4
subarachnoid G06.2
   brain G06.0
   spinal cord G06.1
subareolar —*see* Abscess, breast
subcecal K35.3
subcutaneous —*see also* Abscess, by site
   pheomycotic (chromomycotic) B43.2
subdiaphragmatic K65.1
subdural G06.2
   brain G06.0
      sequelae G09
   spinal cord G06.1
subgaleal L02.811
subhepatic K65.1
sublingual K12.2
   gland K11.3
submammary —*see* Abscess, breast
submandibular (region) (space) (triangle) K12.2
   gland K11.3
submaxillary (region) L02.01
   gland K11.3
submental L02.01
   gland K11.3
subperiosteal —*see* Osteomyelitis, specified type NEC
subphrenic K65.1
   postoperative T81.4
suburethral N34.0
sudoriparous L75.8
supraclavicular (fossa) —*see* Abscess, upper limb
suprapelvic, acute N73.0
suprarenal (capsule) (gland) E27.8
sweat gland L74.8
tear duct —*see* Inflammation, lacrimal, passages, acute
temple L02.01
temporal region L02.01
temporosphenoidal G06.0
tendon (sheath) M65.00
   ankle M65.07-
   foot M65.07-
   forearm M65.03-
   hand M65.04-
   lower leg M65.06-
   pelvic region M65.05-
   shoulder region M65.01-
   specified site NEC M65.08
   thigh M65.05-
   upper arm M65.02-
testis N45.4
thigh —*see* Abscess, lower limb
thorax J86.9
   with fistula J86.0
throat J39.1
thumb —*see also* Abscess, hand
   nail —*see* Cellulitis, finger
thymus (gland) E32.1
thyroid (gland) E06.0
toe (any) —*see also* Abscess, foot
   nail —*see* Cellulitis, toe
tongue (staphylococcal) K14.0

Abscess *(Continued)*

tonsil (s) (lingual) J36
tonsillopharyngeal J36
tooth, teeth (root) K04.7
   with sinus (alveolar) K04.6
   supporting structures NEC K05.21
trachea J39.8
trunk L02.219
   abdominal wall L02.211
   back L02.212
   chest wall L02.213
   groin L02.214
   perineum L02.215
   umbilicus L02.216
tubal —*see* Salpingitis
tuberculous —*see* Tuberculosis, abscess
tubo-ovarian —*see* Salpingo-oophoritis
tunica vaginalis N49.1
umbilicus L02.216
upper
   limb L02.41-
   respiratory J39.8
urethral (gland) N34.0
urinary N34.0
uterus, uterine (wall) —*see also* Endometritis
   ligament (*see also* Disease, pelvis, inflammatory) N73.2
   neck —*see* Cervicitis
uvula K12.2
vagina (wall) —*see* Vaginitis
vaginorectal —*see* Vaginitis
vas deferens N49.1
vermiform appendix K35.3
vertebra (column) (tuberculous) A18.01
   nontuberculous —*see* Osteomyelitis, vertebra
vesical —*see* Cystitis, specified type NEC
vesico-uterine pouch —*see* Peritonitis, pelvic, female
vitreous (humor) —*see* Endophthalmitis, purulent
vocal cord J38.3
von Bezold's —*see* Mastoiditis, acute
vulva N76.4
vulvovaginal gland N75.1
web space —*see* Abscess, hand
wound T81.4
wrist —*see* Abscess, upper limb

Absence (of) (organ or part) (complete or partial)
adrenal (gland) (congenital) Q89.1
   acquired E89.6
albumin in blood E88.09
alimentary tract (congenital) Q45.8
   upper Q40.8
alveolar process (acquired) —*see* Anomaly, alveolar
ankle (acquired) Z89.44-
anus (congenital) Q42.3
   with fistula Q42.2
aorta (congenital) Q25.4
appendix, congenital Q42.8
arm (acquired) Z89.20-
   above elbow Z89.22-
      congenital (with hand present) —*see* Agenesis, arm, with hand present and hand —*see* Agenesis, forearm, and hand
   below elbow Z89.21-
      congenital (with hand present) —*see* Agenesis, arm, with hand present and hand —*see* Agenesis, forearm, and hand
   congenital —*see* Defect, reduction, upper limb
   shoulder (following explanation of shoulder joint prosthesis) (joint) (with or without presence of antibiotic-impregnated cement spacer) Z89.23-
      congenital (with hand present) —*see* Agenesis, arm, with hand present

Absence *(Continued)*

artery (congenital) (peripheral) Q27.8
   brain Q28.3
   coronary Q24.5
   pulmonary Q25.79
   specified NEC Q27.8
   umbilical Q27.0
atrial septum (congenital) Q21.1
auditory canal (congenital) (external) Q16.1
auricle (ear), congenital Q16.0
bile, biliary duct, congenital Q44.5
bladder (acquired) Z90.6
   congenital Q64.5
bowel sounds R19.11
brain Q00.0
   part of Q04.3
breast (s) (and nipple (s)) (acquired) Z90.1-
   congenital Q83.8
broad ligament Q50.6
bronchus (congenital) Q32.4
canaliculus lacrimalis, congenital Q10.4
cerebellum (vermis) Q04.3
cervix (acquired) (with uterus) Z90.710
   with remaining uterus Z90.712
   congenital Q51.5
chin, congenital Q18.8
cilia (congenital) Q10.3
   acquired —*see* Madarosis
clitoris (congenital) Q52.6
coccyx, congenital Q76.49
cold sense R20.8
congenital
   lumen —*see* Atresia
   organ or site NEC —*see* Agenesis
   septum —*see* Imperfect, closure
corpus callosum Q04.0
cricoid cartilage, congenital Q31.8
diaphragm (with hernia), congenital Q79.1
digestive organ (s) or tract, congenital Q45.8
   acquired NEC Z90.49
   upper Q40.8
ductus arteriosus Q28.8
duodenum (acquired) Z90.49
   congenital Q41.0
ear, congenital Q16.9
   acquired H93.8-
   auricle Q16.0
   external Q16.0
   inner Q16.5
   lobe, lobule Q17.8
   middle, except ossicles Q16.4
      ossicles Q16.3
   ossicles Q16.3
ejaculatory duct (congenital) Q55.4
endocrine gland (congenital) NEC Q89.2
   acquired E89.89
epididymis (congenital) Q55.4
   acquired Z90.79
epiglottis, congenital Q31.8
esophagus (congenital) Q39.8
   acquired (partial) Z90.49
eustachian tube (congenital) Q16.2
extremity (acquired) Z89.9
   congenital Q73.0
   knee (following explanation of knee joint prosthesis) (joint) (with or without presence of antibiotic-impregnated cement spacer) Z89.52-
   lower (above knee) Z89.619
      below knee Z89.51-
   upper —*see* Absence, arm
eye (acquired) Z90.01
   congenital Q11.1
   muscle (congenital) Q10.3
eyeball (acquired) Z90.01
eyelid (fold) (congenital) Q10.3
   acquired Z90.01
face, specified part NEC Q18.8
fallopian tube (s) (acquired) Z90.79
   congenital Q50.6

◀ New   ⫷ Revised   ~~deleted~~ Deleted

Absence *(Continued)*
  family member (causing problem in home)
      NEC *(see also* Disruption, family)
      Z63.32
  femur, congenital —*see* Defect, reduction,
      lower limb, longitudinal, femur
  fibrinogen (congenital) D68.2
      acquired D65
  finger (s) (acquired) Z89.02-
      congenital —*see* Agenesis, hand
  foot (acquired) Z89.43-
      congenital —*see* Agenesis, foot
  forearm (acquired) —*see* Absence, arm, below
      elbow
  gallbladder (acquired) Z90.49
      congenital Q44.0
  gamma globulin in blood D80.1
      hereditary D80.0
  genital organs
      acquired (female) (male) Z90.79
      female, congenital Q52.8
          external Q52.71
          internal NEC Q52.8
      male, congenital Q55.8
  genitourinary organs, congenital NEC
      female Q52.8
      male Q55.8
  globe (acquired) Z90.01
      congenital Q11.1
  glottis, congenital Q31.8
  hand and wrist (acquired) Z89.11-
      congenital —*see* Agenesis, hand
  head, part (acquired) NEC Z90.09
  heat sense R20.8
  hip (following explantation of hip joint
      prosthesis) (joint) (with or without
      presence of antibiotic-impregnated
      cement spacer) Z89.62-
  hymen (congenital) Q52.4
  ileum (acquired) Z90.49
      congenital Q41.2
  immunoglobulin, isolated NEC D80.3
      IgA D80.2
      IgG D80.3
      IgM D80.4
  incus (acquired) —*see* Loss, ossicles, ear
      congenital Q16.3
  inner ear, congenital Q16.5
  intestine (acquired) (small) Z90.49
      congenital Q41.9
          specified NEC Q41.8
      large Z90.49
          congenital Q42.9
              specified NEC Q42.8
  iris, congenital Q13.1
  jejunum (acquired) Z90.49
      congenital Q41.1
  joint
      acquired
          hip (following explantation of hip
              joint prosthesis) (with or without
              presence of antibiotic-impregnated
              cement spacer) Z89.62-
          knee (following explantation of knee
              joint prosthesis) (with or without
              presence of antibiotic-impregnated
              cement spacer) Z89.52-
          shoulder (following explantation of
              shoulder joint prosthesis) (with
              or without presence of antibiotic-
              impregnated cement spacer)
              Z89.23-
      congenital NEC Q74.8
  kidney (s) (acquired) Z90.5
      congenital Q60.2
          bilateral Q60.1
          unilateral Q60.0
  knee (following explantation of knee joint
      prosthesis) (joint) (with or without
      presence of antibiotic-impregnated
      cement spacer) Z89.52-

Absence *(Continued)*
  labyrinth, membranous Q16.5
  larynx (congenital) Q31.8
      acquired Z90.02
  leg (acquired) (above knee) Z89.61-
      below knee (acquired) Z89.51-
      congenital —*see* Defect, reduction, lower
          limb
  lens (acquired) —*see also* Aphakia
      congenital Q12.3
      post cataract extraction Z98.4-
  limb (acquired) —*see* Absence, extremity
  lip Q38.6
  liver (congenital) Q44.7
  lung (fissure) (lobe) (bilateral) (unilateral)
      (congenital) Q33.3
      acquired (any part) Z90.2
  menstruation —*see* Amenorrhea
  muscle (congenital) (pectoral) Q79.8
      ocular Q10.3
  neck, part Q18.8
  neutrophil —*see* Agranulocytosis
  nipple (s) (with breast (s)) (acquired)
      Z90.1-
      congenital Q83.2
  nose (congenital) Q30.1
      acquired Z90.09
  organ
      of Corti, congenital Q16.5
      or site, congenital NEC Q89.8
          acquired NEC Z90.89
  osseous meatus (ear) Q16.4
  ovary (acquired)
      bilateral Z90.722
      congenital
          bilateral Q50.02
          unilateral Q50.01
      unilateral Z90.721
  oviduct (acquired)
      bilateral Z90.722
      congenital Q50.6
      unilateral Z90.721
  pancreas (congenital) Q45.0
      acquired Z90.410
          complete Z90.410
          partial Z90.411
          total Z90.410
  parathyroid gland (acquired)
      E89.2
      congenital Q89.2
  patella, congenital Q74.1
  penis (congenital) Q55.5
      acquired Z90.79
  pericardium (congenital) Q24.8
  pituitary gland (congenital) Q89.2
      acquired E89.3
  prostate (acquired) Z90.79
      congenital Q55.4
  pulmonary valve Q22.0
  punctum lacrimale (congenital) Q10.4
  radius, congenital —*see* Defect, reduction,
      upper limb, longitudinal, radius
  rectum (congenital) Q42.1
      with fistula Q42.0
      acquired Z90.49
  respiratory organ NOS Q34.9
  rib (acquired) Z90.89
      congenital Q76.6
  sacrum, congenital Q76.49
  salivary gland (s), congenital Q38.4
  scrotum, congenital Q55.29
  seminal vesicles (congenital) Q55.4
      acquired Z90.79
  septum
      atrial (congenital) Q21.1
      between aorta and pulmonary artery
          Q21.4
      ventricular (congenital) Q20.4
  sex chromosome
      female phenotype Q97.8
      male phenotype Q98.8

Absence *(Continued)*
  skull bone (congenital) Q75.8
      with
          anencephaly Q00.0
          encephalocele —*see* Encephalocele
          hydrocephalus Q03.9
              with spina bifida —*see* Spina
                  bifida, by site, with
                  hydrocephalus
          microcephaly Q02
  spermatic cord, congenital Q55.4
  spine, congenital Q76.49
  spleen (congenital) Q89.01
      acquired Z90.81
  sternum, congenital Q76.7
  stomach (acquired) (partial) Z90.3
      congenital Q40.2
  superior vena cava, congenital
      Q26.8
  teeth, tooth (congenital) K00.0
      acquired (complete) K08.109
          class I K08.101
          class II K08.102
          class III K08.103
          class IV K08.104
          due to
              caries K08.139
                  class I K08.131
                  class II K08.132
                  class III K08.133
                  class IV K08.134
              periodontal disease K08.129
                  class I K08.121
                  class II K08.122
                  class III K08.123
                  class IV K08.124
          specified NEC K08.199
              class I K08.191
              class II K08.192
              class III K08.193
              class IV K08.194
          trauma K08.119
              class I K08.111
              class II K08.112
              class III K08.113
              class IV K08.114
      partial K08.409
          class I K08.401
          class II K08.402
          class III K08.403
          class IV K08.404
          due to
              caries K08.439
                  class I K08.431
                  class II K08.432
                  class III K08.433
                  class IV K08.434
              periodontal disease K08.429
                  class I K08.421
                  class II K08.422
                  class III K08.423
                  class IV K08.424
          specified NEC K08.499
              class I K08.491
              class II K08.492
              class III K08.493
              class IV K08.494
          trauma K08.419
              class I K08.411
              class II K08.412
              class III K08.413
              class IV K08.414
  tendon (congenital) Q79.8
  testis (congenital) Q55.0
      acquired Z90.79
  thumb (acquired) Z89.01-
      congenital —*see* Agenesis, hand
  thymus gland Q89.2
  thyroid (gland) (acquired) E89.0
      cartilage, congenital Q31.8
      congenital E03.1

A

Absence *(Continued)*
 toe (s) (acquired) Z89.42-
  with foot —*see* Absence, foot and
    ankle
  congenital —*see* Agenesis, foot
  great Z89.41-
 tongue, congenital Q38.3
 trachea (cartilage), congenital Q32.1
 transverse aortic arch, congenital
   Q25.4
 tricuspid valve Q22.4
 umbilical artery, congenital Q27.0
 upper arm and forearm with hand present,
    congenital —*see* Agenesis, arm, with
    hand present
 ureter (congenital) Q62.4
  acquired Z90.6
 urethra, congenital Q64.5
 uterus (acquired) Z90.710
  with cervix Z90.710
  with remaining cervical stump
    Z90.711
  congenital Q51.0
 uvula, congenital Q38.5
 vagina, congenital Q52.0
 vas deferens (congenital) Q55.4
  acquired Z90.79
 vein (peripheral) congenital NEC
   Q27.8
  cerebral Q28.3
  digestive system Q27.8
  great Q26.8
  lower limb Q27.8
  portal Q26.5
  precerebral Q28.1
  specified site NEC Q27.8
  upper limb Q27.8
 vena cava (inferior) (superior), congenital
   Q26.8
 ventricular septum Q20.4
 vertebra, congenital Q76.49
 vulva, congenital Q52.71
 wrist (acquired) Z89.12-
Absorbent system disease I87.8
Absorption
 carbohydrate, disturbance K90.4
 chemical —*see* Table of ᵈDrugs and
   ᶜChemicals ◀▥▥
  through placenta (newborn) P04.9
   environmental substance P04.6
   nutritional substance P04.5
   obstetric anesthetic or analgesic drug
     P04.0
 drug NEC —*see* Table of ᵈDrugs and
   ᶜChemicals ◀▥▥
  addictive
   through placenta (newborn) P04.49
    cocaine P04.41
  medicinal
   through placenta (newborn) P04.1
  through placenta (newborn) P04.1
   obstetric anesthetic or analgesic drug
     P04.0
 fat, disturbance K90.4
  pancreatic K90.3
 noxious substance —*see* Table of ᵈDrugs and
   ᶜChemicals ◀▥▥
 protein, disturbance K90.4
 starch, disturbance K90.4
 toxic substance —*see* Table of ᵈDrugs and
   ᶜChemicals ◀▥▥
 uremic —*see* Uremia
Abstinence symptoms, syndrome
 alcohol F10.239
  with delirium F10.231
 cocaine F14.23
 neonatal P96.1
 nicotine —*see* Dependence, drug, nicotine,
   with, withdrawal
 opioid F11.93
  with dependence F11.23

Abstinence symptoms, syndrome *(Continued)*
 psychoactive NEC F19.939
  with
   delirium F19.931
   dependence F19.239
    with
     delirium F19.231
     perceptual disturbance F19.232
    uncomplicated F19.230
   perceptual disturbance F19.932
  uncomplicated F19.930
 sedative F13.939
  with
   delirium F13.931
   dependence F13.239
    with
     delirium F13.231
     perceptual disturbance F13.232
    uncomplicated F13.230
   perceptual disturbance F13.932
  uncomplicated F13.930
 stimulant NEC F15.93
  with dependence F15.23
Abulia R68.89
Abulomania F60.7
Abuse
 adult —*see* Maltreatment, adult
  as reason for
   couple seeking advice (including
     offender) Z63.0
 alcohol (non-dependent) F10.10
  with
   anxiety disorder F10.180
   intoxication F10.129
    with delirium F10.121
    uncomplicated F10.120
   mood disorder F10.14
   other specified disorder F10.188
   psychosis F10.159
    delusions F10.150
    hallucinations F10.151
   sexual dysfunction F10.181
   sleep disorder F10.182
   unspecified disorder F10.19
  counseling and surveillance Z71.41
 amphetamine (or related substance) —*see*
    Abuse, drug, stimulant NEC
 analgesics (non-prescribed) (over the counter)
    F55.8
 antacids F55.0
 antidepressants —*see* Abuse, drug,
    psychoactive NEC
 anxiolytic —*see* Abuse, drug, sedative
 barbiturates —*see* Abuse, drug, sedative
 caffeine —*see* Abuse, drug, stimulant NEC
 cannabis, cannabinoids —*see* Abuse, drug,
    cannabis
 child —*see* Maltreatment, child
 cocaine —*see* Abuse, drug, cocaine
 drug NEC (non-dependent) F19.10
  with sleep disorder F19.182
  amphetamine type —*see* Abuse, drug,
    stimulant NEC
  analgesics (non-prescribed) (over the
    counter) F55.8
  antacids F55.0
  antidepressants —*see* Abuse, drug,
    psychoactive NEC
  anxiolytics —*see* Abuse, drug, sedative
  barbiturates —*see* Abuse, drug, sedative
  caffeine —*see* Abuse, drug, stimulant NEC
  cannabis F12.10
   with
    anxiety disorder F12.180
    intoxication F12.129
     with
      delirium F12.121
      perceptual disturbance
        F12.122
     uncomplicated F12.120
    other specified disorder F12.188

Abuse *(Continued)*
 drug NEC *(Continued)*
  cannabis *(Continued)*
   with *(Continued)*
    psychosis F12.159
     delusions F12.150
     hallucinations F12.151
    unspecified disorder F12.19
  cocaine F14.10
   with
    anxiety disorder F14.180
    intoxication F14.129
     with
      delirium F14.121
      perceptual disturbance F14.122
     uncomplicated F14.120
    mood disorder F14.14
    other specified disorder F14.188
    psychosis F14.159
     delusions F14.150
     hallucinations F14.151
    sexual dysfunction F14.181
    sleep disorder F14.182
    unspecified disorder F14.19
   counseling and surveillance Z71.51
  hallucinogen F16.10
   with
    anxiety disorder F16.180
    flashbacks F16.183
    intoxication F16.129
     with
      delirium F16.121
      perceptual disturbance F16.122
     uncomplicated F16.120
    mood disorder F16.14
    other specified disorder F16.188
    perception disorder, persisting F16.183
    psychosis F16.159
     delusions F16.150
     hallucinations F16.151
    unspecified disorder F16.19
  hashish —*see* Abuse, drug, cannabis
  herbal or folk remedies F55.1
  hormones F55.3
  hypnotics —*see* Abuse, drug, sedative
  inhalant F18.10
   with
    anxiety disorder F18.180
    dementia, persisting F18.17
    intoxication F18.129
     with delirium F18.121
     uncomplicated F18.120
    mood disorder F18.14
    other specified disorder F18.188
    psychosis F18.159
     delusions F18.150
     hallucinations F18.151
    unspecified disorder F18.19
  laxatives F55.2
  LSD —*see* Abuse, drug, hallucinogen
  marihuana —*see* Abuse, drug, cannabis
  morphine type (opioids) —*see* Abuse, drug,
    opioid
  opioid F11.10
   with
    intoxication F11.129
     with
      delirium F11.121
      perceptual disturbance F11.122
     uncomplicated F11.120
    mood disorder F11.14
    other specified disorder F11.188
    psychosis F11.159
     delusions F11.150
     hallucinations F11.151
    sexual dysfunction F11.181
    sleep disorder F11.182
    unspecified disorder F11.19
  PCP (phencyclidine) (or related
    substance) —*see* Abuse, drug,
    hallucinogen

◀ New   ◀▥▥ Revised   ~~deleted~~ Deleted

Abuse *(Continued)*
  drug NEC *(Continued)*
    psychoactive NEC F19.10
      with
        amnestic disorder F19.16
        anxiety disorder F19.180
        dementia F19.17
        intoxication F19.129
          with
            delirium F19.121
            perceptual disturbance
              F19.122
          uncomplicated F19.120
        mood disorder F19.14
        other specified disorder F19.188
        psychosis F19.159
          delusions F19.150
          hallucinations F19.151
        sexual dysfunction F19.181
        sleep disorder F19.182
        unspecified disorder F19.19
    sedative, hypnotic or anxiolytic F13.10
      with
        anxiety disorder F13.180
        intoxication F13.129
          with delirium F13.121
          uncomplicated F13.120
        mood disorder F13.14
        other specified disorder F13.188
        psychosis F13.159
          delusions F13.150
          hallucinations F13.151
        sexual dysfunction F13.181
        sleep disorder F13.182
        unspecified disorder F13.19
    solvent —*see* Abuse, drug, inhalant
    steroids F55.3
    stimulant NEC F15.10
      with
        anxiety disorder F15.180
        intoxication F15.129
          with
            delirium F15.121
            perceptual disturbance F15.122
          uncomplicated F15.120
        mood disorder F15.14
        other specified disorder F15.188
        psychosis F15.159
          delusions F15.150
          hallucinations F15.151
        sexual dysfunction F15.181
        sleep disorder F15.182
        unspecified disorder F15.19
    tranquilizers —*see* Abuse, drug, sedative
    vitamins F55.4
  hallucinogens —*see* Abuse, drug,
      hallucinogen
  hashish —*see* Abuse, drug, cannabis
  herbal or folk remedies F55.1
  hormones F55.3
  hypnotic —*see* Abuse, drug, sedative
  inhalant —*see* Abuse, drug, inhalant
  laxatives F55.2
  LSD —*see* Abuse, drug, hallucinogen
  marihuana —*see* Abuse, drug, cannabis
  morphine type (opioids) —*see* Abuse, drug,
      opioid
  non-psychoactive substance NEC F55.8
    antacids F55.0
    folk remedies F55.1
    herbal remedies F55.1
    hormones F55.3
    laxatives F55.2
    steroids F55.3
    vitamins F55.4
  opioids —*see* Abuse, drug, opioid
  PCP (phencyclidine) (or related substance) —
      see Abuse, drug, hallucinogen
  physical (adult) (child) —*see* Maltreatment
  psychoactive substance —*see* Abuse, drug,
      psychoactive NEC

Abuse *(Continued)*
  psychological (adult) (child) —*see*
      Maltreatment
  sedative —*see* Abuse, drug, sedative
  sexual —*see* Maltreatment
  solvent —*see* Abuse, drug, inhalant
  steroids F55.3
  vitamins F55.4
Acalculia R48.8
  developmental F81.2
Acanthamebiasis (with) B60.10
  conjunctiva B60.12
  keratoconjunctivitis B60.13
  meningoencephalitis B60.11
  other specified B60.19
Acanthocephaliasis B83.8
Acanthocheilonemiasis B74.4
Acanthocytosis E78.6
Acantholysis L11.9
Acanthosis (acquired) (nigricans) L83
  benign Q82.8
  congenital Q82.8
  seborrheic L82.1
    inflamed L82.0
  tongue K14.3
Acapnia E87.3
Acarbia E87.2
Acardia, acardius Q89.8
Acardiacus amorphus Q89.8
Acardiotrophia I51.4
Acariasis B88.0
  scabies B86
Acarodermatitis (urticarioides) B88.0
Acarophobia F40.218
Acatalasemia, acatalasia E80.3
Acathisia (drug induced) G25.71
Accelerated atrioventricular conduction
    I45.6
Accentuation of personality traits (type A)
    Z73.1
Accessory (congenital)
  adrenal gland Q89.1
  anus Q43.4
  appendix Q43.4
  atrioventricular conduction I45.6
  auditory ossicles Q16.3
  auricle (ear) Q17.0
  biliary duct or passage Q44.5
  bladder Q64.79
  blood vessels NEC Q27.9
    coronary Q24.5
  bone NEC Q79.8
  breast tissue, axilla Q83.1
  carpal bones Q74.0
  cecum Q43.4
  chromosome (s) NEC (nonsex) Q92.9
    with complex rearrangements NEC
        Q92.5
      seen only at prometaphase
          Q92.8
    13 —*see* Trisomy, 13
    18 —*see* Trisomy, 18
    21 —*see* Trisomy, 21
    partial Q92.9
    sex
      female phenotype Q97.8
  coronary artery Q24.5
  cusp (s), heart valve NEC Q24.8
    pulmonary Q22.3
  cystic duct Q44.5
  digit (s) Q69.9
  ear (auricle) (lobe) Q17.0
  endocrine gland NEC Q89.2
  eye muscle Q10.3
  eyelid Q10.3
  face bone (s) Q75.8
  fallopian tube (fimbria) (ostium)
      Q50.6
  finger (s) Q69.0
  foreskin N47.8
  frontonasal process Q75.8

Accessory *(Continued)*
  gallbladder Q44.1
  genital organ (s)
    female Q52.8
      external Q52.79
      internal NEC Q52.8
    male Q55.8
  genitourinary organs NEC Q89.8
    female Q52.8
    male Q55.8
  hallux Q69.2
  heart Q24.8
    valve NEC Q24.8
      pulmonary Q22.3
  hepatic ducts Q44.5
  hymen Q52.4
  intestine (large) (small) Q43.4
  kidney Q63.0
  lacrimal canal Q10.6
  leaflet, heart valve NEC Q24.8
  ligament, broad Q50.6
  liver Q44.7
    duct Q44.5
  lobule (ear) Q17.0
  lung (lobe) Q33.1
  muscle Q79.8
  navicular of carpus Q74.0
  nervous system, part NEC Q07.8
  nipple Q83.3
  nose Q30.8
  organ or site not listed —*see* Anomaly,
      by site
  ovary Q50.31
  oviduct Q50.6
  pancreas Q45.3
  parathyroid gland Q89.2
  parotid gland (and duct) Q38.4
  pituitary gland Q89.2
  preauricular appendage Q17.0
  prepuce N47.8
  renal arteries (multiple) Q27.2
  rib Q76.6
    cervical Q76.5
  roots (teeth) K00.2
  salivary gland Q38.4
  sesamoid bones Q74.8
    foot Q74.2
    hand Q74.0
  skin tags Q82.8
  spleen Q89.09
  sternum Q76.7
  submaxillary gland Q38.4
  tarsal bones Q74.2
  teeth, tooth K00.1
  tendon Q79.8
  thumb Q69.1
  thymus gland Q89.2
  thyroid gland Q89.2
  toes Q69.2
  tongue Q38.3
  tooth, teeth K00.1
  tragus Q17.0
  ureter Q62.5
  urethra Q64.79
  urinary organ or tract NEC Q64.8
  uterus Q51.2
  vagina Q52.10
  valve, heart NEC Q24.8
    pulmonary Q22.3
  vertebra Q76.49
  vocal cords Q31.8
  vulva Q52.79
Accident
  birth —*see* Birth, injury
  cardiac —*see* Infarct, myocardium
  cerebral I63.9
  cerebrovascular (embolic) (ischemic)
      (thrombotic) I63.9
    aborted I63.9
    hemorrhagic —*see* Hemorrhage,
        intracranial, intracerebral

Accident *(Continued)*
  cerebrovascular *(Continued)*
    old (without sequelae) Z86.73
      with sequelae (of) —*see* Sequelae,
        infarction, cerebral
    coronary —*see* Infarct, myocardium
    craniovascular I63.9
    vascular, brain I63.9
Accidental —*see* condition
Accommodation (disorder) —*see also* condition
  hysterical paralysis of F44.89
  insufficiency of H52.4
  paresis —*see* Paresis, of accommodation
  spasm —*see* Spasm, of accommodation
Accouchement —*see* Delivery
Accreta placenta O43.21-
Accretio cordis (nonrheumatic) I31.0
Accretions, tooth, teeth K03.6
Acculturation difficulty Z60.3
Accumulation secretion, prostate N42.89
Acephalia, acephalism, acephalus, acephaly
  Q00.0
Acephalobrachia monster Q89.8
Acephalochirus monster Q89.8
Acephalogaster Q89.8
Acephalostomus monster Q89.8
Acephalothorax Q89.8
Acerophobia F40.298
Acetonemia R79.89
  in Type 1 diabetes E10.10
    with coma E10.11
Acetonuria R82.4
Achalasia (cardia) (esophagus) K22.0
  congenital Q39.5
  pylorus Q40.0
  sphincteral NEC K59.8
Ache (s) —*see* Pain
Acheilia Q38.6
Achillobursitis —*see* Tendinitis, Achilles
Achillodynia —*see* Tendinitis, Achilles
Achlorhydria, achlorhydric (neurogenic)
  K31.83
  anemia D50.8
  diarrhea K31.83
  psychogenic F45.8
  secondary to vagotomy K91.1
Achluophobia F40.228
Acholia K82.8
Acholuric jaundice (familial)
  (splenomegalic) —*see also* Spherocytosis
  acquired D59.8
Achondrogenesis Q77.0
Achondroplasia (osteosclerosis congenita)
  Q77.4
Achroma, cutis L80
Achromat (ism), achromatopsia (acquired)
  (congenital) H53.51
Achromia, congenital —*see* Albinism
Achromia parasitica B36.0
Achylia gastrica K31.89
  psychogenic F45.8
Acid
  burn —*see* Corrosion
  deficiency
    amide nicotinic E52
    ascorbic E54
    folic E53.8
    nicotinic E52
    pantothenic E53.8
  intoxication E87.2
  peptic disease K30
  phosphatase deficiency E83.39
  stomach K30
    psychogenic F45.8
Acidemia E87.2
  argininosuccinic E72.22
  isovaleric E71.110
  metabolic (newborn) P19.9
    first noted before onset of labor P19.0
    first noted during labor P19.1
    noted at birth P19.2

Acidemia *(Continued)*
  methylmalonic E71.120
  pipecolic E72.3
  propionic E71.121
Acidity, gastric (high) K30
  psychogenic F45.8
Acidocytopenia —*see* Agranulocytosis
Acidocytosis D72.1
Acidopenia —*see* Agranulocytosis
Acidosis (lactic) (respiratory) E87.2
  in Type 1 diabetes E10.10
    with coma E10.11
  kidney, tubular N25.89
  lactic E87.2
  metabolic NEC E87.2
    with respiratory acidosis E87.4
    late, of newborn P74.0
  mixed metabolic and respiratory,
    newborn P84
  newborn P84
  renal (hyperchloremic) (tubular)
    N25.89
  respiratory E87.2
    complicated by
      metabolic
        acidosis E87.4
        alkalosis E87.4
Aciduria
  argininosuccinic E72.22
  glutaric (type I) E72.3
    type II E71.313
    type III E71.5-
  orotic (congenital) (hereditary) (pyrimidine
    deficiency) E79.8
    anemia D53.0
Acladiosis (skin) B36.0
Aclasis, diaphyseal Q78.6
Acleistocardia Q21.1
Aclusion —*see* Anomaly, dentofacial,
  malocclusion
Acne L70.9
  artificialis L70.8
  atrophica L70.2
  cachecticorum (Hebra) L70.8
  conglobata L70.1
  cystic L70.0
  decalvans L66.2
  excoriée des jeunes filles L70.5
  frontalis L70.2
  indurata L70.0
  infantile L70.4
  keloid L73.0
  lupoid L70.2
  necrotic, necrotica (miliaris) L70.2
  neonatal L70.4
  nodular L70.0
  occupational L70.8
  picker's L70.5
  pustular L70.0
  rodens L70.2
  rosacea L71.9
  specified NEC L70.8
  tropica L70.3
  varioliformis L70.2
  vulgaris L70.0
Acnitis (primary) A18.4
Acosta's disease T70.29
Acoustic —*see* condition
Acousticophobia F40.298
Acquired —*see also* condition
  immunodeficiency syndrome
    (AIDS) B20
Acrania Q00.0
Acroangiodermatitis I78.9
Acroasphyxia, chronic I73.89
Acrobystitis N47.7
Acrocephalopolysyndactyly Q87.0
Acrocephalosyndactyly Q87.0
Acrocephaly Q75.0
Acrochondrohyperplasia —*see* Syndrome,
  Marfan's

Acrocyanosis I73.8
  newborn P28.2
    meaning transient blue hands and feet -
      omit code
Acrodermatitis L30.8
  atrophicans (chronica) L90.4
  continua (Hallopeau) L40.2
  enteropathica (hereditary) E83.2
  Hallopeau's L40.2
  infantile papular L44.4
  perstans L40.2
  pustulosa continua L40.2
  recalcitrant pustular L40.2
Acrodynia —*see* Poisoning, mercury
Acromegaly, acromegalia E22.0
Acromelalgia I73.81
Acromicria, acromikria Q79.8
Acronyx L60.0
Acropachy, thyroid —*see* Thyrotoxicosis
Acroparesthesia (simple) (vasomotor)
  I73.89
Acropathy, thyroid —*see* Thyrotoxicosis
Acrophobia F40.241
Acroposthitis N47.7
Acroscleriasis, acroscleroderma,
  acrosclerosis —*see* Sclerosis, systemic
Acrosphacelus I96
Acrospiroma, eccrine —*see* Neoplasm, skin,
  benign
Acrostealgia —*see* Osteochondropathy
Acrotrophodynia —*see* Immersion
ACTH ectopic syndrome E24.3
Actinic —*see* condition
Actinobacillosis, actinobacillus A28.8
  mallei A24.0
  muris A25.1
Actinomyces israelii (infection) —*see*
  Actinomycosis
Actinomycetoma (foot) B47.1
Actinomycosis, actinomycotic A42.9
  with pneumonia A42.0
  abdominal A42.1
  cervicofacial A42.2
  cutaneous A42.89
  gastrointestinal A42.1
  pulmonary A42.0
  sepsis A42.7
  specified site NEC A42.89
Actinoneuritis G62.82
Action, heart
  disorder I49.9
  irregular I49.9
    psychogenic F45.8
Activated protein C resistance D68.51
Active —*see* condition
Acute —*see also* condition
  abdomen R10.0
  gallbladder —*see* Cholecystitis, acute
Acyanotic heart disease (congenital) Q24.9
Acystia Q64.5
Adair-Dighton syndrome (brittle bones and
  blue sclera, deafness) Q78.0
Adamantinoblastoma —*see* Ameloblastoma
Adamantinoma —*see also* Cyst, calcifying
  odontogenic
  long bones C40.90
    lower limb C40.2-
    upper limb C40.0-
  malignant C41.1
    jaw (bone) (lower) C41.1
      upper C41.0
  tibial C40.2-
Adamantoblastoma —*see* Ameloblastoma
Adams-Stokes (-Morgagni) disease or
  syndrome I45.9
Adaption reaction —*see* Disorder, adjustment
Addiction (*see also* Dependence) F19.20
  alcohol, alcoholic (ethyl) (methyl) (wood)
    (without remission) F10.20
    with remission F10.21
  drug —*see* Dependence, drug

Addiction (Continued)
  ethyl alcohol (without remission) F10.20
    with remission F10.21
  heroin —see Dependence, drug, opioid
  methyl alcohol (without remission) F10.20
    with remission F10.21
  methylated spirit (without remission) F10.20
    with remission F10.21
  morphine(-like substances) —see
    Dependence, drug, opioid
  nicotine —see Dependence, drug, nicotine
  opium and opioids —see Dependence, drug,
    opioid
  tobacco —see Dependence, drug, nicotine
Addisonian crisis E27.2
Addison's
  anemia (pernicious) D51.0
  disease (bronze) or syndrome E27.1
    tuberculous A18.7
  keloid L94.0
Addison-Biermer anemia (pernicious) D51.0
Addison-Schilder complex E71.528
Additional —see also Accessory
  chromosome (s) Q99.8
    21 —see Trisomy, 21
    sex —see Abnormal, chromosome, sex
Adduction contracture, hip or other joint —see
    Contraction, joint
Adenitis —see also Lymphadenitis
  acute, unspecified site L04.9
  axillary I88.9
    acute L04.2
    chronic or subacute I88.1
  Bartholin's gland N75.8
  bulbourethral gland —see Urethritis
  cervical I88.9
    acute L04.0
    chronic or subacute I88.1
  chancroid (Hemophilus ducreyi) A57
  chronic, unspecified site I88.1
  Cowper's gland —see Urethritis
  due to Pasteurella multocida (p. septica)
    A28.0
  epidemic, acute B27.09
  gangrenous L04.9
  gonorrheal NEC A54.89
  groin I88.9
    acute L04.1
    chronic or subacute I88.1
  infectious (acute) (epidemic) B27.09
  inguinal I88.9
    acute L04.1
    chronic or subacute I88.1
  lymph gland or node, except mesenteric
    I88.9
    acute —see Lymphadenitis, acute
    chronic or subacute I88.1
  mesenteric (acute) (chronic) (nonspecific)
    (subacute) I88.0
  parotid gland (suppurative) —see
    Sialoadenitis
  salivary gland (any) (suppurative) —see
    Sialoadenitis
  scrofulous (tuberculous) A18.2
  Skene's duct or gland —see Urethritis
  strumous, tuberculous A18.2
  subacute, unspecified site I88.1
  sublingual gland (suppurative) —see
    Sialoadenitis
  submandibular gland (suppurative) —see
    Sialoadenitis
  submaxillary gland (suppurative) —see
    Sialoadenitis
  tuberculous —see Tuberculosis, lymph gland
  urethral gland —see Urethritis
  Wharton's duct (suppurative) —see
    Sialoadenitis
Adenoacanthoma —see Neoplasm, malignant,
  by site
Adenoameloblastoma —see Cyst, calcifying
  odontogenic

Adenocarcinoid (tumor) —see Neoplasm,
  malignant, by site
Adenocarcinoma —see also Neoplasm,
  malignant, by site
  acidophil
    specified site —see Neoplasm, malignant,
      by site
    unspecified site C75.1
  adrenal cortical C74.0-
  alveolar —see Neoplasm, lung, malignant
  apocrine
    breast —see Neoplasm, breast, malignant
    in situ
      breast D05.8-
      specified site NEC —see Neoplasm, skin,
        in situ
      unspecified site D04.9
    specified site NEC —see Neoplasm, skin,
      malignant
    unspecified site C44.99
  basal cell
    specified site —see Neoplasm, skin,
      malignant
    unspecified site C08.9
  basophil
    specified site —see Neoplasm, malignant,
      by site
    unspecified site C75.1
  bile duct type C22.1
    liver C22.1
    specified site NEC —see Neoplasm,
      malignant, by site
    unspecified site C22.1
  bronchiolar —see Neoplasm, lung, malignant
  bronchioloalveolar —see Neoplasm, lung,
    malignant
  ceruminous C44.29-
  cervix, in situ (see also Carcinoma, cervix
    uteri, in situ) D06.9
  chromophobe
    specified site —see Neoplasm, malignant,
      by site
    unspecified site C75.1
  diffuse type
    specified site —see Neoplasm, malignant,
      by site
    unspecified site C16.9
  duct
    infiltrating
      with Paget's disease —see Neoplasm,
        breast, malignant
      specified site —see Neoplasm,
        malignant, by site
      unspecified site (female) C50.91-
        male C50.92-
    specified site —see Neoplasm, malignant,
      by site
    unspecified site
      female C56.9
      male C61
  eosinophil
    specified site —see Neoplasm, malignant,
      by site
    unspecified site C75.1
  follicular
    with papillary C73
    moderately differentiated C73
    specified site —see Neoplasm, malignant,
      by site
    trabecular C73
    unspecified site C73
    well differentiated C73
  Hurthle cell C73
  in
    adenomatous
      polyposis coli C18.9
  infiltrating duct
    with Paget's disease —see Neoplasm,
      breast, malignant
    specified site —see Neoplasm, malignant,
      by site

Adenocarcinoma (Continued)
  infiltrating duct (Continued)
    unspecified site (female) C50.91-
      male C50.92-
    inflammatory
      specified site —see Neoplasm, malignant,
        by site
      unspecified site (female) C50.91-
        male C50.92-
    intestinal type
      specified site —see Neoplasm, malignant,
        by site
      unspecified site C16.9
    intracystic papillary
    intraductal
      breast D05.1-
      noninfiltrating
        breast D05.1-
      papillary
        with invasion
          specified site —see Neoplasm,
            malignant, by site
          unspecified site (female)
            C50.91-
            male C50.92-
        breast D05.1-
        specified site NEC —see Neoplasm, in
          situ, by site
        unspecified site D05.1-
      specified site NEC —see Neoplasm, in
        situ, by site
      unspecified site D05.1-
    papillary
      with invasion
        specified site —see Neoplasm,
          malignant, by site
        unspecified site (female) C50.91-
          male C50.92-
      breast D05.1-
      specified site —see Neoplasm, in situ,
        by site
      unspecified site D05.1-
    specified site NEC —see Neoplasm, in situ,
      by site
    unspecified site D05.1-
  islet cell
    with exocrine, mixed
      specified site —see Neoplasm,
        malignant, by site
      unspecified site C25.9
    pancreas C25.4
    specified site NEC —see Neoplasm,
      malignant, by site
    unspecified site C25.4
  lobular
    in situ
      breast D05.0-
      specified site NEC —see Neoplasm, in
        situ, by site
      unspecified site D05.0-
    specified site —see Neoplasm, malignant,
      by site
    unspecified site (female) C50.91-
      male C50.92-
  mucoid —see also Neoplasm, malignant, by
    site
    cell
      specified site —see Neoplasm,
        malignant, by site
      unspecified site C75.1
  nonencapsulated sclerosing C73
  papillary
    with follicular C73
    follicular variant C73
    intraductal (noninfiltrating)
      with invasion
        specified site —see Neoplasm,
          malignant, by site
        unspecified site (female) C50.91-
          male C50.92-
      breast D05.1-

Adenocarcinoma *(Continued)*
  papillary *(Continued)*
    intraductal *(Continued)*
      specified site NEC —*see* Neoplasm, in
        situ, by site
      unspecified site D05.1-
    serous
      specified site —*see* Neoplasm,
        malignant, by site
      unspecified site C56.9
  papillocystic
    specified site —*see* Neoplasm, malignant,
      by site
    unspecified site C56.9
  pseudomucinous
    specified site —*see* Neoplasm, malignant,
      by site
    unspecified site C56.9
  renal cell C64-
  sebaceous —*see* Neoplasm, skin, malignant,
    by site
  serous —*see also* Neoplasm, malignant, by site
    papillary
      specified site —*see* Neoplasm,
        malignant, by site
      unspecified site C56.9
  sweat gland —*see* Neoplasm, skin, malignant
  water-clear cell C75.0
Adenocarcinoma-in-situ —*see also* Neoplasm,
  in situ, by site
  breast D05.9-
Adenofibroma
  clear cell —*see* Neoplasm, benign, by site
  endometrioid D27.9
    borderline malignancy D39.10
    malignant C56-
  mucinous
    specified site —*see* Neoplasm, benign, by
      site
    unspecified site D27.9
  papillary
    specified site —*see* Neoplasm, benign, by
      site
    unspecified site D27.9
  prostate —*see* Enlargement, enlarged,
    prostate
  serous
    specified site —*see* Neoplasm, benign, by
      site
    unspecified site D27.9
  specified site —*see* Neoplasm, benign,
    by site
  unspecified site D27.9
Adenofibrosis
  breast —*see* Fibroadenosis, breast
  endometrioid N80.0
Adenoiditis (chronic) J35.02
  with tonsillitis J35.03
  acute J03.90
    recurrent J03.91
    specified organism NEC J03.80
      recurrent J03.81
    staphylococcal J03.80
      recurrent J03.81
    streptococcal J03.00
      recurrent J03.01
Adenoids —*see* condition
Adenolipoma —*see* Neoplasm, benign, by site
Adenolipomatosis, Launois-Bensaude E88.89
Adenolymphoma
  specified site —*see* Neoplasm, benign, by site
  unspecified site D11.9
Adenoma —*see also* Neoplasm, benign, by site
  acidophil
    specified site —*see* Neoplasm, benign, by
      site
    unspecified site D35.2
  acidophil-basophil, mixed
    specified site —*see* Neoplasm, benign, by
      site
    unspecified site D35.2

Adenoma *(Continued)*
  adrenal (cortical) D35.00
    clear cell D35.00
    compact cell D35.00
    glomerulosa cell D35.00
    heavily pigmented variant D35.00
    mixed cell D35.00
  alpha-cell
    pancreas D13.7
    specified site NEC —*see* Neoplasm, benign,
      by site
    unspecified site D13.7
  alveolar D14.30
  apocrine
    breast D24-
    specified site NEC —*see* Neoplasm, skin,
      benign, by site
    unspecified site D23.9
  basal cell D11.9
  basophil
    specified site —*see* Neoplasm, benign, by
      site
    unspecified site D35.2
  basophil-acidophil, mixed
    specified site —*see* Neoplasm, benign, by
      site
    unspecified site D35.2
  beta-cell
    pancreas D13.7
    specified site NEC —*see* Neoplasm, benign,
      by site
    unspecified site D13.7
  bile duct D13.4
    common D13.5
    extrahepatic D13.5
    intrahepatic D13.4
    specified site NEC —*see* Neoplasm, benign,
      by site
    unspecified site D13.4
  black D35.00
  bronchial D38.1
    cylindroid type —*see* Neoplasm, lung,
      malignant
  ceruminous D23.2-
  chief cell D35.1
  chromophobe
    specified site —*see* Neoplasm, benign, by
      site
    unspecified site D35.2
  colloid
    specified site —*see* Neoplasm, benign, by
      site
    unspecified site D34
  duct
  eccrine, papillary —*see* Neoplasm, skin,
    benign
  endocrine, multiple
    single specified site —*see* Neoplasm,
      uncertain behavior, by site
    two or more specified sites D44-
    unspecified site D44.9
  endometrioid —*see also* Neoplasm, benign
    borderline malignancy —*see* Neoplasm,
      uncertain behavior, by site
  eosinophil
    unspecified site D35.2
  fetal
    specified site —*see* Neoplasm, benign, by
      site
    unspecified site D34
  follicular
    specified site —*see* Neoplasm, benign, by
      site
    unspecified site D34
  hepatocellular D13.4
  Hurthle cell D34
  islet cell
    pancreas D13.7
    specified site NEC —*see* Neoplasm, benign,
      by site
    unspecified site D13.7

Adenoma *(Continued)*
  liver cell D13.4
  macrofollicular
    specified site —*see* Neoplasm, benign, by
      site
    unspecified site D34
  malignant, malignum —*see* Neoplasm,
    malignant, by site
  microcystic
    pancreas D13.7
    specified site NEC —*see* Neoplasm, benign,
      by site
    unspecified site D13.7
  microfollicular
    specified site —*see* Neoplasm, benign, by
      site
    unspecified site D34
  mucoid cell
    specified site —*see* Neoplasm, benign, by
      site
    unspecified site D35.2
  multiple endocrine
    single specified site —*see* Neoplasm,
      uncertain behavior, by site
    two or more specified sites D44-
    unspecified site D44.9
  nipple D24-
  papillary —*see also* Neoplasm, benign, by site
    eccrine —*see* Neoplasm, skin, benign, by
      site
  Pick's tubular
    specified site —*see* Neoplasm, benign, by
      site
    unspecified site
      female D27.9
      male D29.20
  pleomorphic
    carcinoma in —*see* Neoplasm, salivary
      gland, malignant
    specified site —*see* Neoplasm,
      malignant, by site
    unspecified site C08.9
  polypoid —*see also* Neoplasm, benign
    adenocarcinoma in —*see* Neoplasm,
      malignant, by site
    adenocarcinoma in situ —*see* Neoplasm, in
      situ, by site
  prostate —*see* Neoplasm, benign, prostate
  rete cell D29.20
  sebaceous —*see* Neoplasm, skin, benign
  Sertoli cell
    specified site —*see* Neoplasm, benign, by
      site
    unspecified site
      female D27.9
      male D29.20
  skin appendage —*see* Neoplasm, skin,
    benign
  sudoriferous gland —*see* Neoplasm, skin,
    benign
  sweat gland —*see* Neoplasm, skin, benign
  testicular
    unspecified site
      female D27.9
      male D29.20
  tubular —*see also* Neoplasm, benign, by site
    adenocarcinoma in —*see* Neoplasm,
      malignant, by site
    adenocarcinoma in situ —*see* Neoplasm, in
      situ, by site
    Pick's
      specified site —*see* Neoplasm, benign
      unspecified site
        female D27.9
        male D29.20
  tubulovillous —*see also* Neoplasm, benign,
    by site
    adenocarcinoma in —*see* Neoplasm,
      malignant, by site
    adenocarcinoma in situ —*see* Neoplasm, in
      situ, by site

◀ New   ◀▥ Revised   ~~deleted~~ Deleted

Adenoma *(Continued)*
  villous —*see* Neoplasm, uncertain behavior, by site
    adenocarcinoma in —*see* Neoplasm, malignant, by site
    adenocarcinoma in situ —*see* Neoplasm, in situ, by site
    water-clear cell D35.1
Adenomatosis
  endocrine (multiple) E31.20
    single specified site —*see* Neoplasm, uncertain behavior, by site
  erosive of nipple D24-
  pluriendocrine —*see* Adenomatosis, endocrine
  pulmonary D38.1
    malignant —*see* Neoplasm, lung, malignant
  specified site —*see* Neoplasm, benign, by site
  unspecified site D12.6
Adenomatous
  goiter (nontoxic) E04.9
    with hyperthyroidism —*see* Hyperthyroidism, with, goiter, nodular
    toxic —*see* Hyperthyroidism, with, goiter, nodular
Adenomyoma —*see also* Neoplasm, benign, by site
  prostate —*see* Enlarged, prostate
Adenomyometritis N80.0
Adenomyosis N80.0
Adenopathy (lymph gland) R59.9
  generalized R59.1
  inguinal R59.0
  localized R59.0
  mediastinal R59.0
  mesentery R59.0
  syphilitic (secondary) A51.49
  tracheobronchial R59.0
    tuberculous A15.4
      primary (progressive) A15.7
  tuberculous —*see also* Tuberculosis, lymph gland
    tracheobronchial A15.4
      primary (progressive) A15.7
Adenosalpingitis —*see* Salpingitis
Adenosarcoma —*see* Neoplasm, malignant, by site
Adenosclerosis I88.8
Adenosis (sclerosing) breast —*see* Fibroadenosis, breast
Adenovirus, as cause of disease classified elsewhere B97.0
Adentia (complete) (partial) —*see* Absence, teeth
Adherent —*see also* Adhesions
  labia (minora) N90.89
  pericardium (nonrheumatic) I31.0
    rheumatic I09.2
  placenta (with hemorrhage) O72.0
    without hemorrhage O73.0
  prepuce, newborn N47.0
  scar (skin) L90.5
  tendon in scar L90.5
Adhesions, adhesive (postinfective) K66.0
  with intestinal obstruction K56.5
  abdominal (wall) —*see* Adhesions, peritoneum
  appendix K38.8
  bile duct (common) (hepatic) K83.8
  bladder (sphincter) N32.89
  bowel —*see* Adhesions, peritoneum
  cardiac I31.0
    rheumatic I09.2
  cecum —*see* Adhesions, peritoneum
  cervicovaginal N88.1
    congenital Q52.8
    postpartal O90.89
      old N88.1
  cervix N88.1
  ciliary body NEC —*see* Adhesions, iris

Adhesions, adhesive *(Continued)*
  clitoris N90.89
  colon —*see* Adhesions, peritoneum
  common duct K83.8
  congenital —*see also* Anomaly, by site
    fingers —*see* Syndactylism, complex, fingers
    omental, anomalous Q43.3
    peritoneal Q43.3
    tongue (to gum or roof of mouth) Q38.3
  conjunctiva (acquired) H11.21-
    congenital Q15.8
  cystic duct K82.8
  diaphragm —*see* Adhesions, peritoneum
  due to foreign body —*see* Foreign body
  duodenum —*see* Adhesions, peritoneum
  ear
    middle H74.1-
  epididymis N50.8
  epidural —*see* Adhesions, meninges
  epiglottis J38.7
  eyelid H02.59
  female pelvis N73.6
  gallbladder K82.8
  globe H44.89
  heart I31.0
    rheumatic I09.2
  ileocecal (coil) —*see* Adhesions, peritoneum
  ileum —*see* Adhesions, peritoneum
  intestine —*see also* Adhesions, peritoneum
    with obstruction K56.5
  intra-abdominal —*see* Adhesions, peritoneum
  iris H21.50-
    anterior H21.51-
    goniosynechiae H21.52-
    posterior H21.54-
    to corneal graft T85.89
  joint —*see* Ankylosis
    knee M23.8X
    temporomandibular M26.61
  labium (majus) (minus), congenital Q52.5
  liver —*see* Adhesions, peritoneum
  lung J98.4
  mediastinum J98.5
  meninges (cerebral) (spinal) G96.12
    congenital Q07.8
    tuberculous (cerebral) (spinal) A17.0
  mesenteric —*see* Adhesions, peritoneum
  nasal (septum) (to turbinates) J34.89
  ocular muscle —*see* Strabismus, mechanical
  omentum —*see* Adhesions, peritoneum
  ovary N73.6
    congenital (to cecum, kidney or omentum) Q50.39
  paraovarian N73.6
  pelvic (peritoneal)
    female N73.6
      postprocedural N99.4
    male —*see* Adhesions, peritoneum
    postpartal (old) N73.6
    tuberculous A18.17
  penis to scrotum (congenital) Q55.8
  periappendiceal —*see also* Adhesions, peritoneum
  pericardium (nonrheumatic) I31.0
    focal I31.8
    rheumatic I09.2
    tuberculous A18.84
  pericholecystic K82.8
  perigastric —*see* Adhesions, peritoneum
  periovarian N73.6
  periprostatic N42.89
  perirectal —*see* Adhesions, peritoneum
  perirenal N28.89
  peritoneum, peritoneal (postinfective) (postprocedural) K66.0
    with obstruction (intestinal) K56.5
    congenital Q43.3
    pelvic, female N73.6
      postprocedural N99.4

Adhesions, adhesive *(Continued)*
  peritoneum, peritoneal *(Continued)*
    postpartal, pelvic N73.6
    to uterus N73.6
  peritubal N73.6
  periureteral N28.89
  periuterine N73.6
  perivesical N32.89
  perivesicular (seminal vesicle) N50.8
  pleura, pleuritic J94.8
    tuberculous NEC A15.6
  pleuropericardial J94.8
  postoperative (gastrointestinal tract) K66.0
    with obstruction K91.3
    due to foreign body accidentally left in wound —*see* Foreign body, accidentally left during a procedure
    pelvic peritoneal N99.4
    urethra —*see* Stricture, urethra, postprocedural
    vagina N99.2
  postpartal, old (vulva or perineum) N90.89
  preputial, prepuce N47.5
  pulmonary J98.4
  pylorus —*see* Adhesions, peritoneum
  sciatic nerve —*see* Lesion, nerve, sciatic
  seminal vesicle N50.8
  shoulder (joint) —*see* Capsulitis, adhesive
  sigmoid flexure —*see* Adhesions, peritoneum
  spermatic cord (acquired) N50.8
    congenital Q55.4
  spinal canal G96.12
  stomach —*see* Adhesions, peritoneum
  subscapular —*see* Capsulitis, adhesive
  temporomandibular M26.61
  tendinitis —*see also* Tenosynovitis, specified type NEC
    shoulder —*see* Capsulitis, adhesive
  testis N44.8
  tongue, congenital (to gum or roof of mouth) Q38.3
    acquired K14.8
  trachea J39.8
  tubo-ovarian N73.6
  tunica vaginalis N44.8
  uterus N73.6
    internal N85.6
    to abdominal wall N73.6
  vagina (chronic) N89.5
    postoperative N99.2
  vitreomacular H43.82-
  vitreous H43.89
  vulva N90.89
Adiaspiromycosis B48.8
Adie (-Holmes) pupil or syndrome —*see* Anomaly, pupil, function, tonic pupil
Adiponecrosis neonatorum P83.8
Adiposis —*see also* Obesity
  cerebralis E23.6
  dolorosa E88.2
Adiposity —*see also* Obesity
  heart —*see* Degeneration, myocardial
  localized E65
Adiposogenital dystrophy E23.6
Adjustment
  disorder —*see* Disorder, adjustment
  implanted device —*see* Encounter (for), adjustment (of)
  prosthesis, external —*see* Fitting
  reaction —*see* Disorder, adjustment
Administration of tPA (rtPA) in a different facility within the last 24 hours prior to admission to current facility Z92.82
Admission (for) —*see also* Encounter (for)
  adjustment (of)
    artificial
      arm Z44.00-
        complete Z44.01-
        partial Z44.02-
      eye Z44.2

Admission *(Continued)*
  adjustment *(Continued)*
    artificial *(Continued)*
      leg Z44.10-
        complete Z44.11-
        partial Z44.12-
    brain neuropacemaker Z46.2
      implanted Z45.42
    breast
      implant Z45.81
      prosthesis (external) Z44.3
    colostomy belt Z46.89
    contact lenses Z46.0
    cystostomy device Z46.6
    dental prosthesis Z46.3
    device NEC
      abdominal Z46.89
      implanted Z45.89
        cardiac Z45.09
          defibrillator (with synchronous
            cardiace pacemaker) Z45.02
          pacemaker Z45.018
            pulse generator Z45.010
        hearing device Z45.328
          bone conduction Z45.320
          cochlear Z45.321
        infusion pump Z45.1
        nervous system Z45.49
          CSF drainage Z45.41
          hearing device —*see* Admission,
            adjustment, device, implanted,
            hearing device
          neuropacemaker Z45.42
          visual substitution Z45.31
        specified NEC Z45.89
        vascular access Z45.2
        visual substitution Z45.31
      nervous system Z46.2
        implanted —*see* Admission,
          adjustment, device, implanted,
          nervous system
      orthodontic Z46.4
      prosthetic Z44.9
        arm —*see* Admission, adjustment,
          artificial, arm
        breast Z44.3
        dental Z46.3
        eye Z44.2
        leg —*see* Admission, adjustment,
          artificial, leg
        specified type NEC Z44.8
      substitution
        auditory Z46.2
          implanted —*see* Admission,
            adjustment, device, implanted,
            hearing device
        nervous system Z46.2
          implanted —*see* Admission,
            adjustment, device, implanted,
            nervous system
        visual Z46.2
          implanted Z45.31
        urinary Z46.6
    hearing aid Z46.1
      implanted —*see* Admission, adjustment,
        device, implanted, hearing device
    ileostomy device Z46.89
    intestinal appliance or device NEC
      Z46.89
    neuropacemaker (brain) (peripheral nerve)
      (spinal cord) Z46.2
      implanted Z45.42
    orthodontic device Z46.4
    orthopedic (brace) (cast) (device) (shoes)
      Z46.89
    pacemaker
      cardiac Z45.018
        pulse generator Z45.010
      nervous system Z46.2
        implanted Z45.42
    portacath (port-a-cath) Z45.2

Admission *(Continued)*
  adjustment *(Continued)*
    prosthesis Z44.9
      arm —*see* Admission, adjustment,
        artificial, arm
      breast Z44.3
      dental Z46.3
      eye Z44.2
      leg —*see* Admission, adjustment,
        artificial, leg
      specified NEC Z44.8
    spectacles Z46.0
  aftercare (*see also* Aftercare) Z51.89
    postpartum
      immediately after delivery Z39.0
      routine follow-up Z39.2
    radiation therapy (antineoplastic) Z51.0
  attention to artificial opening (of) Z43.9
    artificial vagina Z43.7
    colostomy Z43.3
    cystostomy Z43.5
    enterostomy Z43.4
    gastrostomy Z43.1
    ileostomy Z43.2
    jejunostomy Z43.4
    nephrostomy Z43.6
    specified site NEC Z43.8
      intestinal tract Z43.4
      urinary tract Z43.6
    tracheostomy Z43.0
    ureterostomy Z43.6
    urethrostomy Z43.6
  breast augmentation or reduction Z41.1
  breast reconstruction following mastectomy
    Z42.1
  change of
    dressing (nonsurgical) Z48.00
    neuropacemaker device (brain) (peripheral
      nerve) (spinal cord) Z46.2
      implanted Z45.42
    surgical dressing Z48.01
  circumcision, ritual or routine (in absence of
    diagnosis) Z41.2
  clinical research investigation (control)
    (normal comparison) (participant)
    Z00.6
  contraceptive management Z30.9
  cosmetic surgery NEC Z41.1
  counseling (*see also* Counseling)
    dietary Z71.3
    HIV Z71.7
    human immunodeficiency virus Z71.7
    nonattending third party Z71.0
    procreative management NEC Z31.69
  delivery, full-term, uncomplicated O80
    cesarean, without indication O82
  dietary surveillance and counseling Z71.3
  ear piercing Z41.3
  examination at health care facility (adult) (*see
    also* Examination) Z00.00
    with abnormal findings Z00.01
    clinical research investigation (control)
      (normal comparison) (participant)
      Z00.6
    dental Z01.20
      with abnormal findings Z01.21
    donor (potential) Z00.5
    ear Z01.10
      with abnormal findings NEC
        Z01.118
    eye Z01.00
      with abnormal findings Z01.01
    general, specified reason NEC Z00.8
    hearing Z01.10
      with abnormal findings NEC
        Z01.118
    postpartum checkup Z39.2
    psychiatric (general) Z00.8
      requested by authority Z04.6
    vision Z01.00
      with abnormal findings Z01.01

Admission *(Continued)*
  fitting (of)
    artificial
      arm —*see* Admission, adjustment,
        artificial, arm
      eye Z44.2
      leg —*see* Admission, adjustment,
        artificial, leg
    brain neuropacemaker Z46.2
      implanted Z45.42
    breast prosthesis (external) Z44.3
    colostomy belt Z46.89
    contact lenses Z46.0
    cystostomy device Z46.6
    dental prosthesis Z46.3
    dentures Z46.3
    device NEC
      abdominal Z46.89
      nervous system Z46.2
        implanted —*see* Admission,
          adjustment, device, implanted,
          nervous system
      orthodontic Z46.4
      prosthetic Z44.9
        breast Z44.3
        dental Z46.3
        eye Z44.2
      substitution
        auditory Z46.2
          implanted —*see* Admission,
            adjustment, device, implanted,
            hearing device
        nervous system Z46.2
          implanted —*see* Admission,
            adjustment, device, implanted,
            nervous system
        visual Z46.2
          implanted Z45.31
    hearing aid Z46.1
    ileostomy device Z46.89
    intestinal appliance or device NEC
      Z46.89
    neuropacemaker (brain) (peripheral nerve)
      (spinal cord) Z46.2
      implanted Z45.42
    orthodontic device Z46.4
    orthopedic device (brace) (cast) (shoes)
      Z46.89
    prosthesis Z44.9
      arm —*see* Admission, adjustment,
        artificial, arm
      breast Z44.3
      dental Z46.3
      eye Z44.2
      leg —*see* Admission, adjustment,
        artificial, leg
      specified type NEC Z44.8
    spectacles Z46.0
  follow-up examination Z09
  intrauterine device management Z30.431
    initial prescription Z30.014
  mental health evaluation Z00.8
    requested by authority Z04.6
  observation —*see* Observation
  Papanicolaou smear, cervix Z12.4
    for suspected malignant neoplasm
      Z12.4
  plastic and reconstructive surgery following
    medical procedure or healed injury
    NEC Z42.8
  plastic surgery, cosmetic NEC Z41.1
  postpartum observation
    immediately after delivery Z39.0
    routine follow-up Z39.2
  poststerilization (for restoration) Z31.0
    aftercare Z31.42
  procreative management Z31.9
  prophylactic (measure)
    organ removal Z40.00
      breast Z40.01
      ovary Z40.02

◀ New   ◀▦ Revised   ~~deleted~~ Deleted

Admission *(Continued)*
  prophylactic *(Continued)*
    organ removal *(Continued)*
      specified organ NEC Z40.09
      testes Z40.09
      vaccination Z23
  psychiatric examination (general) Z00.8
    requested by authority Z04.6
  radiation therapy (antineoplastic) Z51.0
  reconstructive surgery following medical procedure or healed injury NEC Z42.8
  removal of
    cystostomy catheter Z43.5
    drains Z48.03
    dressing (nonsurgical) Z48.00
    intrauterine contraceptive device Z30.432
    neuropacemaker (brain) (peripheral nerve) (spinal cord) Z46.2
      implanted Z45.42
    staples Z48.02
    surgical dressing Z48.01
    sutures Z48.02
    ureteral stent Z46.6
  respirator [ventilator] use during power failure Z99.12
  restoration of organ continuity (poststerilization) Z31.0
    aftercare Z31.42
  sensitivity test —*see also* Test, skin
    allergy NEC Z01.82
    Mantoux Z11.1
  tuboplasty following previous sterilization Z31.0
    aftercare Z31.42
  vasoplasty following previous sterilization Z31.0
    aftercare Z31.42
  vision examination Z01.00
    with abnormal findings Z01.01
  waiting period for admission to other facility Z75.1
Adnexitis (suppurative) —*see* Salpingo-oophoritis
Adolescent X-linked adrenoleukodystrophy E71.521
Adrenal (gland) —*see* condition
Adrenalism, tuberculous A18.7
Adrenalitis, adrenitis E27.8
  autoimmune E27.1
  meningococcal, hemorrhagic A39.1
Adrenarche, premature E27.0
Adrenocortical syndrome —*see* Cushing's, syndrome
Adrenogenital syndrome E25.9
  acquired E25.8
  congenital E25.0
  salt loss E25.0
Adrenogenitalism, congenital E25.0
Adrenoleukodystrophy E71.529
  neonatal E71.511
  X-linked E71.529
    Addison only phenotype E71.528
    Addison-Schilder E71.528
    adolescent E71.521
    adrenomyeloneuropathy E71.522
    childhood cerebral E71.520
    other specified E71.528
Adrenomyeloneuropathy E71.522
Adventitious bursa —*see* Bursopathy, specified type NEC
Adverse effect —*see* Table of Drugs and Chemicals, categories T36-T50, with 6th character 5 ◀▥▥
Advice —*see* Counseling
Adynamia (episodica) (hereditary) (periodic) G72.3
Aeration lung imperfect, newborn —*see* Atelectasis
Aerobullosis T70.3
Aerocele —*see* Embolism, air

Aerodermectasia
  subcutaneous (traumatic) T79.7
Aerodontalgia T70.29
Aeroembolism T70.3
Aerogenes capsulatus infection A48.0
Aero-otitis media T70.0
Aerophagy, aerophagia (psychogenic) F45.8
Aerophobia F40.228
Aerosinusitis T70.1
Aerotitis T70.0
Affection —*see* Disease
Afibrinogenemia (*see also* Defect, coagulation) D68.8
  acquired D65
  congenital D68.2
  following ectopic or molar pregnancy O08.1
  in abortion —*see* Abortion, by type, complicated by, afibrinogenemia
  puerperal O72.3
African
  sleeping sickness B56.9
  tick fever A68.1
  trypanosomiasis B56.9
    gambian B56.0
    rhodesian B56.1
Aftercare (*see also* Care) Z51.89
  following surgery (for) (on)
    amputation Z47.81
    attention to
      drains Z48.03
      dressings (nonsurgical) Z48.00
        surgical Z48.01
      sutures Z48.02
    circulatory system Z48.812
    delayed (planned) wound closure Z48.1
    digestive system Z48.815
    explantation of joint prosthesis (staged procedure)
      hip Z47.32
      knee Z47.33
      shoulder Z47.31
    genitourinary system Z48.816
    joint replacement Z47.1
    neoplasm Z48.3
    nervous system Z48.811
    oral cavity Z48.814
    organ transplant
      bone marrow Z48.290
      heart Z48.21
      heart-lung Z48.280
      kidney Z48.22
      liver Z48.23
      lung Z48.24
      multiple organs NEC Z48.288
      specified NEC Z48.298
    orthopedic NEC Z47.89
    planned wound closure Z48.1
    removal of internal fixation device Z47.2
    respiratory system Z48.813
    scoliosis Z47.82
    sense organs Z48.810
    skin and subcutaneous tissue Z48.817
    specified body system
      circulatory Z48.812
      digestive Z48.815
      genitourinary Z48.816
      nervous Z48.811
      oral cavity Z48.814
      respiratory Z48.813
      sense organs Z48.810
      skin and subcutaneous tissue Z48.817
      teeth Z48.814
    specified NEC Z48.89
    spinal Z48.89
    teeth Z48.814
    fracture — code to fracture with seventh character D
  involving
    removal of
      drains Z48.03
      dressings (nonsurgical) Z48.00

Aftercare *(Continued)*
  involving *(Continued)*
    removal of *(Continued)*
      staples Z48.02
      surgical dressings Z48.01
      sutures Z48.02
    neuropacemaker (brain) (peripheral nerve) (spinal cord) Z46.2
      implanted Z45.42
    orthopedic NEC Z47.89
    postprocedural —*see* Aftercare, following surgery
After-cataract —*see* Cataract, secondary
Agalactia (primary) O92.3
  elective, secondary or therapeutic O92.5
Agammaglobulinemia (acquired (secondary)) (nonfamilial) D80.1
  with
    immunoglobulin-bearing B-lymphocytes D80.1
    lymphopenia D81.9
  autosomal recessive (Swiss type) D80.0
  Bruton's X-linked D80.0
  common variable (CVAgamma) D80.1
  congenital sex-linked D80.0
  hereditary D80.0
  lymphopenic D81.9
  Swiss type (autosomal recessive) D80.0
  X-linked (with growth hormone deficiency) (Bruton) D80.0
Aganglionosis (bowel) (colon) Q43.1
Age (old) —*see* Senility
Agenesis
  adrenal (gland) Q89.1
  alimentary tract (complete) (partial) NEC Q45.8
    upper Q40.8
  anus, anal (canal) Q42.3
    with fistula Q42.2
  aorta Q25.4
  appendix Q42.8
  arm (complete) Q71.0-
    with hand present Q71.1-
  artery (peripheral) Q27.9
    brain Q28.3
    coronary Q24.5
    pulmonary Q25.79
    specified NEC Q27.8
    umbilical Q27.0
  auditory (canal) (external) Q16.1
  auricle (ear) Q16.0
  bile duct or passage Q44.5
  bladder Q64.5
  bone Q79.9
  brain Q00.0
    part of Q04.3
  breast (with nipple present) Q83.8
    with absent nipple Q83.0
  bronchus Q32.4
  canaliculus lacrimalis Q10.4
  carpus —*see* Agenesis, hand
  cartilage Q79.9
  cecum Q42.8
  cerebellum Q04.3
  cervix Q51.5
  chin Q18.8
  cilia Q10.3
  circulatory system, part NOS Q28.9
  clavicle Q74.0
  clitoris Q52.6
  coccyx Q76.49
  colon Q42.9
    specified NEC Q42.8
  corpus callosum Q04.0
  cricoid cartilage Q31.8
  diaphragm (with hernia) Q79.1
  digestive organ (s) or tract (complete) (partial) NEC Q45.8
    upper Q40.8
  ductus arteriosus Q28.8
  duodenum Q41.0

Agenesis *(Continued)*
ear Q16.9
auricle Q16.0
lobe Q17.8
ejaculatory duct Q55.4
endocrine (gland) NEC Q89.2
epiglottis Q31.8
esophagus Q39.8
eustachian tube Q16.2
eye Q11.1
adnexa Q15.8
eyelid (fold) Q10.3
face
bones NEC Q75.8
specified part NEC Q18.8
fallopian tube Q50.6
femur —*see* Defect, reduction, lower limb,
longitudinal, femur
fibula —*see* Defect, reduction, lower limb,
longitudinal, fibula
finger (complete) (partial) —*see* Agenesis,
hand
foot (and toes) (complete) (partial) Q72.3-
forearm (with hand present) —*see* Agenesis,
arm, with hand present
and hand Q71.2-
gallbladder Q44.0
gastric Q40.2
genitalia, genital (organ (s))
female Q52.8
external Q52.71
internal NEC Q52.8
male Q55.8
glottis Q31.8
hair Q84.0
hand (and fingers) (complete) (partial) Q71.3-
heart Q24.8
valve NEC Q24.8
pulmonary Q22.0
hepatic Q44.7
humerus —*see* Defect, reduction, upper limb
hymen Q52.4
ileum Q41.2
incus Q16.3
intestine (small) Q41.9
large Q42.9
specified NEC Q42.8
iris (dilator fibers) Q13.1
jaw M26.09
jejunum Q41.1
kidney (s) (partial) Q60.2
bilateral Q60.1
unilateral Q60.0
labium (majus) (minus) Q52.71
labyrinth, membranous Q16.5
lacrimal apparatus Q10.4
larynx Q31.8
leg (complete) Q72.0-
with foot present Q72.1-
lower leg (with foot present) —*see*
Agenesis, leg, with foot present
and foot Q72.2-
lens Q12.3
limb (complete) Q73.0
lower —*see* Agenesis, leg
upper —*see* Agenesis, arm
lip Q38.0
liver Q44.7
lung (fissure) (lobe) (bilateral) (unilateral)
Q33.3
mandible, maxilla M26.09
metacarpus —*see* Agenesis, hand
metatarsus —*see* Agenesis, foot
muscle Q79.8
eyelid Q10.3
ocular Q15.8
musculoskeletal system NEC Q79.8
nail (s) Q84.3
neck, part Q18.8
nerve Q07.8
nervous system, part NEC Q07.8

Agenesis *(Continued)*
nipple Q83.2
nose Q30.1
nuclear Q07.8
~~oesophagus Q39.8~~
organ
of Corti Q16.5
or site not listed —*see* Anomaly, by site
osseous meatus (ear) Q16.1
ovary
bilateral Q50.02
unilateral Q50.01
oviduct Q50.6
pancreas Q45.0
parathyroid (gland) Q89.2
parotid gland (s) Q38.4
patella Q74.1
pelvic girdle (complete) (partial) Q74.2
penis Q55.5
pericardium Q24.8
pituitary (gland) Q89.2
prostate Q55.4
punctum lacrimale Q10.4
radioulnar —*see* Defect, reduction, upper
limb
radius —*see* Defect, reduction, upper limb,
longitudinal, radius
rectum Q42.1
with fistula Q42.0
renal Q60.2
bilateral Q60.1
unilateral Q60.0
respiratory organ NEC Q34.8
rib Q76.6
roof of orbit Q75.8
round ligament Q52.8
sacrum Q76.49
salivary gland Q38.4
scapula Q74.0
scrotum Q55.29
seminal vesicles Q55.4
septum
atrial Q21.1
between aorta and pulmonary artery Q21.4
ventricular Q20.4
shoulder girdle (complete) (partial) Q74.0
skull (bone) Q75.8
with
anencephaly Q00.0
encephalocele —*see* Encephalocele
hydrocephalus Q03.9
with spina bifida —*see* Spina bifida, by
site, with hydrocephalus
microcephaly Q02
spermatic cord Q55.4
spinal cord Q06.0
spine Q76.49
spleen Q89.01
sternum Q76.7
stomach Q40.2
submaxillary gland (s) (congenital) Q38.4
tarsus —*see* Agenesis, foot
tendon Q79.8
testicle Q55.0
thymus (gland) Q89.2
thyroid (gland) E03.1
cartilage Q31.8
tibia —*see* Defect, reduction, lower limb,
longitudinal, tibia
tibiofibular —*see* Defect, reduction, lower
limb, specified type NEC
toe (and foot) (complete) (partial) —*see*
Agenesis, foot
tongue Q38.3
trachea (cartilage) Q32.1
ulna —*see* Defect, reduction, upper limb,
longitudinal, ulna
upper limb —*see* Agenesis, arm
ureter Q62.4
urethra Q64.5
urinary tract NEC Q64.8

Agenesis *(Continued)*
uterus Q51.0
uvula Q38.5
vagina Q52.0
vas deferens Q55.4
vein (s) (peripheral) Q27.9
brain Q28.3
great NEC Q26.8
portal Q26.5
vena cava (inferior) (superior) Q26.8
vermis of cerebellum Q04.3
vertebra Q76.49
vulva Q52.71
Ageusia R43.2
Agitated —*see* condition
Agitation R45.1
Aglossia (congenital) Q38.3
Aglossia-adactylia syndrome Q87.0
Aglycogenosis E74.00
Agnosia (body image) (other senses) (tactile)
R48.1
developmental F88
verbal R48.1
auditory R48.1
developmental F80.2
developmental F80.2
visual (object) R48.3
Agoraphobia F40.00
with panic disorder F40.01
without panic disorder F40.02
Agrammatism R48.8
Agranulocytopenia —*see* Agranulocytosis
Agranulocytosis (chronic) (cyclical) (genetic)
(infantile) (periodic) (pernicious) (*see also*
Neutropenia) D70.9
congenital D70.0
cytoreductive cancer chemotherapy sequela
D70.1
drug-induced D70.2
due to cytoreductive cancer chemotherapy
D70.1
due to infection D70.3
secondary D70.4
drug-induced D70.2
due to cytoreductive cancer
chemotherapy D70.1
Agraphia (absolute) R48.8
with alexia R48.0
developmental F81.81
Ague (dumb) —*see* Malaria
Agyria Q04.3
Ahumada-del Castillo syndrome E23.0
Aichomophobia F40.298
AIDS (related complex) B20
Ailment heart —*see* Disease, heart
Ailurophobia F40.218
Ainhum (disease) L94.6
AIPHI (acute idiopathic pulmonary hemorrhage
in infants (over 28 days old)) R04.81
Air
anterior mediastinum J98.2
compressed, disease T70.3
conditioner lung or pneumonitis J67.7
embolism (artery) (cerebral) (any site) T79.0
with ectopic or molar pregnancy O08.2
due to implanted device NEC —*see*
Complications, by site and type,
specified NEC
following
abortion —*see* Abortion by type,
complicated by, embolism
ectopic or molar pregnancy O08.2
infusion, therapeutic injection or
transfusion T80.0
in pregnancy, childbirth or puerperium —
see Embolism, obstetric
traumatic T79.0
hunger, psychogenic F45.8
rarefied, effects of —*see* Effect, adverse, high
altitude
sickness T75.3

◀ New ◀▥▥ Revised ~~deleted~~ Deleted

Airplane sickness T75.3
Akathisia (drug-induced) (treatment- induced)
   G25.71
   neuroleptic induced (acute) G25.71
Akinesia R29.898
Akinetic mutism R41.89
Akureyri's disease G93.3
Alactasia, congenital E73.0
Alagille's syndrome Q44.7
Alastrim B03
Albers-Schönberg syndrome Q78.2
Albert's syndrome —see Tendinitis, Achilles
Albinism, albino E70.30
   with hematologic abnormality E70.339
      Chédiak-Higashi syndrome E70.330
      Hermansky-Pudlak syndrome E70.331
      other specified E70.338
   I E70.320
   II E70.321
   ocular E70.319
      autosomal recessive E70.311
      other specified E70.318
      X-linked E70.310
   oculocutaneous E70.329
      other specified E70.328
      tyrosinase (ty) negative E70.320
      tyrosinase (ty) positive E70.321
   other specified E70.39
Albinismus E70.30
Albright (-McCune)(-Sternberg) syndrome
   Q78.1
Albuminous —see condition
Albuminuria, albuminuric (acute) (chronic)
   (subacute) (see also Proteinuria) R80.9
   complicating pregnancy —see Proteinuria,
      gestational
   with
      gestational hypertension —see
         Pre-eclampsia
      pre-existing hypertension —see
         Hypertension, complicating
         pregnancy, pre-existing, with,
         pre-eclampsia
   gestational —see Proteinuria, gestational
   with
      gestational hypertension —see
         Pre-eclampsia
      pre-existing hypertension —see
         Hypertension, complicating
         pregnancy, pre-existing, with,
         pre-eclampsia
   orthostatic R80.2
   postural R80.2
   pre-eclamptic —see Pre-eclampsia
   scarlatinal A38.8
Albuminurophobia F40.298
Alcaptonuria E70.29
Alcohol, alcoholic, alcohol-induced
   addiction (without remission) F10.20
      with remission F10.21
   amnestic disorder, persisting F10.96
      with dependence F10.26
   brain syndrome, chronic F10.97
      with dependence F10.27
   cardiopathy I42.6
   counseling and surveillance Z71.41
      family member Z71.42
   delirium (acute) (tremens) (withdrawal)
      F10.231
      with intoxication F10.921
         in
            abuse F10.121
            dependence F10.221
   dementia F10.97
      with dependence F10.27
   deterioration F10.97
      with dependence F10.27
   hallucinosis (acute) F10.951
      in
         abuse F10.151
         dependence F10.251

Alcohol, alcoholic, alcohol-induced (Continued)
   insanity F10.959
   intoxication (acute) (without dependence)
      F10.129
      with
         delirium F10.121
         dependence F10.229
            with delirium F10.221
            uncomplicated F10.220
         uncomplicated F10.120
   jealousy F10.988
   Korsakoff's, Korsakov's, Korsakow's
      F10.26
   liver K70.9
      acute —see Disease, liver, alcoholic,
         hepatitis
   mania (acute) (chronic) F10.959
   paranoia, paranoid (type) psychosis F10.950
   pellagra E52
   poisoning, accidental (acute) NEC —see Table
      of ⌐Drugs and ⌐Chemicals, alcohol,
      poisoning ◄▥
   psychosis —see Psychosis, alcoholic
   withdrawal (without convulsions) F10.239
      with delirium F10.231
Alcoholism (chronic) (without remission)
   F10.20
   with
      psychosis —see Psychosis, alcoholic
      remission F10.21
   Korsakov's F10.96
      with dependence F10.26
Alder (-Reilly) anomaly or syndrome
   (leukocyte granulation) D72.0
Aldosteronism E26.9
   familial (type I) E26.02
   glucocorticoid-remediable E26.02
   primary (due to (bilateral) adrenal
      hyperplasia) E26.09
   primary NEC E26.09
   secondary E26.1
   specified NEC E26.89
Aldosteronoma D44.10
Aldrich(-Wiskott) syndrome (eczema-
   thrombocytopenia) D82.0
Alektorophobia F40.218
Aleppo boil B55.1
Aleukemic —see condition Aleukia
   congenital D70.0
   hemorrhagica D61.9
      congenital D61.09
   splenica D73.1
Alexia R48.0
   developmental F81.0
   secondary to organic lesion R48.0
Algoneurodystrophy M89.00
   ankle M89.07-
   foot M89.07-
   forearm M89.03-
   hand M89.04-
   lower leg M89.06-
   multiple sites M89.0-
   shoulder M89.01-
   specified site NEC M89.08
   thigh M89.05-
   upper arm M89.02-
Algophobia F40.298
Alienation, mental —see Psychosis
Alkalemia E87.3
Alkalosis E87.3
   metabolic E87.3
      with respiratory acidosis E87.4
   respiratory E87.3
Alkaptonuria E70.29
Allen-Masters syndrome N83.8
Allergy, allergic (reaction) (to) T78.40
   air-borne substance NEC (rhinitis) J30.89
   alveolitis (extrinsic) J67.9
      due to
         Aspergillus clavatus J67.4
         Cryptostroma corticale J67.6 ◄▥

Allergy, allergic (Continued)
   alveolitis (Continued)
      due to (Continued)
         organisms (fungal, thermophilic
            actinomycete) growing in
            ventilation (air conditioning)
            systems J67.7
         specified type NEC J67.8
   anaphylactic reaction or shock T78.2
   angioneurotic edema T78.3
   animal (dander) (epidermal) (hair) (rhinitis)
      J30.81
   bee sting (anaphylactic shock) —see Toxicity,
      venom, arthropod, bee
   biological —see Allergy, drug
   colitis K52.2
   dander (animal) (rhinitis) J30.81
   dandruff (rhinitis) J30.81
   dental restorative material (existing) K08.55
   dermatitis —see Dermatitis, contact, allergic
   diathesis —see History, allergy
   drug, medicament & biological (any)
      (external) (internal) T78.40
      correct substance properly administered —
         see Table of ⌐Drugs and ⌐Chemicals,
         by drug, adverse effect ◄▥
      wrong substance given or taken NEC (by
         accident) —see Table of ⌐Drugs and
         ⌐Chemicals, by drug, poisoning ◄▥
   due to pollen J30.1
   dust (house) (stock) (rhinitis) J30.89
      with asthma —see Asthma, allergic
         extrinsic
   eczema —see Dermatitis, contact, allergic
   epidermal (animal) (rhinitis) J30.81
   feathers (rhinitis) J30.89
   food (any) (ingested) NEC T78.1
      anaphylactic shock —see Shock,
         anaphylactic, due to food
      dermatitis —see Dermatitis, due to,
         food
      dietary counseling and surveillance
         Z71.3
      in contact with skin L23.6
      rhinitis J30.5
   status (without reaction) Z91.018
      eggs Z91.012
      milk products Z91.011
      peanuts Z91.010
      seafood Z91.013
      specified NEC Z91.018
   gastrointestinal K52.2
   grain J30.1
   grass (hay fever) (pollen) J30.1
      asthma —see Asthma, allergic extrinsic
   hair (animal) (rhinitis) J30.81
   history (of) —see History, allergy
   horse serum —see Allergy, serum
   inhalant (rhinitis) J30.89
      pollen J30.1
   kapok (rhinitis) J30.89
   medicine —see Allergy, drug
   milk protein K52.2
   nasal, seasonal due to pollen J30.1
   pneumonia J82
   pollen (any) (hay fever) J30.1
      asthma —see Asthma, allergic extrinsic
   primrose J30.1
   primula J30.1
   purpura D69.0
   ragweed (hay fever) (pollen) J30.1
      asthma —see Asthma, allergic extrinsic
   rose (pollen) J30.1
   seasonal NEC J30.2
   Senecio jacobae (pollen) J30.1
   serum (see also Reaction, serum) T80.69
      anaphylactic shock T80.59
   shock (anaphylactic) T78.2
      due to
         administration of blood and blood
            products T80.51

Allergy, allergic *(Continued)*
shock *(Continued)*
due to *(Continued)*
adverse effect of correct medicinal
substance properly administered
T88.6
immunization T80.52
serum NEC T80.59
vaccination T80.52
specific NEC T78.49
tree (any) (hay fever) (pollen) J30.1
asthma —*see* Asthma, allergic extrinsic
upper respiratory J30.9
urticaria L50.0
vaccine —*see* Allergy, serum
wheat —*see* Allergy, food ◀
Allescheriasis B48.2
Alligator skin disease Q80.9
Allocheiria, allochiria R20.8
Almeida's disease —*see*
Paracoccidioidomycosis
Alopecia (hereditaria) (seborrheica) L65.9
androgenic L64.9
drug-induced L64.0
specified NEC L64.8
areata L63.9
ophiasis L63.2
specified NEC L63.8
totalis L63.0
universalis L63.1
cicatricial L66.9
specified NEC L66.8
circumscripta L63.9
congenital, congenitalis Q84.0
due to cytotoxic drugs NEC L65.8
mucinosa L65.2
postinfective NEC L65.8
postpartum L65.0
premature L64.8
specific (syphilitic) A51.32
specified NEC L65.8
syphilitic (secondary) A51.32
totalis (capitis) L63.0
universalis (entire body) L63.1
X-ray L58.1
Alpers' disease G31.81
Alpine sickness T70.29
Alport syndrome Q87.81
ALTE (apparent life threatening event) in
newborn and infant R68.13
Alteration (of), **Altered**
awareness, transient R40.4
mental status R41.82
pattern of family relationships affecting child
Z62.898
sensation
following
cerebrovascular disease I69.998
cerebral infarction I69.398
intracerebral hemorrhage I69.198
nontraumatic intracranial hemorrhage
NEC I69.298
specified disease NEC I69.898
subarachnoid hemorrhage I69.098
Alternating —*see* condition
Altitude, high (effects) —*see* Effect, adverse,
high altitude
Aluminosis (of lung) J63.0
Alveolitis
allergic (extrinsic) —*see* Pneumonitis,
hypersensitivity
due to
Aspergillus clavatus J67.4
Cryptostroma corticale J67.6
fibrosing (cryptogenic) (idiopathic) J84.112
jaw M27.3
sicca dolorosa M27.3
Alveolus, alveolar —*see* condition
Alymphocytosis D72.810 ⬅
thymic (with immunodeficiency) D82.1
Alymphoplasia, thymic D82.1

Alzheimer's disease or sclerosis —*see* Disease,
Alzheimer's
Amastia (with nipple present) Q83.8
with absent nipple Q83.0
Amathophobia F40.228
Amaurosis (acquired) (congenital) —*see also*
Blindness
fugax G45.3
hysterical F44.6
Leber's congenital H35.50
uremic —*see* Uremia
Amaurotic idiocy (infantile) (juvenile) (late) E75.4
Amaxophobia F40.248
Ambiguous genitalia Q56.4
Amblyopia (congenital) (ex anopsia) (partial)
(suppression) H53.00-
anisometropic —*see* Amblyopia, refractive
deprivation H53.01-
hysterical F44.6
nocturnal —*see also* Blindness, night
vitamin A deficiency E50.5
refractive H53.02-
strabismic H53.03-
tobacco H53.8
toxic NEC H53.8
uremic —*see* Uremia
Ameba, amebic (histolytica) —*see also*
Amebiasis
abscess (liver) A06.4
Amebiasis A06.9
with abscess —*see* Abscess, amebic
acute A06.0
chronic (intestine) A06.1
with abscess —*see* Abscess, amebic
cutaneous A06.7
cutis A06.7
cystitis A06.81
genitourinary tract NEC A06.82
hepatic —*see* Abscess, liver, amebic
intestine A06.0
nondysenteric colitis A06.2
skin A06.7
specified site NEC A06.89
Ameboma (of intestine) A06.3
Amelia Q73.0
lower limb —*see* Agenesis, leg
upper limb —*see* Agenesis, arm
Ameloblastoma —*see also* Cyst, calcifying
odontogenic
long bones C40.9-
lower limb C40.2-
upper limb C40.0-
malignant C41.1
jaw (bone) (lower) C41.1
upper C41.0
tibial C40.2-
Amelogenesis imperfecta K00.5
nonhereditaria (segmentalis) K00.4
Amenorrhea N91.2
hyperhormonal E28.8
primary N91.0
secondary N91.1
Amentia —*see* Disability, intellectual
Meynert's (nonalcoholic) F04
American
leishmaniasis B55.2
mountain tick fever A93.2
Ametropia —*see* Disorder, refraction
Amianthosis J61
Amimia R48.8
Amino-acid disorder E72.9
anemia D53.0
Aminoacidopathy E72.9
Aminoaciduria E72.9
Amnes (t)ic **syndrome** (post-traumatic) F04
induced by
alcohol F10.96
with dependence F10.26
psychoactive NEC F19.96
with
abuse F19.16
dependence F19.26

Amnes (t)ic **syndrome** *(Continued)*
induced by *(Continued)*
sedative F13.96
with dependence F13.26
Amnesia R41.3
anterograde R41.1
auditory R48.8
dissociative F44.0
hysterical F44.0
postictal in epilepsy —*see* Epilepsy
psychogenic F44.0
retrograde R41.2
transient global G45.4
Amnion, amniotic —*see* condition
Amnionitis —*see* Pregnancy, complicated by
Amok F68.8
Amoral traits F60.89
Ampulla
lower esophagus K22.8
phrenic K22.8
Amputation —*see also* Absence, by site,
acquired
neuroma (postoperative) (traumatic) —*see*
Complications, amputation stump,
neuroma
stump (surgical)
abnormal, painful, or with complication
(late) —*see* Complications,
amputation stump
healed or old NOS Z89.9
traumatic (complete) (partial)
arm (upper) (complete) S48.91-
at
elbow S58.01-
partial S58.02-
shoulder joint (complete) S48.01-
partial S48.02-
between
elbow and wrist (complete) S58.11-
partial S58.12-
shoulder and elbow (complete) S48.11-
partial S48.12-
partial S48.92-
breast (complete) S28.21-
partial S28.22-
clitoris (complete) S38.211
partial S38.212
ear (complete) S08.11-
partial S08.12-
finger (complete) (metacarpophalangeal)
S68.11-
index S68.11-
little S68.11-
middle S68.11-
partial S68.12-
index S68.12-
little S68.12-
middle S68.12-
ring S68.12-
ring S68.11-
thumb —*see* Amputation, traumatic,
thumb
transphalangeal (complete) S68.61-
index S68.61-
little S68.61-
middle S68.61-
partial S68.62-
index S68.62-
little S68.62-
middle S68.62-
ring S68.62-
ring S68.61-
foot (complete) S98.91-
at ankle level S98.01-
partial S98.02-
midfoot S98.31-
partial S98.32-
partial S98.92-
forearm (complete) S58.91-
at elbow level (complete) S58.01-
partial S58.02-

◀ New ⬅ Revised ~~deleted~~ Deleted

Amputation (Continued)
  traumatic (Continued)
    forearm (Continued)
      between elbow and wrist (complete) S58.11-
        partial S58.12-
      partial S58.92-
    genital organ (s) (external)
      female (complete) S38.211
        partial S38.212
      male
        penis (complete) S38.221
          partial S38.222
        scrotum (complete) S38.231
          partial S38.232
        testes (complete) S38.231
          partial S38.232
    hand (complete) (wrist level) S68.41-
      finger (s) alone —see Amputation, traumatic, finger
      partial S68.42-
      thumb alone —see Amputation, traumatic, thumb
      transmetacarpal (complete) S68.71-
        partial S68.72-
    head
      ear —see Amputation, traumatic, ear
      nose (partial) S08.812
        complete S08.811
      part S08.89
        scalp S08.0
    hip (and thigh) (complete) S78.91-
      at hip joint (complete) S78.01-
        partial S78.02-
      between hip and knee (complete) S78.11-
        partial S78.12-
      partial S78.92-
    labium (majus) (minus) (complete) S38.21-
      partial S38.21-
    leg (lower) S88.91-
      at knee level S88.01-
        partial S88.02-
      between knee and ankle S88.11-
        partial S88.12-
      partial S88.92-
    nose (partial) S08.812
      complete S08.811
    penis (complete) S38.221
      partial S38.222
    scrotum (complete) S38.231
      partial S38.232
    shoulder —see Amputation, traumatic, arm
    at shoulder joint —see Amputation, traumatic, arm, at shoulder joint
    testes (complete) S38.231
      partial S38.232
    thigh —see Amputation, traumatic, hip
    thorax, part of S28.1
      breast —see Amputation, traumatic, breast
    thumb (complete) (metacarpophalangeal) S68.01-
      partial S68.02-
      transphalangeal (complete) S68.51-
        partial S68.52-
    toe (lesser) S98.13-
      great S98.11-
        partial S98.12-
      more than one S98.21-
        partial S98.22-
      partial S98.14-
    vulva (complete) S38.211
      partial S38.212
Amputee (bilateral) (old) Z89.9
Amsterdam dwarfism Q87.1
Amusia R48.8
  developmental F80.89
Amyelencephalus, amyelencephaly Q00.0
Amyelia Q06.0
Amygdalitis —see Tonsillitis
Amygdalolith J35.8

Amyloid heart (disease) E85.4 [I43]
Amyloidosis (generalized) (primary) E85.9
  with lung involvement E85.4 [J99]
  familial E85.2
  genetic E85.2
  heart E85.4 [I43]
  hemodialysis-associated E85.3
  liver E85.4 [K77]
  localized E85.4
  neuropathic heredofamilial E85.1
  non-neuropathic heredofamilial E85.0
  organ limited E85.4
  Portuguese E85.1
  pulmonary E85.4 [J99]
  secondary systemic E85.3
  skin (lichen) (macular) E85.4 [L99]
  specified NEC E85.8
  subglottic E85.4 [J99]
Amylopectinosis (brancher enzyme deficiency) E74.03
Amylophagia —see Pica
Amyoplasia congenita Q79.8
Amyotonia M62.89
  congenita G70.2
Amyotrophia, amyotrophy, amyotrophic G71.8
  congenita Q79.8
  diabetic —see Diabetes, amyotrophy
  lateral sclerosis G12.21
  neuralgic G54.5
  spinal progressive G12.21
Anacidity, gastric K31.83
  psychogenic F45.8
Anaerosis of newborn P28.89
Analbuminemia E88.09
Analgesia —see Anesthesia
Analphalipoproteinemia E78.6
Anaphylactic
  purpura D69.0
  shock or reaction —see Shock, anaphylactic
Anaphylactoid shock or reaction —see Shock, anaphylactic
Anaphylactoid syndrome of pregnancy O88.01-
Anaphylaxis —see Shock, anaphylactic
Anaplasia cervix (see also Dysplasia, cervix) N87.9
Anaplasmosis, human A77.49
Anarthria R47.1
Anasarca R60.1
  cardiac —see Failure, heart, congestive
  lung J18.2
  newborn P83.2
  nutritional E43
  pulmonary J18.2
  renal N04.9
Anastomosis
  aneurysmal —see Aneurysm
  arteriovenous ruptured brain I60.8
  intestinal K63.89
    complicated NEC K91.89
      involving urinary tract N99.89
  retinal and choroidal vessels (congenital) Q14.8
Anatomical narrow angle H40.03-
Ancylostoma, ancylostomiasis (braziliense) (caninum) (ceylanicum) (duodenale) B76.0
  Necator americanus B76.1
Andersen's disease (glycogen storage) E74.09
Anderson-Fabry disease E75.21
Andes disease T70.29
Andrews' disease (bacterid) L08.89
Androblastoma
  benign
    specified site —see Neoplasm, benign, by site
    unspecified site
      female D27.9
      male D29.20

Androblastoma (Continued)
  malignant
    specified site —see Neoplasm, malignant, by site
    unspecified site
      female C56.9
      male C62.90
  specified site —see Neoplasm, uncertain behavior, by site
  tubular
    with lipid storage
      specified site —see Neoplasm, benign, by site
      unspecified site
        female D27.9
        male D29.20
    specified site —see Neoplasm, benign, by site
    unspecified site
      female D27.9
      male D29.20
  unspecified site
    female D39.10
    male D40.10
Androgen insensitivity syndrome (see also Syndrome, androgen insensitivity) E34.50
Androgen resistance syndrome (see also Syndrome, androgen insensitivity) E34.50
Android pelvis Q74.2
  with disproportion (fetopelvic) O33.3
    causing obstructed labor O65.3
Androphobia F40.290
Anectasis, pulmonary (newborn) —see Atelectasis
Anemia (essential) (general) (hemoglobin deficiency) (infantile) (primary) (profound) D64.9
  with (due to) (in)
    disorder of
      anaerobic glycolysis D55.2
      pentose phosphate pathway D55.1
    koilonychia D50.9
  achlorhydric D50.8
  achrestic D53.1
  Addison (-Biermer) (pernicious) D51.0
  agranulocytic —see Agranulocytosis
  amino-acid-deficiency D53.0
  aplastic D61.9
    congenital D61.09
    drug-induced D61.1
    due to
      drugs D61.1
      external agents NEC D61.2
      infection D61.2
      radiation D61.2
    idiopathic D61.3
    red cell (pure) D60.9
      chronic D60.0
      congenital D61.01
      specified type NEC D60.8
      transient D60.1
    specified type NEC D61.89
    toxic D61.2
  aregenerative
    congenital D61.09
  asiderotic D50.9
  atypical (primary) D64.9
  Baghdad spring D55.0
  Balantidium coli A07.0
  Biermer's (pernicious) D51.0
  blood loss (chronic) D50.0
    acute D62
  bothriocephalus B70.0 [D63.8]
  brickmaker's B76.9 [D63.8]
  cerebral I67.89
  childhood D58.9
  chlorotic D50.8
  chronic
    blood loss D50.0
    hemolytic D58.9
      idiopathic D59.9
    simple D53.9

Anemia *(Continued)*
chronica congenita aregenerativa D61.09
combined system disease NEC D51.0 *[G32.0]*
  due to dietary vitamin B12 deficiency
    D51.3 *[G32.0]*
complicating pregnancy, childbirth
    or puerperium —*see* Pregnancy,
    complicated by (management affected
    by), anemia
congenital P61.4
  aplastic D61.09
  due to isoimmunization NOS P55.9
  dyserythropoietic, dyshematopoietic
    D64.4
  following fetal blood loss P61.3
  Heinz body D58.2
  hereditary hemolytic NOS D58.9
  pernicious D51.0
  spherocytic D58.0
Cooley's (erythroblastic) D56.1
cytogenic D51.0
deficiency D53.9
  2, 3 diphosphoglycurate mutase D55.2
  2, 3 PG D55.2
  6 phosphogluconate dehydrogenase
    D55.1
  6-PGD D55.1
  amino-acid D53.0
  combined B12 and folate D53.1
  enzyme D55.9
    drug-induced (hemolytic) D59.2
    glucose-6-phosphate dehydrogenase
      (G6PD) D55.0
    glycolytic D55.2
    nucleotide metabolism D55.3
    related to hexose monophosphate
      (HMP) shunt pathway NEC D55.1
    specified type NEC D55.8
  erythrocytic glutathione D55.1
  folate D52.9
    dietary D52.0
    drug-induced D52.1
  folic acid D52.9
    dietary D52.0
    drug-induced D52.1
  G SH D55.1
  G6PD D55.0
  GGS-R D55.1
  glucose-6-phosphate dehydrogenase D55.0
  glutathione reductase D55.1
  glyceraldehyde phosphate dehydrogenase
    D55.2
  hexokinase D55.2
  iron D50.9
    secondary to blood loss (chronic) D50.0
  nutritional D53.9
    with
      poor iron absorption D50.8
      specified deficiency NEC D53.8
  phosphofructo-aldolase D55.2
  phosphoglycerate kinase D55.2
  PK D55.2
  protein D53.0
  pyruvate kinase D55.2
  transcobalamin II D51.2
  triose-phosphate isomerase D55.2
  vitamin B12 NOS D51.9
    dietary D51.3
    due to
      intrinsic factor deficiency D51.0
      selective vitamin B12 malabsorption
        with proteinuria D51.1
    pernicious D51.0
    specified type NEC D51.8
Diamond-Blackfan (congenital hypoplastic)
    D61.01
dibothriocephalus B70.0 *[D63.8]*
dimorphic D53.1
diphasic D53.1
Diphyllobothrium (Dibothriocephalus) B70.0
    [D63.8]

Anemia *(Continued)*
due to (in) (with)
  antineoplastic chemotherapy D64.81
  blood loss (chronic) D50.0
    acute D62
  chemotherapy, antineoplastic D64.81
  chronic disease classified elsewhere NEC
    D63.8
  chronic kidney disease D63.1
  deficiency
    amino-acid D53.0
    copper D53.8
    folate (folic acid) D52.9
      dietary D52.0
      drug-induced D52.1
    molybdenum D53.8
    protein D53.0
    zinc D53.8
  dietary vitamin B12 deficiency D51.3
  disorder of
    glutathione metabolism D55.1
    nucleotide metabolism D55.3
  drug —*see* Anemia, by type —*see also* Table
    of Drugs and Chemicals
  end stage renal disease D63.1
  enzyme disorder D55.9
  fetal blood loss P61.3
  fish tapeworm (D latum) infestation B70.0
    [D63.8]
  hemorrhage (chronic) D50.0
    acute D62
  impaired absorption D50.9
  loss of blood (chronic) D50.0
    acute D62
  myxedema E03.9 *[D63.8]*
  Necator americanus B76.1 *[D63.8]*
  prematurity P61.2
  selective vitamin B12 malabsorption with
    proteinuria D51.1
  transcobalamin II deficiency D51.2
Dyke-Young type (secondary) (symptomatic)
    D59.1
dyserythropoietic (congenital) D64.4
dyshematopoietic (congenital) D64.4
Egyptian B76.9 *[D63.8]*
elliptocytosis —*see* Elliptocytosis
enzyme-deficiency, drug-induced D59.2
epidemic (*see also* Ancylostomiasis) B76.9
    [D63.8]
erythroblastic
  familial D56.1
  newborn (*see also* Disease, hemolytic) P55.9
  of childhood D56.1
erythrocytic glutathione deficiency D55.1
erythropoietin-resistant anemia (EPO
    resistant anemia) D63.1
Faber's (achlorhydric anemia) D50.9
factitious (self-induced blood letting) D50.0
familial erythroblastic D56.1
Fanconi's (congenital pancytopenia) D61.09
favism D55.0
fish tapeworm (D. latum) infestation B70.0
    [D63.8]
folate (folic acid) deficiency D52.9
glucose-6-phosphate dehydrogenase (G6PD)
    deficiency D55.0
glutathione-reductase deficiency D55.1
goat's milk D52.0
granulocytic —*see* Agranulocytosis
Heinz body, congenital D58.2
hemolytic D58.9
  acquired D59.9
    with hemoglobinuria NEC D59.6
    autoimmune NEC D59.1
    infectious D59.4
    specified type NEC D59.8
    toxic D59.4
  acute D59.9
    due to enzyme deficiency specified type
      NEC D55.8
    Lederer's D59.1

Anemia *(Continued)*
hemolytic *(Continued)*
  autoimmune D59.1
    drug-induced D59.0
  chronic D58.9
    idiopathic D59.9
  cold type (secondary) (symptomatic) D59.1
  congenital (spherocytic) —*see*
    Spherocytosis
  due to
    cardiac conditions D59.4
    drugs (nonautoimmune) D59.2
      autoimmune D59.0
    enzyme disorder D55.9
      drug-induced D59.2
    presence of shunt or other internal
      prosthetic device D59.4
  familial D58.9
  hereditary D58.9
    due to enzyme disorder D55.9
      specified type NEC D55.8
    specified type NEC D58.8
  idiopathic (chronic) D59.9
  mechanical D59.4
  microangiopathic D59.4
  nonautoimmune D59.4
    drug-induced D59.2
  nonspherocytic
    congenital or hereditary NEC D55.8
      glucose-6-phosphate dehydrogenase
        deficiency D55.0
      pyruvate kinase deficiency D55.2
      type
        I D55.1
        II D55.2
    type
      I D55.1
      II D55.2
  secondary D59.4
    autoimmune D59.1
  specified (hereditary) type NEC D58.8
  Stransky-Regala type (*see also*
    Hemoglobinopathy) D58.8
  symptomatic D59.4
    autoimmune D59.1
  toxic D59.4
  warm type (secondary) (symptomatic)
    D59.1
hemorrhagic (chronic) D50.0
  acute D62
Herrick's D57.1
hexokinase deficiency D55.2
hookworm B76.9 *[D63.8]*
hypochromic (idiopathic) (microcytic)
    (normoblastic) D50.9
  due to blood loss (chronic) D50.0
    acute D62
  familial sex-linked D64.0
  pyridoxine-responsive D64.3
  sideroblastic, sex-linked D64.0
hypoplasia, red blood cells D61.9
  congenital or familial D61.01
hypoplastic (idiopathic) D61.9
  congenital or familial (of childhood)
    D61.01
hypoproliferative (refractive) D61.9
idiopathic D64.9
  aplastic D61.3
  hemolytic, chronic D59.9
in (due to) (with)
  chronic kidney disease D63.1
  end stage renal disease D63.1
  failure, kidney (renal) D63.1
  neoplastic disease (*see also* Neoplasm)
    D63.0
intertropical (*see also* Ancylostomiasis)
    D63.8
iron deficiency D50.9
  secondary to blood loss (chronic) D50.0
    acute D62
  specified type NEC D50.8

Anemia (Continued)
  Joseph-Diamond-Blackfan (congenital
    hypoplastic) D61.01
  Lederer's (hemolytic) D59.1
  leukoerythroblastic D61.82
  macrocytic D53.9
    nutritional D52.0
    tropical D52.8
  malarial (see also Malaria) B54 [D63.8]
  malignant (progressive) D51.0
  malnutrition D53.9
  marsh (see also Malaria) B54 [D63.8]
  Mediterranean (with other
    hemoglobinopathy) D56.9
  megaloblastic D53.1
    combined B12 and folate deficiency
      D53.1
    hereditary D51.1
    nutritional D52.0
    orotic aciduria D53.0
    refractory D53.1
    specified type NEC D53.1
  megalocytic D53.1
  microcytic (hypochromic) D50.9
    due to blood loss (chronic) D50.0
      acute D62
    familial D56.8
  microdrepanocytosis D57.40
  microelliptopoikilocytic (Rietti-Greppi-
    Micheli) D56.9
  miner's B76.9 [D63.0]
  myelodysplastic D46.9
  myelofibrosis D75.81
  myelogenous D64.89
  myelopathic D64.89
  myelophthisic D61.82
  myeloproliferative D47.Z9
  newborn P61.4
    due to
      ABO (antibodies, isoimmunization,
        maternal/fetal incompatibility)
        P55.1
      Rh (antibodies, isoimmunization,
        maternal/fetal incompatibility)
        P55.0
    following fetal blood loss P61.3
    posthemorrhagic (fetal) P61.3
  nonspherocytic hemolytic —see Anemia,
    hemolytic, nonspherocytic
  normocytic (infectional) D64.9
    due to blood loss (chronic) D50.0
      acute D62
    myelophthisic D61.82
  nutritional (deficiency) D53.9
    with
      poor iron absorption D50.8
      specified deficiency NEC D53.8
    megaloblastic D52.0
  of prematurity P61.2
  orotaciduric (congenital) (hereditary) D53.0
  osteosclerotic D64.89
  ovalocytosis (hereditary) —see Elliptocytosis
  paludal (see also Malaria) B54 [D63.8]
  pernicious (congenital) (malignant)
    (progressive) D51.0
  pleochromic D64.89
    of sprue D52.8
  posthemorrhagic (chronic) D50.0
    acute D62
    newborn P61.3
  postoperative (postprocedural)
    due to (acute) blood loss D62
      chronic blood loss D50.0
    specified NEC D64.9
  postpartum O90.81
  pressure D64.89
  progressive D64.9
    malignant D51.0
    pernicious D51.0
  protein-deficiency D53.0
  pseudoleukemica infantum D64.89

Anemia (Continued)
  pure red cell D60.9
    congenital D61.01
  pyridoxine-responsive D64.3
  pyruvate kinase deficiency D55.2
  refractory D46.4
    with
      excess of blasts D46.20
        1 (RAEB 1) D46.21
        2 (RAEB 2) D46.22
        in transformation (RAEB T) —see
          Leukemia, acute myeloblastic
      hemochromatosis D46.1
      sideroblasts (ring) (RARS) D46.1
    without ring sideroblasts, so stated D46.0
    without sideroblasts without excess of
      blasts D46.0
    megaloblastic D53.1
    sideroblastic D46.1
    sideropenic D50.9 ◄▥
  Rietti-Greppi-Micheli D56.9
  scorbutic D53.2
  secondary to
    blood loss (chronic) D50.0
      acute D62
    hemorrhage (chronic) D50.0
      acute D62
  semiplastic D61.89
  sickle-cell —see Disease, sickle-cell
  sideroblastic D64.3
    hereditary D64.0
    hypochromic, sex-linked D64.0
    pyridoxine-responsive NEC D64.3
    refractory D46.1
    secondary (due to)
      disease D64.1
      drugs and toxins D64.2
    specified type NEC D64.3
  sideropenic (refractory) D50.9
    due to blood loss (chronic) D50.0
      acute D62
  simple chronic D53.9
  specified type NEC D64.89
  spherocytic (hereditary) —see Spherocytosis
  splenic D64.89
  splenomegalic D64.89
  stomatocytosis D58.8
  syphilitic (acquired) (late) A52.79 [D63.8]
  target cell D64.89
  thalassemia D56.9
  thrombocytopenic —see Thrombocytopenia
  toxic D61.2
  tropical B76.9 [D63.8]
    macrocytic D52.8
  tuberculous A18.89 [D63.8]
  vegan D51.3
  vitamin
    B6-responsive D64.3
    B12 deficiency (dietary) pernicious D51.0
  von Jaksch's D64.89
  Witts' (achlorhydric anemia) D50.8
Anemophobia F40.228
Anencephalus, anencephaly Q00.0
Anergasia —see Psychosis, organic
Anesthesia, anesthetic R20.0
  complication or reaction NEC (see also
    Complications, anesthesia) T88.59
  due to
    correct substance properly
      administered —see Table of ‡Drugs
      and ‡Chemicals, by drug, adverse
      effect ◄▥
    overdose or wrong substance given —see
      Table of ‡Drugs and ‡Chemicals,
      by drug, poisoning ◄▥
  cornea H18.81-
  dissociative F44.6
  functional (hysterical) F44.6
  hyperesthetic, thalamic G89.0
  hysterical F44.6
  local skin lesion R20.0

Anesthesia, anesthetic (Continued)
  sexual (psychogenic) F52.1
  shock (due to) T88.2
  skin R20.0
  testicular N50.9
Anetoderma (maculosum) (of) L90.8
  Jadassohn-Pellizzari L90.2
  Schweniger-Buzzi L90.1
Aneurin deficiency E51.9
Aneurysm (anastomotic) (artery) (cirsoid)
    (diffuse) (false) (fusiform) (multiple)
    (saccular) I72.9
  abdominal (aorta) I71.4
    ruptured I71.3
    syphilitic A52.01
  aorta, aortic (nonsyphilitic) I71.9
    abdominal I71.4
      ruptured I71.3
    arch I71.2
      ruptured I71.1
    arteriosclerotic I71.9
      ruptured I71.8
    ascending I71.2
      ruptured I71.1
    congenital Q25.4
    descending I71.9
      abdominal I71.4
        ruptured I71.3
      ruptured I71.8
      thoracic I71.2
        ruptured I71.1
    ruptured I71.8
    sinus, congenital Q25.4
    syphilitic A52.01
    thoracic I71.2
      ruptured I71.1
    thoracoabdominal I71.6
      ruptured I71.5
    thorax, thoracic (arch) I71.2
      ruptured I71.1
    transverse I71.2
      ruptured I71.1
    valve (heart) (see also Endocarditis, aortic)
      I35.8
  arteriosclerotic I72.9
    cerebral I67.1
      ruptured —see Hemorrhage, intracranial,
        subarachnoid
  arteriovenous (congenital) —see also
    Malformation, arteriovenous
    acquired I77.0
      brain I67.1
      coronary I25.41
      pulmonary I28.0
    brain Q28.2
      ruptured I60.8
    peripheral —see Malformation,
      arteriovenous, peripheral
    precerebral vessels Q28.0
    specified site NEC —see also Malformation,
      arteriovenous
      acquired I77.0
  basal —see Aneurysm, brain
  berry (congenital) (nonruptured) I67.1
    ruptured I60.7
  brain I67.1
    arteriosclerotic I67.1
      ruptured —see Hemorrhage, intracranial,
        subarachnoid
    arteriovenous (congenital) (nonruptured)
      Q28.2
      acquired I67.1
        ruptured I60.8
      ruptured I60.8
    berry (congenital) (nonruptured) I67.1
      ruptured (see also Hemorrhage,
        intracranial, subarachnoid) I60.7
    congenital Q28.3
      ruptured I60.7
    meninges I67.1
      ruptured I60.8

Aneurysm *(Continued)*
  brain *(Continued)*
    miliary (congenital) (nonruptured) I67.1
      ruptured *(see also* Hemorrhage,
        intracranial, subarachnoid) I60.7
    mycotic I33.0
    ruptured *—see* Hemorrhage, intracranial,
      subarachnoid
    syphilitic (hemorrhage) A52.05
  cardiac (false) *(see also* Aneurysm, heart)
    I25.3
  carotid artery (common) (external) I72.0
    internal (intracranial) I67.1
      extracranial portion I72.0
      ruptured into brain I60.0-
      syphilitic A52.09
        intracranial A52.05
  cavernous sinus I67.1
    arteriovenous (congenital) (nonruptured)
      Q28.3
      ruptured I60.8
  celiac I72.8
  central nervous system, syphilitic A52.05
  cerebral *—see* Aneurysm, brain
  chest *—see* Aneurysm, thorax
  circle of Willis I67.1
    congenital Q28.3
      ruptured I60.6
    ruptured I60.6
  common iliac artery I72.3
  congenital (peripheral) Q27.8
    brain Q28.3
      ruptured I60.7
    coronary Q24.5
    digestive system Q27.8
    lower limb Q27.8
    pulmonary Q25.79
    retina Q14.1
    specified site NEC Q27.8
    upper limb Q27.8
  conjunctiva *—see* Abnormality, conjunctiva,
    vascular
  conus arteriosus *—see* Aneurysm, heart
  coronary (arteriosclerotic) (artery) I25.41
    arteriovenous, congenital Q24.5
    congenital Q24.5
    ruptured *—see* Infarct, myocardium
    syphilitic A52.06
    vein I25.89
  cylindroid (aorta) I71.9
    ruptured I71.8
    syphilitic A52.01
  ductus arteriosus Q25.0
  endocardial, infective (any valve) I33.0
  femoral (artery) (ruptured) I72.4
  gastroduodenal I72.8
  gastroepiploic I72.8
  heart (wall) (chronic or with a stated duration
    of over 4 weeks) I25.3
    valve *—see* Endocarditis
  hepatic I72.8
  iliac (common) (artery) (ruptured) I72.3
  infective I72.9
    endocardial (any valve) I33.0
  innominate (nonsyphilitic) I72.8
    syphilitic A52.09
  interauricular septum *—see* Aneurysm, heart
  interventricular septum *—see* Aneurysm,
    heart
  intrathoracic (nonsyphilitic) I71.2
    ruptured I71.1
    syphilitic A52.01
  lower limb I72.4
  lung (pulmonary artery) I28.1
  mediastinal (nonsyphilitic) I72.8
    syphilitic A52.09
  miliary (congenital) I67.1
    ruptured *—see* Hemorrhage, intracerebral,
      subarachnoid, intracranial
  mitral (heart) (valve) I34.8
  mural *—see* Aneurysm, heart

Aneurysm *(Continued)*
  mycotic I72.9
    endocardial (any valve) I33.0
    ruptured, brain *—see* Hemorrhage,
      intracerebral, subarachnoid
  myocardium *—see* Aneurysm, heart
  neck I72.0
  pancreaticoduodenal I72.8
  patent ductus arteriosus Q25.0
  peripheral NEC I72.8
    congenital Q27.8
      digestive system Q27.8
      lower limb Q27.8
      specified site NEC Q27.8
      upper limb Q27.8
  popliteal (artery) (ruptured) I72.4
  precerebral, congenital (nonruptured)
    Q28.1
  pulmonary I28.1
    arteriovenous Q25.72
      acquired I28.0
    syphilitic A52.09
    valve (heart) *—see* Endocarditis,
      pulmonary
  racemose (peripheral) I72.9
    congenital *—see* Aneurysm,
      congenital
  radial I72.1
  Rasmussen NEC A15.0
  renal (artery) I72.2
  retina *—see also* Disorder, retina,
    microaneurysms
    congenital Q14.1
    diabetic *—see* Diabetes, microaneurysms,
      retinal
  sinus of Valsalva Q25.4
  specified NEC I72.8
  spinal (cord) I72.8
    syphilitic (hemorrhage) A52.09
  splenic I72.8
  subclavian (artery) (ruptured)
    I72.8
    syphilitic A52.09
  superior mesenteric I72.8
  syphilitic (aorta) A52.01
    central nervous system A52.05
    congenital (late) A50.54 *[I79.0]*
    spine, spinal A52.09
  thoracoabdominal (aorta) I71.6
    ruptured I71.5
    syphilitic A52.01
  thorax, thoracic (aorta) (arch) (nonsyphilitic)
    I71.2
    ruptured I71.1
    syphilitic A52.01
  traumatic (complication) (early),
    specified site *—see* Injury,
      blood vessel
  tricuspid (heart) (valve) I07.8
  ulnar I72.1
  upper limb (ruptured) I72.1
  valve, valvular *—see* Endocarditis
  visceral NEC I72.8
  venous *(see also* Varix) I86.8
    congenital Q27.8
      digestive system Q27.8
      lower limb Q27.8
      specified site NEC Q27.8
      upper limb Q27.8
  ventricle *—see* Aneurysm, heart
  visceral NEC I72.8
Angelman syndrome Q93.5
Anger R45.4
Angiectasis, angiectopia I99.8
Angiitis I77.6
  allergic granulomatous M30.1
  hypersensitivity M31.0
  necrotizing M31.9
    specified NEC M31.8
  nervous system, granulomatous
    I67.7

Angina (attack) (cardiac) (chest) (heart)
    (pectoris) (syndrome) (vasomotor)
    I20.9
  with
    atherosclerotic heart disease *—see*
      Arteriosclerosis, coronary
      (artery)
    documented spasm I20.1
  abdominal K55.1
  accelerated *—see* Angina, unstable
  agranulocytic *—see* Agranulocytosis
  angiospastic *—see* Angina, with documented
    spasm
  aphthous B08.5
  crescendo *—see* Angina, unstable
  croupous J05.0
  cruris I73.9
  de novo effort *—see* Angina, unstable
  diphtheritic, membranous A36.0
  equivalent I20.8
  exudative, chronic J37.0
  following acute myocardial infarction
    I23.7
  gangrenous diphtheritic A36.0
  intestinal K55.1
  Ludovici K12.2
  Ludwig's K12.2
  malignant diphtheritic A36.0
  membranous J05.0
    diphtheritic A36.0
    Vincent's A69.1
  mesenteric K55.1
  monocytic *—see* Mononucleosis, infectious
  of effort *—see* Angina, specified NEC
  phlegmonous J36
    diphtheritic A36.0
  post-infarctional I23.7
  pre-infarctional *—see* Angina, unstable
  Prinzmetal *—see* Angina, with documented
    spasm
  progressive *—see* Angina, unstable
  pseudomembranous A69.1
  pultaceous, diphtheritic A36.0
  spasm-induced *—see* Angina, with
    documented spasm
  specified NEC I20.8
  stable I20.9
  stenocardia *—see* Angina, specified NEC
  stridulous, diphtheritic A36.2
  tonsil J36
  trachealis J05.0
  unstable I20.0
  variant *—see* Angina, with documented
    spasm
  Vincent's A69.1
  worsening effort *—see* Angina, unstable
Angioblastoma *—see* Neoplasm, connective
  tissue, uncertain behavior
Angiocholecystitis *—see* Cholecystitis, acute
Angiocholitis *(see also* Cholecystitis, acute)
  K83.0
Angiodysgenesis spinalis G95.19
Angiodysplasia (cecum) (colon) K55.20
  with bleeding K55.21
  duodenum (and stomach) K31.819
    with bleeding K31.811
  stomach (and duodenum) K31.819
    with bleeding K31.811
Angioedema (allergic) (any site) (with urticaria)
  T78.3
  hereditary D84.1
Angioendothelioma *—see* Neoplasm, uncertain
  behavior, by site
  benign D18.00
    intra-abdominal D18.03
    intracranial D18.02
    skin D18.01
    specified site NEC D18.09
  bone *—see* Neoplasm, bone, malignant
  Ewing's *—see* Neoplasm, bone, malignant
Angioendotheliomatosis C85.8-

◀ New   ◀▓ Revised   ~~deleted~~ Deleted

Angiofibroma —*see also* Neoplasm, benign, by
  site
  juvenile
    specified site —*see* Neoplasm, benign, by
      site
    unspecified site D10.6
Angiohemophilia (A) (B) D68.0
Angioid streaks (choroid) (macula) (retina)
  H35.33
Angiokeratoma —*see* Neoplasm, skin, benign
  corporis diffusum E75.21
Angioleiomyoma —*see* Neoplasm, connective
  tissue, benign
Angiolipoma —*see also* Lipoma
  infiltrating —*see* Lipoma
Angioma —*see also* Hemangioma, by site
  capillary I78.1
  hemorrhagicum hereditaria I78.0
  intra-abdominal D18.03
  intracranial D18.02
  malignant —*see* Neoplasm, connective tissue,
    malignant
  plexiform D18.00
    intra-abdominal D18.03
    intracranial D18.02
    skin D18.01
    specified site NEC D18.09
  senile I78.1
  serpiginosum L81.7
  skin D18.01
  specified site NEC D18.09
  spider I78.1
  stellate I78.1
  venous Q28.3
Angiomatosis Q82.8
  bacillary A79.89
  encephalotrigeminal Q85.8
  hemorrhagic familial I78.0
  hereditary familial I78.0
  liver K76.4
Angiomyolipoma —*see* Lipoma
Angiomyoliposarcoma —*see* Neoplasm,
  connective tissue, malignant
Angiomyoma —*see* Neoplasm, connective
  tissue, benign
Angiomyosarcoma —*see* Neoplasm, connective
  tissue, malignant
Angiomyxoma —*see* Neoplasm, connective
  tissue, uncertain behavior
Angioneurosis F45.8
Angioneurotic edema (allergic) (any site) (with
  urticaria) T78.3
  hereditary D84.1
Angiopathia, angiopathy I99.9
  cerebral I67.9
    amyloid E85.4 [I68.0]
  diabetic (peripheral) —*see* Diabetes,
    angiopathy
  peripheral I73.9
    diabetic —*see* Diabetes, angiopathy
    specified type NEC I73.89
  retinae syphilitica A52.05
  retinalis (juvenilis)
    diabetic —*see* Diabetes, retinopathy
    proliferative —*see* Retinopathy,
      proliferative
Angiosarcoma —*see also* Neoplasm, connective
  tissue, malignant
  liver C22.3
Angiosclerosis —*see* Arteriosclerosis
Angiospasm (peripheral) (traumatic) (vessel)
  I73.9
  brachial plexus G54.0
  cerebral G45.9
  cervical plexus G54.2
  nerve
    arm —*see* Mononeuropathy, upper limb
      axillary G54.0
      median —*see* Lesion, nerve, median
      ulnar —*see* Lesion, nerve, ulnar
    axillary G54.0

Angiospasm (Continued)
  nerve (Continued)
    leg —*see* Mononeuropathy, lower limb
    median —*see* Lesion, nerve, median
    plantar —*see* Lesion, nerve, plantar
    ulnar —*see* Lesion, nerve, ulnar
Angiospastic disease or edema I73.9
Angiostrongyliasis
  due to
    Parastrongylus
      cantonensis B83.2
      costaricensis B81.3
  intestinal B81.3
Anguillulosis —*see* Strongyloidiasis
Angulation
  cecum —*see* Obstruction, intestine
  coccyx (acquired) (*see also* subcategory) M43.8
    congenital NEC Q76.49
  femur (acquired) —*see also* Deformity, limb,
    specified type NEC, thigh
    congenital Q74.2
  intestine (large) (small) —*see* Obstruction,
    intestine
  sacrum (acquired) (*see also* subcategory)
    M43.8
    congenital NEC Q76.49
  sigmoid (flexure) —*see* Obstruction, intestine
  spine —*see* Dorsopathy, deforming, specified
    NEC
  tibia (acquired) —*see also* Deformity, limb,
    specified type NEC, lower leg
    congenital Q74.2
  ureter N13.5
    with infection N13.6
  wrist (acquired) —*see also* Deformity, limb,
    specified type NEC, forearm
    congenital Q74.0
Angulus infectiosus (lips) K13.0
Anhedonia R45.84
Anhidrosis L74.4
Anhydration, anhydremia E86.0
  with
    hypernatremia E87.0
    hyponatremia E87.1
Anhydremia E86.0
  with
    hypernatremia E87.0
    hyponatremia E87.1
Anidrosis L74.4
Aniridia (congenital) Q13.1
Anisakiasis (infection) (infestation) B81.0
Anisakis larvae infestation B81.0
Aniseikonia H52.32
Anisocoria (pupil) H57.02
  congenital Q13.2
Anisocytosis R71.8
Anisometropia (congenital) H52.31
Ankle —*see* condition
Ankyloblepharon (eyelid) (acquired) —*see also*
  Blepharophimosis
  filiforme (adnatum) (congenital) Q10.3
  total Q10.3
Ankyloglossia Q38.1
Ankylosis (fibrous) (osseous) (joint) M24.60
  ankle M24.67-
  arthrodesis status Z98.1
  cricoarytenoid (cartilage) (joint) (larynx) J38.7
  dental K03.5
  ear ossicles H74.31-
  elbow M24.62-
  foot M24.67-
  hand M24.64-
  hip M24.65-
  incostapedial joint (infectional) —*see*
    Ankylosis, ear ossicles
  jaw (temporomandibular) M26.61
  knee M24.66-
  lumbosacral (joint) M43.27
  postoperative (status) Z98.1
  produced by surgical fusion, status Z98.1
  sacro-iliac (joint) M43.28

Ankylosis (Continued)
  shoulder M24.61-
  spine (joint) —*see also* Fusion, spine
    spondylitic —*see* Spondylitis, ankylosing
  surgical Z98.1
  temporomandibular M26.61
  tooth, teeth (hard tissues) K03.5
  wrist M24.63-
Ankylostoma —*see* Ancylostoma
Ankylostomiasis —*see* Ancylostomiasis
Ankylurethria —*see* Stricture, urethra
Annular —*see also* condition
  detachment, cervix N88.8
  organ or site, congenital NEC —*see* Distortion
  pancreas (congenital) Q45.1
Anodontia (complete) (partial) (vera) K00.0
  acquired K08.10
Anomaly, anomalous (congenital) (unspecified
  type) Q89.9
  abdominal wall NEC Q79.59
  acoustic nerve Q07.8
  adrenal (gland) Q89.1
  Alder (-Reilly) (leukocyte granulation) D72.0
  alimentary tract Q45.9
    upper Q40.9
  alveolar M26.70
    hyperplasia M26.79
      mandibular M26.72
      maxillary M26.71
    hypoplasia M26.79
      mandibular M26.74
      maxillary M26.73
    ridge (process) M26.79
    specified NEC M26.79
  ankle (joint) Q74.2
  anus Q43.9
  aorta (arch) NEC Q25.4
    coarctation (preductal) (postductal) Q25.1
  aortic cusp or valve Q23.9
  appendix Q43.8
  apple peel syndrome Q41.1
  aqueduct of Sylvius Q03.0
    with spina bifida —*see* Spina bifida, with
      hydrocephalus
  arm Q74.0
  arteriovenous NEC
    coronary Q24.5
    gastrointestinal Q27.33
      acquired —*see* Angiodysplasia
  artery (peripheral) Q27.9
    basilar NEC Q28.1
    cerebral Q28.3
    coronary Q24.5
    digestive system Q27.8
    eye Q15.8
    great Q25.9
      specified NEC Q25.8
    lower limb Q27.8
    peripheral Q27.9
      specified NEC Q27.8
    pulmonary NEC Q25.79
    renal Q27.2
    retina Q14.1
    specified site NEC Q27.8
    subclavian Q27.8
    umbilical Q27.0
    upper limb Q27.8
    vertebral NEC Q28.1
  aryteno-epiglottic folds Q31.8
  atrial
    bands or folds Q20.8
    septa Q21.1
  atrioventricular
    excitation I45.6
    septum Q21.0
  auditory canal Q17.8
  auricle
    ear Q17.8
      causing impairment of hearing Q16.9
    heart Q20.8
  Axenfeld's Q15.0

Anomaly, anomalous (*Continued*)
back Q89.9
band
  atrial Q20.8
  heart Q24.8
  ventricular Q24.8
Bartholin's duct Q38.4
biliary duct or passage Q44.5
bladder Q64.70
  absence Q64.5
  diverticulum Q64.6
  exstrophy Q64.10
    cloacal Q64.12
    extroversion Q64.19
    specified type NEC Q64.19
    supravesical fissure Q64.11
  neck obstruction Q64.31
  specified type NEC Q64.79
bone Q79.9
  arm Q74.0
  face Q75.9
  leg Q74.2
  pelvic girdle Q74.2
  shoulder girdle Q74.0
  skull Q75.9
    with
      anencephaly Q00.0
      encephalocele —*see* Encephalocele
      hydrocephalus Q03.9
        with spina bifida —*see* Spina bifida,
          by site, with hydrocephalus
      microcephaly Q02
brain (multiple) Q04.9
  vessel Q28.3
breast Q83.9
broad ligament Q50.6
bronchus Q32.4
bulbus cordis Q21.9
bursa Q79.9
canal of Nuck Q52.4
canthus Q10.3
capillary Q27.9
cardiac Q24.9
  chambers Q20.9
    specified NEC Q20.8
  septal closure Q21.9
    specified NEC Q21.8
  valve NEC Q24.8
    pulmonary Q22.3
cardiovascular system Q28.8
carpus Q74.0
caruncle, lacrimal Q10.6
cascade stomach Q40.2
cauda equina Q06.3
cecum Q43.9
cerebral Q04.9
  vessels Q28.3
cervix Q51.9
Chédiak-Higashi(-Steinbrinck) (congenital
  gigantism of peroxidase granules)
  E70.330
cheek Q18.9
chest wall Q67.8
  bones Q76.9
chin Q18.9
chordae tendineae Q24.8
choroid Q14.3
  plexus Q07.8
chromosomes, chromosomal Q99.9
  D (1) —*see* condition, chromosome 13
  E (3) —*see* condition, chromosome 18
  G —*see* condition, chromosome 21
  sex
    female phenotype Q97.8
    gonadal dysgenesis (pure) Q99.1
    Klinefelter's Q98.4
    male phenotype Q98.9
    Turner's Q96.9
  specified NEC Q99.8
cilia Q10.3
circulatory system Q28.9

Anomaly, anomalous (*Continued*)
clavicle Q74.0
clitoris Q52.6
coccyx Q76.49
colon Q43.9
common duct Q44.5
communication
  coronary artery Q24.5
  left ventricle with right atrium Q21.0
concha (ear) Q17.3
connection
  portal vein Q26.5
  pulmonary venous Q26.4
    partial Q26.3
    total Q26.2
  renal artery with kidney Q27.2
cornea (shape) Q13.4
coronary artery or vein Q24.5
cranium —*see* Anomaly, skull
cricoid cartilage Q31.8
cystic duct Q44.5
dental
  alveolar —*see* Anomaly, alveolar
  arch relationship M26.20
    specified NEC M26.29
dentofacial M26.9
  alveolar —*see* Anomaly, alveolar
  dental arch relationship M26.20
    specified NEC M26.29
  functional M26.50
    specified NEC M26.59
  jaw-cranial base relationship M26.10
    asymmetry M26.12
      maxillary M26.11
    specified type NEC M26.19
  jaw size M26.00
    macrogenia M26.05
    mandibular
      hyperplasia M26.03
      hypoplasia M26.04
    maxillary
      hyperplasia M26.01
      hypoplasia M26.02
    microgenia M26.06
    specified type NEC M26.09
  malocclusion M26.4
    dental arch relationship NEC M26.29
    jaw-cranial base relationship —*see*
      Anomaly, dentofacial, jaw-cranial
      base relationship
    jaw size —*see* Anomaly, dentofacial, jaw
      size
  specified type NEC M26.89
  temporomandibular joint M26.60
    adhesions M26.61
    ankylosis M26.61
    arthralgia M26.62
    articular disc M26.63
    specified type NEC M26.69
  tooth position, fully erupted M26.30
    specified NEC M26.39
dermatoglyphic Q82.8
diaphragm (apertures) NEC Q79.1
digestive organ (s) or tract Q45.9
  lower Q43.9
  upper Q40.9
distance, interarch (excessive) (inadequate)
  M26.25
distribution, coronary artery Q24.5
ductus
  arteriosus Q25.0
  botalli Q25.0
duodenum Q43.9
dura (brain) Q04.9
  spinal cord Q06.9
ear (external) Q17.9
  causing impairment of hearing Q16.9
  inner Q16.5
  middle (causing impairment of hearing)
    Q16.4
  ossicles Q16.3

Anomaly, anomalous (*Continued*)
Ebstein's (heart) (tricuspid valve) Q22.5
ectodermal Q82.9
Eisenmenger's (ventricular septal defect)
  Q21.8
ejaculatory duct Q55.4
elbow Q74.0
endocrine gland NEC Q89.2
epididymis Q55.4
epiglottis Q31.8
esophagus Q39.9
eustachian tube Q17.8
eye Q15.9
  anterior segment Q13.9
    specified NEC Q13.89
  posterior segment Q14.9
    specified NEC Q14.8
  ptosis (eyelid) Q10.0
  specified NEC Q15.8
eyebrow Q18.8
eyelid Q10.3
  ptosis Q10.0
face Q18.9
  bone (s) Q75.9
fallopian tube Q50.6
fascia Q79.9
femur NEC Q74.2
fibula NEC Q74.2
finger Q74.0
fixation, intestine Q43.3
flexion (joint) NOS Q74.9
  hip or thigh Q65.89
foot NEC Q74.2
  varus (congenital) Q66.3
foramen
  Botalli Q21.1
  ovale Q21.1
forearm Q74.0
forehead Q75.8
form, teeth K00.2
fovea centralis Q14.1
frontal bone —*see* Anomaly, skull
gallbladder (position) (shape) (size)
  Q44.1
Gartner's duct Q52.4
gastrointestinal tract Q45.9
genitalia, genital organ (s) or system
  female Q52.9
    external Q52.70
    internal NOS Q52.9
  male Q55.9
    hydrocele P83.5
    specified NEC Q55.8
genitourinary NEC
  female Q52.9
  male Q55.9
Gerbode Q21.0
glottis Q31.8
granulation or granulocyte, genetic
  (constitutional) (leukocyte) D72.0
gum Q38.6
gyri Q07.9
hair Q84.2
hand Q74.0
hard tissue formation in pulp K04.3
head —*see* Anomaly, skull
heart Q24.9
  auricle Q20.8
  bands or folds Q24.8
  fibroelastosis cordis I42.4
  obstructive NEC Q22.6
  patent ductus arteriosus (Botalli) Q25.0
  septum Q21.9
    auricular Q21.1
    interatrial Q21.1
    interventricular Q21.0
      with pulmonary stenosis or atresia,
        dextraposition of aorta and
        hypertrophy of right ventricle
        Q21.3
    specified NEC Q21.8

◀ New   ◀▬▬ Revised   ~~deleted~~ Deleted

Anomaly, anomalous *(Continued)*
  heart *(Continued)*
    septum *(Continued)*
      ventricular Q21.0
        with pulmonary stenosis or atresia,
          dextraposition of aorta and
          hypertrophy of right ventricle
          Q21.3
    tetralogy of Fallot Q21.3
    valve NEC Q24.8
      aortic
        bicuspid valve Q23.1
        insufficiency Q23.1
        stenosis Q23.0
          subaortic Q24.4
      mitral
        insufficiency Q23.3
        stenosis Q23.2
      pulmonary Q22.3
        atresia Q22.0
        insufficiency Q22.2
        stenosis Q22.1
          infundibular Q24.3
          subvalvular Q24.3
      tricuspid
        atresia Q22.4
        stenosis Q22.4
    ventricle Q20.8
  heel NEC Q74.2
  Hegglin's D72.0
  hemianencephaly Q00.0
  hemicephaly Q00.0
  hemicrania Q00.0
  hepatic duct Q44.5
  hip NEC Q74.2
  hourglass stomach Q40.2
  humerus Q74.0
  hydatid of Morgagni
    female Q50.5
    male (epididymal) Q55.4
      testicular Q55.29
  hymen Q52.4
  hypersegmentation of neutrophils, hereditary
    D72.0
  hypophyseal Q89.2
  ileocecal (coil) (valve) Q43.9
  ileum Q43.9
  ilium NEC Q74.2
  integument Q84.9
    specified NEC Q84.8
  interarch distance (excessive) (inadequate)
    M26.25
  intervertebral cartilage or disc Q76.49
  intestine (large) (small) Q43.9
    with anomalous adhesions, fixation or
      malrotation Q43.3
  iris Q13.2
  ischium NEC Q74.2
  jaw —*see* Anomaly, dentofacial
    alveolar —*see* Anomaly, alveolar
  jaw-cranial base relationship —*see* Anomaly,
    dentofacial, jaw-cranial base relationship
  jejunum Q43.8
  joint Q74.9
    specified NEC Q74.8
  Jordan's D72.0
  kidney (s) (calyx) (pelvis) Q63.9
    artery Q27.2
    specified NEC Q63.8
  Klippel-Feil (brevicollis) Q76.1
  knee Q74.1
  labium (majus) (minus) Q52.70
  labyrinth, membranous Q16.5
  lacrimal apparatus or duct Q10.6
  larynx, laryngeal (muscle) Q31.9
    web (bed) Q31.0
  lens Q12.9
  ~~leucocytes, genetic D72.0~~
    ~~granulation (constitutional) D72.0~~
  leukocytes, genetic D72.0 ◄
    granulation (constitutional) D72.0 ◄
  lid (fold) Q10.3

Anomaly, anomalous *(Continued)*
  ligament Q79.9
    broad Q50.6
    round Q52.8
  limb Q74.9
    lower NEC Q74.2
      reduction deformity —*see* Defect,
        reduction, lower limb
    upper Q74.0
  lip Q38.0
  liver Q44.7
    duct Q44.5
  lower limb NEC Q74.2
  lumbosacral (joint) (region) Q76.49
    kyphosis —*see* Kyphosis, congenital
    lordosis —*see* Lordosis, congenital
  lung (fissure) (lobe) Q33.9
  mandible —*see* Anomaly, dentofacial
  maxilla —*see* Anomaly, dentofacial
  May (-Hegglin) D72.0
  meatus urinarius NEC Q64.79
  meningeal bands or folds Q07.9
    constriction of Q07.8
    spinal Q06.9
  meninges Q07.9
    cerebral Q04.8
    spinal Q06.9
  meningocele Q05.9
  mesentery Q45.9
  metacarpus Q74.0
  metatarsus NEC Q74.2
  middle ear Q16.4
    ossicles Q16.3
  mitral (leaflets) (valve) Q23.9
    insufficiency Q23.3
    specified NEC Q23.8
    stenosis Q23.2
  mouth Q38.6
  Müllerian —*see also* Anomaly, by site
    uterus NEC Q51.818
  multiple NEC Q89.7
  muscle Q79.9
    eyelid Q10.3
  musculoskeletal system, except limbs Q79.9
  myocardium Q24.8
  nail Q84.6
  narrowness, eyelid Q10.3
  nasal sinus (wall) Q30.9
  neck (any part) Q18.9
  nerve Q07.9
    acoustic Q07.8
    optic Q07.8
  nervous system (central) Q07.9
  nipple Q83.9
  nose, nasal (bones) (cartilage) (septum)
      (sinus) Q30.9
    specified NEC Q30.8
  ocular muscle Q15.8
  omphalomesenteric duct Q43.0
  opening, pulmonary veins Q26.4
  optic
    disc Q14.2
    nerve Q07.8
  opticociliary vessels Q13.2
  orbit (eye) Q10.7
  organ Q89.9
    of Corti Q16.5
  origin
    artery
      innominate Q25.8
      pulmonary Q25.79
      renal Q27.2
      subclavian Q25.8
  osseous meatus (ear) Q16.1
  ovary Q50.39
  oviduct Q50.6
  palate (hard) (soft) NEC Q38.5
  pancreas or pancreatic duct Q45.3
  papillary muscles Q24.8
  parathyroid gland Q89.2
  paraurethral ducts Q64.79

Anomaly, anomalous *(Continued)*
  parotid (gland) Q38.4
  patella Q74.1
  Pelger-Huët (hereditary hyposegmentation)
    D72.0
  pelvic girdle NEC Q74.2
  pelvis (bony) NEC Q74.2
    rachitic E64.3
  penis (glans) Q55.69
  pericardium Q24.8
  peripheral vascular system Q27.9
  Peter's Q13.4
  pharynx Q38.8
  pigmentation L81.9
    congenital Q82.8
  pituitary (gland) Q89.2
  pleural (folds) Q34.0
  portal vein Q26.5
    connection Q26.5
  position, tooth, teeth, fully erupted
    M26.30
    specified NEC M26.39
  precerebral vessel Q28.1
  prepuce Q55.69
  prostate Q55.4
  pulmonary Q33.9
    artery NEC Q25.79
    valve Q22.3
      atresia Q22.0
      insufficiency Q22.2
      specified type NEC Q22.3
      stenosis Q22.1
        infundibular Q24.3
        subvalvular Q24.3
    venous connection Q26.4
      partial Q26.3
      total Q26.2
  pupil Q13.2
    function H57.00
      anisocoria H57.02
      Argyll Robertson pupil H57.01
      miosis H57.03
      mydriasis H57.04
      specified type NEC H57.09
      tonic pupil H57.05-
  pylorus Q40.3
  radius Q74.0
  rectum Q43.9
  reduction (extremity) (limb)
    femur (longitudinal) —*see* Defect,
      reduction, lower limb, longitudinal,
      femur
    fibula (longitudinal) —*see* Defect,
      reduction, lower limb, longitudinal,
      fibula
    lower limb —*see* Defect, reduction, lower
      limb
    radius (longitudinal) —*see* Defect,
      reduction, upper limb, longitudinal,
      radius
    tibia (longitudinal) —*see* Defect, reduction,
      lower limb, longitudinal, tibia
    ulna (longitudinal) —*see* Defect, reduction,
      upper limb, longitudinal, ulna
    upper limb —*see* Defect, reduction, upper
      limb
  refraction —*see* Disorder, refraction
  renal Q63.9
    artery Q27.2
    pelvis Q63.9
      specified NEC Q63.8
  respiratory system Q34.9
    specified NEC Q34.8
  retina Q14.1
  rib Q76.6
    cervical Q76.5
  Rieger's Q13.81
  rotation —*see* Malrotation
    hip or thigh Q65.89
  round ligament Q52.8
  sacroiliac (joint) NEC Q74.2

Anomaly, anomalous (Continued)
  sacrum NEC Q76.49
    kyphosis —see Kyphosis, congenital
    lordosis —see Lordosis, congenital
  saddle nose, syphilitic A50.57
  salivary duct or gland Q38.4
  scapula Q74.0
  scrotum —see Malformation, testis and
    scrotum
  sebaceous gland Q82.9
  seminal vesicles Q55.4
  sense organs NEC Q07.8
  sex chromosomes NEC —see also Anomaly,
    chromosomes
    female phenotype Q97.8
    male phenotype Q98.9
  shoulder (girdle) (joint) Q74.0
  sigmoid (flexure) Q43.9
  simian crease Q82.8
  sinus of Valsalva Q25.4
  skeleton generalized Q78.9
  skin (appendage) Q82.9
  skull Q75.9
    with
      anencephaly Q00.0
      encephalocele —see Encephalocele
      hydrocephalus Q03.9
        with spina bifida —see Spina bifida, by
          site, with hydrocephalus
      microcephaly Q02
  specified organ or site NEC Q89.8
  spermatic cord Q55.4
  spine, spinal NEC Q76.49
    column NEC Q76.49
      kyphosis —see Kyphosis, congenital
      lordosis —see Lordosis, congenital
    cord Q06.9
    nerve root Q07.8
  spleen Q89.09
    agenesis Q89.01
  stenonian duct Q38.4
  sternum NEC Q76.7
  stomach Q40.3
  submaxillary gland Q38.4
  tarsus NEC Q74.2
  tendon Q79.9
  testis —see Malformation, testis and
    scrotum
  thigh NEC Q74.2
  thorax (wall) Q67.8
    bony Q76.9
  throat Q38.8
  thumb Q74.0
  thymus gland Q89.2
  thyroid (gland) Q89.2
    cartilage Q31.8
  tibia NEC Q74.2
    saber A50.56
  toe Q74.2
  tongue Q38.3
  tooth, teeth K00.9
    eruption K00.6
    position, fully erupted M26.30
    spacing, fully erupted M26.30
  trachea (cartilage) Q32.1
  tragus Q17.9
  tricuspid (leaflet) (valve) Q22.9
    atresia or stenosis Q22.4
    Ebstein's Q22.5
  Uhl's (hypoplasia of myocardium, right
    ventricle) Q24.8
  ulna Q74.0
  umbilical artery Q27.0
  union
    cricoid cartilage and thyroid cartilage
      Q31.8
    thyroid cartilage and hyoid bone
      Q31.8
    trachea with larynx Q31.8
  upper limb Q74.0
  urachus Q64.4

Anomaly, anomalous (Continued)
  ureter Q62.8
    obstructive NEC Q62.39
      cecoureterocele Q62.32
      orthotopic ureterocele Q62.31
  urethra Q64.70
    absence Q64.5
    double Q64.74
    fistula to rectum Q64.73
    obstructive Q64.39
      stricture Q64.32
    prolapse Q64.71
    specified type NEC Q64.79
  urinary tract Q64.9
  uterus Q51.9
    with only one functioning horn
      Q51.4
  uvula Q38.5
  vagina Q52.4
  valleculae Q31.8
  valve (heart) NEC Q24.8
    coronary sinus Q24.5
    inferior vena cava Q24.8
    pulmonary Q22.3
    sinus coronario Q24.5
    venae cavae inferioris Q24.8
  vas deferens Q55.4
  vascular Q27.9
    brain Q28.3
    ring Q25.4
  vein (s) (peripheral) Q27.9
    brain Q28.3
    cerebral Q28.3
    coronary Q24.5
    developmental Q28.3
    great Q26.9
      specified NEC Q26.8
  vena cava (inferior) (superior) Q26.9
  venous —see Anomaly, vein (s)
  venous return Q26.8
  ventricular
    bands or folds Q24.8
    septa Q21.0
  vertebra Q76.49
    kyphosis —see Kyphosis, congenital
    lordosis —see Lordosis, congenital
  vesicourethral orifice Q64.79
  vessel (s) Q27.9
    optic papilla Q14.2
    precerebral Q28.1
  vitelline duct Q43.0
  vitreous body or humor Q14.0
  vulva Q52.70
  wrist (joint) Q74.0
Anomia R48.8
Anonychia (congenital) Q84.3
  acquired L60.8
Anophthalmos, anophthalmus (congenital)
  (globe) Q11.1
  acquired Z90.01
Anopia, anopsia H53.46-
  quadrant H53.46-
Anorchia, anorchism, anorchidism Q55.0
Anorexia R63.0
  hysterical F44.89
  nervosa F50.00
    atypical F50.9
    binge-eating type F50.2
      with purging F50.02
    restricting type F50.01
Anorgasmy, psychogenic (female)
  F52.31
  male F52.32
Anosmia R43.0
  hysterical F44.6
  postinfectional J39.8
Anosognosia R41.89
Anosteoplasia Q78.9
Anovulatory cycle N97.0
Anoxemia R09.02
  newborn P84

Anoxia (pathological) R09.02
  altitude T70.29
  cerebral G93.1
    complicating
      anesthesia (general) (local) or other
        sedation T88.59
        in labor and delivery O74.3
        in pregnancy O29.21-
        postpartum, puerperal O89.2
      delivery (cesarean) (instrumental)
        O75.4
    during a procedure G97.81
    newborn P84
    resulting from a procedure G97.82
  due to
    drowning T75.1
    high altitude T70.29
  heart —see Insufficiency, coronary
  intrauterine P84
  myocardial —see Insufficiency, coronary
  newborn P84
  spinal cord G95.11
  systemic (by suffocation) (low content in
    atmosphere) —see Asphyxia,
    traumatic
Anteflexion —see Anteversion
Antenatal
  care (normal pregnancy) Z34.90
  screening (encounter for) of mother
    Z36
Antepartum —see condition
Anterior —see condition
Antero-occlusion M26.220
Anteversion
  cervix —see Anteversion, uterus
  femur (neck), congenital Q65.89
  uterus, uterine (cervix) (postinfectional)
    (postpartal, old) N85.4
    congenital Q51.818
    in pregnancy or childbirth —see Pregnancy,
      complicated by
Anthophobia F40.228
Anthracosilicosis J60
Anthracosis (lung) (occupational) J60
  lingua K14.3
Anthrax A22.9
  with pneumonia A22.1
  cerebral A22.8
  colitis A22.2
  cutaneous A22.0
  gastrointestinal A22.2
  inhalation A22.1
  intestinal A22.2
  meningitis A22.8
  pulmonary A22.1
  respiratory A22.1
  sepsis A22.7
  specified manifestation NEC A22.8
Anthropoid pelvis Q74.2
  with disproportion (fetopelvic) O33.0
Anthropophobia F40.10
  generalized F40.11
Antibodies, maternal (blood group) —see
  Isoimmunization, affecting management
  of pregnancy
  anti-D —see Isoimmunization, affecting
    management of pregnancy, Rh
  newborn P55.0
Antibody
  anticardiolipin R76.0
    with
      hemorrhagic disorder D68.312
      hypercoagulable state D68.61
  antiphosphatidylglycerol R76.0
    with
      hemorrhagic disorder D68.312
      hypercoagulable state D68.61
  antiphosphatidylinositol R76.0
    with
      hemorrhagic disorder D68.312
      hypercoagulable state D68.61

◀ New   ◀ Revised   ~~deleted~~ Deleted

Antibody (Continued)
antiphosphatidylserine R76.0
with
hemorrhagic disorder D68.312
hypercoagulable state D68.61
antiphospholipid R76.0
with
hemorrhagic disorder D68.312
hypercoagulable state D68.61
Anticardiolipin syndrome D68.61
Anticoagulant, circulating (intrinsic) (see also -
Disorder, hemorrhagic) D68.318
drug-induced (extrinsic) (see also - Disorder,
hemorrhagic) D68.32
Antidiuretic hormone syndrome E22.2
Antimonial cholera —see Poisoning, antimony
Antiphospholipid
antibody
with hemorrhagic disorder D68.312
syndrome D68.61
Antisocial personality F60.2
Antithrombinemia —see Circulating
anticoagulants
Antithromboplastinemia D68.318
Antithromboplastinogenemia D68.318
Antitoxin complication or reaction —see
Complications, vaccination
Antlophobia F40.228
Antritis J32.0
maxilla J32.0
acute J01.00
recurrent J01.01
stomach K29.60
with bleeding K29.61
Antrum, antral —see condition
Anuria R34
calculus (impacted) (recurrent) (see also
Calculus, urinary) N20.9
following
abortion —see Abortion by type
complicated by, renal failure
ectopic or molar pregnancy O08.4
newborn P96.0
postprocedural N99.0
postrenal N13.8
traumatic (following crushing) T79.5
Anus, anal —see condition
Anusitis K62.89
Anxiety F41.9
depression F41.8
episodic paroxysmal F41.0
generalized F41.1
hysteria F41.8
neurosis F41.1
panic type F41.0
reaction F41.1
separation, abnormal (of childhood) F93.0
specified NEC F41.8
state F41.1
Aorta, aortic —see condition
Aortectasia —see Ectasia, aorta
with aneurysm —see Aneurysm, aorta
Aortitis (nonsyphilitic) (calcific) I77.6
arteriosclerotic I70.0
Doehle-Heller A52.02
luetic A52.02
rheumatic —see Endocarditis, acute, rheumatic
specific (syphilitic) A52.02
syphilitic A52.02
congenital A50.54 [I79.1]
Apathetic thyroid storm —see Thyrotoxicosis
Apathy R45.3
Apeirophobia F40.228
Apepsia K30
psychogenic F45.8
Aperistalsis, esophagus K22.0
Apertognathia M26.29
Apert's syndrome Q87.0
Aphagia R13.0
psychogenic F50.9
Aphakia (acquired) (postoperative) H27.0-
congenital Q12.3

Aphasia (amnestic) (global) (nominal)
(semantic) (syntactic) R47.01
acquired, with epilepsy (Landau-Kleffner
syndrome) —see Epilepsy, specified
NEC
auditory (developmental) F80.2
developmental (receptive type) F80.2
expressive type F80.1
Wernicke's F80.2
following
cerebrovascular disease I69.920
cerebral infarction I69.320
intracerebral hemorrhage I69.120
nontraumatic intracranial hemorrhage
NEC I69.220
specified disease NEC I69.820
subarachnoid hemorrhage I69.020
primary progressive G31.01 [F02.80]
with behavioral disturbance G31.01
[F02.81]
progressive isolated G31.01 [F02.80]
with behavioral disturbance G31.01
[F02.81]
sensory F80.2
syphilis, tertiary A52.19
Wernicke's (developmental) F80.2
Aphonia (organic) R49.1
hysterical F44.4
psychogenic F44.4
Aphthae, aphthous —see also condition
Bednar's K12.0
cachectic K14.0
epizootic B08.8
fever B08.8
oral (recurrent) K12.0
stomatitis (major) (minor) K12.0
thrush B37.0
ulcer (oral) (recurrent) K12.0
genital organ (s) NEC
female N76.6
male N50.8
larynx J38.7
Apical —see condition
Apiphobia F40.218
Aplasia —see also Agenesis
abdominal muscle syndrome Q79.4
alveolar process (acquired) —see Anomaly,
alveolar
congenital Q38.6
aorta (congenital) Q25.4
axialis extracorticalis (congenita) E75.29
bone marrow (myeloid) D61.9
congenital D61.01
brain Q00.0
part of Q04.3
bronchus Q32.4
cementum K00.4
cerebellum Q04.3
cervix (congenital) Q51.5
congenital pure red cell D61.01
corpus callosum Q04.0
cutis congenita Q84.8
erythrocyte congenital D61.01
extracortical axial E75.29
eye Q11.1
fovea centralis (congenital) Q14.1
gallbladder, congenital Q44.0
iris Q13.1
labyrinth, membranous Q16.5
limb (congenital) Q73.8
lower —see Defect, reduction, lower limb
upper —see Agenesis, arm
lung, congenital (bilateral) (unilateral) Q33.3
pancreas Q45.0
parathyroid-thymic D82.1
Pelizaeus-Merzbacher E75.29
penis Q55.5
prostate Q55.4
red cell (with thymoma) D60.9
acquired D60.9
due to drugs D60.9
adult D60.9

Aplasia (Continued)
red cell (Continued)
chronic D60.0
congenital D61.01
constitutional D61.01
due to drugs D60.9
hereditary D61.01
of infants D61.01
primary D61.01
pure D61.01
due to drugs D60.9
specified type NEC D60.8
transient D60.1
round ligament Q52.8
skin Q84.8
spermatic cord Q55.4
spleen Q89.01
testicle Q55.0
thymic, with immunodeficiency D82.1
thyroid (congenital) (with myxedema) E03.1
uterus Q51.0
ventral horn cell Q06.1
Apnea, apneic (of) (spells) R06.81
newborn NEC P28.4
obstructive P28.4
sleep (central) (obstructive) (primary) P28.3
prematurity P28.4
sleep G47.30
central (primary) G47.31
in conditions classified elsewhere G47.37
obstructive (adult) (pediatric) G47.33
primary central G47.31
specified NEC G47.39
Apneumatosis, newborn P28.0
Apocrine metaplasia (breast) —see Dysplasia,
mammary, specified type NEC
Apophysitis (bone) —see also
Osteochondropathy
calcaneus M92.8
juvenile M92.9
Apoplectiform convulsions (cerebral ischemia)
I67.82
Apoplexia, apoplexy, apoplectic
adrenal A39.1
heart (auricle) (ventricle) —see Infarct,
myocardium
heat T67.0
hemorrhagic (stroke) —see Hemorrhage,
intracranial
meninges, hemorrhagic —see Hemorrhage,
intracranial, subarachnoid
uremic N18.9 [I68.8]
Appearance
bizarre R46.1
specified NEC R46.89
very low level of personal hygiene R46.0
Appendage
epididymal (organ of Morgagni) Q55.4
intestine (epiploic) Q43.8
preauricular Q17.0
testicular (organ of Morgagni) Q55.29
Appendicitis (pneumococcal) (retrocecal) K37
with
perforation or rupture K35.2
peritoneal abscess K35.3
with peritonitis K35.2
peritonitis K35.2
with perforation or rupture K35.2
generalized K35.2
localized K35.3
peritonitis NEC K35.3 ◀
generalized (with perforation or
rupture) K35.2 ◀
localized (with perforation or rupture)
K35.3 ◀
acute (catarrhal) (fulminating) (gangrenous)
(obstructive) (retrocecal) (suppurative)
K35.80
with
perforation or rupture K35.2
peritoneal abscess K35.3
with peritonitis K35.2

Appendicitis (Continued)
  acute (Continued)
    with (Continued)
      ~~peritonitis K35.2~~
        ~~with perforation or rupture K35.2~~
        ~~generalized K35.2~~
        ~~localized K35.3~~
      peritonitis NEC K35.3 ◀
        generalized (with perforation or
          rupture) K35.2 ◀
        localized (with perforation or rupture)
          K35.3 ◀
      specified NEC K35.89
  amebic A06.89
  chronic (recurrent) K36
  exacerbation —see Appendicitis, acute
  gangrenous —see Appendicitis, acute
  healed (obliterative) K36
  interval K36
  neurogenic K36
  obstructive K36
  recurrent K36
  relapsing K36
  subacute (adhesive) K36
  subsiding K36
  suppurative —see Appendicitis, acute
  tuberculous A18.32
Appendicopathia oxyurica B80
Appendix, appendicular —see also condition
  epididymis Q55.4
  Morgagni
    female Q50.5
    male (epididymal) Q55.4
      testicular Q55.29
  testis Q55.29
Appetite
  depraved —see Pica
  excessive R63.2
  lack or loss (see also Anorexia) R63.0
    nonorganic origin F50.8
    psychogenic F50.8
  perverted (hysterical) —see Pica
Apple peel syndrome Q41.1
Apprehension state F41.1
Apprehensiveness, abnormal F41.9
Approximal wear K03.0
Apraxia (classic) (ideational) (ideokinetic)
  (ideomotor) (motor) (verbal) R48.2
  following
    cerebrovascular disease I69.990
      cerebral infarction I69.390
      intracerebral hemorrhage I69.190
      nontraumatic intracranial hemorrhage
        NEC I69.290
      specified disease NEC I69.890
      subarachnoid hemorrhage I69.090
  oculomotor, congenital H51.8
Aptyalism K11.7
Apudoma —see Neoplasm, uncertain behavior,
  by site
Aqueous misdirection H40.83-
Arabicum elephantiasis —see Infestation, filarial
Arachnitis —see Meningitis
Arachnodactyly —see Syndrome, Marfan's
Arachnoiditis (acute) (adhesive) (basal) (brain)
  (cerebrospinal) —see Meningitis
Arachnophobia F40.210
Arboencephalitis, Australian A83.4
Arborization block (heart) I45.5
ARC (AIDS-related complex) B20
Arches —see condition
Arcuate uterus Q51.810
Arcuatus uterus Q51.810
Arcus (cornea) senilis —see Degeneration,
  cornea, senile
Arc-welder's lung J63.4
Areflexia R29.2
Areola —see condition
Argentaffinoma —see also Neoplasm, uncertain
  behavior, by site
  malignant —see Neoplasm, malignant, by site
  syndrome E34.0

Argininemia E72.21
Arginosuccinic aciduria E72.22
Argyll Robertson phenomenon, pupil or
  syndrome (syphilitic) A52.19
  atypical H57.09
  nonsyphilitic H57.09
Argyria, argyriasis
  conjunctival H11.13-
  from drug or medicament —see Table of
    ~~d~~Drugs and ~~c~~Chemicals, by substance ◀▥
Argyrosis, conjunctival H11.13-
Arhinencephaly Q04.1
Ariboflavinosis E53.0
Arm —see condition
Arnold-Chiari disease, obstruction or
  syndrome (type II) Q07.00
  with
    hydrocephalus Q07.02
      with spina bifida Q07.03
    spina bifida Q07.01
      with hydrocephalus Q07.03
  type III —see Encephalocele
  type IV Q04.8
Aromatic amino-acid metabolism disorder
  E70.9
  specified NEC E70.8
Arousals, confusional G47.51
Arrest, arrested
  cardiac I46.9
    complicating
      abortion —see Abortion, by type,
        complicated by, cardiac arrest
      anesthesia (general) (local) or other
        sedation —see Table of ~~d~~Drugs and
        ~~c~~Chemicals, by drug ◀▥
      in labor and delivery O74.2
      in pregnancy O29.11-
        postpartum, puerperal O89.1
      delivery (cesarean) (instrumental) O75.4
    due to
      cardiac condition I46.2
      specified condition NEC I46.8
    intraoperative I97.71-
    newborn P29.81
    postprocedural I97.12-
      obstetric procedure O75.4
  cardiorespiratory —see Arrest, cardiac
  circulatory —see Arrest, cardiac
  deep transverse O64.0
  development or growth
    bone —see Disorder, bone, development or
      growth
    child R62.50
    tracheal rings Q32.1
  epiphyseal
    complete
      femur M89.15-
      humerus M89.12-
      tibia M89.16-
      ulna M89.13-
      forearm M89.13-
        specified NEC M89.13-
        ulna —see Arrest, epiphyseal, by type,
          ulna
      lower leg M89.16-
        specified NEC M89.168
        tibia —see Arrest, epiphyseal, by type,
          tibia
    partial
      femur M89.15-
      humerus M89.12-
      tibia M89.16-
      ulna M89.13-
      specified NEC M89.18
    granulopoiesis —see Agranulocytosis
    growth plate —see Arrest, epiphyseal
  heart —see Arrest, cardiac
  legal, anxiety concerning Z65.3
  physeal —see Arrest, epiphyseal
  respiratory R09.2
    newborn P28.81
  sinus I45.5

Arrest, arrested (Continued)
  spermatogenesis (complete) —see
    Azoospermia
    incomplete —see Oligospermia
  transverse (deep) O64.0
Arrhenoblastoma
  benign
    specified site —see Neoplasm, benign, by
      site
    unspecified site
      female D27.9
      male D29.20
  malignant
    specified site —see Neoplasm, malignant,
      by site
    unspecified site
      female C56.9
      male C62.90
  specified site —see Neoplasm, uncertain
    behavior, by site
  unspecified site
    female D39.10
    male D40.10
Arrhythmia (auricle) (cardiac) (juvenile)
  (nodal) (reflex) (sinus) (supraventricular)
  (transitory) (ventricle) I49.9
  block I45.9
  extrasystolic I49.49
  newborn
    bradycardia P29.12
    occurring before birth P03.819
      before onset of labor P03.810
      during labor P03.811
    tachycardia P29.11
  psychogenic F45.8
  specified NEC I49.8
  vagal R55
  ventricular re-entry I47.0
Arrillaga-Ayerza syndrome (pulmonary
  sclerosis with pulmonary hypertension)
  I27.0
Arsenical pigmentation L81.8
  from drug or medicament —see Table of
    ~~d~~Drugs and ~~medicaments~~Chemicals ◀▥
Arsenism —see Poisoning, arsenic
Arterial —see condition
Arteriofibrosis —see Arteriosclerosis
Arteriolar sclerosis —see Arteriosclerosis
Arteriolith —see Arteriosclerosis
Arteriolitis I77.6
  necrotizing, kidney I77.5
  renal —see Hypertension, kidney
Arteriolosclerosis —see Arteriosclerosis
Arterionephrosclerosis —see Hypertension,
  kidney
Arteriopathy I77.9
Arteriosclerosis, arteriosclerotic (diffuse)
  (obliterans) (of) (senile) (with calcification)
  I70.90
  aorta I70.0
  arteries of extremities —see Arteriosclerosis,
    extremities
  brain I67.2
  bypass graft
    coronary —see Arteriosclerosis, coronary,
      bypass graft
    extremities —see Arteriosclerosis,
      extremities, bypass graft
  cardiac —see Disease, heart, ischemic,
    atherosclerotic
  cardiopathy —see Disease, heart, ischemic,
    atherosclerotic
  cardiorenal —see Hypertension,
    cardiorenal
  cardiovascular —see Disease, heart,
    ischemic, atherosclerotic
  carotid (see also Occlusion, artery, carotid)
    I65.2-
  central nervous system I67.2
  cerebral I67.2
  cerebrovascular I67.2

◀ New   ◀▥ Revised   ~~deleted~~ Deleted

Arteriosclerosis, arteriosclerotic *(Continued)*
  coronary (artery) I25.10
    bypass graft I25.810
      with
        angina pectoris I25.709
          with documented spasm I25.701
          specified type NEC I25.708
          unstable I25.700
        ischemic chest pain I25.709
      autologous artery I25.810
        with
          angina pectoris I25.729
            with documented spasm
              I25.721
            specified type I25.728
            unstable I25.720
          ischemic chest pain I25.729
      autologous vein I25.810
        with
          angina pectoris I25.719
            with documented spasm
              I25.711
            specified type I25.718
            unstable I25.710
          ischemic chest pain I25.719
      nonautologous biological I25.810
        with
          angina pectoris I25.739
            with documented spasm
              I25.731
            specified type I25.738
            unstable I25.730
          ischemic chest pain I25.739
      specified type NEC I25.810
        with
          angina pectoris I25.799
            with documented spasm
              I25.791
            specified type I25.798
            unstable I25.790
          ischemic chest pain I25.799
    due to
      calcified coronary lesion (severely)
        I25.84
      lipid rich plaque I25.83
    native vessel
      with
        angina pectoris I25.119
          with documented spasm I25.111
          specified type NEC I25.118
          unstable I25.110
        ischemic chest pain I25.119
    transplanted heart I25.811
      bypass graft I25.812
        with
          angina pectoris I25.769
            with documented spasm
              I25.761
            specified type I25.768
            unstable I25.760
          ischemic chest pain I25.769
      native coronary artery I25.811
        with
          angina pectoris I25.759
            with documented spasm
              I25.751
            specified type I25.758
            unstable I25.750
          ischemic chest pain I25.759
  extremities (native arteries) I70.209
    bypass graft I70.309
      autologous vein graft I70.409
        leg I70.409
          with
            gangrene (and intermittent
              claudication, rest pain and
              ulcer) I70.469
            intermittent claudication
              I70.419
            rest pain (and intermittent
              claudication) I70.429

Arteriosclerosis, arteriosclerotic *(Continued)*
  extremities *(Continued)*
    bypass graft *(Continued)*
      autologous vein graft *(Continued)*
        leg *(Continued)*
          bilateral I70.403
            with
              gangrene (and intermittent
                claudication, rest pain
                and ulcer) I70.463
              intermittent claudication
                I70.413
              rest pain (and intermittent
                claudication) I70.423
            specified type NEC I70.493
          left I70.402
            with
              gangrene (and intermittent
                claudication, rest pain
                and ulcer) I70.462
              intermittent claudication
                I70.412
              rest pain (and intermittent
                claudication) I70.422
              ulceration (and intermittent
                claudication and rest
                pain) I70.449
              ankle I70.443
              calf I70.442
              foot site NEC I70.445
              heel I70.444
              lower leg NEC I70.448
              midfoot I70.444
              thigh I70.441
            specified type NEC I70.492
          right I70.401
            with
              gangrene (and intermittent
                claudication, rest pain
                and ulcer) I70.461
              intermittent claudication
                I70.411
              rest pain (and intermittent
                claudication) I70.421
              ulceration (and intermittent
                claudication and rest
                pain) I70.439
              ankle I70.433
              calf I70.432
              foot site NEC I70.435
               heel I70.434
              lower leg NEC I70.438
              midfoot I70.434
              thigh I70.431
            specified type NEC I70.491
          specified type NEC I70.499
        specified NEC I70.408
          with
            gangrene (and intermittent
              claudication, rest pain and
              ulcer) I70.468
            intermittent claudication I70.418
            rest pain (and intermittent
              claudication) I70.428
            ulceration (and intermittent
              claudication and rest pain)
             I70.45
          specified type NEC I70.498
      leg I70.309
        with
          gangrene (and intermittent
            claudication, rest pain and
            ulcer) I70.369
          intermittent claudication I70.319
          rest pain (and intermittent
            claudication) I70.329
        bilateral I70.303
          with
            gangrene (and intermittent
             claudication, rest pain and
             ulcer) I70.363

Arteriosclerosis, arteriosclerotic *(Continued)*
  extremities *(Continued)*
    bypass graft *(Continued)*
      leg *(Continued)*
        bilateral *(Continued)*
          with *(Continued)*
            intermittent claudication
              I70.313
            rest pain (and intermittent
              claudication) I70.323
            specified type NEC I70.393
          left I70.302
            with
              gangrene (and intermittent
                claudication, rest pain and
                ulcer) I70.362
              intermittent claudication I70.312
              rest pain (and intermittent
                claudication) I70.322
              ulceration (and intermittent
                claudication and rest pain)
                I70.349
              ankle I70.343
              calf I70.342
              foot site NEC I70.345
              heel I70.344
              lower leg NEC I70.348
              midfoot I70.344
              thigh I70.341
            specified type NEC I70.392
          right I70.301
            with
              gangrene (and intermittent
                claudication, rest pain and
                ulcer) I70.361
              intermittent claudication
                I70.311
              rest pain (and intermittent
                claudication) I70.321
              ulceration (and intermittent
                claudication and rest pain)
                I70.339
              ankle I70.333
              calf I70.332
              foot site NEC I70.335
              heel I70.334
              lower leg NEC I70.338
              midfoot I70.334
              thigh I70.331
            specified type NEC I70.391
          specified type NEC I70.399
      nonautologous biological graft I70.509
        leg I70.509
          with
            gangrene (and intermittent
             claudication, rest pain and
             ulcer) I70.569
            intermittent claudication
              I70.519
            rest pain (and intermittent
              claudication) I70.529
          bilateral I70.503
            with
              gangrene (and intermittent
                claudication, rest pain
                and ulcer) I70.563
              intermittent claudication
                I70.513
              rest pain (and intermittent
                claudication) I70.523
            specified type NEC I70.593
          left I70.502
            with
              gangrene (and intermittent
                claudication, rest pain
                and ulcer) I70.562
              intermittent claudication
                I70.512
              rest pain (and intermittent
                claudication)
                I70.522

Arteriosclerosis, arteriosclerotic (Continued)
  extremities (Continued)
    bypass graft (Continued)
      nonautologous biological graft
        (Continued)
        leg (Continued)
          left (Continued)
            with (Continued)
              ulceration (and intermittent
                claudication and rest
                pain) I70.549
              ankle I70.543
              calf I70.542
              foot site NEC I70.545
              heel I70.544
              lower leg NEC I70.548
              midfoot I70.544
              thigh I70.541
            specified type NEC I70.592
          right I70.501
            with
              gangrene (and intermittent
                claudication, rest pain
                and ulcer) I70.561
              intermittent claudication
                I70.511
              rest pain (and intermittent
                claudication) I70.521
              ulceration (and intermittent
                claudication and rest
                pain) I70.539
              ankle I70.533
              calf I70.532
              foot site NEC I70.535
               heel I70.534
              lower leg NEC I70.538
              midfoot I70.534
              thigh I70.531
            specified type NEC I70.591
          specified type NEC I70.599
        specified NEC I70.508
          with
            gangrene (and intermittent
              claudication, rest pain and
              ulcer) I70.568
            intermittent claudication I70.518
            rest pain (and intermittent
              claudication) I70.528
            ulceration (and intermittent
              claudication and rest pain)
              I70.55
          specified type NEC I70.598
      nonbiological graft I70.609
        leg I70.609
          with
            gangrene (and intermittent
              claudication, rest pain and
              ulcer) I70.669
            intermittent claudication
              I70.619
            rest pain (and intermittent
              claudication) I70.629
        bilateral I70.603
          with
            gangrene (and intermittent
              claudication, rest pain
              and ulcer) I70.663
            intermittent claudication
              I70.613
            rest pain (and intermittent
              claudication) I70.623
            specified type NEC I70.693
        left I70.602
          with
            gangrene (and intermittent
              claudication, rest pain
              and ulcer) I70.662
            intermittent claudication
              I70.612
            rest pain (and intermittent
              claudication) I70.622

Arteriosclerosis, arteriosclerotic (Continued)
  extremities (Continued)
    bypass graft (Continued)
      nonbiological graft (Continued)
        leg (Continued)
          left (Continued)
            with (Continued)
              ulceration (and intermittent
                claudication and rest
                pain) I70.649
              ankle I70.643
              calf I70.642
              foot site NEC I70.645
              heel I70.644
              lower leg NEC I70.648
              midfoot I70.644
              thigh I70.641
            specified type NEC I70.692
          right I70.601
            with
              gangrene (and intermittent
                claudication, rest pain
                and ulcer) I70.661
              intermittent claudication
                I70.611
              rest pain (and intermittent
                claudication) I70.621
              ulceration (and intermittent
                claudication and rest
                pain) I70.639
              ankle I70.633
              calf I70.632
              foot site NEC I70.635
              heel I70.634
              lower leg NEC I70.638
              midfoot I70.634
              thigh I70.631
            specified type NEC I70.691
          specified type NEC I70.699
        specified NEC I70.608
          with
            gangrene (and intermittent
              claudication, rest pain and
              ulcer) I70.668
            intermittent claudication
              I70.618
            rest pain (and intermittent
              claudication) I70.628
            ulceration (and intermittent
              claudication and rest pain)
              I70.65
          specified type NEC I70.698
      specified graft NEC I70.709
        leg I70.709
          with
            gangrene (and intermittent
              claudication, rest pain and
              ulcer) I70.769
            intermittent claudication
              I70.719
            rest pain (and intermittent
              claudication) I70.729
        bilateral I70.703
          with
            gangrene (and intermittent
              claudication, rest pain
              and ulcer) I70.763
            intermittent claudication
              I70.713
            rest pain (and intermittent
              claudication) I70.723
            specified type NEC I70.793
        left I70.702
          with
            gangrene (and intermittent
              claudication, rest pain
              and ulcer) I70.762
            intermittent claudication
              I70.712
            rest pain (and intermittent
              claudication) I70.722

Arteriosclerosis, arteriosclerotic (Continued)
  extremities (Continued)
    bypass graft (Continued)
      specified graft NEC (Continued)
        leg (Continued)
          left (Continued)
            with (Continued)
              ulceration (and intermittent
                claudication and rest
                pain) I70.749
              ankle I70.743
              calf I70.742
              foot site NEC I70.745
              heel I70.744
              lower leg NEC I70.748
              midfoot I70.744
              thigh I70.741
            specified type NEC I70.792
          right I70.701
            with
              gangrene (and intermittent
                claudication, rest pain
                and ulcer) I70.761
              intermittent claudication
                I70.711
              rest pain (and intermittent
                claudication) I70.721
              ulceration (and intermittent
                claudication and rest
                pain) I70.739
              ankle I70.733
              calf I70.732
              foot site NEC I70.735
              heel I70.734
              lower leg NEC I70.738
              midfoot I70.734
              thigh I70.731
            specified type NEC I70.791
          specified type NEC I70.799
        specified NEC I70.708
          with
            gangrene (and intermittent
              claudication, rest pain and
              ulcer) I70.768
            intermittent claudication
              I70.718
            rest pain (and intermittent
              claudication) I70.728
            ulceration (and intermittent
              claudication and rest pain)
              I70.75
          specified type NEC I70.798
        specified NEC I70.308
         with
           gangrene (and intermittent
             claudication, rest pain and
             ulcer) I70.368
          intermittent claudication I70.318
          rest pain (and intermittent
            claudication) I70.328
          ulceration (and intermittent
            claudication and rest pain)
            I70.35
        specified type NEC I70.398
      leg I70.209
        with
          gangrene (and intermittent
            claudication, rest pain and ulcer)
           I70.269
         intermittent claudication I70.219
         rest pain (and intermittent
          claudication) I70.229
      bilateral I70.203
        with
          gangrene (and intermittent
            claudication, rest pain and
            ulcer) I70.263
         intermittent claudication I70.213
         rest pain (and intermittent
          claudication) I70.223
        specified type NEC I70.293

◄ New   ◄▌▌ Revised   ~~deleted~~ Deleted

Arteriosclerosis, arteriosclerotic *(Continued)*
  extremities *(Continued)*
    leg *(Continued)*
      left I70.202
        with
          gangrene (and intermittent
            claudication, rest pain and
            ulcer) I70.262
          intermittent claudication I70.212
          rest pain (and intermittent
            claudication) I70.222
          ulceration (and intermittent
            claudication and rest pain)
            I70.249
            ankle I70.243
            calf I70.242
            foot site NEC I70.245
            heel I70.244
            lower leg NEC I70.248
            midfoot I70.244
            thigh I70.241
          specified type NEC I70.292
      right I70.201
        with
          gangrene (and intermittent
            claudication, rest pain and
            ulcer) I70.261
          intermittent claudication I70.211
          rest pain (and intermittent
            claudication) I70.221
          ulceration (and intermittent
            claudication and rest pain)
            I70.239
            ankle I70.233
            calf I70.232
            foot site NEC I70.235
            heel I70.234
            lower leg NEC I70.238
            midfoot I70.234
            thigh I70.231
          specified type NEC I70.291
      specified type NEC I70.299
    specified site NEC I70.208
      with
        gangrene (and intermittent
          claudication, rest pain and ulcer)
          I70.268
        intermittent claudication I70.218
        rest pain (and intermittent
          claudication) I70.228
        ulceration (and intermittent
          claudication and rest pain)
          I70.25
      specified type NEC I70.298
  generalized I70.91
  heart (disease) —*see* Arteriosclerosis,
    coronary (artery)
  kidney —*see* Hypertension, kidney
  medial —*see* Arteriosclerosis, extremities
  mesenteric (artery) K55.1
  Mönckeberg's —*see* Arteriosclerosis,
    extremities
  myocarditis I51.4
  peripheral (of extremities) —*see*
    Arteriosclerosis, extremities
  pulmonary (idiopathic) I27.0
  renal (arterioles) —*see also* Hypertension,
    kidney
    artery I70.1
  retina (vascular) I70.8 *[H35.0-]*
  specified artery NEC I70.8
  spinal (cord) G95.19
  vertebral (artery) I67.2
Arteriospasm I73.9
Arteriovenous —*see* condition
Arteritis I77.6
  allergic M31.0
  aorta (nonsyphilitic) I77.6
    syphilitic A52.02
  aortic arch M31.4
  brachiocephalic M31.4

Arteritis *(Continued)*
  brain I67.7
    syphilitic A52.04
  cerebral I67.7
    in
      diseases classified elsewhere I68.2
      systemic lupus erythematosus M32.19
    listerial A32.89
    syphilitic A52.04
    tuberculous A18.89
  coronary (artery) I25.89
    rheumatic I01.8
      chronic I09.89
    syphilitic A52.06
  cranial (left) (right), giant cell M31.6
  deformans —*see* Arteriosclerosis
  giant cell NEC M31.6
    with polymyalgia rheumatica M31.5
  necrosing or necrotizing M31.9
    specified NEC M31.8
  nodosa M30.0
  obliterans —*see* Arteriosclerosis
  pulmonary I28.8
  rheumatic —*see* Fever, rheumatic
  senile —*see* Arteriosclerosis
  suppurative I77.2
  syphilitic (general) A52.09
    brain A52.04
    coronary A52.06
    spinal A52.09
  temporal, giant cell M31.6
  young female aortic arch syndrome M31.4
Artery, arterial —*see also* condition
  abscess I77.89
  single umbilical Q27.0
Arthralgia (allergic) —*see also* Pain, joint
  in caisson disease T70.3
  temporomandibular M26.62
Arthritis, arthritic (acute) (chronic)
    (nonpyogenic) (subacute) M19.90
  allergic —*see* Arthritis, specified form NEC
  ankylosing (crippling) (spine) —*see also*
    Spondylitis, ankylosing
    sites other than spine —*see* Arthritis,
      specified form NEC
  atrophic —*see* Osteoarthritis
    spine —*see* Spondylitis, ankylosing
  back —*see* Spondylopathy, inflammatory
  blennorrhagic (gonococcal) A54.42
  Charcot's —*see* Arthropathy, neuropathic
    diabetic —*see* Diabetes, arthropathy,
      neuropathic
    syringomyelic G95.0
  chylous (filarial) (*see also* category M01) B74.9
  climacteric (any site) NEC —*see* Arthritis,
    specified form NEC
  crystal (-induced) —*see* Arthritis, in, crystals
  deformans —*see* Osteoarthritis
  degenerative —*see* Osteoarthritis
  due to or associated with
    acromegaly E22.0
    brucellosis —*see* Brucellosis
    caisson disease T70.3
    diabetes —*see* Diabetes, arthropathy
    dracontiasis (*see also* category M01) B72
    enteritis NEC
      regional —*see* Enteritis, regional
    erysipelas (*see also* category M01) A46
    erythema
      epidemic A25.1
      nodosum L52
    filariasis NOS B74.9
    glanders A24.0
    helminthiasis (*see also* category M01) B83.9
    hemophilia D66 *[M36.2]*
    Henoch-(Schönlein) purpura D69.0 *[M36.4]*
    human parvovirus (*see also* category M01)
      B97.6
    infectious disease NEC —*see* category M01
    leprosy (*see also* category M01) (*see also*
      Leprosy) A30.9

Arthritis, arthritic *(Continued)*
  due to or associated with *(Continued)*
    Lyme disease A69.23
    mycobacteria (*see also* category M01)
      A31.8
    parasitic disease NEC (*see also* category
      M01) B89
    paratyphoid fever (*see also* category M01)
      (*see also* Fever, paratyphoid) A01.4
    rat bite fever (*see also* category M01)
      A25.1
    regional enteritis —*see* Enteritis, regional
    respiratory disorder NOS J98.9
    serum sickness (*see also* Reaction, serum)
      T80.69
    syringomyelia G95.0
    typhoid fever A01.04
  epidemic erythema A25.1
  febrile —*see* Fever, rheumatic
  gonococcal A54.42
  gouty (acute) —*see* Gout, idiopathic
  in (due to)
    acromegaly (*see also* subcategory M14.8-)
      E22.0
    amyloidosis (*see also* subcategory M14.8-)
      E85.4
    bacterial disease (*see also* subcategory M01)
      A49.9
    Behçet's syndrome M35.2
    caisson disease (*see also* subcategory
      M14.8-) T70.3
    coliform bacilli (Escherichia coli) —*see*
      Arthritis, in, pyogenic organism NEC
    crystals M11.9
      dicalcium phosphate —*see* Arthritis, in,
        crystals, specified type NEC
      hydroxyapatite M11.0-
      pyrophosphate —*see* Arthritis, in,
        crystals, specified type NEC
      specified type NEC M11.80
        ankle M11.87-
        elbow M11.82-
        foot joint M11.87-
        hand joint M11.84-
        hip M11.85-
        knee M11.86-
        multiple sites M11.8-
        shoulder M11.81-
        vertebrae M11.88
        wrist M11.83-
    dermatoarthritis, lipoid E78.81
    dracontiasis (dracunculiasis) (*see also*
      category M01) B72
    endocrine disorder NEC (*see also*
      subcategory M14.8-) E34.9
    enteritis, infectious NEC (*see also* category
      M01) A09
      specified organism NEC (*see also*
        category M01) A08.8
    erythema
      multiforme (*see also* subcategory M14.8-)
        L51.9
      nodosum (*see also* subcategory M14.8-)
        L52
    gout —*see* Gout, idiopathic
    helminthiasis NEC (*see also* category M01)
      B83.9
    hemochromatosis (*see also* subcategory
      M14.8-) E83.118
    hemoglobinopathy NEC D58.2 *[M36.3]*
    hemophilia NEC D66 *[M36.2]*
    Hemophilus influenzae M00.8- *[B96.3]*
    Henoch(-Schönlein) purpura D69.0 *[M36.4]*
    hyperparathyroidism NEC (*see also*
      subcategory M14.8-) E21.3
    hypersensitivity reaction NEC T78.49
      [M36.4]
    hypogammaglobulinemia (*see also*
      subcategory M14.8-) D80.1
    hypothyroidism NEC (*see also* subcategory
      M14.8-) E03.9

Arthritis, arthritic *(Continued)*
 in *(Continued)*
  infection —*see* Arthritis, pyogenic or
   pyemic
  spine —*see* Spondylopathy, infective
  infectious disease NEC —*see* category
   M01
  leprosy *(see also* category M01) A30.9
  leukemia NEC C95.9- *[M36.1]*
  lipoid dermatoarthritis E78.81
  Lyme disease A69.23
  Mediterranean fever, familial *(see also*
   subcategory M14.8-) E85.0
  Meningococcus A39.83
  metabolic disorder NEC *(see also*
   subcategory M14.8-) E88.9
  multiple myelomatosis C90.0- *[M36.1]*
  mumps B26.85
  mycosis NEC *(see also* category M01)
   B49
  myelomatosis (multiple) C90.0- *[M36.1]*
  neurological disorder NEC G98.0
  ochronosis *(see also* subcategory M14.8-)
   E70.29
  O'nyong-nyong *(see also* category M01)
   A92.1
  parasitic disease NEC *(see also* category
   M01) B89
  paratyphoid fever *(see also* category M01)
   A01.4
  Pseudomonas —*see* Arthritis, pyogenic,
   bacterial NEC
  psoriasis L40.50
  pyogenic organism NEC —*see* Arthritis,
   pyogenic, bacterial NEC
  Reiter's disease —*see* Reiter's disease
  respiratory disorder NEC *(see also*
   subcategory M14.8-) J98.9
  reticulosis, malignant *(see also* subcategory
   M14.8-) C86.0
  rubella B06.82
  Salmonella (arizonae) (cholerae-suis)
   (enteritidis) (typhimurium)
   A02.23
  sarcoidosis D86.86
  specified bacteria NEC —*see* Arthritis,
   pyogenic, bacterial NEC
  sporotrichosis B42.82
  syringomyelia G95.0
  thalassemia NEC D56.9 *[M36.3]*
  tuberculosis —*see* Tuberculosis, arthritis
  typhoid fever A01.04
  urethritis, Reiter's —*see* Reiter's disease
  viral disease NEC *(see also* category M01)
   B34.9
 infectious or infective —*see also* Arthritis,
  pyogenic or pyemic
  spine —*see* Spondylopathy, infective
 juvenile M08.90
  with systemic onset —*see* Still's disease
  ankle M08.97-
  elbow M08.92-
  foot joint M08.97-
  hand joint M08.94-
  hip M08.95-
  knee M08.96-
  multiple site M08.99
  pauciarticular M08.40
   ankle M08.47-
   elbow M08.42-
   foot joint M08.47-
   hand joint M08.44-
   hip M08.45-
   knee M08.46-
   shoulder M08.41-
   vertebrae M08.48
   wrist M08.43-
  psoriatic L40.54
  rheumatoid —*see* Arthritis, rheumatoid,
   juvenile
  shoulder M08.91-

Arthritis, arthritic *(Continued)*
 juvenile *(Continued)*
  specified type NEC M08.80
   ankle M08.87-
   elbow M08.82-
   foot joint M08.87-
   hand joint M08.84-
   hip M08.85-
   knee M08.86-
   multiple site M08.89
   shoulder M08.81-
   specified joint NEC M08.88
   vertebrae M08.88 ◀
   wrist M08.83-
  vertebra M08.98
  wrist M08.93-
 meaning osteoarthritis —*see* Osteoarthritis
 meningococcal A39.83
 menopausal (any site) NEC —*see* Arthritis,
  specified form NEC
 mutilans (psoriatic) L40.52
 mycotic NEC *(see also* category M01) B49
 neuropathic (Charcot) —*see* Arthropathy,
  neuropathic
  diabetic —*see* Diabetes, arthropathy,
   neuropathic
  nonsyphilitic NEC G98.0
  syringomyelic G95.0
 ochronotic *(see also* subcategory M14.8-) E70.29
 palindromic (any site) —*see* Rheumatism,
  palindromic
 pneumococcal M00.10
  ankle M00.17-
  elbow M00.12-
  foot joint —*see* Arthritis, pneumococcal,
   ankle
  hand joint M00.14-
  hip M00.15-
  knee M00.16-
  multiple site M00.19
  shoulder M00.11-
  vertebra M00.18
  wrist M00.13-
 postdysenteric —*see* Arthropathy,
  postdysenteric
 postmeningococcal A39.84
 postrheumatic, chronic —*see* Arthropathy,
  postrheumatic, chronic
 primary progressive —*see also* Arthritis,
  specified form NEC
  spine —*see* Spondylitis, ankylosing
 psoriatic L40.50
 purulent (any site except spine) —*see*
  Arthritis, pyogenic or pyemic
  spine —*see* Spondylopathy, infective
 pyogenic or pyemic (any site except spine)
  M00.9
  bacterial NEC M00.80
   ankle M00.87-
   elbow M00.82-
   foot joint —*see* Arthritis, pyogenic,
    bacterial NEC, ankle
   hand joint M00.84-
   hip M00.85-
   knee M00.86-
   multiple site M00.89
   shoulder M00.81-
   vertebra M00.88
   wrist M00.83-
  pneumococcal —*see* Arthritis,
   pneumococcal
  spine —*see* Spondylopathy, infective
  staphylococcal —*see* Arthritis,
   staphylococcal
  streptococcal —*see* Arthritis, streptococcal
   NEC
   pneumococcal —*see* Arthritis,
    pneumococcal
 reactive —*see* Reiter's disease
 rheumatic —*see also* Arthritis, rheumatoid
  acute or subacute —*see* Fever, rheumatic

Arthritis, arthritic *(Continued)*
 rheumatoid M06.9
  with
   carditis —*see* Rheumatoid, carditis
   endocarditis —*see* Rheumatoid, carditis
   heart involvement NEC —*see*
    Rheumatoid, carditis
   lung involvement —*see* Rheumatoid,
    lung
   myocarditis —*see* Rheumatoid, carditis
   myopathy —*see* Rheumatoid, myopathy
   pericarditis —*see* Rheumatoid, carditis
   polyneuropathy —*see* Rheumatoid,
    polyneuropathy
   rheumatoid factor —*see* Arthritis,
    rheumatoid, seropositive
   splenoadenomegaly and leukopenia —
    see Felty's syndrome
   vasculitis —*see* Rheumatoid, vasculitis
   visceral involvement NEC —*see*
    Rheumatoid, arthritis, with
    involvement of organs NEC
  juvenile (with or without rheumatoid
   factor) M08.00
   ankle M08.07-
   elbow M08.02-
   foot joint M08.07-
   hand joint M08.04-
   hip M08.05-
   knee M08.06-
   multiple site M08.09
   shoulder M08.01-
   vertebra M08.08
   wrist M08.03-
  seronegative M06.00
   ankle M06.07-
   elbow M06.02-
   foot joint M06.07-
   hand joint M06.04-
   hip M06.05-
   knee M06.06-
   multiple sites M06.09
   shoulder M06.01-
   vertebra M06.08
   wrist M06.03-
  seropositive M05.9
   without organ involvement M05.70
    ankle M05.77-
    elbow M05.72-
    foot joint M05.77-
    hand joint M05.74-
    hip M05.75-
    knee M05.76-
    multiple sites M05.79
    shoulder M05.71-
    vertebra —*see* Spondylitis, ankylosing
    wrist M05.73-
   specified NEC M05.80
    ankle M05.87-
    elbow M05.82-
    foot joint M05.87-
    hand joint M05.84-
    hip M05.85-
    knee M05.86-
    multiple sites M05.89
    shoulder M05.81-
    vertebra —*see* Spondylitis, ankylosing
    wrist M05.83-
  specified type NEC M06.80
   ankle M06.87-
   elbow M06.82-
   foot joint M06.87-
   hand joint M06.84-
   hip M06.85-
   knee M06.86-
   multiple site M06.89
   shoulder M06.81-
   vertebra M06.88
   wrist M06.83-
  spine —*see* Spondylitis, ankylosing
 rubella B06.82

◀ New ◀◀◀ Revised ~~deleted~~ Deleted

Arthritis, arthritic *(Continued)*
  scorbutic *(see also* subcategory M14.8-) E54
  senile or senescent —*see* Osteoarthritis
  septic (any site except spine) —*see* Arthritis,
    pyogenic or pyemic
    spine —*see* Spondylopathy, infective
  serum (nontherapeutic) (therapeutic) —*see*
    Arthropathy, postimmunization
  specified form NEC M13.80
    ankle M13.87-
    elbow M13.82-
    foot joint M13.87-
    hand joint M13.84-
    hip M13.85-
    knee M13.86-
    multiple site M13.89
    shoulder M13.81-
    specified joint NEC M13.88
    wrist M13.83-
  spine —*see also* Spondylopathy,
      inflammatory
    infectious or infective NEC —*see*
        Spondylopathy, infective
    Marie-Strümpell —*see* Spondylitis,
        ankylosing
    pyogenic —*see* Spondylopathy, infective
    rheumatoid —*see* Spondylitis, ankylosing
    traumatic (old) —*see* Spondylopathy,
        traumatic
    tuberculous A18.01
  staphylococcal M00.00
    ankle M00.07-
    elbow M00.02-
    foot joint —*see* Arthritis, staphylococcal,
        ankle
    hand joint M00.04-
    hip M00.05-
    knee M00.06-
    multiple site M00.09
    shoulder M00.01-
    vertebra M00.08
    wrist M00.03-
  streptococcal NEC M00.20
    ankle M00.27-
    elbow M00.22-
    foot joint —*see* Arthritis, streptococcal,
        ankle
    hand joint M00.24-
    hip M00.25-
    knee M00.26-
    multiple site M00.29
    shoulder M00.21-
    vertebra M00.28
    wrist M00.23-
  suppurative —*see* Arthritis, pyogenic or
      pyemic
  syphilitic (late) A52.16
    congenital A50.55 *[M12.80]*
  syphilitica deformans (Charcot) A52.16
  temporomandibular M26.69
  toxic of menopause (any site) —*see* Arthritis,
      specified form NEC
  transient —*see* Arthropathy, specified form
      NEC
  traumatic (chronic) —*see* Arthropathy,
      traumatic
  tuberculous A18.02
    spine A18.01
  uratic —*see* Gout, idiopathic
  urethritica (Reiter's) —*see* Reiter's disease
  vertebral —*see* Spondylopathy, inflammatory
  villous (any site) —*see* Arthropathy, specified
      form NEC
Arthrocele —*see* Effusion, joint
Arthrodesis status Z98.1
Arthrodynia —*see also* Pain, joint
Arthrodysplasia Q74.9
Arthrofibrosis, joint —*see* Ankylosis
Arthrogryposis (congenital) Q68.8
  multiplex congenita Q74.3
Arthrokatadysis M24.7

Arthropathy *(see also* Arthritis) M12.9
  Charcot's —*see* Arthropathy, neuropathic
    diabetic —*see* Diabetes, arthropathy,
        neuropathic
    syringomyelic G95.0
  cricoarytenoid J38.7
  crystal(-induced) —*see* Arthritis, in, crystals
  diabetic NEC —*see* Diabetes, arthropathy
  distal interphalangeal, psoriatic L40.51
  enteropathic M07.60
    ankle M07.67-
    elbow M07.62-
    foot joint M07.67-
    hand joint M07.64-
    hip M07.65-
    knee M07.66-
    multiple site M07.69
    shoulder M07.61-
    vertebra M07.68
    wrist M07.63-
  following intestinal bypass M02.00
    ankle M02.07-
    elbow M02.02-
    foot joint M02.07-
    hand joint M02.04-
    hip M02.05-
    knee M02.06-
    multiple site M02.09
    shoulder M02.01-
    vertebra M02.08
    wrist M02.03-
  gouty —*see also* Gout, idiopathic
    in (due to)
      Lesch-Nyhan syndrome E79.1 *[M14.8-]*
      sickle-cell disorders D57- *[M14.8-]*
  hemophilic NEC D66 *[M36.2]*
    in (due to)
      hyperparathyroidism NEC E21.3
          [M14.8-]
      metabolic disease NOS E88.9 *[M14.8-]*
  in (due to)
    acromegaly E22.0 *[M14.8-]*
    amyloidosis E85.4 *[M14.8-]*
    blood disorder NOS D75.9 *[M36.3]*
    diabetes —*see* Diabetes, arthropathy
    endocrine disease NOS E34.9 *[M14.8-]*
    erythema
      multiforme L51.9 *[M14.8-]*
      nodosum L52 *[M14.8-]*
    hemochromatosis E83.118 *[M14.8-]*
    hemoglobinopathy NEC D58.2 *[M36.3]*
    hemophilia NEC D66 *[M36.2]*
    Henoch-Schönlein purpura D69.0
        [M36.4]
    hyperthyroidism E05.90 *[M14.8-]*
    hypothyroidism E03.9 *[M14.8-]*
    infective endocarditis I33.0 *[M12.80]*
    leukemia NEC C95.9- *[M36.1]*
    malignant histiocytosis C96.A *[M36.1]*
    metabolic disease NOS E88.9 *[M14.8-]*
    multiple myeloma C90.0- *[M36.1]*
    neoplastic disease NOS *(see also* Neoplasm)
        D49.9 *[M36.1]*
    nutritional deficiency *(see also* subcategory
        M14.8-) E63.9
    psoriasis NOS L40.50
    sarcoidosis D86.86
    syphilis (late) A52.77
      congenital A50.55 *[M12.80]*
    thyrotoxicosis *(see also* subcategory M14.8-)
        E05.90
    ulcerative colitis K51.90 *[M07.60]*
    viral hepatitis (postinfectious) NEC B19.9
        [M12.80]
    Whipple's disease *(see also* subcategory
        M14.8-) K90.81
  Jaccoud —*see* Arthropathy, postrheumatic,
      chronic
  juvenile —*see* Arthritis, juvenile
    psoriatic L40.54
  mutilans (psoriatic) L40.52

Arthropathy *(Continued)*
  neuropathic (Charcot) M14.60
    ankle M14.67-
    diabetic —*see* Diabetes, arthropathy,
        neuropathic
    elbow M14.62-
    foot joint M14.67-
    hand joint M14.64-
    hip M14.65-
    knee M14.66-
    multiple site M14.69
    nonsyphilitic NEC G98.0
    shoulder M14.61-
    syringomyelic G95.0
    vertebra M14.68
    wrist M14.63-
  osteopulmonary —*see* Osteoarthropathy,
      hypertrophic, specified NEC
  postdysenteric M02.10
    ankle M02.17-
    elbow M02.12-
    foot joint M02.17-
    hand joint M02.14-
    hip M02.15-
    knee M02.16-
    multiple site M02.19
    shoulder M02.11-
    vertebra M02.18
    wrist M02.13-
  postimmunization M02.20
    ankle M02.27-
    elbow M02.22-
    foot joint M02.27-
    hand joint M02.24-
    hip M02.25-
    knee M02.26-
    multiple site M02.29
    shoulder M02.21-
    vertebra M02.28
    wrist M02.23-
  postinfectious NEC B99 *[M12.80]*
    in (due to)
      enteritis due to Yersinia enterocolitica
          A04.6 *[M12.80]*
      syphilis A52.77
      viral hepatitis NEC B19.9 *[M12.80]*
  postrheumatic, chronic (Jaccoud) M12.00
    ankle M12.07-
    elbow M12.02-
    foot joint M12.07-
    hand joint M12.04-
    hip M12.05-
    knee M12.06-
    multiple site M12.09
    shoulder M12.01-
    specified joint NEC M12.08
    vertebrae M12.08 ◀
    wrist M12.03-
  psoriatic NEC L40.59
    interphalangeal, distal L40.51
  reactive M02.9
    in (due to)
      infective endocarditis I33.0 *[M02.9]*
    specified type NEC M02.80
      ankle M02.87-
      elbow M02.82-
      foot joint M02.87-
      hand joint M02.84-
      hip M02.85-
      knee M02.86-
      multiple site M02.89
      shoulder M02.81-
      vertebra M02.88
      wrist M02.83-
  specified form NEC M12.80
    ankle M12.87-
    elbow M12.82-
    foot joint M12.87-
    hand joint M12.84-
    hip M12.85-
    knee M12.86-
    multiple site M12.89

Arthropathy (Continued)
  specified form NEC (Continued)
    shoulder M12.81-
    specified joint NEC M12.88
    vertebrae M12.88 ◄
    wrist M12.83-
  syringomyelic G95.0
  tabes dorsalis A52.16
  tabetic A52.16
  transient —see Arthropathy, specified form
    NEC
  traumatic M12.50
    ankle M12.57-
    elbow M12.52-
    foot joint M12.57-
    hand joint M12.54-
    hip M12.55-
    knee M12.56-
    multiple site M12.59
    shoulder M12.51-
    specified joint NEC M12.58
    vertebrae M12.58 ◄
    wrist M12.53-
Arthropyosis —see Arthritis, pyogenic or pyemic
Arthrosis (deformans) (degenerative) (localized)
  (see also Osteoarthritis) M19.90
  spine —see Spondylosis
Arthus' phenomenon or reaction T78.41
  due to
    drug —see Table of ᵈDrugs and
      ᶜChemicals, by drug ◄▥
Articular —see condition
Articulation, reverse (teeth) M26.24
Artificial
  insemination complication —see
    Complications, artificial, fertilization
  opening status (functioning) (without
    complication) Z93.9
    anus (colostomy) Z93.3
    colostomy Z93.3
    cystostomy Z93.50
      appendico-vesicostomy Z93.52
      cutaneous Z93.51
      specified NEC Z93.59
    enterostomy Z93.4
    gastrostomy Z93.1
    ileostomy Z93.2
    intestinal tract NEC Z93.4
    jejunostomy Z93.4
    nephrostomy Z93.6
    specified site NEC Z93.8
    tracheostomy Z93.0
    ureterostomy Z93.6
    urethrostomy Z93.6
    urinary tract NEC Z93.6
    vagina Z93.8
  vagina status Z93.8
Arytenoid —see condition
Asbestosis (occupational) J61
ASC-H (atypical squamous cells cannot exclude
  high grade squamous intraepithelial lesion
  on cytologic smear)
  anus R85.611
  cervix R87.611
  vagina R87.621
ASC-US (atypical squamous cells of
  undetermined significance on cytologic
  smear)
  anus R85.610
  cervix R87.610
  vagina R87.620
Ascariasis B77.9
  with
    complications NEC B77.89
    intestinal complications B77.0
    pneumonia, pneumonitis B77.81
Ascaridosis, ascaridiasis —see Ascariasis
Ascaris (infection) (infestation)
  (lumbricoides) —see Ascariasis
Ascending —see condition
Aschoff's bodies —see Myocarditis, rheumatic

Ascites (abdominal) R18.8
  cardiac I50.9
  chylous (nonfilarial) I89.8
    filarial —see Infestation, filarial
  due to
    cirrhosis, alcoholic K70.31
    hepatitis
      alcoholic K70.11
      chronic active K71.51
    S. japonicum B65.2
  heart I50.9
  malignant R18.0
  pseudochylous R18.8
  syphilitic A52.74
  tuberculous A18.31
Aseptic —see condition
Asherman's syndrome N85.6
Asialia K11.7
Asiatic cholera —see Cholera
Asimultagnosia (simultanagnosia) R48.3
Askin's tumor —see Neoplasm, connective
  tissue, malignant
Asocial personality F60.2
Asomatognosia R41.4
Aspartylglucosaminuria E77.1
Asperger's disease or syndrome F84.5
Aspergilloma —see Aspergillosis
Aspergillosis (with pneumonia) B44.9
  bronchopulmonary, allergic B44.81
  disseminated B44.7
  generalized B44.7
  pulmonary NEC B44.1
    allergic B44.81
    invasive B44.0
  specified NEC B44.89
  tonsillar B44.2
Aspergillus (flavus) (fumigatus) (infection)
  (terreus) —see Aspergillosis
Aspermatogenesis —see Azoospermia
Aspermia (testis) —see Azoospermia
Asphyxia, asphyxiation (by) R09.01
  antenatal P84
  birth P84
  bunny bag —see Asphyxia, due to,
    mechanical threat to breathing, trapped
    in bed clothes
  crushing S28.0
  drowning T75.1
  gas, fumes, or vapor —see Table of ᵈDrugs
    and ᶜChemicals ◄▥
  inhalation —see Inhalation
  intrauterine P84
  local I73.00
    with gangrene I73.01
  mucus —see also Foreign body, respiratory
    tract, causing asphyxia
  newborn P84
  pathological R09.01
  postnatal P84
    mechanical —see Asphyxia, due to,
      mechanical threat to breathing
  prenatal P84
  reticularis R23.1
  strangulation —see Asphyxia, due to,
    mechanical threat to breathing
  submersion T75.1
  traumatic T71.9
    due to
      crushed chest S28.0
      foreign body (in) —see Foreign body,
        respiratory tract, causing asphyxia
      low oxygen content of ambient air T71.20
      due to
        being trapped in
          low oxygen environment T71.29
          in car trunk T71.221
            circumstances undetermined
              T71.224
            done with intent to harm by
              another person T71.223
            self T71.222

Asphyxia, asphyxiation (Continued)
  traumatic (Continued)
    due to (Continued)
      low oxygen content of ambient air
        (Continued)
        due to (Continued)
          being trapped in (Continued)
            low oxygen environment
              (Continued)
              in refrigerator T71.231
                circumstances undetermined
                  T71.234
                done with intent to harm by
                  another person T71.233
                self T71.232
        cave-in T71.21
      mechanical threat to breathing
        (accidental) T71.191
      circumstances undetermined T71.194
      done with intent to harm by
        another person T71.193
        self T71.192
      hanging T71.161
        circumstances undetermined
          T71.164
        done with intent to harm by
          another person T71.163
        self T71.162
      plastic bag T71.121
        circumstances undetermined
          T71.124
        done with intent to harm by
          another person T71.123
        self T71.122
      smothering
        in furniture T71.151
          circumstances undetermined
            T71.154
          done with intent to harm by
            another person T71.153
          self T71.152
        under
          another person's body T71.141
            circumstances undetermined
              T71.144
            done with intent to harm
              T71.143
          pillow T71.111
            circumstances undetermined
              T71.114
            done with intent to harm by
              another person T71.113
              self T71.112
      trapped in bed clothes T71.131
        circumstances undetermined
          T71.134
        done with intent to harm by
          another person T71.133
        self T71.132
  vomiting, vomitus —see Foreign body,
    respiratory tract, causing asphyxia
Aspiration
  amniotic (clear) fluid (newborn) P24.10
    with
      pneumonia (pneumonitis) P24.11
      respiratory symptoms P24.11
  blood
    newborn (without respiratory symptoms)
      P24.20
      with
        pneumonia (pneumonitis) P24.21
        respiratory symptoms P24.21
    specified age NEC —see Foreign body,
      respiratory tract
  bronchitis J69.0
  food or foreign body (with asphyxiation) —
    see Asphyxia, food ◄▥
  liquor (amnii) (newborn) P24.10
    with
      pneumonia (pneumonitis) P24.11
      respiratory symptoms P24.11

◄ New   ▥ Revised   ~~deleted~~ Deleted

Aspiration *(Continued)*
  meconium (newborn) (without respiratory symptoms) P24.00
    with
      pneumonitis (pneumonitis) P24.01
      respiratory symptoms P24.01
  milk (newborn) (without respiratory symptoms) P24.30
    with
      pneumonia (pneumonitis) P24.31
      respiratory symptoms P24.31
    specified age NEC —*see* Foreign body, respiratory tract
  mucus —*see also* Foreign body, by site, causing asphyxia
    newborn P24.10
      with
        pneumonia (pneumonitis) P24.11
        respiratory symptoms P24.11
    neonatal P24.9
      specific NEC (without respiratory symptoms) P24.80
        with
          pneumonia (pneumonitis) P24.81
          respiratory symptoms P24.81
    newborn P24.9
      specific NEC (without respiratory symptoms) P24.80
        with
          pneumonia (pneumonitis) P24.81
          respiratory symptoms P24.81
  pneumonia J69.0
  pneumonitis J69.0
  syndrome of newborn —*see* Aspiration, by substance, with pneumonia
  vernix caseosa (newborn) P24.80
    with
      pneumonia (pneumonitis) P24.81
      respiratory symptoms P24.81
  vomitus —*see also* Foreign body, respiratory tract
    newborn (without respiratory symptoms) P24.30
      with
        pneumonia (pneumonitis) P24.31
        respiratory symptoms P24.31
Asplenia (congenital) Q89.01
  postsurgical Z90.81
Assam fever B55.0
Assault, sexual —*see* Maltreatment
Assmann's focus NEC A15.0
Astasia (-abasia) (hysterical) F44.4
Asteatosis cutis L85.3
Astereognosia, astereognosis R48.1
Asterixis R27.8
  in liver disease K71.3
Asteroid hyalitis —*see* Deposit, crystalline
Asthenia, asthenic R53.1
  cardiac (*see also* Failure, heart) I50.9
    psychogenic F45.8
  cardiovascular (*see also* Failure, heart) I50.9
    psychogenic F45.8
  heart (*see also* Failure, heart) I50.9
    psychogenic F45.8
  hysterical F44.4
  myocardial (*see also* Failure, heart) I50.9
    psychogenic F45.8
  nervous F48.8
  neurocirculatory F45.8
  neurotic F48.8
  psychogenic F48.8
  psychoneurotic F48.8
  psychophysiologic F48.8
  reaction (psychophysiologic) F48.8
  senile R54
Asthenopia —*see also* Discomfort, visual
  hysterical F44.6
  psychogenic F44.6

Asthenospermia —*see* Abnormal, specimen, male genital organs
Asthma, asthmatic (bronchial) (catarrh) (spasmodic) J45.909
  with
    chronic obstructive bronchitis J44.9
      with
        acute lower respiratory infection J44.0
        exacerbation (acute) J44.1
    chronic obstructive pulmonary disease J44.9
      with
        acute lower respiratory infection J44.0
        exacerbation (acute) J44.1
    exacerbation (acute) J45.901
    hay fever —*see* Asthma, allergic extrinsic
    rhinitis, allergic —*see* Asthma, allergic extrinsic
    status asthmaticus J45.902
  allergic extrinsic J45.909
    with
      exacerbation (acute) J45.901
      status asthmaticus J45.902
  atopic —*see* Asthma, allergic extrinsic
  cardiac —*see* Failure, ventricular, left
  cardiobronchial I50.1
  childhood J45.909
    with
      exacerbation (acute) J45.901
      status asthmaticus J45.902
  chronic obstructive J44.9
    with
      acute lower respiratory infection J44.0
      exacerbation (acute) J44.1
  collier's J60
  cough variant J45.991
  detergent J69.8
  due to
    detergent J69.8
    inhalation of fumes J68.3
  eosinophilic J82
  extrinsic, allergic —*see* Asthma, allergic extrinsic
  grinder's J62.8
  hay —*see* Asthma, allergic extrinsic
  heart I50.1
  idiosyncratic —*see* Asthma, nonallergic
  intermittent (mild) J45.20
    with
      exacerbation (acute) J45.21
      status asthmaticus J45.22
  intrinsic, nonallergic —*see* Asthma, nonallergic
  Kopp's E32.8
  late-onset J45.909
    with
      exacerbation (acute) J45.901
      status asthmaticus J45.902
  mild intermittent J45.20
    with
      exacerbation (acute) J45.21
      status asthmaticus J45.22
  mild persistent J45.30
    with
      exacerbation (acute) J45.31
      status asthmaticus J45.32
  Millar's (laryngismus stridulus) J38.5
  miner's J60
  mixed J45.909
    with
      exacerbation (acute) J45.901
      status asthmaticus J45.902
  moderate persistent J45.40
    with
      exacerbation (acute) J45.41
      status asthmaticus J45.42

Asthma, asthmatic *(Continued)*
  nervous —*see* Asthma, nonallergic
  nonallergic (intrinsic) J45.909
    with
      exacerbation (acute) J45.901
      status asthmaticus J45.902
  persistent
    mild J45.30
      with
        exacerbation (acute) J45.31
        status asthmaticus J45.32
    moderate J45.40
      with
        exacerbation (acute) J45.41
        status asthmaticus J45.42
    severe J45.50
      with
        exacerbation (acute) J45.51
        status asthmaticus J45.52
  platinum J45.998
  pneumoconiotic NEC J64
  potter's J62.8
  predominantly allergic J45.909
  psychogenic F54
  pulmonary eosinophilic J82
  red cedar J67.8
  Rostan's I50.1
  sandblaster's J62.8
  sequoiosis J67.8
  severe persistent J45.50
    with
      exacerbation (acute) J45.51
      status asthmaticus J45.52
  specified NEC J45.998
  stonemason's J62.8
  thymic E32.8
  tuberculous —*see* Tuberculosis, pulmonary
  Wichmann's (laryngismus stridulus) J38.5
  wood J67.8
Astigmatism (compound) (congenital) H52.20-
  irregular H52.21-
  regular H52.22-
Astraphobia F40.220
Astroblastoma
  specified site —*see* Neoplasm, malignant, by site
  unspecified site C71.9
Astrocytoma (cystic)
  anaplastic
    specified site —*see* Neoplasm, malignant, by site
    unspecified site C71.9
  fibrillary
    specified site —*see* Neoplasm, malignant, by site
    unspecified site C71.9
  fibrous
    specified site —*see* Neoplasm, malignant, by site
    unspecified site C71.9
  gemistocytic
    specified site —*see* Neoplasm, malignant, by site
    unspecified site C71.9
  juvenile
    specified site —*see* Neoplasm, malignant, by site
    unspecified site C71.9
  pilocytic
    specified site —*see* Neoplasm, malignant, by site
    unspecified site C71.9
  piloid
    specified site —*see* Neoplasm, malignant, by site
    unspecified site C71.9
  protoplasmic
    specified site —*see* Neoplasm, malignant, by site
    unspecified site C71.9

Astrocytoma (Continued)
  specified site NEC —see Neoplasm,
    malignant, by site
  subependymal D43.2
    giant cell
      specified site —see Neoplasm, uncertain
        behavior, by site
      unspecified site D43.2
    specified site —see Neoplasm, uncertain
      behavior, by site
    unspecified site D43.2
  unspecified site C71.9
Astroglioma
  specified site —see Neoplasm, malignant, by
    site
  unspecified site C71.9
Asymbolia R48.8
Asymmetry —see also Distortion
  between native and reconstructed breast N65.1
  face Q67.0
  jaw (lower) —see Anomaly, dentofacial, jaw-
    cranial base relationship, asymmetry
Asynergia, asynergy R27.8
  ventricular I51.89
Asystole (heart) —see Arrest, cardiac
At risk
  for falling Z91.81
Ataxia, ataxy, ataxic R27.0
  acute R27.8
  brain (hereditary) G11.9
  cerebellar (hereditary) G11.9
    with defective DNA repair G11.3
    alcoholic G31.2
    early-onset G11.1
    in
      alcoholism G31.2
      myxedema E03.9 [G13.2]
      neoplastic disease (see also Neoplasm)
        D49.9 [G13.1]
      specified disease NEC G32.81
    late-onset (Marie's) G11.2
  cerebral (hereditary) G11.9
  congenital nonprogressive G11.0
  family, familial —see Ataxia, hereditary
  following
    cerebrovascular disease I69.993
      cerebral infarction I69.393
      intracerebral hemorrhage I69.193
      nontraumatic intracranial hemorrhage
        NEC I69.293
      specified disease NEC I69.893
      subarachnoid hemorrhage I69.093
  Friedreich's (heredofamilial) (cerebellar)
    (spinal) G11.1
  gait R26.0
    hysterical F44.4
  general R27.8
  gluten M35.9 [G32.81] ◀
    with celiac disease K90.0 [G32.81] ◀
  hereditary G11.9
    with neuropathy G60.2
    cerebellar —see Ataxia, cerebellar
    spastic G11.4
    specified NEC G11.8
    spinal (Friedreich's) G11.1
  heredofamilial —see Ataxia, hereditary
  Hunt's G11.1
  hysterical F44.4
  locomotor (progressive) (syphilitic) (partial)
    (spastic) A52.11
    diabetic —see Diabetes, ataxia
  Marie's (cerebellar) (heredofamilial) (late-
    onset) G11.2
  nonorganic origin F44.4
  nonprogressive, congenital G11.0
  psychogenic F44.4
  Roussy-Lévy G60.0
  Sanger-Brown's (hereditary) G11.2
  spastic hereditary G11.4
  spinal
    hereditary (Friedreich's) G11.1
    progressive (syphilitic) A52.11

Ataxia, ataxy, ataxic (Continued)
  spinocerebellar, X-linked recessive G11.1
  telangiectasia (Louis-Bar) G11.3
Ataxia-telangiectasia (Louis-Bar) G11.3
Atelectasis (massive) (partial) (pressure)
  (pulmonary) J98.11
  newborn P28.10
    due to resorption P28.11
    partial P28.19
    primary P28.0
    secondary P28.19
  primary (newborn) P28.0
  tuberculous —see Tuberculosis, pulmonary
Atelocardia Q24.9
Atelomyelia Q06.1
Atheroembolism
  of
    extremities
      lower I75.02-
      upper I75.01-
    kidney I75.81
    specified NEC I75.89
Atheroma, atheromatous (see also
  Arteriosclerosis) I70.90
  aorta, aortic I70.0
    valve (see also Endocarditis, aortic) I35.8
  aorto-iliac I70.0
  artery —see Arteriosclerosis
  basilar (artery) I67.2
  carotid (artery) (common) (internal) I67.2
  cerebral (arteries) I67.2
  coronary (artery) I25.10
    with angina pectoris —see Arteriosclerosis,
      coronary (artery)
  degeneration —see Arteriosclerosis
  heart, cardiac —see Disease, heart, ischemic,
    atherosclerotic
  mitral (valve) I34.8
  myocardium, myocardial —see Disease, heart,
    ischemic, atherosclerotic
  pulmonary valve (heart) (see also
    Endocarditis, pulmonary) I37.8
  tricuspid (heart) (valve) I36.8
  valve, valvular —see Endocarditis
  vertebral (artery) I67.2
Atheromatosis —see Arteriosclerosis
Atherosclerosis —see also Arteriosclerosis
  coronary
    artery I25.10
      with angina pectoris —see
        Arteriosclerosis, coronary (artery),
      due to
        calcified coronary lesion (severely)
          I25.84
        lipid rich plaque I25.83
    transplanted heart I25.811
      bypass graft I25.812
        with angina pectoris —see
          Arteriosclerosis, coronary (artery)
      native coronary artery I25.811
        with angina pectoris —see
          Arteriosclerosis, coronary (artery)
Athetosis (acquired) R25.8
  bilateral (congenital) G80.3
  congenital (bilateral) (double) G80.3
  double (congenital) G80.3
  unilateral R25.8
Athlete's
  foot B35.3
  heart I51.7
Athrepsia E41
Athyrea (acquired) —see also Hypothyroidism
  congenital E03.1
Atonia, atony, atonic
  bladder (sphincter) (neurogenic) N31.2
  capillary I78.8
  cecum K59.8
    psychogenic F45.8
  colon —see Atony, intestine
  congenital P94.2
  esophagus K22.8

Atonia, atony, atonic (Continued)
  intestine K59.8
    psychogenic F45.8
  stomach K31.89
    neurotic or psychogenic F45.8
  uterus (during labor) O62.2
    with hemorrhage (postpartum) O72.1
    postpartum (with hemorrhage) O72.1
      without hemorrhage O75.89
Atopy —see History, allergy
Atransferrinemia, congenital E88.09
Atresia, atretic
  alimentary organ or tract NEC Q45.8
    upper Q40.8
  ani, anus, anal (canal) Q42.3
    with fistula Q42.2
  aorta (arch) (ring) Q25.2
  aortic (orifice) (valve) Q23.0
    arch Q25.2
    congenital with hypoplasia of ascending
      aorta and defective development of
      left ventricle (with mitral stenosis)
      Q23.4
    in hypoplastic left heart syndrome Q23.4
  aqueduct of Sylvius Q03.0
    with spina bifida —see Spina bifida, with
      hydrocephalus
  artery NEC Q27.8
    cerebral Q28.3
    coronary Q24.5
    digestive system Q27.8
    eye Q15.8
    lower limb Q27.8
    pulmonary Q25.5
    specified site NEC Q27.8
    umbilical Q27.0
    upper limb Q27.8
  auditory canal (external) Q16.1
  bile duct (common) (congenital) (hepatic)
    Q44.2
    acquired —see Obstruction, bile duct
  bladder (neck) Q64.39
    obstruction Q64.31
  bronchus Q32.4
  cecum Q42.8
  cervix (acquired) N88.2
    congenital Q51.828
    in pregnancy or childbirth —see Anomaly,
      cervix, in pregnancy or childbirth
    causing obstructed labor O65.5
  choana Q30.0
  colon Q42.9
    specified NEC Q42.8
  common duct Q44.2
  cricoid cartilage Q31.8
  cystic duct Q44.2
    acquired K82.8
      with obstruction K82.0
  digestive organs NEC Q45.8
  duodenum Q41.0
  ear canal Q16.1
  ejaculatory duct Q55.4
  epiglottis Q31.8
  esophagus Q39.0
    with tracheoesophageal fistula Q39.1
  eustachian tube Q17.8
  fallopian tube (congenital) Q50.6
    acquired N97.1
  follicular cyst N83.0
  foramen of
    Luschka Q03.1
      with spina bifida —see Spina bifida, with
        hydrocephalus
    Magendie Q03.1
      with spina bifida —see Spina bifida, with
        hydrocephalus
  gallbladder Q44.1
  genital organ
    external
      female Q52.79
      male Q55.8

◀ New   ◀▥ Revised   ~~deleted~~ Deleted

Atresia, atretic *(Continued)*
  genital organ *(Continued)*
    internal
      female Q52.8
      male Q55.8
  glottis Q31.8
  gullet Q39.0
    with tracheoesophageal fistula Q39.1
  heart valve NEC Q24.8
    pulmonary Q22.0
    tricuspid Q22.4
  hymen Q52.3
    acquired (postinfective) N89.6
  ileum Q41.2
  intestine (small) Q41.9
    large Q42.9
      specified NEC Q42.8
  iris, filtration angle Q15.0
  jejunum Q41.1
  lacrimal apparatus Q10.4
  larynx Q31.8
  meatus urinarius Q64.33
  mitral valve Q23.2
    in hypoplastic left heart syndrome Q23.4
  nares (anterior) (posterior) Q30.0
  nasopharynx Q34.8
  nose, nostril Q30.0
    acquired J34.89
  ~~oesophagus Q39.0~~
    ~~with tracheoesophageal fistula Q39.1~~
  organ or site NEC Q89.8
  osseous meatus (ear) Q16.1
  oviduct (congenital) Q50.6
    acquired N97.1
  parotid duct Q38.4
    acquired K11.8
  pulmonary (artery) Q25.5
    valve Q22.0
  pulmonic Q22.0
  pupil Q13.2
  rectum Q42.1
    with fistula Q42.0
  salivary duct Q38.4
    acquired K11.8
  sublingual duct Q38.4
    acquired K11.8
  submandibular duct Q38.4
    acquired K11.8
  submaxillary duct Q38.4
    acquired K11.8
  thyroid cartilage Q31.8
  trachea Q32.1
  tricuspid valve Q22.4
  ureter Q62.10
    pelvic junction Q62.11
    vesical orifice Q62.12
  ureteropelvic junction Q62.11
  ureterovesical orifice Q62.12
  urethra (valvular) Q64.39
    stricture Q64.32
  urinary tract NEC Q64.8
  uterus Q51.818
    acquired N85.8
  vagina (congenital) Q52.4
    acquired (postinfectional) (senile) N89.5
  vas deferens Q55.3
  vascular NEC Q27.8
    cerebral Q28.3
    digestive system Q27.8
    lower limb Q27.8
    specified site NEC Q27.8
    upper limb Q27.8
  vein NEC Q27.8
    digestive system Q27.8
    great Q26.8
    lower limb Q27.8
    portal Q26.5
    pulmonary Q26.3
    specified site NEC Q27.8
    upper limb Q27.8
  vena cava (inferior) (superior) Q26.8

Atresia, atretic *(Continued)*
  vesicourethral orifice Q64.31
  vulva Q52.79
    acquired N90.5
Atrichia, atrichosis —*see* Alopecia
Atrophia —*see also* Atrophy
  cutis senilis L90.8
    due to radiation L57.8
  gyrata of choroid and retina H31.23
  senilis R54
    dermatological L90.8
      due to radiation (nonionizing) (solar) L57.8
  unguium L60.3
    congenita Q84.6
Atrophie blanche (en plaque) (de Milian) L95.0
Atrophoderma, atrophodermia (of) L90.9
  diffusum (idiopathic) L90.4
  maculatum L90.8
    et striatum L90.8
      due to syphilis A52.79
    syphilitic A51.39
  neuriticum L90.8
  Pasini and Pierini L90.3
  pigmentosum Q82.1
  reticulatum symmetricum faciei L66.4
  senile L90.8
    due to radiation (nonionizing) (solar) L57.8
  vermiculata (cheeks) L66.4
Atrophy, atrophic (of)
  adrenal (capsule) (gland) E27.49
    primary (autoimmune) E27.1
  alveolar process or ridge (edentulous) K08.20
  anal sphincter (disuse) N81.84
  appendix K38.8
  arteriosclerotic —*see* Arteriosclerosis
  bile duct (common) (hepatic) K83.8
  bladder N32.89
    neurogenic N31.8
  blanche (en plaque) (of Milian) L95.0
  bone (senile) NEC —*see also* Disorder, bone,
      specified type NEC
    due to
      tabes dorsalis (neurogenic) A52.11
  brain (cortex) (progressive) G31.9
    frontotemporal circumscribed G31.01
      [F02.80]
      with behavioral disturbance G31.01
        [F02.81]
    senile NEC G31.1
  breast N64.2
    obstetric —*see* Disorder, breast, specified
        type NEC
  buccal cavity K13.79
  cardiac —*see* Degeneration, myocardial
  cartilage (infectional) (joint) —*see* Disorder,
      cartilage, specified NEC
  cerebellar —*see* Atrophy, brain
  cerebral —*see* Atrophy, brain
  cervix (mucosa) (senile) (uteri) N88.8
    menopausal N95.8
  Charcot-Marie-Tooth G60.0
  choroid (central) (macular) (myopic) (retina)
      H31.10-
    diffuse secondary H31.12-
    gyrate H31.23
    senile H31.11-
  ciliary body —*see* Atrophy, iris
  conjunctiva (senile) H11.89
  corpus cavernosum N48.89
  cortical —*see* Atrophy, brain
  cystic duct K82.8
  Déjérine-Thomas G23.8
  disuse NEC —*see* Atrophy, muscle
  Duchenne-Aran G12.21
  ear H93.8-
  edentulous alveolar ridge K08.20
  endometrium (senile) N85.8
    cervix N88.8
  enteric K63.89
  epididymis N50.8

Atrophy, atrophic *(Continued)*
  eyeball —*see* Disorder, globe, degenerated
      condition, atrophy
  eyelid (senile) —*see* Disorder, eyelid,
      degenerative
  facial (skin) L90.9
  fallopian tube (senile) N83.32
    with ovary N83.33
  fascioscapulohumeral (Landouzy- Déjérine)
      G71.0
  fatty, thymus (gland) E32.8
  gallbladder K82.8
  gastric K29.40
    with bleeding K29.41
  gastrointestinal K63.89
  glandular I89.8
  globe H44.52-
  gum K06.0
  hair L67.8
  heart (brown) —*see* Degeneration, myocardial
  hemifacial Q67.4
    Romberg G51.8
  infantile E41
    paralysis, acute —*see* Poliomyelitis,
        paralytic
  intestine K63.89
  iris (essential) (progressive) H21.26-
    specified NEC H21.29
  kidney (senile) (terminal) (*see also* Sclerosis,
      renal) N26.1
    congenital or infantile Q60.5
      bilateral Q60.4
      unilateral Q60.3
    hydronephrotic —*see* Hydronephrosis
  lacrimal gland (primary) H04.14-
    secondary H04.15-
  Landouzy-Déjérine G71.0
  laryngitis, infective J37.0
  larynx J38.7
  Leber's optic (hereditary) H47.22
  lip K13.0
  liver (yellow) K72.90
    with coma K72.91
    acute, subacute K72.00
      with coma K72.01
    chronic K72.10
      with coma K72.11
  lung (senile) J98.4
  macular (dermatological) L90.8
    syphilitic, skin A51.39
      striated A52.79
  mandible (edentulous) K08.20
    minimal K08.21
    moderate K08.22
    severe K08.23
  maxilla K08.20
    minimal K08.24
    moderate K08.25
    severe K08.26
  muscle, muscular (diffuse) (general)
      (idiopathic) (primary) M62.50
    ankle M62.57-
    Duchenne-Aran G12.21
    foot M62.57-
    forearm M62.53-
    hand M62.54-
    infantile spinal G12.0
    lower leg M62.56-
    multiple sites M62.59
    myelopathic —*see* Atrophy, muscle, spinal
    myotonic G71.11
    neuritic G58.9
    neuropathic (peroneal) (progressive) G60.0
    pelvic (disuse) N81.84
    peroneal G60.0
    progressive (bulbar) G12.21
      adult G12.1
      infantile (spinal) G12.0
      spinal G12.9
        adult G12.1
        infantile G12.0

Atrophy, atrophic *(Continued)*
  muscle, muscular *(Continued)*
    pseudohypertrophic G71.0
    shoulder region M62.51-
    specified site NEC M62.58
    spinal G12.9
      adult form G12.1
      Aran-Duchenne G12.21
      childhood form, type II G12.1
      distal G12.1
      hereditary NEC G12.1
      infantile, type I (Werdnig- Hoffmann) G12.0
      juvenile form, type III (Kugelberg-Welander) G12.1
      progressive G12.21
      scapuloperoneal form G12.1
      specified NEC G12.8
    syphilitic A52.78
    thigh M62.55-
    upper arm M62.52-
  myocardium —*see* Degeneration, myocardial
  myometrium (senile) N85.8
    cervix N88.8
  myopathic NEC —*see* Atrophy, muscle
  myotonia G71.11
  nail L60.3
  nasopharynx J31.1
  nerve —*see also* Disorder, nerve
    abducens —*see* Strabismus, paralytic, sixth nerve
    accessory G52.8
    acoustic or auditory —*see* subcategory H93.3
    cranial G52.9
      eighth (auditory) —*see* subcategory H93.3
      eleventh (accessory) G52.8
      fifth (trigeminal) G50.8
      first (olfactory) G52.0
      fourth (trochlear) —*see* Strabismus, paralytic, fourth nerve
      second (optic) H47.20
      sixth (abducens) —*see* Strabismus, paralytic, sixth nerve
      tenth (pneumogastric) (vagus) G52.2
      third (oculomotor) —*see* Strabismus, paralytic, third nerve
      twelfth (hypoglossal) G52.3
    hypoglossal G52.3
    oculomotor —*see* Strabismus, paralytic, third nerve
    olfactory G52.0
    optic (papillomacular bundle)
      syphilitic (late) A52.15
        congenital A50.44
    pneumogastric G52.2
    trigeminal G50.8
    trochlear —*see* Strabismus, paralytic, fourth nerve
    vagus (pneumogastric) G52.2
  neurogenic, bone, tabetic A52.11
  nutritional E41
  old age R54
  olivopontocerebellar G23.8
  optic (nerve) H47.20
    glaucomatous H47.23-
    hereditary H47.22
    primary H47.21-
    specified type NEC H47.29-
    syphilitic (late) A52.15
      congenital A50.44
  orbit H05.31-
  ovary (senile) N83.31
    with fallopian tube N83.33
  oviduct (senile) —*see* Atrophy, fallopian tube
  palsy, diffuse (progressive) G12.22
  pancreas (duct) (senile) K86.8
  parotid gland K11.0
  pelvic muscle N81.84
  penis N48.89

Atrophy, atrophic *(Continued)*
  pharynx J39.2
  pluriglandular E31.8
    autoimmune E31.0
  polyarthritis M15.9
  prostate N42.89
  pseudohypertrophic (muscle) G71.0
  renal (*see also* Sclerosis, renal) N26.1
  retina, retinal (postinfectional) H35.89
  rhinitis J31.0
  salivary gland K11.0
  scar L90.5
  sclerosis, lobar (of brain) G31.09 *[F02.80]*
    with behavioral disturbance G31.09 *[F02.81]*
  scrotum N50.8
  seminal vesicle N50.8
  senile R54
    due to radiation (nonionizing) (solar) L57.8
  skin (patches) (spots) L90.9
    degenerative (senile) L90.8
    due to radiation (nonionizing) (solar) L57.8
    senile L90.8
  spermatic cord N50.8
  spinal (acute) (cord) G95.89
    muscular —*see* Atrophy, muscle, spinal
    paralysis G12.20
      acute —*see* Poliomyelitis, paralytic
      meaning progressive muscular atrophy G12.21
  spine (column) —*see* Spondylopathy, specified NEC
  spleen (senile) D73.0
  stomach K29.40
    with bleeding K29.41
  striate (skin) L90.6
    syphilitic A52.79
  subcutaneous L90.9
  sublingual gland K11.0
  submandibular gland K11.0
  submaxillary gland K11.0
  Sudeck's —*see* Algoneurodystrophy
  suprarenal (capsule) (gland) E27.49
    primary E27.1
  systemic affecting central nervous system in
      myxedema E03.9 *[G13.2]*
      neoplastic disease (*see also* Neoplasm) D49.9 *[G13.1]*
      specified disease NEC G13.8
  tarso-orbital fascia, congenital Q10.3
  testis N50.0
  thenar, partial —*see* Syndrome, carpal tunnel
  thymus (fatty) E32.8
  thyroid (gland) (acquired) E03.4
    with cretinism E03.1
    congenital (with myxedema) E03.1
  tongue (senile) K14.8
    papillae K14.4
  trachea J39.8
  tunica vaginalis N50.8
  turbinate J34.89
  tympanic membrane (nonflaccid) H73.82-
    flaccid H73.81-
  upper respiratory tract J39.8
  uterus, uterine (senile) N85.8
    cervix N88.8
    due to radiation (intended effect) N85.8
      adverse effect or misadventure N99.89
  vagina (senile) N95.2
  vas deferens N50.8
  vascular I99.8
  vertebra (senile) —*see* Spondylopathy, specified NEC
  vulva (senile) N90.5
  Werdnig-Hoffmann G12.0
  yellow —*see* Failure, hepatic

Attack, attacks
  with alteration of consciousness (with automatisms) —*see* Epilepsy, localization-related, symptomatic, with complex partial seizures
  without alteration of consciousness — *see* Epilepsy, localization-related, symptomatic, with simple partial seizures
  Adams-Stokes I45.9
  akinetic —*see* Epilepsy, generalized, specified NEC
  angina —*see* Angina
  atonic —*see* Epilepsy, generalized, specified NEC
  benign shuddering G25.83
  cataleptic —*see* Catalepsy
  coronary —*see* Infarct, myocardium
  cyanotic, newborn P28.2
  drop NEC R55
  epileptic —*see* Epilepsy
  heart —*see* infarct, myocardium
  hysterical F44.9
  jacksonian —*see* Epilepsy, localization-related, symptomatic, with simple partial seizures
  myocardium, myocardial —*see* Infarct, myocardium
  myoclonic —*see* Epilepsy, generalized, specified NEC
  panic F41.0
  psychomotor —*see* Epilepsy, localization-related, symptomatic, with complex partial seizures
  salaam —*see* Epilepsy, spasms
  schizophreniform, brief F23
  shuddering, benign G25.83
  Stokes-Adams I45.9
  syncope R55
  transient ischemic (TIA) G45.9
    specified NEC G45.8
  unconsciousness R55
    hysterical F44.89
  vasomotor R55
  vasovagal (paroxysmal) (idiopathic) R55
Attention (to)
  artificial
    opening (of) Z43.9
      digestive tract NEC Z43.4
        colon Z43.3
        ilium Z43.2
        stomach Z43.1
      specified NEC Z43.8
      trachea Z43.0
      urinary tract NEC Z43.6
        cystostomy Z43.5
        nephrostomy Z43.6
        ureterostomy Z43.6
        urethrostomy Z43.6
      vagina Z43.7
    colostomy Z43.3
    cystostomy Z43.5
  deficit disorder or syndrome F98.8
    with hyperactivity —*see* Disorder, attention-deficit hyperactivity
  gastrostomy Z43.1
  ileostomy Z43.2
  jejunostomy Z43.4
  nephrostomy Z43.6
  surgical dressings Z48.01
  sutures Z48.02
  tracheostomy Z43.0
  ureterostomy Z43.6
  urethrostomy Z43.6
Attrition
  gum K06.0
  tooth, teeth (excessive) (hard tissues) K03.0
Atypical, atypism —*see also* condition
  cells (on cytolgocial smear) (endocervical) (endometrial) (glandular)
    cervix R87.619
    vagina R87.629

◀ New   ◀▦ Revised   ~~deleted~~ Deleted

Atypical, atypism (Continued)
 cervical N87.9
 endometrium N85.9
  hyperplasia N85.00
 parenting situation Z62.9
Auditory —see condition
Aujeszky's disease B33.8
Aurantiasis, cutis E67.1
Auricle, auricular —see also condition
 cervical Q18.2
Auriculotemporal syndrome G50.8
Austin Flint murmur (aortic insufficiency) I35.1
Australian
 Q fever A78
 X disease A83.4
Autism, autistic (childhood) (infantile) F84.0
 atypical F84.9
Autodigestion R68.89
Autoerythrocyte sensitization (syndrome)
 D69.2
Autographism L50.3
Autoimmune
 disease (systemic) M35.9
 inhibitors to clotting factors D68.311
 lymphoproliferative syndrome [ALPS]
  D89.82
 thyroiditis E06.3
Autointoxication R68.89
Automatism G93.89
 with temporal sclerosis G93.81
 epileptic —see Epilepsy, localization- related,
  symptomatic, with complex partial
  seizures
 paroxysmal, idiopathic —see Epilepsy,
  localization-related, symptomatic, with
  complex partial seizures
Autonomic, autonomous
 bladder (neurogenic) N31.2
 hysteria seizure F44.5
Autosensitivity, erythrocyte D69.2
Autosensitization, cutaneous L30.2
Autosome —see condition by chromosome
 involved

Autotopagnosia R48.1
Autotoxemia R68.89
Autumn —see condition
Avellis' syndrome G46.8
Aversion
 oral R63.3
  newborn P92.-
  nonorganic origin F98.2
 sexual F52.1
Aviator's
 disease or sickness —see Effect, adverse, high
  altitude
 ear T70.0
Avitaminosis (multiple) (see also Deficiency,
 vitamin) E56.9
 B E53.9
  with
   beriberi E51.11
   pellagra E52
 B2 E53.0
 B6 E53.1
 B12 E53.8
 D E55.9
  with rickets E55.0
 G E53.0
 K E56.1
 nicotinic acid E52
AVNRT (atrioventricular nodal re-entrant
 tachycardia) I47.1
AVRT (atrioventricular nodal re-entrant
 tachycardia) I47.1
Avulsion (traumatic)
 blood vessel —see Injury, blood vessel
 bone —see Fracture, by site
 cartilage —see also Dislocation, by site
  symphyseal (inner), complicating delivery
   O71.6
 external site other than limb —see Wound,
  open, by site
 eye S05.7-
 head (intracranial)
  external site NEC S08.89
  scalp S08.0

Avulsion (Continued)
 internal organ or site —see Injury, by site
 joint —see also Dislocation, by site
  capsule —see Sprain, by site
 kidney S37.06-
 ligament —see Sprain, by site
 limb —see also Amputation, traumatic, by site
  skin and subcutaneous tissue —see Wound,
   open, by site
 muscle —see Injury, muscle
 nerve (root) —see Injury, nerve
 scalp S08.0
 skin and subcutaneous tissue —see Wound,
  open, by site
 spleen S36.032
 symphyseal cartilage (inner), complicating
  delivery O71.6
 tendon —see Injury, muscle
 tooth S03.2
Awareness of heart beat R00.2
Axenfeld's
 anomaly or syndrome Q15.0
 degeneration (calcareous) Q13.4
Axilla, axillary —see also condition
 breast Q83.1
Axonotmesis —see Injury, nerve
Ayerza's disease or syndrome (pulmonary
 artery sclerosis with pulmonary
 hypertension) I27.0
Azoospermia (organic) N46.01
 due to
  drug therapy N46.021
  efferent duct obstruction N46.023
  infection N46.022
  radiation N46.024
  specified cause NEC N46.029
  systemic disease N46.025
Azotemia R79.89
 meaning uremia N19
Aztec ear Q17.3
Azygos
 continuation inferior vena cava Q26.8
 lobe (lung) Q33.1

B

Baastrup's disease —*see* Kissing spine
Babesiosis B60.0
Babington's disease (familial hemorrhagic telangiectasia) I78.0
Babinski's syndrome A52.79
Baby
  crying constantly R68.11
  floppy (syndrome) P94.2
Bacillary —*see* condition
Bacilluria N39.0
Bacillus —*see also* Infection, bacillus
  abortus infection A23.1
  anthracis infection A22.9
  coli infection (*see also* Escherichia coli) B96.20
  Flexner's A03.1
  mallei infection A24.0
  Shiga's A03.0
  suipestifer infection —*see* Infection, salmonella
Back —*see* condition
Backache (postural) M54.9
  sacroiliac M53.3
  specified NEC M54.89
Backflow —*see* Reflux
Backward reading (dyslexia) F81.0
Bacteremia R78.81
  with sepsis —*see* Sepsis
Bactericholia —*see* Cholecystitis, acute
Bacterid, bacteride (pustular) L40.3
Bacterium, bacteria, bacterial
  agent NEC, as cause of disease classified elsewhere B96.89
  in blood —*see* Bacteremia
  in urine —*see* Bacteriuria
Bacteriuria, bacteruria N39.0
  asymptomatic N39.0
Bacteroides
  fragilis, as cause of disease classified elsewhere B96.6
Bad
  heart —*see* Disease, heart
  trip
    due to drug abuse —*see* Abuse, drug, hallucinogen
    due to drug dependence —*see* Dependence, drug, hallucinogen
Baelz's disease (cheilitis glandularis apostematosa) K13.0
Baerensprung's disease (eczema marginatum) B35.6
Bagasse disease or pneumonitis J67.1
Bagassosis J67.1
Baker's cyst —*see* Cyst, Baker's
Bakwin-Krida syndrome (craniometaphyseal dysplasia) Q78.5
Balancing side interference M26.56
Balanitis (circinata) (erosiva) (gangrenosa) (phagedenic) (vulgaris) N48.1
  amebic A06.82
  candidal B37.42
  due to Haemophilus ducreyi A57
  gonococcal (acute) (chronic) A54.09
  xerotica obliterans N48.0
Balanoposthitis N47.6
  gonococcal (acute) (chronic) A54.09
  ulcerative (specific) A63.8
Balanorrhagia —*see* Balanitis
Balantidiasis, balantidiosis A07.0
Bald tongue K14.4
Baldness —*see also* Alopecia
  male-pattern —*see* Alopecia, androgenic
Balkan grippe A78
Balloon disease —*see* Effect, adverse, high altitude
Balo's disease (concentric sclerosis) G37.5
Bamberger-Marie disease —*see* Osteoarthropathy, hypertrophic, specified type NEC
Bancroft's filariasis B74.0

Band (s)
  adhesive —*see* Adhesions, peritoneum
  anomalous or congenital —*see also* Anomaly, by site
    heart (atrial) (ventricular) Q24.8
    intestine Q43.3
    omentum Q43.3
  cervix N88.1
  constricting, congenital Q79.8
  gallbladder (congenital) Q44.1
  intestinal (adhesive) —*see* Adhesions, peritoneum
  obstructive
    intestine K56.5
    peritoneum K56.5
  periappendiceal, congenital Q43.3
  peritoneal (adhesive) —*see* Adhesions, peritoneum
  uterus N73.6
    internal N85.6
  vagina N89.5
Bandemia D72.825
Bandl's ring (contraction), complicating delivery O62.4
Bangkok hemorrhagic fever A91
Bang's disease (brucella abortus) A23.1
Bankruptcy, anxiety concerning Z59.8
Bannister's disease T78.3
  hereditary D84.1
Banti's disease or syndrome (with cirrhosis) (with portal hypertension) K76.6
Bar, median, prostate —*see* Enlargement, enlarged, prostate
Barcoo disease or rot —*see* Ulcer, skin
Barlow's disease E54
Barodontalgia T70.29
Baron Münchausen syndrome —*see* Disorder, factitious
Barosinusitis T70.1
Barotitis T70.0
Barotrauma T70.29
  odontalgia T70.29
  otitic T70.0
  sinus T70.1
Barraquer (-Simons) disease or syndrome (progressive lipodystrophy) E88.1
Barré-Guillain disease or syndrome G61.0
Barré-Liéou syndrome (posterior cervical sympathetic) M53.0
Barrel chest M95.4
Barrett's
  disease —*see* Barrett's, esophagus
  esophagus K22.70
    with dysplasia K22.719
      high grade K22.711
      low grade K22.710
    without dysplasia K22.70
  syndrome —*see* Barrett's, esophagus
  ulcer K22.10
    with bleeding K22.11
    without bleeding K22.10
Barth syndrome E78.71
Bársony (-Polgár) (-Teschendorf) syndrome (corkscrew esophagus) K22.4
Bartholinitis (suppurating) N75.8
  gonococcal (acute) (chronic) (with abscess) A54.1
Bartonellosis A44.9
  cutaneous A44.1
  mucocutaneous A44.1
  specified NEC A44.8
  systemic A44.0
Barton's fracture S52.56-
Bartter's syndrome E26.81
Basal —*see* condition
Basan's (hidrotic) ectodermal dysplasia Q82.4
Baseball finger —*see* Dislocation, finger
Basedow's disease (exophthalmic goiter) —*see* Hyperthyroidism, with, goiter
Basic —*see* condition
Basilar —*see* condition

Bason's (hidrotic) ectodermal dysplasia Q82.4
Basopenia —*see* Agranulocytosis
Basophilia D72.824
Basophilism (cortico-adrenal) (Cushing's) (pituitary) E24.0
Bassen-Kornzweig disease or syndrome E78.6
Bat ear Q17.5
Bateman's
  disease B08.1
  purpura (senile) D69.2
Bathing cramp T75.1
Bathophobia F40.248
Batten (-Mayou) disease E75.4
  retina E75.4 [*H36*]
Batten-Steinert syndrome G71.11
Battered —*see* Maltreatment
Battey Mycobacterium infection A31.0
Battle exhaustion F43.0
Battledore placenta O43.19-
Baumgarten-Cruveilhier cirrhosis, disease or syndrome K74.69
Bauxite fibrosis (of lung) J63.1
Bayle's disease (general paresis) A52.17
Bazin's disease (primary) (tuberculous) A18.4
Beach ear —*see* Swimmer's, ear
Beaded hair (congenital) Q84.1
Béal conjunctivitis or syndrome B30.2
Beard's disease (neurasthenia) F48.8
Beat (s)
  atrial, premature I49.1
  ectopic I49.49
  elbow —*see* Bursitis, elbow
  escaped, heart I49.49
  hand —*see* Bursitis, hand
  knee —*see* Bursitis, knee
  premature I49.40
    atrial I49.1
    auricular I49.1
    supraventricular I49.1
Beau's
  disease or syndrome —*see* Degeneration, myocardial
  lines (transverse furrows on fingernails) L60.4
Bechterev's syndrome —*see* Spondylitis, ankylosing
Beck's syndrome (anterior spinal artery occlusion) I65.8
Becker's
  cardiomyopathy I42.8
  disease
    idiopathic mural endomyocardial disease I42.3
    myotonia congenita, recessive form G71.12
  dystrophy G71.0
  pigmented hairy nevus D22.5
Beckwith-Wiedemann syndrome Q87.3
Bed confinement status Z74.01
Bed sore —*see* Ulcer, pressure, by site
Bedbug bite (s) —*see* Bite (s), by site, superficial, insect
Bedclothes, asphyxiation or suffocation by —*see* Asphyxia, traumatic, due to, mechanical, trapped
Bednar's
  aphthae K12.0
  tumor —*see* Neoplasm, malignant, by site
Bedridden Z74.01
Bedsore —*see* Ulcer, pressure, by site
Bedwetting —*see* Enuresis
Bee sting (with allergic or anaphylactic shock) —*see* Toxicity, venom, arthropod, bee
Beer drinker's heart (disease) I42.6
Begbie's disease (exophthalmic goiter) —*see* Hyperthyroidism, with, goiter
Behavior
  antisocial
    adult Z72.811
    child or adolescent Z72.810
  disorder, disturbance —*see* Disorder, conduct
  disruptive —*see* Disorder, conduct

◀ New ◀◀ Revised ~~deleted~~ Deleted

Behavior *(Continued)*
  drug seeking Z72.89
  inexplicable R46.2
  marked evasiveness R46.5
  obsessive-compulsive R46.81
  overactivity R46.3
  poor responsiveness R46.4
  self-damaging (life-style) Z72.89
  sleep-incompatible Z72.821
  slowness R46.4
  specified NEC R46.89
  strange (and inexplicable) R46.2
  suspiciousness R46.5
  type A pattern Z73.1
  undue concern or preoccupation with
    stressful events R46.6
  verbosity and circumstantial detail obscuring
    reason for contact R46.7
Behcet's disease or syndrome M35.2
Behr's disease —*see* Degeneration, macula
Beigel's disease or morbus (white piedra)
  B36.2
Bejel A65
Bekhterev's syndrome —*see* Spondylitis,
  ankylosing
Belching —*see* Eructation
Bell's
  mania F30.8
  palsy, paralysis G51.0
    infant or newborn P11.3
  spasm G51.3
Bence Jones albuminuria or proteinuria NEC
  R80.3
Bends T70.3
Benedikt's paralysis or syndrome G46.3
Benign (*see also* condition)
  prostatic hyperplasia —*see* Hyperplasia,
    prostate
Bennett's fracture (displaced) S62.21-
Benson's disease —*see* Deposit, crystalline
Bent
  back (hysterical) F44.4
  nose M95.0
    congenital Q67.4
Bereavement (uncomplicated) Z63.4
Bergeron's disease (hysterical chorea) F44.4
Berger's disease —*see* Nephropathy, IgA
Beriberi (dry) E51.11
  heart (disease) E51.12
  polyneuropathy E51.11
  wet E51.12
    involving circulatory system E51.11
Berlin's disease or edema (traumatic) S05.8X-
Berlock (berloque) dermatitis L56.2
Bernard-Horner syndrome G90.2
Bernard-Soulier disease or thrombopathia
  D69.1
Bernhardt (-Roth) disease —*see*
  Mononeuropathy, lower limb, meralgia
  paresthetica
Bernheim's syndrome —*see* Failure, heart,
  congestive
Bertielliasis B71.8
Berylliosis (lung) J63.2
Besnier-Boeck (-Schaumann) disease —*see*
  Sarcoidosis
Besnier's
  lupus pernio D86.3
  prurigo L20.0
Bestiality F65.89
Best's disease H35.50
Beta-mercaptolactate-cysteine disulfiduria
  E72.09
Betalipoproteinemia, broad or floating E78.2
Betting and gambling Z72.6
  pathological (compulsive) F63.0
Bezoar T18.9
  intestine T18.3
  stomach T18.2
Bezold's abscess —*see* Mastoiditis, acute
Bianchi's syndrome R48.8

Bicornate or bicornis uterus Q51.3
  in pregnancy or childbirth O34.59-
    causing obstructed labor O65.5
Bicuspid aortic valve Q23.1
Biedl-Bardet syndrome Q87.89
Bielschowsky (-Jansky) disease E75.4
Biermer's (pernicious) anemia or disease D51.0
Biett's disease L93.0
Bifid (congenital)
  apex, heart Q24.8
  clitoris Q52.6
  kidney Q63.8
  nose Q30.2
  patella Q74.1
  scrotum Q55.29
  toe NEC Q74.2
  tongue Q38.3
  ureter Q62.8
  uterus Q51.3
  uvula Q35.7
Biforis uterus (suprasimplex) Q51.3
Bifurcation (congenital)
  gallbladder Q44.1
  kidney pelvis Q63.8
  renal pelvis Q63.8
  rib Q76.6
  tongue, congenital Q38.3
  trachea Q32.1
  ureter Q62.8
  urethra Q64.74
  vertebra Q76.49
Big spleen syndrome D73.1
Bigeminal pulse R00.8
Bilateral —*see* condition
Bile
  duct —*see* condition
  pigments in urine R82.2
Bilharziasis —*see also* Schistosomiasis
  chyluria B65.0
  cutaneous B65.3
  galacturia B65.0
  hematochyluria B65.0
  intestinal B65.1
  lipemia B65.9
  lipuria B65.0
  oriental B65.2
  piarhemia B65.9
  pulmonary NOS B65.9 *[J99]*
    pneumonia B65.9 *[J17]*
  tropical hematuria B65.0
  vesical B65.0
Biliary —*see* condition
Bilirubin metabolism disorder E80.7
  specified NEC E80.6
Bilirubinemia, familial nonhemolytic E80.4
Bilirubinuria R82.2
Biliuria R82.2
Bilocular stomach K31.2
Binswanger's disease I67.3
Biparta, bipartite
  carpal scaphoid Q74.0
  patella Q74.1
  vagina Q52.10
Bird
  face Q75.8
  fancier's disease or lung J67.2
Birt-Hogg-Dube syndrome Q87.89
Birth
  complications in mother —*see* Delivery,
    complicated
  compression during NOS P15.9
  defect —*see* Anomaly
  immature (less than 37 completed weeks) —
    see Preterm, newborn
    extremely (less than 28 completed
      weeks) —*see* Immaturity, extreme
  inattention, at or after —*see* Maltreatment,
    child, neglect
  injury NOS P15.9
    basal ganglia P11.1
    brachial plexus NEC P14.3

Birth *(Continued)*
  injury NOS *(Continued)*
    brain (compression) (pressure)
      P11.2
    central nervous system NOS P11.9
    cerebellum P11.1
    cerebral hemorrhage P10.1
    external genitalia P15.5
    eye P15.3
    face P15.4
    fracture
      bone P13.9
        specified NEC P13.8
      clavicle P13.4
      femur P13.2
      humerus P13.3
      long bone, except femur P13.3
      radius and ulna P13.3
      skull P13.0
      spine P11.5
      tibia and fibula P13.3
    intracranial P11.2
      laceration or hemorrhage P10.9
        specified NEC P10.8
    intraventricular hemorrhage P10.2
    laceration
      brain P10.1
      by scalpel P15.8
      peripheral nerve P14.9
    liver P15.0
    meninges
      brain P11.1
      spinal cord P11.5
    nerve
      brachial plexus P14.3
      cranial NEC (except facial) P11.4
      facial P11.3
      peripheral P14.9
      phrenic (paralysis) P14.2
    paralysis
      facial nerve P11.3
      spinal P11.5
    penis P15.5
    rupture
      spinal cord P11.5
    scalp P12.9
    scalpel wound P15.8
    scrotum P15.5
    skull NEC P13.1
      fracture P13.0
    specified type NEC P15.8
    spinal cord P11.5
    spine P11.5
    spleen P15.1
    sternomastoid (hematoma) P15.2
    subarachnoid hemorrhage P10.3
    subcutaneous fat necrosis P15.6
    subdural hemorrhage P10.0
    tentorial tear P10.4
    testes P15.5
    vulva P15.5
  lack of care, at or after —*see* Maltreatment,
    child, neglect
  neglect, at or after —*see* Maltreatment, child,
    neglect
  palsy or paralysis, newborn, NOS (birth
    injury) P14.9
  premature (infant) —*see* Preterm,
    newborn
  shock, newborn P96.89
  trauma —*see* Birth, injury
  weight
    4000 grams to 4499 grams P08.1
    4500 grams or more P08.0
    low (2499 grams or less) —*see* Low,
      birthweight
      extremely (999 grams or less) —*see* Low,
        birthweight, extreme
Birthmark Q82.5
Bisalbuminemia E88.09
Biskra's button B55.1

Bite (s) (animal) (human)
abdomen, abdominal
    wall S31.159
        with penetration into peritoneal cavity
            S31.659
        epigastric region S31.152
            with penetration into peritoneal cavity
                S31.652
        left
            lower quadrant S31.154
                with penetration into peritoneal
                    cavity S31.654
            upper quadrant S31.151
                with penetration into peritoneal
                    cavity S31.651
        periumbilic region S31.155
            with penetration into peritoneal cavity
                S31.655
        right
            lower quadrant S31.153
                with penetration into peritoneal
                    cavity S31.653
            upper quadrant S31.150
                with penetration into peritoneal
                    cavity S31.650
        superficial NEC S30.871
            insect S30.861
alveolar (process) —see Bite, oral cavity
amphibian (venomous) —see Venom, bite,
    amphibian
animal —see also Bite, by site
    venomous —see Venom
ankle S91.05-
    superficial NEC S90.57-
        insect S90.56-
antecubital space —see Bite, elbow
anus S31.835
    superficial NEC S30.877
        insect S30.867
arm (upper) S41.15-
    lower —see Bite, forearm
    superficial NEC S40.87-
        insect S40.86-
arthropod NEC —see Venom, bite,
    arthropod
auditory canal (external) (meatus) —
    see Bite, ear
auricle, ear —see Bite, ear
axilla —see Bite, arm
back —see also Bite, thorax, back
    lower S31.050
        with penetration into retroperitoneal
            space S31.051
        superficial NEC S30.870
            insect S30.860
bedbug —see Bite (s), by site, superficial,
    insect
breast S21.05-
    superficial NEC S20.17-
        insect S20.16-
brow —see Bite, head, specified site NEC
buttock S31.805
    left S31.825
    right S31.815
    superficial NEC S30.870
        insect S30.860
calf —see Bite, leg
canaliculus lacrimalis —see Bite, eyelid
canthus, eye —see Bite, eyelid
centipede —see Toxicity, venom, arthropod,
    centipede
cheek (external) S01.45-
    internal —see Bite, oral cavity
    superficial NEC S00.87
        insect S00.86
chest wall —see Bite, thorax
chigger B88.0
chin —see Bite, head, specified site
    NEC
clitoris —see Bite, vulva
costal region —see Bite, thorax

Bite (Continued)
digit (s)
    hand —see Bite, finger
    toe —see Bite, toe
ear (canal) (external) S01.35-
    superficial NEC S00.47-
        insect S00.46-
elbow S51.05-
    superficial NEC S50.37-
        insect S50.36-
epididymis —see Bite, testis
epigastric region —see Bite, abdomen
epiglottis —see Bite, neck, specified site
    NEC
esophagus, cervical S11.25
    superficial NEC S10.17
        insect S10.16
eyebrow —see Bite, eyelid
eyelid S01.15-
    superficial NEC S00.27-
        insect S00.26-
face NEC —see Bite, head, specified site
    NEC
finger (s) S61.259
    with
        damage to nail S61.359
    index S61.258
        with
            damage to nail S61.358
        left S61.251
            with
                damage to nail S61.351
        right S61.250
            with
                damage to nail S61.350
        superficial NEC S60.478
            insect S60.46-
    little S61.25-
        with
            damage to nail S61.35-
        superficial NEC S60.47-
            insect S60.46-
    middle S61.25-
        with
            damage to nail S61.35-
        superficial NEC S60.47-
            insect S60.46-
    ring S61.25-
        with
            damage to nail S61.35-
        superficial NEC S60.47-
            insect S60.46-
    superficial NEC S60.479
        insect S60.469
    thumb —see Bite, thumb
flank —see Bite, abdomen, wall
flea —see Bite, by site, superficial,
    insect
foot (except toe (s) alone) S91.35-
    superficial NEC S90.87-
        insect S90.86-
    toe —see Bite, toe
forearm S51.85-
    elbow only —see Bite, elbow
    superficial NEC S50.87-
        insect S50.86-
forehead —see Bite, head, specified site
    NEC
genital organs, external
    female S31.552
        superficial NEC S30.876
            insect S30.866
        vagina and vulva —see Bite, vulva
    male S31.551
        penis —see Bite, penis
        scrotum —see Bite, scrotum
        superficial NEC S30.875
            insect S30.865
        testes —see Bite, testis
groin —see Bite, abdomen, wall
gum —see Bite, oral cavity

Bite (Continued)
hand S61.45-
    finger —see Bite, finger
    superficial NEC S60.57-
        insect S60.56-
    thumb —see Bite, thumb
head S01.95
    cheek —see Bite, cheek
    ear —see Bite, ear
    eyelid —see Bite, eyelid
    lip —see Bite, lip
    nose —see Bite, nose
    oral cavity —see Bite, oral cavity
    scalp —see Bite, scalp
    specified site NEC S01.85
        superficial NEC S00.87
            insect S00.86
    superficial NEC S00.97
        insect S00.96
    temporomandibular area —see Bite, cheek
heel —see Bite, foot
hip S71.05-
    superficial NEC S70.27-
        insect S70.26-
hymen S31.45
hypochondrium —see Bite, abdomen, wall
hypogastric region —see Bite, abdomen, wall
inguinal region —see Bite, abdomen, wall
insect —see Bite, by site, superficial, insect
instep —see Bite, foot
interscapular region —see Bite, thorax, back
jaw —see Bite, head, specified site NEC
knee S81.05-
    superficial NEC S80.27-
        insect S80.26-
labium (majus) (minus) —see Bite, vulva
lacrimal duct —see Bite, eyelid
larynx S11.015
    superficial NEC S10.17
        insect S10.16
leg (lower) S81.85-
    ankle —see Bite, ankle
    foot —see Bite, foot
    knee —see Bite, knee
    superficial NEC S80.87-
        insect S80.86-
    toe —see Bite, toe
    upper —see Bite, thigh
lip S01.551
    superficial NEC S00.571
        insect S00.561
lizard (venomous) —see Venom, bite, reptile
loin —see Bite, abdomen, wall
lower back —see Bite, back, lower
lumbar region —see Bite, back, lower
malar region —see Bite, head, specified site
    NEC
mammary —see Bite, breast
marine animals (venomous) —see Toxicity,
    venom, marine animal
mastoid region —see Bite, head, specified site
    NEC
mouth —see Bite, oral cavity
nail
    finger —see Bite, finger
    toe —see Bite, toe
nape —see Bite, neck, specified site NEC
nasal (septum) (sinus) —see Bite, nose
nasopharynx —see Bite, head, specified site
    NEC
neck S11.95
    involving
        cervical esophagus —see Bite,
            esophagus, cervical
        larynx —see Bite, larynx
        pharynx —see Bite, pharynx
        thyroid gland S11.15
        trachea —see Bite, trachea
    specified site NEC S11.85
        superficial NEC S10.87
            insect S10.86

◀ New   ◀═ Revised   ~~deleted~~ Deleted

Bite *(Continued)*
  neck *(Continued)*
    superficial NEC S10.97
      insect S10.96
    throat S11.85
      superficial NEC S10.17
        insect S10.16
  nose (septum) (sinus) S01.25
    superficial NEC S00.37
      insect S00.36
  occipital region —*see* Bite, scalp
  oral cavity S01.552
    superficial NEC S00.572
      insect S00.562
  orbital region —*see* Bite, eyelid
  palate —*see* Bite, oral cavity
  palm —*see* Bite, hand
  parietal region —*see* Bite, scalp
  pelvis S31.050
    with penetration into retroperitoneal space S31.051
    superficial NEC S30.870
      insect S30.860
  penis S31.25
    superficial NEC S30.872
      insect S30.862
  perineum
    female —*see* Bite, vulva
    male —*see* Bite, pelvis
  periocular area (with or without lacrimal passages) —*see* Bite, eyelid
  phalanges
    finger —*see* Bite, finger
    toe —*see* Bite, toe
  pharynx S11.25
    superficial NEC S10.17
      insect S10.16
  pinna —*see* Bite, ear
  poisonous —*see* Venom
  popliteal space —*see* Bite, knee
  prepuce —*see* Bite, penis
  pubic region —*see* Bite, abdomen, wall
  rectovaginal septum —*see* Bite, vulva
  red bug B88.0
  reptile NEC —*see also* Venom, bite, reptile
    nonvenomous —*see* Bite, by site
    snake —*see* Venom, bite, snake
  sacral region —*see* Bite, back, lower
  sacroiliac region —*see* Bite, back, lower
  salivary gland —*see* Bite, oral cavity
  scalp S01.05
    superficial NEC S00.07
      insect S00.06
  scapular region —*see* Bite, shoulder
  scrotum S31.35
    superficial NEC S30.873
      insect S30.863
  sea-snake (venomous) —*see* Toxicity, venom, snake, sea snake
  shin —*see* Bite, leg
  shoulder S41.05-
    superficial NEC S40.27-
      insect S40.26-
  snake —*see also* Venom, bite, snake
    nonvenomous —*see* Bite, by site
  spermatic cord —*see* Bite, testis
  spider (venomous) —*see* Toxicity, venom, spider
    nonvenomous —*see* Bite, by site, superficial, insect
  sternal region —*see* Bite, thorax, front
  submaxillary region —*see* Bite, head, specified site NEC
  submental region —*see* Bite, head, specified site NEC
  subungual
    finger (s) —*see* Bite, finger
    toe —*see* Bite, toe
  superficial —*see* Bite, by site, superficial
  supraclavicular fossa S11.85

Bite *(Continued)*
  supraorbital —*see* Bite, head, specified site NEC
  temple, temporal region —*see* Bite, head, specified site NEC
  temporomandibular area —*see* Bite, cheek
  testis S31.35
    superficial NEC S30.873
      insect S30.863
  thigh S71.15-
    superficial NEC S70.37-
      insect S70.36-
  thorax, thoracic (wall) S21.95
    back S21.25-
      with penetration into thoracic cavity S21.45-
    breast —*see* Bite, breast
    front S21.15-
      with penetration into thoracic cavity S21.35-
    superficial NEC S20.97
      back S20.47-
      front S20.37-
      insect S20.96
        back S20.46-
        front S20.36-
  throat —*see* Bite, neck, throat
  thumb S61.05-
    with
      damage to nail S61.15-
    superficial NEC S60.37-
      insect S60.36-
  thyroid S11.15
    superficial NEC S10.87
      insect S10.86
  toe (s) S91.15-
    with
      damage to nail S91.25-
    great S91.15-
      with
        damage to nail S91.25-
    lesser S91.15-
      with
        damage to nail S91.25-
    superficial NEC S90.47-
      great S90.47-
      insect S90.46-
        great S90.46-
  tongue S01.552
  trachea S11.025
    superficial NEC S10.17
      insect S10.16
  tunica vaginalis —*see* Bite, testis
  tympanum, tympanic membrane —*see* Bite, ear
  umbilical region S31.155
  uvula —*see* Bite, oral cavity
  vagina —*see* Bite, vulva
  venomous —*see* Venom
  vocal cords S11.035
    superficial NEC S10.17
      insect S10.16
  vulva S31.45
    superficial NEC S30.874
      insect S30.864
  wrist S61.55-
    superficial NEC S60.87-
      insect S60.86-
Biting, cheek or lip K13.1
Biventricular failure (heart) I50.9
Björck (-Thorson) syndrome (malignant carcinoid) E34.0
Black
  death A20.9
  eye S00.1-
  hairy tongue K14.3
  heel (foot) S90.3-
  lung (disease) J60
  palm (hand) S60.22-
Blackfan-Diamond anemia or syndrome (congenital hypoplastic anemia) D61.01

Blackhead L70.0
Blackout R55
Bladder —*see* condition
Blast (air) (hydraulic) (immersion) (underwater)
  blindness S05.8X-
  injury
    abdomen or thorax —*see* Injury, by site
    ear (acoustic nerve trauma) —*see* Injury, nerve, acoustic, specified type NEC
    syndrome NEC T70.8
Blastoma —*see* Neoplasm, malignant, by site
  pulmonary —*see* Neoplasm, lung, malignant
Blastomycosis, blastomycotic B40.9
  Brazilian —*see* Paracoccidioidomycosis
  cutaneous B40.3
  disseminated B40.7
  European —*see* Cryptococcosis
  generalized B40.7
  keloidal B48.0
  North American B40.9
  primary pulmonary B40.0
  pulmonary B40.2
    acute B40.0
    chronic B40.1
  skin B40.3
  South American —*see* Paracoccidioidomycosis
  specified NEC B40.89
Bleb (s) R23.8
  emphysematous (lung) (solitary) J43.9
  endophthalmitis H59.43
  filtering (vitreous), after glaucoma surgery Z98.83
  inflamed (infected), postprocedural H59.40
    stage 1 H59.41
    stage 2 H59.42
    stage 3 H59.43
  lung (ruptured) J43.9
    congenital —*see* Atelectasis
    newborn P25.8
  subpleural (emphysematous) J43.9
Blebitis, postprocedural H59.40
  stage 1 H59.41
  stage 2 H59.42
  stage 3 H59.43
Bleeder (familial) (hereditary) —*see* Hemophilia
Bleeding —*see also* Hemorrhage
  anal K62.5
  anovulatory N97.0
  atonic, following delivery O72.1
  capillary I78.8
    puerperal O72.2
  contact (postcoital) N93.0
  due to uterine subinvolution N85.3
  ear —*see* Otorrhagia
  excessive, associated with menopausal onset N92.4
  familial —*see* Defect, coagulation
  following intercourse N93.0
  gastrointestinal K92.2
  hemorrhoids —*see* Hemorrhoids
  intermenstrual (regular) N92.3
    irregular N92.1
  intraoperative —*see* Complication, intraoperative, hemorrhage
  irregular N92.6
  menopausal N92.4
  newborn, intraventricular —*see* Newborn, affected by, hemorrhage, intraventricular
  nipple N64.59
  nose R04.0
  ovulation N92.3
  postclimacteric N95.0
  postcoital N93.0
  postmenopausal N95.0
  postoperative —*see* Complication, postprocedural, hemorrhage ◀▦
  preclimacteric N92.4
  puberty (excessive, with onset of menstrual periods) N92.2

Bleeding (Continued)
rectum, rectal K62.5
newborn P54.2
tendencies —*see* Defect, coagulation
throat R04.1
tooth socket (post-extraction) K91.840
umbilical stump P51.9
uterus, uterine NEC N93.9
climacteric N92.4
dysfunctional of functional N93.8
menopausal N92.4
preclimacteric or premenopausal N92.4
unrelated to menstrual cycle N93.9
vagina, vaginal (abnormal) N93.9
dysfunctional or functional N93.8
newborn P54.6
vicarious N94.89
Blennorrhagia, blennorrhagic —*see* Gonorrhea
Blennorrhea (acute) (chronic) —*see also* Gonorrhea
inclusion (neonatal) (newborn) P39.1
lower genitourinary tract (gonococcal) A54.00
neonatorum (gonococcal ophthalmia) A54.31
Blepharelosis —*see* Entropion
Blepharitis (angularis) (ciliaris) (eyelid) (marginal) (nonulcerative) H01.009
herpes zoster B02.39
left H01.006
lower H01.005
upper H01.004
right H01.003
lower H01.002
upper H01.001
squamous H01.029
left H01.026
lower H01.025
upper H01.024
right H01.023
lower H01.022
upper H01.021
ulcerative H01.019
left H01.016
lower H01.015
upper H01.014
right H01.013
lower H01.012
upper H01.011
Blepharochalasis H02.30
congenital Q10.0
left H02.36
lower H02.35
upper H02.34
right H02.33
lower H02.32
upper H02.31
Blepharoclonus H02.59
Blepharoconjunctivitis H10.50-
angular H10.52-
contact H10.53-
ligneous H10.51-
Blepharophimosis (eyelid) H02.529
congenital Q10.3
left H02.526
lower H02.525
upper H02.524
right H02.523
lower H02.522
upper H02.521
Blepharoptosis H02.40-
congenital Q10.0
mechanical H02.41-
myogenic H02.42-
neurogenic H02.43-
paralytic H02.43-
Blepharopyorrhea, gonococcal A54.39
Blepharospasm G24.5
drug induced G24.01
Blighted ovum O02.0

Blind —*see also* Blindness
bronchus (congenital) Q32.4
loop syndrome K90.2
congenital Q43.8
sac, fallopian tube (congenital) Q50.6
spot, enlarged —*see* Defect, visual field, localized, scotoma, blind spot area
tract or tube, congenital NEC —*see* Atresia, by site
Blindness (acquired) (congenital) (both eyes) H54.0
blast S05.8X-
color —*see* Deficiency, color vision
concussion S05.8X-
cortical H47.619
left brain H47.612
right brain H47.611
day H53.11
due to injury (current episode) S05.9-
sequelae — code to injury with seventh character S
eclipse (total) —*see* Retinopathy, solar
emotional (hysterical) F44.6
face H53.16
hysterical F44.6
legal (both eyes) (USA definition) H54.8
mind R48.8
night H53.60
abnormal dark adaptation curve H53.61
acquired H53.62
congenital H53.63
specified type NEC H53.69
vitamin A deficiency E50.5
one eye (other eye normal) H54.40
left (normal vision on right) H54.42
low vision on right H54.12
low vision, other eye H54.10
right (normal vision on left) H54.41
low vision on left H54.11
psychic R48.8
river B73.01
snow —*see* Photokeratitis
sun, solar —*see* Retinopathy, solar
transient —*see* Disturbance, vision, subjective, loss, transient
traumatic (current episode) S05.9-
word (developmental) F81.0
acquired R48.0
secondary to organic lesion R48.0
Blister (nonthermal)
abdominal wall S30.821
alveolar process S00.522
ankle S90.52-
antecubital space —*see* Blister, elbow
anus S30.827
arm (upper) S40.82-
auditory canal —*see* Blister, ear
auricle —*see* Blister, ear
axilla —*see* Blister, arm
back, lower S30.820
beetle dermatitis L24.89
breast S20.12-
brow S00.82
calf —*see* Blister, leg
canthus —*see* Blister, eyelid
cheek S00.82
internal S00.522
chest wall —*see* Blister, thorax
chin S00.82
costal region —*see* Blister, thorax
digit (s)
foot —*see* Blister, toe
hand —*see* Blister, finger
due to burn —*see* Burn, by site, second degree
ear S00.42-
elbow S50.32-
epiglottis S10.12
esophagus, cervical S10.12
eyebrow —*see* Blister, eyelid
eyelid S00.22-
face S00.82

Blister (Continued)
fever B00.1
finger (s) S60.429
index S60.42-
little S60.42-
middle S60.42-
ring S60.42-
foot (except toe (s) alone) S90.82-
toe —*see* Blister, toe
forearm S50.82-
elbow only —*see* Blister, elbow
forehead S00.82
fracture - omit code
genital organ
female S30.826
male S30.825
gum S00.522
hand S60.52-
head S00.92
ear —*see* Blister, ear
eyelid —*see* Blister, eyelid
lip S00.521
nose S00.32
oral cavity S00.522
scalp S00.02
specified site NEC S00.82
heel —*see* Blister, foot
hip S70.22-
interscapular region S20.429
jaw S00.82
knee S80.22-
larynx S10.12
leg (lower) S80.82-
knee —*see* Blister, knee
upper —*see* Blister, thigh
lip S00.521
malar region S00.82
mammary —*see* Blister, breast
mastoid region S00.82
mouth S00.522
multiple, skin, nontraumatic R23.8
nail
finger —*see* Blister, finger
toe —*see* Blister, toe
nasal S00.32
neck S10.92
specified site NEC S10.82
throat S10.12
nose S00.32
occipital region S00.02
oral cavity S00.522
orbital region —*see* Blister, eyelid
palate S00.522
palm —*see* Blister, hand
parietal region S00.02
pelvis S30.820
penis S30.822
periocular area —*see* Blister, eyelid
phalanges
finger —*see* Blister, finger
toe —*see* Blister, toe
pharynx S10.12
pinna —*see* Blister, ear
popliteal space —*see* Blister, knee
scalp S00.02
scapular region —*see* Blister, shoulder
scrotum S30.823
shin —*see* Blister, leg
shoulder S40.22-
sternal region S20.329
submaxillary region S00.82
submental region S00.82
subungual
finger (s) —*see* Blister, finger
toe (s) —*see* Blister, toe
supraclavicular fossa S10.82
supraorbital S00.82
temple S00.82
temporal region S00.82
testis S30.823
thermal —*see* Burn, second degree, by site

◀ New   ◀▥ Revised   ~~deleted~~ Deleted

Blister *(Continued)*
thigh S70.32-
thorax, thoracic (wall) S20.92
back S20.42-
front S20.32-
throat S10.12
thumb S60.32-
toe (s) S90.42-
great S90.42-
tongue S00.522
trachea S10.12
tympanum, tympanic membrane —*see* Blister, ear
upper arm —*see* Blister, arm (upper)
uvula S00.522
vagina S30.824
vocal cords S10.12
vulva S30.824
wrist S60.82-
Bloating R14.0
Bloch-Sulzberger disease or syndrome Q82.3
Block, blocked
alveolocapillary J84.10
arborization (heart) I45.5
arrhythmic I45.9
atrioventricular (incomplete) (partial) I44.30
with atrioventricular dissociation I44.2
complete I44.2
congenital Q24.6
congenital Q24.6
first degree I44.0
second degree (types I and II) I44.1
specified NEC I44.39
third degree I44.2
types I and II I44.1
auriculoventricular —*see* Block, atrioventricular
bifascicular (cardiac) I45.2
bundle-branch (complete) (false) (incomplete) I45.4
bilateral I45.2
left I44.7
with right bundle branch block I45.2
hemiblock I44.60
anterior I44.4
posterior I44.5
incomplete I44.7
with right bundle branch block I45.2
right I45.10
with
left bundle branch block I45.2
left fascicular block I45.2
specified NEC I45.19
Wilson's type I45.19
cardiac I45.9
conduction I45.9
complete I44.2
fascicular (left) I44.60
anterior I44.4
posterior I44.5
right I45.0
specified NEC I44.69
foramen Magendie (acquired) G91.1
congenital Q03.1
with spina bifida —*see* Spina bifida, by site, with hydrocephalus
heart I45.9
bundle branch I45.4
bilateral I45.2
complete (atrioventricular) I44.2
congenital Q24.6
first degree (atrioventricular) I44.0
second degree (atrioventricular) I44.1
specified type NEC I45.5
third degree (atrioventricular) I44.2
hepatic vein I82.0
intraventricular (nonspecific) I45.4
bundle branch
bilateral I45.2
kidney N28.9
postcystoscopic or postprocedural N99.0

Block, blocked *(Continued)*
Mobitz (types I and II) I44.1
myocardial —*see* Block, heart
nodal I45.5
organ or site, congenital NEC —*see* Atresia, by site
portal (vein) I81
second degree (types I and II) I44.1
sinoatrial I45.5
sinoauricular I45.5
third degree I44.2
trifascicular I45.3
tubal N97.1
vein NOS I82.90
Wenckebach (types I and II) I44.1
Blockage —*see* Obstruction
Blocq's disease F44.4
Blood
constituents, abnormal R78.9
disease D75.9
donor —*see* Donor, blood
dyscrasia D75.9
with
abortion —*see* Abortion, by type, complicated by, hemorrhage
ectopic pregnancy O08.1
molar pregnancy O08.1
following ectopic or molar pregnancy O08.1
newborn P61.9
puerperal, postpartum O72.3
flukes NEC —*see* Schistosomiasis
in
feces K92.1
occult R19.5
urine —*see* Hematuria
mole O02.0
occult in feces R19.5
pressure
decreased, due to shock following injury T79.4
examination only Z01.30
fluctuating I99.8
high —*see* Hypertension
borderline R03.0
incidental reading, without diagnosis of hypertension R03.0
low —*see also* Hypotension
incidental reading, without diagnosis of hypotension R03.1
spitting —*see* Hemoptysis
staining cornea —*see* Pigmentation, cornea, stromal
transfusion
reaction or complication —*see* Complications, transfusion
type
A (Rh positive) Z67.10
Rh negative Z67.11
AB (Rh positive) Z67.30
Rh negative Z67.31
B (Rh positive) Z67.20
Rh negative Z67.21
O (Rh positive) Z67.40
Rh negative Z67.41
Rh (positive) Z67.90
negative Z67.91
vessel rupture —*see* Hemorrhage
vomiting —*see* Hematemesis
Blood-forming organs, disease D75.9
Bloodgood's disease —*see* Mastopathy, cystic
Bloom (-Machacek)(-Torre) syndrome Q82.8
Blount's disease or osteochondrosis —*see* Osteochondrosis, juvenile, tibia
Blue
baby Q24.9
diaper syndrome E72.09
dome cyst (breast) —*see* Cyst, breast
dot cataract Q12.0

Blue *(Continued)*
nevus D22.9
sclera Q13.5
with fragility of bone and deafness Q78.0
toe syndrome I75.02-
Blueness —*see* Cyanosis
Blues, postpartal O90.6
baby O90.6
Blurring, visual H53.8
Blushing (abnormal) (excessive) R23.2
BMI —*see* Body, mass index
Boarder, hospital NEC Z76.4
accompanying sick person Z76.3
healthy infant or child Z76.2
foundling Z76.1
Bockhart's impetigo L01.02
Bodechtel-Guttman disease (subacute sclerosing panencephalitis) A81.1
Boder-Sedgwick syndrome (ataxia-telangiectasia) G11.3
Body, bodies
Aschoff's —*see* Myocarditis, rheumatic
asteroid, vitreous —*see* Deposit, crystalline
cytoid (retina) —*see* Occlusion, artery, retina
drusen (degenerative) (macula) (retinal) —*see also* Degeneration, macula, drusen
optic disc —*see* Drusen, optic disc
foreign —*see* Foreign body
loose
joint, except knee —*see* Loose, body, joint
knee M23.4-
sheath, tendon —*see* Disorder, tendon, specified type NEC
mass index (BMI)
adult
19 or less Z68.1
20.0-20.9 Z68.20
21.0-21.9 Z68.21
22.0-22.9 Z68.22
23.0-23.9 Z68.23
24.0-24.9 Z68.24
25.0-25.9 Z68.25
26.0-26.9 Z68.26
27.0-27.9 Z68.27
28.0-28.9 Z68.28
29.0-29.9 Z68.29
30.0-30.9 Z68.30
31.0-31.9 Z68.31
32.0-32.9 Z68.32
33.0-33.9 Z68.33
34.0-34.9 Z68.34
35.0-35.9 Z68.35
36.0-36.9 Z68.36
37.0-37.9 Z68.37
38.0-38.9 Z68.38
39.0-39.9 Z68.39
40.0-44.9 Z68.41
45.0-49.9 Z68.42
50.0-59.9 Z68.43
60.0-69.9 Z68.44
70 and over Z68.45
pediatric
5th percentile to less than 85th percentile for age Z68.52
85th percentile to less than 95th percentile for age Z68.53
greater than or equal to ninety-fifth percentile for age Z68.54
less than fifth percentile for age Z68.51
Mooser's A75.2
rice —*see also* Loose, body, joint
knee M23.4-
rocking F98.4
Boeck's
disease or sarcoid —*see* Sarcoidosis
lupoid (miliary) D86.3
Boerhaave's syndrome (spontaneous esophageal rupture) K22.3
Boggy
cervix N88.8
uterus N85.8

Boil —*see also* Furuncle, by site
  Aleppo B55.1
  Baghdad B55.1
  Delhi B55.1
  lacrimal
    gland —*see* Dacryoadenitis
    passages (duct) (sac) —*see* Inflammation,
      lacrimal, passages, acute
  Natal B55.1
  orbit, orbital —*see* Abscess, orbit
  tropical B55.1
Bold hives —*see* Urticaria
Bombé, iris —*see* Membrane, pupillary
Bone —*see* condition
Bonnevie-Ullrich syndrome Q87.1
Bonnier's syndrome —*see* subcategory
  H81.8
Bonvale dam fever T73.3
Bony block of joint —*see* Ankylosis
BOOP (bronchiolitis obliterans organized
  pneumonia) J84.89
Borderline
  diabetes mellitus R73.09
  hypertension R03.0
  osteopenia M85.8-
  pelvis, with obstruction during labor
    O65.1
  personality F60.3
Borna disease A83.9
Bornholm disease B33.0
Boston exanthem A88.0
Botalli, ductus (patent) (persistent) Q25.0
Bothriocephalus latus infestation B70.0
Botulism (foodborne intoxication) A05.1
  infant A48.51
  non-foodborne A48.52
  wound A48.52
Bouba —*see* Yaws
Bouchard's nodes (with arthropathy) M15.2
Bouffée délirante F23
Bouillaud's disease or syndrome (rheumatic
  heart disease) I01.9
Bourneville's disease Q85.1
Boutonniere deformity (finger) —*see*
  Deformity, finger, boutonniere
Bouveret (-Hoffmann) syndrome (paroxysmal
  tachycardia) I47.9
Bovine heart —*see* Hypertrophy, cardiac
Bowel —*see* condition
Bowen's
  dermatosis (precancerous) —*see* Neoplasm,
    skin, in situ ◄▥
  disease —*see* Neoplasm, skin, in situ
  epithelioma —*see* Neoplasm, skin, in situ
  type
    epidermoid carcinoma-in-situ —*see*
      Neoplasm, skin, in situ ◄▥
    intraepidermal squamous cell carcinoma —
      see Neoplasm, skin, in situ
Bowing
  femur —*see also* Deformity, limb, specified
    type NEC, thigh
    congenital Q68.3
  fibula —*see also* Deformity, limb, specified
    type NEC, lower leg
    congenital Q68.4
  forearm —*see* Deformity, limb, specified type
    NEC, forearm
  leg (s), long bones, congenital Q68.5
  radius —*see* Deformity, limb, specified type
    NEC, forearm
  tibia —*see also* Deformity, limb, specified type
    NEC, lower leg
    congenital Q68.4
Bowleg (s) (acquired) M21.16-
  congenital Q68.5
  rachitic E64.3
Boyd's dysentery A03.2
Brachial —*see* condition
Brachycardia R00.1
Brachycephaly Q75.0

Bradley's disease A08.19
Bradyarrhythmia, cardiac I49.8
Bradycardia (sinoatrial) (sinus) (vagal) R00.1
  neonatal P29.12
  reflex G90.09
  tachycardia syndrome I49.5
Bradykinesia R25.8
Bradypnea R06.89
Bradytachycardia I49.5
Brailsford's disease or osteochondrosis —*see*
  Osteochondrosis, juvenile, radius
Brain —*see also* condition
  death G93.82
  syndrome —*see* Syndrome, brain
Branched-chain amino-acid disorder E71.2
Branchial —*see* condition
  cartilage, congenital Q18.2
Branchiogenic remnant (in neck) Q18.0
Brandt's syndrome (acrodermatitis
  enteropathica) E83.2
Brash (water) R12
Bravais-jacksonian epilepsy —*see* Epilepsy,
  localization-related, symptomatic, with
  simple partial seizures
Braxton Hicks contractions —*see* False, labor
Brazilian leishmaniasis B55.2
BRBPR K62.5
Break, retina (without detachment) H33.30-
  with retinal detachment —*see* Detachment,
    retina
  horseshoe tear H33.31-
  multiple H33.33-
  round hole H33.32-
Breakdown
  device, graft or implant (*see also*
    Complications, by site and type,
    mechanical) T85.618
    arterial graft NEC —*see* Complication,
      cardiovascular device, mechanical,
      vascular
    breast (implant) T85.41
    catheter NEC T85.618
      cystostomy T83.010
      dialysis (renal) T82.41
        intraperitoneal T85.611
      infusion NEC T82.514
        spinal (epidural) (subdural) T85.610
      urinary (indwelling) T83.018
    electronic (electrode) (pulse generator)
      (stimulator)
      bone T84.310
      cardiac T82.119
        electrode T82.110
          pulse generator T82.111
          specified type NEC T82.118
      nervous system —*see* Complication,
        prosthetic device, mechanical,
        electronic nervous system
        stimulator
      urinary —*see* Complication,
        genitourinary, device, urinary,
        mechanical
    fixation, internal (orthopedic) NEC —*see*
      Complication, fixation device,
      mechanical
    gastrointestinal —*see* Complications,
      prosthetic device, mechanical,
      gastrointestinal device
    genital NEC T83.418
      intrauterine contraceptive device T83.31
      penile prosthesis T83.410
    heart NEC —*see* Complication,
      cardiovascular device, mechanical
    joint prosthesis —*see* Complications...,
      joint prosthesis, internal, mechanical,
      by site
    ocular NEC —*see* Complications, prosthetic
      device, mechanical, ocular device
    orthopedic NEC —*see* Complication,
      orthopedic, device, mechanical
    specified NEC T85.618

Breakdown (*Continued*)
  device, graft or implant (*Continued*)
    sutures, permanent T85.612
      used in bone repair —*see* Complications,
        fixation device, internal
        (orthopedic), mechanical
    urinary NEC —*see also* Complication,
      genitourinary, device, urinary,
      mechanical
      graft T83.21
    vascular NEC —*see* Complication,
      cardiovascular device, mechanical
    ventricular intracranial shunt T85.01
  nervous F48.8
  perineum O90.1
  respirator J95.850
    specified NEC J95.859
  ventilator J95.850
    specified NEC J95.859
Breast —*see also* condition
  buds E30.1
    in newborn P96.89
  dense R92.2
  nodule N63
Breath
  foul R19.6
  holder, child R06.89
  holding spell R06.89
  shortness R06.02
Breathing
  labored —*see* Hyperventilation
  mouth R06.5
    causing malocclusion M26.5
  periodic R06.3
    high altitude G47.32
Breathlessness R06.81
Breda's disease —*see* Yaws
Breech presentation (mother) O32.1
  causing obstructed labor O64.1
  footling O32.8
    causing obstructed labor O64.8
  incomplete O32.8
    causing obstructed labor O64.8
Breisky's disease N90.4
Brennemann's syndrome I88.0
Brenner
  tumor (benign) D27.9
    borderline malignancy D39.1-
    malignant C56
    proliferating D39.1
Bretonneau's disease or angina A36.0
Breus' mole O02.0
Brevicollis Q76.49
Brickmakers' anemia B76.9 [D63.8] ◄▥
Bridge, myocardial Q24.5
Bright red blood per rectum (BRBPR) K62.5
Bright's disease —*see also* Nephritis
  arteriosclerotic —*see* Hypertension, kidney
Brill (-Zinsser) disease (recrudescent typhus)
  A75.1
  flea-borne A75.2
  louse-borne A75.1
Brill-Symmers' disease C82.90
Brion-Kayser disease —*see* Fever, parathyroid
Briquet's disorder or syndrome F45.0
Brissaud's
  infantilism or dwarfism E23.0
  motor-verbal tic F95.2
Brittle
  bones disease Q78.0
  nails L60.3
    congenital Q84.6
Broad —*see also* condition
  beta disease E78.2
  ligament laceration syndrome N83.8
Broad- or floating-betalipoproteinemia
  E78.2
Brock's syndrome (atelectasis due to enlarged
  lymph nodes) J98.19
Brocq-Duhring disease (dermatitis
  herpetiformis) L13.0

◄ New   ◄▥ Revised   ~~deleted~~ Deleted

Brodie's abscess or disease M86.8X-
Broken
  arches —*see also* Deformity, limb, flat foot
  arm (meaning upper limb) —*see* Fracture, arm
  back —*see* Fracture, vertebra
  bone —*see* Fracture
  implant or internal device —*see* Complications, by site and type, mechanical
  leg (meaning lower limb) —*see* Fracture, leg
  nose S02.2
  tooth, teeth —*see* Fracture, tooth
Bromhidrosis, bromidrosis L75.0
Bromidism, bromism G92
  chronic (dependence) F13.20
  due to
    correct substance properly administered —*see* Table of dDrugs and cChemicals, by drug, adverse effect
    overdose or wrong substance given or taken —*see* Table of dDrugs and cChemicals, by drug, poisoning
Bromidrosiphobia F40.298
Bronchi, bronchial —*see* condition
Bronchiectasis (cylindrical) (diffuse) (fusiform) (localized) (saccular) J47.9
  with
    acute
      bronchitis J47.0
      lower respiratory infection J47.0
    exacerbation (acute) J47.1
  congenital Q33.4
  tuberculous NEC —*see* Tuberculosis, pulmonary
Bronchiolectasis —*see* Bronchiectasis
Bronchiolitis (acute) (infective) (subacute) J21.9
  with
    bronchospasm or obstruction J21.9
    influenza, flu or grippe —*see* Influenza, with, respiratory manifestations NEC
  chemical (chronic) J68.4
    acute J68.0
  chronic (fibrosing) (obliterative) J44.9
  due to
    external agent —*see* Bronchitis, acute, due to
    human metapneumovirus J21.1
    respiratory syncytial virus J21.0
    specified organism NEC J21.8
  fibrosa obliterans J44.9
  influenzal —*see* Influenza, with, respiratory manifestations NEC
  obliterans J42
    with organizing pneumonia (BOOP) J84.89
  obliterative (chronic) (subacute) J44.9
    due to chemicals, gases, fumes or vapors (inhalation) J68.4
    due to fumes or vapors J68.4
  respiratory, interstitial lung disease J84.115
Bronchitis (diffuse) (fibrinous) (hypostatic) (infective) (membranous) J40
  with
    influenza, flu or grippe —*see* Influenza, with, respiratory manifestations NEC
    obstruction (airway) (lung) J44.9
    tracheitis (15 years of age and above) J40
      acute or subacute J20.9
      chronic J42
      under 15 years of age J20.9
  acute or subacute (with bronchospasm or obstruction) J20.9
    with
      bronchiectasis J47.0
      chronic obstructive pulmonary disease J44.0
    chemical (due to gases, fumes or vapors) J68.0

Bronchitis (Continued)
  acute or subacute (Continued)
    due to
      fumes or vapors J68.0
      Haemophilus influenzae J20.1
      Mycoplasma pneumoniae J20.0
      radiation J70.0
      specified organism NEC J20.8
      Streptococcus J20.2
      virus
        coxsackie J20.3
        echovirus J20.7
        parainfluenzae J20.4
        respiratory syncytial J20.5
        rhinovirus J20.6
      viral NEC J20.8
  allergic (acute) J45.909
    with
      exacerbation (acute) J45.901
      status asthmaticus J45.902
  arachidic T17.528
  aspiration (due to fumes or vapors) J68.0
  asthmatic J45.9
    chronic J44.9
      with
        acute lower respiratory infection J44.0
        exacerbation (acute) J44.1
  capillary —*see* Pneumonia, broncho
  caseous (tuberculous) A15.5
  Castellani's A69.8
  catarrhal (15 years of age and above) J40
    acute —*see* Bronchitis, acute
    chronic J41.0
    under 15 years of age J20.9
  chemical (acute) (subacute) J68.0
    chronic J68.4
    due to fumes or vapors J68.0
      chronic J68.4
  chronic J42
    with
      airways obstruction J44.9
      tracheitis (chronic) J42
    asthmatic (obstructive) J44.9
    catarrhal J41.0
    chemical (due to fumes or vapors) J68.4
    due to
      chemicals, gases, fumes or vapors (inhalation) J68.4
      radiation J70.1
      tobacco smoking J41.0
    emphysematous J44.9
    mucopurulent J41.1
    non-obstructive J41.0
    obliterans J44.9
    obstructive J44.9
    purulent J41.1
    simple J41.0
  croupous —*see* Bronchitis, acute
  due to gases, fumes or vapors (chemical) J68.0
  emphysematous (obstructive) J44.9
  exudative —*see* Bronchitis, acute
  fetid J41.1
  grippal —*see* Influenza, with, respiratory manifestations NEC
  in those under 15 years age —*see* Bronchitis, acute
    chronic —*see* Bronchitis, chronic
  influenzal —*see* Influenza, with, respiratory manifestations NEC
  mixed simple and mucopurulent J41.8
  moulder's J62.8
  mucopurulent (chronic) (recurrent) J41.1
    acute or subacute J20.9
    simple (mixed) J41.8
  obliterans (chronic) J44.9
  obstructive (chronic) (diffuse) J44.9
  pituitous J41.1
  pneumococcal, acute or subacute J20.2
  pseudomembranous, acute or subacute —*see* Bronchitis, acute

Bronchitis (Continued)
  purulent (chronic) (recurrent) J41.1
    acute or subacute —*see* Bronchitis, acute
  putrid J41.1
  senile (chronic) J42
  simple and mucopurulent (mixed) J41.8
  smokers' J41.0
  spirochetal NEC A69.8
  subacute —*see* Bronchitis, acute
  suppurative (chronic) J41.1
    acute or subacute —*see* Bronchitis, acute
  tuberculous A15.5
  under 15 years of age —*see* Bronchitis, acute
    chronic —*see* Bronchitis, chronic
  viral NEC, acute or subacute (*see also* Bronchitis, acute) J20.8
Bronchoalveolitis J18.0
Bronchoaspergillosis B44.1
Bronchocele meaning goiter E04.0
Broncholithiasis J98.09
  tuberculous NEC A15.5
Bronchomalacia J98.09
  congenital Q32.2
Bronchomycosis NOS B49 *[J99]*
  candidal B37.1
Bronchopleuropneumonia —*see* Pneumonia, broncho
Bronchopneumonia —*see* Pneumonia, broncho
Bronchopneumonitis —*see* Pneumonia, broncho
Bronchopulmonary —*see* condition
Bronchopulmonitis —*see* Pneumonia, broncho
Bronchorrhagia (*see* Hemoptysis)
Bronchorrhea J98.09
  acute J20.9
  chronic (infective) (purulent) J42
Bronchospasm (acute) J98.01
  with
    bronchiolitis, acute J21.9
    bronchitis, acute (conditions in J20) —*see* Bronchitis, acute
  due to external agent —*see* condition, respiratory, acute, due to
  exercise induced J45.990
Bronchospirochetosis A69.8
  Castellani A69.8
Bronchostenosis J98.09
Bronchus —*see* condition
Brontophobia F40.220
Bronze baby syndrome P83.8
Brooke's tumor —*see* Neoplasm, skin, benign
Brown enamel of teeth (hereditary) K00.5
Brown's sheath syndrome H50.61-
Brown-Séquard disease, paralysis or syndrome G83.81
Bruce sepsis A23.0
Brucellosis (infection) A23.9
  abortus A23.1
  canis A23.3
  dermatitis A23.9
  melitensis A23.0
  mixed A23.8
  sepsis A23.9
    melitensis A23.0
    specified NEC A23.8
  suis A23.2
Bruck-de Lange disease Q87.1
Bruck's disease —*see* Deformity, limb
Brugsch's syndrome Q82.8
Bruise (skin surface intact) —*see also* Contusion
  with
    open wound —*see* Wound, open
    internal organ —*see* Injury, by site
  newborn P54.5
  scalp, due to birth injury, newborn P12.3
  umbilical cord O69.5
Bruit (arterial) R09.89
  cardiac R01.1
Brush burn —*see* Abrasion, by site
Bruton's X-linked agammaglobulinemia D80.0

◄ New   ◄▥ Revised   ~~deleted~~ Deleted

Burn *(Continued)*
  extent *(Continued)*
    30-39 percent *(Continued)*
      with 20-29 percent third degree burns T31.32
      with 30-39 percent third degree burns T31.33
    40-49 percent T31.40
      with 0-9 percent third degree burns T31.40
      with 10-19 percent third degree burns T31.41
      with 20-29 percent third degree burns T31.42
      with 30-39 percent third degree burns T31.43
      with 40-49 percent third degree burns T31.44
    50-59 percent T31.50
      with 0-9 percent third degree burns T31.50
      with 10-19 percent third degree burns T31.51
      with 20-29 percent third degree burns T31.52
      with 30-39 percent third degree burns T31.53
      with 40-49 percent third degree burns T31.54
      with 50-59 percent third degree burns T31.55
    60-69 percent T31.60
      with 0-9 percent third degree burns T31.60
      with 10-19 percent third degree burns T31.61
      with 20-29 percent third degree burns T31.62
      with 30-39 percent third degree burns T31.63
      with 40-49 percent third degree burns T31.64
      with 50-59 percent third degree burns T31.65
      with 60-69 percent third degree burns T31.66
    70-79 percent T31.70
      with 0-9 percent third degree burns T31.70
      with 10-19 percent third degree burns T31.71
      with 20-29 percent third degree burns T31.72
      with 30-39 percent third degree burns T31.73
      with 40-49 percent third degree burns T31.74
      with 50-59 percent third degree burns T31.75
      with 60-69 percent third degree burns T31.76
      with 70-79 percent third degree burns T31.77
    80-89 percent T31.80
      with 0-9 percent third degree burns T31.80
      with 10-19 percent third degree burns T31.81
      with 20-29 percent third degree burns T31.82
      with 30-39 percent third degree burns T31.83
      with 40-49 percent third degree burns T31.84
      with 50-59 percent third degree burns T31.85
      with 60-69 percent third degree burns T31.86
      with 70-79 percent third degree burns T31.87
      with 80-89 percent third degree burns T31.88
    90 percent or more T31.90
      with 0-9 percent third degree burns T31.90
      with 10-19 percent third degree burns T31.91

Burn *(Continued)*
  extent *(Continued)*
    90 percent or more *(Continued)*
      with 20-29 percent third degree burns T31.92
      with 30-39 percent third degree burns T31.93
      with 40-49 percent third degree burns T31.94
      with 50-59 percent third degree burns T31.95
      with 60-69 percent third degree burns T31.96
      with 70-79 percent third degree burns T31.97
      with 80-89 percent third degree burns T31.98
      with 90 percent or more third degree burns T31.99
  extremity —*see* Burn, limb
  eye (s) and adnexa T26.4-
    with resulting rupture and destruction of eyeball T26.2-
    conjunctival sac —*see* Burn, cornea
    cornea —*see* Burn, cornea
    lid —*see* Burn, eyelid
    periocular area —*see* Burn, eyelid
    specified site NEC T26.3-
  eyeball —*see* Burn, eye
  eyelid (s) T26.0-
    chemical —*see* Corrosion, eyelid
  face —*see* Burn, head
  finger T23.029
    first degree T23.129
    left T23.022
      first degree T23.122
      second degree T23.222
      third degree T23.322
    multiple sites (without thumb) T23.039
      with thumb T23.049
        first degree T23.149
        left T23.042
          first degree T23.142
          second degree T23.242
          third degree T23.342
        right T23.041
          first degree T23.141
          second degree T23.241
          third degree T23.341
        second degree T23.249
        third degree T23.349
      first degree T23.139
      left T23.032
        first degree T23.132
        second degree T23.232
        third degree T23.332
      right T23.031
        first degree T23.131
        second degree T23.231
        third degree T23.331
      second degree T23.239
      third degree T23.339
    right T23.021
      first degree T23.121
      second degree T23.221
      third degree T23.321
    second degree T23.229
    third degree T23.329
  flank —*see* Burn, abdominal wall
  foot T25.029
    first degree T25.129
    left T25.022
      first degree T25.122
      second degree T25.222
      third degree T25.322
    multiple with ankle —*see* Burn, lower, limb, multiple, ankle and foot
    right T25.021
      first degree T25.121
      second degree T25.221
      third degree T25.321

Burn *(Continued)*
  foot *(Continued)*
    second degree T25.229
    third degree T25.329
  forearm T22.019
    first degree T22.119
    left T22.012
      first degree T22.112
      second degree T22.212
      third degree T22.312
    right T22.011
      first degree T22.111
      second degree T22.211
      third degree T22.311
    second degree T22.219
    third degree T22.319
  forehead T20.06
    first degree T20.16
    second degree T20.26
    third degree T20.36
  fourth degree - code as Burn, third degree, by site
  friction —*see* Burn, by site
  from swallowing caustic or corrosive substance NEC —*see* Corrosion, by site
  full thickness skin loss - code as Burn, third degree, by site
  gastrointestinal tract NEC T28.2
    from swallowing caustic or corrosive substance T28.7
  genital organs
    external
      female T21.07
        first degree T21.17
        second degree T21.27
        third degree T21.37
      male T21.06
        first degree T21.16
        second degree T21.26
        third degree T21.36
    internal T28.3
      from caustic or corrosive substance T28.8
  groin —*see* Burn, abdominal wall
  hand (s) T23.009
    back —*see* Burn, dorsum of hand
    finger —*see* Burn, finger
    first degree T23.109
    left T23.002
      first degree T23.102
      second degree T23.202
      third degree T23.302
    multiple sites with wrist T23.099
      first degree T23.199
      left T23.092
        first degree T23.192
        second degree T23.292
        third degree T23.392
      right T23.091
        first degree T23.191
        second degree T23.291
        third degree T23.391
      second degree T23.299
      third degree T23.399
    palm —*see* Burn, palm
    right T23.001
      first degree T23.101
      second degree T23.201
      third degree T23.301
    second degree T23.209
    third degree T23.309
    thumb —*see* Burn, thumb
  head (and face) (and neck) T20.00
    cheek —*see* Burn, cheek
    chin —*see* Burn, chin
    ear —*see* Burn, ear
    eye (s) only —*see* Burn, eye
    first degree T20.10
    forehead —*see* Burn, forehead
    lip —*see* Burn, lip

◀ New   ◀▥ Revised   ~~deleted~~ Deleted

Burn *(Continued)*
  tongue T28.0
  tonsil (s) T28.0
  trachea T27.0
    with lung T27.1
  trunk T21.00
    abdominal wall —*see* Burn, abdominal wall
    anus —*see* Burn, buttock
    axilla —*see* Burn, upper limb
    back —*see* Burn, back
    breast —*see* Burn, chest wall
    buttock —*see* Burn, buttock
    chest wall —*see* Burn, chest wall
    first degree T21.10
    flank —*see* Burn, abdominal wall
    genital
      female —*see* Burn, genital organs, external, female
      male —*see* Burn, genital organs, external, male
    groin —*see* Burn, abdominal wall
    interscapular region —*see* Burn, back, upper
    labia —*see* Burn, genital organs, external, female
    lower back —*see* Burn, back
    penis —*see* Burn, genital organs, external, male
    perineum
      female —*see* Burn, genital organs, external, female
      male —*see* Burn, genital organs, external, male
    scapula region —*see* Burn, scapular region
    scrotum —*see* Burn, genital organs, external, male
    second degree T21.20
    specified site NEC T21.09
      first degree T21.19
      second degree T21.29
      third degree T21.39
    testes —*see* Burn, genital organs, external, male
    third degree T21.30
    upper back —*see* Burn, back, upper
    vulva —*see* Burn, genital organs, external, female
  unspecified site with extent of body surface involved specified
    less than 10 percent T31.0
    10-19 percent (0-9 percent third degree) T31.10
      with 10-19 percent third degree T31.11
    20-29 percent (0-9 percent third degree) T31.20
      with
        10-19 percent third degree T31.21
        20-29 percent third degree T31.22
    30-39 percent (0-9 percent third degree) T31.30
      with
        10-19 percent third degree T31.31
        20-29 percent third degree T31.32
        30-39 percent third degree T31.33
    40-49 percent (0-9 percent third degree) T31.40
      with
        10-19 percent third degree T31.41
        20-29 percent third degree T31.42
        30-39 percent third degree T31.43
        40-49 percent third degree T31.44
    50-59 percent (0-9 percent third degree) T31.50
      with
        10-19 percent third degree T31.51
        20-29 percent third degree T31.52
        30-39 percent third degree T31.53
        40-49 percent third degree T31.54
        50-59 percent third degree T31.55

Burn *(Continued)*
  unspecified site with extent of body surface involved specified *(Continued)*
    60-69 percent (0-9 percent third degree) T31.60
      with
        10-19 percent third degree T31.61
        20-29 percent third degree T31.62
        30-39 percent third degree T31.63
        40-49 percent third degree T31.64
        50-59 percent third degree T31.65
        60-69 percent third degree T31.66
    70-79 percent (0-9 percent third degree) T31.70
      with
        10-19 percent third degree T31.71
        20-29 percent third degree T31.72
        30-39 percent third degree T31.73
        40-49 percent third degree T31.74
        50-59 percent third degree T31.75
        60-69 percent third degree T31.76
        70-79 percent third degree T31.77
    80-89 percent (0-9 percent third degree) T31.80
      with
        10-19 percent third degree T31.81
        20-29 percent third degree T31.82
        30-39 percent third degree T31.83
        40-49 percent third degree T31.84
        50-59 percent third degree T31.85
        60-69 percent third degree T31.86
        70-79 percent third degree T31.87
        80-89 percent third degree T31.88
    90 percent or more (0-9 percent third degree) T31.90
      with
        10-19 percent third degree T31.91
        20-29 percent third degree T31.92
        30-39 percent third degree T31.93
        40-49 percent third degree T31.94
        50-59 percent third degree T31.95
        60-69 percent third degree T31.96
        70-79 percent third degree T31.97
        80-89 percent third degree T31.98
        90-99 percent third degree T31.99
  upper limb T22.00
    above elbow —*see* Burn, above elbow
    axilla —*see* Burn, axilla
    elbow —*see* Burn, elbow
    first degree T22.10
    forearm —*see* Burn, forearm
    hand —*see* Burn, hand
    interscapular region —*see* Burn, back, upper
    multiple sites T22.099
      first degree T22.199
      left T22.092
        first degree T22.192
        second degree T22.292
        third degree T22.392
      right T22.091
        first degree T22.191
        second degree T22.291
        third degree T22.391
      second degree T22.299
      third degree T22.399
    scapular region —*see* Burn, scapular region
    second degree T22.20
    shoulder —*see* Burn, shoulder
    third degree T22.30
    wrist —*see* Burn, wrist
  uterus T28.3
  vagina T28.3
  vulva —*see* Burn, genital organs, external, female
  wrist T23.079
    first degree T23.179
    left T23.072
      first degree T23.172
      second degree T23.272
      third degree T23.372

Burn *(Continued)*
  wrist *(Continued)*
    multiple sites with hand T23.099
      first degree T23.199
      left T23.092
        first degree T23.192
        second degree T23.292
        third degree T23.392
      right T23.091
        first degree T23.191
        second degree T23.291
        third degree T23.391
      second degree T23.299
      third degree T23.399
    right T23.071
      first degree T23.171
      second degree T23.271
      third degree T23.371
    second degree T23.279
    third degree T23.379
Burnett's syndrome E83.52
Burning
  feet syndrome E53.9
  sensation R20.8
  tongue K14.6
Burn-out (state) Z73.0
Burns' disease or osteochondrosis —*see* Osteochondrosis, juvenile, ulna
Bursa —*see* condition
Bursitis M71.9
  Achilles —*see* Tendinitis, Achilles
  adhesive —*see* Bursitis, specified NEC
  ankle —*see* Enthesopathy, lower limb, ankle, specified type NEC
  calcaneal —*see* Enthesopathy, foot, specified type NEC
  collateral ligament, tibial —*see* Bursitis, tibial collateral
  due to use, overuse, pressure —*see also* Disorder, soft tissue, due to use, specified type NEC
    specified NEC —*see* Disorder, soft tissue, due to use, specified NEC
  Duplay's M75.0
  elbow NEC M70.3-
    olecranon M70.2-
  finger —*see* Disorder, soft tissue, due to use, specified type NEC, hand
  foot —*see* Enthesopathy, foot, specified type NEC
  gonococcal A54.49
  gouty —*see* Gout, idiopathic
  hand M70.1-
  hip NEC M70.7-
    trochanteric M70.6-
  infective NEC M71.10
    abscess —*see* Abscess, bursa
    ankle M71.17-
    elbow M71.12-
    foot M71.17-
    hand M71.14-
    hip M71.15-
    knee M71.16-
    multiple sites M71.19
    shoulder M71.11-
    specified site NEC M71.18
    wrist M71.13-
  ischial —*see* Bursitis, hip
  knee NEC M70.5-
    prepatellar M70.4-
  occupational NEC —*see also* Disorder, soft tissue, due to, use
  olecranon —*see* Bursitis, elbow, olecranon
  pharyngeal J39.1
  popliteal —*see* Bursitis, knee
  prepatellar M70.4-
  radiohumeral M77.8
  rheumatoid M06.20
    ankle M06.27-
    elbow M06.22-
    foot joint M06.27-

Bursitis *(Continued)*
  rheumatoid *(Continued)*
    hand joint M06.24-
    hip M06.25-
    knee M06.26-
    multiple site M06.29
    shoulder M06.21-
    vertebra M06.28
    wrist M06.23-
  scapulohumeral —*see* Bursitis, shoulder
  semimembranous muscle (knee) —*see*
    Bursitis, knee
  shoulder M75.5-
    adhesive —*see* Capsulitis, adhesive
  specified NEC M71.50
    ankle M71.57-
    due to use, overuse or pressure —*see*
      Disorder, soft tissue, due to, use
    elbow M71.52-
    foot M71.57-
    hand M71.54-
    hip M71.55-
    knee M71.56-
    shoulder —*see* Bursitis, shoulder
    specified site NEC M71.58

Bursitis *(Continued)*
  specified NEC *(Continued)*
    tibial collateral M76.4-
    wrist M71.53-
  subacromial —*see* Bursitis, shoulder
  subcoracoid —*see* Bursitis, shoulder
  subdeltoid —*see* Bursitis, shoulder
  syphilitic A52.78
  Thornwaldt, Tornwaldt J39.2
  tibial collateral —*see* Bursitis, tibial collateral
  toe —*see* Enthesopathy, foot, specified type
    NEC
  trochanteric (area) —*see* Bursitis, hip,
    trochanteric
  wrist —*see* Bursitis, hand
Bursopathy M71.9
  specified type NEC M71.80
    ankle M71.87-
    elbow M71.82-
    foot M71.87-
    hand M71.84-
    hip M71.85-
    knee M71.86-
    multiple sites M71.89
    shoulder M71.81-

Bursopathy *(Continued)*
  specified type NEC *(Continued)*
    specified site NEC M71.88
    wrist M71.83-
Burst stitches or sutures (complication of
  surgery) T81.31
  external operation wound T81.31
  internal operation wound T81.32
Buruli ulcer A31.1
Bury's disease L95.1
Buschke's
  disease B45.3
  scleredema —*see* Sclerosis, systemic
Busse-Buschke disease B45.3
Buttock —*see* condition
Button
  Biskra B55.1
  Delhi B55.1
  oriental B55.1
Buttonhole deformity (finger) —*see* Deformity,
  finger, boutonniere
Bwamba fever A92.8
Byssinosis J66.0
Bywaters' syndrome T79.5

B

C

Cachexia R64
  cancerous R64
  cardiac —see Disease, heart
  dehydration E86.0
    with
      hypernatremia E87.0
      hyponatremia E87.1
  due to malnutrition R64
  exophthalmic —see Hyperthyroidism
  heart —see Disease, heart
  hypophyseal E23.0
  hypopituitary E23.0
  lead —see Poisoning, lead
  malignant R64
  marsh —see Malaria
  nervous F48.8
  old age R54
  paludal —see Malaria
  pituitary E23.0
  renal N28.9
  saturnine —see Poisoning, lead
  senile R54
  Simmonds' E23.0
  splenica D73.0
  strumipriva E03.4
  tuberculous NEC —see Tuberculosis
Café au lait spots L81.3
Caffey's syndrome Q78.8
Caisson disease T70.3
Cake kidney Q63.1
Caked breast (puerperal, postpartum) O92.79
Calabar swelling B74.3
Calcaneal spur —see Spur, bone, calcaneal
Calcaneo-apophysitis M92.8
Calcareous —see condition
Calcicosis J62.8
Calciferol (vitamin D) deficiency E55.9
  with rickets E55.0
Calcification
  adrenal (capsule) (gland) E27.49
    tuberculous B90.8 [E35]E35 [B90.8] ◀▥▥▥
  aorta I70.0
  artery (annular) —see Arteriosclerosis
  auricle (ear) —see Disorder, pinna, specified type NEC
  basal ganglia G23.8
  bladder N32.89
    due to Schistosoma hematobium B65.0
  brain (cortex) —see Calcification, cerebral
  bronchus J98.09
  bursa M71.40
    ankle M71.47-
    elbow M71.42-
    foot M71.47-
    hand M71.44-
    hip M71.45-
    knee M71.46-
    multiple sites M71.49
    shoulder M75.3-
    specified site NEC M71.48
    wrist M71.43-
  cardiac —see Degeneration, myocardial
  cerebral (cortex) G93.89
    artery I67.2
  cervix (uteri) N88.8
  choroid plexus G93.89
  conjunctiva —see Concretion, conjunctiva
  corpora cavernosa (penis) N48.89
  cortex (brain) —see Calcification, cerebral
  dental pulp (nodular) K04.2
  dentinal papilla K00.4
  fallopian tube N83.8
  falx cerebri G96.19
  gallbladder K82.8
  general E83.59
  heart —see also Degeneration, myocardial
    valve —see Endocarditis
  idiopathic infantile arterial (IIAC) Q28.8

Calcification (Continued)
  intervertebral cartilage or disc (postinfective) —see Disorder, disc, specified NEC
  intracranial —see Calcification, cerebral
  joint —see Disorder, joint, specified type NEC
  kidney N28.89
    tuberculous B90.1 [N29]N29 [B90.1] ◀▥▥▥
  larynx (senile) J38.7
  lens —see Cataract, specified NEC
  lung (active) (postinfectional) J98.4
    tuberculous B90.9
  lymph gland or node (postinfectional) I89.8
    tuberculous (see also Tuberculosis, lymph gland) B90.8
  mammographic R92.1
  massive (paraplegic) —see Myositis, ossificans, in, quadriplegia
  medial —see Arteriosclerosis, extremities
  meninges (cerebral) (spinal) G96.19
  metastatic E83.59
  Mönckeberg's —see Arteriosclerosis, extremities
  muscle M61.9
    due to burns —see Myositis, ossificans, in, burns
    paralytic —see Myositis, ossificans, in, quadriplegia
    specified type NEC M61.40
      ankle M61.47-
      foot M61.47-
      forearm M61.43-
      hand M61.44-
      lower leg M61.46-
      multiple sites M61.49
      pelvic region M61.45-
      shoulder region M61.41-
      specified site NEC M61.48
      thigh M61.45-
      upper arm M61.42-
  myocardium, myocardial —see Degeneration, myocardial
  ovary N83.8
  pancreas K86.8
  penis N48.89
  periarticular —see Disorder, joint, specified type NEC
  pericardium (see also Pericarditis) I31.1
  pineal gland E34.8
  pleura J94.8
    postinfectional J94.8
    tuberculous NEC B90.9
  pulpal (dental) (nodular) K04.2
  sclera H15.89
  spleen D73.89
  subcutaneous L94.2
  suprarenal (capsule) (gland) E27.49
  tendon (sheath) —see also Tenosynovitis, specified type NEC
    with bursitis, synovitis or tenosynovitis —see Tendinitis, calcific
  trachea J39.8
  ureter N28.89
  vitreous —see Deposit, crystalline
Calcified —see Calcification
Calcinosis (interstitial) (tumoral) (universalis) E83.59
  with Raynaud's phenomenon, esophageal dysfunction, sclerodactyly, telangiectasia (CREST syndrome) M34.1
  circumscripta (skin) L94.2
  cutis L94.2
Calciphylaxis (see also Calcification, by site) E83.59
Calcium
  deposits —see Calcification, by site
  metabolism disorder E83.50
  salts or soaps in vitreous —see Deposit, crystalline

Calciuria R82.99
Calculi —see Calculus
Calculosis, intrahepatic —see Calculus, bile duct
Calculus, calculi, calculous
  ampulla of Vater —see Calculus, bile duct
  anuria (impacted) (recurrent) (see also Calculus, urinary) N20.9
  appendix K38.1
  bile duct (common) (hepatic) K80.50
    with
      calculus of gallbladder —see Calculus, gallbladder and bile duct
      cholangitis K80.30
        with
          cholecystitis —see Calculus, bile duct, with cholecystitis
          obstruction K80.31
        acute K80.32
          with
            chronic cholangitis K80.36
              with obstruction K80.37
            obstruction K80.33
        chronic K80.34
          with
            acute cholangitis K80.36
              with obstruction K80.37
            obstruction K80.35
      cholecystitis (with cholangitis) K80.40
        with obstruction K80.41
        acute K80.42
          with
            chronic cholecystitis K80.46
              with obstruction K80.47
            obstruction K80.43
        chronic K80.44
          with
            acute cholecystitis K80.46
              with obstruction K80.47
            obstruction K80.45
      obstruction K80.51
  biliary —see also Calculus, gallbladder
    specified NEC K80.80
      with obstruction K80.81
  bilirubin, multiple —see Calculus, gallbladder
  bladder (encysted) (impacted) (urinary) (diverticulum) N21.0
  bronchus J98.09
  calyx (kidney) (renal) —see Calculus, kidney
  cholesterol (pure) (solitary) —see Calculus, gallbladder
  common duct (bile) —see Calculus, bile duct
  conjunctiva —see Concretion, conjunctiva
  cystic N21.0
    duct —see Calculus, gallbladder
  dental (subgingival) (supragingival) K03.6
  diverticulum
    bladder N21.0
    kidney N20.0
  epididymis N50.8
  gallbladder K80.20
    with
      bile duct calculus —see Calculus, gallbladder and bile duct
      cholecystitis K80.10
        with obstruction K80.11
        acute K80.00
          with
            chronic cholecystitis K80.12
              with obstruction K80.13
            obstruction K80.01
        chronic K80.10
          with
            acute cholecystitis K80.12
              with obstruction K80.13
            obstruction K80.11
      specified NEC K80.18
        with obstruction K80.19
      obstruction K80.21

Calculus, calculi, calculous *(Continued)*
- gallbladder and bile duct K80.70
  - with
    - cholecystitis K80.60
      - with obstruction K80.61
      - acute K80.62
        - with
          - chronic cholecystitis K80.66
            - with obstruction K80.67
          - obstruction K80.63
        - chronic K80.64
          - with
            - acute cholecystitis K80.66
              - with obstruction K80.67
            - obstruction K80.65
      - obstruction K80.71
- hepatic (duct) —*see* Calculus, bile duct
- hepatobiliary K80.80
  - with obstruction K80.81
- ileal conduit N21.8
- intestinal (impaction) (obstruction) K56.49
- kidney (impacted) (multiple) (pelvis) (recurrent) (staghorn) N20.0
  - with calculus, ureter N20.2
  - congenital Q63.8
- lacrimal passages —*see* Dacryolith
- liver (impacted) —*see* Calculus, bile duct
- lung J98.4
- mammographic R92.1
- nephritic (impacted) (recurrent) —*see* Calculus, kidney
- nose J34.89
- pancreas (duct) K86.8
- parotid duct or gland K11.5
- pelvis, encysted —*see* Calculus, kidney
- prostate N42.0
- pulmonary J98.4
- pyelitis (impacted) (recurrent) N20.0
  - with hydronephrosis N13.2
- pyelonephritis (impacted) (recurrent) —*see* category N20
  - with hydronephrosis N13.2
- renal (impacted) (recurrent) —*see* Calculus, kidney
- salivary (duct) (gland) K11.5
- seminal vesicle N50.8
- staghorn —*see* Calculus, kidney
- Stensen's duct K11.5
- stomach K31.89
- sublingual duct or gland K11.5
  - congenital Q38.4
- submandibular duct, gland or region K11.5
- submaxillary duct, gland or region K11.5
- suburethral N21.8
- tonsil J35.8
- tooth, teeth (subgingival) (supragingival) K03.6
- tunica vaginalis N50.8
- ureter (impacted) (recurrent) N20.1
  - with calculus, kidney N20.2
    - with hydronephrosis N13.2
      - with infection N13.6
- urethra (impacted) N21.1
- urinary (duct) (impacted) (passage) (tract) N20.9
  - with hydronephrosis N13.2
    - with infection N13.6
  - in (due to)
  - lower N21.9
    - specified NEC N21.8
- vagina N89.8
- vesical (impacted) N21.0
- Wharton's duct K11.5
- xanthine E79.8 [N22]

Calicectasis N28.89
Caliectasis N28.89
California
- disease B38.9
- encephalitis A83.5
Caligo cornea —*see* Opacity, cornea, central
Callositas, callosity (infected) L84

Callus (infected) L84
- bone —*see* Osteophyte
- excessive, following fracture - code as Sequelae of fracture
Calorie deficiency or malnutrition *(see also* Malnutrition) E46
Calvé-Perthes disease —*see* Legg-Calve-Perthes disease
Calvé's disease —*see* Osteochondrosis, juvenile, spine
Calvities —*see* Alopecia, androgenic
Cameroon fever —*see* Malaria
Camptocormia (hysterical) F44.4
Camurati-Engelmann syndrome Q78.3
Canal —*see also* condition
- atrioventricular common Q21.2
Canaliculitis (lacrimal) (acute) (subacute) H04.33-
- Actinomyces A42.89
- chronic H04.42-
Canavan's disease E75.29
Canceled procedure (surgical) Z53.9
- because of
  - contraindication Z53.09
    - smoking Z53.01
  - left against medical advice (AMA) Z53.21
  - patient's decision Z53.20
    - for reasons of belief or group pressure Z53.1
    - specified reason NEC Z53.29
  - specified reason NEC Z53.8
Cancer —*see also* Neoplasm, by site, malignant
- bile duct type, liver C22.1
- blood —*see* Leukemia
- breast *(see also* Neoplasm, breast, malignant) C50.91-
- hepatocellular C22.0
- lung *(see also* Neoplasm, lung, malignant) C34.90- ◀▦
- ovarian *(see also* Neoplasm, ovary, malignant) C56.9- ◀▦
- unspecified site (primary) C80.1
Cancer (o)phobia F45.29
Cancerous —*see* Neoplasm, malignant, by site
Cancrum oris A69.0
Candidiasis, candidal B37.9
- balanitis B37.42
- bronchitis B37.1
- cheilitis B37.83
- congenital P37.5
- cystitis B37.41
- disseminated B37.7
- endocarditis B37.6
- enteritis B37.82
- esophagitis B37.81
- intertrigo B37.2
- lung B37.1
- meningitis B37.5
- mouth B37.0
- nails B37.2
- neonatal P37.5
- onychia B37.2
- oral B37.0
- osteomyelitis B37.89
- otitis externa B37.84
- paronychia B37.2
- perionyxis B37.2
- pneumonia B37.1
- proctitis B37.82
- pulmonary B37.1
- pyelonephritis B37.49
- sepsis B37.7
- skin B37.2
- specified site NEC B37.89
- stomatitis B37.0
- systemic B37.7
- urethritis B37.41
- urogenital site NEC B37.49
- vagina B37.3
- vulva B37.3
- vulvovaginitis B37.3

Candidid L30.2
Candidosis —*see* Candidiasis
Candiru infection or infestation B88.8
Canities (premature) L67.1
- congenital Q84.2
Canker (mouth) (sore) K12.0
- rash A38.9
Cannabinosis J66.2
Canton fever A75.9
Cantrell's syndrome Q87.89
Capillariasis (intestinal) B81.1
- hepatic B83.8
Capillary —*see* condition
Caplan's syndrome —*see* Rheumatoid, lung
Capsule —*see* condition
Capsulitis (joint) —*see also* Enthesopathy
- adhesive (shoulder) M75.0-
- hepatic K65.8
- labyrinthine —*see* Otosclerosis, specified NEC
- thyroid E06.9
Caput
- crepitus Q75.8
- medusae I86.8
- succedaneum P12.81
Car sickness T75.3
Carapata (disease) A68.0
Carate —*see* Pinta
Carbon lung J60
Carbuncle L02.93
- abdominal wall L02.231
- anus K61.0
- auditory canal, external —*see* Abscess, ear, external
- auricle ear —*see* Abscess, ear, external
- axilla L02.43-
- back (any part) L02.232
- breast N61
- buttock L02.33
- cheek (external) L02.03
- chest wall L02.233
- chin L02.03
- corpus cavernosum N48.21
- ear (any part) (external) (middle) —*see* Abscess, ear, external
- external auditory canal —*see* Abscess, ear, external
- eyelid —*see* Abscess, eyelid
- face NEC L02.03
- femoral (region) —*see* Carbuncle, lower limb
- finger —*see* Carbuncle, hand
- flank L02.231
- foot L02.63-
- forehead L02.03
- genital —*see* Abscess, genital
- gluteal (region) L02.33
- groin L02.234
- hand L02.53-
- head NEC L02.831
- heel —*see* Carbuncle, foot
- hip —*see* Carbuncle, lower limb
- kidney —*see* Abscess, kidney
- knee —*see* Carbuncle, lower limb
- labium (majus) (minus) N76.4
- lacrimal
  - gland —*see* Dacryoadenitis
  - passages (duct) (sac) —*see* Inflammation, lacrimal, passages, acute
- leg —*see* Carbuncle, lower limb
- lower limb L02.43-
- malignant A22.0
- navel L02.236
- neck L02.13
- nose (external) (septum) J34.0
- orbit, orbital —*see* Abscess, orbit
- palmar (space) —*see* Carbuncle, hand
- partes posteriores L02.33
- pectoral region L02.233
- penis N48.21
- perineum L02.235
- pinna —*see* Abscess, ear, external
- popliteal —*see* Carbuncle, lower limb

Carbuncle *(Continued)*
  scalp L02.831
  seminal vesicle N49.0
  shoulder —*see* Carbuncle, upper limb
  specified site NEC L02.838
  temple (region) L02.03
  thumb —*see* Carbuncle, hand
  toe —*see* Carbuncle, foot
  trunk L02.239
    abdominal wall L02.231
    back L02.232
    chest wall L02.233
    groin L02.234
    perineum L02.235
    umbilicus L02.236
  umbilicus L02.236
  upper limb L02.43-
  urethra N34.0
  vulva N76.4
Carbunculus —*see* Carbuncle
Carcinoid (tumor) —*see* Tumor, carcinoid
Carcinoidosis E34.0
Carcinoma (malignant) —*see also* Neoplasm, by
    site, malignant
  acidophil
    specified site —*see* Neoplasm, malignant,
      by site
    unspecified site C75.1
  acidophil-basophil, mixed
    specified site —*see* Neoplasm, malignant,
      by site
    unspecified site C75.1
  adnexal (skin) —*see* Neoplasm, skin,
    malignant
  adrenal cortical C74.0-
  alveolar —*see* Neoplasm, lung, malignant
    cell —*see* Neoplasm, lung, malignant
  ameloblastic C41.1
    upper jaw (bone) C41.0
  apocrine
    breast —*see* Neoplasm, breast, malignant
    specified site NEC —*see* Neoplasm, skin,
      malignant
    unspecified site C44.99
  basal cell (pigmented) (*see also* Neoplasm,
    skin, malignant) C44.91
    fibro-epithelial —*see* Neoplasm, skin,
      malignant
    morphea —*see* Neoplasm, skin, malignant
    multicentric —*see* Neoplasm, skin,
      malignant
  basaloid
  basal-squamous cell, mixed —*see* Neoplasm,
    skin, malignant ◀▦
  basophil
    specified site —*see* Neoplasm, malignant,
      by site
    unspecified site C75.1
  basophil-acidophil, mixed
    specified site —*see* Neoplasm, malignant,
      by site
    unspecified site C75.1
  basosquamous —*see* Neoplasm, skin,
    malignant
  bile duct
    with hepatocellular, mixed C22.0
    liver C22.1
    specified site NEC —*see* Neoplasm,
      malignant, by site
    unspecified site C22.1
  branchial or branchiogenic C10.4
  bronchial or bronchogenic —*see* Neoplasm,
    lung, malignant
  bronchiolar —*see* Neoplasm, lung, malignant
  bronchioloalveolar —*see* Neoplasm, lung,
    malignant
  C cell
    specified site —*see* Neoplasm, malignant,
      by site
    unspecified site C73
  ceruminous C44.29-

Carcinoma *(Continued)*
  cervix uteri
    in situ D06.9
      endocervix D06.0
      exocervix D06.1
      specified site NEC D06.7
  chorionic
    specified site —*see* Neoplasm, malignant,
      by site
    unspecified site
      female C58
      male C62.90
  chromophobe
    specified site —*see* Neoplasm, malignant,
      by site
    unspecified site C75.1
  cloacogenic
    specified site —*see* Neoplasm, malignant,
      by site
    unspecified site C21.2
  diffuse type
    specified site —*see* Neoplasm, malignant,
      by site
    unspecified site C16.9
  duct (cell)
    with Paget's disease —*see* Neoplasm,
      breast, malignant
    infiltrating
      with lobular carcinoma (in situ)
        specified site —*see* Neoplasm,
          malignant, by site
        unspecified site (female) C50.91-
          male C50.92-
      specified site —*see* Neoplasm,
        malignant, by site
      unspecified site (female) C50.91-
        male C50.92-
  ductal
    with lobular
      specified site —*see* Neoplasm,
        malignant, by site
      unspecified site (female) C50.91-
        male C50.92-
  ductular, infiltrating
    specified site —*see* Neoplasm, malignant,
      by site
    unspecified site (female) C50.91-
      male C50.92-
  embryonal
    liver C22.7
  endometrioid
    specified site —*see* Neoplasm, malignant,
      by site
    unspecified site
      female C56.9
      male C61
  eosinophil
    specified site —*see* Neoplasm, malignant,
      by site
    unspecified site C75.1
  epidermoid —*see also* ~~Carcinoma, squamous~~
    ~~cell~~ Neoplasm, skin malignant ◀▦
    in situ, Bowen's type —*see* Neoplasm, skin,
      in situ
  fibroepithelial, basal cell —*see* Neoplasm,
    skin, malignant
  follicular
    with papillary (mixed) C73
    moderately differentiated C73
    pure follicle C73
    specified site —*see* Neoplasm, malignant,
      by site
    trabecular C73
    unspecified site C73
    well differentiated C73
  generalized, with unspecified primary site
    C80.0
  glycogen-rich —*see* Neoplasm, breast,
    malignant
  granulosa cell C56-
  hepatic cell C22.0

Carcinoma *(Continued)*
  hepatocellular C22.0
    with bile duct, mixed C22.0
    fibrolamellar C22.0
  hepatocholangiolitic C22.0
  Hurthle cell C73
  in
    adenomatous
      polyposis coli C18.9
    pleomorphic adenoma —*see* Neoplasm,
      salivary glands, malignant
    situ —*see* Carcinoma-in-situ
  infiltrating
    duct
      with lobular
        specified site —*see* Neoplasm,
          malignant, by site
        unspecified site (female) C50.91-
          male C50.92-
      with Paget's disease —*see* Neoplasm,
        breast, malignant
      specified site —*see* Neoplasm,
        malignant
      unspecified site (female) C50.91-
        male C50.92-
    ductular
      specified site —*see* Neoplasm,
        malignant
      unspecified site (female) C50.91-
        male C50.92-
    lobular
      specified site —*see* Neoplasm,
        malignant
      unspecified site (female) C50.91-
        male C50.92-
  inflammatory
    specified site —*see* Neoplasm, malignant
    unspecified site (female) C50.91-
      male C50.92-
  intestinal type
    specified site —*see* Neoplasm, malignant,
      by site
    unspecified site C16.9
  intracystic
    noninfiltrating —*see* Neoplasm, in situ,
      by site
  intraductal (noninfiltrating)
    with Paget's disease —*see* Neoplasm,
      breast, malignant
    breast D05.1-
    papillary
      with invasion
        specified site —*see* Neoplasm,
          malignant, by site
        unspecified site (female) C50.91-
          male C50.92-
      breast D05.1-
      specified site NEC —*see* Neoplasm,
        in situ, by site
      unspecified site (female) D05.1-
    specified site NEC —*see* Neoplasm,
      in situ, by site
    unspecified site (female) D05.1-
  intraepidermal —*see* Neoplasm, in situ
    squamous cell, Bowen's type —*see*
      Neoplasm, skin, in situ
  intraepithelial —*see* Neoplasm, in situ,
      by site
    squamous cell —*see* Neoplasm, in situ,
      by site
  intraosseous C41.1
    upper jaw (bone) C41.0
  islet cell
    with exocrine, mixed
      specified site —*see* Neoplasm,
        malignant, by site
      unspecified site C25.9
    pancreas C25.4
    specified site NEC —*see* Neoplasm,
      malignant, by site
    unspecified site C25.4

Carcinoma *(Continued)*
    juvenile, breast —*see* Neoplasm, breast,
        malignant
    large cell
        small cell
            specified site —*see* Neoplasm,
                malignant, by site
            unspecified site C34.90
    Leydig cell (testis)
        specified site —*see* Neoplasm, malignant,
            by site
        unspecified site
            female C56.9
            male C62.90
    lipid-rich (female) C50.91-
        male C50.92-
    liver cell C22.0
    liver NEC C22.7
    lobular (infiltrating)
        with intraductal
            specified site —*see* Neoplasm,
                malignant, by site
            unspecified site (female) C50.91-
                male C50.92-
        noninfiltrating
            breast D05.0-
            specified site NEC —*see* Neoplasm, in
                situ, by site
            unspecified site D05.0-
        specified site —*see* Neoplasm, malignant,
            by site
        unspecified site (female) C50.91-
            male C50.92-
    medullary
        with
            amyloid stroma
                specified site —*see* Neoplasm,
                    malignant, by site
                unspecified site C73
            lymphoid stroma
                specified site —*see* Neoplasm,
                    malignant, by site
                unspecified site (female) C50.91-
                    male C50.92-
    Merkel cell C4A.9
        anal margin C4A.51
        anal skin C4A.51
        canthus C4A.1-
        ear and external auricular canal C4A.2-
        external auricular canal C4A.2-
        eyelid, including canthus C4A.1-
        face C4A.30
            specified NEC C4A.39
        hip C4A.7-
        lip C4A.0
        lower limb, including hip C4A.7-
        neck C4A.4
        nodal presentation C7B.1
        nose C4A.31
        overlapping sites C4A.8
        perianal skin C4A.51
        scalp C4A.4
        secondary C7B.1
        shoulder C4A.6-
        skin of breast C4A.52
        trunk NEC C4A.59
        upper limb, including shoulder C4A.6-
        visceral metastatic C7B.1
    metastatic —*see* Neoplasm, secondary
    metatypical —*see* Neoplasm, skin, malignant
    morphea, basal cell —*see* Neoplasm, skin,
        malignant
    mucoid
        cell
            specified site —*see* Neoplasm,
                malignant, by site
            unspecified site C75.1
    neuroendocrine —*see also* Tumor,
        neuroendocrine
        high grade, any site C7A.1
        poorly differentiated, any site C7A.1

Carcinoma *(Continued)*
    nonencapsulated sclerosing C73
    noninfiltrating
        intracystic —*see* Neoplasm, in situ, by site
        intraductal
            breast D05.1-
            papillary
                breast D05.1-
                specified site NEC —*see* Neoplasm, in
                    situ, by site
                unspecified site D05.1-
            specified site —*see* Neoplasm, in situ,
                by site
            unspecified site D05.1-
        lobular
            breast D05.0-
            specified site NEC —*see* Neoplasm, in
                situ, by site
            unspecified site (female) D05.0-
    oat cell
        specified site —*see* Neoplasm, malignant,
            by site
        unspecified site C34.90
    odontogenic C41.1
        upper jaw (bone) C41.0
    papillary
        with follicular (mixed) C73
        follicular variant C73
        intraductal (noninfiltrating)
            with invasion
                specified site —*see* Neoplasm,
                    malignant, by site
                unspecified site (female) C50.91-
                    male C50.92-
            breast D05.1-
            specified site NEC —*see* Neoplasm, in
                situ, by site
            unspecified site D05.1-
        serous
            specified site —*see* Neoplasm,
                malignant, by site
            surface
                specified site —*see* Neoplasm,
                    malignant, by site
                unspecified site C56.9
            unspecified site C56.9
    papillocystic
        specified site —*see* Neoplasm, malignant,
            by site
        unspecified site C56.9
    parafollicular cell
        specified site —*see* Neoplasm, malignant,
            by site
        unspecified site C73
    pilomatrix —*see* Neoplasm, skin, malignant
    pseudomucinous
        specified site —*see* Neoplasm, malignant,
            by site
        unspecified site C56.9
    renal cell C64-
    Schmincke —*see* Neoplasm, nasopharynx,
        malignant
    Schneiderian
        specified site —*see* Neoplasm, malignant,
            by site
        unspecified site C30.0
    sebaceous —*see* Neoplasm, skin, malignant
    secondary —*see also* Neoplasm, secondary,
        by site
        Merkel cell C7B.1
    secretory, breast —*see* Neoplasm, breast,
        malignant
    serous
        papillary
            specified site —*see* Neoplasm,
                malignant, by site
            unspecified site C56.9
        surface, papillary
            specified site —*see* Neoplasm,
                malignant, by site
            unspecified site C56.9

Carcinoma *(Continued)*
    Sertoli cell
        specified site —*see* Neoplasm, malignant,
            by site
        unspecified site C62.90
            female C56.9
            male C62.90
    skin appendage —*see* Neoplasm, skin,
        malignant
    small cell
        fusiform cell
            specified site —*see* Neoplasm,
                malignant, by site
            unspecified site C34.90
        intermediate cell
            specified site —*see* Neoplasm,
                malignant, by site
            unspecified site C34.90
        large cell
            specified site —*see* Neoplasm,
                malignant, by site
            unspecified site C34.90
    solid
        with amyloid stroma
            specified site —*see* Neoplasm,
                malignant, by site
            unspecified site C73
        microinvasive
            specified site —*see* Neoplasm,
                malignant, by site
            unspecified site C53.9
    sweat gland —*see* Neoplasm, skin,
        malignant
    theca cell C56.-
    thymic C37
    unspecified site (primary) C80.1
    water-clear cell C75.0
Carcinoma-in-situ —*see also* Neoplasm, in situ,
    by site
    breast NOS D05.9-
        specified type NEC D05.8-
    epidermoid —*see also* Neoplasm, in situ, by
        site
        with questionable stromal invasion
            cervix D06.9
        specified site NEC —*see* Neoplasm, in
            situ, by site
        unspecified site D06.9
    Bowen's type —*see* Neoplasm, skin,
        in situ
    intraductal
        breast D05.1-
        specified site NEC —*see* Neoplasm, in situ,
            by site
        unspecified site D05.1-
    lobular
        with
            infiltrating duct
                breast (female) C50.91-
                    male C50.92-
                specified site NEC —*see* Neoplasm,
                    malignant
                unspecified site (female) C50.91-
                    male C50.92-
            intraductal
                breast D05.8-
                specified site NEC —*see* Neoplasm, in
                    situ, by site
                unspecified site (female) D05.8-
        breast D05.0-
        specified site NEC —*see* Neoplasm, in situ,
            by site
        unspecified site D05.0-
    squamous cell —*see also* Neoplasm, in situ,
        by site
        with questionable stromal invasion
            cervix D06.9
        specified site NEC —*see* Neoplasm, in
            situ, by site
        unspecified site D06.9
Carcinomaphobia F45.29

◀ New   ◀▦ Revised   ~~deleted~~ Deleted

Carcinomatosis C80.0
  peritonei C78.6
  unspecified site (primary) (secondary) C80.0
Carcinosarcoma —*see* Neoplasm, malignant, by site
  embryonal —*see* Neoplasm, malignant, by site
Cardia, cardial —*see* condition
Cardiac —*see also* condition
  death, sudden —*see* Arrest, cardiac
  pacemaker
    in situ Z95.0
      management or adjustment Z45.018
  tamponade I31.4
Cardialgia —*see* Pain, precordial
Cardiectasis —*see* Hypertrophy, cardiac
Cardiochalasia K21.9
Cardiomalacia I51.5
Cardiomegalia glycogenica diffusa E74.02 [*143*]
Cardiomegaly —*see also* Hypertrophy, cardiac
  congenital Q24.8
  glycogen E74.02 [*143*]
  idiopathic I51.7
Cardiomyoliposis I51.5
Cardiomyopathy (familial) (idiopathic) I42.9
  alcoholic I42.6
  amyloid E85.4 [*143*]
  arteriosclerotic —*see* Disease, heart, ischemic, atherosclerotic
  beriberi E51.12
  cobalt-beer I42.6
  congenital I42.4
  congestive I42.0
  constrictive NOS I42.5
  dilated I42.0
  due to
    alcohol I42.6
    beriberi E51.12
    cardiac glycogenosis E74.02 [*143*]
    drugs I42.7
    external agents NEC I42.7
    Friedreich's ataxia G11.1
    myotonia atrophica G71.11 [*143*]
    progressive muscular dystrophy G71.0
  glycogen storage E74.02 [*143*]
  hypertensive —*see* Hypertension, heart
  hypertrophic (nonobstructive) I42.2
    obstructive I42.1
      congenital Q24.8
  in
    Chagas' disease (chronic) B57.2
      acute B57.0
    sarcoidosis D86.85
  ischemic I25.5
  metabolic E88.9 [*143*]
    thyrotoxic E05.90 [*143*]
      with thyroid storm E05.91 [*143*]
  newborn I42.8
    congenital I42.4
  nutritional E63.9 [*143*]
    beriberi E51.12
  obscure of Africa I42.8
  peripartum O90.3
  postpartum O90.3
  restrictive NEC I42.5
  rheumatic I09.0
  secondary I42.9
  stress induced I51.81
  takotsubo I51.81
  thyrotoxic E05.90 [*143*]
    with thyroid storm E05.91 [*143*]
  toxic NEC I42.7
  tuberculous A18.84
  viral B33.24
Cardionephritis —*see* Hypertension, cardiorenal
Cardionephropathy —*see* Hypertension, cardiorenal
Cardionephrosis —*see* Hypertension, cardiorenal
Cardiopathia nigra I27.0

Cardiopathy (*see also* Disease, heart) I51.9
  idiopathic I42.9
  mucopolysaccharidosis E76.3 [*152*]
Cardiopericarditis —*see* Pericarditis
Cardiophobia F45.29
Cardiorenal —*see* condition
Cardiorrhexis —*see* Infarct, myocardium
Cardiosclerosis —*see* Disease, heart, ischemic, atherosclerotic
Cardiosis —*see* Disease, heart
Cardiospasm (esophagus) (reflex) (stomach) K22.0
  congenital Q39.5
    with megaesophagus Q39.5
Cardiostenosis —*see* Disease, heart
Cardiosymphysis I31.0
Cardiovascular —*see* condition
Carditis (acute) (bacterial) (chronic) (subacute) I51.89
  meningococcal A39.50
  rheumatic —*see* Disease, heart, rheumatic
  rheumatoid —*see* Rheumatoid, carditis
  viral B33.20
Care (of) (for) (following)
  child (routine) Z76.2
  family member (handicapped) (sick)
    creating problem for family Z63.6
    provided away from home for holiday relief Z75.5
    unavailable, due to
      absence (person rendering care) (sufferer) Z74.2
      inability (any reason) of person rendering care Z74.2
  foundling Z76.1
  holiday relief Z75.5
  improper —*see* Maltreatment
  lack of (at or after birth) (infant) —*see* Maltreatment, child, neglect
  lactating mother Z39.1
  palliative Z51.5
  postpartum
    immediately after delivery Z39.0
    routine follow-up Z39.2
  respite Z75.5
  unavailable, due to
    absence of person rendering care Z74.2
    inability (any reason) of person rendering care Z74.2
  well-baby Z76.2
Caries
  bone NEC A18.03
  dental K02.9
    arrested (coronal) (root) K02.3
    chewing surface
      limited to enamel K02.51
      penetrating into dentin K02.52
      penetrating into pulp K02.53
    coronal surface
      chewing surface
        limited to enamel K02.51
        penetrating into dentin K02.52
        penetrating into pulp K02.53
      pit and fissure surface
        limited to enamel K02.51
        penetrating into dentin K02.52
        penetrating into pulp K02.53
      smooth surface
        limited to enamel K02.61
        penetrating into dentin K02.62
        penetrating into pulp K02.63
    pit and fissure surface
      limited to enamel K02.51
      penetrating into dentin K02.52
      penetrating into pulp K02.53
    root K02.7
    smooth surface
      limited to enamel K02.61
      penetrating into dentin K02.62
      penetrating into pulp K02.63

Caries (Continued)
  external meatus —*see* Disorder, ear, external, specified type NEC
  hip (tuberculous) A18.02
  initial (tooth)
    chewing surface K02.51
    pit and fissure surface K02.51
    smooth surface K02.61
  knee (tuberculous) A18.02
  labyrinth —*see* subcategory H83.8
  limb NEC (tuberculous) A18.03
  mastoid process (chronic) —*see* Mastoiditis, chronic
    tuberculous A18.03
  middle ear —*see* subcategory H74.8
  nose (tuberculous) A18.03
  orbit (tuberculous) A18.03
  ossicles, ear —*see* Abnormal, ear ossicles
  petrous bone —*see* Petrositis
  root (dental) (tooth) K02.7
  sacrum (tuberculous) A18.01
  spine, spinal (column) (tuberculous) A18.01
  syphilitic A52.77
    congenital (early) A50.02 [*M90.80*]
  tooth, teeth —*see* Caries, dental
  tuberculous A18.03
  vertebra (column) (tuberculous) A18.01
Carious teeth —*see* Caries, dental
Carneous mole O02.0
Carnitine insufficiency E71.40
Carotid body or sinus syndrome G90.01
Carotidynia G90.01
Carotinemia (dietary) E67.1
Carotinosis (cutis) (skin) E67.1
Carpal tunnel syndrome —*see* Syndrome, carpal tunnel
Carpenter's syndrome Q87.0
Carpopedal spasm —*see* Tetany
Carr-Barr-Plunkett syndrome Q97.1
Carrier (suspected) of
  amebiasis Z22.1
  bacterial disease NEC Z22.39
    diphtheria Z22.2
    intestinal infectious NEC Z22.1
      typhoid Z22.0
    meningococcal Z22.31
    sexually transmitted Z22.4
    specified NEC Z22.39
    staphylococcal (Methicillin susceptible) Z22.321
      Methicillin resistant Z22.322
    streptococcal Z22.338
      group B Z22.330
    typhoid Z22.0
  cholera Z22.1
  diphtheria Z22.2
  gastrointestinal pathogens NEC Z22.1
  genetic Z14.8
    cystic fibrosis Z14.1
    hemophilia A (asymptomatic) Z14.01
      symptomatic Z14.02
  gonorrhea Z22.4
  HAA (hepatitis Australian-antigen) Z22.59
  HB (c)(s)-AG Z22.51
  hepatitis (viral) Z22.50
    Australia-antigen (HAA) Z22.59
    B surface antigen (HBsAg) Z22.51
      with acute delta- (super)infection B17.0
    C Z22.52
    specified NEC Z22.59
  human T-cell lymphotropic virus type-1 (HTLV-1) infection Z22.6
  infectious organism Z22.9
    specified NEC Z22.8
  meningococci Z22.31
  Salmonella typhosa Z22.0
  serum hepatitis —*see* Carrier, hepatitis
  staphylococci (Methicillin susceptible) Z22.321
    Methicillin resistant Z22.322

Carrier of (Continued)
- streptococci Z22.338
  - group B Z22.330
- syphilis Z22.4
- typhoid Z22.0
- venereal disease NEC Z22.4

Carrion's disease A44.0

Carter's relapsing fever (Asiatic) A68.1

Cartilage —see condition

Caruncle (inflamed)
- conjunctiva (acute) —see Conjunctivitis, acute
- labium (majus) (minus) N90.89
- lacrimal —see Inflammation, lacrimal, passages
- myrtiform N89.8
- urethral (benign) N36.2

Cascade stomach K31.2

Caseation lymphatic gland (tuberculous) A18.2

Cassidy (-Scholte) syndrome (malignant carcinoid) E34.0

Castellani's disease A69.8

Castration, traumatic, male S38.231

Casts in urine R82.99

Cat
- cry syndrome Q93.4
- ear Q17.3
- eye syndrome Q92.8

Catabolism, senile R54

Catalepsy (hysterical) F44.2
- schizophrenic F20.2

Cataplexy (idiopathic) —see - Narcolepsy

Cataract (cortical) (immature) (incipient) H26.9
- with
  - neovascularization —see Cataract, complicated
- age-related —see Cataract, senile
- anterior
  - and posterior axial embryonal Q12.0
  - pyramidal Q12.0
- associated with
  - galactosemia E74.21 [H28]
  - myotonic disorders G71.19 [H28]
- blue Q12.0
- central Q12.0
- cerulean Q12.0
- complicated H26.20
  - with
    - neovascularization H26.21-
    - ocular disorder H26.22-
    - glaucomatous flecks H26.23-
- congenital Q12.0
- coraliform Q12.0
- coronary Q12.0
- crystalline Q12.0
- diabetic —see Diabetes, cataract
- drug-induced H26.3-
- due to
  - ocular disorder —see Cataract, complicated
  - radiation H26.8
- electric H26.8
- extraction status Z98.4-
- glass-blower's H26.8
- heat ray H26.8
- heterochromic —see Cataract, complicated
- hypermature —see Cataract, senile, morgagnian type
- in (due to)
  - chronic iridocyclitis —see Cataract, complicated
  - diabetes —see Diabetes, cataract
  - endocrine disease E34.9 [H28]
  - eye disease —see Cataract, complicated
  - hypoparathyroidism E20.9 [H28]
  - malnutrition-dehydration E46 [H28]
  - metabolic disease E88.9 [H28]
  - myotonic disorders G71.19 [H28]
  - nutritional disease E63.9 [H28]
- infantile —see Cataract, presenile
- irradiational —see Cataract, specified NEC
- juvenile —see Cataract, presenile
- malnutrition-dehydration E46 [H28]

Cataract (Continued)
- morgagnian —see Cataract, senile, morgagnian type
- myotonic G71.19 [H28]
- myxedema E03.9 [H28]
- nuclear
  - embryonal Q12.0
  - sclerosis —see Cataract, senile, nuclear
- presenile H26.00-
  - combined forms H26.06-
  - cortical H26.01-
  - lamellar —see Cataract, presenile, cortical
  - nuclear H26.03-
  - specified NEC H26.09
  - subcapsular polar (anterior) H26.04-
    - posterior H26.05-
  - zonular —see Cataract, presenile, cortical
- secondary H26.40
  - Soemmering's ring H26.41-
  - specified NEC H26.49-
  - to eye disease —see Cataract, complicated
- senile H25.9
  - brunescens —see Cataract, senile, nuclear
  - combined forms H25.81-
  - coronary —see Cataract, senile, incipient
  - cortical H25.01-
  - hypermature —see Cataract, senile, morgagnian type
  - incipient (mature) (total) H25.09-
    - cortical —see Cataract, senile, cortical
    - subcapsular —see Cataract, senile, subcapsular
  - morgagnian type (hypermature) H25.2-
  - nuclear (sclerosis) H25.1-
  - polar subcapsular (anterior) (posterior) — see Cataract, senile, incipient
  - punctate —see Cataract, senile, incipient
  - specified NEC H25.89
  - subcapsular polar (anterior) H25.03-
    - posterior H25.04-
- snowflake —see Diabetes, cataract
- specified NEC H26.8
- toxic —see Cataract, drug-induced
- traumatic H26.10-
  - localized H26.11-
  - partially resolved H26.12-
  - total H26.13-
- zonular (perinuclear) Q12.0

Cataracta —see also Cataract
- brunescens —see Cataract, senile, nuclear
- centralis pulverulenta Q12.0
- cerulea Q12.0
- complicata —see Cataract, complicated
- congenita Q12.0
- coralliformis Q12.0
- coronaria Q12.0
- diabetic —see Diabetes, cataract
- membranacea
  - accreta —see Cataract, secondary
  - congenita Q12.0
- nigra —see Cataract, senile, nuclear
- sunflower —see Cataract, complicated

Catarrh, catarrhal (acute) (febrile) (infectious) (inflammation) (see also condition) J00
- bronchial —see Bronchitis
- chest —see Bronchitis
- chronic J31.0
- due to congenital syphilis A50.03
- enteric —see Enteritis
- eustachian H68.009
- fauces —see Pharyngitis
- gastrointestinal —see Enteritis
- gingivitis K05.00
  - nonplaque induced K05.01
  - plaque induced K05.00
- hay —see Fever, hay
- intestinal —see Enteritis
- larynx, chronic J37.0
- liver B15.9
  - with hepatic coma B15.0
- lung —see Bronchitis

Catarrh, catarrhal (Continued)
- middle ear, chronic —see Otitis, media, nonsuppurative, chronic, serous
- mouth K12.1
- nasal (chronic) —see Rhinitis
- nasobronchial J31.1
- nasopharyngeal (chronic) J31.1
  - acute J00
- pulmonary —see Bronchitis
- spring (eye) (vernal) —see Conjunctivitis, acute, atopic
- summer (hay) —see Fever, hay
- throat J31.2
- tubotympanal —see also Otitis, media, nonsuppurative
  - chronic —see Otitis, media, nonsuppurative, chronic, serous

Catatonia (schizophrenic) F20.2

Catatonic
- disorder due to known physiologic condition F06.1
- schizophrenia F20.2
- stupor R40.1

Cat-scratch —see also Abrasion
- disease or fever A28.1

Cauda equina —see condition

Cauliflower ear M95.1-

Causalgia (upper limb) G56.4-
- lower limb G57.7-

Cause
- external, general effects T75.89

Caustic burn —see Corrosion, by site

Cavare's disease (familial periodic paralysis) G72.3

Cave-in, injury
- crushing (severe) —see Crush
- suffocation —see Asphyxia, traumatic, due to low oxygen, due to cave-in

Cavernitis (penis) N48.29

Cavernositis N48.29

Cavernous —see condition

Cavitation of lung —see also Tuberculosis, pulmonary
- nontuberculous J98.4

Cavities, dental —see Caries, dental

Cavity
- lung —see Cavitation of lung
- optic papilla Q14.2
- pulmonary —see Cavitation of lung

Cavovarus foot, congenital Q66.1

Cavus foot (congenital) Q66.7
- acquired —see Deformity, limb, foot, specified NEC

Cazenave's disease L10.2

Cecitis K52.9
- with perforation, peritonitis, or rupture K65.8

Cecum —see condition

Celiac
- artery compression syndrome I77.4
- disease K90.0
- infantilism K90.0

Cell (s), cellular —see also condition
- in urine R82.99

Cellulitis (diffuse) (phlegmonous) (septic) (suppurative) L03.90
- abdominal wall L03.311
- anaerobic A48.0
- ankle —see Cellulitis, lower limb
- anus K61.0
- arm —see Cellulitis, upper limb
- auricle (ear) —see Cellulitis, ear
- axilla L03.11-
- back (any part) L03.312
- broad ligament
  - acute N73.0
- buttock L03.317
- cervical (meaning neck) L03.221
- cervix (uteri) —see Cervicitis
- cheek (external) L03.211
  - internal K12.2
- chest wall L03.313

◀ New ◀ Revised ~~deleted~~ Deleted

Cellulitis *(Continued)*
　chronic L03.90
　clostridial A48.0
　corpus cavernosum N48.22
　digit
　　finger —*see* Cellulitis, finger
　　toe —*see* Cellulitis, toe
　Douglas' cul-de-sac or pouch
　　acute N73.0
　drainage site (following operation) T81.4
　ear (external) H60.1-
　eosinophilic (granulomatous) L98.3
　erysipelatous —*see* Erysipelas
　external auditory canal —*see* Cellulitis, ear
　eyelid —*see* Abscess, eyelid
　face NEC L03.211
　finger (intrathecal) (periosteal)
　　(subcutaneous) (subcuticular) L03.01-
　foot —*see* Cellulitis, lower limb
　gangrenous —*see* Gangrene
　genital organ NEC
　　female (external) N76.4
　　male N49.9
　　　multiple sites N49.8
　　　specified NEC N49.8
　gluteal (region) L03.317
　gonococcal A54.89
　groin L03.314
　hand —*see* Cellulitis, upper limb
　head NEC L03.811
　　face (any part, except ear, eye and nose)
　　　L03.211
　heel —*see* Cellulitis, lower limb
　hip —*see* Cellulitis, lower limb
　jaw (region) L03.211
　knee —*see* Cellulitis, lower limb
　labium (majus) (minus) —*see* Vulvitis
　lacrimal passages —*see* Inflammation,
　　lacrimal, passages
　larynx J38.7
　leg —*see* Cellulitis, lower limb
　lip K13.0
　lower limb L03.11-
　　toe —*see* Cellulitis, toe
　mouth (floor) K12.2
　multiple sites, so stated L03.90
　nasopharynx J39.1
　navel L03.316
　　newborn P38.9
　　　with mild hemorrhage P38.1
　　　without hemorrhage P38.9
　neck (region) L03.221
　nose (septum) (external) J34.0
　orbit, orbital H05.01-
　palate (soft) K12.2
　pectoral (region) L03.313
　pelvis, pelvic (chronic)
　　female *(see also* Disease, pelvis,
　　　inflammatory) N73.2
　　　acute N73.0
　　　following ectopic or molar pregnancy
　　　　O08.0
　　male K65.0
　penis N48.22
　perineal, perineum L03.315
　perirectal K61.1
　peritonsillar J36
　periurethral N34.0
　periuterine *(see also* Disease, pelvis,
　　inflammatory) N73.2
　　acute N73.0
　pharynx J39.1
　rectum K61.1
　retroperitoneal K68.9
　round ligament
　　acute N73.0
　scalp (any part) L03.811
　scrotum N49.2
　seminal vesicle N49.0
　shoulder —*see* Cellulitis, upper limb
　specified site NEC L03.818

Cellulitis *(Continued)*
　submandibular (region) (space) (triangle)
　　K12.2
　　gland K11.3
　submaxillary (region) K12.2
　　gland K11.3
　thigh —*see* Cellulitis, lower limb
　thumb (intrathecal) (periosteal)
　　(subcutaneous) (subcuticular) —*see*
　　Cellulitis, finger
　toe (intrathecal) (periosteal) (subcutaneous)
　　(subcuticular) L03.03-
　tonsil J36
　trunk L03.319
　　abdominal wall L03.311
　　back (any part) L03.312
　　buttock L03.317
　　chest wall L03.313
　　groin L03.314
　　perineal, perineum L03.315
　　umbilicus L03.316
　tuberculous (primary) A18.4
　umbilicus L03.316
　upper limb L03.11-
　　axilla —*see* Cellulitis, axilla
　　finger —*see* Cellulitis, finger
　　thumb —*see* Cellulitis, finger
　vaccinal T88.0
　vocal cord J38.3
　vulva —*see* Vulvitis
　wrist —*see* Cellulitis, upper limb
Cementoblastoma, benign —*see* Cyst,
　calcifying odontogenic
Cementoma —*see* Cyst, calcifying odontogenic
Cementoperiostitis —*see* Periodontitis
Cementosis K03.4
Central auditory processing disorder H93.25
Central pain syndrome G89.0
Cephalematocele, cephal (o)hematocele
　newborn P52.8
　　birth injury P10.8
　traumatic —*see* Hematoma, brain
Cephalematoma, cephalhematoma (calcified)
　newborn (birth injury) P12.0
　traumatic —*see* Hematoma, brain
Cephalgia, cephalalgia —*see also* Headache
　histamine G44.009
　　intractable G44.001
　　not intractable G44.009
　trigeminal autonomic (TAC) NEC G44.099
　　intractable G44.091
　　not intractable G44.099
Cephalic —*see* condition
Cephalitis —*see* Encephalitis
Cephalocele —*see* Encephalocele
Cephalomenia N94.89
Cephalopelvic —*see* condition
Cerclage (with cervical incompetence) in
　pregnancy —*see* Incompetence, cervix, in
　pregnancy
Cerebellitis —*see* Encephalitis
Cerebellum, cerebellar —*see* condition
Cerebral —*see* condition
Cerebritis —*see* Encephalitis
Cerebro-hepato-renal syndrome Q87.89
Cerebromalacia —*see* Softening, brain
　sequelae of cerebrovascular disease I69.398
Cerebroside lipidosis E75.22
Cerebrospasticity (congenital) G80.1
Cerebrospinal —*see* condition
Cerebrum —*see* condition
Ceroid-lipofuscinosis, neuronal E75.4
Cerumen (accumulation) (impacted) H61.2-
Cervical —*see also* condition
　auricle Q18.2
　dysplasia in pregnancy —*see* Abnormal,
　　cervix, in pregnancy or childbirth
　erosion in pregnancy —*see* Abnormal, cervix,
　　in pregnancy or childbirth
　fibrosis in pregnancy —*see* Abnormal, cervix,
　　in pregnancy or childbirth

Cervical *(Continued)*
　fusion syndrome Q76.1
　rib Q76.5
　shortening (complicating pregnancy)
　　O26.87-
Cervicalgia M54.2
Cervicitis (acute) (chronic) (nonvenereal)
　　(senile (atrophic)) (subacute) (with
　　ulceration) N72
　with
　　abortion —*see* Abortion, by type
　　complicated by genital tract and
　　　pelvic infection
　　ectopic pregnancy O08.0
　　molar pregnancy O08.0
　chlamydial A56.09
　gonococcal A54.03
　herpesviral A60.03
　puerperal (postpartum) O86.11
　syphilitic A52.76
　trichomonal A59.09
　tuberculous A18.16
Cervicocolpitis (emphysematosa) *(see also*
　Cervicitis) N72
Cervix —*see* condition
Cesarean delivery, previous, affecting
　management of pregnancy O34.21
Céstan (-Chenais) paralysis or syndrome
　G46.3
Céstan-Raymond syndrome I65.8
Cestode infestation B71.9
　specified type NEC B71.8
Cestodiasis B71.9
Chabert's disease A22.9
Chacaleh E53.8
Chafing L30.4
Chagas' (-Mazza) disease (chronic) B57.2
　with
　　cardiovascular involvement NEC B57.2
　　digestive system involvement B57.30
　　　megacolon B57.32
　　　megaesophagus B57.31
　　　other specified B57.39
　　megacolon B57.32
　　megaesophagus B57.31
　　myocarditis B57.2
　　nervous system involvement B57.40
　　　meningitis B57.41
　　　meningoencephalitis B57.42
　　　other specified B57.49
　　specified organ involvement NEC B57.5
　acute (with) B57.1
　　cardiovascular NEC B57.0
　　myocarditis B57.0
Chagres fever B50.9
Chairridden Z74.09
Chalasia (cardiac sphincter) K21.9
Chalazion H00.19
　left H00.16
　　lower H00.15
　　upper H00.14
　right H00.13
　　lower H00.12
　　upper H00.11
Chalcosis —*see also* Disorder, globe,
　degenerative, chalcosis
　cornea —*see* Deposit, cornea
　crystalline lens —*see* Cataract, complicated
　retina H35.89
Chalicosis (pulmonum) J62.8
Chancre (any genital site) (hard) (hunterian)
　　(mixed) (primary) (seronegative)
　　(seropositive) (syphilitic) A51.0
　congenital A50.07
　conjunctiva NEC A51.2
　Ducrey's A57
　extragenital A51.2
　eyelid A51.2
　lip A51.2
　nipple A51.2
　Nisbet's A57

Chancre *(Continued)*
of
carate A67.0
pinta A67.0
yaws A66.0
palate, soft A51.2
phagedenic A57
simple A57
soft A57
bubo A57
palate A51.2
urethra A51.0
yaws A66.0
Chancroid (anus) (genital) (penis) (perineum)
(rectum) (urethra) (vulva) A57
Chandler's disease (osteochondritis dissecans,
hip) —*see* Osteochondritis, dissecans, hip
Change (s) (in) (of) —*see also* Removal
arteriosclerotic —*see* Arteriosclerosis
bone —*see also* Disorder, bone
diabetic —*see* Diabetes, bone change
bowel habit R19.4
cardiorenal (vascular) —*see* Hypertension,
cardiorenal
cardiovascular —*see* Disease, cardiovascular
circulatory I99.9
cognitive (mild) (organic) R41.89
color, tooth, teeth
during formation K00.8
posteruptive K03.7
contraceptive device Z30.433
corneal membrane H18.30
Bowman's membrane fold or rupture
H18.31-
Descemet's membrane
fold H18.32-
rupture H18.33-
coronary —*see* Disease, heart, ischemic
degenerative, spine or vertebra —*see*
Spondylosis
dental pulp, regressive K04.2
dressing (nonsurgical) Z48.00
surgical Z48.01
heart —*see* Disease, heart
hip joint —*see* Derangement, joint, hip
hyperplastic larynx J38.7
hypertrophic
nasal sinus J34.89
turbinate, nasal J34.3
upper respiratory tract J39.8
indwelling catheter Z46.6
inflammatory —*see also* Inflammation
sacroiliac M46.1
job, anxiety concerning Z56.1
joint —*see* Derangement, joint
life —*see* Menopause
mental status R41.82
minimal (glomerular) (*see also* N00-N07 with
fourth character .0) N05.0
myocardium, myocardial —*see* Degeneration,
myocardial - of life —*see* Menopause
pacemaker Z45.018
pulse generator Z45.010
personality (enduring) F68.8
due to (secondary to)
general medical condition F07.0
secondary (nonspecific) F60.89
regressive, dental pulp K04.2
renal —*see* Disease, renal
retina H35.9
myopic H44.2-
sacroiliac joint M53.3
senile (*see also* condition) R54
sensory R20.8
skin R23.9
acute, due to ultraviolet radiation L56.9
specified NEC L56.8
chronic, due to nonionizing radiation L57.9
specified NEC L57.8
cyanosis R23.0
flushing R23.2

Change *(Continued)*
skin *(Continued)*
pallor R23.1
petechiae R23.3
specified change NEC R23.8
swelling —*see* Mass, localized
texture R23.4
trophic
arm —*see* Mononeuropathy, upper limb
leg —*see* Mononeuropathy, lower limb
vascular I99.9
vasomotor I73.9
voice R49.9
psychogenic F44.4
specified NEC R49.8
Changing sleep-work schedule, affecting sleep
G47.26
Changuinola fever A93.1
Chapping skin T69.8
Charcot-Marie-Tooth disease, paralysis or
syndrome G60.0
Charcot's
arthropathy —*see* Arthropathy, neuropathic
cirrhosis K74.3
disease (tabetic arthropathy) A52.16
joint (disease) (tabetic) A52.16
diabetic —*see* Diabetes, with, arthropathy
syringomyelic G95.0
syndrome (intermittent claudication) I73.9
CHARGE association Q89.8
Charley-horse (quadriceps) M62.831
traumatic (quadriceps) S76.11-
Charlouis' disease —*see* Yaws
Cheadle's disease E54
Checking (of)
cardiac pacemaker (battery) (electrode (s))
Z45.018
pulse generator Z45.010
intrauterine contraceptive device Z30.431
Check-up —*see* Examination
Chédiak-Higashi (-Steinbrinck) syndrome
(congenital gigantism of peroxidase
granules) E70.330
Cheek —*see* condition
Cheese itch B88.0
Cheese-washer's lung J67.8
Cheese-worker's lung J67.8
Cheilitis (acute) (angular) (catarrhal) (chronic)
(exfoliative) (gangrenous) (glandular)
(infectional) (suppurative) (ulcerative)
(vesicular) K13.0
actinic (due to sun) L56.8
other than from sun L59.8
candidal B37.83
Cheilodynia K13.0
Cheiloschisis —*see* Cleft, lip
Cheilosis (angular) K13.0
with pellagra E52
due to
vitamin B2 (riboflavin) deficiency E53.0
Cheiromegaly M79.89
Cheiropompholyx L30.1
Cheloid —*see* Keloid
Chemical burn —*see* Corrosion, by site
Chemodectoma —*see* Paraganglioma,
nonchromaffin
Chemosis, conjunctiva —*see* Edema,
conjunctiva
Chemotherapy (session) (for)
cancer Z51.11
neoplasm Z51.11
Cherubism M27.8
Chest —*see* condition
Cheyne-Stokes breathing (respiration) R06.3
Chiari's
disease or syndrome (hepatic vein
thrombosis) I82.0
malformation
type I G93.5
type II —*see* Spina bifida
net Q24.8

Chicago disease B40.9
Chickenpox —*see* Varicella
Chiclero ulcer or sore B55.1
Chigger (infestation) B88.0
Chignon (disease) B36.8
newborn (from vacuum extraction) (birth
injury) P12.1
Chilaiditi's syndrome (subphrenic
displacement, colon) Q43.3
Chilblain (s) (lupus) T69.1
Child
custody dispute Z65.3
Childbirth —*see* Delivery
Childhood
cerebral X-linked adrenoleukodystrophy
E71.520
period of rapid growth Z00.2
Chill (s) R68.83
with fever R50.9
without fever R68.83
congestive in malarial regions B54
Chilomastigiasis A07.8
Chimera 46,XX/46,XY Q99.0
Chin —*see* condition
Chinese dysentery A03.9
Chionophobia F40.228
Chitral fever A93.1
Chlamydia, chlamydial A74.9
cervicitis A56.09
conjunctivitis A74.0
cystitis A56.01
endometritis A56.11
epididymitis A56.19
female
pelvic inflammatory disease A56.11
pelviperitonitis A56.11
orchitis A56.19
peritonitis A74.81
pharyngitis A56.4
proctitis A56.3
psittaci (infection) A70
salpingitis A56.11
sexually-transmitted infection NEC
A56.8
specified NEC A74.89
urethritis A56.01
vulvovaginitis A56.02
Chlamydiosis —*see* Chlamydia
Chloasma (skin) (idiopathic) (symptomatic)
L81.1
eyelid H02.719
hyperthyroid E05.90 *[H02.719]*
with thyroid storm E05.91 *[H02.719]*
left H02.716
lower H02.715
upper H02.714
right H02.713
lower H02.712
upper H02.711
Chloroma C92.3-
Chlorosis D50.9
Egyptian's B76.9 *[D63.8]*
miner's B76.9 *[D63.8]*
Chlorotic anemia D50.8
Chocolate cyst (ovary) N80.1
Choked
disc or disk —*see* Papilledema
on food, phlegm, or vomitus NOS —*see*
Foreign body, by site
while vomiting NOS —*see* Foreign body, by
site
Chokes (resulting from bends) T70.3
Choking sensation R09.89
Cholangiectasis K83.8
Cholangiocarcinoma
with hepatocellular carcinoma, combined
C22.0
liver C22.1
specified site NEC —*see* Neoplasm,
malignant, by site
unspecified site C22.1

◀ New ◀▥ Revised ~~deleted~~ Deleted

Cholangiohepatitis K83.8
  due to fluke infestation B66.1
Cholangiohepatoma C22.0
Cholangiolitis (acute) (chronic) (extrahepatic)
    (gangrenous) (intrahepatic) K83.0
  paratyphoidal —see Fever, paratyphoid
  typhoidal A01.09
Cholangioma D13.4
  malignant —see Cholangiocarcinoma
Cholangitis (ascending) (primary) (recurrent)
    (sclerosing) (secondary) (stenosing)
    (suppurative) K83.0
  with calculus, bile duct —see Calculus, bile
      duct, with cholangitis
  chronic nonsuppurative destructive K74.3
Cholecystectasia K82.8
Cholecystitis K81.9
  with
    calculus, stones in
      bile duct (common) (hepatic) —
          see Calculus, bile duct, with
          cholecystitis
      cystic duct —see Calculus, gallbladder,
          with cholecystitis
      gallbladder —see Calculus, gallbladder,
          with cholecystitis
      choledocholithiasis —see Calculus, bile
          duct, with cholecystitis
      cholelithiasis —see Calculus, gallbladder,
          with cholecystitis
  acute (emphysematous) (gangrenous)
      (suppurative) K81.0
    with
      calculus, stones in
        cystic duct —see Calculus,
            gallbladder, with cholecystitis,
            acute
        gallbladder —see Calculus,
            gallbladder, with cholecystitis,
            acute
        choledocholithiasis —see Calculus, bile
            duct, with cholecystitis, acute
        cholelithiasis —see Calculus,
            gallbladder, with cholecystitis,
            acute
      chronic cholecystitis K81.2
        with gallbladder calculus K80.12
          with obstruction K80.13
  chronic K81.1
    with acute cholecystitis K81.2
      with gallbladder calculus K80.12
        with obstruction K80.13
  emphysematous (acute) —see Cholecystitis,
      acute
  gangrenous —see Cholecystitis, acute
  paratyphoidal, current A01.4
  suppurative —see Cholecystitis, acute
  typhoidal A01.09
Cholecystolithiasis —see Calculus, gallbladder
Choledochitis (suppurative) K83.0
Choledocholith —see Calculus, bile duct
Choledocholithiasis (common duct) (hepatic
    duct) —see Calculus, bile duct
  cystic —see Calculus, gallbladder
  typhoidal A01.09
Cholelithiasis (cystic duct) (gallbladder)
    (impacted) (multiple) —see Calculus,
    gallbladder
  bile duct (common) (hepatic) —see Calculus,
      bile duct
  hepatic duct —see Calculus, bile duct
  specified NEC K80.80
    with obstruction K80.81
Cholemia —see also Jaundice
  familial (simple) (congenital) E80.4
  Gilbert's E80.4
Choleperitoneum, choleperitonitis K65.3
Cholera (Asiatic) (epidemic) (malignant)
    A00.9
  antimonial —see Poisoning, antimony
  classical A00.0

Cholera (Continued)
  due to Vibrio cholerae 01 A00.9
    biovar cholerae A00.0
    biovar eltor A00.1
    el tor A00.1
  el tor A00.1
Cholerine —see Cholera
Cholestasis NEC K83.1
  with hepatocyte injury K71.0
  due to total parenteral nutrition (TPN) K76.89
  pure K71.0
Cholesteatoma (ear) (middle) (with reaction)
    H71.9-
  attic H71.0-
  external ear (canal) H60.4-
  mastoid H71.2-
  postmastoidectomy cavity (recurrent) —see
      Complications, postmastoidectomy,
      recurrent cholesteatoma
  recurrent (postmastoidectomy) —see
      Complications, postmastoidectomy,
      recurrent cholesteatoma
  tympanum H71.1-
Cholesteatosis, diffuse H71.3-
Cholesteremia E78.0
Cholesterin in vitreous —see Deposit,
    crystalline
Cholesterol
  deposit
    retina H35.89
    vitreous —see Deposit, crystalline
  elevated (high) E78.0
    with elevated (high) triglycerides E78.2
    screening for Z13.220
  imbibition of gallbladder K82.4
Cholesterolemia (essential) (familial)
    (hereditary) (pure) E78.0
Cholesterolosis, cholesterosis (gallbladder)
    K82.4
  cerebrotendinous E75.5
Cholocolic fistula K82.3
Choluria R82.2
Chondritis M94.8X9
  aurical H61.03-
  costal (Tietze's) M94.0
  external ear H61.03-
  patella, posttraumatic —see Chondromalacia,
      patella
  pinna H61.03-
  purulent M94.8X-
  tuberculous NEC A18.02
    intervertebral A18.01
Chondroblastoma —see also Neoplasm, bone,
    benign
  malignant —see Neoplasm, bone, malignant
Chondrocalcinosis M11.20
  ankle M11.27-
  elbow M11.22-
  familial M11.10
    ankle M11.17-
    elbow M11.12-
    foot joint M11.17-
    hand joint M11.14-
    hip M11.15-
    knee M11.16-
    multiple site M11.19
    shoulder M11.11-
    vertebrae M11.18
    wrist M11.13-
  foot joint M11.27-
  hand joint M11.24-
  hip M11.25-
  knee M11.26-
  multiple site M11.29
  shoulder M11.21-
  specified type NEC M11.20
    ankle M11.27-
    elbow M11.22-
    foot joint M11.27-
    hand joint M11.24-
    hip M11.25-

Chondrocalcinosis (Continued)
  specified type NEC (Continued)
    knee M11.26-
    multiple site M11.29
    shoulder M11.21-
    vertebrae M11.28
    wrist M11.23-
  vertebrae M11.28
  wrist M11.23-
Chondrodermatitis nodularis helicis or
    anthelicis —see Perichondritis, ear
Chondrodysplasia Q78.9
  with hemangioma Q78.4
  calcificans congenita Q77.3
  fetalis Q77.4
  metaphyseal (Jansen's) (McKusick's)
      (Schmid's) Q78.5
  punctata Q77.3
Chondrodystrophy, chondrodystrophia
    (familial) (fetalis) (hypoplastic) Q78.9
  calcificans congenita Q77.3
  myotonic (congenital) G71.13
  punctata Q77.3
Chondroectodermal dysplasia Q77.6
Chondrogenesis imperfecta Q77.4
Chondrolysis M94.35-
Chondroma —see also Neoplasm, cartilage,
    benign
  juxtacortical —see Neoplasm, bone, benign
  periosteal —see Neoplasm, bone, benign
Chondromalacia (systemic) M94.20
  acromioclavicular joint M94.21-
  ankle M94.27-
  elbow M94.22-
  foot joint M94.27-
  glenohumeral joint M94.21-
  hand joint M94.24-
  hip M94.25-
  knee M94.26-
    patella M22.4-
  multiple sites M94.29
  patella M22.4-
  rib M94.28
  sacroiliac joint M94.259
  shoulder M94.21-
  sternoclavicular joint M94.21-
  vertebral joint M94.28
  wrist M94.23-
Chondromatosis —see also Neoplasm, cartilage,
    uncertain behavior
  internal Q78.4
Chondromyxosarcoma —see Neoplasm,
    cartilage, malignant
Chondro-osteodysplasia (Morquio-Brailsford
    type) E76.219
Chondro-osteodystrophy E76.29
Chondro-osteoma —see Neoplasm, bone,
    benign
Chondropathia tuberosa M94.0
Chondrosarcoma —see Neoplasm, cartilage,
    malignant
  juxtacortical —see Neoplasm, bone, malignant
  mesenchymal —see Neoplasm, connective
      tissue, malignant
  myxoid —see Neoplasm, cartilage, malignant
Chordee (nonvenereal) N48.89
  congenital Q54.4
  gonococcal A54.09
Chorditis (fibrinous) (nodosa) (tuberosa) J38.2
Chordoma —see Neoplasm, vertebral (column),
    malignant
Chorea (chronic) (gravis) (posthemiplegic)
    (senile) (spasmodic) G25.5
  with
    heart involvement I02.0
      active or acute (conditions in I01-) I02.0
      rheumatic I02.9
        with valvular disorder I02.0
    rheumatic heart disease (chronic) (inactive)
        (quiescent) — code to rheumatic heart
        condition involved

Chorea (Continued)
   drug-induced G25.4
   habit F95.8
   hereditary G10
   Huntington's G10
   hysterical F44.4
   minor I02.9
      with heart involvement I02.0
   progressive G25.5
      hereditary G10
   rheumatic (chronic) I02.9
      with heart involvement I02.0
   Sydenham's I02.9
      with heart involvement —see Chorea, with
         rheumatic heart disease
      nonrheumatic G25.5
Choreoathetosis (paroxysmal) G25.5
Chorioadenoma (destruens) D39.2
Chorioamnionitis O41.12-
Chorioangioma D26.7
Choriocarcinoma —see Neoplasm, malignant,
      by site
   combined with
      embryonal carcinoma —see Neoplasm,
         malignant, by site
      other germ cell elements —see Neoplasm,
         malignant, by site
      teratoma —see Neoplasm, malignant, by
         site
   specified site —see Neoplasm, malignant, by
      site
   unspecified site
      female C58
      male C62.90
Chorioencephalitis (acute) (lymphocytic)
      (serous) A87.2
Chorioepithelioma —see Choriocarcinoma
Choriomeningitis (acute) (lymphocytic)
      (serous) A87.2
Chorionepithelioma —see Choriocarcinoma
Chorioretinitis —see also Inflammation,
      chorioretinal
   disseminated —see also Inflammation,
         chorioretinal, disseminated
      in neurosyphilis A52.19
   Egyptian B76.9 [D63.8]
   focal —see also Inflammation, chorioretinal,
         focal
   histoplasmic B39.9 [H32]
   in (due to)
      histoplasmosis B39.9 [H32]
      syphilis (secondary) A51.43
         late A52.71
      toxoplasmosis (acquired) B58.01
         congenital (active) P37.1 [H32]
      tuberculosis A18.53
   juxtapapillary, juxtapapillaris —see
         Inflammation, chorioretinal, focal,
         juxtapapillary
   leprous A30.9 [H32]
   miner's B76.9 [D63.8]
   progressive myopia (degeneration) H44.2-
   syphilitic (secondary) A51.43
      congenital (early) A50.01 [H32]
         late A50.32
      late A52.71
   tuberculous A18.53
Chorioretinopathy, central serous H35.71-
Choroid —see condition
Choroideremia H31.21
Choroiditis —see Chorioretinitis
Choroidopathy —see Disorder, choroid
Choroidoretinitis —see Chorioretinitis
Choroidoretinopathy, central serous —see
      Chorioretinopathy, central serous
Christian-Weber disease M35.6
Christmas disease D67
Chromaffinoma —see also Neoplasm, benign,
      by site
   malignant —see Neoplasm, malignant, by site
Chromatopsia —see Deficiency, color vision

Chromhidrosis, chromidrosis L75.1
Chromoblastomycosis —see Chromomycosis
Chromoconversion R82.91
Chromomycosis B43.9
   brain abscess B43.1
   cerebral B43.1
   cutaneous B43.0
   skin B43.0
   specified NEC B43.8
   subcutaneous abscess or cyst B43.2
Chromophytosis B36.0
Chromosome —see condition by chromosome
      involved
   D (1) —see condition, chromosome 13
   E (3) —see condition, chromosome 18
   G —see condition, chromosome 21
Chromotrichomycosis B36.8
Chronic —see condition
   fracture —see Fracture, pathological
Churg-Strauss syndrome M30.1
Chyle cyst, mesentery I89.8
Chylocele (nonfilarial) I89.8
   filarial (see also Infestation, filarial) B74.9
      [N51]
   tunica vaginalis N50.8
      filarial (see also Infestation, filarial) B74.9
         [N51]
Chylomicronemia (fasting) (with
      hyperprebetalipoproteinemia) E78.3
Chylopericardium I31.3
   acute I30.9
Chylothorax (nonfilarial) I89.8
   filarial (see also Infestation, filarial) B74.9
      [J91.8]
Chylous —see condition
Chyluria (nonfilarial) R82.0
   due to
      bilharziasis B65.0
      Brugia (malayi) B74.1
         timori B74.2
      schistosomiasis (bilharziasis) B65.0
      Wuchereria (bancrofti) B74.0
   filarial —see Infestation, filarial
Cicatricial (deformity) —see Cicatrix
Cicatrix (adherent) (contracted) (painful)
      (vicious) (see also Scar) L90.5
   adenoid (and tonsil) J35.8
   alveolar process M26.79
   anus K62.89
   auricle —see Disorder, pinna, specified type
      NEC
   bile duct (common) (hepatic) K83.8
   bladder N32.89
   bone —see Disorder, bone, specified type
      NEC
   brain G93.89
   cervix (postoperative) (postpartal) N88.1
   common duct K83.8
   cornea H17.9
      tuberculous A18.59
   duodenum (bulb), obstructive K31.5
   esophagus K22.2
   eyelid —see Disorder, eyelid function
   hypopharynx J39.2
   lacrimal passages —see Obstruction, lacrimal
   larynx J38.7
   lung J98.4
   middle ear —see subcategory H74.8
   mouth K13.79
   muscle M62.89
      with contracture —see Contraction, muscle
         NEC
   nasopharynx J39.2
   palate (soft) K13.79
   penis N48.89
   pharynx J39.2
   prostate N42.89
   rectum K62.89
   retina —see Scar, chorioretinal
   semilunar cartilage —see Derangement,
      meniscus

Cicatrix (Continued)
   seminal vesicle N50.8
   skin L90.5
      infected L08.89
      postinfective L90.5
      tuberculous B90.8
   specified site NEC L90.5
   throat J39.2
   tongue K14.8
   tonsil (and adenoid) J35.8
   trachea J39.8
   tuberculous NEC B90.9
   urethra N36.8
   uterus N85.8
   vagina N89.8
      postoperative N99.2
   vocal cord J38.3
   wrist, constricting (annular) L90.5
CIDP (chronic inflammatory demyelinating
      polyneuropathy) G61.81
CIN —see Neoplasia, intraepithelial, cervix
Cinchonism —see Deafness, ototoxic
   correct substance properly administered —see
         Table of Drugs and Chemicals, by
         drug, adverse effect ◄▦▦
   overdose or wrong substance given or
         taken —see Table of Drugs and
         Chemicals, by drug, poisoning ◄▦▦
Circle of Willis —see condition
Circular —see condition
Circulating anticoagulants (see also - Disorder,
      hemorrhagic) D68.318
   due to drugs (see also - Disorder,
      hemorrhagic) D68.32
   following childbirth O72.3
Circulation
   collateral, any site I99.8
   defective (lower extremity) I99.8
      congenital Q28.9
   embryonic Q28.9
   failure (peripheral) R57.9
      newborn P29.89
   fetal, persistent P29.3
   heart, incomplete Q28.9
Circulatory system —see condition
Circulus senilis (cornea) —see Degeneration,
      cornea, senile
Circumcision (in absence of medical indication)
      (ritual) (routine) Z41.2
Circumscribed —see condition
Circumvallate placenta O43.11-
Cirrhosis, cirrhotic (hepatic) (liver) K74.60
   alcoholic K70.30
      with ascites K70.31
   atrophic —see Cirrhosis, liver
   Baumgarten-Cruveilhier K74.69
   biliary (cholangiolitic) (cholangitic)
         (hypertrophic) (obstructive)
         (pericholangiolitic) K74.5
      due to
         Clonorchiasis B66.1
         flukes B66.3
      primary K74.3
      secondary K74.4
   cardiac (of liver) K76.1
   Charcot's K74.3
   cholangiolitic, cholangitic, cholostatic
         (primary) K74.3
   congestive K76.1
   Cruveilhier-Baumgarten K74.69
   cryptogenic (liver) K74.69
   due to
      hepatolenticular degeneration E83.01
      Wilson's disease E83.01
      xanthomatosis E78.2
   fatty K76.0
      alcoholic K70.0
   Hanot's (hypertrophic) K74.3
   hepatic —see Cirrhosis, liver
   hypertrophic K74.3
   Indian childhood K74.69

◄ New   ◄▦▦ Revised   ~~deleted~~ Deleted

Cirrhosis, cirrhotic *(Continued)*
  kidney —*see* Sclerosis, renal
  Laennec's K70.30
    with ascites K70.31
    alcoholic K70.30
      with ascites K70.31
    nonalcoholic K74.69
  liver K74.60
    alcoholic K70.30
      with ascites K70.31
      fatty K70.0
    congenital P78.81
    syphilitic A52.74
  lung (chronic) J84.10
  macronodular K74.69
    alcoholic K70.30
      with ascites K70.31
  micronodular K74.69
    alcoholic K70.30
      with ascites K70.31
  mixed type K74.69
  monolobular K74.3
  nephritis —*see* Sclerosis, renal
  nutritional K74.69
    alcoholic K70.30
      with ascites K70.31
  obstructive —*see* Cirrhosis, biliary
  ovarian N83.8
  pancreas (duct) K86.8
  pigmentary E83.110
  portal K74.69
    alcoholic K70.30
      with ascites K70.31
  postnecrotic K74.69
    alcoholic K70.30
      with ascites K70.31
  pulmonary J84.10
  renal —*see* Sclerosis, renal
  spleen D73.2
  stasis K76.1
  Todd's K74.3
  unilobar K74.3
  xanthomatous (biliary) K74.5
    due to xanthomatosis (familial) (metabolic)
      (primary) E78.2
Cistern, subarachnoid R93.0
Citrullinemia E72.23
Citrullinuria E72.23
Civatte's disease or poikiloderma
  L57.3
Clam digger's itch B65.3
Clammy skin R23.1
Clap —*see* Gonorrhea
Clarke-Hadfield syndrome (pancreatic
  infantilism) K86.8
Clark's paralysis G80.9
Clastothrix L67.8
Claude Bernard-Horner syndrome
  G90.2
  traumatic —*see* Injury, nerve, cervical
    sympathetic
Claude's disease or syndrome G46.3
Claudicatio venosa intermittens I87.8
Claudication, intermittent I73.9
  cerebral (artery) G45.9
  spinal cord (arteriosclerotic) G95.19
    syphilitic A52.09
  venous (axillary) I87.8
Claustrophobia F40.240
Clavus (infected) L84
Clawfoot (congenital) Q66.89
  acquired —*see* Deformity, limb, clawfoot
Clawhand (acquired) —*see also* Deformity, limb,
  clawhand
  congenital Q68.1
Clawtoe (congenital) Q66.89
  acquired —*see* Deformity, toe, specified
    NEC
Clay eating —*see* Pica
Cleansing of artificial opening —*see* Attention
  to, artificial, opening

Cleft (congenital) —*see also* Imperfect,
  closure
  alveolar process M26.79
  branchial (cyst) (persistent) Q18.2
  cricoid cartilage, posterior Q31.8
  lip (unilateral) Q36.9
    with cleft palate Q37.9
      hard Q37.1
        with soft Q37.5
      soft Q37.3
        with hard Q37.5
    bilateral Q36.0
      with cleft palate Q37.8
        hard Q37.0
          with soft Q37.4
        soft Q37.2
          with hard Q37.4
    median Q36.1
  nose Q30.2
  palate Q35.9
    with cleft lip (unilateral) Q37.9
      bilateral Q37.8
    hard Q35.1
      with
        cleft lip (unilateral) Q37.1
          bilateral Q37.0
        soft Q35.5
          with cleft lip (unilateral) Q37.5
            bilateral Q37.4
    medial Q35.5
    soft Q35.3
      with
        cleft lip (unilateral) Q37.3
          bilateral Q37.2
        hard Q35.5
          with cleft lip (unilateral) Q37.5
            bilateral Q37.4
  penis Q55.69
  scrotum Q55.29
  thyroid cartilage Q31.8
  uvula Q35.7
Cleidocranial dysostosis Q74.0
Cleptomania F63.2
Clicking hip (newborn) R29.4
Climacteric (female) —*see also* Menopause
  arthritis (any site) NEC —*see* Arthritis,
    specified form NEC
  depression (single episode) F32.8
  male (symptoms) (syndrome) NEC N50.8
  paranoid state F22
  polyarthritis NEC —*see* Arthritis, specified
    form NEC
  symptoms (female) N95.1
Clinical research investigation (clinical trial)
  (control subject) (normal comparison)
  (participant) Z00.6
Clitoris —*see* condition Cloaca (persistent)
  Q43.7
Clonorchiasis, clonorchis infection (liver)
  B66.1
Clonus R25.8
Closed bite M26.29
Clostridium (C.) perfringens, as cause of
  disease classified elsewhere B96.7
Closure
  congenital, nose Q30.0
  cranial sutures, premature Q75.0
  defective or imperfect NEC —*see* Imperfect,
    closure
  fistula, delayed —*see* Fistula
  foramen ovale, imperfect Q21.1
  hymen N89.6
  interauricular septum, defective Q21.1
  interventricular septum, defective Q21.0
  lacrimal duct —*see also* Stenosis, lacrimal,
    duct
    congenital Q10.5
  nose (congenital) Q30.0
    acquired M95.0
  of artificial opening —*see* Attention to,
    artificial, opening

Closure *(Continued)*
  primary angle, without glaucoma damage
    H40.06-
  vagina N89.5
  valve —*see* Endocarditis
  vulva N90.5
Clot (blood) —*see also* Embolism
  artery (obstruction) (occlusion) —*see*
    Embolism
  bladder N32.89
  brain (intradural or extradural) —*see*
    Occlusion, artery, cerebral
  circulation I74.9
  heart —*see also* Infarct, myocardium
    not resulting in infarction I24.0
  vein —*see* Thrombosis
Clouded state R40.1
  epileptic —*see* Epilepsy, specified NEC
  paroxysmal —*see* Epilepsy, specified NEC
Cloudy antrum, antra J32.0
Clouston's (hidrotic) ectodermal dysplasia
  Q82.4
Clubbed nail pachydermoperiostosis M89.40
  [L62]
Clubbing of finger (s) (nails) R68.3
Clubfinger R68.3
  congenital Q68.1
Clubfoot (congenital) Q66.89
  acquired —*see* Deformity, limb, clubfoot
  equinovarus Q66.0
  paralytic —*see* Deformity, limb, clubfoot
Clubhand (congenital) (radial) Q71.4-
  acquired —*see* Deformity, limb, clubhand
Clubnail R68.3
  congenital Q84.6
Clump, kidney Q63.1
Clumsiness, clumsy child syndrome F82
Cluttering F98.81
Clutton's joints A50.51 [M12.80]
Coagulation, intravascular (diffuse)
  (disseminated) —*see also* Defibrination
    syndrome
  complicating abortion —*see* Abortion, by
    type, complicated by, intravascular
    coagulation
  following ectopic or molar pregnancy O08.1
Coagulopathy —*see also* Defect, coagulation
  consumption D65
  intravascular D65
  newborn P60
Coalition
  calcaneo-scaphoid Q66.89
  tarsal Q66.89
Coalminer's
  elbow —*see* Bursitis, elbow, olecranon
  lung or pneumoconiosis J60
Coalworker's lung or pneumoconiosis J60
Coarctation
  aorta (preductal) (postductal) Q25.1
  pulmonary artery Q25.71
Coated tongue K14.3
Coats' disease (exudative retinopathy) —*see*
  Retinopathy, exudative
Cocainism —*see* Dependence, drug, cocaine
Coccidioidomycosis B38.9
  cutaneous B38.3
  disseminated B38.7
  generalized B38.7
  meninges B38.4
  prostate B38.81
  pulmonary B38.2
    acute B38.0
    chronic B38.1
  skin B38.3
  specified NEC B38.89
Coccidioidosis —*see* Coccidioidomycosis
Coccidiosis (intestinal) A07.3
Coccydynia, coccygodynia M53.3
Coccyx —*see* condition
Cochin-China diarrhea K90.1
Cockayne's syndrome Q87.1

Cocked up toe —see Deformity, toe, specified NEC
Cock's peculiar tumor L72.3
Codman's tumor —see Neoplasm, bone, benign
Coenurosis B71.8
Coffee-worker's lung J67.8
Cogan's syndrome H16.32-
    oculomotor apraxia H51.8
Coitus, painful (female) N94.1
    male N53.12
    psychogenic F52.6
Cold J00
    with influenza, flu, or grippe —see Influenza,
        with, respiratory manifestations NEC
    agglutinin disease or hemoglobinuria
        (chronic) D59.1
    bronchial —see Bronchitis
    chest —see Bronchitis
    common (head) J00
    effects of T69.9
        specified effect NEC T69.8
    excessive, effects of T69.9
        specified effect NEC T69.8
    exhaustion from T69.8
    exposure to T69.9
        specified effect NEC T69.8
    head J00
    injury syndrome (newborn) P80.0
    on lung —see Bronchitis
    rose J30.1
    sensitivity, auto-immune D59.1
    virus J00
Coldsore B00.1
Colibacillosis A49.8
    as the cause of other disease (see also
        Escherichia coli) B96.20
    generalized A41.50
Colic (bilious) (infantile) (intestinal) (recurrent)
        (spasmodic) R10.83
    abdomen R10.83
        psychogenic F45.8
    appendix, appendicular K38.8
    bile duct —see Calculus, bile duct
    biliary —see Calculus, bile duct
    common duct —see Calculus, bile duct
    cystic duct —see Calculus, gallbladder
    Devonshire NEC —see Poisoning, lead
    gallbladder —see Calculus, gallbladder
    gallstone —see Calculus, gallbladder
        gallbladder or cystic duct —see Calculus,
            gallbladder
    hepatic (duct) —see Calculus, bile duct
    hysterical F45.8
    kidney N23
    lead NEC —see Poisoning, lead
    mucous K58.9
        with diarrhea K58.0
        psychogenic F54
    nephritic N23
    painter's NEC —see Poisoning, lead
    pancreas K86.8
    psychogenic F45.8
    renal N23
    saturnine NEC —see Poisoning, lead
    ureter N23
    urethral N36.8
        due to calculus N21.1
    uterus NEC N94.89
        menstrual —see Dysmenorrhea
    worm NOS B83.9
Colicystitis —see Cystitis
Colitis (acute) (catarrhal) (chronic)
        (noninfective) (hemorrhagic) (see also
        Enteritis) K52.9
    allergic K52.2
    amebic (acute) (see also Amebiasis) A06.0
        nondysenteric A06.2
    anthrax A22.2
    bacillary —see Infection, Shigella
    balantidial A07.0
    Clostridium difficile A04.7

Colitis (Continued)
    coccidial A07.3
    collagenous K52.89
    cystica superficialis K52.89
    dietary counseling and surveillance (for)
        Z71.3
    dietetic K52.2
    drug-induced K52.1
    due to radiation K52.0
    eosinophilic K52.82
    food hypersensitivity K52.2
    giardial A07.1
    granulomatous —see Enteritis, regional, large
        intestine
    infectious —see Enteritis, infectious
    ischemic K55.9
        acute (fulminant) (subacute) K55.0
        chronic K55.1
        due to mesenteric artery insufficiency
            K55.1
        fulminant (acute) K55.0
    left sided K51.50
        with
            abscess K51.514
            complication K51.519
                specified NEC K51.518
            fistula K51.513
            obstruction K51.512
            rectal bleeding K51.511
    lymphocytic K52.89
    membranous
        psychogenic F54
    microscopic (collagenous) (lymphocytic)
        K52.89
    mucous —see Syndrome, irritable, bowel
        psychogenic F54
    noninfective K52.9
        specified NEC K52.89
    polyposa —see Polyps, colon, inflammatory ◄▥▥
    protozoal A07.9
    pseudomembranous A04.7
    pseudomucinous —see Syndrome, irritable,
        bowel
    regional —see Enteritis, regional, large
        intestine
    segmental —see Enteritis, regional, large
        intestine
    septic —see Enteritis, infectious
    spastic K58.9
        with diarrhea K58.0
        psychogenic F54
    staphylococcal A04.8
        foodborne A05.0
    subacute ischemic K55.0
    thromboulcerative K55.0
    toxic NEC K52.1
        due to Clostridium difficile A04.7
    transmural —see Enteritis, regional, large
        intestine
    trichomonal A07.8
    tuberculous (ulcerative) A18.32
    ulcerative (chronic) K51.90
        with
            complication K51.919
                abscess K51.914
                fistula K51.913
                obstruction K51.912
                rectal bleeding K51.911
                specified complication NEC
                    K51.918
        enterocolitis —see Enterocolitis,
            ulcerative
        ileocolitis —see Ileocolitis, ulcerative
        mucosal proctocolitis —see Proctocolitis,
            mucosal
        proctitis —see Proctitis, ulcerative
        pseudopolyposis —see Polyps, colon,
            inflammatory ◄▥▥
        psychogenic F54
        rectosigmoiditis —see Rectosigmoiditis,
            ulcerative

Colitis (Continued)
    ulcerative (Continued)
        specified type NEC K51.80
            with
                complication K51.819
                    abscess K51.814
                    fistula K51.813
                    obstruction K51.812
                    rectal bleeding K51.811
                    specified complication NEC
                        K51.818
Collagenosis, collagen disease (nonvascular)
        (vascular) M35.9
    cardiovascular I42.8
    reactive perforating L87.1
    specified NEC M35.8
Collapse R55
    adrenal E27.2
    cardiorespiratory R57.0
    cardiovascular R57.0
        newborn P29.89
    circulatory (peripheral) R57.9
        during or after labor and delivery O75.1
        following ectopic or molar pregnancy
            O08.3
        newborn P29.89
    during or
        after labor and delivery O75.1
        resulting from a procedure, not elsewhere
            classified T81.10
    external ear canal —see Stenosis, external ear
        canal
    general R55
    heart —see Disease, heart
    heat T67.1
    hysterical F44.89
    labyrinth, membranous (congenital) Q16.5
    lung (massive) (see also Atelectasis) J98.19
        pressure due to anesthesia (general) (local)
            or other sedation T88.2
            during labor and delivery O74.1
            in pregnancy O29.02-
            postpartum, puerperal O89.09
    myocardial —see Disease, heart
    nervous F48.8
    neurocirculatory F45.8
    nose M95.0
    postoperative (cardiovascular) T81.10 ◄▥▥
    pulmonary (see also Atelectasis) J98.19
        newborn —see Atelectasis
    trachea J39.8
    tracheobronchial J98.09
    valvular —see Endocarditis
    vascular (peripheral) R57.9
        during or after labor and delivery O75.1
        following ectopic or molar pregnancy
            O08.3
        newborn P29.89
    vertebra M48.50-
        cervical region M48.52-
        cervicothoracic region M48.53-
        in (due to)
            metastasis —see Collapse, vertebra, in,
                specified disease NEC
            osteoporosis (see also Osteoporosis)
                M80.88
                cervical region M80.88
                cervicothoracic region M80.88
                lumbar region M80.88
                lumbosacral region M80.88
                multiple sites M80.88
                occipito-atlanto-axial region M80.88
                sacrococcygeal region M80.88
                thoracic region M80.88
                thoracolumbar region M80.88
            specified disease NEC M48.50-
                cervical region M48.52-
                cervicothoracic region M48.53-
                lumbar region M48.56-
                lumbosacral region M48.57-
                occipito-atlanto-axial region M48.51-

◄ New   ◄▥▥ Revised   ~~deleted~~ Deleted

Collapse *(Continued)*
  vertebra *(Continued)*
    in *(Continued)*
      specified disease NEC *(Continued)*
        sacrococcygeal region M48.58-
        thoracic region M48.54-
        thoracolumbar region M48.55-
      lumbar region M48.56-
      lumbosacral region M48.57-
      occipito-atlanto-axial region M48.51-
      sacrococcygeal region M48.58-
      thoracic region M48.54-
      thoracolumbar region M48.55-
Collateral —*see also* condition
  circulation (venous) I87.8
  dilation, veins I87.8
Colles' fracture S52.53-
Collet (-Sicard) syndrome G52.7
Collier's asthma or lung J60
Collodion baby Q80.2
Colloid nodule (of thyroid) (cystic) E04.1
Coloboma (iris) Q13.0
  eyelid Q10.3
  fundus Q14.8
  lens Q12.2
  optic disc (congenital) Q14.2
    acquired H47.31-
Coloenteritis —*see* Enteritis
Colon —*see* condition
Colonization
  MRSA (Methicillin resistant Staphylococcus
    aureus) Z22.322
  MSSA (Methicillin susceptible
    Staphylococcus aureus) Z22.321
  status —*see* Carrier (suspected) of
Coloptosis K63.4
Color blindness —*see* Deficiency, color vision
Colostomy
  attention to Z43.3
  fitting or adjustment Z46.89
  malfunctioning K94.03
  status Z93.3
Colpitis (acute) —*see* Vaginitis
Colpocele N81.5
Colpocystitis —*see* Vaginitis
Colpospasm N94.2
Column, spinal, vertebral —*see* condition
Coma R40.20
  with
    motor response (none) R40.231
      abnormal R40.233
      extension R40.232
      flexion withdrawal R40.234
      localizes pain R40.235
      obeys commands R40.236
    opening of eyes (never) R40.211
      in response to
        pain R40.212
        sound R40.213
      spontaneous R40.214
    verbal response (none) R40.221
      confused conversation R40.224
      inappropriate words R40.223
      incomprehensible words R40.222
      oriented R40.225
  eclamptic —*see* Eclampsia
  epileptic —*see* Epilepsy
  Glascow, scale score —*see* Glasgow coma scale
  Glasgow, scale score —*see* Glasgow coma
    scale ◀
  hepatic —*see* Failure, hepatic, by type, with
    coma
  hyperglycemic (diabetic) —*see* Diabetes, coma
  hyperosmolar (diabetic) —*see* Diabetes, coma
  hypoglycemic (diabetic) —*see* Diabetes, coma,
    hypoglycemic
    nondiabetic E15
  in diabetes —*see* Diabetes, coma
  insulin-induced —*see* Coma, hypoglycemic
  myxedematous E03.5
  newborn P91.5

Coma *(Continued)*
  persistent vegetative state R40.3
  ~~specified NEC, without documented Glasgow~~
    ~~coma scale score, or with partial Glasgow~~
    ~~coma scale score reported R40.244~~
  specified NEC, without documented Glasgow
    coma scale score, or with partial Glasgow
    coma scale score reported R40.244 ◀
Comatose —*see* Coma
Combat fatigue F43.0
Combined —*see* condition
Comedo, comedones (giant) L70.0
Comedocarcinoma —*see also* Neoplasm, breast,
  malignant
  noninfiltrating
    breast D05.8-
    specified site —*see* Neoplasm, in situ, by site
    unspecified site D05.8-
Comedomastitis —*see* Ectasia, mammary duct
Comminuted fracture - code as Fracture, closed
Common
  arterial trunk Q20.0
  atrioventricular canal Q21.2
  atrium Q21.1
  cold (head) J00
  truncus (arteriosus) Q20.0
  variable immunodeficiency —*see*
    Immunodeficiency, common variable
  ventricle Q20.4
Commotio, commotion (current)
  brain —*see* Injury, intracranial, concussion
  cerebri —*see* Injury, intracranial, concussion
  retinae S05.8X-
  spinal cord —*see* Injury, spinal cord, by region
  spinalis —*see* Injury, spinal cord, by region
Communication
  between
    base of aorta and pulmonary artery Q21.4
    left ventricle and right atrium Q20.5
    pericardial sac and pleural sac Q34.8
    pulmonary artery and pulmonary vein,
      congenital Q25.72
  congenital between uterus and digestive or
    urinary tract Q51.7
Compartment syndrome (deep) (posterior)
  (traumatic) T79.A0
  abdomen T79.A3
  lower extremity (hip, buttock, thigh, leg, foot,
    toes) T79.A2
  nontraumatic
    abdomen M79.A3
    lower extremity (hip, buttock, thigh, leg,
      foot, toes) M79.A2-
    specified site NEC M79.A9
    upper extremity (shoulder, arm, forearm,
      wrist, hand, fingers) M79.A1- ◀⫶⫶
  specified site NEC T79.A9
  upper extremity (shoulder, arm, forearm,
    wrist, hand, fingers) T79.A1
Compensation
  failure —*see* Disease, heart
  neurosis, psychoneurosis —*see* Disorder,
    factitious
Complaint —*see also* Disease
  bowel, functional K59.9
    psychogenic F45.8
  intestine, functional K59.9
    psychogenic F45.8
  kidney —*see* Disease, renal
  miners' J60
Complete —*see* condition
Complex
  Addison-Schilder E71.528
  cardiorenal —*see* Hypertension, cardiorenal
  Costen's M26.69
  disseminated mycobacterium avium-
    intracellulare (DMAC) A31.2
  Eisenmenger's (ventricular septal defect) I27.89
  hypersexual F52.8
  jumped process, spine —*see* Dislocation,
    vertebra

Complex *(Continued)*
  primary, tuberculous A15.7
  Schilder-Addison E71.528
  subluxation (vertebral) M99.19
    abdomen M99.19
    acromioclavicular M99.17
    cervical region M99.11
    cervicothoracic M99.11
    costochondral M99.18
    costovertebral M99.18
    head region M99.10
    hip M99.15
    lower extremity M99.16
    lumbar region M99.13
    lumbosacral M99.13
    occipitocervical M99.10
    pelvic region M99.15
    pubic M99.15
    rib cage M99.18
    sacral region M99.14
    sacrococcygeal M99.14
    sacroiliac M99.14
    specified NEC M99.19
    sternochondral M99.18
    sternoclavicular M99.17
    thoracic region M99.12
    thoracolumbar M99.12
    upper extremity M99.17
  Taussig-Bing (transposition, aorta and
    overriding pulmonary artery)
    Q20.1
Complication (s) (from) (of)
  accidental puncture or laceration during a
    procedure (of) —*see* Complications,
    intraoperative (intraprocedural),
    puncture or laceration
  amputation stump (surgical) (late) NEC
    T87.9
    dehiscence T87.81
    infection or inflammation T87.40
      lower limb T87.4-
      upper limb T87.4-
    necrosis T87.50
      lower limb T87.5-
      upper limb T87.5-
    neuroma T87.30
      lower limb T87.3-
      upper limb T87.3-
    specified type NEC T87.89
  anastomosis (and bypass) —*see also*
    Complications, prosthetic device or
    implant
    intestinal (internal) NEC K91.89
      involving urinary tract N99.89
    urinary tract (involving intestinal tract)
      N99.89
    vascular —*see* Complications,
      cardiovascular device or
      implant
  anesthesia, anesthetic (see also Anesthesia,
    complication) T88.59
    brain, postpartum, puerperal
      O89.2
    cardiac
      in
        labor and delivery O74.2
        pregnancy O29.19-
      postpartum, puerperal O89.1
    central nervous system
      in
        labor and delivery O74.3
        pregnancy O29.29-
      postpartum, puerperal O89.2
    difficult or failed intubation T88.4
      in pregnancy O29.6-
    failed sedation (conscious) (moderate)
      during procedure T88.52
    hyperthermia, malignant T88.3
    hypothermia T88.51
    intubation failure T88.4
    malignant hyperthermia T88.3

Complication *(Continued)*
anesthesia, anesthetic *(Continued)*
pulmonary
in
labor and delivery O74.1
pregnancy NEC O29.09-
postpartum, puerperal O89.09
shock T88.2
spinal and epidural
in
labor and delivery NEC O74.6
headache O74.5
pregnancy NEC O29.5X-
postpartum, puerperal NEC O89.5
headache O89.4
anti-reflux device —*see* Complications,
esophageal anti-reflux device
aortic (bifurcation) graft —*see* Complications,
graft, vascular
aortocoronary (bypass) graft —*see*
Complications, coronary artery (bypass)
graft
aortofemoral (bypass) graft —*see*
Complications, extremity artery
(bypass) graft
arteriovenous
fistula, surgically created T82.9
embolism T82.818
fibrosis T82.828
hemorrhage T82.838
infection or inflammation T82.7
mechanical
breakdown T82.510
displacement T82.520
leakage T82.530
malposition T82.520
obstruction T82.590
perforation T82.590
protrusion T82.590
pain T82.848
specified type NEC T82.898
stenosis T82.858
thrombosis T82.868
shunt, surgically created T82.9
embolism T82.818
fibrosis T82.828
hemorrhage T82.838
infection or inflammation T82.7
mechanical
breakdown T82.511
displacement T82.521
leakage T82.531
malposition T82.521
obstruction T82.591
perforation T82.591
protrusion T82.591
pain T82.848
specified type NEC T82.898
stenosis T82.858
thrombosis T82.868
arthroplasty —*see* Complications, joint
prosthesis
artificial
fertilization or insemination N98.9
attempted introduction (of)
embryo in embryo transfer N98.3
ovum following in vitro fertilization
N98.2
hyperstimulation of ovaries N98.1
infection N98.0
specified NEC N98.8
heart T82.9
embolism T82.817
fibrosis T82.827
hemorrhage T82.837
infection or inflammation T82.7
mechanical
breakdown T82.512
displacement T82.522
leakage T82.532
malposition T82.522

Complication *(Continued)*
artificial *(Continued)*
heart *(Continued)*
mechanical *(Continued)*
obstruction T82.592
perforation T82.592
protrusion T82.592
pain T82.847
specified type NEC T82.897
stenosis T82.857
thrombosis T82.867
opening
cecostomy —*see* Complications,
colostomy
colostomy —*see* Complications,
colostomy
cystostomy —*see* Complications,
cystostomy
enterostomy —*see* Complications,
enterostomy
gastrostomy —*see* Complications,
gastrostomy
ileostomy —*see* Complications,
enterostomy
jejunostomy —*see* Complications,
enterostomy
nephrostomy —*see* Complications,
stoma, urinary tract
tracheostomy —*see* Complications,
tracheostomy
ureterostomy —*see* Complications,
stoma, urinary tract
urethrostomy —*see* Complications,
stoma, urinary tract
balloon implant or device
gastrointestinal T85.9
embolism T85.81
fibrosis T85.82
hemorrhage T85.83
infection and inflammation
T85.79
pain T85.84
specified type NEC T85.89
stenosis T85.85
thrombosis T85.86
vascular (counterpulsation) T82.9
embolism T82.818
fibrosis T82.828
hemorrhage T82.838
infection or inflammation T82.7
mechanical
breakdown T82.513
displacement T82.523
leakage T82.533
malposition T82.523
obstruction T82.593
perforation T82.593
protrusion T82.593
pain T82.848
specified type NEC T82.898
stenosis T82.858
thrombosis T82.868
bariatric procedure
gastric band procedure K95.09
infection K95.01
specified procedure NEC K95.89
infection K95.81
bile duct implant (prosthetic) T85.9
embolism T85.81
fibrosis T85.82
hemorrhage T85.83
infection and inflammation T85.79
mechanical
breakdown T85.510
displacement T85.520
malfunction T85.510
malposition T85.520
obstruction T85.590
perforation T85.590
protrusion T85.590
specified NEC T85.590

Complication *(Continued)*
bile duct implant *(Continued)*
pain T85.84
specified type NEC T85.89
stenosis T85.85
thrombosis T85.86
bladder device (auxiliary) —*see*
Complications, genitourinary, device or
implant, urinary system
bleeding (postoperative) —*see* Complication,
postoperative, hemorrhage
intraoperative —*see* Complication,
intraoperative, hemorrhage
blood vessel graft —*see* Complications, graft,
vascular
bone
device NEC T84.9
embolism T84.81
fibrosis T84.82
hemorrhage T84.83
infection or inflammation T84.7
mechanical
breakdown T84.318
displacement T84.328
malposition T84.328
obstruction T84.398
perforation T84.398
protrusion T84.398
pain T84.84
specified type NEC T84.89
stenosis T84.85
thrombosis T84.86
graft —*see* Complications, graft, bone
growth stimulator (electrode) —*see*
Complications, electronic stimulator
device, bone
marrow transplant —*see* Complications,
transplant, bone, marrow
brain neurostimulator (electrode) —*see*
Complications, electronic stimulator
device, brain
breast implant (prosthetic) T85.9
capsular contracture T85.44
embolism T85.81
fibrosis T85.82
hemorrhage T85.83
infection and inflammation
T85.79
mechanical
breakdown T85.41
displacement T85.42
leakage T85.43
malposition T85.42
obstruction T85.49
perforation T85.49
protrusion T85.49
specified NEC T85.49
pain T85.84
specified type NEC T85.89
stenosis T85.85
thrombosis T85.86
bypass —*see also* Complications, prosthetic
device or implant
aortocoronary —*see* Complications,
coronary artery (bypass) graft
arterial —*see also* Complications, graft,
vascular
extremity —*see* Complications, extremity
artery (bypass) graft
cardiac —*see also* Disease, heart
device, implant or graft T82.9
embolism T82.817
fibrosis T82.827
hemorrhage T82.837
infection or inflammation T82.7
valve prosthesis T82.6
mechanical
breakdown T82.519
specified device NEC T82.518
displacement T82.529
specified device NEC T82.528

◀ New ◀▥ Revised ~~deleted~~ Deleted

Complication (Continued)
  cardiac (Continued)
    device, implant or graft (Continued)
      mechanical (Continued)
        leakage T82.539
          specified device NEC T82.538
        malposition T82.529
          specified device NEC T82.528
        obstruction T82.599
          specified device NEC T82.598
        perforation T82.599
          specified device NEC T82.598
        protrusion T82.599
          specified device NEC T82.598
      pain T82.847
      specified type NEC T82.897
      stenosis T82.857
      thrombosis T82.867
  cardiovascular device, graft or implant
      T82.9
    aortic graft —see Complications, graft,
        vascular
    arteriovenous
      fistula, artificial —see Complication,
          arteriovenous, fistula, surgically
          created
      shunt —see Complication, arteriovenous,
          shunt, surgically created
    artificial heart —see Complication,
        artificial, heart
    balloon (counterpulsation) device —see
        Complication, balloon implant,
        vascular
    carotid artery graft —see Complications,
        graft, vascular
    coronary bypass graft —see Complication,
        coronary artery (bypass) graft
    dialysis catheter (vascular) —see
        Complication, catheter, dialysis
    electronic T82.9
      electrode T82.9
        embolism T82.817
        fibrosis T82.827
        hemorrhage T82.837
        infection T82.7
        mechanical
          breakdown T82.110
          displacement T82.120
          leakage T82.190
          obstruction T82.190
          perforation T82.190
          protrusion T82.190
          specified type NEC T82.190
        pain T82.847
        specified NEC T82.897
        stenosis T82.857
        thrombosis T82.867
      embolism T82.817
      fibrosis T82.827
      hemorrhage T82.837
      infection T82.7
      mechanical
        breakdown T82.119
        displacement T82.129
        leakage T82.199
        obstruction T82.199
        perforation T82.199
        protrusion T82.199
        specified type NEC T82.199
      pain T82.847
      pulse generator T82.9
        embolism T82.817
        fibrosis T82.827
        hemorrhage T82.837
        infection T82.7
        mechanical
          breakdown T82.111
          displacement T82.121
          leakage T82.191
          obstruction T82.191
          perforation T82.191

Complication (Continued)
  cardiovascular device, graft or implant
      (Continued)
    electronic (Continued)
      pulse generator (Continued)
        mechanical (Continued)
          protrusion T82.191
          specified type NEC T82.191
        pain T82.847
        specified NEC T82.897
        stenosis T82.857
        thrombosis T82.867
    specified condition NEC T82.897
    specified device NEC T82.9
      embolism T82.817
      fibrosis T82.827
      hemorrhage T82.837
      infection T82.7
      mechanical
        breakdown T82.118
        displacement T82.128
        leakage T82.198
        obstruction T82.198
        perforation T82.198
        protrusion T82.198
        specified type NEC T82.198
      pain T82.847
      specified NEC T82.897
      stenosis T82.857
      thrombosis T82.867
    stenosis T82.857
    thrombosis T82.867
    extremity artery graft —see Complication,
        extremity artery (bypass) graft
    femoral artery graft —see Complication,
        extremity artery (bypass) graft
    heart
      transplant —see Complication,
          transplant, heart
      valve —see Complication, prosthetic
          device, heart valve
        graft —see Complication, heart, valve,
            graft
    heart-lung transplant —see Complication,
        transplant, heart, with lung
    infection or inflammation T82.7
    umbrella device —see Complication,
        umbrella device, vascular
    vascular graft (or anastomosis) —see
        Complication, graft, vascular
  carotid artery (bypass) graft —see
      Complications, graft, vascular
  catheter (device) NEC —see also
      Complications, prosthetic device or
      implant
    cystostomy T83.9
      embolism T83.81
      fibrosis T83.82
      hemorrhage T83.83
      infection and inflammation
          T83.59
      mechanical
        breakdown T83.010
        displacement T83.020
        leakage T83.030
        malposition T83.020
        obstruction T83.090
        perforation T83.090
        protrusion T83.090
        specified NEC T83.090
      pain T83.84
      specified type NEC T83.89
      stenosis T83.85
      thrombosis T83.86
    dialysis (vascular) T82.9
      embolism T82.818
      fibrosis T82.828
      hemorrhage T82.838
      infection and inflammation T82.7
      intraperitoneal —see Complications,
          catheter, intraperitoneal

Complication (Continued)
  catheter NEC (Continued)
    dialysis (Continued)
      mechanical
        breakdown T82.41
        displacement T82.42
        leakage T82.43
        malposition T82.42
        obstruction T82.49
        perforation T82.49
        protrusion T82.49
      pain T82.848
      specified type NEC T82.898
      stenosis T82.858
      thrombosis T82.868
    epidural infusion T85.9
      embolism T85.81
      fibrosis T85.82
      hemorrhage T85.83
      infection and inflammation T85.79
      mechanical
        breakdown T85.610
        displacement T85.620
        leakage T85.630
        malfunction T85.610
        malposition T85.620
        obstruction T85.690
        perforation T85.690
        protrusion T85.690
        specified NEC T85.690
      pain T85.84
      specified type NEC T85.89
      stenosis T85.85
      thrombosis T85.86
    intraperitoneal dialysis T85.9
      embolism T85.81
      fibrosis T85.82
      hemorrhage T85.83
      infection and inflammation T85.71
      mechanical
        breakdown T85.611
        displacement T85.621
        leakage T85.631
        malfunction T85.611
        malposition T85.621
        obstruction T85.691
        perforation T85.691
        protrusion T85.691
        specified NEC T85.691
      pain T85.84
      specified type NEC T85.89
      stenosis T85.85
      thrombosis T85.86
    intravenous infusion T82.9
      embolism T82.818
      fibrosis T82.828
      hemorrhage T82.838
      infection or inflammation T82.7
      mechanical
        breakdown T82.514
        displacement T82.524
        leakage T82.534
        malposition T82.524
        obstruction T82.594
        perforation T82.594
        protrusion T82.594
      pain T82.848
      specified type NEC T82.898
      stenosis T82.858
      thrombosis T82.868
    subdural infusion T85.9
      embolism T85.81
      fibrosis T85.82
      hemorrhage T85.83
      infection and inflammation T85.79
      mechanical
        breakdown T85.610
        displacement T85.620
        leakage T85.630
        malfunction T85.610
        malposition T85.620

Complication (Continued)

catheter NEC (Continued)

subdural infusion (Continued)

mechanical (Continued)

obstruction T85.690

perforation T85.690

protrusion T85.690

specified NEC T85.690

pain T85.84

specified type NEC T85.89

stenosis T85.85

thrombosis T85.86

urethral, indwelling T83.9

displacement T83.028

embolism T83.81

fibrosis T83.82

hemorrhage T83.83

infection and inflammation T83.51

leakage T83.038

malposition T83.028

mechanical

breakdown T83.018

obstruction (mechanical) T83.098

pain T83.84

perforation T83.098

protrusion T83.098

specified type NEC T83.098

stenosis T83.85

thrombosis T83.86

urinary (indwelling) —see Complications, catheter, urethral, indwelling

cecostomy (stoma) —see Complications, colostomy

cesarean delivery wound NEC O90.89

disruption O90.0

hematoma O90.2

infection (following delivery) O86.0

chemotherapy (antineoplastic) NEC T88.7

chin implant (prosthetic) —see Complication, prosthetic device or implant, specified NEC

circulatory system I99.8

intraoperative I97.88

postprocedural I97.89

following cardiac surgery I97.19-

postcardiotomy syndrome I97.0

hypertension I97.3

lymphedema after mastectomy I97.2

postcardiotomy syndrome I97.0

specified NEC I97.89

colostomy (stoma) K94.00

hemorrhage K94.01

infection K94.02

malfunction K94.03

mechanical K94.03

specified complication NEC K94.09

contraceptive device, intrauterine — see Complications, intrauterine, contraceptive device

cord (umbilical) —see Complications, umbilical cord

corneal graft —see Complications, graft, cornea

coronary artery (bypass) graft T82.9

atherosclerosis —see Arteriosclerosis, coronary (artery)

embolism T82.818

fibrosis T82.828

hemorrhage T82.838

infection and inflammation T82.7

mechanical

breakdown T82.211

displacement T82.212

leakage T82.213

malposition T82.212

obstruction T82.218

perforation T82.218

protrusion T82.218

specified NEC T82.218

pain T82.848

specified type NEC T82.897

Complication (Continued)

coronary artery graft (Continued)

stenosis T82.858

thrombosis T82.868

counterpulsation device (balloon), intra-aortic —see Complications, balloon implant, vascular

cystostomy (stoma) N99.518

catheter —see Complications, catheter, cystostomy

hemorrhage N99.510

infection N99.511

malfunction N99.512

specified type NEC N99.518

delivery (see also Complications, obstetric) O75.9

procedure (instrumental) (manual) (surgical) O75.4

specified NEC O75.89

dialysis (peritoneal) (renal) —see also Complications, infusion

catheter (vascular) —see Complication, catheter, dialysis

peritoneal, intraperitoneal —see Complications, catheter, intraperitoneal

dorsal column (spinal) neurostimulator —see Complications, electronic stimulator device, spinal cord

drug NEC T88.7

ear procedure —see also Disorder, ear

intraoperative H95.88-

hematoma —see Complications, intraoperative, hemorrhage (hematoma) (of), ear

hemorrhage —see Complications, intraoperative, hemorrhage (hematoma) (of), ear

laceration —see Complications, intraoperative, puncture or laceration..., ear

specified NEC H95.88-

postoperative H95.89-

external ear canal stenosis H95.81-

hematoma —see Complications, postprocedural, hemorrhage (hematoma) (of), ear

hemorrhage —see Complications, postprocedural, hemorrhage (hematoma) (of), ear

postmastoidectomy —see Complications, postmastoidectomy

specified NEC H95.89-

ectopic pregnancy O08.9

damage to pelvic organs O08.6

embolism O08.2

genital infection O08.0

hemorrhage (delayed) (excessive) O08.1

metabolic disorder O08.5

renal failure O08.4

shock O08.3

specified type NEC O08.0

venous complication NEC O08.7

electronic stimulator device

bladder (urinary) —see Complications, electronic stimulator device, urinary

bone T84.9

breakdown T84.310

displacement T84.320

embolism T84.81

fibrosis T84.82

hemorrhage T84.83

infection or inflammation T84.7

malfunction T84.310

malposition T84.320

mechanical NEC T84.390

obstruction T84.390

pain T84.84

perforation T84.390

protrusion T84.390

specified type NEC T84.89

Complication (Continued)

electronic stimulator device (Continued)

bone (Continued)

stenosis T84.85

thrombosis T84.86

brain T85.9

embolism T85.81

fibrosis T85.82

hemorrhage T85.83

infection and inflammation T85.79

mechanical

breakdown T85.110

displacement T85.120

leakage T85.190

malposition T85.120

obstruction T85.190

perforation T85.190

protrusion T85.190

specified NEC T85.190

pain T85.84

specified type NEC T85.89

stenosis T85.85

thrombosis T85.86

cardiac (defibrillator) (pacemaker) —see Complications, cardiovascular device or implant, electronic

muscle T84.9

breakdown T84.418

displacement T84.428

embolism T84.81

fibrosis T84.82

hemorrhage T84.83

infection or inflammation T84.7

mechanical NEC T84.498

pain T84.84

specified type NEC T84.89

stenosis T84.85

thrombosis T84.86

nervous system T85.9

brain —see Complications, electronic stimulator device, brain

embolism T85.81

fibrosis T85.82

hemorrhage T85.83

infection and inflammation T85.79

mechanical

breakdown T85.118

displacement T85.128

leakage T85.199

malposition T85.128

obstruction T85.199

perforation T85.199

protrusion T85.199

specified NEC T85.199

pain T85.84

peripheral nerve —see Complications, electronic stimulator device, peripheral nerve

specified type NEC T85.89

spinal cord —see Complications, electronic stimulator device, spinal cord

stenosis T85.85

thrombosis T85.86

peripheral nerve T85.9

embolism T85.81

fibrosis T85.82

hemorrhage T85.83

infection and inflammation T85.79

mechanical

breakdown T85.111

displacement T85.121

leakage T85.191

malposition T85.121

obstruction T85.191

perforation T85.191

protrusion T85.191

specified NEC T85.191

pain T85.84

specified type NEC T85.89

stenosis T85.85

thrombosis T85.86

Complication *(Continued)*
  electronic stimulator device *(Continued)*
    spinal cord T85.9
      embolism T85.81
      fibrosis T85.82
      hemorrhage T85.83
      infection and inflammation
        T85.79
      mechanical
        breakdown T85.112
        displacement T85.122
        leakage T85.192
        malposition T85.122
        obstruction T85.192
        perforation T85.192
        protrusion T85.192
        specified NEC T85.192
      pain T85.84
      specified type NEC T85.89
      stenosis T85.85
      thrombosis T85.86
    urinary T83.9
      embolism T83.81
      fibrosis T83.82
      hemorrhage T83.83
      infection and inflammation T83.59
      mechanical
        breakdown T83.110
        displacement T83.120
        malposition T83.120
        perforation T83.190
        protrusion T83.190
        specified NEC T83.190
      pain T83.84
      specified type NEC T83.89
      stenosis T83.85
      thrombosis T83.86
  electroshock therapy T88.9
    specified NEC T88.8
  endocrine E34.9
    postprocedural
      adrenal hypofunction E89.6
      hypoinsulinemia E89.1
      hypoparathyroidism E89.2
      hypopituitarism E89.3
      hypothyroidism E89.0
      ovarian failure E89.40
        asymptomatic E89.40
        symptomatic E89.41
      specified NEC E89.89
      testicular hypofunction E89.5
  endodontic treatment NEC M27.59
  enterostomy (stoma) K94.10
    hemorrhage K94.11
    infection K94.12
    malfunction K94.13
    mechanical K94.13
    specified complication NEC K94.19
  episiotomy, disruption O90.1
  esophageal anti-reflux device T85.9
    embolism T85.81
    fibrosis T85.82
    hemorrhage T85.83
    infection and inflammation T85.79
    mechanical
      breakdown T85.511
      displacement T85.521
      malfunction T85.511
      malposition T85.521
      obstruction T85.591
      perforation T85.591
      protrusion T85.591
      specified NEC T85.591
    pain T85.84
    specified type NEC T85.89
    stenosis T85.85
    thrombosis T85.86
  esophagostomy K94.30
    hemorrhage K94.31
    infection K94.32
    malfunction K94.33

Complication *(Continued)*
  esophagostomy *(Continued)*
    mechanical K94.33
    specified complication NEC K94.39
  extracorporeal circulation T80.90
  extremity artery (bypass) graft T82.9
    arteriosclerosis —*see* Arteriosclerosis,
      extremities, bypass graft
    embolism T82.818
    fibrosis T82.828
    hemorrhage T82.838
    infection and inflammation T82.7
    mechanical
      breakdown T82.318
        femoral artery T82.312
      displacement T82.328
        femoral artery T82.322
      leakage T82.338
        femoral artery T82.332
      malposition T82.328
        femoral artery T82.322
      obstruction T82.398
        femoral artery T82.392
      perforation T82.398
        femoral artery T82.392
      protrusion T82.398
        femoral artery T82.392
    pain T82.848
    specified type NEC T82.898
    stenosis T82.858
    thrombosis T82.868
  eye H57.9
    corneal graft —*see* Complications, graft,
      cornea
    implant (prosthetic) T85.9
      embolism T85.81
      fibrosis T85.82
      hemorrhage T85.83
      infection and inflammation T85.79
      mechanical
        breakdown T85.318
        displacement T85.328
        leakage T85.398
        malposition T85.328
        obstruction T85.398
        perforation T85.398
        protrusion T85.398
        specified NEC T85.398
      pain T85.84
      specified type NEC T85.89
      stenosis T85.85
      thrombosis T85.86
    intraocular lens —*see* Complications,
      intraocular lens
    orbital prosthesis —*see* Complications,
      orbital prosthesis
  female genital N94.9
    device, implant or graft NEC —*see*
      Complications, genitourinary, device
      or implant, genital tract
  femoral artery (bypass) graft —*see*
    Complication, extremity artery (bypass)
    graft
  fixation device, internal (orthopedic) T84.9
    infection and inflammation T84.60
      arm T84.61-
        humerus T84.61-
        radius T84.61-
        ulna T84.61-
      leg T84.629
        femur T84.62-
        fibula T84.62-
        tibia T84.62-
      specified site NEC T84.69
      spine T84.63
    mechanical
      breakdown
        limb T84.119
          carpal T84.210
          femur T84.11-
          fibula T84.11-

Complication *(Continued)*
  fixation device, internal *(Continued)*
    mechanical *(Continued)*
      breakdown *(Continued)*
        limb *(Continued)*
          humerus T84.11-
          metacarpal T84.210
          metatarsal T84.213
          phalanx
            foot T84.213
            hand T84.210
          radius T84.11-
          tarsal T84.213
          tibia T84.11-
          ulna T84.11-
          specified bone NEC T84.218
        spine T84.216
      displacement
        limb T84.129
          carpal T84.220
          femur T84.12-
          fibula T84.12-
          humerus T84.12-
          metacarpal T84.220
          metatarsal T84.223
          phalanx
            foot T84.223
            hand T84.220
          radius T84.12-
          tarsal T84.223
          tibia T84.12-
          ulna T84.12-
          specified bone NEC T84.228
        spine T84.226
      malposition —*see* Complications,
        fixation device, internal,
        mechanical, displacement
      obstruction —*see* Complications, fixation
        device, internal, mechanical,
        specified type NEC
      perforation —*see* Complications, fixation
        device, internal, mechanical,
        specified type NEC
      protrusion —*see* Complications, fixation
        device, internal, mechanical,
        specified type NEC
      specified type NEC
        limb T84.199
          carpal T84.290
          femur T84.19-
          fibula T84.19-
          humerus T84.19-
          metacarpal T84.290
          metatarsal T84.293
          phalanx
            foot T84.293
            hand T84.290
          radius T84.19-
          tarsal T84.293
          tibia T84.19-
          ulna T84.19-
          specified bone NEC T84.298
        vertebra T84.296
    specified type NEC T84.89 ◀▥
      embolism T84.81
      fibrosis T84.82
      hemorrhage T84.83
      pain T84.84
      specified complication NEC T84.89
      stenosis T84.85
      thrombosis T84.86
  following
    acute myocardial infarction NEC I23.8
      aneurysm (false) (of cardiac wall) (of
        heart wall) (ruptured) I23.3
      angina I23.7
      atrial
        septal defect I23.1
        thrombosis I23.6
      cardiac wall rupture I23.3
      chordae tendinae rupture I23.4

Complication (Continued)
 following (Continued)
  acute myocardial infarction NEC
    (Continued)
   defect
    septal
     atrial (heart) I23.1
     ventricular (heart) I23.2
   hemopericardium I23.0
   papillary muscle rupture I23.5
   rupture
    cardiac wall I23.3
     with hemopericardium
       I23.0
    chordae tendineae I23.4
    papillary muscle I23.5
   specified NEC I23.8
   thrombosis
    atrium I23.6
    auricular appendage I23.6
    ventricle (heart) I23.6
   ventricular
    septal defect I23.2
    thrombosis I23.6
  ectopic or molar pregnancy O08.9
   cardiac arrest O08.81
   sepsis O08.82
   specified type NEC O08.89
   urinary tract infection O08.83
  termination of pregnancy —see Abortion
 gastrointestinal K92.9
  bile duct prosthesis —see Complications,
    bile duct implant
  esophageal anti-reflux device —see
    Complications, esophageal
    anti-reflux device
  postoperative
   colostomy —see Complications,
     colostomy
   dumping syndrome K91.1
   enterostomy —see Complications,
     enterostomy
   gastrostomy —see Complications,
     gastrostomy
   malabsorption NEC K91.2
   obstruction K91.3
   postcholecystectomy syndrome
     K91.5
   specified NEC K91.89
   vomiting after GI surgery K91.0
  prosthetic device or implant
   bile duct prosthesis —see Complications,
     bile duct implant
   esophageal anti-reflux device —see
     Complications, esophageal anti-
     reflux device
   specified type NEC
    embolism T85.81
    fibrosis T85.82
    hemorrhage T85.83
    mechanical
     breakdown T85.518
     displacement T85.528
     malfunction T85.518
     malposition T85.528
     obstruction T85.598
     perforation T85.598
     protrusion T85.598
     specified NEC T85.598
    pain T85.84
    specified complication NEC
      T85.89
    stenosis T85.85
    thrombosis T85.86
 gastrostomy (stoma) K94.20
  hemorrhage K94.21
  infection K94.22
  malfunction K94.23
  mechanical K94.23
  specified complication NEC
    K94.29

Complication (Continued)
 genitourinary
  device or implant T83.9
   genital tract T83.9
    infection or inflammation T83.6
    intrauterine contraceptive device —see
      Complications, intrauterine,
      contraceptive device
    mechanical —see Complications, by
      device, mechanical
    mesh —see Complications, mesh
    penile prosthesis —see Complications,
      prosthetic device, penile
    specified type NEC T83.89
     embolism T83.81
     fibrosis T83.82
     hemorrhage T83.83
     pain T83.84
     specified complication NEC T83.89
     stenosis T83.85
     thrombosis T83.86
    vaginal mesh —see Complications,
      mesh
   urinary system T83.9
    cystostomy catheter —see
      Complication, catheter,
      cystostomy
    electronic stimulator —see
      Complications, electronic
      stimulator device, urinary
    indwelling urethral catheter —see
      Complications, catheter, urethral,
      indwelling
    infection or inflammation T83.59
     indwelling urinary catheter T83.51
    kidney transplant —see Complication,
      transplant, kidney
    organ graft —see Complication, graft,
      urinary organ
    specified type NEC T83.89
     embolism T83.81
     fibrosis T83.82
     hemorrhage T83.83
     mechanical T83.198
      breakdown T83.118
      displacement T83.128
      malfunction T83.118
      malposition T83.128
      obstruction T83.198
      perforation T83.198
      protrusion T83.198
      specified NEC T83.198
     pain T83.84
     specified complication NEC
       T83.89
     stenosis T83.85
     thrombosis T83.86
    sphincter implant —see
      Complications, implant, urinary
      sphincter
  postprocedural
   pelvic peritoneal adhesions N99.4
   renal failure N99.0
   specified NEC N99.89
   stoma —see Complications, stoma,
     urinary tract
   urethral stricture —see Stricture, urethra,
     postprocedural
   vaginal
    adhesions N99.2
    vault prolapse N99.3
 graft (bypass) (patch) —see also
   Complications, prosthetic device or
   implant
  aorta —see Complications, graft,
    vascular
  arterial —see Complication, graft,
    vascular
  bone T86.839
   failure T86.831
   infection T86.832

Complication (Continued)
 graft (Continued)
  bone (Continued)
   mechanical T84.318
    breakdown T84.318
    displacement T84.328
    protrusion T84.398
    specified type NEC T84.398
   rejection T86.830
   specified type NEC T86.838
  carotid artery —see Complications, graft,
    vascular
  cornea T86.849
   failure T86.841
   infection T86.842
   mechanical T85.398
    breakdown T85.318
    displacement T85.328
    protrusion T85.398
    specified type NEC T85.398
   rejection T86.840
   retroprosthetic membrane T85.398
   specified type NEC T86.848
  femoral artery (bypass) —see Complication,
    extremity artery (bypass) graft
  genital organ or tract —see Complications,
    genitourinary, device or implant,
    genital tract
  muscle T84.9
   breakdown T84.410
   displacement T84.420
   embolism T84.81
   fibrosis T84.82
   hemorrhage T84.83
   infection and inflammation T84.7
   mechanical NEC T84.490
   pain T84.84
   specified type NEC T84.89
   stenosis T84.85
   thrombosis T84.86
  nerve —see Complication, prosthetic device
    or implant, specified NEC
  skin —see Complications, prosthetic device
    or implant, skin graft
  tendon T84.9
   breakdown T84.410
   displacement T84.420
   embolism T84.81
   fibrosis T84.82
   hemorrhage T84.83
   infection and inflammation T84.7
   mechanical NEC T84.490
   pain T84.84
   specified type NEC T84.89
   stenosis T84.85
   thrombosis T84.86
  urinary organ T83.9
   embolism T83.81
   fibrosis T83.82
   hemorrhage T83.83
   infection and inflammation T83.59
    indwelling urinary catheter T83.51
   mechanical
    breakdown T83.21
    displacement T83.22
    leakage T83.23
    malposition T83.22
    obstruction T83.29
    perforation T83.29
    protrusion T83.29
    specified NEC T83.29
   pain T83.84
   specified type NEC T83.89
   stenosis T83.85
   thrombosis T83.86
  vascular T82.9
   embolism T82.818
   femoral artery —see Complication,
     extremity artery (bypass) graft
   fibrosis T82.828
   hemorrhage T82.838

◀ New   ◀ Revised   ~~deleted~~ Deleted

Complication (Continued)
  graft (Continued)
    vascular (Continued)
      mechanical
        breakdown T82.319
          aorta (bifurcation) T82.310
          carotid artery T82.311
          specified vessel NEC T82.318
        displacement T82.329
          aorta (bifurcation) T82.320
          carotid artery T82.321
          specified vessel NEC T82.328
        leakage T82.339
          aorta (bifurcation) T82.330
          carotid artery T82.331
          specified vessel NEC T82.338
        malposition T82.329
          aorta (bifurcation) T82.320
          carotid artery T82.321
          specified vessel NEC T82.328
        obstruction T82.399
          aorta (bifurcation) T82.390
          carotid artery T82.391
          specified vessel NEC T82.398
        perforation T82.399
          aorta (bifurcation) T82.390
          carotid artery T82.391
          specified vessel NEC T82.398
        protrusion T82.399
          aorta (bifurcation) T82.390
          carotid artery T82.391
          specified vessel NEC T82.398
      pain T82.848
      specified complication NEC
          T82.898
      stenosis T82.858
      thrombosis T82.868
  heart I51.9
    assist device
      infection and inflammation T82.7
    following acute myocardial infarction —
        see Complications, following, acute
        myocardial infarction ◀▮▮▮
    postoperative —see Complications,
        circulatory system
    transplant —see Complication, transplant,
        heart
      and lung (s) —see Complications,
          transplant, heart, with lung
    valve
      graft (biological) T82.9
        embolism T82.817
        fibrosis T82.827
        hemorrhage T82.837
        infection and inflammation
            T82.7
        mechanical T82.228
          breakdown T82.221
          displacement T82.222
          leakage T82.223
          malposition T82.222
          obstruction T82.228
          perforation T82.228
          protrusion T82.228
        pain T82.847
        specified type NEC T82.897
        stenosis T82.857
        thrombosis T82.867
      prosthesis T82.9
        embolism T82.817
        fibrosis T82.827
        hemorrhage T82.837
        infection or inflammation T82.6
        mechanical T82.09
          breakdown T82.01
          displacement T82.02
          leakage T82.03
          malposition T82.02
          obstruction T82.09
          perforation T82.09
          protrusion T82.09

Complication (Continued)
  heart (Continued)
    valve (Continued)
      prosthesis (Continued)
        pain T82.847
        specified type NEC T82.897
          mechanical T82.09
        stenosis T82.857
        thrombosis T82.867
  hematoma
    intraoperative —see Complication,
        intraoperative, hemorrhage
    postprocedural —see Complication,
        postprocedural, hemorrhage
  hemodialysis —see Complications,
      dialysis
  hemorrhage
    intraoperative —see Complication,
        intraoperative, hemorrhage
    postprocedural —see Complication,
        postprocedural, hemorrhage
  ileostomy (stoma) —see Complications,
      enterostomy
  immunization (procedure) —see
      Complications, vaccination
  implant —see also Complications, by site and
      type
    urinary sphincter T83.9
      embolism T83.81
      fibrosis T83.82
      hemorrhage T83.83
      infection and inflammation T83.59
      mechanical
        breakdown T83.111
        displacement T83.121
        leakage T83.191
        malposition T83.121
        obstruction T83.191
        perforation T83.191
        protrusion T83.191
        specified NEC T83.191
      pain T83.84
      specified type NEC T83.89
      stenosis T83.85
      thrombosis T83.86
  infusion (procedure) T80.90
    air embolism T80.0
    blood —see Complications, transfusion
    catheter —see Complications, catheter
    infection T80.29
    pump —see Complications, cardiovascular,
        device or implant
    sepsis T80.29
    serum reaction (see also Reaction, serum)
        T80.69
      anaphylactic shock (see also Shock,
          anaphylactic) T80.59
    specified type NEC T80.89
  inhalation therapy NEC T81.81
  injection (procedure) T80.90
    drug reaction —see Reaction, drug
    infection T80.29
    sepsis T80.29
    serum (prophylactic) (therapeutic) —see
        Complications, vaccination
    specified type NEC T80.89
    vaccine (any) —see Complications,
        vaccination
  inoculation (any) —see Complications,
      vaccination
  insulin pump
    infection and inflammation T85.72
    mechanical
      breakdown T85.614
      displacement T85.624
      leakage T85.633
      malposition T85.624
      obstruction T85.694
      perforation T85.694
      protrusion T85.694
      specified NEC T85.694

Complication (Continued)
  intestinal pouch NEC K91.858
  intraocular lens (prosthetic) T85.9
    embolism T85.81
    fibrosis T85.82
    hemorrhage T85.83
    infection and inflammation T85.79
    mechanical
      breakdown T85.21
      displacement T85.22
      malposition T85.22
      obstruction T85.29
      perforation T85.29
      protrusion T85.29
      specified NEC T85.29
    pain T85.84
    specified type NEC T85.89
    stenosis T85.85
    thrombosis T85.86
  intraoperative (intraprocedural)
    cardiac arrest
      during cardiac surgery I97.710
      during other surgery I97.711
    cardiac functional disturbance NEC
      during cardiac surgery I97.790
      during other surgery I97.791
    hemorrhage (hematoma) (of)
      circulatory system organ or structure
        during cardiac bypass I97.411
        during cardiac catheterization I97.410
        during other circulatory system
            procedure I97.418
        during other procedure I97.42
      digestive system organ
        during procedure on digestive system
            K91.61
        during procedure on other organ
            K91.62
      ear
        during procedure on ear and mastoid
            process H95.21
        during procedure on other organ
            H95.22
      endocrine system organ or structure
        during procedure on endocrine
            system organ or structure E36.01
        during procedure on other organ
            E36.02
      eye and adnexa
        during ophthalmic procedure H59.11-
        during other procedure H59.12-
      genitourinary organ or structure
        during procedure on genitourinary
            organ or structure N99.61
        during procedure on other organ
            N99.62
      mastoid process
        during procedure on ear and mastoid
            process H95.21
        during procedure on other organ
            H95.22
      musculoskeletal structure
        during musculoskeletal surgery
            M96.810
        during non-orthopedic surgery
            M96.811
        during orthopedic surgery M96.810
      nervous system
        during a nervous system procedure
            G97.31
        during other procedure G97.32
      respiratory system
        during other procedure J95.62
        during procedure on respiratory
            system organ or structure
            J95.61
      skin and subcutaneous tissue
        during a dermatologic procedure
            L76.01
        during a procedure on other organ
            L76.02

◀ New　◀▥ Revised　~~deleted~~ Deleted

Complication (*Continued*)
musculoskeletal system —*see also*
    Complication, intraoperative
    (intraprocedural), by site
  device, implant or graft NEC —*see*
    Complications, orthopedic, device or
    implant
  internal fixation (nail) (plate) (rod) —*see*
    Complications, fixation device,
    internal
  joint prosthesis —*see* Complications, joint
    prosthesis
  postoperative (postprocedural) M96.89
    with osteoporosis —*see* Osteoporosis
    fracture following insertion of device —
      see Fracture, following insertion of
      orthopedic implant, joint prosthesis
      or bone plate
    joint instability after prosthesis removal
      M96.89
    lordosis M96.4
    postlaminectomy syndrome NEC
      M96.1
      kyphosis M96.3
    pseudarthrosis M96.0
    specified complication NEC M96.89
  post radiation M96.89
    kyphosis M96.3
    scoliosis M96.5
    specified complication NEC M96.89
nephrostomy (stoma) —*see* Complications,
  stoma, urinary tract, external NEC
nervous system G98.8
  central G96.9
  device, implant or graft —*see also*
    Complication, prosthetic device or
    implant, specified NEC
    electronic stimulator (electrode (s)) —
      see Complications, electronic
      stimulator device
    ventricular shunt —*see* Complications,
      ventricular shunt
  electronic stimulator (electrode (s)) —*see*
    Complications, electronic stimulator
    device
  postprocedural G97.82
    intracranial hypotension G97.2
    specified NEC G97.82
    spinal fluid leak G97.0
newborn, due to intrauterine (fetal)
  procedure P96.5
nonabsorbable (permanent) sutures —*see*
  Complication, sutures, permanent
obstetric O75.9
  procedure (instrumental) (manual)
    (surgical) specified NEC O75.4
  specified NEC O75.89
  surgical wound NEC O90.89
    hematoma O90.2
    infection O86.0
ocular lens implant —*see* Complications,
  intraocular lens
ophthalmologic
  postprocedural bleb —*see* Blebitis
orbital prosthesis T85.9
  embolism T85.81
  fibrosis T85.82
  hemorrhage T85.83
  infection and inflammation T85.79
  mechanical
    breakdown T85.31-
    displacement T85.32-
    malposition T85.32-
    obstruction T85.39-
    perforation T85.39-
    protrusion T85.39-
    specified NEC T85.39-
  pain T85.84
  specified type NEC T85.89
  stenosis T85.85
  thrombosis T85.86

Complication (*Continued*)
organ or tissue transplant (partial) (total) —
  see Complications, transplant
orthopedic —*see also* Disorder, soft tissue
  device or implant T84.9
    bone
      device or implant —*see* Complication,
        bone, device NEC
      graft —*see* Complication, graft, bone
    breakdown T84.418
    displacement T84.428
    electronic bone stimulator —*see*
      Complications, electronic
      stimulator device, bone
    embolism T84.81
    fibrosis T84.82
    fixation device —*see* Complication,
      fixation device, internal
    hemorrhage T84.83
    infection or inflammation T84.7
    joint prosthesis —*see* Complication, joint
      prosthesis, internal
    malfunction T84.418
    malposition T84.428
    mechanical NEC T84.498
    muscle graft —*see* Complications, graft,
      muscle
    obstruction T84.498
    pain T84.84
    perforation T84.498
    protrusion T84.498
    specified complication NEC T84.89
    stenosis T84.85
    tendon graft —*see* Complications, graft,
      tendon
    thrombosis T84.86
  fracture (following insertion of device) —
    see Fracture, following insertion of
    orthopedic implant, joint prosthesis
    or bone plate
  postprocedural M96.89
    fracture —*see* Fracture, following
      insertion of orthopedic implant,
      joint prosthesis or bone plate
    postlaminectomy syndrome NEC
      M96.1
      kyphosis M96.3
      lordosis M96.4
    postradiation
      kyphosis M96.2
      scoliosis M96.5
    pseudarthrosis post-fusion M96.0
    specified type NEC M96.89
pacemaker (cardiac) —*see* Complications,
  cardiovascular device or implant,
  electronic
pancreas transplant —*see* Complications,
  transplant, pancreas
penile prosthesis (implant) —*see*
  Complications, prosthetic device, penile
perfusion NEC T80.90
perineal repair (obstetrical) NEC O90.89
  disruption O90.1
  hematoma O90.2
  infection (following delivery) O86.0
phototherapy T88.9
  specified NEC T88.8
postmastoidectomy NEC H95.19-
  cyst, mucosal H95.13-
  granulation H95.12-
  inflammation, chronic H95.11-
  recurrent cholesteatoma H95.0-
postoperative —*see* Complications,
  postprocedural
  circulatory —*see* Complications, circulatory
    system
  ear —*see* Complications, ear
  endocrine —*see* Complications, endocrine
  eye —*see* Complications, eye
  lumbar puncture G97.1
    cerebrospinal fluid leak G97.0

Complication (*Continued*)
postoperative (*Continued*)
  nervous system (central) (peripheral) —*see*
    Complications, nervous system
  respiratory system —*see* Complications,
    respiratory system
postprocedural —*see also* Complications,
  surgical procedure
  cardiac arrest
    following cardiac surgery I97.120
    following other surgery I97.121
  cardiac functional disturbance NEC
    following cardiac surgery I97.190
    following other surgery I97.191
  cardiac insufficiency
    following cardiac surgery I97.110
    following other surgery I97.111
  chorioretinal scars following retinal
    surgery H59.81-
  following cataract surgery
    cataract (lens) fragments H59.02-
    cystoid macular edema H59.03-
    specified NEC H59.09-
    vitreous (touch) syndrome H59.01-
  heart failure
    following cardiac surgery I97.130
    following other surgery I97.131
  hemorrhage (hematoma) (of)
    circulatory system organ or structure
      following a cardiac bypass I97.611
      following a cardiac catheterization
        I97.610
      following other circulatory system
        procedure I97.618
      following other procedure I97.62
    digestive system
      following procedure on digestive
        system K91.840
      following procedure on other organ
        K91.841
    ear
      following other procedure H95.42
      following procedure on ear and
        mastoid process H95.41
    endocrine system
      following endocrine system procedure
        E89.810
      following other procedure E89.811
    eye and adnexa
      following ophthalmic procedure
        H59.31-
      following other procedure H59.32-
    genitourinary organ or structure
      following procedure on genitourinary
        organ or structure N99.820
      following procedure on other organ
        N99.821
    mastoid process
      following other procedure H95.42
      following procedure on ear and
        mastoid process H95.41
    musculoskeletal structure
      following musculoskeletal surgery
        M96.830
      following non-orthopedic surgery
        M96.831
      following orthopedic surgery M96.830
    nervous system
      ~~during a nervous system procedure G97.51~~
      ~~during other procedure G97.52~~
      following a nervous system procedure
        G97.51 ◄
      following other procedure G97.52 ◄
    respiratory system
      ~~during other procedure J95.831~~
      ~~during procedure on respiratory system organ or structure J95.830~~
      following other procedure J95.831 ◄
      following procedure on respiratory
        system organ or structure
        J95.830 ◄

Complication (Continued)
  postprocedural (Continued)
    hemorrhage (Continued)
      skin and subcutaneous tissue
        following a dermatologic procedure
          L76.21
        following a procedure on other organ
          L76.22
      spleen
        following procedure on other organ
          D78.22
        following procedure on the spleen
          D78.21
    specified NEC
      circulatory system I97.89
      digestive K91.89
      ear H95.89
      endocrine E89.89
      eye and adnexa H59.89
      genitourinary N99.89
      mastoid process H95.89
      metabolic E89.89
      musculoskeletal structure M96.89
      nervous system G97.82
      respiratory system J95.89
      skin and subcutaneous tissue L76.82
      spleen D78.89
  pregnancy NEC —see Pregnancy,
    complicated by
  prosthetic device or implant T85.9
    bile duct —see Complications, bile duct
      implant
    breast —see Complications, breast implant
    cardiac and vascular NEC —see
      Complications, cardiovascular
      device or implant
    corneal transplant —see Complications,
      graft, cornea
    electronic nervous system stimulator —see
      Complications, electronic stimulator
      device
    epidural infusion catheter —see
      Complications, catheter, epidural
    esophageal anti-reflux device —see
      Complications, esophageal anti-reflux
      device
    genital organ or tract —see Complications,
      genitourinary, device or implant,
      genital tract
    heart valve —see Complications, heart,
      valve, prosthesis
    infection or inflammation T85.79
      intestine transplant T86.892
      liver transplant T86.43
      lung transplant T86.812
      pancreas transplant T86.892
      skin graft T86.822
    intraocular lens —see Complications,
      intraocular lens
    intraperitoneal (dialysis) catheter —
      see Complications, catheter,
      intraperitoneal
    joint —see Complications, joint prosthesis,
      internal
    mechanical NEC T85.698
      dialysis catheter (vascular) —see also
        Complication, catheter, dialysis,
        mechanical
        peritoneal —see Complication,
          catheter, intraperitoneal,
          mechanical
      gastrointestinal device T85.598
      ocular device T85.398
      subdural (infusion) catheter T85.690
      suture, permanent T85.692
        that for bone repair —see
          Complications, fixation device,
          internal (orthopedic), mechanical
      ventricular shunt
        breakdown T85.01
        displacement T85.02
        leakage T85.03

Complication (Continued)
  prosthetic device or implant (Continued)
    mechanical NEC (Continued)
      ventricular shunt (Continued)
        malposition T85.02
        obstruction T85.09
        perforation T85.09
        protrusion T85.09
        specified NEC T85.09
    mesh
      erosion (to surrounding organ or tissue)
        T83.718
        vaginal (into pelvic floor muscles)
          T83.711
      exposure (into surrounding organ or
        tissue) T83.728
        vaginal (into vagina) (through vaginal
          wall) T83.721
    orbital —see Complications, orbital
      prosthesis
    penile T83.9
      embolism T83.81
      fibrosis T83.82
      hemorrhage T83.83
      infection and inflammation T83.6
      mechanical
        breakdown T83.410
        displacement T83.420
        leakage T83.490
        malposition T83.420
        obstruction T83.490
        perforation T83.490
        protrusion T83.490
        specified NEC T83.490
      pain T83.84
      specified type NEC T83.89
      stenosis T83.85
      thrombosis T83.86
    prosthetic materials NEC
      erosion (to surrounding organ or tissue)
        T83.718
        vaginal (into pelvic floor muscles)
          T83.711
      exposure (into surrounding organ or
        tissue) T83.728
        vaginal (into vagina) (through vaginal
          wall) T83.721
    skin graft T86.829
      artificial skin or decellularized
        allodermis
        embolism T85.81
        fibrosis T85.82
        hemorrhage T85.83
        infection and inflammation T85.79
        mechanical
          breakdown T85.613
          displacement T85.623
          malfunction T85.613
          malposition T85.623
          obstruction T85.693
          perforation T85.693
          protrusion T85.693
          specified NEC T85.693
        pain T85.84
        specified type NEC T85.89
        stenosis T85.85
        thrombosis T85.86
      failure T86.821
      infection T86.822
      rejection T86.820
      specified NEC T86.828
    specified NEC T85.9
      embolism T85.81
      fibrosis T85.82
      hemorrhage T85.83
      infection and inflammation T85.79
      mechanical
        breakdown T85.618
        displacement T85.628
        leakage T85.638
        malfunction T85.618
        malposition T85.628

Complication (Continued)
  prosthetic device or implant (Continued)
    specified NEC (Continued)
      mechanical (Continued)
        obstruction T85.698
        perforation T85.698
        protrusion T85.698
        specified NEC T85.698
      pain T85.84
      specified type NEC T85.89
      stenosis T85.85
      thrombosis T85.86
    subdural infusion catheter —see
      Complications, catheter, subdural
    sutures —see Complications, sutures
    urinary organ or tract NEC —see
      Complications, genitourinary, device
      or implant, urinary system
    vascular —see Complications,
      cardiovascular device or implant
    ventricular shunt —see Complications,
      ventricular shunt (device)
  puerperium —see Puerperal
  puncture, spinal G97.1
    cerebrospinal fluid leak G97.0
    headache or reaction G97.1
  pyelogram N99.89
  radiation
    kyphosis M96.2
    scoliosis M96.5
  reattached
    extremity (infection) (rejection)
      lower T87.1X-
      upper T87.0X-
    specified body part NEC T87.2
  reconstructed breast
    asymmetry between native and
      reconstructed breast N65.1
    deformity N65.0
    disproportion between native and
      reconstructed breast N65.1
    excess tissue N65.0
    misshappen N65.0
  reimplant NEC —see also Complications,
    prosthetic device or implant
    limb (infection) (rejection) —see
      Complications, reattached,
      extremity
    organ (partial) (total) —see Complications,
      transplant
    prosthetic device NEC —see Complications,
      prosthetic device
  renal N28.9
    allograft —see Complications, transplant,
      kidney
    dialysis —see Complications, dialysis
  respirator
    mechanical J95.850
      specified NEC J95.859
  respiratory system J98.9
    device, implant or graft —see
      Complication, prosthetic device or
      implant, specified NEC
    lung transplant —see Complications,
      prosthetic device or implant, lung
      transplant
    postoperative J95.89
      air leak J95.812
      Mendelson's syndrome (chemical
        pneumonitis) J95.4
      pneumothorax J95.811
      pulmonary insufficiency (acute) (after
        nonthoracic surgery) J95.2
        chronic J95.3
        following thoracic surgery J95.1
      respiratory failure (acute) J95.821
        acute and chronic J95.822
      specified NEC J95.89
      subglottic stenosis J95.5
      tracheostomy complication —see
        Complications, tracheostomy
  therapy T81.89

◀ New   ◀▥ Revised   ~~deleted~~ Deleted

Complication (Continued)

sedation during labor and delivery O74.9
  cardiac O74.2
  central nervous system O74.3
  pulmonary NEC O74.1
shunt —see also Complications, prosthetic device or implant
  arteriovenous —see Complications, arteriovenous, shunt
  ventricular (communicating) —see Complications, ventricular shunt
skin
  graft T86.829
    failure T86.821
    infection T86.822
    rejection T86.820
    specified type NEC T86.828
spinal
  anesthesia —see Complications, anesthesia, spinal
  catheter (epidural) (subdural) —see Complications, catheter
  puncture or tap G97.1
    cerebrospinal fluid leak G97.0
    headache or reaction G97.1
stent
  bile duct —see Complications, bile duct prosthesis
  urinary T83.9
    embolism T83.81
    fibrosis T83.82
    hemorrhage T83.83
    infection and inflammation T83.59
    mechanical
      breakdown T83.112
      displacement T83.122
      leakage T83.192
      malposition T83.122
      obstruction T83.192
      perforation T83.192
      protrusion T83.192
      specified NEC T83.192
    pain T83.84
    specified type NEC T83.89
    stenosis T83.85
    thrombosis T83.86
stoma
  digestive tract
    colostomy —see Complications, colostomy
    enterostomy —see Complications, enterostomy
    esophagostomy —see Complications, esophagostomy
    gastrostomy —see Complications, gastrostomy
  urinary tract N99.538
    cystostomy —see Complications, cystostomy
    external NOS N99.528
      hemorrhage N99.520
      infection N99.521
      malfunction N99.522
      specified type NEC N99.528
    hemorrhage N99.530
    infection N99.531
    malfunction N99.532
    specified type NEC N99.538
stomach banding —see Complication (s), bariatric procedure
stomach stapling —see Complication (s), bariatric procedure
surgical material, nonabsorbable —see Complication, suture, permanent
surgical procedure (on) T81.9
  amputation stump (late) —see Complications, amputation stump
  cardiac —see Complications, circulatory system

Complication (Continued)

surgical procedure (Continued)
  cholesteatoma, recurrent —see Complications, postmastoidectomy, recurrent cholesteatoma
  circulatory (early) —see Complications, circulatory system
  digestive system —see Complications, gastrointestinal
  dumping syndrome (postgastrectomy) K91.1
  ear —see Complications, ear
  elephantiasis or lymphedema I97.89
    postmastectomy I97.2
  emphysema (surgical) T81.82
  endocrine —see Complications, endocrine
  eye —see Complications, eye
  fistula (persistent postoperative) T81.83
  foreign body inadvertently left in wound (sponge) (suture) (swab) —see Foreign body, accidentally left during a procedure
  gastrointestinal —see Complications, gastrointestinal
  genitourinary NEC N99.89
  hematoma
    intraoperative —see Complication, intraoperative, hemorrhage
    postprocedural —see Complication, postprocedural, hemorrhage
  hemorrhage
    intraoperative —see Complication, intraoperative, hemorrhage
    postprocedural —see Complication, postprocedural, hemorrhage
  hepatic failure K91.82
  hyperglycemia (postpancreatectomy) E89.1
  hypoinsulinemia (postpancreatectomy) E89.1
  hypoparathyroidism (postparathyroidectomy) E89.2
  hypopituitarism (posthypophysectomy) E89.3
  hypothyroidism (post-thyroidectomy) E89.0
  intestinal obstruction K91.3
  intracranial hypotension following ventricular shunting (ventriculostomy) G97.2
  lymphedema I97.89
    postmastectomy I97.2
  malabsorption (postsurgical) NEC K91.2
    osteoporosis —see Osteoporosis, postsurgical malabsorption
  mastoidectomy cavity NEC —see Complications, postmastoidectomy
  metabolic E89.89
    specified NEC E89.89
  musculoskeletal —see Complications, musculoskeletal system
  nervous system (central) (peripheral) —see Complications, nervous system
  ovarian failure E89.40
    asymptomatic E89.40
    symptomatic E89.41
  peripheral vascular —see Complications, surgical procedure, vascular
  postcardiotomy syndrome I97.0
  postcholecystectomy syndrome K91.5
  postcommissurotomy syndrome I97.0
  postgastrectomy dumping syndrome K91.1
  postlaminectomy syndrome NEC M96.1
    kyphosis M96.3
  postmastectomy lymphedema syndrome I97.2
  postmastoidectomy cholesteatoma —see Complications, postmastoidectomy, recurrent cholesteatoma
  postvagotomy syndrome K91.1
  postvalvulotomy syndrome I97.0

Complication (Continued)

surgical procedure (Continued)
  pulmonary insufficiency (acute) J95.2
    chronic J95.3
    following thoracic surgery J95.1
  reattached body part —see Complications, reattached
  respiratory —see Complications, respiratory system
  shock (hypovolemic) T81.19
  spleen (postoperative) D78.89
    intraoperative D78.81
  stitch abscess T81.4
  subglottic stenosis (postsurgical) J95.5
  testicular hypofunction E89.5
  transplant —see Complications, organ or tissue transplant
  urinary NEC N99.89
  vaginal vault prolapse (posthysterectomy) N99.3
  vascular (peripheral)
    artery T81.719
      mesenteric T81.710
      renal T81.711
      specified NEC T81.718
    vein T81.72
  wound infection T81.4
suture, permanent (wire) NEC T85.9
  with repair of bone —see Complications, fixation device, internal
  embolism T85.81
  fibrosis T85.82
  hemorrhage T85.83
  infection and inflammation T85.79
  mechanical
    breakdown T85.612
    displacement T85.622
    malfunction T85.612
    malposition T85.622
    obstruction T85.692
    perforation T85.692
    protrusion T85.692
    specified NEC T85.692
  pain T85.84
  specified type NEC T85.89
  stenosis T85.85
  thrombosis T85.86
tracheostomy J95.00
  granuloma J95.09
  hemorrhage J95.01
  infection J95.02
  malfunction J95.03
  mechanical J95.03
  obstruction J95.03
  specified type NEC J95.09
  tracheo-esophageal fistula J95.04
transfusion (blood) (lymphocytes) (plasma) T80.92
  air embolism T80.0
  circulatory overload E87.71
  febrile nonhemolytic transfusion reaction R50.84
  hemochromatosis E83.111
  hemolysis T80.89
  hemolytic reaction (antigen unspecified) T80.919
  incompatibility reaction (antigen unspecified) T80.919
    ABO T80.30
      delayed serologic (DSTR) T80.39
      hemolytic transfusion reaction (HTR) (unspecified time after transfusion) T80.319
        acute (AHTR) (less than 24 hours after transfusion) T80.310
        delayed (DHTR) (24 hours or more after transfusion) T80.311
      specified NEC T80.39
    acute (antigen unspecified) T80.910
    delayed (antigen unspecified) T80.911
    delayed serologic (DSTR) T80.89

Complication *(Continued)*
  transfusion *(Continued)*
    incompatibility reaction *(Continued)*
      Non-ABO (minor antigens (Duffy) (Kell)
        (Kidd) (Lewis) (M) (N) (P) (S)) T80.
        A0
        delayed serologic (DSTR) T80.A9
        hemolytic transfusion reaction
          (HTR) (unspecified time after
          transfusion) T80.A19
          acute (AHTR) (less than 24 hours
            after transfusion) T80.A10
          delayed (DHTR) (24 hours or more
            after transfusion) T80.A11
        specified NEC T80.A9
      Rh (antigens (C) (c) (D) (E) (e)) (factor)
        T80.40
        delayed serologic (DSTR) T80.49
        hemolytic transfusion reaction
          (HTR) (unspecified time after
          transfusion) T80.419
          acute (AHTR) (less than 24 hours
            after transfusion) T80.410
          delayed (DHTR) (24 hours or more
            after transfusion) T80.411
        specified NEC T80.49
    infection T80.29
      acute T80.22
    reaction NEC T80.89
    sepsis T80.29
    shock T80.89
  transplant T86.90
    bone T86.839
      failure T86.831
      infection T86.832
      rejection T86.830
      specified type NEC T86.838
    bone marrow T86.00
      failure T86.02
      infection T86.03
      rejection T86.01
      specified type NEC T86.09
    cornea T86.849
      failure T86.841
      infection T86.842
      rejection T86.840
      specified type NEC T86.848
    failure T86.92
    heart T86.20
      with lung T86.30
      cardiac allograft vasculopathy T86.290
        failure T86.32
        infection T86.33
        rejection T86.31
        specified type NEC T86.39
      failure T86.22
      infection T86.23
      rejection T86.21
      specified type NEC T86.298
    infection T86.93
    intestine T86.859
      failure T86.851
      infection T86.852
      rejection T86.850
      specified type NEC T86.858
    kidney T86.10
      failure T86.12
      infection T86.13
      rejection T86.11
      specified type NEC T86.19
    liver T86.40
      failure T86.42
      infection T86.43
      rejection T86.41
      specified type NEC T86.49
    lung T86.819
      with heart T86.30
        failure T86.32
        infection T86.33
        rejection T86.31
        specified type NEC T86.39

Complication *(Continued)*
  transplant *(Continued)*
    lung *(Continued)*
      failure T86.811
      infection T86.812
      rejection T86.810
      specified type NEC T86.818
    malignant neoplasm C80.2
    pancreas T86.899
      failure T86.891
      infection T86.892
      rejection T86.890
      specified type NEC T86.898
    peripheral blood stem cells T86.5
    post-transplant lymphoproliferative
      disorder (PTLD) D47.Z1
    rejection T86.91
    skin T86.829
      failure T86.821
      infection T86.822
      rejection T86.820
      specified type NEC T86.828
    specified
      tissue T86.899
        failure T86.891
        infection T86.892
        rejection T86.890
        specified type NEC T86.898
      type NEC T86.99
    stem cell (from peripheral blood) (from
      umbilical cord) T86.5
    umbilical cord stem cells T86.5
  trauma (early) T79.9
    specified NEC T79.8
  ultrasound therapy NEC T88.9
  umbilical cord NEC
    complicating delivery O69.9
      specified NEC O69.89
  umbrella device, vascular T82.9
    embolism T82.818
    fibrosis T82.828
    hemorrhage T82.838
    infection or inflammation T82.7
    mechanical
      breakdown T82.515
      displacement T82.525
      leakage T82.535
      malposition T82.525
      obstruction T82.595
      perforation T82.595
      protrusion T82.595
    pain T82.848
    specified type NEC T82.898
    stenosis T82.858
    thrombosis T82.868
  urethral catheter —*see* Complications,
    catheter, urethral, indwelling
  vaccination T88.1
    anaphylaxis NEC T80.52
    arthropathy —*see* Arthropathy,
      postimmunization
    cellulitis T88.0
    encephalitis or encephalomyelitis
      G04.02
    infection (general) (local) NEC T88.0
    meningitis G03.8
    myelitis G04.89
    protein sickness T80.62
    rash T88.1
    reaction (allergic) T88.1
      serum T80.62
    sepsis T88.0
    serum intoxication, sickness, rash,
      or other serum reaction NEC
      T80.62
      anaphylactic shock T80.52
    shock (allergic) (anaphylactic) T80.52
    vaccinia (generalized) (localized) T88.1
  vas deferens device or implant —*see*
    Complications, genitourinary, device or
    implant, genital tract

Complication *(Continued)*
  vascular I99.9
    device or implant T82.9
      embolism T82.818
      fibrosis T82.828
      hemorrhage T82.838
      infection or inflammation T82.7
      mechanical
        breakdown T82.519
          specified device NEC T82.518
        displacement T82.529
          specified device NEC T82.528
        leakage T82.539
          specified device NEC T82.538
        malposition T82.529
          specified device NEC T82.528
        obstruction T82.599
          specified device NEC T82.598
        perforation T82.599
          specified device NEC T82.598
        protrusion T82.599
          specified device NEC T82.598
      pain T82.848
      specified type NEC T82.898
      stenosis T82.858
      thrombosis T82.868
    dialysis catheter —*see* Complication,
      catheter, dialysis
    following infusion, therapeutic injection or
      transfusion T80.1
    graft T82.9
      embolism T82.818
      fibrosis T82.828
      hemorrhage T82.838
      mechanical
        breakdown T82.319
          aorta (bifurcation) T82.310
          carotid artery T82.311
          specified vessel NEC T82.318
        displacement T82.329
          aorta (bifurcation) T82.320
          carotid artery T82.321
          specified vessel NEC T82.328
        leakage T82.339
          aorta (bifurcation) T82.330
          carotid artery T82.331
          specified vessel NEC T82.338
        malposition T82.329
          aorta (bifurcation) T82.320
          carotid artery T82.321
          specified vessel NEC T82.328
        obstruction T82.399
          aorta (bifurcation) T82.390
          carotid artery T82.391
          specified vessel NEC T82.398
        perforation T82.399
          aorta (bifurcation) T82.390
          carotid artery T82.391
          specified vessel NEC T82.398
        protrusion T82.399
          aorta (bifurcation) T82.390
          carotid artery T82.391
          specified vessel NEC T82.398
      pain T82.848
      specified complication NEC T82.898
      stenosis T82.858
      thrombosis T82.868
    postoperative —*see* Complications,
      postoperative, circulatory
  vena cava device (filter) (sieve) (umbrella) —
    see Complications, umbrella device,
    vascular
  ventilation therapy NEC T81.81
  ventilator
    mechanical J95.850
      specified NEC J95.859
  ventricular (communicating) shunt (device)
    T85.9
    embolism T85.81
    fibrosis T85.82
    hemorrhage T85.83

◄ New   ◄═ Revised   ~~deleted~~ Deleted

Complication (*Continued*)
  ventricular shunt (*Continued*)
    infection and inflammation T85.79
    mechanical
      breakdown T85.01
      displacement T85.02
      leakage T85.03
      malposition T85.02
      obstruction T85.09
      perforation T85.09
      protrusion T85.09
      specified NEC T85.09
    pain T85.84
    specified type NEC T85.89
    stenosis T85.85
    thrombosis T85.86
  wire suture, permanent (implanted) —*see* Complications, suture, permanent
Compressed air disease T70.3
Compression
  with injury - code by Nature of injury
  artery I77.1
    celiac, syndrome I77.4
  brachial plexus G54.0
  brain (stem) G93.5
    due to
      contusion (diffuse) —*see* Injury, intracranial, diffuse
        focal —*see* Injury, intracranial, focal
      injury NEC —*see* Injury, intracranial, diffuse
      traumatic —*see* Injury, intracranial, diffuse
  bronchus J98.09
  cauda equina G83.4
  celiac (artery) (axis) I77.4
  cerebral —*see* Compression, brain
  cervical plexus G54.2
  cord
    spinal —*see* Compression, spinal
    umbilical —*see* Compression, umbilical cord
  cranial nerve G52.9
    eighth —*see* subcategory H93.3
    eleventh G52.8
    fifth G50.8
    first G52.0
    fourth —*see* Strabismus, paralytic, fourth nerve
    ninth G52.1
    second —*see* Disorder, nerve, optic
    seventh G52.8
    sixth —*see* Strabismus, paralytic, sixth nerve
    tenth G52.2
    third —*see* Strabismus, paralytic, third nerve
    twelfth G52.3
  diver's squeeze T70.3
  during birth (newborn) P15.9
  esophagus K22.2
  eustachian tube —*see* Obstruction, eustachian tube, cartilaginous
  facies Q67.1
  fracture —*see* Fracture
  heart —*see* Disease, heart
  intestine —*see* Obstruction, intestine
  laryngeal nerve, recurrent G52.2
    with paralysis of vocal cords and larynx J38.00
      bilateral J38.02
      unilateral J38.01
  lumbosacral plexus G54.1
  lung J98.4
  lymphatic vessel I89.0
  medulla —*see* Compression, brain
  nerve (*see also* Disorder, nerve) G58.9
    arm NEC —*see* Mononeuropathy, upper limb
    axillary G54.0
    cranial —*see* Compression, cranial nerve

Compression (*Continued*)
  nerve (*Continued*)
    leg NEC —*see* Mononeuropathy, lower limb
    median (in carpal tunnel) —*see* Syndrome, carpal tunnel
    optic —*see* Disorder, nerve, optic
    plantar —*see* Lesion, nerve, plantar
    posterior tibial (in tarsal tunnel) —*see* Syndrome, tarsal tunnel
    root or plexus NOS (in) G54.9
      intervertebral disc disorder NEC —*see* Disorder, disc, with, radiculopathy
        with myelopathy —*see* Disorder, disc, with, myelopathy
      neoplastic disease (*see also* Neoplasm) D49.9 [G55]
      spondylosis —*see* Spondylosis, with radiculopathy
    sciatic (acute) —*see* Lesion, nerve, sciatic
    sympathetic G90.8
    traumatic —*see* Injury, nerve
    ulnar —*see* Lesion, nerve, ulnar
    upper extremity NEC —*see* Mononeuropathy, upper limb
  spinal (cord) G95.20
    by displacement of intervertebral disc NEC —*see also* Disorder, disc, with, myelopathy
    nerve root NOS G54.9
      due to displacement of intervertebral disc NEC —*see* Disorder, disc, with, radiculopathy
        with myelopathy —*see* Disorder, disc, with, myelopathy
    specified NEC G95.29
    spondylogenic (cervical) (lumbar, lumbosacral) (thoracic) —*see* Spondylosis, with myelopathy NEC
    anterior —*see* Syndrome, anterior, spinal artery, compression
    traumatic —*see* Injury, spinal cord, by region
  subcostal nerve (syndrome) —*see* Mononeuropathy, upper limb, specified NEC
  sympathetic nerve NEC G90.8
  syndrome T79.5
  trachea J39.8
  ulnar nerve (by scar tissue) —*see* Lesion, nerve, ulnar
  umbilical cord
    complicating delivery O69.2
      cord around neck O69.1
      prolapse O69.0
      specified NEC O69.2
  ureter N13.5
  vein I87.1
  vena cava (inferior) (superior) I87.1
Compulsion, compulsive
  gambling F63.0
  neurosis F42
  personality F60.5
  states F42
  swearing F42
    in Gilles de la Tourette's syndrome F95.2
  tics and spasms F95.9
Concato's disease (pericardial polyserositis) A19.9
  nontubercular I31.1
  pleural —*see* Pleurisy, with effusion
Concavity chest wall M95.4
Concealed penis Q55.69
Concern (normal) **about sick person in family** Z63.6
Concrescence (teeth) K00.2
Concretio cordis I31.1
  rheumatic I09.2

Concretion —*see also* Calculus
  appendicular K38.1
  canaliculus —*see* Dacryolith
  clitoris N90.89
  conjunctiva H11.12-
  eyelid —*see* Disorder, eyelid, specified type NEC
  lacrimal passages —*see* Dacryolith
  prepuce (male) N47.8
  salivary gland (any) K11.5
  seminal vesicle N50.8
  tonsil J35.8
Concussion (brain) (cerebral) (current) S06.0X-
  blast (air) (hydraulic) (immersion) (underwater)
    abdomen or thorax —*see* Injury, blast, by site
    ear with acoustic nerve injury —*see* Injury, nerve, acoustic, specified type NEC
  cauda equina S34.3
  conus medullaris S34.02 ◀▥
  ocular S05.8X-
  spinal (cord)
    cervical S14.0
    lumbar S34.01
    sacral S34.02
    thoracic S24.0
  syndrome F07.81
Condition —*see* Disease
Conditions arising in the perinatal period —*see* Newborn, affected by
Conduct disorder —*see* Disorder, conduct
Condyloma A63.0
  acuminatum A63.0
  gonorrheal A54.09
  latum A51.31
  syphilitic A51.31
    congenital A50.07
  venereal, syphilitic A51.31
Conflagration —*see also* Burn
  asphyxia (by inhalation of gases, fumes or vapors) —*see also* Table of ͏Drugs and ͏Chemicals T59.9- ◀▥
Conflict (with) —*see also* Discord
  family Z73.9
  marital Z63.0
    involving divorce or estrangement Z63.5
  parent-child Z62.820
    parent-adopted child Z62.821
    parent-biological child Z62.820
    parent-foster child Z62.822
  social role NEC Z73.5
Confluent —*see* condition
Confusion, confused R41.0
  epileptic F05
  mental state (psychogenic) F44.89
  psychogenic F44.89
  reactive (from emotional stress, psychological trauma) F44.89
Confusional arousals G47.51
Congelation T69.9
Congenital —*see also* condition
  aortic septum Q25.4
  intrinsic factor deficiency D51.0
  malformation —*see* Anomaly
Congestion, congestive
  bladder N32.89
  bowel K63.89
  brain G93.89
  breast N64.59
  bronchial J98.09
  catarrhal J31.0
  chest R09.89
  chill, malarial —*see* Malaria
  circulatory NEC I99.8
  duodenum K31.89
  eye —*see* Hyperemia, conjunctiva
  facial, due to birth injury P15.4
  general R68.89
  glottis J37.0
  heart —*see* Failure, heart, congestive

Congestion, congestive *(Continued)*
  hepatic K76.1
  hypostatic (lung) —*see* Edema, lung
  intestine K63.89
  kidney N28.89
  labyrinth —*see* subcategory H83.8
  larynx J37.0
  liver K76.1
  lung R09.89
    active or acute —*see* Pneumonia
  malaria, malarial —*see* Malaria
  nasal R09.81
  nose R09.81
  orbit, orbital —*see also* Exophthalmos
    inflammatory (chronic) —*see* Inflammation, orbit
  ovary N83.8
  pancreas K86.8
  pelvic, female N94.89
  pleural J94.8
  prostate (active) N42.1
  pulmonary —*see* Congestion, lung
  renal N28.89
  retina H35.81
  seminal vesicle N50.1
  spinal cord G95.19
  spleen (chronic) D73.2
  stomach K31.89
  trachea —*see* Tracheitis
  urethra N36.8
  uterus N85.8
    with subinvolution N85.3
  venous (passive) I87.8
  viscera R68.89
Congestive —*see* Congestion
Conical
  cervix (hypertrophic elongation) N88.4
  cornea —*see* Keratoconus
  teeth K00.2
Conjoined twins Q89.4
Conjugal maladjustment Z63.0
  involving divorce or estrangement Z63.5
Conjunctiva —*see* condition
Conjunctivitis (staphylococcal) (streptococcal)
    NOS H10.9
  Acanthamoeba B60.12
  acute H10.3-
    atopic H10.1-
    chemical (*see also* Corrosion, cornea) H10.21-
    mucopurulent H10.02-
      follicular H10.01-
    pseudomembranous H10.22-
    serous except viral H10.23-
      viral —*see* Conjunctivitis, viral
    toxic H10.21-
  adenoviral (acute) (follicular) B30.1
  allergic (acute) —*see* Conjunctivitis, acute, atopic
    chronic H10.45
      vernal H10.44
  anaphylactic —*see* Conjunctivitis, acute, atopic
  Apollo B30.3
  atopic (acute) —*see* Conjunctivitis, acute, atopic
  Béal's B30.2
  blennorrhagic (gonococcal) (neonatorum) A54.31
  chemical (acute) (*see also* Corrosion, cornea) H10.21-
  chlamydial A74.0
    due to trachoma A71.1
    neonatal P39.1
  chronic (nodosa) (petrificans) (phlyctenular) H10.40-
    allergic H10.45
      vernal H10.44
    follicular H10.43-
    giant papillary H10.41-
    simple H10.42-
    vernal H10.44

Conjunctivitis *(Continued)*
  coxsackievirus 24 B30.3
  diphtheritic A36.86
  due to
    dust —*see* Conjunctivitis, acute, atopic
    filariasis B74.9
    mucocutaneous leishmaniasis B55.2
  enterovirus type 70 (hemorrhagic) B30.3
  epidemic (viral) B30.9
    hemorrhagic B30.3
  gonococcal (neonatorum) A54.31
  granular (trachomatous) A71.1
    sequelae (late effect) B94.0
  hemorrhagic (acute) (epidemic) B30.3
  herpes zoster B02.31
  in (due to)
    Acanthamoeba B60.12
    adenovirus (acute) (follicular) B30.1
    Chlamydia A74.0
    coxsackievirus 24 B30.3
    diphtheria A36.86
    enterovirus type 70 (hemorrhagic) B30.3
    filariasis B74.9
    gonococci A54.31
    herpes (simplex) virus B00.53
      zoster B02.31
    infectious disease NEC B99
    meningococci A39.89
    mucocutaneous leishmaniasis B55.2
    rosacea L71.9
    syphilis (late) A52.71
    zoster B02.31
  inclusion A74.0
  infantile P39.1
    gonococcal A54.31
  Koch-Weeks' —*see* Conjunctivitis, acute, mucopurulent
  light —*see* Conjunctivitis, acute, atopic
  ligneous —*see* Blepharoconjunctivitis, ligneous
  meningococcal A39.89
  mucopurulent —*see* Conjunctivitis, acute, mucopurulent
  neonatal P39.1
    gonococcal A54.31
  Newcastle B30.8
  of Béal B30.2
  parasitic
    filariasis B74.9
    mucocutaneous leishmaniasis B55.2
  Parinaud's H10.89
  petrificans H10.89
  rosacea L71.9
  specified NEC H10.89
  swimming-pool B30.1
  trachomatous A71.1
    acute A71.0
    sequelae (late effect) B94.0
  traumatic NEC H10.89
  tuberculous A18.59
  tularemic A21.1
  tularensis A21.1
  viral B30.9
    due to
      adenovirus B30.1
      enterovirus B30.3
    specified NEC B30.8
Conjunctivochalasis H11.82-
Connective tissue —*see* condition
Conn's syndrome E26.01
Conradi (-Hunermann) disease Q77.3
Consanguinity Z84.3
  counseling Z71.89
Conscious simulation (of illness) Z76.5
Consecutive —*see* condition
Consolidation lung (base) —*see* Pneumonia, lobar
Constipation (atonic) (neurogenic) (simple) (spastic) K59.00
  drug-induced —*see* Table of ◁Drugs and ◁Chemicals ◀▥

Constipation *(Continued)*
  outlet dysfunction K59.02
  psychogenic F45.8
  slow transit K59.01
  specified NEC K59.09
Constitutional —*see also* condition
  substandard F60.7
Constitutionally substandard F60.7
Constriction —*see also* Stricture
  auditory canal —*see* Stenosis, external ear canal
  bronchial J98.09
  duodenum K31.5
  esophagus K22.2
  external
    abdomen, abdominal (wall) S30.841
    alveolar process S00.542
    ankle S90.54-
    antecubital space —*see* Constriction, external, forearm
    arm (upper) S40.84-
    auricle —*see* Constriction, external, ear
    axilla —*see* Constriction, external, arm
    back, lower S30.840
    breast S20.14-
    brow S00.84
    buttock S30.840
    calf —*see* Constriction, external, leg
    canthus —*see* Constriction, external, eyelid
    cheek S00.84
      internal S00.542
    chest wall —*see* Constriction, external, thorax
    chin S00.84
    clitoris S30.844
    costal region —*see* Constriction, external, thorax
    digit (s)
      foot —*see* Constriction, external, toe
      hand —*see* Constriction, external, finger
    ear S00.44-
    elbow S50.34-
    epididymis S30.843
    epigastric region S30.841
    esophagus, cervical S10.14
    eyebrow —*see* Constriction, external, eyelid
    eyelid S00.24-
    face S00.84
    finger (s) S60.44-
      index S60.44-
      little S60.44-
      middle S60.44-
      ring S60.44-
    flank S30.841
    foot (except toe (s) alone) S90.84-
      toe —*see* Constriction, external, toe
    forearm S50.84-
      elbow only —*see* Constriction, external, elbow
    forehead S00.84
    genital organs, external
      female S30.846
      male S30.845
    groin S30.841
    gum S00.542
    hand S60.54-
    head S00.94
      ear —*see* Constriction, external, ear
      eyelid —*see* Constriction, external, eyelid
      lip S00.541
      nose S00.34
      oral cavity S00.542
      scalp S00.04
      specified site NEC S00.84
    heel —*see* Constriction, external, foot
    hip S70.24-
    inguinal region S30.841
    interscapular region S20.449
    jaw S00.84
    knee S80.24-
    labium (majus) (minus) S30.844

◀ New   ◀▥ Revised   ~~deleted~~ Deleted

Constriction *(Continued)*
external *(Continued)*
larynx S10.14
leg (lower) S80.84-
knee —*see* Constriction, external, knee
upper —*see* Constriction, external, thigh
lip S00.541
lower back S30.840
lumbar region S30.840
malar region S00.84
mammary —*see* Constriction, external, breast
mastoid region S00.84
mouth S00.542
nail
finger —*see* Constriction, external, finger
toe —*see* Constriction, external, toe
nasal S00.34
neck S10.94
specified site NEC S10.84
throat S10.14
nose S00.34
occipital region S00.04
oral cavity S00.542
orbital region —*see* Constriction, external, eyelid
palate S00.542
palm —*see* Constriction, external, hand
parietal region S00.04
pelvis S30.840
penis S30.842
perineum
female S30.844
male S30.840
periocular area —*see* Constriction, external, eyelid
phalanges
finger —*see* Constriction, external, finger
toe —*see* Constriction, external, toe
pharynx S10.14
pinna —*see* Constriction, external, ear
popliteal space —*see* Constriction, external, knee
prepuce S30.842
pubic region S30.840
pudendum
female S30.846
male S30.845
sacral region S30.840
scalp S00.04
scapular region —*see* Constriction, external, shoulder
scrotum S30.843
shin —*see* Constriction, external, leg
shoulder S40.24-
sternal region S20.349
submaxillary region S00.84
submental region S00.84
subungual
finger (s) —*see* Constriction, external, finger
toe (s) —*see* Constriction, external, toe
supraclavicular fossa S10.84
supraorbital S00.84
temple S00.84
temporal region S00.84
testis S30.843
thigh S70.34-
thorax, thoracic (wall) S20.94
back S20.44-
front S20.34-
throat S10.14
thumb S60.34-
toe (s) (lesser) S90.44-
great S90.44-
tongue S00.542
trachea S10.14
tunica vaginalis S30.843
uvula S00.542

Constriction *(Continued)*
external *(Continued)*
vagina S30.844
vulva S30.844
wrist S60.84-
gallbladder —*see* Obstruction, gallbladder
intestine —*see* Obstruction, intestine
larynx J38.6
congenital Q31.8
specified NEC Q31.8
subglottic Q31.1
organ or site, congenital NEC —*see* Atresia, by site
prepuce (acquired) (congenital) N47.1
pylorus (adult hypertrophic) K31.1
congenital or infantile Q40.0
newborn Q40.0
ring dystocia (uterus) O62.4
spastic —*see also* Spasm
ureter N13.5
ureter N13.5
with infection N13.6
urethra —*see* Stricture, urethra
visual field (peripheral) (functional) —*see* Defect, visual field
Constrictive —*see* condition
Consultation
without complaint or sickness Z71.9
feared complaint unfounded Z71.1
specified reason NEC Z71.89
medical —*see* Counseling, medical
religious Z71.81
specified reason NEC Z71.89
spiritual Z71.81
Consumption —*see* Tuberculosis
Contact (with) —*see also* Exposure (to) ◀▮▮▮
acariasis Z20.7
AIDS virus Z20.6
air pollution Z77.110
algae and algae toxins Z77.121
algae bloom Z77.121
anthrax Z20.810
aromatic (hazardous) compounds NEC Z77.028
aromatic amines Z77.020
aromatic dyes NOS Z77.028
arsenic Z77.010
asbestos Z77.090
bacterial disease NEC Z20.818
benzene Z77.021
blue-green algae bloom Z77.121
body fluids (potentially hazardous) Z77.21
brown tide Z77.121
chemicals (chiefly nonmedicinal) (hazardous) NEC Z77.098
cholera Z20.09
chromium compounds Z77.018
communicable disease Z20.9
bacterial NEC Z20.818
specified NEC Z20.89
viral NEC Z20.828
cyanobacteria bloom Z77.121
dyes Z77.098
Escherichia coli (E. coli) Z20.01
fiberglass —*see* Table of ~~d~~Drugs and ~~c~~Chemicals, fiberglass ▮▮▮▶
German measles Z20.4
gonorrhea Z20.2
hazardous metals NEC Z77.018
hazardous substances NEC Z77.29
hazards in the physical environment NEC Z77.128
hazards to health NEC Z77.9
HIV Z20.6
HTLV-III/LAV Z20.6
human immunodeficiency virus (HIV) Z20.6
infection Z20.9
specified NEC Z20.89
infestation (parasitic) NEC Z20.7
intestinal infectious disease NEC Z20.09
Escherichia coli (E. coli) Z20.01

Contact *(Continued)*
lead Z77.011
meningococcus Z20.811
mold (toxic) Z77.120
nickel dust Z77.018
noise Z77.122
parasitic disease Z20.7
pediculosis Z20.7
pfiesteria piscicida Z77.121
poliomyelitis Z20.89
pollution
air Z77.110
environmental NEC Z77.118
soil Z77.112
water Z77.111
polycyclic aromatic hydrocarbons Z77.028
rabies Z20.3
radiation, naturally occurring NEC Z77.123
radon Z77.123
red tide (Florida) Z77.121
rubella Z20.4
sexually-transmitted disease Z20.2
smallpox (laboratory) Z20.89
syphilis Z20.2
tuberculosis Z20.1
uranium Z77.012
varicella Z20.820
venereal disease Z20.2
viral disease NEC Z20.828
viral hepatitis Z20.5
water pollution Z77.111
Contamination, food —*see* Intoxication, foodborne
Contraception, contraceptive
advice Z30.09
counseling Z30.09
device (intrauterine) (in situ) Z97.5
causing menorrhagia T83.83
checking Z30.431
complications —*see* Complications, intrauterine, contraceptive device
in place Z97.5
initial prescription Z30.014
reinsertion Z30.433
removal Z30.432
replacement Z30.433
emergency (postcoital) Z30.012
initial prescription Z30.019
injectable Z30.013
intrauterine device Z30.014
pills Z30.011
postcoital (emergency) Z30.012
specified type NEC Z30.018
subdermal implantable Z30.019
maintenance Z30.40
examination Z30.8
injectable Z30.42
intrauterine device Z30.431
pills Z30.41
specified type NEC Z30.49
subdermal implantable Z30.49
management Z30.9
specified NEC Z30.8
postcoital (emergency) Z30.012
prescription Z30.019
repeat Z30.40
sterilization Z30.2
surveillance (drug) —*see* Contraception, maintenance
Contraction (s), contracture, contracted
Achilles tendon —*see also* Short, tendon, Achilles
congenital Q66.89
amputation stump (surgical) (flexion) (late) next proximal joint T87.89
anus K59.8
bile duct (common) (hepatic) K83.8
bladder N32.89
neck or sphincter N32.0
bowel, cecum, colon or intestine, any part — *see* Obstruction, intestine

Contraction, contracture, contracted
(Continued)
Braxton Hicks —see False, labor
breast implant, capsular T85.44
bronchial J98.09
burn (old) —see Cicatrix
cervix —see Stricture, cervix
cicatricial —see Cicatrix
conjunctiva, trachomatous, active A71.1
  sequelae (late effect) B94.0
Dupuytren's M72.0
eyelid —see Disorder, eyelid function
fascia (lata) (postural) M72.8
  Dupuytren's M72.0
  palmar M72.0
  plantar M72.2
finger NEC —see also Deformity, finger
  congenital Q68.1
  joint —see Contraction, joint, hand
flaccid —see Contraction, paralytic
gallbladder K82.0
heart valve —see Endocarditis
hip —see Contraction, joint, hip
hourglass
  bladder N32.89
    congenital Q64.79
  gallbladder K82.0
    congenital Q44.1
  stomach K31.89
    congenital Q40.2
    psychogenic F45.8
  uterus (complicating delivery) O62.4
hysterical F44.4
internal os —see Stricture, cervix
joint (abduction) (acquired) (adduction)
  (flexion) (rotation) M24.50
  ankle M24.57-
  congenital NEC Q68.8
    hip Q65.89
  elbow M24.52-
  foot joint M24.57-
  hand joint M24.54-
  hip M24.55-
    congenital Q65.89
  hysterical F44.4
  knee M24.56-
  shoulder M24.51-
  wrist M24.53-
kidney (granular) (secondary) N26.9
  congenital Q63.8
  hydronephritic —see Hydronephrosis
  Page N26.2
  pyelonephritic —see Pyelitis, chronic
  tuberculous A18.11
ligament —see also Disorder, ligament
  congenital Q79.8
muscle (postinfective) (postural) NEC M62.40
  with contracture of joint —see Contraction,
    joint
  ankle M62.47-
  congenital Q79.8
    sternocleidomastoid Q68.0
  extraocular —see Strabismus
  eye (extrinsic) —see Strabismus
  foot M62.47-
  forearm M62.43-
  hand M62.44-
  hysterical F44.4
  ischemic (Volkmann's) T79.6
  lower leg M62.46-
  multiple sites M62.49
  pelvic region M62.45-
  posttraumatic —see Strabismus, paralytic
  psychogenic F45.8
    conversion reaction F44.4
  shoulder region M62.41-
  specified site NEC M62.48
  thigh M62.45-
  upper arm M62.42-
neck —see Torticollis
ocular muscle —see Strabismus

Contraction, contracture, contracted
(Continued)
organ or site, congenital NEC —see Atresia,
  by site
outlet (pelvis) —see Contraction, pelvis
palmar fascia M72.0
paralytic
  joint —see Contraction, joint
  muscle —see also Contraction, muscle NEC
    ocular —see Strabismus, paralytic
pelvis (acquired) (general) M95.5
  with disproportion (fetopelvic) O33.1
    causing obstructed labor O65.1
    inlet O33.2
    mid-cavity O33.3
    outlet O33.3
plantar fascia M72.2
premature
  atrium I49.1
  auriculoventricular I49.49
  heart I49.49
  junctional I49.2
  supraventricular I49.1
  ventricular I49.3
prostate N42.89
pylorus NEC —see also Pylorospasm
  psychogenic F45.8
rectum, rectal (sphincter) K59.8
ring (Bandl's) (complicating delivery) O62.4
scar —see Cicatrix
spine —see Dorsopathy, deforming
sternocleidomastoid (muscle), congenital
  Q68.0
stomach K31.89
  hourglass K31.89
    congenital Q40.2
    psychogenic F45.8
  psychogenic F45.8
tendon (sheath) M62.40
  with contracture of joint —see Contraction,
    joint
  Achilles —see Short, tendon, Achilles
  ankle M62.47-
    Achilles —see Short, tendon, Achilles
  foot M62.47-
  forearm M62.43-
  hand M62.44-
  lower leg M62.46-
  multiple sites M62.49
  neck M62.48
  pelvic region M62.45-
  shoulder region M62.41-
  specified site NEC M62.48
  thigh M62.45-
  thorax M62.48
  trunk M62.48
  upper arm M62.42-
toe —see Deformity, toe, specified NEC
ureterovesical orifice (postinfectional) N13.5
  with infection N13.6
urethra —see also Stricture, urethra
  orifice N32.0
uterus N85.8
  abnormal NEC O62.9
  clonic (complicating delivery) O62.4
  dyscoordinate (complicating delivery) O62.4
  hourglass (complicating delivery) O62.4
  hypertonic O62.4
  hypotonic NEC O62.2
  inadequate
    primary O62.0
    secondary O62.1
  incoordinate (complicating delivery) O62.4
  poor O62.2
  tetanic (complicating delivery) O62.4
vagina (outlet) N89.5
vesical N32.89
  neck or urethral orifice N32.0
visual field —see Defect, visual field,
  generalized
Volkmann's (ischemic) T79.6

Contusion (skin surface intact) T14.8
abdomen, abdominal (muscle) (wall) S30.1
adnexa, eye NEC S05.8X-
adrenal gland S37.812
alveolar process S00.532
ankle S90.0-
antecubital space —see Contusion, forearm
anus S30.3
arm (upper) S40.02-
  lower (with elbow) —see Contusion,
    forearm
auditory canal —see Contusion, ear
auricle —see Contusion, ear
axilla —see Contusion, arm, upper
back —see also Contusion, thorax, back
  lower S30.0
bile duct S36.13
bladder S37.22
bone NEC T14.8
brain (diffuse) —see Injury, intracranial, diffuse
  focal —see Injury, intracranial, focal
brainstem S06.38-
breast S20.0-
broad ligament S37.892
brow S00.83
buttock S30.0
canthus, eye S00.1-
cauda equina S34.3
cerebellar, traumatic S06.37-
cerebral S06.33-
  left side S06.32-
  right side S06.31-
cheek S00.83
  internal S00.532
chest (wall) —see Contusion, thorax
chin S00.83
clitoris S30.23
colon —see Injury, intestine, large, contusion
common bile duct S36.13
conjunctiva S05.1-
  with foreign body (in conjunctival sac) —
    see Foreign body, conjunctival sac
conus medullaris (spine) S34.139
cornea —see Contusion, eyeball
  with foreign body —see Foreign body,
    cornea
corpus cavernosum S30.21
cortex (brain) (cerebral) —see Injury,
  intracranial, diffuse
  focal —see Injury, intracranial, focal
costal region —see Contusion, thorax
cystic duct S36.13
diaphragm S27.802
duodenum S36.420
ear S00.43-
elbow S50.0-
  with forearm —see Contusion, forearm
epididymis S30.22
epigastric region S30.1
epiglottis S10.0
esophagus (thoracic) S27.812
  cervical S10.0
eyeball S05.1-
eyebrow S00.1-
eyelid (and periocular area) S00.1-
face NEC S00.83
fallopian tube S37.529
  bilateral S37.522
  unilateral S37.521
femoral triangle S30.1
finger (s) S60.00
  with damage to nail (matrix) S60.10
  index S60.02-
    with damage to nail S60.12-
  little S60.05-
    with damage to nail S60.15-
  middle S60.03-
    with damage to nail S60.13-
  ring S60.04-
    with damage to nail S60.14-
  thumb —see Contusion, thumb

◀ New   ⬅ Revised   ~~deleted~~ Deleted

Contusion *(Continued)*
  flank S30.1
  foot (except toe (s) alone) S90.3-
    toe —*see* Contusion, toe
  forearm S50.1-
    elbow only —*see* Contusion, elbow
  forehead S00.83
  gallbladder S36.122
  genital organs, external
    female S30.202
    male S30.201
  globe (eye) —*see* Contusion, eyeball
  groin S30.1
  gum S00.532
  hand S60.22-
    finger (s) —*see* Contusion, finger
    wrist —*see* Contusion, wrist
  head S00.93
    ear —*see* Contusion, ear
    eyelid —*see* Contusion, eyelid
    lip S00.531
    nose S00.33
    oral cavity S00.532
    scalp S00.03
    specified part NEC S00.83
  heel —*see* Contusion, foot
  hepatic duct S36.13
  hip S70.0-
  ileum S36.428
  iliac region S30.1
  inguinal region S30.1
  interscapular region S20.229
  intra-abdominal organ S36.92
    colon —*see* Injury, intestine, large, contusion
    liver S36.112
    pancreas —*see* Contusion, pancreas
    rectum S36.62
    small intestine —*see* Injury, intestine, small, contusion
    specified organ NEC S36.892
    spleen —*see* Contusion, spleen
    stomach S36.32
  iris (eye) —*see* Contusion, eyeball
  jaw S00.83
  jejunum S36.428
  kidney S37.01-
    major (greater than 2 cm) S37.02-
    minor (less than 2 cm) S37.01-
  knee S80.0-
  labium (majus) (minus) S30.23
  lacrimal apparatus, gland or sac S05.8X-
  larynx S10.0
  leg (lower) S80.1-
    knee —*see* Contusion, knee
  lens —*see* Contusion, eyeball
  lip S00.531
  liver S36.112
  lower back S30.0
  lumbar region S30.0
  lung S27.329
    bilateral S27.322
    unilateral S27.321
  malar region S00.83
  mastoid region S00.83
  membrane, brain —*see* Injury, intracranial, diffuse
    focal —*see* Injury, intracranial, focal
  mesentery S36.892
  mesosalpinx S37.892 ◀▬
    ~~bilateral S37.522~~
    ~~unilateral S37.521~~
  mouth S00.532
  muscle —*see* Contusion, by site
  nail
    finger —*see* Contusion, finger, with damage to nail
    toe —*see* Contusion, toe, with damage to nail
  nasal S00.33

Contusion *(Continued)*
  neck S10.93
    specified site NEC S10.83
    throat S10.0
  nerve —*see* Injury, nerve
  newborn P54.5
  nose S00.33
  occipital
    lobe (brain) —*see* Injury, intracranial, diffuse
      focal —*see* Injury, intracranial, focal
    region (scalp) S00.03
  orbit (region) (tissues) S05.1-
  ovary S37.429
    bilateral S37.422
    unilateral S37.421
  palate S00.532
  pancreas S36.229
    body S36.221
    head S36.220
    tail S36.222
  parietal
    lobe (brain) —*see* Injury, intracranial, diffuse
      focal —*see* Injury, intracranial, focal
    region (scalp) S00.03
  pelvic organ S37.92
    adrenal gland S37.812
    bladder S37.22
    fallopian tube —*see* Contusion, fallopian tube
    kidney —*see* Contusion, kidney
    ovary —*see* Contusion, ovary
    prostate S37.822 ◀▬
    specified organ NEC S37.892
    ureter S37.12
    urethra S37.32
    uterus S37.62
  pelvis S30.0
  penis S30.21
  perineum
    female S30.23
    male S30.0
  periocular area S00.1-
  peritoneum S36.81
  periurethral tissue —*see* Contusion, urethra
  pharynx S10.0
  pinna —*see* Contusion, ear
  popliteal space —*see* Contusion, knee
  prepuce S30.21
  prostate S37.822
  pubic region S30.1
  pudendum
    female S30.202
    male S30.201
  quadriceps femoris —*see* Contusion, thigh
  rectum S36.62
  retroperitoneum S36.892
  round ligament S37.892
  sacral region S30.0
  scalp S00.03
    due to birth injury P12.3
  scapular region —*see* Contusion, shoulder
  sclera —*see* Contusion, eyeball
  scrotum S30.22
  seminal vesicle S37.892
  shoulder S40.01-
  skin NEC T14.8
  small intestine —*see* Injury, intestine, small, contusion
  spermatic cord S30.22
  spinal cord —*see* Injury, spinal cord, by region
    cauda equina S34.3
    conus medullaris S34.139
  spleen S36.029
    major S36.021
    minor S36.020
  sternal region S20.219
  stomach S36.32
  subconjunctival S05.1-
  subcutaneous NEC T14.8

Contusion *(Continued)*
  submaxillary region S00.83
  submental region S00.83
  subperiosteal NEC T14.8
  subungual
    finger —*see* Contusion, finger, with damage to nail
    toe —*see* Contusion, toe, with damage to nail
  supraclavicular fossa S10.83
  supraorbital S00.83
  suprarenal gland S37.812
  temple (region) S00.83
  temporal
    lobe (brain) —*see* Injury, intracranial, diffuse
      focal —*see* Injury, intracranial, focal
    region S00.83
  testis S30.22
  thigh S70.1-
  thorax (wall) S20.20
    back S20.22-
    front S20.21-
  throat S10.0
  thumb S60.01-
    with damage to nail S60.11-
  toe (s) (lesser) S90.12-
    with damage to nail S90.22-
    great S90.11-
      with damage to nail S90.21-
      specified type NEC S90.221
  tongue S00.532
  trachea (cervical) S10.0
    thoracic S27.52
  tunica vaginalis S30.22
  tympanum, tympanic membrane —*see* Contusion, ear
  ureter S37.12
  urethra S37.32
  urinary organ NEC S37.892
  uterus S37.62
  uvula S00.532
  vagina S30.23
  vas deferens S37.892
  vesical S37.22
  vocal cord (s) S10.0
  vulva S30.23
  wrist S60.21-
Conus (congenital) (any type) Q14.8
  cornea —*see* Keratoconus
  medullaris syndrome G95.81
Conversion hysteria, neurosis or reaction F44.9
Converter, tuberculosis (test reaction) R76.11
Conviction (legal), **anxiety concerning** Z65.0
  with imprisonment Z65.1
Convulsions (idiopathic) (*see also* Seizure (s)) R56.9 ◀▬
  apoplectiform (cerebral ischemia) I67.82
  benign neonatal (familial) —*see* Epilepsy, generalized, idiopathic
  dissociative F44.5
  epileptic —*see* Epilepsy
  epileptiform, epileptoid —*see* Seizure, epileptiform
  ether (anesthetic) —*see* Table of ~~d~~Drugs and ~~c~~Chemicals, by drug ◀▬
  febrile R56.00
    with status epilepticus G40.901
    complex R56.01
      with status epilepticus G40.901
    simple R56.00
  hysterical F44.5
  infantile P90
    epilepsy —*see* Epilepsy
  jacksonian —*see* Epilepsy, localization-related, symptomatic, with simple partial seizures
  myoclonic G25.3
  neonatal, benign (familial) —*see* Epilepsy, generalized, idiopathic
  newborn P90

Convulsions (*Continued*)
    obstetrical (nephritic) (uremic) —*see*
        Eclampsia
    paretic A52.17
    post traumatic R56.1
    psychomotor —*see* Epilepsy, localization-
        related, symptomatic, with complex
        partial seizures
    recurrent R56.9
    reflex R25.8
    scarlatinal A38.8
    tetanus, tetanic —*see* Tetanus
    thymic E32.8
Convulsive —*see also* Convulsions
Cooley's anemia D56.1
Coolie itch B76.9
Cooper's
    disease —*see* Mastopathy, cystic
    hernia —*see* Hernia, abdomen, specified site
        NEC
Copra itch B88.0
Coprophagy F50.8
Coprophobia F40.298
Coproporphyria, hereditary E80.29
Cor
    biloculare Q20.8
    bovis, bovinum —*see* Hypertrophy, cardiac
    pulmonale (chronic) I27.81
        acute I26.09
    triatriatum, triatrium Q24.2
    triloculare Q20.8
        biatrium Q20.4
        biventriculare Q21.1
Corbus' disease (gangrenous balanitis) N48.1
Cord —*see also* condition
    around neck (tightly) (with compression)
        complicating delivery O69.1
    bladder G95.89
        tabetic A52.19
Cordis ectopia Q24.8
Corditis (spermatic) N49.1
Corectopia Q13.2
Cori's disease (glycogen storage) E74.03
Corkhandler's disease or lung J67.3
Corkscrew esophagus K22.4
Corkworker's disease or lung J67.3
Corn (infected) L84
Cornea —*see also* condition
    donor Z52.5
    plana Q13.4
Cornelia de Lange syndrome Q87.1
Cornu cutaneum L85.8
Cornual gestation or pregnancy O00.8
Coronary (artery) —*see* condition
Coronavirus, as cause of disease classified
        elsewhere B97.29
    SARS-associated B97.21
Corpora —*see also* condition
    amylacea, prostate N42.89
    cavernosa —*see* condition
Corpulence —*see* Obesity
Corpus —*see* condition
Corrected transposition Q20.5
Corrosion (injury) (acid) (caustic) (chemical)
        (lime) (external) (internal) T30.4
    abdomen, abdominal (muscle) (wall) T21.42
        first degree T21.52
        second degree T21.62
        third degree T21.72
    above elbow T22.439
        first degree T22.539
        left T22.432
            first degree T22.532
            second degree T22.632
            third degree T22.732
        right T22.431
            first degree T22.531
            second degree T22.631
            third degree T22.731
        second degree T22.639
        third degree T22.739

Corrosion (*Continued*)
    alimentary tract NEC T28.7
    ankle T25.419
        first degree T25.519
        left T25.412
            first degree T25.512
            second degree T25.612
            third degree T25.712
        multiple with foot —*see* Corrosion,
            lower, limb, multiple, ankle
            and foot
        right T25.411
            first degree T25.511
            second degree T25.611
            third degree T25.711
        second degree T25.619
        third degree T25.719
    anus —*see* Corrosion, buttock
    arm (s) (meaning upper limb (s)) —*see*
        Corrosion, upper limb
    axilla T22.449
        first degree T22.549
        left T22.442
            first degree T22.542
            second degree T22.642
            third degree T22.742
        right T22.441
            first degree T22.541
            second degree T22.641
            third degree T22.741
        second degree T22.649
        third degree T22.749
    back (lower) T21.44
        first degree T21.54
        second degree T21.64
        third degree T21.74
        upper T21.43
            first degree T21.53
            second degree T21.63
            third degree T21.73
    blisters - code as Corrosion, second degree,
        by site
    breast (s) —*see* Corrosion, chest wall
    buttock (s) T21.45
        first degree T21.55
        second degree T21.65
        third degree T21.75
    calf T24.439
        first degree T24.539
        left T24.432
            first degree T24.532
            second degree T24.632
            third degree T24.732
        right T24.431
            first degree T24.531
            second degree T24.631
            third degree T24.731
        second degree T24.639
        third degree T24.739
    canthus (eye) —*see* Corrosion,
        eyelid
    cervix T28.8
    cheek T20.46
        first degree T20.56
        second degree T20.66
        third degree T20.76
    chest wall T21.41
        first degree T21.51
        second degree T21.61
        third degree T21.71
    chin T20.43
        first degree T20.53
        second degree T20.63
        third degree T20.73
    colon T28.7
    conjunctiva (and cornea) —*see* Corrosion,
        cornea
    cornea (and conjunctiva) T26.6-
    deep necrosis of underlying tissue -
        code as Corrosion, third degree,
        by site

Corrosion (*Continued*)
    dorsum of hand T23.469
        first degree T23.569
        left T23.462
            first degree T23.562
            second degree T23.662
            third degree T23.762
        right T23.461
            first degree T23.561
            second degree T23.661
            third degree T23.761
        second degree T23.669
        third degree T23.769
    ear (auricle) (external) (canal)
        T20.41
        drum T28.91
        first degree T20.51
        second degree T20.61
        third degree T20.71
    elbow T22.429
        first degree T22.529
        left T22.422
            first degree T22.522
            second degree T22.622
            third degree T22.722
        right T22.421
            first degree T22.521
            second degree T22.621
            third degree T22.721
        second degree T22.629
        third degree T22.729
    entire body —*see* Corrosion, multiple
        body regions
    epidermal loss - code as Corrosion,
        second degree, by site
    epiglottis T27.4
    erythema, erythematous - code
        as Corrosion, first degree,
        by site
    esophagus T28.6
    extent (percentage of body surface)
        less than 10 percent T32.0
        10-19 percent (0-9 percent third degree)
            T32.10
            with 10-19 percent third degree
                T32.11
        20-29 percent (0-9 percent third degree)
            T32.20
            with
                10-19 percent third degree T32.21
                20-29 percent third degree T32.22
        30-39 percent (0-9 percent third degree)
            T32.30
            with
                10-19 percent third degree T32.31
                20-29 percent third degree T32.32
                30-39 percent third degree T32.33
        40-49 percent (0-9 percent third degree)
            T32.40
            with
                10-19 percent third degree T32.41
                20-29 percent third degree T32.42
                30-39 percent third degree T32.43
                40-49 percent third degree T32.44
        50-59 percent (0-9 percent third degree)
            T32.50
            with
                10-19 percent third degree T32.51
                20-29 percent third degree T32.52
                30-39 percent third degree T32.53
                40-49 percent third degree T32.54
                50-59 percent third degree T32.55
        60-69 percent (0-9 percent third degree)
            T32.60
            with
                10-19 percent third degree T32.61
                20-29 percent third degree T32.62
                30-39 percent third degree T32.63
                40-49 percent third degree T32.64
                50-59 percent third degree T32.65
                60-69 percent third degree T32.66

◀ New   ◀═ Revised   ~~deleted~~ Deleted

Corrosion *(Continued)*
  lower *(Continued)*
    limb *(Continued)*
      multiple sites, except ankle and foot
        (Continued)
        ankle and foot *(Continued)*
          right T25.491
            first degree T25.591
            second degree T25.691
            third degree T25.791
          second degree T25.699
          third degree T25.799
        first degree T24.599
        left T24.492
          first degree T24.592
          second degree T24.692
          third degree T24.792
        right T24.491
          first degree T24.591
          second degree T24.691
          third degree T24.791
        second degree T24.699
        third degree T24.799
      right T24.401
        first degree T24.501
        second degree T24.601
        third degree T24.701
      second degree T24.609
      thigh —*see* Corrosion, thigh
      third degree T24.709
  lung (with larynx and trachea)
    T27.5
  mouth T28.5
  neck T20.47
    first degree T20.57
    second degree T20.67
    third degree T20.77
  nose (septum) T20.44
    first degree T20.54
    second degree T20.64
    third degree T20.74
  ocular adnexa —*see* Corrosion,
    eye
  orbit region —*see* Corrosion,
    eyelid
  palm T23.459
    first degree T23.559
    left T23.452
      first degree T23.552
      second degree T23.652
      third degree T23.752
    right T23.451
      first degree T23.551
      second degree T23.651
      third degree T23.751
    second degree T23.659
    third degree T23.759
  partial thickness - code as Corrosion,
    unspecified degree, by site
  pelvis —*see* Corrosion, trunk
  penis —*see* Corrosion, genital organs,
    external, male
  perineum
    female —*see* Corrosion, genital organs,
      external, female
    male —*see* Corrosion, genital organs,
      external, male
  periocular area —*see* Corrosion,
    eyelid
  pharynx T28.5
  rectum T28.7
  respiratory tract T27.7
    larynx —*see* Corrosion, larynx
    specified part NEC T27.6
    trachea —*see* Corrosion, larynx
  sac, lacrimal —*see* Corrosion, eye,
    specified site NEC
  scalp T20.45
    first degree T20.55
    second degree T20.65
    third degree T20.75

Corrosion *(Continued)*
  scapular region T22.469
    first degree T22.569
    left T22.462
      first degree T22.562
      second degree T22.662
      third degree T22.762
    right T22.461
      first degree T22.561
      second degree T22.661
      third degree T22.761
    second degree T22.669
    third degree T22.769
  sclera —*see* Corrosion, eye, specified site
    NEC
  scrotum —*see* Corrosion, genital organs,
    external, male
  shoulder T22.459
    first degree T22.559
    left T22.452
      first degree T22.552
      second degree T22.652
      third degree T22.752
    right T22.451
      first degree T22.551
      second degree T22.651
      third degree T22.751
    second degree T22.659
    third degree T22.759
  stomach T28.7
  temple —*see* Corrosion, head
  testis —*see* Corrosion, genital organs,
    external, male
  thigh T24.419
    first degree T24.519
    left T24.412
      first degree T24.512
      second degree T24.612
      third degree T24.712
    right T24.411
      first degree T24.511
      second degree T24.611
      third degree T24.711
    second degree T24.619
    third degree T24.719
  thorax (external) —*see* Corrosion, trunk
  throat (meaning pharynx) T28.5
  thumb (s) T23.419
    first degree T23.519
    left T23.412
      first degree T23.512
      second degree T23.612
      third degree T23.712
  multiple sites with fingers T23.449
    first degree T23.549
    left T23.442
      first degree T23.542
      second degree T23.642
      third degree T23.742
    right T23.441
      first degree T23.541
      second degree T23.641
      third degree T23.741
    second degree T23.649
    third degree T23.749
  right T23.411
    first degree T23.511
    second degree T23.611
    third degree T23.711
  second degree T23.619
  third degree T23.719
  toe T25.439
    first degree T25.539
    left T25.432
      first degree T25.532
      second degree T25.632
      third degree T25.732
    right T25.431
      first degree T25.531
      second degree T25.631
      third degree T25.731

Corrosion *(Continued)*
  toe *(Continued)*
    second degree T25.639
    third degree T25.739
  tongue T28.5
  tonsil (s) T28.5
  total body —*see* Corrosion, multiple body
    regions
  trachea T27.4
    with lung T27.5
  trunk T21.40
    abdominal wall —*see* Corrosion,
      abdominal wall
    anus —*see* Corrosion, buttock
    axilla —*see* Corrosion, upper limb
    back —*see* Corrosion, back
    breast —*see* Corrosion, chest wall
    buttock —*see* Corrosion, buttock
    chest wall —*see* Corrosion, chest wall
    first degree T21.50
    flank —*see* Corrosion, abdominal wall
    genital
      female —*see* Corrosion, genital organs,
        external, female
      male —*see* Corrosion, genital organs,
        external, male
    groin —*see* Corrosion, abdominal
      wall
    interscapular region —*see* Corrosion,
      back, upper
    labia —*see* Corrosion, genital organs,
      external, female
    lower back —*see* Corrosion, back
    penis —*see* Corrosion, genital organs,
      external, male
    perineum
      female —*see* Corrosion, genital organs,
        external, female
      male —*see* Corrosion, genital organs,
        external, male
    scapular region —*see* Corrosion, upper
      limb
    scrotum —*see* Corrosion, genital organs,
      external, male
    second degree T21.60
    shoulder —*see* Corrosion, upper limb
    specified site NEC T21.49
      first degree T21.59
      second degree T21.69
      third degree T21.79
    testes —*see* Corrosion, genital organs,
      external, male
    third degree T21.70
    upper back —*see* Corrosion, back, upper
    vagina T28.8
    vulva —*see* Corrosion, genital organs,
      external, female
  unspecified site with extent of body surface
    involved specified
    less than 10 percent T32.0
    10-19 percent (0-9 percent third degree)
      T32.10
      with 10-19 percent third degree T32.11
    20-29 percent (0-9 percent third degree)
      T32.20
      with
        10-19 percent third degree T32.21
        20-29 percent third degree T32.22
    30-39 percent (0-9 percent third degree)
      T32.30
      with
        10-19 percent third degree T32.31
        20-29 percent third degree T32.32
        30-39 percent third degree T32.33
    40-49 percent (0-9 percent third degree)
      T32.40
      with
        10-19 percent third degree T32.41
        20-29 percent third degree T32.42
        30-39 percent third degree T32.43
        40-49 percent third degree T32.44

◀ New   ◀⋘ Revised   ~~deleted~~ Deleted

Corrosion *(Continued)*
  unspecified site with extent of body surface
      involved specified *(Continued)*
    50-59 percent (0-9 percent third degree)
        T32.50
      with
        10-19 percent third degree T32.51
        20-29 percent third degree T32.52
        30-39 percent third degree T32.53
        40-49 percent third degree T32.54
        50-59 percent third degree T32.55
    60-69 percent (0-9 percent third degree)
        T32.60
      with
        10-19 percent third degree T32.61
        20-29 percent third degree T32.62
        30-39 percent third degree T32.63
        40-49 percent third degree T32.64
        50-59 percent third degree T32.65
        60-69 percent third degree T32.66
    70-79 percent (0-9 percent third degree)
        T32.70
      with
        10-19 percent third degree T32.71
        20-29 percent third degree T32.72
        30-39 percent third degree T32.73
        40-49 percent third degree T32.74
        50-59 percent third degree T32.75
        60-69 percent third degree T32.76
        70-79 percent third degree T32.77
    80-89 percent (0-9 percent third degree)
        T32.80
      with
        10-19 percent third degree T32.81
        20-29 percent third degree T32.82
        30-39 percent third degree T32.83
        40-49 percent third degree T32.84
        50-59 percent third degree T32.85
        60-69 percent third degree T32.86
        70-79 percent third degree T32.87
        80-89 percent third degree T32.88
    90 percent or more (0-9 percent third
        degree) T32.90
      with
        10-19 percent third degree T32.91
        20-29 percent third degree T32.92
        30-39 percent third degree T32.93
        40-49 percent third degree T32.94
        50-59 percent third degree T32.95
        60-69 percent third degree T32.96
        70-79 percent third degree T32.97
        80-89 percent third degree T32.98
        90-99 percent third degree T32.99
  upper limb (axilla) (scapular region) T22.40
    above elbow —*see* Corrosion, above
        elbow
    axilla —*see* Corrosion, axilla
    elbow —*see* Corrosion, elbow
    first degree T22.50
    forearm —*see* Corrosion, forearm
    hand —*see* Corrosion, hand
    interscapular region —*see* Corrosion, back,
        upper
    multiple sites T22.499
      first degree T22.599
      left T22.492
        first degree T22.592
        second degree T22.692
        third degree T22.792
      right T22.491
        first degree T22.591
        second degree T22.691
        third degree T22.791
      second degree T22.699
      third degree T22.799
    scapular region —*see* Corrosion, scapular
        region
    second degree T22.60
    shoulder —*see* Corrosion, shoulder
    third degree T22.70
    wrist —*see* Corrosion, hand

Corrosion *(Continued)*
  uterus T28.8
  vagina T28.8
  vulva —*see* Corrosion, genital organs,
      external, female
  wrist T23.479
    first degree T23.579
    left T23.472
      first degree T23.572
      second degree T23.672
      third degree T23.772
    multiple sites with hand T23.499
      first degree T23.599
      left T23.492
        first degree T23.592
        second degree T23.692
        third degree T23.792
      right T23.491
        first degree T23.591
        second degree T23.691
        third degree T23.791
      second degree T23.699
      third degree T23.799
    right T23.471
      first degree T23.571
      second degree T23.671
      third degree T23.771
    second degree T23.679
    third degree T23.779
Corrosive burn —*see* Corrosion
Corsican fever —*see* Malaria
Cortical —*see* condition
Cortico-adrenal —*see* condition
Coryza (acute) J00
  with grippe or influenza —*see* Influenza,
      with, respiratory manifestations
      NEC
  syphilitic
    congenital (chronic) A50.05
Costen's syndrome or complex M26.69
Costiveness —*see* Constipation
Costochondritis M94.0
Cot death R99
Cotard's syndrome F22
Cotia virus B08.8
Cotton wool spots (retinal) H35.81
Cotungo's disease —*see* Sciatica
Cough (affected) (chronic) (epidemic) (nervous)
    R05
  with hemorrhage —*see* Hemoptysis
  bronchial R05
    with grippe or influenza —*see* Influenza,
        with, respiratory manifestations
        NEC
  functional F45.8
  hysterical F45.8
  laryngeal, spasmodic R05
  psychogenic F45.8
  smokers' J41.0
  tea taster's B49
Counseling (for) Z71.9
  abuse NEC
    perpetrator Z69.82
    victim Z69.81
  alcohol abuser Z71.41
    family Z71.42
  child abuse
    nonparental
      perpetrator Z69.021
      victim Z69.020
    parental
      perpetrator Z69.011
      victim Z69.010
  consanguinity Z71.89
  contraceptive Z30.09
  dietary Z71.3
  drug abuser Z71.51
    family member Z71.52
  family Z71.89
  fertility preservation (prior to cancer therapy)
      (prior to removal of gonads) Z31.62

Counseling *(Continued)*
  for non-attending third party Z71.0
    related to sexual behavior or orientation
        Z70.2
  genetic NEC Z31.5
  health (advice) (education) (instruction) —*see*
      Counseling, medical
  human immunodeficiency virus (HIV)
      Z71.7
  impotence Z70.1
  insulin pump use Z46.81
  medical (for) Z71.9
    boarding school resident Z59.3
    consanguinity Z71.89
    feared complaint and no disease found
        Z71.1
    human immunodeficiency virus (HIV)
        Z71.7
    institutional resident Z59.3
    on behalf of another Z71.0
      related to sexual behavior or orientation
          Z70.2
    person living alone Z60.2
    specified reason NEC Z71.89
  natural family planning
    procreative Z31.61
    to avoid pregnancy Z30.02
  perpetrator (of)
    abuse NEC Z69.82
    child abuse
      non-parental Z69.021
      parental Z69.011
    rape NEC Z69.82
    spousal abuse Z69.12
  procreative NEC Z31.69
    fertility preservation (prior to cancer
        therapy) (prior to removal of
        gonads) Z31.62
    using natural family planning
        Z31.61
  promiscuity Z70.1
  rape victim Z69.81
  religious Z71.81
  sex, sexual (related to) Z70.9
    attitude (s) Z70.0
    behavior or orientation Z70.1
    combined concerns Z70.3
    non-responsiveness Z70.1
    on behalf of third party Z70.2
    specified reason NEC Z70.8
  specified reason NEC Z71.89
  spiritual Z71.81
  spousal abuse (perpetrator) Z69.12
    victim Z69.11
  substance abuse Z71.89
    alcohol Z71.41
    drug Z71.51
    tobacco Z71.6
  tobacco use Z71.6
  use (of)
    insulin pump Z46.81
  victim (of)
    abuse Z69.81
    child abuse
      by parent Z69.010
      non-parental Z69.020
    rape NEC Z69.81
Coupled rhythm R00.8
Couvelaire syndrome or uterus (complicating
    delivery) O45.8X-
Cowperitis —*see* Urethritis
Cowper's gland —*see* condition
Cowpox B08.010
  due to vaccination T88.1
Coxa
  magna M91.4-
  plana M91.2-
  valga (acquired) —*see also* Deformity, limb,
      specified type NEC, thigh
    congenital Q65.81
    sequelae (late effect) of rickets E64.3

Coxa *(Continued)*
  vara (acquired) —*see also* Deformity, limb,
    specified type NEC, thigh
     congenital Q65.82
     sequelae (late effect) of rickets E64.3
Coxalgia, coxalgic (nontuberculous) —*see also*
  Pain, joint, hip
  tuberculous A18.02
Coxitis —*see* Monoarthritis, hip
Coxsackie (virus) (infection) B34.1
  as cause of disease classified elsewhere B97.11
  carditis B33.20
  central nervous system NEC A88.8
  endocarditis B33.21
  enteritis A08.39
  meningitis (aseptic) A87.0
  myocarditis B33.22
  pericarditis B33.23
  pharyngitis B08.5
  pleurodynia B33.0
  specific disease NEC B33.8
Crabs, meaning pubic lice B85.3
Crack baby P04.41
Cracked nipple N64.0
  associated with
    lactation O92.13
    pregnancy O92.11-
    puerperium O92.12 ◀
Cracked tooth K03.81
Cradle cap L21.0
Craft neurosis F48.8
Cramp (s) R25.2
  abdominal —*see* Pain, abdominal
  bathing T75.1
  colic R10.83
    psychogenic F45.8
  due to immersion T75.1
  fireman T67.2
  heat T67.2
  immersion T75.1
  intestinal —*see* Pain, abdominal
    psychogenic F45.8
  leg, sleep related G47.62
  limb (lower) (upper) NEC R25.2
    sleep related G47.62
  linotypist's F48.8
    organic G25.89
  muscle (limb) (general) R25.2
    due to immersion T75.1
    psychogenic F45.8
  occupational (hand) F48.8
    organic G25.89
  salt-depletion E87.1
  sleep related, leg G47.62
  stoker's T67.2
  swimmer's T75.1
  telegrapher's F48.8
    organic G25.89
  typist's F48.8
    organic G25.89
  uterus N94.89
    menstrual —*see* Dysmenorrhea
  writer's F48.8
    organic G25.89
Cranial —*see* condition
Craniocleidodysostosis Q74.0
Craniofenestria (skull) Q75.8
Craniolacunia (skull) Q75.8
Craniopagus Q89.4
Craniopathy, metabolic M85.2
Craniopharyngeal —*see* condition
Craniopharyngioma D44.4
Craniorachischisis (totalis) Q00.1
Cranioschisis Q75.8
Craniostenosis Q75.0
Craniosynostosis Q75.0
Craniotabes (cause unknown) M83.8
  neonatal P96.3
  rachitic E64.3
  syphilitic A50.56
Cranium —*see* condition

Craw-craw —*see* Onchocerciasis
Creaking joint —*see* Derangement, joint,
  specified type NEC
Creeping
  eruption B76.9
  palsy or paralysis G12.22
Crenated tongue K14.8
Creotoxism A05.9
Crepitus
  caput Q75.8
  joint —*see* Derangement, joint, specified type
    NEC
Crescent or conus choroid, congenital Q14.3
CREST syndrome M34.1
Cretin, cretinism (congenital) (endemic)
  (nongoitrous) (sporadic) E00.9
  pelvis
    with disproportion (fetopelvic) O33.0
     causing obstructed labor O65.0
  type
    hypothyroid E00.1
    mixed E00.2
    myxedematous E00.1
    neurological E00.0
Creutzfeldt-Jakob disease or syndrome (with
  dementia) A81.00
  familial A81.09
  iatrogenic A81.09
  specified NEC A81.09
  sporadic A81.09
  variant (vCJD) A81.01
Crib death R99
Cribriform hymen Q52.3
Cri-du-chat syndrome Q93.4
Crigler-Najjar disease or syndrome E80.5
Crime, victim of Z65.4
Crimean hemorrhagic fever A98.0
Criminalism F60.2
Crisis
  abdomen R10.0
  acute reaction F43.0
  addisonian E27.2
  adrenal (cortical) E27.2
  celiac K90.0
  Dietl's N13.8
  emotional —*see also* Disorder, adjustment
    acute reaction to stress F43.0
    specific to childhood and adolescence
     F93.8
  glaucomatocyclitic —*see* Glaucoma,
    secondary, inflammation
  heart —*see* Failure, heart
  nitritoid I95.2
    correct substance properly administered —
     see Table of Drugs and Chemicals,
     by drug, adverse effect ◀▥
    overdose or wrong substance given or
     taken —*see* Table of Drugs and
     Chemicals, by drug, poisoning ◀▥
  oculogyric H51.8
    psychogenic F45.8
  Pel's (tabetic) A52.11
  psychosexual identity F64.2
  renal N28.0
  sickle-cell D57.00
    with
     acute chest syndrome D57.01
     splenic sequestration D57.02
  state (acute reaction) F43.0
  tabetic A52.11
  thyroid —*see* Thyrotoxicosis with thyroid
    storm
  thyrotoxic —*see* Thyrotoxicosis with thyroid
    storm
Crocq's disease (acrocyanosis) I73.89
Crohn's disease —*see* Enteritis, regional
Crooked septum, nasal J34.2
Cross syndrome E70.328
Crossbite (anterior) (posterior) M26.24
Cross-eye —*see* Strabismus, convergent
  concomitant

Croup, croupous (catarrhal) (infectious)
  (inflammatory) (nondiphtheritic) J05.0
  bronchial J20.9
  diphtheritic A36.2
  false J38.5
  spasmodic J38.5
    diphtheritic A36.2
  stridulous J38.5
    diphtheritic A36.2
Crouzon's disease Q75.1
Crowding, tooth, teeth, fully erupted M26.31
CRST syndrome M34.1
Cruchet's disease A85.8
Cruelty in children —*see also* Disorder,
  conduct
Crural ulcer —*see* Ulcer, lower limb
Crush, crushed, crushing T14.8
  abdomen S38.1
  ankle S97.0-
  arm (upper) (and shoulder) S47.-
  axilla —*see* Crush, arm
  back, lower S38.1
  buttock S38.1
  cheek S07.0
  chest S28.0
  cranium S07.1
  ear S07.0
  elbow S57.0-
  extremity
    lower
     ankle —*see* Crush, ankle
     below knee —*see* Crush, leg
     foot —*see* Crush, foot
     hip —*see* Crush, hip
     knee —*see* Crush, knee
     thigh —*see* Crush, thigh
     toe —*see* Crush, toe
    upper
     below elbow S67.9-
     elbow —*see* Crush, elbow
     finger —*see* Crush, finger
     forearm —*see* Crush, forearm
     hand —*see* Crush, hand
     thumb —*see* Crush, thumb
     upper arm —*see* Crush, arm
     wrist —*see* Crush, wrist
  face S07.0
  finger (s) S67.1-
    with hand (and wrist) —*see* Crush, hand,
     specified site NEC
    index S67.19-
    little S67.19-
    middle S67.19-
    ring S67.19-
    thumb —*see* Crush, thumb
  foot S97.8-
    toe —*see* Crush, toe
  forearm S57.8-
  genitalia, external
    female S38.002
     vagina S38.03
     vulva S38.03
    male S38.001
     penis S38.01
     scrotum S38.02
     testis S38.02
  hand (except fingers alone) S67.2-
    with wrist S67.4-
  head S07.9
    specified NEC S07.8
  heel —*see* Crush, foot
  hip S77.0-
    with thigh S77.2-
  internal organ (abdomen, chest, or pelvis)
    NEC T14.8
  knee S87.0-
  labium (majus) (minus) S38.03
  larynx S17.0
  leg (lower) S87.8-
    knee —*see* Crush, knee
  lip S07.0

◀ New   ◀▥ Revised   ~~deleted~~ Deleted

Crush, crushed, crushing *(Continued)*
  lower
    back S38.1
    leg —*see* Crush, leg
  neck S17.9
  nerve —*see* Injury, nerve
  nose S07.0
  pelvis S38.1
  penis S38.01
  scalp S07.8
  scapular region —*see* Crush, arm
  scrotum S38.02
  severe, unspecified site T14.8
  shoulder (and upper arm) —*see* Crush, arm
  skull S07.1
  syndrome (complication of trauma) T79.5
  testis S38.02
  thigh S77.1-
    with hip S77.2-
  throat S17.8
  thumb S67.0-
    with hand (and wrist) —*see* Crush, hand, specified site NEC
  toe (s) S97.10-
    great S97.11-
    lesser S97.12-
  trachea S17.0
  vagina S38.03
  vulva S38.03
  wrist S67.3-
    with hand S67.4-
Crusta lactea L21.0
Crusts R23.4
Crutch paralysis —*see* Injury, brachial plexus
Cruveilhier-Baumgarten cirrhosis, disease or syndrome K74.69
Cruveilhier's atrophy or disease G12.8
Crying (constant) (continuous) (excessive)
  child, adolescent, or adult R45.83
  infant (baby) (newborn) R68.11
Cryofibrinogenemia D89.2
Cryoglobulinemia (essential) (idiopathic) (mixed) (primary) (purpura) (secondary) (vasculitis) D89.1
  with lung involvement D89.1 *[J99]*
Cryptitis (anal) (rectal) K62.89
Cryptococcosis, cryptococcus (infection) (neoformans) B45.9
  bone B45.3
  cerebral B45.1
  cutaneous B45.2
  disseminated B45.7
  generalized B45.7
  meningitis B45.1
  meningocerebralis B45.1
  osseous B45.3
  pulmonary B45.0
  skin B45.2
  specified NEC B45.8
Cryptopapillitis (anus) K62.89
Cryptophthalmos Q11.2
  syndrome Q87.0
Cryptorchid, cryptorchism, cryptorchidism Q53.9
  bilateral Q53.20
    abdominal Q53.21
    perineal Q53.22
  unilateral Q53.10
    abdominal Q53.11
    perineal Q53.12
Cryptosporidiosis A07.2
  hepatobiliary B88.8
  respiratory B88.8
Cryptostromosis J67.6
Crystalluria R82.99
Cubitus
  congenital Q68.8
  valgus (acquired) M21.0-
    congenital Q68.8
    sequelae (late effect) of rickets E64.3

Cubitus *(Continued)*
  varus (acquired) M21.1-
    congenital Q68.8
    sequelae (late effect) of rickets E64.3
Cultural deprivation or shock Z60.3
Curling esophagus K22.4
Curling's ulcer —*see* Ulcer, peptic, acute
Curschmann (-Batten) (-Steinert) disease or syndrome G71.11
Curse, Ondine's —*see* Apnea, sleep
Curvature
  organ or site, congenital NEC —*see* Distortion
  penis (lateral) Q55.61
  Pott's (spinal) A18.01
  radius, idiopathic, progressive (congenital) Q74.0
  spine (acquired) (angular) (idiopathic) (incorrect) (postural) —*see* Dorsopathy, deforming
    congenital Q67.5
    due to or associated with
      Charcot-Marie-Tooth disease (see also subcategory M49.8) G60.0
      osteitis
        deformans M88.88
        fibrosa cystica (see also subcategory M49.8) E21.0
      tuberculosis (Pott's curvature) A18.01
    sequelae (late effect) of rickets E64.3
    tuberculous A18.01
Cushingoid due to steroid therapy E24.2
  correct substance properly administered —*see* Table of ~~d~~Drugs and ~~c~~Chemicals, by drug, adverse effect ◀▥
  overdose or wrong substance given or taken —*see* Table of ~~d~~Drugs and ~~c~~Chemicals, by drug, poisoning ◀▥
Cushing's
  syndrome or disease E24.9
    drug-induced E24.2
    iatrogenic E24.2
    pituitary-dependent E24.0
    specified NEC E24.8
  ulcer —*see* Ulcer, peptic, acute
Cusp, Carabelli - omit code
Cut (external) —*see also* Laceration
  muscle —*see* Injury, muscle
Cutaneous —*see also* condition
  hemorrhage R23.3
  larva migrans B76.9
Cutis —*see also* condition
  hyperelastica Q82.8
    acquired L57.4
  laxa (hyperelastica) —*see* Dermatolysis
  marmorata R23.8
  osteosis L94.2
  pendula —*see* Dermatolysis
  rhomboidalis nuchae L57.2
  verticis gyrata Q82.8
    acquired L91.8
Cyanosis R23.0
  due to
    patent foramen botalli Q21.1
    persistent foramen ovale Q21.1
  enterogenous D74.8
  paroxysmal digital —*see* Raynaud's disease
    with gangrene I73.01
  retina, retinal H35.89
Cyanotic heart disease I24.9
  congenital Q24.9
Cycle
  anovulatory N97.0
  menstrual, irregular N92.6
Cyclencephaly Q04.9
Cyclical vomiting (see also Vomiting, cyclical) G43.A0
  psychogenic F50.8
Cyclitis (see also Iridocyclitis) H20.9
  chronic —*see* Iridocyclitis, chronic
  Fuchs' heterochromic H20.81-
  granulomatous —*see* Iridocyclitis, chronic

Cyclitis *(Continued)*
  lens-induced —*see* Iridocyclitis, lens-induced
  posterior H30.2-
Cycloid personality F34.0
Cyclophoria H50.54
Cyclopia, cyclops Q87.0
Cyclopism Q87.0
Cyclosporiasis A07.4
Cyclothymia F34.0
Cyclothymic personality F34.0
Cyclotropia H50.41-
Cylindroma —*see also* Neoplasm, malignant, by site
  eccrine dermal —*see* Neoplasm, skin, benign
  skin —*see* Neoplasm, skin, benign
Cylindruria R82.99
Cynanche
  diphtheritic A36.2
  tonsillaris J36
Cynophobia F40.218
Cynorexia R63.2
Cyphosis —*see* Kyphosis
Cyprus fever —*see* Brucellosis
Cyst (colloid) (mucous) (simple) (retention)
  adenoid (infected) J35.8
  adrenal gland E27.8
    congenital Q89.1
  air, lung J98.4
  allantoic Q64.4
  alveolar process (jaw bone) M27.40
  amnion, amniotic O41.8X-
  anterior
    chamber (eye) —*see* Cyst, iris
    nasopalatine K09.1
  antrum J34.1
  anus K62.89
  apical (tooth) (periodontal) K04.8
  appendix K38.8
  arachnoid, brain (acquired) G93.0
    congenital Q04.6
  arytenoid J38.7
  Baker's M71.2-
    ruptured M66.0
    tuberculous A18.02
  Bartholin's gland N75.0
  bile duct (common) (hepatic) K83.5
  bladder (multiple) (trigone) N32.89
  blue dome (breast) —*see* Cyst, breast
  bone (local) NEC M85.60
    aneurysmal M85.50
      ankle M85.57-
      foot M85.57-
      forearm M85.53-
      hand M85.54-
      jaw M27.49
      lower leg M85.56-
      multiple site M85.59
      neck M85.58
      rib M85.58
      shoulder M85.51-
      skull M85.58
      specified site NEC M85.58
      thigh M85.55-
      toe M85.57-
      upper arm M85.52-
      vertebra M85.58
    solitary M85.40
      ankle M85.47-
      fibula M85.46-
      foot M85.47-
      hand M85.44-
      humerus M85.42-
      jaw M27.49
      neck M85.48
      pelvis M85.45-
      radius M85.43-
      rib M85.48
      shoulder M85.41-
      skull M85.48
      specified site NEC M85.48

Cyst (Continued)
  bone NEC (Continued)
    solitary (Continued)
      tibia M85.46-
      toe M85.47-
      ulna M85.43-
      vertebra M85.48
      specified type NEC M85.60
        ankle M85.67-
        foot M85.67-
        forearm M85.63-
        hand M85.64-
        jaw M27.40
          developmental (nonodontogenic)
            K09.1
            odontogenic K09.0
          latent M27.0
        lower leg M85.66-
        multiple site M85.69
        neck M85.68
        rib M85.68
        shoulder M85.61-
        skull M85.68
        specified site NEC M85.68
        thigh M85.65-
        toe M85.67-
        upper arm M85.62-
        vertebra M85.68
  brain (acquired) G93.0
    congenital Q04.6
    hydatid B67.99 [G94]
    third ventricle (colloid), congenital Q04.6
  branchial (cleft) Q18.0
  branchiogenic Q18.0
  breast (benign) (blue dome) (pedunculated)
    (solitary) N60.0-
    involution —see Dysplasia, mammary,
      specified type NEC
    sebaceous —see Dysplasia, mammary,
      specified type NEC
  broad ligament (benign) N83.8
  bronchogenic (mediastinal) (sequestration)
    J98.4
    congenital Q33.0
  buccal K09.8
  bulbourethral gland N36.8
  bursa, bursal NEC M71.30
    with rupture —see Rupture, synovium
    ankle M71.37-
    elbow M71.32-
    foot M71.37-
    hand M71.34-
    hip M71.35-
    multiple sites M71.39
    pharyngeal J39.2
    popliteal space —see Cyst, Baker's
    shoulder M71.31-
    specified site NEC M71.38
    wrist M71.33-
  calcifying odontogenic D16.5
    upper jaw (bone) (maxilla) D16.4
  canal of Nuck (female) N94.89
    congenital Q52.4
  canthus —see Cyst, conjunctiva
  carcinomatous —see Neoplasm, malignant,
    by site
  cauda equina G95.89
  cavum septi pellucidi —see Cyst, brain
  celomic (pericardium) Q24.8
  cerebellopontine (angle) —see Cyst, brain
  cerebellum —see Cyst, brain
  cerebral —see Cyst, brain
  cervical lateral Q18.1
  cervix NEC N88.8
    embryonic Q51.6
    nabothian N88.8
  chiasmal optic NEC —see Disorder, optic,
    chiasm
  chocolate (ovary) N80.1
  choledochus, congenital Q44.4
  chorion O41.8X-

Cyst (Continued)
  choroid plexus G93.0
  ciliary body —see Cyst, iris
  clitoris N90.7
  colon K63.89
  common (bile) duct K83.5
  congenital NEC Q89.8
    adrenal gland Q89.1
    epiglottis Q31.8
    esophagus Q39.8
    fallopian tube Q50.4
    kidney Q61.00
      more than one (multiple) Q61.02
        specified as polycystic Q61.3
          adult type Q61.2
          infantile type NEC Q61.19
            collecting duct dilation Q61.11
      solitary Q61.01
    larynx Q31.8
    liver Q44.6
    lung Q33.0
    mediastinum Q34.1
    ovary Q50.1
    oviduct Q50.4
    periurethral (tissue) Q64.79
    prepuce Q55.69
    salivary gland (any) Q38.4
    sublingual Q38.6
    submaxillary gland Q38.6
    thymus (gland) Q89.2
    tongue Q38.3
    ureterovesical orifice Q62.8
    vulva Q52.79
  conjunctiva H11.44-
  cornea H18.89-
  corpora quadrigemina G93.0
  corpus
    albicans N83.29
    luteum (hemorrhagic) (ruptured) N83.1
  Cowper's gland (benign) (infected) N36.8
  cranial meninges G93.0
  craniobuccal pouch E23.6
  craniopharyngeal pouch E23.6
  cystic duct K82.8
  Cysticercus —see Cysticercosis
  Dandy-Walker Q03.1
    with spina bifida —see Spina bifida
  dental (root) K04.8
    developmental K09.0
    eruption K09.0
    primordial K09.0
  dentigerous (mandible) (maxilla) K09.0
  dermoid —see Neoplasm, benign, by site
    with malignant transformation C56.-
    implantation
      external area or site (skin) NEC L72.0
      iris —see Cyst, iris, implantation
      vagina N89.8
      vulva N90.7
    mouth K09.8
    oral soft tissue K09.8
    sacrococcygeal —see Cyst, pilonidal
  developmental K09.1
    odontogenic K09.0
    oral region (nonodontogenic) K09.1
    ovary, ovarian Q50.1
  dura (cerebral) G93.0
    spinal G96.19
  ear (external) Q18.1
  echinococcal —see Echinococcus
  embryonic
    cervix uteri Q51.6
    fallopian tube Q50.4
    vagina Q51.6
  endometrium, endometrial (uterus) N85.8
    ectopic —see Endometriosis
  enterogenous Q43.8
  epidermal, epidermoid (inclusion) (see also
    Cyst, skin) L72.0
    mouth K09.8
    oral soft tissue K09.8

Cyst (Continued)
  epididymis N50.3
  epiglottis J38.7
  epiphysis cerebri E34.8
  epithelial (inclusion) L72.0
  epoophoron Q50.5
  eruption K09.0
  esophagus K22.8
  ethmoid sinus J34.1
  external female genital organs NEC
    N90.7
  eye NEC H57.8
    congenital Q15.8
  eyelid (sebaceous) H02.829
    infected —see Hordeolum
    left H02.826
      lower H02.825
      upper H02.824
    right H02.823
      lower H02.822
      upper H02.821
  fallopian tube N83.8
    congenital Q50.4
  fimbrial (twisted) Q50.4
  fissural (oral region) K09.1
  follicle (graafian) (hemorrhagic) N83.0
    nabothian N88.8
  follicular (atretic) (hemorrhagic) (ovarian)
    N83.0
    dentigerous K09.0
    odontogenic K09.0
    skin L72.9
    specified NEC L72.8
  frontal sinus J34.1
  gallbladder K82.8
  ganglion —see Ganglion
  Gartner's duct Q52.4
  gingiva K09.0
  gland of Moll —see Cyst, eyelid
  globulomaxillary K09.1
  graafian follicle (hemorrhagic) N83.0
  granulosal lutein (hemorrhagic) N83.1
  hemangiomatous D18.00
    intra-abdominal D18.03
    intracranial D18.02
    skin D18.01
    specified site NEC D18.09
  hydatid (see also Echinococcus) B67.90
    brain B67.99 [G94]
    liver (see also Cyst, liver, hydatid) B67.8
    lung NEC B67.99 [J99]
    Morgagni
      female Q50.5
      male (epididymal) Q55.4
        testicular Q55.29
    specified site NEC B67.99
  hymen N89.8
    embryonic Q52.4
  hypopharynx J39.2
  hypophysis, hypophyseal (duct) (recurrent)
    E23.6
    cerebri E23.6
  implantation (dermoid)
    external area or site (skin) NEC L72.0
    iris —see Cyst, iris, implantation
    vagina N89.8
    vulva N90.7
  incisive canal K09.1
  inclusion (epidermal) (epithelial)
    (epidermoid) (squamous) L72.0
    not of skin - code under Cyst, by site
  intestine (large) (small) K63.89
  intracranial —see Cyst, brain
  intraligamentous —see also Disorder,
    ligament
    knee —see Derangement, knee
  intrasellar E23.6
  iris H21.309
    exudative H21.31-
    idiopathic H21.30-
    implantation H21.32-

Cyst (Continued)
  iris (Continued)
    parasitic H21.33-
    pars plana (primary) H21.34-
      exudative H21.35-
  jaw (bone) ~~(aneurysmal) (hemorrhagic) (traumatic)~~M27.40 ◀▥
    aneurysmal M27.49 ◀
    developmental (odontogenic) K09.0
    fissural K09.1
    hemorrhagic M27.49 ◀
    traumatic M27.49 ◀
  joint NEC —see Disorder, joint, specified type NEC
  kidney (acquired) N28.1
    calyceal —see Hydronephrosis
    congenital Q61.00
    more than one (multiple) Q61.02
      specified as polycystic Q61.3
        adult type (autosomal dominant) Q61.2
        infantile type (autosomal recessive) NEC Q61.19
          collecting duct dilation Q61.11
    pyelogenic —see Hydronephrosis
    simple N28.1
    solitary (single) Q61.01
      acquired N28.1
  labium (majus) (minus) N90.7
    sebaceous N90.7
  lacrimal —see also Disorder, lacrimal system, specified NEC
    gland H04.13-
    passages or sac —see Disorder, lacrimal system, specified NEC
  larynx J38.7
  lateral periodontal K09.0
  lens H27.8
    congenital Q12.8
  lip (gland) K13.0
  liver (idiopathic) (simple) K76.89
    congenital Q44.6
    hydatid B67.8
      granulosus B67.0
      multilocularis B67.5
  lung J98.4
    congenital Q33.0
    giant bullous J43.9
  lutein N83.1
  lymphangiomatous D18.1
  lymphoepithelial, oral soft tissue K09.8
  macula —see Degeneration, macula, hole
  malignant —see Neoplasm, malignant, by site
  mammary gland —see Cyst, breast
  mandible M27.40
    dentigerous K09.0
    radicular K04.8
  maxilla M27.40
    dentigerous K09.0
    radicular K04.8
  medial, face and neck Q18.8
  median
    anterior maxillary K09.1
    palatal K09.1
  mediastinum, congenital Q34.1
  meibomian (gland) —see Chalazion
    infected —see Hordeolum
  membrane, brain G93.0
  meninges (cerebral) G93.0
    spinal G96.19
  meniscus, knee —see Derangement, knee, meniscus, cystic
  mesentery, mesenteric K66.8
    chyle I89.8
  mesonephric duct
    female Q50.5
    male Q55.4
  milk N64.89
  Morgagni (hydatid)
    female Q50.5
    male (epididymal) Q55.4
      testicular Q55.29
  mouth K09.8

Cyst (Continued)
  Müllerian duct Q50.4
    appendix testis Q55.29
    cervix Q51.6
    fallopian tube Q50.4
    female Q50.4
    male Q55.29
    prostatic utricle Q55.4
    vagina (embryonal) Q52.4
  multilocular (ovary) D39.10
    benign —see Neoplasm, benign, by site
  myometrium N85.8
  nabothian (follicle) (ruptured) N88.8
  nasoalveolar K09.1
  nasolabial K09.1
  nasopalatine (anterior) (duct) K09.1
  nasopharynx J39.2
  neoplastic —see Neoplasm, uncertain behavior, by site
    benign —see Neoplasm, benign, by site
  nervous system NEC G96.8
  neuroenteric (congenital) Q06.8
  nipple —see Cyst, breast
  nose (turbinates) J34.1
    sinus J34.1
  odontogenic, developmental K09.0
  omentum (lesser) K66.8
    congenital Q45.8
  ora serrata —see Cyst, retina, ora serrata
  oral
    region K09.9
      developmental (nonodontogenic) K09.1
      specified NEC K09.8
    soft tissue K09.9
      specified NEC K09.8
  orbit H05.81-
  ovary, ovarian (twisted) N83.20
    adherent N83.20
    chocolate N80.1
    corpus
      albicans N83.29
      luteum (hemorrhagic) N83.1
    dermoid D27.9
    developmental Q50.1
    due to failure of involution NEC N83.20
    endometrial N80.1
    follicular (graafian) (hemorrhagic) N83.0
    hemorrhagic N83.20
    in pregnancy or childbirth O34.8-
      with obstructed labor O65.5
    multilocular D39.10
    pseudomucinous D27.9
    retention N83.29
    serous N83.20
    specified NEC N83.29
    theca lutein (hemorrhagic) N83.1
    tuberculous A18.18
  oviduct N83.8
  palate (median) (fissural) K09.1
  palatine papilla (jaw) K09.1
  pancreas, pancreatic (hemorrhagic) (true) K86.2
    congenital Q45.2
    false K86.3
  paralabral
    hip M24.85-
    shoulder S43.43-
  paramesonephric duct Q50.4
    female Q50.4
    male Q55.29
  paranephric N28.1
  paraphysis, cerebri, congenital Q04.6
  parasitic B89
  parathyroid (gland) E21.4
  paratubal N83.8
  paraurethral duct N36.8
  paroophoron Q50.5
  parotid gland K11.6
  parovarian Q50.5
  pelvis, female N94.89
    in pregnancy or childbirth O34.8-
      causing obstructed labor O65.5

Cyst (Continued)
  penis (sebaceous) N48.89
  periapical K04.8
  pericardial (congenital) Q24.8
    acquired (secondary) I31.8
  pericoronal K09.0
  periodontal K04.8
    lateral K09.0
  peripelvic (lymphatic) N28.1
  peritoneum K66.8
    chylous I89.8
  periventricular, acquired, newborn P91.1
  pharynx (wall) J39.2
  pilar L72.11
  pilonidal (infected) (rectum) L05.91
    with abscess L05.01
    malignant C44.59-
  pituitary (duct) (gland) E23.6
  placenta O43.19-
  pleura J94.8
  popliteal —see Cyst, Baker's
  porencephalic Q04.6
    acquired G93.0
  postanal (infected) —see Cyst, pilonidal
  postmastoidectomy cavity (mucosal) —see Complications, postmastoidectomy, cyst
  preauricular Q18.1
  prepuce N47.4
    congenital Q55.69
  primordial (jaw) K09.0
  prostate N42.83
  pseudomucinous (ovary) D27.9
  pupillary, miotic H21.27-
  radicular (residual) K04.8
  radiculodental K04.8
  ranular K11.8
  Rathke's pouch E23.6
  rectum (epithelium) (mucous) K62.89
  renal —see Cyst, kidney
  residual (radicular) K04.8
  retention (ovary) N83.29
    salivary gland K11.6
  retina H33.19-
    ora serrata H33.11-
    parasitic H33.12-
  retroperitoneal K68.9
  sacrococcygeal (dermoid) —see Cyst, pilonidal
  salivary gland or duct (mucous extravasation or retention) K11.6
  Sampson's N80.1
  sclera H15.89
  scrotum L72.9
    sebaceous L72.3
  sebaceous (duct) (gland) L72.3
    breast —see Dysplasia, mammary, specified type NEC
    eyelid —see Cyst, eyelid
    genital organ NEC
      female N94.89
      male N50.8
    scrotum L72.3
  semilunar cartilage (knee) (multiple) —see Derangement, knee, meniscus, cystic
  seminal vesicle N50.8
  serous (ovary) N83.20
  sinus (accessory) (nasal) J34.1
  Skene's gland N36.8
  skin L72.9
    breast —see Dysplasia, mammary, specified type NEC
    epidermal, epidermoid L72.0
    epithelial L72.0
    eyelid —see Cyst, eyelid
    genital organ NEC
      female N90.7
      male N50.8
    inclusion L72.0
    scrotum L72.9
    sebaceous L72.3
    sweat gland or duct L74.8

Cyst *(Continued)*
  solitary
    bone —*see* Cyst, bone, solitary
      jaw M27.40
      kidney N28.1
  spermatic cord N50.8
  sphenoid sinus J34.1
  spinal meninges G96.19
  spleen NEC D73.4
    congenital Q89.09
    hydatid *(see also* Echinococcus) B67.99
      [D77]
  Stafne's M27.0
  subarachnoid intrasellar R93.0
  subcutaneous, pheomycotic (chromomycotic)
    B43.2
  subdural (cerebral) G93.0
    spinal cord G96.19
  sublingual gland K11.6
  submandibular gland K11.6
  submaxillary gland K11.6
  suburethral N36.8
  suprarenal gland E27.8
  suprasellar —*see* Cyst, brain
  sweat gland or duct L74.8
  synovial —*see also* Cyst, bursa
    ruptured —*see* Rupture, synovium
  tarsal —*see* Chalazion
  tendon (sheath) —*see* Disorder, tendon,
    specified type NEC
  testis N44.2
    tunica albuginea N44.1
  theca lutein (ovary) N83.1
  Thornwaldt's J39.2
  thymus (gland) E32.8
  thyroglossal duct (infected) (persistent) Q89.2
  thyroid (gland) E04.1
  thyrolingual duct (infected) (persistent) Q89.2
  tongue K14.8
  tonsil J35.8
  tooth —*see* Cyst, dental
  Tornwaldt's J39.2
  trichilemmal (proliferating) L72.12
  trichodermal L72.12
  tubal (fallopian) N83.8
    inflammatory —*see* Salpingitis, chronic
  tubo-ovarian N83.8
    inflammatory N70.13
  tunica
    albuginea testis N44.1
    vaginalis N50.8
  turbinate (nose) J34.1
  Tyson's gland N48.89
  urachus, congenital Q64.4
  ureter N28.89
  ureterovesical orifice N28.89
  urethra, urethral (gland) N36.8
  uterine ligament N83.8
  uterus (body) (corpus) (recurrent) N85.8
    embryonic Q51.818
      cervix Q51.6
  vagina, vaginal (implantation) (inclusion)
    (squamous cell) (wall) N89.8
    embryonic Q52.4
  vallecula, vallecular (epiglottis) J38.7
  vesical (orifice) N32.89
  vitreous body H43.89
  vulva (implantation) (inclusion) N90.7
    congenital Q52.79
    sebaceous gland N90.7
  vulvovaginal gland N90.7
  wolffian
    female Q50.5
    male Q55.4
Cystadenocarcinoma —*see* Neoplasm,
    malignant, by site
  bile duct C22.1
  endometrioid —*see* Neoplasm, malignant,
    by site
    specified site —*see* Neoplasm, malignant,
      by site

Cystadenocarcinoma *(Continued)*
  endometrioid *(Continued)*
    unspecified site
      female C56.9
      male C61
  mucinous
    papillary
      specified site —*see* Neoplasm,
        malignant, by site
      unspecified site C56.9
    specified site —*see* Neoplasm, malignant,
      by site
    unspecified site C56.9
  papillary
    mucinous
      specified site —*see* Neoplasm,
        malignant, by site
      unspecified site C56.9
    pseudomucinous
      specified site —*see* Neoplasm,
        malignant, by site
      unspecified site C56.9
    serous
      specified site —*see* Neoplasm,
        malignant, by site
      unspecified site C56.9
    specified site —*see* Neoplasm, malignant,
      by site
    unspecified site C56.9
  pseudomucinous
    papillary
      specified site —*see* Neoplasm,
        malignant, by site
      unspecified site C56.9
    specified site —*see* Neoplasm, malignant,
      by site
    unspecified site C56.9
  serous
    papillary
      specified site —*see* Neoplasm,
        malignant, by site
      unspecified site C56.9
    specified site —*see* Neoplasm, malignant,
      by site
    unspecified site C56.9
Cystadenofibroma
  clear cell —*see* Neoplasm, benign, by site
  endometrioid D27.9
    borderline malignancy D39.1-
    malignant C56.-
  mucinous
    specified site —*see* Neoplasm, benign, by site
    unspecified site D27.9
  serous
    specified site —*see* Neoplasm, benign, by site
    unspecified site D27.9
  specified site —*see* Neoplasm, benign, by site
  unspecified site D27.9
Cystadenoma —*see also* Neoplasm, benign, by
    site
  bile duct D13.4
  endometrioid —*see* Neoplasm, benign, by site
    borderline malignancy —*see* Neoplasm,
      uncertain behavior, by site
  malignant —*see* Neoplasm, malignant,
    by site
  mucinous
    borderline malignancy
      ovary C56.-
      specified site NEC —*see* Neoplasm,
        uncertain behavior, by site
      unspecified site C56.9
    papillary
      borderline malignancy
        ovary C56.-
        specified site NEC —*see* Neoplasm,
          uncertain behavior, by site
        unspecified site C56.9
      specified site —*see* Neoplasm, benign,
        by site
      unspecified site D27.9

Cystadenoma *(Continued)*
  mucinous *(Continued)*
    specified site —*see* Neoplasm, benign, by
      site
    unspecified site D27.9
  papillary
    borderline malignancy
      ovary C56-
      specified site NEC —*see* Neoplasm,
        uncertain behavior, by site
      unspecified site C56.9
    lymphomatosum
      specified site —*see* Neoplasm, benign,
        by site
      unspecified site D11.9
    mucinous
      borderline malignancy
        ovary C56.-
        specified site NEC —*see* Neoplasm,
          uncertain behavior, by site
        unspecified site C56.9
      specified site —*see* Neoplasm, benign,
        by site
      unspecified site D27.9
    pseudomucinous
      borderline malignancy
        ovary C56.-
        specified site NEC —*see* Neoplasm,
          uncertain behavior, by site
        unspecified site C56.9
      specified site —*see* Neoplasm, benign,
        by site
      unspecified site D27.9
    serous
      borderline malignancy
        ovary C56.-
        specified site NEC —*see* Neoplasm,
          uncertain behavior, by site
        unspecified site C56.9
      specified site —*see* Neoplasm, benign,
        by site
      unspecified site D27.9
    specified site —*see* Neoplasm, benign, by
      site
    unspecified site D27.9
  pseudomucinous
    borderline malignancy
      ovary C56.-
      specified site NEC —*see* Neoplasm,
        uncertain behavior, by site
      unspecified site C56.9
    papillary
      borderline malignancy
        ovary C56.-
        specified site NEC —*see* Neoplasm,
          uncertain behavior, by site
        unspecified site C56.9
      specified site —*see* Neoplasm, benign,
        by site
      unspecified site D27.9
    specified site —*see* Neoplasm, benign, by
      site
    unspecified site D27.9
  serous
    borderline malignancy
      ovary C56.-
      specified site NEC —*see* Neoplasm,
        uncertain behavior, by site
      unspecified site C56.9
    papillary
      borderline malignancy
        ovary C56.-
        specified site NEC —*see* Neoplasm,
          uncertain behavior, by site
        unspecified site C56.9
      specified site —*see* Neoplasm, benign,
        by site
      unspecified site D27.9
    specified site —*see* Neoplasm, benign, by
      site
    unspecified site D27.9

Cystathionine synthase deficiency E72.11
Cystathioninemia E72.19
Cystathioninuria E72.19
Cystic —*see also* condition
  breast (chronic) —*see* Mastopathy, cystic
  corpora lutea (hemorrhagic) N83.1
  duct —*see* condition
  eyeball (congenital) Q11.0
  fibrosis —*see* Fibrosis, cystic
  kidney (congenital) Q61.9
    adult type Q61.2
    infantile type NEC Q61.19
      collecting duct dilatation Q61.11
    medullary Q61.5
  liver, congenital Q44.6
  lung disease J98.4
    congenital Q33.0
  mastitis, chronic —*see* Mastopathy, cystic
  medullary, kidney Q61.5
  meniscus —*see* Derangement, knee,
      meniscus, cystic
  ovary N83.20
Cysticercosis, cysticerciasis B69.9
  with
    epileptiform fits B69.0
    myositis B69.81
  brain B69.0
  central nervous system B69.0
  cerebral B69.0
  ocular B69.1
  specified NEC B69.89
Cysticercus cellulose infestation —*see*
      Cysticercosis
Cystinosis (malignant) E72.04
Cystinuria E72.01
Cystitis (exudative) (hemorrhagic) (septic)
      (suppurative) N30.90
  with
    fibrosis —*see* Cystitis, chronic, interstitial
    hematuria N30.91
    leukoplakia —*see* Cystitis, chronic,
        interstitial
    malakoplakia —*see* Cystitis, chronic,
        interstitial
    metaplasia —*see* Cystitis, chronic,
        interstitial
    prostatitis N41.3
  acute N30.00
    with hematuria N30.01
    of trigone N30.30
      with hematuria N30.31
  allergic —*see* Cystitis, specified type NEC
  amebic A06.81
  bilharzial B65.9 [*N33*]

Cystitis (*Continued*)
  blennorrhagic (gonococcal) A54.01
  bullous —*see* Cystitis, specified type NEC
  calculous N21.0
  chlamydial A56.01
  chronic N30.20
    with hematuria N30.21
    interstitial N30.10
      with hematuria N30.11
    of trigone N30.30
      with hematuria N30.31
    specified NEC N30.20
      with hematuria N30.21
  cystic (a) —*see* Cystitis, specified type NEC
  diphtheritic A36.85
  echinococcal
    granulosus B67.39
    multilocularis B67.69
  emphysematous —*see* Cystitis, specified type
      NEC
  encysted —*see* Cystitis, specified type NEC
  eosinophilic —*see* Cystitis, specified type
      NEC
  follicular —*see* Cystitis, of trigone
  gangrenous —*see* Cystitis, specified type NEC
  glandularis —*see* Cystitis, specified type NEC
  gonococcal A54.01
  incrusted —*see* Cystitis, specified type NEC
  interstitial (chronic) —*see* Cystitis, chronic,
      interstitial
  irradiation N30.40
    with hematuria N30.41
  irritation —*see* Cystitis, specified type NEC
  malignant —*see* Cystitis, specified type NEC
  of trigone N30.30
    with hematuria N30.31
  panmural —*see* Cystitis, chronic, interstitial
  polyposa —*see* Cystitis, specified type NEC
  prostatic N41.3
  puerperal (postpartum) O86.22
  radiation —*see* Cystitis, irradiation
  specified type NEC N30.80
    with hematuria N30.81
  subacute —*see* Cystitis, chronic
  submucous —*see* Cystitis, chronic, interstitial
  syphilitic (late) A52.76
  trichomonal A59.03
  tuberculous A18.12
  ulcerative —*see* Cystitis, chronic, interstitial
Cystocele (-urethrocele)
  female N81.10
    with prolapse of uterus —*see* Prolapse,
        uterus
    lateral N81.12

Cystocele (*Continued*)
  female (*Continued*)
    midline N81.11
    paravaginal N81.12
    in pregnancy or childbirth O34.8-
      causing obstructed labor O65.5
  male N32.89
Cystolithiasis N21.0
Cystoma —*see also* Neoplasm, benign, by site
  endometrial, ovary N80.1
  mucinous
    specified site —*see* Neoplasm, benign, by
        site
    unspecified site D27.9
  serous
    specified site —*see* Neoplasm, benign, by
        site
    unspecified site D27.9
  simple (ovary) N83.29
Cystoplegia N31.2
Cystoptosis N32.89
Cystopyelitis —*see* Pyelonephritis
Cystorrhagia N32.89
Cystosarcoma phyllodes D48.6-
  benign D24-
  malignant —*see* Neoplasm, breast, malignant
Cystostomy
  attention to Z43.5
  complication —*see* Complications,
      cystostomy
  status Z93.50
    appendico-vesicostomy Z93.52
    cutaneous Z93.51
    specified NEC Z93.59
Cystourethritis —*see* Urethritis
Cystourethrocele —*see also* Cystocele
  female N81.10
    with uterine prolapse —*see* Prolapse,
        uterus
    lateral N81.12
    midline N81.11
    paravaginal N81.12
  male N32.89
Cytomegalic inclusion disease
  congenital P35.1
Cytomegalovirus infection B25.9
Cytomycosis (reticuloendothelial) B39.4
Cytopenia D75.9
  refractory
    with multilineage dysplasia D46.A
      and ring sideroblasts (RCMD RS) D46.B
Czerny's disease (periodic hydrarthrosis of the
      knee) —*see* Effusion, joint, knee

D

Daae (-Finsen) disease (epidemic pleurodynia) B33.0
Dabney's grip B33.0
Da Costa's syndrome F45.8
Dacryoadenitis, dacryadenitis H04.00-
  acute H04.01-
  chronic H04.02-
Dacryocystitis H04.30-
  acute H04.32-
  chronic H04.41-
  neonatal P39.1
  phlegmonous H04.31-
  syphilitic A52.71
    congenital (early) A50.01
  trachomatous, active A71.1
    sequelae (late effect) B94.0
Dacryocystoblenorrhea —see Inflammation, lacrimal, passages, chronic
Dacryocystocele —see Disorder, lacrimal system, changes
Dacryolith, dacryolithiasis H04.51-
Dacryoma —see Disorder, lacrimal system, changes
Dacryopericystitis —see Dacryocystitis
Dacryops H04.11-
Dacryostenosis —see also Stenosis, lacrimal
  congenital Q10.5
Dactylitis
  bone —see Osteomyelitis
  sickle-cell D57.00
    Hb C D57.219
    Hb SS D57.00
    specified NEC D57.819
  skin L08.9
  syphilitic A52.77
  tuberculous A18.03
Dactylolysis spontanea (ainhum) L94.6
Dactylosymphysis Q70.9
  fingers —see Syndactylism, complex, fingers
  toes —see Syndactylism, complex, toes
Damage
  arteriosclerotic —see Arteriosclerosis
  brain (nontraumatic) G93.9
    anoxic, hypoxic G93.1
      resulting from a procedure G97.82
    child NEC G80.9
    due to birth injury P11.2
  cardiorenal (vascular) —see Hypertension, cardiorenal
  cerebral NEC —see Damage, brain
  coccyx, complicating delivery O71.6
  coronary —see Disease, heart, ischemic
  eye, birth injury P15.3
  liver (nontraumatic) K76.9
    alcoholic K70.9
    due to drugs —see Disease, liver, toxic
    toxic —see Disease, liver, toxic
  medication T88.7
  pelvic
    joint or ligament, during delivery O71.6
    organ NEC
      during delivery O71.5
      following ectopic or molar pregnancy O08.6
  renal —see Disease, renal
  subendocardium, subendocardial —see Degeneration, myocardial
  vascular I99.9
Dana-Putnam syndrome (subacute combined sclerosis with pernicious anemia) —see Degeneration, combined
Danbolt (-Cross) syndrome (acrodermatitis enteropathica) E83.2
Dandruff L21.0
Dandy-Walker syndrome Q03.1
  with spina bifida —see Spina bifida
Danlos' syndrome Q79.6

Darier (-White) disease (congenital) Q82.8
  meaning erythema annulare centrifugum L53.1
Darier-Roussy sarcoid D86.3
Darling's disease or histoplasmosis B39.4
Darwin's tubercle Q17.8
Dawson's (inclusion body) encephalitis A81.1
De Beurmann (-Gougerot) disease B42.1
De la Tourette's syndrome F95.2
De Lange's syndrome Q87.1
De Morgan's spots (senile angiomas) I78.1
De Quervain's
  disease (tendon sheath) M65.4
  syndrome E34.51
  thyroiditis (subacute granulomatous thyroiditis) E06.1
De Toni-Fanconi (-Debré) syndrome E72.09
  with cystinosis E72.04
Dead
  fetus, retained (mother) O36.4
    early pregnancy O02.1
  labyrinth —see subcategory H83.2
  ovum, retained O02.0
Deaf nonspeaking NEC H91.3
Deafmutism (acquired) (congenital) NEC H91.3
  hysterical F44.6
  syphilitic, congenital (see also subcategory H94.8) A50.09
Deafness (acquired) (complete) (hereditary) (partial) H91.9-
  with blue sclera and fragility of bone Q78.0
  auditory fatigue —see Deafness, specified type NEC
  aviation T70.0
    nerve injury —see Injury, nerve, acoustic, specified type NEC
  boilermaker's —see subcategory H83.3
  central —see Deafness, sensorineural
  conductive H90.2
    and sensorineural, mixed H90.8
      bilateral H90.6
    bilateral H90.0
    unilateral H90.1-
  congenital H90.5
    with blue sclera and fragility of bone Q78.0
  due to toxic agents —see Deafness, ototoxic
  emotional (hysterical) F44.6
  functional (hysterical) F44.6
  high frequency H91.9-
  hysterical F44.6
  low frequency H91.9-
  mental R48.8
  mixed conductive and sensorineural H90.8
    bilateral H90.6
    unilateral H90.7-
  nerve —see Deafness, sensorineural
  neural —see Deafness, sensorineural
  noise-induced —see also subcategory H83.3
    nerve injury —see Injury, nerve, acoustic, specified type NEC
  nonspeaking H91.3
  ototoxic —see subcategory H91.0
  perceptive —see Deafness, sensorineural
  psychogenic (hysterical) F44.6
  sensorineural H90.5
    and conductive, mixed H90.8
      bilateral H90.6
    bilateral H90.3
    unilateral H90.4-
  sensory —see Deafness, sensorineural
  specified type NEC —see subcategory H91.8
  sudden (idiopathic) H91.2-
  syphilitic A52.15
  transient ischemic H93.01-
  traumatic —see Injury, nerve, acoustic, specified type NEC
  word (developmental) H93.25

Death (cause unknown) (of) (unexplained) (unspecified cause) R99
  brain G93.82
  cardiac (sudden) (with successful resuscitation) — code to underlying disease
    family history of Z82.41
    personal history of Z86.74
  family member (assumed) Z63.4
Debility (chronic) (general) (nervous) R53.81
  congenital or neonatal NOS P96.9
  nervous R53.81
  old age R54
  senile R54
Débove's disease (splenomegaly) R16.1
Decalcification
  bone —see Osteoporosis
  teeth K03.89
Decapsulation, kidney N28.89
Decay
  dental —see Caries, dental
  senile R54
  tooth, teeth —see Caries, dental
Deciduitis (acute)
  following ectopic or molar pregnancy O08.0
Decline (general) —see Debility
  cognitive, age-associated R41.81
Decompensation
  cardiac (acute) (chronic) —see Disease, heart
  cardiovascular —see Disease, cardiovascular
  heart —see Disease, heart
  hepatic —see Failure, hepatic
  myocardial (acute) (chronic) —see Disease, heart
  respiratory J98.8
Decompression sickness T70.3
Decrease (d)
  absolute neutrophile count —see Neutropenia
  blood
    platelets —see Thrombocytopenia
    pressure R03.1
      due to shock following
        injury T79.4
        operation T81.19
  estrogen E28.39
    postablative E89.40
      asymptomatic E89.40
      symptomatic E89.41
  fragility of erythrocytes D58.8
  function
    lipase (pancreatic) K90.3
    ovary in hypopituitarism E23.0
    parenchyma of pancreas K86.8
    pituitary (gland) (anterior) (lobe) E23.0
      posterior (lobe) E23.0
  functional activity R68.89
  glucose R73.09
  hematocrit R71.0
  hemoglobin R71.0
  leukocytes D72.819
    specified NEC D72.818
  libido R68.82
  lymphocytes D72.810
  platelets D69.6
  respiration, due to shock following injury T79.4
  sexual desire R68.82
  tear secretion NEC —see Syndrome, dry eye
  tolerance
    fat K90.4
    glucose R73.09
    pancreatic K90.3
    salt and water E87.8
  vision NEC H54.7
  white blood cell count D72.819
    specified NEC D72.818
Decubitus (ulcer) —see Ulcer, pressure, by site
  cervix N86
Deepening acetabulum —see Derangement, joint, specified type NEC, hip

◀ New ◀▦ Revised ~~deleted~~ Deleted

Defect, defective Q89.9
 3-beta-hydroxysteroid dehydrogenase E25.0
 11-hydroxylase E25.0
 21-hydroxylase E25.0
 abdominal wall, congenital Q79.59
 antibody immunodeficiency D80.9
 aorticopulmonary septum Q21.4
 atrial septal (ostium secundum type) Q21.1
  following acute myocardial infarction
    (current complication) I23.1
  ostium primum type Q21.2
 atrioventricular
  canal Q21.2
  septum Q21.2
 auricular septal Q21.1
 bilirubin excretion NEC E80.6
 biosynthesis, androgen (testicular) E29.1
 bulbar septum Q21.0
 catalase E80.3
 cell membrane receptor complex (CR3) D71
 circulation I99.9
  congenital Q28.9
  newborn Q28.9
 coagulation (factor) (see also Deficiency,
    factor) D68.9
  with
   ectopic pregnancy O08.1
   molar pregnancy O08.1
  acquired D68.4
  antepartum with hemorrhage —see
    Hemorrhage, antepartum, with
    coagulation defect
  due to
   liver disease D68.4
   vitamin K deficiency D68.4
  hereditary NEC D68.2
  intrapartum O67.0
  newborn, transient P61.6
  postpartum O72.3
  specified type NEC D68.8
 complement system D84.1
 conduction (heart) I45.9
  bone —see Deafness, conductive
 congenital, organ or site not listed —see
    Anomaly, by site
 coronary sinus Q21.1
 cushion, endocardial Q21.2
 degradation, glycoprotein E77.1
 dental bridge, crown, fillings —see Defect,
    dental restoration
 dental restoration K08.50
  specified NEC K08.59
 dentin (hereditary) K00.5
 Descemet's membrane, congenital Q13.89
 developmental —see also Anomaly
  cauda equina Q06.3
 diaphragm
  with elevation, eventration or hernia —see
    Hernia, diaphragm ◀▥
  congenital Q79.1
   with hernia Q79.0
   gross (with hernia) Q79.0
 ectodermal, congenital Q82.9
 Eisenmenger's Q21.8
 enzyme
  catalase E80.3
  peroxidase E80.3
 esophagus, congenital Q39.9
 extensor retinaculum M62.89
 fibrin polymerization D68.2
 filling
  bladder R93.4
  kidney R93.4
  stomach R93.3
  ureter R93.4
 Gerbode Q21.0
 glycoprotein degradation E77.1
 Hageman (factor) D68.2
 hearing —see Deafness
 high grade F70
 interatrial septal Q21.1

Defect, defective (Continued)
 interauricular septal Q21.1
 interventricular septal Q21.0
  with dextroposition of aorta, pulmonary
    stenosis and hypertrophy of right
    ventricle Q21.3
  in tetralogy of Fallot Q21.3
 learning (specific) —see Disorder, learning
 lymphocyte function antigen-1 (LFA-1) D84.0
 lysosomal enzyme, post-translational
    modification E77.0
 major osseous M89.70
  ankle M89.77-
  carpus M89.74-
  clavicle M89.71-
  femur M89.75-
  fibula M89.76-
  fingers M89.74-
  foot M89.77-
  forearm M89.73-
  hand M89.74-
  humerus M89.72-
  lower leg M89.76-
  metacarpus M89.74-
  metatarsus M89.77-
  multiple sites M89.79
  pelvic region M89.75-
  pelvis M89.75-
  radius M89.73-
  scapula M89.71-
  shoulder region M89.71-
  specified NEC M89.78
  tarsus M89.77-
  thigh M89.75-
  tibia M89.76-
  toes M89.77-
  ulna M89.73-
 mental —see Disability, intellectual
 modification, lysosomal enzymes, post-
    translational E77.0
 obstructive, congenital
  renal pelvis Q62.39
  ureter Q62.39
   atresia —see Atresia, ureter
   cecoureterocele Q62.32
   megaureter Q62.2
   orthotopic ureterocele Q62.31
 osseous, major M89.70
  ankle M89.77-
  carpus M89.74-
  clavicle M89.71-
  femur M89.75-
  fibula M89.76-
  fingers M89.74-
  foot M89.77-
  forearm M89.73-
  hand M89.74-
  humerus M89.72-
  lower leg M89.76-
  metacarpus M89.74-
  metatarsus M89.77-
  multiple sites M89.9
  pelvic region M89.75-
  pelvis M89.75-
  radius M89.73-
  scapula M89.71-
  shoulder region M89.71-
  specified NEC M89.78
  tarsus M89.77-
  thigh M89.75-
  tibia M89.76-
  toes M89.77-
  ulna M89.73-
 osteochondral NEC (see also Deformity)
    M95.8-
 ostium
  primum Q21.2
  secundum Q21.1
 peroxidase E80.3
 placental blood supply —see Insufficiency,
    placental

Defect, defective (Continued)
 platelets, qualitative D69.1
  constitutional D68.0
 postural NEC, spine —see Dorsopathy,
    deforming
 reduction
  limb Q73.8
   lower Q72.9-
    absence —see Agenesis, leg
     foot —see Agenesis, foot
    longitudinal
     femur Q72.4-
     fibula Q72.6-
     tibia Q72.5-
     specified type NEC Q72.89-
    split foot Q72.7-
    specified type NEC Q73.8
   upper Q71.9-
    absence —see Agenesis, arm
     forearm —see Agenesis, forearm
     hand —see Agenesis, hand
    lobster-claw hand Q71.6-
    longitudinal
     radius Q71.4-
     ulna Q71.5-
    specified type NEC Q71.89-
  renal pelvis Q63.8
   obstructive Q62.39
  respiratory system, congenital Q34.9
  restoration, dental K08.50
   specified NEC K08.59
  retinal nerve bundle fibers H35.89
  septal (heart) NOS Q21.9
   acquired (atrial) (auricular) (ventricular)
     (old) I51.0
   atrial Q21.1
    concurrent with acute myocardial
      infarction —see Infarct,
      myocardium
    following acute myocardial infarction
      (current complication) I23.1
   ventricular (see also Defect, ventricular
     septal) Q21.0
  sinus venosus Q21.1
  speech R47.9
   developmental F80.9
   specified NEC R47.89
  Taussig-Bing (aortic transposition and
    overriding pulmonary artery) Q20.1
  teeth, wedge K03.1
  vascular (local) I99.9
   congenital Q27.9
  ventricular septal Q21.0
   concurrent with acute myocardial
     infarction —see Infarct, myocardium
   following acute myocardial infarction
     (current complication) I23.2
   in tetralogy of Fallot Q21.3
  vision NEC H54.7
  visual field H53.40
   bilateral
    heteronymous H53.47
    homonymous H53.46-
   generalized contraction H53.48-
   localized
    arcuate H53.43-
    scotoma (central area) H53.41-
     blind spot area H53.42-
    sector H53.43-
    specified type NEC H53.45-
  voice R49.9
   specified NEC R49.8
  wedge, tooth, teeth (abrasion) K03.1
Deferentitis N49.1
 gonorrheal (acute) (chronic) A54.23
Defibrination (syndrome) D65
 antepartum —see Hemorrhage, antepartum,
    with coagulation defect, disseminated
    intravascular coagulation
 following ectopic or molar pregnancy O08.1
 intrapartum O67.0

Defibrination (Continued)
  newborn P60
  postpartum O72.3
Deficiency, deficient
  3-beta hydroxysteroid dehydrogenase E25.0
  11-hydroxylase E25.0
  21-hydroxylase E25.0
  5-alpha reductase (with male
    pseudohermaphroditism) E29.1
  abdominal muscle syndrome Q79.4
  AC globulin (congenital) (hereditary) D68.2
    acquired D68.4
  accelerator globulin (Ac G) (blood) D68.2
  acid phosphatase E83.39
  activating factor (blood) D68.2
  adenosine deaminase (ADA) D81.3
  aldolase (hereditary) E74.19
  alpha-1-antitrypsin E88.01
  amino-acids E72.9
  anemia —see Anemia
  aneurin E51.9
  antibody with
    hyperimmunoglobulinemia D80.6
    near-normal immunoglobins D80.6
  antidiuretic hormone E23.2
  anti-hemophilic
    factor (A) D66
      B D67
      C D68.1
    globulin (AHG) NEC D66
  antithrombin (antithrombin III) D68.59
  ascorbic acid E54
  attention (disorder) (syndrome) F98.8
    with hyperactivity —see Disorder,
      attention-deficit hyperactivity
  autoprothrombin
    I D68.2
    II D67
    C D68.2
  beta-glucuronidase E76.29
  biotin E53.8
  biotin-dependent carboxylase D81.819
  biotinidase D81.810
  brancher enzyme (amylopectinosis) E74.03
  C1 esterase inhibitor (C1-INH) D84.1
  calciferol E55.9
    with
      adult osteomalacia M83.8
      rickets —see Rickets
  calcium (dietary) E58
  calorie, severe E43
    with marasmus E41
      and kwashiorkor E42
  cardiac —see Insufficiency, myocardial
  carnitine E71.40
    due to
      hemodialysis E71.43
      inborn errors of metabolism E71.42
      Valproic acid therapy E71.43
    iatrogenic E71.43
    muscle palmityltransferase E71.314
    primary E71.41
    secondary E71.448
  carotene E50.9
  central nervous system G96.8
  ceruloplasmin (Wilson) E83.01
  choline E53.8
  Christmas factor D67
  chromium E61.4
  clotting (blood) (see also Deficiency,
    coagulation factor) D68.9
  clotting factor NEC (hereditary) (see also
    Deficiency, factor) D68.2
  coagulation NOS D68.9
    with
      ectopic pregnancy O08.1
      molar pregnancy O08.1
    acquired (any) D68.4
    antepartum hemorrhage —see
      Hemorrhage, antepartum, with
      coagulation defect

Deficiency, deficient (Continued)
  coagulation NOS (Continued)
    clotting factor NEC (see also Deficiency,
      factor) D68.2
    due to
      hyperprothrombinemia D68.4
      liver disease D68.4
      vitamin K deficiency D68.4
    newborn, transient P61.6
    postpartum O72.3
    specified NEC D68.8
  cognitive F09
  color vision H53.50
    achromatopsia H53.51
    acquired H53.52
    deuteranomaly H53.53
    protanomaly H53.54
    specified type NEC H53.59
    tritanomaly H53.55
  combined glucocorticoid and
    mineralocorticoid E27.49
  contact factor D68.2
  copper (nutritional) E61.0
  corticoadrenal E27.40
    primary E27.1
  craniofacial axis Q75.0
  cyanocobalamin E53.8
  debrancher enzyme (limit dextrinosis) E74.03
  dehydrogenase
    long chain/very long chain acyl CoA
      E71.310
    medium chain acyl CoA E71.311
    short chain acyl CoA E71.312
  diet E63.9
  dihydropyrimidine dehydrogenase (DPD)
    E88.89
  disaccharidase E73.9
  edema —see Malnutrition, severe
  endocrine E34.9
  energy-supply —see Malnutrition
  enzymes, circulating NEC E88.09
  ergosterol E55.9
    with
      adult osteomalacia M83.8
      rickets —see Rickets
  essential fatty acid (EFA) E63.0
  factor —see also Deficiency, coagulation
    Hageman D68.2
    I (congenital) (hereditary) D68.2
    II (congenital) (hereditary) D68.2
    IX (congenital) (functional) (hereditary)
      (with functional defect) D67
    multiple (congenital) D68.8
      acquired D68.4
    V (congenital) (hereditary) D68.2
    VII (congenital) (hereditary) D68.2
    VIII (congenital) (functional) (hereditary)
      (with functional defect) D66
      with vascular defect D68.0
    X (congenital) (hereditary) D68.2
    XI (congenital) (hereditary) D68.1
    XII (congenital) (hereditary) D68.2
    XIII (congenital) (hereditary) D68.2
  femoral, proximal focal (congenital) —
    see Defect, reduction, lower limb,
    longitudinal, femur
  fibrin-stabilizing factor (congenital)
    (hereditary) D68.2
    acquired D68.4
  fibrinase D68.2
  fibrinogen (congenital) (hereditary) D68.2
    acquired D65
  folate E53.8
  folic acid E53.8
  foreskin N47.3
  fructokinase E74.11
  fructose 1,6-diphosphatase E74.19
  fructose-1-phosphate aldolase E74.19
  galactokinase E74.29
  galactose-1-phosphate uridyl transferase
    E74.29

Deficiency, deficient (Continued)
  gammaglobulin in blood D80.1
    hereditary D80.0
  glass factor D68.2
  glucocorticoid E27.49
    mineralocorticoid E27.49
  glucose-6-phosphatase E74.01
  glucose-6-phosphate dehydrogenase anemia
    D55.0
  glucuronyl transferase E80.5
  glycogen synthetase E74.09
  gonadotropin (isolated) E23.0
  growth hormone (idiopathic) (isolated) E23.0
  Hageman factor D68.2
  hemoglobin D64.9
  hepatophosphorylase E74.09
  homogentisate 1,2-dioxygenase E70.29
  hormone
    anterior pituitary (partial) NEC E23.0
      growth E23.0
    growth (isolated) E23.0
    pituitary E23.0
    testicular E29.1
  hypoxanthine-(guanine)-
    phosphoribosyltransferase (HG-PRT)
    (total HG-PRT) E79.1
  immunity D84.9
    cell-mediated D84.8
      with thrombocytopenia and eczema
        D82.0
    combined D81.9
    humoral D80.9
    IgA (secretory) D80.2
    IgG D80.3
    IgM D80.4
  immuno —see Immunodeficiency
  immunoglobulin, selective
    A (IgA) D80.2
    G (IgG) (subclasses) D80.3
    M (IgM) D80.4
  inositol (B complex) E53.8
  intrinsic
    factor (congenital) D51.0
    sphincter N36.42
      with urethral hypermobility N36.43
  iodine E61.8
    congenital syndrome —see Syndrome,
      iodine-deficiency, congenital
  iron E61.1
    anemia D50.9
  kalium E87.6
  kappa-light chain D80.8
  labile factor (congenital) (hereditary) D68.2
    acquired D68.4
  lacrimal fluid (acquired) —see also Syndrome,
    dry eye
    congenital Q10.6
  lactase
    congenital E73.0
    secondary E73.1
  Laki-Lorand factor D68.2
  lecithin cholesterol acyltransferase E78.6
  lipocaic K86.8
  lipoprotein (familial) (high density) E78.6
  liver phosphorylase E74.09
  lysosomal alpha-1, 4 glucosidase E74.02
  magnesium E61.2
  major histocompatibility complex
    class I D81.6
    class II D81.7
  manganese E61.3
  menadione (vitamin K) E56.1
    newborn P53
  mental (familial) (hereditary) —see Disability,
    intellectual
  methylenetetrahydrofolate reductase
    (MTHFR) E72.12
  mineral NEC E61.8
  mineralocorticoid E27.49
    with glucocorticoid E27.49
  molybdenum (nutritional) E61.5

◀ New   ⬅ Revised   ~~deleted~~ Deleted

Deficiency, deficient *(Continued)*
moral F60.2
multiple nutrient elements E61.7
muscle
 carnitine (palmityltransferase) E71.314
 phosphofructokinase E74.09
myoadenylate deaminase E79.2
myocardial —*see* Insufficiency, myocardial
myophosphorylase E74.04
NADH diaphorase or reductase (congenital) D74.0
NADH-methemoglobin reductase (congenital) D74.0
natrium E87.1
niacin (amide) (-tryptophan) E52
nicotinamide E52
nicotinic acid E52
number of teeth —*see* Anodontia
nutrient element E61.9
 multiple E61.7
 specified NEC E61.8
nutrition, nutritional E63.9
 sequelae —*see* Sequelae, nutritional deficiency
 specified NEC E63.8
ornithine transcarbamylase E72.4
ovarian E28.39
oxygen —*see* Anoxia
pantothenic acid E53.8
parathyroid (gland) E20.9
perineum (female) N81.89
phenylalanine hydroxylase E70.1
phosphoenolpyruvate carboxykinase E74.4
phosphofructokinase E74.19
phosphomannomutase E74.8
phosphomannose isomerase E74.8
phosphomannosyl mutase E74.8
phosphorylase kinase, liver E74.09
pituitary hormone (isolated) E23.0
plasma thromboplastin
 antecedent (PTA) D68.1
 component (PTC) D67
platelet NEC D69.1
 constitutional D68.0
polyglandular E31.8
 autoimmune E31.0
potassium (K) E87.6
prepuce N47.3
proaccelerin (congenital) (hereditary) D68.2
 acquired D68.4
proconvertin factor (congenital) (hereditary) D68.2
 acquired D68.4
protein (*see also* Malnutrition) E46
 anemia D53.0
 C D68.59
 S D68.59
prothrombin (congenital) (heredItary) D68.2
 acquired D68.4
Prower factor D68.2
pseudocholinesterase E88.09
PTA (plasma thromboplastin antecedent) D68.1
PTC (plasma thromboplastin component) D67
purine nucleoside phosphorylase (PNP) D81.5
pyracin (alpha) (beta) E53.1
pyridoxal E53.1
pyridoxamine E53.1
pyridoxine (derivatives) E53.1
pyruvate
 carboxylase E74.4
 dehydrogenase E74.4
riboflavin (vitamin B2) E53.0
salt E87.1
secretion
 ovary E28.39
 salivary gland (any) K11.7
 urine R34
selenium (dietary) E59
serum antitrypsin, familial E88.01

Deficiency, deficient *(Continued)*
short stature homeobox gene (SHOX)
 with
  dyschondrosteosis Q78.8
  short stature (idiopathic) E34.3
  Turner's syndrome Q96.9
sodium (Na) E87.1
SPCA (factor VII) D68.2
sphincter, intrinsic N36.42
 with urethral hypermobility N36.43
stable factor (congenital) (hereditary) D68.2
 acquired D68.4
Stuart-Prower (factor X) D68.2
sucrase E74.39
sulfatase E75.29
sulfite oxidase E72.19
thiamin, thiaminic (chloride) E51.9
 beriberi (dry) E51.11
  wet E51.12
thrombokinase D68.2
 newborn P53
thyroid (gland) —*see* Hypothyroidism
tocopherol E56.0
tooth bud K00.0
transcobalamine II (anemia) D51.2
vanadium E61.6
vascular I99.9
vasopressin E23.2
viosterol —*see* Deficiency, calciferol
vitamin (multiple) NOS E56.9
 A E50.9
  with
   Bitot's spot (corneal) E50.1
   follicular keratosis E50.8
   keratomalacia E50.4
   manifestations NEC E50.8
   night blindness E50.5
   scar of cornea, xerophthalmic E50.6
   xeroderma E50.8
   xerophthalmia E50.7
   xerosis
    conjunctival E50.0
     and Bitot's spot E50.1
    cornea E50.2
     and ulceration E50.3
  sequelae E64.1
 B (complex) NOS E53.9
  with
   beriberi (dry) E51.11
    wet E51.12
   pellagra E52
 B1 NOS E51.9
  beriberi (dry) E51.11
   with circulatory system manifestations E51.11
   wet E51.12
 B12 E53.8
 B2 (riboflavin) E53.0
 B6 E53.1
 C E54
  sequelae E64.2
 D E55.9
  with
   adult osteomalacia M83.8
   rickets —*see* Rickets
  25-hydroxylase E83.32
 E E56.0
 folic acid E53.8
 G E53.0
 group B E53.9
  specified NEC E53.8
 H (biotin) E53.8
 K E56.1
  of newborn P53
 nicotinic E52
 P E56.8
 PP (pellagra-preventing) E52
 specified NEC E56.8
 thiamin E51.9
  beriberi —*see* Beriberi
zinc, dietary E60

Deficit —*see also* Deficiency
attention and concentration R41.840
 disorder —*see* Attention, deficit
cognitive communication R41.841
cognitive NEC R41.89
 following
  cerebral infarction I69.31
  cerebrovascular disease I69.91
   specified disease NEC I69.81
  intracerebral hemorrhage I69.11
  nontraumatic intracranial hemorrhage NEC I69.21
  subarachnoid hemorrhage I69.01
concentration R41.840
executive function R41.844
frontal lobe R41.844
neurologic NEC R29.818
 ischemic
  reversible (RIND) I63.9
  prolonged (PRIND) I63.9
oxygen R09.02
prolonged reversible ischemic neurologic (PRIND) I63.9
psychomotor R41.843
visuospatial R41.842

Deflection
radius —*see* Deformity, limb, specified type NEC, forearm
septum (acquired) (nasal) (nose) J34.2
spine —*see* Curvature, spine
turbinate (nose) J34.2

Defluvium
capillorum —*see* Alopecia
ciliorum —*see* Madarosis
unguium L60.8

Deformity Q89.9
abdomen, congenital Q89.9
abdominal wall
 acquired M95.8
 congenital Q79.59
acquired (unspecified site) M95.9
adrenal gland Q89.1
alimentary tract, congenital Q45.9
 upper Q40.9
ankle (joint) (acquired) —*see also* Deformity, limb, lower leg
 abduction —*see* Contraction, joint, ankle
 congenital Q68.8
 contraction —*see* Contraction, joint, ankle
 specified type NEC —*see* Deformity, limb, foot, specified NEC
anus (acquired) K62.89
 congenital Q43.9
aorta (arch) (congenital) Q25.4
 acquired I77.89
aortic
 arch, acquired I77.89
 cusp or valve (congenital) Q23.8
  acquired (*see also* Endocarditis, aortic) I35.8
arm (acquired) (upper) —*see also* Deformity, limb, upper arm
 congenital Q68.8
 forearm —*see* Deformity, limb, forearm
artery (congenital) (peripheral) NOS Q27.9
 acquired I77.89
 coronary (acquired) I25.9
  congenital Q24.5
 umbilical Q27.0
atrial septal Q21.1
auditory canal (external) (congenital) —*see also* Malformation, ear, external
 acquired —*see* Disorder, ear, external, specified type NEC
auricle
 ear (congenital) —*see also* Malformation, ear, external
  acquired —*see* Disorder, pinna, deformity
back —*see* Dorsopathy, deforming

Deformity *(Continued)*
bile duct (common) (congenital) (hepatic) Q44.5
  acquired K83.8
biliary duct or passage (congenital) Q44.5
  acquired K83.8
bladder (neck) (trigone) (sphincter) (acquired) N32.89
  congenital Q64.79
bone (acquired) NOS M95.9
  congenital Q79.9
  turbinate M95.0
brain (congenital) Q04.9
  acquired G93.89
  reduction Q04.3
breast (acquired) N64.89
  congenital Q83.9
  reconstructed N65.0
bronchus (congenital) Q32.4
  acquired NEC J98.09
bursa, congenital Q79.9
canaliculi (lacrimalis) (acquired) —*see also* Disorder, lacrimal system, changes
  congenital Q10.6
canthus, acquired —*see* Disorder, eyelid, specified type NEC
capillary (acquired) I78.8
cardiovascular system, congenital Q28.9
caruncle, lacrimal (acquired) —*see also* Disorder, lacrimal system, changes
  congenital Q10.6
cascade, stomach K31.2
cecum (congenital) Q43.9
  acquired K63.89
cerebral, acquired G93.89
  congenital Q04.9
cervix (uterus) (acquired) NEC N88.8
  congenital Q51.9
cheek (acquired) M95.2
  congenital Q18.9
chest (acquired) (wall) M95.4
  congenital Q67.8
  sequelae (late effect) of rickets E64.3
chin (acquired) M95.2
  congenital Q18.9
choroid (congenital) Q14.3
  acquired H31.8
  plexus Q07.8
    acquired G96.19
cicatricial —*see* Cicatrix
cilia, acquired —*see* Disorder, eyelid, specified type NEC
clavicle (acquired) M95.8
  congenital Q68.8
clitoris (congenital) Q52.6
  acquired N90.89
clubfoot —*see* Clubfoot
coccyx (acquired) —*see* subcategory M43.8
colon (congenital) Q43.9
  acquired K63.89
concha (ear), congenital —*see also* Malformation, ear, external
  acquired —*see* Disorder, pinna, deformity
cornea (acquired) H18.70
  congenital Q13.4
  descemetocele —*see* Descemetocele
  ectasia —*see* Ectasia, cornea
  specified NEC H18.79-
  staphyloma —*see* Staphyloma, cornea
coronary artery (acquired) I25.9
  congenital Q24.5
cranium (acquired) —*see* Deformity, skull
cricoid cartilage (congenital) Q31.8
  acquired J38.7
cystic duct (congenital) Q44.5
  acquired K82.8
Dandy-Walker Q03.1
  with spina bifida —*see* Spina bifida
diaphragm (congenital) Q79.1
  acquired J98.6
digestive organ NOS Q45.9

Deformity *(Continued)*
ductus arteriosus Q25.0
duodenal bulb K31.89
duodenum (congenital) Q43.9
  acquired K31.89
dura —*see* Deformity, meninges
ear (acquired) —*see also* Disorder, pinna, deformity
  congenital (external) Q17.9
    internal Q16.5
    middle Q16.4
      ossicles Q16.3
    ossicles Q16.3
ectodermal (congenital) NEC Q84.9
ejaculatory duct (congenital) Q55.4
  acquired N50.8
elbow (joint) (acquired) —*see also* Deformity, limb, upper arm
  congenital Q68.8
  contraction —*see* Contraction, joint, elbow
endocrine gland NEC Q89.2
epididymis (congenital) Q55.4
  acquired N50.8 ◄▥
epiglottis (congenital) Q31.8
  acquired J38.7
esophagus (congenital) Q39.9
  acquired K22.8
eustachian tube (congenital) NEC Q17.8
eye, congenital Q15.9
eyebrow (congenital) Q18.8
eyelid (acquired) —*see also* Disorder, eyelid, specified type NEC
  congenital Q10.3
face (acquired) M95.2
  congenital Q18.9
fallopian tube, acquired N83.8
femur (acquired) —*see* Deformity, limb, specified type NEC, thigh
fetal
  with fetopelvic disproportion O33.7
  causing obstructed labor O66.3
finger (acquired) M20.00-
  boutonniere M20.02-
  congenital Q68.1
  flexion contracture —*see* Contraction, joint, hand
  mallet finger M20.01-
  specified NEC M20.09-
  swan-neck M20.03-
flexion (joint) (acquired) (*see also* Deformity, limb, flexion) M21.20
  congenital NOS Q74.9
  hip Q65.89
foot (acquired) —*see also* Deformity, limb, lower leg
  cavovarus (congenital) Q66.1
  congenital NOS Q66.9
    specified type NEC Q66.89
  specified type NEC —*see* Deformity, limb, foot, specified NEC
  valgus (congenital) Q66.6
    acquired —*see* Deformity, valgus, ankle
  varus (congenital) NEC Q66.3
    acquired —*see* Deformity, varus, ankle
forearm (acquired) —*see also* Deformity, limb, forearm
  congenital Q68.8
forehead (acquired) M95.2
  congenital Q75.8
frontal bone (acquired) M95.2
  congenital Q75.8
gallbladder (congenital) Q44.1
  acquired K82.8
gastrointestinal tract (congenital) NOS Q45.9
  acquired K63.89
genitalia, genital organ (s) or system NEC
  female (congenital) Q52.9
    acquired N94.89
    external Q52.70
  male (congenital) Q55.9
    acquired N50.8

Deformity *(Continued)*
globe (eye) (congenital) Q15.8
  acquired H44.89
gum, acquired NEC K06.8
hand (acquired) —*see* Deformity, limb, hand
  congenital Q68.1
head (acquired) M95.2
  congenital Q75.8
heart (congenital) Q24.9
  septum Q21.9
    auricular Q21.1
    ventricular Q21.0
  valve (congenital) NEC Q24.8
    acquired —*see* Endocarditis
heel (acquired) —*see* Deformity, foot
hepatic duct (congenital) Q44.5
  acquired K83.8
hip (joint) (acquired) —*see also* Deformity, limb, thigh
  congenital Q65.9
  due to (previous) juvenile osteochondrosis —*see* Coxa, plana
  flexion —*see* Contraction, joint, hip
hourglass —*see* Contraction, hourglass
humerus (acquired) M21.82-
  congenital Q74.0
hypophyseal (congenital) Q89.2
ileocecal (coil) (valve) (acquired) K63.89
  congenital Q43.9
ileum (congenital) Q43.9
  acquired K63.89
ilium (acquired) M95.5
  congenital Q74.2
integument (congenital) Q84.9
intervertebral cartilage or disc (acquired) — *see* Disorder, disc, specified NEC ◄▥
intestine (large) (small) (congenital) NOS Q43.9
  acquired K63.89
intrinsic minus or plus (hand) —*see* Deformity, limb, specified type NEC, forearm
iris (acquired) H21.89
  congenital Q13.2
ischium (acquired) M95.5
  congenital Q74.2
jaw (acquired) (congenital) M26.9
joint (acquired) NEC M21.90
  congenital Q68.8
  elbow M21.92-
  hand M21.94-
  hip M21.95-
  knee M21.96-
  shoulder M21.92-
  wrist M21.93-
kidney (s) (calyx) (pelvis) (congenital) Q63.9
  acquired N28.89
  artery (congenital) Q27.2
    acquired I77.89
Klippel-Feil (brevicollis) Q76.1
knee (acquired) NEC —*see also* Deformity, limb, lower leg
  congenital Q68.2
labium (majus) (minus) (congenital) Q52.79
  acquired N90.89
lacrimal passages or duct (congenital) NEC Q10.6
  acquired —*see* Disorder, lacrimal system, changes
larynx (muscle) (congenital) Q31.8
  acquired J38.7
  web (glottic) Q31.0
leg (upper) (acquired) NEC —*see also* Deformity, limb, thigh
  congenital Q68.8
  lower leg —*see* Deformity, limb, lower leg
lens (acquired) H27.8
  congenital Q12.9
lid (fold) (acquired) —*see also* Disorder, eyelid, specified type NEC
  congenital Q10.3

◄ New   ◄▥ Revised   ~~deleted~~ Deleted

Deformity (Continued)

ligament (acquired) —see Disorder, ligament
   congenital Q79.9
limb (acquired) M21.90
   clawfoot M21.53-
   clawhand M21.51-
   clubfoot M21.54-
   clubhand M21.52-
   congenital, except reduction deformity
      Q74.9
   flat foot M21.4-
   flexion M21.20
      ankle M21.27-
      elbow M21.22-
      finger M21.24-
      hip M21.25-
      knee M21.26-
      shoulder M21.21-
      toe M21.27-
      wrist M21.23-
   foot
      claw —see Deformity, limb, clawfoot
      club —see Deformity, limb, clubfoot
      drop M21.37-
      flat —see Deformity, limb, flat foot
      specified NEC M21.6X-
   forearm M21.93-
   hand M21.94-
   lower leg M21.96-
   specified type NEC M21.80
      forearm M21.83-
      lower leg M21.86-
      thigh M21.85-
      upper arm M21.82-
   thigh M21.95-
   unequal length M21.70
      short site is
         femur M21.75-
         fibula M21.76-
         humerus M21.72-
         radius M21.73-
         tibia M21.76-
         ulna M21.73-
   upper arm M21.92-
   valgus —see Deformity, valgus
   varus —see Deformity, varus
   wrist drop M21.33-
lip (acquired) NEC K13.0
   congenital Q38.0
liver (congenital) Q44.7
   acquired K76.89
lumbosacral (congenital) (joint) (region)
      Q76.49
   acquired —see subcategory M43.8
   kyphosis —see Kyphosis, congenital
   lordosis —see Lordosis, congenital
lung (congenital) Q33.9
   acquired J98.4
lymphatic system, congenital Q89.9
Madelung's (radius) Q74.0
mandible (acquired) (congenital) M26.9
maxilla (acquired) (congenital) M26.9
meninges or membrane (congenital) Q07.9
   cerebral Q04.8
      acquired G96.19
   spinal cord (congenital) G96.19
      acquired G96.19
metacarpus (acquired) —see Deformity, limb,
      forearm
   congenital Q74.0
metatarsus (acquired) —see Deformity,
      foot
   congenital Q66.9
middle ear (congenital) Q16.4
   ossicles Q16.3
mitral (leaflets) (valve) I05.8
   parachute Q23.2
   stenosis, congenital Q23.2
mouth (acquired) K13.79
   congenital Q38.6
multiple, congenital NEC Q89.7

Deformity (Continued)

muscle (acquired) M62.89
   congenital Q79.9
   sternocleidomastoid Q68.0
musculoskeletal system (acquired) M95.9
   congenital Q79.9
   specified NEC M95.8
nail (acquired) L60.8
   congenital Q84.6
nasal —see Deformity, nose
neck (acquired) M95.3
   congenital Q18.9
   sternocleidomastoid Q68.0
nervous system (congenital) Q07.9
nipple (congenital) Q83.9
   acquired N64.89
nose (acquired) (cartilage) M95.0
   bone (turbinate) M95.0
   congenital Q30.9
      bent or squashed Q67.4
   saddle M95.0
      syphilitic A50.57
   septum (acquired) J34.2
      congenital Q30.8
   sinus (wall) (congenital) Q30.8
      acquired M95.0
   syphilitic (congenital) A50.57
      late A52.73
ocular muscle (congenital) Q10.3
   acquired —see Strabismus, mechanical
opticociliary vessels (congenital) Q13.2
orbit (eye) (acquired) H05.30
   atrophy —see Atrophy, orbit
   congenital Q10.7
   due to
      bone disease NEC H05.32-
      trauma or surgery H05.33-
   enlargement —see Enlargement, orbit
   exostosis —see Exostosis, orbit
organ of Corti (congenital) Q16.5
ovary (congenital) Q50.39
   acquired N83.8
oviduct, acquired N83.8
palate (congenital) Q38.5
   acquired M27.8
   cleft (congenital) —see Cleft, palate
pancreas (congenital) Q45.3
   acquired K86.8
parathyroid (gland) Q89.2
parotid (gland) (congenital) Q38.4
   acquired K11.8
patella (acquired) —see Disorder, patella,
      specified NEC
pelvis, pelvic (acquired) (bony) M95.5
   with disproportion (fetopelvic) O33.0
      causing obstructed labor O65.0
   congenital Q74.2
   rachitic sequelae (late effect) E64.3
penis (glans) (congenital) Q55.69
   acquired N48.89
pericardium (congenital) Q24.8
   acquired —see Pericarditis
pharynx (congenital) Q38.8
   acquired J39.2
pinna, acquired —see also Disorder, pinna,
      deformity
   congenital Q17.9
pituitary (congenital) Q89.2
posture —see Dorsopathy, deforming
prepuce (congenital) Q55.69
   acquired N47.8
prostate (congenital) Q55.4
   acquired N42.89
pupil (congenital) Q13.2
   acquired —see Abnormality, pupillary
pylorus (congenital) Q40.3
   acquired K31.89
rachitic (acquired), old or healed E64.3
radius (acquired) —see also Deformity, limb,
      forearm
   congenital Q68.8

Deformity (Continued)

rectum (congenital) Q43.9
   acquired K62.89
reduction (extremity) (limb), congenital (see
      also condition and site) Q73.8
   brain Q04.3
   lower —see Defect, reduction, lower limb
   upper —see Defect, reduction, upper limb
renal —see Deformity, kidney
respiratory system (congenital) Q34.9
rib (acquired) M95.4
   congenital Q76.6
   cervical Q76.5
rotation (joint) (acquired) —see Deformity,
      limb, specified site NEC
   congenital Q74.9
   hip —see Deformity, limb, specified type
      NEC, thigh
      congenital Q65.89
sacroiliac joint (congenital) Q74.2
   acquired —see subcategory M43.8
sacrum (acquired) —see subcategory
      M43.8
saddle
   back —see Lordosis
   nose M95.0
      syphilitic A50.57
salivary gland or duct (congenital) Q38.4
   acquired K11.8
scapula (acquired) M95.8
   congenital Q68.8
scrotum (congenital) —see also Malformation,
      testis and scrotum
   acquired N50.8
seminal vesicles (congenital) Q55.4
   acquired N50.8
septum, nasal (acquired) J34.2
shoulder (joint) (acquired) —see Deformity,
      limb, upper arm
   congenital Q74.0
   contraction —see Contraction, joint,
      shoulder
sigmoid (flexure) (congenital) Q43.9
   acquired K63.89
skin (congenital) Q82.9
skull (acquired) M95.2
   congenital Q75.8
      with
         anencephaly Q00.0
         encephalocele —see Encephalocele
         hydrocephalus Q03.9
            with spina bifida —see Spina bifida,
               by site, with hydrocephalus
         microcephaly Q02
soft parts, organs or tissues (of pelvis)
   in pregnancy or childbirth NEC O34.8-
   causing obstructed labor O65.5
spermatic cord (congenital) Q55.4
   acquired N50.8
   torsion —see Torsion, spermatic cord
spinal —see Dorsopathy, deforming
   column (acquired) —see Dorsopathy,
      deforming
   congenital Q67.5
   cord (congenital) Q06.9
      acquired G95.89
   nerve root (congenital) Q07.9
spine (acquired) —see also Dorsopathy,
      deforming
   congenital Q67.5
   rachitic E64.3
   specified NEC —see Dorsopathy,
      deforming, specified NEC
spleen
   acquired D73.89
   congenital Q89.09
Sprengel's (congenital) Q74.0
sternocleidomastoid (muscle), congenital
      Q68.0
sternum (acquired) M95.4
   congenital NEC Q76.7

Deformity (Continued)

stomach (congenital) Q40.3
  acquired K31.89
submandibular gland (congenital) Q38.4
submaxillary gland (congenital) Q38.4
  acquired K11.8
talipes —see Talipes
testis (congenital) —see also Malformation,
    testis and scrotum
  acquired N44.8
    torsion —see Torsion, testis
thigh (acquired) —see also Deformity, limb,
    thigh
  congenital NEC Q68.8
thorax (acquired) (wall) M95.4
  congenital Q67.8
  sequelae of rickets E64.3
thumb (acquired) —see also Deformity, finger
  congenital NEC Q68.1
thymus (tissue) (congenital) Q89.2
thyroid (gland) (congenital) Q89.2
  cartilage Q31.8
    acquired J38.7
tibia (acquired) —see also Deformity, limb,
    specified type NEC, lower leg
  congenital NEC Q68.8
  saber (syphilitic) A50.56
toe (acquired) M20.6-
  congenital Q66.9
  hallux rigidus M20.2-
  hallux valgus M20.1-
  hallux varus M20.3-
  hammer toe M20.4-
  specified NEC M20.5X-
tongue (congenital) Q38.3
  acquired K14.8
tooth, teeth K00.2
trachea (rings) (congenital) Q32.1
  acquired J39.8
transverse aortic arch (congenital) Q25.4
tricuspid (leaflets) (valve) I07.8
  atresia or stenosis Q22.4
  Ebstein's Q22.5
trunk (acquired) M95.8
  congenital Q89.9
ulna (acquired) —see also Deformity, limb,
    forearm
  congenital NEC Q68.8
urachus, congenital Q64.4
ureter (opening) (congenital) Q62.8
  acquired N28.89
urethra (congenital) Q64.79
  acquired N36.8
urinary tract (congenital) Q64.9
  urachus Q64.4
uterus (congenital) Q51.9
  acquired N85.8
uvula (congenital) Q38.5
vagina (acquired) N89.8
  congenital Q52.4
valgus NEC M21.00
  ankle M21.07-
  elbow M21.02-
  hip M21.05-
  knee M21.06-
valve, valvular (congenital) (heart) Q24.8
  acquired —see Endocarditis
varus NEC M21.10
  ankle M21.17-
  elbow M21.12-
  hip M21.15
  knee M21.16-
  tibia —see Osteochondrosis, juvenile, tibia
vas deferens (congenital) Q55.4
  acquired N50.8
vein (congenital) Q27.9
  great Q26.9
vertebra —see Dorsopathy, deforming
vertical talus (congenital) Q66.80
  left foot Q66.82
  right foot Q66.81

Deformity (Continued)

vesicourethral orifice (acquired) N32.89
  congenital NEC Q64.79
vessels of optic papilla (congenital) Q14.2
visual field (contraction) —see Defect, visual
    field
vitreous body, acquired H43.89
vulva (congenital) Q52.79
  acquired N90.89
wrist (joint) (acquired) —see also Deformity,
    limb, forearm
  congenital Q68.8
  contraction —see Contraction, joint, wrist

Degeneration, degenerative

adrenal (capsule) (fatty) (gland) (hyaline)
    (infectional) E27.8
amyloid (see also Amyloidosis) E85.9
anterior cornua, spinal cord G12.29
anterior labral S43.49-
aorta, aortic I70.0
  fatty I77.89
aortic valve (heart) —see Endocarditis, aortic
arteriovascular —see Arteriosclerosis
artery, arterial (atheromatous) (calcareous) —
    see also Arteriosclerosis
  cerebral, amyloid E85.4 [I68.0]
  medial —see Arteriosclerosis, extremities
articular cartilage NEC —see Derangement,
    joint, articular cartilage, by site
atheromatous —see Arteriosclerosis
basal nuclei or ganglia G23.9
  specified NEC G23.8
bone NEC —see Disorder, bone, specified
    type NEC
brachial plexus G54.0
brain (cortical) (progressive) G31.9
  alcoholic G31.2
  arteriosclerotic I67.2
  childhood G31.9
    specified NEC G31.89
  cystic G31.89
    congenital Q04.6
  in
    alcoholism G31.2
    beriberi E51.2
    cerebrovascular disease I67.9
    congenital hydrocephalus Q03.9
      with spina bifida —see also Spina
        bifida
    Fabry-Anderson disease E75.21
    Gaucher's disease E75.22
    Hunter's syndrome E76.1
    lipidosis
      cerebral E75.4
      generalized E75.6
    mucopolysaccharidosis —see
      Mucopolysaccharidosis
    myxedema E03.9 [G32.89]
    neoplastic disease (see also Neoplasm)
      D49.6 [G32.89]
    Niemann-Pick disease E75.249 [G32.89]
    sphingolipidosis E75.3 [G32.89]
    vitamin B12 deficiency E53.8 [G32.89]
  senile NEC G31.1
breast N64.89
Bruch's membrane —see Degeneration,
    choroid
capillaries (fatty) I78.8
  amyloid E85.8 [I79.8]
cardiac —see also Degeneration, myocardial
  valve, valvular —see Endocarditis
cardiorenal —see Hypertension, cardiorenal
cardiovascular —see also Disease,
    cardiovascular
  renal —see Hypertension, cardiorenal
cerebellar NOS G31.9
  alcoholic G31.2
  primary (hereditary) (sporadic) G11.9
cerebral —see Degeneration, brain
cerebrovascular I67.9
  due to hypertension I67.4

Degeneration, degenerative (Continued)

cervical plexus G54.2
cervix N88.8
  due to radiation (intended effect) N88.8
    adverse effect or misadventure N99.89
chamber angle H21.21-
changes, spine or vertebra —see Spondylosis
chorioretinal —see also Degeneration, choroid
  hereditary H31.20
choroid (colloid) (drusen) H31.10-
  atrophy —see Atrophy, choroidal
  hereditary —see Dystrophy, choroidal,
    hereditary
ciliary body H21.22-
cochlear —see subcategory H83.8
combined (spinal cord) (subacute) E53.8
    [G32.0]
  with anemia (pernicious) D51.0 [G32.0]
    due to dietary vitamin B12 deficiency
      D51.3 [G32.0]
  in (due to)
    vitamin B12 deficiency E53.8 [G32.0]
    anemia D51.9 [G32.0]
conjunctiva H11.10
  concretions —see Concretion, conjunctiva
  deposits —see Deposit, conjunctiva
  pigmentations —see Pigmentation,
    conjunctiva
  pinguecula —see Pinguecula
  xerosis —see Xerosis, conjunctiva
cornea H18.40
  calcerous H18.43
    band keratopathy H18.42-
  familial, hereditary —see Dystrophy, cornea
  hyaline (of old scars) H18.49
  keratomalacia —see Keratomalacia
  nodular H18.45-
  peripheral H18.46-
  senile H18.41-
  specified type NEC H18.49
cortical (cerebellar) (parenchymatous) G31.89
  alcoholic G31.2
  diffuse, due to arteriopathy I67.2
corticobasal G31.85
cutis L98.8
  amyloid E85.4 [L99]
dental pulp K04.2
disc disease —see Degeneration,
    intervertebral disc NEC
dorsolateral (spinal cord) —see Degeneration,
    combined
extrapyramidal G25.9
eye, macular —see also Degeneration, macula
  congenital or hereditary —see Dystrophy,
    retina
facet joints —see Spondylosis
fatty
  liver NEC K76.0
    alcoholic K70.0
grey matter (brain) (Alpers') G31.81
heart —see also Degeneration, myocardial
  amyloid E85.4 [I43]
  atheromatous —see Disease, heart,
    ischemic, atherosclerotic
  ischemic —see Disease, heart, ischemic
hepatolenticular (Wilson's) E83.01
hepatorenal K76.7
hyaline (diffuse) (generalized)
  localized —see Degeneration, by site
infrapatellar fat pad M79.4
intervertebral disc NOS
  with
    myelopathy —see Disorder, disc, with,
      myelopathy
    radiculitis or radiculopathy —see
      Disorder, disc, with, radiculopathy
  cervical, cervicothoracic —see Disorder,
    disc, cervical, degeneration
    with
      myelopathy —see Disorder, disc,
        cervical, with myelopathy

◄ New   ⬅ Revised   ~~deleted~~ Deleted

Degeneration, degenerative *(Continued)*
  intervertebral disc NOS *(Continued)*
    cervical, cervicothoracic *(Continued)*
      with *(Continued)*
        neuritis, radiculitis or
          radiculopathy —*see* Disorder,
          disc, cervical, with neuritis
    lumbar region M51.36
      with
        myelopathy M51.06
        neuritis, radiculitis, radiculopathy or
          sciatica M51.16
    lumbosacral region M51.37
      with
        ~~myelopathy M51.07~~
        neuritis, radiculitis, radiculopathy or
          sciatica M51.17
    sacrococcygeal region M53.3
    thoracic region M51.34
      with
        myelopathy M51.04
        neuritis, radiculitis, radiculopathy
          M51.14
    thoracolumbar region M51.35
      with
        myelopathy M51.05
        neuritis, radiculitis, radiculopathy
          M51.15
  intestine, amyloid E85.4
  iris (pigmentary) H21.23-
  ischemic —*see* Ischemia
  joint disease —*see* Osteoarthritis
  kidney N28.89
    amyloid E85.4 *[N29]*
    cystic, congenital Q61.9
    fatty N28.89
    polycystic Q61.3
      adult type (autosomal dominant) Q61.2
      infantile type (autosomal recessive) NEC
        Q61.19
        collecting duct dilatation Q61.11
  Kuhnt-Junius (*see also* Degeneration, macula)
    H35.32
  lens —*see* Cataract
  lenticular (familial) (progressive) (Wilson's)
    (with cirrhosis of liver) E83.01
  liver (diffuse) NEC K76.89
    amyloid E85.4 *[K77]*
    cystic K76.89
      congenital Q44.6
    fatty NEC K76.0
      alcoholic K70.0
    hypertrophic K76.89
    parenchymatous, acute or subacute K72.00
      with coma K72.01
    pigmentary K76.89
    toxic (acute) K71.9
  lung J98.4
  lymph gland I89.8
    hyaline I89.8
  macula, macular (acquired) (age-related)
    (senile) H35.30
    angioid streaks H35.33
    atrophic age-related H35.31
    congenital or hereditary —*see* Dystrophy,
      retina
    cystoid H35.35-
    drusen H35.36-
    exudative H35.32
    hole H35.34-
    nonexudative H35.31
    puckering H35.37-
    toxic H35.38-
  membranous labyrinth, congenital (causing
    impairment of hearing) Q16.5
  meniscus —*see* Derangement, meniscus
  mitral —*see* Insufficiency, mitral
  Mönckeberg's —*see* Arteriosclerosis,
    extremities
  motor centers, senile G31.1
  multi-system G90.3

Degeneration, degenerative *(Continued)*
  mural —*see* Degeneration, myocardial
  muscle (fatty) (fibrous) (hyaline)
    (progressive) M62.89
    heart —*see* Degeneration, myocardial
  myelin, central nervous system G37.9
  myocardial, myocardium (fatty) (hyaline)
    (senile) I51.5
    with rheumatic fever (conditions in I00)
      I09.0
      active, acute or subacute I01.2
        with chorea I02.0
      inactive or quiescent (with chorea)
        I09.0
    hypertensive —*see* Hypertension, heart
    rheumatic —*see* Degeneration, myocardial,
      with rheumatic fever
    syphilitic A52.06
  nasal sinus (mucosa) J32.9
    frontal J32.1
    maxillary J32.0
  nerve —*see* Disorder, nerve
  nervous system G31.9
    alcoholic G31.2
    amyloid E85.4 *[G99.8]*
    autonomic G90.9
    fatty G31.89
    specified NEC G31.89
  nipple N64.89
  olivopontocerebellar (hereditary) (familial)
    G23.8
  osseous labyrinth —*see* subcategory H83.8
  ovary N83.8
    cystic N83.20
    microcystic N83.20
  pallidal pigmentary (progressive) G23.0
  pancreas K86.8
    tuberculous A18.83
  penis N48.89
  pigmentary (diffuse) (general)
    localized —*see* Degeneration, by site
    pallidal (progressive) G23.0
  pineal gland E34.8
  pituitary (gland) E23.6
  popliteal fat pad M79.4
  posterolateral (spinal cord) —*see*
    Degeneration, combined
  pulmonary valve (heart) I37.8
  pulp (tooth) K04.2
  pupillary margin H21.24-
  renal —*see* Degeneration, kidney
  retina H35.9
    hereditary (cerebroretinal) (congenital)
      (juvenile) (macula) (peripheral)
      (pigmentary) —*see* Dystrophy, retina
    Kuhnt-Junius (*see also* Degeneration,
      macula) H35.32
    macula (cystic) (exudative) (hole)
      (nonexudative) (pseudohole) (senile)
      (toxic) —*see* Degeneration, macula
    peripheral H35.40
      lattice H35.41-
      microcystoid H35.42-
      paving stone H35.43-
      secondary
        pigmentary H35.45-
        vitreoretinal H35.46-
      senile reticular H35.44-
    pigmentary (primary) —*see also* Dystrophy,
      retina
    secondary —*see* Degeneration, retina,
      peripheral, secondary
    posterior pole —*see* Degeneration, macula
  saccule, congenital (causing impairment of
    hearing) Q16.5
  senile R54
    brain G31.1
    cardiac, heart or myocardium —*see*
      Degeneration, myocardial
    motor centers G31.1
    vascular —*see* Arteriosclerosis

Degeneration, degenerative *(Continued)*
  sinus (cystic) —*see also* Sinusitis
    polypoid J33.1
  skin L98.8
    amyloid E85.4 *[L99]*
    colloid L98.8
  spinal (cord) G31.89
    amyloid E85.4 *[G32.89]*
    combined (subacute) —*see* Degeneration,
      combined
    dorsolateral —*see* Degeneration, combined
    familial NEC G31.89
    fatty G31.89
    funicular —*see* Degeneration, combined
    posterolateral —*see* Degeneration,
      combined
    subacute combined —*see* Degeneration,
      combined
    tuberculous A17.81
  spleen D73.0
    amyloid E85.4 *[D77]*
  stomach K31.89
  striatonigral G23.2
  suprarenal (capsule) (gland) E27.8
  synovial membrane (pulpy) —*see* Disorder,
    synovium, specified type NEC
  tapetoretinal —*see* Dystrophy, retina
  thymus (gland) E32.8
    fatty E32.8
  thyroid (gland) E07.89
  tricuspid (heart) (valve) I07.9
  tuberculous NEC —*see* Tuberculosis
  turbinate J34.89
  uterus (cystic) N85.8
  vascular (senile) —*see* Arteriosclerosis
    hypertensive —*see* Hypertension
  vitreoretinal, secondary —*see* Degeneration,
    retina, peripheral, secondary,
    vitreoretinal
  vitreous (body) H43.81-
  Wallerian —*see* Disorder, nerve
  Wilson's hepatolenticular E83.01
Deglutition
  paralysis R13.0
    hysterical F44.4
  pneumonia J69.0
Degos' disease I77.89
Dehiscence (of)
  amputation stump T87.81
  cesarean wound O90.0
  closure of
    cornea T81.31
    craniotomy T81.32
    fascia (muscular) (superficial) T81.32
    internal organ or tissue T81.32
    laceration (external) (internal) T81.33
    ligament T81.32
    mucosa T81.31
    muscle or muscle flap T81.32
    ribs or rib cage T81.32
    skin and subcutaneous tissue (full-
      thickness) (superficial) T81.31
    skull T81.32
    sternum (sternotomy) T81.32
    tendon T81.32
    traumatic laceration (external) (internal)
      T81.33
  episiotomy O90.1
  operation wound NEC T81.31
    external operation wound (superficial)
      T81.31
    internal operation wound (deep)
      T81.32
  perineal wound (postpartum) O90.1
  traumatic injury wound repair T81.33
  wound T81.30
    traumatic repair T81.33
Dehydration E86.0
  hypertonic E87.0
  hypotonic E87.1
  newborn P74.1

Déjérine-Roussy syndrome G93.89
Déjérine-Sottas disease or neuropathy
(hypertrophic) G60.0
Déjérine-Thomas atrophy G23.8
Delay, delayed
any plane in pelvis
complicating delivery O66.9
birth or delivery NOS O63.9
closure, ductus arteriosus (Botalli) P29.3
coagulation —see Defect, coagulation
conduction (cardiac) (ventricular) I45.9
delivery, second twin, triplet, etc O63.2
development R62.50
global F88
intellectual (specific) F81.9
language F80.9
due to hearing loss F80.4
learning F81.9
pervasive F84.9
physiological R62.50
specified stage NEC R62.0
reading F81.0
sexual E30.0
speech F80.9
due to hearing loss F80.4
spelling F81.81
gastric emptying K30
menarche E30.0
menstruation (cause unknown) N91.0
milestone R62.0
passage of meconium (newborn) P76.0
primary respiration P28.9
puberty (constitutional) E30.0
separation of umbilical cord P96.82
sexual maturation, female E30.0
sleep phase syndrome G47.21
union, fracture —see Fracture, by site
vaccination Z28.9
Deletion (s)
autosome Q93.9
identified by fluorescence in situ
hybridization (FISH) Q93.89
identified by in situ hybridization (ISH)
Q93.89
chromosome
with complex rearrangements NEC Q93.7
part of NEC Q93.5
seen only at prometaphase Q93.89
short arm
4 Q93.3
5p Q93.4
22q11.2 Q93.81
specified NEC Q93.89
long arm chromosome 18 or 21 Q93.89
with complex rearrangements NEC
Q93.7
microdeletions NEC Q93.88
Delhi boil or button B55.1
Delinquency (juvenile) (neurotic) F91.8
group Z72.810
Delinquent immunization status Z28.3
Delirium, delirious (acute or subacute) (not
alcohol or drug-induced) (with dementia)
R41.0
alcoholic (acute) (tremens) (withdrawal)
F10.921
with intoxication F10.921
in
abuse F10.121
dependence F10.221
due to (secondary to)
alcohol
intoxication F10.921
in
abuse F10.121
dependence F10.221
withdrawal F10.231
amphetamine intoxication F15.921
in
abuse F15.121
dependence F15.221

Delirium, delirious (Continued)
due to (Continued)
anxiolytic
intoxication F13.921
in
abuse F13.121
dependence F13.221
withdrawal F13.231
cannabis intoxication (acute) F12.921
in
abuse F12.121
dependence F12.221
cocaine intoxication (acute) F14.921
in
abuse F14.121
dependence F14.221
general medical condition F05
hallucinogen intoxication F16.921
in
abuse F16.121
dependence F16.221
hypnotic
intoxication F13.921
in
abuse F13.121
dependence F13.221
withdrawal F13.231
inhalant intoxication (acute) F18.921
in
abuse F18.121
dependence F18.221
multiple etiologies F05
opioid intoxication (acute) F11.921
in
abuse F11.121
dependence F11.221
phencyclidine intoxication (acute) F16.921
in
abuse F16.121
dependence F16.221
psychoactive substance NEC intoxication
(acute) F19.921
in
abuse F19.121
dependence F19.221
sedative
intoxication F13.921
in
abuse F13.121
dependence F13.221
withdrawal F13.231
unknown etiology F05
exhaustion F43.0
hysterical F44.89
postprocedural (postoperative) F05
puerperal F05
thyroid —see Thyrotoxicosis with thyroid
storm
traumatic —see Injury, intracranial
tremens (alcohol-induced) F10.231
sedative-induced F13.231
Delivery (childbirth) (labor)
arrested active phase O62.1
cesarean (for)
without indication O82
abnormal
pelvis (bony) (deformity) (major) NEC
with disproportion (fetopelvic)
O33.0
with obstructed labor O65.0
presentation or position O32.9
abruptio placentae (see also Abruptio
placentae) 045.9-
acromion presentation O32.2
atony, uterus O62.2
breech presentation O32.1
incomplete O32.8
brow presentation O32.3
cephalopelvic disproportion O33.9
cerclage O34.3-
chin presentation O32.3

Delivery (Continued)
cesarean (Continued)
cicatrix of cervix O34.4-
contracted pelvis (general)
inlet O33.2
outlet O33.3
cord presentation or prolapse O69.0
cystocele O34.8-
deformity (acquired) (congenital)
pelvic organs or tissues NEC O34.8-
pelvis (bony) NEC O33.0
disproportion NOS O33.9
eclampsia —see Eclampsia
face presentation O32.3
failed
forceps O66.5
induction of labor O61.9
instrumental O61.1
mechanical O61.1
medical O61.0
specified NEC O61.8
surgical O61.1
trial of labor NOS O66.40
following previous cesarean delivery
O66.41
vacuum extraction O66.5
ventouse O66.5
fetal-maternal hemorrhage O43.01-
hemorrhage (intrapartum) O67.9
with coagulation defect O67.0
specified cause NEC O67.8
high head at term O32.4
hydrocephalic fetus O33.6
incarceration of uterus O34.51-
incoordinate uterine action O62.4
increased size, fetus O33.5
inertia, uterus O62.2
primary O62.0
secondary O62.1
lateroversion, uterus O34.59-
mal lie O32.9
malposition
fetus O32.9
pelvic organs or tissues NEC O34.8-
uterus NEC O34.59-
malpresentation NOS O32.9
oblique presentation O32.2
occurring after 37 completed weeks of
gestation but before 39 completed
weeks gestation due to (spontaneous)
onset of labor O75.82
oversize fetus O33.5
pelvic tumor NEC O34.8-
placenta previa O44.1-
without hemorrhage O44.0-
placental insufficiency O36.51-
planned, occurring after 37 completed
weeks of gestation but before 39
completed weeks gestation due to
(spontaneous) onset of labor O75.82
polyp, cervix O34.4-
causing obstructed labor O65.5
poor dilatation, cervix O62.0
pre-eclampsia O14.9-
mild O14.0-
moderate O14.0-
severe
with hemolysis, elevated liver
enzymes and low platelet count
(HELLP) O14.2-
previous
cesarean delivery O34.21
surgery (to)
cervix O34.4-
gynecological NEC O34.8-
rectum O34.7-
uterus O34.29
vagina O34.6-
prolapse
arm or hand O32.2
uterus O34.52-

◀ New ◀▦ Revised ~~deleted~~ Deleted

Delivery (Continued)
  complicated (Continued)
    by (Continued)
      laceration (Continued)
        rectovaginal (septum) (without
            perineal laceration) O71.4
          with perineum O70.2
            with anal or rectal mucosa
                O70.3
        specified NEC O71.89
        sphincter ani —see Delivery,
            complicated, by, laceration, anus
            (sphincter)
        urethra O71.5
        uterus O71.81
          before labor O71.81
        vagina, vaginal (deep) (high) (without
            perineal laceration) O71.4
          with perineum O70.0
            muscles, with perineum O70.1
        vulva O70.0
      liver disorder O26.62
      malignancy O9A.12
      malnutrition O25.2
      malposition, malpresentation
        without obstruction O32.9 —see
            also Delivery, complicated by,
            obstruction
        breech O32.1
        compound O32.6
        face (brow) (chin) O32.3
        footling O38.8
        high head O32.4
        oblique O32.2
        specified NEC O32.8
        transverse O32.2
        unstable lie O32.0
      placenta (with hemorrhage) O44.1-
        without hemorrhage O44.0-
      uterus or cervix O65.5
      meconium in amniotic fluid O77.0
      mental disorder NEC O99.344
      metrorrhexis —see Delivery, complicated
          by, rupture, uterus
      nervous system disorder O99.354
      obesity (pre-existing) O99.214
      obesity surgery status O99.844
      obstetric trauma O71.9
        specified NEC O71.89
      obstructed labor
        due to
          breech (complete) (frank)
              presentation O64.1
            incomplete O64.8
          brow presenation O64.3
          buttock presentation O64.1
          chin presentation O64.2
          compound presentation O64.5
          contracted pelvis O65.1
          deep transverse arrest O64.0
          deformed pelvis O65.0
          dystocia (fetal) O66.9
            due to
              conjoined twins O66.3
              fetal
                abnormality NEC O66.3
                ascites O66.3
                hydrops O66.3
                meningomyelocele O66.3
                sacral teratoma O66.3
                tumor O66.3
              hydrocephalic fetus O66.3
              shoulder O66.0
          face presentation O64.2
          fetopelvic disproportion O65.4
          footling presentation O64.8
          impacted shoulders O66.0
          incomplete rotation of fetal head
              O64.0
          large fetus O66.2
          locked twins O66.1

Delivery (Continued)
  complicated (Continued)
    by (Continued)
      obstructed labor (Continued)
        due to (Continued)
          malposition O64.9
            specified NEC O64.8
          malpresentation O64.9
            specified NEC O64.8
          multiple fetuses NEC O66.6
          pelvic
            abnormality (maternal) O65.9
              organ O65.5
                specified NEC O65.8
            contraction
              inlet O65.2
              mid-cavity O65.3
              outlet O65.3
          persistent (position)
            occipitoiliac O64.0
            occipitoposterior O64.0
            occipitosacral O64.0
            occipitotransverse O64.0
          prolapsed arm O64.4
          shoulder presentation O64.4
        specified NEC O66.8
      pathological retraction ring, uterus
          O62.4
      penetration, pregnant uterus by
          instrument O71.1
      perforation —see Delivery, complicated
          by, laceration
      placenta, placental
        ablatio (see also Abruptio placentae)
            O45.9-
        abnormality O43.9-
          specified NEC O43.89-
        abruptio (see also Abruptio placentae)
            O45.9-
        accreta O43.21-
        adherent (with hemorrhage) O72.0
          without hemorrhage O73.0
        detachment (premature) (see also
            Abruptio placentae) O45.9-
        disorder O43.9-
          specified NEC O43.89-
        hemorrhage NEC O67.8
        increta O43.22- ◄▥
        low (implantation) O44.1-
          without hemorrhage O44.0-
        malformation O43.10-
        malposition O44.1-
          without hemorrhage O44.0-
        percreta O43.23- ◄▥
        previa (central) (lateral) (low)
            (marginal) (partial) (total) O44.1-
          without hemorrhage O44.0-
        retained (with hemorrhage) O72.0
          without hemorrhage O73.0
        separation (premature) O45.9-
          specified NEC O45.8X-
        vicious insertion O44.1-
      precipitate labor O62.3
      premature rupture, membranes (see
          also Pregnancy, complicated by,
          premature rupture of membranes)
          O42.90
      prolapse
        arm or hand O32.2
        cord (umbilical) O69.0
        foot or leg O32.8
        uterus O34.52-
      prolonged labor O63.9
        first stage O63.0
        second stage O63.1
      protozoal disease (maternal) O98.62
      respiratory disease NEC O99.52
      retained membranes or portions of
          placenta O72.2
        without hemorrhage O73.1
      retarded birth O63.9

Delivery (Continued)
  complicated (Continued)
    by (Continued)
      retention of secundines (with
          hemorrhage) O72.0
        without hemorrhage O73.0
        partial O72.2
          without hemorrhage O73.1
      rupture
        bladder (urinary) O71.5
        cervix O71.3
        pelvic organ NEC O71.5
        urethra O71.5
        uterus (during or after labor) O71.1
          before labor O71.0-
      separation, pubic bone (symphysis
          pubis) O71.6
      shock O75.1
      shoulder presentation O64.4
      skin disorder NEC O99.72
      spasm, cervix O62.4
      stenosis or stricture, cervix O65.5
      streptococcus B carrier state O99.824
      subluxation of symphysis (pubis) O26.72
      syphilis (maternal) O98.12
      tear —see Delivery, complicated by,
          laceration
      tetanic uterus O62.4
      trauma (obstetrical) (see also Delivery,
          complicated, by, damage to) O71.9
        non-obstetric O9A.22
        periurethral O71.82
        specified NEC O71.89
      tuberculosis (maternal) O98.02
      tumor, pelvic organs or tissues NEC
          O65.5
      umbilical cord around neck
        with compression O69.1
        without compression O69.81
      uterine inertia O62.2
        during latent phase of labor O62.0
        primary O62.0
        secondary O62.1
      vasa previa O69.4
      velamentous insertion of cord O43.12-
    specified complication NEC O75.89
  delayed NOS O63.9
    following rupture of membranes
        artificial O75.5
    second twin, triplet, etc. O63.2
  forceps, low following failed vacuum
      extraction O66.5
  missed (at or near term) O36.4
  normal O80
  obstructed —see Delivery, complicated by,
      obstruction
  precipitate O62.3
  preterm (see also Pregnancy, complicated by,
      preterm labor) O60.10
  spontaneous O80
  term pregnancy NOS O80
  uncomplicated O80
  vaginal, following previous cesarean delivery
      O34.21
Delusions (paranoid) —see Disorder, delusional
Dementia (degenerative (primary)) (old age)
    (persisting) F03.90
  with
    aggressive behavior F03.91
    behavioral disturbance F03.91
    combative behavior F03.91
    Lewy bodies G31.83 [F02.80]
      with behavioral disturbance G31.83
          [F02.81]
    Parkinson's disease G20 [F02.80]
      with behavioral disturbance G20
          [F02.81]
    Parkinsonism G31.83 [F02.80]
      with behavioral disturbance G31.83
          [F02.81]
    violent behavior F03.91

D

◄ New   ◄▥ Revised   ~~deleted~~ Deleted

Dementia *(Continued)*
 alcoholic F10.97
  with dependence F10.27
 Alzheimer's type —*see* Disease, Alzheimer's
 arteriosclerotic —*see* Dementia, vascular
 atypical, Alzheimer's type —*see* Disease,
  Alzheimer's, specified NEC
 congenital —*see* Disability, intellectual
 frontal (lobe) G31.09 *[F02.80]*
  with behavioral disturbance G31.09
   [F02.81]
 frontotemporal G31.09 *[F02.80]*
  with behavioral disturbance G31.09
   [F02.81]
  specified NEC G31.09 *[F02.80]*
   with behavioral disturbance G31.09
    [F02.81]
 in (due to)
  alcohol F10.97
   with dependence F10.27
  Alzheimer's disease —*see* Disease,
   Alzheimer's
  arteriosclerotic brain disease —*see*
   Dementia, vascular
  cerebral lipidoses E75.- *[F02.80]*
   with behavioral disturbance
    E75.- *[F02.81]*
  Creutzfeldt-Jakob disease *(see also*
   Creutzfeldt-Jakob disease or
   syndrome (with dementia))* A81.00 ◄▥
  epilepsy G40.- *[F02.80]*
   with behavioral disturbance
    G40.- *[F02.81]*
  hepatolenticular degeneration E83.01
   [F02.80]
   with behavioral disturbance E83.01
    [F02.81]
  human immunodeficiency virus (HIV)
   disease B20 *[F02.80]*
   with behavioral disturbance B20
    [F02.81]
  Huntington's disease or chorea G10
  hypercalcemia E83.52 *[F02.80]*
   with behavioral disturbance E83.52
    [F02.81]
  hypothyroidism, acquired E03.9 *[F02.80]*
   with behavioral disturbance E03.9
    [F02.81]
   due to iodine deficiency E01.8
    [F02.80]
    with behavioral disturbance E01.8
     [F02.81]
  inhalants F18.97
   with dependence F18.27
  multiple
   etiologies F03
   sclerosis G35 *[F02.80]*
    with behavioral disturbance G35
     [F02.81]
  neurosyphilis A52.17 *[F02.80]*
   with behavioral disturbance A52.17
    [F02.81]
   juvenile A50.49 *[F02.80]*
    with behavioral disturbance A50.49
     [F02.81]
  niacin deficiency E52 *[F02.80]*
   with behavioral disturbance E52
    [F02.81]
  paralysis agitans G20 *[F02.80]*
   with behavioral disturbance G20
    [F02.81]
  Parkinson's disease G20 *[F02.80]*
  pellagra E52 *[F02.80]*
   with behavioral disturbance E52
    [F02.81]
  Pick's G31.01 *[F02.80]*
   with behavioral disturbance G31.01
    [F02.81]
  polyarteritis nodosa M30.0 *[F02.80]*
   with behavioral disturbance M30.0
    [F02.81]

Dementia *(Continued)*
 in *(Continued)*
  psychoactive drug F19.97
   with dependence F19.27
   inhalants F18.97
    with dependence F18.27
   sedatives, hypnotics or anxiolytics
    F13.97
    with dependence F13.27
  sedatives, hypnotics or anxiolytics F13.97
   with dependence F13.27
  systemic lupus erythematosus
   M32.- *[F02.80]*
   with behavioral disturbance
    M32.- *[F02.81]*
  trypanosomiasis
   African B56.9 *[F02.80]*
    with behavioral disturbance B56.9
     [F02.81]
  unknown etiology F03
  vitamin B12 deficiency E53.8 *[F02.80]*
   with behavioral disturbance E53.8
    [F02.81]
  volatile solvents F18.97
   with dependence F18.27
 infantile, infantilis F84.3
 Lewy body G31.83 *[F02.80]*
  with behavioral disturbance G31.83
   [F02.81]
 multi-infarct —*see* Dementia, vascular
 paralytica, paralytic (syphilitic) A52.17
  [F02.80]
  with behavioral disturbance A52.17
   [F02.81]
  juvenilis A50.45
 paretic A52.17
 praecox —*see* Schizophrenia
 presenile F03
  Alzheimer's type —*see* Disease,
   Alzheimer's, early onset
 primary degenerative F03
 progressive, syphilitic A52.17
 senile F03
  with acute confusional state F05
  Alzheimer's type —*see* Disease,
   Alzheimer's, late onset
  depressed or paranoid type F03
 vascular (acute onset) (mixed) (multi-infarct)
  (subcortical) F01.50
  with behavioral disturbance F01.51
Demineralization, bone —*see* Osteoporosis
Demodex folliculorum (infestation) B88.0
Demophobia F40.248
Demoralization R45.3
Demyelination, demyelinization
 central nervous system G37.9
  specified NEC G37.8
 corpus callosum (central) G37.1
 disseminated, acute G36.9
  specified NEC G36.8
 global G35
 in optic neuritis G36.0
Dengue (classical) (fever) A90
 hemorrhagic A91
 sandfly A93.1
Dennie-Marfan syphilitic syndrome
 A50.45
Dens evaginatus, in dente or invaginatus
 K00.2
Dense breasts R92.2
Density
 increased, bone (disseminated) (generalized)
  (spotted) —*see* Disorder, bone, density
  and structure, specified type NEC
 lung (nodular) J98.4
Dental —*see also* condition
 examination Z01.20
  with abnormal findings Z01.21
 restoration
  aesthetically inadequate or displeasing
   K08.56

Dental *(Continued)*
 restoration *(Continued)*
  defective K08.50
   specified NEC K08.59
  failure of marginal integrity K08.51
  failure of periodontal anatomical integrity
   K08.54
Dentia praecox K00.6
Denticles (pulp) K04.2
Dentigerous cyst K09.0
Dentin
 irregular (in pulp) K04.3
 opalescent K00.5
 secondary (in pulp) K04.3
 sensitive K03.89
Dentinogenesis imperfecta K00.5
Dentinoma —*see* Cyst, calcifying odontogenic
Dentition (syndrome) K00.7
 delayed K00.6
 difficult K00.7
 precocious K00.6
 premature K00.6
 retarded K00.6
Dependence (on) (syndrome) F19.20
 with remission F19.21
 alcohol (ethyl) (methyl) (without remission)
  F10.20
  with
   amnestic disorder, persisting F10.26
   anxiety disorder F10.280
   dementia, persisting F10.27
   intoxication F10.229
    with delirium F10.221
    uncomplicated F10.220
   mood disorder F10.24
   psychotic disorder F10.259
    with
     delusions F10.250
     hallucinations F10.251
   remission F10.21
   sexual dysfunction F10.281
   sleep disorder F10.282
   specified disorder NEC F10.288
   withdrawal F10.239
    with
     delirium F10.231
     perceptual disturbance F10.232
    uncomplicated F10.230
  counseling and surveillance Z71.41
 amobarbital —*see* Dependence, drug,
  sedative
 amphetamine (s) (type) —*see* Dependence,
  drug, stimulant NEC
 amytal (sodium) —*see* Dependence, drug,
  sedative
 analgesic NEC F55.8
 anesthetic (agent) (gas) (general) (local)
  NEC —*see* Dependence, drug,
  psychoactive NEC
 anxiolytic NEC —*see* Dependence, drug,
  sedative
 barbital (s) —*see* Dependence, drug, sedative
 barbiturate (s) (compounds) (drugs
  classifiable to T42) —*see* Dependence,
  drug, sedative
 benzedrine —*see* Dependence, drug,
  stimulant NEC
 bhang —*see* Dependence, drug, cannabis
 bromide (s) NEC —*see* Dependence, drug,
  sedative
 caffeine —*see* Dependence, drug, stimulant
  NEC
 cannabis (sativa) (indica) (resin) (derivatives)
  (type) —*see* Dependence, drug, cannabis
 chloral (betaine) (hydrate) —*see* Dependence,
  drug, sedative
 chlordiazepoxide —*see* Dependence, drug,
  sedative
 coca (leaf) (derivatives) —*see* Dependence,
  drug, cocaine
 cocaine —*see* Dependence, drug, cocaine

Dependence *(Continued)*
  codeine —*see* Dependence, drug, opioid
  combinations of drugs F19.20
  dagga —*see* Dependence, drug, cannabis
  demerol —*see* Dependence, drug, opioid
  dexamphetamine —*see* Dependence, drug, stimulant NEC
  dexedrine —*see* Dependence, drug, stimulant NEC
  dextromethorphan —*see* Dependence, drug, opioid
  dextromoramide —*see* Dependence, drug, opioid
  dextro-nor-pseudo-ephedrine —*see* Dependence, drug, stimulant NEC
  dextrorphan —*see* Dependence, drug, opioid
  diazepam —*see* Dependence, drug, sedative
  dilaudid —*see* Dependence, drug, opioid
  D-lysergic acid diethylamide —*see* Dependence, drug, hallucinogen
  drug NEC F19.20
    with sleep disorder F19.282
    cannabis F12.20
      with
        anxiety disorder F12.280
        intoxication F12.229
          with
            delirium F12.221
            perceptual disturbance F12.222
          uncomplicated F12.220
        other specified disorder F12.288
        psychosis F12.259
          delusions F12.250
          hallucinations F12.251
        unspecified disorder F12.29
      in remission F12.21
    cocaine F14.20
      with
        anxiety disorder F14.280
        intoxication F14.229
          with
            delirium F14.221
            perceptual disturbance F14.222
          uncomplicated F14.220
        mood disorder F14.24
        other specified disorder F14.288
        psychosis F14.259
          delusions F14.250
          hallucinations F14.251
        sexual dysfunction F14.281
        sleep disorder F14.282
        unspecified disorder F14.29
        withdrawal F14.23
      in remission F14.21
      withdrawal symptoms in newborn P96.1
    counseling and surveillance Z71.51
    hallucinogen F16.20
      with
        anxiety disorder F16.280
        flashbacks F16.283
        intoxication F16.229
          with delirium F16.221
          uncomplicated F16.220
        mood disorder F16.24
        other specified disorder F16.288
        perception disorder, persisting F16.283
        psychosis F16.259
          delusions F16.250
          hallucinations F16.251
        unspecified disorder F16.29
      in remission F16.21
    in remission F19.21
    inhalant F18.20
      with
        anxiety disorder F18.280
        dementia, persisting F18.27
        intoxication F18.229
          with delirium F18.221
          uncomplicated F18.220
        mood disorder F18.24
        other specified disorder F18.288

Dependence *(Continued)*
  drug NEC *(Continued)*
    inhalant *(Continued)*
      with *(Continued)*
        psychosis F18.259
          delusions F18.250
          hallucinations F18.251
        unspecified disorder F18.29
      in remission F18.21
    nicotine F17.200
      with disorder F17.209
        remission F17.201
        specified disorder NEC F17.208
        withdrawal F17.203
      chewing tobacco F17.220
        with disorder F17.229
          remission F17.221
          specified disorder NEC F17.228
          withdrawal F17.223
      cigarettes F17.210
        with disorder F17.219
          remission F17.211
          specified disorder NEC F17.218
          withdrawal F17.213
      specified product NEC F17.290
        with disorder F17.299
          remission F17.291
          specified disorder NEC F17.298
          withdrawal F17.293
    opioid F11.20
      with
        intoxication F11.229
          with
            delirium F11.221
            perceptual disturbance F11.222
          uncomplicated F11.220
        mood disorder F11.24
        other specified disorder F11.288
        psychosis F11.259
          delusions F11.250
          hallucinations F11.251
        sexual dysfunction F11.281
        sleep disorder F11.282
        unspecified disorder F11.29
        withdrawal F11.23
      in remission F11.21
    psychoactive NEC F19.20
      with
        amnestic disorder F19.26
        anxiety disorder F19.280
        dementia F19.27
        intoxication F19.229
          with
            delirium F19.221
            perceptual disturbance F19.222
          uncomplicated F19.220
        mood disorder F19.24
        other specified disorder F19.288
        psychosis F19.259
          delusions F19.250
          hallucinations F19.251
        sexual dysfunction F19.281
        sleep disorder F19.282
        unspecified disorder F19.29
        withdrawal F19.239
          with
            delirium F19.231
            perceptual disturbance F19.232
          uncomplicated F19.230
    sedative, hypnotic or anxiolytic F13.20
      with
        amnestic disorder F13.26
        anxiety disorder F13.280
        dementia, persisting F13.27
        intoxication F13.229
          with delirium F13.221
          uncomplicated F13.220
        mood disorder F13.24
        other specified disorder F13.288

Dependence *(Continued)*
  drug NEC *(Continued)*
    sedative, hypnotic or anxiolytic *(Continued)*
      with *(Continued)*
        psychosis F13.259
          delusions F13.250
          hallucinations F13.251
        sexual dysfunction F13.281
        sleep disorder F13.282
        unspecified disorder F13.29
        withdrawal F13.239
          with
            delirium F13.231
            perceptual disturbance F13.232
          uncomplicated F13.230
      in remission F13.21
    stimulant NEC F15.20
      with
        anxiety disorder F15.280
        intoxication F15.229
          with
            delirium F15.221
            perceptual disturbance F15.222
          uncomplicated F15.220
        mood disorder F15.24
        other specified disorder F15.288
        psychosis F15.259
          delusions F15.250
          hallucinations F15.251
        sexual dysfunction F15.281
        sleep disorder F15.282
        unspecified disorder F15.29
        withdrawal F15.23
      in remission F15.21
    ethyl
      alcohol (without remission) F10.20
        with remission F10.21
      bromide —*see* Dependence, drug, sedative
      carbamate F19.20
      chloride F19.20
      morphine —*see* Dependence, drug, opioid
    ganja —*see* Dependence, drug, cannabis
    glue (airplane) (sniffing) —*see* Dependence, drug, inhalant
    glutethimide —*see* Dependence, drug, sedative
    hallucinogenics —*see* Dependence, drug, hallucinogen
    hashish —*see* Dependence, drug, cannabis
    hemp —*see* Dependence, drug, cannabis
    heroin (salt) (any) —*see* Dependence, drug, opioid
    hypnotic NEC —*see* Dependence, drug, sedative
    Indian hemp —*see* Dependence, drug, cannabis
    inhalants —*see* Dependence, drug, inhalant
    khat —*see* Dependence, drug, stimulant NEC
    laudanum —*see* Dependence, drug, opioid
    LSD (-25) (derivatives) —*see* Dependence, drug, hallucinogen
    luminal —*see* Dependence, drug, sedative
    lysergic acid —*see* Dependence, drug, hallucinogen
    maconha —*see* Dependence, drug, cannabis
    marihuana —*see* Dependence, drug, cannabis
    meprobamate —*see* Dependence, drug, sedative
    mescaline —*see* Dependence, drug, hallucinogen
    methadone —*see* Dependence, drug, opioid
    methamphetamine (s) —*see* Dependence, drug, stimulant NEC
    methaqualone —*see* Dependence, drug, sedative
    methyl
      alcohol (without remission) F10.20
        with remission F10.21
      bromide —*see* Dependence, drug, sedative
      morphine —*see* Dependence, drug, opioid

◄ New ◄▪▪▪ Revised ~~deleted~~ Deleted

Dependence *(Continued)*
  methyl *(Continued)*
    phenidate —*see* Dependence, drug,
      stimulant NEC
    sulfonal —*see* Dependence, drug, sedative
  morphine (sulfate) (sulfite) (type) —*see*
    Dependence, drug, opioid
  narcotic (drug) NEC —*see* Dependence, drug,
    opioid
  nembutal —*see* Dependence, drug, sedative
  neraval —*see* Dependence, drug, sedative
  neravan —*see* Dependence, drug, sedative
  neurobarb —*see* Dependence, drug, sedative
  nicotine —*see* Dependence, drug, nicotine
  nitrous oxide F19.20
  nonbarbiturate sedatives and tranquilizers
    with similar effect —*see* Dependence,
    drug, sedative
  on
    artificial heart (fully implantable)
      (mechanical) Z95.812 ◀
    aspirator Z99.0
    care provider (because of) Z74.9
      impaired mobility Z74.09
      need for
        assistance with personal care Z74.1
        continuous supervision Z74.3
      no other household member able to
        render care Z74.2
      specified reason NEC Z74.8
    machine Z99.89
      enabling NEC Z99.89
      specified type NEC Z99.89
    renal dialysis (hemodialysis) (peritoneal)
      Z99.2
    respirator Z99.11
    ventilator Z99.11
    wheelchair Z99.3
  opiate —*see* Dependence, drug, opioid
  opioids —*see* Dependence, drug, opioid
  opium (alkaloids) (derivatives) (tincture) —
    see Dependence, drug, opioid
  oxygen (long-term) (supplemental) Z99.81
  paraldehyde —*see* Dependence, drug,
    sedative
  paregoric —*see* Dependence, drug, opioid
  PCP (phencyclidine) (*see also* Abuse, drug,
    hallucinogen) F16.20
  pentobarbital —*see* Dependence, drug,
    sedative
  pentobarbitone (sodium) —*see* Dependence,
    drug, sedative
  pentothal —*see* Dependence, drug, sedative
  peyote —*see* Dependence, drug, hallucinogen
  phencyclidine (PCP) (and related substances)
    (*see also* Abuse, drug, hallucinogen) F16.20
  phenmetrazine —*see* Dependence, drug,
    stimulant NEC
  phenobarbital —*see* Dependence, drug,
    sedative
  polysubstance F19.20
  psilocibin, psilocin, psilocyn, psilocyline —*see*
    Dependence, drug, hallucinogen
  psychostimulant NEC —*see* Dependence,
    drug, stimulant NEC
  secobarbital —*see* Dependence, drug, sedative
  seconal —*see* Dependence, drug, sedative
  sedative NEC —*see* Dependence, drug,
    sedative
  specified drug NEC —*see* Dependence, drug
  stimulant NEC —*see* Dependence, drug,
    stimulant NEC
  substance NEC —*see* Dependence, drug
  supplemental oxygen Z99.81
  tobacco —*see* Dependence, drug, nicotine
    counseling and surveillance Z71.6
  tranquilizer NEC —*see* Dependence, drug,
    sedative
  vitamin B6 E53.1
  volatile solvents —*see* Dependence, drug,
    inhalant

Dependency
  care-provider Z74.9
  passive F60.7
  reactions (persistent) F60.7
Depersonalization (in neurotic state) (neurotic)
  (syndrome) F48.1
Depletion
  extracellular fluid E86.9
  plasma E86.1
  potassium E87.6
    nephropathy N25.89
  salt or sodium E87.1
    causing heat exhaustion or prostration
      T67.4
    nephropathy N28.9
  volume NOS E86.9
Deployment (current) (military) status Z56.82
  in theater or in support of military war,
    peacekeeping and humanitarian
    operations Z56.82
  personal history of Z91.82
    military war, peacekeeping and
      humanitarian deployment (current or
      past conflict) Z91.82
  returned from Z91.82
Depolarization, premature I49.40
  atrial I49.1
  junctional I49.2
  specified NEC I49.49
  ventricular I49.3
Deposit
  bone in Boeck's sarcoid D86.89
  calcareous, calcium —*see* Calcification
  cholesterol
    retina H35.89
    vitreous (body) (humor) —*see* Deposit,
      crystalline
  conjunctiva H11.11-
  cornea H18.00-
    argentous H18.02-
    due to metabolic disorder H18.03-
    Kayser-Fleischer ring H18.04-
    pigmentation —*see* Pigmentation, cornea
  crystalline, vitreous (body) (humor) H43.2-
  hemosiderin in old scars of cornea —*see*
    Pigmentation, cornea, stromal
  metallic in lens —*see* Cataract, specified NEC
  skin R23.8
  tooth, teeth (betel) (black) (green) (materia
    alba) (orange) (tobacco) K03.6
  urate, kidney —*see* Calculus, kidney
Depraved appetite —*see* Pica
Depressed
  HDL cholesterol E78.6
Depression (acute) (mental) F32.9
  agitated (single episode) F32.2
  anaclitic —*see* Disorder, adjustment
  anxiety F41.8
    persistent F34.1
  arches —*see also* Deformity, limb, flat foot
  atypical (single episode) F32.8
  basal metabolic rate R94.8
  bone marrow D75.89
  central nervous system R09.2
  cerebral R29.818
    newborn P91.4
  cerebrovascular I67.9
  chest wall M95.4
  climacteric (single episode) F32.8
  endogenous (without psychotic symptoms)
    F33.2
    with psychotic symptoms F33.3
  functional activity R68.89
  hysterical F44.89
  involutional (single episode) F32.8
  major F32.9
    with psychotic symptoms F32.3
    recurrent —*see* Disorder, depressive,
      recurrent
  manic-depressive —*see* Disorder, depressive,
    recurrent

Depression *(Continued)*
  masked (single episode) F32.8
  medullary G93.89
  menopausal (single episode) F32.8
  metatarsus —*see* Depression, arches
  monopolar F33.9
  nervous F34.1
  neurotic F34.1
  nose M95.0
  postnatal F53
  postpartum F53
  post-psychotic of schizophrenia F32.8
  post-schizophrenic F32.8
  psychogenic (reactive) (single episode)
    F32.9
  psychoneurotic F34.1
  psychotic (single episode) F32.3
    recurrent F33.3
  reactive (psychogenic) (single episode)
    F32.9
    psychotic (single episode) F32.3
  recurrent —*see* Disorder, depressive,
    recurrent
  respiratory center G93.89
  seasonal —*see* Disorder, depressive, recurrent
  senile F03

  severe, single episode F32.2
  situational F43.21
  skull Q67.4
  specified NEC (single episode) F32.8
  sternum M95.4
  visual field —*see* Defect, visual field
  vital (recurrent) (without psychotic
    symptoms) F33.2
    with psychotic symptoms F33.3
    single episode F32.2
Deprivation
  cultural Z60.3
  effects NOS T73.9
    specified NEC T73.8
  emotional NEC Z65.8
    affecting infant or child —*see*
      Maltreatment, child, psychological
  food T73.0
  protein —*see* Malnutrition
  sleep Z72.820
  social Z60.4
    affecting infant or child —*see*
      Maltreatment, child, psychological
  specified NEC T73.8
  vitamins —*see* Deficiency, vitamin
  water T73.1
Derangement
  ankle (internal) —*see* Derangement, joint,
    ankle
  cartilage (articular) NEC —*see* Derangement,
    joint, articular cartilage, by site
    recurrent —*see* Dislocation, recurrent
  cruciate ligament, anterior, current injury —
    see Sprain, knee, cruciate, anterior
  elbow (internal) —*see* Derangement, joint,
    elbow
  hip (joint) (internal) (old) —*see* Derangement,
    joint, hip
  joint (internal) M24.9
    ankylosis —*see* Ankylosis
    articular cartilage M24.10
      ankle M24.17-
      elbow M24.12-
      foot M24.17-
      hand M24.14-
      hip M24.15-
      knee NEC M23.9-
      loose body —*see* Loose, body
      shoulder M24.11-
      wrist M24.13-
    contracture —*see* Contraction, joint
    current injury —*see also* Dislocation
      knee, meniscus or cartilage —*see* Tear,
      meniscus

Derangement *(Continued)*
joint *(Continued)*
dislocation
pathological —*see* Dislocation,
pathological
recurrent —*see* Dislocation, recurrent
knee —*see* Derangement, knee
ligament —*see* Disorder, ligament
loose body —*see* Loose, body
recurrent —*see* Dislocation, recurrent
specified type NEC M24.80
ankle M24.87-
elbow M24.82-
foot joint M24.87-
hand joint M24.84-
hip M24.85-
shoulder M24.81-
wrist M24.83-
temporomandibular M26.69
knee (recurrent) M23.9-
ligament disruption, spontaneous
M23.60-
anterior cruciate M23.61-
capsular M23.67-
instability, chronic M23.5-
lateral collateral M23.64-
medial collateral M23.63-
posterior cruciate M23.62-
loose body M23.4-
meniscus M23.30-
cystic M23.00-
lateral M23.002 ◀▥
anterior horn M23.04-
posterior horn M23.05-
specified NEC M23.06-
medial M23.005 ◀▥
anterior horn M23.01-
posterior horn M23.02-
specified NEC M23.03-
degenerate —*see* Derangement, knee,
meniscus, specified NEC
detached —*see* Derangement, knee,
meniscus, specified NEC
due to old tear or injury M23.20-
lateral M23.20-
anterior horn M23.24-
posterior horn M23.25-
specified NEC M23.26-
medial M23.20-
anterior horn M23.21-
posterior horn M23.22-
specified NEC M23.23-
retained —*see* Derangement, knee,
meniscus, specified NEC
specified NEC M23.30-
lateral M23.30-
anterior horn M23.34-
posterior horn M23.35-
specified NEC M23.36-
medial M23.30-
anterior horn M23.31-
posterior horn M23.32-
specified NEC M23.33-
old M23.8X-
specified NEC —*see* subcategory M23.8
low back NEC —*see* Dorsopathy, specified
NEC
meniscus —*see* Derangement, knee,
meniscus
mental —*see* Psychosis
patella, specified NEC —*see* Disorder,
patella, derangement NEC
semilunar cartilage (knee) —*see*
Derangement, knee, meniscus,
specified NEC
shoulder (internal) —*see* Derangement,
joint, shoulder
Dercum's disease E88.2
Derealization (neurotic) F48.1
Dermal —*see* condition
Dermaphytid —*see* Dermatophytosis

Dermatitis (eczematous) L30.9
ab igne L59.0
acarine B88.0
actinic (due to sun) L57.8
other than from sun L59.8
allergic —*see* Dermatitis, contact, allergic
ambustionis, due to burn or scald —*see* Burn
amebic A06.7
ammonia L22
arsenical (ingested) L27.8
artefacta L98.1
psychogenic F54
atopic L20.9
psychogenic F54
specified NEC L20.89
autoimmune progesterone L30.8
berlock, berloque L56.2
blastomycotic B40.3
blister beetle L24.89
bullous, bullosa L13.9
mucosynechial, atrophic L12.1
seasonal L30.8
specified NEC L13.8
calorica L59.0
due to burn or scald —*see* Burn
caterpillar L24.89
cercarial B65.3
combustionis L59.0
due to burn or scald —*see* Burn
congelationis T69.1
contact (occupational) L25.9
allergic L23.9
due to
adhesives L23.1
cement L23.5
chemical products NEC L23.5
chromium L23.0
cosmetics L23.2
dander (cat) (dog) L23.81
drugs in contact with skin L23.3
dyes L23.4
food in contact with skin L23.6
hair (cat) (dog) L23.81
insecticide L23.5
metals L23.0
nickel L23.0
plants, non-food L23.7
plastic L23.5
rubber L23.5
specified agent NEC L23.89
due to
cement L25.3 ◀
chemical products NEC L25.3
cosmetics L25.0
dander (cat) (dog) L23.81
drugs in contact with skin L25.1
dyes L25.2
food in contact with skin L25.4
hair (cat) (dog) L23.81
plants, non-food L25.5
specified agent NEC L25.8
irritant L24.9
due to
cement L25.3 ◀
chemical products NEC L24.5
cosmetics L24.3
detergents L24.0
drugs in contact with skin L24.4
food in contact with skin L24.6
oils and greases L24.1
plants, non-food L24.7
solvents L24.2
specified agent NEC L24.89
contusiformis L52
diabetic —*see* E08-E13 with .620
diaper L22
diphtheritica A36.3
dry skin L85.3
due to
acetone (contact) (irritant) L24.2
acids (contact) (irritant) L24.5

Dermatitis *(Continued)*
due to *(Continued)*
adhesive (s) (allergic) (contact) (plaster)
L23.1
irritant L24.5
alcohol (irritant) (skin contact) (substances in
~~T51.00-T51.93~~category T51) L24.2 ◀▥
taken internally L27.8
alkalis (contact) (irritant) L24.5
arsenic (ingested) L27.8
carbon disulfide (contact) (irritant) L24.2
caustics (contact) (irritant) L24.5
cement (contact) L25.3 ◀▥
cereal (ingested) L27.2
chemical (s) NEC L25.3 ◀▥
taken internally L27.8
chlorocompounds L24.2
chromium (contact) (irritant) L24.81
coffee (ingested) L27.2
cold weather L30.8
cosmetics (contact) L25.0
allergic L23.2
irritant L24.3
cyclohexanes L24.2
dander (cat) (dog) L23.81
Demodex species B88.0
Dermanyssus gallinae B88.0
detergents (contact) (irritant) L24.0
dichromate L24.81
drugs and medicaments (generalized)
(internal use) L27.0
external —*see* Dermatitis, due to, drugs,
in contact with skin
in contact with skin L25.1
allergic L23.3
irritant L24.4
localized skin eruption L27.1
specified substance —*see* Table of
₊Drugs and ₊Chemicals ◀▥
dyes (contact) L25.2
allergic L23.4
irritant L24.89
epidermophytosis —*see* Dermatophytosis
esters L24.2
external irritant NEC L24.9
fish (ingested) L27.2
flour (ingested) L27.2
food (ingested) L27.2
in contact with skin L25.4
fruit (ingested) L27.2
furs (allergic) (contact) L23.81
glues —*see* Dermatitis, due to, adhesives
glycols L24.2
greases NEC (contact) (irritant) L24.1
hair (cat) (dog) L23.81
hot
objects and materials —*see* Burn
weather or places L59.0
hydrocarbons L24.2
infrared rays L59.8
ingestion, ingested substance L27.9
chemical NEC L27.8
drugs and medicaments —*see*
Dermatitis, due to, drugs
food L27.2
specified NEC L27.8
insecticide in contact with skin L24.5
internal agent L27.9
drugs and medicaments (generalized) —
see Dermatitis, due to, drugs
food L27.2
irradiation —*see* Dermatitis, due to,
radioactive substance
ketones L24.2
lacquer tree (allergic) (contact) L23.7
light (sun) NEC L57.8
acute L56.8
other L59.8
Liponyssoides sanguineus B88.0
low temperature L30.8
meat (ingested) L27.2

◀ New   ◀▥ Revised   ~~deleted~~ Deleted

Dermatitis *(Continued)*
  due to *(Continued)*
    metals, metal salts (contact) (irritant)
      L24.81
    milk (ingested) L27.2
    nickel (contact) (irritant) L24.81
    nylon (contact) (irritant) L24.5
    oils NEC (contact) (irritant) L24.1
    paint solvent (contact) (irritant) L24.2
    petroleum products (contact) (irritant)
      (substances in T52) L24.2
    plants NEC (contact) L25.5
      allergic L23.7
      irritant L24.7
    plasters (adhesive) (any) (allergic) (contact)
      L23.1
      irritant L24.5
    plastic (contact) L25.3 ◀▥
    preservatives (contact) —*see* Dermatitis,
      due to, chemical, in contact with
      skin
    primrose (allergic) (contact) L23.7
    primula (allergic) (contact) L23.7
    radiation L59.8
      nonionizing (chronic exposure) L57.8
      sun NEC L57.8
        acute L56.8
    radioactive substance L58.9
      acute L58.0
      chronic L58.1
    radium L58.9
      acute L58.0
      chronic L58.1
    ragweed (allergic) (contact) L23.7
    Rhus (allergic) (contact) (diversiloba)
      (radicans) (toxicodendron) (venenata)
      (verniciflua) L23.7
    rubber (contact) L24.5
    Senecio jacobaea (allergic) (contact)
      L23.7
    solvents (contact) (irritant) (substances in
      ~~T52.00-T52.93~~categories T52) L24.2 ◀▥
    specified agent NEC (contact) L25.8
      allergic L23.89
      irritant L24.89
    sunshine NEC L57.8
      acute L56.8
    tetrachlorethylene (contact) (irritant)
      L24.2
    toluene (contact) (irritant) L24.2
    turpentine (contact) L24.2
    ultraviolet rays (sun NEC) (chronic
      exposure) L57.8
      acute L56.8
    vaccine or vaccination L27.0
      specified substance —*see* Table of
        ~~d~~Drugs and ~~c~~Chemicals ◀▥
    varicose veins —*see* Varix, leg, with,
      inflammation
    X-rays L58.9
      acute L58.0
      chronic L58.1
  dyshydrotic L30.1
  dysmenorrheica N94.6
  escharotica —*see* Burn
  exfoliative, exfoliativa (generalized) L26
    neonatorum L00
  eyelid —*see also* Dermatosis, eyelid
    allergic H01.119
      left H01.116
        lower H01.115
        upper H01.114
      right H01.113
        lower H01.112
        upper H01.111
    contact —*see* Dermatitis, eyelid,
      allergic
    due to
      Demodex species B88.0
      herpes (zoster) B02.39
        simplex B00.59

Dermatitis *(Continued)*
  eyelid *(Continued)*
    eczematous H01.139
      left H01.136
        lower H01.135
        upper H01.134
      right H01.133
        lower H01.132
        upper H01.131
    facta, factitia, factitial L98.1
      psychogenic F54
    flexural NEC L20.82
    friction L30.4
    fungus B36.9
      specified type NEC B36.8
    gangrenosa, gangrenous infantum
      L08.0
    harvest mite B88.0
    heat L59.0
    herpesviral, vesicular (ear) (lip) B00.1
    herpetiformis (bullous) (erythematous)
      (pustular) (vesicular) L13.0
      juvenile L12.2
      senile L12.0
    hiemalis L30.8
    hypostatic, hypostatica —*see* Varix, leg, with,
      inflammation
    infectious eczematoid L30.3
    infective L30.3
    irritant —*see* Dermatitis, contact, irritant
    Jacquet's (diaper dermatitis) L22
    Leptus B88.0
    lichenified NEC L28.0
    medicamentosa (generalized) (internal
      use) —*see* Dermatitis, due to drugs
    mite B88.0
    multiformis L13.0
      juvenile L12.2
    napkin L22
    neurotica L13.0
    nummular L30.0
    papillaris capillitii L73.0
    pellagrous E52
    perioral L71.0
    photocontact L56.2
    polymorpha dolorosa L13.0
    pruriginosa L13.0
    pruritic NEC L30.8
    psychogenic F54
    purulent L08.0
    pustular
      contagious B08.02
      subcorneal L13.1
    pyococcal L08.0
    pyogenica L08.0
    repens L40.2
    Ritter's (exfoliativa) L00
    Schamberg's L81.7
    schistosome B65.3
    seasonal bullous L30.8
    seborrheic L21.9
      infantile L21.1
      specified NEC L21.8
    sensitization NOS L23.9
    septic L08.0
    solare L57.8
    specified NEC L30.8
    stasis I87.2
      with varicose ulcer —*see* Varix, leg, with
        ulcer, with inflammation
      due to postthrombotic syndrome —*see*
        Syndrome, postthrombotic
    suppurative L08.0
    traumatic NEC L30.4
    trophoneurotica L13.0
    ultraviolet (sun) (chronic exposure) L57.8
      acute L56.8
    varicose —*see* Varix, leg, with, inflammation
    vegetans L10.1
    verrucosa B43.0
    vesicular, herpesviral B00.1

Dermatoarthritis, lipoid E78.81
Dermatochalasis, eyelid H02.839
  left H02.836
    lower H02.835
    upper H02.834
  right H02.833
    lower H02.832
    upper H02.831
Dermatofibroma (lenticulare) —*see* Neoplasm,
  skin, benign ◀▥
  protuberans —*see* Neoplasm, skin, uncertain
    behavior
Dermatofibrosarcoma (pigmented)
  (protuberans) —*see* Neoplasm, skin,
  malignant
Dermatographia L50.3
Dermatolysis (exfoliativa) (congenital)
  Q82.8
  acquired L57.4
  eyelids —*see* Blepharochalasis
  palpebrarum —*see* Blepharochalasis
  senile L57.4
Dermatomegaly NEC Q82.8
Dermatomucosomyositis M33.10
  with
    myopathy M33.12
    respiratory involvement M33.11
    specified organ involvement NEC
      M33.19
Dermatomycosis B36.9
  furfuracea B36.0
  specified type NEC B36.8
Dermatomyositis (acute) (chronic) —*see also*
  Dermatopolymyositis
  in (due to) neoplastic disease (*see also*
    Neoplasm) D49.9 *[M36.0]*
Dermatoneuritis of children —*see* Poisoning,
  mercury
Dermatophilosis A48.8
Dermatophytid L30.2
Dermatophytide —*see* Dermatophytosis
Dermatophytosis (epidermophyton) (infection)
  (Microsporum) (tinea) (Trichophyton)
  B35.9
  beard B35.0
  body B35.4
  capitis B35.0
  corporis B35.4
  deep-seated B35.8
  disseminated B35.8
  foot B35.3
  granulomatous B35.8
  groin B35.6
  hand B35.2
  nail B35.1
  perianal (area) B35.6
  scalp B35.0
  specified NEC B35.8
Dermatopolymyositis M33.90
  with
    myopathy M33.92
    respiratory involvement M33.91
    specified organ involvement NEC
      M33.99
  in neoplastic disease (*see also* Neoplasm)
    D49.9 *[M36.0]*
  juvenile M33.00
    with
      myopathy M33.02
      respiratory involvement M33.01
      specified organ involvement NEC
        M33.09
  specified NEC M33.10
    myopathy M33.12
    respiratory involvement M33.11
    specified organ involvement NEC M33.19
Dermatopolyneuritis —*see* Poisoning, mercury
Dermatorrhexis Q79.6
  acquired L57.4
Dermatosclerosis —*see also* Scleroderma
  localized L94.0

Dermatosis L98.9
  Andrews' L08.89
  Bowen's —see Neoplasm, skin, in situ
  bullous L13.9
    specified NEC L13.8
  exfoliativa L26
  eyelid (noninfectious)
    dermatitis —see Dermatitis, eyelid
    discoid lupus erythematosus —see Lupus,
      erythematosus, eyelid
    xeroderma —see Xeroderma, acquired,
      eyelid
  factitial L98.1
  febrile neutrophilic L98.2
  gonococcal A54.89
  herpetiformis L13.0
    juvenile L12.2
  linear IgA L13.8
  menstrual NEC L98.8
  neutrophilic, febrile L98.2
  occupational —see Dermatitis, contact
  papulosa nigra L82.1
  pigmentary L81.9
    progressive L81.7
    Schamberg's L81.7
  psychogenic F54
  purpuric, pigmented L81.7
  pustular, subcorneal L13.1
  transient acantholytic L11.1
Dermographia, dermographism L50.3
Dermoid (cyst) —see also Neoplasm, benign,
    by site
  with malignant transformation C56-
  due to radiation (nonionizing) L57.8
Dermopathy
  infiltrative with thyrotoxicosis —see
    Thyrotoxicosis
  nephrogenic fibrosing L90.8
Dermophytosis —see Dermatophytosis
Descemetocele H18.73-
Descemet's membrane —see condition
Descending —see condition
Descensus uteri —see Prolapse, uterus
Desert
  rheumatism B38.0
  sore —see Ulcer, skin
Desertion (newborn) —see Maltreatment
Desmoid (extra-abdominal) (tumor) —see
    Neoplasm, connective tissue, uncertain
    behavior
  abdominal D48.1
Despondency F32.9
Desquamation, skin R23.4
Destruction, destructive —see also Damage
  articular facet —see also Derangement, joint,
      specified type NEC
    knee M23.8X-
    vertebra —see Spondylosis
  bone —see also Disorder, bone, specified type
      NEC
    syphilitic A52.77
  joint —see also Derangement, joint, specified
      type NEC
    sacroiliac M53.3
  rectal sphincter K62.89
  septum (nasal) J34.89
  tuberculous NEC —see Tuberculosis
  tympanum, tympanic membrane
      (nontraumatic) —see Disorder,
      tympanic membrane, specified
      NEC
  vertebral disc —see Degeneration,
      intervertebral disc
Destructiveness —see also Disorder, conduct
  adjustment reaction —see Disorder,
      adjustment
Desultory labor O62.2
Detachment
  cartilage —see Sprain
  cervix, annular N88.8
    complicating delivery O71.3

Detachment (Continued)
  choroid (old) (postinfectional) (simple)
      (spontaneous) H31.40-
    hemorrhagic H31.41-
    serous H31.42-
  ligament —see Sprain
  meniscus (knee) —see also Derangement,
      knee, meniscus, specified NEC
    current injury —see Tear, meniscus
    due to old tear or injury —see
        Derangement, knee, meniscus, due
        to old tear
  retina (without retinal break) (serous) H33.2-
    with retinal:
      break H33.00-
        giant H33.03-
        multiple H33.02-
        single H33.01-
      dialysis H33.04-
    pigment epithelium —see Degeneration,
        retina, separation of layers, pigment
        epithelium detachment
    rhegmatogenous —see Detachment, retina,
        with retinal, break
    specified NEC H33.8
    total H33.05-
    traction H33.4-
  vitreous (body) H43.81
Detergent asthma J69.8
Deterioration
  epileptic F06.8
  general physical R53.81
  heart, cardiac —see Degeneration, myocardial
  mental —see Psychosis
  myocardial, myocardium —see Degeneration,
      myocardial
  senile (simple) R54
Deuteranomaly (anomalous trichromat) H53.53
Deuteranopia (complete) (incomplete) H53.53
Development
  abnormal, bone Q79.9
  arrested R62.50
    bone —see Arrest, development or growth,
        bone
    child R62.50
    due to malnutrition E45
  defective, congenital —see also Anomaly, by
      site
    cauda equina Q06.3
    left ventricle Q24.8
      in hypoplastic left heart syndrome
          Q23.4
    valve Q24.8
      pulmonary Q22.3
  delayed (see also Delay, development) R62.50
    arithmetical skills F81.2
    language (skills) (expressive) F80.1
    learning skill F81.9
    mixed skills F88
    motor coordination F82
    reading F81.0
    specified learning skill NEC F81.89
    speech F80.9
    spelling F81.81
    written expression F81.81
  imperfect, congenital —see also Anomaly, by
      site
    heart Q24.9
    lungs Q33.6
  incomplete
    bronchial tree Q32.4
    organ or site not listed —see Hypoplasia,
        by site
    respiratory system Q34.9
    sexual, precocious NEC E30.1
  tardy, mental (see also Disability, intellectual)
      F79
Developmental —see condition
  testing, child —see Examination, child
Devergie's disease (pityriasis rubra pilaris)
    L44.0

Deviation (in)
  conjugate palsy (eye) (spastic) H51.0
  esophagus (acquired) K22.8
  eye, skew H51.8
  midline (jaw) (teeth) (dental arch) M26.29
    specified site NEC —see Malposition
  nasal septum J34.2
    congenital Q67.4
  opening and closing of the mandible M26.53
  organ or site, congenital NEC —see
      Malposition, congenital
  septum (nasal) (acquired) J34.2
    congenital Q67.4
  sexual F65.9
    bestiality F65.89
    erotomania F52.8
    exhibitionism F65.2
    fetishism, fetishistic F65.0
      transvestism F65.1
    frotteurism F65.81
    masochism F65.51
    multiple F65.89
    necrophilia F65.89
    nymphomania F52.8
    pederosis F65.4
    pedophilia F65.4
    sadism, sadomasochism F65.52
    satyriasis F52.8
    specified type NEC F65.89
    transvestism F64.1
    voyeurism F65.3
  teeth, midline M26.29
  trachea J39.8
  ureter, congenital Q62.61
Device
  cerebral ventricle (communicating) in situ
      Z98.2
  contraceptive —see Contraceptive, device
  drainage, cerebrospinal fluid, in situ Z98.2
Devic's disease G36.0
Devil's
  grip B33.0
  pinches (purpura simplex) D69.2
Devitalized tooth K04.99
Devonshire colic —see Poisoning, lead
Dextraposition, aorta Q20.3
  in tetralogy of Fallot Q21.3
Dextrinosis, limit (debrancher enzyme
    deficiency) E74.03
Dextrocardia (true) Q24.0
  with
    complete transposition of viscera Q89.3
    situs inversus Q89.3
Dextrotransposition, aorta Q20.3
d-glycericacidemia E72.59
Dhat syndrome F48.8
Dhobi itch B35.6
Di George's syndrome D82.1
Di Guglielmo's disease C94.0-
Diabetes, diabetic (mellitus) (sugar) E11.9
  with
    amyotrophy E11.44
    arthropathy NEC E11.618
    autonomic (poly)neuropathy E11.43
    cataract E11.36
    Charcot's joints E11.610
    chronic kidney disease E11.22
    circulatory complication NEC E11.59
    complication E11.8
      specified NEC E11.69
    dermatitis E11.620
    foot ulcer E11.621
    gangrene E11.52
    gastroparesis E11.43
    glomerulonephrosis, intracapillary E11.21
    glomerulosclerosis, intercapillary E11.21
    hyperglycemia E11.65
    hyperosmolarity E11.00
      with coma E11.01
    hypoglycemia E11.649
      with coma E11.641

◀ New   ◀▦ Revised   ~~deleted~~ Deleted

Diabetes, diabetic (Continued)
  with (Continued)
    kidney complications NEC E11.29
    Kimmelstiel-Wilson disease E11.21
    loss of protective sensation (LOPS) —see
      Diabetes, by type, with neuropathy
    mononeuropathy E11.41
    myasthenia E11.44
    necrobiosis lipoidica E11.620
    nephropathy E11.21
    neuralgia E11.42
    neurologic complication NEC E11.49
    neuropathic arthropathy E11.610
    neuropathy E11.40
    ophthalmic complication NEC E11.39
    oral complication NEC E11.638
    periodontal disease E11.630
    peripheral angiopathy E11.51
      with gangrene E11.52
    polyneuropathy E11.42
    renal complication NEC E11.29
    renal tubular degeneration E11.29
    retinopathy E11.319
      with macular edema E11.311
      nonproliferative E11.329
        with macular edema E11.321
        mild E11.329
          with macular edema E11.321
        moderate E11.339
          with macular edema E11.331
        severe E11.349
          with macular edema E11.341
      proliferative E11.359
        with macular edema E11.351
    skin complication NEC E11.628
    skin ulcer NEC E11.622
  bronzed E83.110
  complicating pregnancy —see Pregnancy,
    complicated by, diabetes
  dietary counseling and surveillance Z71.3
  due to drug or chemical E09.9
    with
      amyotrophy E09.44
      arthropathy NEC E09.618
      autonomic (poly)neuropathy E09.43
      cataract E09.36
      Charcot's joints E09.610
      chronic kidney disease E09.22
      circulatory complication NEC E09.59
      complication E09.8
        specified NEC E09.69
      dermatitis E09.620
      foot ulcer E09.621
      gangrene E09.52
      gastroparesis E09.43
      glomerulonephrosis, intracapillary
        E09.21
      glomerulosclerosis, intercapillary E09.21
      hyperglycemia E09.65
      hyperosmolarity E09.00
        with coma E09.01
      hypoglycemia E09.649
        with coma E09.641
      ketoacidosis E09.10
        with coma E09.11
      kidney complications NEC E09.29
      Kimmelstiel-Wilson disease E09.21
      mononeuropathy E09.41
      myasthenia E09.44
      necrobiosis lipoidica E09.620
      nephropathy E09.21
      neuralgia E09.42
      neurologic complication NEC E09.49
      neuropathic arthropathy E09.610
      neuropathy E09.40
      ophthalmic complication NEC E09.39
      oral complication NEC E09.638
      periodontal disease E09.630
      peripheral angiopathy E09.51
        with gangrene E09.52
      polyneuropathy E09.42

Diabetes, diabetic (Continued)
  due to drug or chemical (Continued)
    with (Continued)
      renal complication NEC E09.29
      renal tubular degeneration E09.29
      retinopathy E09.319
        with macular edema E09.311
        nonproliferative E09.329
          with macular edema E09.321
          mild E09.329
            with macular edema E09.321
          moderate E09.339
            with macular edema E09.331
          severe E09.349
            with macular edema E09.341
        proliferative E09.359
          with macular edema E09.351
      skin complication NEC E09.628
      skin ulcer NEC E09.622
  due to underlying condition E08.9
    with
      amyotrophy E08.44
      arthropathy NEC E08.618
      autonomic (poly)neuropathy E08.43
      cataract E08.36
      Charcot's joints E08.610
      chronic kidney disease E08.22
      circulatory complication NEC E08.59
      complication E08.8
        specified NEC E08.69
      dermatitis E08.620
      foot ulcer E08.621
      gangrene E08.52
      gastroparesis E08.43
      glomerulonephrosis, intracapillary
        E08.21
      glomerulosclerosis, intercapillary
        E08.21
      hyperglycemia E08.69
      hyperosmolarity E08.00
        with coma E08.01
      hypoglycemia E08.649
        with coma E08.641
      ketoacidosis E08.10
        with coma E08.11
      kidney complications NEC E08.29
      Kimmelstiel-WIlson disease E08.21
      mononeuropathy E08.41
      myasthenia E08.44
      necrobiosis lipoidica E08.620
      nephropathy E08.21
      neuralgia E08.42
      neurologic complication NEC E08.49
      neuropathic arthropathy E08.610
      neuropathy E08.40
      ophthalmic complication NEC
        E08.39
      oral complication NEC E08.638
      periodontal disease E08.630
      peripheral angiopathy E08.51
        with gangrene E08.52
      polyneuropathy E08.42
      renal complication NEC E08.29
      renal tubular degeneration E08.29
      retinopathy E08.319
        with macular edema E08.311
        nonproliferative E08.329
          with macular edema E08.321
          mild E08.329
            with macular edema E08.321
          moderate E08.339
            with macular edema E08.331
          severe E08.349
            with macular edema E08.341
        proliferative E08.359
          with macular edema E08.351
      skin complication NEC E08.628
      skin ulcer NEC E08.622
  gestational (in pregnancy) O24.419
    affecting newborn P70.0
    diet-controlled O24.410

Diabetes, diabetic (Continued)
  gestational (Continued)
    in childbirth O24.429
      diet-controlled O24.420
      insulin (and diet) controlled
        O24.424
    insulin (and diet) controlled
      O24.414
    puerperal O24.439
      diet-controlled O24.430
      insulin (and diet) controlled O24.434
  hepatogenous E13.9
  inadequately controlled — code to Diabetes,
    by type, with hyperglycemia
  insipidus E23.2
    nephrogenic N25.1
    pituitary E23.2
    vasopressin resistant N25.1
  insulin dependent — code to type of
    diabetes
  juvenile-onset —see Diabetes, type 1
  ketosis-prone —see Diabetes, type 1
  latent R73.09
  neonatal (transient) P70.2
  non-insulin dependent — code to type of
    diabetes
  out of control — code to Diabetes, by type,
    with hyperglycemia
  phosphate E83.39
  poorly controlled — code to Diabetes, by
    type, with hyperglycemia
  postpancreatectomy —see Diabetes, specified
    type NEC
  postprocedural —see Diabetes, specified type
    NEC
  secondary diabetes mellitus NEC —see
    Diabetes, specified type NEC
  specified type NEC E13.9
    with
      amyotrophy E13.44
      arthropathy NEC E13.618
      autonomic (poly)neuropathy E13.43
      cataract E13.36
      Charcot's joints E13.610
      chronic kidney disease E13.22
      circulatory complication NEC E13.59
      complication E13.8
        specified NEC E13.69
      dermatitis E13.620
      foot ulcer E13.621
      gangrene E13.52
      gastroparesis E13.43
      glomerulonephrosis, intracapillary
        E13.21
      glomerulosclerosis, intercapillary
        E13.21
      hyperglycemia E13.65
      hyperosmolarity E13.00
        with coma E13.01
      hypoglycemia E13.649
        with coma E13.641
      ketoacidosis E13.10
        with coma E13.11
      kidney complications NEC E13.29
      Kimmelstiel-Wilson disease E13.21
      mononeuropathy E13.41
      myasthenia E13.44
      necrobiosis lipoidica E13.620
      nephropathy E13.21
      neuralgia E13.42
      neurologic complication NEC E13.49
      neuropathic arthropathy E13.610
      neuropathy E13.40
      ophthalmic complication NEC E13.39
      oral complication NEC E13.638
      periodontal disease E13.630
      peripheral angiopathy E13.51
        with gangrene E13.52
      polyneuropathy E13.42
      renal complication NEC E13.29
      renal tubular degeneration E13.29

Diabetes, diabetic (Continued)
  specified type NEC (Continued)
    with (Continued)
      retinopathy E13.319
        with macular edema E13.311
        nonproliferative E13.329
          with macular edema E13.321
          mild E13.329
            with macular edema E13.321
          moderate E13.339
            with macular edema E13.331
          severe E13.349
            with macular edema E13.341
        proliferative E13.359
          with macular edema E13.351
      skin complication NEC E13.628
      skin ulcer NEC E13.622
    steroid-induced —see Diabetes, due to, drug
      or chemical
  type 1 E10.9
    with
      amyotrophy E10.44
      arthropathy NEC E10.618
      autonomic (poly)neuropathy E10.43
      cataract E10.36
      Charcot's joints E10.610
      chronic kidney disease E10.22
      circulatory complication NEC E10.59
      complication E10.8
        specified NEC E10.69
      dermatitis E10.620
      foot ulcer E10.621
      gangrene E10.52
      gastroparesis E10.43
      glomerulonephrosis, intracapillary
        E10.21
      glomerulosclerosis, intercapillary E10.21
      hyperglycemia E10.65
      hypoglycemia E10.649
        with coma E10.641
      ketoacidosis E10.10
        with coma E10.11
      kidney complications NEC E10.29
      Kimmelstiel-Wilson disease E10.21
      mononeuropathy E10.41
      myasthenia E10.44
      necrobiosis lipoidica E10.620
      nephropathy E10.21
      neuralgia E10.42
      neurologic complication NEC E10.49
      neuropathic arthropathy E10.610
      neuropathy E10.40
      ophthalmic complication NEC E10.39
      oral complication NEC E10.638
      periodontal disease E10.630
      peripheral angiopathy E10.51
        with gangrene E10.52
      polyneuropathy E10.42
      renal complication NEC E10.29
      renal tubular degeneration E10.29
      retinopathy E10.319
        with macular edema E10.311
        nonproliferative E10.329
          with macular edema E10.321
          mild E10.329
            with macular edema E10.321
          moderate E10.339
            with macular edema E10.331
          severe E10.349
            with macular edema E10.341
        proliferative E10.359
          with macular edema E10.351
      skin complication NEC E10.628
      skin ulcer NEC E10.622
  type 2 E11.9
    with
      amyotrophy E11.44
      arthropathy NEC E11.618
      autonomic (poly)neuropathy E11.43
      cataract E11.36
      Charcot's joints E11.610

Diabetes, diabetic (Continued)
  type 2 (Continued)
    with (Continued)
      chronic kidney disease E11.22
      circulatory complication NEC E11.59
      complication E11.8
        specified NEC E11.69
      dermatitis E11.620
      foot ulcer E11.621
      gangrene E11.52
      gastroparesis E11.43
      glomerulonephrosis, intracapillary
        E11.21
      glomerulosclerosis, intercapillary E11.21
      hyperglycemia E11.65
      hyperosmolarity E11.00
        with coma E11.01
      hypoglycemia E11.649
        with coma E11.641
      kidney complications NEC E11.29
      Kimmelstiel-Wilson disease E11.21
      mononeuropathy E11.41
      myasthenia E11.44
      necrobiosis lipoidica E11.620
      nephropathy E11.21
      neuralgia E11.42
      neurologic complication NEC E11.49
      neuropathic arthropathy E11.610
      neuropathy E11.40
      ophthalmic complication NEC E11.39
      oral complication NEC E11.638
      periodontal disease E11.630
      peripheral angiopathy E11.51
        with gangrene E11.52
      polyneuropathy E11.42
      renal complication NEC E11.29
      renal tubular degeneration E11.29
      retinopathy E11.319
        with macular edema E11.311
        nonproliferative E11.329
          with macular edema E11.321
          mild E11.329
            with macular edema E11.321
          moderate E11.339
            with macular edema E11.331
          severe E11.349
            with macular edema E11.341
        proliferative E11.359
          with macular edema E11.351
      skin complication NEC E11.628
      skin ulcer NEC E11.622
Diacyclothrombopathia D69.1
Diagnosis deferred R69
Dialysis (intermittent) (treatment)
  noncompliance (with) Z91.15
  renal (hemodialysis) (peritoneal), status Z99.2
  retina, retinal —see Detachment, retina, with
    retinal, dialysis
Diamond-Blackfan anemia (congenital
    hypoplastic) D61.01
Diamond-Gardener syndrome
    (autoerythrocyte sensitization) D69.2
Diaper rash L22
Diaphoresis (excessive) R61
Diaphragm —see condition
Diaphragmalgia R07.1
Diaphragmatitis, diaphragmitis J98.6
Diaphysial aclasis Q78.6
Diaphysitis —see Osteomyelitis, specified type
    NEC
Diarrhea, diarrheal (disease) (infantile)
    (inflammatory) R19.7
  achlorhydric K31.83
  allergic K52.2
  amebic (see also Amebiasis) A06.0
    with abscess —see Abscess, amebic
    acute A06.0
    chronic A06.1
    nondysenteric A06.2
  bacillary —see Dysentery, bacillary
  balantidial A07.0

Diarrhea, diarrheal (Continued)
  cachectic NEC K52.89
  Chilomastix A07.8
  choleriformis A00.1
  chronic (noninfectious) K52.9
  coccidial A07.3
  Cochin-China K90.1
    strongyloidiasis B78.0
  Dientamoeba A07.8
  dietetic K52.2
  drug-induced K52.1
  due to
    bacteria A04.9
      specified NEC A04.8
    Campylobacter A04.5
    Capillaria philippinensis B81.1
    Clostridium difficile A04.7
    Clostridium perfringens (C) (F) A04.8
    Cryptosporidium A07.2
    drugs K52.1
    Escherichia coli A04.4
      enteroaggregative A04.4
      enterohemorrhagic A04.3
      enteroinvasive A04.2
      enteropathogenic A04.0
      enterotoxigenic A04.1
      specified NEC A04.4
    food hypersensitivity K52.2
    Necator americanus B76.1
    S. japonicum B65.2
    specified organism NEC A08.8
      bacterial A04.8
      viral A08.39
    Staphylococcus A04.8
    Trichuris trichiuria B79
    virus —see Enteritis, viral
    Yersinia enterocolitica A04.6
  dysenteric A09
  endemic A09
  epidemic A09
  flagellate A07.9
  Flexner's (ulcerative) A03.1
  functional K59.1
    following gastrointestinal surgery K91.89
    psychogenic F45.8
  Giardia lamblia A07.1
  giardial A07.1
  hill K90.1
  infectious A09
  malarial —see Malaria
  mite B88.0
  mycotic NEC B49
  neonatal (noninfectious) P78.3
  nervous F45.8
  neurogenic K59.1
  noninfectious K52.9
  postgastrectomy K91.1
  postvagotomy K91.1
  protozoal A07.9
    specified NEC A07.8
  psychogenic F45.8
  specified
    bacterium NEC A04.8
    virus NEC A08.39
  strongyloidiasis B78.0
  toxic K52.1
  trichomonal A07.8
  tropical K90.1
  tuberculous A18.32
  viral —see Enteritis, viral
Diastasis
  cranial bones M84.88
    congenital NEC Q75.8
  joint (traumatic) —see Dislocation
  muscle M62.00
    ankle M62.07-
    congenital Q79.8
    foot M62.07-
    forearm M62.03-
    hand M62.04-
    lower leg M62.06-

◀ New   ◀▥▥ Revised   ~~deleted~~ Deleted

Diastasis (Continued)
  muscle (Continued)
    pelvic region M62.05-
    shoulder region M62.01-
    specified site NEC M62.08
    thigh M62.05-
    upper arm M62.02-
  recti (abdomen)
    complicating delivery O71.89
    congenital Q79.59
Diastema, tooth, teeth, fully erupted M26.32
Diastematomyelia Q06.2
Diataxia, cerebral G80.4
Diathesis
  allergic —see History, allergy
  bleeding (familial) D69.9
  cystine (familial) E72.00
  gouty —see Gout
  hemorrhagic (familial) D69.9
    newborn NEC P53
  spasmophilic R29.0
Diaz's disease or osteochondrosis (juvenile)
  (talus) —see Osteochondrosis, juvenile,
  tarsus
Dibothriocephalus, dibothriocephaliasis
  (latus) (infection) (infestation) B70.0
  larval B70.1
Dicephalus, dicephaly Q89.4
Dichotomy, teeth K00.2
Dichromat, dichromatopsia (congenital) —see
  Deficiency, color vision
Dichuchwa A65
Dicroceliasis B66.2
Didelphia, didelphys —see Double uterus
Didymytis N45.1
  with orchitis N45.3
Dietary
  inadequacy or deficiency E63.9
  surveillance and counseling Z71.3
Dietl's crisis N13.8
Dieulafoy lesion (hemorrhagic)
  duodenum K31.82
  esophagus K22.8
  intestine (colon) K63.81
  stomach K31.82
Difficult, difficulty (in)
  acculturation Z60.3
  feeding R63.3
    newborn P92.9
      breast P92.5
      specified NEC P92.8
    nonorganic (infant or child) F98.29
  intubation, in anesthesia T88.4
  mechanical, gastroduodenal stoma K91.89
    causing obstruction K91.3
  reading (developmental) F81.0
    secondary to emotional disorders F93.9
  spelling (specific) F81.81
    with reading disorder F81.89
    due to inadequate teaching Z55.8
  swallowing —see Dysphagia
  walking R26.2
  work
    conditions NEC Z56.5
    schedule Z56.3
Diffuse —see condition
DiGeorge's syndrome (thymic hypoplasia)
  D82.1
Digestive —see condition
Dihydropyrimidine dehydrogenase disease
  (DPD) E88.89
Diktyoma —see Neoplasm, malignant, by site
Dilaceration, tooth K00.4
Dilatation
  anus K59.8
    venule —see Hemorrhoids
  aorta (focal) (general) —see Ectasia, aorta
    with aneurysm —see Aneurysm, aorta
  artery —see Aneurysm
  bladder (sphincter) N32.89
    congenital Q64.79

Dilatation (Continued)
  blood vessel I99.8
  bronchial J47.9
    with
      exacerbation (acute) J47.1
      lower respiratory infection J47.0
  calyx (due to obstruction) —see
    Hydronephrosis
  capillaries I78.8
  cardiac (acute) (chronic) —see also
    Hypertrophy, cardiac
    congenital Q24.8
      valve NEC Q24.8
        pulmonary Q22.3
    valve —see Endocarditis
  cavum septi pellucidi Q06.8
  cervix (uteri) —see also Incompetency,
    cervix
    incomplete, poor, slow complicating
      delivery O62.0
  colon K59.3
    congenital Q43.1
    psychogenic F45.8
  common duct (acquired) K83.8
    congenital Q44.5
  cystic duct (acquired) K82.8
    congenital Q44.5
  duct, mammary —see Ectasia, mammary
    duct
  duodenum K59.8
  esophagus K22.8
    congenital Q39.5
    due to achalasia K22.0
  eustachian tube, congenital Q17.8
  gallbladder K82.8
  gastric —see Dilatation, stomach
  heart (acute) (chronic) —see also Hypertrophy,
    cardiac
    congenital Q24.8
    valve —see Endocarditis
  ileum K59.8
    psychogenic F45.8
  jejunum K59.8
    psychogenic F45.8
  kidney (calyx) (collecting structures) (cystic)
    (parenchyma) (pelvis) (idiopathic)
    N28.89
  lacrimal passages or duct —see Disorder,
    lacrimal system, changes
  lymphatic vessel I89.0
  mammary duct —see Ectasia, mammary
    duct
  Meckel's diverticulum (congenital) Q43.0
    malignant —see Table of Neoplasms, small
      intestine, malignant
  myocardium (acute) (chronic) —see
    Hypertrophy, cardiac organ or site,
    congenital NEC —see Distortion
  pancreatic duct K86.8
  pericardium —see Pericarditis
  pharynx J39.2
  prostate N42.89
  pulmonary
    artery (idiopathic) I28.8
    valve, congenital Q22.3
  pupil H57.04
  rectum K59.3
  saccule, congenital Q16.5
  salivary gland (duct) K11.8
  sphincter ani K62.89
  stomach K31.89
    acute K31.0
    psychogenic F45.8
  submaxillary duct K11.8
  trachea, congenital Q32.1
  ureter (idiopathic) N28.82
    congenital Q62.2
    due to obstruction N13.4
  urethra (acquired) N36.8
  vasomotor I73.9
  vein I86.8

Dilatation (Continued)
  ventricular, ventricle (acute) (chronic) —see
    also Hypertrophy, cardiac
    cerebral, congenital Q04.8
  venule NEC I86.8
  vesical orifice N32.89
Dilated, dilation —see Dilatation
Diminished, diminution
  hearing (acuity) —see Deafness
  sense or sensation (cold) (heat) (tactile)
    (vibratory) R20.8
  vision NEC H54.7
  vital capacity R94.2
Diminuta taenia B71.0
Dimitri-Sturge-Weber disease Q85.8
Dimple
  parasacral, pilonidal or postanal —see Cyst,
    pilonidal
Dioctophyme renalis (infection) (infestation)
  B83.8
Dipetalonemiasis B74.4
Diphallus Q55.69
Diphtheria, diphtheritic (gangrenous)
  (hemorrhagic) A36.9
  carrier (suspected) Z22.2
  cutaneous A36.3
  faucial A36.0
  infection of wound A36.3
  laryngeal A36.2
  myocarditis A36.81
  nasal, anterior A36.89
  nasopharyngeal A36.1
  neurological complication A36.89
  pharyngeal A36.0
  specified site NEC A36.89
  tonsillar A36.0
Diphyllobothriasis (intestine) B70.0
  larval B70.1
Diplacusis H93.22-
Diplegia (upper limbs) G83.0
  congenital (cerebral) G80.8
  facial G51.0
  lower limbs G82.20
  spastic G80.1
Diplococcus, diplococcal —see condition
Diplopia H53.2
Dipsomania F10.20
  with
    psychosis —see Psychosis, alcoholic
    remission F10.21
Dipylidiasis B71.1
Direction, teeth, abnormal, fully erupted
  M26.30
Dirofilariasis B74.8
Dirt-eating child F98.3
Disability, disabilities
  heart —see Disease, heart
  intellectual F79
    with
      autistic features F84.9
    mild (I.Q. 50-69) F70 ◀▥
    moderate (I.Q. 35-49) F71 ◀▥
    profound (I.Q. under 20) F73
    severe (I.Q. 20-34) F72 ◀▥
    specified level NEC F78
  knowledge acquisition F81.9
  learning F81.9
  limiting activities Z73.6
  spelling, specific F81.81
Disappearance of family member Z63.4
Disarticulation —see Amputation
  meaning traumatic amputation —see
    Amputation, traumatic
Discharge (from)
  abnormal finding in —see Abnormal,
    specimen
  breast (female) (male) N64.52
  diencephalic autonomic idiopathic —see
    Epilepsy, specified NEC
  ear —see also Otorrhea
    blood —see Otorrhagia

Discharge (Continued)
  excessive urine R35.8
  nipple N64.52
  penile R36.9
  postnasal R09.82
  prison, anxiety concerning Z65.2
  urethral R36.9
    without blood R36.0
    hematospermia R36.1
  vaginal N89.8
Discitis, diskitis M46.40
  cervical region M46.42
  cervicothoracic region M46.43
  lumbar region M46.46
  lumbosacral region M46.47
  multiple sites M46.49
  occipito-atlanto-axial region M46.41
  pyogenic —see Infection, intervertebral
    disc, pyogenic
  sacrococcygeal region M46.48
  thoracic region M46.44
  thoracolumbar region M46.45
Discoid
  meniscus (congenital) Q68.6
  semilunar cartilage (congenital) —see
    Derangement, knee, meniscus,
    specified NEC
Discoloration
  nails L60.8
  teeth (posteruptive) K03.7
    during formation K00.8
Discomfort
  chest R07.89
  visual H53.14-
Discontinuity, ossicles, ear
  H74.2-
Discord (with)
  boss Z56.4
  classmates Z55.4
  counselor Z64.4
  employer Z56.4
  family Z63.8
  fellow employees Z56.4
  in-laws Z63.1
  landlord Z59.2
  lodgers Z59.2
  neighbors Z59.2
  probation officer Z64.4
  social worker Z64.4
  teachers Z55.4
  workmates Z56.4
Discordant connection
  atrioventricular (congenital) Q20.5
  ventriculoarterial Q20.3
Discrepancy
  centric occlusion maximum intercuspation
    M26.55
  leg length (acquired) —see Deformity, limb,
    unequal length
    congenital —see Defect, reduction, lower
      limb
  uterine size date O26.84-
Discrimination
  ethnic Z60.5
  political Z60.5
  racial Z60.5
  religious Z60.5
  sex Z60.5
Disease, diseased —see also Syndrome
  absorbent system I87.8
  acid-peptic K30
  Acosta's T70.29
  Adams-Stokes (-Morgagni) (syncope with
    heart block) I45.9
  Addison's anemia (pernicious) D51.0
  adenoids (and tonsils) J35.9
  adrenal (capsule) (cortex) (gland) (medullary)
    E27.9
    hyperfunction E27.0
    specified NEC E27.8
  ainhum L94.6

Disease, diseased (Continued)
  airway
    obstructive, chronic J44.9
      due to
        cotton dust J66.0
        specific organic dusts NEC J66.8
    reactive —see Asthma
  akamushi (scrub typhus) A75.3
  Albers-Schönberg (marble bones) Q78.2
  Albert's —see Tendinitis, Achilles
  alimentary canal K63.9
  alligator-skin Q80.9
    acquired L85.0
  alpha heavy chain C88.3
  alpine T70.29
  altitude T70.20
  alveolar ridge
    edentulous K06.9
      specified NEC K06.8
  alveoli, teeth K08.9
  Alzheimer's G30.9 [F02.80]
    with behavioral disturbance G30.9
      [F02.81]
    early onset G30.0 [F02.80]
      with behavioral disturbance G30.0
        [F02.81]
    late onset G30.1 [F02.80]
      with behavioral disturbance G30.1
        [F02.81]
    specified NEC G30.8 [F02.80]
      with behavioral disturbance G30.8
        [F02.81]
  amyloid —see Amyloidosis
  Andersen's (glycogenosis IV) E74.09
  Andes T70.29
  Andrews' (bacterid) L08.89
  angiospastic I73.9
    cerebral G45.9
    vein I87.8
  anterior
    chamber H21.9
    horn cell G12.29
  antiglomerular basement membrane
    (anti-GBM) antibody M31.0
    tubulo-interstitial nephritis N12
  antral —see Sinusitis, maxillary
  anus K62.9
    specified NEC K62.89
  aorta (nonsyphilitic) I77.9
    syphilitic NEC A52.02
  aortic (heart) (valve) I35.9
    rheumatic I06.9
  Apollo B30.3
  aponeuroses —see Enthesopathy
  appendix K38.9
    specified NEC K38.8
  aqueous (chamber) H21.9
  Arnold-Chiari —see Arnold-Chiari disease
  arterial I77.9
    occlusive —see Occlusion, by site
    due to stricture or stenosis I77.1
  arteriocardiorenal —see Hypertension,
    cardiorenal
  arteriolar (generalized) (obliterative)
    I77.9
  arteriorenal —see Hypertension, kidney
  arteriosclerotic —see also Arteriosclerosis
    cardiovascular —see Disease, heart,
      ischemic, atherosclerotic
    coronary (artery) —see Disease, heart,
      ischemic, atherosclerotic
    heart —see Disease, heart, ischemic,
      atherosclerotic
  artery I77.9
    cerebral I67.9
    coronary I25.10
      with angina pectoris —see
        Arteriosclerosis, coronary
        (artery)
  arthropod-borne NOS (viral) A94
    specified type NEC A93.8

Disease, diseased (Continued)
  atticoantral, chronic H66.20
    left H66.22
      with right H66.23
    right H66.21
      with left H66.23
  auditory canal —see Disorder, ear, external
  auricle, ear NEC —see Disorder, pinna
  Australian X A83.4
  autoimmune (systemic) NOS M35.9
    hemolytic (cold type) (warm type) D59.1
      drug-induced D59.0
    thyroid E06.3
  aviator's —see Effect, adverse, high altitude
  Ayala's Q78.5
  Ayerza's (pulmonary artery sclerosis with
    pulmonary hypertension) I27.0
  Babington's (familial hemorrhagic
    telangiectasia) I78.0
  bacterial A49.9
    specified NEC A48.8
    zoonotic A28.9
      specified type NEC A28.8
  Baelz's (cheilitis glandularis apostematosa)
    K13.0
  bagasse J67.1
  balloon —see Effect, adverse, high altitude
  Bang's (brucella abortus) A23.1
  Bannister's T78.3
  barometer makers' —see Poisoning, mercury
  Barraquer (-Simons') (progressive
    lipodystrophy) E88.1
  Barrett's —see Barrett's, esophagus
  Bartholin's gland N75.9
  basal ganglia G25.9
    degenerative G23.9
      specified NEC G23.8
    specified NEC G25.89
  Basedow's (exophthalmic goiter) —see
    Hyperthyroidism, with, goiter (diffuse)
  Bateman's B08.1
  Batten-Steinert G71.11
  Battey A31.0
  Beard's (neurasthenia) F48.8
  Becker
    idiopathic mural endomyocardial I42.3
    myotonia congenita G71.12
  Begbie's (exophthalmic goiter) —see
    Hyperthyroidism, with, goiter (diffuse)
  behavioral, organic F07.9
  Beigel's (white piedra) B36.2
  Benson's —see Deposit, crystalline
  Bernard-Soulier (thrombopathy) D69.1
  Bernhardt (-Roth) —see Mononeuropathy,
    lower limb, meralgia paresthetica
  Biermer's (pernicious anemia) D51.0
  bile duct (common) (hepatic) K83.9
    with calculus, stones —see Calculus, bile
      duct
    specified NEC K83.8
  biliary (tract) K83.9
    specified NEC K83.8
  Billroth's —see Spina bifida
  bird fancier's J67.2
  black lung J60
  bladder N32.9
    in (due to)
      schistosomiasis (bilharziasis) B65.0 [N33]
    specified NEC N32.89
  bleeder's D66
  blood D75.9
    forming organs D75.9
    vessel I99.9
  Bloodgood's —see Mastopathy, cystic
  Bodechtel-Guttmann (subacute sclerosing
    panencephalitis) A81.1
  bone —see also Disorder, bone
    aluminum M83.4
    fibrocystic NEC
      jaw M27.49
    bone-marrow D75.9

◀ New   ◀═ Revised   ~~deleted~~ Deleted

Disease, diseased (Continued)
Borna A83.9
Bornholm (epidemic pleurodynia) B33.0
Bouchard's (myopathic dilatation of the
stomach) K31.0
Bouillaud's (rheumatic heart disease) I01.9
Bourneville (-Brissaud) (tuberous sclerosis)
Q85.1
Bouveret (-Hoffmann) (paroxysmal
tachycardia) I47.9
bowel K63.9
functional K59.9
psychogenic F45.8
brain G93.9
arterial, artery I67.9
arteriosclerotic I67.2
congenital Q04.9
degenerative —see Degeneration, brain
inflammatory —see Encephalitis
organic G93.9
arteriosclerotic I67.2
parasitic NEC B71.9 [G94]
senile NEC G31.1
specified NEC G93.89
breast (see also Disorder, breast) N64.9
cystic (chronic) —see Mastopathy, cystic
fibrocystic —see Mastopathy, cystic
Paget's
female, unspecified side C50.91-
male, unspecified side C50.92-
specified NEC N64.89
Breda's —see Yaws
Bretonneau's (diphtheritic malignant angina)
A36.0
Bright's —see Nephritis
arteriosclerotic —see Hypertension, kidney
Brill's (recrudescent typhus) A75.1
Brill-Zinsser (recrudescent typhus) A75.1
Brion-Kayser —see Fever, paratyphoid
broad
beta E78.2
ligament (noninflammatory) N83.9
inflammatory —see Disease, pelvis,
inflammatory
specified NEC N83.8
Brocq-Duhring (dermatitis herpetiformis)
L13.0
Brocq's
meaning
dermatitis herpetiformis L13.0
prurigo L28.2
bronchopulmonary J98.4
bronchus NEC J98.09
bronze Addison's E27.1
tuberculous A18.7
budgerigar fancier's J67.2
Buerger's (thromboangiitis obliterans)
I73.1
bullous L13.9
chronic of childhood L12.2
specified NEC L13.8
Bürger-Grütz (essential familial
hyperlipemia) E78.3
bursa —see Bursopathy
caisson T70.3
California —see Coccidioidomycosis
capillaries I78.9
specified NEC I78.8
Carapata A68.0
cardiac —see Disease, heart
cardiopulmonary, chronic I27.9
cardiorenal (hepatic) (hypertensive)
(vascular) —see Hypertension,
cardiorenal
cardiovascular (atherosclerotic) I25.10
with angina pectoris —see Arteriosclerosis,
coronary (artery),
congenital Q28.9
hypertensive —see Hypertension, heart
newborn P29.9
specified NEC P29.89

Disease, diseased (Continued)
cardiovascular (Continued)
renal (hypertensive) —see Hypertension,
cardiorenal
syphilitic (asymptomatic) A52.00
cartilage —see Disorder, cartilage
Castellani's A69.8
cat-scratch A28.1
Cavare's (familial periodic paralysis)
G72.3
cecum K63.9
celiac (adult) (infantile) K90.0
cellular tissue L98.9
central core G71.2
cerebellar, cerebellum —see Disease, brain
cerebral —see also Disease, brain
degenerative —see Degeneration, brain
cerebrospinal G96.9
cerebrovascular I67.9
acute I67.89
embolic I63.4-
thrombotic I63.3-
arteriosclerotic I67.2
specified NEC I67.89
cervix (uteri) (noninflammatory) N88.9
inflammatory —see Cervicitis
specified NEC N88.8
Chabert's A22.9
Chandler's (osteochondritis dissecans, hip) —
see Osteochondritis, dissecans, hip
Charlouis —see Yaws
Chédiak-Steinbrinck (-Higashi) (congenital
gigantism of peroxidase granules)
E70.330
chest J98.9
Chiari's (hepatic vein thrombosis) I82.0
Chicago B40.9
Chignon B36.8
chigo, chigoe B88.1
childhood granulomatous D71
Chinese liver fluke B66.1
chlamydial A74.9
specified NEC A74.89
cholecystic K82.9
choroid H31.9
specified NEC H31.8
Christmas D67
chronic bullous of childhood L12.2
chylomicron retention E78.3
ciliary body H21.9
specified NEC H21.89
circulatory (system) NEC I99.8
newborn P29.9
syphilitic A52.00
congenital A50.54
coagulation factor deficiency (congenital) —
see Defect, coagulation
coccidioidal —see Coccidioidomycosis
cold
agglutinin or hemoglobinuria D59.1
paroxysmal D59.6
hemagglutinin (chronic) D59.1
collagen NOS (nonvascular) (vascular)
M35.9
specified NEC M35.8
colon K63.9
functional K59.9
congenital Q43.2
ischemic K55.0
combined system —see Degeneration,
combined
compressed air T70.3
Concato's (pericardial polyserositis)
A19.9
nontubercular I31.1
pleural —see Pleurisy, with effusion
conjunctiva H11.9
chlamydial A74.0
specified NEC H11.89
viral B30.9
specified NEC B30.8

Disease, diseased (Continued)
connective tissue, systemic (diffuse) M35.9
in (due to)
hypogammaglobulinemia D80.1 [M36.8]
ochronosis E70.29 [M36.8]
specified NEC M35.8
Conor and Bruch's (boutonneuse fever) A77.1
Cooper's —see Mastopathy, cystic
Cori's (glycogenosis III) E74.03
corkhandler's or corkworker's J67.3
cornea H18.9
specified NEC H18.89-
coronary (artery) —see Disease, heart,
ischemic, atherosclerotic
congenital Q24.5
ostial, syphilitic (aortic) (mitral)
(pulmonary) A52.03
corpus cavernosum N48.9
specified NEC N48.89
Cotugno's —see Sciatica
coxsackie (virus) NEC B34.1
cranial nerve NOS G52.9
Creutzfeldt-Jakob —see Creutzfeldt- Jakob
disease or syndrome
Crocq's (acrocyanosis) I73.89
Crohn's —see Enteritis, regional
Curschmann G71.11
cystic
breast (chronic) —see Mastopathy, cystic
kidney, congenital Q61.9
liver, congenital Q44.6
lung J98.4
congenital Q33.0
cytomegalic inclusion (generalized) B25.9
with pneumonia B25.0
congenital P35.1
cytomegaloviral B25.9
specified NEC B25.8
Czerny's (periodic hydrarthrosis of the
knee) —see Effusion, joint, knee
Daae (-Finsen) (epidemic pleurodynia) B33.0
Darling's —see Histoplasmosis capsulati
Débove's (splenomegaly) R16.1
deer fly —see Tularemia
Degos' I77.8
demyelinating, demyelinizating (nervous
system) G37.9
multiple sclerosis G35
specified NEC G37.8
dense deposit (see also N00-N07 with fourth
character .6) N05.6
deposition, hydroxyapatite —see Disease,
hydroxyapatite deposition
de Quervain's (tendon sheath) M65.4
thyroid (subacute granulomatous
thyroiditis) E06.1
Devergie's (pityriasis rubra pilaris) L44.0
Devic's G36.0
diaphorase deficiency D74.0
diaphragm J98.6
diarrheal, infectious NEC A09
digestive system K92.9
specified NEC K92.89
disc, degenerative —see Degeneration,
intervertebral disc
discogenic —see also Displacement,
intervertebral disc NEC
with myelopathy —see Disorder, disc, with,
myelopathy
diverticular —see Diverticula
Dubois (thymus) A50.59 [E35]
Duchenne-Griesinger G71.0
Duchenne's
muscular dystrophy G71.0
pseudohypertrophy, muscles G71.0
ductless glands E34.9
Duhring's (dermatitis herpetiformis) L13.0
duodenum K31.9
specified NEC K31.89
Dupré's (meningism) R29.1
Dupuytren's (muscle contracture) M72.0

Disease, diseased *(Continued)*
  Durand-Nicholas-Favre (climatic bubo) A55
  Duroziez's (congenital mitral stenosis) Q23.2
  ear —*see* Disorder, ear
  Eberth's —*see* Fever, typhoid
  Ebola (virus) A98.4
  Ebstein's heart Q22.5
  Echinococcus —*see* Echinococcus
  echovirus NEC B34.1
  Eddowes' (brittle bones and blue sclera)
    Q78.0
  edentulous (alveolar) ridge K06.9
    specified NEC K06.8
  Edsall's T67.2
  Eichstedt's (pityriasis versicolor) B36.0
  Ellis-van Creveld (chondroectodermal
    dysplasia) Q77.6
  end stage renal (ESRD) N18.6
    due to hypertension I12.0
  endocrine glands or system NEC E34.9
  endomyocardial (eosinophilic) I42.3
  English (rickets) E55.0
  enteroviral, enterovirus NEC B34.1
    central nervous system NEC A88.8
  epidemic B99.9
    specified NEC B99.8
  epididymis N50.9
  Erb (-Landouzy) G71.0
  Erdheim-Chester (ECD) E88.89
  esophagus K22.9
    functional K22.4
    psychogenic F45.8
    specified NEC K22.8
  Eulenburg's (congenital paramyotonia)
    G71.19
  eustachian tube —*see* Disorder, eustachian
    tube
  external
    auditory canal —*see* Disorder, ear, external
    ear —*see* Disorder, ear, external
  extrapyramidal G25.9
    specified NEC G25.89
  eye H57.9
    anterior chamber H21.9
    inflammatory NEC H57.8
    muscle (external) —*see* Strabismus
    specified NEC H57.8
    syphilitic —*see* Oculopathy, syphilitic
  eyeball H44.9
    specified NEC H44.89
  eyelid —*see* Disorder, eyelid
    specified NEC —*see* Disorder, eyelid,
      specified type NEC
  eyeworm of Africa B74.3
  facial nerve (seventh) G51.9
    newborn (birth injury) P11.3
  Fahr (of brain) G23.8
  Fahr Volhard (of kidney) I12.-
  fallopian tube (noninflammatory) N83.9
    inflammatory —*see* Salpingo-oophoritis
    specified NEC N83.8
  familial periodic paralysis G72.3
  Fanconi's (congenital pancytopenia) D61.09
  fascia NEC —*see also* Disorder, muscle
    inflammatory —*see* Myositis
    specified NEC M62.89
  Fauchard's (periodontitis) —*see* Periodontitis
  Favre-Durand-Nicolas (climatic bubo) A55
  Fede's K14.0
  Feer's —*see* Poisoning, mercury
  female pelvic inflammatory (*see also* Disease,
    pelvis, inflammatory) N73.9
    syphilitic (secondary) A51.42
    tuberculous A18.17
  Fernels' (aortic aneurysm) I71.9
  fibrocaseous of lung —*see* Tuberculosis,
    pulmonary
  fibrocystic —*see* Fibrocystic disease
  Fiedler's (leptospiral jaundice) A27.0
  fifth B08.3
  file-cutter's —*see* Poisoning, lead

Disease, diseased *(Continued)*
  fish-skin Q80.9
    acquired L85.0
  Flajani (-Basedow) (exophthalmic goiter) —
    see Hyperthyroidism, with, goiter
    (diffuse)
  flax-dresser's J66.1
  fluke —*see* Infestation, fluke
  foot and mouth B08.8
  foot process N04.9
  Forbes' (glycogenosis III) E74.03
  Fordyce-Fox (apocrine miliaria) L75.2
  Fordyce's (ectopic sebaceous glands) (mouth)
    Q38.6
  Forestier's (rhizomelic pseudopolyarthritis)
    M35.3
    meaning ankylosing hyperostosis —*see*
      Hyperostosis, ankylosing
  Fothergill's
    neuralgia —*see* Neuralgia, trigeminal
    scarlatina anginosa A38.9
  Fournier (gangrene) N49.3
    female N76.89
  fourth B08.8
  Fox (-Fordyce) (apocrine miliaria) L75.2
  Francis' —*see* Tularemia
  Franklin C88.2
  Frei's (climatic bubo) A55
  Friedreich's
    combined systemic or ataxia G11.1
    myoclonia G25.3
  frontal sinus —*see* Sinusitis, frontal
  fungus NEC B49
  Gaisböck's (polycythemia hypertonica) D75.1
  gallbladder K82.9
    calculus —*see* Calculus, gallbladder
    cholecystitis —*see* Cholecystitis
    cholesterolosis K82.4
    fistula —*see* Fistula, gallbladder
    hydrops K82.1
    obstruction —*see* Obstruction, gallbladder
    perforation K82.2
    specified NEC K82.8
  gamma heavy chain C88.2
  Gamna's (siderotic splenomegaly) D73.2
  Gamstorp's (adynamia episodica hereditaria)
    G72.3
  Gandy-Nanta (siderotic splenomegaly) D73.2
  ganister J62.8
  gastric —*see* Disease, stomach
  gastroesophageal reflux (GERD) K21.9
    with esophagitis K21.0
  gastrointestinal (tract) K92.9
    amyloid E85.4
    functional K59.9
      psychogenic F45.8
    specified NEC K92.89
  Gee (-Herter) (-Heubner) (-Thaysen)
    (nontropical sprue) K90.0
  genital organs
    female N94.9
    male N50.9
  Gerhardt's (erythromelalgia) I73.81
  Gibert's (pityriasis rosea) L42
  Gierke's (glycogenosis I) E74.01
  Gilles de la Tourette's (motor-verbal tic) F95.2
  gingiva K06.9
    specified NEC K06.8
  gland (lymph) I89.9
  Glanzmann's (hereditary hemorrhagic
    thrombasthenia) D69.1
  glass-blower's (cataract) —*see* Cataract,
    specified NEC
    salivary gland hypertrophy K11.1
  Glisson's —*see* Rickets
  globe H44.9
    specified NEC H44.89
  glomerular —*see also* Glomerulonephritis
    with edema —*see* Nephrosis
    acute —*see* Nephritis, acute
    chronic —*see* Nephritis, chronic

Disease, diseased *(Continued)*
  glomerular *(Continued)*
    minimal change N05.0
    rapidly progressive N01.9
  glycogen storage E74.00
    Andersen's E74.09
    Cori's E74.03
    Forbes' E74.03
    generalized E74.00
    glucose-6-phosphatase deficiency E74.01
    heart E74.02 *[143]*
    hepatorenal E74.09
    Hers' E74.09
    liver and kidney E74.09
    McArdle's E74.04
    muscle phosphofructokinase E74.09
    myocardium E74.02 *[143]*
    Pompe's E74.02
    Tauri's E74.09
    type 0 E74.09
    type I E74.01
    type II E74.02
    type III E74.03
    type IV E74.09
    type V E74.04
    type VI-XI E74.09
    Von Gierke's E74.01
  Goldstein's (familial hemorrhagic
    telangiectasia) I78.0
  gonococcal NOS A54.9
  graft-versus-host (GVH) D89.813
    acute D89.810
    acute on chronic D89.812
    chronic D89.811
  grainhandler's J67.8
  granulomatous (childhood) (chronic) D71
  Graves' (exophthalmic goiter) —*see*
    Hyperthyroidism, with, goiter
    (diffuse)
  Griesinger's —*see* Ancylostomiasis
  Grisel's M43.6
  Gruby's (tinea tonsurans) B35.0
  Guillain-Barré G61.0 ◀▥
  Guinon's (motor-verbal tic) F95.2
  gum K06.9
  gynecological N94.9
  H (Hartnup's) E72.02
  Haff —*see* Poisoning, mercury
  Hageman (congenital factor XII deficiency)
    D68.2
  hair (color) (shaft) L67.9
    follicles L73.9
      specified NEC L73.8
  Hamman's (spontaneous mediastinal
    emphysema) J98.2
  hand, foot and mouth B08.4
  Hansen's —*see* Leprosy
  Hantavirus, with pulmonary manifestations
    B33.4
    with renal manifestations A98.5
  Harada's H30.81-
  Hartnup (pellagra-cerebellar ataxia-renal
    aminoaciduria) E72.02
  Hart's (pellagra-cerebellar ataxia-renal
    aminoaciduria) E72.02
  Hashimoto's (struma lymphomatosa)
    E06.3
  Hb —*see* Disease, hemoglobin
  heart (organic) I51.9
    with
      pulmonary edema (acute) (*see also*
        Failure, ventricular, left) I50.1
      rheumatic fever (conditions in I00)
        active I01.9
          with chorea I02.0
          specified NEC I01.8
        inactive or quiescent (with chorea)
          I09.9
          specified NEC I09.89
    amyloid E85.4 *[143]*
    aortic (valve) I35.9

Disease, diseased (Continued)
heart (Continued)
arteriosclerotic or sclerotic (senile) —
see Disease, heart, ischemic,
atherosclerotic
artery, arterial —see Disease, heart,
ischemic, atherosclerotic
beer drinkers' I42.6
beriberi (wet) E51.12
black I27.0
congenital Q24.9
cyanotic Q24.9
specified NEC Q24.8
coronary —see Disease, heart, ischemic
cryptogenic I51.9
fibroid —see Myocarditis
functional I51.89
psychogenic F45.8
glycogen storage E74.02 [I43]
gonococcal A54.83
hypertensive —see Hypertension, heart
hyperthyroid (see also Hyperthyroidism)
E05.90 [I43]
with thyroid storm E05.91 [I43]
ischemic (chronic or with a stated duration
of over 4 weeks) I25.9
atherosclerotic (of) I25.10
with angina pectoris —see
Arteriosclerosis, coronary
(artery)
coronary artery bypass graft —see
Arteriosclerosis, coronary
(artery),
cardiomyopathy I25.5
diagnosed on ECG or other special
investigation, but currently
presenting no symptoms I25.6
silent I25.6
specified form NEC I25.89
kyphoscoliotic I27.1
meningococcal A39.50
endocarditis A39.51
myocarditis A39.52
pericarditis A39.53
mitral I05.9
specified NEC I05.8
muscular —see Degeneration,
myocardial
psychogenic (functional) F45.8
pulmonary (chronic) I27.9
in schistosomiasis B65.9 [I52]
specified NEC I27.89
rheumatic (chronic) (inactive) (old)
(quiescent) (with chorea) I09.9
active or acute I01.9
with chorea (acute) (rheumatic)
(Sydenham's) I02.0
specified NEC I09.89
senile —see Myocarditis
syphilitic A52.06
aortic A52.03
aneurysm A52.01
congenital A50.54 [I52]
thyrotoxic (see also Thyrotoxicosis) E05.90
[I43]
with thyroid storm E05.91 [I43]
valve, valvular (obstructive)
(regurgitant) —see also Endocarditis
congenital NEC Q24.8
pulmonary Q22.3
vascular —see Disease, cardiovascular
heavy chain NEC C88.2
alpha C88.3
gamma C88.2
mu C88.2
Hebra's
pityriasis
maculata et circinata L42
rubra pilaris L44.0
prurigo L28.2
hematopoietic organs D75.9

Disease, diseased (Continued)
hemoglobin or Hb
abnormal (mixed) NEC D58.2
with thalassemia D56.9
AS genotype D57.3
Bart's D56.0
C (Hb-C) D58.2
with other abnormal hemoglobin NEC
D58.2
elliptocytosis D58.1
Hb-S D57.2-
sickle-cell D57.2-
thalassemia D56.8
Constant Spring D58.2
D (Hb-D) D58.2
E (Hb-E) D58.2
E-beta thalassemia D56.5
elliptocytosis D58.1
H (Hb-H) (thalassemia) D56.0
with other abnormal hemoglobin NEC
D56.9
Constant Spring D56.0
I thalassemia D56.9
M D74.0
S or SS D57.1
SC D57.2-
SD D57.8-
SE D57.8-
spherocytosis D58.0
unstable, hemolytic D58.2
hemolytic (newborn) P55.9
autoimmune (cold type) (warm type) D59.1
drug-induced D59.0
due to or with
incompatibility
ABO (blood group) P55.1
blood (group) (Duffy) (K(ell)) (Kidd)
(Lewis) (M) (S) NEC P55.8
Rh (blood group) (factor) P55.0
Rh negative mother P55.0
specified type NEC P55.8
unstable hemoglobin D58.2
hemorrhagic D69.9
newborn P53
Henoch (-Schönlein) (purpura nervosa) D69.0
hepatic —see Disease, liver
hepatobiliary K83.9
toxic K71.9
hepatolenticular E83.01
heredodegenerative NEC
spinal cord G95.89
herpesviral, disseminated B00.7
Hers' (glycogenosis VI) E74.09
Herter (-Gee) (-Heubner) (nontropical sprue)
K90.0
Heubner-Herter (nontropical sprue) K90.0
high fetal gene or hemoglobin thalassemia
D56.9
Hildenbrand's —see Typhus
hip (joint) M25.9
congenital Q65.89
suppurative M00.9
tuberculous A18.02
His (-Werner) (trench fever) A79.0
Hodgson's I71.2
ruptured I71.1
Holla —see Spherocytosis
hookworm B76.9
specified NEC B76.8
host-versus-graft D89.813
acute D89.810
acute on chronic D89.812
chronic D89.811
human immunodeficiency virus (HIV) B20
Huntington's G10
Hutchinson's (cheiropompholyx) —see
Hutchinson's disease
hyaline (diffuse) (generalized)
membrane (lung) (newborn) P22.0
adult J80
hydatid —see Echinococcus

Disease, diseased (Continued)
hydroxyapatite deposition M11.00
ankle M11.07-
elbow M11.02-
foot joint M11.07-
hand joint M11.04-
hip M11.05-
knee M11.06-
multiple site M11.09
shoulder M11.01-
vertebra M11.08
wrist M11.03-
hyperkinetic —see Hyperkinesia
hypertensive —see Hypertension
hypophysis E23.7
Iceland G93.3
I-cell E77.0
immune D89.9
immunoproliferative (malignant) C88.9
small intestinal C88.3
specified NEC C88.8
inclusion B25.9
salivary gland B25.9
infectious, infective B99.9
congenital P37.9
specified NEC P37.8
viral P35.9 ◀▦▦
specified type NEC P35.8 ◀
specified NEC B99.8
inflammatory
penis N48.29
abscess N48.21
cellulitis N48.22
prepuce N47.7
balanoposthitis N47.6
tubo-ovarian —see Salpingo-oophoritis
intervertebral disc —see also Disorder, disc
with myelopathy —see Disorder, disc, with,
myelopathy
cervical, cervicothoracic —see Disorder,
disc, cervical
with
myelopathy —see Disorder, disc,
cervical, with myelopathy
neuritis, radiculitis or
radiculopathy —see Disorder,
disc, cervical, with neuritis
specified NEC —see Disorder, disc,
cervical, specified type NEC
lumbar (with)
myelopathy M51.06
neuritis, radiculitis, radiculopathy or
sciatica M51.16
specified NEC M51.86
lumbosacral (with)
myelopathy M51.07
neuritis, radiculitis, radiculopathy or
sciatica M51.17
specified NEC M51.87
specified NEC —see Disorder, disc,
specified NEC
thoracic (with)
myelopathy M51.04
neuritis, radiculitis or radiculopathy
M51.14
specified NEC M51.84
thoracolumbar (with)
myelopathy M51.05
neuritis, radiculitis or radiculopathy
M51.15
specified NEC M51.85
intestine K63.9
functional K59.9
psychogenic F45.8
specified NEC K59.8
organic K63.9
protozoal A07.9
specified NEC K63.89
iris H21.9
specified NEC H21.89
iron metabolism or storage E83.10

Disease, diseased *(Continued)*
  island (scrub typhus) A75.3
  itai-itai —*see* Poisoning, cadmium
  Jakob-Creutzfeldt —*see* Creutzfeldt- Jakob
    disease or syndrome
  jaw M27.9
    fibrocystic M27.49
    specified NEC M27.8
  jigger B88.1
  joint —*see also* Disorder, joint
    Charcot's —*see* Arthropathy, neuropathic
      (Charcot)
    degenerative —*see* Osteoarthritis
      multiple M15.9
      spine —*see* Spondylosis
    hypertrophic —*see* Osteoarthritis
    sacroiliac M53.3
    specified NEC —*see* Disorder, joint,
      specified type NEC
    spine NEC —*see* Dorsopathy
    suppurative —*see* Arthritis, pyogenic or
      pyemic
  Jourdain's (acute gingivitis) K05.00
    nonplaque induced K05.01
    plaque induced K05.00
  Kaschin-Beck (endemic polyarthritis) M12.10
    ankle M12.17-
    elbow M12.12-
    foot joint M12.17-
    hand joint M12.14-
    hip M12.15-
    knee M12.16-
    multiple site M12.19
    shoulder M12.11-
    vertebra M12.18
    wrist M12.13-
  Katayama B65.2
  Kedani (scrub typhus) A75.3
  Keshan E59
  kidney (functional) (pelvis) N28.9
    chronic N18.9
      hypertensive —*see* Hypertension, kidney
      stage 1 N18.1
      stage 2 (mild) N18.2
      stage 3 (moderate) N18.3
      stage 4 (severe) N18.4
      stage 5 N18.5
    complicating pregnancy —*see* Pregnancy,
      complicated by, renal disease
    cystic (congenital) Q61.9
    diabetic - see E08-E13 with .22
    fibrocystic (congenital) Q61.8
    hypertensive —*see* Hypertension, kidney
    in (due to)
      schistosomiasis (bilharziasis) B65.9 *[N29]*
    multicystic Q61.4
    polycystic Q61.3
      adult type Q61.2
      childhood type NEC Q61.19
        collecting duct dilatation Q61.11
  Kimmelstiel (-Wilson) (intercapillary polycystic
    (congenital) glomerulosclerosis) —*see*
    E08-E13 with .21
  Kimura D21.9
    specified site (see Neoplasm, connective
      tissue benign)
  Kinnier Wilson's (hepatolenticular
    degeneration) E83.01
  kissing —*see* Mononucleosis, infectious
  Klebs' (*see also* Glomerulonephritis) N05.-
  Klippel-Feil (brevicollis) Q76.1
  Köhler-Pellegrini-Stieda (calcification, knee
    joint) —*see* Bursitis, tibial collateral
  Kok Q89.8
  König's (osteochondritis dissecans) —*see*
    Osteochondritis, dissecans
  Korsakoff's (nonalcoholic) F04
    alcoholic F10.96
      with dependence F10.26
  Kostmann's (infantile genetic
    agranulocytosis) D70.0

Disease, diseased *(Continued)*
  kuru A81.81
  Kyasanur Forest A98.2
  labyrinth, ear —*see* Disorder, ear, inner
  lacrimal system —*see* Disorder, lacrimal
    system
  Lafora's —*see* Epilepsy, generalized,
    idiopathic
  Lancereaux-Mathieu (leptospiral jaundice)
    A27.0
  Landry's G61.0
  Larrey-Weil (leptospiral jaundice) A27.0
  larynx J38.7
  legionnaires' A48.1
    nonpneumonic A48.2
  Lenegre's I44.2
  lens H27.9
    specified NEC H27.8
  Lev's (acquired complete heart block) I44.2
  Lewy body (dementia) G31.83 *[F02.80]*
    with behavioral disturbance G31.83
      [F02.81]
  Lichtheim's (subacute combined sclerosis
    with pernicious anemia) D51.0
  Lightwood's (renal tubular acidosis) N25.89
  Lignac's (cystinosis) E72.04
  lip K13.0
  lipid-storage E75.6
    specified NEC E75.5
  Lipschütz's N76.6
  liver (chronic) (organic) K76.9
    alcoholic (chronic) K70.9
      acute —*see* Disease, liver, alcoholic,
        hepatitis
      cirrhosis K70.30
        with ascites K70.31
      failure K70.40
        with coma K70.41
      fatty liver K70.0
      fibrosis K70.2
      hepatitis K70.10
        with ascites K70.11
      sclerosis K70.2
    cystic, congenital Q44.6
    drug-induced (idiosyncratic) (toxic)
      (predictable) (unpredictable) —*see*
      Disease, liver, toxic
    end stage K72.90
      due to hepatitis —*see* Hepatitis
    fatty, nonalcoholic (NAFLD) K76.0
      alcoholic K70.0
    fibrocystic (congenital) Q44.6
    fluke
      Chinese B66.1
      oriental B66.1
      sheep B66.3
    glycogen storage E74.09 *[K77]*
    in (due to)
      schistosomiasis (bilharziasis) B65.9 *[K77]*
    inflammatory K75.9
      alcoholic K70.1
      specified NEC K75.89
    polycystic (congenital) Q44.6
    toxic K71.9
      with
        cholestasis K71.0
        cirrhosis (liver) K71.7
        fibrosis (liver) K71.7
        focal nodular hyperplasia K71.8
        hepatic granuloma K71.8
        hepatic necrosis K71.10
          with coma K71.11
        hepatitis NEC K71.6
          acute K71.2
          chronic
            active K71.50
              with ascites K71.51
            lobular K71.4
            persistent K71.3
          lupoid K71.50
            with ascites K71.51

Disease, diseased *(Continued)*
  liver *(Continued)*
    toxic *(Continued)*
      with *(Continued)*
        peliosis hepatis K71.8
        veno-occlusive disease (VOD) of liver
          K71.8
      veno-occlusive K76.5
  Lobo's (keloid blastomycosis) B48.0
  Lobstein's (brittle bones and blue sclera)
    Q78.0
  Ludwig's (submaxillary cellulitis) K12.2
  lumbosacral region M53.87
  lung J98.4
    black J60
    congenital Q33.9
    cystic J98.4
      congenital Q33.0
    fibroid (chronic) —*see* Fibrosis, lung
    fluke B66.4
      oriental B66.4
    in
      amyloidosis E85.4 *[J99]*
      sarcoidosis D86.0
      Sjögren's syndrome M35.02
      systemic
        lupus erythematosus M32.13
        sclerosis M34.81
    interstitial J84.9
      of childhood, specified NEC J84.848
      respiratory bronchiolitis J84.115
      specified NEC J84.89
    obstructive (chronic) J44.9
      with
        acute
          bronchitis J44.0
          exacerbation NEC J44.1
          lower respiratory infection J44.0
        alveolitis, allergic J67.9
        asthma J44.9
        bronchiectasis J47.9
          with
            exacerbation (acute) J47.1
            lower respiratory infection J47.0
        bronchitis J44.9
          with
            exacerbation (acute) J44.1
            lower respiratory infection J44.0
        emphysema J44.9
        hypersensitivity pneumonitis J67.9
      decompensated J44.1
        with
          exacerbation (acute) J44.1
    polycystic J98.4
      congenital Q33.0
    rheumatoid (diffuse) (interstitial) —*see*
      Rheumatoid, lung
  Lutembacher's (atrial septal defect with
    mitral stenosis) Q21.1
  Lyme A69.20
  lymphatic (gland) (system) (channel) (vessel)
    I89.9
  lymphoproliferative D47.9
    specified NEC D47.Z9
    T-gamma D47.Z9
    X-linked D82.3
  Magitot's M27.2
  malarial —*see* Malaria
  malignant —*see also* Neoplasm, malignant,
    by site
  Manson's B65.1
  maple bark J67.6
  maple-syrup-urine E71.0
  Marburg (virus) A98.3
  Marion's (bladder neck obstruction) N32.0
  Marsh's (exophthalmic goiter) —*see*
    Hyperthyroidism, with, goiter (diffuse)
  mastoid (process) —*see* Disorder, ear,
    middle
  Mathieu's (leptospiral jaundice) A27.0
  Maxcy's A75.2

Disease, diseased *(Continued)*
McArdle (-Schmid-Pearson) (glycogenosis V) E74.04
mediastinum J98.5
medullary center (idiopathic) (respiratory) G93.89
Meige's (chronic hereditary edema) Q82.0
meningococcal —*see* Infection, meningococcal
mental F99
  organic F09
mesenchymal M35.9
mesenteric embolic K55.0
metabolic, metabolism E88.9
  bilirubin E80.7
metal-polisher's J62.8
metastatic *(see also* Neoplasm, secondary, by site) C79.9
microvascular — code to condition
microvillus
  atrophy Q43.8
  inclusion (MVD) Q43.8
middle ear —*see* Disorder, ear, middle
Mikulicz' (dryness of mouth, absent or decreased lacrimation) K11.8
Milroy's (chronic hereditary edema) Q82.0
Minamata —*see* Poisoning, mercury
minicore G71.2
Minor's G95.19
Minot's (hemorrhagic disease, newborn) P53
Minot-von Willebrand-Jürgens (angiohemophilia) D68.0
Mitchell's (erythromelalgia) I73.81
mitral (valve) I05.9
  nonrheumatic I34.9
mixed connective tissue M35.1
moldy hay J67.0
Monge's T70.29
Morgagni-Adams-Stokes (syncope with heart block) I45.9
Morgagni's (syndrome) (hyperostosis frontalis interna) M85.2
Morton's (with metatarsalgia) —*see* Lesion, nerve, plantar
Morvan's G60.8
motor neuron (bulbar) (familial) (mixed type) (spinal) G12.20
  amyotrophic lateral sclerosis G12.21
  progressive bulbar palsy G12.22
  specified NEC G12.29
moyamoya I67.5
mu heavy chain disease C88.2
multicore G71.2
muscle —*see also* Disorder, muscle
  inflammatory —*see* Myositis
  ocular (external) —*see* Strabismus
musculoskeletal system, soft tissue —*see also* Disorder, soft tissue
  specified NEC —*see* Disorder, soft tissue, specified type NEC
mushroom workers' J67.5
mycotic B49
myelodysplastic, not classified C94.6
myeloproliferative, not classified C94.6
  chronic D47.1
myocardium, myocardial *(see also* Degeneration, myocardial) I51.5
  primary (idiopathic) I42.9
myoneural G70.9
Naegeli's D69.1
nails L60.9
  specified NEC L60.8
Nairobi (sheep virus) A93.8
nasal J34.9
nemaline body G71.2
nerve —*see* Disorder, nerve
nervous system G98.8
  autonomic G90.9
  central G96.9
    specified NEC G96.8
  congenital Q07.9
  parasympathetic G90.9

Disease, diseased *(Continued)*
nervous system *(Continued)*
  specified NEC G98.8
  sympathetic G90.9
  vegetative G90.9
neuromuscular system G70.9
Newcastle B30.8
Nicolas (-Durand)-Favre (climatic bubo) A55
nipple N64.9
  Paget's C50.01-
    female C50.01-
    male C50.02-
Nishimoto (-Takeuchi) I67.5
nonarthropod-borne NOS (viral) B34.9
  enterovirus NEC B34.1
nonautoimmune hemolytic D59.4
  drug-induced D59.2
Nonne-Milroy-Meige (chronic hereditary edema) Q82.0
nose J34.9
nucleus pulposus —*see* Disorder, disc
nutritional E63.9
oast-house-urine E72.19
  ocular
    herpesviral B00.50
    zoster B02.30
obliterative vascular I77.1
Ohara's —*see* Tularemia
Opitz's (congestive splenomegaly) D73.2
Oppenheim-Urbach (necrobiosis lipoidica diabeticorum) —*see* E08-E13 with .620
optic nerve NEC —*see* Disorder, nerve, optic
  orbit —*see* Disorder, orbit
Oriental liver fluke B66.1
Oriental lung fluke B66.4
Ormond's N13.5
Oropouche virus A93.0
Osler-Rendu (familial hemorrhagic telangiectasia) I78.0
osteofibrocystic E21.0
Otto's M24.7
outer ear —*see* Disorder, ear, external
ovary (noninflammatory) N83.9
  cystic N83.20
  inflammatory —*see* Salpingo-oophoritis
  polycystic E28.2
  specified NEC N83.8
Owren's (congenital) —*see* Defect, coagulation
pancreas K86.9
  cystic K86.2
  fibrocystic E84.9
  specified NEC K86.8
panvalvular I08.9
  specified NEC I08.8
parametrium (noninflammatory) N83.9
parasitic B89
  cerebral NEC B71.9 *[G94]*
  intestinal NOS B82.9
  mouth B37.0
  skin NOS B88.9
  specified type —*see* Infestation
  tongue B37.0
parathyroid (gland) E21.5
  specified NEC E21.4
Parkinson's G20
parodontal K05.6
Parrot's (syphilitic osteochondritis) A50.02
Parry's (exophthalmic goiter) —*see* Hyperthyroidism, with, goiter (diffuse)
Parson's (exophthalmic goiter) —*see* Hyperthyroidism, with, goiter (diffuse)
Paxton's (white piedra) B36.2
pearl-worker's —*see* Osteomyelitis, specified type NEC
Pellegrini-Stieda (calcification, knee joint) — *see* Bursitis, tibial collateral
pelvis, pelvic
  female NOS N94.9
    specified NEC N94.89
  gonococcal (acute) (chronic) A54.24

Disease, diseased *(Continued)*
pelvis, pelvic *(Continued)*
  inflammatory (female) N73.9
    acute N73.0
    chronic N73.1
    specified NEC N73.8
    syphilitic (secondary) A51.42
      late A52.76
    tuberculous A18.17
  organ, female N94.9
  peritoneum, female NEC N94.89
penis N48.9
  inflammatory N48.29
    abscess N48.21
    cellulitis N48.22
  specified NEC N48.89
periapical tissues NOS K04.90
periodontal K05.6
  specified NEC K05.5
periosteum —*see* Disorder, bone, specified type NEC
peripheral
  arterial I73.9
  autonomic nervous system G90.9
  nerves —*see* Polyneuropathy
  vascular NOS I73.9
peritoneum K66.9
  pelvic, female NEC N94.89
  specified NEC K66.8
persistent mucosal (middle ear) H66.20
  left H66.22
    with right H66.23
  right H66.21
    with left H66.23
Petit's —*see* Hernia, abdomen, specified site NEC
pharynx J39.2
  specified NEC J39.2
Phocas' —*see* Mastopathy, cystic
photochromogenic (acid-fast bacilli) (pulmonary) A31.0
  nonpulmonary A31.9
Pick's G31.01 *[F02.80]*
  with behavioral disturbance G31.01 *[F02.81]*
pigeon fancier's J67.2
pineal gland E34.8
pink —*see* Poisoning, mercury
Pinkus' (lichen nitidus) L44.1
pinworm B80
Piry virus A93.8
pituitary (gland) E23.7
pituitary-snuff-taker's J67.8
pleura (cavity) J94.9
  specified NEC J94.8
pneumatic drill (hammer) T75.21
Pollitzer's (hidradenitis suppurativa) L73.2
polycystic
  kidney or renal Q61.3
    adult type Q61.2
    childhood type NEC Q61.19
      collecting duct dilatation Q61.11
  liver or hepatic Q44.6
  lung or pulmonary J98.4
    congenital Q33.0
  ovary, ovaries E28.2
  spleen Q89.09
polyethylene T84.05-
Pompe's (glycogenosis II) E74.02
Posadas-Wernicke B38.9
Potain's (pulmonary edema) —*see* Edema, lung
prepuce N47.8
  inflammatory N47.7
    balanoposthitis N47.6
Pringle's (tuberous sclerosis) Q85.1
prion, central nervous system A81.9
  specified NEC A81.89
prostate N42.9
  specified NEC N42.89

Disease, diseased (Continued)
  protozoal B64
    acanthamebiasis —see Acanthamebiasis
    African trypanosomiasis —see African
      trypanosomiasis
    babesiosis B60.0
    Chagas disease —see Chagas disease
    intestine, intestinal A07.9
    leishmaniasis —see Leishmaniasis
    malaria —see Malaria
    naegleriasis B60.2
    pneumocystosis B59
    specified organism NEC B60.8
    toxoplasmosis —see Toxoplasmosis
  pseudo-Hurler's E77.0
  psychiatric F99
  psychotic —see Psychosis
  Puente's (simple glandular cheilitis)
    K13.0
  puerperal (see also Puerperal) O90.89
  pulmonary —see also Disease, lung
    artery I28.9
    chronic obstructive J44.9
      with
        acute bronchitis J44.0
        exacerbation (acute) J44.1
        lower respiratory infection (acute)
          J44.0
      decompensated J44.1
        with
          exacerbation (acute) J44.1
    heart I27.9
      specified NEC I27.89
    hypertensive (vascular) I27.0
    valve I37.9
      rheumatic I09.89
  pulp (dental) NOS K04.90
  pulseless M31.4
  Putnam's (subacute combined sclerosis with
    pernicious anemia) D51.0
  Pyle (-Cohn) (craniometaphyseal dysplasia)
    Q78.5
  ragpicker's or ragsorter's A22.1
  Raynaud's —see Raynaud's disease
  reactive airway —see Asthma
  Reclus' (cystic) —see Mastopathy,
    cystic
  rectum K62.9
    specified NEC K62.89
  Refsum's (heredopathia atactica
    polyneuritiformis) G60.1
  renal (functional) (pelvis) (see also Disease,
    kidney) N28.9
    with
      edema —see Nephrosis
      glomerular lesion —see
        Glomerulonephritis
        with edema —see Nephrosis
      interstitial nephritis N12
    acute N28.9
    chronic (see also Disease, kidney, chronic)
      N18.9
    cystic, congenital Q61.9
    diabetic —see E08-E13 with .22
    end-stage (failure) N18.6
      due to hypertension I12.0
    fibrocystic (congenital) Q61.8
    hypertensive —see Hypertension,
      kidney
    lupus M32.14
    phosphate-losing (tubular) N25.0
    polycystic (congenital) Q61.3
      adult type Q61.2
      childhood type NEC Q61.19
        collecting duct dilatation Q61.11
    rapidly progressive N01.9
    subacute N01.9
  Rendu-Osler-Weber (familial hemorrhagic
    telangiectasia) I78.0
  renovascular (arteriosclerotic) —see
    Hypertension, kidney

Disease, diseased (Continued)
  respiratory (tract) J98.9
    acute or subacute NOS J06.9
      due to
        chemicals, gases, fumes or vapors
          (inhalation) J68.3
        external agent J70.9
          specified NEC J70.8
        radiation J70.0
        smoke inhalation J70.5
      noninfectious J39.8
    chronic NOS J98.9
      due to
        chemicals, gases, fumes or vapors
          J68.4
        external agent J70.9
          specified NEC J70.8
        radiation J70.1
    newborn P27.9
      specified NEC P27.8
    due to
      chemicals, gases, fumes or vapors J68.9
        acute or subacute NEC J68.3
        chronic J68.4
      external agent J70.9
        specified NEC J70.8
    newborn P28.9
      specified type NEC P28.89
    upper J39.9
      acute or subacute J06.9
      noninfectious NEC J39.8
      specified NEC J39.8
      streptococcal J06.9
  retina, retinal H35.9
    Batten's or Batten-Mayou E75.4 [H36]
    specified NEC H35.89
  rheumatoid —see Arthritis, rheumatoid
  rickettsial NOS A79.9
    specified type NEC A79.89
  Riga (-Fede) (cachectic aphthae) K14.0
  Riggs' (compound periodontitis) —see
    Periodontitis
  Ritter's L00
  Rivalta's (cervicofacial actinomycosis)
    A42.2
  Robles' (onchocerciasis) B73.01
  Roger's (congenital interventricular septal
    defect) Q21.0
  Rosenthal's (factor XI deficiency) D68.1
  Ross River B33.1
  Rossbach's (hyperchlorhydria) K30
  Rotes Quérol —see Hyperostosis, ankylosing
  Roth (-Bernhardt) —see Mononeuropathy,
    lower limb, meralgia paresthetica
  Runeberg's (progressive pernicious anemia)
    D51.0
  sacroiliac NEC M53.3
  salivary gland or duct K11.9
    inclusion B25.9
    specified NEC K11.8
    virus B25.9
  sandworm B76.9
  Schimmelbusch's —see Mastopathy, cystic
  Schmorl's —see Schmorl's disease or nodes
  Schönlein (-Henoch) (purpura rheumatica)
    D69.0
  Schottmüller's —see Fever, paratyphoid
  Schultz's (agranulocytosis) —see
    Agranulocytosis
  Schwalbe-Ziehen-Oppenheim G24.1
  Schwartz-Jampel G71.13
  sclera H15.9
    specified NEC H15.89
  scrofulous (tuberculous) A18.2
  scrotum N50.9
  sebaceous glands L73.9
  semilunar cartilage, cystic —see also
    Derangement, knee, meniscus, cystic
  seminal vesicle N50.9
  serum NEC (see also Reaction, serum)
    T80.69

Disease, diseased (Continued)
  sexually transmitted A64
    anogenital
      herpesviral infection —see Herpes,
        anogenital
      warts A63.0
    chancroid A57
    chlamydial infection —see Chlamydia
    gonorrhea —see Gonorrhea
    granuloma inguinale A58
    specified organism NEC A63.8
    syphilis —see Syphilis
    trichomoniasis —see Trichomoniasis ◄▦
  Sézary C84.1-
  shimamushi (scrub typhus) A75.3
  shipyard B30.0
  sickle-cell D57.1
    with crisis (vasoocclusive pain) D57.00
      with
        acute chest syndrome D57.01
        splenic sequestration D57.02
    elliptocytosis D57.8-
    Hb-C D57.20
      with crisis (vasoocclusive pain) D57.219
        with
          acute chest syndrome D57.211
          splenic sequestration D57.212
      without crisis D57.20
    Hb-SD D57.80
      with crisis D57.819
        with
          acute chest syndrome D57.811
          splenic sequestration D57.812
    Hb-SE D57.80
      with crisis D57.819
        with
          acute chest syndrome D57.811
          splenic sequestration D57.812
    specified NEC D57.80
      with crisis D57.819
        with
          acute chest syndrome D57.811
          splenic sequestration D57.812
    spherocytosis D57.80
      with crisis D57.819
        with
          acute chest syndrome D57.811
          splenic sequestration D57.812
    thalassemia D57.40
      with crisis (vasoocclusive pain) D57.419
        with
          acute chest syndrome D57.411
          splenic sequestration D57.412
      without crisis D57.40
  silo-filler's J68.8
    bronchitis J68.0
    pneumonitis J68.0
    pulmonary edema J68.1
  simian B B00.4
  Simons' (progressive lipodystrophy) E88.1
  sin nombre virus B33.4
  sinus —see Sinusitis
  Sirkari's B55.0
  sixth B08.20
    due to human herpesvirus 6 B08.21
    due to human herpesvirus 7 B08.22
  skin L98.9
    due to metabolic disorder NEC E88.9
      [L99]
    specified NEC L98.8
  slim (HIV) B20
  small vessel I73.9
  Sneddon-Wilkinson (subcorneal pustular
    dermatosis) L13.1
  South African creeping B88.0
  spinal (cord) G95.9
    congenital Q06.9
    specified NEC G95.89
  spine —see also Spondylopathy
    joint —see Dorsopathy
    tuberculous A18.01

Disease, diseased (*Continued*)
spinocerebellar (hereditary) G11.9
   specified NEC G11.8
spleen D73.9
   amyloid E85.4 [*D77*]
   organic D73.9
   polycystic Q89.09
   postinfectional D73.89
sponge-diver's —*see* Toxicity, venom, marine
      animal, sea anemone
Startle Q89.8
Steinert's G71.11
Sticker's (erythema infectiosum) B08.3
Stieda's (calcification, knee joint) —*see*
      Bursitis, tibial collateral
Stokes' (exophthalmic goiter) —*see*
      Hyperthyroidism, with, goiter (diffuse)
Stokes-Adams (syncope with heart block)
      I45.9
stomach K31.9
   functional, psychogenic F45.8
   specified NEC K31.89
stonemason's J62.8
storage
   glycogen —*see* Disease, glycogen storage
   mucopolysaccharide —*see*
      Mucopolysaccharidosis
striatopallidal system NEC G25.89
Stuart-Prower (congenital factor X deficiency)
      D68.2
Stuart's (congenital factor X deficiency) D68.2
subcutaneous tissue —*see* Disease, skin
supporting structures of teeth K08.9
   specified NEC K08.8
suprarenal (capsule) (gland) E27.9
   hyperfunction E27.0
   specified NEC E27.8
sweat glands L74.9
   specified NEC L74.8
Sweeley-Klionsky E75.21
Swift (-Feer) —*see* Poisoning, mercury
swimming-pool granuloma A31.1
Sylvest's (epidemic pleurodynia) B33.0
sympathetic nervous system G90.9
synovium —*see* Disorder, synovium
syphilitic —*see* Syphilis
systemic tissue mast cell C96.2
tanapox (virus) B08.71
Tangier E78.6
Tarral-Besnier (pityriasis rubra pilaris) L44.0
Tauri's E74.09
tear duct —*see* Disorder, lacrimal system
tendon, tendinous —*see also* Disorder, tendon
   nodular —*see* Trigger finger
terminal vessel I73.9
testis N50.9
thalassemia Hb-S —*see* Disease, sickle-cell,
      thalassemia
Thaysen-Gee (nontropical sprue) K90.0
Thomsen G71.12
throat J39.2
   septic J02.0
thromboembolic —*see* Embolism
thymus (gland) E32.9
   specified NEC E32.8
thyroid (gland) E07.9
   heart (*see also* Hyperthyroidism) E05.90
      [*I43*]
      with thyroid storm E05.91 [*I43*]
   specified NEC E07.89
Tietze's M94.0
tongue K14.9
   specified NEC K14.8
tonsils, tonsillar (and adenoids) J35.9
tooth, teeth K08.9
   hard tissues K03.9
      specified NEC K03.89
   pulp NEC K04.99
   specified NEC K08.8
Tourette's F95.2
trachea NEC J39.8

Disease, diseased (*Continued*)
tricuspid I07.9
   nonrheumatic I36.9
triglyceride-storage E75.5
trophoblastic —*see* Mole, hydatidiform
tsutsugamushi A75.3
tube (fallopian) (noninflammatory) N83.9
   inflammatory —*see* Salpingitis
   specified NEC N83.8
tuberculous NEC —*see* Tuberculosis
tubo-ovarian (noninflammatory) N83.9
   inflammatory —*see* Salpingo-oophoritis
   specified NEC N83.8
tubotympanic, chronic —*see* Otitis, media,
      suppurative, chronic, tubotympanic
tubulo-interstitial N15.9
   specified NEC N15.8
tympanum —*see* Disorder, tympanic
      membrane
Uhl's Q24.8
Underwood's (sclerema neonatorum)
      P83.0
Unverricht (-Lundborg) —*see* Epilepsy,
      generalized, idiopathic
Urbach-Oppenheim (necrobiosis lipoidica
      diabeticorum) —*see* E08-E13 with
      .620
ureter N28.9
   in (due to)
      schistosomiasis (bilharziasis) B65.0
         [*N29*]
urethra N36.9
   specified NEC N36.8
urinary (tract) N39.9
   bladder N32.9
      specified NEC N32.89
   specified NEC N39.8
uterus (noninflammatory) N85.9
   infective —*see* Endometritis
   inflammatory —*see* Endometritis
   specified NEC N85.8
uveal tract (anterior) H21.9
   posterior H31.9
vagabond's B85.1
vagina, vaginal (noninflammatory) N89.9
   inflammatory NEC N76.89
   specified NEC N89.8
valve, valvular I38
   multiple I08.9
      specified NEC I08.8
van Creveld-von Gierke (glycogenosis I)
      E74.01
vas deferens N50.9
vascular I99.9
   arteriosclerotic —*see* Arteriosclerosis
   ciliary body NEC —*see* Disorder, iris,
      vascular
   hypertensive —*see* Hypertension
   iris NEC —*see* Disorder, iris, vascular
   obliterative I77.1
      peripheral I73.9
   occlusive I99.8
   peripheral (occlusive) I73.9
      in diabetes mellitus —*see* E08-E13 with
         .51
vasomotor I73.9
vasospastic I73.9
vein I87.9
venereal (*see also* Disease, sexually
      transmitted) A64
   chlamydial NEC A56.8
      anus A56.3
      genitourinary NOS A56.2
      pharynx A56.4
      rectum A56.3
   fifth A55
   sixth A55
   specified nature or type NEC A63.8
vertebra, vertebral —*see* Spondylopathy
   disc —*see* Disorder, disc
vibration —*see* Vibration, adverse effects

Disease, diseased (*Continued*)
viral, virus (*see also* Disease, by type of virus)
      B34.9
   arbovirus NOS A94
   arthropod-borne NOS A94
   congenital P35.9
      specified NEC P35.8
   Hanta (with renal manifestations)
      (Dobrava) (Puumala) (Seoul) A98.5
      with pulmonary manifestations (Andes)
         (Bayou) (Bermejo) (Black Creek
         Canal) (Choclo) (Juquitiba)
         (Laguna negra) (Lechiguanas)
         (New York) (Oran) (Sin nombre)
         B33.4
   Hantaan (Korean hemorrhagic fever) A98.5
   human immunodeficiency (HIV) B20
   Kunjin A83.4
   nonarthropod-borne NOS B34.9
   Powassan A84.8
   Rocio (encephalitis) A83.6
   Sin nombre (Hantavirus) (cardio)-
      pulmonary syndrome B33.4
   Tahyna B33.8
   vesicular stomatitis A93.8
vitreous H43.9
   specified NEC H43.89
vocal cord J38.3
Volkmann's, acquired T79.6
von Eulenburg's (congenital paramyotonia)
      G71.19
von Gierke's (glycogenosis I) E74.01
von Graefe's —*see* Strabismus, paralytic,
      ophthalmoplegia, progressive
von Willebrand (-Jürgens) (angiohemophilia)
      D68.0
Vrolik's (osteogenesis imperfecta) Q78.0
vulva (noninflammatory) N90.9
   inflammatory NEC N76.89
   specified NEC N90.89
Wallgren's (obstruction of splenic vein with
      collateral circulation) I87.8
Wassilieff's (leptospiral jaundice) A27.0
wasting NEC R64
   due to malnutrition E41
Waterhouse-Friderichsen A39.1
Wegner's (syphilitic osteochondritis) A50.02
Weil's (leptospiral jaundice of lung) A27.0
Weir Mitchell's (erythromelalgia) I73.81
Werdnig-Hoffmann G12.0
Wermer's E31.21
Werner-His (trench fever) A79.0
Werner-Schultz (neutropenic splenomegaly)
      D73.81
Wernicke-Posadas B38.9
whipworm B79
white blood cells D72.9
   specified NEC D72.89
white matter R90.82
white-spot, meaning lichen sclerosus et
      atrophicus L90.0
   penis N48.0
   vulva N90.4
Wilkie's K55.1
Wilkinson-Sneddon (subcorneal pustular
      dermatosis) L13.1
Willis' —*see* Diabetes
Wilson's (hepatolenticular degeneration)
      E83.01
woolsorter's A22.1
yaba monkey tumor B08.72
yaba pox (virus) B08.72
zoonotic, bacterial A28.9
   specified type NEC A28.8
Disfigurement (due to scar) L90.5
Disgerminoma —*see* Dysgerminoma
DISH (diffuse idiopathic skeletal
      hyperostosis) —*see* Hyperostosis,
      ankylosing
Disinsertion, retina —*see* Detachment, retina
Dislocatable hip, congenital Q65.6

Dislocation (articular)
  with fracture —see Fracture
  acromioclavicular (joint) S43.10-
    with displacement
      100%-200% S43.12-
      more than 200% S43.13-
    inferior S43.14-
    posterior S43.15-
  ankle S93.0-
  astragalus —see Dislocation, ankle
  atlantoaxial S13.121
  atlantooccipital S13.111
  atloidooccipital S13.111
  breast bone S23.29
  capsule, joint code by site under Dislocation
  carpal (bone) —see Dislocation, wrist
  carpometacarpal (joint) NEC S63.05-
    thumb S63.04-
  cartilage (joint) - code by site under
      Dislocation
  cervical spine (vertebra) —see Dislocation,
      vertebra, cervical
  chronic —see Dislocation, recurrent
  clavicle —see Dislocation, acromioclavicular
      joint
  coccyx S33.2
  congenital NEC Q68.8
  coracoid —see Dislocation, shoulder
  costal cartilage S23.29
  costochondral S23.29
  cricoarytenoid articulation S13.29
  cricothyroid articulation S13.29
  dorsal vertebra —see Dislocation, vertebra,
      thoracic
  ear ossicle —see Discontinuity, ossicles, ear
  elbow S53.10-
    congenital Q68.8
    pathological —see Dislocation, pathological
        NEC, elbow
    radial head alone —see Dislocation, radial
        head
    recurrent —see Dislocation, recurrent,
        elbow
    traumatic S53.10-
      anterior S53.11-
      lateral S53.14-
      medial S53.13-
      posterior S53.12-
      specified type NEC S53.19-
  eye, nontraumatic —see Luxation, globe
  eyeball, nontraumatic —see Luxation, globe
  femur
    distal end —see Dislocation, knee
    proximal end —see Dislocation, hip
  fibula
    distal end —see Dislocation, ankle
    proximal end —see Dislocation, knee
  finger S63.25-
    index S63.25-
    interphalangeal S63.27-
      distal S63.29-
        index S63.29-
        little S63.29-
        middle S63.29-
        ring S63.29-
      index S63.27-
      little S63.27-
      middle S63.27-
      proximal S63.28-
        index S63.28-
        little S63.28-
        middle S63.28-
        ring S63.28-
      ring S63.27-
    little S63.25-
    metacarpophalangeal S63.26-
      index S63.26-
      little S63.26-
      middle S63.26-
      ring S63.26-
    middle S63.25-

Dislocation (Continued)
  finger (Continued)
    recurrent —see Dislocation, recurrent,
        finger
    ring S63.25-
    thumb —see Dislocation, thumb
  foot S93.30-
    recurrent —see Dislocation, recurrent,
        foot
    specified site NEC S93.33-
    tarsal joint S93.31-
    tarsometatarsal joint S93.32-
    toe —see Dislocation, toe
  fracture —see Fracture
  glenohumeral (joint) —see Dislocation,
      shoulder
  glenoid —see Dislocation, shoulder
  habitual —see Dislocation, recurrent
  hip S73.00-
    anterior S73.03-
      obturator S73.02-
    central S73.04-
    congenital (total) Q65.2
      bilateral Q65.1
      partial Q65.5
        bilateral Q65.4
        unilateral Q65.3-
      unilateral Q65.0-
    developmental M24.85-
    pathological —see Dislocation, pathological
        NEC, hip
    posterior S73.01-
    recurrent —see Dislocation, recurrent, hip
  humerus, proximal end —see Dislocation,
      shoulder
  incomplete —see Subluxation, by site
  incus —see Discontinuity, ossicles, ear
  infracoracoid —see Dislocation, shoulder
  innominate (pubic junction) (sacral junction)
      S33.39
    acetabulum —see Dislocation, hip
  interphalangeal (joint (s))
    finger S63.279
      distal S63.29-
        index S63.29-
        little S63.29-
        middle S63.29-
        ring S63.29-
      index S63.27-
      little S63.27-
      middle S63.27-
      proximal S63.28-
        index S63.28-
        little S63.28-
        middle S63.28-
        ring S63.28-
      ring S63.27-
    foot or toe —see Dislocation, toe
    thumb S63.12-
      distal joint S63.14-
      proximal joint S63.13-
  jaw (cartilage) (meniscus) S03.0
  joint prosthesis —see Complications, joint
      prosthesis, mechanical, displacement,
      by site
  knee S83.106
    cap —see Dislocation, patella
    congenital Q68.2
    old M23.8X-
    patella —see Dislocation, patella
    pathological —see Dislocation, pathological
        NEC, knee
    proximal tibia
      anteriorly S83.11-
      laterally S83.14-
      medially S83.13-
      posteriorly S83.12-
    recurrent —see also Derangement, knee,
        specified NEC
    specified type NEC S83.19-
  lacrimal gland H04.16-

Dislocation (Continued)
  lens (complete) H27.10-
    anterior H27.12-
    congenital Q12.1
    ocular implant —see Complications,
        intraocular lens
    partial H27.11-
    posterior H27.13-
    traumatic S05.8X-
  ligament code by site under Dislocation
  lumbar (vertebra) —see Dislocation, vertebra,
      lumbar
  lumbosacral (vertebra) —see also Dislocation,
      vertebra, lumbar
    congenital Q76.49
  mandible S03.0
  meniscus (knee) —see Tear, meniscus
    other sites code by site under Dislocation
  metacarpal (bone)
    distal end —see Dislocation, finger
    proximal end S63.06-
  metacarpophalangeal (joint)
    finger S63.26-
      index S63.26-
      little S63.26-
      middle S63.26-
      ring S63.26-
    thumb S63.11-
  metatarsal (bone) —see Dislocation, foot
  metatarsophalangeal (joint (s)) —see
      Dislocation, toe
  midcarpal (joint) S63.03-
  midtarsal (joint) —see Dislocation, foot
  neck S13.20
    specified site NEC S13.29
    vertebra —see Dislocation, vertebra,
        cervical
  nose (septal cartilage) S03.1
  occipitoatloid S13.111
  old —see Derangement, joint, specified type
      NEC
  ossicles, ear —see Discontinuity, ossicles,
      ear
  partial —see Subluxation, by site
  patella S83.006
    congenital Q74.1
    lateral S83.01-
    recurrent (nontraumatic) M22.0-
      incomplete M22.1-
    specified type NEC S83.09-
  pathological NEC M24.30
    ankle M24.37-
    elbow M24.32-
    foot joint M24.37-
    hand joint M24.34-
    hip M24.35-
    knee M24.36-
    lumbosacral joint —see subcategory
        M53.2
    pelvic region —see Dislocation,
        pathological, hip
    sacroiliac —see subcategory M53.2
    shoulder M24.31-
    wrist M24.33-
  pelvis NEC S33.30
    specified NEC S33.39
  phalanx
    finger or hand —see Dislocation, finger
    foot or toe —see Dislocation, toe
  prosthesis, internal —see Complications,
      prosthetic device, by site, mechanical
  radial head S53.006
    anterior S53.01-
    posterior S53.02-
    specified type NEC S53.09-
  radiocarpal (joint) S63.02-
  radiohumeral (joint) —see Dislocation, radial
      head
  radioulnar (joint)
    distal S63.01-
    proximal —see Dislocation, elbow

◀ New   ◀◀◀ Revised   ~~deleted~~ Deleted

Dislocation *(Continued)*
  radius
    distal end —*see* Dislocation, wrist
    proximal end —*see* Dislocation, radial
      head
  recurrent M24.40
    ankle M24.47-
    elbow M24.42-
    finger M24.44-
    foot joint M24.47-
    hand joint M24.44-
    hip M24.45-
    knee M24.46-
      patella —*see* Dislocation, patella,
        recurrent
    patella —*see* Dislocation, patella, recurrent
    sacroiliac —*see* subcategory M53.2
    shoulder M24.41-
    toe M24.47-
    vertebra *(see also* subcategory) M43.5
      atlantoaxial M43.4
        with myelopathy M43.3
    wrist M24.43-
  rib (cartilage) S23.29
  sacrococcygeal S33.2
  sacroiliac (joint) (ligament) S33.2
    congenital Q74.2
    recurrent —*see* subcategory M53.2
  sacrum S33.2
  scaphoid (bone) (hand) (wrist) —*see*
    Dislocation, wrist
  foot —*see* Dislocation, foot
  scapula —*see* Dislocation, shoulder, girdle,
    scapula
  semilunar cartilage, knee —*see* Tear, meniscus
  septal cartilage (nose) S03.1
  septum (nasal) (old) J34.2
  sesamoid bone code by site under Dislocation
  shoulder (blade) (ligament) (joint) (traumatic)
    S43.006
    acromioclavicular —*see* Dislocation,
      acromioclavicular
    chronic —*see* Dislocation, recurrent,
      shoulder
    congenital Q68.8
    girdle S43.30-
      scapula S43.31-
      specified site NEC S43.39-
    humerus S43.00-
      anterior S43.01-
      inferior S43.03-
      posterior S43.02-
    pathological —*see* Dislocation, pathological
      NEC, shoulder
    recurrent —*see* Dislocation, recurrent,
      shoulder
    specified type NEC S43.08-
  spine
    cervical —*see* Dislocation, vertebra, cervical
    congenital Q76.49
    due to birth trauma P11.5
    lumbar —*see* Dislocation, vertebra, lumbar
    thoracic —*see* Dislocation, vertebra,
      thoracic
  spontaneous —*see* Dislocation, pathological
  sternoclavicular (joint) S43.206
    anterior S43.21-
    posterior S43.22-
  sternum S23.29
  subglenoid —*see* Dislocation, shoulder
  symphysis pubis S33.4
  talus —*see* Dislocation, ankle
  tarsal (bone (s)) (joint (s)) —*see* Dislocation,
    foot
  tarsometatarsal (joint (s)) —*see* Dislocation,
    foot
  temporomandibular (joint) S03.0
  thigh, proximal end —*see* Dislocation, hip
  thorax S23.20
    specified site NEC S23.29
    vertebra —*see* Dislocation, vertebra

Dislocation *(Continued)*
  thumb S63.10-
    interphalangeal joint —*see* Dislocation,
      interphalangeal (joint), thumb
    metacarpophalangeal joint —*see*
      Dislocation, metacarpophalangeal
      (joint), thumb
  thyroid cartilage S13.29
  tibia
    distal end —*see* Dislocation, ankle
    proximal end —*see* Dislocation, knee
  tibiofibular (joint)
    distal —*see* Dislocation, ankle
    superior —*see* Dislocation, knee
  toe (s) S93.106
    great S93.10-
      interphalangeal joint S93.11-
      metatarsophalangeal joint S93.12-
    interphalangeal joint S93.119
    lesser S93.106
      interphalangeal joint S93.11-
      metatarsophalangeal joint S93.12-
    metatarsophalangeal joint S93.12-
  tooth S03.2
  trachea S23.29
  ulna
    distal end S63.07-
    proximal end —*see* Dislocation, elbow
  ulnohumeral (joint) —*see* Dislocation, elbow
  vertebra (articular process) (body)
    (traumatic)
    cervical S13.101
      atlantoaxial joint S13.121
      atlantooccipital joint S13.111
      atloidooccipital joint S13.111
      joint between
        C0 and C1 S13.111
        C1 and C2 S13.121
        C2 and C3 S13.131
        C3 and C4 S13.141
        C4 and C5 S13.151
        C5 and C6 S13.161
        C6 and C7 S13.171
        C7 and T1 S13.181
      occipitoatloid joint S13.111
    congenital Q76.49
    lumbar S33.101
      joint between
        L1 and L2 S33.111
        L2 and L3 S33.121
        L3 and L4 S33.131
        L4 and L5 S33.141
    nontraumatic —*see* Displacement,
      intervertebral disc
    partial —*see* Subluxation, by site
    recurrent NEC —*see* subcategory
      M43.5
    thoracic S23.101
      joint between
        T1 and T2 S23.111
        T2 and T3 S23.121
        T3 and T4 S23.123
        T4 and T5 S23.131
        T5 and T6 S23.133
        T6 and T7 S23.141
        T7 and T8 S23.143
        T8 and T9 S23.151
        T9 and T10 S23.153
        T10 and T11 S23.161
        T11 and T12 S23.163
        T12 and L1 S23.171
  wrist (carpal bone) S63.006
    carpometacarpal joint —*see* Dislocation,
      carpometacarpal (joint)
    distal radioulnar joint —*see* Dislocation,
      radioulnar (joint), distal
    metacarpal bone, proximal —*see*
      Dislocation, metacarpal (bone),
      proximal end
    midcarpal —*see* Dislocation, midcarpal
      (joint)

Dislocation *(Continued)*
  wrist *(Continued)*
    radiocarpal joint —*see* Dislocation,
      radiocarpal (joint)
    recurrent —*see* Dislocation, recurrent,
      wrist
    specified site NEC S63.09-
    ulna —*see* Dislocation, ulna, distal end
  xiphoid cartilage S23.29
Disorder (of) —*see also* Disease
  acantholytic L11.9
    specified NEC L11.8
  acute
    psychotic —*see* Psychosis, acute
    stress F43.0
  adjustment (grief) F43.20
    with
      anxiety F43.22
        with depressed mood F43.23
      conduct disturbance F43.24
        with emotional disturbance
          F43.25
      depressed mood F43.21
        with anxiety F43.23
      other specified symptom F43.29
  adrenal (capsule) (gland) (medullary)
    E27.9
    specified NEC E27.8
  adrenogenital E25.9
    drug-induced E25.8
    iatrogenic E25.8
    idiopathic E25.8
  adult personality (and behavior) F69
    specified NEC F68.8
  affective (mood) —*see* Disorder, mood
  aggressive, unsocialized F91.1
  alcohol-related F10.99
    with
      amnestic disorder, persisting
        F10.96
      anxiety disorder F10.980
      dementia, persisting F10.97
      intoxication F10.929
        with delirium F10.921
        uncomplicated F10.920
      mood disorder F10.94
      other specified F10.988
      psychotic disorder F10.959
        with
          delusions F10.950
          hallucinations F10.951
      sexual dysfunction F10.981
      sleep disorder F10.982
  allergic —*see* Allergy
  alveolar NEC J84.09
  amino-acid
    cystathioninuria E72.19
    cystinosis E72.04
    cystinuria E72.01
    glycinuria E72.09
    homocystinuria E72.11
    metabolism —*see* Disturbance,
      metabolism, amino-acid
    specified NEC E72.8
    neonatal, transitory P74.8
    renal transport NEC E72.09
    transport NEC E72.09
  amnesic, amnestic
    alcohol-induced F10.96
      with dependence F10.26
    due to (secondary to) general medical
      condition F04
    psychoactive NEC-induced F19.96
      with
        abuse F19.16
        dependence F19.26
    sedative, hypnotic or anxiolytic-
      induced F13.96
      with dependence F13.26
  anaerobic glycolysis with anemia
    D55.2

Disorder *(Continued)*
anxiety F41.9
  due to (secondary to)
    alcohol F10.980
    amphetamine F15.980
      in
        abuse F15.180
        dependence F15.280
    anxiolytic F13.980
      in
        abuse F13.180
        dependence F13.280
    caffeine F15.980
      in
        abuse F15.180
        dependence F15.280
    cannabis F12.980
      in
        abuse F12.180
        dependence F12.280
    cocaine F14.980
      in
        abuse F14.180
        dependence F14.180
    general medical condition F06.4
    hallucinogen F16.980
      in
        abuse F16.180
        dependence F16.280
    hypnotic F13.980
      in
        abuse F13.180
        dependence F13.280
    inhalant F18.980
      in
        abuse F18.180
        dependence F18.280
    phencyclidine F16.980
      in
        abuse F16.180
        dependence F16.280
    psychoactive substance NEC
        F19.980
      in
        abuse F19.180
        dependence F19.280
    sedative F13.980
      in
        abuse F13.180
        dependence F13.280
    volatile solvents F18.980
      in
        abuse F18.180
        dependence F18.280
  generalized F41.1
  mixed
    with depression (mild) F41.8
    specified NEC F41.3
  organic F06.4
  phobic F40.9
    of childhood F40.8
  specified NEC F41.8
aortic valve —*see* Endocarditis, aortic
aromatic amino-acid metabolism E70.9
  specified NEC E70.8
arteriole NEC I77.89
artery NEC I77.89
articulation —*see* Disorder, joint
attachment (childhood)
  disinhibited F94.2
  reactive F94.1
attention-deficit hyperactivity (adolescent)
    (adult) (child) F90.9
  combined type F90.2
  hyperactive type F90.1
  inattentive type F90.0
  specified type NEC F90.8
attention-deficit without hyperactivity
    (adolescent) (adult) (child) F90.0
auditory processing (central) H93.25
autistic F84.0

Disorder *(Continued)*
autonomic nervous system G90.9
  specified NEC G90.8
avoidant, child or adolescent F40.10
balance
  acid-base E87.8
    mixed E87.4
  electrolyte E87.8
  fluid NEC E87.8
behavioral (disruptive) —*see* Disorder,
    conduct
beta-amino-acid metabolism E72.8
bile acid and cholesterol metabolism
    E78.70
  Barth syndrome E78.71
  other specified E78.79
  Smith-Lemli-Opitz syndrome E78.72
bilirubin excretion E80.6
binocular
  movement H51.9
    convergence
      excess H51.12
      insufficiency H51.11
    internuclear ophthalmoplegia —*see*
        Ophthalmoplegia, internuclear
    palsy of conjugate gaze H51.0
    specified type NEC H51.8
  vision NEC —*see* Disorder, vision,
      binocular
bipolar (I) F31.9
  current episode
    depressed F31.9
      with psychotic features F31.5
      without psychotic features
          F31.30
        mild F31.31
        moderate F31.32
        severe (without psychotic features)
            F31.4
          with psychotic features
              F31.5
    hypomanic F31.0
    manic F31.9
      with psychotic features F31.2
      without psychotic features F31.10
        mild F31.11
        moderate F31.12
        severe (without psychotic features)
            F31.13
          with psychotic features F31.2
    mixed F31.60
      mild F31.61
      moderate F31.62
      severe (without psychotic features)
          F31.63
        with psychotic features F31.64
      severe depression (without psychotic
          features) F31.4
        with psychotic features F31.5
  II F31.81
  in remission (currently) F31.70
    in full remission
      most recent episode
        depressed F31.76
        hypomanic F31.72
        manic F31.74
        mixed F31.78
    in partial remission
      most recent episode
        depressed F31.75
        hypomanic F31.71
        manic F31.73
        mixed F31.77
  organic F06.30
  single manic episode F30.9
    mild F30.11
    moderate F30.12
    severe (without psychotic symptoms)
        F30.13
      with psychotic symptoms F30.2
  specified NEC F31.89

Disorder *(Continued)*
bladder N32.9
  functional NEC N31.9
  in schistosomiasis B65.0 [N33]
  specified NEC N32.89
bleeding D68.9
blood D75.9
  in congenital early syphilis A50.09 [D77]
body dysmorphic F45.22
bone M89.9
  continuity M84.9
    specified type NEC M84.80
      ankle M84.87-
      fibula M84.86-
      foot M84.87-
      hand M84.84-
      humerus M84.82-
      neck M84.88
      pelvis M84.859
      radius M84.83-
      rib M84.88
      shoulder M84.81-
      skull M84.88
      thigh M84.85-
      tibia M84.86-
      ulna M84.83-
      vertebra M84.88
  density and structure M85.9
    cyst —*see also* Cyst, bone, specified type
        NEC
      aneurysmal —*see* Cyst, bone,
          aneurysmal
      solitary —*see* Cyst, bone, solitary
    diffuse idiopathic skeletal
        hyperostosis —*see* Hyperostosis,
        ankylosing
    fibrous dysplasia (monostotic) —*see*
        Dysplasia, fibrous, bone
    fluorosis —*see* Fluorosis, skeletal
    hyperostosis of skull M85.2
    osteitis condensans —*see* Osteitis,
        condensans
    specified type NEC M85.8-
      ankle M85.87-
      foot M85.87-
      forearm M85.83-
      hand M85.84-
      lower leg M85.86-
      multiple sites M85.89
      neck M85.88
      rib M85.88
      shoulder M85.81-
      skull M85.88
      thigh M85.85-
      upper arm M85.82-
      vertebra M85.88
  development and growth NEC
      M89.20
    carpus M89.24-
    clavicle M89.21-
    femur M89.25-
    fibula M89.26-
    finger M89.24-
    humerus M89.22-
    ilium M89.259
    ischium M89.259
    metacarpus M89.24-
    metatarsus M89.27-
    multiple sites M89.29
    neck M89.28
    radius M89.23-
    rib M89.28
    scapula M89.21-
    skull M89.28
    tarsus M89.27-
    tibia M89.26-
    toe M89.27-
    ulna M89.23-
    vertebra M89.28
  specified type NEC M89.8X-
brachial plexus G54.0

◀ New   ◀▥▥ Revised   ~~deleted~~ Deleted

Disorder *(Continued)*
branched-chain amino-acid metabolism E71.2
   specified NEC E71.19
breast N64.9
   agalactia —*see* Agalactia
   associated with
     lactation O92.70
      specified NEC O92.79
     pregnancy O92.20
      specified NEC O92.29
     puerperium O92.20
      specified NEC O92.29
   cracked nipple —*see* Cracked nipple
   galactorrhea —*see* Galactorrhea
   hypogalactia O92.4
   lactation disorder NEC O92.79
   mastitis —*see* Mastitis
   nipple infection —*see* Infection, nipple
   retracted nipple —*see* Retraction, nipple
   specified type NEC N64.89
Briquet's F45.0
bullous, in diseases classified elsewhere L14
cannabis use
   due to drug abuse —*see* Abuse, drug, cannabis
   due to drug dependence —*see* Dependence, drug, cannabis ◄▦
carbohydrate
   absorption, intestinal NEC E74.39
   metabolism (congenital) E74.9
     specified NEC E74.8
cardiac, functional I51.89
carnitine metabolism E71.40
cartilage M94.9
   articular NEC —*see* Derangement, joint, articular cartilage
   chondrocalcinosis —*see* Chondrocalcinosis
   specified type NEC M94.8X-
     articular —*see* Derangement, joint, articular cartilage
     multiple sites M94.8X0
catatonic
   due to (secondary to) known physiological condition F06.1
   organic F06.1
central auditory processing H93.25
cervical
   region NEC M53.82
   root (nerve) NEC G54.2
character NOS F60.9
childhood disintegrative NEC F84.3
cholesterol and bile acid metabolism E78.70
   Barth syndrome E78.71
   other specified E78.79
   Smith-Lemli-Opitz syndrome E78.72
choroid H31.9
   atrophy —*see* Atrophy, choroid
   degeneration —*see* Degeneration, choroid
   detachment —*see* Detachment, choroid
   dystrophy —*see* Dystrophy, choroid
   hemorrhage —*see* Hemorrhage, choroid
   rupture —*see* Rupture, choroid
   scar —*see* Scar, chorioretinal
   solar retinopathy —*see* Retinopathy, solar
   specified type NEC H31.8
ciliary body —*see* Disorder, iris
   degeneration —*see* Degeneration, ciliary body
coagulation (factor) (*see also* Defect, coagulation) D68.9
   newborn, transient P61.6
coccyx NEC M53.3
cognitive F09
   due to (secondary to) general medical condition F09
   persisting R41.89
     due to
      alcohol F10.97
       with dependence F10.27

Disorder *(Continued)*
cognitive *(Continued)*
   persisting *(Continued)*
     due to *(Continued)*
      anxiolytics F13.97
       with dependence F13.27
      hypnotics F13.97
       with dependence F13.27
      sedatives F13.97
       with dependence F13.27
      specified substance NEC F19.97
       with
        abuse F19.17
        dependence F19.27
communication F80.9
conduct (childhood) F91.9
   adjustment reaction —*see* Disorder, adjustment
   adolescent onset type F91.2
   childhood onset type F91.1
   compulsive F63.9
   confined to family context F91.0
   depressive F91.8
   group type F91.2
   hyperkinetic —*see* Disorder, attention-deficit hyperactivity
   oppositional defiance F91.3
   socialized F91.2
   solitary aggressive type F91.1
   specified NEC F91.8
   unsocialized (aggressive) F91.1
conduction, heart I45.9
congenital glycosylation (CDG) E74.8
conjunctiva H11.9
   infection —*see* Conjunctivitis
connective tissue, localized L94.9
   specified NEC L94.8
conversion —*see* Disorder, dissociative
convulsive (secondary) —*see* Convulsions
cornea H18.9
   deformity —*see* Deformity, cornea
   degeneration —*see* Degeneration, cornea
   deposits —*see* Deposit, cornea
   due to contact lens H18.82-
     specified as edema —*see* Edema, cornea
   edema —*see* Edema, cornea
   keratitis —*see* Keratitis
   keratoconjunctivitis —*see* Keratoconjunctivitis
   membrane change —*see* Change, corneal membrane
   neovascularization —*see* Neovascularization, cornea
   scar —*see* Opacity, cornea
   specified type NEC H18.89-
   ulcer —*see* Ulcer, cornea
corpus cavernosum N48.9
cranial nerve —*see* Disorder, nerve, cranial
cyclothymic F34.0
defiant oppositional F91.3
delusional (persistent) (systematized) F22
   induced F24
depersonalization F48.1
depressive F32.9
   major F32.9
     with psychotic symptoms F32.3
     in remission (full) F32.5
      partial F32.4
     recurrent F33.9
     single episode F32.9
      mild F32.0
      moderate F32.1
      severe (without psychotic symptoms) F32.2
       with psychotic symptoms F32.3
   organic F06.31
   recurrent F33.9
     current episode
      mild F33.0
      moderate F33.1

Disorder *(Continued)*
depressive *(Continued)*
   recurrent *(Continued)*
     current episode *(Continued)*
      severe (without psychotic symptoms) F33.2
       with psychotic symptoms F33.3
     in remission F33.40
      full F33.42
      partial F33.41
     specified NEC F33.8
   single episode —*see* Episode, depressive
developmental F89
   arithmetical skills F81.2
   coordination (motor) F82
   expressive writing F81.81
   language F80.9
     expressive F80.1
     mixed receptive and expressive F80.2
     receptive type F80.2
     specified NEC F80.89
   learning F81.9
     arithmetical F81.2
     reading F81.0
   mixed F88
   motor coordination or function F82
   pervasive F84.9
     specified NEC F84.8
   phonological F80.0
   reading F81.0
   scholastic skills —*see also* Disorder, learning
     mixed F81.89
   specified NEC F88
   speech F80.9
     articulation F80.0
     specified NEC F80.89
   written expression F81.81
diaphragm J98.6
digestive (system) K92.9
   newborn P78.9
     specified NEC P78.89
   postprocedural —*see* Complication, gastrointestinal
   psychogenic F45.8
disc (intervertebral) M51.9
   with
     myelopathy
      cervical region M50.00
      cervicothoracic region M50.03
      high cervical region M50.01 ◄
      lumbar region M51.06
      ~~lumbosacral region M51.07~~
      mid-cervical region M50.02
      ~~occipito-atlanto-axial region M50.01~~
      sacrococcygeal region M53.3
      thoracic region M51.04
      thoracolumbar region M51.05
     radiculopathy
      cervical region M50.10
      cervicothoracic region M50.13
      high cervical region M50.11 ◄
      lumbar region M51.16
      lumbosacral region M51.17
      mid-cervical region M50.12
      ~~occipito-atlanto-axial region M50.11~~
      sacrococcygeal region M53.3
      thoracic region M51.14
      thoracolumbar region M51.15
   cervical M50.90
     with
      myelopathy M50.00
       C2-C3 M50.01 ◄
       C3-C4 M50.01 ◄
       C4-C5 M50.02 ◄
       C5-C6 M50.02 ◄
       C6-C7 M50.02 ◄
       C7-T1 M50.03 ◄
      cervicothoracic region M50.03
      high cervical region M50.01 ◄
      mid-cervical region M50.02
      ~~occipito-atlanto-axial region M50.01~~

Disorder (Continued)
 disc (Continued)
  cervical (Continued)
   with (Continued)
    neuritis, radiculitis or radiculopathy
      M50.10
     C2-C3 M50.11 ◄
     C3-C4 M50.11 ◄
     C4-C5 M50.12 ◄
     C5-C6 M50.12 ◄
     C6-C7 M50.12 ◄
     C7-T1 M50.13 ◄
     cervicothoracic region M50.13
     high cervical region M50.11 ◄
     mid-cervical region M50.12
     occipito-atlanto-axial region M50.11
    C2-C3 M50.91 ◄
    C3-C4 M50.91 ◄
    C4-C5 M50.92 ◄
    C5-C6 M50.92 ◄
    C6-C7 M50.92 ◄
    C7-T1 M50.93 ◄
    cervicothoracic region M50.93
   degeneration M50.30
    C2-C3 M50.31 ◄
    C3-C4 M50.31 ◄
    C4-C5 M50.32 ◄
    C5-C6 M50.32 ◄
    C6-C7 M50.32 ◄
    C7-T1 M50.33 ◄
    cervicothoracic region M50.33
    high cervical region M50.31 ◄
    mid-cervical region M50.32
    occipito-atlanto-axial region M50.31
   displacement M50.20
    C2-C3 M50.21 ◄
    C3-C4 M50.21 ◄
    C4-C5 M50.22 ◄
    C5-C6 M50.22 ◄
    C6-C7 M50.22 ◄
    C7-T1 M50.23 ◄
    cervicothoracic region M50.23
    high cervical region M50.21 ◄
    mid-cervical region M50.22
    occipito-atlanto-axial region M50.21
   high cervical region M50.91 ◄
   mid-cervical region M50.92
   occipito-atlanto-axial region M50.91
   specified type NEC M50.80
    C2-C3 M50.81 ◄
    C3-C4 M50.81 ◄
    C4-C5 M50.82 ◄
    C5-C6 M50.82 ◄
    C6-C7 M50.82 ◄
    C7-T1 M50.83 ◄
    cervicothoracic region M50.83
    high cervical region M50.81 ◄
    mid-cervical region M50.82
    occipito-atlanto-axial region M50.81
  specified NEC
   lumbar region M51.86
   lumbosacral region M51.87
   sacrococcygeal region M53.3
   thoracic region M51.84
   thoracolumbar region M51.85
 disinhibited attachment (childhood) F94.2
 disintegrative, childhood NEC F84.3
 disruptive behavior F98.9
 dissocial personality F60.2
 dissociative F44.9
  affecting
   motor function F44.4
    and sensation F44.7
   sensation F44.6
    and motor function F44.7
  brief reactive F43.0
  due to (secondary to) general medical
    condition F06.8
  mixed F44.7
  organic F06.8
  other specified NEC F44.89

Disorder (Continued)
 double heterozygous sickling —see Disease,
   sickle-cell
 dream anxiety F51.5
 drug induced hemorrhagic D68.32
 drug related F19.99
  abuse —see Abuse, drug
  dependence —see Dependence, drug
 dysmorphic body F45.1
 dysthymic F34.1
 ear H93.9-
  bleeding —see Otorrhagia
  deafness —see Deafness
  degenerative H93.09-
  discharge —see Otorrhea
  external H61.9-
   auditory canal stenosis —see Stenosis,
     external ear canal
   exostosis —see Exostosis, external ear
     canal
   impacted cerumen —see Impaction,
     cerumen
   otitis —see Otitis, externa
   perichondritis —see Perichondritis,
     ear
   pinna —see Disorder, pinna
   specified type NEC H61.89-
    in diseases classified elsewhere
      H62.8X-
  inner H83.9-
   vestibular dysfunction —see Disorder,
     vestibular function
  middle H74.9-
   adhesive H74.1-
   ossicle —see Abnormal, ear ossicles
   polyp —see Polyp, ear (middle)
   specified NEC, in diseases classified
     elsewhere H75.8-
  postprocedural —see Complications, ear,
    procedure
  specified NEC, in diseases classified
    elsewhere H94.8-
 eating (adult) (psychogenic) F50.9
  anorexia —see Anorexia
  bulimia F50.2
  child F98.29
   pica F98.3
   rumination disorder F98.21
  pica F50.8
   childhood F98.3
 electrolyte (balance) NEC E87.8
  with
   abortion —see Abortion by type
     complicated by specified condition
       NEC
   ectopic pregnancy O08.5
   molar pregnancy O08.5
  acidosis (metabolic) (respiratory) E87.2
  alkalosis (metabolic) (respiratory)
    E87.3
 elimination, transepidermal L87.9
  specified NEC L87.8
 emotional (persistent) F34.9
  of childhood F93.9
   specified NEC F93.8
 endocrine E34.9
  postprocedural E89.89
  specified NEC E89.89
 erectile (male) (organic) (see also Dysfunction,
   sexual, male, erectile) N52.9
  nonorganic F52.21
 erythematous —see Erythema
 esophagus K22.9
  functional K22.4
  psychogenic F45.8
 eustachian tube H69.9-
  infection —see Salpingitis, eustachian
  obstruction —see Obstruction, eustachian
    tube
  patulous —see Patulous, eustachian tube
  specified NEC H69.8-

Disorder (Continued)
 extrapyramidal G25.9
  in diseases classified elsewhere —see
    category G26 ◄
  specified type NEC G25.89
 eye H57.9
  postprocedural —see Complication,
    postprocedural, eye
 eyelid H02.9
  cyst —see Cyst, eyelid
  degenerative H02.70
   chloasma —see Chloasma, eyelid
   madarosis —see Madarosis
   specified type NEC H02.79
   vitiligo —see Vitiligo, eyelid
   xanthelasma —see Xanthelasma
  dermatochalasis —see Dermato-chalasis
  edema —see Edema, eyelid
  elephantiasis —see Elephantiasis, eyelid
  foreign body, retained —see Foreign body,
    retained, eyelid
  function H02.59
   abnormal innervation syndrome —see
     Syndrome, abnormal innervation
   blepharochalasis —see Blepharochalasis
   blepharoclonus —see Blepharoclonus
   blepharophimosis —see
     Blepharophimosis
   blepharoptosis —see Blepharoptosis
   lagophthalmos —see Lagophthalmos
   lid retraction —see Retraction, lid
  hypertrichosis —see Hypertrichosis, eyelid
  specified type NEC H02.89
  vascular H02.879
   left H02.876
    lower H02.875
    upper H02.874
   right H02.873
    lower H02.872
    upper H02.871
 factitious F68.10
  with predominantly
   physical symptoms F68.12
    with psychological symptoms F68.13
   psychological symptoms F68.11
    with physical symptoms F68.13
 factor, coagulation —see Defect, coagulation
 fatty acid
  metabolism E71.30
   specified NEC E71.39
  oxidation
   LCAD E71.310
   MCAD E71.311
   SCAD E71.312
   specified deficiency NEC E71.318
 feeding (infant or child) (see also Disorder,
   eating) R63.3-
 feigned (with obvious motivation) Z76.5
  without obvious motivation —see Disorder,
    factitious
 female
  hypoactive sexual desire F52.0
  orgasmic F52.31
  sexual arousal F52.22
 fibroblastic M72.9
  specified NEC M72.8
 fluency
  adult onset F98.5
  childhood onset F80.81
  following
   cerebral infarction I69.323
   cerebrovascular disease I69.923
    specified disease NEC I69.823
   intracerebral hemorrhage I69.123
   nontraumatic intracranial hemorrhage
     NEC I69.223
   subarachnoid hemorrhage I69.023
  in conditions classified elsewhere R47.82
 fluid balance E87.8
 follicular (skin) L73.9
  specified NEC L73.8

◄ New   ◄▪▪ Revised   ~~deleted~~ Deleted

Disorder *(Continued)*
  fructose metabolism E74.10
    essential fructosuria E74.11
    fructokinase deficiency E74.11
    fructose-1, 6-diphosphatase deficiency
      E74.19
    hereditary fructose intolerance E74.12
    other specified E74.19
  functional polymorphonuclear neutrophils
    D71
  gallbladder, biliary tract and pancreas in
    diseases classified elsewhere K87
  gamma-glutamyl cycle E72.8
  gastric (functional) K31.9
    motility K30
    psychogenic F45.8
    secretion K30
  gastrointestinal (functional) NOS K92.9
    newborn P78.9
    psychogenic F45.8
  gender-identity or -role F64.9
    childhood F64.2
    effect on relationship F66
    of adolescence or adulthood
      (nontranssexual) F64.1
    specified NEC F64.8
    uncertainty F66
  genitourinary system
    female N94.9
    male N50.9
    psychogenic F45.8
  globe H44.9
    degenerated condition H44.50
      absolute glaucoma H44.51-
      atrophy H44.52-
      leucocoria H44.53-
    degenerative H44.30
      chalcosis H44.31-
      myopia H44.2-
      siderosis H44.32-
      specified type NEC H44.39-
    endophthalmitis —*see* Endophthalmitis
    foreign body, retained —*see* Foreign body,
      intraocular, old, retained
    hemophthalmos —*see* Hemophthalmos
    hypotony H44.40
      due to
        ocular fistula H44.42-
        specified disorder NEC H44.43-
      flat anterior chamber H44.41-
      primary H44.44-
    luxation —*see* Luxation, globe
    specified type NEC H44.89
  glomerular (in) N05.9
    amyloidosis E85.4 *[N08]*
    cryoglobulinemia D89.1 *[N08]*
    disseminated intravascular coagulation
      D65 *[N08]*
    Fabry's disease E75.21 *[N08]*
    familial lecithin cholesterol acyltransferase
      deficiency E78.6 *[N08]*
    Goodpasture's syndrome M31.0
    hemolytic-uremic syndrome D59.3
    Henoch (-Schönlein) purpura D69.0 *[N08]*
    malariae malaria B52.0
    microscopic polyangiitis M31.7 *[N08]*
    multiple myeloma C90.0- *[N08]*
    mumps B26.83
    schistosomiasis B65.9 *[N08]*
    sepsis NEC A41.- *[N08]*
      streptococcal A40.- *[N08]*
    sickle-cell disorders D57.- *[N08]*
    strongyloidiasis B78.9 *[N08]*
    subacute bacterial endocarditis I33.0 *[N08]*
    syphilis A52.75
    systemic lupus erythematosus M32.14
    thrombotic thrombocytopenic purpura
      M31.1 *[N08]*
    Waldenström macroglobulinemia C88.0
      [N08]
    Wegener's granulomatosis M31.31

Disorder *(Continued)*
  gluconeogenesis E74.4
  glucosaminoglycan metabolism —
    see Disorder, metabolism,
    glucosaminoglycan
  glycine metabolism E72.50
    d-glycericacidemia E72.59
    hyperhydroxyprolinemia E72.59
    hyperoxaluria E72.53
    hyperprolinemia E72.59
    non-ketotic hyperglycinemia E72.51
    oxalosis E72.53
    oxaluria E72.53
    sarcosinemia E72.59
    trimethylaminuria E72.52
  glycoprotein metabolism E77.9
    specified NEC E77.8
  habit (and impulse) F63.9
    involving sexual behavior NEC F65.9
    specified NEC F63.89
  heart action I49.9
  hematological D75.9
    newborn (transient) P61.9
      specified NEC P61.8
  hematopoietic organs D75.9
  hemorrhagic NEC D69.9
    drug-induced D68.32
    due to
      extrinsic circulating anticoagulants D68.32
      increase in
        anti-IIa D68.32
        anti-Xa D68.32
      intrinsic
        circulating anticoagulants D68.318
        increase in
          antithrombin D68.318
          anti-VIIIa D68.318
          anti-IXa D68.318
          anti-XIa D68.318
    following childbirth O72.3
  hemostasis —*see* Defect, coagulation
  histidine metabolism E70.40
    histidinemia E70.41
    other specified E70.49
  hyperkinetic —*see* Disorder, attention-deficit
    hyperactivity
  hyperleucine-isoleucinemia E71.19
  hypervalinemia E71.19
  hypoactive sexual desire F52.0
  hypochondriacal F45.20
    body dysmorphic F45.22
    neurosis F45.21
    other specified F45.29
  identity
    dissociative F44.81
    of childhood F93.8
  immune mechanism (immunity) D89.9
    specified type NEC D89.89
  impaired renal tubular function N25.9
    specified NEC N25.89
  impulse (control) F63.9
  inflammatory
    pelvic, in diseases classified elsewhere —
      see category N74 ◀
    penis N48.29
      abscess N48.21
      cellulitis N48.22
  integument, newborn P83.9
    specified NEC P83.8
  intermittent explosive F63.81
  internal secretion pancreas —*see* Increased,
    secretion, pancreas, endocrine
  intestine, intestinal
    carbohydrate absorption NEC E74.39
      postoperative K91.2
    functional NEC K59.9
      postoperative K91.89
      psychogenic F45.8
    vascular K55.9
      chronic K55.1
      specified NEC K55.8

Disorder *(Continued)*
  intraoperative (intraprocedural) —*see*
    Complications, intraoperative
  involuntary emotional expression (IEED)
    F48.2
  iris H21.9
    adhesions —*see* Adhesions, iris
    atrophy —*see* Atrophy, iris
    chamber angle recession —*see* Recession,
      chamber angle
    cyst —*see* Cyst, iris
    degeneration —*see* Degeneration, iris
    in diseases classified elsewhere H22
    iridodialysis —*see* Iridodialysis
    iridoschisis —*see* Iridoschisis
    miotic pupillary cyst —*see* Cyst, pupillary
    pupillary
      abnormality —*see* Abnormality,
        pupillary
      membrane —*see* Membrane, pupillary
    specified type NEC H21.89
    vascular NEC H21.1X-
  iron metabolism E83.10
    specified NEC E83.19
  isovaleric acidemia E71.110
  jaw, developmental M27.0
    temporomandibular —*see* Anomaly,
      dentofacial, temporomandibular joint
  joint M25.9
    derangement —*see* Derangement, joint
    effusion —*see* Effusion, joint
    fistula —*see* Fistula, joint
    hemarthrosis —*see* Hemarthrosis
    instability —*see* Instability, joint
    osteophyte —*see* Osteophyte
    pain —*see* Pain, joint
    psychogenic F45.8
    specified type NEC M25.80
      ankle M25.87-
      elbow M25.82-
      foot joint M25.87-
      hand joint M25.84-
      hip M25.85-
      knee M25.86-
      shoulder M25.81-
      wrist M25.83-
    stiffness —*see* Stiffness, joint
  ketone metabolism E71.32
  kidney N28.9
    functional (tubular) N25.9
    in
      schistosomiasis B65.9 *[N29]*
    tubular function N25.9
      specified NEC N25.89
  lacrimal system H04.9
    changes H04.69
    fistula —*see* Fistula, lacrimal
    gland H04.19
      atrophy —*see* Atrophy, lacrimal gland
      cyst —*see* Cyst, lacrimal, gland
      dacryops —*see* Dacryops
      dislocation —*see* Dislocation, lacrimal
        gland
      dry eye syndrome —*see* Syndrome, dry
        eye
      infection —*see* Dacryoadenitis
      granuloma —*see* Granuloma, lacrimal
      inflammation —*see* Inflammation, lacrimal
      obstruction —*see* Obstruction, lacrimal
      specified NEC H04.89
  lactation NEC O92.79
  language (developmental) F80.9
    expressive F80.1
    mixed receptive and expressive F80.2
    receptive F80.2
  late luteal phase dysphoric N94.89
  learning (specific) F81.9
    acalculia R48.8
    alexia R48.0
    mathematics F81.2
    reading F81.0

◄ New   ⬤ Revised   ~~deleted~~ Deleted

Disorder (Continued)
  mixed
    anxiety and depressive F41.8
    of scholastic skills (developmental)
        F81.89
    receptive expressive language F80.2
  mood F39
    bipolar —see Disorder, bipolar
    depressive —see Disorder, depressive
    due to (secondary to)
      alcohol F10.94
      amphetamine F15.94
        in
          abuse F15.14
          dependence F15.24
      anxiolytic F13.94
        in
          abuse F13.14
          dependence F13.24
      cocaine F14.94
        in
          abuse F14.14
          dependence F14.24
      general medical condition F06.30
      hallucinogen F16.94
        in
          abuse F16.14
          dependence F16.24
      hypnotic F13.94
        in
          abuse F13.14
          dependence F13.24
      inhalant F18.94
        in
          abuse F18.14
          dependence F18.24
      opioid F11.94
        in
          abuse F11.14
          dependence F11.24
      phencyclidine (PCP) F16.94
        in
          abuse F16.14
          dependence F16.24
      physiological condition F06.30
        with
          depressive features F06.31
          major depressive-like episode
              F06.32
          manic features F06.33
          mixed features F06.34
      psychoactive substance NEC F19.94
        in
          abuse F19.14
          dependence F19.24
      sedative F13.94
        in
          abuse F13.14
          dependence F13.24
      volatile solvents F18.94
        in
          abuse F18.14
          dependence F18.24
    manic episode F30.9
      with psychotic symptoms F30.2
      without psychotic symptoms
          F30.10
        mild F30.11
        moderate F30.12
        severe F30.13
      in remission (full) F30.4
        partial F30.3
      specified type NEC F30.8
    organic F06.30
      right hemisphere F07.89
    persistent F34.9
      cyclothymia F34.0
      dysthymia F34.1
      specified type NEC F34.8
    recurrent F39
    right hemisphere organic F07.89

Disorder (Continued)
  movement G25.9
    drug-induced G25.70
      akathisia G25.71
      specified NEC G25.79
    hysterical F44.4
    in diseases classified elsewhere —see
        category G26 ◀
    periodic limb G47.61
      sleep related G47.61
    sleep related NEC G47.69
    specified NEC G25.89
    stereotyped F98.4
    treatment-induced G25.9
  multiple personality F44.81
  muscle M62.9
    attachment, spine —see Enthesopathy,
        spinal
    in trichinellosis —see Trichinellosis, with
        muscle disorder
    psychogenic F45.8
    specified type NEC M62.89
    tone, newborn P94.9
      specified NEC P94.8
  muscular
    attachments —see also Enthesopathy
      spine —see Enthesopathy, spinal
    urethra N36.44
  musculoskeletal system, soft tissue —see
      Disorder, soft tissue
    postprocedural M96.89
    psychogenic F45.8
  myoneural G70.9
    due to lead G70.1
    specified NEC G70.89
    toxic G70.1
  myotonic NEC G71.19
  nail, in diseases classified elsewhere L62
  neck region NEC —see Dorsopathy, specified
      NEC
  nerve G58.9
    abducent NEC —see Strabismus, paralytic,
        sixth nerve
    accessory G52.8
    acoustic —see subcategory H93.3
    auditory —see subcategory H93.3
    auriculotemporal G50.8
    axillary G54.0
    cerebral —see Disorder, nerve, cranial
    cranial G52.9
      eighth —see subcategory H93.3
      eleventh G52.8
      fifth G50.9
      first G52.0
      fourth NEC —see Strabismus, paralytic,
          fourth nerve
      multiple G52.7
      ninth G52.1
      second NEC —see Disorder, nerve, optic
      seventh NEC G51.8
      sixth NEC —see Strabismus, paralytic,
          sixth nerve
      specified NEC G52.8
      tenth G52.2
      third NEC —see Strabismus, paralytic,
          third nerve
      twelfth G52.3
    entrapment —see Neuropathy, entrapment
    facial G51.9
      specified NEC G51.8
    femoral —see Lesion, nerve, femoral
    glossopharyngeal NEC G52.1
    hypoglossal G52.3
    intercostal G58.0
    lateral
      cutaneous of thigh —see
          Mononeuropathy, lower limb,
          meralgia paresthetica
      popliteal —see Lesion, nerve, popliteal
    lower limb —see Mononeuropathy, lower
        limb

Disorder (Continued)
  nerve (Continued)
    medial popliteal —see Lesion, nerve,
        popliteal, medial
    median NEC —see Lesion, nerve, median
    multiple G58.7
    oculomotor NEC —see Strabismus,
        paralytic, third nerve
    olfactory G52.0
    optic NEC H47.09-
      hemorrhage into sheath —see
          Hemorrhage, optic nerve
      ischemic H47.01-
    peroneal —see Lesion, nerve, popliteal
    phrenic G58.8
    plantar —see Lesion, nerve, plantar
    pneumogastric G52.2
    posterior tibial —see Syndrome, tarsal
        tunnel
    radial —see Lesion, nerve, radial
    recurrent laryngeal G52.2
    root G54.9
      cervical G54.2
      lumbosacral G54.1
      specified NEC G54.8
      thoracic G54.3
    sciatic NEC —see Lesion, nerve, sciatic
    specified NEC G58.8
      lower limb —see Mononeuropathy,
          lower limb, specified NEC
      upper limb —see Mononeuropathy,
          upper limb, specified NEC
    sympathetic G90.9
    tibial —see Lesion, nerve, popliteal,
        medial
    trigeminal G50.9
      specified NEC G50.8
    trochlear NEC —see Strabismus, paralytic,
        fourth nerve
    ulnar —see Lesion, nerve, ulnar
    upper limb —see Mononeuropathy, upper
        limb
    vagus G52.2
  nervous system G98.8
    autonomic (peripheral) G90.9
      specified NEC G90.8
    central G96.9
      specified NEC G96.8
    parasympathetic G90.9
    specified NEC G98.8
    sympathetic G90.9
    vegetative G90.9
  neurohypophysis NEC E23.3
  neurological NEC R29.818
  neuromuscular G70.9
    hereditary NEC G71.9
    specified NEC G70.89
    toxic G70.1
  neurotic F48.9
    specified NEC F48.8
  neutrophil, polymorphonuclear D71
  nicotine use —see Dependence, drug,
      nicotine
  nightmare F51.5
  nose J34.9
    specified NEC J34.89
  obsessive-compulsive F42
  odontogenesis NOS K00.9
  oesophagus —see Disorder, esophagus
  opioid use
    with
      opioid-induced psychotic disorder
          F11.959 ◀
        with ◀
          delusions F11.950 ◀
          hallucinations F11.951 ◀
      due to drug abuse —see Abuse, drug,
          opioid
      due to drug dependence —see Dependence,
          drug, opioid
  oppositional defiant F91.3

Disorder (Continued)
optic
  chiasm H47.49
    due to
      inflammatory disorder H47.41
      neoplasm H47.42
      vascular disorder H47.43
  disc H47.39-
    coloboma —see Coloboma, optic disc
    drusen —see Drusen, optic disc
    pseudopapilledema —see
      Pseudopapilledema
  radiations —see Disorder, visual, pathway
  tracts —see Disorder, visual, pathway
orbit H05.9
  cyst —see Cyst, orbit
  deformity —see Deformity, orbit
  edema —see Edema, orbit
  enophthalmos —see Enophthalmos
  exophthalmos —see Exophthalmos
  hemorrhage —see Hemorrhage, orbit
  inflammation —see Inflammation, orbit
  myopathy —see Myopathy, extraocular
    muscles
  retained foreign body —see Foreign body,
    orbit, old
  specified type NEC H05.89
organic
  anxiety F06.4
  catatonic F06.1
  delusional F06.2
  dissociative F06.8
  emotionally labile (asthenic) F06.8
  mood (affective) F06.30
  schizophrenia-like F06.2
orgasmic (female) F52.31
  male F52.32
ornithine metabolism E72.4
overanxious F41.1
  of childhood F93.8
pain
  with related psychological factors F45.42
  exclusively related to psychological factors
    F45.41
pancreatic internal secretion E16.9
  specified NEC E16.8
panic F41.0
  with agoraphobia F40.01
papulosquamous L44.9
  in diseases classified elsewhere L45
  specified NEC L44.8
paranoid F22
  induced F24
  shared F24
parathyroid (gland) E21.5
  specified NEC E21.4
parietoalveolar NEC J84.09
paroxysmal, mixed R56.9
patella M22.9-
  chondromalacia —see Chondromalacia,
    patella
  derangement NEC M22.3X-
  recurrent
    dislocation —see Dislocation, patella,
      recurrent
    subluxation —see Dislocation, patella,
      recurrent, incomplete
  specified NEC M22.8X-
patellofemoral M22.2X-
pentose phosphate pathway with anemia
  D55.1
perception, due to hallucinogens F16.983
  in
    abuse F16.183
    dependence F16.283
peripheral nervous system NEC G64
peroxisomal E71.50
  biogenesis
    neonatal adrenoleukodystrophy E71.511
    specified disorder NEC E71.518
    Zellweger syndrome E71.510

Disorder (Continued)
peroxisomal (Continued)
  rhizomelic chondrodysplasia punctata
    E71.540
    specified form NEC E71.548
      group 1 E71.518
      group 2 E71.53
      group 3 E71.542
  X-linked adrenoleukodystrophy
    E71.529
    adolescent E71.521
    adrenomyeloneuropathy E71.522
    childhood E71.520
    specified form NEC E71.528
  Zellweger-like syndrome E71.541
persistent
  (somatoform) pain F45.41
  affective (mood) F34.9
personality (see also Personality) F60.9
  affective F34.0
  aggressive F60.3
  amoral F60.2
  anankastic F60.5
  antisocial F60.2
  anxious F60.6
  asocial F60.2
  asthenic F60.7
  avoidant F60.6
  borderline F60.3
  change (secondary) due to general medical
    condition F07.0
  compulsive F60.5
  cyclothymic F34.0
  dependent (passive) F60.7
  depressive F34.1
  dissocial F60.2
  emotional instability F60.3
  expansive paranoid F60.0
  explosive F60.3
  following organic brain damage
    F07.9
  histrionic F60.4
  hyperthymic F34.0
  hypothymic F34.1
  hysterical F60.4
  immature F60.89
  inadequate F60.7
  labile F60.3
  mixed (nonspecific) F60.89
  moral deficiency F60.2
  narcissistic F60.81
  negativistic F60.89
  obsessional F60.5
  obsessive (-compulsive) F60.5
  organic F07.9
  overconscientious F60.5
  paranoid F60.0
  passive (-dependent) F60.7
  passive-aggressive F60.89
  pathological NEC F60.9
  pseudosocial F60.2
  psychopathic F60.2
  schizoid F60.1
  schizotypal F21
  self-defeating F60.7
  specified NEC F60.89
  type A F60.5
  unstable (emotional) F60.3
pervasive, developmental F84.9
phobic anxiety, childhood F40.8
phosphate-losing tubular N25.0
pigmentation L81.9
  choroid, congenital Q14.3
  diminished melanin formation L81.6
  iron L81.8
  specified NEC L81.8
pinna (noninfective) H61.10-
  deformity, acquired H61.11-
  hematoma H61.12-
  perichondritis —see Perichondritis, ear
  specified type NEC H61.19-

Disorder (Continued)
pituitary gland E23.7
  iatrogenic (postprocedural) E89.3
  specified NEC E23.6
platelets D69.1
plexus G54.9
  specified NEC G54.8
polymorphonuclear neutrophils D71
porphyrin metabolism —see Porphyria
postconcussional F07.81
posthallucinogen perception F16.983
  in
    abuse F16.183
    dependence F16.283
postmenopausal N95.9
  specified NEC N95.8
postprocedural (postoperative) —see
  Complications, postprocedural
post-transplant lymphoproliferative D47.z1
post-traumatic stress (PTSD) F43.10
  acute F43.11
  chronic F43.12
premenstrual dysphoric (PMDD) N94.3
prepuce N47.8
propionic acidemia E71.121
prostate N42.9
  specified NEC N42.89
psychogenic NOS (see also condition) F45.9
  anxiety F41.8
  appetite F50.9
  asthenic F48.8
  cardiovascular (system) F45.8
  compulsive F42
  cutaneous F54
  depressive F32.9
  digestive (system) F45.8
  dysmenorrheic F45.8
  dyspneic F45.8
  endocrine (system) F54
  eye NEC F45.8
  feeding —see Disorder, eating
  functional NEC F45.8
  gastric F45.8
  gastrointestinal (system) F45.8
  genitourinary (system) F45.8
  heart (function) (rhythm) F45.8
  hyperventilatory F45.8
  hypochondriacal —see Disorder,
    hypochondriacal
  intestinal F45.8
  joint F45.8
  learning F81.9
  limb F45.8
  lymphatic (system) F45.8
  menstrual F45.8
  micturition F45.8
  monoplegic NEC F44.4
  motor F44.4
  muscle F45.8
  musculoskeletal F45.8
  neurocirculatory F45.8
  obsessive F42
  occupational F48.8
  organ or part of body NEC F45.8
  paralytic NEC F44.4
  phobic F40.9
  physical NEC F45.8
  rectal F45.8
  respiratory (system) F45.8
  rheumatic F45.8
  sexual (function) F52.9
  skin (allergic) (eczematous) F54
  sleep F51.9
  specified part of body NEC F45.8
  stomach F45.8
psychological F99
  associated with
    disease classified elsewhere F54
    sexual
      development F66
      relationship F66
      uncertainty about gender identity F66

Disorder *(Continued)*
  psychomotor NEC F44.4
    hysterical F44.4
  psychoneurotic —*see also* Neurosis
    mixed NEC F48.8
  psychophysiologic —*see* Disorder,
      somatoform
  psychosexual F65.9
    development F66
    identity of childhood F64.2
  psychosomatic NOS —*see* Disorder,
      somatoform
    multiple F45.0
    undifferentiated F45.1
  psychotic —*see* Psychosis
    transient (acute) F23
  puberty E30.9
    specified NEC E30.8
  pulmonary (valve) —*see* Endocarditis,
      pulmonary
  purine metabolism E79.9
  pyrimidine metabolism E79.9
  pyruvate metabolism E74.4
  reactive attachment (childhood) F94.1
  reading R48.0
    developmental (specific) F81.0
  receptive language F80.2
  receptor, hormonal, peripheral *(see also*
      Syndrome, androgen insensitivity)
      E34.50
  recurrent brief depressive F33.8
  reflex R29.2
  refraction H52.7
    aniseikonia H52.32
    anisometropia H52.31
    astigmatism —*see* Astigmatism
    hypermetropia —*see* Hypermetropia
    myopia —*see* Myopia
    presbyopia H52.4
    specified NEC H52.6
  relationship F68.8
    due to sexual orientation F66
  REM sleep behavior G47.52
  renal function, impaired (tubular) N25.9
  resonance R49.9
    specified NEC R49.8
  respiratory function, impaired —*see also*
      Failure, respiration
    postprocedural —*see* Complication,
        postoperative, respiratory system
    psychogenic F45.8
  retina H35.9
    angioid streaks H35.33
    changes in vascular appearance H35.01-
    degeneration —*see* Degeneration, retina
    dystrophy (hereditary) —*see* Dystrophy,
        retina
    edema H35.81
    hemorrhage —*see* Hemorrhage, retina
    ischemia H35.82
    macular degeneration —*see* Degeneration,
        macula
    microaneurysms H35.04-
    microvascular abnormality NEC
        H35.09
    neovascularization —*see*
        Neovascularization, retina
    retinopathy —*see* Retinopathy
    separation of layers H35.70
      central serous chorioretinopathy
          H35.71-
      pigment epithelium detachment (serous)
          H35.72-
      hemorrhagic H35.73-
    specified type NEC H35.89
    telangiectasis —*see* Telangiectasis, retina
    vasculitis —*see* Vasculitis, retina
  retroperitoneal K68.9
  right hemisphere organic affective F07.89
  rumination (infant or child) F98.21
  sacrum, sacrococcygeal NEC M53.3

Disorder *(Continued)*
  schizoaffective F25.9
    bipolar type F25.0
    depressive type F25.1
    manic type F25.0
    mixed type F25.0
    specified NEC F25.8
  schizoid of childhood F84.5
  schizophreniform F20.81
    brief F23
  schizotypal (personality) F21
  secretion, thyrocalcitonin E07.0
  seizure *(see also* Epilepsy) G40.909
    intractable G40.919
      with status epilepticus G40.911
  semantic pragmatic F80.89
    with autism F84.0
  sense of smell R43.1
    psychogenic F45.8
  separation anxiety, of childhood F93.0
  sexual
    arousal, female F52.22
    aversion F52.1
    function, psychogenic F52.9
    maturation F66
    nonorganic F52.9
    preference *(see also* Deviation, sexual) F65.9
      fetishistic transvestism F65.1
    relationship F66
  shyness, of childhood and adolescence
      F40.10
  sibling rivalry F93.8
  sickle-cell (sickling) (homozygous) —*see*
      Disease, sickle-cell
    heterozygous D57.3
    specified type NEC D57.8-
    trait D57.3
  sinus (nasal) J34.9
    specified NEC J34.89
  skin L98.9
    atrophic L90.9
      specified NEC L90.8
    granulomatous L92.9
      specified NEC L92.8
    hypertrophic L91.9
      specified NEC L91.8
    infiltrative NEC L98.6
    newborn P83.9
      specified NEC P83.8
    psychogenic (allergic) (eczematous)
        F54
  sleep G47.9
    breathing-related —*see* Apnea, sleep
    circadian rhythm G47.20
      advance sleep phase type G47.22
      delayed sleep phase type G47.21
      due to
        alcohol
          abuse F10.182
          dependence F10.282
          use F10.982
        amphetamines
          abuse F15.182
          dependence F15.282
          use F15.982
        caffeine
          abuse F15.182
          dependence F15.282
          use F15.982
        cocaine
          abuse F14.182
          dependence F14.282
          use F14.982
        drug NEC
          abuse F19.182
          dependence F19.282
          use F19.982
        opioid
          abuse F11.182
          dependence F11.282
          use F11.982

Disorder *(Continued)*
  sleep *(Continued)*
    circadian rhythm *(Continued)*
      due to *(Continued)*
        psychoactive substance NEC
          abuse F19.182
          dependence F19.282
          use F19.982
        sedative, hypnotic, or anxiolytic
          abuse F13.182
          dependence F13.282
          use F13.982
        stimulant NEC
          abuse F15.182
          dependence F15.282
          use F15.982
      free running type G47.24
      in conditions classified elsewhere
          G47.27
      irregular sleep wake type G47.23
      jet lag type G47.25
      shift work type G47.26
      specified NEC G47.29
    due to
      alcohol
        abuse F10.182
        dependence F10.282
        use F10.982
      amphetamine
        abuse F15.182
        dependence F15.282
        use F15.982
      anxiolytic
        abuse F13.182
        dependence F13.282
        use F13.982
      caffeine
        abuse F15.182
        dependence F15.282
        use F15.982
      cocaine
        abuse F14.182
        dependence F14.282
        use F14.982
      drug NEC
        abuse F19.182
        dependence F19.282
        use F19.982
      hypnotic
        abuse F13.182
        dependence F13.282
        use F13.982
      opioid
        abuse F11.182
        dependence F11.282
        use F11.982
      psychoactive substance NEC
        abuse F19.182
        dependence F19.282
        use F19.982
      sedative
        abuse F13.182
        dependence F13.282
        use F13.982
      stimulant NEC
        abuse F15.182
        dependence F15.282
        use F15.982
    emotional F51.9
    excessive somnolence —*see* Hypersomnia
    hypersomnia type —*see* Hypersomnia
    initiating or maintaining —*see* Insomnia
    nightmares F51.5
    nonorganic F51.9
      specified NEC F51.8
    parasomnia type G47.50
    specified NEC G47.8
    terrors F51.4
    walking F51.3
  sleep-wake pattern or schedule —*see*
      Disorder, sleep, circadian rhythm

Disorder (Continued)

social

anxiety of childhood F40.10

functioning in childhood F94.9

specified NEC F94.8

soft tissue M79.9

ankle M79.9

due to use, overuse and pressure M70.90

ankle M70.97-

bursitis —see Bursitis

foot M70.97-

forearm M70.93-

hand M70.94-

lower leg M70.96-

multiple sites M70.99

pelvic region M70.95-

shoulder region M70.91-

specified site NEC M70.98

specified type NEC M70.80

ankle M70.87-

foot M70.87-

forearm M70.83-

hand M70.84-

lower leg M70.86-

multiple sites M70.89

pelvic region M70.85-

shoulder region M70.81-

specified site NEC M70.88

thigh M70.85-

upper arm M70.82-

thigh M70.95-

upper arm M70.92-

foot M79.9

forearm M79.9

hand M79.9

lower leg M79.9

multiple sites M79.9

occupational —see Disorder, soft tissue, due to use, overuse and pressure

pelvic region M79.9

shoulder region M79.9

specified type NEC M79.89

thigh M79.9

upper arm M79.9

somatization F45.0

somatoform F45.9

pain (persistent) F45.41

somatization (multiple) (long-lasting) F45.0

specified NEC F45.8

undifferentiated F45.1

somnolence, excessive —see Hypersomnia

specific

arithmetical F81.2

developmental, of motor F82

reading F81.0

speech and language F80.9

spelling F81.81

written expression F81.81

speech R47.9

articulation (functional) (specific) F80.0

developmental F80.9

specified NEC R47.89

spelling (specific) F81.81

spine —see also Dorsopathy

ligamentous or muscular attachments, peripheral —see Enthesopathy, spinal

specified NEC —see Dorsopathy, specified NEC

stereotyped, habit or movement F98.4

stomach (functional) —see Disorder, gastric

stress F43.9

post-traumatic F43.10

acute F43.11

chronic F43.12

sulfur-bearing amino-acid metabolism E72.10

sweat gland (eccrine) L74.9

apocrine L75.9

specified NEC L75.8

specified NEC L74.8

Disorder (Continued)

synovium M67.90

acromioclavicular M67.91-

ankle M67.97-

elbow M67.92-

foot M67.97-

forearm M67.93-

hand M67.94-

hip M67.95-

knee M67.96-

multiple sites M67.99

rupture —see Rupture, synovium

shoulder M67.91-

specified type NEC M67.80

acromioclavicular M67.81-

ankle M67.87-

elbow M67.82-

foot M67.87-

hand M67.84-

hip M67.85-

knee M67.86-

multiple sites M67.89

wrist M67.83-

synovitis —see Synovitis

upper arm M67.92-

wrist M67.93-

temperature regulation, newborn P81.9

specified NEC P81.8

temporomandibular joint —see Anomaly, dentofacial, temporomandibular joint

tendon M67.90

acromioclavicular M67.91-

ankle M67.97-

contracture —see Contracture, tendon

elbow M67.92-

foot M67.97-

forearm M67.93-

hand M67.94-

hip M67.95-

knee M67.96-

multiple sites M67.99

rupture —see Rupture, tendon

shoulder M67.91-

specified type NEC M67.80

acromioclavicular M67.81-

ankle M67.87-

elbow M67.82-

foot M67.87-

hand M67.84-

hip M67.85-

knee M67.86-

multiple sites M67.89

trunk M67.88

wrist M67.83-

synovitis —see Synovitis

tendinitis —see Tendinitis

tenosynovitis —see Tenosynovitis

trunk M67.98

upper arm M67.92-

wrist M67.93-

thoracic root (nerve) NEC G54.3

thyrocalcitonin hypersecretion E07.0

thyroid (gland) E07.9

function NEC, neonatal, transitory P72.2

iodine-deficiency related E01.8

specified NEC E07.89

tic —see Tic

tooth K08.9

development K00.9

specified NEC K00.8

eruption K00.6

Tourette's F95.2

trance and possession F44.89

tricuspid (valve) —see Endocarditis, tricuspid

tryptophan metabolism E70.5

tubular, phosphate-losing N25.0

tubulo-interstitial (in)

brucellosis A23.9 [N16]

cystinosis E72.04

diphtheria A36.84

Disorder (Continued)

tubulo-interstitial (Continued)

glycogen storage disease E74.00 [N16]

leukemia NEC C95.9- [N16]

lymphoma NEC C85.9- [N16]

mixed cryoglobulinemia D89.1 [N16]

multiple myeloma C90.0- [N16]

Salmonella infection A02.25

sarcoidosis D86.84

sepsis A41.9 [N16]

streptococcal A40.9 [N16]

systemic lupus erythematosus M32.15

toxoplasmosis B58.83

transplant rejection T86.91 [N16]

Wilson's disease E83.01 [N16]

tubulo-renal function, impaired N25.9

specified NEC N25.89

tympanic membrane H73.9-

atrophy —see Atrophy, tympanic membrane

infection —see Myringitis

perforation —see Perforation, tympanum

specified NEC H73.89-

unsocialized aggressive F91.1

urea cycle metabolism E72.20

argininemia E72.21

arginosuccinic aciduria E72.22

citrullinemia E72.23

ornithine transcarbamylase deficiency E72.4

other specified E72.29

ureter (in) N28.9

schistosomiasis B65.0 [N29]

tuberculosis A18.11

urethra N36.9

specified NEC N36.8

urinary system N39.9

specified NEC N39.8

valve, heart

aortic —see Endocarditis, aortic

mitral —see Endocarditis, mitral

pulmonary —see Endocarditis, pulmonary

rheumatic

aortic —see Endocarditis, aortic, rheumatic

mitral —see Endocarditis, mitral

pulmonary —see Endocarditis, pulmonary, rheumatic

tricuspid —see Endocarditis, tricuspid

tricuspid —see Endocarditis, tricuspid

vestibular function H81.9-

specified NEC —see subcategory H81.8

in diseases classified elsewhere H82.-

vertigo —see Vertigo

vision, binocular H53.30

abnormal retinal correspondence H53.31

diplopia H53.2

fusion with defective stereopsis H53.32

simultaneous perception H53.33

suppression H53.34

visual

cortex

blindness H47.619

left brain H47.612

right brain H47.611

due to

inflammatory disorder H47.629

left brain H47.622

right brain H47.621

neoplasm H47.639

left brain H47.632

right brain H47.631

vascular disorder H47.649

left brain H47.642

right brain H47.641

pathway H47.9

due to

inflammatory disorder H47.51-

neoplasm H47.52-

vascular disorder H47.53-

optic chiasm —see Disorder, optic, chiasm

Disorder (Continued)
  vitreous body H43.9
    crystalline deposits —see Deposit,
      crystalline
    degeneration —see Degeneration, vitreous
    hemorrhage —see Hemorrhage, vitreous
    opacities —see Opacity, vitreous
    prolapse —see Prolapse, vitreous
    specified type NEC H43.89
  voice R49.9
    specified type NEC R49.8
  volatile solvent use
    due to drug abuse —see Abuse, drug,
      inhalant
    due to drug dependence —see Dependence,
      drug, inhalant
  white blood cells D72.9
    specified NEC D72.89
  withdrawing, child or adolescent F40.10
Disorientation R41.0
Displacement, displaced
  acquired traumatic of bone, cartilage, joint,
    tendon NEC —see Dislocation
  adrenal gland (congenital) Q89.1
  appendix, retrocecal (congenital) Q43.8
  auricle (congenital) Q17.4
  bladder (acquired) N32.89
    congenital Q64.19
  brachial plexus (congenital) Q07.8
  brain stem, caudal (congenital) Q04.8
  canaliculus (lacrimalis), congenital Q10.6
  cardia through esophageal hiatus (congenital)
    Q40.1
  cerebellum, caudal (congenital) Q04.8
  cervix —see Malposition, uterus
  colon (congenital) Q43.3
  device, implant or graft (see also
    Complications, by site and type,
    mechanical) T85.628
    arterial graft NEC —see Complication,
      cardiovascular device, mechanical,
      vascular
    breast (implant) T85.42
    catheter NEC T85.628
      dialysis (renal) T82.42
        intraperitoneal T85.621
      infusion NEC T82.524
        spinal (epidural) (subdural)
          T85.620
      urinary (indwelling) T83.028
        cystostomy T83.020
    electronic (electrode) (pulse generator)
      (stimulator) —see Complication,
      electronic stimulator
    fixation, internal (orthopedic) NEC —see
      Complication, fixation device,
      mechanical
    gastrointestinal —see Complications,
      prosthetic device, mechanical,
      gastrointestinal device
    genital NEC T83.428
      intrauterine contraceptive device
        T83.32
      penile prosthesis T83.420
    heart NEC —see Complication,
      cardiovascular device, mechanical
    joint prosthesis —see Complications, joint
      prosthesis, mechanical
    ocular —see Complications, prosthetic
      device, mechanical, ocular device
    orthopedic NEC —see Complication,
      orthopedic, device or graft,
      mechanical
    specified NEC T85.628
    urinary NEC —see also Complication,
      genitourinary, device, urinary,
      mechanical
      graft T83.22
    vascular NEC —see Complication,
      cardiovascular device, mechanical
    ventricular intracranial shunt T85.02

Displacement, displaced (Continued)
  electronic stimulator
    bone T84.320
    cardiac —see Complications, cardiac
      device, electronic
    nervous system —see Complication,
      prosthetic device, mechanical,
      electronic nervous system stimulator
    urinary —see Complications, electronic
      stimulator, urinary
  esophageal mucosa into cardia of stomach,
    congenital Q39.8
  esophagus (acquired) K22.8
    congenital Q39.8
  eyeball (acquired) (lateral) (old) —see
    Displacement, globe
    congenital Q15.8
    current —see Avulsion, eye
  fallopian tube (acquired) N83.4
    congenital Q50.6
    opening (congenital) Q50.6
  gallbladder (congenital) Q44.1
  gastric mucosa (congenital) Q40.2
  globe (acquired) (old) (lateral) H05.21-
    current —see Avulsion, eye
  heart (congenital) Q24.8
    acquired I51.89
  hymen (upward) (congenital) Q52.4
  intervertebral disc NEC
    with myelopathy —see Disorder, disc, with,
      myelopathy
    cervical, cervicothoracic (with) M50.20
      myelopathy —see Disorder, disc,
        cervical, with myelopathy
      neuritis, radiculitis or radiculopathy —
        see Disorder, disc, cervical, with
        neuritis
    due to trauma —see Dislocation, vertebra
    lumbar region M51.26
      with
        myelopathy M51.06
        neuritis, radiculitis, radiculopathy or
          sciatica M51.16
    lumbosacral region M51.27
      with
        myelopathy M51.07
        neuritis, radiculitis, radiculopathy or
          sciatica M51.17
    sacrococcygeal region M53.3
    thoracic region M51.24
      with
        myelopathy M51.04
        neuritis, radiculitis, radiculopathy
          M51.14
    thoracolumbar region M51.25
      with
        myelopathy M51.05
        neuritis, radiculitis, radiculopathy
          M51.15
  intrauterine device T83.32
  kidney (acquired) N28.83
    congenital Q63.2
  lachrymal, lacrimal apparatus or duct
    (congenital) Q10.6
  lens, congenital Q12.1
  macula (congenital) Q14.1
  Meckel's diverticulum Q43.0
    malignant —see Table of Neoplasms, small
      intestine, malignant
  nail (congenital) Q84.6
    acquired L60.8
  oesophagus (acquired) —see Displacement,
    esophagus
  opening of Wharton's duct in mouth Q38.4
  organ or site, congenital NEC —see
    Malposition, congenital
  ovary (acquired) N83.4
    congenital Q50.39
    free in peritoneal cavity (congenital)
      Q50.39
    into hernial sac N83.4

Displacement, displaced (Continued)
  oviduct (acquired) N83.4
    congenital Q50.6
  parathyroid (gland) E21.4
  parotid gland (congenital) Q38.4
  punctum lacrimale (congenital) Q10.6
  sacro-iliac (joint) (congenital) Q74.2
    current injury S33.2
    old —see subcategory M53.2
  salivary gland (any) (congenital) Q38.4
  spleen (congenital) Q89.09
  stomach, congenital Q40.2
  sublingual duct Q38.4
  tongue (downward) (congenital) Q38.3
  tooth, teeth, fully erupted M26.30
    horizontal M26.33
    vertical M26.34
  trachea (congenital) Q32.1
  ureter or ureteric opening or orifice
    (congenital) Q62.62
  uterine opening of oviducts or fallopian tubes
    Q50.6
  uterus, uterine —see Malposition, uterus
  ventricular septum Q21.0
    with rudimentary ventricle Q20.4
Disproportion
  between native and reconstructed breast
    N65.1
  fiber-type G71.2
Disruptio uteri —see Rupture, uterus
Disruption (of)
  ciliary body NEC H21.89
  closure of
    cornea T81.31
    craniotomy T81.32
    fascia (muscular) (superficial) T81.32
    internal organ or tissue T81.32
    laceration (external) (internal) T81.33
    ligament T81.32
    mucosa T81.31
    muscle or muscle flap T81.32
    ribs or rib cage T81.32
    skin and subcutaneous tissue (full-
      thickness) (superficial) T81.31
    skull T81.32
    sternum (sternotomy) T81.32
    tendon T81.32
    traumatic laceration (external) (internal)
      T81.33
  family Z63.8
    due to
      absence of family member due to
        military deployment Z63.31
      absence of family member NEC
        Z63.32
      alcoholism and drug addiction in
        family Z63.72
      bereavement Z63.4
      death (assumed) or disappearance of
        family member Z63.4
      divorce or separation Z63.5
      drug addiction in family Z63.72
      return of family member from military
        deployment (current or past
        conflict) Z63.71
      stressful life events NEC Z63.79
  iris NEC H21.89
  ligament (s) —see also Sprain
    knee
      current injury —see Dislocation,
        knee
      old (chronic) —see Derangement,
        knee, ligament, instability,
        chronic
      spontaneous NEC —see Derangement,
        knee, disruption ligament
  ossicular chain —see Discontinuity, ossicles,
    ear
  pelvic ring (stable) S32.810
    unstable S32.811
  traumatic injury wound repair T81.33

Disruption (Continued)
wound T81.30
  episiotomy O90.1
  operation T81.31
    cesarean O90.0
    external operation wound (superficial) T81.31
    internal operation wound (deep) T81.32
  perineal (obstetric) O90.1
  traumatic injury repair T81.33

Dissatisfaction with
employment Z56.9
school environment Z55.4

Dissecting —see condition

Dissection
aorta I71.00
  abdominal I71.02
  thoracic I71.01
  thoracoabdominal I71.03
artery
  carotid I77.71
  cerebral (nonruptured) I67.0
    ruptured —see Hemorrhage, intracranial, subarachnoid
  coronary I25.42
  iliac I77.72
  renal I77.73
  specified NEC I77.79
  vertebral I77.74
  traumatic —see Wound, open, by site
vascular I99.8
wound —see Wound, open

Disseminated —see condition

Dissociation
auriculoventricular or atrioventricular (AV) (any degree) (isorhythmic) I45.89
  with heart block I44.2
interference I45.89

Dissociative reaction, state F44.9

Dissolution, vertebra —see Osteoporosis

Distension, distention
abdomen R14.0
bladder N32.89
cecum K63.89
colon K63.89
gallbladder K82.8
intestine K63.89
kidney N28.89
liver K76.89
seminal vesicle N50.8
stomach K31.89
  acute K31.0
  psychogenic F45.8
ureter —see Dilatation, ureter
uterus N85.8

Distoma hepaticum infestation B66.3

Distomiasis B66.9
bile passages B66.3
hemic B65.9
hepatic B66.3
  due to Clonorchis sinensis B66.1
intestinal B66.5
liver B66.3
  due to Clonorchis sinensis B66.1
lung B66.4
pulmonary B66.4

Distomolar (fourth molar) K00.1

Disto-occlusion (Division I) (Division II) M26.212

Distortion (s) (congenital)
adrenal (gland) Q89.1
arm NEC Q68.8
bile duct or passage Q44.5
bladder Q64.79
brain Q04.9
cervix (uteri) Q51.9
chest (wall) Q67.8
  bones Q76.8
clavicle Q74.0
clitoris Q52.6

Distortion (Continued)
coccyx Q76.49
common duct Q44.5
coronary Q24.5
cystic duct Q44.5
ear (auricle) (external) Q17.3
  inner Q16.5
  middle Q16.4
    ossicles Q16.3
endocrine NEC Q89.2
eustachian tube Q17.8
eye (adnexa) Q15.8
face bone (s) NEC Q75.8
fallopian tube Q50.6
femur NEC Q68.8
fibula NEC Q68.8
finger (s) Q68.1
foot Q66.9
genitalia, genital organ (s)
  female Q52.8
    external Q52.79
    internal NEC Q52.8
gyri Q04.8
hand bone (s) Q68.1
heart (auricle) (ventricle) Q24.8
  valve (cusp) Q24.8
hepatic duct Q44.5
humerus NEC Q68.8
hymen Q52.4
intrafamilial communications Z63.8
jaw NEC M26.89
labium (majus) (minus) Q52.79
leg NEC Q68.8
lens Q12.8
liver Q44.7
lumbar spine Q76.49
  with disproportion O33.8
    causing obstructed labor O65.0
lumbosacral (joint) (region) Q76.49
  kyphosis —see Kyphosis, congenital
  lordosis —see Lordosis, congenital
nerve Q07.8
nose Q30.8
organ
  of Corti Q16.5
  or site not listed —see Anomaly, by site
    ossicles, ear Q16.3
oviduct Q50.6
pancreas Q45.3
parathyroid (gland) Q89.2
pituitary (gland) Q89.2
radius NEC Q68.8
sacroiliac joint Q74.2
sacrum Q76.49
scapula Q74.0
shoulder girdle Q74.0
skull bone (s) NEC Q75.8
  with
    anencephalus Q00.0
    encephalocele —see Encephalocele
    hydrocephalus Q03.9
      with spina bifida —see Spina bifida, with hydrocephalus
    microcephaly Q02
spinal cord Q06.8
spine Q76.49
  kyphosis —see Kyphosis, congenital
  lordosis —see Lordosis, congenital
spleen Q89.09
sternum NEC Q76.7
thorax (wall) Q67.8
  bony Q76.8
thymus (gland) Q89.2
thyroid (gland) Q89.2
tibia NEC Q68.8
toe (s) Q66.9
tongue Q38.3
trachea (cartilage) Q32.1
ulna NEC Q68.8
ureter Q62.8

Distortion (Continued)
urethra Q64.79
  causing obstruction Q64.39
uterus Q51.9
vagina Q52.4
vertebra Q76.49
  kyphosis —see Kyphosis, congenital
  lordosis —see Lordosis, congenital
visual —see also Disturbance, vision
  shape and size H53.15
vulva Q52.79
wrist (bones) (joint) Q68.8

Distress
abdomen —see Pain, abdominal
acute respiratory (adult) (child) J80
epigastric R10.13
fetal P84
  complicating pregnancy —see Stress, fetal
gastrointestinal (functional) K30
  psychogenic F45.8
intestinal (functional) NOS K59.9
  psychogenic F45.8
maternal, during labor and delivery O75.0
respiratory R06.00
  adult J80
  child J80
  newborn P22.9
    specified NEC P22.8
  orthopnea R06.01
  psychogenic F45.8
  shortness of breath R06.02
  specified type NEC R06.09

Distribution vessel, atypical Q27.9
coronary artery Q24.5
precerebral Q28.1

Districhiasis L68.8

Disturbance (s) —see also Disease
absorption K90.9
  calcium E58
  carbohydrate K90.4
  fat K90.4
    pancreatic K90.3
  protein K90.4
  starch K90.4
  vitamin —see Deficiency, vitamin
acid-base equilibrium E87.8
  mixed E87.4
activity and attention (with hyperkinesis) — see Disorder, attention-deficit hyperactivity
amino acid transport E72.00
assimilation, food K90.9
auditory nerve, except deafness —see subcategory H93.3
behavior —see Disorder, conduct
blood clotting (mechanism) (see also Defect, coagulation) D68.9
cerebral
  nerve —see Disorder, nerve, cranial
  status, newborn P91.9
    specified NEC P91.8
circulatory I99.9
conduct (see also Disorder, conduct) F91.9
  adjustment reaction —see Disorder, adjustment
  compulsive F63.9
  disruptive F91.9
  hyperkinetic —see Disorder, attention-deficit hyperactivity
  socialized F91.2
  specified NEC F91.8
  unsocialized F91.1
coordination R27.8
cranial nerve —see Disorder, nerve, cranial
deep sensibility —see Disturbance, sensation
digestive K30
  psychogenic F45.8

◀ New   ◀▥ Revised   ~~deleted~~ Deleted

Disturbance (Continued)
  electrolyte —see also Imbalance, electrolyte
    newborn, transitory P74.4
      hyperammonemia P74.6
      potassium balance P74.3
      sodium balance P74.2
      specified type NEC P74.4
  emotions specific to childhood and
      adolescence F93.9
    with
      anxiety and fearfulness NEC F93.8
      elective mutism F94.0
      oppositional disorder F91.3
      sensitivity (withdrawal) F40.10
      shyness F40.10
      social withdrawal F40.10
    involving relationship problems F93.8
    mixed F93.8
    specified NEC F93.8
  endocrine (gland) E34.9
    neonatal, transitory P72.9
      specified NEC P72.8
  equilibrium R42
  fructose metabolism E74.10
  gait —see Gait
    hysterical F44.4
    psychogenic F44.4
  gastrointestinal (functional) K30
    psychogenic F45.8
  habit, child F98.9
  hearing, except deafness and tinnitus —see
      Abnormal, auditory perception
  heart, functional (conditions in I44-I50)
    due to presence of (cardiac) prosthesis
        I97.19-
    postoperative I97.89
      cardiac surgery I97.19-
  hormones E34.9
  innervation uterus (parasympathetic)
      (sympathetic) N85.8
  keratinization NEC
    gingiva K05.10
      nonplaque induced K05.11
      plaque induced K05.10
    lip K13.0
    oral (mucosa) (soft tissue) K13.29
    tongue K13.29
  learning (specific) —see Disorder,
      learning
  memory —see Amnesia
    mild, following organic brain damage
        F06.8
  mental F99
    associated with diseases classified
        elsewhere F54
  metabolism E88.9
    with
      abortion —see Abortion, by type with
          other specified complication
      ectopic pregnancy O08.5
      molar pregnancy O08.5
    amino-acid E72.9
      aromatic E70.9
      branched-chain E71.2
      straight-chain E72.8
      sulfur-bearing E72.10
    ammonia E72.20
    arginine E72.21
    arginosuccinic acid E72.22
    carbohydrate E74.9
    cholesterol E78.9
    citrulline E72.23
    cystathionine E72.19
    general E88.9
    glutamine E72.8
    histidine E70.40
    homocystine E72.19
    hydroxylysine E72.3
    in labor or delivery O75.89
    iron E83.10
    lipoid E78.9

Disturbance (Continued)
  metabolism (Continued)
    lysine E72.3
    methionine E72.19
    neonatal, transitory P74.9
      calcium and magnesium P71.9
        specified type NEC P71.8
      carbohydrate metabolism P70.9
        specified type NEC P70.8
      specified NEC P74.8
    ornithine E72.4
    phosphate E83.39
    sodium NEC E87.8
    threonine E72.8
    tryptophan E70.5
    tyrosine E70.20
    urea cycle E72.20
  motor R29.2
  nervous, functional R45.0
  neuromuscular mechanism (eye), due to
      syphilis A52.15
  nutritional E63.9
    nail L60.3
  ocular motion H51.9
    psychogenic F45.8
  oculogyric H51.8
    psychogenic F45.8
  oculomotor H51.9
    psychogenic F45.8
  olfactory nerve R43.1
  optic nerve NEC —see Disorder, nerve,
      optic
  oral epithelium, including tongue NEC
      K13.29
  perceptual due to
    alcohol withdrawal F10.232
    amphetamine intoxication F15.922
      in
        abuse F15.122
        dependence F15.222
    anxiolytic withdrawal F13.232
    cannabis intoxication (acute) F12.922
      in
        abuse F12.122
        dependence F12.222
    cocaine intoxication (acute) F14.922
      in
        abuse F14.122
        dependence F14.222
    hypnotic withdrawal F13.232
    opioid intoxication (acute) F11.922
      in
        abuse F11.122
        dependence F11.222
    phencyclidine intoxication (acute)
        F19.922
      in
        abuse F19.122
        dependence F19.222
    sedative withdrawal F13.232
  personality (pattern) (trait) (see also Disorder,
      personality) F60.9
    following organic brain damage
        F07.9
  polyglandular E31.9
    specified NEC E31.8
  potassium balance, newborn P74.3
  psychogenic F45.9
  psychomotor F44.4
  psychophysical visual H53.16
  pupillary —see Anomaly, pupil, function
  reflex R29.2
  rhythm, heart I49.9
  salivary secretion K11.7
  sensation (cold) (heat) (localization) (tactile
      discrimination) (texture) (vibratory)
      NEC R20.9
    hysterical F44.6
    skin R20.9
      anesthesia R20.0
      hyperesthesia R20.3

Disturbance (Continued)
  sensation (Continued)
    skin (Continued)
      hypoesthesia R20.1
      paresthesia R20.2
      specified type NEC R20.8
    smell R43.9
      and taste (mixed) R43.8
      anosmia R43.0
      parosmia R43.1
      specified NEC R43.8
    taste R43.9
      and smell (mixed) R43.8
      parageusia R43.2
      specified NEC R43.8
  sensory —see Disturbance, sensation
  situational (transient) —see also Disorder,
      adjustment
    acute F43.0
  sleep G47.9
    nonorganic origin F51.9
  smell —see Disturbance, sensation,
      smell
  sociopathic F60.2
  sodium balance, newborn P74.2
  speech R47.9
    developmental F80.9
    specified NEC R47.89
  stomach (functional) K31.9
  sympathetic (nerve) G90.9
  taste —see Disturbance, sensation,
      taste
  temperature
    regulation, newborn P81.9
      specified NEC P81.8
    sense R20.8
      hysterical F44.6
  tooth
    eruption K00.6
    formation K00.4
    structure, hereditary NEC K00.5
  touch —see Disturbance, sensation
  vascular I99.9
    arteriosclerotic —see Arteriosclerosis
  vasomotor I73.9
  vasospastic I73.9
  vision, visual H53.9
    following
      cerebral infarction I69.398
      cerebrovascular disease I69.998
        specified NEC I69.898
      intracerebral hemorrhage I69.198
      nontraumatic intracranial hemorrhage
          NEC I69.298
      specified disease NEC I69.898
      subarachnoid hemorrhage I69.098
    psychophysical H53.16
    specified NEC H53.8
    subjective H53.10
      day blindness H53.11
      discomfort H53.14-
      distortions of shape and size H53.15
      loss
        sudden H53.13-
        transient H53.12-
      specified type NEC H53.19
  voice R49.9
    psychogenic F44.4
    specified NEC R49.8
Diuresis R35.8
Diver's palsy, paralysis or squeeze T70.3
Diverticulitis (acute) K57.92
  bladder —see Cystitis
  ileum —see Diverticulitis, intestine, small
  intestine K57.92
    with
      abscess, perforation or peritonitis
          K57.80
        with bleeding K57.81
      bleeding K57.93
    congenital Q43.8

Diverticulitis *(Continued)*
  intestine *(Continued)*
    large K57.32
      with
        abscess, perforation or peritonitis
          K57.20
          with bleeding K57.21
        bleeding K57.33
        small intestine K57.52
          with
            abscess, perforation or peritonitis
              K57.40
              with bleeding K57.41
              bleeding K57.53
    small K57.12
      with
        abscess, perforation or peritonitis
          K57.00
          with bleeding K57.01
        bleeding K57.13
        large intestine K57.52
          with
            abscess, perforation or peritonitis
              K57.40
              with bleeding K57.41
              bleeding K57.53
Diverticulosis K57.90
  with bleeding K57.91
  large intestine K57.30
    with
      bleeding K57.31
      small intestine K57.50
        with bleeding K57.51
  small intestine K57.10
    with
      bleeding K57.11
      large intestine K57.50
        with bleeding K57.51
Diverticulum, diverticula (multiple) K57.90
  appendix (noninflammatory) K38.2
  bladder (sphincter) N32.3
    congenital Q64.6
  bronchus (congenital) Q32.4
    acquired J98.09
  calyx, calyceal (kidney) N28.89
  cardia (stomach) K31.4
  cecum —*see* Diverticulosis, intestine, large
    congenital Q43.8
  colon —*see* Diverticulosis, intestine, large
    congenital Q43.8
  duodenum —*see* Diverticulosis, intestine,
    small
    congenital Q43.8
  epiphrenic (esophagus) K22.5
  esophagus (congenital) Q39.6
    acquired (epiphrenic) (pulsion) (traction)
      K22.5
  eustachian tube —*see* Disorder, eustachian
    tube, specified NEC
  fallopian tube N83.8
  gastric K31.4
  heart (congenital) Q24.8
  ileum —*see* Diverticulosis, intestine, small
  jejunum —*see* Diverticulosis, intestine, small
  kidney (pelvis) (calyces) N28.89
    with calculus —*see* Calculus, kidney
  Meckel's (displaced) (hypertrophic) Q43.0
    malignant —*see* Table of Neoplasms, small
      intestine, malignant
  midthoracic K22.5
  organ or site, congenital NEC —*see* Distortion
  pericardium (congenital) (cyst) Q24.8
    acquired I31.8
  pharyngoesophageal (congenital) Q39.6
    acquired K22.5
  pharynx (congenital) Q38.7
  rectosigmoid —*see* Diverticulosis, intestine,
    large
    congenital Q43.8
  rectum —*see* Diverticulosis, intestine, large
  Rokitansky's K22.5

Diverticulum, diverticula *(Continued)*
  seminal vesicle N50.8
  sigmoid —*see* Diverticulosis, intestine, large
    congenital Q43.8
  stomach (acquired) K31.4
    congenital Q40.2
  trachea (acquired) J39.8
  ureter (acquired) N28.89
    congenital Q62.8
  ureterovesical orifice N28.89
  urethra (acquired) N36.1
    congenital Q64.79
  ventricle, left (congenital) Q24.8
  vesical N32.3
    congenital Q64.6
  Zenker's (esophagus) K22.5
Division
  cervix uteri (acquired) N88.8
  glans penis Q55.69
  labia minora (congenital) Q52.79
  ligament (partial or complete) (current) —*see*
    also Sprain
    with open wound —*see* Wound, open
  muscle (partial or complete) (current) —*see*
    also Injury, muscle
    with open wound —*see* Wound, open
  nerve (traumatic) —*see* Injury, nerve
  spinal cord —*see* Injury, spinal cord,
    by region
  vein I87.8
Divorce, causing family disruption Z63.5
Dix-Hallpike neurolabyrinthitis —*see*
    Neuronitis, vestibular
Dizziness R42
  hysterical F44.89
  psychogenic F45.8
DMAC (disseminated mycobacterium avium-
    intracellulare complex) A31.2
DNR (do not resuscitate) Z66
Doan-Wiseman syndrome (primary splenic
    neutropenia) —*see* Agranulocytosis
Doehle-Heller aortitis A52.02
Dog bite —*see* Bite
Dohle body panmyelopathic syndrome
    D72.0
Dolichocephaly Q67.2
Dolichocolon Q43.8
Dolichostenomelia —*see* Syndrome, Marfan's
Donohue's syndrome E34.8
Donor (organ or tissue) Z52.9
  blood (whole) Z52.000
    autologous Z52.010
    specified component (lymphocytes)
      (platelets) NEC Z52.008
      autologous Z52.018
      specified donor NEC Z52.098
    specified donor NEC Z52.090
    stem cells Z52.001
      autologous Z52.011
      specified donor NEC Z52.091
  bone Z52.20
    autologous Z52.21
    marrow Z52.3
    specified type NEC Z52.29
  cornea Z52.5
  egg (Oocyte) Z52.819
    age 35 and over Z52.812
      anonymous recipient Z52.812
      designated recipient Z52.813
    under age 35 Z52.810
      anonymous recipient Z52.810
      designated recipient Z52.811
  kidney Z52.4
  liver Z52.6
  lung Z52.89
  lymphocyte —*see* Donor, blood, specified
    components NEC
  Oocyte —*see* Donor, egg
  platelets Z52.008
  potential, examination of Z00.5
  semen Z52.89

Donor *(Continued)*
  skin Z52.10
    autologous Z52.11
    specified type NEC Z52.19
  specified organ or tissue NEC Z52.89
  sperm Z52.89
Donovanosis A58
Dorsalgia M54.9
  psychogenic F45.41
  specified NEC M54.89
Dorsopathy M53.9
  deforming M43.9
    specified NEC —*see* subcategory M43.8
  specified NEC M53.80
    cervical region M53.82
    cervicothoracic region M53.83
    lumbar region M53.86
    lumbosacral region M53.87
    occipito-atlanto-axial region M53.81
    sacrococcygeal region M53.88
    thoracic region M53.84
    thoracolumbar region M53.85
Double
  albumin E88.09
  aortic arch Q25.4
  auditory canal Q17.8
  auricle (heart) Q20.8
  bladder Q64.79
  cervix Q51.820
    with doubling of uterus (and vagina)
      Q51.10
      with obstruction Q51.11
  inlet ventricle Q20.4
  kidney with double pelvis (renal) Q63.0
  meatus urinarius Q64.75
  monster Q89.4
  outlet
    left ventricle Q20.2
    right ventricle Q20.1
  pelvis (renal) with double ureter Q62.5
  tongue Q38.3
  ureter (one or both sides) Q62.5
    with double pelvis (renal) Q62.5
  urethra Q64.74
  urinary meatus Q64.75
  uterus Q51.2
    with
      doubling of cervix (and vagina)
        Q51.10
        with obstruction Q51.11
      in pregnancy or childbirth O34.59-
        causing obstructed labor O65.5
  vagina Q52.10
    with doubling of uterus (and cervix)
      Q51.10
      with obstruction Q51.11
  vision H53.2
  vulva Q52.79
Douglas' pouch, cul-de-sac —*see* condition
Down syndrome Q90.9
  meiotic nondisjunction Q90.0
  mitotic nondisjunction Q90.1
  mosaicism Q90.1
  translocation Q90.2
DPD (dihydropyrimidine dehydrogenase
    deficiency) E88.89
Dracontiasis B72
Dracunculiasis, dracunculosis B72
Dream state, hysterical F44.89
Drepanocytic anemia —*see* Disease, sickle-cell
Dresbach's syndrome (elliptocytosis) D58.1
Dreschlera (hawaiiensis) (infection) B43.8
Dressler's syndrome I24.1
Drift, ulnar —*see* Deformity, limb, specified
    type NEC, forearm
Drinking (alcohol)
  excessive, to excess NEC (without
    dependence) F10.10
    habitual (continual) (without remission)
      F10.20
      with remission F10.21

◀ New   ◀▮▮▮ Revised   ~~deleted~~ Deleted

Drip, postnasal (chronic) R09.82
  due to
    allergic rhinitis —*see* Rhinitis, allergic
    common cold J00
    gastroesophageal reflux —*see* Reflux,
      gastroesophageal
    nasopharyngitis —*see* Nasopharyngitis
    other known condition — code to
      condition
    sinusitis —*see* Sinusitis
Droop
  facial R29.810
    cerebrovascular disease I69.992
      cerebral infarction I69.392
      intracerebral hemorrhage I69.192
      nontraumatic intracranial hemorrhage
        NEC I69.292
      specified disease NEC I69.892
      subarachnoid hemorrhage I69.092
Drop (in)
  attack NEC R55
  finger —*see* Deformity, finger
  foot —*see* Deformity, limb, foot, drop
  hematocrit (precipitous) R71.0
  hemoglobin R71.0
  toe —*see* Deformity, toe, specified NEC
  wrist —*see* Deformity, limb, wrist drop
Dropped heart beats I45.9
Dropsy, dropsical —*see also* Hydrops
  abdomen R18.8
  brain —*see* Hydrocephalus
  cardiac, heart —*see* Failure, heart, congestive
  gangrenous —*see* Gangrene
  heart —*see* Failure, heart, congestive
  kidney —*see* Nephrosis
  lung —*see* Edema, lung
  newborn due to isoimmunization P56.0
  pericardium —*see* Pericarditis
Drowned, drowning (near) T75.1
Drowsiness R40.0
Drug
  abuse counseling and surveillance Z71.51
  addiction —*see* Dependence
  dependence —*see* Dependence
  habit —*see* Dependence
  harmful use —*see* Abuse, drug
  induced fever R50.2
  overdose —*see* Table of dDrugs and
    eChemicals, by drug, poisoning ◀▥
  poisoning —*see* Table of dDrugs and
    eChemicals, by drug, poisoning ◀▥
  resistant organism infection (*see also*
    Resistant, organism, to, drug) Z16.30
  therapy
    long term (current) (prophylactic) —*see*
      Therapy, drug long-term (current)
      (prophylactic)
    short term - omit code
  wrong substance given or taken in error —*see*
    Table of dDrugs and eChemicals, by
    drug, poisoning ◀▥
Drunkenness (without dependence) F10.129
  acute in alcoholism F10.229
  chronic (without remission) F10.20
    with remission F10.21
  pathological (without dependence) F10.129
    with dependence F10.229
  sleep F51.9
Drusen
  macula (degenerative) (retina) —*see*
    Degeneration, macula, drusen
  optic disc H47.32-
Dry, dryness —*see also* condition
  larynx J38.7
  mouth R68.2
    due to dehydration E86.0
  nose J34.89
  socket (teeth) M27.3
  throat J39.2
DSAP L56.5
Duane's syndrome H50.81-

Dubin-Johnson disease or syndrome E80.6
Dubois' disease (thymus gland) A50.59 *[E35]*
Dubowitz' syndrome Q87.1
Duchenne-Aran muscular atrophy G12.21
Duchenne-Griesinger disease G71.0
Duchenne's
  disease or syndrome
    motor neuron disease G12.22
    muscular dystrophy G71.0
  locomotor ataxia (syphilitic) A52.11
  paralysis
    birth injury P14.0
    due to or associated with
      motor neuron disease G12.22
      muscular dystrophy G71.0
Ducrey's chancre A57
Duct, ductus —*see* condition
Duhring's disease (dermatitis herpetiformis)
  L13.0
Dullness, cardiac (decreased) (increased) R01.2
Dumb ague —*see* Malaria
Dumbness —*see* Aphasia
Dumdum fever B55.0
Dumping syndrome (postgastrectomy) K91.1
Duodenitis (nonspecific) (peptic) K29.80
  with bleeding K29.81
Duodenocholangitis —*see* Cholangitis
Duodenum, duodenal —*see* condition
Duplay's bursitis or periarthritis —*see*
  Tendinitis, calcific, shoulder
Duplication, duplex —*see also* Accessory
  alimentary tract Q45.8
  anus Q43.4
  appendix (and cecum) Q43.4
  biliary duct (any) Q44.5
  bladder Q64.79
  cecum (and appendix) Q43.4
  cervix Q51.820
  chromosome NEC
    with complex rearrangements NEC Q92.5
    seen only at prometaphase Q92.8
  cystic duct Q44.5
  digestive organs Q45.8
  esophagus Q39.8
  frontonasal process Q75.8
  intestine (large) (small) Q43.4
  kidney Q63.0
  liver Q44.7
  ~~oesophagus Q39.8~~
  pancreas Q45.3
  penis Q55.69
  respiratory organs NEC Q34.8
  salivary duct Q38.4
  spinal cord (incomplete) Q06.2
  stomach Q40.2
Dupré's disease (meningism) R29.1
Dupuytren's contraction or disease M72.0
Durand-Nicolas-Favre disease A55
Durotomy (inadvertent) (incidental) G97.41
Duroziez's disease (congenital mitral stenosis)
  Q23.2
Dutton's relapsing fever (West African) A68.1
Dwarfism E34.3
  achondroplastic Q77.4
  congenital E34.3
  constitutional E34.3
  hypochondroplastic Q77.4
  hypophyseal E23.0
  infantile E34.3
  Laron-type E34.3
  Lorain (-Levi) type E23.0
  metatropic Q77.8
  nephrotic-glycosuric (with
    hypophosphatemic rickets) E72.09
  nutritional E45
  pancreatic K86.8
  pituitary E23.0
  renal N25.0
  thanatophoric Q77.1
Dyke-Young anemia (secondary)
  (symptomatic) D59.1

Dysacusis —*see* Abnormal, auditory
  perception
Dysadrenocortism E27.9
  hyperfunction E27.0
Dysarthria R47.1
  following
    cerebral infarction I69.322
    cerebrovascular disease I69.922
      specified disease NEC I69.822
    intracerebral hemorrhage I69.122
    nontraumatic intracranial hemorrhage
      NEC I69.222
    subarachnoid hemorrhage I69.022
Dysautonomia (familial) G90.1
Dysbarism T70.3
Dysbasia R26.2
  angiosclerotica intermittens I73.9
  hysterical F44.4
  lordotica (progressiva) G24.1
  nonorganic origin F44.4
  psychogenic F44.4
Dysbetalipoproteinemia (familial) E78.2
Dyscalculia R48.8
  developmental F81.2
Dyschezia K59.00
Dyschondroplasia (with hemangiomata)
  Q78.4
Dyschromia (skin) L81.9
Dyscollagenosis M35.9
Dyscranio-pygo-phalangy Q87.0
Dyscrasia
  blood (with) D75.9
    antepartum hemorrhage —*see*
      Hemorrhage, antepartum, with
      coagulation defect
    intrapartum hemorrhage O67.0
    newborn P61.9
      specified type NEC P61.8
    puerperal, postpartum O72.3
  polyglandular, pluriglandular E31.9
Dysendocrinism E34.9
Dysentery, dysenteric (catarrhal) (diarrhea)
  (epidemic) (hemorrhagic) (infectious)
  (sporadic) (tropical) A09
  abscess, liver A06.4
  amebic (*see also* Amebiasis) A06.0
    with abscess —*see* Abscess, amebic
    acute A06.0
    chronic A06.1
  arthritis (*see also* category M01) A09
  bacillary (*see also* category M01) A03.9
  bacillary A03.9
    arthritis (*see also* category M01)
      A03.9
    Boyd A03.2
    Flexner A03.1
    Schmitz (-Stutzer) A03.0
    Shiga (-Kruse) A03.0
    Shigella A03.9
      boydii A03.2
      dysenteriae A03.0
      flexneri A03.1
      group A A03.0
      group B A03.1
      group C A03.2
      group D A03.3
      sonnei A03.3
      specified type NEC A03.8
    Sonne A03.3
    specified type NEC A03.8
  balantidial A07.0
  Balantidium coli A07.0
  Boyd's A03.2
  candidal B37.82
  Chilomastix A07.8
  Chinese A03.9
  coccidial A07.3
  Dientamoeba (fragilis) A07.8
  Embadomonas A07.8
  Entamoeba, entamebic —*see* Dysentery,
    amebic

Dysentery, dysenteric (Continued)
Flexner-Boyd A03.2
Flexner's A03.1
Giardia lamblia A07.1
Hiss-Russell A03.1
Lamblia A07.1
leishmanial B55.0
malarial —see Malaria
metazoal B82.0
monilial B37.82
protozoal A07.9
Salmonella A02.0
schistosomal B65.1
Schmitz (-Stutzer) A03.0
Shiga (-Kruse) A03.0
Shigella NOS —see Dysentery, bacillary
Sonne A03.3
strongyloidiasis B78.0
trichomonal A07.8
viral (see also Enteritis, viral) A08.4
Dysequilibrium R42
Dysesthesia R20.8
hysterical F44.6
Dysfibrinogenemia (congenital) D68.2
Dysfunction
adrenal E27.9
hyperfunction E27.0
autonomic
due to alcohol G31.2
somatoform F45.8
bladder N31.9
neurogenic NOS —see Dysfunction,
bladder, neuromuscular
neuromuscular NOS N31.9
atonic (motor) (sensory) N31.2
autonomous N31.2
flaccid N31.2
nonreflex N31.2
reflex N31.1
specified NEC N31.8
uninhibited N31.0
bleeding, uterus N93.8
cerebral G93.89
colon K59.9
psychogenic F45.8
colostomy K94.03
cystic duct K82.8
cystostomy (stoma) —see Complications,
cystostomy
ejaculatory N53.19
anejaculatory orgasm N53.13
painful N53.12
premature F52.4
retarded N53.11
endocrine NOS E34.9
endometrium N85.8
enterostomy K94.13
gallbladder K82.8
gastrostomy (stoma) K94.23
gland, glandular NOS E34.9
heart I51.89
hemoglobin D75.89
hepatic K76.89
hypophysis E23.7
hypothalamic NEC E23.3
ileostomy (stoma) K94.13
jejunostomy (stoma) K94.13
kidney —see Disease, renal
labyrinthine —see subcategory H83.2
left ventricular, following sudden emotional
stress I51.81
liver K76.89
male —see Dysfunction, sexual, male
orgasmic (female) F52.31
male F52.32
ovary E28.9
specified NEC E28.8
papillary muscle I51.89
parathyroid E21.4
physiological NEC R68.89
psychogenic F59

Dysfunction (Continued)
pineal gland E34.8
pituitary (gland) E23.3
platelets D69.1
polyglandular E31.9
specified NEC E31.8
psychophysiologic F59
psychosexual F52.9
with
dyspareunia F52.6
premature ejaculation F52.4
vaginismus F52.5
pylorus K31.9
rectum K59.9
psychogenic F45.8
reflex (sympathetic) —see Syndrome, pain,
complex regional I
segmental —see Dysfunction, somatic
senile R54
sexual (due to) R37
alcohol F10.981
amphetamine F15.981
in
abuse F15.181
dependence F15.281
anxiolytic F13.981
in
abuse F13.181
dependence F13.281
cocaine F14.981
in
abuse F14.181
dependence F14.281
excessive sexual drive F52.8
failure of genital response (male)
F52.21
female F52.22
female N94.9
aversion F52.1
dyspareunia N94.1
psychogenic F52.6
frigidity F52.22
nymphomania F52.8
orgasmic F52.31
psychogenic F52.9
aversion F52.1
dyspareunia F52.6
frigidity F52.22
nymphomania F52.8
orgasmic F52.31
vaginismus F52.5
vaginismus N94.2
psychogenic F52.5
hypnotic F13.981
in
abuse F13.181
dependence F13.281
inhibited orgasm (female) F52.31
male F52.32
lack
of sexual enjoyment F52.1
or loss of sexual desire F52.0
male N53.9
anejaculatory orgasm N53.13
ejaculatory N53.19
painful N53.12
premature F52.4
retarded N53.11
erectile N52.9
drug induced N52.2
due to
disease classified elsewhere N52.1
drug N52.2
postoperative (postprocedural) N52.39
following
prostatectomy N52.34
radical N52.31
radical cystectomy N52.32
urethral surgery N52.33
psychogenic F52.21
specified cause NEC N52.8

Dysfunction (Continued)
sexual (Continued)
male (Continued)
erectile (Continued)
vasculogenic
arterial insufficiency N52.01
with corporo-venous occlusive
N52.03
corporo-venous occlusive N52.02
with arterial insufficiency
N52.03
impotence —see Dysfunction, sexual,
male, erectile
psychogenic F52.9
aversion F52.1
erectile F52.21
orgasmic F52.32
premature ejaculation F52.4
satyriasis F52.8
specified type NEC F52.8
specified type NEC N53.8
nonorganic F52.9
specified NEC F52.8
opioid F11.981
in
abuse F11.181
dependence F11.281
orgasmic dysfunction (female) F52.31
male F52.32
premature ejaculation F52.4
psychoactive substances NEC F19.981
in
abuse F19.181
dependence F19.281
psychogenic F52.9
sedative F13.981
in
abuse F13.181
dependence F13.281
sexual aversion F52.1
vaginismus (nonorganic) (psychogenic)
F52.5
sinoatrial node I49.5
somatic M99.09
abdomen M99.09
acromioclavicular M99.07
cervical region M99.01
cervicothoracic M99.01
costochondral M99.08
costovertebral M99.08
head region M99.00
hip M99.05
lower extremity M99.06
lumbar region M99.03
lumbosacral M99.03
occipitocervical M99.00
pelvic region M99.05
pubic M99.05
rib cage M99.08
sacral region M99.04
sacrococcygeal M99.04
sacroiliac M99.04
specified NEC M99.09
sternochondral M99.08
sternoclavicular M99.07
thoracic region M99.02
thoracolumbar M99.02
upper extremity M99.07
somatoform autonomic F45.8
stomach K31.89
psychogenic F45.8
suprarenal E27.9
hyperfunction E27.0
symbolic R48.9
specified type NEC R48.8
temporomandibular (joint) M26.69
joint-pain syndrome M26.62
testicular (endocrine) E29.9
specified NEC E29.8
thymus E32.9
thyroid E07.9

◀ New ◀▬ Revised ~~deleted~~ Deleted

Dysfunction *(Continued)*
  ureterostomy (stoma) —*see* Complications,
    stoma, urinary tract
  urethrostomy (stoma) —*see* Complications,
    stoma, urinary tract
  uterus, complicating delivery O62.9
    hypertonic O62.4
    hypotonic O62.2
      primary O62.0
      secondary O62.1
  ventricular I51.9
    with congestive heart failure I50.9-
      left, reversible, following sudden
        emotional stress I51.81
Dysgenesis
  gonadal (due to chromosomal anomaly)
    Q96.9
    pure Q99.1
  renal Q60.5
    bilateral Q60.4
    unilateral Q60.3
  reticular D72.0
  tidal platelet D69.3
Dysgerminoma
  specified site —*see* Neoplasm, malignant,
    by site
  unspecified site
    female C56.9
    male C62.90
Dysgeusia R43.2
Dysgraphia R27.8
Dyshidrosis, dysidrosis L30.1
Dyskaryotic cervical smear R87.619
Dyskeratosis L85.8
  cervix —*see* Dysplasia, cervix
  congenital Q82.8
  uterus NEC N85.8
Dyskinesia G24.9
  biliary (cystic duct or gallbladder)
    K82.8
  drug induced
    orofacial G24.01
  esophagus K22.4
  hysterical F44.4
  intestinal K59.8
  nonorganic origin F44.4
  orofacial (idiopathic) G24.4
    drug induced G24.01
  psychogenic F44.4
  subacute, drug induced G24.01
  tardive G24.01
    neuroleptic induced G24.01
  trachea J39.8
  tracheobronchial J98.09
Dyslalia (developmental) F80.0
Dyslexia R48.0
  developmental F81.0
Dyslipidemia E78.5
  depressed HDL cholesterol E78.6
  elevated fasting triglycerides E78.1
Dysmaturity —*see also* Light for dates
  pulmonary (newborn) (Wilson-Mikity)
    P27.0
Dysmenorrhea (essential) (exfoliative)
  N94.6
  congestive (syndrome) N94.6
  primary N94.4
  psychogenic F45.8
  secondary N94.5
Dysmetabolic syndrome X E88.81
Dysmetria R27.8
Dysmorphism (due to)
  alcohol Q86.0
  exogenous cause NEC Q86.8
  hydantoin Q86.1
  warfarin Q86.2
Dysmorphophobia (nondelusional) F45.22
  delusional F22
Dysnomia R47.01
Dysorexia R63.0
  psychogenic F50.8

Dysostosis
  cleidocranial, cleidocranialis Q74.0
  craniofacial Q75.1
  Fairbank's (idiopathic familial generalized
    osteophytosis) Q78.9
  mandibulofacial (incomplete) Q75.4
  multiplex E76.01
  oculomandibular Q75.5
Dyspareunia (female) N94.1
  male N53.12
  nonorganic F52.6
  psychogenic F52.6
  secondary N94.1
Dyspepsia R10.13
  atonic K30
  functional (allergic) (congenital)
    (gastrointestinal) (occupational) (reflex)
    K30
  intestinal K59.8
  nervous F45.8
  neurotic F45.8
  psychogenic F45.8
Dysphagia R13.10
  cervical R13.19
  following
    cerebral infarction I69.391
    cerebrovascular disease I69.991
      specified NEC I69.891
    intracerebral hemorrhage I69.191
    nontraumatic intracranial hemorrhage
      NEC I69.291
    specified disease NEC I69.891
    subarachnoid hemorrhage I69.091
  functional (hysterical) F45.8
  hysterical F45.8
  nervous (hysterical) F45.8
  neurogenic R13.19
  oral phase R13.11
  oropharyngeal phase R13.12
  pharyneal phase R13.13
  pharyngoesophageal phase R13.14
  psychogenic F45.8
  sideropenic D50.1
  spastica K22.4
  specified NEC R13.19
Dysphagocytosis, congenital D71
Dysphasia R47.02
  developmental
    expressive type F80.1
    receptive type F80.2
  following
    cerebrovascular disease I69.921
      cerebral infarction I69.321
      intracerebral hemorrhage I69.121
    nontraumatic intracranial hemorrhage NEC
      I69.221
    specified disease NEC I69.821
    subarachnoid hemorrhage I69.021
Dysphonia R49.0
  functional F44.4
  hysterical F44.4
  psychogenic F44.4
  spastica J38.3
Dysphoria, postpartal O90.6
Dyspituitarism E23.3
Dysplasia —*see also* Anomaly
  acetabular, congenital Q65.89
  alveolar capillary, with vein misalignment
    J84.843
  anus (histologically confirmed) (mild)
    (moderate) K62.82
    severe D01.3
  arrhythmogenic right ventricular I42.8
  arterial, fibromuscular I77.3
  asphyxiating thoracic (congenital) Q77.2
  brain Q07.9
  bronchopulmonary, perinatal P27.1
  cervix (uteri) N87.9
    mild N87.0
    moderate N87.1
    severe D06.9

Dysplasia *(Continued)*
  chondroectodermal Q77.6
  colon D12.6
  craniometaphyseal Q78.5
  dentinal K00.5
  diaphyseal, progressive Q78.3
  dystrophic Q77.5
  ectodermal (anhidrotic) (congenital)
    (hereditary) Q82.4
    hydrotic Q82.8
  epithelial, uterine cervix —*see* Dysplasia,
    cervix
  eye (congenital) Q11.2
  fibrous
    bone NEC (monostotic) M85.00
      ankle M85.07-
      foot M85.07-
      forearm M85.03-
      hand M85.04-
      lower leg M85.06-
      multiple site M85.09
      neck M85.08
      rib M85.08
      shoulder M85.01-
      skull M85.08
      specified site NEC M85.08
      thigh M85.05-
      toe M85.07-
      upper arm M85.02-
      vertebra M85.08
    diaphyseal, progressive Q78.3
    jaw M27.8
    polyostotic Q78.1
  florid osseous —*see also* Cyst, calcifying
    odontogenic
  high grade, focal D12.6
  hip, congenital Q65.89
  joint, congenital Q74.8
  kidney Q61.4
    multicystic Q61.4
  leg Q74.2
  lung, congenital (not associated with short
    gestation) Q33.6
  mammary (gland) (benign) N60.9-
    cyst (solitary) —*see* Cyst, breast
    cystic —*see* Mastopathy, cystic
    duct ectasia —*see* Ectasia, mammary
      duct
    fibroadenosis —*see* Fibroadenosis, breast
    fibrosclerosis —*see* Fibrosclerosis, breast
    specified type NEC N60.8-
  metaphyseal (Jansen's) (McKusick's)
    (Schmid's) Q78.5
  muscle Q79.8
  oculodentodigital Q87.0
  periapical (cemental) (cemento-osseous) —*see*
    Cyst, calcifying odontogenic
  periosteum —*see* Disorder, bone, specified
    type NEC
  polyostotic fibrous Q78.1
  prostate (*see also* Neoplasia, intraepithelial,
    prostate) N42.3
    severe D07.5
  renal Q61.4
    multicystic Q61.4
  retinal, congenital Q14.1
  right ventricular, arrhythmogenic I42.8
  septo-optic Q04.4
  skin L98.8
  spinal cord Q06.1
  spondyloepiphyseal Q77.7
  thymic, with immunodeficiency
    D82.1
  vagina N89.3
    mild N89.0
    moderate N89.1
    severe NEC D07.2
  vulva N90.3
    mild N90.0
    moderate N90.1
    severe NEC D07.1

Dyspnea (nocturnal) (paroxysmal) R06.00
  asthmatic (bronchial) J45.909
    with
      bronchitis J45.909
        with
          exacerbation (acute) J45.901
          status asthmaticus J45.902
        chronic J44.9
      exacerbation (acute) J45.901
      status asthmaticus J45.902
    cardiac —see Failure, ventricular, left
  cardiac —see Failure, ventricular, left
  functional F45.8
  hyperventilation R06.4
  hysterical F45.8
  newborn P28.89
  psychogenic F45.8
  shortness of breath R06.02
  specified type NEC R06.09
Dyspraxia R27.8
  developmental (syndrome) F82
Dysproteinemia E88.09
Dysreflexia, autonomic G90.4
Dysrhythmia
  cardiac I49.9
    newborn
      bradycardia P29.12
      occurring before birth P03.819
        before onset of labor P03.810
        during labor P03.811
      tachycardia P29.11
    postoperative I97.89
  cerebral or cortical —see Epilepsy
Dyssomnia —see Disorder, sleep
Dyssynergia
  biliary K83.8
  bladder sphincter N36.44
  cerebellaris myoclonica (Hunt's ataxia)
    G11.1
Dysthymia F34.1
Dysthyroidism E07.9
Dystocia O66.9
  affecting newborn P03.1
  cervical (hypotonic) O62.2
    affecting newborn P03.6
    primary O62.0
    secondary O62.1
  contraction ring O62.4
  fetal O66.9
    abnormality NEC O66.3
    conjoined twins O66.3
    oversize O66.2
  maternal O66.9
  positional O64.9
  shoulder (girdle) O66.0
    causing obstructed labor O66.0
  uterine NEC O62.4

Dystonia G24.9
  deformans progressiva G24.1
  drug induced NEC G24.09
    acute G24.02
    specified NEC G24.09
  familial G24.1
  idiopathic G24.1
    familial G24.1
    nonfamilial G24.2
    orofacial G24.4
  lenticularis G24.8
  musculorum deformans G24.1
  neuroleptic induced (acute) G24.02
  orofacial (idiopathic) G24.4
  oromandibular G24.4
    due to drug G24.01
  specified NEC G24.8
  torsion (familial) (idiopathic) G24.1
    acquired G24.8
    genetic G24.1
    symptomatic (nonfamilial) G24.2
Dystonic movements R25.8
Dystrophy, dystrophia
  adiposogenital E23.6
  Becker's type G71.0
  cervical sympathetic G90.2
  choroid (hereditary) H31.20
    central areolar H31.22
    choroideremia H31.21
    gyrate atrophy H31.23
    specified type NEC H31.29
  cornea (hereditary) H18.50
    endothelial H18.51
    epithelial H18.52
    granular H18.53
    lattice H18.54
    macular H18.55
    specified type NEC H18.59
  Duchenne's type G71.0
  due to malnutrition E45
  Erb's G71.0
  Fuchs' H18.51
  Gower's muscular G71.0
  hair L67.8
  infantile neuraxonal G31.89
  Landouzy-Déjérine G71.0
  Leyden-Möbius G71.0
  muscular G71.0
    benign (Becker type) G71.0
    congenital (hereditary) (progressive)
      (with specific morphological
      abnormalities of the muscle fiber)
      G71.0
      myotonic G71.11
    distal G71.0
    Duchenne type G71.0
    Emery-Dreifuss G71.0

Dystrophy, dystrophia (Continued)
  muscular (Continued)
    Erb type G71.0
    facioscapulohumeral G71.0
    Gower's G71.0
    hereditary (progressive) G71.0
    Landouzy-Déjérine type G71.0
    limb-girdle G71.0
    myotonic G71.11
    progressive (hereditary) G71.0
      Charcot-Marie (-Tooth) type
      G60.0
    pseudohypertrophic (infantile)
      G71.0
    severe (Duchenne type) G71.0
  myocardium, myocardial —see
    Degeneration, myocardial
  ~~myotonic, myotonica G71.11~~
  nail L60.3
    congenital Q84.6
  nutritional E45
  ocular G71.0
  oculocerebrorenal E72.03
  oculopharyngeal G71.0
  ovarian N83.8
  polyglandular E31.8
  reflex (neuromuscular) (sympathetic) —
    see Syndrome, pain, complex
    regional I
  retinal (hereditary) H35.50
    in
      lipid storage disorders E75.6
      [H36]
      systemic lipidoses E75.6 [H36]
    involving
      pigment epithelium H35.54
      sensory area H35.53
    pigmentary H35.52
    vitreoretinal H35.51
  Salzmann's nodular —see Degeneration,
    cornea, nodular
  scapuloperoneal G71.0
  skin NEC L98.8
  sympathetic (reflex) —see Syndrome, pain,
    complex regional I
    cervical G90.2
  tapetoretinal H35.54
  thoracic, asphyxiating Q77.2
  unguium L60.3
    congenital Q84.6
  vitreoretinal H35.51
  vulva N90.4
  yellow (liver) —see Failure, hepatic
Dysuria R30.0
  psychogenic F45.8

◀ New   ◀◀ Revised   ~~deleted~~ Deleted

E

Eales' disease H35.06-
Ear —*see also* condition
  piercing Z41.3
  tropical B36.8
  wax (impacted) H61.20
    left H61.22
      with right H61.23
    right H61.21
      with left H61.23
Earache —*see* subcategory H92.0
Early satiety R68.81
Eaton-Lambert syndrome—*see* Syndrome,
    Lambert-Eaton
Eberth's disease (typhoid fever) A01.00
Ebola virus disease A98.4
Ebstein's anomaly or syndrome (heart) Q22.5
Eccentro-osteochondrodysplasia E76.29
Ecchondroma —*see* Neoplasm, bone, benign
Ecchondrosis D48.0
Ecchymosis R58
  conjunctiva —*see* Hemorrhage, conjunctiva
  eye (traumatic) —*see* Contusion, eyeball
  eyelid (traumatic) —*see* Contusion, eyelid ◀▥
  newborn P54.5
  spontaneous R23.3
  traumatic —*see* Contusion
Echinococciasis —*see* Echinococcus
Echinococcosis —*see* Echinococcus
Echinococcus (infection) B67.90
  granulosus B67.4
    bone B67.2
    liver B67.0
    lung B67.1
    multiple sites B67.32
    specified site NEC B67.39
    thyroid B67.31 [E35]
  liver NOS B67.8
    granulosus B67.0
    multilocularis B67.5
  lung NEC B67.99
    granulosus B67.1
    multilocularis B67.69
  multilocularis B67.7
    liver B67.5
    multiple sites B67.61
    specified site NEC B67.69
  specified site NEC B67.99
    granulosus B67.39
    multilocularis B67.69
  thyroid NEC B67.99
    granulosus B67.31 [E35]
    multilocularis B67.69 [E35]
Echinorhynchiasis B83.8
Echinostomiasis B66.8
Echolalia R48.8
Echovirus, as cause of disease classified
    elsewhere B97.12
Eclampsia, eclamptic (coma) (convulsions)
    (delirium) (with hypertension) NEC O15.9
  during labor and delivery O15.1
  postpartum O15.2
  pregnancy O15.0-
  puerperal O15.2
Economic circumstances affecting care Z59.9
Economo's disease A85.8
Ectasia, ectasis
  annuloaortic I35.8
  aorta I77.819
    with aneurysm —*see* Aneurysm, aorta
    abdominal I77.811
    thoracic I77.810
    thoracoabdominal I77.812
  breast —*see* Ectasia, mammary duct
  capillary I78.8
  cornea H18.71-
  gastric antral vascular (GAVE) K31.819
    with hemorrhage K31.811
    without hemorrhage K31.819
  mammary duct N60.4-

Ectasia, ectasis (Continued)
  salivary gland (duct) K11.8
  sclera —*see* Sclerectasia
Ecthyma L08.0
  contagiosum B08.02
  gangrenosum L08.0
  infectiosum B08.02
Ectocardia Q24.8
Ectodermal dysplasia (anhidrotic) Q82.4
Ectodermosis erosiva pluriorificialis
    L51.1
Ectopic, ectopia (congenital)
  abdominal viscera Q45.8
    due to defect in anterior abdominal wall
      Q79.59
  ACTH syndrome E24.3
  adrenal gland Q89.1
  anus Q43.5
  atrial beats I49.1
  beats I49.49
    atrial I49.1
    ventricular I49.3
  bladder Q64.10
  bone and cartilage in lung Q33.5
  brain Q04.8
  breast tissue Q83.8
  cardiac Q24.8
  cerebral Q04.8
  cordis Q24.8
  endometrium —*see* Endometriosis
  gastric mucosa Q40.2
  gestation —*see* Pregnancy, by site
  heart Q24.8
  hormone secretion NEC E34.2
  kidney (crossed) (pelvis) Q63.2
  lens, lentis Q12.1
  mole —*see* Pregnancy, by site
  organ or site NEC —*see* Malposition,
    congenital
  pancreas Q45.3
  pregnancy —*see* Pregnancy, ectopic
  pupil —*see* Abnormality, pupillary
  renal Q63.2
  sebaceous glands of mouth Q38.6
  spleen Q89.09
  testis Q53.00
    bilateral Q53.02
    unilateral Q53.01
  thyroid Q89.2
  tissue in lung Q33.5
  ureter Q62.63
  ventricular beats I49.3
  vesicae Q64.10
Ectromelia Q73.8
  lower limb —*see* Defect, reduction, limb,
    lower, specified type NEC
  upper limb —*see* Defect, reduction, limb,
    upper, specified type NEC
Ectropion H02.109
  cervix N86
    with cervicitis N72
  congenital Q10.1
  eyelid (paralytic) H02.109
    cicatricial H02.119
      left H02.116
        lower H02.115
        upper H02.114
      right H02.113
        lower H02.112
        upper H02.111
    congenital Q10.1
    left H02.106
      lower H02.105
      upper H02.104
    mechanical H02.129
      left H02.126
        lower H02.125
        upper H02.124
      right H02.123
        lower H02.122
        upper H02.121

Ectropion (Continued)
  eyelid (Continued)
    right H02.103
      lower H02.102
      upper H02.101
    senile H02.139
      left H02.136
        lower H02.135
        upper H02.134
      right H02.133
        lower H02.132
        upper H02.131
    spastic H02.149
      left H02.146
        lower H02.145
        upper H02.144
      right H02.143
        lower H02.142
        upper H02.141
  iris H21.89
  lip (acquired) K13.0
    congenital Q38.0
  urethra N36.8
  uvea H21.89
Eczema (acute) (chronic) (erythematous)
    (fissum) (rubrum) (squamous) (*see also*
    Dermatitis) L30.9
  contact —*see* Dermatitis, contact
  dyshydrotic L30.1
  external ear —*see* Otitis, externa, acute,
    eczematoid
  flexural L20.82
  herpeticum B00.0
  hypertrophicum L28.0
  hypostatic —*see* Varix, leg, with,
    inflammation
  impetiginous L01.1
  infantile (due to any substance)
    L20.83
    intertriginous L21.1
    seborrheic L21.1
  intertriginous NEC L30.4
    infantile L21.1
  intrinsic (allergic) L20.84
  lichenified NEC L28.0
  marginatum (hebrae) B35.6
  pustular L30.3
  stasis —*see* Varix, leg, with, inflammation
  vaccination, vaccinatum T88.1
  varicose —*see* Varix, leg, with,
    inflammation
Eczematid L30.2
Eddowes (-Spurway) syndrome Q78.0
Edema, edematous (infectious) (pitting)
    (toxic) R60.9
  with nephritis —*see* Nephrosis
  allergic T78.3
  amputation stump (surgical) (sequelae)
    (late effect) T87.89
  angioneurotic (allergic) (any site) (with
    urticaria) T78.3
    hereditary D84.1
  angiospastic I73.9
  Berlin's (traumatic) S05.8X-
  brain (cytotoxic) (vasogenic) G93.6
    due to birth injury P11.0
    newborn (anoxia or hypoxia) P52.4
      birth injury P11.0
    traumatic —*see* Injury, intracranial,
      cerebral edema
  cardiac —*see* Failure, heart, congestive
  cardiovascular —*see* Failure, heart,
    congestive
  cerebral —*see* Edema, brain
  cerebrospinal —*see* Edema, brain
  cervix (uteri) (acute) N88.8
    puerperal, postpartum O90.89
  chronic hereditary Q82.0
  circumscribed, acute T78.3
    hereditary D84.1
  conjunctiva H11.42-

Edema, edematous (Continued)
cornea H18.2-
idiopathic H18.22-
secondary H18.23-
due to contact lens H18.21-
due to
lymphatic obstruction I89.0
salt retention E87.0
epiglottis —see Edema, glottis
essential, acute T78.3
hereditary D84.1
extremities, lower —see Edema, legs
eyelid NEC H02.849
left H02.846
lower H02.845
upper H02.844
right H02.843
lower H02.842
upper H02.841
familial, hereditary Q82.0
famine —see Malnutrition, severe
generalized R60.1
glottis, glottic, glottidis (obstructive) (passive)
J38.4
allergic T78.3
hereditary D84.1
heart —see Failure, heart, congestive
heat T67.7
hereditary Q82.0
inanition —see Malnutrition, severe
intracranial G93.6
iris H21.89
joint —see Effusion, joint
larynx —see Edema, glottis
legs R60.0
due to venous obstruction I87.1
hereditary Q82.0
localized R60.0
due to venous obstruction I87.1
lower limbs —see Edema, legs
lung J81.1
with heart condition or failure —see
Failure, ventricular, left
acute J81.0
chemical (acute) J68.1
chronic J68.1
chronic J81.1
due to
chemicals, gases, fumes or vapors
(inhalation) J68.1
external agent J70.9
specified NEC J70.8
radiation J70.1
due to
chemicals, fumes or vapors (inhalation)
J68.1
external agent J70.9
specified NEC J70.8
high altitude T70.29
near drowning T75.1
radiation J70.0
meaning failure, left ventricle I50.1
lymphatic I89.0
due to mastectomy I97.2
macula H35.81
cystoid, following cataract surgery —see
Complications, postprocedural,
following cataract surgery
diabetic —see Diabetes, by type, with,
retinopathy, with macular edema ◄▬
malignant —see Gangrene, gas
Milroy's Q82.0
nasopharynx J39.2
newborn P83.30
hydrops fetalis —see Hydrops, fetalis
specified NEC P83.39
nutritional —see also Malnutrition, severe
with dyspigmentation, skin and hair E40
optic disc or nerve —see Papilledema
orbit H05.22-
pancreas K86.8

Edema, edematous (Continued)
papilla, optic —see Papilledema
penis N48.89
periodic T78.3
hereditary D84.1
pharynx J39.2
pulmonary —see Edema, lung
Quincke's T78.3
hereditary D84.1
renal —see Nephrosis
retina H35.81
diabetic —see Diabetes, by type, with,
retinopathy, with macular edema ◄▬
salt E87.0
scrotum N50.8
seminal vesicle N50.8
spermatic cord N50.8
spinal (cord) (vascular) (nontraumatic) G95.19
starvation —see Malnutrition, severe
stasis —see Hypertension, venous, (chronic)
subglottic —see Edema, glottis
supraglottic —see Edema, glottis
testis N44.8
tunica vaginalis N50.8
vas deferens N50.8
vulva (acute) N90.89
Edentulism —see Absence, teeth, acquired
Edsall's disease T67.2
Educational handicap Z55.9
specified NEC Z55.8
Edward's syndrome —see Trisomy, 18
Effect, adverse
abnormal gravitational (G) forces or states
T75.81
abuse —see Maltreatment
air pressure T70.9
specified NEC T70.8
altitude (high) —see Effect, adverse, high
altitude
anesthesia (see also Anesthesia) T88.59
in labor and delivery O74.9
in pregnancy NEC O29.3-
local, toxic
in labor and delivery O74.4-
postpartum, puerperal O89.3
postpartum, puerperal O89.9
specified NEC T88.59
in labor and delivery O74.8
postpartum, puerperal O89.8
spinal and epidural T88.59
headache T88.59
in labor and delivery O74.5
postpartum, puerperal O89.4
specified NEC
in labor and delivery O74.6
postpartum, puerperal O89.5
antitoxin —see Complications, vaccination
atmospheric pressure T70.9
due to explosion T70.8
high T70.3
low —see Effect, adverse, high altitude
specified effect NEC T70.8
biological, correct substance properly
administered —see Effect, adverse, drug
blood (derivatives) (serum) (transfusion) —
see Complications, transfusion ◄▬
chemical substance —see Table of Drugs and
Chemicals ◄▬
cold (temperature) (weather) T69.9
chilblains T69.1
frostbite —see Frostbite
specified effect NEC T69.8
drugs and medicaments T88.7
specified drug —see Table of Drugs and
Chemicals, by drug, adverse effect ◄▬
specified effect — code to condition
electric current, electricity (shock) T75.4
burn —see Burn
exertion (excessive) T73.3
exposure —see Exposure
external cause NEC T75.89

Effect, adverse (Continued)
foodstuffs T78.1
allergic reaction —see Allergy, food
causing anaphylaxis —see Shock,
anaphylactic, due to food
noxious —see Poisoning, food, noxious
gases, fumes, or vapors T59.9-
specified agent —see Table of Drugs and
Chemicals ◄▬
glue (airplane) sniffing
due to drug abuse —see Abuse, drug,
inhalant
due to drug dependence —see Dependence,
drug, inhalant
heat —see Heat
high altitude NEC T70.29
anoxia T70.29
on
ears T70.0
sinuses T70.1
polycythemia D75.1
high pressure fluids T70.4
hot weather —see Heat
hunger T73.0
immersion, foot —see Immersion
immunization —see Complications,
vaccination
immunological agents —see Complications,
vaccination
infrared (radiation) (rays) NOS T66
dermatitis or eczema L59.8
infusion —see Complications, infusion
lack of care of infants —see Maltreatment,
child
lightning —see Lightning
medical care T88.9
specified NEC T88.8
medicinal substance, correct, properly
administered —see Effect, adverse, drug
motion T75.3
noise, on inner ear —see subcategory H83.3
overheated places —see Heat
psychosocial, of work environment Z56.5
radiation (diagnostic) (infrared) (natural
source) (therapeutic) (ultraviolet)
(X-ray) NOS T66
dermatitis or eczema —see Dermatitis, due
to, radiation
fibrosis of lung J70.1
pneumonitis J70.0
pulmonary manifestations
acute J70.0
chronic J70.1
skin L59.9
radioactive substance NOS
dermatitis or eczema —see Radiodermatitis
reduced temperature T69.9
immersion foot or hand —see Immersion
specified effect NEC T69.8
serum NEC (see also Reaction, serum)
T80.69
specified NEC T78.8
external cause NEC T75.89
strangulation —see Asphyxia, traumatic
submersion T75.1
thirst T73.1
toxic —see Toxicity
transfusion —see Complications, transfusion
ultraviolet (radiation) (rays) NOS T66
burn —see Burn
dermatitis or eczema —see Dermatitis, due
to, ultraviolet rays
acute L56.8
vaccine (any) —see Complications,
vaccination
vibration —see Vibration, adverse effects
water pressure NEC T70.9
specified NEC T70.8
weightlessness T75.82
whole blood —see Complications, transfusion
work environment Z56.5

◄ New ◄▬ Revised ~~deleted~~ Deleted

Effect (s) (of) (from) —*see* Effect, adverse NEC
Effects, late —*see* Sequelae
Effluvium
    anagen L65.1
    telogen L65.0
Effort syndrome (psychogenic) F45.8
Effusion
    amniotic fluid —*see* Pregnancy, complicated
        by, prematue rupture of membranes
    brain (serous) G93.6
    bronchial —*see* Bronchitis
    cerebral G93.6
    cerebrospinal —*see also* Meningitis
        vessel G93.6
    chest —*see* Effusion, pleura
    chylous, chyliform (pleura) J94.0
    intracranial G93.6
    joint M25.40
        ankle M25.47-
        elbow M25.42-
        foot joint M25.47-
        hand joint M25.44-
        hip M25.45-
        knee M25.46-
        shoulder M25.41-
        specified joint NEC M25.48
        wrist M25.43-
    malignant pleural J91.0
    meninges —*see* Meningitis
    pericardium, pericardial (noninflammatory)
        I31.3
        acute —*see* Pericarditis, acute
    peritoneal (chronic) R18.8
    pleura, pleurisy, pleuritic, pleuropericardial
        J90
        chylous, chyliform J94.0
        due to systemic lupus erythematosis
            M32.13
        influenzal —*see* Influenza, with, respiratory
            manifestations NEC
        malignant J91.0
        newborn P28.89
        tuberculous NEC A15.6
            primary (progressive) A15.7
    spinal —*see* Meningitis
    thorax, thoracic —*see* Effusion, pleura
Egg shell nails L60.3
    congenital Q84.6
Egyptian splenomegaly B65.1
Ehlers-Danlos syndrome Q79.6
Ehrlichiosis A77.40
    due to
        E. chafeensis A77.41
        E. sennetsu A79.81
        specified organism NEC A77.49
Eichstedt's disease B36.0
Eisenmenger's
    complex or syndrome I27.89
    defect Q21.8
Ejaculation
    painful N53.12
    premature F52.4
    retarded N53.11
    retrograde N53.14
    semen, painful N53.12
        psychogenic F52.6
Ekbom's syndrome (restless legs) G25.81
Ekman's syndrome (brittle bones and blue
    sclera) Q78.0
Elastic skin Q82.8
    acquired L57.4
Elastofibroma —*see* Neoplasm, connective
    tissue, benign
Elastoma (juvenile) Q82.8
    Miescher's L87.2
Elastomyofibrosis I42.4
Elastosis
    actinic, solar L57.8
    atrophicans (senile) L57.4
    perforans serpiginosa L87.2
    senilis L57.4

Elbow —*see* condition
Electric current, electricity, effects (concussion)
    (fatal) (nonfatal) (shock) T75.4
    burn —*see* Burn
Electric feet syndrome E53.8
Electrocution T75.4
    from electroshock gun (taser) T75.4
Electrolyte imbalance E87.8
    with
        abortion —*see* Abortion by type,
            complicated by, electrolyte imbalance
        ectopic pregnancy O08.5
        molar pregnancy O08.5
Elephantiasis (nonfilarial) I89.0
    arabicum —*see* Infestation, filarial
    bancroftian B74.0
    congenital (any site) (hereditary) Q82.0
    due to
        Brugia (malayi) B74.1
            timori B74.2
        mastectomy I97.2
        Wuchereria (bancrofti) B74.0
    eyelid H02.859
        left H02.856
            lower H02.855
            upper H02.854
        right H02.853
            lower H02.852
            upper H02.851
    filarial, filariensis —*see* Infestation, filarial
    glandular I89.0
    graecorum A30.9
    lymphangiectatic I89.0
    lymphatic vessel I89.0
        due to mastectomy I97.2
    scrotum (nonfilarial) I89.0
    streptococcal I89.0
    surgical I97.89
        postmastectomy I97.2
    telangiectodes I89.0
    vulva (nonfilarial) N90.89
Elevated, elevation
    antibody titer R76.0
    basal metabolic rate R94.8
    blood pressure —*see also* Hypertension
        reading (incidental) (isolated) (nonspecific),
            no diagnosis of hypertension R03.0
    blood sugar R73.9
    body temperature (of unknown origin) R50.9
    C-reactive protein (CRP) R79.82
    cancer antigen 125 [CA 125] R97.1
    carcinoembryonic antigen [CEA] R97.0
    cholesterol E78.0
        with triglycerides E78.2
    conjugate, eye H51.0
    diaphragm, congenital Q79.1
    erythrocyte sedimentation rate R70.0
    fasting glucose R73.01
    fasting triglycerides E78.1
    finding on laboratory examination —*see*
        Findings, abnormal, inconclusive,
        without diagnosis, by type of exam
    GFR (glomerular filtration rate) —*see*
        Findings, abnormal, inconclusive,
        without diagnosis, by type of exam
    glucose tolerance (oral) R73.02
    immunoglobulin level R76.8
    indoleacetic acid R82.5
    lactic acid dehydrogenase (LDH) level R74.0
    leukocytes D72.829
    lipoprotein a level E78.8
    liver function
        study R94.5
        test R79.89
            alkaline phosphatase R74.8
            aminotransferase R74.0
            bilirubin R17
            hepatic enzyme R74.8
            lactate dehydrogenase R74.0
    lymphocytes D72.820
    prostate specific antigen [PSA] R97.2

Elevated, elevation (*Continued*)
    Rh titer —*see* Complication (s), transfusion,
        incompatibility reaction, Rh (factor)
    scapula, congenital Q74.0
    sedimentation rate R70.0
    SGOT R74.0
    SGPT R74.0
    transaminase level R74.0
    triglycerides E78.1
        with high cholesterol E78.2
    tumor associated antigens [TAA] NEC
        R97.8
    tumor specific antigens [TSA] NEC R97.8
    urine level of
        17-ketosteroids R82.5
        catecholamine R82.5
        indoleacetic acid R82.5
        steroids R82.5
        vanillylmandelic acid (VMA) R82.5
    venous pressure I87.8
    white blood cell count D72.829
        specified NEC D72.828
Elliptocytosis (congenital) (hereditary) D58.1
    Hb C (disease) D58.1
    hemoglobin disease D58.1
    sickle-cell (disease) D57.8-
        trait D57.3
Ellison-Zollinger syndrome E16.4
Ellis-van Creveld syndrome
    (chondroectodermal dysplasia) Q77.6
Elongated, elongation (congenital) —*see also*
    Distortion
    bone Q79.9
    cervix (uteri) Q51.828
        acquired N88.4
        hypertrophic N88.4
    colon Q43.8
    common bile duct Q44.5
    cystic duct Q44.5
    frenulum, penis Q55.69
    labia minora (acquired) N90.6
    ligamentum patellae Q74.1
    petiolus (epiglottidis) Q31.8
    tooth, teeth K00.2
    uvula Q38.6
Eltor cholera A00.1
Emaciation (due to malnutrition) E41
Embadomoniasis A07.8
Embedded tooth, teeth K01.0
    root only K08.3
Embolic —*see* condition
Embolism (multiple) (paradoxical) I74.9
    air (any site) (traumatic) T79.0
        following
            abortion —*see* Abortion by type
                complicated by embolism
            ectopic pregnancy O08.2
            infusion, therapeutic injection or
                transfusion T80.0
            molar pregnancy O08.2
            procedure NEC
                artery T81.719
                    mesenteric T81.710
                    renal T81.711
                    specified NEC T81.718
                vein T81.72
        in pregnancy, childbirth or puerperium —
            see Embolism, obstetric
    amniotic fluid (pulmonary) —*see also*
        Embolism, obstetric
        following
            abortion —*see* Abortion by type
                complicated by embolism
            ectopic pregnancy O08.2
            molar pregnancy O08.2
    aorta, aortic I74.10
        abdominal I74.09
            saddle I74.01
        bifurcation I74.09
            saddle I74.01
        thoracic I74.11

◄ New   ◄═ Revised   ~~deleted~~ Deleted

Embolism (Continued)
  vein (Continued)
    deep (Continued)
      upper leg I82.4Y
        chronic I82.5y--
      femoral I82.41-
        chronic I82.51-
      iliac (iliofemoral) I82.42-
        chronic I82.52-
      innominate I82.290
        chronic I82.291
      internal jugular I82.C1-
        chronic I82.C2-
      lower extremity
        deep I82.40-
          chronic I82.50-
          specified NEC I82.49-
            chronic NEC I82.59-
        distal
          deep I82.4Z-
        proximal
          deep I82.4Y-
            chronic I82.5Y-
        superficial I82.81-
      popliteal I82.43-
        chronic I82.53-
      radial I82.62-
        chronic I82.72-
      renal I82.3
      saphenous (greater) (lesser) I82.81-
      specified NEC I82.890
        chronic NEC I82.891
      subclavian I82.B1-
        chronic I82.B2-
      thoracic NEC I82.290
        chronic I82.291
      tibial I82.44-
        chronic I82.54-
      ulnar I82.62-
        chronic I82.72-
      upper extremity I82.60-
        chronic I82.70-
        deep I82.62-
          chronic I82.72-
        superficial I82.61-
          chronic I82.71-
  vena cava
    inferior (acute) I82.220
      chronic I82.221
    superior (acute) I82.210
      chronic I82.211
  venous sinus G08
  vessels of brain —see Occlusion, artery, cerebral
Embolus —see Embolism
Embryoma —see also Neoplasm, uncertain behavior, by site
  benign —see Neoplasm, benign, by site
  kidney C64.-
  liver C22.0
  malignant —see also Neoplasm, malignant, by site
    kidney C64.-
    liver C22.0
    testis C62.9-
      descended (scrotal) C62.1-
      undescended C62.0-
  testis C62.9-
    descended (scrotal) C62.1-
    undescended C62.0-
Embryonic
  circulation Q28.9
  heart Q28.9
  vas deferens Q55.4
Embryopathia NOS Q89.9
Embryotoxon Q13.4
Emesis —see Vomiting
Emotional lability R45.86
Emotionality, pathological F60.3
Emotogenic disease —see Disorder, psychogenic

Emphysema (atrophic) (bullous) (chronic) (interlobular) (lung) (obstructive) (pulmonary) (senile) (vesicular) J43.9
  cellular tissue (traumatic) T79.7
    surgical T81.82
  centrilobular J43.2
  compensatory J98.3
  congenital (interstitial) P25.0
  conjunctiva H11.89
  connective tissue (traumatic) T79.7
    surgical T81.82
  due to chemicals, gases, fumes or vapors J68.4
  eyelid (s) —see Disorder, eyelid, specified type NEC
    surgical T81.82
    traumatic T79.7
  interstitial J98.2
    congenital P25.0
    perinatal period P25.0
  laminated tissue T79.7
    surgical T81.82
  mediastinal J98.2
    newborn P25.2
  orbit, orbital —see Disorder, orbit, specified type NEC
  panacinar J43.1
  panlobular J43.1
  specified NEC J43.8
  subcutaneous (traumatic) T79.7
    nontraumatic J98.2
    postprocedural T81.82
    surgical T81.82
  surgical T81.82
  thymus (gland) (congenital) E32.8
  traumatic (subcutaneous) T79.7
  unilateral J43.0
Empty nest syndrome Z60.0
Empyema (acute) (chest) (double) (pleura) (supradiaphragmatic) (thorax) J86.9
  with fistula J86.0
  accessory sinus (chronic) —see Sinusitis
  antrum (chronic) —see Sinusitis, maxillary
  brain (any part) —see Abscess, brain
  ethmoidal (chronic) (sinus) —see Sinusitis, ethmoidal
  extradural —see Abscess, extradural
  frontal (chronic) (sinus) —see Sinusitis, frontal
  gallbladder K81.0
  mastoid (process) (acute) —see Mastoiditis, acute
  maxilla, maxillary M27.2
    sinus (chronic) —see Sinusitis, maxillary
  nasal sinus (chronic) —see Sinusitis
  sinus (accessory) (chronic) (nasal) —see Sinusitis
  sphenoidal (sinus) (chronic) —see Sinusitis, sphenoidal
  subarachnoid —see Abscess, extradural
  subdural —see Abscess, subdural
  tuberculous A15.6
  ureter —see Ureteritis
  ventricular —see Abscess, brain
En coup de sabre lesion L94.1
Enamel pearls K00.2
Enameloma K00.2
Enanthema, viral B09
Encephalitis (chronic) (hemorrhagic) (idiopathic) (nonepidemic) (spurious) (subacute) G04.90
  acute (see also Encephalitis, viral) A86
    disseminated G04.00
      infectious G04.01
      noninfectious G04.81
      postimmunization (postvaccination) G04.02
      postinfectious G04.01
    inclusion body A85.8

Encephalitis (Continued)
  acute (Continued)
    necrotizing hemorrhagic G04.30
      postimmunization G04.32
      postinfectious G04.31
      specified NEC G04.39
  arboviral, arbovirus NEC A85.2
  arthropod-borne NEC (viral) A85.2
  Australian A83.4
  California (virus) A83.5
  Central European (tick-borne) A84.1
  Czechoslovakian A84.1
  Dawson's (inclusion body) A81.1
  diffuse sclerosing A81.1
  disseminated, acute G04.00
  due to
    cat scratch disease A28.1
    human immunodeficiency virus (HIV) disease B20 [G05.3] ◀
    malaria —see Malaria
    rickettsiosis —see Rickettsiosis
    smallpox inoculation G04.02
    typhus —see Typhus
  Eastern equine A83.2
  endemic (viral) A86
  epidemic NEC (viral) A86
  equine (acute) (infectious) (viral) A83.9
    Eastern A83.2
    Venezuelan A92.2
    Western A83.1
  Far Eastern (tick-borne) A84.0
  following vaccination or other immunization procedure G04.02
  herpes zoster B02.0
  herpesviral B00.4
    due to herpesvirus 6 B10.01
    due to herpesvirus 7 B10.09
    specified NEC B10.09
  Ilheus (virus) A83.8
  in (due to)
    actinomycosis A42.82
    adenovirus A85.1
    African trypanosomiasis B56.9 [G05.3]
    Chagas' disease (chronic) B57.42
    cytomegalovirus B25.8
    enterovirus A85.0
    herpes (simplex) virus B00.4
      due to herpesvirus 6 B10.01
      due to herpesvirus 7 B10.09
      specified NEC B10.09
    infectious disease NEC B99 [G05.3]
    influenza —see Influenza, with, encephalopathy
    listeriosis A32.12
    measles B05.0
    mumps B26.2
    naegleriasis B60.2
    parasitic disease NEC B89 [G05.3]
    poliovirus A80.9 [G05.3]
    rubella B06.01
    syphilis
      congenital A50.42
      late A52.14
    systemic lupus erythematosus M32.19
    toxoplasmosis (acquired) B58.2
      congenital P37.1
    tuberculosis A17.82
    zoster B02.0
  inclusion body A81.1
  infectious (acute) (virus) NEC A86
  Japanese (B type) A83.0
  La Crosse A83.5
  lead —see Poisoning, lead
  lethargica (acute) (infectious) A85.8
  louping ill A84.8
  lupus erythematosus, systemic M32.19
  lymphatica A87.2
  Mengo A85.8
  meningococcal A39.81
  Murray Valley A83.4
  otitic NEC H66.40 [G05.3]

Encephalitis *(Continued)*
  parasitic NOS B71.9
  periaxial G37.0
  periaxialis (concentrica) (diffuse) G37.5
  postchickenpox B01.11
  postexanthematous NEC B09
  postimmunization G04.02
  postinfectious NEC G04.01
  postmeasles B05.0
  postvaccinal G04.02
  postvaricella B01.11
  postviral NEC A86
  Powassan A84.8
  Rasmussen G04.81
  Rio Bravo A85.8
  Russian
    autumnal A83.0
    spring-summer (taiga) A84.0
  saturnine —*see* Poisoning, lead
  specified NEC G04.81
  St. Louis A83.3
  subacute sclerosing A81.1
  summer A83.0
  suppurative G04.81
  tick-borne A84.9
  Torula, torular (cryptococcal) B45.1
  toxic NEC G92
  trichinosis B75 *[G05.3]*
  type
    B A83.0
    C A83.3
  van Bogaert's A81.1
  Venezuelan equine A92.2
  Vienna A85.8
  viral, virus A86
    arthropod-borne NEC A85.2
      mosquito-borne A83.9
        Australian X disease A83.4
        California virus A83.5
        Eastern equine A83.2
        Japanese (B type) A83.0
        Murray Valley A83.4
        specified NEC A83.8
        St. Louis A83.3
        type B A83.0
        type C A83.3
        Western equine A83.1
      tick-borne A84.9
        biundulant A84.1
        central European A84.1
        Czechoslovakian A84.1
        diphasic meningoencephalitis A84.1
        Far Eastern A84.0
        Russian spring-summer (taiga) A84.0
        specified NEC A84.8
      specified type NEC A85.8
    Western equine A83.1
Encephalocele Q01.9
  frontal Q01.0
  nasofrontal Q01.1
  occipital Q01.2
  specified NEC Q01.8
Encephalocystocele —*see* Encephalocele
Encephaloduroarteriomyosynangiosis (EDAMS) I67.5
Encephalomalacia (brain) (cerebellar) (cerebral) —*see* Softening, brain
Encephalomeningitis —*see* Meningoencephalitis
Encephalomeningocele —*see* Encephalocele
Encephalomeningomyelitis —*see* Meningoencephalitis
Encephalomyelitis *(see also* Encephalitis) G04.90
  acute disseminated G04.00
    infectious G04.01
    noninfectious G04.81
    postimmunization G04.02
    postinfectious G04.01

Encephalomyelitis *(Continued)*
  acute necrotizing hemorrhagic G04.30
    postimmunization G04.32
    postinfectious G04.31
    specified NEC G04.39
  benign myalgic G93.3
  equine A83.9
    Eastern A83.2
    Venezuelan A92.2
    Western A83.1
  in diseases classified elsewhere G05.3
  myalgic, benign G93.3
  postchickenpox B01.11
  postinfectious NEC G04.01
  postmeasles B05.0
  postvaccinal G04.02
  postvaricella B01.11
  rubella B06.01
  specified NEC G04.81
  Venezuelan equine A92.2
Encephalomyelocele —*see* Encephalocele
Encephalomyelomeningitis —*see* Meningoencephalitis
Encephalomyelopathy G96.9
Encephalomyeloradiculitis (acute) G61.0
Encephalomyeloradiculoneuritis (acute) (Guillain-Barré) G61.0
Encephalomyeloradiculopathy G96.9
Encephalopathia hyperbilirubinemica, newborn P57.9
  due to isoimmunization (conditions in P55) P57.0
Encephalopathy (acute) G93.40
  acute necrotizing hemorrhagic G04.30
    postimmunization G04.32
    postinfectious G04.31
    specified NEC G04.39
  alcoholic G31.2
  anoxic —*see* Damage, brain, anoxic
  arteriosclerotic I67.2
  centrolobar progressive (Schilder) G37.0
  congenital Q07.9
  degenerative, in specified disease NEC G32.89
  due to
    drugs *(see also* Table of Drugs and Chemicals) G92
  demyelinating callosal G37.1
  hepatic —*see* Failure, hepatic
  hyperbilirubinemic, newborn P57.9
    due to isoimmunization (conditions in P55) P57.0
  hypertensive I67.4
  hypoglycemic E16.2
  hypoxic —*see* Damage, brain, anoxic
  hypoxic ischemic P91.60
    mild P91.61
    moderate P91.62
    severe P91.63
  in (due to) (with)
    birth injury P11.1
    hyperinsulinism E16.1 *[G94]*
    influenza —*see* Influenza, with, encephalopathy
    lack of vitamin *(see also* Deficiency, vitamin) E56.9 *[G32.89]*
    neoplastic disease *(see also* Neoplasm) D49.9 *[G13.1]*
    serum *(see also* Reaction, serum) T80.69
    syphilis A52.17
    trauma (postconcussional) F07.81
      current injury —*see* Injury, intracranial
    vaccination G04.02
  lead —*see* Poisoning, lead
  metabolic G93.41
    drug induced G92
    toxic G92
  myoclonic, early, symptomatic —*see* Epilepsy, generalized, specified NEC
  necrotizing, subacute (Leigh) G31.82
  pellagrous E52 *[G32.89]*

Encephalopathy *(Continued)*
  portosystemic —*see* Failure, hepatic
  postcontusional F07.81
    current injury —*see* Injury, intracranial, diffuse
  posthypoglycemic (coma) E16.1 *[G94]*
  postradiation G93.89
  saturnine —*see* Poisoning, lead
  septic G93.41
  specified NEC G93.49
  spongioform, subacute (viral) A81.09
  toxic G92
    metabolic G92
  traumatic (postconcussional) F07.81
    current injury —*see* Injury, intracranial
  vitamin B deficiency NEC E53.9 *[G32.89]*
    vitamin B1 E51.2
  Wernicke's E51.2
Encephalorrhagia —*see* Hemorrhage, intracranial, intracerebral
Encephalosis, posttraumatic F07.81
Enchondroma —*see also* Neoplasm, bone, benign
Enchondromatosis (cartilaginous) (multiple) Q78.4
Encopresis R15.9
  functional F98.1
  nonorganic origin F98.1
  psychogenic F98.1
Encounter (with health service) (for) Z76.89
  adjustment and management (of)
    breast implant Z45.81
    implanted device NEC Z45.89
    myringotomy device (stent) (tube) Z45.82
  administrative purpose only Z02.9
    examination for
      adoption Z02.82
      armed forces Z02.3
      disability determination Z02.71
      driving license Z02.4
      employment Z02.1
      insurance Z02.6
      medical certificate NEC Z02.79
      paternity testing Z02.81
      residential institution admission Z02.2
      school admission Z02.0
      sports Z02.5
      specified reason NEC Z02.89
  aftercare —*see* Aftercare
  antenatal screening Z36
  assisted reproductive fertility procedure cycle Z31.83
  blood typing Z01.83
    Rh typing Z01.83
  breast augmentation or reduction Z41.1
  breast implant exchange (different material) (different size) Z45.81
  breast reconstruction following mastectomy Z42.1
  check-up —*see* Examination
  chemotherapy for neoplasm Z51.11
  colonoscopy, screening Z12.11
  counseling —*see* Counseling
  delivery, full-term, uncomplicated O80
    cesarean, without indication O82
  ear piercing Z41.3
  examination —*see* Examination
  expectant parent (s) (adoptive) pre-birth pediatrician visit Z76.81
  fertility preservation procedure (prior to cancer therapy) (prior to removal of gonads) Z31.84
  fitting (of) —*see* Fitting (and adjustment) (of)
  genetic
    counseling Z31.5
    testing —*see* Test, genetic
  hearing conservation and treatment Z01.12
  immunotherapy for neoplasm Z51.12
  in vitro fertilization cycle Z31.83

◄ New ◄ Revised deleted Deleted

Encounter *(Continued)*
  instruction (in)
    child care (postpartal) (prenatal) Z32.3
    childbirth Z32.2
    natural family planning
      procreative Z31.61
      to avoid pregnancy Z30.02
  insulin pump titration Z46.81
  joint prosthesis insertion following prior
      explantation of joint prosthesis (staged
      procedure)
    hip Z47.32
    knee Z47.33
    shoulder Z47.31
  laboratory (as part of a general medical
      examination) Z00.00
    with abnormal findings Z00.01
  mental health services (for)
    abuse NEC
      perpetrator Z69.82
      victim Z69.81
    child abuse
      nonparental
        perpetrator Z69.021
        victim Z69.020
      parental
        perpetrator Z69.011
        victim Z69.010
    spousal or partner abuse
      perpetrator Z69.12
      victim Z69.11
  observation (for) (ruled out)
    exposure to (suspected)
      anthrax Z03.810
      biological agent NEC Z03.818
  pediatrician visit, by expectant parent (s)
      (adoptive) Z76.81
  plastic and reconstructive surgery following
      medical procedure or healed injury
      NEC Z42.8
  pregnancy
    supervision of —*see* Pregnancy,
        supervision of
    test Z32.00
      result negative Z32.02
      result positive Z32.01
  radiation therapy (antineoplastic) Z51.0
  radiological (as part of a general medical
      examination) Z00.00
    with abnormal findings Z00.01
  reconstructive surgery following medical
      procedure or healed injury NEC Z42.8
  removal (of) —*see also* Removal
    artificial
      arm Z44.00-
        complete Z44.01-
        partial Z44.02-
      eye Z44.2-
      leg Z44.10-
        complete Z44.11-
        partial Z44.12-
    breast implant Z45.81
      tissue expander (without synchronous
          insertion of permanent implant)
          Z45.81
    device Z46.9
      specified NEC Z46.89
    external
      fixation device — code to fracture with
          seventh character D
      prosthesis, prosthetic device Z44.9
        breast Z44.3-
        specified NEC Z44.8
    implanted device NEC Z45.89
    insulin pump Z46.81
    internal fixation device Z47.2
    myringotomy device (stent) (tube) Z45.82
    nervous system device NEC Z46.2
      brain neuropacemaker Z46.2
      visual substitution device Z46.2
        implanted Z45.31

Encounter *(Continued)*
  removal *(Continued)*
    non-vascular catheter Z46.82
    orthodontic device Z46.4
    stent
      ureteral Z46.6
    urinary device Z46.6
  repeat cervical smear to confirm findings of
      recent normal smear following initial
      abnormal smear Z01.42
  respirator [ventilator] use during power
      failure (Z99.12)
  Rh typing Z01.83
  screening —*see* Screening
  specified NEC Z76.89
  sterilization Z30.2
  suspected condition, ruled out
    amniotic cavity and membrane Z03.71
    cervical shortening Z03.75
    fetal anomaly Z03.73
    fetal growth Z03.74
    maternal and fetal conditions NEC Z03.79
    oligohydramnios Z03.71
    placental problem Z03.72
    polyhydramnios Z03.71
  suspected exposure (to), ruled out
    anthrax Z03.810
    biological agents NEC Z03.818
  termination of pregnancy, elective Z33.2
  testing —*see* Test
  therapeutic drug level monitoring Z51.81
  titration, insulin pump Z46.81
  to determine fetal viability of pregnancy
      O36.80
  training
    insulin pump Z46.81
  X-ray of chest (as part of a general medical
      examination Z00.00)
    with abnormal findings Z00.01
Encystment —*see* Cyst
Endarteritis (bacterial, subacute) (infective)
    I77.6
  brain I67.7
  cerebral or cerebrospinal I67.7
  deformans —*see* Arteriosclerosis
  embolic —*see* Embolism
  obliterans —*see also* Arteriosclerosis
    pulmonary I28.8
  pulmonary I28.8
  retina —*see* Vasculitis, retina
  senile —*see* Arteriosclerosis
  syphilitic A52.09
    brain or cerebral A52.04
    congenital A50.54 *[I79.8]*
  tuberculous A18.89
Endemic —*see* condition
Endocarditis (chronic) (marantic) (nonbacterial)
    (thrombotic) (valvular) I38
  with rheumatic fever (conditions in I00)
    active —*see* Endocarditis, acute, rheumatic
    inactive or quiescent (with chorea) I09.1
  acute or subacute I33.9
    infective I33.0
    rheumatic (aortic) (mitral) (pulmonary)
        (tricuspid) I01.1
      with chorea (acute) (rheumatic)
          (Sydenham's) I02.0
  aortic (heart) (nonrheumatic) (valve) I35.8
    with
      mitral disease I08.0
        with tricuspid (valve) disease I08.3
        active or acute I01.1
          with chorea (acute) (rheumatic)
              (Sydenham's) I02.0
      rheumatic fever (conditions in I00)
        active —*see* Endocarditis, acute,
            rheumatic
        inactive or quiescent (with chorea)
            I06.9
      tricuspid (valve) disease I08.2
        with mitral (valve) disease I08.3

Endocarditis *(Continued)*
  aortic *(Continued)*
    acute or subacute I33.9
    arteriosclerotic I35.8
    rheumatic I06.9
      with mitral disease I08.0
        with tricuspid (valve) disease I08.3
        active or acute I01.1
          with chorea (acute) (rheumatic)
              (Sydenham's) I02.0
      active or acute I01.1
        with chorea (acute) (rheumatic)
            (Sydenham's) I02.0
      specified NEC I06.8
    specified cause NEC I35.8
    syphilitic A52.03
  arteriosclerotic I38
  atypical verrucous (Libman-Sacks) M32.11
  bacterial (acute) (any valve) (subacute) I33.0
  candidal B37.6
  congenital Q24.8
  constrictive I33.0
  Coxiella burnetii A78 *[I39]*
  Coxsackie B33.21
  due to
    prosthetic cardiac valve T82.6
    Q fever A78 *[I39]*
    Serratia marcescens I33.0
    typhoid (fever) A01.02
  gonococcal A54.83
  infectious or infective (acute) (any valve)
      (subacute) I33.0
  lenta (acute) (any valve) (subacute) I33.0
  Libman-Sacks M32.11
  listerial A32.82
  Löffler's I42.3
  malignant (acute) (any valve) (subacute) I33.0
  meningococcal A39.51
  mitral (chronic) (double) (fibroid) (heart)
      (inactive) (valve) (with chorea) I05.9
    with
      aortic (valve) disease I08.0
        with tricuspid (valve) disease I08.3
        active or acute I01.1
          with chorea (acute) (rheumatic)
              (Sydenham's) I02.0
      rheumatic fever (conditions in I00)
        active —*see* Endocarditis, acute,
            rheumatic
        inactive or quiescent (with chorea)
            I05.9
      tricuspid (valve) disease I08.1
        with aortic (valve) disease I08.3
    active or acute I01.1
      with chorea (acute) (rheumatic)
          (Sydenham's) I02.0
    bacterial I33.0
    arteriosclerotic I34.8
    nonrheumatic I34.8
      acute or subacute I33.9
    specified NEC I05.8
  monilial B37.6
  multiple valves I08.9
    specified disorders I08.8
  mycotic (acute) (any valve) (subacute) I33.0
  pneumococcal (acute) (any valve) (subacute)
      I33.0
  pulmonary (chronic) (heart) (valve) I37.8
    with rheumatic fever (conditions in I00)
      active —*see* Endocarditis, acute,
          rheumatic
      inactive or quiescent (with chorea)
          I09.89
        with aortic, mitral or tricuspid disease
            I08.8
    acute or subacute I33.9
      rheumatic I01.1
        with chorea (acute) (rheumatic)
            (Sydenham's) I02.0
    arteriosclerotic I37.8
    congenital Q22.2

Endocarditis *(Continued)*
  pulmonary *(Continued)*
    rheumatic (chronic) (inactive) (with chorea)
        I09.89
      active or acute I01.1
        with chorea (acute) (rheumatic)
            (Sydenham's) I02.0
    syphilitic A52.03
  purulent (acute) (any valve) (subacute) I33.0
  Q fever A78 [I39]
  rheumatic (chronic) (inactive) (with chorea)
        I09.1
    active or acute (aortic) (mitral)
        (pulmonary) (tricuspid) I01.1
      with chorea (acute) (rheumatic)
          (Sydenham's) I02.0
  rheumatoid —*see* Rheumatoid, carditis
  septic (acute) (any valve) (subacute) I33.0
  streptococcal (acute) (any valve) (subacute)
        I33.0
  subacute —*see* Endocarditis, acute
  suppurative (acute) (any valve) (subacute)
        I33.0
  syphilitic A52.03
  toxic I33.9
  tricuspid (chronic) (heart) (inactive)
        (rheumatic) (valve) (with chorea) I07.9
    with
      aortic (valve) disease I08.2
        mitral (valve) disease I08.3
      mitral (valve) disease I08.1
        aortic (valve) disease I08.3
      rheumatic fever (conditions in I00)
        active —*see* Endocarditis, acute,
            rheumatic
        inactive or quiescent (with chorea)
            I07.8
    active or acute I01.1
      with chorea (acute) (rheumatic)
          (Sydenham's) I02.0
  arteriosclerotic I36.8
  nonrheumatic I36.8
    acute or subacute I33.9
    specified cause, except rheumatic I36.8
  tuberculous —*see* Tuberculosis, endocarditis
  typhoid A01.02
  ulcerative (acute) (any valve) (subacute) I33.0
  vegetative (acute) (any valve) (subacute) I33.0
  verrucous (atypical) (nonbacterial)
        (nonrheumatic) M32.11
Endocardium, endocardial —*see also* condition
  cushion defect Q21.2
Endocervicitis —*see also* Cervicitis
  due to intrauterine (contraceptive) device
        T83.6
  hyperplastic N72
Endocrine —*see* condition
Endocrinopathy, pluriglandular E31.9
Endodontic
  overfill M27.52
  underfill M27.53
Endodontitis K04.0
Endomastoiditis —*see* Mastoiditis
Endometrioma N80.9
Endometriosis N80.9
  appendix N80.5
  bladder N80.8
  bowel N80.5
  broad ligament N80.3
  cervix N80.0
  colon N80.5
  cul-de-sac (Douglas') N80.3
  exocervix N80.0
  fallopian tube N80.2
  female genital organ NEC N80.8
  gallbladder N80.8
  in scar of skin N80.6
  internal N80.0
  intestine N80.5
  lung N80.8
  myometrium N80.0

Endometriosis *(Continued)*
  ovary N80.1
  parametrium N80.3
  pelvic peritoneum N80.3
  peritoneal (pelvic) N80.3
  rectovaginal septum N80.4
  rectum N80.5
  round ligament N80.3
  skin (scar) N80.6
  specified site NEC N80.8
  stromal D39.0
  umbilicus N80.8
  uterus (internal) N80.0
  vagina N80.4
  vulva N80.8
Endometritis (decidual) (nonspecific)
        (purulent) (senile (atrophic) (suppurative)
        N71.9
  with ectopic pregnancy O08.0
  acute N71.0
  blenorrhagic (gonococcal) (acute) (chronic)
        A54.24
  cervix, cervical (with erosion or ectropion) —
        see also Cervicitis
    hyperplastic N72
  chlamydial A56.11
  chronic N71.1
  following
    abortion —*see* Abortion by type
        complicated by genital infection
    ectopic or molar pregnancy O08.0
  gonococcal, gonorrheal (acute) (chronic)
        A54.24
  hyperplastic (*see also* Hyperplasia,
        endometrial) N85.00- ◄▥
    cervix N72
  puerperal, postpartum, childbirth O86.12
  subacute N71.0
  tuberculous A18.17
Endometrium —*see* condition
Endomyocardiopathy, South African I42.3
Endomyocarditis —*see* Endocarditis
Endomyofibrosis I42.3
Endomyometritis —*see* Endometritis
Endopericarditis —*see* Endocarditis
Endoperineuritis —*see* Disorder, nerve
Endophlebitis —*see* Phlebitis
Endophthalmia —*see* Endophthalmitis,
        purulent
Endophthalmitis (acute) (infective) (metastatic)
        (subacute) H44.009
  bleb associated H59.4 —*see also* Bleb,
        inflamed (infected), postprocedural
  gonorrheal A54.39
  in (due to)
    cysticercosis B69.1
    onchocerciasis B73.01
    toxocariasis B83.0
  panuveitis —*see* Panuveitis
  parasitic H44.12-
  purulent H44.00-
    panophthalmitis —*see* Panophthalmitis
    vitreous abscess H44.02-
  specified NEC H44.19
  sympathetic —*see* Uveitis, sympathetic
Endosalpingioma D28.2
Endosalpingiosis N94.89
Endosteitis —*see* Osteomyelitis
Endothelioma, bone —*see* Neoplasm, bone,
        malignant
Endotheliosis (hemorrhagic infectional) D69.8
Endotoxemia — code to condition
Endotrachelitis —*see* Cervicitis
Engelmann (-Camurati) syndrome Q78.3
English disease —*see* Rickets
Engman's disease L30.3
Engorgement
  breast N64.59
    newborn P83.4
    puerperal, postpartum O92.79
  lung (passive) —*see* Edema, lung

Engorgement *(Continued)*
  pulmonary (passive) —*see* Edema, lung
  stomach K31.89
  venous, retina —*see* Occlusion, retina, vein,
        engorgement
Enlargement, enlarged —*see also* Hypertrophy
  adenoids J35.2
    with tonsils J35.3
  alveolar ridge K08.8
    congenital —*see* Anomaly, alveolar
  apertures of diaphragm (congenital) Q79.1
  gingival K06.1
  heart, cardiac —*see* Hypertrophy, cardiac
  lacrimal gland, chronic H04.03-
  liver —*see* Hypertrophy, liver
  lymph gland or node R59.9
    generalized R59.1
    localized R59.0
  orbit H05.34-
  organ or site, congenital NEC —*see* Anomaly,
        by site
  parathyroid (gland) E21.0
  pituitary fossa R93.0
  prostate N40.0
    with lower urinary tract symptoms (LUTS)
        N40.1
    without lower urinary tract symptoms
        (LUTS) N40.0
  sella turcica R93.0
  spleen —*see* Splenomegaly
  thymus (gland) (congenital) E32.0
  thyroid (gland) —*see* Goiter
  tongue K14.8
  tonsils J35.1
    with adenoids J35.3
  uterus N85.2
Enophthalmos H05.40-
  due to
    orbital tissue atrophy H05.41-
    trauma or surgery H05.42-
Enostosis M27.8
Entamebic, entamebiasis —*see* Amebiasis
Entanglement
  umbilical cord (s) O69.2
    with compression O69.2
      without compression O69.82
    around neck (with compression) O69.1
      without compression O69.81
    of twins in monoamniotic sac O69.2
Enteralgia —*see* Pain, abdominal
Enteric —*see* condition
Enteritis (acute) (diarrheal) (hemorrhagic)
        (noninfective) (septic) K52.9
  adenovirus A08.2
  aertrycke infection A02.0
  allergic K52.2
  amebic (acute) A06.0
    with abscess —*see* Abscess, amebic
    chronic A06.1
      with abscess —*see* Abscess, amebic
      nondysenteric A06.2
    nondysenteric A06.2
  astrovirus A08.32
  bacillary NOS A03.9
  bacterial A04.9
    specified NEC A04.8
  calicivirus A08.31
  candidal B37.82
  Chilomastix A07.8
  choleriformis A00.1
  chronic (noninfectious) K52.9
    ulcerative —*see* Colitis, ulcerative
  cicatrizing (chronic) —*see* Enteritis, regional,
        small intestine
  Clostridium
    botulinum (food poisoning) A05.1
    difficile A04.7
  coccidial A07.3
  coxsackie virus A08.39
  dietetic K52.2
  drug-induced K52.1

◄ New   ◄▥ Revised   ~~deleted~~ Deleted

Enteritis *(Continued)*
  due to
    astrovirus A08.32
    calicivirus A08.31
    coxsackie virus A08.39
    drugs K52.1
    echovirus A08.39
    enterovirus NEC A08.39
    food hypersensitivity K52.2
    infectious organism (bacterial) (viral) —*see* Enteritis, infectious ◄═
    torovirus A08.39
    Yersinia enterocolitica A04.6
  echovirus A08.39
  eltor A00.1
  enterovirus NEC A08.39
  eosinophilic K52.81
  epidemic (infectious) A09
  fulminant K55.0
  gangrenous —*see* Enteritis, infectious
  giardial A07.1
  infectious NOS A09
    due to
      adenovirus A08.2
      Aerobacter aerogenes A04.8
      Arizona (bacillus) A02.0
      bacteria NOS A04.9
        specified NEC A04.8
      Campylobacter A04.5
      Clostridium difficile A04.7
      Clostridium perfringens A04.8
      Enterobacter aerogenes A04.8
      enterovirus A08.39
      Escherichia coli A04.4
        enteroaggregative A04.4
        enterohemorrhagic A04.3
        enteroinvasive A04.2
        enteropathogenic A04.0
        enterotoxigenic A04.1
        specified NEC A04.4
      specified
        bacteria NEC A04.8
        virus NEC A08.39
      Staphylococcus A04.8
      virus NEC A08.4
        specified type NEC A08.39
      Yersinia enterocolitica A04.6
    specified organism NEC A08.8
  influenzal —*see* Influenza, with, digestive manifestations
  ischemic K55.9
    acute K55.0
    chronic K55.1
  microsporidial A07.8
  mucomembranous, myxomembranous —*see* Syndrome, irritable bowel ◄═
  mucous —*see* Syndrome, irritable bowel
  necroticans A05.2
  necrotizing of newborn —*see* Enterocolitis, necrotizing, in newborn
  neurogenic —*see* Syndrome, irritable bowel
  newborn necrotizing —*see* Enterocolitis, necrotizing, in newborn
  noninfectious K52.9
  norovirus A08.11
  parasitic NEC B82.9
  paratyphoid (fever) —*see* Fever, paratyphoid
  protozoal A07.9
    specified NEC A07.8
  radiation K52.0
  regional (of) K50.90
    with
      complication K50.919
        abscess K50.914
        fistula K50.913
        intestinal obstruction K50.912
        rectal bleeding K50.911
        specified complication NEC K50.918
    colon —*see* Enteritis, regional, large intestine

Enteritis *(Continued)*
  regional *(Continued)*
    duodenum —*see* Enteritis, regional, small intestine
    ileum —*see* Enteritis, regional, small intestine
    jejunum —*see* Enteritis, regional, small intestine
    large bowel —*see* Enteritis, regional, large intestine
    large intestine (colon) (rectum) K50.10
      with
        complication K50.119
          abscess K50.114
          fistula K50.113
          intestinal obstruction K50.112
          rectal bleeding K50.111
          small intestine (duodenum) (ileum) (jejunum) involvement K50.80
            with
              complication K50.819
                abscess K50.814
                fistula K50.813
                intestinal obstruction K50.812
                rectal bleeding K50.811
                specified complication NEC K50.818
          specified complication NEC K50.118
    rectum —*see* Enteritis, regional, large intestine
    small intestine (duodenum) (ileum) (jejunum) K50.00
      with
        complication K50.019
          abscess K50.014
          fistula K50.013
          intestinal obstruction K50.012
          large intestine (colon) (rectum) involvement K50.80
            with
              complication K50.819
                abscess K50.814
                fistula K50.813
                intestinal obstruction K50.812
                rectal bleeding K50.811
                specified complication NEC K50.818
          rectal bleeding K50.011
          specified complication NEC K50.018
  rotaviral A08.0
  Salmonella, salmonellosis (arizonae) (cholerae-suis) (enteritidis) (typhimurium) A02.0
  segmental —*see* Enteritis, regional
  septic A09
  Shigella —*see* Infection, Shigella
  small round structured NEC A08.19
  spasmodic, spastic —*see* Syndrome, irritable bowel
  staphylococcal A04.8
    due to food A05.0
  torovirus A08.39
  toxic NEC K52.1
    due to Clostridium difficile A04.7
  trichomonal A07.8
  tuberculous A18.32
  typhosa A01.00
  ulcerative (chronic) —*see* Colitis, ulcerative
  viral A08.4
    adenovirus A08.2
    enterovirus A08.39
    Rotavirus A08.0
    small round structured NEC A08.19
    specified NEC A08.39
    virus specified NEC A08.39
Enterobiasis B80
Enterobius vermicularis (infection) (infestation) B80

Enterocele —*see also* Hernia, abdomen
  pelvic, pelvis (acquired) (congenital) N81.5
  vagina, vaginal (acquired) (congenital) NEC N81.5
Enterocolitis *(see also* Enteritis) K52.9
  due to Clostridium difficile A04.7
  fulminant ischemic K55.0
  granulomatous —*see* Enteritis, regional
  hemorrhagic (acute) K55.0
    chronic K55.1
  infectious NEC A09
  ischemic K55.9
  necrotizing
    due to Clostridium difficile A04.7
    in newborn P77.9
      stage 1 (without pneumatosis, without perforation) P77.1
      stage 2 (with pneumatosis, without perforation) P77.2
      stage 3 (with pneumatosis, with perforation) P77.3
  noninfectious K52.9
    newborn —*see* Enterocolitis, necrotizing, in newborn
  pseudomembranous (newborn) A04.7
  radiation K52.0
    newborn —*see* Enterocolitis, necrotizing, in newborn
  ulcerative (chronic) —*see* Pancolitis, ulcerative (chronic)
Enterogastritis —*see* Enteritis
Enteropathy K63.9
  gluten-sensitive K90.0
  hemorrhagic, terminal K55.0
  protein-losing K90.4
Enteroperitonitis —*see* Peritonitis
Enteroptosis K63.4
Enterorrhagia K92.2
Enterospasm —*see also* Syndrome, irritable, bowel
  psychogenic F45.8
Enterostenosis —*see also* Obstruction, intestine K56.69 ◄═
Enterostomy
  complication —*see* Complication, enterostomy
  status Z93.4
Enterovirus, as cause of disease classified elsewhere B97.10
  coxsackievirus B97.11
  echovirus B97.12
  other specified B97.19
Enthesopathy (peripheral) M77.9
  Achilles tendinitis —*see* Tendinitis, Achilles
  ankle and tarsus M77.9
    specified type NEC —*see* Enthesopathy, foot, specified type NEC
  anterior tibial syndrome M76.81-
  calcaneal spur —*see* Spur, bone, calcaneal
  elbow region M77.8
    lateral epicondylitis —*see* Epicondylitis, lateral
    medial epicondylitis —*see* Epicondylitis, medial
  foot NEC M77.9
    metatarsalgia —*see* Metatarsalgia
    specified type NEC M77.5-
  forearm M77.9
  gluteal tendinitis —*see* Tendinitis, gluteal
  hand M77.9
  hip —*see* Enthesopathy, lower limb, specified type NEC
  iliac crest spur —*see* Spur, bone, iliac crest
  iliotibial band syndrome —*see* Syndrome, iliotibial band
  knee —*see* Enthesopathy, lower limb, lower leg, specified type NEC
  lateral epicondylitis —*see* Epicondylitis, lateral

Enthesopathy (Continued)
  lower limb (excluding foot) M76.9
    Achilles tendinitis —see Tendinitis, Achilles
    anterior tibial syndrome M76.81-
    gluteal tendinitis —see Tendinitis, gluteal
    iliac crest spur —see Spur, bone, iliac crest
    iliotibial band syndrome —see Syndrome,
      iliotibial band
    patellar tendinitis —see Tendinitis, patellar
    pelvic region —see Enthesopathy, lower
      limb, specified type NEC
    peroneal tendinitis —see Tendinitis,
      peroneal
    posterior tibial syndrome M76.82-
    psoas tendinitis —see Tendinitis, psoas
    shoulder M77.9
    specified type NEC M76.89-
    tibial collateral bursitis —see Bursitis, tibial
      collateral
  medial epicondylitis —see Epicondylitis,
    medial
  multiple sites M77.9
  patellar tendinitis —see Tendinitis, patellar
  pelvis M77.9
  periarthritis of wrist —see Periarthritis,
    wrist
  peroneal tendinitis —see Tendinitis,
    peroneal
  posterior tibial syndrome M76.82-
  psoas tendinitis —see Tendinitis, psoas
  shoulder region —see Lesion, shoulder
  specified site NEC M77.9
  specified type NEC M77.8
  spinal M46.00
    cervical region M46.02
    cervicothoracic region M46.03
    lumbar region M46.06
    lumbosacral region M46.07
    multiple sites M46.09
    occipito-atlanto-axial region M46.01
    sacrococcygeal region M46.08
    thoracic region M46.04
    thoracolumbar region M46.05
  tibial collateral bursitis —see Bursitis, tibial
    collateral
  upper arm M77.9
  wrist and carpus NEC M77.8
    calcaneal spur —see Spur, bone, calcaneal
    periarthritis of wrist —see Periarthritis,
      wrist
Entomophobia F40.218
Entomophthoromycosis B46.8
Entrance, air into vein —see Embolism, air
Entrapment, nerve —see Neuropathy,
  entrapment
Entropion (eyelid) (paralytic) H02.009
  cicatricial H02.019
    left H02.016
      lower H02.015
      upper H02.014
    right H02.013
      lower H02.012
      upper H02.011
  congenital Q10.2
  left H02.006
    lower H02.005
    upper H02.004
  mechanical H02.029
    left H02.026
      lower H02.025
      upper H02.024
    right H02.023
      lower H02.022
      upper H02.021
  right H02.003
    lower H02.002
    upper H02.001
  senile H02.039
    left H02.036
      lower H02.035
      upper H02.034

Entropion (Continued)
  senile (Continued)
    right H02.033
      lower H02.032
      upper H02.031
  spastic H02.049
    left H02.046
      lower H02.045
      upper H02.044
    right H02.043
      lower H02.042
      upper H02.041
Enucleated eye (traumatic, current) S05.7-
Enuresis R32
  functional F98.0
  habit disturbance F98.0
  nocturnal N39.44
    psychogenic F98.0
  nonorganic origin F98.0
  psychogenic F98.0
Eosinopenia —see Agranulocytosis
Eosinophilia (allergic) (hereditary) (idiopathic)
    (secondary) D72.1
  with
    angiolymphoid hyperplasia (ALHE)
      D18.01
    infiltrative J82
    Löffler's J82
  peritoneal —see Peritonitis, eosinophilic
  pulmonary NEC J82
  tropical (pulmonary) J82
Eosinophilia-myalgia syndrome M35.8
Ependymitis (acute) (cerebral) (chronic)
    (granular) —see Encephalomyelitis
Ependymoblastoma
  specified site —see Neoplasm, malignant, by
    site
  unspecified site C71.9
Ependymoma (epithelial) (malignant)
  anaplastic
    specified site —see Neoplasm, malignant,
      by site
    unspecified site C71.9
  benign
    specified site —see Neoplasm, benign, by
      site
    unspecified site D33.2
  myxopapillary D43.2
    specified site —see Neoplasm, uncertain
      behavior, by site
    unspecified site D43.2
  papillary D43.2
    specified site —see Neoplasm, uncertain
      behavior, by site
    unspecified site D43.2
  specified site —see Neoplasm, malignant, by
    site
  unspecified site C71.9
Ependymopathy G93.89
Ephelis, ephelides L81.2
Epiblepharon (congenital) Q10.3
Epicanthus, epicanthic fold (eyelid)
    (congenital) Q10.3
Epicondylitis (elbow)
  lateral M77.1-
  medial M77.0-
Epicystitis —see Cystitis
Epidemic —see condition
Epidermidalization, cervix —see Dysplasia,
  cervix
Epidermis, epidermal —see condition
Epidermodysplasia verruciformis B07.8
Epidermolysis
  bullosa (congenital) Q81.9
    acquired L12.30
      drug-induced L12.31
      specified cause NEC L12.35
    dystrophica Q81.2
    letalis Q81.1
    simplex Q81.0
    specified NEC Q81.8

Epidermolysis (Continued)
  necroticans combustiformis L51.2
    due to drug —see Table of Drugs and
      Chemicals, by drug ◀◀◀◀
Epidermophytid —see Dermatophytosis
Epidermophytosis (infected) —see
  Dermatophytosis
Epididymis —see condition
Epididymitis (acute) (nonvenereal) (recurrent)
    (residual) N45.1
  with orchitis N45.3
  blennorrhagic (gonococcal) A54.23
  caseous (tuberculous) A18.15
  chlamydial A56.19
  filarial (see also Infestation, filarial) B74.9
    [N51] ◀◀◀◀
  gonococcal A54.23
  syphilitic A52.76
  tuberculous A18.15
Epididymo-orchitis (see also Epididymitis) N45.3
Epidural —see condition
Epigastrium, epigastric —see condition
Epigastrocele —see Hernia, ventral
Epiglottis —see condition
Epiglottitis, epiglottiditis (acute) J05.10
  with obstruction J05.11
  chronic J37.0
Epignathus Q89.4
Epilepsia partialis continua (see also
  Kozhevnikof's epilepsy) G40.1-
Epilepsy, epileptic, epilepsia (attack) (cerebral)
    (convulsion) (fit) (seizure) G40.909

> Note: the following terms are to be
> considered equivalent to intractable:
> pharmacoresistant (pharmacologically
> resistant), treatment resistant, refractory
> (medically) and poorly controlled

  with
    complex partial seizures —see Epilepsy,
      localization-related, symptomatic,
      with complex partial seizures
    grand mal seizures on awakening —see
      Epilepsy, generalized, specified NEC
    myoclonic absences —see Epilepsy,
      generalized, specified NEC
    myoclonic-astatic seizures —see Epilepsy,
      generalized, specified NEC
    simple partial seizures —see Epilepsy,
      localization-related, symptomatic,
      with simple partial seizures
  akinetic —see Epilepsy, generalized, specified
    NEC
  benign childhood with centrotemporal EEG
    spikes —see Epilepsy, localization-
    related, idiopathic
  benign myoclonic in infancy G40.80-
  Bravais-jacksonian —see Epilepsy,
    localization-related, symptomatic,
    with simple partial seizures
  ~~childhood with occipital EEG paroxysms —see~~
    ~~Epilepsy, localization-related, idiopathic~~
  ~~childhood absence G40.A09~~
    ~~intractable G40.A19~~
      ~~with status epilepticus G40.A11~~
      ~~without status epilepticus G40.A19~~
    ~~not intractable G40.A09~~
      ~~with status epilepticus G40.A01~~
      ~~without status epilepticus G40.A09~~
  childhood ◀
    with occipital EEG paroxysms —see
      Epilepsy, localization-related,
      idiopathic
    absence G40.A09 ◀
      intractable G40.A19 ◀
        with status epilepticus G40.A11 ◀
        without status epilepticus G40.A19 ◀
      not intractable G40.A09 ◀
        with status epilepticus G40.A01 ◀
        without status epilepticus G40.A09 ◀

◀ New   ◀◀◀◀ Revised   ~~deleted~~ Deleted

Epilepsy, epileptic, epilepsia *(Continued)*
  climacteric —*see* Epilepsy, specified NEC
  cysticercosis B69.0
  deterioration (mental) F06.8
  due to syphilis A52.19
  focal —*see* Epilepsy, localization-related,
    symptomatic, with simple partial
    seizures
  generalized
    idiopathic G40.309
      intractable G40.319
        with status epilepticus G40.311
        without status epilepticus G40.319
      not intractable G40.309
        with status epilepticus G40.301
        without status epilepticus G40.309
    specified NEC G40.409
      intractable G40.419
        with status epilepticus G40.411
        without status epilepticus G40.419
      not intractable G40.409
        with status epilepticus G40.401
        without status epilepticus G40.409
  impulsive petit mal —*see* Epilepsy, juvenile
    myoclonic
  intractable G40.919
    with status epilepticus G40.911
    without status epilepticus G40.919
  juvenile absence G40.A09
    intractable G40.A19
      with status epilepticus G40.A11
      without status epilepticus G40.A19
    not intractable G40.A09
      with status epilepticus G40.A01
      without status epilepticus G40.A09
  juvenile myoclonic G40.B11
    intractable G40.B19
      with status epilepticus G40.B11
      without status epilepticus G40.B19
    not intractable G40.B09
      with status epilepticus G40.B01
      without status epilepticus G40.B09
  localization-related (focal) (partial)
    idiopathic G40.009
      with seizures of localized onset G40.009
        intractable G40.019
          with status epilepticus G40.011
          without status epilepticus G40.019
        not intractable G40.009
          with status epilepticus G40.001
          without status epilepticus G40.009
    symptomatic
      with complex partial seizures G40.209
        intractable G40.219
          with status epilepticus G40.211
          without status epilepticus G40.219
        not intractable G40.209
          with status epilepticus G40.201
          without status epilepticus G40.209
      with simple partial seizures G40.109
        intractable G40.119
          with status epilepticus G40.111
          without status epilepticus G40.119
        not intractable G40.109
          with status epilepticus G40.101
          without status epilepticus G40.109
  myoclonus, myoclonic (progressive) —*see*
    Epilepsy, generalized, specified NEC
  not intractable G40.909
    with status epilepticus G40.901
    without status epilepticus G40.909
  on awakening —*see* Epilepsy, generalized,
    specified NEC
  parasitic NOS B71.9 *[G94]*
  partialis continua (*see also* Kozhevnikof's
    epilepsy) G40.1-
  peripheral —*see* Epilepsy, specified NEC
  procursiva —*see* Epilepsy, localization-
    related, symptomatic, with simple
    partial seizures
  progressive (familial) myoclonic —*see*
    Epilepsy, generalized, idiopathic

Epilepsy, epileptic, epilepsia *(Continued)*
  reflex —*see* Epilepsy, specified NEC
  related to
    alcohol G40.509
      not intractable G40.509
        with status epilepticus G40.501
        without status eplilepticus G40.509
    drugs G40.509
      not intractable G40.509
        with status epilepticus G40.501
        without status epilepticus G40.509
    external causes G40.509
      not intractable G40.509
        with status epilepticus G40.501
        without status epilepticus G40.509
    hormonal changes G40.509
      not intractable G40.509
        with status epilepticus G40.501
        without status eplilepticus G40.509
    sleep deprivation G40.509
      not intractable G40.509
        with status epilepticus G40.501
        without status eplilepticus G40.509
    stress G40.509
      not intractable G40.509
        with status epilepticus G40.501
        without status epilepticus G40.509
  somatomotor —*see* Epilepsy, localization-
    related, symptomatic, with simple
    partial seizures
  somatosensory —*see* Epilepsy, localization-
    related, symptomatic, with simple
    partial seizures
  spasms G40.822
    intractable G40.824
      with status epilepticus G40.823
      without status epilepticus G40.824
    not intractable G40.822
      with status epilepticus G40.821
      without status epilepticus G40.822
  specified NEC G40.802
    intractable G40.804
      with status epilepticus G40.803
      without status epilepticus G40.804
    not intractable G40.802
      with status epilepticus G40.801
      without status epilepticus G40.802
  syndromes
    generalized
      idiopathic G40.309
        intractable G40.319
          with status epilepticus G40.311
          without status epilepticus G40.319
        not intractable G40.309
          with status epilepticus G40.301
          without status epilepticus G40.309
      specified NEC G40.409
        intractable G40.419
          with status epilepticus G40.411
          without status epilepticus G40.419
        not intractable G40.409
          with status epilepticus G40.401
          without status epilepticus G40.409
    localization-related (focal) (partial)
      idiopathic G40.009
        with seizures of localized onset
          G40.009
          intractable G40.019
            with status epilepticus G40.011
            without status epilepticus
              G40.019
          not intractable G40.009
            with status epilepticus G40.001
            without status epilepticus G40.009
      symptomatic
        with complex partial seizures
          G40.209
          intractable G40.219
            with status epilepticus G40.211
            without status epilepticus
              G40.219

Epilepsy, epileptic, epilepsia *(Continued)*
  syndromes *(Continued)*
    localization-related *(Continued)*
      symptomatic *(Continued)*
        with complex partial seizures
          (Continued)
          not intractable G40.209
            with status epilepticus G40.201
            without status epilepticus G40.209
        with simple partial seizures G40.109
          intractable G40.119
            with status epilepticus G40.111
            without status epilepticus G40.119
          not intractable G40.109
            with status epilepticus G40.101
            without status epilepticus G40.109
    specified NEC G40.802
      intractable G40.804
        with status epilepticus G40.803
        without status epilepticus G40.804
      not intractable G40.802
        with status epilepticus G40.801
        without status epilepticus G40.802
  tonic (-clonic) —*see* Epilepsy, generalized,
    specified NEC
  twilight F05
  uncinate (gyrus) —*see* Epilepsy, localization-
    related, symptomatic, with complex
    partial seizures
  Unverricht (-Lundborg) (familial
    myoclonic) —*see* Epilepsy, generalized,
    idiopathic
  visceral —*see* Epilepsy, specified NEC
  visual —*see* Epilepsy, specified NEC
Epiloia Q85.1
Epimenorrhea N92.0
Epipharyngitis —*see* Nasopharyngitis
Epiphora H04.20-
  due to
    excess lacrimation H04.21-
    insufficient drainage H04.22-
Epiphyseal arrest —*see* Arrest, epiphyseal
Epiphyseolysis, epiphysiolysis —*see*
  Osteochondropathy
Epiphysitis —*see also* Osteochondropathy
  juvenile M92.9
  syphilitic (congenital) A50.02
Epiplocele —*see* Hernia, abdomen
Epiploitis —*see* Peritonitis
Epiplosarcomphalocele —*see* Hernia, umbilicus
Episcleritis (suppurative) H15.10-
  in (due to)
    syphilis A52.71
    tuberculosis A18.51
  nodular H15.12-
  periodica fugax H15.11-
    angioneurotic —*see* Edema, angioneurotic
  syphilitic (late) A52.71
  tuberculous A18.51
Episode
  affective, mixed F39
  depersonalization (in neurotic state) F48.1
  depressive F32.9
    major F32.9
      mild F32.0
      moderate F32.1
      severe (without psychotic symptoms)
        F32.2
        with psychotic symptoms F32.3
    recurrent F33.9
      brief F33.8
    specified NEC F32.8
  hypomanic F30.8
  manic F30.9
    with
      psychotic symptoms F30.2
      remission (full) F30.4
        partial F30.3
    without psychotic symptoms F30.10
      mild F30.11
      moderate F30.12

Episode (Continued)
  manic (Continued)
    without psychotic symptoms (Continued)
      severe (without psychotic symptoms)
        F30.13
        with psychotic symptoms F30.2
      other specified F30.8
      recurrent F31.89
    psychotic F23
      organic F06.8
    schizophrenic (acute) NEC, brief F23
Epispadias (female) (male) Q64.0
Episplenitis D73.89
Epistaxis (multiple) R04.0
  hereditary I78.0
  vicarious menstruation N94.89
Epithelioma (malignant) —see also Neoplasm,
  malignant, by site
  adenoides cysticum —see Neoplasm, skin,
    benign
  basal cell —see Neoplasm, skin, malignant
  benign —see Neoplasm, benign, by site
  Bowen's —see Neoplasm, skin, in situ
  calcifying, of Malherbe —see Neoplasm, skin,
    benign
  external site —see Neoplasm, skin, malignant
  intraepidermal, Jadassohn —see Neoplasm,
    skin, benign ◄▦
  squamous cell —see Neoplasm, malignant,
    by site
Epitheliomatosis pigmented Q82.1
Epitheliopathy, multifocal placoid pigment
  H30.14-
Epithelium, epithelial —see condition
Epituberculosis (with atelectasis) (allergic) A15.7
Eponychia Q84.6
Epstein's
  nephrosis or syndrome —see Nephrosis
  pearl K09.8
Epulis (gingiva) (fibrous) (giant cell) K06.8
Equinia A24.0
Equinovarus (congenital) (talipes) Q66.0
  acquired —see Deformity, limb, clubfoot
Equivalent
  convulsive (abdominal) —see Epilepsy,
    specified NEC
  epileptic (psychic) —see Epilepsy,
    localization-related, symptomatic, with
    complex partial seizures
Erb (-Duchenne) paralysis (birth injury)
  (newborn) P14.0
Erb's
  disease G71.0
  palsy, paralysis (brachial) (birth) (newborn)
    P14.0
    spinal (spastic) syphilitic A52.17
  pseudohypertrophic muscular dystrophy
    G71.0
Erb-Goldflam disease or syndrome
  G70.00
  with exacerbation (acute) G70.01
  in crisis G70.01
Erdheim's syndrome (acromegalic
  macrospondylitis) E22.0
Erection, painful (persistent) —see Priapism
Ergosterol deficiency (vitamin D) E55.9
  with
    adult osteomalacia M83.8
    rickets —see Rickets
Ergotism —see also Poisoning, food, noxious,
  plant
  from ergot used as drug (migraine
    therapy) —see Table of Drugs and
    Chemicals
Erosio interdigitalis blastomycetica B37.2
Erosion
  artery I77.2
    without rupture I77.89
  bone —see Disorder, bone, density and
    structure, specified NEC
  bronchus J98.09

Erosion (Continued)
  cartilage (joint) —see Disorder, cartilage,
    specified type NEC
  cervix (uteri) (acquired) (chronic) (congenital)
    N86
    with cervicitis N72
  cornea (nontraumatic) —see Ulcer, cornea
    recurrent H18.83-
    traumatic —see Abrasion, cornea
  dental (idiopathic) (occupational) (due to
    diet, drugs or vomiting) K03.2
  duodenum, postpyloric —see Ulcer,
    duodenum
  esophagus K22.10
    with bleeding K22.11
  gastric —see Ulcer, stomach
  gastrojejunal —see Ulcer, gastrojejunal
  implanted mesh —see Complications, mesh
  intestine K63.3
  lymphatic vessel I89.8
  pylorus, pyloric (ulcer) —see Ulcer, stomach
  spine, aneurysmal A52.09
  stomach —see Ulcer, stomach
  teeth (idiopathic) (occupational) (due to diet,
    drugs or vomiting) K03.2
  urethra N36.8
  uterus N85.8
Erotomania F52.8
Error
  metabolism, inborn —see Disorder,
    metabolism
  refractive —see Disorder, refraction
Eructation R14.2
  nervous or psychogenic F45.8
Eruption
  creeping B76.9
  drug (generalized) (taken internally) L27.0
    fixed L27.1
    in contact with skin —see Dermatitis, due
      to drugs
    localized L27.1
  Hutchinson, summer L56.4
  Kaposi's varicelliform B00.0
  napkin L22
  polymorphous light (sun) L56.4
  recalcitrant pustular L13.8
  ringed R23.8
  skin (nonspecific) R21
    creeping (meaning hookworm) B76.9
    due to inoculation/vaccination
      (generalized) (see also Dermatitis, due
      to, vaccine) L27.0
      localized L27.1
    erysipeloid A26.0
    feigned L98.1
    Kaposi's varicelliform B00.0
    lichenoid L28.0
    meaning dermatitis —see Dermatitis
    toxic NEC L53.0
  tooth, teeth, abnormal (incomplete) (late)
    (premature) (sequence) K00.6
  vesicular R23.8
Erysipelas (gangrenous) (infantile) (newborn)
  (phlegmonous) (suppurative) A46
  external ear A46 [H62.40]
  puerperal, postpartum O86.89
Erysipeloid A26.9
  cutaneous (Rosenbach's) A26.0
  disseminated A26.8
  sepsis A26.7
  specified NEC A26.8
Erythema, erythematous (infectional)
  (inflammation) L53.9
  ab igne L59.0
  annulare (centrifugum) (rheumaticum) L53.1
  arthriticum epidemicum A25.1
  brucellum —see Brucellosis
  chronic figurate NEC L53.3
  chronicum migrans (Borrelia burgdorferi)
    A69.20
  diaper L22

Erythema, erythematous (Continued)
  due to
    chemical NEC L53.0
      in contact with skin L24.5
    drug (internal use) —see Dermatitis, due
      to, drugs
  elevatum diutinum L95.1
  endemic E52
  epidemic, arthritic A25.1
  figuratum perstans L53.3
  gluteal L22
  heat - code by site under Burn, first degree
  ichthyosiforme congenitum bullous Q80.3
  in diseases classified elsewhere L54
  induratum (nontuberculous) L52
    tuberculous A18.4
  infectiosum B08.3
  intertrigo L30.4
  iris L51.9
  marginatum L53.2
    in (due to) acute rheumatic fever I00
  medicamentosum —see Dermatitis, due to,
    drugs
  migrans A26.0
    chronicum A69.20
    tongue K14.1
  multiforme (major) (minor) L51.9
    bullous, bullosum L51.1
    conjunctiva L51.1
    nonbullous L51.0
    pemphigoides L12.0
    specified NEC L51.8
  napkin L22
  neonatorum P83.8
    toxic P83.1
  nodosum L52
    tuberculous A18.4
  palmar L53.8
  pernio T69.1
  rash, newborn P83.8
  scarlatiniform (recurrent) (exfoliative)
    L53.8
  solare L55.0
  specified NEC L53.8
  toxic, toxicum NEC L53.0
    newborn P83.1
  tuberculous (primary) A18.4
Erythematous, erythematosus —see condition
Erythermalgia (primary) I73.81
Erythralgia I73.81
Erythrasma L08.1
Erythredema (polyneuropathy) —see Poisoning,
  mercury
Erythremia (acute) C94.0-
  chronic D45
  secondary D75.1
Erythroblastopenia (see also Aplasia, red cell)
  D60.9
  congenital D61.01
Erythroblastophthisis D61.09
Erythroblastosis (fetalis) (newborn) P55.9
  due to
    ABO (antibodies) (incompatibility)
      (isoimmunization) P55.1
    Rh (antibodies) (incompatibility)
      (isoimmunization) P55.0
Erythrocyanosis (crurum) I73.89
Erythrocythemia —see Erythremia
Erythrocytosis (megalosplenic) (secondary)
  D75.1
  familial D75.0
  oval, hereditary —see Elliptocytosis
  secondary D75.1
  stress D75.1
Erythroderma (secondary) (see also Erythema)
  L53.9
  bullous ichthyosiform, congenital Q80.3
  desquamativum L21.1
  ichthyosiform, congenital (bullous) Q80.3
  neonatorum P83.8
  psoriaticum L40.8

◄ New   ◄▦ Revised   ~~deleted~~ Deleted

Erythrodysesthesia, palmar plantar (PPE) L27.1
Erythrogenesis imperfecta D61.09
Erythroleukemia C94.0-
Erythromelalgia I73.81
Erythrophagocytosis D75.89
Erythrophobia F40.298
Erythroplakia, oral epithelium, and tongue K13.29
Erythroplasia (Queyrat) D07.4
  specified site —see Neoplasm, skin, in situ
  unspecified site D07.4
Escherichia coli (E. coli), as cause of disease classified elsewhere B96.20
  non-O157 Shiga toxin-producing (with known O group) B96.22
  non-Shiga toxin-producing B96.29
  O157 with confirmation of Shiga toxin when H antigen is unknown, or is not H7 B96.21
  O157:H- (nonmotile) with confirmation of Shiga toxin B96.21
  O157:H7 with or without confirmation of Shiga toxin-production B96.21
  Shiga toxin-producing (with unspecified O group) (STEC) B96.23
  O157 B96.21 ◀▥▥
  O157:H7 with or without confirmation of Shiga toxin-production B96.21 ◀▥▥
    specified NEC B96.22
    specified NEC B96.29
Esophagismus K22.4
Esophagitis (acute) (alkaline) (chemical) (chronic) (infectional) (necrotic) (peptic) (postoperative) K20.9
  candidal B37.81
  due to gastrointestinal reflux disease K21.0
  eosinophilic K20.0
  reflux K21.0
  specified NEC K20.8
  tuberculous A18.83
  ulcerative K22.10
    with bleeding K22.11
Esophagocele K22.5
Esophagomalacia K22.8
Esophagospasm K22.4
Esophagostenosis K22.2
Esophagostomiasis B81.8
Esophagotracheal —see condition
Esophagus —see condition
Esophoria H50.51
  convergence, excess H51.12
  divergence, insufficiency H51.8
Esotropia —see Strabismus, convergent concomitant
Espundia B55.2
Essential —see condition
Esthesioneuroblastoma C30.0
Esthesioneurocytoma C30.0
Esthesioneuroepithelioma C30.0
Esthiomene A55
Estivo-autumnal malaria (fever) B50.9
Estrangement (marital) Z63.5
  parent-child NEC Z62.890
Estriasis —see Myiasis
Ethanolism —see Alcoholism
Etherism —see Dependence, drug, inhalant
Ethmoid, ethmoidal —see condition
Ethmoiditis (chronic) (nonpurulent) (purulent) —see also Sinusitis, ethmoidal
  influenzal —see Influenza, with, respiratory manifestations NEC
  Woakes' J33.1
Ethylism —see Alcoholism
Eulenburg's disease (congenital paramyotonia) G71.19
Eumycetoma B47.0
Eunuchoidism E29.1
  hypogonadotropic E23.0
European blastomycosis —see Cryptococcosis
Eustachian —see condition

Evaluation (for) (of)
  development state
    adolescent Z00.3
    period of
      delayed growth in childhood Z00.70
        with abnormal findings Z00.71
      rapid growth in childhood Z00.2
    puberty Z00.3
  growth and developmental state (period of rapid growth) Z00.2
    delayed growth Z00.70
      with abnormal findings Z00.71
  mental health (status) Z00.8
    requested by authority Z04.6
  period of
    delayed growth in childhood Z00.70
      with abnormal findings Z00.71
    rapid growth in childhood Z00.2
  suspected condition —see Observation
Evans syndrome D69.41
Event, apparent life threatening in newborn and infant (ALTE) R68.13
Eventration —see also Hernia, ventral
  colon into chest —see Hernia, diaphragm
  diaphragm (congenital) Q79.1
Eversion
  bladder N32.89
  cervix (uteri) N86
    with cervicitis N72
  foot NEC —see also Deformity, valgus, ankle
    congenital Q66.6
  punctum lacrimale (postinfectional) (senile) H04.52-
  ureter (meatus) N28.89
  urethra (meatus) N36.8
  uterus N81.4
Evidence
  cytologic
    of malignancy on anal smear R85.614
    of malignancy on cervical smear R87.614
    of malignancy on vaginal smear R87.624
Evisceration
  birth injury P15.8
  traumatic NEC
    eye —see Enucleated eye
Evulsion —see Avulsion
Ewing's sarcoma or tumor —see Neoplasm, bone, malignant
Examination (for) (following) (general) (of) (routine) Z00.00
  with abnormal findings Z00.01
  abuse, physical (alleged), ruled out
    adult Z04.71
    child Z04.72
  adolescent (development state) Z00.3
  alleged rape or sexual assault (victim), ruled out
    adult Z04.41
    child Z04.42
  allergy Z01.82
  annual (adult) (periodic) (physical) Z00.00
    with abnormal findings Z00.01
    gynecological Z01.419
      with abnormal findings Z01.411
  antibody response Z01.84
  blood —see Examination, laboratory
  blood pressure Z01.30
    with abnormal findings Z01.31
  cancer staging —see Neoplasm, malignant, by site
  cervical Papanicolaou smear Z12.4
    as part of routine gynecological examination Z01.419
      with abnormal findings Z01.411
  child (over 28 days old) Z00.129
    with abnormal findings Z00.121
    under 28 days old —see Newborn, examination
  clinical research control or normal comparison (control) (participant) Z00.6

Examination (Continued)
  contraceptive (drug) maintenance (routine) Z30.8
  device (intrauterine) Z30.431
  dental Z01.20
    with abnormal findings Z01.21
  developmental —see Examination, child
  donor (potential) Z00.5
  ear Z01.10
    with abnormal findings NEC Z01.118
  eye Z01.00
    with abnormal findings Z01.01
  following
    accident NEC Z04.3
      transport Z04.1
      work Z04.2
    assault, alleged, ruled out
      adult Z04.71
      child Z04.72
    motor vehicle accident Z04.1
    treatment (for) Z09
      combined NEC Z09
        fracture Z09
        malignant neoplasm Z08
      malignant neoplasm Z08
      mental disorder Z09
      specified condition NEC Z09
  follow-up (routine) (following) Z09
    chemotherapy NEC Z09
      malignant neoplasm Z08
    fracture Z09
    malignant neoplasm Z08
    postpartum Z39.2
    psychotherapy Z09
    radiotherapy NEC Z09
      malignant neoplasm Z08
    surgery NEC Z09
      malignant neoplasm Z08
  gynecological Z01.419
    with abnormal findings Z01.411
    for contraceptive maintenance Z30.8
  health —see Examination, medical
  hearing Z01.10
    with abnormal findings NEC Z01.118
    following failed hearing screening Z01.110
  immunity status testing Z01.84
  laboratory (as part of a general medical examination) Z00.00
    with abnormal findings Z00.01
    preprocedural Z01.812
  lactating mother Z39.1
  medical (adult) (for) (of) Z00.00
    with abnormal findings Z00.01
    administrative purpose only Z02.9
      specified NEC Z02.89
    admission to
      armed forces Z02.3
      old age home Z02.2
      prison Z02.89
      residential institution Z02.2
      school Z02.0
        following illness or medical treatment Z02.0
      summer camp Z02.89
    adoption Z02.82
    blood alcohol or drug level Z02.83
    camp (summer) Z02.89
    clinical research, normal subject (control) (participant) Z00.6
    control subject in clinical research (normal comparison) (participant) Z00.6
    donor (potential) Z00.5
    driving license Z02.4
    general (adult) Z00.00
      with abnormal findings Z00.01
    immigration Z02.89
    insurance purposes Z02.6
    marriage Z02.89
    medicolegal reasons NEC Z04.8
    naturalization Z02.89
    participation in sport Z02.5

Examination *(Continued)*
  medical *(Continued)*
    paternity testing Z02.81
    population survey Z00.8
    pre-employment Z02.1
    pre-operative —*see* Examination,
      pre-procedural
    pre-procedural
      cardiovascular Z01.810
      respiratory Z01.811
      specified NEC Z01.818
    preschool children
      for admission to school Z02.0
    prisoners
      for entrance into prison Z02.89
    recruitment for armed forces Z02.3
    specified NEC Z00.8
    sport competition Z02.5
  medicolegal reason NEC Z04.8
  newborn —*see* Newborn, examination
  pelvic (annual) (periodic) Z01.419
    with abnormal findings Z01.411
  period of rapid growth in childhood Z00.2
  periodic (adult) (annual) (routine) Z00.00
    with abnormal findings Z00.01
  physical (adult) —*see also* Examination,
    medical Z00.00 ◄▥
    sports Z02.5
  postpartum
    immediately after delivery Z39.0
    routine follow-up Z39.2
  pre-chemotherapy (antineoplastic) Z01.818
  prenatal (normal pregnancy) (*see also*
    Pregnancy, normal) Z34.9-
  pre-procedural (pre-operative)
    cardiovascular Z01.810
    laboratory Z01.812
    respiratory Z01.811
    specified NEC Z01.818
  prior to chemotherapy (antineoplastic)
    Z01.818
  psychiatric NEC Z00.8
    follow-up not needing further care Z09
    requested by authority Z04.6
  radiological (as part of a general medical
    examination) Z00.00
    with abnormal findings Z00.01
  repeat cervical smear to confirm findings of
    recent normal smear following initial
    abnormal smear Z01.42
  skin (hypersensitivity) Z01.82
  special (*see also* Examination, by type) Z01.89
    specified type NEC Z01.89
  specified type or reason NEC Z04.8
  teeth Z01.20
    with abnormal findings Z01.21
  urine —*see* Examination, laboratory
  vision Z01.00
    with abnormal findings Z01.01
Exanthem, exanthema —*see also* Rash
  with enteroviral vesicular stomatitis B08.4
  Boston A88.0
  epidemic with meningitis A88.0 *[G02]*
  subitum B08.20
    due to human herpesvirus 6 B08.21
    due to human herpesvirus 7 B08.22
  viral, virus B09
    specified type NEC B08.8
Excess, excessive, excessively
  alcohol level in blood R78.0
  androgen (ovarian) E28.1
  attrition, tooth, teeth K03.0
  carotene, carotin (dietary) E67.1
  cold, effects of T69.9
    specified effect NEC T69.8
  convergence H51.12
  crying
    in child, adolescent, or adult R45.83
    in infant R68.11
  development, breast N62
  divergence H51.8

Excess, excessive, excessively *(Continued)*
  drinking (alcohol) NEC (without
    dependence) F10.10
    habitual (continual) (without remission)
      F10.20
  eating R63.2
  estrogen E28.0
  fat —*see also* Obesity
    in heart —*see* Degeneration, myocardial
    localized E65
  foreskin N47.8
  gas R14.0
  glucagon E16.3
  heat —*see* Heat
  intermaxillary vertical dimension of fully
    erupted teeth M26.37
  interocclusal distance of fully erupted teeth
    M26.37
  kalium E87.5
  large
    colon K59.3
      congenital Q43.8
    infant P08.1
    organ or site, congenital NEC —*see*
      Anomaly, by site
  long
    organ or site, congenital NEC —*see*
      Anomaly, by site
  menstruation (with regular cycle) N92.0
    with irregular cycle N92.1
  napping Z72.821
  natrium E87.0
  number of teeth K00.1
  nutrient (dietary) NEC R63.2
  potassium (K) E87.5
  salivation K11.7
  secretion —*see also* Hypersecretion
    milk O92.6
    sputum R09.3
    sweat R61
  sexual drive F52.8
  short
    organ or site, congenital NEC —*see*
      Anomaly, by site
    umbilical cord in labor or delivery O69.3
  skin, eyelid (acquired) —*see* Blepharochalasis
    congenital Q10.3
  sodium (Na) E87.0
  spacing of fully erupted teeth M26.32
  sputum R09.3
  sweating R61
  thirst R63.1
    due to deprivation of water T73.1
  tuberosity of jaw M26.07
  vitamin
    A (dietary) E67.0
      administered as drug (prolonged
        intake) —*see* Table of ⊣Drugs and
        ⊢Chemicals, vitamins, adverse
        effect ◄▥
      overdose or wrong substance given or
        taken —*see* Table of ⊣Drugs and
        ⊢Chemicals, vitamins, poisoning ◄▥
    D (dietary) E67.3
      administered as drug (prolonged
        intake) —*see* Table of ⊣Drugs and
        ⊢Chemicals, vitamins, adverse
        effect ◄▥
      overdose or wrong substance given or
        taken —*see* Table of ⊣Drugs and
        ⊢Chemicals, vitamins, poisoning ◄▥
  weight
    gain R63.5
    loss R63.4
Excitability, abnormal, under minor stress
  (personality disorder) F60.3
Excitation
  anomalous atrioventricular I45.6
  psychogenic F30.8
  reactive (from emotional stress, psychological
    trauma) F30.8

Excitement
  hypomanic F30.8
  manic F30.9
  mental, reactive (from emotional stress,
    psychological trauma) F30.8
  state, reactive (from emotional stress,
    psychological trauma) F30.8
Excoriation (traumatic) —*see also* Abrasion
  neurotic L98.1
Exfoliation
  due to erythematous conditions according to
    extent of body surface involved L49.0
    10-19 percent of body surface L49.1
    20-29 percent of body surface L49.2
    30-39 percent of body surface L49.3
    40-49 percent of body surface L49.4
    50-59 percent of body surface L49.5
    60-69 percent of body surface L49.6
    70-79 percent of body surface L49.7
    80-89 percent of body surface L49.8
    90-99 percent of body surface L49.9
    less than 10 percent of body surface L49.0
  teeth, due to systemic causes K08.0
Exfoliative —*see* condition
Exhaustion, exhaustive (physical NEC) R53.83
  battle F43.0
  cardiac —*see* Failure, heart
  delirium F43.0
  due to
    cold T69.8
    excessive exertion T73.3
    exposure T73.2
    neurasthenia F48.8
  heart —*see* Failure, heart
  heat (*see also* Heat, exhaustion) T67.5
    due to
      salt depletion T67.4
      water depletion T67.3
  maternal, complicating delivery O75.81
  mental F48.8
  myocardium, myocardial —*see* Failure, heart
  nervous F48.8
  old age R54
  psychogenic F48.8
  psychosis F43.0
  senile R54
  vital NEC Z73.0
Exhibitionism F65.2
Exocervicitis —*see* Cervicitis
Exomphalos Q79.2
  meaning hernia —*see* Hernia, umbilicus
Exophoria H50.52
  convergence, insufficiency H51.11
  divergence, excess H51.8
Exophthalmos H05.2-
  congenital Q15.8
  constant NEC H05.24-
  displacement, globe —*see* Displacement,
    globe
  due to thyrotoxicosis (hyperthyroidism) —*see*
    Hyperthyroidism, with, goiter (diffuse)
  dysthyroid —*see* Hyperthyroidism, with,
    goiter (diffuse)
  goiter —*see* Hyperthyroidism, with, goiter
    (diffuse)
  intermittent NEC H05.25-
  malignant —*see* Hyperthyroidism, with,
    goiter (diffuse)
  orbital
    edema —*see* Edema, orbit
    hemorrhage —*see* Hemorrhage, orbit
  pulsating NEC H05.26-
  thyrotoxic, thyrotropic —*see*
    Hyperthyroidism, with, goiter (diffuse)
Exostosis —*see also* Disorder, bone
  cartilaginous —*see* Neoplasm, bone, benign
  congenital (multiple) Q78.6
  external ear canal H61.81-
  gonococcal A54.49
  jaw (bone) M27.8
  multiple, congenital Q78.6

Exostosis *(Continued)*
    orbit H05.35-
    osteocartilaginous —*see* Neoplasm, bone,
        benign
    syphilitic A52.77
Exotropia —*see* Strabismus, divergent
    concomitant
Explanation of
    investigation finding Z71.2
    medication Z71.89
Exposure (to) *(see also* Contact, with) T75.89
    acariasis Z20.7
    AIDS virus Z20.6
    air pollution Z77.110
    algae and algae toxins Z77.121
    algae bloom Z77.121
    anthrax Z20.810
    aromatic amines Z77.020
    aromatic (hazardous) compounds NEC
        Z77.028
    aromatic dyes NOS Z77.028
    arsenic Z77.010
    asbestos Z77.090
    bacterial disease NEC Z20.818
    benzene Z77.021
    blue-green algae bloom Z77.121
    body fluids (potentially hazardous) Z77.21
    brown tide Z77.121
    chemicals (chiefly nonmedicinal) (hazardous)
        NEC Z77.098
    cholera Z20.09
    chromium compounds Z77.018
    cold, effects of T69.9
        specified effect NEC T69.8
    communicable disease Z20.9
        bacterial NEC Z20.818
        specified NEC Z20.89
        viral NEC Z20.828
    cyanobacteria bloom Z77.121
    disaster Z65.5
    discrimination Z60.5
    dyes Z77.098
    effects of T73.9
    environmental tobacco smoke (acute)
        (chronic) Z77.22
    Escherichia coli (E. coli) Z20.01
    exhaustion due to T73.2
    fiberglass —*see* Table of ~~d~~Drugs and
        ~~c~~Chemicals, fiberglass ◀‖‖
    German measles Z20.4
    gonorrhea Z20.2
    hazardous metals NEC Z77.018
    hazardous substances NEC Z77.29
    hazards in the physical environment NEC
        Z77.128
    hazards to health NEC Z77.9
    human immunodeficiency virus (HIV) Z20.6
    human T-lymphotropic virus type-1 (HTLV-1)
        Z20.89

Exposure *(Continued)*
    implanted
        mesh —*see* Complications, mesh
        prosthetic materials NEC —*see*
            Complications, prosthetic materials
            NEC
    infestation (parasitic) NEC Z20.7
    intestinal infectious disease NEC Z20.09
        Escherichia coli (E. coli) Z20.01
    lead Z77.011
    meningococcus Z20.811
    mold (toxic) Z77.120
    nickel dust Z77.018
    noise Z77.122
    occupational
        air contaminants NEC Z57.39
        dust Z57.2
        environmental tobacco smoke Z57.31
        extreme temperature Z57.6
        noise Z57.0
        radiation Z57.1
        risk factors Z57.9
            specified NEC Z57.8
        toxic agents (gases) (liquids) (solids)
            (vapors) in agriculture Z57.4
        toxic agents (gases) (liquids) (solids)
            (vapors) in industry NEC Z57.5
        vibration Z57.7
    parasitic disease NEC Z20.7
    pediculosis Z20.7
    persecution Z60.5
    pfiesteria piscicida Z77.121
    poliomyelitis Z20.89
    pollution
        air Z77.110
        environmental NEC Z77.118
        soil Z77.112
        water Z77.111
    polycyclic aromatic hydrocarbons Z77.028
    prenatal (drugs) (toxic chemicals) —*see*
        Newborn, affected by (suspected to
        be), noxious substances transmitted via
        placenta or breast milk
    rabies Z20.3
    radiation, naturally occurring NEC Z77.123
    radon Z77.123
    red tide (Florida) Z77.121
    rubella Z20.4
    second hand tobacco smoke (acute) (chronic)
        Z77.22
        in the perinatal period P96.81
    sexually-transmitted disease Z20.2
    smallpox (laboratory) Z20.89
    syphilis Z20.2
    terrorism Z65.4
    torture Z65.4
    tuberculosis Z20.1
    uranium Z77.012
    varicella Z20.820

Exposure *(Continued)*
    venereal disease Z20.2
    viral disease NEC Z20.828
    war Z65.5
    water pollution Z77.111
Exsanguination —*see* Hemorrhage
Exstrophy
    abdominal contents Q45.8
    bladder Q64.10
        cloacal Q64.12
        specified type NEC Q64.19
        supravesical fissure Q64.11
Extensive —*see* condition
Extra —*see also* Accessory
    marker chromosomes (normal individual)
        Q92.61
        in abnormal individual Q92.62
    rib Q76.6
        cervical Q76.5
Extrasystoles (supraventricular) I49.49
    atrial I49.1
    auricular I49.1
    junctional I49.2
    ventricular I49.3
Extrauterine gestation or pregnancy —*see*
    Pregnancy, by site
Extravasation
    blood R58
    chyle into mesentery I89.8
    pelvicalyceal N13.8
    pyelosinus N13.8
    urine (from ureter) R39.0
    vesicant agent
        antineoplastic chemotherapy T80.810
        other agent NEC T80.818
Extremity —*see* condition, limb
Extrophy —*see* Exstrophy
Extroversion
    bladder Q64.19
    uterus N81.4
        complicating delivery O71.2
        postpartal (old) N81.4
Extruded tooth (teeth) M26.34
Extrusion
    breast implant (prosthetic) T85.42
    eye implant (globe) (ball) T85.328
    intervertebral disc —*see* Displacement,
        intervertebral disc
    ocular lens implant (prosthetic) —*see*
        Complications, intraocular lens
    vitreous —*see* Prolapse, vitreous
Exudate
    pleural —*see* Effusion, pleura
    retina H35.89
Exudative —*see* condition
Eye, eyeball, eyelid —*see* condition
Eyestrain —*see* Disturbance, vision, subjective
Eyeworm disease of Africa B74.3

F

Faber's syndrome (achlorhydric anemia) D50.9
Fabry (-Anderson) disease E75.21
Faciocephalalgia, autonomic (see also
    Neuropathy, peripheral, autonomic)
    G90.09
Factor (s)
  psychic, associated with diseases classified
    elsewhere F54
  psychological
    affecting physical conditions F54
    or behavioral
      affecting general medical condition F54
      associated with disorders or diseases
        classified elsewhere F54
Fahr disease (of brain) G23.8
Fahr Volhard disease (of kidney) I12.-
Failure, failed
  abortion —see Abortion, attempted
  aortic (valve) I35.8
    rheumatic I06.8
  attempted abortion —see Abortion, attempted
  biventricular I50.9
  bone marrow —see Anemia, aplastic
  cardiac —see Failure, heart
  cardiorenal (chronic) I50.9
    hypertensive I13.2
  cardiorespiratory (see also Failure, heart)
    R09.2
  cardiovascular (chronic) —see Failure, heart
  cerebrovascular I67.9
  cervical dilatation in labor O62.0
  circulation, circulatory (peripheral) R57.9
    newborn P29.89
  compensation —see Disease, heart
  compliance with medical treatment or
    regimen —see Noncompliance
  congestive —see Failure, heart, congestive
  dental implant (endosseous) M27.69
    due to
      failure of dental prosthesis M27.63
      lack of attached gingiva M27.62
      occlusal trauma (poor prosthetic design)
        M27.62
      parafunctional habits M27.62
      periodontal infection (peri-implantitis)
        M27.62
      poor oral hygiene M27.62
    osseointegration M27.61
      due to
        complications of systemic disease
          M27.61
          poor bone quality M27.61
      iatrogenic M27.61
    post-osseointegration
      biological M27.62
      due to complications of systemic disease
        M27.62
      iatrogenic M27.62
      mechanical M27.63
    pre-integration M27.61
    pre-osseointegration M27.61
    specified NEC M27.69
  descent of head (at term) of pregnancy
    (mother) O32.4
  endosseous dental implant —see Failure,
    dental implant
  engagement of head (term of pregnancy)
    (mother) O32.4
  erection (penile) (see also Dysfunction, sexual,
    male, erectile) N52.9
    nonorgqanic F52.21
  examination (s), anxiety concerning Z55.2
  expansion terminal respiratory units
    (newborn) (primary) P28.0
  forceps NOS (with subsequent cesarean
    delivery) O66.5
  gain weight (child over 28 days old) R62.51
    adult R62.7
    newborn P92.6

Failure, failed (Continued)
  genital response (male) F52.21
    female F52.22
  heart (acute) (senile) (sudden) I50.9
    with
      acute pulmonary edema —see Failure,
        ventricular, left
      decompensation —see Failure, heart,
        congestive
      dilatation —see Disease, heart
    arteriosclerotic I70.90
    biventricular I50.9
    combined left-right sided I50.9
    compensated I50.9
    complicating
      anesthesia (general) (local) or other
        sedation
        in labor and delivery O74.2
        in pregnancy O29.12-
        postpartum, puerperal O89.1
      delivery (cesarean) (instrumental) O75.4
    congestive (compensated)
      (decompensated) I50.9
      with rheumatic fever (conditions in I00)
        active I01.8
        inactive or quiescent (with chorea)
          I09.81
      newborn P29.0
      rheumatic (chronic) (inactive) (with
        chorea) I09.81
        active or acute I01.8
          with chorea I02.0
    decompensated I50.9
    degenerative —see Degeneration,
      myocardial
    diastolic (congestive) I50.30
      acute (congestive) I50.31
        and (on) chronic (congestive) I50.33
      chronic (congestive) I50.32
        and (on) acute (congestive) I50.33
      combined with systolic (congestive)
        I50.40
      acute (congestive) I50.41
        and (on) chronic (congestive)
          I50.43
      chronic (congestive) I50.42
        and (on) acute (congestive) I50.43
    due to presence of cardiac prosthesis
      I97.13-
    following cardiac surgery I97.13-
    high output NOS I50.9
    hypertensive —see Hypertension, heart
    left (ventricular) —see Failure, ventricular,
      left
    low output (syndrome) NOS I50.9
    newborn P29.0
    organic —see Disease, heart
    peripartum O90.3
    postprocedural I97.13-
    rheumatic (chronic) (inactive) I09.9
    right (ventricular) (secondary to left
      heart failure) —see Failure, heart,
      congestive
    systolic (congestive) I50.20
      acute (congestive) I50.21
        and (on) chronic (congestive)
          I50.23
      chronic (congestive) I50.22
        and (on) acute (congestive) I50.23
      combined with diastolic (congestive)
        I50.40
      acute (congestive) I50.41
        and (on) chronic (congestive)
          I50.43
      chronic (congestive) I50.42
        and (on) acute (congestive)
          I50.43
    thyrotoxic (see also Thyrotoxicosis)
      E05.90 [143]
      with thyroid storm E05.91 [143]
    valvular —see Endocarditis

Failure, failed (Continued)
  hepatic K72.90
    with coma K72.91
    acute or subacute K72.00
      with coma K72.01
      due to drugs K71.10
        with coma K71.11
    alcoholic (acute) (chronic) (subacute)
      K70.40
      with coma K70.41
    chronic K72.10
      with coma K72.11
      due to drugs (acute) (subacute) (chronic)
        K71.10
        with coma K71.11
    due to drugs (acute) (subacute) (chronic)
      K71.10
      with coma K71.11
    postprocedural K91.82
  hepatorenal K76.7
  induction (of labor) O61.9
    abortion —see Abortion, attempted
    by
      oxytocic drugs O61.0
      prostaglandins O61.0
    instrumental O61.1
    mechanical O61.1
    medical O61.0
    specified NEC O61.8
    surgical O61.1
  intubation during anesthesia T88.4
    in pregnancy O29.6-
    labor and delivery O74.7
    postpartum, puerperal O89.6
  involution, thymus (gland) E32.0
  kidney (see also Disease, kidney, chronic) N19
    acute (see also Failure, renal, acute) N17.9- ◀
    diabetic - see E08-E13 with .22
  lactation (complete) O92.3
    partial O92.4
  Leydig's cell, adult E29.1
  liver —see Failure, hepatic
  menstruation at puberty N91.0
  mitral I05.8
  myocardial, myocardium (see also Failure,
    heart) I50.9
    chronic (see also Failure, heart, congestive)
      I50.9
    congestive (see also Failure, heart,
      congestive) I50.9
  orgasm (female) (psychogenic) F52.31
    male F52.32
  ovarian (primary) E28.39
    iatrogenic E89.40
      asymptomatic E89.40
      symptomatic E89.41
    postprocedural (postablative)
      (postirradiation) (postsurgical)
      E89.40
      asymptomatic E89.40
      symptomatic E89.41
  ovulation causing infertility N97.0
  polyglandular, autoimmune E31.0
  prosthetic joint implant —see Complications,
    joint prosthesis, mechanical,
    breakdown, by site
  renal N19
    with
      tubular necrosis (acute) N17.0
    acute N17.9
      with
        cortical necrosis N17.1
        medullary necrosis N17.2
        tubular necrosis N17.0
      specified NEC N17.8
    chronic N18.9
      hypertensive —see Hypertension,
        kidney
    congenital P96.0
    end stage (chronic) N18.6
      due to hypertension I12.0

◀ New   ◀▦ Revised,   ~~deleted~~ Deleted

Failure, failed *(Continued)*
  renal *(Continued)*
    following
      abortion —*see* Abortion by type
        complicated by specified
        condition NEC
      crushing T79.5
      ectopic or molar pregnancy O08.4
      labor and delivery (acute) O90.4
    hypertensive —*see* Hypertension,
      kidney ◄
    postprocedural N99.0
  respiration, respiratory J96.9
    with
      hypercapnia J96.92
      hypoxia J96.91
    acute J96.00
      with
        hypercapnia J96.02
        hypoxia J96.01
    acute and (on) chronic J96.20
      with
        hypercapnia J96.22
        hypoxia J96.21
    center G93.89
    chronic J96.10
      with
        hypercapnia J96.12
        hypoxia J96.11
    newborn P28.5
    postprocedural (acute) J95.821
      acute and chronic J95.822
  rotation
    cecum Q43.3
    colon Q43.3
    intestine Q43.3
    kidney Q63.2
  sedation (conscious) (moderate) during
    procedure T88.52
    history of Z92.83
  segmentation —*see also* Fusion
    fingers —*see* Syndactylism, complex,
      fingers
    vertebra Q76.49
      with scoliosis Q76.3
  seminiferous tubule, adult E29.1
  senile (general) R54
  sexual arousal (male) F52.21
    female F52.22
  testicular endocrine function E29.1
  to thrive (child over 28 days old)
    R62.51
    adult R62.7
    newborn P92.6
  transplant T86.92
    bone T86.831
      marrow T86.02
    cornea T86.841
    heart T86.22
      with lung (s) T86.32
    intestine T86.851
    kidney T86.12
    liver T86.42
    lung (s) T86.811
      with heart T86.32
    pancreas T86.891
    skin (allograft) (autograft) T86.821
    specified organ or tissue NEC T86.891
    stem cell (peripheral blood) (umbilical
      cord) T86.5
  trial of labor (with subsequent cesarean
    delivery) O66.40
    following previous cesarean delivery
      O66.41
  tubal ligation N99.89
  urinary —*see* Disease, kidney, chronic
  vacuum extraction NOS (with subsequent
    cesarean delivery) O66.5
  vasectomy N99.89
  ventouse NOS (with subsequent cesarean
    delivery) O66.5

Failure, failed *(Continued)*
  ventricular (*see also* Failure, heart) I50.9
    left I50.1
      with rheumatic fever (conditions in I00)
        active I01.8
          with chorea I02.0
        inactive or quiescent (with chorea)
          I09.81
      rheumatic (chronic) (inactive) (with
        chorea) I09.81
        active or acute I01.8
          with chorea I02.0
    right (*see also* Failure, heart, congestive)
      I50.9
  vital centers, newborn P91.8
Fainting (fit) R55
Fallen arches —*see* Deformity, limb, flat foot
Falling, falls (repeated) R29.6
  any organ or part —*see* Prolapse
Fallopian
  insufflation Z31.41
  tube —*see* condition
Fallot's
  pentalogy Q21.8
  tetrad or tetralogy Q21.3
  triad or trilogy Q22.3
False —*see also* condition
  croup J38.5
  joint —*see* Nonunion, fracture
  labor (pains) O47.9
    at or after 37 completed weeks of gestation
      O47.1
    before 37 completed weeks of gestation
      O47.0-
  passage, urethra (prostatic) N36.5
  pregnancy F45.8
Family, familial —*see also* condition
  disruption Z63.8
    involving divorce or separation Z63.5
  Li-Fraumeni (syndrome) Z15.01
  planning advice Z30.09
  problem Z63.9
    specified NEC Z63.8
  retinoblastoma C69.2-
Famine (effects of) T73.0
  edema —*see* Malnutrition, severe
Fanconi (-de Toni)(-Debré) syndrome E72.09
  with cystinosis E72.04
Fanconi's anemia (congenital pancytopenia)
  D61.09
Farber's disease or syndrome E75.29
Farcy A24.0
Farmer's
  lung J67.0
  skin L57.8
Farsightedness —*see* Hypermetropia
Fascia —*see* condition
Fasciculation R25.3
Fasciitis M72.9
  diffuse (eosinophilic) M35.4
  infective M72.8
    necrotizing M72.6
  necrotizing M72.6
  nodular M72.4
  perirenal (with ureteral obstruction)
    N13.5
    with infection N13.6
  plantar M72.2
  specified NEC M72.8
  traumatic (old) M72.8
    current - code by site under Sprain
Fascioliasis B66.3
Fasciolopsis, fasciolopsiasis (intestinal)
  B66.5
Fascioscapulohumeral myopathy G71.0
Fast pulse R00.0
Fat
  embolism —*see* Embolism, fat
  excessive —*see also* Obesity
    in heart —*see* Degeneration, myocardial
  in stool R19.5

Fat *(Continued)*
  localized (pad) E65
    heart —*see* Degeneration, myocardial
    knee M79.4
    retropatellar M79.4
  necrosis
    breast N64.1
    mesentery K65.4
    omentum K65.4
  pad E65
    knee M79.4
Fatigue R53.83
  auditory deafness —*see* Deafness
  chronic R53.82
  combat F43.0
  general R53.83
    psychogenic F48.8
  heat (transient) T67.6
  muscle M62.89
  myocardium —*see* Failure, heart
  neoplasm-related R53.0
  nervous, neurosis F48.8
  operational F48.8
  psychogenic (general) F48.8
  senile R54
  voice R49.8
Fatness —*see* Obesity
Fatty —*see also* condition
  apron E65
  degeneration —*see* Degeneration, fatty
  heart (enlarged) —*see* Degeneration,
    myocardial
  liver NEC K76.0
    alcoholic K70.0
    nonalcoholic K76.0
  necrosis —*see* Degeneration, fatty
Fauces —*see* condition
Fauchard's disease (periodontitis) —*see*
  Periodontitis
Faucitis J02.9
Favism (anemia) D55.0
Favus —*see* Dermatophytosis
Fazio-Londe disease or syndrome
  G12.1
Fear complex or reaction F40.9
Fear of —*see* Phobia
Feared complaint unfounded Z71.1
Febris, febrile —*see also* Fever
  flava (*see also* Fever, yellow) A95.9
  melitensis A23.0
  pestis —*see* Plague
  recurrens —*see* Fever, relapsing
  rubra A38.9
Fecal
  incontinence R15.9
  smearing R15.1
  soiling R15.1
  urgency R15.2
Fecalith (impaction) K56.41
  appendix K38.1
  congenital P76.8
Fede's disease K14.0
Feeble rapid pulse due to shock following
  injury T79.4
Feeble-minded F70
Feeding
  difficulties R63.3
  problem R63.3
    newborn P92.9
      specified NEC P92.8
    nonorganic (adult) —*see* Disorder,
      eating
Feeling (of)
  foreign body in throat R09.89
Feer's disease —*see* Poisoning, mercury
Feet —*see* condition
Feigned illness Z76.5
Feil-Klippel syndrome (brevicollis) Q76.1
Feinmesser's (hidrotic) ectodermal dysplasia
  Q82.4
Felinophobia F40.218

Felon —see also Cellulitis, digit
  with lymphangitis —see Lymphangitis, acute,
    digit
Felty's syndrome M05.00
  ankle M05.07-
  elbow M05.02-
  foot joint M05.07-
  hand joint M05.04-
  hip M05.05-
  knee M05.06-
  multiple site M05.09
  shoulder M05.01-
  vertebra —see Spondylitis, ankylosing
  wrist M05.03-
Female genital cutting status —see Female
  genital mutilation status (FGM) ◀▥
Female genital mutilation status (FGM) N90.810
  specified NEC N90.818
  type I (clitorectomy status) N90.811
  type II (clitorectomy with excision of labia
    minora status) N90.812
  type III (infibulation status) N90.813
  type IV N90.818
Femur, femoral —see condition
Fenestration, fenestrated —see also Imperfect,
  closure
  aortico-pulmonary Q21.4
  cusps, heart valve NEC Q24.8
    pulmonary Q22.3
  pulmonic cusps Q22.3
Fernell's disease (aortic aneurysm) I71.9
Fertile eunuch syndrome E23.0
Fetid
  breath R19.6
  sweat L75.0
Fetishism F65.0
  transvestic F65.1
Fetus, fetal —see also condition
  alcohol syndrome (dysmorphic) Q86.0
  compressus O31.0-
  hydantoin syndrome Q86.1
  lung tissue P28.0
  papyraceous O31.0-
Fever (inanition) (of unknown origin)
    (persistent) (with chills) (with rigor) R50.9
  abortus A23.1
  Aden (dengue) A90
  African tick-borne A68.1
  American
    mountain (tick) A93.2
    spotted A77.0
  aphthous B08.8
  arbovirus, arboviral A94
    hemorrhagic A94
    specified NEC A93.8
  Argentinian hemorrhagic A96.0
  Assam B55.0
  Australian Q A78
  Bangkok hemorrhagic A91
  Barmah forest A92.8
  Bartonella A44.0
  bilious, hemoglobinuric B50.8
  blackwater B50.8
  blister B00.1
  Bolivian hemorrhagic A96.1
  Bonvale dam T73.3
  boutonneuse A77.1
  brain —see Encephalitis
  Brazilian purpuric A48.4
  breakbone A90
  Bullis A77.0
  Bunyamwera A92.8
  Burdwan B55.0
  Bwamba A92.8
  Cameroon —see Malaria
  Canton A75.9
  catarrhal (acute) J00
    chronic J31.0
  cat-scratch A28.1
  Central Asian hemorrhagic A98.0
  cerebral —see Encephalitis

Fever (Continued)
  cerebrospinal meningococcal A39.0
  Chagres B50.9
  Chandipura A92.8
  Changuinola A93.1
  Charcot's (biliary) (hepatic) (intermittent) —
    see Calculus, bile duct
  Chikungunya (viral) (hemorrhagic) A92.0
  Chitral A93.1
  Colombo —see Fever, paratyphoid
  Colorado tick (virus) A93.2
  congestive (remittent) —see Malaria
  Congo virus A98.0
  continued malarial B50.9
  Corsican —see Malaria
  Crimean-Congo hemorrhagic A98.0
  Cyprus —see Brucellosis
  dandy A90
  deer fly —see Tularemia
  dengue (virus) A90
    hemorrhagic A91
    sandfly A93.1
  desert B38.0
  drug induced R50.2
  ~~due to conditions classified elsewhere R50.81~~
  ~~due to heat T67.0~~
  due to ◀
    conditions classified elsewhere R50.81 ◀
    heat T67.0 ◀
  enteric A01.00
  enteroviral exanthematous (Boston
    exanthem) A88.0
  ephemeral (of unknown origin) R50.9
  epidemic hemorrhagic A98.5
  erysipelatous —see Erysipelas
  estivo-autumnal (malarial) B50.9
  famine A75.0
  five day A79.0
  following delivery O86.4
  Fort Bragg A27.89
  gastroenteric A01.00
  gastromalarial —see Malaria
  Gibraltar —see Brucellosis
  glandular —see Mononucleosis, infectious
  Guama (viral) A92.8
  Haverhill A25.1
  hay (allergic) J30.1
    with asthma (bronchial) J45.909
      with
        exacerbation (acute) J45.901
        status asthmaticus J45.902
      due to
        allergen other than pollen J30.89
        pollen, any plant or tree J30.1
  heat (effects) T67.0
  hematuric, bilious B50.8
  hemoglobinuric (malarial) (bilious) B50.8
  hemorrhagic (arthropod-borne) NOS A94
    with renal syndrome A98.5
    arenaviral A96.9
      specified NEC A96.8
    Argentinian A96.0
    Bangkok A91
    Bolivian A96.1
    Central Asian A98.0
    Chikungunya A92.0
    Crimean-Congo A98.0
    dengue (virus) A91
    epidemic A98.5
    Junin (virus) A96.0
    Korean A98.5
    Kyasanur forest A98.2
    Machupo (virus) A96.1
    mite-borne A93.8
    mosquito-borne A92.8
    Omsk A98.1
    Philippine A91
    Russian A98.5
    Singapore A91
    Southeast Asia A91
    Thailand A91

Fever (Continued)
  hemorrhagic NOS (Continued)
    tick-borne NEC A93.8
    viral A99
      specified NEC A98.8
  hepatic —see Cholecystitis
  herpetic —see Herpes
  icterohemorrhagic A27.0
  Indiana A93.8
  infective B99.9
    specified NEC B99.8
  intermittent (bilious) —see also Malaria
    of unknown origin R50.9
    pernicious B50.9
  iodide R50.2
  Japanese river A75.3
  jungle —see also Malaria
    yellow A95.0
  Junin (virus) hemorrhagic A96.0
  Katayama B65.2
  kedani A75.3
  Kenya (tick) A77.1
  Kew Garden A79.1
  Korean hemorrhagic A98.5
  Lassa A96.2
  Lone Star A77.0
  Machupo (virus) hemorrhagic A96.1
  malaria, malarial —see Malaria
  Malta A23.9
  Marseilles A77.1
  marsh —see Malaria
  Mayaro (viral) A92.8
  Mediterranean (see also Brucellosis) A23.9
    familial E85.0
    tick A77.1
  meningeal —see Meningitis
  Meuse A79.0
  Mexican A75.2
  mianeh A68.1
  miasmatic —see Malaria
  mosquito-borne (viral) A92.9
    hemorrhagic A92.8
  mountain —see also Brucellosis
    meaning Rocky Mountain spotted fever
      A77.0
    tick (American) (Colorado) (viral) A93.2
  Mucambo (viral) A92.8
  mud A27.9
  Neapolitan —see Brucellosis
  neutropenic D70.9
  newborn P81.9
    environmental P81.0
  Nine-Mile A78
  non-exanthematous tick A93.2
  North Asian tick-borne A77.2
  Omsk hemorrhagic A98.1
  O'nyong-nyong (viral) A92.1
  Oropouche (viral) A93.0
  Oroya A44.0
  paludal —see Malaria
  Panama (malarial) B50.9
  Pappataci A93.1
  paratyphoid A01.4
    A A01.1
    B A01.2
    C A01.3
  parrot A70
  periodic (Mediterranean) E85.0
  persistent (of unknown origin) R50.9
  petechial A39.0
  pharyngoconjunctival B30.2
  Philippine hemorrhagic A91
  phlebotomus A93.1
  Piry (virus) A93.8
  Pixuna (viral) A92.8
  Plasmodium ovale B53.0
  polioviral (nonparalytic) A80.4
  Pontiac A48.2
  postimmunization R50.83
  postoperative R50.82
    due to infection T81.4

◀ New   ◀▥ Revised   ~~deleted~~ Deleted

Fever *(Continued)*
 posttransfusion R50.84
 postvaccination R50.83
 presenting with conditions classified
   elsewhere R50.81
 pretibial A27.89
 puerperal O86.4
 Q A78
 quadrilateral A78
 quartan (malaria) B52.9
 Queensland (coastal) (tick) A77.3
 quintan A79.0
 rabbit —*see* Tularemia
 rat-bite A25.9
   due to
     Spirillum A25.0
     Streptobacillus moniliformis A25.1
 recurrent —*see* Fever, relapsing
 relapsing (Borrelia) A68.9
   Carter's (Asiatic) A68.1
   Dutton's (West African) A68.1
   Koch's A68.9
   louse-borne A68.0
   Novy's
     louse-borne A68.0
     tick-borne A68.1
   Obermeyer's (European) A68.0
   tick-borne A68.1
 remittent (bilious) (congestive) (gastric) —*see*
   Malaria
 rheumatic (active) (acute) (chronic) (subacute)
   I00
   with central nervous system involvement
     I02.9
   active with heart involvement *(see*
     category) I01
   inactive or quiescent with
     cardiac hypertrophy I09.89
     carditis I09.9
     endocarditis I09.1
       aortic (valve) I06.9
         with mitral (valve) disease I08.0
       mitral (valve) I05.9
         with aortic (valve) disease I08.0
       pulmonary (valve) I09.89
       tricuspid (valve) I07.8
     heart disease NEC I09.89
     heart failure (congestive) (conditions in
       I50.9) I09.81
     left ventricular failure (conditions in
       I50.1) I09.81
     myocarditis, myocardial degeneration
       (conditions in I51.4) I09.0
     pancarditis I09.9
     pericarditis I09.2
 Rift Valley (viral) A92.4
 Rocky Mountain spotted A77.0
 rose J30.1
 Ross River B33.1
 Russian hemorrhagic A98.5
 San Joaquin (Valley) B38.0
 sandfly A93.1
 Sao Paulo A77.0
 scarlet A38.9
 seven day (leptospirosis) (autumnal)
   (Japanese) A27.89
   dengue A90
 shin-bone A79.0
 Singapore hemorrhagic A91
 solar A90
 Songo A98.5
 sore B00.1
 South African tick-bite A68.1
 Southeast Asia hemorrhagic A91
 spinal —*see* Meningitis
 spirillary A25.0
 splenic —*see* Anthrax
 spotted A77.9
   American A77.0
   Brazilian A77.0
   cerebrospinal meningitis A39.0

Fever *(Continued)*
 spotted *(Continued)*
   Colombian A77.0
   due to Rickettsia
     australis A77.3
     conorii A77.1
     rickettsii A77.0
     sibirica A77.2
     specified type NEC A77.8
   Ehrlichiosis A77.40
     due to
       E. chafeensis A77.41
       specified organism NEC A77.49
     Rocky Mountain A77.0
 steroid R50.2
 streptobacillary A25.1
 subtertian B50.9
 Sumatran mite A75.3
 sun A90
 swamp A27.9
 swine A02.8
 sylvatic, yellow A95.0
 Tahyna B33.8
 tertian —*see* Malaria, tertian
 Thailand hemorrhagic A91
 thermic T67.0
 three-day A93.1
 tick
   American mountain A93.2
   Colorado A93.2
   Kemerovo A93.8
   Mediterranean A77.1
   mountain A93.2
   nonexanthematous A93.2
   Quaranfil A93.8
 tick-bite NEC A93.8
 tick-borne (hemorrhagic) NEC A93.8
 trench A79.0
 tsutsugamushi A75.3
 typhogastric A01.00
 typhoid (abortive) (hemorrhagic)
   (intermittent) (malignant) A01.00
   complicated by
     arthritis A01.04
     heart involvement A01.02
     meningitis A01.01
     osteomyelitis A01.05
     pneumonia A01.03
     specified NEC A01.09
 typhomalarial —*see* Malaria
 typhus —*see* Typhus (fever)
 undulant —*see* Brucellosis
 unknown origin R50.9
 uveoparotid D86.89
 valley B38.0
 Venezuelan equine A92.2
 vesicular stomatitis A93.8
 viral hemorrhagic —*see* Fever, hemorrhagic,
   by type of virus
 Volhynian A79.0
 Wesselsbron (viral) A92.8
 West
   African B50.8
   Nile (viral) A92.30
     with
       complications NEC A92.39
       cranial nerve disorders A92.32
       encephalitis A92.31
       encephalomyelitis A92.31
       neurologic manifestation NEC
         A92.32
       optic neuritis A92.32
       polyradiculitis A92.32
 Whitmore's —*see* Melioidosis
 Wolhynian A79.0
 worm B83.9
 yellow A95.9
   jungle A95.0
   sylvatic A95.0
   urban A95.1
 Zika (viral) A92.8

Fibrillation
 atrial or auricular (established) I48.91
   chronic I48.2
   paroxysmal I48.0
   permanent I48.2
   persistent I48.1
 cardiac I49.8
 heart I49.8
 muscular M62.89
 ventricular I49.01
Fibrin
 ball or bodies, pleural (sac) J94.1
 chamber, anterior (eye) (gelatinous
   exudate) —*see* Iridocyclitis, acute
Fibrinogenolysis —*see* Fibrinolysis
Fibrinogenopenia D68.8
 acquired D65
 congenital D68.2
Fibrinolysis (hemorrhagic) (acquired) D65
 antepartum hemorrhage —*see* Hemorrhage,
   antepartum, with coagulation defect
 following
   abortion —*see* Abortion by type
     complicated by hemorrhage
   ectopic or molar pregnancy O08.1
 intrapartum O67.0
 newborn, transient P60
 postpartum O72.3
Fibrinopenia (hereditary) D68.2
 acquired D68.4
Fibrinopurulent —*see* condition
Fibrinous —*see* condition
Fibroadenoma
 cellular intracanalicular D24-
 giant D24-
 intracanalicular
   cellular D24-
   giant D24-
   specified site —*see* Neoplasm, benign, by
     site
   unspecified site D24-
 juvenile D24-
 pericanalicular
   specified site —*see* Neoplasm, benign, by
     site
   unspecified site D24-
 phyllodes D24-
 prostate D29.1
 specified site NEC —*see* Neoplasm, benign,
   by site
 unspecified site D24-
Fibroadenosis, breast (chronic) (cystic) (diffuse)
 (periodic) (segmental) N60.2-
Fibroangioma —*see also* Neoplasm, benign, by
 site
 juvenile
   specified site —*see* Neoplasm, benign, by
     site
   unspecified site D10.6
Fibrochondrosarcoma —*see* Neoplasm,
 cartilage, malignant
Fibrocystic
 disease —*see also* Fibrosis, cystic
   breast —*see* Mastopathy, cystic
   jaw M27.49
   kidney (congenital) Q61.8
   liver Q44.6
   pancreas E84.9
 kidney (congenital) Q61.8
Fibrodysplasia ossificans progressiva —*see*
 Myositis, ossificans, progressiva
Fibroelastosis (cordis) (endocardial)
 (endomyocardial) I42.4
Fibroid (tumor) —*see also* Neoplasm, connective
 tissue, benign
 disease, lung (chronic) —*see* Fibrosis, lung
 heart (disease) —*see* Myocarditis
 in pregnancy or childbirth O34.1-
   causing obstructed labor O65.5
 induration, lung (chronic) —*see* Fibrosis, lung
 lung —*see* Fibrosis, lung

Fibroid *(Continued)*
  pneumonia (chronic) —*see* Fibrosis, lung
  uterus D25.9
Fibrolipoma —*see* Lipoma
Fibroliposarcoma —*see* Neoplasm, connective
    tissue, malignant
Fibroma —*see also* Neoplasm, connective tissue,
    benign
  ameloblastic —*see* Cyst, calcifying
    odontogenic
  bone (nonossifying) —*see* Disorder, bone,
    specified type NEC
    ossifying —*see* Neoplasm, bone,
      benign
  cementifying —*see* Neoplasm, bone,
    benign
  chondromyxoid —*see* Neoplasm, bone,
    benign
  desmoplastic —*see* Neoplasm, connective
    tissue, uncertain behavior
  durum —*see* Neoplasm, connective tissue,
    benign
  fascial —*see* Neoplasm, connective tissue,
    benign
  invasive —*see* Neoplasm, connective tissue,
    uncertain behavior
  molle —*see* Lipoma
  myxoid —*see* Neoplasm, connective tissue,
    benign
  nasopharynx, nasopharyngeal (juvenile)
    D10.6
  nonosteogenic (nonossifying) —*see* Dysplasia,
    fibrous
  odontogenic (central) —*see* Cyst, calcifying
    odontogenic
  ossifying —*see* Neoplasm, bone, benign
  periosteal —*see* Neoplasm, bone, benign
  soft —*see* Lipoma
Fibromatosis M72.9
  abdominal —*see* Neoplasm, connective tissue,
    uncertain behavior
  aggressive —*see* Neoplasm, connective tissue,
    uncertain behavior
  congenital generalized —*see* Neoplasm,
    connective tissue, uncertain behavior
  Dupuytren's M72.0
  gingival K06.1
  palmar (fascial) M72.0
  plantar (fascial) M72.2
  pseudosarcomatous (proliferative)
    (subcutaneous) M72.4
  retroperitoneal D48.3
  specified NEC M72.8
Fibromyalgia M79.7
Fibromyoma —*see also* Neoplasm, connective
    tissue, benign
  uterus (corpus) —*see also* Leiomyoma, uterus
    in pregnancy or childbirth —*see* Fibroid, in
      pregnancy or childbirth
    causing obstructed labor O65.5
Fibromyositis M79.7
Fibromyxolipoma D17.9
Fibromyxoma —*see* Neoplasm, connective
    tissue, benign
Fibromyxosarcoma —*see* Neoplasm, connective
    tissue, malignant
Fibro-odontoma, ameloblastic —*see* Cyst,
    calcifying odontogenic
Fibro-osteoma —*see* Neoplasm, bone, benign
Fibroplasia, retrolental H35.17
Fibropurulent —*see* condition
Fibrosarcoma —*see also* Neoplasm, connective
    tissue, malignant
  ameloblastic C41.1
    upper jaw (bone) C41.0
  congenital —*see* Neoplasm, connective tissue,
    malignant
  fascial —*see* Neoplasm, connective tissue,
    malignant
  infantile —*see* Neoplasm, connective tissue,
    malignant

Fibrosarcoma *(Continued)*
  odontogenic C41.1
    upper jaw (bone) C41.0
  periosteal —*see* Neoplasm, bone, malignant
Fibrosclerosis
  breast N60.3-
  multifocal M35.5
  penis (corpora cavernosa) N48.6
Fibrosis, fibrotic
  adrenal (gland) E27.8
  amnion O41.8X-
  anal papillae K62.89
  arteriocapillary —*see* Arteriosclerosis
  bladder N32.89
    interstitial —*see* Cystitis, chronic,
      interstitial
    localized submucosal —*see* Cystitis,
      chronic, interstitial
    panmural —*see* Cystitis, chronic,
      interstitial
  breast —*see* Fibrosclerosis, breast
  capillary (*see also* Arteriosclerosis) I70.90
    lung (chronic) —*see* Fibrosis, lung
  cardiac —*see* Myocarditis
  cervix N88.8
  chorion O41.8X-
  corpus cavernosum (sclerosing) N48.6
  cystic (of pancreas) E84.9
    with
      distal intestinal obstruction syndrome
        E84.19
      fecal impaction E84.19
      intestinal manifestations NEC E84.19
      pulmonary manifestations E84.0
      specified manifestations NEC E84.8
  due to device, implant or graft (*see also*
    Complications, by site and type,
    specified NEC) T85.82
    arterial graft NEC T82.828
    breast (implant) T85.82
    catheter NEC T85.82
      dialysis (renal) T82.828
        intraperitoneal T85.82
      infusion NEC T82.828
        spinal (epidural) (subdural) T85.82
      urinary (indwelling) T83.82
    electronic (electrode) (pulse generator)
      (stimulator)
      bone T84.82
      cardiac T82.827
      nervous system (brain) (peripheral
        nerve) (spinal) T85.82
      urinary T83.82
    fixation, internal (orthopedic) NEC T84.82
    gastrointestinal (bile duct) (esophagus)
      T85.82
    genital NEC T83.82
    heart NEC T82.827
    joint prosthesis T84.82
    ocular (corneal graft) (orbital implant)
      NEC T85.82
    orthopedic NEC T84.82
    specified NEC T85.82
    urinary NEC T83.82
    vascular NEC T82.828
    ventricular intracranial shunt T85.82
  ejaculatory duct N50.8
  endocardium —*see* Endocarditis
  endomyocardial (tropical) I42.3
  epididymis N50.8
  eye muscle —*see* Strabismus, mechanical
  heart —*see* Myocarditis
  hepatic —*see* Fibrosis, liver
  hepatolienal (portal hypertension) K76.6
  hepatosplenic (portal hypertension) K76.6
  infrapatellar fat pad M79.4
  intrascrotal N50.8
  kidney N26.9
  liver K74.0
    with sclerosis K74.2
    alcoholic K70.2

Fibrosis, fibrotic *(Continued)*
  lung (atrophic) (chronic) (confluent)
    (massive) (perialveolar) (peribronchial)
    J84.10
    with
      anthracosilicosis J60
      anthracosis J60
      asbestosis J61
      bagassosis J67.1
      bauxite J63.1
      berylliosis J63.2
      byssinosis J66.0
      calcicosis J62.8
      chalicosis J62.8
      dust reticulation J64
      farmer's lung J67.0
      ganister disease J62.8
      graphite J63.3
      pneumoconiosis NOS J64
      siderosis J63.4
      silicosis J62.8
    capillary J84.10
    congenital P27.8
    diffuse (idiopathic) J84.10
      chemicals, gases, fumes or vapors
        (inhalation) J68.4
      interstitial J84.10
        acute J84.114
      talc J62.0
    following radiation J70.1
    idiopathic J84.112
    postinflammatory J84.10
    silicotic J62.8
    tuberculous —*see* Tuberculosis, pulmonary
  lymphatic gland I89.8
  median bar —*see* Hyperplasia, prostate
  mediastinum (idiopathic) J98.5
  meninges G96.19
  myocardium, myocardial —*see* Myocarditis
  ovary N83.8
  oviduct N83.8
  pancreas K86.8
  penis NEC N48.6
  pericardium I31.0
  perineum, in pregnancy or childbirth O34.7-
    causing obstructed labor O65.5
  pleura J94.1
  popliteal fat pad M79.4
  prostate (chronic) —*see* Hyperplasia, prostate
  pulmonary (*see also* Fibrosis, lung) J84.10
    congenital P27.8
    idiopathic J84.112
  rectal sphincter K62.89
  retroperitoneal, idiopathic (with ureteral
    obstruction) N13.5
    with infection N13.6
  sclerosing mesenteric (idiopathic) K65.4
  scrotum N50.8
  seminal vesicle N50.8
  senile R54
  skin L90.5
  spermatic cord N50.8
  spleen D73.89
    in schistosomiasis (bilharziasis) B65.9
      [D77]
  subepidermal nodular —*see* Neoplasm, skin,
    benign
  submucous (oral) (tongue) K13.5
  testis N44.8
    chronic, due to syphilis A52.76
  thymus (gland) E32.8
  tongue, submucous K13.5
  tunica vaginalis N50.8
  uterus (non-neoplastic) N85.8
  vagina N89.8
  valve, heart —*see* Endocarditis
  vas deferens N50.8
  vein I87.8
Fibrositis (periarticular) M79.7
  nodular, chronic (Jaccoud's) (rheumatoid) —
    see Arthropathy, postrheumatic, chronic

◀ New   ◀▥ Revised   ~~deleted~~ Deleted

Fibrothorax J94.1
Fibrotic —*see* Fibrosis
Fibrous —*see* condition
Fibroxanthoma —*see also* Neoplasm, connective
  tissue, benign
  atypical —*see* Neoplasm, connective tissue,
    uncertain behavior
  malignant —*see* Neoplasm, connective tissue,
    malignant
Fibroxanthosarcoma —*see* Neoplasm,
  connective tissue, malignant
Fiedler's
  disease (icterohemorrhagic leptospirosis)
    A27.0
  myocarditis (acute) I40.1
Fifth disease B08.3
  venereal A55
Filaria, filarial, filariasis —*see* Infestation,
  filarial
Filatov's disease —*see* Mononucleosis,
  infectious
File-cutter's disease —*see* Poisoning, lead
Filling defect
  biliary tract R93.2
  bladder R93.4
  duodenum R93.3
  gallbladder R93.2
  gastrointestinal tract R93.3
  intestine R93.3
  kidney R93.4
  stomach R93.3
  ureter R93.4
Fimbrial cyst Q50.4
Financial problem affecting care NOS Z59.9
  bankruptcy Z59.8
  foreclosure on loan Z59.8
Findings, abnormal, inconclusive, without
  diagnosis —*see also* Abnormal
  17-ketosteroids, elevated R82.5
  acetonuria R82.4
  alcohol in blood R78.0
  anisocytosis R71.8
  antenatal screening of mother O28.9
    biochemical O28.1
    chromosomal O28.5
    cytological O28.2
    genetic O28.5
    hematological O28.0
    radiological O28.4
    specified NEC O28.8
    ultrasonic O28.3
  antibody titer, elevated R76.0
  anticardiolipin antibody R76.0
  antiphosphatidylglycerol antibody R76.0
  antiphosphatidylinositol antibody R76.0
  antiphosphatidylserine antibody R76.0
  antiphospholipid antibody R76.0
  bacteriuria N39.0
  bicarbonate E87.8
  bile in urine R82.2
  blood sugar R73.09
    high R73.9
    low (transient) E16.2
  body fluid or substance, specified NEC R88.8
  casts, urine R82.99
  catecholamines R82.5
  cells, urine R82.99
  chloride E87.8
  cholesterol E78.9
    high E78.0
      with high triglycerides E78.2
  chyluria R82.0
  cloudy
    dialysis effluent R88.0
    urine R82.90
  creatinine clearance R94.4
  crystals, urine R82.99
  culture
    blood R78.81
    positive —*see* Positive, culture
  echocardiogram R93.1

Findings, abnormal, inconclusive, without
  diagnosis (*Continued*)
  electrolyte level, urinary R82.99
  function study NEC R94.8
    bladder R94.8
    endocrine NEC R94.7
      thyroid R94.6
    kidney R94.4
    liver R94.5
    pancreas R94.8
    placenta R94.8
    pulmonary R94.2
    spleen R94.8
  gallbladder, nonvisualization R93.2
  glucose (tolerance test) (non-fasting)
    R73.09
  glycosuria R81
  heart
    shadow R93.1
    sounds R01.2
  hematinuria R82.3
  hematocrit drop (precipitous) R71.0
  hemoglobinuria R82.3
  human papillomavirus (HPV) DNA test
    positive
    cervix
      high risk R87.810
      low risk R87.820
    vagina
      high risk R87.811
      low risk R87.821
  in blood (of substance not normally found in
    blood) R78.9
    addictive drug NEC R78.4
    alcohol (excessive level) R78.0
    cocaine R78.2
    hallucinogen R78.3
    heavy metals (abnormal level) R78.79
    lead R78.71
    lithium (abnormal level) R78.89
    opiate drug R78.1
    psychotropic drug R78.5
    specified substance NEC R78.89
    steroid agent R78.6
  indoleacetic acid, elevated R82.5
  ketonuria R82.4
  lactic acid dehydrogenase (LDH) R74.0
  liver function test R79.89
  mammogram NEC R92.8
    calcification (calculus) R92.1
    inconclusive result (due to dense breasts)
      R92.2
    microcalcification R92.0
  mediastinal shift R93.8
  melanin, urine R82.99
  myoglobinuria R82.1
  neonatal screening P09
  nonvisualization of gallbladder R93.2
  odor of urine NOS R82.90
  Papanicolaou cervix R87.619
    non-atypical endometrial cells R87.618
  pneumoencephalogram R93.0
  poikilocytosis R71.8
  potassium (deficiency) E87.6
    excess E87.5
  PPD R76.11
  radiologic (X-ray) R93.8
    abdomen R93.5
    biliary tract R93.2
    breast R92.8
    gastrointestinal tract R93.3
    genitourinary organs R93.8
    head R93.0
    inconclusive due to excess body fat of
      patient R93.9
    intrathoracic organs NEC R93.1
    placenta R93.8
    retroperitoneum R93.5
    skin R93.8
    skull R93.0
    subcutaneous tissue R93.8

Findings, abnormal, inconclusive, without
  diagnosis (*Continued*)
  red blood cell (count) (morphology) (sickling)
    (volume) R71.8
  scan NEC R94.8
    bladder R94.8
    bone R94.8
    kidney R94.4
    liver R93.2
    lung R94.2
    pancreas R94.8
    placental R94.8
    spleen R94.8
    thyroid R94.6
  sedimentation rate, elevated R70.0
  SGOT R74.0
  SGPT R74.0
  sodium (deficiency) E87.1
    excess E87.0
  specified body fluid NEC R88.8
  stress test R94.39
  thyroid (function) (metabolic rate) (scan)
    (uptake) R94.6
  transaminase (level) R74.0
  triglycerides E78.9
    high E78.1
      with high cholesterol E78.2
  tuberculin skin test (without active
    tuberculosis) R76.11
  urine R82.90
    acetone R82.4
    bacteria N39.0
    bile R82.2
    casts or cells R82.99
    chyle R82.0
    culture positive R82.7
    glucose R81
    hemoglobin R82.3
    ketone R82.4
    sugar R81
  vanillylmandelic acid (VMA), elevated
    R82.5
  vectorcardiogram (VCG) R94.39
  ventriculogram R93.0
  white blood cell (count) (differential)
    (morphology) D72.9
  xerography R92.8
Finger —*see* condition
Fire, Saint Anthony's —*see* Erysipelas
Fire-setting
  pathological (compulsive) F63.1
Fish hook stomach K31.89
Fishmeal-worker's lung J67.8
Fissure, fissured
  anus, anal K60.2
    acute K60.0
    chronic K60.1
    congenital Q43.8
  ear, lobule, congenital Q17.8
  epiglottis (congenital) Q31.8
  larynx J38.7
    congenital Q31.8
  lip K13.0
    congenital —*see* Cleft, lip
  nipple N64.0
    associated with
      lactation O92.13
      pregnancy O92.11-
      puerperium O92.12
  nose Q30.2
  palate (congenital) —*see* Cleft, palate
  skin R23.4
  spine (congenital) —*see also* Spina bifida
    with hydrocephalus —*see* Spina bifida, by
      site, with hydrocephalus
  tongue (acquired) K14.5
    congenital Q38.3
Fistula (cutaneous) L98.8
  abdomen (wall) K63.2
    bladder N32.2
    intestine NEC K63.2

Fistula *(Continued)*
  abdomen *(Continued)*
    ureter N28.89
    uterus N82.5
  abdominorectal K63.2
  abdominosigmoidal K63.2
  abdominothoracic J86.0
  abdominouterine N82.5
    congenital Q51.7
  abdominovesical N32.2
  accessory sinuses —*see* Sinusitis
  actinomycotic —*see* Actinomycosis
  alveolar antrum —*see* Sinusitis, maxillary
  alveolar process K04.6
  anorectal K60.5
  antrobuccal —*see* Sinusitis, maxillary
  antrum —*see* Sinusitis, maxillary
  anus, anal (recurrent) (infectional) K60.3
    congenital Q43.6
      with absence, atresia and stenosis Q42.2
    tuberculous A18.32
  aorta-duodenal I77.2
  appendix, appendicular K38.3
  arteriovenous (acquired) (nonruptured) I77.0
    brain I67.1
      congenital Q28.2
        ruptured I60.8
      ruptured I60.8
    cerebral —*see* Fistula, arteriovenous, brain
    congenital (peripheral) —*see also*
      Malformation, arteriovenous
      brain Q28.2
        ruptured I60.8
      coronary Q24.5
      pulmonary Q25.72
    coronary I25.41
      congenital Q24.5
    pulmonary I28.0
      congenital Q25.72
    surgically created (for dialysis) Z99.2
      complication —*see* Complication,
        arteriovenous, fistula, surgically
        created
    traumatic —*see* Injury, blood vessel
  artery I77.2
  aural (mastoid) —*see* Mastoiditis, chronic
  auricle —*see also* Disorder, pinna, specified
    type NEC
    congenital Q18.1
  Bartholin's gland N82.8
  bile duct (common) (hepatic) K83.3
    with calculus, stones —*see* Calculus, bile
      duct
  biliary (tract) —*see* Fistula, bile duct
  bladder (sphincter) NEC *(see also* Fistula,
    vesico-) N32.2
    into seminal vesicle N32.2
  bone —*see also* Disorder, bone, specified type
    NEC
    with osteomyelitis, chronic —*see*
      Osteomyelitis, chronic, with draining
      sinus
  brain G93.89
    arteriovenous (acquired) I67.1
      congenital Q28.2
  branchial (cleft) Q18.0
  branchiogenous Q18.0
  breast N61
    puerperal, postpartum or gestational, due
      to mastitis (purulent) —*see* Mastitis,
      obstetric, purulent
  bronchial J86.0
  bronchocutaneous, bronchomediastinal,
    bronchopleural,
    bronchopleuromediastinal (infective)
    J86.0
    tuberculous NEC A15.5
  bronchoesophageal J86.0
    congenital Q39.2
      with atresia of esophagus Q39.1
  bronchovisceral J86.0

Fistula *(Continued)*
  buccal cavity (infective) K12.2
  cecosigmoidal K63.2
  cecum K63.2
  cerebrospinal (fluid) G96.0
  cervical, lateral Q18.1
  cervicoaural Q18.1
  cervicosigmoidal N82.4
  cervicovesical N82.1
  cervix N82.8
  chest (wall) J86.0
  cholecystenteric —*see* Fistula, gallbladder
  cholecystocolic —*see* Fistula, gallbladder
  cholecystocolonic —*see* Fistula, gallbladder
  cholecystoduodenal —*see* Fistula,
    gallbladder
  cholecystogastric —*see* Fistula, gallbladder
  cholecystointestinal —*see* Fistula,
    gallbladder
  choledochoduodenal —*see* Fistula,
    bile duct
  cholocolic K82.3
  coccyx —*see* Sinus, pilonidal
  colon K63.2
  colostomy K94.09
  common duct —*see* Fistula, bile duct
  congenital, site not listed —*see* Anomaly, by
    site
  coronary, arteriovenous I25.41
    congenital Q24.5
  costal region J86.0
  cul-de-sac, Douglas' N82.8
  cystic duct —*see also* Fistula, gallbladder
    congenital Q44.5
  dental K04.6
  diaphragm J86.0
  duodenum K31.6
  ear (external) (canal) —*see* Disorder, ear,
    external, specified type NEC
  enterocolic K63.2
  enterocutaneous K63.2
  enterouterine N82.4
    congenital Q51.7
  enterovaginal N82.4
    congenital Q52.2
    large intestine N82.3
    small intestine N82.2
  enterovesical N32.1
  epididymis N50.8
    tuberculous A18.15
  esophagobronchial J86.0
    congenital Q39.2
      with atresia of esophagus Q39.1
  esophagocutaneous K22.8
  esophagopleural-cutaneous J86.0
  esophagotracheal J86.0
    congenital Q39.2
      with atresia of esophagus Q39.1
  esophagus K22.8
    congenital Q39.2
      with atresia of esophagus Q39.1
  ethmoid —*see* Sinusitis, ethmoidal
  eyeball (cornea) (sclera) —*see* Disorder, globe,
    hypotony
  eyelid H01.8
  fallopian tube, external N82.5
  fecal K63.2
    congenital Q43.6
  from periapical abscess K04.6
  frontal sinus —*see* Sinusitis, frontal
  gallbladder K82.3
    with calculus, cholelithiasis, stones —*see*
      Calculus, gallbladder
  gastric K31.6
  gastrocolic K31.6
    congenital Q40.2
    tuberculous A18.32
  gastroenterocolic K31.6
  gastroesophageal K31.6
  gastrojejunal K31.6
  gastrojejunocolic K31.6

Fistula *(Continued)*
  genital tract (female) N82.9
    specified NEC N82.8
    to intestine NEC N82.4
    to skin N82.5
  hepatic artery-portal vein, congenital Q26.6
  hepatopleural J86.0
  hepatopulmonary J86.0
  ileorectal or ileosigmoidal K63.2
  ileovaginal N82.2
  ileovesical N32.1
  ileum K63.2
  in ano K60.3
    tuberculous A18.32
  inner ear (labyrinth) —*see* subcategory H83.1
  intestine NEC K63.2
  intestinocolonic (abdominal) K63.2
  intestinoureteral N28.89
  intestinouterine N82.4
  intestinovaginal N82.4
    large intestine N82.3
    small intestine N82.2
  intestinovesical N32.1
  ischiorectal (fossa) K61.3
  jejunum K63.2
  joint M25.10
    ankle M25.17-
    elbow M25.12-
    foot joint M25.17-
    hand joint M25.14-
    hip M25.15-
    knee M25.16-
    shoulder M25.11-
    specified joint NEC M25.18
    tuberculous —*see* Tuberculosis, joint
    vertebrae M25.18 ◀
    wrist M25.13-
  kidney N28.89
  labium (majus) (minus) N82.8
  labyrinth —*see* subcategory H83.1
  lacrimal (gland) (sac) H04.61-
  lacrimonasal duct —*see* Fistula, lacrimal
  laryngotracheal, congenital Q34.8
  larynx J38.7
  lip K13.0
    congenital Q38.0
  lumbar, tuberculous A18.01
  lung J86.0
  lymphatic I89.8
  mammary (gland) N61
  mastoid (process) (region) —*see* Mastoiditis,
    chronic
  maxillary J32.0
  medial, face and neck Q18.8
  mediastinal J86.0
  mediastinobronchial J86.0
  mediastinocutaneous J86.0
  middle ear —*see* subcategory H74.8
  mouth K12.2
  nasal J34.89
    sinus —*see* Sinusitis
  nasopharynx J39.2
  nipple N64.0
  nose J34.89
  oral (cutaneous) K12.2
    maxillary J32.0
    nasal (with cleft palate) —*see* Cleft, palate
  orbit, orbital —*see* Disorder, orbit, specified
    type NEC
  oroantral J32.0
  oviduct, external N82.5
  palate (hard) M27.8
  pancreatic K86.8
  pancreaticoduodenal K86.8
  parotid (gland) K11.4
    region K12.2
  penis N48.89
  perianal K60.3
  pericardium (pleura) (sac) —*see* Pericarditis
  pericecal K63.2
  perineorectal K60.4
  perineosigmoidal K63.2

Fistula (Continued)
  perineum, perineal (with urethral
      involvement) NEC N36.0
    tuberculous A18.13
    ureter N28.89
  perirectal K60.4
    tuberculous A18.32
  peritoneum K65.9
  pharyngoesophageal J39.2
  pharynx J39.2
    branchial cleft (congenital) Q18.0
  pilonidal (infected) (rectum) —see Sinus,
      pilonidal
  pleura, pleural, pleurocutaneous,
      pleuroperitoneal J86.0
    tuberculous NEC A15.6
  pleuropericardial I31.8
  portal vein-hepatic artery, congenital Q26.6
  postauricular H70.81-
  postoperative, persistent T81.83
    specified site —see Fistula, by site
  preauricular (congenital) Q18.1
  prostate N42.89
  pulmonary J86.0
    arteriovenous I28.0
      congenital Q25.72
    tuberculous —see Tuberculosis, pulmonary
  pulmonoperitoneal J86.0
  rectolabial N82.4
  rectosigmoid (intercommunicating) K63.2
  rectoureteral N28.89
  rectourethral N36.0
    congenital Q64.73
  rectouterine N82.4
    congenital Q51.7
  rectovaginal N82.3
    congenital Q52.2
    tuberculous A18.18
  rectovesical N32.1
    congenital Q64.79
  rectovesicovaginal N82.3
  rectovulval N82.4
    congenital Q52.79
  rectum (to skin) K60.4
    congenital Q43.6
      with absence, atresia and stenosis Q42.0
    tuberculous A18.32
  renal N28.89
  retroauricular —see Fistula, postauricular
  salivary duct or gland (any) K11.4
    congenital Q38.4
  scrotum (urinary) N50.8
    tuberculous A18.15
  semicircular canals —see subcategory H83.1
  sigmoid K63.2
    to bladder N32.1
  sinus —see Sinusitis
  skin L98.8
    to genital tract (female) N82.5
  splenocolic D73.89
  stercoral K63.2
  stomach K31.6
  sublingual gland K11.4
  submandibular gland K11.4
  submaxillary (gland) K11.4
    region K12.2
  thoracic J86.0
    duct I89.8
  thoracoabdominal J86.0
  thoracogastric J86.0
  thoracointestinal J86.0
  thorax J86.0
  thyroglossal duct Q89.2
  thyroid E07.89
  trachea, congenital (external) (internal) Q32.1
  tracheoesophageal J86.0
    congenital Q39.2
      with atresia of esophagus Q39.1
    following tracheostomy J95.04
  traumatic arteriovenous —see Injury, blood
      vessel, by site

Fistula (Continued)
  tuberculous - code by site under
      Tuberculosis
  typhoid A01.09
  umbilicourinary Q64.8
  urachus, congenital Q64.4
  ureter (persistent) N28.89
  ureteroabdominal N28.89
  ureterorectal N28.89
  ureterosigmoido-abdominal N28.89
  ureterovaginal N82.1
  ureterovesical N32.2
  urethra N36.0
    congenital Q64.79
    tuberculous A18.13
  urethroperineal N36.0
  urethroperineovesical N32.2
  urethrorectal N36.0
    congenital Q64.73
  urethroscrotal N50.8
  urethrovaginal N82.1
  urethrovesical N32.2
  urinary (tract) (persistent) (recurrent)
      N36.0
  uteroabdominal N82.5
    congenital Q51.7
  uteroenteric, uterointestinal N82.4
    congenital Q51.7
  uterorectal N82.4
    congenital Q51.7
  uteroureteric N82.1
  uterourethral Q51.7
  uterovaginal N82.8
  uterovesical N82.1
    congenital Q51.7
  uterus N82.8
  vagina (postpartal) (wall) N82.8
  vaginocutaneous (postpartal) N82.5
  vaginointestinal NEC N82.4
    large intestine N82.3
    small intestine N82.2
  vaginoperineal N82.5
  vasocutaneous, congenital Q55.7
  vesical NEC N32.2
  vesicoabdominal N32.2
  vesicocervicovaginal N82.1
  vesicocolic N32.1
  vesicocutaneous N32.2
  vesicoenteric N32.1
  vesicointestinal N32.1
  vesicometrorectal N82.4
  vesicoperineal N32.2
  vesicorectal N32.1
    congenital Q64.79
  vesicosigmoidal N32.1
  vesicosigmoidovaginal N82.3
  vesicoureteral N32.2
  vesicoureterovaginal N82.1
  vesicourethral N32.2
  vesicourethrorectal N32.1
  vesicouterine N82.1
    congenital Q51.7
  vesicovaginal N82.0
  vulvorectal N82.4
    congenital Q52.79
Fit R56.9
  epileptic —see Epilepsy
  fainting R55
  hysterical F44.5
  newborn P90
Fitting (and adjustment) (of)
  artificial
    arm —see Admission, adjustment, artificial,
        arm
    breast Z44.3
    eye Z44.2
    leg —see Admission, adjustment, artificial,
        leg
  automatic implantable cardiac defibrillator
      (with synchronous cardiac pacemaker)
      Z45.02

Fitting (Continued)
  brain neuropacemaker Z46.2
    implanted Z45.42
  cardiac defibrillator —see Fitting (and
      adjustment) (of), automatic implantable
      cardiac defibrillator
  catheter, non-vascular Z46.82
  colostomy belt Z46.89
  contact lenses Z46.0
  cystostomy device Z46.6
  defibrillator, cardiac —see Fitting (and
      adjustment) (of), automatic implantable
      cardiac defibrillator
  dentures Z46.3
  device NOS Z46.9
    abdominal Z46.89
    gastrointestinal NEC Z46.59
    implanted NEC Z45.89
    nervous system Z46.2
      implanted —see Admission, adjustment,
          device, implanted, nervous
          system
    orthodontic Z46.4
    orthoptic Z46.0
    orthotic Z46.89
    prosthetic (external) Z44.9
      breast Z44.3
      dental Z46.3
      eye Z44.2
      specified NEC Z44.8
    specified NEC Z46.89
    substitution
      auditory Z46.2
        implanted —see Admission,
            adjustment, device, implanted,
            hearing device
      nervous system Z46.2
        implanted —see Admission,
            adjustment, device, implanted,
            nervous system
      visual Z46.2
        implanted Z45.31
    urinary Z46.6
  gastric lap band Z46.51
  gastrointestinal appliance NEC Z46.59
  glasses (reading) Z46.0
  hearing aid Z46.1
  ileostomy device Z46.89
  insulin pump Z46.81
  intestinal appliance NEC Z46.89
  myringotomy device (stent) (tube) Z45.82
  neuropacemaker Z46.2
    implanted Z45.42
  non-vascular catheter Z46.82
  orthodontic device Z46.4
  orthopedic device (brace) (cast) (corset)
      (shoes) Z46.89
  pacemaker (cardiac) Z45.018
    nervous system (brain) (peripheral nerve)
        (spinal cord) Z46.2
      implanted Z45.42
    pulse generator Z45.010
  portacath (port-a-cath) Z45.2
  prosthesis (external) Z44.9
    arm —see Admission, adjustment, artificial,
        arm
    breast Z44.3
    dental Z46.3
    eye Z44.2
    leg —see Admission, adjustment, artificial,
        leg
    specified NEC Z44.8
  spectacles Z46.0
  wheelchair Z46.89
Fitzhugh-Curtis syndrome
  due to
    Chlamydia trachomatis A74.81
    Neisseria gonorrhorea (gonococcal
        peritonitis) A54.85
Fitz's syndrome (acute hemorrhagic
    pancreatitis) K85.8

Fixation
    joint —*see* Ankylosis
    larynx J38.7
    stapes —*see* Ankylosis, ear ossicles
        deafness —*see* Deafness, conductive
    uterus (acquired) —*see* Malposition, uterus
    vocal cord J38.3
Flabby ridge K06.8
Flaccid —*see also* condition
    palate, congenital Q38.5
Flail
    chest S22.5-
        newborn (birth injury) P13.8
    joint (paralytic) M25.20
        ankle M25.27-
        elbow M25.22-
        foot joint M25.27-
        hand joint M25.24-
        hip M25.25-
        knee M25.26-
        shoulder M25.21-
        specified joint NEC M25.28
        wrist M25.23-
Flajani's disease —*see* Hyperthyroidism, with,
        goiter (diffuse)
Flap, liver K71.3
Flashbacks (residual to hallucinogen use)
        F16.283
Flat
    chamber (eye) —*see* Disorder, globe,
        hypotony, flat anterior chamber
    chest, congenital Q67.8
    foot (acquired) (fixed type) (painful)
        (postural) —*see also* Deformity, limb,
        flat foot
        congenital (rigid) (spastic (everted))
            Q66.5-
            rachitic sequelae (late effect) E64.3
    organ or site, congenital NEC —*see* Anomaly,
        by site
    pelvis M95.5
        with disproportion (fetopelvic) O33.0
            causing obstructed labor O65.0
        congenital Q74.2
Flatau-Schilder disease G37.0
Flatback syndrome M40.30
    lumbar region M40.36
    lumbosacral region M40.37
    thoracolumbar region M40.35
Flattening
    head, femur M89.8X5
    hip —*see* Coxa, plana
    lip (congenital) Q18.8
    nose (congenital) Q67.4
        acquired M95.0
Flatulence R14.3
    psychogenic F45.8
Flatus R14.3
    vaginalis N89.8
Flax-dresser's disease J66.1
Flea bite —*see* Injury, bite, by site, superficial,
        insect
Flecks, glaucomatous (subcapsular) —*see*
        Cataract, complicated
Fleischer (-Kayser) **ring** (cornea) H18.04-
Fleshy mole O02.0
Flexibilitas cerea —*see* Catalepsy
Flexion
    amputation stump (surgical) T87.89
    cervix —*see* Malposition, uterus
    contracture, joint —*see* Contraction, joint
    deformity, joint (*see also* Deformity, limb,
        flexion) M21.20
        hip, congenital Q65.89
    uterus —*see also* Malposition, uterus
        lateral —*see* Lateroversion, uterus
Flexner-Boyd dysentery A03.2
Flexner's dysentery A03.1
Flexure —*see* Flexion
Flint murmur (aortic insufficiency) I35.1
Floater, vitreous —*see* Opacity, vitreous

Floating
    cartilage (joint) —*see also* Loose, body, joint
        knee —*see* Derangement, knee, loose body
    gallbladder, congenital Q44.1
    kidney N28.89
        congenital Q63.8
    spleen D73.89
Flooding N92.0
Floor —*see* condition
Floppy
    baby syndrome (nonspecific) P94.2
    iris syndrome (intraoperative) (IFIS)
        H21.81
    nonrheumatic mitral valve syndrome I34.1
Flu —*see also* Influenza
    avian (*see also* Influenza, due to, identified
        novel influenza A virus) J09.X2
    bird (*see also* Influenza, due to, identified
        novel influenza A virus) J09.X2
    intestinal NEC A08.4
    swine (viruses that normally cause infections
        in pigs) (*see also* Influenza, due to,
        identified novel influenza A virus)
        J09.X2
Fluctuating blood pressure I99.8
Fluid
    abdomen R18.8
    chest J94.8
    heart —*see* Failure, heart, congestive
    joint —*see* Effusion, joint
    loss (acute) E86.9
        with
            hypernatremia E87.0
            hyponatremia E87.1
    lung —*see* Edema, lung
    overload E87.70
        specified NEC E87.79
    peritoneal cavity R18.8
    pleural cavity J94.8
    retention R60.9
Flukes NEC —*see also* Infestation, fluke
    blood NEC —*see* Schistosomiasis
    liver B66.3
Fluor (vaginalis) N89.8
    trichomonal or due to Trichomonas
        (vaginalis) A59.00
Fluorosis
    dental K00.3
    skeletal M85.10
        ankle M85.17-
        foot M85.17-
        forearm M85.13-
        hand M85.14-
        lower leg M85.16-
        multiple site M85.19
        neck M85.18
        rib M85.18
        shoulder M85.11-
        skull M85.18
        specified site NEC M85.18
        thigh M85.15-
        toe M85.17-
        upper arm M85.12-
        vertebra M85.18
Flush syndrome E34.0
Flushing R23.2
    menopausal N95.1
Flutter
    atrial or auricular I48.92
        atypical I48.4
        type I I48.3
        type II I48.4
        typical I48.3
    heart I49.8
        atrial or auricular I48.92
            atypical I48.4
            type I I48.3
            type II I48.4
            typical I48.3
        ventricular I49.02
    ventricular I49.02

FNHTR (febrile nonhemolytic transfusion
        reaction) R50.84
Fochier's abscess - code by site under Abscess
Focus, Assmann's —*see* Tuberculosis,
        pulmonary
Fogo selvagem L10.3
Foix-Alajouanine syndrome G95.19
Fold, folds (anomalous) —*see also* Anomaly,
        by site
    Descemet's membrane —*see* Change, corneal
        membrane, Descemet's, fold
    epicanthic Q10.3
    heart Q24.8
Folie à deux F24
Follicle
    cervix (nabothian) (ruptured) N88.8
    graafian, ruptured, with hemorrhage N83.0
    nabothian N88.8
Follicular —*see* condition
Folliculitis (superficial) L73.9
    abscedens et suffodiens L66.3
    cyst N83.0
    decalvans L66.2
    deep —*see* Furuncle, by site
    gonococcal (acute) (chronic) A54.01
    keloid, keloidalis L73.0
    pustular L01.02
    ulerythematosa reticulata L66.4
Folliculome lipidique
    specified site —*see* Neoplasm, benign, by site
    unspecified site
        female D27.9
        male D29.20
Følling's disease E70.0
Follow-up —*see* Examination, follow-up
Fong's syndrome (hereditary osteo-
        onychodysplasia) Q78.5
Food
    allergy L27.2
    asphyxia (from aspiration or inhalation) —*see*
        Foreign body, by site
    choked on —*see* Foreign body, by site
    deprivation T73.0
        specified kind of food NEC E63.8
    intoxication —*see* Poisoning, food
    lack of T73.0
    poisoning —*see* Poisoning, food
    rejection NEC —*see* Disorder, eating
    strangulation or suffocation —*see* Foreign
        body, by site
    toxemia —*see* Poisoning, food
Foot —*see* condition
Foramen ovale (nonclosure) (patent)
        (persistent) Q21.1
Forbes' glycogen storage disease E74.03
Fordyce-Fox disease L75.2
Fordyce's disease (mouth) Q38.6
Forearm —*see* condition
Foreign body
    with
        laceration —*see* Laceration, by site, with
            foreign body
        puncture wound —*see* Puncture, by site,
            with foreign body
    accidentally left following a procedure
        T81.509
        aspiration T81.506
            resulting in
                adhesions T81.516
                obstruction T81.526
                perforation T81.536
                specified complication NEC T81.596
        cardiac catheterization T81.505
            resulting in
                acute reaction T81.60
                    aseptic peritonitis T81.61
                    specified NEC T81.69
                adhesions T81.515
                obstruction T81.525
                perforation T81.535
                specified complication NEC T81.595

◀ New   ◀▥ Revised   ~~deleted~~ Deleted

Foreign body (Continued)
  accidentally left following a procedure
      (Continued)
    causing
      acute reaction T81.60
        aseptic peritonitis T81.61
        specified complication NEC T81.69
      adhesions T81.519
      aseptic peritonitis T81.61
      obstruction T81.529
      perforation T81.539
      specified complication NEC T81.599
    endoscopy T81.504
      resulting in
        adhesions T81.514
        obstruction T81.524
        perforation T81.534
        specified complication NEC T81.594
    immunization T81.503
      resulting in
        adhesions T81.513
        obstruction T81.523
        perforation T81.533
        specified complication NEC T81.593
    infusion T81.501
      resulting in
        adhesions T81.511
        obstruction T81.521
        perforation T81.531
        specified complication NEC T81.591
    injection T81.503
      resulting in
        adhesions T81.513
        obstruction T81.523
        perforation T81.533
        specified complication NEC T81.593
    kidney dialysis T81.502
      resulting in
        adhesions T81.512
        obstruction T81.522
        perforation T81.532
        specified complication NEC T81.592
    packing removal T81.507
      resulting in
        acute reaction T81.60
          aseptic peritonitis T81.61
          specified NEC T81.69
        adhesions T81.517
        obstruction T81.527
        perforation T81.537
        specified complication NEC T81.597
    puncture T81.506
      resulting in
        adhesions T81.516
        obstruction T81.526
        perforation T81.536
        specified complication NEC T81.596
    specified procedure NEC T81.508
      resulting in
        acute reaction T81.60
          aseptic peritonitis T81.61
          specified NEC T81.69
        adhesions T81.518
        obstruction T81.528
        perforation T81.538
        specified complication NEC T81.598
    surgical operation T81.500
      resulting in
        acute reaction T81.60
          aseptic peritonitis T81.61
          specified NEC T81.69
        adhesions T81.510
        obstruction T81.520
        perforation T81.530
        specified complication NEC T81.590
    transfusion T81.501
      resulting in
        adhesions T81.511
        obstruction T81.521
        perforation T81.531
        specified complication NEC T81.591

Foreign body (Continued)
  alimentary tract T18.9
    anus T18.5
    colon T18.4
    esophagus —see Foreign body, esophagus
    mouth T18.0
    multiple sites T18.8
    rectosigmoid (junction) T18.5
    rectum T18.5
    small intestine T18.3
    specified site NEC T18.8
    stomach T18.2
  anterior chamber (eye) S05.5-
  auditory canal —see Foreign body, entering
      through orifice, ear
  bronchus T17.508
    causing
      asphyxiation T17.500
        food (bone) (seed) T17.520
        gastric contents (vomitus) T17.510
        specified type NEC T17.590
      injury NEC T17.508
        food (bone) (seed) T17.528
        gastric contents (vomitus) T17.518
        specified type NEC T17.598
  canthus —see Foreign body, conjunctival sac
  ciliary body (eye) S05.5-
  conjunctival sac T15.1-
  cornea T15.0-
  entering through orifice
    accessory sinus T17.0
    alimentary canal T18.9
      multiple parts T18.8
      specified part NEC T18.8
    alveolar process T18.0
    antrum (Highmore's) T17.0
    anus T18.5
    appendix T18.4
    auditory canal —see Foreign body, entering
        through orifice, ear
    auricle —see Foreign body, entering
        through orifice, ear
    bladder T19.1
    bronchioles —see Foreign body, respiratory
        tract, specified site NEC
    bronchus (main) —see Foreign body,
        bronchus
    buccal cavity T18.0
    canthus (inner) —see Foreign body,
        conjunctival sac
    cecum T18.4
    cervix (canal) (uteri) T19.3
    colon T18.4
    conjunctival sac —see Foreign body,
        conjunctival sac
    cornea —see Foreign body, cornea
    digestive organ or tract NOS T18.9
      multiple parts T18.8
      specified part NEC T18.8
    duodenum T18.3
    ear (external) T16.-
    esophagus —see Foreign body, esophagus
    eye (external) NOS T15.9-
      conjunctival sac —see Foreign body,
          conjunctival sac
      cornea —see Foreign body, cornea
      specified part NEC T15.8-
      eyeball —see also Foreign body, entering
          through orifice, eye, specified part
          NEC
        with penetrating wound —see Puncture,
            eyeball
      eyelid —see also Foreign body, conjunctival
          sac
        with
          laceration —see Laceration, eyelid,
              with foreign body
          puncture —see Puncture, eyelid, with
              foreign body
          superficial injury —see Foreign body,
              superficial, eyelid

Foreign body (Continued)
  entering through orifice (Continued)
    gastrointestinal tract T18.9
      multiple parts T18.8
      specified part NEC T18.8
    genitourinary tract T19.9
      multiple parts T19.8
      specified part NEC T19.8
    globe —see Foreign body, entering through
        orifice, eyeball
    gum T18.0
    Highmore's antrum T17.0
    hypopharynx —see Foreign body, pharynx
    ileum T18.3
    intestine (small) T18.3
      large T18.4
    lacrimal apparatus (punctum) —see
        Foreign body, entering through
        orifice, eye, specified part NEC
    large intestine T18.4
    larynx —see Foreign body, larynx
    lung —see Foreign body, respiratory tract,
        specified site NEC
    maxillary sinus T17.0
    mouth T18.0
    nasal sinus T17.0
    nasopharynx —see Foreign body, pharynx
    nose (passage) T17.1
    nostril T17.1
    oral cavity T18.0
    palate T18.0
    penis T19.4
    pharynx —see Foreign body, pharynx
    piriform sinus —see Foreign body, pharynx
    rectosigmoid (junction) T18.5
    rectum T18.5
    respiratory tract —see Foreign body,
        respiratory tract
    sinus (accessory) (frontal) (maxillary)
        (nasal) T17.0
      piriform —see Foreign body, pharynx
    small intestine T18.3
    stomach T18.2
    suffocation by —see Foreign body, by site
    tear ducts or glands —see Foreign body,
        entering through orifice, eye,
        specified part NEC
    throat —see Foreign body, pharynx
    tongue T18.0
    tonsil, tonsillar (fossa) —see Foreign body,
        pharynx
    trachea —see Foreign body, trachea
    ureter T19.8
    urethra T19.0
    uterus (any part) T19.3
    vagina T19.2
    vulva T19.2
  esophagus T18.108
    causing
      injury NEC T18.108
        food (bone) (seed) T18.128
        gastric contents (vomitus) T18.118
        specified type NEC T18.198
      tracheal compression T18.100
        food (bone) (seed) T18.120
        gastric contents (vomitus) T18.110
        specified type NEC T18.190
  felling of, in throat R09.89
  fragment —see Retained, foreign body
      fragments (type of)
  genitourinary tract T19.9
    bladder T19.1
    multiple parts T19.8
    penis T19.4
    specified site NEC T19.8
    urethra T19.0
    uterus T19.3
      IUD Z97.5
    vagina T19.2
      contraceptive device Z97.5
    vulva T19.2

Foreign body *(Continued)*
 granuloma (old) (soft tissue) —*see also*
  Granuloma, foreign body
  skin L92.3
 in
  laceration —*see* Laceration, by site, with
   foreign body
  puncture wound —*see* Puncture, by site,
   with foreign body
  soft tissue (residual) M79.5
 inadvertently left in operation wound —*see*
  Foreign body, accidentally left during a
  procedure
 ingestion, ingested NOS T18.9
 inhalation or inspiration —*see* Foreign body,
  by site
 internal organ, not entering through a natural
  orifice - code as specific injury with
  foreign body
 intraocular S05.5-
  old, retained (nonmagnetic) H44.70-
   anterior chamber H44.71-
   ciliary body H44.72-
   iris H44.72-
   lens H44.73-
   magnetic H44.60-
    anterior chamber H44.61-
    ciliary body H44.62-
    iris H44.62-
    lens H44.63-
    posterior wall H44.64-
    specified site NEC H44.69-
    vitreous body H44.65-
   posterior wall H44.74-
   specified site NEC H44.79-
   vitreous body H44.75-
  iris —*see* Foreign body, intraocular
 lacrimal punctum —*see* Foreign body,
  entering through orifice, eye, specified
  part NEC
 larynx T17.308
  causing
   asphyxiation T17.300
    food (bone) (seed) T17.320
    gastric contents (vomitus) T17.310
    specified type NEC T17.390
   injury NEC T17.308
    food (bone) (seed) T17.328
    gastric contents (vomitus) T17.318
    specified type NEC T17.398
 lens —*see* Foreign body, intraocular
 ocular muscle S05.4-
  old, retained —*see* Foreign body, orbit, old
 old or residual
  soft tissue (residual) M79.5
 operation wound, left accidentally —*see*
  Foreign body, accidentally left during a
  procedure
 orbit S05.4-
  old, retained H05.5-
 pharynx T17.208
  causing
   asphyxiation T17.200
    food (bone) (seed) T17.220
    gastric contents (vomitus)
     T17.210
    specified type NEC T17.290
   injury NEC T17.208
    food (bone) (seed) T17.228
    gastric contents (vomitus)
     T17.218
    specified type NEC T17.298
 respiratory tract T17.908
  bronchioles —*see* Foreign body, respiratory
   tract, specified site NEC
  bronchus —*see* Foreign body, bronchus
  causing
   asphyxiation T17.900
    food (bone) (seed) T17.920
    gastric contents (vomitus) T17.910
    specified type NEC T17.990

Foreign body *(Continued)*
 respiratory tract *(Continued)*
  causing *(Continued)*
   injury NEC T17.908
    food (bone) (seed) T17.928
    gastric contents (vomitus) T17.918
    specified type NEC T17.998
  larynx —*see* Foreign body, larynx
  lung —*see* Foreign body, respiratory tract,
   specified site NEC
  multiple parts —*see* Foreign body,
   respiratory tract, specified site NEC
  nasal sinus T17.0
  nasopharynx —*see* Foreign body, pharynx
  nose T17.1
  nostril T17.1
  pharynx —*see* Foreign body, pharynx
  specified site NEC T17.808
   causing
    asphyxiation T17.800
     food (bone) (seed) T17.820
     gastric contents (vomitus)
      T17.810
     specified type NEC T17.890
    injury NEC T17.808
     food (bone) (seed) T17.828
     gastric contents (vomitus)
      T17.818
     specified type NEC T17.898
  throat —*see* Foreign body, pharynx
  trachea —*see* Foreign body, trachea
 retained (old) (nonmagnetic) (in)
  anterior chamber (eye) —*see* Foreign body,
   intraocular, old, retained, anterior
   chamber
   magnetic —*see* Foreign body, intraocular,
    old, retained, magnetic, anterior
    chamber
  ciliary body —*see* Foreign body,
   intraocular, old, retained, ciliary
   body
   magnetic —*see* Foreign body, intraocular,
    old, retained, magnetic, ciliary
    body
  eyelid H02.819
   left H02.816
    lower H02.815
    upper H02.814
   right H02.813
    lower H02.812
    upper H02.811
  fragments —*see* Retained, foreign body
   fragments (type of)
  globe —*see* Foreign body, intraocular, old,
   retained
   magnetic —*see* Foreign body, intraocular,
    old, retained, magnetic
  intraocular —*see* Foreign body, intraocular,
   old, retained
   magnetic —*see* Foreign body, intraocular,
    old, retained, magnetic
  iris —*see* Foreign body, intraocular, old,
   retained, iris
   magnetic —*see* Foreign body, intraocular,
    old, retained, magnetic, iris
  lens —*see* Foreign body, intraocular, old,
   retained, lens
   magnetic —*see* Foreign body, intraocular,
    old, retained, magnetic, lens
  muscle —*see* Foreign body, retained, soft
   tissue
  orbit —*see* Foreign body, orbit, old
  posterior wall of globe —*see* Foreign body,
   intraocular, old, retained, posterior
   wall
   magnetic —*see* Foreign body, intraocular,
    old, retained, magnetic, posterior
    wall
  retrobulbar —*see* Foreign body, orbit, old,
   retrobulbar
  soft tissue M79.5

Foreign body *(Continued)*
 retained *(Continued)*
  vitreous —*see* Foreign body, intraocular,
   old, retained, vitreous body
  magnetic —*see* Foreign body, intraocular,
   old, retained, magnetic, vitreous
   body
 retina S05.5-
 superficial, without open wound
  abdomen, abdominal (wall) S30.851
  alveolar process S00.552
  ankle S90.55-
  antecubital space —*see* Foreign body,
   superficial, forearm
  anus S30.857
  arm (upper) S40.85-
  auditory canal —*see* Foreign body,
   superficial, ear
  auricle —*see* Foreign body, superficial, ear
  axilla —*see* Foreign body, superficial, arm
  back, lower S30.850
  breast S20.15-
  brow S00.85
  buttock S30.850
  calf —*see* Foreign body, superficial, leg
  canthus —*see* Foreign body, superficial,
   eyelid
  cheek S00.85
   internal S00.552
  chest wall —*see* Foreign body, superficial,
   thorax
  chin S00.85
  clitoris S30.854
  costal region —*see* Foreign body,
   superficial, thorax
  digit (s)
   foot —*see* Foreign body, superficial, toe
   hand —*see* Foreign body, superficial,
    finger
  ear S00.45-
  elbow S50.35-
  epididymis S30.853
  epigastric region S30.851
  epiglottis S10.15
  esophagus, cervical S10.15
  eyebrow —*see* Foreign body, superficial,
   eyelid
  eyelid S00.25-
  face S00.85
  finger (s) S60.459
   index S60.45-
   little S60.45-
   middle S60.45-
   ring S60.45-
  flank S30.851
  foot (except toe (s) alone) S90.85-
   toe —*see* Foreign body, superficial, toe
  forearm S50.85-
   elbow only —*see* Foreign body,
    superficial, elbow
  forehead S00.85
  genital organs, external
   female S30.856
   male S30.855
  groin S30.851
  gum S00.552
  hand S60.55-
  head S00.95
   ear —*see* Foreign body, superficial, ear
   eyelid —*see* Foreign body, superficial,
    eyelid
   lip S00.551
   nose S00.35
   oral cavity S00.552
   scalp S00.05
   specified site NEC S00.85
  heel —*see* Foreign body, superficial, foot
  hip S70.25-
  inguinal region S30.851
  interscapular region S20.459
  jaw S00.85

◄ New ◄▬ Revised ~~deleted~~ Deleted

Foreign body (Continued)
  superficial, without open wound (Continued)
    knee S80.25-
    labium (majus) (minus) S30.854
    larynx S10.15
    leg (lower) S80.85-
      knee —see Foreign body, superficial, knee
      upper —see Foreign body, superficial, thigh
    lip S00.551
    lower back S30.850
    lumbar region S30.850
    malar region S00.85
    mammary —see Foreign body, superficial, breast
    mastoid region S00.85
    mouth S00.552
    nail
      finger —see Foreign body, superficial, finger
      toe —see Foreign body, superficial, toe
    nape S10.85
    nasal S00.35
    neck S10.95
      specified site NEC S10.85
      throat S10.15
    nose S00.35
    occipital region S00.05
    oral cavity S00.552
    orbital region —see Foreign body, superficial, eyelid
    palate S00.552
    palm —see Foreign body, superficial, hand
    parietal region S00.05
    pelvis S30.850
    penis S30.852
    perineum
      female S30.854
      male S30.850
    periocular area —see Foreign body, superficial, eyelid
    phalanges
      finger —see Foreign body, superficial, finger
      toe —see Foreign body, superficial, toe
    pharynx S10.15
    pinna —see Foreign body, superficial, ear
    popliteal space —see Foreign body, superficial, knee
    prepuce S30.852
    pubic region S30.850
    pudendum
      female S30.856
      male S30.855
    sacral region S30.850
    scalp S00.05
    scapular region —see Foreign body, superficial, shoulder
    scrotum S30.853
    shin —see Foreign body, superficial, leg
    shoulder S40.25-
    sternal region S20.359
    submaxillary region S00.85
    submental region S00.85
    subungual
      finger (s) —see Foreign body, superficial, finger
      toe (s) —see Foreign body, superficial, toe
    supraclavicular fossa S10.85
    supraorbital S00.85
    temple S00.85
    temporal region S00.85
    testis S30.853
    thigh S70.35-
    thorax, thoracic (wall) S20.95
      back S20.45-
      front S20.35-
    throat S10.15
    thumb S60.35-

Foreign body (Continued)
  superficial, without open wound (Continued)
    toe (s) (lesser) S90.456
      great S90.45-
    tongue S00.552
    trachea S10.15
    tunica vaginalis S30.853
    tympanum, tympanic membrane —see Foreign body, superficial, ear
    uvula S00.552
    vagina S30.854
    vocal cords S10.15
    vulva S30.854
    wrist S60.85-
  swallowed T18.9
  trachea T17.408
    causing
      asphyxiation T17.400
        food (bone) (seed) T17.420
        gastric contents (vomitus) T17.410
        specified type NEC T17.490
      injury NEC T17.408
        food (bone) (seed) T17.428
        gastric contents (vomitus) T17.418
        specified type NEC T17.498
  type of fragment —see Retained, foreign body fragments (type of)
  vitreous (humor) S05.5-
Forestier's disease (rhizomelic pseudopolyarthritis) M35.3-
  meaning ankylosing hyperostosis —see Hyperostosis, ankylosing
Formation
  hyalin in cornea —see Degeneration, cornea
  sequestrum in bone (due to infection) —see Osteomyelitis, chronic
  valve
    colon, congenital Q43.8
    ureter (congenital) Q62.39
Formication R20.2
Fort Bragg fever A27.89
Fossa —see also condition
  pyriform —see condition
Foster-Kennedy syndrome H47.14-
Fothergill's
  disease (trigeminal neuralgia) —see also Neuralgia, trigeminal
  scarlatina anginosa A38.9
Foul breath R19.6
Foundling Z76.1
Fournier disease or gangrene N49.3
  female N76.89
Fourth
  cranial nerve —see condition
  molar K00.1
Foville's (peduncular) disease or syndrome G46.3
Fox (-Fordyce) disease (apocrine miliaria) L75.2
Fracture, burst —see Fracture, traumatic, by site
Fracture, chronic —see Fracture, pathological
Fracture, insufficiency —see Fracture, pathologic, by site
Fracture, pathological (pathologic) —see also Fracture, traumatic M84.40 ◀▥
  ankle M84.47-
  carpus M84.44-
  clavicle M84.41-
  dental implant M27.63
  dental restorative material K08.539
    with loss of material K08.531
    without loss of material K08.530
  due to
    neoplastic disease NEC (see also Neoplasm) M84.50
      ankle M84.57-
      carpus M84.54-
      clavicle M84.51-
      femur M84.55-
      fibula M84.56-
      finger M84.54-
      hip M84.559

Fracture, pathological (Continued)
  due to (Continued)
    neoplastic disease NEC (Continued)
      humerus M84.52-
      ilium M84.550
      ischium M84.550
      metacarpus M84.54-
      metatarsus M84.57-
      neck M84.58
      pelvis M84.550
      radius M84.53-
      rib M84.58
      scapula M84.51-
      skull M84.58
      specified site NEC M84.58 ◀
      tarsus M84.57-
      tibia M84.56-
      toe M84.57-
      ulna M84.53-
      vertebra M84.58
    osteoporosis M80.80
      disuse —see Osteoporosis, specified type NEC, with pathological fracture
      drug-induced —see Osteoporosis, drug induced, with pathological fracture
      idiopathic —see Osteoporosis, specified type NEC, with pathological fracture
      postmenopausal —see Osteoporosis, postmenopausal, with pathological fracture
      postoophorectomy —see Osteoporosis, postoophorectomy, with pathological fracture
      postsurgical malabsorption —see Osteoporosis, specified type NEC, with pathological fracture
      specified cause NEC —see Osteoporosis, specified type NEC, with pathological fracture
    specified disease NEC M84.60
      ankle M84.67-
      carpus M84.64-
      clavicle M84.61-
      femur M84.65-
      fibula M84.66-
      finger M84.64-
      hip M84.65-
      humerus M84.62-
      ilium M84.650
      ischium M84.650
      metacarpus M84.64-
      metatarsus M84.67-
      neck M84.68
      radius M84.63-
      rib M84.68
      scapula M84.61-
      skull M84.68
      tarsus M84.67-
      tibia M84.66-
      toe M84.67-
      ulna M84.63-
      vertebra M84.68
  femur M84.45-
  fibula M84.46-
  finger M84.44-
  hip M84.459
  humerus M84.42-
  ilium M84.454
  ischium M84.454
  joint prosthesis —see Complications, joint prosthesis, mechanical, breakdown, by site
  periprosthetic —see Complications, joint prosthesis, mechanical, periprosthesis, fracture, by site
  metacarpus M84.44-
  metatarsus M84.47-
  neck M84.48
  pelvis M84.454
  radius M84.43-

◀ New   ⬅ Revised   ~~deleted~~ Deleted

Fracture, traumatic (*Continued*)
  femur, femoral (*Continued*)
    shaft (*Continued*)
      spiral (displaced) S72.34-
        nondisplaced S72.34-
      transverse (displaced) S72.32-
        nondisplaced S72.32-
      specified site NEC —*see* subcategory S72.8
    subcapital (displaced) S72.01-
    subtrochanteric (region) (section)
        (displaced) S72.2-
      nondisplaced S72.2-
    transcervical —*see* Fracture, femur, upper
        end, neck
    transtrochanteric —*see* Fracture, femur,
        trochanteric
    trochanteric S72.10-
      apophyseal (displaced) S72.13-
        nondisplaced S72.13-
      greater trochanter (displaced) S72.11-
        nondisplaced S72.11-
      intertrochanteric (displaced) S72.14-
        nondisplaced S72.14-
      lesser trochanter (displaced) S72.12-
        nondisplaced S72.12-
    upper end S72.00-
      apophyseal (displaced) S72.13-
        nondisplaced S72.13-
      cervicotrochanteric —*see* Fracture,
          femur, upper end, neck, base
      epiphysis (displaced) S72.02-
        nondisplaced S72.02-
      head S72.05-
        articular (displaced) S72.06-
          nondisplaced S72.06-
        specified NEC S72.09-
      intertrochanteric (displaced) S72.14-
        nondisplaced S72.14-
      intracapsular S72.01-
      midcervical (displaced) S72.03-
        nondisplaced S72.03-
      neck S72.00-
        base (displaced) S72.04-
          nondisplaced S72.04-
        specified NEC S72.09-
      pertrochanteric —*see* Fracture, femur,
          upper end, trochanteric
      physeal S79.00-
        Salter-Harris type I S79.01-
        specified NEC S79.09-
      subcapital (displaced) S72.01-
      subtrochanteric (displaced) S72.2-
        nondisplaced S72.2-
      transcervical —*see* Fracture, femur,
          upper end, midcervical
      trochanteric S72.10-
        greater (displaced) S72.11-
          nondisplaced S72.11-
        lesser (displaced) S72.12-
          nondisplaced S72.12-
  fibula (shaft) (styloid) S82.40-
    comminuted (displaced) S82.45-
      nondisplaced S82.45-
    following insertion of implant, prosthesis
        or plate M96.67-
    involving ankle or malleolus —*see*
        Fracture, fibula, lateral malleolus
    lateral malleolus (displaced) S82.6-
      nondisplaced S82.6-
    lower end
      physeal S89.30-
        Salter-Harris
          Type I S89.31-
          Type II S89.32-
        specified NEC S89.39-
      specified NEC S82.83-
      torus S82.82-
    oblique (displaced) S82.43-
      nondisplaced S82.43-
    segmental (displaced) S82.46-
      nondisplaced S82.46-

Fracture, traumatic (*Continued*)
  fibula (*Continued*)
    specified NEC S82.49-
    spiral (displaced) S82.44-
      nondisplaced S82.44-
    transverse (displaced) S82.42-
      nondisplaced S82.42-
    upper end
      physeal S89.20-
        Salter-Harris
          Type I S89.21-
          Type II S89.22-
        specified NEC S89.29-
      specified NEC S82.83-
      torus S82.81-
  finger (except thumb) S62.60-
    distal phalanx (displaced) S62.63-
      nondisplaced S62.66-
    index S62.60-
      distal phalanx (displaced) S62.63-
        nondisplaced S62.66-
      medial phalanx (displaced) S62.62-
        nondisplaced S62.65-
      proximal phalanx (displaced) S62.61-
        nondisplaced S62.64-
    little S62.60-
      distal phalanx (displaced) S62.63-
        nondisplaced S62.66-
      medial phalanx (displaced) S62.62-
        nondisplaced S62.65-
      proximal phalanx (displaced) S62.61-
        nondisplaced S62.64-
    medial phalanx (displaced) S62.62-
      nondisplaced S62.65-
    middle S62.60-
      distal phalanx (displaced) S62.63-
        nondisplaced S62.66-
      medial phalanx (displaced) S62.62-
        nondisplaced S62.65-
      proximal phalanx (displaced) S62.61-
        nondisplaced S62.64-
    proximal phalanx (displaced) S62.61-
      nondisplaced S62.64-
    ring S62.60-
      distal phalanx (displaced) S62.63-
        nondisplaced S62.66-
      medial phalanx (displaced) S62.62-
        nondisplaced S62.65-
      proximal phalanx (displaced) S62.61-
        nondisplaced S62.64-
    thumb —*see* Fracture, thumb
  following insertion (intraoperative)
      (postoperative) of orthopedic implant,
      joint prosthesis or bone plate M96.69
    femur M96.66-
    fibula M96.67-
    humerus M96.62-
    pelvis M96.65
    radius M96.63-
    specified bone NEC M96.69
    tibia M96.67-
    ulna M96.63-
  foot S92.90-
    astragalus —*see* Fracture, tarsal, talus
    calcaneus —*see* Fracture, tarsal, calcaneus
    cuboid —*see* Fracture, tarsal, cuboid
    cuneiform —*see* Fracture, tarsal, cuneiform
    metatarsal —*see* Fracture, metatarsal
    navicular —*see* Fracture, tarsal, navicular
    talus —*see* Fracture, tarsal, talus
    tarsal —*see* Fracture, tarsal
    toe —*see* Fracture, toe
  forearm S52.9-
    radius —*see* Fracture, radius
    ulna —*see* Fracture, ulna
  fossa (anterior) (middle) (posterior) S02.19
  frontal (bone) (skull) S02.0
    sinus S02.19
  glenoid (cavity) (scapula) —*see* Fracture,
      scapula, glenoid cavity
  greenstick —*see* Fracture, by site

Fracture, traumatic (*Continued*)
  hallux —*see* Fracture, toe, great
  hand S62.9-
    carpal —*see* Fracture, carpal bone
    finger (except thumb) —*see* Fracture, finger
    metacarpal —*see* Fracture, metacarpal
    navicular (scaphoid) (hand) —*see* Fracture,
        carpal bone, navicular
    thumb —*see* Fracture, thumb
  healed or old
    with complications - code by Nature of the
        complication
  heel bone —*see* Fracture, tarsal, calcaneus
  Hill-Sachs S42.29-
  hip —*see* Fracture, femur, neck
  humerus S42.30-
    anatomical neck —*see* Fracture, humerus,
        upper end
    articular process —*see* Fracture, humerus,
        lower end
    capitellum —*see* Fracture, humerus, lower
        end, condyle, lateral
    distal end —*see* Fracture, humerus, lower
        end
    epiphysis
      lower —*see* Fracture, humerus, lower
          end, physeal
      upper —*see* Fracture, humerus, upper
          end, physeal
    external condyle —*see* Fracture, humerus,
        lower end, condyle, lateral
    following insertion of implant, prosthesis
        or plate M96.62-
    great tuberosity —*see* Fracture, humerus,
        upper end, greater tuberosity
    intercondylar —*see* Fracture, humerus,
        lower end
    internal epicondyle —*see* Fracture,
        humerus, lower end, epicondyle,
        medial
    lesser tuberosity —*see* Fracture, humerus,
        upper end, lesser tuberosity
    lower end S42.40-
      condyle
        lateral (displaced) S42.45-
          nondisplaced S42.45-
        medial (displaced) S42.46-
          nondisplaced S42.46-
      epicondyle
        lateral (displaced) S42.43-
          nondisplaced S42.43-
        medial (displaced) S42.44-
          incarcerated S42.44-
          nondisplaced S42.44-
      physeal S49.10-
        Salter-Harris
          Type I S49.11-
          Type II S49.12-
          Type III S49.13-
          Type IV S49.14-
        specified NEC S49.19-
      specified NEC (displaced) S42.49-
        nondisplaced S42.49-
      supracondylar (simple) (displaced)
          S42.41-
        comminuted (displaced) S42.42-
          nondisplaced S42.42-
        nondisplaced S42.41-
      torus S42.48-
      transcondylar (displaced) S42.47-
        nondisplaced S42.47-
    proximal end —*see* Fracture, humerus,
        upper end
    shaft S42.30-
      comminuted (displaced) S42.35-
        nondisplaced S42.35-
      greenstick S42.31-
      oblique (displaced) S42.33-
        nondisplaced S42.33-
      segmental (displaced) S42.36-
        nondisplaced S42.36-

Fracture, traumatic (Continued)
  humerus (Continued)
    shaft (Continued)
      specified NEC S42.39-
      spiral (displaced) S42.34-
        nondisplaced S42.34-
      transverse (displaced) S42.32-
        nondisplaced S42.32-
    supracondylar —see Fracture, humerus,
      lower end
    surgical neck —see Fracture, humerus,
      upper end, surgical neck
    trochlea —see Fracture, humerus, lower
      end, condyle, medial
    tuberosity —see Fracture, humerus, upper
      end
    upper end S42.20-
      anatomical neck —see Fracture, humerus,
        upper end, specified NEC
      articular head —see Fracture, humerus,
        upper end, specified NEC
      epiphysis —see Fracture, humerus,
        upper end, physeal
      greater tuberosity (displaced) S42.25-
        nondisplaced S42.25-
      lesser tuberosity (displaced) S42.26-
        nondisplaced S42.26-
      physeal S49.00-
        Salter-Harris
          Type I S49.01-
          Type II S49.02-
          Type III S49.03-
          Type IV S49.04-
        specified NEC S49.09-
      specified NEC (displaced) S42.29-
        nondisplaced S42.29-
      surgical neck (displaced) S42.21-
        four-part S42.24-
        nondisplaced S42.21-
        three-part S42.23-
        two-part (displaced) S42.22-
        nondisplaced S42.22-
      torus S42.27-
      transepiphyseal —see Fracture, humerus,
        upper end, physeal
  hyoid bone S12.8
  ilium S32.30-
    with disruption of pelvic ring —see
      Disruption, pelvic ring
    avulsion (displaced) S32.31-
      nondisplaced S32.31-
    specified NEC S32.39-
  impaction, impacted - code as Fracture, by
    site
  innominate bone —see Fracture, ilium
  instep —see Fracture, foot
  ischium S32.60-
    with disruption of pelvic ring —see
      Disruption, pelvic ring
    avulsion (displaced) S32.61-
      nondisplaced S32.61-
    specified NEC S32.69-
  jaw (bone) (lower) —see Fracture, mandible
    upper —see Fracture, maxilla
  joint prosthesis —see Complications, joint
    prosthesis, mechanical, breakdown, by
    site
    periprosthetic —see Complications,
      joint prosthesis, mechanical,
      periprosthesis, fracture, by site
  knee cap —see Fracture, patella
  larynx S12.8
  late effects —see Sequelae, fracture
  leg (lower) S82.9-
    ankle —see Fracture, ankle
    femur —see Fracture, femur
    fibula —see Fracture, fibula
    malleolus —see Fracture, ankle
    patella —see Fracture, patella
    specified site NEC S82.89-
    tibia —see Fracture, tibia

Fracture, traumatic (Continued)
  lumbar spine —see Fracture, vertebra, lumbar
  lumbosacral spine S32.9
  Maisonneuve's (displaced) S82.86-
    nondisplaced S82.86-
  malar bone (see also Fracture, maxilla) S02.400
  malleolus —see Fracture, ankle
  malunion —see Fracture, by site
  mandible (lower jawbone) S02.609
    alveolus S02.67
    angle (of jaw) S02.65
    body, unspecified S02.600
    condylar process S02.61
    coronoid process S02.63
    ramus, unspecified S02.64
    specified site NEC S02.69
    subcondylar process S02.62
    symphysis S02.66
  manubrium (sterni) S22.21
    dissociation from sternum S22.23
  march —see Fracture, traumatic, stress, by site
  maxilla, maxillary (bone) (sinus) (superior)
    (upper jaw) S02.401
    alveolus S02.42
    inferior —see Fracture, mandible
    LeFort I S02.411
    LeFort II S02.412
    LeFort III S02.413
  metacarpal S62.309
    base (displaced) S62.319
      nondisplaced S62.349
    fifth S62.30-
      base (displaced) S62.31-
        nondisplaced S62.34-
      neck (displaced) S62.33-
        nondisplaced S62.36-
      shaft (displaced) S62.32-
        nondisplaced S62.35-
      specified NEC S62.398
    first S62.20-
      base NEC (displaced) S62.23-
        nondisplaced S62.23-
      Bennett's —see Bennett's fracture
      neck (displaced) S62.25-
        nondisplaced S62.25-
      shaft (displaced) S62.24-
        nondisplaced S62.24-
      specified NEC S62.29-
    fourth S62.30-
      base (displaced) S62.31-
        nondisplaced S62.34-
      neck (displaced) S62.33-
        nondisplaced S62.36-
      shaft (displaced) S62.32-
        nondisplaced S62.35-
      specified NEC S62.39-
    neck (displaced) S62.33-
      nondisplaced S62.36-
    Rolando's —see Rolando's fracture
    second S62.30-
      base (displaced) S62.31-
        nondisplaced S62.34-
      neck (displaced) S62.33-
        nondisplaced S62.36-
      shaft (displaced) S62.32-
        nondisplaced S62.35-
      specified NEC S62.39-
    shaft (displaced) S62.32-
      nondisplaced S62.35-
    specified NEC S62.399
    third S62.30-
      base (displaced) S62.31-
        nondisplaced S62.34-
      neck (displaced) S62.33-
        nondisplaced S62.36-
      shaft (displaced) S62.32-
        nondisplaced S62.35-
      specified NEC S62.39-
  metastatic —see Fracture, pathological,
    due to, neoplastic disease —see also
    Neoplasm

Fracture, traumatic (Continued)
  metatarsal bone S92.30-
    fifth (displaced) S92.35-
      nondisplaced S92.35-
    first (displaced) S92.31-
      nondisplaced S92.31-
    fourth (displaced) S92.34-
      nondisplaced S92.34-
    second (displaced) S92.32-
      nondisplaced S92.32-
    third (displaced) S92.33-
      nondisplaced S92.33-
  Monteggia's —see Monteggia's fracture
  multiple
    hand (and wrist) NEC —see Fracture, by
      site
    ribs —see Fracture, rib, multiple
  nasal (bone (s)) S02.2
  navicular (scaphoid) (foot) —see also Fracture,
    tarsal, navicular
    hand —see Fracture, carpal, navicular
  neck S12.9
    cervical vertebra S12.9
      fifth (displaced) S12.400
        nondisplaced S12.401
        specified type NEC (displaced)
          S12.490
          nondisplaced S12.491
      first (displaced) S12.000
        burst (stable) S12.01
          unstable S12.02
        lateral mass (displaced) S12.040
          nondisplaced S12.041
        nondisplaced S12.001
        posterior arch (displaced) S12.030
          nondisplaced S12.031
        specified type NEC (displaced)
          S12.090
          nondisplaced S12.091
      fourth (displaced) S12.300
        nondisplaced S12.301
        specified type NEC (displaced)
          S12.390
          nondisplaced S12.391
      second (displaced) S12.100
        dens (anterior) (displaced) (type II)
          S12.110
          nondisplaced S12.112
          posterior S12.111
        specified type NEC (displaced)
          S12.120
          nondisplaced S12.121
        nondisplaced S12.101
        specified type NEC (displaced)
          S12.190
          nondisplaced S12.191
      seventh (displaced) S12.600
        nondisplaced S12.601
        specified type NEC (displaced)
          S12.690
          displaced S12.691
      sixth (displaced) S12.500
        nondisplaced S12.501
        specified type NEC (displaced)
          S12.590
          displaced S12.591
      third (displaced) S12.200
        nondisplaced S12.201
        specified type NEC (displaced)
          S12.290
          displaced S12.291
    hyoid bone S12.8
    larynx S12.8
    specified site NEC S12.8
    thyroid cartilage S12.8
    trachea S12.8
  neoplastic NEC —see Fracture, pathological,
    due to, neoplastic disease
  neural arch —see Fracture, vertebra
  newborn —see Birth, injury, fracture
  nontraumatic —see Fracture, pathological

◀ New   ◀▥ Revised   ~~deleted~~ Deleted

Fracture, traumatic *(Continued)*
  nonunion —*see* Nonunion, fracture
  nose, nasal (bone) (septum) S02.2
  occiput —*see* Fracture, skull, base, occiput
  odontoid process —*see* Fracture, neck, cervical vertebra, second
  olecranon (process) (ulna) —*see* Fracture, ulna, upper end, olecranon process
  orbit, orbital (bone) (region) S02.8
    floor (blow-out) S02.3
    roof S02.19
  os
    calcis —*see* Fracture, tarsal, calcaneus
    magnum —*see* Fracture, carpal, capitate
    pubis —*see* Fracture, pubis
  palate S02.8
  parietal bone (skull) S02.0
  patella S82.00-
    comminuted (displaced) S82.04-
      nondisplaced S82.04-
    longitudinal (displaced) S82.02-
      nondisplaced S82.02-
    osteochondral (displaced) S82.01-
      nondisplaced S82.01-
    specified NEC S82.09-
    transverse (displaced) S82.03-
      nondisplaced S82.03-
  pedicle (of vertebral arch) —*see* Fracture, vertebra
  pelvis, pelvic (bone) S32.9
    acetabulum —*see* Fracture, acetabulum
    circle —*see* Disruption, pelvic ring
    following insertion of implant, prosthesis or plate M96.65
    ilium —*see* Fracture, ilium
    ischium —*see* Fracture, ischium
    multiple
      with disruption of pelvic ring (circle) — *see* Disruption, pelvic ring
      without disruption of pelvic ring (circle) S32.82
    pubis —*see* Fracture, pubis
    sacrum —*see* Fracture, sacrum
    specified site NEC S32.89
  phalanx
    foot —*see* Fracture, toe
    hand —*see* Fracture, finger
  pisiform —*see* Fracture, carpal, pisiform
  pond —*see* Fracture, skull
  prosthetic device, internal —*see* Complications, prosthetic device, by site, mechanical
  pubis S32.50-
    with disruption of pelvic ring —*see* Disruption, pelvic ring
    specified site NEC S32.59-
    superior rim S32.59-
  radius S52.9-
    distal end —*see* Fracture, radius, lower end
    following insertion of implant, prosthesis or plate M96.63-
    head —*see* Fracture, radius, upper end, head
    lower end S52.50-
      Barton's —*see* Barton's fracture
      Colles' —*see* Colles' fracture
      extraarticular NEC S52.55-
      intraarticular NEC S52.57-
      physeal S59.20-
        Salter-Harris
          Type I S59.21-
          Type II S59.22-
          Type III S59.23-
          Type IV S59.24-
        specified NEC S59.29-
      Smith's —*see* Smith's fracture
      specified NEC S52.59-
      styloid process (displaced) S52.51-
        nondisplaced S52.51-
      torus S52.52-

Fracture, traumatic *(Continued)*
  radius *(Continued)*
    neck —*see* Fracture, radius, upper end
    proximal end —*see* Fracture, radius, upper end
    shaft S52.30-
      bent bone S52.38-
      comminuted (displaced) S52.35-
        nondisplaced S52.35-
      Galeazzi's —*see* Galeazzi's fracture
      greenstick S52.31-
      oblique (displaced) S52.33-
        nondisplaced S52.33-
      segmental (displaced) S52.36-
        nondisplaced S52.36-
      specified NEC S52.39-
      spiral (displaced) S52.34-
        nondisplaced S52.34-
      transverse (displaced) S52.32-
        nondisplaced S52.32-
    upper end S52.10-
      head (displaced) S52.12-
        nondisplaced S52.12-
      neck (displaced) S52.13-
        nondisplaced S52.13-
      physeal S59.10-
        Salter-Harris
          Type I S59.11-
          Type II S59.12-
          Type III S59.13-
          Type IV S59.14-
        specified NEC S59.19-
      specified NEC S52.18-
      torus S52.11-
  ramus
    inferior or superior, pubis —*see* Fracture, pubis
    mandible —*see* Fracture, mandible
  restorative material (dental) K08.539
    with loss of material K08.531
    without loss of material K08.530
  rib S22.3-
    with flail chest —*see* Flail, chest
    multiple S22.4-
      with flail chest —*see* Flail, chest
  root, tooth —*see* Fracture, tooth
  sacrum S32.10
    specified NEC S32.19
    Type
      1 S32.14
      2 S32.15
      3 S32.16
      4 S32.17
    Zone
      I S32.119
        displaced (minimally) S32.111
          severely S32.112
        nondisplaced S32.110
      II S32.129
        displaced (minimally) S32.121
          severely S32.122
        nondisplaced S32.120
      III S32.139
        displaced (minimally) S32.131
          severely S32.132
        nondisplaced S32.130
  scaphoid (hand) —*see also* Fracture, carpal, navicular
    foot —*see* Fracture, tarsal, navicular
  scapula S42.10-
    acromial process (displaced) S42.12-
      nondisplaced S42.12-
    body (displaced) S42.11-
      nondisplaced S42.11-
    coracoid process (displaced) S42.13-
      nondisplaced S42.13-
    glenoid cavity (displaced) S42.14-
      nondisplaced S42.14-
    neck (displaced) S42.15-
      nondisplaced S42.15-
    specified NEC S42.19-

Fracture, traumatic *(Continued)*
  semilunar bone, wrist —*see* Fracture, carpal, lunate
  sequelae —*see* Sequelae, fracture
  sesamoid bone
    hand —*see* Fracture, carpal
    other - code by site under Fracture
  shepherd's —*see* Fracture, tarsal, talus
  shoulder (girdle) S42.9-
    blade —*see* Fracture, scapula
  sinus (ethmoid) (frontal) S02.19
  skull S02.91
    base S02.10
      occiput S02.119
        condyle S02.113
        type I S02.110
        type II S02.111
        type III S02.112
        specified NEC S02.118
      specified NEC S02.19
    birth injury P13.0
    frontal bone S02.0
    parietal bone S02.0
    specified site NEC S02.8
    temporal bone S02.19
    vault S02.0
  Smith's —*see* Smith's fracture
  sphenoid (bone) (sinus) S02.19
  spine —*see* Fracture, vertebra
  spinous process —*see* Fracture, vertebra
  spontaneous (cause unknown) —*see* Fracture, pathological
  stave (of thumb) —*see* Fracture, metacarpal, first
  sternum S22.20
    with flail chest —*see* Flail, chest
    body S22.22
    manubrium S22.21
    xiphoid (process) S22.24
  stress M84.30
    ankle M84.37-
    carpus M84.34-
    clavicle M84.31-
    femoral neck M84.359
    femur M84.35-
    fibula M84.36-
    finger M84.34-
    hip M84.359
    humerus M84.32-
    ilium M84.350
    ischium M84.350
    metacarpus M84.34-
    metatarsus M84.37-
    neck —*see* Fracture, fatigue, vertebra
    pelvis M84.350
    radius M84.33-
    rib M84.38
    scapula M84.31-
    skull M84.38
    tarsus M84.37-
    tibia M84.36-
    toe M84.37-
    ulna M84.33-
    vertebra —*see* Fracture, fatigue, vertebra
  supracondylar, elbow —*see* Fracture, humerus, lower end, supracondylar
  symphysis pubis —*see* Fracture, pubis
  talus (ankle bone) —*see* Fracture, tarsal, talus
  tarsal bone (s) S92.20-
    astragalus —*see* Fracture, tarsal, talus
    calcaneus S92.00-
      anterior process (displaced) S92.02-
        nondisplaced S92.02-
      body (displaced) S92.01-
        nondisplaced S92.01-
      extraarticular NEC (displaced) S92.05-
        nondisplaced S92.05-
      intraarticular (displaced) S92.06-
        nondisplaced S92.06-

Fracture, traumatic *(Continued)*
  tarsal bone *(Continued)*
    calcaneus *(Continued)*
      tuberosity (displaced) S92.04-
        avulsion (displaced) S92.03-
          nondisplaced S92.03-
        nondisplaced S92.04-
    cuboid (displaced) S92.21-
      nondisplaced S92.21-
    cuneiform
      intermediate (displaced) S92.23-
        nondisplaced S92.23-
      lateral (displaced) S92.22-
        nondisplaced S92.22-
      medial (displaced) S92.24-
        nondisplaced S92.24-
    navicular (displaced) S92.25-
      nondisplaced S92.25-
    scaphoid —*see* Fracture, tarsal,
        navicular
    talus S92.10-
      avulsion (displaced) S92.15-
        nondisplaced S92.15-
      body (displaced) S92.12-
        nondisplaced S92.12-
      dome (displaced) S92.14-
        nondisplaced S92.14-
      head (displaced) S92.12-
        nondisplaced S92.12-
      lateral process (displaced) S92.14-
        nondisplaced S92.14-
      neck (displaced) S92.11-
        nondisplaced S92.11-
      posterior process (displaced)
          S92.13-
        nondisplaced S92.13-
      specified NEC S92.19-
  temporal bone (styloid) S02.19
  thorax (bony) S22.9
    with flail chest —*see* Flail, chest
    rib S22.3-
      multiple S22.4-
        with flail chest —*see* Flail, chest
    sternum S22.20
      body S22.22
      manubrium S22.21
      xiphoid process S22.24
    vertebra (displaced) S22.009
      burst (stable) S22.001
        unstable S22.002
      eighth S22.069
        burst (stable) S22.061
          unstable S22.062
        specified type NEC S22.068
        wedge compression S22.060
      eleventh S22.089
        burst (stable) S22.081
          unstable S22.082
        specified type NEC S22.088
        wedge compression S22.080
      fifth S22.059
        burst (stable) S22.051
          unstable S22.052
        specified type NEC S22.058
        wedge compression S22.050
      first S22.019
        burst (stable) S22.011
          unstable S22.012
        specified type NEC S22.018
        wedge compression S22.010
      fourth S22.049
        burst (stable) S22.041
          unstable S22.042
        specified type NEC S22.048
        wedge compression S22.040
      ninth S22.079
        burst (stable) S22.071
          unstable S22.072
        specified type NEC S22.078
        wedge compression S22.070
      nondisplaced S22.001

Fracture, traumatic *(Continued)*
  thorax *(Continued)*
    vertebra *(Continued)*
      second S22.029
        burst (stable) S22.021
          unstable S22.022
        specified type NEC S22.028
        wedge compression S22.020
      seventh S22.069
        burst (stable) S22.061
          unstable S22.062
        specified type NEC S22.068
        wedge compression S22.060
      sixth S22.059
        burst (stable) S22.051
          unstable S22.052
        specified type NEC S22.058
        wedge compression S22.050
      specified type NEC S22.008
      tenth S22.079
        burst (stable) S22.071
          unstable S22.072
        specified type NEC S22.078
        wedge compression S22.070
      third S22.039
        burst (stable) S22.031
          unstable S22.032
        specified type NEC S22.038
        wedge compression S22.030
      twelfth S22.089
        burst (stable) S22.081
          unstable S22.082
        specified type NEC S22.088
        wedge compression S22.080
      wedge compression S22.000
    thumb S62.50-
      distal phalanx (displaced) S62.52-
        nondisplaced S62.52-
      proximal phalanx (displaced) S62.51-
        nondisplaced S62.51-
    thyroid cartilage S12.8
    tibia (shaft) S82.20-
      comminuted (displaced) S82.25-
        nondisplaced S82.25-
      condyles —*see* Fracture, tibia, upper end
      distal end —*see* Fracture, tibia, lower end
      epiphysis
        lower —*see* Fracture, tibia, lower end
        upper —*see* Fracture, tibia, upper end
      following insertion of implant, prosthesis
          or plate M96.67-
      head (involving knee joint) —*see* Fracture,
          tibia, upper end
      intercondyloid eminence —*see* Fracture,
          tibia, upper end
      involving ankle or malleolus —*see*
          Fracture, ankle, medial malleolus
      lower end S82.30-
        physeal S89.10-
          Salter-Harris
            Type I S89.11-
            Type II S89.12-
            Type III S89.13-
            Type IV S89.14-
            specified NEC S89.19-
        pilon (displaced) S82.87-
          nondisplaced S82.87-
        specified NEC S82.39-
        torus S82.31-
      malleolus —*see* Fracture, ankle, medial
          malleolus
      oblique (displaced) S82.23-
        nondisplaced S82.23-
      pilon —*see* Fracture, tibia, lower end,
          pilon
      proximal end —*see* Fracture, tibia, upper
          end
      segmental (displaced) S82.26-
        nondisplaced S82.26-
      specified NEC S82.29-
      spine —*see* Fracture, upper end, spine

Fracture, traumatic *(Continued)*
  tibia *(Continued)*
    spiral (displaced) S82.24-
      nondisplaced S82.24-
    transverse (displaced) S82.22-
      nondisplaced S82.22-
    tuberosity —*see* Fracture, tibia, upper end,
        tuberosity
    upper end S82.10-
      bicondylar (displaced) S82.14-
        nondisplaced S82.14-
      lateral condyle (displaced) S82.12-
        nondisplaced S82.12-
      medial condyle (displaced) S82.13-
        nondisplaced S82.13-
      physeal S89.00-
        Salter-Harris
          Type I S89.01-
          Type II S89.02-
          Type III S89.03-
          Type IV S89.04-
          specified NEC S89.09-
      plateau —*see* Fracture, tibia, upper end,
          bicondylar
      specified NEC S82.19-
      spine (displaced) S82.11-
        nondisplaced S82.11-
      torus S82.16-
      tuberosity (displaced) S82.15-
        nondisplaced S82.15-
  toe S92.91-
    great (displaced) S92.40-
      distal phalanx (displaced) S92.42-
        nondisplaced S92.42-
      nondisplaced S92.40-
      proximal phalanx (displaced) S92.41-
        nondisplaced S92.41-
      specified NEC S92.49-
    lesser (displaced) S92.50-
      distal phalanx (displaced) S92.53-
        nondisplaced S92.53-
      medial phalanx (displaced) S92.52-
        nondisplaced S92.52-
      nondisplaced S92.50-
      proximal phalanx (displaced) S92.51-
        nondisplaced S92.51-
      specified NEC S92.59-
  tooth (root) S02.5
  trachea (cartilage) S12.8
  transverse process —*see* Fracture, vertebra
  trapezium or trapezoid bone —*see* Fracture,
      carpal
  trimalleolar —*see* Fracture, ankle, trimalleolar
  triquetrum (cuneiform of carpus) —*see*
      Fracture, carpal, triquetrum
  trochanter —*see* Fracture, femur,
      trochanteric
  tuberosity (external) - code by site under
      Fracture
  ulna (shaft) S52.20-
    bent bone S52.28-
    coronoid process —*see* Fracture, ulna,
        upper end, coronoid process
    distal end —*see* Fracture, ulna, lower end
    following insertion of implant, prosthesis
        or plate M96.63-
    head S52.00-
    lower end S52.60-
      physeal S59.00-
        Salter-Harris
          Type I S59.01-
          Type II S59.02-
          Type III S59.03-
          Type IV S59.04-
          specified NEC S59.09-
      specified NEC S52.69-
      styloid process (displaced) S52.61-
        nondisplaced S52.61-
      torus S52.62-
    proximal end —*see* Fracture, ulna, upper
        end

◀ New   ◀▥ Revised   ~~deleted~~ Deleted

Fracture, traumatic *(Continued)*
  ulna *(Continued)*
    shaft S52.20-
      comminuted (displaced) S52.25-
        nondisplaced S52.25-
      greenstick S52.21-
      Monteggia's —*see* Monteggia's fracture
      oblique (displaced) S52.23-
        nondisplaced S52.23-
      segmental (displaced) S52.26-
        nondisplaced S52.26-
      specified NEC S52.29-
      spiral (displaced) S52.24-
        nondisplaced S52.24-
      transverse (displaced) S52.22-
        nondisplaced S52.22-
    upper end S52.00-
      coronoid process (displaced) S52.04-
        nondisplaced S52.04-
      olecranon process (displaced)
        S52.02-
        with intraarticular extension
          S52.03-
        nondisplaced S52.02-
          with intraarticular extension
            S52.03-
      specified NEC S52.09-
      torus S52.01-
    unciform —*see* Fracture, carpal, hamate
  vault of skull S02.0
  vertebra, vertebral (arch) (body) (column)
    (neural arch) (pedicle) (spinous process)
    (transverse process)
    atlas —*see* Fracture, neck, cervical vertebra,
      first
    axis —*see* Fracture, neck, cervical vertebra,
      second
    cervical (teardrop) S12.9
      axis —*see* Fracture, neck, cervical
        vertebra, second
      first (atlas) —*see* Fracture, neck, cervical
        vertebra, first
      second (axis) —*see* Fracture, neck,
        cervical vertebra, second
    chronic M84.48
    coccyx S32.2
    dorsal —*see* Fracture, thorax, vertebra
    lumbar S32.009
      burst (stable) S32.001
        unstable S32.002
      fifth S32.059
        burst (stable) S32.051
          unstable S32.052
        specified type NEC S32.058
        wedge compression S32.050
      first S32.019
        burst (stable) S32.011
          unstable S32.012
        specified type NEC S32.018
        wedge compression S32.010
      fourth S32.049
        burst (stable) S32.041
          unstable S32.042
        specified type NEC S32.048
        wedge compression S32.040
      second S32.029
        burst (stable) S32.021
          unstable S32.022
        specified type NEC S32.028
        wedge compression S32.020
      specified type NEC S32.008
      third S32.039
        burst (stable) S32.031
          unstable S32.032
        specified type NEC S32.038
        wedge compression S32.030
      wedge compression S32.000
    metastatic —*see* Collapse, vertebra, in,
      specified disease NEC —*see also*
      Neoplasm
    newborn (birth injury) P11.5

Fracture, traumatic *(Continued)*
  vertebra, vertebral *(Continued)*
    sacrum S32.10
      specified NEC S32.19
      Type
        1 S32.14
        2 S32.15
        3 S32.16
        4 S32.17
      Zone
        I S32.119
          displaced (minimally) S32.111
            severely S32.112
          nondisplaced S32.110
        II S32.129
          displaced (minimally) S32.121
            severely S32.122
          nondisplaced S32.120
        III S32.139
          displaced (minimally) S32.131
            severely S32.132
          nondisplaced S32.130
    thoracic —*see* Fracture, thorax, vertebra
    vertex S02.0
    vomer (bone) S02.2
    wrist S62.10-
      carpal —*see* Fracture, carpal bone
      navicular (scaphoid) (hand) —*see* Fracture,
        carpal, navicular
    xiphisternum, xiphoid (process) S22.24
    zygoma S02.442
Fragile, fragility
  autosomal site Q95.5
  bone, congenital (with blue sclera) Q78.0
  capillary (hereditary) D69.8
  hair L67.8
  nails L60.3
  non-sex chromosome site Q95.5
  X chromosome Q99.2
Fragilitas
  crinium L67.8
  ossium (with blue sclerae) (hereditary)
    Q78.0
  unguium L60.3
    congenital Q84.6
Fragments, cataract (lens), following cataract
    surgery H59.02-
  retained foreign body —*see* Retained, foreign
    body fragments (type of)
Frailty (frail) R54
  mental R41.81
Frambesia, frambesial (tropica) —*see also* Yaws
  initial lesion or ulcer A66.0
  primary A66.0
Frambeside
  gummatous A66.4
  of early yaws A66.2
Frambesioma A66.1
Franceschetti-Klein (-Wildervanck) disease or
    syndrome Q75.4
Francis' disease —*see* Tularemia
Franklin disease C88.2
Frank's essential thrombocytopenia D69.3
Fraser's syndrome Q87.0
Freckle (s) L81.2
  malignant melanoma in —*see* Melanoma
  melanotic (Hutchinson's) —*see* Melanoma,
    in situ
  retinal D49.81
Frederickson's hyperlipoproteinemia, type
    I and V E78.3
    IIA E78.0
    IIB and III E78.2
    IV E78.1
Freeman Sheldon syndrome Q87.0
Freezing —*see also* Effect, adverse, cold T69.9
Freiberg's disease (infraction of metatarsal
    head or osteochondrosis) —*see*
    Osteochondrosis, juvenile, metatarsus
Frei's disease A55
Fremitus, friction, cardiac R01.2

Frenum, frenulum
  external os Q51.828
  tongue (shortening) (congenital) Q38.1
Frequency micturition (nocturnal) R35.0
  psychogenic F45.8
Frey's syndrome
  auriculotemporal G50.8
  hyperhidrosis L74.52
Friction
  burn —*see* Burn, by site
  fremitus, cardiac R01.2
  precordial R01.2
  sounds, chest R09.89
Friderichsen-Waterhouse syndrome or disease
  A39.1
Friedländer's B (bacillus) NEC *(see also*
  condition) A49.8
Friedreich's
  ataxia G11.1
  combined systemic disease G11.1
  facial hemihypertrophy Q67.4
  sclerosis (cerebellum) (spinal cord)
    G11.1
Frigidity F52.22
Fröhlich's syndrome E23.6
Frontal —*see also* condition
  lobe syndrome F07.0
Frostbite (superficial) T33.90
  with
    partial thickness skin loss —*see* Frostbite
      (superficial), by site
    tissue necrosis T34.90
  abdominal wall T33.3
    with tissue necrosis T34.3
  ankle T33.81-
    with tissue necrosis T34.81-
  arm T33.4-
    with tissue necrosis T34.4-
    finger (s) —*see* Frostbite, finger
    hand —*see* Frostbite, hand
    wrist —*see* Frostbite, wrist
  ear T33.01-
    with tissue necrosis T34.01-
  face T33.09
    with tissue necrosis T34.09
  finger T33.53-
    with tissue necrosis T34.53-
  foot T33.82-
    with tissue necrosis T34.82-
  hand T33.52-
    with tissue necrosis T34.52-
  head T33.09
    with tissue necrosis T34.09
    ear —*see* Frostbite, ear
    nose —*see* Frostbite, nose
  hip (and thigh) T33.6-
    with tissue necrosis T34.6-
  knee T33.7-
    with tissue necrosis T34.7-
  leg T33.9-
    with tissue necrosis T34.9-
    ankle —*see* Frostbite, ankle
    foot —*see* Frostbite, foot
    knee —*see* Frostbite, knee
    lower T33.7-
      with tissue necrosis T34.7-
    thigh —*see* Frostbite, hip
    toe —*see* Frostbite, toe
  limb
    lower T33.99
      with tissue necrosis T34.99
    upper —*see* Frostbite, arm
  neck T33.1
    with tissue necrosis T34.1
  nose T33.02
    with tissue necrosis T34.02
  pelvis T33.3
    with tissue necrosis T34.3
  specified site NEC T33.99
    with tissue necrosis T34.99
  thigh —*see* Frostbite, hip

Frostbite *(Continued)*
  thorax T33.2
    with tissue necrosis T34.2
  toes T33.83-
    with tissue necrosis T34.83-
  trunk T33.99
    with tissue necrosis T34.99
  wrist T33.51-
    with tissue necrosis T34.51-
Frotteurism F65.81
Frozen *(see also* Effect, adverse, cold) T69.9
  pelvis (female) N94.89
    male K66.8
  shoulder —*see* Capsulitis, adhesive
Fructokinase deficiency E74.11
Fructose 1,6 diphosphatase deficiency E74.19
Fructosemia (benign) (essential) E74.12
Fructosuria (benign) (essential) E74.11
Fuchs'
  black spot (myopic) H44.2-
  dystrophy (corneal endothelium) H18.51
  heterochromic cyclitis —*see* Cyclitis, Fuchs'
    heterochromic
Fucosidosis E77.1
Fugue R68.89
  dissociative F44.1
  hysterical (dissociative) F44.1
  postictal in epilepsy —*see* Epilepsy
  reaction to exceptional stress (transient)
    F43.0
Fulminant, fulminating —*see* condition
Functional —*see also* condition
  bleeding (uterus) N93.8
Functioning, intellectual, borderline R41.83
Fundus —*see* condition
Fungemia NOS B49
Fungus, fungous
  cerebral G93.89
  disease NOS B49
  infection —*see* Infection, fungus
Funiculitis (acute) (chronic) (endemic) N49.1
  gonococcal (acute) (chronic) A54.23
  tuberculous A18.15
Funnel
  breast (acquired) M95.4
    congenital Q67.6
    sequelae (late effect) of rickets E64.3
  chest (acquired) M95.4
    congenital Q67.6
    sequelae (late effect) of rickets E64.3
  pelvis (acquired) M95.5
    with disproportion (fetopelvic) O33.3
      causing obstructed labor O65.3
    congenital Q74.2
FUO (fever of unknown origin) R50.9
Furfur L21.0
  microsporon B36.0
Furrier's lung J67.8
Furrowed K14.5
  nail (s) (transverse) L60.4
    congenital Q84.6
  tongue K14.5
    congenital Q38.3
Furuncle L02.92
  abdominal wall L02.221
  ankle —*see* Furuncle, lower limb
  antecubital space —*see* Furuncle, upper limb
  anus K61.0
  arm —*see* Furuncle, upper limb

Furuncle *(Continued)*
  auditory canal, external —*see* Abscess, ear,
    external
  auricle (ear) —*see* Abscess, ear, external
  axilla (region) L02.42-
  back (any part) L02.222
  breast N61
  buttock L02.32
  cheek (external) L02.02
  chest wall L02.223
  chin L02.02
  corpus cavernosum N48.21
  ear, external —*see* Abscess, ear, external
  external auditory canal —*see* Abscess, ear,
    external
  eyelid —*see* Abscess, eyelid
  face L02.02
  femoral (region) —*see* Furuncle, lower limb
  finger —*see* Furuncle, hand
  flank L02.221
  foot L02.62-
  forehead L02.02
  gluteal (region) L02.32
  groin L02.224
  hand L02.52-
  head L02.821
    face L02.02
  hip —*see* Furuncle, lower limb
  kidney —*see* Abscess, kidney
  knee —*see* Furuncle, lower limb
  labium (majus) (minus) N76.4
  lacrimal
    gland —*see* Dacryoadenitis
    passages (duct) (sac) —*see* Inflammation,
      lacrimal, passages, acute
  leg (any part) —*see* Furuncle, lower limb
  lower limb L02.42-
  malignant A22.0
  mouth K12.2
  navel L02.226
  neck L02.12
  nose J34.0
  orbit, orbital —*see* Abscess, orbit
  palmar (space) —*see* Furuncle, hand
  partes posteriores L02.32
  pectoral region L02.223
  penis N48.21
  perineum L02.225
  pinna —*see* Abscess, ear, external
  popliteal —*see* Furuncle, lower limb
  prepatellar —*see* Furuncle, lower limb
  scalp L02.821
  seminal vesicle N49.0
  shoulder —*see* Furuncle, upper limb
  specified site NEC L02.828
  submandibular K12.2
  temple (region) L02.02
  thumb —*see* Furuncle, hand
  toe —*see* Furuncle, foot
  trunk L02.229
    abdominal wall L02.221
    back L02.222
    chest wall L02.223
    groin L02.224
    perineum L02.225
    umbilicus L02.226
  umbilicus L02.226
  upper limb L02.42-
  vulva N76.4

Furunculosis —*see* Furuncle
Fused —*see* Fusion, fused
Fusion, fused (congenital)
  astragaloscaphoid Q74.2
  atria Q21.1
  auditory canal Q16.1
  auricles, heart Q21.1
  binocular with defective stereopsis H53.32
  bone Q79.8
  cervical spine M43.22
  choanal Q30.0
  commissure, mitral valve Q23.2
  cusps, heart valve NEC Q24.8
    mitral Q23.2
    pulmonary Q22.1
    tricuspid Q22.4
  ear ossicles Q16.3
  fingers Q70.0- ◀▥
  hymen Q52.3
  joint (acquired) —*see also* Ankylosis
    congenital Q74.8
  kidneys (incomplete) Q63.1
  labium (majus) (minus) Q52.5
  larynx and trachea Q34.8
  limb, congenital Q74.8
    lower Q74.2
    upper Q74.0
  lobes, lung Q33.8
  lumbosacral (acquired) M43.27
    arthrodesis status Z98.1
    congenital Q76.49
    postprocedural status Z98.1
  nares, nose, nasal, nostril (s) Q30.0
  organ or site not listed —*see* Anomaly,
    by site
  ossicles Q79.9
    auditory Q16.3
  pulmonic cusps Q22.1
  ribs Q76.6
  sacroiliac (joint) (acquired) M43.28
    arthrodesis status Z98.1
    congenital Q74.2
    postprocedural status Z98.1
  spine (acquired) NEC M43.20
    arthrodesis status Z98.1
    cervical region M43.22
    cervicothoracic region M43.23
    congenital Q76.49
    lumbar M43.26
    lumbosacral region M43.27
    occipito-atlanto-axial region M43.21
    postoperative status Z98.1
    sacrococcygeal region M43.28
    thoracic region M43.24
    thoracolumbar region M43.25
  sublingual duct with submaxillary duct at
    opening in mouth Q38.4
  testes Q55.1
  toes Q70.2
  tooth, teeth K00.2
  trachea and esophagus Q39.8
  twins Q89.4
  vagina Q52.4
  ventricles, heart Q21.0
  vertebra (arch) —*see* Fusion, spine
  vulva Q52.5
Fusospirillosis (mouth) (tongue) (tonsil)
  A69.1
Fussy baby R68.12

G

Gain in weight (abnormal) (excessive) —*see also* Weight, gain
Gaisböck's disease (polycythemia hypertonica) D75.1
Gait abnormality R26.9
　ataxic R26.0
　falling R29.6
　hysterical (ataxic) (staggering) F44.4
　paralytic R26.1
　spastic R26.1
　specified type NEC R26.89
　staggering R26.0
　unsteadiness R26.81
　walking difficulty NEC R26.2
Galactocele (breast) N64.89
　puerperal, postpartum O92.79
Galactokinase deficiency E74.29
Galactophoritis N61
　gestational, puerperal, postpartum O91.2-
Galactorrhea O92.6
　not associated with childbirth N64.3
Galactosemia (classic) (congenital) E74.21
Galactosuria E74.29
Galacturia R82.0
　schistosomiasis (bilharziasis) B65.0
Galeazzi's fracture S52.37-
Galen's vein —*see* condition
Galeophobia F40.218
Gall duct —*see* condition
Gallbladder —*see also* condition
　acute K81.0
Gallop rhythm R00.8
Gallstone (colic) (cystic duct) (gallbladder) (impacted) (multiple) —*see also* Calculus, gallbladder
　with
　　cholecystitis —*see* Calculus, gallbladder, with cholecystitis
　　bile duct (common) (hepatic) —*see* Calculus, bile duct
　　causing intestinal obstruction K56.3
　specified NEC K80.80
　　with obstruction K80.81
Gambling Z72.6
　pathological (compulsive) F63.0
Gammopathy (of undetermined significance [MGUS]) D47.2
　associated with lymphoplasmacytic dyscrasia D47.2
　monoclonal D47.2
　polyclonal D89.0
Gamna's disease (siderotic splenomegaly) D73.1
Gamophobia F40.298
Gampsodactylia (congenital) Q66.7
Gamstorp's disease (adynamia episodica hereditaria) G72.3
Gandy-Nanta disease (siderotic splenomegaly) D73.1
Gang
　membership offenses Z72.810
Gangliocytoma D36.10
Ganglioglioma —*see* Neoplasm, uncertain behavior, by site
Ganglion (compound) (diffuse) (joint) (tendon) (sheath) M67.40
　ankle M67.47-
　foot M67.47-
　forearm M67.43-
　hand M67.44-
　lower leg M67.46-
　multiple sites M67.49
　of yaws (early) (late) A66.6
　pelvic region M67.45-
　periosteal —*see* Periostitis
　shoulder region M67.41-
　specified site NEC M67.48
　thigh region M67.45-
　tuberculous A18.09
　upper arm M67.42-
　wrist M67.43-

Ganglioneuroblastoma —*see* Neoplasm, nerve, malignant
Ganglioneuroma D36.10
　malignant —*see* Neoplasm, nerve, malignant
Ganglioneuromatosis D36.10
Ganglionitis
　fifth nerve —*see* Neuralgia, trigeminal
　gasserian (postherpetic) (postzoster) B02.21
　geniculate G51.1
　　newborn (birth injury) P11.3
　　postherpetic, postzoster B02.21
　herpes zoster B02.21
　postherpetic geniculate B02.21
Gangliosidosis E75.10
　GM1 E75.19
　GM2 E75.00
　　other specified E75.09
　　Sandhoff disease E75.01
　　Tay-Sachs disease E75.02
　GM3 E75.19
　mucolipidosis IV E75.11
Gangosa A66.5
Gangrene, gangrenous (connective tissue) (dropsical) (dry) (moist) (skin) (ulcer) (*see also* Necrosis) I96
　with diabetes (mellitus) —*see* Diabetes, gangrene
　abdomen (wall) I96
　alveolar M27.3
　appendix K35.80 ◀▥
　　with
　　　perforation or rupture K35.2
　　　peritoneal abscess K35.3
　　　~~peritonitis, localized K35.3~~
　　　　~~with perforation or rupture K35.2~~
　　　　~~generalized K35.2~~
　　　peritonitis NEC K35.3 ◀
　　　　generalized (with perforation or rupture) K35.2 ◀
　　　　localized (with perforation or rupture) K35.3 ◀
　arteriosclerotic (general) (senile) —*see* Arteriosclerosis, extremities, with, gangrene
　auricle I96
　Bacillus welchii A48.0
　bladder (infectious) —*see* Cystitis, specified type NEC
　bowel, cecum, or colon —*see* Gangrene, intestine
　Clostridium perfringens or welchii A48.0
　cornea H18.89-
　corpora cavernosa N48.29
　　noninfective N48.89
　cutaneous, spreading I96
　decubital —*see* Ulcer, pressure, by site
　diabetic (any site) —*see* Diabetes, gangrene
　emphysematous —*see* Gangrene, gas
　epidemic —*see* Poisoning, food, noxious, plant
　epididymis (infectional) N45.1
　erysipelas —*see* Erysipelas
　extremity (lower) (upper) I96
　Fournier N49.3
　　female N76.89
　fusospirochetal A69.0
　gallbladder —*see* Cholecystitis, acute
　gas (bacillus) A48.0
　　following
　　　abortion —*see* Abortion by type complicated by infection
　　　ectopic or molar pregnancy O08.0
　glossitis K14.0
　hernia —*see* Hernia, by site, with gangrene
　intestine, intestinal (hemorrhagic) (massive) K55.0
　　with
　　　mesenteric embolism K55.0
　　　obstruction —*see* Obstruction, intestine
　laryngitis J04.0

Gangrene, gangrenous (*Continued*)
　limb (lower) (upper) I96
　lung J85.0
　　spirochetal A69.8
　lymphangitis I89.1
　Meleney's (synergistic) —*see* Ulcer, skin
　mesentery K55.0
　　with
　　　embolism K55.0
　　　intestinal obstruction —*see* Obstruction, intestine
　mouth A69.0
　ovary —*see* Oophoritis
　pancreas K85.9
　penis N48.29
　　noninfective N48.89
　perineum I96
　pharynx —*see also* Pharyngitis
　　Vincent's A69.1
　presenile I73.1
　progressive synergistic —*see* Ulcer, skin
　pulmonary J85.0
　pulpal (dental) K04.1
　quinsy J36
　Raynaud's (symmetric gangrene) I73.01
　retropharyngeal J39.2
　scrotum N49.3
　　noninfective N50.8
　senile (atherosclerotic) —*see* Arteriosclerosis, extremities, with, gangrene
　spermatic cord N49.1
　　noninfective N50.8
　spine I96
　spirochetal NEC A69.8
　spreading cutaneous I96
　stomatitis A69.0
　symmetrical I73.01
　testis (infectional) N45.2
　　noninfective N44.8
　throat —*see also* Pharyngitis
　　diphtheritic A36.0
　　Vincent's A69.1
　thyroid (gland) E07.89
　tooth (pulp) K04.1
　tuberculous NEC —*see* Tuberculosis
　tunica vaginalis N49.1
　　noninfective N50.8
　umbilicus I96
　uterus —*see* Endometritis
　uvulitis K12.2
　vas deferens N49.1
　　noninfective N50.8
　vulva N76.89
Ganister disease J62.8
Ganser's syndrome (hysterical) F44.89
Gardner-Diamond syndrome (autoerythrocyte sensitization) D69.2
Gargoylism E76.01
Garré's disease, osteitis (sclerosing), osteomyelitis —*see* Osteomyelitis, specified type NEC
Garrod's pad, knuckle M72.1
Gartner's duct
　cyst Q52.4
　persistent Q50.6
Gas R14.3
　asphyxiation, inhalation, poisoning, suffocation NEC —*see* Table of ~~d~~Drugs and ~~c~~Chemicals ◀▥
　excessive R14.0
　gangrene A48.0
　　following
　　　abortion —*see* Abortion by type complicated by infection
　　　ectopic or molar pregnancy O08.0
　on stomach R14.0
　pains R14.1
Gastralgia —*see also* Pain, abdominal
Gastrectasis K31.0
　psychogenic F45.8
Gastric —*see* condition

Gastrinoma
  malignant
    pancreas C25.4
    specified site NEC —*see* Neoplasm,
      malignant, by site
    unspecified site C25.4
  specified site —*see* Neoplasm, uncertain
    behavior
  unspecified site D37.9
Gastritis (simple) K29.70
  with bleeding K29.71
  acute (erosive) K29.00
    with bleeding K29.01
  alcoholic K29.20
    with bleeding K29.21
  allergic K29.60
    with bleeding K29.61
  atrophic (chronic) K29.40
    with bleeding K29.41
  chronic (antral) (fundal) K29.50
    with bleeding K29.51
    atrophic K29.40
      with bleeding K29.41
    superficial K29.30
      with bleeding K29.31
  dietary counseling and surveillance Z71.3
  due to diet deficiency E63.9
  eosinophilic K52.81
  giant hypertrophic K29.60
    with bleeding K29.61
  granulomatous K29.60
    with bleeding K29.61
  hypertrophic (mucosa) K29.60
    with bleeding K29.61
  nervous F54
  spastic K29.60
    with bleeding K29.61
  specified NEC K29.60
    with bleeding K29.61
  superficial chronic K29.30
    with bleeding K29.31
  tuberculous A18.83
  viral NEC A08.4
Gastrocarcinoma —*see* Neoplasm, malignant,
    stomach
Gastrocolic —*see* condition
Gastrodisciasis, gastrodiscoidiasis B66.8
Gastroduodenitis K29.90
  with bleeding K29.91
  virus, viral A08.4
    specified type NEC A08.39
Gastrodynia —*see* Pain, abdominal
Gastroenteritis (acute) (chronic) (noninfectious)
    (*see also* Enteritis) K52.9
  allergic K52.2
  dietetic K52.2
  drug-induced K52.1
  due to
    Cryptosporidium A07.2
    drugs K52.1
    food poisoning —*see* Intoxication, foodborne
    radiation K52.0
  eosinophilic K52.81
  epidemic (infectious) A09
  food hypersensitivity K52.2
  infectious —*see* Enteritis, infectious
  influenzal —*see* Influenza, with
    gastroenteritis
  noninfectious K52.9
    specified NEC K52.89
  rotaviral A08.0
  Salmonella A02.0
  toxic K52.1
  viral NEC A08.4
    acute infectious A08.39
      type Norwalk A08.11
    infantile (acute) A08.39
    Norwalk agent A08.11
    rotaviral A08.0
    severe of infants A08.39
    specified type NEC A08.39

Gastroenteropathy (*see also* Gastroenteritis)
    K52.9
  acute, due to Norovirus A08.11
  acute, due to Norwalk agent A08.11
  infectious A09
Gastroenteroptosis K63.4
Gastroesophageal laceration-hemorrhage
    syndrome K22.6
Gastrointestinal —*see* condition
Gastrojejunal —*see* condition
Gastrojejunitis (*see also* Enteritis) K52.9
Gastrojejunocolic —*see* condition
Gastroliths K31.89
Gastromalacia K31.89
Gastroparalysis K31.84
  diabetic —*see* Diabetes, gastroparalysis
Gastroparesis K31.84
  diabetic —*see* Diabetes, by type, with
    gastroparesis
Gastropathy K31.9
  congestive portal K31.89
  erythematous K29.70
  exudative K90.89
  portal hypertensive K31.89
Gastroptosis K31.89
Gastrorrhagia K92.2
  psychogenic F45.8
Gastroschisis (congenital) Q79.3
Gastrospasm (neurogenic) (reflex) K31.89
  neurotic F45.8
  psychogenic F45.8
Gastrostaxis —*see* Gastritis, with bleeding
Gastrostenosis K31.89
Gastrostomy
  attention to Z43.1
  status Z93.1
Gastrosuccorrhea (continuous) (intermittent)
    K31.89
  neurotic F45.8
  psychogenic F45.8
Gatophobia F40.218
Gaucher's disease or splenomegaly (adult)
    (infantile) E75.22
Gee (-Herter)(-Thaysen) disease (nontropical
    sprue) K90.0
Gélineau's syndrome G47.419
  with cataplexy G47.411
Gemination, tooth, teeth K00.2
Gemistocytoma
  specified site —*see* Neoplasm, malignant, by
    site
  unspecified site C71.9
General, generalized —*see* condition
Genetic
  carrier (status)
    cystic fibrosis Z14.1
    hemophilia A (asymptomatic) Z14.01
      symptomatic Z14.02
    specified NEC Z14.8
  susceptibility to disease NEC Z15.89
    malignant neoplasm Z15.09
      breast Z15.01
      endometrium Z15.04
      ovary Z15.02
      prostate Z15.03
      specified NEC Z15.09
    multiple endocrine neoplasia Z15.81
Genital —*see* condition
Genito-anorectal syndrome A55
Genitourinary system —*see* condition
Genu
  congenital Q74.1
  extrorsum (acquired) —*see also* Deformity,
    varus, knee
    congenital Q74.1
    sequelae (late effect) of rickets E64.3
  introrsum (acquired) —*see also* Deformity,
    valgus, knee
    congenital Q74.1
    sequelae (late effect) of rickets E64.3
  rachitic (old) E64.3

Genu (*Continued*)
  recurvatum (acquired) —*see also* Deformity,
    limb, specified type NEC, lower leg
    congenital Q68.2
    sequelae (late effect) of rickets E64.3
  valgum (acquired) (knock-knee) M21.06-
    congenital Q74.1
    sequelae (late effect) of rickets E64.3
  varum (acquired) (bowleg) M21.16-
    congenital Q74.1
    sequelae (late effect) of rickets E64.3
Geographic tongue K14.1
Geophagia —*see* Pica
Geotrichosis B48.3
  stomatitis B48.3
Gephyrophobia F40.242
Gerbode defect Q21.0
GERD (gastroesophageal reflux disease)
    K21.9
Gerhardt's
  disease (erythromelalgia) I73.81
  syndrome (vocal cord paralysis)
    J38.00
    bilateral J38.02
    unilateral J38.01
German measles —*see also* Rubella
  exposure to Z20.4
Germinoblastoma (diffuse) C85.9-
  follicular C82.9-
Germinoma —*see* Neoplasm, malignant,
    by site
Gerontoxon —*see* Degeneration, cornea, senile
Gerstmann-Sträussler-Scheinker syndrome
    (GSS) A81.82
Gerstmann's syndrome R48.8
  developmental F81.2
Gestation (period) —*see also* Pregnancy
  ectopic —*see* Pregnancy, by site
  multiple O30.9-
    greater than quadruplets —*see* Pregnancy,
      multiple (gestation), specified NEC
    specified NEC —*see* Pregnancy, multiple
      (gestation), specified NEC
Gestational
  mammary abscess O91.11-
  purulent mastitis O91.11-
  subareolar abscess O91.11-
Ghon tubercle, primary infection A15.7
Ghost
  teeth K00.4
  vessels (cornea) H16.41-
Ghoul hand A66.3
Gianotti-Crosti disease L44.4
Giant
  cell
    epulis K06.8
    peripheral granuloma K06.8
  esophagus, congenital Q39.5
  kidney, congenital Q63.3
  oesophagus, congenital Q39.5
  urticaria T78.3
    hereditary D84.1
Giardiasis A07.1
Gibert's disease or pityriasis L42
Giddiness R42
  hysterical F44.89
  psychogenic F45.8
Gierke's disease (glycogenosis I) E74.01
Gigantism (cerebral) (hypophyseal) (pituitary)
    E22.0
  constitutional E34.4
Gilbert's disease or syndrome E80.4
Gilchrist's disease B40.9
Gilford-Hutchinson disease E34.8
Gilles de la Tourette's disease or syndrome
    (motor-verbal tic) F95.2
Gingivitis K05.10
  acute (catarrhal) K05.00
    necrotizing A69.1
    nonplaque induced K05.01
    plaque induced K05.00

Gingivitis (Continued)
  chronic (desquamative) (hyperplastic)
    (simple marginal) (ulcerative) K05.10
    nonplaque induced K05.11
    plaque induced K05.10
  expulsiva —see Periodontitis
  necrotizing ulcerative (acute) A69.1
  pellagrous E52
    acute necrotizing A69.1
  Vincent's A69.1
Gingivoglossitis K14.0
Gingivopericementitis —see Periodontitis
Gingivosis —see Gingivitis, chronic
Gingivostomatitis K05.10
  herpesviral B00.2
  necrotizing ulcerative (acute) A69.1
Gland, glandular —see condition
Glanders A24.0
Glanzmann (-Naegeli) disease or
  thrombasthenia D69.1
Glasgow~~cow~~ coma scale ◀║▌
  total score
    3-8 R40.243
    9-12 R40.242
    13-15 R40.241
Glass-blower's disease (cataract) —see
  Cataract, specified NEC
Glaucoma H40.9
  with
    increased episcleral venous pressure
      H40.81-
    pseudoexfoliation of lens —see Glaucoma,
      open angle, primary, capsular
  absolute H44.51-
  angle-closure (primary) H40.20-
    acute (attack) (crisis) H40.21-
    chronic H40.22-
    intermittent H40.23-
    residual stage H40.24-
  borderline H40.00-
  capsular (with pseudoexfoliation of lens) —
    see Glaucoma, open angle, primary,
    capsular
  childhood Q15.0
  closed angle —see Glaucoma, angle-closure
  congenital Q15.0
  corticosteroid-induced —see Glaucoma,
    secondary, drugs
  hypersecretion H40.82-
  in (due to)
    amyloidosis E85.4 [H42]
    aniridia Q13.1 [H42]
    concussion of globe —see Glaucoma,
      secondary, trauma
    dislocation of lens —see Glaucoma,
      secondary
    disorder of lens NEC —see Glaucoma,
      secondary
    drugs —see Glaucoma, secondary, drugs
    endocrine disease NOS E34.9 [H42]
    eye
      inflammation —see Glaucoma,
        secondary, inflammation
      trauma —see Glaucoma, secondary,
        trauma
    hypermature cataract —see Glaucoma,
      secondary
    iridocyclitis —see Glaucoma, secondary,
      inflammation
    lens disorder —see Glaucoma, secondary,
      Lowe's syndrome E72.03 [H42]
    metabolic disease NOS E88.9 [H42]
    ocular disorders NEC —see Glaucoma,
      secondary
    onchocerciasis B73.02
    pupillary block —see Glaucoma, secondary
    retinal vein occlusion —see Glaucoma,
      secondary
    Rieger's anomaly Q13.81 [H42]
    rubeosis of iris —see Glaucoma, secondary
    tumor of globe —see Glaucoma, secondary

Glaucoma (Continued)
  infantile Q15.0
  low tension —see Glaucoma, open angle,
    primary, low-tension
  malignant H40.83-
  narrow angle —see Glaucoma, angle-closure
  newborn Q15.0
  noncongestive (chronic) —see Glaucoma,
    open angle
  nonobstructive —see Glaucoma, open
    angle
  obstructive —see also Glaucoma,
    angle-closure
    due to lens changes —see Glaucoma,
      secondary
  open angle H40.10-
    primary H40.11-
      capsular (with pseudoexfoliation of lens)
        H40.14-
      low-tension H40.12-
      pigmentary H40.13-
      residual stage H40.15-
  phacolytic —see Glaucoma, secondary
  pigmentary —see Glaucoma, open angle,
    primary, pigmentary
  postinfectious —see Glaucoma, secondary,
    inflammation
  secondary (to) H40.5-
    drugs H40.6-
    inflammation H40.4-
    trauma H40.3-
  simple (chronic) H40.11
  simplex H40.11
  specified type NEC H40.89
  suspect H40.00-
  syphilitic A52.71
  traumatic —see also Glaucoma, secondary,
    trauma
    newborn (birth injury) P15.3
  tuberculous A18.59
Glaucomatous flecks (subcapsular) —see
  Cataract, complicated
Glazed tongue K14.4
Gleet (gonococcal) A54.01
Glénard's disease K63.4
Glioblastoma (multiforme)
  with sarcomatous component
    specified site —see Neoplasm, malignant,
      by site
    unspecified site C71.9
  giant cell
    specified site —see Neoplasm, malignant,
      by site
    unspecified site C71.9
  specified site —see Neoplasm, malignant, by
    site
  unspecified site C71.9
Glioma (malignant)
  astrocytic
    specified site —see Neoplasm, malignant,
      by site
    unspecified site C71.9
  mixed
    specified site —see Neoplasm, malignant,
      by site
    unspecified site C71.9
  nose Q30.8
  specified site NEC —see Neoplasm,
    malignant, by site
  subependymal D43.2
    specified site —see Neoplasm, uncertain
      behavior, by site
    unspecified site D43.2
  unspecified site C71.9
Gliomatosis cerebri C71.0
Glioneuroma —see Neoplasm, uncertain
  behavior, by site
Gliosarcoma
  specified site —see Neoplasm, malignant, by
    site
  unspecified site C71.9

Gliosis (cerebral) G93.89
  spinal G95.89
Glisson's disease —see Rickets
Globinuria R82.3
Globus (hystericus) F45.8
Glomangioma D18.00
  intra-abdominal D18.03
  intracranial D18.02
  skin D18.01
  specified site NEC D18.09
Glomangiomyoma D18.00
  intra-abdominal D18.03
  intracranial D18.02
  skin D18.01
  specified site NEC D18.09
Glomangiosarcoma —see Neoplasm, connective
  tissue, malignant
Glomerular
  disease in syphilis A52.75
  nephritis —see Glomerulonephritis
Glomerulitis —see Glomerulonephritis
Glomerulonephritis (see also Nephritis)
  N05.9
  with
    edema —see Nephrosis
    minimal change N05.0
    minor glomerular abnormality N05.0
  acute N00.9
  chronic N03.9
  crescentic (diffuse) NEC (see also N00-N07
    with fourth character .7) N05.7
  dense deposit (see also N00-N07 with fourth
    character .6) N05.6
  diffuse
    crescentic (see also N00-N07 with fourth
      character .7) N05.7
    endocapillary proliferative (see also
      N00N07 with fourth character .4)
      N05.4
    membranous (see also N00-N07 with fourth
      character .2) N05.2
    mesangial proliferative (see also N00N07
      with fourth character .3) N05.3
    mesangiocapillary (see also N00-N07 with
      fourth character .5) N05.5
    sclerosing N05.8
  endocapillary proliferative (diffuse) NEC (see
    also N00-N07 with fourth character .4)
    N05.4
  extracapillary NEC (see also N00-N07 with
    fourth character .7) N05.7
  focal (and segmental) (see also N00-N07 with
    fourth character .1) N05.1
  hypocomplementemic —see
    Glomerulonephritis,
    membranoproliferative
  IgA —see Nephropathy, IgA
  immune complex (circulating) NEC
    N05.8
  in (due to)
    amyloidosis E85.4 [N08]
    bilharziasis B65.9 [N08]
    cryoglobulinemia D89.1 [N08]
    defibrination syndrome D65 [N08]
    diabetes mellitus —see Diabetes,
      glomerulosclerosis
    disseminated intravascular coagulation
      D65 [N08]
    Fabry (-Anderson) disease E75.21 [N08]
    Goodpasture's syndrome M31.0
    hemolytic-uremic syndrome D59.3
    Henoch (-Schönlein) purpura D69.0
      [N08]
    lecithin cholesterol acyltransferase
      deficiency E78.6 [N08]
    microscopic polyangiitis M31.7 [N08]
    multiple myeloma C90.0- [N08]
    Plasmodium malariae B52.0
    schistosomiasis B65.9 [N08]
    sepsis A41.9- [N08]
      streptococcal A40- [N08]

Glomerulonephritis (Continued)
in (Continued)
    sickle-cell disorders D57.- [N08]
    strongyloidiasis B78.9 [N08]
    subacute bacterial endocarditis I33.0
      [N08]
    syphilis (late) congenital A50.59 [N08]
    systemic lupus erythematosus M32.14
    thrombotic thrombocytopenic purpura
      M31.1 [N08]
    typhoid fever A01.09
    Waldenström macroglobulinemia C88.0
      [N08]
    Wegener's granulomatosis M31.31
latent or quiescent N03.9
lobular, lobulonodular —see
    Glomerulonephritis,
    membranoproliferative
membranoproliferative (diffuse) (type 1
    or 3) (see also N00-N07 with fourth
    character .5) N05.5
    dense deposit (type 2) NEC (see also
      N00-N07 with fourth character .6)
      N05.6
membranous (diffuse) NEC (see also N00-N07
    with fourth character .2) N05.2
mesangial
    IgA/IgG —see Nephropathy, IgA
    proliferative (diffuse) NEC (see also
      N00-N07 with fourth character .3)
      N05.3
mesangiocapillary (diffuse) NEC (see also
    N00-N07 with fourth character .5)
    N05.5
necrotic, necrotizing NEC (see also N00-N07
    with fourth character .8) N05.8 ◄▥
nodular —see Glomerulonephritis,
    membranoproliferative
poststreptococcal NEC N05.9
    acute N00.9
    chronic N03.9
    rapidly progressive N01.9
proliferative NEC (see also N00-N07 with
    fourth character .8) N05.8
    diffuse (lupus) M32.14
rapidly progressive N01.9
sclerosing, diffuse N05.8
specified pathology NEC (see also N00-N07
    with fourth character .8) N05.8 ◄▥
subacute N01.9
Glomerulopathy —see Glomerulonephritis
Glomerulosclerosis —see also Sclerosis,
    renal
intercapillary (nodular) (with diabetes) —see
    Diabetes, glomerulosclerosis
intracapillary —see Diabetes,
    glomerulosclerosis
Glossagra K14.6
Glossalgia K14.6
Glossitis (chronic superficial) (gangrenous)
    (Moeller's) K14.0
areata exfoliativa K14.1
atrophic K14.4
benign migratory K14.1
cortical superficial, sclerotic K14.0
Hunter's D51.0
interstitial, sclerous K14.0
median rhomboid K14.2
pellagrous E52
superficial, chronic K14.0
Glossocele K14.8
Glossodynia K14.6
exfoliativa K14.4
Glossoncus K14.8
Glossopathy K14.9
Glossophytia K14.3
Glossoplegia K14.8
Glossoptosis K14.8
Glossopyrosis K14.6
Glossotrichia K14.3
Glossy skin L90.8

Glottis —see condition
Glottitis (see also Laryngitis) J04.0
Glucagonoma
pancreas
    benign D13.7
    malignant C25.4
    uncertain behavior D37.8
specified site NEC
    benign —see Neoplasm, benign, by site
    malignant —see Neoplasm, malignant, by
      site
    uncertain behavior —see Neoplasm,
      uncertain behavior, by site
unspecified site
    benign D13.7
    malignant C25.4
    uncertain behavior D37.8
Glucoglycinuria E72.51
Glucose-galactose malabsorption E74.39
Glue
ear —see Otitis, media, nonsuppurative,
    chronic, mucoid
sniffing (airplane) —see Abuse, drug,
    inhalant
    dependence —see Dependence, drug,
      inhalant
Glutaric aciduria E72.3
Glycinemia E72.51
Glycinuria (renal) (with ketosis) E72.09
Glycogen
infiltration —see Disease, glycogen storage
storage disease —see Disease, glycogen
    storage
Glycogenosis (diffuse) (generalized) —see also
    Disease, glycogen storage
cardiac E74.02 [I43]
diabetic, secondary —see Diabetes,
    glycogenosis, secondary
pulmonary interstitial J84.842
Glycopenia E16.2
Glycosuria R81
renal E74.8
Gnathostoma spinigerum (infection)
    (infestation), gnathostomiasis (wandering
    swelling) B83.1
Goiter (plunging) (substernal) E04.9
with
    hyperthyroidism (recurrent) —see
      Hyperthyroidism, with, goiter
    thyrotoxicosis —see Hyperthyroidism,
      with, goiter
adenomatous —see Goiter, nodular
cancerous C73
congenital (nontoxic) E03.0
    diffuse E03.0
    parenchymatous E03.0
    transitory, with normal functioning
      P72.0
cystic E04.2
    due to iodine-deficiency E01.1
due to
    enzyme defect in synthesis of thyroid
      hormone E07.1
    iodine-deficiency (endemic) E01.2
dyshormonogenetic (familial) E07.1
endemic (iodine-deficiency) E01.2
    diffuse E01.0
    multinodular E01.1
exophthalmic —see Hyperthyroidism, with,
    goiter
iodine-deficiency (endemic) E01.2
    diffuse E01.0
    multinodular E01.1
    nodular E01.1
lingual Q89.2
lymphadenoid E06.3
malignant C73
multinodular (cystic) (nontoxic) E04.2
    toxic or with hyperthyroidism E05.20
      with thyroid storm E05.21
neonatal NEC P72.0

Goiter (Continued)
nodular (nontoxic) (due to) E04.9
with
    hyperthyroidism E05.20
      with thyroid storm E05.21
    thyrotoxicosis E05.20
      with thyroid storm E05.21
endemic E01.1
iodine-deficiency E01.1
sporadic E04.9
toxic E05.20
    with thyroid storm E05.21
nontoxic E04.9
    diffuse (colloid) E04.0
    multinodular E04.2
    simple E04.0
    specified NEC E04.8
    uninodular E04.1
simple E04.0
toxic —see Hyperthyroidism, with, goiter
uninodular (nontoxic) E04.1
    toxic or with hyperthyroidism E05.10
      with thyroid storm E05.11
Goiter-deafness syndrome E07.1
Goldberg syndrome Q89.8
Goldberg-Maxwell syndrome E34.51
Goldblatt's hypertension or kidney I70.1
Goldenhar (-Gorlin) syndrome Q87.0
Goldflam-Erb disease or syndrome G70.00
    with exacerbation (acute) G70.01
    in crisis G70.01
Goldscheider's disease Q81.8
Goldstein's disease (familial hemorrhagic
    telangiectasia) I78.0
Golfer's elbow —see Epicondylitis, medial
Gonadoblastoma
specified site —see Neoplasm, uncertain
    behavior, by site
unspecified site
    female D39.10
    male D40.10
Gonecystitis —see Vesiculitis
Gongylonemiasis B83.8
Goniosynechiae —see Adhesions, iris,
    goniosynechiae
Gonococcemia A54.86
Gonococcus, gonococcal (disease) (infection)
    (see also condition) A54.9
anus A54.6
bursa, bursitis A54.49
conjunctiva, conjunctivitis (neonatorum)
    A54.31
endocardium A54.83
eye A54.30
    conjunctivitis A54.31
    iridocyclitis A54.32
    keratitis A54.33
    newborn A54.31
    other specified A54.39
fallopian tubes (acute) (chronic) A54.24
genitourinary (organ) (system) (tract) (acute)
    lower A54.00
      with abscess (accessory gland)
        (periurethral) A54.1
    upper (see also condition) A54.29
heart A54.83
iridocyclitis A54.32
joint A54.42
lymphatic (gland) (node) A54.89
meninges, meningitis A54.81
musculoskeletal A54.40
    arthritis A54.42
    osteomyelitis A54.43
    other specified A54.49
    spondylopathy A54.41
pelviperitonitis A54.24
pelvis (acute) (chronic) A54.24
pharynx A54.5
proctitis A54.6
pyosalpinx (acute) (chronic) A54.24
rectum A54.6

◄ New   ◀▥ Revised   ~~deleted~~ Deleted

Gonococcus, gonococcal (Continued)
  skin A54.89
  specified site NEC A54.89
  tendon sheath A54.49
  throat A54.5
  urethra (acute) (chronic) A54.01
    with abscess (accessory gland)
        (periurethral) A54.1
  vulva (acute) (chronic) A54.02
Gonocytoma
  specified site —see Neoplasm, uncertain
      behavior, by site
  unspecified site
    female D39.10
    male D40.10
Gonorrhea (acute) (chronic) A54.9
  Bartholin's gland (acute) (chronic) (purulent)
      A54.02
    with abscess (accessory gland)
        (periurethral) A54.1
  bladder A54.01
  cervix A54.03
  conjunctiva, conjunctivitis (neonatorum)
      A54.31
  contact Z20.2
  Cowper's gland (with abscess) A54.1
  exposure to Z20.2
  fallopian tube (acute) (chronic) A54.24
  kidney (acute) (chronic) A54.21
  lower genitourinary tract A54.00
    with abscess (accessory gland)
        (periurethral) A54.1
  ovary (acute) (chronic) A54.24
  pelvis (acute) (chronic) A54.24
    female pelvic inflammatory disease A54.24
  penis A54.09
  prostate (acute) (chronic) A54.22
  seminal vesicle (acute) (chronic) A54.23
  specified site not listed (see also Gonococcus)
      A54.89
  spermatic cord (acute) (chronic) A54.23
  urethra A54.01
    with abscess (accessory gland)
        (periurethral) A54.1
  vagina A54.02
  vas deferens (acute) (chronic) A54.23
  vulva A54.02
Goodall's disease A08.19
Goodpasture's syndrome M31.0
Gopalan's syndrome (burning feet) E53.0
Gorlin-Chaudry-Moss syndrome Q87.0
Gottron's papules L94.4
Gougerot's syndrome (trisymptomatic) L81.7
Gougerot-Blum syndrome (pigmented
    purpuric lichenoid dermatitis) L81.7
Gougerot-Carteaud disease or syndrome
    (confluent reticulate papillomatosis) L83
Gouley's syndrome (constrictive pericarditis)
    I31.1
Goundou A66.6
Gout, chronic (see also Gout, gouty) M1A.9-
  drug-induced M1A.20
    ankle M1A.27-
    elbow M1A.22-
    foot joint M1A.27-
    hand joint M1A.24-
    hip M1A.25-
    knee M1A.26-
    multiple site M1A.29-
    shoulder M1A.21-
    vertebrae M1A.28
    wrist M1A.23-
  idiopathic M1A.00
    ankle M1A.07-
    elbow M1A.02-
    foot joint M1A.07-
    hand joint M1A.04-
    hip M1A.05-
    knee M1A.06-
    multiple site M1A.09
    shoulder M1A.01-

Gout, chronic (Continued)
  idiopathic (Continued)
    vertebrae M1A.08
    wrist M1A.03-
  in (due to) renal impairment M1A.30
    ankle M1A.37-
    elbow M1A.32-
    foot joint M1A.37-
    hand joint M1A.34-
    hip M1A.35-
    knee M1A.36-
    multiple site M1A.39
    shoulder M1A.31-
    vertebrae M1A.38
    wrist M1A.33-
  lead-induced M1A.10
    ankle M1A.17-
    elbow M1A.12-
    foot joint M1A.17-
    hand joint M1A.14-
    hip M1A.15-
    knee M1A.16-
    multiple site M1A.19
    shoulder M1A.11-
    vertebrae M1A.18
    wrist M1A.13-
  primary —see Gout, chronic, idiopathic
  saturnine —see Gout, chronic, lead-induced
  secondary NEC M1A.40
    ankle M1A.47-
    elbow M1A.42-
    foot joint M1A.47-
    hand joint M1A.44-
    hip M1A.45-
    knee M1A.46-
    multiple site M1A.49
    shoulder M1A.41-
    vertebrae M1A.48
    wrist M1A.43-
  syphilitic (see also subcategory M14.8-) A52.77
  tophi —see Gout by type M1A.9 ◀▥
Gout, gouty (acute) (attack) (flare) (see also
    Gout, chronic) M10.9-
  drug-induced M10.20
    ankle M10.27-
    elbow M10.22-
    foot joint M10.27-
    hand joint M10.24-
    hip M10.25-
    knee M10.26-
    multiple site M10.29
    shoulder M10.21-
    vertebrae M10.28
    wrist M10.23-
  idiopathic M10.00
    ankle M10.07-
    elbow M10.02-
    foot joint M10.07-
    hand joint M10.04-
    hip M10.05-
    knee M10.06-
    multiple site M10.09
    shoulder M10.01-
    vertebrae M10.08
    wrist M10.03-
  in (due to) renal impairment M10.30
    ankle M10.37-
    elbow M10.32-
    foot joint M10.37-
    hand joint M10.34-
    hip M10.35-
    knee M10.36-
    multiple site M10.39
    shoulder M10.31-
    vertebrae M10.38
    wrist M10.33-
  lead-induced M10.10
    ankle M10.17-
    elbow M10.12-
    foot joint M10.17-
    hand joint M10.14-

Gout, gouty (Continued)
  lead-induced (Continued)
    hip M10.15-
    knee M10.16-
    multiple site M10.19
    shoulder M10.11-
    vertebrae M10.18
    wrist M10.13-
  primary —see Gout, idiopathic
  saturnine —see Gout, lead-induced
  secondary NEC M10.40
    ankle M10.47-
    elbow M10.42-
    foot joint M10.47-
    hand joint M10.44-
    hip M10.45-
    knee M10.46-
    multiple site M10.49
    shoulder M10.41-
    vertebrae M10.48
    wrist M10.43-
  syphilitic (see also subcategory M14.8-) A52.77
  tophi NEC —see Gout by type, chronic ◀▥
Gower's
  muscular dystrophy G71.0
  syndrome (vasovagal attack) R55
Gradenigo's syndrome —see Otitis, media,
    suppurative, acute
Graefe's disease —see Strabismus, paralytic,
    ophthalmoplegia, progressive
Graft-versus-host disease D89.813
  acute D89.810
  acute on chronic D89.812
  chronic D89.811
Grain mite (itch) B88.0
Grainhandler's disease or lung J67.8
Grand mal —see Epilepsy, generalized,
    specified NEC
Grand multipara status only (not pregnant)
    Z64.1
  pregnant —see Pregnancy, complicated by,
      grand multiparity
Granite worker's lung J62.8
Granular —see also condition
  inflammation, pharynx J31.2
  kidney (contracting) —see Sclerosis, renal
  liver K74.69
Granulation tissue (abnormal) (excessive)
    L92.9
  postmastoidectomy cavity —see
      Complications, postmastoidectomy,
      granulation
Granulocytopenia (primary) (malignant) —see
    Agranulocytosis
Granuloma L92.9
  abdomen K66.8
    from residual foreign body L92.3
    pyogenicum L98.0
  actinic L57.5
  annulare (perforating) L92.0
  apical K04.5
  aural —see Otitis, externa, specified NEC
  beryllium (skin) L92.3
  bone
    eosinophilic C96.6
    from residual foreign body —see
        Osteomyelitis, specified type NEC
    lung C96.6
  brain (any site) G06.0
    schistosomiasis B65.9 [G07]
  canaliculus lacrimalis —see Granuloma,
      lacrimal
  candidal (cutaneous) B37.2
  cerebral (any site) G06.0
  coccidioidal (primary) (progressive) B38.7
    lung B38.1
    meninges B38.4
  colon K63.89
  conjunctiva H11.22-
  dental K04.5
  ear, middle —see Cholesteatoma

Granuloma *(Continued)*
eosinophilic C96.6
  bone C96.6
  lung C96.6
  oral mucosa K13.4
  skin L92.2
eyelid H01.8
facial (e) L92.2
foreign body (in soft tissue) NEC M60.20
  ankle M60.27-
  foot M60.27-
  forearm M60.23-
  hand M60.24-
  in operation wound —*see* Foreign body,
      accidentally left during a procedure
  lower leg M60.26-
  pelvic region M60.25-
  shoulder region M60.21-
  skin L92.3
  specified site NEC M60.28
  subcutaneous tissue L92.3
  thigh M60.25-
  upper arm M60.22-
gangraenescens M31.2
genito-inguinale A58
giant cell (central) (reparative) (jaw) M27.1
  gingiva (peripheral) K06.8
gland (lymph) I88.8
hepatic NEC K75.3
  in (due to)
    berylliosis J63.2 [K77]
    sarcoidosis D86.89
Hodgkin C81.9
ileum K63.89
infectious B99.9
  specified NEC B99.8
inguinale (Donovan) (venereal) A58
intestine NEC K63.89
intracranial (any site) G06.0
intraspinal (any part) G06.1
iridocyclitis —*see* Iridocyclitis, chronic
jaw (bone) (central) M27.1
  reparative giant cell M27.1
kidney (*see also* Infection, kidney) N15.8
lacrimal H04.81-
larynx J38.7
lethal midline (faciale (e)) M31.2
liver NEC —*see* Granuloma, hepatic
lung (infectious) —*see also* Fibrosis, lung
  coccidioidal B38.1
  eosinophilic C96.6
Majocchi's B35.8
malignant (facial (e)) M31.2
mandible (central) M27.1
midline (lethal) M31.2
monilial (cutaneous) B37.2
nasal sinus —*see* Sinusitis
operation wound T81.89
  foreign body —*see* Foreign body,
      accidentally left during a procedure
  stitch T81.89
  talc —*see* Foreign body, accidentally left
      during a procedure
oral mucosa K13.4
orbit, orbital H05.11-
paracoccidioidal B41.8
penis, venereal A58
periapical K04.5
peritoneum K66.8
  due to ova of helminths NOS (*see also*
      Helminthiasis) B83.9 [K67]
postmastoidectomy cavity —*see*
      Complications, postmastoidectomy,
      recurrent cholesteatoma
prostate N42.89
pudendi (ulcerating) A58
pulp, internal (tooth) K03.3
pyogenic, pyogenicum (of) (skin) L98.0
  gingiva K06.8
  maxillary alveolar ridge K04.5
  oral mucosa K13.4

Granuloma *(Continued)*
rectum K62.89
reticulohistiocytic D76.3
rubrum nasi L74.8
Schistosoma —*see* Schistosomiasis
septic (skin) L98.0
silica (skin) L92.3
sinus (accessory) (infective) (nasal) —*see*
      Sinusitis
skin L92.9
  from residual foreign body L92.3
  pyogenicum L98.0
spine
  syphilitic (epidural) A52.19
  tuberculous A18.01
stitch (postoperative) T81.89
suppurative (skin) L98.0
swimming pool A31.1
talc —*see also* Granuloma, foreign body
  in operation wound —*see* Foreign body,
      accidentally left during a procedure
telangiectaticum (skin) L98.0
tracheostomy J95.09
trichophyticum B35.8
tropicum A66.4
umbilicus L92.9
urethra N36.8
uveitis —*see* Iridocyclitis, chronic
vagina A58
venereum A58
vocal cord J38.3
Granulomatosis L92.9
lymphoid C83.8-
miliary (listerial) A32.89
necrotizing, respiratory M31.30
progressive septic D71
specified NEC L92.8
Wegener's M31.30
  with renal involvement M31.31
Granulomatous tissue (abnormal) (excessive)
      L92.9
Granulosis rubra nasi L74.8
Graphite fibrosis (of lung) J63.3
Graphospasm F48.8
organic G25.89
Grating scapula M89.8X1
Gravel (urinary) —*see* Calculus, urinary
Graves' disease —*see* Hyperthyroidism, with,
      goiter
Gravis —*see* condition
Grawitz tumor C64.-
Gray syndrome (newborn) P93.0
Grayness, hair (premature) L67.1
congenital Q84.2
Green sickness D50.8
Greenfield's disease
meaning
  concentric sclerosis (encephalitis periaxialis
      concentrica) G37.5
  metachromatic leukodystrophy E75.25
Greenstick fracture - code as Fracture,
      by site
Grey syndrome (newborn) P93.0
Grief F43.21
prolonged F43.29
reaction (*see also* Disorder, adjustment)
      F43.20
Griesinger's disease B76.9
Grinder's lung or pneumoconiosis J62.8
Grinding, teeth
psychogenic F45.8
sleep related G47.63
Grip
Dabney's B33.0
devil's B33.0
Grippe, grippal —*see also* Influenza
Balkan A78
summer, of Italy A93.1
Grisel's disease M43.6
Groin —*see* condition
Grooved tongue K14.5

Ground itch B76.9
Grover's disease or syndrome L11.1
Growing pains, children R29.898
Growth (fungoid) (neoplastic) (new) —*see also*
      Neoplasm
adenoid (vegetative) J35.8
benign —*see* Neoplasm, benign, by site
malignant —*see* Neoplasm, malignant, by site
rapid, childhood Z00.2
secondary —*see* Neoplasm, secondary, by site
Gruby's disease B35.0
Gubler-Millard paralysis or syndrome G46.3
Guerin-Stern syndrome Q74.3
Guidance, insufficient anterior (occlusal)
      M26.54
Guillain-Barré disease or syndrome G61.0
sequelae G65.0
Guinea worms (infection) (infestation) B72
Guinon's disease (motor-verbal tic) F95.2
Gull's disease E03.4
Gum —*see* condition
Gumboil K04.7
with sinus K04.6
Gumma (syphilitic) A52.79
artery A52.09
  cerebral A52.04
bone A52.77
  of yaws (late) A66.6
brain A52.19
cauda equina A52.19
central nervous system A52.3
ciliary body A52.71
congenital A50.59
eyelid A52.71
heart A52.06
intracranial A52.19
iris A52.71
kidney A52.75
larynx A52.73
leptomeninges A52.19
liver A52.74
meninges A52.19
myocardium A52.06
nasopharynx A52.73
neurosyphilitic A52.3
nose A52.73
orbit A52.71
palate (soft) A52.79
penis A52.76
pericardium A52.06
pharynx A52.73
pituitary A52.79
scrofulous (tuberculous) A18.4
skin A52.79
specified site NEC A52.79
spinal cord A52.19
tongue A52.79
tonsil A52.73
trachea A52.73
tuberculous A18.4
ulcerative due to yaws A66.4
ureter A52.75
yaws A66.4
  bone A66.6
Gunn's syndrome Q07.8
Gunshot wound —*see also* Wound, open
fracture - code as Fracture, by site
internal organs —*see* Injury, by site
Gynandrism Q56.0
Gynandroblastoma
specified site —*see* Neoplasm, uncertain
      behavior, by site
unspecified site
  female D39.10
  male D40.10
Gynecological examination (periodic) (routine)
      Z01.419
with abnormal findings Z01.411
Gynecomastia N62
Gynephobia F40.291
Gyrate scalp Q82.8

◀ New   ◀▥ Revised   ~~deleted~~ Deleted

H

H (Hartnup's) disease E72.02
Haas' disease or osteochondrosis (juvenile) (head of humerus) —see Osteochondrosis, juvenile, humerus
Habit, habituation
  bad sleep Z72.821
  chorea F95.8
  disturbance, child F98.9
  drug —see Dependence, drug
  irregular sleep Z72.821
  laxative F55.2
  spasm —see Tic
  tic —see Tic
Haemophilus (H.) influenzae, as cause of disease classified elsewhere B96.3
Haff disease —see Poisoning, mercury
Hageman's factor defect, deficiency or disease D68.2
Haglund's disease or osteochondrosis (juvenile) (os tibiale externum) —see Osteochondrosis, juvenile, tarsus
Hailey-Hailey disease Q82.8
Hair —see also condition
  plucking F63.3
    in stereotyped movement disorder F98.4
  tourniquet syndrome —see also Constriction, external, by site
    finger S60.44-
    penis S30.842
    thumb S60.34-
    toe S90.44-
Hairball in stomach T18.2
Hair-pulling, pathological (compulsive) F63.3
Hairy black tongue K14.3
Half vertebra Q76.49
Halitosis R19.6
Hallerman-Streiff syndrome Q87.0
Hallervorden-Spatz disease G23.0
Hallopeau's acrodermatitis or disease L40.2
Hallucination R44.3
  auditory R44.0
  gustatory R44.2
  olfactory R44.2
  specified NEC R44.2
  tactile R44.2
  visual R44.1
Hallucinosis (chronic) F28
  alcoholic (acute) F10.951
    in
      abuse F10.151
      dependence F10.251
  drug-induced F19.951
    cannabis F12.951
    cocaine F14.951
    hallucinogen F16.151
      in
        abuse F19.151
          cannabis F12.151
          cocaine F14.151
          hallucinogen F16.151
          inhalant F18.151
          opioid F11.151
          sedative, anxiolytic or hypnotic F13.151
          stimulant NEC F15.151
        dependence F19.251
          cannabis F12.251
          cocaine F14.251
          hallucinogen F16.251
          inhalant F18.251
          opioid F11.251
          sedative, anxiolytic or hypnotic F13.251
          stimulant NEC F15.251
      inhalant F18.951
      opioid F11.951
      sedative, anxiolytic or hypnotic F13.951
      stimulant NEC F15.951
    organic F06.0

Hallux
  deformity (acquired) NEC M20.5X-
  limitus M20.5X-
  malleus (acquired) NEC M20.3-
  rigidus (acquired) M20.2-
    congenital Q74.2
    sequelae (late effect) of rickets E64.3
  valgus (acquired) M20.1-
    congenital Q66.6
  varus (acquired) M20.3-
    congenital Q66.3
Halo, visual H53.19
Hamartoma, hamartoblastoma Q85.9
  epithelial (gingival), odontogenic, central or peripheral —see Cyst, calcifying odontogenic
Hamartosis Q85.9
Hamman-Rich syndrome J84.114
Hammer toe (acquired) NEC —see also Deformity, toe, hammer toe
  congenital Q66.89
  sequelae (late effect) of rickets E64.3
Hand —see condition
Hand-foot syndrome L27.1
Handicap, handicapped
  educational Z55.9
    specified NEC Z55.8
Hand-Schüller-Christian disease or syndrome C96.5
Hanging (asphyxia) (strangulation) (suffocation) —see Asphyxia, traumatic, due to mechanical threat
Hangnail —see also Cellulitis, digit
  with lymphangitis —see Lymphangitis, acute, digit
Hangover (alcohol) F10.129
Hanhart's syndrome Q87.0
Hanot-Chauffard (-Troisier) syndrome E83.19
Hanot's cirrhosis or disease K74.3
Hansen's disease —see Leprosy
Hantaan virus disease (Korean hemorrhagic fever) A98.5
Hantavirus disease (with renal manifestations) (Dobrava) (Puumala) (Seoul) A98.5
  with pulmonary manifestations (Andes) (Bayou) (Bermejo) (Black Creek Canal) (Choclo) (Juquitiba) (Laguna negra) (Lechiguanas) (New York) (Oran) (Sin nombre) B33.4
Happy puppet syndrome Q93.5
Harada's disease or syndrome H30.81-
Hardening
  artery —see Arteriosclerosis
  brain G93.89
Harelip (complete) (incomplete) —see Cleft, lip
Harlequin (newborn) Q80.4
Harley's disease D59.6
Harmful use (of)
  alcohol F10.10
  anxiolytics —see Abuse, drug, sedative
  cannabinoids —see Abuse, drug, cannabis
  cocaine —see Abuse, drug, cocaine
  drug —see Abuse, drug
  hallucinogens —see Abuse, drug, hallucinogen
  hypnotics —see Abuse, drug, sedative -
    opioids —see Abuse, drug, opioid
  PCP (phencyclidine) —see Abuse, drug, hallucinogen
  sedatives —see Abuse, drug, sedative
  stimulants NEC —see Abuse, drug, stimulant
Harris' lines —see Arrest, epiphyseal
Hartnup's disease E72.02
Harvester's lung J67.0
Harvesting ovum for in vitro fertilization Z31.83
Hashimoto's disease or thyroiditis E06.3
Hashitoxicosis (transient) E06.3
Hassal-Henle bodies or warts (cornea) H18.49
Haut mal —see Epilepsy, generalized, specified NEC

Haverhill fever A25.1
Hay fever (see also Fever, hay) J30.1
Hayem-Widal syndrome D59.8
Haygarth's nodes M15.8
Haymaker's lung J67.0
Hb (abnormal)
  Bart's disease D56.0
  disease —see Disease, hemoglobin
  trait —see Trait
Head —see condition
Headache R51
  allergic NEC G44.89
  associated with sexual activity G44.82
  chronic daily R51
  cluster G44.009
    chronic G44.029
      intractable G44.021
      not intractable G44.029
    episodic G44.019
      intractable G44.011
      not intractable G44.019
    intractable G44.001
    not intractable G44.009
  cough (primary) G44.83
  daily chronic R51
  drug-induced NEC G44.40
    intractable G44.41
    not intractable G44.40
  exertional (primary) G44.84
  histamine G44.009
    intractable G44.001
    not intractable G44.009
  hypnic G44.81
  lumbar puncture G97.1
  medication overuse G44.40
    intractable G44.41
    not intractable G44.40
  menstrual —see Migraine, menstrual
  migraine (type) (see also Migraine) G43.909
  nasal septum R51
  neuralgiform, short lasting unilateral, with conjunctival injection and tearing (SUNCT) G44.059
    intractable G44.051
    not intractable G44.059
  new daily persistent (NDPH) G44.52
  orgasmic G44.82
  periodic syndromes in adults and children G43.C0
    with refractory migraine G43.C1
    intractable G43.C1
    not intractable G43.C0
    without refractory migraine G43.C0
  postspinal puncture G97.1
  post-traumatic G44.309
    acute G44.319
      intractable G44.311
      not intractable G44.319
    chronic G44.329
      intractable G44.321
      not intractable G44.329
    intractable G44.301
    not intractable G44.309
  pre-menstrual —see Migraine, menstrual
  preorgasmic G44.82
  primary
    cough G44.83
    exertional G44.84
    stabbing G44.85
    thunderclap G44.53
  rebound G44.40
    intractable G44.41
    not intractable G44.40
  short lasting unilateral neuralgiform, with conjunctival injection and tearing (SUNCT) G44.059
    intractable G44.051
    not intractable G44.059
  specified syndrome NEC G44.89

Headache (Continued)
  spinal and epidural anesthesia - induced T88.59
    in labor and delivery O74.5
    in pregnancy O29.4-
    postpartum, puerperal O89.4
  spinal fluid loss (from puncture) G97.1
  stabbing (primary) G44.85
  tension (-type) G44.209
    chronic G44.229
      intractable G44.221
      not intractable G44.229
    episodic G44.219
      intractable G44.211
      not intractable G44.219
    intractable G44.201
    not intractable G44.209
  thunderclap (primary) G44.53
  vascular NEC G44.1
Healthy
  infant
    accompanying sick mother Z76.3
    receiving care Z76.2
  person accompanying sick person Z76.3
Hearing examination Z01.10
  with abnormal findings NEC Z01.118
  following failed hearing screening Z01.110
  for hearing conservation and treatment Z01.12
Heart —see condition
Heart beat
  abnormality R00.9
    specified NEC R00.8
  awareness R00.2
  rapid R00.0
  slow R00.1
Heartburn R12
  psychogenic F45.8
Heat (effects) T67.9
  apoplexy T67.0
  burn (see also Burn) L55.9
  collapse T67.1
  cramps T67.2
  dermatitis or eczema L59.0
  edema T67.7
  erythema - code by site under Burn, first degree
  excessive T67.9
    specified effect NEC T67.8
  exhaustion T67.5
    anhydrotic T67.3
    due to
      salt (and water) depletion T67.4
      water depletion T67.3
        with salt depletion T67.4
  fatigue (transient) T67.6
  fever T67.0
  hyperpyrexia T67.0
  prickly L74.0
  prostration —see Heat, exhaustion
  pyrexia T67.0
  rash L74.0
  specified effect NEC T67.8
  stroke T67.0
  sunburn —see Sunburn
  syncope T67.1
Heavy-for-dates NEC (infant) (4000g to 4499g) P08.1
  exceptionally (4500g or more) P08.0
Hebephrenia, hebephrenic (schizophrenia) F20.1
Heberden's disease or nodes (with arthropathy) M15.1
Hebra's
  pityriasis L26
  prurigo L28.2
Heel —see condition
Heerfordt's disease D86.89
Hegglin's anomaly or syndrome D72.0
Heilmeyer-Schoner disease D45
Heine-Medin disease A80.9

Heinz body anemia, congenital D58.2
Heliophobia F40.228
Heller's disease or syndrome F84.3
HELLP syndrome (hemolysis, elevated liver enzymes and low platelet count) O14.2-
Helminthiasis —see also Infestation, helminth
  Ancylostoma B76.0
  intestinal B82.0
    mixed types (types classifiable to more than one of the titles B65.0-B81.3 and B81.8) B81.4
    specified type NEC B81.8
  mixed types (intestinal) (types classifiable to more than one of the titles B65.0-B81.3 and B81.8) B81.4
  Necator (americanus) B76.1
  specified type NEC B83.8
Heloma L84
Hemangioblastoma —see Neoplasm, connective tissue, uncertain behavior
  malignant —see Neoplasm, connective tissue, malignant
Hemangioendothelioma —see also Neoplasm, uncertain behavior, by site
  benign D18.00
    intra-abdominal D18.03
    intracranial D18.02
    skin D18.01
    specified site NEC D18.09
  bone (diffuse) —see Neoplasm, bone, malignant
  epithelioid —see also Neoplasm, uncertain behavior, by site
    malignant —see Neoplasm, malignant, by site
  malignant —see Neoplasm, connective tissue, malignant
Hemangiofibroma —see Neoplasm, benign, by site
Hemangiolipoma —see Lipoma
Hemangioma D18.00
  arteriovenous D18.00
    intra-abdominal D18.03
    intracranial D18.02
    skin D18.01
    specified site NEC D18.09
  capillary D18.00
    intra-abdominal D18.03
    intracranial D18.02
    skin D18.01
    specified site NEC D18.09
  cavernous D18.00
    intra-abdominal D18.03
    intracranial D18.02
    skin D18.01
    specified site NEC D18.09
  epithelioid D18.00
    intra-abdominal D18.03
    intracranial D18.02
    skin D18.01
    specified site NEC D18.09
  histiocytoid D18.00
    intra-abdominal D18.03
    intracranial D18.02
    skin D18.01
    specified site NEC D18.09
  infantile D18.00
    intra-abdominal D18.03
    intracranial D18.02
    skin D18.01
    specified site NEC D18.09
  intra-abdominal D18.03
  intracranial D18.02
  intramuscular D18.00
    intra-abdominal D18.03
    intracranial D18.02
    skin D18.01
    specified site NEC D18.09
  juvenile D18.00
  malignant —see Neoplasm, connective tissue, malignant

Hemangioma (Continued)
  plexiform D18.00
    intra-abdominal D18.03
    intracranial D18.02
    skin D18.01
    specified site NEC D18.09
  racemose D18.00
    intra-abdominal D18.03
    intracranial D18.02
    skin D18.01
    specified site NEC D18.09
  sclerosing —see Neoplasm, skin, benign
  simplex D18.00
    intra-abdominal D18.03
    intracranial D18.02
    skin D18.01
    specified site NEC D18.09
  skin D18.01
  specified site NEC D18.09
  venous D18.00
    intra-abdominal D18.03
    intracranial D18.02
    skin D18.01
    specified site NEC D18.09
  verrucous keratotic D18.00
    intra-abdominal D18.03
    intracranial D18.02
    skin D18.01
    specified site NEC D18.09
Hemangiomatosis (systemic) I78.8
  involving single site —see Hemangioma
Hemangiopericytoma —see also Neoplasm, connective tissue, uncertain behavior
  benign —see Neoplasm, connective tissue, benign
  malignant —see Neoplasm, connective tissue, malignant
Hemangiosarcoma —see Neoplasm, connective tissue, malignant
Hemarthrosis (nontraumatic) M25.00
  ankle M25.07-
  elbow M25.02-
  foot joint M25.07-
  hand joint M25.04-
  hip M25.05-
  in hemophilic arthropathy —see Arthropathy, hemophilic
  knee M25.06-
  shoulder M25.01-
  specified joint NEC M25.08
  traumatic —see Sprain, by site
  vertebrae M25.08 ◀
  wrist M25.03-
Hematemesis K92.0
  with ulcer - code by site under Ulcer, with hemorrhage K27.4
  newborn, neonatal P54.0
    due to swallowed maternal blood P78.2
Hematidrosis L74.8
Hematinuria —see also Hemoglobinuria
  malarial B50.8
Hematobilia K83.8
Hematocele
  female NEC N94.89
    with ectopic pregnancy O00.9
    ovary N83.8
  male N50.1
Hematochezia (see also Melena) K92.1
Hematochyluria —see also Infestation, filarial schistosomiasis (bilharziasis) B65.0
Hematocolpos (with hematometra or hematosalpinx) N89.7
Hematocornea —see Pigmentation, cornea, stromal
Hematogenous —see condition
Hematoma (traumatic) (skin surface intact) — see also Contusion
  with
    injury of internal organs —see Injury, by site
    open wound —see Wound, open
  amputation stump (surgical) (late) T87.89

◀ New   ◀|||| Revised   ~~deleted~~ Deleted

Hematoma *(Continued)*
  aorta, dissecting I71.00
    abdominal I71.02
    thoracic I71.01
    thoracoabdominal I71.03
  aortic intramural —*see* Dissection, aorta
  arterial (complicating trauma) —*see* Injury,
      blood vessel, by site
  auricle —*see* Contusion, ear
    nontraumatic —*see* Disorder, pinna,
      hematoma
  birth injury NEC P15.8
  brain (traumatic)
    with
      cerebral laceration or contusion
          (diffuse) —*see* Injury, intracranial,
          diffuse
        focal —*see* Injury, intracranial, focal
    cerebellar, traumatic S06.37-
    intracerebral, traumatic —*see* Injury,
        intracranial, intracerebral hemorrhage
    newborn NEC P52.4
      birth injury P10.1
    nontraumatic —*see* Hemorrhage,
        intracranial
    subarachnoid, arachnoid, traumatic —*see*
        Injury, intracranial, subarachnoid
        hemorrhage
    subdural, traumatic —*see* Injury,
        intracranial, subdural hemorrhage
  breast (nontraumatic) N64.89
  broad ligament (nontraumatic) N83.7
    traumatic S37.892
  cerebellar, traumatic S06.37-
  cerebral —*see* Hematoma, brain
  cerebrum S06.36-
    left S06.35-
    right S06.34-
  cesarean delivery wound O90.2
  complicating delivery (perineal) (pelvic)
      (vagina) (vulva) O71.7
  corpus cavernosum (nontraumatic) N48.89
  epididymis (nontraumatic) N50.1
  epidural (traumatic) —*see* Injury, intracranial,
      epidural hemorrhage
    spinal —*see* Injury, spinal cord, by region
  episiotomy O90.2
  face, birth injury P15.4
  genital organ NEC (nontraumatic)
    female (nonobstetric) N94.89
      traumatic S30.202
    male N50.1
      traumatic S30.201
  internal organs —*see* Injury, by site
  intracerebral, traumatic —*see* Injury,
      intracranial, intracerebral hemorrhage
  intraoperative —*see* Complications,
      intraoperative, hemorrhage
  labia (nontraumatic) (nonobstetric) N90.8
  liver (subcapsular) (nontraumatic) K76.89
    birth injury P15.0
  mediastinum —*see* Injury, intrathoracic
  mesosalpinx (nontraumatic) N83.7
    traumatic S37.898 ◄▥
      bilateral S37.522
      unilateral S37.521
  muscle - code by site under Contusion
  nontraumatic
    muscle M79.81
    soft tissue M79.81
  obstetrical surgical wound O90.2
  orbit, orbital (nontraumatic) —*see also*
      Hemorrhage, orbit
    traumatic —*see* Contusion, orbit
  pelvis (female) (nontraumatic) (nonobstetric)
      N94.89
    obstetric O71.7
    traumatic —*see* Injury, by site
  penis (nontraumatic) N48.89
    birth injury P15.5
  perianal (nontraumatic) K64.5

Hematoma *(Continued)*
  perineal S30.23
    complicating delivery O71.7
  perirenal —*see* Injury, kidney
  pinna —*see* Contusion, ear
    nontraumatic —*see* Disorder, pinna,
      hematoma
  placenta O43.89-
  postoperative (postprocedural) —*see*
      Complication, postprocedural,
      hemorrhage
  retroperitoneal (nontraumatic) K66.1
    traumatic S36.892
  scrotum, superficial S30.22
    birth injury P15.5
  seminal vesicle (nontraumatic) N50.1
    traumatic S37.892
  spermatic cord (traumatic) S37.892
    nontraumatic N50.1
  spinal (cord) (meninges) —*see also* Injury,
      spinal cord, by region
    newborn (birth injury) P11.5
  spleen D73.5
    intraoperative —*see* Complications,
        intraoperative, hemorrhage, spleen
    postprocedural (postoperative) —*see*
        Complications, postprocedural,
        hemorrhage, spleen
  sternocleidomastoid, birth injury P15.2
  sternomastoid, birth injury P15.2
  subarachnoid (traumatic) —*see* Injury,
      intracranial, subarachnoid hemorrhage
    newborn (nontraumatic) P52.5
      due to birth injury P10.3
    nontraumatic —*see* Hemorrhage,
        intracranial, subarachnoid
  subdural (traumatic) —*see* Injury, intracranial,
      subdural hemorrhage
    newborn (localized) P52.8
      birth injury P10.0
    nontraumatic —*see* Hemorrhage,
        intracranial, subdural
  superficial, newborn P54.5
  testis (nontraumatic) N50.1
    birth injury P15.5
  tunica vaginalis (nontraumatic) N50.1
  umbilical cord, complicating delivery
      O69.5
  uterine ligament (broad) (nontraumatic)
      N83.7
    traumatic S37.892 ◄▥
  vagina (ruptured) (nontraumatic) N89.8
    complicating delivery O71.7
  vas deferens (nontraumatic) N50.1
    traumatic S37.892
  vitreous —*see* Hemorrhage, vitreous
  vulva (nontraumatic) (nonobstetric)
      N90.89
    complicating delivery O71.7
    newborn (birth injury) P15.5
Hematometra N85.7
  with hematocolpos N89.7
Hematomyelia (central) G95.19
  newborn (birth injury) P11.5
  traumatic T14.8
Hematomyelitis G04.90
Hematoperitoneum —*see* Hemoperitoneum
Hematophobia F40.230
Hematopneumothorax *(see* Hemothorax)
Hematopoiesis, cyclic D70.4
Hematoporphyria —*see* Porphyria
Hematorachis, hematorrhachis G95.19
  newborn (birth injury) P11.5
Hematosalpinx N83.6
  with
    hematocolpos N89.7
    hematometra N85.7
      with hematocolpos N89.7
    infectional —*see* Salpingitis
Hematospermia R36.1
Hematothorax *(see* Hemothorax)

Hematuria R31.9
  benign (familial) (of childhood) —*see also*
      Hematuria, idiopathic
    essential microscopic R31.1
  due to sulphonamide, sulfonamide —*see* Table
      of Drugs and Chemicals, by drug ◄▥
  endemic *(see also* Schistosomiasis) B65.0
  gross R31.0
  idiopathic N02.9
    with glomerular lesion
      crescentic (diffuse) glomerulonephritis
          N02.7
        dense deposit disease N02.6
        endocapillary proliferative
            glomerulonephritis N02.4
        focal and segmental hyalinosis or
            sclerosis N02.1
        membranoproliferative (diffuse) N02.5
        membranous (diffuse) N02.2
        mesangial proliferative (diffuse) N02.3
        mesangiocapillary (diffuse) N02.5
        minor abnormality N02.0
        proliferative NEC N02.8
        specified pathology NEC N02.8
  intermittent —*see* Hematuria, idiopathic
  malarial B50.8
  microscopic NEC R31.2
    benign essential R31.1
  paroxysmal —*see also* Hematuria, idiopathic
    nocturnal D59.5
  persistent —*see* Hematuria, idiopathic
  recurrent —*see* Hematuria, idiopathic
  tropical *(see also* Schistosomiasis) B65.0
  tuberculous A18.13
Hemeralopia (day blindness) H53.11
  vitamin A deficiency E50.5
Hemi-akinesia R41.4
Hemianalgesia R20.0
Hemianencephaly Q00.0
Hemianesthesia R20.0
Hemianopia, hemianopsia (heteronymous)
    H53.47
  homonymous H53.46-
  syphilitic A52.71
Hemiathetosis R25.8
Hemiatrophy R68.89
  cerebellar G31.9
  face, facial, progressive (Romberg) G51.8
  tongue K14.8
Hemiballism (us) G25.5
Hemicardia Q24.8
Hemicephalus, hemicephaly Q00.0
Hemichorea G25.5
Hemicolitis, left —*see* Colitis, left sided
Hemicrania
  congenital malformation Q00.0
  continua G44.51
  meaning migraine *(see also* Migraine) G43.909
  paroxysmal G44.039
    chronic G44.049
      intractable G44.041
      not intractable G44.049
    episodic G44.039
      intractable G44.031
      not intractable G44.039
    intractable G44.031
    not intractable G44.039
Hemidystrophy —*see* Hemiatrophy
Hemiectromelia Q73.8
Hemihypalgesia R20.8
Hemihypesthesia R20.1
Hemi-inattention R41.4
Hemimelia Q73.8
  lower limb —*see* Defect, reduction, lower
      limb, specified type NEC
  upper limb —*see* Defect, reduction, upper
      limb, specified type NEC
Hemiparalysis —*see* Hemiplegia
Hemiparesis —*see* Hemiplegia
Hemiparesthesia R20.2
Hemiparkinsonism G20

Hemiplegia G81.9-
- alternans facialis G83.89
- ascending NEC G81.90
  - spinal G95.89
- congenital (cerebral) G80.8
  - spastic G80.2
- embolic (current episode) I63.4-
- flaccid G81.0-
- following
  - cerebrovascular disease I69.959
    - cerebral infarction I69.35-
    - intracerebral hemorrhage I69.15-
    - nontraumatic intracranial hemorrhage NEC I69.25-
    - specified disease NEC I69.85-
    - stroke NOS I69.35-
    - subarachnoid hemorrhage I69.05-
- hysterical F44.4
- newborn NEC P91.8
  - birth injury P11.9
- spastic G81.1-
  - congenital G80.2
- thrombotic (current episode) I63.3

Hemisection, spinal cord —see Injury, spinal cord, by region

Hemispasm (facial) R25.2

Hemisporosis B48.8

Hemitremor R25.1

Hemivertebra Q76.49
- failure of segmentation with scoliosis Q76.3
- fusion with scoliosis Q76.3

Hemochromatosis E83.119
- with refractory anemia D46.1
- due to repeated red blood cell transfusion E83.111
- hereditary (primary) E83.110
- primary E83.110
- specified NEC E83.118

Hemoglobin —see also condition
- abnormal (disease) —see Disease, hemoglobin
- AS genotype D57.3
- Constant Spring D58.2
- E-beta thalassemia D56.5
- fetal, hereditary persistence (HPFH) D56.4
- H Constant Spring D56.0
- low NOS D64.9
- S (Hb S), heterozygous D57.3

Hemoglobinemia D59.9
- due to blood transfusion T80.89
- paroxysmal D59.6
  - nocturnal D59.5

Hemoglobinopathy (mixed) D58.2
- with thalassemia D56.8
- sickle-cell D57.1
  - with thalassemia D57.40
    - with crisis (vasoocclusive pain) D57.419
      - with
        - acute chest syndrome D57.411
        - splenic sequestration D57.412
      - without crisis D57.40

Hemoglobinuria R82.3
- with anemia, hemolytic, acquired (chronic) NEC D59.6
- cold (agglutinin) (paroxysmal) (with Raynaud's syndrome) D59.6
- due to exertion or hemolysis NEC D59.6
- intermittent D59.6
- malarial B50.8
- march D59.6
- nocturnal (paroxysmal) D59.5
- paroxysmal (cold) D59.6
  - nocturnal D59.5

Hemolymphangioma D18.1

Hemolysis
- intravascular
  - with
    - abortion —see Abortion, by type, complicated by, hemorrhage
    - ectopic or molar pregnancy O08.1

Hemolysis (Continued)
- intravascular (Continued)
  - with (Continued)
    - hemorrhage
      - antepartum —see Hemorrhage, antepartum, with coagulation defect
      - intrapartum (see also Hemorrhage, complicating, delivery) O67.0
    - postpartum O72.3
- neonatal (excessive) P58.9
  - specified NEC P58.8

Hemolytic —see condition

Hemopericardium I31.2
- following acute myocardial infarction (current complication) I23.0
- newborn P54.8
- traumatic —see Injury, heart, with hemopericardium

Hemoperitoneum K66.1
- infectional K65.9
- traumatic S36.899
  - with open wound —see Wound, open, with penetration into peritoneal cavity

Hemophilia (classical) (familial) (hereditary) D66
- A D66
- B D67
- C D68.1
- acquired D68.311
- autoimmune D68.311
- calcipriva (see also Defect, coagulation) D68.4
- nonfamilial (see also Defect, coagulation) D68.4
- secondary D68.311
- vascular D68.0

Hemophthalmos H44.81-

Hemopneumothorax —see also Hemothorax
- traumatic S27.2

Hemoptysis R04.2
- newborn P26.9
- tuberculous —see Tuberculosis, pulmonary

Hemorrhage, hemorrhagic (concealed) R58
- abdomen R58
- accidental antepartum —see Hemorrhage, antepartum
- acute idiopathic pulmonary, in infants R04.81
- adenoid J35.8
- adrenal (capsule) (gland) E27.49
  - medulla E27.8
  - newborn P54.4
- after delivery —see Hemorrhage, postpartum
- alveolar
  - lung, newborn P26.8
  - process K08.8
- alveolus K08.8
- amputation stump (surgical) T87.89
- anemia (chronic) D50.0
  - acute D62
- antepartum (with) O46.90
  - with coagulation defect O46.00-
    - afibrinogenemia O46.01-
    - disseminated intravascular coagulation O46.02-
    - hypofibrinogenemia O46.01-
    - specified defect NEC O46.09-
  - before 20 weeks gestation O20.9
    - specified type NEC O20.8
    - threatened abortion O20.0
  - due to
    - abruptio placenta (see also Abruptio placentae) O45.9-
    - leiomyoma, uterus —see Hemorrhage, antepartum, specified cause NEC
    - placenta previa O44.1-
  - specified cause NEC —see subcategory O46.8X-
- anus (sphincter) K62.5
- apoplexy (stroke) —see Hemorrhage, intracranial, intracerebral

Hemorrhage, hemorrhagic (Continued)
- arachnoid —see Hemorrhage, intracranial, subarachnoid
- artery R58
  - brain —see Hemorrhage, intracranial, intracerebral
  - basilar (ganglion) I61.0
- bladder N32.89
- bowel K92.2
  - newborn P54.3
- brain (miliary) (nontraumatic) —see Hemorrhage, intracranial, intracerebral
  - due to
    - birth injury P10.1
    - syphilis A52.05
  - epidural or extradural (traumatic) — see Injury, intracranial, epidural hemorrhage
  - newborn P52.4
    - birth injury P10.1
  - subarachnoid —see Hemorrhage, intracranial, subarachnoid
  - subdural —see Hemorrhage, intracranial, subdural
- brainstem (nontraumatic) I61.3
  - traumatic S06.38-
- breast N64.59
- bronchial tube —see Hemorrhage, lung
- bronchopulmonary —see Hemorrhage, lung
- bronchus —see Hemorrhage, lung
- bulbar I61.5
- capillary I78.8
  - primary D69.8
- cecum K92.2
- cerebellar, cerebellum (nontraumatic) I61.4
  - newborn P52.6
  - traumatic S06.37-
- cerebral, cerebrum —see also Hemorrhage, intracranial, intracerebral
  - lobe I61.1
  - newborn (anoxic) P52.4
    - birth injury P10.1
- cerebromeningeal I61.8
- cerebrospinal —see Hemorrhage, intracranial, intracerebral
- cervix (uteri) (stump) NEC N88.8
- chamber, anterior (eye) —see Hyphema
- childbirth —see Hemorrhage, complicating, delivery
- choroid H31.30-
  - expulsive H31.31-
- ciliary body —see Hyphema
- cochlea —see subcategory H83.8
- colon K92.2
- complicating
  - abortion —see Abortion, by type, complicated by, hemorrhage
  - delivery O67.9
    - associated with coagulation defect (afibrinogenemia) (DIC) (hyperfibrinolysis) O67.0
    - specified cause NEC O67.8
  - surgical procedure —see Hemorrhage, intraoperative
- conjunctiva H11.3-
  - newborn P54.8
- cord, newborn (stump) P51.9
- corpus luteum (ruptured) cyst N83.1
- cortical (brain) I61.1
- cranial —see Hemorrhage, intracranial
- cutaneous R23.3
  - due to autosensitivity, erythrocyte D69.2
  - newborn P54.5
- delayed
  - following ectopic or molar pregnancy O08.1
  - postpartum O72.2
- diathesis (familial) D69.9
- disease D69.9
  - newborn P53
  - specified type NEC D69.8

Hemorrhage, hemorrhagic *(Continued)*
  due to or associated with
    afibrinogenemia or other coagulation
      defect (conditions in categories
      D65-D69) ◄▥
      antepartum —*see* Hemorrhage,
        antepartum, with coagulation
        defect
      intrapartum O67.0
    dental implant M27.61
    device, implant or graft *(see also*
      Complications, by site and type,
      specified NEC) T85.83
      arterial graft NEC T82.838
      breast T85.83
      catheter NEC T85.83
        dialysis (renal) T82.838
          intraperitoneal T85.83
        infusion NEC T82.838
          spinal (epidural) (subdural) T85.83
        urinary (indwelling) T83.83
      electronic (electrode) (pulse generator)
        (stimulator)
        bone T84.83
        cardiac T82.837
        nervous system (brain) (peripheral
          nerve) (spinal) T85.83
        urinary T83.83
      fixation, internal (orthopedic) NEC T84.83
      gastrointestinal (bile duct) (esophagus)
        T85.83
      genital NEC T83.83
      heart NEC T82.837
      joint prosthesis T84.83
      ocular (corneal graft) (orbital implant)
        NEC T85.83
      orthopedic NEC T84.83
        bone graft T86.838
      specified NEC T85.83
      urinary NEC T83.83
      vascular NEC T82.838
      ventricular intracranial shunt T85.83
  duodenum, duodenal K92.2
    ulcer —*see* Ulcer, duodenum, with
      hemorrhage
  dura mater —*see* Hemorrhage, intracranial,
    subdural
  endotracheal —*see* Hemorrhage, lung
  epicranial subaponeurotic (massive), birth
    injury P12.2
  epidural (traumatic) —*see also* Injury,
    intracranial, epidural hemorrhage
    nontraumatic I62.1
  esophagus K22.8
    varix I85.01
      secondary I85.11
  excessive, following ectopic gestation
    (subsequent episode) O08.1
  extradural (traumatic) —*see* Injury,
    intracranial, epidural hemorrhage
    birth injury P10.8
    newborn (anoxic) (nontraumatic) P52.8
    nontraumatic I62.1
  eye NEC H57.8
    fundus —*see* Hemorrhage, retina
    lid —*see* Disorder, eyelid, specified type
      NEC
  fallopian tube N83.6
  fibrinogenolysis —*see* Fibrinolysis
  fibrinolytic (acquired) —*see* Fibrinolysis
  from
    ear (nontraumatic) —*see* Otorrhagia
    tracheostomy stoma J95.01
  fundus, eye —*see* Hemorrhage, retina
  funis —*see* Hemorrhage, umbilicus, cord
  gastric —*see* Hemorrhage, stomach
  gastroenteric K92.2
    newborn P54.3
  gastrointestinal (tract) K92.2
    newborn P54.3
  genital organ, male N50.1

Hemorrhage, hemorrhagic *(Continued)*
  genitourinary (tract) NOS R31.9
  gingiva K06.8
  globe (eye) —*see* Hemophthalmos
  graafian follicle cyst (ruptured) N83.0
  gum K06.8
  heart I51.89
  hypopharyngeal (throat) R04.1
  intermenstrual (regular) N92.3
    irregular N92.1
  internal (organs) NEC R58
    capsule I61.0
    ear —*see* subcategory H83.8
    newborn P54.8
  intestine K92.2
    newborn P54.3
  intra-abdominal R58
  intra-alveolar (lung), newborn P26.8
  intracerebral (nontraumatic) —*see*
    Hemorrhage, intracranial,
    intracerebral
  intracranial (nontraumatic) I62.9
    birth injury P10.9
    epidural, nontraumatic I62.1
    extradural, nontraumatic I62.1
    intracerebral (nontraumatic) (in) I61.9
      brain stem I61.3
      cerebellum I61.4
      hemisphere I61.2
        cortical (superficial) I61.1
        subcortical (deep) I61.0
      intraoperative
        during a nervous system procedure
          G97.31
        during other procedure G97.32
      intraventricular I61.5
      multiple localized I61.6
      newborn P52.4
        birth injury P10.1
      postprocedural
        ~~during a nervous system procedure~~
          ~~G97.51~~
        ~~during other procedure G97.52~~
        following a nervous system procedure
          G97.51 ◄
        following other procedure G97.52 ◄
      specified NEC I61.8
      superficial I61.1
      traumatic (diffuse) —*see* Injury,
        intracranial, diffuse
        focal —*see* Injury, intracranial, focal
    newborn P52.9
      specified NEC P52.8
    subarachnoid (nontraumatic) (from) I60.9
      intracranial (cerebral) artery I60.7
        anterior communicating I60.2-
        basilar I60.4
        carotid siphon and bifurcation I60.0-
        communicating I60.7
          anterior I60.2-
          posterior I60.3-
        middle cerebral I60.1-
        posterior communicating I60.3-
        specified artery NEC I60.6
        vertebral I60.5-
      newborn P52.5
        birth injury P10.3
      specified NEC I60.8
      traumatic S06.6X-
    subdural (nontraumatic) I62.00
      acute I62.01
      birth injury P10.0
      chronic I62.03
      newborn (anoxic) (hypoxic) P52.8
        birth injury P10.0
      spinal G95.19
      subacute I62.02
      traumatic —*see* Injury, intracranial,
        subdural hemorrhage
    traumatic —*see* Injury, intracranial, focal
      brain injury

Hemorrhage, hemorrhagic *(Continued)*
  intramedullary NEC G95.19
  intraocular —*see* Hemophthalmos
  intraoperative, intraprocedural —*see*
    Complication, hemorrhage (hematoma),
    intraoperative (intraprocedural), by site
  intrapartum —*see* Hemorrhage, complicating,
    delivery
  intrapelvic
    female N94.89
    male K66.1
  intraperitoneal K66.1
  intrapontine I61.3
  intraprocedural —*see* Complication,
    hemorrhage (hematoma), intraoperative
    (intraprocedural), by site
  intrauterine N85.7
    complicating delivery *(see also* Hemorrhage,
      complicating, delivery) O67.9
    postpartum —*see* Hemorrhage, postpartum
  intraventricular I61.5
    newborn (nontraumatic) *(see also* Newborn,
      affected by, hemorrhage) P52.3
      due to birth injury P10.2
      grade
        1 P52.0
        2 P52.1
        3 P52.21
        4 P52.22
  intravesical N32.89
  iris (postinfectional) (postinflammatory)
    (toxic) —*see* Hyphema
  joint (nontraumatic) —*see* Hemarthrosis
  kidney N28.89
  knee (joint) (nontraumatic) —*see*
    Hemarthrosis, knee
  labyrinth —*see* subcategory H83.8
  lenticular striate artery I61.0
  ligature, vessel —*see* Hemorrhage,
    postoperative
  liver K76.89
  lung R04.89
    newborn P26.9
      massive P26.1
      specified NEC P26.8
    tuberculous —*see* Tuberculosis, pulmonary
  massive umbilical, newborn P51.0
  mediastinum —*see* Hemorrhage, lung
  medulla I61.3
  membrane (brain) I60.8
    spinal cord —*see* Hemorrhage, spinal cord
  meninges, meningeal (brain) (middle) I60.8
    spinal cord —*see* Hemorrhage, spinal cord
  mesentery K66.1
  metritis —*see* Endometritis
  mouth K13.79
  mucous membrane NEC R58
    newborn P54.8
  muscle M62.89
  nail (subungual) L60.8
  nasal turbinate R04.0
    newborn P54.8
  navel, newborn P51.9
  newborn P54.9
    specified NEC P54.8
  nipple N64.59
  nose R04.0
    newborn P54.8
  omentum K66.1
  optic nerve (sheath) H47.02-
  orbit, orbital H05.23-
  ovary NEC N83.8
  oviduct N83.6
  pancreas K86.8
  parathyroid (gland) (spontaneous) E21.4
  parturition —*see* Hemorrhage, complicating,
    delivery
  penis N48.89
  pericardium, pericarditis I31.2
  peritoneum, peritoneal K66.1
  peritonsillar tissue J35.8
    due to infection J36

Hemorrhage, hemorrhagic *(Continued)*
 petechial R23.3
  due to autosensitivity, erythrocyte D69.2
 pituitary (gland) E23.6
 pleura —*see* Hemorrhage, lung
 polioencephalitis, superior E51.2
 polymyositis —*see* Polymyositis
 pons, pontine I61.3
 posterior fossa (nontraumatic) I61.8
  newborn P52.6
 postmenopausal N95.0
 postnasal R04.0
 postoperative —*see* Complications,
   postprocedural, hemorrhage, by site
 postpartum NEC (following delivery of
   placenta) O72.1
  delayed or secondary O72.2
  retained placenta O72.0
  third stage O72.0
 pregnancy —*see* Hemorrhage, antepartum
 preretinal —*see* Hemorrhage, retina
 prostate N42.1
 puerperal —*see* Hemorrhage, postpartum
  delayed or secondary O72.2
 pulmonary R04.89
  newborn P26.9
   massive P26.1
   specified NEC P26.8
  tuberculous —*see* Tuberculosis, pulmonary
 purpura (primary) D69.3
 rectum (sphincter) K62.5
  newborn P54.2
 recurring, following initial hemorrhage at
   time of injury T79.2
 renal N28.89
 respiratory passage or tract R04.9
  specified NEC R04.89
 retina, retinal (vessels) H35.6-
  diabetic —*see* Diabetes, retinal, hemorrhage
 retroperitoneal R58
 scalp R58
 scrotum N50.1
 secondary (nontraumatic) R58
  following initial hemorrhage at time of
   injury T79.2
 seminal vesicle N50.1
 skin R23.3
  newborn P54.5
 slipped umbilical ligature P51.8
 spermatic cord N50.1
 spinal (cord) G95.19
  newborn (birth injury) P11.5
 spleen D73.5
  intraoperative —*see* Complications,
   intraoperative, hemorrhage, spleen
  postprocedural —*see* Complications,
   postprocedural, hemorrhage, spleen
 stomach K92.2
  newborn P54.3
  ulcer —*see* Ulcer, stomach, with
   hemorrhage
 subarachnoid (nontraumatic) —*see*
   Hemorrhage, intracranial, subarachnoid
 subconjunctival —*see also* Hemorrhage,
   conjunctiva
  birth injury P15.3
 subcortical (brain) I61.0
 subcutaneous R23.3
 subdiaphragmatic R58
 subdural (acute) (nontraumatic) —*see*
   Hemorrhage, intracranial, subdural
 subependymal
  newborn P52.0
   with intraventricular extension P52.1
    and intracerebral extension P52.22
 subgaleal P12.1 ◀
 subhyaloid —*see* Hemorrhage, retina
 subperiosteal —*see* Disorder, bone, specified
   type NEC
 subretinal —*see* Hemorrhage, retina
 subtentorial —*see* Hemorrhage, intracranial,
   subdural

Hemorrhage, hemorrhagic *(Continued)*
 subungual L60.8
 suprarenal (capsule) (gland) E27.49
  newborn P54.4
 tentorium (traumatic) NEC —*see*
   Hemorrhage, brain
  newborn (birth injury) P10.4
 testis N50.1
 third stage (postpartum) O72.0
 thorax —*see* Hemorrhage, lung
 throat R04.1
 thymus (gland) E32.8
 thyroid (cyst) (gland) E07.89
 tongue K14.8
 tonsil J35.8
 trachea —*see* Hemorrhage, lung
 tracheobronchial R04.89
  newborn P26.0
 traumatic — code to specific injury
  cerebellar —*see* Hemorrhage, brain
  intracranial —*see* Hemorrhage, brain
  recurring or secondary (following initial
    hemorrhage at time of injury)
    T79.2
 tuberculous NEC (*see also* Tuberculosis,
   pulmonary) A15.0
 tunica vaginalis N50.1
 ulcer - code by site under Ulcer, with
   hemorrhage K27.4
 umbilicus, umbilical
  cord
   after birth, newborn P51.9
   complicating delivery O69.5
  newborn P51.9
   massive P51.0
   slipped ligature P51.8
  stump P51.9
 urethra (idiopathic) N36.8
 uterus, uterine (abnormal) N93.9
  climacteric N92.4
  complicating delivery —*see* Hemorrhage,
   complicating, delivery
  dysfunctional or functional N93.8
  intermenstrual (regular) N92.3
   irregular N92.1
  postmenopausal N95.0
  postpartum —*see* Hemorrhage,
   postpartum
  preclimacteric or premenopausal N92.4
  prepubertal N93.8
  pubertal N92.2
 vagina (abnormal) N93.9
  newborn P54.6
 vas deferens N50.1
 vasa previa O69.4
 ventricular I61.5
 vesical N32.89
 viscera NEC R58
  newborn P54.8
 vitreous (humor) (intraocular) H43.1-
 vulva N90.89
Hemorrhoids (bleeding) (without mention of
   degree) K64.9
 1st degree (grade/stage I) (without prolapse
    outside of anal canal) K64.0
 2nd degree (grade/stage II) (that
    prolapse with straining but retract
    spontaneously) K64.1
 3rd degree (grade/stage III) (that prolapse
    with straining and require manual
    replacement back inside anal canal)
    K64.2
 4th degree (grade/stage IV) (with prolapsed
    tissue that cannot be manually replaced)
    K64.3
 complicating
  pregnancy O22.4
  puerperium O87.2
 external K64.4
  with
   thrombosis K64.5

Hemorrhage, hemorrhagic *(Continued)*
 internal (without mention of degree) K64.8
 prolapsed K64.8
 skin tags
  anus K64.4
  residual K64.4
 specified NEC K64.8
 strangulated (*see also* Hemorrhoids, by
   degree) K64.8
 thrombosed (*see also* Hemorrhoids, by degree)
   K64.5
 ulcerated (*see also* Hemorrhoids, by degree)
   K64.8
Hemosalpinx N83.6
 with
  hematocolpos N89.7
  hematometra N85.7
   with hematocolpos N89.7
Hemosiderosis (dietary) E83.19
 pulmonary, idiopathic E83.1 *[J84.03]*
 transfusion T80.89
Hemothorax (bacterial) (nontuberculous)
   J94.2
 newborn P54.8
 traumatic S27.1
  with pneumothorax S27.2
 tuberculous NEC A15.6
Henoch (-Schönlein) disease or syndrome
   (purpura) D69.0
Henpue, henpuye A66.6
Hepar lobatum (syphilitic) A52.74
Hepatalgia K76.89
Hepatitis K75.9
 acute B17.9
  with coma K72.01
  with hepatic failure —*see* Failure, hepatic
  alcoholic —*see* Hepatitis, alcoholic
  infectious B15.9
   with hepatic coma B15.0
  viral B17.9
 alcoholic (acute) (chronic) K70.10
  with ascites K70.11
 amebic —*see* Abscess, liver, amebic
 anicteric (viral) —*see* Hepatitis, viral
 antigen-associated (HAA) —*see* Hepatitis, B
 Australia-antigen (positive) —*see* Hepatitis, B
 autoimmune K75.4
 B B19.10
  with hepatic coma B19.11
  acute B16.9
   with
    delta-agent (coinfection) (without
      hepatic coma) B16.1
     with hepatic coma B16.0
    hepatic coma (without delta-agent
      coinfection) B16.2
  chronic B18.1
   with delta-agent B18.0
 bacterial NEC K75.89
 C (viral) B19.20
  with hepatic coma B19.21
  acute B17.10
   with hepatic coma B17.11
  chronic B18.2
 catarrhal (acute) B15.9
  with hepatic coma B15.0
 cholangiolitic K75.89
 cholestatic K75.89
 chronic K73.9
  active NEC K73.2
  lobular NEC K73.1
  persistent NEC K73.0
  specified NEC K73.8
 cytomegaloviral B25.1
 due to ethanol (acute) (chronic) —*see*
   Hepatitis, alcoholic
 epidemic B15.9
  with hepatic coma B15.0
 fulminant NEC (viral) —*see* Hepatitis, viral
 granulomatous NEC K75.3
 herpesviral B00.81

◀ New   ◀▥ Revised   ~~deleted~~ Deleted

Hepatitis *(Continued)*
history of
  B Z86.19
  C Z86.19
homologous serum —*see* Hepatitis, viral,
    type B
in (due to)
  mumps B26.81
  toxoplasmosis (acquired) B58.1
    congenital (active) P37.1 *[K77]*
infectious, infective (acute) (chronic)
  (subacute) B15.9
  with hepatic coma B15.0
inoculation —*see* Hepatitis, viral, type B
interstitial (chronic) K74.69
lupoid NEC K75.2
malignant NEC (with hepatic failure)
  K72.90
  with coma K72.91
neonatal giant cell P59.29
neonatal (idiopathic) (toxic) P59.29
newborn P59.29
postimmunization —*see* Hepatitis, viral,
  type B
post-transfusion —*see* Hepatitis, viral, type B
reactive, nonspecific K75.2
serum —*see* Hepatitis, viral, type B
specified type NEC
  with hepatic failure —*see* Failure, hepatic
syphilitic (late) A52.74
  congenital (early) A50.08 *[K77]*
    late A50.59 *[K77]*
  secondary A51.45
toxic (*see also* Disease, liver, toxic) K71.6
tuberculous A18.83
viral, virus B19.9
  with hepatic coma B19.0
  acute B17.9
  chronic B18.9
    specified NEC B18.8
    type
      B B18.1
        with delta-agent B18.0
      C B18.2
  congenital P35.3
  coxsackie B33.8 *[K77]*
  cytomegalic inclusion B25.1
  in remission, any type — code to Hepatitis,
    chronic, by type
  non-A, non-B B17.8
  specified type NEC (with or without coma)
    B17.8
  type
    A B15.9
      with hepatic coma B15.0
    B B19.10
      with hepatic coma B19.11
      acute B16.9
      with
        delta-agent (coinfection) (without
          hepatic coma) B16.1
          with hepatic coma B16.0
        hepatic coma (without delta-
          agent coinfection) B16.2
      chronic B18.1
        with delta-agent B18.0
    C B19.20
      with hepatic coma B19.21
      acute B17.10
        with hepatic coma B17.11
      chronic B18.2
    E B17.2
    non-A, non-B B17.8
Hepatization lung (acute) —*see* Pneumonia,
  lobar
Hepatoblastoma C22.2
Hepatocarcinoma C22.0
Hepatocholangiocarcinoma C22.0
Hepatocholangioma, benign D13.4
Hepatocholangitis K75.89
Hepatolenticular degeneration E83.01

Hepatoma (malignant) C22.0
benign D13.4
embryonal C22.0
Hepatomegaly —*see also* Hypertrophy, liver
with splenomegaly R16.2
congenital Q44.7
in mononucleosis
  gammaherpesviral B27.09
  infectious specified NEC B27.89
Hepatoptosis K76.89
Hepatorenal syndrome following labor and
  delivery O90.4
Hepatosis K76.89
Hepatosplenomegaly R16.2
hyperlipemic (Bürger-Grütz type) E78.3 *[K77]*
Hereditary —*see* condition
Heredodegeneration, macular —*see* Dystrophy,
  retina
Heredopathia atactica polyneuritiformis G60.1
Heredosyphilis —*see* Syphilis, congenital
Herlitz' syndrome Q81.1
Hermansky-Pudlak syndrome E70.331
Hermaphrodite, hermaphroditism (true) Q56.0
46,XX with streak gonads Q99.1
46,XX/46,XY Q99.0
46,XY with streak gonads Q99.1
chimera 46,XX/46,XY Q99.0
Hernia, hernial (acquired) (recurrent) K46.9
with
  gangrene —*see* Hernia, by site, with,
    gangrene
  incarceration —*see* Hernia, by site, with,
    obstruction
  irreducible —*see* Hernia, by site, with,
    obstruction
  obstruction —*see* Hernia, by site, with,
    obstruction
  strangulation —*see* Hernia, by site, with,
    obstruction
abdomen, abdominal K46.9
  with
    gangrene (and obstruction) K46.1
    obstruction K46.0
  femoral —*see* Hernia, femoral
  incisional —*see* Hernia, incisional
  inguinal —*see* Hernia, inguinal
  specified site NEC K45.8
    with
      gangrene (and obstruction) K45.1
      obstruction K45.0
  umbilical —*see* Hernia, umbilical
  wall —*see* Hernia, ventral
appendix —*see* Hernia, abdomen
bladder (mucosa) (sphincter)
  congenital (female) (male) Q79.51
  female —*see* Cystocele
  male N32.89
brain, congenital —*see* Encephalocele
cartilage, vertebra —*see* Displacement,
  intervertebral disc
cerebral, congenital —*see also* Encephalocele
  endaural Q01.8
ciliary body (traumatic) S05.2-
colon —*see* Hernia, abdomen
Cooper's —*see* Hernia, abdomen, specified
  site NEC
crural —*see* Hernia, femoral
diaphragm, diaphragmatic K44.9
  with
    gangrene (and obstruction) K44.1
    obstruction K44.0
  congenital Q79.0
direct (inguinal) —*see* Hernia, inguinal
diverticulum, intestine —*see* Hernia,
  abdomen
double (inguinal) —*see* Hernia, inguinal,
  bilateral
due to adhesions (with obstruction) K56.5
epigastric (*see also* Hernia, ventral) K43.9
esophageal hiatus —*see* Hernia, hiatal
external (inguinal) —*see* Hernia, inguinal

Hernia, hernial *(Continued)*
fallopian tube N83.4
fascia M62.89
femoral K41.90
  with
    gangrene (and obstruction) K41.40
      not specified as recurrent K41.40
      recurrent K41.41
    obstruction K41.30
      not specified as recurrent K41.30
      recurrent K41.31
  bilateral K41.20
    with
      gangrene (and obstruction) K41.10
        not specified as recurrent K41.10
        recurrent K41.11
      obstruction K41.00
        not specified as recurrent K41.00
        recurrent K41.01
    not specified as recurrent K41.20
    recurrent K41.21
  not specified as recurrent K41.90
  recurrent K41.91
  unilateral K41.90
    with
      gangrene (and obstruction) K41.40
        not specified as recurrent K41.40
        recurrent K41.41
      obstruction K41.30
        not specified as recurrent K41.30
        recurrent K41.31
    not specified as recurrent K41.90
    recurrent K41.91
foramen magnum G93.5
  congenital Q01.8
funicular (umbilical) —*see also* Hernia,
  umbilicus
  spermatic (cord) —*see* Hernia, inguinal
gastrointestinal tract —*see* Hernia, abdomen
Hesselbach's —*see* Hernia, femoral, specified
  site NEC
hiatal (esophageal) (sliding) K44.9
  with
    gangrene (and obstruction) K44.1
    obstruction K44.0
  congenital Q40.1
hypogastric —*see* Hernia, ventral
incarcerated —*see also* Hernia, by site, with
  obstruction
  with gangrene —*see* Hernia, by site, with
    gangrene
incisional K43.92
  with
    gangrene (and obstruction) K43.1
    obstruction K43.0
indirect (inguinal) —*see* Hernia, inguinal
inguinal (direct) (external) (funicular)
  (indirect) (internal) (oblique) (scrotal)
  (sliding) K40.90
  with
    gangrene (and obstruction) K40.40
      not specified as recurrent K40.40
      recurrent K40.41
    obstruction K40.30
      not specified as recurrent K40.30
      recurrent K40.31
  bilateral K40.20
    with
      gangrene (and obstruction)
        K40.10
        not specified as recurrent
          K40.10
        recurrent K40.11
      obstruction K40.00
        not specified as recurrent
          K40.00
        recurrent K40.01
    not specified as recurrent K40.20
    recurrent K40.21
  not specified as recurrent K40.90
  recurrent K40.91

Hernia, hernial (Continued)
  inguinal (Continued)
    unilateral K40.90
      with
        gangrene (and obstruction) K40.40
          not specified as recurrent K40.40
          recurrent K40.41
        obstruction K40.30
          not specified as recurrent K40.30
          recurrent K40.31
      not specified as recurrent K40.90
      recurrent K40.91
  internal —see also Hernia, abdomen
    inguinal —see Hernia, inguinal
  interstitial —see Hernia, abdomen
  intervertebral cartilage or disc —see
    Displacement, intervertebral disc
  intestine, intestinal —see Hernia, by site
  intra-abdominal —see Hernia, abdomen
  iris (traumatic) S05.2-
  irreducible —see also Hernia, by site, with
    obstruction
    with gangrene —see Hernia, by site, with
      gangrene
  ischiatic —see Hernia, abdomen, specified
    site NEC
  ischiorectal —see Hernia, abdomen, specified
    site NEC
  lens (traumatic) S05.2-
  linea (alba) (semilunaris) —see Hernia,
    ventral
  Littre's —see Hernia, abdomen
  lumbar —see Hernia, abdomen, specified site
    NEC
  lung (subcutaneous) J98.4
  mediastinum J98.5
  mesenteric (internal) —see Hernia, abdomen
  midline —see Hernia, ventral
  muscle (sheath) M62.89
  nucleus pulposus —see Displacement,
    intervertebral disc
  oblique (inguinal) —see Hernia, inguinal
  obstructive —see also Hernia, by site, with
    obstruction
    with gangrene —see Hernia, by site, with
      gangrene
  obturator —see Hernia, abdomen, specified
    site NEC
  omental —see Hernia, abdomen
  ovary N83.4
  oviduct N83.4
  paraesophageal —see also Hernia, diaphragm
    congenital Q40.1
  parastomal K43.5
    with
      gangrene (and obstruction) K43.4
      obstruction K43.3
  paraumbilical —see Hernia, umbilicus
  perineal —see Hernia, abdomen, specified
    site NEC
  Petit's —see Hernia, abdomen, specified site
    NEC
  postoperative —see Hernia, incisional
  pregnant uterus —see Abnormal, uterus in
    pregnancy or childbirth
  prevesical N32.89
  properitoneal —see Hernia, abdomen,
    specified site NEC
  pudendal —see Hernia, abdomen, specified
    site NEC
  rectovaginal N81.6
  retroperitoneal —see Hernia, abdomen,
    specified site NEC
  Richter's —see Hernia, abdomen, with
    obstruction
  Rieux's, Riex's —see Hernia, abdomen,
    specified site NEC
  sac condition (adhesion) (dropsy)
    (inflammation) (laceration)
    (suppuration) - code by site under
    Hernia

Hernia, hernial (Continued)
  sciatic —see Hernia, abdomen, specified site
    NEC
  scrotum, scrotal —see Hernia, inguinal
  sliding (inguinal) —see also Hernia,
    inguinal
    hiatus —see Hernia, hiatal
  spigelian —see Hernia, ventral
  spinal —see Spina bifida
  strangulated —see also Hernia, by site, with
    obstruction
    with gangrene —see Hernia, by site, with
      gangrene
  subxiphoid —see Hernia, ventral
  supra-umbilicus —see Hernia, ventral
  tendon —see Disorder, tendon, specified type
    NEC
  Treitz's (fossa) —see Hernia, abdomen,
    specified site NEC
  tunica vaginalis Q55.29
  umbilicus, umbilical K42.9
    with
      gangrene (and obstruction) K42.1
      obstruction K42.0
  ureter N28.89
  urethra, congenital Q64.79
  urinary meatus, congenital Q64.79
  uterus N81.4
    pregnant —see Abnormal, uterus in
      pregnancy or childbirth
  vaginal (anterior) (wall) —see Cystocele
  Velpeau's —see Hernia, femoral
  ventral K43.90
    with
      gangrene (and obstruction) K43.7
      obstruction K43.6
    incisional K43.2
      with
        gangrene (and obstruction) K43.1
        obstruction K43.0
      recurrent —see Hernia, incisional
    specified NEC K43.9
      with
        gangrene (and obstruction) K43.7
        obstruction K43.6
  vesical
    congenital (female) (male) Q79.51
    female —see Cystocele
    male N32.89
  vitreous (into wound) S05.2-
    into anterior chamber —see Prolapse,
      vitreous
Herniation —see also Hernia
  brain (stem) G93.5
  cerebral G93.5
  mediastinum J98.5
  nucleus pulposus —see Displacement,
    intervertebral disc
Herpangina B08.5
Herpes, herpesvirus, herpetic B00.9
  anogenital A60.9
    perianal skin A60.1
    rectum A60.1
    urogenital tract A60.00
      cervix A60.03
      male genital organ NEC A60.02
      penis A60.01
      specified site NEC A60.09
      vagina A60.04
      vulva A60.04
  blepharitis (zoster) B02.39
    simplex B00.59
  circinatus B35.4
    bullosus L12.0
  conjunctivitis (simplex) B00.53
    zoster B02.31
  cornea B02.33
  encephalitis B00.4
    due to herpesvirus 6 B10.01
    due to herpesvirus 7 B10.09
    specified NEC B10.09

Herpes, herpesvirus, herpetic (Continued)
  eye (zoster) B02.30
    simplex B00.50
  eyelid (zoster) B02.39
    simplex B00.59
  facialis B00.1
  febrilis B00.1
  geniculate ganglionitis B02.21
  genital, genitalis A60.00
    female A60.09
    male A60.02
  gestational, gestationis O26.4-
  gingivostomatitis B00.2
  human B00.9
    1 —see Herpes, simplex
    2 —see Herpes, simplex
    3 —see Varicella
    4 —see Mononucleosis, Epstein-Barr (virus)
    5 —see Disease, cytomegalic inclusion
      (generalized)
    6
      encephalitis B10.01
      specified NEC B10.81
    7
      encephalitis B10.09
      specified NEC B10.82
    8 B10.89
  infection NEC B10.89
    Kaposi's sarcoma associated B10.89
  iridocyclitis (simplex) B00.51
    zoster B02.32
  iris (vesicular erythema multiforme) L51.9
  iritis (simplex) B00.51
  Kaposi's sarcoma associated B10.89
  keratitis (simplex) (dendritic) (disciform)
    (interstitial) B00.52
    zoster (interstitial) B02.33
  keratoconjunctivitis (simplex) B00.52
    zoster B02.33
  labialis B00.1
  lip B00.1
  meningitis (simplex) B00.3
    zoster B02.1
  ophthalmicus (zoster) NEC B02.30
    simplex B00.50
  penis A60.01
  perianal skin A60.1
  pharyngitis, pharyngotonsillitis B00.2
  rectum A60.1
  scrotum A60.02
  sepsis B00.7
  simplex B00.9
    complicated NEC B00.89
    congenital P35.2
    conjunctivitis B00.53
    external ear B00.1
    eyelid B00.59
    hepatitis B00.81
    keratitis (interstitial) B00.52
    myelitis B00.82
    specified complication NEC B00.89
    visceral B00.89
  stomatitis B00.2
  tonsurans B35.0
  visceral B00.89
  vulva A60.04
  whitlow B00.89
  zoster (see also condition) B02.9
    auricularis B02.21
    complicated NEC B02.8
    conjunctivitis B02.31
    disseminated B02.7
    encephalitis B02.0
    eye(lid) B02.39
    geniculate ganglionitis B02.21
    keratitis (interstitial) B02.33
    meningitis B02.1
    myelitis B02.24
    neuritis, neuralgia B02.29
    ophthalmicus NEC B02.30
    oticus B02.21

Herpes, herpesvirus, herpetic *(Continued)*
  zoster *(Continued)*
    polyneuropathy B02.23
    specified complication NEC B02.8
    trigeminal neuralgia B02.22
Herpesvirus (human) —*see* Herpes
Herpetophobia F40.218
Herrick's anemia —*see* Disease, sickle-cell
Hers' disease E74.09
Herter-Gee syndrome K90.0
Herxheimer's reaction R68.89
Hesitancy
  of micturition R39.11
  urinary R39.11
Hesselbach's hernia —*see* Hernia, femoral,
    specified site NEC
Heterochromia (congenital) Q13.2
  cataract —*see* Cataract, complicated
  cyclitis (Fuchs) —*see* Cyclitis, Fuchs'
    heterochromic
  hair L67.1
  iritis —*see* Cyclitis, Fuchs' heterochromic
  retained metallic foreign body
      (nonmagnetic) —*see* Foreign body,
      intraocular, old, retained
    magnetic —*see* Foreign body, intraocular,
      old, retained, magnetic
  uveitis —*see* Cyclitis, Fuchs' heterochromic
Heterophoria —*see* Strabismus, heterophoria
Heterophyes, heterophyiasis (small intestine)
    B66.8
Heterotopia, heterotopic —*see also* Malposition,
    congenital
  cerebralis Q04.8
Heterotropia —*see* Strabismus
Heubner-Herter disease K90.0
Hexadactylism Q69.9
HGSIL (cytology finding) (high grade
    squamous intraepithelial lesion on
    cytologic smear) (Pap smear finding)
  anus R85.613
  cervix R87.613
    biopsy (histology) finding — code to CIN
      II or CIN III
  vagina R87.623
    biopsy (histology) finding — code to VAIN
      II or VAIN III
Hibernoma —*see* Lipoma
Hiccup, hiccough R06.6
  epidemic B33.0
  psychogenic F45.8
Hidden penis (congenital) Q55.64
  acquired N48.83
Hidradenitis (axillaris) (suppurative) L73.2
Hidradenoma (nodular) —*see also* Neoplasm,
    skin, benign
  clear cell —*see* Neoplasm, skin, benign
  papillary —*see* Neoplasm, skin, benign
Hidrocystoma —*see* Neoplasm, skin, benign
High
  altitude effects T70.20
    anoxia T70.29
    on
      ears T70.0
      sinuses T70.1
    polycythemia D75.1
  arch
    foot Q66.7
    palate, congenital Q38.5
  arterial tension —*see* Hypertension
  basal metabolic rate R94.8
  blood pressure —*see also* Hypertension
    borderline R03.0
    reading (incidental) (isolated)
      (nonspecific), without diagnosis of
      hypertension R03.0
  cholesterol E78.0
    with high triglycerides E78.2
  diaphragm (congenital) Q79.1
  expressed emotional level within family
    Z63.8

High *(Continued)*
  head at term O32.4
  palate, congenital Q38.5
  risk
    infant NEC Z76.2
    sexual behavior (heterosexual) Z72.51
      bisexual Z72.53
      homosexual Z72.52
  temperature (of unknown origin) R50.9
  thoracic rib Q76.6
  triglycerides E78.1
    with high cholesterol E78.2
Hildenbrand's disease A75.0
Hilum —*see* condition Hip —*see* condition
Hippel's disease Q85.8
Hippophobia F40.218
Hippus H57.09
Hirschsprung's disease or megacolon Q43.1
Hirsutism, hirsuties L68.0
Hirudiniasis
  external B88.3
  internal B83.4
Hiss-Russell dysentery A03.1
Histidinemia, histidinuria E70.41
Histiocytoma —*see also* Neoplasm, skin, benign
  fibrous —*see also* Neoplasm, skin, benign
    atypical —*see* Neoplasm, connective tissue,
      uncertain behavior
    malignant —*see* Neoplasm, connective
      tissue, malignant
Histiocytosis D76.3
  acute differentiated progressive C96.0
  Langerhans' cell NEC C96.6
    multifocal X
      multisystemic (disseminated) C96.0
      unisystemic C96.5
    pulmonary, adult (adult PLCH) J84.82
    unifocal (X) C96.6
  lipid, lipoid D76.3
    essential E75.29
  malignant C96.A
  mononuclear phagocytes NEC D76.1
    Langerhans' cells C96.6
  non-Langerhans cell D76.3
  polyostotic sclerosing D76.3
  sinus, with massive lymphadenopathy D76.3
  syndrome NEC D76.3
  X NEC C96.6
    acute (progressive) C96.0
    chronic C96.6
    multifocal C96.5
    multisystemic C96.0
    unifocal C96.6
Histoplasmosis B39.9
  with pneumonia NEC B39.2[J17] ◀▥▥
  African B39.5
  American —*see* Histoplasmosis, capsulati
  capsulati B39.4
    disseminated B39.3
    generalized B39.3
    pulmonary B39.2
      acute B39.0
      chronic B39.1
  Darling's B39.4
  duboisii B39.5
  lung NEC B39.2
History
  family (of) —*see also* History, personal (of)
    alcohol abuse Z81.1
    allergy NEC Z84.89
    anemia Z83.2
    arthritis Z82.61
    asthma Z82.5
    blindness Z82.1
    cardiac death (sudden) Z82.41
    carrier of genetic disease Z84.81
    chromosomal anomaly Z82.79
    chronic
      disabling disease NEC Z82.8
      lower respiratory disease Z82.5
    colonic polyps Z83.71

History *(Continued)*
  family *(Continued)*
    congenital malformations and
      deformations Z82.79
      polycystic kidney Z82.71
    consanguinity Z84.3
    deafness Z82.2
    diabetes mellitus Z83.3
    disability NEC Z82.8
    disease or disorder (of)
      allergic NEC Z84.89
      behavioral NEC Z81.8
      blood and blood-forming organs Z83.2
      cardiovascular NEC Z82.49
      chronic disabling NEC Z82.8
      digestive Z83.79
      ear NEC Z83.52
      endocrine NEC Z83.49
      eye NEC Z83.518
        glaucoma Z83.511
      genitourinary NEC Z84.2
      glaucoma Z83.511
      hematological Z83.2
      immune mechanism Z83.2
      infectious NEC Z83.1
      ischemic heart Z82.49
      kidney Z84.1
      mental NEC Z81.8
      metabolic Z83.49
      musculoskeletal NEC Z82.69
      neurological NEC Z82.0
      nutritional Z83.49
      parasitic NEC Z83.1
      psychiatric NEC Z81.8
      respiratory NEC Z83.6
      skin and subcutaneous tissue NEC Z84.0
      specified NEC Z84.89
    drug abuse NEC Z81.3
    epilepsy Z82.0
    genetic disease carrier Z84.81
    glaucoma Z83.511
    hearing loss Z82.2
    human immunodeficiency virus (HIV)
      infection Z83.0
    Huntington's chorea Z82.0
    intellectual disability Z81.0
    leukemia Z80.6
    malignant neoplasm (of) NOS Z80.9
      bladder Z80.52
      breast Z80.3
      bronchus Z80.1
      digestive organ Z80.0
      gastrointestinal tract Z80.0
      genital organ Z80.49
        ovary Z80.41
        prostate Z80.42
        specified organ NEC Z80.49
        testis Z80.43
      hematopoietic NEC Z80.7
      intrathoracic organ NEC Z80.2
      kidney Z80.51
      lung Z80.1
      lymphatic NEC Z80.7
      ovary Z80.41
      prostate Z80.42
      respiratory organ NEC Z80.2
      specified site NEC Z80.8
      testis Z80.43
      trachea Z80.1
      urinary organ or tract Z80.59
        bladder Z80.52
        kidney Z80.51
    mental
      disorder NEC Z81.8
    multiple endocrine neoplasia (MEN)
      syndrome Z83.41
    osteoporosis Z82.62
    polycystic kidney Z82.71
    polyps (colon) Z83.71
    psychiatric disorder Z81.8
    psychoactive substance abuse NEC Z81.3

◀ New   ◀▥ Revised   ~~deleted~~ Deleted

History *(Continued)*
  personal *(Continued)*
    malignant neoplasm *(Continued)*
      genital organ
        female Z85.40
          specified NEC Z85.44
        male Z85.45
          specified NEC Z85.49
      hematopoietic NEC Z85.79
      intrathoracic organ Z85.20-
      kidney NEC Z85.528
        carcinoid Z85.520
      large intestine NEC Z85.038
        carcinoid Z85.030
      larynx Z85.21
      liver Z85.05
      lung NEC Z85.118
        carcinoid Z85.110
      mediastinum Z85.29
      Merkel cell Z85.821
      middle ear Z85.22
      nasal cavities Z85.22
      nervous system NEC Z85.848
      oral cavity Z85.819
        specified site NEC Z85.818
      ovary Z85.43
      pancreas Z85.07
      pelvis Z85.53
      pharynx Z85.819
        specified site NEC Z85.818
      pleura Z85.29
      prostate Z85.46
      rectosigmoid junction NEC Z85.048
        carcinoid Z85.040
      rectum NEC Z85.048
        carcinoid Z85.040
      respiratory organ Z85.20
      sinuses, accessory Z85.22
      skin NEC Z85.828
        melanoma Z85.820
        Merkel cell Z85.821
      small intestine NEC Z85.068
        carcinoid Z85.060
      soft tissue Z85.831
      specified site NEC Z85.89
      stomach NEC Z85.028
        carcinoid Z85.020
      testis Z85.47
      thymus NEC Z85.238
        carcinoid Z85.230
      thyroid Z85.850
      tongue Z85.810
      trachea Z85.12
      ureter Z85.54
      urinary organ or tract Z85.50
        specified NEC Z85.59
      uterus Z85.42
    maltreatment Z91.89
    medical treatment NEC Z92.89
    melanoma (malignant) (skin) Z85.820
    meningitis Z86.61
    mental disorder Z86.59
    Merkel cell carcinoma (skin) Z85.821
    Methicillin resistant Staphylococcus aureus
      (MRSA) Z86.14
    military deployment Z91.82
    military war, peacekeeping and
      humanitarian deployment (current or
      past conflict) Z91.82
    myocardial infarction (old) I25.2
    neglect (in)
      adult Z91.412
      childhood Z62.812
    neoplasm
      benign Z86.018
        brain Z86.011
        colon polyp Z86.010
      in situ
        breast Z86.000
        cervix uteri Z86.001
        specified NEC Z86.008

History *(Continued)*
  personal *(Continued)*
    neoplasm *(Continued)*
      malignant —*see* History of, malignant
        neoplasm
      uncertain behavior Z86.03
    nephrotic syndrome Z87.441
    nicotine dependence Z87.891
    noncompliance with medical treatment or
      regimen —*see* Noncompliance
    nutritional deficiency Z86.39
    obstetric complications Z87.59
      childbirth Z87.59
      pregnancy Z87.59
      pre-term labor Z87.51
      puerperium Z87.59
    osteoporosis fractures Z87.31
    parasuicide (attempt) Z91.5
    physical trauma NEC Z87.828
      self-harm or suicide attempt Z91.5
    pneumonia (recurrent) Z87.01
    poisoning NEC Z91.89
      self-harm or suicide attempt Z91.5
    poor personal hygiene Z91.89
    preterm labor Z87.51
    procedure during pregnancy Z98.870
    procedure while a fetus Z98.871
    prolonged reversible ischemic neurologic
      deficit (PRINO) Z86.73
    prostatic dysplasia Z87.430
    psychiatric disorder NEC Z87.89
    psychological
      abuse
        adult Z91.411
        child Z62.811
      trauma, specified NEC Z91.49
    radiation therapy Z92.3
    removal
      implant
        breast Z98.86
    renal calculi Z87.442
    respiratory condition NEC Z87.09
    retained foreign body fully removed
      Z87.821
    risk factors NEC Z91.89
    self-harm Z91.5
    self-poisoning attempt Z91.5
    sex reassignment Z87.890
    sleep-wake cycle problem Z72.821
    specified NEC Z87.898
    steroid therapy (systemic) Z92.241
      inhaled Z92.240
    stroke without residual deficits
      Z86.73
    substance abuse NEC F10-F19 with
      fifth character 1 ◄▥
    sudden cardiac arrest Z86.74
    sudden cardiac death successfully
      resuscitated Z86.74
    suicide attempt Z91.5
    surgery NEC Z98.89
      sex reassignment Z87.890
      transplant —*see* Transplant
    thrombophlebitis Z86.72
    thrombosis (venous) Z86.718
      pulmonary Z86.711
    tobacco dependence Z87.891
    transient ischemic attack (TIA) without
      residual deficits Z86.73
    trauma (physical) NEC Z87.828
      psychological NEC Z91.49
      self-harm Z91.5
    traumatic brain injury Z87.820
    unhealthy sleep-wake cycle Z72.821
    urinary (recurrent) (tract) infection (s)
      Z87.440
    urinary calculi Z87.42
    vaginal dysplasia Z87.411
    venous thrombosis or embolism Z86.718
      pulmonary Z86.711
    vulvar dysplasia Z87.412

His-Werner disease A79.0
HIV (*see also* Human, immunodeficiency virus)
  B20
  laboratory evidence (nonconclusive) R75
  nonconclusive test (in infants) R75
  positive, seropositive Z21
Hives (bold) —*see* Urticaria
Hoarseness R49.0
Hobo Z59.0
Hodgkin disease —*see* Lymphoma,
  Hodgkin
Hodgson's disease I71.2
  ruptured I71.1
Hoffa-Kastert disease E88.89
Hoffa's disease E88.89
Hoffmann-Bouveret syndrome I47.9
Hoffmann's syndrome E03.9 *[G73.7]*
Hole (round)
  macula H35.34-
  retina (without detachment) —*see* Break,
    retina, round hole
    with detachment —*see* Detachment, retina,
      with retinal, break
Holiday relief care Z75.5
Hollenhorst's plaque —*see* Occlusion, artery,
  retina
Hollow foot (congenital) Q66.7
  acquired —*see* Deformity, limb, foot, specified
    NEC
Holoprosencephaly Q04.2
Holt-Oram syndrome Q87.2
Homelessness Z59.0
Homesickness —*see* Disorder, adjustment
Homocystinemia, homocystinuria E72.11
Homogentisate 1,2-dioxygenase deficiency
  E70.29
Homologous serum hepatitis (prophylactic)
  (therapeutic) —*see* Hepatitis, viral,
  type B
Honeycomb lung J98.4
  congenital Q33.0
Hooded
  clitoris Q52.6
  penis Q55.69
Hookworm (anemia) (disease) (infection)
  (infestation) B76.9
  specified NEC B76.8
Hordeolum (eyelid) (externum) (recurrent)
  H00.019
  internum H00.029
    left H00.026
      lower H00.025
      upper H00.024
    right H00.023
      lower H00.022
      upper H00.021
  left H00.016
    lower H00.015
    upper H00.014
  right H00.013
    lower H00.012
    upper H00.011
Horn
  cutaneous L85.8
  nail L60.2
    congenital Q84.6
Horner (-Claude Bernard) syndrome G90.2
  traumatic —*see* Injury, nerve, cervical
    sympathetic
Horseshoe kidney (congenital) Q63.1
Horton's headache or neuralgia G44.099
  intractable G44.091
  not intractable G44.099
Hospital hopper syndrome —*see* Disorder,
  factitious
Hospitalism in children —*see* Disorder,
  adjustment
Hostility R45.5
  towards child Z62.3
Hot flashes
  menopausal N95.1

Hourglass (contracture) —*see also* Contraction, hourglass
  stomach K31.89
    congenital Q40.2
    stricture K31.2
Household, housing circumstance affecting care Z59.9
  specified NEC Z59.8
Housemaid's knee —*see* Bursitis, prepatellar
Hudson (-Stähli) line (cornea) —*see* Pigmentation, cornea, anterior
Human
  bite (open wound) —*see also* Bite
    intact skin surface —*see* Bite, superficial
  herpesvirus —*see* Herpes
  immunodeficiency virus (HIV) disease (infection) B20
    asymptomatic status Z21
    contact Z20.6
    counseling Z71.7
    dementia B20 [F02.80]
      with behavioral disturbance B20 [F02.81]
    exposure to Z20.6
    laboratory evidence R75
    type-2 (HIV 2) as cause of disease classified elsewhere B97.35
  papillomavirus (HPV)
    DNA test positive
      high risk
        cervix R87.810
        vagina R87.811
      low risk
        cervix R87.820
        vagina R87.821
    screening for Z11.51
  T-cell lymphotropic virus
    type-1 (HTLV-I) infection B33.3
      as cause of disease classified elsewhere B97.33
      carrier Z22.6
    type-2 (HTLV-II) as cause of disease classified elsewhere B97.34
Humidifier lung or pneumonitis J67.7
Humiliation (experience) in childhood Z62.898
Humpback (acquired) —*see* Kyphosis
Hunchback (acquired) —*see* Kyphosis
Hunger T73.0
  air, psychogenic F45.8
Hungry bone syndrome E83.81
Hunner's ulcer —*see* Cystitis, chronic, interstitial
Hunter's
  glossitis D51.0
  syndrome E76.1
Huntington's disease or chorea G10
  with dementia G10 [F02.80]
    with behavioral disturbance G10 [F02.81]
Hunt's
  disease or syndrome (herpetic geniculate ganglionitis) B02.21
    dyssynergia cerebellaris myoclonica G11.1
  neuralgia B02.21
Hurler (-Scheie) disease or syndrome E76.02
Hurst's disease G36.1
Hurthle cell
  adenocarcinoma C73
  adenoma D34
  carcinoma C73
  tumor D34
Hutchinson-Boeck disease or syndrome —*see* Sarcoidosis
Hutchinson-Gilford disease or syndrome E34.8
Hutchinson's
  disease, meaning
    angioma serpiginosum L81.7
    pompholyx (cheiropompholyx) L30.1
    prurigo estivalis L56.4
    summer eruption or summer prurigo L56.4
  melanotic freckle —*see* Melanoma, in situ
    malignant melanoma in —*see* Melanoma

Hutchinson's (*Continued*)
  teeth or incisors (congenital syphilis) A50.52
  triad (congenital syphilis) A50.53
Hyalin plaque, sclera, senile H15.89
Hyaline membrane (disease) (lung) (pulmonary) (newborn) P22.0
Hyalinosis
  cutis (et mucosae) E78.89
  focal and segmental (glomerular) (*see also* N00-N07 with fourth character .1) N05.1
Hyalitis, hyalosis, asteroid —*see also* Deposit, crystalline
  syphilitic (late) A52.71
Hydatid
  cyst or tumor —*see* Echinococcus
  mole —*see* Hydatidiform mole
  Morgagni
    female Q50.5
    male (epididymal) Q55.4
      testicular Q55.29
Hydatidiform mole (benign) (complicating pregnancy) (delivered) (undelivered) O01.9
  classical O01.0
  complete O01.0
  incomplete O01.1
  invasive D39.2
  malignant D39.2
  partial O01.1
Hydatidosis —*see* Echinococcus
Hydradenitis (axillaris) (suppurative) L73.2
Hydradenoma —*see* Hidradenoma
Hydramnios O40.-
Hydrancephaly, hydranencephaly Q04.3
  with spina bifida —*see* Spina bifida, with hydrocephalus
Hydrargyrism NEC —*see* Poisoning, mercury
Hydrarthrosis —*see also* Effusion, joint
  gonococcal A54.42
  intermittent M12.40
    ankle M12.47-
    elbow M12.42-
    foot joint M12.47-
    hand joint M12.44-
    hip M12.45-
    knee M12.46-
    multiple site M12.49
    shoulder M12.41-
    specified joint NEC M12.48
    wrist M12.43-
  of yaws (early) (late) (*see also* subcategory M14.8-) A66.6
  syphilitic (late) A52.77
    congenital A50.55 [M12.80]
Hydremia D64.89
Hydrencephalocele (congenital) —*see* Encephalocele
Hydrencephalomeningocele (congenital) —*see* Encephalocele
Hydroa R23.8
  aestivale L56.4
  vacciniforme L56.4
Hydroadenitis (axillaris) (suppurative) L73.2
Hydrocalycosis —*see* Hydronephrosis
Hydrocele (spermatic cord) (testis) (tunica vaginalis) N43.3
  canal of Nuck N94.89
  communicating N43.2
    congenital P83.5
  congenital P83.5
  encysted N43.0
  female NEC N94.89
  infected N43.1
  newborn P83.5
  round ligament N94.89
  specified NEC N43.2
  spinalis —*see* Spina bifida
  vulva N90.89

Hydrocephalus (acquired) (external) (internal) (malignant) (recurrent) G91.9
  aqueduct Sylvius stricture Q03.0
  causing disproportion O33.6
    with obstructed labor O66.3
  communicating G91.0
  congenital (external) (internal) Q03.9
    with spina bifida Q05.4
      cervical Q05.0
      dorsal Q05.1
      lumbar Q05.2
      lumbosacral Q05.2
      sacral Q05.3
      thoracic Q05.1
      thoracolumbar Q05.1
    specified NEC Q03.8
  due to toxoplasmosis (congenital) P37.1
  foramen Magendie block (acquired) G91.1
    congenital (*see also* Hydrocephalus, congenital) Q03.1
  in (due to)
    infectious disease NEC B89 [G91.4]
    neoplastic disease NEC (*see also* Neoplasm) G91.4
    parasitic disease B89 [G91.4]
  newborn Q03.9
    with spina bifida —*see* Spina bifida, with hydrocephalus
  noncommunicating G91.1
  normal pressure G91.2
    secondary G91.0
  obstructive G91.1
  otitic G93.2
  post-traumatic NEC G91.3
  secondary G91.4
    post-traumatic G91.3
  specified NEC G91.8
  syphilitic, congenital A50.49
Hydrocolpos (congenital) N89.8
Hydrocystoma —*see* Neoplasm, skin, benign
Hydroencephalocele (congenital) —*see* Encephalocele
Hydroencephalomeningocele (congenital) —*see* Encephalocele
Hydrohematopneumothorax —*see* Hemothorax
Hydromeningitis —*see* Meningitis
Hydromeningocele (spinal) —*see also* Spina bifida
  cranial —*see* Encephalocele
Hydrometra N85.8
Hydrometrocolpos N89.8
Hydromicrocephaly Q02
Hydromphalos (since birth) Q45.8
Hydromyelia Q06.4
Hydromyelocele —*see* Spina bifida
Hydronephrosis (atrophic) (early) (functionless) (intermittent) (primary) (secondary) NEC N13.30
  with
    infection N13.6
    obstruction (by) (of)
      renal calculus N13.2
        with infection N13.6
      ureteral NEC N13.1
        with infection N13.6
        calculus N13.2
          with infection N13.6
      ureteropelvic junction (congenital) Q62.0
        with infection N13.6
      ureteral stricture NEC N13.1
        with infection N13.6
  congenital Q62.0
  specified type NEC N13.39
  tuberculous A18.11
Hydropericarditis —*see* Pericarditis
Hydropericardium —*see* Pericarditis
Hydroperitoneum R18.8
Hydrophobia —*see* Rabies
Hydrophthalmos Q15.0
Hydropneumohemothorax —*see* Hemothorax
Hydropneumopericarditis —*see* Pericarditis

Hydropneumopericardium —*see* Pericarditis
Hydropneumothorax J94.8
  traumatic —*see* Injury, intrathoracic, lung
  tuberculous NEC A15.6
Hydrops R60.9
  abdominis R18.8
  articulorum intermittens —*see* Hydrarthrosis,
    intermittent
  cardiac —*see* Failure, heart, congestive
  causing obstructed labor (mother) O66.3
  endolymphatic H81.0-
  fetal —*see* Pregnancy, complicated by,
    hydrops, fetalis
  fetalis P83.2
    due to
      ABO isoimmunization P56.0
      alpha thalassemia D56.0
      hemolytic disease P56.90
        specified NEC P56.99
      isoimmunization (ABO) (Rh) P56.0
      other specified nonhemolytic disease
        NEC P83.2
      Rh incompatibility P56.0
    during pregnancy —*see* Pregnancy,
      complicated by, hydrops, fetalis
  gallbladder K82.1
  joint —*see* Effusion, joint
  labyrinth H81.0
  newborn (idiopathic) P83.2
    due to
      ABO isoimmunization P56.0
      alpha thalassemia D56.0
      hemolytic disease P56.90
        specified NEC P56.99
      isoimmunization (ABO) (Rh) P56.0
      Rh incompatibility P56.0
  nutritional —*see* Malnutrition, severe
  pericardium —*see* Pericarditis
  pleura —*see* Hydrothorax
  spermatic cord —*see* Hydrocele
Hydropyonephrosis N13.6
Hydrorachis Q06.4
Hydrorrhea (nasal) J34.89
  pregnancy —*see* Rupture, membranes,
    premature
Hydrosadenitis (axillaris) (suppurative) L73.2
Hydrosalpinx (fallopian tube) (follicularis)
  N70.11
Hydrothorax (double) (pleura) J94.8
  chylous (nonfilarial) I89.8
    filarial (*see also* Infestation, filarial) B74.9
      [J91.8]
  traumatic —*see* Injury, intrathoracic
  tuberculous NEC (non primary) A15.6
Hydroureter (*see also* Hydronephrosis) N13.4
  with infection N13.6
  congenital Q62.39
Hydroureteronephrosis —*see* Hydronephrosis
Hydrourethra N36.8
Hydroxykynureninuria E70.8
Hydroxylysinemia E72.3
Hydroxyprolinemia E72.59
Hygiene, sleep
  abuse Z72.821
  inadequate Z72.821
  poor Z72.821
Hygroma (congenital) (cystic) D18.1
  praepatellare, prepatellar —*see* Bursitis,
    prepatellar
Hymen —*see* condition
Hymenolepis, hymenolepiasis (diminuta)
  (infection) (infestation) (nana) B71.0
Hypalgesia R20.8
Hyperacidity (gastric) K31.89
  psychogenic F45.8
Hyperactive, hyperactivity F90.9
  basal cell, uterine cervix —*see* Dysplasia,
    cervix
  bowel sounds R19.12
  cervix epithelial (basal) —*see* Dysplasia,
    cervix

Hyperactive, hyperactivity (*Continued*)
  child F90.9
    attention deficit —*see* Disorder, attention-
      deficit hyperactivity
  detrusor muscle N32.81
  gastrointestinal K31.89
    psychogenic F45.8
  nasal mucous membrane J34.3
  stomach K31.89
  thyroid (gland) —*see* Hyperthyroidism
Hyperacusis H93.23-
Hyperadrenalism E27.5
Hyperadrenocorticism E24.9
  congenital E25.0
  iatrogenic E24.2
    correct substance properly administered —
      see Table of ɖDrugs and ɕChemicals,
      by drug, adverse effect ◀▥
    overdose or wrong substance given or
      taken —*see* Table of ɖDrugs and
      ɕChemicals, by drug, poisoning ◀▥
  not associated with Cushing's syndrome
    E27.0
  pituitary-dependent E24.0
Hyperaldosteronism E26.9
  familial (type I) E26.02
  glucocorticoid-remediable E26.02
  primary (due to (bilateral) adrenal
    hyperplasia) E26.09
  primary NEC E26.09
  secondary E26.1
  specified NEC E26.89
Hyperalgesia R20.8
Hyperalimentation R63.2
  carotene, carotin E67.1
  specified NEC E67.8
  vitamin
    A E67.0
    D E67.3
Hyperaminoaciduria
  arginine E72.21
  cystine E72.01
  lysine E72.3
  ornithine E72.4
Hyperammonemia (congenital) E72.20
Hyperazotemia —*see* Uremia
Hyperbetalipoproteinemia (familial) E78.0
  with prebetalipoproteinemia E78.2
Hyperbilirubinemia
  constitutional E80.6
  familial conjugated E80.6
  neonatal (transient) —*see* Jaundice, newborn
Hypercalcemia, hypocalciuric, familial E83.52
Hypercalciuria, idiopathic E83.52
Hypercapnia R06.89
  newborn P84
Hypercarotenemia, hypercarotinemia (dietary)
  E67.1
Hypercementosis K03.4
Hyperchloremia E87.8
Hyperchlorhydria K31.89
  neurotic F45.8
  psychogenic F45.8
Hypercholesterinemia —*see*
  Hypercholesterolemia
Hypercholesterolemia (essential) (familial)
  (hereditary) (primary) (pure) E78.0
  with hyperglyceridemia, endogenous E78.2
  dietary counseling and surveillance Z71.3
Hyperchylia gastrica, psychogenic F45.8
Hyperchylomicronemia (familial) (primary)
  E78.3
  with hyperbetalipoproteinemia E78.3
Hypercoagulable (state) D68.59
  activated protein C resistance D68.51
  antithrombin (III) deficiency D68.59
  factor V Leiden mutation D68.51
  primary NEC D68.59
  protein C deficiency D68.59
  protein S deficiency D68.59
  prothrombin gene mutation D68.52

Hypercoagulable (*Continued*)
  secondary D68.69
  specified NEC D68.69
Hypercoagulation (state) D68.59
Hypercorticalism, pituitary-dependent E24.0
Hypercorticosolism —*see* Cushing's, syndrome
Hypercorticosteronism E24.2
  correct substance properly administered —*see*
    Table of ɖDrugs and ɕChemicals, by
    drug, adverse effect ◀▥
  overdose or wrong substance given or
    taken —*see* Table of ɖDrugs and
    ɕChemicals, by drug, poisoning ◀▥
Hypercortisonism E24.2
  correct substance properly administered —*see*
    Table of ɖDrugs and ɕChemicals, by
    drug, adverse effect ◀▥
  overdose or wrong substance given or
    taken —*see* Table of ɖDrugs and
    ɕChemicals, by drug, poisoning ◀▥
Hyperekplexia Q89.8
Hyperelectrolytemia E87.8
Hyperemesis R11.10
  with nausea R11.2
  gravidarum (mild) O21.0
    with
      carbohydrate depletion O21.1
      dehydration O21.1
      electrolyte imbalance O21.1
      metabolic disturbance O21.1
      severe (with metabolic disturbance) O21.1
  projectile R11.12
  psychogenic F45.8
Hyperemia (acute) (passive) R68.89
  anal mucosa K62.89
  bladder N32.89
  cerebral I67.89
  conjunctiva H11.43-
  ear internal, acute —*see* subcategory
    H83.0
  enteric K59.8
  eye —*see* Hyperemia, conjunctiva
  eyelid (active) (passive) —*see* Disorder,
    eyelid, specified type NEC
  intestine K59.8
  iris —*see* Disorder, iris, vascular
  kidney N28.89
  labyrinth —*see* subcategory H83.0
  liver (active) K76.89
  lung (passive) —*see* Edema, lung
  pulmonary (passive) —*see* Edema, lung
  renal N28.89
  retina H35.89
  stomach K31.89
Hyperesthesia (body surface) R20.3
  larynx (reflex) J38.7
    hysterical F44.89
  pharynx (reflex) J39.2
    hysterical F44.89
Hyperestrogenism (drug-induced) (iatrogenic)
  E28.0
Hyperexplexia Q89.8
Hyperfibrinolysis —*see* Fibrinolysis
Hyperfructosemia E74.19
Hyperfunction
  adrenal cortex, not associated with Cushing's
    syndrome E27.0
  medulla E27.5
    adrenomedullary E27.5
  virilism E25.9
    congenital E25.0
  ovarian E28.8
  pancreas K86.8
  parathyroid (gland) E21.3
  pituitary (gland) (anterior) E22.9
    specified NEC E22.8
  polyglandular E31.1
  testicular E29.0
Hypergammaglobulinemia D89.2
  polyclonal D89.0
  Waldenström D89.0

Hypergastrinemia E16.4
Hyperglobulinemia R77.1
Hyperglycemia, hyperglycemic (transient)
    R73.9
    coma —see Diabetes, by type, with coma
    postpancreatectomy E89.1
Hyperglyceridemia (endogenous) (essential)
    (familial) (hereditary) (pure) E78.1
    mixed E78.3
Hyperglycinemia (non-ketotic) E72.51
Hypergonadism
    ovarian E28.8
    testicular (primary) (infantile) E29.0
Hyperheparinemia D68.32
Hyperhidrosis, hyperidrosis R61
    focal
        primary L74.519
            axilla L74.510
            face L74.511
            palms L74.512
            soles L74.513
        secondary L74.52
    generalized R61
    localized
        primary L74.519
            axilla L74.510
            face L74.511
            palms L74.512
            soles L74.513
        secondary L74.52
    psychogenic F45.8
    secondary R61
        focal L74.52
Hyperhistidinemia E70.41
Hyperhomocysteinemia E72.11
Hyperhydroxyprolinemia E72.59
Hyperinsulinism (functional) E16.1
    with
        coma (hypoglycemic) E15
        encephalopathy E16.1 [G94]
    ectopic E16.1
    therapeutic misadventure (from
        administration of insulin) —see
        subcategory T38.3
Hyperkalemia E87.5
Hyperkeratosis (see also Keratosis) L85.9
    cervix N88.0
    due to yaws (early) (late) (palmar or plantar)
        A66.3
    follicularis Q82.8
        penetrans (in cutem) L87.0
    palmoplantaris climacterica L85.1
    pinta A67.1
    senile (with pruritus) L57.0
    universalis congenita Q80.8
    vocal cord J38.3
    vulva N90.4
Hyperkinesia, hyperkinetic (disease) (reaction)
        (syndrome) (childhood) (adolescence) —
        see also Disorder, attention-deficit
        hyperactivity
    heart I51.89
Hyperleucine-isoleucinemia E71.19
Hyperlipemia, hyperlipidemia E78.5
    combined E78.2
        familial E78.4
    group
        A E78.0
        B E78.1
        C E78.2
        D E78.3
    mixed E78.2
    specified NEC E78.4
Hyperlipidosis E75.6
    hereditary NEC E75.5
Hyperlipoproteinemia E78.5
    Fredrickson's type
        I E78.3
        IIa E78.0
        IIb E78.2
        III E78.2

Hyperlipoproteinemia (Continued)
    Fredrickson's type (Continued)
        IV E78.1
        V E78.3
    low-density-lipoprotein-type (LDL) E78.0
    very-low-density-lipoprotein-type (VLDL)
        E78.1
Hyperlucent lung, unilateral J43.0
Hyperlysinemia E72.3
Hypermagnesemia E83.41
    neonatal P71.8
Hypermenorrhea N92.0
Hypermethioninemia E72.19
Hypermetropia (congenital) H52.0-
Hypermobility, hypermotility
    cecum —see Syndrome, irritable bowel
    coccyx —see subcategory M53.2
    colon —see Syndrome, irritable bowel
        psychogenic F45.8
    ileum K58.9
    intestine (see also Syndrome, irritable bowel)
        K58.9
        psychogenic F45.8
    meniscus (knee) —see Derangement, knee,
        meniscus
    scapula —see Instability, joint, shoulder
    stomach K31.89
        psychogenic F45.8
    syndrome M35.7
    urethra N36.41
        with intrinsic sphincter deficiency N36.43
Hypernasality R49.21
Hypernatremia E87.0
Hypernephroma C64.-
Hyperopia —see Hypermetropia
Hyperorexia nervosa F50.2
Hyperornithinemia E72.4
Hyperosmia R43.1
Hyperosmolality E87.0
Hyperostosis (monomelic) —see also Disorder,
        bone, density and structure, specified NEC
    ankylosing (spine) M48.10
        cervical region M48.12
        cervicothoracic region M48.13
        lumbar region M48.16
        lumbosacral region M48.17
        multiple sites M48.19
        occipito-atlanto-axial region M48.11
        sacrococcygeal region M48.18
        thoracic region M48.14
        thoracolumbar region M48.15
    cortical (skull) M85.2
        infantile M89.8X-
    frontal, internal of skull M85.2
    interna frontalis M85.2
    skeletal, diffuse idiopathic —see
        Hyperostosis, ankylosing
    skull M85.2
        congenital Q75.8
    vertebral, ankylosing —see Hyperostosis,
        ankylosing
Hyperovarism E28.8
Hyperoxaluria (primary) E72.53
Hyperparathyroidism E21.3
    primary E21.0
    secondary (renal) N25.81
        non-renal E21.1
    specified NEC E21.2
    tertiary E21.2
Hyperpathia R20.8
Hyperperistalsis R19.2
    psychogenic F45.8
Hyperpermeability, capillary I78.8
Hyperphagia R63.2
Hyperphenylalaninemia NEC E70.1
Hyperphoria (alternating) H50.53
Hyperphosphatemia E83.39
Hyperpiesis, hyperpiesia —see Hypertension
Hyperpigmentation —see also Pigmentation
    melanin NEC L81.4
    postinflammatory L81.0

Hyperpinealism E34.8
Hyperpituitarism E22.9
Hyperplasia, hyperplastic
    adenoids J35.2
    adrenal (capsule) (cortex) (gland) E27.8
        with
            sexual precocity (male) E25.9
                congenital E25.0
            virilism, adrenal E25.9
                congenital E25.0
            virilization (female) E25.9
                congenital E25.0
        congenital E25.0
        salt-losing E25.0
    adrenomedullary E27.5
    angiolymphoid, eosinophilia (ALHE) D18.01
    appendix (lymphoid) K38.0
    artery, fibromuscular I77.3
    bone —see also Hypertrophy, bone
        marrow D75.89
    breast —see also Hypertrophy, breast
        ductal (atypical) N60.9-
    C-cell, thyroid E07.0
    cementation (tooth) (teeth) K03.4
    cervical gland R59.0
    cervix (uteri) (basal cell) (endometrium)
        (polypoid) —see also Dysplasia, cervix
        congenital Q51.828
    clitoris, congenital Q52.6
    denture K06.2
    endocervicitis N72
    endometrium, endometrial (adenomatous)
        (benign) (cystic) (glandular) (glandular-
        cystic) (polypoid) N85.00
        with atypia N85.02
        cervix —see Dysplasia, cervix
        complex (without atypia) N85.01
        simple (without atypia) N85.01
    epithelial L85.9
        focal, oral, including tongue K13.29
        nipple N62
        skin L85.9
        tongue K13.29
        vaginal wall N89.3
    erythroid D75.89
    fibromuscular of artery (carotid) (renal) I77.3
    genital
        female NEC N94.89
        male N50.8
    gingiva K06.1
    glandularis cystica uteri (interstitialis) (see also
        Hyperplasia, endometrial) N85.00- ◀
    gum K06.1
    hymen, congenital Q52.4
    irritative, edentulous (alveolar) K06.2
    jaw M26.09
        alveolar M26.79
        lower M26.03
            alveolar M26.72
        upper M26.01
            alveolar M26.71
    kidney (congenital) Q63.3
    labia N90.6
        epithelial N90.3
    liver (congenital) Q44.7
        nodular, focal K76.89
    lymph gland or node R59.9
    mandible, mandibular M26.03
        alveolar M26.72
        unilateral condylar M27.8
    maxilla, maxillary M26.01
        alveolar M26.71
    myometrium, myometrial N85.2
    neuroendocrine cell, of infancy J84.841
    nose
        lymphoid J34.89
        polypoid J33.9
    oral mucosa (irritative) K13.6
    organ or site, congenital NEC —see Anomaly,
        by site
    ovary N83.8

◀ New   ◀▬▬ Revised   ~~deleted~~ Deleted

Hyperplasia, hyperplastic *(Continued)*
  palate, papillary (irritative) K13.6
  pancreatic islet cells E16.9
    alpha E16.8
      with excess
        gastrin E16.4
        glucagon E16.3
    beta E16.1
  parathyroid (gland) E21.0
  pharynx (lymphoid) J39.2
  prostate (adenofibromatous) (nodular)
    N40.0
    with lower urinary tract symptoms (LUTS)
      N40.1
    without lower urinary tract symptoms
      (LUTS) N40.0
  renal artery I77.89
  reticulo-endothelial (cell) D75.89
  salivary gland (any) K11.1
  Schimmelbusch's —*see* Mastopathy,
    cystic
  suprarenal capsule (gland) E27.8
  thymus (gland) (persistent) E32.0
  thyroid (gland) —*see* Goiter
  tonsils (faucial) (infective) (lingual)
    (lymphoid) J35.1
    with adenoids J35.3
  unilateral condylar M27.8
  uterus, uterine N85.2
    endometrium (glandular) *(see also*
      Hyperplasia, endometrial)
      N85.00- ◀▥
  vulva N90.6
    epithelial N90.3
Hyperpnea —*see* Hyperventilation
Hyperpotassemia E87.5
Hyperprebetalipoproteinemia (familial)
  E78.1
Hyperprolactinemia E22.1
Hyperprolinemia (type I) (type II) E72.59
Hyperproteinemia E88.09
Hyperprothrombinemia, causing coagulation
  factor deficiency D68.4
Hyperpyrexia R50.9
  heat (effects) T67.0
  malignant, due to anesthetic T88.3
  rheumatic —*see* Fever, rheumatic
  unknown origin R50.9
Hyper-reflexia R29.2
Hypersalivation K11.7
Hypersecretion
  ACTH (not associated with Cushing's
    syndrome) E27.0
    pituitary E24.0
  adrenaline E27.5
  adrenomedullary E27.5
  androgen (testicular) E29.0
    ovarian (drug-induced) (iatrogenic)
      E28.1
  calcitonin E07.0
  catecholamine E27.5
  corticoadrenal E24.9
  cortisol E24.9
  epinephrine E27.5
  estrogen E28.0
  gastric K31.89
    psychogenic F45.8
  gastrin E16.4
  glucagon E16.3
  hormone (s)
    ACTH (not associated with Cushing's
      syndrome) E27.0
      pituitary E24.0
    antidiuretic E22.2
    growth E22.0
    intestinal NEC E34.1
    ovarian androgen E28.1
    pituitary E22.9
    testicular E29.0
    thyroid stimulating E05.80
      with thyroid storm E05.81

Hypersecretion *(Continued)*
  insulin —*see* Hyperinsulinism
  lacrimal glands —*see* Epiphora
  medulloadrenal E27.5
  milk O92.6
  ovarian androgens E28.1
  salivary gland (any) K11.7
  thyrocalcitonin E07.0
  upper respiratory J39.8
Hypersegmentation, leukocytic, hereditary
  D72.0
Hypersensitive, hypersensitiveness,
  hypersensitivity —*see also* Allergy
  carotid sinus G90.01
  colon —*see* Irritable, colon
  drug T88.7
  gastrointestinal K52.2
    psychogenic F45.8
  labyrinth —*see* subcategory H83.2
  pain R20.8
  pneumonitis —*see* Pneumonitis,
    allergic
  reaction T78.40
    upper respiratory tract NEC J39.3
Hypersomnia (organic) G47.10
  due to
    alcohol
      abuse F10.182
      dependence F10.282
      use F10.982
    amphetamines
      abuse F15.182
      dependence F15.282
      use F15.982
    caffeine
      abuse F15.182
      dependence F15.282
      use F15.982
    cocaine
      abuse F14.182
      dependence F14.282
      use F14.982
    drug NEC
      abuse F19.182
      dependence F19.282
      use F19.982
    medical condition G47.14
    mental disorder F51.13
    opioid
      abuse F11.182
      dependence F11.282
      use F11.982
    psychoactive substance NEC
      abuse F19.182
      dependence F19.282
      use F19.982
    sedative, hypnotic, or anxiolytic
      abuse F13.182
      dependence F13.282
      use F13.982
    stimulant NEC
      abuse F15.182
      dependence F15.282
      use F15.982
  idiopathic G47.11
    with long sleep time G47.11
    without long sleep time G47.12
  menstrual related G47.13
  nonorganic origin F51.11
    specified NEC F51.19
  not due to a substance or known
    physiological condition F51.11
    specified NEC F51.19
  primary F51.11
  recurrent G47.13
  specified NEC G47.19
Hypersplenia, hypersplenism D73.1
Hyperstimulation, ovaries (associated with
  induced ovulation) N98.1
Hypersusceptibility —*see* Allergy
Hypertelorism (ocular) (orbital) Q75.2

Hypertension, hypertensive (accelerated)
  (benign) (essential) (idiopathic)
  (malignant) (systemic) I10
  with
    heart involvement (conditions in
      I51.4-I51.9 due to hypertension) —*see*
      Hypertension, heart ◀▥
    kidney involvement —*see* Hypertension,
      kidney
  benign, intracranial G93.2
  borderline R03.0
  cardiorenal (disease) I13.10
    with heart failure I13.0
      with stage 1 through stage 4 chronic
        kidney disease I13.0
      with stage 5 or end stage renal disease
        I13.2
    without heart failure I13.10
      with stage 1 through stage 4 chronic
        kidney disease I13.10
      with stage 5 or end stage renal disease
        I13.11
  cardiovascular
    disease (arteriosclerotic) (sclerotic) —*see*
      Hypertension, heart
    renal (disease) —*see* Hypertension,
      cardiorenal
  chronic venous —*see* Hypertension, venous
    (chronic)
  complicating
    childbirth (labor) O10.92
      with
        heart disease O10.12
          with renal disease O10.32
        renal disease O10.22
          with heart disease O10.32
        essential O10.02
        secondary O10.42
    pregnancy O16.-
      with edema *(see also* Pre-eclampsia) O14.9-
      gestational (pregnancy induced)
        (transient) (without proteinuria)
        O13.-
        with proteinuria O14.9-
          mild pre-eclampsia O14.0-
          moderate pre-eclampsia O14.0-
          severe pre-eclampsia O14.1-
            with hemolysis, elevated liver
              enzymes and low platelet
              count (HELLP) O14.2-
      pre-existing O10.91-
        with
          heart disease O10.11-
            with renal disease O10.31-
          pre-eclampsia O11.-
          renal disease O10.21-
            with heart disease O10.31-
          essential O10.01-
          secondary O10.41-
      puerperium pre-existing O10.93 ◀▥
        with
          heart disease O10.13
            with renal disease O10.33
          renal disease O10.23
            with heart disease O10.33
          essential O10.03
          pregnancy-induced O13.9 ◀
          secondary O10.43
  due to
    endocrine disorders I15.2
    pheochromocytoma I15.2
    renal disorders NEC I15.1
      arterial I15.0
    renovascular disorders I15.0
    specified disease NEC I15.8
  encephalopathy I67.4
  gestational (without significant proteinuria)
    (pregnancy-induced) (transient) O13.-
    with significant proteinuria —*see*
      Pre-eclampsia
  Goldblatt's I70.1

Hypertension, hypertensive *(Continued)*
  heart (disease) (conditions in I51.4-I51.9 due to hypertension) I11.9
    with
      heart failure (congestive) I11.0
      kidney disease (chronic) —*see* Hypertension, cardiorenal
  intracranial (benign) G93.2
  kidney I12.9
    with
      heart disease —*see* Hypertension, cardiorenal
      stage 1 through stage 4 chronic kidney disease I12.9
      stage 5 chronic kidney disease (CKD) or end stage renal disease (ESRD) I12.0
  lesser circulation I27.0
  newborn P29.2
    pulmonary (persistent) P29.3
  ocular H40.05-
  pancreatic duct — code to underlying condition
    with chronic pancreatitis K86.1
  portal (due to chronic liver disease) (idiopathic) K76.6
    gastropathy K31.89
    in (due to) schistosomiasis (bilharziasis) B65.9 [K77]
  postoperative I97.3
  psychogenic F45.8
  pulmonary (artery) (secondary) NEC I27.2
    with
      cor pulmonale (chronic) I27.2
        acute I26.09
      right heart ventricular strain/failure I27.2
        acute I26.09
    of newborn (persistent) P29.3
    primary (idiopathic) I27.0
  renal —*see* Hypertension, kidney
  renovascular I15.0
  secondary NEC I15.9
    due to
      endocrine disorders I15.2
      pheochromocytoma I15.2
      renal disorders NEC I15.1
        arterial I15.0
      renovascular disorders I15.0
    specified NEC I15.8
  venous (chronic)
    due to
      deep vein thrombosis —*see* Syndrome, postthrombotic
    idiopathic I87.309
      with
        inflammation I87.32-
          with ulcer I87.33-
        specified complication NEC I87.39-
        ulcer I87.31-
          with inflammation I87.33-
      asymptomatic I87.30-
Hypertensive urgency —*see* Hypertension
Hyperthecosis ovary E28.8
Hyperthermia (of unknown origin) —*see also* Hyperpyrexia
  malignant, due to anesthesia T88.3
  newborn P81.9
    environmental P81.0
Hyperthyroid (recurrent) —*see* Hyperthyroidism
Hyperthyroidism (latent) (pre-adult) (recurrent) E05.90
  with
    goiter (diffuse) E05.00
      with thyroid storm E05.01
      nodular (multinodular) E05.20
        with thyroid storm E05.21
        uninodular E05.10
          with thyroid storm E05.11
    storm E05.91

Hyperthyroidism *(Continued)*
  due to ectopic thyroid tissue E05.30
    with thyroid storm E05.31
  neonatal, transitory P72.1
  specified NEC E05.80
    with thyroid storm E05.81
Hypertony, hypertonia, hypertonicity
  bladder N31.8
  congenital P94.1
  stomach K31.89
    psychogenic F45.8
  uterus, uterine (contractions) (complicating delivery) O62.4
Hypertrichosis L68.9
  congenital Q84.2
  eyelid H02.869
    left H02.866
      lower H02.865
      upper H02.864
    right H02.863
      lower H02.862
      upper H02.861
  lanuginosa Q84.2
    acquired L68.1
  localized L68.2
  specified NEC L68.8
Hypertriglyceridemia, essential E78.1
Hypertrophy, hypertrophic
  adenofibromatous, prostate —*see* Enlargement, enlarged, prostate
  adenoids (infective) J35.2
    with tonsils J35.3
  adrenal cortex E27.8
  alveolar process or ridge —*see* Anomaly, alveolar
  anal papillae K62.89
  artery I77.89
    congenital NEC Q27.8
      digestive system Q27.8
      lower limb Q27.8
      specified site NEC Q27.8
      upper limb Q27.8
  auricular —*see* Hypertrophy, cardiac
  Bartholin's gland N75.8
  bile duct (common) (hepatic) K83.8
  bladder (sphincter) (trigone) N32.89
  bone M89.30
    carpus M89.34-
    clavicle M89.31-
    femur M89.35-
    fibula M89.36-
    finger M89.34-
    humerus M89.32-
    ilium M89.359
    ischium M89.359
    metacarpus M89.34-
    metatarsus M89.37-
    multiple sites M89.39
    neck M89.38
    radius M89.33-
    rib M89.38
    scapula M89.31-
    skull M89.38
    tarsus M89.37-
    tibia M89.36-
    toe M89.37-
    ulna M89.33-
    vertebra M89.38
  brain G93.89
  breast N62
    cystic —*see* Mastopathy, cystic
    newborn P83.4
    pubertal, massive N62
    puerperal, postpartum —*see* Disorder, breast, specified type NEC
    senile (parenchymatous) N62
  cardiac (chronic) (idiopathic) I51.7
    with rheumatic fever (conditions in I00)
      active I01.8
      inactive or quiescent (with chorea) I09.89
    congenital NEC Q24.8

Hypertrophy, hypertrophic *(Continued)*
  cardiac *(Continued)*
    fatty —*see* Degeneration, myocardial
    hypertensive —*see* Hypertension, heart
    rheumatic (with chorea) I09.89
      active or acute I01.8
        with chorea I02.0
    valve —*see* Endocarditis
  cartilage —*see* Disorder, cartilage, specified type NEC
  cecum —*see* Megacolon
  cervix (uteri) N88.8
    congenital Q51.828
    elongation N88.4
  clitoris (cirrhotic) N90.89
    congenital Q52.6
  colon —*see also* Megacolon
    congenital Q43.2
  conjunctiva, lymphoid H11.89
  corpora cavernosa N48.89
  cystic duct K82.8
  duodenum K31.89
  endometrium (glandular) (see also Hyperplasia, endometrial) N85.00- ◀▥
    cervix N88.8
  epididymis N50.8
  esophageal hiatus (congenital) Q79.1
    with hernia —*see* Hernia, hiatal
  eyelid —*see* Disorder, eyelid, specified type NEC
  fat pad E65
    knee (infrapatellar) (popliteal) (prepatellar) (retropatellar) M79.4
  foot (congenital) Q74.2
  frenulum, frenum (tongue) K14.8
    lip K13.0
  gallbladder K82.8
  gastric mucosa K29.60
    with bleeding K29.61
  gland, glandular R59.9
    generalized R59.1
    localized R59.0
  gum (mucous membrane) K06.1
  heart (idiopathic) —*see also* Hypertrophy, cardiac
    valve (see also Endocarditis) I38
  hemifacial Q67.4
  hepatic —*see* Hypertrophy, liver
  hiatus (esophageal) Q79.1
  hilus gland R59.0
  hymen, congenital Q52.4
  ileum K63.89
  intestine NEC K63.89
  jejunum K63.89
  kidney (compensatory) N28.81
    congenital Q63.3
  labium (majus) (minus) N90.6
  ligament —*see* Disorder, ligament
  lingual tonsil (infective) J35.1
    with adenoids J35.3
  lip K13.0
    congenital Q18.6
  liver R16.0
    acute K76.89
    cirrhotic —*see* Cirrhosis, liver
    congenital Q44.7
    fatty —*see* Fatty, liver
  lymph, lymphatic gland R59.9
    generalized R59.1
    localized R59.0
    tuberculous —*see* Tuberculosis, lymph gland
  mammary gland —*see* Hypertrophy, breast
  Meckel's diverticulum (congenital) Q43.0
    malignant —*see* Table of Neoplasms, small intestine, malignant
  median bar —*see* Hyperplasia, prostate
  meibomian gland —*see* Chalazion
  meniscus, knee, congenital Q74.1
  metatarsal head —*see* Hypertrophy, bone, metatarsus

◀ New   ◀▥ Revised   ~~deleted~~ Deleted

Hypertrophy, hypertrophic *(Continued)*
  metatarsus —*see* Hypertrophy, bone,
      metatarsus
  mucous membrane
    alveolar ridge K06.2
    gum K06.1
    nose (turbinate) J34.3
  muscle M62.89
  muscular coat, artery I77.89
  myocardium —*see also* Hypertrophy, cardiac
    idiopathic I42.2
  myometrium N85.2
  nail L60.2
    congenital Q84.5
  nasal J34.89
    alae J34.89
    bone J34.89
    cartilage J34.89
    mucous membrane (septum) J34.3
    sinus J34.89
    turbinate J34.3
  nasopharynx, lymphoid (infectional) (tissue)
      (wall) J35.2
  nipple N62
  organ or site, congenital NEC —*see* Anomaly,
      by site - ovary N83.8
  palate (hard) M27.8
    soft K13.79
  pancreas, congenital Q45.3
  parathyroid (gland) E21.0
  parotid gland K11.1
  penis N48.89
  pharyngeal tonsil J35.2
  pharynx J39.2
    lymphoid (infectional) (tissue) (wall)
        J35.2
  pituitary (anterior) (fossa) (gland) E23.6
  prepuce (congenital) N47.8
    female N90.89
  prostate —*see* Enlargement, enlarged,
      prostate
    congenital Q55.4
  pseudomuscular G71.0
  pylorus (adult) (muscle) (sphincter) K31.1
    congenital or infantile Q40.0
  rectal, rectum (sphincter) K62.89
  rhinitis (turbinate) J31.0
  salivary gland (any) K11.1
    congenital Q38.4
  scaphoid (tarsal) —*see* Hypertrophy, bone,
      tarsus
  scar L91.0
  scrotum N50.8
  seminal vesicle N50.8
  sigmoid —*see* Megacolon
  skin L91.9
    specified NEC L91.8
  spermatic cord N50.8
  spleen —*see* Splenomegaly
  spondylitis —*see* Spondylosis
  stomach K31.89
  sublingual gland K11.1
  submandibular gland K11.1
  suprarenal cortex (gland) E27.8
  synovial NEC M67.20
    acromioclavicular M67.21-
    ankle M67.27-
    elbow M67.22-
    foot M67.27-
    hand M67.24-
    hip M67.25-
    knee M67.26-
    multiple sites M67.29
    specified site NEC M67.28
    wrist M67.23-
  tendon —*see* Disorder, tendon, specified type
      NEC
  testis N44.8
    congenital Q55.29
  thymic, thymus (gland) (congenital)
      E32.0

Hypertrophy, hypertrophic *(Continued)*
  thyroid (gland) —*see* Goiter
  toe (congenital) Q74.2
    acquired —*see also* Deformity, toe, specified
        NEC
  tongue K14.8
    congenital Q38.2
    papillae (foliate) K14.3
  tonsils (faucial) (infective) (lingual)
      (lymphoid) J35.1
    with adenoids J35.3
  tunica vaginalis N50.8
  ureter N28.89
  urethra N36.8
  uterus N85.2
    neck (with elongation) N88.4
    puerperal O90.89
  uvula K13.79
  vagina N89.8
  vas deferens N50.8
  vein I87.8
  ventricle, ventricular (heart) —*see also*
      Hypertrophy, cardiac
    congenital Q24.8
    in tetralogy of Fallot Q21.3
  verumontanum N36.8
  vocal cord J38.3
  vulva N90.6
    stasis (nonfilarial) N90.6
Hypertropia H50.2-
Hypertyrosinemia E70.21
Hyperuricemia (asymptomatic) E79.0
Hypervalinemia E71.19
Hyperventilation (tetany) R06.4
  hysterical F45.8
  psychogenic F45.8
  syndrome F45.8
Hypervitaminosis (dietary) NEC E67.8
  A E67.0
    administered as drug (prolonged intake) —
        see Table of Drugs and Chemicals,
        vitamins, adverse effect ◄▥
    overdose or wrong substance given or
        taken —*see* Table of Drugs and
        Chemicals, vitamins, poisoning ◄▥
  B6 E67.2
  D E67.3
    administered as drug (prolonged intake) —
        see Table of Drugs and Chemicals,
        vitamins, adverse effect ◄▥
    overdose or wrong substance given or
        taken —*see* Table of Drugs and
        Chemicals, vitamins, poisoning ◄▥
  K E67.8
    administered as drug (prolonged intake) —
        see Table of Drugs and Chemicals,
        vitamins, adverse effect ◄▥
    overdose or wrong substance given or
        taken —*see* Table of Drugs and
        Chemicals, vitamins, poisoning ◄▥
Hypervolemia E87.70
  specified NEC E87.79
Hypesthesia R20.1
  cornea —*see* Anesthesia, cornea
Hyphema H21.0-
  traumatic S05.1-
Hypoacidity, gastric K31.89
  psychogenic F45.8
Hypoadrenalism, hypoadrenia E27.40
  primary E27.1
  tuberculous A18.7
Hypoadrenocorticism E27.40
  pituitary E23.0
  primary E27.1
Hypoalbuminemia E88.09
Hypoaldosteronism E27.40
Hypoalphalipoproteinemia E78.6
Hypobarism T70.29
Hypobaropathy T70.29
Hypobetalipoproteinemia (familial)
    E78.6

Hypocalcemia E83.51
  dietary E58
  neonatal P71.1
    due to cow's milk P71.0
    phosphate-loading (newborn) P71.1
Hypochloremia E87.8
Hypochlorhydria K31.89
  neurotic F45.8
  psychogenic F45.8
Hypochondria, hypochondriac,
    hypochondriasis (reaction) F45.21
  sleep F51.03
Hypochondrogenesis Q77.0
Hypochondroplasia Q77.4
Hypochromasia, blood cells D50.8
Hypodontia —*see* Anodontia
Hypoeosinophilia D72.89
Hypoesthesia R20.1
Hypofibrinogenemia D68.8
  acquired D65
  congenital (hereditary) D68.2
Hypofunction
  adrenocortical E27.40
    drug-induced E27.3
    postprocedural E89.6
    primary E27.1
  adrenomedullary, postprocedural E89.6
  cerebral R29.818
  corticoadrenal NEC E27.40
  intestinal K59.8
  labyrinth —*see* subcategory H83.2
  ovary E28.39
  pituitary (gland) (anterior) E23.0
  testicular E29.1
    postprocedural (postsurgical)
        (postirradiation) (iatrogenic) E89.5
Hypogalactia O92.4
Hypogammaglobulinemia (*see also*
    Agammaglobulinemia) D80.1
  hereditary D80.0
  nonfamilial D80.1
  transient, of infancy D80.7
Hypogenitalism (congenital) —*see*
    Hypogonadism
Hypoglossia Q38.3
Hypoglycemia (spontaneous) E16.2
  coma E15
    diabetic —*see* Diabetes, coma
  diabetic —*see* Diabetes, hypoglycemia
  dietary counseling and surveillance Z71.3
  drug-induced E16.0
    with coma (nondiabetic) E15
  due to insulin E16.0
    with coma (nondiabetic) E15
      therapeutic misadventure —*see*
          subcategory T38.3
  functional, nonhyperinsulinemic E16.1
  iatrogenic E16.0
    with coma (nondiabetic) E15
  in infant of diabetic mother P70.1
    gestational diabetes P70.0
  infantile E16.1
  leucine-induced E71.19
  neonatal (transitory) P70.4
    iatrogenic P70.3
  reactive (not drug-induced) E16.1
  transitory neonatal P70.4
Hypogonadism
  female E28.39
  hypogonadotropic E23.0
  male E29.1
  ovarian (primary) E28.39
  pituitary E23.0
  testicular (primary) E29.1
Hypohidrosis, hypoidrosis L74.4
Hypoinsulinemia, postprocedural E89.1
Hypokalemia E87.6
Hypoleukocytosis —*see* Agranulocytosis
Hypolipoproteinemia (alpha) (beta) E78.6
Hypomagnesemia E83.42
  neonatal P71.2

Hypomania, hypomanic reaction F30.8
Hypomenorrhea —*see* Oligomenorrhea
Hypometabolism R63.8
Hypomotility
 gastrointestinal (tract) K31.89
  psychogenic F45.8
 intestine K59.8
  psychogenic F45.8
 stomach K31.89
  psychogenic F45.8
Hyponasality R49.22
Hyponatremia E87.1
Hypo-osmolality E87.1
Hypo-ovarianism, hypo-ovarism E28.39
Hypoparathyroidism E20.9
 familial E20.8
 idiopathic E20.0
 neonatal, transitory P71.4
 postprocedural E89.2
 specified NEC E20.8
Hypoperfusion (in)
 newborn P96.89
Hypopharyngitis —*see* Laryngopharyngitis
Hypophoria H50.53
Hypophosphatemia, hypophosphatasia
  (acquired) (congenital) (renal) E83.39
 familial E83.31
Hypophyseal, hypophysis —*see also* condition
 dwarfism E23.0
 gigantism E22.0
Hypopiesis —*see* Hypotension
Hypopinealism E34.8
Hypopituitarism (juvenile) E23.0
 drug-induced E23.1
 due to
  hypophysectomy E89.3
  radiotherapy E89.3
 iatrogenic NEC E23.1
 postirradiation E89.3
 postpartum E23.0
 postprocedural E89.3
Hypoplasia, hypoplastic
 adrenal (gland), congenital Q89.1
 alimentary tract, congenital Q45.8
  upper Q40.8
 anus, anal (canal) Q42.3
  with fistula Q42.2
 aorta, aortic Q25.4
  ascending, in hypoplastic left heart
   syndrome Q23.4
  valve Q23.1
   in hypoplastic left heart syndrome
    Q23.4
 areola, congenital Q83.8
 arm (congenital) —*see* Defect, reduction,
  upper limb
 artery (peripheral) Q27.8
  brain (congenital) Q28.3
  coronary Q24.5
  digestive system Q27.8
  lower limb Q27.8
  pulmonary Q25.79
   functional, unilateral J43.0
  retinal (congenital) Q14.1
  specified site NEC Q27.8
  umbilical Q27.0
  upper limb Q27.8
 auditory canal Q17.8
  causing impairment of hearing Q16.9
 biliary duct or passage Q44.5
 bone NOS Q79.9
  face Q75.8
  marrow D61.9
   megakaryocytic D69.49
  skull —*see* Hypoplasia, skull
 brain Q02
  gyri Q04.3
  part of Q04.3
 breast (areola) N64.82
 bronchus Q32.4
 cardiac Q24.8

Hypoplasia, hypoplastic (*Continued*)
 carpus —*see* Defect, reduction, upper limb,
  specified type NEC
 cartilage hair Q78.5
 cecum Q42.8
 cementum K00.4
 cephalic Q02
 cerebellum Q04.3
 cervix (uteri), congenital Q51.821
 clavicle (congenital) Q74.0
 coccyx Q76.49
 colon Q42.9
  specified NEC Q42.8
 corpus callosum Q04.0
 cricoid cartilage Q31.2
 digestive organ (s) or tract NEC Q45.8
  upper (congenital) Q40.8
 ear (auricle) (lobe) Q17.2
  middle Q16.4
 enamel of teeth (neonatal) (postnatal)
   (prenatal) K00.4
 endocrine (gland) NEC Q89.2
 endometrium N85.8
 epididymis (congenital) Q55.4
 epiglottis Q31.2
 erythroid, congenital D61.01
 esophagus (congenital) Q39.8
 eustachian tube Q17.8
 eye Q11.2
 eyelid (congenital) Q10.3
 face Q18.8
  bone (s) Q75.8
 femur (congenital) —*see* Defect,
   reduction, lower limb, specified
   type NEC
 fibula (congenital) —*see* Defect,
   reduction, lower limb, specified
   type NEC
 finger (congenital) —*see* Defect,
   reduction, upper limb, specified
   type NEC
 focal dermal Q82.8
 foot —*see* Defect, reduction, lower limb,
  specified type NEC
 gallbladder Q44.0
 genitalia, genital organ (s)
  female, congenital Q52.8
   external Q52.79
   internal NEC Q52.8
  in adiposogenital dystrophy E23.6
 glottis Q31.2
 hair Q84.2
 hand (congenital) —*see* Defect, reduction,
  upper limb, specified type NEC
 heart Q24.8
 humerus (congenital) —*see* Defect,
   reduction, upper limb, specified
   type NEC
 intestine (small) Q41.9
  large Q42.9
   specified NEC Q42.8
 jaw M26.09
  alveolar M26.79
  lower M26.04
   alveolar M26.74
  upper M26.02
   alveolar M26.73
 kidney (s) Q60.5
  bilateral Q60.4
  unilateral Q60.3
 labium (majus) (minus), congenital Q52.79
 larynx Q31.2
 left heart syndrome Q23.4
 leg (congenital) —*see* Defect, reduction, lower
  limb
 limb Q73.8
  lower (congenital) —*see* Defect, reduction,
   lower limb
  upper (congenital) —*see* Defect, reduction,
   upper limb
 liver Q44.7

Hypoplasia, hypoplastic (*Continued*)
 lung (lobe) (not associated with short
   gestation) Q33.6
  associated with immaturity, low birth
   weight, prematurity, or short
   gestation P28.0
 mammary (areola), congenital Q83.8
 mandible, mandibular M26.04
  alveolar M26.74
  unilateral condylar M27.8
 maxillary M26.02
  alveolar M26.73
 medullary D61.9
 megakaryocytic D69.49
 metacarpus —*see* Defect, reduction, upper
  limb, specified type NEC
 metatarsus —*see* Defect, reduction, lower
  limb, specified type NEC
 muscle Q79.8
 nail (s) Q84.6
 nose, nasal Q30.1
 optic nerve H47.03-
 osseous meatus (ear) Q17.8
 ovary, congenital Q50.39
 pancreas Q45.0
 parathyroid (gland) Q89.2
 parotid gland Q38.4
 patella Q74.1
 pelvis, pelvic girdle Q74.2
 penis (congenital) Q55.62
 peripheral vascular system Q27.8
  digestive system Q27.8
  lower limb Q27.8
  specified site NEC Q27.8
  upper limb Q27.8
 pituitary (gland) (congenital) Q89.2
 pulmonary (not associated with short
   gestation) Q33.6
  artery, functional J43.0
  associated with short gestation P28.0
 radioulnar —*see* Defect, reduction, upper
  limb, specified type NEC
 radius —*see* Defect, reduction, upper limb
 rectum Q42.1
  with fistula Q42.0
 respiratory system NEC Q34.8
 rib Q76.6
 right heart syndrome Q22.6
 sacrum Q76.49
 scapula Q74.0
 scrotum Q55.1
 shoulder girdle Q74.0
 skin Q82.8
 skull (bone) Q75.8
  with
   anencephaly Q00.0
   encephalocele —*see* Encephalocele
   hydrocephalus Q03.9
    with spina bifida —*see* Spina bifida, by
     site, with hydrocephalus
   microcephaly Q02
 spinal (cord) (ventral horn cell) Q06.1
 spine Q76.49
 sternum Q76.7
 tarsus —*see* Defect, reduction, lower limb,
  specified type NEC
 testis Q55.1
 thymic, with immunodeficiency D82.1
 thymus (gland) Q89.2
  with immunodeficiency D82.1
 thyroid (gland) E03.1
  cartilage Q31.2
 tibiofibular (congenital) —*see* Defect,
   reduction, lower limb, specified type
   NEC
 toe —*see* Defect, reduction, lower limb,
  specified type NEC
 tongue Q38.3
 Turner's K00.4
 ulna (congenital) —*see* Defect, reduction,
  upper limb

◀ New   ◀▦ Revised   ~~deleted~~ Deleted

Hypoplasia, hypoplastic *(Continued)*
  umbilical artery Q27.0
  unilateral condylar M27.8
  ureter Q62.8
  uterus, congenital Q51.811
  vagina Q52.4
  vascular NEC peripheral Q27.8
    brain Q28.3
    digestive system Q27.8
    lower limb Q27.8
    specified site NEC Q27.8
    upper limb Q27.8
  vein (s) (peripheral) Q27.8
    brain Q28.3
    digestive system Q27.8
    great Q26.8
    lower limb Q27.8
    specified site NEC Q27.8
    upper limb Q27.8
  vena cava (inferior) (superior) Q26.8
  vertebra Q76.49
  vulva, congenital Q52.79
  zonule (ciliary) Q12.8
Hypopotassemia E87.6
Hypoproconvertinemia, congenital (hereditary) D68.2
Hypoproteinemia E77.8
Hypoprothrombinemia (congenital) (hereditary) (idiopathic) D68.2
  acquired D68.4
  newborn, transient P61.6
Hypoptyalism K11.7
Hypopyon (eye) (anterior chamber) —*see* Iridocyclitis, acute, hypopyon
Hypopyrexia R68.0
Hyporeflexia R29.2
Hyposecretion
  ACTH E23.0
  antidiuretic hormone E23.2
  ovary E28.39
  salivary gland (any) K11.7
  vasopressin E23.2
Hyposegmentation, leukocytic, hereditary D72.0
Hyposiderinemia D50.9
Hypospadias Q54.9
  balanic Q54.0
  coronal Q54.0
  glandular Q54.0
  penile Q54.1
  penoscrotal Q54.2

Hypospadias *(Continued)*
  perineal Q54.3
  specified NEC Q54.8
Hypospermatogenesis —*see* Oligospermia
Hyposplenism D73.0
Hypostasis pulmonary, passive —*see* Edema, lung
Hypostatic —*see* condition
Hyposthenuria N28.89
Hypotension (arterial) (constitutional) I95.9
  chronic I95.89
  drug-induced I95.2
  due to (of) hemodialysis I95.3
  iatrogenic I95.89
  idiopathic (permanent) I95.0
  intracranial, following ventricular shunting (ventriculostomy) G97.2
  intra-dialytic I95.3
  maternal, syndrome (following labor and delivery) O26.5-
  neurogenic, orthostatic G90.3
  orthostatic (chronic) I95.1
    due to drugs I95.2
    neurogenic G90.3
  postoperative I95.81
  postural I95.1
  specified NEC I95.89
Hypothermia (accidental) T68
  due to anesthesia, anesthetic T88.51
  low environmental temperature T68
  neonatal P80.9
    environmental (mild) NEC P80.8
    mild P80.8
    severe (chronic) (cold injury syndrome) P80.0
    specified NEC P80.8
  not associated with low environmental temperature R68.0
Hypothyroidism (acquired) E03.9
  congenital (without goiter) E03.1
    with goiter (diffuse) E03.0
  due to
    exogenous substance NEC E03.2
    iodine-deficiency, acquired E01.8
      subclinical E02
    irradiation therapy E89.0
    medicament NEC E03.2
    P-aminosalicylic acid (PAS) E03.2
    phenylbutazone E03.2
    resorcinol E03.2
    sulfonamide E03.2

Hypothyroidism *(Continued)*
  due to *(Continued)*
    surgery E89.0
    thiourea group drugs E03.2
  iatrogenic NEC E03.2
  iodine-deficiency (acquired) E01.8
    congenital —*see* Syndrome, iodine-deficiency, congenital
    subclinical E02
  neonatal, transitory P72.2
  postinfectious E03.3
  postirradiation E89.0
  postprocedural E89.0
  postsurgical E89.0
  specified NEC E03.8
  subclinical, iodine-deficiency related E02
Hypotonia, hypotonicity, hypotony
  bladder N31.2
  congenital (benign) P94.2
  eye —*see* Disorder, globe, hypotony
Hypotrichosis —*see* Alopecia
Hypotropia H50.2-
Hypoventilation R06.89
  congenital central alveolar G47.35
  sleep related
    idiopathic nonobstructive alveolar G47.34
    in conditions classified elsewhere G47.36
Hypovitaminosis —*see* Deficiency, vitamin
Hypovolemia E86.1
  surgical shock T81.19
  traumatic (shock) T79.4
Hypoxemia R09.02
  newborn P84
  sleep related, in conditions classified elsewhere G47.36
Hypoxia (see also Anoxia) R09.02
  cerebral, during a procedure NEC G97.81
    postprocedural NEC G97.82
  intrauterine P84
  myocardial —*see* Insufficiency, coronary
  newborn P84
  sleep-related G47.34
Hypsarhythmia —*see* Epilepsy, generalized, specified NEC
Hysteralgia, pregnant uterus O26.89-
Hysteria, hysterical (conversion) (dissociative state) F44.9
  anxiety F41.8
  convulsions F44.5
  psychosis, acute F44.9
Hysteroepilepsy F44.5

I

Ichthyoparasitism due to Vandellia cirrhosa B88.8
Ichthyosis (congenital) Q80.9
  acquired L85.0
  fetalis Q80.4
  hystrix Q80.8
  lamellar Q80.2
  lingual K13.29
  palmaris and plantaris Q82.8
  simplex Q80.0
  vera Q80.8
  vulgaris Q80.0
  X-linked Q80.1
Ichthyotoxism —see Poisoning, fish
  bacterial —see Intoxication, foodborne
Icteroanemia, hemolytic (acquired) D59.9
  congenital —see Spherocytosis
Icterus —see also Jaundice
  conjunctiva R17
  gravis, newborn P55.0
  hematogenous (acquired) D59.9
  hemolytic (acquired) D59.9
    congenital —see Spherocytosis
  hemorrhagic (acute) (leptospiral)
    (spirochetal) A27.0
    newborn P53
  infectious B15.9
    with hepatic coma B15.0
    leptospiral A27.0
    spirochetal A27.0
  neonatorum —see Jaundice, newborn
  newborn P59.9
  spirochetal A27.0
Ictus solaris, solis T67.0
Ideation
  homicidal R45.850
  suicidal R45.851
Identity disorder (child) F64.9
  gender role F64.2
  psychosexual F64.2
Idioglossia F80.0
Idiopathic —see condition
Idiot, idiocy (congenital) F73
  amaurotic (Bielschowsky(-Jansky)) (family)
    (infantile (late)) (juvenile (late)) (Vogt-
    Spielmeyer) E75.4
  microcephalic Q02
Id reaction (due to bacteria) L30.2
IgE asthma J45.909
IIAC (idiopathic infantile arterial calcification)
  Q28.8
Ileitis (chronic) (noninfectious) (see also
  Enteritis) K52.9
  backwash —see Pancolitis, ulcerative
    (chronic)
  infectious A09
  regional (ulcerative) —see Enteritis, regional,
    small intestine
  segmental —see Enteritis, regional
  terminal (ulcerative) —see Enteritis, regional,
    small intestine
Ileocolitis (see also Enteritis) K52.9
  infectious A09
  regional —see Enteritis, regional
Ileostomy
  attention to Z43.2
  malfunctioning K94.13
  status Z93.2
    with complication —see Complications,
    enterostomy
Ileotyphus —see Typhoid
Ileum —see condition
Ileus (bowel) (colon) (inhibitory) (intestine)
  K56.7
  adynamic K56.0
  due to gallstone (in intestine) K56.3
  duodenal (chronic) K31.5
  gallstone K56.3
  mechanical NEC K56.69

Ileus (Continued)
  meconium P76.0
    in cystic fibrosis E84.11
    meaning meconium plug (without cystic
      fibrosis) P76.0
  myxedema K59.8
  neurogenic K56.0
    Hirschsprung's disease or megacolon
      Q43.1
  newborn
    due to meconium P76.0
      in cystic fibrosis E84.11
      meaning meconium plug (without cystic
        fibrosis) P76.0
    transitory P76.1
  obstructive K56.69
  paralytic K56.0
Iliac —see condition
Iliotibial band syndrome M76.3-
Illiteracy Z55.0
Illness (see also Disease) R69
  manic-depressive —see Disorder, bipolar
Imbalance R26.89
  autonomic G90.8
  constituents of food intake E63.1
  electrolyte E87.8
    with
      abortion —see Abortion by type,
        complicated by, electrolyte
        imbalance
      molar pregnancy O08.5
    due to hyperemesis gravidarum O21.1
    following ectopic or molar pregnancy
      O08.5
    neonatal, transitory NEC P74.4
      potassium P74.3
      sodium P74.2
  endocrine E34.9
  eye muscle NOS H50.9
  hormone E34.9
  hysterical F44.4
  labyrinth —see subcategory H83.2
  posture R29.3
  protein-energy —see Malnutrition
  sympathetic G90.8
Imbecile, imbecility (I.Q. 35-49) F71 ◀▥
Imbedding, intrauterine device T83.39
Imbibition, cholesterol (gallbladder) K82.4
Imbrication, teeth, fully erupted M26.30
Imerslund (-Gräsbeck) syndrome D51.1
Immature —see also Immaturity
  birth (less than 37 completed weeks) —see
    Preterm, newborn
  extremely (less than 28 completed
    weeks) —see Immaturity, extreme
  personality F60.89
Immaturity (less than 37 completed weeks) —
  see also Preterm, newborn
  extreme of newborn (less than 28 completed
    weeks of gestation) (less than
    196 completed days of gestation)
    (unspecified weeks of gestation) P07.20
    gestational age
      23 completed weeks (23 weeks, 0 days
        through 23 weeks, 6 days) P07.22
      24 completed weeks (24 weeks, 0 days
        through 24 weeks, 6 days) P07.23
      25 completed weeks (25 weeks, 0 days
        through 25 weeks, 6 days) P07.24
      26 completed weeks (26 weeks, 0 days
        through 26 weeks, 6 days) P07.25
      27 completed weeks (27 weeks, 0 days
        through 27 weeks, 6 days) P07.26
    less than 23 completed weeks P07.21
  fetus or infant light-for-dates —see
    Light-for-dates
  lung, newborn P28.0
  organ or site NEC —see Hypoplasia
  pulmonary, newborn P28.0
  reaction F60.89
  sexual (female) (male), after puberty E30.0

Immersion T75.1
  foot T69.02-
  hand T69.01-
Immobile, immobility
  complete, due to severe physical disability or
    frailty R53.2
  intestine K59.8
  syndrome (paraplegic) M62.3
Immune reconstitution (inflammatory)
  syndrome [IRIS] D89.3
Immunization —see also Vaccination
  ABO —see Incompatibility, ABO
    in newborn P55.1
  complication —see Complications,
    vaccination
  encounter for Z23
  not done (not carried out) Z28.9
    because (of)
      acute illness of patient Z28.01
      allergy to vaccine (or component) Z28.04
      caregiver refusal Z28.82
      chronic illness of patient Z28.02
      contraindication NEC Z28.09
      group pressure Z28.1
      guardian refusal Z28.82
      immune compromised state of patient
        Z28.03
      parent refusal Z28.82
      patient's belief Z28.1
      patient had disease being vaccinated
        against Z28.81
      patient refusal Z28.21
      religious beliefs of patient Z28.1
      specified reason NEC Z28.89
        of patient Z28.29
      unspecified patient reason Z28.20
  Rh factor
    affecting management of pregnancy NEC
      O36.09-
      anti-D antibody O36.01-
    from transfusion —see Complication (s),
      transfusion, incompatibility reaction,
      Rh (factor)
Immunocytoma C83.0-
Immunodeficiency D84.9
  with
    adenosine-deaminase deficiency D81.3
    antibody defects D80.9
      specified type NEC D80.8
    hyperimmunoglobulinemia D80.6
    increased immunoglobulin M (IgM) D80.5
    major defect D82.9
      specified type NEC D82.8
    partial albinism D82.8
    short-limbed stature D82.2
    thrombocytopenia and eczema D82.0
  antibody with
    hyperimmunoglobulinemia D80.6
    near-normal immunoglobulins D80.6
  autosomal recessive, Swiss type D80.0
  combined D81.9
    biotin-dependent carboxylase D81.819
      biotinidase D81.810
      holocarboxylase synthetase D81.818
      specified type NEC D81.818
    severe (SCID) D81.9
      with
        low or normal B-cell numbers D81.2
        low T- and B-cell numbers D81.1
        reticular dysgenesis D81.0
    specified type NEC D81.89
  common variable D83.9
    with
      abnormalities of B-cell numbers and
        function D83.0
      autoantibodies to B- or T-cells D83.2
      immunoregulatory T-cell disorders
        D83.1
    specified type NEC D83.8
  following hereditary defective response to
    Epstein-Barr virus (EBV) D82.3

◀ New   ⬅▥ Revised   ~~deleted~~ Deleted

Immunodeficiency *(Continued)*
  selective, immunoglobulin
    A (IgA) D80.2
    G (IgG) (subclasses) D80.3
    M (IgM) D80.4
  severe combined (SCID) D81.9
  specified type NEC D84.8
  X-linked, with increased IgM D80.5
Immunotherapy (encounter for)
  antineoplastic Z51.12
Impaction, impacted
  bowel, colon, rectum *(see also* Impaction, fecal) K56.49
    by gallstone K56.3
  calculus —*see* Calculus
  cerumen (ear) (external) H61.2-
  cuspid —*see* Impaction, tooth
  dental (same or adjacent tooth) K01.1
  fecal, feces K56.41
  fracture —*see* Fracture, by site
  gallbladder —*see* Calculus, gallbladder
  gallstone (s) —*see* Calculus, gallbladder
    bile duct (common) (hepatic) —*see* Calculus, bile duct
    cystic duct —*see* Calculus, gallbladder
    in intestine, with obstruction (any part) K56.3
  intestine (calculous) NEC *(see also* Impaction, fecal) K56.49
    gallstone, with ileus K56.3
  intrauterine device (IUD) T83.39
  molar —*see* Impaction, tooth
  shoulder, causing obstructed labor O66.0
  tooth, teeth K01.1
  turbinate J34.89
Impaired, impairment (function)
  auditory discrimination —*see* Abnormal, auditory perception
  cognitive, mild, so stated G31.84
  dual sensory Z73.82
  fasting glucose R73.01
  glucose tolerance (oral) R73.02
  hearing —*see* Deafness
  heart —*see* Disease, heart
  kidney N28.9
    disorder resulting from N25.9
      specified NEC N25.89
  liver K72.90
    with coma K72.91
  mastication K08.8
  mild cognitive, so stated G31.84
  mobility
    ear ossicles —*see* Ankylosis, ear ossicles
    requiring care provider Z74.09
  myocardium, myocardial —*see* Insufficiency, myocardial
  rectal sphincter R19.8
  renal (acute) (chronic) N28.9
    disorder resulting from N25.9
      specified NEC N25.89
  vision NEC H54.7
    both eyes H54.3
Impediment, speech R47.9
  psychogenic (childhood) F98.8
  slurring R47.81
  specified NEC R47.89
Impending
  coronary syndrome I20.0
  delirium tremens F10.239
  myocardial infarction I20.0
Imperception auditory (acquired) —*see also* Deafness
  congenital H93.25
Imperfect
  aeration, lung (newborn) NEC —*see* Atelectasis
  closure (congenital)
    alimentary tract NEC Q45.8
      lower Q43.8
      upper Q40.8
    atrioventricular ostium Q21.2

Imperfect *(Continued)*
  closure *(Continued)*
    atrium (secundum) Q21.1
    branchial cleft or sinus Q18.0
    choroid Q14.3
    cricoid cartilage Q31.8
    cusps, heart valve NEC Q24.8
      pulmonary Q22.3
    ductus
      arteriosus Q25.0
      Botalli Q25.0
    ear drum (causing impairment of hearing) Q16.4
    esophagus with communication to bronchus or trachea Q39.1
    eyelid Q10.3
    foramen
      botalli Q21.1
      ovale Q21.1
    genitalia, genital organ (s) or system
      female Q52.8
        external Q52.79
        internal NEC Q52.8
      male Q55.8
    glottis Q31.8
    interatrial ostium or septum Q21.1
    interauricular ostium or septum Q21.1
    interventricular ostium or septum Q21.0
    larynx Q31.8
    lip —*see* Cleft, lip
    nasal septum Q30.3
    nose Q30.2
    omphalomesenteric duct Q43.0
    optic nerve entry Q14.2
    organ or site not listed —*see* Anomaly, by site
    ostium
      interatrial Q21.1
      interauricular Q21.1
      interventricular Q21.0
    palate —*see* Cleft, palate
    preauricular sinus Q18.1
    retina Q14.1
    roof of orbit Q75.8
    sclera Q13.5
    septum
      aorticopulmonary Q21.4
      atrial (secundum) Q21.1
      between aorta and pulmonary artery Q21.4
      heart Q21.9
      interatrial (secundum) Q21.1
      interauricular (secundum) Q21.1
      interventricular Q21.0
        in tetralogy of Fallot Q21.3
      nasal Q30.3
      ventricular Q21.0
        with pulmonary stenosis or atresia, dextraposition of aorta, and hypertrophy of right ventricle Q21.3
        in tetralogy of Fallot Q21.3
    skull Q75.0
      with
        anencephaly Q00.0
        encephalocele —*see* Encephalocele
        hydrocephalus Q03.9
          with spina bifida —*see* Spina bifida, by site, with hydrocephalus
        microcephaly Q02
    spine (with meningocele) —*see* Spina bifida
    trachea Q32.1
    tympanic membrane (causing impairment of hearing) Q16.4
    uterus Q51.818
    vitelline duct Q43.0
  erection —*see* Dysfunction, sexual, male, erectile
  fusion —*see* Imperfect, closure
  inflation, lung (newborn) —*see* Atelectasis

Imperfect *(Continued)*
  posture R29.3
  rotation, intestine Q43.3
  septum, ventricular Q21.0
Imperfectly descended testis —*see* Cryptorchid
Imperforate (congenital) —*see also* Atresia
  anus Q42.3
    with fistula Q42.2
  cervix (uteri) Q51.828
  esophagus Q39.0
    with tracheoesophageal fistula Q39.1
  hymen Q52.3
  jejunum Q41.1
  pharynx Q38.8
  rectum Q42.1
    with fistula Q42.0
  urethra Q64.39
  vagina Q52.4
Impervious (congenital) —*see also* Atresia
  anus Q42.3
    with fistula Q42.2
  bile duct Q44.2
  esophagus Q39.0
    with tracheoesophageal fistula Q39.1
  intestine (small) Q41.9
    large Q42.9
      specified NEC Q42.8
  rectum Q42.1
    with fistula Q42.0
  ureter —*see* Atresia, ureter
  urethra Q64.39
Impetiginization of dermatoses L01.1
Impetigo (any organism) (any site) (circinate) (contagiosa) (simplex) (vulgaris) L01.00
  Bockhart's L01.02
  bullous, bullosa L01.03
  external ear L01.00 *[H62.40]*
  follicularis L01.02
  furfuracea L30.5
  herpetiformis L40.1
    nonobstetrical L40.1
  neonatorum L01.03
  nonbullous L01.01
  specified type NEC L01.09
  ulcerative L01.09
Impingement (on teeth)
  soft tissue
    anterior M26.81
    posterior M26.82
Implant, endometrial N80.9
Implantation
  anomalous —*see* Anomaly, by site
    ureter Q62.63
  cyst
    external area or site (skin) NEC L72.0
    iris —*see* Cyst, iris, implantation
    vagina N89.8
    vulva N90.7
  dermoid (cyst) —*see* Implantation, cyst
Impotence (sexual) N52.9
  counseling Z70.1
  organic origin *(see also* Dysfunction, sexual, male, erectile) N52.9
  psychogenic F52.21
Impression, basilar Q75.8
Imprisonment, anxiety concerning Z65.1
Improper care (child) (newborn) —*see* Maltreatment
Improperly tied umbilical cord (causing hemorrhage) P51.8
Impulsiveness (impulsive) R45.87
Inability to swallow —*see* Aphagia
Inaccessible, inaccessibility
  health care NEC Z75.3
    due to
      waiting period Z75.2
        for admission to facility elsewhere Z75.1
    other helping agencies Z75.4
Inactive —*see* condition

Inadequate, inadequacy

aesthetics of dental restoration K08.56
biologic, constitutional, functional, or social F60.7
development
  child R62.50
  genitalia
    after puberty NEC E30.0
    congenital
      female Q52.8
        external Q52.79
        internal Q52.8
      male Q55.8
  lungs Q33.6
    associated with short gestation P28.0
  organ or site not listed —see Anomaly, by site
diet (causing nutritional deficiency) E63.9
eating habits Z72.4
environment, household Z59.1
family support Z63.8
food (supply) NEC Z59.4
  hunger effects T73.0
functional F60.7
household care, due to
  family member
    handicapped or ill Z74.2
    on vacation Z75.5
    temporarily away from home Z74.2
  technical defects in home Z59.1
  temporary absence from home of person rendering care Z74.2
housing (heating) (space) Z59.1
income (financial) Z59.6
intrafamilial communication Z63.8
material resources Z59.9
mental —see Disability, intellectual
parental supervision or control of child Z62.0
personality F60.7
pulmonary
  function R06.89
    newborn P28.5
  ventilation, newborn P28.5
sample of cytologic smear
  anus R85.615
  cervix R87.615
  vagina R87.625
social F60.7
  insurance Z59.7
  skills NEC Z73.4
supervision of child by parent Z62.0
teaching affecting education Z55.8
welfare support Z59.7

Inanition R64

with edema —see Malnutrition, severe
due to
  deprivation of food T73.0
  malnutrition —see Malnutrition
fever R50.9

Inappropriate

change in quantitative human chorionic gonadotropin (hCG) in early pregnancy O02.81
diet or eating habits Z72.4
level of quantitative human chorionic gonadotropin (hCG) for gestational age in early pregnancy O02.81
secretion
  antidiuretic hormone (ADH) (excessive) E22.2
    deficiency E23.2
  pituitary (posterior) E22.2

Inattention at or after birth —see Neglect

Incarceration, incarcerated

enterocele K46.0
  gangrenous K46.1
epiplocele K46.0
  gangrenous K46.1
exophthalmos K42.0
  gangrenous K42.1

Incarceration, incarcerated (Continued)

hernia —see also Hernia, by site, with obstruction
  with gangrene —see Hernia, by site, with gangrene
iris, in wound —see Injury, eye, laceration, with prolapse
lens, in wound —see Injury, eye, laceration, with prolapse
omphalocele K42.0
prison, anxiety concerning Z65.1
rupture —see Hernia, by site
sarcoepiplocele K46.0
  gangrenous K46.1
sarcoepiplomphalocele K42.0
  with gangrene K42.1
uterus N85.8
  gravid O34.51-
    causing obstructed labor O65.5

Incised wound

external —see Laceration
internal organs —see Injury, by site

Incision, incisional

hernia K43.2
  with
    gangrene (and obstruction) K43.1
    obstruction K43.0
surgical, complication —see Complications, surgical procedure
traumatic
  external —see Laceration
  internal organs —see Injury, by site

Inclusion

azurophilic leukocytic D72.0
blennorrhea (neonatal) (newborn) P39.1
gallbladder in liver (congenital) Q44.1

Incompatibility

ABO
  affecting management of pregnancy O36.11-
    anti-A sensitization O36.11-
    anti-B sensitization O36.19-
    specified NEC O36.19-
  infusion or transfusion reaction —see Complication (s), transfusion, incompatibility reaction, ABO
  newborn P55.1
blood (group) (Duffy) (K(ell)) (Kidd) (Lewis) (M) (S) NEC
  affecting management of pregnancy O36.11-
    anti-A sensitization O36.11-
    anti-B sensitization O36.19-
  infusion or transfusion reaction T80.89
  newborn P55.8
divorce or estrangement Z63.5
Rh (blood group) (factor) Z31.82
  affecting management of pregnancy NEC O36.09-
    anti-D antibody O36.01-
  infusion or transfusion reaction —see Complication (s), transfusion, incompatibility reaction, Rh (factor)
  newborn P55.0
rhesus —see Incompatibility, Rh

Incompetency, incompetent, incompetence

annular
  aortic (valve) —see Insufficiency, aortic
  mitral (valve) I34.0
  pulmonary valve (heart) I37.1
aortic (valve) —see Insufficiency, aortic
cardiac valve —see Endocarditis
cervix, cervical (os) N88.3
  in pregnancy O34.3-
chronotropic I45.89
  with
    autonomic dysfunction G90.8
    ischemic heart disease I25.89
    left ventricular dysfunction I51.89
    sinus node dysfunction I49.8
esophagogastric (junction) (sphincter) K22.0

Incompetency, incompetent, incompetence (Continued)

mitral (valve) —see Insufficiency, mitral
pelvic fundus N81.89
pubocervical tissue N81.82
pulmonary valve (heart) I37.1
  congenital Q22.3
rectovaginal tissue N81.83
tricuspid (annular) (valve) —see Insufficiency, tricuspid
valvular —see Endocarditis
  congenital Q24.8
vein, venous (saphenous) (varicose) —see Varix, leg

Incomplete —see also condition

bladder, emptying R33.9
defecation R15.0
expansion lungs (newborn) NEC —see Atelectasis
rotation, intestine Q43.3

Inconclusive

diagnostic imaging due to excess body fat of patient R93.9
findings on diagnostic imaging of breast NEC R92.8
mammogram (due to dense breasts) R92.2

Incontinence R32

anal sphincter R15.9
feces R15.9
  nonorganic origin F98.1
overflow N39.490
psychogenic F45.8
rectal R15.9
reflex N39.498
stress (female) (male) N39.3
  and urge N39.46
urethral sphincter R32
urge N39.41
  and stress (female) (male) N39.46
urine (urinary) R32
  continuous N39.45
  due to cognitive impairment, or severe physical disability or immobility R39.81
  functional R39.81
  mixed (stress and urge) N39.46
  nocturnal N39.44
  nonorganic origin F98.0
  overflow N39.490
  post dribbling N39.43
  reflex N39.498
  specified NEC N39.498
  stress (female) (male) N39.3
    and urge N39.46
  total N39.498
  unaware N39.42
  urge N39.41
    and stress (female) (male) N39.46

Incontinentia pigmenti Q82.3

Incoordinate, incoordination

esophageal-pharyngeal (newborn) —see Dysphagia
muscular R27.8
uterus (action) (contractions) (complicating delivery) O62.4

Increase, increased

abnormal, in development R63.8
androgens (ovarian) E28.1
anticoagulants (antithrombin) (anti-VIIIa) (anti-IXa) (anti-Xa) (anti-XIa) —see Circulating anticoagulants)
cold sense R20.8
estrogen E28.0
function
  adrenal
    cortex —see Cushing's, syndrome
    medulla E27.5
  pituitary (gland) (anterior) (lobe) E22.9
    posterior E22.2
heat sense R20.8
intracranial pressure (benign) G93.2

Increase, increased (Continued)
 permeability, capillaries I78.8
 pressure, intracranial G93.2
 secretion
  gastrin E16.4
  glucagon E16.3
  pancreas, endocrine E16.9
   growth hormone-releasing hormone
    E16.8
   pancreatic polypeptide E16.8
   somatostatin E16.8
   vasoactive-intestinal polypeptide
    E16.8
 sphericity, lens Q12.4
 splenic activity D73.1
 venous pressure I87.8
  portal K76.6
Increta placenta O43.22-
Incrustation, cornea, foreign body (lead)
  (zinc) —see Foreign body, cornea
Incyclophoria H50.54
Incyclotropia —see Cyclotropia
Indeterminate sex Q56.4
India rubber skin Q82.8
Indigestion (acid) (bilious) (functional) K30
 catarrhal K31.89
 due to decomposed food NOS A05.9
 nervous F45.8
 psychogenic F45.8
Indirect —see condition
Induratio penis plastica N48.6
Induration, indurated
 brain G93.89
 breast (fibrous) N64.51
  puerperal, postpartum O92.29
 broad ligament N83.8
 chancre
  anus A51.1
   congenital A50.07
  extragenital NEC A51.2
 corpora cavernosa (penis) (plastic) N48.6
 liver (chronic) K76.89
 lung (black) (chronic) (fibroid) (see also
   Fibrosis, lung) J84.10
  essential brown J84.03
 penile (plastic) N48.6
 phlebitic —see Phlebitis
 skin R23.4
Inebriety (without dependence) —see Alcohol,
  intoxication
Inefficiency, kidney N28.9
Inelasticity, skin R23.4
Inequality, leg (length) (acquired) —see also
  Deformity, limb, unequal length
 congenital —see Defect, reduction, lower
   limb
 lower leg —see Deformity, limb, unequal
   length
Inertia
 bladder (neurogenic) N31.2
 stomach K31.89
  psychogenic F45.8
 uterus, uterine during labor O62.2
  during latent phase of labor O62.0
  primary O62.0
  secondary O62.1
 vesical (neurogenic) N31.2
Infancy, infantile, infantilism —see also
  condition
 celiac K90.0
 genitalia, genitals (after puberty) E30.0
 Herter's (nontropical sprue) K90.0
 intestinal K90.0
 Lorain E23.0
 pancreatic K86.8
 pelvis M95.5
  with disproportion (fetopelvic) O33.1
   causing obstructed labor O65.1
 pituitary E23.0
 renal N25.0
 uterus —see Infantile, genitalia

Infant (s) —see also Infancy
 excessive crying R68.11
 irritable child R68.12
 lack of care —see Neglect
 liveborn (singleton) Z38.2
  born in hospital Z38.00
   by cesarean Z38.01
  born outside hospital Z38.1
  multiple NEC Z38.8
   born in hospital Z38.68
    by cesarean Z38.69
   born outside hospital Z38.7
  quadruplet Z38.8
   born in hospital Z38.63
    by cesarean Z38.64
   born outside hospital Z38.7
  quintuplet Z38.8
   born in hospital Z38.65
    by cesarean Z38.66
   born outside hospital Z38.7
  triplet Z38.8
   born in hospital Z38.61
    by cesarean Z38.62
   born outside hospital Z38.7
  twin Z38.5
   born in hospital Z38.30
    by cesarean Z38.31
   born outside hospital Z38.4
  of diabetic mother (syndrome of) P70.1
   gestational diabetes P70.0
Infantile —see also condition
 genitalia, genitals E30.0
 os, uterine E30.0
 penis E30.0
 testis E29.1
 uterus E30.0
Infantilism —see Infancy
Infarct, infarction
 adrenal (capsule) (gland) E27.49
 appendices epiploicae K55.0
 bowel K55.0
 brain (stem) —see Infarct, cerebral
 breast N64.89
 brewer's (kidney) N28.0
 cardiac —see Infarct, myocardium
 cerebellar —see Infarct, cerebral
 cerebral (see also Occlusion, artery cerebral or
   precerebral, with infarction) I63.9- ◄▥▥
  aborted I63.9
  cortical I63.9
  due to
   cerebral venous thrombosis,
    nonpyogenic I63.6
   embolism
    cerebral arteries I63.4-
    precerebral arteries I63.1-
   occlusion NEC
    cerebral arteries I63.5-
    precerebral arteries I63.2-
   stenosis NEC
    cerebral arteries I63.5-
    precerebral arteries I63.2-
   thrombosis
    cerebral artery I63.3-
    precerebral artery I63.0-
  intraoperative
   during cardiac surgery I97.810
   during other surgery I97.811
  postprocedural
   following cardiac surgery I97.820
   following other surgery I97.821
  specified NEC I63.8
 colon (acute) (agnogenic) (embolic)
   (hemorrhagic) (nonocclusive)
   (nonthrombotic) (occlusive) (segmental)
   (thrombotic) (with gangrene) K55.0
 coronary artery —see Infarct, myocardium
 embolic —see Embolism
 fallopian tube N83.8
 gallbladder K82.8
 heart —see Infarct, myocardium

Infarct, infarction (Continued)
 hepatic K76.3
 hypophysis (anterior lobe) E23.6
 impending (myocardium) I20.0
 intestine (acute) (agnogenic) (embolic)
   (hemorrhagic) (nonocclusive)
   (nonthrombotic) (occlusive)
   (thrombotic) (with gangrene) K55.0
 kidney N28.0
 liver K76.3
 lung (embolic) (thrombotic) —see Embolism,
   pulmonary
 lymph node I89.8
 mesentery, mesenteric (embolic) (thrombotic)
   (with gangrene) K55.0
 muscle (ischemic) M62.20
  ankle M62.27-
  foot M62.27-
  forearm M62.23-
  hand M62.24-
  lower leg M62.26-
  pelvic region M62.25-
  shoulder region M62.21-
  specified site NEC M62.28
  thigh M62.25-
  upper arm M62.22-
 myocardium, myocardial (acute) (with stated
   duration of 4 weeks or less) I21.3
  diagnosed on ECG, but presenting no
    symptoms I25.2
  healed or old I25.2
  intraoperative
   during cardiac surgery I97.790
   during other surgery I97.791
  non-Q wave I21.4
  non-ST elevation (NSTEMI) I21.4
   subsequent I22.2
  nontransmural I21.4
  past (diagnosed on ECG or other
    investigation, but currently
    presenting no symptoms) I25.2
  postprocedural
   following cardiac surgery I97.190
   following other surgery I97.191
  Q wave (see also, Infarct, myocardium, by
    site) I21.3
  ST elevation (STEMI) I21.3
   anterior (anteroapical) (anterolateral)
     (anteroseptal) (Q wave) (wall)
     I21.09
    subsequent I22.0
   inferior (diaphragmatic) (inferolateral)
     (inferoposterior) (wall) NEC
     I21.19
    subsequent I22.1
   inferoposterior transmural (Q wave)
     I21.11
   involving
    coronary artery of anterior wall NEC
      I21.09
    coronary artery of inferior wall NEC
      I21.19
    diagonal coronary artery I21.02
    left anterior descending coronary
      artery I21.02
    left circumflex coronary artery I21.21
    left main coronary artery I21.01
    oblique marginal coronary artery
      I21.21
    right coronary artery I21.11
   lateral (apical-lateral) (basal-lateral)
     (high) I21.29
    subsequent I22.8
   posterior (posterobasal) (posterolateral)
     (posteroseptal) (true) I21.29
    subsequent I22.8
   septal I21.29
    subsequent I22.8
   specified NEC I21.29
    subsequent I22.8
    subsequent I22.9

Infarct, infarction (Continued)
  myocardium, myocardial (Continued)
    subsequent (recurrent) (reinfarction) I22.9
      anterior (anteroapical) (anterolateral)
          (anteroseptal) (wall) I22.0
      diaphragmatic (wall) I22.1
      inferior (diaphragmatic) (inferolateral)
          (inferoposterior) (wall) I22.1
      lateral (apical-lateral) (basal-lateral)
          (high) I22.8
      non-ST elevation (NSTEMI) I22.2
      posterior (posterobasal) (posterolateral)
          (posteroseptal) (true) I22.8
      septal I22.8
      specified NEC I22.8
      ST elevation I22.9
        anterior (anteroapical) (anterolateral)
            (anteroseptal) (wall) I22.0
        inferior (diaphragmatic) (inferolateral)
            (inferoposterior) (wall) I22.1
        specified NEC I22.8
    subendocardial I22.2
    transmural I22.9
      anterior (anteroapical) (anterolateral)
          (anteroseptal) (wall) I22.0
      diaphragmatic (wall) I22.1
      inferior (diaphragmatic) (inferolateral)
          (inferoposterior) (wall) I22.1
      lateral (apical-lateral) (basal-lateral)
          (high) I22.8
      posterior (posterobasal)
          (posterolateral) (posteroseptal)
          (true) I22.8
      specified NEC I22.8
  syphilitic A52.06
  transmural I21.3
    anterior (anteroapical) (anterolateral)
        (anteroseptal) (Q wave) (wall) NEC
        I21.09
    inferior (diaphragmatic) (inferolateral)
        (inferoposterior) (Q wave) (wall)
        NEC I21.19
    inferoposterior (Q wave) I21.11
    lateral (apical-lateral) (basal-lateral)
        (high) NEC I21.29
    posterior (posterobasal) (posterolateral)
        (posteroseptal) (true) NEC I21.29
    septal NEC I21.29
    specified NEC I21.29
  nontransmural I21.4
  omentum K55.0
  ovary N83.8
  pancreas K86.8 ◄▥
  papillary muscle —see Infarct, myocardium
  parathyroid gland E21.4
  pituitary (gland) E23.6
  placenta O43.81-
  prostate N42.89
  pulmonary (artery) (vein) (hemorrhagic) —
      see Embolism, pulmonary
  renal (embolic) (thrombotic) N28.0
  retina, retinal (artery) —see Occlusion, artery,
      retina
  spinal (cord) (acute) (embolic) (nonembolic)
      G95.11
  spleen D73.5
    embolic or thrombotic I74.8
  subendocardial (acute) (nontransmural) I21.4
  suprarenal (capsule) (gland) E27.49
  testis N50.1
  thrombotic —see also Thrombosis
    artery, arterial —see Embolism
  thyroid (gland) E07.89
  ventricle (heart) —see Infarct, myocardium
Infecting —see condition
Infection, infected, infective (opportunistic)
    B99.9
  with
    drug resistant organism —see Resistance
        (to), drug —see also specific organism
    lymphangitis —see Lymphangitis

Infection, infected, infective (Continued)
  with (Continued)
    organ dysfunction (acute) R65.20
      with septic shock R65.21
    abscess (skin) - code by site under Abscess
  Absidia —see Mucormycosis
  Acanthamoeba —see Acanthamebiasis
  Acanthocheilonema (perstans) (streptocerca)
      B74.4
  accessory sinus (chronic) —see Sinusitis
  achorion —see Dermatophytosis
  Acremonium falciforme B47.0
  acromioclavicular M00.9
  Actinobacillus (actinomycetem-comitans)
      A28.8
    mallei A24.0
    muris A25.1
  Actinomadura B47.1
  Actinomyces (israelii) (see also Actinomycosis)
      A42.9
  Actinomycetales —see Actinomycosis
  actinomycotic NOS —see Actinomycosis
  adenoid (and tonsil) J03.90
    chronic J35.02
  adenovirus NEC
    as cause of disease classified elsewhere
        B97.0
    unspecified nature or site B34.0
  aerogenes capsulatus A48.0
  aertrycke —see Infection, salmonella
  alimentary canal NOS —see Enteritis,
      infectious
  Allescheria boydii B48.2
  Alternaria B48.8
  alveolus, alveolar (process) K04.7
  Ameba, amebic (histolytica) —see Amebiasis
  amniotic fluid, sac or cavity O41.10-
    chorioamnionitis O41.12-
    placentitis O41.14-
  amputation stump (surgical) —see
      Complication, amputation stump,
      infection
  Ancylostoma (duodenalis) B76.0
  Anisakiasis, Anisakis larvae B81.0
  anthrax —see Anthrax
  antrum (chronic) —see Sinusitis, maxillary
  anus, anal (papillae) (sphincter) K62.89
  arbovirus (arbor virus) A94
    specified type NEC A93.8
  artificial insemination N98.0
  Ascaris lumbricoides —see Ascariasis
  Ascomycetes B47.0
  Aspergillus (flavus) (fumigatus) (terreus) —
      see Aspergillosis
  atypical
    acid-fast (bacilli) —see Mycobacterium,
        atypical
    mycobacteria —see Mycobacterium,
        atypical
    virus A81.9
      specified type NEC A81.89
  auditory meatus (external) —see Otitis,
      externa, infective
  auricle (ear) —see Otitis, externa, infective
  axillary gland (lymph) L04.2
  Bacillus A49.9
    abortus A23.1
    anthracis —see Anthrax
    Ducrey's (any location) A57
    Flexner's A03.1
    Friedländer's NEC A49.8
    gas (gangrene) A48.0
    mallei A24.0
    melitensis A23.0
    paratyphoid, paratyphosus A01.4
      A A01.1
      B A01.2
      C A01.3
    Shiga (-Kruse) A03.0
    suipestifer —see Infection, salmonella
    swimming pool A31.1

Infection, infected, infective (Continued)
  Bacillus (Continued)
    typhosa A01.00
    welchii —see Gangrene, gas
  bacterial NOS A49.9
    as cause of disease classified elsewhere
        B96.89
      Bacteroides fragilis [B. fragilis] B96.6
      Clostridium perfringens [C. perfringens]
          B96.7
      Enterobacter sakazakii B96.89
      Enterococcus B95.2
      Escherichia coli [E. coli] (see also
          Escherichia coli) B96.20
      Helicobacter pylori [H.pylori] B96.81
      Hemophilus influenzae [H. influenzae]
          B96.3
      Klebsiella pneumoniae [K. pneumoniae]
          B96.1
      Mycoplasma pneumoniae [M.
          pneumoniae] B96.0
      Proteus (mirabilis) (morganii) B96.4
      Pseudomonas (aeruginosa) (mallei)
          (pseudomallei) B96.5
      Staphylococcus B95.8
        aureus (methicillin susceptible)
            (MSSA) B95.61
          methicillin resistant (MRSA) B95.62
        specified NEC B95.7
      Streptococcus B95.5
        group A B95.0
        group B B95.1
        pneumoniae B95.3
        specified NEC B95.4
      Vibrio vulnificus B96.82
    specified NEC A48.8
  Bacterium
    paratyphosum A01.4
      A A01.1
      B A01.2
      C A01.3
    typhosum A01.00
  Bacteroides NEC A49.8
    fragilis, as cause of disease classified
        elsewhere B96.6
  Balantidium coli A07.0
  Bartholin's gland N75.8
  Basidiobolus B46.8
  bile duct (common) (hepatic) —see
      Cholangitis
  bladder —see Cystitis
  Blastomyces, blastomycotic —see also
      Blastomycosis
    brasiliensis —see Paracoccidioidomycosis
    dermatitidis —see Blastomycosis
    European —see Cryptococcosis
    Loboi B48.0
    North American B40.9
    South American —see
        Paracoccidioidomycosis
  bleb, postprocedure —see Blebitis
  bone —see Osteomyelitis
  Bordetella —see Whooping cough
  Borrelia bergdorfi A69.20
  brain (see also Encephalitis) G04.90
    membranes —see Meningitis
    septic G06.0
    meninges —see Meningitis, bacterial
  branchial cyst Q18.0
  breast —see Mastitis
  bronchus —see Bronchitis
  Brucella A23.9
    abortus A23.1
    canis A23.3
    melitensis A23.0
    mixed A23.8
    specified NEC A23.8
    suis A23.2
  Brugia (malayi) B74.1
    timori B74.2
  bursa —see Bursitis, infective

◄ New   ◄▥ Revised   ~~deleted~~ Deleted

Infection, infected, infective (Continued)
buttocks (skin) L08.9
Campylobacter, intestinal A04.5
   as cause of disease classified elsewhere
      B96.81
Candida (albicans) (tropicalis) —see
   Candidiasis
candiru B88.8
Capillaria (intestinal) B81.1
   hepatica B83.8
   philippinensis B81.1
cartilage —see Disorder, cartilage, specified
   type NEC
catheter-related bloodstream (CRBSI) T80.211
cat liver fluke B66.0
cellulitis - code by site under Cellulitis
central line-associated T80.219
   bloodstream (CLABSI) T80.211
   specified NEC T80.218
Cephalosporium falciforme B47.0
cerebrospinal —see Meningitis
cervical gland (lymph) L04.0
cervix —see Cervicitis
cesarean delivery wound (puerperal) O86.0
cestodes —see Infestation, cestodes
chest J22
Chilomastix (intestinal) A07.8
Chlamydia, chlamydial A74.9
   anus A56.3
   genitourinary tract A56.2
      lower A56.00
      specified NEC A56.19
   lymphogranuloma A55
   pharynx A56.4
   psittaci A70
   rectum A56.3
   sexually transmitted NEC A56.8
cholera —see Cholera
Cladosporium
   bantianum (brain abscess) B43.1
   carrionii B43.0
   castellanii B36.1
   trichoides (brain abscess) B43.1
   werneckii B36.1
Clonorchis (sinensis) (liver) B66.1
Clostridium NEC
   bifermentans A48.0
   botulinum (food poisoning) A05.1
      infant A48.51
      wound A48.52
   difficile
      as cause of disease classified elsewhere
         B96.89
      foodborne (disease) A04.7
      gas gangrene A48.0
      necrotizing enterocolitis A04.7
      sepsis A41.4
   gas-forming NEC A48.0
   histolyticum A48.0
   novyi, causing gas gangrene A48.0
   oedematiens A48.0
   perfringens
      as cause of disease classified elsewhere
         B96.7
      due to food A05.2
      foodborne (disease) A05.2
      gas gangrene A48.0
      sepsis A41.4
   septicum, causing gas gangrene A48.0
   sordellii, causing gas gangrene A48.0
   welchii
      as cause of disease classified elsewhere
         B96.7
      foodborne (disease) A05.2
      gas gangrene A48.0
      necrotizing enteritis A05.2
      sepsis A41.4
Coccidioides (immitis) —see
   Coccidioidomycosis
colon —see Enteritis, infectious
colostomy K94.02

Infection, infected, infective (Continued)
common duct —see Cholangitis
congenital P39.9
   Candida (albicans) P37.5
   cytomegalovirus P35.1
   hepatitis, viral P35.3
   herpes simplex P35.2
   infectious or parasitic disease P37.9
      specified NEC P37.8
   listeriosis (disseminated) P37.2
   malaria NEC P37.4
      falciparum P37.3
   Plasmodium falciparum P37.3
   poliomyelitis P35.8
   rubella P35.0
   skin P39.4
   toxoplasmosis (acute) (subacute) (chronic)
      P37.1
   tuberculosis P37.0
   urinary (tract) P39.3
   vaccinia P35.8
   virus P35.9
      specified type NEC P35.8
Conidiobolus B46.8
coronavirus NEC B34.2
   as cause of disease classified elsewhere
      B97.29
   severe acute respiratory syndrome (SARS
      associated) B97.21
corpus luteum —see Salpingo-oophoritis
Corynebacterium diphtheriae —see
   Diphtheria
cotia virus B08.8
Coxiella burnetii A78
coxsackie —see Coxsackie
Cryptococcus neoformans —see
   Cryptococcosis
Cryptosporidium A07.2
Cunninghamella —see Mucormycosis
cyst —see Cyst
cystic duct (see also Cholecystitis) K81.9
Cysticercus cellulosae —see Cysticercosis
cytomegalovirus, cytomegaloviral B25.9
   congenital P35.1
   maternal, maternal care for (suspected)
      damage to fetus O35.3
   mononucleosis B27.10
      with
         complication NEC B27.19
         meningitis B27.12
         polyneuropathy B27.11
delta-agent (acute), in hepatitis B carrier
   B17.0
dental (pulpal origin) K04.7
Deuteromycetes B47.0
Dicrocoelium dendriticum B66.2
Dipetalonema (perstans) (streptocerca) B74.4
diphtherial —see Diphtheria
Diphyllobothrium (adult) (latum) (pacificum)
   B70.0
   larval B70.1
Diplogonoporus (grandis) B71.8
Dipylidium caninum B67.4
Dirofilaria B74.8
Dracunculus medinensis B72
Drechslera (hawaiiensis) B43.8
Ducrey Haemophilus (any location) A57
due to or resulting from
   artificial insemination N98.0
   central venous catheter T80.219
      bloodstream T80.211
      exit or insertion site T80.212
      localized T80.212
      port or reservoir T80.212
      specified NEC T80.218
      tunnel T80.212
   device, implant or graft (see also
      Complications, by site and type,
      infection or inflammation) T85.79
      arterial graft NEC T82.7
      breast (implant) T85.79

Infection, infected, infective (Continued)
due to or resulting from (Continued)
   device, implant or graft (Continued)
      catheter NEC T85.79
         dialysis (renal) T82.7
            intraperitoneal T85.71
         infusion NEC T82.7
            spinal (epidural) (subdural)
               T85.79
         urinary (indwelling) T83.51
      electronic (electrode) (pulse generator)
         (stimulator)
         bone T84.7
         cardiac T82.7
         nervous system (brain) (peripheral
            nerve) (spinal) T85.79
         urinary T83.59
      fixation, internal (orthopedic) NEC —see
         Complication, fixation device,
         infection
      gastrointestinal (bile duct) (esophagus)
         T85.79
      genital NEC T83.6
      heart NEC T82.7
         valve (prosthesis) T82.6
            graft T82.7
      joint prosthesis —see Complication, joint
         prosthesis, infection
      ocular (corneal graft) (orbital implant)
         NEC T85.79
      orthopedic NEC T84.7
      specified NEC T85.79
      urinary NEC T83.59
      vascular NEC T82.7
      ventricular intracranial shunt
         T85.79
   Hickman catheter T80.219
      bloodstream T80.211
      localized T80.212
      specified NEC T80.218
   immunization or vaccination T88.0
   infusion, injection or transfusion NEC
      T80.29
      acute T80.22
   injury NEC - code by site under Wound,
      open
   peripherally inserted central catheter
      (PICC) T80.219
      bloodstream T80.211
      localized T80.212
      specified NEC T80.218
   portacath (port-a-cath) T80.219
      bloodstream T80.211
      localized T80.212
      specified NEC T80.218
   surgery T81.4
   triple lumen catheter T80.219
      bloodstream T80.211
      localized T80.212
      specified NEC T80.218
   umbilical venous catheter T80.219
      bloodstream T80.211
      localized T80.212
      specified NEC T80.218
during labor NEC O75.3
ear (middle) —see also Otitis media
   external —see Otitis, externa, infective
   inner —see subcategory H83.0
Eberthella typhosa A01.00
Echinococcus —see Echinococcus
echovirus
   as cause of disease classified elsewhere
      B97.12
   unspecified nature or site B34.1
endocardium I33.0
endocervix —see Cervicitis
Entamoeba —see Amebiasis
enteric —see Enteritis, infectious
Enterobacter sakazakii B96.89
Enterobius vermicularis B80
enterostomy K94.12

◀ New   ◀▥ Revised   ~~deleted~~ Deleted

Infection, infected, infective *(Continued)*
- mammary gland N61
- Mansonella (ozzardi) (perstans) (streptocerca) B74.4
- mastoid —*see* Mastoiditis
- maxilla, maxillary M27.2
  - sinus (chronic) —*see* Sinusitis, maxillary
- mediastinum J98.5
- Medina (worm) B72
- meibomian cyst or gland —*see* Hordeolum
- meninges —*see* Meningitis, bacterial
- meningococcal (*see also* condition) A39.9
  - adrenals A39.1
  - brain A39.81
  - cerebrospinal A39.0
  - conjunctiva A39.89
  - endocardium A39.51
  - heart A39.50
    - endocardium A39.51
    - myocardium A39.52
    - pericardium A39.53
  - joint A39.83
  - meninges A39.0
  - meningococcemia A39.4
    - acute A39.2
    - chronic A39.3
  - myocardium A39.52
  - pericardium A39.53
  - retrobulbar neuritis A39.82
  - specified site NEC A39.89
- mesenteric lymph nodes or glands NEC I88.0
- Metagonimus B66.8
- metatarsophalangeal M00.9
- methicillin
  - resistant Staphylococcus aureus (MRSA) A49.02
  - susceptible Staphylococcus aureus (MSSA) A49.01
- Microsporum, microsporic —*see* Dermatophytosis
- mixed flora (bacterial) NEC A49.8
- Monilia —*see* Candidiasis
- Monosporium apiospermum B48.2
- mouth, parasitic B37.0
- Mucor —*see* Mucormycosis
- muscle NEC —*see* Myositis, infective
- mycelium NOS B49
- mycetoma B47.9
  - actinomycotic NEC B47.1
  - mycotic NEC B47.0
- Mycobacterium, mycobacterial —*see* Mycobacterium
- Mycoplasma NEC A49.3
  - pneumoniae, as cause of disease classified elsewhere B96.0
- mycotic NOS B49
  - pathogenic to compromised host only B48.8
  - skin NOS B36.9
- myocardium NEC I40.0
- nail (chronic)
  - with lymphangitis —*see* Lymphangitis, acute, digit
  - finger L03.01-
    - fungus B35.1
  - ingrowing L60.0
  - toe L03.03-
    - fungus B35.1
- nasal sinus (chronic) —*see* Sinusitis
- nasopharynx —*see* Nasopharyngitis
- navel L08.82
- Necator americanus B76.1
- Neisseria —*see* Gonococcus
- Neotestudina rosatii B47.0
- newborn P39.9
  - intra-amniotic NEC P39.2
  - skin P39.4
  - specified type NEC P39.8

Infection, infected, infective *(Continued)*
- nipple N61
  - associated with
    - lactation O91.03
    - pregnancy O91.01-
    - puerperium O91.02
- Nocardia —*see* Nocardiosis
- obstetrical surgical wound (puerperal) O86.0
- Oesophagostomum (apiostomum) B81.8
- Oestrus ovis —*see* Myiasis
- Oidium albicans B37.9
- Onchocerca (volvulus) —*see* Onchocerciasis - oncovirus, as cause of disease classified elsewhere B97.32
- operation wound T81.4
- Opisthorchis (felineus) (viverrini) B66.0
- orbit, orbital —*see* Inflammation, orbit
- orthopoxvirus NEC B08.09
- ovary —*see* Salpingo-oophoritis
- Oxyuris vermicularis B80
- pancreas (acute) K85.9
  - abscess —*see* Pancreatitis, acute
  - specified NEC K85.8
- papillomavirus, as cause of disease classified elsewhere B97.7
- papovavirus NEC B34.4
- Paracoccidioides brasiliensis —*see* Paracoccidioidomycosis
- Paragonimus (westermani) B66.4
- parainfluenza virus B34.8
- parameningococcus NOS A39.9
- parapoxvirus B08.60
  - specified NEC B08.69
- parasitic B89
- Parastrongylus
  - cantonensis B83.2
  - costaricensis B81.3
  - paratyphoid A01.4
    - Type A A01.1
    - Type B A01.2
    - Type C A01.3
- paraurethral ducts N34.2
- parotid gland —*see* Sialoadenitis
- parvovirus NEC B34.3
  - as cause of disease classified elsewhere B97.6
- Pasteurella NEC A28.0
  - multocida A28.0
  - pestis —*see* Plague
  - pseudotuberculosis A28.0
  - septica (cat bite) (dog bite) A28.0
  - tularensis —*see* Tularemia
- pelvic, female —*see* Disease, pelvis, inflammatory
- Penicillium (marneffei) B48.4
- penis (glans) (retention) NEC N48.29
- periapical K04.5
- peridental, periodontal K05.20
  - generalized K05.22
  - localized K05.21
- perinatal period P39.9
  - specified type NEC P39.8
- perineal repair (puerperal) O86.0
- periorbital —*see* Inflammation, orbit
- perirectal K62.89
- perirenal —*see* Infection, kidney
- peritoneal —*see* Peritonitis
- periureteral N28.89
- Petriellidium boydii B48.2
- pharynx —*see also* Pharyngitis
  - coxsackievirus B08.5
  - posterior, lymphoid (chronic) J35.03
- Phialophora
  - gougerotii (subcutaneous abscess or cyst) B43.2
  - jeanselmei (subcutaneous abscess or cyst) B43.2
  - verrucosa (skin) B43.0
- Piedraia hortae B36.3

Infection, infected, infective *(Continued)*
- pinta A67.9
  - intermediate A67.1
  - late A67.2
  - mixed A67.3
  - primary A67.0
- pinworm B80
- pityrosporum furfur B36.0
- pleuro-pneumonia-like organism (PPLO) NEC A49.3
  - as cause of disease classified elsewhere B96.0
- pneumococcus, pneumococcal NEC A49.1
  - as cause of disease classified elsewhere B95.3
  - generalized (purulent) A40.3
    - with pneumonia J13
- Pneumocystis carinii (pneumonia) B59
- Pneumocystis jiroveci (pneumonia) B59
- port or reservoir T80.212
- postoperative T81.4
- postoperative wound T81.4
- postprocedural T81.4
- postvaccinal T88.0
- prepuce NEC N47.7
  - with penile inflammation N47.6
- prion —*see* Disease, prion, central nervous system
- prostate (capsule) —*see* Prostatitis
- Proteus (mirabilis) (morganii) (vulgaris) NEC A49.8
  - as cause of disease classified elsewhere B96.4
- protozoal NEC B64
  - intestinal A07.9
    - specified NEC A07.8
  - specified NEC B60.8
- Pseudoallescheria boydii B48.2
- Pseudomonas NEC A49.8
  - as cause of disease classified elsewhere B96.5
  - mallei A24.0
  - pneumonia J15.1
  - pseudomallei —*see* Melioidosis
- puerperal O86.4
  - genitourinary tract NEC O86.89
  - major or generalized O85
  - minor O86.4
  - specified NEC O86.89
- pulmonary —*see* Infection, lung
- purulent —*see* Abscess
- Pyrenochaeta romeroi B47.0
- Q fever A78
- rectum (sphincter) K62.89
- renal —*see also* Infection, kidney
  - pelvis and ureter (cystic) N28.85
- reovirus, as cause of disease classified elsewhere B97.5
- respiratory (tract) NEC J98.8
  - acute J22
  - chronic J98.8
  - influenzal (upper) (acute) —*see* Influenza, with, respiratory manifestations NEC
  - lower (acute) J22
    - chronic —*see* Bronchitis, chronic
  - rhinovirus J00
  - syncytial virus, as cause of disease classified elsewhere B97.4
  - upper (acute) NOS J06.9
    - chronic J39.8
    - streptococcal J06.9
    - viral NOS J06.9
- resulting from
  - presence of internal prosthesis, implant, graft —*see* Complications, by site and type, infection
- retortamoniasis A07.8
- retroperitoneal NEC K68.9

Infection, infected, infective *(Continued)*
  retrovirus B33.3
    as cause of disease classified elsewhere
      B97.30
      human
        immunodeficiency, type 2 (HIV 2)
          B97.35
        T-cell lymphotropic
          type I (HTLV-I) B97.33
          type II (HTLV-II) B97.34
      lentivirus B97.31
      oncovirus B97.32
      specified NEC B97.39
  Rhinosporidium (seeberi) B48.1
  rhinovirus
    as cause of disease classified elsewhere
      B97.89
    unspecified nature or site B34.8
  Rhizopus —*see* Mucormycosis
  rickettsial NOS A79.9
  roundworm (large) NEC B82.0
    Ascariasis (*see also* Ascariasis) B77.9
  rubella —*see* Rubella
  Saccharomyces —*see* Candidiasis
  salivary duct or gland (any) —*see*
    Sialoadenitis
  Salmonella (aertrycke) (arizonae)
    (callinarum) (cholerae-suis) (enteritidis)
    (suipestifer) (typhimurium) A02.9
    with
      (gastro) enteritis A02.0
      sepsis A02.1
      specified manifestation NEC A02.8
    due to food (poisoning) A02.9
    hirschfeldii A01.3
    localized A02.20
      arthritis A02.23
      meningitis A02.21
      osteomyelitis A02.24
      pneumonia A02.22
      pyelonephritis A02.25
      specified NEC A02.29
    paratyphi A01.4
      A A01.1
      B A01.2
      C A01.3
    schottmuelleri A01.2
    typhi, typhosa —*see* Typhoid
  Sarcocystis A07.8
  scabies B86
  Schistosoma —*see* Infestation, Schistosoma
  scrotum (acute) NEC N49.2
  seminal vesicle —*see* Vesiculitis
  septic
    localized, skin —*see* Abscess
  sheep liver fluke B66.3
  Shigella A03.9
    boydii A03.2
    dysenteriae A03.0
    flexneri A03.1
    group
      A A03.0
      B A03.1
      C A03.2
      D A03.3
    Schmitz (-Stutzer) A03.0
    schmitzii A03.0
    shigae A03.0
    sonnei A03.3
    specified NEC A03.8
  shoulder (joint) NEC M00.9
    due to internal joint prosthesis T84.59
    skin NEC L08.9
  sinus (accessory) (chronic) (nasal) —*see also*
    Sinusitis
    pilonidal —*see* Sinus, pilonidal
    skin NEC L08.89
  Skene's duct or gland —*see* Urethritis
  skin (local) (staphylococcal) (streptococcal)
    L08.9
    abscess - code by site under Abscess

Infection, infected, infective *(Continued)*
  skin *(Continued)*
    cellulitis - code by site under Cellulitis
    due to fungus B36.9
      specified type NEC B36.8
    mycotic B36.9
      specified type NEC B36.8
    newborn P39.4
    ulcer —*see* Ulcer, skin
  slow virus A81.9
    specified NEC A81.89
  Sparganum (mansoni) (proliferum) (baxteri)
    B70.1
  specific —*see also* Syphilis
    to perinatal period —*see* Infection,
      congenital
  specified NEC B99.8
  spermatic cord NEC N49.1
  sphenoidal (sinus) —*see* Sinusitis,
    sphenoidal
  spinal cord NOS (*see also* Myelitis)
    G04.91
    abscess G06.1
    meninges —*see* Meningitis
    streptococcal G04.89
  Spirillum A25.0
  spirochetal NOS A69.9
    lung A69.8
    specified NEC A69.8
  Spirometra larvae B70.1
  spleen D73.89
  Sporotrichum, Sporothrix (schenckii) —*see*
    Sporotrichosis
  staphylococcal, unspecified site
    aureus (methicillin susceptible) (MSSA)
      A49.01
      methicillin resistant (MRSA) A49.02
    as cause of disease classified elsewhere
      B95.8
      aureus (methicillin susceptible) (MSSA)
        B95.61
        methicillin resistant (MRSA)
          B95.62
      specified NEC B95.7
    food poisoning A05.0
    generalized (purulent) A41.2
    pneumonia —*see* Pneumonia,
      staphylococcal
  Stellantchasmus falcatus B66.8
  streptobacillus moniliformis A25.1
  streptococcal NEC A49.1
    as cause of disease classified elsewhere
      B95.5
    B genitourinary complicating
      childbirth O98.82
      pregnancy O98.81-
      puerperium O98.83
    congenital
      sepsis P36.10
        group B P36.0
        specified NEC P36.19
    generalized (purulent) A40.9
  Streptomyces B47.1
  Strongyloides (stercoralis) —*see*
    Strongyloidiasis
  stump (amputation) (surgical) —*see*
    Complication, amputation stump,
    infection
  subcutaneous tissue, local L08.9
  suipestifer —*see* Infection, salmonella
  swimming pool bacillus A31.1
  Taenia —*see* Infestation, Taenia
  Taeniarhynchus saginatus B68.1
  tapeworm —*see* Infestation, tapeworm
  tendon (sheath) —*see* Tenosynovitis, infective
    NEC
  Ternidens diminutus B81.8
  testis —*see* Orchitis
  threadworm B80
  throat —*see* Pharyngitis
  thyroglossal duct K14.8

Infection, infected, infective *(Continued)*
  toe (skin) L08.9
    cellulitis L03.03-
      fungus B35.1
    nail L03.03-
      fungus B35.1
  tongue NEC K14.0
    parasitic B37.0
  tonsil (and adenoid) (faucial) (lingual)
    (pharyngeal) —*see* Tonsillitis
  tooth, teeth K04.7
    periapical K04.7
    peridental, periodontal K05.20
      generalized K05.22
      localized K05.21
    pulp K04.0
    socket M27.3
  TORCH —*see* Infection, congenital
    without active infection P00.2
  Torula histolytica —*see* Cryptococcosis
  Toxocara (canis) (cati) (felis) B83.0
  Toxoplasma gondii —*see* Toxoplasma
  trachea, chronic J42
  trematode NEC —*see* Infestation, fluke
  trench fever A79.0
  Treponema pallidum —*see* Syphilis
  Trichinella (spiralis) B75
  Trichomonas A59.9
    cervix A59.09
    intestine A07.8
    prostate A59.02
    specified site NEC A59.8
    urethra A59.03
    urogenitalis A59.00
    vagina A59.01
    vulva A59.01
  Trichophyton, trichophytic —*see*
    Dermatophytosis
  Trichosporon (beigelii) cutaneum B36.2
  Trichostrongylus B81.2
  Trichuris (trichiura) B79
  Trombicula (irritans) B88.0
  Trypanosoma
    brucei
      gambiense B56.0
      rhodesiense B56.1
    cruzi —*see* Chagas' disease
  tubal —*see* Salpingo-oophoritis
  tuberculous NEC —*see* Tuberculosis
  tubo-ovarian —*see* Salpingo-oophoritis
  tunica vaginalis N49.1
  tunnel T80.212
  tympanic membrane NEC —*see* Myringitis
  typhoid (abortive) (ambulant) (bacillus) —*see*
    Typhoid
  typhus A75.9
    flea-borne A75.2
    mite-borne A75.3
    recrudescent A75.1
    tick-borne A77.9
      African A77.1
      North Asian A77.2
  umbilicus L08.82
  ureter N28.86
  urethra —*see* Urethritis
  urinary (tract) N39.0
    bladder —*see* Cystitis
    complicating
      pregnancy O23.4-
        specified type NEC O23.3-
    kidney —*see* Infection, kidney
    newborn P39.3
    puerperal (postpartum) O86.20
    tuberculous A18.13
    urethra —*see* Urethritis
  uterus, uterine —*see* Endometritis
  vaccination T88.0
  vaccinia not from vaccination B08.011
  vagina (acute) —*see* Vaginitis
  varicella B01.9
  varicose veins —*see* Varix

◀ New   ◀◀◀ Revised   ~~deleted~~ Deleted

Infection, infected, infective (Continued)
vas deferens NEC N49.1
vesical —see Cystitis
Vibrio
cholerae A00.0
El Tor A00.1
parahaemolyticus (food poisoning) A05.3
vulnificus
as cause of disease classified elsewhere
B96.82
foodborne intoxication A05.5
Vincent's (gum) (mouth) (tonsil) A69.1
virus, viral NOS B34.9
adenovirus
as cause of disease classified elsewhere
B97.0
unspecified nature or site B34.0
arborvirus, arbovirus arthropod-borne A94
as cause of disease classified elsewhere
B97.89
adenovirus B97.0
coronavirus B97.29
SARS-associated B97.21
coxsackievirus B97.11
echovirus B97.12
enterovirus B97.10
coxsackievirus B97.11
echovirus B97.12
specified NEC B97.19
human
immunodeficiency, type 2 (HIV 2)
B97.35
metapneumovirus B97.81
T-cell lymphotropic,
type I (HTLV-I) B97.33
type II (HTLV-II) B97.34
papillomavirus B97.7
parvovirus B97.6
reovirus B97.5
respiratory syncytial B97.4
retrovirus B97.30
human
immunodeficiency, type 2 (HIV 2)
B97.35
T-cell lymphotropic,
type I (HTLV-I) B97.33
type II (HTLV-II) B97.34
lentivirus B97.31
oncovirus B97.32
specified NEC B97.39
specified NEC B97.89
central nervous system A89
atypical A81.9
specified NEC A81.89
enterovirus NEC A88.8
meningitis A87.0
slow virus A81.9
specified NEC A81.89
specified NEC A88.8
chest J98.8
cotia B08.8
coxsackie (see also Infection, coxsackie)
B34.1
as cause of disease classified elsewhere
B97.11
ECHO
as cause of disease classified elsewhere
B97.12
unspecified nature or site B34.1
encephalitis, tick-borne A84.9
enterovirus, as cause of disease classified
elsewhere B97.10
coxsackievirus B97.11
echovirus B97.12
specified NEC B97.19
exanthem NOS B09
human metapneumovirus as cause of
disease classified elsewhere B97.81
human papilloma as cause of disease
classified elsewhere B97.7
intestine —see Enteritis, viral

Infection, infected, infective (Continued)
virus, viral NOS (Continued)
respiratory syncytial
as cause of disease classified elsewhere
B97.4
bronchopneumonia J12.1
common cold syndrome J00
nasopharyngitis (acute) J00
rhinovirus
as cause of disease classified elsewhere
B97.89
unspecified nature or site B34.8
slow A81.9
specified NEC A81.89
specified type NEC B33.8
as cause of disease classified elsewhere
B97.89
unspecified nature or site B34.8
unspecified nature or site B34.9
West Nile —see Virus, West Nile
vulva (acute) —see Vulvitis
West Nile —see Virus, West Nile
whipworm B79
worms B83.9
specified type NEC B83.8
Wuchereria (bancrofti) B74.0
malayi B74.1
yatapoxvirus B08.70
specified NEC B08.79
yeast (see also Candidiasis) B37.9
yellow fever —see Fever, yellow
Yersinia
enterocolitica (intestinal) A04.6
pestis —see Plague
pseudotuberculosis A28.2
Zeis' gland —see Hordeolum
zoonotic bacterial NOS A28.9
Zopfia senegalensis B47.0
Infective, infectious —see condition
Infertility
female N97.9
age-related N97.8
associated with
anovulation N97.0
cervical (mucus) disease or anomaly
N88.3
congenital anomaly
cervix N88.3
fallopian tube N97.1
uterus N97.2
vagina N97.8
dysmucorrhea N88.3
fallopian tube disease or anomaly N97.1
pituitary-hypothalamic origin E23.0
specified origin NEC N97.8
Stein-Leventhal syndrome E28.2
uterine disease or anomaly N97.2
vaginal disease or anomaly N97.8
due to
cervical anomaly N88.3
fallopian tube anomaly N97.1
ovarian failure E28.39
Stein-Leventhal syndrome E28.2
uterine anomaly N97.2
vaginal anomaly N97.8
nonimplantation N97.2
origin
cervical N88.3
tubal (block) (occlusion) (stenosis)
N97.1
uterine N97.2
vaginal N97.8
male N46.9
azoospermia N46.01
extratesticular cause N46.029
drug therapy N46.021
efferent duct obstruction N46.023
infection N46.022
radiation N46.024
specified cause NEC N46.029
systemic disease N46.025

Infertility (Continued)
male (Continued)
oligospermia N46.11
extratesticular cause N46.129
drug therapy N46.121
efferent duct obstruction N46.123
infection N46.122
radiation N46.124
specified cause NEC N46.129
systemic disease N46.125
specified type NEC N46.8
Infestation B88.9
Acanthocheilonema (perstans) (streptocerca)
B74.4
Acariasis B88.0
demodex folliculorum B88.0
sarcoptes scabiei B86
trombiculae B88.0
Agamofilaria streptocerca B74.4
Ancylostoma, ankylostoma (braziliense)
(caninum) (ceylanicum) (duodenale)
B76.0
americanum B76.1
new world B76.1
Anisakis larvae, anisakiasis B81.0
arthropod NEC B88.2
Ascaris lumbricoides —see Ascariasis
Balantidium coli A07.0
beef tapeworm B68.1
Bothriocephalus (latus) B70.0
larval B70.1
broad tapeworm B70.0
larval B70.1
Brugia (malayi) B74.1
timori B74.2
candiru B88.8
Capillaria
hepatica B83.8
philippinensis B81.1
cat liver fluke B66.0
cestodes B71.9
diphyllobothrium —see Infestation,
diphyllobothrium
dipylidiasis B71.1
hymenolepiasis B71.0
specified type NEC B71.8
chigger B88.0
chigo, chigoe B88.1
Clonorchis (sinensis) (liver) B66.1
coccidial A07.3
crab-lice B85.3
Cysticercus cellulosae —see Cysticercosis
Demodex (folliculorum) B88.0
Dermanyssus gallinae B88.0
Dermatobia (hominis) —see Myiasis
Dibothriocephalus (latus) B70.0
larval B70.1
Dicrocoelium dendriticum B66.2
Diphyllobothrium (adult) (latum) (intestinal)
(pacificum) B70.0
larval B70.1
Diplogonoporus (grandis) B71.8
Dipylidium caninum B67.4
Distoma hepaticum B66.3
dog tapeworm B67.4
Dracunculus medinensis B72
dragon worm B72
dwarf tapeworm B71.0
Echinococcus —see Echinococcus
Echinostomum ilocanum B66.8
Entamoeba (histolytica) —see Infection,
Ameba
Enterobius vermicularis B80
eyelid
in (due to)
leishmaniasis B55.1
loiasis B74.3
onchocerciasis B73.09
phthriasis B85.3
parasitic NOS B89
eyeworm B74.3

Infiltrate, infiltration *(Continued)*
 liver K76.89
  fatty —*see* Fatty, liver NEC
  glycogen *(see also* Disease, glycogen
   storage) E74.03 *[K77]*
 lung R91.8
  eosinophilic J82
 lymphatic *(see also* Leukemia, lymphatic)
   C91.9-
  gland I88.9
 muscle, fatty M62.89
 myocardium, myocardial
  fatty —*see* Degeneration, myocardial
  glycogenic E74.02 *[I43]*
 on chest x-ray R91.8
 pulmonary R91.8
  with eosinophilia J82
 skin (lymphocytic) L98.6
 thymus (gland) (fatty) E32.8
 urine R39.0
 vesicant agent
  antineoplastic chemotherapy T80.810
  other agent NEC T80.818
 vitreous body H43.89
Infirmity R68.89
 senile R54
Inflammation, inflamed, inflammatory (with
  exudation)
 abducent (nerve) —*see* Strabismus, paralytic,
   sixth nerve
 accessory sinus (chronic) —*see* Sinusitis
 adrenal (gland) E27.8
 alveoli, teeth M27.3
  scorbutic E54
 anal canal, anus K62.89
 antrum (chronic) —*see* Sinusitis, maxillary
 appendix —*see* Appendicitis
 arachnoid —*see* Meningitis
 areola N61
  puerperal, postpartum or gestational —*see*
    Infection, nipple
 areolar tissue NOS L08.9
 artery —*see* Arteritis
 auditory meatus (external) —*see* Otitis,
   externa
 Bartholin's gland N75.8
 bile duct (common) (hepatic) or passage —*see*
   Cholangitis
 bladder —*see* Cystitis
 bone —*see* Osteomyelitis
 brain —*see also* Encephalitis
  membrane —*see* Meningitis
 breast N61
  puerperal, postpartum, gestational —*see*
    Mastitis, obstetric
 broad ligament —*see* Disease, pelvis,
   inflammatory
 bronchi —*see* Bronchitis
 catarrhal J00
 cecum —*see* Appendicitis
 cerebral —*see also* Encephalitis
  membrane —*see* Meningitis
 cerebrospinal
  meningococcal A39.0
 cervix (uteri) —*see* Cervicitis
 chest J98.8
 chorioretinal H30.9-
  cyclitis —*see* Cyclitis
  disseminated H30.10-
   generalized H30.13-
   peripheral H30.12-
   posterior pole H30.11-
  epitheliopathy —*see* Epitheliopathy
  focal H30.00-
   juxtapapillary H30.01-
   macular H30.04-
   paramacular —*see* Inflammation,
     chorioretinal, focal, macular
   peripheral H30.03-
   posterior pole H30.02-
  specified type NEC H30.89-

Inflammation, inflamed, inflammatory
  (Continued)
 choroid —*see* Inflammation, chorioretinal
 chronic, postmastoidectomy cavity —*see*
   Complications, postmastoidectomy,
   inflammation
 colon —*see* Enteritis
 connective tissue (diffuse) NEC —*see*
   Disorder, soft tissue, specified type NEC
 cornea —*see* Keratitis
 corpora cavernosa N48.29
 cranial nerve —*see* Disorder, nerve, cranial
 Douglas' cul-de-sac or pouch (chronic) N73.0
 due to device, implant or graft —*see also*
   Complications, by site and type,
   infection or inflammation
  arterial graft T82.7
  breast (implant) T85.79
  catheter T85.79
   dialysis (renal) T82.7
    intraperitoneal T85.71
   infusion T82.7
    spinal (epidural) (subdural) T85.79
   urinary (indwelling) T83.51
  electronic (electrode) (pulse generator)
    (stimulator)
   bone T84.7
   cardiac T82.7
   nervous system (brain) (peripheral
     nerve) (spinal) T85.79
   urinary T83.59
  fixation, internal (orthopedic) NEC —*see*
    Complication, fixation device,
    infection
  gastrointestinal (bile duct) (esophagus)
    T85.79
  genital NEC T83.6
  heart NEC T82.7
   valve (prosthesis) T82.6
    graft T82.7
  joint prosthesis —*see* Complication, joint
    prosthesis, infection
  ocular (corneal graft) (orbital implant)
    NEC T85.79
  orthopedic NEC T84.7
  specified NEC T85.79
  urinary NEC T83.59
  vascular NEC T82.7
  ventricular intracranial shunt T85.79
 duodenum K29.80
  with bleeding K29.81
 dura mater —*see* Meningitis
 ear (middle) —*see also* Otitis, media
  external —*see* Otitis, externa
  inner —*see* subcategory H83.0
 epididymis —*see* Epididymitis
 esophagus K20.9
 ethmoidal (sinus) (chronic) —*see* Sinusitis,
   ethmoidal
 eustachian tube (catarrhal) —*see* Salpingitis,
   eustachian
 eyelid H01.9
  abscess —*see* Abscess, eyelid
  blepharitis —*see* Blepharitis
  chalazion —*see* Chalazion
  dermatosis (noninfectious) —*see*
    Dermatosis, eyelid
  hordeolum —*see* Hordeolum
  specified NEC H01.8
 fallopian tube —*see* Salpingo-oophoritis
 fascia —*see* Myositis
 follicular, pharynx J31.2
 frontal (sinus) (chronic) —*see* Sinusitis, frontal
 gallbladder —*see* Cholecystitis
 gastric —*see* Gastritis
 gastrointestinal —*see* Enteritis
 genital organ (internal) (diffuse)
  female —*see* Disease, pelvis, inflammatory
  male N49.9
   multiple sites N49.8
   specified NEC N49.8

Inflammation, inflamed, inflammatory
  (Continued)
 gland (lymph) —*see* Lymphadenitis
 glottis —*see* Laryngitis
 granular, pharynx J31.2
 gum K05.10
  nonplaque induced K05.11
  plaque induced K05.10
 heart —*see* Carditis
 hepatic duct —*see* Cholangitis
 ileoanal (internal) pouch K91.850
 ileum —*see also* Enteritis
  regional or terminal —*see* Enteritis,
    regional
 intestinal pouch K91.850
 intestine (any part) —*see* Enteritis
 jaw (acute) (bone) (chronic) (lower)
   (suppurative) (upper) M27.2
 joint NEC —*see* Arthritis
  sacroiliac M46.1
 kidney —*see* Nephritis
 knee (joint) M13.169
  tuberculous A18.02
 labium (majus) (minus) —*see* Vulvitis
 lacrimal
  gland —*see* Dacryoadenitis
  passages (duct) (sac) —*see also*
    Dacryocystitis
   canaliculitis —*see* Canaliculitis, lacrimal
 larynx —*see* Laryngitis
 leg NOS L08.9
 lip K13.0
 liver (capsule) —*see also* Hepatitis
  chronic K73.9
  suppurative K75.0
 lung (acute) —*see also* Pneumonia
  chronic J98.4
 lymphatic vessel —*see* Lymphangitis
 lymph gland or node —*see* Lymphadenitis
 maxilla, maxillary M27.2
  sinus (chronic) —*see* Sinusitis, maxillary
 membranes of brain or spinal cord —*see*
   Meningitis
 meninges —*see* Meningitis
 mouth K12.1
 muscle —*see* Myositis
 myocardium —*see* Myocarditis
 nasal sinus (chronic) —*see* Sinusitis
 nasopharynx —*see* Nasopharyngitis
 navel L08.82
 nerve NEC —*see* Neuralgia
 nipple N61
  puerperal, postpartum or gestational —*see*
    Infection, nipple
 nose —*see* Rhinitis
 oculomotor (nerve) —*see* Strabismus,
   paralytic, third nerve
 optic nerve —*see* Neuritis, optic
 orbit (chronic) H05.10
  acute H05.00
   abscess —*see* Abscess, orbit
   cellulitis —*see* Cellulitis, orbit
   osteomyelitis —*see* Osteomyelitis,
     orbit
   periostitis —*see* Periostitis, orbital
   tenonitis —*see* Tenonitis, eye
  granuloma —*see* Granuloma, orbit
  myositis —*see* Myositis, orbital
 ovary —*see* Salpingo-oophoritis
 oviduct —*see* Salpingo-oophoritis
 pancreas (acute) —*see* Pancreatitis
 parametrium N73.0
 parotid region L08.9
 pelvis, female —*see* Disease, pelvis,
   inflammatory
 penis (corpora cavernosa) N48.29
 perianal K62.89
 pericardium —*see* Pericarditis
 perineum (female) (male) L08.9
 perirectal K62.89
 peritoneum —*see* Peritonitis

Inflammation, inflamed, inflammatory
(Continued)
periuterine —*see* Disease, pelvis, inflammatory
perivesical —*see* Cystitis
petrous bone (acute) (chronic) —*see* Petrositis
pharynx (acute) —*see* Pharyngitis
pia mater —*see* Meningitis
pleura —*see* Pleurisy
polyp, colon (*see also* Polyp, colon, inflammatory) K51.40
prostate —*see also* Prostatitis
specified type NEC N41.8
rectosigmoid —*see* Rectosigmoiditis
rectum (*see also* Proctitis) K62.89
respiratory, upper (*see also* Infection, respiratory, upper) J06.9
acute, due to radiation J70.0
chronic, due to external agent —*see* condition, respiratory, chronic, due to
due to
chemicals, gases, fumes or vapors (inhalation) J68.2
radiation J70.1
retina —*see* Chorioretinitis
retrocecal —*see* Appendicitis
retroperitoneal —*see* Peritonitis
salivary duct or gland (any) (suppurative) —*see* Sialoadenitis
scorbutic, alveoli, teeth E54
scrotum N49.2
seminal vesicle —*see* Vesiculitis
sigmoid —*see* Enteritis
sinus —*see* Sinusitis
Skene's duct or gland —*see* Urethritis
skin L08.9
spermatic cord N49.1
sphenoidal (sinus) —*see* Sinusitis, sphenoidal
spinal
cord —*see* Encephalitis
membrane —*see* Meningitis
nerve —*see* Disorder, nerve
spine —*see* Spondylopathy, inflammatory
spleen (capsule) D73.89
stomach —*see* Gastritis
subcutaneous tissue L08.9
suprarenal (gland) E27.8
synovial —*see* Tenosynovitis
tendon (sheath) NEC —*see* Tenosynovitis
testis —*see* Orchitis
throat (acute) —*see* Pharyngitis
thymus (gland) E32.8
thyroid (gland) —*see* Thyroiditis
tongue K14.0
tonsil —*see* Tonsillitis
trachea —*see* Tracheitis
trochlear (nerve) —*see* Strabismus, paralytic, fourth nerve
tubal —*see* Salpingo-oophoritis
tuberculous NEC —*see* Tuberculosis
tubo-ovarian —*see* Salpingo-oophoritis
tunica vaginalis N49.1
tympanic membrane —*see* Tympanitis
umbilicus, umbilical L08.82
uterine ligament —*see* Disease, pelvis, inflammatory
uterus (catarrhal) —*see* Endometritis
uveal tract (anterior) NOS —*see also* Iridocyclitis
posterior —*see* Chorioretinitis
vagina —*see* Vaginitis
vas deferens N49.1
vein —*see also* Phlebitis
intracranial or intraspinal (septic) G08
thrombotic I80.9
leg —*see* Phlebitis, leg
lower extremity —*see* Phlebitis, leg
vocal cord J38.3
vulva —*see* Vulvitis
Wharton's duct (suppurative) —*see* Sialoadenitis

Inflation, lung, imperfect (newborn) —*see* Atelectasis
Influenza (bronchial) (epidemic) (respiratory (upper)) (unidentified influenza virus) J11.1
with
digestive manifestations J11.2
encephalopathy J11.81
enteritis J11.2
gastroenteritis J11.2
gastrointestinal manifestations J11.2
laryngitis J11.1
myocarditis J11.82
otitis media J11.83
pharyngitis J11.1
pneumonia J11.00
specified type J11.08
respiratory manifestations NEC J11.1
specified manifestation NEC J11.89
A/H5N1 —*see also* Influenza, due to, identified novel influenza A virus J09.X2
avian —*see also* Influenza, due to, identified novel influenza A virus J09.X2
bird (*see also* Influenza, due to, identified novel influenza A virus) J09.X2
novel (2009) H1N1 influenza (*see also* Influenza, due to, identified influenza virus NEC) J10.1
novel influenza A/H1N1 (*see also* Influenza, due to, identified influenza virus NEC) J10.1
due to
avian (*see also* Influenza, due to, identified novel influenza A virus) J09.X2
identified influenza virus NEC J10.1
with
digestive manifestations J10.2
encephalopathy J10.81
enteritis J10.2
gastroenteritis J10.2
gastrointestinal manifestations J10.2
laryngitis J10.1
myocarditis J10.82
otitis media J10.83
pharyngitis J10.1
pneumonia (unspecified type) J10.00
with same identified influenza virus J10.01
specified type NEC J10.08
respiratory manifestations NEC J10.1
specified manifestation NEC J10.89
identified novel influenza A virus J09.X2
with
digestive manifestations J09.X3
encephalopathy J09.X9
enteritis J09.X3
gastroenteritis J09.X3
gastrointestinal manifestations J09.X3
laryngitis J09.X2
myocarditis J09.X9
otitis media J09.X9
pharyngitis J09.X2
pneumonia J09.X1
respiratory manifestations NEC J09.X2
specified manifestation NEC J09.X9
upper respiratory symptoms J09.X2
of other animal origin, not bird or swine (*see also* Influenza, due to, identified novel influenza A virus) J09.X2
swine (viruses that normally cause infections in pigs) (*see also* Influenza, due to, identified novel influenza A virus) J09.X2
Influenza-like disease —*see* Influenza
Influenzal —*see* Influenza
Infraction, Freiberg's (metatarsal head) —*see* Osteochondrosis, juvenile, metatarsus
Infraeruption of tooth (teeth) M26.34
Infusion complication, misadventure, or reaction —*see* Complications, infusion

Ingestion
chemical —*see* Table of ⊕Drugs and ⊕Chemicals, by substance, poisoning ◀◁
drug or medicament
correct substance properly administered —*see* Table of ⊕Drugs and ⊕Chemicals, by drug, adverse effect ◀◁
overdose or wrong substance given or taken —*see* Table of ⊕Drugs and ⊕Chemicals, by drug, poisoning ◀◁
foreign body —*see* Foreign body, alimentary tract
tularemia A21.3
Ingrowing
hair (beard) L73.1
nail (finger) (toe) L60.0
Inguinal —*see also* condition
testicle Q53.9
bilateral Q53.21
unilateral Q53.11
Inhalation
anthrax A22.1
flame T27.3
food or foreign body —*see* Foreign body, by site
gases, fumes, or vapors NEC T59.9-
specified agent —*see* Table of ⊕Drugs and ⊕Chemicals, by substance ◀◁
liquid or vomitus —*see* Asphyxia
meconium (newborn) P24.00
with
with respiratory symptoms P24.01
pneumonia (pneumonitis) P24.01
mucus —*see* Asphyxia, mucus
oil or gasoline (causing suffocation) —*see* Foreign body, by site
smoke J70.5
due to chemicals, gases, fumes and vapors J68.9
steam —*see* Toxicity, vapors
stomach contents or secretions —*see* Foreign body, by site
due to anesthesia (general) (local) or other sedation T88.59
in labor and delivery O74.0
in pregnancy O29.01-
postpartum, puerperal O89.01
Inhibition, orgasm
female F52.31
male F52.32
Inhibitor, systemic lupus erythematosus (presence of) D68.62
Iniencephalus, iniencephaly Q00.2
Injection, traumatic jet (air) (industrial) (water) (paint or dye) T70.4
Injury (*see also* specified injury type) T14.90
abdomen, abdominal S39.91
blood vessel —*see* Injury, blood vessel, abdomen
cavity —*see* Injury, intra-abdominal
contusion S30.1
internal —*see* Injury, intra-abdominal
intra-abdominal organ —*see* Injury, intra-abdominal
nerve —*see* Injury, nerve, abdomen
open —*see* Wound, open, abdomen
specified NEC S39.81
superficial —*see* Injury, superficial, abdomen
Achilles tendon S86.00-
laceration S86.02-
specified type NEC S86.09-
strain S86.01-
acoustic, resulting in deafness —*see* Injury, nerve, acoustic
adrenal (gland) S37.819
contusion S37.812
laceration S37.813
specified type NEC S37.818
alveolar (process) S09.93

◀ New   ◀◁ Revised   ~~deleted~~ Deleted

Injury (Continued)
  ankle S99.91-
    contusion —see Contusion, ankle
    dislocation —see Dislocation, ankle
    fracture —see Fracture, ankle
    nerve —see Injury, nerve, ankle
    open —see Wound, open, ankle
    specified type NEC S99.81-
    sprain —see Sprain, ankle
    superficial —see Injury, superficial, ankle
  anterior chamber, eye —see Injury, eye,
      specified site NEC
  anus —see Injury, abdomen
  aorta (thoracic) S25.00
    abdominal S35.00
      laceration (minor) (superficial) S35.01
        major S35.02
      specified type NEC S35.09
    laceration (minor) (superficial) S25.01
      major S25.02
    specified type NEC S25.09
  arm (upper) S49.9-
    blood vessel —see Injury, blood vessel,
        arm
    contusion —see Contusion, arm, upper
    fracture —see Fracture, humerus
    lower —see Injury, forearm
    muscle —see Injury, muscle, shoulder
    nerve —see Injury, nerve, arm
    open —see Wound, open, arm
    specified type NEC S49.8-
    superficial —see Injury, superficial, arm
  artery (complicating trauma) —see also Injury,
      blood vessel, by site
    cerebral or meningeal —see Injury,
        intracranial
  auditory canal (external) (meatus) S09.91
  auricle, auris, ear S09.91
  axilla —see Injury, shoulder
  back —see Injury, back, lower
  bile duct —see Injury, gallbladder S36.13 ◀▥
  birth —see also Birth, injury P15.9
  bladder (sphincter) S37.20
    at delivery O71.5
    contusion S37.22
    laceration S37.23
    obstetrical trauma O71.5
    specified type NEC S37.29
  blast (air) (hydraulic) (immersion)
      (underwater) NEC T14.8
    acoustic nerve trauma —see Injury, nerve,
        acoustic
    bladder —see Injury, bladder, blast injury ◀▥
    brain —see Concussion
    colon —see Injury, intestine, large, blast
        injury
    ear (primary) S09.31-
      secondary S09.39-
    generalized T70.8
    lung —see Injury, intrathoracic, lung, blast
        injury
    multiple body organs T70.8
    peritoneum S36.81
    rectum S36.61
    retroperitoneum S36.898
    small intestine S36.419
      duodenum S36.410
      specified site NEC S36.418
    specified
      intra-abdominal organ NEC S36.898
      pelvic organ NEC S37.899
  blood vessel NEC T14.8
    abdomen S35.9- ◀▥
      aorta —see Injury, aorta, abdominal
      celiac artery —see Injury, blood vessel,
          celiac artery
      iliac vessel —see Injury, blood vessel,
          iliac
      laceration S35.91
      mesenteric vessel —see Injury,
          mesenteric

Injury (Continued)
  blood vessel NEC (Continued)
    abdomen (Continued)
      portal vein —see Injury, blood vessel,
          portal vein
      renal vessel —see Injury, blood vessel,
          renal
      specified T14.8
        site NEC —see subcategory S35.8
        type NEC S35.99
      specified vessel NEC S35.8X- ◀
      splenic vessel —see Injury, blood vessel,
          splenic
      vena cava —see Injury, vena cava,
          inferior
    ankle —see Injury, blood vessel, foot
    aorta (abdominal) (thoracic) —see Injury,
        aorta
    arm (upper) NEC S45.90-
      forearm —see Injury, blood vessel,
          forearm
      laceration S45.91
      specified
        site NEC S45.80-
          laceration S45.81-
          specified type NEC S45.89-
        type NEC S45.99-
      superficial vein S45.30-
        laceration S45.31-
        specified type NEC S45.39-
    axillary
      artery S45.00-
        laceration S45.01-
        specified type NEC S45.09-
      vein S45.20-
        laceration S45.21-
        specified type NEC S45.29-
    azygos vein —see Injury, blood vessel,
        thoracic, specified site NEC
    brachial
      artery S45.10-
        laceration S45.11-
        specified type NEC S45.19-
      vein S45.20-
        laceration S45.219
        specified type NEC S45.29-
    carotid artery (common) (external)
        (internal, extracranial) S15.00-
      internal, intracranial S06.8-
      laceration (minor) (superficial) S15.01-
        major S15.02-
      specified type NEC S15.09-
    celiac artery S35.219
      branch S35.299
        laceration (minor) (superficial) S35.291
          major S35.292
        specified NEC S35.298
      laceration (minor) (superficial) S35.211
        major S35.212
      specified type NEC S35.218
    cerebral —see Injury, intracranial
    deep plantar —see Injury, nerve, medial
        plantar blood vessel, plantar artery ◀▥
    digital (hand) —see Injury, blood vessel,
        finger
    dorsal
      artery (foot) S95.00-
        laceration S95.01-
        specified type NEC S95.09-
      vein (foot) S95.20-
        laceration S95.21-
        specified type NEC S95.29-
    due to accidental laceration during
        procedure —see Laceration, accidental
        complicating surgery
    extremity —see Injury, blood vessel, limb
    femoral
      artery (common) (superficial) S75.00-
        laceration (minor) (superficial) S75.01-
          major S75.02-
        specified type NEC S75.09-

Injury (Continued)
  blood vessel NEC (Continued)
    femoral (Continued)
      vein (hip level) (thigh level) S75.10-
        laceration (minor) (superficial) S75.11-
          major S75.12-
        specified type NEC S75.19-
    finger S65.50-
      index S65.50-
        laceration S65.51-
        specified type NEC S65.59-
      laceration S65.51-
      little S65.50-
        laceration S65.51-
        specified type NEC S65.59-
      middle S65.50-
        laceration S65.51-
        specified type NEC S65.59-
      specified type NEC S65.59-
      thumb —see Injury, blood vessel, thumb
    foot S95.90-
      dorsal
        artery —see Injury, blood vessel,
            dorsal, artery
        vein —see Injury, blood vessel, dorsal,
            vein
      laceration S95.91-
      plantar artery —see Injury, blood vessel,
          plantar artery
      specified
        site NEC S95.80-
          laceration S95.81-
          specified type NEC S95.89-
        specified type NEC S95.99-
    forearm S55.90-
      laceration S55.91-
      radial artery —see Injury, blood vessel,
          radial artery
      specified
        site NEC S55.80-
          laceration S55.81-
          specified type NEC S55.89-
        type NEC S55.99-
      ulnar artery —see Injury, blood vessel,
          ulnar artery
      vein S55.20-
        laceration S55.21-
        specified type NEC S55.29-
    gastric
      artery —see Injury, mesenteric, artery,
          branch
      vein —see Injury, blood vessel, abdomen
    gastroduodenal artery —see Injury,
        mesenteric, artery, branch
    greater saphenous vein (lower leg level)
        S85.30-
      hip (and thigh) level S75.20-
        laceration (minor) (superficial) S75.21-
          major S75.22-
        specified type NEC S75.29-
      laceration S85.31-
      specified type NEC S85.39-
    hand (level) S65.90-
      finger —see Injury, blood vessel, finger
      laceration S65.91-
      palmar arch —see Injury, blood vessel,
          palmar arch
      radial artery —see Injury, blood vessel,
          radial artery, hand
      specified
        site NEC S65.80-
          laceration S65.81-
          specified type NEC S65.89-
        type NEC S65.99-
      thumb —see Injury, blood vessel,
          thumb
      ulnar artery —see Injury, blood vessel,
          ulnar artery, hand
    head S09.0
      intracranial —see Injury, intracranial
      multiple S09.0

Injury (Continued)
  blood vessel NEC (Continued)
    hepatic
      artery —see Injury, mesenteric, artery
      vein —see Injury, vena cava, inferior
    hip S75.90-
      femoral artery —see Injury, blood vessel,
        femoral, artery
      femoral vein —see Injury, blood vessel,
        femoral, vein
      greater saphenous vein —see Injury,
        blood vessel, greater saphenous,
        hip level
      laceration S75.91-
      specified
        site NEC S75.80-
          laceration S75.81-
            specified type NEC S75.89-
          type NEC S75.99-
    hypogastric (artery) (vein) —see Injury,
      blood vessel, iliac
    iliac S35.5-
      artery S35.51-
      specified vessel NEC S35.5-
      uterine vessel —see Injury, blood vessel,
        uterine
      vein S35.51-
    innominate —see Injury, blood vessel,
      thoracic, innominate
    intercostal (artery) (vein) —see Injury,
      blood vessel, thoracic, intercostal
    jugular vein (external) S15.20-
      internal S15.30-
        laceration (minor) (superficial)
          S15.31-
          major S15.32-
        specified type NEC S15.39-
      laceration (minor) (superficial) S15.21-
        major S15.22-
      specified type NEC S15.29-
    leg (level) (lower) S85.90-
      greater saphenous —see Injury, blood
        vessel, greater saphenous
      laceration S85.91-
      lesser saphenous —see Injury, blood
        vessel, lesser saphenous
      peroneal artery —see Injury, blood
        vessel, peroneal artery
      popliteal
        artery —see Injury, blood vessel,
          popliteal, artery
        vein —see Injury, blood vessel,
          popliteal, vein
      specified
        site NEC S85.80-
          laceration S85.81-
            specified type NEC S85.89-
          type NEC S85.99-
      thigh —see Injury, blood vessel, hip
      tibial artery —see Injury, blood vessel,
        tibial artery
    lesser saphenous vein (lower leg level)
      S85.40-
      laceration S85.41-
      specified type NEC S85.49-
    limb
      lower —see Injury, blood vessel, leg
      upper —see Injury, blood vessel, arm
    lower back —see Injury, blood vessel,
      abdomen
      specified NEC —see Injury, blood vessel,
        abdomen, specified, site NEC
    mammary (artery) (vein) —see Injury,
      blood vessel, thoracic, specified site
      NEC
    mesenteric (inferior) (superior)
      artery —see Injury, mesenteric, artery
      vein —see Injury, blood vessel,
        portalmesenteric, vein ◄▪▪▪
    neck S15.9
      specified site NEC S15.8

Injury (Continued)
  blood vessel NEC (Continued)
    ovarian (artery) (vein) —see subcategory
      S35.8
    palmar arch (superficial) S65.20-
      deep S65.30-
        laceration S65.31-
        specified type NEC S65.39-
      laceration S65.21-
      specified type NEC S65.29-
    pelvis —see Injury, blood vessel, abdomen
      specified NEC —see Injury, blood vessel,
        abdomen, specified, site NEC
    peroneal artery S85.20-
      laceration S85.21-
      specified type NEC S85.29-
    plantar artery (deep) (foot) S95.10-
      laceration S95.11-
      specified type NEC S95.19-
    popliteal
      artery S85.00-
        laceration S85.01-
        specified type NEC S85.09-
      vein S85.50-
        laceration S85.51-
        specified type NEC S85.59-
    portal vein S35.319
      laceration S35.311
      specified type NEC S35.318
    precerebral —see Injury, blood vessel, neck
    pulmonary (artery) (vein) —see Injury,
      blood vessel, thoracic, pulmonary
    radial artery (forearm level) S55.10-
      hand and wrist (level) S65.10-
        laceration S65.11-
        specified type NEC S65.19-
      laceration S55.11-
      specified type NEC S55.19-
    renal
      artery S35.40-
        laceration S35.41-
        specified NEC S35.49-
      vein S35.40-
        laceration S35.41-
        specified NEC S35.49-
    saphenous vein (greater) (lower leg
      level) (vein) —see Injury, blood vessel,
      greater saphenous
      hip and thigh level —see Injury, blood
        vessel, greater saphenous, hip level
      lesser —see Injury, blood vessel, lesser
        saphenous
    shoulder
      specified NEC —see Injury, blood vessel,
        arm, specified site NEC
      superficial vein —see Injury, blood
        vessel, arm, superficial vein
    specified NEC T14.8 ◄▪▪▪
    splenic
      artery —see Injury, blood vessel, celiac
        artery, branch
      vein S35.329
        laceration S35.321
        specified NEC S35.328
    subclavian —see Injury, blood vessel,
      thoracic, innominate
    thigh —see Injury, blood vessel, hip
    thoracic S25.90
      aorta S25.00
        laceration (minor) (superficial)
          S25.01
          major S25.02
        specified type NEC S25.09
      azygos vein —see Injury, blood vessel,
        thoracic, specified, site NEC
      innominate
        artery S25.10-
          laceration (minor) (superficial)
            S25.11-
            major S25.12-
          specified type NEC S25.19-

Injury (Continued)
  blood vessel NEC (Continued)
    thoracic (Continued)
      innominate (Continued)
        vein S25.30-
          laceration (minor) (superficial)
            S25.31-
            major S25.32-
          specified type NEC S25.39-
      intercostal S25.50-
        laceration S25.51-
        specified type NEC S25.59-
      laceration S25.91
      mammary vessel —see Injury, blood
        vessel, thoracic, specified, site NEC
      pulmonary S25.40-
        laceration (minor) (superficial) S25.41-
          major S25.42-
        specified type NEC S25.49-
        specified
          site NEC S25.80-
            laceration S25.81-
              specified type NEC S25.89-
            type NEC S25.99
      subclavian —see Injury, blood vessel,
        thoracic, innominate
      vena cava (superior) S25.20
        laceration (minor) (superficial) S25.21-
          major S25.22-
        specified type NEC S25.29-
    thumb S65.40-
      laceration S65.41-
      specified type NEC S65.49-
    tibial artery S85.10-
      anterior S85.13-
        laceration S85.14-
        specified injury NEC S85.15-
      laceration S85.11-
      posterior S85.16-
        laceration S85.17-
        specified injury NEC S85.18-
      specified injury NEC S85.12-
    ulnar artery (forearm level) S55.00-
      hand and wrist (level) S65.00-
        laceration S65.01-
        specified type NEC S65.09-
      laceration S55.01-
      specified type NEC S55.09-
    upper arm (level) —see Injury, blood vessel,
      arm
      superficial vein —see Injury, blood
        vessel, arm, superficial vein
    uterine S35.5-
      artery S35.53-
      vein S35.53-
    vena cava —see Injury, vena cava
    vertebral artery S15.10-
      laceration (minor) (superficial) S15.11-
        major S15.12-
      specified type NEC S15.19-
    wrist (level) —see Injury, blood vessel,
      hand
  brachial plexus S14.3
    newborn P14.3
  brain (traumatic) S06.9-
    diffuse (axonal) S06.2X-
    focal S06.30-
    traumatic —see category S06
  brainstem S06.38-
  breast NOS S29.9
  broad ligament —see Injury, pelvic organ,
    specified site NEC
  bronchus, bronchi —see Injury, intrathoracic,
    bronchus
  brow S09.90
  buttock S39.92
  canthus, eye S05.90
  cardiac plexus —see Injury, nerve, thorax,
    sympathetic
  cauda equina S34.3
  cavernous sinus —see Injury, intracranial

Injury *(Continued)*

cecum —*see* Injury, colon

celiac ganglion or plexus —*see* Injury, nerve, lumbosacral, sympathetic

cerebellum —*see* Injury, intracranial

cerebral —*see* Injury, intracranial

cervix (uteri) —*see* Injury, uterus

cheek (wall) S09.93

chest —*see* Injury, thorax

childbirth (newborn) —*see also* Birth, injury maternal NEC O71.9

chin S09.93

choroid (eye) —*see* Injury, eye, specified site NEC

clitoris S39.94

coccyx —*see also* Injury, back, lower complicating delivery O71.6

colon —*see* Injury, intestine, large

common bile duct —*see* Injury, liver

conjunctiva (superficial) —*see* Injury, eye, conjunctiva

conus medullaris —*see* Injury, spinal, sacral cord

spermatic (pelvic region) S37.898
scrotal region S39.848
spinal —*see* Injury, spinal cord, by region

cornea —*see* Injury, eye, specified site NEC
abrasion —*see* Injury, eye, cornea, abrasion

cortex (cerebral) —*see also* Injury, intracranial
visual —*see* Injury, nerve, optic

costal region NEC S29.9

costochondral NEC S29.9

cranial
cavity —*see* Injury, intracranial
nerve —*see* Injury, nerve, cranial

crushing —*see* Crush

cutaneous sensory nerve

cystic duct —*see* Injury, liver

deep tissue —*see* Contusion, by site
meaning pressure ulcer —*see* Ulcer, pressure, unstageable, by site

delivery (newborn) P15.9
maternal NEC O71.9

Descemet's membrane —*see* Injury, eyeball, penetrating

diaphragm —*see* Injury, intrathoracic, diaphragm

duodenum —*see* Injury, intestine, small, duodenum

ear (auricle) (external) (canal) S09.91
abrasion —*see* Abrasion, ear
bite —*see* Bite, ear
blister —*see* Blister, ear
bruise —*see* Contusion, ear
contusion —*see* Contusion, ear
external constriction —*see* Constriction, external, ear
hematoma —*see* Hematoma, ear
inner —*see* Injury, ear, middle
laceration —*see* Laceration, ear
middle S09.30-
blast —*see* Injury, blast, ear
specified NEC S09.39-
puncture —*see* Puncture, ear
superficial —*see* Injury, superficial, ear

eighth cranial nerve (acoustic or auditory) — *see* Injury, nerve, acoustic

elbow S59.90-
contusion —*see* Contusion, elbow
dislocation —*see* Dislocation, elbow
fracture —*see* Fracture, ulna, upper end
open —*see* Wound, open, elbow
specified NEC S59.80-
sprain —*see* Sprain, elbow
superficial —*see* Injury, superficial, elbow

eleventh cranial nerve (accessory) — *see* Injury, nerve, accessory

epididymis S39.94

epigastric region S39.91

epiglottis NEC S19.89

Injury *(Continued)*

esophageal plexus —*see* Injury, nerve, thorax, sympathetic

esophagus (thoracic part) —*see also* Injury, intrathoracic, esophagus
cervical NEC S19.85

eustachian tube S09.30- ◀▥

eye S05.9-
avulsion S05.7-
ball —*see* Injury, eyeball
conjunctiva S05.0-
cornea
abrasion S05.0-
laceration S05.3-
with prolapse S05.2-
lacrimal apparatus S05.8X-
orbit penetration S05.4-
specified site NEC S05.8X-

eyeball S05.8X-
contusion S05.1-
penetrating S05.6-
with
foreign body S05.5-
prolapse or loss of intraocular tissue S05.2-
without prolapse or loss of intraocular tissue S05.3-
specified type NEC S05.8-

eyebrow S09.93

eyelid S09.93
abrasion —*see* Abrasion, eyelid
contusion —*see* Contusion, eyelid
open —*see* Wound, open, eyelid

face S09.93

fallopian tube S37.509
bilateral S37.502
blast injury S37.512
contusion S37.522
laceration S37.532
specified type NEC S37.592
blast injury (primary) S37.519
bilateral S37.512
secondary —*see* Injury, fallopian tube, specified type NEC
unilateral S37.511
contusion S37.529
bilateral S37.522
unilateral S37.521
laceration S37.539
bilateral S37.532
unilateral S37.531
specified type NEC S37.599
bilateral S37.592
unilateral S37.591
unilateral S37.501
blast injury S37.511
contusion S37.521
laceration S37.531
specified type NEC S37.591

fascia —*see* Injury, muscle

fifth cranial nerve (trigeminal) —*see* Injury, nerve, trigeminal

finger (nail) S69.9-
blood vessel —*see* Injury, blood vessel, finger
contusion —*see* Contusion, finger
dislocation —*see* Dislocation, finger
fracture —*see* Fracture, finger
muscle —*see* Injury, muscle, finger
nerve —*see* Injury, nerve, digital, finger
open —*see* Wound, open, finger
specified NEC S69.8-
sprain —*see* Sprain, finger
superficial —*see* Injury, superficial, finger

first cranial nerve (olfactory) —*see* Injury, nerve, olfactory

flank —*see* Injury, abdomen

foot S99.92-
blood vessel —*see* Injury, blood vessel, foot
contusion —*see* Contusion, foot
dislocation —*see* Dislocation, foot

Injury *(Continued)*

foot *(Continued)*
fracture —*see* Fracture, foot
muscle —*see* Injury, muscle, foot
open —*see* Wound, open, foot
specified type NEC S99.82-
sprain —*see* Sprain, foot
superficial —*see* Injury, superficial, foot

forceps NOS P15.9

forearm S59.91-
blood vessel —*see* Injury, blood vessel, forearm
contusion —*see* Contusion, forearm
fracture —*see* Fracture, forearm
muscle —*see* Injury, muscle, forearm
nerve —*see* Injury, nerve, forearm
open —*see* Wound, open, forearm
specified NEC S59.81-
superficial —*see* Injury, superficial, forearm

forehead S09.90

fourth cranial nerve (trochlear) —*see* Injury, nerve, trochlear

gallbladder S36.129
contusion S36.122
laceration S36.123
specified NEC S36.128

ganglion
celiac, coeliac —*see* Injury, nerve, lumbosacral, sympathetic
gasserian —*see* Injury, nerve, trigeminal
stellate —*see* Injury, nerve, thorax, sympathetic
thoracic sympathetic —*see* Injury, nerve, thorax, sympathetic

gasserian ganglion —*see* Injury, nerve, trigeminal

gastric artery —*see* Injury, blood vessel, celiac artery, branch

gastroduodenal artery —*see* Injury, blood vessel, celiac artery, branch

gastrointestinal tract —*see* Injury, intra-abdominal
with open wound into abdominal cavity — *see* Wound, open, with penetration into peritoneal cavity
colon —*see* Injury, intestine, large
rectum —*see* Injury, intestine, large, rectum
with open wound into abdominal cavity S36.61
small intestine —*see* Injury, intestine, small
specified site NEC —*see* Injury, intra-abdominal, specified, site NEC
stomach —*see* Injury, stomach

genital organ (s)
external S39.94
specified NEC S39.848
internal S37.90
fallopian tube —*see* Injury, fallopian tube
ovary —*see* Injury, ovary
prostate —*see* Injury, prostate
seminal vesicle —*see* Injury, pelvis, organ, specified site NEC
uterus —*see* Injury, uterus
vas deferens —*see* Injury, pelvis, organ, specified site NEC
obstetrical trauma O71.9

gland
lacrimal laceration —*see* Injury, eye, specified site NEC
salivary S09.90
thyroid NEC S19.84

globe (eye) S05.90
specified NEC S05.8X-

groin —*see* Injury, abdomen

gum S09.90

hand S69.9-
blood vessel —*see* Injury, blood vessel, hand
contusion —*see* Contusion, hand
fracture —*see* Fracture, hand
muscle —*see* Injury, muscle, hand

Injury (Continued)
  hand (Continued)
    nerve —see Injury, nerve, hand
    open —see Wound, open, hand
    specified NEC S69.8-
    sprain —see Sprain, hand
    superficial —see Injury, superficial, hand
  head S09.90
    with loss of consciousness S06.9-
    specified NEC S09.8-
  heart S26.90
    with hemopericardium S26.00
      contusion S26.01
      laceration (mild) S26.020
        major S26.022
        moderate S26.021
      specified type NEC S26.09
    without hemopericardium S26.10
      contusion S26.11
      laceration S26.12
      specified type NEC S26.19
    contusion S26.91
    laceration S26.92
    specified type NEC S26.99
  heel —see Injury, foot
  hepatic
    artery —see Injury, blood vessel, celiac
      artery, branch
    duct —see Injury, liver
    vein —see Injury, vena cava, inferior
  hip S79.91-
    blood vessel —see Injury, blood vessel, hip
    contusion —see Contusion, hip
    dislocation —see Dislocation, hip
    fracture —see Fracture, femur, neck
    muscle —see Injury, muscle, hip
    nerve —see Injury, nerve, hip
    open —see Wound, open, hip
    specified NEC S79.81-
    sprain —see Sprain, hip
    superficial —see Injury, superficial, hip
  hymen S39.94
  hypogastric
    blood vessel —see Injury, blood vessel, iliac
    plexus —see Injury, nerve, lumbosacral,
      sympathetic
  ileum —see Injury, intestine, small
  iliac region S39.91
  instrumental (during surgery) —see
    Laceration, accidental complicating
    surgery
    birth injury —see Birth, injury
    nonsurgical —see Injury, by site
    obstetrical O71.9
      bladder O71.5
      cervix O71.3
      high vaginal O71.4
      perineal NOS O70.9
      urethra O71.5
      uterus O71.5
        with rupture or perforation O71.1
  internal T14.8
    aorta —see Injury, aorta
    bladder (sphincter) —see Injury, bladder
    with
      ectopic or molar pregnancy O08.6
      following ectopic or molar pregnancy
        O08.6
      obstetrical trauma O71.5
    bronchus, bronchi —see Injury,
      intrathoracic, bronchus
    cecum —see Injury, intestine, large
    cervix (uteri) —see also Injury, uterus
      with ectopic or molar pregnancy O08.6
      following ectopic or molar pregnancy
        O08.6
      obstetrical trauma O71.3
    chest —see Injury, intrathoracic
    gastrointestinal tract —see Injury,
      intra-abdominal
    heart —see Injury, heart

Injury (Continued)
  internal (Continued)
    intestine NEC —see Injury, intestine
    intrauterine —see Injury, uterus
    mesentery —see Injury, intra-abdominal,
      specified, site NEC
    pelvis, pelvic (organ) S37.90
      following ectopic or molar pregnancy
        (subsequent episode) O08.6
      obstetrical trauma NEC O71.5
        rupture or perforation O71.1
      specified NEC S39.83
    rectum —see Injury, intestine, large,
      rectum
    stomach —see Injury, stomach
    ureter —see Injury, ureter
    urethra (sphincter) following ectopic or
      molar pregnancy O08.6
    uterus —see Injury, uterus
  interscapular area —see Injury, thorax
  intestine
    large S36.509
      ascending (right) S36.500
        blast injury (primary) S36.510
          secondary S36.590
        contusion S36.520
        laceration S36.530
        specified type NEC S36.590
      blast injury (primary) S36.519
        ascending (right) S36.510
        descending (left) S36.512
        rectum S36.61
        sigmoid S36.513
        specified site NEC S36.518
        transverse S36.511
      contusion S36.529
        ascending (right) S36.520
        descending (left) S36.522
        rectum S36.62
        sigmoid S36.523
        specified site NEC S36.528
        transverse S36.521
      descending (left) S36.502
        blast injury (primary) S36.512
          secondary S36.592
        contusion S36.522
        laceration S36.532
        specified type NEC S36.592
      laceration S36.539
        ascending (right) S36.530
        descending (left) S36.532
        rectum S36.63
        sigmoid S36.533
        specified site NEC S36.538
        transverse S36.531
      rectum S36.60
        blast injury (primary) S36.61
          secondary S36.69
        contusion S36.62
        laceration S36.63
        specified type NEC S36.69
      sigmoid S36.503
        blast injury (primary) S36.513
          secondary S36.593
        contusion S36.523
        laceration S36.533
        specified type NEC S36.593
      specified
        site NEC S36.508
          blast injury (primary) S36.518
            secondary S36.598
          contusion S36.528
          laceration S36.538
          specified type NEC S36.598
        type NEC S36.599
          ascending (right) S36.590
          descending (left) S36.592
          rectum S36.69
          sigmoid S36.593
          specified site NEC S36.598
          transverse S36.591

Injury (Continued)
  intestine (Continued)
    large (Continued)
      transverse S36.501
        blast injury (primary) S36.511
          secondary S36.591
        contusion S36.521
        laceration S36.531
        specified type NEC S36.591
    small S36.409
      blast injury (primary) S36.419
        duodenum S36.410
        secondary S36.499
          duodenum S36.490
          specified site NEC S36.498
        specified site NEC S36.418
      contusion S36.429
        duodenum S36.420
        specified site NEC S36.428
      duodenum S36.400
        blast injury (primary) S36.410
          secondary S36.490
        contusion S36.420
        laceration S36.430
        specified NEC S36.490
      laceration S36.439
        duodenum S36.430
        specified site NEC S36.438
      specified
        site NEC S36.408
        type NEC S36.499
          duodenum S36.490
          specified site NEC S36.498
  intra-abdominal S36.90
    adrenal gland —see Injury, adrenal gland
    bladder —see Injury, bladder
    colon —see Injury, intestine, large
    contusion S36.92
    fallopian tube —see Injury, fallopian tube
    gallbladder —see Injury, gallbladder
    intestine —see Injury, intestine
    kidney —see Injury, kidney
    laceration S36.93
    liver —see Injury, liver
    ovary —see Injury, ovary
    pancreas —see Injury, pancreas
    pelvic NOS S37.90
    peritoneum —see Injury, intra-abdominal,
      specified, site NEC
    prostate —see Injury, prostate
    rectum —see Injury, intestine, large, rectum
    retroperitoneum —see Injury, intra-
      abdominal, specified, site NEC
    seminal vesicle —see Injury, pelvis, organ,
      specified site NEC
    small intestine —see Injury, intestine, small
    specified
      pelvic S37.90
        specified
          site NEC S37.899
            specified type NEC S37.898
          type NEC S37.99
      site NEC S36.899
        contusion S36.892
        laceration S36.893
        specified type NEC S36.898
      type NEC S36.99
    spleen —see Injury, spleen
    stomach —see Injury, stomach
    ureter —see Injury, ureter
    urethra —see Injury, urethra
    uterus —see Injury, uterus
    vas deferens —see Injury, pelvis, organ,
      specified site NEC
  intracranial (traumatic) S06.9-
    cerebellar hemorrhage, traumatic —see
      Injury, intracranial, focal
    cerebral edema, traumatic S06.1X-
      diffuse S06.1X-
      focal S06.1X-
    diffuse (axonal) S06.2X-

◀ New   ◀▥ Revised   ~~deleted~~ Deleted

Injury (Continued)
  intracranial (Continued)
    epidural hemorrhage (traumatic) S06.4X-
    focal brain injury S06.30-
      contusion —see Contusion, cerebral
      laceration —see Laceration, cerebral
    intracerebral hemorrhage, traumatic
      S06.36-
      left side S06.35-
      right side S06.34-
    subarachnoid hemorrhage, traumatic
      S06.6X-
    subdural hemorrhage, traumatic S06.5X-
  intraocular —see Injury, eyeball, penetrating
  intrathoracic S27.9
    bronchus S27.409
      bilateral S27.402
      blast injury (primary) S27.419
        bilateral S27.412
        secondary —see Injury, intrathoracic,
          bronchus, specified type NEC
        unilateral S27.411
      contusion S27.429
        bilateral S27.422
        unilateral S27.421
      laceration S27.439
        bilateral S27.432
        unilateral S27.431
      specified type NEC S27.499
        bilateral S27.492
        unilateral S27.491
      unilateral S27.401
    diaphragm S27.809
      contusion S27.802
      laceration S27.803
      specified type NEC S27.808
    esophagus (thoracic) S27.819
      contusion S27.812
      laceration S27.813
      specified type NEC S27.818
    heart —see Injury, heart
    hemopneumothorax S27.2
    hemothorax S27.1
    lung S27.309
      aspiration J69.0
      bilateral S27.302
      blast injury (primary) S27.319
        bilateral S27.312
        secondary —see Injury, intrathoracic,
          lung, specified type NEC
        unilateral S27.311
      contusion S27.329
        bilateral S27.322
        unilateral S27.321
      laceration S27.339
        bilateral S27.332
        unilateral S27.331
      specified type NEC S27.399
        bilateral S27.392
        unilateral S27.391
      unilateral S27.301
    pleura S27.60
      laceration S27.63
      specified type NEC S27.69
    pneumothorax S27.0
    specified organ NEC S27.899
      contusion S27.892
      laceration S27.893
      specified type NEC S27.898
    thoracic duct —see Injury, intrathoracic,
      specified organ NEC
    thymus gland —see Injury, intrathoracic,
      specified organ NEC
    trachea, thoracic S27.50
      blast (primary) S27.51
      contusion S27.52
      laceration S27.53
      specified type NEC S27.59
  iris —see Injury, eye, specified site NEC
    penetrating —see Injury, eyeball,
      penetrating

Injury (Continued)
  jaw S09.93
  jejunum —see Injury, intestine, small
  joint NOS T14.8
    old or residual —see Disorder, joint,
      specified type NEC
  kidney S37.00-
    acute (nontraumatic) N17.9 ◀
    contusion —see Contusion, kidney
    laceration —see Laceration, kidney
    specified NEC S37.09-
  knee S89.9-
    contusion —see Contusion, knee
    dislocation —see Dislocation, knee
    meniscus (lateral) (medial) —see Sprain,
      knee, specified site NEC
      old injury or tear —see Derangement,
        knee, meniscus, due to old injury
    open —see Wound, open, knee
    specified NEC S89.8-
    sprain —see Sprain, knee
    superficial —see Injury, superficial, knee
  labium (majus) (minus) S39.94
  labyrinth, ear S09.30- ◀║
  lacrimal apparatus, duct, gland, or sac —see
    Injury, eye, specified site NEC
  larynx NEC S19.81
  leg (lower) S89.9-
    blood vessel —see Injury, blood vessel, leg
    contusion —see Contusion, leg
    fracture —see Fracture, leg
    muscle —see Injury, muscle, leg
    nerve —see Injury, nerve, leg
    open —see Wound, open, leg
    specified NEC S89.8-
    superficial —see Injury, superficial, leg
  lens, eye —see Injury, eye, specified site NEC
    penetrating —see Injury, eyeball,
      penetrating
  limb NEC T14.8
  lip S09.93
  liver S36.119
    contusion S36.112
    laceration S36.113
      major (stellate) S36.116
      minor S36.114
      moderate S36.115
      specified NEC S36.118
  lower back S39.92
    specified NEC S39.82
  lumbar, lumbosacral (region) S39.92
    plexus —see Injury, lumbosacral plexus
  lumbosacral plexus S34.4
  lung —see also Injury, intrathoracic, lung
    aspiration J69.0
    transfusion-related (TRALI) J95.84
  lymphatic thoracic duct —see Injury,
    intrathoracic, specified organ NEC
  malar region S09.93
  mastoid region S09.90
  maxilla S09.93
  mediastinum —see Injury, intrathoracic,
    specified organ NEC
  membrane, brain —see Injury, intracranial
  meningeal artery —see Injury, intracranial,
    subdural hemorrhage
  meninges (cerebral) —see Injury, intracranial
  mesenteric
    artery
      branch S35.299
        laceration (minor) (superficial) S35.291
        major S35.292
        specified NEC S35.298
      inferior S35.239
        laceration (minor) (superficial) S35.231
        major S35.232
        specified NEC S35.238
      superior S35.229
        laceration (minor) (superficial) S35.221
        major S35.222
        specified NEC S35.228

Injury (Continued)
  mesenteric (Continued)
    plexus (inferior) (superior) —see Injury,
      nerve, lumbosacral, sympathetic
    vein
      inferior S35.349
        laceration S35.341
        specified NEC S35.348
      superior S35.339
        laceration S35.331
        specified NEC S35.338
  mesentery —see Injury, intra-abdominal,
    specified site NEC
  mesosalpinx —see Injury, pelvic organ,
    specified site NEC
  middle ear S09.30- ◀║
  midthoracic region NOS S29.9
  mouth S09.93
  multiple NOS T07
  muscle (and fascia) (and tendon)
    abdomen S39.001
      laceration S39.021
      specified type NEC S39.091
      strain S39.011
    abductor
      thumb, forearm level —see Injury,
        muscle, thumb, abductor
    adductor
      thigh S76.20-
        laceration S76.22-
        specified type NEC S76.29-
        strain S76.21-
    ankle —see Injury, muscle, foot
    anterior muscle group, at leg level (lower)
      S86.20-
      laceration S86.22-
      specified type NEC S86.29-
      strain S86.21-
    arm (upper) —see Injury, muscle,
      shoulder
    biceps (parts NEC) S46.20-
      laceration S46.22-
      long head S46.10-
        laceration S46.12-
        specified type NEC S46.19-
        strain S46.11-
      specified type NEC S46.29-
      strain S46.21-
    extensor
      finger (s) (other than thumb) —see Injury,
        muscle, finger by site, extensor
      forearm level, specified NEC —see
        Injury, muscle, forearm, extensor
      thumb —see Injury, muscle, thumb,
        extensor
      toe (large) (ankle level) (foot level) —see
        Injury, muscle, toe, extensor
    finger
      extensor (forearm level) S56.40-
        hand level S66.309
          laceration S66.329
          specified type NEC S66.399
          strain S66.319
        laceration S56.429
        specified type NEC S56.499
        strain S56.419
      flexor (forearm level) S56.10-
        hand level S66.109
          laceration S66.129
          specified type NEC S66.199
          strain S66.119
        laceration S56.129
        specified type NEC S56.199
        strain S56.119
      index
        extensor (forearm level)
          hand level S66.308
            laceration S66.32-
            specified type NEC S66.39-
            strain S66.31-
          specified type NEC S56.492-

Injury *(Continued)*
  muscle *(Continued)*
    finger *(Continued)*
      index *(Continued)*
        flexor (forearm level)
          hand level S66.108
            laceration S66.12-
            specified type NEC
              S66.19-
            strain S66.11-
          specified type NEC S56.19-
          strain S56.11-
        intrinsic S66.50-
          laceration S66.52-
          specified type NEC S66.59-
          strain S66.51-
      intrinsic S66.509
        laceration S66.529
        specified type NEC S66.599
        strain S66.519
      little
        extensor (forearm level)
          hand level S66.30-
            laceration S66.32-
            specified type NEC S66.39-
            strain S66.31-
          laceration S56.42-
          specified type NEC S56.49-
          strain S56.41-
        flexor (forearm level)
          hand level S66.10-
            laceration S66.12-
            specified type NEC S66.19-
            strain S66.11-
          laceration S56.12-
          specified type NEC S56.19-
          strain S56.11-
        intrinsic S66.50-
          laceration S66.52-
          specified type NEC S66.59-
          strain S66.51-
      middle
        extensor (forearm level)
          hand level S66.30-
            laceration S66.32-
            specified type NEC
              S66.39-
            strain S66.31-
          laceration S56.42-
          specified type NEC S56.49-
          strain S56.41-
        flexor (forearm level)
          hand level S66.10-
            laceration S66.12-
            specified type NEC
              S66.19-
            strain S66.11-
          laceration S56.12-
          specified type NEC S56.19-
          strain S56.11-
        intrinsic S66.50-
          laceration S66.52-
          specified type NEC S66.59-
          strain S66.51-
      ring
        extensor (forearm level)
          hand level S66.30-
            laceration S66.32-
            specified type NEC S66.39-
            strain S66.31-
          laceration S56.42-
          specified type NEC S56.49-
          strain S56.41-
        flexor (forearm level)
          hand level S66.10-
            laceration S66.12-
            specified type NEC S66.19-
            strain S66.11-
          laceration S56.12-
          specified type NEC S56.19-
          strain S56.11-

Injury *(Continued)*
  muscle *(Continued)*
    finger *(Continued)*
      ring *(Continued)*
        intrinsic S66.50-
          laceration S66.52-
          specified type NEC S66.59-
          strain S66.51-
      flexor
        finger (s) (other than thumb) — *see*
          Injury, muscle, finger
        forearm level, specified NEC — *see*
          Injury, muscle, forearm, flexor
        thumb —*see* Injury, muscle, thumb,
          flexor
        toe (long) (ankle level) (foot level) —*see*
          Injury, muscle, toe, flexor
    foot S96.90-
      intrinsic S96.20-
        laceration S96.22-
        specified type NEC S96.29-
        strain S96.21-
      laceration S96.92-
      long extensor, toe —*see* Injury, muscle,
        toe, extensor
      long flexor, toe —*see* Injury, muscle, toe,
        flexor
      specified
        site NEC S96.80-
          laceration S96.82-
          specified type NEC S96.89-
          strain S96.81-
        type NEC S96.99-
      strain S96.91-
    forearm (level) S56.90-
      extensor S56.50-
        laceration S56.52-
        specified type NEC S56.59-
        strain S56.51-
      flexor S56.20-
        laceration S56.22-
        specified type NEC S56.29-
        strain S56.21-
      laceration S56.92-
      specified S56.99-
        site NEC S56.80-
          laceration S56.82-
          strain S56.81-
        type NEC S56.89-
      strain S56.91-
    hand (level) S66.90-
      laceration S66.92-
      specified
        site NEC S66.80-
          laceration S66.82-
          specified type NEC S66.89-
          strain S66.81-
        type NEC S66.99-
      strain S66.91-
    head S09.10
      laceration S09.12
      specified type NEC S09.19
      strain S09.11
    hip NEC S76.00-
      laceration S76.02-
      specified type NEC S76.09-
      strain S76.01-
    intrinsic
      ankle and foot level —*see* Injury, muscle,
        foot, intrinsic
      finger (other than thumb) —*see* Injury,
        muscle, finger by site, intrinsic
      foot (level) —*see* Injury, muscle, foot,
        intrinsic
      thumb —*see* Injury, muscle, thumb,
        intrinsic
    leg (level) (lower) S86.90-
      Achilles tendon —*see* Injury, Achilles
        tendon
      anterior muscle group —*see* Injury,
        muscle, anterior muscle group

Injury *(Continued)*
  muscle *(Continued)*
    leg *(Continued)*
      laceration S86.92-
      peroneal muscle group —*see* Injury,
        muscle, peroneal muscle group
      posterior muscle group —*see* Injury,
        muscle, posterior muscle group,
        leg level
      specified
        site NEC S86.80-
          laceration S86.82-
          specified type NEC S86.89-
          strain S86.81-
        type NEC S86.99-
      strain S86.91-
    long
      extensor toe, at ankle and foot level —*see*
        Injury, muscle, toe, extensor
      flexor, toe, at ankle and foot level —*see*
        Injury, muscle, toe, flexor
      head, biceps —*see* Injury, muscle, biceps,
        long head
    lower back S39.002
      laceration S39.022
      specified type NEC S39.092
      strain S39.012
    neck (level) S16.9
      laceration S16.2
      specified type NEC S16.8
      strain S16.1
    pelvis S39.003
      laceration S39.023
      specified type NEC S39.093
      strain S39.013
    peroneal muscle group, at leg level (lower)
      S86.30-
      laceration S86.32-
      specified type NEC S86.39-
      strain S86.31-
    posterior muscle (group)
      leg level (lower) S86.10-
        laceration S86.12-
        specified type NEC S86.19-
        strain S86.11-
      thigh level S76.30-
        laceration S76.32-
        specified type NEC S76.39-
        strain S76.31-
    quadriceps (thigh) S76.10-
      laceration S76.12-
      specified type NEC S76.19-
      strain S76.11-
    shoulder S46.90-
      laceration S46.92-
      rotator cuff —*see* Injury, rotator cuff
      specified site NEC S46.80-
        laceration S46.82-
        specified type NEC S46.89-
        strain S46.81-
      specified type NEC S46.99-
      strain S46.91-
    thigh NEC (level) S76.90-
      adductor —*see* Injury, muscle, adductor,
        thigh
      laceration S76.92-
      posterior muscle (group) —*see* Injury,
        muscle, posterior muscle, thigh
        level
      quadriceps —*see* Injury, muscle,
        quadriceps
      specified
        site NEC S76.80-
          laceration S76.82-
          specified type NEC S76.89-
          strain S76.81-
        type NEC S76.99-
      strain S76.91-
    thorax (level) S29.009
      back wall S29.002
      front wall S29.001

◀ New   ◀╍╍ Revised   ~~deleted~~ Deleted

Injury (Continued)
  muscle (Continued)
    thorax (Continued)
      laceration S29.029
        back wall S29.022
        front wall S29.021
      specified type NEC S29.099
        back wall S29.092
        front wall S29.091
      strain S29.019
        back wall S29.012
        front wall S29.011
    thumb
      abductor (forearm level) S56.30-
        laceration S56.32-
        specified type NEC S56.39-
        strain S56.31-
      extensor (forearm level) S56.30-
        hand level S66.20-
          laceration S66.22-
          specified type NEC S66.29-
          strain S66.21-
        laceration S56.32-
        specified type NEC S56.39-
        strain S56.31-
      flexor (forearm level) S56.00-
        hand level S66.00-
          laceration S66.02-
          specified type NEC S66.09-
          strain S66.01-
        laceration S56.02-
        specified type NEC S56.09-
        strain S56.01-
        wrist level —see Injury, muscle,
          thumb, flexor, hand level
      intrinsic S66.40-
        laceration S66.42-
        specified type NEC S66.49-
        strain S66.41-
    toe —see also Injury, muscle, foot
      extensor, long S96.10-
        laceration S96.12-
        specified type NEC S96.19-
        strain S96.11-
      flexor, long S96.00-
        laceration S96.02-
        specified type NEC S96.09-
        strain S96.01-
    triceps S46.30-
      laceration S46.32-
      specified type NEC S46.39-
      strain S46.31-
    wrist (and hand) level —see Injury, muscle,
      hand
  musculocutaneous nerve —see Injury, nerve,
    musculocutaneous
  myocardium —see Injury, heart
  nape —see Injury, neck
  nasal (septum) (sinus) S09.92
  nasopharynx S09.92
  neck S19.9
    specified NEC S19.80
    specified site NEC S19.89
  nerve NEC T14.8
    abdomen S34.9
      peripheral S34.6
      specified site NEC S34.8
    abducens S04.4-
      contusion S04.4-
      laceration S04.4-
      specified type NEC S04.4-
    abducent —see Injury, nerve,
      abducens
    accessory S04.7-
      contusion S04.7-
      laceration S04.7-
      specified type NEC S04.7-
    acoustic S04.6-
      contusion S04.6-
      laceration S04.6-
      specified type NEC S04.6-

Injury (Continued)
  nerve NEC (Continued)
    ankle S94.9-
      cutaneous sensory S94.3-
      specified site NEC —see subcategory
        S94.8
    anterior crural, femoral —see Injury, nerve,
      femoral
    arm (upper) S44.9-
      axillary —see Injury, nerve, axillary
      cutaneous —see Injury, nerve, cutaneous,
        arm
      median —see Injury, nerve, median,
        upper arm
      musculocutaneous —see Injury, nerve,
        musculocutaneous
      radial —see Injury, nerve, radial, upper
        arm
      specified site NEC —see subcategory
        S44.8
      ulnar —see Injury, nerve, ulnar, arm
    auditory —see Injury, nerve, acoustic
    axillary S44.3-
    brachial plexus —see Injury, brachial plexus
    cervical sympathetic S14.5
    cranial S04.9
      contusion S04.9
      eighth (acoustic or auditory) —see Injury,
        nerve, acoustic
      eleventh (accessory) —see Injury, nerve,
        accessory
      fifth (trigeminal) —see Injury, nerve,
        trigeminal
      first (olfactory) —see Injury, nerve,
        olfactory
      fourth (trochlear) —see Injury, nerve,
        trochlear
      laceration S04.9
      ninth (glossopharyngeal) —see Injury,
        nerve, glossopharyngeal
      second (optic) —see Injury, nerve, optic
      seventh (facial) —see Injury, nerve, facial
      sixth (abducent) —see Injury, nerve,
        abducens
      specified
        nerve NEC S04.89-
          contusion S04.89-
          laceration S04.89-
          specified type NEC S04.89-
        type NEC S04.9
      tenth (pneumogastric or vagus) —see
        Injury, nerve, vagus
      third (oculomotor) —see Injury, nerve,
        oculomotor
      twelfth (hypoglossal) —see Injury, nerve,
        hypoglossal
    cutaneous sensory
      ankle (level) S94.3-
      arm (upper) (level) S44.5-
      foot (level) —see Injury, nerve, cutaneous
        sensory, ankle
      forearm (level) S54.3-
      hip (level) S74.2-
      leg (lower level) S84.2-
      shoulder (level) —see Injury, nerve,
        cutaneous sensory, arm
      thigh (level) —see Injury, nerve,
        cutaneous sensory, hip
    deep peroneal —see Injury, nerve, peroneal,
      foot
    digital
      finger S64.4-
        index S64.49-
        little S64.49-
        middle S64.49-
        ring S64.49-
        thumb S64.3-
      toe —see Injury, nerve, ankle, specified
        site NEC
    eighth cranial (acoustic or auditory) —see
      Injury, nerve, acoustic

Injury (Continued)
  nerve NEC (Continued)
    eleventh cranial (accessory) —see Injury,
      nerve, accessory
    facial S04.5-
      contusion S04.5-
      laceration S04.5-
      newborn P11.3
      specified type NEC S04.5-
    femoral (hip level) (thigh level) S74.1-
    fifth cranial (trigeminal) —see Injury, nerve,
      trigeminal
    finger (digital) —see Injury, nerve, digital,
      finger
    first cranial (olfactory) —see Injury, nerve,
      olfactory
    foot S94.9-
      cutaneous sensory S94.3-
      deep peroneal S94.2-
      lateral plantar S94.0-
      medial plantar S94.1-
      specified site NEC —see subcategory
        S94.8
    forearm (level) S54.9-
      cutaneous sensory —see Injury, nerve,
        cutaneous sensory, forearm
      median —see Injury, nerve, median
      radial —see Injury, nerve, radial
      specified site NEC —see subcategory
        S54.8
      ulnar —see Injury, nerve, ulnar
    fourth cranial (trochlear) —see Injury,
      nerve, trochlear
    glossopharyngeal S04.89-
      specified type NEC S04.89-
    hand S64.9-
      median —see Injury, nerve, median,
        hand
      radial —see Injury, nerve, radial, hand
      specified NEC —see subcategory
        S64.8
      ulnar —see Injury, nerve, ulnar, hand
    hip (level) S74.9-
      cutaneous sensory —see Injury, nerve,
        cutaneous sensory, hip
      femoral —see Injury, nerve, femoral
      sciatic —see Injury, nerve, sciatic
      specified site NEC —see subcategory
        S74.8
    hypoglossal S04.89-
      specified type NEC S04.89-
    lateral plantar S94.0-
    leg (lower) S84.9-
      cutaneous sensory —see Injury, nerve,
        cutaneous sensory, leg
      peroneal —see Injury, nerve, peroneal
      specified site NEC —see subcategory
        S84.8
      tibial —see Injury, nerve, tibial
      upper —see Injury, nerve, thigh
    lower
      back —see Injury, nerve, abdomen,
        specified site NEC
        peripheral —see Injury, nerve,
          abdomen, peripheral
      limb —see Injury, nerve, leg
    lumbar plexus —see Injury, nerve,
      lumbosacral, sympathetic
    lumbar spinal —see Injury, nerve, spinal,
      lumbar
    lumbosacral
      plexus —see Injury, nerve, lumbosacral,
        sympathetic
      sympathetic S34.5
    medial plantar S94.1-
    median (forearm level) S54.1-
      hand (level) S64.1-
      upper arm (level) S44.1-
      wrist (level) —see Injury, nerve, median,
        hand
    musculocutaneous S44.4-

Injury (Continued)
  nerve NEC (Continued)
    musculospiral (upper arm level) —see
        Injury, nerve, radial, upper arm
    neck S14.9
      peripheral S14.4
      specified site NEC S14.8
      sympathetic S14.5
    ninth cranial (glossopharyngeal) —see
        Injury, nerve, glossopharyngeal
    oculomotor S04.1-
      contusion S04.1-
      laceration S04.1-
      specified type NEC S04.1-
    olfactory S04.81-
      specified type NEC S04.81-
    optic S04.01-
      contusion S04.01-
      laceration S04.01-
      specified type NEC S04.01-
    pelvic girdle —see Injury, nerve, hip
    pelvis —see Injury, nerve, abdomen,
        specified site NEC
      peripheral —see Injury, nerve, abdomen,
          peripheral
    peripheral NEC T14.8
      abdomen —see Injury, nerve, abdomen,
          peripheral
      lower back —see Injury, nerve, abdomen,
          peripheral
      neck —see Injury, nerve, neck,
          peripheral
      pelvis —see Injury, nerve, abdomen,
          peripheral
      specified NEC T14.8
    peroneal (lower leg level) S84.1-
      foot S94.2-
    plexus
      brachial —see Injury, brachial
          plexus
      celiac, coeliac —see Injury, nerve,
          lumbosacral, sympathetic
      mesenteric, inferior —see Injury, nerve,
          lumbosacral, sympathetic
      sacral —see Injury, lumbosacral
          plexus
      spinal
        brachial —see Injury, brachial
            plexus
        lumbosacral —see Injury, lumbosacral
            plexus
    pneumogastric —see Injury, nerve,
        vagus
    radial (forearm level) S54.2-
      hand (level) S64.2-
      upper arm (level) S44.2-
      wrist (level) —see Injury, nerve, radial,
          hand
    root —see Injury, nerve, spinal, root
    sacral plexus —see Injury, lumbosacral
        plexus
    sacral spinal —see Injury, nerve, spinal,
        sacral
    sciatic (hip level) (thigh level) S74.0-
    second cranial (optic) —see Injury, nerve,
        optic
    seventh cranial (facial) —see Injury, nerve,
        facial
    shoulder —see Injury, nerve, arm
    sixth cranial (abducent) —see Injury, nerve,
        abducens
    spinal
      plexus —see Injury, nerve, plexus,
          spinal
      root
        cervical S14.2
        dorsal S24.2
        lumbar S34.21
        sacral S34.22
          thoracic —see Injury, nerve, spinal,
              root, dorsal

Injury (Continued)
  nerve NEC (Continued)
    splanchnic —see Injury, nerve, lumbosacral,
        sympathetic
    sympathetic NEC —see Injury, nerve,
        lumbosacral, sympathetic
      cervical —see Injury, nerve, cervical
          sympathetic
      tenth cranial (pneumogastric or vagus) —
          see Injury, nerve, vagus
    thigh (level) —see Injury, nerve, hip
      cutaneous sensory —see Injury, nerve,
          cutaneous sensory, hip
      femoral —see Injury, nerve, femoral
      sciatic —see Injury, nerve, sciatic
      specified NEC —see Injury, nerve, hip
    third cranial (oculomotor) —see Injury,
        nerve, oculomotor
    thorax S24.9
      peripheral S24.3
      specified site NEC S24.8
      sympathetic S24.4
    thumb, digital —see Injury, nerve, digital,
        thumb
    tibial (lower leg level) (posterior)
        S84.0-
    toe —see Injury, nerve, ankle
    trigeminal S04.3-
      contusion S04.3-
      laceration S04.3-
      specified type NEC S04.3-
    trochlear S04.2-
      contusion S04.2-
      laceration S04.2-
      specified type NEC S04.2-
    twelfth cranial (hypoglossal) —see Injury,
        nerve, hypoglossal
    ulnar (forearm level) S54.0-
      arm (upper) (level) S44.0-
      hand (level) S64.0-
      wrist (level) —see Injury, nerve, ulnar,
          hand
    vagus S04.89-
      specified type NEC S04.89-
    wrist (level) —see Injury, nerve, hand
  ninth cranial nerve (glossopharyngeal) —see
      Injury, nerve, glossopharyngeal
  nose (septum) S09.92
  obstetrical O71.9
    specified NEC O71.89
  occipital (region) (scalp) S09.90
    lobe —see Injury, intracranial
  optic chiasm S04.02
  optic radiation S04.03-
  optic tract and pathways S04.03-
  orbit, orbital (region) —see Injury, eye
    penetrating (with foreign body) —see
        Injury, eye, orbit, penetrating
    specified NEC —see Injury, eye, specified
        site NEC
  ovary, ovarian S37.409
    bilateral S37.402
      contusion S37.422
      laceration S37.432
      specified type NEC S37.492
    blood vessel —see Injury, blood vessel,
        ovarian
    contusion S37.429
      bilateral S37.422
      unilateral S37.421
    laceration S37.439
      bilateral S37.432
      unilateral S37.431
    specified type NEC S37.499
      bilateral S37.492
      unilateral S37.491
    unilateral S37.401
      contusion S37.421
      laceration S37.431
      specified type NEC S37.491
  palate (hard) (soft) S09.93

Injury (Continued)
  pancreas S36.209
    body S36.201
      contusion S36.221
      laceration S36.231
        major S36.261
        minor S36.241
        moderate S36.251
      specified type NEC S36.291
    contusion S36.229
    head S36.200
      contusion S36.220
      laceration S36.230
        major S36.260
        minor S36.240
        moderate S36.250
      specified type NEC S36.290
    laceration S36.239
      major S36.269
      minor S36.249
      moderate S36.259
    specified type NEC S36.299
    tail S36.202
      contusion S36.222
      laceration S36.232
        major S36.262
        minor S36.242
        moderate S36.252
      specified type NEC S36.292
  parietal (region) (scalp) S09.90
    lobe —see Injury, intracranial
  patellar ligament (tendon) S76.10-
    laceration S76.12-
    specified NEC S76.19-
    strain S76.11-
  pelvis, pelvic (floor) S39.93
    complicating delivery O70.1
    joint or ligament, complicating delivery
        O71.6
    organ S37.90
      with ectopic or molar pregnancy O08.6
      complication of abortion —see Abortion
      contusion S37.92
      following ectopic or molar pregnancy
          O08.6
      laceration S37.93
      obstetrical trauma NEC O71.5
      specified
        site NEC S37.899
          contusion S37.892
          laceration S37.893
          specified type NEC S37.898
        type NEC S37.99
    specified NEC S39.83
  penis S39.94
  perineum S39.94
  peritoneum —see Injury, intra-
      abdominal, specified site NEC S36.81 ◀═
    laceration S36.893 ◀
  periurethral tissue —see Injury, urethra
    complicating delivery O71.82
  phalanges
    foot —see Injury, foot
    hand —see Injury, hand
  pharynx NEC S19.85
  pleura —see Injury, intrathoracic, pleura
  plexus
    brachial —see Injury, brachial plexus
    cardiac —see Injury, nerve, thorax,
        sympathetic
    celiac, coeliac —see Injury, nerve,
        lumbosacral, sympathetic
    esophageal —see Injury, nerve, thorax,
        sympathetic
    hypogastric —see Injury, nerve,
        lumbosacral, sympathetic
    lumbar, lumbosacral —see Injury,
        lumbosacral plexus
    mesenteric —see Injury, nerve, lumbosacral,
        sympathetic
    pulmonary —see Injury, nerve, thorax,
        sympathetic

◀ New   ◀═ Revised   ~~deleted~~ Deleted

Injury *(Continued)*
  postcardiac surgery (syndrome) I97.0
  prepuce S39.94
  prostate S37.829
    contusion S37.822
    laceration S37.823
    specified type NEC S37.828
  pubic region S39.94
  pudendum S39.94
  pulmonary plexus —*see* Injury, nerve, thorax, sympathetic
  rectovaginal septum NEC S39.83
  rectum —*see* Injury, intestine, large, rectum
  retina —*see* Injury, eye, specified site NEC
    penetrating —*see* Injury, eyeball, penetrating
  retroperitoneal —*see* Injury, intra-abdominal, specified site NEC
  rotator cuff (muscle (s)) (tendon (s)) S46.00-
    laceration S46.02-
    specified type NEC S46.09-
    strain S46.01-
  round ligament —*see* Injury, pelvic organ, specified site NEC
  sacral plexus —*see* Injury, lumbosacral plexus
  salivary duct or gland S09.93
  scalp S09.90
    newborn (birth injury) P12.9
      due to monitoring (electrode) (sampling incision) P12.4
      specified NEC P12.89
        caput succedaneum P12.81
  scapular region —*see* Injury, shoulder
  sclera —*see* Injury, eye, specified site NEC
    penetrating —*see* Injury, eyeball, penetrating
  scrotum S39.94
  second cranial nerve (optic) —*see* Injury, nerve, optic
  seminal vesicle —*see* Injury, pelvic organ, specified site NEC
  seventh cranial nerve (facial) —*see* Injury, nerve, facial
  shoulder S49.9-
    blood vessel —*see* Injury, blood vessel, arm
    contusion —*see* Contusion, shoulder
    dislocation —*see* Dislocation, shoulder
    fracture —*see* Fracture, shoulder
    muscle —*see* Injury, muscle, shoulder
    nerve —*see* Injury, nerve, shoulder
    open —*see* Wound, open, shoulder
    specified type NEC S49.8-
    sprain —*see* Sprain, shoulder girdle
    superficial —*see* Injury, superficial, shoulder
  sinus
    cavernous —*see* Injury, intracranial
    nasal S09.92
  sixth cranial nerve (abducent) —*see* Injury, nerve, abducens
  skeleton, birth injury P13.9
    specified part NEC P13.8
  skin NEC T14.8
    surface intact —*see* Injury, superficial
  skull NEC S09.90
  specified NEC T14.8
  spermatic cord (pelvic region) S37.898
    scrotal region S39.848
  spinal (cord)
    cervical (neck) S14.109
      anterior cord syndrome S14.139
        C1 level S14.131
        C2 level S14.132
        C3 level S14.133
        C4 level S14.134
        C5 level S14.135
        C6 level S14.136
        C7 level S14.137
        C8 level S14.138

Injury *(Continued)*
  spinal *(Continued)*
    cervical *(Continued)*
      Brown-Séquard syndrome S14.149
        C1 level S14.141
        C2 level S14.142
        C3 level S14.143
        C4 level S14.144
        C5 level S14.145
        C6 level S14.146
        C7 level S14.147
        C8 level S14.148
      C1 level S14.101
      C2 level S14.102
      C3 level S14.103
      C4 level S14.104
      C5 level S14.105
      C6 level S14.106
      C7 level S14.107
      C8 level S14.108
      central cord syndrome S14.129
        C1 level S14.121
        C2 level S14.122
        C3 level S14.123
        C4 level S14.124
        C5 level S14.125
        C6 level S14.126
        C7 level S14.127
        C8 level S14.128
      complete lesion S14.119
        C1 level S14.111
        C2 level S14.112
        C3 level S14.113
        C4 level S14.114
        C5 level S14.115
        C6 level S14.116
        C7 level S14.117
        C8 level S14.118
      concussion S14.0
      edema S14.0
      incomplete lesion specified NEC S14.159
        C1 level S14.151
        C2 level S14.152
        C3 level S14.153
        C4 level S14.154
        C5 level S14.155
        C6 level S14.156
        C7 level S14.157
        C8 level S14.158
      posterior cord syndrome S14.159
        C1 level S14.151
        C2 level S14.152
        C3 level S14.153
        C4 level S14.154
        C5 level S14.155
        C6 level S14.156
        C7 level S14.157
        C8 level S14.158
    dorsal —*see* Injury, spinal, thoracic
    lumbar S34.109
      complete lesion S34.119
        L1 level S34.111
        L2 level S34.112
        L3 level S34.113
        L4 level S34.114
        L5 level S34.115
      concussion S34.01
      edema S34.01
      incomplete lesion S34.129
        L1 level S34.121
        L2 level S34.122
        L3 level S34.123
        L4 level S34.124
        L5 level S34.125
      L1 level S34.101
      L2 level S34.102
      L3 level S34.103
      L4 level S34.104
      L5 level S34.105

Injury *(Continued)*
  spinal *(Continued)*
    nerve root NEC
      cervical —*see* Injury, nerve, spinal, root, cervical
      dorsal —*see* Injury, nerve, spinal, root, dorsal
      lumbar S34.21
      sacral S34.22
      thoracic —*see* Injury, nerve, spinal, root, dorsal
    plexus
      brachial —*see* Injury, brachial plexus
      lumbosacral —*see* Injury, lumbosacral plexus
    sacral S34.139
      complete lesion S34.131
      incomplete lesion S34.132
    thoracic S24.109
      anterior cord syndrome S24.139
        T1 level S24.131
        T2-T6 level S24.132
        T7-T10 level S24.133
        T11-T12 level S24.134
      Brown-Séquard syndrome S24.149
        T1 level S24.141
        T2-T6 level S24.142
        T7-T10 level S24.143
        T11-T12 level S24.144
      complete lesion S24.119
        T1 level S24.111
        T2-T6 level S24.112
        T7-T10 level S24.113
        T11-T12 level S24.114
      concussion S24.0
      edema S24.0
      incomplete lesion specified NEC S24.159
        T1 level S24.151
        T2-T6 level S24.152
        T7-T10 level S24.153
        T11-T12 level S24.154
      posterior cord syndrome S24.159
        T1 level S24.151
        T2-T6 level S24.152
        T7-T10 level S24.153
        T11-T12 level S24.154
      T1 level S24.101
      T2-T6 level S24.102
      T7-T10 level S24.103
      T11-T12 level S24.104
  splanchnic nerve —*see* Injury, nerve, lumbosacral, sympathetic
  spleen S36.00
    contusion S36.029
      major S36.021
      minor S36.020
    laceration S36.039
      major (massive) (stellate) S36.032
      moderate S36.031
      superficial (capsular) (minor) S36.030
    specified type NEC S36.09
  splenic artery —*see* Injury, blood vessel, celiac artery, branch
  stellate ganglion —*see* Injury, nerve, thorax, sympathetic
  sternal region S29.9
  stomach S36.30
    contusion S36.32
    laceration S36.33
    specified type NEC S36.39
  subconjunctival —*see* Injury, eye, conjunctiva
  subcutaneous NEC T14.8
  submaxillary region S09.93
  submental region S09.93
  subungual
    fingers —*see* Injury, hand
    toes —*see* Injury, foot

Injury (Continued)
superficial NEC T14.8
abdomen, abdominal (wall) S30.92
abrasion S30.811
bite S30.871
insect S30.861
contusion S30.1
external constriction S30.841
foreign body S30.851
abrasion —see Abrasion, by site
adnexa, eye NEC —see Injury, eye,
specified site NEC
alveolar process —see Injury, superficial,
oral cavity
ankle S90.91-
abrasion —see Abrasion, ankle
bite —see Bite, ankle
blister —see Blister, ankle
contusion —see Contusion, ankle
external constriction —see Constriction,
external, ankle
foreign body —see Foreign body,
superficial, ankle
anus S30.98
arm (upper) S40.92-
abrasion —see Abrasion, arm
bite —see Bite, superficial, arm
blister —see Blister, arm (upper)
contusion —see Contusion, arm
external constriction —see Constriction,
external, arm
foreign body —see Foreign body,
superficial, arm
auditory canal (external) (meatus) —see
Injury, superficial, ear
auricle —see Injury, superficial, ear
axilla —see Injury, superficial, arm
back —see also Injury, superficial, thorax,
back
lower S30.91
abrasion S30.810
contusion S30.0
external constriction S30.840
superficial
bite NEC S30.870
insect S30.860
foreign body S30.850
bite NEC —see Bite, superficial NEC, by
site
blister —see Blister, by site
breast S20.10-
abrasion —see Abrasion, breast
bite —see Bite, superficial, breast
contusion —see Contusion, breast
external constriction —see Constriction,
external, breast
foreign body —see Foreign body,
superficial, breast
brow —see Injury, superficial, head,
specified NEC
buttock S30.91
calf —see Injury, superficial, leg
canthus, eye —see Injury, superficial,
periocular area
cheek (external) —see Injury, superficial,
head, specified NEC
internal —see Injury, superficial, oral
cavity
chest wall —see Injury, superficial,
thorax
chin —see Injury, superficial, head NEC
clitoris S30.95
conjunctiva —see Injury, eye, conjunctiva
with foreign body (in conjunctival
sac) —see Foreign body,
conjunctival sac
contusion —see Contusion, by site
costal region —see Injury, superficial,
thorax
digit (s)
hand —see Injury, superficial, finger

Injury (Continued)
superficial NEC (Continued)
ear (auricle) (canal) (external) S00.40-
abrasion —see Abrasion, ear
bite —see Bite, superficial, ear
contusion —see Contusion, ear
external constriction —see Constriction,
external, ear
foreign body —see Foreign body,
superficial, ear
elbow S50.90-
abrasion —see Abrasion, elbow
bite —see Bite, superficial, elbow
blister —see Blister, elbow
contusion —see Contusion, elbow
external constriction —see Constriction,
external, elbow
foreign body —see Foreign body,
superficial, elbow
epididymis S30.94
epigastric region S30.92
epiglottis —see Injury, superficial, throat
esophagus
cervical —see Injury, superficial, throat
external constriction —see Constriction,
external, by site
extremity NEC T14.8
eyeball NEC —see Injury, eye, specified
site NEC
eyebrow —see Injury, superficial,
periocular area
eyelid S00.20-
abrasion —see Abrasion, eyelid
bite —see Bite, superficial, eyelid
contusion —see Contusion, eyelid
external constriction —see Constriction,
external, eyelid
foreign body —see Foreign body,
superficial, eyelid
face NEC —see Injury, superficial, head,
specified NEC
finger (s) S60.949
abrasion —see Abrasion, finger
bite —see Bite, superficial, finger
blister —see Blister, finger
contusion —see Contusion, finger
external constriction —see Constriction,
external, finger
foreign body —see Foreign body,
superficial, finger
index S60.94-
insect bite —see Bite, by site, superficial,
insect
little S60.94-
middle S60.94-
ring S60.94-
flank S30.92
foot S90.92-
abrasion —see Abrasion, foot
bite —see Bite, foot
blister —see Blister, foot
contusion —see Contusion, foot
external constriction —see Constriction,
external, foot
foreign body —see Foreign body,
superficial, foot
forearm S50.91-
abrasion —see Abrasion, forearm
bite —see Bite, forearm, superficial
blister —see Blister, forearm
contusion —see Contusion, forearm
elbow only —see Injury, superficial,
elbow
external constriction —see Constriction,
external, forearm
foreign body —see Foreign body,
superficial, forearm
forehead —see Injury, superficial, head
NEC
foreign body —see Foreign body,
superficial

Injury (Continued)
superficial NEC (Continued)
genital organs, external
female S30.97
male S30.96
globe (eye) —see Injury, eye, specified site
NEC
groin S30.92
gum —see Injury, superficial, oral cavity
hand S60.92-
abrasion —see Abrasion, hand
bite —see Bite, superficial, hand
contusion —see Contusion, hand
external constriction —see Constriction,
external, hand
foreign body —see Foreign body,
superficial, hand
head S00.90
ear —see Injury, superficial, ear
eyelid —see Injury, superficial, eyelid
nose S00.30
oral cavity S00.502
scalp S00.00
specified site NEC S00.80
heel —see Injury, superficial, foot
hip S70.91-
abrasion —see Abrasion, hip
bite —see Bite, superficial, hip
blister —see Blister, hip
contusion —see Contusion, hip
external constriction —see Constriction,
external, hip
foreign body —see Foreign body,
superficial, hip
iliac region —see Injury, superficial,
abdomen
inguinal region —see Injury, superficial,
abdomen
insect bite —see Bite, by site, superficial,
insect
interscapular region —see Injury,
superficial, thorax, back
jaw —see Injury, superficial, head, specified
NEC
knee S80.91-
abrasion —see Abrasion, knee
bite —see Bite, superficial, knee
blister —see Blister, knee
contusion —see Contusion, knee
external constriction —see Constriction,
external, knee
foreign body —see Foreign body,
superficial, knee
labium (majus) (minus) S30.95
lacrimal (apparatus) (gland) (sac) —see
Injury, eye, specified site NEC
larynx —see Injury, superficial, throat
leg (lower) S80.92-
abrasion —see Abrasion, leg
bite —see Bite, superficial, leg
contusion —see Contusion, leg
external constriction —see Constriction,
external, leg
foreign body —see Foreign body,
superficial, leg
knee —see Injury, superficial, knee
limb NEC T14.8
lip S00.501
lower back S30.91
lumbar region S30.91
malar region —see Injury, superficial, head,
specified NEC
mammary —see Injury, superficial, breast
mastoid region —see Injury, superficial,
head, specified NEC
mouth —see Injury, superficial, oral
cavity
muscle NEC T14.8
nail NEC T14.8
finger —see Injury, superficial, finger
toe —see Injury, superficial, toe

Injury (Continued)
  superficial NEC (Continued)
    nasal (septum) —see Injury, superficial, nose
    neck S10.90
      specified site NEC S10.80
    nose (septum) S00.30
    occipital region —see Injury, superficial, scalp
    oral cavity S00.502
    orbital region —see Injury, superficial, periocular area
    palate —see Injury, superficial, oral cavity
    palm —see Injury, superficial, hand
    parietal region —see Injury, superficial, scalp
    pelvis S30.91
      girdle —see Injury, superficial, hip
    penis S30.93
    perineum
      female S30.95
      male S30.91
    periocular area S00.20-
      abrasion —see Abrasion, eyelid
      bite —see Bite, superficial, eyelid
      contusion —see Contusion, eyelid
      external constriction —see Constriction, external, eyelid
      foreign body —see Foreign body, superficial, eyelid
    phalanges
      finger —see Injury, superficial, finger
      toe —see Injury, superficial, toe
    pharynx —see Injury, superficial, throat
    pinna —see Injury, superficial, ear
    popliteal space —see Injury, superficial, knee
    prepuce S30.93
    pubic region S30.91
    pudendum
      female S30.97
      male S30.96
    sacral region S30.91
    scalp S00.00
    scapular region —see Injury, superficial, shoulder
    sclera —see Injury, eye, specified site NEC
    scrotum S30.94
    shin —see Injury, superficial, leg
    shoulder S40.91-
      abrasion —see Abrasion, shoulder
      bite —see Bite, superficial, shoulder
      blister —see Blister, shoulder
      contusion —see Contusion, shoulder
      external constriction —see Constriction, external, shoulder
      foreign body —see Foreign body, superficial, shoulder
    skin NEC T14.8
    sternal region —see Injury, superficial, thorax, front
    subconjunctival —see Injury, eye, specified site NEC
    subcutaneous NEC T14.8
    submaxillary region —see Injury, superficial, head, specified NEC
    submental region —see Injury, superficial, head, specified NEC
    subungual
      finger (s) —see Injury, superficial, finger
      toe (s) —see Injury, superficial, toe
    supraclavicular fossa —see Injury, superficial, neck
    supraorbital —see Injury, superficial, head, specified NEC
    temple —see Injury, superficial, head, specified NEC
    temporal region —see Injury, superficial, head, specified NEC
    testis S30.94

Injury (Continued)
  superficial NEC (Continued)
    thigh S70.92-
      abrasion —see Abrasion, thigh
      bite —see Bite, superficial, thigh
      blister —see Blister, thigh
      contusion —see Contusion, thigh
      external constriction —see Constriction, external, thigh
      foreign body —see Foreign body, superficial, thigh
    thorax, thoracic (wall) S20.90
      abrasion —see Abrasion, thorax
      back S20.40-
      bite —see Bite, thorax, superficial
      blister —see Blister, thorax
      contusion —see Contusion, thorax
      external constriction —see Constriction, external, thorax
      foreign body —see Foreign body, superficial, thorax
      front S20.30-
    throat S10.10
      abrasion S10.11
      bite S10.17
        insect S10.16
      blister S10.12
      contusion S10.0
      external constriction S10.14
      foreign body S10.15
    thumb S60.93-
      abrasion —see Abrasion, thumb
      bite —see Bite, superficial, thumb
      blister —see Blister, thumb
      contusion —see Contusion, thumb
      external constriction —see Constriction, external, thumb
      foreign body —see Foreign body, superficial, thumb
      insect bite —see Bite, by site, superficial, insect
      specified type NEC S60.391
      specified type NEC S60.392
      specified type NEC S60.39- ◂▥
    toe (s) S90.93-
      abrasion —see Abrasion, toe
      bite —see Bite, toe
      blister —see Blister, toe
      contusion —see Contusion, toe
      external constriction —see Constriction, external, toe
      foreign body —see Foreign body, superficial, toe
      great S90.93-
    tongue —see Injury, superficial, oral cavity
    tooth, teeth —see Injury, superficial, oral cavity
    trachea S10.10
    tunica vaginalis S30.94
    tympanum, tympanic membrane —see Injury, superficial, ear
    uvula —see Injury, superficial, oral cavity
    vagina S30.95
    vocal cords —see Injury, superficial, throat
    vulva S30.95
    wrist S60.91-
  supraclavicular region —see Injury, neck
  supraorbital S09.93
  suprarenal gland (multiple) —see Injury, adrenal
  surgical complication (external or internal site) —see Laceration, accidental complicating surgery
  temple S09.90
  temporal region S09.90
  tendon —see also Injury, muscle, by site
    abdomen —see Injury, muscle, abdomen
    Achilles —see Injury, Achilles tendon
    lower back —see Injury, muscle, lower back
    pelvic organs —see Injury, muscle, pelvis

Injury (Continued)
  tenth cranial nerve (pneumogastric or vagus) —see Injury, nerve, vagus
  testis S39.94
  thigh S79.92-
    blood vessel —see Injury, blood vessel, hip
    contusion —see Contusion, thigh
    fracture —see Fracture, femur
    muscle —see Injury, muscle, thigh
    nerve —see Injury, nerve, thigh
    open —see Wound, open, thigh
    specified NEC S79.82-
    superficial —see Injury, superficial, thigh
  third cranial nerve (oculomotor) —see Injury, nerve, oculomotor
  thorax, thoracic S29.9
    blood vessel —see Injury, blood vessel, thorax
    cavity —see Injury, intrathoracic
    dislocation —see Dislocation, thorax
    external (wall) S29.9
      contusion —see Contusion, thorax
      nerve —see Injury, nerve, thorax
      open —see Wound, open, thorax
      specified NEC S29.8
      sprain —see Sprain, thorax
      superficial —see Injury, superficial, thorax
    fracture —see Fracture, thorax
    internal —see Injury, intrathoracic
    intrathoracic organ —see Injury, intrathoracic
    sympathetic ganglion —see Injury, nerve, thorax, sympathetic
  throat (see also Injury, neck) S19.9
  thumb S69.9-
    blood vessel —see Injury, blood vessel, thumb
    contusion —see Contusion, thumb
    dislocation —see Dislocation, thumb
    fracture —see Fracture, thumb
    muscle —see Injury, muscle, thumb
    nerve —see Injury, nerve, digital, thumb
    open —see Wound, open, thumb
    specified NEC S69.8-
    sprain —see Sprain, thumb
    superficial —see Injury, superficial, thumb
  thymus (gland) —see Injury, intrathoracic, specified organ NEC
  thyroid (gland) NEC S19.84
  toe S99.92-
    contusion —see Contusion, toe
    dislocation —see Dislocation, toe
    fracture —see Fracture, toe
    muscle —see Injury, muscle, toe
    open —see Wound, open, toe
    specified type NEC S99.82-
    sprain —see Sprain, toe
    superficial —see Injury, superficial, toe
  tongue S09.93
  tonsil S09.93
  tooth S09.93
  trachea (cervical) NEC S19.82
    thoracic —see Injury, intrathoracic, trachea, thoracic
  transfusion-related acute lung (TRALI) J95.84
  tunica vaginalis S39.94
  twelfth cranial nerve (hypoglossal) —see Injury, nerve, hypoglossal
  ureter S37.10
    contusion S37.12
    laceration S37.13
    specified type NEC S37.19
  urethra (sphincter) S37.30
    at delivery O71.5
    contusion S37.32
    laceration S37.33
    specified type NEC S37.38

Injury (Continued)
  urinary organ S37.899
    contusion S37.92
    laceration S37.93
    specified
      site NEC S37.899
        contusion S37.892
        laceration S37.893
        specified type NEC S37.898
      type NEC S37.99
  uterus, uterine S37.60
    with ectopic or molar pregnancy O08.6
    blood vessel —see Injury, blood vessel, iliac
    contusion S37.62
    laceration S37.63
      cervix at delivery O71.3
    rupture associated with obstetrics —see
        Rupture, uterus
    specified type NEC S37.69
  uvula S09.93
  vagina S39.93
    abrasion S30.814
    bite S31.45
      insect S30.864
      superficial NEC S30.874
    contusion S30.23
    crush S38.03
    during delivery —see Laceration, vagina,
        during delivery
    external constriction S30.844
    insect bite S30.864
    laceration S31.41
      with foreign body S31.42
    open wound S31.40
    puncture S31.43
      with foreign body S31.44
    superficial S30.95
      foreign body S30.854
  vas deferens —see Injury, pelvic organ,
      specified site NEC
  vascular NEC T14.8
  vein —see Injury, blood vessel
  vena cava (superior) S25.20
    inferior S35.10
      laceration (minor) (superficial) S35.11
        major S35.12
      specified type NEC S35.19
    laceration (minor) (superficial) S25.21
      major S25.22
    specified type NEC S25.29
  vesical (sphincter) —see Injury, bladder
  visual cortex S04.04-
  vitreous (humor) S05.90
    specified NEC S05.8X-
  vocal cord NEC S19.83
  vulva S39.94
    abrasion S30.814
    bite S31.45
      insect S30.864
      superficial NEC S30.874
    contusion S30.23
    crush S38.03
    during delivery —see Laceration,
        perineum, female, during delivery
    external constriction S30.844
    insect bite S30.864
    laceration S31.41
      with foreign body S31.42
    open wound S31.40
    puncture S31.43
      with foreign body S31.44
    superficial S30.95
      foreign body S30.854
  whiplash (cervical spine) S13.4
  wrist S69.9-
    blood vessel —see Injury, blood vessel,
        hand
    contusion —see Contusion, wrist
    dislocation —see Dislocation, wrist
    fracture —see Fracture, wrist
    muscle —see Injury, muscle, hand

Injury (Continued)
  wrist (Continued)
    nerve —see Injury, nerve, hand
    open —see Wound, open, wrist
    specified NEC S69.8-
    sprain —see Sprain, wrist
    superficial —see Injury, superficial, wrist
Inoculation —see also Vaccination
  complication or reaction —see Complications,
      vaccination
Insanity, insane —see also Psychosis
  adolescent —see Schizophrenia
  confusional F28
    acute or subacute F05
  delusional F22
  senile F03
Insect
  bite —see Bite, by site, superficial, insect
  venomous, poisoning NEC (by) —see Venom,
      arthropod
Insensitivity
  adrenocorticotropin hormone (ACTH) E27.49
  androgen E34.50
    complete E34.51
    partial E34.52
Insertion
  cord (umbilical) lateral or velamentous
      O43.12-
  intrauterine contraceptive device (encounter
      for) —see Intrauterine contraceptive
      device
Insolation (sunstroke) T67.0
Insomnia (organic) G47.00
  without objective findings F51.02
  adjustment F51.02
  adjustment disorder F51.02
  behavioral, of childhood Z73.819
    combined type Z73.812
    limit setting type Z73.811
    sleep-onset association type Z73.810
  childhood Z73.819
  chronic F51.04
    somatized tension F51.04
  conditioned F51.04
  due to
    alcohol
      abuse F10.182
      dependence F10.282
      use F10.982
    amphetamines
      abuse F15.182
      dependence F15.282
      use F15.982
    anxiety disorder F51.05
    caffeine
      abuse F15.182
      dependence F15.282
      use F15.982
    cocaine
      abuse F14.182
      dependence F14.282
      use F14.982
    depression F51.05
    drug NEC
      abuse F19.182
      dependence F19.282
      use F19.982
    medical condition G47.01
    mental disorder NEC F51.05
    opioid
      abuse F11.182
      dependence F11.282
      use F11.982
    psychoactive substance NEC
      abuse F19.182
      dependence F19.282
      use F19.982
    sedative, hypnotic, or anxiolytic
      abuse F13.182
      dependence F13.282
      use F13.982

Insomnia (Continued)
  due to (Continued)
    stimulant NEC
      abuse F15.182
      dependence F15.282
      use F15.982
    fatal familial (FFI) A81.83
    idiopathic F51.01
    learned F51.3
    nonorganic origin F51.01
    not due to a substance or known
        physiological condition F51.01
      specified NEC F51.09
    paradoxical F51.03
    primary F51.01
    psychiatric F51.05
    psychophysiologic F51.04
    related to psychopathology F51.05
    short-term F51.02
    specified NEC G47.09
    stress-related F51.02
    transient F51.02
Inspiration
  food or foreign body —see Foreign body, by
      site
  mucus —see Asphyxia, mucus
Inspissated bile syndrome (newborn)
    P59.1
Instability
  emotional (excessive) F60.3
  joint (post-traumatic) M25.30
    ankle M25.37-
    due to old ligament injury —see Disorder,
        ligament
    elbow M25.32-
    flail —see Flail, joint
    foot M25.37-
    hand M25.34-
    hip M25.35-
    knee M25.36-
    lumbosacral —see subcategory M53.2
    prosthesis —see Complications, joint
        prosthesis, mechanical, displacement,
        by site
    sacroiliac —see subcategory M53.2
    secondary to
      old ligament injury —see Disorder,
          ligament
      removal of joint prosthesis M96.89
    shoulder (region) M25.31-
    spine —see subcategory M53.2
    wrist M25.33-
  knee (chronic) M23.5-
  lumbosacral —see subcategory M53.2
  nervous F48.8
  personality (emotional) F60.3
  spine —see Instability, joint, spine
  vasomotor R55
Institutional syndrome (childhood) F94.2
Institutionalization, affecting child
    Z62.22
  disinhibited attachment F94.2
Insufficiency, insufficient
  accommodation, old age H52.4
  adrenal (gland) E27.40
    primary E27.1
  adrenocortical E27.40
    drug-induced E27.3
    iatrogenic E27.3
    primary E27.1
  anterior (occlusal) guidance M26.54
  anus K62.89
  aortic (valve) I35.1
    with
      mitral (valve) disease I08.0
        with tricuspid (valve) disease
            I08.3
      stenosis I35.2
      tricuspid (valve) disease I08.2
        with mitral (valve) disease I08.3
    congenital Q23.1

◀ New   ◀◀ Revised   ~~deleted~~ Deleted

Insufficiency, insufficient (Continued)
  aortic (Continued)
    rheumatic I06.1
      with
        mitral (valve) disease I08.0
          with tricuspid (valve) disease
            I08.3
        stenosis I06.2
          with mitral (valve) disease I08.0
            with tricuspid (valve) disease
              I08.3
          tricuspid (valve) disease I08.2
            with mitral (valve) disease I08.3
    specified cause NEC I35.1
    syphilitic A52.03
  arterial I77.1
    basilar G45.0
    carotid (hemispheric) G45.1
    cerebral I67.81
    coronary (acute or subacute) I24.8
    mesenteric K55.1
    peripheral I73.9
    precerebral (multiple) (bilateral) G45.2
    vertebral G45.0
  arteriovenous I99.8
  biliary K83.8
  cardiac —see also Insufficiency, myocardial
    due to presence of (cardiac) prosthesis
      I97.11-
    postprocedural I97.11-
  cardiorenal, hypertensive I13.2
  cardiovascular —see Disease, cardiovascular
  cerebrovascular (acute) I67.81
    with transient focal neurological signs and
      symptoms G45.8
  circulatory NEC I99.8
    newborn P29.89
  convergence H51.11
  coronary (acute or subacute) I24.8
    chronic or with a stated duration of over 4
      weeks I25.89
  corticoadrenal E27.40
    primary E27.1
  dietary E63.9
  divergence H51.8
  food T73.0
  gastroesophageal K22.8
  gonadal
    ovary E28.39
    testis E29.1
  heart —see also Insufficiency, myocardial
    newborn P29.0
    valve —see Endocarditis
  hepatic —see Failure, hepatic
  idiopathic autonomic G90.09
  interocclusal distance of fully erupted teeth
    (ridge) M26.36
  kidney N28.9
    acute N28.9
    chronic N18.9
  lacrimal (secretion) H04.12-
    passages —see Stenosis, lacrimal
  liver —see Failure, hepatic
  lung —see Insufficiency, pulmonary
  mental (congenital) —see Disability,
    intellectual
  mesenteric K55.1
  mitral (valve) I34.0
    with
      aortic valve disease I08.0
        with tricuspid (valve) disease
          I08.3
      obstruction or stenosis I05.2
        with aortic valve disease I08.0
        tricuspid (valve) disease I08.1
          with aortic (valve) disease I08.3
    congenital Q23.3
    rheumatic I05.1
      with
        aortic valve disease I08.0
          with tricuspid (valve) disease I08.3

Insufficiency, insufficient (Continued)
  mitral (Continued)
    rheumatic (Continued)
      with (Continued)
        obstruction or stenosis I05.2
          with aortic valve disease I08.0
            with tricuspid (valve) disease
              I08.3
          tricuspid (valve) disease I08.1
            with aortic (valve) disease I08.3
        active or acute I01.1
          with chorea, rheumatic (Sydenham's)
            I02.0
      specified cause, except rheumatic
        I34.0
  muscle —see also Disease, muscle
    heart —see Insufficiency, myocardial
    ocular NEC H50.9
  myocardial, myocardium (with
    arteriosclerosis) I50.9
    with
      rheumatic fever (conditions in I00)
        I09.0
        active, acute or subacute I01.2
          with chorea I02.0
        inactive or quiescent (with chorea)
          I09.0
    congenital Q24.8
    hypertensive —see Hypertension, heart
    newborn P29.0
    rheumatic I09.0
      active, acute, or subacute I01.2
    syphilitic A52.06
  nourishment T73.0
  pancreatic K86.8
  parathyroid (gland) E20.9
  peripheral vascular (arterial) I73.9
  pituitary E23.0
  placental (mother) O36.51-
  platelets D69.6
  prenatal care affecting management of
    pregnancy O09.3-
  progressive pluriglandular E31.0
  pulmonary J98.4
    acute, following surgery (nonthoracic)
      J95.2
      thoracic J95.1
    chronic, following surgery J95.3
    following
      shock J98.4 ◀▥
      trauma J98.4 ◀▥
    newborn P28.5
    valve I37.1
      with stenosis I37.2
      congenital Q22.2
      rheumatic I09.89
        with aortic, mitral or tricuspid (valve)
          disease I08.8
  pyloric K31.89
  renal (acute) N28.9
    chronic N18.9
  respiratory R06.89
    newborn P28.5
  rotation —see Malrotation
  sleep syndrome F51.12
  social insurance Z59.7
  suprarenal E27.40
    primary E27.1
  tarso-orbital fascia, congenital Q10.3
  testis E29.1
  thyroid (gland) (acquired) E03.9
    congenital E03.1
  tricuspid (valve) (rheumatic) I07.1
    with
      aortic (valve) disease I08.2
        with mitral (valve) disease I08.3
      mitral (valve) disease I08.1
        with aortic (valve) disease I08.3
      obstruction or stenosis I07.2
        with aortic (valve) disease I08.2
          with mitral (valve) disease I08.3

Insufficiency, insufficient (Continued)
  tricuspid (Continued)
    congenital Q22.8
    nonrheumatic I36.1
      with stenosis I36.2
  urethral sphincter R32
  valve, valvular (heart) —see Endocarditis
    congenital Q24.8
  vascular I99.8
    intestine K55.9
      acute K55.0
    mesenteric K55.1
    peripheral I73.9
    renal —see Hypertension, kidney
  velopharyngeal
    acquired K13.79
    congenital Q38.8
  venous (chronic) (peripheral) I87.2
  ventricular —see Insufficiency, myocardial
  welfare support Z59.7
Insufflation, fallopian Z31.41
Insular —see condition
Insulinoma
  pancreas
    benign D13.7
    malignant C25.4
    uncertain behavior D37.8
  specified site
    benign —see Neoplasm, by site, benign
    malignant —see Neoplasm, by site,
      malignant
    uncertain behavior —see Neoplasm, by site,
      uncertain behavior
  unspecified site
    benign D13.7
    malignant C25.4
    uncertain behavior D37.8
Insuloma —see Insulinoma
Interference
  balancing side M26.56
  non-working side M26.56
Intermenstrual —see condition
Intermittent —see condition
Internal —see condition
Interrogation
  cardiac defibrillator (automatic) (implantable)
    Z45.02
  cardiac pacemaker Z45.018
  cardiac (event) (loop) recorder Z45.09
  infusion pump (implanted) (intrathecal)
    Z45.1
  neurostimulator Z46.2
Interruption
  phase-shift, sleep cycle —see Disorder, sleep,
    circadian rhythm
  sleep phase-shift, or 24 hour sleep-wake
    cycle —see Disorder, sleep, circadian
    rhythm
Interstitial —see condition
Intertrigo L30.4
  labialis K13.0
Intervertebral disc —see condition
Intestine, intestinal —see condition
Intolerance
  carbohydrate K90.4
  disaccharide, hereditary E73.0
  fat NEC K90.4
    pancreatic K90.3
  food K90.4
    dietary counseling and surveillance
      Z71.3
  fructose E74.10
    hereditary E74.12
  glucose(-galactose) E74.39
  gluten K90.0
  lactose E73.9
    specified NEC E73.8
  lysine E72.3
  milk NEC K90.4
    lactose E73.9
  protein K90.4

Intolerance *(Continued)*
  starch NEC K90.4
  sucrose (-isomaltose) E74.31
Intoxicated NEC (without dependence) —*see*
  Alcohol, intoxication
Intoxication
  acid E87.2
  alcoholic (acute) (without dependence) —*see*
    Alcohol, intoxication
  alimentary canal K52.1
  amphetamine (without dependence) —
    see Abuse, drug, stimulant, with
    intoxication
    with dependence —*see* Dependence, drug,
      stimulant, with intoxication
  anxiolytic (acute) (without dependence) —*see*
    Abuse, drug, sedative, with intoxication
    with dependence —*see* Dependence, drug,
      sedative, with intoxication
  caffeine (acute) (without dependence) —
    see Abuse, drug, stimulant, with
    intoxication
    with dependence —*see* Dependence, drug,
      stimulant, with intoxication
  cannabinoids (acute) (without dependence) —
    see Abuse, drug, cannabis, with
    intoxication
    with dependence —*see* Dependence, drug,
      cannabis, with intoxication
  chemical —*see* Table of ⊞Drugs and
    eChemicals ◀▥
    via placenta or breast milk —*see* -
      Absorption, chemical, through
      placenta
  cocaine (acute) (without dependence) —*see*
    Abuse, drug, cocaine, with intoxication
    with dependence —*see* Dependence, drug,
      cocaine, with intoxication
  drug
    acute (without dependence) —*see* Abuse,
      drug, by type with intoxication
      with dependence —*see* Dependence,
        drug, by type with intoxication
    addictive
      via placenta or breast milk —*see*
        Absorption, drug, addictive,
        through placenta
    newborn P93.8
      gray baby syndrome P93.0
    overdose or wrong substance given or
      taken —*see* Table of ⊞Drugs and
      eChemicals, by drug, poisoning ◀▥
  enteric K52.1
  foodborne A05.9
    bacterial A05.9
    classical (Clostridium botulinum) A05.1
    due to
      Bacillus cereus A05.4
      bacterium A05.9
        specified NEC A05.8
      Clostridium
        botulinum A05.1
        perfringens A05.2
        welchii A05.2
      Salmonella A02.9
        with
          (gastro) enteritis A02.0
          localized infection (s) A02.20
            arthritis A02.23
            meningitis A02.21
            osteomyelitis A02.24
            pneumonia A02.22
            pyelonephritis A02.25
            specified NEC A02.29
          sepsis A02.1
          specified manifestation NEC A02.8
      Staphylococcus A05.0
      Vibrio
        parahaemolyticus A05.3
        vulnificus A05.5
    enterotoxin, staphylococcal A05.0
    noxious —*see* Poisoning, food, noxious

Intoxication *(Continued)*
  gastrointestinal K52.1
  hallucinogenic (without dependence) —*see*
    Abuse, drug, hallucinogen, with
    intoxication
    with dependence —*see* Dependence, drug,
      hallucinogen, with intoxication
  hypnotic (acute) (without dependence) —*see*
    Abuse, drug, sedative, with intoxication
    with dependence —*see* Dependence, drug,
      sedative, with intoxication
  inhalant (acute) (without dependence) —*see*
    Abuse, drug, inhalant, with intoxication
    with dependence —*see* Dependence, drug,
      inhalant, with intoxication
  meaning
    inebriation —*see* category F10
    poisoning —*see* Table of ⊞Drugs and
      eChemicals ◀▥
  methyl alcohol (acute) (without
    dependence) —*see* Alcohol, intoxication
  opioid (acute) (without dependence) —*see*
    Abuse, drug, opioid, with intoxication
    with dependence —*see* Dependence, drug,
      opioid, with intoxication
  pathologic NEC (without dependence) —*see*
    Alcohol, intoxication
  phencyclidine (without dependence) —*see*
    Abuse, drug, psychoactive NEC, with
    intoxication
    with dependence —*see* Dependence, drug,
      psychoactive NEC, with intoxication
  potassium (K) E87.5
  psychoactive substance NEC (without
    dependence) —*see* Abuse, drug,
    psychoactive NEC, with intoxication
    with dependence —*see* Dependence, drug,
      psychoactive NEC, with intoxication
  sedative (acute) (without dependence) —*see*
    Abuse, drug, sedative, with intoxication
    with dependence —*see* Dependence, drug,
      sedative, with intoxication
  serum (*see also* Reaction, serum) T80.69
  uremic —*see* Uremia
  volatile solvents (acute) (without
    dependence) —*see* Abuse, drug, inhalant,
    with intoxication
    with dependence —*see* Dependence, drug,
      inhalant, with intoxication
  water E87.79
Intracranial —*see* condition
Intrahepatic gallbladder Q44.1
Intraligamentous —*see* condition
Intrathoracic —*see also* condition
  kidney Q63.2
Intrauterine contraceptive device
  checking Z30.431
  in situ Z97.5
  insertion Z30.430
    immediately following removal Z30.433
  management Z30.431
  reinsertion Z30.433
  removal Z30.432
  replacement Z30.433
  retention in pregnancy O26.3-
Intraventricular —*see* condition
Intrinsic deformity —*see* Deformity
Intubation, difficult or failed T88.4
Intumescence, lens (eye) (cataract) —*see* Cataract
Intussusception (bowel) (colon) (enteric)
    (ileocecal) (ileocolic) (intestine) (rectum)
    K56.1
  appendix K38.8
  congenital Q43.8
  ureter (with obstruction) N13.5
Invagination (bowel, colon, intestine or rectum)
    K56.1
Inversion
  albumin-globulin (A-G) ratio E88.09
  bladder N32.89
  cecum —*see* Intussusception
  cervix N88.8

Inversion *(Continued)*
  chromosome in normal individual Q95.1
  circadian rhythm —*see* Disorder, sleep,
    circadian rhythm
  nipple N64.59
    congenital Q83.8
    gestational —*see* Retraction, nipple
    puerperal, postpartum —*see* Retraction,
      nipple
  nyctohemeral rhythm —*see* Disorder, sleep,
    circadian rhythm
  optic papilla Q14.2
  organ or site, congenital NEC —*see* Anomaly,
    by site
  sleep rhythm —*see* Disorder, sleep, circadian
    rhythm
  testis (congenital) Q55.29
  uterus (chronic) (postinfectional) (postpartal,
    old) N85.5
    postpartum O71.2
  vagina (posthysterectomy) N99.3
  ventricular Q20.5
Investigation (*see also* Examination) Z04.9
  clinical research subject (control) (normal
    comparison) (participant) Z00.6
Involuntary movement, abnormal R25.9
Involution, involutional —*see also* condition
  breast, cystic —*see* Dysplasia, mammary,
    specified type NEC
  depression (single episode) F32.8
    recurrent episode F33.9
  melancholia (recurrent episode) (single
    episode) F32.8
  ovary, senile —*see* Atrophy, ovary
  thymus failure E32.8
I.Q.
  under 20 F73
  20-34 F72
  35-49 F71
  50-69 F70
IRDS (type I) P22.0
  type II P22.1
Irideremia Q13.1
Iridis rubeosis —*see* Disorder, iris, vascular
Iridochoroiditis (panuveitis) —*see* Panuveitis
Iridocyclitis H20.9-
  acute H20.0-
    hypopyon H20.05-
    primary H20.01-
    recurrent H20.02-
    secondary (noninfectious) H20.04-
      infectious H20.03-
  chronic H20.1-
  due to allergy —*see* Iridocyclitis, acute,
    secondary
  endogenous —*see* Iridocyclitis, acute, primary
  Fuchs' —*see* Cyclitis, Fuchs' heterochromic
  gonococcal A54.32
  granulomatous —*see* Iridocyclitis, chronic
  herpes, herpetic (simplex) B00.51
    zoster B02.32
  hypopyon —*see* Iridocyclitis, acute, hypopyon
  in (due to)
    ankylosing spondylitis M45.9
    gonococcal infection A54.32
    herpes (simplex) virus B00.51
      zoster B02.32
    infectious disease NOS B99
    parasitic disease NOS B89 [H22]
    sarcoidosis D86.83
    syphilis A51.43
    tuberculosis A18.54
    zoster B02.32
  lens-induced H20.2-
  nongranulomatous —*see* Iridocyclitis, acute
  recurrent —*see* Iridocyclitis, acute, recurrent
  rheumatic —*see* Iridocyclitis, chronic
  subacute —*see* Iridocyclitis, acute
  sympathetic —*see* Uveitis, sympathetic
  syphilitic (secondary) A51.43
  tuberculous (chronic) A18.54
  Vogt-Koyanagi H20.82-

◀ New   ◀▥ Revised   ~~deleted~~ Deleted

Iridocyclochoroiditis (panuveitis) —*see* Panuveitis
Iridodialysis H21.53-
Iridodonesis H21.89
Iridoplegia (complete) (partial) (reflex) H57.09
Iridoschisis H21.25-
Iris —*see also* condition
  bombé —*see* Membrane, pupillary
Iritis —*see also* Iridocyclitis
  chronic —*see* Iridocyclitis, chronic
  diabetic —*see* E08-E13 with .39
  due to
    herpes simplex B00.51
    leprosy A30.9 [H22]
  gonococcal A54.32
  gouty M10.9
  granulomatous —*see* Iridocyclitis, chronic
  lens induced —*see* Iridocyclitis, lens-induced
  papulosa (syphilitic) A52.71
  rheumatic —*see* Iridocyclitis, chronic
  syphilitic (secondary) A51.43
    congenital (early) A50.01
    late A52.71
  tuberculous A18.54
Iron —*see* condition
Iron-miner's lung J63.4
Irradiated enamel (tooth, teeth) K03.89
Irradiation effects, adverse T66
Irreducible, irreducibility —*see* condition
Irregular, irregularity
  action, heart I49.9
  alveolar process K08.8
  bleeding N92.6
  breathing R06.89
  contour of cornea (acquired) —*see* Deformity, cornea
    congenital Q13.4
  contour, reconstructed breast N65.0
  dentin (in pulp) K04.3
  eye movements H55.89
    nystagmus —*see* Nystagmus
    saccadic H55.81
  labor O62.2
  menstruation (cause unknown) N92.6
  periods N92.6
  prostate N42.9
  pupil —*see* Abnormality, pupillary
  reconstructed breast N65.0
  respiratory R06.89
  septum (nasal) J34.2
  shape, organ or site, congenital NEC —*see* Distortion
  sleep-wake pattern (rhythm) G47.23
Irritable, irritability R45.4
  bladder N32.89
  bowel (syndrome) K58.9
    with diarrhea K58.0
    psychogenic F45.8
  bronchial —*see* Bronchitis
  cerebral, in newborn P91.3
  colon K58.9
    with diarrhea K58.0
    psychogenic F45.8
  duodenum K59.8
  heart (psychogenic) F45.8
  hip —*see* Derangement, joint, specified type NEC, hip
  ileum K59.8
  infant R68.12
  jejunum K59.8
  rectum K59.8
  stomach K31.89
    psychogenic F45.8
  sympathetic G90.8
  urethra N36.8
Irritation
  anus K62.89
  axillary nerve G54.0
  bladder N32.89
  brachial plexus G54.0
  bronchial —*see* Bronchitis
  cervical plexus G54.2

Irritation (*Continued*)
  cervix —*see* Cervicitis
  choroid, sympathetic —*see* Endophthalmitis
  cranial nerve —*see* Disorder, nerve, cranial
  gastric K31.89
    psychogenic F45.8
  globe, sympathetic —*see* Uveitis, sympathetic
  labyrinth —*see* subcategory H83.2
  lumbosacral plexus G54.1
  meninges (traumatic) —*see* Injury, intracranial
    nontraumatic —*see* Meningismus
  nerve —*see* Disorder, nerve
  nervous R45.0
  penis N48.89
  perineum NEC L29.3
  peripheral autonomic nervous system G90.8
  peritoneum —*see* Peritonitis
  pharynx J39.2
  plantar nerve —*see* Lesion, nerve, plantar
  spinal (cord) (traumatic) —*see also* Injury, spinal cord, by region
    nerve G58.9
      root NEC —*see* Radiculopathy
    nontraumatic —*see* Myelopathy
  stomach K31.89
    psychogenic F45.8
  sympathetic nerve NEC G90.8
  ulnar nerve —*see* Lesion, nerve, ulnar
  vagina N89.8
Ischemia, ischemic I99.8
  bowel (transient)
    acute K55.0
    chronic K55.1
    due to mesenteric artery insufficiency K55.1
  brain —*see* Ischemia, cerebral
  cardiac (*see* Disease, heart, ischemic)
  cardiomyopathy I25.5
  cerebral (chronic) (generalized) I67.82
    arteriosclerotic I67.2
    intermittent G45.9
    newborn P91.0
    recurrent focal G45.8
    transient G45.9
  colon chronic (due to mesenteric artery insufficiency) K55.1
  coronary —*see* Disease, heart, ischemic
  demand (coronary) (*see also* Angina) I24.8
  heart (chronic or with a stated duration of over 4 weeks) I25.9
    acute or with a stated duration of 4 weeks or less I24.9
    subacute I24.9
  infarction, muscle —*see* Infarct, muscle
  intestine (large) (small) (transient) K55.9
    acute K55.0
    chronic K55.1
    due to mesenteric artery insufficiency K55.1
  kidney N28.0
  mesenteric, acute K55.0
  muscle, traumatic T79.6
  myocardium, myocardial (chronic or with a stated duration of over 4 weeks) I25.9
    acute, without myocardial infarction I24.0
    silent (asymptomatic) I25.6
    transient of newborn P29.4
  renal N28.0
  retina, retinal —*see* Occlusion, artery, retina
  small bowel
    acute K55.0
    chronic K55.1
    due to mesenteric artery insufficiency K55.1
  spinal cord G95.11
  subendocardial —*see* Insufficiency, coronary
  supply (coronary) (*see also* Angina) I25.9
    due to vasospasm I20.1
Ischial spine —*see* condition
Ischialgia —*see* Sciatica
Ischiopagus Q89.4
Ischium, ischial —*see* condition

Ischuria R34
Iselin's disease or osteochondrosis —*see* Osteochondrosis, juvenile, metatarsus
Islands of
  parotid tissue in
    lymph nodes Q38.6
    neck structures Q38.6
  submaxillary glands in
    fascia Q38.6
    lymph nodes Q38.6
    neck muscles Q38.6
Islet cell tumor, pancreas D13.7
Isoimmunization NEC —*see also* Incompatibility
  affecting management of pregnancy (ABO) (with hydrops fetalis) O36.11-
    anti-A sensitization O36.11-
    anti-B sensitization O36.19-
    anti-c sensitization O36.09-
    anti-C sensitization O36.09-
    anti-e sensitization O36.09-
    anti-E sensitization O36.09-
    Rh NEC O36.09-
      anti-D antibody O36.01-
    specified NEC O36.19-
  newborn P55.9
    with
      hydrops fetalis P56.0
      kernicterus P57.0
    ABO (blood groups) P55.1
    Rhesus (Rh) factor P55.0
    specified type NEC P55.8
Isolation, isolated
  dwelling Z59.8
  family Z63.79
  social Z60.4
Isoleucinosis E71.19
Isomerism atrial appendages (with asplenia or polysplenia) Q20.6
Isosporiasis, isosporosis A07.3
Isovaleric acidemia E71.110
Issue of
  medical certificate Z02.79
    for disability determination Z02.71
  repeat prescription (appliance) (glasses) (medicinal substance, medicament, medicine) Z76.0
  contraception —*see* Contraception
Itch, itching —*see also* Pruritus
  baker's L23.6
  barber's B35.0
  bricklayer's L24.5
  cheese B88.0
  clam digger's B65.3
  coolie B76.9
  copra B88.0
  dew B76.9
  dhobi B35.6
  filarial —*see* Infestation, filarial
  grain B88.0
  grocer's B88.0
  ground B76.9
  harvest B88.0
  jock B35.6
  Malabar B35.5
    beard B35.0
    foot B35.3
    scalp B35.0
  meaning scabies B86
  Norwegian B86
  perianal L29.0
  poultrymen's B88.0
  sarcoptic B86
  scabies B86
  scrub B88.0
  straw B88.0
  swimmer's B65.3
  water B76.9
  winter L29.8
Ivemark's syndrome (asplenia with congenital heart disease) Q89.01
Ivory bones Q78.2
Ixodiasis NEC B88.8

J

Jaccoud's syndrome —see Arthropathy, postrheumatic, chronic
Jackson's
  membrane Q43.3
  paralysis or syndrome G83.89
  veil Q43.3
Jacquet's dermatitis (diaper dermatitis) L22
Jadassohn-Pellizari's disease or anetoderma L90.2
Jadassohn's
  blue nevus —see Nevus
  intraepidermal epithelioma —see Neoplasm, skin, benign
Jaffe-Lichtenstein (-Uehlinger) syndrome —see Dysplasia, fibrous, bone NEC
Jakob-Creutzfeldt disease or syndrome —see Creutzfeldt-Jakob disease or syndrome
Jaksch-Luzet disease D64.89
Jamaican
  neuropathy G92
  paraplegic tropical ataxic-spastic syndrome G92
Janet's disease F48.8
Janiceps Q89.4
Jansky-Bielschowsky amaurotic idiocy E75.4
Japanese
  B-type encephalitis A83.0
  river fever A75.3
Jaundice (yellow) R17
  acholuric (familial) (splenomegalic) —see also Spherocytosis
    acquired D59.8
  breast-milk (inhibitor) P59.3
  catarrhal (acute) B15.9
    with hepatic coma B15.0
  cholestatic (benign) R17
  due to or associated with
    delayed conjugation P59.8
      associated with (due to) preterm delivery P59.0
    preterm delivery P59.0
  epidemic (catarrhal) B15.9
    with hepatic coma B15.0
    leptospiral A27.0
    spirochetal A27.0
  familial nonhemolytic (congenital) (Gilbert) E80.4
    Crigler-Najjar E80.5
  febrile (acute) B15.9
    with hepatic coma B15.0
    leptospiral A27.0
    spirochetal A27.0
  hematogenous D59.9
  hemolytic (acquired) D59.9
    congenital —see Spherocytosis

Jaundice (Continued)
  hemorrhagic (acute) (leptospiral) (spirochetal) A27.0
  infectious (acute) (subacute) B15.9
    with hepatic coma B15.0
    leptospiral A27.0
    spirochetal A27.0
  leptospiral (hemorrhagic) A27.0
  malignant (without coma) K72.90
    with coma K72.91
  neonatal —see Jaundice, newborn
  newborn P59.9
    due to or associated with
      ABO
        antibodies P55.1
        incompatibility, maternal/fetal P55.1
        isoimmunization P55.1
      absence or deficiency of enzyme system for bilirubin conjugation (congenital) P59.8
      bleeding P58.1
      breast milk inhibitors to conjugation P59.3
        associated with preterm delivery P59.0
      bruising P58.0
      Crigler-Najjar syndrome E80.5
      delayed conjugation P59.8
        associated with preterm delivery P59.0
      drugs or toxins
        given to newborn P58.42
        transmitted from mother P58.41
      excessive hemolysis P58.9
        due to
          bleeding P58.1
          bruising P58.0
          drugs or toxins
            given to newborn P58.42
            transmitted from mother P58.41
          infection P58.2
          polycythemia P58.3
          swallowed maternal blood P58.5
        specified type NEC P58.8
      galactosemia E74.21
      Gilbert syndrome E80.4
      hemolytic disease P55.9
        ABO isoimmunization P55.1
        Rh isoimmunization P55.0
        specified NEC P55.8
      hepatocellular damage P59.20
        specified NEC P59.29
      hereditary hemolytic anemia P58.8
      hypothyroidism, congenital E03.1
      incompatibility, maternal/fetal NOS P55.9
      infection P58.2

Jaundice (Continued)
  newborn (Continued)
    due to or associated with (Continued)
      inspissated bile syndrome P59.1
      isoimmunization NOS P55.9
      mucoviscidosis E84.9
      polycythemia P58.3
      preterm delivery P59.0
      Rh
        antibodies P55.0
        incompatibility, maternal/fetal P55.0
        isoimmunization P55.0
      specified cause NEC P59.8
      swallowed maternal blood P58.5
      spherocytosis (congenital) D58.0
  nonhemolytic congenital familial (Gilbert) E80.4
  nuclear, newborn (see also Kernicterus of newborn) P57.9
  obstructive (see also Obstruction, bile duct) K83.1
  post-immunization —see Hepatitis, viral, type, B
  post-transfusion —see Hepatitis, viral, type, B
  regurgitation (see also Obstruction, bile duct) K83.1
  serum (homologous) (prophylactic) (therapeutic) —see Hepatitis, viral, type, B
  spirochetal (hemorrhagic) A27.0
  symptomatic R17
    newborn P59.9
Jaw —see condition
Jaw-winking phenomenon or syndrome Q07.8
Jealousy
  alcoholic F10.988
  childhood F93.8
  sibling F93.8
Jejunitis —see Enteritis
Jejunostomy status Z93.4
Jejunum, jejunal —see condition
Jensen's disease —see Inflammation, chorioretinal, focal, juxtapapillary
Jerks, myoclonic G25.3
Jervell-Lange-Nielsen syndrome I45.81
Jeune's disease Q77.2
Jigger disease B88.1
Job's syndrome (chronic granulomatous disease) D71
Joint —see also condition
  mice —see Loose, body, joint
    knee M23.4-
Jordan's anomaly or syndrome D72.0
Joseph-Diamond-Blackfan anemia (congenital hypoplastic) D61.01
Jungle yellow fever A95.0
Jüngling's disease —see Sarcoidosis
Juvenile —see condition

◄ New   ◄▦ Revised   ~~deleted~~ Deleted

K

Kahler's disease C90.0-
Kakke E51.11
Kala-azar B55.0
Kallmann's syndrome E23.0
Kanner's syndrome (autism) —see Psychosis, childhood
Kaposi's
  dermatosis (xeroderma pigmentosum) Q82.1
  lichen ruber L44.0
    acuminatus L44.0
  sarcoma
    colon C46.4
    connective tissue C46.1
    gastrointestinal organ C46.4
    lung C46.5-
    lymph node (multiple) C46.3
    palate (hard) (soft) C46.2
    rectum C46.4
    skin (multiple sites) C46.0
    specified site NEC C46.7
    stomach C46.4
    unspecified site C46.9
  varicelliform eruption B00.0
    vaccinia T88.1
Kartagener's syndrome or triad (sinusitis, bronchiectasis, situs inversus) Q89.3
Karyotype
  with abnormality except iso (Xq) Q96.2
  45,X Q96.0
  46,X
    iso (Xq) Q96.1
  46,XX Q98.3
    with streak gonads Q50.32
    hermaphrodite (true) Q99.1
    male Q98.3
  46,XY
    with streak gonads Q56.1
    female Q97.3
    hermaphrodite (true) Q99.1
  47,XXX Q97.0
  47,XXY Q98.0
  47,XYY Q98.5
Kaschin-Beck disease —see Disease, Kaschin-Beck
Katayama's disease or fever B65.2
Kawasaki's syndrome M30.3
Kayser-Fleischer ring (cornea) (pseudosclerosis) H18.04-
Kaznelson's syndrome (congenital hypoplastic anemia) D61.01
Kearns-Sayre syndrome H49.81-
Kedani fever A75.3
Kelis L91.0
Kelly (-Patterson) syndrome (sideropenic dysphagia) D50.1
Keloid, cheloid L91.0
  acne L73.0
  Addison's L94.0
  cornea —see Opacity, cornea
  Hawkin's L91.0
  scar L91.0
Keloma L91.0
Kenya fever A77.1
Keratectasia —see also Ectasia, cornea
  congenital Q13.4
Keratinization of alveolar ridge mucosa
  excessive K13.23
  minimal K13.22
Keratinized residual ridge mucosa
  excessive K13.23
  minimal K13.22
Keratitis (nodular) (nonulcerative) (simple) (zonular) H16.9
  with ulceration (central) (marginal) (perforated) (ring) —see Ulcer, cornea
  actinic —see Photokeratitis
  arborescens (herpes simplex) B00.52
  areolar H16.11-
  bullosa H16.8

Keratitis (Continued)
  deep H16.309
    specified type NEC H16.399
  dendritic (a) (herpes simplex) B00.52
  disciform (is) (herpes simplex) B00.52
    varicella B01.81
  filamentary H16.12-
  gonococcal (congenital or prenatal) A54.33
  herpes, herpetic (simplex) B00.52
    zoster B02.33
  in (due to)
    acanthamebiasis B60.13
    adenovirus B30.0
    exanthema (see also Exanthem) B09
    herpes (simplex) virus B00.52
    measles B05.81
    syphilis A50.31
    tuberculosis A18.52
    zoster B02.33
  interstitial (nonsyphilitic) H16.30-
    diffuse H16.32-
    herpes, herpetic (simplex) B00.52
      zoster B02.33
    sclerosing H16.33-
    specified type NEC H16.39-
    syphilitic (congenital) (late) A50.31
    tuberculous A18.52
  macular H16.11-
  nummular H16.11-
  oyster shuckers' H16.8
  parenchymatous —see Keratitis, interstitial
  petrificans H16.8
  postmeasles B05.81
  punctata
    leprosa A30.9 [H16.14-]
    syphilitic (profunda) A50.31
  punctate H16.14-
  purulent H16.8
  rosacea L71.8
  sclerosing H16.33-
  specified type NEC H16.8
  stellate H16.11-
  striate H16.11-
  superficial H16.10-
    with conjunctivitis —see Keratoconjunctivitis
    due to light —see Photokeratitis
  suppurative H16.8
  syphilitic (congenital) (prenatal) A50.31
  trachomatous A71.1
    sequelae B94.0
  tuberculous A18.52
  vesicular H16.8
  xerotic (see also Keratomalacia) H16.8
    vitamin A deficiency E50.4
Keratoacanthoma L85.8
Keratocele —see Descemetocele
Keratoconjunctivitis H16.20-
  Acanthamoeba B60.13
  adenoviral B30.0
  epidemic B30.0
  exposure H16.21-
  herpes, herpetic (simplex) B00.52
    zoster B02.33
  in exanthema (see also Exanthem) B09
  infectious B30.0
  lagophthalmic —see Keratoconjunctivitis, specified type NEC
  neurotrophic H16.23-
  phlyctenular H16.25-
  postmeasles B05.81
  shipyard B30.0
  sicca (Sjogren's) M35.0-
    not Sjogren's H16.22-
  specified type NEC H16.29-
  tuberculous (phlyctenular) A18.52
  vernal H16.26-
Keratoconus H18.60-
  congenital Q13.4
  stable H18.61-
  unstable H18.62-

Keratocyst (dental) (odontogenic) —see Cyst, calcifying odontogenic
Keratoderma, keratodermia (congenital) (palmaris et plantaris) (symmetrical) Q82.8
  acquired L85.1
    in diseases classified elsewhere L86
  climactericum L85.1
  gonococcal A54.89
  gonorrheal A54.89
  punctata L85.2
  Reiter's —see Reiter's disease
Keratodermatocele —see Descemetocele
Keratoglobus H18.79
  congenital Q15.8
    with glaucoma Q15.0
Keratohemia —see Pigmentation, cornea, stromal
Keratoiritis —see also Iridocyclitis
  syphilitic A50.39
  tuberculous A18.54
Keratoma L57.0
  palmaris and plantaris hereditarium Q82.8
  senile L57.0
Keratomalacia H18.44-
  vitamin A deficiency E50.4
Keratomegaly Q13.4
Keratomycosis B49
  nigrans, nigricans (palmaris) B36.1
Keratopathy H18.9
  band H18.42-
  bullous H18.1-
  bullous (aphakic), following cataract surgery H59.01-
Keratoscleritis, tuberculous A18.52
Keratosis L57.0
  actinic L57.0
  arsenical L85.8
  congenital, specified NEC Q80.8
  female genital NEC N94.89
  follicularis Q82.8
    acquired L11.0
    congenita Q82.8
    et parafollicularis in cutem penetrans L87.0
    spinulosa (decalvans) Q82.8
    vitamin A deficiency E50.8
  gonococcal A54.89
  male genital (external) N50.8
  nigricans L83
  obturans, external ear (canal) —see Cholesteatoma, external ear
  palmaris et plantaris (inherited) (symmetrical) Q82.8
    acquired L85.1
  penile N48.89
  pharynx J39.2
  pilaris, acquired L85.8
  punctata (palmaris et plantaris) L85.2
  scrotal N50.8
  seborrheic L82.1
    inflamed L82.0
  senile L57.0
  solar L57.0
  tonsillaris J35.8
  vagina N89.4
  vegetans Q82.8
  vitamin A deficiency E50.8
  vocal cord J38.3
Kerato-uveitis —see Iridocyclitis
Kerion (celsi) B35.0
Kernicterus of newborn (not due to isoimmunization) P57.9
  due to isoimmunization (conditions in P55.0-P55.9) P57.0
  specified type NEC P57.8
Kerunoparalysis T75.09
Keshan disease E59
Ketoacidosis E87.2
  diabetic —see Diabetes, by type, with ketoacidosis
Ketonuria R82.4

Ketosis NEC E88.89
  diabetic —*see* Diabetes, by type, with
    ketoacidosis
Kew Garden fever A79.1
Kidney —*see* condition
Kienböck's disease —*see also* Osteochondrosis,
    juvenile, hand, carpal lunate
  adult M93.1
Kimmelstiel (-Wilson) disease —*see* Diabetes,
    Kimmelstiel (-Wilson) disease
Kimura disease D21.9
  specified site (see Neoplasm, connective
    tissue benign)
Kink, kinking
  artery I77.1
  hair (acquired) L67.8
  ileum or intestine —*see* Obstruction,
    intestine
  Lane's —*see* Obstruction, intestine
  organ or site, congenital NEC —*see* Anomaly,
    by site
  ureter (pelvic junction) N13.5
    with
      hydronephrosis N13.1
        with infection N13.6
      pyelonephritis (chronic) N11.1
    congenital Q62.39
  vein (s) I87.8
    caval I87.1
    peripheral I87.1
Kinnier Wilson's disease (hepatolenticular
    degeneration) E83.01
Kissing spine M48.20
  cervical region M48.22
  cervicothoracic region M48.23
  lumbar region M48.26
  lumbosacral region M48.27
  occipito-atlanto-axial region M48.21
  thoracic region M48.24
  thoracolumbar region M48.25
Klatskin's tumor C24.0
Klauder's disease A26.8
Klebs' disease (see also Glomerulonephritis)
    N05.-
Klebsiella (K.) pneumoniae, as cause of
    disease classified elsewhere B96.1
Klein (e)-Levin syndrome G47.13
Kleptomania F63.2
Klinefelter's syndrome Q98.4
  karyotype 47,XXY Q98.0
  male with more than two X chromosomes
    Q98.1
Klippel-Feil deficiency, disease, or syndrome
    (brevicollis) Q76.1
Klippel's disease I67.2
Klippel-Trenaunay (-Weber) syndrome
    Q87.2
Klumpke (-Déjerine) palsy, paralysis (birth)
    (newborn) P14.1
Knee —*see* condition
Knock knee (acquired) M21.06-
  congenital Q74.1

Knot (s)
  intestinal, syndrome (volvulus) K56.2
  surfer S89.8-
  umbilical cord (true) O69.2
Knotting (of)
  hair L67.8
  intestine K56.2
Knuckle pad (Garrod's) M72.1
Koch's
  infection —*see* Tuberculosis
  relapsing fever A68.9
Koch-Weeks' conjunctivitis —*see*
    Conjunctivitis, acute, mucopurulent
Köebner's syndrome Q81.8
Köenig's disease (osteochondritis dissecans) —
    see Osteochondritis, dissecans
Köhler-Pellegrini-Steida disease or syndrome
    (calcification, knee joint) —*see* Bursitis,
    tibial collateral
Köhler's disease
  patellar —*see* Osteochondrosis, juvenile,
    patella
  tarsal navicular —*see* Osteochondrosis,
    juvenile, tarsus
Koilonychia L60.3
  congenital Q84.6
Kojevnikov's, epilepsy —*see* Kozhevnikof's
    epilepsy
Koplik's spots B05.9
Kopp's asthma E32.8
Korsakoff's (Wernicke) disease, psychosis or
    syndrome (alcoholic) F10.96
  with dependence F10.26
  drug-induced
    due to drug abuse —*see* Abuse, drug, by
      type, with amnestic disorder
    due to drug dependence —*see* Dependence,
      drug, by type, with amnestic disorder
  nonalcoholic F04
Korsakov's disease, psychosis or syndrome —
    see Korsakoff's disease
Korsakow's disease, psychosis or syndrome —
    see Korsakoff's disease
Kostmann's disease or syndrome (infantile
    genetic agranulocytosis) —*see*
    Agranulocytosis
Kozhevnikof's epilepsy G40.109
  intractable G40.119
    with status epilepticus G40.111
    without status epilepticus G40.119
  not intractable G40.109
    with status epilepticus G40.101
    without status epilepticus G40.109
Krabbe's
  disease E75.23
  syndrome, congenital muscle hypoplasia
    Q79.8
Kraepelin-Morel disease —*see* Schizophrenia
Kraft-Weber-Dimitri disease Q85.8
Kraurosis
  ani K62.89
  penis N48.0

Kraurosis (Continued)
  vagina N89.8
  vulva N90.4
Kreotoxism A05.9
Krukenberg's
  spindle —*see* Pigmentation, cornea, posterior
  tumor C79.6-
Kufs' disease E75.4
Kugelberg-Welander disease G12.1
Kuhnt-Junius degeneration (see also
    Degeneration, macula) H35.32
Kümmell's disease or spondylitis —*see*
    Spondylopathy, traumatic
Kupffer cell sarcoma C22.3
Kuru A81.81
Kussmaul's
  disease M30.0
  respiration E87.2
    in diabetic acidosis —*see* Diabetes, by type,
      with ketoacidosis
Kwashiorkor E40
  marasmic, marasmus type E42
Kyasanur Forest disease A98.2
Kyphoscoliosis, kyphoscoliotic (acquired) (see
    also Scoliosis) M41.9
  congenital Q67.5
  heart (disease) I27.1
  sequelae of rickets E64.3
  tuberculous A18.01
Kyphosis, kyphotic (acquired) M40.209
  cervical region M40.202
  cervicothoracic region M40.203
  congenital Q76.419
    cervical region Q76.412
    cervicothoracic region Q76.413
    occipito-atlanto-axial region Q76.411
    thoracic region Q76.414
    thoracolumbar region Q76.415
  Morquio-Brailsford type (spinal) (see also
    subcategory M49.8) E76.219
  postlaminectomy M96.3
  postradiation therapy M96.2
  postural (adolescent) M40.00
    cervicothoracic region M40.03
    thoracic region M40.04
    thoracolumbar region M40.05
  secondary NEC M40.10
    cervical region M40.12
    cervicothoracic region M40.13
    thoracic region M40.14
    thoracolumbar region M40.15
  sequelae of rickets E64.3
  specified type NEC M40.299
    cervical region M40.292
    cervicothoracic region M40.293
    thoracic region M40.294
    thoracolumbar region M40.295
  syphilitic, congenital A50.56
  thoracic region M40.204
  thoracolumbar region M40.205
  tuberculous A18.01
Kyrle disease L87.0

◀ New ◀◀◀ Revised ~~deleted~~ Deleted

L

Labia, labium —*see* condition
Labile
blood pressure R09.89
vasomotor system I73.9
Labioglossal paralysis G12.29
Labium leporinum —*see* Cleft, lip
Labor —*see* Delivery
Labored breathing —*see* Hyperventilation
Labyrinthitis (circumscribed) (destructive)
(diffuse) (inner ear) (latent) (purulent)
(suppurative) (*see also* subcategory)
H83.0
syphilitic A52.79
Laceration
with abortion —*see* Abortion, by type,
complicated by laceration of pelvic
organs
abdomen, abdominal
wall S31.119
with
foreign body S31.129
penetration into peritoneal cavity
S31.619
with foreign body S31.629
epigastric region S31.112
with
foreign body S31.122
penetration into peritoneal cavity
S31.612
with foreign body S31.622
left
lower quadrant S31.114
with
foreign body S31.124
penetration into peritoneal cavity
S31.614
with foreign body S31.624
upper quadrant S31.111
with
foreign body S31.121
penetration into peritoneal cavity
S31.611
with foreign body S31.621
periumbilic region S31.115
with
foreign body S31.125
penetration into peritoneal cavity
S31.615
with foreign body S31.625
right
lower quadrant S31.113
with
foreign body S31.123
penetration into peritoneal cavity
S31.613
with foreign body S31.623
upper quadrant S31.110
with
foreign body S31.120
penetration into peritoneal cavity
S31.610
with foreign body S31.620
accidental, complicating surgery —*see*
Complications, surgical, accidental
puncture or laceration
Achilles tendon S86.02-
adrenal gland S37.813
alveolar (process) —*see* Laceration, oral cavity
ankle S91.01-
with
foreign body S91.02-
antecubital space —*see* Laceration, elbow
anus (sphincter) S31.831
with
ectopic or molar pregnancy O08.6
foreign body S31.832
complicating delivery —*see* Delivery,
complicated, by, laceration, anus
(sphincter)

Laceration (*Continued*)
anus (*Continued*)
following ectopic or molar pregnancy
O08.6
nontraumatic, nonpuerperal —*see* Fissure,
anus
arm (upper) S41.11-
with foreign body S41.12-
lower —*see* Laceration, forearm
auditory canal (external) (meatus) —*see*
Laceration, ear
auricle, ear —*see* Laceration, ear
axilla —*see* Laceration, arm
back —*see also* Laceration, thorax, back
lower S31.010
with
foreign body S31.020
with penetration into
retroperitoneal space S31.021
penetration into retroperitoneal space
S31.011
bile duct S36.13
bladder S37.23
with ectopic or molar pregnancy O08.6
following ectopic or molar pregnancy
O08.6
obstetrical trauma O71.5
blood vessel —*see* Injury, blood vessel
bowel —*see also* Laceration, intestine
with ectopic or molar pregnancy O08.6
complicating abortion —*see* Abortion,
by type, complicated by, specified
condition NEC
following ectopic or molar pregnancy
O08.6
obstetrical trauma O71.5
brain (any part) (cortex) (diffuse)
(membrane) —*see also* Injury,
intracranial, diffuse
during birth P10.8
with hemorrhage P10.1
focal —*see* Injury, intracranial, focal brain
injury
brainstem S06.38-
breast S21.01-
with foreign body S21.02-
broad ligament S37.893
with ectopic or molar pregnancy O08.6
following ectopic or molar pregnancy
O08.6
laceration syndrome N83.8
obstetrical trauma O71.6
syndrome (laceration) N83.8
buttock S31.801
with foreign body S31.802
left S31.821
with foreign body S31.822
right S31.811
with foreign body S31.812
calf —*see* Laceration, leg
canaliculus lacrimalis —*see* Laceration,
eyelid
canthus, eye —*see* Laceration, eyelid
capsule, joint —*see* Sprain
causing eversion of cervix uteri (old) N86
central (perineal), complicating delivery
O70.9
cerebellum, traumatic S06.37-
cerebral S06.33-
during birth P10.8
with hemorrhage P10.1
left side S06.32-
right side S06.31-
cervix (uteri)
with ectopic or molar pregnancy O08.6
following ectopic or molar pregnancy
O08.6
nonpuerperal, nontraumatic N88.1
obstetrical trauma (current) O71.3
old (postpartal) N88.1
traumatic S37.63

Laceration (*Continued*)
cheek (external) S01.41-
with foreign body S01.42-
internal —*see* Laceration, oral cavity
chest wall —*see* Laceration, thorax
chin —*see* Laceration, head, specified site
NEC
chordae tendinae NEC I51.1
concurrent with acute myocardial
infarction —*see* Infarct, myocardium
following acute myocardial infarction
(current complication) I23.4
clitoris —*see* Laceration, vulva
colon —*see* Laceration, intestine, large,
colon
common bile duct S36.13
cortex (cerebral) —*see* Injury, intracranial,
diffuse
costal region —*see* Laceration, thorax
cystic duct S36.13
diaphragm S27.803
digit (s)
foot —*see* Laceration, toe
hand —*see* Laceration, finger
duodenum S36.430
ear (canal) (external) S01.31-
with foreign body S01.32-
drum S09.2-
elbow S51.01-
with
foreign body S51.02-
epididymis —*see* Laceration, testis
epigastric region —*see* Laceration, abdomen,
wall, epigastric region
esophagus K22.8
traumatic
cervical S11.21
with foreign body S11.22
thoracic S27.813
eye (ball) S05.3-
with prolapse or loss of intraocular tissue
S05.2-
penetrating S05.6-
eyebrow —*see* Laceration, eyelid
eyelid S01.11-
with foreign body S01.12-
face NEC —*see* Laceration, head, specified
site NEC
fallopian tube S37.539
bilateral S37.532
unilateral S37.531
finger (s) S61.219
with
damage to nail S61.319
with
foreign body S61.329
foreign body S61.229
index S61.218
with
damage to nail S61.318
with
foreign body S61.328
foreign body S61.228
left S61.211
with
damage to nail S61.311
with
foreign body S61.321
foreign body S61.221
right S61.210
with
damage to nail S61.310
with
foreign body S61.320
foreign body S61.220
little S61.218
with
damage to nail S61.318
with
foreign body S61.328
foreign body S61.228

Laceration (Continued)
  finger (Continued)
    little (Continued)
      left S61.217
        with
          damage to nail S61.317
            with
              foreign body S61.327
          foreign body S61.227
      right S61.216
        with
          damage to nail S61.316
            with
              foreign body S61.326
          foreign body S61.226
    middle S61.218
      with
        damage to nail S61.318
          with
            foreign body S61.328
        foreign body S61.228
    left S61.213
      with
        damage to nail S61.313
          with
            foreign body S61.323
        foreign body S61.223
    right S61.212
      with
        damage to nail S61.312
          with
            foreign body S61.322
        foreign body S61.222
  ring S61.218
    with
      damage to nail S61.318
        with
          foreign body S61.328
      foreign body S61.228
    left S61.215
      with
        damage to nail S61.315
          with
            foreign body S61.325
        foreign body S61.225
    right S61.214
      with
        damage to nail S61.314
          with
            foreign body S61.324
        foreign body S61.224
  flank S31.119
    with foreign body S31.129
  foot (except toe (s) alone) S91.319
    with foreign body S91.329
    left S91.312
      with foreign body S91.322
    right S91.311
      with foreign body S91.321
    toe —see Laceration, toe
  forearm S51.819
    with
      foreign body S51.829
    elbow only —see Laceration,
      elbow
    left S51.812
      with
        foreign body S51.822
    right S51.811
      with
        foreign body S51.821
  forehead S01.81
    with foreign body S01.82
  fourchette O70.0
    with ectopic or molar pregnancy
      O08.6
    complicating delivery O70.0
    following ectopic or molar pregnancy
      O08.6
  gallbladder S36.123

Laceration (Continued)
  genital organs, external
    female S31.512
      with foreign body S31.522
      vagina —see Laceration, vagina
      vulva —see Laceration, vulva
    male S31.511
      with foreign body S31.521
      penis —see Laceration, penis
      scrotum —see Laceration, scrotum
      testis —see Laceration, testis
  groin —see Laceration, abdomen, wall
  gum —see Laceration, oral cavity
  hand S61.419
    with
      foreign body S61.429
    finger —see Laceration, finger
    left S61.412
      with
        foreign body S61.422
    right S61.411
      with
        foreign body S61.421
    thumb —see Laceration, thumb
  head S01.91
    with foreign body S01.92
    cheek —see Laceration, cheek
    ear —see Laceration, ear
    eyelid —see Laceration, eyelid
    lip —see Laceration, lip
    nose —see Laceration, nose
    oral cavity —see Laceration, oral
      cavity
    scalp S01.01
      with foreign body S01.02
    specified site NEC S01.81
      with foreign body S01.82
    temporomandibular area —see Laceration,
      cheek
  heart —see Injury, heart, laceration
  heel —see Laceration, foot
  hepatic duct S36.13
  hip S71.019
    with foreign body S71.029
    left S71.012
      with foreign body S71.022
    right S71.011
      with foreign body S71.021
  hymen —see Laceration, vagina
  hypochondrium —see Laceration, abdomen,
    wall
  hypogastric region —see Laceration,
    abdomen, wall
  ileum S36.438
  inguinal region —see Laceration, abdomen,
    wall
  instep —see Laceration, foot
  internal organ —see Injury, by site
  interscapular region —see Laceration, thorax,
    back
  intestine
    large
      colon S36.539
        ascending S36.530
        descending S36.532
        sigmoid S36.533
        specified site NEC S36.538
        rectum S36.63
        transverse S36.531
      small S36.439
        duodenum S36.430
        specified site NEC S36.438
  intra-abdominal organ S36.93
    intestine —see Laceration, intestine
    liver —see Laceration, liver
    pancreas —see Laceration, pancreas
    peritoneum S36.81
    specified site NEC S36.893
    spleen —see Laceration, spleen
    stomach —see Laceration, stomach

Laceration (Continued)
  intracranial NEC —see also Injury,
    intracranial, diffuse
    birth injury P10.9
  jaw —see Laceration, head, specified site NEC
  jejunum S36.438
  joint capsule —see Sprain, by site
  kidney S37.03-
    major (greater than 3 cm) (massive)
      (stellate) S37.06-
    minor (less than 1 cm) S37.04-
    moderate (1 to 3 cm) S37.05-
    multiple S37.06-
  knee S81.01-
    with foreign body S81.02-
  labium (majus) (minus) —see Laceration,
    vulva
  lacrimal duct —see Laceration, eyelid
  large intestine —see Laceration, intestine,
    large
  larynx S11.011
    with foreign body S11.012
  leg (lower) S81.819
    with foreign body S81.829
    foot —see Laceration, foot
    knee —see Laceration, knee
    left S81.812
      with foreign body S81.822
    right S81.811
      with foreign body S81.821
    upper —see Laceration, thigh
  ligament —see Sprain
  lip S01.511
    with foreign body S01.521
  liver S36.113
    major (stellate) S36.116
    minor S36.114
    moderate S36.115
  loin —see Laceration, abdomen, wall
  lower back —see Laceration, back, lower
  lumbar region —see Laceration, back, lower
  lung S27.339
    bilateral S27.332
    unilateral S27.331
  malar region —see Laceration, head, specified
    site NEC
  mammary —see Laceration, breast
  mastoid region —see Laceration, head,
    specified site NEC
  meninges —see Injury, intracranial, diffuse
  meniscus —see Tear, meniscus
  mesentery S36.893
  mesosalpinx S37.893 ◀▥▥
    ~~bilateral S37.532~~
    ~~unilateral S37.531~~
  mouth —see Laceration, oral cavity
  muscle —see Injury, muscle, by site, laceration
  nail
    finger —see Laceration, finger, with
      damage to nail
    toe —see Laceration, toe, with damage to
      nail
  nasal (septum) (sinus) —see Laceration, nose
  nasopharynx —see Laceration, head, specified
    site NEC
  neck S11.91
    with foreign body S11.92
    involving
      cervical esophagus S11.21
        with foreign body S11.22
      larynx —see Laceration, larynx
      pharynx —see Laceration, pharynx
      thyroid gland —see Laceration, thyroid
        gland
      trachea —see Laceration, trachea
    specified site NEC S11.81
      with foreign body S11.82
  nerve —see Injury, nerve
  nose (septum) (sinus) S01.21
    with foreign body S01.22

Laceration *(Continued)*
ocular NOS S05.3-
  adnexa NOS S01.11-
oral cavity S01.512
  with foreign body S01.522
orbit (eye) —*see* Wound, open, ocular, orbit
ovary S37.439
  bilateral S37.432
  unilateral S37.431
palate —*see* Laceration, oral cavity
palm —*see* Laceration, hand
pancreas S36.239
  body S36.231
    major S36.261
    minor S36.241
    moderate S36.251
  head S36.230
    major S36.260
    minor S36.240
    moderate S36.250
  major S36.269
  minor S36.249
  moderate S36.259
  tail S36.232
    major S36.262
    minor S36.242
    moderate S36.252
pelvic S31.010
  with
    foreign body S31.020
      penetration into retroperitoneal cavity S31.021
    penetration into retroperitoneal cavity S31.011
  floor —*see also* Laceration, back, lower
    with ectopic or molar pregnancy O08.6
    complicating delivery O70.1
    following ectopic or molar pregnancy O08.6
    old (postpartal) N81.89
  organ S37.93
    with ectopic or molar pregnancy O08.6
    adrenal gland S37.813
    bladder S37.23
    fallopian tube —*see* Laceration, fallopian tube
    following ectopic or molar pregnancy O08.6
    kidney —*see* Laceration, kidney
    obstetrical trauma O71.5
    ovary —*see* Laceration, ovary
    prostate S37.823
    specified site NEC S37.893
    ureter S37.13
    urethra S37.33
    uterus S37.63
penis S31.21
  with foreign body S31.22
perineum
  female S31.41
    with
      ectopic or molar pregnancy O08.6
      foreign body S31.42
    during delivery O70.9
      first degree O70.0
      fourth degree O70.3
      second degree O70.1
      third degree O70.2
    old (postpartal) N81.89
    postpartal N81.89
    secondary (postpartal) O90.1
  male S31.119
    with foreign body S31.129
periocular area (with or without lacrimal passages) —*see* Laceration, eyelid
peritoneum S36.893
periumbilic region —*see* Laceration, abdomen, wall, periumbilic
periurethral tissue —*see* Laceration, urethra

Laceration *(Continued)*
phalanges
  finger —*see* Laceration, finger
  toe —*see* Laceration, toe
pharynx S11.21
  with foreign body S11.22
pinna —*see* Laceration, ear
popliteal space —*see* Laceration, knee
prepuce —*see* Laceration, penis
prostate S37.823
pubic region S31.119
  with foreign body S31.129
pudendum —*see* Laceration, genital organs, external
rectovaginal septum —*see* Laceration, vagina
rectum S36.63
retroperitoneum S36.893
round ligament S37.893
sacral region —*see* Laceration, back, lower
sacroiliac region —*see* Laceration, back, lower
salivary gland —*see* Laceration, oral cavity
scalp S01.01
  with foreign body S01.02
scapular region —*see* Laceration, shoulder
scrotum S31.31
  with foreign body S31.32
seminal vesicle S37.893
shin —*see* Laceration, leg
shoulder S41.019
  with foreign body S41.029
  left S41.012
    with foreign body S41.022
  right S41.011
    with foreign body S41.021
small intestine —*see* Laceration, intestine, small
spermatic cord —*see* Laceration, testis
spinal cord (meninges) —*see also* Injury, spinal cord, by region
  due to injury at birth P11.5
  newborn (birth injury) P11.5
spleen S36.039
  major (massive) (stellate) S36.032
  moderate S36.031
  superficial (minor) S36.030
sternal region —*see* Laceration, thorax, front
stomach S36.33
submaxillary region —*see* Laceration, head, specified site NEC
submental region —*see* Laceration, head, specified site NEC
subungual
  finger (s) —*see* Laceration, finger, with damage to nail
  toe (s) —*see* Laceration, toe, with damage to nail
suprarenal gland —*see* Laceration, adrenal gland
temple, temporal region —*see* Laceration, head, specified site NEC
temporomandibular area —*see* Laceration, cheek
tendon —*see* Injury, muscle, by site, laceration
  Achilles S86.02-
tentorium cerebelli —*see* Injury, intracranial, diffuse
testis S31.31
  with foreign body S31.32
thigh S71.11-
  with foreign body S71.12-
thorax, thoracic (wall) S21.91
  with foreign body S21.92
  back S21.22-
    with penetration into thoracic cavity S21.42-
  front S21.12-
    with penetration into thoracic cavity S21.32-

Laceration *(Continued)*
thorax, thoracic *(Continued)*
  back S21.21-
    with
      foreign body S21.22-
        with penetration into thoracic cavity S21.42-
      penetration into thoracic cavity S21.41-
  breast —*see* Laceration, breast
  front S21.11-
    with
      foreign body S21.12-
        with penetration into thoracic cavity S21.32-
      penetration into thoracic cavity S21.31-
thumb S61.019
  with
    damage to nail S61.119
      with foreign body S61.129
    foreign body S61.029
  left S61.012
    with
      damage to nail S61.112
        with foreign body S61.122
      foreign body S61.022
  right S61.011
    with
      damage to nail S61.111
        with foreign body S61.121
      foreign body S61.021
thyroid gland S11.11
  with foreign body S11.12
toe (s) S91.119
  with
    damage to nail S91.219
      with foreign body S91.229
    foreign body S91.129
  great S91.113
    with
      damage to nail S91.213
        with foreign body S91.223
      foreign body S91.123
    left S91.112
      with
        damage to nail S91.212
          with foreign body S91.222
        foreign body S91.122
    right S91.111
      with
        damage to nail S91.211
          with foreign body S91.221
        foreign body S91.121
  lesser S91.116
    with
      damage to nail S91.216
        with foreign body S91.226
      foreign body S91.126
    left S91.115
      with
        damage to nail S91.215
          with foreign body S91.225
        foreign body S91.125
    right S91.114
      with
        damage to nail S91.214
          with foreign body S91.224
        foreign body S91.124
tongue —*see* Laceration, oral cavity

Laceration (Continued)
  trachea S11.021
    with foreign body S11.022
  tunica vaginalis —see Laceration, testis
  tympanum, tympanic membrane —see
    Laceration, ear, drum
  umbilical region S31.115
    with foreign body S31.125
  ureter S37.13
  urethra S37.33
    with or following ectopic or molar
      pregnancy O08.6
    obstetrical trauma O71.5
  urinary organ NEC S37.893
  uterus S37.63
    with ectopic or molar pregnancy O08.6
    following ectopic or molar pregnancy
      O08.6
    nonpuerperal, nontraumatic N85.8
    obstetrical trauma NEC O71.81
    old (postpartal) N85.8
  uvula —see Laceration, oral cavity
  vagina S31.41
    with
      ectopic or molar pregnancy O08.6
      foreign body S31.42
    during delivery O71.4
      with perineal laceration —see Laceration,
        perineum, female, during delivery
    following ectopic or molar pregnancy
      O08.6
    nonpuerperal, nontraumatic N89.8
    old (postpartal) N89.8
  vas deferens S37.893
  vesical —see Laceration, bladder
  vocal cords S11.031
    with foreign body S11.032
  vulva S31.41
    with
      ectopic or molar pregnancy O08.6
      foreign body S31.42
    complicating delivery O70.0
    following ectopic or molar pregnancy
      O08.6
    nonpuerperal, nontraumatic N90.89
    old (postpartal) N90.89
  wrist S61.519
    with
      foreign body S61.529
    left S61.512
      with
        foreign body S61.522
    right S61.511
      with
        foreign body S61.521
Lack of
  achievement in school Z55.3
  adequate
    food Z59.4
    intermaxillary vertical dimension of fully
      erupted teeth M26.36
    sleep Z72.820
  appetite (see Anorexia) R63.0
  awareness R41.9
  care
    in home Z74.2
    of infant (at or after birth) T76.02
      confirmed T74.02
  cognitive functions R41.9
  coordination R27.9
    ataxia R27.0
    specified type NEC R27.8
  development (physiological) R62.50
    failure to thrive (child over 28 days old)
      R62.51
    adult R62.7
    newborn P92.6
    short stature R62.52
    specified type NEC R62.59
  energy R53.83
  financial resources Z59.6

Lack of (Continued)
  food T73.0
  growth R62.52
  heating Z59.1
  housing (permanent) (temporary) Z59.0
    adequate Z59.1
  learning experiences in childhood Z62.898
  leisure time (affecting life-style) Z73.2
  material resources Z59.9
  memory —see also Amnesia
    mild, following organic brain damage
      F06.8
  ovulation N97.0
  parental supervision or control of child
    Z62.0
  person able to render necessary care Z74.2
  physical exercise Z72.3
  play experience in childhood Z62.898
  posterior occlusal support M26.57
  relaxation (affecting life-style) Z73.2
  sexual
    desire F52.0
    enjoyment F52.1
  shelter Z59.0
  sleep (adequate) Z72.820
  supervision of child by parent Z62.0
  support, posterior occlusal M26.57
  water T73.1
Lacrimal —see condition
Lacrimation, abnormal —see Epiphora
Lacrimonasal duct —see condition
Lactation, lactating (breast) (puerperal,
    postpartum)
  associated
    cracked nipple O92.13
    retracted nipple O92.03
  defective O92.4
  disorder NEC O92.79
  excessive O92.6
  failed (complete) O92.3
    partial O92.4
  mastitis NEC —see Mastitis, obstetric
  mother (care and/or examination) Z39.1
  nonpuerperal N64.3
Lacticemia, excessive E87.2
Lacunar skull Q75.8
Laennec's cirrhosis K74.69
  alcoholic K70.30
    with ascites K70.31
Lafora's disease —see Epilepsy, generalized,
    idiopathic
Lag, lid (nervous) —see Retraction, lid
Lagophthalmos (eyelid) (nervous) H02.209
  cicatricial H02.219
    left H02.216
      lower H02.215
      upper H02.214
    right H02.213
      lower H02.212
      upper H02.211
  keratoconjunctivitis —see Keratoconjunctivitis
  left H02.206
    lower H02.205
    upper H02.204
  mechanical H02.229
    left H02.226
      lower H02.225
      upper H02.224
    right H02.223
      lower H02.222
      upper H02.221
  paralytic H02.239
    left H02.236
      lower H02.235
      upper H02.234
    right H02.233
      lower H02.232
      upper H02.231
  right H02.203
    lower H02.202
    upper H02.201

Laki-Lorand factor deficiency —see Defect,
    coagulation, specified type NEC
Lalling F80.0
Lambert-Eaton syndrome —see Syndrome,
    Lambert-Eaton
Lambliasis, lambliosis A07.1
Landau-Kleffner syndrome —see Epilepsy,
    specified NEC
Landouzy-Déjérine dystrophy or
    facioscapulohumeral atrophy G71.0
Landouzy's disease (icterohemorrhagic
    leptospirosis) A27.0
Landry-Guillain-Barré, syndrome or paralysis
    G61.0
Landry's disease or paralysis G61.0
Lane's
  band Q43.3
  kink —see Obstruction, intestine
  syndrome K90.2
Langdon Down's syndrome —see Trisomy, 21
Lapsed immunization schedule status Z28.3
Large
  baby (regardless of gestational age) (4000g to
    4499g) P08.1
  ear, congenital Q17.1
  physiological cup Q14.2
  stature R68.89
Large-for-dates NEC (infant) (4000g to 4499g)
    P08.1
  affecting management of pregnancy O36.6-
  exceptionally (4500g or more) P08.0
Larsen-Johansson disease
    orosteochondrosis —see Osteochondrosis,
    juvenile, patella
Larsen's syndrome (flattened facies and
    multiple congenital dislocations) Q74.8
Larva migrans
  cutaneous B76.9
    Ancylostoma B76.0
  visceral B83.0
Laryngeal —see condition
Laryngismus (stridulus) J38.5
  congenital P28.89
  diphtheritic A36.2
Laryngitis (acute) (edematous) (fibrinous)
    (infective) (infiltrative) (malignant)
    (membranous) (phlegmonous)
    (pneumococcal) (pseudomembranous)
    (septic) (subglottic) (suppurative)
    (ulcerative) J04.0
  with
    influenza, flu, or grippe —see Influenza,
      with, laryngitis
    tracheitis (acute) —see Laryngotracheitis
  atrophic J37.0
  catarrhal J37.0
  chronic J37.0
    with tracheitis (chronic) J37.1
  diphtheritic A36.2
  due to external agent —see Inflammation,
    respiratory, upper, due to
  Hemophilus influenzae J04.0
  H. influenzae J04.0
  hypertrophic J37.0
  influenzal —see Influenza, with, respiratory
    manifestations NEC
  obstructive J05.0
  sicca J37.0
  spasmodic J05.0
    acute J04.0
  streptococcal J04.0
  stridulous J05.0
  syphilitic (late) A52.73
    congenital A50.59 [J99]
    early A50.03 [J99]
  tuberculous A15.5
  Vincent's A69.1
Laryngocele (congenital) (ventricular) Q31.3
Laryngofissure J38.7
  congenital Q31.8
Laryngomalacia (congenital) Q31.5

◀ New   ⬛ Revised   ~~deleted~~ Deleted

Laryngopharyngitis (acute) J06.0
  chronic J37.0
  due to external agent —*see* Inflammation,
    respiratory, upper, due to
Laryngoplegia J38.00
  bilateral J38.02
  unilateral J38.01
Laryngoptosis J38.7
Laryngospasm J38.5
Laryngostenosis J38.6
Laryngotracheitis (acute) (Infectional)
    (infective) (viral) J04.2
  atrophic J37.1
  catarrhal J37.1
  chronic J37.1
  diphtheritic A36.2
  due to external agent —*see* Inflammation,
    respiratory, upper, due to
  Hemophilus influenzae J04.2
  hypertrophic J37.1
  influenzal —*see* Influenza, with, respiratory
    manifestations NEC
  pachydermic J38.7
  sicca J37.1
  spasmodic J38.5
    acute J05.0
  streptococcal J04.2
  stridulous J38.5
  syphilitic (late) A52.73
    congenital A50.59 *[J99]*
    early A50.03 *[J99]*
  tuberculous A15.5
  Vincent's A69.1
Laryngotracheobronchitis —*see* Bronchitis
Larynx, laryngeal —*see* condition
Lassa fever A96.2
Lassitude —*see* Weakness
Late
  talker R62.0
  walker R62.0
Late effect (s) —*see* Sequelae
Latent —*see* condition
Laterocession —*see* Lateroversion
Lateroflexion —*see* Lateroversion
Lateroversion
  cervix —*see* Lateroversion, uterus
  uterus, uterine (cervix) (postinfectional)
    (postpartal, old) N85.4
    congenital Q51.818
    in pregnancy or childbirth O34.59-
Lathyrism —*see* Poisoning, food, noxious, plant
Launois' syndrome (pituitary gigantism) E22.0
Launois-Bensaude adenolipomatosis E88.89
Laurence-Moon (-Bardet)-Biedl syndrome
    Q87.89
Lax, laxity —*see also* Relaxation
  ligament (ous) —*see also* Disorder, ligament
    familial M35.7
    knee —*see* Derangement, knee
  skin (acquired) L57.4
    congenital Q82.8
Laxative habit F55.2
Lazy leukocyte syndrome D70.8
Lead miner's lung J63.6
Leak, leakage
  air NEC J93.82
    postprocedural J95.812
  amniotic fluid —*see* Rupture, membranes,
    premature
  blood (microscopic), fetal, into maternal
    circulation affecting management of
    pregnancy —*see* Pregnancy, complicated
    by
  cerebrospinal fluid G96.0
    from spinal (lumbar) puncture G97.0
  device, implant or graft —*see also*
    Complications, by site and type,
    mechanical
  arterial graft NEC —*see* Complication,
    cardiovascular device, mechanical,
    vascular

Leak, leakage *(Continued)*
  device, implant or graft *(Continued)*
    breast (implant) T85.43
    catheter NEC T85.638
      dialysis (renal) T82.43
        intraperitoneal T85.631
      infusion NEC T82.534
        spinal (epidural) (subdural) T85.630
      urinary, indwelling T83.038
        cystostomy T83.030
    gastrointestinal —*see* Complications,
      prosthetic device, mechanical,
      gastrointestinal device
    genital NEC T83.498
      penile prosthesis T83.490
    heart NEC —*see* Complication,
      cardiovascular device, mechanical
    joint prosthesis —*see* Complications, joint
      prosthesis, mechanical, specified
      NEC, by site
    ocular NEC —*see* Complications,
      prosthetic device, mechanical, ocular
      device
    orthopedic NEC —*see* Complication,
      orthopedic, device, mechanical
    persistent air J93.82
    specified NEC T85.638
    urinary NEC —*see also* Complication,
      genitourinary, device, urinary,
      mechanical
      graft T83.23
    vascular NEC —*see* Complication,
      cardiovascular device, mechanical
    ventricular intracranial shunt T85.03
  urine —*see* Incontinence
Leaky heart —*see* Endocarditis
Learning defect (specific) F81.9
Leather bottle stomach C16.9
Leber's
  congenital amaurosis H35.50
  optic atrophy (hereditary) H47.22
Lederer's anemia D59.1
Leeches (external) —*see* Hirudiniasis
Leg —*see* condition
Legg (-Calvé)-Perthes disease, syndrome or
    osteochondrosis M91.1-
Legionellosis A48.1
  nonpneumonic A48.2
Legionnaires'
  disease A48.1
    nonpneumonic A48.2
  pneumonia A48.1
Leigh's disease G31.82
Leiner's disease L21.1
Leiofibromyoma —*see* Leiomyoma
Leiomyoblastoma —*see* Neoplasm, connective
    tissue, benign
Leiomyofibroma —*see also* Neoplasm,
    connective tissue, benign
  uterus (cervix) (corpus) D25.9
Leiomyoma —*see also* Neoplasm, connective
    tissue, benign
  bizarre —*see* Neoplasm, connective tissue,
    benign
  cellular —*see* Neoplasm, connective tissue,
    benign
  epithelioid —*see* Neoplasm, connective
    tissue, benign
  uterus (cervix) (corpus) D25.9
    intramural D25.1
    submucous D25.0
    subserosal D25.2
  vascular —*see* Neoplasm, connective tissue,
    benign
Leiomyoma, leiomyomatosis (intravascular) —
    see Neoplasm, connective tissue, uncertain
    behavior
Leiomyosarcoma —*see also* Neoplasm,
    connective tissue, malignant
  epithelioid —*see* Neoplasm, connective
    tissue, malignant

Leiomyosarcoma *(Continued)*
  myxoid —*see* Neoplasm, connective tissue,
    malignant
Leishmaniasis B55.9
  American (mucocutaneous) B55.2
    cutaneous B55.1
  Asian Desert B55.1
  Brazilian B55.2
  cutaneous (any type) B55.1
    dermal —*see also* Leishmaniasis, cutaneous
      post-kala-azar B55.0
    eyelid B55.1
    infantile B55.0
    Mediterranean B55.0
    mucocutaneous (American) (New World)
      B55.2
    naso-oral B55.2
    nasopharyngeal B55.2
    old world B55.1
    tegumentaria diffusa B55.1
    visceral B55.0
Leishmanoid, dermal —*see also* Leishmaniasis,
    cutaneous
  post-kala-azar B55.0
Lenegre's disease I44.2
Lengthening, leg —*see* Deformity, limb,
    unequal length
Lennert's lymphoma —*see* Lymphoma,
    Lennert's
Lennox-Gastaut syndrome G40.812
  intractable G40.814
    with status epilepticus G40.813
    without status epilepticus G40.814
  not intractable G40.812
    with status epilepticus G40.811
    without status epilepticus G40.812
Lens —*see* condition
Lenticonus (anterior) (posterior) (congenital)
    Q12.8
Lenticular degeneration, progressive E83.01
Lentiglobus (posterior) (congenital) Q12.8
Lentigo (congenital) L81.4
  maligna —*see also* Melanoma, in situ
    melanoma —*see* Melanoma
Lentivirus, as cause of disease classified
    elsewhere B97.31
Leontiasis
  ossium M85.2
  syphilitic (late) A52.78
    congenital A50.59
Lepothrix A48.8
Lepra —*see* Leprosy
Leprechaunism E34.8
Leprosy A30.-
  with muscle disorder A30.9 *[M63.80]*
    ankle A30.9 *[M63.87-]*
    foot A30.9 *[M63.87-]*
    forearm A30.9 *[M63.83-]*
    hand A30.9 *[M63.84-]*
    lower leg A30.9 *[M63.86-]*
    multiple sites A30.9 *[M63.89]*
    pelvic region A30.9 *[M63.85-]*
    shoulder region A30.9 *[M63.81-]*
    specified site NEC A30.9 *[M63.88]*
    thigh A30.9 *[M63.85-]*
    upper arm A30.9 *[M63.82-]*
  anesthetic A30.9
  BB A30.3
  BL A30.4
  borderline (infiltrated) (neuritic) A30.3
    lepromatous A30.4
    tuberculoid A30.2
  BT A30.2
  dimorphous (infiltrated) (neuritic) A30.3
  I A30.0
  indeterminate (macular) (neuritic) A30.0
  lepromatous (diffuse) (infiltrated) (macular)
    (neuritic) (nodular) A30.5
  LL A30.5
  macular (early) (neuritic) (simple) A30.9
  maculoanesthetic A30.9

Leprosy *(Continued)*
 mixed A30.3
 neural A30.9
 nodular A30.5
 primary neuritic A30.3
 specified type NEC A30.8
 TT A30.1
 tuberculoid (major) (minor) A30.1
Leptocytosis, hereditary D56.9
Leptomeningitis (chronic) (circumscribed)
  (hemorrhagic) (nonsuppurative) —*see*
  Meningitis
Leptomeningopathy G96.19
Leptospiral —*see* condition
Leptospirochetal —*see* condition
Leptospirosis A27.9
 canicola A27.89
 due to Leptospira interrogans serovar
  icterohaemorrhagiae A27.0
 icterohemorrhagica A27.0
 pomona A27.89
 Weil's disease A27.0
Leptus dermatitis B88.0
Leriche's syndrome (aortic bifurcation
  occlusion) I74.09
Leri's pleonosteosis Q78.8
Leri-Weill syndrome Q77.8
Lermoyez' syndrome —*see* Vertigo, peripheral
  NEC
Lesch-Nyhan syndrome E79.1
Leser-Trélat disease L82.1
 inflamed L82.0
Lesion (s) (nontraumatic)
 abducens nerve —*see* Strabismus, paralytic,
  sixth nerve
 alveolar process K08.9
 angiocentric immunoproliferative D47.Z9
 anorectal K62.9
 aortic (valve) I35.9
 auditory nerve —*see* subcategory H93.3
 basal ganglion G25.9
 bile duct —*see* Disease, bile duct
 biomechanical M99.9
  specified type NEC M99.89
   abdomen M99.89
   acromioclavicular M99.87
   cervical region M99.81
   cervicothoracic M99.81
   costochondral M99.88
   costovertebral M99.88
   head region M99.80
   hip M99.85
   lower extremity M99.86
   lumbar region M99.83
   lumbosacral M99.83
   occipitocervical M99.80
   pelvic region M99.85
   pubic M99.85
   rib cage M99.88
   sacral region M99.84
   sacrococcygeal M99.84
   sacroiliac M99.84
   specified NEC M99.89
   sternochondral M99.88
   sternoclavicular M99.87
   thoracic region M99.82
   thoracolumbar M99.82
   upper extremity M99.87
 bladder N32.9
 bone —*see* Disorder, bone
 brachial plexus G54.0
 brain G93.9
  congenital Q04.9
  vascular I67.9
   degenerative I67.9
   hypertensive I67.4
 buccal cavity K13.79
 calcified —*see* Calcification
 canthus —*see* Disorder, eyelid
 carate —*see* Pinta, lesions
 cardia K22.9

Lesion *(Continued)*
 cardiac (*see also* Disease, heart) I51.9
  congenital Q24.9
  valvular —*see* Endocarditis
 cauda equina G83.4
 cecum K63.9
 cerebral —*see* Lesion, brain
 cerebrovascular I67.9
  degenerative I67.9
  hypertensive I67.4
 cervical (nerve) root NEC G54.2
 chiasmal —*see* Disorder, optic, chiasm
 chorda tympani G51.8
 coin, lung R91.1
 colon K63.9
 congenital —*see* Anomaly, by site
 conjunctiva H11.9
 conus medullaris —*see* Injury, conus
  medullaris
 coronary artery —*see* Ischemia, heart
 cranial nerve G52.9
  eighth —*see* Disorder, ear
  eleventh G52.9
  fifth G50.9
  first G52.0
  fourth —*see* Strabismus, paralytic, fourth
   nerve
  seventh G51.9
  sixth —*see* Strabismus, paralytic, sixth
   nerve
  tenth G52.2
  twelfth G52.3
 cystic —*see* Cyst
 degenerative —*see* Degeneration
 duodenum K31.9
 edentulous (alveolar) ridge, associated with
  trauma, due to traumatic occlusion
  K06.2
 en coup de sabre L94.1
 eyelid —*see* Disorder, eyelid
 gasserian ganglion G50.8
 gastric K31.9
 gastroduodenal K31.9
 gastrointestinal K63.9
 gingiva, associated with trauma K06.2
 glomerular
  focal and segmental (*see also* N00-N07 with
   fourth character .1) N05.1
  minimal change (*see also* N00-N07 with
   fourth character .0) N05.0
 heart (organic) —*see* Disease, heart
 hyperchromic, due to pinta (carate)
  A67.1
 hyperkeratotic —*see* Hyperkeratosis
 hypothalamic E23.7
 ileocecal K63.9
 ileum K63.9
 iliohypogastric nerve G57.8-
 inflammatory —*see* Inflammation
 intestine K63.9
 intracerebral —*see* Lesion, brain
 intrachiasmal (optic) —*see* Disorder, optic,
  chiasm
 intracranial, space-occupying R90.0
 joint —*see* Disorder, joint
  sacroiliac (old) M53.3
 keratotic —*see* Keratosis
 kidney —*see* Disease, renal
 laryngeal nerve (recurrent) G52.2
 lip K13.0
 liver K76.9
 lumbosacral
  plexus G54.1
  root (nerve) NEC G54.4
 lung (coin) R91.1
 maxillary sinus J32.0
 mitral I05.9
 Morel-Lavallée —*see* Hematoma,
  by site
 motor cortex NEC G93.89
 mouth K13.79

Lesion *(Continued)*
 nerve G58.9
  femoral G57.2-
  median G56.1-
   carpal tunnel syndrome —*see* Syndrome,
    carpal tunnel
  plantar G57.6-
  popliteal (lateral) G57.3-
   medial G57.4-
  radial G56.3-
  sciatic G57.0-
  spinal —*see* Injury, nerve, spinal
  ulnar G56.2-
 nervous system, congenital Q07.9
 nonallopathic —*see* Lesion, biomechanical
 nose (internal) J34.89
 obstructive —*see* Obstruction
 obturator nerve G57.8-
 oral mucosa K13.70
 organ or site NEC —*see* Disease, by site
 osteolytic —*see* Osteolysis
 peptic K27.9
 periodontal, due to traumatic occlusion
  K05.5
 pharynx J39.2
 pigment, pigmented (skin) L81.9
 pinta —*see* Pinta, lesions
 polypoid —*see* Polyp
 prechiasmal (optic) —*see* Disorder, optic,
  chiasm
 primary (*see also* Syphilis, primary) A51.0
  carate A67.0
  pinta A67.0
  yaws A66.0
 pulmonary J98.4
  valve I37.9
 pylorus K31.9
 rectosigmoid K63.9
 retina, retinal H35.9
 sacroiliac (joint) (old) M53.3
 salivary gland K11.9
  benign lymphoepithelial K11.8
 saphenous nerve G57.8-
 sciatic nerve G57.0-
 secondary —*see* Syphilis, secondary
 shoulder (region) M75.9-
  specified NEC M75.8-
 sigmoid K63.9
 sinus (accessory) (nasal) J34.89
 skin L98.9
  suppurative L08.0
 SLAP S43.43-
 spinal cord G95.9
  congenital Q06.9
 spleen D73.89
 stomach K31.9
 superior glenoid labrum S43.43-
 syphilitic —*see* Syphilis
 tertiary —*see* Syphilis, tertiary
 thoracic root (nerve) NEC G54.3
 tonsillar fossa J35.9
 tooth, teeth K08.9
  white spot
   chewing surface K02.51
   pit and fissure surface K02.51
   smooth surface K02.61
 traumatic —*see* specific type of injury
  by site
 tricuspid (valve) I07.9
  nonrheumatic I36.9
 trigeminal nerve G50.9
 ulcerated or ulcerative —*see* Ulcer, skin
 uterus N85.9
 vagus nerve G52.2
 valvular —*see* Endocarditis
 vascular I99.9
  affecting central nervous system I67.9
  following trauma NEC T14.8
  umbilical cord, complicating delivery
   O69.5
 warty —*see* Verruca

Lesion (Continued)
  white spot (tooth)
    chewing surface K02.51
    pit and fissure surface K02.51
    smooth surface K02.61
Lethargic —see condition
Lethargy R53.83
Letterer-Siwe's disease C96.0
Leuc (o) —see Leuk (o)
Leukemia, leukemic C95.9-
  acute basophilic C94.8-
  acute bilineal C95.0-
  acute erythroid C94.0-
  acute lymphoblastic C91.0-
  acute megakaryoblastic C94.2-
  acute megakaryocytic C94.2-
  acute mixed lineage C95.0-
  acute monoblastic (monoblastic/monocytic)
    C93.0-
  acute monocytic (monoblastic/monocytic)
    C93.0-
  acute myeloblastic (minimal differentiation)
    (with maturation) C92.0-
  acute myeloid
    with
      11q23-abnormality C92.6-
      dysplasia of remaining hematopoesis
        and/or myelodysplastic disease in
        its history C92.A-
      multilineage dysplasia C92.A-
      variation of MLL-gene C92.6-
      M6 (a)(b) C94.0-
      M7 C94.2-
  acute myelomonocytic C92.5-
  acute promyelocytic C92.4-
  adult T-cell (HTLV-1-associated)
    (acute variant) (chronic variant)
    (lymphomatoid variant) (smouldering
    variant) C91.5-
  aggressive NK-cell C94.8-
  AML (1/ETO) (M0) (M1) (M2) (without a
    FAB classification) C92.0-
  AML M3 C92.4-
  AML M4 (Eo with inv(16) or t(16;16)) C92.5-
  AML M5 C93.0-
  AML M5a C93.0-
  AML M5b C93.0-
  AML Me with t (15;17) and variants C92.4-
  atypical chronic myeloid, BCR/ABL-negative
    C92.2-
  biphenotypic acute C95.0-
  blast cell C95.0-
  Burkitt-type, mature B-cell C91.A-
  chronic lymphocytic, of B-cell type C91.1-
  chronic monocytic C93.1-
  chronic myelogenous (Philadelphia
    chromosome (Ph1) positive) (t(9;22))
    (q34;q11) (with crisis of blast cells)
    C92.1-
  chronic myeloid, BCR/ABL-positive C92.1-
    atypical, BCR/ABL-negative C92.2-
  chronic myelomonocytic C93.1-
  chronic neutrophilic D47.1
  CMML (-1) (-2) (with eosinophilia) C93.1-
  granulocytic (see also Category C92) C92.9-
  hairy-cell C91.4-
  juvenile myelomonocytic C93.3-
  lymphoid C91.9-
    specified NEC C91.Z-
  mast cell C94.3-
  mature B-cell, Burkitt-type C91.A-
  monocytic (subacute) C93.9-
    specified NEC C93.Z-
  myelogenous (see also Category C92) C92.9-
  myeloid C92.9-
    specified NEC C92.Z-
  plasma cell C90.1-
  plasmacytic C90.1-
  prolymphocytic
    of B-cell type C91.3-
    of T-cell type C91.6-

Leukemia, leukemic (Continued)
  specified NEC C94.8-
  stem cell, of unclear lineage C95.0-
  subacute lymphocytic C91.9-
  T-cell large granular lymphocytic C91.Z-
  unspecified cell type C95.9-
    acute C95.0-
    chronic C95.1-
Leukemoid reaction (see also Reaction,
    leukemoid) D72.823- ◀▦
Leukoaraiosis (hypertensive) I67.81
Leukoariosis —see Leukoaraiosis
Leukocoria —see Disorder, globe, degenerated
    condition, leucocoria
Leukocytopenia D72.819
Leukocytosis D72.829
  eosinophilic D72.1
Leukoderma, leukodermia NEC L81.5
  syphilitic A51.39
    late A52.79
Leukodystrophy E75.29
Leukoedema, oral epithelium K13.29
Leukoencephalitis G04.81
  acute (subacute) hemorrhagic G36.1
    postimmunization or postvaccinal G04.02
  postinfectious G04.01
  subacute sclerosing A81.1
  van Bogaert's (sclerosing) A81.1
Leukoencephalopathy (see also
    Encephalopathy) G93.49
  Binswanger's I67.3
  heroin vapor G92
  metachromatic E75.25
  multifocal (progressive) A81.2
  postimmunization and postvaccinal G04.02
  progressive multifocal A81.2
  reversible, posterior G93.6
  van Bogaert's (sclerosing) A81.1
  vascular, progressive I67.3
Leukoerythroblastosis D75.9
Leukokeratosis —see also Leukoplakia
  mouth K13.21
  nicotina palati K13.24
  oral mucosa K13.21
  tongue K13.21
  vocal cord J38.3
Leukokraurosis vulva (e) N90.4
Leukoma (cornea) —see also Opacity, cornea
  adherent H17.0-
  interfering with central vision —see Opacity,
    cornea, central
Leukomalacia, cerebral, newborn P91.2
  periventricular P91.2
Leukomelanopathy, hereditary D72.0
Leukonychia (punctata) (striata) L60.8
  congenital Q84.4
Leukopathia unguium L60.8
  congenital Q84.4
Leukopenia D72.819
  basophilic D72.818
  chemotherapy (cancer) induced D70.1
  congenital D70.0
  cyclic D70.0
  drug induced NEC D70.2
    due to cytoreductive cancer chemotherapy
      D70.1
  eosinophilic D72.818
  familial D70.0
  infantile genetic D70.0
  malignant D70.9
  periodic D70.0
  transitory neonatal P61.5
Leukopenic —see condition
Leukoplakia
  anus K62.89
  bladder (postinfectional) N32.89
  buccal K13.21
  cervix (uteri) N88.0
  esophagus K22.8
  gingiva K13.21
  hairy (oral mucosa) (tongue) K13.3

Leukoplakia (Continued)
  kidney (pelvis) N28.89
  larynx J38.7
  lip K13.21
  mouth K13.21
  oral epithelium, including tongue (mucosa)
    K13.21
  palate K13.21
  pelvis (kidney) N28.89
  penis (infectional) N48.0
  rectum K62.89
  syphilitic (late) A52.79
  tongue K13.21
  ureter (postinfectional) N28.89
  urethra (postinfectional) N36.8
  uterus N85.8
  vagina N89.4
  vocal cord J38.3
  vulva N90.4
Leukorrhea N89.8
  due to Trichomonas (vaginalis)
    A59.00
  trichomonal A59.00
Leukosarcoma C85.9
Levocardia (isolated) Q24.1
  with situs inversus Q89.3
Levotransposition Q20.5
Lev's disease or syndrome (acquired complete
    heart block) I44.2
Levulosuria —see Fructosuria
Levurid L30.2
Lewy body (ies) (dementia) (disease)
    G31.83
Leyden-Moebius dystrophy G71.0
Leydig cell
  carcinoma
    specified site —see Neoplasm, malignant,
      by site
    unspecified site
      female C56.9-
      male C62.9-
  tumor
    benign
      specified site —see Neoplasm, benign,
        by site
      unspecified site
        female D27.-
        male D29.2-
    malignant
      specified site —see Neoplasm,
        malignant, by site
      unspecified site
        female C56.-
        male C62.9-
    specified site —see Neoplasm, uncertain
      behavior, by site
    unspecified site
      female D39.1-
      male D40.1-
Leydig-Sertoli cell tumor
  specified site —see Neoplasm, benign,
    by site
  unspecified site
    female D27.-
    male D29.2-
LGSIL (Low grade squamous intraepithelial
    lesion on cytologic smear of)
  anus R85.612
  cervix R87.612
  vagina R87.622
Liar, pathologic F60.2
Libido
  decreased R68.82
Libman-Sacks disease M32.11
Lice (infestation) B85.2
  body (Pediculus corporis) B85.1
  crab B85.3
  head (Pediculus capitis) B85.0
  mixed (classifiable to more than one of the
    titles B85.0-B85.3) B85.4
  pubic (Phthirus pubis) B85.3

Lichen L28.0
albus L90.0
  penis N48.0
  vulva N90.4
amyloidosis E85.4 [L99]
atrophicus L90.0
  penis N48.0
  vulva N90.4
congenital Q82.8
myxedematosus L98.5
nitidus L44.1
pilaris Q82.8
  acquired L85.8
planopilaris L66.1
planus (chronicus) L43.9
  annularis L43.8
  bullous L43.1
  follicular L66.1
  hypertrophic L43.0
  moniliformis L44.3
  of Wilson L43.9
  specified NEC L43.8
  subacute (active) L43.3
  tropicus L43.3
ruber
  acuminatus L44.0
  moniliformis L44.3
  planus L43.9
sclerosus (et atrophicus) L90.0
  penis N48.0
  vulva N90.4
scrofulosus (primary) (tuberculous) A18.4
simplex (chronicus) (circumscriptus) L28.0
striatus L44.2
urticatus L28.2
Lichenification L28.0
Lichenoides tuberculosis (primary) A18.4
Lichtheim's disease or syndrome —see
    Degeneration, combined
Lien migrans D73.89
Ligament —see condition
Light
for gestational age —see Light for dates
headedness R42
Light-for-dates (infant) P05.00
with weight of
  499 grams or less P05.01
  500-749 grams P05.02
  750-999 grams P05.03
  1000-1249 grams P05.04
  1250-1499 grams P05.05
  1500-1749 grams P05.06
  1750-1999 grams P05.07
  2000-2499 grams P05.08
affecting management of pregnancy O36.59-
and small-for-dates —see Small for dates
Lightning (effects) (stroke) (struck by) T75.00
burn —see Burn
foot E53.8
shock T75.01
specified effect NEC T75.09
Lightwood-Albright syndrome N25.89
Lightwood's disease or syndrome (renal
    tubular acidosis) N25.89
Lignac (-de Toni) (-Fanconi) (-Debré) disease or
    syndrome E72.09
with cystinosis E72.04
Ligneous thyroiditis E06.5
Likoff's syndrome I20.8
Limb —see condition
Limbic epilepsy personality syndrome F07.0
Limitation, limited
activities due to disability Z73.6
cardiac reserve —see Disease, heart
eye muscle duction, traumatic —see
    Strabismus, mechanical
mandibular range of motion M26.52
Lindau (-von Hippel) disease Q85.8
Line (s)
Beau's L60.4
Harris' —see Arrest, epiphyseal

Line (Continued)
Hudson's (cornea) —see Pigmentation,
    cornea, anterior
Stähli's (cornea) —see Pigmentation, cornea,
    anterior
Linea corneae senilis —see Change, cornea,
    senile
Lingua
geographica K14.1
nigra (villosa) K14.3
plicata K14.5
tylosis K13.29
Lingual —see condition
Linguatulosis B88.8
Linitis (gastric) plastica C16.9
Lip —see condition
Lipedema —see Edema
Lipemia —see also Hyperlipidemia
retina, retinalis E78.3
Lipidosis E75.6
cerebral (infantile) (juvenile) (late) E75.4
cerebroretinal E75.4
cerebroside E75.22
cholesterol (cerebral) E75.5
glycolipid E75.21
hepatosplenomegalic E78.3
sphingomyelin —see Niemann-Pick disease
    or syndrome
sulfatide E75.29
Lipoadenoma —see Neoplasm, benign,
    by site
Lipoblastoma —see Lipoma
Lipoblastomatosis —see Lipoma
Lipochondrodystrophy E76.01
Lipochrome histiocytosis (familial) D71
Lipodermatosclerosis —see Varix, leg, with,
    inflammation
ulcerated —see Varix, leg, with, ulcer, with
    inflammation by site
Lipodystrophia progressiva E88.1
Lipodystrophy (progressive) E88.1
insulin E88.1
intestinal K90.81
mesenteric K65.4
Lipofibroma —see Lipoma
Lipofuscinosis, neuronal (with ceroidosis)
    E75.4
Lipogranuloma, sclerosing L92.8
Lipogranulomatosis E78.89
Lipoid —see also condition
histiocytosis D76.3
  essential E75.29
nephrosis N04.9
proteinosis of Urbach E78.89
Lipoidemia —see Hyperlipidemia
Lipoidosis —see Lipidosis
Lipoma D17.9
fetal D17.9
fat cell D17.9
infiltrating D17.9
intramuscular D17.9
pleomorphic D17.9
site classification
  arms (skin) (subcutaneous) D17.2-
  connective tissue D17.30
    intra-abdominal D17.5
    intrathoracic D17.4
    peritoneum D17.79
    retroperitoneum D17.79
    specified site NEC D17.39
    spermatic cord D17.6
  face (skin) (subcutaneous) D17.0
  genitourinary organ NEC D17.72
  head (skin) (subcutaneous) D17.0
  intra-abdominal D17.5
  intrathoracic D17.4
  kidney D17.71
  legs (skin) (subcutaneous) D17.2-
  neck (skin) (subcutaneous) D17.0
  peritoneum D17.79
  retroperitoneum D17.79

Lipoma (Continued)
site classification (Continued)
  skin D17.30
    specified site NEC D17.39
  specified site NEC D17.79
  spermatic cord D17.6
  subcutaneous D17.30
    specified site NEC D17.39
  trunk (skin) (subcutaneous) D17.1
  unspecified D17.9
spindle cell D17.9
Lipomatosis E88.2
dolorosa (Dercum) E88.2
fetal —see Lipoma
Launois-Bensaude E88.89
Lipomyoma —see Lipoma
Lipomyxoma —see Lipoma
Lipomyxosarcoma —see Neoplasm, connective
    tissue, malignant
Lipoprotein metabolism disorder E78.9
Lipoproteinemia E78.5
broad-beta E78.2
floating-beta E78.2
hyper-pre-beta E78.1
Liposarcoma —see also Neoplasm, connective
    tissue, malignant
dedifferentiated —see Neoplasm, connective
    tissue, malignant
differentiated type —see Neoplasm,
    connective tissue, malignant
embryonal —see Neoplasm, connective tissue,
    malignant
mixed type —see Neoplasm, connective
    tissue, malignant
myxoid —see Neoplasm, connective tissue,
    malignant
pleomorphic —see Neoplasm, connective
    tissue, malignant
round cell —see Neoplasm, connective tissue,
    malignant
well differentiated type —see Neoplasm,
    connective tissue, malignant
Liposynovitis prepatellaris E88.89
Lipping, cervix N86
Lipschütz disease or ulcer N76.6
Lipuria R82.0
schistosomiasis (bilharziasis) B65.0
Lisping F80.0
Lissauer's paralysis A52.17
Lissencephalia, lissencephaly Q04.3
Listeriosis, listerellosis A32.9
congenital (disseminated) P37.2
cutaneous A32.0
neonatal, newborn (disseminated) P37.2
oculoglandular A32.81
specified NEC A32.89
Lithemia E79.0
Lithiasis —see Calculus
Lithosis J62.8
Lithuria R82.99
Litigation, anxiety concerning Z65.3
Little leaguer's elbow —see Epicondylitis,
    medial
Little's disease G80.9
Littre's
gland —see condition
hernia —see Hernia, abdomen
Littritis —see Urethritis
Livedo (annularis) (racemosa) (reticularis) R23.1
Liver —see condition
Living alone (problems with) Z60.2
with handicapped person Z74.2
Lloyd's syndrome —see Adenomatosis,
    endocrine
Loa loa, loaiasis, loasis B74.3
Lobar —see condition
Lobomycosis B48.0
Lobo's disease B48.0
Lobotomy syndrome F07.0
Lobstein (-Ekman) disease or syndrome Q78.0
Lobster-claw hand Q71.6-

◀ New ◀ Revised ~~deleted~~ Deleted

Lobulation (congenital) —see also Anomaly,
    by site
  kidney, Q63.1
  liver, abnormal Q44.7
  spleen Q89.09
Lobule, lobular —see condition
Local, localized —see condition
Locked twins causing obstructed labor
    O66.1
Locked-in state G83.5
Locking
  joint —see Derangement, joint, specified type
    NEC
    knee —see Derangement, knee
Lockjaw —see Tetanus
Löffler's
  endocarditis I42.3
  eosinophilia J82
  pneumonia J82
  syndrome (eosinophilic pneumonitis) J82
Loiasis (with conjunctival infestation) (eyelid)
    B74.3
Lone Star fever A77.0
Long
  labor O63.9
    first stage O63.0
    second stage O63.1
  QT syndrome I45.81
Long-term (current) (prophylactic) drug
    therapy (use of)
  agents affecting estrogen receptors and
    estrogen levels NEC Z79.818
  anastrozole (Arimidex) Z79.811
  antibiotics Z79.2
    short-term use - omit code
  anticoagulants Z79.01
  anti-inflammatory, non-steroidal (NSAID)
    Z79.1
  antiplatelet Z79.02
  antithrombotics Z79.02
  aromatase inhibitors Z79.811
  aspirin Z79.82
  birth control pill or patch Z79.3
  bisphosphonates Z79.83
  contraceptive, oral Z79.3
  drug, specified NEC Z79.899
  estrogen receptor downregulators Z79.818
  Evista Z79.810
  exemestane (Aromasin) Z79.811
  Fareston Z79.810
  fulvestrant (Faslodex) Z79.818
  gonadotropin-releasing hormone (GnRH)
    agonist Z79.818
  goserelin acetate (Zoladex) Z79.818
  hormone replacement (postmenopausal)
    Z79.890
  insulin Z79.4
  letrozole (Femara) Z79.811
  leuprolide acetate (leuprorelin) (Lupron)
    Z79.818
  megestrol acetate (Megace) Z79.818
  methadone for pain management Z79.891
  Nolvadex Z79.810
  non-steroidal anti-inflammatories (NSAID)
    Z79.1
  opiate analgesic Z79.891
  oral contraceptive Z79.3
  raloxifene (Evista) Z79.810
  selective estrogen receptor modulators
    (SERMs) Z79.810
  steroids
    inhaled Z79.51
    systemic Z79.52
  tamoxifen (Nolvadex) Z79.810
  toremifene (Fareston) Z79.810
Longitudinal stripes or grooves, nails
    L60.8
  congenital Q84.6
Loop
  intestine —see Volvulus
  vascular on papilla (optic) Q14.2

Loose —see also condition
  body
    joint M24.00
      ankle M24.07-
      elbow M24.02-
      hand M24.04-
      hip M24.05-
      knee M23.4-
      shoulder (region) M24.01-
      specified site NEC M24.08
      toe M24.07-
      vertebra M24.08
      wrist M24.03-
    knee M23.4-
    sheath, tendon —see Disorder, tendon,
      specified type NEC
  cartilage —see Loose, body, joint
  tooth, teeth K08.8
Loosening
  aseptic
    joint prosthesis —see Complications, joint
      prosthesis, mechanical, loosening,
      by site
    epiphysis —see Osteochondropathy
  mechanical
    joint prosthesis —see Complications, joint
      prosthesis, mechanical, loosening,
      by site
Looser-Milkman (-Debray) syndrome M83.8
Lop ear (deformity) Q17.3
Lorain (-Levi) short stature syndrome E23.0
Lordosis M40.50
  acquired —see Lordosis, specified type
    NEC
  congenital Q76.429
    lumbar region Q76.426
    lumbosacral region Q76.427
    sacral region Q76.428
    sacrococcygeal region Q76.428
    thoracolumbar region Q76.425
  lumbar region M40.56
  lumbosacral region M40.57
  postsurgical M96.4
  postural —see Lordosis, specified type NEC
  rachitic (late effect) (sequelae) E64.3
  sequelae of rickets E64.3
  specified type NEC M40.40
    lumbar region M40.46
    lumbosacral region M40.47
    thoracolumbar region M40.45
  thoracolumbar region M40.55
  tuberculous A18.01
Loss (of)
  appetite (see Anorexia) R63.0
    hysterical F50.8
    nonorganic origin F50.8
    psychogenic F50.8
  blood —see Hemorrhage
  consciousness, transient R55
    traumatic —see Injury, intracranial
  control, sphincter, rectum R15.9
    nonorganic origin F98.1
  elasticity, skin R23.4
  family (member) in childhood Z62.898
  fluid (acute) E86.9
    with
      hypernatremia E87.0
      hyponatremia E87.1
  function of labyrinth —see subcategory
    H83.2
  hair, nonscarring —see Alopecia
  hearing —see also Deafness
    central NOS H90.5
    neural NOS H90.5
    perceptive NOS H90.5
    sensorineural NOS H90.5
    sensory NOS H90.5
  height R29.890
  limb or member, traumatic, current —see
    Amputation, traumatic
  love relationship in childhood Z62.898

Loss (Continued)
  memory —see also Amnesia
    mild, following organic brain damage
      F06.8
  mind —see Psychosis
  occlusal vertical dimension of fully erupted
    teeth M26.37
  organ or part —see Absence, by site, acquired
  ossicles, ear (partial) H74.32-
  parent in childhood Z63.4
  pregnancy, recurrent N96
    without current pregnancy N96
    care in current pregnancy O26.2-
  recurrent pregnancy —see Loss, pregnancy,
    recurrent
  self-esteem, in childhood Z62.898
  sense of
    smell —see Disturbance, sensation, smell
    taste —see Disturbance, sensation, taste
    touch R20.8
  sensory R44.9
    dissociative F44.6
  sexual desire F52.0
  sight (acquired) (complete) (congenital) —see
    Blindness
  substance of
    bone —see Disorder, bone, density and
      structure, specified NEC
    cartilage —see Disorder, cartilage, specified
      type NEC
    auricle (ear) —see Disorder, pinna,
      specified type NEC
    vitreous (humor) H15.89
  tooth, teeth —see Absence, teeth, acquired
  vision, visual H54.7
    both eyes H54.3
    one eye H54.60
      left (normal vision on right) H54.62
      right (normal vision on left) H54.61
    specified as blindness —see Blindness
    subjective
      sudden H53.13-
      transient H53.12-
  vitreous —see Prolapse, vitreous
  voice —see Aphonia
  weight (abnormal) (cause unknown) R63.4
Louis-Bar syndrome (ataxia-telangiectasia)
    G11.3
Louping ill (encephalitis) A84.8
Louse, lousiness —see Lice
Low
  achiever, school Z55.3
  back syndrome M54.5
  basal metabolic rate R94.8
  birthweight (2499 grams or less) P07.10
    with weight of
      1000-1249 grams P07.14
      1250-1499 grams P07.15
      1500-1749 grams P07.16
      1750-1999 grams P07.17
      2000-2499 grams P07.18
    extreme (999 grams or less) P07.00
      with weight of
        499 grams or less P07.01
        500-749 grams P07.02
        750-999 grams P07.03
    for gestational age —see Light for dates
  blood pressure —see also Hypotension
    reading (incidental) (isolated) (nonspecific)
      R03.1
  cardiac reserve —see Disease, heart
  function —see also Hypofunction
    kidney N28.9
  hematocrit D64.9
  hemoglobin D64.9
  income Z59.6
  level of literacy Z55.0
  lying
    kidney N28.89
    organ or site, congenital —see Malposition,
      congenital

Low (*Continued*)
  output syndrome (cardiac) —*see* Failure,
      heart
  platelets (blood) —*see* Thrombocytopenia
  reserve, kidney N28.89
  salt syndrome E87.1
  self esteem R45.81
  set ears Q17.4
  vision H54.2
      one eye (other eye normal) H54.50
          left (normal vision on right) H54.52
          other eye blind —*see* Blindness
          right (normal vision on left) H54.51
Low-density-lipoprotein-type (LDL)
      hyperlipoproteinemia E78.0
Lowe's syndrome E72.03
Lown-Ganong-Levine syndrome I45.6
LSD reaction (acute) (without dependence)
      F16.90
  with dependence F16.20
L-shaped kidney Q63.8
Ludwig's angina or disease K12.2
Lues (venerea), luetic —*see* Syphilis
Luetscher's syndrome (dehydration) E86.0
Lumbago, lumbalgia M54.5
  with sciatica M54.4-
      due to intervertebral disc disorder M51.17
  due to displacement, intervertebral disc
      M51.27
      with sciatica M51.17
Lumbar —*see* condition
Lumbarization, vertebra, congenital Q76.49
Lumbermen's itch B88.0
Lump —*see* Mass
Lunacy —*see* Psychosis
Lung —*see* condition
Lupoid (miliary) of Boeck D86.3
Lupus
  anticoagulant D68.62
      with
          hemorrhagic disorder D68.312
          hypercoagulable state D68.62
      finding without diagnosis R76.0
  discoid (local) L93.0
  erythematosus (discoid) (local) L93.0
      disseminated —*see* Lupus, erythematosus,
          systemic
      eyelid H01.129
          left H01.126
              lower H01.125
              upper H01.124
          right H01.123
              lower H01.122
              upper H01.121
      profundus L93.2
      specified NEC L93.2
      subacute cutaneous L93.1
      systemic M32.9
          with organ or system involvement M32.10
              endocarditis M32.11
              lung M32.13
              pericarditis M32.12
              renal (glomerular) M32.14
                  tubulo-interstitial M32.15
              specified organ or system NEC
                  M32.19
          drug-induced M32.0
          inhibitor (presence of) D68.62
              with
                  hemorrhagic disorder D68.312
                  hypercoagulable state D68.62
              finding without diagnosis R76.0
          specified NEC M32.8
  exedens A18.4
  hydralazine M32.0
      correct substance properly administered —
          see Table of Drugs and Chemicals,
          by drug, adverse effect ◀▥
      overdose or wrong substance given or
          taken —*see* Table of Drugs and
          Chemicals, by drug, poisoning ◀▥

Lupus (*Continued*)
  nephritis (chronic) M32.14
  nontuberculous, not disseminated L93.0
  panniculitis L93.2
  pernio (Besnier) D86.3
  systemic —*see* Lupus, erythematosus,
      systemic
  tuberculous A18.4
      eyelid A18.4
  vulgaris A18.4
      eyelid A18.4
Luteinoma D27.-
Lutembacher's disease or syndrome (atrial
      septal defect with mitral stenosis) Q21.1
Luteoma D27.-
Lutz (-Splendore-de Almeida) **disease** —*see*
      Paracoccidioidomycosis
Luxation —*see also* Dislocation
  eyeball (nontraumatic) —*see* Luxation, globe
      birth injury P15.3
  globe, nontraumatic H44.82-
  lacrimal gland —*see* Dislocation, lacrimal
      gland
  lens (old) (partial) (spontaneous)
      congenital Q12.1
      syphilitic A50.39
Lycanthropy F22
Lyell's syndrome L51.2
  due to drug L51.2
      correct substance properly administered —
          see Table of Drugs and Chemicals,
          by drug, adverse effect ◀▥
      overdose or wrong substance given or
          taken —*see* Table of Drugs and
          Chemicals, by drug, poisoning ◀▥
Lyme disease A69.20
Lymph
  gland or node —*see* condition
  scrotum —*see* Infestation, filarial
Lymphadenitis I88.9
  with ectopic or molar pregnancy O08.0
  acute L04.9
      axilla L04.2
      face L04.0
      head L04.0
      hip L04.3
      limb
          lower L04.3
          upper L04.2
      neck L04.0
      shoulder L04.2
      specified site NEC L04.8
      trunk L04.1
  anthracosis (occupational) J60
  any site, except mesenteric I88.9
      chronic I88.1
      subacute I88.1
  breast
      gestational —*see* Mastitis, obstetric
      puerperal, postpartum (nonpurulent)
          O91.22
  chancroidal (congenital) A57
  chronic I88.1
      mesenteric I88.0
  due to
      Brugia (malayi) B74.1
          timori B74.2
      chlamydial lymphogranuloma A55
      diphtheria (toxin) A36.89
      lymphogranuloma venereum A55
      Wuchereria bancrofti B74.0
  following ectopic or molar pregnancy O08.0
  gonorrheal A54.89
  infective —*see* Lymphadenitis, acute
  mesenteric (acute) (chronic) (nonspecific)
      (subacute) I88.0
      due to Salmonella typhi A01.09
      tuberculous A18.39
  mycobacterial A31.8
  purulent —*see* Lymphadenitis, acute
  pyogenic —*see* Lymphadenitis, acute

Lymphadenitis (*Continued*)
  regional, nonbacterial I88.8
  septic —*see* Lymphadenitis, acute
  subacute, unspecified site I88.1
  suppurative —*see* Lymphadenitis, acute
  syphilitic (early) (secondary) A51.49
      late A52.79
  tuberculous —*see* Tuberculosis, lymph gland
  venereal (chlamydial) A55
Lymphadenoid goiter E06.3
Lymphadenopathy (generalized) R59.1
  angioimmunoblastic, with dysproteinemia
      (AILD) C86.5
  due to toxoplasmosis (acquired) B58.89
      congenital (acute) (subacute) (chronic)
          P37.1
  localized R59.0
  syphilitic (early) (secondary) A51.49
Lymphadenosis R59.1
Lymphangiectasis I89.0
  conjunctiva H11.89
  postinfectional I89.0
  scrotum I89.0
Lymphangiectatic elephantiasis, nonfilarial
      I89.0
Lymphangioendothelioma D18.1
  malignant —*see* Neoplasm, connective tissue,
      malignant
Lymphangioleiomyomatosis J84.81
Lymphangioma D18.1
  capillary D18.1
  cavernous D18.1
  cystic D18.1
  malignant —*see* Neoplasm, connective tissue,
      malignant
Lymphangiomyoma D18.1
Lymphangiomyomatosis J84.81
Lymphangiosarcoma —*see* Neoplasm,
      connective tissue, malignant
Lymphangitis I89.1
  with
      abscess - code by site under Abscess
      cellulitis - code by site under Cellulitis
      ectopic or molar pregnancy O08.0
  acute L03.91
      abdominal wall L03.321
      ankle —*see* Lymphangitis, acute, lower
          limb
      arm —*see* Lymphangitis, acute, upper limb
      auricle (ear) —*see* Lymphangitis, acute, ear
      axilla L03.12-
      back (any part) L03.322
      buttock L03.327
      cervical (meaning neck) L03.222
      cheek (external) L03.212
      chest wall L03.323
      digit
          finger —*see* Lymphangitis, acute, finger
          toe —*see* Lymphangitis, acute, toe
      ear (external) H60.1-
      external auditory canal —*see*
          Lymphangitis, acute, ear
      eyelid —*see* Abscess, eyelid
      face NEC L03.212
      finger (intrathecal) (periosteal)
          (subcutaneous) (subcuticular) L03.02-
      foot —*see* Lymphangitis, acute, lower limb
      gluteal (region) L03.327
      groin L03.324
      hand —*see* Lymphangitis, acute, upper
          limb
      head NEC L03.891
          face (any part, except ear, eye and nose)
              L03.212
      heel —*see* Lymphangitis, acute, lower limb
      hip —*see* Lymphangitis, acute, lower limb
      jaw (region) L03.212
      knee —*see* Lymphangitis, acute, lower limb
      leg —*see* Lymphangitis, acute, lower limb
      lower limb L03.12-
          toe —*see* Lymphangitis, acute, toe

Lymphangitis *(Continued)*
  acute *(Continued)*
    navel L03.326
    neck (region) L03.222
    orbit, orbital —*see* Cellulitis, orbit
    pectoral (region) L03.323
    perineal, perineum L03.325
    scalp (any part) L03.891
    shoulder —*see* Lymphangitis, acute, upper
      limb
    specified site NEC L03.898
    thigh —*see* Lymphangitis, acute, lower
      limb
    thumb (intrathecal) (periosteal)
      (subcutaneous) (subcuticular) —*see*
      Lymphangitis, acute, finger
    toe (intrathecal) (periosteal) (subcutaneous)
      (subcuticular) L03.04-
    trunk L03.329
      abdominal wall L03.321
      back (any part) L03.322
      buttock L03.327
      chest wall L03.323
      groin L03.324
      perineal, perineum L03.325
      umbilicus L03.326
    umbilicus L03.326
    upper limb L03.12-
      axilla —*see* Lymphangitis, acute, axilla
      finger —*see* Lymphangitis, acute, finger
      thumb —*see* Lymphangitis, acute, finger
      wrist —*see* Lymphangitis, acute, upper
        limb
  breast
    gestational —*see* Mastitis, obstetric
  chancroidal A57
  chronic (any site) I89.1
  due to
    Brugia (malayi) B74.1
      timori B74.2
    Wuchereria bancrofti B74.0
  following ectopic or molar pregnancy O08.89
  penis
    acute N48.29
    gonococcal (acute) (chronic) A54.09
  puerperal, postpartum, childbirth O86.89
  strumous, tuberculous A18.2
  subacute (any site) I89.1
  tuberculous —*see* Tuberculosis, lymph gland
Lymphatic (vessel) —*see* condition
Lymphatism E32.8
Lymphectasia I89.0
Lymphedema (acquired) —*see also* Elephantiasis
  congenital Q82.0
  hereditary (chronic) (idiopathic) Q82.0
  postmastectomy I97.2
  praecox I89.0
  secondary I89.0
  surgical NEC I97.89
    postmastectomy (syndrome) I97.2
Lymphoblastic —*see* condition
Lymphoblastoma (diffuse) —*see* Lymphoma,
    lymphoblastic (diffuse)
  giant follicular —*see* Lymphoma,
    lymphoblastic (diffuse)
  macrofollicular —*see* Lymphoma,
    lymphoblastic (diffuse)
Lymphocele I89.8
Lymphocytic
  chorioencephalitis (acute) (serous) A87.2
  choriomeningitis (acute) (serous) A87.2
  meningoencephalitis A87.2

Lymphocytoma, benign cutis L98.8
Lymphocytopenia D72.810
Lymphocytosis (symptomatic)
    D72.820
  infectious (acute) B33.8
Lymphoepithelioma —*see* Neoplasm,
    malignant, by site
Lymphogranuloma (malignant) —*see also*
    Lymphoma, Hodgkin
  chlamydial A55
  inguinale A55
  venereum (any site) (chlamydial) (with
    stricture of rectum) A55
Lymphogranulomatosis (malignant) —*see also*
    Lymphoma, Hodgkin
  benign (Boeck's sarcoid) (Schaumann's)
    D86.1
Lymphohistiocytosis, hemophagocytic
    (familial) D76.1
Lymphoid —*see* condition
Lymphoma (of) (malignant) C85.90
  adult T-cell (HTLV-1-associated)
      (acute variant) (chronic variant)
      (lymphomatoid variant) (smouldering
      variant) C91.5-
  anaplastic large cell
    ALK-negative C84.7-
    ALK-positive C84.6-
    CD30-positive C84.6-
    primary cutaneous C86.6
  angioimmunoblastic T-cell C86.5
  BALT C88.4
  B-cell C85.1-
  B-precursor C83.5-
  blastic NK-cell C86.4
  bronchial-associated lymphoid tissue
    [BALT-lymphoma] C88.4
  Burkitt (atypical) C83.7-
  Burkitt-like C83.7-
  centrocytic C83.1-
  cutaneous follicle center C82.6-
  cutaneous T-cell C84.A-
  diffuse follicle center C82.5-
  diffuse large cell C83.3-
    anaplastic C83.3-
    B-cell C83.3-
    CD30-positive C83.3-
    centroblastic C83.3-
    immunoblastic C83.3-
    plasmablastic C83.3-
    subtype not specified C83.3-
    T-cell rich C83.3-
  enteropathy-type (associated) (intestinal)
    T-cell C86.2
  extranodal marginal zone B-cell
    lymphoma of mucosa-associated
    lymphoid tissue [MALT-lymphoma]
    C88.4
  extranodal NK/T-cell, nasal type
    C86.0
  follicular C82.9-
    grade
      I C82.0-
      II C82.1-
      III C82.2-
      IIIa C82.3-
      IIIb C82.4-
    specified NEC C82.8-
  hepatosplenic T-cell (alpha-beta)
    (gamma-delta) C86.1
  histiocytic C85.9-
    true C96.A

Lymphoma *(Continued)*
  Hodgkin C81.9
    classical C81.7-
      lymphocyte-rich C81.4-
      lymphocytic depletion C81.3-
      mixed cellularity C81.2-
      nodular sclerosis C81.1-
      specified NEC C81.7-
    lymphocyte-rich classical C81.4-
    lymphocyte depleted classical C81.3-
    mixed cellularity classical C81.2-
    nodular
      lymphocyte predominant C81.0-
      sclerosis classical C81.1-
  intravascular large B-cell C83.8-
  Lennert's C84.4-
  lymphoblastic (diffuse) C83.5-
  lymphoblastic B-cell C83.5-
  lymphoblastic T-cell C83.5-
  lymphoepithelioid C84.4-
  lymphoplasmacytic C83.0-
    with IgM-production C88.0
  MALT C88.4
  mantle cell C83.1-
  mature T-cell NEC C84.4-
  mature T/NK-cell C84.9-
    specified NEC C84.Z-
  mediastinal (thymic) large B-cell
    C85.2-
  Mediterranean C88.3
  mucosa-associated lymphoid tissue
    [MALT-lymphoma] C88.4
  NK/T cell C84.9-
  nodal marginal zone C83.0-
  non-follicular (diffuse) C83.9-
    specified NEC C83.8-
  non-Hodgkin (*see also* Lymphoma, by type)
    C85.9-
    specified NEC C85.8-
  non-leukemic variant of B-CLL C83.0-
  peripheral T-cell, not classified C84.4-
  primary cutaneous
    anaplastic large cell C86.6
    CD30-positive large T-cell C86.6
  primary effusion B-cell C83.8-
  SALT C88.4
  skin-associated lymphoid tissue [SALT-
    lymphoma] C88.4
  small cell B-cell C83.0-
  splenic marginal zone C83.0-
  subcutaneous panniculitis-like T-cell
    C86.3
  T-precursor C83.5-
  true histiocytic C96.A
Lymphomatosis —*see* Lymphoma
Lymphopathia venereum, veneris A55
Lymphopenia D72.810
Lymphoplasmacytic leukemia —*see* Leukemia,
    chronic lymphocytic, B-cell type
Lymphoproliferation, X-linked disease
    D82.3
Lymphoreticulosis, benign (of inoculation)
    A28.1
Lymphorrhea I89.8
Lymphosarcoma (diffuse) (*see also* Lymphoma)
    C85.9-
Lymphostasis I89.8
Lypemania —*see* Melancholia
Lysine and hydroxylysine metabolism
    disorder E72.3
Lyssa —*see* Rabies

M

Macacus ear Q17.3
Maceration, wet feet, tropical (syndrome) T69.02-
MacLeod's syndrome J43.0
Macrocephalia, macrocephaly Q75.3
Macrocheilia, macrochilia (congenital)Q18.6
Macrocolon (see also Megacolon) Q43.1
Macrocornea Q15.8
  with glaucoma Q15.0
Macrocytic —see condition
Macrocytosis D75.89
Macrodactylia, macrodactylism (fingers) (thumbs) Q74.0
  toes Q74.2
Macrodontia K00.2
Macrogenia M26.05
Macrogenitosomia (adrenal) (male) (praecox) E25.9
  congenital E25.0
Macroglobulinemia (idiopathic) (primary) C88.0
  monoclonal (essential) D47.2
  Waldenström C88.0
Macroglossia (congenital) Q38.2
  acquired K14.8
Macrognathia, macrognathism (congenital) (mandibular) (maxillary) M26.09
Macrogyria (congenital) Q04.8
Macrohydrocephalus —see Hydrocephalus
Macromastia —see Hypertrophy, breast
Macrophthalmos Q11.3
  in congenital glaucoma Q15.0
Macropsia H53.15
Macrosigmoid K59.3
  congenital Q43.2
Macrospondylitis, acromegalic E22.0
Macrostomia (congenital) Q18.4
Macrotia (external ear) (congenital) Q17.1
Macula
  cornea, corneal —see Opacity, cornea
  degeneration (atrophic) (exudative) (senile) —see also Degeneration, macula
    hereditary —see Dystrophy, retina
Maculae ceruleae — B85.1
Maculopathy, toxic —see Degeneration, macula, toxic
Madarosis (eyelid) H02.729
  left H02.726
    lower H02.725
    upper H02.724
  right H02.723
    lower H02.722
    upper H02.721
Madelung's
  deformity (radius) Q74.0
  disease
    radial deformity Q74.0
    symmetrical lipomas, neck E88.89
Madness —see Psychosis
Madura
  foot B47.9
    actinomycotic B47.1
    mycotic B47.0
Maduromycosis B47.0
Maffucci's syndrome Q78.4
Magnesium metabolism disorder —see Disorder, metabolism, magnesium
Main en griffe (acquired) —see also Deformity, limb, clawhand
  congenital Q74.0
Maintenance (encounter for)
  antineoplastic chemotherapy Z51.11
  antineoplastic radiation therapy Z51.0
  methadone F11.20
Majocchi's
  disease L81.7
  granuloma B35.8
Major —see condition
Malabar itch (any site) B35.5

Malabsorption K90.9
  calcium K90.89
  carbohydrate K90.4
  disaccharide E73.9
  fat K90.4
  galactose E74.20
  glucose(-galactose) E74.39
  intestinal K90.9
    specified NEC K90.89
  isomaltose E74.31
  lactose E73.9
  methionine E72.19
  monosaccharide E74.39
  postgastrectomy K91.2
  postsurgical K91.2
  protein K90.4
  starch K90.4
  sucrose E74.39
  syndrome K90.9
    postsurgical K91.2
Malacia, bone (adult) M83.9
  juvenile —see Rickets
Malacoplakia
  bladder N32.89
  pelvis (kidney) N28.89
  ureter N28.89
  urethra N36.8
Malacosteon, juvenile —see Rickets
Maladaptation —see Maladjustment
Maladie de Roger Q21.0
Maladjustment
  conjugal Z63.0
    involving divorce or estrangement Z63.5
  educational Z55.4
  family Z63.9
  marital Z63.0
    involving divorce or estrangement Z63.5
  occupational NEC Z56.89
  simple, adult —see Disorder, adjustment
  situational —see Disorder, adjustment
  social Z60.9
    due to
      acculturation difficulty Z60.3
      discrimination and persecution (perceived) Z60.5
      exclusion and isolation Z60.4
      life-cycle (phase of life) transition Z60.0
      rejection Z60.4
      specified reason NEC Z60.8
Malaise R53.81
Malakoplakia —see Malacoplakia
Malaria, malarial (fever) B54
  with
    blackwater fever B50.8
      hemoglobinuric (bilious) B50.8
    hemoglobinuria B50.8
  accidentally induced (therapeutically) - code by type under Malaria
  algid B50.9
  cerebral B50.0 [G94]
  clinically diagnosed (without parasitological confirmation) B54
  congenital NEC P37.4
    falciparum P37.3
  congestion, congestive B54
  continued (fever) B50.9
  estivo-autumnal B50.9
  falciparum B50.9
    with complications NEC B50.8
      cerebral B50.0 [G94]
    severe B50.8
  hemorrhagic B54
  malariae B52.9
    with
      complications NEC B52.8
      glomerular disorder B52.0
  malignant (tertian) —see Malaria, falciparum
  mixed infections — code to first listed type in B50-B53
  ovale B53.0
  parasitologically confirmed NEC B53.8

Malaria, malarial (Continued)
  pernicious, acute —see Malaria, falciparum
  Plasmodium (P.)
    falciparum NEC —see Malaria, falciparum
    malariae NEC B52.9
      with Plasmodium
        falciparum (and or vivax) —see Malaria, falciparum
        vivax —see also Malaria, vivax
          and falciparum —see Malaria, falciparum
    ovale B53.0
      with Plasmodium malariae —see also Malaria, malariae
        and vivax —see also Malaria, vivax
          and falciparum —see Malaria, falciparum
    simian B53.1
      with Plasmodium malariae —see also Malaria, malariae
        and vivax —see also Malaria, vivax
          and falciparum —see Malaria, falciparum
    vivax NEC B51.9
      with Plasmodium falciparum —see Malaria, falciparum
  quartan —see Malaria, malariae
  quotidian —see Malaria, falciparum
  recurrent B54
  remittent B54
  specified type NEC (parasitologically confirmed) B53.8
  spleen B54
  subtertian (fever) —see Malaria, falciparum
  tertian (benign) —see also Malaria, vivax
    malignant B50.9
  tropical B50.9
  typhoid B54
  vivax B51.9
    with
      complications NEC B51.8
      ruptured spleen B51.0
Malassez's disease (cystic) N50.8
Malassimilation K90.9
Mal de los pintos —see Pinta
Mal de mer T75.3
Maldescent, testis Q53.9
  bilateral Q53.20
    abdominal Q53.21
    perineal Q53.22
  unilateral Q53.10
    abdominal Q53.11
    perineal Q53.12
Maldevelopment —see also Anomaly
  brain Q07.9
  colon Q43.9
  hip Q74.2
    congenital dislocation Q65.2
      bilateral Q65.1
      unilateral Q65.0-
  mastoid process Q75.8
  middle ear Q16.4
    except ossicles Q16.4
    ossicles Q16.3
  ossicles Q16.3
  spine Q76.49
  toe Q74.2
Male type pelvis Q74.2
  with disproportion (fetopelvic) O33.3
    causing obstructed labor O65.3
Malformation (congenital) —see also Anomaly
  adrenal gland Q89.1
  affecting multiple systems with skeletal changes NEC Q87.5
  alimentary tract Q45.9
    specified type NEC Q45.8
    upper Q40.9
      specified type NEC Q40.8
  aorta Q25.9
    atresia Q25.2
    coarctation (preductal) (postductal) Q25.1

Malformation (Continued)
aorta (Continued)
patent ductus arteriosus Q25.0
specified type NEC Q25.4
stenosis (supravalvular) Q25.3
aortic valve Q23.9
specified NEC Q23.8
arteriovenous, aneurysmatic (congenital) Q27.30
brain Q28.2
cerebral Q28.2
peripheral Q27.30
digestive system Q27.33
lower limb Q27.32
other specified site Q27.39
renal vessel Q27.34
upper limb Q27.31
precerebral vessels (nonruptured) Q28.0
auricle
ear (congenital) Q17.3
acquired H61.119
left H61.112
with right H61.113
right H61.111
with left H61.113
bile duct Q44.5
bladder Q64.79
aplasia Q64.5
diverticulum Q64.6
exstrophy —see Exstrophy, bladder
neck obstruction Q64.31
bone Q79.9
face Q75.9
specified type NEC Q75.8
skull Q75.9
specified type NEC Q75.8
brain (multiple) Q04.9
arteriovenous Q28.2
specified type NEC Q04.8
branchial cleft Q18.2
breast Q83.9
specified type NEC Q83.8
broad ligament Q50.6
bronchus Q32.4
bursa Q79.9
cardiac
chambers Q20.9
specified type NEC Q20.8
septum Q21.9
specified type NEC Q21.8
cerebral Q04.9
vessels Q28.3
cervix uteri Q51.9
specified type NEC Q51.828
Chiari
Type I G93.5
Type II Q07.01
choroid (congenital) Q14.3
plexus Q07.8
circulatory system Q28.9
cochlea Q16.5
cornea Q13.4
coronary vessels Q24.5
corpus callosum (congenital) Q04.0
diaphragm Q79.1
digestive system NEC, specified type NEC Q45.8
dura Q07.9
brain Q04.9
spinal Q06.9
ear Q17.9
causing impairment of hearing Q16.9
external Q17.9
accessory auricle Q17.0
causing impairment of hearing Q16.9
absence of
auditory canal Q16.1
auricle Q16.0
macrotia Q17.1
microtia Q17.2
misplacement Q17.4

Malformation (Continued)
ear (Continued)
external (Continued)
misshapen NEC Q17.3
prominence Q17.5
specified type NEC Q17.8
inner Q16.5
middle Q16.4
absence of eustachian tube Q16.2
ossicles (fusion) Q16.3
ossicles Q16.3
specified type NEC Q17.8
epididymis Q55.4
esophagus Q39.9
specified type NEC Q39.8
eye Q15.9
lid Q10.3
specified NEC Q15.8
fallopian tube Q50.6
genital organ —see Anomaly, genitalia
great
artery Q25.9
aorta —see Malformation, aorta
pulmonary artery —see Malformation, pulmonary, artery
specified type NEC Q25.8
vein Q26.9
anomalous
portal venous connection Q26.5
pulmonary venous connection Q26.4
partial Q26.3
total Q26.2
persistent left superior vena cava Q26.1
portal vein-hepatic artery fistula Q26.6
specified type NEC Q26.8
vena cava stenosis, congenital Q26.0
gum Q38.6
hair Q84.2
heart Q24.9
specified type NEC Q24.8
integument Q84.9
specified type NEC Q84.8
internal ear Q16.5
intestine Q43.9
specified type NEC Q43.8
iris Q13.2
joint Q74.9
ankle Q74.2
lumbosacral Q76.49
sacroiliac Q74.2
specified type NEC Q74.8
kidney Q63.9
accessory Q63.0
giant Q63.3
horseshoe Q63.1
hydronephrosis Q62.0
malposition Q63.2
specified type NEC Q63.8
lacrimal apparatus Q10.6
lingual Q38.3
lip Q38.0
liver Q44.7
lung Q33.9
meninges or membrane (congenital) Q07.9
cerebral Q04.8
spinal (cord) Q06.9
middle ear Q16.4
ossicles Q16.3
mitral valve Q23.9
specified NEC Q23.8
Mondini's (congenital) (malformation, cochlea) Q16.5
mouth (congenital) Q38.6
multiple types NEC Q89.7
musculoskeletal system Q79.9
myocardium Q24.8
nail Q84.6
nervous system (central) Q07.9
nose Q30.9
specified type NEC Q30.8
optic disc Q14.2

Malformation (Continued)
orbit Q10.7
ovary Q50.39
palate Q38.5
parathyroid gland Q89.2
pelvic organs or tissues NEC
in pregnancy or childbirth O34.8-
causing obstructed labor O65.5
penis Q55.69
aplasia Q55.5
curvature (lateral) Q55.61
hypoplasia Q55.62
pericardium Q24.8
peripheral vascular system Q27.9
specified type NEC Q27.8
pharynx Q38.8
precerebral vessels Q28.1
prostate Q55.4
pulmonary
arteriovenous Q25.72
artery Q25.9
atresia Q25.5
specified type NEC Q25.79
stenosis Q25.6
valve Q22.3
renal artery Q27.2
respiratory system Q34.9
retina Q14.1
scrotum —see Malformation, testis and scrotum
seminal vesicles Q55.4
sense organs NEC Q07.9
skin Q82.9
specified NEC Q89.8
spinal
cord Q06.9
nerve root Q07.8
spine Q76.49
kyphosis —see Kyphosis, congenital
lordosis —see Lordosis, congenital
spleen Q89.09
stomach Q40.3
specified type NEC Q40.2
teeth, tooth K00.9
tendon Q79.9
testis and scrotum Q55.20
aplasia Q55.0
hypoplasia Q55.1
polyorchism Q55.21
retractile testis Q55.22
scrotal transposition Q55.23
specified NEC Q55.29
thorax, bony Q76.9
throat Q38.8
thyroid gland Q89.2
tongue (congenital) Q38.3
hypertrophy Q38.2
tie Q38.1
trachea Q32.1
tricuspid valve Q22.9
specified type NEC Q22.8
umbilical cord NEC (complicating delivery) O69.89
umbilicus Q89.9
ureter Q62.8
agenesis Q62.4
duplication Q62.5
malposition —see Malposition, congenital, ureter
obstructive defect —see Defect, obstructive, ureter
vesico-uretero-renal reflux Q62.7
urethra Q64.79
aplasia Q64.5
duplication Q64.74
posterior valves Q64.2
prolapse Q64.71
stricture Q64.32
urinary system Q64.9
uterus Q51.9
specified type NEC Q51.818

Malformation (*Continued*)
vagina Q52.4
vascular system, peripheral Q27.9
vas deferens Q55.4
atresia Q55.3
venous —*see* Anomaly, vein (s)
vulva Q52.70
Malfunction —*see also* Dysfunction
cardiac electronic device T82.119
electrode T82.110
pulse generator T82.111
specified type NEC T82.118
catheter device NEC T85.618
cystostomy T83.010
dialysis (renal) (vascular) T82.41
intraperitoneal T85.611
infusion NEC T82.514
spinal (epidural) (subdural) T85.610
urinary, indwelling T83.018
colostomy K94.03
valve K94.03
cystostomy (stoma) N99.512
catheter T83.010
enteric stoma K94.13
enterostomy K94.13
esophagostomy K94.33
gastroenteric K31.89
gastrostomy K94.23
ileostomy K94.13
valve K94.13
jejunostomy K94.13
pacemaker —*see* Malfunction, cardiac
electronic device
prosthetic device, internal —*see*
Complications, prosthetic device, by
site, mechanical
tracheostomy J95.03
urinary device NEC —*see* Complication,
genitourinary, device, urinary,
mechanical
valve
colostomy K94.03
heart T82.09
ileostomy K94.13
vascular graft or shunt NEC —*see*
Complication, cardiovascular device,
mechanical, vascular
ventricular (communicating shunt) T85.01
Malherbe's tumor —*see* Neoplasm, skin, benign
Malibu disease L98.8-
Malignancy —*see also* Neoplasm, malignant,
by site
unspecified site (primary) C80.1
Malignant —*see* condition
Malingerer, malingering Z76.5
Mallet finger (acquired) —*see* Deformity, finger,
mallet finger
congenital Q74.0
sequelae of rickets E64.3
Malleus A24.0
Mallory's bodies R89.7
Mallory-Weiss syndrome K22.6
Malnutrition E46
degree
first E44.1
mild (protein) E44.1
moderate (protein) E44.0
second E44.0
severe (protein-energy) E43
intermediate form E42
with
kwashiorkor (and marasmus) E42
marasmus E41
third E43
following gastrointestinal surgery K91.2
intrauterine
light-for-dates —*see* Light for dates
small-for-dates —*see* Small for dates
lack of care, or neglect (child) (infant) T76.02
confirmed T74.02
malignant E40

Malnutrition (*Continued*)
protein E46
calorie E46
mild E44.1
moderate E44.0
severe E43
intermediate form E42
with
kwashiorkor (and marasmus)
E42
marasmus E41
energy E46
mild E44.1
moderate E44.0
severe E43
intermediate form E42
with
kwashiorkor (and marasmus)
E42
marasmus E41
severe (protein-energy) E43
with
kwashiorkor (and marasmus) E42
marasmus E41
Malocclusion (teeth) M26.4
Angle's M26.219
class I M26.211
class II M26.212
class III M26.213
due to
abnormal swallowing M26.59
mouth breathing M26.59
tongue, lip or finger habits M26.59
temporomandibular (joint) M26.69
Malposition
cervix —*see* Malposition, uterus
congenital
adrenal (gland) Q89.1
alimentary tract Q45.8
lower Q43.8
upper Q40.8
aorta Q25.4
appendix Q43.8
arterial trunk Q20.0
artery (peripheral) Q27.8
coronary Q24.5
digestive system Q27.8
lower limb Q27.8
pulmonary Q25.79
specified site NEC Q27.8
upper limb Q27.8
auditory canal Q17.8
causing impairment of hearing Q16.9
auricle (ear) Q17.4
causing impairment of hearing Q16.9
cervical Q18.2
biliary duct or passage Q44.5
bladder (mucosa) —*see* Exstrophy, bladder
brachial plexus Q07.8
brain tissue Q04.8
breast Q83.8
bronchus Q32.4
cecum Q43.8
clavicle Q74.0
colon Q43.8
digestive organ or tract NEC Q45.8
lower Q43.8
upper Q40.8
ear (auricle) (external) Q17.4
ossicles Q16.3
endocrine (gland) NEC Q89.2
epiglottis Q31.8
eustachian tube Q17.8
eye Q15.8
facial features Q18.8
fallopian tube Q50.6
finger (s) Q68.1
supernumerary Q69.0
foot Q66.9
gallbladder Q44.1
gastrointestinal tract Q45.8

Malposition (*Continued*)
congenital (*Continued*)
genitalia, genital organ (s) or tract
female Q52.8
external Q52.79
internal NEC Q52.8
male Q55.8
glottis Q31.8
hand Q68.1
heart Q24.8
dextrocardia Q24.0
with complete transposition of viscera
Q89.3
hepatic duct Q44.5
hip (joint) Q65.89
intestine (large) (small) Q43.8
with anomalous adhesions, fixation or
malrotation Q43.3
joint NEC Q68.8
kidney Q63.2
larynx Q31.8
limb Q68.8
lower Q68.8
upper Q68.8
liver Q44.7
lung (lobe) Q33.8
nail (s) Q84.6
nerve Q07.8
nervous system NEC Q07.8
nose, nasal (septum) Q30.8
organ or site not listed —*see* Anomaly,
by site
ovary Q50.39
pancreas Q45.3
parathyroid (gland) Q89.2
patella Q74.1
peripheral vascular system Q27.8
pituitary (gland) Q89.2
respiratory organ or system NEC
Q34.8
rib (cage) Q76.6
supernumerary in cervical region
Q76.5
scapula Q74.0
shoulder Q74.0
spinal cord Q06.8
spleen Q89.09
sternum NEC Q76.7
stomach Q40.2
symphysis pubis Q74.2
thymus (gland) Q89.2
thyroid (gland) (tissue) Q89.2
cartilage Q31.8
toe (s) Q66.9
supernumerary Q69.2
tongue Q38.3
trachea Q32.1
ureter Q62.60
deviation Q62.61
displacement Q62.62
ectopia Q62.63
specified type NEC Q62.69
uterus Q51.818
vein (s) (peripheral) Q27.8
great Q26.8
vena cava (inferior) (superior) Q26.8
device, implant or graft (*see also*
Complications, by site and type,
mechanical) T85.628
arterial graft NEC —*see* Complication,
cardiovascular device, mechanical,
vascular
breast (implant) T85.42
catheter NEC T85.628
cystostomy T83.020
dialysis (renal) T82.42
intraperitoneal T85.621
infusion NEC T82.524
spinal (epidural) (subdural)
T85.620
urinary, indwelling T83.028

◀ New   ◀‖‖ Revised   ~~deleted~~ Deleted

Malposition *(Continued)*
  device, implant or graft *(Continued)*
    electronic (electrode) (pulse generator)
        (stimulator)
      bone T84.320
      cardiac T82.129
        electrode T82.120
        pulse generator T82.121
        specified type NEC T82.128
      nervous system —*see* Complication,
          prosthetic device, mechanical,
          electronic nervous system
          stimulator
      urinary —*see* Complication,
          genitourinary, device, urinary,
          mechanical
    fixation, internal (orthopedic) NEC —*see*
        Complication, fixation device,
        mechanical
    gastrointestinal —*see* Complications,
        prosthetic device, mechanical,
        gastrointestinal device
    genital NEC T83.428
      intrauterine contraceptive device T83.32
      penile prosthesis T83.420
    heart NEC —*see* Complication,
        cardiovascular device, mechanical
    joint prosthesis —*see* Complication, joint
        prosthesis, mechanical
    ocular NEC —*see* Complications, prosthetic
        device, mechanical, ocular device
    orthopedic NEC —*see* Complication,
        orthopedic, device, mechanical
    specified NEC T85.628
    urinary NEC —*see also* Complication,
        genitourinary, device, urinary,
        mechanical
      graft T83.22
    vascular NEC —*see* Complication,
        cardiovascular device, mechanical
    ventricular intracranial shunt T85.02
  fetus —*see* Pregnancy, complicated by
      (management affected by), presentation,
      fetal
  gallbladder K82.8
  gastrointestinal tract, congenital Q45.8
  heart, congenital NEC Q24.8
  joint prosthesis —*see* Complications, joint
      prosthesis, mechanical, displacement,
      by site
  stomach K31.89
    congenital Q40.2
  tooth, teeth, fully erupted M26.30
  uterus (acute) (acquired) (adherent)
      (asymptomatic) (postinfectional)
      (postpartal, old) N85.4
    anteflexion or anteversion N85.4
      congenital Q51.818
    flexion N85.4
      lateral —*see* Lateroversion, uterus
    inversion N85.5
    lateral (flexion) (version) —*see*
        Lateroversion, uterus
    in pregnancy or childbirth —*see*
        subcategory O34.5
    retroflexion or retroversion —*see*
        Retroversion, uterus
Malposture R29.3
Malrotation
  cecum Q43.3
  colon Q43.3
  intestine Q43.3
  kidney Q63.2
Malta fever —*see* Brucellosis
Maltreatment
  adult
    abandonment
      confirmed T74.01
      suspected T76.01
    confirmed T74.91
    history of Z91.419

Maltreatment *(Continued)*
  adult *(Continued)*
    neglect
      confirmed T74.01
      suspected T76.01
    physical abuse
      confirmed T74.11
      suspected T76.11
    psychological abuse
      confirmed T74.31
      history of Z91.411
      suspected T76.31
    sexual abuse
      confirmed T74.21
      suspected T76.21
    suspected T76.91
  child
    abandonment
      confirmed T74.02
      suspected T76.02
    confirmed T74.92
    history of —*see* History, personal (of),
        abuse
    neglect
      confirmed T74.02
      history of —*see* History, personal (of),
          abuse
      suspected T76.02
    physical abuse
      confirmed T74.12
      history of —*see* History, personal (of),
          abuse
      suspected T76.12
    psychological abuse
      confirmed T74.32
      history of —*see* History, personal (of),
          abuse
      suspected T76.32
    sexual abuse
      confirmed T74.22
      history of —*see* History, personal (of),
          abuse
      suspected T76.22
    suspected T76.92
    personal history of Z91.89
Maltworker's lung J67.4
Malunion, fracture —*see* Fracture, by site
Mammillitis N61
  puerperal, postpartum O91.02
Mammitis —*see* Mastitis
Mammogram (examination) Z12.39
  routine Z12.31
Mammoplasia N62
Management (of)
  bone conduction hearing device (implanted)
      Z45.320
  cardiac pacemaker NEC Z45.018
  cerebrospinal fluid drainage device Z45.41
  cochlear device (implanted) Z45.321
  contraceptive Z30.9
    specified NEC Z30.8
  implanted device Z45.9
    specified NEC Z45.89
  infusion pump Z45.1
  procreative Z31.9
    male factor infertility in female Z31.81
    specified NEC Z31.89
  prosthesis (external) (*see also* Fitting)
      Z44.9
    implanted Z45.9
      specified NEC Z45.89
  renal dialysis catheter Z49.01
  vascular access device Z45.2
Mangled —*see* specified injury by site
Mania (monopolar) —*see also* Disorder, mood,
    manic episode
  with psychotic symptoms F30.2
  without psychotic symptoms F30.10
    mild F30.11
    moderate F30.12
    severe F30.13

Mania *(Continued)*
  Bell's F30.8
  chronic (recurrent) F31.89
  hysterical F44.89
  puerperal F30.8
  recurrent F31.89
Manic-depressive insanity, psychosis, or
    syndrome —*see* Disorder, bipolar
Mannosidosis E77.1
Mansonelliasis, mansonellosis B74.4
Manson's
  disease B65.1
  schistosomiasis B65.1
Manual —*see* condition
Maple-bark-stripper's lung (disease) J67.6
Maple-syrup-urine disease E71.0
Marable's syndrome (celiac artery
    compression) I77.4
Marasmus E41
  due to malnutrition E41
  intestinal E41
  nutritional E41
  senile R54
  tuberculous NEC —*see* Tuberculosis
Marble
  bones Q78.2
  skin R23.8
Marburg virus disease A98.3
March
  fracture —*see* Fracture, traumatic, stress, by
      site
  hemoglobinuria D59.6
Marchesani (-Weill) syndrome Q87.0
Marchiafava (-Bignami) syndrome or disease
    G37.1
Marchiafava-Micheli syndrome D59.5
Marcus Gunn's syndrome Q07.8
Marfan's syndrome —*see* Syndrome, Marfan's
Marie-Bamberger disease —*see*
    Osteoarthropathy, hypertrophic, specified
    NEC
Marie-Charcot-Tooth neuropathic muscular
    atrophy G60.0
Marie's
  cerebellar ataxia (late-onset) G11.2
  disease or syndrome (acromegaly) E22.0
Marie-Strümpell arthritis, disease or
    spondylitis —*see* Spondylitis, ankylosing
Marion's disease (bladder neck obstruction)
    N32.0
Marital conflict Z63.0
Mark
  port wine Q82.5
  raspberry Q82.5
  strawberry Q82.5
  stretch L90.6
  tattoo L81.8
Marker heterochromatin —*see* Extra, marker
    chromosomes
Maroteaux-Lamy syndrome (mild) (severe)
    E76.29
Marrow (bone)
  arrest D61.9
  poor function D75.89
Marseilles fever A77.1
Marsh fever —*see* Malaria
Marshall's (hidrotic) ectodermal dysplasia
    Q82.4
Marsh's disease (exophthalmic goiter) E05.00
  with storm E05.01
Masculinization (female) with adrenal
    hyperplasia E25.9
  congenital E25.0
Masculinovoblastoma D27.-
Masochism (sexual) F65.51
Mason's lung J62.8
Mass
  abdominal R19.00
    epigastric R19.06
    generalized R19.07
    left lower quadrant R19.04

M

Mass *(Continued)*
  abdominal *(Continued)*
    left upper quadrant R19.02
    periumbilic R19.05
    right lower quadrant R19.03
    right upper quadrant R19.01
    specified site NEC R19.09
  breast N63
  chest R22.2
  cystic —*see* Cyst
  ear H93.8-
  head R22.0
  intra-abdominal (diffuse) (generalized) —*see*
    Mass, abdominal
  kidney N28.89
  liver R16.0
  localized (skin) R22.9
    chest R22.2
    head R22.0
    limb
      lower R22.4-
      upper R22.3-
    neck R22.1
    trunk R22.2
  lung R91.8
  malignant —*see* Neoplasm, malignant,
    by site
  neck R22.1
  pelvic (diffuse) (generalized) —*see* Mass,
    abdominal
  specified organ NEC —*see* Disease, by site
  splenic R16.1
  substernal thyroid —*see* Goiter
  superficial (localized) R22.9
  umbilical (diffuse) (generalized) R19.09
Massive —*see* condition
Mast cell
  disease, systemic tissue D47.0
  leukemia C94.3-
  sarcoma C96.2
  tumor D47.0
    malignant C96.2
Mastalgia N64.4
Masters-Allen syndrome N83.8
Mastitis (acute) (diffuse) (nonpuerperal)
    (subacute) N61
  chronic (cystic) —*see* Mastopathy, cystic
  cystic (Schimmelbusch's type) —*see*
    Mastopathy, cystic
  fibrocystic —*see* Mastopathy, cystic
  infective N61
    newborn P39.0
  interstitial, gestational or puerperal —*see*
    Mastitis, obstetric
  neonatal (noninfective) P83.4
    infective P39.0
  obstetric (interstitial) (nonpurulent)
    associated with
      lactation O91.23
      pregnancy O91.21-
      puerperium O91.22
    purulent
      associated with
        lactation O91.13
        pregnancy O91.11-
        puerperium O91.12
  periductal —*see* Ectasia, mammary duct
  phlegmonous —*see* Mastopathy, cystic
  plasma cell —*see* Ectasia, mammary duct
Mastocytoma D47.0
  malignant C96.2
Mastocytosis Q82.2
  aggressive systemic C96.2
  indolent systemic D47.0
  malignant C96.2
  systemic, associated with clonal hematopoetic
    non-mast-cell disease (SM-AHNMD)
    D47.0
Mastodynia N64.4
Mastoid —*see* condition
Mastoidalgia —*see* subcategory H92.0

Mastoiditis (coalescent) (hemorrhagic)
    (suppurative) H70.9-
  acute, subacute H70.00-
    complicated NEC H70.09-
    subperiosteal H70.01-
  chronic (necrotic) (recurrent) H70.1-
  in (due to)
    infectious disease NEC B99 [H75.0-]
    parasitic disease NEC B89 [H75.0-]
    tuberculosis A18.03
  petrositis —*see* Petrositis
  postauricular fistula —*see* Fistula,
    postauricular
  specified NEC H70.89-
  tuberculous A18.03
Mastopathy, mastopathia N64.9
  chronica cystica —*see* Mastopathy, cystic
  cystic (chronic) (diffuse) N60.1
    with epithelial proliferation N60.3-
  diffuse cystic —*see* Mastopathy, cystic
  estrogenic, oestrogenica N64.89
  ovarian origin N64.89
Mastoplasia, mastoplastia N62
Masturbation (excessive) F98.8
Maternal care (for) —*see* Pregnancy
    (complicated by) (management
    affected by)
Matheiu's disease (leptospiral jaundice)
    A27.0
Mauclaire's disease or osteochondrosis —
    see Osteochondrosis, juvenile, hand,
    metacarpal
Maxcy's disease A75.2
Maxilla, maxillary —*see* condition
May (-Hegglin) anomaly or syndrome
    D72.0
McArdle (-Schmid)(-Pearson) disease
    (glycogen storage) E74.04
McCune-Albright syndrome Q78.1
McQuarrie's syndrome (idiopathic familial
    hypoglycemia) E16.2
Meadow's syndrome Q86.1
Measles (black) (hemorrhagic) (suppressed)
    B05.9
  with
    complications NEC B05.89
    encephalitis B05.0
    intestinal complications B05.4
    keratitis (keratoconjunctivitis) B05.81
    meningitis B05.1
    otitis media B05.3
    pneumonia B05.2
  French —*see* Rubella
  German —*see* Rubella
  Liberty —*see* Rubella
Meatitis, urethral —*see* Urethritis
Meatus, meatal —*see* condition
Meat-wrappers' asthma J68.9
Meckel-Gruber syndrome Q61.9
Meckel's diverticulitis, diverticulum
    (displaced) (hypertrophic) Q43.0
Meconium
  ileus, newborn P76.0
    in cystic fibrosis E84.11
    meaning meconium plug (without cystic
      fibrosis) P76.0
  obstruction, newborn P76.0
    due to fecaliths P76.0
    in mucoviscidosis E84.11
  peritonitis P78.0
  plug syndrome (newborn) NEC P76.0
Median —*see also* condition
  arcuate ligament syndrome I77.4
  bar (prostate) (vesical orifice) —*see*
    Hyperplasia, prostate
  rhomboid glossitis K14.2
Mediastinal shift R93.8
Mediastinitis (acute) (chronic)
    J98.5
  syphilitic A52.73
  tuberculous A15.8

Mediastinopericarditis —*see also* Pericarditis
  acute I30.9
  adhesive I31.0
  chronic I31.8
  rheumatic I09.2
Mediastinum, mediastinal —*see* condition
~~Medical services provided for —see Health,~~
    ~~services provided because (of)~~
Medicine poisoning —*see* Table of ~~d~~Drugs and
    ~~c~~Chemicals, by drug, poisoning ◀
Mediterranean
  fever —*see* Brucellosis
    familial E85.0
    tick A77.1
  kala-azar B55.0
  leishmaniasis B55.0
  tick fever A77.1
Medulla —*see* condition
Medullary cystic kidney Q61.5
Medullated fibers
  optic (nerve) Q14.8
  retina Q14.1
Medulloblastoma
  desmoplastic C71.6
  specified site —*see* Neoplasm, malignant, by
    site
  unspecified site C71.6
Medulloepithelioma —*see also* Neoplasm,
    malignant, by site
  teratoid —*see* Neoplasm, malignant, by site
Medullomyoblastoma
  specified site —*see* Neoplasm, malignant, by
    site
  unspecified site C71.6
Meekeren-Ehlers-Danlos syndrome Q79.6
Megacolon (acquired) (functional) (not
    Hirschsprung's disease) (in) K59.3
  Chagas' disease B57.32
  congenital, congenitum (aganglionic) Q43.1
  Hirschsprung's (disease) Q43.1
  toxic NEC K59.3
    due to Clostridium difficile A04.7
Megaesophagus (functional) K22.0
  congenital Q39.5
  in (due to) Chagas' disease B57.31
Megalencephaly Q04.5
Megalerythema (epidemic) B08.3
Megaloappendix Q43.8
Megalocephalus, megalocephaly NEC Q75.3
Megalocornea Q15.8
  with glaucoma Q15.0
Megalocytic anemia D53.1
Megalodactylia (fingers) (thumbs) (congenital)
    Q74.0
  toes Q74.2
Megaloduodenum Q43.8
Megaloesophagus (functional) K22.0
  congenital Q39.5
Megalogastria (acquired) K31.89
  congenital Q40.2
Megalophthalmos Q11.3
Megalopsia H53.15
Megalosplenia —*see* Splenomegaly
Megaloureter N28.82
  congenital Q62.2
Megarectum K62.89
Megasigmoid K59.3
  congenital Q43.2
Megaureter N28.82
  congenital Q62.2
Megavitamin-B6 syndrome E67.2
Megrim —*see* Migraine
Meibomian
  cyst, infected —*see* Hordeolum
  gland —*see* condition
  sty, stye —*see* Hordeolum
Meibomitis —*see* Hordeolum
Meige-Milroy disease (chronic hereditary
    edema) Q82.0
Meige's syndrome Q82.0
Melalgia, nutritional E53.8

◀ New   ◀▥ Revised   ~~deleted~~ Deleted

Melancholia F32.9
  climacteric (single episode) F32.8
    recurrent episode F33.9
  hypochondriac F45.29
  intermittent (single episode) F32.8
    recurrent episode F33.9
  involutional (single episode) F32.8
    recurrent episode F33.9
  menopausal (single episode) F32.8
    recurrent episode F33.9
  puerperal F32.8
  reactive (emotional stress or trauma) F32.3
  recurrent F33.9
  senile F03
  stuporous (single episode) F32.8
    recurrent episode F33.9
Melanemia R79.89
Melanoameloblastoma —see Neoplasm, bone,
    benign
Melanoblastoma —see Melanoma
Melanocarcinoma —see Melanoma
Melanocytoma, eyeball D31.4-
Melanocytosis, neurocutaneous Q82.8
Melanoderma, melanodermia L81.4
Melanodontia, infantile K03.89
Melanodontoclasia K03.89
Melanoepithelioma —see Melanoma
Melanoma (malignant) C43.9
  acral lentiginous, malignant —see Melanoma,
    skin, by site
  amelanotic —see Melanoma, skin, by site
  balloon cell —see Melanoma, skin, by site
  benign —see Nevus
  desmoplastic, malignant —see Melanoma,
    skin, by site
  epithelioid cell —see Melanoma, skin, by site
    with spindle cell, mixed —see Melanoma,
      skin, by site
  in
    giant pigmented nevus —see Melanoma,
      skin, by site
    Hutchinson's melanotic freckle —see
      Melanoma, skin, by site
    junctional nevus —see Melanoma, skin,
      by site
    precancerous melanosis —see Melanoma,
      skin, by site
  in situ D03.9
    abdominal wall D03.59
    ala nasi D03.39
    ankle D03.7-
    anus, anal (margin) (skin) D03.51
    arm D03.6-
    auditory canal D03.2-
    auricle (ear) D03.2-
    auricular canal (external) D03.2-
    axilla, axillary fold D03.59
    back D03.59
    breast D03.52
    brow D03.39
    buttock D03.59
    canthus (eye) D03.1-
    cheek (external) D03.39
    chest wall D03.59
    chin D03.39
    choroid D03.8
    conjunctiva D03.8
    ear (external) D03.2-
    external meatus (ear) D03.2-
    eye D03.8
    eyebrow D03.39
    eyelid (lower) (upper) D03.1-
    face D03.30
      specified NEC D03.39
    female genital organ (external) NEC D03.8
    finger D03.6-
    flank D03.59
    foot D03.7-
    forearm D03.6-
    forehead D03.39
    foreskin D03.8

Melanoma (Continued)
  in situ (Continued)
    gluteal region D03.59
    groin D03.59
    hand D03.6-
    heel D03.7-
    helix D03.2-
    hip D03.7-
    interscapular region D03.59
    iris D03.8
    jaw D03.39
    knee D03.7-
    labium (majus) (minus) D03.8
    lacrimal gland D03.8
    leg D03.7-
    lip (lower) (upper) D03.0
    lower limb NEC D03.7-
    male genital organ (external) NEC
      D03.8
    nail D03.9
      finger D03.6-
      toe D03.7-
    neck D03.4
    nose (external) D03.39
    orbit D03.8
    penis D03.8
    perianal skin D03.51
    perineum D03.51
    pinna D03.2-
    popliteal fossa or space D03.7-
    prepuce D03.8
    pudendum D03.8
    retina D03.8
    retrobulbar D03.8
    scalp D03.4
    scrotum D03.8
    shoulder D03.6-
    specified site NEC D03.8
    submammary fold D03.52
    temple D03.39
    thigh D03.7-
    toe D03.7-
    trunk NEC D03.59
    umbilicus D03.59
    upper limb NEC D03.6-
    vulva D03.8
  juvenile —see Nevus
  malignant, of soft parts except skin —see
      Neoplasm, connective tissue,
      malignant
  metastatic
    breast C79.81
    genital organ C79.82
    specified site NEC C79.89
  neurotropic, malignant —see Melanoma, skin,
      by site
  nodular —see Melanoma, skin, by site
  regressing, malignant —see Melanoma, skin,
      by site
  skin C43.9
    abdominal wall C43.59
    ala nasi C43.31
    ankle C43.7-
    anus, anal (skin) C43.51
    arm C43.6-
    auditory canal (external) C43.2-
    auricle (ear) C43.2-
    auricular canal (external) C43.2-
    axilla, axillary fold C43.59
    back C43.59
    breast (female) (male) C43.52
    brow C43.39
    buttock C43.59
    canthus (eye) C43.1-
    cheek (external) C43.39
    chest wall C43.59
    chin C43.39
    ear (external) C43.2-
    elbow C43.6-
    external meatus (ear) C43.2-
    eyebrow C43.39

Melanoma (Continued)
  skin (Continued)
    eyelid (lower) (upper) C43.1-
    face C43.30
      specified NEC C43.39
    female genital organ (external) NEC C51.9
    finger C43.6-
    flank C43.59
    foot C43.7-
    forearm C43.6-
    forehead C43.39
    foreskin C60.0
    glabella C43.39
    gluteal region C43.59
    groin C43.59
    hand C43.6-
    heel C43.7-
    helix C43.2-
    hip C43.7-
    interscapular region C43.59
    jaw (external) C43.39
    knee C43.7-
    labium C51.9
      majus C51.0
      minus C51.1
    leg C43.7-
    lip (lower) (upper) C43.0
    lower limb NEC C43.7-
    male genital organ (external) NEC C63.9
    nail
      finger C43.6-
      toe C43.7-
    nasolabial groove C43.39
    nates C43.59
    neck C43.4
    nose (external) C43.31
    overlapping site C43.8
    palpebra C43.1-
    penis C60.9
    perianal skin C43.51
    perineum C43.51
    pinna C43.2-
    popliteal fossa or space C43.7-
    prepuce C60.0
    pudendum C51.9
    scalp C43.4
    scrotum C63.2
    shoulder C43.6-
    skin NEC C43.9
    submammary fold C43.52
    temple C43.39
    thigh C43.7-
    toe C43.7-
    trunk NEC C43.59
    umbilicus C43.59
    upper limb NEC C43.6-
    vulva C51.9
      overlapping sites C51.8
  spindle cell
    with epithelioid, mixed —see Melanoma,
      skin, by site
    type A C69.4-
    type B C69.4-
  superficial spreading —see Melanoma, skin,
      by site
Melanosarcoma —see also Melanoma
  epithelioid cell —see Melanoma
Melanosis L81.4
  addisonian E27.1
    tuberculous A18.7
  adrenal E27.1
  colon K63.89
  conjunctiva —see Pigmentation, conjunctiva
    congenital Q13.89
  cornea (presenile) (senile) —see also
      Pigmentation, cornea
    congenital Q13.4
  eye NEC H57.8
    congenital Q15.8
  lenticularis progressiva Q82.1
  liver K76.89

Melanosis *(Continued)*
  precancerous —*see also* Melanoma, in situ
    malignant melanoma in —*see* Melanoma
  Riehl's L81.4
  sclera H15.89
    congenital Q13.89
  suprarenal E27.1
  tar L81.4
  toxic L81.4
Melanuria R82.99
MELAS syndrome E88.41
Melasma L81.1
  adrenal (gland) E27.1
  suprarenal (gland) E27.1
Melena K92.1
  with ulcer - code by site under Ulcer, with
    hemorrhage K27.4
  due to swallowed maternal blood P78.2
  newborn, neonatal P54.1
    due to swallowed maternal blood P78.2
Meleney's
  gangrene (cutaneous) —*see* Ulcer, skin
  ulcer (chronic undermining) —*see* Ulcer, skin
Melioidosis A24.9
  acute A24.1
  chronic A24.2
  fulminating A24.1
  pneumonia A24.1
  pulmonary (chronic) A24.2
    acute A24.1
    subacute A24.2
  sepsis A24.1
  specified NEC A24.3
  subacute A24.2
Melitensis, febris A23.0
Melkersson (-Rosenthal) syndrome G51.2
Mellitus, diabetes —*see* Diabetes
Melorheostosis (bone) —*see* Disorder, bone,
    density and structure, specified NEC
Meloschisis Q18.4
Melotia Q17.4
Membrana
  capsularis lentis posterior Q13.89
  epipapillaris Q14.2
Membranacea placenta O43.19-
Membranaceous uterus N85.8
Membrane (s), membranous —*see also*
    condition
  cyclitic —*see* Membrane, pupillary
  folds, congenital —*see* Web
  Jackson's Q43.3
  over face of newborn P28.9
  premature rupture —*see* Rupture,
    membranes, premature
  pupillary H21.4-
    persistent Q13.89
  retained (with hemorrhage) (complicating
    delivery) O72.2
    without hemorrhage O73.1
  secondary cataract —*see* Cataract, secondary
  unruptured (causing asphyxia) —*see*
    Asphyxia, newborn
  vitreous —*see* Opacity, vitreous, membranes
    and strands
Membranitis —*see* Chorioamnionitis
Memory disturbance, lack or loss —*see also*
    Amnesia
  mild, following organic brain damage F06.8
Menadione deficiency E56.1
Menarche
  delayed E30.0
  precocious E30.1
Mendacity, pathologic F60.2
Mendelson's syndrome (due to anesthesia)
    J95.4
  in labor and delivery O74.0
  in pregnancy O29.01-
  obstetric O74.0
  postpartum, puerperal O89.01
Ménétrier's disease or syndrome K29.60
  with bleeding K29.61

Ménière's disease, syndrome or vertigo H81.0-
Meninges, meningeal —*see* condition
Meningioma —*see also* Neoplasm, meninges,
    benign
  angioblastic —*see* Neoplasm, meninges,
    benign
  angiomatous —*see* Neoplasm, meninges,
    benign
  endotheliomatous —*see* Neoplasm, meninges,
    benign
  fibroblastic —*see* Neoplasm, meninges,
    benign
  fibrous —*see* Neoplasm, meninges, benign
  hemangioblastic —*see* Neoplasm, meninges,
    benign
  hemangiopericytic —*see* Neoplasm,
    meninges, benign
  malignant —*see* Neoplasm, meninges,
    malignant
  meningiothelial —*see* Neoplasm, meninges,
    benign
  meningotheliomatous —*see* Neoplasm,
    meninges, benign
  mixed —*see* Neoplasm, meninges, benign
  multiple —*see* Neoplasm, meninges,
    uncertain behavior
  papillary —*see* Neoplasm, meninges,
    uncertain behavior
  psammomatous —*see* Neoplasm, meninges,
    benign
  syncytial —*see* Neoplasm, meninges, benign
  transitional —*see* Neoplasm, meninges,
    benign
Meningiomatosis (diffuse) —*see* Neoplasm,
    meninges, uncertain behavior
Meningism —*see* Meningismus
Meningismus (infectional) (pneumococcal)
    R29.1
  due to serum or vaccine R29.1
  influenzal —*see* Influenza, with,
    manifestations NEC
Meningitis (basal) (basic) (brain) (cerebral)
    (cervical) (congestive) (diffuse)
    (hemorrhagic) infantile) (membranous)
    (metastatic) (nonspecific) (pontine)
    (progressive) (simple) (spinal) (subacute)
    (sympathetic) (toxic) G03.9
  abacterial G03.0
  actinomycotic A42.81
  adenoviral A87.1
  arbovirus A87.8
  aseptic (acute) G03.0
  bacterial G00.9
    Escherichia coli (E. coli) G00.8
    Friedländer (bacillus) G00.8
    gram-negative G00.9
    H. influenzae G00.0
    Klebsiella G00.8
    pneumococcal G00.1
    specified organism NEC G00.8
    staphylococcal G00.3
    streptococcal (acute) G00.2
  benign recurrent (Mollaret) G03.2
  candidal B37.5
  caseous (tuberculous) A17.0
  cerebrospinal A39.0
  chronic NEC G03.1
  clear cerebrospinal fluid NEC G03.0
  coxsackievirus A87.0
  cryptococcal B45.1
  diplococcal (gram positive) A39.0
  echovirus A87.0
  enteroviral A87.0
  eosinophilic B83.2
  epidemic NEC A39.0
  Escherichia coli (E. coli) G00.8
  fibrinopurulent G00.9
    specified organism NEC G00.8
  Friedländer (bacillus) G00.8
  gonococcal A54.81
  gram-negative cocci G00.9

Meningitis *(Continued)*
  gram-positive cocci G00.9
  Haemophilus (influenzae) G00.0
  H. influenzae G00.0
  in (due to)
    adenovirus A87.1
    African trypanosomiasis B56.9 *[G02]*
    anthrax A22.8
    bacterial disease NEC A48.8 *[G01]*
    Chagas' disease (chronic) B57.41
    chickenpox B01.0
    coccidioidomycosis B38.4
    Diplococcus pneumoniae G00.1
    enterovirus A87.0
    herpes (simplex) virus B00.3
      zoster B02.1
    infectious mononucleosis B27.92
    leptospirosis A27.81
    Listeria monocytogenes A32.11
    Lyme disease A69.21
    measles B05.1
    mumps (virus) B26.1
    neurosyphilis (late) A52.13
    parasitic disease NEC B89 *[G02]*
    poliovirus A80.9 *[G02]*
    preventive immunization, inoculation or
      vaccination G03.8
    rubella B06.02
    Salmonella infection A02.21
    specified cause NEC G03.8
    typhoid fever A01.01
    varicella B01.0
    viral disease NEC A87.8
    whooping cough A37.90
    zoster B02.1
  infectious G00.9
  influenzal (H. influenzae) G00.0
  Klebsiella G00.8
  leptospiral (aseptic) A27.81
  lymphocytic (acute) (benign) (serous)
    A87.2
  meningococcal A39.0
  Mima polymorpha G00.8
  Mollaret (benign recurrent) G03.2
  monilial B37.5
  mycotic NEC B49 *[G02]*
  Neisseria A39.0
  nonbacterial G03.0
  nonpyogenic NEC G03.0
  ossificans G96.19
  pneumococcal G00.1
  poliovirus A80.9 *[G02]*
  postmeasles B05.1
  purulent G00.9
    specified organism NEC G00.8
  pyogenic G00.9
    specified organism NEC G00.8
  Salmonella (arizonae) (Cholerae-Suis)
    (enteritidis) (typhimurium) A02.21
  septic G00.9
    specified organism NEC G00.8
  serosa circumscripta NEC G03.0
  serous NEC G93.2
  specified organism NEC G00.8
  sporotrichosis B42.81
  staphylococcal G00.3
  sterile G03.0
  streptococcal (acute) G00.2
  suppurative G00.9
    specified organism NEC G00.8
  syphilitic (late) (tertiary) A52.13
    acute A51.41
    congenital A50.41
    secondary A51.41
  Torula histolytica (cryptococcal) B45.1
  traumatic (complication of injury)
    T79.8
  tuberculous A17.0
  typhoid A01.01
  viral NEC A87.9
  Yersinia pestis A20.3

◀ New   ◀▥ Revised   ~~deleted~~ Deleted

Mesothelioma *(Continued)*
  epithelioid C45.9
    benign
      mesentery D19.1
      mesocolon D19.1
      omentum D19.1
      peritoneum D19.1
      pleura D19.0
      specified site NEC D19.7
      unspecified site D19.9
  fibrous C45.9
    benign
      mesentery D19.1
      mesocolon D19.1
      omentum D19.1
      peritoneum D19.1
      pleura D19.0
      specified site NEC D19.7
      unspecified site D19.9
  site classification
    liver C45.7
    lung C45.7
    mediastinum C45.7
    mesentery C45.1
    mesocolon C45.1
    omentum C45.1
    pericardium C45.2
    peritoneum C45.1
    pleura C45.0
      parietal C45.0
    retroperitoneum C45.7
    specified site NEC C45.7
    unspecified C45.9
Metabolic syndrome E88.81
Metagonimiasis B66.8
Metagonimus infestation (intestine) B66.8
Metal
  pigmentation L81.8
  polisher's disease J62.8
Metamorphopsia H53.15
Metaplasia
  apocrine (breast) —*see* Dysplasia, mammary,
    specified type NEC
  cervix (squamous) —*see* Dysplasia, cervix
  endometrium (squamous) (uterus) N85.8
  esophagus
  kidney (pelvis) (squamous) N28.89
  myelogenous D73.1
  myeloid (agnogenic) (megakaryocytic) D73.1
  spleen D73.1
  squamous cell, bladder N32.89
Metastasis, metastatic
  abscess —*see* Abscess
  calcification E83.59
  cancer
    from specified site —*see* Neoplasm,
      malignant, by site
    to specified site —*see* Neoplasm, secondary,
      by site
  deposits (in) —*see* Neoplasm, secondary, by
    site
  disease (*see also* Neoplasm, secondary, by site)
    C79.9
  spread (to) —*see* Neoplasm, secondary, by site
Metastrongyliasis B83.8
Metatarsalgia M77.4-
  anterior G57.6-
  Morton's G57.6-
Metatarsus, metatarsal —*see also* condition
  valgus (abductus), congenital Q66.6
  varus (adductus) (congenital) Q66.2
Methadone use F11.20
Methemoglobinemia D74.9
  acquired (with sulfhemoglobinemia) D74.8
  congenital D74.0
  enzymatic (congenital) D74.0
  Hb M disease D74.0
  hereditary D74.0
  toxic D74.8
Methemoglobinuria —*see* Hemoglobinuria
Methioninemia E72.19

Methylmalonic acidemia E71.120
Metritis (catarrhal) (hemorrhagic) (septic)
  (suppurative) —*see also* Endometritis
  cervical —*see* Cervicitis
Metropathia hemorrhagica N93.8
Metroperitonitis —*see* Peritonitis, pelvic, female
Metrorrhagia N92.1
  climacteric N92.4
  menopausal N92.4
  postpartum NEC (atonic) (following delivery
    of placenta) O72.1
    delayed or secondary O72.2
  preclimacteric or premenopausal N92.4
  psychogenic F45.8
Metrorrhexis —*see* Rupture, uterus
Metrosalpingitis N70.91
Metrostaxis N93.8
Metrovaginitis —*see* Endometritis
Meyer-Schwickerath and Weyers syndrome
  Q87.0
Meynert's amentia (nonalcoholic) F04
  alcoholic F10.96
    with dependence F10.26
Mibelli's disease (porokeratosis) Q82.8
Mice, joint —*see* Loose, body, joint
  knee M23.4
Micrencephalon, micrencephaly Q02
Microalbuminuria R80.9
Microaneurysm, retinal —*see also* Disorder,
  retina, microaneurysms
  diabetic —*see* E08-E13 with .31
Microangiopathy (peripheral) I73.9
  thrombotic M31.1
Microcalcifications, breast R92.0
Microcephalus, microcephalic, microcephaly
  Q02
  due to toxoplasmosis (congenital) P37.1
Microcheilia Q18.7
Microcolon (congenital) Q43.8
Microcornea (congenital) Q13.4
Microcytic —*see* condition D57.40
Microdeletions NEC Q93.88
Microdontia K00.2
Microdrepanocytosis D57.40
  ~~with sickle-cell crisis D57.41~~
  with crisis (vasoocclusive pain) D57.419 ◀
    with
      acute chest syndrome D57.411 ◀
      splenic sequestration D57.412 ◀
Microembolism
  atherothrombotic —*see* Atheroembolism
  retinal —*see* Occlusion, artery, retina
Microencephalon Q02
Microfilaria streptocerca infestation —*see*
  Onchocerciasis
Microgastria (congenital) Q40.2
Microgenia M26.06
Microgenitalia, congenital
  female Q52.8
  male Q55.8
Microglioma —*see* Lymphoma, non-Hodgkin,
  specified NEC
Microglossia (congenital) Q38.3
Micrognathia, micrognathism (congenital)
  (mandibular) (maxillary) M26.09
Microgyria (congenital) Q04.3
Microinfarct of heart —*see* Insufficiency,
  coronary
Microlentia (congenital) Q12.8
Microlithiasis, alveolar, pulmonary J84.02
Micromastia N64.82
Micromyelia (congenital) Q06.8
Micropenis Q55.62
Microphakia (congenital) Q12.8
Microphthalmos, microphthalmia (congenital)
  Q11.2
  due to toxoplasmosis P37.1
Micropsia H53.15
Microscopic polyangiitis (polyarteritis) M31.7
Microsporidiosis B60.8
  intestinal A07.8

Microsporon furfur infestation B36.0
Microsporosis —*see also* Dermatophytosis
  nigra B36.1
Microstomia (congenital) Q18.5
Microtia (congenital) (external ear) Q17.2
Microtropia H50.40
Microvillus inclusion disease (MVD) (MVID)
  Q43.8
Micturition
  disorder NEC R39.19
    psychogenic F45.8
  frequency R35.0
    psychogenic F45.8
  hesitancy R39.11
  incomplete emptying R39.14
  nocturnal R35.1
  painful R30.9
    dysuria R30.0
    psychogenic F45.8
    tenesmus R30.1
  poor stream R39.12
  split stream R39.13
  straining R39.16
  urgency R39.15
Mid plane —*see* condition
Middle
  ear —*see* condition
  lobe (right) syndrome J98.19
Miescher's elastoma L87.2
Mietens' syndrome Q87.2
Migraine (idiopathic) G43.909
  with refractory migraine G43.919
    with status migrainosus G43.911
    without status migrainosus G43.919
  with aura (acute-onset) (prolonged) (typical)
    (without headache) G43.109
    with refractory migraine G43.119
      with status migrainosus G43.111
      without status migrainosus G43.119
    intractable G43.119
      with status migrainosus G43.111
      without status migrainosus G43.119
    not intractable G43.109
      with status migrainosus G43.101
      without status migrainosus G43.109
    persistent G43.509
      with cerebral infarction G43.609
        with refractory migraine G43.619
          with status migrainosus G43.611
          without status migrainosus G43.619
        intractable G43.619
          with status migrainosus G43.611
          without status migrainosus G43.619
        not intractable G43.609
          with status migrainosus G43.601
          without status migrainosus G43.609
        without refractory migraine G43.609
          with status migrainosus G43.601
          without status migrainosus G43.609
      without cerebral infarction G43.509
        with refractory migraine G43.519
          with status migrainosus G43.511
          without status migrainosus G43.519
        intractable G43.519
          with status migrainosus G43.511
          without status migrainosus G43.519
        not intractable G43.509
          with status migrainosus G43.501
          without status migrainosus G43.509
        without refractory migraine G43.509
          with status migrainosus G43.501
          without status migrainosus G43.509
    without mention of refractory migraine
      G43.109
      with status migrainosus G43.101
      without status migrainosus G43.109
  abdominal G43.D0
    with refractory migraine G43.D1
    intractable G43.D1
    not intractable G43.D0
    without refractory migraine G43.D0

Migraine (Continued)
  basilar —see Migraine, with aura
  classical —see Migraine, with aura
  common —see Migraine, without aura
  complicated G43.109
  equivalents —see Migraine, with aura
  familiar —see Migraine, hemiplegic
  hemiplegic G43.409
    with refractory migraine G43.419
      with status migrainosus G43.411
      without status migrainosus G43.419
    intractable G43.419
      with status migrainosus G43.411
      without status migrainosus G43.419
    not intractable G43.409
      with status migrainosus G43.401
      without status migrainosus G43.409
    without refractory migraine G43.409
      with status migrainosus G43.401
      without status migrainosus G43.409
  intractable G43.919
    with status migrainosus G43.911
    without status migrainosus G43.919
  menstrual G43.829
    with refractory migraine G43.839
      with status migrainosus G43.831
      without status migrainosus G43.839
    intractable G43.839
      with status migrainosus G43.831
      without status migrainosus G43.839
    not intractable G43.829
      with status migrainosus G43.821
      without status migrainosus G43.829
    without refractory migraine G43.829
      with status migrainosus G43.821
      without status migrainosus G43.829
  menstrually related —see Migraine,
    menstrual
  not intractable G43.909
    with status migrainosus G43.901
    without status migrainosus G43.919
  ophthalmoplegic G43.B0
    with refractory migraine G43.B1
    intractable G43.B1
    not intractable G43.B0
    without refractory migraine G43.B0
  persistent aura (with, without) cerebral
    infarction —see Migraine, with aura,
    persistent
  preceded or accompanied by transient
    focal neurological phenomena —see
    Migraine, with aura
  pre-menstrual —see Migraine, menstrual
  pure menstrual —see Migraine, menstrual
  retinal —see Migraine, with aura
  specified NEC G43.809
    intractable G43.819
      with status migrainosus G43.811
      without status migrainosus G43.819
    not intractable G43.809
      with status migrainosus G43.801
      without status migrainosus G43.809
  sporadic —see Migraine, hemiplegic
  transformed —see Migraine, without aura,
    chronic
  triggered seizures —see Migraine, with
    aura
  without aura G43.009
    with refractory migraine G43.019
      with status migrainosus G43.011
      without status migrainosus G43.019
    chronic G43.709
      with refractory migraine G43.719
        with status migrainosus G43.711
        without status migrainosus G43.719
      intractable
        with status migrainosus G43.711
        without status migrainosus G43.719
      not intractable
        with status migrainosus G43.701
        without status migrainosus G43.709

Migraine (Continued)
  without aura (Continued)
    chronic (Continued)
      without refractory migraine G43.709
        with status migrainosus G43.701
        without status migrainosus
          G43.709
    intractable
      with status migrainosus G43.011
      without status migrainosus G43.019
    not intractable
      with status migrainosus G43.001
      without status migrainosus G43.009
    without mention of refractory migraine
      G43.009
      with status migrainosus G43.001
      without status migrainosus G43.009
    without refractory migraine G43.909
      with status migrainosus G43.901
      without status migrainosus G43.919
Migrant, social Z59.0
Migration, anxiety concerning Z60.3
Migratory, migrating —see also condition
  person Z59.0
  testis Q55.29
Mikity-Wilson disease or syndrome P27.0
Mikulicz' disease or syndrome K11.8
Miliaria L74.3
  alba L74.1
  apocrine L75.2
  crystallina L74.1
  profunda L74.2
  rubra L74.0
  tropicalis L74.2
Miliary —see condition
Milium L72.0
  colloid L57.8
Milk
  crust L21.0
  excessive secretion O92.6
  poisoning —see Poisoning, food, noxious
  retention O92.79
  sickness —see Poisoning, food, noxious
  spots I31.0
Milk-alkali disease or syndrome E83.52
Milk-leg (deep vessels) (nonpuerperal) —see
  Embolism, vein, lower extremity
  complicating pregnancy O22.3-
  puerperal, postpartum, childbirth O87.1
Milkman's disease or syndrome M83.8
Milky urine —see Chyluria
Millard-Gubler (-Foville) paralysis or
  syndrome G46.3
Millar's asthma J38.5
Miller-Fisher syndrome G61.0
Mills' disease —see Hemiplegia
Millstone maker's pneumoconiosis J62.8
Milroy's disease (chronic hereditary edema)
  Q82.0
Minamata disease T26.1
Miners' asthma or lung J60
Minkowski-Chauffard syndrome —see
  Spherocytosis
Minor —see condition
Minor's disease (hematomyelia) G95.19
Minot's disease (hemorrhagic disease),
  newborn P53
Minot-von Willebrand-Jurgens disease or
  syndrome (angiohemophilia) D68.0
Minus (and plus) hand (intrinsic) —see
  Deformity, limb, specified type NEC,
  forearm
Miosis (pupil) H57.03
Mirizzi's syndrome (hepatic duct stenosis)
  K83.1
Mirror writing F81.0
Misadventure (of) (prophylactic) (therapeutic)
  (see also Complications) T88.9
  administration of insulin (by accident) —see
    subcategory T38.3
  infusion —see Complications, infusion

Misadventure (Continued)
  local applications (of fomentations, plasters,
    etc.) T88.9
    burn or scald —see Burn
    specified NEC T88.8
  medical care (early) (late) T88.9
    adverse effect of drugs or chemicals —see
      Table of Drugs and Chemicals ◄▬▬
  medical care (early) (late)
    burn or scald —see Burn
    specified NEC T88.8
  specified NEC T88.8
  surgical procedure (early) (late) —see
    Complications, surgical procedure
  transfusion —see Complications, transfusion
  vaccination or other immunological
    procedure —see Complications,
    vaccination
Miscarriage O03.9
Misdirection, aqueous H40.83-
Misperception, sleep state F51.02
Misplaced, misplacement
  ear Q17.4
  kidney (acquired) N28.89
    congenital Q63.2
  organ or site, congenital NEC —see
    Malposition, congenital
Missed
  abortion O02.1
  delivery O36.4
Missing —see Absence
Misuse of drugs F19.99
Mitchell's disease (erythromelalgia) I73.81
Mite (s) (infestation) B88.9
  diarrhea B88.0
  grain (itch) B88.0
  hair follicle (itch) B88.0
  in sputum B88.0
Mitral —see condition
Mittelschmerz N94.0
Mixed —see condition
MNGIE (Mitochondrial Neurogastrointestinal
  Encephalopathy) syndrome E88.49
Mobile, mobility
  cecum Q43.3
  excessive —see Hypermobility
  gallbladder, congenital Q44.1
  kidney N28.89
  organ or site, congenital NEC —see
    Malposition, congenital
Mobitz heart block (atrioventricular) I44.1
Moebius, Möbius
  disease (ophthalmoplegic migraine) —see
    Migraine, ophthalmoplegic
  syndrome Q87.0
    congenital oculofacial paralysis (with other
      anomalies) Q87.0
    ophthalmoplegic migraine —see Migraine,
      ophthalmoplegic
Moeller's glossitis K14.0
Mohr's syndrome (Types I and II) Q87.0
Mola destruens D39.2
Molar pregnancy O02.0
Molarization of premolars K00.2
Molding, head (during birth) - omit code
Mole (pigmented) —see also Nevus
  blood O02.0
  Breus' O02.0
  cancerous —see Melanoma
  carneous O02.0
  destructive D39.2
  fleshy O02.0
  hydatid, hydatidiform (benign) (complicating
    pregnancy) (delivered) (undelivered)
    O01.9
    classical O01.0
    complete O01.0
    incomplete O01.1
    invasive D39.2
    malignant D39.2
    partial O01.1

Mole *(Continued)*
  intrauterine O02.0
  invasive (hydatidiform) D39.2
  malignant
    meaning
      malignant hydatidiform mole D39.2
      melanoma —*see* Melanoma
  nonhydatidiform O02.0
  nonpigmented —*see* Nevus
  pregnancy NEC O02.0
  skin —*see* Nevus
  tubal O00.1
  vesicular —*see* Mole, hydatidiform
Molimen, molimina (menstrual) N94.3
Molluscum contagiosum (epitheliale) B08.1
Mönckeberg's arteriosclerosis, disease, or
  sclerosis —*see* Arteriosclerosis, extremities
Mondini's malformation (cochlea) Q16.5
Mondor's disease I80.8
Monge's disease T70.29
Monilethrix (congenital) Q84.1
Moniliasis (*see also* Candidiasis) B37.9
  neonatal P37.5
Monitoring (encounter for)
  therapeutic drug level Z51.81
Monkey malaria B53.1
Monkeypox B04
Monoarthritis M13.10
  ankle M13.17-
  elbow M13.12-
  foot joint M13.17-
  hand joint M13.14-
  hip M13.15-
  knee M13.16-
  shoulder M13.11-
  wrist M13.13-
Monoblastic —*see* condition
Monochromat (ism), monochromatopsia
  (acquired) (congenital) H53.51
Monocytic —*see* condition
Monocytopenia D72.818
Monocytosis (symptomatic) D72.821
Monomania —*see* Psychosis
Mononeuritis G58.9
  cranial nerve —*see* Disorder, nerve,
    cranial
  femoral nerve G57.2-
  lateral
    cutaneous nerve of thigh G57.1-
    popliteal nerve G57.3-
  lower limb G57.9-
    specified nerve NEC G57.8-
  medial popliteal nerve G57.4-
  median nerve G56.1-
  multiplex G58.7
  plantar nerve G57.6-
  posterior tibial nerve G57.5-
  radial nerve G56.3-
  sciatic nerve G57.0-
  specified NEC G58.8
  tibial nerve G57.4-
  ulnar nerve G56.2-
  upper limb G56.9-
    specified nerve NEC G56.8-
  vestibular —*see* subcategory H93.3
Mononeuropathy G58.9
  carpal tunnel syndrome —*see* Syndrome,
    carpal tunnel
  diabetic NEC —*see* E08-E13 with .41
  femoral nerve —*see* Lesion, nerve, femoral
  ilioinguinal nerve G57.8-
  in diseases classified elsewhere —*see* category
    G59 ◄
  intercostal G58.0
  lower limb G57.9-
    causalgia —*see* Causalgia, lower limb
    femoral nerve —*see* Lesion, nerve, femoral
    meralgia paresthetica G57.1-
    plantar nerve —*see* Lesion, nerve, plantar
    popliteal nerve —*see* Lesion, nerve,
      popliteal

Mononeuropathy *(Continued)*
  lower limb *(Continued)*
    sciatic nerve —*see* Lesion, nerve, sciatic
    specified NEC G57.8-
    tarsal tunnel syndrome —*see* Syndrome,
      tarsal tunnel
  median nerve —*see* Lesion, nerve, median
  multiplex G58.7
  obturator nerve G57.8-
  popliteal nerve —*see* Lesion, nerve, popliteal
  radial nerve —*see* Lesion, nerve, radial
  saphenous nerve G57.8-
  specified NEC G58.8
  tarsal tunnel syndrome —*see* Syndrome,
    tarsal tunnel
  tuberculous A17.83
  ulnar nerve —*see* Lesion, nerve, ulnar
  upper limb G56.9-
    carpal tunnel syndrome —*see* Syndrome,
      carpal tunnel
    causalgia —*see* Causalgia
    median nerve —*see* Lesion, nerve, median
    radial nerve —*see* Lesion, nerve, radial
    specified site NEC G56.8-
    ulnar nerve —*see* Lesion, nerve, ulnar
Mononucleosis, infectious B27.90
  with
    complication NEC B27.99
    meningitis B27.92
    polyneuropathy B27.91
  cytomegaloviral B27.10
    with
      complication NEC B27.19
      meningitis B27.12
      polyneuropathy B27.11
  Epstein-Barr (virus) B27.00
    with
      complication NEC B27.09
      meningitis B27.02
      polyneuropathy B27.01
  gammaherpesviral B27.00
    with
      complication NEC B27.09
      meningitis B27.02
      polyneuropathy B27.01
  specified NEC B27.80
    with
      complication NEC B27.89
      meningitis B27.82
      polyneuropathy B27.81
Monoplegia G83.3-
  congenital (cerebral) G80.8
    spastic G80.1
  embolic (current episode) I63.4
  following
    cerebrovascular disease
      cerebral infarction
        lower limb I69.34-
        upper limb I69.33-
      intracerebral hemorrhage
        lower limb I69.14-
        upper limb I69.13-
      lower limb I69.94-
      nontraumatic intracranial hemorrhage
        NEC
        lower limb I69.24-
        upper limb I69.23-
      specified disease NEC
        lower limb I69.84-
        upper limb I69.83-
      stroke NOS
        lower limb I69.34-
        upper limb I69.33-
      subarachnoid hemorrhage
        lower limb I69.04-
        upper limb I69.03-
      upper limb I69.93-
  hysterical (transient) F44.4
  lower limb G83.1-
  psychogenic (conversion reaction) F44.4
  thrombotic (current episode) I63.3

Monoplegia *(Continued)*
  transient R29.818
  upper limb G83.2-
Monorchism, monorchidism Q55.0
Monosomy (*see also* Deletion, chromosome)
  Q93.9
  specified NEC Q93.89
  whole chromosome
    meiotic nondisjunction Q93.0
    mitotic nondisjunction Q93.1
    mosaicism Q93.1
  X Q96.9
Monster, monstrosity (single) Q89.7
  acephalic Q00.0
  twin Q89.4
Monteggia's fracture (-dislocation) S52.27-
Mooren's ulcer (cornea) —*see* Ulcer, cornea,
  Mooren's
Moore's syndrome —*see* Epilepsy, specified
  NEC
Mooser-Neill reaction A75.2
Mooser's bodies A75.2
Morbidity not stated or unknown R69
Morbilli —*see* Measles
Morbus —*see also* Disease
  angelicus, anglorum E55.0
  Beigel B36.2
  caducus —*see* Epilepsy
  celiacus K90.0
  comitialis —*see* Epilepsy
  cordis (*see also* Disease, heart) I51.9
    valvulorum —*see* Endocarditis
  coxae senilis M16.9
    tuberculous A18.02
  hemorrhagicus neonatorum P53
  maculosus neonatorum P54.5
Morel (-Stewart)(-Morgagni) syndrome M85.2
Morel-Kraepelin disease —*see* Schizophrenia
Morel-Moore syndrome M85.2
Morgagni's
  cyst, organ, hydatid, or appendage
    female Q50.5
    male (epididymal) Q55.4
      testicular Q55.29
  syndrome M85.2
Morgagni-Stewart-Morel syndrome M85.2
Morgagni-Stokes-Adams syndrome I45.9
Morgagni-Turner (-Albright) syndrome Q96.9
Moria F07.0
Moron (I.Q. 50-69) F70 ◄▥
Morphea L94.0
Morphinism (without remission) F11.20
  with remission F11.21
Morphinomania (without remission) F11.20
  with remission F11.21
Morquio (-Ullrich)(-Brailsford) disease or
  syndrome —*see* Mucopolysaccharidosis
Mortification (dry) (moist) —*see* Gangrene
Morton's metatarsalgia (neuralgia)(neuroma)
  (syndrome) G57.6
Morvan's disease or syndrome G60.8
Mosaicism, mosaic (autosomal) (chromosomal)
  45,X/46,XX Q96.3
  45,X/other cell lines NEC with abnormal sex
    chromosome Q96.4
  sex chromosome
    female Q97.8
    lines with various numbers of X
      chromosomes Q97.2
    male Q98.7
  XY Q96.3
Moschowitz' disease M31.1
Mother yaw A66.0
Motion sickness (from travel, any vehicle)
  (from roundabouts or swings) T75.3
Mottled, mottling, teeth (enamel) (endemic)
  (nonendemic) K00.3
Mounier-Kuhn syndrome Q32.4
  with bronchiectasis J47.9
    exacerbation (acute) J47.1
    lower respiratory infection J47.0

Mounier-Kuhn syndrome *(Continued)*
  acquired J98.09
    with bronchiectasis J47.9
      with
        exacerbation (acute) J47.1
        lower respiratory infection J47.0
Mountain
  sickness T70.29
    with polycythemia , acquired (acute) D75.1
  tick fever A93.2
Mouse, joint —*see* Loose, body, joint
  knee M23.4-
Mouth —*see* condition
Movable
  coccyx —*see* subcategory M53.2
  kidney N28.89
    congenital Q63.8
  spleen D73.89
Movements, dystonic R25.8
Moyamoya disease I67.5
MRSA (Methicillin resistant Staphylococcus
    aureus)
  infection A49.02
    as the cause of diseases classified
      elsewhere B95.62
  sepsis A41.02
MSSA (Methicillin susceptible Staphylococcus
    aureus)
  infection A49.01
    as the cause of diseases classified
      elsewhere B95.61
  sepsis A41.01
Mucha-Habermann disease L41.0
Mucinosis (cutaneous) (focal) (papular)
    (reticular erythematous) (skin) L98.5
  oral K13.79
Mucocele
  appendix K38.8
  buccal cavity K13.79
  gallbladder K82.1
  lacrimal sac, chronic H04.43-
  nasal sinus J34.1
  nose J34.1
  salivary gland (any) K11.6
  sinus (accessory) (nasal) J34.1
  turbinate (bone) (middle) (nasal) J34.1
  uterus N85.8
Mucolipidosis
  I E77.1
  II, III E77.0
  IV E75.11
Mucopolysaccharidosis E76.3
  beta-gluduronidase deficiency E76.29
  cardiopathy E76.3 *[152]*
  Hunter's syndrome E76.1
  Hurler's syndrome E76.01
  Hurler-Scheie syndrome E76.02
  Maroteaux-Lamy syndrome E76.29
  Morquio syndrome E76.219
    A E76.210
    B E76.211
    classic E76.210
  Sanfilippo syndrome E76.22
  Scheie's syndrome E76.03
  specified NEC E76.29
  type
    I
      Hurler's syndrome E76.01
      Hurler-Scheie syndrome E76.02
      Scheie's syndrome E76.03
    II E76.1
    III E76.22
    IV E76.219
    IVA E76.210
    IVB E76.211
    VI E76.29
    VII E76.29
Mucormycosis B46.5
  cutaneous B46.3
  disseminated B46.4
  gastrointestinal B46.2

Mucormycosis *(Continued)*
  generalized B46.4
  pulmonary B46.0
  rhinocerebral B46.1
  skin B46.3
  subcutaneous B46.3
Mucositis (ulcerative) K12.30
  due to drugs NEC K12.32
  gastrointestinal K92.81
  mouth (oral) (oropharyngeal) K12.30
    due to antineoplastic therapy K12.31
    due to drugs NEC K12.32
    due to radiation K12.33
    specified NEC K12.39
    viral K12.39
  nasal J34.81
  oral cavity —*see* Mucositis, mouth
  oral soft tissues —*see* Mucositis, mouth
  vagina and vulva N76.81
Mucositis necroticans agranulocytica —*see*
    Agranulocytosis
Mucous —*see also* condition
  patches (syphilitic) A51.39
    congenital A50.07
Mucoviscidosis E84.9
  with meconium obstruction E84.11
Mucus
  asphyxia or suffocation —*see* Asphyxia,
    mucus
  in stool R19.5
  plug —*see* Asphyxia, mucus
Muguet B37.0
Mulberry molars (congenital syphilis) A50.52
Müllerian mixed tumor
  specified site —*see* Neoplasm, malignant, by
    site
  unspecified site C54.9
Multicystic kidney (development) Q61.4
Multiparity (grand) Z64.1
  affecting management of pregnancy, labor
    and delivery (supervision only)
    O09.4-
  requiring contraceptive management —*see*
    Contraception
Multipartita placenta O43.19-
Multiple, multiplex —*see also* condition
  digits (congenital) Q69.9
  endocrine neoplasia —*see* Neoplasia,
    endocrine, multiple [MEN]
  personality F44.81
Mumps B26.9
  arthritis B26.85
  complication NEC B26.89
  encephalitis B26.2
  hepatitis B26.81
  meningitis (aseptic) B26.1
  meningoencephalitis B26.2
  myocarditis B26.82
  oophoritis B26.89
  orchitis B26.0
  pancreatitis B26.3
  polyneuropathy B26.84
Mumu (see also Infestation, filarial) B74.9 *[N51]*
Münchhausen's syndrome —*see* Disorder,
    factitious
Münchmeyer's syndrome —*see* Myositis,
    ossificans, progressiva
Mural —*see* condition
Murmur (cardiac) (heart) (organic) R01.1
  abdominal R19.15
  aortic (valve) —*see* Endocarditis, aortic
  benign R01.0
  diastolic —*see* Endocarditis
  Flint I35.1
  functional R01.0
  Graham Steell I37.1
  innocent R01.0
  mitral (valve) —*see* Insufficiency, mitral
  nonorganic R01.0
  presystolic, mitral —*see* Insufficiency, mitral
  pulmonic (valve) I37.8

Murmur *(Continued)*
  systolic (valvular) —*see* Endocarditis
  tricuspid (valve) I07.9
  valvular —*see* Endocarditis
Murri's disease (intermittent hemoglobinuria)
    D59.6
Muscle, muscular —*see also* condition
  carnitine (palmityltransferase) deficiency
    E71.314
Musculoneuralgia —*see* Neuralgia
Mushroom-workers' (pickers') disease or lung
    J67.5
Mushrooming hip —*see* Derangement, joint,
    specified NEC, hip
Mutation (s)
  factor V Leiden D68.51
  surfactant, of lung J84.83
  prothrombin gene D68.52
Mutism —*see also* Aphasia
  deaf (acquired) (congenital) NEC H91.3
  elective (adjustment reaction) (childhood)
    F94.0
  hysterical F44.4
  selective (childhood) F94.0
MVD (microvillus inclusion disease) Q43.8
MVID (microvillus inclusion disease) Q43.8
Myalgia M79.1
  epidemic (cervical) B33.0
  traumatic NEC T14.8
Myasthenia G70.9
  congenital G70.2
  cordis —*see* Failure, heart
  developmental G70.2
  gravis G70.00
    with exacerbation (acute) G70.01
    in crisis G70.01
  neonatal, transient P94.0
  pseudoparalytica G70.00
    with exacerbation (acute) G70.01
    in crisis G70.01
  stomach, psychogenic F45.8
  syndrome
    in
      diabetes mellitus —*see* E08-E13 with .44
      neoplastic disease (see also Neoplasm)
        D49.9 *[G73.3]*
      pernicious anemia D51.0 *[G73.3]*
      thyrotoxicosis E05.90 *[G73.3]*
        with thyroid storm E05.91 *[G73.3]*
Myasthenic M62.81
Mycelium infection B49
Mycetismus —*see* Poisoning, food, noxious,
    mushroom
Mycetoma B47.9
  actinomycotic B47.1
  bone (mycotic) B47.9 *[M90.80]*
  eumycotic B47.0
  foot B47.9
    actinomycotic B47.1
    mycotic B47.0
  madurae NEC B47.9
    mycotic B47.0
  maduromycotic B47.0
  mycotic B47.0
  nocardial B47.1
Mycobacteriosis —*see* Mycobacterium
Mycobacterium, mycobacterial (infection)
    A31.9
  anonymous A31.9
  atypical A31.9
    cutaneous A31.1
    pulmonary A31.0
      tuberculous —*see* Tuberculosis,
        pulmonary
    specified site NEC A31.8
  avium (intracellulare complex) A31.0
  balnei A31.1
  Battey A31.0
  chelonei A31.8
  cutaneous A31.1
  extrapulmonary systemic A31.8

◀ New　◀═ Revised　~~deleted~~ Deleted

Myocarditis *(Continued)*
meningococcal A39.52
mumps B26.82
nonrheumatic, active I40.9
parenchymatous I40.9
pneumococcal I40.0
rheumatic (chronic) (inactive) (with chorea)
I09.0
active or acute I01.2
with chorea (acute) (rheumatic)
(Sydenham's) I02.0
rheumatoid —*see* Rheumatoid, carditis
septic I40.0
staphylococcal I40.0
suppurative I40.0
syphilitic (chronic) A52.06
toxic I40.8
rheumatic —*see* Myocarditis, acute,
rheumatic
tuberculous A18.84
typhoid A01.02
valvular —*see* Endocarditis
virus, viral I40.0
of newborn (Coxsackie) B33.22
Myocardium, myocardial —*see* condition
Myocardosis —*see* Cardiomyopathy
Myoclonus, myoclonic, myoclonia (familial)
(essential) (multifocal) (simplex) G25.3
drug-induced G25.3
epilepsy (*see also* Epilepsy, generalized,
specified NEC) G40.4-
familial (progressive) G25.3
epileptica G40.409
with status epilepticus G40.401
facial G51.3
familial progressive G25.3
Friedreich's G25.3
jerks G25.3
massive G25.3
palatal G25.3
pharyngeal G25.3
Myocytolysis I51.5
Myodiastasis —*see* Diastasis, muscle
Myoendocarditis —*see* Endocarditis
Myoepithelioma —*see* Neoplasm, benign, by
site
Myofasciitis (acute) —*see* Myositis
Myofibroma —*see also* Neoplasm, connective
tissue, benign
uterus (cervix) (corpus) —*see* Leiomyoma
Myofibromatosis D48.1
infantile Q89.8
Myofibrosis M62.89
heart —*see* Myocarditis
scapulohumeral —*see* Lesion, shoulder,
specified NEC
Myofibrositis M79.7
scapulohumeral —*see* Lesion, shoulder,
specified NEC
Myoglobulinuria, myoglobinuria (primary)
R82.1
Myokymia, facial G51.4
Myolipoma —*see* Lipoma
Myoma —*see also* Neoplasm, connective tissue,
benign
malignant —*see* Neoplasm, connective tissue,
malignant
prostate D29.1
uterus (cervix) (corpus) —*see* Leiomyoma
Myomalacia M62.89
Myometritis —*see* Endometritis
Myometrium —*see* condition
Myonecrosis, clostridial A48.0
Myopathy G72.9
acute
necrotizing G72.81
quadriplegic G72.81
alcoholic G72.1
benign congenital G71.2
central core G71.2
centronuclear G71.2

Myopathy *(Continued)*
congenital (benign) G71.2
critical illness G72.81
distal G71.0
drug-induced G72.0
endocrine NEC E34.9 *[G73.7]*
extraocular muscles H05.82-
facioscapulohumeral G71.0
hereditary G71.9
specified NEC G71.8
immune NEC G72.49
in (due to)
Addison's disease E27.1 *[G73.7]*
alcohol G72.1
amyloidosis E85.0 *[G73.7]*
cretinism E00.9 *[G73.7]*
Cushing's syndrome E24.9 *[G73.7]*
drugs G72.0
endocrine disease NEC E34.9 *[G73.7]*
giant cell arteritis M31.6 *[G73.7]*
glycogen storage disease E74.00 *[G73.7]*
hyperadrenocorticism E24.9 *[G73.7]*
hyperparathyroidism NEC E21.3 *[G73.7]*
hypoparathyroidism E20.9 *[G73.7]*
hypopituitarism E23.0 *[G73.7]*
hypothyroidism E03.9 *[G73.7]*
infectious disease NEC B99 *[G73.7]*
lipid storage disease E75.6 *[G73.7]*
metabolic disease NEC E88.9 *[G73.7]*
myxedema E03.9 *[G73.7]*
parasitic disease NEC B89 *[G73.7]*
polyarteritis nodosa M30.0 *[G73.7]*
rheumatoid arthritis —*see* Rheumatoid,
myopathy
sarcoidosis D86.87
scleroderma M34.82
sicca syndrome M35.03
Sjögren's syndrome M35.03
systemic lupus erythematosus M32.19
thyrotoxicosis (hyperthyroidism) E05.90
[G73.7]
with thyroid storm E05.91 *[G73.7]*
toxic agent NEC G72.2
inflammatory NEC G72.49
intensive care (ICU) G72.81
limb-girdle G71.0
mitochondrial NEC G71.3
myotubular G71.2
mytonic, proximal (PROMM) G71.11
nemaline G71.2
ocular G71.0
oculopharyngeal G71.0
of critical illness G72.81
primary G71.9
specified NEC G71.8
progressive NEC G72.89
proximal myotonic (PROMM) G71.11
rod G71.2
scapulohumeral G71.0
specified NEC G72.89
toxic G72.2
Myopericarditis —*see also* Pericarditis
chronic rheumatic I09.2
Myopia (axial) (congenital) H52.1-
degenerative (malignant) H44.2-
malignant H44.2-
pernicious H44.2-
progressive high (degenerative) H44.2-
Myosarcoma —*see* Neoplasm, connective tissue,
malignant
Myosis (pupil) H57.03
stromal (endolymphatic) D39.0
Myositis M60.9
clostridial A48.0
due to posture —*see* Myositis, specified type
NEC
epidemic B33.0
fibrosa or fibrous (chronic), Volkmann's
T79.6
foreign body granuloma —*see* Granuloma,
foreign body

Myositis *(Continued)*
in (due to)
bilharziasis B65.9 *[M63.8-]*
cysticercosis B69.81
leprosy A30.9 *[M63.8-]*
mycosis B49 *[M63.8-]*
sarcoidosis D86.87
schistosomiasis B65.9 *[M63.8-]*
syphilis
late A52.78
secondary A51.49
toxoplasmosis (acquired) B58.82
trichinellosis B75 *[M63.8-]*
tuberculosis A18.09
inclusion body [IBM] G72.41
infective M60.009
arm M60.002
left M60.001
right M60.000
leg M60.005
left M60.004
right M60.003
lower limb M60.005
ankle M60.07-
foot M60.07-
lower leg M60.06-
thigh M60.05-
toe M60.07-
multiple sites M60.09
specified site NEC M60.08
upper limb M60.002
finger M60.04-
forearm M60.03-
hand M60.04-
shoulder region M60.01-
upper arm M60.02-
interstitial M60.10
ankle M60.17-
foot M60.17-
forearm M60.13-
hand M60.14-
lower leg M60.16-
multiple sites M60.19
shoulder region M60.11-
specified site NEC M60.18
thigh M60.15-
upper arm M60.12-
mycotic B49 *[M63.8-]*
ossificans or ossifying (circumscripta) —*see
also* Ossification, muscle, specified NEC
in (due to)
burns M61.30
ankle M61.37-
foot M61.37-
forearm M61.33-
hand M61.34-
lower leg M61.36-
multiple sites M61.39
pelvic region M61.35-
shoulder region M61.31-
specified site NEC M61.38
thigh M61.35-
upper arm M61.32-
quadriplegia or paraplegia M61.20
ankle M61.27-
foot M61.27-
forearm M61.23-
hand M61.24-
lower leg M61.26-
multiple sites M61.29
pelvic region M61.25-
shoulder region M61.21-
specified site NEC M61.28
thigh M61.25-
upper arm M61.22-
progressiva M61.10
ankle M61.17-
finger M61.14-
foot M61.17-
forearm M61.13-
hand M61.14-

Myositis *(Continued)*
　ossificans or ossifying *(Continued)*
　　progressiva *(Continued)*
　　　lower leg M61.16-
　　　multiple sites M61.19
　　　pelvic region M61.15-
　　　shoulder region M61.11-
　　　specified site NEC M61.18
　　　thigh M61.15-
　　　toe M61.17-
　　　upper arm M61.12-
　　traumatica M61.00
　　　ankle M61.07-
　　　foot M61.07-
　　　forearm M61.03-
　　　hand M61.04-
　　　lower leg M61.06-
　　　multiple sites M61.09
　　　pelvic region M61.05-
　　　shoulder region M61.01-
　　　specified site NEC M61.08
　　　thigh M61.05-
　　　upper arm M61.02-
　purulent —*see* Myositis, infective
　specified type NEC M60.80
　　ankle M60.87-
　　foot M60.87-
　　forearm M60.83-
　　hand M60.84-
　　lower leg M60.86-
　　multiple sites M60.89
　　pelvic region M60.85-

Myositis *(Continued)*
　specified type NEC *(Continued)*
　　shoulder region M60.81-
　　specified site NEC M60.88
　　thigh M60.85-
　　upper arm M60.82-
　suppurative —*see* Myositis, infective
　traumatic (old) —*see* Myositis, specified type
　　NEC
Myospasia impulsiva F95.2
Myotonia (acquisita) (intermittens) M62.89
　atrophica G71.11
　chondrodystrophic G71.13
　congenita (acetazolamide responsive)
　　(dominant) (recessive) G71.12
　drug-induced G71.14
　dystrophica G71.11
　fluctuans G71.19
　levior G71.12
　permanens G71.19
　symptomatic G71.19
Myotonic pupil —*see* Anomaly, pupil, function,
　tonic pupil
Myriapodiasis B88.2
Myringitis H73.2-
　with otitis media —*see* Otitis, media
　acute H73.00-
　　bullous H73.01-
　　specified NEC H73.09-
　bullous —*see* Myringitis, acute, bullous
　chronic H73.1-
Mysophobia F40.228

Mytilotoxism —*see* Poisoning, fish
Myxadenitis labialis K13.0
Myxedema (adult) (idiocy) (infantile) (juvenile)
　(*see also* Hypothyroidism) E03.9
　circumscribed E05.90
　　with storm E05.91
　coma E03.5
　congenital E00.1
　cutis L98.5
　localized (pretibial) E05.90
　　with storm E05.91
　papular L98.5
Myxochondrosarcoma —*see* Neoplasm,
　cartilage, malignant
Myxofibroma —*see* Neoplasm, connective
　tissue, benign
　odontogenic —*see* Cyst, calcifying
　　odontogenic
Myxofibrosarcoma —*see* Neoplasm, connective
　tissue, malignant
Myxolipoma D17.9
Myxoliposarcoma —*see* Neoplasm, connective
　tissue, malignant
Myxoma —*see also* Neoplasm, connective tissue,
　benign
　nerve sheath —*see* Neoplasm, nerve,
　　benign
　odontogenic —*see* Cyst, calcifying
　　odontogenic
Myxosarcoma —*see* Neoplasm, connective
　tissue, malignant

M

◄ New　◄▥▥ Revised　~~deleted~~ Deleted

N

Naegeli's
  disease Q82.8
  leukemia, monocytic C93.1-
Naegleriasis (with meningoencephalitis) B60.2
Naffziger's syndrome G54.0
Naga sore —see Ulcer, skin
Nägele's pelvis M95.5
  with disproportion (fetopelvic) O33.0
    causing obstructed labor O65.0
Nail —see also condition
  biting F98.8
  patella syndrome Q87.2
Nanism, nanosomia —see Dwarfism
Nanophyetiasis B66.8
Nanukayami A27.89
Napkin rash L22
Narcolepsy G47.419
  with cataplexy G47.411
  in conditions classified elsewhere G47.429
    with cataplexy G47.421
Narcosis R06.89
Narcotism —see Dependence
NARP (Neuropathy, Ataxia and Retinitis
    pigmentosa) syndrome E88.49
Narrow
  anterior chamber angle H40.03-
  pelvis —see Contraction, pelvis
Narrowing —see also Stenosis
  artery I77.1
    auditory, internal I65.8
    basilar —see Occlusion, artery, basilar
    carotid —see Occlusion, artery, carotid
    cerebellar —see Occlusion, artery, cerebellar
    cerebral —see Occlusion artery, cerebral
    choroidal —see Occlusion, artery, cerebral,
      specified NEC
    communicating posterior —see Occlusion,
      artery, cerebral, specified NEC
    coronary —see also Disease, heart, ischemic,
      atherosclerotic
      congenital Q24.5
      syphilitic A50.54 [I52]
      due to syphilis NEC A52.06
    hypophyseal —see Occlusion, artery,
      cerebral, specified NEC
    pontine —see Occlusion, artery, cerebral,
      specified NEC
    precerebral —see Occlusion, artery,
      precerebral
    vertebral —see Occlusion, artery, vertebral
  auditory canal (external) —see Stenosis,
    external ear canal
  eustachian tube —see Obstruction, eustachian
    tube
  eyelid —see Disorder, eyelid function
  larynx J38.6
  mesenteric artery K55.0
  palate M26.89
  palpebral fissure —see Disorder, eyelid
    function
  ureter N13.5
    with infection N13.6
  urethra —see Stricture, urethra
Narrowness, abnormal, eyelid Q10.3
Nasal —see condition
Nasolachrymal, nasolacrimal —see condition
Nasopharyngeal —see also condition
  pituitary gland Q89.2
  torticollis M43.6
Nasopharyngitis (acute) (infective)
    (streptococcal) (subacute) J00
  chronic (suppurative) (ulcerative) J31.1
Nasopharynx, nasopharyngeal —see condition
Natal tooth, teeth K00.6
Nausea (without vomiting) R11.0
  with vomiting R11.2
  gravidarum —see Hyperemesis, gravidarum
  marina T75.3
  navalis T75.3

Navel —see condition
Neapolitan fever —see Brucellosis
Near drowning T75.1
Nearsightedness —see Myopia
Near-syncope R55
Nebula, cornea —see Opacity, cornea
Necator americanus infestation B76.1
Necatoriasis B76.1
Neck —see condition
Necrobiosis R68.89
  lipoidica NEC L92.1
    with diabetes —see E08-E13 with .620
Necrolysis, toxic epidermal L51.2
  due to drug
    correct substance properly administered —
      see Table of Drugs and Chemicals,
      by drug, adverse effect
    overdose or wrong substance given or
      taken —see Table of Drugs and
      Chemicals, by drug, poisoning
Necrophilia F65.89
Necrosis, necrotic (ischemic) —see also
    Gangrene
  adrenal (capsule) (gland) E27.49
  amputation stump (surgical) (late)
    T87.50
    arm T87.5-
    leg T87.5-
  antrum J32.0
  aorta (hyaline) —see also Aneurysm, aorta
    cystic medial —see Dissection, aorta
  artery I77.5
  bladder (aseptic) (sphincter) N32.89
  bone (see also Osteonecrosis) M87.9
    aseptic or avascular —see Osteonecrosis
      idiopathic M87.00
    ethmoid J32.2
    jaw M27.2
    tuberculous —see Tuberculosis, bone
  brain I67.89
  breast (aseptic) (fat) (segmental) N64.1
  bronchus J98.09
  central nervous system NEC I67.89
  cerebellar I67.89
  cerebral I67.89
  colon K55.0
  cornea H18.40
  cortical (acute) (renal) N17.1
  cystic medial (aorta) —see Dissection, aorta
  dental pulp K04.1
  esophagus K22.8
  ethmoid (bone) J32.2
  eyelid —see Disorder, eyelid, degenerative
  fat, fatty (generalized) —see also Disorder, soft
    tissue, specified type NEC
    abdominal wall K65.4
    breast (aseptic) (segmental) N64.1
    localized —see Degeneration, by site,
      fatty
    mesentery K65.4
    omentum K65.4
    pancreas K86.8
    peritoneum K65.4
    skin (subcutaneous), newborn P83.0
    subcutaneous, due to birth injury P15.6
  gallbladder —see Cholecystitis, acute
  heart —see Infarct, myocardium
  hip, aseptic or avascular —see Osteonecrosis,
    by type, femur
  intestine (acute) (hemorrhagic) (massive)
    K55.0
  jaw M27.2
  kidney (bilateral) N28.0
    acute N17.9
    cortical (acute) (bilateral) N17.1
      with ectopic or molar pregnancy
        O08.4
    medullary (bilateral) (in acute renal
      failure) (papillary) N17.2
    papillary (bilateral) (in acute renal
      failure) N17.2

Necrosis, necrotic (Continued)
  kidney (Continued)
    tubular N17.0
      with ectopic or molar pregnancy O08.4
      complicating
        abortion —see Abortion, by type,
          complicated by, tubular necrosis
        ectopic or molar pregnancy O08.4
        pregnancy —see Pregnancy,
          complicated by, diseases of,
          specified type or system NEC
      following ectopic or molar pregnancy
        O08.4
      traumatic T79.5
  larynx J38.7
  liver (with hepatic failure) (cell) —see Failure,
    hepatic
    hemorrhagic, central K76.2
  lung J85.0
  lymphatic gland —see Lymphadenitis, acute
  mammary gland (fat) (segmental) N64.1
  mastoid (chronic) —see Mastoiditis, chronic
  medullary (acute) (renal) N17.2
  mesentery K55.0
    fat K65.4
  mitral valve —see Insufficiency, mitral
  myocardium, myocardial —see Infarct,
    myocardium
  nose J34.0
  omentum (with mesenteric infarction)
    K55.0
    fat K65.4
  orbit, orbital —see Osteomyelitis, orbit
  ossicles, ear —see Abnormal, ear ossicles
  ovary N70.92
  pancreas (aseptic) (duct) (fat) K86.8
    acute (infective) —see Pancreatitis, acute
    infective —see Pancreatitis, acute
  papillary (acute) (renal) N17.2
  perineum N90.89
  peritoneum (with mesenteric infarction)
    K55.0
    fat K65.4
  pharynx J02.9
    in granulocytopenia —see Neutropenia
    Vincent's A69.1
  phosphorus —see subcategory T54.2
  pituitary (gland) (postpartum) (Sheehan)
    E23.0
  pressure —see Ulcer, pressure, by site
  pulmonary J85.0
  pulp (dental) K04.1
  radiation —see Necrosis, by site
  radium —see Necrosis, by site
  renal —see Necrosis, kidney
  sclera H15.89
  scrotum N50.8
  skin or subcutaneous tissue NEC I96
  spine, spinal (column) —see also
    Osteonecrosis, by type, vertebra
    cord G95.19
  spleen D73.5
  stomach K31.89
  stomatitis (ulcerative) A69.0
  subcutaneous fat, newborn P83.8
  subendocardial (acute) I21.4
    chronic I25.89
  suprarenal (capsule) (gland) E27.49
  testis N50.8
  thymus (gland) E32.8
  tonsil J35.8
  trachea J39.8
  tuberculous NEC —see Tuberculosis
  tubular (acute) (anoxic) (renal) (toxic) N17.0
    postprocedural N99.0
  vagina N89.8
  vertebra —see also Osteonecrosis, by type,
    vertebra
    tuberculous A18.01
  vulva N90.89
  X-ray —see Necrosis, by site

Necrospermia —*see* Infertility, male
Need (for)
  care provider because (of)
    assistance with personal care Z74.1
    continuous supervision required Z74.3
    impaired mobility Z74.09
    no other household member able to render
      care Z74.2
    specified reason NEC Z74.8
  immunization —*see* Vaccination
  vaccination —*see* Vaccination
Neglect
  adult
    confirmed T74.01
    history of Z91.412
    suspected T76.01
  child (childhood)
    confirmed T74.02
    history of Z62.812
    suspected T76.02
  emotional, in childhood Z62.898
  hemispatial R41.4
  left-sided R41.4
  sensory R41.4
  visuospatial R41.4
Neisserian infection NEC —*see* Gonococcus
Nelaton's syndrome G60.8
Nelson's syndrome E24.1
Nematodiasis (intestinal) B82.0
  Ancylostoma B76.0
Neonatal —*see also* Newborn
  acne L70.4
  bradycardia P29.12
  screening, abnormal findings on P09
  tachycardia P29.11
  tooth, teeth K00.6
Neonatorum —*see* condition
Neoplasia
  endocrine, multiple (MEN) E31.20
    type I E31.21
    type IIA E31.22
    type IIB E31.23
  intraepithelial (histologically confirmed)
    anal (AIN) (histologically confirmed)
      K62.82
      grade I K62.82
      grade II K62.82
      severe D01.3
    cervical glandular (histologically
      confirmed) D06.9
    cervix (uteri) (CIN) (histologically
      confirmed) N87.9
      glandular D06.9
      grade I N87.0
      grade II N87.1
      grade III (severe dysplasia) —*see also*
        Carcinoma, cervix uteri, in situ
        D06.9
    prostate (histologically confirmed) (PIN I)
      (PIN II) N42.3
      grade I N42.3
      grade II N42.3
      severe D07.5
    vagina (histologically confirmed) (VAIN)
      N89.3
      grade I N89.0
      grade II N89.1
      grade III (severe dysplasia) D07.2
    vulva (histologically confirmed) (VIN)
      N90.3
      grade I N90.0
      grade II N90.1
      grade III (severe dysplasia) D07.1
Neoplasm, neoplastic —*see also* Table of
  Neoplasms
  lipomatous, benign —*see* Lipoma
Neovascularization
  ciliary body —*see* Disorder, iris, vascular
  cornea H16.40-
    deep H16.44-
      ghost vessels —*see* Ghost, vessels

Neovascularization (Continued)
  cornea (Continued)
    localized H16.43-
    pannus —*see* Pannus
  iris —*see* Disorder, iris, vascular
  retina H35.05-
Nephralgia N23
Nephritis, nephritic (albuminuric) (azotemic)
    (congenital) (disseminated) (epithelial)
    (familial) (focal) (granulomatous)
    (hemorrhagic) (infantile) (nonsuppurative,
    excretory) (uremic) N05.9
  with
    dense deposit disease N05.6
    diffuse
      crescentic glomerulonephritis N05.7
      endocapillary proliferative
        glomerulonephritis N05.4
      membranous glomerulonephritis
        N05.2
      mesangial proliferative
        glomerulonephritis N05.3
      mesangiocapillary glomerulonephritis
        N05.5
    edema —*see* Nephrosis
    focal and segmental glomerular lesions
      N05.1
    foot process disease N04.9
    glomerular lesion
      diffuse sclerosing N05.8
      hypocomplementemic —*see* Nephritis,
        membranoproliferative
      IgA —*see* Nephropathy, IgA
      lobular, lobulonodular —*see* Nephritis,
        membranoproliferative
      nodular —*see* Nephritis,
        membranoproliferative
    lesion of
      glomerulonephritis, proliferative
        N05.8
      renal necrosis N05.9
    minor glomerular abnormality N05.0
    specified morphological changes NEC
      N05.8
  acute N00.9
    with
      dense deposit disease N00.6
      diffuse
        crescentic glomerulonephritis
          N00.7
        endocapillary proliferative
          glomerulonephritis N00.4
        membranous glomerulonephritis
          N00.2
        mesangial proliferative
          glomerulonephritis N00.3
        mesangiocapillary glomerulonephritis
          N00.5
      focal and segmental glomerular lesions
        N00.1
      minor glomerular abnormality N00.0
      specified morphological changes NEC
        N00.8
    amyloid E85.4 [N08]
    antiglomerular basement membrane (anti-
      GBM) antibody NEC
      in Goodpasture's syndrome M31.0
    antitubular basement membrane
      (tubulo-interstitial) NEC N12
      toxic —*see* Nephropathy, toxic
    arteriolar —*see* Hypertension, kidney
    arteriosclerotic —*see* Hypertension,
      kidney
    ascending —*see* Nephritis, tubulo-interstitial
    atrophic N03.9
    Balkan (endemic) N15.0
    calculous, calculus —*see* Calculus,
      kidney
    cardiac —*see* Hypertension, kidney
    cardiovascular —*see* Hypertension,
      kidney

Nephritis, nephritic (Continued)
  chronic N03.9
    with
      dense deposit disease N03.6
      diffuse
        crescentic glomerulonephritis
          N03.7
        endocapillary proliferative
          glomerulonephritis N03.4
        membranous glomerulonephritis
          N03.2
        mesangial proliferative
          glomerulonephritis N03.3
        mesangiocapillary glomerulonephritis
          N03.5
      focal and segmental glomerular lesions
        N03.1
      minor glomerular abnormality
        N03.0
      specified morphological changes
        NEC N03.8
    arteriosclerotic —*see* Hypertension,
      kidney
  cirrhotic N26.9
  complicating pregnancy O26.83-
  croupous N00.9
  degenerative —*see* Nephrosis
  diffuse sclerosing N05.8
  due to
    diabetes mellitus —*see* E08-E13 with .21
    subacute bacterial endocarditis I33.0
    systemic lupus erythematosus (chronic)
      M32.14
    typhoid fever A01.09
  gonococcal (acute) (chronic) A54.21
  hypocomplementemic —*see* Nephritis,
    membranoproliferative
  IgA —*see* Nephropathy, IgA
  immune complex (circulating) NEC N05.8
  infective —*see* Nephritis, tubulo-interstitial
  interstitial —*see* Nephritis, tubulo-interstitial
  lead N14.3
  membranoproliferative (diffuse) (type 1 or 3)
    (*see also* N00-N07 with fourth character
    .5) N05.5
    type 2 (*see also* N00-N07 with fourth
      character .6) N05.6
  minimal change N05.0
  necrotic, necrotizing NEC (*see also*
    N00-N07 with fourth character .8)
    N05.8
  nephrotic —*see* Nephrosis
  nodular —*see* Nephritis,
    membranoproliferative
  polycystic Q61.3
    adult type Q61.2
    autosomal
      dominant Q61.2
      recessive NEC Q61.19
    childhood type NEC Q61.19
    infantile type NEC Q61.19
  poststreptococcal N05.9
    acute N00.9
    chronic N03.9
  rapidly progressive N01.9
  proliferative NEC (*see also* N00-N07 with
    fourth character .8) N05.8
  purulent —*see* Nephritis, tubulo-interstitial
  rapidly progressive N01.9
    with
      dense deposit disease N01.6
      diffuse
        crescentic glomerulonephritis N01.7
        endocapillary proliferative
          glomerulonephritis N01.4
        membranous glomerulonephritis
          N01.2
        mesangial proliferative
          glomerulonephritis N01.3
        mesangiocapillary glomerulonephritis
          N01.5

◀ New   ◀ Revised   ~~deleted~~ Deleted

Nephritis, nephritic *(Continued)*
  rapidly progressive *(Continued)*
    with *(Continued)*
      focal and segmental glomerular lesions
        N01.1
      minor glomerular abnormality N01.0
      specified morphological changes NEC
        N01.8
  salt losing or wasting NEC N28.89
  saturnine N14.3
  sclerosing, diffuse N05.8
  septic —*see* Nephritis, tubulo-interstitial
  specified pathology NEC *(see also* N00-N07
    with fourth character .8) N05.8
  subacute N01.9
  suppurative —*see* Nephritis,
    tubulo-interstitial
  syphilitic (late) A52.75
    congenital A50.59 *[N08]*
    early (secondary) A51.44
  toxic —*see* Nephropathy, toxic
  tubal, tubular —*see* Nephritis,
    tubulo-interstitial
  tuberculous A18.11
  tubulo-interstitial (in) N12
    acute (infectious) N10
    chronic (infectious) N11.9
      nonobstructive N11.8
        reflux-associated N11.0
      obstructive N11.1
      specified NEC N11.8
    due to
      brucellosis A23.9 *[N16]*
      cryoglobulinemia D89.1 *[N16]*
      glycogen storage disease E74.00
        [N16]
      Sjögren's syndrome M35.04
  vascular —*see* Hypertension, kidney
  war N00.9
Nephroblastoma (epithelial) (mesenchymal)
  C64-
Nephrocalcinosis E83.59 *[N29]*
Nephrocystitis, pustular —*see* Nephritis,
  tubulo-interstitial
Nephrolithiasis (congenital) (pelvis)
  (recurrent) —*see also* Calculus, kidney
Nephroma C64-
  mesoblastic D41.0-
Nephronephritis —*see* Nephrosis
Nephronophthisis Q61.5
Nephropathia epidemica A98.5
Nephropathy *(see also* Nephritis) N28.9
  with
    edema —*see* Nephrosis
    glomerular lesion —*see*
      Glomerulonephritis
  amyloid, hereditary E85.0
  analgesic N14.0
    with medullary necrosis, acute N17.2
  Balkan (endemic) N15.0
  chemical —*see* Nephropathy, toxic
  diabetic —*see* E08-E13 with .21
  drug-induced N14.2
    specified NEC N14.1
  focal and segmental hyalinosis or sclerosis
    N02.1
  heavy metal-induced N14.3
  hereditary NEC N07.9
    with
      dense deposit disease N07.6
      diffuse
        crescentic glomerulonephritis
          N07.7
        endocapillary proliferative
          glomerulonephritis N07.4
        membranous glomerulonephritis
          N07.2
        mesangial proliferative
          glomerulonephritis N07.3
        mesangiocapillary glomerulonephritis
          N07.5

Nephropathy *(Continued)*
  hereditary NEC *(Continued)*
    with *(Continued)*
      focal and segmental glomerular lesions
        N07.1
      minor glomerular abnormality N07.0
      specified morphological changes NEC
        N07.8
  hypercalcemic N25.89
  hypertensive —*see* Hypertension, kidney
  hypokalemic (vacuolar) N25.89
  IgA N02.8
    with glomerular lesion N02.9
      focal and segmental hyalinosis or
        sclerosis N02.1
      membranoproliferative (diffuse) N02.5
      membranous (diffuse) N02.2
      mesangial proliferative (diffuse) N02.3
      mesangiocapillary (diffuse) N02.5
      proliferative NEC N02.8
      specified pathology NEC N02.8
  lead N14.3
  membranoproliferative (diffuse) N02.5
  membranous (diffuse) N02.2
  mesangial (IgA/IgG) —*see* Nephropathy, IgA
    proliferative (diffuse) N02.3
  mesangiocapillary (diffuse) N02.5
  obstructive N13.8
  phenacetin N17.2
  phosphate-losing N25.0
  potassium depletion N25.89
  pregnancy-related O26.83-
  proliferative NEC *(see also* N00-N07 with
    fourth character .8) N05.8
  protein-losing N25.89
  saturnine N14.3
  sickle-cell D57.- *[N08]*
  toxic NEC N14.4
    due to
      drugs N14.2
        analgesic N14.0
        specified NEC N14.1
      heavy metals N14.3
  vasomotor N17.0
  water-losing N25.89
Nephroptosis N28.83
Nephropyosis —*see* Abscess, kidney
Nephrorrhagia N28.89
Nephrosclerosis (arteriolar) (arteriosclerotic)
  (chronic) (hyaline) —*see also* Hypertension,
  kidney
  hyperplastic —*see* Hypertension, kidney
  senile N26.9
Nephrosis, nephrotic (Epstein's) (syndrome)
  (congenital) N04.9
  with
    foot process disease N04.9
    glomerular lesion N04.1
    hypocomplementemic N04.5
  acute N04.9
  anoxic —*see* Nephrosis, tubular
  chemical —*see* Nephrosis, tubular
  cholemic K76.7
  diabetic —*see* E08-E13 with .21
  Finnish type (congenital) Q89.8
  hemoglobin N10
  hemoglobinuric —*see* Nephrosis, tubular
  in
    amyloidosis E85.4 *[N08]*
    diabetes mellitus —*see* E08-E13 with .21
    epidemic hemorrhagic fever A98.5
    malaria (malariae) B52.0
  ischemic —*see* Nephrosis, tubular
  lipoid N04.9
  lower nephron —*see* Nephrosis, tubular
  malarial (malariae) B52.0
  minimal change N04.0
  myoglobin N10
  necrotizing —*see* Nephrosis, tubular
  osmotic (sucrose) N25.89
  radiation N04.9

Nephrosis, nephrotic *(Continued)*
  syphilitic (late) A52.75
  toxic —*see* Nephrosis, tubular
  tubular (acute) N17.0
    postprocedural N99.0
    radiation N04.9
Nephrosonephritis, hemorrhagic (endemic)
  A98.5
Nephrostomy
  attention to Z43.6
  status Z93.6
Nerve —*see also* condition
  injury —*see* Injury, nerve, by body site
Nerves R45.0
Nervous *(see also* condition) R45.0
  heart F45.8
  stomach F45.8
  tension R45.0
Nervousness R45.0
Nesidioblastoma
  pancreas D13.7
  specified site NEC —*see* Neoplasm, benign,
    by site
  unspecified site D13.7
Nettleship's syndrome Q82.2
Neumann's disease or syndrome L10.1
Neuralgia, neuralgic (acute) M79.2
  accessory (nerve) G52.8
  acoustic (nerve) —*see* subcategory
    H93.3
  auditory (nerve) —*see* subcategory
    H93.3
  ciliary G44.009
    intractable G44.001
    not intractable G44.009
  cranial
    nerve —*see also* Disorder, nerve, cranial
      fifth or trigeminal —*see* Neuralgia,
        trigeminal
      postherpetic, postzoster B02.29
  ear —*see* subcategory H92.0
  facialis vera G51.1
  Fothergill's —*see* Neuralgia, trigeminal
  glossopharyngeal (nerve) G52.1
  Horton's G44.099
    intractable G44.091
    not intractable G44.099
  Hunt's B02.21
  hypoglossal (nerve) G52.3
  infraorbital —*see* Neuralgia, trigeminal
  malarial —*see* Malaria
  migrainous G44.009
    intractable G44.001
    not intractable G44.009
  Morton's G57.6-
  nerve, cranial —*see* Disorder, nerve,
    cranial
  nose G52.0
  occipital M54.81
  olfactory G52.0
  penis N48.9
  perineum R10.2
  postherpetic NEC B02.29
    trigeminal B02.22
  pubic region R10.2
  scrotum R10.2
  Sluder's G44.89
  specified nerve NEC G58.8
  spermatic cord R10.2
  sphenopalatine (ganglion) G90.09
  trifacial —*see* Neuralgia, trigeminal
  trigeminal G50.0
    postherpetic, postzoster B02.22
  vagus (nerve) G52.2
  writer's F48.8
    organic G25.89
Neurapraxia —*see* Injury, nerve
Neurasthenia F48.8
  cardiac F45.8
  gastric F45.8
  heart F45.8

Neurilemmoma —see also Neoplasm, nerve, benign
  acoustic (nerve) D33.3
  malignant —see also Neoplasm, nerve, malignant
    acoustic (nerve) C72.4
Neurilemmosarcoma —see Neoplasm, nerve, malignant
Neurinoma —see Neoplasm, nerve, benign
Neurinomatosis —see Neoplasm, nerve, uncertain behavior
Neuritis (rheumatoid) M79.2
  abducens (nerve) —see Strabismus, paralytic, sixth nerve
  accessory (nerve) G52.8
  acoustic (nerve) (see also subcategory) H93.3
    in (due to)
      infectious disease NEC B99 [H94.0-]
      parasitic disease NEC B89 [H94.0-]
    syphilitic A52.15
  alcoholic G62.1
    with psychosis —see Psychosis, alcoholic
  amyloid, any site E85.4 [G63]
  auditory (nerve) —see subcategory H93.3
  brachial —see Radiculopathy
    due to displacement, intervertebral disc —see Disorder, disc, cervical, with neuritis
  cranial nerve
    due to Lyme disease A69.22
    eighth or acoustic or auditory —see subcategory H93.3
    eleventh or accessory G52.8
    fifth or trigeminal G51.0
    first or olfactory G52.0
    fourth or trochlear —see Strabismus, paralytic, fourth nerve
    second or optic —see Neuritis, optic
    seventh or facial G51.8
      newborn (birth injury) P11.3
    sixth or abducent —see Strabismus, paralytic, sixth nerve
    tenth or vagus G52.2
    third or oculomotor —see Strabismus, paralytic, third nerve
    twelfth or hypoglossal G52.3
  Déjérine-Sottas G60.0
  diabetic (mononeuropathy) —see E08-E13 with .41
    polyneuropathy —see E08-E13 with .42
  due to
    beriberi E51.11
    displacement, prolapse or rupture, intervertebral disc —see Disorder, disc, with, radiculopathy
    herniation, nucleus pulposus M51.9 [G55]
  endemic E51.11
  facial G51.8
    newborn (birth injury) P11.3
  general —see Polyneuropathy
  geniculate ganglion G51.1
    due to herpes (zoster) B02.21
  gouty M10.00 [G63]
  hypoglossal (nerve) G52.3
  ilioinguinal (nerve) G57.9-
  infectious (multiple) NEC G61.0
  interstitial hypertrophic progressive G60.0
  lumbar M54.16
  lumbosacral M54.17
  multiple —see also Polyneuropathy
    endemic E51.11
    infective, acute G61.0
    multiplex endemica E51.11
  nerve root —see Radiculopathy
  oculomotor (nerve) —see Strabismus, paralytic, third nerve
  olfactory nerve G52.0
  optic (nerve) (hereditary) (sympathetic) H46.9
    with demyelination G36.0
    in myelitis G36.0
    nutritional H46.2

Neuritis (Continued)
  optic (Continued)
    papillitis —see Papillitis, optic
    retrobulbar H46.1-
      specified type NEC H46.8
      toxic H46.3
  peripheral (nerve) G62.9
    multiple —see Polyneuropathy
    single —see Mononeuritis
  pneumogastric (nerve) G52.2
  postherpetic, postzoster B02.29
  progressive hypertrophic interstitial G60.0
  retrobulbar —see also Neuritis, optic, retrobulbar
    in (due to)
      late syphilis A52.15
      meningococcal infection A39.82
    meningococcal A39.82
    syphilitic A52.15
  sciatic (nerve) —see also Sciatica
    due to displacement of intervertebral disc —see Disorder, disc, with, radiculopathy
  serum (see also Reaction, serum) T80.69
  shoulder-girdle G54.5
  specified nerve NEC G58.8
  spinal (nerve) root —see Radiculopathy
  syphilitic A52.15
  thenar (median) G56.1-
  thoracic M54.14
  toxic NEC G62.2
  trochlear (nerve) —see Strabismus, paralytic, fourth nerve
  vagus (nerve) G52.2
Neuroastrocytoma —see Neoplasm, uncertain behavior, by site
Neuroavitaminosis E56.9 [G99.8]
Neuroblastoma
  olfactory C30.0
  specified site —see Neoplasm, malignant, by site
  unspecified site C74.90
Neurochorioretinitis —see Chorioretinitis
Neurocirculatory asthenia F45.8
Neurocysticercosis B69.0
Neurocytoma —see Neoplasm, benign, by site
Neurodermatitis (circumscribed) (circumscripta) (local) L28.0
  atopic L20.81
  diffuse (Brocq) L20.81
  disseminated L20.81
Neuroencephalomyelopathy, optic G36.0
Neuroepithelioma —see also Neoplasm, malignant, by site
  olfactory C30.0
Neurofibroma —see also Neoplasm, nerve, benign
  melanotic —see Neoplasm, nerve, benign
  multiple —see Neurofibromatosis
  plexiform —see Neoplasm, nerve, benign
Neurofibromatosis (multiple) (nonmalignant) Q85.00
  acoustic Q85.02
  malignant —see Neoplasm, nerve, malignant
  specified NEC Q85.09
  type 1 (von Recklinghausen) Q85.01
  type 2 Q85.02
Neurofibrosarcoma —see Neoplasm, nerve, malignant
Neurogenic —see also condition
  bladder (see also Dysfunction, bladder, neuromuscular) N31.9
    cauda equina syndrome G83.4
  bowel NEC K59.2
  heart F45.8
Neuroglioma —see Neoplasm, uncertain behavior, by site
Neurolabyrinthitis (of Dix and Hallpike) —see Neuronitis, vestibular
Neurolathyrism —see Poisoning, food, noxious, plant

Neuroleprosy A30.9
Neuroma —see also Neoplasm, nerve, benign
  acoustic (nerve) D33.3
  amputation (stump) (traumatic) (surgical complication) (late) T87.3-
    arm T87.3-
    leg T87.3-
  digital (toe) G57.6-
  interdigital (toe) G58.8
    lower limb G57.8-
    upper limb G56.8-
  intermetatarsal G57.8-
  Morton's G57.6-
  nonneoplastic
    arm G56.9-
    leg G57.9-
    lower extremity G57.9-
    upper extremity G56.9-
  optic (nerve) D33.3
  plantar G57.6-
  plexiform —see Neoplasm, nerve, benign
  surgical (nonneoplastic)
    arm G56.9-
    leg G57.9-
    lower extremity G57.9-
    upper extremity G56.9-
Neuromyalgia —see Neuralgia
Neuromyasthenia (epidemic) (postinfectious) G93.3
Neuromyelitis G36.9
  ascending G61.0
  optica G36.0
Neuromyopathy G70.9
  paraneoplastic D49.9 [G13.0]
Neuromyotonia (Isaacs) G71.19
Neuronevus —see Nevus
Neuronitis G58.9
  ascending (acute) G57.2-
  vestibular H81.2-
Neuroparalytic —see condition
Neuropathy, neuropathic G62.9
  acute motor G62.81
  alcoholic G62.1
    with psychosis —see Psychosis, alcoholic
  arm G56.9-
  autonomic, peripheral —see Neuropathy, peripheral, autonomic
  axillary G56.9-
  bladder N31.9
    atonic (motor) (sensory) N31.2
    autonomous N31.2
    flaccid N31.2
    nonreflex N31.2
    reflex N31.1
    uninhibited N31.0
  brachial plexus G54.0
  cervical plexus G54.2
  chronic
    progressive segmentally demyelinating G62.89
    relapsing demyelinating G62.89
  Déjérine-Sottas G60.0
  diabetic —see E08-E13 with .40
    mononeuropathy —see E08-E13 with .41
    polyneuropathy —see E08-E13 with .42
  entrapment G58.9
    iliohypogastric nerve G57.8-
    ilioinguinal nerve G57.8-
    lateral cutaneous nerve of thigh G57.1-
    median nerve G56.0-
    obturator nerve G57.8-
    peroneal nerve G57.3-
    posterior tibial nerve G57.5-
    saphenous nerve G57.8-
    ulnar nerve G56.2-
  facial nerve G51.9
  hereditary G60.9
    motor and sensory (types I-IV) G60.0
    sensory G60.8
    specified NEC G60.8

◀ New ◀◀◀ Revised ~~deleted~~ Deleted

Neuropathy, neuropathic (Continued)
- hypertrophic G60.0
  - Charcot-Marie-Tooth G60.0
  - Déjérine-Sottas G60.0
  - interstitial progressive G60.0
  - of infancy G60.0
  - Refsum G60.1
- idiopathic G60.9
  - progressive G60.3
  - specified NEC G60.8
- in association with hereditary ataxia G60.2
- intercostal G58.0
- ischemic —see Disorder, nerve
- Jamaica (ginger) G62.2
- leg NEC G57.9-
- lower extremity G57.9-
- lumbar plexus G54.1
- median nerve G56.1-
- motor and sensory —see also Polyneuropathy
  - hereditary (types I-IV) G60.0
- multiple (acute) (chronic) —see Polyneuropathy
- optic (nerve) —see also Neuritis, optic
  - ischemic H47.01-
- paraneoplastic (sensorial) (Denny Brown) D49.9 [G13.0]
- peripheral (nerve) (see also Polyneuropathy) G62.9
  - autonomic G90.9
    - idiopathic G90.09
    - in (due to)
      - amyloidosis E85.4 [G99.0]
      - diabetes mellitus —see E08-E13 with .43
      - endocrine disease NEC E34.9 [G99.0]
      - gout M10.00 [G99.0]
      - hyperthyroidism E05.90 [G99.0]
        - with thyroid storm E05.91 [G99.0]
      - metabolic disease NEC E88.9 [G99.0]
  - idiopathic G60.9
    - progressive G60.3
  - in (due to)
    - antitetanus serum G62.0
    - arsenic G62.2
    - drugs NEC G62.0
    - lead G62.2
    - organophosphate compounds G62.2
    - toxic agent NEC G62.2
- plantar nerves G57.6-
- progressive
  - hypertrophic interstitial G60.0
  - inflammatory G62.81
- radicular NEC —see Radiculopathy
- sacral plexus G54.1
- sciatic G57.0-
- serum G61.1
- toxic NEC G62.2
- trigeminal sensory G50.8
- ulnar nerve G56.2-
- uremic N18.9 [G63]
- vitamin B12 E53.8 [G63]
  - with anemia (pernicious) D51.0 [G63]
  - due to dietary deficiency D51.3 [G63]

Neurophthisis —see also Disorder, nerve
- peripheral, diabetic —see E08-E13 with .42

Neuroretinitis —see Chorioretinitis
Neuroretinopathy, hereditary optic H47.22
Neurosarcoma —see Neoplasm, nerve, malignant
Neurosclerosis —see Disorder, nerve
Neurosis, neurotic F48.9
- anankastic F42
- anxiety (state) F41.1
  - panic type F41.0
- asthenic F48.8
- bladder F45.8
- cardiac (reflex) F45.8
- cardiovascular F45.8
- character F60.9
- colon F45.8
- compensation F68.1

Neurosis, neurotic (Continued)
- compulsive, compulsion F42
- conversion F44.9
- craft F48.8
- cutaneous F45.8
- depersonalization F48.1
- depressive (reaction) (type) F34.1
- environmental F48.8
- excoriation L98.1
- fatigue F48.8
- functional —see Disorder, somatoform
- gastric F45.8
- gastrointestinal F45.8
- heart F45.8
- hypochondriacal F45.21
- hysterical F44.9
- incoordination F45.8
  - larynx F45.8
  - vocal cord F45.8
- intestine F45.8
- larynx (sensory) F45.8
  - hysterical F44.4
- mixed NEC F48.8
- musculoskeletal F45.8
- obsessional F42
- obsessive-compulsive F42
- occupational F48.8
- ocular NEC F45.8
- organ —see Disorder, somatoform
- pharynx F45.8
- phobic F40.9
- posttraumatic (situational) F43.10
  - acute F43.11
  - chronic F43.12
- psychasthenic (type) F48.8
- railroad F48.8
- rectum F45.8
- respiratory F45.8
- rumination F45.8
- sexual F65.9
- situational F48.8
- social F40.10
  - generalized F40.11
- specified type NEC F48.8
- state F48.9
  - with depersonalization episode F48.1
- stomach F45.8
- traumatic F43.10
  - acute F43.11
  - chronic F43.12
- vasomotor F45.8
- visceral F45.8
- war F48.8

Neurospongioblastosis diffusa Q85.1
Neurosyphilis (arrested) (early) (gumma) (late) (latent) (recurrent) (relapse) A52.3
- with ataxia (cerebellar) (locomotor) (spastic) (spinal) A52.19
- aneurysm (cerebral) A52.05
- arachnoid (adhesive) A52.13
- arteritis (any artery) (cerebral) A52.04
- asymptomatic A52.2
- congenital A50.40
- dura (mater) A52.13
- general paresis A52.17
- hemorrhagic A52.05
- juvenile (asymptomatic) (meningeal) A50.40
- leptomeninges (aseptic) A52.13
- meningeal, meninges (adhesive) A52.13
- meningitis A52.13
- meningovascular (diffuse) A52.13
- optic atrophy A52.15
- parenchymatous (degenerative) A52.19
- paresis, paretic A52.17
  - juvenile A50.45
- remission in (sustained) A52.3
- serological (without symptoms) A52.2
- specified nature or site NEC A52.19
- tabes, tabetic (dorsalis) A52.11
  - juvenile A50.45

Neurosyphilis (Continued)
- taboparesis A52.17
  - juvenile A50.45
- thrombosis (cerebral) A52.05
- vascular (cerebral) NEC A52.05

Neurothekeoma —see Neoplasm, nerve, benign
Neurotic —see Neurosis
Neurotoxemia —see Toxemia
Neutroclusion M26.211
Neutropenia, neutropenic (chronic) (genetic) (idiopathic) (immune) (infantile) (malignant) (pernicious) (splenic) D70.9
- congenital (primary) D70.0
- cyclic D70.4
- cytoreductive cancer chemotherapy sequela D70.1
- drug-induced D70.2
  - due to cytoreductive cancer chemotherapy D70.1
- due to infection D70.3
- fever D70.9
- neonatal, transitory (isoimmune) (maternal transfer) P61.5
- periodic D70.4
- secondary (cyclic) (periodic) (splenic) D70.4
  - drug-induced D70.2
    - due to cytoreductive cancer chemotherapy D70.1
- toxic D70.8

Neutrophilia, hereditary giant D72.0
Nevocarcinoma —see Melanoma
Nevus D22.9
- achromic —see Neoplasm, skin, benign
- amelanotic —see Neoplasm, skin, benign
- angiomatous D18.00
  - intra-abdominal D18.03
  - intracranial D18.02
  - skin D18.01
  - specified site NEC D18.09
- araneus I78.1
- balloon cell —see Neoplasm, skin, benign
- bathing trunk D48.5
- blue —see Neoplasm, skin, benign
  - cellular —see Neoplasm, skin, benign
  - giant —see Neoplasm, skin, benign
  - Jadassohn's —see Neoplasm, skin, benign
  - malignant —see Melanoma
- capillary D18.00
  - intra-abdominal D18.03
  - intracranial D18.02
  - skin D18.01
  - specified site NEC D18.09
- cavernous D18.00
  - intra-abdominal D18.03
  - intracranial D18.02
  - skin D18.01
  - specified site NEC D18.09
- cellular —see Neoplasm, skin, benign
  - blue —see Neoplasm, skin, benign
- choroid D31.3-
- comedonicus Q82.5
- conjunctiva D31.0-
- dermal —see Neoplasm, skin, benign
  - with epidermal nevus —see Neoplasm, skin, benign
- dysplastic —see Neoplasm, skin, benign
- eye D31.9-
- flammeus Q82.5
- hemangiomatous D18.00
  - intra-abdominal D18.03
  - intracranial D18.02
  - skin D18.01
  - specified site NEC D18.09
- iris D31.4-
- lacrimal gland D31.5-
- lymphatic D18.1
- magnocellular
  - specified site —see Neoplasm, benign, by site
  - unspecified site D31.40
- malignant —see Melanoma

Nevus *(Continued)*
  meaning hemangioma D18.00
    intra-abdominal D18.03
    intracranial D18.02
    skin D18.01
    specified site NEC D18.09
  mouth (mucosa) D10.30
    specified site NEC D10.39
    white sponge Q38.6
  multiplex Q85.1
  non-neoplastic I78.1
  oral mucosa D10.30
    specified site NEC D10.39
    white sponge Q38.6
  orbit D31.6-
  pigmented
    giant *(see also* Neoplasm, skin, uncertain behavior) D48.5
      malignant melanoma in —*see* Melanoma
  portwine Q82.5
  retina D31.2-
  retrobulbar D31.6-
  sanguineous Q82.5
  senile I78.1
  skin D22.9
    abdominal wall D22.5
    ala nasi D22.39
    ankle D22.7-
    anus, anal D22.5
    arm D22.6-
    auditory canal (external) D22.2-
    auricle (ear) D22.2-
    auricular canal (external) D22.2-
    axilla, axillary fold D22.5
    back D22.5
    breast D22.5
    brow D22.39
    buttock D22.5
    canthus (eye) D22.1-
    cheek (external) D22.39
    chest wall D22.5
    chin D22.39
    ear (external) D22.2-
    external meatus (ear) D22.2-
    eyebrow D22.39
    eyelid (lower) (upper) D22.1-
    face D22.30
      specified NEC D22.39
    female genital organ (external) NEC D28.0
    finger D22.6-
    flank D22.5
    foot D22.7-
    forearm D22.6-
    forehead D22.39
    foreskin D29.0
    genital organ (external) NEC
      female D28.0
      male D29.9
    gluteal region D22.5
    groin D22.5
    hand D22.6-
    heel D22.7-
    helix D22.2-
    hip D22.7-
    interscapular region D22.5
    jaw D22.39
    knee D22.7-
    labium (majus) (minus) D28.0
    leg D22.7-
    lip (lower) (upper) D22.0
    lower limb D22.7-
    male genital organ (external) D29.9
    nail D22.9
      finger D22.6-
      toe D22.7-
    nasolabial groove D22.39
    nates D22.5
    neck D22.4
    nose (external) D22.39
    palpebra D22.1-

Nevus *(Continued)*
  skin *(Continued)*
    penis D29.0
    perianal skin D22.5
    perineum D22.5
    pinna D22.2-
    popliteal fossa or space D22.7-
    prepuce D29.0
    pudendum D28.0
    scalp D22.4
    scrotum D29.4
    shoulder D22.6-
    submammary fold D22.5
    temple D22.39
    thigh D22.7-
    toe D22.7-
    trunk NEC D22.5
    umbilicus D22.5
    upper limb D22.6-
    vulva D28.0
  specified site NEC —*see* Neoplasm, benign, by site
  spider I78.1
  stellar I78.1
  strawberry Q82.5
  Sutton's —*see* Neoplasm, skin, benign
  unius lateris Q82.5
  Unna's Q82.5
  vascular Q82.5
  verrucous Q82.5

Newborn (infant) (liveborn) (singleton) Z38.2
  abstinence syndrome P96.1
  acne L70.4
  affected by (suspected to be)
    abnormalities of membranes P02.9
      specified NEC P02.8
    abruptio placenta P02.1
    amino-acid metabolic disorder, transitory P74.8
    amniocentesis (while in utero) P00.6
    amnionitis P02.7
    apparent life threatening event (ALTE) R68.13
    bleeding (into)
      cerebral cortex P52.22
      germinal matrix P52.0
      ventricles P52.1
    breech delivery P03.0
    cardiac arrest P29.81
    cardiomyopathy I42.8
      congenital I42.4
    cerebral ischemia P91.0
    Cesarean delivery P03.4
    chemotherapy agents P04.1
    chorioamnionitis P02.7
    cocaine (crack) P04.41
    complications of labor and delivery P03.9
      specified NEC P03.89
    compression of umbilical cord NEC P02.5
    contracted pelvis P03.1
    delivery P03.9
      Cesarean P03.4
      forceps P03.2
      vacuum extractor P03.3
    entanglement (knot) in umbilical cord P02.5
    environmental chemicals P04.6
    fetal (intrauterine)
      growth retardation P05.9
      malnutrition not light or small for gestational age P05.2
    forceps delivery P03.2
    heart rate abnormalities
      bradycardia P29.12
      intrauterine P03.819
        before onset of labor P03.810
        during labor P03.811
      tachycardia P29.11

Newborn *(Continued)*
  affected by *(Continued)*
    hemorrhage (antepartum) P02.1
      cerebellar (nontraumatic) P52.6
      intracerebral (nontraumatic) P52.4
      intracranial (nontraumatic) P52.9
        specified NEC P52.8
      intraventricular (nontraumatic) P52.3
        grade 1 P52.0
        grade 2 P52.1
        grade 3 P52.21
        grade 4 P52.22
      posterior fossa (nontraumatic) P52.6
      subarachnoid (nontraumatic) P52.5
      subependymal P52.0
        with intracerebral extension P52.22
        with intraventricular extension P52.1
          with enlargment of ventricles P52.21
        without intraventricular extension P52.0
    hypoxic ischemic encephalopathy [HIE] P91.60
      mild P91.61
      moderate P91.62
      severe P91.63
    induction of labor P03.89
    intestinal perforation P78.0
    intrauterine (fetal) blood loss P50.9
      due to (from)
        cut end of co-twin cord P50.5
        hemorrhage into
          co-twin P50.3
          maternal circulation P50.4
        placenta P50.2
        ruptured cord blood P50.1
        vasa previa P50.0
        specified NEC P50.8
    intrauterine (fetal) hemorrhage P50.9
    intrauterine (in utero) procedure P96.5
    malpresentation (malposition) NEC P03.1
    maternal (complication of) (use of)
      alcohol P04.3
      analgesia (maternal) P04.0
      anesthesia (maternal) P04.0
      blood loss P02.1
      circulatory disease P00.3
      condition P00.9
        specified NEC P00.89
      delivery P03.9
        Cesarean P03.4
        forceps P03.2
        vacuum extractor P03.3
      diabetes mellitus (pre-existing) P70.1
      disorder P00.9
        specified NEC P00.89
      drugs (addictive) (illegal) NEC P04.49
      ectopic pregnancy P01.4
      gestational diabetes P70.0
      hemorrhage P02.1
      hypertensive disorder P00.0
      incompetent cervix P01.0
      infectious disease P00.2
      injury P00.5
      labor and delivery P03.9
      malpresentation before labor P01.7
      maternal death P01.6
      medical procedure P00.7
      medication P04.1
      multiple pregnancy P01.5
      nutritional disorder P00.4
      oligohydramnios P01.2
      parasitic disease P00.2
      periodontal disease P00.81
      placenta previa P02.0
      polyhydramnios P01.3
      precipitate delivery P03.5
      pregnancy P01.9
        specified P01.8
      premature rupture of membranes P01.1
      renal disease P00.1

◀ New   ◀▦ Revised   ~~deleted~~ Deleted

Newborn *(Continued)*
 affected by *(Continued)*
  maternal *(Continued)*
   respiratory disease P00.3
   surgical procedure P00.6
   urinary tract disease P00.1
   uterine contraction (abnormal) P03.6
  meconium peritonitis P78.0
  medication (legal) (maternal use)
    (prescribed) P04.1
  membrane abnormalities P02.9
   specified NEC P02.8
  membranitis P02.7
  methamphetamine (s) P04.49
  mixed metabolic and respiratory acidosis
    P84
  neonatal abstinence syndrome P96.1
  noxious substances transmitted via
    placenta or breast milk P04.9
   specified NEC P04.8
  nutritional supplements P04.5
  placenta previa P02.0
  placental
   abnormality (functional)
     (morphological) P02.20
    specified NEC P02.29
   dysfunction P02.29
   infarction P02.29
   insufficiency P02.29
   separation NEC P02.1
   transfusion syndromes P02.3
  placentitis P02.7
  precipitate delivery P03.5
  prolapsed cord P02.4
  respiratory arrest P28.81
  slow intrauterine growth P05.9
  tobacco P04.2
  twin to twin transplacental transfusion
    P02.3
  umbilical cord (tightly) around neck
    P02.5
  umbilical cord condition P02.60
   short cord P02.69
   specified NEC P02.69
  uterine contractions (abnormal) P03.6
  vasa previa P02.69
   from intrauterine blood loss P50.0
 apnea P28.3
  obstructive P28.4
  primary P28.3
  specified P28.4
 born in hospital Z38.00
  by cesarean Z38.01
 born outside hospital Z38.1
 breast buds P96.89
 breast engorgement P83.4
 check-up —*see* Newborn, examination
 convulsion P90
 dehydration P74.1
 examination
  8 to 28 days old Z00.111
  under 8 days old Z00.110
 fever P81.9
  environmentally-induced P81.0
 hyperbilirubinemia P59.9
  of prematurity P59.0
 hypernatremia P74.2
 hyponatremia P74.2
 infection P39.9
  candidal P37.5
  specified NEC P39.8
  urinary tract P39.3
 jaundice P59.8
  due to
   breast milk inhibitor P59.3
   hepatocellular damage P59.20
    specified NEC P59.29
   preterm delivery P59.0
  of prematurity P59.0
  specified NEC P59.8
 late metabolic acidosis P74.0

Newborn *(Continued)*
 mastitis P39.0
  infective P39.0
  noninfective P83.4
 multiple born NEC Z38.8
  born in hospital Z38.68
   by cesarean Z38.69
  born outside hospital Z38.7
 omphalitis P38.9
  with mild hemorrhage P38.1
  without hemorrhage P38.9
 post-term P08.21
 prolonged gestation (over 42 completed
   weeks) P08.22
 quadruplet Z38.8
  born in hospital Z38.63
   by cesarean Z38.64
  born outside hospital Z38.7
 quintuplet Z38.8
  born in hospital Z38.65
   by cesarean Z38.66
  born outside hospital Z38.7
 seizure P90
 sepsis (congenital) P36.9
  due to
   anaerobes NEC P36.5
   Escherichia coli P36.4
   Staphylococcus P36.30
    aureus P36.2
    specified NEC P36.39
   Streptococcus P36.10
    group B P36.0
    specified NEC P36.19
   specified NEC P36.8
 triplet Z38.8
  born in hospital Z38.61
   by cesarean Z38.62
  born outside hospital Z38.7
 twin Z38.5
  born in hospital Z38.30
   by cesarean Z38.31
  born outside hospital Z38.4
 vomiting P92.09
  bilious P92.01
 weight check Z00.111
Newcastle conjunctivitis or disease B30.8
Nezelof's syndrome (pure alymphocytosis)
  D81.4
Niacin (amide) deficiency E52
Nicolas (-Durand)-Favre disease A55
Nicotine —*see* Tobacco
Nicotinic acid deficiency E52
Niemann-Pick disease or syndrome E75.249
 specified NEC E75.248
 type
  A E75.240
  B E75.241
  C E75.242
  D E75.243
Night
 blindness —*see* Blindness, night
 sweats R61
 terrors (child) F51.4
Nightmares (REM sleep type) F51.5
Nipple —*see* condition
Nisbet's chancre A57
Nishimoto (-Takeuchi) disease I67.5
Nitritoid crisis or reaction —*see* Crisis,
  nitritoid
Nitrosohemoglobinemia D74.8
Njovera A65
Nocardiosis, nocardiasis A43.9
 cutaneous A43.1
 lung A43.0
 pneumonia A43.0
 pulmonary A43.0
 specified site NEC A43.8
Nocturia R35.1
 psychogenic F45.8
Nocturnal —*see* condition
Nodal rhythm I49.8

Node (s) —*see also* Nodule
 Bouchard's (with arthropathy) M15.2
 Haygarth's M15.8
 Heberden's (with arthropathy) M15.1
 larynx J38.7
 lymph —*see* condition
 milker's B08.03
 Osler's I33.0
 Schmorl's —*see* Schmorl's disease
 singer's J38.2
 teacher's J38.2
 tuberculous —*see* Tuberculosis, lymph
   gland
 vocal cord J38.2
Nodule (s), nodular
 actinomycotic —*see* Actinomycosis
 breast NEC N63
 colloid (cystic), thyroid E04.1
 cutaneous —*see* Swelling, localized
 endometrial (stromal) D26.1
 Haygarth's M15.8
 inflammatory —*see* Inflammation
 juxta-articular
  syphilitic A52.77
  yaws A66.7
 larynx J38.7
 lung, solitary (subsegmental branch of the
   bronchial tree) R91.1
  multiple R91.8
 milker's B08.03
 prostate N40.2
  with lower urinary tract symptoms (LUTS)
    N40.3
  without lower urinary tract symptoms
    (LUTS) N40.2
 pulmonary, solitary (subsegmental branch of
   the bronchial tree) R91.1
 retrocardiac R09.89
 rheumatoid M06.30
  ankle M06.37-
  elbow M06.32-
  foot joint M06.37-
  hand joint M06.34-
  hip M06.35-
  knee M06.36-
  multiple site M06.39
  shoulder M06.31-
  vertebra M06.38
  wrist M06.33-
 scrotum (inflammatory) N49.2
 singer's J38.2
 solitary, lung (subsegmental branch of the
   bronchial tree) R91.1
  multiple R91.8
 subcutaneous —*see* Swelling, localized
 teacher's J38.2
 thyroid (cold) (gland) (nontoxic) E04.1
  with thyrotoxicosis E05.20
   with thyroid storm E05.21
  toxic or with hyperthyroidism E05.20
   with thyroid storm E05.21
 vocal cord J38.2
Noma (gangrenous) (hospital) (infective)
  A69.0
 auricle I96
 mouth A69.0
 pudendi N76.89
 vulvae N76.89
Nomad, nomadism Z59.0
Nonautoimmune hemolytic anemia D59.4
 drug-induced D59.2
Nonclosure —*see also* Imperfect, closure
 ductus arteriosus (Botallo's) Q25.0
 foramen
  botalli Q21.1
  ovale Q21.1
Noncompliance Z91.19
 with
  dialysis Z91.15
  dietary regimen Z91.11
  medical treatment Z91.19

Noncompliance *(Continued)*
　with *(Continued)*
　　medication regimen NEC Z91.14
　　　underdosing *(see also* Table of Drugs
　　　　and Chemicals, categories T36-T50,
　　　　with final character 6) Z91.14 ◀▥
　　　　intentional NEC Z91.128
　　　　　due to financial hardship of patient
　　　　　　Z91.120
　　　　unintentional NEC Z91.138
　　　　　due to patient's age related debility
　　　　　　Z91.130
　　renal dialysis Z91.15
Nondescent (congenital) —*see also* Malposition,
　congenital
　cecum Q43.3
　colon Q43.3
　testicle Q53.9
　　bilateral Q53.20
　　　abdominal Q53.21
　　　perineal Q53.22
　　unilateral Q53.10
　　　abdominal Q53.11
　　　perineal Q53.12
Nondevelopment
　brain Q02
　　part of Q04.3
　heart Q24.8
　organ or site, congenital NEC —*see*
　　Hypoplasia
Nonengagement
　head NEC O32.4
　　in labor, causing obstructed labor O64.8
Nonexanthematous tick fever A93.2
Nonexpansion, lung (newborn) P28.0
Nonfunctioning
　cystic duct *(see also* Disease, gallbladder)
　　K82.8
　gallbladder *(see also* Disease, gallbladder)
　　K82.8
　kidney N28.9
　labyrinth —*see* subcategory H83.2

Non-Hodgkin lymphoma NEC —*see*
　Lymphoma, non-Hodgkin
Nonimplantation, ovum N97.2
Noninsufflation, fallopian tube N97.1
Non-ketotic hyperglycinemia E72.51
Nonne-Milroy syndrome Q82.0
Nonovulation N97.0
Nonpatent fallopian tube N97.1
Nonpneumatization, lung NEC P28.0
Nonrotation —*see* Malrotation
Nonsecretion, urine —*see* Anuria
Nonunion
　fracture —*see* Fracture, by site
　organ or site, congenital NEC —*see* Imperfect,
　　closure
　symphysis pubis, congenital Q74.2
Nonvisualization, gallbladder R93.2
Nonvital, nonvitalized tooth K04.99
Non-working side interference
　M26.56
Noonan's syndrome Q87.1
Normocytic anemia (infectional) due to blood
　loss (chronic) D50.0
　acute D62
Norrie's disease (congenital) Q15.8
North American blastomycosis B40.9
Norwegian itch B86
Nose, nasal —*see* condition
Nosebleed R04.0
Nose-picking F98.8
Nosomania F45.21
Nosophobia F45.22
Nostalgia F43.20
Notch of iris Q13.2
Notching nose, congenital (tip) Q30.2
Nothnagel's
　syndrome —*see* Strabismus, paralytic, third
　　nerve
　vasomotor acroparesthesia I73.89
Novy's relapsing fever A68.9
　louse-borne A68.0
　tick-borne A68.1

Noxious
　foodstuffs, poisoning by —*see* Poisoning,
　　food, noxious, plant
　substances transmitted through placenta or
　　breast milk P04.9
Nucleus pulposus —*see* condition
Numbness R20.0
Nuns' knee —*see* Bursitis, prepatellar
Nursemaid's elbow S53.03-
Nutcracker esophagus K22.4
Nutmeg liver K76.1
Nutrient element deficiency E61.9
　specified NEC E61.8
Nutrition deficient or insufficient *(see also*
　Malnutrition) E46
　due to
　　insufficient food T73.0
　　lack of
　　　care (child) T76.02
　　　　adult T76.01
　　　food T73.0
Nutritional stunting E45
Nyctalopia (night blindness) —*see* Blindness,
　night
Nycturia R35.1
　psychogenic F45.8
Nymphomania F52.8
Nystagmus H55.00
　benign paroxysmal —*see* Vertigo, benign
　　paroxysmal
　central positional H81.4-
　congenital H55.01
　dissociated H55.04
　latent H55.02
　miners' H55.09
　positional
　　benign paroxysmal H81.4-
　　central H81.4-
　specified form NEC H55.09
　visual deprivation H55.03

◀ New　◀▥ Revised　~~deleted~~ Deleted

O

Obermeyer's relapsing fever (European) A68.0
Obesity E66.9
  with alveolar hyperventilation E66.2
  adrenal E27.8
  complicating
    childbirth O99.214
    pregnancy O99.21-
    puerperium O99.215
  constitutional E66.8
  dietary counseling and surveillance Z71.3
  drug-induced E66.1
  due to
    drug E66.1
    excess calories E66.09
      morbid E66.01
      severe E66.01
  endocrine E66.8
  endogenous E66.8
  familial E66.8
  glandular E66.8
  hypothyroid —see Hypothyroidism
  morbid E66.01
    with alveolar hypoventilation E66.2
    due to excess calories E66.01
  nutritional E66.09
  pituitary E23.6
  severe E66.01
  specified type NEC E66.8
Oblique —see condition
Obliteration
  appendix (lumen) K38.8
  artery I77.1
  bile duct (noncalculous) K83.1
  common duct (noncalculous) K83.1
  cystic duct —see Obstruction, gallbladder
  disease, arteriolar I77.1
  endometrium N85.8
  eye, anterior chamber —see Disorder, globe, hypotony
  fallopian tube N97.1
  lymphatic vessel I89.0
    due to mastectomy I97.2
  organ or site, congenital NEC —see Atresia, by site
  ureter N13.5
    with infection N13.6
  urethra —see Stricture, urethra
  vein I87.8
  vestibule (oral) K08.8
Observation (following) (for) (without need for further medical care) Z04.9
  accident NEC Z04.3
    at work Z04.2
    transport Z04.1
  adverse effect of drug Z03.6
  alleged rape or sexual assault (victim), ruled out
    adult Z04.41
    child Z04.42
  criminal assault Z04.8
  development state
    adolescent Z00.3
    period of rapid growth in childhood Z00.2
    puberty Z00.3
  disease, specified NEC Z03.89
  following work accident Z04.2
  growth and development state —see Observation, development state
  injuries (accidental) NEC —see also Observation, accident
  newborn (for suspected condition, ruled out) —see Newborn, affected by (suspected to be), maternal (complication of) (use of)
  postpartum
    immediately after delivery Z39.0
    routine follow-up Z39.2

Observation (Continued)
  pregnancy (normal) (without complication) Z34.9-
    high risk O09.9-
  suicide attempt, alleged NEC Z03.89
    self-poisoning Z03.6
  suspected, ruled out —see also Suspected condition, ruled out
    abuse, physical
      adult Z04.71
      child Z04.72
    accident at work Z04.2
    adult battering victim Z04.71
    child battering victim Z04.72
    condition NEC Z03.89
      newborn —see Newborn, affected by (suspected to be), maternal (complication of) (use of)
    drug poisoning or adverse effect Z03.6
    exposure (to)
      anthrax Z03.810
      biological agent NEC Z03.818
    inflicted injury NEC Z04.8
    suicide attempt, alleged Z03.89
      self-poisoning Z03.6
    toxic effects from ingested substance (drug) (poison) Z03.6
  toxic effects from ingested substance (drug) (poison) Z03.6
Obsession, obsessional state F42
Obsessive-compulsive neurosis or reaction F42
Obstetric embolism, septic —see Embolism, obstetric, septic
Obstetrical trauma (complicating delivery) O71.9
  with or following ectopic or molar pregnancy O08.6
  specified type NEC O71.89
Obstipation —see Constipation
Obstruction, obstructed, obstructive
  airway J98.8
    with
      allergic alveolitis J67.9
      asthma J45.909
        with
          exacerbation (acute) J45.901
          status asthmaticus J45.902
      bronchiectasis J47.9
        with
          exacerbation (acute) J47.1
          lower respiratory infection J47.0
      bronchitis (chronic) J44.9
      emphysema J43.9
    chronic J44.9
      with
        allergic alveolitis —see Pneumonitis, hypersensitivity
        bronchiectasis J47.9
          with
            exacerbation (acute) J47.1
            lower respiratory infection J47.0
    due to
      foreign body —see Foreign body, by site, causing asphyxia
      inhalation of fumes or vapors J68.9
      laryngospasm J38.5
  ampulla of Vater K83.1
  aortic (heart) (valve) —see Stenosis, aortic
  aortoiliac I74.09
  aqueduct of Sylvius G91.1
    congenital Q03.0
      with spina bifida —see Spina bifida, by site, with hydrocephalus
  Arnold-Chiari —see Arnold-Chiari disease
  artery (see also Embolism, artery) I74.9
    basilar (complete) (partial) —see Occlusion, artery, basilar
    carotid (complete) (partial) —see Occlusion, artery, carotid
    cerebellar —see Occlusion, artery, cerebellar

Obstruction, obstructed, obstructive (Continued)
  artery (Continued)
    cerebral (anterior) (middle) (posterior) —see Occlusion, artery, cerebral
    precerebral —see Occlusion, artery, precerebral
    renal N28.0
    retinal NEC —see Occlusion, artery, retina
    vertebral (complete) (partial) —see Occlusion, artery, vertebral
  band (intestinal) K56.69
  bile duct or passage (common) (hepatic) (noncalculous) K83.1
    with calculus K80.51
    congenital (causing jaundice) Q44.3
  biliary (duct) (tract) K83.1
    gallbladder K82.0
  bladder-neck (acquired) N32.0
    congenital Q64.31
    due to hyperplasia (hypertrophy) of prostate —see Hyperplasia, prostate
  bowel —see Obstruction, intestine
  bronchus J98.09
  canal, ear —see Stenosis, external ear canal
  cardia K22.2
  caval veins (inferior) (superior) I87.1
  cecum —see Obstruction, intestine
  circulatory I99.8
  colon —see Obstruction, intestine
  common duct (noncalculous) K83.1
  coronary (artery) —see Occlusion, coronary
  cystic duct —see also Obstruction, gallbladder
    with calculus K80.21
  device, implant or graft (see also Complications, by site and type, mechanical) T85.698
    arterial graft NEC —see Complication, cardiovascular device, mechanical, vascular
    catheter NEC T85.628
      cystostomy T83.090
      dialysis (renal) T82.49
        intraperitoneal T85.691
      infusion NEC T82.594
        spinal (epidural) (subdural) T85.690
      urinary, indwelling T83.098
    due to infection T85.79
    gastrointestinal —see Complications, prosthetic device, mechanical, gastrointestinal device
    genital NEC T83.498
      intrauterine contraceptive device T83.39
      penile prosthesis T83.490
    heart NEC —see Complication, cardiovascular device, mechanical
    joint prosthesis —see Complications, joint prosthesis, mechanical, specified NEC, by site
    orthopedic NEC —see Complication, orthopedic, device, mechanical
    specified NEC T85.628
    urinary NEC —see also Complication, genitourinary, device, urinary, mechanical
      graft T83.29
    vascular NEC —see Complication, cardiovascular device, mechanical
    ventricular intracranial shunt T85.09
  due to foreign body accidentally left in operative wound T81.529
  duodenum K31.5
  ejaculatory duct N50.8
  esophagus K22.2
  eustachian tube (complete) (partial) H68.10-
    cartilagenous (extrinsic) H68.13-
      intrinsic H68.12-
    osseous H68.11-
  fallopian tube (bilateral) N97.1

Obstruction, obstructed, obstructive
(Continued)
fecal K56.41
    with hernia —see Hernia, by site, with
        obstruction
foramen of Monro (congenital) Q03.8
    with spina bifida —see Spina bifida,
        by site, with hydrocephalus
foreign body —see Foreign body
gallbladder K82.0
    with calculus, stones K80.21
    congenital Q44.1
gastric outlet K31.1
gastrointestinal —see Obstruction, intestine
hepatic K76.89
    duct (noncalculous) K83.1
hepatobiliary K83.1
ileum —see Obstruction, intestine
iliofemoral (artery) I74.5
intestine K56.60
    with
        adhesions (intestinal) (peritoneal)
            K56.5
    adynamic K56.0
    by gallstone K56.3
    congenital (small) Q41.9
        large Q42.9
            specified part NEC Q42.8
    neurogenic K56.0
        Hirschsprung's disease or megacolon
            Q43.1
    newborn P76.9
        due to
            fecaliths P76.8
            inspissated milk P76.2
            meconium (plug) P76.0
                in mucoviscidosis E84.11
            specified NEC P76.8
    postoperative K91.3
    reflex K56.0
    specified NEC K56.69
    volvulus K56.2
intracardiac ball valve prosthesis T82.09
jejunum —see Obstruction, intestine
joint prosthesis —see Complications, joint
    prosthesis, mechanical, specified NEC,
    by site
kidney (calices) N28.89
labor —see Delivery
lacrimal (passages) (duct)
    by
        dacryolith —see Dacryolith
        stenosis —see Stenosis, lacrimal
    congenital Q10.5
    neonatal H04.53-
lacrimonasal duct —see Obstruction,
    lacrimal
lacteal, with steatorrhea K90.2
laryngitis —see Laryngitis
larynx NEC J38.6
    congenital Q31.8
lung J98.4
    disease, chronic J44.9
lymphatic I89.0
meconium (plug)
    newborn P76.0
        due to fecaliths P76.0
        in mucoviscidosis E84.11
mitral —see Stenosis, mitral
nasal J34.89
nasolacrimal duct —see also Obstruction,
    lacrimal
    congenital Q10.5
nasopharynx J39.2
nose J34.89
organ or site, congenital NEC —see Atresia,
    by site
pancreatic duct K86.8
parotid duct or gland K11.8
pelviureteral junction N13.5
    congenital Q62.39

Obstruction, obstructed, obstructive
(Continued)
pharynx J39.2
portal (circulation) (vein) I81
prostate —see also Hyperplasia, prostate
    valve (urinary) N32.0
pulmonary valve (heart) I37.0
pyelonephritis (chronic) N11.1
pylorus
    adult K31.1
    congenital or infantile Q40.0
rectosigmoid —see Obstruction,
    intestine
rectum K62.4
renal N28.89
    outflow N13.8
    pelvis, congenital Q62.39
respiratory J98.8
    chronic J44.9
retinal (vessels) H34.9
salivary duct (any) K11.8
    with calculus K11.5
sigmoid —see Obstruction, intestine
sinus (accessory) (nasal) J34.89
Stensen's duct K11.8
stomach NEC K31.89
    acute K31.0
    congenital Q40.2
    due to pylorospasm K31.3
submandibular duct K11.8
submaxillary gland K11.8
    with calculus K11.5
thoracic duct I89.0
thrombotic —see Thrombosis
trachea J39.8
tracheostomy airway J95.03
tricuspid (valve) —see Stenosis,
    tricuspid
upper respiratory, congenital Q34.8
ureter (functional) (pelvic junction) NEC
    N13.5
    with
        hydronephrosis N13.1
            with infection N13.6
        pyelonephritis (chronic) N11.1
    congenital Q62.39
    due to calculus —see Calculus, ureter
urethra NEC N36.8
    congenital Q64.39
urinary (moderate) N13.9
    due to hyperplasia (hypertrophy) of
        prostate —see Hyperplasia,
        prostate
    organ or tract (lower) N13.9
    prostatic valve N32.0
    specified NEC N13.8
uropathy N13.9
uterus N85.8
vagina N89.5
valvular —see Endocarditis
vein, venous I87.1
    caval (inferior) (superior) I87.1
    thrombotic —see Thrombosis
vena cava (inferior) (superior) I87.1
vesical NEC N32.0
vesicourethral orifice N32.0
    congenital Q64.31
vessel NEC I99.8
Obturator —see condition
Occlusal wear, teeth K03.0
Occlusio pupillae —see Membrane,
    pupillary
Occlusion, occluded
anus K62.4
    congenital Q42.3
        with fistula Q42.2
aortoiliac (chronic) I74.09
aqueduct of Sylvius G91.1
    congenital Q03.0
        with spina bifida —see Spina bifida, by
            site, with hydrocephalus

Occlusion, occluded (Continued)
artery (see also Embolism, artery) I74.9
    auditory, internal I65.8
    basilar I65.1
        with
            infarction I63.22
            due to
                embolism I63.12
                thrombosis I63.02
    brain or cerebral I66.9
        with infarction (due to) I63.5
            embolism I63.4
            thrombosis I63.3
    carotid I65.2-
        with
            infarction I63.23-
            due to
                embolism I63.13-
                thrombosis I63.03-
    cerebellar (anterior inferior) (posterior
        inferior) (superior) I66.3
        with infarction I63.54-
            due to
                embolism I63.44-
                thrombosis I63.34-
    cerebral I66.9
        with infarction I63.50
            due to
                embolism I63.40
                    specified NEC I63.49
                thrombosis I63.30
                    specified NEC I63.39
        anterior I66.1-
            with infarction I63.52-
            due to
                embolism I63.42-
                thrombosis I63.32-
        middle I66.0-
            with infarction I63.51-
            due to
                embolism I63.41-
                thrombosis I63.31-
        posterior I66.2-
            with infarction I63.53-
            due to
                embolism I63.43-
                thrombosis I63.33-
        specified NEC I66.8
            with infarction I63.59
            due to
                embolism I63.4
                thrombosis I63.3
    choroidal (anterior) —see Occlusion,
        artery, cerebral, specified NEC
    communicating posterior —see
        Occlusion, artery, precerebral,
        specified NEC
    complete
        coronary I25.82
        extremities I70.92
    coronary (acute) (thrombotic) (without
        myocardial infarction) I24.0
        with myocardial infarction —see
            Infarction, myocardium
        chronic total I25.82
        complete I25.82
        healed or old I25.2
        total (chronic) I25.82
    hypophyseal —see Occlusion, artery,
        precerebral, specified NEC
    iliac I74.5
    lower extremities due to stenosis or
        stricture I77.1
    mesenteric (embolic) (thrombotic)
        K55.0
    perforating —see Occlusion, artery,
        cerebral, specified NEC
    peripheral I77.9
        thrombotic or embolic I74.4
    pontine —see Occlusion, artery, cerebral,
        specified NEC

Occlusion, occluded (*Continued*)
 artery (*Continued*)
  precerebral I65.9
   with infarction I63.20
    due to
     embolism I63.10
      specified NEC I63.19
     thrombosis I63.00
      specified NEC I63.09
    specified NEC I63.29
   basilar —*see* Occlusion, artery, basilar
   carotid —*see* Occlusion, artery, carotid
   puerperal O88.23
   specified NEC I65.8
    with infarction I63.29
     due to
      embolism I63.19
      thrombosis I63.00
   vertebral —*see* Occlusion, artery, vertebral
  renal N28.0
  retinal
   branch H34.23-
   central H34.1-
   partial H34.21-
   transient H34.0-
  spinal —*see* Occlusion, artery, precerebral, vertebral
  total (chronic)
   coronary I25.82
   extremities I70.92
  vertebral I65.0-
   with
    infarction I63.21-
     due to
      embolism I63.11-
      thrombosis I63.01-
 basilar artery —*see* Occlusion, artery, basilar
 bile duct (common) (hepatic) (noncalculous) K83.1
 bowel —*see* Obstruction, intestine
 carotid (artery) (common) (internal) —*see* Occlusion, artery, carotid
 centric (of teeth) M26.59
  maximum intercuspation discrepancy M26.55
 cerebellar (artery) —*see* Occlusion, artery, cerebellar
 cerebral (artery) —*see* Occlusion, artery, cerebral
 cerebrovascular —*see also* Occlusion, artery, cerebral
  with infarction I63.5
 cervical canal —*see* Stricture, cervix
 cervix (uteri) —*see* Stricture, cervix
 choanal Q30.0
 choroidal (artery) —*see* Occlusion, artery, precerebral, specified NEC
 colon —*see* Obstruction, intestine
 communicating posterior artery —*see* Occlusion, artery, precerebral, specified NEC
 coronary (artery) (vein) (thrombotic) —*see also* Infarct, myocardium
  chronic total I25.82
  healed or old I25.2
  not resulting in infarction I24.0
  total (chronic) I25.82
 cystic duct —*see* Obstruction, gallbladder
 embolic —*see* Embolism
 fallopian tube N97.1
  congenital Q50.6
 gallbladder —*see also* Obstruction, gallbladder
  congenital (causing jaundice) Q44.1
 gingiva, traumatic K06.2
 hymen N89.6
  congenital Q52.3
 hypophyseal (artery) —*see* Occlusion, artery, precerebral, specified NEC
 iliac artery I74.5

Occlusion, occluded (*Continued*)
 intestine —*see* Obstruction, intestine
 lacrimal passages —*see* Obstruction, lacrimal
 lung J98.4
 lymph or lymphatic channel I89.0
 mammary duct N64.89
 mesenteric artery (embolic) (thrombotic) K55.0
 nose J34.89
  congenital Q30.0
 organ or site, congenital NEC —*see* Atresia, by site
 oviduct N97.1
  congenital Q50.6
 peripheral arteries
  due to stricture or stenosis I77.1
  upper extremity I74.2
 pontine (artery) —*see* Occlusion, artery, precerebral, specified NEC
 posterior lingual, of mandibular teeth M26.29
 precerebral artery —*see* Occlusion, artery, precerebral
 punctum lacrimale —*see* Obstruction, lacrimal
 pupil —*see* Membrane, pupillary
 pylorus, adult (*see also* Stricture, pylorus) K31.1
 renal artery N28.0
 retina, retinal
  artery —*see* Occlusion, artery, retinal
  vein (central) H34.81-
   engorgement H34.82-
   tributary H34.83-
   vessels H34.9
 spinal artery —*see* Occlusion, artery, precerebral, vertebral
 teeth (mandibular) (posterior lingual) M26.29
 thoracic duct I89.0
 thrombotic —*see* Thrombosis, artery
 traumatic
  edentulous (alveolar) ridge K06.2
  gingiva K06.2
  periodontal K05.5
 tubal N97.1
 ureter (complete) (partial) N13.5
  congenital Q62.10
 ureteropelvic junction N13.5
  congenital Q62.11
 ureterovesical orifice N13.5
  congenital Q62.12
 urethra —*see* Stricture, urethra
 uterus N85.8
 vagina N89.5
 vascular NEC I99.8
 vein —*see* Thrombosis
  retinal —*see* Occlusion, retinal, vein
 vena cava (inferior) (superior) —*see* Embolism, vena cava
 ventricle (brain) NEC G91.1
 vertebral (artery) —*see* Occlusion, artery, vertebral
 vessel (blood) I99.8
 vulva N90.5
Occult
 blood in feces (stools) R19.5
Occupational
 problems NEC Z56.89
Ochlophobia —*see* Agoraphobia
Ochronosis (endogenous) E70.29
Ocular muscle —*see* condition
Oculogyric crisis or disturbance H51.8
 psychogenic F45.8
Oculomotor syndrome H51.9
Oculopathy
 syphilitic NEC A52.71
  congenital
   early A50.01
   late A50.30
  early (secondary) A51.43
  late A52.71

Oddi's sphincter spasm K83.4
Odontalgia K08.8
Odontoameloblastoma —*see* Cyst, calcifying odontogenic
Odontoclasia K03.89
Odontodysplasia, regional K00.4
Odontogenesis imperfecta K00.5
Odontoma (ameloblastic) (complex) (compound) (fibroameloblastic) —*see* Cyst, calcifying odontogenic
Odontomyelitis (closed) (open) K04.0
Odontorrhagia K08.8
Odontosarcoma, ameloblastic C41.1
 upper jaw (bone) C41.0
~~Oedema, oedematous —see Edema~~
~~Oesophag (o) —see Esophag (o)~~
Oestriasis —*see* Myiasis
Oguchi's disease H53.63
Ohara's disease —*see* Tularemia
Oidiomycosis —*see* Candidiasis
Oidium albicans infection —*see* Candidiasis
Old (previous) myocardial infarction I25.2
Old age (without mention of debility) R54-
 dementia F03
Olfactory —*see* condition
Oligemia —*see* Anemia
Oligoastrocytoma
 specified site —*see* Neoplasm, malignant, by site
 unspecified site C71.9
Oligocythemia D64.9
Oligodendroblastoma
 specified site —*see* Neoplasm, malignant
 unspecified site C71.9
Oligodendroglioma
 anaplastic type
  specified site —*see* Neoplasm, malignant, by site
  unspecified site C71.9
 specified site —*see* Neoplasm, malignant, by site
 unspecified site C71.9
Oligodontia —*see* Anodontia
Oligoencephalon Q02
Oligohidrosis L74.4
Oligohydramnios O41.0-
Oligohydrosis L74.4
Oligomenorrhea N91.5
 primary N91.3
 secondary N91.4
Oligophrenia —*see also* Disability, intellectual
 phenylpyruvic E70.0
Oligospermia N46.11
 due to
  drug therapy N46.121
  efferent duct obstruction N46.123
  infection N46.122
  radiation N46.124
  specified cause NEC N46.129
  systemic disease N46.125
Oligotrichia —*see* Alopecia
Oliguria R34
 with, complicating or following ectopic or molar pregnancy O08.4
 postprocedural N99.0
Ollier's disease Q78.4
Omenotocele —*see* Hernia, abdomen, specified site NEC
Omentitis —*see* Peritonitis
Omentum, omental —*see* condition
Omphalitis (congenital) (newborn) P38.9
 with mild hemorrhage P38.1
 without hemorrhage P38.9
 not of newborn L08.82
 tetanus A33
Omphalocele Q79.2
Omphalomesenteric duct, persistent Q43.0
Omphalorrhagia, newborn P51.9
Omsk hemorrhagic fever A98.1
Onanism (excessive) F98.8

Onchocerciasis, onchocercosis B73.1
  with
    eye disease B73.00
      endophthalmitis B73.01
      eyelid B73.09
      glaucoma B73.02
      specified NEC B73.09
    eye NEC B73.00
    eyelid B73.09
Oncocytoma —*see* Neoplasm, benign, by site
Oncovirus, as cause of disease classified
  elsewhere B97.32
Ondine's curse —*see* Apnea, sleep
Oneirophrenia F23
Onychauxis L60.2
  congenital Q84.5
Onychia —*see also* Cellulitis, digit
  with lymphangitis —*see* Lymphangitis, acute,
    digit
  candidal B37.2
  dermatophytic B35.1
Onychitis —*see also* Cellulitis, digit
  with lymphangitis —*see* Lymphangitis, acute,
    digit
Onychocryptosis L60.0
Onychodystrophy L60.3
  congenital Q84.6
Onychogryphosis, onychogryposis L60.2
Onycholysis L60.1
Onychomadesis L60.8
Onychomalacia L60.3
Onychomycosis (finger) (toe) B35.1
Onycho-osteodysplasia Q79.8
Onychophagia F98.8
Onychophosis L60.8
Onychoptosis L60.8
Onychorrhexis L60.3
  congenital Q84.6
Onychoschizia L60.3
Onyxis (finger) (toe) L60.0
Onyxitis —*see also* Cellulitis, digit
  with lymphangitis —*see* Lymphangitis, acute,
    digit
Oophoritis (cystic) (infectional) (interstitial)
  N70.92
  with salpingitis N70.93
  acute N70.02
    with salpingitis N70.03
  chronic N70.12
    with salpingitis N70.13
  complicating abortion —*see* Abortion, by
    type, complicated by, oophoritis
Oophorocele N83.4
Opacity, opacities
  cornea H17.-
    central H17.1-
    congenital Q13.3
    degenerative —*see* Degeneration, cornea
    hereditary —*see* Dystrophy, cornea
    inflammatory —*see* Keratitis
    minor H17.81-
    peripheral H17.82-
    sequelae of trachoma (healed) B94.0
    specified NEC H17.89
  enamel (teeth) (fluoride) (nonfluoride)
    K00.3
  lens —*see* Cataract
  snowball —*see* Deposit, crystalline
  vitreous (humor) NEC H43.39-
    congenital Q14.0
    membranes and strands H43.31-
Opalescent dentin (hereditary) K00.5
Open, opening
  abnormal, organ or site, congenital —*see*
    Imperfect, closure
  angle with
    borderline
      findings
        high risk H40.02-
        low risk H40.01-
        intraocular pressure H40.00-

Open, opening (Continued)
  angle with (Continued)
    cupping of discs H40.01-
    glaucoma (primary) —*see* Glaucoma, open
      angle
  bite
    anterior M26.220
    posterior M26.221
  false —*see* Imperfect, closure
  margin on tooth restoration K08.51
  restoration margins of tooth K08.51
  wound —*see* Wound, open
Operational fatigue F48.8
Operative —*see* condition
Operculitis —*see* Periodontitis
Operculum —*see* Break, retina
Ophiasis L63.2
Ophthalmia (*see also* Conjunctivitis) H10.9
  actinic rays —*see* Photokeratitis
  allergic (acute) —*see* Conjunctivitis, acute,
    atopic
  blennorrhagic (gonococcal) (neonatorum)
    A54.31
  diphtheritic A36.86
  Egyptian A71.1
  electrica —*see* Photokeratitis
  gonococcal (neonatorum) A54.31
  metastatic —*see* Endophthalmitis, purulent
  migraine —*see* Migraine, ophthalmoplegic
  neonatorum, newborn P39.1
    gonococcal A54.31
  nodosa H16.24-
  purulent —*see* Conjunctivitis, acute,
    mucopurulent
  spring —*see* Conjunctivitis, acute, atopic
  sympathetic —*see* Uveitis, sympathetic
Ophthalmitis —*see* Ophthalmia
Ophthalmocele (congenital) Q15.8
Ophthalmoneuromyelitis G36.0
Ophthalmoplegia —*see also* Strabismus,
  paralytic
  anterior internuclear —*see* Ophthalmoplegia,
    internuclear
  ataxia-areflexia G61.0
  diabetic —*see* E08-E13 with .39
  exophthalmic E05.00
    with thyroid storm E05.01
  external H49.88-
    progressive H49.4-
      with pigmentary retinopathy —*see*
        Kearns-Sayre syndrome
    total H49.3-
  internal (complete) (total) H52.51-
  internuclear H51.2-
  migraine —*see* Migraine, ophthalmoplegic
  Parinaud's H49.88-
  progressive external —*see* Ophthalmoplegia,
    external, progressive
  supranuclear, progressive G23.1
  total (external) —*see* Ophthalmoplegia,
    external, total
Opioid (s)
  abuse —*see* Abuse, drug, opioids
  dependence —*see* Dependence, drug, opioids
Opisthognathism M26.09
Opisthorchiasis (felineus) (viverrini) B66.0
Opitz' disease D73.2
Opiumism —*see* Dependence, drug, opioid
Oppenheim's disease G70.2
Oppenheim-Urbach disease (necrobiosis
  lipoidica diabeticorum) —*see* E08-E13 with
  .620
Optic nerve —*see* condition
Orbit —*see* condition
Orchioblastoma C62.9-
Orchitis (gangrenous) (nonspecific) (septic)
  (suppurative) N45.2
  blennorrhagic (gonococcal) (acute) (chronic)
    A54.23
  chlamydial A56.19
  filarial (*see also* Infestation, filarial) B74.9
    [N51] ◀

Orchitis (Continued)
  gonococcal (acute) (chronic) A54.23
  mumps B26.0
  syphilitic A52.76
  tuberculous A18.15
Orf (virus disease) B08.02
Organic —*see also* condition
  brain syndrome F09
  heart —*see* Disease, heart
  mental disorder F09
  psychosis F09
Orgasm
  anejaculatory N53.13
Oriental
  bilharziasis B65.2
  schistosomiasis B65.2
Orifice —*see* condition
Origin of both great vessels from right
  ventricle Q20.1
Ormond's disease (with ureteral obstruction)
  N13.5
  with infection N13.6
Ornithine metabolism disorder E72.4
Ornithinemia (Type I) (Type II) E72.4
Ornithosis A70
Orotaciduria, oroticaciduria (congenital)
  (hereditary) (pyrimidine deficiency) E79.8
  anemia D53.0
Orthodontics
  adjustment Z46.4
  fitting Z46.4
Orthopnea R06.01
Orthopoxvirus B08.09
  specified NEC B08.09
Os, uterus —*see* condition
Osgood-Schlatter disease or
  osteochondrosis —*see* Osteochondrosis,
  juvenile, tibia
Osler (-Weber)-Rendu disease I78.0
Osler's nodes I33.0
Osmidrosis L75.0
Osseous —*see* condition
Ossification
  artery —*see* Arteriosclerosis
  auricle (ear) —*see* Disorder, pinna, specified
    type NEC
  bronchial J98.09
  cardiac —*see* Degeneration, myocardial
  cartilage (senile) —*see* Disorder, cartilage,
    specified type NEC
  coronary (artery) —*see* Disease, heart,
    ischemic, atherosclerotic
  diaphragm J98.6
  ear, middle —*see* Otosclerosis
  falx cerebri G96.19
  fontanel, premature Q75.0
  heart —*see also* Degeneration, myocardial
    valve —*see* Endocarditis
  larynx J38.7
  ligament —*see* Disorder, tendon, specified
    type NEC
    posterior longitudinal —*see*
      Spondylopathy, specified NEC
  meninges (cerebral) (spinal) G96.19
  multiple, eccentric centers —*see* Disorder,
    bone, development or growth
  muscle —*see also* Calcification, muscle
    due to burns —*see* Myositis, ossificans, in,
      burns
    paralytic —*see* Myositis, ossificans, in,
      quadriplegia
    progressive —*see* Myositis, ossificans,
      progressiva
    specified NEC M61.50
      ankle M61.57-
      foot M61.57-
      forearm M61.53-
      hand M61.54-
      lower leg M61.56-
      multiple sites M61.59
      pelvic region M61.55-

Ossification (Continued)
   muscle (Continued)
      specified NEC (Continued)
         shoulder region M61.51-
         specified site NEC M61.58
         thigh M61.55-
         upper arm M61.52-
      traumatic —see Myositis, ossificans, traumatica
   myocardium, myocardial —see Degeneration, myocardial
   penis N48.89
   periarticular —see Disorder, joint, specified type NEC
   pinna —see Disorder, pinna, specified type NEC
   rider's bone —see Ossification, muscle, specified NEC
   sclera H15.89
   subperiosteal, post-traumatic M89.8X-
   tendon —see Disorder, tendon, specified type NEC
   trachea J39.8
   tympanic membrane —see Disorder, tympanic membrane, specified NEC
   vitreous (humor) —see Deposit, crystalline
Osteitis —see also Osteomyelitis
   alveolar M27.3
   condensans M85.30
      ankle M85.37-
      foot M85.37-
      forearm M85.33-
      hand M85.34-
      lower leg M85.36-
      multiple site M85.39
      neck M85.38
      rib M85.38
      shoulder M85.31-
      skull M85.38
      specified site NEC M85.38
      thigh M85.35-
      toe M85.37-
      upper arm M85.32-
      vertebra M85.38
   deformans M88.9
      in (due to)
         malignant neoplasm of bone C41.9 [M90.60]
         neoplastic disease (see also Neoplasm) D49.9 [M90.60]
            carpus D49.9 [M90.64-]
            clavicle D49.9 [M90.61-]
            femur D49.9 [M90.65-]
            fibula D49.9 [M90.66-]
            finger D49.9 [M90.64-]
            humerus D49.9 [M90.62-]
            ilium D49.9 [M90.65-]
            ischium D49.9 [M90.65-]
            metacarpus D49.9 [M90.64-]
            metatarsus D49.9 [M90.67-]
            multiple sites D49.9 [M90.69]
            neck D49.9 [M90.68]
            radius D49.9 [M90.63-]
            rib D49.9 [M90.68]
            scapula D49.9 [M90.61-]
            skull D49.9 [M90.68]
            tarsus D49.9 [M90.67-]
            tibia D49.9 [M90.66-]
            toe D49.9 [M90.67-]
            ulna D49.9 [M90.63-]
            vertebra D49.9 [M90.68]
      skull M88.0
      specified NEC —see Paget's disease, bone, by site
      vertebra M88.1
   due to yaws A66.6
   fibrosa NEC —see Cyst, bone, by site
      circumscripta —see Dysplasia, fibrous, bone NEC

Osteitis (Continued)
   fibrosa NEC (Continued)
      cystica (generalisata) E21.0
      disseminata Q78.1
      osteoplastica E21.0
   fragilitans Q78.0
   Garr's (sclerosing) —see Osteomyelitis, specified type NEC
   jaw (acute) (chronic) (lower) (suppurative) (upper) M27.2
   parathyroid E21.0
   petrous bone (acute) (chronic) —see Petrositis
   sclerotic, nonsuppurative —see Osteomyelitis, specified type NEC
   tuberculosa A18.09
      cystica D86.89
      multiplex cystoides D86.89
Osteoarthritis M19.90
   ankle M19.07-
   elbow M19.02-
   foot joint M19.07-
   generalized M15.9
      erosive M15.4
      primary M15.0
      specified NEC M15.8
   hand joint M19.04-
      first carpometacarpal joint M18.9-
   hip M16.1-
      bilateral M16.0
      due to hip dysplasia (unilateral) M16.3-
         bilateral M16.2
   interphalangeal
      distal (Heberden) M15.1
      proximal (Bouchard) M15.2
   knee M17.9-
      bilateral M17.0
   post-traumatic NEC M19.92
      ankle M19.17-
      elbow M19.12-
      foot joint M19.17-
      hand M19.14-
         first carpometacarpal joint M18.3-
            bilateral M18.2
      hip M16.5-
         bilateral M16.4
      knee M17.3-
         bilateral M17.2
      shoulder M19.11-
      wrist M19.13-
   primary M19.91
      ankle M19.07-
      elbow M19.02-
      foot joint M19.07-
      hand joint M19.04-
         first carpometacarpal joint M18.1-
            bilateral M18.0
      hip M16.1-
         bilateral M16.0
      knee M17.1-
         bilateral M17.0
      shoulder M19.01-
      spine —see Spondylosis
      wrist M19.03-
   secondary M19.93
      ankle M19.27-
      elbow M19.22-
      foot joint M19.27-
      hand joint M19.24-
         first carpometacarpal joint M18.5-
            bilateral M18.4
      hip M16.7
         bilateral M16.6
      knee M17.5
         bilateral M17.4
      multiple M15.3
      shoulder M19.21-
      spine —see Spondylosis
      wrist M19.23-
   shoulder M19.01-
   spine —see Spondylosis
   wrist M19.03-

Osteoarthropathy (hypertrophic) M19.90
   ankle —see Osteoarthritis, primary, ankle
   elbow —see Osteoarthritis, primary, elbow
   foot joint —see Osteoarthritis, primary, foot
   hand joint —see Osteoarthritis, primary, hand joint
   knee joint —see Osteoarthritis, primary, knee
   multiple site —see Osteoarthritis, primary, multiple joint
   pulmonary —see also Osteoarthropathy, specified type NEC
      hypertrophic —see Osteoarthropathy, hypertrophic, specified type NEC
   secondary —see Osteoarthropathy, specified type NEC
   secondary hypertrophic —see Osteoarthropathy, specified type NEC
   shoulder —see Osteoarthritis, primary, shoulder
   specified joint NEC —see Osteoarthritis, primary, specified joint NEC
   specified type NEC M89.40
      carpus M89.44-
      clavicle M89.41-
      femur M89.45-
      fibula M89.46-
      finger M89.44-
      humerus M89.42-
      ilium M89.459
      ischium M89.459
      metacarpus M89.44-
      metatarsus M89.47-
      multiple sites M89.49
      neck M89.48
      radius M89.43-
      rib M89.48
      scapula M89.41-
      skull M89.48
      tarsus M89.47-
      tibia M89.46-
      toe M89.47-
      ulna M89.43-
      vertebra M89.48
   spine —see Spondylosis
   wrist —see Osteoarthritis, primary, wrist
Osteoarthrosis (degenerative) (hypertrophic) (joint) —see also Osteoarthritis
   deformans alkaptonurica E70.29 [M36.8]
   erosive M15.4
   generalized M15.9
      primary M15.0
   polyarticular M15.9
   spine —see Spondylosis
Osteoblastoma —see Neoplasm, bone, benign
   aggressive —see Neoplasm, bone, uncertain behavior
Osteochondroarthrosis deformans endemica —see Disease, Kaschin-Beck
Osteochondritis —see also Osteochondropathy, by site
   Brailsford's —see Osteochondrosis, juvenile, radius
   dissecans M93.20
      ankle M93.27-
      elbow M93.22-
      foot M93.27-
      hand M93.24-
      hip M93.25-
      knee M93.26-
      multiple sites M93.29
      shoulder joint M93.21-
      specified site NEC M93.28
      wrist M93.23-
   juvenile M92.9
      patellar —see Osteochondrosis, juvenile, patella
   syphilitic (congenital) (early) A50.02 [M90.80]
      ankle A50.02 [M90.87-]
      elbow A50.02 [M90.82-]
      foot A50.02 [M90.87-]
      forearm A50.02 [M90.83-]

Osteochondritis (Continued)
  syphilitic (Continued)
    hand A50.02 [M90.84-]
    hip A50.02 [M90.85-]
    knee A50.02 [M90.86-]
    multiple sites A50.02 [M90.89]
    shoulder joint A50.02 [M90.81-]
    specified site NEC A50.02 [M90.88]
Osteochondrodysplasia Q78.9
  with defects of growth of tubular bones and
    spine Q77.9
    specified NEC Q77.8
  specified NEC Q78.8
Osteochondrodystrophy E78.9
Osteochondrolysis —see Osteochondritis,
  dissecans
Osteochondroma —see Neoplasm, bone, benign
Osteochondromatosis D48.0
  syndrome Q78.4
Osteochondromyxosarcoma —see Neoplasm,
  bone, malignant
Osteochondropathy M93.90
  ankle M93.97-
  elbow M93.92-
  foot M93.97-
  hand M93.94-
  hip M93.95-
  Kienböck's disease of adults M93.1
  knee M93.96-
  multiple joints M93.99
  osteochondritis dissecans —see
    Osteochondritis, dissecans
  osteochondrosis —see Osteochondrosis
  shoulder region M93.91-
  slipped upper femoral epiphysis —see
    Slipped, epiphysis, upper femoral
  specified joint NEC M93.98
  specified type NEC M93.80
    ankle M93.87-
    elbow M93.82-
    foot M93.87-
    hand M93.84-
    hip M93.85-
    knee M93.86-
    multiple joints M93.89
    shoulder region M93.81-
    specified joint NEC M93.88
    wrist M93.83-
  syphilitic, congenital
    early A50.02 [M90.80]
    late A50.56 [M90.80]
  wrist M93.93-
Osteochondrosarcoma —see Neoplasm, bone,
  malignant
Osteochondrosis —see also Osteochondropathy,
  by site
  acetabulum (juvenile) M91.0
  adult —see Osteochondropathy, specified
    type NEC, by site
  astragalus (juvenile) —see Osteochondrosis,
    juvenile, tarsus
  Blount's —see Osteochondrosis, juvenile, tibia
  Buchanan's M91.0
  Burns' —see Osteochondrosis, juvenile, ulna
  calcaneus (juvenile) —see Osteochondrosis,
    juvenile, tarsus
  capitular epiphysis (femur) (juvenile) —see
    Legg-Calvé-Perthes disease
  carpal (juvenile) (lunate) (scaphoid) —see
    Osteochondrosis, juvenile, hand, carpal
    lunate
    adult M93.1
  coxae juvenilis —see Legg-Calvé-Perthes
    disease
  deformans juvenilis, coxae —see Legg-Calvé-
    Perthes disease
  Diaz's —see Osteochondrosis, juvenile, tarsus
  dissecans (knee) (shoulder) —see
    Osteochondritis, dissecans
  femoral capital epiphysis (juvenile) —see
    Legg-Calvé-Perthes disease

Osteochondrosis (Continued)
  femur (head), juvenile —see Legg-Calvé-
    Perthes disease
  fibula (juvenile) —see Osteochondrosis,
    juvenile, fibula
  foot NEC (juvenile) M92.8
  Freiberg's —see Osteochondrosis, juvenile,
    metatarsus
  Haas' (juvenile) —see Osteochondrosis,
    juvenile, humerus
  Haglund's —see Osteochondrosis, juvenile,
    tarsus
  hip (juvenile) —see Legg-Calvé-Perthes
    disease
  humerus (capitulum) (head) (juvenile) —see
    Osteochondrosis, juvenile, humerus
  ilium, iliac crest (juvenile) M91.0
  ischiopubic synchondrosis M91.0
  Iselin's —see Osteochondrosis, juvenile,
    metatarsus
  juvenile, juvenilis M92.9
    after congenital dislocation of hip
      reduction —see Osteochondrosis,
      juvenile, hip, specified NEC
    arm —see Osteochondrosis, juvenile, upper
      limb NEC
    capitular epiphysis (femur) —see Legg-
      Calvé-Perthes disease
    clavicle, sternal epiphysis —see
      Osteochondrosis, juvenile, upper
      limb NEC
    coxae —see Legg-Calvé-Perthes
      disease
    deformans M92.9
    fibula M92.5-
    foot NEC M92.8
    hand M92.20-
      carpal lunate M92.21-
      metacarpal head M92.22-
      specified site NEC M92.29-
    head of femur —see Legg-Calvé-Perthes
      disease
    hip and pelvis M91.9-
      coxa plana —see Coxa, plana
      femoral head —see Legg-Calvé-Perthes
        disease
      pelvis M91.0
      pseudocoxalgia —see Pseudocoxalgia
      specified NEC M91.8-
    humerus M92.0-
    limb
      lower NEC M92.8
      upper NEC —see Osteochondrosis,
        juvenile, upper limb NEC
    medial cuneiform bone —see
      Osteochondrosis, juvenile, tarsus
    metatarsus M92.7-
    patella M92.4-
    radius M92.1-
    specified site NEC M92.8
    spine M42.00
      cervical region M42.02
      cervicothoracic region M42.03
      lumbar region M42.06
      lumbosacral region M42.07
      multiple sites M42.09
      occipito-atlanto-axial region
        M42.01
      sacrococcygeal region M42.08
      thoracic region M42.04
      thoracolumbar region M42.05
    tarsus M92.6-
    tibia M92.5-
    ulna M92.1-
    upper limb NEC M92.3-
    vertebra (body) (epiphyseal plates)
      (Calvé's) (Scheuermann's) —see
      Osteochondrosis, juvenile, spine
  Kienböck's —see Osteochondrosis, juvenile,
    hand, carpal lunate
    adult M93.1

Osteochondrosis (Continued)
  Köhler's
    patellar —see Osteochondrosis, juvenile,
      patella
    tarsal navicular —see Osteochondrosis,
      juvenile, tarsus
  Legg-Perthes (-Calvé's) (-Waldenström) —see
    Legg-Calvé-Perthes disease
  limb
    lower NEC (juvenile) M92.8
    upper NEC (juvenile) —see
      Osteochondrosis, juvenile, upper
      limb NEC
  lunate bone (carpal) (juvenile) —see also
    Osteochondrosis, juvenile, hand, carpal
    lunate
    adult M93.1
  Mauclaire's —see Osteochondrosis, juvenile,
    hand, metacarpal
  metacarpal (head) (juvenile) —see
    Osteochondrosis, juvenile, hand,
    metacarpal
  metatarsus (fifth) (head) (juvenile)
    (second) —see Osteochondrosis,
    juvenile, metatarsus
  navicular (juvenile) —see Osteochondrosis,
    juvenile, tarsus
  os
    calcis (juvenile) —see Osteochondrosis,
      juvenile, tarsus
    tibiale externum (juvenile) —see
      Osteochondrosis, juvenile, tarsus
  Osgood-Schlatter —see Osteochondrosis,
    juvenile, tibia
  Panner's —see Osteochondrosis, juvenile,
    humerus
  patellar center (juvenile) (primary)
    (secondary) —see Osteochondrosis,
    juvenile, patella
  pelvis (juvenile) M91.0
  Pierson's M91.0
  radius (head) (juvenile) —see
    Osteochondrosis, juvenile, radius
  Scheuermann's —see Osteochondrosis,
    juvenile, spine
  Sever's —see Osteochondrosis, juvenile,
    tarsus
  Sinding-Larsen —see Osteochondrosis,
    juvenile, patella
  spine M42.9
    adult M42.10
      cervical region M42.12
      cervicothoracic region M42.13
      lumbar region M42.16
      lumbosacral region M42.17
      multiple sites M42.19
      occipito-atlanto-axial region M42.11
      sacrococcygeal region M42.18
      thoracic region M42.14
      thoracolumbar region M42.15
    juvenile —see Osteochondrosis, juvenile,
      spine
  symphysis pubis (juvenile) M91.0
  syphilitic (congenital) A50.02
  talus (juvenile) —see Osteochondrosis,
    juvenile, tarsus
  tarsus (navicular) (juvenile) —see
    Osteochondrosis, juvenile, tarsus
  tibia (proximal) (tubercle) (juvenile) —see
    Osteochondrosis, juvenile, tibia
  tuberculous —see Tuberculosis, bone
  ulna (lower) (juvenile) —see Osteochondrosis,
    juvenile, ulna
  van Neck's M91.0
  vertebral —see Osteochondrosis,
    spine
Osteoclastoma D48.0
  malignant —see Neoplasm, bone,
    malignant
Osteodynia —see Disorder, bone,
    specified type NEC

◀ New   ◀◀◀ Revised   ~~deleted~~ Deleted

Osteodystrophy Q78.9
  azotemic N25.0
  congenital Q78.9
  parathyroid, secondary E21.1
  renal N25.0
Osteofibroma —*see* Neoplasm, bone,
  benign
Osteofibrosarcoma —*see* Neoplasm,
  bone, malignant
Osteogenesis imperfecta Q78.0
Osteogenic —*see* condition
Osteolysis M89.50
  carpus M89.54-
  clavicle M89.51-
  femur M89.55-
  fibula M89.56-
  finger M89.54-
  humerus M89.52-
  ilium M89.559
  ischium M89.559
  joint prosthesis (periprosthetic) —*see*
    Complications, joint prosthesis,
    mechanical, periprosthetic, osteolysis,
    by site
  metacarpus M89.54-
  metatarsus M89.57-
  multiple sites M89.59
  neck M89.58
  periprosthetic —*see* Complications, joint
    prosthesis, mechanical, periprosthetic,
    osteolysis, by site
  radius M89.53-
  rib M89.58
  scapula M89.51-
  skull M89.58
  tarsus M89.57-
  tibia M89.56-
  toe M89.57-
  ulna M89.53-
  vertebra M89.58
Osteoma —*see also* Neoplasm, bone, benign
  osteoid —*see also* Neoplasm, bone, benign
    giant —*see* Neoplasm, bone, benign
Osteomalacia M83.9
  adult M83.9
    drug-induced NEC M83.5
    due to
      malabsorption (postsurgical)
        M83.2
      malnutrition M83.3
    specified NEC M83.8
  aluminium-induced M83.4
  infantile —*see* Rickets
  juvenile —*see* Rickets
  oncogenic E83.89
  pelvis M83.8
  puerperal M83.0
  senile M83.1
  vitamin-D-resistant in adults E83.31
    [M90.8-]
    carpus E83.31 *[M90.84-]*
    clavicle E83.31 *[M90.81-]*
    femur E83.31 *[M90.85-]*
    fibula E83.31 *[M90.86-]*
    finger E83.31 *[M90.84-]*
    humerus E83.31 *[M90.82-]*
    ilium E83.31 *[M90.859]*
    ischium E83.31 *[M90.859]*
    metacarpus E83.31 *[M90.84-]*
    metatarsus E83.31 *[M90.87-]*
    multiple sites E83.31 *[M90.89]*
    neck E83.31 *[M90.88]*
    radius E83.31 *[M90.83-]*
    rib E83.31 *[M90.88]*
    scapula E83.31 *[M90.819]*
    skull E83.31 *[M90.88]*
    tarsus E83.31 *[M90.879]*
    tibia E83.31 *[M90.869]*
    toe E83.31 *[M90.879]*
    ulna E83.31 *[M90.839]*
    vertebra E83.31 *[M90.88]*

Osteomyelitis (general) (infective)
    (localized) (neonatal) (purulent)
    (septic) (staphylococcal) (streptococcal)
    (suppurative) (with periostitis) M86.9
  acute M86.10
    carpus M86.14-
    clavicle M86.11-
    femur M86.15-
    fibula M86.16-
    finger M86.14-
    hematogenous M86.00
      carpus M86.04-
      clavicle M86.01-
      femur M86.05-
      fibula M86.06-
      finger M86.04-
      humerus M86.02-
      ilium M86.059
      ischium M86.059
      mandible M27.2
      metacarpus M86.04-
      metatarsus M86.07-
      multiple sites M86.09
      neck M86.08
      orbit H05.02-
      petrous bone —*see* Petrositis
      radius M86.03-
      rib M86.08
      scapula M86.01-
      skull M86.08
      tarsus M86.07-
      tibia M86.06-
      toe M86.07-
      ulna M86.03-
      vertebra —*see* Osteomyelitis, vertebra
    humerus M86.12-
    ilium M86.159
    ischium M86.159
    mandible M27.2
    metacarpus M86.14-
    metatarsus M86.17-
    multiple sites M86.19
    neck M86.18
    orbit H05.02-
    petrous bone —*see* Petrositis
    radius M86.13-
    rib M86.18
    scapula M86.11-
    skull M86.18
    tarsus M86.17-
    tibia M86.16-
    toe M86.17-
    ulna M86.13-
    vertebra —*see* Osteomyelitis, vertebra
  chronic (or old) M86.60
    with draining sinus M86.40
      carpus M86.44-
      clavicle M86.41-
      femur M86.45-
      fibula M86.46-
      finger M86.44-
      humerus M86.42-
      ilium M86.459
      ischium M86.459
      mandible M27.2
      metacarpus M86.44-
      metatarsus M86.47-
      multiple sites M86.49
      neck M86.48
      orbit H05.02-
      petrous bone —*see* Petrositis
      radius M86.43-
      rib M86.48
      scapula M86.41-
      skull M86.48
      tarsus M86.47-
      tibia M86.46-
      toe M86.47-
      ulna M86.43-
      vertebra —*see* Osteomyelitis, vertebra
    carpus M86.64-

Osteomyelitis (*Continued*)
  chronic (*Continued*)
    clavicle M86.61-
    femur M86.65-
    fibula M86.66-
    finger M86.64-
    hematogenous NEC M86.50
      carpus M86.54-
      clavicle M86.51-
      femur M86.55-
      fibula M86.56-
      finger M86.54-
      humerus M86.52-
      ilium M86.559
      ischium M86.559
      mandible M27.2
      metacarpus M86.54-
      metatarsus M86.57-
      multifocal M86.30
        carpus M86.34-
        clavicle M86.31-
        femur M86.35-
        fibula M86.36-
        finger M86.34-
        humerus M86.32-
        ilium M86.359
        ischium M86.359
        metacarpus M86.34-
        metatarsus M86.37-
        multiple sites M86.39
        neck M86.38
        radius M86.33-
        rib M86.38
        scapula M86.31-
        skull M86.38
        tarsus M86.37-
        tibia M86.36-
        toe M86.37-
        ulna M86.33-
        vertebra —*see* Osteomyelitis, vertebra
      multiple sites M86.59
      neck M86.58
      orbit H05.02-
      petrous bone —*see* Petrositis
      radius M86.53-
      rib M86.58
      scapula M86.51-
      skull M86.58
      tarsus M86.57-
      tibia M86.56-
      toe M86.57-
      ulna M86.53-
      vertebra —*see* Osteomyelitis, vertebra
    humerus M86.62-
    ilium M86.659
    ischium M86.659
    mandible M27.2
    metacarpus M86.64-
    metatarsus M86.67-
    multifocal —*see* Osteomyelitis, chronic,
      hematogenous, multifocal
    multiple sites M86.69
    neck M86.68
    orbit H05.02-
    petrous bone —*see* Petrositis
    radius M86.63-
    rib M86.68
    scapula M86.61-
    skull M86.68
    tarsus M86.67-
    tibia M86.66-
    toe M86.67-
    ulna M86.63-
    vertebra —*see* Osteomyelitis, vertebra
  echinococcal B67.2
  Garr's —*see* Osteomyelitis, specified type
    NEC
  jaw (acute) (chronic) (lower) (neonatal)
    (suppurative) (upper) M27.2
  nonsuppurating —*see* Osteomyelitis,
    specified type NEC

Osteomyelitis (Continued)
  orbit H05.02-
  petrous bone —see Petrositis
  Salmonella (arizonae) (cholerae-suis)
      (enteritidis) (typhimurium) A02.24
  sclerosing, nonsuppurative —see
      Osteomyelitis, specified type NEC
  specified type NEC (see also subcategory)
      M86.8X-
    mandible M27.2
    orbit H05.02-
    petrous bone —see Petrositis
    vertebra —see Osteomyelitis, vertebra
  subacute M86.20
    carpus M86.24-
    clavicle M86.21-
    femur M86.25-
    fibula M86.26-
    finger M86.24-
    humerus M86.22-
    mandible M27.2
    metacarpus M86.24-
    metatarsus M86.27-
    multiple sites M86.29
    neck M86.28
    orbit H05.02-
    petrous bone —see Petrositis
    radius M86.23-
    rib M86.28
    scapula M86.21-
    skull M86.28
    tarsus M86.27-
    tibia M86.26-
    toe M86.27-
    ulna M86.23-
    vertebra —see Osteomyelitis, vertebra
  syphilitic A52.77
    congenital (early) A50.02 [M90.80]
  tuberculous —see Tuberculosis, bone
  typhoid A01.05
  vertebra M46.20
    cervical region M46.22
    cervicothoracic region M46.23
    lumbar region M46.26
    lumbosacral region M46.27
    occipito-atlanto-axial region M46.21
    sacrococcygeal region M46.28
    thoracic region M46.24
    thoracolumbar region M46.25
Osteomyelofibrosis D75.89
Osteomyelosclerosis D75.89
Osteonecrosis M87.9
  due to
    drugs —see Osteonecrosis, secondary, due
        to, drugs
    trauma —see Osteonecrosis, secondary, due
        to, trauma
  idiopathic aseptic M87.00
    ankle M87.07-
    carpus M87.03-
    clavicle M87.01-
    femur M87.05-
    fibula M87.06-
    finger M87.04-
    humerus M87.02-
    ilium M87.050
    ischium M87.050
    metacarpus M87.04-
    metatarsus M87.07-
    multiple sites M87.09
    neck M87.08
    pelvis M87.050
    radius M87.03-
    rib M87.08
    scapula M87.01-
    skull M87.08
    tarsus M87.07-
    tibia M87.06-
    toe M87.07-
    ulna M87.03-
    vertebra M87.08

Osteonecrosis (Continued)
  secondary NEC M87.30
    carpus M87.33-
    clavicle M87.31-
    due to
      drugs M87.10
        carpus M87.13-
        clavicle M87.11-
        femur M87.15-
        fibula M87.16-
        finger M87.14-
        humerus M87.12-
        ilium M87.159
        ischium M87.159
        jaw M87.180
        metacarpus M87.14-
        metatarsus M87.17-
        multiple sites M87.19
        neck M87.18
        radius M87.13-
        rib M87.18
        scapula M87.11-
        skull M87.18
        tarsus M87.17-
        tibia M87.16-
        toe M87.17-
        ulna M87.13-
        vertebra M87.18
      hemoglobinopathy NEC D58.2 [M90.50]
        carpus D58.2 [M90.54-]
        clavicle D58.2 [M90.51-]
        femur D58.2 [M90.55-]
        fibula D58.2 [M90.56-]
        finger D58.2 [M90.54-]
        humerus D58.2 [M90.52-]
        ilium D58.2 [M90.55-]
        ischium D58.2 [M90.55-]
        metacarpus D58.2 [M90.54-]
        metatarsus D58.2 [M90.57-]
        multiple sites D58.2 [M90.58]
        neck D58.2 [M90.58]
        radius D58.2 [M90.53-]
        rib D58.2 [M90.58]
        scapula D58.2 [M90.51-]
        skull D58.2 [M90.58]
        tarsus D58.2 [M90.57-]
        tibia D58.2 [M90.56-]
        toe D58.2 [M90.57-]
        ulna D58.2 [M90.53-]
        vertebra D58.2 [M90.58]
      trauma (previous) M87.20
        carpus M87.23-
        clavicle M87.21-
        femur M87.25-
        fibula M87.26-
        finger M87.24-
        humerus M87.22-
        ilium M87.25-
        ischium M87.25-
        metacarpus M87.24-
        metatarsus M87.27-
        multiple sites M87.29
        neck M87.28
        radius M87.23-
        rib M87.28
        scapula M87.21-
        skull M87.28
        tarsus M87.27-
        tibia M87.26-
        toe M87.27-
        ulna M87.23-
        vertebra M87.28
    femur M87.35-
    fibula M87.36-
    finger M87.34-
    humerus M87.32
    ilium M87.350
    in
      caisson disease T70.3 [M90.50]
        carpus T70.3 [M90.54-]
        clavicle T70.3 [M90.51-]

Osteonecrosis (Continued)
  secondary NEC (Continued)
    in (Continued)
      caisson disease (Continued)
        femur T70.3 [M90.55-]
        fibula T70.3 [M90.56-]
        finger T70.3 [M90.54-]
        humerus T70.3 [M90.52-]
        ilium T70.3 [M90.55-]
        ischium T70.3 [M90.55-]
        metacarpus T70.3 [M90.54-]
        metatarsus T70.3 [M90.57-]
        multiple sites T70.3 [M90.59]
        neck T70.3 [M90.58]
        radius T70.3 [M90.53-]
        rib T70.3 [M90.58]
        scapula T70.3 [M90.51-]
        skull T70.3 [M90.58]
        tarsus T70.3 [M90.57-]
        tibia T70.3 [M90.56-]
        toe T70.3 [M90.57-]
        ulna T70.3 [M90.53-]
        vertebra T70.3 [M90.58]
    ischium M87.350
    metacarpus M87.34-
    metatarsus M87.37-
    multiple site M87.39
    neck M87.38
    radius M87.33-
    rib M87.38
    scapula M87.319
    skull M87.38
    tarsus M87.379
    tibia M87.366
    toe M87.379
    ulna M87.33-
    vertebra M87.38
  specified type NEC M87.80
    carpus M87.83-
    clavicle M87.81-
    femur M87.85-
    fibula M87.86-
    finger M87.84-
    humerus M87.82-
    ilium M87.85-
    ischium M87.85-
    metacarpus M87.84-
    metatarsus M87.87-
    multiple sites M87.89
    neck M87.88
    radius M87.83-
    rib M87.88-
    scapula M87.81-
    skull M87.88
    tarsus M87.87-
    tibia M87.86-
    toe M87.87-
    ulna M87.83-
    vertebra M87.88
Osteo-onycho-arthro-dysplasia Q79.8
Osteo-onychodysplasia, hereditary Q79.8
Osteopathia condensans disseminata Q78.8
Osteopathy —see also Osteomyelitis,
    Osteonecrosis, Osteoporosis
  after poliomyelitis M89.60
    carpus M89.64-
    clavicle M89.61-
    femur M89.65-
    fibula M89.66-
    finger M89.64-
    humerus M89.62-
    ilium M89.659
    ischium M89.659
    metacarpus M89.64-
    metatarsus M89.67-
    multiple sites M89.69
    neck M89.68
    radius M89.63-
    rib M89.68
    scapula M89.61-
    skull M89.68

Otitis (Continued)
  media (Continued)
    chronic (Continued)
      catarrhal —see Otitis, media,
        nonsuppurative, chronic, serous
      exudative —see Otitis, media,
        nonsuppurative, chronic
      mucinous —see Otitis, media,
        nonsuppurative, chronic, mucoid
      mucoid —see Otitis, media,
        nonsuppurative, chronic, mucoid
      nonsuppurative NEC —see Otitis, media,
        nonsuppurative, chronic
      purulent —see Otitis, media,
        suppurative, chronic
      secretory —see Otitis, media,
        nonsuppurative, chronic, mucoid
      seromucinous —see Otitis, media,
        nonsuppurative, chronic
      serous —see Otitis, media,
        nonsuppurative, chronic, serous
      suppurative —see Otitis, media,
        suppurative, chronic
      transudative —see Otitis, media,
        nonsuppurative, chronic, mucoid
    exudative —see Otitis, media,
      nonsuppurative
    in (due to) (with)
      influenza —see Influenza, with, otitis
        media
      measles B05.3
      scarlet fever A38.0
      tuberculosis A18.6
      viral disease NEC B34.- [H67.-]
    mucoid —see Otitis, media,
      nonsuppurative
    nonsuppurative H65.9-
      acute or subacute NEC H65.19-
        allergic H65.11-
          recurrent H65.11-
        recurrent H65.19-
        secretory —see Otitis, media,
          nonsuppurative, serous
        serous H65.0-
          recurrent H65.0-
      chronic H65.49-
        allergic H65.41-
        mucoid H65.3-
        serous H65.2-
    postmeasles B05.3
    purulent —see Otitis, media, suppurative
    secretory —see Otitis, media,
      nonsuppurative
    seromucinous —see Otitis, media,
      nonsuppurative
    serous —see Otitis, media, nonsuppurative
    suppurative H66.4-
      acute H66.00-
        with rupture of ear drum H66.01-
        recurrent H66.00-
          with rupture of ear drum H66.01-
      chronic (see also subcategory) H66.3
        atticoantral H66.2-
        benign —see Otitis, media,
          suppurative, chronic,
          tubotympanic
        tubotympanic H66.1-
    transudative —see Otitis, media,
      nonsuppurative
    tuberculous A18.6

Otocephaly Q18.2
Otolith syndrome —see subcategory H81.8
Otomycosis (diffuse) NEC B36.9 [H62.40]
  in
    aspergillosis B44.89
    candidiasis B37.84
    moniliasis B37.84
Otoporosis —see Otosclerosis
Otorrhagia (nontraumatic) H92.2-
  traumatic - code by Type of injury
Otorrhea H92.1-
  cerebrospinal G96.0
Otosclerosis (general) H80.9-
  cochlear (endosteal) H80.2-
  involving
    otic capsule —see Otosclerosis, cochlear
    oval window
      nonobliterative H80.0-
        obliterative H80.1-
    round window —see Otosclerosis, cochlear
  nonobliterative —see Otosclerosis, involving,
    oval window, nonobliterative
  obliterative —see Otosclerosis, involving, oval
    window, obliterative
  specified NEC H80.8-
Otospongiosis —see Otosclerosis
Otto's disease or pelvis M24.7
Outcome of delivery Z37.9
  multiple births Z37.9
    all liveborn Z37.50
      quadruplets Z37.52
      quintuplets Z37.53
      sextuplets Z37.54
      specified number NEC Z37.59
      triplets Z37.51
    all stillborn Z37.7
    some liveborn Z37.60
      quadruplets Z37.62
      quintuplets Z37.63
      sextuplets Z37.64
      specified number NEC Z37.69
      triplets Z37.61
  single NEC Z37.9
    liveborn Z37.0
    stillborn Z37.1
  twins NEC Z37.9
    both liveborn Z37.2
    both stillborn Z37.4
    one liveborn, one stillborn Z37.3
Outlet —see condition
Ovalocytosis (congenital) (hereditary) —see
  Elliptocytosis
Ovarian —see Condition
Ovariocele N83.4
Ovaritis (cystic) —see Oophoritis
Ovary, ovarian —see also condition
  resistant syndrome E28.39
  vein syndrome N13.8
Overactive —see also Hyperfunction
  adrenal cortex NEC E27.0
  bladder N32.81
  hypothalamus E23.3
  thyroid —see Hyperthyroidism
Overactivity R46.3
  child —see Disorder, attention-deficit
    hyperactivity
Overbite (deep) (excessive) (horizontal)
  (vertical) M26.29
Overbreathing —see Hyperventilation
Overconscientious personality F60.5

Overdevelopment —see Hypertrophy
Overdistension —see Distension
Overdose, overdosage (drug) —see Table
  of Drugs and Chemicals, by drug,
  poisoning
Overeating R63.2
  nonorganic origin F50.8
  psychogenic F50.8
Overexertion (effects) (exhaustion) T73.3
Overexposure (effects) T73.9
  exhaustion T73.2
Overfeeding —see Overeating
  newborn P92.4
Overfill, endodontic M27.52
Overgrowth, bone —see Hypertrophy, bone
Overhanging of dental restorative material
  (unrepairable) K08.52
Overheated (places) (effects) —see Heat
Overjet (excessive horizontal) M26.23
Overlaid, overlying (suffocation) —see Asphyxia,
  traumatic, due to mechanical threat
Overlap, excessive horizontal (teeth) M26.23
Overlapping toe (acquired) —see also
  Deformity, toe, specified NEC
  congenital (fifth toe) Q66.89
Overload
  circulatory, due to transfusion (blood) (blood
    components) (TACO) E87.71
  fluid E87.70
    due to transfusion (blood) (blood
      components) E87.71
    specified NEC E87.79
  iron, due to repeated red blood cell
    transfusions E83.111
  potassium (K) E87.5
  sodium (Na) E87.0
Overnutrition —see Hyperalimentation
Overproduction —see also Hypersecretion
  ACTH E27.0
  catecholamine E27.5
  growth hormone E22.0
Overprotection, child by parent Z62.1
Overriding
  aorta Q25.4
  finger (acquired) —see Deformity, finger
    congenital Q68.1
  toe (acquired) —see also Deformity, toe,
    specified NEC
    congenital Q66.89
Overstrained R53.83
  heart —see Hypertrophy, cardiac
Overuse, muscle NEC M70.8-
Overweight E66.3
Overworked R53.83
Oviduct —see condition
Ovotestis Q56.0
Ovulation (cycle)
  failure or lack of N97.0
  pain N94.0
Ovum —see condition
Owren's disease or syndrome (parahemophilia)
  D68.2
Ox heart —see Hypertrophy, cardiac
Oxalosis E72.53
Oxaluria E72.53
Oxycephaly, oxycephalic Q75.0
  syphilitic, congenital A50.02
Oxyuriasis B80
Oxyuris vermicularis (infestation) B80
Ozena J31.0

P

Pachyderma, pachydermia L85.9
 larynx (verrucosa) J38.7
Pachydermatocele (congenital) Q82.8
Pachydermoperiostosis —*see also*
  Osteoarthropathy, hypertrophic, specified
  type NEC
 clubbed nail M89.40 *[L62]*
Pachygyria Q04.3
Pachymeningitis (adhesive) (basal) (brain)
  (cervical) (chronic) (circumscribed)
  (external) (fibrous) (hemorrhagic)
  (hypertrophic) (internal) (purulent)
  (spinal) (suppurative) —*see* Meningitis
Pachyonychia (congenital) Q84.5
Pacinian tumor —*see* Neoplasm, skin, benign
Pad, knuckle or Garrod's M72.1
Paget-Schroetter syndrome I82.890
Paget's disease
 with infiltrating duct carcinoma —*see*
  Neoplasm, breast, malignant
 bone M88.9
  carpus M88.84-
  clavicle M88.81-
  femur M88.85-
  fibula M88.86-
  finger M88.84-
  humerus M88.82-
  ilium M88.85-
  in neoplastic disease —*see* Osteitis,
   deformans, in neoplastic disease
  ischium M88.85-
  metacarpus M88.84-
  metatarsus M88.87-
  multiple sites M88.89
  neck M88.88
  radius M88.83-
  rib M88.88
  scapula M88.81-
  skull M88.0
  tarsus M88.87-
  tibia M88.86-
  toe M88.87-
  ulna M88.83-
  vertebra M88.88
 breast (female) C50.01-
  male C50.02-
 extramammary —*see also* Neoplasm, skin,
   malignant
  anus C21.0
   margin C44.590
   skin C44.590
 intraductal carcinoma —*see* Neoplasm,
   breast, malignant
 malignant —*see* Neoplasm, skin, malignant
  breast (female) C50.01-
   male C50.02-
  unspecified site (female) C50.01-
   male C50.02-
 mammary —*see* Paget's disease, breast
 nipple —*see* Paget's disease, breast
 osteitis deformans —*see* Paget's disease, bone
Pain (s) (*see also* Painful) R52
 abdominal R10.9
  colic R10.83
  generalized R10.84
   with acute abdomen R10.0
  lower R10.30
   left quadrant R10.32
   pelvic or perineal R10.2
   periumbilical R10.33
   right quadrant R10.31
  rebound —*see* Tenderness, abdominal,
    rebound
  severe with abdominal rigidity R10.0
  tenderness —*see* Tenderness, abdominal
  upper R10.10
   epigastric R10.13
   left quadrant R10.12
   right quadrant R10.11

Pain *(Continued)*
 acute R52
  due to trauma G89.11
  neoplasm related G89.3
  postprocedural NEC G89.18
  post-thoracotomy G89.12
  specified by site — code to Pain, by site
 adnexa (uteri) R10.2
 anginoid —*see* Pain, precordial
 anus K62.89
 arm —*see* Pain, limb, upper
 axillary (axilla) M79.62-
 back (postural) M54.9
 bladder R39.89
  associated with micturition —*see*
    Micturition, painful
 bone —*see* Disorder, bone, specified type
    NEC
 breast N64.4
 broad ligament R10.2
 cancer associated (acute) (chronic) G89.3
 cecum —*see* Pain, abdominal
 cervicobrachial M53.1
 chest (central) R07.9
  anterior wall R07.89
  atypical R07.89
  ischemic I20.9
  musculoskeletal R07.89
  non-cardiac R07.89
  on breathing R07.1
  pleurodynia R07.81
  precordial R07.2
  wall (anterior) R07.89
 chronic G89.29
  associated with significant psychosocial
    dysfunction G89.4
  due to trauma G89.21
  neoplasm related G89.3
  postoperative NEC G89.28
  postprocedural NEC G89.28
  post-thoracotomy G89.22
  specified NEC G89.29
 coccyx M53.3
 colon —*see* Pain, abdominal
 coronary —*see* Angina
 costochondral R07.1
 diaphragm R07.1
 due to cancer G89.3
 due to device, implant or graft (*see also*
    Complications, by site and type,
    specified NEC) T85.84
  arterial graft NEC T82.848
  breast (implant) T85.84
  catheter NEC T85.84
   dialysis (renal) T82.848
    intraperitoneal T85.84
   infusion NEC T82.848
    spinal (epidural) (subdural) T85.84
   urinary (indwelling) T83.84
  electronic (electrode) (pulse generator)
    (stimulator)
   bone T84.84
   cardiac T82.847
   nervous system (brain) (peripheral
     nerve) (spinal) T85.84
   urinary T83.84
  fixation, internal (orthopedic) NEC
    T84.84
  gastrointestinal (bile duct) (esophagus)
    T85.84
  genital NEC T83.84
  heart NEC T82.847
  infusion NEC T85.84
  joint prosthesis T84.84
  ocular (corneal graft) (orbital implant)
    NEC T85.84
  orthopedic NEC T84.84
  specified NEC T85.84
  urinary NEC T83.84
  vascular NEC T82.848
  ventricular intracranial shunt T85.84

Pain *(Continued)*
 due to malignancy (primary) (secondary)
    G89.3
 ear —*see* subcategory H92.0
 epigastric, epigastrium R10.13
 eye —*see* Pain, ocular
 face, facial R51
  atypical G50.1
 female genital organs NEC N94.89
 finger —*see* Pain, limb, upper
 flank —*see* Pain, abdominal
 foot —*see* Pain, limb, lower
 gallbladder K82.9
 gas (intestinal) R14.1
 gastric —*see* Pain, abdominal
 generalized NOS R52
 genital organ
  female N94.89
  male N50.8
 groin —*see* Pain, abdominal, lower
 hand —*see* Pain, limb, upper
 head —*see* Headache
 heart —*see* Pain, precordial
 infra-orbital —*see* Neuralgia, trigeminal
 intercostal R07.82
 intermenstrual N94.0
 jaw R68.84
 joint M25.50
  ankle M25.57-
  elbow M25.52-
  finger M79.64-
  foot M25.57-
  hand M79.64-
  hip M25.55-
  knee M25.56-
  shoulder M25.51-
  toe M25.57-
  wrist M25.53-
 kidney N23
 laryngeal R07.0
 leg —*see* Pain, limb, lower
 limb M79.609
  lower M79.60-
   foot M79.67-
   lower leg M79.66-
   thigh M79.65-
   toe M79.67-
  upper M79.60-
   axilla M79.62-
   finger M79.64-
   forearm M79.63-
   hand M79.64-
   upper arm M79.62-
 loin M54.5
 low back M54.5
 lumbar region M54.5
 mandibular R68.84
 mastoid —*see* subcategory H92.0
 maxilla R68.84
 menstrual (*see also* Dysmenorrhea) N94.6
 metacarpophalangeal (joint) —*see* Pain, joint,
    hand
 metatarsophalangeal (joint) —*see* Pain, joint,
    foot
 mouth K13.79
 muscle —*see* Myalgia
 musculoskeletal (*see also* Pain, by site) M79.1
 myofascial M79.1
 nasal J34.89
 nasopharynx J39.2
 neck NEC M54.2
 nerve NEC —*see* Neuralgia
 neuromuscular —*see* Neuralgia
 nose J34.89
 ocular H57.1-
 ophthalmic —*see* Pain, ocular
 orbital region —*see* Pain, ocular
 ovary N94.89
 over heart —*see* Pain, precordial
 ovulation N94.0
 pelvic (female) R10.2

Pain (Continued)
  penis N48.89
  pericardial —see Pain, precordial
  perineal, perineum R10.2
  pharynx J39.2
  pleura, pleural, pleuritic R07.81 ◀▥▥
  postoperative NOS G89.18
  postprocedural NOS G89.18
  post-thoracotomy G89.12
  precordial (region) R07.2
  premenstrual N94.3
  psychogenic (persistent) (any site) F45.41
  radicular (spinal) —see Radiculopathy
  rectum K62.89
  respiration R07.1
  retrosternal R07.2
  rheumatoid, muscular —see Myalgia
  rib R07.81
  root (spinal) —see Radiculopathy
  round ligament (stretch) R10.2
  sacroiliac M53.3
  sciatic —see Sciatica
  scrotum N50.8
  seminal vesicle N50.8
  shoulder M25.51-
  spermatic cord N50.8
  spinal root —see Radiculopathy
  spine M54.9
    cervical M54.2
    low back M54.5
      with sciatica M54.4-
    thoracic M54.6
  stomach —see Pain, abdominal
  substernal R07.2
  temporomandibular (joint) M26.62
  testis N50.8
  thoracic spine M54.6
    with radicular and visceral pain
        M54.14
  throat R07.0
  tibia —see Pain, limb, lower
  toe —see Pain, limb, lower
  tongue K14.6
  tooth K08.8
  trigeminal —see Neuralgia, trigeminal
  tumor associated G89.3
  ureter N23
  urinary (organ) (system) N23
  uterus NEC N94.89
  vagina R10.2
  vertebrogenic (syndrome) M54.89
  vesical R39.89
    associated with micturition —see
        Micturition, painful
  vulva R10.2
Painful —see also Pain
  coitus
    female N94.1
    male N53.12
    psychogenic F52.6
  ejaculation (semen) N53.12
    psychogenic F52.6
  erection —see Priapism
  feet syndrome E53.8
  joint replacement (hip) (knee) T84.84
  menstruation —see Dysmenorrhea
    psychogenic F45.8
  micturition —see Micturition, painful
  respiration R07.1
  scar NEC L90.5
  wire sutures T81.89
Painter's colic —see subcategory T56.0
Palate —see condition
Palatoplegia K13.79
Palatoschisis —see Cleft, palate
Palilalia R48.8
Palliative care Z51.5
Pallor R23.1
  optic disc, temporal —see Atrophy, optic
Palmar —see also condition
  fascia —see condition

Palpable
  cecum K63.89
  kidney N28.89
  ovary N83.8
  prostate N42.9
  spleen —see Splenomegaly
Palpitations (heart) R00.2
  psychogenic F45.8
Palsy (see also Paralysis) G83.9
  atrophic diffuse (progressive) G12.22
  Bell's —see also Palsy, facial
    newborn P11.3
  brachial plexus NEC G54.0
    newborn (birth injury) P14.3
  brain —see Palsy, cerebral
  bulbar (progressive) (chronic) G12.22
    of childhood (Fazio-Londe) G12.1
    pseudo NEC G12.29
    supranuclear (progressive) G23.1
  cerebral (congenital) G80.9
    ataxic G80.4
    athetoid G80.3
    choreathetoid G80.3
    diplegic G80.8
      spastic G80.1
    dyskinetic G80.3
      athetoid G80.3
      choreathetoid G80.3
      distonic G80.3
    dystonic G80.3
    hemiplegic G80.8
      spastic G80.2
    mixed G80.8
    monoplegic G80.8
      spastic G80.1
    paraplegic G80.8
      spastic G80.1
    quadriplegic G80.8
      spastic G80.0
    spastic G80.1
      diplegic G80.1
      hemiplegic G80.2
      monoplegic G80.1
      quadriplegic G80.0
      specified NEC G80.1
      tetrapelgic G80.0
    specified NEC G80.8
    syphilitic A52.12
      congenital A50.49
    tetraplegic G80.8
      spastic G80.0
  cranial nerve —see also Disorder, nerve,
      cranial
  multiple G52.7
    in
      infectious disease B99 [G53]
      neoplastic disease (see also Neoplasm)
          D49.9 [G53]
      parasitic disease B89 [G53]
      sarcoidosis D86.82
  creeping G12.22
  diver's T70.3
  Erb's P14.0
  facial G51.0
    newborn (birth injury) P11.3
  glossopharyngeal G52.1
  Klumpke (-Déjérine) P14.1
  lead —see subcategory T56.0
  median nerve (tardy) G56.1-
  nerve G58.9
    specified NEC G58.8
  peroneal nerve (acute) (tardy) G57.3-
  progressive supranuclear G23.1
  pseudobulbar NEC G12.29
  radial nerve (acute) G56.3-
  seventh nerve —see also Palsy, facial
    newborn P11.3
  shaking —see Parkinsonism
  spastic (cerebral) (spinal) G80.1
  ulnar nerve (tardy) G56.2-
  wasting G12.29

Paludism —see Malaria
Panangiitis M30.0
Panaris, panaritium —see also Cellulitis, digit
  with lymphangitis —see Lymphangitis, acute,
      digit
Panarteritis nodosa M30.0
  brain or cerebral I67.7
Pancake heart R93.1
  with cor pulmonale (chronic) I27.81
Pancarditis (acute) (chronic) I51.89
  rheumatic I09.89
    active or acute I01.8
Pancoast's syndrome or tumor C34.1-
Pancolitis, ulcerative (chronic) K51.00
  with
    abscess K51.014
    complication K51.019
    fistula K51.013
    obstruction K51.012
    rectal bleeding K51.011
    specified complication NEC K51.018
Pancreas, pancreatic —see condition
Pancreatitis (annular) (apoplectic) (calcareous)
      (edematous) (hemorrhagic) (malignant)
      (recurrent) (subacute) (suppurative) K85.9
  acute K85.9
    alcohol induced K85.2
    biliary K85.1
    drug induced K85.3
    gallstone K85.1
    idiopathic K85.0
    specified NEC K85.8
  chronic (infectious) K86.1
    alcohol-induced K86.0
    recurrent K86.1
    relapsing K86.1
  cystic (chronic) K86.1
  cytomegaloviral B25.2
  fibrous (chronic) K86.1
  gallstone K85.1
  gangrenous K85.8
  interstitial (chronic) K86.1
    acute K85.8
  mumps B26.3
  recurrent (chronic) K86.1
  relapsing, chronic K86.1
  syphilitic A52.74
Pancreatoblastoma —see Neoplasm, pancreas,
    malignant
Pancreolithiasis K86.8
Pancytolysis D75.89
Pancytopenia (acquired) D61.818
  with
    malformations D61.09
    myelodysplastic syndrome —see
        Syndrome, myelodysplastic
    antineoplastic chemotherapy induced
        D61.810
    congenital D61.09
    drug-induced NEC D61.811
Panencephalitis, subacute, sclerosing
    A81.1
Panhematopenia D61.9
  congenital D61.09
  constitutional D61.09
  splenic, primary D73.1
Panhemocytopenia D61.9
  congenital D61.09
  constitutional D61.09
Panhypogonadism E29.1
Panhypopituitarism E23.0
  prepubertal E23.0
Panic (attack) (state) F41.0
  reaction to exceptional stress (transient)
      F43.0
Panmyelopathy, familial, constitutional
    D61.09
Panmyelophthisis D61.82
  congenital D61.09
Panmyelosis (acute) (with myelofibrosis)
    C94.4-

Panner's disease —see Osteochondrosis, juvenile, humerus
Panneuritis endemica E51.11
Panniculitis (nodular) (nonsuppurative) M79.3
  back M54.00
    cervical region M54.02
    cervicothoracic region M54.03
    lumbar region M54.06
    lumbosacral region M54.07
    multiple sites M54.09
    occipito-atlanto-axial region M54.01
    sacrococcygeal region M54.08
    thoracic region M54.04
    thoracolumbar region M54.05
  lupus L93.2
  mesenteric K65.4
  neck M54.02
    cervicothoracic region M54.03
    occipito-atlanto-axial region M54.01
  relapsing M35.6
Panniculus adiposus (abdominal) E65
Pannus (allergic) (cornea) (degenerativus) (keratic) H16.42-
  abdominal (symptomatic) E65
  trachomatosus, trachomatous (active) A71.1
Panophthalmitis H44.01-
Pansinusitis (chronic) (hyperplastic) (nonpurulent) (purulent) J32.4
  acute J01.40
    recurrent J01.41
  tuberculous A15.8
Panuveitis (sympathetic) H44.11-
Panvalvular disease I08.9
  specified NEC I08.8
Papanicolaou smear, cervix Z12.4
  as part of routine gynecological examination Z01.419
    with abnormal findings Z01.411
  for suspected neoplasm Z12.4
  nonspecific abnormal finding R87.619
  routine Z01.419
    with abnormal findings Z01.411
Papilledema (choked disc) H47.10
  associated with
    decreased ocular pressure H47.12
    increased intracranial pressure H47.11
    retinal disorder H47.13
  Foster-Kennedy syndrome H47.14-
Papillitis H46.00
  anus K62.89
  chronic lingual K14.4
  necrotizing, kidney N17.2
  optic H46.0-
  rectum K62.89
  renal, necrotizing N17.2
  tongue K14.0
Papilloma —see also Neoplasm, benign, by site
  acuminatum (female) (male) (anogenital) A63.0
  benign pinta (primary) A67.0
  bladder (urinary) (transitional cell) D41.4
  choroid plexus (lateral ventricle) (third ventricle) D33.0
    anaplastic C71.5
    fourth ventricle D33.1
    malignant C71.5
  renal pelvis (transitional cell) D41.1-
    benign D30.1-
  Schneiderian
    specified site —see Neoplasm, benign, by site
    unspecified site D14.0
  serous surface
    borderline malignancy
      specified site —see Neoplasm, uncertain behavior, by site
      unspecified site D39.10
    specified site —see Neoplasm, benign, by site
    unspecified site D27.9

Papilloma (Continued)
  transitional (cell)
    bladder (urinary) D41.4
      inverted type —see Neoplasm, uncertain behavior, by site
    renal pelvis D41.1-
    ureter D41.2-
  ureter (transitional cell) D41.2-
    benign D30.2-
  urothelial —see Neoplasm, uncertain behavior, by site
  villous —see Neoplasm, uncertain behavior, by site
    adenocarcinoma in —see Neoplasm, malignant, by site
    in situ —see Neoplasm, in situ
  yaws, plantar or palmar A66.1
Papillomata, multiple, of yaws A66.1
Papillomatosis —see also Neoplasm, benign, by site
  confluent and reticulated L83
  cystic, breast —see Mastopathy, cystic
  ductal, breast —see Mastopathy, cystic
  intraductal (diffuse) —see Neoplasm, benign, by site
  subareolar duct D24-
Papillomavirus, as cause of disease classified elsewhere B97.7
Papillon-Léage and Psaume syndrome Q87.0
Papule (s) R23.8
  carate (primary) A67.0
  fibrous, of nose D22.39
  Gottron's L94.4
  pinta (primary) A67.0
Papulosis
  lymphomatoid C86.6
  malignant I77.89
Papyraceous fetus O31.0-
Para-albuminemia E88.09
Paracephalus Q89.7
Parachute mitral valve Q23.2
Paracoccidioidomycosis B41.9
  disseminated B41.7
  generalized B41.7
  mucocutaneous-lymphangitic B41.8
  pulmonary B41.0
  specified NEC B41.8
  visceral B41.8
Paradentosis K05.4
Paraffinoma T88.8
Paraganglioma D44.7
  adrenal D35.0-
    malignant C74.1-
  aortic body D44.7
    malignant C75.5
  carotid body D44.6
    malignant C75.4
  chromaffin —see also Neoplasm, benign, by site
    malignant —see Neoplasm, malignant, by site
  extra-adrenal D44.7
    malignant C75.5
      specified site —see Neoplasm, malignant, by site
      unspecified site C75.5
    specified site —see Neoplasm, uncertain behavior, by site
    unspecified site D44.7
  gangliocytic D13.2
    specified site —see Neoplasm, benign, by site
    unspecified site D13.2
  glomus jugulare D44.7
    malignant C75.5
  jugular D44.7
  malignant C75.5
    specified site —see Neoplasm, malignant, by site
    unspecified site C75.5

Paraganglioma (Continued)
  nonchromaffin D44.7
    malignant C75.5
      specified site —see Neoplasm, malignant, by site
      unspecified site C75.5
    specified site —see Neoplasm, uncertain behavior, by site
    unspecified site D44.7
  parasympathetic D44.7
    specified site —see Neoplasm, uncertain behavior, by site
    unspecified site D44.7
  specified site —see Neoplasm, uncertain behavior, by site
  sympathetic D44.7
    specified site —see Neoplasm, uncertain behavior, by site
    unspecified site D44.7
  unspecified site D44.7
Parageusia R43.2
  psychogenic F45.8
Paragonimiasis B66.4
Paragranuloma, Hodgkin —see Lymphoma, Hodgkin, classical, specified NEC
Parahemophilia (see also Defect, coagulation) D68.2
Parakeratosis R23.4
  variegata L41.0
Paralysis, paralytic (complete) (incomplete) G83.9
  with
    syphilis A52.17
  abducens, abducent (nerve) —see Strabismus, paralytic, sixth nerve
  abductor, lower extremity G57.9-
  accessory nerve G52.8
  accommodation —see also Paresis, of accommodation
    hysterical F44.89
  acoustic nerve (except Deafness) —see subcategory H93.3
  agitans (see also Parkinsonism) G20
    arteriosclerotic G21.4
  alternating (oculomotor) G83.89
  amyotrophic G12.21
  ankle G57.9-
  anus (sphincter) K62.89
  arm —see Monoplegia, upper limb
  ascending (spinal), acute G61.0
  association G12.29
  asthenic bulbar G70.00
    with exacerbation (acute) G70.01
    in crisis G70.01
  ataxic (hereditary) G11.9
    general (syphilitic) A52.17
  atrophic G58.9
    infantile, acute —see Poliomyelitis, paralytic
    progressive G12.22
    spinal (acute) —see Poliomyelitis, paralytic
  axillary G54.0
  Babinski-Nageotte's G83.89
  Bell's G51.0
    newborn P11.3
  Benedikt's G46.3
  birth injury P14.9
    spinal cord P11.5
  bladder (neurogenic) (sphincter) N31.2
  bowel, colon or intestine K56.0
  brachial plexus G54.0
    birth injury P14.3
    newborn (birth injury) P14.3
  brain G83.9
    diplegia G83.0
    triplegia G83.89
  bronchial J98.09
  Brown-Séquard G83.81

Paralysis, paralytic (Continued)
  bulbar (chronic) (progressive) G12.22
    infantile —see Poliomyelitis, paralytic
    poliomyelitic —see Poliomyelitis, paralytic
    pseudo G12.29
  bulbospinal G70.00
    with exacerbation (acute) G70.01
    in crisis G70.01
  cardiac (see also Failure, heart) I50.9
  cerebrocerebellar, diplegic G80.1
  cervical
    plexus G54.2
    sympathetic G90.09
  Céstan-Chenais G46.3
  Charcot-Marie-Tooth type G60.0
  Clark's G80.9
  colon K56.0
  compressed air T70.3
  compression
    arm G56.9-
    leg G57.9-
    lower extremity G57.9-
    upper extremity G56.9-
  congenital (cerebral) —see Palsy, cerebral
  conjugate movement (gaze) (of eye) H51.0
    cortical (nuclear) (supranuclear) H51.0
  cordis —see Failure, heart
  cranial or cerebral nerve G52.9
  creeping G12.22
  crossed leg G83.89
  crutch —see Injury, brachial plexus
  deglutition R13.0
    hysterical F44.4
  dementia A52.17
  descending (spinal) NEC G12.29
  diaphragm (flaccid) J98.6
    due to accidental dissection of phrenic
        nerve during procedure —see
        Puncture, accidental complicating
        surgery
  digestive organs NEC K59.8
  diplegic —see Diplegia
  divergence (nuclear) H51.8
  diver's T70.3
  Duchenne's
    birth injury P14.0
    due to or associated with
        motor neuron disease G12.22
        muscular dystrophy G71.0
    due to intracranial or spinal birth injury —see
        Palsy, cerebral
  embolic (current episode) I63.4
  Erb (-Duchenne) (birth) (newborn) P14.0
  Erb's syphilitic spastic spinal A52.17
  esophagus K22.8
  eye muscle (extrinsic) H49.9
    intrinsic —see also Paresis, of
        accommodation
  facial (nerve) G51.0
    birth injury P11.3
    congenital P11.3
    following operation NEC —see Puncture,
        accidental complicating surgery
    newborn (birth injury) P11.3
  familial (recurrent) (periodic) G72.3
    spastic G11.4
  fauces J39.2
  finger G56.9-
  gait R26.1
  gastric nerve (nondiabetic) G52.2
  gaze, conjugate H51.0
  general (progressive) (syphilitic) A52.17
    juvenile A50.45
  glottis J38.00
    bilateral J38.02
    unilateral J38.01
  gluteal G54.1
  Gubler (-Millard) G46.3
  hand —see Monoplegia, upper limb
  heart —see Arrest, cardiac
  hemiplegic —see Hemiplegia

Paralysis, paralytic (Continued)
  hyperkalemic periodic (familial) G72.3
  hypoglossal (nerve) G52.3
  hypokalemic periodic G72.3
  hysterical F44.4
  ileus K56.0
  infantile (see also Poliomyelitis, paralytic)
      A80.30
    bulbar —see Poliomyelitis, paralytic
    cerebral —see Palsy, cerebral
    spastic —see Palsy, cerebral, spastic
  infective —see Poliomyelitis, paralytic
  inferior nuclear G83.9
  internuclear —see Ophthalmoplegia,
      internuclear
  intestine K56.0
  iris H57.09
    due to diphtheria (toxin) A36.89
  ischemic, Volkmann's (complicating trauma)
      T79.6
  Jackson's G83.89
  jake —see Poisoning, food, noxious, plant
  Jamaica ginger (jake) G62.2
  juvenile general A50.45
  Klumpke (-Déjérine) (birth) (newborn) P14.1
  labioglossal (laryngeal) (pharyngeal) G12.29
  Landry's G61.0
  laryngeal nerve (recurrent) (superior)
      (unilateral) J38.00
    bilateral J38.02
    unilateral J38.01
  larynx J38.00
    bilateral J38.02
    due to diphtheria (toxin) A36.2
    unilateral J38.01
  lateral G12.21
  lead —see subcategory T56.0
  left side —see Hemiplegia
  leg G83.1-
    both —see Paraplegia
    crossed G83.89
    hysterical F44.4
    psychogenic F44.4
    transient or transitory R29.818
      traumatic NEC —see Injury, nerve, leg
  levator palpebrae superioris —see
      Blepharoptosis, paralytic
  limb —see Monoplegia
  lip K13.0
  Lissauer's A52.17
  lower limb —see Monoplegia, lower limb
    both —see Paraplegia
  lung J98.4
  median nerve G56.1-
  medullary (tegmental) G83.89
  mesencephalic NEC G83.89
    tegmental G83.89
  middle alternating G83.89
  Millard-Gubler-Foville G46.3
  monoplegic —see Monoplegia
  motor G83.9
  muscle, muscular NEC G72.89
    due to nerve lesion G58.9
    eye (extrinsic) H49.9
      intrinsic —see Paresis, of accommodation
      oblique —see Strabismus, paralytic,
          fourth nerve
    iris sphincter H21.9
    ischemic (Volkmann's) (complicating
        trauma) T79.6
    progressive G12.21
    pseudohypertrophic G71.0
  musculocutaneous nerve G56.9-
  musculospiral G56.9-
  nerve —see also Disorder, nerve
    abducent —see Strabismus, paralytic, sixth
        nerve
    accessory G52.8
    auditory (except Deafness) —see
        subcategory H93.3
    birth injury P14.9

Paralysis, paralytic (Continued)
  nerve (Continued)
    cranial or cerebral G52.9
    facial G51.0
      birth injury P11.3
      congenital P11.3
      newborn (birth injury) P11.3
    fourth or trochlear —see Strabismus,
        paralytic, fourth nerve
    newborn (birth injury) P14.9
    oculomotor —see Strabismus, paralytic,
        third nerve
    phrenic (birth injury) P14.2
    radial G56.3-
    seventh or facial G51.0
      newborn (birth injury) P11.3
    sixth or abducent —see Strabismus,
        paralytic, sixth nerve
    syphilitic A52.15
    third or oculomotor —see Strabismus,
        paralytic, third nerve
    trigeminal G50.9
    trochlear —see Strabismus, paralytic,
        fourth nerve
    ulnar G56.2-
  normokalemic periodic G72.3
  ocular H49.9
    alternating G83.89
  oculofacial, congenital (Moebius) Q87.0
  oculomotor (external bilateral) (nerve) —see
      Strabismus, paralytic, third nerve
  palate (soft) K13.79
  paratrigeminal G50.9
  periodic (familial) (hyperkalemic)
      (hypokalemic) (myotonic)
      (normokalemic) (potassium sensitive)
      (secondary) G72.3
  peripheral autonomic nervous system —see
      Neuropathy, peripheral, autonomic
  peroneal (nerve) G57.3-
  pharynx J39.2
  phrenic nerve G56.8-
  plantar nerve (s) G57.6-
  pneumogastric nerve G52.2
  poliomyelitis (current) —see Poliomyelitis,
      paralytic
  popliteal nerve G57.3-
  postepileptic transitory G83.84
  progressive (atrophic) (bulbar) (spinal)
      G12.22
    general A52.17
    infantile acute —see Poliomyelitis, paralytic
    supranuclear G23.1
  pseudobulbar G12.29
  pseudohypertrophic (muscle) G71.0
  psychogenic F44.4
  quadriceps G57.9-
  quadriplegic —see Tetraplegia
  radial nerve G56.3-
  rectus muscle (eye) H49.9
  recurrent isolated sleep G47.53
  respiratory (muscle) (system) (tract) R06.81
    center NEC G93.89
    congenital P28.89
    newborn P28.89
  right side —see Hemiplegia
  saturnine —see subcategory T56.0
  sciatic nerve G57.0-
  senile G83.9
  shaking —see Parkinsonism
  shoulder G56.9-
  sleep, recurrent isolated G47.53
  spastic G83.9
    cerebral —see Palsy, cerebral, spastic
    congenital (cerebral) —see Palsy, cerebral,
        spastic
    familial G11.4
    hereditary G11.4
    quadriplegic G80.0
    syphilitic (spinal) A52.17
  sphincter, bladder —see Paralysis, bladder

◀ New   ◀|||| Revised   ~~deleted~~ Deleted

Paralysis, paralytic (Continued)
  spinal (cord) G83.9
    accessory nerve G52.8
    acute —see Poliomyelitis, paralytic
    ascending acute G61.0
    atrophic (acute) —see also Poliomyelitis,
      paralytic
      spastic, syphilitic A52.17
    congenital NEC —see Palsy, cerebral
    hereditary G95.89
    infantile —see Poliomyelitis, paralytic
    progressive G12.21
    sequelae NEC G83.89
  sternomastoid G52.8
  stomach K31.84
    diabetic —see Diabetes, by type, with
      gastroparesis
    nerve G52.2
      diabetic —see Diabetes, by type, with
        gastroparesis
  stroke —see Infarct, brain
  subcapsularis G56.8-
  supranuclear (progressive) G23.1
  sympathetic G90.8
    cervical G90.09
    nervous system —see Neuropathy,
      peripheral, autonomic
  syndrome G83.9
    specified NEC G83.89
  syphilitic spastic spinal (Erb's) A52.17
  thigh G57.9-
  throat J39.2
    diphtheritic A36.0
    muscle J39.2
  thrombotic (current episode) I63.3
  thumb G56.9-
  tick —see Toxicity, venom, arthropod,
    specified NEC
  Todd's (postepileptic transitory paralysis)
    G83.84
  toe G57.6-
  tongue K14.8
  transient R29.5
    arm or leg NEC R29.818
    traumatic NEC —see Injury, nerve
  trapezius G52.8
  traumatic, transient NEC —see Injury,
    nerve
  trembling —see Parkinsonism
  triceps brachii G56.9-
  trigeminal nerve G50.9
  trochlear (nerve) —see Strabismus, paralytic,
    fourth nerve
  ulnar nerve G56.2-
  upper limb —see Monoplegia, upper limb
  uremic N18.9 [G99.8]
  uveoparotitic D86.89
  uvula K13.79
    postdiphtheritic A36.0
  vagus nerve G52.2
  vasomotor NEC G90.8
  velum palati K13.79
  vesical —see Paralysis, bladder
  vestibular nerve (except Vertigo) —see
    subcategory H93.3
  vocal cords J38.00
    bilateral J38.02
    unilateral J38.01
  Volkmann's (complicating trauma) T79.6
  wasting G12.29
  Weber's G46.3
  wrist G56.9-
Paramedial urethrovesical orifice Q64.79
Paramenia N92.6
Parametritis (see also Disease, pelvis,
  inflammatory) N73.2
  acute N73.0
  complicating abortion —see Abortion, by
    type, complicated by, parametritis
Parametrium, parametric —see condition
Paramnesia —see Amnesia

Paramolar K00.1
Paramyloidosis E85.8
Paramyoclonus multiplex G25.3
Paramyotonia (congenita) G71.19
Parangi —see Yaws
Paranoia (querulans) F22
  senile F03
Paranoid
  dementia (senile) F03
    praecox —see Schizophrenia
  personality F60.0
  psychosis (climacteric) (involutional)
    (menopausal) F22
    psychogenic (acute) F23
    senile F03
  reaction (acute) F23
    chronic F22
  schizophrenia F20.0
  state (climacteric) (involutional)
    (menopausal) (simple) F22
    senile F03
  tendencies F60.0
  traits F60.0
  trends F60.0
  type, psychopathic personality F60.0
Paraparesis —see Paraplegia
Paraphasia R47.02
Paraphilia F65.9
Paraphimosis (congenital) N47.2
  chancroidal A57
Paraphrenia, paraphrenic (late) F22
  schizophrenia F20.0
Paraplegia (lower) G82.20
  ataxic —see Degeneration, combined, spinal
    cord
  complete G82.21
  congenital (cerebral) G80.8
    spastic G80.1
  familial spastic G11.4
  functional (hysterical) F44.4
  hereditary, spastic G11.4
  hysterical F44.4
  incomplete G82.22
  Pott's A18.01
  psychogenic F44.4
  spastic
    Erb's spinal, syphilitic A52.17
    hereditary G11.4
    tropical G04.1
  syphilitic (spastic) A52.17
  tropical spastic G04.1
Parapoxvirus B08.60
  specified NEC B08.69
Paraproteinemia D89.2
  benign (familial) D89.2
  monoclonal D47.2
  secondary to malignant disease D47.2
Parapsoriasis L41.9
  en plaques L41.4
  guttata L41.1
  large plaque L41.4
  retiform, retiformis L41.5
  small plaque L41.3
  specified NEC L41.8
  varioliformis (acuta) L41.0
Parasitic —see also condition
  disease NEC B89
  stomatitis B37.0
  sycosis (beard) (scalp) B35.0
  twin Q89.4
Parasitism B89
  intestinal B82.9
  skin B88.9
  specified —see Infestation
Parasitophobia F40.218
Parasomnia G47.50
  due to
    alcohol
      abuse F10.182
      dependence F10.282
      use F10.982

Parasomnia (Continued)
  due to (Continued)
    amphetamines
      abuse F15.182
      dependence F15.282
      use F15.982
    caffeine
      abuse F15.182
      dependence F15.282
      use F15.982
    cocaine
      abuse F14.182
      dependence F14.282
      use F14.982
    drug NEC
      abuse F19.182
      dependence F19.282
      use F19.982
    opioid
      abuse F11.182
      dependence F11.282
      use F11.982
    psychoactive substance NEC
      abuse F19.182
      dependence F19.282
      use F19.982
    sedative, hypnotic, or anxiolytic
      abuse F13.182
      dependence F13.282
      use F13.982
    stimulant NEC
      abuse F15.182
      dependence F15.282
      use F15.982
  in conditions classified elsewhere G47.54
  nonorganic origin F51.8
  organic G47.50
  specified NEC G47.59
Paraspadias Q54.9
Paraspasmus facialis G51.8
Parasuicide (attempt)
  history of (personal) Z91.5
    in family Z81.8
Parathyroid gland —see condition
Parathyroid tetany E20.9
Paratrachoma A74.0
Paratyphilitis —see Appendicitis
Paratyphoid (fever) —see Fever, paratyphoid
Paratyphus —see Fever, paratyphoid
Paraurethral duct Q64.79
  nonorganic origin F51.5
Paraurethritis —see also Urethritis
  gonococcal (acute) (chronic) (with abscess)
    A54.1
Paravaccinia NEC B08.04
Paravaginitis —see Vaginitis
Parencephalitis —see also Encephalitis
  sequelae G09
Parent-child conflict —see Conflict, parent-child
  estrangement NEC Z62.890
Paresis —see also Paralysis
  accommodation —see Paresis, of
    accommodation
  Bernhardt's G57.1-
  bladder (sphincter) —see also Paralysis,
    bladder
    tabetic A52.17
  bowel, colon or intestine K56.0
  extrinsic muscle, eye H49.9
  general (progressive) (syphilitic) A52.17
    juvenile A50.45
  heart —see Failure, heart
  insane (syphilitic) A52.17
  juvenile (general) A50.45
  of accommodation H52.52-
  peripheral progressive (idiopathic) G60.3
  pseudohypertrophic G71.0
  senile G83.9
  syphilitic (general) A52.17
    congenital A50.45
  vesical NEC N31.2

Paresthesia —*see also* Disturbance, sensation
   Bernhardt G57.1-
Paretic —*see* condition
Parinaud's
   conjunctivitis H10.89
   oculoglandular syndrome H10.89
   ophthalmoplegia H49.88
Parkinsonism (idiopathic) (primary) G20
   with neurogenic orthostatic hypotension
      (symptomatic) G90.3
   arteriosclerotic G21.4
   dementia G31.83 *[F02.80]*
      with behavioral disturbance G31.83
         [F02.81]
   due to
      drugs NEC G21.19
         neuroleptic G21.11
   neuroleptic induced G21.11
   postencephalitic G21.3
   secondary G21.9
      due to
         arteriosclerosis G21.4
         drugs NEC G21.19
            neuroleptic G21.11
         encephalitis G21.3
         external agents NEC G21.2
         syphilis A52.19
      specified NEC G21.8
   syphilitic A52.19
   treatment-induced NEC G21.19
   vascular G21.4
Parkinson's disease, syndrome or tremor —*see*
   Parkinsonism
Parodontitis —*see* Periodontitis
Parodontosis K05.4
Paronychia —*see also* Cellulitis, digit
   with lymphangitis —*see* Lymphangitis, acute,
      digit
   candidal (chronic) B37.2
   tuberculous (primary) A18.4
Parorexia (psychogenic) F50.8
Parosmia R43.1
   psychogenic F45.8
Parotid gland —*see* condition
Parotitis, parotiditis (allergic) (nonspecific
      toxic) (purulent) (septic) (suppurative) —
      see also Sialoadenitis
   epidemic —*see* Mumps
   infectious —*see* Mumps
   postoperative K91.89
   surgical K91.89
Parrot fever A70
Parrot's disease (early congenital syphilitic
      pseudoparalysis) A50.02
Parry-Romberg syndrome G51.8
Parry's disease or syndrome E05.00
   with thyroid storm E05.01
Pars planitis —*see* Cyclitis
Parsonage (-Aldren)-Turner syndrome G54.5
Parson's disease (exophthalmic goiter)
      E05.00
   with thyroid storm E05.01
Particolored infant Q82.8
Parturition —*see* Delivery
Parulis K04.7
   with sinus K04.6
Parvovirus, as cause of disease classified
      elsewhere B97.6
Pasini and Pierini's atrophoderma L90.3
Passage
   false, urethra N36.5
   meconium (newborn) during delivery
      P03.82
   of sounds or bougies —*see* Attention to,
      artificial, opening
Passive —*see* condition
   smoking Z77.22
Pasteurella septica A28.0
Pasteurellosis —*see* Infection, Pasteurella
PAT (paroxysmal atrial tachycardia) I47.1
Patau's syndrome —*see* Trisomy, 13

Patches
   mucous (syphilitic) A51.39
      congenital A50.07
   smokers' (mouth) K13.24
Patellar —*see* condition
Patent —*see also* Imperfect, closure
   canal of Nuck Q52.4
   cervix N88.3
   ductus arteriosus or Botallo's Q25.0
   foramen
      botalli Q21.1
      ovale Q21.1
   interauricular septum Q21.1
   interventricular septum Q21.0
   omphalomesenteric duct Q43.0
   os (uteri) —*see* Patent, cervix
   ostium secundum Q21.1
   urachus Q64.4
   vitelline duct Q43.0
Paterson (-Brown)(-Kelly) syndrome or web
      D50.1
Pathologic, pathological —*see also* condition
   asphyxia R09.01
   fire-setting F63.1
   gambling F63.0
   ovum O02.0
   resorption, tooth K03.3
   stealing F63.2
Pathology (of) —*see* Disease
   periradicular, associated with previous
      endodontic treatment NEC M27.59
Pattern, sleep-wake, irregular G47.23
Patulous —*see also* Imperfect, closure
      (congenital)
   alimentary tract Q45.8
      lower Q43.8
      upper Q40.8
   eustachian tube H69.0-
Pause, sinoatrial I49.5
Paxton's disease B36.2
Pearl (s)
   enamel K00.2
   Epstein's K09.8
Pearl-worker's disease —*see* Osteomyelitis,
      specified type NEC
Pectenosis K62.4
Pectoral —*see* condition
Pectus
   carinatum (congenital) Q67.7
      acquired M95.4
      rachitic sequelae (late effect) E64.3
   excavatum (congenital) Q67.6
      acquired M95.4
      rachitic sequelae (late effect) E64.3
   recurvatum (congenital) Q67.6
Pedatrophia E41
Pederosis F65.4
Pediculosis (infestation) B85.2
   capitis (head-louse) (any site) B85.0
   corporis (body-louse) (any site) B85.1
   eyelid B85.0
   mixed (classifiable to more than one of the
      titles B85.0-B85.3) B85.4
   pubis (pubic louse) (any site) B85.3
   vestimenti B85.1
   vulvae B85.3
Pediculus (infestation) —*see* Pediculosis
Pedophilia F65.4
Peg-shaped teeth K00.2
Pelade —*see* Alopecia, areata
Pelger-Huët anomaly or syndrome D72.0
Peliosis (rheumatica) D69.0
   hepatis K76.4
      with toxic liver disease K71.8
Pelizaeus-Merzbacher disease E75.29
Pellagra (alcoholic) (with polyneuropathy) E52
Pellagra-cerebellar-ataxia-renal aminoaciduria
      syndrome E72.02
Pellegrini (-Stieda) disease or syndrome —*see*
      Bursitis, tibial collateral
Pellizzi's syndrome E34.8

Pel's crisis A52.11
Pelvic —*see also* condition
   examination (periodic) (routine) Z01.419
      with abnormal findings Z01.411
   kidney, congenital Q63.2
Pelviolithiasis —*see* Calculus, kidney
Pelviperitonitis —*see also* Peritonitis, pelvic
   gonococcal A54.24
   puerperal O85
Pelvis —*see* condition or type
Pemphigoid L12.9
   benign, mucous membrane L12.1
   bullous L12.0
   cicatricial L12.1
   juvenile L12.2
   ocular L12.1
   specified NEC L12.8
Pemphigus L10.9
   benign familial (chronic) Q82.8
   Brazilian L10.3
   circinatus L13.0
   conjunctiva L12.1
   drug-induced L10.5
   erythematosus L10.4
   foliaceous L10.2
   gangrenous —*see* Gangrene
   neonatorum L01.03
   ocular L12.1
   paraneoplastic L10.81
   specified NEC L10.89
   syphilitic (congenital) A50.06
   vegetans L10.1
   vulgaris L10.0
   wildfire L10.3
Pendred's syndrome E07.1
Pendulous
   abdomen, in pregnancy —*see* Pregnancy,
      complicated by, abnormal, pelvic organs
      or tissues NEC
   breast N64.89
Penetrating wound —*see also* Puncture
   with internal injury —*see* Injury, by site
   eyeball —*see* Puncture, eyeball
   orbit (with or without foreign body) —*see*
      Puncture, orbit
   uterus by instrument with or following
      ectopic or molar pregnancy O08.6
Penicillosis B48.4
Penis —*see* condition
Penitis N48.29
Pentalogy of Fallot Q21.8
Pentasomy X syndrome Q97.1
Pentosuria (essential) E74.8
Percreta placenta O43.23- ◀▥
Peregrinating patient —*see* Disorder, factitious
Perforation, perforated (nontraumatic) (of)
   accidental during procedure (blood vessel)
      (nerve) (organ) —*see* Complication,
      accidental puncture or laceration
   antrum —*see* Sinusitis, maxillary
   appendix K35.2
   atrial septum, multiple Q21.1
   attic, ear —*see* Perforation, tympanum, attic
   bile duct (common) (hepatic) K83.2
      cystic K82.2
   bladder (urinary)
      with or following ectopic or molar
         pregnancy O08.6
      obstetrical trauma O71.5
      traumatic S37.29
         at delivery O71.5
   bowel K63.1
      with or following ectopic or molar
         pregnancy O08.6
      newborn P78.0
      obstetrical trauma O71.5
      traumatic —*see* Laceration, intestine
   broad ligament N83.8
      with or following ectopic or molar
         pregnancy O08.6
      obstetrical trauma O71.6

Perforation, perforated (Continued)
  by
    device, implant or graft (see also
      Complications, by site and type,
      mechanical) T85.628
     arterial graft NEC —see Complication,
      cardiovascular device, mechanical,
      vascular
     breast (implant) T85.49
     catheter NEC T85.698
      cystostomy T83.090
      dialysis (renal) T82.49
       intraperitoneal T85.691
      infusion NEC T82.594
       spinal (epidural) (subdural)
        T85.690
     electronic (electrode) (pulse generator)
      (stimulator)
      bone T84.390
      cardiac T82.199
       electrode T82.190
       pulse generator T82.191
       specified type NEC T82.198
      nervous system —see Complication,
       prosthetic device, mechanical,
       electronic nervous system
       stimulator
      urinary —see Complication,
       genitourinary, device, urinary,
       mechanical
     fixation, internal (orthopedic) NEC —see
      Complication, fixation device,
      mechanical
     gastrointestinal —see Complications,
      prosthetic device, mechanical,
      gastrointestinal device
     genital NEC T83.498
      intrauterine contraceptive device
       T83.39
      penile prosthesis T83.490
     heart NEC —see Complication,
      cardiovascular device,
      mechanical
     joint prosthesis —see Complications,
      joint prosthesis, mechanical,
      specified NEC, by site
     ocular NEC —see Complications,
      prosthetic device, mechanical,
      ocular device
     orthopedic NEC —see Complication,
      orthopedic, device, mechanical
     specified NEC T85.628
     urinary NEC —see also Complication,
      genitourinary, device, urinary,
      mechanical
      graft T83.29
      urinary, indwelling T83.098
     vascular NEC —see Complication,
      cardiovascular device,
      mechanical
     ventricular intracranial shunt
      T85.09
  foreign body left accidentally in
    operative wound T81.539
  instrument (any) during a procedure,
    accidental —see Puncture, accidental
    complicating surgery
  cecum K35.2
  cervix (uteri) N88.8
   with or following ectopic or molar
    pregnancy O08.6
   obstetrical trauma O71.3
  colon K63.1
   newborn P78.0
   obstetrical trauma O71.5
   traumatic —see Laceration, intestine,
    large
  common duct (bile) K83.2
  cornea (due to ulceration) —see Ulcer,
    cornea, perforated
  cystic duct K82.2

Perforation, perforated (Continued)
  diverticulum (intestine) K57.80
   with bleeding K57.81
   large intestine K57.20
    with
     bleeding K57.21
     small intestine K57.40
      with bleeding K57.41
   small intestine K57.00
    with
     bleeding K57.01
     large intestine K57.40
      with bleeding K57.41
  ear drum —see Perforation, tympanum
  esophagus K22.3
  ethmoidal sinus —see Sinusitis, ethmoidal
  frontal sinus —see Sinusitis, frontal
  gallbladder K82.2
  heart valve —see Endocarditis
  ileum K63.1
   newborn P78.0
   obstetrical trauma O71.5
   traumatic —see Laceration, intestine, small
  instrumental, surgical (accidental) (blood
    vessel) (nerve) (organ) —see Puncture,
    accidental complicating surgery
  intestine NEC K63.1
   with ectopic or molar pregnancy O08.6
   newborn P78.0
   obstetrical trauma O71.5
   traumatic —see Laceration, intestine
   ulcerative NEC K63.1
    newborn P78.0
  jejunum, jejunal K63.1
   obstetrical trauma O71.5
   traumatic —see Laceration, intestine, small
   ulcer —see Ulcer, gastrojejunal, with
    perforation
  joint prosthesis —see Complications, joint
    prosthesis, mechanical, specified NEC,
    by site
  mastoid (antrum) (cell) —see Disorder,
    mastoid, specified NEC
  maxillary sinus —see Sinusitis, maxillary
  membrana tympani —see Perforation,
    tympanum
  nasal
   septum J34.89
    congenital Q30.3
    syphilitic A52.73
   sinus J34.89
    congenital Q30.8
    due to sinusitis —see Sinusitis
  palate (see also Cleft, palate) Q35.9
   syphilitic A52.79
  palatine vault (see also Cleft, palate, hard)
    Q35.1
   syphilitic A52.79
   congenital A50.59
  pars flaccida (ear drum) —see Perforation,
    tympanum, attic
  pelvic
   floor S31.030
    with
     ectopic or molar pregnancy O08.6
     penetration into retroperitoneal space
      S31.031
     retained foreign body S31.040
      with penetration into
       retroperitoneal space S31.041
    following ectopic or molar pregnancy
     O08.6
    obstetrical trauma O70.1
   organ S37.99
    adrenal gland S37.818
    bladder —see Perforation, bladder
    fallopian tube S37.599
     bilateral S37.592
     unilateral S37.591
    kidney S37.09-
    obstetrical trauma O71.5

Perforation, perforated (Continued)
  pelvic (Continued)
   organ (Continued)
    ovary S37.499
     bilateral S37.492
     unilateral S37.491
    prostate S37.828
    specified organ NEC S37.898
    ureter —see Perforation, ureter
    urethra —see Perforation, urethra
    uterus —see Perforation, uterus
  perineum —see Laceration, perineum
  pharynx J39.2
  rectum K63.1
   newborn P78.0
   obstetrical trauma O71.5
   traumatic S36.63
  root canal space due to endodontic treatment
    M27.51
  sigmoid K63.1
   newborn P78.0
   obstetrical trauma O71.5
   traumatic S36.533
  sinus (accessory) (chronic) (nasal) J34.89
  sphenoidal sinus —see Sinusitis, sphenoidal
  surgical (accidental) (by instrument) (blood
    vessel) (nerve) (organ) —see Puncture,
    accidental complicating surgery
  traumatic
   external —see Puncture
   eye —see Puncture, eyeball
   internal organ —see Injury, by site
  tympanum, tympanic (membrane) (persistent
    post-traumatic) (postinflammatory)
    H72.9-
   attic H72.1-
    multiple —see Perforation, tympanum,
     multiple
    total —see Perforation, tympanum, total
   central H72.0-
    multiple —see Perforation, tympanum,
     multiple
    total —see Perforation, tympanum, total
   marginal NEC —see subcategory H72.2
   multiple H72.81-
    pars flaccida —see Perforation, tympanum,
     attic
   total H72.82-
   traumatic, current episode S09.2-
  typhoid, gastrointestinal —see Typhoid
  ulcer —see Ulcer, by site, with perforation
  ureter N28.89
   traumatic S37.19
  urethra N36.8
   with ectopic or molar pregnancy O08.6
   following ectopic or molar pregnancy
    O08.6
   obstetrical trauma O71.5
   traumatic S37.39
    at delivery O71.5
  uterus
   with ectopic or molar pregnancy O08.6
   by intrauterine contraceptive device T83.39
   following ectopic or molar pregnancy
    O08.6
   obstetrical trauma O71.1
   traumatic S37.69
    obstetric O71.1
  uvula K13.79
   syphilitic A52.79
  vagina (see also Puncture, vagina) O71.4 ◄▥
   obstetrical trauma O71.4 ◄
   other trauma - see Puncture, vagina ◄
Periadenitis mucosa necrotica recurrens K12.0
Periappendicitis (acute) —see Appendicitis
Periarteritis nodosa (disseminated) (infectious)
  (necrotizing) M30.0
Periarthritis (joint) —see also Enthesopathy
  Duplay's M75.0-
  gonococcal A54.42
  humeroscapularis —see Capsulitis, adhesive

Periarthritis (Continued)
  scapulohumeral —see Capsulitis, adhesive
  shoulder —see Capsulitis, adhesive
  wrist M77.2-
Periarthrosis (angioneural) —see
    Enthesopathy
Pericapsulitis, adhesive (shoulder) —see
    Capsulitis, adhesive
Pericarditis (with decompensation) (with
      effusion) I31.9
  with rheumatic fever (conditions in I00)
    active —see Pericarditis, rheumatic
    inactive or quiescent I09.2
  acute (hemorrhagic) (nonrheumatic) (Sicca)
      I30.9
    with chorea (acute) (rheumatic)
        (Sydenham's) I02.0
    benign I30.8
    nonspecific I30.0
    rheumatic I01.0
      with chorea (acute) (Sydenham's)
          I02.0
  adhesive or adherent (chronic) (external)
      (internal) I31.0
    acute —see Pericarditis, acute
    rheumatic I09.2
  bacterial (acute) (subacute) (with serous or
      seropurulent effusion) I30.1
  calcareous I31.1
  cholesterol (chronic) I31.8
    acute I30.9
  chronic (nonrheumatic) I31.9
    rheumatic I09.2
  constrictive (chronic) I31.1
  coxsackie B33.23
  fibrinocaseous (tuberculous) A18.84
  fibrinopurulent I30.1
  fibrinous I30.8
  fibrous I31.0
  gonococcal A54.83
  idiopathic I30.0
  in systemic lupus erythematosus M32.12
  infective I30.1
  meningococcal A39.53
  neoplastic (chronic) I31.8
    acute I30.9
  obliterans, obliterating I31.0
  plastic I31.0
  pneumococcal I30.1
  postinfarction I24.1
  purulent I30.1
  rheumatic (active) (acute) (with effusion)
      (with pneumonia) I01.0
    with chorea (acute) (rheumatic)
        (Sydenham's) I02.0
    chronic or inactive (with chorea) I09.2
  rheumatoid —see Rheumatoid, carditis
  septic I30.1
  serofibrinous I30.8
  staphylococcal I30.1
  streptococcal I30.1
  suppurative I30.1
  syphilitic A52.06
  tuberculous A18.84
  uremic N18.9 [I32]
  viral I30.1
Pericardium, pericardial —see condition
Pericellulitis —see Cellulitis
Pericementitis (chronic) (suppurative) —see also
    Periodontitis
  acute K05.20
    generalized K05.22
    localized K05.21
Perichondritis
  auricle —see Perichondritis, ear
  bronchus J98.09
  ear (external) H61.00-
    acute H61.01-
    chronic H61.02-
  external auditory canal —see Perichondritis,
      ear

Perichondritis (Continued)
  larynx J38.7
    syphilitic A52.73
    typhoid A01.09
  nose J34.89
  pinna —see Perichondritis, ear
  trachea J39.8
Periclasia K05.4
Pericoronitis —see Periodontitis
Pericystitis N30.90
  with hematuria N30.91
Peridiverticulitis (intestine) K57.92
  cecum —see Diverticulitis, intestine, large
  colon —see Diverticulitis, intestine, large
  duodenum —see Diverticulitis, intestine,
      small
  intestine —see Diverticulitis, intestine
  jejunum —see Diverticulitis, intestine, small
  rectosigmoid —see Diverticulitis, intestine,
      large
  rectum —see Diverticulitis, intestine, large
  sigmoid —see Diverticulitis, intestine, large
Periendocarditis —see Endocarditis
Periepididymitis N45.1
Perifolliculitis L01.02
  abscedens, caput, scalp L66.3
  capitis, abscedens (et suffodiens) L66.3
  superficial pustular L01.02
Perihepatitis K65.8
Perilabyrinthitis (acute) —see subcategory
    H83.0
Perimeningitis —see Meningitis
Perimetritis —see Endometritis
Perimetrosalpingitis —see Salpingo-oophoritis
Perineocele N81.81
Perinephric, perinephritic —see condition
Perinephritis —see also Infection, kidney
  purulent —see Abscess, kidney
Perineum, perineal —see condition
Perineuritis NEC —see Neuralgia
Periodic —see condition
Periodontitis (chronic) (complex) (compound)
      (local) (simplex) K05.30
  acute K05.20
    generalized K05.22
    localized K05.21
  apical K04.5
    acute (pulpal origin) K04.4
  generalized K05.32
  localized K05.31
Periodontoclasia K05.4
Periodontosis (juvenile) K05.4
Periods —see also Menstruation
  heavy N92.0
  irregular N92.6
  shortened intervals (irregular) N92.1
Perionychia —see also Cellulitis, digit
  with lymphangitis —see Lymphangitis, acute,
      digit
Perioophoritis —see Salpingo-oophoritis
Periorchitis N45.2
Periosteum, periosteal —see condition
Periostitis (albuminosa) (circumscribed)
      (diffuse) (infective) (monomelic) —see also
    Osteomyelitis
  alveolar M27.3
  alveolodental M27.3
  dental M27.3
  gonorrheal A54.43
  jaw (lower) (upper) M27.2
  orbit H05.03-
  syphilitic A52.77
    congenital (early) A50.02 [M90.80]
    secondary A51.46
  tuberculous —see Tuberculosis, bone
  yaws (hypertrophic) (early) (late) A66.6
      [M90.80]
Periostosis (hyperplastic) —see also Disorder,
    bone, specified type NEC
  with osteomyelitis —see Osteomyelitis,
      specified type NEC

Peripartum
  cardiomyopathy O90.3
Periphlebitis —see Phlebitis
Periproctitis K62.89
Periprostatitis —see Prostatitis
Perirectal —see condition
Perirenal —see condition
Perisalpingitis —see Salpingo-oophoritis
Perisplenitis (infectional) D73.89
Peristalsis, visible or reversed R19.2
Peritendinitis —see Enthesopathy
Peritoneum, peritoneal —see condition
Peritonitis (adhesive) (bacterial) (fibrinous)
      (hemorrhagic) (idiopathic) (localized)
      (perforative) (primary) (with adhesions)
      (with effusion) K65.9
  with or following
    abscess K65.1
    appendicitis K35.2
      with perforation or rupture K35.2
      generalized K35.2
      localized K35.3
    diverticular disease (intestine) K57.80
      with bleeding K57.81
    ectopic or molar pregnancy O08.0
    large intestine K57.20
      with
        bleeding K57.21
        small intestine K57.40
          with bleeding K57.41
    small intestine K57.00
      with
        bleeding K57.01
        large intestine K57.40
          with bleeding K57.41
  acute (generalized) K65.0
  aseptic T81.61
  bile, biliary K65.3
  chemical T81.61
  chlamydial A74.81
  chronic proliferative K65.8
  complicating abortion —see Abortion, by
      type, complicated by, pelvic peritonitis
  congenital P78.1
  diaphragmatic K65.0
  diffuse K65.0
  diphtheritic A36.89
  disseminated K65.0
  due to
    bile K65.3
    foreign
      body or object accidentally left during
          a procedure (instrument) (sponge)
          (swab) T81.599
      substance accidentally left during a
          procedure (chemical) (powder)
          (talc) T81.61
    talc T81.61
    urine K65.8
  eosinophilic K65.8
    acute K65.0
  fibrocaseous (tuberculous) A18.31
  fibropurulent K65.0
  following ectopic or molar pregnancy O08.0
  general (ized) K65.0
  gonococcal A54.85
  meconium (newborn) P78.0
  neonatal P78.1
    meconium P78.0
  pancreatic K65.0
  paroxysmal, familial E85.0
    benign E85.0
  pelvic
    female N73.5
      acute N73.3
      chronic N73.4
        with adhesions N73.6
    male K65.0
  periodic, familial E85.0
  proliferative, chronic K65.8
  puerperal, postpartum, childbirth O85

◀ New   ◀▥ Revised   ~~deleted~~ Deleted

Peritonitis *(Continued)*
  purulent K65.0
  septic K65.0
  specified NEC K65.8
  spontaneous bacterial K65.2
  subdiaphragmatic K65.0
  subphrenic K65.0
  suppurative K65.0
  syphilitic A52.74
    congenital (early) A50.08 [K67]
  talc T81.61
  tuberculous A18.31
  urine K65.8
Peritonsillar —*see* condition
Peritonsillitis J36
Perityphlitis K37
Periureteritis N28.89
Periurethral —*see* condition
Periurethritis (gangrenous) —*see* Urethritis
Periuterine —*see* condition
Perivaginitis —*see* Vaginitis
Perivasculitis, retinal H35.06-
Perivasitis (chronic) N49.1
Perivesiculitis (seminal) —*see* Vesiculitis
Perlèche NEC K13.0
  due to
    candidiasis B37.83
    moniliasis B37.83
    riboflavin deficiency E53.0
    vitamin B2 (riboflavin) deficiency E53.0
Pernicious —*see* condition
Pernio, perniosis T69.1
Perpetrator (of abuse) —*see* Index to External
  Causes of Injury, Perpetrator ◀▥
Persecution
  delusion F22
  social Z60.5
Perseveration (tonic) R48.8
Persistence, persistent (congenital)
  anal membrane Q42.3
    with fistula Q42.2
  arteria stapedia Q16.3
  atrioventricular canal Q21.2
  branchial cleft Q18.0
  bulbus cordis in left ventricle Q21.8
  canal of Cloquet Q14.0
  capsule (opaque) Q12.8
  cilioretinal artery or vein Q14.8
  cloaca Q43.7
  communication —*see* Fistula, congenital
  convolutions
    aortic arch Q25.4
    fallopian tube Q50.6
    oviduct Q50.6
    uterine tube Q50.6
  double aortic arch Q25.4
  ductus arteriosus (Botalli) Q25.0
  fetal
    circulation P29.3
    form of cervix (uteri) Q51.828
    hemoglobin, hereditary (HPFH) D56.4
  foramen
    Botalli Q21.1
    ovale Q21.1
  Gartner's duct Q52.4
  hemoglobin, fetal (hereditary) (HPFH)
    D56.4
  hyaloid
    artery (generally incomplete) Q14.0
    system Q14.8
  hymen, in pregnancy or childbirth —*see*
    Pregnancy, complicated by, abnormal,
    vulva
  lanugo Q84.2
  left
    posterior cardinal vein Q26.8
    root with right arch of aorta Q25.4
    superior vena cava Q26.1
  Meckel's diverticulum Q43.0
    malignant —*see* Table of Neoplasms, small
      intestine, malignant

Persistence, persistent *(Continued)*
  mucosal disease (middle ear) —*see*
    Otitis, media, suppurative, chronic,
    tubotympanic
  nail (s), anomalous Q84.6
  omphalomesenteric duct Q43.0
  organ or site not listed —*see* Anomaly, by site
  ostium
    atrioventriculare commune Q21.2
    primum Q21.2
    secundum Q21.1
  ovarian rests in fallopian tube Q50.6
  pancreatic tissue in intestinal tract Q43.8
  primary (deciduous)
    teeth K00.6
    vitreous hyperplasia Q14.0
  pupillary membrane Q13.89
  rhesus (Rh)titer —*see* Complication (s),
    transfusion, incompatibility reaction,
    Rh (factor)
  right aortic arch Q25.4
  sinus
    urogenitalis
      female Q52.8
      male Q55.8
    venosus with imperfect incorporation in
      right auricle Q26.8
  thymus (gland) (hyperplasia) E32.0
  thyroglossal duct Q89.2
  thyrolingual duct Q89.2
  truncus arteriosus or communis Q20.0
  tunica vasculosa lentis Q12.2
  umbilical sinus Q64.4
  urachus Q64.4
  vitelline duct Q43.0
Person (with)
  admitted for clinical research, as a control
    subject (normal comparison)
    (participant) Z00.6
  awaiting admission to adequate facility
    elsewhere Z75.1
  concern (normal) about sick person in family
    Z63.6
  consulting on behalf of another Z71.0
  feigning illness Z76.5
  living (in)
    without
      adequate housing (heating) (space) Z59.1
      housing (permanent) (temporary) Z59.0
      person able to render necessary care
        Z74.2
      shelter Z59.0
    alone Z60.2
    boarding school Z59.3
    residential institution Z59.3
  on waiting list Z75.1
  sick or handicapped in family Z63.6
Personality (disorder) F60.9
  accentuation of traits (type A pattern) Z73.1
  affective F34.0
  aggressive F60.3
  amoral F60.2
  anacastic, anankastic F60.5
  antisocial F60.2
  anxious F60.6
  asocial F60.2
  asthenic F60.7
  avoidant F60.6
  borderline F60.3
  change due to organic condition (enduring)
    F07.0
  compulsive F60.5
  cycloid F34.0
  cyclothymic F34.0
  dependent F60.7
  depressive F34.1
  dissocial F60.2
  dual F44.81
  eccentric F60.89
  emotionally unstable F60.3
  expansive paranoid F60.0

Personality *(Continued)*
  explosive F60.3
  fanatic F60.0
  haltlose type F60.89
  histrionic F60.4
  hyperthymic F34.0
  hypothymic F34.1
  hysterical F60.4
  immature F60.89
  inadequate F60.7
  labile (emotional) F60.3
  mixed (nonspecific) F60.81
  morally defective F60.2
  multiple F44.81
  narcissistic F60.81
  obsessional F60.5
  obsessive (-compulsive) F60.5
  organic F07.0
  overconscientious F60.5
  paranoid F60.0
  passive (-dependent) F60.7
  passive-aggressive F60.89
  pathologic F60.9
  pattern defect or disturbance F60.9
  pseudopsychopathic (organic) F07.0
  pseudoretarded (organic) F07.0
  psychoinfantile F60.4
  psychoneurotic NEC F60.89
  psychopathic F60.2
  querulant F60.0
  sadistic F60.89
  schizoid F60.1
  self-defeating F60.7
  sensitive paranoid F60.0
  sociopathic (amoral) (antisocial) (asocial)
    (dissocial) F60.2
  specified NEC F60.89
  type A Z73.1
  unstable (emotional) F60.3
Perthes' disease —*see* Legg-Calvé-Perthes
  disease
Pertussis (see also Whooping cough)
  A37.90
Perversion, perverted
  appetite F50.8
    psychogenic F50.8
  function
    pituitary gland E23.2
      posterior lobe E22.2
  sense of smell and taste R43.8
    psychogenic F45.8
  sexual —*see* Deviation, sexual
Pervious, congenital —*see also* Imperfect,
  closure
  ductus arteriosus Q25.0
Pes (congenital) —*see also* Talipes
  acquired —*see also* Deformity, limb, foot,
    specified NEC
    planus —*see* Deformity, limb, flat foot
  adductus Q66.89
  cavus Q66.7
  deformity NEC, acquired —*see* Deformity,
    limb, foot, specified NEC
  planus (acquired) (any degree) —*see also*
    Deformity, limb, flat foot
    rachitic sequelae (late effect) E64.3
  valgus Q66.6
Pest, pestis —*see* Plague
Petechia, petechiae R23.3
  newborn P54.5
Petechial typhus A75.9
Peter's anomaly Q13.4
Petit mal seizure —*see* Epilepsy, generalized,
  specified NEC
Petit's hernia —*see* Hernia, abdomen, specified
  site NEC
Petrellidosis B48.2
Petrositis H70.20-
  acute H70.21-
  chronic H70.22-
Peutz-Jeghers disease or syndrome Q85.8

Peyronie's disease N48.6
Pfeiffer's disease —see Mononucleosis, infectious
Phagedena (dry) (moist) (sloughing) —see also Gangrene
  geometric L88
  penis N48.29
  tropical —see Ulcer, skin
  vulva N76.6
Phagedenic —see condition
Phakoma H35.89
Phakomatosis (see also specific eponymous syndromes) Q85.9
  Bourneville's Q85.1
  specified NEC Q85.8
Phantom limb syndrome (without pain) G54.7
  with pain G54.6
Pharyngeal pouch syndrome D82.1
Pharyngitis (acute) (catarrhal) (gangrenous) (infective) (malignant) (membranous) (phlegmonous) (pseudomembranous) (simple) (subacute) (suppurative) (ulcerative) (viral) J02.9
  with influenza, flu, or grippe —see Influenza, with, pharyngitis
  aphthous B08.5
  atrophic J31.2
  chlamydial A56.4
  chronic (atrophic) (granular) (hypertrophic) J31.2
  coxsackievirus B08.5
  diphtheritic A36.0
  enteroviral vesicular B08.5
  follicular (chronic) J31.2
  fusospirochetal A69.1
  gonococcal A54.5
  granular (chronic) J31.2
  herpesviral B00.2
  hypertrophic J31.2
  infectional, chronic J31.2
  influenzal —see Influenza, with, respiratory manifestations NEC
  lymphonodular, acute (enteroviral) B08.8
  pneumococcal J02.8
  purulent J02.9
  putrid J02.9
  septic J02.0
  sicca J31.2
  specified organism NEC J02.8
  staphylococcal J02.8
  streptococcal J02.0
  syphilitic, congenital (early) A50.03
  tuberculous A15.8
  vesicular, enteroviral B08.5
  viral NEC J02.8
Pharyngoconjunctivitis, viral B30.2
Pharyngolaryngitis (acute) J06.0
  chronic J37.0
Pharyngoplegia J39.2
Pharyngotonsillitis, herpesviral B00.2
Pharyngotracheitis, chronic J42
Pharynx, pharyngeal —see condition
Phenomenon
  Arthus' —see Arthus' phenomenon
  jaw-winking Q07.8
  lupus erythematosus (LE) cell M32.9
  Raynaud's (secondary) I73.00
    with gangrene I73.01
  vasomotor R55
  vasospastic I73.9
  vasovagal R55
  Wenckebach's I44.1
Phenylketonuria E70.1
  classical E70.0
  maternal E70.1
Pheochromoblastoma
  specified site —see Neoplasm, malignant, by site
  unspecified site C74.10

Pheochromocytoma
  malignant
    specified site —see Neoplasm, malignant, by site
    unspecified site C74.10
  specified site —see Neoplasm, benign, by site
  unspecified site D35.00
Pheohyphomycosis —see Chromomycosis
Pheomycosis —see Chromomycosis
Phimosis (congenital) (due to infection) N47.1
  chancroidal A57
Phlebectasia (see also Varix
  congenital Q27.4
Phlebitis (infective) (pyemic) (septic) (suppurative) I80.9
  antepartum —see Thrombophlebitis, antepartum
  blue —see Phlebitis, leg, deep
  breast, superficial I80.8
  cavernous (venous) sinus —see Phlebitis, intracranial (venous) sinus
  cerebral (venous) sinus —see Phlebitis, intracranial (venous) sinus
  chest wall, superficial I80.8
  cranial (venous) sinus —see Phlebitis, intracranial (venous) sinus
  deep (vessels) —see Phlebitis, leg, deep
  due to implanted device —see Complications, by site and type, specified NEC
  during or resulting from a procedure T81.72
  femoral vein (superficial) I80.1-
  femoropopliteal vein I80.0-
  gestational —see Phlebopathy, gestational
  hepatic veins I80.8
  iliofemoral —see Phlebitis, femoral vein
  intracranial (venous) sinus (any) G08
    nonpyogenic I67.6
  intraspinal venous sinuses and veins G08
    nonpyogenic G95.19
  lateral (venous) sinus —see Phlebitis, intracranial (venous) sinus
  leg I80.3
    antepartum —see Thrombophlebitis, antepartum
    deep (vessels) NEC I80.20-
      iliac I80.21-
      popliteal vein I80.22-
      specified vessel NEC I80.29-
      tibial vein I80.23-
    femoral vein (superficial) I80.1-
    superficial (vessels) I80.0-
  longitudinal sinus —see Phlebitis, intracranial (venous) sinus
  lower limb —see Phlebitis, leg
  migrans, migrating (superficial) I82.1
  pelvic
    with ectopic or molar pregnancy O08.0
    following ectopic or molar pregnancy O08.0
    puerperal, postpartum O87.1
  popliteal vein —see Phlebitis, leg, deep, popliteal
  portal (vein) K75.1
  postoperative T81.72
  pregnancy —see Thrombophlebitis, antepartum
  puerperal, postpartum, childbirth O87.0
    deep O87.1
    pelvic O87.1
    superficial O87.0
  retina —see Vasculitis, retina
  saphenous (accessory) (great) (long) (small) —see Phlebitis, leg, superficial
  sinus (meninges) —see Phlebitis, intracranial (venous) sinus
  specified site NEC I80.8
  syphilitic A52.09
  tibial vein —see Phlebitis, leg, deep, tibial
  ulcerative I80.9
    leg —see Phlebitis, leg
  umbilicus I80.8

Phlebitis (Continued)
  uterus (septic) —see Endometritis
  varicose (leg) (lower limb) —see Varix, leg, with, inflammation
Phlebofibrosis I87.8
Phleboliths I87.8
Phlebopathy
  gestational O22.9-
  puerperal O87.9
Phlebosclerosis I87.8
Phlebothrombosis —see also Thrombosis
  antepartum —see Thrombophlebitis, antepartum
  pregnancy —see Thrombophlebitis, antepartum
  puerperal —see Thrombophlebitis, puerperal
Phlebotomus fever A93.1
Phlegmasia
  alba dolens O87.1
    nonpuerperal —see Phlebitis, femoral vein
  cerulea dolens —see Phlebitis, leg, deep
Phlegmon —see Abscess
Phlegmonous —see condition
Phlyctenulosis (allergic) (keratoconjunctivitis) (nontuberculous) —see also Keratoconjunctivitis
  cornea —see Keratoconjunctivitis
  tuberculous A18.52
Phobia, phobic F40.9
  animal F40.218
    spiders F40.210
  examination F40.298
  reaction F40.9
  simple F40.298
  social F40.10
    generalized F40.11
  specific (isolated) F40.298
    animal F40.218
      spiders F40.210
    blood F40.230
    injection F40.231
    injury F40.233
    men F40.290
    natural environment F40.228
      thunderstorms F40.220
    situational F40.248
      bridges F40.242
      closed in spaces F40.240
      flying F40.243
      heights F40.241
    specified focus NEC F40.298
    transfusion F40.231
    women F40.291
  specified NEC F40.8
    medical care NEC F40.232
  state F40.9
Phocas' disease —see Mastopathy, cystic
Phocomelia Q73.1
  lower limb —see Agenesis, leg, with foot present
  upper limb —see Agenesis, arm, with hand present
Phoria H50.50
Phosphate-losing tubular disorder N25.0
Phosphatemia E83.39
Phosphaturia E83.39
Photodermatitis (sun) L56.8
  chronic L57.8
  due to drug L56.8
  light other than sun L59.8
Photokeratitis H16.13-
Photophobia H53.14-
Photophthalmia —see Photokeratitis
Photopsia H53.19
Photoretinitis —see Retinopathy, solar
Photosensitivity, photosensitization (sun) skin L56.8
  light other than sun L59.8
Phrenitis —see Encephalitis
Phrynoderma (vitamin A deficiency) E50.8

Phthiriasis (pubis) B85.3
  with any infestation classifiable to
    B85.0-B85.2 B85.4
Phthirus infestation —*see* Phthiriasis
Phthisis —*see also* Tuberculosis
  bulbi (infectional) —*see* Disorder, globe,
    degenerated condition, atrophy
  eyeball (due to infection) —*see* Disorder,
    globe, degenerated condition, atrophy
Phycomycosis —*see* Zygomycosis
Physalopteriasis B81.8
Physical restraint status Z78.1
Phytobezoar T18.9
  intestine T18.3
  stomach T18.2
Pian —*see* Yaws
Pianoma A66.1
Pica F50.8
  in adults F50.8
  infant or child F98.3
Picking, nose F98.8
Pick-Niemann disease —*see* Niemann-Pick
    disease or syndrome
Pick's
  cerebral atrophy G31.01 *[F02.80]*
    with behavioral disturbance G31.01
      [F02.81]
  disease or syndrome (brain) G31.01 *[F02.80]*
    with behavioral disturbance G31.01
      [F02.81]
Pickwickian syndrome E66.2
Piebaldism E70.39
Piedra (beard) (scalp) B36.8
  black B36.3
  white B36.2
Pierre Robin deformity or syndrome Q87.0
Pierson's disease or osteochondrosis M91.0
Pig-bel A05.2
Pigeon
  breast or chest (acquired) M95.4
    congenital Q67.7
      rachitic sequelae (late effect) E64.3
  breeder's disease or lung J67.2
  fancier's disease or lung J67.2
  toe —*see* Deformity, toe, specified NEC
Pigmentation (abnormal) (anomaly) L81.9
  conjunctiva H11.13-
  cornea (anterior) H18.01-
    posterior H18.05-
    stromal H18.06-
  diminished melanin formation NEC L81.6
  iron L81.8
  lids, congenital Q82.8
  limbus corneae —*see* Pigmentation, cornea
  metals L81.8
  optic papilla, congenital Q14.2
  retina, congenital (grouped) (nevoid) Q14.1
  scrotum, congenital Q82.8
  tattoo L81.8
Piles (*see also* Hemorrhoids) K64.9
Pili
  annulati or torti (congenital) Q84.1
  incarnati L73.1
Pill roller hand (intrinsic) —*see* Parkinsonism
Pilomatrixoma —*see* Neoplasm, skin, benign
  malignant —*see* Neoplasm, skin, malignant
Pilonidal —*see* condition
Pimple R23.8
Pinched nerve —*see* Neuropathy, entrapment
Pindborg tumor —*see* Cyst, calcifying
    odontogenic
Pineal body or gland —*see* condition
Pinealoblastoma C75.3
Pinealoma D44.5
  malignant C75.3
Pineoblastoma C75.3
Pineocytoma D44.5
Pinguecula H11.15-
Pingueculitis H10.81-
Pinhole meatus (*see also* Stricture, urethra)
    N35.9

Pink
  disease —*see* subcategory T56.1
  eye —*see* Conjunctivitis, acute, mucopurulent
Pinkus' disease (lichen nitidus) L44.1
Pinpoint
  meatus —*see* Stricture, urethra
  os (uteri) —*see* Stricture, cervix
Pins and needles R20.2
Pinta A67.9
  cardiovascular lesions A67.2
  chancre (primary) A67.0
  erythematous plaques A67.1
  hyperchromic lesions A67.1
  hyperkeratosis A67.1
  lesions A67.9
    cardiovascular A67.2
    hyperchromic A67.1
    intermediate A67.1
    late A67.2
    mixed A67.3
    primary A67.0
    skin (achromic) (cicatricial) (dyschromic)
      A67.2
      hyperchromic A67.1
      mixed (achromic and hyperchromic)
        A67.3
  papule (primary) A67.0
  skin lesions (achromic) (cicatricial)
    (dyschromic) A67.2
    hyperchromic A67.1
    mixed (achromic and hyperchromic) A67.3
  vitiligo A67.2
Pintids A67.1
Pinworm (disease) (infection) (infestation) B80
Piroplasmosis B60.0
Pistol wound —*see* Gunshot wound
Pitchers' elbow —*see* Derangement, joint,
    specified type NEC, elbow
Pithecoid pelvis Q74.2
  with disproportion (fetopelvic) O33.0
    causing obstructed labor O65.0
Pithiatism F48.8
Pitted —*see* Pitting
Pitting —*see also* Edema R60.9
  lip R60.0
  nail L60.8
  teeth K00.4
Pituitary gland —*see* condition
Pituitary-snuff-taker's disease J67.8
Pityriasis (capitis) L21.0
  alba L30.5
  circinata (et maculata) L42
  furfuracea L21.0
  Hebra's L26
  lichenoides L41.0
    chronica L41.1
    et varioliformis (acuta) L41.0
  maculata (et circinata) L30.5
  nigra B36.1
  pilaris, Hebra's L44.0
  rosea L42
  rotunda L44.8
  rubra (Hebra) pilaris L44.0
  simplex L30.5
  specified type NEC L30.5
  streptogenes L30.5
  versicolor (scrotal) B36.0
Placenta, placental —*see* Pregnancy,
    complicated by (care of) (management
    affected by), specified condition
Placentitis O41.14-
Plagiocephaly Q67.3
Plague A20.9
  abortive A20.8
  ambulatory A20.8
  asymptomatic A20.8
  bubonic A20.0
  cellulocutaneous A20.1
  cutaneobubonic A20.1
  lymphatic gland A20.0
  meningitis A20.3

Plague (*Continued*)
  pharyngeal A20.8
  pneumonic (primary) (secondary) A20.2
  pulmonary, pulmonic A20.2
  septicemic A20.7
  tonsillar A20.8
    septicemic A20.7
Planning, family
  contraception Z30.9
  procreation Z31.69
Plaque (s)
  artery, arterial —*see* Arteriosclerosis
  calcareous —*see* Calcification
  coronary, lipid rich I25.83
  epicardial I31.8
  erythematous, of pinta A67.1
  Hollenhorst's —*see* Occlusion, artery, retina
  lipid rich, coronary I25.83
  pleural (without asbestos) J92.9
    with asbestos J92.0
  tongue K13.29
Plasmacytoma C90.3-
  extramedullary C90.2-
  medullary C90.0-
  solitary C90.3-
Plasmacytopenia D72.818
Plasmacytosis D72.822
Plaster ulcer —*see* Ulcer, pressure, by site
Plateau iris syndrome (post-iridectomy)
    (postprocedural) (without glaucoma)
    H21.82
  with glaucoma H40.22-
Platybasia Q75.8
Platyonychia (congenital) Q84.6
  acquired L60.8
Platypelloid pelvis M95.5
  with disproportion (fetopelvic) O33.0
    causing obstructed labor O65.0
  congenital Q74.2
Platyspondylisis Q76.49
Plaut (-Vincent) disease (*see also* Vincent's)
    A69.1
Plethora R23.2
  newborn P61.1
Pleura, pleural —*see* condition
Pleuralgia R07.81 ◀▥
Pleurisy (acute) (adhesive) (chronic) (costal)
    (diaphragmatic) (double) (dry) (fibrinous)
    (fibrous) (interlobar) (latent) (plastic)
    (primary) (residual) (sicca) (sterile)
    (subacute) (unresolved) R09.1
  with
    adherent pleura J86.0
    effusion J90
      chylous, chyliform J94.0
      tuberculous (non primary) A15.6
        primary (progressive) A15.7
      tuberculosis —*see* Pleurisy, tuberculous
        (non primary)
  encysted —*see* Pleurisy, with effusion
  exudative —*see* Pleurisy, with effusion
  fibrinopurulent, fibropurulent —*see*
    Pyothorax
  hemorrhagic —*see* Hemothorax
  pneumococcal J90
  purulent —*see* Pyothorax
  septic —*see* Pyothorax
  serofibrinous —*see* Pleurisy, with effusion
  seropurulent —*see* Pyothorax
  serous —*see* Pleurisy, with effusion
  staphylococcal J86.9
  streptococcal J90
  suppurative —*see* Pyothorax
  traumatic (post) (current) —*see* Injury,
    intrathoracic, pleura
  tuberculous (with effusion) (non primary)
    A15.6
    primary (progressive) A15.7
Pleuritis sicca —*see* Pleurisy
Pleurobronchopneumonia —*see* Pneumonia,
    broncho

Pleurodynia R07.81
　epidemic B33.0
　viral B33.0
Pleuropericarditis —see also Pericarditis
　acute I30.9
Pleuropneumonia (acute) (bilateral) (double)
　　(septic) (see also Pneumonia) J18.8
　chronic —see Fibrosis, lung
Pleuro-pneumonia-like-organism (PPLO),
　　as cause of disease classified elsewhere
　　B96.0
Pleurorrhea —see Pleurisy, with effusion
Plexitis, brachial G54.0
Plica
　polonica B85.0
　syndrome, knee M67.5
　tonsil J35.8
Plicated tongue K14.5
Plug
　bronchus NEC J98.09
　meconium (newborn) NEC syndrome P76.0
　mucus —see Asphyxia, mucus
Plumbism —see subcategory T56.0
Plummer's disease E05.20
　with thyroid storm E05.21
Plummer-Vinson syndrome D50.1
Pluricarential syndrome of infancy E40
Plus (and minus) hand (intrinsic) —see
　　Deformity, limb, specified type NEC,
　　forearm
Pneumathemia —see Air, embolism
Pneumatic hammer (drill) syndrome T75.21
Pneumatocele (lung) J98.4
　intracranial G93.89
　tension J44.9
Pneumatosis
　cystoides intestinalis K63.89
　intestinalis K63.89
　peritonei K66.8
Pneumaturia R39.89
Pneumoblastoma —see Neoplasm, lung,
　　malignant
Pneumocephalus G93.89
Pneumococcemia A40.3
Pneumococcus, pneumococcal —see condition
Pneumoconiosis (due to) (inhalation of) J64
　with tuberculosis (any type in A15) J65
　aluminum J63.0
　asbestos J61
　bagasse, bagassosis J67.1
　bauxite J63.1
　beryllium J63.2
　coal miners' (simple) J60
　coalworkers' (simple) J60
　collier's J60
　cotton dust J66.0
　diatomite (diatomaceous earth) J62.8
　dust
　　inorganic NEC J63.6
　　lime J62.8
　　marble J62.8
　　organic NEC J66.8
　fumes or vapors (from silo) J68.9
　graphite J63.3
　grinder's J62.8
　kaolin J62.8
　mica J62.8
　millstone maker's J62.8
　mineral fibers NEC J61
　miner's J60
　moldy hay J67.0
　potter's J62.8
　rheumatoid —see Rheumatoid, lung
　sandblaster's J62.8
　silica, silicate NEC J62.8
　　with carbon J60
　stonemason's J62.8
　talc (dust) J62.0
Pneumocystis carinii pneumonia B59
Pneumocystis jiroveci (pneumonia) B59
Pneumocystosis (with pneumonia) B59

Pneumohemopericardium I31.2
Pneumohemothorax J94.2
　traumatic S27.2
Pneumohydropericardium —see Pericarditis
Pneumohydrothorax —see Hydrothorax
Pneumomediastinum J98.2
　congenital or perinatal P25.2
Pneumomycosis B49 [J99]
Pneumonia (acute) (double) (migratory)
　　(purulent) (septic) (unresolved) J18.9
　with
　　influenza —see Influenza, with, pneumonia
　　lung abscess J85.1
　　　due to specified organism —see
　　　　Pneumonia, in (due to)
　adenoviral J12.0
　adynamic J18.2
　alba A50.04
　allergic (eosinophilic) J82
　alveolar —see Pneumonia, lobar
　anaerobes J15.8
　anthrax A22.1
　apex, apical —see Pneumonia, lobar
　Ascaris B77.81
　aspiration J69.0
　　due to
　　　aspiration of microorganisms
　　　　bacterial J15.9
　　　　viral J12.9
　　　food (regurgitated) J69.0
　　　gastric secretions J69.0
　　　milk (regurgitated) J69.0
　　　oils, essences J69.1
　　　solids, liquids NEC J69.8
　　　vomitus J69.0
　　newborn P24.81
　　　amniotic fluid (clear) P24.11
　　　blood P24.21
　　　food (regurgitated) P24.31
　　　liquor (amnii) P24.11
　　　meconium P24.01
　　　milk P24.31
　　　mucus P24.11
　　　specified NEC P24.81
　　　stomach contents P24.31
　　postprocedural J95.4
　atypical NEC J18.9
　bacillus J15.9
　　specified NEC J15.8
　bacterial J15.9
　　specified NEC J15.8
　Bacteroides (fragilis) (oralis)
　　(melaninogenicus) J15.8
　basal, basic, basilar —see Pneumonia, by type
　bronchiolitis obliterans organized (BOOP)
　　J84.89
　broncho-, bronchial (confluent) (croupous)
　　(diffuse) (disseminated) (hemorrhagic)
　　(involving lobes) (lobar) (terminal) J18.0
　　allergic (eosinophilic) J82
　　aspiration —see Pneumonia, aspiration
　　bacterial J15.9
　　　specified NEC J15.8
　　chronic —see Fibrosis, lung
　　diplococcal J13
　　Eaton's agent J15.7
　　Escherichia coli (E. coli) J15.5
　　Friedländer's bacillus J15.0
　　Hemophilus influenzae J14
　　hypostatic J18.2
　　inhalation (see also Pneumonia, aspiration
　　　due to fumes or vapors (chemical) J68.0
　　　of oils or essences J69.1
　　Klebsiella (pneumoniae) J15.0
　　lipid, lipoid J69.1
　　　endogenous J84.89
　　Mycoplasma (pneumoniae) J15.7
　　pleuro-pneumonia-like-organisms (PPLO)
　　　J15.7
　　pneumococcal J13
　　Proteus J15.6

Pneumonia (Continued)
　broncho-, bronchial (Continued)
　　Pseudomonas J15.1
　　Serratia marcescens J15.6
　　specified organism NEC J16.8
　　staphylococcal —see Pneumonia,
　　　staphylococcal
　　streptococcal NEC J15.4
　　　group B J15.3
　　　pneumoniae J13
　　viral, virus —see Pneumonia, viral
　Butyrivibrio (fibriosolvens) J15.8
　Candida B37.1
　caseous —see Tuberculosis, pulmonary
　catarrhal —see Pneumonia, broncho
　chlamydial J16.0
　　congenital P23.1
　cholesterol J84.89
　cirrhotic (chronic) —see Fibrosis, lung
　Clostridium (haemolyticum) (novyi) J15.8
　confluent —see Pneumonia, broncho
　congenital (infective) P23.9
　　due to
　　　bacterium NEC P23.6
　　　Chlamydia P23.1
　　　Escherichia coli P23.4
　　　Haemophilus influenzae P23.6
　　　infective organism NEC P23.8
　　　Klebsiella pneumoniae P23.6
　　　Mycoplasma P23.6
　　　Pseudomonas P23.5
　　　Staphylococcus P23.2
　　　Streptococcus (except group B) P23.6
　　　　group B P23.3
　　　viral agent P23.0
　　specified NEC P23.8
　croupous —see Pneumonia, lobar
　cryptogenic organizing J84.116
　cytomegalic inclusion B25.0
　cytomegaloviral B25.0
　deglutition —see Pneumonia, aspiration
　desquamative interstitial J84.117
　diffuse —see Pneumonia, broncho
　diplococcal, diplococcus (broncho-) (lobar)
　　J13
　disseminated (focal) —see Pneumonia,
　　broncho
　Eaton's agent J15.7
　embolic, embolism —see Embolism,
　　pulmonary
　Enterobacter J15.6
　eosinophilic J82
　Escherichia coli (E. coli) J15.5
　Eubacterium J15.8
　fibrinous —see Pneumonia, lobar
　fibroid, fibrous (chronic) —see Fibrosis, lung
　Friedländer's bacillus J15.0
　Fusobacterium (nucleatum) J15.8
　gangrenous J85.0
　giant cell (measles) B05.2
　gonococcal A54.84
　gram-negative bacteria NEC J15.6
　　anaerobic J15.8
　Hemophilus influenzae (broncho) (lobar) J14
　human metapneumovirus J12.3
　hypostatic (broncho) (lobar) J18.2
　in (due to)
　　actinomycosis A42.0
　　adenovirus J12.0
　　anthrax A22.1
　　ascariasis B77.81
　　aspergillosis B44.9
　　Bacillus anthracis A22.1
　　Bacterium anitratum J15.6
　　candidiasis B37.1
　　chickenpox B01.2
　　Chlamydia J16.0
　　　neonatal P23.1
　　coccidioidomycosis B38.2
　　　acute B38.0
　　　chronic B38.1

Pneumonia *(Continued)*
  in *(Continued)*
    cytomegalovirus disease B25.0
    Diplococcus (pneumoniae) J13
    Eaton's agent J15.7
    Enterobacter J15.6
    Escherichia coli (E. coli) J15.5
    Friedländer's bacillus J15.0
    fumes and vapors (chemical) (inhalation) J68.0
    gonorrhea A54.84
    Hemophilus influenzae (H. influenzae) J14
    Herellea J15.6
    histoplasmosis B39.2
      acute B39.0
      chronic B39.1
    human metapneumovirus J12.3
    Klebsiella (pneumoniae) J15.0
    measles B05.2
    Mycoplasma (pneumoniae) J15.7
    nocardiosis, nocardiasis A43.0
    ornithosis A70
    parainfluenza virus J12.2
    pleuro-pneumonia-like-organism (PPLO) J15.7
    pneumococcus J13
    pneumocystosis (Pneumocystis carinii) (Pneumocystis jiroveci) B59
    Proteus J15.6
    Pseudomonas NEC J15.1
      pseudomallei A24.1
    psittacosis A70
    Q fever A78
    respiratory syncytial virus J12.1
    rheumatic fever I00 *[J17]*
    rubella B06.81
    Salmonella (infection) A02.22
      typhi A01.03
    schistosomiasis B65.9 *[[17]*
    Serratia marcescens J15.6
    specified
      bacterium NEC J15.8
      organism NEC J16.8
      spirochetal NEC A69.8
    Staphylococcus J15.20
      aureus (methicillin susceptible) (MSSA) J15.211
        methicillin resistant (MRSA) J15.212
      specified NEC J15.29
    Streptococcus J15.4
      group B J15.3
      pneumoniae J13
      specified NEC J15.4
    toxoplasmosis B58.3
    tularemia A21.2
    typhoid (fever) A01.03
    varicella B01.2
    virus —*see* Pneumonia, viral
    whooping cough A37.91
      due to
        Bordetella parapertussis A37.11
        Bordetella pertussis A37.01
        specified NEC A37.81
    Yersinia pestis A20.2
  inhalation of food or vomit —*see* Pneumonia, aspiration
  interstitial J84.9
    chronic J84.111
    desquamative J84.117
    due to
      collagen vascular disease J84.17
      known underlying cause J84.17
    idiopathic NOS J84.111
    in disease classified elsewhere J84.17
    lymphocytic (due to collagen vascular disease) (in diseases classified elsewhere) J84.17
    lymphoid J84.2

Pneumonia *(Continued)*
  interstitial *(Continued)*
    non-specific J84.89
      due to
        collagen vascular disease J84.17
        known underlying cause J84.17
      idiopathic J84.113
      in diseases classified elsewhere J84.17
    plasma cell B59
    pseudomonas J15.1
    usual J84.112
      due to collagen vascular disease J84.17
      idiopathic J84.112
      in diseases classified elsewhere J84.17
  Klebsiella (pneumoniae) J15.0
  lipid, lipoid (exogenous) J69.1
    endogenous J84.89
  lobar (disseminated) (double) (interstitial) J18.1
    bacterial J15.9
      specified NEC J15.8
    chronic —*see* Fibrosis, lung
    Escherichia coli (E. coli) J15.5
    Friedländer's bacillus J15.0
    Hemophilus influenzae J14
    hypostatic J18.2
    Klebsiella (pneumoniae) J15.0
    pneumococcal J13
    Proteus J15.6
    Pseudomonas J15.1
    specified organism NEC J16.8
    staphylococcal —*see* Pneumonia, staphylococcal
    streptococcal NEC J15.4
    Streptococcus pneumoniae J13
    viral, virus —*see* Pneumonia, viral
  lobular —*see* Pneumonia, broncho
  Löffler's J82
  lymphoid interstitial J84.2
  massive —*see* Pneumonia, lobar
  meconium P24.01
  MSSA (methicillin susceptible Staphylococcus aureus) J15.211
  multilobar —*see* Pneumonia, by type
  Mycoplasma (pneumoniae) J15.7
  necrotic J85.0
  neonatal P23.9
    aspiration —*see* Aspiration, by substance, with pneumonia
  nitrogen dioxide J68.9
  organizing J84.89
    due to
      collagen vascular disease J84.17
      known underlying cause J84.17
    in diseases classified elsewhere J84.17
  orthostatic J18.2
  parainfluenza virus J12.2
  parenchymatous —*see* Fibrosis, lung
  passive J18.2
  patchy —*see* Pneumonia, broncho
  Peptococcus J15.8
  Peptostreptococcus J15.8
  plasma cell (of infants) B59
  pleurolobar —*see* Pneumonia, lobar
  pleuro-pneumonia-like organism (PPLO) J15.7
  pneumococcal (broncho) (lobar) J13
  Pneumocystis (carinii) (jiroveci) B59
  postinfectional NEC B99 *[J17]*
  postmeasles B05.2
  Proteus J15.6
  Pseudomonas J15.1
  psittacosis A70
  radiation J70.0
  respiratory syncytial virus J12.1
  resulting from a procedure J95.89
  rheumatic I00 *[J17]*
  Salmonella (arizonae) (cholerae-suis) (enteritidis) (typhimurium) A02.22
    typhi A01.03
    typhoid fever A01.03

Pneumonia *(Continued)*
  SARS-associated coronavirus J12.81
  segmented, segmental —*see* Pneumonia, broncho-
  Serratia marcescens J15.6
  specified NEC J18.8
    bacterium NEC J15.8
    organism NEC J16.8
    virus NEC J12.89
  spirochetal NEC A69.8
  staphylococcal (broncho) (lobar) J15.20
    aureus (methicillin susceptible) (MSSA) J15.211
      methicillin resistant (MRSA) J15.212
    specified NEC J15.29
  static, stasis J18.2
  streptococcal NEC (broncho) (lobar) J15.4
    group
      A J15.4
      B J15.3
    specified NEC J15.4
  Streptococcus pneumoniae J13
  syphilitic, congenital (early) A50.04
  traumatic (complication) (early) (secondary) T79.8
  tuberculous (any) —*see* Tuberculosis, pulmonary
  tularemic A21.2
  varicella B01.2
  Veillonella J15.8
  ventilator associated J95.851
  viral, virus (broncho) (interstitial) (lobar) J12.9
    adenoviral J12.0
    congenital P23.0
    human metapneumovirus J12.3
    parainfluenza J12.2
    respiratory syncytial J12.1
    SARS-associated coronavirus J12.81
    specified NEC J12.89
  white (congenital) A50.04
Pneumonic —*see* condition
Pneumonitis (acute) (primary) —*see also* Pneumonia
  air-conditioner J67.7
  allergic (due to) J67.9
    organic dust NEC J67.8
    red cedar dust J67.8
    sequoiosis J67.8
    wood dust J67.8
  aspiration J69.0
    due to
      anesthesia J95.4
        during
          labor and delivery O74.0
          pregnancy O29.01-
          puerperium O89.01
      fumes or gases J68.0
      obstetric O74.0
  chemical (due to gases, fumes or vapors) (inhalation) J68.0
    due to anesthesia J95.4
  cholesterol J84.89
  chronic —*see* Fibrosis, lung
  congenital rubella P35.0
  crack (cocaine) J68.0
  due to
    beryllium J68.0
    cadmium J68.0
    crack (cocaine) J68.0
    detergent J69.8
    fluorocarbon-polymer J68.0
    food, vomit (aspiration) J69.0
    fumes or vapors J68.0
    gases, fumes or vapors (inhalation) J68.0
    inhalation
      blood J69.8
      essences J69.1
      food (regurgitated), milk, vomit J69.0
      oils, essences J69.1
      saliva J69.0
      solids, liquids NEC J69.8

Pneumonitis (Continued)
  due to (Continued)
    manganese J68.0
    nitrogen dioxide J68.0
    oils, essences J69.1
    solids, liquids NEC J69.8
    toxoplasmosis (acquired) B58.3
      congenital P37.1
    vanadium J68.0
    ventilator J95.851
  eosinophilic J82
  hypersensitivity J67.9
    air conditioner lung J67.7
    bagassosis J67.1
    bird fancier's lung J67.2
    farmer's lung J67.0
    maltworker's lung J67.4
    maple bark-stripper's lung J67.6
    mushroom worker's lung J67.5
    specified organic dust NEC J67.8
    suberosis J67.3
  interstitial (chronic) J84.89
    acute J84.114
    lymphoid J84.2
    non-specific J84.89
      idiopathic J84.113
  lymphoid, interstitial J84.2
  meconium P24.01
  postanesthetic J95.4
    correct substance properly administered —
      see Table of Drugs and Chemcials,
      by drug, adverse effect ◀▥
    in labor and delivery O74.0
    in pregnancy O29.01-
    obstetric O74.0
    overdose or wrong substance given or
      taken (by accident) —see Table of
      Drugs and Chemicals, by drug,
      poisoning ◀▥
    postpartum, puerperal O89.01
  postoperative J95.4
    obstetric O74.0
  radiation J70.0
  rubella, congenital P35.0
  ventilation (air-conditioning) J67.7
  ventilator associated J95.851
  wood-dust J67.8
Pneumonoconiosis —see Pneumoconiosis
Pneumoparotid K11.8
Pneumopathy NEC J98.4
  alveolar J84.09
  due to organic dust NEC J66.8
  parietoalveolar J84.09
Pneumopericarditis —see also Pericarditis
  acute I30.9
Pneumopericardium —see also Pericarditis
  congenital P25.3
  newborn P25.3
  traumatic (post) —see Injury, heart
Pneumophagia (psychogenic) F45.8
Pneumopleurisy, pneumopleuritis (see also
  Pneumonia) J18.8
Pneumopyopericardium I30.1
Pneumopyothorax —see Pyopneumothorax
  with fistula J86.0
Pneumorrhagia —see also Hemorrhage, lung
  tuberculous —see Tuberculosis, pulmonary
Pneumothorax NOS J93.9
  acute J93.83
  chronic J93.81
  congenital P25.1
  perinatal period P25.1
  postprocedural J95.811
  specified NEC J93.83
  spontaneous NOS J93.83
    newborn P25.1
    primary J93.11
    secondary J93.12
    tension J93.0
  tense valvular, infectional J93.0
  tension (spontaneous) J93.0

Pneumothorax NOS (Continued)
  traumatic S27.0
    with hemothorax S27.2
  tuberculous —see Tuberculosis, pulmonary
Podagra (see also Gout) M10.9
Podencephalus Q01.9
Poikilocytosis R71.8
Poikiloderma L81.6
  Civatte's L57.3
  congenital Q82.8
  vasculare atrophicans L94.5
Poikilodermatomyositis M33.10
  with
    myopathy M33.12
    respiratory involvement M33.11
    specified organ involvement NEC M33.19
Pointed ear (congenital) Q17.3
Poison ivy, oak, sumac or other plant
  dermatitis (allergic) (contact) L23.7
Poisoning (acute) —see also Table of Drugs
  and Chemicals ◀▥
  algae and toxins T65.82-
  Bacillus B (aertrycke) (cholerae (suis))
    (paratyphosus) (suipestifer) A02.9
    botulinus A05.1
  bacterial toxins A05.9
  berries, noxious —see Poisoning, food,
    noxious, berries
  botulism A05.1
  ciguatera fish T61.0-
  Clostridium botulinum A05.1
  death-cap (Amanita phalloides) (Amanita
    verna) —see Poisoning, food, noxious,
    mushrooms
  drug —see Table of Drugs and Chemicals,
    by drug, poisoning ◀▥
  epidemic, fish (noxious) —see Poisoning,
    seafood
    bacterial A05.9
  fava bean D55.0
  fish (noxious) T61.9-
    bacterial —see Intoxication, foodborne, by
      agent
    ciguatera fish —see Poisoning, ciguatera
      fish
    scombroid fish —see Poisoning, scombroid
      fish
    specified type NEC T61.77-
  food (acute) (diseased) (infected) (noxious)
    NEC T62.9-
    bacterial —see Intoxication, foodborne, by
      agent
    due to
      Bacillus (aertrycke) (choleraesuis)
        (paratyphosus) (suipestifer) A02.9
        botulinus A05.1
      Clostridium (perfringens) (Welchii)
        A05.2
      salmonella (aertrycke) (callinarum)
        (choleraesuis) (enteritidis)
        (paratyphi) (suipestifer) A02.9
        with
          gastroenteritis A02.0
          sepsis A02.1
        staphylococcus A05.0
      Vibrio
        parahaemolyticus A05.3
        vulnificus A05.5
    noxious or naturally toxic T62.9-
      berries —see subcategory T62.1-
      fish —see Poisoning, seafood
      mushrooms —see subcategory T62.0X-
      plants NEC —see subcategory T62.2X-
      seafood —see Poisoning, seafood
      specified NEC —see subcategory T62.8X-
  ichthyotoxism —see Poisoning, seafood
  kreotoxism, food A05.9
  latex T65.81-
  lead T56.0-
  mushroom —see Poisoning, food, noxious,
    mushroom

Poisoning (Continued)
  mussels —see also Poisoning, shellfish
    bacterial —see Intoxication, foodborne, by
      agent
  nicotine (tobacco) T65.2-
  noxious foodstuffs —see Poisoning, food,
    noxious
  plants, noxious —see Poisoning, food,
    noxious, plants NEC
  ptomaine —see Poisoning, food
  radiation J70.0
  Salmonella (arizonae) (cholerae-suis)
    (enteritidis) (typhimurium) A02.9
  scombroid fish T61.1-
  seafood (noxious) T61.9-
    bacterial —see Intoxication, foodborne, by
      agent
    fish —see Poisoning, fish
    shellfish —see Poisoning, shellfish
    specified NEC —see subcategory T61.8X-
  shellfish (amnesic) (azaspiracid) (diarrheic)
    (neurotoxic) (noxious) (paralytic)
    T61.78-
    bacterial —see Intoxication, foodborne, by
      agent
    ciguatera mollusk —see Poisoning,
      ciguatera fish
  specified substance NEC T65.891
  Staphylococcus, food A05.0
  tobacco (nicotine) T65.2-
  water E87.79
Poker spine —see Spondylitis, ankylosing
Poland syndrome Q79.8
Polioencephalitis (acute) (bulbar) A80.9
  inferior G12.22
  influenzal —see Influenza, with,
    encephalopathy
  superior hemorrhagic (acute) (Wernicke's)
    E51.2
  Wernicke's E51.2
Polioencephalomyelitis (acute) (anterior)
  A80.9
  with beriberi E51.2
Polioencephalopathy, superior hemorrhagic
  E51.2
  with
    beriberi E51.11
    pellagra E52
Poliomeningoencephalitis —see
  Meningoencephalitis
Poliomyelitis (acute) (anterior) (epidemic)
  A80.9
  with paralysis (bulbar) —see Poliomyelitis,
    paralytic
  abortive A80.4
  ascending (progressive) —see Poliomyelitis,
    paralytic
  bulbar (paralytic) —see Poliomyelitis,
    paralytic
  congenital P35.8
  nonepidemic A80.9
  nonparalytic A80.4
  paralytic A80.30
    specified NEC A80.39
    vaccine-associated A80.0
    wild virus
      imported A80.1
      indigenous A80.2
  spinal, acute A80.9
Poliosis (eyebrow) (eyelashes) L67.1
  circumscripta, acquired L67.1
Pollakiuria R35.0
  psychogenic F45.8
Pollinosis J30.1
Pollitzer's disease L73.2
Polyadenitis —see also Lymphadenitis
  malignant A20.0
Polyalgia M79.89
Polyangiitis M30.0
  microscopic M31.7
  overlap syndrome M30.8

◀ New   ◀▥ Revised   ~~deleted~~ Deleted

Polyarteritis
  microscopic M31.7
  nodosa M30.0
    with lung involvement M30.1
    juvenile M30.2
    related condition NEC M30.8
Polyarthralgia —*see* Pain, joint
Polyarthritis, polyarthropathy (*see also*
    Arthritis) M13.0
  due to or associated with other specified
    conditions —*see* Arthritis
  epidemic (Australian) (with exanthema)
    B33.1
  infective —*see* Arthritis, pyogenic or pyemic
  inflammatory M06.4
  juvenile (chronic) (seronegative) M08.3
  migratory —*see* Fever, rheumatic
  rheumatic, acute —*see* Fever, rheumatic
Polyarthrosis M15.9
  post-traumatic M15.3
  primary M15.0
  specified NEC M15.8
Polycarential syndrome of infancy E40
Polychondritis (atrophic) (chronic) —*see also*
    Disorder, cartilage, specified type NEC
  relapsing M94.1
Polycoria Q13.2
Polycystic (disease)
  degeneration, kidney Q61.3
    autosomal dominant (adult type) Q61.2
    autosomal recessive (infantile type) NEC
      Q61.19
  kidney Q61.3
    autosomal
      dominant Q61.2
      recessive NEC Q61.19
    autosomal dominant (adult type) Q61.2
    autosomal recessive (childhood type) NEC
      Q61.19
    infantile type NEC Q61.19
  liver Q44.6
  lung J98.4
    congenital Q33.0
  ovary, ovaries E28.2
  spleen Q89.09
Polycythemia (secondary) D75.1
  acquired D75.1
  benign (familial) D75.0
  due to
    donor twin P61.1
    erythropoietin D75.1
    fall in plasma volume D75.1
    high altitude D75.1
    maternal-fetal transfusion P61.1
    stress D75.1
  emotional D75.1
  erythropoietin D75.1
  familial (benign) D75.0
  Gaisböck's (hypertonica) D75.1
  high altitude D75.1
  hypertonica D75.1
  hypoxemic D75.1
  neonatorum P61.1
  nephrogenous D75.1
  relative D75.1
  secondary D75.1
  spurious D75.1
  stress D75.1
  vera D45
Polycytosis cryptogenica D75.1
Polydactylism, polydactyly Q69.9
  toes Q69.2
Polydipsia R63.1
Polydystrophy, pseudo-Hurler E77.0
Polyembryoma —*see* Neoplasm, malignant,
    by site
Polyglandular
  deficiency E31.0
  dyscrasia E31.9
  dysfunction E31.9
  syndrome E31.8

Polyhydramnios O40.-
Polymastia Q83.1
Polymenorrhea N92.0
Polymyalgia M35.3
  arteritica, giant cell M31.5
  rheumatica M35.3
    with giant cell arteritis M31.5
Polymyositis (acute) (chronic) (hemorrhagic)
    M33.20
  with
    myopathy M33.22
    respiratory involvement M33.21
    skin involvement —*see*
      Dermatopolymyositis
  specified organ involvement NEC M33.29
  ossificans (generalisata) (progressiva) —*see*
    Myositis, ossificans, progressiva
Polyneuritis, polyneuritic —*see also*
    Polyneuropathy
  acute (post-)infective G61.0
  alcoholic G62.1
  cranialis G52.7
  demyelinating, chronic inflammatory (CIDP)
    G61.81
  diabetic —*see* Diabetes, polyneuropathy
  diphtheritic A36.83
  due to lack of vitamin NEC E56.9 [G63]
  endemic E51.11
  erythredema —*see* subcategory T56.1
  febrile, acute G61.0
  hereditary ataxic G60.1
  idiopathic, acute G61.0
  infective (acute) G61.0
  inflammatory, chronic demyelinating (CIDP)
    G61.81
  nutritional E63.9 [G63]
  postinfective (acute) G61.0
  specified NEC G62.89
Polyneuropathy (peripheral) G62.9
  alcoholic G62.1
  amyloid (Portuguese) E85.1 [G63]
  arsenical G62.2
  critical illness G62.81
  demyelinating, chronic inflammatory (CIDP)
    G61.81
  diabetic —*see* Diabetes, polyneuropathy
  drug-induced G62.0
  hereditary G60.9
    specified NEC G60.8
  idiopathic G60.9
    progressive G60.3
  in (due to)
    alcohol G62.1
      sequelae G65.2
    amyloidosis, familial (Portuguese) E85.1
      [G63]
    antitetanus serum G61.1
    arsenic G62.2
      sequelae G65.2
    avitaminosis NEC E56.9 [G63]
    beriberi E51.11
    collagen vascular disease NEC M35.9 [G63]
    deficiency (of)
      B (-complex) vitamins E53.9 [G63]
      vitamin B6 E53.1 [G63]
    diabetes —*see* Diabetes, polyneuropathy
    diphtheria A36.83
    drug or medicament G62.0
      correct substance properly
        administered —*see* Table of ɟDrugs
        and ɕChemicals, by drug, adverse
        effect ◀▦▦
      overdose or wrong substance given or
        taken —*see* Table of ɟDrugs and
        ɕChemicals, by drug, poisoning ◀▦▦
    endocrine disease NEC E34.9 [G63]
    herpes zoster B02.23
    hypoglycemia E16.2 [G63]
    infectious
      disease NEC B99 [G63]
      mononucleosis B27.91

Polyneuropathy (*Continued*)
  in (*Continued*)
    lack of vitamin NEC E56.9 [G63]
    lead G62.2
      sequelae G65.2
    leprosy A30.9 [G63]
    Lyme disease A69.22
    metabolic disease NEC E88.9 [G63]
    microscopic polyangiitis M31.7 [G63]
    mumps B26.84
    neoplastic disease (*see also* Neoplasm)
      D49.9 [G63]
    nutritional deficiency NEC E63.9 [G63]
    organophosphate compounds G62.2
      sequelae G65.2
    parasitic disease NEC B89 [G63]
    pellagra E52 [G63]
    polyarteritis nodosa M30.0
    porphyria E80.20 [G63]
    radiation G62.82
    rheumatoid arthritis —*see* Rheumatoid,
      polyneuropathy
    sarcoidosis D86.89
    serum G61.1
    syphilis (late) A52.15
      congenital A50.43
    systemic
      connective tissue disorder M35.9
        [G63]
      lupus erythematosus M32.19
    toxic agent NEC G62.2
      sequelae G65.2
    triorthocresyl phosphate G62.2
      sequelae G65.2
    tuberculosis A17.89
    uremia N18.9 [G63]
    vitamin B12 deficiency E53.8 [G63]
      with anemia (pernicious) D51.0
        [G63]
      due to dietary deficiency D51.3
        [G63]
    zoster B02.23
  inflammatory G61.9
    chronic demyelinating (CIDP) G61.81
    sequelae G65.1
    specified NEC G61.89
  lead G62.2
    sequelae G65.2
  nutritional NEC E63.9 [G63]
  postherpetic (zoster) B02.23
  progressive G60.3
  radiation-induced G62.82
  sensory (hereditary) (idiopathic) G60.8
  specified NEC G62.89
  syphilitic (late) A52.15
    congenital A50.43
Polyopia H53.8
Polyorchism, polyorchidism Q55.21
Polyosteoarthritis (*see also* Osteoarthritis,
    generalized) M15.9- ◀▦▦
  post-traumatic M15.3
  specified NEC M15.8
Polyostotic fibrous dysplasia Q78.1
Polyotia Q17.0
Polyp, polypus
  accessory sinus J33.8
  adenocarcinoma in —*see* Neoplasm,
    malignant, by site
  adenocarcinoma in situ in —*see* Neoplasm, in
    situ, by site
  adenoid tissue J33.0
  adenomatous —*see also* Neoplasm, benign,
    by site
    adenocarcinoma in —*see* Neoplasm,
      malignant, by site
    adenocarcinoma in situ in —*see* Neoplasm,
      in situ, by site
    carcinoma in —*see* Neoplasm, malignant,
      by site
    carcinoma in situ in —*see* Neoplasm, in
      situ, by site

Polyp, polypus *(Continued)*
  adenomatous *(Continued)*
    multiple —*see* Neoplasm, benign
      adenocarcinoma in —*see* Neoplasm,
        malignant, by site
      adenocarcinoma in situ in —*see*
        Neoplasm, in situ, by site
  antrum J33.8
  anus, anal (canal) K62.0
  Bartholin's gland N84.3
  bladder D41.4
  carcinoma in —*see* Neoplasm, malignant, by
    site
  carcinoma in situ in —*see* Neoplasm, in situ,
    by site
  cecum D12.0
  cervix (uteri) N84.1
    in pregnancy or childbirth —*see* Pregnancy,
      complicated by, abnormal, cervix
    mucous N84.1
    nonneoplastic N84.1
  choanal J33.0
  cholesterol K82.4
  clitoris N84.3
  colon K63.5
    adenomatous D12.6
    ascending D12.2
    cecum D12.0
    descending D12.4
    inflammatory K51.40
      with
        abscess K51.414
        complication K51.419
          specified NEC K51.418
        fistula K51.413
        intestinal obstruction K51.412
        rectal bleeding K51.411
    sigmoid D12.5
    transverse D12.3
  corpus uteri N84.0
  dental K04.0
  duodenum K31.7
  ear (middle) H74.4-
  endometrium N84.0
  ethmoidal (sinus) J33.8
  fallopian tube N84.8
  female genital tract N84.9
    specified NEC N84.8
  frontal (sinus) J33.8
  gallbladder K82.4
  gingiva, gum K06.8
  labia, labium (majus) (minus) N84.3
  larynx (mucous) J38.1
    adenomatous D14.1
  malignant —*see* Neoplasm, malignant, by site
  maxillary (sinus) J33.8
  middle ear —*see* Polyp, ear (middle)
  myometrium N84.0
  nares
    anterior J33.9
    posterior J33.0
  nasal (mucous) J33.9
    cavity J33.0
    septum J33.0
  nasopharyngeal J33.0
  nose (mucous) J33.9
  oviduct N84.8
  pharynx J39.2
  placenta O90.89
  prostate —*see* Enlargement, enlarged,
    prostate
  pudenda, pudendum N84.3
  pulpal (dental) K04.0
  rectum (nonadenomatous) K62.1
    adenomatous —*see* Polyp, adenomatous
  septum (nasal) J33.0
  sinus (accessory) (ethmoidal) (frontal)
    (maxillary) (sphenoidal) J33.8
  sphenoidal (sinus) J33.8
  stomach K31.7
    adenomatous D13.1

Polyp, polypus *(Continued)*
  tube, fallopian N84.8
  turbinate, mucous membrane J33.8
  umbilical, newborn P83.6
  ureter N28.89
  urethra N36.2
  uterus (body) (corpus) (mucous) N84.0
    cervix N84.1
    in pregnancy or childbirth —*see* Pregnancy,
      complicated by, tumor, uterus
  vagina N84.2
  vocal cord (mucous) J38.1
  vulva N84.3
Polyphagia R63.2
Polyploidy Q92.7
Polypoid —*see* condition
Polyposis —*see also* Polyp
  coli (adenomatous) D12.6
    adenocarcinoma in C18.9
    adenocarcinoma in situ in —*see* Neoplasm,
      in situ, by site
    carcinoma in C18.9
  colon (adenomatous) D12.6
  familial D12.6
    adenocarcinoma in situ in —*see* Neoplasm,
      in situ, by site
  intestinal (adenomatous) D12.6
  malignant lymphomatous C83.1
  multiple, adenomatous *(see also* Neoplasm,
    benign) D36.9
Polyradiculitis —*see* Polyneuropathy
Polyradiculoneuropathy (acute) (postinfective)
  (segmentally demyelinating) G61.0
Polyserositis
  due to pericarditis I31.1
  pericardial I31.1
  periodic, familial E85.0
  tuberculous A19.9
    acute A19.1
    chronic A19.8
Polysplenia syndrome Q89.09
Polysyndactyly *(see also* Syndactylism,
  syndactyly) Q70.4
Polytrichia L68.3
Polyunguia Q84.6
Polyuria R35.8
  nocturnal R35.1
  psychogenic F45.8
Pompe's disease (glycogen storage) E74.02
Pompholyx L30.1
Poncet's disease (tuberculous rheumatism)
  A18.09
Pond fracture —*see* Fracture, skull
Ponos B55.0
Pons, pontine —*see* condition
Poor
  aesthetic of existing restoration of tooth
    K08.56
  contractions, labor O62.2
  gingival margin to tooth restoration K08.51
  personal hygiene R46.0
  prenatal care, affecting management of
    pregnancy —*see* Pregnancy, complicated
    by, insufficient, prenatal care
  sucking reflex (newborn) R29.2
  urinary stream R39.12
  vision NEC H54.7
Poradenitis, nostras inguinalis or venerea A55
Porencephaly (congenital) (developmental)
  (true) Q04.6
  acquired G93.0
  nondevelopmental G93.0
  traumatic (post) F07.89
Porocephaliasis B88.8
Porokeratosis Q82.8
Poroma, eccrine —*see* Neoplasm, skin, benign
Porphyria (South African) E80.20
  acquired E80.20
  acute intermittent (hepatic) (Swedish) E80.21
  cutanea tarda (hereditary) (symptomatic)
    E80.1

Porphyria *(Continued)*
  due to drugs E80.20
    correct substance properly administered —
      see Table of Drugs and Chemicals,
      by drug, adverse effect ◄▥
    overdose or wrong substance given or
      taken —*see* Table of Drugs and
      Chemicals, by drug, poisoning ◄▥
  erythropoietic (congenital) (hereditary)
    E80.0
  hepatocutaneous type E80.1
  secondary E80.20
  toxic NEC E80.20
  variegata E80.20
Porphyrinuria —*see* Porphyria
Porphyruria —*see* Porphyria
Portal —*see* condition
Port wine nevus, mark, or stain Q82.5
Posadas-Wernicke disease B38.9
Positive
  culture (nonspecific)
    blood R78.81
    bronchial washings R84.5
    cerebrospinal fluid R83.5
    cervix uteri R87.5
    nasal secretions R84.5
    nipple discharge R89.5
    nose R84.5
      staphylococcus (Methicillin susceptible)
        Z22.321
        Methicillin resistant Z22.322
    peritoneal fluid R85.5
    pleural fluid R84.5
    prostatic secretions R86.5
    saliva R85.5
    seminal fluid R86.5
    sputum R84.5
    synovial fluid R89.5
    throat scrapings R84.5
    urine R82.7
    vagina R87.5
    vulva R87.5
    wound secretions R89.5
  PPD (skin test) R76.11
  serology for syphilis A53.0
    with signs or symptoms - code as Syphilis,
      by site and stage
    false R76.8
  skin test, tuberculin (without active
    tuberculosis) R76.11
  test, human immunodeficiency virus (HIV)
    R75
  VDRL A53.0
    with signs or symptoms - code by site and
      stage under Syphilis A53.9
  Wassermann reaction A53.0
Postcardiotomy syndrome I97.0
Postcaval ureter Q62.62
Postcholecystectomy syndrome K91.5
Postclimacteric bleeding N95.0
Postcommissurotomy syndrome I97.0
Postconcussional syndrome F07.81
Postcontusional syndrome F07.81
Postcricoid region —*see* condition
Post-dates (40-42 weeks) (pregnancy) (mother)
  O48.0
  more than 42 weeks gestation O48.1
Postencephalitic syndrome F07.89
Posterior —*see* condition
Posterolateral sclerosis (spinal cord) —*see*
  Degeneration, combined
Postexanthematous —*see* condition
Postfebrile —*see* condition
Postgastrectomy dumping syndrome K91.1
Posthemiplegic chorea —*see* Monoplegia
Posthemorrhagic anemia (chronic) D50.0
  acute D62
  newborn P61.3
Postherpetic neuralgia (zoster) B02.29
  trigeminal B02.22
Posthitis N47.7

◄ New ◄▥ Revised ~~deleted~~ Deleted

Postimmunization complication or reaction — *see* Complications, vaccination
Postinfectious —*see* condition
Postlaminectomy syndrome NEC M96.1
Postleukotomy syndrome F07.0
Postmastectomy lymphedema (syndrome) I97.2
Postmaturity, postmature (over 42 weeks)
  maternal (over 42 weeks gestation) O48.1
  newborn P08.22
Postmeasles complication NEC (*see also* condition) B05.89
Postmenopausal
  endometrium (atrophic) N95.8
    suppurative (*see also* Endometritis) N71.9
  osteoporosis —*see* Osteoporosis, postmenopausal
Postnasal drip R09.82
  due to
    allergic rhinitis —*see* Rhinitis, allergic
    common cold J00
    gastroesophageal reflux —*see* Reflux, gastroesophageal
    nasopharyngitis —*see* Nasopharyngitis
    other know condition — code to condition
    sinusitis —*see* Sinusitis
Postnatal —*see* condition
Postoperative (postprocedural) —*see* Complication, postoperative
  pneumothorax, therapeutic Z98.3
  state NEC Z98.89
Postpancreatectomy hyperglycemia E89.1
Postpartum —*see* Puerperal
Postphlebitic syndrome —*see* Syndrome, postthrombotic
Postpolio (myelitic) syndrome G14
Postpoliomyelitic —*see also* condition
  osteopathy —*see* Osteopathy, after poliomyelitis
Postprocedural —*see also* Postoperative
  hypoinsulinemia E89.1
Postschizophrenic depression F32.8
Postsurgery status —*see also* Status (post)
  pneumothorax, therapeutic Z98.3
Post-term (40-42 weeks) (pregnancy) (mother) O48.0
  infant P08.21
  more than 42 weeks gestation (mother) O48.1
Post-traumatic brain syndrome, nonpsychotic F07.81
Post-typhoid abscess A01.09
Postures, hysterical F44.2
Postvaccinal reaction or complication —*see* Complications, vaccination
Postvalvulotomy syndrome I97.0
Potain's
  disease (pulmonary edema) —*see* Edema, lung
  syndrome (gastrectasis with dyspepsia) K31.0
Potter's
  asthma J62.8
  facies Q60.6
  lung J62.8
  syndrome (with renal agenesis) Q60.6
Pott's
  curvature (spinal) A18.01
  disease or paraplegia A18.01
  spinal curvature A18.01
  tumor, puffy —*see* Osteomyelitis, specified type NEC
Pouch
  bronchus Q32.4
  Douglas' —*see* condition
  esophagus, esophageal, congenital Q39.6
    acquired K22.5
  gastric K31.4
  Hartmann's K82.8
  pharynx, pharyngeal (congenital) Q38.7
Pouchitis K91.850
Poultrymen's itch B88.0
Poverty NEC Z59.6
  extreme Z59.5

Poxvirus NEC B08.8
Prader-Willi syndrome Q87.1
Preauricular appendage or tag Q17.0
Prebetalipoproteinemia (acquired) (essential) (familial) (hereditary) (primary) (secondary) E78.1
  with chylomicronemia E78.3
Precipitate labor or delivery O62.3
Preclimacteric bleeding (menorrhagia) N92.4
Precocious
  adrenarche E30.1
  menarche E30.1
  menstruation E30.1
  pubarche E30.1
  puberty E30.1
    central E22.8
  sexual development NEC E30.1
  thelarche E30.8
Precocity, sexual (constitutional) (cryptogenic) (female) (idiopathic) (male) E30.1
  with adrenal hyperplasia E25.9
    congenital E25.0
Precordial pain R07.2
Predeciduous teeth K00.2
Prediabetes, prediabetic R73.09
  complicating
    pregnancy —*see* Pregnancy, complicated by, diseases of, specified type or system NEC
    puerperium O99.89
Predislocation status of hip at birth Q65.6
Pre-eclampsia O14.9-
  with pre-existing hypertension —*see* Hypertension, complicating pregnancy, pre-existing, with, pre-eclampsia
  mild O14.0-
  moderate O14.0-
  severe O14.1-
    with hemolysis, elevated liver enzymes and low platelet count (HELLP) O14.2-
Pre-eruptive color change, teeth, tooth K00.8
Pre-excitation atrioventricular conduction I45.6
Preglaucoma H40.00-
Pregnancy (single) (uterine) —*see also* Delivery and Puerperal

---

Note: The Tabular must be reviewed for assignment of the appropriate character indicating the trimester of the pregnancy

Note: The Tabular must be reviewed for assignment of appropriate seventh character for multiple gestation codes in Chapter 15

---

  abdominal (ectopic) O00.0
    with viable fetus O36.7-
  ampullar O00.1
  biochemical O02.81
  broad ligament O00.8
  cervical O00.8
  chemical O02.81
  complicated NOS O26.9-
  complicated by (care of) (management affected by)
    abnormal, abnormality
      cervix O34.4-
        causing obstructed labor O65.5
      cord (umbilical) O69.9
      findings on antenatal screening of mother O28.9
        biochemical O28.1
        chromosomal O28.5
        cytological O28.2
        genetic O28.5
        hematological O28.0
        radiological O28.4
        specified NEC O28.8
        ultrasonic O28.3
      glucose (tolerance) NEC O99.810

Pregnancy (*Continued*)
  complicated by (*Continued*)
    abnormal, abnormality (*Continued*)
      pelvic organs O34.9-
        specified NEC O34.8-
          causing obstructed labor O65.5
      pelvis (bony) (major) NEC O33.0
      perineum O34.7-
      position
        placenta O44.1-
          without hemorrhage O44.0-
        uterus O34.59-
      uterus O34.59-
        causing obstructed labor O65.5
        congenital O34.0-
      vagina O34.6-
        causing obstructed labor O65.5
      vulva O34.7-
        causing obstructed labor O65.5
    abruptio placentae —*see* Abruptio placentae
    abscess or cellulitis
      bladder O23.1-
      breast O91.11-
      genital organ or tract O23.9-
    abuse
      physical O9A.31- ◀▥
      psychological O9A.51- ◀▥
      sexual O9A.41- ◀▥
    adverse effect anesthesia O29.9-
      aspiration pneumonitis O29.01-
      cardiac arrest O29.11-
      cardiac complication NEC O29.19-
      cardiac failure O29.12-
      central nervous system complication NEC O29.29-
      cerebral anoxia O29.21-
      failed or difficult intubation O29.6-
      inhalation of stomach contents or secretions NOS O29.01-
      local, toxic reaction O29.3X
      Mendelson's syndrome O29.01-
      pressure collapse of lung O29.02-
      pulmonary complications NEC O29.09-
      specified NEC O29.8X
      spinal and epidural type NEC O29.5X
        induced headache O29.4-
    albuminuria O12.1-
    alcohol use O99.31-
    amnionitis O41.12-
    anaphylactoid syndrome of pregnancy O88.01-
    anemia (conditions in D50-D64) (pre-existing) O99.01-
      complicating the puerperium O99.03
    antepartum hemorrhage O46.9-
      with coagulation defect —*see* Hemorrhage, antepartum, with coagulation defect
      specified NEC O46.8X-
    appendicitis O99.61-
    atrophy (yellow) (acute) liver (subacute) O26.61-
    bariatric surgery status O99.84-
    bicornis or bicornuate uterus O34.59-
    biliary tract problems O26.61-
    breech presentation O32.1
    cardiovascular diseases (conditions in I00-I09, I20-I52, I70-I99) O99.41-
    cerebrovascular disorders (conditions in I60-I69) O99.41-
    cervical shortening O26.87-
    cervicitis O23.51-
    chloasma (gravidarum) O26.89-
    cholecystitis O99.61-
    cholestasis (intrahepatic) O26.61-
    chorioamnionitis O41.12-
    circulatory system disorder (conditions in I00-I09, I20-I99, O99.41-)
    compound presentation O32.6
    conjoined twins O30.02-

Pregnancy (Continued)
  complicated by (Continued)
    connective system disorders (conditions in M00-M99) O99.89
    contracted pelvis (general) O33.1
      inlet O33.2
      outlet O33.3
    convulsions (eclamptic) (uremic) (see also Eclampsia) O15.9- ◄▪▪▪
    cracked nipple O92.11-
    cystitis O23.1-
    cystocele O34.8-
    death of fetus (near term) O36.4
      early pregnancy O02.1
      of one fetus or more in multiple gestation O31.2-
    deciduitis O41.14-
    decreased fetal movement O36.81-
    dental problems O99.61-
    diabetes (mellitus) O24.91-
      gestational (pregnancy induced) —see Diabetes, gestational
      pre-existing O24.31-
        specified NEC O24.81-
        type 1 O24.01-
        type 2 O24.11-
    digestive system disorders (conditions in K00-K93) O99.61-
    diseases of —see Pregnancy, complicated by, specified body system disease
      biliary tract O26.61-
      blood NEC (conditions in D65-D77) O99.11-
      liver O26.61-
      specified NEC O99.89
    disorders of —see Pregnancy, complicated by, specified body system disorder
      amniotic fluid and membranes O41.9-
        specified NEC O41.8X-
      biliary tract O26.61-
      ear and mastoid process (conditions in H60-H95) O99.89
      eye and adnexa (conditions in H00-H59) O99.89
      liver O26.61-
      skin (conditions in L00-L99) O99.71-
      specified NEC O99.89
    displacement, uterus NEC O34.59-
      causing obstructed labor O65.5
    disproportion (due to) O33.9
      fetal deformities NEC O33.7
      generally contracted pelvis O33.1
      hydrocephalic fetus O33.6
      inlet contraction of pelvis O33.2
      mixed maternal and fetal origin O33.4
      specified NEC O33.8
    double uterus O34.59-
      causing obstructed labor O65.5
    drug use (conditions in F11-F19) O99.32-
    eclampsia, eclamptic (coma) (convulsions) (delirium) (nephritis) (uremia) (see also Eclampsia) O15-
    ectopic pregnancy —see Pregnancy, ectopic
    edema O12.0-
      with
        gestational hypertension, mild (see also Pre-eclampsia) O14.0- ◄▪▪▪
        proteinuria O12.2-
    effusion, amniotic fluid —see Pregnancy, complicated by, premature rupture of membranes
    elderly
      multigravida O09.52-
      primigravida O09.51-
    embolism (see also Embolism, obstetric, pregnancy) O88.-
    endocrine diseases NEC O99.28-
    endometritis O86.12
    excessive weight gain O26.0-
    exhaustion O26.81-
      during labor and delivery O75.81

Pregnancy (Continued)
  complicated by (Continued)
    face presentation O32.3
    failed induction of labor O61.9
    failed or difficult intubation for anesthesia O29.6- ◄▪▪▪
      instrumental O61.1
      mechanical O61.1
      medical O61.0
      specified NEC O61.8
      surgical O61.1
    false labor (pains) O47.9
      at or after 37 completed weeks of pregnancy O47.1
      before 37 completed weeks of pregnancy O47.0-
    fatigue O26.81-
      during labor and delivery O75.81
    fatty metamorphosis of liver O26.61-
    female genital mutilation O34.8- [N90.81-]
    fetal (maternal care for)
      abnormality or damage O35.9
        acid-base balance O68
        specified type NEC O35.8
      acidemia O68
      acidosis O68
      alkalosis O68
      anemia and thrombocytopenia O36.82-
      anencephaly O35.0
      chromosomal abnormality (conditions in Q90-Q99) O35.1
      conjoined twins O30.02-
      damage from
        amniocentesis O35.7
        biopsy procedures O35.7
        drug addiction O35.5
        hematological investigation O35.7
        intrauterine contraceptive device O35.7
        maternal
          alcohol addiction O35.4
          cytomegalovirus infection O35.3
          disease NEC O35.8
          drug addiction O35.5
          listeriosis O35.8
          rubella O35.3
          toxoplasmosis O35.8
          viral infection O35.3
        medical procedure NEC O35.7
        radiation O35.6
      death (near term) O36.4
        early pregnancy O02.1
      decreased movement O36.81-
      disproportion due to deformity (fetal) O33.7
      excessive growth (large for dates) O36.6-
      growth retardation O36.59-
        light for dates O36.59-
        small for dates O36.59-
      heart rate irregularity (bradycardia) (decelerations) (tachycardia) O76
      hereditary disease O35.2
      hydrocephalus O35.0
      intrauterine death O36.4
      poor growth O36.59-
        light for dates O36.59-
        small for dates O36.59-
      problem O36.9-
        specified NEC O36.89-
      reduction (elective) O31.3-
      selective termination O31.3-
      spina bifida O35.0
      thrombocytopenia O36.82-
    fibroid (tumor) (uterus) O34.1-
    fissure of nipple O92.11-
    gallstones O99.61-
    gastric banding status O99.84-
    gastric bypass status O99.84-
    genital herpes (asymptomatic) (history of) (inactive) O98.51-
    genital tract infection O23.9-

Pregnancy (Continued)
  complicated by (Continued)
    glomerular diseases (conditions in N00-N07) O26.83-
      with hypertension, pre-existing —see Hypertension, complicating, pregnancy, pre-existing, with, renal disease
    gonorrhea O98.21-
    grand multiparity O09.4
    habitual aborter —see Pregnancy, complicated by, recurrent pregnancy loss
    HELLP syndrome (hemolysis, elevated liver enzymes and low platelet count) O14.2-
    hemorrhage
      antepartum —see Hemorrhage, antepartum
      before 20 completed weeks gestation O20.9
        specified NEC O20.8
      due to premature separation, placenta (see also Abruptio placentae) O45.9-
      early O20.9
        specified NEC O20.8
      threatened abortion O20.0
    hemorrhoids O22.4-
    hepatitis (viral) O98.41-
    herniation of uterus O34.59-
    high
      head at term O32.4
      risk —see Supervision (of) (for), high-risk
    history of in utero procedure during previous pregnancy O09.82-
    HIV O98.71-
    human immunodeficiency virus (HIV) disease O98.71-
    hydatidiform mole (see also Mole, hydatidiform) O01.9- ◄▪▪▪
    hydramnios O40.-
    hydrocephalic fetus (disproportion) O33.6
    hydrops
      amnii O40.-
      fetalis O36.2-
        associated with isoimmunization (see also Pregnancy, complicated by, isoimmunization) O36.11-
    hydrorrhea O42.90
    hyperemesis (gravidarum) (mild) (see also Hyperemesis, gravidarum) O21.0- ◄▪▪▪
    hypertension —see Hypertension, complicating pregnancy
    hypertensive
      heart and renal disease, pre-existing —see Hypertension, complicating, pregnancy, pre-existing, with, heart disease, with renal disease
      heart disease, pre-existing —see Hypertension, complicating, pregnancy, pre-existing, with, heart disease
      renal disease, pre-existing —see Hypertension, complicating, pregnancy, pre-existing, with, renal disease
    hypotension O26.5-
    immune disorders NEC (conditions in D80-D89) O99.11-
    incarceration, uterus O34.51-
    incompetent cervix O34.3-
    inconclusive fetal viability O36.80
    infection (s) O98.91-
      amniotic fluid or sac O41.10-
      bladder O23.1-
      carrier state NEC O99.830
        streptococcus B O99.820
      genital organ or tract O23.9-
        specified NEC O23.59-
      genitourinary tract O23.9-

◄ New   ◄▪▪▪ Revised   ~~deleted~~ Deleted

Pregnancy *(Continued)*
  complicated by *(Continued)*
    infection *(Continued)*
      gonorrhea O98.21-
      hepatitis (viral) O98.41-
      HIV O98.71-
      human immunodeficiency virus (HIV)
        O98.71-
      kidney O23.0-
      nipple O91.01-
      parasitic disease O98.91-
        specified NEC O98.81-
      protozoal disease O98.61-
      sexually transmitted NEC O98.31-
      specified type NEC O98.81-
      syphilis O98.11-
      tuberculosis O98.01-
      urethra O23.2-
      urinary (tract) O23.4-
        specified NEC O23.3-
      viral disease O98.51-
    injury or poisoning (conditions in S00-T88)
      O9A.21-
      due to abuse
        physical O9A.31-
        psychological O9A.51-
        sexual O9A.41-
    insufficient
      prenatal care O09.3-
      weight gain O26.1-
    insulin resistance O26.89
    intrauterine fetal death (near term) O36.4
      early pregnancy O02.1
      multiple gestation (one fetus or more)
        O31.2-
    isoimmunization O36.11-
      anti-A sensitization O36.11-
      anti-B sensitization O36.19-
      Rh O36.09-
        anti-D antibody O36.01-
      specified NEC O36.19-
    laceration of uterus NEC O71.81
    malformation
      placenta, placental (vessel) O43.10-
        specified NEC O43.19-
      uterus (congenital) O34.0-
    malnutrition (conditions in E40-E46) O25.1-
    maternal hypotension syndrome O26.5-
    mental disorders (conditions in F01-F09,
      F20-F99) O99.34-
      alcohol use O99.31-
      drug use O99.32-
      smoking O99.33-
    mentum presentation O32.3
    metabolic disorders O99.28-
    missed
      abortion O02.1
      delivery O36.4
    multiple gestations O30.9-
      conjoined twins O30.02-
      quadruplet —*see* Pregnancy, quadruplet
      specified complication NEC O31.8X-
      specified number of multiples NEC —*see*
        Pregnancy, multiple (gestation),
        specified NEC
      triplet —*see* Pregnancy, triplet
      twin —*see* Pregnancy, twin
    musculoskeletal condition (conditions is
      M00-M99) O99.89
    necrosis, liver (conditions in K72) O26.61-
    neoplasm
      benign
        cervix O34.4-
        corpus uteri O34.1-
        uterus O34.1-
      malignant O9A.11-
    nephropathy NEC O26.83-
    nervous system condition (conditions in
      G00-G99) O99.35-
    nutritional diseases NEC O99.28-
    obesity (pre-existing) O99.21-

Pregnancy *(Continued)*
  complicated by *(Continued)*
    obesity surgery status O99.84-
    oblique lie or presentation O32.2
    older mother —*see* Pregnancy, complicated
      by, elderly
    oligohydramnios O41.0-
      with premature rupture of membranes
        (*see also* Pregnancy, complicated by,
        premature rupture of membranes)
        O42-
    onset (spontaneous) of labor after 37
      completed weeks of gestation but
      before 39 completed weeks gestation,
      with delivery by (planned) cesarean
      section O75.82
    oophoritis O23.52-
    overdose, drug (*see also* Table of ᵈDrugs
      and ᶜChemicals, by drug, poisoning)
      O9A.21- ◄▦
    oversize fetus O33.5
    papyraceous fetus O31.0-
    pelvic inflammatory disease O99.89
    periodontal disease O99.61-
    peripheral neuritis O26.82-
    peritoneal (pelvic) adhesions O99.89
    phlebitis O22.9-
    phlebopathy O22.9-
    phlebothrombosis (superficial) O22.2-
      deep O22.3-
    placenta accreta O43.21-
    placenta increta O43.22-
    placenta percreta O43.23-
    placenta previa O44.1-
      without hemorrhage O44.0-
    placental disorder O43.9-
      specified NEC O43.89-
    placental dysfunction O43.89-
    placental infarction O43.81-
    placental insufficiency O36.51-
    placental transfusion syndromes
      fetomaternal O43.01-
      fetus to fetus O43.02-
      maternofetal O43.01-
    placentitis O41.14-
    pneumonia O99.51-
    poisoning (*see also* Table of ᵈDrugs and
      ᶜChemicals) O9A.21- ◄▦
    polyhydramnios O40-
    polymorphic eruption of pregnancy
      O26.86
    poor obstetric history NEC O09.29-
    postmaturity (post-term) (40 to 42 weeks)
      O48.0
      more than 42 completed weeks gestation
        (prolonged) O48.1
    pre-eclampsia O14.9-
      mild O14.0-
      moderate O14.0-
      severe O14.1-
        with hemolysis, elevated liver
          enzymes and low platelet count
          (HELLP) O14.2-
    premature labor —*see* Pregnancy,
      complicated by, preterm labor
    premature rupture of membranes O42.90
      with onset of labor
        within 24 hours O42.00
          after 37 weeks gestation O42.02
          pre-term (before 37 completed
            weeks of gestation) O42.01-
        after 24 hours O42.10
          after 37 weeks gestation O42.12
          pre-term (before 37 completed
            weeks of gestation) O42.11-
      after 37 weeks gestation O42.92
      full-term O42.92
      pre-term (before 37 completed weeks of
        gestation) O42.91-
    premature separation of placenta - (*see also*
      Abruptio placentae) O45.9-

Pregnancy *(Continued)*
  complicated by *(Continued)*
    presentation, fetal —*see* Delivery(childbirth)
      (labor) (complicated by), complicated
      by, malposition ◄▦
    preterm delivery O60.10
    preterm labor
      with delivery O60.10
        preterm O60.10
        term O60.20
      second trimester
        with preterm delivery
          second trimester O60.12
          third trimester O60.13
        with term delivery O60.22
        without delivery O60.02
      third trimester
        with term delivery O60.23
        with third trimester preterm delivery
          O60.14
        without delivery O60.03
      without delivery O60.00
        second trimester O60.02
        third trimester O60.03
    previous history of —*see* Pregnancy,
      supervision of, high-risk
    prolapse, uterus O34.52-
    proteinuria (gestational) O12.1-
      with edema O12.2-
    pruritic urticarial papules and plaques of
      pregnancy (PUPPP) O26.86
    pruritus (neurogenic) O26.89-
    psychosis or psychoneurosis (puerperal) F53
    ptyalism O26.89-
    PUPPP (pruritic urticarial papules and
      plaques of pregnancy) O26.86
    pyelitis O23.0-
    recurrent pregnancy loss O26.2-
    renal disease or failure NEC O26.83-
      with secondary hypertension,
        pre-existing —*see* Hypertension,
        complicating, pregnancy,
        pre-existing, secondary
      hypertensive, pre-existing —*see*
        Hypertension, complicating,
        pregnancy, pre-existing, with, renal
        disease
    respiratory condition (conditions in
      J00-J99) O99.51-
    retained, retention
      dead ovum O02.0
      intrauterine contraceptive device
        O26.3-
    retroversion, uterus O34.53-
    Rh immunization, incompatibility or
      sensitization NEC O36.09-
      anti-D antibody O36.01-
    rupture
      amnion (premature) (*see also* Pregnancy,
        complicated by, premature rupture
        of membranes) O42-
      membranes (premature) (*see also*
        Pregnancy, complicated by,
        premature rupture of membranes)
        O42-
      uterus (during labor) O71.1
        before onset of labor O71.0-
    salivation (excessive) O26.89-
    salpingitis O23.52-
    salpingo-oophoritis O23.52-
    sepsis (conditions in A40, A41) O98.81-
    size date discrepancy (uterine) O26.84-
    skin condition (conditions in L00-L99)
      O99.71-
    smoking (tobacco) O99.33-
    social problem O09.7-
    specified condition NEC O26.89-
    spotting O26.85-
    streptococcus B carrier state O99.820
    subluxation of symphysis (pubis) O26.71-
    syphilis (conditions in A50-A53) O98.11-

Pregnancy *(Continued)*
  complicated by *(Continued)*
    threatened
      abortion O20.0
      labor O47.9
        at or after 37 completed weeks of
          gestation O47.1
        before 37 completed weeks of
          gestation O47.0-
    thrombophlebitis (superficial) O22.2-
    thrombosis O22.9-
      cerebral venous O22.5-
      cerebrovenous sinus O22.5-
      deep O22.3-
    torsion of uterus O34.59-
    toxemia O14.9-
    transverse lie or presentation O32.2
    tuberculosis (conditions in A15-A19) O98.01-
    tumor (benign)
      cervix O34.4-
      malignant O9A.11- ◄▬
      uterus O34.1-
    unstable lie O32.0
    upper respiratory infection O99.51-
    urethritis O23.2-
    uterine size date discrepancy O26.84-
    vaginitis or vulvitis O23.59-
    varicose veins (lower extremities) O22.0-
      genitals O22.1-
      legs O22.0-
      perineal O22.1-
      vaginal or vulval O22.1-
    venereal disease NEC (conditions in A63.8)
      O98.31-
    venous disorders O22.9-
      specified NEC O22.8X-
    very young mother —*see* Pregnancy,
      complicated by, young mother
    viral diseases (conditions in A80-B09,
      B25-B34) O98.51-
    vomiting O21.9
      due to diseases classified elsewhere O21.8
      hyperemesis gravidarum (mild) *(see
        also* Hyperemesis, gravidarum)
        O21.0- ◄▬
      late (occurring after 20 weeks of
        gestation) O21.2
    young mother
      multigravida O09.62-
      primigravida O09.61-
  concealed O09.3-
  continuing following
    elective fetal reduction of one or more fetus
      O31.3-
    intrauterine death of one or more fetus
      O31.2-
    spontaneous abortion of one or more fetus
      O31.1-
  cornual O00.8
  ectopic (ruptured) O00.9
    abdominal O00.0
      with viable fetus O36.7-
    cervical O00.8
    complicated (by) O08.9 ◄▬
      afibrinogenemia O08.1 ◄▬
      cardiac arrest O08.81 ◄▬
      chemical damage of pelvic organ (s)
        O08.6 ◄▬
      circulatory collapse O08.3 ◄▬
      defibrination syndrome O08.1 ◄▬
      electrolyte imbalance O08.5 ◄▬
      embolism (amniotic fluid) (blood clot)
        (pulmonary) (septic) O08.2 ◄▬
      endometritis O08.0 ◄▬
      genital tract and pelvic infection
        O08.0 ◄▬
      hemorrhage (delayed) (excessive)
        O08.1 ◄▬
      infection
        genital tract or pelvic O08.0 ◄▬
        kidney 008.83 ◄
        urinary tract O08.83 ◄▬

Pregnancy *(Continued)*
  ectopic *(Continued)*
    complicated *(Continued)*
      intravascular coagulation O08.1 ◄▬
      laceration of pelvic organ (s)
        O08.6 ◄▬
      metabolic disorder O08.5 ◄▬
      oliguria O08.4 ◄▬
      oophoritis O08.0 ◄▬
      parametritis O08.0 ◄▬
      pelvic peritonitis O08.0 ◄▬
      perforation of pelvic organ (s)
        O08.6 ◄▬
      renal failure or shutdown O08.4 ◄▬
      salpingitis or salpingo-oophoritis
        O08.0 ◄▬
      sepsis O08.82 ◄▬
      shock O08.83 ◄▬
        septic O08.82 ◄▬
      specified condition NEC O08.89 ◄▬
      tubular necrosis (renal) O08.4 ◄▬
      uremia O08.4 ◄▬
      urinary infection O08.83 ◄▬
      venous complication NEC O08.7 ◄▬
        embolism O08.2 ◄▬
    cornual O00.8
    intraligamentous O00.8
    mural O00.8
    ovarian O00.2
    specified site NEC O00.8
    tubal (ruptured) O00.1
  examination (normal) Z34.9-
    first Z34.0-
    high-risk —*see* Pregnancy, supervision of,
      high-risk
    specified Z34.8-
  extrauterine —*see* Pregnancy, ectopic
  fallopian O00.1
  false F45.8
  hidden O09.3-
  high-risk —*see* Pregnancy, supervision of,
    high-risk
  incidental finding Z33.1
  interstitial O00.8
  intraligamentous O00.8
  intramural O00.8
  intraperitoneal O00.0
  isthmian O00.1
  mesometric (mural) O00.8
  molar NEC O02.0
    complicated (by) O08.9 ◄▬
      afibrinogenemia O08.1 ◄▬
      cardiac arrest O08.81 ◄▬
      chemical damage of pelvic organ (s)
        O08.6 ◄▬
      circulatory collapse O08.3 ◄▬
      defibrination syndrome O08.1 ◄▬
      electrolyte imbalance O08.5 ◄▬
      embolism (amniotic fluid) (blood clot)
        (pulmonary) (septic) O08.2 ◄▬
      endometritis O08.0 ◄▬
      genital tract and pelvic infection
        O08.0 ◄▬
      hemorrhage (delayed) (excessive)
        O08.1 ◄▬
      infection
        genital tract or pelvic O08.0 ◄▬
        kidney O08.83 ◄▬
        urinary tract O08.83 ◄▬
      intravascular coagulation O08.1 ◄▬
      laceration of pelvic organ (s)
        O08.6 ◄▬
      metabolic disorder O08.5 ◄▬
      oliguria O08.4 ◄▬
      oophoritis O08.0 ◄▬
      parametritis O08.0 ◄▬
      pelvic peritonitis O08.0 ◄▬
      perforation of pelvic organ (s)
        O08.6 ◄▬
      renal failure or shutdown O08.4 ◄▬
      salpingitis or salpingo-oophoritis
        O08.0 ◄▬

Pregnancy *(Continued)*
  molar NEC *(Continued)*
    complicated *(Continued)*
      sepsis O08.82 ◄▬
      shock O08.3 ◄▬
        septic O08.82 ◄▬
      specified condition NEC O08.89 ◄▬
      tubular necrosis (renal) O08.4 ◄▬
      uremia O08.4 ◄▬
      urinary infection O08.83 ◄▬
      venous complication NEC O08.7 ◄▬
        embolism O08.2 ◄▬
  hydatidiform *(see also* Mole, hydatidiform)
    O01.9- ◄▬
  multiple (gestation) O30.9-
    greater than quadruplets —*see* Pregnancy,
      multiple (gestation), specified NEC
    specified NEC O30.80-
      with
        two or more monoamniotic fetuses
          O30.82-
        two or more monochorionic fetuses
          O30.81-
      two or more monoamniotic fetuses
        O30.82-
      two or more monochorionic fetuses
        O30.81-
      unable to determine number of placenta
        and number of amniotic sacs
        O30.89-
      unspecified number of placenta and
        unspecified number of amniotic
        sacs O30.80-
  mural O00.8
  normal (supervision of) Z34.9-
    first Z34.0-
    high-risk —*see* Pregnancy, supervision of,
      high-risk
    specified Z34.8-
  ovarian O00.2
  postmature (40 to 42 weeks) O48.0
    more than 42 weeks gestation O48.1
  post-term (40 to 42 weeks) O48.0
  prenatal care only Z34.9-
    first Z34.0-
    high-risk —*see* Pregnancy, supervision of,
      high-risk
    specified Z34.8-
  prolonged (more than 42 weeks gestation)
    O48.1
  quadruplet O30.20-
    with
      two or more monoamniotic fetuses
        O30.22-
      two or more monochorionic fetuses
        O30.21-
    two or more monoamniotic fetuses O30.22-
    two or more monochorionic fetuses
      O30.21-
    unable to determine number of placenta
      and number of amniotic sacs O30.29-
    unspecified number of placenta and
      unspecified number of amniotic sacs
      O30.20-
  quintuplet —*see* Pregnancy, multiple
    (gestation), specified NEC
  sextuplet —*see* Pregnancy, multiple
    (gestation), specified NEC
  supervision of
    concealed pregnancy O09.3-
    elderly mother
      multigravida O09.52-
      primigravida O09.51-
    hidden pregnancy O09.3-
    high-risk O09.9-
      due to (history of)
        ectopic pregnancy O09.1-
        elderly —*see* Pregnancy, supervision,
          elderly mother
        grand multiparity O09.4
        infertility O09.0-
        insufficient prenatal care O09.3-

◄ New   ◄▬ Revised   ~~deleted~~ Deleted

Pregnancy *(Continued)*
  supervision of *(Continued)*
    high-risk *(Continued)*
      due to *(Continued)*
        in utero procedure during previous
          pregnancy O09.82-
        in vitro fertilization O09.81-
        molar pregnancy O09.1-
        multiple previous pregnancies O09.4-
        older mother —*see* Pregnancy,
          supervision of, elderly mother
        poor reproductive or obstetric history
          NEC O09.29-
        pre-term labor O09.21-
        previous
          neonatal death O09.29-
        social problems O09.7-
        specified NEC O09.89-
        very young mother —*see* Pregnancy,
          supervision, young mother
    resulting from in vitro fertilization
      O09.81-
    normal Z34.9-
      first Z34.0-
      specified NEC Z34.8-
    young mother
      multigravida O09.62-
      primigravida O09.61-
  triplet O30.10-
    with
      two or more monoamniotic fetuses
        O30.12-
      two or more monochorionic fetuses
        O30.11-
    two or more monoamniotic fetuses O30.12-
    two or more monochorionic fetuses O30.11-
    unable to determine number of placenta
      and number of amniotic sacs O30.19-
    unspecified number of placenta and
      unspecified number of amniotic sacs
      O30.10-
  tubal (with abortion) (with rupture) O00.1
  twin O30.00-
    conjoined O30.02-
    dichorionic/diamniotic (two placenta, two
      amniotic sacs) O30.04-
    monochorionic/diamniotic (one placenta,
      two amniotic sacs) O30.03-
    monochorionic/monoamniotic (one
      placenta, one amniotic sac) O30.01-
    unable to determine number of placenta
      and number of amniotic sacs O30.09-
    unspecified number of placenta and
      unspecified number of amniotic sacs
      O30.00-
  unwanted Z64.0
  weeks of gestation
    8 weeks E3A.08
    9 weeks Z3A.09
    10 weeks Z3A.10
    11 weeks Z3A.11
    12 weeks Z3A.12
    13 weeks Z3A.13
    14 weeks Z3A.14
    15 weeks Z3A.15
    16 weeks Z3A.16
    17 weeks Z3A.17
    18 weeks Z3A.18
    19 weeks Z3A.19
    20 weeks Z3A.20
    21 weeks Z3A.21
    22 weeks Z3A.22
    23 weeks Z3A.23
    24 weeks Z3A.24
    25 weeks Z3A.25
    26 weeks Z3A.26
    27 weeks Z3A.27
    28 weeks Z3A.28
    29 weeks Z3A.29
    30 weeks Z3A.30
    31 weeks Z3A.31
    32 weeks Z3A.32

Pregnancy *(Continued)*
  weeks of gestation *(Continued)*
    33 weeks Z3A.33
    34 weeks Z3A.34
    35 weeks Z3A.35
    36 weeks Z3A.36
    37 weeks Z3A.37
    38 weeks Z3A.38
    39 weeks Z3A.39
    40 weeks Z3A.40
    41 weeks Z3A.41
    42 weeks Z3A.42
    greater than 42 weeks Z3A.49
    less than 8 weeks Z3A.01
    not specified Z3A.00
Preiser's disease —*see* Osteonecrosis,
  secondary, due to, trauma, metacarpus
Pre-kwashiorkor —*see* Malnutrition, severe
Preleukemia (syndrome) D46.9
Preluxation, hip, congenital Q65.6
Premature —*see also* condition
  adrenarche E27.0
  aging E34.8
  beats I49.40
    atrial I49.1
    auricular I49.1
    supraventricular I49.1
  birth NEC —*see* Preterm, newborn
  closure, foramen ovale Q21.8
  contraction
    atrial I49.1
    atrioventricular I49.49
    auricular I49.1
    auriculoventricular I49.2
    heart (extrasystole) I49.49
    junctional I49.2
    ventricular I49.3
  delivery (*see also* Pregnancy, complicated by,
    preterm labor) O60.10
  ejaculation F52.4
  infant NEC —*see* Preterm, newborn
    light-for-dates —*see* Light for dates
  labor —*see* Pregnancy, complicated by,
    preterm labor
  lungs P28.0
  menopause E28.319
    asymptomatic E28.319
    symptomatic E28.310
  newborn
    extreme (less than 28 completed weeks) —
      see Immaturity, extreme
    less than 37 completed weeks —*see*
      Preterm, newborn
  puberty E30.1
  rupture membranes or amnion —*see*
    Pregnancy, complicated by, premature
    rupture of membranes
  senility E34.8
  thelarche E30.8
  ventricular systole I49.3
Prematurity NEC (less than 37 completed
  weeks) —*see* Preterm, newborn
  extreme (less than 28 completed weeks) —*see*
    Immaturity, extreme
Premenstrual
  dysphoric disorder (PMDD) N94.3
  tension (syndrome) N94.3
Premolarization, cuspids K00.2
Prenatal
  care, normal pregnancy —*see* Pregnancy,
    normal
  screening of mother Z36
  teeth K00.6
Preparatory care for subsequent treatment
  NEC
  for dialysis Z49.01
    peritoneal Z49.02
Prepartum —*see* condition
Preponderance, left or right ventricular I51.7
Prepuce —*see* condition
PRES (posterior reversible encephalopathy
  syndrome) I67.83

Presbycardia R54
Presbycusis, presbyacusia H91.1-
Presbyesophagus K22.8
Presbyophrenia F03
Presbyopia H52.4
Prescription of contraceptives (initial) Z30.019
  emergency (postcoital) Z30.012
  implantable subdermal Z30.019
  injectable Z30.013
  intrauterine contraceptive device Z30.014
  pills Z30.011
  postcoital (emergency) Z30.012
  repeat Z30.40
    implantable subdermal Z30.49
    injectable Z30.42
    pills Z30.41
    specified type NEC Z30.49
  specified type NEC Z30.018
Presence (of)
  ankle-joint implant (functional) (prosthesis)
    Z96.66-
  aortocoronary (bypass) graft Z95.1
  arterial-venous shunt (dialysis) Z99.2
  artificial
    eye (globe) Z97.0
    heart (fully implantable) (mechanical)
      Z95.812
    valve Z95.2
    larynx Z96.3
    lens (intraocular) Z96.1
    limb (complete) (partial) Z97.1-
      arm Z97.1-
        bilateral Z97.15
      leg Z97.1-
        bilateral Z97.16
  audiological implant (functional) Z96.29
  bladder implant (functional) Z96.0
  bone
    conduction hearing device Z96.29
    implant (functional) NEC Z96.7
    joint (prosthesis) —*see* Presence, joint
      implant
  cardiac
    defibrillator (functional) (with synchronous
      cardiac pacemaker)Z95.810
    implant or graft Z95.9
      specified type NEC Z95.818
    pacemaker Z95.0
  cerebrospinal fluid drainage device Z98.2
  cochlear implant (functional) Z96.21
  contact lens (es) Z97.3
  coronary artery graft or prosthesis Z95.5
  CSF shunt Z98.2
  dental prosthesis device Z97.2
  dentures Z97.2
  device (external) NEC Z97.8
    cardiac NEC Z95.818
    heart assist Z95.811
    implanted (functional) Z96.9
      specified NEC Z96.89
    prosthetic Z97.8
  ear implant Z96.20
    cochlear implant Z96.21
    myringotomy tube Z96.22
    specified type NEC Z96.29
  elbow-joint implant (functional) (prosthesis)
    Z96.62-
  endocrine implant (functional) NEC Z96.49
  eustachian tube stent or device (functional)
    Z96.29
  external hearing-aid or device Z97.4
  finger-joint implant (functional) (prosthetic)
    Z96.69-
  functional implant Z96.9
    specified NEC Z96.89
  graft
    cardiac NEC Z95.818
    vascular NEC Z95.828
  hearing-aid or device (external) Z97.4
    implant (bone) (cochlear) (functional)
      Z96.21
  heart assist device Z95.811

Presence *(Continued)*
 heart valve implant (functional) Z95.2
  prosthetic Z95.2
  specified type NEC Z95.4
  xenogenic Z95.3
 hip-joint implant (functional) (prosthesis)
  Z96.64-
 implanted device (artificial) (functional)
  (prosthetic) Z96.9
  automatic cardiac defibrillator (with
   synchronous cardiac pacemaker)
   Z95.810
  cardiac pacemaker Z95.0
  cochlear Z96.21
  dental Z96.5
  heart Z95.812
  heart valve Z95.2
   prosthetic Z95.2
   specified NEC Z95.4
   xenogenic Z95.3
  insulin pump Z96.41
  intraocular lens Z96.1
  joint Z96.60
   ankle Z96.66-
   elbow Z96.62-
   finger Z96.69-
   hip Z96.64-
   knee Z96.65-
   shoulder Z96.61-
   specified NEC Z96.698
   wrist Z96.63-
  larynx Z96.3
  myringotomy tube Z96.22
  otological Z96.20
   cochlear Z96.21
   eustachian stent Z96.29
   myringotomy Z96.22
   specified NEC Z96.29
   stapes Z96.29
  skin Z96.81
  skull plate Z96.7
  specified NEC Z96.89
  urogenital Z96.0
 insulin pump (functional) Z96.41
 intestinal bypass or anastomosis Z98.0
 intraocular lens (functional) Z96.1
 intrauterine contraceptive device (IUD) Z97.5
 intravascular implant (functional) (prosthetic)
  NEC Z95.9
  coronary artery Z95.5
  defibrillator (with synchronous cardiac
   pacemaker) Z95.810
  peripheral vessel (with angioplasty)
   Z95.820
 joint implant (prosthetic) (any) Z96.60
  ankle —*see* Presence, ankle joint implant
  elbow —*see* Presence, elbow joint implant
  finger —*see* Presence, finger joint implant
  hip —*see* Presence, hip joint implant
  knee —*see* Presence, knee joint implant
  shoulder —*see* Presence, shoulder joint
   implant
  specified joint NEC Z96.698
  wrist —*see* Presence, wrist joint implant
 knee-joint implant (functional) (prosthesis)
  Z96.65-
 laryngeal implant (functional) Z96.3
 mandibular implant (dental) Z96.5
 myringotomy tube (s) Z96.22
 orthopedic-joint implant (prosthetic) (any) —
  see Presence, joint implant
 otological implant (functional) Z96.29
 shoulder-joint implant (functional)
  (prosthesis) Z96.61-
 skull-plate implant Z96.7
 spectacles Z97.3
 stapes implant (functional) Z96.29
 systemic lupus erythematosus [SLE] inhibitor
  D68.62
 tendon implant (functional) (graft) Z96.7
 tooth root (s) implant Z96.5

Presence *(Continued)*
 ureteral stent Z96.0
 urethral stent Z96.0
 urogenital implant (functional) Z96.0
 vascular implant or device Z95.9
  access port device Z95.828
  specified type NEC Z95.828
 wrist-joint implant (functional) (prosthesis)
  Z96.63-
Presenile —*see also* condition
 dementia F03
 premature aging E34.8
Presentation, fetal —*see* Delivery (childbirth)
 (labor) (complicated by), malposition,
 malpresentation, complicated by,
 malposition ◄▥
Prespondylolisthesis (congenital) Q76.2
Pressure
 area, skin —*see* Ulcer, pressure, by site
 brachial plexus G54.0
 brain G93.5
  injury at birth NEC P11.1
 cerebral —*see* Pressure, brain
 chest R07.89
 cone, tentorial G93.5
 hyposystolic —*see also* Hypotension
  incidental reading, without diagnosis of
   hypotension R03.1
 increased
  intracranial (benign) G93.2
   injury at birth P11.0
  intraocular H40.05-
 lumbosacral plexus G54.1
 mediastinum J98.5
 necrosis (chronic) —*see* Ulcer, pressure, by site
 parental, inappropriate (excessive) Z62.6
 sore (chronic) —*see* Ulcer, pressure, by site
 spinal cord G95.20
 ulcer (chronic) —*see* Ulcer, pressure,
  by site
 venous, increased I87.8
Pre-syncope R55
Preterm
 delivery (*see also* Pregnancy, complicated by,
  preterm labor) O60.10
 labor —*see* Pregnancy, complicated by,
  preterm labor
 newborn (infant) P07.30
  gestational age
   28 completed weeks (28 weeks, 0 days
    through 28 weeks, 6 days) P07.31
   29 completed weeks (29 weeks, 0 days
    through 29 weeks, 6 days) P07.32
   30 completed weeks (30 weeks, 0 days
    through 30 weeks, 6 days) P07.33
   31 completed weeks (31 weeks, 0 days
    through 31 weeks, 6 days) P07.34
   32 completed weeks (32 weeks, 0 days
    through 32 weeks, 6 days) P07.35
   33 completed weeks (33 weeks, 0 days
    through 33 weeks, 6 days) P07.36
   34 completed weeks (34 weeks, 0 days
    through 34 weeks, 6 days) P07.37
   35 completed weeks (35 weeks, 0 days
    through 35 weeks, 6 days) P07.38
   36 completed weeks (36 weeks, 0 days
    through 36 weeks, 6 days) P07.39
Previa
 placenta (low) (marginal) (partial) (total)
  (with hemorrhage) O44.1-
  without hemorrhage O44.0-
 vasa O69.4
Priapism N48.30
 due to
  disease classified elsewhere N48.32
  drug N48.33
  specified cause NEC N48.39
  trauma N48.31
Prickling sensation (skin) R20.2
Prickly heat L74.0
Primary —*see* condition

Primigravida
 elderly, affecting management of pregnancy,
  labor and delivery (supervision only) —
  see Pregnancy, complicated by, elderly,
  primigravida
 older, affecting management of pregnancy,
  labor and delivery (supervision only) —
  see Pregnancy, complicated by, elderly,
  primigravida
 very young, affecting management of
  pregnancy, labor and delivery
  (supervision only) —*see* Pregnancy,
  complicated by, young mother,
  primigravida
Primipara
 elderly, affecting management of pregnancy,
  labor and delivery (supervision only) —
  see Pregnancy, complicated by, elderly,
  primigravida
 older, affecting management of pregnancy,
  labor and delivery (supervision only) —
  see Pregnancy, complicated by, elderly,
  primigravida
 very young, affecting management of
  pregnancy, labor and delivery
  (supervision only) —*see* Pregnancy,
  complicated by, young mother,
  primigravida
Primus varus (bilateral) Q66.2
PRIND (Prolonged reversible ischemic
 neurologic deficit) I63.9
Pringle's disease (tuberous sclerosis)Q85.1
Prinzmetal angina I20.1
Prizefighter ear —*see* Cauliflower ear
Problem (with) (related to)
 academic Z55.8
 acculturation Z60.3
 adjustment (to)
  change of job Z56.1
  life-cycle transition Z60.0
  pension Z60.0
  retirement Z60.0
 adopted child Z62.821
 alcoholism in family Z63.72
 atypical parenting situation Z62.9
 bankruptcy Z59.8
 behavioral (adult) F69
  drug seeking Z72.89
 birth of sibling affecting child Z62.898
 care (of)
  provider dependency Z74.9
   specified NEC Z74.8
  sick or handicapped person in family or
   household Z63.6
 child
  abuse (affecting the child) —*see*
   Maltreatment, child
  custody or support proceedings Z65.3
  in care of non-parental family member
   Z62.21
  in foster care Z62.21
  in welfare custody Z62.21
  living in orphanage or group home Z62.22
 child-rearing Z62.9
  specified NEC Z62.898
 communication (developmental) F80.9
 conflict or discord (with)
  boss Z56.4
  classmates Z55.4
  counselor Z64.4
  employer Z56.4
  family Z63.9
   specified NEC Z63.8
  probation officer Z64.4
  social worker Z64.4
  teachers Z55.4
  workmates Z56.4
 conviction in legal proceedings Z65.0
  with imprisonment Z65.1
 counselor Z64.4
 creditors Z59.8

◄ New ◄▥ Revised ~~deleted~~ Deleted

Problem *(Continued)*
  digestive K92.9
  drug addict in family Z63.72
  ear —*see* Disorder, ear
  economic Z59.9
    affecting care Z59.9
    specified NEC Z59.8
  education Z55.9
    specified NEC Z55.8
  employment Z56.9
    change of job Z56.1
    discord Z56.4
    environment Z56.5
    sexual harassment Z56.81
    specified NEC Z56.89
    stress NEC Z56.6
    stressful schedule Z56.3
    threat of job loss Z56.2
    unemployment Z56.0
  enuresis, child F98.0
  eye H57.9
  failed examinations (school) Z55.2
  falling Z91.81
  family *(see also* Disruption, family) Z63.9- ◄▥
    specified NEC Z63.8
  feeding (elderly) (infant) R63.3
    newborn P92.9
      breast P92.5
      overfeeding P92.4
      slow P92.2
      specified NEC P92.8
      underfeeding P92.3
    nonorganic F50.8
  finance Z59.9
    specified NEC Z59.8
  foreclosure on loan Z59.8
  foster child Z62.822
  frightening experience (s) in childhood Z62.898
  genital NEC
    female N94.9
    male N50.9
  health care Z75.9
    specified NEC Z75.8
  hearing —*see* Deafness
  homelessness Z59.0
  housing Z59.9
    inadequate Z59.1
    isolated Z59.8
    specified NEC Z59.8
  identity (of childhood) F93.8
  illegitimate pregnancy (unwanted) Z64.0
  illiteracy Z55.0
  impaired mobility Z74.09
  imprisonment or incarceration Z65.1
  inadequate teaching affecting education Z55.8
  inappropriate (excessive) parental pressure Z62.6
  influencing health status NEC Z78.9
  in-law Z63.1
  institutionalization, affecting child Z62.22
  intrafamilial communication Z63.8
  jealousy, child F93.8
  landlord Z59.2
  language (developmental) F80.9
  learning (developmental) F81.9
  legal Z65.3
    conviction without imprisonment Z65.0
    imprisonment Z65.1
    release from prison Z65.2
  life-management Z73.9
    specified NEC Z73.89
  life-style Z72.9
    gambling Z72.6
    high-risk sexual behavior (heterosexual) Z72.51
      bisexual Z72.53
      homosexual Z72.52
    inappropriate eating habits Z72.4

Problem *(Continued)*
  life-style *(Continued)*
    self-damaging behavior NEC Z72.89
    specified NEC Z72.89
    tobacco use Z72.0
  literacy Z55.9
    low level Z55.0
    specified NEC Z55.8
  living alone Z60.2
  lodgers Z59.2
  loss of love relationship in childhood Z62.898
  marital Z63.0
    involving
      divorce Z63.5
      estrangement Z63.5
      gender identity F66
  mastication K08.8
  medical
    care, within family Z63.6
    facilities Z75.9
      specified NEC Z75.8
  mental F48.9
  multiparity Z64.1
  negative life events in childhood Z62.9
    altered pattern of family relationships Z62.898
    frightening experience Z62.898
    loss of
      love relationship Z62.898
      self-esteem Z62.898
    physical abuse (alleged) —*see* Maltreatment, child
    removal from home Z62.29
    specified event NEC Z62.898
  neighbor Z59.2
  neurological NEC R29.818
  new step-parent affecting child Z62.898
  none (feared complaint unfounded) Z71.1
  occupational NEC Z56.89
  parent-child —*see* Conflict, parent-child
  personal hygiene Z91.89
  personality F69
  phase-of-life transition, adjustment Z60.0
  presence of sick or disabled person in family or household Z63.79
    needing care Z63.6
  primary support group (family) Z63.9
    specified NEC Z63.8
  probation officer Z64.4
  psychiatric F99
  psychosexual (development) F66
  psychosocial Z65.9
    specified NEC Z65.8
  relationship Z63.9
    childhood F93.8
  release from prison Z65.2
  removal from home affecting child Z62.29
  seeking and accepting known hazardous and harmful
    behavioral or psychological interventions Z65.8
    chemical, nutritional or physical interventions Z65.8
  sexual function (nonorganic) F52.9
  sight H54.7
  sleep disorder, child F51.9
  smell —*see* Disturbance, sensation, smell
  social
    environment Z60.9
      specified NEC Z60.8
    exclusion and rejection Z60.4
    worker Z64.4
  speech R47.9
    developmental F80.9
    specified NEC R47.89
  swallowing —*see* Dysphagia
  taste —*see* Disturbance, sensation, taste
  tic, child F95.0
  underachievement in school Z55.3
  unemployment Z56.0
    threatened Z56.2

Problem *(Continued)*
  unwanted pregnancy Z64.0
  upbringing Z62.9
    specified NEC Z62.898
  urinary N39.9
  voice production R47.89
  work schedule (stressful) Z56.3
Procedure (surgical)
  for purpose other than remedying health state Z41.9
    specified NEC Z41.8
  not done Z53.9
    because of
      administrative reasons Z53.8
      contraindication Z53.09
        smoking Z53.01
      patient's decision Z53.20
        for reasons of belief or group pressure Z53.1
        left against medical advice (AMA) Z53.21
        specified reason NEC Z53.29
      specified reason NEC Z53.8
Procidentia (uteri) N81.3
Proctalgia K62.89
  fugax K59.4
  spasmodic K59.4
Proctitis K62.89
  amebic (acute) A06.0
  chlamydial A56.3
  gonococcal A54.6
  granulomatous —*see* Enteritis, regional, large intestine
  herpetic A60.1
  radiation K62.7
  tuberculous A18.32
  ulcerative (chronic) K51.20
    with
      complication K51.219
        abscess K51.214
        fistula K51.213
        obstruction K51.212
        rectal bleeding K51.211
        specified NEC K51.218
Proctocele
  female (without uterine prolapse) N81.6
    with uterine prolapse N81.2
      complete N81.3
  male K62.3
Proctocolitis, mucosal —*see* Rectosigmoiditis, ulcerative
Proctoptosis K62.3
Proctorrhagia K62.5
Proctosigmoiditis K63.89
  ulcerative (chronic) —*see* Rectosigmoiditis, ulcerative
Proctospasm K59.4
  psychogenic F45.8
Profichet's disease —*see* Disorder, soft tissue, specified type NEC
Progeria E34.8
Prognathism (mandibular) (maxillary) M26.19
Progonoma (melanotic) —*see* Neoplasm, benign, by site
Progressive —*see* condition
Prolactinoma
  specified site —*see* Neoplasm, benign, by site
  unspecified site D35.2
Prolapse, prolapsed
  anus, anal (canal) (sphincter) K62.2
  arm or hand O32.2
    causing obstructed labor O64.4
  bladder (mucosa) (sphincter) (acquired)
    congenital Q79.4
    female —*see* Cystocele
    male N32.89
  breast implant (prosthetic) T85.49
  cecostomy K94.09
  cecum K63.4

P

Prolapse, prolapsed *(Continued)*
  cervix, cervical (hypertrophied) N81.2
    anterior lip, obstructing labor O65.5
    congenital Q51.828
    postpartal, old N81.2
    stump N81.85
  ciliary body (traumatic) —*see* Laceration, eye(ball), with prolapse or loss of interocular tissue
  colon (pedunculated) K63.4
  colostomy K94.09
  disc (intervertebral) —*see* Displacement, intervertebral disc
  eye implant (orbital) T85.398
    lens (ocular) —*see* Complications, intraocular lens
  fallopian tube N83.4
  gastric (mucosa) K31.89
  genital, female N81.9
    specified NEC N81.89
  globe, nontraumatic —*see* Luxation, globe
  ileostomy bud K94.19
  intervertebral disc —*see* Displacement, intervertebral disc
  intestine (small) K63.4
  iris (traumatic) —*see* Laceration, eye(ball), with prolapse or loss of interocular tissue
    nontraumatic H21.89
  kidney N28.83
    congenital Q63.2
  laryngeal muscles or ventricle J38.7
  liver K76.89
  meatus urinarius N36.8
  mitral (valve) I34.1
  ocular lens implant —*see* Complications, intraocular lens
  organ or site, congenital NEC —*see* Malposition, congenital
  ovary N83.4
  pelvic floor, female N81.89
  perineum, female N81.89
  rectum (mucosa) (sphincter) K62.3
    due to trichuris trichuria B79
  spleen D73.89
  stomach K31.89
  umbilical cord
    complicating delivery O69.0
  urachus, congenital Q64.4
  ureter N28.89
    with obstruction N13.5
      with infection N13.6
  ureterovesical orifice N28.89
  urethra (acquired) (infected) (mucosa) N36.8
    congenital Q64.71
  urinary meatus N36.8
    congenital Q64.72
  uterovaginal N81.4
    complete N81.3
    incomplete N81.2
  uterus (with prolapse of vagina) N81.4
    complete N81.3
    congenital Q51.818
    first degree N81.2
    in pregnancy or childbirth —*see* Pregnancy, complicated by, abnormal, uterus
    incomplete N81.2
    postpartal (old) N81.4
    second degree N81.2
    third degree N81.3
  uveal (traumatic) —*see* Laceration, eye(ball), with prolapse or loss of interocular tissue
  vagina (anterior) (wall) —*see* Cystocele
    with prolapse of uterus N81.4
      complete N81.3
      incomplete N81.2
    posterior wall N81.6
    posthysterectomy N99.3

Prolapse, prolapsed *(Continued)*
  vitreous (humor) H43.0-
    in wound —*see* Laceration, eye(ball), with prolapse or loss of interocular tissue
  womb —*see* Prolapse, uterus
Prolapsus, female N81.9
  specified NEC N81.89
Proliferation (s)
  primary cutaneous CD30-positive large T-cell C86.6
Proliferative —*see* condition
Prolonged, prolongation (of)
  bleeding (time) (idiopathic) R79.1
  coagulation (time) R79.1
  gestation (over 42 completed weeks)
    mother O48.1
    newborn P08.22
  interval I44.0
  labor O63.9
    first stage O63.0
    second stage O63.1
  partial thromboplastin time (PTT) R79.1
  pregnancy (more than 42 weeks gestation) O48.1
  prothrombin time R79.1
  QT interval I45.81
  uterine contractions in labor O62.4
Prominence, prominent
  with disproportion (fetopelvic) O33.0
    causing obstructed labor O65.0
  auricle (congenital) (ear) Q17.5
  ischial spine or sacral promontory
  nose (congenital) acquired M95.0
Promiscuity —*see* High, risk, sexual behavior
Pronation
  ankle —*see* Deformity, limb, foot, specified NEC
  foot —*see also* Deformity, limb, foot, specified NEC
    congenital Q74.2
Prophylactic
  administration of
    antibiotics, long-term Z79.2
      short-term use - omit code
    drug (*see also* Long-term (current) drug therapy (use of)) Z79.899-
    medication Z79.899
    organ removal (for neoplasia management) Z40.00
      breast Z40.01
      ovary Z40.02
      specified site NEC Z40.09
    surgery Z40.9
      for risk factors related to malignant neoplasm —*see* Prophylactic, organ removal
      specified NEC Z40.8
    vaccination Z23
Propionic acidemia E71.121
Proptosis (ocular) —*see also* Exophthalmos
  thyroid —*see* Hyperthyroidism, with goiter
Prosecution, anxiety concerning Z65.3
Prosopagnosia R48.3
Prostadynia N42.81
Prostate, prostatic —*see* condition
Prostatism —*see* Hyperplasia, prostate
Prostatitis (congestive) (suppurative) (with cystitis) N41.9
  acute N41.0
  cavitary N41.8
  chronic N41.1
  diverticular N41.8
  due to Trichomonas (vaginalis) A59.02
  fibrous N41.1
  gonococcal (acute) (chronic) A54.22
  granulomatous N41.4
  hypertrophic N41.1
  subacute N41.1
  trichomonal A59.02
  tuberculous A18.14
Prostatocystitis N41.3

Prostatorrhea N42.89
Prostatosis N42.82
Prostration R53.83
  heat —*see also* Heat, exhaustion
    anhydrotic T67.3
    due to
      salt (and water) depletion T67.4
      water depletion T67.3
  nervous F48.8
  senile R54
Protanomaly (anomalous trichromat) H53.54
Protanopia (complete) (incomplete) H53.54
Protection (against) (from) —*see* Prophylactic
Protein
  deficiency NEC —*see* Malnutrition
  malnutrition —*see* Malnutrition
  sickness (*see also* Reaction, serum) T80.69
Proteinemia R77.9
Proteinosis
  alveolar (pulmonary) J84.01
  lipid or lipoid (of Urbach) E78.89
Proteinuria R80.9
  Bence Jones R80.3
  complicating pregnancy —*see* Proteinuria, gestational
  gestational O12.1-
    with edema O12.2-
  idiopathic R80.0
  isolated R80.0
    with glomerular lesion N06.9
      dense deposit disease N06.6
      diffuse
        crescentic glomerulonephritis N06.7
        endocapillary proliferative glomerulonephritis N06.4
        mesangiocapillary glomerulonephritis N06.5
      focal and segmental hyalinosis or sclerosis N06.1
      membranous (diffuse) N06.2
      mesangial proliferative (diffuse) N06.3
      minimal change N06.0
      specified pathology NEC N06.8
  orthostatic R80.2
    with glomerular lesion —*see* Proteinuria, isolated, with glomerular lesion
  persistent R80.1
    with glomerular lesion —*see* Proteinuria, isolated, with glomerular lesion
  postural R80.2
    with glomerular lesion —*see* Proteinuria, isolated, with glomerular lesion
  pre-eclamptic —*see* Pre-eclampsia
  specified type NEC R80.8
Proteolysis, pathologic D65
Proteus (mirabilis) (morganii), as cause of disease classified elsewhere B96.4
Prothrombin gene mutation D68.52
Protoporphyria, erythropoietic E80.0
Protozoal —*see also* condition
  disease B64
    specified NEC B60.8
Protrusion, protrusio
  acetabuli M24.7
  acetabulum (into pelvis) M24.7
  device, implant or graft (*see also* Complications, by site and type, mechanical) T85.698
    arterial graft NEC —*see* Complication, cardiovascular device, mechanical, vascular
    breast (implant) T85.49
    catheter NEC T85.698
      cystostomy T83.090
      dialysis (renal) T82.49
        intraperitoneal T85.691
      infusion NEC T82.594
        spinal (epidural) (subdural) T85.690
      urinary, indwelling T83.098

◀ New   ◀◀ Revised   ~~deleted~~ Deleted

Protrusion, protrusio *(Continued)*
  device, implant or graft *(Continued)*
    electronic (electrode) (pulse generator)
        (stimulator)
      bone T84.390
      nervous system —*see* Complication,
          prosthetic device, mechanical,
          electronic nervous system
          stimulator
    fixation, internal (orthopedic) NEC —*see*
        Complication, fixation device,
        mechanical
    gastrointestinal —*see* Complications,
        prosthetic device, mechanical,
        gastrointestinal device
    genital NEC T83.498
      intrauterine contraceptive device
          T83.39
      penile prosthesis T83.490
    heart NEC —*see* Complication,
        cardiovascular device, mechanical
    joint prosthesis —*see* Complications, joint
        prosthesis, mechanical, specified
        NEC, by site
    ocular NEC —*see* Complications, prosthetic
        device, mechanical, ocular device
    orthopedic NEC —*see* Complication,
        orthopedic, device, mechanical
    specified NEC T85.628
    urinary NEC —*see also* Complication,
        genitourinary, device, urinary,
        mechanical
      graft T83.29
    vascular NEC —*see* Complication,
        cardiovascular device, mechanical
    ventricular intracranial shunt T85.09
  intervertebral disc —*see* Displacement,
      intervertebral disc
  joint prosthesis —*see* Complications, joint
      prosthesis, mechanical, specified NEC,
      by site
  nucleus pulposus —*see* Displacement,
      intervertebral disc
Prune belly (syndrome) Q79.4
Prurigo (ferox) (gravis) (Hebrae) (Hebra's)
    (mitis) (simplex) L28.2
  Besnier's L20.0
  estivalis L56.4
  nodularis L28.1
  psychogenic F45.8
Pruritus, pruritic (essential) L29.9
  ani, anus L29.0
    psychogenic F45.8
  anogenital L29.3
    psychogenic F45.8
  due to onchocerca volvulus B73.1
  gravidarum —*see* Pregnancy, complicated by,
      specified pregnancy-related condition
      NEC
  hiemalis L29.8
  neurogenic (any site) F45.8
  perianal L29.0
  psychogenic (any site) F45.8
  scroti, scrotum L29.1
    psychogenic F45.8
  senile, senilis L29.8
  specified NEC L29.8
    psychogenic F45.8
  Trichomonas A59.9
  vulva, vulvae L29.2
    psychogenic F45.8
Pseudarthrosis, pseudoarthrosis (bone) —*see*
    Nonunion, fracture
  clavicle, congenital Q74.0
  joint, following fusion or arthrodesis
      M96.0
Pseudoaneurysm —*see* Aneurysm
Pseudoangina (pectoris) —*see* Angina
Pseudoangioma I81
Pseudoarteriosus Q28.8
Pseudoarthrosis —*see* Pseudarthrosis

Pseudobulbar affect (PBA) F48.2
Pseudochromhidrosis L67.8
Pseudocirrhosis, liver, pericardial I31.1
Pseudocowpox B08.03
Pseudocoxalgia M91.3-
Pseudocroup J38.5
Pseudo-Cushing's syndrome, alcohol-induced
    E24.4
Pseudocyesis F45.8
Pseudocyst
  lung J98.4
  pancreas K86.3
  retina —*see* Cyst, retina
Pseudoelephantiasis neuroarthritica
    Q82.0
Pseudoexfoliation, capsule (lens) —*see*
    Cataract, specified NEC
Pseudofolliculitis barbae L73.1
Pseudoglioma H44.89
Pseudohemophilia (Bernuth's) (hereditary)
    (type B) D68.0
  Type A D69.8
  vascular D69.8
Pseudohermaphroditism Q56.3
  adrenal E25.8
  female Q56.2
    with adrenocortical disorder E25.8
    without adrenocortical disorder
        Q56.2
    adrenal, congenital E25.0
  male Q56.1
    with
      adrenocortical disorder E25.8
      androgen resistance E34.51
      cleft scrotum Q56.1
      feminizing testis E34.51
      5-alpha-reductase deficiency E29.1
    without gonadal disorder Q56.1
    adrenal E25.8
Pseudo-Hurler's polydystrophy E77.0
Pseudohydrocephalus G93.2
Pseudohypertrophic muscular dystrophy
    (Erb's) G71.0
Pseudohypertrophy, muscle G71.0
Pseudohypoparathyroidism E20.1
Pseudoinsomnia F51.03
Pseudoleukemia, infantile D64.89
Pseudomembranous —*see* condition
Pseudomeningocele (cerebral) (infective)
    (post-traumatic) G96.19
  postprocedural (spinal) G97.82
Pseudomenses (newborn) P54.6
Pseudomenstruation (newborn) P54.6
Pseudomonas
  aeruginosa, as cause of disease classified
      elsewhere B96.5
  mallei infection A24.0
    as cause of disease classified elsewhere
        B96.5
  pseudomallei, as cause of disease classified
      elsewhere B96.5
Pseudomyotonia G71.19
Pseudomyxoma peritonei C78.6
Pseudoneuritis, optic (nerve) (disc) (papilla),
    congenital Q14.2
Pseudo-obstruction intestine (acute) (chronic)
    (idiopathic) (intermittent secondary)
    (primary) K59.8
Pseudopapilledema H47.33-
  congenital Q14.2
Pseudoparalysis
  arm or leg R29.818
  atonic, congenital P94.2
Pseudopelade L66.0
Pseudophakia Z96.1
Pseudopolyarthritis, rhizomelic M35.3
Pseudopolycythemia D75.1
Pseudopseudohypoparathyroidism
    E20.1
Pseudopterygium H11.81-
Pseudoptosis (eyelid) —*see* Blepharochalasis

Pseudopuberty, precocious
  female heterosexual E25.8
  male isosexual E25.8
Pseudorickets (renal) N25.0
Pseudorubella B08.20
Pseudosclerema, newborn P83.8
Pseudosclerosis (brain)
  Jakob's —*see* Creutzfeldt-Jakob disease or
      syndrome
  of Westphal (Strümpell) E83.01
  spastic —*see* Creutzfeldt-Jakob disease or
      syndrome
Pseudotetanus —*see* Convulsions
Pseudotetany R29.0
  hysterical F44.5
Pseudotruncus arteriosus Q25.4
Pseudotuberculosis A28.2
  enterocolitis A04.8
  pasteurella (infection) A28.0
Pseudotumor
  cerebri G93.2
  orbital —*see Inflammation, orbit* H05.11- ◄▮▮
Pseudoxanthoma elasticum Q82.8
Psilosis (sprue) (tropical) K90.1
  nontropical K90.0
Psittacosis A70
Psoitis M60.88
Psoriasis L40.9
  arthropathic L40.50
    arthritis mutilans L40.52
    distal interphalangeal L40.51
    juvenile L40.54
    other specified L40.59
    spondylitis L40.53
  buccal K13.29
  flexural L40.8
  guttate L40.4
  mouth K13.29
  nummular L40.0
  plaque L40.0
  psychogenic F54
  pustular (generalized) L40.1
    palmaris et plantaris L40.3
  specified NEC L40.8
  vulgaris L40.0
Psychasthenia F48.8
Psychiatric disorder or problem F99
Psychogenic —*see also* condition
  factors associated with physical conditions
      F54
Psychological and behavioral factors affecting
    medical condition F59
Psychoneurosis, psychoneurotic —*see also*
    Neurosis
  anxiety (state) F41.1
  depersonalization F48.1
  hypochondriacal F45.21
  hysteria F44.9
  neurasthenic F48.8
  personality NEC F60.89
Psychopathy, psychopathic
  affectionless F94.2
  autistic F84.5
  constitution, post-traumatic F07.81
  personality —*see* Disorder, personality
  sexual —*see* Deviation, sexual
  state F60.2
Psychosexual identity disorder of childhood
    F64.2
Psychosis, psychotic F29
  acute (transient) F23
    hysterical F44.9
  affective —*see* Disorder, mood
  alcoholic F10.959
    with
      abuse F10.159
      anxiety disorder F10.980
        with
          abuse F10.180
          dependence F10.280
      delirium tremens F10.231

◄ New   ◄▮▮ Revised   ~~deleted~~ Deleted

Psychosis, psychotic (Continued)
 alcoholic (Continued)
  with (Continued)
   delusions F10.950
    with
     abuse F10.150
     dependence F10.250
   dementia F10.97
    with dependence F10.27
   dependence F10.259
   hallucinosis F10.951
    with
     abuse F10.151
     dependence F10.251
   mood disorder F10.94
    with
     abuse F10.14
     dependence F10.24
   paranoia F10.950
    with
     abuse F10.150
     dependence F10.250
   persisting amnesia F10.96
    with dependence F10.26
  amnestic confabulatory F10.96
   with dependence F10.26
  delirium tremens F10.231
  Korsakoff's, Korsakov's, Korsakow's F10.26
  paranoid type F10.950
   with
    abuse F10.150
    dependence F10.250
 anergastic —see Psychosis, organic
 arteriosclerotic (simple type) (uncomplicated)
  F01.50
  with behavioral disturbance F01.51
 childhood F84.0
  atypical F84.8
 climacteric —see Psychosis, involutional
 confusional F29
  acute or subacute F05
  reactive F23
 cycloid F23
 depressive —see Disorder, depressive
 disintegrative (childhood) F84.3
 drug-induced —see F11-F19 with .x59
  paranoid and hallucinatory states —see
   F11-F19 with .x50 or .x51
 due to or associated with
  addiction, drug —see F11-F19 with
   .X59 ◄▦
  dependence
   alcohol F10.259
   drug —see F11-F19 with .x59
  epilepsy F06.8
  Huntington's chorea F06.8
  ischemia, cerebrovascular (generalized)
   F06.8
  multiple sclerosis F06.8
  physical disease F06.8
  presenile dementia F03
  senile dementia F03
  vascular disease (arteriosclerotic) (cerebral)
   F01.50
   with behavioral disturbance F01.51
 epileptic F06.8
 episode F23
  due to or associated with physical
   condition F06.8
 exhaustive F43.0
 hallucinatory, chronic F28
 hypomanic F30.8
 hysterical (acute) F44.9
 induced F24
 infantile F84.0
  atypical F84.8
 infective (acute) (subacute) F05
 involutional F28
  depressive —see Disorder, depressive
  melancholic —see Disorder, depressive
  paranoid (state) F22

Psychosis, psychotic (Continued)
 Korsakoff's, Korsakov's, Korsakow's
  (nonalcoholic) F04
  alcoholic F10.96
   in dependence F10.26
  induced by other psychoactive
   substance —see categories F11-F19
    with .x5x
 mania, manic (single episode) F30.2
  recurrent type F31.89
 manic-depressive —see Disorder, mood
 menopausal —see Psychosis, involutional
 mixed schizophrenic and affective F25.8
 multi-infarct (cerebrovascular) F01.50
  with behavioral disturbance F01.51
 nonorganic F29
  specified NEC F28
 organic F09
  due to or associated with
   arteriosclerosis (cerebral) —see
    Psychosis, arteriosclerotic
   cerebrovascular disease,
    arteriosclerotic —see Psychosis,
    arteriosclerotic
   childbirth —see Psychosis, puerperal
   Creutzfeldt-Jakob disease or
    syndrome —see Creutzfeldt-Jakob
    disease or syndrome
   dependence, alcohol F10.259
   disease
    alcoholic liver F10.259
    brain, arteriosclerotic —see Psychosis,
     arteriosclerotic
    cerebrovascular F01.50
     with behavioral disturbance
      F01.51
    Creutzfeldt-Jakob —see Creutzfeldt-
     Jakob disease or syndrome
    endocrine or metabolic F06.8
     acute or subacute F05
    liver, alcoholic F10.259
   epilepsy transient (acute) F05
   infection
    brain (intracranial) F06.8
    acute or subacute F05
   intoxication
    alcoholic (acute) F10.259
    drug F19 with .X59 F11- ◄▦
   ischemia, cerebrovascular (generalized) —
    see Psychosis, arteriosclerotic
   puerperium —see Psychosis, puerperal
   trauma, brain (birth) (from electric
    current) (surgical) F06.8
   acute or subacute F05
  infective F06.8
   acute or subacute F05
  post-traumatic F06.8
   acute or subacute F05
 paranoiac F22
 paranoid (climacteric) (involutional)
  (menopausal) F22
  psychogenic (acute) F23
  schizophrenic F20.0
  senile F03
 postpartum F53
 presbyophrenic (type) F03
 presenile F03
 psychogenic (paranoid) F23
  depressive F32.3
 puerperal F53
  specified type —see Psychosis, by type
 reactive (brief) (transient) (emotional stress)
  (psychological trauma) F23
  depressive F32.3
   recurrent F33.3
  excitative type F30.8
 schizoaffective F25.9
  depressive type F25.1
  manic type F25.0
 schizophrenia, schizophrenic —see
  Schizophrenia

Psychosis, psychotic (Continued)
 schizophrenia-like, in epilepsy F06.2
 schizophreniform F20.81
  affective type F25.9
  brief F23
  confusional type F23
  depressive type F25.1
  manic type F25.0
  mixed type F25.0
  senile NEC F03
  depressed or paranoid type F03
  simple deterioration F03
  specified type — code to condition
 shared F24
 situational (reactive) F23
 symbiotic (childhood) F84.3
 symptomatic F09
Psychosomatic —see Disorder, psychosomatic
Psychosyndrome, organic F07.9
Psychotic episode due to or associated with
 physical condition F06.8
Pterygium (eye) H11.00-
 amyloid H11.01-
 central H11.02-
 colli Q18.3
 double H11.03-
 peripheral
  progressive H11.05-
  stationary H11.04-
 recurrent H11.06-
Ptilosis (eyelid) —see Madarosis
Ptomaine (poisoning) —see Poisoning, food
Ptosis —see also Blepharoptosis
 adiposa (false) —see Blepharoptosis
 breast N64.81
 cecum K63.4
 colon K63.4
 congenital (eyelid) Q10.0
  specified site NEC —see Anomaly,
   by site
 eyelid —see Blepharoptosis
  congenital Q10.0
 gastric K31.89
 intestine K63.4
 kidney N28.83
 liver K76.89
 renal N28.83
 splanchnic K63.4
 spleen D73.89
 stomach K31.89
 viscera K63.4
PTP D69.51
Ptyalism (periodic) K11.7
 hysterical F45.8
 pregnancy —see Pregnancy, complicated by,
  specified pregnancy-related condition
  NEC
 psychogenic F45.8
Ptyalolithiasis K11.5
Pubarche, precocious E30.1
Pubertas praecox E30.1
Puberty (development state) Z00.3
 bleeding (excessive) N92.2
 delayed E30.0
 precocious (constitutional) (cryptogenic)
  (idiopathic) E30.1
  central E22.8
  due to
   ovarian hyperfunction E28.1
    estrogen E28.0
   testicular hyperfunction E29.0
 premature E30.1
  due to
   adrenal cortical hyperfunction E25.8
   pineal tumor E34.8
   pituitary (anterior) hyperfunction E22.8
Puckering, macula —see Degeneration, macula,
 puckering
Pudenda, pudendum —see condition
Puente's disease (simple glandular cheilitis)
 K13.0

Puerperal, puerperium (complicated by, complications)
 abnormal glucose (tolerance test) O99.815
 abscess
  areola O91.02
   associated with lactation O91.03
  Bartholin's gland O86.19
  breast O91.12
   associated with lactation O91.13
  cervix (uteri) O86.11
  genital organ NEC O86.19
  kidney O86.21
  mammary O91.12
   associated with lactation O91.13
  nipple O91.02
   associated with lactation O91.03
  peritoneum O85
  subareolar O91.12
   associated with lactation O91.13
  urinary tract —see Puerperal, infection, urinary
  uterus O86.12
  vagina (wall) O86.13
  vaginorectal O86.13
  vulvovaginal gland O86.13
 adnexitis O86.19
 afibrinogenemia, or other coagulation defect O72.3
 albuminuria (acute) (subacute) —see Proteinuria, gestational
 alcohol use O99.315
 anemia O90.81
  pre-existing (pre-pregnancy) O99.03
 anesthetic death O89.8
 apoplexy O99.43
 bariatric surgery status O99.845
 blood disorder NEC O99.13
 blood dyscrasia O72.3
 cardiomyopathy O90.3
 cerebrovascular disorder (conditions in I60-I69) O99.43
 cervicitis O86.11
 circulatory system disorder O99.43
 coagulopathy (any) O72.3
 complications O90.9
  specified NEC O90.89
 convulsions —see Eclampsia
 cystitis O86.22
 cystopyelitis O86.29
 delirium NEC F05
 diabetes O24.93
  gestational —see Puerperal, gestational diabetes
  pre-existing O24.33
   specified NEC O24.83
   type 1 O24.03
   type 2 O24.13
 digestive system disorder O99.63
 disease O90.9
  breast NEC O92.29
  cerebrovascular (acute) O99.43
  nonobstetric NEC O99.89
  tubo-ovarian O86.19
  Valsuani's O99.03
 disorder O90.9
  biliary tract O26.63
  lactation O92.70 ◄▥
  liver O26.63
  nonobstetric NEC O99.89
 disruption
  cesarean wound O90.0
  episiotomy wound O90.1
  perineal laceration wound O90.1
 drug use O99.325
 eclampsia (with pre-existing hypertension) O15.2
 embolism (pulmonary) (blood clot) —see Embolism, obstetric, puerperal
 endocrine, nutritional or metabolic disease NEC O99.285
 endophlebitis —see Puerperal, phlebitis

Puerperal, puerperium (Continued)
 endotrachelitis O86.11 ◄▥
 failure
  lactation (complete) O92.3
   partial O92.4
  renal, acute O90.4
 fever (of unknown origin) O86.4
  septic O85
 fissure, nipple O92.12
  associated with lactation O92.13
 fistula
  breast (due to mastitis) O91.12
   associated with lactation O91.13
  nipple O91.02
   associated with lactation O91.03
 galactophoritis O91.22
  associated with lactation O91.23
 galactorrhea O92.6
 gastric banding status O99.845
 gastric bypass status O99.845
 gastrointestinal disease NEC O99.63
 gestational diabetes O24.439
  diet controlled O24.430
  insulin (and diet) controlled O24.434
 gonorrhea O98.23
 hematoma, subdural O99.43
 hemiplegia, cerebral O99.355-
  due to cerebrovascular disorder O99.43
 hemorrhage O72.1
  brain O99.43
  bulbar O99.43
  cerebellar O99.43
  cerebral O99.43
  cortical O99.43
  delayed or secondary O72.2
  extradural O99.43
  internal capsule O99.43
  intracranial O99.43
  intrapontine O99.43
  meningeal O99.43
  pontine O99.43
  retained placenta O72.0
  subarachnoid O99.43
  subcortical O99.43
  subdural O99.43
  third stage O72.0
  uterine, delayed O72.2
  ventricular O99.43
 hemorrhoids O87.2
 hepatorenal syndrome O90.4
 hypertension —see Hypertension, complicating, puerperium
 hypertrophy, breast O92.29
 induration breast (fibrous) O92.29
 infection O86.4
  cervix O86.11
  generalized O85
  genital tract NEC O86.19
   obstetric surgical wound O86.0
  kidney (bacillus coli) O86.21
  maternal O98.93
   carrier state NEC O99.835
   gonorrhea O98.23
   human immunodeficiency virus (HIV) O98.73
   protozoal O98.63
   sexually transmitted NEC O98.33
   specified NEC O98.83
   streptococcus B carrier state O99.825
   syphilis O98.13
   tuberculosis O98.03
   viral hepatitis O98.43
   viral NEC O98.53
  nipple O91.02
   associated with lactation O91.03
  peritoneum O85
  renal O86.21
  specified NEC O86.89

Puerperal, puerperium (Continued)
 infection (Continued)
  urinary (asymptomatic) (tract) NEC O86.20
   bladder O86.22
   kidney O86.21
   specified site NEC O86.29
   urethra O86.22
   vagina O86.13
   vein —see Puerperal, phlebitis
 ischemia, cerebral O99.43
 lymphangitis O86.89
  breast O91.22
   associated with lactation O91.23
 malignancy O9A.13
 malnutrition O25.3
 mammillitis O91.02
  associated with lactation O91.03
 mammitis O91.22
  associated with lactation O91.23
 mania F30.8
 mastitis O91.22
  associated with lactation O91.23
  purulent O91.12
   associated with lactation O91.13
 melancholia —see Disorder, depressive
 mental disorder NEC O99.345
 metroperitonitis O85
 metrorrhagia —see Hemorrhage, postpartum
 metrosalpingitis O86.19
 metrovaginitis O86.13
 milk leg O87.1
 monoplegia, cerebral O99.43
 mood disturbance O90.6
 necrosis, liver (acute) (subacute) (conditions in subcategory K72.0) O26.63
  with renal failure O90.4
 nervous system disorder O99.355
 neuritis O90.89
 obesity (pre-existing prior to pregnancy) O99.215
 obesity surgery status O99.845
 occlusion, precerebral artery O99.43
 paralysis
  bladder (sphincter) O90.89
  cerebral O99.43
 paralytic stroke O99.43
 parametritis O85
 paravaginitis O86.13
 pelviperitonitis O85
 perimetritis O86.12 ◄▥
 perimetrosalpingitis O86.19
 perinephritis O86.21
 periphlebitis —see Puerperal phlebitis
 peritoneal infection O85
 peritonitis (pelvic) O85
 perivaginitis O86.13
 phlebitis O87.0
  deep O87.1
  pelvic O87.1
  superficial O87.0
 phlebothrombosis, deep O87.1
 phlegmasia alba dolens O87.1
 placental polyp O90.89
 pneumonia, embolic —see Embolism, obstetric, puerperal
 pre-eclampsia —see Pre-eclampsia
 psychosis F53
 pyelitis O86.21
 pyelocystitis O86.29
 pyelonephritis O86.21
 pyelonephrosis O86.21
 pyemia O85
 pyocystitis O86.29
 pyohemia O85
 pyometra O86.12 ◄▥
 pyonephritis O86.21
 pyosalpingitis O86.19
 pyrexia (of unknown origin) O86.4
 renal
  disease NEC O90.89
  failure O90.4

Puerperal, puerperium (Continued)
  respiratory disease NEC O99.53
  retention
    decidua —see Retention, decidua
    placenta O72.0
    secundines —see Retention, secundines
  retrated nipple O92.02
  salpingo-ovaritis O86.19
  salpingoperitonitis O85
  secondary perineal tear O90.1
  sepsis O85
  sepsis (pelvic) O85
  septic thrombophlebitis O86.81
  skin disorder NEC O99.73
  specified condition NEC O99.89
  stroke O99.43
  subinvolution (uterus) O90.89
  subluxation of symphysis (pubis) O26.73
  suppuration —see Puerperal, abscess
  tetanus A34
  thelitis O91.02
    associated with lactation O91.03
  thrombocytopenia O72.3
  thrombophlebitis (superficial) O87.0
    deep O87.1
    pelvic O87.1
    septic O86.81
  thrombosis (venous) —see Thrombosis, puerperal
  thyroiditis O90.5
  toxemia (eclamptic) (pre-eclamptic) (with convulsions) O15.2
  trauma, non-obstetric O9A.23
    caused by abuse (physical) (suspected) O9A.33
      confirmed O9A.33
    psychological (suspected) O9A.53
      confirmed O9A.53
    sexual (suspected) O9A.43
      confirmed O9A.43
  uremia (due to renal failure) O90.4
  urethritis O86.22
  vaginitis O86.13
  varicose veins (legs) O87.4
    vulva or perineum O87.8
  venous O87.9
  vulvitis O86.19
  vulvovaginitis O86.13
  white leg O87.1
Puerperium —see Puerperal
Pulmolithiasis J98.4
Pulmonary —see condition
Pulpitis (acute) (anachoretic) (chronic) (hyperplastic) (irreversible) (putrescent) (reversible) (suppurative) (ulcerative) K04.0
Pulpless tooth K04.99
Pulse
  alternating R00.8
  bigeminal R00.8
  fast R00.0
  feeble, rapid due to shock following injury T79.4
  rapid R00.0
  weak R09.89
Pulsus alternans or trigeminus R00.8
Punch drunk F07.81
Punctum lacrimale occlusion —see Obstruction, lacrimal
Puncture
  abdomen, abdominal
    wall S31.139
      with
        foreign body S31.149
        penetration into peritoneal cavity S31.639
          with foreign body S31.649

Puncture (Continued)
  abdomen, abdominal (Continued)
    wall (Continued)
      epigastric region S31.132
        with
          foreign body S31.142
          penetration into peritoneal cavity S31.632
            with foreign body S31.642
      left
        lower quadrant S31.134
          with
            foreign body S31.144
            penetration into peritoneal cavity S31.634
              with foreign body S31.644
        upper quadrant S31.131
          with
            foreign body S31.141
            penetration into peritoneal cavity S31.631
              with foreign body S31.641
      periumbilic region S31.135
        with
          foreign body S31.145
          penetration into peritoneal cavity S31.635
            with foreign body S31.645
      right
        lower quadrant S31.133
          with
            foreign body S31.143
            penetration into peritoneal cavity S31.633
              with foreign body S31.643
        upper quadrant S31.130
          with
            foreign body S31.140
            penetration into peritoneal cavity S31.630
              with foreign body S31.640
    accidental, complicating surgery —see Complication, accidental puncture or laceration
    alveolar (process) —see Puncture, oral cavity
  ankle S91.039
    with
      foreign body S91.049
    left S91.032
      with
        foreign body S91.042
    right S91.031
      with
        foreign body S91.041
  anus S31.833
    with foreign body S31.834
  arm (upper) S41.139
    with foreign body S41.149
    left S41.132
      with foreign body S41.142
    lower —see Puncture, forearm
    right S41.131
      with foreign body S41.141
  auditory canal (external) (meatus) —see Puncture, ear
  auricle, ear —see Puncture, ear
  axilla —see Puncture, arm
  back —see also Puncture, thorax, back
    lower S31.030
      with
        foreign body S31.040
          with penetration into retroperitoneal space S31.041
        penetration into retroperitoneal space S31.031
  bladder (traumatic) S37.29
    nontraumatic N32.89
  breast S21.039
    with foreign body S21.049
    left S21.032
      with foreign body S21.042

Puncture (Continued)
  breast (Continued)
    right S21.031
      with foreign body S21.041
  buttock S31.803
    with foreign body S31.804
    left S31.823
      with foreign body S31.824
    right S31.813
      with foreign body S31.814
  by
    device, implant or graft —see Complications, by site and type, mechanical
    foreign body left accidentally in operative wound T81.539
    instrument (any) during a procedure, accidental —see Puncture, accidental complicating surgery
  calf —see Puncture, leg
  canaliculus lacrimalis —see Puncture, eyelid
  canthus, eye —see Puncture, eyelid
  cervical esophagus S11.23
    with foreign body S11.24
  cheek (external) S01.439
    with foreign body S01.449
    internal —see Puncture, oral cavity
    left S01.432
      with foreign body S01.442
    right S01.431
      with foreign body S01.441
  chest wall —see Puncture, thorax
  chin —see Puncture, head, specified site NEC
  clitoris —see Puncture, vulva
  costal region —see Puncture, thorax
  digit (s)
    foot —see Puncture, toe
    hand —see Puncture, finger
  ear (canal) (external) S01.339
    with foreign body S01.349
    drum S09.2-
    left S01.332
      with foreign body S01.342
    right S01.331
      with foreign body S01.341
  elbow S51.039
    with
      foreign body S51.049
    left S51.032
      with
        foreign body S51.042
    right S51.031
      with
        foreign body S51.041
  epididymis —see Puncture, testis
  epigastric region —see Puncture, abdomen, wall, epigastric
  epiglottis S11.83
    with foreign body S11.84
  esophagus
    cervical S11.23
      with foreign body S11.24
    thoracic S27.818
  eyeball S05.6-
    with foreign body S05.5-
  eyebrow —see Puncture, eyelid
  eyelid S01.13-
    with foreign body S01.14-
    left S01.132
      with foreign body S01.142
    right S01.131
      with foreign body S01.141
  face NEC —see Puncture, head, specified site NEC
  finger (s) S61.239
    with
      damage to nail S61.339
        with
          foreign body S61.349
      foreign body S61.249

Puncture (Continued)
  finger (Continued)
    index S61.238
      with
        damage to nail S61.338
          with
            foreign body S61.348
        foreign body S61.248
      left S61.231
        with
          damage to nail S61.331
            with
              foreign body S61.341
          foreign body S61.241
      right S61.230
        with
          damage to nail S61.330
            with
              foreign body S61.340
          foreign body S61.240
    little S61.238
      with
        damage to nail S61.338
          with
            foreign body S61.348
        foreign body S61.248
      left S61.237
        with
          damage to nail S61.337
            with
              foreign body S61.347
          foreign body S61.247
      right S61.236
        with
          damage to nail S61.336
            with
              foreign body S61.346
          foreign body S61.246
    middle S61.238
      with
        damage to nail S61.338
          with
            foreign body S61.348
        foreign body S61.248
      left S61.233
        with
          damage to nail S61.333
            with
              foreign body S61.343
          foreign body S61.243
      right S61.232
        with
          damage to nail S61.332
            with
              foreign body S61.342
          foreign body S61.242
    ring S61.238
      with
        damage to nail S61.338
          with
            foreign body S61.348
        foreign body S61.248
      left S61.235
        with
          damage to nail S61.335
            with
              foreign body S61.345
          foreign body S61.245
      right S61.234
        with
          damage to nail S61.334
            with
              foreign body
                S61.344
          foreign body S61.244
  flank S31.139
    with foreign body S31.149
  foot (except toe (s) alone) S91.339
    with foreign body S91.349
    left S91.332
      with foreign body S91.342

Puncture (Continued)
  foot (Continued)
    right S91.331
      with foreign body S91.341
    toe —see Puncture, toe
  forearm S51.839
    with
      foreign body S51.849
    elbow only —see Puncture, elbow
    left S51.832
      with
        foreign body S51.842
    right S51.831
      with
        foreign body S51.841
  forehead —see Puncture, head, specified site
    NEC
  genital organs, external
    female S31.532
      with foreign body S31.542
      vagina —see Puncture, vagina
      vulva —see Puncture, vulva
    male S31.531
      with foreign body S31.541
      penis —see Puncture, penis
      scrotum —see Puncture, scrotum
      testis —see Puncture, testis
  groin —see Puncture, abdomen, wall
  gum —see Puncture, oral cavity
  hand S61.439
    with
      foreign body S61.449
    finger —see Puncture, finger
    left S61.432
      with
        foreign body S61.442
    right S61.431
      with
        foreign body S61.441
    thumb —see Puncture, thumb
  head S01.93
    with foreign body S01.94
    cheek —see Puncture, cheek
    ear —see Puncture, ear
    eyelid —see Puncture, eyelid
    lip —see Puncture, oral cavity
    nose —see Puncture, nose
    oral cavity —see Puncture, oral cavity
    scalp S01.03
      with foreign body S01.04
    specified site NEC S01.83
      with foreign body S01.84
    temporomandibular area —see Puncture,
      cheek
  heart S26.99
    with hemopericardium S26.09
    without hemopericardium S26.19
  heel —see Puncture, foot
  hip S71.039
    with foreign body S71.049
    left S71.032
      with foreign body S71.042
    right S71.031
      with foreign body S71.041
  hymen —see Puncture, vagina
  hypochondrium —see Puncture, abdomen,
    wall
  hypogastric region —see Puncture, abdomen,
    wall
  inguinal region —see Puncture, abdomen,
    wall
  instep —see Puncture, foot
  internal organs —see Injury, by site
  interscapular region —see Puncture, thorax,
    back
  intestine
    large
      colon S36.599
        ascending S36.590
        descending S36.592
        sigmoid S36.593

Puncture (Continued)
  intestine (Continued)
    large (Continued)
      colon (Continued)
        specified site NEC S36.598
        transverse S36.591
      rectum S36.69
    small S36.499
      duodenum S36.490
      specified site NEC S36.498
  intra-abdominal organ S36.99
    gallbladder S36.128
    intestine —see Puncture, intestine
    liver S36.118
    pancreas —see Puncture, pancreas
    peritoneum S36.81
    specified site NEC S36.898
    spleen S36.09
    stomach S36.39
  jaw —see Puncture, head, specified site
    NEC
  knee S81.039
    with foreign body S81.049
    left S81.032
      with foreign body S81.042
    right S81.031
      with foreign body S81.041
  labium (majus) (minus) —see Puncture,
    vulva
  lacrimal duct —see Puncture, eyelid
  larynx S11.013
    with foreign body S11.014
  leg (lower) S81.839
    with foreign body S81.849
    foot —see Puncture, foot
    knee —see Puncture, knee
    left S81.832
      with foreign body S81.842
    right S81.831
      with foreign body S81.841
    upper —see Puncture, thigh
  lip S01.531
    with foreign body S01.541
  loin —see Puncture, abdomen, wall
  lower back —see Puncture, back, lower
  lumbar region —see Puncture, back, lower
  malar region —see Puncture, head, specified
    site NEC
  mammary —see Puncture, breast
  mastoid region —see Puncture, head,
    specified site NEC
  mouth —see Puncture, oral cavity
  nail
    finger —see Puncture, finger, with damage
      to nail
    toe —see Puncture, toe, with damage to
      nail
  nasal (septum) (sinus) —see Puncture,
    nose
  nasopharynx —see Puncture, head, specified
    site NEC
  neck S11.93
    with foreign body S11.94
    involving
      cervical esophagus —see Puncture,
        cervical esophagus
      larynx —see Puncture, larynx
      pharynx —see Puncture, pharynx
      thyroid gland —see Puncture, thyroid
        gland
      trachea —see Puncture, trachea
    specified site NEC S11.83
      with foreign body S11.84
  nose (septum) (sinus) S01.23
    with foreign body S01.24
  ocular —see Puncture, eyeball - oral cavity
    S01.532
    with foreign body S01.542
  orbit S05.4-
  palate —see Puncture, oral cavity
  palm —see Puncture, hand

Puncture *(Continued)*
 pancreas S36.299
  body S36.291
  head S36.290
  tail S36.292
 pelvis —*see* Puncture, back, lower
 penis S31.23
  with foreign body S31.24
 perineum
  female S31.43
   with foreign body S31.44
  male S31.139
   with foreign body S31.149
 periocular area (with or without lacrimal
   passages) —*see* Puncture, eyelid
 phalanges
  finger —*see* Puncture, finger
  toe —*see* Puncture, toe
 pharynx S11.23
  with foreign body S11.24
 pinna —*see* Puncture, ear
 popliteal space —*see* Puncture, knee
 prepuce —*see* Puncture, penis
 pubic region S31.139
  with foreign body S31.149
 pudendum —*see* Puncture, genital organs,
   external
 rectovaginal septum —*see* Puncture,
   vagina
 sacral region —*see* Puncture, back,
   lower
 sacroiliac region —*see* Puncture, back,
   lower
 salivary gland —*see* Puncture, oral
   cavity
 scalp S01.03
  with foreign body S01.04
 scapular region —*see* Puncture,
   shoulder
 scrotum S31.33
  with foreign body S31.34
 shin —*see* Puncture, leg
 shoulder S41.039
  with foreign body S41.049
  left S41.032
   with foreign body S41.042
  right S41.031
   with foreign body S41.041
 spermatic cord —*see* Puncture, testis
 sternal region —*see* Puncture, thorax, front
 submaxillary region —*see* Puncture, head,
   specified site NEC
 submental region —*see* Puncture, head,
   specified site NEC
 subungual
  finger (s) —*see* Puncture, finger, with
    damage to nail
  toe —*see* Puncture, toe, with damage to
    nail
 supraclavicular fossa —*see* Puncture, neck,
   specified site NEC
 temple, temporal region —*see* Puncture, head,
   specified site NEC
 temporomandibular area —*see* Puncture,
   cheek
 testis S31.33
  with foreign body S31.34
 thigh S71.139
  with foreign body S71.149
  left S71.132
   with foreign body S71.142
  right S71.131
   with foreign body S71.141
 thorax, thoracic (wall) S21.93
  with foreign body S21.94
  back S21.23-
   with
    foreign body S21.24-
     with penetration S21.44
    penetration S21.43
   breast —*see* Puncture, breast

Puncture *(Continued)*
 thorax, thoracic *(Continued)*
  front S21.13-
   with
    foreign body S21.14-
     with penetration S21.34
    penetration S21.33
 throat —*see* Puncture, neck
 thumb S61.039
  with
   damage to nail S61.139
    with
     foreign body S61.149
   foreign body S61.049
  left S61.032
   with
    damage to nail S61.132
     with
      foreign body S61.142
    foreign body S61.042
  right S61.031
   with
    damage to nail S61.131
     with
      foreign body S61.141
    foreign body S61.041
 thyroid gland S11.13
  with foreign body S11.14
 toe (s) S91.139
  with
   damage to nail S91.239
    with
     foreign body S91.249
   foreign body S91.149
  great S91.133
   with
    damage to nail S91.233
     with
      foreign body S91.243
    foreign body S91.143
   left S91.132
    with
     damage to nail S91.232
      with
       foreign body S91.242
     foreign body S91.142
   right S91.131
    with
     damage to nail S91.231
      with
       foreign body S91.241
     foreign body S91.141
  lesser S91.136
   with
    damage to nail S91.236
     with
      foreign body S91.246
    foreign body S91.146
   left S91.135
    with
     damage to nail S91.235
      with
       foreign body S91.245
     foreign body S91.145
   right S91.134
    with
     damage to nail S91.234
      with
       foreign body S91.244
     foreign body S91.144
 tongue —*see* Puncture, oral cavity
 trachea S11.023
  with foreign body S11.024
 tunica vaginalis —*see* Puncture, testis
 tympanum, tympanic membrane
   S09.2-
 umbilical region S31.135
  with foreign body S31.145
 uvula —*see* Puncture, oral cavity
 vagina S31.43
  with foreign body S31.44

Puncture *(Continued)*
 vocal cords S11.033
  with foreign body S11.034
 vulva S31.43
  with foreign body S31.44
 wrist S61.539
  with
   foreign body S61.549
  left S61.532
   with
    foreign body S61.542
  right S61.531
   with
    foreign body S61.541
PUO (pyrexia of unknown origin) R50.9
Pupillary membrane (persistent) Q13.89
Pupillotonia —*see* Anomaly, pupil, function,
   tonic pupil
Purpura D69.2
 abdominal D69.0
 allergic D69.0
 anaphylactoid D69.0
 annularis telangiectodes L81.7
 arthritic D69.0
 autoerythrocyte sensitization D69.2
 autoimmune D69.0
 bacterial D69.0
 Bateman's (senile) D69.2
 capillary fragility (hereditary) (idiopathic)
   D69.8
 cryoglobulinemic D89.1
 Devil's pinches D69.2
 fibrinolytic —*see* Fibrinolysis
 fulminans, fulminous D65
 gangrenous D65
 hemorrhagic, hemorrhagica D69.3
  not due to thrombocytopenia D69.0
 Henoch (-Schönlein) (allergic) D69.0
 hypergammaglobulinemic (benign)
   (Waldenström's) D89.0
 idiopathic (thrombocytopenic) D69.3
  nonthrombocytopenic D69.0
 immune thrombocytopenic D69.3
 infectious D69.0
 malignant D69.0
 neonatorum P54.5
 nervosa D69.0
 newborn P54.5
 nonthrombocytopenic D69.2
  hemorrhagic D69.0
  idiopathic D69.0
 nonthrombopenic D69.2
 peliosis rheumatica D69.0
 posttransfusion (post-transfusion) (from
   (fresh) whole blood or blood products)
   D69.51
 primary D69.49
 red cell membrane sensitivity D69.2
 rheumatica D69.0
 Schönlein (-Henoch) (allergic) D69.0
 scorbutic E54 *[D77]*
 senile D69.2
 simplex D69.2
 symptomatica D69.0
 telangiectasia annularis L81.7
 thrombocytopenic D69.49
  congenital D69.42
  hemorrhagic D69.3
  hereditary D69.42
  idiopathic D69.3
  immune D69.3
  neonatal, transitory P61.0
  thrombotic M31.1
 thrombohemolytic —*see* Fibrinolysis
 thrombolytic —*see* Fibrinolysis
 thrombopenic D69.49
 thrombotic, thrombocytopenic M31.1
 toxic D69.0
 vascular D69.0
 visceral symptoms D69.0
Purpuric spots R23.3

◀ New ◀▥ Revised ~~deleted~~ Deleted

Purulent —*see* condition
Pus
  in
    stool R19.5
    urine N39.0
  tube (rupture) —*see* Salpingo-oophoritis
Pustular rash L08.0
Pustule (nonmalignant) L08.9
  malignant A22.0
Pustulosis palmaris et plantaris L40.3
Putnam (-Dana) disease or syndrome —*see*
    Degeneration, combined
Putrescent pulp (dental) K04.1
Pyarthritis, pyarthrosis —*see* Arthritis,
    pyogenic or pyemic
  tuberculous —*see* Tuberculosis, joint
Pyelectasis —*see* Hydronephrosis
Pyelitis (congenital) (uremic) —*see also*
    Pyelonephritis
  with
    calculus —*see* category N20
      with hydronephrosis N13.2
    contracted kidney N11.9
  acute N10
  chronic N11.9
    with calculus —*see* category N20
      with hydronephrosis N13.2
  cystica N28.84
  puerperal (postpartum) O86.21
  tuberculous A18.11
Pyelocystitis —*see* Pyelonephritis
Pyelonephritis —*see also* Nephritis,
    tubulo-interstitial
  with
    calculus —*see* category N20
      with hydronephrosis N13.2
    contracted kidney N11.9
  acute N10
  calculus —*see* category N20
    with hydronephrosis N13.2
  chronic N11.9
    with calculus —*see* category N20
      with hydronephrosis N13.2
    associated with ureteral obstruction or
        stricture N11.1
    nonobstructive N11.8
      with reflux (vesicoureteral) N11.0
    obstructive N11.1
    specified NEC N11.8
  in (due to)
    brucellosis A23.9 *[N16]*
    cryoglobulinemia (mixed) D89.1 *[N16]*
    cystinosis E72.04
    diphtheria A36.84

Pyelonephritis (*Continued*)
  in (*Continued*)
    glycogen storage disease E74.09 *[N16]*
    leukemia NEC C95.9- *[N16]*
    lymphoma NEC C85.90 *[N16]*
    multiple myeloma C90.0- *[N16]*
    obstruction N11.1
    Salmonella infection A02.25
    sarcoidosis D86.84
    sepsis A41.9 *[N16]*
    Sjögren's disease M35.04
    toxoplasmosis B58.83
    transplant rejection T86.91 *[N16]*
    Wilson's disease E83.01 *[N16]*
  nonobstructive N12
    with reflux (vesicoureteral) N11.0
    chronic N11.8
  syphilitic A52.75
Pyelonephrosis (obstructive) N11.1
  chronic N11.9
Pyelophlebitis I80.8
Pyeloureteritis cystica N28.85
Pyemia, pyemic (fever) (infection) (purulent) —
    see also Sepsis
  joint —*see* Arthritis, pyogenic or pyemic
  liver K75.1
  pneumococcal A40.3
  portal K75.1
  postvaccinal T88.0
  puerperal, postpartum, childbirth O85
  specified organism NEC A41.89
  tuberculous —*see* Tuberculosis, miliary
Pygopagus Q89.4
Pyknoepilepsy (idiopathic) —*see* Pyknolepsy
Pyknolepsy G40.A09
  intractable G40.A19
    with status epilepticus G40.A11
    without status epilepticus G40.A19
  not intractable G40.A09
    with status epilepticus G40.A01
    without status epilepticus G40.A09
Pylephlebitis K75.1
Pyle's syndrome Q78.5
Pylethrombophlebitis K75.1
Pylethrombosis K75.1
Pyloritis K29.90
  with bleeding K29.91
Pylorospasm (reflex) NEC K31.3
  congenital or infantile Q40.0
  neurotic F45.8
  newborn Q40.0
  psychogenic F45.8
Pylorus, pyloric —*see* condition

Pyoarthrosis —*see* Arthritis, pyogenic or
    pyemic
Pyocele
  mastoid —*see* Mastoiditis, acute
  sinus (accessory) —*see* Sinusitis
  turbinate (bone) J32.9
  urethra (*see also* Urethritis) N34.0
Pyocolpos —*see* Vaginitis
Pyocystitis N30.80
  with hematuria N30.81
Pyoderma, pyodermia L08.0
  gangrenosum L88
  newborn P39.4
  phagedenic L88
  vegetans L08.81
Pyodermatitis L08.0
  vegetans L08.81
Pyogenic —*see* condition
Pyohydronephrosis N13.6
Pyometra, pyometrium, pyometritis —*see*
    Endometritis
Pyomyositis (tropical) —*see* Myositis, infective
Pyonephritis N12
Pyonephrosis N13.6
  tuberculous A18.11
Pyo-oophoritis —*see* Salpingo-oophoritis
Pyo-ovarium —*see* Salpingo-oophoritis
Pyopericarditis, pyopericardium I30.1
Pyophlebitis —*see* Phlebitis
Pyopneumopericardium I30.1
Pyopneumothorax (infective) J86.9
  with fistula J86.0
  tuberculous NEC A15.6
Pyosalpinx, pyosalpingitis —*see also*
    Salpingo-oophoritis
Pyothorax J86.9
  with fistula J86.0
  tuberculous NEC A15.6
Pyoureter N28.89
  tuberculous A18.11
Pyramidopallidonigral syndrome G20
Pyrexia (of unknown origin) R50.9
  atmospheric T67.0
  during labor NEC O75.2
  heat T67.0
  newborn P81.9
    environmentally-induced P81.0
  persistent R50.9
  puerperal O86.4
Pyroglobulinemia NEC E88.09
Pyromania F63.1
Pyrosis R12
Pyuria (bacterial) N39.0

Q

Q fever A78
 with pneumonia A78
Quadricuspid aortic valve Q23.8
Quadrilateral fever A78
Quadriparesis —*see* Quadriplegia
 meaning muscle weakness M62.81
Quadriplegia G82.50-
 complete
  C1-C4 level G82.51
  C5-C7 level G82.53
 congenital (cerebral) (spinal) G80.8
  spastic G80.0

Quadriplegia (*Continued*)
 embolic (current episode) I63.4
 functional R53.2
 incomplete
  C1-C4 level G82.52
  C5-C7 level G82.54
 thrombotic (current episode) I63.3
 traumatic — code to injury with seventh
  character S
  current episode —*see* Injury, spinal (cord),
   cervical
Quadruplet, pregnancy —*see* Pregnancy,
 quadruplet
Quarrelsomeness F60.3

Queensland fever A77.3
Quervain's disease M65.4
 thyroid E06.1
Queyrat's erythroplasia D07.4
 penis D07.4
 specified site —*see* Neoplasm, skin,
  in situ
 unspecified site D07.4
Quincke's disease or edema T78.3
 hereditary D84.1
Quinsy (gangrenous) J36
Quintan fever A79.0
Quintuplet, pregnancy —*see* Pregnancy,
 quintuplet

◀ New   ◀▥ Revised   ~~deleted~~ Deleted

R

Rabbit fever —*see* Tularemia
Rabies A82.9
  contact Z20.3
  exposure to Z20.3
  inoculation reaction —*see* Complications,
    vaccination
  sylvatic A82.0
  urban A82.1
Rachischisis —*see* Spina bifida
Rachitic —*see also* condition
  deformities of spine (late effect) (sequelae)
    E64.3
  pelvis (late effect) (sequelae) E64.3
    with disproportion (fetopelvic) O33.0
      causing obstructed labor O65.0
Rachitis, rachitism (acute) (tarda) —*see also*
    Rickets
  renalis N25.0
  sequelae E64.3
Radial nerve —*see* condition
Radiation
  burn —*see* Burn
  effects NOS T66
  sickness NOS T66
  therapy, encounter for Z51.0
Radiculitis (pressure) (vertebrogenic) —*see*
    Radiculopathy
Radiculomyelitis —*see also* Encephalitis
  toxic, due to
    Clostridium tetani A35
    Corynebacterium diphtheriae A36.82
Radiculopathy M54.10
  cervical region M54.12
  cervicothoracic region M54.13
  due to displacement of intervertebral disc —
    see Disorder, disc, with, radiculopathy
  due to ◀
    disc disorder ◀
      C3 M50.11 ◀
      C4 M50.11 ◀
      C5 M50.12 ◀
      C6 M50.12 ◀
      C7 M50.12 ◀
      C8 M50.13 ◀
    displacement of intervertebral disc —*see*
      Disorder, disc, with, radiculopathy ◀
  leg M54.1-
  lumbar region M54.16
  lumbosacral region M54.17
  occipito-atlanto-axial region M54.11
  postherpetic B02.29
  sacrococcygeal region M54.18
  syphilitic A52.11
  thoracic region (with visceral pain)
    M54.14
  thoracolumbar region M54.15
Radiodermal burns (acute, chronic, or
    occupational) —*see* Burn
Radiodermatitis L58.9
  acute L58.0
  chronic L58.1
Radiotherapy session Z51.0
Rage, meaning rabies —*see* Rabies
Ragpicker's disease A22.1
Ragsorter's disease A22.1
Raillietiniasis B71.8
Railroad neurosis F48.8
Railway spine F48.8
Raised —*see also* Elevated
  antibody titer R76.0
Rake teeth, tooth M26.39
Rales R09.89
Ramifying renal pelvis Q63.8
Ramsay-Hunt disease or syndrome (*see also*
    Hunt's disease) B02.21
  meaning dyssynergia cerebellaris myoclonica
    G11.1
Ranula K11.6
  congenital Q38.4

Rape
  adult
    confirmed T74.21
    suspected T76.21
  alleged, observation or examination, ruled out
    adult Z04.41
    child Z04.42
  child
    confirmed T74.22
    suspected T76.22
Rapid
  feeble pulse, due to shock, following injury
    T79.4
  heart (beat) R00.0
    psychogenic F45.8
  second stage (delivery) O62.3
  time-zone change syndrome —*see* Disorder,
    sleep, circadian rhythm, psychogenic
Rarefaction, bone —*see* Disorder, bone, density
    and structure, specified NEC
Rash (toxic) R21
  canker A38.9
  diaper L22
  drug (internal use) L27.0
    contact (*see also* Dermatitis, due to, drugs,
      external) L25.1
  following immunization T88.1
  food —*see* Dermatitis, due to, food
  heat L74.0
  napkin (psoriasiform) L22
  nettle —*see* Urticaria
  pustular L08.0
  rose R21
    epidemic B06.9
  scarlet A38.9
  serum (*see also* Reaction, serum) T80.69
  wandering tongue K14.1
Rasmussen aneurysm —*see* Tuberculosis,
    pulmonary
Rasmussen encephalitis G04.81
Rat-bite fever A25.9
  due to Streptobacillus moniliformis A25.1
  spirochetal (morsus muris) A25.0
Rathke's pouch tumor D44.3
Raymond (-Céstan) syndrome I65.8
Raynaud's disease, phenomenon or syndrome
    (secondary) I73.00
  with gangrene (symmetric) I73.01
RDS (newborn) (type I) P22.0
  type II P22.1
Reaction —*see also* Disorder
  adaptation —*see* Disorder, adjustment
  adjustment (anxiety) (conduct disorder)
    (depressiveness) (distress) —*see*
      Disorder, adjustment
    with
      mutism, elective (child) (adolescent) F94.0
  adverse
    food (any) (ingested) NEC T78.1
      anaphylactic —*see* Shock, anaphylactic,
        due to food
  anaphylactoid —*see* Shock, anaphylactic
  affective —*see* Disorder, mood
  allergic —*see* Allergy
  anaphylactic —*see* Shock, anaphylactic
  anesthesia —*see* Anesthesia, complication
  antitoxin (prophylactic) (therapeutic) —*see*
    Complications, vaccination
  anxiety F41.1
  Arthus —*see* Arthus' phenomenon
  asthenic F48.8
  combat and operational stress F43.0
  compulsive F42
  conversion F44.9
  crisis, acute F43.0
  deoxyribonuclease (DNA) (DNase)
    hypersensitivity D69.2
  depressive (single episode) F32.9
    affective (single episode) F31.4
      recurrent episode F33.9
    neurotic F34.1
    psychoneurotic F34.1

Reaction (*Continued*)
  depressive (*Continued*)
    psychotic F32.3
    recurrent —*see* Disorder, depressive,
      recurrent
  dissociative F44.9
  drug NEC T88.7
    addictive —*see* Dependence, drug
      transmitted via placenta or breast
        milk —*see* Absorption, drug,
        addictive, through placenta
    allergic —*see* Allergy, drug
    lichenoid L43.2
    newborn P93.8
      gray baby syndrome P93.0
    overdose or poisoning (by accident) —*see*
      Table of d̶Drugs and c̶Chemicals, by
      drug, poisoning ◀||||
    photoallergic L56.1
    phototoxic L56.0
    withdrawal —*see* Dependence, by drug,
      with, withdrawal
      infant of dependent mother P96.1
      newborn P96.1
    wrong substance given or taken (by
      accident) —*see* Table of d̶Drugs and
      c̶Chemicals, by drug, poisoning ◀||||
  fear F40.9
    child (abnormal) F93.8
  febrile nonhemolytic transfusion (FNHTR)
    R50.84
  fluid loss, cerebrospinal G97.1
  foreign
    body NEC —*see* Granuloma, foreign body
      in operative wound (inadvertently
        left) —*see* Foreign body,
        accidentally left during a
        procedure
    substance accidentally left during a
      procedure (chemical) (powder) (talc)
      T81.60
        aseptic peritonitis T81.61
        body or object (instrument) (sponge)
          (swab) —*see* Foreign body,
          accidentally left during a
          procedure
        specified reaction NEC T81.69
  grief —*see* Disorder, adjustment
  Herxheimer's R68.89
  hyperkinetic —*see* Hyperkinesia
  hypochondriacal F45.20
  hypoglycemic, due to insulin E16.0
    with coma (diabetic) —*see* Diabetes, coma
      nondiabetic E15
    therapeutic misadventure —*see*
      subcategory T38.3
  hypomanic F30.8
  hysterical F44.9
  immunization —*see* Complications, vaccination
  incompatibility
    ABO blood group (infusion) (transfusion) —
      see Complication (s), transfusion,
      incompatibility reaction, ABO
    delayed serologic T80.39
    minor blood group (Duffy) (E) (K(ell))
      (Kidd) (Lewis) (M) (N) (P) (S) T80.89
    Rh (factor) (infusion) (transfusion) —*see*
      Complication (s), transfusion,
      incompatibility reaction, Rh (factor)
  inflammatory —*see* Infection
  infusion —*see* Complications, infusion
  inoculation (immune serum) —*see*
    Complications, vaccination
  insulin T38.3-
  involutional psychotic —*see* Disorder,
    depressive
  leukemoid D72.823
    basophilic D72.823
    lymphocytic D72.823
    monocytic D72.823
    myelocytic D72.823
    neutrophilic D72.823

Reaction *(Continued)*
  LSD (acute)
    due to drug abuse —*see* Abuse, drug,
      hallucinogen
    due to drug dependence —*see* Dependence,
      drug, hallucinogen
  lumbar puncture G97.1
  manic-depressive —*see* Disorder, bipolar
  neurasthenic F48.8
  neurogenic —*see* Neurosis
  neurotic F48.9
  neurotic-depressive F34.1
  nitritoid —*see* Crisis, nitritoid - obsessive-
    compulsive F42
  nonspecific
    to
      cell mediated immunity measurement
        of gamma interferon antigen
        response without active
        tuberculosis R76.12
      QuantiFERON-TB test (QFT) without
        active tuberculosis R76.12
      tuberculin test (*see also* Reaction,
        tuberculin skin test) R76.11
  obsessive-compulsive F42
  organic, acute or subacute —*see* Delirium
  paranoid (acute) F23
    chronic F22
    senile F03
  passive dependency F60.7
  phobic F40.9
  post-traumatic stress, uncomplicated
    Z73.3
  psychogenic F99
  psychoneurotic —*see also* Neurosis
    compulsive F42
    depersonalization F48.1
    depressive F34.1
    hypochondriacal F45.20
    neurasthenic F48.8
    obsessive F42
  psychophysiologic —*see* Disorder,
    somatoform
  psychosomatic —*see* Disorder, somatoform
  psychotic —*see* Psychosis
  scarlet fever toxin —*see* Complications,
    vaccination
  schizophrenic F23
    acute (brief) (undifferentiated) F23
    latent F21
    undifferentiated (acute) (brief) F23
  serological for syphilis —*see* Serology for
    syphilis
  serum T80.69
    anaphylactic (immediate) (*see also* Shock,
      anaphylactic) T80.59
    specified reaction NEC
      due to
        administration of blood and blood
          products T80.61
        immunization T80.62
        serum specified NEC T80.69
        vaccination T80.62
  situational —*see* Disorder, adjustment
  somatization —*see* Disorder, somatoform
  spinal puncture G97.1
  stress (severe) F43.9
    acute (agitation) ("daze") (disorientation)
      (disturbance of consciousness) (flight
      reaction) (fugue) F43.0
    specified NEC F43.8
  surgical procedure —*see* Complications,
    surgical procedure
  tetanus antitoxin —*see* Complications,
    vaccination
  toxic, to local anesthesia T81.89
    in labor and delivery O74.4
    in pregnancy O29.3X-
    postpartum, puerperal O89.3
  toxin-antitoxin —*see* Complications,
    vaccination

Reaction *(Continued)*
  transfusion (blood) (bone marrow)
    (lymphocytes) (allergic) —*see*
    Complications, transfusion
  tuberculin skin test, abnormal R76.11
  vaccination (any) —*see* Complications,
    vaccination
  withdrawing, child or adolescent F93.8
Reactive airway disease —*see* Asthma
Reactive depression —*see* Reaction, depressive
Rearrangement
  chromosomal
    balanced (in) Q95.9
      abnormal individual (autosomal) Q95.2
      non-sex (autosomal) chromosomes
        Q95.2
      sex/non-sex chromosomes Q95.3
      specified NEC Q95.8
Recalcitrant patient —*see* Noncompliance
Recanalization, thrombus —*see* Thrombosis
Recession, receding
  chamber angle (eye) H21.55-
  chin M26.09
  gingival (generalized) (localized)
    (postinfective) (postoperative) K06.0
Recklinghausen's disease Q85.01
  bones E21.0
Reclus' disease (cystic) —*see* Mastopathy, cystic
Recrudescent typhus (fever) A75.1
Recruitment, auditory H93.21-
Rectalgia K62.89
Rectitis K62.89
Rectocele
  female (without uterine prolapse) N81.6
    with uterine prolapse N81.4
      incomplete N81.2
  in pregnancy —*see* Pregnancy, complicated
    by, abnormal, pelvic organs or tissues
    NEC
  male K62.3
Rectosigmoid junction —*see* condition
Rectosigmoiditis K63.89
  ulcerative (chronic) K51.30
    with
      complication K51.319
        abscess K51.314
        fistula K51.313
        obstruction K51.312
        rectal bleeding K51.311
        specified NEC K51.318
Rectourethral —*see* condition
Rectovaginal —*see* condition
Rectovesical —*see* condition
Rectum, rectal —*see* condition
Recurrent —*see* condition
  pregnancy loss —*see* Loss (of), pregnancy,
    recurrent
Red bugs B88.0
Red-cedar lung or pneumonitis J67.8
Red tide (*see also* Table of Drugs and Chemicals)
  T65.82-
Reduced
  mobility Z74.09
  ventilatory or vital capacity R94.2
Redundant, redundancy
  anus (congenital) Q43.8
  clitoris N90.89
  colon (congenital) Q43.8
  foreskin (congenital) N47.8
  intestine (congenital) Q43.8
  labia N90.6
  organ or site, congenital NEC —*see* Accessory
  panniculus (abdominal) E65
  prepuce (congenital) N47.8
  pylorus K31.89
  rectum (congenital) Q43.8
  scrotum N50.8
  sigmoid (congenital) Q43.8
  skin (of face) L57.4
    eyelids —*see* Blepharochalasis
  stomach K31.89

Reduplication —*see* Duplication
Reflex R29.2
  hyperactive gag J39.2
  pupillary, abnormal —*see* Anomaly, pupil,
    function
  vasoconstriction I73.9
  vasovagal R55
Reflux K21.9
  acid K21.9
  esophageal K21.9
    with esophagitis K21.0
    newborn P78.83
  gastroesophageal K21.9
    with esophagitis K21.0
  mitral —*see* Insufficiency, mitral
  ureteral —*see* Reflux, vesicoureteral
  vesicoureteral (with scarring) N13.70
    with
      nephropathy N13.729
        with hydroureter N13.739
          bilateral N13.732
          unilateral N13.731
        without hydroureter N13.729
          bilateral N13.722
          unilateral N13.721
      bilateral N13.722
      unilateral N13.721
      pyelonephritis (chronic) N11.0
    without nephropathy N13.71
    congenital Q62.7
Reforming, artificial openings —*see* Attention
  to, artificial, opening
Refractive error —*see* Disorder, refraction
Refsum's disease or syndrome G60.1
Refusal of
  food, psychogenic F50.8
  treatment (because of) Z53.20
    left against medical advice (AMA) Z53.21
    patient's decision NEC Z53.29
    reasons of belief or group pressure Z53.1
Regional —*see* condition
Regurgitation R11.10
  aortic (valve) —*see* Insufficiency, aortic
  food —*see also* Vomiting
    with reswallowing —*see* Rumination
    newborn P92.1
  gastric contents —*see* Vomiting
  heart —*see* Endocarditis
  mitral (valve) —*see* Insufficiency, mitral
    congenital Q23.3
  myocardial —*see* Endocarditis
  pulmonary (valve) (heart) I37.1
    congenital Q22.2
    syphilitic A52.03
  tricuspid —*see* Insufficiency, tricuspid
  valve, valvular —*see* Endocarditis
    congenital Q24.8
  vesicoureteral —*see* Reflux, vesicoureteral
Reichmann's disease or syndrome K31.89
Reifenstein syndrome E34.52
Reinsertion, contraceptive device Z30.433
Reiter's disease, syndrome, or urethritis
  M02.30
  ankle M02.37-
  elbow M02.32-
  foot joint M02.37-
  hand joint M02.34-
  hip M02.35-
  knee M02.36-
  multiple site M02.39
  shoulder M02.31-
  vertebra M02.38
  wrist M02.33-
Rejection
  food, psychogenic F50.8
  transplant T86.91
    bone T86.830
      marrow T86.01
    cornea T86.840
    heart T86.21
      with lung (s) T86.31

◀ New   ◀▥ Revised   ~~deleted~~ Deleted

Rejection (Continued)
  transplant (Continued)
    intestine T86.850
    kidney T86.11
    liver T86.41
    lung (s) T86.810
      with heart T86.31
    organ (immune or nonimmune cause)
        T86.91
    pancreas T86.890
    skin (allograft) (autograft) T86.820
    specified NEC T86.890
    stem cell (peripheral blood) (umbilical
        cord) T86.5
Relapsing fever A68.9
  Carter's (Asiatic) A68.1
  Dutton's (West African) A68.1
  Koch's A68.9
  louse-borne (epidemic) A68.0
  Novy's (American) A68.1
  Obermeyers's (European) A68.0
  Spirillum A68.9
  tick-borne (endemic) A68.1
Relationship
  occlusal
    open anterior M26.220
    open posterior M26.221
Relaxation
  anus (sphincter) K62.89
    psychogenic F45.8
  arch (foot) —see also Deformity, limb, flat
      foot
  back ligaments —see Instability, joint, spine
  bladder (sphincter) N31.2
  cardioesophageal K21.9
  cervix —see Incompetency, cervix
  diaphragm J98.6
  joint (capsule) (ligament) (paralytic) —see
      Flail, joint
    congenital NEC Q74.8
  lumbosacral (joint) —see subcategory M53.2
  pelvic floor N81.89
  perineum N81.89
  posture R29.3
  rectum (sphincter) K62.89
  sacroiliac (joint) —see subcategory M53.2
  scrotum N50.8
  urethra (sphincter) N36.44
  vesical N31.2
Release from prison, anxiety concerning
    Z65.2
Remains
  canal of Cloquet Q14.0
  capsule (opaque) Q14.8
Remittent fever (malarial) B54
Remnant
  canal of Cloquet Q14.0
  capsule (opaque) Q14.8
  cervix, cervical stump (acquired)
      (postoperative) N88.8
  cystic duct, postcholecystectomy K91.5
  fingernail L60.8
    congenital Q84.6
  meniscus, knee —see Derangement, knee,
      meniscus, specified NEC
  thyroglossal duct Q89.2
  tonsil J35.8
    infected (chronic) J35.01
  urachus Q64.4
Removal (from) (of)
  artificial
    arm Z44.00-
      complete Z44.01-
      partial Z44.02-
    eye Z44.2-
    leg Z44.10-
      complete Z44.11-
      partial Z44.12-
  breast implant Z45.81
  cardiac pulse generator (battery) (end-of-life)
      Z45.010

Removal (Continued)
  catheter (urinary) (indwelling) Z46.6
    from artificial opening —see Attention to,
        artificial, opening
    non-vascular Z46.82
    vascular NEC Z45.2
  device Z46.9
    contraceptive Z30.432
    implanted NEC Z45.89
    specified NEC Z46.89
  drains Z48.03
  dressing (nonsurgical) Z48.00
    surgical Z48.01
  external
    fixation device — code to fracture with
        seventh character D
    prosthesis, prosthetic device Z44.9
      breast Z44.3-
      specified NEC Z44.8
  home in childhood (to foster home or
      institution) Z62.29
  ileostomy Z43.2
  insulin pump Z46.81
  myringotomy device (stent) (tube) Z45.82
  nervous system device NEC Z46.2
    brain neuropacemaker Z46.2
    visual substitution device Z46.2
      implanted Z45.31
  non-vascular catheter Z46.82
  organ, prophylactic (for neoplasia
      management) —see Prophylactic, organ
      removal
  orthodontic device Z46.4
  staples Z48.02
  stent
    ureteral Z46.6
  suture Z48.02
  urinary device Z46.6
  vascular access device or catheter Z45.2
Ren
  arcuatus Q63.1
  mobile, mobilis N28.89
    congenital Q63.8
  unguliformis Q63.1
Renal —see condition
Rendu-Osler-Weber disease or syndrome I78.0
Reninoma D41.0-
Renon-Delille syndrome E23.3
Reovirus, as cause of disease classified
    elsewhere B97.5
Repeated falls NEC R29.6
Replaced chromosome by dicentric ring Q93.2
Replacement by artificial or mechanical device
    or prosthesis of
  bladder Z96.0
  blood vessel NEC Z95.828
  bone NEC Z96.7
  cochlea Z96.21
  coronary artery Z95.5
  eustachian tube Z96.29
  eye globe Z97.0
  heart Z95.812
    valve Z95.2
      prosthetic Z95.2
      specified NEC Z95.4
      xenogenic Z95.3
  intestine Z96.89
  joint Z96.60
    hip —see Presence, hip joint implant
    knee —see Presence, knee joint implant
    specified site NEC Z96.698
  larynx Z96.3
  lens Z96.1
  limb (s) —see Presence, artificial, limb
  mandible NEC (for tooth root implant (s))
      Z96.5
  organ NEC Z96.89
  peripheral vessel NEC Z95.828
  stapes Z96.29
  teeth Z97.2
  tendon Z96.7

Replacement by artificial or mechanical device
    or prosthesis of (Continued)
  tissue NEC Z96.89
  tooth root (s) Z96.5
  vessel NEC Z95.828
    coronary (artery) Z95.5
Request for expert evidence Z04.8
Reserve, decreased or low
  cardiac —see Disease, heart
  kidney N28.89
Residual —see also condition
  ovary syndrome N99.83
  state, schizophrenic F20.5
  urine R39.19
Resistance, resistant (to)
  activated protein C D68.51
  complicating pregnancy O26.89
  insulin E88.81
  organism (s)
    to
      drug
        aminoglycosides Z16.29
        amoxicillin Z16.11
        ampicillin Z16.11
        antibiotic (s) Z16.20
          multiple Z16.24
          specified NEC Z16.29
        antifungal Z16.32
        antimicrobial (single) Z16.30
          multiple Z16.35
          specified NEC Z16.39
        antimycbacterial (single) Z16.341
          multiple Z16.342
        antiparasitic Z16.31
        antiviral Z16.33
        beta lactam antibiotics Z16.10
          specified NEC Z16.19
        cephalosporins Z16.19
        extended beta lactamase (ESBL)
            Z16.12
        fluoroquinolones Z16.23
        macrolides Z16.29
        methicillin —see MRSA
        multiple drugs (MDRO)
          antibiotics Z16.24
        penicillins Z16.11
        quinine (and related compounds)
            Z16.31
        quinolones Z16.23
        sulfonamides Z16.29
        tetracyclines Z16.29
        tuberculostatics (single) Z16.341
          multiple Z16.342
        vancomycin Z16.21
          related antibiotics Z16.22
  thyroid hormone E07.89
Resorption
  dental (roots) K03.3
    alveoli M26.79
  teeth (external) (internal) (pathological)
      (roots) K03.3
Respiration
  Cheyne-Stokes R06.3
  decreased due to shock, following injury
      T79.4
  disorder of, psychogenic F45.8
  insufficient, or poor R06.89
    newborn P28.5
  painful R07.1
  sighing, psychogenic F45.8
Respiratory —see also condition
  distress syndrome (newborn) (type I)
      P22.0
    type II P22.1
  syncytial virus, as cause of disease classified
      elsewhere B97.4
Respite care Z75.5
Response (drug)
  photoallergic L56.1
  phototoxic L56.0
Restless legs (syndrome) G25.81

Restlessness R45.1
Restoration (of)
  dental
    aesthetically inadequate or displeasing
      K08.56
    defective K08.50
      specified NEC K08.59
    failure of marginal integrity K08.51
    failure of periodontal anatomical intergrity
      K08.54
  organ continuity from previous sterilization
    (tuboplasty) (vasoplasty) Z31.0
    aftercare Z31.42
  tooth (existing)
    contours biologically incompatible with
      oral health K08.54
    open margins K08.51
    overhanging K08.52
    poor aesthetic K08.56
    poor gingival margins K08.51
  unsatisfactory, of tooth K08.50
    specified NEC K08.59
Restorative material (dental)
  allergy to K08.55
  fractured K08.539
    with loss of material K08.531
    without loss of material K08.530
  unrepairable overhanging of K08.52
Restriction of housing space Z59.1
Rests, ovarian, in fallopian tube Q50.6
Restzustand (schizophrenic) F20.5
Retained —see also Retention
  cholelithiasis following cholecystectomy
    K91.86
  foreign body fragments (type of) Z18.9
    acrylics Z18.2
    animal quill (s) or spines Z18.31
    cement Z18.83
    concrete Z18.83
    crystalline Z18.83
    depleted isotope Z18.09
    depleted uranium Z18.01
    diethylhexylphthalates Z18.2
    glass Z18.81
    isocyanate Z18.2
    magnetic metal Z18.11
    metal Z18.10
    nonmagnetic metal Z18.12
    nontherapeutic radioactive Z18.09
    organic NEC Z18.39
    plastic Z18.2
    quill (s) (animal) Z18.31
    radioactive (nontherapeutic) NEC
      Z18.09
    specified NEC Z18.89
    spine (s) (animal) Z18.31
    stone Z18.83
    tooth (teeth) Z18.32
    wood Z18.33
  fragments (type of) Z18.9
    acrylics Z18.2
    animal quill (s) or spines Z18.31
    cement Z18.83
    concrete Z18.83
    crystalline Z18.83
    depleted isotope Z18.09
    depleted uranium Z18.01
    diethylhexylphthalates Z18.2
    glass Z18.81
    isocyanate Z18.2
    magnetic metal Z18.11
    metal Z18.10
    nonmagnectic metal Z18.12
    nontherapeutic radioactive Z18.09
    organic NEC Z18.39
    plastic Z18.2
    quill (s) (animal) Z18.31
    radioactive (nontherapeutic) NEC
      Z18.09
    specified NEC Z18.89
    spine (s) (animal) Z18.31

Retained (Continued)
  fragments (Continued)
    stone Z18.83
    tooth (teeth) Z18.32
    wood Z18.33
  gallstones, following cholecystectomy K91.86
Retardation
  development, developmental, specific —see
    Disorder, developmental
  endochondral bone growth —see Disorder,
    bone, development or growth
  growth R62.50
    due to malnutrition E45
  mental —see Disability, intellectual
  motor function, specific F82
  physical (child) R62.52
    due to malnutrition E45
  reading (specific) F81.0
  spelling (specific) (without reading disorder)
    F81.81
Retching —see Vomiting
Retention —see also Retained
  bladder —see Retention, urine
  carbon dioxide E87.2
  cholelithiasis following cholecystectomy
    K91.86
  cyst —see Cyst
  dead
    fetus (at or near term) (mother) O36.4
      early fetal death O02.1
    ovum O02.0
  decidua (fragments) (following delivery)
    (with hemorrhage) O72.2
    without hemorrhage O73.1
  deciduous tooth K00.6
  dental root K08.3
  fecal —see Constipation
  fetus
    dead O36.4
    early O02.1
  fluid R60.9
  foreign body —see also Foreign body, retained
    current trauma - code as Foreign body, by
      site or type
  gallstones, following cholecystectomy
    K91.86
  gastric K31.89
  intrauterine contraceptive device, in
    pregnancy —see Pregnancy, complicated
    by, retention, intrauterine device
  membranes (complicating delivery) (with
    hemorrhage) O72.2
    with abortion —see Abortion, by type
    without hemorrhage O73.1
  meniscus —see Derangement, meniscus
  menses N94.89
  milk (puerperal, postpartum) O92.79
  nitrogen, extrarenal R39.2
  ovary syndrome N99.83
  placenta (total) (with hemorrhage) O72.0
    without hemorrhage O73.0
    portions or fragments (with hemorrhage)
      O72.2
    without hemorrhage O73.1
  products of conception
    early pregnancy (dead fetus) O02.1
    following
      delivery (with hemorrhage) O72.2
        without hemorrhage O73.1
  secundines (following delivery) (with
    hemorrhage) O72.0
    without hemorrhage O73.0
    complicating puerperium (delayed
      hemorrhage) O72.2
    partial O72.2
      without hemorrhage O73.1
  smegma, clitoris N90.89
  urine R33.9
    drug-induced R33.0
    due to hyperplasia (hypertrophy) of
      prostate —see Hyperplasia, prostate

Retention (Continued)
  urine (Continued)
    organic R33.8
      drug-induced R33.0
    psychogenic F45.8
    specified NEC R33.8
  water (in tissues) —see Edema
Reticular erythematous mucinosis L98.5
Reticulation, dust —see Pneumoconiosis
Reticulocytosis R70.1
Reticuloendotheliosis
  acute infantile C96.0
  leukemic C91.4-
  malignant C96.9
  nonlipid C96.0
Reticulohistiocytoma (giant-cell) D76.3
Reticuloid, actinic L57.1
Reticulosis (skin)
  acute of infancy C96.0
  hemophagocytic, familial D76.1
  histiocytic medullary C96.9
  lipomelanotic I89.8
  malignant (midline) C86.0
  nonlipid C96.0
  polymorphic C86.0
  Sézary —see Sézary disease
Retina, retinal —see also condition
  dark area D49.81
Retinitis —see also Inflammation, chorioretinal
  albuminurica N18.9 [H32]
  diabetic —see Diabetes, retinitis
  disciformis —see Degeneration, macula
  focal —see Inflammation, chorioretinal,
    focal
  gravidarum —see Pregnancy, complicated by,
    specified pregnancy-related condition
    NEC
  juxtapapillaris —see Inflammation,
    chorioretinal, focal, juxtapapillary
  luetic —see Retinitis, syphilitic
  pigmentosa H35.52
  proliferans —see Disorder, globe,
    degenerative, specified type NEC
  proliferating —see Disorder, globe,
    degenerative, specified type NEC
  renal N18.9 [H32]
  syphilitic (early) (secondary) A51.43
    central, recurrent A52.71
    congenital (early) A50.01 [H32]
    late A52.71
  tuberculous A18.53
Retinoblastoma C69.2-
  differentiated C69.2-
  undifferentiated C69.2-
Retinochoroiditis —see also Inflammation,
  chorioretinal
  disseminated —see Inflammation,
    chorioretinal, disseminated
    syphilitic A52.71
  focal —see Inflammation, chorioretinal
  juxtapapillaris —see Inflammation,
    chorioretinal, focal, juxtapapillary
Retinopathy (background) H35.00
  arteriosclerotic I70.8 [H35.0-]
  atherosclerotic I70.8 [H35.0-]
  central serous —see Chorioretinopathy,
    central serous
  Coats H35.02-
  diabetic —see Diabetes, retinopathy
  exudative H35.02-
  hypertensive H35.03-
  in (due to)
    diabetes —see Diabetes, retinopathy
    sickle-cell disorders D57.- [H36]
  of prematurity H35.10-
    stage 0 H35.11-
    stage 1 H35.12-
    stage 2 H35.13-
    stage 3 H35.14-
    stage 4 H35.15-
    stage 5 H35.16-

◀ New   ◀▦ Revised   ~~deleted~~ Deleted

Retinopathy (Continued)
  pigmentary, congenital —see Dystrophy, retina
  proliferative NEC H35.2-
    diabetic —see Diabetes, retinopathy, proliferative
    sickle-cell D57.- [H36]
  solar H31.02-
Retinoschisis H33.10-
  congenital Q14.1
  specified type NEC H33.19-
Retortamoniasis A07.8
Retractile testis Q55.22
Retraction
  cervix —see Retroversion, uterus
  drum (membrane) —see Disorder, tympanic membrane, specified NEC
  finger —see Deformity, finger
  lid H02.539
    left H02.536
      lower H02.535
      upper H02.534
    right H02.533
      lower H02.532
      upper H02.531
  lung J98.4
  mediastinum J98.5
  nipple N64.53
    associated with
      lactation O92.03
      pregnancy O92.01-
      puerperium O92.02
    congenital Q83.8
  palmar fascia M72.0
  pleura —see Pleurisy
  ring, uterus (Bandl's) (pathological) O62.4
  sternum (congenital) Q76.7
    acquired M95.4
  uterus —see Retroversion, uterus
  valve (heart) —see Endocarditis
Retrobulbar —see condition
Retrocecal —see condition
Retrocession —see Retroversion
Retrodisplacement —see Retroversion
Retroflection, retroflexion —see Retroversion
Retrognathia, retrognathism (mandibular) (maxillary) M26.19
Retrograde menstruation N92.5
Retroperineal —see condition
Retroperitoneal —see condition
Retroperitonitis K68.9
Retropharyngeal —see condition
Retroplacental —see condition
Retroposition —see Retroversion
Retroprosthetic membrane T85.398
Retrosternal thyroid (congenital) Q89.2
Retroversion, retroverted
  cervix —see Retroversion, uterus
  female NEC —see Retroversion, uterus
  iris H21.89
  testis (congenital) Q55.29
  uterus (acquired) (acute) (any degree) (asymptomatic) (cervix) (postinfectional) (postpartal, old) N85.4
    congenital Q51.818
    in pregnancy O34.53-
Retrovirus, as cause of disease classified elsewhere B97.30
  human
    immunodeficiency, type 2 (HIV 2) B97.35
    T-cell lymphotropic
      type I (HTLV-I) B97.33
      type II (HTLV-II) B97.34
  lentivirus B97.31
  oncovirus B97.32
  specified NEC B97.39
Retrusion, premaxilla (developmental) M26.09
Rett's disease or syndrome F84.2
Reverse peristalsis R19.2

Reye's syndrome G93.7
Rh (factor)
  hemolytic disease (newborn) P55.0
  incompatibility, immunization or sensitization
    affecting management of pregnancy NEC O36.09-
      anti-D antibody O36.01-
    newborn P55.0
    transfusion reaction —see Complication (s), transfusion, incompatibility reaction, Rh (factor)
  negative mother affecting newborn P55.0
  titer elevated —see Complication (s), transfusion, incompatibility reaction, Rh (factor)
  transfusion reaction —see Complication (s), transfusion, incompatibility reaction, Rh (factor)
Rhabdomyolysis (idiopathic) NEC M62.82
  traumatic T79.6
Rhabdomyoma —see also Neoplasm, connective tissue, benign
  adult —see Neoplasm, connective tissue, benign
  fetal —see Neoplasm, connective tissue, benign
  glycogenic —see Neoplasm, connective tissue, benign
Rhabdomyosarcoma (any type) —see Neoplasm, connective tissue, malignant
Rhabdosarcoma —see Rhabdomyosarcoma
Rhesus (factor) incompatibility —see Rh, incompatibility
Rheumatic (acute) (subacute) (chronic)
  adherent pericardium I09.2
  coronary arteritis I01.9
  degeneration, myocardium I09.0
  fever (acute) —see Fever, rheumatic
  heart —see Disease, heart, rheumatic
  myocardial degeneration —see Degeneration, myocardium
  myocarditis (chronic) (inactive) (with chorea) I09.0
    with chorea (acute) (rheumatic) (Sydenham's) I02.0
    active or acute I01.2
  pancarditis, acute I01.8
    with chorea (acute (rheumatic) Sydenham's) I02.0
  pericarditis (active) (acute) (with effusion) (with pneumonia) I01.0
    with chorea (acute) (rheumatic) (Sydenham's) I02.0
    chronic or inactive I09.2
  pneumonia I00 [J17]
  torticollis M43.6
  typhoid fever A01.09
Rheumatism (articular) (neuralgic) (nonarticular) M79.0
  gout —see Arthritis, rheumatoid
  intercostal, meaning Tietze's disease M94.0
  palindromic (any site) M12.30
    ankle M12.37-
    elbow M12.32-
    foot joint M12.37-
    hand joint M12.34-
    hip M12.35-
    knee M12.36-
    multiple site M12.39
    shoulder M12.31-
    specified joint NEC M12.38
    vertebrae M12.38 ◀
    wrist M12.33-
  sciatic M54.4-
Rheumatoid —see also condition
  arthritis —see also Arthritis, rheumatoid
    with involvement of organs NEC M05.60
      ankle M05.67-
      elbow M05.62-
      foot joint M05.67-
      hand joint M05.64-

Rheumatoid (Continued)
  arthritis (Continued)
    with involvement of organs NEC (Continued)
      hip M05.65-
      knee M05.66-
      multiple site M05.69
      shoulder M05.61-
      vertebra —see Spondylitis, ankylosing
      wrist M05.63-
    seronegative —see Arthritis, rheumatoid, seronegative
    seropositive —see Arthritis, rheumatoid, seropositive
  carditis M05.30
    ankle M05.37-
    elbow M05.32-
    foot joint M05.37-
    hand joint M05.34-
    hip M05.35-
    knee M05.36-
    multiple site M05.39
    shoulder M05.31-
    vertebra —see Spondylitis, ankylosing
    wrist M05.33-
  endocarditis —see Rheumatoid, carditis
  lung (disease) M05.10
    ankle M05.17-
    elbow M05.12-
    foot joint M05.17-
    hand joint M05.14-
    hip M05.15-
    knee M05.16-
    multiple site M05.19
    shoulder M05.11-
    vertebra —see Spondylitis, ankylosing
    wrist M05.13-
  myocarditis —see Rheumatoid, carditis
  myopathy M05.40
    ankle M05.47-
    elbow M05.42-
    foot joint M05.47-
    hand joint M05.44-
    hip M05.45-
    knee M05.46-
    multiple site M05.49
    shoulder M05.41-
    vertebra —see Spondylitis, ankylosing
    wrist M05.43-
  pericarditis —see Rheumatoid, carditis
  polyarthritis —see Arthritis, rheumatoid
  polyneuropathy M05.50
    ankle M05.57-
    elbow M05.52-
    foot joint M05.57-
    hand joint M05.54-
    hip M05.55-
    knee M05.56-
    multiple site M05.59
    shoulder M05.51-
    vertebra —see Spondylitis, ankylosing
    wrist M05.53-
  vasculitis M05.20
    ankle M05.27-
    elbow M05.22-
    foot joint M05.27-
    hand joint M05.24-
    hip M05.25-
    knee M05.26-
    multiple site M05.29
    shoulder M05.21-
    vertebra —see Spondylitis, ankylosing
    wrist M05.23-
Rhinitis (atrophic) (catarrhal) (chronic) (croupous) (fibrinous) (granulomatous) (hyperplastic) (hypertrophic) (membranous) (obstructive) (purulent) (suppurative) (ulcerative) J31.0
  with
    sore throat —see Nasopharyngitis
  acute J00

Rhinitis *(Continued)*
  allergic J30.9
    with asthma J45.909
      with
        exacerbation (acute) J45.901
        status asthmaticus J45.902
      due to
        food J30.5
        pollen J30.1
      nonseasonal J30.89
      perennial J30.89
      seasonal NEC J30.2
      specified NEC J30.89
  infective J00
  pneumococcal J00
  syphilitic A52.73
    congenital A50.05 *[J99]*
  tuberculous A15.8
  vasomotor J30.0
Rhinoantritis (chronic) —*see* Sinusitis,
    maxillary
Rhinodacryolith —*see* Dacryolith
Rhinolith (nasal sinus) J34.89
Rhinomegaly J34.89
Rhinopharyngitis (acute) (subacute) —*see also*
    Nasopharyngitis
  chronic J31.1
  destructive ulcerating A66.5
  mutilans A66.5
Rhinophyma L71.1
Rhinorrhea J34.89
  cerebrospinal (fluid) G96.0
  paroxysmal —*see* Rhinitis, allergic
  spasmodic —*see* Rhinitis, allergic
Rhinosalpingitis —*see* Salpingitis,
    eustachian
Rhinoscleroma A48.8
Rhinosporidiosis B48.1
Rhinovirus infection NEC B34.8
Rhizomelic chondrodysplasia punctata
    E71.540
Rhythm
  atrioventricular nodal I49.8
  disorder I49.9
    coronary sinus I49.8
    ectopic I49.8
    nodal I49.8
  escape I49.9
  heart, abnormal I49.9
  idioventricular I44.2
  nodal I49.8
  sleep, inversion G47.2-
    nonorganic origin —*see* Disorder, sleep,
        circadian rhythm, psychogenic
Rhytidosis facialis L98.8
Rib —*see also* condition
  cervical Q76.5
Riboflavin deficiency E53.0
Rice bodies —*see also* Loose, body, joint
  knee M23.4-
Richter syndrome —*see* Leukemia, chronic
    lymphocytic, B-cell type
Richter's hernia —*see* Hernia, abdomen, with
    obstruction
Ricinism —*see* Poisoning, food, noxious,
    plant
Rickets (active) (acute) (adolescent) (chest
    wall) (congenital) (current) (infantile)
    (intestinal) E55.0
  adult —*see* Osteomalacia
  celiac K90.0
  hypophosphatemic with nephrotic-glycosuric
    dwarfism E72.09
  inactive E64.3
  kidney N25.0
  renal N25.0
  sequelae, any E64.3
  vitamin-D-resistant E83.31 *[M90.80]*
Rickettsial disease A79.9
  specified type NEC A79.89
Rickettsialpox (Rickettsia akari) A79.1

Rickettsiosis A79.9
  due to
    Ehrlichia sennetsu A79.81
    Rickettsia akari (rickettsialpox) A79.1
  specified type NEC A79.89
  tick-borne A77.9
  vesicular A79.1
Rider's bone —*see* Ossification, muscle,
    specified NEC
Ridge, alveolus —*see also* condition
  flabby K06.8
Ridged ear, congenital Q17.3
Riedel's
  lobe, liver Q44.7
  struma, thyroiditis or disease E06.5
Rieger's anomaly or syndrome Q13.81
Riehl's melanosis L81.4
Rietti-Greppi-Micheli anemia D56.9
Rieux's hernia —*see* Hernia, abdomen, specified
    site NEC
Riga (-Fede) disease K14.0
Riggs' disease —*see* Periodontitis
Right middle lobe syndrome J98.11
Rigid, rigidity —*see also* condition
  abdominal R19.30
    with severe abdominal pain R10.0
      epigastric R19.36
      generalized R19.37
      left lower quadrant R19.34
      left upper quadrant R19.32
      periumbilic R19.35
      right lower quadrant R19.33
      right upper quadrant R19.31
  articular, multiple, congenital Q68.8
  cervix (uteri) in pregnancy —*see* Pregnancy,
    complicated by, abnormal, cervix
  hymen (acquired) (congenital) N89.6
  nuchal R29.1
  pelvic floor in pregnancy —*see* Pregnancy,
    complicated by, abnormal, pelvic organs
    or tissues NEC
  perineum or vulva in pregnancy —*see*
    Pregnancy, complicated by, abnormal,
    vulva
  spine —*see* Dorsopathy, specified NEC
  vagina in pregnancy —*see* Pregnancy,
    complicated by, abnormal, vagina
Rigors R68.89
  with fever R50.9
Riley-Day syndrome G90.1
RIND (reversible ischemic neurologic deficit)
    I63.9
Ring (s)
  aorta (vascular) Q25.4
  Bandl's O62.4
  contraction, complicating delivery O62.4
  esophageal, lower (muscular) K22.2
  Fleischer's (cornea) H18.04-
  hymenal, tight (acquired) (congenital)
    N89.6
  Kayser-Fleischer (cornea) H18.04-
  retraction, uterus, pathological O62.4
  Schatzki's (esophagus) (lower) K22.2
    congenital Q39.3
  Soemmerring's —*see* Cataract, secondary
  vascular (congenital) Q25.8
    aorta Q25.4
Ringed hair (congenital) Q84.1
Ringworm B35.9
  beard B35.0
  black dot B35.0
  body B35.4
  Burmese B35.5
  corporeal B35.4
  foot B35.3
  groin B35.6
  hand B35.2
  honeycomb B35.0
  nails B35.1
  perianal (area) B35.6
  scalp B35.0

Ringworm *(Continued)*
  specified NEC B35.8
  Tokelau B35.5
Rise, venous pressure I87.8
Risk, suicidal
  meaning personal history of attempted
    suicide Z91.5
  meaning suicidal ideation —*see* Ideation,
    suicidal
Ritter's disease L00
Rivalry, sibling Z62.891
Rivalta's disease A42.2
River blindness B73.01
Robert's pelvis Q74.2
  with disproportion (fetopelvic) O33.0
    causing obstructed labor O65.0
Robin (-Pierre) syndrome Q87.0
Robinow-Silvermann-Smith syndrome Q87.1
Robinson's (hidrotic) ectodermal dysplasia or
    syndrome Q82.4
Robles' disease B73.01
Rocky Mountain (spotted) fever A77.0
Roetheln —*see* Rubella
Roger's disease Q21.0
Rokitansky-Aschoff sinuses (gallbladder)
    K82.8
Rolando's fracture (displaced) S62.22-
    nondisplaced S62.22-
Romano-Ward (prolonged QT interval)
    syndrome I45.81
Romberg's disease or syndrome G51.8
Roof, mouth —*see* condition
Rosacea L71.9
  acne L71.9
  keratitis L71.8
  specified NEC L71.8
Rosary, rachitic E55.0
Rose
  cold J30.1
  fever J30.1
  rash R21
    epidemic B06.9
Rosenbach's erysipeloid A26.0
Rosenthal's disease or syndrome D68.1
Roseola B09
  infantum B08.20
    due to human herpesvirus 6 B08.21
    due to human herpesvirus 7 B08.22
Ross River disease or fever B33.1
Rossbach's disease K31.89
  psychogenic F45.8
Rostan's asthma (cardiac) —*see* Failure,
    ventricular, left
Rotation
  anomalous, incomplete or insufficient,
    intestine Q43.3
  cecum (congenital) Q43.3
  colon (congenital) Q43.3
  spine, incomplete or insufficient —*see*
    Dorsopathy, deforming, specified NEC
  tooth, teeth, fully erupted M26.35
  vertebra, incomplete or insufficient —*see*
    Dorsopathy, deforming, specified NEC
Rotes Quérol disease or syndrome —*see*
    Hyperostosis, ankylosing
Roth (-Bernhardt) disease or syndrome —*see*
    Meralgia paraesthetica
Rothmund (-Thomson) syndrome Q82.8
Rotor's disease or syndrome E80.6
Round
  back (with wedging of vertebrae) —*see*
    Kyphosis
  sequelae (late effect) of rickets E64.3
  worms (large) (infestation) NEC B82.0
    Ascariasis *(see also* Ascariasis) B77.9
Roussy-Lévy syndrome G60.0
Rubella (German measles) B06.9
  complication NEC B06.09
    neurological B06.00
  congenital P35.0
  contact Z20.4

Rubella *(Continued)*
  exposure to Z20.4
  maternal
    care for (suspected) damage to fetus O35.3
    manifest rubella in infant P35.0
    suspected damage to fetus affecting
      management of pregnancy O35.3
  specified complications NEC B06.89
Rubeola (meaning measles) —*see* Measles
  meaning rubella —*see* Rubella
Rubeosis, iris —*see* Disorder, iris, vascular
Rubinstein-Taybi syndrome Q87.2
Rudimentary (congenital) —*see also* Agenesis
  arm —*see* Defect, reduction, upper limb
  bone Q79.9
  cervix uteri Q51.828
  eye Q11.2
  lobule of ear Q17.3
  patella Q74.1
  respiratory organs in thoracopagus Q89.4
  tracheal bronchus Q32.4
  uterus Q51.818
    in male Q56.1
  vagina Q52.0
Ruled out condition —*see* Observation,
  suspected
Rumination R11.10
  with nausea R11.2
  disorder of infancy F98.21
  neurotic F42
  newborn P92.1
  obsessional F42
  psychogenic F42
Runeberg's disease D51.0
Runny nose R09.89
Rupia (syphilitic) A51.39
  congenital A50.06
  tertiary A52.79
Rupture, ruptured
  abscess (spontaneous) - code by site under
    Abscess
  aneurysm —*see* Aneurysm
  anus (sphincter) —*see* Laceration, anus
  aorta, aortic I71.8
    abdominal I71.3
    arch I71.1
    ascending I71.1
    descending I71.8
      abdominal I71.3
      thoracic I71.1
    syphilitic A52.01
    thoracoabdominal I71.5
    thorax, thoracic I71.1
    transverse I71.1
    traumatic —*see* Injury, aorta, laceration,
      major
    valve or cusp (*see also* Endocarditis, aortic)
      I35.8
  appendix (with peritonitis) K35.2
  arteriovenous fistula, brain I60.8
  artery I77.2
    brain —*see* Hemorrhage, intracranial,
      intracerebral
    coronary —*see* Infarct, myocardium
    heart —*see* Infarct, myocardium
    pulmonary I28.8
    traumatic (complication) —*see* Injury,
      blood vessel
  bile duct (common) (hepatic) K83.2
    cystic K82.2
  bladder (sphincter) (nontraumatic)
    (spontaneous) N32.89
    following ectopic or molar pregnancy
      O08.6
    obstetrical trauma O71.5
    traumatic S37.29
  blood vessel —*see also* Hemorrhage
    brain —*see* Hemorrhage, intracranial,
      intracerebral
    heart —*see* Infarct, myocardium
    traumatic (complication) —*see* Injury,
      blood vessel, laceration, major, by site

Rupture, ruptured *(Continued)*
  bone —*see* Fracture
  bowel (nontraumatic) K63.1
  brain
    aneurysm (congenital) —*see also*
      Hemorrhage, intracranial,
      subarachnoid
      syphilitic A52.05
    hemorrhagic —*see* Hemorrhage,
      intracranial, intracerebral
  capillaries I78.8
  cardiac (auricle) (ventricle) (wall) I23.3
    with hemopericardium I23.0
    infectional I40.9
    traumatic —*see* Injury, heart
  cartilage (articular) (current) —*see also* Sprain
    knee S83.3-
    semilunar —*see* Tear, meniscus
  cecum (with peritonitis) K65.0
    with peritoneal abscess K35.3
    traumatic S36.598
  celiac artery, traumatic —*see* Injury, blood
    vessel, celiac artery, laceration, major
  cerebral aneurysm (congenital) (*see*
    Hemorrhage, intracranial,
    subarachnoid)
  cervix (uteri)
    with ectopic or molar pregnancy O08.6
    following ectopic or molar pregnancy
      O08.6
    obstetrical trauma O71.3
    traumatic S37.69
  chordae tendineae NEC I51.1
    concurrent with acute myocardial
      infarction —*see* Infarct, myocardium
    following acute myocardial infarction
      (current complication) I23.4
  choroid (direct) (indirect) (traumatic) H31.32-
  circle of Willis I60.6
  colon (nontraumatic) K63.1
    traumatic —*see* Injury, intestine, large
  cornea (traumatic) —*see* Injury, eye, laceration
  coronary (artery) (thrombotic) —*see* Infarct,
    myocardium
  corpus luteum (infected) (ovary) N83.1
  cyst —*see* Cyst
  cystic duct K82.2
  Descemet's membrane —*see* Change, corneal
    membrane, Descemet's, rupture
    traumatic —*see* Injury, eye, laceration
  diaphragm, traumatic —*see* Injury,
    intrathoracic, diaphragm
  disc —*see* Rupture, intervertebral disc
  diverticulum (intestine) K57.80
    with bleeding K57.81
    bladder N32.3
    large intestine K57.20
      with
        bleeding K57.21
        small intestine K57.40
          with bleeding K57.41
    small intestine K57.00
      with
        bleeding K57.01
        large intestine K57.40
          with bleeding K57.41
  duodenal stump K31.89
  ear drum (nontraumatic) —*see also*
    Perforation, tympanum
    traumatic S09.2-
      due to blast injury —*see* Injury, blast, ear
  esophagus K22.3
  eye (without prolapse or loss of intraocular
    tissue) —*see* Injury, eye, laceration
  fallopian tube NEC (nonobstetric)
    (nontraumatic) N83.8
    due to pregnancy O00.1
  fontanel P13.1
  gallbladder K82.2
    traumatic S36.128
  gastric —*see also* Rupture, stomach
    vessel K92.2

Rupture, ruptured *(Continued)*
  globe (eye) (traumatic) —*see* Injury, eye,
    laceration
  graafian follicle (hematoma) N83.0
  heart —*see* Rupture, cardiac
  hymen (nontraumatic) (nonintentional)
    N89.8
  internal organ, traumatic —*see* Injury, by site
  intervertebral disc —*see* Displacement,
    intervertebral disc
    traumatic —*see* Rupture, traumatic,
      intervertebral disc
  intestine NEC (nontraumatic) K63.1
    traumatic —*see* Injury, intestine
  iris —*see also* Abnormality, pupillary
    traumatic —*see* Injury, eye, laceration
  joint capsule, traumatic —*see* Sprain
  kidney (traumatic) S37.06-
    birth injury P15.8
    nontraumatic N28.89
  lacrimal duct (traumatic) —*see* Injury, eye,
    specified site NEC
  lens (cataract) (traumatic) —*see* Cataract,
    traumatic
  ligament, traumatic —*see* Rupture, traumatic,
    ligament, by site
  liver S36.116
    birth injury P15.0
  lymphatic vessel I89.8
  marginal sinus (placental) (with
    hemorrhage) —*see* Hemorrhage,
    antepartum, specified cause NEC
  membrana tympani (nontraumatic) —*see*
    Perforation, tympanum
  membranes (spontaneous)
    artificial
      delayed delivery following O75.5
    delayed delivery following —*see*
      Pregnancy, complicated by,
      premature rupture of membranes
  meningeal artery I60.8
  meniscus (knee) —*see also* Tear, meniscus
    old —*see* Derangement, meniscus
    site other than knee - code as Sprain
  mesenteric artery, traumatic —*see* Injury,
    mesenteric, artery, laceration, major
  mesentery (nontraumatic) K66.8
    traumatic —*see* Injury, intra-abdominal,
      specified, site NEC
  mitral (valve) I34.8
  muscle (traumatic) —*see also* Strain
    diastasis —*see* Diastasis, muscle
    nontraumatic M62.10
      ankle M62.17-
      foot M62.17-
      forearm M62.13-
      hand M62.14-
      lower leg M62.16-
      pelvic region M62.15-
      shoulder region M62.11-
      specified site NEC M62.18
      thigh M62.15-
      upper arm M62.12-
    traumatic —*see* Strain, by site
  musculotendinous junction NEC,
    nontraumatic —*see* Rupture, tendon,
    spontaneous
  mycotic aneurysm causing cerebral
    hemorrhage —*see* Hemorrhage,
    intracranial, subarachnoid
  myocardium, myocardial —*see* Rupture,
    cardiac
    traumatic —*see* Injury, heart
  nontraumatic, meaning hernia —*see* Hernia
  obstructed —*see* Hernia, by site, obstructed
  operation wound —*see* Disruption, wound,
    operation
  ovary, ovarian N83.8
    corpus luteum cyst N83.1
    follicle (graafian) N83.0
  oviduct (nonobstetric) (nontraumatic) N83.8
    due to pregnancy O00.1

Rupture, ruptured *(Continued)*
  pancreas (nontraumatic) K86.8
    traumatic S36.299
  papillary muscle NEC I51.2
    following acute myocardial infarction
      (current complication) I23.5
  pelvic
    floor, complicating delivery O70.1
    organ NEC, obstetrical trauma O71.5
  perineum (nonobstetric) (nontraumatic)
    N90.89
    complicating delivery —*see* Delivery,
      complicated, by, laceration, anus
      (sphincter)
  postoperative wound —*see* Disruption,
    wound, operation
  prostate (traumatic) S37.828
  pulmonary
    artery I28.8
    valve (heart) I37.8
    vein I28.8
    vessel I28.8
  pus tube —*see* Salpingitis
  pyosalpinx —*see* Salpingitis
  rectum (nontraumatic) K63.1
    traumatic S36.69
  retina, retinal (traumatic) (without
    detachment) —*see also* Break, retina
    with detachment —*see* Detachment, retina,
      with retinal, break
  rotator cuff (nontraumatic) M75.10-
    complete M75.12-
    incomplete M75.11-
  sclera —*see* Injury, eye, laceration
  sigmoid (nontraumatic) K63.1
    traumatic S36.593
  spinal cord —*see also* Injury, spinal cord, by
    region
    due to injury at birth P11.5
    newborn (birth injury) P11.5
  spleen (traumatic) S36.09
    birth injury P15.1
    congenital (birth injury) P15.1
    due to P. vivax malaria B51.0
    nontraumatic D73.5
    spontaneous D73.5
  splenic vein R58
    traumatic —*see* Injury, blood vessel,
      ~~portal~~splenic vein ◀
  stomach (nontraumatic) (spontaneous)
    K31.89
    traumatic S36.39
  supraspinatus (complete) (incomplete)
    (nontraumatic) —*see* Tear, rotator
    cuff
  symphysis pubis
    obstetric O71.6
    traumatic S33.4
  synovium (cyst) M66.10
    ankle M66.17-
    elbow M66.12-
    finger M66.14-
    foot M66.17-
    forearm M66.13-
    hand M66.14-
    pelvic region M66.15-
    shoulder region M66.11-
    specified site NEC M66.18
    thigh M66.15-
    toe M66.17-
    upper arm M66.12-
    wrist M66.13-
  tendon (traumatic) —*see* Strain
    nontraumatic (spontaneous) M66.9
      ankle M66.87-
      extensor M66.20
        ankle M66.27-
        foot M66.27-
        forearm M66.23-
        hand M66.24-
        lower leg M66.26-
        multiple sites M66.29

Rupture, ruptured *(Continued)*
  tendon *(Continued)*
    nontraumatic *(Continued)*
      extensor *(Continued)*
        pelvic region M66.25-
        shoulder region M66.21-
        specified site NEC M66.28
        thigh M66.25-
        upper arm M66.22-
      flexor M66.30
        ankle M66.37-
        foot M66.37-
        forearm M66.33-
        hand M66.34-
        lower leg M66.36-
        multiple sites M66.39
        pelvic region M66.35-
        shoulder region M66.31-
        specified site NEC M66.38
        thigh M66.35-
        upper arm M66.32-
      foot M66.87-
      forearm M66.83-
      hand M66.84-
      lower leg M66.86-
      multiple sites M66.89
      pelvic region M66.85-
      shoulder region M66.81-
      specified
        site NEC M66.88
        tendon M66.80
      thigh M66.85-
      upper arm M66.82-
  thoracic duct I89.8
  tonsil J35.8
  traumatic
    aorta —*see* Injury, aorta, laceration, major
    diaphragm —*see* Injury, intrathoracic,
      diaphragm
    external site —*see* Wound, open, by site
    eye —*see* Injury, eye, laceration
    internal organ —*see* Injury, by site
    intervertebral disc
      cervical S13.0
      lumbar S33.0
      thoracic S23.0
    kidney S37.06-
    ligament —*see also* Sprain
      ankle —*see* Sprain, ankle
      carpus —*see* Rupture, traumatic,
        ligament, wrist
      collateral (hand) —*see* Rupture,
        traumatic, ligament, finger,
        collateral
      finger (metacarpophalangeal)
        (interphalangeal) S63.40-
        collateral S63.41-
          index S63.41-
          little S63.41-
          middle S63.41-
          ring S63.41-
        index S63.40-
        little S63.40-
        middle S63.40-
        palmar S63.42-
          index S63.42-
          little S63.42-
          middle S63.42-
          ring S63.42-
        ring S63.40-
        specified site NEC S63.499
          index S63.49-
          little S63.49-
          middle S63.49-
          ring S63.49-
        volar plate S63.43-
          index S63.43-
          little S63.43-
          middle S63.43-
          ring S63.43-
      foot —*see* Sprain, foot
      radial collateral S53.2-

Rupture, ruptured *(Continued)*
  traumatic *(Continued)*
    ligament *(Continued)*
      radiocarpal —*see* Rupture, traumatic,
        ligament, wrist, radiocarpal
      ulnar collateral S53.3-
      ulnocarpal —*see* Rupture, traumatic,
        ligament, wrist, ulnocarpal
      wrist S63.30-
        collateral S63.31-
        radiocarpal S63.32-
        specified site NEC S63.39-
        ulnocarpal (palmar) S63.33-
    liver S36.116
    membrana tympani —*see* Rupture, ear
      drum, traumatic
    muscle or tendon —*see* Strain
    myocardium —*see* Injury, heart
    pancreas S36.299
    rectum S36.69
    sigmoid S36.593
    spleen S36.09
    stomach S36.39
    symphysis pubis S33.4
    tympanum, tympanic (membrane) —*see*
      Rupture, ear drum, traumatic
    ureter S37.19
    uterus S37.69
    vagina —*see* Injury, vagina
    vena cava —*see* Injury, vena cava,
      laceration, major
  tricuspid (heart) (valve) I07.8
  tube, tubal (nonobstetric) (nontraumatic)
    N83.8
    abscess —*see* Salpingitis
    due to pregnancy O00.1
  tympanum, tympanic (membrane)
    (nontraumatic) (*see also* Perforation,
    tympanic membrane) H72.9-
    traumatic —*see* Rupture, ear drum,
      traumatic
  umbilical cord, complicating delivery
    O69.89
  ureter (traumatic) S37.19
    nontraumatic N28.89
  urethra (nontraumatic) N36.8
    with ectopic or molar pregnancy
      O08.6
    following ectopic or molar pregnancy
      O08.6
    obstetrical trauma O71.5
    traumatic S37.39
  uterosacral ligament (nonobstetric)
    (nontraumatic) N83.8
  uterus (traumatic) S37.69
    before labor O71.0-
    during or after labor O71.1
    nonpuerperal, nontraumatic N85.8
    pregnant (during labor) O71.1
      before labor O71.0-
  vagina —*see* Injury, vagina
  valve, valvular (heart) —*see* Endocarditis
  varicose vein —*see* Varix
  varix —*see* Varix
  vena cava R58
    traumatic —*see* Injury, vena cava,
      laceration, major
  vesical (urinary) N32.89
  vessel (blood) R58
    pulmonary I28.8
    traumatic —*see* Injury, blood vessel
  viscus R19.8
  vulva complicating delivery O70.0
Russell-Silver syndrome Q87.1
Russian spring-summer type encephalitis
  A84.0
Rust's disease (tuberculous cervical spondylitis)
  A18.01
Ruvalcaba-Myhre-Smith syndrome
  E71.440
Rytand-Lipsitch syndrome I44.2

◀ New   ◀≡ Revised   ~~deleted~~ Deleted

S

Saber, sabre shin or tibia (syphilitic) A50.56
  [M90.8-]
Sac lacrimal —see condition
Saccharomyces infection B37.9
Saccharopinuria E72.3
Saccular —see condition
Sacculation
  aorta (nonsyphilitic) —see Aneurysm,
    aorta
  bladder N32.3
  intralaryngeal (congenital) (ventricular)
    Q31.3
  larynx (congenital) (ventricular) Q31.3
  organ or site, congenital —see Distortion
  pregnant uterus —see Pregnancy, complicated
    by, abnormal, uterus
  ureter N28.89
  urethra N36.1
  vesical N32.3
Sachs' amaurotic familial idiocy or disease
    E75.02
Sachs-Tay disease E75.02
Sacks-Libman disease M32.11
Sacralgia M53.3
Sacralization Q76.49
Sacrodynia M53.3
Sacroiliac joint —see condition
Sacroiliitis NEC M46.1
Sacrum —see condition
Saddle
  back —see Lordosis
  embolus
    abdominal aorta I74.01
    pulmonary artery I26.92
      with acute cor pulmonale I26.02
  injury — code to condition
  nose M95.0
    due to syphilis A50.57
Sadism (sexual) F65.52
Sadness, postpartal O90.6
Sadomasochism F65.50
Saemisch's ulcer (cornea) —see Ulcer, cornea,
    central
Sahib disease B55.0
Sailors' skin L57.8
Saint
  Anthony's fire —see Erysipelas
  triad —see Hernia, diaphragm
  Vitus' dance —see Chorea, Sydenham's
Salaam
  attack (s) —see Epilepsy, spasms
  tic R25.8
Salicylism
  abuse F55.8
  overdose or wrong substance given —see
    Table of dDrugs and cChemicals, by
    drug, poisoning ◀▥▥
Salivary duct or gland —see condition
Salivation, excessive K11.7
Salmonella —see Infection, Salmonella
Salmonellosis A02.0
Salpingitis (catarrhal) (fallopian tube) (nodular)
    (pseudofollicular) (purulent) (septic)
    N70.91
  with oophoritis N70.93
  acute N70.01
    with oophoritis N70.03
  chlamydial A56.11
  chronic N70.11
    with oophoritis N70.13
  complicating abortion —see Abortion, by
    type, complicated by, salpingitis
  ear —see Salpingitis, eustachian
  eustachian (tube) H68.00-
    acute H68.01-
    chronic H68.02-
  follicularis N70.11
    with oophoritis N70.13
  gonococcal (acute) (chronic) A54.24

Salpingitis (Continued)
  interstitial, chronic N70.11
    with oophoritis N70.13
  isthmica nodosa N70.11
    with oophoritis N70.13
  specific (gonococcal) (acute) (chronic) A54.24
  tuberculous (acute) (chronic) A18.17
  venereal (gonococcal) (acute) (chronic) A54.24
Salpingocele N83.4
Salpingo-oophoritis (catarrhal) (purulent)
    (ruptured) (septic) (suppurative) N70.93
  acute N70.03
    with ectopic or molar pregnancy O08.0
    following ectopic or molar pregnancy
      O08.0
    gonococcal A54.24
  chronic N70.13
  following ectopic or molar pregnancy O08.0
  gonococcal (acute) (chronic) A54.24
  puerperal O86.19
  specific (gonococcal) (acute) (chronic) A54.24
  subacute N70.03
  tuberculous (acute) (chronic) A18.17
  venereal (gonococcal) (acute) (chronic)
    A54.24
Salpingo-ovaritis —see Salpingo-oophoritis
Salpingoperitonitis —see Salpingo-oophoritis
Salzmann's nodular dystrophy —see
    Degeneration, cornea, nodular
Sampson's cyst or tumor N80.1
San Joaquin (Valley) fever B38.0
Sandblaster's asthma, lung or pneumoconiosis
    J62.8
Sander's disease (paranoia) F22
Sandfly fever A93.1
Sandhoff's disease E75.01
Sanfilippo (Type B) (Type C) (Type D)
    syndrome E76.22
Sanger-Brown ataxia G11.2
Sao Paulo fever or typhus A77.0
Saponification, mesenteric K65.8
Sarcocele (benign)
  syphilitic A52.76
    congenital A50.59
Sarcocystosis A07.8
Sarcoepiplocele —see Hernia
Sarcoepiplomphalocele Q79.2
Sarcoid —see also Sarcoidosis
  arthropathy D86.86
  Boeck's D86.9
  Darier-Roussy D86.3
  iridocyclitis D86.83
  meningitis D86.81
  myocarditis D86.85
  myositis D86.87
  pyelonephritis D86.84
  Spiegler-Fendt L08.89
Sarcoidosis D86.9
  with
    cranial nerve palsies D86.82
    hepatic granuloma D86.89
    polyarthritis D86.86
    tubulo-interstitial nephropathy D86.84
  combined sites NEC D86.89
  lung D86.0
    and lymph nodes D86.2
  lymph nodes D86.1
    and lung D86.2
  meninges D86.81
  skin D86.3
  specified type NEC D86.89
Sarcoma (of) —see also Neoplasm, connective
    tissue, malignant
  alveolar soft part —see Neoplasm, connective
    tissue, malignant
  ameloblastic C41.1
    upper jaw (bone) C41.0
  botryoid —see Neoplasm, connective tissue,
    malignant
  botryoides —see Neoplasm, connective tissue,
    malignant

Sarcoma (Continued)
  cerebellar C71.6
    circumscribed (arachnoidal) C71.6
  circumscribed (arachnoidal) cerebellar
    C71.6
  clear cell —see also Neoplasm, connective
    tissue, malignant
    kidney C64.-
  dendritic cells (accessory cells) C96.4
  embryonal —see Neoplasm, connective tissue,
    malignant
  endometrial (stromal) C54.1
    isthmus C54.0
  epithelioid (cell) —see Neoplasm, connective
    tissue, malignant
  Ewing's —see Neoplasm, bone, malignant
  follicular dendritic cell C96.4
  germinoblastic (diffuse) —see Lymphoma,
    diffuse, large cell
    follicular —see Lymphoma, follicular,
      specified NEC
  giant cell (except of bone) —see also Neoplasm,
    connective tissue, malignant
    bone —see Neoplasm, bone, malignant
  glomoid —see Neoplasm, connective tissue,
    malignant
  granulocytic C92.3-
  hemangioendothelial —see Neoplasm,
    connective tissue, malignant
  hemorrhagic, multiple —see Sarcoma,
    Kaposi's
  histiocytic C96.A
  Hodgkin —see Lymphoma, Hodgkin
  immunoblastic (diffuse) —see Lymphoma,
    diffuse large cell
  interdigitating dendritic cell C96.4
  Kaposi's
    colon C46.4
    connective tissue C46.1
    gastrointestinal organ C46.4
    lung C46.5-
    lymph node (s) C46.3
    palate (hard) (soft) C46.2
    rectum C46.4
    skin C46.0
    specified site NEC C46.7
    stomach C46.4
    unspecified site C46.9
  Kupffer cell C22.3
  Langerhans cell C96.4
  leptomeningeal —see Neoplasm, meninges,
    malignant
  liver NEC C22.4
  lymphangioendothelial —see Neoplasm,
    connective tissue, malignant
  lymphoblastic —see Lymphoma,
    lymphoblastic (diffuse)
  lymphocytic —see Lymphoma, small cell
    B-cell
  mast cell C96.2
  melanotic —see Melanoma
  meningeal —see Neoplasm, meninges,
    malignant
  meningothelial —see Neoplasm, meninges,
    malignant
  mesenchymal —see also Neoplasm,
    connective tissue, malignant
    mixed —see Neoplasm, connective tissue,
      malignant
  mesothelial —see Mesothelioma
  monstrocellular
    specified site —see Neoplasm, malignant,
      by site
    unspecified site C71.9
  myeloid C92.3-
  neurogenic —see Neoplasm, nerve,
    malignant
  odontogenic C41.1
    upper jaw (bone) C41.0
  osteoblastic —see Neoplasm, bone,
    malignant

Sarcoma (*Continued*)
  osteogenic —*see also* Neoplasm, bone,
    malignant
    juxtacortical —*see* Neoplasm, bone,
      malignant
    periosteal —*see* Neoplasm, bone,
      malignant
  periosteal —*see also* Neoplasm, bone,
    malignant
    osteogenic —*see* Neoplasm, bone,
      malignant
  pleomorphic cell —*see* Neoplasm, connective
    tissue, malignant
  reticulum cell (diffuse) —*see* Lymphoma,
    diffuse large cell
    nodular —*see* Lymphoma, follicular
    pleomorphic cell type —*see* Lymphoma,
      diffuse large cell
  rhabdoid —*see* Neoplasm, malignant,
    by site
  round cell —*see* Neoplasm, connective tissue,
    malignant
  small cell —*see* Neoplasm, connective tissue,
    malignant
  soft tissue —*see* Neoplasm, connective tissue,
    malignant
  spindle cell —*see* Neoplasm, connective
    tissue, malignant
  stromal (endometrial) C54.1
    isthmus C54.0
  synovial —*see also* Neoplasm, connective
    tissue, malignant
    biphasic —*see* Neoplasm, connective tissue,
      malignant
    epithelioid cell —*see* Neoplasm, connective
      tissue, malignant
    spindle cell —*see* Neoplasm, connective
      tissue, malignant
Sarcomatosis
  meningeal —*see* Neoplasm, meninges,
    malignant
  specified site NEC —*see* Neoplasm,
    connective tissue, malignant
  unspecified site C80.1
Sarcosinemia E72.59
Sarcosporidiosis (intestinal) A07.8
Satiety, early R68.81
Saturnine —*see* condition
Saturnism
  overdose or wrong substance given or
    taken —*see* Table of ~~d~~Drugs and
    ~~c~~Chemicals, by drug, poisoning ◀▥
Satyriasis F52.8
Sauriasis —*see* Ichthyosis
SBE (subacute bacterial endocarditis) I33.0
Scabies (any site) B86
Scabs R23.4
Scaglietti-Dagnini syndrome E22.0
Scald —*see* Burn
Scalenus anticus (anterior) syndrome G54.0
Scales R23.4
Scaling, skin R23.4
Scalp —*see* condition
Scapegoating affecting child Z62.3
Scaphocephaly Q75.0
Scapulalgia M89.8X1
Scapulohumeral myopathy G71.0
Scar, scarring (*see also* Cicatrix) L90.5
  adherent L90.5
  atrophic L90.5
  cervix
    in pregnancy or childbirth —*see* Pregnancy,
      complicated by, abnormal cervix
  cheloid L91.0
  chorioretinal H31.00-
    posterior pole macula H31.01-
    postsurgical H59.81-
    solar retinopathy H31.02-
    specified type NEC H31.09-
  choroid —*see* Scar, chorioretinal
  conjunctiva H11.24-

Scar, scarring (*Continued*)
  cornea H17.9
    xerophthalmic —*see also* Opacity, cornea
      vitamin A deficiency E50.6
  duodenum, obstructive K31.5
  hypertrophic L91.0
  keloid L91.0
  labia N90.89
  lung (base) J98.4
  macula —*see* Scar, chorioretinal, posterior
    pole
  muscle M62.89
  myocardium, myocardial I25.2
  painful L90.5
  posterior pole (eye) —*see* Scar, chorioretinal,
    posterior pole
  retina —*see* Scar, chorioretinal
  trachea J39.8
  uterus N85.8
    in pregnancy O34.29
  vagina N89.8
    postoperative N99.2
  vulva N90.89
Scarabiasis B88.2
Scarlatina (anginosa) (maligna) (ulcerosa)
  A38.9
  myocarditis (acute) A38.1
    old —*see* Myocarditis
  otitis media A38.0
Scarlet fever (albuminuria) (angina) A38.9
Schamberg's disease (progressive pigmentary
  dermatosis) L81.7
Schatzki's ring (acquired) (esophagus) (lower)
  K22.2
  congenital Q39.3
Schaufenster krankheit I20.8
Schaumann's
  benign lymphogranulomatosis D86.1
  disease or syndrome —*see* Sarcoidosis
Scheie's syndrome E76.03
Schenck's disease B42.1
Scheuermann's disease or osteochondrosis —
  see Osteochondrosis, juvenile, spine
Schilder (-Flatau) disease G37.0
Schilling-type monocytic leukemia C93.0-
Schimmelbusch's disease, cystic mastitis, or
  hyperplasia —*see* Mastopathy, cystic
Schistosoma infestation —*see* Infestation,
  Schistosoma
Schistosomiasis B65.9
  with muscle disorder B65.9 [*M63.80*]
    ankle B65.9 [*M63.87-*]
    foot B65.9 [*M63.87-*]
    forearm B65.9 [*M63.83-*]
    hand B65.9 [*M63.84-*]
    lower leg B65.9 [*M63.86-*]
    multiple sites B65.9 [*M63.89*]
    pelvic region B65.9 [*M63.85-*]
    shoulder region B65.9 [*M63.81-*]
    specified site NEC B65.9 [*M63.88*]
    thigh B65.9 [*M63.85-*]
    upper arm B65.9 [*M63.82-*]
  Asiatic B65.2
  bladder B65.0
  chestermani B65.8
  colon B65.1
  cutaneous B65.3
  due to
    S. haematobium B65.0
    S. japonicum B65.2
    S. mansoni B65.1
    S. mattheii B65.8
  Eastern B65.2
  genitourinary tract B65.0
  intestinal B65.1
  lung NEC B65.9 [*J99*]
    pneumonia B65.9 [*J17*]
  Manson's (intestinal) B65.1
  oriental B65.2
  pulmonary NEC B65.9 [*J99*]
    pneumonia B65.9

Schistosomiasis (*Continued*)
  Schistosoma
    haematobium B65.0
    japonicum B65.2
    mansoni B65.1
  specified type NEC B65.8
  urinary B65.0
  vesical B65.0
Schizencephaly Q04.6
Schizoaffective psychosis F25.9
Schizodontia K00.2
Schizoid personality F60.1
Schizophrenia, schizophrenic F20.9
  acute (brief) (undifferentiated) F23
  atypical (form) F20.3
  borderline F21
  catalepsy F20.2
  catatonic (type) (excited) (withdrawn) F20.2
  cenesthopathic, cenesthesiopathic F20.89
  childhood type F84.5
  chronic undifferentiated F20.5
  cyclic F25.0
  disorganized (type) F20.1
  flexibilitas cerea F20.2
  hebephrenic (type) F20.1
  incipient F21
  latent F21
  negative type F20.5
  paranoid (type) F20.0
  paraphrenic F20.0
  post-psychotic depression F32.8
  prepsychotic F21
  prodromal F21
  pseudoneurotic F21
  pseudopsychopathic F21
  reaction F23
  residual (state) (type) F20.5
  restzustand F20.5
  schizoaffective (type) —*see* Psychosis,
    schizoaffective
  simple (type) F20.89
  simplex F20.89
  specified type NEC F20.89
  stupor F20.2
  syndrome of childhood F84.5
  undifferentiated (type) F20.3
    chronic F20.5
Schizothymia (persistent) F60.1
Schlatter-Osgood disease or
  osteochondrosis —*see* Osteochondrosis,
  juvenile, tibia
Schlatter's tibia —*see* Osteochondrosis,
  juvenile, tibia
Schmidt's syndrome (polyglandular,
  autoimmune) E31.0
Schmincke's carcinoma or tumor —*see*
  Neoplasm, nasopharynx, malignant
Schmitz (-Stutzer) dysentery A03.0
Schmorl's disease or nodes
  lumbar region M51.46
  lumbosacral region M51.47
  sacrococcygeal region M53.3
  thoracic region M51.44
  thoracolumbar region M51.45
Schneiderian
  papilloma —*see* Neoplasm, nasopharynx
    benign
      specified site —*see* Neoplasm, benign, by
        site
      unspecified site D14.0
    specified site —*see* Neoplasm, malignant, by
      site
    unspecified site C30.0
Scholte's syndrome (malignant carcinoid) E34.0
Scholz (-Bielchowsky-Henneberg) disease or
  syndrome E75.25
Schönlein (-Henoch) disease or purpura
  (primary) (rheumatic) D69.0
Schottmuller's disease A01.4
Schroeder's syndrome (endocrine
  hypertensive) E27.0

◀ New   ◀▥ Revised   ~~deleted~~ Deleted

Schüller-Christian disease or syndrome C96.5
Schultze's type acroparesthesia, simple I73.89
Schultz's disease or syndrome —*see*
    Agranulocytosis
Schwalbe-Ziehen-Oppenheim disease G24.1
Schwannoma —*see also* Neoplasm, nerve,
    benign
    malignant —*see also* Neoplasm, nerve,
        malignant
        with rhabdomyoblastic differentiation —
          see Neoplasm, nerve, malignant
    melanocytic —*see* Neoplasm, nerve, benign
    pigmented —*see* Neoplasm, nerve, benign
Schwannomatosis Q85.03
Schwartz (-Jampel) syndrome G71.13
Schwartz-Bartter syndrome E22.2
Schweniger-Buzzi anetoderma L90.1
Sciatic —*see* condition
Sciatica (infective)
    with lumbago M54.4-
        due to intervertebral disc disorder —*see*
          Disorder, disc, with, radiculopathy
    due to displacement of intervertebral disc
        (with lumbago) —*see* Disorder, disc,
        with, radiculopathy
    wallet M54.3-
Scimitar syndrome Q26.8
Sclera —*see* condition
Sclerectasia H15.84-
Scleredema
    adultorum —*see* Sclerosis, systemic
    Buschke's —*see* Sclerosis, systemic
    newborn P83.0
Sclerema (adiposum) (edematosum)
    (neonatorum) (newborn) P83.0
    adultorum —*see* Sclerosis, systemic
Scleriasis —*see* Scleroderma
Scleritis H15.00-
    with corneal involvement H15.04-
    anterior H15.01-
    brawny H15.02-
    in (due to) zoster B02.34
    posterior H15.03-
    specified type NEC H15.09-
    syphilitic A52.71
    tuberculous (nodular) A18.51
Sclerochoroiditis H31.8
Scleroconjunctivitis —*see* Scleritis
Sclerocystic ovary syndrome E28.2
Sclerodactyly, sclerodactylia L94.3
Scleroderma, sclerodermia (acrosclerotic)
    (diffuse) (generalized) (progressive)
    (pulmonary) (*see also* Sclerosis, systemic)
    M34.9- ◀|||
    circumscribed L94.0
    linear L94.1
    localized L94.0
    newborn P83.8
    systemic M34.9
Sclerokeratitis H16.8
    tuberculous A18.52
Scleroma nasi A48.8
Scleromalacia (perforans) H15.05-
Scleromyxedema L98.5
Sclérose en plaques G35
Sclerosis, sclerotic
    adrenal (gland) E27.8
    Alzheimer's —*see* Disease, Alzheimer's
    amyotrophic (lateral) G12.21
    aorta, aortic I70.0
        valve —*see* Endocarditis, aortic
    artery, arterial, arteriolar, arteriovascular —
        see Arteriosclerosis
    ascending multiple G35
    brain (generalized) (lobular) G37.9
        artery, arterial I67.2
        diffuse G37.0
        disseminated G35
        insular G35
        Krabbe's E75.23
        miliary G35

Sclerosis, sclerotic *(Continued)*
    brain *(Continued)*
        multiple G35
        presenile (Alzheimer's) —*see* Disease,
          Alzheimer's, early onset
        senile (arteriosclerotic) I67.2
        stem, multiple G35
        tuberous Q85.1
    bulbar, multiple G35
    bundle of His I44.39
    cardiac —*see* Disease, heart, ischemic,
        atherosclerotic
    cardiorenal —*see* Hypertension, cardiorenal
    cardiovascular —*see also* Disease,
        cardiovascular
        renal —*see* Hypertension, cardiorenal
    cerebellar —*see* Sclerosis, brain
    cerebral —*see* Sclerosis, brain
    cerebrospinal (disseminated) (multiple) G35
    cerebrovascular I67.2
    choroid —*see* Degeneration, choroid
    combined (spinal cord) —*see also*
        Degeneration, combined
        multiple G35
    concentric (Balo) G37.5
    cornea —*see* Opacity, cornea
    coronary (artery) I25.10
        with angina pectoris —*see* Arteriosclerosis,
          coronary (artery),
    corpus cavernosum
        female N90.89
        male N48.6
    diffuse (brain) (spinal cord) G37.0
    disseminated G35
    dorsal G35
    dorsolateral (spinal cord) —*see* Degeneration,
        combined
    endometrium N85.5
    extrapyramidal G25.9
    eye, nuclear (senile) —*see* Cataract, senile,
        nuclear
    focal and segmental (glomerular) (*see also*
        N00-N07 with fourth character .1)
        N05.1
    Friedreich's (spinal cord) G11.1
    funicular (spermatic cord) N50.8
    general (vascular) —*see* Arteriosclerosis
    gland (lymphatic) I89.8
    hepatic K74.1
        alcoholic K70.2
    hereditary
        cerebellar G11.9
        spinal (Friedreich's ataxia) G11.1
    hippocampal G93.81
    insular G35
    kidney —*see* Sclerosis, renal
    larynx J38.7
    lateral (amyotrophic) (descending) (primary)
        (spinal) G12.21
    lens, senile nuclear —*see* Cataract, senile,
        nuclear
    liver K74.1
        with fibrosis K74.2
          alcoholic K70.2
        alcoholic K70.2
        cardiac K76.1
    lung —*see* Fibrosis, lung
    mastoid —*see* Mastoiditis, chronic
    mesial temporal G93.81
    mitral I05.8
    Mönckeberg's (medial) —*see* Arteriosclerosis,
        extremities
    multiple (brain stem) (cerebral) (generalized)
        (spinal cord) G35
    myocardium, myocardial —*see* Disease, heart,
        ischemic, atherosclerotic
    nuclear (senile), eye —*see* Cataract, senile,
        nuclear
    ovary N83.8
    pancreas K86.8
    penis N48.6

Sclerosis, sclerotic *(Continued)*
    peripheral arteries —*see* Arteriosclerosis,
        extremities
    plaques G35
    pluriglandular E31.8
    polyglandular E31.8
    posterolateral (spinal cord) —*see*
        Degeneration, combined
    presenile (Alzheimer's) —*see* Disease,
        Alzheimer's, early onset
    primary, lateral G12.29
    progressive, systemic M34.0
    pulmonary —*see* Fibrosis, lung
        artery I27.0
        valve (heart) —*see* Endocarditis,
          pulmonary
    renal N26.9
        with
          cystine storage disease E72.09
          hypertensive heart disease (conditions
            in I11) —*see* Hypertension,
            cardiorenal
          arteriolar (hyaline) (hyperplastic) —*see*
            Hypertension, kidney
    retina (senile) (vascular) H35.00
    senile (vascular) —*see* Arteriosclerosis
    spinal (cord) (progressive) G95.89
        ascending G61.0
        combined —*see also* Degeneration,
          combined
          multiple G35
          syphilitic A52.11
        disseminated G35
        dorsolateral —*see* Degeneration, combined
        hereditary (Friedreich's) (mixed form)
          G11.1
        lateral (amyotrophic) G12.21
        multiple G35
        posterior (syphilitic) A52.11
    stomach K31.89
    subendocardial, congenital I42.4
    systemic M34.9
        with
          lung involvement M34.81
          myopathy M34.82
          polyneuropathy M34.83
        drug-induced M34.2
        due to chemicals NEC M34.2
        progressive M34.0
        specified NEC M34.89
    temporal (mesial) G93.81
    tricuspid (heart) (valve) I07.8
    tuberous (brain) Q85.1
    tympanic membrane —*see* Disorder,
        tympanic membrane, specified NEC
    valve, valvular (heart) —*see* Endocarditis
    vascular —*see* Arteriosclerosis
    vein I87.8
Scoliosis (acquired) (postural) M41.9
    adolescent (idiopathic) —*see* Scoliosis,
        idiopathic, juvenile
    congenital Q67.5
        due to bony malformation Q76.3
        failure of segmentation (hemivertebra)
          Q76.3
        hemivertebra fusion Q76.3
        postural Q67.5
    idiopathic M41.20
        adolescent M41.129
          cervical region M41.122
          cervicothoracic region M41.123
          lumbar region M41.126
          lumbosacral region M41.127
          thoracic region M41.124
          thoracolumbar region M41.125
        cervical region M41.22
        cervicothoracic region M41.23
        infantile M41.00
          cervical region M41.02
          cervicothoracic region M41.03
          lumbar region M41.06

Scoliosis (Continued)
  idiopathic (Continued)
    infantile (Continued)
      lumbosacral region M41.07
      sacrococcygeal region M41.08
      thoracic region M41.04
      thoracolumbar region M41.05
    juvenile M41.119
      cervical region M41.112
      cervicothoracic region M41.113
      lumbar region M41.116
      lumbosacral region M41.117
      thoracic region M41.114
      thoracolumbar region M41.115
    lumbar region M41.26
    lumbosacral region M41.27
    thoracic region M41.24
    thoracolumbar region M41.25
  neuromuscular M41.40
    cervical region M41.42
    cervicothoracic region M41.43
    lumbar region M41.46
    lumbosacral region M41.47
    occipito-atlanto-axial region M41.41
    thoracic region M41.44
    thoracolumbar region M41.45
  paralytic —see Scoliosis, neuromuscular
  postradiation therapy M96.5
  rachitic (late effect or sequelae) E64.3
      [M49.80]
    cervical region E64.3 [M49.82]
    cervicothoracic region E64.3 [M49.83]
    lumbar region E64.3 [M49.86]
    lumbosacral region E64.3 [M49.87]
    multiple sites E64.3 [M49.89]
    occipito-atlanto-axial region E64.3 [M49.81]
    sacrococcygeal region E64.3 [M49.88]
    thoracic region E64.3 [M49.84]
    thoracolumbar region E64.3 [M49.85]
  sciatic M54.4-
  secondary (to) NEC M41.50
    cerebral palsy, Friedreich's ataxia,
        poliomyelitis, neuromuscular
        disorders —see Scoliosis,
        neuromuscular
    cervical region M41.52
    cervicothoracic region M41.53
    lumbar region M41.56
    lumbosacral region M41.57
    thoracic region M41.54
    thoracolumbar region M41.55
  specified form NEC M41.80
    cervical region M41.82
    cervicothoracic region M41.83
    lumbar region M41.86
    lumbosacral region M41.87
    thoracic region M41.84
    thoracolumbar region M41.85
  thoracogenic M41.30
    thoracic region M41.34
    thoracolumbar region M41.35
  tuberculous A18.01
Scoliotic pelvis
  with disproportion (fetopelvic) O33.0
    causing obstructed labor O65.0
Scorbutus, scorbutic —see also Scurvy
  anemia D53.2
Scotoma (arcuate) (Bjerrum) (central) (ring) —
    see also Defect, visual field, localized,
    scotoma
  scintillating H53.19
Scratch —see Abrasion
Scratchy throat R09.89
Screening (for) Z13.9
  alcoholism Z13.89
  anemia Z13.0
  anomaly, congenital Z13.89
  antenatal, of mother Z36
  arterial hypertension Z13.6
  arthropod-borne viral disease NEC Z11.59
  bacteriuria, asymptomatic Z13.89

Screening (Continued)
  behavioral disorder Z13.89
  brain injury, traumatic Z13.850
  bronchitis, chronic Z13.83
  brucellosis Z11.2
  cardiovascular disorder Z13.6
  cataract Z13.5
  chlamydial diseases Z11.8
  cholera Z11.0
  chromosomal abnormalities (nonprocreative)
      NEC Z13.79
  colonoscopy Z12.11
  congenital
    dislocation of hip Z13.89
    eye disorder Z13.5
    malformation or deformation Z13.89
  contamination NEC Z13.88
  cystic fibrosis Z13.228
  dengue fever Z11.59
  dental disorder Z13.84
  depression Z13.89
  developmental handicap Z13.4
    in early childhood Z13.4
  diabetes mellitus Z13.1
  diphtheria Z11.2
  disability, intellectual Z13.4
  disease or disorder Z13.9
    bacterial NEC Z11.2
      intestinal infectious Z11.0
      respiratory tuberculosis Z11.1
    blood or blood-forming organ Z13.0
    cardiovascular Z13.6
    Chagas' Z11.6
    chlamydial Z11.8
    dental Z13.89
    developmental Z13.4
    digestive tract NEC Z13.818
      lower GI Z13.811
      upper GI Z13.810
    ear Z13.5
    endocrine Z13.29
    eye Z13.5
    genitourinary Z13.89
    heart Z13.6
    human immunodeficiency virus (HIV)
        infection Z11.4
    immunity Z13.0
    infection
      intestinal Z11.0
        specified NEC Z11.6
    infectious Z11.9
    mental Z13.89
    metabolic Z13.228
    neurological Z13.89
    nutritional Z13.21
      metabolic Z13.228
        lipid disorders Z13.220
    protozoal Z11.6
      intestinal Z11.0
    respiratory Z13.83
    rheumatic Z13.828
    rickettsial Z11.8
    sexually-transmitted NEC Z11.3
      human immunodeficiency virus (HIV)
          Z11.4
    sickle-cell (trait) Z13.0
    skin Z13.89
    specified NEC Z13.89
    spirochetal Z11.8
    thyroid Z13.29
    vascular Z13.6
    venereal Z11.3
    viral NEC Z11.59
      human immunodeficiency virus (HIV)
          Z11.4
      intestinal Z11.0
  elevated titer Z13.89
  emphysema Z13.83
  encephalitis, viral (mosquito- or tick-borne)
      Z11.59
  exposure to contaminants (toxic) Z13.88

Screening (Continued)
  fever
    dengue Z11.59
    hemorrhagic Z11.59
    yellow Z11.59
  filariasis Z11.6
  galactosemia Z13.228
  gastrointestinal condition Z13.818
  genetic (nonprocreative)- for procreative
      management —see Testing, genetic, for
      procreative management
    disease carrier status (nonprocreative)
        Z13.71
    specified NEC (nonprocreative) Z13.79
  genitourinary condition Z13.89
  glaucoma Z13.5
  gonorrhea Z11.3
  gout Z13.89
  helminthiasis (intestinal) Z11.6
  hematopoietic malignancy Z12.89
  hemoglobinopathies NEC Z13.0
  hemorrhagic fever Z11.59
  Hodgkin disease Z12.89
  human immunodeficiency virus (HIV)
      Z11.4
  human papillomavirus Z11.51
  hypertension Z13.6
  immunity disorders Z13.0
  infection
    mycotic Z11.8
    parasitic Z11.8
  ingestion of radioactive substance Z13.88
  intellectual disability Z13.4
  intestinal
    helminthiasis Z11.6
    infectious disease Z11.0
  leishmaniasis Z11.6
  leprosy Z11.2
  leptospirosis Z11.8
  leukemia Z12.89
  lymphoma Z12.89
  malaria Z11.6
  malnutrition Z13.29
    metabolic Z13.228
    nutritional Z13.21
  measles Z11.59
  mental disorder Z13.89
  metabolic errors, inborn Z13.228
  multiphasic Z13.89
  musculoskeletal disorder Z13.828
    osteoporosis Z13.820
  mycoses Z11.8
  myocardial infarction (acute) Z13.6
  neoplasm (malignant) (of) Z12.9
    bladder Z12.6
    blood Z12.89
    breast Z12.39
      routine mammogram Z12.31
    cervix Z12.4
    colon Z12.11
    genitourinary organs NEC Z12.79
      bladder Z12.6
      cervix Z12.4
      ovary Z12.73
      prostate Z12.5
      testis Z12.71
      vagina Z12.72
    hematopoietic system Z12.89
    intestinal tract Z12.10
      colon Z12.11
      rectum Z12.12
      small intestine Z12.13
    lung Z12.2
    lymph (glands) Z12.89
    nervous system Z12.82
    oral cavity Z12.81
    prostate Z12.5
    rectum Z12.12
    respiratory organs Z12.2
    skin Z12.83
    small intestine Z12.13

◀ New   ◀▥ Revised   deleted Deleted

Screening *(Continued)*
  neoplasm *(Continued)*
    specified site NEC Z12.89
    stomach Z12.0
  nephropathy Z13.89
  nervous system disorders NEC Z13.858
  neurological condition Z13.89
  osteoporosis Z13.820
  parasitic infestation Z11.9
    specified NEC Z11.8
  phenylketonuria Z13.228
  plague Z11.2
  poisoning (chemical) (heavy metal)
    Z13.88
  poliomyelitis Z11.59
  postnatal, chromosomal abnormalities
    Z13.89
  prenatal, of mother Z36
  protozoal disease Z11.6
    intestinal Z11.0
  pulmonary tuberculosis Z11.1
  radiation exposure Z13.88
  respiratory condition Z13.83
  respiratory tuberculosis Z11.1
  rheumatoid arthritis Z13.828
  rubella Z11.59
  schistosomiasis Z11.6
  sexually-transmitted disease NEC Z11.3
    human immunodeficiency virus (HIV)
      Z11.4
  sickle-cell disease or trait Z13.0
  skin condition Z13.89
  sleeping sickness Z11.6
  special Z13.9
    specified NEC Z13.89
  syphilis Z11.3
  tetanus Z11.2
  trachoma Z11.8
  traumatic brain injury Z13.850
  trypanosomiasis Z11.6
  tuberculosis, respiratory Z11.1
  venereal disease Z11.3
  viral encephalitis (mosquito- or tick-borne)
    Z11.59
  whooping cough Z11.2
  worms, intestinal Z11.6
  yaws Z11.8
  yellow fever Z11.59
Scrofula, scrofulosis (tuberculosis of cervical
  lymph glands) A18.2
Scrofulide (primary) (tuberculous) A18.4
Scrofuloderma, scrofulodermia (any site)
  (primary) A18.4
Scrofulosus lichen (primary) (tuberculous)
  A18.4
Scrofulous —*see* condition
Scrotal tongue K14.5
Scrotum —*see* condition
Scurvy, scorbutic E54
  anemia D53.2
  gum E54
  infantile E54
  rickets E55.0 [M90.80]
Sealpox B08.62
Seasickness T75.3
Seatworm (infection) (infestation) B80
Sebaceous —*see also* condition
  cyst —*see* Cyst, sebaceous
Seborrhea, seborrheic L21.9
  capillitii R23.8
  capitis L21.0
  dermatitis L21.9
    infantile L21.1
  eczema L21.9
    infantile L21.1
  sicca L21.0
Seckel's syndrome Q87.1
Seclusion, pupil —*see* Membrane, pupillary
Second hand tobacco smoke exposure (acute)
  (chronic) Z77.22
  in the perinatal period P96.81

Secondary
  dentin (in pulp) K04.3
  neoplasm, secondaries —*see* Table of
    Neoplasms, secondary
Secretion
  antidiuretic hormone, inappropriate E22.2
  catecholamine, by pheochromocytoma
    E27.5
  hormone
    antidiuretic, inappropriate (syndrome)
      E22.2
    by
      carcinoid tumor E34.0
      pheochromocytoma E27.5
    ectopic NEC E34.2
  urinary
    excessive R35.8
    suppression R34
Section
  nerve, traumatic —*see* Injury, nerve
Segmentation, incomplete (congenital) —*see
  also* Fusion
  bone NEC Q78.8
  lumbosacral (joint) (vertebra) Q76.49
Seitelberger's syndrome (infantile neuraxonal
  dystrophy) G31.89
Seizure (s) (*see also* Convulsions) R56.9
  akinetic —*see* Epilepsy, generalized, specified
    NEC
  atonic —*see* Epilepsy, generalized, specified
    NEC
  autonomic (hysterical) F44.5
  convulsive —*see* Convulsions
  cortical (focal) (motor) —*see* Epilepsy,
    localization-related, symptomatic, with
    simple partial seizures
  disorder (*see also* Epilepsy) G40.909
  due to stroke —*see* Sequelae (of), disease,
    cerebrovascular, by type, specified
    NEC
  epileptic —*see* Epilepsy
  febrile (simple) R56.00
    with status epilepticus G40.901
    complex (atypical) (complicated)
      R56.01
      with status epilepticus G40.901
  grand mal G40.409
    intractable G40.419
      with status epilepticus G40.411
      without status epilepticus G40.419
    not intractable G40.409
      with status epilepticus G40.401
      without status epilepticus G40.409
  heart —*see* Disease, heart
  hysterical F44.5
  intractable G40.919
    with status epilepticus G40.911
  Jacksonian (focal) (motor type) (sensory
    type) —*see* Epilepsy, localization-
    related, symptomatic, with simple
    partial seizures
  newborn P90
  nonspecific epileptic
    atonic —*see* Epilepsy, generalized, specified
      NEC
    clonic —*see* Epilepsy, generalized, specified
      NEC
    myoclonic —*see* Epilepsy, generalized,
      specified NEC
    tonic —*see* Epilepsy, generalized, specified
      NEC
    tonic-clonic —*see* Epilepsy, generalized,
      specified NEC
  partial, developing into secondarily
    generalized seizures
    complex —*see* Epilepsy, localization-
      related, symptomatic, with complex
      partial seizures
    simple —*see* Epilepsy, localization-related,
      symptomatic, with simple partial
      seizures

Seizure *(Continued)*
  petit mal G40.409
    intractable G40.419
      with status epilepticus G40.411
      without status epilepticus G40.419
    not intractable G40.409
      with status epilepticus G40.401
      without status epilepticus G40.409
  post traumatic R56.1
  recurrent G40.909
  specified NEC G40.89
  uncinate —*see* Epilepsy, localization-related,
    symptomatic, with complex partial
    seizures
Selenium deficiency, dietary E59
Self-damaging behavior (life-style) Z72.89
Self-harm (attempted)
  history (personal) Z91.5
  in family Z81.8
Self-mutilation (attempted)
  history (personal) Z91.5
  in family Z81.8
Self-poisoning
  history (personal) Z91.5
  in family Z81.8
  observation following (alleged) attempt Z03.6
Semicoma R40.1
Seminal vesiculitis N49.0
Seminoma C62.9-
  specified site —*see* Neoplasm, malignant, by
    site
Senear-Usher disease or syndrome L10.4
Senectus R54
Senescence (without mention of psychosis) R54
Senile, senility (*see also* condition) R41.81
  with
    acute confusional state F05
    mental changes NOS F03
    psychosis NEC —*see* Psychosis, senile
  asthenia R54
  cervix (atrophic) N88.8
  debility R54
  endometrium (atrophic) N85.8
  fallopian tube (atrophic) —*see* Atrophy,
    fallopian tube
  heart (failure) R54
  ovary (atrophic) —*see* Atrophy, ovary
  premature E34.8
  vagina, vaginitis (atrophic) N95.2
  wart L82.1
Sensation
  burning (skin) R20.8
    tongue K14.6
  loss of R20.8
  prickling (skin) R20.2
  tingling (skin) R20.2
Sense loss
  smell —*see* Disturbance, sensation, smell
  taste —*see* Disturbance, sensation, taste
  touch R20.8
Sensibility disturbance (cortical) (deep)
  (vibratory) R20.9
Sensitive, sensitivity —*see also* Allergy
  carotid sinus G90.01
  child (excessive) F93.8
  cold, autoimmune D59.1
  dentin K03.89
  latex Z91.040
  methemoglobin D74.8
  tuberculin, without clinical or radiological
    symptoms R76.11
  visual
    glare H53.71
    impaired contrast H53.72
Sensitiver Beziehungswahn F22
Sensitization, auto-erythrocytic D69.2
Separation
  anxiety, abnormal (of childhood) F93.0
  apophysis, traumatic - code as Fracture, by
    site
  choroid —*see* Detachment, choroid

Separation *(Continued)*
 epiphysis, epiphyseal
  nontraumatic —*see also*
    Osteochondropathy, specified type
     NEC
   upper femoral —*see* Slipped, epiphysis,
     upper femoral
  traumatic - code as Fracture, by site
 fracture —*see* Fracture
 infundibulum cardiac from right ventricle by
   a partition Q24.3
 joint (traumatic) (current) - code by site under
   Dislocation
 pubic bone, obstetrical trauma O71.6
 retina, retinal —*see* Detachment, retina
 symphysis pubis, obstetrical trauma O71.6
 tracheal ring, incomplete, congenital Q32.1
Sepsis (generalized) (unspecified organism)
  A41.9
 with
  organ dysfunction (acute) (multiple) R65.20
   with septic shock R65.21
 actinomycotic A42.7
 adrenal hemorrhage syndrome
   (meningococcal) A39.1
 anaerobic A41.4
 Bacillus anthracis A22.7
 Brucella (*see also* Brucellosis) A23.9
 candidal B37.7
 cryptogenic A41.9
 due to device, implant or graft T85.79
  arterial graft NEC T82.8
  breast (implant) T85.79
  catheter NEC T85.79
   dialysis (renal) T82.7
    intraperitoneal T85.71
   infusion NEC T82.7
    spinal (epidural) (subdural) T85.79
   urinary (indwelling) T83.51
  ectopic or molar pregnancy O08.82
  electronic (electrode) (pulse generator)
    (stimulator)
   bone T84.7
   cardiac T82.7
   nervous system (brain) (peripheral
     nerve) (spinal) T85.79
   urinary T83.59
  fixation, internal (orthopedic) —*see*
    Complication, fixation device,
    infection
  gastrointestinal (bile duct) (esophagus)
    T85.79
  genital T83.6
  heart NEC T82.7
   valve (prosthesis) T82.6
    graft T82.7
  joint prosthesis —*see* Complication, joint
    prosthesis, infection
  ocular (corneal graft) (orbital implant)
    T85.79
  orthopedic NEC T84.7
   fixation device, internal —*see*
     Complication, fixation device,
     infection
  specified NEC T85.79
  vascular T82.7
  ventricular intracranial shunt T85.79
 during labor O75.3
 Enterococcus A41.81
 Erysipelothrix (rhusiopathiae) (erysipeloid)
   A26.7
 Escherichia coli (E. coli) A41.5
 extraintestinal yersiniosis A28.2
 following
  abortion (subsequent episode) O08.0
   current episode —*see* Abortion
  ectopic or molar pregnancy O08.82
  immunization T88.0
  infusion, therapeutic injection or
    transfusion NEC T80.29
 gangrenous A41.9

Sepsis *(Continued)*
 gonococcal A54.86
 Gram-negative (organism) A41.5
  anaerobic A41.4
 Haemophilus influenzae A41.3
 herpesviral B00.7
 intra-abdominal K65.1
 intraocular —*see* Endophthalmitis, purulent
 Listeria monocytogenes A32.7
 localized — code to specific localized
   infection
  in operation wound T81.4
  skin —*see* Abscess
 malleus A24.0
 melioidosis A24.1
 meningeal —*see* Meningitis
 meningococcal A39.4
  acute A39.2
  chronic A39.3
 MSSA (Methicillin susceptible
   Staphylococcus aureus) A41.01
 newborn P36.9
  due to
   anaerobes NEC P36.5
   Escherichia coli P36.4
   Staphylococcus P36.30
    aureus P36.2
    specified NEC P36.39
   Streptococcus P36.10
    group B P36.0
    specified NEC P36.19
  specified NEC P36.8
 Pasteurella multocida A28.0
 pelvic, puerperal, postpartum, childbirth O85
 pneumococcal A40.3
 postprocedural T81.4
 puerperal, postpartum, childbirth (pelvic)
   O85
 Salmonella (arizonae) (cholerae-suis)
   (enteritidis) (typhimurium) A02.1
 severe R65.20
  with septic shock R65.21
 Shigella (*see also* Dysentery, bacillary) A03.9
 skin, localized —*see* Abscess
 specified organism NEC A41.89
 Staphylococcus, staphylococcal A41.2
  aureus (methicillin susceptible) (MSSA)
    A41.01
   methicillin resistant (MRSA) A41.02
  coagulase-negative A41.1
  specified NEC A41.1
 Streptococcus, streptococcal A40.9
  agalactiae A40.1
  group
   A A40.0
   B A40.1
   D A41.81
  neonatal P36.10
   group B P36.0
   specified NEC P36.19
  pneumoniae A40.3
  pyogenes A40.0
  specified NEC A40.8
 tracheostomy stoma J95.02
 tularemic A21.7
 umbilical, umbilical cord (newborn) —*see*
   Sepsis, newborn
 Yersinia pestis A20.7
Septate —*see* Septum
Septic —*see* condition
 arm —*see* Cellulitis, upper limb
  with lymphangitis —*see* Lymphangitis,
    acute, upper limb
 embolus —*see* Embolism
 finger —*see* Cellulitis, digit
  with lymphangitis —*see* Lymphangitis,
    acute, digit
 foot —*see* Cellulitis, lower limb
  with lymphangitis —*see* Lymphangitis,
    acute, lower limb
 gallbladder (acute) K81.0

Septic *(Continued)*
 hand —*see* Cellulitis, upper limb
  with lymphangitis —*see* Lymphangitis,
    acute, upper limb
 joint —*see* Arthritis, pyogenic or pyemic
 leg —*see* Cellulitis, lower limb
  with lymphangitis —*see* Lymphangitis,
    acute, lower limb
 nail —*see also* Cellulitis, digit
  with lymphangitis —*see* Lymphangitis,
    acute, digit
 sore —*see also* Abscess
  throat J02.0
   streptococcal J02.0
 spleen (acute) D73.89
 teeth, tooth (pulpal origin) K04.4
 throat —*see* Pharyngitis
 thrombus —*see* Thrombosis
 toe —*see* Cellulitis, digit
  with lymphangitis —*see* Lymphangitis,
    acute, digit
 tonsils, chronic J35.01
  with adenoiditis J35.03
 uterus —*see* Endometritis
Septicemia A41.9
 meaning sepsis —*see* Sepsis
Septum, septate (congenital) —*see also*
  Anomaly, by site
 anal Q42.3
  with fistula Q42.2
 aqueduct of Sylvius Q03.0
  with spina bifida —*see* Spina bifida, by site,
    with hydrocephalus
 uterus (complete) (partial) Q51.2
 vagina Q52.10
  in pregnancy —*see* Pregnancy, complicated
    by, abnormal vagina
   causing obstructed labor O65.5
  longitudinal (with or without obstruction)
    Q52.12
  transverse Q52.11
Sequelae (of) —*see also* condition
 abscess, intracranial or intraspinal (conditions
   in G06) G09
 amputation — code to injury with seventh
   character S
 burn and corrosion — code to injury with
   seventh character S
 calcium deficiency E64.8
 cerebrovascular disease —*see* Sequelae,
   disease, cerebrovascular
 childbirth O94
 contusion — code to injury with seventh
   character S
 corrosion —*see* Sequelae, burn and
   corrosion
 crushing injury — code to injury with
   seventh character S
 disease
  cerebrovascular I69.90
   alteration of sensation I69.998
   aphasia I69.920
   apraxia I69.990
   ataxia I69.993
   cognitive deficits I69.91
   disturbance of vision I69.998
   dysarthria I69.922
   dysphagia I69.991
   dysphasia I69.921
   facial droop I69.992
   facial weakness I69.992
   fluency disorder I69.923
   hemiplegia I69.95-
   hemorrhage
    intracerebral —*see* Sequelae,
      hemorrhage, intracerebral
    intracranial, nontraumatic NEC —
      see Sequelae, hemorrhage,
      intracranial, nontraumatic
    subarachnoid —*see* Sequelae,
      hemorrhage, subarachnoid

Sequelae *(Continued)*
  disease *(Continued)*
    cerebrovascular *(Continued)*
      language deficit I69.928
      monoplegia
        lower limb I69.84-
        upper limb I69.93-
      paralytic syndrome I69.96-
      specified effect NEC I69.998
      specified type NEC I69.80
        alteration of sensation I69.898
        aphasia I69.820
        apraxia I69.890
        ataxia I69.893
        cognitive deficits I69.81
        disturbance of vision I69.898
        dysarthria I69.822
        dysphagia I69.891
        dysphasia I69.821
        facial droop I69.892
        facial weakness I69.892
        fluency disorder I69.823
        hemiplegia I69.85-
        language deficit I69.828
        monoplegia
          lower limb I69.84-
          upper limb I69.83-
        paralytic syndrome I69.86-
        specified effect NEC I69.898
      speech deficit I69.928
      speech deficit I69.828
      stroke NOS —*see* Sequelae, stroke
          NOS
  dislocation — code to injury with seventh
      character S
  encephalitis or encephalomyelitis (conditions
      in G04) G09
    in infectious disease NEC B94.8
    viral B94.1
  external cause — code to injury with seventh
      character S
  foreign body entering natural orifice — code
      to injury with seventh character S
  fracture — code to injury with seventh
      character S
  frostbite — code to injury with seventh
      character S
  Hansen's disease B92
  hemorrhage
    intracerebral I69.10
      alteration of sensation I69.198
      aphasia I69.120
      apraxia I69.190
      ataxia I69.193
      cognitive deficits I69.11
      disturbance of vision I69.198
      dysarthria I69.122
      dysphagia I69.191
      dysphasia I69.121
      facial droop I69.192
      facial weakness I69.192
      fluency disorder I69.123
      hemiplegia I69.15-
      language deficit NEC I69.128
      monoplegia
        lower limb I69.14-
        upper limb I69.13-
      paralytic syndrome I69.16-
      specified effect NEC I69.198
      speech deficit NEC I69.128
    intracranial, nontraumatic NEC I69.20
      alteration of sensation I69.298
      aphasia I69.220
      apraxia I69.290
      ataxia I69.293
      cognitive deficits I69.21
      disturbance of vision I69.298
      dysarthria I69.222
      dysphagia I69.291
      dysphasia I69.221
      facial droop I69.292

Sequelae *(Continued)*
  hemorrhage *(Continued)*
    intracranial, nontraumatic NEC
        (Continued)
      facial weakness I69.292
      fluency disorder I69.223
      hemiplegia I69.25-
      language deficit NEC I69.228
      monoplegia
        lower limb I69.24-
        upper limb I69.23-
      paralytic syndrome I69.26-
      specified effect NEC I69.298
      speech deficit NEC I69.228
    subarachnoid I69.00
      alteration of sensation I69.098
      aphasia I69.020
      apraxia I69.090
      ataxia I69.093
      cognitive deficits I69.01
      disturbance of vision I69.098
      dysarthria I69.022
      dysphagia I69.091
      dysphasia I69.021
      facial droop I69.092
      facial weakness I69.092
      fluency disorder I69.023
      hemiplegia I69.05-
      language deficit NEC I69.028
      monoplegia
        lower limb I69.04-
        upper limb I69.03-
      paralytic syndrome I69.06-
      specified effect NEC I69.098
      speech deficit NEC I69.028
  hepatitis, viral B94.2
  hyperalimentation E68
  infarction
    cerebral I69.30
      alteration of sensation I69.398
      aphasia I69.320
      apraxia I69.390
      ataxia I69.393
      cognitive deficits I69.31
      disturbance of vision I69.398
      dysarthria I69.322
      dysphagia I69.391
      dysphasia I69.321
      facial droop I69.392
      facial weakness I69.392
      fluency disorder I69.323
      hemiplegia I69.35-
      language deficit NEC I69.328
      monoplegia
        lower limb I69.34-
        upper limb I69.33-
      paralytic syndrome I69.36-
      specified effect NEC I69.398
      speech deficit NEC I69.328
  infection, pyogenic, intracranial or intraspinal
      G09
  infectious disease B94.9
    specified NEC B94.8
  injury — code to injury with seventh
      character S
  leprosy B92
  meningitis
    bacterial (conditions in G00) G09
    other or unspecified cause (conditions in
        G03) G09
  muscle (and tendon) injury — code to injury
      with seventh character S
  myelitis —*see* Sequelae, encephalitis
  niacin deficiency E64.8
  nutritional deficiency E64.9
    specified NEC E64.8
  obstetrical condition O94
  parasitic disease B94.9
  phlebitis or thrombophlebitis of intracranial
      or intraspinal venous sinuses and veins
      (conditions in G08) G09

Sequelae *(Continued)*
  poisoning — code to poisoning with seventh
      character S
    nonmedicinal substance —*see* Sequelae,
        toxic effect, nonmedicinal substance
  poliomyelitis (acute) B91
  pregnancy O94
  protein-energy malnutrition E64.0
  puerperium O94
  rickets E64.3
  selenium deficiency E64.8
  sprain and strain — code to injury with
      seventh character S
  stroke NOS I69.30
    alteration in sensation I69.398
    aphasia I69.320
    apraxia I69.390
    ataxia I69.393
    cognitive deficits I69.31
    disturbance of vision I69.398
    dysarthria I69.322
    dysphagia I69.391
    dysphasia I69.321
    facial droop I69.392
    facial weakness I69.392
    hemiplegia I69.35-
    language deficit NEC I69.328
    monoplegia
      lower limb I69.34-
      upper limb I69.33-
    paralytic syndrome I69.36-
    specified effect NEC I69.398
    speech deficit NEC I69.328
  tendon and muscle injury — code to injury
      with seventh character S
  thiamine deficiency E64.8
  trachoma B94.0
  tuberculosis B90.9
    bones and joints B90.2
    central nervous system B90.0
    genitourinary B90.1
    pulmonary (respiratory) B90.9
    specified organs NEC B90.8
  viral
    encephalitis B94.1
    hepatitis B94.2
  vitamin deficiency NEC E64.8
    A E64.1
    B E64.8
    C E64.2
  wound, open — code to injury with seventh
      character S
Sequestration —*see also* Sequestrum
  lung, congenital Q33.2
Sequestrum
  bone —*see* Osteomyelitis, chronic
  dental M27.2
  jaw bone M27.2
  orbit —*see* Osteomyelitis, orbit
  sinus (accessory) (nasal) —*see* Sinusitis
Sequoiosis lung or pneumonitis J67.8
Serology for syphilis
  doubtful
    with signs or symptoms - code by site and
        stage under Syphilis
    follow-up of latent syphilis —*see* Syphilis,
        latent
  negative, with signs or symptoms — code by
      site and stage under Syphilis
  positive A53.0
    with signs or symptoms - code by site and
        stage under Syphilis
  reactivated A53.0
Seroma —*see also* Hematoma
  traumatic, secondary and recurrent
      T79.2
Seropurulent —*see* condition
Serositis, multiple K65.8
  pericardial I31.1
  peritoneal K65.8
Serous —*see* condition

Sertoli cell
　adenoma
　　specified site —see Neoplasm, benign, by
　　　site
　　unspecified site
　　　female D27.9
　　　male D29.20
　carcinoma
　　specified site —see Neoplasm, malignant,
　　　by site
　　unspecified site (male) C62.9-
　　　female C56.9
　tumor
　　with lipid storage
　　　specified site —see Neoplasm, benign,
　　　　by site
　　　unspecified site
　　　　female D27.9
　　　　male D29.20
　　specified site —see Neoplasm, benign, by
　　　site
　　unspecified site
　　　female D27.9
　　　male D29.20
Sertoli-Leydig cell tumor —see Neoplasm,
　benign, by site
　specified site —see Neoplasm, benign,
　　by site
　unspecified site
　　female D27.9
　　male D29.20
Serum
　allergy, allergic reaction (see also Reaction,
　　serum) T80.69
　　shock (see also Shock, anaphylactic) T80.59
　arthritis (see also Reaction, serum) T80.69
　complication or reaction NEC (see also
　　Reaction, serum) T80.69
　disease NEC (see also Reaction, serum) T80.69
　hepatitis —see also Hepatitis, viral, type B
　　carrier (suspected) of Z22.51
　intoxication (see also Reaction, serum) T80.69
　neuritis (see also Reaction, serum) T80.69
　neuropathy G61.1
　poisoning NEC (see also Reaction, serum)
　　T80.69
　rash NEC (see also Reaction, serum) T80.69
　reaction NEC (see also Reaction, serum)
　　T80.69
　sickness NEC (see also Reaction, serum)
　　T80.69
　urticaria (see also Reaction, serum) T80.69
Sesamoiditis ~~—see Osteomyelitis, specified type~~
　~~NEC~~M25.8- ◄▥
Sever's disease or osteochondrosis —see
　Osteochondrosis, juvenile, tarsus
Severe sepsis R65.20
　with septic shock R65.21
Sex
　chromosome mosaics Q97.8
　　lines with various numbers of
　　　X chromosomes Q97.2
　education Z70.8
　reassignment surgery status Z87.890
Sextuplet pregnancy —see Pregnancy, sextuplet
Sexual
　function, disorder of (psychogenic) F52.9
　immaturity (female) E30.0
　impotence (psychogenic) organic origin
　　NEC —see Dysfunction, sexual, male
　precocity (constitutional) (cryptogenic)
　　(female) (idiopathic) (male) E30.1
Sexuality, pathologic —see Deviation, sexual
Sézary disease C84.1-
Shadow, lung R91.8
Shaking palsy or paralysis —see Parkinsonism
Shallowness, acetabulum —see Derangement,
　joint, specified type NEC, hip
Shaver's disease J63.1
Sheath (tendon) —see condition
Sheathing, retinal vessels H35.01-

Shedding
　nail L60.8
　premature, primary (deciduous) teeth K00.6
Sheehan's disease or syndrome E23.0
Shelf, rectal K62.89
Shell teeth K00.5
Shellshock (current) F43.0
　lasting state —see Disorder, post-traumatic
　　stress
Shield kidney Q63.1
Shift
　auditory threshold (temporary) H93.24-
　mediastinal R93.8
Shifting sleep-work schedule (affecting sleep)
　G47.26
Shiga (-Kruse) dysentery A03.0
Shiga's bacillus A03.0
Shigella (dysentery) —see Dysentery, bacillary
Shigellosis A03.9
　Group A A03.0
　Group B A03.1
　Group C A03.2
　Group D A03.3
Shin splints S86.89 ◄▥
Shingles —see Herpes, zoster
Shipyard disease or eye B30.0
Shirodkar suture, in pregnancy —see
　Pregnancy, complicated by, incompetent
　cervix
Shock R57.9
　with ectopic or molar pregnancy O08.3
　adrenal (cortical) (Addisonian) E27.2
　adverse food reaction (anaphylactic) —see
　　Shock, anaphylactic, due to food
　allergic —see Shock, anaphylactic
　anaphylactic T78.2
　　chemical —see Table of dDrugs and
　　　eChemicals ◄▥
　　due to drug or medicinal substance
　　　correct substance properly administered
　　　　T88.6
　　　overdose or wrong substance given or
　　　　taken (by accident) —see Table of
　　　　dDrugs and eChemicals, by drug,
　　　　poisoning ◄▥
　　due to food (nonpoisonous) T78.00
　　　additives T78.06
　　　dairy products T78.07
　　　eggs T78.08
　　　fish T78.03
　　　　shellfish T78.02
　　　fruit T78.04
　　　milk T78.07
　　　nuts T78.05
　　　　peanuts T78.01
　　　peanuts T78.01
　　　seeds T78.05
　　　specified type NEC T78.09
　　　vegetable T78.04
　　following sting (s) —see Venom
　　immunization T80.52
　　serum T80.59
　　　blood and blood products T80.51
　　　immunization T80.52
　　　specified NEC T80.59
　　　vaccination T80.52
　anaphylactoid —see Shock, anaphylactic
　anesthetic
　　correct substance properly administered
　　　T88.2
　　overdose or wrong substance given or
　　　taken —see Table of dDrugs and
　　　eChemicals, by drug, poisoning ◄▥
　　specified anesthetic —see Table of
　　　dDrugs and eChemicals, by drug,
　　　poisoning ◄▥
　cardiogenic R57.0
　chemical substance —see Table of dDrugs and
　　eChemicals ◄▥
　complicating ectopic or molar pregnancy O08.3
　culture —see Disorder, adjustment

Shock (Continued)
　drug
　　due to correct substance properly
　　　administered T88.6
　　overdose or wrong substance given or
　　　taken (by accident) —see Table of
　　　dDrugs and eChemicals, by drug,
　　　poisoning ◄▥
　during or after labor and delivery O75.1
　electric T75.4
　　(taser) T75.4
　endotoxic R65.21
　　postprocedural (during or resulting from a
　　　procedure, not elsewhere classified)
　　　T81.12
　following
　　ectopic or molar pregnancy O08.3
　　injury (immediate) (delayed) T79.4
　　labor and delivery O75.1
　food (anaphylactic) —see Shock, anaphylactic,
　　due to food
　from electroshock gun (taser) T75.4
　gram-negative R65.21
　　postprocedural (during or resulting from a
　　　procedure, not elsewhere classified)
　　　T81.12
　hematologic R57.8
　hemorrhagic
　　surgery (intraoperative) (postoperative)
　　　T81.19
　　trauma T79.4
　hypovolemic R57.1
　　surgical T81.19
　　traumatic T79.4
　insulin E15
　　therapeutic misadventure —see
　　　subcategory T38.3
　kidney N17.0
　　traumatic (following crushing) T79.5
　lightning T75.01
　lung J80
　obstetric O75.1
　　with ectopic or molar pregnancy O08.3
　　following ectopic or molar pregnancy
　　　O08.3
　pleural (surgical) T81.19
　　due to trauma T79.4
　postprocedural (postoperative) T81.10
　　with ectopic or molar pregnancy O08.3
　　cardiogenic T81.11
　　endotoxic T81.12
　　following ectopic or molar pregnancy
　　　O08.3
　　gram-negative T81.12
　　hypovolemic T81.19
　　septic T81.12
　　specified type NEC T81.19
　psychic F43.0
　septic (due to severe sepsis) R65.21
　specified NEC R57.8
　surgical T81.10
　taser gun (taser) T75.4
　therapeutic misadventure NEC T81.10
　thyroxin
　　overdose or wrong substance given or
　　　taken —see Table of dDrugs and
　　　eChemicals, by drug, poisoning ◄▥
　toxic, syndrome A48.3
　transfusion —see Complications, transfusion
　traumatic (immediate) (delayed) T79.4
Shoemaker's chest M95.4
Short, shortening, shortness
　arm (acquired) —see also Deformity, limb,
　　unequal length
　　congenital Q71.81-
　　forearm —see Deformity, limb, unequal
　　　length
　bowel syndrome K91.2
　breath R06.02
　cervical (complicating pregnancy) O26.87-
　　non-gravid uterus N88.3

◄ New　◄▥ Revised　~~deleted~~ Deleted

Short, shortening, shortness *(Continued)*
  common bile duct, congenital Q44.5
  cord (umbilical), complicating delivery O69.3
  cystic duct, congenital Q44.5
  esophagus (congenital) Q39.8
  femur (acquired) —*see* Deformity, limb, unequal length, femur
    congenital —*see* Defect, reduction, lower limb, longitudinal, femur
  frenum, frenulum, linguae (congenital) Q38.1
  hip (acquired) —*see also* Deformity, limb, unequal length
    congenital Q65.89
  leg (acquired) —*see also* Deformity, limb, unequal length
    congenital Q72.81-
    lower leg —*see also* Deformity, limb, unequal length
  limbed stature, with immunodeficiency D82.2
  lower limb (acquired) —*see also* Deformity, limb, unequal length
    congenital Q72.81-
  organ or site, congenital NEC —*see* Distortion
  palate, congenital Q38.5
  radius (acquired) —*see also* Deformity, limb, unequal length
    congenital —*see* Defect, reduction, upper limb, longitudinal, radius
  rib syndrome Q77.2
  stature (child) (hereditary) (idiopathic) NEC R62.52
    constitutional E34.3
    due to endocrine disorder E34.3
    Laron-type E34.3
  tendon —*see also* Contraction, tendon
    with contracture of joint —*see* Contraction, joint
    Achilles (acquired) M67.0-
      congenital Q66.89
    congenital Q79.8
  thigh (acquired) —*see also* Deformity, limb, unequal length, femur
    congenital —*see* Defect, reduction, lower limb, longitudinal, femur
  tibialis anterior (tendon) —*see* Contraction, tendon
  umbilical cord
    complicating delivery O69.3
  upper limb, congenital —*see* Defect, reduction, upper limb, specified type NEC
  urethra N36.8
  uvula, congenital Q38.5
  vagina (congenital) Q52.4
Shortsightedness —*see* Myopia
Shoshin (acute fulminating beriberi) E51.11
Shoulder —*see* condition
Shovel-shaped incisors K00.2
Shower, thromboembolic —*see* Embolism
Shunt
  arterial-venous (dialysis) Z99.2
  arteriovenous, pulmonary (acquired) I28.0
    congenital Q25.72
  cerebral ventricle (communicating) in situ Z98.2
  surgical, prosthetic, with complications —*see* Complications, cardiovascular, device or implant Shutdown, renal N28.9
Shutdown, renal N28.9
Shy-Drager syndrome G90.3
Sialadenitis, sialadenosis (any gland) (chronic) (periodic) (suppurative) —*see* Sialoadenitis
Sialectasia K11.8
Sialidosis E77.1
Sialitis, silitis (any gland) (chronic) (suppurative) —*see* Sialoadenitis
Sialoadenitis (any gland) (periodic) (suppurative) K11.20
  acute K11.21
    recurrent K11.22
  chronic K11.23

Sialoadenopathy K11.9
Sialoangitis —*see* Sialoadenitis
Sialodochitis (fibrinosa) —*see* Sialoadenitis
Sialodocholithiasis K11.5
Sialolithiasis K11.5
Sialometaplasia, necrotizing K11.8
Sialorrhea —*see also* Ptyalism
  periodic —*see* Sialoadenitis
Sialosis K11.7
Siamese twin Q89.4
Sibling rivalry Z62.891
Sicard's syndrome G52.7
Sicca syndrome M35.00
  with
    keratoconjunctivitis M35.01
    lung involvement M35.02
    myopathy M35.03
    renal tubulo-interstitial disorders M35.04
    specified organ involvement NEC M35.09
Sick R69
  or handicapped person in family Z63.79
    needing care at home Z63.6
  sinus (syndrome) I49.5
Sick-euthyroid syndrome E07.81
Sickle-cell
  anemia —*see* Disease, sickle-cell
  trait D57.3
Sicklemia —*see also* Disease, sickle-cell
  trait D57.3
Sickness
  air (travel) T75.3
  airplane T75.3
  alpine T70.29
  altitude T70.20
  Andes T70.29
  aviator's T70.29
  balloon T70.29
  car T75.3
  compressed air T70.3
  decompression T70.3
  green D50.8
  milk —*see* Poisoning, food, noxious
  motion T75.3
  mountain T70.29
    acute D75.1
  protein *(see also* Reaction, serum) T80.69
  radiation T66
  roundabout (motion) T75.3
  sea T75.3
  serum NEC *(see also* Reaction, serum) T80.69
  sleeping (African) B56.9
    by Trypanosoma B56.9
      brucei
        gambiense B56.0
        rhodesiense B56.1
    East African B56.1
    Gambian B56.0
    Rhodesian B56.1
    West African B56.0
  swing (motion) T75.3
  train (railway) (travel) T75.3
  travel (any vehicle) T75.3
Sideropenia —*see* Anemia, iron deficiency
Siderosilicosis J62.8
Siderosis (lung) J63.4
  eye (globe) —*see* Disorder, globe, degenerative, siderosis
Siemens' syndrome (ectodermal dysplasia) Q82.8
Sighing R06.89
  psychogenic F45.8
Sigmoid —*see also* condition
  flexure —*see* condition
  kidney Q63.1
Sigmoiditis *(see also* Enteritis) K52.9
  infectious A09
  noninfectious K52.9
Silfversköld's syndrome Q78.9
Silicosiderosis J62.8
Silicosis, silicotic (simple) (complicated) J62.8
  with tuberculosis J65
Silicotuberculosis J65

Silo-fillers' disease J68.8
  bronchitis J68.0
  pneumonitis J68.0
  pulmonary edema J68.1
Silver's syndrome Q87.1
Simian malaria B53.1
Simmonds' cachexia or disease E23.0
Simons' disease or syndrome (progressive lipodystrophy) E88.1
Simple, simplex —*see* condition
Simulation, conscious (of illness) Z76.5
Simultanagnosia (asimultagnosia) R48.3
Sin Nombre virus disease (Hantavirus) (cardio)-pulmonary syndrome B33.4
Sinding-Larsen disease or osteochondrosis — *see* Osteochondrosis, juvenile, patella
Singapore hemorrhagic fever A91
Singer's node or nodule J38.2
Single
  atrium Q21.2
  coronary artery Q24.5
  umbilical artery Q27.0
  ventricle Q20.4
Singultus R06.6
  epidemicus B33.0
Sinus —*see also* Fistula
  abdominal K63.89
  arrest I45.5
  arrhythmia I49.8
  bradycardia R00.1
  branchial cleft (internal) (external) Q18.0
  coccygeal —*see* Sinus, pilonidal
  dental K04.6
  dermal (congenital) Q06.8
    with abscess Q06.8
    coccygeal, pilonidal —*see* Sinus, coccygeal
  infected, skin NEC L08.89
  marginal, ruptured or bleeding —*see* Hemorrhage, antepartum, specified cause NEC
  medial, face and neck Q18.8
  pause I45.5
  pericranii Q01.9
  pilonidal (infected) (rectum) L05.92
    with abscess L05.02
  preauricular Q18.1
  rectovaginal N82.3
  Rokitansky-Aschoff (gallbladder) K82.8
  sacrococcygeal (dermoid) (infected) —*see* Sinus, pilonidal
  tachycardia R00.0
    paroxysmal I47.1
  tarsi syndrome —*see* Syndrome, tarsal tunnel M25.57- ◄⫶⫶⫶
  testis N50.8
  tract (postinfective) —*see* Fistula
  urachus Q64.4
Sinusitis (accessory) (chronic) (hyperplastic) (nasal) (nonpurulent) (purulent) J32.9
  acute J01.90
    ethmoidal J01.20
      recurrent J01.21
    frontal J01.10
      recurrent J01.11
    involving more than one sinus, other than pansinusitis J01.80
      recurrent J01.81
    maxillary J01.00
      recurrent J01.01
    pansinusitis J01.40
      recurrent J01.41
    recurrent J01.91
    specified NEC J01.80
      recurrent J01.81
    sphenoidal J01.30
      recurrent J01.31
  allergic —*see* Rhinitis, allergic
  due to high altitude T70.1
  ethmoidal J32.2
    acute J01.20
      recurrent J01.21

Sinusitis (Continued)
  frontal J32.1
    acute J01.10
      recurrent J01.11
  influenzal —see Influenza, with, respiratory
    manifestations NEC
  involving more than one sinus but not
    pansinusitis J32.8
    acute J01.80
      recurrent J01.81
  maxillary J32.0
    acute J01.00
      recurrent J01.01
  sphenoidal J32.3
    acute J01.30
      recurrent J01.31
  tuberculous, any sinus A15.8
Sinusitis-bronchiectasis-situs inversus
  (syndrome) (triad) Q89.3
Sipple's syndrome E31.22
Sirenomelia (syndrome) Q87.2
Siriasis T67.0
Sirkari's disease B55.0
Siti A65
Situation, psychiatric F99
Situational
  disturbance (transient) —see Disorder,
    adjustment
    acute F43.0
  maladjustment —see Disorder, adjustment
  reaction —see Disorder, adjustment
    acute F43.0
Situs inversus or transversus (abdominalis)
  (thoracis) Q89.3
Sixth disease B08.20
  due to human herpesvirus 6 B08.21
  due to human herpesvirus 7 B08.22
Sjögren-Larsson syndrome Q87.1
Sjögren's syndrome or disease —see Sicca
  syndrome
Skeletal —see condition
Skene's gland —see condition
Skenitis —see Urethritis
Skerljevo A65
Skevas-Zerfus disease —see Toxicity, venom,
  marine animal, sea anemone
Skin —see also condition
  clammy R23.1
  donor —see Donor, skin
  hidebound M35.9
Slate-dressers' or slate-miners' lung J62.8
Sleep
  apnea —see Apnea, sleep
  deprivation Z72.820
  disorder or disturbance G47.9
    child F51.9
    nonorganic origin F51.9
    specified NEC G47.8
  disturbance G47.9
    nonorganic origin F51.9
  drunkenness F51.9
  rhythm inversion G47.2-
  terrors F51.4
  walking F51.3
    hysterical F44.89
Sleep hygiene
  abuse Z72.821
  inadequate Z72.821
  poor Z72.821
Sleeping sickness —see Sickness, sleeping
Sleeplessness —see Insomnia
  menopausal N95.11
Sleep-wake schedule disorder G47.20
Slim disease (in HIV infection) B20
Slipped, slipping
  epiphysis (traumatic) —see also
    Osteochondropathy, specified type
    NEC
    capital femoral (traumatic)
      acute (on chronic) S79.01-
      current traumatic - code as Fracture, by site

Slipped, slipping (Continued)
  epiphysis (Continued)
    upper femoral (nontraumatic) M93.00-
      acute M93.01-
        on chronic M93.03-
      chronic M93.02-
  intervertebral disc —see Displacement,
    intervertebral disc
  ligature, umbilical P51.8
  patella —see Disorder, patella, derangement
    NEC
  rib M89.8X8
  sacroiliac joint —see subcategory M53.2
  tendon —see Disorder, tendon
  ulnar nerve, nontraumatic —see Lesion,
    nerve, ulnar
  vertebra NEC —see Spondylolisthesis
Slocumb's syndrome E27.0
Sloughing (multiple) (phagedena) (skin) —see
  also Gangrene
  abscess —see Abscess
  appendix K38.8
  fascia —see Disorder, soft tissue, specified
    type NEC
  scrotum N50.8
  tendon —see Disorder, tendon
  transplanted organ —see Rejection, transplant
  ulcer —see Ulcer, skin
Slow
  feeding, newborn P92.2
  flow syndrome, coronary I20.8
  heart(beat) R00.1
Slowing, urinary stream R39.19
Sluder's neuralgia (syndrome) G44.89
Slurred, slurring speech R47.81
Small (ness)
  for gestational age —see Small for dates
  introitus, vagina N89.6
  kidney (unknown cause) N27.9
    bilateral N27.1
    unilateral N27.0
  ovary (congenital) Q50.39
  pelvis
    with disproportion (fetopelvic) O33.1
      causing obstructed labor O65.1
  uterus N85.8
  white kidney N03.9
Small-and-light-for-dates —see Small for
  dates
Small-for-dates (infant) P05.10
  with weight of
    499 grams or less P05.11
    500-749 grams P05.12
    750-999 grams P05.13
    1000-1249 grams P05.14
    1250-1499 grams P05.15
    1500-1749 grams P05.16
    1750-1999 grams P05.17
    2000-2499 grams P05.18
Smallpox B03
Smearing, fecal R15.1
Smith-Lemli-Opitz syndrome E78.72
Smith's fracture S52.54-
Smoker —see Dependence, drug, nicotine
Smoker's
  bronchitis J41.0
  cough J41.0
  palate K13.24
  throat J31.2
  tongue K13.24
Smoking
  passive Z77.22
Smothering spells R06.81
Snaggle teeth, tooth M26.39
Snapping
  finger —see Trigger finger
  hip —see Derangement, joint, specified type
    NEC, hip
    involving the iliotibial band M76.3-
  knee —see Derangement, knee
    involving the iliotibial band M76.3-

Sneddon-Wilkinson disease or syndrome (sub-
  corneal pustular dermatosis) L13.1
Sneezing (intractable) R06.7
Sniffing
  cocaine
    abuse —see Abuse, drug, cocaine
    dependence —see Dependence, drug,
      cocaine
  gasoline
    abuse —see Abuse, drug, inhalant
    dependence —see Dependence, drug,
      inhalant
  glue (airplane)
    abuse —see Abuse, drug, inhalant
    drug dependence —see Dependence, drug,
      inhalant
Sniffles
  newborn P28.89
Snoring R06.83
Snow blindness —see Photokeratitis
Snuffles (non-syphilitic) R06.5
  newborn P28.89
  syphilitic (infant) A50.05 [99]
Social
  exclusion Z60.4
    due to discrimination or persecution
      (perceived) Z60.5
  migrant Z59.0
    acculturation difficulty Z60.3
  rejection Z60.4
    due to discrimination or persecution
      Z60.5
  role conflict NEC Z73.5
  skills inadequacy NEC Z73.4
  transplantation Z60.3
Sodoku A25.0
Soemmerring's ring —see Cataract, secondary
Soft —see also condition
  nails L60.3
Softening
  bone —see Osteomalacia
  brain (necrotic) (progressive) G93.89
    congenital Q04.8
    embolic I63.4
    hemorrhagic —see Hemorrhage,
      intracranial, intracerebral
    occlusive I63.5
    thrombotic I63.3
  cartilage M94.2-
    patella M22.4-
  cerebellar —see Softening, brain
  cerebral —see Softening, brain
  cerebrospinal —see Softening, brain
  myocardial, heart —see Degeneration,
    myocardial
  spinal cord G95.89
  stomach K31.89
Soldier's
  heart F45.8
  patches I31.0
Solitary
  cyst, kidney N28.1
  kidney, congenital Q60.0
Solvent abuse —see Abuse, drug, inhalant
  dependence —see Dependence, drug,
    inhalant
Somatization reaction, somatic reaction —see
  Disorder, somatoform
Somnambulism F51.3
  hysterical F44.89
Somnolence R40.0
  nonorganic origin F51.11
Sonne dysentery A03.3
Soor B37.0
Sore
  bed —see Ulcer, pressure, by site
  chiclero B55.1
  Delhi B55.1
  desert —see Ulcer, skin
  eye H57.1-
  Lahore B55.1

◀ New   ◀▦ Revised   ~~deleted~~ Deleted

Sore *(Continued)*
 mouth K13.79
  canker K12.0
 muscle M79.1
 Naga —*see* Ulcer, skin
 of skin —*see* Ulcer, skin - oriental B55.1
 pressure —*see* Ulcer, pressure, by site
 skin L98.9
 soft A57
 throat (acute) —*see also* Pharyngitis
  with influenza, flu, or grippe —*see*
    Influenza, with, respiratory
    manifestations NEC
  chronic J31.2
  coxsackie (virus) B08.5
  diphtheritic A36.0
  herpesviral B00.2
  influenzal —*see* Influenza, with, respiratory
    manifestations NEC
  septic J02.0
  streptococcal (ulcerative) J02.0
  viral NEC J02.8
   coxsackie B08.5
  tropical —*see* Ulcer, skin
  veldt —*see* Ulcer, skin
Soto's syndrome (cerebral gigantism) Q87.3
South African cardiomyopathy syndrome I42.8
Southeast Asian hemorrhagic fever A91
Spacing
 abnormal, tooth, teeth, fully erupted M26.30
 excessive, tooth, fully erupted M26.32
Spade-like hand (congenital) Q68.1
Spading nail L60.8
 congenital Q84.6
Spanish collar N47.1
Sparganosis B70.1
Spasm (s), spastic, spasticity *(see also* condition)
  R25.2
 accommodation —*see* Spasm, of
   accommodation
 ampulla of Vater K83.4
 anus, ani (sphincter) (reflex) K59.4
  psychogenic F45.8
 artery I73.9
  cerebral G45.9
 Bell's G51.3
 bladder (sphincter, external or internal)
   N32.89
  psychogenic F45.8
 bronchus, bronchiole J98.01
 cardia K22.0
 cardiac I20.1
 carpopedal —*see* Tetany
 cerebral (arteries) (vascular) G45.9
 cervix, complicating delivery O62.4
 ciliary body (of accommodation) —*see* Spasm,
   of accommodation
 colon K58.9
  with diarrhea K58.0
  psychogenic F45.8
 common duct K83.8
 compulsive —*see* Tic
 conjugate H51.8
 coronary (artery) I20.1
 diaphragm (reflex) R06.6
  epidemic B33.0
  psychogenic F45.8
 duodenum K59.8
 epidemic diaphragmatic (transient) B33.0
 esophagus (diffuse) K22.4
  psychogenic F45.8
 facial G51.3
 fallopian tube N83.8
 gastrointestinal (tract) K31.89
  psychogenic F45.8
 glottis J38.5
  hysterical F44.4
  psychogenic F45.8
   conversion reaction F44.4
  reflex through recurrent laryngeal nerve
    J38.5

Spasm (s), spastic, spasticity *(Continued)*
 habit —*see* Tic
 heart I20.1
 hemifacial (clonic) G51.3
 hourglass —*see* Contraction, hourglass
 hysterical F44.4
 infantile —*see* Epilepsy, spasms
 inferior oblique, eye H51.8
 intestinal *(see also* Syndrome, irritable bowel)
   K58.9
  psychogenic F45.8
 larynx, laryngeal J38.5
  hysterical F44.4
  psychogenic F45.8
   conversion reaction F44.4
 levator palpebrae superioris —*see* Disorder,
   eyelid function
 muscle NEC M62.838
  back M62.830
 nerve, trigeminal G51.0
 nervous F45.8
 nodding F98.4
 occupational F48.8
 oculogyric H51.8
  psychogenic F45.8
 of accommodation H52.53-
 ophthalmic artery —*see* Occlusion, artery,
   retina
 perineal, female N94.89
 peroneo-extensor —*see also* Deformity, limb,
   flat foot
 pharynx (reflex) J39.2
  hysterical F45.8
  psychogenic F45.8
 psychogenic F45.8
 pylorus NEC K31.3
  adult hypertrophic K31.89
  congenital or infantile Q40.0
  psychogenic F45.8
 rectum (sphincter) K59.4
  psychogenic F45.8
 retinal (artery) —*see* Occlusion, artery, retina
 sigmoid *(see also* Syndrome, irritable bowel)
   K58.9
  psychogenic F45.8
 sphincter of Oddi K83.4
 stomach K31.89
  neurotic F45.8
 throat J39.2
  hysterical F45.8
  psychogenic F45.8
 tic F95.9
  chronic F95.1
  transient of childhood F95.0
 tongue K14.8
 torsion (progressive) G24.1
 trigeminal nerve —*see* Neuralgia, trigeminal
 ureter N13.5
 urethra (sphincter) N35.9
 uterus N85.8
  complicating labor O62.4
 vagina N94.2
  psychogenic F52.5
 vascular I73.9
 vasomotor I73.9
 vein NEC I87.8
 viscera —*see* Pain, abdominal
Spasmodic —*see* condition
Spasmophilia —*see* Tetany
Spasmus nutans F98.4
Spastic, spasticity —*see also* Spasm
 child (cerebral) (congenital) (paralysis) G80.1
Speaker's throat R49.8
Specific, specified —*see* condition
Speech
 defect, disorder, disturbance, impediment
   R47.9
  psychogenic, in childhood and adolescence
    F98.8
  slurring R47.81
  specified NEC R47.89

Spencer's disease A08.19
Spens' syndrome (syncope with heart block)
  I45.9
Sperm counts (fertility testing) Z31.41
 postvasectomy Z30.8
  reversal Z31.42
Spermatic cord —*see* condition
Spermatocele N43.40
 congenital Q55.4
 multiple N43.42
 single N43.41
Spermatocystitis N49.0
Spermatocytoma C62.9-
 specified site —*see* Neoplasm, malignant, by
   site
Spermatorrhea N50.8
Sphacelus —*see* Gangrene
Sphenoidal —*see* condition
Sphenoiditis (chronic) —*see* Sinusitis,
   sphenoidal
Sphenopalatine ganglion neuralgia
   G90.09
Sphericity, increased, lens (congenital)
   Q12.4
Spherocytosis (congenital) (familial)
   (hereditary) D58.0
 hemoglobin disease D58.0
 sickle-cell (disease) D57.8-
Spherophakia Q12.4
Sphincter —*see* condition
Sphincteritis, sphincter of Oddi —*see*
   Cholangitis
Sphingolipidosis E75.3
 specified NEC E75.29
Sphingomyelinosis E75.3
Spicule tooth K00.2
Spider
 bite —*see* Toxicity, venom, spider
 fingers —*see* Syndrome, Marfan's
 nevus I78.1
 toes —*see* Syndrome, Marfan's
 vascular I78.1
Spiegler-Fendt
 benign lymphocytoma L98.8
 sarcoid L08.89
Spielmeyer-Vogt disease E75.4
Spina bifida (aperta) Q05.9
 with hydrocephalus NEC Q05.4
 cervical Q05.5
  with hydrocephalus Q05.0
 dorsal Q05.6
  with hydrocephalus Q05.1
 lumbar Q05.7
  with hydrocephalus Q05.2
 lumbosacral Q05.7
  with hydrocephalus Q05.2
 occulta Q76.0
 sacral Q05.8
  with hydrocephalus Q05.3
 thoracic Q05.6
  with hydrocephalus Q05.1
 thoracolumbar Q05.6
  with hydrocephalus Q05.1
Spindle, Krukenberg's —*see* Pigmentation,
   cornea, posterior
Spine, spinal —*see* condition
Spiradenoma (eccrine) —*see* Neoplasm, skin,
   benign
Spirillosis A25.0
Spirillum
 minus A25.0
 obermeieri infection A68.0
Spirochetal —*see* condition
Spirochetosis A69.9
 arthritic, arthritica A69.9
 bronchopulmonary A69.8
 icterohemorrhagic A27.0
 lung A69.8
Spirometrosis B70.1
Spitting blood —*see* Hemoptysis
Splanchnoptosis K63.4

Spleen, splenic —see condition
Splenectasis —see Splenomegaly
Splenitis (interstitial) (malignant) (nonspecific) D73.89
  malarial (see also Malaria) B54 [D77] ◀▥
  tuberculous A18.85
Splenocele D73.89
Splenomegaly, splenomegalia (Bengal) (cryptogenic) (idiopathic) (tropical) R16.1
  with hepatomegaly R16.2
  cirrhotic D73.2
  congenital Q89.09
  congestive, chronic D73.2
  Egyptian B65.1
  Gaucher's E75.22
  malarial (see also Malaria) B54 [D77]
  neutropenic D73.81
  Niemann-Pick —see Niemann-Pick disease or syndrome
  siderotic D73.2
  syphilitic A52.79
    congenital (early) A50.08 [D77]
Splenopathy D73.9
Splenoptosis D73.89
Splenosis D73.89
Splinter —see Foreign body, superficial, by site
Split, splitting
  foot Q72.7-
  heart sounds R01.2
  lip, congenital —see Cleft, lip
  nails L60.3
  urinary stream R39.13
Spondylarthrosis —see Spondylosis
Spondylitis (chronic) —see also Spondylopathy, inflammatory
  ankylopoietica —see Spondylitis, ankylosing
  ankylosing (chronic) M45.9
    with lung involvement M45.9 [J99]
    cervical region M45.2
    cervicothoracic region M45.3
    juvenile M08.1
    lumbar region M45.6
    lumbosacral region M45.7
    multiple sites M45.0
    occipito-atlanto-axial region M45.1
    sacrococcygeal region M45.8
    thoracic region M45.4
    thoracolumbar region M45.5
  atrophic (ligamentous) —see Spondylitis, ankylosing
  deformans (chronic) —see Spondylosis
  gonococcal A54.41
  gouty M10.08
  in (due to)
    brucellosis A23.9 [M49.80]
      cervical region A23.9 [M49.82]
      cervicothoracic region A23.9 [M49.83]
      lumbar region A23.9 [M49.86]
      lumbosacral region A23.9 [M49.87]
      multiple sites A23.9 [M49.89]
      occipito-atlanto-axial region A23.9 [M49.81]
      sacrococcygeal region A23.9 [M49.88]
      thoracic region A23.9 [M49.84]
      thoracolumbar region A23.9 [M49.85]
    enterobacteria (see also subcategory M49.8) A04.9
    tuberculosis A18.01
  infectious NEC —see Spondylopathy, infective
  juvenile ankylosing (chronic) M08.1
  Kümmell's —see Spondylopathy, traumatic
  Marie-Strümpell —see Spondylitis, ankylosing
  muscularis —see Spondylopathy, specified NEC
  psoriatic L40.53
  rheumatoid —see Spondylitis, ankylosing
  rhizomelica —see Spondylitis, ankylosing
  sacroiliac NEC M46.1
  senescent, senile —see Spondylosis

Spondylitis (Continued)
  traumatic (chronic) or post-traumatic —see Spondylopathy, traumatic
  tuberculous A18.01
  typhosa A01.05
Spondylolisthesis (acquired) (degenerative) M43.10
  with disproportion (fetopelvic) O33.0
    causing obstructed labor O65.0
  cervical region M43.12
  cervicothoracic region M43.13
  congenital Q76.2
  lumbar region M43.16
  lumbosacral region M43.17
  multiple sites M43.19
  occipito-atlanto-axial region M43.11
  sacrococcygeal region M43.18
  thoracic region M43.14
  thoracolumbar region M43.15
  traumatic (old) M43.10
    acute
      fifth cervical (displaced) S12.430
        nondisplaced S12.431
        specified type NEC (displaced) S12.450
          nondisplaced S12.451
        type III S12.44
      fourth cervical (displaced) S12.330
        nondisplaced S12.331
        specified type NEC (displaced) S12.350
          nondisplaced S12.351
        type III S12.34
      second cervical (displaced) S12.130
        nondisplaced S12.131
        specified type NEC (displaced) S12.150
          nondisplaced S12.151
        type III S12.14
      seventh cervical (displaced) S12.630
        nondisplaced S12.631
        specified type NEC (displaced) S12.650
          nondisplaced S12.651
        type III S12.64
      sixth cervical (displaced) S12.530
        nondisplaced S12.531
        specified type NEC (displaced) S12.550
          nondisplaced S12.551
        type III S12.54
      third cervical (displaced) S12.230
        nondisplaced S12.231
        specified type NEC (displaced) S12.250
          nondisplaced S12.251
        type III S12.24
Spondylolysis (acquired) M43.00
  cervical region M43.02
  cervicothoracic region M43.03
  congenital Q76.2
  lumbar region M43.06
  lumbosacral region M43.07
    with disproportion (fetopelvic) O33.0
    causing obstructed labor O65.8
  multiple sites M43.09
  occipito-atlanto-axial region M43.01
  sacrococcygeal region M43.08
  thoracic region M43.04
  thoracolumbar region M43.05
Spondylopathy M48.9
  infective NEC M46.50
    cervical region M46.52
    cervicothoracic region M46.53
    lumbar region M46.56
    lumbosacral region M46.57
    multiple sites M46.59
    occipito-atlanto-axial region M46.51
    sacrococcygeal region M46.58
    thoracic region M46.54
    thoracolumbar region M46.55

Spondylopathy (Continued)
  inflammatory M46.90
    cervical region M46.92
    cervicothoracic region M46.93
    lumbar region M46.96
    lumbosacral region M46.97
    multiple sites M46.99
    occipito-atlanto-axial region M46.91
    sacrococcygeal region M46.98
    specified type NEC M46.80
      cervical region M46.82
      cervicothoracic region M46.83
      lumbar region M46.86
      lumbosacral region M46.87
      multiple sites M46.89
      occipito-atlanto-axial region M46.81
      sacrococcygeal region M46.88
      thoracic region M46.84
      thoracolumbar region M46.85
    thoracic region M46.94
    thoracolumbar region M46.95
  neuropathic, in
    syringomyelia and syringobulbia G95.0
    tabes dorsalis A52.11
  specified NEC —see subcategory M48.8
  traumatic M48.30
    cervical region M48.32
    cervicothoracic region M48.33
    lumbar region M48.36
    lumbosacral region M48.37
    occipito-atlanto-axial region M48.31
    sacrococcygeal region M48.38
    thoracic region M48.34
    thoracolumbar region M48.35
Spondylosis M47.9
  with
    disproportion (fetopelvic) O33.0
      causing obstructed labor O65.0
    myelopathy NEC M47.10
      cervical region M47.12
      cervicothoracic region M47.13
      lumbar region M47.16
      ~~lumbosacral region M47.17~~
      occipito-atlanto-axial region M47.11
      ~~sacrococcygeal region M47.18~~
      thoracic region M47.14
      thoracolumbar region M47.15
    radiculopathy M47.20
      cervical region M47.22
      cervicothoracic region M47.23
      lumbar region M47.26
      lumbosacral region M47.27
      occipito-atlanto-axial region M47.21
      sacrococcygeal region M47.28
      thoracic region M47.24
      thoracolumbar region M47.25
  without myelopathy or radiculopathy M47.819
    cervical region M47.812
    cervicothoracic region M47.813
    lumbar region M47.816
    lumbosacral region M47.817
    occipito-atlanto-axial region M47.811
    sacrococcygeal region M47.818
    thoracic region M47.814
    thoracolumbar region M47.815
  specified NEC M47.899
    cervical region M47.892
    cervicothoracic region M47.893
    lumbar region M47.896
    lumbosacral region M47.897
    occipito-atlanto-axial region M47.891
    sacrococcygeal region M47.898
    thoracic region M47.894
    thoracolumbar region M47.895
  traumatic —see Spondylopathy, traumatic
Sponge
  inadvertently left in operation wound —see Foreign body, accidentally left during a procedure
  kidney (medullary) Q61.5

◀ New   ◀▥ Revised   ~~deleted~~ Deleted

Sponge-diver's disease —*see* Toxicity, venom, marine animal, sea anemone
Spongioblastoma (any type) —*see* Neoplasm, malignant, by site
  specified site —*see* Neoplasm, malignant, by site
  unspecified site C71.9
Spongioneuroblastoma —*see* Neoplasm, malignant, by site
Spontaneous —*see also* condition
  fracture (cause unknown) —*see* Fracture, pathological
Spoon nail L60.3
  congenital Q84.6
Sporadic —*see* condition
Sporothrix schenckii infection —*see* Sporotrichosis
Sporotrichosis B42.9
  arthritis B42.82
  disseminated B42.7
  generalized B42.7
  lymphocutaneous (fixed) (progressive) B42.1
  pulmonary B42.0
  specified NEC B42.89
Spots, spotting (in) (of)
  Bitot's —*see also* Pigmentation, conjunctiva
    in the young child E50.1
      vitamin A deficiency E50.1
  café, au lait L81.3
  Cayenne pepper I78.1
  cotton wool, retina —*see* Occlusion, artery, retina
  de Morgan's (senile angiomas) I78.1
  Fuchs' black (myopic) H44.2-
  intermenstrual (regular) N92.0
    irregular N92.1
  Koplik's B05.9
  liver L81.4
  pregnancy O26.85-
  purpuric R23.3
  ruby I78.1
Spotted fever (see Fever, spotted) N92.3
Sprain (joint) (ligament)
  acromioclavicular joint or ligament S43.5-
  ankle S93.40-
    calcaneofibular ligament S93.41-
    deltoid ligament S93.42-
    internal collateral ligament —*see* Sprain, ankle, specified ligament NEC
    specified ligament NEC S93.49-
    talofibular ligament —*see* Sprain, ankle, specified ligament NEC
    tibiofibular ligament S93.43-
  anterior longitudinal, cervical S13.4
  atlas, atlanto-axial, atlanto-occipital S13.4
  breast bone —*see* Sprain, sternum
  calcaneofibular —*see* Sprain, ankle
  carpal —*see* Sprain, wrist
  carpometacarpal —*see* Sprain, hand, specified site NEC
  cartilage
    costal S23.41
    semilunar (knee) —*see* Sprain, knee, specified site NEC
      with current tear —*see* Tear, meniscus
    thyroid region S13.5
    xiphoid —*see* Sprain, sternum
  cervical, cervicodorsal, cervicothoracic S13.4
  chondrosternal S23.421
  coracoclavicular S43.8-
  coracohumeral S43.41-
  coronary, knee —*see* Sprain, knee, specified site NEC
  costal cartilage S23.41
  cricoarytenoid articulation or ligament S13.5
  cricothyroid articulation S13.5
  cruciate, knee —*see* Sprain, knee, cruciate
  deltoid, ankle —*see* Sprain, ankle
  dorsal (spine) S23.3

Sprain *(Continued)*
  elbow S53.40-
    radial collateral ligament S53.43-
    radiohumeral S53.41-
    rupture
      radial collateral ligament —*see* Rupture, traumatic, ligament, radial collateral
      ulnar collateral ligament —*see* Rupture, traumatic, ligament, ulnar collateral
    specified type NEC S53.49-
    ulnar collateral ligament S53.44-
    ulnohumeral S53.42-
  femur, head —*see* Sprain, hip
  fibular collateral, knee —*see* Sprain, knee, collateral
  fibulocalcaneal —*see* Sprain, ankle
  finger (s) S63.61-
    index S63.61-
    interphalangeal (joint) S63.63-
      index S63.63-
      little S63.63-
      middle S63.63-
      ring S63.63-
    little S63.61-
    metacarpophalangeal (joint) S63.65-
    middle S63.61-
    ring S63.61-
    specified site NEC S63.69-
      index S63.69-
      little S63.69-
      middle S63.69-
      ring S63.69-
  foot S93.60-
    specified ligament NEC S93.69-
    tarsal ligament S93.61-
    tarsometatarsal ligament S93.62-
    toe —*see* Sprain, toe
  hand S63.9-
    finger —*see* Sprain, finger
    specified site NEC —*see* subcategory S63.8
    thumb —*see* Sprain, thumb
  head S03.9
  hip S73.10-
    iliofemoral ligament S73.11-
    ischiocapsular (ligament) S73.12-
    specified NEC S73.19-
  iliofemoral —*see* Sprain, hip
  innominate
    acetabulum —*see* Sprain, hip
    sacral junction S33.6
  internal
    collateral, ankle —*see* Sprain, ankle
    semilunar cartilage —*see* Sprain, knee, specified site NEC
  interphalangeal
    finger —*see* Sprain, finger, interphalangeal (joint)
    toe —*see* Sprain, toe, interphalangeal joint
  ischiocapsular —*see* Sprain, hip
  ischiofemoral —*see* Sprain, hip
  jaw (articular disc) (cartilage) (meniscus) S03.4
    old M26.69
  knee S83.9-
    collateral ligament S83.40-
      lateral (fibular) S83.42-
      medial (tibial) S83.41-
    cruciate ligament S83.50-
      anterior S83.51-
      posterior S83.52-
    lateral (fibular) collateral ligament S83.42-
    medial (tibial) collateral ligament S83.41-
    patellar ligament S76.11-
    specified site NEC S83.8X-
    superior tibiofibular joint (ligament) S83.6-
  lateral collateral, knee —*see* Sprain, knee, collateral
  lumbar (spine) S33.5
  lumbosacral S33.9

Sprain *(Continued)*
  mandible (articular disc) S03.4
    old M26.69
  medial collateral, knee —*see* Sprain, knee, collateral
  meniscus
    jaw S03.4
      old M26.69
    knee —*see* Sprain, knee, specified site NEC
      with current tear —*see* Tear, meniscus
        old —*see* Derangement, knee, meniscus, due to old tear
    mandible S03.4
      old M26.69
  metacarpal (distal) (proximal) —*see* Sprain, hand, specified site NEC
  metacarpophalangeal —*see* Sprain, finger, metacarpophalangeal (joint)
  metatarsophalangeal —*see* Sprain, toe, metatarsophalangeal joint
  midcarpal —*see* Sprain, hand, specified site NEC
  midtarsal —*see* Sprain, foot, specified site NEC
  neck S13.9
    anterior longitudinal cervical ligament S13.4
    atlanto-axial joint S13.4
    atlanto-occipital joint S13.4
    cervical spine S13.4
    cricoarytenoid ligament S13.5
    cricothyroid ligament S13.5
    specified site NEC S13.8
    thyroid region (cartilage) S13.5
  nose S03.8
  orbicular, hip —*see* Sprain, hip
  patella —*see* Sprain, knee, specified site NEC
  patellar ligament S76.11-
  pelvis NEC S33.8
  phalanx
    finger —*see* Sprain, finger
    toe —*see* Sprain, toe
  pubofemoral —*see* Sprain, hip
  radiocarpal —*see* Sprain, wrist
  radiohumeral —*see* Sprain, elbow
  radius, collateral —*see* Rupture, traumatic, ligament, radial collateral
  rib (cage) S23.41
  rotator cuff (capsule) S43.42-
  sacroiliac (region)
    chronic or old —*see* subcategory M53.2
    joint S33.6
  scaphoid (hand) —*see* Sprain, hand, specified site NEC
  scapula (r) —*see* Sprain, shoulder girdle, specified site NEC
  semilunar cartilage (knee) —*see* Sprain, knee, specified site NEC
    with current tear —*see* Tear, meniscus
      old —*see* Derangement, knee, meniscus, due to old tear
  shoulder joint S43.40-
    acromioclavicular joint (ligament) —*see* Sprain, acromioclavicular joint
    blade —*see* Sprain, shoulder, girdle, specified site NEC
    coracoclavicular joint (ligament) —*see* Sprain, coracoclavicular joint
    coracohumeral ligament —*see* Sprain, coracohumeral joint
    girdle S43.9-
      specified site NEC S43.8-
    rotator cuff —*see* Sprain, rotator cuff
    specified site NEC S43.49-
    sternoclavicular joint (ligament) —*see* Sprain, sternoclavicular joint
  spine
    cervical S13.4
    lumbar S33.5
    thoracic S23.3
  sternoclavicular joint S43.6-

Sprain (Continued)
  sternum S23.429
    chondrosternal joint S23.421
    specified site NEC S23.428
    sternoclavicular (joint) (ligament)
        S23.420
  symphysis
    jaw S03.4
      old M26.69
    mandibular S03.4
      old M26.69
  talofibular —see Sprain, ankle
  tarsal —see Sprain, foot, specified site NEC
  tarsometatarsal —see Sprain, foot, specified
      site NEC
  temporomandibular S03.4
    old M26.69
  thorax S23.9
    ribs S23.41
    specified site NEC S23.8
    spine S23.3
    sternum —see Sprain, sternum
  thumb S63.60-
    interphalangeal (joint) S63.62-
    metacarpophalangeal (joint) S63.64-
    specified site NEC S63.68-
  thyroid cartilage or region S13.5
  tibia (proximal end) —see Sprain, knee,
      specified site NEC
  tibial collateral, knee —see Sprain, knee,
      collateral
  tibiofibular
    distal —see Sprain, ankle
    superior —see Sprain, knee, specified site
        NEC
  toe (s) S93.50-
    great S93.50-
    interphalangeal joint S93.51-
      great S93.51-
      lesser S93.51-
    lesser S93.50-
    metatarsophalangeal joint S93.52-
      great S93.52-
      lesser S93.52-
  ulna, collateral —see Rupture, traumatic,
      ligament, ulnar collateral
  ulnohumeral —see Sprain, elbow
  wrist S63.50-
    carpal S63.51-
    radiocarpal S63.52-
    specified site NEC S63.59-
  xiphoid cartilage —see Sprain, sternum
Sprengel's deformity (congenital) Q74.0
Sprue (tropical) K90.1
  celiac K90.0
  idiopathic K90.0
  meaning thrush B37.0
  nontropical K90.0
Spur, bone —see also Enthesopathy
  calcaneal M77.3-
  iliac crest M76.2-
  nose (septum) J34.89
Spurway's syndrome Q78.0
Sputum
  abnormal (amount) (color) (odor) (purulent)
      R09.3
  blood-stained R04.2
  excessive (cause unknown) R09.3
Squamous —see also condition
  epithelium in
    cervical canal (congenital) Q51.828
    uterine mucosa (congenital) Q51.818
Squashed nose M95.0
  congenital Q67.4
Squeeze, diver's T70.3
Squint —see also Strabismus
  accommodative —see Strabismus, convergent
      concomitant
St. Hubert's disease A82.9
Stab —see also Laceration
  internal organs —see Injury, by site

Stafne's cyst or cavity M27.0
Staggering gait R26.0
  hysterical F44.4
Staghorn calculus —see Calculus, kidney
Stähli's line (cornea) (pigment) —see
    Pigmentation, cornea, anterior
Stain, staining
  meconium (newborn) P96.83
  port wine Q82.5
  tooth, teeth (hard tissues) (extrinsic) K03.6
    due to
      accretions K03.6
      deposits (betel) (black) (green) (materia
          alba) (orange) (soft) (tobacco) K03.6
      metals (copper) (silver) K03.7
      nicotine K03.6
      pulpal bleeding K03.7
      tobacco K03.6
    intrinsic K00.8
Stammering (see also Disorder, fluency) F80.81
Standstill
  auricular I45.5
  cardiac —see Arrest, cardiac
  sinoatrial I45.5
  ventricular —see Arrest, cardiac
Stannosis J63.5
Stanton's disease —see Melioidosis
Staphylitis (acute) (catarrhal) (chronic)
    (gangrenous) (membranous) (suppurative)
    (ulcerative) K12.2
Staphylococcal scalded skin syndrome L00
Staphylococcemia A41.2
Staphylococcus, staphylococcal —see also
    condition
  as cause of disease classified elsewhere
      B95.8
    aureus (methicillin susceptible) (MSSA)
        B95.61
      methicillin resistant (MRSA) B95.62
  specified NEC, as cause of disease classified
      elsewhere B95.7
Staphyloma (sclera)
  cornea H18.72-
  equatorial H15.81-
  localized (anterior) H15.82-
  posticum H15.83-
  ring H15.85-
Stargardt's disease —see Dystrophy, retina
Starvation (inanition) (due to lack of food)
    T73.0
  edema —see Malnutrition, severe
Stasis
  bile (noncalculous) K83.1
  bronchus J98.09
    with infection —see Bronchitis
  cardiac —see Failure, heart, congestive
  cecum K59.8
  colon K59.8
  dermatitis —see Varix, leg, with,
      inflammation
  duodenal K31.5
  eczema —see Varix, leg, with, inflammation
  edema —see Hypertension, venous (chronic),
      idiopathic
  foot T69.0-
  ileocecal coil K59.8
  ileum K59.8
  intestinal K59.8
  jejunum K59.8
  kidney N19
  liver (cirrhotic) K76.1
  lymphatic I89.8
  pneumonia J18.2
  pulmonary —see Edema, lung
  rectal K59.8
  renal N19
    tubular N17.0
  ulcer —see Varix, leg, with, ulcer
    without varicose veins I87.2
  urine —see Retention, urine
  venous I87.8

State (of)
  affective and paranoid, mixed, organic
      psychotic F06.8
  agitated R45.1
    acute reaction to stress F43.0
  anxiety (neurotic) F41.1
  apprehension F41.1
  burn-out Z73.0
  climacteric, female Z78.0
    symptomatic N95.1
  compulsive F42
    mixed with obsessional thoughts
        F42
  confusional (psychogenic) F44.89
    acute —see also Delirium
      with
        arteriosclerotic dementia F01.50
          with behavioral disturbance
              F01.51
        senility or dementia F05
    alcoholic F10.231
    epileptic F05
    reactive (from emotional stress,
        psychological trauma) F44.89
    subacute —see Delirium
  convulsive —see Convulsions
  crisis F43.0
  depressive F32.9
    neurotic F34.1
  dissociative F44.9
  emotional shock (stress) R45.7
  hypercoagulation —see Hypercoagulable
  locked-in G83.5
  menopausal Z78.0
    symptomatic N95.1
  neurotic F48.9
    with depersonalization F48.1
  obsessional F42
  oneiroid (schizophrenia-like) F23
  organic
    hallucinatory (nonalcoholic) F06.0
    paranoid (-hallucinatory) F06.2
  panic F41.0
  paranoid F22
    climacteric F22
    involutional F22
    menopausal F22
    organic F06.2
    senile F03
    simple F22
  persistent vegetative R40.3
  phobic F40.9
  postleukotomy F07.0
  pregnant, incidental Z33.1
  psychogenic, twilight F44.89
  psychopathic (constitutional) F60.2
  psychotic, organic —see also Psychosis,
      organic
    mixed paranoid and affective F06.8
    senile or presenile F03
    transient NEC F06.8
      with
        depression F06.31
        hallucinations F06.0
  residual schizophrenic F20.5
  restlessness R45.1
  stress (emotional) R45.7
  tension (mental) F48.9
    specified NEC F48.8
  transient organic psychotic NEC F06.8
    depressive type F06.31
    hallucinatory type F06.30
  twilight
    epileptic F05
    psychogenic F44.89
  vegetative, persistent R40.3
  vital exhaustion Z73.0
  withdrawal —see Withdrawal, state
Status (post) —see also Presence (of)
  absence, epileptic —see Epilepsy, by type,
      with status epilepticus

◀ New   ◀ Revised   deleted Deleted

Status *(Continued)*
  administration of tPA (rtPA) in a different
    facility within the last 24 hours prior to
    admission to the current facility
    Z92.82
  adrenalectomy (unilateral) (bilateral) E89.6
  anastomosis Z98.0
  anginosus I20.9
  angioplasty (peripheral) Z98.62
    with implant Z95.820
    coronary artery Z98.61
      with implant Z95.5
  aortocoronary bypass Z95.1
  arthrodesis Z98.1
  artificial opening (of) Z93.9
    gastrointestinal tract Z93.4
    specified NEC Z93.8
    urinary tract Z93.6
    vagina Z93.8
  asthmaticus —*see* Asthma, by type, with
    status asthmaticus
  awaiting organ transplant Z76.82
  bariatric surgery Z98.84
  bed confinement Z74.01
  bleb, filtering (vitreous), after glaucoma
    surgery Z98.83
  breast implant Z98.82
    removal Z98.86
  cataract extraction Z98.4-
  cholecystectomy Z90.49
  clitorectomy N90.811
    with excision of labia minora N90.812
  colectomy (complete) (partial) Z90.49
  colonization —*see* Carrier (suspected) of
  colostomy Z93.3
  convulsivus idiopathicus —*see* Epilepsy, by
    type, with status epilepticus
  coronary artery angioplasty —*see* Status,
    angioplasty, coronary artery
  cystectomy (urinary bladder) Z90.6
  cystostomy Z93.50
    appendico-vesicostomy Z93.52
    cutaneous Z93.51
    specified NEC Z93.59
  delinquent immunization Z28.3
  dental Z98.818
    crown Z98.811
    fillings Z98.811
    restoration Z98.811
    sealant Z98.810
    specified NEC Z98.818
  deployment (current) (military) Z56.82
  dialysis (hemodialysis) (peritoneal) Z99.2
  do not resuscitate (DNR) Z66
  donor —*see* Donor
  embedded fragments —*see* Retained, foreign
    body fragments (type of)
  embedded splinter —*see* Retained, foreign
    body fragments (type of)
  enterostomy Z93.4
  epileptic, epilepticus (*see also* Epilepsy, by
    type, with status epilepticus) G40.901
  estrogen receptor
    negative Z17.1 ◀▥
    positive Z17.0 ◀▥
  female genital cutting —*see* Female genital
    mutilation status
  female genital mutilation —*see* Female genital
    mutilation status
  filtering (vitreous) bleb after glaucoma
    surgery Z98.83
  gastrectomy (complete) (partial) Z90.3
  gastric banding Z98.84
  gastric bypass for obesity Z98.84
  gastrostomy Z93.1
  human immunodeficiency virus (HIV)
    infection, asymptomatic Z21
  hysterectomy (complete) (total) Z90.710
    partial (with remaining cervial stump)
    Z90.711
  ileostomy Z93.2

Status *(Continued)*
  implant
    breast Z98.82
  infibulation N90.813
  intestinal bypass Z98.0
  jejunostomy Z93.4
  lapsed immunization schedule Z28.3
  laryngectomy Z90.02
  lymphaticus E32.8
  marmoratus G80.3
  mastectomy (unilateral) (bilateral) Z90.1-
  military deployment status (current)
    Z56.82
    in theater or in support of military war,
      peacekeeping and humanitarian
      operations Z56.82
  nephrectomy (unilateral) (bilateral) Z90.5
  nephrostomy Z93.6
  obesity surgery Z98.84
  oophorectomy
    bilateral Z90.722
    unilateral Z90.721
  organ replacement
    by artificial or mechanical device or
      prosthesis of
      artery Z95.828
      bladder Z96.0
      blood vessel Z95.828
      breast Z97.8
      eye globe Z97.0
      heart Z95.812
        valve Z95.2
      intestine Z97.8
      joint Z96.60
        hip —*see* Presence, hip joint implant
        knee —*see* Presence, knee joint
          implant
        specified site NEC Z96.698
      kidney Z97.8
      larynx Z96.3
      lens Z96.1
      limbs —*see* Presence, artificial, limb
      liver Z97.8
      lung Z97.8
      pancreas Z97.8
    by organ transplant (heterologous)
      (homologous) —*see* Transplant
  pacemaker
    brain Z96.89
    cardiac Z95.0
    specified NEC Z96.89
  pancreatectomy Z90.410
    complete Z90.410
    partial Z90.411
    total Z90.410
  pneumonectomy (complete) (partial) Z90.2
  pneumothorax, therapeutic Z98.3
  postcommotio cerebri F07.81
  postoperative (postprocedural) NEC
    Z98.89
    breast implant Z98.82
    dental Z98.818
      crown Z98.811
      fillings Z98.811
      restoration Z98.811
      sealant Z98.810
      specified NEC Z98.818
    pneumothorax, therapeutic Z98.3
  postpartum (routine follow-up) Z39.2
    care immediately after delivery Z39.0
  postsurgical (postprocedural) NEC Z98.89
    pneumothorax, therapeutic Z98.3
  pregnancy, incidental Z33.1
  prosthesis coronary angioplasty Z95.5
  pseudophakia Z96.1
  renal dialysis (hemodialysis) (peritoneal)
    Z99.2
  retained foreign body —*see* Retained, foreign
    body fragments (type of)
  reversed jejunal transposition (for bypass)
    Z98.0

Status *(Continued)*
  salpingo-oophorectomy
    bilateral Z90.722
    unilateral Z90.721
  sex reassignment surgery status Z87.890
  shunt
    arteriovenous (for dialysis) Z99.2
    cerebrospinal fluid Z98.2
    ventricular (communicating) (for
      drainage) Z98.2
  splenectomy Z90.81
  thymicolymphaticus E32.8
  thymicus E32.8
  thymolymphaticus E32.8
  thyroidectomy (hypothyroidism) E89.0
  tooth (teeth) extraction (*see also* Absence,
    teeth, acquired) K08.409
  tPA (rtPA) administration in a different
    facility within the last 24 hours prior to
    admission to current facility Z92.82
  tracheostomy Z93.0
  transplant —*see* Transplant
    organ removed Z98.85
  tubal ligation Z98.51
  underimmunization Z28.3
  ureterostomy Z93.6
  urethrostomy Z93.6
  vagina, artificial Z93.8
  vasectomy Z98.52
  wheelchair confinement Z99.3
Stealing
  child problem F91.8
    in company with others Z72.810
  pathological (compulsive) F63.2
Steam burn —*see* Burn
Steatocystoma multiplex L72.2
Steatohepatitis (nonalcoholic) (NASH)
  K75.81
Steatoma L72.3
  eyelid (cystic) —*see* Dermatosis, eyelid
  infected —*see* Hordeolum
Steatorrhea (chronic) K90.4
  with lacteal obstruction K90.2
  idiopathic (adult) (infantile) K90.0
  pancreatic K90.3
  primary K90.0
  tropical K90.1
Steatosis E88.89
  heart —*see* Degeneration, myocardial
  kidney N28.89
  liver NEC K76.0
Steele-Richardson-Olszewski disease or
  syndrome G23.1
Steinbrocker's syndrome G90.8
Steinert's disease G71.11
Stein-Leventhal syndrome E28.2
Stein's syndrome E28.2
STEMI (*see also* - Infarct, myocardium, ST
  elevation) I21.3
Stenocardia I20.8
Stenocephaly Q75.8
Stenosis, stenotic (cicatricial) —*see also* Stricture
  ampulla of Vater K83.1
  anus, anal (canal) (sphincter) K62.4
    and rectum K62.4
    congenital Q42.3
      with fistula Q42.2
  aorta (ascending) (supraventricular)
    (congenital) Q25.3
    arteriosclerotic I70.0
    calcified I70.0
  aortic (valve) I35.0
    with insufficiency I35.2
    congenital Q23.0
    rheumatic I06.0
      with
        incompetency, insufficiency or
          regurgitation I06.2
        with mitral (valve) disease I08.0
        with tricuspid (valve) disease
          I08.3

Stenosis, stenotic *(Continued)*
  aortic *(Continued)*
    rheumatic *(Continued)*
      with *(Continued)*
        mitral (valve) disease I08.0
          with tricuspid (valve) disease
            I08.3
        tricuspid (valve) disease I08.2
          with mitral (valve) disease I08.3
    specified cause NEC I35.0
    syphilitic A52.03
  aqueduct of Sylvius (congenital) Q03.0
    with spina bifida —*see* Spina bifida,
      by site, with hydrocephalus
    acquired G91.1
  artery NEC *(see also* Arteriosclerosis)
    I77.1
    celiac I77.4
    cerebral —*see* Occlusion, artery, cerebral
    extremities —*see* Arteriosclerosis,
      extremities
    precerebral —*see* Occlusion, artery,
      precerebral
    pulmonary (congenital) Q25.6
      acquired I28.8
    renal I70.1
  bile duct (common) (hepatic) K83.1
    congenital Q44.3
  bladder-neck (acquired) N32.0
    congenital Q64.31
  brain G93.89
  bronchus J98.09
    congenital Q32.3
    syphilitic A52.72
  cardia (stomach) K22.2
    congenital Q39.3
  cardiovascular —*see* Disease, cardiovascular
  caudal M48.08
  cervix, cervical (canal) N88.2
    congenital Q51.828
    in pregnancy or childbirth —*see* Pregnancy,
      complicated by, abnormal cervix
  colon —*see also* Obstruction, intestine
    congenital Q42.9
      specified NEC Q42.8
  colostomy K94.03
  common (bile) duct K83.1
    congenital Q44.3
  coronary (artery) —*see* Disease, heart,
    ischemic, atherosclerotic
  cystic duct —*see* Obstruction, gallbladder
  due to presence of device, implant or graft
    (see also Complications, by site and type,
      specified NEC) T85.85
    arterial graft NEC T82.858
    breast (implant) T85.85
    catheter T85.85
      dialysis (renal) T82.858
        intraperitoneal T85.85
      infusion NEC T82.858
        spinal (epidural) (subdural) T85.85
      urinary (indwelling) T83.85
    fixation, internal (orthopedic) NEC
      T84.85
    gastrointestinal (bile duct) (esophagus)
      T85.85
    genital NEC T83.85
    heart NEC T82.857
    joint prosthesis T84.85
    ocular (corneal graft) (orbital implant)
      NEC T85.85
    orthopedic NEC T84.85
    specified NEC T85.85
    urinary NEC T83.85
    vascular NEC T82.858
    ventricular intracranial shunt T85.85
  duodenum K31.5
    congenital Q41.0
  ejaculatory duct NEC N50.8
  endocervical os —*see* Stenosis, cervix
  enterostomy K94.13

Stenosis, stenotic *(Continued)*
  esophagus K22.2
    congenital Q39.3
    syphilitic A52.79
    congenital A50.59 *[K23]*
  eustachian tube —*see* Obstruction, eustachian
    tube
  external ear canal (acquired) H61.30-
    congenital Q16.1
    due to
      inflammation H61.32-
      trauma H61.31-
    postprocedural H95.81-
    specified cause NEC H61.39-
  gallbladder —*see* Obstruction, gallbladder
  glottis J38.6
  heart valve (congenital) Q24.8
    aortic Q23.0
    mitral Q23.2
    pulmonary Q22.1
    tricuspid Q22.4
  hepatic duct K83.1
  hymen N89.6
  hypertrophic subaortic (idiopathic) I42.1
  ileum K56.69
    congenital Q41.2
  infundibulum cardia Q24.3
  intervertebral foramina —*see also* Lesion,
    biomechanical, specified NEC
    connective tissue M99.79
      abdomen M99.79
      cervical region M99.71
      cervicothoracic M99.71
      head region M99.70
      lumbar region M99.73
      lumbosacral M99.73
      occipitocervical M99.70
      sacral region M99.74
      sacrococcygeal M99.74
      sacroiliac M99.74
      specified NEC M99.79
      thoracic region M99.72
      thoracolumbar M99.72
    disc M99.79
      abdomen M99.79
      cervical region M99.71
      cervicothoracic M99.71
      head region M99.70
      lower extremity M99.76
      lumbar region M99.73
      lumbosacral M99.73
      occipitocervical M99.70
      pelvic M99.75
      rib cage M99.78
      sacral region M99.74
      sacrococcygeal M99.74
      sacroiliac M99.74
      specified NEC M99.79
      thoracic region M99.72
      thoracolumbar M99.72
      upper extremity M99.77
    osseous M99.69
      abdomen M99.69
      cervical region M99.61
      cervicothoracic M99.61
      head region M99.60
      lower extremity M99.66
      lumbar region M99.63
      lumbosacral M99.63
      occipitocervical M99.60
      pelvic M99.65
      rib cage M99.68
      sacral region M99.64
      sacrococcygeal M99.64
      sacroiliac M99.64
      specified NEC M99.69
      thoracic region M99.62
      thoracolumbar M99.62
      upper extremity M99.67
    subluxation —*see* Stenosis, intervertebral
      foramina, osseous

Stenosis, stenotic *(Continued)*
  intestine —*see also* Obstruction, intestine
    congenital (small) Q41.9
      large Q42.9
        specified NEC Q42.8
      specified NEC Q41.8
  jejunum K56.69
    congenital Q41.1
  lacrimal (passage)
    canaliculi H04.54-
    congenital Q10.5
    duct H04.55-
    punctum H04.56-
    sac H04.57-
  lacrimonasal duct —*see* Stenosis, lacrimal,
    duct
    congenital Q10.5
  larynx J38.6
    congenital NEC Q31.8
      subglottic Q31.1
    syphilitic A52.73
      congenital A50.59 *[J99]*
  mitral (chronic) (inactive) (valve) I05.0
    with
      aortic valve disease I08.0
      incompetency, insufficiency or
        regurgitation I05.2
    active or acute I01.1
      with rheumatic or Sydenham's chorea
        I02.0
    congenital Q23.2
    specified cause, except rheumatic I34.2
    syphilitic A52.03
  myocardium, myocardial —*see also*
    Degeneration, myocardial
    hypertrophic subaortic (idiopathic) I42.1
  nares (anterior) (posterior) J34.89
    congenital Q30.0
  nasal duct —*see also* Stenosis, lacrimal, duct
    congenital Q10.5
  nasolacrimal duct —*see also* Stenosis, lacrimal,
    duct
    congenital Q10.5
  neural canal —*see also* Lesion, biomechanical,
    specified NEC
    connective tissue M99.49
      abdomen M99.49
      cervical region M99.41
      cervicothoracic M99.41
      head region M99.40
      lower extremity M99.46
      lumbar region M99.43
      lumbosacral M99.43
      occipitocervical M99.40
      pelvic M99.45
      rib cage M99.48
      sacral region M99.44
      sacrococcygeal M99.44
      sacroiliac M99.44
      specified NEC M99.49
      thoracic region M99.42
      thoracolumbar M99.42
      upper extremity M99.47
    intervertebral disc M99.59
      abdomen M99.59
      cervical region M99.51
      cervicothoracic M99.51
      head region M99.50
      lower extremity M99.56
      lumbar region M99.53
      lumbosacral M99.53
      occipitocervical M99.50
      pelvic M99.55
      rib cage M99.58
      sacral region M99.54
      sacrococcygeal M99.54
      sacroiliac M99.54
      specified NEC M99.59
      thoracic region M99.52
      thoracolumbar M99.52
      upper extremity M99.57

Stenosis, stenotic (Continued)
  neural canal (Continued)
    osseous M99.39
      abdomen M99.39
      cervical region M99.31
      cervicothoracic M99.31
      head region M99.30
      lower extremity M99.36
      lumbar region M99.33
      lumbosacral M99.33
      occipitocervical M99.30
      pelvic M99.35
      rib cage M99.38
      sacral region M99.34
      sacrococcygeal M99.34
      sacroiliac M99.34
      specified NEC M99.39
      thoracic region M99.32
      thoracolumbar M99.32
      upper extremity M99.37
    subluxation M99.29
      cervical region M99.21
      cervicothoracic M99.21
      head region M99.20
      lower extremity M99.26
      lumbar region M99.23
      lumbosacral M99.23
      occipitocervical M99.20
      pelvic M99.25
      rib cage M99.28
      sacral region M99.24
      sacrococcygeal M99.24
      sacroiliac M99.24
      specified NEC M99.29
      thoracic region M99.22
      thoracolumbar M99.22
      upper extremity M99.27
  oesophagus —see Stenosis, esophagus
  organ or site, congenital NEC —see Atresia,
    by site
  papilla of Vater K83.1
  pulmonary (artery) (congenital) Q25.6
    with ventricular septal defect,
      transposition of aorta, and
      hypertrophy of right ventricle
      Q21.3
    acquired I28.8
    in tetralogy of Fallot Q21.3
    infundibular Q24.3
    subvalvular Q24.3
    supravalvular Q25.6
    valve I37.0
      with insufficiency I37.2
      congenital Q22.1
      rheumatic I09.89
        with aortic, mitral or tricuspid (valve)
        disease I08.8
    vein, acquired I28.8
    vessel NEC I28.8
  pulmonic (congenital) Q22.1
    infundibular Q24.3
    subvalvular Q24.3
  pylorus (hypertrophic) (acquired) K31.1
    adult K31.1
    congenital Q40.0
    infantile Q40.0
  rectum (sphincter) —see Stricture, rectum
  renal artery I70.1
    congenital Q27.1
  salivary duct (any) K11.8
  sphincter of Oddi K83.1
  spinal M48.00
    cervical region M48.02
    cervicothoracic region M48.03
    lumbar region M48.06
    lumbosacral region M48.07
    occipito-atlanto-axial region M48.01
    sacrococcygeal region M48.08
    thoracic region M48.04
    thoracolumbar region M48.05
  stomach, hourglass K31.2

Stenosis, stenotic (Continued)
  subaortic (congenital) Q24.4
    hypertrophic (idiopathic) I42.1
  subglottic J38.6
    congenital Q31.1
    postprocedural J95.5
  trachea J39.8
    congenital Q32.1
    syphilitic A52.73
    tuberculous NEC A15.5
  tracheostomy J95.03
  tricuspid (valve) I07.0
    with
      aortic (valve) disease I08.2
      incompetency, insufficiency or
        regurgitation I07.2
        with aortic (valve) disease I08.2
          with mitral (valve) disease I08.3
      mitral (valve) disease I08.1
        with aortic (valve) disease I08.3
    congenital Q22.4
    nonrheumatic I36.0
      with insufficiency I36.2
  tubal N97.1
  ureter —see Atresia, ureter
  ureteropelvic junction, congenital Q62.11
  ureterovesical orifice, congenital Q62.12
  urethra (valve) —see also Stricture, urethra
    congenital Q64.32
  urinary meatus, congenital Q64.33
  vagina N89.5
    congenital Q52.4
    in pregnancy —see Pregnancy, complicated
      by, abnormal vagina
      causing obstructed labor O65.5
  valve (cardiac) (heart) (see also Endocarditis)
    I38
    congenital Q24.8
      aortic Q23.0
      mitral Q23.2
      pulmonary Q22.1
      tricuspid Q22.4
  vena cava (inferior) (superior) I87.1
    congenital Q26.0
  vesicourethral orifice Q64.31
  vulva N90.5
Stent jail T82.897
Stercolith (impaction) K56.41
  appendix K38.1
Stercoraceous, stercoral ulcer K63.3
  anus or rectum K62.6
Stereotypies NEC F98.4
Sterility —see Infertility
Sterilization —see Encounter (for), sterilization
Sternalgia —see Angina
Sternopagus Q89.4
Sternum bifidum Q76.7
Steroid
  effects (adverse) (adrenocortical) (iatrogenic)
    cushingoid E24.2
      correct substance properly
        administered —see Table of Drugs
        and Chemicals, by drug, adverse
        effect ◀▥▥
      overdose or wrong substance given or
        taken —see Table of Drugs and
        Chemicals, by drug, poisoning ◀▥▥
    diabetes —see category E09
      correct substance properly
        administered —see Table of Drugs
        and Chemicals, by drug, adverse
        effect ◀▥▥
      overdose or wrong substance given or
        taken —see Table of Drugs and
        Chemicals, by drug, poisoning ◀▥▥
    fever R50.2
    insufficiency E27.3
      correct substance properly
        administered —see Table of Drugs
        and Chemicals, by drug, adverse
        effect ◀▥▥

Steroid (Continued)
  effects (Continued)
    insufficiency (Continued)
      overdose or wrong substance given or
        taken —see Table of Drugs and
        Chemicals, by drug, poisoning ◀▥▥
    responder H40.04-
Stevens-Johnson disease or syndrome L51.1
  toxic epidermal necrolysis overlap L51.3
Stewart-Morel syndrome M85.2
Sticker's disease B08.3
Sticky eye —see Conjunctivitis, acute,
  mucopurulent
Stieda's disease —see Bursitis, tibial collateral
Stiff neck —see Torticollis
Stiff-man syndrome G25.82
Stiffness, joint NEC M25.60- ◀▥▥
  ankle M25.67-
  ankylosis —see Ankylosis, joint
  contracture —see Contraction, joint
  elbow M25.62- ◀▥▥
  foot M25.67- ◀▥▥
  hand M25.64- ◀▥▥
  hip M25.65- ◀▥▥
  knee M25.66- ◀▥▥
  shoulder M25.61- ◀▥▥
  wrist M25.63- ◀▥▥
Stigmata congenital syphilis A50.59
Stillbirth P95
Still-Felty syndrome —see Felty's syndrome
Still's disease or syndrome (juvenile) M08.20
  adult-onset M06.1
  ankle M08.27-
  elbow M08.22-
  foot joint M08.27-
  hand joint M08.24-
  hip M08.25-
  knee M08.26-
  multiple site M08.29
  shoulder M08.21-
  vertebra M08.28
  wrist M08.23-
Stimulation, ovary E28.1
Sting (venomous) (with allergic or anaphylactic
  shock) —see Table of Drugs and
  Chemicals, by animal or substance,
  poisoning ◀▥▥
Stippled epiphyses Q78.8
Stitch
  abscess T81.4
  burst (in operation wound) —see Disruption,
    wound, operation
Stokes-Adams disease or syndrome I45.9
Stokes' disease E05.00
  with thyroid storm E05.01
Stokvis (-Talma) disease D74.8 ◀▥▥
Stoma malfunction
  colostomy K94.03
  enterostomy K94.13
  gastrostomy K94.23
  ileostomy K94.13
  tracheostomy J95.03
Stomach —see condition
Stomatitis (denture) (ulcerative) K12.1
  angular K13.0
    due to dietary or vitamin deficiency E53.0
  aphthous K12.0
  bovine B08.61
  candidal B37.0
  catarrhal K12.1
  diphtheritic A36.89
  due to
    dietary deficiency E53.0
    thrush B37.0
    vitamin deficiency
      B group NEC E53.9
      B2 (riboflavin) E53.0
  epidemic B08.8
  epizootic B08.8
  follicular K12.1
  gangrenous A69.0
  Geotrichum B48.3

Stomatitis *(Continued)*
  herpesviral, herpetic B00.2
  herpetiformis K12.0
  malignant K12.1
  membranous acute K12.1
  monilial B37.0
  mycotic B37.0
  necrotizing ulcerative A69.0
  parasitic B37.0
  septic K12.1
  spirochetal A69.1
  suppurative (acute) K12.2
  ulceromembranous A69.1
  vesicular K12.1
    with exanthem (enteroviral) B08.4
    virus disease A93.8
  Vincent's A69.1
Stomatocytosis D58.8
Stomatomycosis B37.0
Stomatorrhagia K13.79
Stone (s) —*see also* Calculus
  bladder (diverticulum) N21.0
  cystine E72.09
  heart syndrome I50.1
  kidney N20.0
  prostate N42.0
  pulpal (dental) K04.2
  renal N20.0
  salivary gland or duct (any) K11.5
  urethra (impacted) N21.1
  urinary (duct) (impacted) (passage) N20.9
    bladder (diverticulum) N21.0
    lower tract N21.9
    specified NEC N21.8
  xanthine E79.8 *[N22]*
Stonecutter's lung J62.8
Stonemason's asthma, disease, lung or
    pneumoconiosis J62.8
Stoppage
  heart —*see* Arrest, cardiac
  urine —*see* Retention, urine
Storm, thyroid —*see* Thyrotoxicosis
Strabismus (congenital) (nonparalytic) H50.9
  concomitant H50.40
    convergent —*see* Strabismus, convergent
      concomitant
    divergent —*see* Strabismus, divergent
      concomitant
  convergent concomitant H50.00
    accommodative component H50.43
    alternating H50.05
      with
        A pattern H50.06
        specified nonconcomitances NEC
          H50.08
        V pattern H50.07
    monocular H50.01-
      with
        A pattern H50.02-
        specified nonconcomitances NEC
          H50.04-
        V pattern H50.03-
      intermittent H50.31-
        alternating H50.32
  cyclotropia H50.1-
  divergent concomitant H50.10
    alternating H50.15
      with
        A pattern H50.16
        specified nonconcomitances NEC
          H50.18
        V pattern H50.17
    monocular H50.11-
      with
        A pattern H50.12-
        specified nonconcomitances NEC
          H50.14-
        V pattern H50.13-
      intermittent H50.33-
        alternating H50.34
  Duane's syndrome H50.81-

Strabismus *(Continued)*
  due to adhesions, scars H50.69
  heterophoria H50.50
    alternating H50.55
    cyclophoria H50.54
    esophoria H50.51
    exophoria H50.52
    vertical H50.53
  heterotropia H50.40
    intermittent H50.30
  hypertropia H50.2-
  hypotropia —*see* Hypertropia
  latent H50.50
  mechanical H50.60
    Brown's sheath syndrome H50.61-
    specified type NEC H50.69
  monofixation syndrome H50.42
  paralytic H49.9
    abducens nerve H49.2-
    fourth nerve H49.1-
    Kearns-Sayre syndrome H49.81-
    ophthalmoplegia (external)
      progressive H49.4-
        with pigmentary retinopathy
          H49.81-
      total H49.3-
    sixth nerve H49.2-
    specified type NEC H49.88-
    third nerve H49.0-
    trochlear nerve H49.1-
  specified type NEC H50.89
  vertical H50.2-
Strain
  back S39.012
  cervical S16.1
  eye NEC —*see* Disturbance, vision,
    subjective
  heart —*see* Disease, heart
  low back S39.012
  mental NOS Z73.3
    work-related Z56.6
  muscle (tendon) —*see* Injury, muscle, by site,
    strain
  neck S16.1
  physical NOS Z73.3
    work-related Z56.6
  postural —*see also* Disorder, soft tissue, due
    to use
  psychological NEC Z73.3
  tendon —*see* Injury, muscle, by site, strain
Straining, on urination R39.16
Strand, vitreous —*see* Opacity, vitreous,
    membranes and strands
Strangulation, strangulated —*see also*
    Asphyxia, traumatic
  appendix K38.8
  bladder-neck N32.0
  bowel or colon K56.2
  food or foreign body —*see* Foreign body, by
    site
  hemorrhoids —*see* Hemorrhoids, with
    complication
  hernia —*see also* Hernia, by site, with
    obstruction
    with gangrene —*see* Hernia, by site, with
      gangrene
  intestine (large) (small) K56.2
    with hernia —*see also* Hernia, by site, with
      obstruction
      with gangrene —*see* Hernia, by site, with
        gangrene
  mesentery K56.2
  mucus —*see* Asphyxia, mucus
  omentum K56.2
  organ or site, congenital NEC —*see* Atresia,
    by site
  ovary —*see* Torsion, ovary
  penis N48.89
    foreign body T19.4
  rupture —*see* Hernia, by site, with
    obstruction

Strangulation, strangulated *(Continued)*
  stomach due to hernia —*see also* Hernia, by
    site, with obstruction
    with gangrene —*see* Hernia, by site, with
      gangrene
  vesicourethral orifice N32.0
Strangury R30.0
Straw itch B88.0
Strawberry
  gallbladder K82.4
  mark Q82.5
  tongue (red) (white) K14.3
Streak (s)
  macula, angioid H35.33
  ovarian Q50.32
Strephosymbolia F81.0
  secondary to organic lesion R48.8
Streptobacillary fever A25.1
Streptobacillosis A25.1
Streptobacillus moniliformis A25.1
Streptococcus, streptococcal —*see also*
    condition
  as cause of disease classified elsewhere
    B95.5
  group
    A, as cause of disease classified elsewhere
      B95.0
    B, as cause of disease classified elsewhere
      B95.1
    D, as cause of disease classified elsewhere
      B95.2
  pneumoniae, as cause of disease classified
    elsewhere B95.3
  specified NEC, as cause of disease classified
    elsewhere B95.4
Streptomycosis B47.1
Streptotrichosis A48.8
Stress F43.9
  family —*see* Disruption, family
  fetal P84
    complicating pregnancy O77.9
      due to drug administration O77.1
  mental NEC Z73.3
    work-related Z56.6
  physical NEC Z73.3
    work-related Z56.6
  polycythemia D75.1
  reaction (*see also* Reaction, stress) F43.9
  work schedule Z56.3
Stretching, nerve —*see* Injury, nerve
Striae albicantes, atrophicae or distensae
    (cutis) L90.6
Stricture —*see also* Stenosis
  ampulla of Vater K83.1
  anus (sphincter) K62.4
    congenital Q42.3
      with fistula Q42.2
    infantile Q42.3
      with fistula Q42.2
  aorta (ascending) (congenital) Q25.3
    arteriosclerotic I70.0
    calcified I70.0
    supravalvular, congenital Q25.3
  aortic (valve) —*see* Stenosis, aortic
  aqueduct of Sylvius (congenital) Q03.0
    with spina bifida —*see* Spina bifida, by site,
      with hydrocephalus
    acquired G91.1
  artery I77.1
    basilar —*see* Occlusion, artery, basilar
    carotid —*see* Occlusion, artery, carotid
    celiac I77.4
    congenital (peripheral) Q27.8
      cerebral Q28.3
      coronary Q24.5
      digestive system Q27.8
      lower limb Q27.8
      retinal Q14.1
      specified site NEC Q27.8
      umbilical Q27.0
      upper limb Q27.8

◀ New   ◀ Revised   ~~deleted~~ Deleted

Stricture *(Continued)*
  artery *(Continued)*
    coronary —*see* Disease, heart, ischemic,
      atherosclerotic
      congenital Q24.5
    precerebral —*see* Occlusion, artery,
      precerebral
    pulmonary (congenital) Q25.6
      acquired I28.8
    renal I70.1
    vertebral —*see* Occlusion, artery, vertebral
  auditory canal (external) (congenital)
    acquired —*see* Stenosis, external ear canal
  bile duct (common) (hepatic) K83.1
    congenital Q44.3
    postoperative K91.89
  bladder N32.89
    neck N32.0
  bowel —*see* Obstruction, intestine
  brain G93.89
  bronchus J98.09
    congenital Q32.3
    syphilitic A52.72
  cardia (stomach) K22.2
    congenital Q39.3
  cardiac —*see also* Disease, heart
    orifice (stomach) K22.2
  cecum —*see* Obstruction, intestine
  cervix, cervical (canal) N88.2
    congenital Q51.828
    in pregnancy —*see* Pregnancy, complicated
      by, abnormal cervix
      causing obstructed labor O65.5
  colon —*see also* Obstruction, intestine
    congenital Q42.9
      specified NEC Q42.8
  colostomy K94.03
  common (bile) duct K83.1
  coronary (artery) —*see* Disease, heart,
    ischemic, atherosclerotic
  cystic duct —*see* Obstruction, gallbladder
  digestive organs NEC, congenital Q45.8
  duodenum K31.5
    congenital Q41.0
  ear canal (external) (congenital) Q16.1
    acquired —*see* Stricture, auditory canal,
      acquired
  ejaculatory duct N50.8
  enterostomy K94.13
  esophagus K22.2
    congenital Q39.3
    syphilitic A52.79
      congenital A50.59 *[K23]*
  eustachian tube —*see also* Obstruction,
    eustachian tube
    congenital Q17.8
  fallopian tube N97.1
    gonococcal A54.24
    tuberculous A18.17
  gallbladder —*see* Obstruction, gallbladder
  glottis J38.6
  heart —*see also* Disease, heart
    valve (*see also* Endocarditis) I38
      aortic Q23.0
      mitral Q23.4
      pulmonary Q22.1
      tricuspid Q22.4
  hepatic duct K83.1
  hourglass, of stomach K31.2
  hymen N89.6
  hypopharynx J39.2
  ileum K56.69
    congenital Q41.2
  intestine —*see also* Obstruction, intestine
    congenital (small) Q41.9
      large Q42.9
        specified NEC Q42.8
        specified NEC Q41.8
    ischemic K55.1
  jejunum K56.69
    congenital Q41.1

Stricture *(Continued)*
  lacrimal passages —*see also* Stenosis, lacrimal
    congenital Q10.5
  larynx J38.6
    congenital NEC Q31.8
      subglottic Q31.1
    syphilitic A52.73
      congenital A50.59 *[J99]*
  meatus
    ear (congenital) Q16.1
      acquired —*see* Stricture, auditory canal,
        acquired
    osseous (ear) (congenital) Q16.1
      acquired —*see* Stricture, auditory canal,
        acquired
    urinarius —*see also* Stricture, urethra
      congenital Q64.33
  mitral (valve) —*see* Stenosis, mitral
  myocardium, myocardial I51.5
    hypertrophic subaortic (idiopathic) I42.1
  nares (anterior) (posterior) J34.89
    congenital Q30.0
  nasal duct —*see also* Stenosis, lacrimal, duct
    congenital Q10.5
  nasolacrimal duct —*see also* Stenosis, lacrimal,
    duct
    congenital Q10.5
  nasopharynx J39.2
    syphilitic A52.73
  nose J34.89
    congenital Q30.0
  nostril (anterior) (posterior) J34.89
    congenital Q30.0
    syphilitic A52.73
      congenital A50.59 *[J99]*
  ~~oesophagus —see Stricture, esophagus~~
  organ or site, congenital NEC —*see* Atresia,
    by site
  os uteri —*see* Stricture, cervix
  osseous meatus (ear) (congenital) Q16.1
    acquired —*see* Stricture, auditory canal,
      acquired
  oviduct —*see* Stricture, fallopian tube
  pelviureteric junction (congenital)
    Q62.11
  penis, by foreign body T19.4
  pharynx J39.2
  prostate N42.89
  pulmonary, pulmonic
    artery (congenital) Q25.6
      acquired I28.8
      noncongenital I28.8
    infundibulum (congenital) Q24.3
    valve I37.0
      congenital Q22.1
    vein, acquired I28.8
    vessel NEC I28.8
  punctum lacrimale —*see also* Stenosis,
    lacrimal, punctum
    congenital Q10.5
  pylorus (hypertrophic) K31.1
    adult K31.1
    congenital Q40.0
    infantile Q40.0
  rectosigmoid K56.69
  rectum (sphincter) K62.4
    congenital Q42.1
      with fistula Q42.0
    due to
      chlamydial lymphogranuloma A55
      irradiation K91.89
      lymphogranuloma venereum A55
    gonococcal A54.6
    inflammatory (chlamydial) A55
    syphilitic A52.74
    tuberculous A18.32
  renal artery I70.1
    congenital Q27.1
  salivary duct or gland (any) K11.8
  sigmoid (flexure) —*see* Obstruction, intestine
  spermatic cord N50.8

Stricture *(Continued)*
  stoma (following) (of)
    colostomy K94.03
    enterostomy K94.13
    gastrostomy K94.23
    ileostomy K94.13
    tracheostomy J95.03
  stomach K31.89
    congenital Q40.2
    hourglass K31.2
  subaortic Q24.4
    hypertrophic (acquired) (idiopathic) I42.1
  subglottic J38.6
  syphilitic NEC A52.79
  trachea J39.8
    congenital Q32.1
    syphilitic A52.73
    tuberculous NEC A15.5
  tracheostomy J95.03
  tricuspid (valve) —*see* Stenosis, tricuspid
  tunica vaginalis N50.8
  ureter (postoperative) N13.5
    with
      hydronephrosis N13.1
        with infection N13.6
      pyelonephritis (chronic) N11.1
    congenital —*see* Atresia, ureter
    tuberculous A18.11
  ureteropelvic junction (congenital) Q62.11
  ureterovesical orifice N13.5
    with infection N13.6
  urethra (organic) (spasmodic) N35.9
    associated with schistosomiasis B65.0 *[N37]*
    congenital Q64.39
      valvular (posterior) Q64.2
    due to
      infection —*see* Stricture, urethra,
        postinfective
      trauma —*see* Stricture, urethra,
        post-traumatic
    gonococcal, gonorrheal A54.01
    infective NEC —*see* Stricture, urethra,
      postinfective
    late effect (sequelae) of injury —*see*
      Stricture, urethra, post-traumatic
    postcatheterization —*see* Stricture, urethra,
      postprocedural
    postinfective NEC
      female N35.12
      male N35.119
        anterior urethra N35.114
        bulbous urethra N35.112
        meatal N35.111
        membranous urethra N35.113
    postobstetric N35.021
    postoperative —*see* Stricture, urethra,
      postprocedural
    postprocedural
      female N99.12
      male N99.114
        anterior urethra N99.113
        bulbous urethra N99.111
        meatal N99.110
        membranous urethra N99.112
    post-traumatic
      female N35.028
        due to childbirth N35.021
      male N35.014
        anterior urethra N35.013
        bulbous urethra N35.011
        meatal N35.010
        membranous urethra N35.012
    sequela (late effect) of
      childbirth N35.021
      injury —*see* Stricture, urethra,
        post-traumatic
    specified cause NEC N35.8
    syphilitic A52.76
    traumatic —*see* Stricture, urethra,
      post-traumatic
    valvular (posterior), congenital Q64.2

Stricture (*Continued*)
　urinary meatus —*see* Stricture, urethra
　uterus, uterine (synechiae) N85.6
　　os (external) (internal) —*see* Stricture,
　　　cervix
　vagina (outlet) —*see* Stenosis, vagina
　valve (cardiac) (heart) —*see also* Endocarditis
　　congenital
　　　aortic Q23.0
　　　mitral Q23.2
　　　pulmonary Q22.1
　　　tricuspid Q22.4
　vas deferens N50.8
　　congenital Q55.4
　vein I87.1
　vena cava (inferior) (superior) NEC I87.1
　　congenital Q26.0
　vesicourethral orifice N32.0
　　congenital Q64.31
　vulva (acquired) N90.5
Stridor R06.1
　congenital (larynx) P28.89
Stridulous —*see* condition
Stroke (apoplectic) (brain) (embolic) (ischemic)
　　(paralytic) (thrombotic) I63.9
　epileptic —*see* Epilepsy
　heat T67.0
　in evolution I63.9
　intraoperative
　　during cardiac surgery I97.810
　　during other surgery I97.811
　lightning —*see* Lightning
　meaning
　　cerebral hemorrhage — code to
　　　Hemorrhage, intracranial
　　cerebral infarction — code to Infarction,
　　　cerebral
　postprocedural
　　following cardiac surgery I97.820
　　following other surgery I97.821
　unspecified (NOS) I63.9
Stromatosis, endometrial D39.0
Strongyloidiasis, strongyloidosis B78.9
　cutaneous B78.1
　disseminated B78.7
　intestinal B78.0
Strophulus pruriginosus L28.2
Struck by lightning —*see* Lightning
Struma —*see also* Goiter
　Hashimoto E06.3
　lymphomatosa E06.3
　nodosa (simplex) E04.9
　　endemic E01.2
　　　multinodular E01.1
　　multinodular E04.2
　　　iodine-deficiency related E01.1
　　toxic or with hyperthyroidism E05.20
　　　with thyroid storm E05.21
　　　multinodular E05.20
　　　　with thyroid storm E05.21
　　　uninodular E05.10
　　　　with thyroid storm E05.11
　　toxicosa E05.20
　　　with thyroid storm E05.21
　　　multinodular E05.20
　　　　with thyroid storm E05.21
　　　uninodular E05.10
　　　　with thyroid storm E05.11
　　uninodular E04.1
　ovarii D27.-
　Riedel's E06.5
Strumipriva cachexia E03.4
Strümpell-Marie spine —*see* Spondylitis,
　ankylosing
Strümpell-Westphal pseudosclerosis E83.01
Stuart deficiency disease (factor X) D68.2
Stuart-Prower factor deficiency (factor X)
　D68.2
Student's elbow —*see* Bursitis, elbow,
　olecranon
Stump —*see* Amputation

Stunting, nutritional E45
Stupor (catatonic) R40.1
　depressive F32.8
　dissociative F44.2
　manic F30.2
　manic-depressive F31.89
　psychogenic (anergic) F44.2
　reaction to exceptional stress (transient)
　　F43.0
Sturge (-Weber) (-Dimitri) (-Kalischer) **disease**
　or syndrome Q85.8
Stuttering F80.81
　adult onset F98.5
　childhood onset F80.81
　following cerebrovascular disease —
　　see Disorder, fluency, following
　　cerebrovascular disease
　in conditions classified elsewhere R47.82
Sty, stye (external) (internal) (meibomian)
　(zeisian) —*see* Hordeolum
Subacidity, gastric K31.89
　psychogenic F45.8
Subacute —*see* condition
Subarachnoid —*see* condition
Subcortical —*see* condition
Subcostal syndrome, nerve compression —*see*
　Mononeuropathy, upper limb, specified
　site NEC
Subcutaneous, subcuticular —*see* condition
Subdural —*see* condition
Subendocardium —*see* condition
Subependymoma
　specified site —*see* Neoplasm, uncertain
　　behavior, by site
　unspecified site D43.2
Suberosis J67.3
Subglossitis —*see* Glossitis
Subhemophilia D66
Subinvolution
　breast (postlactational) (postpuerperal)
　　N64.89
　puerperal O90.89
　uterus (chronic) (nonpuerperal) N85.3
　　puerperal O90.89
Sublingual —*see* condition
Sublinguitis —*see* Sialoadenitis
Subluxatable hip Q65.6
Subluxation —*see also* Dislocation
　acromioclavicular S43.11-
　ankle S93.0-
　atlantoaxial, recurrent M43.4
　　with myelopathy M43.3
　carpometacarpal (joint) NEC S63.05-
　　thumb S63.04-
　complex, vertebral —*see* Complex,
　　subluxation
　congenital —*see also* Malposition,
　　congenital
　　hip —*see* Dislocation, hip, congenital,
　　　partial
　　joint (excluding hip)
　　　lower limb Q68.8
　　　shoulder Q68.8
　　　upper limb Q68.8
　elbow (traumatic) S53.10-
　　anterior S53.11-
　　lateral S53.14-
　　medial S53.13-
　　posterior S53.12-
　　specified type NEC S53.19-
　finger S63.20-
　　index S63.20-
　　interphalangeal S63.22-
　　　distal S63.24-
　　　　index S63.24-
　　　　little S63.24-
　　　　middle S63.24-
　　　　ring S63.24-
　　　index S63.22-
　　　little S63.22-
　　　middle S63.22-

Subluxation (*Continued*)
　finger (*Continued*)
　　interphalangeal (*Continued*)
　　　proximal S63.23-
　　　　index S63.23-
　　　　little S63.23-
　　　　middle S63.23-
　　　　ring S63.23-
　　　ring S63.22-
　　little S63.20-
　　metacarpophalangeal S63.21-
　　　index S63.21-
　　　little S63.21-
　　　middle S63.21-
　　　ring S63.21-
　　middle S63.20-
　　ring S63.20-
　foot S93.30-
　　specified site NEC S93.33-
　　tarsal joint S93.31-
　　tarsometatarsal joint S93.32-
　　toe —*see* Subluxation, toe
　hip S73.00-
　　anterior S73.03-
　　　obturator S73.02-
　　central S73.04-
　　posterior S73.01-
　interphalangeal (joint)
　　finger S63.22-
　　　distal joint S63.24-
　　　　index S63.24-
　　　　little S63.24-
　　　　middle S63.24-
　　　　ring S63.24-
　　　index S63.22-
　　　little S63.22-
　　　middle S63.22-
　　　proximal joint S63.23-
　　　　index S63.23-
　　　　little S63.23-
　　　　middle S63.23-
　　　　ring S63.23-
　　　ring S63.22-
　　thumb S63.12-
　　　distal joint S63.14-
　　　proximal joint S63.13-
　　toe S93.13-
　　　great S93.13-
　　　lesser S93.13-
　joint prosthesis —*see* Complications, joint
　　prosthesis, mechanical, displacement,
　　by site
　knee S83.10-
　　cap —*see* Subluxation, patella
　　patella —*see* Subluxation, patella
　　proximal tibia
　　　anteriorly S83.11-
　　　laterally S83.14-
　　　medially S83.13-
　　　posteriorly S83.12-
　　　specified type NEC S83.19-
　lens —*see* Dislocation, lens, partial
　ligament, traumatic —*see* Sprain, by site
　metacarpal (bone)
　　proximal end S63.06-
　metacarpophalangeal (joint)
　　finger S63.21-
　　　index S63.21-
　　　little S63.21-
　　　middle S63.21-
　　　ring S63.21-
　　thumb S63.11-
　metatarsophalangeal joint S93.14-
　　great toe S93.14-
　　lesser toe S93.14-
　midcarpal (joint) S63.03-
　patella S83.00-
　　lateral S83.01-
　　recurrent (nontraumatic) —*see* Dislocation,
　　　patella, recurrent, incomplete
　　specified type NEC S83.09-

◀ New　◀◀ Revised　~~deleted~~ Deleted

Subluxation *(Continued)*
  pathological —*see* Dislocation, pathological
  radial head S53.00-
    anterior S53.01-
    nursemaid's elbow S53.03-
    posterior S53.02-
    specified type NEC S53.09-
  radiocarpal (joint) S63.02-
  radioulnar (joint)
    distal S63.01-
    proximal —*see* Subluxation, elbow
  shoulder
    congenital Q68.8
    girdle S43.30-
      scapula S43.31-
      specified site NEC S43.39-
    traumatic S43.00-
      anterior S43.01-
      inferior S43.03-
      posterior S43.02-
      specified type NEC S43.08-
  sternoclavicular (joint) S43.20-
    anterior S43.21-
    posterior S43.22-
  symphysis (pubis)
  thumb S63.103
    interphalangeal joint —*see* Subluxation,
      interphalangeal (joint), thumb
    metacarpophalangeal joint —*see*
      Subluxation, metacarpophalangeal
      (joint), thumb
  toe (s) S93.10-
    great S93.10-
      interphalangeal joint S93.13-
      metatarsophalangeal joint S93.14-
    interphalangeal joint S93.13-
    lesser S93.10-
      interphalangeal joint S93.13-
      metatarsophalangeal joint S93.14-
    metatarsophalangeal joint S93.149
  ulnohumeral joint —*see* Subluxation, elbow
  vertebral
    recurrent NEC —*see* subcategory M43.5
    traumatic
      cervical S13.100
        atlantoaxial joint S13.120
        atlantooccipital joint S13.110
        atloidooccipital joint S13.110
        joint between
          C0 and C1 S13.110
          C1 and C2 S13.120
          C2 and C3 S13.130
          C3 and C4 S13.140
          C4 and C5 S13.150
          C5 and C6 S13.160
          C6 and C7 S13.170
          C7 and T1 S13.180
        occipitoatloid joint S13.110
      lumbar S33.100
        joint between
          L1 and L2 S33.110
          L2 and L3 S33.120
          L3 and L4 S33.130
          L4 and L5 S33.140
      thoracic S23.100
        joint between
          T1 and T2 S23.110
          T2 and T3 S23.120
          T3 and T4 S23.122
          T4 and T5 S23.130
          T5 and T6 S23.132
          T6 and T7 S23.140
          T7 and T8 S23.142
          T8 and T9 S23.150
          T9 and T10 S23.152
          T10 and T11 S23.160
          T11 and T12 S23.162
          T12 and L1 S23.170
  ulna
    distal end S63.07-
    proximal end —*see* Subluxation, elbow

Subluxation *(Continued)*
  wrist (carpal bone) S63.00-
    carpometacarpal joint —*see* Subluxation,
      carpometacarpal (joint)
    distal radioulnar joint —*see* Subluxation,
      radioulnar (joint), distal
    metacarpal bone, proximal —*see*
      Subluxation, metacarpal (bone),
      proximal end
    midcarpal —*see* Subluxation, midcarpal
      (joint)
    radiocarpal joint —*see* Subluxation,
      radiocarpal (joint)
    recurrent —*see* Dislocation, recurrent, wrist
    specified site NEC S63.09-
    ulna —*see* Subluxation, ulna, distal end
Submaxillary —*see* condition
Submersion (fatal) (nonfatal) T75.1
Submucous —*see* condition
Subnormal, subnormality
  accommodation (old age) H52.4
  mental —*see* Disability, intellectual
  temperature (accidental) T68
Subphrenic —*see* condition
Subscapular nerve —*see* condition
Subseptus uterus Q51.2
Subsiding appendicitis K36
Substernal thyroid E04.9
  congenital Q89.2
Substitution disorder F44.9
Subtentorial —*see* condition
Subthyroidism (acquired) —*see also*
    Hypothyroidism
  congenital E03.1
Succenturiate placenta O43.19-
Sucking thumb, child (excessive) F98.8
Sudamen, sudamina L74.1
Sudanese kala-azar B55.0
Sudden
  hearing loss —*see* Deafness, sudden
  heart failure —*see* Failure, heart
Sudeck's atrophy, disease, or syndrome —*see*
    Algoneurodystrophy
Suffocation —*see* Asphyxia, traumatic
Sugar
  blood
    high (transient) R73.9
    low (transient) E16.2
  in urine R81
Suicide, suicidal (attempted) T14.91
  by poisoning —*see* Table of ~~d~~Drugs and
    ~~c~~Chemicals ◀▬▬
  history of (personal) Z91.5
    in family Z81.8
  ideation —*see* Ideation, suicidal
  risk
    meaning personal history of attempted
      suicide Z91.5
    meaning suicidal ideation —*see* Ideation,
      suicidal
  tendencies
    meaning personal history of attempted
      suicide Z91.5
    meaning suicidal ideation —*see* Ideation,
      suicidal
  trauma —*see* nature of injury by site
Suipestifer infection —*see* Infection, salmonella
Sulfhemoglobinemia, sulphemoglobinemia
    (acquired) (with methemoglobinemia)
    D74.8
Sumatran mite fever A75.3
Summer —*see* condition
Sunburn L55.9
  first degree L55.0
  second degree L55.1
  third degree L55.2
SUNCT (short lasting unilateral neuralgiform
    headache with conjunctival injection and
    tearing) G44.059
  intractable G44.051
  not intractable G44.059

Sunken acetabulum —*see* Derangement, joint,
    specified type NEC, hip
Sunstroke T67.0
Superfecundation —*see* Pregnancy,
    multiple
Superfetation —*see* Pregnancy, multiple
Superinvolution (uterus) N85.8
Supernumerary (congenital)
  aortic cusps Q23.8
  auditory ossicles Q16.3
  bone Q79.8
  breast Q83.1
  carpal bones Q74.0
  cusps, heart valve NEC Q24.8
    aortic Q23.8
    mitral Q23.2
    pulmonary Q22.3
  digit (s) Q69.9
  ear (lobule) Q17.0
  fallopian tube Q50.6
  finger Q69.0
  hymen Q52.4
  kidney Q63.0
  lacrimonasal duct Q10.6
  lobule (ear) Q17.0
  mitral cusps Q23.2
  muscle Q79.8
  nipple (s) Q83.3
  organ or site not listed —*see* Accessory
  ossicles, auditory Q16.3
  ovary Q50.31
  oviduct Q50.6
  pulmonary, pulmonic cusps Q22.3
  rib Q76.6
    cervical or first (syndrome) Q76.5
  roots (of teeth) K00.2
  spleen Q89.09
  tarsal bones Q74.2
  teeth K00.1
  testis Q55.29
  thumb Q69.1
  toe Q69.2
  uterus Q51.2
  vagina Q52.1
  vertebra Q76.49
Supervision (of)
  contraceptive —*see* Prescription,
    contraceptives
  dietary (for) Z71.3
    allergy (food) Z71.3
    colitis Z71.3
    diabetes mellitus Z71.3
    food allergy or intolerance Z71.3
    gastritis Z71.3
    hypercholesterolemia Z71.3
    hypoglycemia Z71.3
    intolerance (food) Z71.3
    obesity Z71.3
    specified NEC Z71.3
  healthy infant or child Z76.2
    foundling Z76.1
  high-risk pregnancy —*see* Pregnancy,
    complicated by, high, risk
  lactation Z39.1
  pregnancy —*see* Pregnancy, supervision of
Supplemental teeth K00.1
Suppression
  binocular vision H53.34
  lactation O92.5
  menstruation N94.89
  ovarian secretion E28.39
  renal N28.9
  urine, urinary secretion R34
Suppuration, suppurative —*see also* condition
  accessory sinus (chronic) —*see* Sinusitis
  adrenal gland
  antrum (chronic) —*see* Sinusitis,
    maxillary
  bladder —*see* Cystitis
  brain G06.0
    sequelae G09

Suppuration, suppurative *(Continued)*
- breast N61
  - puerperal, postpartum or gestational —*see* Mastitis, obstetric, purulent
- dental periosteum M27.3
- ear (middle) —*see also* Otitis, media
  - external NEC —*see* Otitis, externa, infective
  - internal —*see* subcategory H83.0
- ethmoidal (chronic) (sinus) —*see* Sinusitis, ethmoidal
- fallopian tube —*see* Salpingo-oophoritis
- frontal (chronic) (sinus) —*see* Sinusitis, frontal
- gallbladder (acute) K81.0
- gum K05.20
  - generalized K05.22
  - localized K05.21
- intracranial G06.0
- joint —*see* Arthritis, pyogenic or pyemic
- labyrinthine —*see* subcategory H83.0
- lung —*see* Abscess, lung
- mammary gland N61
  - puerperal, postpartum O91.12
    - associated with lactation O91.13
- maxilla, maxillary M27.2
  - sinus (chronic) —*see* Sinusitis, maxillary
- muscle —*see* Myositis, infective
- nasal sinus (chronic) —*see* Sinusitis
- pancreas, acute K85.8
- parotid gland —*see* Sialoadenitis
- pelvis, pelvic
  - female —*see* Disease, pelvis, inflammatory
  - male K65.0
- pericranial —*see* Osteomyelitis
- salivary duct or gland (any) —*see* Sialoadenitis
- sinus (accessory) (chronic) (nasal) —*see* Sinusitis
- sphenoidal sinus (chronic) —*see* Sinusitis, sphenoidal
- thymus (gland) E32.1
- thyroid (gland) E06.0
- tonsil —*see* Tonsillitis
- uterus —*see* Endometritis

Supraeruption of tooth (teeth) M26.34
Supraglottitis J04.30
- with obstruction J04.31
Suprarenal (gland) —*see* condition
Suprascapular nerve —*see* condition
Suprasellar —*see* condition
Surfer's knots or nodules S89.8-
Surgical
- emphysema T81.82
- procedures, complication or misadventure — *see* Complications, surgical procedures
- shock T81.10
Surveillance (of) (for) —*see also* Observation
- alcohol abuse Z71.41
- contraceptive —*see* Prescription, contraceptives
- dietary Z71.3
- drug abuse Z71.51
Susceptibility to disease, genetic Z15.89
- malignant neoplasm Z15.09
  - breast Z15.01
  - endometrium Z15.04
  - ovary Z15.02
  - prostate Z15.03
  - specified NEC Z15.09
- multiple endocrine neoplasia Z15.81
Suspected condition, ruled out —*see also* Observation, suspected
- amniotic cavity and membrane Z03.71
- cervical shortening Z03.75
- fetal anomaly Z03.73
- fetal growth Z03.74
- maternal and fetal conditions NEC Z03.79
- oligohydramnios Z03.71
- placental problem Z03.72
- polyhydramnios Z03.71

Suspended uterus
- in pregnancy or childbirth —*see* Pregnancy, complicated by, abnormal uterus
Sutton's nevus D22.9
Suture
- burst (in operation wound) T81.31
  - external operation wound T81.31
  - internal operation wound T81.32
- inadvertently left in operation wound —*see* Foreign body, accidentally left during a procedure
- removal Z48.02
Swab inadvertently left in operation wound — *see* Foreign body, accidentally left during a procedure
Swallowed, swallowing
- difficulty —*see* Dysphagia
- foreign body —*see* Foreign body, alimentary tract
Swan-neck deformity (finger) —*see* Deformity, finger, swan-neck
Swearing, compulsive F42
- in Gilles de la Tourette's syndrome F95.2
Sweat, sweats
- fetid L75.0
- night R61
Sweating, excessive R61
Sweeley-Klionsky disease E75.21
Sweet's disease or dermatosis L98.2
Swelling (of) R60.9
- abdomen, abdominal (not referable to any particular organ) —*see* Mass, abdominal
- ankle —*see* Effusion, joint, ankle
- arm M79.89
  - forearm M79.89
- breast N63
- Calabar B74.3
- cervical gland R59.0
- chest, localized R22.2
- ear H93.8-
- extremity (lower) (upper) —*see* Disorder, soft tissue, specified type NEC
- finger M79.89
- foot M79.89
- glands R59.9
  - generalized R59.1
  - localized R59.0
- hand M79.89
- head (localized) R22.0
- inflammatory —*see* Inflammation
- intra-abdominal —*see* Mass, abdominal
- joint —*see* Effusion, joint
- leg M79.89
  - lower M79.89
- limb —*see* Disorder, soft tissue, specified type NEC
- localized (skin) R22.9
  - chest R22.2
  - head R22.0
  - limb
    - lower —*see* Mass, localized, limb, lower
    - upper —*see* Mass, localized, limb, upper
  - neck R22.1
  - trunk R22.2
- neck (localized) R22.1
- pelvic —*see* Mass, abdominal
- scrotum N50.8
- splenic —*see* Splenomegaly
- testis N50.8
- toe M79.89
- umbilical R19.09
- wandering, due to Gnathostoma (spinigerum) B83.1
- white —*see* Tuberculosis, arthritis
Swift (-Feer) disease
- overdose or wrong substance given or taken —*see* Table of ~~d~~Drugs and ~~c~~Chemicals, by drug, poisoning ◀︎▥

Swimmer's
- cramp T75.1
- ear H60.33-
- itch B65.3
Swimming in the head R42
Swollen —*see* Swelling
Swyer syndrome Q99.1
Sycosis L73.8
- barbae (not parasitic) L73.8
- contagiosa (mycotic) B35.0
- lupoides L73.8
- mycotic B35.0
- parasitic B35.0
- vulgaris L73.8
Sydenham's chorea —*see* Chorea, Sydenham's
Sylvatic yellow fever A95.0
Sylvest's disease B33.0
Symblepharon H11.23-
- congenital Q10.3
Symond's syndrome G93.2
Sympathetic —*see* condition
Sympatheticotonia G90.8
Sympathicoblastoma
- specified site —*see* Neoplasm, malignant, by site
- unspecified site C74.90
Sympathogonioma —*see* Sympathicoblastoma
Symphalangy (fingers) (toes) Q70.9
Symptoms NEC R68.89
- breast NEC N64.59
- development NEC R63.8
- factitious, self-induced —*see* Disorder, factitious
- genital organs, female R10.2
- involving
  - abdomen NEC R19.8
  - appearance NEC R46.89
  - awareness R41.9
    - altered mental status R41.82
    - amnesia —*see* Amnesia
    - borderline intellectual functioning R41.83
    - coma —*see* Coma
    - disorientation R41.0
    - neurologic neglect syndrome R41.4
    - senile cognitive decline R41.81
    - specified symptom NEC R41.89
  - behavior NEC R46.89
  - cardiovascular system NEC R09.89
  - chest NEC R09.89
  - circulatory system NEC R09.89
  - cognitive functions R41.9
    - altered mental status R41.82
    - amnesia —*see* Amnesia
    - borderline intellectual functioning R41.83
    - coma —*see* Coma
    - disorientation R41.0
    - neurologic neglect syndrome R41.4
    - senile cognitive decline R41.81
    - specified symptom NEC R41.89
  - development NEC R62.50
  - digestive system NEC R19.8
  - emotional state NEC R45.89
    - emotional lability R45.86
  - food and fluid intake R63.8
  - general perceptions and sensations R44.9
    - specified NEC R44.8
  - musculoskeletal system R29.91
    - specified NEC R29.898
  - nervous system R29.90
    - specified NEC R29.818
  - pelvis NEC R19.8
  - respiratory system NEC R09.89
  - skin and integument R23.9
  - urinary system R39.9
- menopausal N95.1
- metabolism NEC R63.8
- neurotic F48.8
- of infancy R68.19

Symptoms NEC *(Continued)*
pelvis NEC, female R10.2
skin and integument NEC R23.9 ◀▬▬
subcutaneous tissue NEC R23.9 ◀▬▬
Sympus Q74.2
Syncephalus Q89.4
Synchondrosis
abnormal (congenital) Q78.8
ischiopubic M91.0
Synchysis (scintillans) (senile) (vitreous body)
H43.89
Syncope (near) (pre-) R55
anginosa I20.8
bradycardia R00.1
cardiac R55
carotid sinus G90.01
due to spinal (lumbar) puncture G97.1
heart R55
heat T67.1
laryngeal R05
psychogenic F48.8
tussive R05
vasoconstriction R55
vasodepressor R55
vasomotor R55
vasovagal R55
Syndactylism, syndactyly Q70.9
complex (with synostosis)
fingers Q70.0-
toes Q70.2-
simple (without synostosis)
fingers Q70.1-
toes Q70.3-
Syndrome *—see also* Disease
5q minus NOS D46.C
48,XXXX Q97.1
49,XXXXX Q97.1
abdominal
acute R10.0
muscle deficiency Q79.4
abnormal innervation H02.519
left H02.516
lower H02.515
upper H02.514
right H02.513
lower H02.512
upper H02.511
abstinence, neonatal P96.1
acid pulmonary aspiration, obstetric O74.0
acquired immunodeficiency *—see* Human,
immunodeficiency virus (HIV)
disease
acute abdominal R10.0
acute respiratory distress (adult) (child) J80
Adair-Dighton Q78.0
Adams-Stokes (-Morgagni) I45.9
adiposogenital E23.6
adrenal
hemorrhage (meningococcal) A39.1
meningococcic A39.1
adrenocortical *—see* Cushing's, syndrome
adrenogenital E25.9
congenital, associated with enzyme
deficiency E25.0
afferent loop NEC K91.89
Alagille's Q44.7
alcohol withdrawal (without convulsions) —
see Dependence, alcohol, with,
withdrawal
Alder's D72.0
Aldrich (-Wiskott) D82.0
alien hand R41.4
Alport Q87.81
alveolar hypoventilation E66.2
alveolocapillary block J84.10
amnesic, amnestic (confabulatory) (due to) —
see Disorder, amnesic
amyostatic (Wilson's disease) E83.01
androgen insensitivity E34.50
complete E34.51
partial E34.52

Syndrome *(Continued)*
androgen resistance (*see also* Syndrome,
androgen insensitivity) E34.50
Angelman Q93.5
anginal *—see* Angina
ankyloglossia superior Q38.1
anterior
chest wall R07.89
cord G83.82
spinal artery G95.19
compression M47.019
cervical region M47.012
cervicothoracic region M47.013
lumbar region M47.016
occipito-atlanto-axial region M47.011
thoracic region M47.014
thoracolumbar region M47.015
tibial M76.81-
antibody deficiency D80.9
agammaglobulinemic D80.1
hereditary D80.0
congenital D80.0
hypogammaglobulinemic D80.1
hereditary D80.0
anticardiolipin (-antibody) D68.61
antiphospholipid (-antibody) D68.61
aortic
arch M31.4
bifurcation I74.09
aortomesenteric duodenum occlusion K31.5
apical ballooning (transient left ventricular)
I51.81
arcuate ligament I77.4
argentaffin, argintaffinoma E34.0
Arnold-Chiari *—see* Arnold-Chiari disease
Arrillaga-Ayerza I27.0
Asherman's N85.6
aspiration, of newborn *—see* Aspiration, by
substance, with pneumonia
meconium P24.01
ataxia-telangiectasia G11.3
auriculotemporal G50.8
autoerythrocyte sensitization (Gardner-
Diamond) D69.2
autoimmune lymphoproliferative [ALPS]
D89.82
autoimmune polyglandular E31.0
autosomal *—see* Abnormal, autosomes
Avellis' G46.8
Ayerza (-Arrillaga) I27.0
Babinski-Nageotte G83.89
Bakwin-Krida Q79.8
bare lymphocyte D81.6
Barré-Guillain G61.0
Barré-Liéou M53.0
Barrett's *—see* Barrett's, esophagus
Barsony-Polgar K22.4
Barsony-Teschendorf K22.4
Barth E78.71
Bartter's E26.81
basal cell nevus Q87.89
Basedow's E05.00
with thyroid storm E05.01
basilar artery G45.0
Batten-Steinert G71.11
battered
baby or child *—see* Maltreatment, child,
physical abuse
spouse *—see* Maltreatment, adult, physical
abuse
Beals Q87.40
Beau's I51.5
Beck's I65.8
Benedikt's G46.3
Béquez César (-Steinbrinck-Chédiak-Higashi)
D70.330
Bernhardt-Roth *—see* Meralgia paresthetica
Bernheim's I50.9
big spleen D73.1
bilateral polycystic ovarian E28.2
Bing-Horton's *—see* Horton's headache

Syndrome *(Continued)*
Birt-Hogg-Dube syndrome Q87.89
Björck (-Thorsen) E34.0
black
lung J60
widow spider bite *—see* Toxicity, venom,
spider, black widow
Blackfan-Diamond D61.01
blind loop K90.2
congenital Q43.8
postsurgical K91.2
blue sclera Q78.0
blue toe I75.02-
Boder-Sedgewick G11.3
Boerhaave's K22.3
Borjeson Forssman Lehmann Q89.8
Bouillaud's I01.9
Bourneville (-Pringle) Q85.1
Bouveret (-Hoffman) I47.9
brachial plexus G54.0
bradycardia-tachycardia I49.5
brain (nonpsychotic) F09
with psychosis, psychotic reaction F09
acute or subacute *—see* Delirium
congenital *—see* Disability, intellectual
organic F09
post-traumatic (nonpsychotic) F07.81
psychotic F09
personality change F07.0
postcontusional F07.81
post-traumatic, nonpsychotic F07.81
psycho-organic F09
psychotic F06.8
brain stem stroke G46.3
Brandt's (acrodermatitis enteropathica) E83.2
broad ligament laceration N83.8
Brock's J98.11
bronze baby P83.8
Brown-Sequard G83.81
bubbly lung P27.0
Buchem's M85.2
Budd-Chiari I82.0
bulbar (progressive) G12.22
Bürger-Grütz E78.3
Burke's K86.8
Burnett's (milk-alkali) E83.52
burning feet E53.9
Bywaters' T79.5
Call-Fleming I67.841
carbohydrate-deficient glycoprotein (CDGS)
E77.8
carcinogenic thrombophlebitis I82.1
carcinoid E34.0
cardiac asthma I50.1
cardiacos negros I27.0
cardiofaciocutaneous Q87.89
cardiopulmonary-obesity E66.2
cardiorenal *—see* Hypertension, cardiorenal
cardiorespiratory distress (idiopathic),
newborn P22.0
cardiovascular renal *—see* Hypertension,
cardiorenal
carotid
artery (hemispheric) (internal) G45.1
body G90.01
sinus G90.01
carpal tunnel G56.0-
Cassidy (-Scholte) E34.0
cat-cry Q93.4
cat eye Q92.8
cauda equina G83.4
causalgia *—see* Causalgia
celiac K90.0
artery compression I77.4
axis I77.4
central pain G89.0
cerebellar
hereditary G11.9
stroke G46.4
cerebellomedullary malformation *—see* Spina
bifida

Syndrome *(Continued)*
  cerebral
    artery
      anterior G46.1
      middle G46.0
      posterior G46.2
    gigantism E22.0
  cervical (root) M53.1
    disc —*see* Disorder, disc, cervical, with
      neuritis
    fusion Q76.1
    posterior, sympathicus M53.0
    rib Q76.5
    sympathetic paralysis G90.2
  cervicobrachial (diffuse) M53.1
  cervicocranial M53.0
  cervicodorsal outlet G54.2
  cervicothoracic outlet G54.0
  Céstan (-Raymond) I65.8
  Charcot's (angina cruris) (intermittent
      claudication) I73.9
  Charcot-Weiss-Baker G90.09
  CHARGE Q89.8
  Chédiak-Higashi (-Steinbrinck) E70.330
  chest wall R07.1
  Chiari's (hepatic vein thrombosis) I82.0
  Chilaiditi's Q43.3
  child maltreatment —*see* Maltreatment,
      child
  chondrocostal junction M94.0
  chondroectodermal dysplasia Q77.6
  chromosome 4 short arm deletion Q93.3
  chromosome 5 short arm deletion Q93.4
  chronic
    pain G89.4
      personality F68.8
  Clarke-Hadfield K86.8
  Clerambault's automatism G93.89
  Clouston's (hidrotic ectodermal dysplasia)
      Q82.4
  clumsiness, clumsy child F82
  cluster headache G44.009
    intractable G44.001
    not intractable G44.009
  Coffin-Lowry Q89.8
  cold injury (newborn) P80.0
  combined immunity deficiency D81.9
  compartment (deep) (posterior) (traumatic)
      T79.A0
    abdomen T79.A3
    lower extremity (hip, buttock, thigh, leg,
        foot, toes) T79.A2
    nontraumatic
      abdomen M79.A3
      lower extremity (hip, buttock, thigh, leg,
          foot, toes) M79.A2-
      specified site NEC M79.A9
      upper extremity (shoulder, arm, forearm,
          wrist, hand, fingers) M79.A1-
    postprocedural —*see* Syndrome
        compartment, nontraumatic
    specified site NEC T79.A9
    upper extremity (shoulder, arm, forearm,
        wrist, hand, fingers) T79.A1
  complex regional pain —*see* Syndrome, pain,
      complex regional
  compression T79.5
    anterior spinal —*see* Syndrome, anterior,
        spinal artery, compression
    cauda equina G83.4
    celiac artery I77.4
    vertebral artery M47.029
      cervical region M47.022
      occipito-atlanto-axial region M47.021
  concussion F07.81
  congenital
    affecting multiple systems NEC Q87.89
    central alveolar hypoventilation G47.35
    facial diplegia Q87.0
    muscular hypertrophy-cerebral Q87.89
    oculo-auriculovertebral Q87.0

Syndrome *(Continued)*
  congenital *(Continued)*
    oculofacial diplegia (Moebius) Q87.0
    rubella (manifest) P35.0
  congestion-fibrosis (pelvic), female N94.89
  congestive dysmenorrhea N94.6
  Conn's E26.01
  connective tissue M35.9
    overlap NEC M35.1
  conus medullaris G95.81
  cord
    anterior G83.82
    posterior G83.83
  coronary
    acute NEC I24.9
    insufficiency or intermediate I20.0
    slow flow I20.8
  Costen's (complex) M26.69
  costochondral junction M94.0
  costoclavicular G54.0
  costovertebral E22.0
  Cowden Q85.8
  craniovertebral M53.0
  Creutzfeldt-Jakob —*see* Creutzfeldt-Jakob
      disease or syndrome
  cri-du-chat Q93.4
  crib death R99
  cricopharyngeal —*see* Dysphagia
  croup J05.0
  CRPS I —*see* Syndrome, pain, complex
      regional I
  crush T79.5
  cryptophthalmos Q87.0
  cubital tunnel —*see* Lesion, nerve, ulnar
  Curschmann (-Batten) (-Steinert) G71.11
  Cushing's E24.9
    alcohol-induced E24.4
    drug-induced E24.2
    due to
      alcohol
        drugs E24.2
      ectopic ACTH E24.3
      overproduction of pituitary ACTH E24.0
    overdose or wrong substance given or
        taken —*see* Table of dDrugs and
        eChemicals, by drug, poisoning ◀▥▥
    pituitary-dependent E24.0
    specified type NEC E24.8
  cystic duct stump K91.5
  Dana-Putnam D51.0
  Danbolt (-Cross) (acrodermatitis
      enteropathica) E83.2
  Dandy-Walker Q03.1
    with spina bifida Q07.01
  Danlos' Q79.8
  defibrination —*see also* Fibrinolysis
    with
      antepartum hemorrhage —*see*
          Hemorrhage, antepartum, with
          coagulation defect
      intrapartum hemorrhage —*see*
          Hemorrhage, complicating,
          delivery
      newborn P60
      postpartum O72.3
  Degos' I77.8
  Déjérine-Roussy G89.0
  delayed sleep phase G47.21
  demyelinating G37.9
  dependence —*see* F10-F19 with fourth
      character .2
  depersonalization (-derealization) F48.1
  De Quervain E34.51
  de Toni-Fanconi (-Debré) E72.09
    with cystinosis E72.04
  diabetes mellitus-hypertension-nephrosis —
      see Diabetes, nephrosis
  diabetes mellitus in newborn infant P70.2
  diabetes-nephrosis —*see* Diabetes, nephrosis
  diabetic amyotrophy —*see* Diabetes,
      amyotrophy

Syndrome *(Continued)*
  Diamond-Blackfan D61.01
  Diamond-Gardener D69.2
  DIC (diffuse or disseminated intravascular
      coagulopathy) D65
  di George's D82.1
  Dighton's Q78.0
  disequilibrium E87.8
  Döhle body-panmyelopathic D72.0
  dorsolateral medullary G46.4
  double athetosis G80.3
  Down (*see also* Down syndrome) Q90.9
  Dresbach's (elliptocytosis) D58.1
  Dressler's (postmyocardial infarction)
      I24.1
    postcardiotomy I97.0
  drug withdrawal, infant of dependent mother
      P96.1
  dry eye H04.12-
  due to abnormality
    chromosomal Q99.9
    sex
      female phenotype Q97.9
      male phenotype Q98.9
      specified NEC Q99.8
  dumping (postgastrectomy) K91.1
    nonsurgical K31.89
  Dupré's (meningism) R29.1
  dysmetabolic X E88.81
  dyspraxia, developmental F82
  Eagle-Barrett Q79.4
  Eaton-Lambert —*see* Syndrome,
      Lambert-Eaton
  Ebstein's Q22.5
  ectopic ACTH E24.3
  eczema-thrombocytopenia D82.0
  Eddowes' Q78.0
  effort (psychogenic) F45.8
  Ehlers-Danlos Q79.6
  Eisenmenger's I27.89
  Ekman's Q78.0
  electric feet E53.8
  Ellis-van Creveld Q77.6
  empty nest Z60.0
  endocrine-hypertensive E27.0
  entrapment —*see* Neuropathy,
      entrapment
  eosinophilia-myalgia M35.8
  epileptic —*see also* Epilepsy, by type
    absence G40.A09
      intractable G40.A19
        with status epilepticus G40.A11
        without status epilepticus G40.A19
      not intractable G40.A09
        with status epilepticus G40.A01
        without status epilepticus G40.A09
  Erdheim-Chester (ECD) E88.89
  Erdheim's E22.0
  erythrocyte fragmentation D59.4
  Evans D69.41
  exhaustion F48.8
  extrapyramidal G25.9
    specified NEC G25.89
  eye retraction —*see* Strabismus
  eyelid-malar-mandible Q87.0
  Faber's D50.9
  facial pain, paroxysmal G50.0
  Fallot's Q21.3
  familial eczema-thrombocytopenia
      (Wiskott-Aldrich) D82.0
  Fanconi (-de Toni) (-Debré) E72.09
    with cystinosis E72.04
  Fanconi's (anemia) (congenital pancytopenia)
      D61.09
  fatigue
    chronic R53.82
    psychogenic F48.8
  faulty bowel habit K59.3
  Feil-Klippel (brevicollis) Q76.1
  Felty's —*see* Felty's syndrome
  fertile eunuch E23.0

◀ New   ◀▥▥ Revised   ~~deleted~~ Deleted

Syndrome *(Continued)*
  fetal
    alcohol (dysmorphic) Q86.0
    hydantoin Q86.1
  Fiedler's I40.1
  first arch Q87.0
  fish odor E72.8
  Fisher's G61.0
  Fitzhugh-Curtis
    due to
      Chlamydia trachomatis A74.81
      Neisseria gonorrhorea (gonococcal
        peritonitis) A54.85
  Fitz's K85.8
  Flajani (-Basedow) E05.00
    with thyroid storm E05.01
  flatback —*see* Flatback syndrome
  floppy
    baby P94.2
    iris (intraoeprative) (IFIS) H21.81
    mitral valve I34.1
  flush E34.0
  Foix-Alajouanine G95.19
  Fong's Q79.8
  foramen magnum G93.5
  Foster-Kennedy H47.14-
  Foville's (peduncular) G46.3
  fragile X Q99.2
  Franceschetti Q75.4
  Frey's
    auriculotemporal G50.8
    hyperhidrosis L74.52
  Friderichsen-Waterhouse A39.1
  Froin's G95.89
  frontal lobe F07.0
  Fukuhara E88.49
  functional
    bowel K59.9
    prepubertal castrate E29.1
  Gaisböck's D75.1
  ganglion (basal ganglia brain) G25.9
    geniculi G51.1
  Gardner-Diamond D69.2
  gastroesophageal
    junction K22.0
    laceration-hemorrhage K22.6
  gastrojejunal loop obstruction K91.89
  Gee-Herter-Heubner K90.0
  Gelineau's G47.419
    with cataplexy G47.411
  genito-anorectal A55
  Gerstmann-Sträussler-Scheinker (GSS)
    A81.82
  Gianotti-Crosti L44.4
  giant platelet (Bernard-Soulier) D69.1
  Gilles de la Tourette's F95.2
  goiter-deafness E07.1
  Goldberg Q89.8
  Goldberg-Maxwell E34.51
  Good's D83.8
  Gopalan' (burning feet) E53.8
  Gorlin's Q87.89
  Gougerot-Blum L81.7
  Gouley's I31.1
  Gower's R55
  gray or grey (newborn) P93.0
    platelet D69.1
  Gubler-Millard G46.3
  Guillain-Barré (-Strohl) G61.0
  gustatory sweating G50.8
  Hadfield-Clarke K86.8
  hair tourniquet —*see* Constriction, external,
    by site
  Hamman's J98.19
  hand-foot L27.1
  hand-shoulder G90.8
  hantavirus (cardio)-pulmonary (HPS) (HCPS)
    B33.4
  happy puppet Q93.5
  Harada's H30.81-
  Hayem-Faber D50.9

Syndrome *(Continued)*
  headache NEC G44.89
    complicated NEC G44.59
  Heberden's I20.8
  Hedinger's E34.0
  Hegglin's D72.0
  HELLP (hemolysis, elevated liver enzymes
    and low platelet count) O14.2-
  hemolytic-uremic D59.3
  hemophagocytic, infection-associated
    D76.2
  Henoch-Schönlein D69.0
  hepatic flexure K59.8
  hepatopulmonary K76.81
  hepatorenal K76.7
    following delivery O90.4
    postoperative or postprocedural K91.83
    postpartum, puerperal O90.4
  hepatourologic K76.7
  Herter (-Gee) (nontropical sprue) K90.0
  Heubner-Herter K90.0
  Heyd's K76.7
  Hilger's G90.09
  histamine-like (fish poisoning) —*see*
    Poisoning, fish
  histiocytic D76.3
  histiocytosis NEC D76.3
  HIV infection, acute B20
  Hoffmann-Werdnig G12.0
  Hollander-Simons E88.1
  Hoppe-Goldflam G70.00
    with exacerbation (acute) G70.01
    in crisis G70.01
  Horner's G90.2
  hungry bone E83.81
  hunterian glossitis D51.0
  Hutchinson's triad A50.53
  hyperabduction G54.0
  hyperammonemia-hyperornithinemia-
    homocitrullinemia E72.4
  hypereosinophilic (idiopathic) D72.1
  hyperimmunoglobulin E (IgE) D82.4
  hyperkalemic E87.5
  hyperkinetic —*see* Hyperkinesia
  hypermobility M35.7
  hypernatremia E87.0
  hyperosmolarity E87.0
  hyperperfusion G97.82
  hypersplenic D73.1
  hypertransfusion, newborn P61.1
  hyperventilation F45.8
  hyperviscosity (of serum)
    polycythemic D75.1
    sclerothymic D58.8
  hypoglycemic (familial) (neonatal) E16.2
  hypokalemic E87.6
  hyponatremic E87.1
  hypopituitarism E23.0
  hypoplastic left-heart Q23.4
  hypopotassemia E87.6
  hyposmolality E87.1
  hypotension, maternal O26.5-
  hypothenar hammer I73.89
  ICF (intravascular coagulation-fibrinolysis)
    D65
  idiopathic
    cardiorespiratory distress, newborn P22.0
    nephrotic (infantile) N04.9
  iliotibial band M76.3-
  immobility, immobilization (paraplegic)
    M62.3
  immune reconstitution D89.3
  immune reconstitution inflammatory [IRIS]
    D89.3
  immunity deficiency, combined D81.9
  immunodeficiency
    acquired —*see* Human, immunodeficiency
      virus (HIV) disease
    combined D81.9
  impending coronary I20.0
  impingement, shoulder M75.4-

Syndrome *(Continued)*
  inappropriate secretion of antidiuretic
    hormone E22.2
  infant
    gestational diabetes P70.0
    of diabetic mother P70.1
  infantilism (pituitary) E23.0
  inferior vena cava I87.1
  inspissated bile (newborn) P59.1
  institutional (childhood) F94.2
  insufficient sleep F51.12
  intermediate coronary (artery) I20.0
  interspinous ligament —*see* Spondylopathy,
    specified NEC
  intestinal
    carcinoid E34.0
    knot K56.2
  intravascular coagulation-fibrinolysis (ICF)
    D65
  iodine-deficiency, congenital E00.9
    type
      mixed E00.2
      myxedematous E00.1
      neurological E00.0
  IRDS (idiopathic respiratory distress,
    newborn) P22.0
  irritable
    bowel K58.9
      with diarrhea K58.0
      psychogenic F45.8
    heart (psychogenic) F45.8
    weakness F48.8
  ischemic bowel (transient) K55.9
    chronic K55.1
    due to mesenteric artery insufficiency
      K55.1
  IVC (intravascular coagulopathy) D65
  Ivemark's Q89.01
  Jaccoud's —*see* Arthropathy, postrheumatic,
    chronic
  Jackson's G83.89
  Jakob-Creutzfeldt —*see* Creutzfeldt-Jakob
    disease or syndrome
  jaw-winking Q07.8
  Jervell-Lange-Nielsen I45.81
  jet lag G47.25
  Job's D71
  Joseph-Diamond-Blackfan D61.01
  jugular foramen G52.7
  Kabuki Q89.8
  Kanner's (autism) F84.0
  Kartagener's Q89.3
  Kelly's D50.1
  Kimmelsteil-Wilson —*see* Diabetes, specified
    type, with Kimmelsteil-Wilson disease
  Klein (e)-Levine G47.13
  Klippel-Feil (brevicollis) Q76.1
  Köhler-Pellegrini-Steida —*see* Bursitis, tibial
    collateral
  König's K59.8
  Korsakoff (-Wernicke) (nonalcoholic) F04
    alcoholic F10.26
  Kostmann's D70.0
  Krabbe's congenital muscle hypoplasia Q79.8
  labyrinthine —*see* subcategory H83.2
  lacunar NEC G46.7
  Lambert-Eaton G70.80
    in
      neoplastic disease G73.1
      specified disease NEC G70.81
  Landau-Kleffner —*see* Epilepsy, specified
    NEC
  Larsen's Q74.8
  lateral
    cutaneous nerve of thigh G57.1-
    medullary G46.4
  Launois' E22.0
  lazy
    leukocyte D70.8
    posture M62.3
  Lemiere I80.8

Syndrome *(Continued)*
   Lennox-Gastaut G40.812
      intractable G40.814
         with status epilepticus G40.813
         without status epilepticus G40.814
      not intractable G40.812
         with status epilepticus G40.811
         without status epilepticus G40.812
   lenticular, progressive E83.01
   Leopold-Levi's E05.90
   Lev's I44.2
   Li-Fraumeni Z15.01
   Lichtheim's D51.0
   Lightwood's N25.89
   Lignac (de Toni) (-Fanconi) (-Debré) E72.09
      with cystinosis E72.04
   Likoff's I20.8
   limbic epilepsy personality F07.0
   liver-kidney K76.7
   lobotomy F07.0
   Loffler's J82
   long arm 18 or 21 deletion Q93.89
   long QT I45.81
   Louis-Barré G11.3
   low
      atmospheric pressure T70.29
      back M54.5
      output (cardiac) I50.9
   lower radicular, newborn (birth injury) P14.8
   Luetscher's (dehydration) E86.0
   Lupus anticoagulant D68.62
   Lutembacher's Q21.1
   macrophage activation D76.1
      due to infection D76.2
   magnesium-deficiency R29.0
   Mal de Debarquement R42
   malabsorption K90.9
      postsurgical K91.2
   malformation, congenital, due to
      alcohol Q86.0
      exogenous cause NEC Q86.8
      hydantoin Q86.1
      warfarin Q86.2
   malignant
      carcinoid E34.0
      neuroleptic G21.0
   Mallory-Weiss K22.6
   mandibulofacial dysostosis Q75.4
   manic-depressive —*see* Disorder, bipolar,
      affective
   maple-syrup-urine E71.0
   Marable's I77.4
   Marfan's Q87.40
      with
         cardiovascular manifestations Q87.418
            aortic dilation Q87.410
         ocular manifestations Q87.42
         skeletal manifestations Q87.43
   Marie's (acromegaly) E22.0
   maternal hypotension —*see* Syndrome,
      hypotension, maternal
   May (-Hegglin) D72.0
   McArdle (-Schmidt) (-Pearson) E74.04
   McQuarrie's E16.2
   meconium plug (newborn) P76.0
   median arcuate ligament I77.4
   Meekeren-Ehlers-Danlos Q79.6
   megavitamin-B6 E67.2
   Meige G24.4
   MELAS E88.41
   Mendelson's O74.0
   MERRF (myoclonic epilepsy associated with
      ragged-red fibers) E88.42
   mesenteric
      artery (superior) K55.1
      vascular insufficiency K55.1
   metabolic E88.81
   metastatic carcinoid E34.0
   micrognathia-glossoptosis Q87.0
   midbrain NEC G93.89
   middle lobe (lung) J98.19

Syndrome *(Continued)*
   middle radicular G54.0
   migraine *(see also* Migraine) G43.909- ⬅
   Mikulicz' K11.8
   milk-alkali E83.52
   Millard-Gubler G46.3
   Miller-Dieker Q93.88
   Miller-Fisher G61.0
   Minkowski-Chauffard D58.0
   Mirizzi's K83.1
   MNGIE (Mitochondrial Neurogastrointestinal
      Encephalopathy) E88.49
   Möbius, ophthalmoplegic migraine —*see*
      Migraine, ophthalmoplegic
   monofixation H50.42
   Morel-Moore M85.2
   Morel-Morgagni M85.2
   Morgagni (-Morel) (-Stewart) M85.2
   Morgagni-Adams-Stokes I45.9
   Mounier-Kuhn Q32.4
      with bronchiectasis J47.9
         with
            exacerbation (acute) J47.1
            lower respiratory infection J47.0
      acquired J98.09
         with bronchiectasis J47.9
            with
               exacerbation (acute) J47.1
               lower respiratory infection J47.0
   mucocutaneous lymph node (acute febrile)
      (MCLS) M30.3
   multiple endocrine neoplasia (MEN) —*see*
      Neoplasia, endocrine, multiple (MEN)
   multiple operations —*see* Disorder, factitious
   myasthenic G70.9
      in
         diabetes mellitus —*see* Diabetes,
            amyotrophy
         endocrine disease NEC E34.9 *[G73.3]*
         neoplastic disease *(see also* Neoplasm)
            D49.9 *[G73.3]*
         thyrotoxicosis (hyperthyroidism) E05.90
            [G73.3]
            with thyroid storm E05.91 *[G73.3]*
   myelodysplastic D46.9
      with
         5q deletion D46.C
         isolated del (5q) chromosomal
            abnormality D46.C
      lesions, low grade D46.20
      specified NEC D46.Z
   myelopathic pain G89.0
   myeloproliferative (chronic) D47.1
   myofascial pain M79.1
   Naffziger's G54.0
   nail patella Q87.2
   NARP (Neuropathy, Ataxia and Retinitis
      pigmentosa) E88.49
   neonatal abstinence P96.1
   nephritic —*see also* Nephritis
      with edema —*see* Nephrosis
      acute N00.9
      chronic N03.9
      rapidly progressive N01.9
   nephrotic (congenital) *(see also* Nephrosis)
      N04.9
      with
         dense deposit disease N04.6
         diffuse
            crescentic glomerulonephritis
               N04.7
            endocapillary proliferative
               glomerulonephritis N04.4
            membranous glomerulonephritis
               N04.2
            mesangial proliferative
               glomerulonephritis N04.3
            mesangiocapillary glomerulonephritis
               N04.5
         focal and segmental glomerular lesions
            N04.1

Syndrome *(Continued)*
   nephrotic *(Continued)*
      with *(Continued)*
         minor glomerular abnormality N04.0
         specified morphological changes NEC
            N04.8
      diabetic —*see* Diabetes, nephrosis
   neurologic neglect R41.4
   Nezelof's D81.4
   Nonne-Milroy-Meige Q82.0
   Nothnagel's vasomotor acroparesthesia
      I73.89
   oculomotor H51.9
   ophthalmoplegia-cerebellar ataxia —*see*
      Strabismus, paralytic, third nerve
   oral-facial-digital Q87.0
   organic
      affective F06.30
      amnesic (not alcohol- or drug-induced) F04
      brain F09
      depressive F06.31
      hallucinosis F06.0
      personality F07.0
   Ormond's N13.5
   oro-facial-digital Q87.0
   os trigonum Q68.8
   Osler-Weber-Rendu I78.0
   osteoporosis-osteomalacia M83.8
   Osterreicher-Turner Q79.8
   otolith —*see* subcategory H81.8
   oto-palatal-digital Q87.0
   outlet (thoracic) G54.0
   ovary
      polycystic E28.2
      resistant E28.39
      sclerocystic E28.2
   Owren's D68.2
   Paget-Schroetter I82.890
   pain —*see also* Pain
      complex regional I G90.50
         lower limb G90.52-
         specified site NEC G90.59
         upper limb G90.51-
      complex regional II —*see* Causalgia
   painful
      bruising D69.2
      feet E53.8
      prostate N42.81
   paralysis agitans —*see* Parkinsonism
   paralytic G83.9
      specified NEC G83.89
   Parinaud's H51.0
   parkinsonian —*see* Parkinsonism
   Parkinson's —*see* Parkinsonism
   paroxysmal facial pain G50.0
   Parry's E05.00
      with thyroid storm E05.01
   Parsonage (-Aldren)-Turner G54.5
   patella clunk M25.86-
   Paterson (-Brown) (-Kelly) D50.1
   pectoral girdle I77.89
   pectoralis minor I77.89
   Pelger-Huet D72.0
   pellagra-cerebellar ataxia-renal
      aminoaciduria E72.02
   pellagroid E52
   Pellegrini-Stieda —*see* Bursitis, tibial
      collateral
   pelvic congestion-fibrosis, female N94.89
   penta X Q97.1
   peptic ulcer —*see* Ulcer, peptic
   perabduction I77.89
   periodic headache, in adults and children —
      see Headache, periodic syndromes in
      adults and children
   periurethral fibrosis N13.5
   phantom limb (without pain) G54.7
      with pain G54.6
   pharyngeal pouch D82.1
   Pick's (heart) (liver) I31.1
   Pickwickian E66.2

Syndrome *(Continued)*
  PIE (pulmonary infiltration with eosinophilia) J82
  pigmentary pallidal degeneration (progressive) G23.0
  pineal E34.8
  pituitary E22.0
  placental transfusion —*see* Pregnancy, complicated by, placental transfusion syndromes
  plantar fascia M72.2
  plateau iris (post-iridectomy) (postprocedural) H21.82
  Plummer-Vinson D50.1
  pluricarential of infancy E40
  plurideficiency E40
  pluriglandular (compensatory) E31.8
    autoimmune E31.0
  pneumatic hammer T75.21
  polyangiitis overlap M30.8
  polycarential of infancy E40
  polyglandular E31.8
    autoimmune E31.0
  polysplenia Q89.09
  pontine NEC G93.89
  popliteal
    artery entrapment I77.89
    web Q87.89
  postcardiac injury
    postcardiotomy I97.0
    postmyocardial infarction I24.1
  postcardiotomy I97.0
  post chemoembolization — code to associated conditions
  postcholecystectomy K91.5
  postcommissurotomy I97.0
  postconcussional F07.81
  postcontusional F07.81
  postencephalitic F07.89
  posterior
    cervical sympathetic M53.0
    cord G83.83
    fossa compression G93.5
    reversible encephalopathy (PRES) I67.83
  postgastrectomy (dumping) K91.1
  postgastric surgery K91.1
  postinfarction I24.1
  postlaminectomy NEC M96.1
  postleukotomy F07.0
  postmastectomy lymphedema I97.2
  postmyocardial infarction I24.1
  postoperative NEC T81.9
    blind loop K90.2
  postpartum panhypopituitary (Sheehan) E23.0
  postpolio (myelitic) G14
  postthrombotic I87.009
    with
      inflammation I87.02-
        with ulcer I87.03-
      specified complication NEC I87.09-
      ulcer I87.01-
        with inflammation I87.03-
    asymptomatic I87.00-
  postvagotomy K91.1
  postvalvulotomy I97.0
  postviral NEC G93.3
    fatigue G93.3
  Potain's K31.0
  potassium intoxication E87.5
  precerebral artery (multiple) (bilateral) G45.2
  preinfarction I20.0
  preleukemic D46.9
  premature senility E34.8
  premenstrual dysphoric N94.3
  premenstrual tension N94.3
  Prinzmetal-Massumi R07.1
  prune belly Q79.4
  pseudocarpal tunnel (sublimis) —*see* Syndrome, carpal tunnel

Syndrome *(Continued)*
  pseudoparalytica G70.00
    with exacerbation (acute) G70.01
    in crisis G70.01
  pseudo -Turner's Q87.1
  psycho-organic (nonpsychotic severity) F07.9
    acute or subacute F05
    depressive type F06.31
    hallucinatory type F06.0
    nonpsychotic severity F07.0
    specified NEC F07.89
  pulmonary
    arteriosclerosis I27.0
    dysmaturity (Wilson-Mikity) P27.0
    hypoperfusion (idiopathic) P22.0
    renal (hemorrhagic) (Goodpasture's) M31.0
  pure
    motor lacunar G46.5
    sensory lacunar G46.6
  Putnam-Dana D51.0
  pyramidopallidonigral G20
  pyriformis —*see* Lesion, nerve, sciatic
  QT interval prolongation I45.81
  radicular NEC —*see* Radiculopathy
    upper limbs, newborn (birth injury) P14.3
  rapid time-zone change G47.25
  Rasmussen G04.81
  Raymond (-Céstan) I65.8
  Raynaud's I73.00
    with gangrene I73.01
  RDS (respiratory distress syndrome, newborn) P22.0
  reactive airways dysfunction J68.3
  Refsum's G60.1
  Reifenstein E34.52
  renal glomerulohyalinosis-diabetic —*see* Diabetes, nephrosis
  Rendu-Osler-Weber I78.0
  residual ovary N99.83
  resistant ovary E28.39
  respiratory
    distress
      acute J80
        adult J80
        child J80
      newborn (idiopathic) (type I) P22.0
      type II P22.1
  restless legs G25.81
  retinoblastoma (familial) C69.2
  retroperitoneal fibrosis N13.5
  retroviral seroconversion (acute) Z21
  Reye's G93.7
  Richter —*see* Leukemia, chronic lymphocytic, B-cell type
  Ridley's I50.1
  right
    heart, hypoplastic Q22.6
    ventricular obstruction —*see* Failure, heart, congestive
  Romano-Ward (prolonged QT interval) I45.81
  rotator cuff, shoulder (*see also* Tear, rotator cuff) M75.10-
  Rotes Quérol —*see* Hyperostosis, ankylosing
  Roth —*see* Meralgia paresthetica
  rubella (congenital) P35.0
  Ruvalcaba-Myhre-Smith E71.440
  Rytand-Lipsitch I44.2
  salt
    depletion E87.1
      due to heat NEC T67.8
        causing heat exhaustion or prostration T67.4
    low E87.1
  salt-losing N28.89
  Scaglietti-Dagnini E22.0
  scalenus anticus (anterior) G54.0
  scapulocostal —*see* Mononeuropathy, upper limb, specified site NEC
  scapuloperoneal G71.0
  schizophrenic, of childhood NEC F84.5
  Schnitzler D47.2

Syndrome *(Continued)*
  Scholte's E34.0
  Schroeder's E27.0
  Schüller-Christian C96.5
  Schwachman's —*see* Syndrome, Shwachman's
  Schwartz (-Jampel) G71.13
  Schwartz-Bartter E22.2
  scimitar Q26.8
  sclerocystic ovary E28.2
  Seitelberger's G31.89
  septicemic adrenal hemorrhage A39.1
  seroconversion, retroviral (acute) Z21
  serous meningitis G93.2
  severe acute respiratory (SARS) J12.81
  shaken infant T74.4
  shock (traumatic) T79.4
    kidney N17.0
      following crush injury T79.5
    toxic A48.3
  shock-lung J80
  Shone's — code to specific anomalies
  short
    bowel K91.2
    rib Q77.2
  shoulder-hand —*see* Algoneurodystrophy
  Shwachman's D70.4
  sicca —*see* Sicca syndrome
  sick
    cell E87.1
    sinus I49.5
  sick-euthyroid E07.81
  sideropenic D50.1
  Siemens' ectodermal dysplasia Q82.4
  Silfversköld's Q78.9
  Simons' E88.1
  sinus tarsi —~~*see* Syndrome, tarsal tunnel~~M25.57- ◀
  sinusitis-bronchiectasis-situs inversus Q89.3
  Sipple's E31.22
  sirenomelia Q87.2
  Slocumb's E27.0
  slow flow, coronary I20.8
  Sluder's G44.89
  Smith-Magenis Q93.88
  Sneddon-Wilkinson L13.1
  Sotos' E22.0
  South African cardiomyopathy I42.8
  spasmodic
    upward movement, eyes H51.8
    winking F95.8
  Spen's I45.9
  splenic
    agenesis Q89.01
    flexure K59.8
    neutropenia D73.81
  Spurway's Q78.0
  staphylococcal scalded skin L00
  Stein-Leventhal E28.2
  Stein's E28.2
  Stevens-Johnson syndrome L51.1
    toxic epidermal necrolysis overlap L51.3
  Stewart-Morel M85.2
  Stickler Q89.8
  stiff baby Q89.8
  stiff man G25.82
  Still-Felty —*see* Felty's syndrome
  Stokes (-Adams) I45.9
  stone heart I50.1
  straight back, congenital Q76.49
  subclavian steal G45.8
  subcoracoid-pectoralis minor G54.0
  subcostal nerve compression I77.89
  subphrenic interposition Q43.3
  superior
    cerebellar artery I63.8
    mesenteric artery K55.1
    semi-circular canal dehiscence H83.8X-
    vena cava I87.1
  supine hypotensive (maternal) —*see* Syndrome, hypotension, maternal

Syndrome (Continued)
suprarenal cortical E27.0
supraspinatus (see also Tear, rotator cuff)
M75.10-
Susac G93.49
swallowed blood P78.2
sweat retention L74.0
Swyer Q99.1
Symond's G93.2
sympathetic
cervical paralysis G90.2
pelvic, female N94.89
systemic inflammatory response (SIRS), of
non-infectious origin (without organ
dysfunction) R65.10
with acute organ dysfunction R65.11
tachycardia-bradycardia I49.5
takotsubo I51.81
TAR (thrombocytopenia with absent radius)
Q87.2
tarsal tunnel G57.5-
teething K00.7
tegmental G93.89
telangiectasic-pigmentation-cataract
Q82.8
temporal pyramidal apex —see Otitis,
media, suppurative, acute
temporomandibular joint-pain-dysfunction
M26.62
Terry's H44.2-
testicular feminization (see also Syndrome,
androgen insensitivity) E34.51
thalamic pain (hyperesthetic) G89.0
thoracic outlet (compression) G54.0
Thorson-Björck E34.0
thrombocytopenia with absent radius (TAR)
Q87.2
thyroid-adrenocortical insufficiency E31.0
tibial
anterior M76.81-
posterior M76.82-
Tietze's M94.0
time-zone (rapid) G47.25
Toni-Fanconi E72.09
with cystinosis E72.04
Touraine's Q79.8
tourniquet —see Constriction, external,
by site
toxic shock A48.3
transient left ventricular apical ballooning
I51.81
traumatic vasospastic T75.22
Treacher Collins Q75.4
triple X, female Q97.0
trisomy Q92.9
13 Q91.7
meiotic nondisjunction Q91.4
mitotic nondisjunction Q91.5
mosaicism Q91.5
translocation Q91.6
18 Q91.3
meiotic nondisjunction Q91.0
mitotic nondisjunction Q91.1
mosaicism Q91.1
translocation Q91.2
20 (q)(p) Q92.8
21 Q90.9
meiotic nondisjunction Q90.0
mitotic nondisjunction Q90.1
mosaicism Q90.1
translocation Q90.2
22 Q92.8
tropical wet feet T69.0-
Trousseau's I82.1
tumor lysis (following antineoplastic
chemotherapy) (spontaneous) NEC
E88.3
Twiddler's (due to)
automatic implantable defibrillator
T82.198
cardiac pacemaker T82.198

Syndrome (Continued)
Unverricht (-Lundborg) —see Epilepsy,
generalized, idiopathic
upward gaze H51.8
uremia, chronic (see also Disease, kidney,
chronic) N18.9
urethral N34.3
urethro-oculo-articular —see Reiter's disease
urohepatic K76.7
vago-hypoglossal G52.7
van Buchem's M85.2
van der Hoeve's Q78.0
vascular NEC in cerebrovascular disease
G46.8
vasoconstriction, reversible cerebrovascular
I67.841
vasomotor I73.9
vasospastic (traumatic) T75.22
vasovagal R55
VATER Q87.2
velo-cardio-facial Q93.81
vena cava (inferior) (superior) (obstruction)
I87.1
vertebral
artery G45.0
compression —see Syndrome, anterior,
spinal artery, compression
steal G45.0
vertebro-basilar artery G45.0
vertebrogenic (pain) M54.89
vertiginous —see Disorder, vestibular
function
Vinson-Plummer D50.1
virus B34.9
visceral larva migrans B83.0
visual disorientation H53.8
vitamin B6 deficiency E53.1
vitreal corneal H59.01-
vitreous (touch) H59.01-
Vogt-Koyanagi H20.82-
Volkmann's T79.6
von Schroetter's I82.890
von Willebrand (-Jürgen) D68.0
Waldenström-Kjellberg D50.1
Wallenberg's G46.3
water retention E87.79
Waterhouse (-Friderichsen) A39.1
Weber-Gubler G46.3
Weber-Leyden G46.3
Weber's G46.3
Wegener's M31.30
with
kidney involvement M31.31
lung involvement M31.30
with kidney involvement M31.31
Weingarten's (tropical eosinophilia) J82
Weiss-Baker G90.09
Werdnig-Hoffman G12.0
Wermer's E31.21
Werner's E34.8
Wernicke-Korsakoff (nonalcoholic) F04
alcoholic F10.26
West's —see Epilepsy, spasms
Westphal-Strümpell E83.01
wet
feet (maceration) (tropical) T69.0-
lung, newborn P22.1
whiplash S13.4
whistling face Q87.0
Wilkie's K55.1
Wilkinson-Sneddon L13.1
Willebrand (-Jürgens) D68.0
Wilson's (hepatolenticular degeneration)
E83.01
Wiskott-Aldrich D82.0
withdrawal —see Withdrawal, state
drug
infant of dependent mother P96.1
therapeutic use, newborn P96.2
Woakes' (ethmoiditis) J33.1
Wright's (hyperabduction) I77.89

Syndrome (Continued)
X I20.9
XXXX Q97.1
XXXXX Q97.1
XXXXY Q98.1
XXY Q98.0
yellow nail L60.5
Zahorsky's B08.5
Zellweger syndrome E71.510
Zellweger-like syndrome E71.541
Synechia (anterior) (iris) (posterior) (pupil) —
see also Adhesions, iris
intra-uterine (traumatic) N85.6
Synesthesia R20.8
Syngamiasis, syngamosis B83.3
Synodontia K00.2
Synorchidism, synorchism Q55.1
Synostosis (congenital) Q78.8
astragalo-scaphoid Q74.2
radioulnar Q74.0
Synovial sarcoma —see Neoplasm, connective
tissue, malignant
Synovioma (malignant) —see also Neoplasm,
connective tissue, malignant
benign —see Neoplasm, connective tissue,
benign
Synoviosarcoma —see Neoplasm, connective
tissue, malignant
Synovitis —see also Tenosynovitis
crepitant
hand M70.0-
wrist M70.03-
gonococcal A54.49
gouty —see Gout, idiopathic
in (due to)
crystals M65.8-
gonorrhea A54.49
syphilis (late) A52.78
use, overuse, pressure —see Disorder, soft
tissue, due to use
infective NEC —see Tenosynovitis, infective
NEC
specified NEC —see Tenosynovitis, specified
type NEC
syphilitic A52.78
congenital (early) A50.02
toxic —see Synovitis, transient
transient M67.3-
ankle M67.37-
elbow M67.32-
foot joint M67.37-
hand joint M67.34-
hip M67.35-
knee M67.36-
multiple site M67.39
pelvic region M67.35-
shoulder M67.31-
specified joint NEC M67.38
wrist M67.33-
traumatic, current —see Sprain
tuberculous —see Tuberculosis, synovitis
villonodular (pigmented) M12.2-
ankle M12.27-
elbow M12.22-
foot joint M12.27-
hand joint M12.24-
hip M12.25-
knee M12.26-
multiple site M12.29
pelvic region M12.25-
shoulder M12.21-
specified joint NEC M12.28
vertebrae M12.28 ◀
wrist M12.23-
Syphilid A51.39
congenital A50.06
newborn A50.06
tubercular (late) A52.79
Syphilis, syphilitic (acquired) A53.9
abdomen (late) A52.79
acoustic nerve A52.15

Syphilis, syphilitic *(Continued)*
  adenopathy (secondary) A51.49
  adrenal (gland) (with cortical hypofunction)
    A52.79
  age under 2 years NOS —*see also* Syphilis,
    congenital, early
    acquired A51.9
  alopecia (secondary) A51.32
  anemia (late) A52.79 *[D63.8]*
  aneurysm (aorta) (ruptured) A52.01
    central nervous system A52.05
    congenital A50.54 *[I79.0]*
  anus (late) A52.74
    primary A51.1
    secondary A51.39
  aorta (arch) (abdominal) (thoracic) A52.02
    aneurysm A52.01
  aortic (insufficiency) (regurgitation)
    (stenosis) A52.03
    aneurysm A52.01
  arachnoid (adhesive) (cerebral) (spinal)
    A52.13
  asymptomatic —*see* Syphilis, latent
  ataxia (locomotor) A52.11
  atrophoderma maculatum A51.39
  auricular fibrillation A52.06
  bladder (late) A52.76
  bone A52.77
    secondary A51.46
  brain A52.17
  breast (late) A52.79
  bronchus (late) A52.72
  bubo (primary) A51.0
  bulbar palsy A52.19
  bursa (late) A52.78
  cardiac decompensation A52.06
  cardiovascular A52.00
  central nervous system (late) (recurrent)
    (relapse) (tertiary) A52.3
    with
      ataxia A52.11
      general paralysis A52.17
        juvenile A50.45
      paresis (general) A52.17
        juvenile A50.45
      tabes (dorsalis) A52.11
        juvenile A50.45
      taboparesis A52.17
        juvenile A50.45
    aneurysm A52.05
    congenital A50.40
    juvenile A50.40
    remission in (sustained) A52.3
    serology doubtful, negative, or positive
      A52.3
    specified nature or site NEC A52.19
    vascular A52.05
  cerebral A52.17
    meningovascular A52.13
    nerves (multiple palsies) A52.15
    sclerosis A52.17
    thrombosis A52.05
  cerebrospinal (tabetic type) A52.12
  cerebrovascular A52.05
  cervix (late) A52.76
  chancre (multiple) A51.0
    extragenital A51.2
    Rollet's A51.0
  Charcot's joint A52.16
  chorioretinitis A51.43
    congenital A50.01
    late A52.71
    prenatal A50.01
  choroiditis —*see* Syphilitic chorioretinitis
  choroidoretinitis —*see* Syphilitic
    chorioretinitis
  ciliary body (secondary) A51.43
    late A52.71
  colon (late) A52.74
  combined spinal sclerosis A52.11
  condyloma (latum) A51.31

Syphilis, syphilitic *(Continued)*
  congenital A50.9
    with
      paresis (general) A50.45
      tabes (dorsalis) A50.45
      taboparesis A50.45
    chorioretinitis, choroiditis A50.01 *[H32]*
    early, or less than 2 years after birth NEC
      A50.2
      with manifestations —*see* Syphilis,
        congenital, early, symptomatic
      latent (without manifestations) A50.1
        negative spinal fluid test A50.1
        serology positive A50.1
      symptomatic A50.09
        cutaneous A50.06
        mucocutaneous A50.07
        oculopathy A50.01
        osteochondropathy A50.02
        pharyngitis A50.03
        pneumonia A50.04
        rhinitis A50.05
        visceral A50.08
    interstitial keratitis A50.31
    juvenile neurosyphilis A50.45
    late, or 2 years or more after birth NEC
      A50.7
      chorioretinitis, choroiditis A50.32
      interstitial keratitis A50.31
      juvenile neurosyphilis A50.45
      latent (without manifestations) A50.6
        negative spinal fluid test A50.6
        serology positive A50.6
      symptomatic or with manifestations
        NEC A50.59
        arthropathy A50.55
        cardiovascular A50.54
        Clutton's joints A50.51
        Hutchinson's teeth A50.52
        Hutchinson's triad A50.53
        osteochondropathy A50.56
        saddle nose A50.57
  conjugal A53.9
    tabes A52.11
  conjunctiva (late) A52.71
  contact Z20.2
  cord bladder A52.19
  cornea, late A52.71
  coronary (artery) (sclerosis) A52.06
  coryza, congenital A50.05
  cranial nerve A52.15
    multiple palsies A52.15
  cutaneous —*see* Syphilis, skin
  dacryocystitis (late) A52.71
  degeneration, spinal cord A52.12
  dementia paralytica A52.17
    juvenilis A50.45
  destruction of bone A52.77
  dilatation, aorta A52.01
  due to blood transfusion A53.9
  dura mater A52.13
  ear A52.79
    inner A52.79
      nerve (eighth) A52.15
      neurorecurrence A52.15
  early A51.9
    cardiovascular A52.00
    central nervous system A52.3
    latent (without manifestations) (less
      than 2 years after infection)
      A51.5
      negative spinal fluid test A51.5
      serological relapse after treatment
        A51.5
      serology positive A51.5
    relapse (treated, untreated) A51.9
    skin A51.39
    symptomatic A51.9
      extragenital chancre A51.2
      primary, except extragenital chancre
        A51.0

Syphilis, syphilitic *(Continued)*
  early *(Continued)*
    symptomatic *(Continued)*
      secondary *(see also* Syphilis, secondary)
        A51.39
        relapse (treated, untreated) A51.49
      ulcer A51.39
  eighth nerve (neuritis) A52.15
  endemic A65
  endocarditis A52.03
    aortic A52.03
    pulmonary A52.03
  epididymis (late) A52.76
  epiglottis (late) A52.73
  epiphysitis (congenital) (early) A50.02
  episcleritis (late) A52.71
  esophagus A52.79
  eustachian tube A52.73
  exposure to Z20.2
  eye A52.71
  eyelid (late) (with gumma) A52.71
  fallopian tube (late) A52.76
  fracture A52.77
  gallbladder (late) A52.74
  gastric (polyposis) (late) A52.74
  general A53.9
    paralysis A52.17
      juvenile A50.45
  genital (primary) A51.0
  glaucoma A52.71
  gumma NEC A52.79
    cardiovascular system A52.00
    central nervous system A52.3
    congenital A50.59
  heart (block) (decompensation) (disease)
    (failure) A52.06 *[I52]*
    valve NEC A52.03
  hemianesthesia A52.19
  hemianopsia A52.71
  hemiparesis A52.17
  hemiplegia A52.17
  hepatic artery A52.09
  hepatis A52.74
  hepatomegaly, congenital A50.08
  hereditaria tarda —*see* Syphilis, congenital,
    late
  hereditary —*see* Syphilis, congenital
  Hutchinson's teeth A50.52
  hyalitis A52.71
  inactive —*see* Syphilis, latent
  infantum —*see* Syphilis, congenital
  inherited —*see* Syphilis, congenital
  internal ear A52.79
  intestine (late) A52.74
  iris, iritis (secondary) A51.43
    late A52.71
  joint (late) A52.77
  keratitis (congenital) (interstitial) (late)
    A50.31
  kidney (late) A52.75
  lacrimal passages (late) A52.71
  larynx (late) A52.73
  late A52.9
    cardiovascular A52.00
    central nervous system A52.3
    kidney A52.75
    latent or 2 years or more after infection
      (without manifestations) A52.8
      negative spinal fluid test A52.8
      serology positive A52.8
    paresis A52.17
    specified site NEC A52.79
    symptomatic or with manifestations A52.79
    tabes A52.11
  latent A53.0
    with signs or symptoms - code by site and
      stage under Syphilis
    central nervous system A52.2
    date of infection unspecified A53.0
    early, or less than 2 years after infection
      A51.5

Syphilis, syphilitic *(Continued)*
  latent *(Continued)*
    follow-up of latent syphilis A53.0
      date of infection unspecified A53.0
      late, or 2 years or more after infection
        A52.8
      late, or 2 years or more after infection
        A52.8
    positive serology (only finding) A53.0
      date of infection unspecified A53.0
      early, or less than 2 years after infection
        A51.5
      late, or 2 years or more after infection
        A52.8
  lens (late) A52.71
  leukoderma A51.39
    late A52.79
  lienitis A52.79
  lip A51.39
    chancre (primary) A51.2
    late A52.79
  Lissauer's paralysis A52.17
  liver A52.74
  locomotor ataxia A52.11
  lung A52.72
  lymph gland (early) (secondary) A51.49
    late A52.79
  lymphadenitis (secondary) A51.49
  macular atrophy of skin A51.39
    striated A52.79
  mediastinum (late) A52.73
  meninges (adhesive) (brain) (spinal cord)
    A52.13
  meningitis A52.13
    acute (secondary) A51.41
    congenital A50.41
  meningoencephalitis A52.14
  meningovascular A52.13
    congenital A50.41
  mesarteritis A52.09
    brain A52.04
  middle ear A52.77
  mitral stenosis A52.03
  monoplegia A52.17
  mouth (secondary) A51.39
    late A52.79
  mucocutaneous (secondary) A51.39
    late A52.79
  mucous
    membrane (secondary) A51.39
      late A52.79
    patches A51.39
      congenital A50.07
  mulberry molars A50.52
  muscle A52.78
  myocardium A52.06
  nasal sinus (late) A52.73
  neonatorum —*see* Syphilis, congenital
  nephrotic syndrome (secondary)
    A51.44
  nerve palsy (any cranial nerve) A52.15
    multiple A52.15
  nervous system, central A52.3
  neuritis A52.15
    acoustic A52.15
  neurorecidive of retina A52.19
  neuroretinitis A52.19
  newborn —*see* Syphilis, congenital
  nodular superficial (late) A52.79
  nonvenereal A65
  nose (late) A52.73
    saddle back deformity A50.57
  occlusive arterial disease A52.09
  oculopathy A52.71
  oesophagus (late) A52.79
  ophthalmic (late) A52.71
  optic nerve (atrophy) (neuritis) (papilla)
    A52.15
  orbit (late) A52.71
  organic A53.9
  osseous (late) A52.77

Syphilis, syphilitic *(Continued)*
  osteochondritis (congenital) (early) A50.02
    [M90.80]
  osteoporosis A52.77
  ovary (late) A52.76
  oviduct (late) A52.76
  palate (late) A52.79
  pancreas (late) A52.74
  paralysis A52.17
    general A52.17
      juvenile A50.45
  paresis (general) A52.17
    juvenile A50.45
  paresthesia A52.19
  Parkinson's disease or syndrome A52.19
  paroxysmal tachycardia A52.06
  pemphigus (congenital) A50.06
  penis (chancre) A51.0
    late A52.76
  pericardium A52.06
  perichondritis, larynx (late) A52.73
  periosteum (late) A52.77
    congenital (early) A50.02 *[M90.80]*
    early (secondary) A51.46
  peripheral nerve A52.79
  petrous bone (late) A52.77
  pharynx (late) A52.73
    secondary A51.39
  pituitary (gland) A52.79
  pleura (late) A52.73
  pneumonia, white A50.04
  pontine lesion A52.17
  portal vein A52.09
  primary A51.0
    anal A51.1
    and secondary —*see* Syphilis, secondary
    central nervous system A52.3
    extragenital chancre NEC A51.2
    fingers A51.2
    genital A51.0
    lip A51.2
    specified site NEC A51.2
    tonsils A51.2
  prostate (late) A52.76
  ptosis (eyelid) A52.71
  pulmonary (late) A52.72
    artery A52.09
  pyelonephritis (late) A52.75
  recently acquired, symptomatic A51.9
  rectum (late) A52.74
  respiratory tract (late) A52.73
  retina, late A52.71
  retrobulbar neuritis A52.15
  salpingitis A52.76
  sclera (late) A52.71
  sclerosis
    cerebral A52.17
    coronary A52.06
    multiple A52.11
  scotoma (central) A52.71
  scrotum (late) A52.76
  secondary (and primary) A51.49
    adenopathy A51.49
    anus A51.39
    bone A51.46
    chorioretinitis, choroiditis A51.43
    hepatitis A51.45
    liver A51.45
    lymphadenitis A51.49
    meningitis (acute) A51.41
    mouth A51.39
    mucous membranes A51.39
    periosteum, periostitis A51.46
    pharynx A51.39
    relapse (treated, untreated) A51.49
    skin A51.39
    specified form NEC A51.49
    tonsil A51.39
    ulcer A51.39
    viscera NEC A51.49
    vulva A51.39

Syphilis, syphilitic *(Continued)*
  seminal vesicle (late) A52.76
  seronegative with signs or symptoms -
    code by site and stage under
    Syphilis
  seropositive
    with signs or symptoms - code
      by site and stage under
      Syphilis
    follow-up of latent syphilis —*see* Syphilis,
      latent
    only finding —*see* Syphilis, latent
  seventh nerve (paralysis) A52.15
  sinus, sinusitis (late) A52.73
  skeletal system A52.77
  skin (with ulceration) (early) (secondary)
    A51.39
    late or tertiary A52.79
  small intestine A52.74
  spastic spinal paralysis A52.17
  spermatic cord (late) A52.76
  spinal (cord) A52.12
  spleen A52.79
  splenomegaly A52.79
  spondylitis A52.77
  staphyloma A52.71
  stigmata (congenital) A50.59
  stomach A52.74
  synovium A52.78
  tabes dorsalis (late) A52.11
    juvenile A50.45
  tabetic type A52.11
    juvenile A50.45
  taboparesis A52.17
    juvenile A50.45
  tachycardia A52.06
  tendon (late) A52.78
  tertiary A52.9
    with symptoms NEC A52.79
    cardiovascular A52.00
    central nervous system A52.3
    multiple NEC A52.79
    specified site NEC A52.79
  testis A52.76
  thorax A52.73
  throat A52.73
  thymus (gland) (late) A52.79
  thyroid (late) A52.79
  tongue (late) A52.79
  tonsil (lingual) (late) A52.73
    primary A51.2
    secondary A51.39
  trachea (late) A52.73
  tunica vaginalis (late) A52.76
  ulcer (any site) (early) (secondary)
    A51.39
    late A52.79
    perforating A52.79
      foot A52.11
  urethra (late) A52.76
  urogenital (late) A52.76
  uterus (late) A52.76
  uveal tract (secondary) A51.43
    late A52.71
  uveitis (secondary) A51.43
    late A52.71
  uvula (late) (perforated) A52.79
  vagina A51.0
    late A52.76
  valvulitis NEC A52.03
  vascular A52.00
    brain (cerebral) A52.05
  ventriculi A52.74
  vesicae urinariae (late) A52.76
  viscera (abdominal) (late) A52.74
    secondary A51.49
  vitreous (opacities) (late) A52.71
    hemorrhage A52.71
  vulva A51.0
    late A52.76
    secondary A51.39

◀ New   ◀|||| Revised   ~~deleted~~ Deleted

Syphiloma A52.79
  cardiovascular system A52.00
  central nervous system A52.3
  circulatory system A52.00
  congenital A50.59
Syphilophobia F45.29
Syringadenoma —*see also* Neoplasm, skin,
  benign
  papillary —*see* Neoplasm, skin, benign
Syringobulbia G95.0

Syringocystadenoma —*see* Neoplasm, skin,
  benign
  papillary —*see* Neoplasm, skin, benign
Syringoma —*see also* Neoplasm, skin, benign
  chondroid —*see* Neoplasm, skin, benign
Syringomyelia G95.0
Syringomyelitis —*see* Encephalitis
Syringomyelocele —*see* Spina bifida
Syringopontia G95.0

System, systemic —*see also* condition
  disease, combined —*see* Degeneration,
    combined
  inflammatory response syndrome (SIRS) of
    non-infectious origin (without organ
    dysfunction) R65.10
    with acute organ dysfunction R65.11
  lupus erythematosus M32.9
    inhibitor present D68.62

S

T

Tabacism, tabacosis, tabagism —*see also*
    Poisoning, tobacco ◄▥
  meaning dependence (without remission)
    F17.200
    with
      disorder F17.299
        remission F17.211
        specified disorder NEC F17.298
      withdrawal F17.203
Tabardillo A75.9
  flea-borne A75.2
  louse-borne A75.0
Tabes, tabetic A52.10
  with
    central nervous system syphilis A52.10
    Charcot's joint A52.16
    cord bladder A52.19
    crisis, viscera (any) A52.19
    paralysis, general A52.17
    paresis (general) A52.17
    perforating ulcer (foot) A52.19
  arthropathy (Charcot) A52.16
  bladder A52.19
  bone A52.11
  cerebrospinal A52.12
  congenital A50.45
  conjugal A52.10
  dorsalis A52.11
    juvenile A50.49
  juvenile A50.49
  latent A52.19
  mesenterica A18.39
  paralysis, insane, general A52.17
  spasmodic A52.17
  syphilis (cerebrospinal) A52.12
Taboparalysis A52.17
Taboparesis (remission) A52.17
  juvenile A50.45
TAC (trigeminal autonomic cephalgia) NEC
    G44.099
  intractable G44.091
  not intractable G44.099
Tache noir S60.22-
Tachyalimentation K91.2
Tachyarrhythmia, tachyrhythmia —*see*
    Tachycardia
Tachycardia R00.0
  atrial (paroxysmal) I47.1
  auricular I47.1
  AV nodal re-entry (re-entrant) I47.1
  junctional (paroxysmal) I47.1
  newborn P29.11
  nodal (paroxysmal) I47.1
  non-paroxysmal AV nodal I45.89
  paroxysmal (sustained) (nonsustained)
    I47.9
    with sinus bradycardia I49.5
    atrial (PAT) I47.1
    atrioventricular (AV) (re-entrant) I47.1
      psychogenic F54
    junctional I47.1
      ectopic I47.1
    nodal I47.1
    psychogenic (atrial) (supraventricular)
      (ventricular) F54
    supraventricular (sustained) I47.1
      psychogenic F54
    ventricular I47.2
      psychogenic F54
  psychogenic F45.8
  sick sinus I49.5
  sinoauricular NOS R00.0
    paroxysmal I47.1
  sinus [sinusal] NOS R00.0
    paroxysmal I47.1
  supraventricular I47.1
  ventricular (paroxysmal) (sustained) I47.2
    psychogenic F54
Tachygastria K31.89

Tachypnea R06.82
  hysterical F45.8
  newborn (idiopathic) (transitory) P22.1
  psychogenic F45.8
  transitory, of newborn P22.1
TACO (transfusion associated circulatory
    overload) E87.71
Taenia (infection) (infestation) B68.9
  diminuta B71.0
  echinococcal infestation B67.90
  mediocanellata B68.1
  nana B71.0
  saginata B68.1
  solium (intestinal form) B68.0
    larval form —*see* Cysticercosis
Taeniasis (intestine) —*see* Taenia
Tag (hypertrophied skin) (infected) L91.8
  adenoid J35.8
  anus K64.4
  hemorrhoidal K64.4
  hymen N89.8
  perineal N90.89
  preauricular Q17.0
  sentinel K64.4
  skin L91.8
    accessory (congenital) Q82.8
    anus K64.4
    congenital Q82.8
    preauricular Q17.0
  tonsil J35.8
  urethra, urethral N36.8
  vulva N90.89
Tahyna fever B33.8
Takahara's disease E80.3
Takayasu's disease or syndrome M31.4
Talcosis (pulmonary) J62.0
Talipes (congenital) Q66.89
  acquired, planus —*see* Deformity, limb, flat
    foot
  asymmetric Q66.89
  calcaneovalgus Q66.4
  calcaneovarus Q66.1
  calcaneus Q66.89
  cavus Q66.7
  equinovalgus Q66.6
  equinovarus Q66.0
  equinus Q66.89
  percavus Q66.7
  planovalgus Q66.6
  planus (acquired) (any degree) —*see also*
    Deformity, limb, flat foot
    congenital Q66.5-
    due to rickets (sequelae) E64.3
  valgus Q66.6
  varus Q66.3
Tall stature, constitutional E34.4
Talma's disease M62.89
Talon noir S90.3-
  hand S60.22-
  heel S90.3-
  toe S90.1-
Tamponade, heart I31.4
Tanapox (virus disease) B08.71
Tangier disease E78.6
Tantrum, child problem F91.8
Tapeworm (infection) (infestation) —*see*
    Infestation, tapeworm
Tapia's syndrome G52.7
TAR (thrombocytopenia with absent radius)
    syndrome Q87.2
Tarral-Besnier disease L44.0
Tarsal tunnel syndrome —*see* Syndrome, tarsal
    tunnel
Tarsalgia —*see* Pain, limb, lower
Tarsitis (eyelid) H01.8
  syphilitic A52.71
  tuberculous A18.4
Tartar (teeth) (dental calculus) K03.6
Tattoo (mark) L81.8
Tauri's disease E74.09
Taurodontism K00.2

Taussig-Bing syndrome Q20.1
Taybi's syndrome Q87.2
Tay-Sachs amaurotic familial idiocy or disease
    E75.02
TBI (traumatic brain injury) —*see* category
    S06
Teacher's node or nodule J38.2
Tear, torn (traumatic) —*see also* Laceration
  with abortion —*see* Abortion
  annular fibrosis M51.35
  anus, anal (sphincter) S31.831
    complicating delivery
      with third degree perineal laceration
        O70.2
        with mucosa O70.3
      without third degree perineal laceration
        O70.4
    nontraumatic (healed) (old) K62.81
  articular cartilage, old —*see* Derangement,
    joint, articular cartilage, by site
  bladder
    with ectopic or molar pregnancy O08.6
    following ectopic or molar pregnancy
      O08.6
    obstetrical O71.5
    traumatic —*see* Injury, bladder
  bowel
    with ectopic or molar pregnancy O08.6
    following ectopic or molar pregnancy
      O08.6
    obstetrical trauma O71.5
  broad ligament
    with ectopic or molar pregnancy O08.6
    following ectopic or molar pregnancy
      O08.6
    obstetrical trauma O71.6
  bucket handle (knee) (meniscus) —*see* Tear,
    meniscus
  capsule, joint —*see* Sprain
  cartilage —*see also* Sprain
    articular, old —*see* Derangement, joint,
      articular cartilage, by site
  cervix
    with ectopic or molar pregnancy O08.6
    following ectopic or molar pregnancy
      O08.6
    obstetrical trauma (current) O71.3
    old N88.1
    traumatic —*see* Injury, uterus
  dural G97.41
    nontraumatic G96.11
  internal organ —*see* Injury, by site
  knee cartilage
    articular (current) S83.3-
    old —*see* Derangement, knee, meniscus,
      due to old tear
  ligament —*see* Sprain
  meniscus (knee) (current injury) S83.209
    bucket-handle S83.20-
    lateral
      bucket-handle S83.25-
      complex S83.27-
      peripheral S83.26-
      specified type NEC S83.28-
    medial
      bucket-handle S83.21-
      complex S83.23-
      peripheral S83.22-
      specified type NEC S83.24-
    old —*see* Derangement, knee, meniscus,
      due to old tear
    site other than knee - code as Sprain
    specified type NEC S83.20-
  muscle —*see* Strain
  pelvic
    floor, complicating delivery O70.1
    organ NEC, obstetrical trauma O71.5
      with ectopic or molar pregnancy O08.6
      following ectopic or molar pregnancy
        O08.6
  perineal, secondary O90.1

◄ New   ◄▥ Revised   ~~deleted~~ Deleted

Tear, torn (Continued)
- periurethral tissue, obstetrical trauma O71.82
  - with ectopic or molar pregnancy O08.6
  - following ectopic or molar pregnancy O08.6
- rectovaginal septum —*see* Laceration, vagina
- retina, retinal (without detachment) (horseshoe) —*see also* Break, retina, horseshoe
  - with detachment —*see* Detachment, retina, with retinal, break
- rotator cuff (nontraumatic) M75.10-
  - complete M75.12-
  - incomplete M75.11-
  - traumatic S46.01-
  - capsule S43.42-
- semilunar cartilage, knee —*see* Tear, meniscus
- supraspinatus (complete) (incomplete) (nontraumatic) (*see also* Tear, rotator cuff) M75.10-
- tendon —*see* Strain
- tentorial, at birth P10.4
- umbilical cord
  - complicating delivery O69.89
- urethra
  - with ectopic or molar pregnancy O08.6
  - following ectopic or molar pregnancy O08.6
  - obstetrical trauma O71.5
- uterus —*see* Injury, uterus
- vagina —*see* Laceration, vagina
- vessel, from catheter —*see* Puncture, accidental complicating surgery
- vulva, complicating delivery O70.0

Tear-stone —*see* Dacryolith

Teeth —*see also* condition
- grinding
  - psychogenic F45.8
  - sleep related G47.63

Teething (syndrome) K00.7

Telangiectasia, telangiectasis (verrucous) I78.1
- ataxic (cerebellar) (Louis-Bar) G11.3
- familial I78.0
- hemorrhagic, hereditary (congenital) (senile) I78.0
- hereditary, hemorrhagic (congenital) (senile) I78.0
- juxtafoveal H35.07-
- macular H35.07-
- parafoveal H35.07-
- retinal (idiopathic) (juxtafoveal) (macular) (parafoveal) H35.07-
- spider I78.1

Telephone scatologia F65.89

Telescoped bowel or intestine K56.1
- congenital Q43.8

Temperature
- body, high (of unknown origin) R50.9
- cold, trauma from T69.9
  - newborn P80.0
  - specified effect NEC T69.8

Temple —*see* condition

Temporal —*see* condition

Temporomandibular joint pain-dysfunction syndrome M26.62

Temporosphenoidal —*see* condition

Tendency
- bleeding —*see* Defect, coagulation
- suicide
  - meaning personal history of attempted suicide Z91.5
  - meaning suicidal ideation —*see* Ideation, suicidal
- to fall R29.6

Tenderness, abdominal R10.819
- epigastric R10.816
- generalized R10.817
- left lower quadrant R10.814
- left upper quadrant R10.812
- periumbilic R10.815

Tenderness, abdominal (Continued)
- rebound R10.829
  - epigastric R10.826
  - generalized R10.827
  - left lower quadrant R10.824
  - left upper quadrant R10.822
  - periumbilic R10.825
  - right lower quadrant R10.823
  - right upper quadrant R10.821
- right lower quadrant R10.813
- right upper quadrant R10.811

Tendinitis, tendonitis —*see also* Enthesopathy
- Achilles M76.6-
- adhesive —*see* Tenosynovitis, specified type NEC
  - shoulder —*see* Capsulitis, adhesive
- bicipital M75.2-
- calcific M65.2-
  - ankle M65.27-
  - foot M65.27-
  - forearm M65.23-
  - hand M65.24-
  - lower leg M65.26-
  - multiple sites M65.29
  - pelvic region M65.25-
  - shoulder M75.3-
  - specified site NEC M65.28
  - thigh M65.25-
  - upper arm M65.22-
- due to use, overuse, pressure —*see also* Disorder, soft tissue, due to use
  - specified NEC —*see* Disorder, soft tissue, due to use, specified NEC
- gluteal M76.0-
- patellar M76.5-
- peroneal M76.7-
- psoas M76.1-
- tibial (posterior) M76.82-
  - anterior M76.81-
- trochanteric —*see* Bursitis, hip, trochanteric

Tendon —*see* condition

Tendosynovitis —*see* Tenosynovitis

Tenesmus (rectal) R19.8
- vesical R30.1

Tennis elbow —*see* Epicondylitis, lateral

Tenonitis —*see also* Tenosynovitis
- eye (capsule) H05.04-

Tenontosynovitis —*see* Tenosynovitis

Tenontothecitis —*see* Tenosynovitis

Tenophyte —*see* Disorder, synovium, specified type NEC

Tenosynovitis (*see also* Synovitis) M65.9
- adhesive —*see* Tenosynovitis, specified type NEC
  - shoulder —*see* Capsulitis, adhesive
- bicipital (calcifying) —*see* Tendinitis, bicipital
- gonococcal A54.49
- in (due to)
  - crystals M65.8-
  - gonorrhea A54.49
  - syphilis (late) A52.78
  - use, overuse, pressure —*see also* Disorder, soft tissue, due to use
    - specified NEC —*see* Disorder, soft tissue, due to use, specified NEC
- infective NEC M65.1-
  - ankle M65.17-
  - foot M65.17-
  - forearm M65.13-
  - hand M65.14-
  - lower leg M65.16-
  - multiple sites M65.19
  - pelvic region M65.15-
  - shoulder region M65.11-
  - specified site NEC M65.18
  - thigh M65.15-
  - upper arm M65.12-
- radial styloid M65.4
- shoulder region M65.81-
  - adhesive —*see* Capsulitis, adhesive

Tenosynovitis (Continued)
- specified type NEC M65.88
  - ankle M65.87-
  - foot M65.87-
  - forearm M65.83-
  - hand M65.84-
  - lower leg M65.86-
  - multiple sites M65.89
  - pelvic region M65.85-
  - shoulder region M65.81-
  - specified site NEC M65.88
  - thigh M65.85-
  - upper arm M65.82-
- tuberculous —*see* Tuberculosis, tenosynovitis

Tenovaginitis —*see* Tenosynovitis

Tension
- arterial, high —*see also* Hypertension
  - without diagnosis of hypertension R03.0
- headache G44.209
  - intractable G44.201
  - not intractable G44.209
- nervous R45.0
- pneumothorax J93.0
- premenstrual N94.3
- state (mental) F48.9

Tentorium —*see* condition

Teratencephalus Q89.8

Teratism Q89.7

Teratoblastoma (malignant) —*see* Neoplasm, malignant, by site

Teratocarcinoma —*see also* Neoplasm, malignant, by site
- liver C22.7

Teratoma (solid) —*see also* Neoplasm, uncertain behavior, by site
- with embryonal carcinoma, mixed —*see* Neoplasm, malignant, by site
- with malignant transformation —*see* Neoplasm, malignant, by site
- adult (cystic) —*see* Neoplasm, benign, by site
- benign —*see* Neoplasm, benign, by site
- combined with choriocarcinoma —*see* Neoplasm, malignant, by site
- cystic (adult) —*see* Neoplasm, benign, by site
- differentiated —*see* Neoplasm, benign, by site
- embryonal —*see also* Neoplasm, malignant, by site
  - liver C22.7
- immature —*see* Neoplasm, malignant, by site
- liver C22.7
  - adult, benign, cystic, differentiated type or mature D13.4
- malignant —*see also* Neoplasm, malignant, by site
  - anaplastic —*see* Neoplasm, malignant, by site
  - intermediate —*see* Neoplasm, malignant, by site
  - specified site —*see* Neoplasm, malignant, by site
  - unspecified site C62.90
  - undifferentiated —*see* Neoplasm, malignant, by site
- mature —*see* Neoplasm, uncertain behavior, by site
- malignant —*see* Neoplasm, by site, malignant, by site
- ovary D27.-
  - embryonal, immature or malignant C56-
- solid —*see* Neoplasm, uncertain behavior, by site
- testis C62.9-
  - adult, benign, cystic, differentiated type or mature D29.2-
  - scrotal C62.1-
  - undescended C62.0-

Termination
- anomalous —*see also* Malposition, congenital
  - right pulmonary vein Q26.3
- pregnancy, elective Z33.2

Ternidens diminutus infestation B81.8
Ternidensiasis B81.8
Terror (s) night (child) F51.4
Terrorism, victim of Z65.4
Terry's syndrome H44.2-
Tertiary —see condition
Test, tests, testing (for)
    adequacy (for dialysis)
        hemodialysis Z49.31
        peritoneal Z49.32
    blood pressure Z01.30
        abnormal reading —see Blood, pressure
    blood typing Z01.83
        Rh typing Z01.83
    blood-alcohol Z04.8
        positive —see Findings, abnormal, in
            blood
    blood-drug Z04.8
        positive —see Findings, abnormal, in
            blood
    cardiac pulse generator (battery) Z45.010
    fertility Z31.41
    genetic
        disease carrier status for procreative
            management
            female Z31.430
            male Z31.440
        male partner of patient with recurrent
            pregnancy loss Z31.441
        procreative management NEC
            female Z31.438
            male Z31.448
    hearing Z01.10
        with abnormal findings NEC Z01.118
    HIV (human immunodeficiency virus)
        nonconclusive (in infants) R75
        positive Z21
        seropositive Z21
    immunity status Z01.84
    intelligence NEC Z01.89
    laboratory (as part of a general medical
        examination) Z00.00
        with abnormal finding Z00.01
        for medicolegal reason NEC Z04.8
    male partner of patient with recurrent
        pregnancy loss Z31.441
    Mantoux (for tuberculosis) Z11.1
        abnormal result R76.11
    pregnancy, positive first pregnancy —see
        Pregnancy, normal, first
    procreative Z31.49
        fertility Z31.41
    skin, diagnostic
        allergy Z01.82
            special screening examination —see
                Screening, by name of disease
        Mantoux Z11.1
        tuberculin Z11.1
    specified NEC Z01.89
    tuberculin Z11.1
        abnormal result R76.11
    vision Z01.00
        with abnormal findings Z01.01
    Wassermann Z11.3
        positive —see Serology for syphilis,
            positive
Testicle, testicular, testis —see also condition
    feminization syndrome (see also Syndrome,
        androgen insensitivity) E34.51
    migrans Q55.29
Tetanus, tetanic (cephalic) (convulsions) A35
    with
        abortion A34
        ectopic or molar pregnancy O08.0
    following ectopic or molar pregnancy
        O08.0
    inoculation reaction (due to serum) —see
        Complications, vaccination
    neonatorum A33
    obstetrical A34
    puerperal, postpartum, childbirth A34

Tetany (due to) R29.0
    alkalosis E87.3
    associated with rickets E55.0
    convulsions R29.0
        hysterical F44.5
    functional (hysterical) F44.5
    hyperkinetic R29.0
        hysterical F44.5
    hyperpnea R06.4
        hysterical F44.5
        psychogenic F45.8
    hyperventilation (see also Hyperventilation)
        R06.4
        hysterical F44.5
    neonatal (without calcium or magnesium
        deficiency) P71.3
    parathyroid (gland) E20.9
    parathyroprival E89.2
    post- (para)thyroidectomy E89.2
    postoperative E89.2
    pseudotetany R29.0
    psychogenic (conversion reaction) F44.5
Tetralogy of Fallot Q21.3
Tetraplegia (chronic) (see also Quadriplegia)
    G82.50-
Thailand hemorrhagic fever A91
Thalassanemia —see Thalassemia
Thalassemia (anemia) (disease) D56.9
    with other hemoglobinopathy D56.8
    alpha (major) (severe) (triple gene defect)
        D56.0
        minor D56.3
        silent carrier D56.3
        trait D56.3
    beta (severe) D56.1
        homozygous D56.1
        major D56.1
        minor D56.3
        trait D56.3
    delta-beta (homozygous) D56.2
        minor D56.3
        trait D56.3
    dominant D56.8
    hemoglobin
        C D56.8
        E-beta D56.5
    intermedia D56.1
    major D56.1
    minor D56.3
    mixed D56.8
    sickle-cell —see Disease, sickle-cell,
        thalassemia
    specified type NEC D56.8
    trait D56.3
    variants D56.8
Thanatophoric dwarfism or short stature Q77.1
Thaysen-Gee disease (nontropical sprue) K90.0
Thaysen's disease K90.0
Thecoma D27-
    luteinized D27-
    malignant C56-
Thelarche, premature E30.8
Thelaziasis B83.8
Thelitis N61
    puerperal, postpartum or gestational —see
        Infection, nipple
Therapeutic —see condition
Therapy
    drug, long-term (current) (prophylactic)
        agents affecting estrogen receptors and
            estrogen levels NEC Z79.818
        anastrozole (Arimidex) Z79.811
        antibiotics Z79.2
            short-term use - omit code
        anticoagulants Z79.01
        anti-inflammatory Z79.1
        antiplatelet Z79.02
        antithrombotics Z79.02
        aromatase inhibitors Z79.811
        aspirin Z79.82
        birth control pill or patch Z79.3

Therapy (Continued)
    drug, long-term (Continued)
        bisphosphonates Z79.83
        contraceptive, oral Z79.3
        drug, specified NEC Z79.899
        estrogen receptor downregulators
            Z79.818
        Evista Z79.810
        exemestane (Aromasin) Z79.811
        Fareston Z79.810
        fulvestrant (Faslodex) Z79.818
        gonadotropin-releasing hormone (GnRH)
            agonist Z79.818
        goserelin acetate (Zoladex) Z79.818
        hormone replacement (postmenopausal)
            Z79.890
        insulin Z79.4
        letrozole (Femara) Z79.811
        leuprolide acetate (leuprorelin) (Lupron)
            Z79.818
        megestrol acetate (Megace) Z79.818
        methadone
            for pain management Z79.891
            maintenance therapy F11.20
        Nolvadex Z79.810
        opiate analgesic Z79.891
        oral contraceptive Z79.3
        raloxifene (Evista) Z79.810
        selective estrogen receptor modulators
            (SERMs) Z79.810
        short term - omit code
        steroids
            inhaled Z79.51
            systemic Z79.52
        tamoxifen (Nolvadex) Z79.810
        toremifene (Fareston) Z79.810
Thermic —see condition
Thermography (abnormal) (see also Abnormal,
    diagnostic imaging) R93.8
    breast R92.8
Thermoplegia T67.0
Thesaurismosis, glycogen —see Disease,
    glycogen storage
Thiamin deficiency E51.9
    specified NEC E51.8
Thiaminic deficiency with beriberi E51.11
Thibierge-Weissenbach syndrome —see
    Sclerosis, systemic
Thickening
    bone —see Hypertrophy, bone
    breast N64.59
    endometrium R93.8
    epidermal L85.9
        specified NEC L85.8
    hymen N89.6
    larynx J38.7
    nail L60.2
        congenital Q84.5
    periosteal —see Hypertrophy, bone
    pleura J92.9
        with asbestos J92.0
    skin R23.4
    subepiglottic J38.7
    tongue K14.8
    valve, heart —see Endocarditis
Thigh —see condition
Thinning vertebra —see Spondylopathy,
    specified NEC
Thirst, excessive R63.1
    due to deprivation of water T73.1
Thomsen disease G71.12
Thoracic —see also condition
    kidney Q63.2
    outlet syndrome G54.0
Thoracogastroschisis (congenital) Q79.8
Thoracopagus Q89.4
Thorax —see condition
Thorn's syndrome N28.89
Thorson-Björck syndrome E34.0
Threadworm (infection) (infestation)
    B80

◀ New ◀▬ Revised ~~deleted~~ Deleted

Threatened
abortion O20.0
with subsequent abortion O03.9
job loss, anxiety concerning Z56.2
labor (without delivery) O47.9
after 37 completed weeks of gestation
O47.1
before 37 completed weeks of gestation
O47.0-
loss of job, anxiety concerning Z56.2
miscarriage O20.0
unemployment, anxiety concerning Z56.2
Three-day fever A93.1
Threshers' lung J67.0 ◀
Thrix annulata (congenital) Q84.1
Throat —see condition
Thrombasthenia (Glanzmann) (hemorrhagic)
(hereditary) D69.1
Thromboangiitis I73.1
obliterans (general) I73.1
cerebral I67.89
vessels
brain I67.89
spinal cord I67.89
Thromboarteritis —see Arteritis
Thromboasthenia (Glanzmann) (hemorrhagic)
(hereditary) D69.1
Thrombocytasthenia (Glanzmann) D69.1
Thrombocythemia (essential) (hemorrhagic)
(idiopathic) (primary) D47.3
Thrombocytopathy (dystrophic) (granulopenic)
D69.1
Thrombocytopenia, thrombocytopenic D69.6
with absent radius (TAR) Q87.2
congenital D69.42
dilutional D69.59
due to
drugs D69.59
extracorporeal circulation of blood D69.59
(massive)blood transfusion D69.59
platelet alloimmunization D69.59
essential D69.3
heparin induced (HIT) D75.82
hereditary D69.42
idiopathic D69.3
neonatal, transitory P61.0
due to
exchange transfusion P61.0
idiopathic maternal thrombocytopenia
P61.0
isoimmunization P61.0
primary NEC D69.49
idiopathic D69.3
puerperal, postpartum O72.3
secondary D69.59
transient neonatal P61.0
Thrombocytosis, essential D47.3
primary D47.3
Thromboembolism —see Embolism
Thrombopathy (Bernard-Soulier) D69.1
constitutional D68.0
Willebrand-Jurgens D68.0
Thrombopenia —see Thrombocytopenia
Thrombophilia D68.59
primary NEC D68.59
secondary NEC D68.69
specified NEC D68.69
Thrombophlebitis I80.9
antepartum O22.2-
deep O22.3-
superficial O22.2-
cavernous (venous) sinus G08
complicating pregnancy O22.5-
nonpyogenic I67.6
cerebral (sinus) (vein) G08
nonpyogenic I67.6
sequelae G09
due to implanted device —see Complications,
by site and type, specified NEC
during or resulting from a procedure NEC
T81.72

Thrombophlebitis (Continued)
femoral vein (superficial) I80.1-
femoropopliteal vein I80.0-
hepatic (vein) I80.8
idiopathic, recurrent I82.1
iliofemoral I80.1-
intracranial venous sinus (any) G08
nonpyogenic I67.6
sequelae G09
intraspinal venous sinuses and veins G08
nonpyogenic G95.19
lateral (venous) sinus G08
nonpyogenic I67.6
leg I80.299
superficial I80.0-
longitudinal (venous) sinus G08
nonpyogenic I67.6
lower extremity I80.299
migrans, migrating I82.1
pelvic
with ectopic or molar pregnancy O08.0
following ectopic or molar pregnancy
O08.0
puerperal O87.1
popliteal vein —see Phlebitis, leg, deep,
popliteal
portal (vein) K75.1
postoperative T81.72
pregnancy —see Thrombophlebitis,
antepartum
puerperal, postpartum, childbirth O87.0
deep O87.1
pelvic O87.1
septic O86.81
superficial O87.0
saphenous (greater) (lesser) I80.0-
sinus (intracranial) G08
nonpyogenic I67.6
specified site NEC I80.8
tibial vein I80.23-
Thrombosis, thrombotic (bland) (multiple)
(progressive) (silent) (vessel) I82.90
anal K64.5
antepartum —see Thrombophlebitis,
antepartum
aorta, aortic I74.10
abdominal I74.09
saddle I74.01
bifurcation I74.09
saddle I74.01
specified site NEC I74.19
terminal I74.09
thoracic I74.11
valve —see Endocarditis, aortic
apoplexy I63.3
artery, arteries (postinfectional) I74.9
auditory, internal —see Occlusion, artery,
precerebral, specified NEC
basilar —see Occlusion, artery, basilar
carotid (common) (internal) —see
Occlusion, artery, carotid
cerebellar (anterior inferior) (posterior
inferior) (superior) —see Occlusion,
artery, cerebellar
cerebral —see Occlusion, artery, cerebral
choroidal (anterior) —see Occlusion, artery,
cerebral, specified NEC
communicating, posterior —see Occlusion,
artery, cerebral, specified NEC
coronary —see also Infarct, myocardium
not resulting in infarction I24.0
hepatic I74.8
hypophyseal —see Occlusion, artery,
cerebral, specified NEC
iliac I74.5
limb I74.4
lower I74.3
upper I74.2
meningeal, anterior or posterior —see
Occlusion, artery, cerebral, specified
NEC

Thrombosis, thrombotic (Continued)
artery, arteries (Continued)
mesenteric (with gangrene) K55.0
ophthalmic —see Occlusion, artery, retina
pontine —see Occlusion, artery, cerebral,
specified NEC
precerebral —see Occlusion, artery,
precerebral
pulmonary (iatrogenic) —see Embolism,
pulmonary
renal N28.0
retinal —see Occlusion, artery, retina
spinal, anterior or posterior G95.11
traumatic NEC T14.8
vertebral —see Occlusion, artery, vertebral
atrium, auricular —see also Infarct,
myocardium
following acute myocardial infarction
(current complication) I23.6
not resulting in infarction I24.0
basilar (artery) —see Occlusion, artery,
basilar
brain (artery) (stem) —see also Occlusion,
artery, cerebral
due to syphilis A52.05
puerperal O99.43
sinus —see Thrombosis, intracranial
venous sinus
capillary I78.8
cardiac —see also Infarct, myocardium
not resulting in infarction I24.0
valve —see Endocarditis
carotid (artery) (common) (internal) —see
Occlusion, artery, carotid
cavernous (venous) sinus —see Thrombosis,
intracranial venous sinus
cerebellar artery (anterior inferior) (posterior
inferior) (superior) I66.3
cerebral (artery) —see Occlusion, artery,
cerebral
cerebrovenous sinus —see also Thrombosis,
intracranial venous sinus
puerperium O87.3
chronic I82.91
coronary (artery) (vein) —see also Infarct,
myocardium
not resulting in infarction I24.0
corpus cavernosum N48.89
cortical I66.9
deep —see Embolism, vein, lower extremity
due to device, implant or graft (see also
Complications, by site and type,
specified NEC) T85.86
arterial graft NEC T82.868
breast (implant) T85.86
catheter NEC T85.86
dialysis (renal) T82.868
intraperitoneal T85.86
infusion NEC T82.868
spinal (epidural) (subdural) T85.86
urinary (indwelling) T83.86
electronic (electrode) (pulse generator)
(stimulator)
bone T84.86
cardiac T82.867
nervous system (brain) (peripheral
nerve) (spinal) T85.86
urinary T83.86
fixation, internal (orthopedic) NEC T84.86
gastrointestinal (bile duct) (esophagus)
T85.86
genital NEC T83.86
heart T82.867
joint prosthesis T84.86
ocular (corneal graft) (orbital implant)
NEC T85.86
orthopedic NEC T84.86
specified NEC T85.86
urinary NEC T83.86
vascular NEC T82.868
ventricular intracranial shunt T85.86

Thrombosis, thrombotic *(Continued)*
  during the puerperium —*see* Thrombosis,
      puerperal
  endocardial —*see also* Infarct, myocardium
      not resulting in infarction I24.0
  eye —*see* Occlusion, retina
  genital organ
      female NEC N94.89
          pregnancy —*see* Thrombophlebitis,
              antepartum
      male N50.1
  gestational —*see* Phlebopathy, gestational
  heart (chamber) —*see also* Infarct,
      myocardium
      not resulting in infarction I24.0
  hepatic (vein) I82.0
      artery I74.8
  history (of) Z86.718
  intestine (with gangrene) K55.0
  intracardiac NEC (apical) (atrial) (auricular)
      (ventricular) (old) I51.3
  intracranial (arterial) I66.9
      venous sinus (any) G08
          nonpyogenic origin I67.6
          puerperium O87.3
  intramural —*see also* Infarct, myocardium
      not resulting in infarction I24.0
  intraspinal venous sinuses and veins G08
      nonpyogenic G95.19
  kidney (artery) N28.0
  lateral (venous) sinus —*see* Thrombosis,
      intracranial venous sinus
  leg —*see* Thrombosis, vein, lower
      extremity
      arterial I74.3
  liver (venous) I82.0
      artery I74.8
      portal vein I81
  longitudinal (venous) sinus —*see* Thrombosis,
      intracranial venous sinus
  lower limb —*see* Thrombosis, vein, lower
      extremity
  lung (iatrogenic) (postoperative) —*see*
      Embolism, pulmonary
  meninges (brain) (arterial) I66.8
  mesenteric (artery) (with gangrene) K55.0
      vein (inferior) (superior) I81
  mitral I34.8
  mural —*see also* Infarct, myocardium
      due to syphilis A52.06
      not resulting in infarction I24.0
  omentum (with gangrene) K55.0
  ophthalmic —*see* Occlusion, retina
  pampiniform plexus (male) N50.1
  parietal —*see also* Infarct, myocardium
      not resulting in infarction I24.0
  penis, superficial vein N48.81
  perianal venous K64.5
  peripheral arteries I74.4
      upper I74.2
  personal history (of) Z86.718
  portal I81
      due to syphilis A52.09
  precerebral artery —*see* Occlusion, artery,
      precerebral
  puerperal, postpartum O87.0
      brain (artery) O99.43
          venous (sinus) O87.3
      cardiac O99.43
      cerebral (artery) O99.43
          venous (sinus) O87.3
      superficial O87.0
  pulmonary (artery) (iatrogenic)
      (postoperative) (vein) —*see* Embolism,
      pulmonary
  renal (artery) N28.0
      vein I82.3
  resulting from presence of device, implant or
      graft —*see* Complications, by site and
      type, specified NEC
  retina, retinal —*see* Occlusion, retina

Thrombosis, thrombotic *(Continued)*
  scrotum N50.1
  seminal vesicle N50.1
  sigmoid (venous) sinus —*see* Thrombosis,
      intracranial venous sinus
  sinus, intracranial (any) —*see* Thrombosis,
      intracranial venous sinus
  specified site NEC I82.890
      chronic I82.891
  spermatic cord N50.1
  spinal cord (arterial) G95.11
      due to syphilis A52.09
      pyogenic origin G06.1
  spleen, splenic D73.5
      artery I74.8
  testis N50.1
  traumatic NEC T14.8
  tricuspid I07.8
  tumor —*see* Neoplasm, by site
  tunica vaginalis N50.1
  umbilical cord (vessels), complicating
      delivery O69.5
  vas deferens N50.1
  vein (acute) I82.90
      antecubital I82.61-
          chronic I82.71-
      axillary I82.A1-
          chronic I82.A2-
      basilic I82.61-
          chronic I82.71-
      brachial I82.62-
          chronic I82.72-
      brachiocephalic (innominate) I82.290
          chronic I82.291
      cerebral, nonpyogenic I67.6
      cephalic I82.61-
          chronic I82.71-
      chronic I82.91
      deep (DVT) I82.40-
          calf I82.4Z-
              chronic I82.5Z-
          lower leg I82.4Z-
              chronic I82.5Z-
          thigh I82.4Y-
              chronic I82.5Y-
          upper leg I82.4Y
              chronic I82.5y-
      femoral I82.41-
          chronic I82.51-
      iliac (iliofemoral) I82.42-
          chronic I82.52-
      innominate I82.290
          chronic I82.291
      internal jugular I82.C1-
          chronic I82.C2-
      lower extremity
          deep I82.40-
              chronic I82.50-
              specified NEC I82.49-
                  chronic NEC I82.59-
          distal
              deep I82.4Z-
          proximal
              deep I82.4Y-
                  chronic I82.5Y-
          superficial I82.81-
      perianal K64.5
      popliteal I82.43-
          chronic I82.53-
      radial I82.62-
          chronic I82.72-
      renal I82.3
      saphenous (greater) (lesser) I82.81-
      specified NEC I82.890
          chronic NEC I82.891
      subclavian I82.B1-
          chronic I82.B2-
      thoracic NEC I82.290
          chronic I82.291
      tibial I82.44-
          chronic I82.54-

Thrombosis, thrombotic *(Continued)*
  vein *(Continued)*
      ulnar I82.62-
          chronic I82.72-
      upper extremity I82.60-
          chronic I82.70-
          deep I82.62-
              chronic I82.72-
          superficial I82.61-
              chronic I82.71-
      vena cava
          inferior I82.220
              chronic I82.221
          superior I82.210
              chronic I82.211
      venous, perianal K64.5
      ventricle —*see also* Infarct, myocardium
          following acute myocardial infarction
              (current complication) I23.6
          not resulting in infarction I24.0
Thrombus —*see* Thrombosis
Thrush —*see also* Candidiasis
  newborn P37.5
  oral B37.0
  vaginal B37.3
Thumb —*see also* condition
  sucking (child problem) F98.8
Thymitis E32.8
Thymoma (benign) D15.0
  malignant C37
Thymus, thymic (gland) —*see* condition
Thyrocele —*see* Goiter
Thyroglossal —*see also* condition
  cyst Q89.2
  duct, persistent Q89.2
Thyroid (gland) (body) —*see also* condition
  hormone resistance E07.89
  lingual Q89.2
  nodule (cystic) (nontoxic) (single) E04.1
Thyroiditis E06.9
  acute (nonsuppurative) (pyogenic)
      (suppurative) E06.0
  autoimmune E06.3
  chronic (nonspecific) (sclerosing) E06.5
      with thyrotoxicosis, transient E06.2
      fibrous E06.5
      lymphadenoid E06.3
      lymphocytic E06.3
      lymphoid E06.3
  de Quervain's E06.1
  drug-induced E06.4
  fibrous (chronic) E06.5
  giant-cell (follicular) E06.1
  granulomatous (de Quervain) (subacute)
      E06.1
  Hashimoto's (struma lymphomatosa)
      E06.3
  iatrogenic E06.4
  ligneous E06.5
  lymphocytic (chronic) E06.3
  lymphoid E06.3
  lymphomatous E06.3
  nonsuppurative E06.1
  postpartum, puerperal O90.5
  pseudotuberculous E06.1
  pyogenic E06.0
  radiation E06.4
  Riedel's E06.5
  subacute (granulomatous) E06.1
  suppurative E06.0
  tuberculous A18.81
  viral E06.1
  woody E06.5
Thyrolingual duct, persistent Q89.2
Thyromegaly E01.0
Thyrotoxic
  crisis —*see* Thyrotoxicosis
  heart disease or failure (*see also*
      Thyrotoxicosis) E05.90 *[I43]*
      with thyroid storm E05.91 *[I43]*
  storm —*see* Thyrotoxicosis

◀ New   ◀▥ Revised   ~~deleted~~ Deleted

Thyrotoxicosis (recurrent) E05.90
  with
    goiter (diffuse) E05.00
      with thyroid storm E05.01
      adenomatous uninodular E05.10
        with thyroid storm E05.11
      multinodular E05.20
        with thyroid storm E05.21
      nodular E05.20
        with thyroid storm E05.21
      uninodular E05.10
        with thyroid storm E05.11
    infiltrative
      dermopathy E05.00
        with thyroid storm E05.01
      ophthalmopathy E05.00
        with thyroid storm E05.01
    single thyroid nodule E05.10
      with thyroid storm E05.11
    thyroid storm E05.91
  due to
    ectopic thyroid nodule or tissue E05.30
      with thyroid storm E05.31
    ingestion of (excessive) thyroid material
      E05.40
      with thyroid storm E05.41
    overproduction of thyroid-stimulating
      hormone E05.80
      with thyroid storm E05.81
    specified cause NEC E05.80
      with thyroid storm E05.81
  factitia E05.40
    with thyroid storm E05.41
  heart E05.90 *[I43]*
    with thyroid storm E05.91 *[I43]*
    failure E05.90 *[I43]*
  neonatal (transient) P72.1
  transient with chronic thyroiditis E06.2
Tibia vara —*see* Osteochondrosis, juvenile, tibia
Tic (disorder) F95.9
  breathing F95.8
  child problem F95.8
  compulsive F95.1
  de la Tourette F95.2
  degenerative (generalized) (localized) G25.69
    facial G25.69
  disorder
    chronic
      motor F95.1
      vocal F95.1
    combined vocal and multiple motor F95.2
    transient F95.0
  douloureux G50.0
    atypical G50.1
    postherpetic, postzoster B02.22
  drug-induced G25.61
  eyelid F95.8
  habit F95.9
    chronic F95.1
    transient of childhood F95.0
  lid, transient of childhood F95.0
  motor-verbal F95.2
  occupational F48.8
  orbicularis F95.8
    transient of childhood F95.0
  organic origin G25.69
  postchoreic G25.69
  psychogenic, compulsive F95.1
  salaam R25.8
  spasm (motor or vocal) F95.9
    chronic F95.1
    transient of childhood F95.0
  specified NEC F95.8
Tick-borne —*see* condition
Tietze's disease or syndrome M94.0
Tight, tightness
  anus K62.89
  chest R07.89
  fascia (lata) M62.89
  foreskin (congenital) N47.1
  hymen, hymenal ring N89.6

Tight, tightness *(Continued)*
  introitus (acquired) (congenital) N89.6
  rectal sphincter K62.89
  tendon —*see* Short, tendon
  urethral sphincter N35.9
Tilting vertebra —*see* Dorsopathy, deforming,
    specified NEC
Timidity, child F93.8
Tin-miner's lung J63.5
Tinea (intersecta) (tarsi) B35.9
  amiantacea L44.8
  asbestina B35.0
  barbae B35.0
  beard B35.0
  black dot B35.0
  blanca B36.2
  capitis B35.0
  corporis B35.4
  cruris B35.6
  flava B36.0
  foot B35.3
  furfuracea B36.0
  imbricata (Tokelau) B35.5
  kerion B35.0
  manuum B35.2
  microsporic —*see* Dermatophytosis
  nigra B36.1
  nodosa —*see* Piedra
  pedis B35.3
  scalp B35.0
  specified site NEC B35.8
  sycosis B35.0
  tonsurans B35.0
  trichophytic —*see* Dermatophytosis
  unguium B35.1
  versicolor B36.0
Tingling sensation (skin) R20.2
Tinnitus (audible) (aurium) (subjective) —*see*
    subcategory H93.1
Tipped tooth (teeth) M26.33
Tipping
  pelvis M95.5
    with disproportion (fetopelvic) O33.0
      causing obstructed labor O65.0
  tooth (teeth), fully erupted M26.33
Tiredness R53.83
Tissue —*see* condition
Tobacco (nicotine)
  dependence —*see* Dependence, drug, nicotine
  harmful use Z72.0
  heart —*see* Tobacco, toxic effect
  maternal use, affecting newborn P04.2
  toxic effect —*see* Table of ⊕Drugs and
      ⊖Chemicals, by substance, poisoning ◀▥
    chewing tobacco —*see* Table of ⊕Drugs
        and ⊖Chemicals, by substance,
        poisoning ◀▥
    cigarettes —*see* Table of ⊕Drugs
        and ⊖Chemicals, by substance,
        poisoning ◀▥
  use Z72.0
    complicating
      childbirth O99.334
      pregnancy O99.33-
      puerperium O99.335
    counseling and surveillance Z71.6
  withdrawal state —*see* Dependence, drug,
      nicotine
Tocopherol deficiency E56.0
Todd's
  cirrhosis K74.3
  paralysis (postepileptic) (transitory) G83.84
Toe —*see* condition
Toilet, artificial opening —*see* Attention to,
    artificial, opening
Tokelau (ringworm) B35.5
Tollwut —*see* Rabies
Tommaselli's disease R31.9
  correct substance properly administered —*see*
      Table of ⊕Drugs and ⊖Chemicals, by
      drug, adverse effect ◀▥

Tommaselli's disease *(Continued)*
  overdose or wrong substance given or
      taken —*see* Table of ⊕Drugs and
      ⊖Chemicals, by drug, poisoning ◀▥
Tongue —*see also* condition
  tie Q38.1
Tonic pupil —*see* Anomaly, pupil, function,
    tonic pupil
Toni-Fanconi syndrome (cystinosis) E72.09
  with cystinosis E72.04
Tonsil —*see* condition
Tonsillitis (acute) (catarrhal) (croupous)
      (follicular) (gangrenous) (infective)
      (lacunar) (lingual) (malignant)
      (membranous) (parenchymatous)
      (phlegmonous) (pseudomembranous)
      (purulent) (septic) (subacute)
      (suppurative) (toxic) (ulcerative)
      (vesicular) (viral) J03.90
  chronic J35.01
    with adenoiditis J35.03
  diphtheritic A36.0
  hypertrophic J35.01
    with adenoiditis J35.03
  recurrent J03.91
  specified organism NEC J03.80
    recurrent J03.81
  staphylococcal J03.80
    recurrent J03.81
  streptococcal J03.00
    recurrent J03.01
  tuberculous A15.8
  Vincent's A69.1
Tooth, teeth —*see* condition
Toothache K08.8
Topagnosis R20.8
Tophi —*see* Gout, chronic ◀▥
TORCH infection —*see* Infection, congenital
  without active infection P00.2
Torn —*see* Tear
Tornwaldt's cyst or disease J39.2
Torsion
  accessory tube —*see* Torsion, fallopian tube
  adnexa (female) —*see* Torsion, fallopian tube
  aorta, acquired I77.1
  appendix epididymis N44.04
  appendix testis N44.03
  bile duct (common) (hepatic) K83.8
    congenital Q44.5
  bowel, colon or intestine K56.2
  cervix —*see* Malposition, uterus
  cystic duct K82.8
  dystonia —*see* Dystonia, torsion
  epididymis (appendix) N44.04
  fallopian tube N83.52
    with ovary N83.53
  gallbladder K82.8
    congenital Q44.1
  hydatid of Morgagni
    female N83.52
    male N44.03
  kidney (pedicle) (leading to infarction)
      N28.0
  Meckel's diverticulum (congenital) Q43.0
    malignant —*see* Table of Neoplasms, small
        intestine, malignant
  mesentery K56.2
  omentum K56.2
  organ or site, congenital NEC —*see* Anomaly,
      by site
  ovary (pedicle) N83.51
    with fallopian tube N83.53
    congenital Q50.2
  oviduct —*see* Torsion, fallopian tube
  penis (acquired) N48.82
    congenital Q55.63
  spasm —*see* Dystonia, torsion
  spermatic cord N44.02
    extravaginal N44.01
    intravaginal N44.02
  spleen D73.5

Torsion (Continued)
  testis, testicle N44.00
    appendix N44.03
  tibia —see Deformity, limb, specified type
    NEC, lower leg
  uterus —see Malposition, uterus
Torticollis (intermittent) (spastic) M43.6
  congenital (sternomastoid) Q68.0
  due to birth injury P15.8
  hysterical F44.4
  ocular R29.891
  psychogenic F45.8
    conversion reaction F44.4
  rheumatic M43.6
  rheumatoid M06.88
  spasmodic G24.3
  traumatic, current S13.4
Tortipelvis G24.1
Tortuous
  artery I77.1
  organ or site, congenital NEC —see Distortion
  retinal vessel, congenital Q14.1
  ureter N13.8
  urethra N36.8
  vein —see Varix
Torture, victim of Z65.4
Torula, torular (histolytica) (infection) —see
    Cryptococcosis
Torulosis —see Cryptococcosis
Torus (mandibularis) (palatinus) M27.0
  fracture —see Fracture, by site, torus
Touraine's syndrome Q79.8
Tourette's syndrome F95.2
Tourniquet syndrome —see Constriction,
    external, by site
Tower skull Q75.0
  with exophthalmos Q87.0
Toxemia R68.89
  bacterial —see Sepsis
  burn —see Burn
  eclamptic (with pre-existing hypertension) —
    see Eclampsia
  erysipelatous —see Erysipelas
  fatigue R68.89
  food —see Poisoning, food
  gastrointestinal K52.1
  intestinal K52.1
  kidney —see Uremia
  malarial —see Malaria
  myocardial —see Myocarditis, toxic
  of pregnancy —see Pre-eclampsia
  pre-eclamptic —see Pre-eclampsia
  small intestine K52.1
  staphylococcal, due to food A05.0
  stasis R68.89
  uremic —see Uremia
  urinary —see Uremia
Toxemica cerebropathia psychica
    (nonalcoholic) F04
  alcoholic —see Alcohol, amnestic disorder
Toxic (poisoning) —see also condition T65.91
  effect —see Table of dDrugs and cChemicals,
    by substance, poisoning ◀▥▥
  shock syndrome A48.3
  thyroid (gland) —see Thyrotoxicosis
Toxicemia —see Toxemia
Toxicity —see Table of dDrugs and cChemicals,
    by substance, poisoning ◀▥▥
  fava bean D55.0
  food, noxious —see Poisoning, food
  from drug or nonmedicinal substance —see
    Table of Drugs and Chemicals, by
    drug
Toxicosis —see also Toxemia
  capillary, hemorrhagic D69.0
Toxinfection, gastrointestinal K52.1
Toxocariasis B83.0
Toxoplasma, toxoplasmosis (acquired) B58.9
  with
    hepatitis B58.1
    meningoencephalitis B58.2
    ocular involvement B58.00

Toxoplasma, toxoplasmosis (Continued)
  with (Continued)
    other organ involvement B58.89
    pneumonia, pneumonitis B58.3
  congenital (acute) (subacute) (chronic) P37.1
  maternal, manifest toxoplasmosis in infant
    (acute) (subacute) (chronic) P37.1
tPA (rtPA) administation in a different facility
    within the last 24 hours prior to admission
    to current facility Z92.82
Trabeculation, bladder N32.89
Trachea —see condition
Tracheitis (catarrhal) (infantile) (membranous)
    (plastic) (septal) (suppurative) (viral)
    J04.10
  with
    bronchitis (15 years of age and above) J40
      acute or subacute —see Bronchitis,
        acute
      chronic J42
      tuberculous NEC A15.5
      under 15 years of age J20.9
    laryngitis (acute) J04.2
      chronic J37.1
      tuberculous NEC A15.5
  acute J04.10
    with obstruction J04.11
  chronic J42
    with
      bronchitis (chronic) J42
      laryngitis (chronic) J37.1
  diphtheritic (membranous) A36.89
  due to external agent —see Inflammation,
    respiratory, upper, due to
  syphilitic A52.73
  tuberculous A15.5
Trachelitis (nonvenereal) —see Cervicitis
Tracheobronchial —see condition
Tracheobronchitis (15 years of age and
    above) —see also Bronchitis
  due to
    Bordetella bronchiseptica A37.80
      with pneumonia A37.81
    Francisella tularensis A21.8
Tracheobronchomegaly Q32.4
  with bronchiectasis J47.9
    with
      exacerbation (acute) J47.1
      lower respiratory infection J47.0
  acquired J98.09
    with bronchiectasis J47.9
      with
        exacerbation (acute) J47.1
        lower respiratory infection J47.0
Tracheobronchopneumonitis —see Pneumonia,
    broncho-
Tracheocele (external) (internal) J39.8
  congenital Q32.1
Tracheomalacia J39.8
  congenital Q32.0
Tracheopharyngitis (acute) J06.9
  chronic J42
  due to external agent —see Inflammation,
    respiratory, upper, due to
Tracheostenosis J39.8
Tracheostomy
  complication —see Complication,
    tracheostomy
  status Z93.0
    attention to Z43.0
    malfunctioning J95.03
Trachoma, trachomatous A71.9
  active (stage) A71.1
  contraction of conjunctiva A71.1
  dubium A71.0
  healed or sequelae B94.0
  initial (stage) A71.0
  pannus A71.1
  Türck's J37.0
Traction, vitreomacular H43.82-
Train sickness T75.3

Trait (s)
  Hb-S D57.3
  hemoglobin
    abnormal NEC D58.2
      with thalassemia D56.3
    C —see Disease, hemoglobin C
    S (Hb-S) D57.3
  Lepore D56.3
  personality, accentuated Z73.1
  sickle-cell D57.3
    with elliptocytosis or spherocytosis
      D57.3
  type A personality Z73.1
Tramp Z59.0
Trance R41.89
  hysterical F44.89
Transaminasemia R74.0
Transection
  abdomen (partial) S38.3
  aorta (incomplete) —see also Injury, aorta
    complete —see Injury, aorta, laceration,
      major
  carotid artery (incomplete) —see also Injury,
    blood vessel, carotid, laceration
    complete —see Injury, blood vessel, carotid,
      laceration, major
  celiac artery (incomplete) S35.211
    branch (incomplete) S35.291
      complete S35.292
    complete S35.212
  innominate
    artery (incomplete) —see also Injury, blood
      vessel, thoracic, innominate, artery,
      laceration
      complete —see Injury, blood vessel,
        thoracic, innominate, artery,
        laceration, major
    vein (incomplete) —see also Injury, blood
      vessel, thoracic, innominate, vein,
      laceration
      complete —see Injury, blood vessel,
        thoracic, innominate, vein,
        laceration, major
  jugular vein (external) (incomplete) —see
    also Injury, blood vessel, jugular vein,
    laceration
    complete —see Injury, blood vessel, jugular
      vein, laceration, major
    internal (incomplete) —see also Injury,
      blood vessel, jugular vein, internal,
      laceration
      complete —see Injury, blood vessel,
        jugular vein, internal, laceration,
        major
  mesenteric artery (incomplete) —see also
    Injury, mesenteric, artery, laceration
    complete —see Injury, mesenteric artery,
      laceration, major
  pulmonary vessel (incomplete) —see
    also Injury, blood vessel, thoracic,
    pulmonary, laceration
    complete —see Injury, blood vessel,
      thoracic, pulmonary, laceration,
      major
  subclavian —see Transection, innominate
  vena cava (incomplete) —see also Injury, vena
    cava
    complete —see Injury, vena cava,
      laceration, major
  vertebral artery (incomplete) —see also
    Injury, blood vessel, vertebral,
    laceration
    complete —see Injury, blood vessel,
      vertebral, laceration, major
Transfusion
  associated (red blood cell) hemochromatosis
    E83.111
  blood
    ABO incompatible —see Complication (s),
      transfusion, incompatibility reaction,
      ABO

◀ New   ◀▥▥ Revised   ~~deleted~~ Deleted

Transfusion (Continued)
- blood (Continued)
  - minor blood group (Duffy) (E) (K(ell)) (Kidd) (Lewis) (M) (N) (P) (S) T80.89
  - reaction or complication —see Complications, transfusion
  - fetomaternal (mother) —see Pregnancy, complicated by, placenta, transfusion syndrome
  - maternofetal (mother) —see Pregnancy, complicated by, placenta, transfusion syndrome
  - placental (syndrome) (mother) —see Pregnancy, complicated by, placenta, transfusion syndrome
  - reaction (adverse) —see Complications, transfusion
  - related acute lung injury (TRALI) J95.84
  - twin-to-twin —see Pregnancy, complicated by, placenta, transfusion syndrome, fetus to fetus

Transient (meaning homeless) (see also condition) Z59.0

Translocation
- balanced autosomal Q95.9
  - in normal individual Q95.0
- chromosomes NEC Q99.8
  - balanced and insertion in normal individual Q95.0
- Down's syndrome Q90.2
- trisomy
  - 13 Q91.6
  - 18 Q91.2
  - 21 Q90.2

Translucency, iris —see Degeneration, iris

Transmission of chemical substances through the placenta —see Absorption, chemical, through placenta

Transparency, lung, unilateral J43.0

Transplant (ed) (status) Z94.9
- awaiting organ Z76.82
- bone Z94.6
  - marrow Z94.81
- candidate Z76.82
- complication —see Complication, transplant
- cornea Z94.7
- heart Z94.1
  - and lung (s) Z94.3
  - valve Z95.2
    - prosthetic Z95.2
    - specified NEC Z95.4
    - xenogenic Z95.3
- intestine Z94.82
- kidney Z94.0
- liver Z94.4
- lung (s) Z94.2
  - and heart Z94.3
- organ (failure) (infection) (rejection)Z94.9
  - removal status Z98.85
- pancreas Z94.83
- skin Z94.5
- social Z60.3
- specified organ or tissue NEC Z94.89
- stem cells Z94.84
- tissue Z94.9

Transplants, ovarian, endometrial N80.1

Transposed —see Transposition

Transposition (congenital) —see also Malposition, congenital
- abdominal viscera Q89.3
- aorta (dextra) Q20.3
- appendix Q43.8
- colon Q43.8
- corrected Q20.5
- great vessels (complete) (partial) Q20.3
- heart Q24.0
  - with complete transposition of viscera Q89.3
- intestine (large) (small) Q43.8
- reversed jejunal (for bypass) (status) Z98.0
- scrotum Q55.23

Transposition (Continued)
- stomach Q40.2
  - with general transposition of viscera Q89.3
- tooth, teeth, fully erupted M26.30
- vessels, great (complete) (partial) Q20.3
- viscera (abdominal) (thoracic) Q89.3

Transsexualism F64.1

Transverse —see also condition
- arrest (deep), in labor O64.0
- lie (mother) O32.2
  - causing obstructed labor O64.8

Transvestism, transvestitism (dual-role) F64.1
- fetishistic F65.1

Trapped placenta (with hemorrhage) O72.0
- without hemorrhage O73.0

Trauma, traumatism —see also Injury
- acoustic —see subcategory H83.3
- birth —see Birth, injury
- complicating ectopic or molar pregnancy O08.6
- during delivery O71.9
- following ectopic or molar pregnancy O08.6
- obstetric O71.9
  - specified NEC O71.89

Traumatic —see also condition
- brain injury —see category S06

Treacher Collins syndrome Q75.4

Treitz's hernia —see Hernia, abdomen, specified site NEC

Trematode infestation —see Infestation, fluke

Trematodiasis —see Infestation, fluke

Trembling paralysis —see Parkinsonism

Tremor (s) R25.1
- drug induced G25.1
- essential (benign) G25.0
- familial G25.0
- hereditary G25.0
- hysterical F44.4
- intention G25.2
- medication induced postural G25.1
- mercurial —see subcategory T56.1
- Parkinson's —see Parkinsonism
- psychogenic (conversion reaction) F44.4
- senilis R54
- specified type NEC G25.2

Trench
- fever A79.0
- foot —see Immersion, foot
- mouth A69.1

Treponema pallidum infection —see Syphilis

Treponematosis
- due to
  - T. pallidum —see Syphilis
  - T. pertenue —see Yaws

Triad
- Hutchinson's (congenital syphilis) A50.53
- Kartagener's Q89.3
- Saint's —see Hernia, diaphragm

Trichiasis (eyelid) H02.059
- with entropion —see Entropion
- left H02.056
  - lower H02.055
  - upper H02.054
- right H02.053
  - lower H02.052
  - upper H02.051

Trichinella spiralis (infection) (infestation) B75

Trichinellosis, trichiniasis, trichinelliasis, trichinosis B75
- with muscle disorder B75 [M63.80]
  - ankle B75 [M63.87-]
  - foot B75 [M63.87-]
  - forearm B75 [M63.83-]
  - hand B75 [M63.84-]
  - lower leg B75 [M63.86-]
  - multiple sites B75 [M63.89]
  - pelvic region B75 [M63.85-]
  - shoulder region B75 [M63.81-]
  - specified site NEC B75 [M63.88]
  - thigh B75 [M63.85-]
  - upper arm B75 [M63.82-]

Trichobezoar T18.9
- intestine T18.3
- stomach T18.2

Trichocephaliasis, trichocephalosis B79

Trichocephalus infestation B79

Trichoclasis L67.8

Trichoepithelioma —see also Neoplasm, skin, benign
- malignant —see Neoplasm, skin, malignant

Trichofolliculoma —see Neoplasm, skin, benign

Tricholemmoma —see Neoplasm, skin, benign

Trichomoniasis A59.9
- bladder A59.03
- cervix A59.09
- intestinal A07.8
- prostate A59.02
- seminal vesicles A59.09
- specified site NEC A59.8
- urethra A59.03
- urogenitalis A59.00
- vagina A59.01
- vulva A59.01

Trichomycosis
- axillaris A48.8
- nodosa, nodularis B36.8

Trichonodosis L67.8

Trichophytid, trichophyton infection —see Dermatophytosis

Trichophytobezoar T18.9
- intestine T18.3
- stomach T18.2

Trichophytosis —see Dermatophytosis

Trichoptilosis L67.8

Trichorrhexis (nodosa) (invaginata) L67.0

Trichosis axillaris A48.8

Trichosporosis nodosa B36.2

Trichostasis spinulosa (congenital) Q84.1

Trichostrongyliasis, trichostrongylosis (small intestine) B81.2

Trichostrongylus infection B81.2

Trichotillomania F63.3

Trichromat, trichromatopsia, anomalous (congenital) H53.55

Trichuriasis B79

Trichuris trichiura (infection) (infestation) (any site) B79

Tricuspid (valve) —see condition

Trifid —see also Accessory
- kidney (pelvis) Q63.8
- tongue Q38.3

Trigeminal neuralgia —see Neuralgia, trigeminal

Trigeminy R00.8

Trigger finger (acquired) M65.30
- congenital Q74.0
- index finger M65.32-
- little finger M65.35-
- middle finger M65.33-
- ring finger M65.34-
- thumb M65.31-

Trigonitis (bladder) (chronic) (pseudomembranous) N30.30
- with hematuria N30.31

Trigonocephaly Q75.0

Trilocular heart —see Cor triloculare

Trimethylaminuria E72.52

Tripartite placenta O43.19-

Triphalangeal thumb Q74.0

Triple —see also Accessory
- kidneys Q63.0
- uteri Q51.818
- X, female Q97.0

Triplegia G83.89
- congenital G80.8

Triplet (newborn) —see also Newborn, triplet
- complicating pregnancy —see Pregnancy, triplet

Triplication —see Accessory

Triploidy Q92.7

Trismus R25.2
  neonatorum A33
  newborn A33
Trisomy (syndrome) Q92.9
  13 (partial) Q91.7
    meiotic nondisjunction Q91.4
    mitotic nondisjunction Q91.5
    mosaicism Q91.5
    translocation Q91.6
  18 (partial) Q91.3
    meiotic nondisjunction Q91.0
    mitotic nondisjunction Q91.1
    mosaicism Q91.1
    translocation Q91.2
  20 Q92.8
  21 (partial) Q90.9
    meiotic nondisjunction Q90.0
    mitotic nondisjunction Q90.1
    mosaicism Q90.1
    translocation Q90.2
  22 Q92.8
  autosomes Q92.9
  chromosome specified NEC Q92.8
    partial Q92.2
      due to unbalanced translocation Q92.5
    specified NEC Q92.8
    whole (nonsex chromosome)
      meiotic nondisjunction Q92.0
      mitotic nondisjunction Q92.1
      mosaicism Q92.1
  due to
    dicentrics —see Extra, marker
        chromosomes
    extra rings —see Extra, marker
        chromosomes
    isochromosomes —see Extra, marker
        chromosomes
  specified NEC Q92.8
  whole chromosome Q92.9
    meiotic nondisjunction Q92.0
    mitotic nondisjunction Q92.1
    mosaicism Q92.1
    partial Q92.9
    specified NEC Q92.8
Tritanomaly, tritanopia H53.55
Trombiculosis, trombiculiasis, trombidiosis
    B88.0
Trophedema (congenital) (hereditary) Q82.0
Trophoblastic disease (see also Mole,
    hydatidiform) O01.9
Tropholymphedema Q82.0
Trophoneurosis NEC G96.8
  disseminated M34.9
Tropical —see condition
Trouble —see also Disease
  heart —see Disease, heart
  kidney —see Disease, renal
  nervous R45.0
  sinus —see Sinusitis
Trousseau's syndrome (thrombophlebitis
    migrans) I82.1
Truancy, childhood
  from school Z72.810
Truncus
  arteriosus (persistent) Q20.0
  communis Q20.0
Trunk —see condition
Trypanosomiasis
  African B56.9
    by Trypanosoma brucei
      gambiense B56.0
      rhodesiense B56.1
  American —see Chagas' disease
  Brazilian —see Chagas' disease
  by Trypanosoma
    brucei gambiense B56.0
    brucei rhodesiense B56.1
    cruzi —see Chagas' disease
  gambiensis, Gambian B56.0
  rhodesiensis, Rhodesian B56.1
  South American —see Chagas' disease

Trypanosomiasis (Continued)
  where
    African trypanosomiasis is prevalent B56.9
    Chagas' disease is prevalent B57.2
T-shaped incisors K00.2
Tsutsugamushi (disease) (fever) A75.3
Tube, tubal, tubular —see condition
Tubercle —see also Tuberculosis
  brain, solitary A17.81
  Darwin's Q17.8
  Ghon, primary infection A15.7
Tuberculid, tuberculide (indurating,
    subcutaneous) (lichenoid) (miliary)
    (papulonecrotic) (primary) (skin) A18.4
Tuberculoma —see also Tuberculosis
  brain A17.81
  meninges (cerebral) (spinal) A17.1
  spinal cord A17.81
Tuberculosis, tubercular, tuberculous
    (calcification) (calcified) (caseous)
    (chromogenic acid-fast bacilli)
    (degeneration) (fibrocaseous) (fistula)
    (interstitial) (isolated circumscribed
    lesions) (necrosis) (parenchymatous)
    (ulcerative) A15.9
  with pneumoconiosis (any condition in
    J60-J64) J65
  abdomen (lymph gland) A18.39
  abscess (respiratory) A15.9
    bone A18.03
      hip A18.02
      knee A18.02
      sacrum A18.01
      specified site NEC A18.03
      spinal A18.01
      vertebra A18.01
    brain A17.81
    breast A18.89
    Cowper's gland A18.15
    dura (mater) (cerebral) (spinal) A17.81
    epidural (cerebral) (spinal) A17.81
    female pelvis A18.17
    frontal sinus A15.8
    genital organs NEC A18.10
    genitourinary A18.10
    gland (lymphatic) —see Tuberculosis,
        lymph gland
    hip A18.02
    intestine A18.32
    ischiorectal A18.32
    joint NEC A18.02
      hip A18.02
      knee A18.02
      specified NEC A18.02
      vertebral A18.01
    kidney A18.11
    knee A18.02
    latent R76.11
    lumbar (spine) A18.01
    lung —see Tuberculosis, pulmonary
    meninges (cerebral) (spinal) A17.0
    muscle A18.09
    perianal (fistula) A18.32
    perinephritic A18.11
    perirectal A18.32
    rectum A18.32
    retropharyngeal A15.8
    sacrum A18.01
    scrofulous A18.2
    scrotum A18.15
    skin (primary) A18.4
    spinal cord A17.81
    spine or vertebra (column) A18.01
    subdiaphragmatic A18.31
    testis A18.15
    urinary A18.13
    uterus A18.17
  accessory sinus —see Tuberculosis, sinus
  Addison's disease A18.7
  adenitis —see Tuberculosis, lymph gland
  adenoids A15.8

Tuberculosis, tubercular, tuberculous
    (Continued)
  adenopathy —see Tuberculosis, lymph gland
  adherent pericardium A18.84
  adnexa (uteri) A18.17
  adrenal (capsule) (gland) A18.7
  alimentary canal A18.32
  anemia A18.89
  ankle (joint) (bone) A18.02
  anus A18.32
  apex, apical —see Tuberculosis, pulmonary
  appendicitis, appendix A18.32
  arachnoid A17.0
  artery, arteritis A18.89
    cerebral A18.89
  arthritis (chronic) (synovial) A18.02
    spine or vertebra (column) A18.01
  articular —see Tuberculosis, joint
  ascites A18.31
  asthma —see Tuberculosis, pulmonary
  axilla, axillary (gland) A18.2
  bladder A18.12
  bone A18.03
    hip A18.02
    knee A18.02
    limb NEC A18.03
    sacrum A18.01
    spine or vertebral column A18.01
  bowel (miliary) A18.32
  brain A17.81
  breast A18.89
  broad ligament A18.17
  bronchi, bronchial, bronchus A15.5
    ectasia, ectasis (bronchiectasis) —see
        Tuberculosis, pulmonary
    fistula A15.5
      primary (progressive) A15.7
    gland or node A15.4
      primary (progressive) A15.7
    lymph gland or node A15.4
      primary (progressive) A15.7
  bronchiectasis —see Tuberculosis, pulmonary
  bronchitis A15.5
  bronchopleural A15.6
  bronchopneumonia, bronchopneumonic —see
        Tuberculosis, pulmonary
  bronchorrhagia A15.5
  bronchotracheal A15.5
  bronze disease A18.7
  buccal cavity A18.83
  bulbourethral gland A18.15
  bursa A18.09
  cachexia A15.9
  cardiomyopathy A18.84
  caries —see Tuberculosis, bone
  cartilage A18.02
    intervertebral A18.01
  catarrhal —see Tuberculosis, respiratory
  cecum A18.32
  cellulitis (primary) A18.4
  cerebellum A17.81
  cerebral, cerebrum A17.81
  cerebrospinal A17.81
    meninges A17.0
  cervical (lymph gland or node) A18.2
  cervicitis, cervix (uteri) A18.16
  chest —see Tuberculosis, respiratory
  chorioretinitis A18.53
  choroid, choroiditis A18.53
  ciliary body A18.54
  colitis A18.32
  collier's J65
  colliquativa (primary) A18.4
  colon A18.32
  complex, primary A15.7
  congenital P37.0
  conjunctiva A18.59
  connective tissue (systemic) A18.89
  contact Z20.1
  cornea (ulcer) A18.52
  Cowper's gland A18.15

◀ New   ◀|||| Revised   ~~deleted~~ Deleted

Tuberculosis, tubercular, tuberculous
  (Continued)
  coxae A18.02
  coxalgia A18.02
  cul-de-sac of Douglas A18.17
  curvature, spine A18.01
  cutis (colliquativa) (primary) A18.4
  cyst, ovary A18.18
  cystitis A18.12
  dactylitis A18.03
  diarrhea A18.32
  diffuse —see Tuberculosis, miliary
  digestive tract A18.32
  disseminated —see Tuberculosis, miliary
  duodenum A18.32
  dura (mater) (cerebral) (spinal) A17.0
    abscess (cerebral) (spinal) A17.81
  dysentery A18.32
  ear (inner) (middle) A18.6
    bone A18.03
    external (primary) A18.4
    skin (primary) A18.4
  elbow A18.02
  emphysema —see Tuberculosis, pulmonary
  empyema A15.6
  encephalitis A17.82
  endarteritis A18.89
  endocarditis A18.84
    aortic A18.84
    mitral A18.84
    pulmonary A18.84
    tricuspid A18.84
  endocrine glands NEC A18.82
  endometrium A18.17
  enteric, enterica, enteritis A18.32
  enterocolitis A18.32
  epididymis, epididymitis A18.15
  epidural abscess (cerebral) (spinal) A17.81
  epiglottis A15.5
  episcleritis A18.51
  erythema (induratum) (nodosum) (primary)
    A18.4
  esophagus A18.83
  eustachian tube A18.6
  exposure (to) Z20.1
  exudative —see Tuberculosis, pulmonary
  eye A18.50
  eyelid (primary) (lupus) A18.4
  fallopian tube (acute) (chronic) A18.17
  fascia A18.09
  fauces A15.8
  female pelvic inflammatory disease A18.17
  finger A18.03
  first infection A15.7
  gallbladder A18.83
  ganglion A18.09
  gastritis A18.83
  gastrocolic fistula A18.32
  gastroenteritis A18.32
  gastrointestinal tract A18.32
  general, generalized —see Tuberculosis,
    miliary
  genital organs A18.10
  genitourinary A18.10
  genu A18.02
  glandula suprarenalis A18.7
  glandular, general A18.2
  glottis A15.5
  grinder's J65
  gum A18.83
  hand A18.03
  heart A18.84
  hematogenous —see Tuberculosis, miliary
  hemoptysis —see Tuberculosis, pulmonary
  hemorrhage NEC —see Tuberculosis,
    pulmonary
  hemothorax A15.6
  hepatitis A18.83
  hilar lymph nodes A15.4
    primary (progressive) A15.7
  hip (joint) (disease) (bone) A18.02

Tuberculosis, tubercular, tuberculous
  (Continued)
  hydropneumothorax A15.6
  hydrothorax A15.6
  hypoadrenalism A18.7
  hypopharynx A15.8
  ileocecal (hyperplastic) A18.32
  ileocolitis A18.32
  ileum A18.32
  iliac spine (superior) A18.03
  immunological findings only A15.7
  indurativa (primary) A18.4
  infantile A15.7
  infection A15.9
    without clinical manifestations A15.7
  infraclavicular gland A18.2
  inguinal gland A18.2
  inguinalis A18.2
  intestine (any part) A18.32
  iridocyclitis A18.54
  iris, iritis A18.54
  ischiorectal A18.32
  jaw A18.03
  jejunum A18.32
  joint A18.02
    vertebral A18.01
  keratitis (interstitial) A18.52
  keratoconjunctivitis A18.52
  kidney A18.11
  knee (joint) A18.02
  kyphosis, kyphoscoliosis A18.01
  laryngitis A15.5
  larynx A15.5
  latent R76.11
  leptomeninges, leptomeningitis (cerebral)
    (spinal) A17.0
  lichenoides (primary) A18.4
  linguae A18.83
  lip A18.83
  liver A18.83
  lordosis A18.01
  lung —see Tuberculosis, pulmonary
  lupus vulgaris A18.4
  lymph gland or node (peripheral) A18.2
    abdomen A18.39
    bronchial A15.4
      primary (progressive) A15.7
    cervical A18.2
    hilar A15.4
      primary (progressive) A15.7
    intrathoracic A15.4
      primary (progressive) A15.7
    mediastinal A15.4
      primary (progressive) A15.7
    mesenteric A18.39
    retroperitoneal A18.39
    tracheobronchial A15.4
      primary (progressive) A15.7
  lymphadenitis —see Tuberculosis, lymph
    gland
  lymphangitis —see Tuberculosis, lymph
    gland
  lymphatic (gland) (vessel) —see Tuberculosis,
    lymph gland
  mammary gland A18.89
  marasmus A18.9
  mastoiditis A18.03
  mediastinal lymph gland or node
    A15.4
    primary (progressive) A15.7
  mediastinitis A15.8
    primary (progressive) A15.7
  mediastinum A15.8
    primary (progressive) A15.7
  medulla A17.81
  melanosis, Addisonian A18.7
  meninges, meningitis (basilar) (cerebral)
    (cerebrospinal) (spinal) A17.0
  meningoencephalitis A17.82
  mesentery, mesenteric (gland or node)
    A18.39

Tuberculosis, tubercular, tuberculous
  (Continued)
  miliary A19.9
    acute A19.2
      multiple sites A19.1
      single specified site A19.0
    chronic A19.8
    specified NEC A19.8
  millstone makers' J65
  miner's J65
  molder's J65
  mouth A18.83
  multiple A19.9
    acute A19.1
    chronic A19.8
  muscle A18.09
  myelitis A17.82
  myocardium, myocarditis A18.84
  nasal (passage) (sinus) A15.8
  nasopharynx A15.8
  neck gland A18.2
  nephritis A18.11
  nerve (mononeuropathy) A17.83
  nervous system A17.9
  nose (septum) A15.8
  ocular A18.50
  omentum A18.31
  oophoritis (acute) (chronic) A18.17
  optic (nerve trunk) (papilla) A18.59
  orbit A18.59
  orchitis A18.15
  organ, specified NEC A18.89
  osseous —see Tuberculosis, bone
  osteitis —see Tuberculosis, bone
  osteomyelitis —see Tuberculosis, bone
  otitis media A18.6
  ovary, ovaritis (acute) (chronic) A18.17
  oviduct (acute) (chronic) A18.17
  pachymeningitis A17.0
  palate (soft) A18.83
  pancreas A18.83
  papulonecrotic (a) (primary) A18.4
  parathyroid glands A18.82
  paronychia (primary) A18.4
  parotid gland or region A18.83
  pelvis (bony) A18.03
  penis A18.15
  peribronchitis A15.5
  pericardium, pericarditis A18.84
  perichondritis, larynx A15.5
  periostitis —see Tuberculosis, bone
  perirectal fistula A18.32
  peritoneum NEC A18.31
  peritonitis A18.31
  pharynx, pharyngitis A15.8
  phlyctenulosis (keratoconjunctivitis) A18.52
  phthisis NEC —see Tuberculosis, pulmonary
  pituitary gland A18.82
  pleura, pleural, pleurisy, pleuritis (fibrinous)
    (obliterative) (purulent) (simple plastic)
    (with effusion) A15.6
    primary (progressive) A15.7
  pneumonia, pneumonic —see Tuberculosis,
    pulmonary
  pneumothorax (spontaneous) (tense
    valvular) —see Tuberculosis, pulmonary
  polyneuropathy A17.89
  polyserositis A19.9
    acute A19.1
    chronic A19.8
  potter's J65
  prepuce A18.15
  primary (complex) A15.7
  proctitis A18.32
  prostate, prostatitis A18.14
  pulmonalis —see Tuberculosis, pulmonary
  pulmonary (cavitated) (fibrotic) (infiltrative)
    (nodular) A15.0
    childhood type or first infection A15.7
    primary (complex) A15.7
  pyelitis A18.11

Tuberculosis, tubercular, tuberculous
(Continued)
pyelonephritis A18.11
pyemia —see Tuberculosis, miliary
pyonephrosis A18.11
pyopneumothorax A15.6
pyothorax A15.6
rectum (fistula) (with abscess) A18.32
reinfection stage —see Tuberculosis,
pulmonary
renal A18.11
renis A18.11
respiratory A15.9
primary A15.7
specified site NEC A15.8
retina, retinitis A18.53
retroperitoneal (lymph gland or node)
A18.39
rheumatism NEC A18.09
rhinitis A15.8
sacroiliac (joint) A18.01
sacrum A18.01
salivary gland A18.83
salpingitis (acute) (chronic) A18.17
sandblaster's J65
sclera A18.51
scoliosis A18.01
scrofulous A18.2
scrotum A18.15
seminal tract or vesicle A18.15
senile A15.9
septic —see Tuberculosis, miliary
shoulder (joint) A18.02
blade A18.03
sigmoid A18.32
sinus (any nasal) A15.8
bone A18.03
epididymis A18.15
skeletal NEC A18.03
skin (any site) (primary) A18.4
small intestine A18.32
soft palate A18.83
spermatic cord A18.15
spine, spinal (column) A18.01
cord A17.81
medulla A17.81
membrane A17.0
meninges A17.0
spleen, splenitis A18.85
spondylitis A18.01
sternoclavicular joint A18.02
stomach A18.83
stonemason's J65
subcutaneous tissue (cellular) (primary)
A18.4
subcutis (primary) A18.4
subdeltoid bursa A18.83
submaxillary (region) A18.83
supraclavicular gland A18.2
suprarenal (capsule) (gland) A18.7
swelling, joint (see also category M01) (see also
Tuberculosis, joint) A18.02
symphysis pubis A18.02
synovitis A18.09
articular A18.02
spine or vertebra A18.01
systemic —see Tuberculosis, miliary
tarsitis A18.4
tendon (sheath) —see Tuberculosis,
tenosynovitis
tenosynovitis A18.09
spine or vertebra A18.01
testis A18.15
throat A15.8
thymus gland A18.82
thyroid gland A18.81
tongue A18.83
tonsil, tonsillitis A15.8
trachea, tracheal A15.5
lymph gland or node A15.4
primary (progressive) A15.7

Tuberculosis, tubercular, tuberculous
(Continued)
tracheobronchial A15.5
lymph gland or node A15.4
primary (progressive) A15.7
tubal (acute) (chronic) A18.17
tunica vaginalis A18.15
ulcer (skin) (primary) A18.4
bowel or intestine A18.32
specified NEC - code under Tuberculosis,
by site
unspecified site A15.9
ureter A18.11
urethra, urethral (gland) A18.13
urinary organ or tract A18.13
uterus A18.17
uveal tract A18.54
uvula A18.83
vagina A18.18
vas deferens A18.15
verruca, verrucosa (cutis) (primary)
A18.4
vertebra (column) A18.01
vesiculitis A18.15
vulva A18.18
wrist (joint) A18.02
Tuberculum
Carabelli (see Note at) K00.2
occlusal (see Note at) K00.2
paramolare K00.2
Tuberosity, enitre maxillary M26.07
Tuberous sclerosis (brain) Q85.1
Tubo-ovarian —see condition
Tuboplasty, after previous sterilization
Z31.0
aftercare Z31.42
Tubotympanitis, catarrhal (chronic) —see
Otitis, media, nonsuppurative, chronic,
serous
Tularemia A21.9
with
conjunctivitis A21.1
pneumonia A21.2
abdominal A21.3
bronchopneumonic A21.2
conjunctivitis A21.1
cryptogenic A21.3
enteric A21.3
gastrointestinal A21.3
generalized A21.7
ingestion A21.3
intestinal A21.3
oculoglandular A21.1
ophthalmic A21.1
pneumonia (any), pneumonic A21.2
pulmonary A21.2
sepsis A21.7
specified NEC A21.8
typhoidal A21.7
ulceroglandular A21.0
Tularensis conjunctivitis A21.1
Tumefaction —see also Swelling
liver —see Hypertrophy, liver
Tumor —see also Neoplasm, unspecified
behavior, by site
acinar cell —see Neoplasm, uncertain
behavior, by site
acinic cell —see Neoplasm, uncertain
behavior, by site
adenocarcinoid —see Neoplasm, malignant,
by site
adenomatoid —see also Neoplasm, benign,
by site
odontogenic —see Cyst, calcifying
odontogenic
adnexal (skin) —see Neoplasm, skin, benign,
by site
adrenal
cortical (benign) D35.0-
malignant C74.0-
rest —see Neoplasm, benign, by site

Tumor (Continued)
alpha-cell
malignant
pancreas C25.4
specified site NEC —see Neoplasm,
malignant, by site
unspecified site C25.4
pancreas D13.7
specified site NEC —see Neoplasm, benign,
by site
unspecified site D13.7
aneurysmal —see Aneurysm
aortic body D44.7
malignant C75.5
Askin's —see Neoplasm, connective tissue,
malignant
basal cell (see also Neoplasm, skin, uncertain
behavior) D48.5
Bednar —see Neoplasm, skin, malignant
benign (unclassified) —see Neoplasm, benign,
by site
beta-cell
malignant
pancreas C25.4
specified site NEC —see Neoplasm,
malignant, by site
unspecified site C25.4
pancreas D13.7
specified site NEC —see Neoplasm, benign,
by site
unspecified site D13.7
Brenner D27.9
borderline malignancy D39.1-
malignant C56-
proliferating D39.1
bronchial alveolar, intravascular D38.1
Brooke's —see Neoplasm, skin, benign
brown fat —see Lipoma
Burkitt —see Lymphoma, Burkitt
calcifying epithelial odontogenic —see Cyst,
calcifying odontogenic
carcinoid
benign D3A.00
appendix D3A.020
ascending colon D3A.022
bronchus (lung) D3A.090
cecum D3A.021
colon D3A.029
descending colon D3A.024
duodenum D3A.010
foregut NOS D3A.094
hindgut NOS D3A.096
ileum D3A.012
jejunum D3A.011
kidney D3A.093
large intestine D3A.029
lung (bronchus) D3A.090
midgut NOS D3A.095
rectum D3A.026
sigmoid colon D3A.025
small intestine D3A.019
specified NEC D3A.098
stomach D3A.092
thymus D3A.091
transverse colon D3A.023
malignant C7A.00
appendix C7A.020
ascending colon C7A.022
bronchus (lung) C7A.090
cecum C7A.021
colon C7A.029
descending colon C7A.024
duodenum C7A.010
foregut NOS C7A.094
hindgut NOS C7A.096
ileum C7A.012
jejunum C7A.011
kidney C7A.093
large intestine C7A.029
lung (bronchus) C7A.090
midgut NOS C7A.095

◀ New   ◀▥ Revised   ~~deleted~~ Deleted

Tumor (*Continued*)
  carcinoid (*Continued*)
    malignant (*Continued*)
      rectum C7A.026
      sigmoid colon C7A.025
      small intestine C7A.019
      specified NEC C7A.098
      stomach C7A.092
      thymus C7A.091
      transverse colon C7A.023
    mesentary metastasis C7B.04
    secondary C7B.00
      bone C7B.03
      distant lymph nodes C7B.01
      liver C7B.02
      peritoneum C7B.04
      specified NEC C7B.09
  carotid body D44.6
    malignant C75.4
  cells —*see also* Neoplasm, unspecified
    behavior, by site
    benign —*see* Neoplasm, benign, by site
    malignant —*see* Neoplasm, malignant, by
      site
    uncertain whether benign or malignant —
      see Neoplasm, uncertain behavior,
      by site
  cervix, in pregnancy or childbirth —*see*
    Pregnancy, complicated by, tumor,
    cervix
  chondromatous giant cell —*see* Neoplasm,
    bone, benign
  chromaffin —*see also* Neoplasm, benign, by
    site
    malignant —*see* Neoplasm, malignant, by
      site
  Cock's peculiar L72.3
  Codman's —*see* Neoplasm, bone, benign
  dentigerous, mixed —*see* Cyst, calcifying
    odontogenic
  dermoid —*see* Neoplasm, benign, by site
    with malignant transformation C56-
  desmoid (extra-abdominal) —*see also*
    Neoplasm, connective tissue, uncertain
    behavior
    abdominal —*see* Neoplasm, connective
      tissue, uncertain behavior
  embolus —*see* Neoplasm, secondary,
    by site
  embryonal (mixed) —*see also* Neoplasm,
    uncertain behavior, by site
    liver C22.7
  endodermal sinus
    specified site —*see* Neoplasm, malignant,
      by site
    unspecified site
      female C56.-
      male C62.90
  epithelial
    benign —*see* Neoplasm, benign, by site
    malignant —*see* Neoplasm, malignant, by
      site
  Ewing's —*see* Neoplasm, bone, malignant,
    by site
  fatty —*see* Lipoma
  fibroid —*see* Leiomyoma
  G cell
    malignant
      pancreas C25.4
      specified site NEC —*see* Neoplasm,
        malignant, by site
      unspecified site C25.4
    specified site —*see* Neoplasm, uncertain
      behavior, by site
    unspecified site D37.8
  germ cell —*see also* Neoplasm, malignant,
    by site
    mixed —*see* Neoplasm, malignant,
      by site
  ghost cell, odontogenic —*see* Cyst, calcifying
    odontogenic

Tumor (*Continued*)
  giant cell —*see also* Neoplasm, uncertain
    behavior, by site
    bone D48.0
      malignant —*see* Neoplasm, bone,
        malignant
    chondromatous —*see* Neoplasm, bone,
      benign
    malignant —*see* Neoplasm, malignant, by
      site
    soft parts —*see* Neoplasm, connective
      tissue, uncertain behavior
      malignant —*see* Neoplasm, connective
        tissue, malignant
  glomus D18.00
    intra-abdominal D18.03
    intracranial D18.02
    jugulare D44.7
      malignant C75.5
    skin D18.01
    specified site NEC D18.09
  gonadal stromal —*see* Neoplasm, uncertain
    behavior, by site
  granular cell —*see also* Neoplasm, connective
    tissue, benign
    malignant —*see* Neoplasm, connective
      tissue, malignant
  granulosa cell D39.1-
    juvenile D39.1-
    malignant C56-
  granulosa cell-theca cell D39.1-
    malignant C56-
  Grawitz's C64-
  hemorrhoidal —*see* Hemorrhoids
  hilar cell D27-
  hilus cell D27-
  Hurthle cell (benign) D34
    malignant C73
  hydatid —*see* Echinococcus
  hypernephroid —*see also* Neoplasm,
    uncertain behavior, by site
  interstitial cell —*see also* Neoplasm, uncertain
    behavior, by site
    benign —*see* Neoplasm, benign, by site
    malignant —*see* Neoplasm, malignant, by
      site
  intravascular bronchial alveolar D38.1
  islet cell —*see* Neoplasm, benign, by site
    malignant —*see* Neoplasm, malignant, by
      site
    pancreas C25.4
    specified site NEC —*see* Neoplasm,
      malignant, by site
    unspecified site C25.4
    pancreas D13.7
    specified site NEC —*see* Neoplasm, benign,
      by site
    unspecified site D13.7
  juxtaglomerular D41.0-
  Klatskin's C24.0
  Krukenberg's C79.6-
  Leydig cell —*see* Neoplasm, uncertain
    behavior, by site
    benign —*see* Neoplasm, benign, by site
      specified site —*see* Neoplasm, benign,
        by site
      unspecified site
        female D27.9
        male D29.20
    malignant —*see* Neoplasm, malignant, by
      site
      specified site —*see* Neoplasm,
        malignant, by site
      unspecified site
        female C56.9
        male C62.90
    specified site —*see* Neoplasm, uncertain
      behavior, by site
    unspecified site
      female D39.10
      male D40.10

Tumor (*Continued*)
  lipid cell, ovary D27-
  lipoid cell, ovary D27-
  malignant (*see also* Neoplasm, malignant, by
    site) C80.1
    fusiform cell (type) C80.1
    giant cell (type) C80.1
    localized, plasma cell —*see* Plasmacytoma,
      solitary
    mixed NEC C80.1
    small cell (type) C80.1
    spindle cell (type) C80.1
    unclassified C80.1
  mast cell D47.0
    malignant C96.2
  melanotic, neuroectodermal —*see* Neoplasm,
    benign, by site
  Merkel cell —*see* Carcinoma, Merkel cell
  mesenchymal
    malignant —*see* Neoplasm, connective
      tissue, malignant
    mixed —*see* Neoplasm, connective tissue,
      uncertain behavior
  mesodermal, mixed —*see also* Neoplasm,
    malignant, by site
    liver C22.4
  mesonephric —*see also* Neoplasm, uncertain
    behavior, by site
    malignant —*see* Neoplasm, malignant, by
      site
  metastatic
    from specified site —*see* Neoplasm,
      malignant, by site
    of specified site —*see* Neoplasm,
      malignant, by site
    to specified site —*see* Neoplasm, secondary,
      by site
  mixed NEC —*see also* Neoplasm, benign, by
    site
    malignant —*see* Neoplasm, malignant, by
      site
  mucinous of low malignant potential
    specified site —*see* Neoplasm, malignant,
      by site
    unspecified site C56.9
  mucocarcinoid
    specified site —*see* Neoplasm, malignant,
      by site
    unspecified site C18.1
  mucoepidermoid —*see* Neoplasm, uncertain
    behavior, by site
  Müllerian, mixed
    specified site —*see* Neoplasm, malignant,
      by site
    unspecified site C54.9
  myoepithelial —*see* Neoplasm, benign,
    by site
  neuroectodermal (peripheral) —*see*
    Neoplasm, malignant, by site
  primitive
    specified site —*see* Neoplasm,
      malignant, by site
    unspecified site C71.9
  neuroendocrine D3A.8
    malignant poorly differentiated
      C7A.1
    secondary NEC C7B.8
    specified NEC C7A.8
  neurogenic olfactory C30.0
  nonencapsulated sclerosing C73
  odontogenic (adenomatoid) (benign)
    (calcifying epithelial) (keratocystic)
    (squamous) —*see* Cyst, calcifying
    odontogenic
    malignant C41.1
      upper jaw (bone) C41.0
  ovarian stromal D39.1-
  ovary, in pregnancy —*see* Pregnancy,
    complicated by
  pacinian —*see* Neoplasm, skin, benign
  Pancoast's —*see* Pancoast's syndrome

Tumor *(Continued)*
  papillary —*see also* Papilloma
    cystic D37.9
    mucinous of low malignant potential C56-
      specified site —*see* Neoplasm,
        malignant, by site
      unspecified site C56.9
    serous of low malignant potential
      specified site —*see* Neoplasm,
        malignant, by site
      unspecified site C56.9
  pelvic, in pregnancy or childbirth —*see*
    Pregnancy, complicated by
  phantom F45.8
  phyllodes D48.6-
    benign D24-
    malignant —*see* Neoplasm, breast,
      malignant
  Pindborg —*see* Cyst, calcifying odontogenic
  placental site trophoblastic D39.2
  plasma cell (malignant) (localized) —*see*
    Plasmacytoma, solitary
  polyvesicular vitelline
    specified site —*see* Neoplasm, malignant,
      by site
    unspecified site
      female C56.9
      male C62.90
  Pott's puffy —*see* Osteomyelitis, specified
    NEC
  Rathke's pouch D44.3
  retinal anlage —*see* Neoplasm, benign,
    by site
  salivary gland type, mixed —*see* Neoplasm,
    salivary gland, benign
    malignant —*see* Neoplasm, salivary gland,
      malignant
  Sampson's N80.1
  Schmincke's —*see* Neoplasm, nasopharynx,
    malignant
  sclerosing stromal D27-
  sebaceous —*see* Cyst, sebaceous
  secondary —*see* Neoplasm, secondary,
    by site
    carcinoid C7B.00
      bone C7B.03
      distant lymph nodes C7B.01
      liver C7B.02
      peritoneum C7B.04
      specified NEC C7B.09
    neuroendocrine NEC C7B.8
  serous of low malignant potential
    specified site —*see* Neoplasm, malignant,
      by site
    unspecified site C56.9
  Sertoli cell —*see* Neoplasm, benign, by site
    with lipid storage
      specified site —*see* Neoplasm, benign,
        by site
      unspecified site
        female D27.9
        male D29.20
    specified site —*see* Neoplasm, benign, by
      site
    unspecified site
      female D27.9
      male D29.20
  Sertoli-Leydig cell —*see* Neoplasm, benign,
    by site
    specified site —*see* Neoplasm, benign, by
      site
    unspecified site
      female D27.9
      male D29.20
  sex cord(-stromal) —*see* Neoplasm, uncertain
    behavior, by site
    with annular tubules D39.1-
  skin appendage —*see* Neoplasm, skin,
    benign
  smooth muscle —*see* Neoplasm, connective
    tissue, uncertain behavior

Tumor *(Continued)*
  soft tissue
    benign —*see* Neoplasm, connective tissue,
      benign
    malignant —*see* Neoplasm, connective
      tissue, malignant
  sternomastoid (congenital) Q68.0
  stromal
    endometrial D39.0
    gastric D48.1
      benign D21.4
      malignant C16.9
      uncertain behavior D48.1
    gastrointestinal
      benign D21.4
      malignant C49.4
      uncertain behavior D48.1
    intestine
      benign D21.4
      malignant C49.4
      uncertain behavior D48.1
    ovarian D39.1-
    stomach
      benign D21.4
      malignant C16.9
      uncertain behavior D48.1
  sweat gland —*see also* Neoplasm, skin,
    uncertain behavior
    benign —*see* Neoplasm, skin, benign
    malignant —*see* Neoplasm, skin, malignant
  syphilitic, brain A52.17
  testicular D40.10
  testicular stromal D40.1-
  theca cell D27.-
  theca cell-granulosa cell D39.1-
  Triton, malignant —*see* Neoplasm, nerve,
    malignant
  trophoblastic, placental site D39.2
  turban D23.4
  uterus (body), in pregnancy or childbirth —
    see Pregnancy, complicated by, tumor,
    uterus
  vagina, in pregnancy or childbirth —*see*
    Pregnancy, complicated by
  varicose —*see* Varix
  von Recklinghausen's —*see*
    Neurofibromatosis
  vulva or perineum, in pregnancy or
    childbirth —*see* Pregnancy, complicated
    by
    causing obstructed labor O65.5
  Warthin's —*see* Neoplasm, salivary gland,
    benign
  Wilms' C64-
  yolk sac —*see* Neoplasm, malignant, by site
    specified site —*see* Neoplasm, malignant,
      by site
    unspecified site
      female C56.9
      male C62.90
Tumor lysis syndrome (following
  antineoplastic chemotherapy)
  (spontaneous) NEC E88.3
Tumorlet —*see* Neoplasm, uncertain behavior,
  by site
Tungiasis B88.1
Tunica vasculosa lentis Q12.2
Turban tumor D23.4
Türck's trachoma J37.0
Turner-Kieser syndrome Q79.8
Turner-like syndrome Q87.1
Turner's
  hypoplasia (tooth) K00.4
  syndrome Q96.9
    specified NEC Q96.8
  tooth K00.4
Turner-Ullrich syndrome Q96.9
Tussis convulsiva —*see* Whooping cough
Twiddler's syndrome (due to)
  automatic implantable defibrillator T82.198
  cardiac pacemaker T82.198

Twilight state
  epileptic F05
  psychogenic F44.89
Twin (newborn) —*see also* Newborn, twin
  conjoined Q89.4
  pregnancy —*see* Pregnancy, twin, conjoined
Twinning, teeth K00.2
Twist, twisted
  bowel, colon or intestine K56.2
  hair (congenital) Q84.1
  mesentery K56.2
  omentum K56.2
  organ or site, congenital NEC —*see* Anomaly,
    by site
  ovarian pedicle —*see* Torsion, ovary
Twitching R25.3
Tylosis (acquired) L84
  buccalis K13.29
  linguae K13.29
  palmaris et plantaris (congenital) (inherited)
    Q82.8
    acquired L85.1
Tympanism R14.0
Tympanites (abdominal) (intestinal) R14.0
Tympanitis —*see* Myringitis
Tympanosclerosis —*see* subcategory H74.0
Tympanum —*see* condition
Tympany
  abdomen R14.0
  chest R09.89
Type A behavior pattern Z73.1
Typhlitis —*see* Appendicitis
Typhoenteritis —*see* Typhoid
Typhoid (abortive) (ambulant) (any site)
    (clinical) (fever) (hemorrhagic) (infection)
    (intermittent) (malignant) (rheumatic)
    (Widal negative) A01.00
  with pneumonia A01.03
  abdominal A01.09
  arthritis A01.04
  carrier (suspected) of Z22.0
  cholecystitis (current) A01.09
  endocarditis A01.02
  heart involvement A01.02
  inoculation reaction —*see* Complications,
    vaccination
  meningitis A01.01
  mesenteric lymph nodes A01.09
  myocarditis A01.02
  osteomyelitis A01.05
  perichondritis, larynx A01.09
  pneumonia A01.03
  specified NEC A01.09
  spine A01.05
  ulcer (perforating) A01.09
Typhomalaria (fever) —*see* Malaria
Typhomania A01.00
Typhoperitonitis A01.09
Typhus (fever) A75.9
  abdominal, abdominalis —*see* Typhoid
  African tick A77.1
  amarillic A95.9
  brain A75.9 *[G94]*
  cerebral A75.9 *[G94]*
  classical A75.0
  due to Rickettsia
    prowazekii A75.0
      recrudescent A75.1
    tsutsugamushi A75.3
    typhi A75.2
  endemic (flea-borne) A75.2
  epidemic (louse-borne) A75.0
  exanthematic NEC A75.0
  exanthematicus SAI A75.0
    brillii SAI A75.1
    mexicanus SAI A75.2
    typhus murinus A75.2
  flea-borne A75.2
  India tick A77.1
  Kenya (tick) A77.1
  louse-borne A75.0

◀ New   ◀||| Revised   ~~deleted~~ Deleted

Typhus (Continued)
  Mexican A75.2
  mite-borne A75.3
  murine A75.2
  North Asian tick-borne A77.2
  petechial A75.9
  Queensland tick A77.3
  rat A75.2

Typhus (Continued)
  recrudescent A75.1
  recurrens —see Fever, relapsing
  Sao Paulo A77.0
  scrub (China) (India) (Malaysia) (New
    Guinea) A75.3
  shop (of Malaysia) A75.2
  Siberian tick A77.2

Typhus (Continued)
  tick-borne A77.9
  tropical (mite-borne) A75.3
Tyrosinemia E70.21
  newborn, transitory P74.5
Tyrosinosis E70.21
Tyrosinuria E70.29

U

Uhl's anomaly or disease Q24.8

Ulcer, ulcerated, ulcerating, ulceration, ulcerative
  alveolar process M27.3
  amebic (intestine) A06.1
    skin A06.7
  anastomotic —see Ulcer, gastrojejunal
  anorectal K62.6
  antral —see Ulcer, stomach
  anus (sphincter) (solitary) K62.6
  aorta —see Aneurysm
  aphthous (oral) (recurrent) K12.0
    genital organ (s)
      female N76.6
      male N50.8
  artery I77.2
  atrophic —see Ulcer, skin
    decubitus —see Ulcer, pressure, by site
  back L98.429
    with
      bone necrosis L98.424
      exposed fat layer L98.422
      muscle necrosis L98.423
      skin breakdown only L98.421
  Barrett's (esophagus) K22.10
    with bleeding K22.11
  bile duct (common) (hepatic) K83.8
  bladder (solitary) (sphincter) NEC N32.89
    bilharzial B65.9 [N33]
    in schistosomiasis (bilharzial) B65.9 [N33]
    submucosal —see Cystitis, interstitial
    tuberculous A18.12
  bleeding K27.4
  bone —see Osteomyelitis, specified type NEC
  bowel —see Ulcer, intestine
  breast N61
  bronchus J98.09
  buccal (cavity) (traumatic) K12.1
  Buruli A31.1
  buttock L98.419
    with
      bone necrosis L98.414
      exposed fat layer L98.412
      muscle necrosis L98.413
      skin breakdown only L98.411
  cancerous —see Neoplasm, malignant, by site
  cardia K22.10
    with bleeding K22.11
  cardioesophageal (peptic) K22.10
    with bleeding K22.11
  cecum —see Ulcer, intestine
  cervix (uteri) (decubitus) (trophic) N86
    with cervicitis N72
  chancroidal A57
  chiclero B55.1
  chronic (cause unknown) —see Ulcer, skin
  Cochin-China B55.1
  colon —see Ulcer, intestine
  conjunctiva H10.89
  cornea H16.00-
    with hypopyon H16.03-
    central H16.01-
    dendritic (herpes simplex) B00.52
    marginal H16.04-
    Mooren's H16.05-
    mycotic H16.06-
    perforated H16.07-
    ring H16.02-
    tuberculous (phlyctenular) A18.52
  corpus cavernosum (chronic) N48.5
  crural —see Ulcer, lower limb
  Curling's —see Ulcer, peptic, acute
  Cushing's —see Ulcer, peptic, acute
  cystic duct K82.8
  cystitis (interstitial) —see Cystitis, interstitial
  decubitus —see Ulcer, pressure, by site
  dendritic, cornea (herpes simplex) B00.52
  diabetes, diabetic —see Diabetes, ulcer
  Dieulafoy's K25.0

Ulcer, ulcerated, ulcerating, ulceration, ulcerative (Continued)
  due to
    infection NEC —see Ulcer, skin
    radiation NEC L59.8
    trophic disturbance (any region) —see Ulcer, skin
    X-ray L58.1
  duodenum, duodenal (eroded) (peptic) K26.9
    with
      hemorrhage K26.4
        and perforation K26.6
      perforation K26.5
    acute K26.3
      with
        hemorrhage K26.0
          and perforation K26.2
        perforation K26.1
    chronic K26.7
      with
        hemorrhage K26.4
          and perforation K26.6
        perforation K26.5
  dysenteric A09
  elusive —see Cystitis, interstitial
  endocarditis (acute) (chronic) (subacute) I28.8
  epiglottis J38.7
  esophagus (peptic) K22.10
    with bleeding K22.11
    due to
      aspirin K22.10
        with bleeding K22.11
      gastrointestinal reflux disease K21.0
      ingestion of chemical or medicament K22.10
        with bleeding K22.11
    fungal K22.10
      with bleeding K22.11
    infective K22.10
      with bleeding K22.11
    varicose —see Varix, esophagus
  eyelid (region) H01.8
  fauces J39.2
  Fenwick (-Hunner) (solitary) —see Cystitis, interstitial
  fistulous —see Ulcer, skin
  foot (indolent) (trophic) —see Ulcer, lower limb
  frambesial, initial A66.0
  frenum (tongue) K14.0
  gallbladder or duct K82.8
  gangrenous —see Gangrene
  gastric —see Ulcer, stomach
  gastrocolic —see Ulcer, gastrojejunal
  gastroduodenal —see Ulcer, peptic
  gastroesophageal —see Ulcer, stomach
  gastrointestinal —see Ulcer, gastrojejunal
  gastrojejunal (peptic) K28.9
    with
      hemorrhage K28.4
        and perforation K28.6
      perforation K28.5
    acute K28.3
      with
        hemorrhage K28.0
          and perforation K28.2
        perforation K28.1
    chronic K28.7
      with
        hemorrhage K28.4
          and perforation K28.6
        perforation K28.5
  gastrojejunocolic —see Ulcer, gastrojejunal
  gingiva K06.8
  gingivitis K05.10
    nonplaque induced K05.11
    plaque induced K05.10
  glottis J38.7
  granuloma of pudenda A58
  gum K06.8
  gumma, due to yaws A66.4

Ulcer, ulcerated, ulcerating, ulceration, ulcerative (Continued)
  heel —see Ulcer, lower limb
  hemorrhoid (see also Hemorrhoids, by degree) K64.8
  Hunner's —see Cystitis, interstitial
  hypopharynx J39.2
  hypopyon (chronic) (subacute) —see Ulcer, cornea, with hypopyon
  hypostaticum —see Ulcer, varicose
  ileum —see Ulcer, intestine
  intestine, intestinal K63.3
    with perforation K63.1
    amebic A06.1
    duodenal —see Ulcer, duodenum
    granulocytopenic (with hemorrhage) —see Neutropenia
    marginal —see Ulcer, gastrojejunal
    perforating K63.1
      newborn P78.0
    primary, small intestine K63.3
    rectum K62.6
    stercoraceous, stercoral K63.3
    tuberculous A18.32
    typhoid (fever) —see Typhoid
    varicose I86.8
  jejunum, jejunal —see Ulcer, gastrojejunal
  keratitis —see Ulcer, cornea
  knee —see Ulcer, lower limb
  labium (majus) (minus) N76.6
  laryngitis —see Laryngitis
  larynx (aphthous) (contact) J38.7
    diphtheritic A36.2
  leg —see Ulcer, lower limb
  lip K13.0
  Lipschütz's N76.6
  lower limb (atrophic) (chronic) (neurogenic) (perforating) (pyogenic) (trophic) (tropical) L97.909
    with
      bone necrosis L97.904
      exposed fat layer L97.902
      muscle necrosis L97.903
      skin breakdown only L97.901
    ankle L97.309
      with
        bone necrosis L97.304
        exposed fat layer L97.302
        muscle necrosis L97.303
        skin breakdown only L97.301
      left L97.329
        with
          bone necrosis L97.324
          exposed fat layer L97.322
          muscle necrosis L97.323
          skin breakdown only L97.321
      right L97.319
        with
          bone necrosis L97.314
          exposed fat layer L97.312
          muscle necrosis L97.313
          skin breakdown only L97.311
    calf L97.209
      with
        bone necrosis L97.204
        exposed fat layer L97.202
        muscle necrosis L97.203
        skin breakdown only L97.201
      left L97.229
        with
          bone necrosis L97.224
          exposed fat layer L97.222
          muscle necrosis L97.223
          skin breakdown only L97.221
      right L97.219
        with
          bone necrosis L97.214
          exposed fat layer L97.212
          muscle necrosis L97.213
          skin breakdown only L97.211
    decubitus —see Ulcer, pressure, by site

◀ New   ◀◀ Revised   ~~deleted~~ Deleted

Ulcer, ulcerated, ulcerating, ulceration, ulcerative *(Continued)*
  lower limb *(Continued)*
    foot specified NEC L97.509
      with
        bone necrosis L97.504
        exposed fat layer L97.502
        muscle necrosis L97.503
        skin breakdown only L97.501
      left L97.529
        with
          bone necrosis L97.524
          exposed fat layer L97.522
          muscle necrosis L97.523
          skin breakdown only L97.521
      right L97.519
        with
          bone necrosis L97.514
          exposed fat layer L97.512
          muscle necrosis L97.513
          skin breakdown only L97.511
    heel L97.409
      with
        bone necrosis L97.404
        exposed fat layer L97.402
        muscle necrosis L97.403
        skin breakdown only L97.401
      left L97.429
        with
          bone necrosis L97.424
          exposed fat layer L97.422
          muscle necrosis L97.423
          skin breakdown only L97.421
      right L97.419
        with
          bone necrosis L97.414
          exposed fat layer L97.412
          muscle necrosis L97.413
          skin breakdown only L97.411
    left L97.929
      with
        bone necrosis L97.924
        exposed fat layer L97.922
        muscle necrosis L97.923
        skin breakdown only L97.921
    lower leg NOS L97.909
      with
        bone necrosis L97.904
        exposed fat layer L97.902
        muscle necrosis L97.903
        skin breakdown only L97.901
      left L97.929
        with
          bone necrosis L97.924
          exposed fat layer L97.922
          muscle necrosis L97.923
          skin breakdown only L97.921
      right L97.919
        with
          bone necrosis L97.914
          exposed fat layer L97.912
          muscle necrosis L97.913
          skin breakdown only L97.911
    specified site NEC L97.809
      with
        bone necrosis L97.804
        exposed fat layer L97.802
        muscle necrosis L97.803
        skin breakdown only L97.801
      left L97.829
        with
          bone necrosis L97.824
          exposed fat layer L97.822
          muscle necrosis L97.823
          skin breakdown only L97.821
      right L97.819
        with
          bone necrosis L97.814
          exposed fat layer L97.812
          muscle necrosis L97.813
          skin breakdown only L97.811

Ulcer, ulcerated, ulcerating, ulceration, ulcerative *(Continued)*
  lower limb *(Continued)*
    midfoot L97.409
      with
        bone necrosis L97.404
        exposed fat layer L97.402
        muscle necrosis L97.403
        skin breakdown only L97.401
      left L97.429
        with
          bone necrosis L97.424
          exposed fat layer L97.422
          muscle necrosis L97.423
          skin breakdown only L97.421
      right L97.419
        with
          bone necrosis L97.414
          exposed fat layer L97.412
          muscle necrosis L97.413
          skin breakdown only L97.411
    right L97.919
      with
        bone necrosis L97.914
        exposed fat layer L97.912
        muscle necrosis L97.913
        skin breakdown only L97.911
    thigh L97.109
      with
        bone necrosis L97.104
        exposed fat layer L97.102
        muscle necrosis L97.103
        skin breakdown only L97.101
      left L97.129
        with
          bone necrosis L97.124
          exposed fat layer L97.122
          muscle necrosis L97.123
          skin breakdown only L97.121
      right L97.119
        with
          bone necrosis L97.114
          exposed fat layer L97.112
          muscle necrosis L97.113
          skin breakdown only L97.111
    toe L97.509
      with
        bone necrosis L97.504
        exposed fat layer L97.502
        muscle necrosis L97.503
        skin breakdown only L97.501
      left L97.529
        with
          bone necrosis L97.524
          exposed fat layer L97.522
          muscle necrosis L97.523
          skin breakdown only L97.521
      right L97.519
        with
          bone necrosis L97.514
          exposed fat layer L97.512
          muscle necrosis L97.513
          skin breakdown only L97.511
  leprous A30.1
  syphilitic A52.19
  varicose —*see* Varix, leg, with, ulcer
  luetic —*see* Ulcer, syphilitic
  lung J98.4
    tuberculous —*see* Tuberculosis, pulmonary
  malignant —*see* Neoplasm, malignant, by site
  marginal NEC —*see* Ulcer, gastrojejunal
  meatus (urinarius) N34.2
  Meckel's diverticulum Q43.0
    malignant —*see* Table of Neoplasms, small intestine, malignant
  Meleney's (chronic undermining) —*see* Ulcer, skin
  Mooren's (cornea) —*see* Ulcer, cornea, Mooren's
  mycobacterial (skin) A31.1
  nasopharynx J39.2

Ulcer, ulcerated, ulcerating, ulceration, ulcerative *(Continued)*
  neck, uterus N86
  neurogenic NEC —*see* Ulcer, skin
  nose, nasal (passage) (infective) (septum) J34.0
    skin —*see* Ulcer, skin
    spirochetal A69.8
    varicose (bleeding) I86.8
  oral mucosa (traumatic) K12.1
  palate (soft) K12.1
  penis (chronic) N48.5
  peptic (site unspecified) K27.9
    with
      hemorrhage K27.4
        and perforation K27.6
      perforation K27.5
    acute K27.3
      with
        hemorrhage K27.0
          and perforation K27.2
        perforation K27.1
    chronic K27.7
      with
        hemorrhage K27.4
          and perforation K27.6
        perforation K27.5
    esophagus K22.10
      with bleeding K22.11
    newborn P78.82
  perforating K27.5
    skin —*see* Ulcer, skin
  peritonsillar J35.8
  phagedenic (tropical) —*see* Ulcer, skin
  pharynx J39.2
  phlebitis —*see* Phlebitis
  plaster —*see* Ulcer, pressure, by site
  popliteal space —*see* Ulcer, lower limb
  postpyloric —*see* Ulcer, duodenum
  prepuce N47.7
  prepyloric —*see* Ulcer, stomach
  pressure (pressure area) L89.9-
    ankle L89.5-
    back L89.1-
    buttock L89.3-
    coccyx L89.15-
    contiguous site of back, buttock, hip L89.4-
    elbow L89.0-
    face L89.81-
    head L89.81-
    heel L89.6-
    hip L89.2-
    sacral region (tailbone) L89.15-
    specified site NEC L89.89-
    stage 1 (healing) (pre-ulcer skin changes limited to persistent focal edema)
      ankle L89.5-
      back L89.1-
      buttock L89.3-
      coccyx L89.15-
      contiguous site of back, buttock, hip L89.4-
      elbow L89.0-
      face L89.81-
      head L89.81-
      heel L89.6-
      hip L89.2-
      sacral region (tailbone) L89.15-
      specified site NEC L89.89-
    stage 2 (healing) (abrasion, blister, partial thickness skin loss involving epidermis and/or dermis)
      ankle L89.5-
      back L89.1-
      buttock L89.3-
      coccyx L89.15-
      contiguous site of back, buttock, hip L89.4-
      elbow L89.0-
      face L89.81-
      head L89.81-

Ulcer, ulcerated, ulcerating, ulceration, ulcerative (Continued)
pressure (Continued)
  stage 2 (Continued)
    heel L89.6-
    hip L89.2-
    sacral region (tailbone) L89.15-
    specified site NEC L89.89-
  stage 3 (healing) (full thickness skin loss involving damage or necrosis of subcutaneous tissue)
    ankle L89.5-
    back L89.1-
    buttock L89.3-
    coccyx L89.15-
    contiguous site of back, buttock, hip L89.4-
    elbow L89.0-
    face L89.81-
    head L89.81-
    heel L89.6-
    hip L89.2-
    sacral region (tailbone) L89.15-
    specified site NEC L89.89-
  stage 4 (healing) (necrosis of soft tissues through to underlying muscle, tendon, or bone)
    ankle L89.5-
    back L89.1-
    buttock L89.3-
    coccyx L89.15-
    contiguous site of back, buttock, hip L89.4-
    elbow L89.0-
    face L89.81-
    head L89.81-
    heel L89.6-
    hip L89.2-
    sacral region (tailbone) L89.15-
    specified site NEC L89.89-
  unspecified stage
    ankle L89.5-
    back L89.1-
    buttock L89.3-
    coccyx L89.15-
    contiguous site of back, buttock, hip L89.4-
    elbow L89.0-
    face L89.81-
    head L89.81-
    heel L89.6-
    hip L89.2-
    sacral region (tailbone) L89.15-
    specified site NEC L89.89-
  unstageable
    ankle L89.5-
    back L89.1-
    buttock L89.3-
    coccyx L89.15-
    contiguous site of back, buttock, hip L89.4-
    elbow L89.0-
    face L89.81-
    head L89.81-
    heel L89.6-
    hip L89.2-
    sacral region (tailbone) L89.15-
    specified site NEC L89.89-
primary of intestine K63.3
  with perforation K63.1
prostate N41.9
pyloric —see Ulcer, stomach
rectosigmoid K63.3
  with perforation K63.1
rectum (sphincter) (solitary) K62.6
  stercoraceous, stercoral K62.6
retina —see Inflammation, chorioretinal
rodent —see also Neoplasm, skin, malignant
sclera —see Scleritis
scrofulous (tuberculous) A18.2

Ulcer, ulcerated, ulcerating, ulceration, ulcerative (Continued)
scrotum N50.8
  tuberculous A18.15
  varicose I86.1
seminal vesicle N50.8
sigmoid —see Ulcer, intestine
skin (atrophic) (chronic) (neurogenic) (non-healing) (perforating) (pyogenic) (trophic) (tropical) L98.499
  with gangrene —see Gangrene
  amebic A06.7
  back —see Ulcer, back
  buttock —see Ulcer, buttock
  decubitus —see Ulcer, pressure
  lower limb —see Ulcer, lower limb
  mycobacterial A31.1
  specified site NEC L98.499
    with
      bone necrosis L98.494
      exposed fat layer L98.492
      muscle necrosis L98.493
      skin breakdown only L98.491
  tuberculous (primary) A18.4
  varicose —see Ulcer, varicose
sloughing —see Ulcer, skin
solitary, anus or rectum (sphincter) K62.6
sore throat J02.9
  streptococcal J02.0
spermatic cord N50.8
spine (tuberculous) A18.01
stasis (venous) —see Varix, leg, with, ulcer
  without varicose veins I87.2
stercoraceous, stercoral K63.3
  with perforation K63.1
  anus or rectum K62.6
stoma, stomal —see Ulcer, gastrojejunal
stomach (eroded) (peptic) (round) K25.9
  with
    hemorrhage K25.4
      and perforation K25.6
    perforation K25.5
  acute K25.3
    with
      hemorrhage K25.0
        and perforation K25.2
      perforation K25.1
  chronic K25.7
    with
      hemorrhage K25.4
        and perforation K25.6
      perforation K25.5
stomal —see Ulcer, gastrojejunal
stomatitis K12.1
stress —see Ulcer, peptic
strumous (tuberculous) A18.2
submucosal, bladder —see Cystitis, interstitial
syphilitic (any site) (early) (secondary) A51.39
  late A52.79
  perforating A52.79
    foot A52.11
testis N50.8
thigh —see Ulcer, lower limb
throat J39.2
  diphtheritic A36.0
toe —see Ulcer, lower limb
tongue (traumatic) K14.0
tonsil J35.8
  diphtheritic A36.0
trachea J39.8
trophic —see Ulcer, skin
tropical —see Ulcer, skin
tuberculous —see Tuberculosis, ulcer
tunica vaginalis N50.8
turbinate J34.89
typhoid (perforating) —see Typhoid

Ulcer, ulcerated, ulcerating, ulceration, ulcerative (Continued)
unspecified site —see Ulcer, skin
urethra (meatus) —see Urethritis
uterus N85.8
  cervix N86
    with cervicitis N72
  neck N86
    with cervicitis N72
vagina N76.5
  in Behçet's disease M35.2 [N77.0]
  pessary N89.8
valve, heart I33.0
varicose (lower limb, any part) —see also Varix, leg, with, ulcer
  broad ligament I86.2
  esophagus —see Varix, esophagus
  inflamed or infected —see Varix, leg, with ulcer, with inflammation
  nasal septum I86.8
  perineum I86.3
  scrotum I86.1
  specified site NEC I86.8
  sublingual I86.0
  vulva I86.3
vas deferens N50.8
vulva (acute) (infectional) N76.6
  in (due to)
    Behçet's disease M35.2 [N77.0]
    herpesviral (herpes simplex) infection A60.04
    tuberculosis A18.18
vulvobuccal, recurring N76.6
X-ray L58.1
yaws A66.4
Ulcerosa scarlatina A38.8
Ulcus —see also Ulcer
cutis tuberculosum A18.4
duodeni —see Ulcer, duodenum
durum (syphilitic) A51.0
  extragenital A51.2
gastrojejunale —see Ulcer, gastrojejunal
hypostaticum —see Ulcer, varicose
molle (cutis) (skin) A57
serpens corneae —see Ulcer, cornea, central
ventriculi —see Ulcer, stomach
Ulegyria Q04.8
Ulerythema
ophryogenes, congenital Q84.2
sycosiforme L73.8
Ullrich(-Bonnevie)(-Turner) syndrome Q87.1
Ullrich-Feichtiger syndrome Q87.0
Ulnar —see condition
Ulorrhagia, ulorrhea K06.8
Umbilicus, umbilical —see condition
Unacceptable
contours of tooth K08.54
morphology of tooth K08.54
Unavailability (of)
bed at medical facility Z75.1
health service-related agencies Z75.4
medical facilities (at) Z75.3
  due to
    investigation by social service agency Z75.2
    lack of services at home Z75.0
    remoteness from facility Z75.3
      waiting list Z75.1
  home Z75.0
  outpatient clinic Z75.3
schooling Z55.1
social service agencies Z75.4
Uncinaria americana infestation B76.1
Uncinariasis B76.9
Uncongenial work Z56.5
Unconscious (ness) —see Coma
Underachievement in school Z55.3
Underdevelopment —see also Undeveloped
nose Q30.1
sexual E30.0

◀ New   ◀‖‖ Revised   ~~deleted~~ Deleted

Underdosing (see also Table of Drugs and Chemicals, categories T36-T50, with final character 6) Z91.14 ◄▥
  intentional NEC Z91.128
    due to financial hardship of patient Z91.120
  unintentional NEC Z91.138
    due to patient's age related debility Z91.130
Underfeeding, newborn P92.3
Underfill, endodontic M27.53
Underimmunization status Z28.3
Undernourishment —see Malnutrition
Undernutrition —see Malnutrition
Under observation —see Observation
Underweight R63.6
  for gestational age —see Light for dates
Underwood's disease P83.0
Undescended —see also Malposition, congenital
  cecum Q43.3
  colon Q43.3
  testicle —see Cryptorchid
Undeveloped, undevelopment —see also Hypoplasia
  brain (congenital) Q02
  cerebral (congenital) Q02
  heart Q24.8
  lung Q33.6
  testis E29.1
  uterus E30.0
Undiagnosed (disease) R69
Undulant fever —see Brucellosis
Unemployment, anxiety concerning Z56.0
  threatened Z56.2
Unequal length (acquired) (limb) —see also Deformity, limb, unequal length
  leg —see also Deformity, limb, unequal length
    congenital Q72.9-
Unextracted dental root K08.3
Unguis incarnatus L60.0
Unhappiness R45.2
Unicornate uterus Q51.4
Unilateral —see also condition
  development, breast N64.89
  organ or site, congenital NEC —see Agenesis, by site
Unilocular heart Q20.8
Union, abnormal —see also Fusion
  larynx and trachea Q34.8
Universal mesentery Q43.3
Unrepairable overhanging of dental restorative materials K08.52
Unsatisfactory
  restoration of tooth K08.50
    specified NEC K08.59
  sample of cytologic smear
    anus R85.615
    cervix R87.615
    vagina R87.625
  surroundings Z59.1
  work Z56.5
Unsoundness of mind —see Psychosis
Unstable
  back NEC —see Instability, joint, spine
  hip (congenital) Q65.6
    acquired —see Derangement, joint, specified type NEC, hip
  joint —see Instability, joint
    secondary to removal of joint prosthesis M96.89
  lie (mother) O32.0
  lumbosacral joint (congenital)
    acquired —see subcategory M53.2
  sacroiliac —see subcategory M53.2
  spine NEC —see Instability, joint, spine
Unsteadiness on feet R26.81
Untruthfulness, child problem F91.8
Unverricht(-Lundborg) disease or epilepsy — see Epilepsy, generalized, idiopathic
Unwanted pregnancy Z64.0

Upbringing, institutional Z62.22
  away from parents NEC Z62.29
  in care of non-parental family member Z62.21
  in foster care Z62.21
  in orphanage or group home Z62.22
  in welfare custody Z62.21
Upper respiratory —see condition
Upset
  gastric K30
  gastrointestinal K30
    psychogenic F45.8
  intestinal (large) (small) K59.9
    psychogenic F45.8
  menstruation N93.9
  mental F48.9
  stomach K30
    psychogenic F45.8
Urachus —see also condition
  patent or persistent Q64.4
Urbach-Oppenheim disease (necrobiosis lipoidica diabeticorum) —see E08-E13 with .620
Urbach's lipoid proteinosis E78.89
Urbach-Wiethe disease E78.89
Urban yellow fever A95.1
Urea
  blood, high —see Uremia
  cycle metabolism disorder —see Disorder, urea cycle metabolism
Uremia, uremic N19
  with
    ectopic or molar pregnancy O08.4
    polyneuropathy N18.9 [G63]
  chronic (see also Disease, kidney, chronic) N18.9
    due to hypertension —see Hypertensive, kidney
  complicating
    ectopic or molar pregnancy O08.4
  congenital P96.0
  extrarenal R39.2
  following ectopic or molar pregnancy O08.4
  newborn P96.0
  prerenal R39.2
Ureter, ureteral —see condition
Ureteralgia N23
Ureterectasis —see Hydroureter
Ureteritis N28.89
  cystica N28.86
  due to calculus N20.1
    with calculus, kidney N20.2
      with hydronephrosis N13.2
  gonococcal (acute) (chronic) A54.21
  nonspecific N28.89
Ureterocele N28.89
  congenital (orthotopic) Q62.31
  ectopic Q62.32
Ureterolith, ureterolithiasis —see Calculus, ureter
Ureterostomy
  attention to Z43.6
  status Z93.6
Urethra, urethral —see condition
Urethralgia R39.89
Urethritis (anterior) (posterior) N34.2
  calculous N21.1
  candidal B37.41
  chlamydial A56.01
  diplococcal (gonococcal) A54.01
    with abscess (accessory gland) (periurethral) A54.1
  gonococcal A54.01
    with abscess (accessory gland) (periurethral) A54.1
  nongonococcal N34.1
    Reiter's —see Reiter's disease
  nonspecific N34.1
  nonvenereal N34.1
  postmenopausal N34.2
  puerperal O86.22 ◄▥
  Reiter's —see Reiter's disease

Urethritis (Continued)
  specified NEC N34.2
  trichomonal or due to Trichomonas (vaginalis) A59.03
Urethrocele N81.0
  with
    cystocele —see Cystocele
    prolapse of uterus —see Prolapse, uterus
Urethrolithiasis (with colic or infection) N21.1
Urethrorectal —see condition
Urethrorrhagia N36.8
Urethrorrhea R36.9
Urethrostomy
  attention to Z43.6
  status Z93.6
Urethrotrigonitis —see Trigonitis
Urethrovaginal —see condition
Urgency
  fecal R15.2
  hypertension —see Hypertension
  urinary N39.41
Urhidrosis, uridrosis L74.8
Uric acid in blood (increased) E79.0
Uricacidemia (asymptomatic) E79.0
Uricemia (asymptomatic) E79.0
Uricosuria R82.99
Urinary —see condition
Urination
  frequent R35.0
  painful R30.9
Urine
  blood in —see Hematuria
  discharge, excessive R35.8
  enuresis, nonorganic origin F98.0
  extravasation R39.0
  frequency R35.0
  incontinence R32
    nonorganic origin F98.0
  intermittent stream R39.19
  pus in N39.0
  retention or stasis R33.9
    organic R33.8
      drug-induced R33.0
    psychogenic F45.8
  secretion
    deficient R34
    excessive R35.8
    frequency R35.0
  stream
    intermittent R39.19
    slowing R39.19
    splitting R39.13
    weak R39.12
Urinemia —see Uremia
Urinoma, urethra N36.8
Uroarthritis, infectious (Reiter's) —see Reiter's disease
Urodialysis R34
Urolithiasis —see Calculus, urinary
Uronephrosis —see Hydronephrosis
Uropathy N39.9
  obstructive N13.9
    specified NEC N13.8
  reflux N13.9
    specified NEC N13.8
  vesicoureteral reflux-associated —see Reflux, vesicoureteral
Urosepsis — code to condition
Urticaria L50.9
  with angioneurotic edema T78.3
    hereditary D84.1
  allergic L50.0
  cholinergic L50.5
  chronic L50.8
  cold, familial L50.2
  contact L50.6
  dermatographic L50.3
  due to
    cold or heat L50.2
    drugs L50.0
    food L50.0

Urticaria (Continued)
   due to (Continued)
      inhalants L50.0
      plants L50.6
      serum (see also Reaction, serum) T80.69
   factitial L50.3
   giant T78.3
      hereditary D84.1
   gigantea T78.3
   idiopathic L50.1
   larynx T78.3
      hereditary D84.1
   neonatorum P83.8
   nonallergic L50.1
   papulosa (Hebra) L28.2
   pigmentosa Q82.2
   recurrent periodic L50.8
   serum (see also Reaction, serum) T80.69
   solar L56.3
   specified type NEC L50.8
   thermal (cold) (heat) L50.2
   vibratory L50.4
   xanthelasmoidea Q82.2
Use (of)
   alcohol F10.99
      with sleep disorder F10.982
      harmful —see Abuse, alcohol
   amphetamines —see Use, stimulant NEC
   caffeine —see Use, stimulant NEC
   cannabis F12.90
      with
         anxiety disorder F12.980
         intoxication F12.929
            with
               delirium F12.921
               perceptual disturbance F12.922
            uncomplicated F12.920
         other specified disorder F12.988
         psychosis F12.959
            delusions F12.950
            hallucinations F12.951
         unspecified disorder F12.99
   cocaine F14.90
      with
         anxiety disorder F14.980
         intoxication F14.929
            with
               delirium F14.921
               perceptual disturbance F14.922
            uncomplicated F14.920
         other specified disorder F14.988
         psychosis F14.959
            delusions F14.950
            hallucinations F14.951
         sexual dysfunction F14.981
         sleep disorder F14.982
         unspecified disorder F14.99
      harmful —see Abuse, drug, cocaine
   drug (s) NEC F19.90
      with sleep disorder F19.982
      harmful —see Abuse, drug, by type
   hallucinogen NEC F16.90
      with
         anxiety disorder F16.980
         intoxication F16.929
            with
               delirium F16.921
            uncomplicated F16.920
         mood disorder F16.94
         other specified disorder F16.988
         perception disorder (flashbacks)
               F16.983

Use (Continued)
   hallucinogen NEC (Continued)
      with (Continued)
         psychosis F16.959
            delusions F16.950
            hallucinations F16.951
         unspecified disorder F16.99
      harmful —see Abuse, drug, hallucinogen
            NEC
   inhalants F18.90
      with
         anxiety disorder F18.980
         intoxication F18.929
            with delirium F18.921
            uncomplicated F18.920
         mood disorder F18.94
         other specified disorder F18.988
         persisting dementia F18.97
         psychosis F18.959
            delusions F18.950
            hallucinations F18.951
         unspecified disorder F18.99
      harmful —see Abuse, drug, inhalant
   methadone F11.20
   nonprescribed drugs F19.90
      harmful —see Abuse, non-psychoactive
            substance
   opioid F11.90
      with
         disorder F11.99
            mood F11.94
            sleep F11.982
            specified type NEC F11.988
         intoxication F11.929
            with
               delirium F11.921
               perceptual disturbance
                     F11.922
            uncomplicated F11.920
         withdrawal F11.93
      harmful —see Abuse, drug, opioid
   patent medicines F19.90
      harmful —see Abuse, non-psychoactive
            substance
   psychoactive drug NEC F19.90
      with
         anxiety disorder F19.980
         intoxication F19.929
            with
               delirium F19.921
               perceptual disturbance
                     F19.922
            uncomplicated F19.920
         mood disorder F19.94
         other specified disorder F19.988
         persisting
            amnestic disorder F19.96
            dementia F19.97
         psychosis F19.959
            delusions F19.950
            hallucinations F19.951
         sexual dysfunction F19.981
         sleep disorder F19.982
         unspecified disorder F19.99
         withdrawal F19.939
            with
               delirium F19.931
               perceptual disturbance
                     F19.932
            uncomplicated F19.930
      harmful —see Abuse, drug NEC,
            psychoactive NEC

Use (Continued)
   sedative, hypnotic, or anxiolytic F13.90
      with
         anxiety disorder F13.980
         intoxication F13.929
            with
               delirium F13.921
            uncomplicated F13.920
         other specified disorder F13.988
         persisting
            amnestic disorder F13.96
            dementia F13.97
         psychosis F13.959
            delusions F13.950
            hallucinations F13.951
         sexual dysfunction F13.981
         sleep disorder F13.982
         unspecified disorder F13.99
      harmful —see Abuse, drug, sedative,
            hypnotic, or anxiolytic
   stimulant NEC F15.90
      with
         anxiety disorder F15.980
         intoxication F15.929
            with
               delirium F15.921
               perceptual disturbance F15.922
            uncomplicated F15.920
         mood disorder F15.94
         other specified disorder F15.988
         psychosis F15.959
            delusions F15.950
            hallucinations F15.951
         sexual dysfunction F15.981
         sleep disorder F15.982
         unspecified disorder F15.99
         withdrawal F15.93
      harmful —see Abuse, drug, stimulant NEC
   tobacco Z72.0
      with dependence —see Dependence, drug,
            nicotine
   volatile solvents (see also Use, inhalant) F18.90
      harmful —see Abuse, drug, inhalant
Usher-Senear disease or syndrome L10.4
Uta B55.1
Uteromegaly N85.2
Uterovaginal —see condition
Uterovesical —see condition
Uveal —see condition
Uveitis (anterior) —see also Iridocyclitis
   acute —see Iridocyclitis, acute
   chronic —see Iridocyclitis, chronic
   due to toxoplasmosis (acquired) B58.09
      congenital P37.1
   granulomatous —see Iridocyclitis, chronic
   heterochromic —see Cyclitis, Fuchs'
         heterochromic
   lens-induced —see Iridocyclitis, lens-induced
   posterior —see Chorioretinitis
   sympathetic H44.13-
   syphilitic (secondary) A51.43
      congenital (early) A50.01
      late A52.71
   tuberculous A18.54
Uveoencephalitis —see Inflammation,
      chorioretinal
Uveokeratitis —see Iridocyclitis
Uveoparotitis D86.89
Uvula —see condition
Uvulitis (acute) (catarrhal) (chronic)
      (membranous) (suppurative) (ulcerative)
      K12.2

◀ New   ◀▥▥ Revised   ~~deleted~~ Deleted

V

Vaccination (prophylactic)
  complication or reaction —see Complications, vaccination
  delayed Z28.9
  encounter for Z23
  not done —see Immunization, not done, because (of)
Vaccinia (generalized) (localized) T88.1
  without vaccination B08.011
  congenital P35.8
Vacuum, in sinus (accessory) (nasal) J34.89
Vagabond, vagabondage Z59.0
Vagabond's disease B85.1
Vagina, vaginal —see condition
Vaginalitis (tunica) (testis) N49.1
Vaginismus (reflex) N94.2
  functional F52.5
  nonorganic F52.5
  psychogenic F52.5
  secondary N94.2
Vaginitis (acute) (circumscribed) (diffuse) (emphysematous) (nonvenereal) (ulcerative) N76.0
  with ectopic or molar pregnancy O08.0
  amebic A06.82
  atrophic, postmenopausal N95.2
  bacterial N76.0
  blennorrhagic (gonococcal) A54.02
  candidal B37.3
  chlamydial A56.02
  chronic N76.1
  due to Trichomonas (vaginalis) A59.01
  following ectopic or molar pregnancy O08.0
  gonococcal A54.02
    with abscess (accessory gland) (periurethral) A54.1
  granuloma A58
  in (due to)
    candidiasis B37.3
    herpesviral (herpes simplex) infection A60.04
    pinworm infection B80 [N77.1]
  monilial B37.3
  mycotic (candidal) B37.3
  postmenopausal atrophic N95.2
  puerperal (postpartum) O86.13
  senile (atrophic) N95.2
  subacute or chronic N76.1
  syphilitic (early) A51.0
    late A52.76
  trichomonal A59.01
  tuberculous A18.18
Vaginosis —see Vaginitis
Vagotonia G52.2
Vagrancy Z59.0
VAIN —see Neoplasia, intraepithelial, vagina
Vallecula —see condition
Valley fever B38.0
Valsuani's disease —see Anemia, obstetric
Valve, valvular (formation) —see also condition
  cerebral ventricle (communicating) in situ Z98.2
  cervix, internal os Q51.828
  congenital NEC —see Atresia, by site
  ureter (pelvic junction) (vesical orifice) Q62.39
  urethra (congenital) (posterior) Q64.2
Valvulitis (chronic) —see Endocarditis
Valvulopathy —see Endocarditis
Van Bogaert's leukoencephalopathy (sclerosing) (subacute) A81.1
Van Bogaert-Scherer-Epstein disease or syndrome E75.5
Van Buchem's syndrome M85.2
Van Creveld-von Gierke disease E74.01
Van der Hoeve (-de Kleyn) syndrome Q78.0
Van der Woude's syndrome Q38.0
Van Neck's disease or osteochondrosis M91.0
Vanishing lung J44.9

Vapor asphyxia or suffocation T59.9
  specified agent —see Table of Drugs and Chemicals ◀▥
Variance, lethal ball, prosthetic heart valve T82.09
Variants, thalassemic D56.8
Variations in hair color L67.1
Varicella B01.9
  with
    complications NEC B01.89
    encephalitis B01.11
    encephalomyelitis B01.11
    meningitis B01.0
    myelitis B01.12
    pneumonia B01.2
  congenital P35.8
Varices —see Varix
Varicocele (scrotum) (thrombosed) I86.1
  ovary I86.2
  perineum I86.3
  spermatic cord (ulcerated) I86.1
Varicose
  aneurysm (ruptured) I77.0
  dermatitis —see Varix, leg, with, inflammation
  eczema —see Varix, leg, with, inflammation
  phlebitis —see Varix, with, inflammation
  tumor —see Varix
  ulcer (lower limb, any part) —see also Varix, leg, with, ulcer
    anus (see also Hemorrhoids) K64.8
    esophagus —see Varix, esophagus
    inflamed or infected —see Varix, leg, with ulcer, with inflammation
    nasal septum I86.8
    perineum I86.3
    scrotum I86.1
    specified site NEC I86.8
  vein —see Varix
  vessel —see Varix, leg
Varicosis, varicosities, varicosity —see Varix
Variola (major) (minor) B03
Varioloid B03
Varix (lower limb) (ruptured) I83.90
  with
    edema I83.899
    inflammation I83.10
      with ulcer (venous) I83.209
    pain I83.819
    specified complication NEC I83.899
    stasis dermatitis I83.10
      with ulcer (venous) I83.209
    swelling I83.899
    ulcer I83.009
      with inflammation I83.209
  aneurysmal I77.0
  asymptomatic I83.9-
  bladder I86.2
  broad ligament I86.2
  complicating
    childbirth (lower extremity) O87.4
      anus or rectum O87.2
      genital (vagina, vulva or perineum) O87.8
    pregnancy (lower extremity) O22.0-
      anus or rectum O22.4-
      genital (vagina, vulva or perineum) O22.1-
    puerperium (lower extremity) O87.4
      anus or rectum O87.2
      genital (vagina, vulva, perineum) O87.8
  congenital (any site) Q27.8
  esophagus (idiopathic) (primary) (ulcerated) I85.00
    bleeding I85.01
    congenital Q27.8
    in (due to)
      alcoholic liver disease I85.10
        bleeding I85.11
      cirrhosis of liver I85.10
        bleeding I85.11

Varix (Continued)
  esophagus (Continued)
    in (Continued)
      portal hypertension I85.10
        bleeding I85.11
      schistosomiasis I85.10
        bleeding I85.11
      toxic liver disease I85.10
        bleeding I85.11
    secondary I85.10
      bleeding I85.11
  gastric I86.4
  inflamed or infected I83.10
    ulcerated I83.209
  labia (majora) I86.3
  leg (asymptomatic) I83.90
    with
      edema I83.899
      inflammation I83.10
        with ulcer —see Varix, leg, with, ulcer, with inflammation by site
      pain I83.819
      specified complication NEC I83.899
      swelling I83.899
      ulcer I83.009
        with inflammation I83.209
        ankle I83.003
          with inflammation I83.203
        calf I83.002
          with inflammation I83.202
        foot NEC I83.005
          with inflammation I83.205
        heel I83.004
          with inflammation I83.204
        lower leg NEC I83.008
          with inflammation I83.208
        midfoot I83.004
          with inflammation I83.204
        thigh I83.001
          with inflammation I83.201
    bilateral (asymptomatic) I83.93
      with
        edema I83.893
        pain I83.813
        specified complication NEC I83.893
        swelling I83.893
        ulcer I83.009
          with inflammation I83.209
    left (asymptomatic) I83.92
      with
        edema I83.892
        inflammation I83.12
          with ulcer —see Varix, leg, with, ulcer, with inflammation by site
        pain I83.812
        specified complication NEC I83.892
        swelling I83.892
        ulcer I83.029
          with inflammation I83.229
          ankle I83.023
            with inflammation I83.223
          calf I83.022
            with inflammation I83.222
          foot NEC I83.025
            with inflammation I83.225
          heel I83.024
            with inflammation I83.224
          lower leg NEC I83.028
            with inflammation I83.228
          midfoot I83.024
            with inflammation I83.224
          thigh I83.021
            with inflammation I83.221
    right (asymptomatic) I83.91
      with
        edema I83.891
        inflammation I83.11
          with ulcer —see Varix, leg, with, ulcer, with inflammation by site

Varix (Continued)
  leg (Continued)
    right (Continued)
      with (Continued)
        pain I83.811
        specified complication NEC I83.891
        swelling I83.891
        ulcer I83.019
          with inflammation I83.219
          ankle I83.013
            with inflammation I83.213
          calf I83.012
            with inflammation I83.212
          foot NEC I83.015
            with inflammation I83.215
          heel I83.014
            with inflammation I83.214
          lower leg NEC I83.018
            with inflammation I83.218
          midfoot I83.014
            with inflammation I83.214
          thigh I83.011
            with inflammation I83.211
  nasal septum I86.8
  orbit I86.8
    congenital Q27.8
  ovary I86.2
  papillary I78.1
  pelvis I86.2
  perineum I86.3
  pharynx I86.8
  placenta O43.89-
  renal papilla I86.8
  retina H35.09
  scrotum (ulcerated) I86.1
  sigmoid colon I86.8
  specified site NEC I86.8
  spinal (cord) (vessels) I86.8
  spleen, splenic (vein) (with phlebolith)
    I86.8
  stomach I86.4
  sublingual I86.0
  ulcerated I83.009
    inflamed or infected I83.209
  uterine ligament I86.2
  vagina I86.8
  vocal cord I86.8
  vulva I86.3
Vas deferens —see condition
Vas deferentitis N49.1
Vasa previa O69.4
  hemorrhage from, affecting newborn
    P50.0
Vascular —see also condition
  loop on optic papilla Q14.2
  spasm I73.9
  spider I78.1
Vascularization, cornea —see
    Neovascularization, cornea
Vasculitis I77.6
  allergic D69.0
  cryoglobulinemic D89.1
  disseminated I77.6
  hypocomplementemic M31.8
  kidney I77.89
  livedoid L95.0
  nodular L95.8
  retina H35.06-
  rheumatic —see Fever, rheumatic
  rheumatoid —see Rheumatoid, vasculitis
  skin (limited to) L95.9
    specified NEC L95.8
Vasculopathy, necrotizing M31.9
  cardiac allograft T86.290
  specified NEC M31.8
Vasitis (nodosa) N49.1
  tuberculous A18.15
Vasodilation I73.9
Vasomotor —see condition
Vasoplasty, after previous sterilization Z31.0
  aftercare Z31.42

Vasospasm (vasoconstriction) I73.9
  cerebral (cerebrovascular) (artery)
    I67.848
    reversible I67.841
  coronary I20.1
  nerve
    arm —see Mononeuropathy, upper limb
    brachial plexus G54.0
    cervical plexus G54.2
    leg —see Mononeuropathy, lower limb
  peripheral NOS I73.9
  retina (artery) —see Occlusion, artery,
    retina
Vasospastic —see condition
Vasovagal attack (paroxysmal) R55
  psychogenic F45.8
VATER syndrome Q87.2
Vater's ampulla —see condition
Vegetation, vegetative
  adenoid (nasal fossa) J35.8
  endocarditis (acute) (any valve) (subacute)
    I33.0
  heart (mycotic) (valve) I33.0
Veil
  Jackson's Q43.3
Vein, venous —see condition
Veldt sore —see Ulcer, skin
Velpeau's hernia —see Hernia, femoral
Venereal
  bubo A55
  disease A64
  granuloma inguinale A58
  lymphogranuloma (Durand-Nicolas-Favre)
    A55
Venofibrosis I87.8
Venom, venomous —see Table of ~~d~~Drugs and
    ~~c~~Chemicals, by animal or substance,
    poisoning ◀▥▥
Venous —see condition
Ventilator lung, newborn P27.8
Ventral —see condition
Ventricle, ventricular —see also condition
  escape I49.3
  inversion Q20.5
Ventriculitis (cerebral) (see also Encephalitis)
    G04.90
Ventriculostomy status Z98.2
Vernet's syndrome G52.7
Verneuil's disease (syphilitic bursitis) A52.78
Verruca (due to HPV) (filiformis) (simplex)
    (viral) (vulgaris) B07.9
  acuminata A63.0
  necrogenica (primary) (tuberculosa) A18.4
  plana B07.8
  plantaris B07.0
  seborrheica L82.1
    inflamed L82.0
  senile (seborrheic) L82.1
    inflamed L82.0
  tuberculosa (primary) A18.4
  venereal A63.0
Verrucosities —see Verruca
Verruga peruana, peruviana A44.1
Version
  with extraction
    cervix —see Malposition, uterus
  uterus (postinfectional) (postpartal, old) —see
    Malposition, uterus
Vertebra, vertebral —see condition
Vertical talus (congenital) Q66.80
  left foot Q66.82
  right foot Q66.81
Vertigo R42
  auditory —see Vertigo, aural
  aural H81.31-
  benign paroxysmal (positional) H81.1-
  central (origin) H81.4-
  cerebral H81.4-
  Dix and Hallpike (epidemic) —see Neuronitis,
    vestibular
  due to infrasound T75.23

Vertigo (Continued)
  epidemic A88.1
    Dix and Hallpike —see Neuronitis,
      vestibular
    Pedersen's —see Neuronitis, vestibular
    vestibular neuronitis —see Neuronitis,
      vestibular
  hysterical F44.89
  infrasound T75.23
  labyrinthine —see subcategory H81.0
  laryngeal R05
  malignant positional H81.4-
  Ménière's —see subcategory H81.40
  menopausal N95.11
  otogenic —see Vertigo, aural
  paroxysmal positional, benign —see Vertigo,
    benign paroxysmal
  Pedersen's (epidemic) —see Neuronitis,
    vestibular
  peripheral NEC H81.39-
  positional
    benign paroxysmal —see Vertigo, benign
      paroxysmal
    malignant H81.4-
Very-low-density-lipoprotein-type (VLDL)
    hyperlipoproteinemia E78.1
Vesania —see Psychosis
Vesical —see condition
Vesicle
  cutaneous R23.8
  seminal —see condition
  skin R23.8
Vesicocolic —see condition
Vesicoperineal —see condition
Vesicorectal —see condition
Vesicourethrorectal —see condition
Vesicovaginal —see condition
Vesicular —see condition
Vesiculitis (seminal) N49.0
  amebic A06.82
  gonorrheal (acute) (chronic) A54.23
  trichomonal A59.09
  tuberculous A18.15
Vestibulitis (ear) (see also subcategory)
    H83.0
  nose (external) J34.89
  vulvar N94.810
Vestibulopathy, acute peripheral (recurrent) —
    see Neuronitis, vestibular
Vestige, vestigial —see also Persistence
  branchial Q18.0
  structures in vitreous Q14.0
Vibration
  adverse effects T75.20
    pneumatic hammer syndrome T75.21
    specified effect NEC T75.29
    vasospastic syndrome T75.22
    vertigo from infrasound T75.23
  exposure (occupational) Z57.7
  vertigo T75.23
Vibriosis A28.9
Victim (of)
  crime Z65.4
  disaster Z65.5
  terrorism Z65.4
  torture Z65.4
  war Z65.5
Vidal's disease L28.0
Villaret's syndrome G52.7
Villous —see condition
VIN —see Neoplasia, intraepithelial, vulva
Vincent's infection (angina) (gingivitis)
    A69.1
  stomatitis NEC A69.1
Vinson-Plummer syndrome D50.1
Violence, physical R45.6
Viosterol deficiency —see Deficiency, calciferol
Vipoma —see Neoplasm, malignant, by site
Viremia B34.9
Virilism (adrenal) E25.9
  congenital E25.0

◀ New   ◀▥▥ Revised   ~~deleted~~ Deleted

Virilization (female) (suprarenal) E25.9
  congenital E25.0
  isosexual E28.2
Virulent bubo A57
Virus, viral —*see also* condition
  as cause of disease classified elsewhere
    B97.89
  cytomegalovirus B25.9
  human immunodeficiency (HIV) —*see*
    Human, immunodeficiency virus (HIV)
    disease
  infection —*see* Infection, virus
  specified NEC B34.8
  swine influenza (viruses that normally cause
    infections in pigs) (*see also* Influenza,
    due to, identified novel influenza A
    virus) J09.X2
  West Nile (fever) A92.30
    with
      complications NEC A92.39
      cranial nerve disorders A92.32
      encephalitis A92.31
      encephalomyelitis A92.31
      neurologic manifestation NEC A92.32
      optic neuritis A92.32
      polyradiculitis A92.32
Viscera, visceral —*see* condition
Visceroptosis K63.4
Visible peristalsis R19.2
Vision, visual
  binocular, suppression H53.34
  blurred, blurring H53.8
    hysterical F44.6
  defect, defective NEC H54.7
  disorientation (syndrome) H53.8
  disturbance H53.9
    hysterical F44.6
  double H53.2
  examination Z01.00
    with abnormal findings Z01.01
  field, limitation (defect) —*see* Defect, visual
    field
  hallucinations R44.1
  halos H53.19
  loss —*see* Loss, vision
    sudden —*see* Disturbance, vision,
      subjective, loss, sudden
  low (both eyes) —*see* Low, vision
  perception, simultaneous without fusion
    H53.33
Vitality, lack or want of R53.83
  newborn P96.89
Vitamin deficiency —*see* Deficiency, vitamin
Vitelline duct, persistent Q43.0
Vitiligo L80
  eyelid H02.739
    left H02.736
      lower H02.735
      upper H02.734

Vitiligo (*Continued*)
  eyelid (*Continued*)
    right H02.733
      lower H02.732
      upper H02.731
  pinta A67.2
  vulva N90.89
Vitreal corneal syndrome H59.01-
Vitreoretinopathy, proliferative —*see also*
    Retinopathy, proliferative
  with retinal detachment —*see* Detachment,
    retina, traction
Vitreous —*see also* condition
  touch syndrome —*see* Complication,
    postprocedural, following cataract
    surgery
Vocal cord —*see* condition
Vogt-Koyanagi syndrome H20.82-
Vogt's disease or syndrome G80.3
Vogt-Spielmeyer amaurotic idiocy or disease
    E75.4
Voice
  change R49.9
    specified NEC R49.8
  loss —*see* Aphonia
Volhynian fever A79.0
Volkmann's ischemic contracture or paralysis
    (complicating trauma) T79.6
Volvulus (bowel) (colon) (duodenum)
    (intestine) K56.2
  with perforation K56.2
  congenital Q43.8
  fallopian tube —*see* Torsion, fallopian
    tube
  oviduct —*see* Torsion, fallopian tube
  stomach (due to absence of gastrocolic
    ligament) K31.89
Vomiting R11.10
  with nausea R11.2
  without nausea R11.11
  asphyxia —*see* Foreign body, by site, causing
    asphyxia, gastric contents
  bilious (cause unknown) R11.14
    following gastro-intestinal surgery
      K91.0
    in newborn P92.01
  blood —*see* Hematemesis
  causing asphyxia, choking, or suffocation —
    see Foreign body, by site
  cyclical G43.A0
    with refractory migraine G43.A1
    intractable G43.A1
    not intractable G43.A0
    psychogenic F50.8
    without refractory migraine G43.A0
  fecal mater R11.13
  following gastrointestinal surgery
    K91.0
  psychogenic F50.8

Vomiting (*Continued*)
  functional K31.89
  hysterical F50.8
  nervous F50.8
  neurotic F50.8
  newborn NEC P92.09
    bilious P92.01
  periodic R11.10
    psychogenic F50.8
  projectile R11.12
  psychogenic F50.8
  uremic —*see* Uremia
Vomito negro —*see* Fever, yellow
Von Bezold's abscess —*see* Mastoiditis,
    acute
Von Economo-Cruchet disease A85.8
Von Eulenburg's disease G71.19
Von Gierke's disease E74.01
Von Hippel (-Lindau) disease or syndrome
    Q85.8
Von Jaksch's anemia or disease D64.89
Von Recklinghausen
  disease (neurofibromatosis) Q85.01
    bones E21.0
Von Schroetter's syndrome I82.890
Von Willebrand (-Jurgens)(-Minot) disease or
    syndrome D68.0
Von Zumbusch's disease L40.1
Voyeurism F65.3
Vrolik's disease Q78.0
Vulva —*see* condition
Vulvismus N94.2
Vulvitis (acute) (allergic) (atrophic)
    (hypertrophic) (intertriginous) (senile)
    N76.2
  with ectopic or molar pregnancy O08.0
  adhesive, congenital Q52.79
  blennorrhagic (gonococcal) A54.02
  candidal B37.3
  chlamydial A56.02
  due to Haemophilus ducreyi A57
  following ectopic or molar pregnancy
    O08.0
  gonococcal A54.02
    with abscess (accessory gland)
      (periurethral) A54.1
  herpesviral A60.04
  leukoplakic N90.4
  monilial B37.3
  puerperal (postpartum) O86.19
  subacute or chronic N76.3
  syphilitic (early) A51.0
    late A52.76
  trichomonal A59.01
  tuberculous A18.18
Vulvodynia N94.819
  specified NEC N94.818
Vulvorectal —*see* condition
Vulvovaginitis (acute) —*see* Vaginitis

W

◀ New   ◀||| Revised   ~~deleted~~ Deleted

◀ New ◀◀◀ Revised ~~deleted~~ Deleted

W

Wound, open *(Continued)*
    finger (s) S61.209
        with
            amputation —*see* Amputation,
                traumatic, finger
            damage to nail S61.309
        bite —*see* Bite, finger
        index S61.208
            with
                damage to nail S61.308
            left S61.201
                with
                    damage to nail S61.301
            right S61.200
                with
                    damage to nail S61.300
        laceration —*see* Laceration, finger
        little S61.208
            with
                damage to nail S61.308
            left S61.207
                with damage to nail S61.307
            right S61.206
                with damage to nail S61.306
        middle S61.208
            with
                damage to nail S61.308
            left S61.203
                with damage to nail S61.303
            right S61.202
                with damage to nail S61.302
        puncture —*see* Puncture, finger
        ring S61.208
            with
                damage to nail S61.308
            left S61.205
                with damage to nail S61.305
            right S61.204
                with damage to nail S61.304
    flank —*see* Wound, open, abdomen, wall
    foot (except toe (s) alone) S91.30-
        with amputation —*see* Amputation,
            traumatic, foot
        bite —*see* Bite, foot
        laceration —*see* Laceration, foot
        puncture —*see* Puncture, foot
        toe —*see* Wound, open, toe
    forearm S51.80-
        with
            amputation —*see* Amputation,
                traumatic, forearm
            bite —*see* Bite, forearm
            elbow only —*see* Wound, open, elbow
            laceration —*see* Laceration, forearm
            puncture —*see* Puncture, forearm
    forehead —*see* Wound, open, head, specified
        site NEC
    genital organs, external
        with amputation —*see* Amputation,
            traumatic, genital organs
        bite —*see* Bite, genital organ
        female S31.502
            vagina S31.40
            vulva S31.40
        laceration —*see* Laceration, genital
            organ
        male S31.501
            penis S31.20
            scrotum S31.30
            testes S31.30
        puncture —*see* Puncture, genital organ
    globe (eye) —*see* Wound, open, ocular
    groin —*see* Wound, open, abdomen, wall
    gum —*see* Wound, open, oral cavity
    hand S61.40-
        with
            amputation —*see* Amputation,
                traumatic, hand
        bite —*see* Bite, hand
        finger (s) —*see* Wound, open, finger
        laceration —*see* Laceration, hand

Wound, open *(Continued)*
    hand *(Continued)*
        puncture —*see* Puncture, hand
        thumb —*see* Wound, open, thumb
    head S01.90
        bite —*see* Bite, head
        cheek —*see* Wound, open, cheek
        ear —*see* Wound, open, ear
        eyelid —*see* Wound, open, eyelid
        laceration —*see* Laceration, head
        lip —*see* Wound, open, lip
        nose S01.20
        oral cavity —*see* Wound, open, oral cavity
        puncture —*see* Puncture, head
        scalp —*see* Wound, open, scalp
        specified site NEC S01.80
        temporomandibular area —*see* Wound,
            open, cheek
    heel —*see* Wound, open, foot
    hip S71.00-
        with amputation —*see* Amputation,
            traumatic, hip
        bite —*see* Bite, hip
        laceration —*see* Laceration, hip
        puncture —*see* Puncture, hip
    hymen S31.40
        bite —*see* Bite, vulva
        laceration —*see* Laceration, vagina
        puncture —*see* Puncture, vagina
    hypochondrium S31.109
        bite —*see* Bite, hypochondrium
        laceration —*see* Laceration,
            hypochondrium
        puncture —*see* Puncture, hypochondrium
    hypogastric region S31.109
        bite —*see* Bite, hypogastric region
        laceration —*see* Laceration, hypogastric
            region
        puncture —*see* Puncture, hypogastric
            region
    iliac (region) —*see* Wound, open, inguinal
        region
    inguinal region S31.109
        bite —*see* Bite, abdomen, wall, lower
            quadrant
        laceration —*see* Laceration, inguinal region
        puncture —*see* Puncture, inguinal region
    instep —*see* Wound, open, foot
    interscapular region —*see* Wound, open,
        thorax, back
    intraocular —*see* Wound, open, ocular
    iris —*see* Wound, open, ocular
    jaw —*see* Wound, open, head, specified site
        NEC
    knee S81.00-
        bite —*see* Bite, knee
        laceration —*see* Laceration, knee
        puncture —*see* Puncture, knee
    labium (majus) (minus) —*see* Wound, open,
        vulva
    laceration —*see* Laceration, by site
    lacrimal duct —*see* Wound, open, eyelid
    larynx S11.019
        bite —*see* Bite, larynx
        laceration —*see* Laceration, larynx
        puncture —*see* Puncture, larynx
    left
        lower quadrant S31.104
            with penetration into peritoneal cavity
                S31.604
            bite —*see* Bite, abdomen, wall, left, lower
                quadrant
            laceration —*see* Laceration, abdomen,
                wall, left, lower quadrant
            puncture —*see* Puncture, abdomen, wall,
                left, lower quadrant
        upper quadrant S31.101
            with penetration into peritoneal cavity
                S31.601
            bite —*see* Bite, abdomen, wall, left,
                upper quadrant

Wound, open *(Continued)*
    left *(Continued)*
        upper quadrant *(Continued)*
            laceration —*see* Laceration, abdomen,
                wall, left, upper quadrant
            puncture —*see* Puncture, abdomen, wall,
                left, upper quadrant
    leg (lower) S81.80-
        with amputation —*see* Amputation,
            traumatic, leg
        ankle —*see* Wound, open, ankle
        bite —*see* Bite, leg
        foot —*see* Wound, open, foot
        knee —*see* Wound, open, knee
        laceration —*see* Laceration, leg
        puncture —*see* Puncture, leg
        toe —*see* Wound, open, toe
        upper —*see* Wound, open, thigh
    lip S01.501
        bite —*see* Bite, lip
        laceration —*see* Laceration, lip
        puncture —*see* Puncture, lip
    loin S31.109
        bite —*see* Bite, abdomen, wall
        laceration —*see* Laceration, loin
        puncture —*see* Puncture, loin
    lower back —*see* Wound, open, back,
        lower
    lumbar region —*see* Wound, open, back,
        lower
    malar region —*see* Wound, open, head,
        specified site NEC
    mammary —*see* Wound, open, breast
    mastoid region —*see* Wound, open, head,
        specified site NEC
    mouth —*see* Wound, open, oral cavity
    nail
        finger —*see* Wound, open, finger, with
            damage to nail
        toe —*see* Wound, open, toe, with damage
            to nail
    nape (neck) —*see* Wound, open, neck
    nasal (septum) (sinus) —*see* Wound, open,
        nose
    nasopharynx —*see* Wound, open, head,
        specified site NEC
    neck S11.90
        bite —*see* Bite, neck
        involving
            cervical esophagus S11.20
            larynx —*see* Wound, open, larynx
            pharynx S11.20
            thyroid S11.10
            trachea (cervical) S11.029
                bite —*see* Bite, trachea
                laceration S11.021
                    with foreign body S11.022
                puncture S11.023
                    with foreign body S11.024
        laceration —*see* Laceration, neck
        puncture —*see* Puncture, neck
        specified site NEC S11.80
            specified type NEC S11.89
    nose (septum) (sinus) S01.20
        with amputation —*see* Amputation,
            traumatic, nose
        bite —*see* Bite, nose
        laceration —*see* Laceration, nose
        puncture —*see* Puncture, nose
    ocular S05.90
        avulsion (traumatic enucleation) S05.7-
        eyeball S05.6-
            with foreign body S05.5-
        eyelid —*see* Wound, open, eyelid
        laceration and rupture S05.3-
            with prolapse or loss of intraocular
                tissue S05.2-
        orbit (penetrating) (with or without foreign
            body) S05.4-
        periocular area —*see* Wound, open, eyelid
        specified NEC S05.8X-

◀ New   ◀▥ Revised   ~~deleted~~ Deleted

Wound, open (Continued)
oral cavity S01.502
bite S01.552
laceration —see Laceration, oral cavity
puncture —see Puncture, oral cavity
orbit —see Wound, open, ocular, orbit
palate —see Wound, open, oral cavity
palm —see Wound, open, hand
pelvis, pelvic —see also Wound, open, back,
lower
girdle —see Wound, open, hip
penetrating —see Puncture, by site
penis S31.20
with amputation —see Amputation,
traumatic, penis
bite S31.25
laceration —see Laceration, penis
puncture —see Puncture, penis
perineum
bite —see Bite, perineum
female S31.502
laceration —see Laceration, perineum
male S31.501
puncture —see Puncture, perineum
periocular area (with or without lacrimal
passages) —see Wound, open, eyelid
periumbilic region S31.105
with penetration into peritoneal cavity
S31.605
bite —see Bite, abdomen, wall, periumbilic
region
laceration —see Laceration, abdomen, wall,
periumbilic region
puncture —see Puncture, abdomen, wall,
periumbilic region
phalanges
finger —see Wound, open, finger
toe —see Wound, open, toe
pharynx S11.20
pinna —see Wound, open, ear
popliteal space —see Wound, open, knee
prepuce —see Wound, open, penis
pubic region —see Wound, open, back,
lower
pudendum —see Wound, open, genital
organs, external
puncture wound —see Puncture
rectovaginal septum —see Wound, open,
vagina
right
lower quadrant S31.103
with penetration into peritoneal cavity
S31.603
bite —see Bite, abdomen, wall, right,
lower quadrant
laceration —see Laceration, abdomen,
wall, right, lower quadrant
puncture —see Puncture, abdomen, wall,
right, lower quadrant
upper quadrant S31.100
with penetration into peritoneal cavity
S31.600
bite —see Bite, abdomen, wall, right,
upper quadrant
laceration —see Laceration, abdomen,
wall, right, upper quadrant
puncture —see Puncture, abdomen, wall,
right, upper quadrant
sacral region —see Wound, open, back,
lower
sacroiliac region —see Wound, open, back,
lower
salivary gland —see Wound, open, oral
cavity

Wound, open (Continued)
scalp S01.00
bite S01.05
laceration —see Laceration, scalp
puncture —see Puncture, scalp
scalpel, newborn (birth injury) P15.8
scapular region —see Wound, open, shoulder
sclera —see Wound, open, ocular
scrotum S31.30
with amputation —see Amputation,
traumatic, scrotum
bite S31.35
laceration —see Laceration, scrotum
puncture —see Puncture, scrotum
shin —see Wound, open, leg
shoulder S41.00-
with amputation —see Amputation,
traumatic, arm
bite —see Bite, shoulder
laceration —see Laceration, shoulder
puncture —see Puncture, shoulder
skin NOS T14.8
spermatic cord —see Wound, open, testis
sternal region —see Wound, open, thorax,
front wall
submaxillary region —see Wound, open,
head, specified site NEC
submental region —see Wound, open, head,
specified site NEC
subungual
finger (s) —see Wound, open, finger
toe (s) —see Wound, open, toe
supraclavicular region —see Wound, open,
neck, specified site NEC
temple, temporal region —see Wound, open,
head, specified site NEC
temporomandibular area —see Wound, open,
cheek
testis S31.30
with amputation —see Amputation,
traumatic, testes
bite S31.35
laceration —see Laceration, testis
puncture —see Puncture, testis
thigh S71.10-
with amputation —see Amputation,
traumatic, hip
bite —see Bite, thigh
laceration —see Laceration, thigh
puncture —see Puncture, thigh
thorax, thoracic (wall) S21.90
back S21.20-
with penetration S21.40
bite —see Bite, thorax
breast —see Wound, open, breast
front S21.10-
with penetration S21.30
laceration —see Laceration, thorax
puncture —see Puncture, thorax
throat —see Wound, open, neck
thumb S61.009
with
amputation —see Amputation,
traumatic, thumb
damage to nail S61.109
bite —see Bite, thumb
laceration —see Laceration, thumb
left S61.002
with
damage to nail S61.102
puncture —see Puncture, thumb
right S61.001
with
damage to nail S61.101

Wound, open (Continued)
thyroid (gland) —see Wound, open, neck,
thyroid
toe (s) S91.109
with
amputation —see Amputation,
traumatic, toe
damage to nail S91.209
bite —see Bite, toe
great S91.103
with
damage to nail S91.203
left S91.102
with
damage to nail S91.202
right S91.101
with
damage to nail S91.201
laceration —see Laceration, toe
lesser S91.106
with
damage to nail S91.206
left S91.105
with
damage to nail S91.205
right S91.104
with
damage to nail S91.204
puncture —see Puncture, toe
tongue —see Wound, open, oral cavity
trachea (cervical region) —see Wound, open,
neck, trachea
tunica vaginalis —see Wound, open, testis
tympanum, tympanic membrane S09.2-
laceration —see Laceration, ear, drum
puncture —see Puncture, tympanum
umbilical region —see Wound, open,
abdomen, wall, periumbilic region
uvula —see Wound, open, oral cavity
vagina S31.40
bite S31.45
laceration —see Laceration, vagina
puncture —see Puncture, vagina
vitreous (humor) —see Wound, open,
ocular
vocal cord S11.039
bite —see Bite, vocal cord
laceration S11.031
with foreign body S11.032
puncture S11.033
with foreign body S11.034
vulva S31.40
with amputation —see Amputation,
traumatic, vulva
bite S31.45
laceration —see Laceration, vulva
puncture —see Puncture, vulva
wrist S61.50-
bite —see Bite, wrist
laceration —see Laceration, wrist
puncture —see Puncture, wrist
Wound, superficial —see Injury (see also
specified injury type)
Wright's syndrome G54.0
Wrist —see condition
Wrong drug (by accident) (given in error) —
see Table of dDrugs and cChemicals, by
drug, poisoning ◀▥
Wry neck —see Torticollis
Wuchereria (bancrofti) infestation B74.0
Wuchereriasis B74.0
Wuchernde Struma Langhans C73

X

Xanthelasma (eyelid) (palpebrarum) H02.60
  left H02.66
    lower H02.65
    upper H02.64
  right H02.63
    lower H02.62
    upper H02.61
Xanthelasmatosis (essential) E78.2
Xanthinuria, hereditary E79.8
Xanthoastrocytoma
  specified site —*see* Neoplasm, malignant, by
    site
  unspecified site C71.9
Xanthofibroma —*see* Neoplasm, connective
  tissue, benign
Xanthogranuloma D76.3
Xanthoma (s), xanthomatosis (primary)
  (familial) (hereditary) E75.5
  with
    hyperlipoproteinemia
      Type I E78.3
      Type III E78.2
      Type IV E78.1
      Type V E78.3
  bone (generalisata) C96.5
  cerebrotendinous E75.5
  cutaneotendinous E75.5

Xanthoma (s), xanthomatosis (Continued)
  disseminatum (skin) E78.2
  eruptive E78.2
  hypercholesterinemic E78.0
  hypercholesterolemic E78.0
  hyperlipidemic E78.5
  joint E75.5
  multiple (skin) E78.2
  tendon (sheath) E75.5
  tuberosum E78.2
  tuberous E78.2
  tubo-eruptive E78.2
  verrucous, oral mucosa K13.4
Xanthosis R23.8
Xenophobia F40.10
Xeroderma —*see also* Ichthyosis
  acquired L85.0
  eyelid H01.149
    left H01.146
      lower H01.145
      upper H01.144
    right H01.143
      lower H01.142
      upper H01.141
  pigmentosum Q82.1
  vitamin A deficiency E50.8
Xerophthalmia (vitamin A deficiency) E50.7
  unrelated to vitamin A deficiency —*see*
    Keratoconjunctivitis

Xerosis
  conjunctiva H11.14-
    with Bitot's spots —*see also* Pigmentation,
      conjunctiva
      vitamin A deficiency E50.1
    vitamin A deficiency E50.0
  cornea H18.89-
    with ulceration —*see* Ulcer, cornea
      vitamin A deficiency E50.3
    vitamin A deficiency E50.2
  cutis L85.3
  skin L85.3
Xerostomia K11.7
Xiphopagus Q89.4
XO syndrome Q96.9
X-ray (of)
  abnormal findings —*see* Abnormal,
    diagnostic imaging
  breast (mammogram) (routine) Z12.31
  chest
    routine (as part of a general medical
      examination) Z00.00
    with abnormal findings Z00.01
  routine (as part of a general medical
    examination) Z00.00
  with abnormal findings Z00.01
XXXXY syndrome Q98.1
XXY syndrome Q98.0

◀ New   ◀▥ Revised   ~~deleted~~ Deleted

Y

Yaba pox virus disease B08.72
Yatapoxvirus B08.70
    specified NEC B08.79
Yawning R06.89
    psychogenic F45.8
Yaws A66.9
    bone lesions A66.6
    butter A66.1
    chancre A66.0
    cutaneous, less than five years after infection
        A66.2
    early (cutaneous) (macular) (maculopapular)
        (micropapular) (papular) A66.2
        frambeside A66.2
        skin lesions NEC A66.2
    eyelid A66.2
    ganglion A66.6
    gangosis, gangosa A66.5
    gumma, gummata A66.4
        bone A66.6
    gummatous
        frambeside A66.4
        osteitis A66.6
        periostitis A66.6
    hydrarthrosis (see also subcategory M14.8-)
        A66.6
    hyperkeratosis (early) (late) A66.3

Yaws (Continued)
    initial lesions A66.0
    joint lesions (see also subcategory M14.8-)
        A66.6
    juxta-articular nodules A66.7
    late nodular (ulcerated) A66.4
    latent (without clinical manifestations) (with
        positive serology) A66.8
    mother A66.0
    mucosal A66.7
    multiple papillomata A66.1
    nodular, late (ulcerated) A66.4
    osteitis A66.6
    papilloma, plantar or palmar A66.1
    periostitis (hypertrophic) A66.6
    specified NEC A66.7
    ulcers A66.4
    wet crab A66.1
Yeast infection (see also Candidiasis) B37.9
Yellow
    atrophy (liver) —see Failure, hepatic
    fever —see Fever, yellow
    jack —see Fever, yellow
    jaundice —see Jaundice
    nail syndrome L60.5
Yersiniosis —see also Infection, Yersinia
    extraintestinal A28.2
    intestinal A04.6

Z

Zahorsky's syndrome (herpangina) B08.5
Zellweger's syndrome Q87.89
Zenker's diverticulum (esophagus) K22.5
Ziehen-Oppenheim disease G24.1
Zieve's syndrome K70.0
Zinc
    deficiency, dietary E60
    metabolism disorder E83.2
Zollinger-Ellison syndrome E16.4
Zona —see Herpes, zoster
Zoophobia F40.218
Zoster (herpes) —see Herpes, zoster
Zygomycosis B46.9
    specified NEC B46.8
Zymotic —see condition

	Malignant Primary	Malignant Secondary	Ca in situ	Benign	Uncertain Behavior	Unspecified Behavior

The list below gives the code numbers for neoplasms by anatomical site. For each site there are six possible code numbers according to whether the neoplasm in question is malignant, benign, in situ, of uncertain behavior, or of unspecified nature. The description of the neoplasm will often indicate which of the six columns is appropriate; e.g., malignant melanoma of skin, benign fibroadenoma of breast, carcinoma in situ of cervix uteri.

Where such descriptors are not present, the remainder of the Index should be consulted where guidance is given to the appropriate column for each morphological (histological) variety listed; e.g., Mesonephroma—*see Neoplasm, malignant;* Embryoma—*see also Neoplasm, uncertain behavior;* Disease, Bowen's—*see Neoplasm, skin, in situ.* However, the guidance in the Index can be overridden if one of the descriptors mentioned above is present; e.g., malignant adenoma of colon is coded to C18.9 and not to D12.6 as the adjective "malignant" overrides the Index entry "Adenoma—*see also Neoplasm, benign.*"

Codes listed with a dash -, following the code have a required additional character for laterality. The tablular must be reviewed for the complete code.

	Malignant Primary	Malignant Secondary	Ca in situ	Benign	Uncertain Behavior	Unspecified Behavior
Neoplasm, neoplastic	C80.1	C79.9	D09.9	D36.9	D48.9	D49.9
abdomen, abdominal	C76.2	C79.8-	D09.8	D36.7	D48.7	D49.89
cavity	C76.2	C79.8-	D09.8	D36.7	D48.7	D49.89
organ	C76.2	C79.8-	D09.8	D36.7	D48.7	D49.89
viscera	C76.2	C79.8-	D09.8	D36.7	D48.7	D49.89
wall—*see also Neoplasm, abdomen, wall, skin*	C44.509	C79.2-	D04.5	D23.5	D48.5	D49.2
connective tissue	C49.4	C79.8-	—	D21.4	D48.1	D49.2
skin	C44.509					
basal cell carcinoma	C44.519	—	—	—	—	—
specified type NEC	C44.599	—	—	—	—	—
squamous cell carcinoma	C44.529	—	—	—	—	—
abdominopelvic	C76.8	C79.8-	—	D36.7	D48.7	D49.89
accessory sinus—*see Neoplasm, sinus*						
acoustic nerve	C72.4-	C79.49	—	D33.3	D43.3	D49.7
adenoid (pharynx) (tissue)	C11.1	C79.89	D00.08	D10.6	D37.05	D49.0
adipose tissue—*see also Neoplasm, connective tissue*	C49.4	C79.89	—	D21.9	D48.1	D49.2
adnexa (uterine)	C57.4	C79.89	D07.39	D28.7	D39.8	D49.5
adrenal	C74.9-	C79.7-	D09.3	D35.0-	D44.1-	D49.7
capsule	C74.9-	C79.7-	D09.3	D35.0-	D44.1-	D49.7
cortex	C74.0-	C79.7-	D09.3	D35.0-	D44.1-	D49.7
gland	C74.9-	C79.7-	D09.3	D35.0-	D44.1-	D49.7
medulla	C74.1-	C79.7-	D09.3	D35.0-	D44.1-	D49.7
ala nasi (external)—*see also Neoplasm, skin, nose*	C44.301	C79.2	D04.39	D23.39	D48.5	D49.2
alimentary canal or tract NEC	C26.9	C78.80	D01.9	D13.9	D37.9	D49.0
alveolar	C03.9	C79.89	D00.03	D10.39	D37.09	D49.0
mucosa	C03.9	C79.89	D00.03	D10.39	D37.09	D49.0
lower	C03.1	C79.89	D00.03	D10.39	D37.09	D49.0
upper	C03.0	C79.89	D00.03	D10.39	D37.09	D49.0
ridge or process	C41.1	C79.51	—	D16.5-	D48.0	D49.2
carcinoma	C03.9	C79.8-	—	—	—	—
lower	C03.1	C79.8-	—	—	—	—
upper	C03.0	C79.8-	—	—	—	—

TABLE OF NEOPLASMS

TABLE OF NEOPLASMS

	Malignant Primary	Malignant Secondary	Ca in situ	Benign	Uncertain Behavior	Unspecified Behavior
alveolar (Continued)						
ridge or process (Continued)						
lower	C41.1	C79.51	—	D16.5-	D48.0	D49.2
mucosa	C03.9	C79.89	D00.03	D10.39	D37.09	D49.0
lower	C03.1	C79.89	D00.03	D10.39	D37.09	D49.0
upper	C03.0	C79.89	D00.03	D10.39	D37.09	D49.0
upper	C41.0	C79.51	—	D16.4-	D48.0	D49.2
sulcus	C06.1	C79.89	D00.02	D10.39	D37.09	D49.0
alveolus	C03.9	C79.89	D00.03	D10.39	D37.09	D49.0
lower	C03.1	C79.89	D00.03	D10.39	D37.09	D49.0
upper	C03.0	C79.89	D00.03	D10.39	D37.09	D49.0
ampulla of Vater	C24.1	C78.89	D01.5	D13.5	D37.6	D49.0
ankle NEC	C76.5-	C79.89	D04.7-	D36.7	D48.7	D49.89
anorectum, anorectal (junction)	C21.8	C78.5	D01.3	D12.9	D37.8	D49.0
antecubital fossa or space	C76.4-	C79.89	D04.6-	D36.7	D48.7	D49.89
antrum (Highmore) (maxillary)	C31.0	C78.39	D02.3	D14.0	D38.5	D49.1
pyloric	C16.3	C78.89	D00.2	D13.1	D37.1	D49.0
tympanicum	C30.1	C78.39	D02.3	D14.0	D38.5	D49.1
anus, anal	C21.0	C78.5	D01.3	D12.9	D37.8	D49.0
canal	C21.1	C78.5	D01.3	D12.9	D37.8	D49.0
cloacogenic zone	C21.2	C78.5	D01.3	D12.9	D37.8	D49.0
margin — see also Neoplasm, anus, skin	C44.500	C79.2	D04.5	D23.5	D48.5	D49.2
overlapping lesion with rectosigmoid junction or rectum	C21.8	—	—	—	—	—
skin	C44.500	C79.2	D04.5	D23.5	D48.5	D49.2
basal cell carcinoma	C44.510	—	—	—	—	—
specified type NEC	C44.590	—	—	—	—	—
squamous cell carcinoma	C44.520	—	—	—	—	—
sphincter	C21.1	C78.5	D01.3	D12.9	D37.8	D49.0
aorta (thoracic)	C49.3	C79.89	—	D21.3	D48.1	D49.2
abdominal	C49.4	C79.89	—	D21.4	D48.1	D49.2
aortic body	C75.5	C79.89	—	D35.6	D44.7	D49.7
aponeurosis	C49.9	C79.89	—	D21.9	D48.1	D49.2
palmar	C49.1-	C79.89	—	D21.1-	D48.1	D49.2
plantar	C49.2-	C79.89	—	D21.2-	D48.1	D49.2
appendix	C18.1	C78.5	D01.0	D12.1	D37.3	D49.0
arachnoid	C70.9	C79.49	—	D32.9	D42.9	D49.7
cerebral	C70.0	C79.32	—	D32.0	D42.0	D49.7
spinal	C70.1	C79.49	—	D32.1	D42.1	D49.7
areola	C50.0-	C79.81	D05.-	D24.-	D48.6-	D49.3
arm NEC	C76.4-	C79.89	D04.6-	D36.7	D48.7	D49.89
artery — see Neoplasm, connective tissue						

◀ New   ◀▦ Revised   ~~deleted~~ Deleted

	Malignant Primary	Malignant Secondary	Ca in situ	Benign	Uncertain Behavior	Unspecified Behavior
aryepiglottic fold	C13.1	C79.89	D00.08	D10.7	D37.05	D49.0
hypopharyngeal aspect	C13.1	C79.89	D00.08	D10.7	D37.05	D49.0
laryngeal aspect	C32.1	C78.39	D02.0	D14.1	D38.0	D49.1
marginal zone	C13.1	C79.89	D00.08	D10.7	D37.05	D49.0
arytenoid (cartilage)	C32.3	C78.39	D02.0	D14.1	D38.0	D49.1
fold — *see Neoplasm, aryepiglottic*						
associated with transplanted organ	C80.2	—	—	—	—	—
atlas	C41.2	C79.51	—	D16.6	D48.0	D49.2
atrium, cardiac	C38.0	C79.89	—	D15.1	D48.7	D49.89
auditory						
canal (external) (skin) A81	C44.20-	C79.2	D04.2-	D23.2-	D48.5	D49.2
internal	C30.1	C78.39	D02.3	D14.0	D38.5	D49.1
nerve	C72.4-	C79.49	—	D33.3	D43.3	D49.7
tube	C30.1	C78.39	D02.3	D14.0	D38.5	D49.1
opening	C11.2	C79.89	D00.08	D10.6	D37.05	D49.0
auricle, ear — *see also Neoplasm, skin, ear*	C44.20-	C79.2	D04.2-	D23.2-	D48.5	D49.2
auricular canal (external) — *see also Neoplasm, skin, ear*	C44.20-	C79.2	D04.2-	D23.2-	D48.5	D49.2
internal	C30.1	C78.39	D02.3	D14.0	D38.5	D49.2
autonomic nerve or nervous system NEC *(see Neoplasm, nerve, peripheral)*						
axilla, axillary	C76.1	C79.89	D09.8	D36.7	D48.7	D49.89
fold — *see also Neoplasm, skin, trunk*	C44.509	C79.2	D04.5	D23.5	D48.5	D49.2
back NEC	C76.8	C79.89	D04.5	D36.7	D48.7	D49.89
Bartholin's gland	C51.0	C79.82	D07.1	D28.0	D39.8	D49.5
basal ganglia	C71.0	C79.31	—	D33.0	D43.0	D49.6
basis pedunculi	C71.7	C79.31	—	D33.1	D43.1	D49.6
bile or biliary (tract)	C24.9	C78.89	D01.5	D13.5	D37.6	D49.0
canaliculi (biliferi) (intrahepatic)	C22.1	C78.7	D01.5	D13.4	D37.6	D49.0
canals, interlobular	C22.1	C78.89	D01.5	D13.4	D37.6	D49.0
duct or passage (common) (cystic) (extrahepatic)	C24.0	C78.89	D01.5	D13.5	D37.6	D49.0
interlobular	C22.1	C78.89	D01.5	D13.4	D37.6	D49.0
intrahepatic	C22.1	C78.7	D01.5	D13.4	D37.6	D49.0
and extrahepatic	C24.8	C78.89	D01.5	D13.5	D37.6	D49.0
bladder (urinary)	C67.9	C79.11	D09.0	D30.3	D41.4	D49.4
dome	C67.1	C79.11	D09.0	D30.3	D41.4	D49.4
neck	C67.5	C79.11	D09.0	D30.3	D41.4	D49.4
orifice	C67.9	C79.11	D09.0	D30.3	D41.4	D49.4
ureteric	C67.6	C79.11	D09.0	D30.3	D41.4	D49.4
urethral	C67.5	C79.11	D09.0	D30.3	D41.4	D49.4
overlapping lesion	C67.8	—	—	—	—	—
sphincter	C67.8	C79.11	D09.0	D30.3	D41.4	D49.4
trigone	C67.0	C79.11	D09.0	D30.3	D41.4	D49.4
urachus	C67.7	C79.11	D09.0	D30.3	D41.4	D49.4

TABLE OF NEOPLASMS

	Malignant Primary	Malignant Secondary	Ca in situ	Benign	Uncertain Behavior	Unspecified Behavior
bladder (urinary) *(Continued)*						
wall	C67.9	C79.11	D09.0	D30.3	D41.4	D49.4
anterior	C67.3	C79.11	D09.0	D30.3	D41.4	D49.4
lateral	C67.2	C79.11	D09.0	D30.3	D41.4	D49.4
posterior	C67.4	C79.11	D09.0	D30.3	D41.4	D49.4
blood vessel — *see Neoplasm, connective tissue*						
bone (periosteum)	C41.9	C79.51	—	D16.9-	D48.0	D49.2
acetabulum	C41.4	C79.51	—	D16.8-	D48.0	D49.2
ankle	C40.3-	C79.51	—	D16.3-	—	—
arm NEC	C40.0-	C79.51	—	D16.0-	—	—
astragalus	C40.3-	C79.51	—	D16.3-	—	—
atlas	C41.2	C79.51	—	D16.6-	D48.0	D49.2
axis	C41.2	C79.51	—	D16.6-	D48.0	D49.2
back NEC	C41.2	C79.51	—	D16.6-	D48.0	D49.2
calcaneus	C40.3-	C79.51	—	D16.3-	—	—
calvarium	C41.0	C79.51	—	D16.4-	D48.0	D49.2
carpus (any)	C40.1-	C79.51	—	D16.1-	—	—
cartilage NEC	C41.9	C79.51	—	D16.9-	D48.0	D49.2
clavicle	C41.3	C79.51	—	D16.7-	D48.0	D49.2
clivus	C41.0	C79.51	—	D16.4-	D48.0	D49.2
coccygeal vertebra	C41.4	C79.51	—	D16.8-	D48.0	D49.2
coccyx	C41.4	C79.51	—	D16.8-	D48.0	D49.2
costal cartilage	C41.3	C79.51	—	D16.7-	D48.0	D49.2
costovertebral joint	C41.3	C79.51	—	D16.7-	D48.0	D49.2
cranial	C41.0	C79.51	—	D16.4-	D48.0	D49.2
cuboid	C40.3-	C79.51	—	D16.3-	—	—
cuneiform	C41.9	C79.51	—	D16.9-	D48.0	D49.2
elbow	C40.0-	C79.51	—	D16.0-	—	—
ethmoid (labyrinth)	C41.0	C79.51	—	D16.4-	D48.0	D49.2
face	C41.0	C79.51	—	D16.4-	D48.0	D49.2
femur (any part)	C40.2-	C79.51	—	D16.2-	—	—
fibula (any part)	C40.2-	C79.51	—	D16.2-	—	—
finger (any)	C40.1-	C79.51	—	D16.1-	—	—
foot	C40.3-	C79.51	—	D16.3-	—	—
forearm	C40.0-	C79.51	—	D16.0-	—	—
frontal	C41.0	C79.51	—	D16.4-	D48.0	D49.2
hand	C40.1-	C79.51	—	D16.1-	—	—
heel	C40.3-	C79.51	—	D16.3-	—	—
hip	C41.4	C79.51	—	D16.8-	D48.0	D49.2
humerus (any part)	C40.0-	C79.51	—	D16.0-	—	—
hyoid	C41.0	C79.51	—	D16.4-	D48.0	D49.2
ilium	C41.4	C79.51	—	D16.8-	D48.0	D49.2
innominate	C41.4	C79.51	—	D16.8-	D48.0	D49.2

	Malignant Primary	Malignant Secondary	Ca in situ	Benign	Uncertain Behavior	Unspecified Behavior
bone *(Continued)*						
intervertebral cartilage or disc	C41.2	C79.51	—	D16.6-	D48.0	D49.2
ischium	C41.4	C79.51	—	D16.8-	D48.0	D49.2
jaw (lower)	C41.1	C79.51	—	D16.5-	D48.0	D49.2
knee	C40.2-	C79.51	—	D16.2-	—	—
leg NEC	C40.2-	C79.51	—	D16.2-	—	—
limb NEC	C40.9-	C79.51	—	D16.9-	—	—
lower (long bones)	C40.2-	C79.51	—	D16.2-	—	—
short bones	C40.3-	C79.51	—	D16.3-	—	—
upper (long bones)	C40.0-	C79.51	—	D16.0-	—	—
short bones	C40.1-	C79.51	—	D16.1-	—	—
malar	C41.0	C79.51	—	D16.4-	D48.0	D49.2
mandible	C41.1	C79.51	—	D16.5-	D48.0	D49.2
marrow NEC (any bone)	C96.9	C79.52	—	—	D47.9	D49.89
mastoid	C41.0	C79.51	—	D16.4-	D48.0	D49.2
maxilla, maxillary (superior)	C41.0	C79.51	—	D16.4-	D48.0	D49.2
inferior	C41.1	C79.51	—	D16.5-	D48.0	D49.2
metacarpus (any)	C40.1-	C79.51	—	D16.1-	—	—
metatarsus (any)	C40.3-	C79.51	—	D16.3-		
overlapping sites	C40.8-	—	—	—	—	—
navicular						
ankle	C40.3-	C79.51	—	—	—	—
hand	C40.1-	C79.51	—	—	—	—
nose, nasal	C41.0	C79.51	—	D16.4-	D48.0	D49.2
occipital	C41.0	C79.51	—	D16.4-	D48.0	D49.2
orbit	C41.0	C79.51	—	D16.4-	D48.0	D49.2
parietal	C41.0	C79.51	—	D16.4-	D48.0	D49.2
patella	C40.2-	C79.51	—	—	—	—
pelvic	C41.4	C79.51	—	D16.8	D48.0	D49.2
phalanges						
foot	C40.3-	C79.51	—	—	—	—
hand	C40.1-	C79.51	—	—	—	—
pubic	C41.4	C79.51	—	D16.8	D48.0	D49.2
radius (any part)	C40.0-	C79.51	—	D16.0-	—	—
rib	C41.3	C79.51	—	D16.7	D48.0	D49.2
sacral vertebra	C41.4	C79.51	—	D16.8	D48.0	D49.2
sacrum	C41.4	C79.51	—	D16.8	D48.0	D49.2
scaphoid					—	—
of ankle	C40.3-	C79.51	—	—	—	—
of hand	C40.1-	C79.51	—	—	—	—
scapula (any part)	C40.0-	C79.51	—	D16.0-	—	—
sella turcica	C41.0	C79.51	—	D16.4-	D48.0	D49.2
shoulder	C40.0-	C79.51	—	D16.0-	—	—

◀ New ◀▦ Revised ~~deleted~~ Deleted

	Malignant Primary	Malignant Secondary	Ca in situ	Benign	Uncertain Behavior	Unspecified Behavior
bone (Continued)						
skull	C41.0	C79.51	—	D16.4-	D48.0	D49.2
sphenoid	C41.0	C79.51	—	D16.4-	D48.0	D49.2
spine, spinal (column)	C41.2	C79.51	—	D16.6	D48.0	D49.2
coccyx	C41.4	C79.51	—	D16.8	D48.0	D49.2
sacrum	C41.4	C79.51	—	D16.8	D48.0	D49.2
sternum	C41.3	C79.51	—	D16.7	D48.0	D49.2
tarsus (any)	C40.3-	C79.51	—	—	—	—
temporal	C41.0	C79.51	—	D16.4-	D48.0	D49.2
thumb	C40.1-	C79.51	—	—	—	—
tibia (any part)	C40.2-	C79.51	—	—	—	—
toe (any)	C40.3-	C79.51	—	—	—	—
trapezium	C40.1-	C79.51	—	—	—	—
trapezoid	C40.1-	C79.51	—	—	—	—
turbinate	C41.0	C79.51	—	D16.4-	D48.0	D49.2
ulna (any part)	C40.0-	C79.51	—	D16.0-	—	—
unciform	C40.1-	C79.51	—	—	—	—
vertebra (column)	C41.2	C79.51	—	D16.6	D48.0	D49.2
coccyx	C41.4	C79.51	—	D16.8	D48.0	D49.2
sacrum	C41.4	C79.51	—	D16.8	D48.0	D49.2
vomer	C41.0	C79.51	—	D16.4-	D48.0	D49.2
wrist	C40.1-	C79.51	—	—	—	—
xiphoid process	C41.3	C79.51	—	D16.7	D48.0	D49.2
zygomatic	C41.0	C79.51	—	D16.4-	D48.0	D49.2
book-leaf (mouth)	C06.89	C79.89	D00.00	D10.39	D37.09	D49.0
bowel — see Neoplasm, intestine						
brachial plexus	C47.1-	C79.89	—	D36.12	D48.2	D49.2
brain NEC	C71.9	C79.31	—	D33.2	D43.2	D49.6
basal ganglia	C71.0	C79.31	—	D33.0	D43.0	D49.6
cerebellopontine angle	C71.6	C79.31	—	D33.1	D43.1	D49.6
cerebellum NOS	C71.6	C79.31	—	D33.1	D43.1	D49.6
cerebrum	C71.0	C79.31	—	D33.0	D43.0	D49.6
choroid plexus	C71.7	C79.31	—	D33.1	D43.1	D49.6
corpus callosum	C71.8	C79.31	—	D33.2	D43.2	D49.6
corpus striatum	C71.0	C79.31	—	D33.0	D43.0	D49.6
cortex (cerebral)	C71.0	C79.31	—	D33.0	D43.0	D49.6
frontal lobe	C71.1	C79.31	—	D33.0	D43.0	D49.6
globus pallidus	C71.0	C79.31	—	D33.0	D43.0	D49.6
hippocampus	C71.2	C79.31	—	D33.0	D43.0	D49.6
hypothalamus	C71.0	C79.31	—	D33.0	D43.0	D49.6
internal capsule	C71.0	C79.31	—	D33.0	D43.0	D49.6
medulla oblongata	C71.7	C79.31	—	D33.1	D43.1	D49.6
meninges	C70.0	C79.32	—	D32.0	D42.0	D49.7

◀ New ◀┉ Revised ~~deleted~~ Deleted

	Malignant Primary	Malignant Secondary	Ca in situ	Benign	Uncertain Behavior	Unspecified Behavior
brain NEC *(Continued)*						
midbrain	C71.7	C79.31	—	D33.1	D43.1	D49.6
occipital lobe	C71.4	C79.31	—	D33.0	D43.0	D49.6
overlapping lesion	C71.8	C79.31	—	—	—	—
parietal lobe	C71.3	C79.31	—	D33.0	D43.0	D49.6
peduncle	C71.7	C79.31	—	D33.1	D43.1	D49.6
pons	C71.7	C79.31	—	D33.1	D43.1	D49.6
stem	C71.7	C79.31	—	D33.1	D43.1	D49.6
tapetum	C71.8	C79.31	—	D33.2	D43.2	D49.6
temporal lobe	C71.2	C79.31	—	D33.0	D43.0	D49.6
thalamus	C71.0	C79.31	—	D33.0	D43.0	D49.6
uncus	C71.2	C79.31	—	D33.0	D43.0	D49.6
ventricle (floor)	C71.5	C79.31	—	D33.0	D43.0	D49.6
fourth	C71.7	C79.31	—	D33.1	D43.1	D49.6
branchial (cleft) (cyst) (vestiges)	C10.4	C79.89	D00.08	D10.5	D37.05	D49.0
breast (connective tissue) (glandular tissue) (soft parts)	C50.9-	C79.81	D05.-	D24.-	D48.6-	D49.3
areola	C50.0-	C79.81	D05.-	D24.-	D48.6-	D49.3
axillary tail	C50.6-	C79.81	D05.-	D24.-	D48.6-	D49.3
central portion	C50.1-	C79.81	D05.-	D24.-	D48.6-	D49.3
inner	C50.8-	C79.81	D05.-	D24.-	D48.6-	D49.3
lower	C50.8-	C79.81	D05.-	D24.-	D48.6-	D49.3
lower-inner quadrant	C50.3-	C79.81	D05.-	D24.-	D48.6-	D49.3
lower-outer quadrant	C50.5-	C79.81	D05.-	D24.-	D48.6-	D49.3
mastectomy site (skin) — *see also Neoplasm, breast, skin*	C44.501	C79.2	—	—	—	—
specified as breast tissue	C50.8-	C79.81	—	—	—	—
midline	C50.8-	C79.81	D05.-	D24.-	D48.6-	D49.3
nipple	C50.0-	C79.81	D05.-	D24.-	D48.6-	D49.3
outer	C50.8-	C79.81	D05.-	D24.-	D48.6-	D49.3
overlapping lesion	C50.8-	—	—	—	—	—
skin	C44.501	C79.2	D04.5	D23.5	D48.5	D49.2
basal cell carcinoma	C44.511	—	—	—	—	—
specified type NEC	C44.591	—	—	—	—	—
squamous cell carcinoma	C44.521	—	—	—	—	—
tail (axillary)	C50.6-	C79.81	D05.-	D24.-	D48.6-	D49.3
upper	C50.8-	C79.81	D05.-	D24.-	D48.6-	D49.3
upper-inner quadrant	C50.2-	C79.81	D05.-	D24.-	D48.6-	D49.3
upper-outer quadrant	C50.4-	C79.81	D05.-	D24.-	D48.6-	D49.3
broad ligament	C57.1	C79.82	D07.39	D28.2	D39.8	D49.5
bronchiogenic, bronchogenic (lung)	C34.9-	C78.0-	D02.2-	D14.3-	D38.1	D49.1
bronchiole	C34.9-	C78.0-	D02.2-	D14.3-	D38.1	D49.1
bronchus	C34.9-	C78.0-	D02.2-	D14.3-	D38.1	D49.1
carina	C34.0-	C78.0-	D02.2-	D14.3-	D38.1	D49.1
lower lobe of lung	C34.3-	C78.0-	D02.2-	D14.3-	D38.1	D49.1

TABLE OF NEOPLASMS

	Malignant Primary	Malignant Secondary	Ca in situ	Benign	Uncertain Behavior	Unspecified Behavior
bronchus *(Continued)*						
main	C34.0-	C78.0-	D02.2-	D14.3-	D38.1	D49.1
middle lobe of lung	C34.2	C78.0-	D02.21	D14.31	D38.1	D49.1
overlapping lesion	C34.8-	—	—	—	—	—
upper lobe of lung	C34.1-	C78.0-	D02.2-	D14.3-	D38.1	D49.1
brow	C44.309	C79.2	D04.39	D23.39	D48.5	D49.2
basal cell carcinoma	C44.319	—	—	—	—	—
specified type NEC	C44.399	—	—	—	—	—
squamous cell carcinoma	C44.329	—	—	—	—	—
buccal (cavity)	C06.9	C79.89	D00.00	D10.39	D37.09	D49.0
commissure	C06.0	C79.89	D00.02	D10.39	D37.09	D49.0
groove (lower) (upper)	C06.1	C79.89	D00.02	D10.39	D37.09	D49.0
mucosa	C06.0	C79.89	D00.02	D10.39	D37.09	D49.0
sulcus (lower) (upper)	C06.1	C79.89	D00.02	D10.39	D37.09	D49.0
bulbourethral gland	C68.0	C79.19	D09.19	D30.4	D41.3	D49.5
bursa — *see Neoplasm, connective tissue*						
buttock NEC	C76.3	C79.89	D04.5	D36.7	D48.7	D49.89
calf	C76.5-	C79.89	D04.7-	D36.7	D48.7	D49.89
calvarium	C41.0	C79.51	—	D16.4-	D48.0	D49.2
calyx, renal	C65.-	C79.0-	D09.19	D30.1-	D41.1-	D49.5
canal						
anal	C21.1	C78.5	D01.3	D12.9	D37.8	D49.0
auditory (external) — *see also Neoplasm, skin, ear*	C44.20-	C79.2	D04.2-	D23.2-	D48.5	D49.2
auricular (external) — *see also Neoplasm, skin, ear*	C44.20-	C79.2	D04.2-	D23.2-	D48.5	D49.2
canaliculi, biliary (biliferi) (intrahepatic)	C22.1	C78.7	D01.5	D13.4	D37.6	D49.0
canthus (eye) (inner) (outer)	C44.10-	C79.2	D04.1-	D23.1-	D48.5	D49.2
basal cell carcinoma	C44.11-	—	—	—	—	—
specified type NEC	C44.19-	—	—	—	—	—
squamous cell carcinoma	C44.12-	—	—	—	—	—
capillary — *see Neoplasm, connective tissue*						
caput coli	C18.0	C78.5	D01.0	D12.0	D37.4	D49.0
carcinoid — *see Tumor, carcinoid*						
cardia (gastric)	C16.0	C78.89	D00.2	D13.1	D37.1	D49.0
cardiac orifice (stomach)	C16.0	C78.89	D00.2	D13.1	D37.1	D49.0
cardio-esophageal junction	C16.0	C78.89	D00.2	D13.1	D37.1	D49.0
cardio-esophagus	C16.0	C78.89	D00.2	D13.1	D37.1	D49.0
carina (bronchus)	C34.0-	C78.0-	D02.2-	D14.3-	D38.1	D49.1
carotid (artery)	C49.0	C79.89	—	D21.0	D48.1	D49.2
body	C75.4	C79.89	—	D35.5	D44.6	D49.7
carpus (any bone)	C40.1-	C79.51	—	D16.1-	—	—
cartilage (articular) (joint) NEC — *see also Neoplasm, bone*	C41.9	C79.51	—	D16.9-	D48.0	D49.2
arytenoid	C32.3	C78.39	D02.0	D14.1	D38.0	D49.1
auricular	C49.0	C79.89	—	D21.0	D48.1	D49.2

◀ New   ◀◀ Revised   ~~deleted~~ Deleted

	Malignant Primary	Malignant Secondary	Ca in situ	Benign	Uncertain Behavior	Unspecified Behavior
cartilage NEC *(Continued)*						
bronchi	C34.0-	C78.39	—	D14.3-	D38.1	D49.1
costal	C41.3	C79.51	—	D16.7	D48.0	D49.2
cricoid	C32.3	C78.39	D02.0	D14.1	D38.0	D49.1
cuneiform	C32.3	C78.39	D02.0	D14.1	D38.0	D49.1
ear (external)	C49.0	C79.89	—	D21.0	D48.1	D49.2
ensiform	C41.3	C79.51	—	D16.7	D48.0	D49.2
epiglottis	C32.1	C78.39	D02.0	D14.1	D38.0	D49.1
anterior surface	C10.1	C79.89	D00.08	D10.5	D37.05	D49.0
eyelid	C49.0	C79.89	—	D21.0	D48.1	D49.2
intervertebral	C41.2	C79.51	—	D16.6	D48.0	D49.2
larynx, laryngeal	C32.3	C78.39	D02.0	D14.1	D38.0	D49.1
nose, nasal	C30.0	C78.39	D02.3	D14.0	D38.5	D49.1
pinna	C49.0	C79.89	—	D21.0	D48.1	D49.2
rib	C41.3	C79.51	—	D16.7	D48.0	D49.2
semilunar (knee)	C40.2-	C79.51	—	D16.2-	D48.0	D49.2
thyroid	C32.3	C78.39	D02.0	D14.1	D38.0	D49.1
trachea	C33	C78.39	D02.1	D14.2	D38.1	D49.1
cauda equina	C72.1	C79.49	—	D33.4	D43.4	D49.7
cavity						
buccal	C06.9	C79.89	D00.00	D10.30	D37.09	D49.0
nasal	C30.0	C78.39	D02.3	D14.0	D38.5	D49.1
oral	C06.9	C79.89	D00.00	D10.30	D37.09	D49.0
peritoneal	C48.2	C78.6	—	D20.1	D48.4	D49.0
tympanic	C30.1	C78.39	D02.3	D14.0	D38.5	D49.1
cecum	C18.0	C78.5	D01.0	D12.0	D37.4	D49.0
central nervous system	C72.9	C79.40	—	—	—	—
cerebellopontine (angle)	C71.6	C79.31	—	D33.1	D43.1	D49.6
cerebellum, cerebellar	C71.6	C79.31	—	D33.1	D43.1	D49.6
cerebrum, cerebral (cortex) (hemisphere) (white matter)	C71.0	C79.31	—	D33.0	D43.0	D49.6
meninges	C70.0	C79.32	—	D32.0	D42.0	D49.7
peduncle	C71.7	C79.31	—	D33.1	D43.1	D49.6
ventricle	C71.5	C79.31	—	D33.0	D43.0	D49.6
fourth	C71.7	C79.31	—	D33.1	D43.1	D49.6
cervical region	C76.0	C79.89	D09.8	D36.7	D48.7	D49.89
cervix (cervical) (uteri) (uterus)	C53.9	C79.82	D06.9	D26.0	D39.0	D49.5
canal	C53.0	C79.82	D06.0	D26.0	D39.0	D49.5
endocervix (canal) (gland)	C53.0	C79.82	D06.0	D26.0	D39.0	D49.5
exocervix	C53.1	C79.82	D06.1	D26.0	D39.0	D49.5
external os	C53.1	C79.82	D06.1	D26.0	D39.0	D49.5
internal os	C53.0	C79.82	D06.0	D26.0	D39.0	D49.5
nabothian gland	C53.0	C79.82	D06.0	D26.0	D39.0	D49.5
overlapping lesion	C53.8	—	—	—	—	—

◀ New   ◀▦ Revised   ~~deleted~~ Deleted

	Malignant Primary	Malignant Secondary	Ca in situ	Benign	Uncertain Behavior	Unspecified Behavior
cervix *(Continued)*						
squamocolumnar junction	C53.8	C79.82	D06.7	D26.0	D39.0	D49.5
stump	C53.8	C79.82	D06.7	D26.0	D39.0	D49.5
cheek	C76.0	C79.89	D09.8	D36.7	D48.7	D49.89
external	C44.309	C79.2	D04.39	D23.39	D48.5	D49.2
basal cell carcinoma	C44.319	—	—	—	—	—
specified type NEC	C44.399	—	—	—	—	—
squamous cell carcinoma	C44.329	—	—	—	—	—
inner aspect	C06.0	C79.89	D00.02	D10.39	D37.09	D49.0
internal	C06.0	C79.89	D00.02	D10.39	D37.09	D49.0
mucosa	C06.0	C79.89	D00.02	D10.39	D37.09	D49.0
chest (wall) NEC	C76.1	C79.89	D09.8	D36.7	D48.7	D49.89
chiasma opticum	C72.3-	C79.49	—	D33.3	D43.3	D49.7
chin	C44.309	C79.2	D04.39	D23.39	D48.5	D49.2
basal cell carcinoma	C44.319	—	—	—	—	—
specified type NEC	C44.399	—	—	—	—	—
squamous cell carcinoma	C44.329	—	—	—	—	—
choana	C11.3	C79.89	D00.08	D10.6	D37.05	D49.0
cholangiole	C22.1	C78.89	D01.5	D13.4	D37.6	D49.0
choledochal duct	C24.0	C78.89	D01.5	D13.5	D37.6	D49.0
choroid	C69.3-	C79.49	D09.2-	D31.3-	D48.7	D49.81
plexus	C71.5	C79.31	—	D33.0	D43.0	D49.6
ciliary body	C69.4-	C79.49	D09.2-	D31.4-	D48.7	D49.89
clavicle	C41.3	C79.51	—	D16.7	D48.0	D49.2
clitoris	C51.2	C79.82	D07.1	D28.0	D39.8	D49.5
clivus	C41.0	C79.51	—	D16.4-	D48.0	D49.2
cloacogenic zone	C21.2	C78.5	D01.3	D12.9	D37.8	D49.0
coccygeal						
body or glomus	C49.5	C79.89	—	D21.5	D48.1	D49.2
vertebra	C41.4	C79.51	—	D16.8	D48.0	D49.2
coccyx	C41.4	C79.51	—	D16.8	D48.0	D49.2
colon — *see also Neoplasm, intestine, large*	C18.9	C78.5	—	—	—	—
with rectum	C19	C78.5	D01.1	D12.7	D37.5	D49.0
column, spinal — *see Neoplasm, spine*						
columnella — *see also Neoplasm, skin, face*	C44.390	C79.2	D04.39	D23.39	D48.5	D49.2
commissure						
labial, lip	C00.6	C79.89	D00.01	D10.39	D37.01	D49.0
laryngeal	C32.0	C78.39	D02.0	D14.1	D38.0	D49.1
common (bile) duct	C24.0	C78.89	D01.5	D13.5	D37.6	D49.0
concha — *see also Neoplasm, skin, ear*	C44.20-	C79.2	D04.2-	D23.2-	D48.5	D49.2
nose	C30.0	C78.39	D02.3	D14.0	D38.5	D49.1
conjunctiva	C69.0-	C79.49	D09.2-	D31.0-	D48.7	D49.89

◄ New ◄ Revised ~~deleted~~ Deleted

	Malignant Primary	Malignant Secondary	Ca in situ	Benign	Uncertain Behavior	Unspecified Behavior
connective tissue NEC	C49.9	C79.89	—	D21.9	D48.1	D49.2

Note: For neoplasms of connective tissue (blood vessel, bursa, fascia, ligament, muscle, peripheral nerves, sympathetic and parasympathetic nerves and ganglia, synovia, tendon, etc.) or of morphological types that indicate connective tissue, code according to the list under "Neoplasm, connective tissue". For sites that do not appear in this list, code to neoplasm of that site; e.g., fibrosarcoma, pancreas (C25.9)

Note: Morphological types that indicate connective tissue appear in their proper place in the alphabetic index with the instruction *"see Neoplasm, connective tissue ...."*

	Malignant Primary	Malignant Secondary	Ca in situ	Benign	Uncertain Behavior	Unspecified Behavior
abdomen	C49.4	C79.89	—	D21.4	D48.1	D49.2
abdominal wall	C49.4	C79.89	—	D21.4	D48.1	D49.2
ankle	C49.2-	C79.89	—	D21.2-	D48.1	D49.2
antecubital fossa or space	C49.1-	C79.89	—	D21.1-	D48.1	D49.2
arm	C49.1-	C79.89	—	D21.1-	D48.1	D49.2
auricle (ear)	C49.0	C79.89	—	D21.0	D48.1	D49.2
axilla	C49.3	C79.89	—	D21.3	D48.1	D49.2
back	C49.6	C79.89	—	D21.6	D48.1	D49.2
breast — *see Neoplasm, breast*						
buttock	C49.5	C79.89	—	D21.5	D48.1	D49.2
calf	C49.2-	C79.89	—	D21.2-	D48.1	D49.2
cervical region	C49.0	C79.89	—	D21.0	D48.1	D49.2
cheek	C49.0	C79.89	—	D21.0	D48.1	D49.2
chest (wall)	C49.3	C79.89	—	D21.3	D48.1	D49.2
chin	C49.0	C79.89	—	D21.0	D48.1	D49.2
diaphragm	C49.3	C79.89	—	D21.3	D48.1	D49.2
ear (external)	C49.0	C79.89	—	D21.0	D48.1	D49.2
elbow	C49.1-	C79.89	—	D21.1-	D48.1	D49.2
extrarectal	C49.5	C79.89	—	D21.5	D48.1	D49.2
extremity	C49.9	C79.89	—	D21.9	D48.1	D49.2
lower	C49.2-	C79.89	—	D21.2-	D48.1	D49.2
upper	C49.1-	C79.89	—	D21.1-	D48.1	D49.2
eyelid	C49.0	C79.89	—	D21.0	D48.1	D49.2
face	C49.0	C79.89	—	D21.0	D48.1	D49.2
finger	C49.1-	C79.89	—	D21.1-	D48.1	D49.2
flank	C49.6	C79.89	—	D21.6	D48.1	D49.2
foot	C49.2-	C79.89	—	D21.2-	D48.1	D49.2
forearm	C49.1-	C79.89	—	D21.1-	D48.1	D49.2
forehead	C49.0	C79.89	—	D21.0	D48.1	D49.2
gastric	C49.4	C79.89	—	D21.4	D48.1	D49.2
gastrointestinal	C49.4	C79.89	—	D21.4	D48.1	D49.2
gluteal region	C49.5	C79.89	—	D21.5	D48.1	D49.2
great vessels NEC	C49.3	C79.89	—	D21.3	D48.1	D49.2
groin	C49.5	C79.89	—	D21.5	D48.1	D49.2
hand	C49.1-	C79.89	—	D21.1-	D48.1	D49.2

◀ New ◀||| Revised ~~deleted~~ Deleted

TABLE OF NEOPLASMS

	Malignant Primary	Malignant Secondary	Ca in situ	Benign	Uncertain Behavior	Unspecified Behavior
connective tissue NEC *(Continued)*						
head	C49.0	C79.89	—	D21.0	D48.1	D49.2
heel	C49.2-	C79.89	—	D21.2-	D48.1	D49.2
hip	C49.2-	C79.89	—	D21.2-	D48.1	D49.2
hypochondrium	C49.4	C79.89	—	D21.4	D48.1	D49.2
iliopsoas muscle	C49.5	C79.89	—	D21.5	D48.1	D49.2
infraclavicular region	C49.3	C79.89	—	D21.3	D48.1	D49.2
inguinal (canal) (region)	C49.5	C79.89	—	D21.5	D48.1	D49.2
intestinal	C49.4	C79.89	—	D21.4	D48.1	D49.2
intrathoracic	C49.3	C79.89	—	D21.3	D48.1	D49.2
ischiorectal fossa	C49.5	C79.89	—	D21.5	D48.1	D49.2
jaw	C03.9	C79.89	D00.03	D10.39	D48.1	D49.0
knee	C49.2-	C79.89	—	D21.2-	D48.1	D49.2
leg	C49.2-	C79.89	—	D21.2-	D48.1	D49.2
limb NEC	C49.9	C79.89	—	D21.9	D48.1	D49.2
lower	C49.2-	C79.89	—	D21.2-	D48.1	D49.2
upper	C49.1-	C79.89	—	D21.1-	D48.1	D49.2
nates	C49.5	C79.89	—	D21.5	D48.1	D49.2
neck	C49.0	C79.89	—	D21.0	D48.1	D49.2
orbit	C69.6-	C79.49	D09.2-	D31.6-	D48.1	D49.89
overlapping lesion	C49.8	—	—	—	—	—
pararectal	C49.5	C79.89	—	D21.5	D48.1	D49.2
para-urethral	C49.5	C79.89	—	D21.5	D48.1	D49.2
paravaginal	C49.5	C79.89	—	D21.5	D48.1	D49.2
pelvis (floor)	C49.5	C79.89	—	D21.5	D48.1	D49.2
pelvo-abdominal	C49.8	C79.89	—	D21.6	D48.1	D49.2
perineum	C49.5	C79.89	—	D21.5	D48.1	D49.2
perirectal (tissue)	C49.5	C79.89	—	D21.5	D48.1	D49.2
periurethral (tissue)	C49.5	C79.89	—	D21.5	D48.1	D49.2
popliteal fossa or space	C49.2-	C79.89	—	D21.2-	D48.1	D49.2
presacral	C49.5	C79.89	—	D21.5	D48.1	D49.2
psoas muscle	C49.4	C79.89	—	D21.4	D48.1	D49.2
pterygoid fossa	C49.0	C79.89	—	D21.0	D48.1	D49.2
rectovaginal septum or wall	C49.5	C79.89	—	D21.5	D48.1	D49.2
rectovesical	C49.5	C79.89	—	D21.5	D48.1	D49.2
retroperitoneum	C48.0	C78.6	—	D20.0	D48.3	D49.0
sacrococcygeal region	C49.5	C79.89	—	D21.5	D48.1	D49.2
scalp	C49.0	C79.89	—	D21.0	D48.1	D49.2
scapular region	C49.3	C79.89	—	D21.3	D48.1	D49.2
shoulder	C49.1-	C79.89	—	D21.1-	D48.1	D49.2
skin (dermis) NEC — *see also Neoplasm, skin, by site*	C44.90	C79.2	D04.9	D23.9	D48.5	D49.2
stomach	C49.4	C79.89	—	D21.4	D48.1	D49.2
submental	C49.0	C79.89	—	D21.0	D48.1	D49.2

◀ New ◀︎ Revised ~~deleted~~ Deleted

	Malignant Primary	Malignant Secondary	Ca in situ	Benign	Uncertain Behavior	Unspecified Behavior
connective tissue NEC *(Continued)*						
supraclavicular region	C49.0	C79.89	—	D21.0	D48.1	D49.2
temple	C49.0	C79.89	—	D21.0	D48.1	D49.2
temporal region	C49.0	C79.89	—	D21.0	D48.1	D49.2
thigh	C49.2-	C79.89	—	D21.2-	D48.1	D49.2
thoracic (duct) (wall)	C49.3	C79.89	—	D21.3	D48.1	D49.2
thorax	C49.3	C79.89	—	D21.3	D48.1	D49.2
thumb	C49.1-	C79.89	—	D21.1-	D48.1	D49.2
toe	C49.2-	C79.89	—	D21.2-	D48.1	D49.2
trunk	C49.6	C79.89	—	D21.6	D48.1	D49.2
umbilicus	C49.4	C79.89	—	D21.4	D48.1	D49.2
vesicorectal	C49.5	C79.89	—	D21.5	D48.1	D49.2
wrist	C49.1-	C79.89	—	D21.1-	D48.1	D49.2
conus medullaris	C72.0	C79.49	—	D33.4	D43.4	D49.7
cord (true) (vocal)	C32.0	C78.39	D02.0	D14.1	D38.0	D49.1
false	C32.1	C78.39	D02.0	D14.1	D38.0	D49.1
spermatic	C63.1-	C79.82	D07.69	D29.8	D40.8	D49.5
spinal (cervical) (lumbar) (thoracic)	C72.0	C79.49	—	D33.4	D43.4	D49.7
cornea (limbus)	C69.1-	C79.49	D09.2-	D31.1-	D48.7	D49.89
corpus						
albicans	C56.-	C79.6-	D07.39	D27.-	D39.1-	D49.5
callosum, brain	C71.0	C79.31	—	D33.2	D43.2	D49.6
cavernosum	C60.2	C79.82	D07.4	D29.0	D40.8	D49.5
gastric	C16.2	C78.89	D00.2	D13.1	D37.1	D49.0
overlapping sites	C54.8	—	—	—	—	—
penis	C60.2	C79.82	D07.4	D29.0	D40.8	D49.5
striatum, cerebrum	C71.0	C79.31	—	D33.0	D43.0	D49.6
uteri	C54.9	C79.82	D07.0	D26.1	D39.0	D49.5
isthmus	C54.0	C79.82	D07.0	D26.1	D39.0	D49.5
cortex						
adrenal	C74.0-	C79.7-	D09.3	D35.0-	D44.1-	D49.7
cerebral	C71.0	C79.31	—	D33.0	D43.0	D49.6
costal cartilage	C41.3	C79.51	—	D16.7	D48.0	D49.2
costovertebral joint	C41.3	C79.51	—	D16.7	D48.0	D49.2
Cowper's gland	C68.0	C79.19	D09.19	D30.4	D41.3	D49.5
cranial (fossa, any)	C71.9	C79.31	—	D33.2	D43.2	D49.6
meninges	C70.0	C79.32	—	D32.0	D42.0	D49.7
nerve	C72.50	C79.49	—	D33.3	D43.3	D49.7
specified NEC	C72.59	C79.49	—	D33.3	D43.3	D49.7
craniobuccal pouch	C75.2	C79.89	D09.3	D35.2	D44.3	D49.7
craniopharyngeal (duct) (pouch)	C75.2	C79.89	D09.3	D35.3	D44.4	D49.7
cricoid	C13.0	C79.89	D00.08	D10.7	D37.05	D49.0
cartilage	C32.3	C78.39	D02.0	D14.1	D38.0	D49.1

TABLE OF NEOPLASMS

TABLE OF NEOPLASMS

	Malignant Primary	Malignant Secondary	Ca in situ	Benign	Uncertain Behavior	Unspecified Behavior
cricopharynx	C13.0	C79.89	D00.08	D10.7	D37.05	D49.0
crypt of Morgagni	C21.8	C78.5	D01.3	D12.9	D37.8	D49.0
crystalline lens	C69.4-	C79.49	D09.2-	D31.4-	D48.7	D49.89
cul-de-sac (Douglas')	C48.1	C78.6	—	D20.1	D48.4	D49.0
cuneiform cartilage	C32.3	C78.39	D02.0	D14.1	D38.0	D49.1
cutaneous — *see Neoplasm, skin*						
cutis — *see Neoplasm, skin*						
cystic (bile) duct (common)	C24.0	C78.89	D01.5	D13.5	D37.6	D49.0
dermis — *see Neoplasm, skin*						
diaphragm	C49.3	C79.89	—	D21.3	D48.1	D49.2
digestive organs, system, tube, or tract NEC	C26.9	C78.89	D01.9	D13.9	D37.9	D49.0
disc, intervertebral	C41.2	C79.51	—	D16.6	D48.0	D49.2
disease, generalized	C80.0	—	—	—	—	—
disseminated	C80.0	—	—	—	—	—
Douglas' cul-de-sac or pouch	C48.1	C78.6	—	D20.1	D48.4	D49.0
duodenojejunal junction	C17.8	C78.4	D01.49	D13.39	D37.2	D49.0
duodenum	C17.0	C78.4	D01.49	D13.2	D37.2	D49.0
dura (cranial) (mater)	C70.9	C79.49	—	D32.9	D42.9	D49.7
cerebral	C70.0	C79.32	—	D32.0	D42.0	D49.7
spinal	C70.1	C79.49	—	D32.1	D42.1	D49.7
ear (external) — *see also Neoplasm, skin, ear*	C44.20-	C79.2	D04.2-	D23.2-	D48.5	D49.2
auricle or auris — *see also Neoplasm, skin, ear*	C44.20-	C79.2	D04.2-	D23.2-	D48.5	D49.2
canal, external — *see also Neoplasm, skin, ear*	C44.20-	C79.2	D04.2-	D23.2-	D48.5	D49.2
cartilage	C49.0	C79.89	—	D21.0	D48.1	D49.2
external meatus — *see also Neoplasm, skin, ear*	C44.20-	C79.2	D04.2-	D23.2-	D48.5	D49.2
inner	C30.1	C78.39	D02.3	D14.0	D38.5	D49.1
lobule — *see also Neoplasm, skin, ear*	C44.20-	C79.2	D04.2-	D23.2-	D48.5	D49.2
middle	C30.1	C78.39	D02.3	D14.0	D38.5	D49.1
overlapping lesion with accessory sinuses	C31.8	—	—	—	—	—
skin	C44.20-	C79.2	D04.2-	D23.2-	D48.5	D49.2
basal cell carcinoma	C44.21-	—	—	—	—	—
specified type NEC	C44.29-	—	—	—	—	—
squamous cell carcinoma	C44.22-	—	—	—	—	—
earlobe	C44.20-	C79.2	D04.2-	D23.2-	D48.5	D49.2
basal cell carcinoma	C44.21-	—	—	—	—	—
specified type NEC	C44.29-	—	—	—	—	—
squamous cell carcinoma	C44.22-	—	—	—	—	—
ejaculatory duct	C63.7	C79.82	D07.69	D29.8	D40.8	D49.5
elbow NEC	C76.4-	C79.89	D04.6-	D36.7	D48.7	D49.89
endocardium	C38.0	C79.89	—	D15.1	D48.7	D49.89
endocervix (canal) (gland)	C53.0	C79.82	D06.0	D26.0	D39.0	D49.5
endocrine gland NEC	C75.9	C79.89	D09.3	D35.9	D44.9	D49.7
pluriglandular	C75.8	C79.89	D09.3	D35.7	D44.9	D49.7

◀ New ◀▥ Revised ~~deleted~~ Deleted

	Malignant Primary	Malignant Secondary	Ca in situ	Benign	Uncertain Behavior	Unspecified Behavior
endometrium (gland) (stroma)	C54.1	C79.82	D07.0	D26.1	D39.0	D49.5
ensiform cartilage	C41.3	C79.51	—	D16.7	D48.0	D49.2
enteric — see Neoplasm, intestine						
ependyma (brain)	C71.5	C79.31	—	D33.0	D43.0	D49.6
fourth ventricle	C71.7	C79.31	—	D33.1	D43.1	D49.6
epicardium	C38.0	C79.89	—	D15.1	D48.7	D49.89
epididymis	C63.0-	C79.82	D07.69	D29.3-	D40.8	D49.5
epidural	C72.9	C79.49	—	D33.9	D43.9	D49.7
epiglottis	C32.1	C78.39	D02.0	D14.1	D38.0	D49.1
anterior aspect or surface	C10.1	C79.89	D00.08	D10.5	D37.05	D49.0
cartilage	C32.3	C78.39	D02.0	D14.1	D38.0	D49.1
free border (margin)	C10.1	C79.89	D00.08	D10.5	D37.05	D49.0
junctional region	C10.8	C79.89	D00.08	D10.5	D37.05	D49.0
posterior (laryngeal) surface	C32.1	C78.39	D02.0	D14.1	D38.0	D49.1
suprahyoid portion	C32.1	C78.39	D02.0	D14.1	D38.0	D49.1
esophagogastric junction	C16.0	C78.89	D00.2	D13.1	D37.1	D49.0
esophagus	C15.9	C78.89	D00.1	D13.0	D37.8	D49.0
abdominal	C15.5	C78.89	D00.1	D13.0	D37.8	D49.0
cervical	C15.3	C78.89	D00.1	D13.0	D37.8	D49.0
distal (third)	C15.5	C78.89	D00.1	D13.0	D37.8	D49.0
lower (third)	C15.5	C78.89	D00.1	D13.0	D37.8	D49.0
middle (third)	C15.4	C78.89	D00.1	D13.0	D37.8	D49.0
overlapping lesion	C15.8	—	—	—	—	—
proximal (third)	C15.3	C78.89	D00.1	D13.0	D37.8	D49.0
thoracic	C15.4	C78.89	D00.1	D13.0	D37.8	D49.0
upper (third)	C15.3	C78.89	D00.1	D13.0	D37.8	D49.0
ethmoid (sinus)	C31.1	C78.39	D02.3	D14.0	D38.5	D49.1
bone or labyrinth	C41.0	C79.51	—	D16.4-	D48.0	D49.2
eustachian tube	C30.1	C78.39	D02.3	D14.0	D38.5	D49.1
exocervix	C53.1	C79.82	D06.1	D26.0	D39.0	D49.5
external						
meatus (ear) — see also Neoplasm, skin, ear	C44.20-	C79.2	D04.2-	D23.2-	D48.5	D49.2
os, cervix uteri	C53.1	C79.82	D06.1	D26.0	D39.0	D49.5
extradural	C72.9	C79.49	—	D33.9	D43.9	D49.7
extrahepatic (bile) duct	C24.0	C78.89	D01.5	D13.5	D37.6	D49.0
overlapping lesion with gallbladder	C24.8	—	—	—	—	—
extraocular muscle	C69.6-	C79.49	D09.2-	D31.6-	D48.7	D49.89
extrarectal	C76.3	C79.89	D09.8	D36.7	D48.7	D49.89
extremity	C76.8	C79.89	D04.8	D36.7	D48.7	D49.89
lower	C76.5-	C79.89	D04.7-	D36.7	D48.7	D49.89
upper	C76.4-	C79.89	D04.6-	D36.7	D48.7	D49.89
eye NEC	C69.9-	C79.49	D09.2	D31.9	D48.7	D49.89
overlapping sites	C69.8	—	—	—	—	—
eyeball	C69.9-	C79.49	D09.2-	D31.9-	D48.7	D49.89

◀ New ◀▥ Revised ~~deleted~~ Deleted

TABLE OF NEOPLASMS

	Malignant Primary	Malignant Secondary	Ca in situ	Benign	Uncertain Behavior	Unspecified Behavior
eyebrow	C44.309	C79.2	D04.39	D23.39	D48.5	D49.2
basal cell carcinoma	C44.319	—	—	—	—	—
specified type NEC	C44.399	—	—	—	—	—
squamous cell carcinoma	C44.329	—	—	—	—	—
eyelid (lower) (skin) (upper)	C44.10-	—	—	—	—	—
basal cell carcinoma	C44.11-	—	—	—	—	—
cartilage	C49.0	C79.89	—	D21.0	D48.1	D49.2
specified type NEC	C44.19-	—	—	—	—	—
squamous cell carcinoma	C44.12-	—	—	—	—	—
face NEC	C76.0	C79.89	D04.39	D36.7	D48.7	D49.89
fallopian tube (accessory)	C57.0-	C79.82	D07.39	D28.2	D39.8	D49.5
falx (cerebella) (cerebri)	C70.0	C79.32	—	D32.0	D42.0	D49.7
fascia — *see also Neoplasm, connective tissue*						
palmar	C49.1-	C79.89	—	D21.1-	D48.1	D49.2
plantar	C49.2-	C79.89	—	D21.2-	D48.1	D49.2
fatty tissue — *see Neoplasm, connective tissue*						
fauces, faucial NEC	C10.9	C79.89	D00.08	D10.5	D37.05	D49.0
pillars	C09.1	C79.89	D00.08	D10.5	D37.05	D49.0
tonsil	C09.9	C79.89	D00.08	D10.4	D37.05	D49.0
femur (any part)	C40.2-	—	—	D16.2-	—	—
fetal membrane	C58	C79.82	D07.0	D26.7	D39.2	D49.5
fibrous tissue — *see Neoplasm, connective tissue*						
fibula (any part)	C40.2-	C79.51	—	D16.2-	—	—
filum terminale	C72.0	C79.49	—	D33.4	D43.4	D49.7
finger NEC	C76.4-	C79.89	D04.6-	D36.7	D48.7	D49.89
flank NEC	C76.8	C79.89	D04.5	D36.7	D48.7	D49.89
follicle, nabothian	C53.0	C79.82	D06.0	D26.0	D39.0	D49.5
foot NEC	C76.5-	C79.89	D04.7-	D36.7	D48.7	D49.89
forearm NEC	C76.4-	C79.89	D04.6-	D36.7	D48.7	D49.89
forehead (skin)	C44.309	C79.2	D04.39	D23.39	D48.5	D49.2
basal cell carcinoma	C44.319	—	—	—	—	—
specified type NEC	C44.399	—	—	—	—	—
squamous cell carcinoma	C44.329	—	—	—	—	—
foreskin	C60.0	C79.82	D07.4	D29.0	D40.8	D49.5
fornix						
pharyngeal	C11.3	C79.89	D00.08	D10.6	D37.05	D49.0
vagina	C52	C79.82	D07.2	D28.1	D39.8	D49.5
fossa (of)						
anterior (cranial)	C71.9	C79.31	—	D33.2	D43.2	D49.6
cranial	C71.9	C79.31	—	D33.2	D43.2	D49.6
ischiorectal	C76.3	C79.89	D09.8	D36.7	D48.7	D49.89
middle (cranial)	C71.9	C79.31	—	D33.2	D43.2	D49.6
piriform	C12	C79.89	D00.08	D10.7	D37.05	D49.0

◀ New   ◀‖ Revised   ~~deleted~~ Deleted

	Malignant Primary	Malignant Secondary	Ca in situ	Benign	Uncertain Behavior	Unspecified Behavior
fossa *(Continued)*						
pituitary	C75.1	C79.89	D09.3	D35.2	D44.3	D49.7
posterior (cranial)	C71.9	C79.31	—	D33.2	D43.2	D49.6
pterygoid	C49.0	C79.89	—	D21.0	D48.1	D49.2
pyriform	C12	C79.89	D00.08	D10.7	D37.05	D49.0
Rosenmuller	C11.2	C79.89	D00.08	D10.6	D37.05	D49.0
tonsillar	C09.0	C79.89	D00.08	D10.5	D37.05	D49.0
fourchette	C51.9	C79.82	D07.1	D28.0	D39.8	D49.5
frenulum						
labii — *see Neoplasm, lip, internal*						
linguae	C02.2	C79.89	D00.07	D10.1	D37.02	D49.0
frontal						
bone	C41.0	C79.51	—	D16.4-	D48.0	D49.2
lobe, brain	C71.1	C79.31	—	D33.0	D43.0	D49.6
pole	C71.1	C79.31	—	D33.0	D43.0	D49.6
sinus	C31.2	C78.39	D02.3	D14.0	D38.5	D49.1
fundus						
stomach	C16.1	C78.89	D00.2	D13.1	D37.1	D49.0
uterus	C54.3	C79.82	D07.0	D26.1	D39.0	D49.5
gall duct (extrahepatic)	C24.0	C78.89	D01.5	D13.5	D37.6	D49.0
intrahepatic	C22.1	C78.7	D01.5	D13.4	D37.6	D49.0
gallbladder	C23	C78.89	D01.5	D13.5	D37.6	D49.0
overlapping lesion with extrahepatic bile ducts	C24.8	—	—	—	—	—
ganglia — *see also Neoplasm, nerve, peripheral*	C47.9	C79.89	—	D36.10	D48.2	D49.2
basal	C71.0	C79.31	—	D33.0	D43.0	D49.6
cranial nerve	C72.50	C79.49	—	D33.3	D43.3	D49.7
Gartner's duct	C52	C79.82	D07.2	D28.1	D39.8	D49.5
gastric — *see Neoplasm, stomach*						
gastrocolic	C26.9	C78.89	D01.9	D13.9	D37.9	D49.0
gastroesophageal junction	C16.0	C78.89	D00.2	D13.1	D37.1	D49.0
gastrointestinal (tract) NEC	C26.9	C78.89	D01.9	D13.9	D37.9	D49.0
generalized	C80.0	—	—	—	—	—
genital organ or tract						
female NEC	C57.9	C79.82	D07.30	D28.9	D39.9	D49.5
overlapping lesion	C57.8	—	—	—	—	—
specified site NEC	C57.7	C79.82	D07.39	D28.7	D39.8	D49.5
male NEC	C63.9	C79.82	D07.60	D29.9	D40.9	D49.5
overlapping lesion	C63.8	—	—	—	—	—
specified site NEC	C63.7	C79.82	D07.69	D29.8	D40.8	D49.5
genitourinary tract						
female	C57.9	C79.82	D07.30	D28.9	D39.9	D49.5
male	C63.9	C79.82	D07.60	D29.9	D40.9	D49.5

TABLE OF NEOPLASMS

	Malignant Primary	Malignant Secondary	Ca in situ	Benign	Uncertain Behavior	Unspecified Behavior
gingiva (alveolar) (marginal)	C03.9	C79.89	D00.03	D10.39	D37.09	D49.0
lower	C03.1	C79.89	D00.03	D10.39	D37.09	D49.0
mandibular	C03.1	C79.89	D00.03	D10.39	D37.09	D49.0
maxillary	C03.0	C79.89	D00.03	D10.39	D37.09	D49.0
upper	C03.0	C79.89	D00.03	D10.39	D37.09	D49.0
gland, glandular (lymphatic) (system) — *see also Neoplasm, lymph gland*						
endocrine NEC	C75.9	C79.89	D09.3	D35.9	D44.9	D49.7
salivary — *see Neoplasm, salivary gland*						
glans penis	C60.1	C79.82	D07.4	D29.0	D40.8	D49.5
globus pallidus	C71.0	C79.31	—	D33.0	D43.0	D49.6
glomus						
coccygeal	C49.5	C79.89	—	D21.5	D48.1	D49.2
jugularis	C75.5	C79.89	—	D35.6	D44.7	D49.7
glosso-epiglottic fold(s)	C10.1	C79.89	D00.08	D10.5	D37.05	D49.0
glossopalatine fold	C09.1	C79.89	D00.08	D10.5	D37.05	D49.0
glossopharyngeal sulcus	C09.0	C79.89	D00.08	D10.5	D37.05	D49.0
glottis	C32.0	C78.39	D02.0	D14.1	D38.0	D49.1
gluteal region	C76.3	C79.89	D04.5	D36.7	D48.7	D49.89
great vessels NEC	C49.3	C79.89	—	D21.3	D48.1	D49.2
groin NEC	C76.3	C79.89	D04.5	D36.7	D48.7	D49.89
gum	C03.9	C79.89	D00.03	D10.39	D37.09	D49.0
lower	C03.1	C79.89	D00.03	D10.39	D37.09	D49.0
upper	C03.0	C79.89	D00.03	D10.39	D37.09	D49.0
hand NEC	C76.4-	C79.89	D04.6-	D36.7	D48.7	D49.89
head NEC	C76.0	C79.89	D04.4	D36.7	D48.7	D49.89
heart	C38.0	C79.89	—	D15.1	D48.7	D49.89
heel NEC	C76.5-	C79.89	D04.7-	D36.7	D48.7	D49.89
helix — *see also Neoplasm, skin, ear*	C44.20-	C79.2	D04.2-	D23.2-	D48.5	D49.2
hematopoietic, hemopoietic tissue NEC	C96.9	—	—	—	—	—
specified NEC	C96.Z	—	—	—	—	—
hemisphere, cerebral	C71.0	C79.31	—	D33.0	D43.0	D49.6
hemorrhoidal zone	C21.1	C78.5	D01.3	D12.9	D37.8	D49.0
hepatic — *see also Index to disease, by histology*	C22.9	C78.7	D01.5	D13.4	D37.6	D49.0
duct (bile)	C24.0	C78.89	D01.5	D13.5	D37.6	D49.0
flexure (colon)	C18.3	C78.5	D01.0	D12.3	D37.4	D49.0
primary	C22.8	C78.7	D01.5	D13.4	D37.6	D49.0
hepatobiliary	C24.9	C79.89	D01.5	D13.5	D37.6	D49.0
hepatoblastoma	C22.2	C78.7	D01.5	D13.4	D37.6	D49.0
hepatoma	C22.0	C78.7	D01.5	D13.4	D37.6	D49.0
hilus of lung	C34.0-	C78.0-	D02.2-	D14.3-	D38.1	D49.1
hip NEC	C76.5-	C79.89	D04.7-	D36.7	D48.7	D49.89
hippocampus, brain	C71.2	C79.31	—	D33.0	D43.0	D49.6
humerus (any part)	C40.0-	C79.51	—	D16.0-	—	—
hymen	C52	C79.82	D07.2	D28.1	D39.8	D49.5

◀ New   ◀ Revised   ~~deleted~~ Deleted

	Malignant Primary	Malignant Secondary	Ca in situ	Benign	Uncertain Behavior	Unspecified Behavior
hypopharynx, hypopharyngeal NEC	C13.9	C79.89	D00.08	D10.7	D37.05	D49.0
overlapping lesion	C13.8	—	—	—	—	—
postcricoid region	C13.0	C79.89	D00.08	D10.7	D37.05	D49.0
posterior wall	C13.2	C79.89	D00.08	D10.7	D37.05	D49.0
pyriform fossa (sinus)	C12	C79.89	D00.08	D10.7	D37.05	D49.0
hypophysis	C75.1	C79.89	D09.3	D35.2	D44.3	D49.7
hypothalamus	C71.0	C79.31	—	D33.0	D43.0	D49.6
ileocecum, ileocecal (coil) (junction) (valve)	C18.0	C78.5	D01.0	D12.0	D37.4	D49.0
ileum	C17.2	C78.4	D01.49	D13.39	D37.2	D49.0
ilium	C41.4	C79.51	—	D16.8	D48.0	D49.2
immunoproliferative NEC	C88.9	—	—	—	—	—
infraclavicular (region)	C76.1	C79.89	D04.5	D36.7	D48.7	D49.89
inguinal (region)	C76.3	C79.89	D04.5	D36.7	D48.7	D49.89
insula	C71.0	C79.31	—	D33.0	D43.0	D49.6
insular tissue (pancreas)	C25.4	C78.89	D01.7	D13.7	D37.8	D49.0
brain	C71.0	C79.31	—	D33.0	D43.0	D49.6
interarytenoid fold	C13.1	C79.89	D00.08	D10.7	D37.05	D49.0
hypopharyngeal aspect	C13.1	C79.89	D00.08	D10.7	D37.05	D49.0
laryngeal aspect	C32.1	C78.39	D02.0	D14.1	D38.0	D49.1
marginal zone	C13.1	C79.89	D00.08	D10.7	D37.05	D49.0
interdental papillae	C03.9	C79.89	D00.03	D10.39	D37.09	D49.0
lower	C03.1	C79.89	D00.03	D10.39	D37.09	D49.0
upper	C03.0	C79.89	D00.03	D10.39	D37.09	D49.0
internal						
capsule	C71.0	C79.31	—	D33.0	D43.0	D49.6
os (cervix)	C53.0	C79.82	D06.0	D26.0	D39.0	D49.5
intervertebral cartilage or disc	C41.2	C79.51	—	D16.6	D48.0	D49.2
intestine, intestinal	C26.0	C78.80	D01.40	D13.9	D37.8	D49.0
large	C18.9	C78.5	D01.0	D12.6	D37.4	D49.0
appendix	C18.1	C78.5	D01.0	D12.1	D37.3	D49.0
caput coli	C18.0	C78.5	D01.0	D12.0	D37.4	D49.0
cecum	C18.0	C78.5	D01.0	D12.0	D37.4	D49.0
colon	C18.9	C78.5	D01.0	D12.6	D37.4	D49.0
and rectum	C19	C78.5	D01.1	D12.7	D37.5	D49.0
ascending	C18.2	C78.5	D01.0	D12.2	D37.4	D49.0
caput	C18.0	C78.5	D01.0	D12.0	D37.4	D49.0
descending	C18.6	C78.5	D01.0	D12.4	D37.4	D49.0
distal	C18.6	C78.5	D01.0	D12.4	D37.4	D49.0
left	C18.6	C78.5	D01.0	D12.4	D37.4	D49.0
overlapping lesion	C18.8	—	—	—	—	—
pelvic	C18.7	C78.5	D01.0	D12.5	D37.4	D49.0
right	C18.2	C78.5	D01.0	D12.2	D37.4	D49.0
sigmoid (flexure)	C18.7	C78.5	D01.0	D12.5	D37.4	D49.0
transverse	C18.4	C78.5	D01.0	D12.3	D37.4	D49.0

TABLE OF NEOPLASMS

TABLE OF NEOPLASMS

	Malignant Primary	Malignant Secondary	Ca in situ	Benign	Uncertain Behavior	Unspecified Behavior
intestine, intestinal (Continued)						
large (Continued)						
hepatic flexure	C18.3	C78.5	D01.0	D12.3	D37.4	D49.0
ileocecum, ileocecal (coil) (valve)	C18.0	C78.5	D01.0	D12.0	D37.4	D49.0
overlapping lesion	C18.8	—	—	—	—	—
sigmoid flexure (lower) (upper)	C18.7	C78.5	D01.0	D12.5	D37.4	D49.0
splenic flexure	C18.5	C78.5	D01.0	D12.3	D37.4	D49.0
small	C17.9	C78.4	D01.40	D13.30	D37.2	D49.0
duodenum	C17.0	C78.4	D01.49	D13.2	D37.2	D49.0
ileum	C17.2	C78.4	D01.49	D13.39	D37.2	D49.0
jejunum	C17.1	C78.4	D01.49	D13.39	D37.2	D49.0
overlapping lesion	C17.8	—	—	—	—	—
tract NEC	C26.0	C78.89	D01.40	D13.9	D37.8	D49.0
intra-abdominal	C76.2	C79.89	D09.8	D36.7	D48.7	D49.89
intracranial NEC	C71.9	C79.31	—	D33.2	D43.2	D49.6
intrahepatic (bile) duct	C22.1	C78.7	D01.5	D13.4	D37.6	D49.0
intraocular	C69.9-	C79.49	D09.2-	D31.9-	D48.7	D49.89
intraorbital	C69.6-	C79.49	D09.2-	D31.6-	D48.7	D49.89
intrasellar	C75.1	C79.89	D09.3	D35.2	D44.3	D49.7
intrathoracic (cavity) (organs)	C76.1	C79.89	D09.8	D15.9	D48.7	D49.89
specified NEC	C76.1	C79.89	D09.8	D15.7	—	—
iris	C69.4-	C79.49	D09.2-	D31.4-	D48.7	D49.89
ischiorectal (fossa)	C76.3	C79.89	D09.8	D36.7	D48.7	D49.89
ischium	C41.4	C79.51	—	D16.8	D48.0	D49.2
island of Reil	C71.0	C79.31	—	D33.0	D43.0	D49.6
islands or islets of Langerhans	C25.4	C78.89	D01.7	D13.7	D37.8	D49.0
isthmus uteri	C54.0	C79.82	D07.0	D26.1	D39.0	D49.5
jaw	C76.0	C79.89	D09.8	D36.7	D48.7	D49.89
bone	C41.1	C79.51	—	D16.5-	D48.0	D49.2
lower	C41.1	C79.51	—	D16.5-	—	—
upper	C41.0	C79.51	—	D16.4-	—	—
carcinoma (any type) (lower) (upper)	C76.0	C79.89	—	—	—	—
skin — see also Neoplasm, skin, face	C44.309	C79.2	D04.39	D23.39	D48.5	D49.2
soft tissues	C03.9	C79.89	D00.03	D10.39	D37.09	D49.0
lower	C03.1	C79.89	D00.03	D10.39	D37.09	D49.0
upper	C03.0	C79.89	D00.03	D10.39	D37.09	D49.0
jejunum	C17.1	C78.4	D01.49	D13.39	D37.2	D49.0
joint NEC — see also Neoplasm, bone	C41.9	C79.51	—	D16.9-	D48.0	D49.2
acromioclavicular	C40.0-	C79.51	—	D16.0-	—	—
bursa or synovial membrane — see Neoplasm, connective tissue						
costovertebral	C41.3	C79.51	—	D16.7	D48.0	D49.2
sternocostal	C41.3	C79.51	—	D16.7	D48.0	D49.2
temporomandibular	C41.1	C79.51	—	D16.5-	D48.0	D49.2

◀ New ◀▥ Revised ~~deleted~~ Deleted

	Malignant Primary	Malignant Secondary	Ca in situ	Benign	Uncertain Behavior	Unspecified Behavior
junction						
anorectal	C21.8	C78.5	D01.3	D12.9	D37.8	D49.0
cardioesophageal	C16.0	C78.89	D00.2	D13.1	D37.1	D49.0
esophagogastric	C16.0	C78.89	D00.2	D13.1	D37.1	D49.0
gastroesophageal	C16.0	C78.89	D00.2	D13.1	D37.1	D49.0
hard and soft palate	C05.9	C79.89	D00.00	D10.39	D37.09	D49.0
ileocecal	C18.0	C78.5	D01.0	D12.0	D37.4	D49.0
pelvirectal	C19	C78.5	D01.1	D12.7	D37.5	D49.0
pelviureteric	C65.-	C79.0-	D09.19	D30.1-	D41.1-	D49.5
rectosigmoid	C19	C78.5	D01.1	D12.7	D37.5	D49.0
squamocolumnar, of cervix	C53.8	C79.82	D06.7	D26.0	D39.0	D49.5
Kaposi's sarcoma — *see Kaposi's, sarcoma*						
kidney (parenchymal)	C64.-	C79.0-	D09.19	D30.0-	D41.0-	D49.5
calyx	C65.-	C79.0-	D09.19	D30.1-	D41.1-	D49.5
hilus	C65.-	C79.0-	D09.19	D30.1-	D41.1-	D49.5
pelvis	C65.-	C79.0-	D09.19	D30.1-	D41.1-	D49.5
knee NEC	C76.5-	C79.89	D04.7-	D36.7	D48.7	D49.89
labia (skin)	C51.9	C79.82	D07.1	D28.0	D39.8	D49.5
majora	C51.0	C79.82	D07.1	D28.0	D39.8	D49.5
minora	C51.1	C79.82	D07.1	D28.0	D39.8	D49.5
labial — *see also Neoplasm, lip*	C00.9	C79.89	D00.01	D10.0	D37.01	D49.0
sulcus (lower) (upper)	C06.1	C79.89	D00.02	D10.39	D37.09	D49.0
labium (skin)	C51.9	C79.82	D07.1	D28.0	D39.8	D49.5
majus	C51.0	C79.82	D07.1	D28.0	D39.8	D49.5
minus	C51.1	C79.82	D07.1	D28.0	D39.8	D49.5
lacrimal						
canaliculi	C69.5-	C79.49	D09.2-	D31.5-	D48.7	D49.89
duct (nasal)	C69.5-	C79.49	D09.2-	D31.5-	D48.7	D49.89
gland	C69.5-	C79.49	D09.2-	D31.5-	D48.7	D49.89
punctum	C69.5-	C79.49	D09.2-	D31.5-	D48.7	D49.89
sac	C69.5-	C79.49	D09.2-	D31.5-	D48.7	D49.89
Langerhans, islands or islets	C25.4	C78.89	D01.7	D13.7	D37.8	D49.0
laryngopharynx	C13.9	C79.89	D00.08	D10.7	D37.05	D49.0
larynx, laryngeal NEC	C32.9	C78.39	D02.0	D14.1	D38.0	D49.1
aryepiglottic fold	C32.1	C78.39	D02.0	D14.1	D38.0	D49.1
cartilage (arytenoid) (cricoid) (cuneiform) (thyroid)	C32.3	C78.39	D02.0	D14.1	D38.0	D49.1
commissure (anterior) (posterior)	C32.0	C78.39	D02.0	D14.1	D38.0	D49.1
extrinsic NEC	C32.1	C78.39	D02.0	D14.1	D38.0	D49.1
meaning hypopharynx	C13.9	C79.89	D00.08	D10.7	D37.05	D49.0
interarytenoid fold	C32.1	C78.39	D02.0	D14.1	D38.0	D49.1
intrinsic	C32.0	C78.39	D02.0	D14.1	D38.0	D49.1
overlapping lesion	C32.8	—	—	—	—	—
ventricular band	C32.1	C78.39	D02.0	D14.1	D38.0	D49.1
leg NEC	C76.5-	C79.89	D04.7-	D36.7	D48.7	D49.89

◀ New ◀ Revised ~~deleted~~ Deleted

TABLE OF NEOPLASMS

TABLE OF NEOPLASMS

	Malignant Primary	Malignant Secondary	Ca in situ	Benign	Uncertain Behavior	Unspecified Behavior
lens, crystalline	C69.4-	C79.49	D09.2-	D31.4-	D48.7	D49.89
lid (lower) (upper)	C44.10-	C79.2	D04.1-	D23.1-	D48.5	D49.2
basal cell carcinoma	C44.11-	—	—	—	—	—
specified type NEC	C44.19-	—	—	—	—	—
squamous cell carcinoma	C44.12-	—	—	—	—	—
ligament — see also Neoplasm, connective tissue						
broad	C57.1	C79.82	D07.39	D28.2	D39.8	D49.5
Mackenrodt's	C57.7	C79.82	D07.39	D28.7	D39.8	D49.5
non-uterine — see Neoplasm, connective tissue						
round	C57.2	C79.82	—	D28.2	D39.8	D49.5
sacro-uterine	C57.3	C79.82	—	D28.2	D39.8	D49.5
uterine	C57.3	C79.82	—	D28.2	D39.8	D49.5
utero-ovarian	C57.7	C79.82	D07.39	D28.2	D39.8	D49.5
uterosacral	C57.3	C79.82	—	D28.2	D39.8	D49.5
limb	C76.8	C79.89	D04.8	D36.7	D48.7	D49.89
lower	C76.5-	C79.89	D04.7-	D36.7	D48.7	D49.89
upper	C76.4-	C79.89	D04.6-	D36.7	D48.7	D49.89
limbus of cornea	C69.1-	C79.49	D09.2-	D31.1-	D48.7	D49.89
lingual NEC — see also Neoplasm, tongue	C02.9	C79.89	D00.07	D10.1	D37.02	D49.0
lingula, lung	C34.1-	C78.0-	D02.2-	D14.3-	D38.1	D49.1
lip	C00.9	C79.89	D00.01	D10.0	D37.01	D49.0
buccal aspect — see Neoplasm, lip, internal						
commissure	C00.6	C79.89	D00.01	D10.0	D37.01	D49.0
external	C00.2	C79.89	D00.01	D10.0	D37.01	D49.0
lower	C00.1	C79.89	D00.01	D10.0	D37.01	D49.0
upper	C00.0	C79.89	D00.01	D10.0	D37.01	D49.0
frenulum — see Neoplasm, lip, internal						
inner aspect — see Neoplasm, lip, internal						
internal	C00.5	C79.89	D00.01	D10.0	D37.01	D49.0
lower	C00.4	C79.89	D00.01	D10.0	D37.01	D49.0
upper	C00.3	C79.89	D00.01	D10.0	D37.01	D49.0
lipstick area	C00.2	C79.89	D00.01	D10.0	D37.01	D49.0
lower	C00.1	C79.89	D00.01	D10.0	D37.01	D49.0
upper	C00.0	C79.89	D00.01	D10.0	D37.01	D49.0
lower	C00.1	C79.89	D00.01	D10.0	D37.01	D49.0
internal	C00.4	C79.89	D00.01	D10.0	D37.01	D49.0
mucosa — see Neoplasm, lip, internal						
oral aspect — see Neoplasm, lip, internal						
overlapping lesion	C00.8	—	—	—	—	—
with oral cavity or pharynx	C14.8	—	—	—	—	—
skin (commissure) (lower) (upper)	C44.00	C79.2	D04.0	D23.0	D48.5	D49.2
basal cell carcinoma	C44.01	—	—	—	—	—
specified type NEC	C44.09	—	—	—	—	—
squamous cell carcinoma	C44.02	—	—	—	—	—

◀ New ◀≣ Revised ~~deleted~~ Deleted

	Malignant Primary	Malignant Secondary	Ca in situ	Benign	Uncertain Behavior	Unspecified Behavior
lip *(Continued)*						
upper	C00.0	C79.89	D00.01	D10.0	D37.01	D49.0
internal	C00.3	C79.89	D00.01	D10.0	D37.01	D49.0
vermilion border	C00.2	C79.89	D00.01	D10.0	D37.01	D49.0
lower	C00.1	C79.89	D00.01	D10.0	D37.01	D49.0
upper	C00.0	C79.89	D00.01	D10.0	D37.01	D49.0
lipomatous — *see Lipoma, by site*						
liver — *see also Index to disease, by histology*	C22.9	C78.7	D01.5	D13.4	D37.6	D49.0
primary	C22.8	C78.7	D01.5	D13.4	D37.6	D49.0
lumbosacral plexus	C47.5	C79.89	—	D36.16	D48.2	D49.2
lung	C34.9-	C78.0-	D02.2-	D14.3-	D38.1	D49.1
azygos lobe	C34.1-	C78.0-	D02.2-	D14.3-	D38.1	D49.1
carina	C34.0-	C78.0-	D02.2-	D14.3-	D38.1	D49.1
hilus	C34.0-	C78.0-	D02.2-	D14.3-	D38.1	D49.1
lingula	C34.1-	C78.0-	D02.2-	D14.3-	D38.1	D49.1
lobe NEC	C34.9-	C78.0-	D02.2-	D14.3-	D38.1	D49.1
lower lobe	C34.3-	C78.0-	D02.2-	D14.3-	D38.1	D49.1
main bronchus	C34.0-	C78.0-	D02.2-	D14.3-	D38.1	D49.1
mesothelioma — *see Mesothelioma*						
middle lobe	C34.2	C78.0-	D02.21	D14.31	D38.1	D49.1
overlapping lesion	C34.8-	—	—	—	—	—
upper lobe	C34.1-	C78.0-	D02.2-	D14.3-	D38.1	D49.1
lymph, lymphatic channel NEC	C49.9	C79.89	—	D21.9	D48.1	D49.2
gland (secondary)	—	C77.9	—	D36.0	D48.7	D49.89
abdominal	—	C77.2	—	D36.0	D48.7	D49.89
aortic	—	C77.2	—	D36.0	D48.7	D49.89
arm	—	C77.3	—	D36.0	D48.7	D49.89
auricular (anterior) (posterior)	—	C77.0	—	D36.0	D48.7	D49.89
axilla, axillary	—	C77.3	—	D36.0	D48.7	D49.89
brachial	—	C77.3	—	D36.0	D48.7	D49.89
bronchial	—	C77.1	—	D36.0	D48.7	D49.89
bronchopulmonary	—	C77.1	—	D36.0	D48.7	D49.89
celiac	—	C77.2	—	D36.0	D48.7	D49.89
cervical	—	C77.0	—	D36.0	D48.7	D49.89
cervicofacial	—	C77.0	—	D36.0	D48.7	D49.89
Cloquet	—	C77.4	—	D36.0	D48.7	D49.89
colic	—	C77.2	—	D36.0	D48.7	D49.89
common duct	—	C77.2	—	D36.0	D48.7	D49.89
cubital	—	C77.3	—	D36.0	D48.7	D49.89
diaphragmatic	—	C77.1	—	D36.0	D48.7	D49.89
epigastric, inferior	—	C77.1	—	D36.0	D48.7	D49.89
epitrochlear	—	C77.3	—	D36.0	D48.7	D49.89
esophageal	—	C77.1	—	D36.0	D48.7	D49.89
face	—	C77.0	—	D36.0	D48.7	D49.89

TABLE OF NEOPLASMS

	Malignant Primary	Malignant Secondary	Ca in situ	Benign	Uncertain Behavior	Unspecified Behavior
lymph, lymphatic channel NEC *(Continued)*						
gland *(Continued)*						
femoral	—	C77.4	—	D36.0	D48.7	D49.89
gastric	—	C77.2	—	D36.0	D48.7	D49.89
groin	—	C77.4	—	D36.0	D48.7	D49.89
head	—	C77.0	—	D36.0	D48.7	D49.89
hepatic	—	C77.2	—	D36.0	D48.7	D49.89
hilar (pulmonary)	—	C77.1	—	D36.0	D48.7	D49.89
splenic	—	C77.2	—	D36.0	D48.7	D49.89
hypogastric	—	C77.5	—	D36.0	D48.7	D49.89
ileocolic	—	C77.2	—	D36.0	D48.7	D49.89
iliac	—	C77.5	—	D36.0	D48.7	D49.89
infraclavicular	—	C77.3	—	D36.0	D48.7	D49.89
inguina, inguinal	—	C77.4	—	D36.0	D48.7	D49.89
innominate	—	C77.1	—	D36.0	D48.7	D49.89
intercostal	—	C77.1	—	D36.0	D48.7	D49.89
intestinal	—	C77.2	—	D36.0	D48.7	D49.89
intrabdominal	—	C77.2	—	D36.0	D48.7	D49.89
intrapelvic	—	C77.5	—	D36.0	D48.7	D49.89
intrathoracic	—	C77.1	—	D36.0	D48.7	D49.89
jugular	—	C77.0	—	D36.0	D48.7	D49.89
leg	—	C77.4	—	D36.0	D48.7	D49.89
limb						
lower	—	C77.4	—	D36.0	D48.7	D49.89
upper	—	C77.3	—	D36.0	D48.7	D49.89
lower limb	—	C77.4	—	D36.0	D48.7	D49.89
lumbar	—	C77.2	—	D36.0	D48.7	D49.89
mandibular	—	C77.0	—	D36.0	D48.7	D49.89
mediastinal	—	C77.1	—	D36.0	D48.7	D49.89
mesenteric (inferior) (superior)	—	C77.2	—	D36.0	D48.7	D49.89
midcolic	—	C77.2	—	D36.0	D48.7	D49.89
multiple sites in categories C77.0 - C77.5	—	C77.8	—	D36.0	D48.7	D49.89
neck	—	C77.0	—	D36.0	D48.7	D49.89
obturator	—	C77.5	—	D36.0	D48.7	D49.89
occipital	—	C77.0	—	D36.0	D48.7	D49.89
pancreatic	—	C77.2	—	D36.0	D48.7	D49.89
para-aortic	—	C77.2	—	D36.0	D48.7	D49.89
paracervical	—	C77.5	—	D36.0	D48.7	D49.89
parametrial	—	C77.5	—	D36.0	D48.7	D49.89
parasternal	—	C77.1	—	D36.0	D48.7	D49.89
parotid	—	C77.0	—	D36.0	D48.7	D49.89
pectoral	—	C77.3	—	D36.0	D48.7	D49.89
pelvic	—	C77.5	—	D36.0	D48.7	D49.89

◀ New ◀▥ Revised ~~deleted~~ Deleted

	Malignant Primary	Malignant Secondary	Ca in situ	Benign	Uncertain Behavior	Unspecified Behavior
lymph, lymphatic channel NEC *(Continued)*						
gland *(Continued)*						
peri-aortic	—	C77.2	—	D36.0	D48.7	D49.89
peripancreatic	—	C77.2	—	D36.0	D48.7	D49.89
popliteal	—	C77.4	—	D36.0	D48.7	D49.89
porta hepatis	—	C77.2	—	D36.0	D48.7	D49.89
portal	—	C77.2	—	D36.0	D48.7	D49.89
preauricular	—	C77.0	—	D36.0	D48.7	D49.89
prelaryngeal	—	C77.0	—	D36.0	D48.7	D49.89
presymphysial	—	C77.5	—	D36.0	D48.7	D49.89
pretracheal	—	C77.0	—	D36.0	D48.7	D49.89
primary (any site) NEC	C96.9	—	—	—	—	—
pulmonary (hiler)	—	C77.1	—	D36.0	D48.7	D49.89
pyloric	—	C77.2	—	D36.0	D48.7	D49.89
retroperitoneal	—	C77.2	—	D36.0	D48.7	D49.89
retropharyngeal	—	C77.0	—	D36.0	D48.7	D49.89
Rosenmuller's	—	C77.4	—	D36.0	D48.7	D49.89
sacral	—	C77.5	—	D36.0	D48.7	D49.89
scalene	—	C77.0	—	D36.0	D48.7	D49.89
site NEC	—	C77.9	—	D36.0	D48.7	D49.89
splenic (hilar)	—	C77.2	—	D36.0	D48.7	D49.89
subclavicular	—	C77.3	—	D36.0	D48.7	D49.89
subinguinal	—	C77.4	—	D36.0	D48.7	D49.89
sublingual	—	C77.0	—	D36.0	D48.7	D49.89
submandibular	—	C77.0	—	D36.0	D48.7	D49.89
submaxillary	—	C77.0	—	D36.0	D48.7	D49.89
submental	—	C77.0	—	D36.0	D48.7	D49.89
subscapular	—	C77.3	—	D36.0	D48.7	D49.89
supraclavicular	—	C77.0	—	D36.0	D48.7	D49.89
thoracic	—	C77.1	—	D36.0	D48.7	D49.89
tibial	—	C77.4	—	D36.0	D48.7	D49.89
tracheal	—	C77.1	—	D36.0	D48.7	D49.89
tracheobronchial	—	C77.1	—	D36.0	D48.7	D49.89
upper limb	—	C77.3	—	D36.0	D48.7	D49.89
Virchow's	—	C77.0	—	D36.0	D48.7	D49.89
node — *see also* Neoplasm, lymph gland						
primary NEC	C96.9	—	—	—	—	—
vessel — *see also* Neoplasm, connective tissue	C49.9	C79.89	—	D21.9	D48.1	D49.2
Mackenrodt's ligament	C57.7	C79.82	D07.39	D28.7	D39.8	D49.5
malar	C41.0	C79.51	—	D16.4-	D48.0	D49.2
region — *see* Neoplasm, cheek						
mammary gland — *see* Neoplasm, breast						

	Malignant Primary	Malignant Secondary	Ca in situ	Benign	Uncertain Behavior	Unspecified Behavior
mandible	C41.1	C79.51	—	D16.5-	D48.0	D49.2
alveolar						
mucosa (carcinoma)	C03.1	C79.89	D00.03	D10.39	D37.09	D49.0
ridge or process	C41.1	C79.51	—	D16.5-	D48.0	D49.2
marrow (bone) NEC	C96.9	C79.52	—	—	D47.9	D49.89
mastectomy site (skin) — see also Neoplasm, breast, skin	C44.501	C79.2	—	—	—	—
specified as breast tissue	C50.8-	C79.81	—	—	—	—
mastoid (air cells) (antrum) (cavity)	C30.1	C78.39	D02.3	D14.0	D38.5	D49.1
bone or process	C41.0	C79.51	—	D16.4-	D48.0	D49.2
maxilla, maxillary (superior)	C41.0	C79.51	—	D16.4-	D48.0	D49.2
alveolar						
mucosa	C03.0	C79.89	D00.03	D10.39	D37.09	D49.0
ridge or process (carcinoma)	C41.0	C79.51	—	D16.4-	D48.0	D49.2
antrum	C31.0	C78.39	D02.3	D14.0	D38.5	D49.1
carcinoma	C03.0	C79.51	—	—	—	—
inferior — see Neoplasm, mandible						
sinus	C31.0	C78.39	D02.3	D14.0	D38.5	D49.1
meatus external (ear) — see also Neoplasm, skin, ear	C44.20-	C79.2	D04.2-	D23.2-	D48.5	D49.2
Meckel diverticulum, malignant	C17.3	C78.4	D01.49	D13.39	D37.2	D49.0
mediastinum, mediastinal	C38.3	C78.1	—	D15.2	D38.3	D49.89
anterior	C38.1	C78.1	—	D15.2	D38.3	D49.89
posterior	C38.2	C78.1	—	D15.2	D38.3	D49.89
medulla						
adrenal	C74.1-	C79.7-	D09.3	D35.0-	D44.1-	D49.7
oblongata	C71.7	C79.31	—	D33.1	D43.1	D49.6
meibomian gland	C44.10-	C79.2	D04.1-	D23.1-	D48.5	D49.2
basal cell carcinoma	C44.11-	—	—	—	—	—
specified type NEC	C44.19-	—	—	—	—	—
squamous cell carcinoma	C44.12-	—	—	—	—	—
melanoma — see Melanoma						
meninges	C70.9	C79.49	—	D32.9	D42.9	D49.7
brain	C70.0	C79.32	—	D32.0	D42.0	D49.7
cerebral	C70.0	C79.32	—	D32.0	D42.0	D49.7
crainial	C70.0	C79.32	—	D32.0	D42.0	D49.7
intracranial	C70.0	C79.32	—	D32.0	D42.0	D49.7
spinal (cord)	C70.1	C79.49	—	D32.1	D42.1	D49.7
meniscus, knee joint (lateral) (medial)	C40.2-	C79.51	—	D16.2-	D48.0	D49.2
Merkel cell — see Carcinoma, Merkel cell						
mesentery, mesenteric	C48.1	C78.6	—	D20.1	D48.4	D49.0
mesoappendix	C48.1	C78.6	—	D20.1	D48.4	D49.0
mesocolon	C48.1	C78.6	—	D20.1	D48.4	D49.0
mesopharynx — see Neoplasm, oropharynx						
mesosalpinx	C57.1	C79.82	D07.39	D28.2	D39.8	D49.5

	Malignant Primary	Malignant Secondary	Ca in situ	Benign	Uncertain Behavior	Unspecified Behavior
mesothelial tissue — *see Mesothelioma*						
mesothelioma — *see Mesothelioma*						
mesovarium	C57.1	C79.82	D07.39	D28.2	D39.8	D49.5
metacarpus (any bone)	C40.1-	C79.51	—	D16.1-	—	—
metastatic NEC — *see also Neoplasm, by site, secondary*	—	C79.9	—	—	—	—
metatarsus (any bone)	C40.3-	C79.51	—	D16.3-	—	—
midbrain	C71.7	C79.31	—	D33.1	D43.1	D49.6
milk duct — *see Neoplasm, breast*						
mons						
pubis	C51.9	C79.82	D07.1	D28.0	D39.8	D49.5
veneris	C51.9	C79.82	D07.1	D28.0	D39.8	D49.5
motor tract	C72.9	C79.49	—	D33.9	D43.9	D49.7
brain	C71.9	C79.31	—	D33.2	D43.2	D49.6
cauda equina	C72.1	C79.49	—	D33.4	D43.4	D49.7
spinal	C72.0	C79.49	—	D33.4	D43.4	D49.7
mouth	C06.9	C79.89	D00.00	D10.30	D37.09	D49.0
book-leaf	C06.89	C79.89	—	—	—	—
floor	C04.9	C79.89	D00.06	D10.2	D37.09	D49.0
anterior portion	C04.0	C79.89	D00.06	D10.2	D37.09	D49.0
lateral portion	C04.1	C79.89	D00.06	D10.2	D37.09	D49.0
overlapping lesion	C04.8	—	—	—	—	—
overlapping NEC	C06.80	—	—	—	—	—
roof	C05.9	C79.89	D00.00	D10.39	D37.09	D49.0
specified part NEC	C06.89	C79.89	D00.00	D10.39	D37.09	D49.0
vestibule	C06.1	C79.89	D00.00	D10.39	D37.09	D49.0
mucosa						
alveolar (ridge or process)	C03.9	C79.89	D00.03	D10.39	D37.09	D49.0
lower	C03.1	C79.89	D00.03	D10.39	D37.09	D49.0
upper	C03.0	C79.89	D00.03	D10.39	D37.09	D49.0
buccal	C06.0	C79.89	D00.02	D10.39	D37.09	D49.0
cheek	C06.0	C79.89	D00.02	D10.39	D37.09	D49.0
lip — *see Neoplasm, lip, internal*						
nasal	C30.0	C78.39	D02.3	D14.0	D38.5	D49.1
oral	C06.0	C79.89	D00.02	D10.39	D37.09	D49.0
Mullerian duct						
female	C57.7	C79.82	D07.39	D28.7	D39.8	D49.5
male	C63.7	C79.82	D07.69	D29.8	D40.8	D49.5
muscle — *see also Neoplasm, connective tissue*						
extraocular	C69.6-	C79.49	D09.2-	D31.6-	D48.7	D49.89
myocardium	C38.0	C79.89	—	D15.1	D48.7	D49.89
myometrium	C54.2	C79.82	D07.0	D26.1	D39.0	D49.5
myopericardium	C38.0	C79.89	—	D15.1	D48.7	D49.89
nabothian gland (follicle)	C53.0	C79.82	D06.0	D26.0	D39.0	D49.5

◀ New   ◀▥ Revised   ~~deleted~~ Deleted

TABLE OF NEOPLASMS

	Malignant Primary	Malignant Secondary	Ca in situ	Benign	Uncertain Behavior	Unspecified Behavior
nail — *see also Neoplasm, skin, limb*	C44.90	C79.2	D04.9	D23.9	D48.5	D49.2
finger — *see also Neoplasm, skin, limb, upper*	C44.60-	C79.2	D04.6-	D23.6-	D48.5	D49.2
toe — *see also Neoplasm, skin, limb, lower*	C44.70-	C79.2	D04.7-	D23.7-	D48.5	D49.2
nares, naris (anterior) (posterior)	C30.0	C78.39	D02.3	D14.0	D38.5	D49.1
nasal — *see Neoplasm, nose*						
nasolabial groove — *see also Neoplasm, skin, face*	C44.309	C79.2	D04.39	D23.39	D48.5	D49.2
nasolacrimal duct	C69.5-	C79.49	D09.2-	D31.5-	D48.7	D49.89
nasopharynx, nasopharyngeal	C11.9	C79.89	D00.08	D10.6	D37.05	D49.0
floor	C11.3	C79.89	D00.08	D10.6	D37.05	D49.0
overlapping lesion	C11.8	—	—	—	—	—
roof	C11.0	C79.89	D00.08	D10.6	D37.05	D49.0
wall	C11.9	C79.89	D00.08	D10.6	D37.05	D49.0
anterior	C11.3	C79.89	D00.08	D10.6	D37.05	D49.0
lateral	C11.2	C79.89	D00.08	D10.6	D37.05	D49.0
posterior	C11.1	C79.89	D00.08	D10.6	D37.05	D49.0
superior	C11.0	C79.89	D00.08	D10.6	D37.05	D49.0
nates — *see also Neoplasm, skin, trunk*	C44.509	C79.2	D04.5	D23.5	D48.5	D49.2
neck NEC	C76.0	C79.89	D09.8	D36.7	D48.7	D49.89
skin	C44.40	—	—	—	—	—
basal cell carcinoma	C44.41	—	—	—	—	—
specified type NEC	C44.49	—	—	—	—	—
squamous cell carcinoma	C44.42	—	—	—	—	—
nerve (ganglion)	C47.9	C79.89	—	D36.10	D48.2	D49.2
abducens	C72.59	C79.49	—	D33.3	D43.3	D49.7
accessory (spinal)	C72.59	C79.49	—	D33.3	D43.3	D49.7
acoustic	C72.4-	C79.49	—	D33.3	D43.3	D49.7
auditory	C72.4-	C79.49	—	D33.3	D43.3	D49.7
autonomic NEC — *see also Neoplasm, nerve, peripheral*	C47.9	C79.89	—	D36.10	D48.2	D49.2
brachial	C47.1-	C79.89	—	D36.12	D48.2	D49.2
cranial	C72.50	C79.49	—	D33.3	D43.3	D49.7
specified NEC	C72.59	C79.49	—	D33.3	D43.3	D49.7
facial	C72.59	C79.49	—	D33.3	D43.3	D49.7
femoral	C47.2-	C79.89	—	D36.13	D48.2	D49.2
ganglion NEC — *see also Neoplasm, nerve, peripheral*	C47.9	C79.89	—	D36.10	D48.2	D49.2
glossopharyngeal	C72.59	C79.49	—	D33.3	D43.3	D49.7
hypoglossal	C72.59	C79.49	—	D33.3	D43.3	D49.7
intercostal	C47.3	C79.89	—	D36.14	D48.2	D49.2
lumbar	C47.6	C79.89	—	D36.17	D48.2	D49.2
median	C47.1-	C79.89	—	D36.12	D48.2	D49.2
obturator	C47.2-	C79.89	—	D36.13	D48.2	D49.2
oculomotor	C72.59	C79.49	—	D33.3	D43.3	D49.7
olfactory	C47.2-	C79.49	—	D33.3	D43.3	D49.7
optic	C72.3-	C79.49	—	D33.3	D43.3	D49.7
parasympathetic NEC	C47.9	C79.89	—	D36.10	D48.2	D49.2

	Malignant Primary	Malignant Secondary	Ca in situ	Benign	Uncertain Behavior	Unspecified Behavior
nerve *(Continued)*						
peripheral NEC	C47.9	C79.89	—	D36.10	D48.2	D49.2
abdomen	C47.4	C79.89	—	D36.15	D48.2	D49.2
abdominal wall	C47.4	C79.89	—	D36.15	D48.2	D49.2
ankle	C47.2-	C79.89	—	D36.13	D48.2	D49.2
antecubital fossa or space	C47.1-	C79.89	—	D36.12	D48.2	D49.2
arm	C47.1-	C79.89	—	D36.12	D48.2	D49.2
auricle (ear)	C47.0	C79.89	—	D36.11	D48.2	D49.2
axilla	C47.3	C79.89	—	D36.12	D48.2	D49.2
back	C47.6	C79.89	—	D36.17	D48.2	D49.2
buttock	C47.5	C79.89	—	D36.16	D48.2	D49.2
calf	C47.2-	C79.89	—	D36.13	D48.2	D49.2
cervical region	C47.0	C79.89	—	D36.11	D48.2	D49.2
cheek	C47.0	C79.89	—	D36.11	D48.2	D49.2
chest (wall)	C47.3	C79.89	—	D36.14	D48.2	D49.2
chin	C47.0	C79.89	—	D36.11	D48.2	D49.2
ear (external)	C47.0	C79.89	—	D36.11	D48.2	D49.2
elbow	C47.1-	C79.89	—	D36.12	D48.2	D49.2
extrarectal	C47.5	C79.89	—	D36.16	D48.2	D49.2
extremity	C47.9	C79.89	—	D36.10	D48.2	D49.2
lower	C47.2-	C79.89	—	D36.13	D48.2	D49.2
upper	C47.1-	C79.89	—	D36.12	D48.2	D49.2
eyelid	C47.0	C79.89	—	D36.11	D48.2	D49.2
face	C47.0	C79.89	—	D36.11	D48.2	D49.2
finger	C47.1-	C79.89	—	D36.12	D48.2	D49.2
flank	C47.6	C79.89	—	D36.17	D48.2	D49.2
foot	C47.2-	C79.89	—	D36.13	D48.2	D49.2
forearm	C47.1-	C79.89	—	D36.12	D48.2	D49.2
forehead	C47.0	C79.89	—	D36.11	D48.2	D49.2
gluteal region	C47.5	C79.89	—	D36.16	D48.2	D49.2
groin	C47.5	C79.89	—	D36.16	D48.2	D49.2
hand	C47.1-	C79.89	—	D36.12	D48.2	D49.2
head	C47.0	C79.89	—	D36.11	D48.2	D49.2
heel	C47.2-	C79.89	—	D36.13	D48.2	D49.2
hip	C47.2-	C79.89	—	D36.13	D48.2	D49.2
infraclavicular region	C47.3	C79.89	—	D36.14	D48.2	D49.2
inguinal (canal) (region)	C47.5	C79.89	—	D36.16	D48.2	D49.2
intrathoracic	C47.3	C79.89	—	D36.14	D48.2	D49.2
ischiorectal fossa	C47.5	C79.89	—	D36.16	D48.2	D49.2
knee	C47.2-	C79.89	—	D36.13	D48.2	D49.2
leg	C47.2-	C79.89	—	D36.13	D48.2	D49.2
limb NEC	C47.9	C79.89	—	D36.10	D48.2	D49.2
lower	C47.2-	C79.89	—	D36.13	D48.2	D49.2
upper	C47.1-	C79.89	—	D36.12	D48.2	D49.2

	Malignant Primary	Malignant Secondary	Ca in situ	Benign	Uncertain Behavior	Unspecified Behavior
nerve *(Continued)*						
peripheral NEC *(Continued)*						
nates	C47.5	C79.89	—	D36.16	D48.2	D49.2
neck	C47.0	C79.89	—	D36.11	D48.2	D49.2
orbit	C69.6-	C79.49	—	D31.6-	D48.7	D49.2
pararectal	C47.5	C79.89	—	D36.16	D48.2	D49.2
paraurethral	C47.5	C79.89	—	D36.16	D48.2	D49.2
paravaginal	C47.5	C79.89	—	D36.16	D48.2	D49.2
pelvis (floor)	C47.5	C79.89	—	D36.16	D48.2	D49.2
pelvoabdominal	C47.8	C79.89		D36.17	D48.2	D49.2
perineum	C47.5	C79.89	—	D36.16	D48.2	D49.2
perirectal (tissue)	C47.5	C79.89	—	D36.16	D48.2	D49.2
periurethral (tissue)	C47.5	C79.89	—	D36.16	D48.2	D49.2
popliteal fossa or space	C47.2-	C79.89	—	D36.13	D48.2	D49.2
presacral	C47.5	C79.89	—	D36.16	D48.2	D49.2
pterygoid fossa	C47.0	C79.89	—	D36.11	D48.2	D49.2
rectovaginal septum or wall	C47.5	C79.89	—	D36.16	D48.2	D49.2
rectovesical	C47.5	C79.89	—	D36.16	D48.2	D49.2
sacrococcygeal region	C47.5	C79.89	—	D36.16	D48.2	D49.2
scalp	C47.0	C79.89	—	D36.11	D48.2	D49.2
scapular region	C47.3	C79.89	—	D36.14	D48.2	D49.2
shoulder	C47.1-	C79.89	—	D36.12	D48.2	D49.2
submental	C47.0	C79.89	—	D36.11	D48.2	D49.2
supraclavicular region	C47.0	C79.89	—	D36.11	D48.2	D49.2
temple	C47.0	C79.89	—	D36.11	D48.2	D49.2
temporal region	C47.0	C79.89	—	D36.11	D48.2	D49.2
thigh	C47.2-	C79.89	—	D36.13	D48.2	D49.2
thoracic (duct) (wall)	C47.3	C79.89	—	D36.14	D48.2	D49.2
thorax	C47.3	C79.89	—	D36.14	D48.2	D49.2
thumb	C47.1-	C79.89	—	D36.12	D48.2	D49.2
toe	C47.2-	C79.89	—	D36.13	D48.2	D49.2
trunk	C47.6	C79.89	—	D36.17	D48.2	D49.2
umbilicus	C47.4	C79.89	—	D36.15	D48.2	D49.2
vesicorectal	C47.5	C79.89	—	D36.16	D48.2	D49.2
wrist	C47.1-	C79.89	—	D36.12	D48.2	D49.2
radial	C47.1-	C79.89	—	D36.12	D48.2	D49.2
sacral	C47.5	C79.89	—	D36.16	D48.2	D49.2
sciatic	C47.2-	C79.89	—	D36.13	D48.2	D49.2
spinal NEC	C47.9	C79.89	—	D36.10	D48.2	D49.2
accessory	C72.59	C79.49	—	D33.3	D43.3	D49.7
sympathetic NEC — *see also Neoplasm, nerve, peripheral*	C47.9	C79.89		D36.10	D48.2	D49.2
trigeminal	C72.59	C79.49	—	D33.3	D43.3	D49.7
trochlear	C72.59	C79.49	—	D33.3	D43.3	D49.7

◀ New ◀▥ Revised ~~deleted~~ Deleted

	Malignant Primary	Malignant Secondary	Ca in situ	Benign	Uncertain Behavior	Unspecified Behavior
nerve *(Continued)*						
ulnar	C47.1-	C79.89	—	D36.12	D48.2	D49.2
vagus	C72.59	C79.49	—	D33.3	D43.3	D49.7
nervous system (central)	C72.9	C79.40	—	D33.9	D43.9	D49.7
autonomic — *see Neoplasm, nerve, peripheral*						
parasympathetic — *see Neoplasm, nerve, peripheral*						
specified site NEC	—	C79.49	—	D33.7	D43.8	—
sympathetic — *see Neoplasm, nerve, peripheral*						
nevus — *see Nevus*						
nipple	C50.0-	C79.81	D05.-	D24.-	—	—
nose, nasal	C76.0	C79.89	D09.8	D36.7	D48.7	D49.89
ala (external) (nasi) — *see also Neoplasm, nose, skin*	C44.301	C79.2	D04.39	D23.39	D48.5	D49.2
bone	C41.0	C79.51	—	D16.4-	D48.0	D49.2
cartilage	C30.0	C78.39	D02.3	D14.0	D38.5	D49.1
cavity	C30.0	C78.39	D02.3	D14.0	D38.5	D49.1
choana	C11.3	C79.89	D00.08	D10.6	D37.05	D49.0
external (skin) — *see also Neoplasm, nose, skin*	C44.301	C79.2	D04.39	D23.39	D48.5	D49.2
fossa	C30.0	C78.39	D02.3	D14.0	D38.5	D49.1
internal	C30.0	C78.39	D02.3	D14.0	D38.5	D49.1
mucosa	C30.0	C78.39	D02.3	D14.0	D38.5	D49.1
septum	C30.0	C78.39	D02.3	D14.0	D38.5	D49.1
posterior margin	C11.3	C79.89	D00.08	D10.6	D37.05	D49.0
sinus — *see Neoplasm, sinus*						
skin	C44.301	C79.2	D04.39	D23.39	D48.5	D49.2
basal cell carcinoma	C44.311	—	—	—	—	—
specified type NEC	C44.391	—	—	—	—	—
squamous cell carcinoma	C44.321	—	—	—	—	—
turbinate (mucosa)	C30.0	C78.39	D02.3	D14.0	D38.5	D49.1
bone	C41.0	C79.51	—	D16.4-	D48.0	D49.2
vestibule	C30.0	C78.39	D02.3	D14.0	D38.5	D49.1
nostril	C30.0	C78.39	D02.3	D14.0	D38.5	D49.1
nucleus pulposus	C41.2	C79.51	—	D16.6	D48.0	D49.2
occipital						
bone	C41.0	C79.51	—	D16.4-	D48.0	D49.2
lobe or pole, brain	C71.4	C79.31	—	D33.0	D43.0	D49.6
odontogenic — *see Neoplasm, jaw bone*						
olfactory nerve or bulb	C72.2-	C79.49	—	D33.3	D43.3	D49.7
olive (brain)	C71.7	C79.31	—	D33.1	D43.1	D49.6
omentum	C48.1	C78.6	—	D20.1	D48.4	D49.0
operculum (brain)	C71.0	C79.31	—	D33.0	D43.0	D49.6
optic nerve, chiasm, or tract	C72.3-	C79.49	—	D33.3	D43.3	D49.7
oral (cavity)	C06.9	C79.89	D00.00	D10.30	D37.09	D49.0
ill-defined	C14.8	C79.89	D00.00	D10.30	D37.09	D49.0
mucosa	C06.0	C79.89	D00.02	D10.39	D37.09	D49.0

◀ New ◀◀ Revised ~~deleted~~ Deleted

TABLE OF NEOPLASMS

	Malignant Primary	Malignant Secondary	Ca in situ	Benign	Uncertain Behavior	Unspecified Behavior
orbit	C69.6-	C79.49	D09.2-	D31.6-	D48.7	D49.89
autonomic nerve	C69.6-	C79.49	—	D31.6-	D48.7	D49.2
bone	C41.0	C79.51	—	D16.4-	D48.0	D49.2
eye	C69.6-	C79.49	D09.2-	D31.6-	D48.7	D49.89
peripheral nerves	C69.6-	C79.49	—	D31.6-	D48.7	D49.2
soft parts	C69.6-	C79.49	D09.2-	D31.6-	D48.7	D49.89
organ of Zuckerkandl	C75.5	C79.89	—	D35.6	D44.7	D49.7
oropharynx	C10.9	C79.89	D00.08	D10.5	D37.05	D49.0
branchial cleft (vestige)	C10.4	C79.89	D00.08	D10.5	D37.05	D49.0
junctional region	C10.8	C79.89	D00.08	D10.5	D37.05	D49.0
lateral wall	C10.2	C79.89	D00.08	D10.5	D37.05	D49.0
overlapping lesion	C10.8	—	—	—	—	—
pillars or fauces	C09.1	C79.89	D00.08	D10.5	D37.05	D49.0
posterior wall	C10.3	C79.89	D00.08	D10.5	D37.05	D49.0
vallecula	C10.0	C79.89	D00.08	D10.5	D37.05	D49.0
os						
external	C53.1	C79.82	D06.1	D26.0	D39.0	D49.5
internal	C53.0	C79.82	D06.0	D26.0	D39.0	D49.5
ovary	C56.-	C79.6-	D07.39	D27.-	D39.1-	D49.5
oviduct	C57.0-	C79.82	D07.39	D28.2	D39.8	D49.5
palate	C05.9	C79.89	D00.00	D10.39	D37.09	D49.0
hard	C05.0	C79.89	D00.05	D10.39	D37.09	D49.0
junction of hard and soft palate	C05.9	C79.89	D00.00	D10.39	D37.09	D49.0
overlapping lesions	C05.8	—	—	—	—	—
soft	C05.1	C79.89	D00.04	D10.39	D37.09	D49.0
nasopharyngeal surface	C11.3	C79.89	D00.08	D10.6	D37.05	D49.0
posterior surface	C11.3	C79.89	D00.08	D10.6	D37.05	D49.0
superior surface	C11.3	C79.89	D00.08	D10.6	D37.05	D49.0
palatoglossal arch	C09.1	C79.89	D00.00	D10.5	D37.09	D49.0
palatopharyngeal arch	C09.1	C79.89	D00.00	D10.5	D37.09	D49.0
pallium	C71.0	C79.31	—	D33.0	D43.0	D49.6
palpebra	C44.10-	C79.2	D04.1-	D23.1-	D48.5	D49.2
basal cell carcinoma	C44.11-	—	—	—	—	—
specified type NEC	C44.19-	—	—	—	—	—
squamous cell carcinoma	C44.12-	—	—	—	—	—
pancreas	C25.9	C78.89	D01.7	D13.6	D37.8	D49.0
body	C25.1	C78.89	D01.7	D13.6	D37.8	D49.0
duct (of Santorini) (of Wirsung)	C25.3	C78.89	D01.7	D13.6	D37.8	D49.0
ectopic tissue	C25.7	C78.89	—	D13.6	D37.8	D49.0
head	C25.0	C78.89	D01.7	D13.6	D37.8	D49.0
islet cells	C25.4	C78.89	D01.7	D13.7	D37.8	D49.0
neck	C25.7	C78.89	D01.7	D13.6	D37.8	D49.0
overlapping lesion	C25.8	—	—	—	—	—
tail	C25.2	C78.89	D01.7	D13.6	D37.8	D49.0

◀ New ◀ Revised ~~deleted~~ Deleted

	Malignant Primary	Malignant Secondary	Ca in situ	Benign	Uncertain Behavior	Unspecified Behavior
para-aortic body	C75.5	C79.89	—	D35.6	D44.7	D49.7
paraganglion NEC	C75.5	C79.89	—	D35.6	D44.7	D49.7
parametrium	C57.3	C79.82	—	D28.2	D39.8	D49.5
paranephric	C48.0	C78.6	—	D20.0	D48.3	D49.0
pararectal	C76.3	C79.89	—	D36.7	D48.7	D49.89
parasagittal (region)	C76.0	C79.89	D09.8	D36.7	D48.7	D49.89
parasellar	C72.9	C79.49	—	D33.9	D43.8	D49.7
parathyroid (gland)	C75.0	C79.89	D09.3	D35.1	D44.2	D49.7
paraurethral	C76.3	C79.89	—	D36.7	D48.7	D49.89
gland	C68.1	C79.19	D09.19	D30.8	D41.8	D49.5
paravaginal	C76.3	C79.89	—	D36.7	D48.7	D49.89
parenchyma, kidney	C64.-	C79.0-	D09.19	D30.0-	D41.0-	D49.5
parietal						
bone	C41.0	C79.51	—	D16.4-	D48.0	D49.2
lobe, brain	C71.3	C79.31	—	D33.0	D43.0	D49.6
paroophoron	C57.1	C79.82	D07.39	D28.2	D39.8	D49.5
parotid (duct) (gland)	C07	C79.89	D00.00	D11.0	D37.030	D49.0
parovarium	C57.1	C79.82	D07.39	D28.2	D39.8	D49.5
patella	C40.20	C79.51	—	—	—	—
peduncle, cerebral	C71.7	C79.31	—	D33.1	D43.1	D49.6
pelvirectal junction	C19	C78.5	D01.1	D12.7	D37.5	D49.0
pelvis, pelvic	C76.3	C79.89	D09.8	D36.7	D48.7	D49.89
bone	C41.4	C79.51	—	D16.8	D48.0	D49.2
floor	C76.3	C79.89	D09.8	D36.7	D48.7	D49.89
renal	C65.-	C79.0-	D09.19	D30.1-	D41.1-	D49.5
viscera	C76.3	C79.89	D09.8	D36.7	D48.7	D49.89
wall	C76.3	C79.89	D09.8	D36.7	D48.7	D49.89
pelvo-abdominal	C76.8	C79.89	D09.8	D36.7	D48.7	D49.89
penis	C60.9	C79.82	D07.4	D29.0	D40.8	D49.5
body	C60.2	C79.82	D07.4	D29.0	D40.8	D49.5
corpus (cavernosum)	C60.2	C79.82	D07.4	D29.0	D40.8	D49.5
glans	C60.1	C79.82	D07.4	D29.0	D40.8	D49.5
overlapping sites	C60.8	—	—	—	—	—
skin NEC	C60.9	C79.82	D07.4	D29.0	D40.8	D49.5
periadrenal (tissue)	C48.0	C78.6	—	D20.0	D48.3	D49.0
perianal (skin) — see also Neoplasm, anus, skin	C44.500	C79.2	D04.5	D23.5	D48.5	D49.2
pericardium	C38.0	C79.89	—	D15.1	D48.7	D49.89
perinephric	C48.0	C78.6	—	D20.0	D48.3	D49.0
perineum	C76.3	C79.89	D09.8	D36.7	D48.7	D49.89
periodontal tissue NEC	C03.9	C79.89	D00.03	D10.39	D37.09	D49.0
periosteum — see Neoplasm, bone						
peripancreatic	C48.0	C78.6	—	D20.0	D48.3	D49.0
peripheral nerve NEC	C47.9	C79.89	—	D36.10	D48.2	D49.2
perirectal (tissue)	C76.3	C79.89	—	D36.7	D48.7	D49.89

	Malignant Primary	Malignant Secondary	Ca in situ	Benign	Uncertain Behavior	Unspecified Behavior
perirenal (tissue)	C48.0	C78.6	—	D20.0	D48.3	D49.0
peritoneum, peritoneal (cavity)	C48.2	C78.6	—	D20.1	D48.4	D49.0
benign mesothelial tissue — *see Mesothelioma, benign*						
overlapping lesion	C48.8	—	—	—	—	—
with digestive organs	C26.9	—	—	—	—	—
parietal	C48.1	C78.6	—	D20.1	D48.4	D49.0
pelvic	C48.1	C78.6	—	D20.1	D48.4	D49.0
specified part NEC	C48.1	C78.6	—	D20.1	D48.4	D49.0
peritonsillar (tissue)	C76.0	C79.89	D09.8	D36.7	D48.7	D49.89
periurethral tissue	C76.3	C79.89		D36.7	D48.7	D49.89
phalanges						
foot	C40.3-	C79.51	—	D16.3-	—	—
hand	C40.1-	C79.51	—	D16.1-	—	—
pharynx, pharyngeal	C14.0	C79.89	D00.08	D10.9	D37.05	D49.0
bursa	C11.1	C79.89	D00.08	D10.6	D37.05	D49.0
fornix	C11.3	C79.89	D00.08	D10.6	D37.05	D49.0
recess	C11.2	C79.89	D00.08	D10.6	D37.05	D49.0
region	C14.0	C79.89	D00.08	D10.9	D37.05	D49.0
tonsil	C11.1	C79.89	D00.08	D10.6	D37.05	D49.0
wall (lateral) (posterior)	C14.0	C79.89	D00.08	D10.9	D37.05	D49.0
pia mater	C70.9	C79.40	—	D32.9	D42.9	D49.7
cerebral	C70.0	C79.32	—	D32.0	D42.0	D49.7
cranial	C70.0	C79.32	—	D32.0	D42.0	D49.7
spinal	C70.1	C79.49	—	D32.1	D42.1	D49.7
pillars of fauces	C09.1	C79.89	D00.08	D10.5	D37.05	D49.0
pineal (body) (gland)	C75.3	C79.89	D09.3	D35.4	D44.5	D49.7
pinna (ear) NEC — *see also Neoplasm, skin, ear*	C44.20-	C79.2	D04.2-	D23.2-	D48.5	D49.2
piriform fossa or sinus	C12	C79.89	D00.08	D10.7	D37.05	D49.0
pituitary (body) (fossa) (gland) (lobe)	C75.1	C79.89	D09.3	D35.2	D44.3	D49.7
placenta	C58	C79.82	D07.0	D26.7	D39.2	D49.5
pleura, pleural (cavity)	C38.4	C78.2	—	D19.0	D38.2	D49.1
overlapping lesion with heart or mediastinum	C38.8	—	—	—	—	—
parietal	C38.4	C78.2	—	D19.0	D38.2	D49.1
visceral	C38.4	C78.2	—	D19.0	D38.2	D49.1
plexus						
brachial	C47.1-	C79.89	—	D36.12	D48.2	D49.2
cervical	C47.0	C79.89	—	D36.11	D48.2	D49.2
choroid	C71.5	C79.31	—	D33.0	D43.0	D49.6
lumbosacral	C47.5	C79.89	—	D36.16	D48.2	D49.2
sacral	C47.5	C79.89	—	D36.16	D48.2	D49.2
pluriendocrine	C75.8	C79.89	D09.3	D35.7	D44.9	D49.7
pole						
frontal	C71.1	C79.31	—	D33.0	D43.0	D49.6
occipital	C71.4	C79.31	—	D33.0	D43.0	D49.6

◀ New   ◀▦ Revised   ~~deleted~~ Deleted

	Malignant Primary	Malignant Secondary	Ca in situ	Benign	Uncertain Behavior	Unspecified Behavior
pons (varolii)	C71.7	C79.31	—	D33.1	D43.1	D49.6
popliteal fossa or space	C76.5-	C79.89	D04.7-	D36.7	D48.7	D49.89
postcricoid (region)	C13.0	C79.89	D00.08	D10.7	D37.05	D49.0
posterior fossa (cranial)	C71.9	C79.31	—	D33.2	D43.2	D49.6
postnasal space	C11.9	C79.89	D00.08	D10.6	D37.05	D49.0
prepuce	C60.0	C79.82	D07.4	D29.0	D40.8	D49.5
prepylorus	C16.4	C78.89	D00.2	D13.1	D37.1	D49.0
presacral (region)	C76.3	C79.89	—	D36.7	D48.7	D49.89
prostate (gland)	C61	C79.82	D07.5	D29.1	D40.0	D49.5
utricle	C68.0	C79.19	D09.19	D30.4	D41.3	D49.5
pterygoid fossa	C49.0	C79.89	—	D21.0	D48.1	D49.2
pubic bone	C41.4	C79.51	—	D16.8	D48.0	D49.2
pudenda, pudendum (femaie)	C51.9	C79.82	D07.1	D28.0	D39.8	D49.5
pulmonary — *see also Neoplasm, lung*	C34.9-	C78.0-	D02.2-	D14.3-	D38.1	D49.1
putamen	C71.0	C79.31	—	D33.0	D43.0	D49.6
pyloric						
antrum	C16.3	C78.89	D00.2	D13.1	D37.1	D49.0
canal	C16.4	C78.89	D00.2	D13.1	D37.1	D49.0
pylorus	C16.4	C78.89	D00.2	D13.1	D37.1	D49.0
pyramid (brain)	C71.7	C79.31	—	D33.1	D43.1	D49.6
pyriform fossa or sinus	C12	C79.89	D00.08	D10.7	D37.05	D49.0
radius (any part)	C40.0-	C79.51	—	D16.0-	—	—
Rathke's pouch	C75.1	C79.89	D09.3	D35.2	D44.3	D49.7
rectosigmoid (junction)	C19	C78.5	D01.1	D12.7	D37.5	D49.0
overlapping lesion with anus or rectum	C21.8	—	—	—	—	—
rectouterine pouch	C48.1	C78.6	—	D20.1	D48.4	D49.0
rectovaginal septum or wall	C76.3	C79.89	D09.8	D36.7	D48.7	D49.89
rectovesical septum	C76.3	C79.89	D09.8	D36.7	D48.7	D49.89
rectum (ampulla)	C20	C78.5	D01.2	D12.8	D37.5	D49.0
and colon	C19	C78.5	D01.1	D12.7	D37.5	D49.0
overlapping lesion with anus or rectosigmoid junction	C21.8	—	—	—	—	—
renal	C64.-	C79.0-	D09.19	D30.0-	D41.0-	D49.5
calyx	C65.-	C79.0-	D09.19	D30.1-	D41.1-	D49.5
hilus	C65.-	C79.0-	D09.19	D30.1-	D41.1-	D49.5
parenchyma	C64.-	C79.0-	D09.19	D30.0-	D41.0-	D49.5
pelvis	C65.-	C79.0-	D09.19	D30.1-	D41.1-	D49.5
respiratory						
organs or system NEC	C39.9	C78.30	D02.4	D14.4	D38.6	D49.1
tract NEC	C39.9	C78.30	D02.4	D14.4	D38.5	D49.1
upper	C39.0	C78.30	D02.4	D14.4	D38.5	D49.1
retina	C69.2-	C79.49	D09.2-	D31.2-	D48.7	D49.81
retrobulbar	C69.6-	C79.49	—	D31.6-	D48.7	D49.89
retrocecal	C48.0	C78.6	—	D20.0	D48.3	D49.0
retromolar (area) (triangle) (trigone)	C06.2	C79.89	D00.00	D10.39	D37.09	D49.0

TABLE OF NEOPLASMS

	Malignant Primary	Malignant Secondary	Ca in situ	Benign	Uncertain Behavior	Unspecified Behavior
retro-orbital	C76.0	C79.89	D09.8	D36.7	D48.7	D49.89
retroperitoneal (space) (tissue)	C48.0	C78.6	—	D20.0	D48.3	D49.0
retroperitoneum	C48.0	C78.6	—	D20.0	D48.3	D49.0
retropharyngeal	C14.0	C79.89	D00.08	D10.9	D37.05	D49.0
retrovesical (septum)	C76.3	C79.89	D09.8	D36.7	D48.7	D49.89
rhinencephalon	C71.0	C79.31	—	D33.0	D43.0	D49.6
rib	C41.3	C79.51	—	D16.7	D48.0	D49.2
Rosenmuller's fossa	C11.2	C79.89	D00.08	D10.6	D37.05	D49.0
round ligament	C57.2	C79.82	—	D28.2	D39.8	D49.5
sacrococcyx, sacrococcygeal	C41.4	C79.51	—	D16.8	D48.0	D49.2
region	C76.3	C79.89	D09.8	D36.7	D48.7	D49.89
sacrouterine ligament	C57.3	C79.82	—	D28.2	D39.8	D49.5
sacrum, sacral (vertebra)	C41.4	C79.51	—	D16.8	D48.0	D49.2
salivary gland or duct (major)	C08.9	C79.89	D00.00	D11.9	D37.039	D49.0
minor NEC	C06.9	C79.89	D00.00	D10.39	D37.04	D49.0
overlapping lesion	C08.9	—	—	—	—	—
parotid	C07	C79.89	D00.00	D11.0	D37.030	D49.0
pluriglandular	C08.9	C79.89	D00.00	D11.9	D37.039	D49.0
sublingual	C08.1	C79.89	D00.00	D11.7	D37.031	D49.0
submandibular	C08.0	C79.89	D00.00	D11.7	D37.032	D49.0
submaxillary	C08.0	C79.89	D00.00	D11.7	D37.032	D49.0
salpinx (uterine)	C57.0-	C79.82	D07.39	D28.2	D39.8	D49.5
Santorini's duct	C25.3	C78.89	D01.7	D13.6	D37.8	D49.0
scalp	C44.40	C79.2	D04.4	D23.4	D48.5	D49.2
basal cell carcinoma	C44.41	—	—	—	—	—
specified type NEC	C44.49	—	—	—	—	—
squamous cell carcinoma	C44.42	—	—	—	—	—
scapula (any part)	C40.0-	C79.51	—	D16.0-	—	—
scapular region	C76.1	C79.89	D09.8	D36.7	D48.7	D49.89
scar NEC — *see also Neoplasm, skin, by site*	C44.90	C79.2	D04.9	D23.9	D48.5	D49.2
sciatic nerve	C47.2-	C79.89	—	D36.13	D48.2	D49.2
sclera	C69.4-	C79.49	D09.2-	D31.4-	D48.7	D49.89
scrotum (skin)	C63.2	C79.82	D07.61	D29.4	D40.8	D49.5
sebaceous gland — *see Neoplasm, skin*						
sella turcica	C75.1	C79.89	D09.3	D35.2	D44.3	D49.7
bone	C41.0	C79.51	—	D16.4-	D48.0	D49.2
semilunar cartilage (knee)	C40.2-	C79.51	—	D16.2-	D48.0	D49.2
seminal vesicle	C63.7	C79.82	D07.69	D29.8	D40.8	D49.5
septum						
nasal	C30.0	C78.39	D02.3	D14.0	D38.5	D49.1
posterior margin	C11.3	C79.89	D00.08	D10.6	D37.05	D49.0
rectovaginal	C76.3	C79.89	D09.8	D36.7	D48.7	D49.89
rectovesical	C76.3	C79.89	D09.8	D36.7	D48.7	D49.89

◀ New   ◀⫶⫶ Revised   ~~deleted~~ Deleted

	Malignant Primary	Malignant Secondary	Ca in situ	Benign	Uncertain Behavior	Unspecified Behavior
septum *(Continued)*						
urethrovaginal	C57.9	C79.82	D07.30	D28.9	D39.9	D49.5
vesicovaginal	C57.9	C79.82	D07.30	D28.9	D39.9	D49.5
shoulder NEC	C76.4-	C79.89	D04.6-	D36.7	D48.7	D49.89
sigmoid flexure (lower) (upper)	C18.7	C78.5	D01.0	D12.5	D37.4	D49.0
sinus (accessory)	C31.9	C78.39	D02.3	D14.0	D38.5	D49.1
bone (any)	C41.0	C79.51	—	D16.4-	D48.0	D49.2
ethmoidal	C31.1	C78.39	D02.3	D14.0	D38.5	D49.1
frontal	C31.2	C78.39	D02.3	D14.0	D38.5	D49.1
maxillary	C31.0	C78.39	D02.3	D14.0	D38.5	D49.1
nasal, paranasal NEC	C31.9	C78.39	D02.3	D14.0	D38.5	D49.1
overlapping lesion	C31.8	—	—	—	—	—
pyriform	C12	C79.89	D00.08	D10.7	D37.05	D49.0
sphenoid	C31.3	C78.39	D02.3	D14.0	D38.5	D49.1
skeleton, skeletal NEC	C41.9	C79.51	—	D16.9-	D48.0	D49.2
Skene's gland	C68.1	C79.19	D09.19	D30.8	D41.8	D49.5
skin NOS	C44.90	C79.2	D04.9	D23.9	D48.5	D49.2
abdominal wall	C44.509	C79.2	D04.5	D23.5	D48.5	D49.2
basal cell carcinoma	C44.519	—	—	—	—	—
specified type NEC	C44.599	—	—	—	—	—
squamous cell carcinoma	C44.529	—	—	—	—	—
ala nasi — *see also Neoplasm, nose, skin*	C44.301	C79.2	D04.39	D23.39	D48.5	D49.2
ankle — *see also Neoplasm, skin, limb, lower*	C44.70-	C79.2	D04.7-	D23.7-	D48.5	D49.2
antecubital space — *see also Neoplasm, skin, limb, upper*	C44.60-	C79.2	D04.6-	D23.6-	D48.5	D49.2
anus	C44.500	C79.2	D04.5	D23.5	D48.5	D49.2
basal cell carcinoma	C44.510	—	—	—	—	—
specified type NEC	C44.590	—	—	—	—	—
squamous cell carcinoma	C44.520	—	—	—	—	—
arm — *see also Neoplasm, skin, limb, upper*	C44.60-	C79.2	D04.6-	D23.6-	D48.5	D49.2
auditory canal (external) — *see also Neoplasm, skin, ear*	C44.20-	C79.2	D04.2-	D23.2-	D48.5	D49.2
auricle (ear) — *see also Neoplasm, skin, ear*	C44.20-	C79.2	D04.2-	D23.2-	D48.5	D49.2
auricular canal (external) — *see also Neoplasm, skin, ear*	C44.20-	C79.2	D04.2-	D23.2-	D48.5	D49.2
axilla, axillary fold — *see also Neoplasm, skin, trunk*	C44.509	C79.2	D04.5	D23.5	D48.5	D49.2
back — *see also Neoplasm, skin, trunk*	C44.509	C79.2	D04.5	D23.5	D48.5	D49.2
basal cell carcinoma	C44.91					
breast	C44.501	C79.2	D04.5	D23.5	D48.5	D49.2
basal cell carcinoma	C44.511	—	—	—	—	—
specified type NEC	C44.591	—	—	—	—	—
squamous cell carcinoma	C44.521	—	—	—	—	—
brow — *see also Neoplasm, skin, face*	C44.309	C79.2	D04.39	D23.39	D48.5	D49.2
buttock — *see also Neoplasm, skin, trunk*	C44.509	C79.2	D04.5	D23.5	D48.5	D49.2
calf — *see also Neoplasm, skin, limb, lower*	C44.70-	C79.2	D04.7-	D23.7-	D48.5	D49.2

TABLE OF NEOPLASMS

TABLE OF NEOPLASMS

	Malignant Primary	Malignant Secondary	Ca in situ	Benign	Uncertain Behavior	Unspecified Behavior
skin NOS *(Continued)*						
canthus (eye) (inner) (outer)	C44.10-	C79.2	D04.1-	D23.1-	D48.5	D49.2
basal cell carcinoma	C44.11-	—	—	—	—	—
specified type NEC	C44.19-	—	—	—	—	—
squamous cell carcinoma	C44.12-	—	—	—	—	—
cervical region — *see also Neoplasm, skin, neck*	C44.40	C79.2	D04.4	D23.4	D48.5	D49.2
cheek (external) — *see also Neoplasm, skin, face*	C44.309	C79.2	D04.39	D23.39	D48.5	D49.2
chest (wall) — *see also Neoplasm, skin, trunk*	C44.509	C79.2	D04.5	D23.5	D48.5	D49.2
chin — *see also Neoplasm, skin, face*	C44.309	C79.2	D04.39	D23.39	D48.5	D49.2
clavicular area — *see also Neoplasm, skin, trunk*	C44.509	C79.2	D04.5	D23.5	D48.5	D49.2
clitoris	C51.2	C79.82	D07.1	D28.0	D39.8	D49.5
columnella — *see also Neoplasm, skin, face*	C44.309	C79.2	D04.39	D23.39	D48.5	D49.2
concha — *see also Neoplasm, skin, ear*	C44.20-	C79.2	D04.2-	D23.2-	D48.5	D49.2
ear (external)	C44.20-	C79.2	D04.2-	D23.2-	D48.5	D49.2
basal cell carcinoma	C44.21-	—	—	—	—	—
specified type NEC	C44.29-	—	—	—	—	—
squamous cell carcinoma	C44.22-	—	—	—	—	—
elbow — *see also Neoplasm, skin, limb, upper*	C44.60-	C79.2	D04.6-	D23.6-	D48.5	D49.2
eyebrow — *see also Neoplasm, skin, face*	C44.309	C79.2	D04.39	D23.39	D48.5	D49.2
eyelid	C44.10-	C79.2	D04.1-	D23.1-	D48.5	D49.2
basal cell carcinoma	C44.11-	—	—	—	—	—
specified type NEC	C44.19-	—	—	—	—	—
squamous cell carcinoma	C44.12-	—	—	—	—	—
face NOS	C44.300	C79.2	D04.30	D23.30	D48.5	D49.2
basal cell carcinoma	C44.310	—	—	—	—	—
specified type NEC	C44.390	—	—	—	—	—
squamous cell carcinoma	C44.320	—	—	—	—	—
female genital organs (external)	C51.9	C79.82	D07.1	D28.0	D39.8	D49.5
clitoris	C51.2	C79.82	D07.1	D28.0	D39.8	D49.5
labium NEC	C51.9	C79.82	D07.1	D28.0	D39.8	D49.5
majus	C51.0	C79.82	D07.1	D28.0	D39.8	D49.5
minus	C51.1	C79.82	D07.1	D28.0	D39.8	D49.5
pudendum	C51.9	C79.82	D07.1	D28.0	D39.8	D49.5
vulva	C51.9	C79.82	D07.1	D28.0	D39.8	D49.5
finger — *see also Neoplasm, skin, limb, upper*	C44.60-	C79.2	D04.6-	D23.6-	D48.5	D49.2
flank — *see also Neoplasm, skin, trunk*	C44.509	C79.2	D04.5	D23.5	D48.5	D49.2
foot — *see also Neoplasm, skin, limb, lower*	C44.70-	C79.2	D04.7-	D23.7-	D48.5	D49.2
forearm — *see also Neoplasm, skin, limb, upper*	C44.60-	C79.2	D04.6-	D23.6-	D48.5	D49.2
forehead — *see also Neoplasm, skin, face*	C44.309	C79.2	D04.39	D23.39	D48.5	D49.2
glabella — *see also Neoplasm, skin, face*	C44.309	C79.2	D04.39	D23.39	D48.5	D49.2
gluteal region — *see also Neoplasm, skin, trunk*	C44.509	C79.2	D04.5	D23.5	D48.5	D49.2
groin — *see also Neoplasm, skin, trunk*	C44.509	C79.2	D04.5	D23.5	D48.5	D49.2
hand — *see also Neoplasm, skin, limb, upper*	C44.60-	C79.2	D04.6-	D23.6-	D48.5	D49.2

◄ New   ◄⫴⫴ Revised   ~~deleted~~ Deleted

	Malignant Primary	Malignant Secondary	Ca in situ	Benign	Uncertain Behavior	Unspecified Behavior
skin NOS *(Continued)*						
head NEC — *see also Neoplasm, skin, scalp*	C44.40	C79.2	D04.4	D23.4	D48.5	D49.2
heel — *see also Neoplasm, skin, limb, lower*	C44.70-	C79.2	D04.7-	D23.7-	D48.5	D49.2
helix — *see also Neoplasm, skin, ear*	C44.20-	C79.2	D04.2-	D23.2-	D48.5	D49.2
hip — *see also Neoplasm, skin, limb, lower*	C44.70-	C79.2	D04.7-	D23.7-	D48.5	D49.2
infraclavicular region — *see also Neoplasm, skin, trunk*	C44.509	C79.2	D04.5	D23.5	D48.5	D49.2
inguinal region — *see also Neoplasm, skin, trunk*	C44.509	C79.2	D04.5	D23.5	D48.5	D49.2
jaw — *see also Neoplasm, skin, face*	C44.309	C79.2	D04.39	D23.39	D48.5	D49.2
Kaposi's sarcoma — *see Kaposi's, sarcoma, skin*						
knee — *see also Neoplasm, skin, limb, lower*	C44.70-	C79.2	D04.7-	D23.7-	D48.5	D49.2
labia						
majora	C51.0	C79.82	D07.1	D28.0	D39.8	D49.5
minora	C51.1	C79.82	D07.1	D28.0	D39.8	D49.5
leg — *see also Neoplasm, skin, limb, lower*	C44.70-	C79.2	D04.7-	D23.7-	D48.5	D49.2
lid (lower) (upper)	C44.10-	C79.2	D04.1-	D23.1-	D48.5	D49.2
basal cell carcinoma	C44.11-	—	—	—	—	—
specified type NEC	C44.19-	—	—	—	—	—
squamous cell carcinoma	C44.12-	—	—	—	—	—
limb NEC	C44.90	C79.2	D04.9	D23.9	D48.5	D49.2
basal cell carcinoma	C44.91					
lower	C44.70-	C79.2	D04.7-	D23.7-	D48.5	D49.2
basal cell carcinoma	C44.71-	—	—	—	—	—
specified type NEC	C44.79-	—	—	—	—	—
squamous cell carcinoma	C44.72-	—	—	—	—	—
upper	C44.60-	C79.2	D04.6-	D23.6-	D48.5	D49.2
basal cell carcinoma	C44.61-	—	—	—	—	—
specified type NEC	C44.69-	—	—	—	—	—
squamous cell carcinoma	C44.62-	—	—	—	—	—
lip (lower) (upper)	C44.00	C79.2	D04.0	D23.0	D48.5	D49.2
basal cell carcinoma	C44.01	—	—	—	—	—
specified type NEC	C44.09	—	—	—	—	—
squamous cell carcinoma	C44.02	—	—	—	—	—
male genital organs	C63.9	C79.82	D07.60	D29.9	D40.8	D49.5
penis	C60.9	C79.82	D07.4	D29.0	D40.8	D49.5
prepuce	C60.0	C79.82	D07.4	D29.0	D40.8	D49.5
scrotum	C63.2	C79.82	D07.61	D29.4	D40.8	D49.5
mastectomy site (skin) — *see also Neoplasm, skin, breast*	C44.501	C79.2	—	—	—	—
specified as breast tissue	C50.8-	C79.81	—	—	—	—
meatus, acoustic (external) — *see also Neoplasm, skin, ear*	C44.20-	C79.2	D04.2-	D23.2-	D48.5	D49.2
melanotic — *see Melanoma*						
Merkel cell — *see Carcinoma, Merkel cell*						
nates — *see also Neoplasm, skin, trunk*	C44.509	C79.2	D04.5	D23.5	D48.5	D49.2

◄ New   ◄▥ Revised   ~~deleted~~ Deleted

TABLE OF NEOPLASMS

	Malignant Primary	Malignant Secondary	Ca in situ	Benign	Uncertain Behavior	Unspecified Behavior
skin NOS *(Continued)*						
neck	C44.40	C79.2	D04.4	D23.4	D48.5	D49.2
basal cell carcinoma	C44.41	—	—	—	—	—
specified type NEC	C44.49	—	—	—	—	—
squamous cell carcinoma	C44.42	—	—	—	—	—
nevus — *see Nevus, skin*						
nose (external) — *see also Neoplasm, nose, skin*	C44.301	C79.2	D04.39	D23.39	D48.5	D49.2
overlapping lesion	C44.80	—	—	—	—	—
basal cell carcinoma	C44.81	—	—	—	—	—
specified type NEC	C44.89	—	—	—	—	—
squamous cell carcinoma	C44.82	—	—	—	—	—
palm — *see also Neoplasm, skin, limb, upper*	C44.60-	C79.2	D04.6-	D23.6-	D48.5	D49.2
palpebra	C44.10-	C79.2	D04.1-	D23.1-	D48.5	D49.2
basal cell carcinoma	C44.11-	—	—	—	—	—
specified type NEC	C44.19-	—	—	—	—	—
squamous cell carcinoma	C44.12-	—	—	—	—	—
penis NEC	C60.9	C79.82	D07.4	D29.0	D40.8	D49.5
perianal — *see also Neoplasm, skin, anus*	C44.500	C79.2	D04.5	D23.5	D48.5	D49.2
perineum — *see also Neoplasm, skin, anus*	C44.500	C79.2	D04.5	D23.5	D48.5	D49.2
pinna — *see also Neoplasm, skin, ear*	C44.20-	C79.2	D04.2-	D23.2-	D48.5	D49.2
plantar — *see also Neoplasm, skin, limb, lower*	C44.70-	C79.2	D04.7-	D23.7-	D48.5	D49.2
popliteal fossa or space — *see also Neoplasm, skin, limb, lower*	C44.70-	C79.2	D04.7-	D23.7-	D48.5	D49.2
prepuce	C60.0	C79.82	D07.4	D29.0	D40.8	D49.5
pubes — *see also Neoplasm, skin, trunk*	C44.509	C79.2	D04.5	D23.5	D48.5	D49.2
sacrococcygeal region — *see also Neoplasm, skin, trunk*	C44.509	C79.2	D04.5	D23.5	D48.5	D49.2
scalp	C44.40	C79.2	D04.4	D23.4	D48.5	D49.2
basal cell carcinoma	C44.41	—	—	—	—	—
specified type NEC	C44.49	—	—	—	—	—
squamous cell carcinoma	C44.42	—	—	—	—	—
scapular region — *see also Neoplasm, skin, trunk*	C44.509	C79.2	D04.5	D23.5	D48.5	D49.2
scrotum	C63.2	C79.82	D07.61	D29.4	D40.8	D49.5
shoulder — *see also Neoplasm, skin, limb, upper*	C44.60-	C79.2	D04.6-	D23.6-	D48.5	D49.2
sole (foot) — *see also Neoplasm, skin, limb, lower*	C44.70-	C79.2	D04.7-	D23.7-	D48.5	D49.2
specified sites NEC	C44.80	C79.2	D04.8	D23.9	D48.5	D49.2
basal cell carcinoma	C44.81	—	—	—	—	—
specified type NEC	C44.89	—	—	—	—	—
squamous cell carcinoma	C44.82	—	—	—	—	—
specified type NEC	C44.99	—	—	—	—	—
squamous cell carcinoma	C44.92	—	—	—	—	—
submammary fold — *see also Neoplasm, skin, trunk*	C44.509	C79.2	D04.5	D23.5	D48.5	D49.2
supraclavicular region — *see also Neoplasm, skin, neck*	C44.40	C79.2	D04.4	D23.4	D48.5	D49.2
temple — *see also Neoplasm, skin, face*	C44.309	C79.2	D04.39	D23.39	D48.5	D49.2
thigh — *see also Neoplasm, skin, limb, lower*	C44.70-	C79.2	D04.7-	D23.7-	D48.5	D49.2
thoracic wall — *see also Neoplasm, skin, trunk*	C44.509	C79.2	D04.5	D23.5	D48.5	D49.2

◀ New   ◀▥ Revised   ~~deleted~~ Deleted

TABLE OF NEOPLASMS

	Malignant Primary	Malignant Secondary	Ca in situ	Benign	Uncertain Behavior	Unspecified Behavior
skin NOS *(Continued)*						
thumb — *see also Neoplasm, skin, limb, upper*	C44.60-	C79.2	D04.6-	D23.6-	D48.5	D49.2
toe — *see also Neoplasm, skin, limb, lower*	C44.70-	C79.2	D04.7-	D23.7-	D48.5	D49.2
tragus — *see also Neoplasm, skin, ear*	C44.20-	C79.2	D04.2-	D23.2-	D48.5	D49.2
trunk	C44.509	C79.2	D04.5	D23.5	D48.5	D49.2
basal cell carcinoma	C44.519	—	—	—	—	—
specified type NEC	C44.599	—	—	—	—	—
squamous cell carcinoma	C44.529	—	—	—	—	—
umbilicus — *see also Neoplasm, skin, trunk*	C44.509	C79.2	D04.5	D23.5	D48.5	D49.2
vulva	C51.9	C79.82	D07.1	D28.0	D39.8	D49.5
overlapping lesion	C51.8	—	—	—	—	—
wrist — *see also Neoplasm, skin, limb, upper*	C44.60-	C79.2	D04.6-	D23.6-	D48.5	D49.2
skull	C41.0	C79.51	—	D16.4-	D48.0	D49.2
soft parts or tissues — *see Neoplasm, connective tissue*						
specified site NEC	C76.8	C79.89	D09.8	D36.7	D48.7	D49.89
spermatic cord	C63.1-	C79.82	D07.69	D29.8	D40.8	D49.5
sphenoid	C31.3	C78.39	D02.3	D14.0	D38.5	D49.1
bone	C41.0	C79.51	—	D16.4-	D48.0	D49.2
sinus	C31.3	C78.39	D02.3	D14.0	D38.5	D49.1
sphincter						
anal	C21.1	C78.5	D01.3	D12.9	D37.8	D49.0
of Oddi	C24.0	C78.89	D01.5	D13.5	D37.6	D49.0
spine, spinal (column)	C41.2	C79.51	—	D16.6	D48.0	D49.2
bulb	C71.7	C79.31	—	D33.1	D43.1	D49.6
coccyx	C41.4	C79.51	—	D16.8	D48.0	D49.2
cord (cervical) (lumbar) (sacral) (thoracic)	C72.0	C79.49	—	D33.4	D43.4	D49.7
dura mater	C70.1	C79.49	—	D32.1	D42.1	D49.7
lumbosacral	C41.2	C79.51	—	D16.6	D48.0	D49.2
marrow NEC	C96.9	C79.52	—	—	D47.9	D49.89
membrane	C70.1	C79.49	—	D32.1	D42.1	D49.7
meninges	C70.1	C79.49	—	D32.1	D42.1	D49.7
nerve (root)	C47.9	C79.89	—	D36.10	D48.2	D49.2
pia mater	C70.1	C79.49	—	D32.1	D42.1	D49.7
root	C47.9	C79.89	—	D36.10	D48.2	D49.2
sacrum	C41.4	C79.51	—	D16.8	D48.0	D49.2
spleen, splenic NEC	C26.1	C78.89	D01.7	D13.9	D37.8	D49.0
flexure (colon)	C18.5	C78.5	D01.0	D12.3	D37.4	D49.0
stem, brain	C71.7	C79.31	—	D33.1	D43.1	D49.6
Stensen's duct	C07	C79.89	D00.00	D11.0	D37.030	D49.0
sternum	C41.3	C79.51	—	D16.7	D48.0	D49.2
stomach	C16.9	C78.89	D00.2	D13.1	D37.1	D49.0
antrum (pyloric)	C16.3	C78.89	D00.2	D13.1	D37.1	D49.0
body	C16.2	C78.89	D00.2	D13.1	D37.1	D49.0
cardia	C16.0	C78.89	D00.2	D13.1	D37.1	D49.0

◀ New   ◀▥ Revised   ~~deleted~~ Deleted

TABLE OF NEOPLASMS

TABLE OF NEOPLASMS

	Malignant Primary	Malignant Secondary	Ca in situ	Benign	Uncertain Behavior	Unspecified Behavior
stomach (Continued)						
cardiac orifice	C16.0	C78.89	D00.2	D13.1	D37.1	D49.0
corpus	C16.2	C78.89	D00.2	D13.1	D37.1	D49.0
fundus	C16.1	C78.89	D00.2	D13.1	D37.1	D49.0
greater curvature NEC	C16.6	C78.89	D00.2	D13.1	D37.1	D49.0
lesser curvature NEC	C16.5	C78.89	D00.2	D13.1	D37.1	D49.0
overlapping lesion	C16.8	—	—	—	—	—
prepylorus	C16.4	C78.89	D00.2	D13.1	D37.1	D49.0
pylorus	C16.4	C78.89	D00.2	D13.1	D37.1	D49.0
wall NEC	C16.9	C78.89	D00.2	D13.1	D37.1	D49.0
anterior NEC	C16.8	C78.89	D00.2	D13.1	D37.1	D49.0
posterior NEC	C16.8	C78.89	D00.2	D13.1	D37.1	D49.0
stroma, endometrial	C54.1	C79.82	D07.0	D26.1	D39.0	D49.5
stump, cervical	C53.8	C79.82	D06.7	D26.0	D39.0	D49.5
subcutaneous (nodule) (tissue) NEC — see Neoplasm, connective tissue						
subdural	C70.9	C79.32	—	D32.9	D42.9	D49.7
subglottis, subglottic	C32.2	C78.39	D02.0	D14.1	D38.0	D49.1
sublingual	C04.9	C79.89	D00.06	D10.2	D37.09	D49.0
gland or duct	C08.1	C79.89	D00.00	D11.7	D37.031	D49.0
submandibular gland	C08.0	C79.89	D00.00	D11.7	D37.032	D49.0
submaxillary gland or duct	C08.0	C79.89	D00.00	D11.7	D37.032	D49.0
submental	C76.0	C79.89	D09.8	D36.7	D48.7	D49.89
subpleural	C34.9-	C78.0-	D02.2-	D14.3-	D38.1	D49.1
substernal	C38.1	C78.1	—	D15.2	D38.3	D49.89
sudoriferous, sudoriparous gland, site unspecified	C44.90	C79.2	D04.9	D23.9	D48.5	D49.2
specified site — see Neoplasm, skin						
supraclavicular region	C76.0	C79.89	D09.8	D36.7	D48.7	D49.89
supraglottis	C32.1	C78.39	D02.0	D14.1	D38.0	D49.1
suprarenal	C74.9-	C79.7-	D09.3	D35.0-	D44.1-	D49.7
capsule	C74.9-	C79.7-	D09.3	D35.0-	D44.1-	D49.7
cortex	C74.0-	C79.7-	D09.3	D35.0-	D44.1-	D49.7
gland	C74.9-	C79.7-	D09.3	D35.0-	D44.1-	D49.7
medulla	C74.1-	C79.7-	D09.3	D35.0-	D44.1-	D49.7
suprasellar (region)	C71.9	C79.31	—	D33.2	D43.2	D49.6
supratentorial (brain) NEC	C71.0	C79.31	—	D33.0	D43.0	D49.6
sweat gland (apocrine) (eccrine), site unspecified	C44.90	C79.2	D04.9	D23.9	D48.5	D49.2
specified site — see Neoplasm, skin						
sympathetic nerve or nervous system NEC	C47.9	C79.89	—	D36.10	D48.2	D49.2
symphysis pubis	C41.4	C79.51	—	D16.8	D48.0	D49.2
synovial membrane — see Neoplasm, connective tissue						
tapetum, brain	C71.8	C79.31	—	D33.2	D43.2	D49.6
tarsus (any bone)	C40.3-	C79.51	—	D16.3-	—	—
temple (skin) — see also Neoplasm, skin, face	C44.309	C79.2	D04.39	D23.39	D48.5	D49.2

◀ New ◀ Revised deleted Deleted

	Malignant Primary	Malignant Secondary	Ca in situ	Benign	Uncertain Behavior	Unspecified Behavior
temporal						
bone	C41.0	C79.51	—	D16.4-	D48.0	D49.2
lobe or pole	C71.2	C79.31	—	D33.0	D43.0	D49.6
region	C76.0	C79.89	D09.8	D36.7	D48.7	D49.89
skin — see also Neoplasm, skin, face	C44.309	C79.2	D04.39	D23.39	D48.5	D49.2
tendon (sheath) — see Neoplasm, connective tissue						
tentorium (cerebelli)	C70.0	C79.32	—	D32.0	D42.0	D49.7
testis, testes	C62.9-	C79.82	D07.69	D29.2-	D40.1-	D49.5
descended	C62.1-	C79.82	D07.69	D29.2-	D40.1-	D49.5
ectopic	C62.0-	C79.82	D07.69	D29.2-	D40.1-	D49.5
retained	C62.0-	C79.82	D07.69	D29.2-	D40.1-	D49.5
scrotal	C62.1-	C79.82	D07.69	D29.2-	D40.1-	D49.5
undescended	C62.0-	C79.82	D07.69	D29.2-	D40.1-	D49.5
unspecified whether descended or undescended	C62.9-	C79.82	D07.69	D29.2-	D40.1-	D49.5
thalamus	C71.0	C79.31	—	D33.0	D43.0	D49.6
thigh NEC	C76.5-	C79.89	D04.7-	D36.7	D48.7	D49.89
thorax, thoracic (cavity) (organs NEC)	C76.1	C79.89	D09.8	D36.7	D48.7	D49.89
duct	C49.3	C79.89	—	D21.3	D48.1	D49.2
wall NEC	C76.1	C79.89	D09.8	D36.7	D48.7	D49.89
throat	C14.0	C79.89	D00.08	D10.9	D37.05	D49.0
thumb NEC	C76.4-	C79.89	D04.6-	D36.7	D48.7	D49.89
thymus (gland)	C37	C79.89	D09.3	D15.0	D38.4	D49.89
thyroglossal duct	C73	C79.89	D09.3	D34	D44.0	D49.7
thyroid (gland)	C73	C79.89	D09.3	D34	D44.0	D49.7
cartilage	C32.3	C78.39	D02.0	D14.1	D38.0	D49.1
tibia (any part)	C40.2-	C79.51	—	D16.2-	—	—
toe NEC	C76.5-	C79.89	D04.7-	D36.7	D48.7	D49.89
tongue	C02.9	C79.89	D00.07	D10.1	D37.02	D49.0
anterior (two-thirds) NEC	C02.3	C79.89	D00.07	D10.1	D37.02	D49.0
dorsal surface	C02.0	C79.89	D00.07	D10.1	D37.02	D49.0
ventral surface	C02.2	C79.89	D00.07	D10.1	D37.02	D49.0
base (dorsal surface)	C01	C79.89	D00.07	D10.1	D37.02	D49.0
border (lateral)	C02.1	C79.89	D00.07	D10.1	D37.02	D49.0
dorsal surface NEC	C02.0	C79.89	D00.07	D10.1	D37.02	D49.0
fixed part NEC	C01	C79.89	D00.07	D10.1	D37.02	D49.0
foreamen cecum	C02.0	C79.89	D00.07	D10.1	D37.02	D49.0
frenulum linguae	C02.2	C79.89	D00.07	D10.1	D37.02	D49.0
junctional zone	C02.8	C79.89	D00.07	D10.1	D37.02	D49.0
margin (lateral)	C02.1	C79.89	D00.07	D10.1	D37.02	D49.0
midline NEC	C02.0	C79.89	D00.07	D10.1	D37.02	D49.0
mobile part NEC	C02.3	C79.89	D00.07	D10.1	D37.02	D49.0
overlapping lesion	C02.8	—	—	—	—	—
posterior (third)	C01	C79.89	D00.07	D10.1	D37.02	D49.0

TABLE OF NEOPLASMS

	Malignant Primary	Malignant Secondary	Ca in situ	Benign	Uncertain Behavior	Unspecified Behavior
tongue *(Continued)*						
root	C01	C79.89	D00.07	D10.1	D37.02	D49.0
surface (dorsal)	C02.0	C79.89	D00.07	D10.1	D37.02	D49.0
base	C01	C79.89	D00.07	D10.1	D37.02	D49.0
ventral	C02.2	C79.89	D00.07	D10.1	D37.02	D49.0
tip	C02.1	C79.89	D00.07	D10.1	D37.02	D49.0
tonsil	C02.4	C79.89	D00.07	D10.1	D37.02	D49.0
tonsil	C09.9	C79.89	D00.08	D10.4	D37.05	D49.0
fauces, faucial	C09.9	C79.89	D00.08	D10.4	D37.05	D49.0
lingual	C02.4	C79.89	D00.07	D10.1	D37.02	D49.0
overlapping sites	C09.8	—	—	—	—	—
palatine	C09.9	C79.89	D00.08	D10.4	D37.05	D49.0
pharyngeal	C11.1	C79.89	D00.08	D10.6	D37.05	D49.0
pillar (anterior) (posterior)	C09.1	C79.89	D00.08	D10.5	D37.05	D49.0
tonsillar fossa	C09.0	C79.89	D00.08	D10.5	D37.05	D49.0
tooth socket NEC	C03.9	C79.89	D00.03	D10.39	D37.09	D49.0
trachea (cartilage) (mucosa)	C33	C78.39	D02.1	D14.2	D38.1	D49.1
overlapping lesion with bronchus or lung	C34.8-	—	—	—	—	—
tracheobronchial	C34.8-	C78.39	D02.1	D14.2	D38.1	D49.1
overlapping lesion with lung	C34.8-	—	—	—	—	—
tragus — *see also Neoplasm, skin, ear*	C44.20-	C79.2	D04.2-	D23.2-	D48.5	D49.2
trunk NEC	C76.8	C79.89	D04.5	D36.7	D48.7	D49.89
tubo-ovarian	C57.8	C79.82	D07.39	D28.7	D39.8	D49.5
tunica vaginalis	C63.7	C79.82	D07.69	D29.8	D40.8	D49.5
turbinate (bone)	C41.0	C79.51	—	D16.4-	D48.0	D49.2
nasal	C30.0	C78.39	D02.3	D14.0	D38.5	D49.1
tympanic cavity	C30.1	C78.39	D02.3	D14.0	D38.5	D49.1
ulna (any part)	C40.0-	C79.51	—	D16.0-	—	—
umbilicus, umbilical — *see also Neoplasm, skin, trunk*	C44.509	C79.2	D04.5	D23.5	D48.5	D49.2
uncus, brain	C71.2	C79.31	—	D33.0	D43.0	D49.6
unknown site or unspecified	C80.1	C79.9	D09.9	D36.9	D48.9	D49.9
urachus	C67.7	C79.11	D09.0	D30.3	D41.4	D49.4
ureter, ureteral	C66.-	C79.19	D09.19	D30.2-	D41.2-	D49.5
orifice (bladder)	C67.6	C79.11	D09.0	D30.3	D41.4	D49.4
ureter-bladder (junction)	C67.6	C79.11	D09.0	D30.3	D41.4	D49.4
urethra, urethral (gland)	C68.0	C79.19	D09.19	D30.4	D41.3	D49.5
orifice, internal	C67.5	C79.11	D09.0	D30.3	D41.4	D49.4
urethrovaginal (septum)	C57.9	C79.82	D07.30	D28.9	D39.8	D49.5
urinary organ or system	C68.9	C79.10	D09.10	D30.9	D41.9	D49.5
bladder — *see Neoplasm, bladder*						
overlapping lesion	C68.8	—	—	—	—	—
specified sites NEC	C68.8	C79.19	D09.19	D30.8	D41.8	D49.5

◄ New ◄▥▥ Revised ~~deleted~~ Deleted

	Malignant Primary	Malignant Secondary	Ca in situ	Benign	Uncertain Behavior	Unspecified Behavior
utero-ovarian	C57.8	C79.82	D07.39	D28.7	D39.8	D49.5
ligament	C57.1	C79.82	D07.39	D28.2	D39.8	D49.5
uterosacral ligament	C57.3	C79.82	—	D28.2	D39.8	D49.5
uterus, uteri, uterine	C55	C79.82	D07.0	D26.9	D39.0	D49.5
adnexa NEC	C57.4	C79.82	D07.39	D28.7	D39.8	D49.5
body	C54.9	C79.82	D07.0	D26.1	D39.0	D49.5
cervix	C53.9	C79.82	D06.9	D26.0	D39.0	D49.5
cornu	C54.9	C79.82	D07.0	D26.1	D39.0	D49.5
corpus	C54.9	C79.82	D07.0	D26.1	D39.0	D49.5
endocervix (canal) (gland)	C53.0	C79.82	D06.0	D26.0	D39.0	D49.5
endometrium	C54.1	C79.82	D07.0	D26.1	D39.0	D49.5
exocervix	C53.1	C79.82	D06.1	D26.0	D39.0	D49.5
external os	C53.1	C79.82	D06.1	D26.0	D39.0	D49.5
fundus	C54.3	C79.82	D07.0	D26.1	D39.0	D49.5
internal os	C53.0	C79.82	D06.0	D26.0	D39.0	D49.5
isthmus	C54.0	C79.82	D07.0	D26.1	D39.0	D49.5
ligament	C57.3	C79.82	—	D28.2	D39.8	D49.5
broad	C57.1	C79.82	D07.39	D28.2	D39.8	D49.5
round	C57.2	C79.82	—	D28.2	D39.8	D49.5
lower segment	C54.0	C79.82	D07.0	D26.1	D39.0	D49.5
myometrium	C54.2	C79.82	D07.0	D26.1	D39.0	D49.5
overlapping sites	C54.8	—	—	—	—	—
squamocolumnar junction	C53.8	C79.82	D06.7	D26.0	D39.0	D49.5
tube	C57.0-	C79.82	D07.39	D28.2	D39.8	D49.5
utricle, prostatic	C68.0	C79.19	D09.19	D30.4	D41.3	D49.5
uveal tract	C69.4-	C79.49	D09.2-	D31.4-	D48.7	D49.89
uvula	C05.2	C79.89	D00.04	D10.39	D37.09	D49.0
vagina, vaginal (fornix) (vault) (wall)	C52	C79.82	D07.2	D28.1	D39.8	D49.5
vaginovesical	C57.9	C79.82	D07.30	D28.9	D39.9	D49.5
septum	C57.9	C79.82	D07.30	D28.9	D39.9	D49.5
vallecula (epigiottis)	C10.0	C79.89	D00.08	D10.5	D37.05	D49.0
vas deferens	C63.1-	C79.82	D07.69	D29.8	D40.8	D49.5
vascular — *see* Neoplasm, connective tissue						
Vater's ampulla	C24.1	C78.89	D01.5	D13.5	D37.6	D49.0
vein, venous — *see* Neoplasm, connective tissue						
vena cava (abdominal) (inferior)	C49.4	C79.89	—	D21.4	D48.1	D49.2
superior	C49.3	C79.89	—	D21.3	D48.1	D49.2
ventricle (cerebral) (floor) (lateral) (third)	C71.5	C79.31	—	D33.0	D43.0	D49.6
cardiac (left) (right)	C38.0	C79.89	—	D15.1	D48.7	D49.89
fourth	C71.7	C79.31	—	D33.1	D43.1	D49.6
ventricular band of larynx	C32.1	C78.39	D02.0	D14.1	D38.0	D49.1
ventriculus — *see* Neoplasm, stomach						

TABLE OF NEOPLASMS

◀ New ◀▭ Revised ~~deleted~~ Deleted

	Malignant Primary	Malignant Secondary	Ca in situ	Benign	Uncertain Behavior	Unspecified Behavior
vermillion border — *see Neoplasm, lip*						
vermis, cerebellum	C71.6	C79.31	—	D33.1	D43.1	D49.6
vertebra (column)	C41.2	C79.51	—	D16.6	D48.0	D49.2
coccyx	C41.4	C79.51	—	D16.8-	D48.0	D49.2
marrow NEC	C96.9	C79.52	—	—	D47.9	D49.89
sacrum	C41.4	C79.51	—	D16.8-	D48.0	D49.2
vesical — *see Neoplasm, bladder*						
vesicle, seminal	C63.7	C79.82	D07.69	D29.8	D40.8	D49.5
vesicocervical tissue	C57.9	C79.82	D07.30	D28.9	D39.9	D49.5
vesicorectal	C76.3	C79.82	D09.8	D36.7	D48.7	D49.89
vesicovaginal	C57.9	C79.82	D07.30	D28.9	D39.9	D49.5
septum	C57.9	C79.82	D07.30	D28.9	D39.8	D49.5
vessel (blood) — *see Neoplasm, connective tissue*						
vestibular gland, greater	C51.0	C79.82	D07.1	D28.0	D39.8	D49.5
vestibule						
mouth	C06.1	C79.89	D00.00	D10.39	D37.09	D49.0
nose	C30.0	C78.39	D02.3	D14.0	D38.5	D49.1
Virchow's gland	C77.0	C77.0	—	D36.0	D48.7	D49.89
viscera NEC	C76.8	C79.89	D09.8	D36.7	D48.7	D49.89
vocal cords (true)	C32.0	C78.39	D02.0	D14.1	D38.0	D49.1
false	C32.1	C78.39	D02.0	D14.1	D38.0	D49.1
vomer	C41.0	C79.51	—	D16.4-	D48.0	D49.2
vulva	C51.9	C79.82	D07.1	D28.0	D39.8	D49.5
vulvovaginal gland	C51.0	C79.82	D07.1	D28.0	D39.8	D49.5
Waldeyer's ring	C14.2	C79.89	D00.08	D10.9	D37.05	D49.0
Wharton's duct	C08.0	C79.89	D00.00	D11.7	D37.032	D49.0
white matter (central) (cerebral)	C71.0	C79.31	—	D33.0	D43.0	D49.6
windpipe	C33	C78.39	D02.1	D14.2	D38.1	D49.1
Wirsung's duct	C25.3	C78.89	D01.7	D13.6	D37.8	D49.0
wolffian (body) (duct)						
female	C57.7	C79.82	D07.39	D28.7	D39.8	D49.5
male	C63.7	C79.82	D07.69	D29.8	D40.8	D49.5
womb — *see Neoplasm, uterus*						
wrist NEC	C76.4-	C79.89	D04.6-	D36.7	D48.7	D49.89
xiphoid process	C41.3	C79.51	—	D16.7	D48.0	D49.2
Zuckerkandl organ	C75.5	C79.89	—	D35.6	D44.7	D49.7

◀ New ◀▮▮ Revised ~~deleted~~ Deleted

Substance	External Cause (T-Code)					
	Poisoning, Accidental (Unintentional)	Poisoning, Intentional Self-Harm	Poisoning, Assault	Poisoning, Undetermined	Adverse Effect	Underdosing
#						
1-propanol	T51.3X1	T51.3X2	T51.3X3	T51.3X4	—	—
2-propanol	T51.2X1	T51.2X2	T51.2X3	T51.2X4	—	—
2,4-D (dichlorophen-oxyacetic acid)	T60.3X1	T60.3X2	T60.3X3	T60.3X4	—	—
2,4-toluene diisocyanate	T65.0X1	T65.0X2	T65.0X3	T65.0X4	—	—
2,4,5-T (trichloro-phenoxyacetic acid)	T60.1X1	T60.1X2	T60.1X3	T60.1X4	—	—
14-hydroxydihydro-morphinone	T40.2X1	T40.2X2	T40.2X3	T40.2X4	T40.2X5	T40.2X6
A						
ABOB	T37.5X1	T37.5X2	T37.5X3	T37.5X4	T37.5X5	T37.5X6
Abrine	T62.2X1	T62.2X2	T62.2X3	T62.2X4	—	—
Abrus (seed)	T62.2X1	T62.2X2	T62.2X3	T62.2X4	—	—
Absinthe	T51.0X1	T51.0X2	T51.0X3	T51.0X4	—	—
beverage	T51.0X1	T51.0X2	T51.0X3	T51.0X4	—	—
Acaricide	T60.8X1	T60.8X2	T60.8X3	T60.8X4	—	—
Acebutolol	T44.7X1	T44.7X2	T44.7X3	T44.7X4	T44.7X5	T44.7X6
Acecarbromal	T42.6X1	T42.6X2	T42.6X3	T42.6X4	T42.6X5	T42.6X6
Aceclidine	T44.1X1	T44.1X2	T44.1X3	T44.1X4	T44.1X5	T44.1X6
Acedapsone	T37.0X1	T37.0X2	T37.0X3	T37.0X4	T37.0X5	T37.0X6
Acefylline piperazine	T48.6X1	T48.6X2	T48.6X3	T48.6X4	T48.6X5	T48.6X6
Acemorphan	T40.2X1	T40.2X2	T40.2X3	T40.2X4	T40.2X5	T40.2X6
Acenocoumarin	T45.511	T45.512	T45.513	T45.514	T45.515	T45.516
Acenocoumarol	T45.511	T45.512	T45.513	T45.514	T45.515	T45.516
Acepifylline	T48.6X1	T48.6X2	T48.6X3	T48.6X4	T48.6X5	T48.6X6
Acepromazine	T43.3X1	T43.3X2	T43.3X3	T43.3X4	T43.3X5	T43.3X6
Acesulfamethoxypyridazine	T37.0X1	T37.0X2	T37.0X3	T37.0X4	T37.0X5	T37.0X6
Acetal	T52.8X1	T52.8X2	T52.8X3	T52.8X4	—	—
Acetaldehyde (vapor)	T52.8X1	T52.8X2	T52.8X3	T52.8X4	—	—
liquid	T65.891	T65.892	T65.893	T65.894	—	—
P-Acetamidophenol	T39.1X1	T39.1X2	T39.1X3	T39.1X4	T39.1X5	T39.1X6
Acetaminophen	T39.1X1	T39.1X2	T39.1X3	T39.1X4	T39.1X5	T39.1X6
Acetaminosalol	T39.1X1	T39.1X2	T39.1X3	T39.1X4	T39.1X5	T39.1X6
Acetanilide	T39.1X1	T39.1X2	T39.1X3	T39.1X4	T39.1X5	T39.1X6
Acetarsol	T37.3X1	T37.3X2	T37.3X3	T37.3X4	T37.3X5	T37.3X6
Acetazolamide	T50.2X1	T50.2X2	T50.2X3	T50.2X4	T50.2X5	T50.2X6
Acetiamine	T45.2X1	T45.2X2	T45.2X3	T45.2X4	T45.2X5	T45.2X6
Acetic						
acid	T54.2X1	T54.2X2	T54.2X3	T54.2X4	—	—
with sodium acetate (ointment)	T49.3X1	T49.3X2	T49.3X3	T49.3X4	T49.3X5	T49.3X6
ester (solvent) (vapor)	T52.8X1	T52.8X2	T52.8X3	T52.8X4	—	—

◀ New ◀▥ Revised ~~deleted~~ Deleted

Substance	External Cause (T-Code)					
	Poisoning, Accidental (Unintentional)	Poisoning, Intentional Self-Harm	Poisoning, Assault	Poisoning, Undetermined	Adverse Effect	Underdosing
Acetic *(Continued)*						
acid *(Continued)*						
irrigating solution	T50.3X1	T50.3X2	T50.3X3	T50.3X4	T50.3X5	T50.3X6
medicinal (lotion)	T49.2X1	T49.2X2	T49.2X3	T49.2X4	T49.2X5	T49.2X6
anhydride	T65.891	T65.892	T65.893	T65.894	—	—
ether (vapor)	T52.8X1	T52.8X2	T52.8X3	T52.8X4	—	—
Acetohexamide	T38.3X1	T38.3X2	T38.3X3	T38.3X4	T38.3X5	T38.3X6
Acetohydroxamic acid	T50.991	T50.992	T50.993	T50.994	T50.995	T50.996
Acetomenaphthone	T45.7X1	T45.7X2	T45.7X3	T45.7X4	T45.7X5	T45.7X6
Acetomorphine	T40.1X1	T40.1X2	T40.1X3	T40.1X4	—	—
Acetone (oils)	T52.4X1	T52.4X2	T52.4X3	T52.4X4	—	—
chlorinated	T52.4X1	T52.4X2	T52.4X3	T52.4X4	—	—
vapor	T52.4X1	T52.4X2	T52.4X3	T52.4X4	—	—
Acetonitrile	T52.8X1	T52.8X2	T52.8X3	T52.8X4	—	—
Acetophenazine	T43.3X1	T43.3X2	T43.3X3	T43.3X4	T43.3X5	T43.3X6
Acetophenetedin	T39.1X1	T39.1X2	T39.1X3	T39.1X4	T39.1X5	T39.1X6
Acetophenone	T52.4X1	T52.4X2	T52.4X3	T52.4X4	—	—
Acetorphine	T40.2X1	T40.2X2	T40.2X3	T40.2X4	—	—
Acetosulfone (sodium)	T37.1X1	T37.1X2	T37.1X3	T37.1X4	T37.1X5	T37.1X6
Acetrizoate (sodium)	T50.8X1	T50.8X2	T50.8X3	T50.8X4	T50.8X5	T50.8X6
Acetylcarbromal	T42.6X1	T42.6X2	T42.6X3	T42.6X4	T42.6X5	T42.6X6
Acetrizoic acid	T50.8X1	T50.8X2	T50.8X3	T50.8X4	T50.8X5	T50.8X6
Acetyl						
bromide	T53.6X1	T53.6X2	T53.6X3	T53.6X4	—	—
chloride	T53.6X1	T53.6X2	T53.6X3	T53.6X4	—	—
Acetylcholine						
chloride	T44.1X1	T44.1X2	T44.1X3	T44.1X4	T44.1X5	T44.1X6
derivative	T44.1X1	T44.1X2	T44.1X3	T44.1X4	T44.1X5	T44.1X6
Acetylcysteine	T48.4X1	T48.4X2	T48.4X3	T48.4X4	T48.4X5	T48.4X6
Acetyldigitoxin	T46.0X1	T46.0X2	T46.0X3	T46.0X4	T46.0X5	T46.0X6
Acetyldigoxin	T46.0X1	T46.0X2	T46.0X3	T46.0X4	T46.0X5	T46.0X6
Acetyldihydrocodeine	T40.2X1	T40.2X2	T40.2X3	T40.2X4	—	—
Acetyldihydrocodeinone	T40.2X1	T40.2X2	T40.2X3	T40.2X4	—	—
Acetylene (gas)	T59.891	T59.892	T59.893	T59.894	—	—
dichloride	T53.6X1	T53.6X2	T53.6X3	T53.6X4	—	—
incomplete combustion of	T58.11	T58.12	T58.13	T58.14	—	—
industrial	T59.891	T59.892	T59.893	T59.894	—	—
tetrachloride	T53.6X1	T53.6X2	T53.6X3	T53.6X4	—	—
vapor	T53.6X1	T53.6X2	T53.6X3	T53.6X4	—	—
Acetylphenylhydrazine	T39.8X1	T39.8X2	T39.8X3	T39.8X4	T39.8X5	T39.8X6

◀ New ◀▥ Revised ~~deleted~~ Deleted

Substance	External Cause (T-Code)					
	Poisoning, Accidental (Unintentional)	Poisoning, Intentional Self-Harm	Poisoning, Assault	Poisoning, Undetermined	Adverse Effect	Underdosing
Acetylpheneturide	T42.6X1	T42.6X2	T42.6X3	T42.6X4	T42.6X5	T42.6X6
Acetylsalicylic acid (salts)	T39.011	T39.012	T39.013	T39.014	T39.015	T39.016
enteric coated	T39.011	T39.012	T39.013	T39.014	T39.015	T39.016
Acetylsulfamethoxypyridazine	T37.0X1	T37.0X2	T37.0X3	T37.0X4	T37.0X5	T37.0X6
Achromycin	T36.4X1	T36.4X2	T36.4X3	T36.4X4	T36.4X5	T36.4X6
ophthalmic preparation	T49.5X1	T49.5X2	T49.5X3	T49.5X4	T49.5X5	T49.5X6
topical NEC	T49.0X1	T49.0X2	T49.0X3	T49.0X4	T49.0X5	T49.0X6
Aciclovir	T37.5X1	T37.5X2	T37.5X3	T37.5X4	T37.5X5	T37.5X6
Acid (corrosive) NEC	T54.2X1	T54.2X2	T54.2X3	T54.2X4	—	—
Acidifying agent NEC	T50.901	T50.902	T50.903	T50.904	T50.905	T50.906
Acipimox	T46.6X1	T46.6X2	T46.6X3	T46.6X4	T46.6X5	T46.6X6
Acitretin	T50.991	T50.992	T50.993	T50.994	T50.995	T50.996
Aclarubicin	T45.1X1	T45.1X2	T45.1X3	T45.1X4	T45.1X5	T45.1X6
Aclatonium napadisilate	T48.1X1	T48.1X2	T48.1X3	T48.1X4	T48.1X5	T48.1X6
Aconite (wild)	T46.991	T46.992	T46.993	T46.994	T46.995	T46.996
Aconitine	T46.991	T46.992	T46.993	T46.994	T46.995	T46.996
Aconitum ferox	T46.991	T46.992	T46.993	T46.994	T46.995	T46.996
Acridine	T65.6X1	T65.6X2	T65.6X3	T65.6X4	—	—
vapor	T59.891	T59.892	T59.893	T59.894	—	—
Acriflavine	T37.91	T37.92	T37.93	T37.94	T37.95	T37.96
Acriflavinium chloride	T49.0X1	T49.0X2	T49.0X3	T49.0X4	T49.0X5	T49.0X6
Acrinol	T49.0X1	T49.0X2	T49.0X3	T49.0X4	T49.0X5	T49.0X6
Acrisorcin	T49.0X1	T49.0X2	T49.0X3	T49.0X4	T49.0X5	T49.0X6
Acrivastine	T45.0X1	T45.0X2	T45.0X3	T45.0X4	T45.0X5	T45.0X6
Acrolein (gas)	T59.891	T59.892	T59.893	T59.894	—	—
liquid	T54.1X1	T54.1X2	T54.1X3	T54.1X4	—	—
Acrylamide	T65.891	T65.892	T65.893	T65.894	—	—
Acrylic resin	T49.3X1	T49.3X2	T49.3X3	T49.3X4	T49.3X5	T49.3X6
Acrylonitrile	T65.891	T65.892	T65.893	T65.894	—	—
Actaea spicata	T62.2X1	T62.2X2	T62.2X3	T62.2X4	—	—
berry	T62.1X1	T62.1X2	T62.1X3	T62.1X4	—	—
Acterol	T37.3X1	T37.3X2	T37.3X3	T37.3X4	T37.3X5	T37.3X6
ACTH	T38.811	T38.812	T38.813	T38.814	T38.815	T38.816
Actinomycin C	T45.1X1	T45.1X2	T45.1X3	T45.1X4	T45.1X5	T45.1X6
Actinomycin D	T45.1X1	T45.1X2	T45.1X3	T45.1X4	T45.1X5	T45.1X6
Activated charcoal — *see also Charcoal, medicinal*	T47.6X1	T47.6X2	T47.6X3	T47.6X4	T47.6X5	T47.6X6
Acyclovir	T37.5X1	T37.5X2	T37.5X3	T37.5X4	T37.5X5	T37.5X6
Adenine	T45.2X1	T45.2X2	T45.2X3	T45.2X4	T45.2X5	T45.2X6
arabinoside	T37.5X1	T37.5X2	T37.5X3	T37.5X4	T37.5X5	T37.5X6
Adenosine (phosphate)	T46.2X1	T46.2X2	T46.2X3	T46.2X4	T46.2X5	T46.2X6

TABLE OF DRUGS AND CHEMICALS

◀ New   ◀‖‖ Revised   ~~deleted~~ Deleted

TABLE OF DRUGS AND CHEMICALS

Substance	External Cause (T-Code)					
	Poisoning, Accidental (Unintentional)	Poisoning, Intentional Self-Harm	Poisoning, Assault	Poisoning, Undetermined	Adverse Effect	Underdosing
ADH	T38.891	T38.892	T38.893	T38.894	T38.895	T38.896
Adhesive NEC	T65.891	T65.892	T65.893	T65.894	—	—
Adicillin	T36.0X1	T36.0X2	T36.0X3	T36.0X4	T36.0X5	T36.0X6
Adiphenine	T44.3X1	T44.3X2	T44.3X3	T44.3X4	T44.3X5	T44.3X6
Adipiodone	T50.8X1	T50.8X2	T50.8X3	T50.8X4	T50.8X5	T50.8X6
Adjunct, pharmaceutical	T50.901	T50.902	T50.903	T50.904	T50.905	T50.906
Adrenal (extract, cortex or medulla) (glucocorticoids) (hormones) (mineralocorticoids)	T38.0X1	T38.0X2	T38.0X3	T38.0X4	T38.0X5	T38.0X6
ENT agent	T49.6X1	T49.6X2	T49.6X3	T49.6X4	T49.6X5	T49.6X6
ophthalmic preparation	T49.5X1	T49.5X2	T49.5X3	T49.5X4	T49.5X5	T49.5X6
topical NEC	T49.0X1	T49.0X2	T49.0X3	T49.0X4	T49.0X5	T49.0X6
Adrenaline	T44.5X1	T44.5X2	T44.5X3	T44.5X4	T44.5X5	T44.5X6
Adrenalin — *see Adrenaline*						
Adrenergic NEC	T44.901	T44.902	T44.903	T44.904	T44.905	T44.906
blocking agent NEC	T44.8X1	T44.8X2	T44.8X3	T44.8X4	T44.8X5	T44.8X6
beta, heart	T44.7X1	T44.7X2	T44.7X3	T44.7X4	T44.7X5	T44.7X6
specified NEC	T44.991	T44.992	T44.993	T44.994	T44.995	T44.996
Adrenochrome						
(mono) semicarbazone	T46.991	T46.992	T46.993	T46.994	T46.995	T46.996
derivative	T46.991	T46.992	T46.993	T46.994	T46.995	T46.996
Adrenocorticotrophic hormone	T38.811	T38.812	T38.813	T38.814	T38.815	T38.816
Adrenocorticotrophin	T38.811	T38.812	T38.813	T38.814	T38.815	T38.816
Adriamycin	T45.1X1	T45.1X2	T45.1X3	T45.1X4	T45.1X5	T45.1X6
Aerosol spray NEC	T65.91	T65.92	T65.93	T65.94	—	—
Aerosporin	T36.8X1	T36.8X2	T36.8X3	T36.8X4	T36.8X5	T36.8X6
ENT agent	T49.6X1	T49.6X2	T49.6X3	T49.6X4	T49.6X5	T49.6X6
ophthalmic preparation	T49.5X1	T49.5X2	T49.5X3	T49.5X4	T49.5X5	T49.5X6
topical NEC	T49.0X1	T49.0X2	T49.0X3	T49.0X4	T49.0X5	T49.0X6
Aethusa cynapium	T62.2X1	T62.2X2	T62.2X3	T62.2X4	—	—
Afghanistan black	T40.7X1	T40.7X2	T40.7X3	T40.7X4	T40.7X5	T40.7X6
Aflatoxin	T64.01	T64.02	T64.03	T64.04	—	—
Afloqualone	T42.8X1	T42.8X2	T42.8X3	T42.8X4	T42.8X5	T42.8X6
African boxwood	T62.2X1	T62.2X2	T62.2X3	T62.2X4	—	—
Agar	T47.4X1	T47.4X2	T47.4X3	T47.4X4	T47.4X5	T47.4X6
Agonist						
predominantly						
alpha-adrenoreceptor	T44.4X1	T44.4X2	T44.4X3	T44.4X4	T44.4X5	T44.4X6
beta-adrenoreceptor	T44.5X1	T44.5X2	T44.5X3	T44.5X4	T44.5X5	T44.5X6
Agricultural agent NEC	T65.91	T65.92	T65.93	T65.94	—	—
Agrypnal	T42.3X1	T42.3X2	T42.3X3	T42.3X4	T42.3X5	T42.3X6

◀ New   ◀▥ Revised   ~~deleted~~ Deleted

Substance	Poisoning, Accidental (Unintentional)	Poisoning, Intentional Self-Harm	Poisoning, Assault	Poisoning, Undetermined	Adverse Effect	Underdosing
			External Cause (T-Code)			
AHLG	T50.Z11	T50.Z12	T50.Z13	T50.Z14	T50.Z15	T50.Z16
Air contaminant(s), source/type NOS	T65.91	T65.92	T65.93	T65.94	—	—
Ajmaline	T46.2X1	T46.2X2	T46.2X3	T46.2X4	T46.2X5	T46.2X6
Akritoin	T37.8X1	T37.8X2	T37.8X3	T37.8X4	T37.8X5	T37.8X6
Akee	T62.1X1	T62.1X2	T62.1X3	T62.1X4	—	—
Akrinol	T49.0X1	T49.0X2	T49.0X3	T49.0X4	T49.0X5	T49.0X6
Alacepril	T46.4X1	T46.4X2	T46.4X3	T46.4X4	T46.4X5	T46.4X6
Alantolactone	T37.4X1	T37.4X2	T37.4X3	T37.4X4	T37.4X5	T37.4X6
Albamycin	T36.8X1	T36.8X2	T36.8X3	T36.8X4	T36.8X5	T36.8X6
Albendazole	T37.4X1	T37.4X2	T37.4X3	T37.4X4	T37.4X5	T37.4X6
Albumin						
bovine	T45.8X1	T45.8X2	T45.8X3	T45.8X4	T45.8X5	T45.8X6
human serum	T45.8X1	T45.8X2	T45.8X3	T45.8X4	T45.8X5	T45.8X6
salt-poor	T45.8X1	T45.8X2	T45.8X3	T45.8X4	T45.8X5	T45.8X6
normal human serum	T45.8X1	T45.8X2	T45.8X3	T45.8X4	T45.8X5	T45.8X6
Albuterol	T48.6X1	T48.6X2	T48.6X3	T48.6X4	T48.6X5	T48.6X6
Albutoin	T42.0X1	T42.0X2	T42.0X3	T42.0X4	T42.0X5	T42.0X6
Alclometasone	T49.0X1	T49.0X2	T49.0X3	T49.0X4	T49.0X5	T49.0X6
Alcohol	T51.91	T51.92	T51.93	T51.94	—	—
absolute	T51.0X1	T51.0X2	T51.0X3	T51.0X4	—	—
beverage	T51.0X1	T51.0X2	T51.0X3	T51.0X4	—	—
allyl	T51.8X1	T51.8X2	T51.8X3	T51.8X4	—	—
amyl	T51.3X1	T51.3X2	T51.3X3	T51.3X4	—	—
antifreeze	T51.1X1	T51.1X2	T51.1X3	T51.1X4	—	—
beverage	T51.0X1	T51.0X2	T51.0X3	T51.0X4	—	—
butyl	T51.3X1	T51.3X2	T51.3X3	T51.3X4	—	—
dehydrated	T51.0X1	T51.0X2	T51.0X3	T51.0X4	—	—
beverage	T51.0X1	T51.0X2	T51.0X3	T51.0X4	—	—
denatured	T51.0X1	T51.0X2	T51.0X3	T51.0X4	—	—
deterrent NEC	T50.6X1	T50.6X2	T50.6X3	T50.6X4	T50.6X5	T50.6X6
diagnostic (gastric function)	T50.8X1	T50.8X2	T50.8X3	T50.8X4	T50.8X5	T50.8X6
ethyl	T51.0X1	T51.0X2	T51.0X3	T51.0X4	—	—
beverage	T51.0X1	T51.0X2	T51.0X3	T51.0X4	—	—
grain	T51.0X1	T51.0X2	T51.0X3	T51.0X4	—	—
beverage	T51.0X1	T51.0X2	T51.0X3	T51.0X4	—	—
industrial	T51.0X1	T51.0X2	T51.0X3	T51.0X4	—	—
isopropyl	T51.2X1	T51.2X2	T51.2X3	T51.2X4	—	—
methyl	T51.1X1	T51.1X2	T51.1X3	T51.1X4	—	—
preparation for consumption	T51.0X1	T51.0X2	T51.0X3	T51.0X4	—	—

TABLE OF DRUGS AND CHEMICALS

Substance	External Cause (T-Code)					
	Poisoning, Accidental (Unintentional)	Poisoning, Intentional Self-Harm	Poisoning, Assault	Poisoning, Undetermined	Adverse Effect	Underdosing
Alcohol *(Continued)*						
propyl	T51.3X1	T51.3X2	T51.3X3	T51.3X4	—	—
secondary	T51.2X1	T51.2X2	T51.2X3	T51.2X4	—	—
radiator	T51.1X1	T51.1X2	T51.1X3	T51.1X4	—	—
rubbing	T51.2X1	T51.2X2	T51.2X3	T51.2X4	—	—
specified type NEC	T51.8X1	T51.8X2	T51.8X3	T51.8X4	—	—
surgical	T51.0X1	T51.0X2	T51.0X3	T51.0X4	—	—
vapor (from any type of Alcohol)	T59.891	T59.892	T59.893	T59.894	—	—
wood	T51.1X1	T51.1X2	T51.1X3	T51.1X4	—	—
Alcuronium (chloride)	T48.1X1	T48.1X2	T48.1X3	T48.1X4	T48.1X5	T48.1X6
Aldactone	T50.0X1	T50.0X2	T50.0X3	T50.0X4	T50.0X5	T50.0X6
Aldesulfone sodium	T37.1X1	T37.1X2	T37.1X3	T37.1X4	T37.1X5	T37.1X6
Aldicarb	T60.0X1	T60.0X2	T60.0X3	T60.0X4	—	—
Aldomet	T46.5X1	T46.5X2	T46.5X3	T46.5X4	T46.5X5	T46.5X6
Aldosterone	T50.0X1	T50.0X2	T50.0X3	T50.0X4	T50.0X5	T50.0X6
Aldrin (dust)	T60.1X1	T60.1X2	T60.1X3	T60.1X4	—	—
Aleve— *see Naproxen*						
Alexitol sodium	T47.1X1	T47.1X2	T47.1X3	T47.1X4	T47.1X5	T47.1X6
Alfacalcidol	T45.2X1	T45.2X2	T45.2X3	T45.2X4	T45.2X5	T45.2X6
Alfadolone	T41.1X1	T41.1X2	T41.1X3	T41.1X4	T41.1X5	T41.1X6
Alfaxalone	T41.1X1	T41.1X2	T41.1X3	T41.1X4	T41.1X5	T41.1X6
Alfentanil	T40.4X1	T40.4X2	T40.4X3	T40.4X4	T40.4X5	T40.4X6
Alfuzosin (hydrochloride)	T44.8X1	T44.8X2	T44.8X3	T44.8X4	T44.8X5	T44.8X6
Algae (harmful) (toxin)	T65.821	T65.822	T65.823	T65.824	—	—
Algeldrate	T47.1X1	T47.1X2	T47.1X3	T47.1X4	T47.1X5	T47.1X6
Algin	T47.8X1	T47.8X2	T47.8X3	T47.8X4	T47.8X5	T47.8X6
Alglucerase	T45.3X1	T45.3X2	T45.3X3	T45.3X4	T45.3X5	T45.3X6
Alidase	T45.3X1	T45.3X2	T45.3X3	T45.3X4	T45.3X5	T45.3X6
Alimemazine	T43.3X1	T43.3X2	T43.3X3	T43.3X4	T43.3X5	T43.3X6
Aliphatic thiocyanates	T65.0X1	T65.0X2	T65.0X3	T65.0X4	—	—
Alizapride	T45.0X1	T45.0X2	T45.0X3	T45.0X4	T45.0X5	T45.0X6
Alkali (caustic)	T54.3X1	T54.3X2	T54.3X3	T54.3X4	—	—
Alkalizing agent NEC	T50.901	T50.902	T50.903	T50.904	T50.905	T50.906
Alkaline antiseptic solution (aromatic)	T49.6X1	T49.6X2	T49.6X3	T49.6X4	T49.6X5	T49.6X6
Alkalinizing agents (medicinal)	T50.901	T50.902	T50.903	T50.904	T50.905	T50.906
Alka-seltzer	T39.011	T39.012	T39.013	T39.014	T39.015	T39.016
Alkavervir	T46.5X1	T46.5X2	T46.5X3	T46.5X4	T46.5X5	T46.5X6
Alkonium (bromide)	T49.0X1	T49.0X2	T49.0X3	T49.0X4	T49.0X5	T49.0X6
Alkylating drug NEC	T45.1X1	T45.1X2	T45.1X3	T45.1X4	T45.1X5	T45.1X6
antimyeloproliferative	T45.1X1	T45.1X2	T45.1X3	T45.1X4	T45.1X5	T45.1X6
lymphatic	T45.1X1	T45.1X2	T45.1X3	T45.1X4	T45.1X5	T45.1X6

◀ New   ◀▥▥ Revised   ~~deleted~~ Deleted

Substance	Poisoning, Accidental (Unintentional)	Poisoning, Intentional Self-Harm	Poisoning, Assault	Poisoning, Undetermined	Adverse Effect	Underdosing
Alkylisocyanate	T65.0X1	T65.0X2	T65.0X3	T65.0X4	—	—
Allantoin	T49.411	T49.412	T49.413	T49.414	T49.415	T49.416
Allegron	T43.0X1	T43.0X2	T43.0X3	T43.0X4	T43.0X5	T43.0X6
Allethrin	T49.0X1	T49.0X2	T49.0X3	T49.0X4	T49.0X5	T49.0X6
Allobarbital	T42.3X1	T42.3X2	T42.3X3	T42.3X4	T42.3X5	T42.3X6
Allopurinol	T50.4X1	T50.4X2	T50.4X3	T50.4X4	T50.4X5	T50.4X6
Allyl						
alcohol	T51.8X1	T51.8X2	T51.8X3	T51.8X4	—	—
disulfide	T46.6X1	T46.6X2	T46.6X3	T46.6X4	T46.6X5	T46.6X6
Allylestrenol	T38.5X1	T38.5X2	T38.5X3	T38.5X4	T38.5X5	T38.5X6
Allylisopropylacetylurea	T42.6X1	T42.6X2	T42.6X3	T42.6X4	T42.6X5	T42.6X6
Allylisopropylmalonylurea	T42.3X1	T42.3X2	T42.3X3	T42.3X4	T42.3X5	T42.3X6
Allylthiourea	T49.3X1	T49.3X2	T49.3X3	T49.3X4	T49.3X5	T49.3X6
Allyltribromide	T42.6X1	T42.6X2	T42.6X3	T42.6X4	T42.6X5	T42.6X6
Allypropymal	T42.3X1	T42.3X2	T42.3X3	T42.3X4	T42.3X5	T42.3X6
Almagate	T47.1X1	T47.1X2	T47.1X3	T47.1X4	T47.1X5	T47.1X6
Almasilate	T47.1X1	T47.1X2	T47.1X3	T47.1X4	T47.1X5	T47.1X6
Almitrine	T50.7X1	T50.7X2	T50.7X3	T50.7X4	T50.7X5	T50.7X6
Aloes	T47.2X1	T47.2X2	T47.2X3	T47.2X4	T47.2X5	T47.2X6
Aloglutamol	T47.1X1	T47.1X2	T47.1X3	T47.1X4	T47.1X5	T47.1X6
Aloin	T47.2X1	T47.2X2	T47.2X3	T47.2X4	T47.2X5	T47.2X6
Aloxidone	T42.2X1	T42.2X2	T42.2X3	T42.2X4	T42.2X5	T42.2X6
Alpha						
acetyldigoxin	T46.0X1	T46.0X2	T46.0X3	T46.0X4	T46.0X5	T46.0X6
adrenergic blocking drug	T44.6X1	T44.6X2	T44.6X3	T44.6X4	T44.6X5	T44.6X6
amylase	T45.3X1	T45.3X2	T45.3X3	T45.3X4	T45.3X5	T45.3X6
tocoferol (acetate)	T45.2X1	T45.2X2	T45.2X3	T45.2X4	T45.2X5	T45.2X6
tocopherol	T45.2X1	T45.2X2	T45.2X3	T45.2X4	T45.2X5	T45.2X6
Alphadolone	T41.1X1	T41.1X2	T41.1X3	T41.1X4	T41.1X5	T41.1X6
Alphaprodine	T40.4X1	T40.4X2	T40.4X3	T40.4X4	T40.4X5	T40.4X6
Alphaxalone	T41.1X1	T41.1X2	T41.1X3	T41.1X4	T41.1X5	T41.1X6
Alprazolam	T42.4X1	T42.4X2	T42.4X3	T42.4X4	T42.4X5	T42.4X6
Alprenolol	T44.7X1	T44.7X2	T44.7X3	T44.7X4	T44.7X5	T44.7X6
Alprostadil	T46.7X1	T46.7X2	T46.7X3	T46.7X4	T46.7X5	T46.7X6
Alsactide	T38.811	T38.812	T38.813	T38.814	T38.815	T38.816
Alseroxylon	T46.5X1	T46.5X2	T46.5X3	T46.5X4	T46.5X5	T46.5X6
Alteplase	T45.611	T45.612	T45.613	T45.614	T45.615	T45.616
Altizide	T50.2X1	T50.2X2	T50.2X3	T50.2X4	T50.2X5	T50.2X6
Altretamine	T45.1X1	T45.1X2	T45.1X3	T45.1X4	T45.1X5	T45.1X6

◀ New ◀ Revised ~~deleted~~ Deleted

Substance	External Cause (T-Code)					
	Poisoning, Accidental (Unintentional)	Poisoning, Intentional Self-Harm	Poisoning, Assault	Poisoning, Undetermined	Adverse Effect	Underdosing
Alum (medicinal)	T49.4X1	T49.4X2	T49.4X3	T49.4X4	T49.4X5	T49.4X6
nonmedicinal (ammonium) (potassium)	T56.891	T56.892	T56.893	T56.894	—	—
Aluminium, aluminum						
acetate	T49.2X1	T49.2X2	T49.2X3	T49.2X4	T49.2X5	T49.2X6
solution	T49.0X1	T49.0X2	T49.0X3	T49.0X4	T49.0X5	T49.0X6
aspirin	T39.011	T39.012	T39.013	T39.014	T39.015	T39.016
bis (acetylsalicylate)	T39.011	T39.012	T39.013	T39.014	T39.015	T39.016
carbonate (gel, basic)	T47.1X1	T47.1X2	T47.1X3	T47.1X4	T47.1X5	T47.1X6
chlorhydroxide-complex	T47.1X1	T47.1X2	T47.1X3	T47.1X4	T47.1X5	T47.1X6
chloride	T49.2X1	T49.2X2	T49.2X3	T49.2X4	T49.2X5	T49.2X6
clofibrate	T46.6X1	T46.6X2	T46.6X3	T46.6X4	T46.6X5	T46.6X6
diacetate	T49.2X1	T49.2X2	T49.2X3	T49.2X4	T49.2X5	T49.2X6
glycinate	T47.1X1	T47.1X2	T47.1X3	T47.1X4	T47.1X5	T47.1X6
hydroxide (gel)	T47.1X1	T47.1X2	T47.1X3	T47.1X4	T47.1X5	T47.1X6
hydroxide-magnesium carb. gel	T47.1X1	T47.1X2	T47.1X3	T47.1X4	T47.1X5	T47.1X6
magnesium silicate	T47.1X1	T47.1X2	T47.1X3	T47.1X4	T47.1X5	T47.1X6
nicotinate	T46.7X1	T46.7X2	T46.7X3	T46.7X4	T46.7X5	T46.7X6
ointment (surgical) (topical)	T49.3X1	T49.3X2	T49.3X3	T49.3X4	T49.3X5	T49.3X6
phosphate	T47.1X1	T47.1X2	T47.1X3	T47.1X4	T47.1X5	T47.1X6
salicylate	T39.091	T39.092	T39.093	T39.094	T39.095	T39.096
silicate	T47.1X1	T47.1X2	T47.1X3	T47.1X4	T47.1X5	T47.1X6
sodium silicate	T47.1X1	T47.1X2	T47.1X3	T47.1X4	T47.1X5	T47.1X6
subacetate	T49.2X1	T49.2X2	T49.2X3	T49.2X4	T49.2X5	T49.2X6
sulfate	T49.0X1	T49.0X2	T49.0X3	T49.0X4	T49.0X5	T49.0X6
tannate	T47.6X1	T47.6X2	T47.6X3	T47.6X4	T47.6X5	T47.6X6
topical NEC	T49.3X1	T49.3X2	T49.3X3	T49.3X4	T49.3X5	T49.3X6
Alurate	T42.3X1	T42.3X2	T42.3X3	T42.3X4	T42.3X5	T42.3X6
Alverine	T44.3X1	T44.3X2	T44.3X3	T44.3X4	T44.3X5	T44.3X6
Alvodine	T40.2X1	T40.2X2	T40.2X3	T40.2X4	T40.2X5	T40.2X6
Amanita phalloides	T62.0X1	T62.0X2	T62.0X3	T62.0X4	—	—
Amanitine	T62.0X1	T62.0X2	T62.0X3	T62.0X4	—	—
Amantadine	T42.8X1	T42.8X2	T42.8X3	T42.8X4	T42.8X5	T42.8X6
Ambazone	T49.6X1	T49.6X2	T49.6X3	T49.6X4	T49.6X5	T49.6X6
Ambenonium (chloride)	T44.0X1	T44.0X2	T44.0X3	T44.0X4	T44.0X5	T44.0X6
Ambroxol	T48.4X1	T48.4X2	T48.4X3	T48.4X4	T48.4X5	T48.4X6
Ambuphylline	T48.6X1	T48.6X2	T48.6X3	T48.6X4	T48.6X5	T48.6X6
Ambutonium bromide	T44.3X1	T44.3X2	T44.3X3	T44.3X4	T44.3X5	T44.3X6
Amcinonide	T49.0X1	T49.0X2	T49.0X3	T49.0X4	T49.0X5	T49.0X6
Amdinocilline	T36.0X1	T36.0X2	T36.0X3	T36.0X4	T36.0X5	T36.0X6

◀ New ◀▥▥ Revised ~~deleted~~ Deleted

	External Cause (T-Code)					
Substance	Poisoning, Accidental (Unintentional)	Poisoning, Intentional Self-Harm	Poisoning, Assault	Poisoning, Undetermined	Adverse Effect	Underdosing
Ametazole	T50.8X1	T50.8X2	T50.8X3	T50.8X4	T50.8X5	T50.8X6
Amethocaine	T41.3X1	T41.3X2	T41.3X3	T41.3X4	T41.3X5	T41.3X6
regional	T41.3X1	T41.3X2	T41.3X3	T41.3X4	T41.3X5	T41.3X6
spinal	T41.3X1	T41.3X2	T41.3X3	T41.3X4	T41.3X5	T41.3X6
Amethopterin	T45.1X1	T45.1X2	T45.1X3	T45.1X4	T45.1X5	T45.1X6
Amezinium metilsulfate	T44.991	T44.992	T44.993	T44.994	T44.995	T44.996
Amfebutamone	T43.291	T43.292	T43.293	T43.294	T43.295	T43.296
Amfepramone	T50.5X1	T50.5X2	T50.5X3	T50.5X4	T50.5X5	T50.5X6
Amfetamine	T43.621	T43.622	T43.623	T43.624	T43.625	T43.626
Amfetaminil	T43.621	T43.622	T43.623	T43.624	T43.625	T43.626
Amfomycin	T36.8X1	T36.8X2	T36.8X3	T36.8X4	T36.8X5	T36.8X6
Amidefrine mesilate	T48.5X1	T48.5X2	T48.5X3	T48.5X4	T48.5X5	T48.5X6
Amidone	T40.3X1	T40.3X2	T40.3X3	T40.3X4	T40.3X5	T40.3X6
Amidopyrine	T39.2X1	T39.2X2	T39.2X3	T39.2X4	T39.2X5	T39.2X6
Amidotrizoate	T50.8X1	T50.8X2	T50.8X3	T50.8X4	T50.8X5	T50.8X6
Amiflamine	T43.1X1	T43.1X2	T43.1X3	T43.1X4	T43.1X5	T43.1X6
Amikacin	T36.5X1	T36.5X2	T36.5X3	T36.5X4	T36.5X5	T36.5X6
Amikhelline	T46.3X1	T46.3X2	T46.3X3	T46.3X4	T46.3X5	T46.3X6
Amiloride	T50.2X1	T50.2X2	T50.2X3	T50.2X4	T50.2X5	T50.2X6
Aminacrine	T49.0X1	T49.0X2	T49.0X3	T49.0X4	T49.0X5	T49.0X6
Amineptine	T43.011	T43.012	T43.013	T43.014	T43.015	T43.016
Aminitrozole	T37.3X1	T37.3X2	T37.3X3	T37.3X4	T37.3X5	T37.3X6
Aminoacetic acid (derivatives)	T50.3X1	T50.3X2	T50.3X3	T50.3X4	T50.3X5	T50.3X6
Amino acids	T50.3X1	T50.3X2	T50.3X3	T50.3X4	T50.3X5	T50.3X6
Aminoacridine	T49.0X1	T49.0X2	T49.0X3	T49.0X4	T49.0X5	T49.0X6
Aminobenzoic acid (-p)	T49.3X1	T49.3X2	T49.3X3	T49.3X4	T49.3X5	T49.3X6
4-Aminobutyric acid	T43.8X1	T43.8X2	T43.8X3	T43.8X4	T43.8X5	T43.8X6
Aminocaproic acid	T45.621	T45.622	T45.623	T45.624	T45.625	T45.626
Aminofenazone	T39.2X1	T39.2X2	T39.2X3	T39.2X4	T39.2X5	T39.2X6
Aminoethylisothiourium	T45.8X1	T45.8X2	T45.8X3	T45.8X4	T45.8X5	T45.8X6
Aminoglutethimide	T45.1X1	T45.1X2	T45.1X3	T45.1X4	T45.1X5	T45.1X6
Aminohippuric acid	T50.8X1	T50.8X2	T50.8X3	T50.8X4	T50.8X5	T50.8X6
Aminomethylbenzoic acid	T45.691	T45.692	T45.693	T45.694	T45.695	T45.696
Aminometradine	T50.2X1	T50.2X2	T50.2X3	T50.2X4	T50.2X5	T50.2X6
Aminopentamide	T44.3X1	T44.3X2	T44.3X3	T44.3X4	T44.3X5	T44.3X6
Aminophenazone	T39.2X1	T39.2X2	T39.2X3	T39.2X4	T39.2X5	T39.2X6
Aminophenol	T54.0X1	T54.0X2	T54.0X3	T54.0X4	—	—
4-Aminophenol derivatives	T39.1X1	T39.1X2	T39.1X3	T39.1X4	T39.1X5	T39.1X6
Aminophenylpyridone	T43.591	T43.592	T43.593	T43.594	T43.595	T43.596

TABLE OF DRUGS AND CHEMICALS

TABLE OF DRUGS AND CHEMICALS

Substance	External Cause (T-Code)					
	Poisoning, Accidental (Unintentional)	Poisoning, Intentional Self-Harm	Poisoning, Assault	Poisoning, Undetermined	Adverse Effect	Underdosing
Aminophylline	T48.6X1	T48.6X2	T48.6X3	T48.6X4	T48.6X5	T48.6X6
Aminopterin sodium	T45.1X1	T45.1X2	T45.1X3	T45.1X4	T45.1X5	T45.1X6
Aminopyrine	T39.2X1	T39.2X2	T39.2X3	T39.2X4	T39.2X5	T39.2X6
8-Aminoquinoline drugs	T37.2X1	T37.2X2	T37.2X3	T37.2X4	T37.2X5	T37.2X6
Aminorex	T50.5X1	T50.5X2	T50.5X3	T50.5X4	T50.5X5	T50.5X6
Aminosalicylic acid	T37.1X1	T37.1X2	T37.1X3	T37.1X4	T37.1X5	T37.1X6
Aminosalylum	T37.1X1	T37.1X2	T37.1X3	T37.1X4	T37.1X5	T37.1X6
Amiodarone	T46.2X1	T46.2X2	T46.2X3	T46.2X4	T46.2X5	T46.2X6
Amiphenazole	T50.7X1	T50.7X2	T50.7X3	T50.7X4	T50.7X5	T50.7X6
Amiquinsin	T46.5X1	T46.5X2	T46.5X3	T46.5X4	T46.5X5	T46.5X6
Amisometradine	T50.2X1	T50.2X2	T50.2X3	T50.2X4	T50.2X5	T50.2X6
Amisulpride	T43.591	T43.592	T43.593	T43.594	T43.595	T43.596
Amitriptyline	T43.021	T43.022	T43.023	T43.024	T43.025	T43.026
Amitriptylinoxide	T43.021	T43.022	T43.023	T43.024	T43.025	T43.026
Amlexanox	T48.6X1	T48.6X2	T48.6X3	T48.6X4	T48.6X5	T48.6X6
Ammonia (fumes) (gas) (vapor)	T59.891	T59.892	T59.893	T59.894	—	—
aromatic spirit	T48.991	T48.992	T48.993	T48.994	T48.995	T48.996
liquid (household)	T54.3X1	T54.3X2	T54.3X3	T54.3X4	—	—
Ammoniated mercury	T49.0X1	T49.0X2	T49.0X3	T49.0X4	T49.0X5	T49.0X6
Ammonium						
acid tartrate	T49.5X1	T49.5X2	T49.5X3	T49.5X4	T49.5X5	T49.5X6
bromide	T42.6X1	T42.6X2	T42.6X3	T42.6X4	T42.6X5	T42.6X6
carbonate	T54.3X1	T54.3X2	T54.3X3	T54.3X4	—	—
chloride	T50.991	T50.992	T50.993	T50.994	T50.995	T50.996
expectorant	T48.4X1	T48.4X2	T48.4X3	T48.4X4	T48.4X5	T48.4X6
compounds (household) NEC	T54.3X1	T54.3X2	T54.3X3	T54.3X4	—	—
fumes (any usage)	T59.891	T59.892	T59.893	T59.894	—	—
industrial	T54.3X1	T54.3X2	T54.3X3	T54.3X4	—	—
ichthyosulronate	T49.4X1	T49.4X2	T49.4X3	T49.4X4	T49.4X5	T49.4X6
mandelate	T37.91	T37.92	T37.93	T37.94	T37.95	T37.96
sulfamate	T60.3X1	T60.3X2	T60.3X3	T60.3X4	—	—
sulfonate resin	T47.8X1	T47.8X2	T47.8X3	T47.8X4	T47.8X5	T47.8X6
Amobarbital (sodium)	T42.3X1	T42.3X2	T42.3X3	T42.3X4	T42.3X5	T42.3X6
Amodiaquine	T37.2X1	T37.2X2	T37.2X3	T37.2X4	T37.2X5	T37.2X6
Amopyroquin(e)	T37.2X1	T37.2X2	T37.2X3	T37.2X4	T37.2X5	T37.2X6
Amoxapine	T43.011	T43.012	T43.013	T43.014	T43.015	T43.016
Amoxicillin	T36.0X1	T36.0X2	T36.0X3	T36.0X4	T36.0X5	T36.0X6
Amperozide	T43.591	T43.592	T43.593	T43.594	T43.595	T43.596
Amphenidone	T43.591	T43.592	T43.593	T43.594	T43.595	T43.596
Amphetamine NEC	T43.621	T43.622	T43.623	T43.624	T43.625	T43.626

◀ New   ◀|||| Revised   ~~deleted~~ Deleted

Substance	External Cause (T-Code)					
	Poisoning, Accidental (Unintentional)	Poisoning, Intentional Self-Harm	Poisoning, Assault	Poisoning, Undetermined	Adverse Effect	Underdosing
Amphomycin	T36.8X1	T36.8X2	T36.8X3	T36.8X4	T36.8X5	T36.8X6
Amphotalide	T37.4X1	T37.4X2	T37.4X3	T37.4X4	T37.4X5	T37.4X6
Amphotericin B	T36.7X1	T36.7X2	T36.7X3	T36.7X4	T36.7X5	T36.7X6
topical	T49.0X1	T49.0X2	T49.0X3	T49.0X4	T49.0X5	T49.0X6
Ampicillin	T36.0X1	T36.0X2	T36.0X3	T36.0X4	T36.0X5	T36.0X6
Amprotropine	T44.3X1	T44.3X2	T44.3X3	T44.3X4	T44.3X5	T44.3X6
Amsacrine	T45.1X1	T45.1X2	T45.1X3	T45.1X4	T45.1X5	T45.1X6
Amygdaline	T62.2X1	T62.2X2	T62.2X3	T62.2X4	—	—
Amyl						
acetate	T52.8X1	T52.8X2	T52.8X3	T52.8X4	—	—
vapor	T59.891	T59.892	T59.893	T59.894	—	—
alcohol	T51.3X1	T51.3X2	T51.3X3	T51.3X4	—	—
chloride	T53.6X1	T53.6X2	T53.6X3	T53.6X4	—	—
formate	T52.8X1	T52.8X2	T52.8X3	T52.8X4	—	—
nitrite	T46.3X1	T46.3X2	T46.3X3	T46.3X4	T46.3X5	T46.3X6
propionate	T65.891	T65.892	T65.893	T65.894	—	—
Amylase	T47.5X1	T47.5X2	T47.5X3	T47.5X4	T47.5X5	T47.5X6
Amyleine, regional	T41.3X1	T41.3X2	T41.3X3	T41.3X4	T41.3X5	T41.3X6
Amylene						
dichloride	T53.6X1	T53.6X2	T53.6X3	T53.6X4	—	—
hydrate	T51.3X1	T51.3X2	T51.3X3	T51.3X4	—	—
Amylmetacresol	T49.6X1	T49.6X2	T49.6X3	T49.6X4	T49.6X5	T49.6X6
Amylobarbitone	T42.3X1	T42.3X2	T42.3X3	T42.3X4	T42.3X5	T42.3X6
Amylocaine, regional	T41.3X1	T41.3X2	T41.3X3	T41.3X4	T41.3X5	T41.3X6
infiltration (subcutaneous)	T41.3X1	T41.3X2	T41.3X3	T41.3X4	T41.3X5	T41.3X6
nerve block (peripheral) (plexus)	T41.3X1	T41.3X2	T41.3X3	T41.3X4	T41.3X5	T41.3X6
spinal	T41.3X1	T41.3X2	T41.3X3	T41.3X4	T41.3X5	T41.3X6
topical (surface)	T41.3X1	T41.3X2	T41.3X3	T41.3X4	T41.3X5	T41.3X6
Amylopectin	T47.6X1	T47.6X2	T47.6X3	T47.6X4	T47.6X5	T47.6X6
Amytal (sodium)	T42.3X1	T42.3X2	T42.3X3	T42.3X4	T42.3X5	T42.3X6
Anabolic steroid	T38.7X1	T38.7X2	T38.7X3	T38.7X4	T38.7X5	T38.7X6
Analeptic NEC	T50.7X1	T50.7X2	T50.7X3	T50.7X4	T50.7X5	T50.7X6
Analgesic	T39.91	T39.92	T39.93	T39.94	T39.95	T39.96
anti-inflammatory NEC	T39.91	T39.92	T39.93	T39.94	T39.95	T39.96
propionic acid derivative	T39.311	T39.312	T39.313	T39.314	T39.315	T39.316
antirheumatic NEC	T39.4X1	T39.4X2	T39.4X3	T39.4X4	T39.4X5	T39.4X6
aromatic NEC	T39.1X1	T39.1X2	T39.1X3	T39.1X4	T39.1X5	T39.1X6
narcotic NEC	T40.601	T40.602	T40.603	T40.604	T40.605	T40.606
combination	T40.601	T40.602	T40.603	T40.604	T40.605	T40.606
obstetric	T40.601	T40.602	T40.603	T40.604	T40.605	T40.606

◀ New   ◀▥ Revised   ~~deleted~~ Deleted

TABLE OF DRUGS AND CHEMICALS

TABLE OF DRUGS AND CHEMICALS

Substance	Poisoning, Accidental (Unintentional)	Poisoning, Intentional Self-Harm	Poisoning, Assault	Poisoning, Undetermined	Adverse Effect	Underdosing
External Cause (T-Code)						
Analgesic *(Continued)*						
non-narcotic NEC	T39.91	T39.92	T39.93	T39.94	T39.95	T39.96
combination	T39.91	T39.92	T39.93	T39.94	T39.95	T39.96
pyrazole	T39.2X1	T39.2X2	T39.2X3	T39.2X4	T39.2X5	T39.2X6
specified NEC	T39.8X1	T39.8X2	T39.8X3	T39.8X4	T39.8X5	T39.8X6
Analgin	T39.2X1	T39.2X2	T39.2X3	T39.2X4	T39.2X5	T39.2X6
Anamirta cocculus	T62.1X1	T62.1X2	T62.1X3	T62.1X4	—	—
Ancillin	T36.0X1	T36.0X2	T36.0X3	T36.0X4	T36.0X5	T36.0X6
Ancrod	T45.691	T45.692	T45.693	T45.694	T45.695	T45.696
Androgen	T38.7X1	T38.7X2	T38.7X3	T38.7X4	T38.7X5	T38.7X6
Androgen-estrogen mixture	T38.7X1	T38.7X2	T38.7X3	T38.7X4	T38.7X5	T38.7X6
Androstalone	T38.7X1	T38.7X2	T38.7X3	T38.7X4	T38.7X5	T38.7X6
Androstanolone	T38.7X1	T38.7X2	T38.7X3	T38.7X4	T38.7X5	T38.7X6
Androsterone	T38.7X1	T38.7X2	T38.7X3	T38.7X4	T38.7X5	T38.7X6
Anemone pulsatilla	T62.2X1	T62.2X2	T62.2X3	T62.2X4	—	—
Anesthesia						
caudal	T41.3X1	T41.3X2	T41.3X3	T41.3X4	T41.3X5	T41.3X6
endotracheal	T41.0X1	T41.0X2	T41.0X3	T41.0X4	T41.0X5	T41.0X6
epidural	T41.3X1	T41.3X2	T41.3X3	T41.3X4	T41.3X5	T41.3X6
inhalation	T41.0X1	T41.0X2	T41.0X3	T41.0X4	T41.0X5	T41.0X6
local	T41.3X1	T41.3X2	T41.3X3	T41.3X4	T41.3X5	T41.3X6
mucosal	T41.3X1	T41.3X2	T41.3X3	T41.3X4	T41.3X5	T41.3X6
muscle relaxation	T48.1X1	T48.1X2	T48.1X3	T48.1X4	T48.1X5	T48.1X6
nerve blocking	T41.3X1	T41.3X2	T41.3X3	T41.3X4	T41.3X5	T41.3X6
plexus blocking	T41.3X1	T41.3X2	T41.3X3	T41.3X4	T41.3X5	T41.3X6
potentiated	T41.201	T41.202	T41.203	T41.204	T41.205	T41.206
rectal	T41.201	T41.202	T41.203	T41.204	T41.205	T41.206
general	T41.201	T41.202	T41.203	T41.204	T41.205	T41.206
local	T41.3X1	T41.3X2	T41.3X3	T41.3X4	T41.3X5	T41.3X6
regional	T41.3X1	T41.3X2	T41.3X3	T41.3X4	T41.3X5	T41.3X6
surface	T41.3X1	T41.3X2	T41.3X3	T41.3X4	T41.3X5	T41.3X6
Anesthetic NEC—*see also Anesthesia*	T41.41	T41.42	T41.43	T41.44	T41.45	T41.46
with muscle relaxant	T41.201	T41.202	T41.203	T41.204	T41.205	T41.206
general	T41.201	T41.202	T41.203	T41.204	T41.205	T41.206
local	T41.3X1	T41.3X2	T41.3X3	T41.3X4	T41.3X5	T41.3X6
gaseous NEC	T41.0X1	T41.0X2	T41.0X3	T41.0X4	T41.0X5	T41.0X6
general NEC	T41.201	T41.202	T41.203	T41.204	T41.205	T41.206
halogenated hydrocarbon derivatives NEC	T41.0X1	T41.0X2	T41.0X3	T41.0X4	T41.0X5	T41.0X6
infiltration NEC	T41.3X1	T41.3X2	T41.3X3	T41.3X4	T41.3X5	T41.3X6
intravenous NEC	T41.1X1	T41.1X2	T41.1X3	T41.1X4	T41.1X5	T41.1X6

◀ New ◀ Revised ~~deleted~~ Deleted

Substance	Poisoning, Accidental (Unintentional)	Poisoning, Intentional Self-Harm	Poisoning, Assault	Poisoning, Undetermined	Adverse Effect	Underdosing
Anesthetic NEC *(Continued)*						
local NEC	T41.3X1	T41.3X2	T41.3X3	T41.3X4	T41.3X5	T41.3X6
rectal	T41.201	T41.202	T41.203	T41.204	T41.205	T41.206
general	T41.201	T41.202	T41.203	T41.204	T41.205	T41.206
local	T41.3X1	T41.3X2	T41.3X3	T41.3X4	T41.3X5	T41.3X6
regional NEC	T41.3X1	T41.3X2	T41.3X3	T41.3X4	T41.3X5	T41.3X6
spinal NEC	T41.3X1	T41.3X2	T41.3X3	T41.3X4	T41.3X5	T41.3X6
thiobarbiturate	T41.1X1	T41.1X2	T41.1X3	T41.1X4	T41.1X5	T41.1X6
topical	T41.3X1	T41.3X2	T41.3X3	T41.3X4	T41.3X5	T41.3X6
Aneurine	T45.2X1	T45.2X2	T45.2X3	T45.2X4	T45.2X5	T45.2X6
Angio-Conray	T50.8X1	T50.8X2	T50.8X3	T50.8X4	T50.8X5	T50.8X6
Angiotensin	T44.5X1	T44.5X2	T44.5X3	T44.5X4	T44.5X5	T44.5X6
Angiotensinamide	T44.991	T44.992	T44.993	T44.994	T44.995	T44.996
Anhydrohydroxy-progesterone	T38.5X1	T38.5X2	T38.5X3	T38.5X4	T38.5X5	T38.5X6
Anhydron	T50.2X1	T50.2X2	T50.2X3	T50.2X4	T50.2X5	T50.2X6
Anileridine	T40.4X1	T40.4X2	T40.4X3	T40.4X4	T40.4X5	T40.4X6
Aniline (dye) (liquid)	T65.3X1	T65.3X2	T65.3X3	T65.3X4	—	—
analgesic	T39.1X1	T39.1X2	T39.1X3	T39.1X4	T39.1X5	T39.1X6
derivatives, therapeutic NEC	T39.1X1	T39.1X2	T39.1X3	T39.1X4	T39.1X5	T39.1X6
vapor	T65.3X1	T65.3X2	T65.3X3	T65.3X4	—	—
Anise oil	T47.5X1	T47.5X2	T47.5X3	T47.5X4	T47.5X5	T47.5X6
Aniscoropine	T44.3X1	T44.3X2	T44.3X3	T44.3X4	T44.3X5	T44.3X6
Anisidine	T65.3X1	T65.3X2	T65.3X3	T65.3X4	—	—
Anisindione	T45.511	T45.512	T45.513	T45.514	T45.515	T45.516
Anisotropine methyl-bromide	T44.3X1	T44.3X2	T44.3X3	T44.3X4	T44.3X5	T44.3X6
Anistreplase	T45.611	T45.612	T45.613	T45.614	T45.615	T45.616
Anorexiant (central)	T50.5X1	T50.5X2	T50.5X3	T50.5X4	T50.5X5	T50.5X6
Anorexic agents	T50.5X1	T50.5X2	T50.5X3	T50.5X4	T50.5X5	T50.5X6
Ansamycin	T36.6X1	T36.6X2	T36.6X3	T36.6X4	T36.6X5	T36.6X6
Ant (bite) (sting)	T63.421	T63.422	T63.423	T63.424	—	—
Antabuse	T50.6X1	T50.6X2	T50.6X3	T50.6X4	T50.6X5	T50.6X6
Ant poison—*see Insecticide*						
Antacid NEC	T47.1X1	T47.1X2	T47.1X3	T47.1X4	T47.1X5	T47.1X6
Antagonist						
Aldosterone	T50.0X1	T50.0X2	T50.0X3	T50.0X4	T50.0X5	T50.0X6
alpha-adrenoreceptor	T44.6X1	T44.6X2	T44.6X3	T44.6X4	T44.6X5	T44.6X6
anticoagulant	T45.7X1	T45.7X2	T45.7X3	T45.7X4	T45.7X5	T45.7X6
beta-adrenoreceptor	T44.7X1	T44.7X2	T44.7X3	T44.7X4	T44.7X5	T44.7X6
extrapyramidal NEC	T44.3X1	T44.3X2	T44.3X3	T44.3X4	T44.3X5	T44.3X6
folic acid	T45.1X1	T45.1X2	T45.1X3	T45.1X4	T45.1X5	T45.1X6

TABLE OF DRUGS AND CHEMICALS

TABLE OF DRUGS AND CHEMICALS

Substance	External Cause (T-Code)					
	Poisoning, Accidental (Unintentional)	Poisoning, Intentional Self-Harm	Poisoning, Assault	Poisoning, Undetermined	Adverse Effect	Underdosing
Antagonist *(Continued)*						
H2 receptor	T47.0X1	T47.0X2	T47.0X3	T47.0X4	T47.0X5	T47.0X6
heavy metal	T45.8X1	T45.8X2	T45.8X3	T45.8X4	T45.8X5	T45.8X6
narcotic analgesic	T50.7X1	T50.7X2	T50.7X3	T50.7X4	T50.7X5	T50.7X6
opiate	T50.7X1	T50.7X2	T50.7X3	T50.7X4	T50.7X5	T50.7X6
pyrimidine	T45.1X1	T45.1X2	T45.1X3	T45.1X4	T45.1X5	T45.1X6
serotonin	T46.5X1	T46.5X2	T46.5X3	T46.5X4	T46.5X5	T46.5X6
Antazolin(e)	T45.0X1	T45.0X2	T45.0X3	T45.0X4	T45.0X5	T45.0X6
Anterior pituitary hormone NEC	T38.811	T38.812	T38.813	T38.814	T38.815	T38.816
Anthelmintic NEC	T37.4X1	T37.4X2	T37.4X3	T37.4X4	T37.4X5	T37.4X6
Anthiolimine	T37.4X1	T37.4X2	T37.4X3	T37.4X4	T37.4X5	T37.4X6
Anthralin	T49.4X1	T49.4X2	T49.4X3	T49.4X4	T49.4X5	T49.4X6
Anthramycin	T45.1X1	T45.1X2	T45.1X3	T45.1X4	T45.1X5	T45.1X6
Antiadrenergic NEC	T44.8X1	T44.8X2	T44.8X3	T44.8X4	T44.8X5	T44.8X6
Antiallergic NEC	T45.0X1	T45.0X2	T45.0X3	T45.0X4	T45.0X5	T45.0X6
Anti-anemic (drug) (preparation)	T45.8X1	T45.8X2	T45.8X3	T45.8X4	T45.8X5	T45.8X6
Antiandrogen NEC	T38.6X1	T38.6X2	T38.6X3	T38.6X4	T38.6X5	T38.6X6
Antianxiety drug NEC	T43.501	T43.502	T43.503	T43.504	T43.505	T43.506
Antiaris toxicaria	T65.891	T65.892	T65.893	T65.894	—	—
Antiarteriosclerotic drug	T46.6X1	T46.6X2	T46.6X3	T46.6X4	T46.6X5	T46.6X6
Antiasthmatic drug NEC	T48.6X1	T48.6X2	T48.6X3	T48.6X4	T48.6X5	T48.6X6
Antibiotic NEC	T36.91	T36.92	T36.93	T36.94	T36.95	T36.96
aminoglycoside	T36.5X1	T36.5X2	T36.5X3	T36.5X4	T36.5X5	T36.5X6
anticancer	T45.1X1	T45.1X2	T45.1X3	T45.1X4	T45.1X5	T45.1X6
antifungal	T36.7X1	T36.7X2	T36.7X3	T36.7X4	T36.7X5	T36.7X6
antimycobacterial	T36.5X1	T36.5X2	T36.5X3	T36.5X4	T36.5X5	T36.5X6
antineoplastic	T45.1X1	T45.1X2	T45.1X3	T45.1X4	T45.1X5	T45.1X6
cephalosporin (group)	T36.1X1	T36.1X2	T36.1X3	T36.1X4	T36.1X5	T36.1X6
chloramphenicol (group)	T36.2X1	T36.2X2	T36.2X3	T36.2X4	T36.2X5	T36.2X6
ENT	T49.6X1	T49.6X2	T49.6X3	T49.6X4	T49.6X5	T49.6X6
eye	T49.5X1	T49.5X2	T49.5X3	T49.5X4	T49.5X5	T49.5X6
fungicidal (local)	T49.0X1	T49.0X2	T49.0X3	T49.0X4	T49.0X5	T49.0X6
intestinal	T36.8X1	T36.8X2	T36.8X3	T36.8X4	T36.8X5	T36.8X6
b-lactam NEC	T36.1X1	T36.1X2	T36.1X3	T36.1X4	T36.1X5	T36.1X6
local	T49.0X1	T49.0X2	T49.0X3	T49.0X4	T49.0X5	T49.0X6
macrolides	T36.3X1	T36.3X2	T36.3X3	T36.3X4	T36.3X5	T36.3X6
polypeptide	T36.8X1	T36.8X2	T36.8X3	T36.8X4	T36.8X5	T36.8X6
specified NEC	T36.8X1	T36.8X2	T36.8X3	T36.8X4	T36.8X5	T36.8X6
tetracycline (group)	T36.4X1	T36.4X2	T36.4X3	T36.4X4	T36.4X5	T36.4X6
throat	T49.6X1	T49.6X2	T49.6X3	T49.6X4	T49.6X5	T49.6X6

◀ New ◀▮▮ Revised ~~deleted~~ Deleted

Substance	External Cause (T-Code)					
	Poisoning, Accidental (Unintentional)	Poisoning, Intentional Self-Harm	Poisoning, Assault	Poisoning, Undetermined	Adverse Effect	Underdosing
Anticancer agents NEC	T45.1X1	T45.1X2	T45.1X3	T45.1X4	T45.1X5	T45.1X6
Anticholesterolemic drug NEC	T46.6X1	T46.6X2	T46.6X3	T46.6X4	T46.6X5	T46.6X6
Anticholinergic NEC	T44.3X1	T44.3X2	T44.3X3	T44.3X4	T44.3X5	T44.3X6
Anticholinesterase	T44.0X1	T44.0X2	T44.0X3	T44.0X4	T44.0X5	T44.0X6
organophosphorus	T44.0X1	T44.0X2	T44.0X3	T44.0X4	T44.0X5	T44.0X6
insecticide	T60.0X1	T60.0X2	T60.0X3	T60.0X4	—	—
nerve gas	T59.891	T59.892	T59.893	T59.894	—	—
reversible	T44.0X1	T44.0X2	T44.0X3	T44.0X4	T44.0X5	T44.0X6
ophthalmological	T49.5X1	T49.5X2	T49.5X3	T49.5X4	T49.5X5	T49.5X6
Anticoagulant NEC	T45.511	T45.512	T45.513	T45.514	T45.515	T45.516
Antagonist	T45.7X1	T45.7X2	T45.7X3	T45.7X4	T45.7X5	T45.7X6
Anti-common-cold drug NEC	T48.5X1	T48.5X2	T48.5X3	T48.5X4	T48.5X5	T48.5X6
Anticonvulsant	T42.71	T42.72	T42.73	T42.74	T42.75	T42.76
barbiturate	T42.3X1	T42.3X2	T42.3X3	T42.3X4	T42.3X5	T42.3X6
combination (with barbiturate)	T42.3X1	T42.3X2	T42.3X3	T42.3X4	T42.3X5	T42.3X6
hydantoin	T42.0X1	T42.0X2	T42.0X3	T42.0X4	T42.0X5	T42.0X6
hypnotic NEC	T42.6X1	T42.6X2	T42.6X3	T42.6X4	T42.6X5	T42.6X6
oxazolidinedione	T42.2X1	T42.2X2	T42.2X3	T42.2X4	T42.2X5	T42.2X6
pyrimidinedione	T42.6X1	T42.6X2	T42.6X3	T42.6X4	T42.6X5	T42.6X6
specified NEC	T42.6X1	T42.6X2	T42.6X3	T42.6X4	T42.6X5	T42.6X6
succinimide	T42.2X1	T42.2X2	T42.2X3	T42.2X4	T42.2X5	T42.2X6
Anti-D immunoglobulin (human)	T50.Z11	T50.Z12	T50.Z13	T50.Z14	T50.Z15	T50.Z16
Antidepressant NEC	T43.201	T43.202	T43.203	T43.204	T43.205	T43.206
monoamine oxidase inhibitor	T43.1X1	T43.1X2	T43.1X3	T43.1X4	T43.1X5	T43.1X6
selective serotonin norepinephrine reuptake inhibitor	T43.211	T43.212	T43.213	T43.214	T43.215	T43.216
selective serotonin reuptake inhibitor	T43.221	T43.222	T43.223	T43.224	T43.225	T43.226
specified NEC	T43.291	T43.292	T43.293	T43.294	T43.295	T43.296
tetracyclic	T43.021	T43.022	T43.023	T43.024	T43.025	T43.026
triazolopyridine	T43.221	T43.222	T43.223	T43.224	T43.225	T43.226
tricyclic	T43.011	T43.012	T43.013	T43.014	T43.015	T43.016
Antidiabetic NEC	T38.3X1	T38.3X2	T38.3X3	T38.3X4	T38.3X5	T38.3X6
biguanide	T38.3X1	T38.3X2	T38.3X3	T38.3X4	T38.3X5	T38.3X6
and sulfonyl combined	T38.3X1	T38.3X2	T38.3X3	T38.3X4	T38.3X5	T38.3X6
combined	T38.3X1	T38.3X2	T38.3X3	T38.3X4	T38.3X5	T38.3X6
sulfonylurea	T38.3X1	T38.3X2	T38.3X3	T38.3X4	T38.3X5	T38.3X6
Antidiarrheal drug NEC	T47.6X1	T47.6X2	T47.6X3	T47.6X4	T47.6X5	T47.6X6
absorbent	T47.6X1	T47.6X2	T47.6X3	T47.6X4	T47.6X5	T47.6X6
Antidiphtheria serum	T50.Z11	T50.Z12	T50.Z13	T50.Z14	T50.Z15	T50.Z16
Antidiuretic hormone	T38.891	T38.892	T38.893	T38.894	T38.895	T38.896

◄ New   ◀ Revised   ~~deleted~~ Deleted

TABLE OF DRUGS AND CHEMICALS

TABLE OF DRUGS AND CHEMICALS

Substance	External Cause (T-Code)					
	Poisoning, Accidental (Unintentional)	Poisoning, Intentional Self-Harm	Poisoning, Assault	Poisoning, Undetermined	Adverse Effect	Underdosing
Antidote NEC	T50.6X1	T50.6X2	T50.6X3	T50.6X4	T50.6X5	T50.6X6
heavy metal	T45.8X1	T45.8X2	T45.8X3	T45.8X4	T45.8X5	T45.8X6
Antidysrhythmic NEC	T46.2X1	T46.2X2	T46.2X3	T46.2X4	T46.2X5	T46.2X6
Antiemetic drug	T45.0X1	T45.0X2	T45.0X3	T45.0X4	T45.0X5	T45.0X6
Antiepilepsy agent	T42.71	T42.72	T42.73	T42.74	T42.75	T42.76
combination	T42.5X1	T42.5X2	T42.5X3	T42.5X4	T42.5X5	T42.5X6
mixed	T42.5X1	T42.5X2	T42.5X3	T42.5X4	T42.5X5	T42.5X6
specified, NEC	T42.6X1	T42.6X2	T42.6X3	T42.6X4	T42.6X5	T42.6X6
Antiestrogen NEC	T38.6X1	T38.6X2	T38.6X3	T38.6X4	T38.6X5	T38.6X6
Antifertility pill	T38.4X1	T38.4X2	T38.4X3	T38.4X4	T38.4X5	T38.4X6
Antifibrinolytic drug	T45.621	T45.622	T45.623	T45.624	T45.625	T45.626
Antifilarial drug	T37.4X1	T37.4X2	T37.4X3	T37.4X4	T37.4X5	T37.4X6
Antiflatulent	T47.5X1	T47.5X2	T47.5X3	T47.5X4	T47.5X5	T47.5X6
Antifreeze	T65.91	T65.92	T65.93	T65.94	—	—
alcohol	T51.1X1	T51.1X2	T51.1X3	T51.1X4	—	—
ethylene glycol	T51.8X1	T51.8X2	T51.8X3	T51.8X4	—	—
Antifungal						
antibiotic (systemic)	T36.7X1	T36.7X2	T36.7X3	T36.7X4	T36.7X5	T36.7X6
anti-infective NEC	T37.91	T37.92	T37.93	T37.94	T37.95	T37.96
disinfectant, local	T49.0X1	T49.0X2	T49.0X3	T49.0X4	T49.0X5	T49.0X6
nonmedicinal (spray)	T60.3X1	T60.3X2	T60.3X3	T60.3X4	—	—
topical	T49.0X1	T49.0X2	T49.0X3	T49.0X4	T49.0X5	T49.0X6
Anti-gastric-secretion drug NEC	T47.1X1	T47.1X2	T47.1X3	T47.1X4	T47.1X5	T47.1X6
Antigonadotrophin NEC	T38.6X1	T38.6X2	T38.6X3	T38.6X4	T38.6X5	T38.6X6
Antihallucinogen	T43.501	T43.502	T43.503	T43.504	T43.505	T43.506
Antihelmintics	T37.4X1	T37.4X2	T37.4X3	T37.4X4	T37.4X5	T37.4X6
Antihemophilic						
factor	T45.8X1	T45.8X2	T45.8X3	T45.8X4	T45.8X5	T45.8X6
fraction	T45.8X1	T45.8X2	T45.8X3	T45.8X4	T45.8X5	T45.8X6
globulin concentrate	T45.7X1	T45.7X2	T45.7X3	T45.7X4	T45.7X5	T45.7X6
human plasma	T45.8X1	T45.8X2	T45.8X3	T45.8X4	T45.8X5	T45.8X6
plasma, dried	T45.7X1	T45.7X2	T45.7X3	T45.7X4	T45.7X5	T45.7X6
Antihemorrhoidal preparation	T49.2X1	T49.2X2	T49.2X3	T49.2X4	T49.2X5	T49.2X6
Antiheparin drug	T45.7X1	T45.7X2	T45.7X3	T45.7X4	T45.7X5	T45.7X6
Antihistamine	T45.0X1	T45.0X2	T45.0X3	T45.0X4	T45.0X5	T45.0X6
Antihookworm drug	T37.4X1	T37.4X2	T37.4X3	T37.4X4	T37.4X5	T37.4X6
Anti-human lymphocytic globulin	T50.Z11	T50.Z12	T50.Z13	T50.Z14	T50.Z15	T50.Z16
Antihyperlipidemic drug	T46.6X1	T46.6X2	T46.6X3	T46.6X4	T46.6X5	T46.6X6
Antihypertensive drug NEC	T46.5X1	T46.5X2	T46.5X3	T46.5X4	T46.5X5	T46.5X6

◀ New   ◀▥ Revised   ~~deleted~~ Deleted

Substance	External Cause (T-Code)					
	Poisoning, Accidental (Unintentional)	Poisoning, Intentional Self-Harm	Poisoning, Assault	Poisoning, Undetermined	Adverse Effect	Underdosing
Anti-infective NEC	T37.91	T37.92	T37.93	T37.94	T37.95	T37.96
anthelmintic	T37.4X1	T37.4X2	T37.4X3	T37.4X4	T37.4X5	T37.4X6
antibiotics	T36.91	T36.92	T36.93	T36.94	T36.95	T36.96
specified NEC	T36.8X1	T36.8X2	T36.8X3	T36.8X4	T36.8X5	T36.8X6
antimalarial	T37.2X1	T37.2X2	T37.2X3	T37.2X4	T37.2X5	T37.2X6
antimycobacterial NEC	T37.1X1	T37.1X2	T37.1X3	T37.1X4	T37.1X5	T37.1X6
antibiotics	T36.5X1	T36.5X2	T36.5X3	T36.5X4	T36.5X5	T36.5X6
antiprotozoal NEC	T37.3X1	T37.3X2	T37.3X3	T37.3X4	T37.3X5	T37.3X6
blood	T37.2X1	T37.2X2	T37.2X3	T37.2X4	T37.2X5	T37.2X6
antiviral	T37.5X1	T37.5X2	T37.5X3	T37.5X4	T37.5X5	T37.5X6
arsenical	T37.8X1	T37.8X2	T37.8X3	T37.8X4	T37.8X5	T37.8X6
bismuth, local	T49.0X1	T49.0X2	T49.0X3	T49.0X4	T49.0X5	T49.0X6
ENT	T49.6X1	T49.6X2	T49.6X3	T49.6X4	T49.6X5	T49.6X6
eye NEC	T49.5X1	T49.5X2	T49.5X3	T49.5X4	T49.5X5	T49.5X6
heavy metals NEC	T37.8X1	T37.8X2	T37.8X3	T37.8X4	T37.8X5	T37.8X6
local NEC	T49.0X1	T49.0X2	T49.0X3	T49.0X4	T49.0X5	T49.0X6
specified NEC	T49.0X1	T49.0X2	T49.0X3	T49.0X4	T49.0X5	T49.0X6
mixed	T37.91	T37.92	T37.93	T37.94	T37.95	T37.96
ophthalmic preparation	T49.5X1	T49.5X2	T49.5X3	T49.5X4	T49.5X5	T49.5X6
topical NEC	T49.0X1	T49.0X2	T49.0X3	T49.0X4	T49.0X5	T49.0X6
Anti-inflammatory drug NEC	T49.0X1	T49.0X2	T49.0X3	T49.0X4	T49.0X5	T49.0X6
local	T49.0X1	T49.0X2	T49.0X3	T49.0X4	T49.0X5	T49.0X6
nonsteroidal NEC	T39.391	T39.392	T39.393	T39.394	T39.395	T39.396
propionic acid derivative	T39.311	T39.312	T39.313	T39.314	T39.315	T39.316
specified NEC	T39.391	T39.392	T39.393	T39.394	T39.395	T39.396
Antikaluretic	T50.3X1	T50.3X2	T50.3X3	T50.3X4	T50.3X5	T50.3X6
Antiknock (tetraethyl lead)	T56.0X1	T56.0X2	T56.0X3	T56.0X4	—	—
Antilipemic drug NEC	T46.6X1	T46.6X2	T46.6X3	T46.6X4	T46.6X5	T46.6X6
Antimalarial	T37.2X1	T37.2X2	T37.2X3	T37.2X4	T37.2X5	T37.2X6
prophylactic NEC	T37.2X1	T37.2X2	T37.2X3	T37.2X4	T37.2X5	T37.2X6
pyrimidine derivative	T37.2X1	T37.2X2	T37.2X3	T37.2X4	T37.2X5	T37.2X6
Antimetabolite	T45.1X1	T45.1X2	T45.1X3	T45.1X4	T45.1X5	T45.1X6
Antimitotic agent	T45.1X1	T45.1X2	T45.1X3	T45.1X4	T45.1X5	T45.1X6
Antimony (compounds) (vapor) NEC	T56.891	T56.892	T56.893	T56.894	—	—
anti-infectives	T37.8X1	T37.8X2	T37.8X3	T37.8X4	T37.8X5	T37.8X6
dimercaptosuccinate	T37.3X1	T37.3X2	T37.3X3	T37.3X4	T37.3X5	T37.3X6
hydride	T56.891	T56.892	T56.893	T56.894	—	—
pesticide (vapor)	T60.8X1	T60.8X2	T60.8X3	T60.8X4	—	—
potassium (sodium) tartrate	T37.8X1	T37.8X2	T37.8X3	T37.8X4	T37.8X5	T37.8X6

◀ New   ◀▥ Revised   ~~deleted~~ Deleted

TABLE OF DRUGS AND CHEMICALS

Substance	External Cause (T-Code)					
	Poisoning, Accidental (Unintentional)	Poisoning, Intentional Self-Harm	Poisoning, Assault	Poisoning, Undetermined	Adverse Effect	Underdosing
Antimony NEC *(Continued)*						
sodium dimercaptosuccinate	T37.3X1	T37.3X2	T37.3X3	T37.3X4	T37.3X5	T37.3X6
tartrated	T37.8X1	T37.8X2	T37.8X3	T37.8X4	T37.8X5	T37.8X6
Antimuscarinic NEC	T44.3X1	T44.3X2	T44.3X3	T44.3X4	T44.3X5	T44.3X6
Antimycobacterial drug NEC	T37.1X1	T37.1X2	T37.1X3	T37.1X4	T37.1X5	T37.1X6
antibiotics	T36.5X1	T36.5X2	T36.5X3	T36.5X4	T36.5X5	T36.5X6
combination	T37.1X1	T37.1X2	T37.1X3	T37.1X4	T37.1X5	T37.1X6
Antinausea drug	T45.0X1	T45.0X2	T45.0X3	T45.0X4	T45.0X5	T45.0X6
Antinematode drug	T37.4X1	T37.4X2	T37.4X3	T37.4X4	T37.4X5	T37.4X6
Antineoplastic NEC	T45.1X1	T45.1X2	T45.1X3	T45.1X4	T45.1X5	T45.1X6
alkaloidal	T45.1X1	T45.1X2	T45.1X3	T45.1X4	T45.1X5	T45.1X6
antibiotics	T45.1X1	T45.1X2	T45.1X3	T45.1X4	T45.1X5	T45.1X6
combination	T45.1X1	T45.1X2	T45.1X3	T45.1X4	T45.1X5	T45.1X6
estrogen	T38.5X1	T38.5X2	T38.5X3	T38.5X4	T38.5X5	T38.5X6
steroid	T38.7X1	T38.7X2	T38.7X3	T38.7X4	T38.7X5	T38.7X6
Antiparasitic drug (systemic)	T37.91	T37.92	T37.93	T37.94	T37.95	T37.96
local	T49.0X1	T49.0X2	T49.0X3	T49.0X4	T49.0X5	T49.0X6
specified NEC	T37.8X1	T37.8X2	T37.8X3	T37.8X4	T37.8X5	T37.8X6
Antiparkinsonism drug NEC	T42.8X1	T42.8X2	T42.8X3	T42.8X4	T42.8X5	T42.8X6
Antiperspirant NEC	T49.2X1	T49.2X2	T49.2X3	T49.2X4	T49.2X5	T49.2X6
Antiphlogistic NEC	T39.4X1	T39.4X2	T39.4X3	T39.4X4	T39.4X5	T39.4X6
Antiplatyhelmintic drug	T37.4X1	T37.4X2	T37.4X3	T37.4X4	T37.4X5	T37.4X6
Antiprotozoal drug NEC	T37.3X1	T37.3X2	T37.3X3	T37.3X4	T37.3X5	T37.3X6
blood	T37.2X1	T37.2X2	T37.2X3	T37.2X4	T37.2X5	T37.2X6
local	T49.0X1	T49.0X2	T49.0X3	T49.0X4	T49.0X5	T49.0X6
Antipruritic drug NEC	T49.1X1	T49.1X2	T49.1X3	T49.1X4	T49.1X5	T49.1X6
Antipsychotic drug	T43.501	T43.502	T43.503	T43.504	T43.505	T43.506
specified NEC	T43.591	T43.592	T43.593	T43.594	T43.595	T43.596
Antipyretic	T39.91	T39.92	T39.93	T39.94	T39.95	T39.96
specified NEC	T39.8X1	T39.8X2	T39.8X3	T39.8X4	T39.8X5	T39.8X6
Antipyrine	T39.2X1	T39.2X2	T39.2X3		T39.2X5	T39.2X6
Antirabies hyperimmune serum	T50.Z11	T50.Z12	T50.Z13	T50.Z14	T50.Z15	T50.Z16
Antirheumatic NEC	T39.4X1	T39.4X2	T39.4X3	T39.4X4	T39.4X5	T39.4X6
Antirigidity drug NEC	T42.8X1	T42.8X2	T42.8X3	T42.8X4	T42.8X5	T42.8X6
Antischistosomal drug	T37.4X1	T37.4X2	T37.4X3	T37.4X4	T37.4X5	T37.4X6
Antiscorpion sera	T50.Z11	T50.Z12	T50.Z13	T50.Z14	T50.Z15	T50.Z16
Antiseborrheics	T49.4X1	T49.4X2	T49.4X3	T49.4X4	T49.4X5	T49.4X6
Antiseptics (external) (medicinal)	T49.0X1	T49.0X2	T49.0X3	T49.0X4	T49.0X5	T49.0X6
Antistine	T45.0X1	T45.0X2	T45.0X3	T45.0X4	T45.0X5	T45.0X6
Antitapeworm drug	T37.4X1	T37.4X2	T37.4X3	T37.4X4	T37.4X5	T37.4X6

◀ New   ◀ⁿⁿ Revised   ~~deleted~~ Deleted

Substance	External Cause (T-Code)					
	Poisoning, Accidental (Unintentional)	Poisoning, Intentional Self-Harm	Poisoning, Assault	Poisoning, Undetermined	Adverse Effect	Underdosing
Antitetanus immunoglobulin	T50.Z11	T50.Z12	T50.Z13	T50.Z14	T50.Z15	T50.Z16
Antithyroid drug NEC	T38.2X1	T38.2X2	T38.2X3	T38.2X4	T38.2X5	T38.2X6
Antitoxin	T50.Z11	T50.Z12	T50.Z13	T50.Z14	T50.Z15	T50.Z16
diphtheria	T50.Z11	T50.Z12	T50.Z13	T50.Z14	T50.Z15	T50.Z16
gas gangrene	T50.Z11	T50.Z12	T50.Z13	T50.Z14	T50.Z15	T50.Z16
tetanus	T50.Z11	T50.Z12	T50.Z13	T50.Z14	T50.Z15	T50.Z16
Antitoxin, any	T50.901	T50.902	T50.903	T50.904	T50.905	T50.906
Antitrichomonal drug	T37.3X1	T37.3X2	T37.3X3	T37.3X4	T37.3X5	T37.3X6
Antituberculars	T37.1X1	T37.1X2	T37.1X3	T37.1X4	T37.1X5	T37.1X6
antibiotics	T36.5X1	T36.5X2	T36.5X3	T36.5X4	T36.5X5	T36.5X6
Antitussive NEC	T48.3X1	T48.3X2	T48.3X3	T48.3X4	T48.3X5	T48.3X6
codeine mixture	T40.2X1	T40.2X2	T40.2X3	T40.2X4	T40.2X5	T40.2X6
opiate	T40.2X1	T40.2X2	T40.2X3	T40.2X4	T40.2X5	T40.2X6
Antivaricose drug	T46.8X1	T46.8X2	T46.8X3	T46.8X4	T46.8X5	T46.8X6
Antivenin, antivenom (sera)	T50.Z11	T50.Z12	T50.Z13	T50.Z14	T50.Z15	T50.Z16
crotaline	T50.Z11	T50.Z12	T50.Z13	T50.Z14	T50.Z15	T50.Z16
spider bite	T50.Z11	T50.Z12	T50.Z13	T50.Z14	T50.Z15	T50.Z16
Antivertigo drug	T45.0X1	T45.0X2	T45.0X3	T45.0X4	T45.0X5	T45.0X6
Antiviral drug NEC	T37.5X1	T37.5X2	T37.5X3	T37.5X4	T37.5X5	T37.5X6
eye	T49.5X1	T49.5X2	T49.5X3	T49.5X4	T49.5X5	T49.5X6
Antiwhipworm drug	T37.4X1	T37.4X2	T37.4X3	T37.4X4	T37.4X5	T37.4X6
Ant poisons — see Pesticides						
Antrol — see also by specific chemical substance	T60.91	T60.92	T60.93	T60.94	—	—
fungicide	T60.91	T60.92	T60.93	T60.94	—	—
ANTU (alpha naphthylthiourea)	T60.4X1	T60.4X2	T60.4X3	T60.4X4	—	—
Apalcillin	T36.0X1	T36.0X2	T36.0X3	T36.0X4	T36.0X5	T36.0X6
APC	T48.5X1	T48.5X2	T48.5X3	T48.5X4	T48.5X5	T48.5X6
Aplonidine	T44.4X1	T44.4X2	T44.4X3	T44.4X4	T44.4X5	T44.4X6
Apomorphine	T47.7X1	T47.7X2	T47.7X3	T47.7X4	T47.7X5	T47.7X6
Appetite depressants, central	T50.5X1	T50.5X2	T50.5X3	T50.5X4	T50.5X5	T50.5X6
Apraclonidine (hydrochloride)	T44.4X1	T44.4X2	T44.4X3	T44.4X4	T44.4X5	T44.4X6
Apresoline	T46.5X1	T46.5X2	T46.5X3	T46.5X4	T46.5X5	T46.5X6
Aprindine	T46.2X1	T46.2X2	T46.2X3	T46.2X4	T46.2X5	T46.2X6
Aprobarbital	T42.3X1	T42.3X2	T42.3X3	T42.3X4	T42.3X5	T42.3X6
Apronalide	T42.6X1	T42.6X2	T42.6X3	T42.6X4	T42.6X5	T42.6X6
Aprotinin	T45.621	T45.622	T45.623	T45.624	T45.625	T45.626
Aptocaine	T41.3X1	T41.3X2	T41.3X3	T41.3X4	T41.3X5	T41.3X6
Aqua fortis	T54.2X1	T54.2X2	T54.2X3	T54.2X4	—	—
Ara-A	T37.5X1	T37.5X2	T37.5X3	T37.5X4	T37.5X5	T37.5X6
Ara-C	T45.1X1	T45.1X2	T45.1X3	T45.1X4	T45.1X5	T45.1X6

TABLE OF DRUGS AND CHEMICALS

Substance	External Cause (T-Code)					
	Poisoning, Accidental (Unintentional)	Poisoning, Intentional Self-Harm	Poisoning, Assault	Poisoning, Undetermined	Adverse Effect	Underdosing
Arachis oil	T49.3X1	T49.3X2	T49.3X3	T49.3X4	T49.3X5	T49.3X6
cathartic	T47.4X1	T47.4X2	T47.4X3	T47.4X4	T47.4X5	T47.4X6
Aralen	T37.2X1	T37.2X2	T37.2X3	T37.2X4	T37.2X5	T37.2X6
Arecoline	T44.1X1	T44.1X2	T44.1X3	T44.1X4	T44.1X5	T44.1X6
Arginine	T50.991	T50.992	T50.993	T50.994	T50.995	T50.996
glutamate	T50.991	T50.992	T50.993	T50.994	T50.995	T50.996
Argyrol	T49.0X1	T49.0X2	T49.0X3	T49.0X4	T49.0X5	T49.0X6
ENT agent	T49.6X1	T49.6X2	T49.6X3	T49.6X4	T49.6X5	T49.6X6
ophthalmic preparation	T49.5X1	T49.5X2	T49.5X3	T49.5X4	T49.5X5	T49.5X6
Aristocort	T38.0X1	T38.0X2	T38.0X3	T38.0X4	T38.0X5	T38.0X6
ENT agent	T49.6X1	T49.6X2	T49.6X3	T49.6X4	T49.6X5	T49.6X6
ophthalmic preparation	T49.5X1	T49.5X2	T49.5X3	T49.5X4	T49.5X5	T49.5X6
topical NEC	T49.0X1	T49.0X2	T49.0X3	T49.0X4	T49.0X5	T49.0X6
Aromatics, corrosive	T54.1X1	T54.1X2	T54.1X3	T54.1X4	—	—
disinfectants	T54.1X1	T54.1X2	T54.1X3	T54.1X4	—	—
Arsenate of lead	T57.0X1	T57.0X2	T57.0X3	T57.0X4	—	—
herbicide	T57.0X1	T57.0X2	T57.0X3	T57.0X4	—	—
Arsenic, arsenicals (compounds) (dust) (vapor) NEC	T57.0X1	T57.0X2	T57.0X3	T57.0X4		
anti-infectives	T37.8X1	T37.8X2	T37.8X3	T37.8X4	T37.8X5	T37.8X6
pesticide (dust) (fumes)	T57.0X1	T57.0X2	T57.0X3	T57.0X4	—	—
Arsine (gas)	T57.0X1	T57.0X2	T57.0X3	T57.0X4	—	—
Arsphenamine (silver)	T37.8X1	T37.8X2	T37.8X3	T37.8X4	T37.8X5	T37.8X6
Arsthinol	T37.3X1	T37.3X2	T37.3X3	T37.3X4	T37.3X5	T37.3X6
Artane	T44.3X1	T44.3X2	T44.3X3	T44.3X4	T44.3X5	T44.3X6
Arthropod (venomous) NEC	T63.481	T63.482	T63.483	T63.484	—	—
Articaine	T41.3X1	T41.3X2	T41.3X3	T41.3X4	T41.3X5	T41.3X6
Asbestos	T57.8X1	T57.8X2	T57.8X3	T57.8X4	—	—
Ascaridole	T37.4X1	T37.4X2	T37.4X3	T37.4X4	T37.4X5	T37.4X6
Ascorbic acid	T45.2X1	T45.2X2	T45.2X3	T45.2X4	T45.2X5	T45.2X6
Asiaticoside	T49.0X1	T49.0X2	T49.0X3	T49.0X4	T49.0X5	T49.0X6
Asparaginase	T45.1X1	T45.1X2	T45.1X3	T45.1X4	T45.1X5	T45.1X6
Aspidium (oleoresin)	T37.4X1	T37.4X2	T37.4X3	T37.4X4	T37.4X5	T37.4X6
Aspirin (aluminum) (soluble)	T39.011	T39.012	T39.013	T39.014	T39.015	T39.016
Aspoxicillin	T36.0X1	T36.0X2	T36.0X4	T36.0X4	T36.0X5	T36.0X6
Astemizole	T45.0X1	T45.0X2	T45.0X3	T45.0X4	T45.0X5	T45.0X6
Astringent (local)	T49.2X1	T49.2X2	T49.2X3	T49.2X4	T49.2X5	T49.2X6
specified NEC	T49.2X1	T49.2X2	T49.2X3	T49.2X4	T49.2X5	T49.2X6
Astromicin	T36.5X1	T36.5X2	T36.5X3	T36.5X4	T36.5X5	T36.5X6
Ataractic drug NEC	T43.501	T43.502	T43.503	T43.504	T43.505	T43.506

◄ New   ◄═ Revised   ~~deleted~~ Deleted

TABLE OF DRUGS AND CHEMICALS

	External Cause (T-Code)					
Substance	Poisoning, Accidental (Unintentional)	Poisoning, Intentional Self-Harm	Poisoning, Assault	Poisoning, Undetermined	Adverse Effect	Underdosing
Atenolol	T44.7X1	T44.7X2	T44.7X3	T44.7X4	T44.7X5	T44.7X6
Atonia drug, intestinal	T47.4X1	T47.4X2	T47.4X3	T47.4X4	T47.4X5	T47.4X6
Atophan	T50.4X1	T50.4X2	T50.4X3	T50.4X4	T50.4X5	T50.4X6
Atracurium besilate	T48.1X1	T48.1X2	T48.1X3	T48.1X4	T48.1X5	T48.1X6
Atropine	T44.3X1	T44.3X2	T44.3X3	T44.3X4	T44.3X5	T44.3X6
derivative	T44.3X1	T44.3X2	T44.3X3	T44.3X4	T44.3X5	T44.3X6
methonitrate	T44.3X1	T44.3X2	T44.3X3	T44.3X4	T44.3X5	T44.3X6
Attapulgite	T47.6X1	T47.6X2	T47.6X3	T47.6X4	T47.6X5	T47.6X6
Attenuvax	T50.991	T50.992	T50.993	T50.994	T50.995	T50.996
Auramine	T65.891	T65.892	T65.893	T65.894	—	—
dye	T65.6X1	T65.6X2	T65.6X3	T65.6X4	—	—
fungicide	T60.3X1	T60.3X2	T60.3X3	T60.3X4	—	—
Auranofin	T39.4X1	T39.4X2	T39.4X3	T39.4X4	T39.4X5	T39.4X6
Aurantiin	T46.991	T46.992	T46.993	T46.994	T46.995	T46.996
Aureomycin	T36.4X1	T36.4X2	T36.4X3	T36.4X4	T36.4X5	T36.4X6
ophthalmic preparation	T49.5X1	T49.5X2	T49.5X3	T49.5X4	T49.5X5	T49.5X6
topical NEC	T49.0X1	T49.0X2	T49.0X3	T49.0X4	T49.0X5	T49.0X6
Aurothioglucose	T39.4X1	T39.4X2	T39.4X3	T39.4X4	T39.4X5	T39.4X6
Aurothioglycanide	T39.4X1	T39.4X2	T39.4X3	T39.4X4	T39.4X5	T39.4X6
Aurothiomalate sodium	T39.4X1	T39.4X2	T39.4X3	T39.4X4	T39.4X5	T39.4X6
Aurotioprol	T39.4X1	T39.4X2	T39.4X3	T39.4X4	T39.4X5	T39.4X6
Automobile fuel	T52.0X1	T52.0X2	T52.0X3	T52.0X4	—	—
Autonomic nervous system agent NEC	T44.901	T44.902	T44.903	T44.904	T44.905	T44.906
Avlosulfon	T37.1X1	T37.1X2	T37.1X3	T37.1X4	T37.1X5	T37.1X6
Avomine	T42.6X1	T42.6X2	T42.6X3	T42.6X4	T42.6X5	T42.6X6
Axerophthol	T45.2X1	T45.2X2	T45.2X3	T45.2X4	T45.2X5	T45.2X6
Azacitidine	T45.1X1	T45.1X2	T45.1X3	T45.1X4	T45.1X5	T45.1X6
Azacyclonol	T43.591	T43.592	T43.593	T43.594	T43.595	T43.596
Azadirachta	T60.2X1	T60.2X2	T60.2X3	T60.2X4	—	—
Azanidazole	T37.3X1	T37.3X2	T37.3X3	T37.3X4	T37.3X5	T37.3X6
Azapetine	T46.7X1	T46.7X2	T46.7X3	T46.7X4	T46.7X5	T46.7X6
Azapropazone	T39.2X1	T39.2X2	T39.2X3	T39.2X4	T39.2X5	T39.2X6
Azaribine	T45.1X1	T45.1X2	T45.1X3	T45.1X4	T45.1X5	T45.1X6
Azaserine	T45.1X1	T45.1X2	T45.1X3	T45.1X4	T45.1X5	T45.1X6
Azatadine	T45.0X1	T45.0X2	T45.0X3	T45.0X4	T45.0X5	T45.0X6
Azatepa	T45.1X1	T45.1X2	T45.1X3	T45.1X4	T45.1X5	T45.1X6
Azathioprine	T45.1X1	T45.1X2	T45.1X3	T45.1X4	T45.1X5	T45.1X6
Azelaic acid	T49.0X1	T49.0X2	T49.0X3	T49.0X4	T49.0X5	T49.0X6
Azelastine	T45.0X1	T45.0X2	T45.0X3	T45.0X4	T45.0X5	T45.0X6

◀ New ◀▥ Revised ~~deleted~~ Deleted

Substance	External Cause (T-Code)					
	Poisoning, Accidental (Unintentional)	Poisoning, Intentional Self-Harm	Poisoning, Assault	Poisoning, Undetermined	Adverse Effect	Underdosing
Azidocillin	T36.0X1	T36.0X2	T36.0X3	T36.0X4	T36.0X5	T36.0X6
Azidothymidine	T37.5X1	T37.5X2	T37.5X3	T37.5X4	T37.5X5	T37.5X6
Azinphos (ethyl) (methyl)	T60.0X1	T60.0X2	T60.0X3	T60.0X4	—	—
Aziridine (chelating)	T54.1X1	T54.1X2	T54.1X3	T54.1X4	—	—
Azithromycin	T36.3X1	T36.3X2	T36.3X3	T36.3X4	T36.3X5	T36.3X6
Azlocillin	T36.01	T36.02	T36.03	T36.04	T36.05	T36.06
Azobenzene smoke	T65.3X1	T65.3X2	T65.3X3	T65.3X4	—	—
acaricide	T60.8X1	T60.8X2	T60.8X3	T60.8X4	—	—
Azosulfamide	T37.0X1	T37.0X2	T37.0X3	T37.0X4	T37.0X5	T37.0X6
AZT	T37.5X1	T37.5X2	T37.5X3	T37.5X4	T37.5X5	T37.5X6
Aztreonam	T36.1X1	T36.1X2	T36.1X3	T36.1X4	T36.1X5	T36.1X6
Azulfidine	T37.0X1	T37.0X2	T37.0X3	T37.0X4	T37.0X5	T37.0X6
Azuresin	T50.8X1	T50.8X2	T50.8X3	T50.8X4	T50.8X5	T50.8X6
B						
Bacampicillin	T36.0X1	T36.0X2	T36.0X3	T36.0X4	T36.0X5	T36.0X6
Bacillus						
lactobacillus	T47.8X1	T47.8X2	T47.8X3	T47.8X4	T47.8X5	T47.8X6
subtilis	T47.6X1	T47.6X2	T47.6X3	T47.6X4	T47.6X5	T47.6X6
Bacimycin	T49.0X1	T49.0X2	T49.0X3	T49.0X4	T49.0X5	T49.0X6
ophthalmic preparation	T49.5X1	T49.5X2	T49.5X3	T49.5X4	T49.5X5	T49.5X6
Bacitracin zinc	T49.0X1	T49.0X2	T49.0X3	T49.0X4	T49.0X5	T49.0X6
with neomycin	T49.0X1	T49.0X2	T49.0X3	T49.0X4	T49.0X5	T49.0X6
ENT agent	T49.6X1	T49.6X2	T49.6X3	T49.6X4	T49.6X5	T49.6X6
ophthalmic preparation	T49.5X1	T49.5X2	T49.5X3	T49.5X4	T49.5X5	T49.5X6
topical NEC	T49.0X1	T49.0X2	T49.0X3	T49.0X4	T49.0X5	T49.0X6
Baclofen	T42.8X1	T42.8X2	T42.8X3	T42.8X4	T42.8X5	T42.8X6
Baking soda	T50.991	T50.992	T50.993	T50.994	T50.995	T50.996
BAL	T45.8X1	T45.8X2	T45.8X3	T45.8X4	T45.8X5	T45.8X6
Bambuterol	T48.6X1	T48.6X2	T48.6X3	T48.6X4	T48.6X5	T48.6X6
Bamethan (sulfate)	T46.7X1	T46.7X2	T46.7X3	T46.7X4	T46.7X5	T46.7X6
Bamifylline	T48.6X1	T48.6X2	T48.6X3	T48.6X4	T48.6X5	T48.6X6
Bamipine	T45.0X1	T45.0X2	T45.0X3	T45.0X4	T45.0X5	T45.0X6
Baneberry — see Actaea spicata						
Banewort — see Belladonna						
Barbenyl	T42.3X1	T42.3X2	T42.3X3	T42.3X4	T42.3X5	T42.3X6
Barbexaclone	T42.6X1	T42.6X2	T42.6X3	T42.6X4	T42.6X5	T42.6X6
Barbital	T42.3X1	T42.3X2	T42.3X3	T42.3X4	T42.3X5	T42.3X6
sodium	T42.3X1	T42.3X2	T42.3X3	T42.3X4	T42.3X5	T42.3X6
Barbitone	T42.3X1	T42.3X2	T42.3X3	T42.3X4	T42.3X5	T42.3X6

◀ New   ◀▥ Revised   ~~deleted~~ Deleted

Substance	Poisoning, Accidental (Unintentional)	Poisoning, Intentional Self-Harm	Poisoning, Assault	Poisoning, Undetermined	Adverse Effect	Underdosing
			External Cause (T-Code)			
Barbiturate NEC	T42.3X1	T42.3X2	T42.3X3	T42.3X4	T42.3X5	T42.3X6
with tranquilizer	T42.3X1	T42.3X2	T42.3X3	T42.3X4	T42.3X5	T42.3X6
anesthetic (intravenous)	T41.1X1	T41.1X2	T41.1X3	T41.1X4	T41.1X5	T41.1X6
Barium (carbonate) (chloride) (sulfite)	T57.8X1	T57.8X2	T57.8X3	T57.8X4	—	—
diagnostic agent	T50.8X1	T50.8X2	T50.8X3	T50.8X4	T50.8X5	T50.8X6
pesticide	T60.4X1	T60.4X2	T60.4X3	T60.4X4	—	—
rodenticide	T60.4X1	T60.4X2	T60.4X3	T60.4X4	—	—
sulfate (medicinal)	T50.8X1	T50.8X2	T50.8X3	T50.8X4	T50.8X5	T50.8X6
Barrier cream	T49.3X1	T49.3X2	T49.3X3	T49.3X4	T49.3X5	T49.3X6
Basic fuchsin	T49.0X1	T49.0X2	T49.0X4	T49.0X4	T49.0X5	T49.0X6
Battery acid or fluid	T54.2X1	T54.2X2	T54.2X3	T54.2X4	—	—
Bay rum	T51.8X1	T51.8X2	T51.8X3	T51.8X4	—	—
BCG (vaccine)	T50.A91	T50.A92	T50.A93	T50.A94	T50.A95	T50.A96
BCNU	T45.1X1	T45.1X2	T45.1X3	T45.1X4	T45.1X5	T45.1X6
Bearsfoot	T62.2X1	T62.2X2	T62.2X3	T62.2X4	—	—
Beclamide	T42.6X1	T42.6X2	T42.6X3	T42.6X4	T42.6X5	T42.6X6
Beclomethasone	T44.5X1	T44.5X2	T44.5X3	T44.5X4	T44.5X5	T44.5X6
Bee (sting) (venom)	T63.441	T63.442	T63.443	T63.444	—	—
Befunolol	T49.5X1	T49.5X2	T49.5X3	T49.5X4	T49.5X5	T49.5X6
Bekanamycin	T36.5X1	T36.5X2	T36.5X3	T36.5X4	T36.5X5	T36.5X6
Belladonna — *see also Nightshade*						
alkaloids	T44.3X1	T44.3X2	T44.3X3	T44.3X4	T44.3X5	T44.3X6
extract	T44.3X1	T44.3X2	T44.3X3	T44.3X4	T44.3X5	T44.3X6
herb	T44.3X1	T44.3X2	T44.3X3	T44.3X4	T44.3X5	T44.3X6
Bemegride	T50.7X1	T50.7X2	T50.7X3	T50.7X4	T50.7X5	T50.7X6
Benactyzine	T44.3X1	T44.3X2	T44.3X3	T44.3X4	T44.3X5	T44.3X6
Benadryl	T45.0X1	T45.0X2	T45.0X3	T45.0X4	T45.0X5	T45.0X6
Benaprizine	T44.3X1	T44.3X2	T44.3X3	T44.3X4	T44.3X5	T44.3X6
Benazepril	T46.4X1	T46.4X2	T46.4X3	T46.4X4	T46.4X5	T46.4X6
Bencyclane	T46.7X1	T46.7X2	T46.7X3	T46.7X4	T46.7X5	T46.7X6
Bendazol	T46.3X1	T46.3X2	T46.3X3	T46.3X4	T46.3X5	T46.3X6
Bendrofluazide	T50.2X1	T50.2X2	T50.2X3	T50.2X4	T50.2X5	T50.2X6
Bendroflumethiazide	T50.2X1	T50.2X2	T50.2X3	T50.2X4	T50.2X5	T50.2X6
Benemid	T50.4X1	T50.4X2	T50.4X3	T50.4X4	T50.4X5	T50.4X6
Benethamine penicillin	T36.0X1	T36.0X2	T36.0X3	T36.0X4	T36.0X5	T36.0X6
Benisone	T49.0X1	T49.0X2	T49.0X3	T49.0X4	T49.0X5	T49.0X6
Benexate	T47.1X1	T47.1X2	T47.1X3	T47.1X4	T47.1X5	T47.1X6
Benfluorex	T46.6X1	T46.6X2	T46.6X3	T46.6X4	T46.6X5	T46.6X6
Benfotiamine	T45.2X1	T45.2X2	T45.2X3	T45.2X4	T45.2X5	T45.2X6
Benomyl	T60.0X1	T60.0X2	T60.0X3	T60.0X4	—	—

TABLE OF DRUGS AND CHEMICALS

Substance	External Cause (T-Code)					
	Poisoning, Accidental (Unintentional)	Poisoning, Intentional Self-Harm	Poisoning, Assault	Poisoning, Undetermined	Adverse Effect	Underdosing
Benoquin	T49.8X1	T49.8X2	T49.8X3	T49.8X4	T49.8X5	T49.8X6
Benoxinate	T41.3X1	T41.3X2	T41.3X3	T41.3X4	T41.3X5	T41.3X6
Benperidol	T43.4X1	T43.4X2	T43.4X3	T43.4X4	T43.4X5	T43.4X6
Benproperine	T48.3X1	T48.3X2	T48.3X3	T48.3X4	T48.3X5	T48.3X6
Benserazide	T42.8X1	T42.8X2	T42.8X3	T42.8X4	T42.8X5	T42.8X6
Bentazepam	T42.4X1	T42.4X2	T42.4X3	T42.4X4	T42.4X5	T42.4X6
Bentiromide	T50.8X1	T50.8X2	T50.8X3	T50.8X4	T50.8X5	T50.8X6
Bentonite	T49.3X1	T49.3X2	T49.3X3	T49.3X4	T49.3X5	T49.3X6
Benzalbutyramide	T46.6X1	T46.6X2	T46.6X3	T46.6X4	T46.6X5	T46.6X6
Benzalkonium (chloride)	T49.0X1	T49.0X2	T49.0X3	T49.0X4	T49.0X5	T49.0X6
ophthalmic preparation	T49.5X1	T49.5X2	T49.5X3	T49.5X4	T49.5X5	T49.5X6
Benzamine	T41.3X1	T41.3X2	T41.3X3	T41.3X4	T41.3X5	T41.3X6
lactate	T49.1X1	T49.1X2	T49.1X3	T49.1X4	T49.1X5	T49.1X6
Benzamidosalicylate (calcium)	T37.1X1	T37.1X2	T37.1X3	T37.1X4	T37.1X5	T37.1X6
Benzamphetamine	T50.5X1	T50.5X2	T50.5X3	T50.5X4	T50.5X5	T50.5X6
Benzapril hydrochloride	T46.5X1	T46.5X2	T46.5X3	T46.5X4	T46.5X5	T46.5X6
Benzathine benzylpenicillin	T36.0X1	T36.0X2	T36.0X3	T36.0X4	T36.0X5	T36.0X6
Benzathine penicillin	T36.0X1	T36.0X2	T36.0X3	T36.0X4	T36.0X5	T36.0X6
Benzatropine	T42.8X1	T42.8X2	T42.8X3	T42.8X4	T42.8X5	T42.8X6
Benzbromarone	T50.4X1	T50.4X2	T50.4X3	T50.4X4	T50.4X5	T50.4X6
Benzcarbimine	T45.1X1	T45.1X2	T45.1X3	T45.1X4	T45.1X5	T45.1X6
Benzedrex	T44.991	T44.992	T44.993	T44.994	T44.995	T44.996
Benzedrine (amphetamine)	T43.621	T43.622	T43.623	T43.624	T43.625	T43.626
Benzenamine	T65.3X1	T65.3X2	T65.3X3	T65.3X4	—	—
Benzene	T52.1X1	T52.1X2	T52.1X3	T52.1X4	—	—
homologues (acetyl) (dimethyl) (methyl) (solvent)	T52.2X1	T52.2X2	T52.2X3	T52.2X4	—	—
Benzethonium (chloride)	T49.0X1	T49.0X2	T49.0X3	T49.0X4	T49.0X5	T49.0X6
Benzfetamine	T50.5X1	T50.5X2	T50.5X3	T50.5X4	T50.5X5	T50.5X6
Benzhexol	T44.3X1	T44.3X2	T44.3X3	T44.3X4	T44.3X5	T44.3X6
Benzhydramine (chloride)	T45.0X1	T45.0X2	T45.0X3	T45.0X4	T45.0X5	T45.0X6
Benzidine	T65.891	T65.892	T65.893	T65.894	—	—
Benzilonium bromide	T44.3X1	T44.3X2	T44.3X3	T44.3X4	T44.3X5	T44.3X6
Benzimidazole	T60.3X1	T60.3X2	T60.3X3	T60.3X4	—	—
Benzin(e) — see Ligroin						
Benziodarone	T46.3X1	T46.3X2	T46.3X3	T46.3X4	T46.3X5	T46.3X6
Benznidazole	T37.3X1	T37.3X2	T37.3X3	T37.3X4	T37.3X5	T37.3X6
Benzocaine	T41.3X1	T41.3X2	T41.3X3	T41.3X4	T41.3X5	T41.3X6
Benzoctamine	T43.0X1	T43.0X2	T43.0X3	T43.0X4	T43.0X5	T43.0X6
Benzodiapin	T42.4X1	T42.4X2	T42.4X3	T42.4X4	T42.4X5	T42.4X6
Benzodiazepine NEC	T42.4X1	T42.4X2	T42.4X3	T42.4X4	T42.4X5	T42.4X6

◀ New ◀◀ Revised ~~deleted~~ Deleted

Substance	External Cause (T-Code)					
	Poisoning, Accidental (Unintentional)	Poisoning, Intentional Self-Harm	Poisoning, Assault	Poisoning, Undetermined	Adverse Effect	Underdosing
Benzoic acid	T49.0X1	T49.0X2	T49.0X3	T49.0X4	T49.0X5	T49.0X6
with salicylic acid	T49.0X1	T49.0X2	T49.0X3	T49.0X4	T49.0X5	T49.0X6
Benzoin (tincture)	T48.5X1	T48.5X2	T48.5X3	T48.5X4	T48.5X5	T48.5X6
Benzol (benzene)	T52.1X1	T52.1X2	T52.1X3	T52.1X4	—	—
vapor	T52.0X1	T52.0X2	T52.0X3	T52.0X4	—	—
Benzomorphan	T40.2X1	T40.2X2	T40.2X3	T40.2X4	T40.2X5	T40.2X6
Benzonatate	T48.3X1	T48.3X2	T48.3X3	T48.3X4	T48.3X5	T48.3X6
Benzophenones	T49.3X1	T49.3X2	T49.3X3	T49.3X4	T49.3X5	T49.3X6
Benzopyrone	T46.991	T46.992	T46.993	T46.994	T46.995	T46.996
Benzothiadiazides	T50.2X1	T50.2X2	T50.2X3	T50.2X4	T50.2X5	T50.2X6
Benzoxonium chloride	T49.0X1	T49.0X2	T49.0X3	T49.0X4	T49.0X5	T49.0X6
Benzoyl peroxide	T49.0X1	T49.0X2	T49.0X3	T49.0X4	T49.0X5	T49.0X6
Benzoylpas calcium	T37.1X1	T37.1X2	T37.1X3	T37.1X4	T37.1X5	T37.1X6
Benzperidin	T43.591	T43.592	T43.593	T43.594	T43.595	T43.596
Benzperidol	T43.591	T43.592	T43.593	T43.594	T43.595	T43.596
Benzphetamine	T50.5X1	T50.5X2	T50.5X3	T50.5X4	T50.5X5	T50.5X6
Benzpyrinium bromide	T44.1X1	T44.1X2	T44.1X3	T44.1X4	T44.1X5	T44.1X6
Benzquinamide	T45.0X1	T45.0X2	T45.0X3	T45.0X4	T45.0X5	T45.0X6
Benzthiazide	T50.2X1	T50.2X2	T50.2X3	T50.2X4	T50.2X5	T50.2X6
Benztropine						
anticholinergic	T44.3X1	T44.3X2	T44.3X3	T44.3X4	T44.3X5	T44.3X6
antiparkinson	T42.8X1	T42.8X2	T42.8X3	T42.8X4	T42.8X5	T42.8X6
Benzydamine	T49.0X1	T49.0X2	T49.0X3	T49.0X4	T49.0X5	T49.0X6
Benzyl						
acetate	T52.8X1	T52.8X2	T52.8X3	T52.8X4	—	—
alcohol	T49.0X1	T49.0X2	T49.0X3	T49.0X4	T49.0X5	T49.0X6
benzoate	T49.0X1	T49.0X2	T49.0X3	T49.0X4	T49.0X5	T49.0X6
Benzoic acid	T49.0X1	T49.0X2	T49.0X3	T49.0X4	T49.0X5	T49.0X6
morphine	T40.2X1	T40.2X2	T40.2X3	T40.2X4	—	—
nicotinate	T46.6X1	T46.6X2	T46.6X3	T46.6X4	T46.6X5	T46.6X6
penicillin	T36.0X1	T36.0X2	T36.0X3	T36.0X4	T36.0X5	T36.0X6
Benzylhydrochlorthia-zide	T50.2X1	T50.2X2	T50.2X3	T50.2X4	T50.2X5	T50.2X6
Benzylpenicillin	T36.0X1	T36.0X2	T36.0X3	T36.0X4	T36.0X5	T36.0X6
Benzylthiouracil	T38.2X1	T38.2X2	T38.2X3	T38.2X4	T38.2X5	T38.2X6
Bephenium hydroxy-naphthoate	T37.4X1	T37.4X2	T37.4X3	T37.4X4	T37.4X5	T37.4X6
Bepridil	T46.1X1	T46.1X2	T46.1X3	T46.1X4	T46.1X5	T46.1X6
Bergamot oil	T65.891	T65.892	T65.893	T65.894	—	—
Bergapten	T50.991	T50.992	T50.993	T50.994	T50.995	T50.996
Berries, poisonous	T62.1X1	T62.1X2	T62.1X3	T62.1X4	—	—
Beryllium (compounds)	T56.7X1	T56.7X2	T56.7X3	T56.7X4	—	—

TABLE OF DRUGS AND CHEMICALS

Substance	Poisoning, Accidental (Unintentional)	Poisoning, Intentional Self-Harm	Poisoning, Assault	Poisoning, Undetermined	Adverse Effect	Underdosing
	External Cause (T-Code)					
b-acetyldigoxin	T46.0X1	T46.0X2	T46.0X3	T46.0X4	T46.0X5	T46.0X6
beta adrenergic blocking agent, heart	T44.7X1	T44.7X2	T44.7X3	T44.7X4	T44.7X5	T44.7X6
b-benzalbutyramide	T46.6X1	T46.6X2	T46.6X3	T46.6X4	T46.6X5	T46.6X6
Betacarotene	T45.2X1	T45.2X2	T45.2X3	T45.2X4	T45.2X5	T45.2X6
b-eucaine	T49.1X1	T49.1X2	T49.1X3	T49.1X4	T49.1X5	T49.1X6
Beta-Chlor	T42.6X1	T42.6X2	T42.6X3	T42.6X4	T42.6X5	T42.6X6
b-galactosidase	T47.5X1	T47.5X2	T47.5X3	T47.5X4	T47.5X5	T47.5X6
Betahistine	T46.7X1	T46.7X2	T46.7X3	T46.7X4	T46.7X5	T46.7X6
Betaine	T47.5X1	T47.5X2	T47.5X3	T47.5X4	T47.5X5	T47.5X6
Betamethasone	T49.0X1	T49.0X2	T49.0X3	T49.0X4	T49.0X5	T49.0X6
topical	T49.0X1	T49.0X2	T49.0X3	T49.0X4	T49.0X5	T49.0X6
Betamicin	T36.8X1	T36.8X2	T36.8X3	T36.8X4	T36.8X5	T36.8X6
Betanidine	T46.5X1	T46.5X2	T46.5X3	T46.5X4	T46.5X5	T46.5X6
b-sitosterol(s)	T46.6X1	T46.6X2	T46.6X3	T46.6X4	T46.6X5	T46.6X6
Betaxolol	T44.7X1	T44.7X2	T44.7X3	T44.7X4	T44.7X5	T44.7X6
Betazole	T50.8X1	T50.8X2	T50.8X3	T50.8X4	T50.8X5	T50.8X6
Bethanechol	T44.1X1	T44.1X2	T44.1X3	T44.1X4	T44.1X5	T44.1X6
chloride	T44.1X1	T44.1X2	T44.1X3	T44.1X4	T44.1X5	T44.1X6
Bethanidine	T46.5X1	T46.5X2	T46.5X3	T46.5X4	T46.5X5	T46.5X6
Betoxycaine	T41.3X1	T41.3X2	T41.3X3	T41.3X4	T41.3X5	T41.3X6
Betula oil	T49.3X1	T49.3X2	T49.3X3	T49.3X4	T49.3X5	T49.3X6
Bevantolol	T44.7X1	T44.7X2	T44.7X3	T44.7X4	T44.7X5	T44.7X6
Bevonium metilsulfate	T44.3X1	T44.3X2	T44.3X3	T44.3X4	T44.3X5	T44.3X6
Bezafibrate	T46.6X1	T46.6X2	T46.6X3	T46.6X4	T46.6X5	T46.6X6
Bezitramide	T40.4X1	T40.4X2	T40.4X3	T40.4X4	T40.4X5	T40.4X6
BHA	T50.991	T50.992	T50.993	T50.994	T50.995	T50.996
Bhang	T40.7X1	T40.7X2	T40.7X3	T40.7X4	T40.7X5	T40.7X6
BHC (medicinal)	T49.0X1	T49.0X2	T49.0X3	T49.0X4	T49.0X5	T49.0X6
nonmedicinal (vapor)	T53.6X1	T53.6X2	T53.6X3	T53.6X4	—	—
Bialamicol	T37.3X1	T37.3X2	T37.3X3	T37.3X4	T37.3X5	T37.3X6
Bibenzonium bromide	T48.3X1	T48.3X2	T48.3X3	T48.3X4	T48.3X5	T48.3X6
Bibrocathol	T49.5X1	T49.5X2	T49.5X3	T49.5X4	T49.5X5	T49.5X6
Bichloride of mercury — see Mercury, chloride						
Bichromates (calcium) (potassium) (sodium) (crystals)	T57.8X1	T57.8X2	T57.8X3	T57.8X4	—	—
fumes	T56.2X1	T56.2X2	T56.2X3	T56.2X4	—	—
Biclotymol	T49.6X1	T49.6X2	T49.6X3	T49.6X4	T49.6X5	T49.6X6
Bicucculine	T50.7X1	T50.7X2	T50.7X3	T50.7X4	T50.7X5	T50.7X6
Bifemelane	T43.291	T43.292	T43.293	T43.294	T43.295	T43.296
Biguanide derivatives, oral	T38.3X1	T38.3X2	T38.3X3	T38.3X4	T38.3X5	T38.3X6

◀ New   ◀▥ Revised   ~~deleted~~ Deleted

TABLE OF DRUGS AND CHEMICALS

Substance	External Cause (T-Code)					
	Poisoning, Accidental (Unintentional)	Poisoning, Intentional Self-Harm	Poisoning, Assault	Poisoning, Undetermined	Adverse Effect	Underdosing
Biligrafin	T50.8X1	T50.8X2	T50.8X3	T50.8X4	T50.8X5	T50.8X6
Bile salts	T47.5X1	T47.5X2	T47.5X3	T47.5X4	T47.5X5	T47.5X6
Bilopaque	T50.8X1	T50.8X2	T50.8X3	T50.8X4	T50.8X5	T50.8X6
Binifibrate	T46.6X1	T46.6X2	T46.6X3	T46.6X4	T46.6X5	T46.6X6
Binitrobenzol	T65.3X1	T65.3X2	T65.3X3	T65.3X4	—	—
Bioflavonoid(s)	T46.991	T46.992	T46.993	T46.994	T46.995	T46.996
Biological substance NEC	T50.901	T50.902	T50.903	T50.904	T50.905	T50.906
Biotin	T45.2X1	T45.2X2	T45.2X3	T45.2X4	T45.2X5	T45.2X6
Biperiden	T44.3X1	T44.3X2	T44.3X3	T44.3X4	T44.3X5	T44.3X6
Bisacodyl	T47.2X1	T47.2X2	T47.2X3	T47.2X4	T47.2X5	T47.2X6
Bisbentiamine	T45.2X1	T45.2X2	T45.2X3	T45.2X4	T45.2X5	T45.2X6
Bisbutiamine	T45.2X1	T45.2X2	T45.2X3	T45.2X4	T45.2X5	T45.2X6
Bisdequalinium (salts) (diacetate)	T49.6X1	T49.6X2	T49.6X3	T49.6X4	T49.6X5	T49.6X6
Bishydroxycoumarin	T45.511	T45.512	T45.513	T45.514	T45.515	T45.516
Bismarsen	T37.8X1	T37.8X2	T37.8X3	T37.8X4	T37.8X5	T37.8X6
Bismuth salts	T47.6X1	T47.6X2	T47.6X3	T47.6X4	T47.6X5	T47.6X6
aluminate	T47.1X1	T47.1X2	T47.1X3	T47.1X4	T47.1X5	T47.1X6
anti-infectives	T37.8X1	T37.8X2	T37.8X3	T37.8X4	T37.8X5	T37.8X6
formic iodide	T49.0X1	T49.0X2	T49.0X3	T49.0X4	T49.0X5	T49.0X6
glycolylarsenate	T49.0X1	T49.0X2	T49.0X3	T49.0X4	T49.0X5	T49.0X6
nonmedicinal (compounds) NEC	T65.91	T65.92	T65.93	T65.94	—	—
subcarbonate	T47.6X1	T47.6X2	T47.6X3	T47.6X4	T47.6X5	T47.6X6
subsalicylate	T37.8X1	T37.8X2	T37.8X3	T37.8X4	T37.8X5	T37.8X6
sulfarsphenamine	T37.8X1	T37.8X2	T37.8X3	T37.8X4	T37.8X5	T37.8X6
Bisoprolol	T44.7X1	T44.7X2	T44.7X3	T44.7X4	T44.7X5	T44.7X6
Bisoxatin	T47.2X1	T47.2X2	T47.2X3	T47.2X4	T47.2X5	T47.2X6
Bisulepin (hydrochloride)	T45.0X1	T45.0X2	T45.0X3	T45.0X4	T45.0X5	T45.0X6
Bithionol	T37.8X1	T37.8X2	T37.8X3	T37.8X4	T37.8X5	T37.8X6
anthelminthic	T37.4X1	T37.4X2	T37.4X3	T37.4X4	T37.4X5	T37.4X6
Bitolterol	T48.6X1	T48.6X2	T48.6X3	T48.6X4	T48.6X5	T48.6X6
Bitoscanate	T37.4X1	T37.4X2	T37.4X3	T37.4X4	T37.4X5	T37.4X6
Bitter almond oil	T62.8X1	T62.8X2	T62.8X3	T62.8X4	—	—
Bittersweet	T62.2X1	T62.2X2	T62.2X3	T62.2X4	—	—
Black						
flag	T60.91	T60.92	T60.93	T60.94	—	—
henbane	T62.2X1	T62.2X2	T62.2X3	T62.2X4	—	—
leaf (40)	T60.91	T60.92	T60.93	T60.94	—	—
widow spider (bite)	T63.311	T63.312	T63.313	T63.314	—	—
antivenin	T50.Z11	T50.Z12	T50.Z13	T50.Z14	T50.Z15	T50.Z16
Blast furnace gas (carbon monoxide from)	T58.8X1	T58.8X2	T58.8X3	T58.8X4		

◀ New   ◀▥ Revised   ~~deleted~~ Deleted

TABLE OF DRUGS AND CHEMICALS

Substance	External Cause (T-Code)					
	Poisoning, Accidental (Unintentional)	Poisoning, Intentional Self-Harm	Poisoning, Assault	Poisoning, Undetermined	Adverse Effect	Underdosing
Bleach	T54.91	T54.92	T54.93	T54.94	—	—
Bleaching agent (medicinal)	T49.4X1	T49.4X2	T49.4X3	T49.4X4	T49.4X5	T49.4X6
Bleomycin	T45.1X1	T45.1X2	T45.1X3	T45.1X4	T45.1X5	T45.1X6
Blockain	T41.3X1	T41.3X2	T41.3X3	T41.3X4	T41.3X5	T41.3X6
infiltration (subcutaneous)	T41.3X1	T41.3X2	T41.3X3	T41.3X4	T41.3X5	T41.3X6
nerve block (peripheral) (plexus)	T41.3X1	T41.3X2	T41.3X3	T41.3X4	T41.3X5	T41.3X6
topical (surface)	T41.3X1	T41.3X2	T41.3X3	T41.3X4	T41.3X5	T41.3X6
Blockers, calcium channel	T46.1X1	T46.1X2	T46.1X3	T46.1X4	T46.1X5	T46.1X6
Blood (derivatives) (natural) (plasma) (whole)	T45.8X1	T45.8X2	T45.8X3	T45.8X4	T45.8X5	T45.8X6
dried	T45.8X1	T45.8X2	T45.8X3	T45.8X4	T45.8X5	T45.8X6
drug affecting NEC	T45.91	T45.92	T45.93	T45.94	T45.95	T45.96
expander NEC	T45.8X1	T45.8X2	T45.8X3	T45.8X4	T45.8X5	T45.8X6
fraction NEC	T45.8X1	T45.8X2	T45.8X3	T45.8X4	T45.8X5	T45.8X6
substitute (macromolecular)	T45.8X1	T45.8X2	T45.8X3	T45.8X4	T45.8X5	T45.8X6
Blue velvet	T40.2X1	T40.2X2	T40.2X3	T40.2X4	—	—
Bone meal	T62.8X1	T62.8X2	T62.8X3	T62.8X4	—	—
Bonine	T45.0X1	T45.0X2	T45.0X3	T45.0X4	T45.0X5	T45.0X6
Bopindolol	T44.7X1	T44.7X2	T44.7X3	T44.7X4	T44.7X5	T44.7X6
Boracic acid	T49.0X1	T49.0X2	T49.0X3	T49.0X4	T49.0X5	T49.0X6
ENT agent	T49.6X1	T49.6X2	T49.6X3	T49.6X4	T49.6X5	T49.6X6
ophthalmic preparation	T49.5X1	T49.5X2	T49.5X3	T49.5X4	T49.5X5	T49.5X6
Borane complex	T57.8X1	T57.8X2	T57.8X3	T57.8X4	—	—
Borate(s)	T57.8X1	T57.8X2	T57.8X3	T57.8X4	—	—
buffer	T50.991	T50.992	T50.993	T50.994	T50.995	T50.996
cleanser	T54.91	T54.92	T54.93	T54.94	—	—
sodium	T57.8X1	T57.8X2	T57.8X3	T57.8X4	—	—
Borax (cleanser)	T54.91	T54.92	T54.93	T54.94	—	—
Bordeaux mixture	T60.3X1	T60.3X2	T60.3X3	T60.3X4	—	—
Boric acid	T49.0X1	T49.0X2	T49.0X3	T49.0X4	T49.0X5	T49.0X6
ENT agent	T49.6X1	T49.6X2	T49.6X3	T49.6X4	T49.6X5	T49.6X6
ophthalmic preparation	T49.5X1	T49.5X2	T49.5X3	T49.5X4	T49.5X5	T49.5X6
Bornaprine	T44.3X1	T44.3X2	T44.3X3	T44.3X4	T44.3X5	T44.3X6
Boron	T57.8X1	T57.8X2	T57.8X3	T57.8X4	—	—
hydride NEC	T57.8X1	T57.8X2	T57.8X3	T57.8X4	—	—
fumes or gas	T57.8X1	T57.8X2	T57.8X3	T57.8X4	—	—
trifluoride	T59.891	T59.892	T59.893	T59.894	—	—
Botox	T48.291	T48.292	T48.293	T48.294	T48.295	T48.296
Botulinus anti-toxin (type A, B)	T50.Z11	T50.Z12	T50.Z13	T50.Z14	T50.Z15	T50.Z16
Brake fluid vapor	T59.891	T59.892	T59.893	T59.894	—	—
Brallobarbital	T42.3X1	T42.3X2	T42.3X3	T42.3X4	T42.3X5	T42.3X6

◀ New ◀ Revised ~~deleted~~ Deleted

Substance	External Cause (T-Code)					
	Poisoning, Accidental (Unintentional)	Poisoning, Intentional Self-Harm	Poisoning, Assault	Poisoning, Undetermined	Adverse Effect	Underdosing
Bran (wheat)	T47.4X1	T47.4X2	T47.4X3	T47.4X4	T47.4X5	T47.4X6
Brass (fumes)	T56.891	T56.892	T56.893	T56.894	—	—
Brasso	T52.0X1	T52.0X2	T52.0X3	T52.0X4	—	—
Bretylium tosilate	T46.2X1	T46.2X2	T46.2X3	T46.2X4	T46.2X5	T46.2X6
Brevital (sodium)	T41.1X1	T41.1X2	T41.1X3	T41.1X4	T41.1X5	T41.1X6
Brinase	T45.3X1	T45.3X2	T45.3X3	T45.3X4	T45.3X5	T45.3X6
British antilewisite	T45.8X1	T45.8X2	T45.8X3	T45.8X4	T45.8X5	T45.8X6
Brodifacoum	T60.4X1	T60.4X2	T60.4X3	T60.4X4	—	—
Bromal (hydrate)	T42.6X1	T42.6X2	T42.6X3	T42.6X4	T42.6X5	T42.6X6
Bromazepam	T42.4X1	T42.4X2	T42.4X3	T42.4X4	T42.4X5	T42.4X6
Bromazine	T45.0X1	T45.0X2	T45.0X3	T45.0X4	T45.0X5	T45.0X6
Brombenzylcyanide	T59.3X1	T59.3X2	T59.3X3	T59.3X4	—	—
Bromelains	T45.3X1	T45.3X2	T45.3X3	T45.3X4	T45.3X5	T45.3X6
Bromethalin	T60.4X1	T60.4X2	T60.4X3	T60.4X4	—	—
Bromhexine	T48.4X1	T48.4X2	T48.4X3	T48.4X4	T48.4X5	T48.4X6
Bromide salts	T42.6X1	T42.6X2	T42.6X3	T42.6X4	T42.6X5	T42.6X6
Bromindione	T45.511	T45.512	T45.513	T45.514	T45.515	T45.516
Bromine						
compounds (medicinal)	T42.6X1	T42.6X2	T42.6X3	T42.6X4	T42.6X5	T42.6X6
sedative	T42.6X1	T42.6X2	T42.6X3	T42.6X4	T42.6X5	T42.6X6
vapor	T59.891	T59.892	T59.893	T59.894	—	—
Bromisovalum	T42.6X1	T42.6X2	T42.6X3	T42.6X4	T42.6X5	T42.6X6
Bromisoval	T42.6X1	T42.6X2	T42.6X3	T42.6X4	T42.6X5	T42.6X6
Bromobenzylcyanide	T59.3X1	T59.3X2	T59.3X3	T59.3X4	—	—
Bromochlorosalicylani-lide	T49.0X1	T49.0X2	T49.0X3	T49.0X4	T49.0X5	T49.0X6
Bromocriptine	T42.8X1	T42.8X2	T42.8X3	T42.8X4	T42.8X5	T42.8X6
Bromodiphenhydramine	T45.0X1	T45.0X2	T45.0X3	T45.0X4	T45.0X5	T45.0X6
Bromoform	T42.6X1	T42.6X2	T42.6X3	T42.6X4	T42.6X5	T42.6X6
Bromophenol blue reagent	T50.991	T50.992	T50.993	T50.994	T50.995	T50.996
Bromopride	T47.8X1	T47.8X2	T47.8X3	T47.8X4	T47.8X5	T47.8X6
Bromosalicylchloranitide	T49.0X1	T49.0X2	T49.0X3	T49.0X4	T49.0X5	T49.0X6
Bromosalicylhydroxamic acid	T37.1X1	T37.1X2	T37.1X3	T37.1X4	T37.1X5	T37.1X6
Bromo-seltzer	T39.1X1	T39.1X2	T39.1X3	T39.1X4	T39.1X5	T39.1X6
Bromoxynil	T60.3X1	T60.3X2	T60.3X3	T60.3X4	—	—
Bromperidol	T43.4X1	T43.4X2	T43.4X3	T43.4X4	T43.4X5	T43.4X6
Brompheniramine	T45.0X1	T45.0X2	T45.0X3	T45.0X4	T45.0X5	T45.0X6
Bromsulfophthalein	T50.8X1	T50.8X2	T50.8X3	T50.8X4	T50.8X5	T50.8X6
Bromural	T42.6X1	T42.6X2	T42.6X3	T42.6X4	T42.6X5	T42.6X6
Bromvaletone	T42.6X1	T42.6X2	T42.6X3	T42.6X4	T42.6X5	T42.6X6
Bronchodilator NEC	T48.6X1	T48.6X2	T48.6X3	T48.6X4	T48.6X5	T48.6X6

◀ New   ◀||| Revised   ~~deleted~~ Deleted

TABLE OF DRUGS AND CHEMICALS

Substance	External Cause (T-Code)					
	Poisoning, Accidental (Unintentional)	Poisoning, Intentional Self-Harm	Poisoning, Assault	Poisoning, Undetermined	Adverse Effect	Underdosing
Brotizolam	T42.4X1	T42.4X2	T42.4X3	T42.4X4	T42.4X5	T42.4X6
Brovincamine	T46.7X1	T46.7X2	T46.7X3	T46.7X4	T46.7X5	T46.7X6
Brown spider (bite) (venom)	T63.391	T63.392	T63.393	T63.394	—	—
Brown recluse spider (bite) (venom)	T63.331	T63.332	T63.333	T63.334	—	—
Broxaterol	T48.6X1	T48.6X2	T48.6X3	T48.6X4	T48.6X5	T48.6X6
Broxuridine	T45.1X1	T45.1X2	T45.1X3	T45.1X4	T45.1X5	T45.1X6
Broxyquinoline	T37.8X1	T37.8X2	T37.8X3	T37.8X4	T37.8X5	T37.8X6
Bruceine	T48.291	T48.292	T48.293	T48.294	T48.295	T48.296
Brucia	T62.2X1	T62.2X2	T62.2X3	T62.2X4	—	—
Brucine	T65.1X1	T65.1X2	T65.1X3	T65.1X4	—	—
Brunswick green — see Copper						
Bruten — see Ibuprofen						
Bryonia	T47.2X1	T47.2X2	T47.2X3	T47.2X4	T47.2X5	T47.2X6
Buclizine	T45.0X1	T45.0X2	T45.0X3	T45.0X4	T45.0X5	T45.0X6
Buclosamide	T49.0X1	T49.0X2	T49.0X3	T49.0X4	T49.0X5	T49.0X6
Budesonide	T44.5X1	T44.5X2	T44.5X3	T44.5X4	T44.5X5	T44.5X6
Budralazine	T46.5X1	T46.5X2	T46.5X3	T46.5X4	T46.5X5	T46.5X6
Bufferin	T39.011	T39.012	T39.013	T39.014	T39.015	T39.016
Buflomedil	T46.7X1	T46.7X2	T46.7X3	T46.7X4	T46.7X5	T46.7X6
Buformin	T38.3X1	T38.3X2	T38.3X3	T38.3X4	T38.3X5	T38.3X6
Bufotenine	T40.991	T40.992	T40.993	T40.994	—	—
Bufrolin	T48.6X1	T48.6X2	T48.6X3	T48.6X4	T48.6X5	T48.6X6
Bufylline	T48.6X1	T48.6X2	T48.6X3	T48.6X4	T48.6X5	T48.6X6
Bulk filler	T50.5X1	T50.5X2	T50.5X3	T50.5X4	T50.5X5	T50.5X6
cathartic	T47.4X1	T47.4X2	T47.4X3	T47.4X4	T47.4X5	T47.4X6
Bumetanide	T50.1X1	T50.1X2	T50.1X3	T50.1X4	T50.1X5	T50.1X6
Bunaftine	T46.2X1	T46.2X2	T46.2X3	T46.2X4	T46.2X5	T46.2X6
Bunamiodyl	T50.8X1	T50.8X2	T50.8X3	T50.8X4	T50.8X5	T50.8X6
Bunazosin	T44.6X1	T44.6X2	T44.6X3	T44.6X4	T44.6X5	T44.6X6
Bunitrolol	T44.7X1	T44.7X2	T44.7X3	T44.7X4	T44.7X5	T44.7X6
Buphenine	T46.7X1	T46.7X2	T46.7X3	T46.7X4	T46.7X5	T46.7X6
Bupivacaine	T41.3X1	T41.3X2	T41.3X3	T41.3X4	T41.3X5	T41.3X6
infiltration (subcutaneous)	T41.3X1	T41.3X2	T41.3X3	T41.3X4	T41.3X5	T41.3X6
nerve block (peripheral) (plexus)	T41.3X1	T41.3X2	T41.3X3	T41.3X4	T41.3X5	T41.3X6
spinal	T41.3X1	T41.3X2	T41.3X3	T41.3X4	T41.3X5	T41.3X6
Bupranolol	T44.7X1	T44.7X2	T44.7X3	T44.7X4	T44.7X5	T44.7X6
Buprenorphine	T40.4X1	T40.4X2	T40.4X3	T40.4X4	T40.4X5	T40.4X6
Bupropion	T43.291	T43.292	T43.293	T43.294	T43.295	T43.296
Burimamide	T47.1X1	T47.1X2	T47.1X3	T47.1X4	T47.1X5	T47.1X6
Buserelin	T38.891	T38.892	T38.893	T38.894	T38.895	T38.896

◀ New ◀||| Revised ~~deleted~~ Deleted

Substance	External Cause (T-Code)					
	Poisoning, Accidental (Unintentional)	Poisoning, Intentional Self-Harm	Poisoning, Assault	Poisoning, Undetermined	Adverse Effect	Underdosing
Buspirone	T43.591	T43.592	T43.593	T43.594	T43.595	T43.596
Busulfan, busulphan	T45.1X1	T45.1X2	T45.1X3	T45.1X4	T45.1X5	T45.1X6
Butabarbital (sodium)	T42.3X1	T42.3X2	T42.3X3	T42.3X4	T42.3X5	T42.3X6
Butabarbitone	T42.3X1	T42.3X2	T42.3X3	T42.3X4	T42.3X5	T42.3X6
Butabarpal	T42.3X1	T42.3X2	T42.3X3	T42.3X4	T42.3X5	T42.3X6
Butacaine	T41.3X1	T41.3X2	T41.3X3	T41.3X4	T41.3X5	T41.3X6
Butalamine	T46.7X1	T46.7X2	T46.7X3	T46.7X4	T46.7X5	T46.7X6
Butalbital	T42.3X1	T42.3X2	T42.3X3	T42.3X4	T42.3X5	T42.3X6
Butallylonal	T42.3X1	T42.3X2	T42.3X3	T42.3X4	T42.3X5	T42.3X6
Butamben	T41.3X1	T41.3X2	T41.3X3	T41.3X4	T41.3X5	T41.3X6
Butamirate	T48.3X1	T48.3X2	T48.3X3	T48.3X4	T48.3X5	T48.3X6
Butane (distributed in mobile container)	T59.891	T59.892	T59.893	T59.894	—	—
distributed through pipes	T59.891	T59.892	T59.893	T59.894	—	—
incomplete combustion	T58.11	T58.12	T58.13	T58.14	—	—
Butanilicaine	T41.3X1	T41.3X2	T41.3X3	T41.3X4	T41.3X5	T41.3X6
Butanol	T51.3X1	T51.3X2	T51.3X3	T51.3X4	—	—
Butanone, 2-butanone	T52.4X1	T52.4X2	T52.4X3	T52.4X4	—	—
Butantrone	T49.4X1	T49.4X2	T49.4X3	T49.4X4	T49.4X5	T49.4X6
Butaperazine	T43.3X1	T43.3X2	T43.3X3	T43.3X4	T43.3X5	T43.3X6
Butazolidin	T39.2X1	T39.2X2	T39.2X3	T39.2X4	T39.2X5	T39.2X6
Butetamate	T48.6X1	T48.6X2	T48.6X3	T48.6X4	T48.6X5	T48.6X6
Butethal	T42.3X1	T42.3X2	T42.3X3	T42.3X4	T42.3X5	T42.3X6
Butethamate	T44.3X1	T44.3X2	T44.3X3	T44.3X4	T44.3X5	T44.3X6
Buthalitone (sodium)	T41.1X1	T41.1X2	T41.1X3	T41.1X4	T41.1X5	T41.1X6
Butisol (sodium)	T42.3X1	T42.3X2	T42.3X3	T42.3X4	T42.3X5	T42.3X6
Butizide	T50.2X1	T50.2X2	T50.2X3	T50.2X4	T50.2X5	T50.2X6
Butobarbital	T42.3X1	T42.3X2	T42.3X3	T42.3X4	T42.3X5	T42.3X6
sodium	T42.3X1	T42.3X2	T42.3X3	T42.3X4	T42.3X5	T42.3X6
Butobarbitone	T42.3X1	T42.3X2	T42.3X3	T42.3X4	T42.3X5	T42.3X6
Butoconazole (nitrate)	T49.0X1	T49.0X2	T49.0X3	T49.0X4	T49.0X5	T49.0X6
Butorphanol	T40.4X1	T40.4X2	T40.4X3	T40.4X4	T40.4X5	T40.4X6
Butriptyline	T43.011	T43.012	T43.013	T43.014	T43.015	T43.016
Butropium bromide	T44.3X1	T44.3X2	T44.3X3	T44.3X4	T44.3X5	T44.3X6
Buttercups	T62.2X1	T62.2X2	T62.2X3	T62.2X4	—	—
Butter of antimony — see Antimony						
Butyl						
acetate (secondary)	T52.8X1	T52.8X2	T52.8X3	T52.8X4	—	—
alcohol	T51.3X1	T51.3X2	T51.3X3	T51.3X4	—	—
aminobenzoate	T41.3X1	T41.3X2	T41.3X3	T41.3X4	T41.3X5	T41.3X6
butyrate	T52.8X1	T52.8X2	T52.8X3	T52.8X4	—	—

◀ New   ◀▥ Revised   deleted Deleted

TABLE OF DRUGS AND CHEMICALS

TABLE OF DRUGS AND CHEMICALS

Substance	External Cause (T-Code)					
	Poisoning, Accidental (Unintentional)	Poisoning, Intentional Self-Harm	Poisoning, Assault	Poisoning, Undetermined	Adverse Effect	Underdosing
Butyl *(Continued)*						
carbinol	T51.3X1	T51.3X2	T51.3X3	T51.3X4	—	—
carbitol	T52.3X1	T52.3X2	T52.3X3	T52.3X4	—	—
cellosolve	T52.3X1	T52.3X2	T52.3X3	T52.3X4	—	—
chloral (hydrate)	T42.6X1	T42.6X2	T42.6X3	T42.6X4	T42.6X5	T42.6X6
formate	T52.8X1	T52.8X2	T52.8X3	T52.8X4	—	—
lactate	T52.8X1	T52.8X2	T52.8X3	T52.8X4	—	—
propionate	T52.8X1	T52.8X2	T52.8X3	T52.8X4	—	—
scopolamine bromide	T44.3X1	T44.3X2	T44.3X3	T44.3X4	T44.3X5	T44.3X6
thiobarbital sodium	T41.1X1	T41.1X2	T41.1X3	T41.1X4	T41.1X5	T41.1X6
Butylated hydroxy-anisole	T50.991	T50.992	T50.993	T50.994	T50.995	T50.996
Butylchloral hydrate	T42.6X1	T42.6X2	T42.6X3	T42.6X4	T42.6X5	T42.6X6
Butyltoluene	T52.2X1	T52.2X2	T52.2X3	T52.2X4	—	—
Butyn	T41.3X1	T41.3X2	T41.3X3	T41.3X4	T41.3X5	T41.3X6
Butyrophenone (-based tranquilizers)	T43.4X1	T43.4X2	T43.4X3	T43.4X4	T43.4X5	T43.4X6
C						
Cabergoline	T42.8X1	T42.8X2	T42.8X3	T42.8X4	T42.8X5	T42.8X6
Cacodyl, cacodylic acid	T57.0X1	T57.0X2	T57.0X3	T57.0X4	—	—
Cactinomycin	T45.1X1	T45.1X2	T45.1X3	T45.1X4	T45.1X5	T45.1X6
Cade oil	T49.4X1	T49.4X2	T49.4X3	T49.4X4	T49.4X5	T49.4X6
Cadexomer iodine	T49.0X1	T49.0X2	T49.0X3	T49.0X4	T49.0X5	T49.0X6
Cadmium (chloride) (fumes) (oxide)	T56.3X1	T56.3X2	T56.3X3	T56.3X4	—	—
sulfide (medicinal) NEC	T49.4X1	T49.4X2	T49.4X3	T49.4X4	T49.4X5	T49.4X6
Cadralazine	T46.5X1	T46.5X2	T46.5X3	T46.5X4	T46.5X5	T46.5X6
Caffeine	T43.611	T43.612	T43.613	T43.614	T43.615	T43.616
Calabar bean	T62.2X1	T62.2X2	T62.2X3	T62.2X4	—	—
Caladium seguinum	T62.2X1	T62.2X2	T62.2X3	T62.2X4	—	—
Calamine (lotion)	T49.3X1	T49.3X2	T49.3X3	T49.3X4	T49.3X5	T49.3X6
Calcifediol	T45.2X1	T45.2X2	T45.2X3	T45.2X4	T45.2X5	T45.2X6
Calciferol	T45.2X1	T45.2X2	T45.2X3	T45.2X4	T45.2X5	T45.2X6
Calcitonin	T50.991	T50.992	T50.993	T50.994	T50.995	T50.996
Calcitriol	T45.2X1	T45.2X2	T45.2X3	T45.2X4	T45.2X5	T45.2X6
Calcium	T50.3X1	T50.3X2	T50.3X3	T50.3X4	T50.3X5	T50.3X6
actylsalicylate	T39.011	T39.012	T39.013	T39.014	T39.015	T39.016
benzamidosalicylate	T37.1X1	T37.1X2	T37.1X3	T37.1X4	T37.1X5	T37.1X6
bromide	T42.6X1	T42.6X2	T42.6X3	T42.6X4	T42.6X5	T42.6X6
bromolactobionate	T42.6X1	T42.6X2	T42.6X3	T42.6X4	T42.6X5	T42.6X6
carbaspirin	T39.011	T39.012	T39.013	T39.014	T39.015	T39.016
carbimide	T50.6X1	T50.6X2	T50.6X3	T50.6X4	T50.6X5	T50.6X6

◄ New ◄ Revised ~~deleted~~ Deleted

Substance	Poisoning, Accidental (Unintentional)	Poisoning, Intentional Self-Harm	Poisoning, Assault	Poisoning, Undetermined	Adverse Effect	Underdosing
Calcium *(Continued)*						
carbonate	T47.1X1	T47.1X2	T47.1X3	T47.1X4	T47.1X5	T47.1X6
chloride	T50.991	T50.992	T50.993	T50.994	T50.995	T50.996
anhydrous	T50.991	T50.992	T50.993	T50.994	T50.995	T50.996
cyanide	T57.8X1	T57.8X2	T57.8X3	T57.8X4	—	—
dioctyl sulfosuccinate	T47.4X1	T47.4X2	T47.4X3	T47.4X4	T47.4X5	T47.4X6
disodium edathamil	T45.8X1	T45.8X2	T45.8X3	T45.8X4	T45.8X5	T45.8X6
disodium edetate	T45.8X1	T45.8X2	T45.8X3	T45.8X4	T45.8X5	T45.8X6
dobesilate	T46.991	T46.992	T46.993	T46.994	T46.995	T46.996
EDTA	T45.8X1	T45.8X2	T45.8X3	T45.8X4	T45.8X5	T45.8X6
ferrous citrate	T45.4X1	T45.4X2	T45.4X3	T45.4X4	T45.4X5	T45.4X6
folinate	T45.8X1	T45.8X2	T45.8X3	T45.8X4	T45.8X5	T45.8X6
glubionate	T50.3X1	T50.3X2	T50.3X3	T50.3X4	T50.3X5	T50.3X6
gluconate	T50.3X1	T50.3X2	T50.3X3	T50.3X4	T50.3X5	T50.3X6
gluconogalactogluconate	T50.3X1	T50.3X2	T50.3X3	T50.3X4	T50.3X5	T50.3X6
hydrate, hydroxide	T54.3X1	T54.3X2	T54.3X3	T54.3X4	—	—
hypochlorite	T54.3X1	T54.3X2	T54.3X3	T54.3X4	—	—
iodide	T48.4X1	T48.4X2	T48.4X3	T48.4X4	T48.4X5	T48.4X6
ipodate	T50.8X1	T50.8X2	T50.8X3	T50.8X4	T50.8X5	T50.8X6
lactate	T50.3X1	T50.3X2	T50.3X3	T50.3X4	T50.3X5	T50.3X6
leucovorin	T45.8X1	T45.8X2	T45.8X3	T45.8X4	T45.8X5	T45.8X6
mandelate	T37.91	T37.92	T37.93	T37.94	T37.95	T37.96
oxide	T54.3X1	T54.3X2	T54.3X3	T54.3X4	—	—
pantothenate	T45.2X1	T45.2X2	T45.2X3	T45.2X4	T45.2X5	T45.2X6
phosphate	T50.3X1	T50.3X2	T50.3X3	T50.3X4	T50.3X5	T50.3X6
salicylate	T39.091	T39.092	T39.093	T39.094	T39.095	T39.096
salts	T50.3X1	T50.3X2	T50.3X3	T50.3X4	T50.3X5	T50.3X6
Calculus-dissolving drug	T50.991	T50.992	T50.993	T50.994	T50.995	T50.996
Calomel	T49.0X1	T49.0X2	T49.0X3	T49.0X4	T49.0X5	T49.0X6
Caloric agent	T50.3X1	T50.3X2	T50.3X3	T50.3X4	T50.3X5	T50.3X6
Calusterone	T38.7X1	T38.7X2	T38.7X3	T38.7X4	T38.7X5	T38.7X6
Camazepam	T42.4X1	T42.4X2	T42.4X3	T42.4X4	T42.4X5	T42.4X6
Camomile	T49.0X1	T49.0X2	T49.0X3	T49.0X4	T49.0X5	T49.0X6
Camoquin	T37.2X1	T37.2X2	T37.2X3	T37.2X4	T37.2X5	T37.2X6
Camphor						
insecticide	T60.2X1	T60.2X2	T60.2X3	T60.2X4	—	—
medicinal	T49.8X1	T49.8X2	T49.8X3	T49.8X4	T49.8X5	T49.8X6
Camylofin	T44.3X1	T44.3X2	T44.3X3	T44.3X4	T44.3X5	T44.3X6
Cancer chemotherapy drug regimen	T45.1X1	T45.1X2	T45.1X3	T45.1X4	T45.1X5	T45.1X6
Candeptin	T49.0X1	T49.0X2	T49.0X3	T49.0X4	T49.0X5	T49.0X6

◀ New   ◀▥ Revised   ~~deleted~~ Deleted

TABLE OF DRUGS AND CHEMICALS

Substance	External Cause (T-Code)					
	Poisoning, Accidental (Unintentional)	Poisoning, Intentional Self-Harm	Poisoning, Assault	Poisoning, Undetermined	Adverse Effect	Underdosing
Candicidin	T49.0X1	T49.0X2	T49.0X3	T49.0X4	T49.0X5	T49.0X6
Cannabinol	T40.7X1	T40.7X2	T40.7X3	T40.7X4	T40.7X5	T40.7X6
Cannabis (derivatives)	T40.7X1	T40.7X2	T40.7X3	T40.7X4	T40.7X5	T40.7X6
Canned heat	T51.1X1	T51.1X2	T51.1X3	T51.1X4	—	—
Canrenoic acid	T50.0X1	T50.0X2	T50.0X3	T50.0X4	T50.0X5	T50.0X6
Canrenone	T50.0X1	T50.0X2	T50.0X3	T50.0X4	T50.0X5	T50.0X6
Cantharides, cantharidin, cantharis	T49.8X1	T49.8X2	T49.8X3	T49.8X4	T49.8X5	T49.8X6
Canthaxanthin	T50.991	T50.992	T50.993	T50.994	T50.995	T50.996
Capillary-active drug NEC	T46.901	T46.902	T46.903	T46.904	T46.905	T46.906
Capreomycin	T36.8X1	T36.8X2	T36.8X3	T36.8X4	T36.8X5	T36.8X6
Capsicum	T49.4X1	T49.4X2	T49.4X3	T49.4X4	T49.4X5	T49.4X6
Captafol	T60.3X1	T60.3X2	T60.3X3	T60.3X4	—	—
Captan	T60.3X1	T60.3X2	T60.3X3	T60.3X4	—	—
Captodiame, captodiamine	T43.591	T43.592	T43.593	T43.594	T43.595	T43.596
Captopril	T46.4X1	T46.4X2	T46.4X3	T46.4X4	T46.4X5	T46.4X6
Caramiphen	T44.3X1	T44.3X2	T44.3X3	T44.3X4	T44.3X5	T44.3X6
Carazolol	T44.7X1	T44.7X2	T44.7X3	T44.7X4	T44.7X5	T44.7X6
Carbachol	T44.1X1	T44.1X2	T44.1X3	T44.1X4	T44.1X5	T44.1X6
Carbacrylamine (resin)	T50.3X1	T50.3X2	T50.3X3	T50.3X4	T50.3X5	T50.3X6
Carbamate (insecticide)	T60.0X1	T60.0X2	T60.0X3	T60.0X4	—	—
Carbamate (sedative)	T42.6X1	T42.6X2	T42.6X3	T42.6X4	T42.6X5	T42.6X6
herbicide	T60.0X1	T60.0X2	T60.0X3	T60.0X4	—	—
insecticide	T60.0X1	T60.0X2	T60.0X3	T60.0X4	—	—
Carbamazepine	T42.1X1	T42.1X2	T42.1X3	T42.1X4	T42.1X5	T42.1X6
Carbamide	T47.3X1	T47.3X2	T47.3X3	T47.3X4	T47.3X5	T47.3X6
peroxide	T49.0X1	T49.0X2	T49.0X3	T49.0X4	T49.0X5	T49.0X6
topical	T49.8X1	T49.8X2	T49.8X3	T49.8X4	T49.8X5	T49.8X6
Carbamylcholine chloride	T44.1X1	T44.1X2	T44.1X3	T44.1X4	T44.1X5	T44.1X6
Carbaril	T60.0X1	T60.0X2	T60.0X3	T60.0X4	—	—
Carbarsone	T37.3X1	T37.3X2	T37.3X3	T37.3X4	T37.3X5	T37.3X6
Carbaryl	T60.0X1	T60.0X2	T60.0X3	T60.0X4	—	—
Carbaspirin	T39.011	T39.012	T39.013	T39.014	T39.015	T39.016
Carbazochrome (salicylate) (sodium sulfonate)	T49.4X1	T49.4X2	T49.4X3	T49.4X4	T49.4X5	T49.4X6
Carbenicillin	T36.0X1	T36.0X2	T36.0X3	T36.0X4	T36.0X5	T36.0X6
Carbenoxolone	T47.1X1	T47.1X2	T47.1X3	T47.1X4	T47.1X5	T47.1X6
Carbetapentane	T48.3X1	T48.3X2	T48.3X3	T48.3X4	T48.3X5	T48.3X6
Carbethyl salicylate	T39.091	T39.092	T39.093	T39.094	T39.095	T39.096
Carbidopa (with levodopa)	T42.8X1	T42.8X2	T42.8X3	T42.8X4	T42.8X5	T42.8X6
Carbimazole	T38.2X1	T38.2X2	T38.2X3	T38.2X4	T38.2X5	T38.2X6

◀ New   ◀▥ Revised   ~~deleted~~ Deleted

Substance	External Cause (T-Code)					
	Poisoning, Accidental (Unintentional)	Poisoning, Intentional Self-Harm	Poisoning, Assault	Poisoning, Undetermined	Adverse Effect	Underdosing
Carbinol	T51.1X1	T51.1X2	T51.1X3	T51.1X4	—	—
Carbinoxamine	T45.0X1	T45.0X2	T45.0X3	T45.0X4	T45.0X5	T45.0X6
Carbiphene	T39.8X1	T39.8X2	T39.8X3	T39.8X4	T39.8X5	T39.8X6
Carbitol	T52.3X1	T52.3X2	T52.3X3	T52.3X4	—	—
Carbocaine	T41.3X1	T41.3X2	T41.3X3	T41.3X4	T41.3X5	T41.3X6
infiltration (subcutaneous)	T41.3X1	T41.3X2	T41.3X3	T41.3X4	T41.3X5	T41.3X6
nerve block (peripheral) (plexus)	T41.3X1	T41.3X2	T41.3X3	T41.3X4	T41.3X5	T41.3X6
topical (surface)	T41.3X1	T41.3X2	T41.3X3	T41.3X4	T41.3X5	T41.3X6
Carbo medicinalis	T47.6X1	T47.6X2	T47.6X3	T47.6X4	T47.6X5	T47.6X6
Carbomycin	T36.8X1	T36.8X2	T36.8X3	T36.8X4	T36.8X5	T36.8X6
Carbocisteine	T48.4X1	T48.4X2	T48.4X3	T48.4X4	T48.4X5	T48.4X6
Carbocromen	T46.3X1	T46.3X2	T46.3X3	T46.3X4	T46.3X5	T46.3X6
Carbol fuchsin	T49.0X1	T49.0X2	T49.0X3	T49.0X4	T49.0X5	T49.0X6
Carbolic acid — *see also Phenol*	T54.0X1	T54.0X2	T54.0X3	T54.0X4	—	—
Carbolonium (bromide)	T48.1X1	T48.1X2	T48.1X3	T48.1X4	T48.1X5	T48.1X6
Carbon						
bisulfide (liquid)	T65.4X1	T65.4X2	T65.4X3	T65.4X4	—	—
vapor	T65.4X1	T65.4X2	T65.4X3	T65.4X4	—	—
dioxide (gas)	T59.7X1	T59.7X2	T59.7X3	T59.7X4	—	—
medicinal	T41.5X1	T41.5X2	T41.5X3	T41.5X4	T41.5X5	T41.5X6
nonmedicinal	T59.7X1	T59.7X2	T59.7X3	T59.7X4	—	—
snow	T49.4X1	T49.4X2	T49.4X3	T49.4X4	T49.4X5	T49.4X6
disulfide (liquid)	T65.4X1	T65.4X2	T65.4X3	T65.4X4	—	—
vapor	T65.4X1	T65.4X2	T65.4X3	T65.4X4	—	—
monoxide (from incomplete combustion)	T58.91	T58.92	T58.93	T58.94	—	—
blast furnace gas	T58.8X1	T58.8X2	T58.8X3	T58.8X4	—	—
butane (distributed in mobile container)	T58.11	T58.12	T58.13	T58.14	—	—
distributed through pipes	T58.11	T58.12	T58.13	T58.14	—	—
charcoal fumes	T58.2X1	T58.2X2	T58.2X3	T58.2X4	—	—
coal	T58.2X1	T58.2X2	T58.2X3	T58.2X4	—	—
coke (in domestic stoves, fireplaces)	T58.2X1	T58.2X2	T58.2X3	T58.2X4	—	—
gas (piped)	T58.11	T58.12	T58.13	T58.14	—	—
solid (in domestic stoves, fireplaces)	T58.2X1	T58.2X2	T58.2X3	T58.2X4	—	—
exhaust gas (motor) not in transit	T58.01	T58.02	T58.03	T58.04	—	—
combustion engine, any not in watercraft	T58.01	T58.02	T58.03	T58.04	—	—
farm tractor, not in transit	T58.01	T58.02	T58.03	T58.04	—	—
gas engine	T58.01	T58.02	T58.03	T58.04	—	—
motor pump	T58.01	T58.02	T58.03	T58.04	—	—
motor vehicle, not in transit	T58.01	T58.02	T58.03	T58.04	—	—

◀ New   ◀▦ Revised   ~~deleted~~ Deleted

TABLE OF DRUGS AND CHEMICALS

Substance	External Cause (T-Code)					
	Poisoning, Accidental (Unintentional)	Poisoning, Intentional Self-Harm	Poisoning, Assault	Poisoning, Undetermined	Adverse Effect	Underdosing
Carbon *(Continued)*						
monoxide *(Continued)*						
fuel (in domestic use)	T58.2X1	T58.2X2	T58.2X3	T58.2X4	—	—
gas (piped)	T58.11	T58.12	T58.13	T58.14	—	—
in mobile container	T58.11	T58.12	T58.13	T58.14	—	—
utility	T58.11	T58.12	T58.13	T58.14	—	—
in mobile container	T58.11	T58.12	T58.13	T58.14	—	—
piped (natural)	T58.11	T58.12	T58.13	T58.14	—	—
illuminating gas	T58.11	T58.12	T58.13	T58.14	—	—
industrial fuels or gases, any	T58.8X1	T58.8X2	T58.8X3	T58.8X4	—	—
kerosene (in domestic stoves, fireplaces)	T58.2X1	T58.2X2	T58.2X3	T58.2X4	—	—
kiln gas or vapor	T58.8X1	T58.8X2	T58.8X3	T58.8X4	—	—
motor exhaust gas, not in transit	T58.01	T58.02	T58.03	T58.04	—	—
piped gas (manufactured) (natural)	T58.11	T58.12	T58.13	T58.14	—	—
producer gas	T58.8X1	T58.8X2	T58.8X3	T58.8X4	—	—
propane (distributed in mobile container)	T58.11	T58.12	T58.13	T58.14	—	—
distributed through pipes	T58.11	T58.12	T58.13	T58.14	—	—
specified source NEC	T58.8X1	T58.8X2	T58.8X3	T58.8X4	—	—
stove gas	T58.11	T58.12	T58.13	T58.14	—	—
piped	T58.11	T58.12	T58.13	T58.14	—	—
utility gas	T58.11	T58.12	T58.13	T58.14	—	—
piped	T58.11	T58.12	T58.13	T58.14	—	—
water gas	T58.11	T58.12	T58.13	T58.14	—	—
wood (in domestic stoves, fireplaces)	T58.2X1	T58.2X2	T58.2X3	T58.2X4	—	—
tetrachloride (vapor) NEC	T53.0X1	T53.0X2	T53.0X3	T53.0X4	—	—
liquid (cleansing agent) NEC	T53.0X1	T53.0X2	T53.0X3	T53.0X4	—	—
solvent	T53.0X1	T53.0X2	T53.0X3	T53.0X4	—	—
Carbonic acid gas	T59.7X1	T59.7X2	T59.7X3	T59.7X4	—	—
anhydrase inhibitor NEC	T50.2X1	T50.2X2	T50.2X3	T50.2X4	T50.2X5	T50.2X6
Carbophenothion	T60.0X1	T60.0X2	T60.0X3	T60.0X4	—	—
Carboplatin	T45.1X1	T45.1X2	T45.1X3	T45.1X4	T45.1X5	T45.1X6
Carboprost	T48.0X1	T48.0X2	T48.0X3	T48.0X4	T48.0X5	T48.0X6
Carboquone	T45.1X1	T45.1X2	T45.1X3	T45.1X4	T45.1X5	T45.1X6
Carbowax	T49.3X1	T49.3X2	T49.3X3	T49.3X4	T49.3X5	T49.3X6
Carboxymethyl-cellulose	T47.4X1	T47.4X2	T47.4X3	T47.4X4	T47.4X5	T47.4X6
S-Carboxymethyl-cysteine	T48.4X1	T48.4X2	T48.4X3	T48.4X4	T48.4X5	T48.4X6
Carbrital	T42.3X1	T42.3X2	T42.3X3	T42.3X4	T42.3X5	T42.3X6
Carbromal	T42.6X1	T42.6X2	T42.6X3	T42.6X4	T42.6X5	T42.6X6
Carbutamide	T38.3X1	T38.3X2	T38.3X3	T38.3X4	T38.3X5	T38.3X6
Carbuterol	T48.6X1	T48.6X2	T48.6X3	T48.6X4	T48.6X5	T48.6X6

◀ New ◀ Revised ~~deleted~~ Deleted

Substance	External Cause (T-Code)					
	Poisoning, Accidental (Unintentional)	Poisoning, Intentional Self-Harm	Poisoning, Assault	Poisoning, Undetermined	Adverse Effect	Underdosing
Cardiac						
depressants	T46.2X1	T46.2X2	T46.2X3	T46.2X4	T46.2X5	T46.2X6
rhythm regulator	T46.2X1	T46.2X2	T46.2X3	T46.2X4	T46.2X5	T46.2X6
specified NEC	T46.2X1	T46.2X2	T46.2X3	T46.2X4	T46.2X5	T46.2X6
Cardiografin	T50.8X1	T50.8X2	T50.8X3	T50.8X4	T50.8X5	T50.8X6
Cardio-green	T50.8X1	T50.8X2	T50.8X3	T50.8X4	T50.8X5	T50.8X6
Cardiotonic (glycoside) NEC	T46.0X1	T46.0X2	T46.0X3	T46.0X4	T46.0X5	T46.0X6
Cardiovascular drug NEC	T46.901	T46.902	T46.903	T46.904	T46.905	T46.906
Cardrase	T50.2X1	T50.2X2	T50.2X3	T50.2X4	T50.2X5	T50.2X6
Carfusin	T49.0X1	T49.0X2	T49.0X3	T49.0X4	T49.0X5	T49.0X6
Carfecillin	T36.0X1	T36.0X2	T36.0X3	T36.0X4	T36.0X5	T36.0X6
Carfenazine	T43.3X1	T43.3X2	T43.3X3	T43.3X4	T43.3X5	T43.3X6
Carindacillin	T36.0X1	T36.0X2	T36.0X3	T36.0X4	T36.0X5	T36.0X6
Carisoprodol	T42.8X1	T42.8X2	T42.8X3	T42.8X4	T42.8X5	T42.8X6
Carmellose	T47.4X1	T47.4X2	T47.4X3	T47.4X4	T47.4X5	T47.4X6
Carminative	T47.5X1	T47.5X2	T47.5X3	T47.5X4	T47.5X5	T47.5X6
Carmofur	T45.1X1	T45.1X2	T45.1X3	T45.1X4	T45.1X5	T45.1X6
Carmustine	T45.1X1	T45.1X2	T45.1X3	T45.1X4	T45.1X5	T45.1X6
Carotene	T45.2X1	T45.2X2	T45.2X3	T45.2X4	T45.2X5	T45.2X6
Carphenazine	T43.3X1	T43.3X2	T43.3X3	T43.3X4	T43.3X5	T43.3X6
Carpipramine	T42.4X1	T42.4X2	T42.4X3	T42.4X4	T42.4X5	T42.4X6
Carprofen	T39.311	T39.312	T39.313	T39.314	T39.315	T39.316
Carpronium chloride	T44.3X1	T44.3X2	T44.3X3	T44.3X4	T44.3X5	T44.3X6
Carrageenan	T47.8X1	T47.8X2	T47.8X3	T47.8X4	T47.8X5	T47.8X6
Carteolol	T44.7X1	T44.7X2	T44.7X3	T44.7X4	T44.7X5	T44.7X6
Carter's Little Pills	T47.2X1	T47.2X2	T47.2X3	T47.2X4	T47.2X5	T47.2X6
Cascara (sagrada)	T47.2X1	T47.2X2	T47.2X3	T47.2X4	T47.2X5	T47.2X6
Cassava	T62.2X1	T62.2X2	T62.2X3	T62.2X4	—	—
Castellani's paint	T49.0X1	T49.0X2	T49.0X3	T49.0X4	T49.0X5	T49.0X6
Castor						
bean	T62.2X1	T62.2X2	T62.2X3	T62.2X4	—	—
oil	T47.2X1	T47.2X2	T47.2X3	T47.2X4	T47.2X5	T47.2X6
Catalase	T45.3X1	T45.3X2	T45.3X3	T45.3X4	T45.3X5	T45.3X6
Caterpillar (sting)	T63.431	T63.432	T63.433	T63.434	—	—
Catha (edulis) (tea)	T43.691	T43.692	T43.693	T43.694	—	—
Cathartic NEC	T47.4X1	T47.4X2	T47.4X3	T47.4X4	T47.4X5	T47.4X6
anthacene derivative	T47.2X1	T47.2X2	T47.2X3	T47.2X4	T47.2X5	T47.2X6
bulk	T47.4X1	T47.4X2	T47.4X3	T47.4X4	T47.4X5	T47.4X6
contact	T47.2X1	T47.2X2	T47.2X3	T47.2X4	T47.2X5	T47.2X6
emollient NEC	T47.4X1	T47.4X2	T47.4X3	T47.4X4	T47.4X5	T47.4X6

TABLE OF DRUGS AND CHEMICALS

TABLE OF DRUGS AND CHEMICALS

Substance	Poisoning, Accidental (Unintentional)	Poisoning, Intentional Self-Harm	Poisoning, Assault	Poisoning, Undetermined	Adverse Effect	Underdosing
Cathartic NEC *(Continued)*						
irritant NEC	T47.2X1	T47.2X2	T47.2X3	T47.2X4	T47.2X5	T47.2X6
mucilage	T47.4X1	T47.4X2	T47.4X3	T47.4X4	T47.4X5	T47.4X6
saline	T47.3X1	T47.3X2	T47.3X3	T47.3X4	T47.3X5	T47.3X6
vegetable	T47.2X1	T47.2X2	T47.2X3	T47.2X4	T47.2X5	T47.2X6
Cathine	T50.5X1	T50.5X2	T50.5X3	T50.5X4	T50.5X5	T50.5X6
Cathomycin	T36.8X1	T36.8X2	T36.8X3	T36.8X4	T36.8X5	T36.8X6
Cation exchange resin	T50.3X1	T50.3X2	T50.3X3	T50.3X4	T50.3X5	T50.3X6
Caustic(s) NEC	T54.91	T54.92	T54.93	T54.94	—	—
alkali	T54.3X1	T54.3X2	T54.3X3	T54.3X4	—	—
hydroxide	T54.3X1	T54.3X2	T54.3X3	T54.3X4	—	—
potash	T54.3X1	T54.3X2	T54.3X3	T54.3X4	—	—
soda	T54.3X1	T54.3X2	T54.3X3	T54.3X4	—	—
specified NEC	T54.91	T54.92	T54.93	T54.94	—	—
Ceepryn	T49.0X1	T49.0X2	T49.0X3	T49.0X4	T49.0X5	T49.0X6
ENT agent	T49.6X1	T49.6X2	T49.6X3	T49.6X4	T49.6X5	T49.6X6
lozenges	T49.6X1	T49.6X2	T49.6X3	T49.6X4	T49.6X5	T49.6X6
Cefacetrile	T36.1X1	T36.1X2	T36.1X3	T36.1X4	T36.1X5	T36.1X6
Cefaclor	T36.1X1	T36.1X2	T36.1X3	T36.1X4	T36.1X5	T36.1X6
Cefadroxil	T36.1X1	T36.1X2	T36.1X3	T36.1X4	T36.1X5	T36.1X6
Cefalexin	T36.1X1	T36.1X2	T36.1X3	T36.1X4	T36.1X5	T36.1X6
Cefaloglycin	T36.1X1	T36.1X2	T36.1X3	T36.1X4	T36.1X5	T36.1X6
Cefaloridine	T36.1X1	T36.1X2	T36.1X3	T36.1X4	T36.1X5	T36.1X6
Cefalosporins	T36.1X1	T36.1X2	T36.1X3	T36.1X4	T36.1X5	T36.1X6
Cefalotin	T36.1X1	T36.1X2	T36.1X3	T36.1X4	T36.1X5	T36.1X6
Cefamandole	T36.1X1	T36.1X2	T36.1X3	T36.1X4	T36.1X5	T36.1X6
Cefamycin antibiotic	T36.1X1	T36.1X2	T36.1X3	T36.1X4	T36.1X5	T36.1X6
Cefapirin	T36.1X1	T36.1X2	T36.1X3	T36.1X4	T36.1X5	T36.1X6
Cefatrizine	T36.1X1	T36.1X2	T36.1X3	T36.1X4	T36.1X5	T36.1X6
Cefazedone	T36.1X1	T36.1X2	T36.1X3	T36.1X4	T36.1X5	T36.1X6
Cefazolin	T36.1X1	T36.1X2	T36.1X3	T36.1X4	T36.1X5	T36.1X6
Cefbuperazone	T36.1X1	T36.1X2	T36.1X3	T36.1X4	T36.1X5	T36.1X6
Cefetamet	T36.1X1	T36.1X2	T36.1X3	T36.1X4	T36.1X5	T36.1X6
Cefixime	T36.1X1	T36.1X2	T36.1X3	T36.1X4	T36.1X5	T36.1X6
Cefmenoxime	T36.1X1	T36.1X2	T36.1X3	T36.1X4	T36.1X5	T36.1X6
Cefmetazole	T36.1X1	T36.1X2	T36.1X3	T36.1X4	T36.1X5	T36.1X6
Cefminox	T36.1X1	T36.1X2	T36.1X3	T36.1X4	T36.1X5	T36.1X6
Cefonicid	T36.1X1	T36.1X2	T36.1X3	T36.1X4	T36.1X5	T36.1X6
Cefoperazone	T36.1X1	T36.1X2	T36.1X3	T36.1X4	T36.1X5	T36.1X6

◀ New   ◀▥ Revised   ~~deleted~~ Deleted

Substance	External Cause (T-Code)					
	Poisoning, Accidental (Unintentional)	Poisoning, Intentional Self-Harm	Poisoning, Assault	Poisoning, Undetermined	Adverse Effect	Underdosing
Ceforanide	T36.1X1	T36.1X2	T36.1X3	T36.1X4	T36.1X5	T36.1X6
Cefotaxime	T36.1X1	T36.1X2	T36.1X3	T36.1X4	T36.1X5	T36.1X6
Cefotetan	T36.1X1	T36.1X2	T36.1X3	T36.1X4	T36.1X5	T36.1X6
Cefotiam	T36.1X1	T36.1X2	T36.1X3	T36.1X4	T36.1X5	T36.1X6
Cefoxitin	T36.1X1	T36.1X2	T36.1X3	T36.1X4	T36.1X5	T36.1X6
Cefpimizole	T36.1X1	T36.1X2	T36.1X3	T36.1X4	T36.1X5	T36.1X6
Cefpiramide	T36.1X1	T36.1X2	T36.1X3	T36.1X4	T36.1X5	T36.1X6
Cefradine	T36.1X1	T36.1X2	T36.1X3	T36.1X4	T36.1X5	T36.1X6
Cefroxadine	T36.1X1	T36.1X2	T36.1X3	T36.1X4	T36.1X5	T36.1X6
Cefsulodin	T36.1X1	T36.1X2	T36.1X3	T36.1X4	T36.1X5	T36.1X6
Ceftazidime	T36.1X1	T36.1X2	T36.1X3	T36.1X4	T36.1X5	T36.1X6
Cefteram	T36.1X1	T36.1X2	T36.1X3	T36.1X4	T36.1X5	T36.1X6
Ceftezole	T36.1X1	T36.1X2	T36.1X3	T36.1X4	T36.1X5	T36.1X6
Ceftizoxime	T36.1X1	T36.1X2	T36.1X3	T36.1X4	T36.1X5	T36.1X6
Ceftriaxone	T36.1X1	T36.1X2	T36.1X3	T36.1X4	T36.1X5	T36.1X6
Cefuroxime	T36.1X1	T36.1X2	T36.1X3	T36.1X4	T36.1X5	T36.1X6
Cefuzonam	T36.1X1	T36.1X2	T36.1X3	T36.1X4	T36.1X5	T36.1X6
Celestone	T38.0X1	T38.0X2	T38.0X3	T38.0X4	T38.0X5	T38.0X6
topical	T49.0X1	T49.0X2	T49.0X3	T49.0X4	T49.0X5	T49.0X6
Celiprolol	T44.7X1	T44.7X2	T44.7X3	T44.7X4	T44.7X5	T44.7X6
Cellosolve	T52.91	T52.92	T52.93	T52.94	—	—
Cell stimulants and proliferants	T49.8X1	T49.8X2	T49.8X3	T49.8X4	T49.8X5	T49.8X6
Cellulose						
cathartic	T47.4X1	T47.4X2	T47.4X3	T47.4X4	T47.4X5	T47.4X6
hydroxyethyl	T47.4X1	T47.4X2	T47.4X3	T47.4X4	T47.4X5	T47.4X6
nitrates (topical)	T49.3X1	T49.3X2	T49.3X3	T49.3X4	T49.3X5	T49.3X6
oxidized	T49.4X1	T49.4X2	T49.4X3	T49.4X4	T49.4X5	T49.4X6
Centipede (bite)	T63.411	T63.412	T63.413	T63.414	—	—
Central nervous system						
depressants	T42.71	T42.72	T42.73	T42.74	T42.75	T42.76
anesthetic (general) NEC	T41.201	T41.202	T41.203	T41.204	T41.205	T41.206
gases NEC	T41.0X1	T41.0X2	T41.0X3	T41.0X4	T41.0X5	T41.0X6
intravenous	T41.1X1	T41.1X2	T41.1X3	T41.1X4	T41.1X5	T41.1X6
barbiturates	T42.3X1	T42.3X2	T42.3X3	T42.3X4	T42.3X5	T42.3X6
benzodiazepines	T42.4X1	T42.4X2	T42.4X3	T42.4X4	T42.4X5	T42.4X6
bromides	T42.6X1	T42.6X2	T42.6X3	T42.6X4	T42.6X5	T42.6X6
cannabis sativa	T40.7X1	T40.7X2	T40.7X3	T40.7X4	T40.7X5	T40.7X6
chloral hydrate	T42.6X1	T42.6X2	T42.6X3	T42.6X4	T42.6X5	T42.6X6
ethanol	T51.0X1	T51.0X2	T51.0X3	T51.0X4	—	—

TABLE OF DRUGS AND CHEMICALS

TABLE OF DRUGS AND CHEMICALS

Substance	External Cause (T-Code)					
	Poisoning, Accidental (Unintentional)	Poisoning, Intentional Self-Harm	Poisoning, Assault	Poisoning, Undetermined	Adverse Effect	Underdosing
Central nervous system *(Continued)*						
depressants *(Continued)*						
hallucinogenics	T40.901	T40.902	T40.903	T40.904	T40.905	T40.906
hypnotics	T42.71	T42.72	T42.73	T42.74	T42.75	T42.76
specified NEC	T42.6X1	T42.6X2	T42.6X3	T42.6X4	T42.6X5	T42.6X6
muscle relaxants	T42.8X1	T42.8X2	T42.8X3	T42.8X4	T42.8X5	T42.8X6
paraldehyde	T42.6X1	T42.6X2	T42.6X3	T42.6X4	T42.6X5	T42.6X6
sedatives; sedative-hypnotics	T42.71	T42.72	T42.73	T42.74	T42.75	T42.76
mixed NEC	T42.6X1	T42.6X2	T42.6X3	T42.6X4	T42.6X5	T42.6X6
specified NEC	T42.6X1	T42.6X2	T42.6X3	T42.6X4	T42.6X5	T42.6X6
muscle-tone depressants	T42.8X1	T42.8X2	T42.8X3	T42.8X4	T42.8X5	T42.8X6
stimulants	T43.601	T43.602	T43.603	T43.604	T43.605	T43.606
amphetamines	T43.621	T43.622	T43.623	T43.624	T43.625	T43.626
analeptics	T50.7X1	T50.7X2	T50.7X3	T50.7X4	T50.7X5	T50.7X6
antidepressants	T43.201	T43.202	T43.203	T43.204	T43.205	T43.206
opiate antagonists	T50.7X1	T50.7X2	T50.7X3	T50.7X4	T50.7X5	T50.7X6
specified NEC	T43.691	T43.692	T43.693	T43.694	T43.695	T43.696
Cephalexin	T36.1X1	T36.1X2	T36.1X3	T36.1X4	T36.1X5	T36.1X6
Cephaloglycin	T36.1X1	T36.1X2	T36.1X3	T36.1X4	T36.1X5	T36.1X6
Cephaloridine	T36.1X1	T36.1X2	T36.1X3	T36.1X4	T36.1X5	T36.1X6
Cephalosporins	T36.1X1	T36.1X2	T36.1X3	T36.1X4	T36.1X5	T36.1X6
N (adicillin)	T36.0X1	T36.0X2	T36.0X3	T36.0X4	T36.0X5	T36.0X6
Cephalothin	T36.1X1	T36.1X2	T36.1X3	T36.1X4	T36.1X5	T36.1X6
Cephalotin	T36.1X1	T36.1X2	T36.1X3	T36.1X4	T36.1X5	T36.1X6
Cephradine	T36.1X1	T36.1X2	T36.1X3	T36.1X4	T36.1X5	T36.1X6
Cerbera (odallam)	T62.2X1	T62.2X2	T62.2X3	T62.2X4	—	—
Cerberin	T46.0X1	T46.0X2	T46.0X3	T46.0X4	T46.0X5	T46.0X6
Cerebral stimulants	T43.601	T43.602	T43.603	T43.604	T43.605	T43.606
psychotherapeutic	T43.601	T43.602	T43.603	T43.604	T43.605	T43.606
specified NEC	T43.691	T43.692	T43.693	T43.694	T43.695	T43.696
Cerium oxalate	T45.0X1	T45.0X2	T45.0X3	T45.0X4	T45.0X5	T45.0X6
Cerous oxalate	T45.0X1	T45.0X2	T45.0X3	T45.0X4	T45.0X5	T45.0X6
Ceruletide	T50.8X1	T50.8X2	T50.8X3	T50.8X4	T50.8X5	T50.8X6
Cetalkonium (chloride)	T49.0X1	T49.0X2	T49.0X3	T49.0X4	T49.0X5	T49.0X6
Cethexonium chloride	T49.0X1	T49.0X2	T49.0X3	T49.0X4	T49.0X5	T49.0X6
Cetiedil	T46.7X1	T46.7X2	T46.7X3	T46.7X4	T46.7X5	T46.7X6
Cetirizine	T45.0X1	T45.0X2	T45.0X3	T45.0X4	T45.0X5	T45.0X6
Cetomacrogol	T50.991	T50.992	T50.993	T50.994	T50.995	T50.996
Cetotiamine	T45.2X1	T45.2X2	T45.2X3	T45.2X4	T45.2X5	T45.2X6

◀ New ◀ Revised ~~deleted~~ Deleted

Substance	External Cause (T-Code)					
	Poisoning, Accidental (Unintentional)	Poisoning, Intentional Self-Harm	Poisoning, Assault	Poisoning, Undetermined	Adverse Effect	Underdosing
Cetoxime	T45.0X1	T45.0X2	T45.0X3	T45.0X4	T45.0X5	T45.0X6
Cetraxate	T47.1X1	T47.1X2	T47.1X3	T47.1X4	T47.1X5	T47.1X6
Cetrimide	T49.0X1	T49.0X2	T49.0X3	T49.0X4	T49.0X5	T49.0X6
Cetrimonium (bromide)	T49.0X1	T49.0X2	T49.0X3	T49.0X4	T49.0X5	T49.0X6
Cetylpyridinium chloride	T49.0X1	T49.0X2	T49.0X3	T49.0X4	T49.0X5	T49.0X6
ENT agent	T49.6X1	T49.6X2	T49.6X3	T49.6X4	T49.6X5	T49.6X6
lozenges	T49.6X1	T49.6X2	T49.6X3	T49.6X4	T49.6X5	T49.6X6
Cevadillasee Sabadilla						
Cevitamic acid	T45.2X1	T45.2X2	T45.2X3	T45.2X4	T45.2X5	T45.2X6
Chalk, precipitated	T47.1X1	T47.1X2	T47.1X3	T47.1X4	T47.1X5	T47.1X6
Chamomile	T49.0X1	T49.0X2	T49.0X3	T49.0X4	T49.0X5	T49.0X6
Ch'an su	T46.0X1	T46.0X2	T46.0X3	T46.0X4	T46.0X5	T46.0X6
Charcoal	T47.6X1	T47.6X2	T47.6X3	T47.6X4	T47.6X5	T47.6X6
activated — see also Charcoal, medicinal	T47.6X1	T47.6X2	T47.6X3	T47.6X4	T47.6X5	T47.6X6
fumes (Carbon monoxide)	T58.2X1	T58.2X2	T58.2X3	T58.2X4	—	—
industrial	T58.8X1	T58.8X2	T58.8X3	T58.8X4	—	—
medicinal (activated)	T47.6X1	T47.6X2	T47.6X3	T47.6X4	T47.6X5	T47.6X6
antidiarrheal	T47.6X1	T47.6X2	T47.6X3	T47.6X4	T47.6X5	T47.6X6
poison control	T47.8X1	T47.8X2	T47.8X3	T47.8X4	T47.8X5	T47.8X6
specified use other than for diarrhea	T47.8X1	T47.8X2	T47.8X3	T47.8X4	T47.8X5	T47.8X6
topical	T49.8X1	T49.8X2	T49.8X3	T49.8X4	T49.8X5	T49.8X6
Chaulmosulfone	T37.1X1	T37.1X2	T37.1X3	T37.1X4	T37.1X5	T37.1X6
Chelating agent NEC	T50.6X1	T50.6X2	T50.6X3	T50.6X4	T50.6X5	T50.6X6
Chelidonium majus	T62.2X1	T62.2X2	T62.2X3	T62.2X4	—	—
Chemical substance NEC	T65.91	T65.92	T65.93	T65.94	—	—
Chenodeoxycholic acid	T47.5X1	T47.5X2	T47.5X3	T47.5X4	T47.5X5	T47.5X6
Chenodiol	T47.5X1	T47.5X2	T47.5X3	T47.5X4	T47.5X5	T47.5X6
Chenopodium	T37.4X1	T37.4X2	T37.4X3	T37.4X4	T37.4X5	T37.4X6
Cherry laurel	T62.2X1	T62.2X2	T62.2X3	T62.2X4	—	—
Chinidin(e)	T46.2X1	T46.2X2	T46.2X3	T46.2X4	T46.2X5	T46.2X6
Chiniofon	T37.8X1	T37.8X2	T37.8X3	T37.8X4	T37.8X5	T37.8X6
Chlophedianol	T48.3X1	T48.3X2	T48.3X3	T48.3X4	T48.3X5	T48.3X6
Chloral	T42.6X1	T42.6X2	T42.6X3	T42.6X4	T42.6X5	T42.6X6
derivative	T42.6X1	T42.6X2	T42.6X3	T42.6X4	T42.6X5	T42.6X6
hydrate	T42.6X1	T42.6X2	T42.6X3	T42.6X4	T42.6X5	T42.6X6
Chloralamide	T42.6X1	T42.6X2	T42.6X3	T42.6X4	T42.6X5	T42.6X6
Chloralodol	T42.6X1	T42.6X2	T42.6X3	T42.6X4	T42.6X5	T42.6X6
Chloralose	T60.4X1	T60.4X2	T60.4X3	T60.4X4	—	—
Chlorambucil	T45.1X1	T45.1X2	T45.1X3	T45.1X4	T45.1X5	T45.1X6

TABLE OF DRUGS AND CHEMICALS

Substance	External Cause (T-Code)					
	Poisoning, Accidental (Unintentional)	Poisoning, Intentional Self-Harm	Poisoning, Assault	Poisoning, Undetermined	Adverse Effect	Underdosing
Chloramine	T57.8X1	T57.8X2	T57.8X3	T57.8X4	—	—
T	T49.0X1	T49.0X2	T49.0X3	T49.0X4	T49.0X5	T49.0X6
topical	T49.0X1	T49.0X2	T49.0X3	T49.0X4	T49.0X5	T49.0X6
Chloramphenicol	T36.2X1	T36.2X2	T36.2X3	T36.2X4	T36.2X5	T36.2X6
ENT agent	T49.6X1	T49.6X2	T49.6X3	T49.6X4	T49.6X5	T49.6X6
ophthalmic preparation	T49.5X1	T49.5X2	T49.5X3	T49.5X4	T49.5X5	T49.5X6
topical NEC	T49.0X1	T49.0X2	T49.0X3	T49.0X4	T49.0X5	T49.0X6
Chlorate (potassium) (sodium) NEC	T60.3X1	T60.3X2	T60.3X3	T60.3X4	—	—
herbicide	T60.3X1	T60.3X2	T60.3X3	T60.3X4	—	—
Chlorazanil	T50.2X1	T50.2X2	T50.2X3	T50.2X4	T50.2X5	T50.2X6
Chlorbenzene, chlorbenzol	T53.7X1	T53.7X2	T53.7X3	T53.7X4	—	—
Chlorbenzoxamine	T44.3X1	T44.3X2	T44.3X3	T44.3X4	T44.3X5	T44.3X6
Chlorbutol	T42.6X1	T42.6X2	T42.6X3	T42.6X4	T42.6X5	T42.6X6
Chlorcyclizine	T45.0X1	T45.0X2	T45.0X3	T45.0X4	T45.0X5	T45.0X6
Chlordan(e) (dust)	T60.1X1	T60.1X2	T60.1X3	T60.1X4	—	—
Chlordantoin	T49.0X1	T49.0X2	T49.0X3	T49.0X4	T49.0X5	T49.0X6
Chlordiazepoxide	T42.4X1	T42.4X2	T42.4X3	T42.4X4	T42.4X5	T42.4X6
Chlordiethyl benzamide	T49.3X1	T49.3X2	T49.3X3	T49.3X4	T49.3X5	T49.3X6
Chloresium	T49.8X1	T49.8X2	T49.8X3	T49.8X4	T49.8X5	T49.8X6
Chlorethiazol	T42.6X1	T42.6X2	T42.6X3	T42.6X4	T42.6X5	T42.6X6
Chlorethyl — see Ethyl chloride						
Chloretone	T42.6X1	T42.6X2	T42.6X3	T42.6X4	T42.6X5	T42.6X6
Chlorex	T53.6X1	T53.6X2	T53.6X3	T53.6X4	—	—
insecticide	T60.1X1	T60.1X2	T60.1X3	T60.1X4	—	—
Chlorfenvinphos	T60.0X1	T60.0X2	T60.0X3	T60.0X4	—	—
Chlorhexadol	T42.6X1	T42.6X2	T42.6X3	T42.6X4	T42.6X5	T42.6X6
Chlorhexamide	T45.1X1	T45.1X2	T45.1X3	T45.1X4	T45.1X5	T45.1X6
Chlorhexidine	T49.0X1	T49.0X2	T49.0X3	T49.0X4	T49.0X5	T49.0X6
Chlorhydroxyquinolin	T49.0X1	T49.0X2	T49.0X3	T49.0X4	T49.0X5	T49.0X6
Chloride of lime (bleach)	T54.3X1	T54.3X2	T54.3X3	T54.3X4	—	—
Chlorimipramine	T43.011	T43.012	T43.013	T43.014	T43.015	T43.016
Chlorinated						
camphene	T53.6X1	T53.6X2	T53.6X3	T53.6X4	—	—
diphenyl	T53.7X1	T53.7X2	T53.7X3	T53.7X4	—	—
hydrocarbons NEC	T53.91	T53.92	T53.93	T53.94	—	—
solvents	T53.91	T53.92	T53.93	T53.94	—	—
lime (bleach)	T54.3X1	T54.3X2	T54.3X3	T54.3X4	—	—
and boric acid solution	T49.0X1	T49.0X2	T49.0X3	T49.0X4	T49.0X5	T49.0X6
naphthalene (insecticide)	T60.1X1	T60.1X2	T60.1X3	T60.1X4	—	—
industrial (non-pesticide)	T53.7X1	T53.7X2	T53.7X3	T53.7X4	—	—

◀ New   ◀▬ Revised   ~~deleted~~ Deleted

Substance	External Cause (T-Code)					
	Poisoning, Accidental (Unintentional)	Poisoning, Intentional Self-Harm	Poisoning, Assault	Poisoning, Undetermined	Adverse Effect	Underdosing
Chlorinated *(Continued)*						
pesticide NEC	T60.8X1	T60.8X2	T60.8X3	T60.8X4	—	—
soda — *see also sodium hypochlorite*						
solution	T49.0X1	T49.0X2	T49.0X3	T49.0X4	T49.0X5	T49.0X6
Chlorine (fumes) (gas)	T59.4X1	T59.4X2	T59.4X3	T59.4X4	—	—
bleach	T54.3X1	T54.3X2	T54.3X3	T54.3X4	—	—
compound gas NEC	T59.4X1	T59.4X2	T59.4X3	T59.4X4	—	—
disinfectant	T59.4X1	T59.4X2	T59.4X3	T59.4X4	—	—
releasing agents NEC	T59.4X1	T59.4X2	T59.4X3	T59.4X4	—	—
Chlorisondamine chloride	T46.991	T46.992	T46.993	T46.994	T46.995	T46.996
Chlormadinone	T38.5X1	T38.5X2	T38.5X3	T38.5X4	T38.5X5	T38.5X6
Chlormephos	T60.0X1	T60.0X2	T60.0X3	T60.0X4	—	—
Chlormerodrin	T50.2X1	T50.2X2	T50.2X3	T50.2X4	T50.2X5	T50.2X6
Chlormethiazole	T42.6X1	T42.6X2	T42.6X3	T42.6X4	T42.6X5	T42.6X6
Chlormethine	T45.1X1	T45.1X2	T45.1X3	T45.1X4	T45.1X5	T45.1X6
Chlormethylenecycline	T36.4X1	T36.4X2	T36.4X3	T36.4X4	T36.4X5	T36.4X6
Chlormezanone	T42.6X1	T42.6X2	T42.6X3	T42.6X4	T42.6X5	T42.6X6
Chloroacetic acid	T60.3X1	T60.3X2	T60.3X3	T60.3X4	—	—
Chloroacetone	T59.3X1	T59.3X2	T59.3X3	T59.3X4	—	—
Chloroacetophenone	T59.3X1	T59.3X2	T59.3X3	T59.3X4	—	—
Chloroaniline	T53.7X1	T53.7X2	T53.7X3	T53.7X4	—	—
Chlorobenzene, chlorobenzol	T53.7X1	T53.7X2	T53.7X3	T53.7X4	—	—
Chlorobromomethane (fire extinguisher)	T53.6X1	T53.6X2	T53.6X3	T53.6X4	—	—
Chlorobutanol	T49.0X1	T49.0X2	T49.0X3	T49.0X4	T49.0X5	T49.0X6
Chlorocresol	T49.0X1	T49.0X2	T49.0X3	T49.0X4	T49.0X5	T49.0X6
Chlorodehydro-methyltestosterone	T38.7X1	T38.7X2	T38.7X3	T38.7X4	T38.7X5	T38.7X6
Chlorodinitrobenzene	T53.7X1	T53.7X2	T53.7X3	T53.7X4	—	—
dust or vapor	T53.7X1	T53.7X2	T53.7X3	T53.7X4	—	—
Chlorodiphenyl	T53.7X1	T53.7X2	T53.7X3	T53.7X4	—	—
Chloroethane — *see Ethyl chloride*						
Chloroethylene	T53.6X1	T53.6X2	T53.6X3	T53.6X4	—	—
Chlorofluorocarbons	T53.5X1	T53.5X2	T53.5X3	T53.5X4	—	—
Chloroform (fumes) (vapor)	T53.1X1	T53.1X2	T53.1X3	T53.1X4	—	—
anesthetic	T41.0X1	T41.0X2	T41.0X3	T41.0X4	T41.0X5	T41.0X6
solvent	T53.1X1	T53.1X2	T53.1X3	T53.1X4	—	—
water, concentrated	T41.0X1	T41.0X2	T41.0X3	T41.0X4	T41.0X5	T41.0X6
Chloroguanide	T37.2X1	T37.2X2	T37.2X3	T37.2X4	T37.2X5	T37.2X6
Chloromycetin	T36.2X1	T36.2X2	T36.2X3	T36.2X4	T36.2X5	T36.2X6
ENT agent	T49.6X1	T49.6X2	T49.6X3	T49.6X4	T49.6X5	T49.6X6
ophthalmic preparation	T49.5X1	T49.5X2	T49.5X3	T49.5X4	T49.5X5	T49.5X6

◀ New   ◀ Revised   ~~deleted~~ Deleted

TABLE OF DRUGS AND CHEMICALS

TABLE OF DRUGS AND CHEMICALS

Substance	External Cause (T-Code)					
	Poisoning, Accidental (Unintentional)	Poisoning, Intentional Self-Harm	Poisoning, Assault	Poisoning, Undetermined	Adverse Effect	Underdosing
Chloromycetin (Continued)						
otic solution	T49.6X1	T49.6X2	T49.6X3	T49.6X4	T49.6X5	T49.6X6
topical NEC	T49.0X1	T49.0X2	T49.0X3	T49.0X4	T49.0X5	T49.0X6
Chloronitrobenzene	T53.7X1	T53.7X2	T53.7X3	T53.7X4	—	—
dust or vapor	T53.7X1	T53.7X2	T53.7X3	T53.7X4	—	—
Chlorophacinone	T60.4X1	T60.4X2	T60.4X3	T60.4X4	—	—
Chlorophenol	T53.7X1	T53.7X2	T53.7X3	T53.7X4	—	—
Chlorophenothane	T60.1X1	T60.1X2	T60.1X3	T60.1X4	—	—
Chlorophyll	T50.991	T50.992	T50.993	T50.994	T50.995	T50.996
Chloropicrin (fumes)	T53.6X1	T53.6X2	T53.6X3	T53.6X4	—	—
fumigant	T60.8X1	T60.8X2	T60.8X3	T60.8X4	—	—
fungicide	T60.3X1	T60.3X2	T60.3X3	T60.3X4	—	—
pesticide	T60.8X1	T60.8X2	T60.8X3	T60.8X4	—	—
Chloroprocaine	T41.3X1	T41.3X2	T41.3X3	T41.3X4	T41.3X5	T41.3X6
infiltration (subcutaneous)	T41.3X1	T41.3X2	T41.3X3	T41.3X4	T41.3X5	T41.3X6
nerve block (peripheral) (plexus)	T41.3X1	T41.3X2	T41.3X3	T41.3X4	T41.3X5	T41.3X6
spinal	T41.3X1	T41.3X2	T41.3X3	T41.3X4	T41.3X5	T41.3X6
Chloroptic	T49.5X1	T49.5X2	T49.5X3	T49.5X4	T49.5X5	T49.5X6
Chloropurine	T45.1X1	T45.1X2	T45.1X3	T45.1X4	T45.1X5	T45.1X6
Chloropyramine	T45.0X1	T45.0X2	T45.0X3	T45.0X4	T45.0X5	T45.0X6
Chloropyrifos	T60.0X1	T60.0X2	T60.0X3	T60.0X4	—	—
Chloropyrilene	T45.0X1	T45.0X2	T45.0X3	T45.0X4	T45.0X5	T45.0X6
Chloroquine	T37.2X1	T37.2X2	T37.2X3	T37.2X4	T37.2X5	T37.2X6
Chlorothalonil	T60.3X1	T60.3X2	T60.3X3	T60.3X4	—	—
Chlorothen	T45.0X1	T45.0X2	T45.0X3	T45.0X4	T45.0X5	T45.0X6
Chlorothiazide	T50.2X1	T50.2X2	T50.2X3	T50.2X4	T50.2X5	T50.2X6
Chlorothymol	T49.4X1	T49.4X2	T49.4X3	T49.4X4	T49.4X5	T49.4X6
Chlorotrianisene	T38.5X1	T38.5X2	T38.5X3	T38.5X4	T38.5X5	T38.5X6
Chlorovinyldichloro-arsine, not in war	T57.0X1	T57.0X2	T57.0X3	T57.0X4	—	—
Chloroxine	T49.4X1	T49.4X2	T49.4X3	T49.4X4	T49.4X5	T49.4X6
Chloroxylenol	T49.0X1	T49.0X2	T49.0X3	T49.0X4	T49.0X5	T49.0X6
Chlorphenamine	T45.0X1	T45.0X2	T45.0X3	T45.0X4	T45.0X5	T45.0X6
Chlorphenesin	T42.8X1	T42.8X2	T42.8X3	T42.8X4	T42.8X5	T42.8X6
topical (antifungal)	T49.0X1	T49.0X2	T49.0X3	T49.0X4	T49.0X5	T49.0X6
Chlorpheniramine	T45.0X1	T45.0X2	T45.0X3	T45.0X4	T45.0X5	T45.0X6
Chlorphenoxamine	T45.0X1	T45.0X2	T45.0X3	T45.0X4	T45.0X5	T45.0X6
Chlorphentermine	T50.5X1	T50.5X2	T50.5X3	T50.5X4	T50.5X5	T50.5X6
Chlorprocaine — see Chloroprocaine						
Chlorproguanil	T37.2X1	T37.2X2	T37.2X3	T37.2X4	T37.2X5	T37.2X6
Chlorpromazine	T43.3X1	T43.3X2	T43.3X3	T43.3X4	T43.3X5	T43.3X6

◀ New ⬅ Revised ~~deleted~~ Deleted

Substance	External Cause (T-Code)					
	Poisoning, Accidental (Unintentional)	Poisoning, Intentional Self-Harm	Poisoning, Assault	Poisoning, Undetermined	Adverse Effect	Underdosing
Chlorpropamide	T38.3X1	T38.3X2	T38.3X3	T38.3X4	T38.3X5	T38.3X6
Chlorprothixene	T43.4X1	T43.4X2	T43.4X3	T43.4X4	T43.4X5	T43.4X6
Chlorquinaldol	T49.0X1	T49.0X2	T49.0X3	T49.0X4	T49.0X5	T49.0X6
Chlorquinol	T49.0X1	T49.0X2	T49.0X3	T49.0X4	T49.0X5	T49.0X6
Chlortalidone	T50.2X1	T50.2X2	T50.2X3	T50.2X4	T50.2X5	T50.2X6
Chlortetracycline	T36.4X1	T36.4X2	T36.4X3	T36.4X4	T36.4X5	T36.4X6
Chlorthalidone	T50.2X1	T50.2X2	T50.2X3	T50.2X4	T50.2X5	T50.2X6
Chlorthiophos	T60.0X1	T60.0X2	T60.0X3	T60.0X4	—	—
Chlorotrianisene	T38.5X1	T38.5X2	T38.5X3	T38.5X4	T38.5X5	T38.5X6
Chlor-Trimeton	T45.0X1	T45.0X2	T45.0X3	T45.0X4	T45.0X5	T45.0X6
Chlorthion	T60.0X1	T60.0X2	T60.0X3	T60.0X4	—	—
Chlorzoxazone	T42.8X1	T42.8X2	T42.8X3	T42.8X4	T42.8X5	T42.8X6
Choke damp	T59.7X1	T59.7X2	T59.7X3	T59.7X4	—	—
Cholagogues	T47.5X1	T47.5X2	T47.5X3	T47.5X4	T47.5X5	T47.5X6
Cholebrine	T50.8X1	T50.8X2	T50.8X3	T50.8X4	T50.8X5	T50.8X6
Cholecalciferol	T45.2X1	T45.2X2	T45.2X3	T45.2X4	T45.2X5	T45.2X6
Cholecystokinin	T50.8X1	T50.8X2	T50.8X3	T50.8X4	T50.8X5	T50.8X6
Cholera vaccine	T50.A91	T50.A92	T50.A93	T50.A94	T50.A95	T50.A96
Choleretic	T47.5X1	T47.5X2	T47.5X3	T47.5X4	T47.5X5	T47.5X6
Cholesterol-lowering agents	T46.6X1	T46.6X2	T46.6X3	T46.6X4	T46.6X5	T46.6X6
Cholestyramine (resin)	T46.6X1	T46.6X2	T46.6X3	T46.6X4	T46.6X5	T46.6X6
Cholic acid	T47.5X1	T47.5X2	T47.5X3	T47.5X4	T47.5X5	T47.5X6
Choline	T48.6X1	T48.6X2	T48.6X3	T48.6X4	T48.6X5	T48.6X6
chloride	T50.991	T50.992	T50.993	T50.994	T50.995	T50.996
dihydrogen citrate	T50.991	T50.992	T50.993	T50.994	T50.995	T50.996
salicylate	T39.091	T39.092	T39.093	T39.094	T39.095	T39.096
theophyllinate	T48.6X1	T48.6X2	T48.6X3	T48.6X4	T48.6X5	T48.6X6
Cholinergic (drug) NEC	T44.1X1	T44.1X2	T44.1X3	T44.1X4	T44.1X5	T44.1X6
muscle tone enhancer	T44.1X1	T44.1X2	T44.1X3	T44.1X4	T44.1X5	T44.1X6
organophosphorus	T44.0X1	T44.0X2	T44.0X3	T44.0X4	T44.0X5	T44.0X6
insecticide	T60.0X1	T60.0X2	T60.0X3	T60.0X4	—	—
nerve gas	T59.891	T59.892	T59.893	T59.894	—	—
trimethyl ammonium propanediol	T44.1X1	T44.1X2	T44.1X3	T44.1X4	T44.1X5	T44.1X6
Cholinesterase reactivator	T50.6X1	T50.6X2	T50.6X3	T50.6X4	T50.6X5	T50.6X6
Cholografin	T50.8X1	T50.8X2	T50.8X3	T50.8X4	T50.8X5	T50.8X6
Chorionic gonadotropin	T38.891	T38.892	T38.893	T38.894	T38.895	T38.896
Chromate	T56.2X1	T56.2X2	T56.2X3	T56.2X4	—	—
dust or mist	T56.2X1	T56.2X2	T56.2X3	T56.2X4	—	—
lead — *see also* lead	T56.0X1	T56.0X2	T56.0X3	T56.0X4	—	—
paint	T56.0X1	T56.0X2	T56.0X3	T56.0X4	—	—

◀ New   ◀||| Revised   ~~deleted~~ Deleted

Substance	External Cause (T-Code)					
	Poisoning, Accidental (Unintentional)	Poisoning, Intentional Self-Harm	Poisoning, Assault	Poisoning, Undetermined	Adverse Effect	Underdosing
Chromic						
acid	T56.2X1	T56.2X2	T56.2X3	T56.2X4	—	—
dust or mist	T56.2X1	T56.2X2	T56.2X3	T56.2X4	—	—
phosphate 32P	T45.1X1	T45.1X2	T45.1X3	T45.1X4	T45.1X5	T45.1X6
Chromium	T56.2X1	T56.2X2	T56.2X3	T56.2X4	—	—
compounds — see Chromate						
sesquioxide	T50.8X1	T50.8X2	T50.8X3	T50.8X4	T50.8X5	T50.8X6
Chromomycin A3	T45.1X1	T45.1X2	T45.1X3	T45.1X4	T45.1X5	T45.1X6
Chromonar	T46.3X1	T46.3X2	T46.3X3	T46.3X4	T46.3X5	T46.3X6
Chromyl chloride	T56.2X1	T56.2X2	T56.2X3	T56.2X4	—	—
Chrysarobin	T49.4X1	T49.4X2	T49.4X3	T49.4X4	T49.4X5	T49.4X6
Chrysazin	T47.2X1	T47.2X2	T47.2X3	T47.2X4	T47.2X5	T47.2X6
Chymar	T45.3X1	T45.3X2	T45.3X3	T45.3X4	T45.3X5	T45.3X6
ophthalmic preparation	T49.5X1	T49.5X2	T49.5X3	T49.5X4	T49.5X5	T49.5X6
Chymopapain	T45.3X1	T45.3X2	T45.3X3	T45.3X4	T45.3X5	T45.3X6
Chymotrypsin	T45.3X1	T45.3X2	T45.3X3	T45.3X4	T45.3X5	T45.3X6
ophthalmic preparation	T49.5X1	T49.5X2	T49.5X3	T49.5X4	T49.5X5	T49.5X6
Cianidanol	T50.991	T50.992	T50.993	T50.994	T50.995	T50.996
Cianopramine	T43.011	T43.012	T43.013	T43.014	T43.015	T43.016
Cibenzoline	T46.2X1	T46.2X2	T46.2X3	T46.2X4	T46.2X5	T46.2X6
Ciclacillin	T36.0X1	T36.0X2	T36.0X3	T36.0X4	T36.0X5	T36.0X6
Ciclobarbital — see Hexobarbital						
Ciclonicate	T46.7X1	T46.7X2	T46.7X3	T46.7X4	T46.7X5	T46.7X6
Ciclopirox (olamine)	T49.0X1	T49.0X2	T49.0X3	T49.0X4	T49.0X5	T49.0X6
Ciclosporin	T45.1X1	T45.1X2	T45.1X3	T45.1X4	T45.1X5	T45.1X6
Cicuta maculata or virosa	T62.2X1	T62.2X2	T62.2X3	T62.2X4	—	—
Cicutoxin	T62.2X1	T62.2X2	T62.2X3	T62.2X4	—	—
Cigarette lighter fluid	T52.0X1	T52.0X2	T52.0X3	T52.0X4	—	—
Cigarettes (tobacco)	T65.221	T65.222	T65.223	T65.224	—	—
Ciguatoxin	T61.01	T61.02	T61.03	T61.04	—	—
Cilazapril	T46.4X1	T46.4X2	T46.4X3	T46.4X4	T46.4X5	T46.4X6
Cimetidine	T47.0X1	T47.0X2	T47.0X3	T47.0X4	T47.0X5	T47.0X6
Cimetropium bromide	T44.3X1	T44.3X2	T44.3X3	T44.3X4	T44.3X5	T44.3X6
Cinchocaine	T41.3X1	T41.3X2	T41.3X3	T41.3X4	T41.3X5	T41.3X6
topical (surface)	T41.3X1	T41.3X2	T41.3X3	T41.3X4	T41.3X5	T41.3X6
Cinchona	T37.2X1	T37.2X2	T37.2X3	T37.2X4	T37.2X5	T37.2X6
Cinchonine alkaloids	T37.2X1	T37.2X2	T37.2X3	T37.2X4	T37.2X5	T37.2X6
Cinchophen	T50.4X1	T50.4X2	T50.4X3	T50.4X4	T50.4X5	T50.4X6
Cinepazide	T46.7X1	T46.7X2	T46.7X3	T46.7X4	T46.7X5	T46.7X6
Cinnamedrine	T48.5X1	T48.5X2	T48.5X3	T48.5X4	T48.5X5	T48.5X6

◀ New ◀━ Revised ~~deleted~~ Deleted

Substance	Poisoning, Accidental (Unintentional)	Poisoning, Intentional Self-Harm	Poisoning, Assault	Poisoning, Undetermined	Adverse Effect	Underdosing
			External Cause (T-Code)			
Cinnarizine	T45.0X1	T45.0X2	T45.0X3	T45.0X4	T45.0X5	T45.0X6
Cinoxacin	T37.8X1	T37.8X2	T37.8X3	T37.8X4	T37.8X5	T37.8X6
Ciprofibrate	T46.6X1	T46.6X2	T46.6X3	T46.6X4	T46.6X5	T46.6X6
Ciprofloxacin	T36.8X1	T36.8X2	T36.8X3	T36.8X4	T36.8X5	T36.8X6
Cisapride	T47.8X1	T47.8X2	T47.8X3	T47.8X4	T47.8X5	T47.8X6
Cisplatin	T45.1X1	T45.1X2	T45.1X3	T45.1X4	T45.1X5	T45.1X6
Citalopram	T43.221	T43.222	T43.223	T43.224	T43.225	T43.226
Citanest	T41.3X1	T41.3X2	T41.3X3	T41.3X4	T41.3X5	T41.3X6
infiltration (subcutaneous)	T41.3X1	T41.3X2	T41.3X3	T41.3X4	T41.3X5	T41.3X6
nerve block (peripheral) (plexus)	T41.3X1	T41.3X2	T41.3X3	T41.3X4	T41.3X5	T41.3X6
Citric acid	T47.5X1	T47.5X2	T47.5X3	T47.5X4	T47.5X5	T47.5X6
Citrovorum (factor)	T45.8X1	T45.8X2	T45.8X3	T45.8X4	T45.8X5	T45.8X6
Claviceps purpurea	T62.2X1	T62.2X2	T62.2X3	T62.2X4	—	—
Clavulanic acid	T36.1X1	T36.1X2	T36.1X3	T36.1X4	T36.1X5	T36.1X6
Cleaner, cleansing agent, type not specified	T65.891	T65.892	T65.893	T65.894	—	—
of paint or varnish	T52.91	T52.92	T52.93	T52.94	—	—
specified type NEC	T65.891	T65.892	T65.893	T65.894	—	—
Clebopride	T47.8X1	T47.8X2	T47.8X3	T47.8X4	T47.8X5	T47.8X6
Clefamide	T37.3X1	T37.3X2	T37.3X3	T37.3X4	T37.3X5	T37.3X6
Clemastine	T45.0X1	T45.0X2	T45.0X3	T45.0X4	T45.0X5	T45.0X6
Clematis vitalba	T62.2X1	T62.2X2	T62.2X3	T62.2X4	—	—
Clemizole	T45.0X1	T45.0X2	T45.0X3	T45.0X4	T45.0X5	T45.0X6
penicillin	T36.0X1	T36.0X2	T36.0X3	T36.0X4	T36.0X5	T36.0X6
Clenbuterol	T48.6X1	T48.6X2	T48.6X3	T48.6X4	T48.6X5	T48.6X6
Clidinium bromide	T44.3X1	T44.3X2	T44.3X3	T44.3X4	T44.3X5	T44.3X6
Clindamycin	T36.8X1	T36.8X2	T36.8X3	T36.8X4	T36.8X5	T36.8X6
Clinofibrate	T46.6X1	T46.6X2	T46.6X3	T46.6X4	T46.6X5	T46.6X6
Clioquinol	T37.8X1	T37.8X2	T37.8X3	T37.8X4	T37.8X5	T37.8X6
Cliradon	T40.2X1	T40.2X2	T40.2X3	T40.2X4	—	—
Clobazam	T42.4X1	T42.4X2	T42.4X3	T42.4X4	T42.4X5	T42.4X6
Clobenzorex	T50.5X1	T50.5X2	T50.5X3	T50.5X4	T50.5X5	T50.5X6
Clobetasol	T49.0X1	T49.0X2	T49.0X3	T49.0X4	T49.0X5	T49.0X6
Clobetasone	T49.0X1	T49.0X2	T49.0X3	T49.0X4	T49.0X5	T49.0X6
Clobutinol	T48.3X1	T48.3X2	T48.3X3	T48.3X4	T48.3X5	T48.3X6
Clocapramine	T43.0X1	T43.0X2	T43.0X3	T43.0X4	T43.0X5	T43.0X6
Clocortolone	T38.0X1	T38.0X2	T38.0X3	T38.0X4	T38.0X5	T38.0X6
Clodantoin	T49.0X1	T49.0X2	T49.0X3	T49.0X4	T49.0X5	T49.0X6
Clodronic acid	T50.991	T50.992	T50.993	T50.994	T50.995	T50.996
Clofazimine	T37.1X1	T37.1X2	T37.1X3	T37.1X4	T37.1X5	T37.1X6
Clofedanol	T48.3X1	T48.3X2	T48.3X3	T48.3X4	T48.3X5	T48.3X6

◀ New   ◀||| Revised   ~~deleted~~ Deleted

TABLE OF DRUGS AND CHEMICALS

Substance	External Cause (T-Code)					
	Poisoning, Accidental (Unintentional)	Poisoning, Intentional Self-Harm	Poisoning, Assault	Poisoning, Undetermined	Adverse Effect	Underdosing
Clofenamide	T50.2X1	T50.2X2	T50.2X3	T50.2X4	T50.2X5	T50.2X6
Clofenotane	T49.0X1	T49.0X2	T49.0X3	T49.0X4	T49.0X5	T49.0X6
Clofezone	T39.2X1	T39.2X2	T39.2X3	T39.2X4	T39.2X5	T39.2X6
Clofibrate	T46.6X1	T46.6X2	T46.6X3	T46.6X4	T46.6X5	T46.6X6
Clofibride	T46.6X1	T46.6X2	T46.6X3	T46.6X4	T46.6X5	T46.6X6
Cloforex	T50.5X1	T50.5X2	T50.5X3	T50.5X4	T50.5X5	T50.5X6
Clomacran	T43.0X1	T43.0X2	T43.0X3	T43.0X4	T43.0X5	T43.0X6
Clomethiazole	T42.6X1	T42.6X2	T42.6X3	T42.6X4	T42.6X5	T42.6X6
Clometocillin	T36.0X1	T36.0X2	T36.0X3	T36.0X4	T36.0X5	T36.0X6
Clomifene	T38.5X1	T38.5X2	T38.5X3	T38.5X4	T38.5X5	T38.5X6
Clomiphene	T38.5X1	T38.5X2	T38.5X3	T38.5X4	T38.5X5	T38.5X6
Clomipramine	T43.011	T43.012	T43.013	T43.014	T43.015	T43.016
Clomocycline	T36.4X1	T36.4X2	T36.4X3	T36.4X4	T36.4X5	T36.4X6
Clonazepam	T42.4X1	T42.4X2	T42.4X3	T42.4X4	T42.4X5	T42.4X6
Clonidine	T46.5X1	T46.5X2	T46.5X3	T46.5X4	T46.5X5	T46.5X6
Clonixin	T39.8X1	T39.8X2	T39.8X3	T39.8X4	T39.8X5	T39.8X6
Clopamide	T50.2X1	T50.2X2	T50.2X3	T50.2X4	T50.2X5	T50.2X6
Clopenthixol	T43.4X1	T43.4X2	T43.4X3	T43.4X4	T43.4X5	T43.4X6
Cloperastine	T48.3X1	T48.3X2	T48.3X3	T48.3X4	T48.3X5	T48.3X6
Clophedianol	T48.3X1	T48.3X2	T48.3X3	T48.3X4	T48.3X5	T48.3X6
Cloponone	T36.2X1	T36.2X2	T36.2X3	T36.2X4	T36.2X5	T36.2X6
Cloprednol	T38.0X1	T38.0X2	T38.0X3	T38.0X4	T38.0X5	T38.0X6
Cloral betaine	T42.6X1	T42.6X2	T42.6X3	T42.6X4	T42.6X5	T42.6X6
Cloramfenicol	T36.2X1	T36.2X2	T36.2X3	T36.2X4	T36.2X5	T36.2X6
Clorazepate (dipotassium)	T42.4X1	T42.4X2	T42.4X3	T42.4X4	T42.4X5	T42.4X6
Clorexolone	T50.2X1	T50.2X2	T50.2X3	T50.2X4	T50.2X5	T50.2X6
Clorox (bleach)	T54.91	T54.92	T54.93	T54.94	—	—
Clorfenamine	T45.0X1	T45.0X2	T45.0X3	T45.0X4	T45.0X5	T45.0X6
Clorgiline	T43.1X1	T43.1X2	T43.1X3	T43.1X4	T43.1X5	T43.1X6
Clorotepine	T44.3X1	T44.3X2	T44.3X3	T44.3X4	T44.3X5	T44.3X6
Clorprenaline	T48.6X1	T48.6X2	T48.6X3	T48.6X4	T48.6X5	T48.6X6
Clortermine	T50.5X1	T50.5X2	T50.5X3	T50.5X4	T50.5X5	T50.5X6
Clotiapine	T43.591	T43.592	T43.593	T43.594	T43.595	T43.596
Clotiazepam	T42.4X1	T42.4X2	T42.4X3	T42.4X4	T42.4X5	T42.4X6
Clotibric acid	T46.6X1	T46.6X2	T46.6X3	T46.6X4	T46.6X5	T46.6X6
Clotrimazole	T49.0X1	T49.0X2	T49.0X3	T49.0X4	T49.0X5	T49.0X6
Cloxacillin	T36.0X1	T36.0X2	T36.0X3	T36.0X4	T36.0X5	T36.0X6
Cloxazolam	T42.4X1	T42.4X2	T42.4X3	T42.4X4	T42.4X5	T42.4X6
Cloxiquine	T49.0X1	T49.0X2	T49.0X3	T49.0X4	T49.0X5	T49.0X6
Clozapine	T42.4X1	T42.4X2	T42.4X3	T42.4X4	T42.4X5	T42.4X6

◄ New   ◄ Revised   ~~deleted~~ Deleted

Substance	External Cause (T-Code)					
	Poisoning, Accidental (Unintentional)	Poisoning, Intentional Self-Harm	Poisoning, Assault	Poisoning, Undetermined	Adverse Effect	Underdosing
Coagulant NEC	T45.7X1	T45.7X2	T45.7X3	T45.7X4	T45.7X5	T45.7X6
Coal (carbon monoxide from) — see also Carbon, monoxide, coal	T58.2X1	T58.2X2	T58.2X3	T58.2X4	—	—
oil — see Kerosene						
tar	T49.1X1	T49.1X2	T49.1X3	T49.1X4	T49.1X5	T49.1X6
fumes	T59.891	T59.892	T59.893	T59.894	—	—
medicinal (ointment)	T49.4X1	T49.4X2	T49.4X3	T49.4X4	T49.4X5	T49.4X6
analgesics NEC	T39.2X1	T39.2X2	T39.2X3	T39.2X4	T39.2X5	T39.2X6
naphtha (solvent)	T52.0X1	T52.0X2	T52.0X3	T52.0X4		
Cobalamine	T45.2X1	T45.2X2	T45.2X3	T45.2X4	T45.2X5	T45.2X6
Cobalt (nonmedicinal) (fumes) (industrial)	T56.891	T56.892	T56.893	T56.894		
medicinal (trace) (chloride)	T45.8X1	T45.8X2	T45.8X3	T45.8X4	T45.8X5	T45.8X6
Cobra (venom)	T63.041	T63.042	T63.043	T63.044		
Coca (leaf)	T40.5X1	T40.5X2	T40.5X3	T40.5X4	T40.5X5	T40.5X6
Cocaine	T40.5X1	T40.5X2	T40.5X3	T40.5X4	T40.5X5	T40.5X6
topical anesthetic	T41.3X1	T41.3X2	T41.3X3	T41.3X4	T41.3X5	T41.3X6
Cocarboxylase	T45.3X1	T45.3X2	T45.3X3	T45.3X4	T45.3X5	T45.3X6
Coccidioidin	T50.8X1	T50.8X2	T50.8X3	T50.8X4	T50.8X5	T50.8X6
Cocculus indicus	T62.1X1	T62.1X2	T62.1X3	T62.1X4		
Cochineal	T65.6X1	T65.6X2	T65.6X3	T65.6X4		
medicinal products	T50.991	T50.992	T50.993	T50.994	T50.995	T50.996
Codeine	T40.2X1	T40.2X2	T40.2X3	T40.2X4	T40.2X5	T40.2X6
Cod-liver oil	T45.2X1	T45.2X2	T45.2X3	T45.2X4	T45.2X5	T45.2X6
Coenzyme A	T50.991	T50.992	T50.993	T50.994	T50.995	T50.996
Coffee	T62.8X1	T62.8X2	T62.8X3	T62.8X4	—	—
Cogalactoisomerase	T50.991	T50.992	T50.993	T50.994	T50.995	T50.996
Cogentin	T44.3X1	T44.3X2	T44.3X3	T44.3X4	T44.3X5	T44.3X6
Coke fumes or gas (carbon monoxide)	T58.2X1	T58.2X2	T58.2X3	T58.2X4	—	—
industrial use	T58.8X1	T58.8X2	T58.8X3	T58.8X4	—	—
Colace	T47.4X1	T47.4X2	T47.4X3	T47.4X4	T47.4X5	T47.4X6
Colaspase	T45.1X1	T45.1X2	T45.1X3	T45.1X4	T45.1X5	T45.1X6
Colchicine	T50.4X1	T50.4X2	T50.4X3	T50.4X4	T50.4X5	T50.4X6
Colchicum	T62.2X1	T62.2X2	T62.2X3	T62.2X4	—	—
Cold cream	T49.3X1	T49.3X2	T49.3X3	T49.3X4	T49.3X5	T49.3X6
Colecalciferol	T45.2X1	T45.2X2	T45.2X3	T45.2X4	T45.2X5	T45.2X6
Colestipol	T46.6X1	T46.6X2	T46.6X3	T46.6X4	T46.6X5	T46.6X6
Colestyramine	T46.6X1	T46.6X2	T46.6X3	T46.6X4	T46.6X5	T46.6X6
Colimycin	T36.8X1	T36.8X2	T36.8X3	T36.8X4	T36.8X5	T36.8X6
Colistimethate	T36.8X1	T36.8X2	T36.8X3	T36.8X4	T36.8X5	T36.8X6
Colistin	T36.8X1	T36.8X2	T36.8X3	T36.8X4	T36.8X5	T36.8X6
sulfate (eye preparation)	T49.5X1	T49.5X2	T49.5X3	T49.5X4	T49.5X5	T49.5X6

◀ New   ◀▥ Revised   ~~deleted~~ Deleted

Substance	External Cause (T-Code)					
	Poisoning, Accidental (Unintentional)	Poisoning, Intentional Self-Harm	Poisoning, Assault	Poisoning, Undetermined	Adverse Effect	Underdosing
Collagen	T50.991	T50.992	T50.993	T50.994	T50.995	T50.996
Collagenase	T49.4X1	T49.4X2	T49.4X3	T49.4X4	T49.4X5	T49.4X6
Collodion	T49.3X1	T49.3X2	T49.3X3	T49.3X4	T49.3X5	T49.3X6
Colocynth	T47.2X1	T47.2X2	T47.2X3	T47.2X4	T47.2X5	T47.2X6
Colophony adhesive	T49.3X1	T49.3X2	T49.3X3	T49.3X4	T49.3X5	T49.3X6
Colorant — see also Dye	T50.991	T50.992	T50.993	T50.994	T50.995	T50.996
Coloring matter — see Dye(s)						
Combustion gas (after combustion) — see Carbon, monoxide						
prior to combustion	T59.891	T59.892	T59.893	T59.894	—	—
Compazine	T43.3X1	T43.3X2	T43.3X3	T43.3X4	T43.3X5	T43.3X6
Compound						
42 (warfarin)	T60.4X1	T60.4X2	T60.4X3	T60.4X4	—	—
269 (endrin)	T60.1X1	T60.1X2	T60.1X3	T60.1X4	—	—
497 (dieldrin)	T60.1X1	T60.1X2	T60.1X3	T60.1X4	—	—
1080 (sodium fluoroacetate)	T60.4X1	T60.4X2	T60.4X3	T60.4X4	—	—
3422 (parathion)	T60.0X1	T60.0X2	T60.0X3	T60.0X4	—	—
3911 (phorate)	T60.0X1	T60.0X2	T60.0X3	T60.0X4	—	—
3956 (toxaphene)	T60.1X1	T60.1X2	T60.1X3	T60.1X4	—	—
4049 (malathion)	T60.0X1	T60.0X2	T60.0X3	T60.0X4	—	—
4069 (malathion)	T60.0X1	T60.0X2	T60.0X3	T60.0X4	—	—
4124 (dicapthon)	T60.0X1	T60.0X2	T60.0X3	T60.0X4	—	—
E (cortisone)	T38.0X1	T38.0X2	T38.0X3	T38.0X4	T38.0X5	T38.0X6
F (hydrocortisone)	T38.0X1	T38.0X2	T38.0X3	T38.0X4	T38.0X5	T38.0X6
Congener, anabolic	T38.7X1	T38.7X2	T38.7X3	T38.7X4	T38.7X5	T38.7X6
Congo red	T50.8X1	T50.8X2	T50.8X3	T50.8X4	T50.8X5	T50.8X6
Coniine, conine	T62.2X1	T62.2X2	T62.2X3	T62.2X4	—	—
Conium (maculatum)	T62.2X1	T62.2X2	T62.2X3	T62.2X4	—	—
Conjugated estrogenic substances	T38.5X1	T38.5X2	T38.5X3	T38.5X4	T38.5X5	T38.5X6
Contac	T48.5X1	T48.5X2	T48.5X3	T48.5X4	T48.5X5	T48.5X6
Contact lens solution	T49.5X1	T49.5X2	T49.5X3	T49.5X4	T49.5X5	T49.5X6
Contraceptive (oral)	T38.4X1	T38.4X2	T38.4X3	T38.4X4	T38.4X5	T38.4X6
vaginal	T49.8X1	T49.8X2	T49.8X3	T49.8X4	T49.8X5	T49.8X6
Contrast medium, radiography	T50.8X1	T50.8X2	T50.8X3	T50.8X4	T50.8X5	T50.8X6
Convallaria glycosides	T46.0X1	T46.0X2	T46.0X3	T46.0X4	T46.0X5	T46.0X6
Convallaria majalis	T62.2X1	T62.2X2	T62.2X3	T62.2X4	—	—
berry	T62.1X1	T62.1X2	T62.1X3	T62.1X4	—	—
Copper (dust) (fumes) (nonmedicinal) NEC	T56.4X1	T56.4X2	T56.4X3	T56.4X4	—	—
arsenate, arsenite	T57.0X1	T57.0X2	T57.0X3	T57.0X4	—	—
insecticide	T60.2X1	T60.2X2	T60.2X3	T60.2X4	—	—

◀ New   ◀▥ Revised   ~~deleted~~ Deleted

TABLE OF DRUGS AND CHEMICALS

Substance	External Cause (T-Code)					
	Poisoning, Accidental (Unintentional)	Poisoning, Intentional Self-Harm	Poisoning, Assault	Poisoning, Undetermined	Adverse Effect	Underdosing
Copper NEC *(Continued)*						
emetic	T47.7X1	T47.7X2	T47.7X3	T47.7X4	T47.7X5	T47.7X6
fungicide	T60.3X1	T60.3X2	T60.3X3	T60.3X4	—	—
gluconate	T49.0X1	T49.0X2	T49.0X3	T49.0X4	T49.0X5	T49.0X6
insecticide	T60.2X1	T60.2X2	T60.2X3	T60.2X4	—	—
medicinal (trace)	T45.8X1	T45.8X2	T45.8X3	T45.8X4	T45.8X5	T45.8X6
oleate	T49.0X1	T49.0X2	T49.0X3	T49.0X4	T49.0X5	T49.0X6
sulfate	T56.4X1	T56.4X2	T56.4X3	T56.4X4	—	—
cupric	T56.4X1	T56.4X2	T56.4X3	T56.4X4	—	—
fungicide	T60.3X1	T60.3X2	T60.3X3	T60.3X4	—	—
medicinal						
ear	T49.6X1	T49.6X2	T49.6X3	T49.6X4	T49.6X5	T49.6X6
emetic	T47.7X1	T47.7X2	T47.7X3	T47.7X4	T47.7X5	T47.7X6
eye	T49.5X1	T49.5X2	T49.5X3	T49.5X4	T49.5X5	T49.5X6
cuprous	T56.4X1	T56.4X2	T56.4X3	T56.4X4	—	—
fungicide	T60.3X1	T60.3X2	T60.3X3	T60.3X4	—	—
medicinal						
ear	T49.6X1	T49.6X2	T49.6X3	T49.6X4	T49.6X5	T49.6X6
emetic	T47.7X1	T47.7X2	T47.7X3	T47.7X4	T47.7X5	T47.7X6
eye	T49.5X1	T49.5X2	T49.5X3	T49.5X4	T49.5X5	T49.5X6
Copperhead snake (bite) (venom)	T63.061	T63.062	T63.063	T63.064	—	—
Coral (sting)	T63.691	T63.692	T63.693	T63.694	—	—
snake (bite) (venom)	T63.021	T63.022	T63.023	T63.024	—	—
Corbadrine	T49.6X1	T49.6X2	T49.6X3	T49.6X4	T49.6X5	T49.6X6
Cordran	T49.0X1	T49.0X2	T49.0X3	T49.0X4	T49.0X5	T49.0X6
Cordite	T65.891	T65.892	T65.893	T65.894	—	—
vapor	T59.891	T59.892	T59.893	T59.894	—	—
Corn cures	T49.4X1	T49.4X2	T49.4X3	T49.4X4	T49.4X5	T49.4X6
Cornhusker's lotion	T49.3X1	T49.3X2	T49.3X3	T49.3X4	T49.3X5	T49.3X6
Corn starch	T49.3X1	T49.3X2	T49.3X3	T49.3X4	T49.3X5	T49.3X6
Coronary vasodilator NEC	T46.3X1	T46.3X2	T46.3X3	T46.3X4	T46.3X5	T46.3X6
Corrosive NEC	T54.91	T54.92	T54.93	T54.94	—	—
acid NEC	T54.2X1	T54.2X2	T54.2X3	T54.2X4	—	—
aromatics	T54.1X1	T54.1X2	T54.1X3	T54.1X4	—	—
disinfectant	T54.1X1	T54.1X2	T54.1X3	T54.1X4	—	—
fumes NEC	T54.91	T54.92	T54.93	T54.94	—	—
specified NEC	T54.91	T54.92	T54.93	T54.94	—	—
sublimate	T56.1X1	T56.1X2	T56.1X3	T56.1X4	—	—
Cortate	T38.0X1	T38.0X2	T38.0X3	T38.0X4	T38.0X5	T38.0X6

TABLE OF DRUGS AND CHEMICALS

◀ New   ◀▥ Revised   ~~deleted~~ Deleted

Substance	External Cause (T-Code)					
	Poisoning, Accidental (Unintentional)	Poisoning, Intentional Self-Harm	Poisoning, Assault	Poisoning, Undetermined	Adverse Effect	Underdosing
Cort-Dome	T38.0X1	T38.0X2	T38.0X3	T38.0X4	T38.0X5	T38.0X6
ENT agent	T49.6X1	T49.6X2	T49.6X3	T49.6X4	T49.6X5	T49.6X6
ophthalmic preparation	T49.5X1	T49.5X2	T49.5X3	T49.5X4	T49.5X5	T49.5X6
topical NEC	T49.0X1	T49.0X2	T49.0X3	T49.0X4	T49.0X5	T49.0X6
Cortef	T38.0X1	T38.0X2	T38.0X3	T38.0X4	T38.0X5	T38.0X6
ENT agent	T49.6X1	T49.6X2	T49.6X3	T49.6X4	T49.6X5	T49.6X6
ophthalmic preparation	T49.5X1	T49.5X2	T49.5X3	T49.5X4	T49.5X5	T49.5X6
topical NEC	T49.0X1	T49.0X2	T49.0X3	T49.0X4	T49.0X5	T49.0X6
Corticosteroid	T38.0X1	T38.0X2	T38.0X3	T38.0X4	T38.0X5	T38.0X6
ENT agent	T49.6X1	T49.6X2	T49.6X3	T49.6X4	T49.6X5	T49.6X6
mineral	T50.0X1	T50.0X2	T50.0X3	T50.0X4	T50.0X5	T50.0X6
ophthalmic	T49.5X1	T49.5X2	T49.5X3	T49.5X4	T49.5X5	T49.5X6
topical NEC	T49.0X1	T49.0X2	T49.0X3	T49.0X4	T49.0X5	T49.0X6
Corticotropin	T38.811	T38.812	T38.813	T38.814	T38.815	T38.816
Cortisol	T49.0X1	T49.0X2	T49.0X3	T49.0X4	T49.0X5	T49.0X6
ENT agent	T49.6X1	T49.6X2	T49.6X3	T49.6X4	T49.6X5	T49.6X6
ophthalmic preparation	T49.5X1	T49.5X2	T49.5X3	T49.5X4	T49.5X5	T49.5X6
topical NEC	T49.0X1	T49.0X2	T49.0X3	T49.0X4	T49.0X5	T49.0X6
Cortisone (acetate)	T38.0X1	T38.0X2	T38.0X3	T38.0X4	T38.0X5	T38.0X6
ENT agent	T49.6X1	T49.6X2	T49.6X3	T49.6X4	T49.6X5	T49.6X6
ophthalmic preparation	T49.5X1	T49.5X2	T49.5X3	T49.5X4	T49.5X5	T49.5X6
topical NEC	T49.0X1	T49.0X2	T49.0X3	T49.0X4	T49.0X5	T49.0X6
Cortivazol	T38.0X1	T38.0X2	T38.0X3	T38.0X4	T38.0X5	T38.0X6
Cortogen	T38.0X1	T38.0X2	T38.0X3	T38.0X4	T38.0X5	T38.0X6
ENT agent	T49.6X1	T49.6X2	T49.6X3	T49.6X4	T49.6X5	T49.6X6
ophthalmic preparation	T49.5X1	T49.5X2	T49.5X3	T49.5X4	T49.5X5	T49.5X6
Cortone	T38.0X1	T38.0X2	T38.0X3	T38.0X4	T38.0X5	T38.0X6
ENT agent	T49.6X1	T49.6X2	T49.6X3	T49.6X4	T49.6X5	T49.6X6
ophthalmic preparation	T49.5X1	T49.5X2	T49.5X3	T49.5X4	T49.5X5	T49.5X6
Cortril	T38.0X1	T38.0X2	T38.0X3	T38.0X4	T38.0X5	T38.0X6
ENT agent	T49.6X1	T49.6X2	T49.6X3	T49.6X4	T49.6X5	T49.6X6
ophthalmic preparation	T49.5X1	T49.5X2	T49.5X3	T49.5X4	T49.5X5	T49.5X6
topical NEC	T49.0X1	T49.0X2	T49.0X3	T49.0X4	T49.0X5	T49.0X6
Corynebacterium parvum	T45.1X1	T45.1X2	T45.1X3	T45.1X4	T45.1X5	T45.1X6
Cosmetic preparation	T49.8X1	T49.8X2	T49.8X3	T49.8X4	T49.8X5	T49.8X6
Cosmetics	T49.8X1	T49.8X2	T49.8X3	T49.8X4	T49.8X5	T49.8X6
Cosyntropin	T38.811	T38.812	T38.813	T38.814	T38.815	T38.816
Cotarnine	T45.7X1	T45.7X2	T45.7X3	T45.7X4	T45.7X5	T45.7X6
Co-trimoxazole	T36.8X1	T36.8X2	T36.8X3	T36.8X4	T36.8X5	T36.8X6
Cottonseed oil	T49.3X1	T49.3X2	T49.3X3	T49.3X4	T49.3X5	T49.3X6

◀ New ◀ Revised ~~deleted~~ Deleted

Substance	Poisoning, Accidental (Unintentional)	Poisoning, Intentional Self-Harm	Poisoning, Assault	Poisoning, Undetermined	Adverse Effect	Underdosing
Cough mixture (syrup)	T48.4X1	T48.4X2	T48.4X3	T48.4X4	T48.4X5	T48.4X6
containing opiates	T40.2X1	T40.2X2	T40.2X3	T40.2X4	T40.2X5	T40.2X6
expectorants	T48.4X1	T48.4X2	T48.4X3	T48.4X4	T48.4X5	T48.4X6
Coumadin	T45.511	T45.512	T45.513	T45.514	T45.515	T45.516
rodenticide	T60.4X1	T60.4X2	T60.4X3	T60.4X4	—	—
Coumaphos	T60.0X1	T60.0X2	T60.0X3	T60.0X4	—	—
Coumarin	T45.511	T45.512	T45.513	T45.514	T45.515	T45.516
Coumetarol	T45.511	T45.512	T45.513	T45.514	T45.515	T45.516
Cowbane	T62.2X1	T62.2X2	T62.2X3	T62.2X4	—	—
Cozyme	T45.2X1	T45.2X2	T45.2X3	T45.2X4	T45.2X5	T45.2X6
Crack	T40.5X1	T40.5X2	T40.5X3	T40.5X4	—	—
Crataegus extract	T46.0X1	T46.0X2	T46.0X3	T46.0X4	T46.0X5	T46.0X6
Creolin	T54.1X1	T54.1X2	T54.1X3	T54.1X4	—	—
disinfectant	T54.1X1	T54.1X2	T54.1X3	T54.1X4	—	—
Creosol (compound)	T49.0X1	T49.0X2	T49.0X3	T49.0X4	T49.0X5	T49.0X6
Creosote (coal tar) (beechwood)	T49.0X1	T49.0X2	T49.0X3	T49.0X4	T49.0X5	T49.0X6
medicinal (expectorant)	T48.4X1	T48.4X2	T48.4X3	T48.4X4	T48.4X5	T48.4X6
syrup	T48.4X1	T48.4X2	T48.4X3	T48.4X4	T48.4X5	T48.4X6
Cresol(s)	T49.0X1	T49.0X2	T49.0X3	T49.0X4	T49.0X5	T49.0X6
and soap solution	T49.0X1	T49.0X2	T49.0X3	T49.0X4	T49.0X5	T49.0X6
Cresyl acetate	T49.0X1	T49.0X2	T49.0X3	T49.0X4	T49.0X5	T49.0X6
Cresylic acid	T49.0X1	T49.0X2	T49.0X3	T49.0X4	T49.0X5	T49.0X6
Crimidine	T60.4X1	T60.4X2	T60.4X3	T60.4X4	—	—
Croconazole	T37.8X1	T37.8X2	T37.8X3	T37.8X4	T37.8X5	T37.8X6
Cromoglicic acid	T48.6X1	T48.6X2	T48.6X3	T48.6X4	T48.6X5	T48.6X6
Cromolyn	T48.6X1	T48.6X2	T48.6X3	T48.6X4	T48.6X5	T48.6X6
Cromonar	T46.3X1	T46.3X2	T46.3X3	T46.3X4	T46.3X5	T46.3X6
Cropropamide	T39.8X1	T39.8X2	T39.8X3	T39.8X4	T39.8X5	T39.8X6
with crotethamide	T50.7X1	T50.7X2	T50.7X3	T50.7X4	T50.7X5	T50.7X6
Crotamiton	T49.0X1	T49.0X2	T49.0X3	T49.0X4	T49.0X5	T49.0X6
Crotethamide	T39.8X1	T39.8X2	T39.8X3	T39.8X4	T39.8X5	T39.8X6
with cropropamide	T50.7X1	T50.7X2	T50.7X3	T50.7X4	T50.7X5	T50.7X6
Croton (oil)	T47.2X1	T47.2X2	T47.2X3	T47.2X4	T47.2X5	T47.2X6
chloral	T42.6X1	T42.6X2	T42.6X3	T42.6X4	T42.6X5	T42.6X6
Crude oil	T52.0X1	T52.0X2	T52.0X3	T52.0X4	—	—
Cryogenine	T39.8X1	T39.8X2	T39.8X3	T39.8X4	T39.8X5	T39.8X6
Cryolite (vapor)	T60.1X1	T60.1X2	T60.1X3	T60.1X4	—	—
insecticide	T60.1X1	T60.1X2	T60.1X3	T60.1X4	—	—
Cryptenamine (tannates)	T46.5X1	T46.5X2	T46.5X3	T46.5X4	T46.5X5	T46.5X6
Crystal violet	T49.0X1	T49.0X2	T49.0X3	T49.0X4	T49.0X5	T49.0X6

TABLE OF DRUGS AND CHEMICALS

TABLE OF DRUGS AND CHEMICALS

Substance	External Cause (T-Code)					
	Poisoning, Accidental (Unintentional)	Poisoning, Intentional Self-Harm	Poisoning, Assault	Poisoning, Undetermined	Adverse Effect	Underdosing
Cuckoopint	T62.2X1	T62.2X2	T62.2X3	T62.2X4	—	—
Cumetharol	T45.511	T45.512	T45.513	T45.514	T45.515	T45.516
Cupric						
acetate	T60.3X1	T60.3X2	T60.3X3	T60.3X4	—	—
acetoarsenite	T57.0X1	T57.0X2	T57.0X3	T57.0X4	—	—
arsenate	T57.0X1	T57.0X2	T57.0X3	T57.0X4	—	—
gluconate	T49.0X1	T49.0X2	T49.0X3	T49.0X4	T49.0X5	T49.0X6
oleate	T49.0X1	T49.0X2	T49.0X3	T49.0X4	T49.0X5	T49.0X6
sulfate	T56.4X1	T56.4X2	T56.4X3	T56.4X4	—	—
Cuprous sulfate—see also Copper sulfate	T56.4X1	T56.4X2	T56.4X3	T56.4X4	—	—
Curare, curarine	T48.1X1	T48.1X2	T48.1X3	T48.1X4	T48.1X5	T48.1X6
Cyamemazine	T43.3X1	T43.3X2	T43.3X3	T43.3X4	T43.3X5	T43.3X6
Cyamopsis tetragono-loba	T46.6X1	T46.6X2	T46.6X3	T46.6X4	T46.6X5	T46.6X6
Cyanacetyl hydrazide	T37.1X1	T37.1X2	T37.1X3	T37.1X4	T37.1X5	T37.1X6
Cyanic acid (gas)	T59.891	T59.892	T59.893	T59.894	—	—
Cyanide(s) (compounds) (potassium) (sodium) NEC	T65.0X1	T65.0X2	T65.0X3	T65.0X4	—	—
dust or gas (inhalation) NEC	T57.3X1	T57.3X2	T57.3X3	T57.3X4	—	—
fumigant	T65.0X1	T65.0X2	T65.0X3	T65.0X4	—	—
hydrogen	T57.3X1	T57.3X2	T57.3X3	T57.3X4	—	—
mercuric—see Mercury						
pesticide (dust) (fumes)	T65.0X1	T65.0X2	T65.0X3	T65.0X4	—	—
Cyanoacrylate adhesive	T49.3X1	T49.3X2	T49.3X3	T49.3X4	T49.3X5	T49.3X6
Cyanocobalamin	T45.8X1	T45.8X2	T45.8X3	T45.8X4	T45.8X5	T45.8X6
Cyanogen (chloride) (gas) NEC	T59.891	T59.892	T59.893	T59.894	—	—
Cyclacillin	T36.0X1	T36.0X2	T36.0X3	T36.0X4	T36.0X5	T36.0X6
Cyclaine	T41.3X1	T41.3X2	T41.3X3	T41.3X4	T41.3X5	T41.3X6
Cyclamate	T50.991	T50.992	T50.993	T50.994	T50.995	T50.996
Cyclamen europaeum	T62.2X1	T62.2X2	T62.2X3	T62.2X4	—	—
Cyclandelate	T46.7X1	T46.7X2	T46.7X3	T46.7X4	T46.7X5	T46.7X6
Cyclazocine	T50.7X1	T50.7X2	T50.7X3	T50.7X4	T50.7X5	T50.7X6
Cyclizine	T45.0X1	T45.0X2	T45.0X3	T45.0X4	T45.0X5	T45.0X6
Cyclobarbital	T42.3X1	T42.3X2	T42.3X3	T42.3X4	T42.3X5	T42.3X6
Cyclobarbitone	T42.3X1	T42.3X2	T42.3X3	T42.3X4	T42.3X5	T42.3X6
Cyclobenzaprine	T48.1X1	T48.1X2	T48.1X3	T48.1X4	T48.1X5	T48.1X6
Cyclodrine	T44.3X1	T44.3X2	T44.3X3	T44.3X4	T44.3X5	T44.3X6
Cycloguanil embonate	T37.2X1	T37.2X2	T37.2X3	T37.2X4	T37.2X5	T37.2X6
Cycloheptadiene	T43.291	T43.292	T43.293	T43.294	T43.295	T43.296
Cyclohexane	T52.8X1	T52.8X2	T52.8X3	T52.8X4	—	—
Cyclohexanol	T51.8X1	T51.8X2	T51.8X3	T51.8X4	—	—
Cyclohexanone	T52.4X1	T52.4X2	T52.4X3	T52.4X4	—	—

◀ New   ◀ Revised   ~~deleted~~ Deleted

Substance	Poisoning, Accidental (Unintentional)	Poisoning, Intentional Self-Harm	Poisoning, Assault	Poisoning, Undetermined	Adverse Effect	Underdosing
Cycloheximide	T60.3X1	T60.3X2	T60.3X3	T60.3X4	—	—
Cyclohexyl acetate	T52.8X1	T52.8X2	T52.8X3	T52.8X4	—	—
Cycloleucin	T45.1X1	T45.1X2	T45.1X3	T45.1X4	T45.1X5	T45.1X6
Cyclomethycaine	T41.3X1	T41.3X2	T41.3X3	T41.3X4	T41.3X5	T41.3X6
Cyclopentamine	T44.4X1	T44.4X2	T44.4X3	T44.4X4	T44.4X5	T44.4X6
Cyclopenthiazide	T50.2X1	T50.2X2	T50.2X3	T50.2X4	T50.2X5	T50.2X6
Cyclopentolate	T44.3X1	T44.3X2	T44.3X3	T44.3X4	T44.3X5	T44.3X6
Cyclophosphamide	T45.1X1	T45.1X2	T45.1X3	T45.1X4	T45.1X5	T45.1X6
Cycloplegic drug	T49.5X1	T49.5X2	T49.5X3	T49.5X4	T49.5X5	T49.5X6
Cyclopropane	T41.291	T41.292	T41.293	T41.294	T41.295	T41.296
Cyclopyrabital	T39.8X1	T39.8X2	T39.8X3	T39.8X4	T39.8X5	T39.8X6
Cycloserine	T37.1X1	T37.1X2	T37.1X3	T37.1X4	T37.1X5	T37.1X6
Cyclosporin	T45.1X1	T45.1X2	T45.1X3	T45.1X4	T45.1X5	T45.1X6
Cyclothiazide	T50.2X1	T50.2X2	T50.2X3	T50.2X4	T50.2X5	T50.2X6
Cycrimine	T44.3X1	T44.3X2	T44.3X3	T44.3X4	T44.3X5	T44.3X6
Cyhalothrin	T60.1X1	T60.1X2	T60.1X3	T60.1X4	—	—
Cymarin	T46.0X1	T46.0X2	T46.0X3	T46.0X4	T46.0X5	T46.0X6
Cypermethrin	T60.1X1	T60.1X2	T60.1X3	T60.1X4	—	—
Cyphenothrin	T60.2X1	T60.2X2	T60.2X3	T60.2X4	—	—
Cyproheptadine	T45.0X1	T45.0X2	T45.0X3	T45.0X4	T45.0X5	T45.0X6
Cyprolidol	T43.291	T43.292	T43.293	T43.294	T43.295	T43.296
Cyproterone	T38.6X1	T38.6X2	T38.6X3	T38.6X4	T38.6X5	T38.6X6
Cysteamine	T50.6X1	T50.6X2	T50.6X3	T50.6X4	T50.6X5	T50.6X6
Cytarabine	T45.1X1	T45.1X2	T45.1X3	T45.1X4	T45.1X5	T45.1X6
Cytisus						
laburnum	T62.2X1	T62.2X2	T62.2X3	T62.2X4	—	—
scoparius	T62.2X1	T62.2X2	T62.2X3	T62.2X4	—	—
Cytochrome C	T47.5X1	T47.5X2	T47.5X3	T47.5X4	T47.5X5	T47.5X6
Cytomel	T38.1X1	T38.1X2	T38.1X3	T38.1X4	T38.1X5	T38.1X6
Cytosine arabinoside	T45.1X1	T45.1X2	T45.1X3	T45.1X4	T45.1X5	T45.1X6
Cytoxan	T45.1X1	T45.1X2	T45.1X3	T45.1X4	T45.1X5	T45.1X6
Cytozyme	T45.7X1	T45.7X2	T45.7X3	T45.7X4	T45.7X5	T45.7X6
2,4-D	T60.3X1	T60.3X2	T60.3X3	T60.3X4	—	—
D						
Dacarbazine	T45.1X1	T45.1X2	T45.1X3	T45.1X4	T45.1X5	T45.1X6
Dactinomycin	T45.1X1	T45.1X2	T45.1X3	T45.1X4	T45.1X5	T45.1X6
DADPS	T37.1X1	T37.1X2	T37.1X3	T37.1X4	T37.1X5	T37.1X6
Dakin's solution	T49.0X1	T49.0X2	T49.0X3	T49.0X4	T49.0X5	T49.0X6
Dalapon (sodium)	T60.3X1	T60.3X2	T60.3X3	T60.3X4	—	—

◀ New   ◀▮▮▮ Revised   ~~deleted~~ Deleted

TABLE OF DRUGS AND CHEMICALS

TABLE OF DRUGS AND CHEMICALS

Substance	External Cause (T-Code)					
	Poisoning, Accidental (Unintentional)	Poisoning, Intentional Self-Harm	Poisoning, Assault	Poisoning, Undetermined	Adverse Effect	Underdosing
Dalmane	T42.4X1	T42.4X2	T42.4X3	T42.4X4	T42.4X5	T42.4X6
Danazol	T38.6X1	T38.6X2	T38.6X3	T38.6X4	T38.6X5	T38.6X6
Danilone	T45.511	T45.512	T45.513	T45.514	T45.515	T45.516
Danthron	T47.2X1	T47.2X2	T47.2X3	T47.2X4	T47.2X5	T47.2X6
Dantrolene	T42.8X1	T42.8X2	T42.8X3	T42.8X4	T42.8X5	T42.8X6
Dantron	T47.2X1	T47.2X2	T47.2X3	T47.2X4	T47.2X5	T47.2X6
Daphne (gnidium) (mezereum)	T62.2X1	T62.2X2	T62.2X3	T62.2X4	—	—
berry	T62.1X1	T62.1X2	T62.1X3	T62.1X4	—	—
Dapsone	T37.1X1	T37.1X2	T37.1X3	T37.1X4	T37.1X5	T37.1X6
Daraprim	T37.2X1	T37.2X2	T37.2X3	T37.2X4	T37.2X5	T37.2X6
Darnel	T62.2X1	T62.2X2	T62.2X3	T62.2X4	—	—
Darvon	T39.8X1	T39.8X2	T39.8X3	T39.8X4	T39.8X5	T39.8X6
Daunomycin	T45.1X1	T45.1X2	T45.1X3	T45.1X4	T45.1X5	T45.1X6
Daunorubicin	T45.1X1	T45.1X2	T45.1X3	T45.1X4	T45.1X5	T45.1X6
DBI	T38.3X1	T38.3X2	T38.3X3	T38.3X4	T38.3X5	T38.3X6
D-Con	T60.91	T60.92	T60.93	T60.94	—	—
insecticide	T60.2X1	T60.2X2	T60.2X3	T60.2X4	—	—
rodenticide	T60.4X1	T60.4X2	T60.4X3	T60.4X4	—	—
DDAVP	T38.891	T38.892	T38.893	T38.894	T38.895	T38.896
DDE (bis(chlorophenyl)-dichloroethylene)	T60.2X1	T60.2X2	T60.2X3	T60.2X4	—	—
DDS	T37.1X1	T37.1X2	T37.1X3	T37.1X4	T37.1X5	T37.1X6
DDT (dust)	T60.1X1	T60.1X2	T60.1X3	T60.1X4	—	—
Deadly nightshade — *see also Belladonna*	T62.2X1	T62.2X2	T62.2X3	T62.2X4	—	—
berry	T62.1X1	T62.1X2	T62.1X3	T62.1X4	—	—
Deamino-D-arginine vasopressin	T38.891	T38.892	T38.893	T38.894	T38.895	T38.896
Deanol (aceglumate)	T50.991	T50.992	T50.993	T50.994	T50.995	T50.996
Debrisoquine	T46.5X1	T46.5X2	T46.5X3	T46.5X4	T46.5X5	T46.5X6
Decaborane	T57.8X1	T57.8X2	T57.8X3	T57.8X4	—	—
fumes	T59.891	T59.892	T59.893	T59.894	—	—
Decadron	T38.0X1	T38.0X2	T38.0X3	T38.0X4	T38.0X5	T38.0X6
ENT agent	T49.6X1	T49.6X2	T49.6X3	T49.6X4	T49.6X5	T49.6X6
ophthalmic preparation	T49.5X1	T49.5X2	T49.5X3	T49.5X4	T49.5X5	T49.5X6
topical NEC	T49.0X1	T49.0X2	T49.0X3	T49.0X4	T49.0X5	T49.0X6
Decahydronaphthalene	T52.8X1	T52.8X2	T52.8X3	T52.8X4	—	—
Decalin	T52.8X1	T52.8X2	T52.8X3	T52.8X4	—	—
Decamethonium (bromide)	T48.1X1	T48.1X2	T48.1X3	T48.1X4	T48.1X5	T48.1X6
Decholin	T47.5X1	T47.5X2	T47.5X3	T47.5X4	T47.5X5	T47.5X6
Declomycin	T36.4X1	T36.4X2	T36.4X3	T36.4X4	T36.4X5	T36.4X6
Decongestant, nasal (mucosa)	T48.5X1	T48.5X2	T48.5X3	T48.5X4	T48.5X5	T48.5X6
combination	T48.5X1	T48.5X2	T48.5X3	T48.5X4	T48.5X5	T48.5X6

◀ New ◀▥ Revised ~~deleted~~ Deleted

Substance	External Cause (T-Code)					
	Poisoning, Accidental (Unintentional)	Poisoning, Intentional Self-Harm	Poisoning, Assault	Poisoning, Undetermined	Adverse Effect	Underdosing
Deet	T60.8X1	T60.8X2	T60.8X3	T60.8X4	—	—
Deferoxamine	T45.8X1	T45.8X2	T45.8X3	T45.8X4	T45.8X5	T45.8X6
Deflazacort	T38.0X1	T38.0X2	T38.0X3	T38.0X4	T38.0X5	T38.0X6
Deglycyrrhizinized extract of licorice	T48.4X1	T48.4X2	T48.4X3	T48.4X4	T48.4X5	T48.4X6
Dehydrocholic acid	T47.5X1	T47.5X2	T47.5X3	T47.5X4	T47.5X5	T47.5X6
Dehydroemetine	T37.3X1	T37.3X2	T37.3X3	T37.3X4	T37.3X5	T37.3X6
Dekalin	T52.8X1	T52.8X2	T52.8X3	T52.8X4	—	—
Delalutin	T38.5X1	T38.5X2	T38.5X3	T38.5X4	T38.5X5	T38.5X6
Delphinium	T62.2X1	T62.2X2	T62.2X3	T62.2X4	—	—
Deltasone	T38.0X1	T38.0X2	T38.0X3	T38.0X4	T38.0X5	T38.0X6
Deltra	T38.0X1	T38.0X2	T38.0X3	T38.0X4	T38.0X5	T38.0X6
Delvinal	T42.3X1	T42.3X2	T42.3X3	T42.3X4	T42.3X5	T42.3X6
Delorazepam	T42.4X1	T42.4X2	T42.4X3	T42.4X4	T42.4X5	T42.4X6
Deltamethrin	T60.1X1	T60.1X2	T60.1X3	T60.1X4	—	—
Demecarium (bromide)	T49.5X1	T49.5X2	T49.5X3	T49.5X4	T49.5X5	T49.5X6
Demeclocycline	T36.4X1	T36.4X2	T36.4X3	T36.4X4	T36.4X5	T36.4X6
Demecolcine	T45.1X1	T45.1X2	T45.1X3	T45.1X4	T45.1X5	T45.1X6
Demegestone	T38.5X1	T38.5X2	T38.5X3	T38.5X4	T38.5X5	T38.5X6
Demelanizing agents	T49.8X1	T49.8X2	T49.8X3	T49.8X4	T49.8X5	T49.8X6
Demephion -0 and -S	T60.0X1	T60.0X2	T60.0X3	T60.0X4	—	—
Demerol	T40.2X1	T40.2X2	T40.2X3	T40.2X4	T40.2X5	T40.2X6
Demethylchlortetracycline	T36.4X1	T36.4X2	T36.4X3	T36.4X4	T36.4X5	T36.4X6
Demethyltetracycline	T36.4X1	T36.4X2	T36.4X3	T36.4X4	T36.4X5	T36.4X6
Demeton -0 and -S	T60.0X1	T60.0X2	T60.0X3	T60.0X4	—	—
Demulcent (external)	T49.3X1	T49.3X2	T49.3X3	T49.3X4	T49.3X5	T49.3X6
specified NEC	T49.3X1	T49.3X2	T49.3X3	T49.3X4	T49.3X5	T49.3X6
Demulen	T38.4X1	T38.4X2	T38.4X3	T38.4X4	T38.4X5	T38.4X6
Denatured alcohol	T51.0X1	T51.0X2	T51.0X3	T51.0X4	—	—
Dendrid	T49.5X1	T49.5X2	T49.5X3	T49.5X4	T49.5X5	T49.5X6
Dental drug, topical application NEC	T49.7X1	T49.7X2	T49.7X3	T49.7X4	T49.7X5	T49.7X6
Dentifrice	T49.7X1	T49.7X2	T49.7X3	T49.7X4	T49.7X5	T49.7X6
Deodorant spray (feminine hygiene)	T49.8X1	T49.8X2	T49.8X3	T49.8X4	T49.8X5	T49.8X6
Deoxycortone	T50.0X1	T50.0X2	T50.0X3	T50.0X4	T50.0X5	T50.0X6
2-Deoxy-5-fluorouridine	T45.1X1	T45.1X2	T45.1X3	T45.1X4	T45.1X5	T45.1X6
5-Deoxy-5-fluorouridine	T45.1X1	T45.1X2	T45.1X3	T45.1X4	T45.1X5	T45.1X6
Deoxyribonuclease (pancreatic)	T45.3X1	T45.3X2	T45.3X3	T45.3X4	T45.3X5	T45.3X6
Depilatory	T49.4X1	T49.4X2	T49.4X3	T49.4X4	T49.4X5	T49.4X6
Deprenalin	T42.8X1	T42.8X2	T42.8X3	T42.8X4	T42.8X5	T42.8X6
Deprenyl	T42.8X1	T42.8X2	T42.8X3	T42.8X4	T42.8X5	T42.8X6

◀ New ◀|||| Revised ~~deleted~~ Deleted

Substance	External Cause (T-Code)					
	Poisoning, Accidental (Unintentional)	Poisoning, Intentional Self-Harm	Poisoning, Assault	Poisoning, Undetermined	Adverse Effect	Underdosing
Depressant, appetite	T50.5X1	T50.5X2	T50.5X3	T50.5X4	T50.5X5	T50.5X6
Depressant						
appetite, central	T50.5X1	T50.5X2	T50.5X3	T50.5X4	T50.5X5	T50.5X6
cardiac	T46.2X1	T46.2X2	T46.2X3	T46.2X4	T46.2X5	T46.2X6
central nervous system (anesthetic) — see also Central nervous system, depressants	T42.71	T42.72	T42.73	T42.74	T42.75	T42.76
general anesthetic	T41.201	T41.202	T41.203	T41.204	T41.205	T41.206
muscle tone	T42.8X1	T42.8X2	T42.8X3	T42.8X4	T42.8X5	T42.8X6
muscle tone, central	T42.8X1	T42.8X2	T42.8X3	T42.8X4	T42.8X5	T42.8X6
psychotherapeutic	T43.501	T43.502	T43.503	T43.504	T43.505	T43.506
Deptropine	T45.0X1	T45.0X2	T45.0X3	T45.0X4	T45.0X5	T45.0X6
Dequalinium (chloride)	T49.0X1	T49.0X2	T49.0X3	T49.0X4	T49.0X5	T49.0X6
Derris root	T60.2X1	T60.2X2	T60.2X3	T60.2X4	—	—
Deserpidine	T43.011	T43.012	T43.013	T43.014	T43.015	T43.016
Desferrioxamine	T45.8X1	T45.8X2	T45.8X3	T45.8X4	T45.8X5	T45.8X6
Desipramine	T43.0X1	T43.0X2	T43.0X3	T43.0X4	T43.0X5	T43.0X6
Deslanoside	T46.0X1	T46.0X2	T46.0X3	T46.0X4	T46.0X5	T46.0X6
Desloughing agent	T49.4X1	T49.4X2	T49.4X3	T49.4X4	T49.4X5	T49.4X6
Desmethylimipramine	T43.011	T43.012	T43.013	T43.014	T43.015	T43.016
Desmopressin	T38.891	T38.892	T38.893	T38.894	T38.895	T38.896
Desocodeine	T40.2X1	T40.2X2	T40.2X3	T40.2X4	T40.2X5	T40.2X6
Desogestrel	T38.5X1	T38.5X2	T38.5X3	T38.5X4	T38.5X5	T38.5X6
Desomorphine	T40.2X1	T40.2X2	T40.2X3	T40.2X4	—	—
Desonide	T49.0X1	T49.0X2	T49.0X3	T49.0X4	T49.0X5	T49.0X6
Desoximetasone	T49.0X1	T49.0X2	T49.0X3	T49.0X4	T49.0X5	T49.0X6
Desoxycorticosteroid	T50.0X1	T50.0X2	T50.0X3	T50.0X4	T50.0X5	T50.0X6
Desoxycortone	T50.0X1	T50.0X2	T50.0X3	T50.0X4	T50.0X5	T50.0X6
Desoxyephedrine	T43.621	T43.622	T43.623	T43.624	T43.625	T43.626
Detaxtran	T46.6X1	T46.6X2	T46.6X3	T46.6X4	T46.6X5	T46.6X6
Detergent	T49.2X1	T49.2X2	T49.2X3	T49.2X4	T49.2X5	T49.2X6
external medication	T49.2X1	T49.2X2	T49.2X3	T49.2X4	T49.2X5	T49.2X6
local	T49.2X1	T49.2X2	T49.2X3	T49.2X4	T49.2X5	T49.2X6
medicinal	T49.2X1	T49.2X2	T49.2X3	T49.2X4	T49.2X5	T49.2X6
nonmedicinal	T55.1X1	T55.1X2	T55.1X3	T55.1X4	—	—
specified NEC	T55.1X1	T55.1X2	T55.1X3	T55.1X4	T55.1X5	T55.1X6
Deterrent, alcohol	T50.6X1	T50.6X2	T50.6X3	T50.6X4	T50.6X5	T50.6X6
Detoxifying agent	T50.6X1	T50.6X2	T50.6X3	T50.6X4	T50.6X5	T50.6X6
Detrothyronine	T38.1X1	T38.1X2	T38.1X3	T38.1X4	T38.1X5	T38.1X6
Dettol (external medication)	T49.0X1	T49.0X2	T49.0X3	T49.0X4	T49.0X5	T49.0X6

◀ New   ◀ Revised   ~~deleted~~ Deleted

TABLE OF DRUGS AND CHEMICALS

Substance	External Cause (T-Code)					
	Poisoning, Accidental (Unintentional)	Poisoning, Intentional Self-Harm	Poisoning, Assault	Poisoning, Undetermined	Adverse Effect	Underdosing
Dexamethasone	T38.0X1	T38.0X2	T38.0X3	T38.0X4	T38.0X5	T38.0X6
ENT agent	T49.6X1	T49.6X2	T49.6X3	T49.6X4	T49.6X5	T49.6X6
ophthalmic preparation	T49.5X1	T49.5X2	T49.5X3	T49.5X4	T49.5X5	T49.5X6
topical NEC	T49.0X1	T49.0X2	T49.0X3	T49.0X4	T49.0X5	T49.0X6
Dexamfetamine	T43.621	T43.622	T43.623	T43.624	T43.625	T43.626
Dexamphetamine	T43.621	T43.622	T43.623	T43.624	T43.625	T43.626
Dexbrompheniramine	T45.0X1	T45.0X2	T45.0X3	T45.0X4	T45.0X5	T45.0X6
Dexchlorpheniramine	T45.0X1	T45.0X2	T45.0X3	T45.0X4	T45.0X5	T45.0X6
Dexedrine	T43.621	T43.622	T43.623	T43.624	T43.625	T43.626
Dexetimide	T44.3X1	T44.3X2	T44.3X3	T44.3X4	T44.3X5	T44.3X6
Dexfenfluramine	T50.5X1	T50.5X2	T50.5X3	T50.5X4	T50.5X5	T50.5X6
Dexpanthenol	T45.2X1	T45.2X2	T45.2X3	T45.2X4	T45.2X5	T45.2X6
Dextran (40) (70) (150)	T45.8X1	T45.8X2	T45.8X3	T45.8X4	T45.8X5	T45.8X6
Dextriferron	T45.4X1	T45.4X2	T45.4X3	T45.4X4	T45.4X5	T45.4X6
Dextroamphetamine	T43.621	T43.622	T43.623	T43.624	T43.625	T43.626
Dextro calcium pantothenate	T45.2X1	T45.2X2	T45.2X3	T45.2X4	T45.2X5	T45.2X6
Dextromethorphan	T48.3X1	T48.3X2	T48.3X3	T48.3X4	T48.3X5	T48.3X6
Dextromoramide	T40.4X1	T40.4X2	T40.4X3	T40.4X4	—	—
topical	T49.8X1	T49.8X2	T49.8X3	T49.8X4	T49.8X5	T49.8X6
Dextro pantothenyl alcohol	T45.2X1	T45.2X2	T45.2X3	T45.2X4	T45.2X5	T45.2X6
Dextropropoxyphene	T40.4X1	T40.4X2	T40.4X3	T40.4X4	T40.4X5	T40.4X6
Dextrorphan	T40.2X1	T40.2X2	T40.2X3	T40.2X4	T40.2X5	T40.2X6
Dextrose	T50.3X1	T50.3X2	T50.3X3	T50.3X4	T50.3X5	T50.3X6
concentrated solution, intravenous	T46.8X1	T46.8X2	T46.8X3	T46.8X4	T46.8X5	T46.8X6
Dextrothyroxin	T38.1X1	T38.1X2	T38.1X3	T38.1X4	T38.1X5	T38.1X6
Dextrothyroxine sodium	T38.1X1	T38.1X2	T38.1X3	T38.1X4	T38.1X5	T38.1X6
DFP	T44.0X1	T44.0X2	T44.0X3	T44.0X4	T44.0X5	T44.0X6
DHE	T37.3X1	T37.3X2	T37.3X3	T37.3X4	T37.3X5	T37.3X6
45	T46.5X1	T46.5X2	T46.5X3	T46.5X4	T46.5X5	T46.5X6
Diabinese	T38.3X1	T38.3X2	T38.3X3	T38.3X4	T38.3X5	T38.3X6
Diacetone alcohol	T52.4X1	T52.4X2	T52.4X3	T52.4X4	—	—
Diacetyl monoxime	T50.991	T50.992	T50.993	T50.994	—	—
Diacetylmorphine	T40.1X1	T40.1X2	T40.1X3	T40.1X4	—	—
Diachylon plaster	T49.4X1	T49.4X2	T49.4X3	T49.4X4	T49.4X5	T49.4X6
Diaethylstilboestrolum	T38.5X1	T38.5X2	T38.5X3	T38.5X4	T38.5X5	T38.5X6
Diagnostic agent NEC	T50.8X1	T50.8X2	T50.8X3	T50.8X4	T50.8X5	T50.8X6
Dial (soap)	T49.2X1	T49.2X2	T49.2X3	T49.2X4	T49.2X5	T49.2X6
sedative	T42.3X1	T42.3X2	T42.3X3	T42.3X4	T42.3X5	T42.3X6
Dialkyl carbonate	T52.91	T52.92	T52.93	T52.94	—	—

◀ New   ◀ Revised   deleted Deleted

TABLE OF DRUGS AND CHEMICALS

TABLE OF DRUGS AND CHEMICALS

Substance	External Cause (T-Code)					
	Poisoning, Accidental (Unintentional)	Poisoning, Intentional Self-Harm	Poisoning, Assault	Poisoning, Undetermined	Adverse Effect	Underdosing
Diallylbarbituric acid	T42.3X1	T42.3X2	T42.3X3	T42.3X4	T42.3X5	T42.3X6
Diallymal	T42.3X1	T42.3X2	T42.3X3	T42.3X4	T42.3X5	T42.3X6
Dialysis solution (intraperitoneal)	T50.3X1	T50.3X2	T50.3X3	T50.3X4	T50.3X5	T50.3X6
Diaminodiphenylsulfone	T37.1X1	T37.1X2	T37.1X3	T37.1X4	T37.1X5	T37.1X6
Diamorphine	T40.1X1	T40.1X2	T40.1X3	T40.1X4	—	—
Diamox	T50.2X1	T50.2X2	T50.2X3	T50.2X4	T50.2X5	T50.2X6
Diamthazole	T49.0X1	T49.0X2	T49.0X3	T49.0X4	T49.0X5	T49.0X6
Dianthone	T47.2X1	T47.2X2	T47.2X3	T47.2X4	T47.2X5	T47.2X6
Diaphenylsulfone	T37.0X1	T37.0X2	T37.0X3	T37.0X4	T37.0X5	T37.0X6
Diasone (sodium)	T37.1X1	T37.1X2	T37.1X3	T37.1X4	T37.1X5	T37.1X6
Diastase	T47.5X1	T47.5X2	T47.5X3	T47.5X4	T47.5X5	T47.5X6
Diatrizoate	T50.8X1	T50.8X2	T50.8X3	T50.8X4	T50.8X5	T50.8X6
Diazepam	T42.4X1	T42.4X2	T42.4X3	T42.4X4	T42.4X5	T42.4X6
Diazinon	T60.0X1	T60.0X2	T60.0X3	T60.0X4	—	—
Diazomethane (gas)	T59.891	T59.892	T59.893	T59.894	—	—
Diazoxide	T46.5X1	T46.5X2	T46.5X3	T46.5X4	T46.5X5	T46.5X6
Dibekacin	T36.5X1	T36.5X2	T36.5X3	T36.5X4	T36.5X5	T36.5X6
Dibenamine	T44.6X1	T44.6X2	T44.6X3	T44.6X4	T44.6X5	T44.6X6
Dibenzepin	T43.011	T43.012	T43.013	T43.014	T43.015	T43.016
Dibenzheptropine	T45.0X1	T45.0X2	T45.0X3	T45.0X4	T45.0X5	T45.0X6
Dibenzyline	T44.6X1	T44.6X2	T44.6X3	T44.6X4	T44.6X5	T44.6X6
Diborane (gas)	T59.891	T59.892	T59.893	T59.894	—	—
Dibromochloropropane	T60.8X1	T60.8X2	T60.8X3	T60.8X4	—	—
Dibromodulcitol	T45.1X1	T45.1X2	T45.1X3	T45.1X4	T45.1X5	T45.1X6
Dibromoethane	T53.6X1	T53.6X2	T53.6X3	T53.6X4	—	—
Dibromomannitol	T45.1X1	T45.1X2	T45.1X3	T45.1X4	T45.1X5	T45.1X6
Dibromopropamidine isethionate	T49.0X1	T49.0X2	T49.0X3	T49.0X4	T49.0X5	T49.0X6
Dibrompropamidine	T49.0X1	T49.0X2	T49.0X3	T49.0X4	T49.0X5	T49.0X6
Dibucaine	T41.3X1	T41.3X2	T41.3X3	T41.3X4	T41.3X5	T41.3X6
topical (surface)	T41.3X1	T41.3X2	T41.3X3	T41.3X4	T41.3X5	T41.3X6
Dibunate sodium	T48.3X1	T48.3X2	T48.3X3	T48.3X4	T48.3X5	T48.3X6
Dibutoline sulfate	T44.3X1	T44.3X2	T44.3X3	T44.3X4	T44.3X5	T44.3X6
Dicamba	T60.3X1	T60.3X2	T60.3X3	T60.3X4	—	—
Dicapthon	T60.0X1	T60.0X2	T60.0X3	T60.0X4	—	—
Dichlobenil	T60.3X1	T60.3X2	T60.3X3	T60.3X4	—	—
Dichlone	T60.3X1	T60.3X2	T60.3X3	T60.3X4	—	—
Dichloralphenozone	T42.6X1	T42.6X2	T42.6X3	T42.6X4	T42.6X5	T42.6X6
Dichlorbenzidine	T65.3X1	T65.3X2	T65.3X3	T65.3X4	—	—
Dichlorhydrin	T52.8X1	T52.8X2	T52.8X3	T52.8X4	—	—
Dichlorhydroxyquinoline	T37.8X1	T37.8X2	T37.8X3	T37.8X4	T37.8X5	T37.8X6

◀ New   ◀▦▦ Revised   ~~deleted~~ Deleted

Substance	Poisoning, Accidental (Unintentional)	Poisoning, Intentional Self-Harm	Poisoning, Assault	Poisoning, Undetermined	Adverse Effect	Underdosing
	External Cause (T-Code)					
Dichlorobenzene	T53.7X1	T53.7X2	T53.7X3	T53.7X4	—	—
Dichlorobenzyl alcohol	T49.6X1	T49.6X2	T49.6X3	T49.6X4	T49.6X5	T49.6X6
Dichlorodifluoromethane	T53.5X1	T53.5X2	T53.5X3	T53.5X4	—	—
Dichloroethane	T52.8X1	T52.8X2	T52.8X3	T52.8X4	—	—
Sym-Dichloroethyl ether	T53.6X1	T53.6X2	T53.6X3	T53.6X4	—	—
Dichloroethyl sulfide, not in war	T59.891	T59.892	T59.893	T59.894	—	—
Dichloroethylene	T53.6X1	T53.6X2	T53.6X3	T53.6X4	—	—
Dichloroformoxine, not in war	T59.891	T59.892	T59.893	T59.894	—	—
Dichlorohydrin, alpha-dichlorohydrin	T52.8X1	T52.8X2	T52.8X3	T52.8X4	—	—
Dichloromethane (solvent)	T53.4X1	T53.4X2	T53.4X3	T53.4X4	—	—
vapor	T53.4X1	T53.4X2	T53.4X3	T53.4X4	—	—
Dichloronaphthoquinone	T60.3X1	T60.3X2	T60.3X3	T60.3X4	—	—
Dichlorophen	T37.4X1	T37.4X2	T37.4X3	T37.4X4	T37.4X5	T37.4X6
2,4-Dichlorophenoxy-acetic acid	T60.3X1	T60.3X2	T60.3X3	T60.3X4	—	—
Dichloropropene	T60.3X1	T60.3X2	T60.3X3	T60.3X4	—	—
Dichloropropionic acid	T60.3X1	T60.3X2	T60.3X3	T60.3X4	—	—
Dichlorphenamide	T50.2X1	T50.2X2	T50.2X3	T50.2X4	T50.2X5	T50.2X6
Dichlorvos	T60.0X1	T60.0X2	T60.0X3	T60.0X4	—	—
Diclofenac	T39.391	T39.392	T39.393	T39.394	T39.395	T39.396
Diclofenamide	T50.2X1	T50.2X2	T50.2X3	T50.2X4	T50.2X5	T50.2X6
Diclofensine	T43.291	T43.292	T43.293	T43.294	T43.295	T43.296
Diclonixine	T39.8X1	T39.8X2	T39.8X3	T39.8X4	T39.8X5	T39.8X6
Dicloxacillin	T36.0X1	T36.0X2	T36.0X3	T36.0X4	T36.0X5	T36.0X6
Dicophane	T49.0X1	T49.0X2	T49.0X3	T49.0X4	T49.0X5	T49.0X6
Dicoumarol, dicoumarin, dicumarol	T45.511	T45.512	T45.513	T45.514	T45.515	T45.516
Dicrotophos	T60.0X1	T60.0X2	T60.0X3	T60.0X4	—	—
Dicyanogen (gas)	T65.0X1	T65.0X2	T65.0X3	T65.0X4	—	—
Dicyclomine	T44.3X1	T44.3X2	T44.3X3	T44.3X4	T44.3X5	T44.3X6
Dicycloverine	T44.3X1	T44.3X2	T44.3X3	T44.3X4	T44.3X5	T44.3X6
Dideoxycytidine	T37.5X1	T37.5X2	T37.5X3	T37.5X4	T37.5X5	T37.5X6
Dideoxyinosine	T37.5X1	T37.5X2	T37.5X3	T37.5X4	T37.5X5	T37.5X6
Dieldrin (vapor)	T60.1X1	T60.1X2	T60.1X3	T60.1X4	—	—
Diemal	T42.3X1	T42.3X2	T42.3X3	T42.3X4	T42.3X5	T42.3X6
Dienestrol	T38.5X1	T38.5X2	T38.5X3	T38.5X4	T38.5X5	T38.5X6
Dienoestrol	T38.5X1	T38.5X2	T38.5X3	T38.5X4	T38.5X5	T38.5X6
Dietetic drug NEC	T50.901	T50.902	T50.903	T50.904	T50.905	T50.906
Diethazine	T42.8X1	T42.8X2	T42.8X3	T42.8X4	T42.8X5	T42.8X6
Diethyl						
barbituric acid	T42.3X1	T42.3X2	T42.3X3	T42.3X4	T42.3X5	T42.3X6
carbamazine	T37.4X1	T37.4X2	T37.4X3	T37.4X4	T37.4X5	T37.4X6

TABLE OF DRUGS AND CHEMICALS

TABLE OF DRUGS AND CHEMICALS

Substance	Poisoning, Accidental (Unintentional)	Poisoning, Intentional Self-Harm	Poisoning, Assault	Poisoning, Undetermined	Adverse Effect	Underdosing
Diethyl *(Continued)*						
carbinol	T51.3X1	T51.3X2	T51.3X3	T51.3X4	—	—
carbonate	T52.8X1	T52.8X2	T52.8X3	T52.8X4	—	—
ether (vapor) — *see also ether*	T41.0X1	T41.0X2	T41.0X3	T41.0X4	T41.0X5	T41.0X6
oxide	T52.8X1	T52.8X2	T52.8X3	T52.8X4	—	—
propion	T50.5X1	T50.5X2	T50.5X3	T50.5X4	T50.5X5	T50.5X6
stilbestrol	T38.5X1	T38.5X2	T38.5X3	T38.5X4	T38.5X5	T38.5X6
toluamide (nonmedicinal)	T60.8X1	T60.8X2	T60.8X3	T60.8X4	—	—
medicinal	T49.3X1	T49.3X2	T49.3X3	T49.3X4	T49.3X5	T49.3X6
Diethylcarbamazine	T37.4X1	T37.4X2	T37.4X3	T37.4X4	T37.4X5	T37.4X6
Diethylene						
dioxide	T52.8X1	T52.8X2	T52.8X3	T52.8X4	—	—
glycol (monoacetate) (monobutyl ether) (monoethyl ether)	T52.3X1	T52.3X2	T52.3X3	T52.3X4	—	—
Diethylhexylphthalate	T65.891	T65.892	T65.893	T65.894	—	—
Diethylpropion	T50.5X1	T50.5X2	T50.5X3	T50.5X4	T50.5X5	T50.5X6
Diethylstilbestrol	T38.5X1	T38.5X2	T38.5X3	T38.5X4	T38.5X5	T38.5X6
Diethylstilboestrol	T38.5X1	T38.5X2	T38.5X3	T38.5X4	T38.5X5	T38.5X6
Diethylsulfone-diethylmethane	T42.6X1	T42.6X2	T42.6X3	T42.6X4	T42.6X5	T42.6X6
Diethyltoluamide	T49.0X1	T49.0X2	T49.0X3	T49.0X4	T49.0X5	T49.0X6
Diethyltryptamine (DET)	T40.991	T40.992	T40.993	T40.994	—	—
Difebarbamate	T42.3X1	T42.3X2	T42.3X3	T42.3X4	T42.3X5	T42.3X6
Difencloxazine	T40.2X1	T40.2X2	T40.2X3	T40.2X4	T40.2X5	T40.2X6
Difenidol	T45.0X1	T45.0X2	T45.0X3	T45.0X4	T45.0X5	T45.0X6
Difenoxin	T47.6X1	T47.6X2	T47.6X3	T47.6X4	T47.6X5	T47.6X6
Difetarsone	T37.3X1	T37.3X2	T37.3X3	T37.3X4	T37.3X5	T37.3X6
Diffusin	T45.3X1	T45.3X2	T45.3X3	T45.3X4	T45.3X5	T45.3X6
Diflorasone	T49.0X1	T49.0X2	T49.0X3	T49.0X4	T49.0X5	T49.0X6
Diflubenzuron	T60.1X1	T60.1X2	T60.1X3	T60.1X4	—	—
Diflos	T44.0X1	T44.0X2	T44.0X3	T44.0X4	T44.0X5	T44.0X6
Diflucortolone	T49.0X1	T49.0X2	T49.0X3	T49.0X4	T49.0X5	T49.0X6
Diflunisal	T39.091	T39.092	T39.093	T39.094	T39.095	T39.096
Difluoromethyldopa	T42.8X1	T42.8X2	T42.8X3	T42.8X4	T42.8X5	T42.8X6
Difluorophate	T44.0X1	T44.0X2	T44.0X3	T44.0X4	T44.0X5	T44.0X6
Digestant NEC	T47.5X1	T47.5X2	T47.5X3	T47.5X4	T47.5X5	T47.5X6
Digitalin(e)	T46.0X1	T46.0X2	T46.0X3	T46.0X4	T46.0X5	T46.0X6
Digitalis (leaf) (glycoside)	T46.0X1	T46.0X2	T46.0X3	T46.0X4	T46.0X5	T46.0X6
lanata	T46.0X1	T46.0X2	T46.0X3	T46.0X4	T46.0X5	T46.0X6
purpurea	T46.0X1	T46.0X2	T46.0X3	T46.0X4	T46.0X5	T46.0X6
Digitoxin	T46.0X1	T46.0X2	T46.0X3	T46.0X4	T46.0X5	T46.0X6

◀ New ◀▥▥ Revised ~~deleted~~ Deleted

Substance	External Cause (T-Code)					
	Poisoning, Accidental (Unintentional)	Poisoning, Intentional Self-Harm	Poisoning, Assault	Poisoning, Undetermined	Adverse Effect	Underdosing
Digitoxose	T46.0X1	T46.0X2	T46.0X3	T46.0X4	T46.0X5	T46.0X6
Digoxin	T46.0X1	T46.0X2	T46.0X3	T46.0X4	T46.0X5	T46.0X6
Digoxine	T46.0X1	T46.0X2	T46.0X3	T46.0X4	T46.0X5	T46.0X6
Dihydralazine	T46.5X1	T46.5X2	T46.5X3	T46.5X4	T46.5X5	T46.5X6
Dihydrazine	T46.5X1	T46.5X2	T46.5X3	T46.5X4	T46.5X5	T46.5X6
Dihydrocodeinone	T40.2X1	T40.2X2	T40.2X3	T40.2X4	T40.2X5	T40.2X6
Dihydroergocornine	T46.7X1	T46.7X2	T46.7X3	T46.7X4	T46.7X5	T46.7X6
Dihydroergocristine (mesilate)	T46.7X1	T46.7X2	T46.7X3	T46.7X4	T46.7X5	T46.7X6
Dihydroergokryptine	T46.7X1	T46.7X2	T46.7X3	T46.7X4	T46.7X5	T46.7X6
Dihydroergotamine	T46.5X1	T46.5X2	T46.5X3	T46.5X4	T46.5X5	T46.5X6
Dihydroergotoxine	T46.7X1	T46.7X2	T46.7X3	T46.7X4	T46.7X5	T46.7X6
mesilate	T46.7X1	T46.7X2	T46.7X3	T46.7X4	T46.7X5	T46.7X6
Dihydrohydroxycodein-one	T40.2X1	T40.2X2	T40.2X3	T40.2X4	T40.2X5	T40.2X6
Dihydrohydroxymorphinone	T40.2X1	T40.2X2	T40.2X3	T40.2X4	T40.2X5	T40.2X6
Dihydroisocodeine	T40.2X1	T40.2X2	T40.2X3	T40.2X4	T40.2X5	T40.2X6
Dihydromorphine	T40.2X1	T40.2X2	T40.2X3	T40.2X4	—	—
Dihydromorphinone	T40.2X1	T40.2X2	T40.2X3	T40.2X4	T40.2X5	T40.2X6
Dihydrostreptomycin	T36.5X1	T36.5X2	T36.5X3	T36.5X4	T36.5X5	T36.5X6
Dihydrotachysterol	T45.2X1	T45.2X2	T45.2X3	T45.2X4	T45.2X5	T45.2X6
Dihydroxyaluminum aminoacetate	T47.1X1	T47.1X2	T47.1X3	T47.1X4	T47.1X5	T47.1X6
Dihydroxyaluminum sodium carbonate	T47.1X1	T47.1X2	T47.1X3	T47.1X4	T47.1X5	T47.1X6
Dihydroxyanthraquinone	T47.2X1	T47.2X2	T47.2X3	T47.2X4	T47.2X5	T47.2X6
Dihydroxycodeinone	T40.2X1	T40.2X2	T40.2X3	T40.2X4	T40.2X5	T40.2X6
Dihydroxypropyl theophylline	T50.2X1	T50.2X2	T50.2X3	T50.2X4	T50.2X5	T50.2X6
Diiodohydroxyquin	T37.8X1	T37.8X2	T37.8X3	T37.8X4	T37.8X5	T37.8X6
topical	T49.0X1	T49.0X2	T49.0X3	T49.0X4	T49.0X5	T49.0X6
Diiodohydroxyquinoline	T37.8X1	T37.8X2	T37.8X3	T37.8X4	T37.8X5	T37.8X6
Diiodotyrosine	T38.2X1	T38.2X2	T38.2X3	T38.2X4	T38.2X5	T38.2X6
Diisopromine	T44.3X1	T44.3X2	T44.3X3	T44.3X4	T44.3X5	T44.3X6
Diisopropylamine	T46.3X1	T46.3X2	T46.3X3	T46.3X4	T46.3X5	T46.3X6
Diisopropylfluorophosphonate	T44.0X1	T44.0X2	T44.0X3	T44.0X4	T44.0X5	T44.0X6
Dilantin	T42.0X1	T42.0X2	T42.0X3	T42.0X4	T42.0X5	T42.0X6
Dilaudid	T40.2X1	T40.2X2	T40.2X3	T40.2X4	T40.2X5	T40.2X6
Dilazep	T46.3X1	T46.3X2	T46.3X3	T46.3X4	T46.3X5	T46.3X6
Dill	T47.5X1	T47.5X2	T47.5X3	T47.5X4	T47.5X5	T47.5X6
Diloxanide	T37.3X1	T37.3X2	T37.3X3	T37.3X4	T37.3X5	T37.3X6
Diltiazem	T46.1X1	T46.1X2	T46.1X3	T46.1X4	T46.1X5	T46.1X6
Dimazole	T49.0X1	T49.0X2	T49.0X3	T49.0X4	T49.0X5	T49.0X6
Dimefline	T50.7X1	T50.7X2	T50.7X3	T50.7X4	T50.7X5	T50.7X6

◄ New   ◄▥ Revised   <s>deleted</s> Deleted

TABLE OF DRUGS AND CHEMICALS

TABLE OF DRUGS AND CHEMICALS

Substance	Poisoning, Accidental (Unintentional)	Poisoning, Intentional Self-Harm	Poisoning, Assault	Poisoning, Undetermined	Adverse Effect	Underdosing
Dimefox	T60.0X1	T60.0X2	T60.0X3	T60.0X4	—	—
Dimemorfan	T48.3X1	T48.3X2	T48.3X3	T48.3X4	T48.3X5	T48.3X6
Dimenhydrinate	T45.0X1	T45.0X2	T45.0X3	T45.0X4	T45.0X5	T45.0X6
Dimercaprol (British anti-lewisite)	T45.8X1	T45.8X2	T45.8X3	T45.8X4	T45.8X5	T45.8X6
Dimercaptopropanol	T45.8X1	T45.8X2	T45.8X3	T45.8X4	T45.8X5	T45.8X6
Dimestrol	T38.5X1	T38.5X2	T38.5X3	T38.5X4	T38.5X5	T38.5X6
Dimetane	T45.0X1	T45.0X2	T45.0X3	T45.0X4	T45.0X5	T45.0X6
Dimethicone	T47.1X1	T47.1X2	T47.1X3	T47.1X4	T47.1X5	T47.1X6
Dimethindene	T45.0X1	T45.0X2	T45.0X3	T45.0X4	T45.0X5	T45.0X6
Dimethisoquin	T49.1X1	T49.1X2	T49.1X3	T49.1X4	T49.1X5	T49.1X6
Dimethisterone	T38.5X1	T38.5X2	T38.5X3	T38.5X4	T38.5X5	T38.5X6
Dimethoate	T60.0X1	T60.0X2	T60.0X3	T60.0X4	—	—
Dimethocaine	T41.3X1	T41.3X2	T41.3X3	T41.3X4	T41.3X5	T41.3X6
Dimethoxanate	T48.3X1	T48.3X2	T48.3X3	T48.3X4	T48.3X5	T48.3X6
Dimethyl						
arsine, arsinic acid	T57.0X1	T57.0X2	T57.0X3	T57.0X4	—	—
carbinol	T51.2X1	T51.2X2	T51.2X3	T51.2X4	—	—
carbonate	T52.8X1	T52.8X2	T52.8X3	T52.8X4	—	—
diguanide	T38.3X1	T38.3X2	T38.3X3	T38.3X4	T38.3X5	T38.3X6
ketone	T52.4X1	T52.4X2	T52.4X3	T52.4X4	—	—
vapor	T52.4X1	T52.4X2	T52.4X3	T52.4X4	—	—
meperidine	T40.2X1	T40.2X2	T40.2X3	T40.2X4	T40.2X5	T40.2X6
parathion	T60.0X1	T60.0X2	T60.0X3	T60.0X4	—	—
phthlate	T49.3X1	T49.3X2	T49.3X3	T49.3X4	T49.3X5	T49.3X6
polysiloxane	T47.8X1	T47.8X2	T47.8X3	T47.8X4	T47.8X5	T47.8X6
sulfate (fumes)	T59.891	T59.892	T59.893	T59.894	—	—
liquid	T65.891	T65.892	T65.893	T65.894	—	—
sulfoxide (nonmedicinal)	T52.8X1	T52.8X2	T52.8X3	T52.8X4	—	—
medicinal	T49.4X1	T49.4X2	T49.4X3	T49.4X4	T49.4X5	T49.4X6
tryptamine	T40.991	T40.992	T40.993	T40.994	—	—
tubocurarine	T48.1X1	T48.1X2	T48.1X3	T48.1X4	T48.1X5	T48.1X6
Dimethylamine sulfate	T49.4X1	T49.4X2	T49.4X3	T49.4X4	T49.4X5	T49.4X6
Dimethylformamide	T52.8X1	T52.8X2	T52.8X3	T52.8X4	—	—
Dimethyltubocurarinium chloride	T48.1X1	T48.1X2	T48.1X3	T48.1X4	T48.1X5	T48.1X6
Dimeticone	T47.1X1	T47.1X2	T47.1X3	T47.1X4	T47.1X5	T47.1X6
Dimetilan	T60.0X1	T60.0X2	T60.0X3	T60.0X4	—	—
Dimetindene	T45.0X1	T45.0X2	T45.0X3	T45.0X4	T45.0X5	T45.0X6
Dimetotiazine	T43.3X1	T43.3X2	T43.3X3	T43.3X4	T43.3X5	T43.3X6

◀ New   ◀◀ Revised   ~~deleted~~ Deleted

Substance	External Cause (T-Code)					
	Poisoning, Accidental (Unintentional)	Poisoning, Intentional Self-Harm	Poisoning, Assault	Poisoning, Undetermined	Adverse Effect	Underdosing
Dimorpholamine	T50.7X1	T50.7X2	T50.7X3	T50.7X4	T50.7X5	T50.7X6
Dimoxyline	T46.3X1	T46.3X2	T46.3X3	T46.3X4	T46.3X5	T46.3X6
Dinitrobenzene	T65.3X1	T65.3X2	T65.3X3	T65.3X4	—	—
vapor	T59.891	T59.892	T59.893	T59.894	—	—
Dinitrobenzol	T65.3X1	T65.3X2	T65.3X3	T65.3X4	—	—
vapor	T59.891	T59.892	T59.893	T59.894	—	—
Dinitrobutylphenol	T65.3X1	T65.3X2	T65.3X3	T65.3X4	—	—
Dinitro (-ortho-)cresol (pesticide) (spray)	T65.3X1	T65.3X2	T65.3X3	T65.3X4	—	—
Dinitrocyclohexylphenol	T65.3X1	T65.3X2	T65.3X3	T65.3X4	—	—
Dinitrophenol	T65.3X1	T65.3X2	T65.3X3	T65.3X4	—	—
Dinoprost	T48.0X1	T48.0X2	T48.0X3	T48.0X4	T48.0X5	T48.0X6
Dinoprostone	T48.0X1	T48.0X2	T48.0X3	T48.0X4	T48.0X5	T48.0X6
Dinoseb	T60.3X1	T60.3X2	T60.3X3	T60.3X4	—	—
Dioctyl sulfosuccinate (calcium) (sodium)	T47.4X1	T47.4X2	T47.4X3	T47.4X4	T47.4X5	T47.4X6
Diodone	T50.8X1	T50.8X2	T50.8X3	T50.8X4	T50.8X5	T50.8X6
Diodoquin	T37.8X1	T37.8X2	T37.8X3	T37.8X4	T37.8X5	T37.8X6
Dionin	T40.2X1	T40.2X2	T40.2X3	T40.2X4	T40.2X5	T40.2X6
Diosmin	T46.991	T46.992	T46.993	T46.994	T46.995	T46.996
Dioxane	T52.8X1	T52.8X2	T52.8X3	T52.8X4	—	—
Dioxathion	T60.0X1	T60.0X2	T60.0X3	T60.0X4	—	—
Dioxin	T53.7X1	T53.7X2	T53.7X3	T53.7X4	—	—
Dioxopromethazine	T43.3X1	T43.3X2	T43.3X3	T43.3X4	T43.3X5	T43.3X6
Dioxyline	T46.3X1	T46.3X2	T46.3X3	T46.3X4	T46.3X5	T46.3X6
Dipentene	T52.8X1	T52.8X2	T52.8X3	T52.8X4	—	—
Diperodon	T41.3X1	T41.3X2	T41.3X3	T41.3X4	T41.3X5	T41.3X6
Diphacinone	T60.4X1	T60.4X2	T60.4X3	T60.4X4	—	—
Diphemanil	T44.3X1	T44.3X2	T44.3X3	T44.3X4	T44.3X5	T44.3X6
metilsulfate	T44.3X1	T44.3X2	T44.3X3	T44.3X4	T44.3X5	T44.3X6
Diphenadione	T45.511	T45.512	T45.513	T45.514	T45.515	T45.516
rodenticide	T60.4X1	T60.4X2	T60.4X3	T60.4X4	—	—
Diphenhydramine	T45.0X1	T45.0X2	T45.0X3	T45.0X4	T45.0X5	T45.0X6
Diphenidol	T45.0X1	T45.0X2	T45.0X3	T45.0X4	T45.0X5	T45.0X6
Diphenoxylate	T47.6X1	T47.6X2	T47.6X3	T47.6X4	T47.6X5	T47.6X6
Diphenylamine	T65.3X1	T65.3X2	T65.3X3	T65.3X4	—	—
Diphenylbutazone	T39.2X1	T39.2X2	T39.2X3	T39.2X4	T39.2X5	T39.2X6
Diphenylchloroarsine, not in war	T57.0X1	T57.0X2	T57.0X3	T57.0X4	—	—
Diphenylhydantoin	T42.0X1	T42.0X2	T42.0X3	T42.0X4	T42.0X5	T42.0X6
Diphenylmethane dye	T52.1X1	T52.1X2	T52.1X3	T52.1X4	—	—

TABLE OF DRUGS AND CHEMICALS

TABLE OF DRUGS AND CHEMICALS

Substance	External Cause (T-Code)					
	Poisoning, Accidental (Unintentional)	Poisoning, Intentional Self-Harm	Poisoning, Assault	Poisoning, Undetermined	Adverse Effect	Underdosing
Diphenylpyraline	T45.0X1	T45.0X2	T45.0X3	T45.0X4	T45.0X5	T45.0X6
Diphtheria						
antitoxin	T50.Z11	T50.Z12	T50.Z13	T50.Z14	T50.Z15	T50.Z16
toxoid	T50.A91	T50.A92	T50.A93	T50.A94	T50.A95	T50.A96
with tetanus toxoid	T50.A21	T50.A22	T50.A23	T50.A24	T50.A25	T50.A26
with pertussis component	T50.A11	T50.A12	T50.A13	T50.A14	T50.A15	T50.A16
vaccine (combination)	T50.A91	T50.A92	T50.A93	T50.A94	T50.A95	T50.A96
combination						
including pertussis	T50.A11	T50.A12	T50.A13	T50.A14	T50.A15	T50.A16
without pertussis	T50.A21	T50.A22	T50.A23	T50.A24	T50.A25	T50.A26
Diphylline	T50.2X1	T50.2X2	T50.2X3	T50.2X4	T50.2X5	T50.2X6
Dipipanone	T40.4X1	T40.4X2	T40.4X3	T40.4X4	—	—
Dipivefrine	T49.5X1	T49.5X2	T49.5X3	T49.5X4	T49.5X5	T49.5X6
Diplovax	T50.B91	T50.B92	T50.B93	T50.B94	T50.B95	T50.B96
Diprophylline	T50.2X1	T50.2X2	T50.2X3	T50.2X4	T50.2X5	T50.2X6
Dipropyline	T48.291	T48.292	T48.293	T48.294	T48.295	T48.296
Dipyridamole	T46.3X1	T46.3X2	T46.3X3	T46.3X4	T46.3X5	T46.3X6
Dipyrone	T39.2X1	T39.2X2	T39.2X3	T39.2X4	T39.2X5	T39.2X6
Diquat (dibromide)	T60.3X1	T60.3X2	T60.3X3	T60.3X4	—	—
Disinfectant	T65.891	T65.892	T65.893	T65.894	—	—
alkaline	T54.3X1	T54.3X2	T54.3X3	T54.3X4	—	—
aromatic	T54.1X1	T54.1X2	T54.1X3	T54.1X4	—	—
intestinal	T37.8X1	T37.8X2	T37.8X3	T37.8X4	T37.8X5	T37.8X6
Disipal	T42.8X1	T42.8X2	T42.8X3	T42.8X4	T42.8X5	T42.8X6
Disodium edetate	T50.6X1	T50.6X2	T50.6X3	T50.6X4	T50.6X5	T50.6X6
Disoprofol	T41.291	T41.292	T41.293	T41.294	T41.295	T41.296
Disopyramide	T46.2X1	T46.2X2	T46.2X3	T46.2X4	T46.2X5	T46.2X6
Distigmine (bromide)	T44.0X1	T44.0X2	T44.0X3	T44.0X4	T44.0X5	T44.0X6
Disulfamide	T50.2X1	T50.2X2	T50.2X3	T50.2X4	T50.2X5	T50.2X6
Disulfanilamide	T37.0X1	T37.0X2	T37.0X3	T37.0X4	T37.0X5	T37.0X6
Disulfiram	T50.6X1	T50.6X2	T50.6X3	T50.6X4	T50.6X5	T50.6X6
Disulfoton	T60.0X1	T60.0X2	T60.0X3	T60.0X4	—	—
Dithiazanine iodide	T37.4X1	T37.4X2	T37.4X3	T37.4X4	T37.4X5	T37.4X6
Dithiocarbamate	T60.0X1	T60.0X2	T60.0X3	T60.0X4	—	—
Dithranol	T49.4X1	T49.4X2	T49.4X3	T49.4X4	T49.4X5	T49.4X6
Diucardin	T50.2X1	T50.2X2	T50.2X3	T50.2X4	T50.2X5	T50.2X6
Diupres	T50.2X1	T50.2X2	T50.2X3	T50.2X4	T50.2X5	T50.2X6
Diuretic NEC	T50.2X1	T50.2X2	T50.2X3	T50.2X4	T50.2X5	T50.2X6
benzothiadiazine	T50.2X1	T50.2X2	T50.2X3	T50.2X4	T50.2X5	T50.2X6
carbonic acid anhydrase inhibitors	T50.2X1	T50.2X2	T50.2X3	T50.2X4	T50.2X5	T50.2X6

◄ New   ◄‖‖ Revised   ~~deleted~~ Deleted

Substance	External Cause (T-Code)					
	Poisoning, Accidental (Unintentional)	Poisoning, Intentional Self-Harm	Poisoning, Assault	Poisoning, Undetermined	Adverse Effect	Underdosing
Diuretic NEC *(Continued)*						
furfuryl NEC	T50.2X1	T50.2X2	T50.2X3	T50.2X4	T50.2X5	T50.2X6
loop (high-ceiling)	T50.1X1	T50.1X2	T50.1X3	T50.1X4	T50.1X5	T50.1X6
mercurial NEC	T50.2X1	T50.2X2	T50.2X3	T50.2X4	T50.2X5	T50.2X6
osmotic	T50.2X1	T50.2X2	T50.2X3	T50.2X4	T50.2X5	T50.2X6
purine NEC	T50.2X1	T50.2X2	T50.2X3	T50.2X4	T50.2X5	T50.2X6
saluretic NEC	T50.2X1	T50.2X2	T50.2X3	T50.2X4	T50.2X5	T50.2X6
sulfonamide	T50.2X1	T50.2X2	T50.2X3	T50.2X4	T50.2X5	T50.2X6
thiazide NEC	T50.2X1	T50.2X2	T50.2X3	T50.2X4	T50.2X5	T50.2X6
xanthine	T50.2X1	T50.2X2	T50.2X3	T50.2X4	T50.2X5	T50.2X6
Diurgin	T50.2X1	T50.2X2	T50.2X3	T50.2X4	T50.2X5	T50.2X6
Diuril	T50.2X1	T50.2X2	T50.2X3	T50.2X4	T50.2X5	T50.2X6
Diuron	T60.3X1	T60.3X2	T60.3X3	T60.3X4	—	—
Divalproex	T42.6X1	T42.6X2	T42.6X3	T42.6X4	T42.6X5	T42.6X6
Divinyl ether	T41.0X1	T41.0X2	T41.0X3	T41.0X4	T41.0X5	T41.0X6
Dixanthogen	T49.0X1	T49.0X2	T49.0X3	T49.0X4	T49.0X5	T49.0X6
Dixyrazine	T43.3X1	T43.3X2	T43.3X3	T43.3X4	T43.3X5	T43.3X6
D-lysergic acid diethylamide	T40.8X1	T40.8X2	T40.8X3	T40.8X4	—	—
DMCT	T36.4X1	T36.4X2	T36.4X3	T36.4X4	T36.4X5	T36.4X6
DMSO — *see Dimethyl sulfoxide*						
DNBP	T60.3X1	T60.3X2	T60.3X3	T60.3X4	—	—
DNOC	T65.3X1	T65.3X2	T65.3X3	T65.3X4	—	—
DOCA	T38.0X1	T38.0X2	T38.0X3	T38.0X4	T38.0X5	T38.0X6
Dobutamine	T44.5X1	T44.5X2	T44.5X3	T44.5X4	T44.5X5	T44.5X6
Docusate sodium	T47.4X1	T47.4X2	T47.4X3	T47.4X4	T47.4X5	T47.4X6
Dodicin	T49.0X1	T49.0X2	T49.0X3	T49.0X4	T49.0X5	T49.0X6
Dofamium chloride	T49.0X1	T49.0X2	T49.0X3	T49.0X4	T49.0X5	T49.0X6
Dolophine	T40.3X1	T40.3X2	T40.3X3	T40.3X4	T40.3X5	T40.3X6
Doloxene	T39.8X1	T39.8X2	T39.8X3	T39.8X4	T39.8X5	T39.8X6
Domestic gas (after combustion) — *see Gas, utility*						
prior to combustion	T59.891	T59.892	T59.893	T59.894	—	—
Domiodol	T48.4X1	T48.4X2	T48.4X3	T48.4X4	T48.4X5	T48.4X6
Domiphen (bromide)	T49.0X1	T49.0X2	T49.0X3	T49.0X4	T49.0X5	T49.0X6
Domperidone	T45.0X1	T45.0X2	T45.0X3	T45.0X4	T45.0X5	T45.0X6
Dopa	T42.8X1	T42.8X2	T42.8X3	T42.8X4	T42.8X5	T42.8X6
Dopamine	T44.991	T44.992	T44.993	T44.994	T44.995	T44.996
Doriden	T42.6X1	T42.6X2	T42.6X3	T42.6X4	T42.6X5	T42.6X6
Dormiral	T42.3X1	T42.3X2	T42.3X3	T42.3X4	T42.3X5	T42.3X6
Dormison	T42.6X1	T42.6X2	T42.6X3	T42.6X4	T42.6X5	T42.6X6
Dornase	T48.4X1	T48.4X2	T48.4X3	T48.4X4	T48.4X5	T48.4X6

Substance	External Cause (T-Code)					
	Poisoning, Accidental (Unintentional)	Poisoning, Intentional Self-Harm	Poisoning, Assault	Poisoning, Undetermined	Adverse Effect	Underdosing
Dorsacaine	T41.3X1	T41.3X2	T41.3X3	T41.3X4	T41.3X5	T41.3X6
Dosulepin	T43.011	T43.012	T43.013	T43.014	T43.015	T43.016
Dothiepin	T43.011	T43.012	T43.013	T43.014	T43.015	T43.016
Doxantrazole	T48.6X1	T48.6X2	T48.6X3	T48.6X4	T48.6X5	T48.6X6
Doxapram	T50.7X1	T50.7X2	T50.7X3	T50.7X4	T50.7X5	T50.7X6
Doxazosin	T44.6X1	T44.6X2	T44.6X3	T44.6X4	T44.6X5	T44.6X6
Doxepin	T43.011	T43.012	T43.013	T43.014	T43.015	T43.016
Doxifluridine	T45.1X1	T45.1X2	T45.1X3	T45.1X4	T45.1X5	T45.1X6
Doxorubicin	T45.1X1	T45.1X2	T45.1X3	T45.1X4	T45.1X5	T45.1X6
Doxycycline	T36.4X1	T36.4X2	T36.4X3	T36.4X4	T36.4X5	T36.4X6
Doxylamine	T45.0X1	T45.0X2	T45.0X3	T45.0X4	T45.0X5	T45.0X6
Dramamine	T45.0X1	T45.0X2	T45.0X3	T45.0X4	T45.0X5	T45.0X6
Drano (drain cleaner)	T54.3X1	T54.3X2	T54.3X3	T54.3X4	—	—
Dressing, live pulp	T49.7X1	T49.7X2	T49.7X3	T49.7X4	T49.7X5	T49.7X6
Drocode	T40.2X1	T40.2X2	T40.2X3	T40.2X4	T40.2X5	T40.2X6
Dromoran	T40.2X1	T40.2X2	T40.2X3	T40.2X4	T40.2X5	T40.2X6
Dromostanolone	T38.7X1	T38.7X2	T38.7X3	T38.7X4	T38.7X5	T38.7X6
Dronabinol	T40.7X1	T40.7X2	T40.7X3	T40.7X4	T40.7X5	T40.7X6
Droperidol	T43.591	T43.592	T43.593	T43.594	T43.595	T43.596
Dropropizine	T48.3X1	T48.3X2	T48.3X3	T48.3X4	T48.3X5	T48.3X6
Drostanolone	T38.7X1	T38.7X2	T38.7X3	T38.7X4	T38.7X5	T38.7X6
Drotaverine	T44.3X1	T44.3X2	T44.3X3	T44.3X4	T44.3X5	T44.3X6
Drotrecogin alfa	T45.511	T45.512	T45.513	T45.514	T45.515	T45.516
Drug NEC	T50.901	T50.902	T50.903	T50.904	T50.905	T50.906
specified NEC	T50.991	T50.992	T50.993	T50.994	T50.995	T50.996
DTIC	T45.1X1	T45.1X2	T45.1X3	T45.1X4	T45.1X5	T45.1X6
Duboisine	T44.3X1	T44.3X2	T44.3X3	T44.3X4	T44.3X5	T44.3X6
Dulcolax	T47.2X1	T47.2X2	T47.2X3	T47.2X4	T47.2X5	T47.2X6
Duponol (C) (EP)	T49.2X1	T49.2X2	T49.2X3	T49.2X4	T49.2X5	T49.2X6
Durabolin	T38.7X1	T38.7X2	T38.7X3	T38.7X4	T38.7X5	T38.7X6
Dyclone	T41.3X1	T41.3X2	T41.3X3	T41.3X4	T41.3X5	T41.3X6
Dyclonine	T41.3X1	T41.3X2	T41.3X3	T41.3X4	T41.3X5	T41.3X6
Dydrogesterone	T38.5X1	T38.5X2	T38.5X3	T38.5X4	T38.5X5	T38.5X6
Dye NEC	T65.6X1	T65.6X2	T65.6X3	T65.6X4	—	—
antiseptic	T49.0X1	T49.0X2	T49.0X3	T49.0X4	T49.0X5	T49.0X6
diagnostic agents	T50.8X1	T50.8X2	T50.8X3	T50.8X4	T50.8X5	T50.8X6
pharmaceutical NEC	T50.901	T50.902	T50.903	T50.904	T50.905	T50.906
Dyflos	T44.0X1	T44.0X2	T44.0X3	T44.0X4	T44.0X5	T44.0X6
Dymelor	T38.3X1	T38.3X2	T38.3X3	T38.3X4	T38.3X5	T38.3X6

◄ New ◄|||| Revised ~~deleted~~ Deleted

Substance	Poisoning, Accidental (Unintentional)	Poisoning, Intentional Self-Harm	Poisoning, Assault	Poisoning, Undetermined	Adverse Effect	Underdosing
Dynamite	T65.3X1	T65.3X2	T65.3X3	T65.3X4	—	—
fumes	T59.891	T59.892	T59.893	T59.894	—	—
Dyphylline	T44.3X1	T44.3X2	T44.3X3	T44.3X4	T44.3X5	T44.3X6
E						
Ear drug NEC	T49.6X1	T49.6X2	T49.6X3	T49.6X4	T49.6X5	T49.6X6
Ear preparations	T49.6X1	T49.6X2	T49.6X3	T49.6X4	T49.6X5	T49.6X6
Econazole	T49.0X1	T49.0X2	T49.0X3	T49.0X4	T49.0X5	T49.0X6
Ecothiopate iodide	T49.5X1	T49.5X2	T49.5X3	T49.5X4	T49.5X5	T49.5X6
Echothiophate, echothiopate, ecothiopate	T49.5X1	T49.5X2	T49.5X3	T49.5X4	T49.5X5	T49.5X6
Ecstasy	T43.621	T43.622	T43.623	T43.624	T43.625	T43.626
Ectylurea	T42.6X1	T42.6X2	T42.6X3	T42.6X4	T42.6X5	T42.6X6
Edathamil disodium	T45.8X1	T45.8X2	T45.8X3	T45.8X4	T45.8X5	T45.8X6
Edecrin	T50.1X1	T50.1X2	T50.1X3	T50.1X4	T50.1X5	T50.1X6
Edetate, disodium (calcium)	T45.8X1	T45.8X2	T45.8X3	T45.8X4	T45.8X5	T45.8X6
Edoxudine	T49.5X1	T49.5X2	T49.5X3	T49.5X4	T49.5X5	T49.5X6
Edrophonium	T44.0X1	T44.0X2	T44.0X3	T44.0X4	T44.0X5	T44.0X6
chloride	T44.0X1	T44.0X2	T44.0X3	T44.0X4	T44.0X5	T44.0X6
EDTA	T50.6X1	T50.6X2	T50.6X3	T50.6X4	T50.6X5	T50.6X6
Eflornithine	T37.2X1	T37.2X2	T37.2X3	T37.2X4	T37.2X5	T37.2X6
Efloxate	T46.3X1	T46.3X2	T46.3X3	T46.3X4	T46.3X5	T46.3X6
Elase	T49.8X1	T49.8X2	T49.8X3	T49.8X4	T49.8X5	T49.8X6
Elastase	T47.5X1	T47.5X2	T47.5X3	T47.5X4	T47.5X5	T47.5X6
Elaterium	T47.2X1	T47.2X2	T47.2X3	T47.2X4	T47.2X5	T47.2X6
Elcatonin	T50.991	T50.992	T50.993	T50.994	T50.995	T50.996
Elder	T62.2X1	T62.2X2	T62.2X3	T62.2X4	—	—
berry (unripe)	T62.1X1	T62.1X2	T62.1X3	T62.1X4	—	—
Electrolyte balance drug	T50.3X1	T50.3X2	T50.3X3	T50.3X4	T50.3X5	T50.3X6
Electrolytes NEC	T50.3X1	T50.3X2	T50.3X3	T50.3X4	T50.3X5	T50.3X6
Electrolytic agent NEC	T50.3X1	T50.3X2	T50.3X3	T50.3X4	T50.3X5	T50.3X6
Elemental diet	T50.901	T50.902	T50.903	T50.904	T50.905	T50.906
Elliptinium acetate	T45.1X1	T45.1X2	T45.1X3	T45.1X4	T45.1X5	T45.1X6
Embramine	T45.0X1	T45.0X2	T45.0X3	T45.0X4	T45.0X5	T45.0X6
Emepronium (salts)	T44.3X1	T44.3X2	T44.3X3	T44.3X4	T44.3X5	T44.3X6
bromide	T44.3X1	T44.3X2	T44.3X3	T44.3X4	T44.3X5	T44.3X6
Emetic NEC	T47.7X1	T47.7X2	T47.7X3	T47.7X4	T47.7X5	T47.7X6
Emetine	T37.3X1	T37.3X2	T37.3X3	T37.3X4	T37.3X5	T37.3X6
Emollient NEC	T49.3X1	T49.3X2	T49.3X3	T49.3X4	T49.3X5	T49.3X6
Emorfazone	T39.8X1	T39.8X2	T39.8X3	T39.8X4	T39.8X5	T39.8X6

TABLE OF DRUGS AND CHEMICALS

◄ New ◄‖‖ Revised ~~deleted~~ Deleted

Substance	External Cause (T-Code)					
	Poisoning, Accidental (Unintentional)	Poisoning, Intentional Self-Harm	Poisoning, Assault	Poisoning, Undetermined	Adverse Effect	Underdosing
Emylcamate	T43.591	T43.592	T43.593	T43.594	T43.595	T43.596
Enalapril	T46.4X1	T46.4X2	T46.4X3	T46.4X4	T46.4X5	T46.4X6
Enalaprilat	T46.4X1	T46.4X2	T46.4X3	T46.4X4	T46.4X5	T46.4X6
Encainide	T46.2X1	T46.2X2	T46.2X3	T46.2X4	T46.2X5	T46.2X6
Endocaine	T41.3X1	T41.3X2	T41.3X3	T41.3X4	T41.3X5	T41.3X6
Endosulfan	T60.2X1	T60.2X2	T60.2X3	T60.2X4	—	—
Endothall	T60.3X1	T60.3X2	T60.3X3	T60.3X4	—	—
Endralazine	T46.5X1	T46.5X2	T46.5X3	T46.5X4	T46.5X5	T46.5X6
Endrin	T60.1X1	T60.1X2	T60.1X3	T60.1X4	—	—
Enflurane	T41.0X1	T41.0X2	T41.0X3	T41.0X4	T41.0X5	T41.0X6
Enhexymal	T42.3X1	T42.3X2	T42.3X3	T42.3X4	T42.3X5	T42.3X6
Enocitabine	T45.1X1	T45.1X2	T45.1X3	T45.1X4	T45.1X5	T45.1X6
Enovid	T38.4X1	T38.4X2	T38.4X3	T38.4X4	T38.4X5	T38.4X6
Enoxacin	T36.8X1	T36.8X2	T36.8X3	T36.8X4	T36.8X5	T36.8X6
Enoxaparin (sodium)	T45.511	T45.512	T45.513	T45.514	T45.515	T45.516
Enpiprazole	T43.591	T43.592	T43.593	T43.594	T43.595	T43.596
Enprofylline	T48.6X1	T48.6X2	T48.6X3	T48.6X4	T48.6X5	T48.6X6
Enprostil	T47.1X1	T47.1X2	T47.1X3	T47.1X4	T47.1X5	T47.1X6
ENT preparations (anti-infectives)	T49.6X1	T49.6X2	T49.6X3	T49.6X4	T49.6X5	T49.6X6
Enviomycin	T36.8X1	T36.8X2	T36.8X3	T36.8X4	T36.8X5	T36.8X6
Enzodase	T45.3X1	T45.3X2	T45.3X3	T45.3X4	T45.3X5	T45.3X6
Enzyme NEC	T45.3X1	T45.3X2	T45.3X3	T45.3X4	T45.3X5	T45.3X6
depolymerizing	T49.8X1	T49.8X2	T49.8X3	T49.8X4	T49.8X5	T49.8X6
fibrolytic	T45.3X1	T45.3X2	T45.3X3	T45.3X4	T45.3X5	T45.3X6
gastric	T47.5X1	T47.5X2	T47.5X3	T47.5X4	T47.5X5	T47.5X6
intestinal	T47.5X1	T47.5X2	T47.5X3	T47.5X4	T47.5X5	T47.5X6
local action	T49.4X1	T49.4X2	T49.4X3	T49.4X4	T49.4X5	T49.4X6
proteolytic	T49.4X1	T49.4X2	T49.4X3	T49.4X4	T49.4X5	T49.4X6
thrombolytic	T45.3X1	T45.3X2	T45.3X3	T45.3X4	T45.3X5	T45.3X6
EPAB	T41.3X1	T41.3X2	T41.3X3	T41.3X4	T41.3X5	T41.3X6
Epanutin	T42.0X1	T42.0X2	T42.0X3	T42.0X4	T42.0X5	T42.0X6
Ephedra	T44.991	T44.992	T44.993	T44.994	T44.995	T44.996
Ephedrine	T44.991	T44.992	T44.993	T44.994	T44.995	T44.996
Epichlorhydrin, epichlorohydrin	T52.8X1	T52.8X2	T52.8X3	T52.8X4	—	—
Epicillin	T36.0X1	T36.0X2	T36.0X3	T36.0X4	T36.0X5	T36.0X6
Epiestriol	T38.5X1	T38.5X2	T38.5X3	T38.5X4	T38.5X5	T38.5X6
Epilim — see Sodium valproate						
Epimestrol	T38.5X1	T38.5X2	T38.5X3	T38.5X4	T38.5X5	T38.5X6
Epinephrine	T44.5X1	T44.5X2	T44.5X3	T44.5X4	T44.5X5	T44.5X6

◀ New   ◀ Revised   ~~deleted~~ Deleted

Substance	Poisoning, Accidental (Unintentional)	Poisoning, Intentional Self-Harm	Poisoning, Assault	Poisoning, Undetermined	Adverse Effect	Underdosing
		External Cause (T-Code)				
Epirubicin	T45.1X1	T45.1X2	T45.1X3	T45.1X4	T45.1X5	T45.1X6
Epitiostanol	T38.7X1	T38.7X2	T38.7X3	T38.7X4	T38.7X5	T38.7X6
Epitizide	T50.2X1	T50.2X2	T50.2X3	T50.2X4	T50.2X5	T50.2X6
EPN	T60.0X1	T60.0X2	T60.0X3	T60.0X4	—	—
EPO	T45.8X1	T45.8X2	T45.8X3	T45.8X4	T45.8X5	T45.8X6
Epoetin alpha	T45.8X1	T45.8X2	T45.8X3	T45.8X4	T45.8X5	T45.8X6
Epomediol	T50.991	T50.992	T50.993	T50.994	T50.995	T50.996
Epoprostenol	T45.521	T45.522	T45.523	T45.524	T45.525	T45.526
Epoxy resin	T65.891	T65.892	T65.893	T65.894	—	—
Eprazinone	T48.4X1	T48.4X2	T48.4X3	T48.4X4	T48.4X5	T48.4X6
Epsilon amino-caproic acid	T45.621	T45.622	T45.623	T45.624	T45.625	T45.626
Epsom salt	T47.3X1	T47.3X2	T47.3X3	T47.3X4	T47.3X5	T47.3X6
Eptazocine	T40.4X1	T40.4X2	T40.4X3	T40.4X4	T40.4X5	T40.4X6
Equanil	T43.591	T43.592	T43.593	T43.594	T43.595	T43.596
Equisetum	T62.2X1	T62.2X2	T62.2X3	T62.2X4	—	—
diuretic	T50.2X1	T50.2X2	T50.2X3	T50.2X4	T50.2X5	T50.2X6
Ergobasine	T48.0X1	T48.0X2	T48.0X3	T48.0X4	T48.0X5	T48.0X6
Ergocalciferol	T45.2X1	T45.2X2	T45.2X3	T45.2X4	T45.2X5	T45.2X6
Ergoloid mesylates	T46.7X1	T46.7X2	T46.7X3	T46.7X4	T46.7X5	T46.7X6
Ergometrine	T48.0X1	T48.0X2	T48.0X3	T48.0X4	T48.0X5	T48.0X6
Ergonovine	T48.0X1	T48.0X2	T48.0X3	T48.0X4	T48.0X5	T48.0X6
Ergot NEC	T64.81	T64.82	T64.83	T64.84	—	—
derivative	T48.0X1	T48.0X2	T48.0X3	T48.0X4	T48.0X5	T48.0X6
medicinal (alkaloids)	T48.0X1	T48.0X2	T48.0X3	T48.0X4	T48.0X5	T48.0X6
prepared	T48.0X1	T48.0X2	T48.0X3	T48.0X4	T48.0X5	T48.0X6
Ergotamine	T46.5X1	T46.5X2	T46.5X3	T46.5X4	T46.5X5	T46.5X6
Ergotocine	T48.0X1	T48.0X2	T48.0X3	T48.0X4	T48.0X5	T48.0X6
Ergotrate	T48.0X1	T48.0X2	T48.0X3	T48.0X4	T48.0X5	T48.0X6
Eritrityl tetranitrate	T46.3X1	T46.3X2	T46.3X3	T46.3X4	T46.3X5	T46.3X6
Erythrityl tetranitrate	T46.3X1	T46.3X2	T46.3X3	T46.3X4	T46.3X5	T46.3X6
Erythrol tetranitrate	T46.3X1	T46.3X2	T46.3X3	T46.3X4	T46.3X5	T46.3X6
Erythromycin (salts)	T36.3X1	T36.3X2	T36.3X3	T36.3X4	T36.3X5	T36.3X6
ophthalmic preparation	T49.5X1	T49.5X2	T49.5X3	T49.5X4	T49.5X5	T49.5X6
topical NEC	T49.0X1	T49.0X2	T49.0X3	T49.0X4	T49.0X5	T49.0X6
Erythropoietin	T45.8X1	T45.8X2	T45.8X3	T45.8X4	T45.8X5	T45.8X6
human	T45.8X1	T45.8X2	T45.8X3	T45.8X4	T45.8X5	T45.8X6
Escin	T46.991	T46.992	T46.993	T46.994	T46.995	T46.996
Esculin	T45.2X1	T45.2X2	T45.2X3	T45.2X4	T45.2X5	T45.2X6
Esculoside	T45.2X1	T45.2X2	T45.2X3	T45.2X4	T45.2X5	T45.2X6

TABLE OF DRUGS AND CHEMICALS

Substance	External Cause (T-Code)					
	Poisoning, Accidental (Unintentional)	Poisoning, Intentional Self-Harm	Poisoning, Assault	Poisoning, Undetermined	Adverse Effect	Underdosing
ESDT (ether-soluble tar distillate)	T49.1X1	T49.1X2	T49.1X3	T49.1X4	T49.1X5	T49.1X6
Eserine	T49.5X1	T49.5X2	T49.5X3	T49.5X4	T49.5X5	T49.5X6
Esflurbiprofen	T39.311	T39.312	T39.313	T39.314	T39.315	T39.316
Eskabarb	T42.3X1	T42.3X2	T42.3X3	T42.3X4	T42.3X5	T42.3X6
Eskalith	T43.8X1	T43.8X2	T43.8X3	T43.8X4	T43.8X5	T43.8X6
Esmolol	T44.7X1	T44.7X2	T44.7X3	T44.7X4	T44.7X5	T44.7X6
Estanozolol	T38.7X1	T38.7X2	T38.7X3	T38.7X4	T38.7X5	T38.7X6
Estazolam	T42.4X1	T42.4X2	T42.4X3	T42.4X4	T42.4X5	T42.4X6
Estradiol	T38.5X1	T38.5X2	T38.5X3	T38.5X4	T38.5X5	T38.5X6
with testosterone	T38.7X1	T38.7X2	T38.7X3	T38.7X4	T38.7X5	T38.7X6
benzoate	T38.5X1	T38.5X2	T38.5X3	T38.5X4	T38.5X5	T38.5X6
Estramustine	T45.1X1	T45.1X2	T45.1X3	T45.1X4	T45.1X5	T45.1X6
Estriol	T38.5X1	T38.5X2	T38.5X3	T38.5X4	T38.5X5	T38.5X6
Estrogen	T38.5X1	T38.5X2	T38.5X3	T38.5X4	T38.5X5	T38.5X6
with progesterone	T38.5X1	T38.5X2	T38.5X3	T38.5X4	T38.5X5	T38.5X6
conjugated	T38.5X1	T38.5X2	T38.5X3	T38.5X4	T38.5X5	T38.5X6
Estrone	T38.5X1	T38.5X2	T38.5X3	T38.5X4	T38.5X5	T38.5X6
Estropipate	T38.5X1	T38.5X2	T38.5X3	T38.5X4	T38.5X5	T38.5X6
Etacrynate sodium	T50.1X1	T50.1X2	T50.1X3	T50.1X4	T50.1X5	T50.1X6
Etacrynic acid	T50.1X1	T50.1X2	T50.1X3	T50.1X4	T50.1X5	T50.1X6
Etafedrine	T48.6X1	T48.6X2	T48.6X3	T48.6X4	T48.6X5	T48.6X6
Etafenone	T46.3X1	T46.3X2	T46.3X3	T46.3X4	T46.3X5	T46.3X6
Etambutol	T37.1X1	T37.1X2	T37.1X3	T37.1X4	T37.1X5	T37.1X6
Etamiphyllin	T48.6X1	T48.6X2	T48.6X3	T48.6X4	T48.6X5	T48.6X6
Etamivan	T50.7X1	T50.7X2	T50.7X3	T50.7X4	T50.7X5	T50.7X6
Etamsylate	T45.7X1	T45.7X2	T45.7X3	T45.7X4	T45.7X5	T45.7X6
Etebenecid	T50.4X1	T50.4X2	T50.4X3	T50.4X4	T50.4X5	T50.4X6
Ethacridine	T49.0X1	T49.0X2	T49.0X3	T49.0X4	T49.0X5	T49.0X6
Ethacrynic acid	T50.1X1	T50.1X2	T50.1X3	T50.1X4	T50.1X5	T50.1X6
Ethadione	T42.2X1	T42.2X2	T42.2X3	T42.2X4	T42.2X5	T42.2X6
Ethambutol	T37.1X1	T37.1X2	T37.1X3	T37.1X4	T37.1X5	T37.1X6
Ethamide	T50.2X1	T50.2X2	T50.2X3	T50.2X4	T50.2X5	T50.2X6
Ethamivan	T50.7X1	T50.7X2	T50.7X3	T50.7X4	T50.7X5	T50.7X6
Ethamsylate	T45.7X1	T45.7X2	T45.7X3	T45.7X4	T45.7X5	T45.7X6
Ethanol	T51.0X1	T51.0X2	T51.0X3	T51.0X4	—	—
beverage	T51.0X1	T51.0X2	T51.0X3	T51.0X4	—	—
Ethanolamine oleate	T46.8X1	T46.8X2	T46.8X3	T46.8X4	T46.8X5	T46.8X6
Ethaverine	T44.3X1	T44.3X2	T44.3X3	T44.3X4	T44.3X5	T44.3X6
Ethchlorvynol	T42.6X1	T42.6X2	T42.6X3	T42.6X4	T42.6X5	T42.6X6
Ethebenecid	T50.4X1	T50.4X2	T50.4X3	T50.4X4	T50.4X5	T50.4X6

◄ New   ◄▥ Revised   ~~deleted~~ Deleted

Substance	External Cause (T-Code)					
	Poisoning, Accidental (Unintentional)	Poisoning, Intentional Self-Harm	Poisoning, Assault	Poisoning, Undetermined	Adverse Effect	Underdosing
Ether (vapor)	T41.0X1	T41.0X2	T41.0X3	T41.0X4	T41.0X5	T41.0X6
anesthetic	T41.0X1	T41.0X2	T41.0X3	T41.0X4	T41.0X5	T41.0X6
divinyl	T41.0X1	T41.0X2	T41.0X3	T41.0X4	T41.0X5	T41.0X6
ethyl (medicinal)	T41.0X1	T41.0X2	T41.0X3	T41.0X4	T41.0X5	T41.0X6
nonmedicinal	T52.8X1	T52.8X2	T52.8X3	T52.8X4	—	—
petroleum — see Ligroin						
solvent	T52.8X1	T52.8X2	T52.8X3	T52.8X4	—	—
Ethiazide	T50.2X1	T50.2X2	T50.2X3	T50.2X4	T50.2X5	T50.2X6
Ethidium chloride (vapor)	T59.891	T59.892	T59.893	T59.894	—	—
Ethinamate	T42.6X1	T42.6X2	T42.6X3	T42.6X4	T42.6X5	T42.6X6
Ethinylestradiol, ethinyloestradiol	T38.5X1	T38.5X2	T38.5X3	T38.5X4	T38.5X5	T38.5X6
with						
levonorgestrel	T38.4X1	T38.4X2	T38.4X3	T38.4X4	T38.4X5	T38.4X6
norethisterone	T38.4X1	T38.4X2	T38.4X3	T38.4X4	T38.4X5	T38.4X6
Ethiodized oil (131 I)	T50.8X1	T50.8X2	T50.8X3	T50.8X4	T50.8X5	T50.8X6
Ethion	T60.0X1	T60.0X2	T60.0X3	T60.0X4	—	—
Ethionamide	T37.1X1	T37.1X2	T37.1X3	T37.1X4	T37.1X5	T37.1X6
Ethioniamide	T37.1X1	T37.1X2	T37.1X3	T37.1X4	T37.1X5	T37.1X6
Ethisterone	T38.5X1	T38.5X2	T38.5X3	T38.5X4	T38.5X5	T38.5X6
Ethobral	T42.3X1	T42.3X2	T42.3X3	T42.3X4	T42.3X5	T42.3X6
Ethocaine (infiltration) (topical)	T41.3X1	T41.3X2	T41.3X3	T41.3X4	T41.3X5	T41.3X6
nerve block (peripheral) (plexus)	T41.3X1	T41.3X2	T41.3X3	T41.3X4	T41.3X5	T41.3X6
spinal	T41.3X1	T41.3X2	T41.3X3	T41.3X4	T41.3X5	T41.3X6
Ethoheptazine	T40.4X1	T40.4X2	T40.4X3	T40.4X4	T40.4X5	T40.4X6
Ethopropazine	T44.3X1	T44.3X2	T44.3X3	T44.3X4	T44.3X5	T44.3X6
Ethosuximide	T42.2X1	T42.2X2	T42.2X3	T42.2X4	T42.2X5	T42.2X6
Ethotoin	T42.0X1	T42.0X2	T42.0X3	T42.0X4	T42.0X5	T42.0X6
Ethoxazene	T37.91	T37.92	T37.93	T37.94	T37.95	T37.96
Ethoxazorutoside	T46.991	T46.992	T46.993	T46.994	T46.995	T46.996
2-Ethoxyethanol	T52.3X1	T52.3X2	T52.3X3	T52.3X4	—	—
Ethoxzolamide	T50.2X1	T50.2X2	T50.2X3	T50.2X4	T50.2X5	T50.2X6
Ethyl						
acetate	T52.8X1	T52.8X2	T52.8X3	T52.8X4	—	—
alcohol	T51.0X1	T51.0X2	T51.0X3	T51.0X4	—	—
beverage	T51.0X1	T51.0X2	T51.0X3	T51.0X4	—	—
aldehyde (vapor)	T59.891	T59.892	T59.893	T59.894	—	—
liquid	T52.8X1	T52.8X2	T52.8X3	T52.8X4	—	—
aminobenzoate	T41.3X1	T41.3X2	T41.3X3	T41.3X4	T41.3X5	T41.3X6
aminophenothiazine	T43.3X1	T43.3X2	T43.3X3	T43.3X4	T43.3X5	T43.3X6
benzoate	T52.8X1	T52.8X2	T52.8X3	T52.8X4	—	—

Substance	External Cause (T-Code)					
	Poisoning, Accidental (Unintentional)	Poisoning, Intentional Self-Harm	Poisoning, Assault	Poisoning, Undetermined	Adverse Effect	Underdosing
Ethyl *(Continued)*						
biscoumacetate	T45.511	T45.512	T45.513	T45.514	T45.515	T45.516
bromide (anesthetic)	T41.0X1	T41.0X2	T41.0X3	T41.0X4	T41.0X5	T41.0X6
carbamate	T45.1X1	T45.1X2	T45.1X3	T45.1X4	T45.1X5	T45.1X6
carbinol	T51.3X1	T51.3X2	T51.3X3	T51.3X4	—	—
carbonate	T52.8X1	T52.8X2	T52.8X3	T52.8X4	—	—
chaulmoograte	T37.1X1	T37.1X2	T37.1X3	T37.1X4	T37.1X5	T37.1X6
chloride (anesthetic)	T41.0X1	T41.0X2	T41.0X3	T41.0X4	T41.0X5	T41.0X6
anesthetic (local)	T41.3X1	T41.3X2	T41.3X3	T41.3X4	T41.3X5	T41.3X6
inhaled	T41.0X1	T41.0X2	T41.0X3	T41.0X4	T41.0X5	T41.0X6
local	T49.4X1	T49.4X2	T49.4X3	T49.4X4	T49.4X5	T49.4X6
solvent	T53.6X1	T53.6X2	T53.6X3	T53.6X4	—	—
dibunate	T48.3X1	T48.3X2	T48.3X3	T48.3X4	T48.3X5	T48.3X6
dichloroarsine (vapor)	T57.0X1	T57.0X2	T57.0X3	T57.0X4	—	—
estranol	T38.7X1	T38.7X2	T38.7X3	T38.7X4	T38.7X5	T38.7X6
ether — *see also ether*	T52.8X1	T52.8X2	T52.8X3	T52.8X4	—	—
formate NEC (solvent)	T52.0X1	T52.0X2	T52.0X3	T52.0X4	—	—
fumarate	T49.4X1	T49.4X2	T49.4X3	T49.4X4	T49.4X5	T49.4X6
hydroxyisobutyrate NEC (solvent)	T52.8X1	T52.8X2	T52.8X3	T52.8X4	—	—
iodoacetate	T59.3X1	T59.3X2	T59.3X3	T59.3X4	—	—
lactate NEC (solvent)	T52.8X1	T52.8X2	T52.8X3	T52.8X4	—	—
loflazepate	T42.4X1	T42.4X2	T42.4X3	T42.4X4	T42.4X5	T42.4X6
mercuric chloride	T56.1X1	T56.1X2	T56.1X3	T56.1X4	—	—
methylcarbinol	T51.8X1	T51.8X2	T51.8X3	T51.8X4	—	—
morphine	T40.2X1	T40.2X2	T40.2X3	T40.2X4	T40.2X5	T40.2X6
noradrenaline	T48.6X1	T48.6X2	T48.6X3	T48.6X4	T48.6X5	T48.6X6
oxybutyrate NEC (solvent)	T52.8X1	T52.8X2	T52.8X3	T52.8X4	—	—
Ethylene (gas)	T59.891	T59.892	T59.893	T59.894	—	—
anesthetic (general)	T41.0X1	T41.0X2	T41.0X3	T41.0X4	T41.0X5	T41.0X6
chlorohydrin	T52.8X1	T52.8X2	T52.8X3	T52.8X4	—	—
vapor	T53.6X1	T53.6X2	T53.6X3	T53.6X4	—	—
dichloride	T52.8X1	T52.8X2	T52.8X3	T52.8X4	—	—
vapor	T53.6X1	T53.6X2	T53.6X3	T53.6X4	—	—
dinitrate	T52.3X1	T52.3X2	T52.3X3	T52.3X4	—	—
glycol(s)	T52.8X1	T52.8X2	T52.8X3	T52.8X4	—	—
dinitrate	T52.3X1	T52.3X2	T52.3X3	T52.3X4	—	—
monobutyl ether	T52.3X1	T52.3X2	T52.3X3	T52.3X4	—	—
imine	T54.1X1	T54.1X2	T54.1X3	T54.1X4	—	—
oxide (fumigant) (nonmedicinal)	T59.891	T59.892	T59.893	T59.894	—	—
medicinal	T49.0X1	T49.0X2	T49.0X3	T49.0X4	T49.0X5	T49.0X6

◀ New ◀▦▦ Revised ~~deleted~~ Deleted

Substance	Poisoning, Accidental (Unintentional)	Poisoning, Intentional Self-Harm	Poisoning, Assault	Poisoning, Undetermined	Adverse Effect	Underdosing
			External Cause (T-Code)			
Ethylenediamine theophylline	T48.6X1	T48.6X2	T48.6X3	T48.6X4	T48.6X5	T48.6X6
Ethylenediaminetetra-acetic acid	T50.6X1	T50.6X2	T50.6X3	T50.6X4	T50.6X5	T50.6X6
Ethylenedinitrilotetra-acetate	T50.6X1	T50.6X2	T50.6X3	T50.6X4	T50.6X5	T50.6X6
Ethylestrenol	T38.7X1	T38.7X2	T38.7X3	T38.7X4	T38.7X5	T38.7X6
Ethylhydroxycellulose	T47.4X1	T47.4X2	T47.4X3	T47.4X4	T47.4X5	T47.4X6
Ethylidene						
chloride NEC	T53.6X1	T53.6X2	T53.6X3	T53.6X4	—	—
diacetate	T60.3X1	T60.3X2	T60.3X3	T60.3X4	—	—
dicoumarin	T45.511	T45.512	T45.513	T45.514	T45.515	T45.516
dicoumarol	T45.511	T45.512	T45.513	T45.514	T45.515	T45.516
diethyl ether	T52.0X1	T52.0X2	T52.0X3	T52.0X4	—	—
Ethylmorphine	T40.2X1	T40.2X2	T40.2X3	T40.2X4	T40.2X5	T40.2X6
Ethylnorepinephrine	T48.6X1	T48.6X2	T48.6X3	T48.6X4	T48.6X5	T48.6X6
Ethylparachlorophen-oxyisobutyrate	T46.6X1	T46.6X2	T46.6X3	T46.6X4	T46.6X5	T46.6X6
Ethynodiol	T38.4X1	T38.4X2	T38.4X3	T38.4X4	T38.4X5	T38.4X6
with mestranol diacetate	T38.4X1	T38.4X2	T38.4X3	T38.4X4	T38.4X5	T38.4X6
Etidocaine	T41.3X1	T41.3X2	T41.3X3	T41.3X4	T41.3X5	T41.3X6
infiltration (subcutaneous)	T41.3X1	T41.3X2	T41.3X3	T41.3X4	T41.3X5	T41.3X6
nerve (peripheral) (plexus)	T41.3X1	T41.3X2	T41.3X3	T41.3X4	T41.3X5	T41.3X6
Etidronate	T50.991	T50.992	T50.993	T50.994	T50.995	T50.996
Etidronic acid (disodium salt)	T50.991	T50.992	T50.993	T50.994	T50.995	T50.996
Etifoxine	T42.6X1	T42.6X2	T42.6X3	T42.6X4	T42.6X5	T42.6X6
Etilefrine	T44.4X1	T44.4X2	T44.4X3	T44.4X4	T44.4X5	T44.4X6
Etilfen	T42.3X1	T42.3X2	T42.3X3	T42.3X4	T42.3X5	T42.3X6
Etinodiol	T38.4X1	T38.4X2	T38.4X3	T38.4X4	T38.4X5	T38.4X6
Etiroxate	T46.6X1	T46.6X2	T46.6X3	T46.6X4	T46.6X5	T46.6X6
Etizolam	T42.4X1	T42.4X2	T42.4X3	T42.4X4	T42.4X5	T42.4X6
Etodolac	T39.391	T39.392	T39.393	T39.394	T39.395	T39.396
Etofamide	T37.3X1	T37.3X2	T37.3X3	T37.3X4	T37.3X5	T37.3X6
Etofibrate	T46.6X1	T46.6X2	T46.6X3	T46.6X4	T46.6X5	T46.6X6
Etofylline	T46.7X1	T46.7X2	T46.7X3	T46.7X4	T46.7X5	T46.7X6
clofibrate	T46.6X1	T46.6X2	T46.6X3	T46.6X4	T46.6X5	T46.6X6
Etoglucid	T45.1X1	T45.1X2	T45.1X3	T45.1X4	T45.1X5	T45.1X6
Etomidate	T41.1X1	T41.1X2	T41.1X3	T41.1X4	T41.1X5	T41.1X6
Etomide	T39.8X1	T39.8X2	T39.8X3	T39.8X4	T39.8X5	T39.8X6
Etomidoline	T44.3X1	T44.3X2	T44.3X3	T44.3X4	T44.3X5	T44.3X6
Etoposide	T45.1X1	T45.1X2	T45.1X3	T45.1X4	T45.1X5	T45.1X6
Etorphine	T40.2X1	T40.2X2	T40.2X3	T40.2X4	T40.2X5	T40.2X6
Etoval	T42.3X1	T42.3X2	T42.3X3	T42.3X4	T42.3X5	T42.3X6
Etozolin	T50.1X1	T50.1X2	T50.1X3	T50.1X4	T50.1X5	T50.1X6

◄ New ◄ Revised ~~deleted~~ Deleted

TABLE OF DRUGS AND CHEMICALS

Substance	Poisoning, Accidental (Unintentional)	Poisoning, Intentional Self-Harm	Poisoning, Assault	Poisoning, Undetermined	Adverse Effect	Underdosing
			External Cause (T-Code)			
Etretinate	T50.991	T50.992	T50.993	T50.994	T50.995	T50.996
Etryptamine	T43.691	T43.692	T43.693	T43.694	T43.695	T43.696
Etybenzatropine	T44.3X1	T44.3X2	T44.3X3	T44.3X4	T44.3X5	T44.3X6
Etynodiol	T38.4X1	T38.4X2	T38.4X3	T38.4X4	T38.4X5	T38.4X6
Eucaine	T41.3X1	T41.3X2	T41.3X3	T41.3X4	T41.3X5	T41.3X6
Eucalyptus oil	T49.7X1	T49.7X2	T49.7X3	T49.7X4	T49.7X5	T49.7X6
Eucatropine	T49.5X1	T49.5X2	T49.5X3	T49.5X4	T49.5X5	T49.5X6
Eucodal	T40.2X1	T40.2X2	T40.2X3	T40.2X4	T40.2X5	T40.2X6
Euneryl	T42.3X1	T42.3X2	T42.3X3	T42.3X4	T42.3X5	T42.3X6
Euphthalmine	T44.3X1	T44.3X2	T44.3X3	T44.3X4	T44.3X5	T44.3X6
Eurax	T49.0X1	T49.0X2	T49.0X3	T49.0X4	T49.0X5	T49.0X6
Euresol	T49.4X1	T49.4X2	T49.4X3	T49.4X4	T49.4X5	T49.4X6
Euthroid	T38.1X1	T38.1X2	T38.1X3	T38.1X4	T38.1X5	T38.1X6
Evans blue	T50.8X1	T50.8X2	T50.8X3	T50.8X4	T50.8X5	T50.8X6
Evipal	T42.3X1	T42.3X2	T42.3X3	T42.3X4	T42.3X5	T42.3X6
sodium	T41.1X1	T41.1X2	T41.1X3	T41.1X4	T41.1X5	T41.1X6
Evipan	T42.3X1	T42.3X2	T42.3X3	T42.3X4	T42.3X5	T42.3X6
sodium	T41.1X1	T41.1X2	T41.1X3	T41.1X4	T41.1X5	T41.1X6
Exalamide	T49.0X1	T49.0X2	T49.0X3	T49.0X4	T49.0X5	T49.0X6
Exalgin	T39.1X1	T39.1X2	T39.1X3	T39.1X4	T39.1X5	T39.1X6
Excipients, pharmaceutical	T50.901	T50.902	T50.903	T50.904	T50.905	T50.906
Exhaust gas (engine) (motor vehicle)	T58.01	T58.02	T58.03	T58.04	—	—
Ex-Lax (phenolphthalein)	T47.2X1	T47.2X2	T47.2X3	T47.2X4	T47.2X5	T47.2X6
Expectorant NEC	T48.4X1	T48.4X2	T48.4X3	T48.4X4	T48.4X5	T48.4X6
Extended insulin zinc suspension	T38.3X1	T38.3X2	T38.3X3	T38.3X4	T38.3X5	T38.3X6
External medications (skin) (mucous membrane)	T49.91	T49.92	T49.93	T49.94	T49.95	T49.96
dental agent	T49.7X1	T49.7X2	T49.7X3	T49.7X4	T49.7X5	T49.7X6
ENT agent	T49.6X1	T49.6X2	T49.6X3	T49.6X4	T49.6X5	T49.6X6
ophthalmic preparation	T49.5X1	T49.5X2	T49.5X3	T49.5X4	T49.5X5	T49.5X6
specified NEC	T49.8X1	T49.8X2	T49.8X3	T49.8X4	T49.8X5	T49.8X6
Extrapyramidal antagonist NEC	T44.3X1	T44.3X2	T44.3X3	T44.3X4	T44.3X5	T44.3X6
Eye agents (anti-infective)	T49.5X1	T49.5X2	T49.5X3	T49.5X4	T49.5X5	T49.5X6
Eye drug NEC	T49.5X1	T49.5X2	T49.5X3	T49.5X4	T49.5X5	T49.5X6
F						
FAC (fluorouracil + doxorubicin + cyclophosphamide)	T45.1X1	T45.1X2	T45.1X3	T45.1X4	T45.1X5	T45.1X6
Factor						
I (fibrinogen)	T45.8X1	T45.8X2	T45.8X3	T45.8X4	T45.8X5	T45.8X6
III (thromboplastin)	T45.8X1	T45.8X2	T45.8X3	T45.8X4	T45.8X5	T45.8X6
VIII (antihemophilic Factor) (Concentrate)	T45.8X1	T45.8X2	T45.8X3	T45.8X4	T45.8X5	T45.8X6

◀ New   ◀▥ Revised   ~~deleted~~ Deleted

Substance	External Cause (T-Code)					
	Poisoning, Accidental (Unintentional)	Poisoning, Intentional Self-Harm	Poisoning, Assault	Poisoning, Undetermined	Adverse Effect	Underdosing
Factor *(Continued)*						
IX complex	T45.7X1	T45.7X2	T45.7X3	T45.7X4	T45.7X5	T45.7X6
human	T45.8X1	T45.8X2	T45.8X3	T45.8X4	T45.8X5	T45.8X6
Famotidine	T47.0X1	T47.0X2	T47.0X3	T47.0X4	T47.0X5	T47.0X6
Fat suspension, intravenous	T50.991	T50.992	T50.993	T50.994	T50.995	T50.996
Fazadinium bromide	T48.1X1	T48.1X2	T48.1X3	T48.1X4	T48.1X5	T48.1X6
Febarbamate	T42.3X1	T42.3X2	T42.3X3	T42.3X4	T42.3X5	T42.3X6
Fecal softener	T47.4X1	T47.4X2	T47.4X3	T47.4X4	T47.4X5	T47.4X6
Fedrilate	T48.3X1	T48.3X2	T48.3X3	T48.3X4	T48.3X5	T48.3X6
Felodipine	T46.1X1	T46.1X2	T46.1X3	T46.1X4	T46.1X5	T46.1X6
Felypressin	T38.891	T38.892	T38.893	T38.894	T38.895	T38.896
Femoxetine	T43.221	T43.222	T43.223	T43.224	T43.225	T43.226
Fenalcomine	T46.3X1	T46.3X2	T46.3X3	T46.3X4	T46.3X5	T46.3X6
Fenamisal	T37.1X1	T37.1X2	T37.1X3	T37.1X4	T37.1X5	T37.1X6
Fenazone	T39.2X1	T39.2X2	T39.2X3	T39.2X4	T39.2X5	T39.2X6
Fenbendazole	T37.4X1	T37.4X2	T37.4X3	T37.4X4	T37.4X5	T37.4X6
Fenbutrazate	T50.5X1	T50.5X2	T50.5X3	T50.5X4	T50.5X5	T50.5X6
Fencamfamine	T43.691	T43.692	T43.693	T43.694	T43.695	T43.696
Fendiline	T46.1X1	T46.1X2	T46.1X3	T46.1X4	T46.1X5	T46.1X6
Fenetylline	T43.691	T43.692	T43.693	T43.694	T43.695	T43.696
Fenflumizole	T39.391	T39.392	T39.393	T39.394	T39.395	T39.396
Fenfluramine	T50.5X1	T50.5X2	T50.5X3	T50.5X4	T50.5X5	T50.5X6
Fenobarbital	T42.3X1	T42.3X2	T42.3X3	T42.3X4	T42.3X5	T42.3X6
Fenofibrate	T46.6X1	T46.6X2	T46.6X3	T46.6X4	T46.6X5	T46.6X6
Fenoprofen	T39.311	T39.312	T39.313	T39.314	T39.315	T39.316
Fenoterol	T48.6X1	T48.6X2	T48.6X3	T48.6X4	T48.6X5	T48.6X6
Fenoverine	T44.3X1	T44.3X2	T44.3X3	T44.3X4	T44.3X5	T44.3X6
Fenoxazoline	T48.5X1	T48.5X2	T48.5X3	T48.5X4	T48.5X5	T48.5X6
Fenproporex	T50.5X1	T50.5X2	T50.5X3	T50.5X4	T50.5X5	T50.5X6
Fenquizone	T50.2X1	T50.2X2	T50.2X3	T50.2X4	T50.2X5	T50.2X6
Fentanyl	T40.4X1	T40.4X2	T40.4X3	T40.4X4	T40.4X5	T40.4X6
Fentazin	T43.3X1	T43.3X2	T43.3X3	T43.3X4	T43.3X5	T43.3X6
Fenthion	T60.0X1	T60.0X2	T60.0X3	T60.0X4	—	—
Fenticlor	T49.0X1	T49.0X2	T49.0X3	T49.0X4	T49.0X5	T49.0X6
Fenylbutazone	T39.2X1	T39.2X2	T39.2X3	T39.2X4	T39.2X5	T39.2X6
Feprazone	T39.2X1	T39.2X2	T39.2X3	T39.2X4	T39.2X5	T39.2X6
Fer de lance (bite) (venom)	T63.061	T63.062	T63.063	T63.064	—	—
Ferric—*see also* Iron						
chloride	T45.4X1	T45.4X2	T45.4X3	T45.4X4	T45.4X5	T45.4X6
citrate	T45.4X1	T45.4X2	T45.4X3	T45.4X4	T45.4X5	T45.4X6

Substance	Poisoning, Accidental (Unintentional)	Poisoning, Intentional Self-Harm	Poisoning, Assault	Poisoning, Undetermined	Adverse Effect	Underdosing
Ferric *(Continued)*						
hydroxide						
colloidal	T45.4X1	T45.4X2	T45.4X3	T45.4X4	T45.4X5	T45.4X6
polymaltose	T45.4X1	T45.4X2	T45.4X3	T45.4X4	T45.4X5	T45.4X6
pyrophosphate	T45.4X1	T45.4X2	T45.4X3	T45.4X4	T45.4X5	T45.4X6
Ferritin	T45.4X1	T45.4X2	T45.4X3	T45.4X4	T45.4X5	T45.4X6
Ferrocholinate	T45.4X1	T45.4X2	T45.4X3	T45.4X4	T45.4X5	T45.4X6
Ferrodextrane	T45.4X1	T45.4X2	T45.4X3	T45.4X4	T45.4X5	T45.4X6
Ferropolimaler	T45.4X1	T45.4X2	T45.4X3	T45.4X4	T45.4X5	T45.4X6
Ferrous — *see also Iron*						
phosphate	T45.4X1	T45.4X2	T45.4X3	T45.4X4	T45.4X5	T45.4X6
salt	T45.4X1	T45.4X2	T45.4X3	T45.4X4	T45.4X5	T45.4X6
with folic acid	T45.4X1	T45.4X2	T45.4X3	T45.4X4	T45.4X5	T45.4X6
Ferrous fumerate, gluconate, lactate, salt NEC, sulfate (medicinal)	T45.4X1	T45.4X2	T45.4X3	T45.4X4	T45.4X5	T45.4X6
Ferrovanadium (fumes)	T59.891	T59.892	T59.893	T59.894	—	—
Ferrum — *see Iron*						
Fertilizers NEC	T65.891	T65.892	T65.893	T65.894	—	—
with herbicide mixture	T60.3X1	T60.3X2	T60.3X3	T60.3X4	—	—
Fetoxilate	T47.6X1	T47.6X2	T47.6X3	T47.6X4	T47.6X5	T47.6X6
Fiber, dietary	T47.4X1	T47.4X2	T47.4X3	T47.4X4	T47.4X5	T47.4X6
Fibrinogen (human)	T45.8X1	T45.8X2	T45.8X3	T45.8X4	T45.8X5	T45.8X6
Fibrinolysin (human)	T45.691	T45.692	T45.693	T45.694	T45.695	T45.696
Fibrinolysis						
affecting drug	T45.601	T45.602	T45.603	T45.604	T45.605	T45.606
inhibitor NEC	T45.621	T45.622	T45.623	T45.624	T45.625	T45.626
Fibrinolytic drug	T45.611	T45.612	T45.613	T45.614	T45.615	T45.616
Filix mas	T37.4X1	T37.4X2	T37.4X3	T37.4X4	T37.4X5	T37.4X6
Filtering cream	T49.3X1	T49.3X2	T49.3X3	T49.3X4	T49.3X5	T49.3X6
Fiorinal	T39.011	T39.012	T39.013	T39.014	T39.015	T39.016
Firedamp	T59.891	T59.892	T59.893	T59.894	—	—
Fish, noxious, nonbacterial	T61.91	T61.92	T61.93	T61.94	—	—
ciguatera	T61.01	T61.02	T61.03	T61.04	—	—
scombroid	T61.11	T61.12	T61.13	T61.14	—	—
shell	T61.781	T61.782	T61.783	T61.784	—	—
specified NEC	T61.771	T61.772	T61.773	T61.774	—	—
Flagyl	T37.3X1	T37.3X2	T37.3X3	T37.3X4	T37.3X5	T37.3X6
Flavine adenine dinucleotide	T45.2X1	T45.2X2	T45.2X3	T45.2X4	T45.2X5	T45.2X6
Flavodic acid	T46.991	T46.992	T46.993	T46.994	T46.995	T46.996
Flavoxate	T44.3X1	T44.3X2	T44.3X3	T44.3X4	T44.3X5	T44.3X6

◀ New   ◀◀◀ Revised   ~~deleted~~ Deleted

Substance	External Cause (T-Code)					
	Poisoning, Accidental (Unintentional)	Poisoning, Intentional Self-Harm	Poisoning, Assault	Poisoning, Undetermined	Adverse Effect	Underdosing
Flaxedil	T48.1X1	T48.1X2	T48.1X3	T48.1X4	T48.1X5	T48.1X6
Flaxseed (medicinal)	T49.3X1	T49.3X2	T49.3X3	T49.3X4	T49.3X5	T49.3X6
Flecainide	T46.2X1	T46.2X2	T46.2X3	T46.2X4	T46.2X5	T46.2X6
Fleroxacin	T36.8X1	T36.8X2	T36.8X3	T36.8X4	T36.8X5	T36.8X6
Floctafenine	T39.8X1	T39.8X2	T39.8X3	T39.8X4	T39.8X5	T39.8X6
Flomax	T44.6X1	T44.6X2	T44.6X3	T44.6X4	T44.6X5	T44.6X6
Flomoxef	T36.1X1	T36.1X2	T36.1X3	T36.1X4	T36.1X5	T36.1X6
Flopropione	T44.3X1	T44.3X2	T44.3X3	T44.3X4	T44.3X5	T44.3X6
Florantyrone	T47.5X1	T47.5X2	T47.5X3	T47.5X4	T47.5X5	T47.5X6
Floraquin	T37.8X1	T37.8X2	T37.8X3	T37.8X4	T37.8X5	T37.8X6
Florinef	T38.0X1	T38.0X2	T38.0X3	T38.0X4	T38.0X5	T38.0X6
ENT agent	T49.6X1	T49.6X2	T49.6X3	T49.6X4	T49.6X5	T49.6X6
ophthalmic preparation	T49.5X1	T49.5X2	T49.5X3	T49.5X4	T49.5X5	T49.5X6
topical NEC	T49.0X1	T49.0X2	T49.0X3	T49.0X4	T49.0X5	T49.0X6
Flowers of sulfur	T49.4X1	T49.4X2	T49.4X3	T49.4X4	T49.4X5	T49.4X6
Floxuridine	T45.1X1	T45.1X2	T45.1X3	T45.1X4	T45.1X5	T45.1X6
Fluanisone	T43.4X1	T43.4X2	T43.4X3	T43.4X4	T43.4X5	T43.4X6
Flubendazole	T37.4X1	T37.4X2	T37.4X3	T37.4X4	T37.4X5	T37.4X6
Fluclorolone acetonide	T49.0X1	T49.0X2	T49.0X3	T49.0X4	T49.0X5	T49.0X6
Flucloxacillin	T36.0X1	T36.0X2	T36.0X3	T36.0X4	T36.0X5	T36.0X6
Fluconazole	T37.8X1	T37.8X2	T37.8X3	T37.8X4	T37.8X5	T37.8X6
Flucytosine	T37.8X1	T37.8X2	T37.8X3	T37.8X4	T37.8X5	T37.8X6
Fludeoxyglucose (18F)	T50.8X1	T50.8X2	T50.8X3	T50.8X4	T50.8X5	T50.8X6
Fludiazepam	T42.4X1	T42.4X2	T42.4X3	T42.4X4	T42.4X5	T42.4X6
Fludrocortisone	T50.0X1	T50.0X2	T50.0X3	T50.0X4	T50.0X5	T50.0X6
ENT agent	T49.6X1	T49.6X2	T49.6X3	T49.6X4	T49.6X5	T49.6X6
ophthalmic preparation	T49.5X1	T49.5X2	T49.5X3	T49.5X4	T49.5X5	T49.5X6
topical NEC	T49.0X1	T49.0X2	T49.0X3	T49.0X4	T49.0X5	T49.0X6
Fludroxycortide	T49.0X1	T49.0X2	T49.0X3	T49.0X4	T49.0X5	T49.0X6
Flufenamic acid	T39.391	T39.392	T39.393	T39.394	T39.395	T39.396
Fluindione	T45.511	T45.512	T45.513	T45.514	T45.515	T45.516
Flumequine	T37.8X1	T37.8X2	T37.8X3	T37.8X4	T37.8X5	T37.8X6
Flumethasone	T49.0X1	T49.0X2	T49.0X3	T49.0X4	T49.0X5	T49.0X6
Flumethiazide	T50.2X1	T50.2X2	T50.2X3	T50.2X4	T50.2X5	T50.2X6
Flumidin	T37.5X1	T37.5X2	T37.5X3	T37.5X4	T37.5X5	T37.5X6
Flunarizine	T46.7X1	T46.7X2	T46.7X3	T46.7X4	T46.7X5	T46.7X6
Flunidazole	T37.8X1	T37.8X2	T37.8X3	T37.8X4	T37.8X5	T37.8X6
Flunisolide	T48.6X1	T48.6X2	T48.6X3	T48.6X4	T48.6X5	T48.6X6
Flunitrazepam	T42.4X1	T42.4X2	T42.4X3	T42.4X4	T42.4X5	T42.4X6

TABLE OF DRUGS AND CHEMICALS

◀ New ◀‖‖ Revised ~~deleted~~ Deleted

Substance	External Cause (T-Code)					
	Poisoning, Accidental (Unintentional)	Poisoning, Intentional Self-Harm	Poisoning, Assault	Poisoning, Undetermined	Adverse Effect	Underdosing
Fluocinolone (acetonide)	T49.0X1	T49.0X2	T49.0X3	T49.0X4	T49.0X5	T49.0X6
Fluocinonide	T49.0X1	T49.0X2	T49.0X3	T49.0X4	T49.0X5	T49.0X6
Fluocortin (butyl)	T49.0X1	T49.0X2	T49.0X3	T49.0X4	T49.0X5	T49.0X6
Fluocortolone	T49.0X1	T49.0X2	T49.0X3	T49.0X4	T49.0X5	T49.0X6
Fluohydrocortisone	T38.0X1	T38.0X2	T38.0X3	T38.0X4	T38.0X5	T38.0X6
ENT agent	T49.6X1	T49.6X2	T49.6X3	T49.6X4	T49.6X5	T49.6X6
ophthalmic preparation	T49.5X1	T49.5X2	T49.5X3	T49.5X4	T49.5X5	T49.5X6
topical NEC	T49.0X1	T49.0X2	T49.0X3	T49.0X4	T49.0X5	T49.0X6
Fluonid	T49.0X1	T49.0X2	T49.0X3	T49.0X4	T49.0X5	T49.0X6
Fluopromazine	T43.3X1	T43.3X2	T43.3X3	T43.3X4	T43.3X5	T43.3X6
Fluoroacetate	T60.8X1	T60.8X2	T60.8X3	T60.8X4	—	—
Fluorescein	T50.8X1	T50.8X2	T50.8X3	T50.8X4	T50.8X5	T50.8X6
Fluorhydrocortisone	T50.0X1	T50.0X2	T50.0X3	T50.0X4	T50.0X5	T50.0X6
Fluoride (nonmedicinal) (pesticide) (sodium) NEC	T60.8X1	T60.8X2	T60.8X3	T60.8X4	—	—
hydrogen — see Hydrofluoric acid						
medicinal NEC	T50.991	T50.992	T50.993	T50.994	T50.995	T50.996
dental use	T49.7X1	T49.7X2	T49.7X3	T49.7X4	T49.7X5	T49.7X6
not pesticide NEC	T54.91	T54.92	T54.93	T54.94	—	—
stannous	T49.7X1	T49.7X2	T49.7X3	T49.7X4	T49.7X5	T49.7X6
Fluorinated corticosteroids	T38.0X1	T38.0X2	T38.0X3	T38.0X4	T38.0X5	T38.0X6
Fluorine (gas)	T59.5X1	T59.5X2	T59.5X3	T59.5X4	—	—
salt — see Fluoride(s)						
Fluoristan	T49.7X1	T49.7X2	T49.7X3	T49.7X4	T49.7X5	T49.7X6
Fluormetholone	T49.0X1	T49.0X2	T49.0X3	T49.0X4	T49.0X5	T49.0X6
Fluoroacetate	T60.8X1	T60.8X2	T60.8X3	T60.8X4	—	—
Fluorocarbon monomer	T53.6X1	T53.6X2	T53.6X3	T53.6X4	—	—
Fluorocytosine	T37.8X1	T37.8X2	T37.8X3	T37.8X4	T37.8X5	T37.8X6
Fluorodeoxyuridine	T45.1X1	T45.1X2	T45.1X3	T45.1X4	T45.1X5	T45.1X6
Fluorometholone	T49.0X1	T49.0X2	T49.0X3	T49.0X4	T49.0X5	T49.0X6
ophthalmic preparation	T49.5X1	T49.5X2	T49.5X3	T49.5X4	T49.5X5	T49.5X6
Fluorophosphate insecticide	T60.0X1	T60.0X2	T60.0X3	T60.0X4	—	—
Fluorosol	T46.3X1	T46.3X2	T46.3X3	T46.3X4	T46.3X5	T46.3X6
Fluorouracil	T45.1X1	T45.1X2	T45.1X3	T45.1X4	T45.1X5	T45.1X6
Fluorphenylalanine	T49.5X1	T49.5X2	T49.5X3	T49.5X4	T49.5X5	T49.5X6
Fluothane	T41.0X1	T41.0X2	T41.0X3	T41.0X4	T41.0X5	T41.0X6
Fluoxetine	T43.221	T43.222	T43.223	T43.224	T43.225	T43.226
Fluoxymesterone	T38.7X1	T38.7X2	T38.7X3	T38.7X4	T38.7X5	T38.7X6
Flupenthixol	T43.4X1	T43.4X2	T43.4X3	T43.4X4	T43.4X5	T43.4X6
Flupentixol	T43.4X1	T43.4X2	T43.4X3	T43.4X4	T43.4X5	T43.4X6
Fluphenazine	T43.3X1	T43.3X2	T43.3X3	T43.3X4	T43.3X5	T43.3X6

◀ New ◀▥ Revised ~~deleted~~ Deleted

Substance	External Cause (T-Code)					
	Poisoning, Accidental (Unintentional)	Poisoning, Intentional Self-Harm	Poisoning, Assault	Poisoning, Undetermined	Adverse Effect	Underdosing
Fluprednidene	T49.0X1	T49.0X2	T49.0X3	T49.0X4	T49.0X5	T49.0X6
Fluprednisolone	T38.0X1	T38.0X2	T38.0X3	T38.0X4	T38.0X5	T38.0X6
Fluradoline	T39.8X1	T39.8X2	T39.8X3	T39.8X4	T39.8X5	T39.8X6
Flurandrenolide	T49.0X1	T49.0X2	T49.0X3	T49.0X4	T49.0X5	T49.0X6
Flurandrenolone	T49.0X1	T49.0X2	T49.0X3	T49.0X4	T49.0X5	T49.0X6
Flurazepam	T42.4X1	T42.4X2	T42.4X3	T42.4X4	T42.4X5	T42.4X6
Flurbiprofen	T39.311	T39.312	T39.313	T39.314	T39.315	T39.316
Flurobate	T49.0X1	T49.0X2	T49.0X3	T49.0X4	T49.0X5	T49.0X6
Flurotyl	T43.291	T43.292	T43.293	T43.294	T43.295	T43.296
Fluroxene	T41.0X1	T41.0X2	T41.0X3	T41.0X4	T41.0X5	T41.0X6
Fluspirilene	T43.591	T43.592	T43.593	T43.594	T43.595	T43.596
Flutamide	T38.6X1	T38.6X2	T38.6X3	T38.6X4	T38.6X5	T38.6X6
Flutazolam	T42.4X1	T42.4X2	T42.4X3	T42.4X4	T42.4X5	T42.4X6
Fluticasone propionate	T49.1X1	T49.1X2	T49.1X3	T49.1X4	T49.1X5	T49.1X6
Flutoprazepam	T42.4X1	T42.4X2	T42.4X3	T42.4X4	T42.4X5	T42.4X6
Flutropium bromide	T48.6X1	T48.6X2	T48.6X3	T48.6X4	T48.6X5	T48.6X6
Fluvoxamine	T43.221	T43.222	T43.223	T43.224	T43.225	T43.226
Folacin	T45.8X1	T45.8X2	T45.8X3	T45.8X4	T45.8X5	T45.8X6
Folic acid	T45.8X1	T45.8X2	T45.8X3	T45.8X4	T45.8X5	T45.8X6
with ferrous salt	T45.2X1	T45.2X2	T45.2X3	T45.2X4	T45.2X5	T45.2X6
antagonist	T45.1X1	T45.1X2	T45.1X3	T45.1X4	T45.1X5	T45.1X6
Folinic acid	T45.8X1	T45.8X2	T45.8X3	T45.8X4	T45.8X5	T45.8X6
Folium stramoniae	T48.6X1	T48.6X2	T48.6X3	T48.6X4	T48.6X5	T48.6X6
Follicle-stimulating hormone, human	T38.811	T38.812	T38.813	T38.814	T38.815	T38.816
Folpet	T60.3X1	T60.3X2	T60.3X3	T60.3X4	—	—
Fominoben	T48.3X1	T48.3X2	T48.3X3	T48.3X4	T48.3X5	T48.3X6
Food, foodstuffs, noxious, nonbacterial, NEC	T62.91	T62.92	T62.93	T62.94	—	—
berries	T62.1X1	T62.1X2	T62.1X3	T62.1X4	—	—
fish — see also Fish	T61.91	T61.92	T61.93	T61.94	—	—
mushrooms	T62.0X1	T62.0X2	T62.0X3	T62.0X4	—	—
plants	T62.2X1	T62.2X2	T62.2X3	T62.2X4	—	—
seafood	T61.91	T61.92	T61.93	T61.94	—	—
specified NEC	T61.8X1	T61.8X2	T61.8X3	T61.8X4	—	—
seeds	T62.2X1	T62.2X2	T62.2X3	T62.2X4	—	—
shellfish	T61.781	T61.782	T61.783	T61.784	—	—
specified NEC	T62.8X1	T62.8X2	T62.8X3	T62.8X4	—	—
Fool's parsley	T62.2X1	T62.2X2	T62.2X3	T62.2X4	—	—
Formaldehyde (solution), gas or vapor	T59.2X1	T59.2X2	T59.2X3	T59.2X4	—	—
fungicide	T60.3X1	T60.3X2	T60.3X3	T60.3X4	—	—

TABLE OF DRUGS AND CHEMICALS

◄ New   ◄ Revised   ~~deleted~~ Deleted

Substance	External Cause (T-Code)					
	Poisoning, Accidental (Unintentional)	Poisoning, Intentional Self-Harm	Poisoning, Assault	Poisoning, Undetermined	Adverse Effect	Underdosing
Formalin	T59.2X1	T59.2X2	T59.2X3	T59.2X4	—	—
fungicide	T60.3X1	T60.3X2	T60.3X3	T60.3X4	—	—
vapor	T59.2X1	T59.2X2	T59.2X3	T59.2X4	—	—
Formic acid	T54.2X1	T54.2X2	T54.2X3	T54.2X4	—	—
vapor	T59.891	T59.892	T59.893	T59.894	—	—
Foscarnet sodium	T37.5X1	T37.5X2	T37.5X3	T37.5X4	T37.5X5	T37.5X6
Fosfestrol	T38.5X1	T38.5X2	T38.5X3	T38.5X4	T38.5X5	T38.5X6
Fosfomycin	T36.8X1	T36.8X2	T36.8X3	T36.8X4	T36.8X5	T36.8X6
Fosfonet sodium	T37.5X1	T37.5X2	T37.5X3	T37.5X4	T37.5X5	T37.5X6
Fosinopril	T46.4X1	T46.4X2	T46.4X3	T46.4X4	T46.4X5	T46.4X6
sodium	T46.4X1	T46.4X2	T46.4X3	T46.4X4	T46.4X5	T46.4X6
Fowler's solution	T57.0X1	T57.0X2	T57.0X3	T57.0X4	—	—
Foxglove	T62.2X1	T62.2X2	T62.2X3	T62.2X4	—	—
Framycetin	T36.5X1	T36.5X2	T36.5X3	T36.5X4	T36.5X5	T36.5X6
Frangula	T47.2X1	T47.2X2	T47.2X3	T47.2X4	T47.2X5	T47.2X6
extract	T47.2X1	T47.2X2	T47.2X3	T47.2X4	T47.2X5	T47.2X6
Frei antigen	T50.8X1	T50.8X2	T50.8X3	T50.8X4	T50.8X5	T50.8X6
Freon	T53.5X1	T53.5X2	T53.5X3	T53.5X4	—	—
Fructose	T50.3X1	T50.3X2	T50.3X3	T50.3X4	T50.3X5	T50.3X6
Frusemide	T50.1X1	T50.1X2	T50.1X3	T50.1X4	T50.1X5	T50.1X6
FSH	T38.811	T38.812	T38.813	T38.814	T38.815	T38.816
Ftorafur	T45.1X1	T45.1X2	T45.1X3	T45.1X4	T45.1X5	T45.1X6
Fuel						
automobile	T52.0X1	T52.0X2	T52.0X3	T52.0X4	—	—
exhaust gas, not in transit	T58.01	T58.02	T58.03	T58.04	—	—
vapor NEC	T52.0X1	T52.0X2	T52.0X3	T52.0X4	—	—
gas (domestic use) — see also Carbon, monoxide, fuel, utility	T59.891	T59.892	T59.893	T59.894	—	—
utility	T59.891	T59.892	T59.893	T59.894	—	—
in mobile container	T59.891	T59.892	T59.893	T59.894	—	—
incomplete combustion of — see Carbon, monoxide, fuel, utility						
piped (natural)	T59.891	T59.892	T59.893	T59.894	—	—
industrial, incomplete combustion	T58.8X1	T58.8X2	T58.8X3	T58.8X4	—	—
Fugillin	T36.8X1	T36.8X2	T36.8X3	T36.8X4	T36.8X5	T36.8X6
Fulminate of mercury	T56.1X1	T56.1X2	T56.1X3	T56.1X4	—	—
Fulvicin	T36.7X1	T36.7X2	T36.7X3	T36.7X4	T36.7X5	T36.7X6
Fumadil	T36.8X1	T36.8X2	T36.8X3	T36.8X4	T36.8X5	T36.8X6
Fumagillin	T36.8X1	T36.8X2	T36.8X3	T36.8X4	T36.8X5	T36.8X6
Fumaric acid	T49.4X1	T49.4X2	T49.4X3	T49.4X4	T49.4X5	T49.4X6
Fumes (from)	T59.91	T59.92	T59.93	T59.94	—	—
carbon monoxide — see Carbon, monoxide						
charcoal (domestic use) — see Charcoal, fumes						

◀ New   ◀▥ Revised   ~~deleted~~ Deleted

Substance	Poisoning, Accidental (Unintentional)	Poisoning, Intentional Self-Harm	Poisoning, Assault	Poisoning, Undetermined	Adverse Effect	Underdosing
Fumes *(Continued)*						
chloroform — *see Chloroform*						
coke (in domestic stoves, fireplaces) — *see Coke, fumes*						
corrosive NEC	T54.91	T54.92	T54.93	T54.94	—	—
ether — *see ether*						
freons	T53.5X1	T53.5X2	T53.5X3	T53.5X4	—	—
hydrocarbons	T59.891	T59.892	T59.893	T59.894	—	—
petroleum (liquefied)	T59.891	T59.892	T59.893	T59.894	—	—
distributed through pipes (pure or mixed with air)	T59.891	T59.892	T59.893	T59.894	—	—
lead — *see lead*						
metal — *see Metals, or the specified metal*						
nitrogen dioxide	T59.0X1	T59.0X2	T59.0X3	T59.0X4	—	—
pesticides — *see Pesticides*						
petroleum (liquefied)	T59.891	T59.892	T59.893	T59.894	—	—
distributed through pipes (pure or mixed with air)	T59.891	T59.892	T59.893	T59.894	—	—
polyester	T59.891	T59.892	T59.893	T59.894	—	—
specified source NEC — *see also substance specified*	T59.891	T59.892	T59.893	T59.894	—	—
sulfur dioxide	T59.1X1	T59.1X2	T59.1X3	T59.1X4	—	—
Fumigant NEC	T60.91	T60.92	T60.93	T60.94	—	—
Fungi, noxious, used as food	T62.0X1	T62.0X2	T62.0X3	T62.0X4	—	—
Fungicide NEC (nonmedicinal)	T60.3X1	T60.3X2	T60.3X3	T60.3X4	—	—
Fungizone	T36.7X1	T36.7X2	T36.7X3	T36.7X4	T36.7X5	T36.7X6
topical	T49.0X1	T49.0X2	T49.0X3	T49.0X4	T49.0X5	T49.0X6
Furacin	T49.0X1	T49.0X2	T49.0X3	T49.0X4	T49.0X5	T49.0X6
Furadantin	T37.91	T37.92	T37.93	T37.94	T37.95	T37.96
Furazolidone	T37.8X1	T37.8X2	T37.8X3	T37.8X4	T37.8X5	T37.8X6
Furazolium chloride	T49.0X1	T49.0X2	T49.0X3	T49.0X4	T49.0X5	T49.0X6
Furfural	T52.8X1	T52.8X2	T52.8X3	T52.8X4	—	—
Furnace (coal burning) (domestic), gas from industrial	T58.2X1	T58.2X2	T58.2X3	T58.2X4	—	—
industrial	T58.8X1	T58.8X2	T58.8X3	T58.8X4	—	—
Furniture polish	T65.891	T65.892	T65.893	T65.894	—	—
Furosemide	T50.1X1	T50.1X2	T50.1X3	T50.1X4	T50.1X5	T50.1X6
Furoxone	T37.91	T37.92	T37.93	T37.94	T37.95	T37.96
Fursultiamine	T45.2X1	T45.2X2	T45.2X3	T45.2X4	T45.2X5	T45.2X6
Fusafungine	T36.8X1	T36.8X2	T36.8X3	T36.8X4	T36.8X5	T36.8X6
Fusel oil (any) (amyl) (butyl) (propyl), vapor	T51.3X1	T51.3X2	T51.3X3	T51.3X4	—	—
Fusidate (ethanolamine) (sodium)	T36.8X1	T36.8X2	T36.8X3	T36.8X4	T36.8X5	T36.8X6
Fusidic acid	T36.8X1	T36.8X2	T36.8X3	T36.8X4	T36.8X5	T36.8X6
Fytic acid, nonasodium	T50.6X1	T50.6X2	T50.6X3	T50.6X4	T50.6X5	T50.6X6

TABLE OF DRUGS AND CHEMICALS

◀ New ◀ Revised ~~deleted~~ Deleted

Substance	External Cause (T-Code)					
	Poisoning, Accidental (Unintentional)	Poisoning, Intentional Self-Harm	Poisoning, Assault	Poisoning, Undetermined	Adverse Effect	Underdosing
G						
GABA	T43.8X1	T43.8X2	T43.8X3	T43.8X4	T43.8X5	T43.8X6
Gadopentetic acid	T50.8X1	T50.8X2	T50.8X3	T50.8X4	T50.8X5	T50.8X6
Galactose	T50.3X1	T50.3X2	T50.3X3	T50.3X4	T50.3X5	T50.3X6
b-Galactosidase	T47.5X1	T47.5X2	T47.5X3	T47.5X4	T47.5X5	T47.5X6
Galantamine	T44.0X1	T44.0X2	T44.0X3	T44.0X4	T44.0X5	T44.0X6
Gallamine (triethiodide)	T48.1X1	T48.1X2	T48.1X3	T48.1X4	T48.1X5	T48.1X6
Gallium citrate	T50.991	T50.992	T50.993	T50.994	T50.995	T50.996
Gallopamil	T46.1X1	T46.1X2	T46.1X3	T46.1X4	T46.1X5	T46.1X6
Gamboge	T47.2X1	T47.2X2	T47.2X3	T47.2X4	T47.2X5	T47.2X6
Gamimune	T50.Z11	T50.Z12	T50.Z13	T50.Z14	T50.Z15	T50.Z16
Gamma-aminobutyric acid	T43.8X1	T43.8X2	T43.8X3	T43.8X4	T43.8X5	T43.8X6
Gamma-benzene hexachloride (medicinal)	T49.0X1	T49.0X2	T49.0X3	T49.0X4	T49.0X5	T49.0X6
nonmedicinal, vapor	T53.6X1	T53.6X2	T53.6X3	T53.6X4	—	—
Gamma-BHC (medicinal) — see also Gamma-benzene hexachloride	T49.0X1	T49.0X2	T49.0X3	T49.0X4	T49.0X5	T49.0X6
Gamma globulin	T50.Z11	T50.Z12	T50.Z13	T50.Z14	T50.Z15	T50.Z16
Gamulin	T50.Z11	T50.Z12	T50.Z13	T50.Z14	T50.Z15	T50.Z16
Ganciclovir (sodium)	T37.5X1	T37.5X2	T37.5X3	T37.5X4	T37.5X5	T37.5X6
Ganglionic blocking drug NEC	T44.2X1	T44.2X2	T44.2X3	T44.2X4	T44.2X5	T44.2X6
specified NEC	T44.2X1	T44.2X2	T44.2X3	T44.2X4	T44.2X5	T44.2X6
Ganja	T40.7X1	T40.7X2	T40.7X3	T40.7X4	T40.7X5	T40.7X6
Garamycin	T36.5X1	T36.5X2	T36.5X3	T36.5X4	T36.5X5	T36.5X6
ophthalmic preparation	T49.5X1	T49.5X2	T49.5X3	T49.5X4	T49.5X5	T49.5X6
topical NEC	T49.0X1	T49.0X2	T49.0X3	T49.0X4	T49.0X5	T49.0X6
Gardenal	T42.3X1	T42.3X2	T42.3X3	T42.3X4	T42.3X5	T42.3X6
Gardepanyl	T42.3X1	T42.3X2	T42.3X3	T42.3X4	T42.3X5	T42.3X6
Gas	T59.91	T59.92	T59.93	T59.94	—	—
acetylene	T59.891	T59.892	T59.893	T59.894	—	—
incomplete combustion of	T58.11	T58.12	T58.13	T58.14	—	—
air contaminants, source or type not specified	T59.91	T59.92	T59.93	T59.94	—	—
anesthetic	T41.0X1	T41.0X2	T41.0X3	T41.0X4	T41.0X5	T41.0X6
blast furnace	T58.8X1	T58.8X2	T58.8X3	T58.8X4	—	—
butane — see butane						
carbon monoxide — see Carbon, monoxide						
chlorine	T59.4X1	T59.4X2	T59.4X3	T59.4X4	—	—
coal	T58.2X1	T58.2X2	T58.2X3	T58.2X4	—	—
cyanide	T57.3X1	T57.3X2	T57.3X3	T57.3X4	—	—
dicyanogen	T65.0X1	T65.0X2	T65.0X3	T65.0X4	—	—
domestic — see Domestic gas	T57.91	T57.92	T57.93	T57.94	—	—

◀ New   ◀▥ Revised   ~~deleted~~ Deleted

TABLE OF DRUGS AND CHEMICALS

Substance	External Cause (T-Code)					
	Poisoning, Accidental (Unintentional)	Poisoning, Intentional Self-Harm	Poisoning, Assault	Poisoning, Undetermined	Adverse Effect	Underdosing
Gas *(Continued)*						
exhaust	T57.91	T57.92	T57.93	T57.94	—	—
from utility (for cooking, heating, or lighting) (after combustion) — *see Carbon, monoxide, fuel, utility*						
prior to combustion	T59.891	T59.892	T59.893	T59.894	—	—
from wood or coal-burning stove or fireplace	T57.91	T57.92	T57.93	T57.94	—	—
fuel (domestic use) (after combustion) — *see also Carbon, monoxide, fuel*	T57.91	T57.92	T57.93	T57.94	—	—
industrial use	T58.8X1	T58.8X2	T58.8X3	T58.8X4	—	—
prior to combustion	T59.891	T59.892	T59.893	T59.894	—	—
utility	T59.891	T59.892	T59.893	T59.894	—	—
in mobile container	T59.891	T59.892	T59.893	T59.894	—	—
incomplete combustion of — *see Carbon, monoxide, fuel, utility*						
piped (natural)	T59.891	T59.892	T59.893	T59.894	—	—
garage	T58.01	T58.02	T58.03	T58.04	—	—
hydrocarbon NEC	T59.891	T59.892	T59.893	T59.894	—	—
incomplete combustion of — *see Carbon, monoxide, fuel, utility*						
liquefied — *see butane*						
piped	T59.891	T59.892	T59.893	T59.894	—	—
hydrocyanic acid	T65.0X1	T65.0X2	T65.0X3	T65.0X4	—	—
illuminating (after combustion)	T58.11	T58.12	T58.13	T58.14	—	—
prior to combustion	T59.891	T59.892	T59.893	T59.894	—	—
incomplete combustion, any — *see Carbon, monoxide*						
kiln	T58.8X1	T58.8X2	T58.8X3	T58.8X4	—	—
lacrimogenic	T59.3X1	T59.3X2	T59.3X3	T59.3X4	—	—
liquefied petroleum — *see butane*						
marsh	T59.891	T59.892	T59.893	T59.894	—	—
motor exhaust, not in transit	T58.01	T58.02	T58.03	T58.04	—	—
mustard, not in war	T59.891	T59.892	T59.893	T59.894	—	—
natural	T59.891	T59.892	T59.893	T59.894	—	—
nerve, not in war	T59.91	T59.92	T59.93	T59.94	—	—
oil	T52.0X1	T52.0X2	T52.0X3	T52.0X4	—	—
petroleum (liquefied) (distributed in mobile containers)	T59.891	T59.892	T59.893	T59.894	—	—
piped (pure or mixed with air)	T59.891	T59.892	T59.893	T59.894	—	—
piped (manufactured) (natural) NEC	T59.891	T59.892	T59.893	T59.894	—	—
producer	T58.8X1	T58.8X2	T58.8X3	T58.8X4	—	—
propane — *see propane*						
refrigerant (chlorofluoro-carbon)	T53.5X1	T53.5X2	T53.5X3	T53.5X4	—	—
not chlorofluoro-carbon	T59.891	T59.892	T59.893	T59.894	—	—
sewer	T59.91	T59.92	T59.93	T59.94	—	—
specified source NEC	T59.91	T59.92	T59.93	T59.94	—	—

◀ New ◀ Revised ~~deleted~~ Deleted

Substance	External Cause (T-Code)					
	Poisoning, Accidental (Unintentional)	Poisoning, Intentional Self-Harm	Poisoning, Assault	Poisoning, Undetermined	Adverse Effect	Underdosing
Gas *(Continued)*						
stove (after combustion)	T58.11	T58.12	T58.13	T58.14	—	—
tear	T59.3X1	T59.3X2	T59.3X3	T59.3X4	—	—
therapeutic	T41.5X1	T41.5X2	T41.5X3	T41.5X4	T41.5X5	T41.5X6
utility (for cooking, heating, or lighting) (piped) NEC	T59.891	T59.892	T59.893	T59.894	—	—
in mobile container	T59.891	T59.892	T59.893	T59.894	—	—
incomplete combustion of—*see Carbon, monoxide, fuel, utilty*						
piped (natural)	T59.891	T59.892	T59.893	T59.894	—	—
water	T58.11	T58.12	T58.13	T58.14	—	—
incomplete combustion of—*see Carbon, monoxide, fuel, utility*						
Gaseous substance—*see Gas*						
Gasoline	T52.0X1	T52.0X2	T52.0X3	T52.0X4	—	—
vapor	T52.0X1	T52.0X2	T52.0X3	T52.0X4	—	—
Gastric enzymes	T47.5X1	T47.5X2	T47.5X3	T47.5X4	T47.5X5	T47.5X6
Gastrografin	T50.8X1	T50.8X2	T50.8X3	T50.8X4	T50.8X5	T50.8X6
Gastrointestinal drug	T47.91	T47.92	T47.93	T47.94	T47.95	T47.96
biological	T47.8X1	T47.8X2	T47.8X3	T47.8X4	T47.8X5	T47.8X6
specified NEC	T47.8X1	T47.8X2	T47.8X3	T47.8X4	T47.8X5	T47.8X6
Gaultheria procumbens	T62.2X1	T62.2X2	T62.2X3	T62.2X4	—	—
Gelatin (intravenous)	T45.8X1	T45.8X2	T45.8X3	T45.8X4	T45.8X5	T45.8X6
absorbable (sponge)	T45.7X1	T45.7X2	T45.7X3	T45.7X4	T45.7X5	T45.7X6
Gefarnate	T44.3X1	T44.3X2	T44.3X3	T44.3X4	T44.3X5	T44.3X6
Gelfilm	T49.8X1	T49.8X2	T49.8X3	T49.8X4	T49.8X5	T49.8X6
Gelfoam	T45.7X1	T45.7X2	T45.7X3	T45.7X4	T45.7X5	T45.7X6
Gelsemine	T50.991	T50.992	T50.993	T50.994	T50.995	T50.996
Gelsemium (sempervirens)	T62.2X1	T62.2X2	T62.2X3	T62.2X4	—	—
Gemeprost	T48.0X1	T48.0X2	T48.0X3	T48.0X4	T48.0X5	T48.0X6
Gemfibrozil	T46.6X1	T46.6X2	T46.6X3	T46.6X4	T46.6X5	T46.6X6
Gemonil	T42.3X1	T42.3X2	T42.3X3	T42.3X4	T42.3X5	T42.3X6
Gentamicin	T36.5X1	T36.5X2	T36.5X3	T36.5X4	T36.5X5	T36.5X6
ophthalmic preparation	T49.5X1	T49.5X2	T49.5X3	T49.5X4	T49.5X5	T49.5X6
topical NEC	T49.0X1	T49.0X2	T49.0X3	T49.0X4	T49.0X5	T49.0X6
Gentian	T47.5X1	T47.5X2	T47.5X3	T47.5X4	T47.5X5	T47.5X6
violet	T49.0X1	T49.0X2	T49.0X3	T49.0X4	T49.0X5	T49.0X6
Gepefrine	T44.4X1	T44.4X2	T44.4X3	T44.4X4	T44.4X5	T44.4X6
Gestonorone caproate	T38.5X1	T38.5X2	T38.5X3	T38.5X4	T38.5X5	T38.5X6
Gexane	T49.0X1	T49.0X2	T49.0X3	T49.0X4	T49.0X5	T49.0X6
Gila monster (venom)	T63.111	T63.112	T63.113	T63.114	—	—
Ginger	T47.5X1	T47.5X2	T47.5X3	T47.5X4	T47.5X5	T47.5X6
Jamaica—*see Jamaica, ginger*						

◄ New ◄▪▪ Revised ~~deleted~~ Deleted

Substance	Poisoning, Accidental (Unintentional)	Poisoning, Intentional Self-Harm	Poisoning, Assault	Poisoning, Undetermined	Adverse Effect	Underdosing
			External Cause (T-Code)			
Gitalin	T46.0X1	T46.0X2	T46.0X3	T46.0X4	T46.0X5	T46.0X6
amorphous	T46.0X1	T46.0X2	T46.0X3	T46.0X4	T46.0X5	T46.0X6
Gitaloxin	T46.0X1	T46.0X2	T46.0X3	T46.0X4	T46.0X5	T46.0X6
Gitoxin	T46.0X1	T46.0X2	T46.0X3	T46.0X4	T46.0X5	T46.0X6
Glafenine	T39.8X1	T39.8X2	T39.8X3	T39.8X4	T39.8X5	T39.8X6
Glandular extract (medicinal) NEC	T50.Z91	T50.Z92	T50.Z93	T50.Z94	T50.Z95	T50.Z96
Glaucarubin	T37.3X1	T37.3X2	T37.3X3	T37.3X4	T37.3X5	T37.3X6
Glibenclamide	T38.3X1	T38.3X2	T38.3X3	T38.3X4	T38.3X5	T38.3X6
Glibornuride	T38.3X1	T38.3X2	T38.3X3	T38.3X4	T38.3X5	T38.3X6
Gliclazide	T38.3X1	T38.3X2	T38.3X3	T38.3X4	T38.3X5	T38.3X6
Glimidine	T38.3X1	T38.3X2	T38.3X3	T38.3X4	T38.3X5	T38.3X6
Glipizide	T38.3X1	T38.3X2	T38.3X3	T38.3X4	T38.3X5	T38.3X6
Gliquidone	T38.3X1	T38.3X2	T38.3X3	T38.3X4	T38.3X5	T38.3X6
Glisolamide	T38.3X1	T38.3X2	T38.3X3	T38.3X4	T38.3X5	T38.3X6
Glisoxepide	T38.3X1	T38.3X2	T38.3X3	T38.3X4	T38.3X5	T38.3X6
Globin zinc insulin	T38.3X1	T38.3X2	T38.3X3	T38.3X4	T38.3X5	T38.3X6
Globulin						
antilymphocytic	T50.Z11	T50.Z12	T50.Z13	T50.Z14	T50.Z15	T50.Z16
antirhesus	T50.Z11	T50.Z12	T50.Z13	T50.Z14	T50.Z15	T50.Z16
antivenin	T50.Z11	T50.Z12	T50.Z13	T50.Z14	T50.Z15	T50.Z16
antiviral	T50.Z11	T50.Z12	T50.Z13	T50.Z14	T50.Z15	T50.Z16
Glucagon	T38.3X1	T38.3X2	T38.3X3	T38.3X4	T38.3X5	T38.3X6
Glucocorticoids	T38.0X1	T38.0X2	T38.0X3	T38.0X4	T38.0X5	T38.0X6
Glucocorticosteroid	T38.0X1	T38.0X2	T38.0X3	T38.0X4	T38.0X5	T38.0X6
Gluconic acid	T50.991	T50.992	T50.993	T50.994	T50.995	T50.996
Glucosamine sulfate	T39.4X1	T39.4X2	T39.4X3	T39.4X4	T39.4X5	T39.4X6
Glucose	T50.3X1	T50.3X2	T50.3X3	T50.3X4	T50.3X5	T50.3X6
with sodium chloride	T50.3X1	T50.3X2	T50.3X3	T50.3X4	T50.3X5	T50.3X6
Glucosulfone sodium	T37.1X1	T37.1X2	T37.1X3	T37.1X4	T37.1X5	T37.1X6
Glucurolactone	T47.8X1	T47.8X2	T47.8X3	T47.8X4	T47.8X5	T47.8X6
Glue NEC	T52.8X1	T52.8X2	T52.8X3	T52.8X4	—	—
Glutamic acid	T47.5X1	T47.5X2	T47.5X3	T47.5X4	T47.5X5	T47.5X6
Glutaral (medicinal)	T49.0X1	T49.0X2	T49.0X3	T49.0X4	T49.0X5	T49.0X6
nonmedicinal	T65.891	T65.892	T65.893	T65.894	—	—
Glutaraldehyde (nonmedicinal)	T65.891	T65.892	T65.893	T65.894	—	—
medicinal	T49.0X1	T49.0X2	T49.0X3	T49.0X4	T49.0X5	T49.0X6
Glutathione	T50.6X1	T50.6X2	T50.6X3	T50.6X4	T50.6X5	T50.6X6
Glutethimide	T42.6X1	T42.6X2	T42.6X3	T42.6X4	T42.6X5	T42.6X6
Glyburide	T38.3X1	T38.3X2	T38.3X3	T38.3X4	T38.3X5	T38.3X6

◄ New   ◀▥ Revised   ~~deleted~~ Deleted

TABLE OF DRUGS AND CHEMICALS

Substance	Poisoning, Accidental (Unintentional)	Poisoning, Intentional Self-Harm	Poisoning, Assault	Poisoning, Undetermined	Adverse Effect	Underdosing
			External Cause (T-Code)			
Glycerin	T47.4X1	T47.4X2	T47.4X3	T47.4X4	T47.4X5	T47.4X6
Glycerol	T47.4X1	T47.4X2	T47.4X3	T47.4X4	T47.4X5	T47.4X6
borax	T49.6X1	T49.6X2	T49.6X3	T49.6X4	T49.6X5	T49.6X6
intravenous	T50.3X1	T50.3X2	T50.3X3	T50.3X4	T50.3X5	T50.3X6
iodinated	T48.4X1	T48.4X2	T48.4X3	T48.4X4	T48.4X5	T48.4X6
Glycerophosphate	T50.991	T50.992	T50.993	T50.994	T50.995	T50.996
Glyceryl						
gualacolate	T48.4X1	T48.4X2	T48.4X3	T48.4X4	T48.4X5	T48.4X6
nitrate	T46.3X1	T46.3X2	T46.3X3	T46.3X4	T46.3X5	T46.3X6
triacetate (topical)	T49.0X1	T49.0X2	T49.0X3	T49.0X4	T49.0X5	T49.0X6
trinitrate	T46.3X1	T46.3X2	T46.3X3	T46.3X4	T46.3X5	T46.3X6
Glycine	T50.3X1	T50.3X2	T50.3X3	T50.3X4	T50.3X5	T50.3X6
Glyclopyramide	T38.3X1	T38.3X2	T38.3X3	T38.3X4	T38.3X5	T38.3X6
Glycobiarsol	T37.3X1	T37.3X2	T37.3X3	T37.3X4	T37.3X5	T37.3X6
Glycols (ether)	T52.3X1	T52.3X2	T52.3X3	T52.3X4	—	—
Glyconiazide	T37.1X1	T37.1X2	T37.1X3	T37.1X4	T37.1X5	T37.1X6
Glycopyrrolate	T44.3X1	T44.3X2	T44.3X3	T44.3X4	T44.3X5	T44.3X6
Glycopyrronium	T44.3X1	T44.3X2	T44.3X3	T44.3X4	T44.3X5	T44.3X6
bromide	T44.3X1	T44.3X2	T44.3X3	T44.3X4	T44.3X5	T44.3X6
Glycoside, cardiac (stimulant)	T46.0X1	T46.0X2	T46.0X3	T46.0X4	T46.0X5	T46.0X6
Glycyclamide	T38.3X1	T38.3X2	T38.3X3	T38.3X4	T38.3X5	T38.3X6
Glycyrrhiza extract	T48.4X1	T48.4X2	T48.4X3	T48.4X4	T48.4X5	T48.4X6
Glycyrrhizic acid	T48.4X1	T48.4X2	T48.4X3	T48.4X4	T48.4X5	T48.4X6
Glycyrrhizinate potassium	T48.4X1	T48.4X2	T48.4X3	T48.4X4	T48.4X5	T48.4X6
Glymidine sodium	T38.3X1	T38.3X2	T38.3X3	T38.3X4	T38.3X5	T38.3X6
Glyphosate	T60.3X1	T60.3X2	T60.3X3	T60.3X4	—	—
Glyphylline	T48.6X1	T48.6X2	T48.6X3	T48.6X4	T48.6X5	T48.6X6
Gold						
colloidal (I98Au)	T45.1X1	T45.1X2	T45.1X3	T45.1X4	T45.1X5	T45.1X6
salts	T39.4X1	T39.4X2	T39.4X3	T39.4X4	T39.4X5	T39.4X6
Golden sulfide of antimony	T56.891	T56.892	T56.893	T56.894	—	—
Goldylocks	T62.2X1	T62.2X2	T62.2X3	T62.2X4	—	—
Gonadal tissue extract	T38.901	T38.902	T38.903	T38.904	T38.905	T38.906
female	T38.5X1	T38.5X2	T38.5X3	T38.5X4	T38.5X5	T38.5X6
male	T38.7X1	T38.7X2	T38.7X3	T38.7X4	T38.7X5	T38.7X6
Gonadorelin	T38.891	T38.892	T38.893	T38.894	T38.895	T38.896
Gonadotropin	T38.891	T38.892	T38.893	T38.894	T38.895	T38.896
chorionic	T38.891	T38.892	T38.893	T38.894	T38.895	T38.896
pituitary	T38.811	T38.812	T38.813	T38.814	T38.815	T38.816
Goserelin	T45.1X1	T45.1X2	T45.1X3	T45.1X4	T45.1X5	T45.1X6

◀ New ◀▥ Revised ~~deleted~~ Deleted

Substance	Poisoning, Accidental (Unintentional)	Poisoning, Intentional Self-Harm	Poisoning, Assault	Poisoning, Undetermined	Adverse Effect	Underdosing
	External Cause (T-Code)					
Grain alcohol	T51.0X1	T51.0X2	T51.0X3	T51.0X4	—	—
Gramicidin	T49.0X1	T49.0X2	T49.0X3	T49.0X4	T49.0X5	T49.0X6
Granisetron	T45.0X1	T45.0X2	T45.0X3	T45.0X4	T45.0X5	T45.0X6
Gratiola officinalis	T62.2X1	T62.2X2	T62.2X3	T62.2X4	—	—
Grease	T65.891	T65.892	T65.893	T65.894	—	—
Green hellebore	T62.2X1	T62.2X2	T62.2X3	T62.2X4	—	—
Green soap	T49.2X1	T49.2X2	T49.2X3	T49.2X4	T49.2X5	T49.2X6
Grifulvin	T36.7X1	T36.7X2	T36.7X3	T36.7X4	T36.7X5	T36.7X6
Griseofulvin	T36.7X1	T36.7X2	T36.7X3	T36.7X4	T36.7X5	T36.7X6
Growth hormone	T38.811	T38.812	T38.813	T38.814	T38.815	T38.816
Guaiacol derivatives	T48.4X1	T48.4X2	T48.4X3	T48.4X4	T48.4X5	T48.4X6
Guaiac reagent	T50.991	T50.992	T50.993	T50.994	T50.995	T50.996
Guaifenesin	T48.4X1	T48.4X2	T48.4X3	T48.4X4	T48.4X5	T48.4X6
Guaimesal	T48.4X1	T48.4X2	T48.4X3	T48.4X4	T48.4X5	T48.4X6
Guaiphenesin	T48.4X1	T48.4X2	T48.4X3	T48.4X4	T48.4X5	T48.4X6
Guamecycline	T36.4X1	T36.4X2	T36.4X3	T36.4X4	T36.4X5	T36.4X6
Guanabenz	T46.5X1	T46.5X2	T46.5X3	T46.5X4	T46.5X5	T46.5X6
Guanacline	T46.5X1	T46.5X2	T46.5X3	T46.5X4	T46.5X5	T46.5X6
Guanadrel	T46.5X1	T46.5X2	T46.5X3	T46.5X4	T46.5X5	T46.5X6
Guanatol	T37.2X1	T37.2X2	T37.2X3	T37.2X4	T37.2X5	T37.2X6
Guanethidine	T46.5X1	T46.5X2	T46.5X3	T46.5X4	T46.5X5	T46.5X6
Guanfacine	T46.5X1	T46.5X2	T46.5X3	T46.5X4	T46.5X5	T46.5X6
Guano	T65.891	T65.892	T65.893	T65.894	—	—
Guanochlor	T46.5X1	T46.5X2	T46.5X3	T46.5X4	T46.5X5	T46.5X6
Guanoclor	T46.5X1	T46.5X2	T46.5X3	T46.5X4	T46.5X5	T46.5X6
Guanoctine	T46.5X1	T46.5X2	T46.5X3	T46.5X4	T46.5X5	T46.5X6
Guanoxabenz	T46.5X1	T46.5X2	T46.5X3	T46.5X4	T46.5X5	T46.5X6
Guanoxan	T46.5X1	T46.5X2	T46.5X3	T46.5X4	T46.5X5	T46.5X6
Guar gum (medicinal)	T46.6X1	T46.6X2	T46.6X3	T46.6X4	T46.6X5	T46.6X6
H						
Hachimycin	T36.7X1	T36.7X2	T36.7X3	T36.7X4	T36.7X5	T36.7X6
Hair						
dye	T49.4X1	T49.4X2	T49.4X3	T49.4X4	T49.4X5	T49.4X6
preparation NEC	T49.4X1	T49.4X2	T49.4X3	T49.4X4	T49.4X5	T49.4X6
Halazepam	T42.4X1	T42.4X2	T42.4X3	T42.4X4	T42.4X5	T42.4X6
Halcinolone	T49.0X1	T49.0X2	T49.0X3	T49.0X4	T49.0X5	T49.0X6
Halcinonide	T49.0X1	T49.0X2	T49.0X3	T49.0X4	T49.0X5	T49.0X6
Halethazole	T49.0X1	T49.0X2	T49.0X3	T49.0X4	T49.0X5	T49.0X6
Hallucinogen NEC	T40.901	T40.902	T40.903	T40.904	T40.905	T40.906

◀ New   ◀ Revised   ~~deleted~~ Deleted

TABLE OF DRUGS AND CHEMICALS

Substance	External Cause (T-Code)					
	Poisoning, Accidental (Unintentional)	Poisoning, Intentional Self-Harm	Poisoning, Assault	Poisoning, Undetermined	Adverse Effect	Underdosing
Halofantrine	T37.2X1	T37.2X2	T37.2X3	T37.2X4	T37.2X5	T37.2X6
Halofenate	T46.6X1	T46.6X2	T46.6X3	T46.6X4	T46.6X5	T46.6X6
Halometasone	T49.0X1	T49.0X2	T49.0X3	T49.0X4	T49.0X5	T49.0X6
Haloperidol	T43.4X1	T43.4X2	T43.4X3	T43.4X4	T43.4X5	T43.4X6
Haloprogin	T49.0X1	T49.0X2	T49.0X3	T49.0X4	T49.0X5	T49.0X6
Halotex	T49.0X1	T49.0X2	T49.0X3	T49.0X4	T49.0X5	T49.0X6
Halothane	T41.0X1	T41.0X2	T41.0X3	T41.0X4	T41.0X5	T41.0X6
Haloxazolam	T42.4X1	T42.4X2	T42.4X3	T42.4X4	T42.4X5	T42.4X6
Halquinols	T49.0X1	T49.0X2	T49.0X3	T49.0X4	T49.0X5	T49.0X6
Hamamelis	T49.2X1	T49.2X2	T49.2X3	T49.2X4	T49.2X5	T49.2X6
Haptendextran	T45.8X1	T45.8X2	T45.8X3	T45.8X4	T45.8X5	T45.8X6
Harmonyl	T46.5X1	T46.5X2	T46.5X3	T46.5X4	T46.5X5	T46.5X6
Hartmann's solution	T50.3X1	T50.3X2	T50.3X3	T50.3X4	T50.3X5	T50.3X6
Hashish	T40.7X1	T40.7X2	T40.7X3	T40.7X4	T40.7X5	T40.7X6
Hawaiian Woodrose seeds	T40.991	T40.992	T40.993	T40.994	—	—
HCB	T60.3X1	T60.3X2	T60.3X3	T60.3X4	—	—
HCH	T53.6X1	T53.6X2	T53.6X3	T53.6X4	—	—
medicinal	T49.0X1	T49.0X2	T49.0X3	T49.0X4	T49.0X5	T49.0X6
HCN	T57.3X1	T57.3X2	T57.3X3	T57.3X4	—	—
Headache cures, drugs, powders NEC	T50.901	T50.902	T50.903	T50.904	T50.905	T50.906
Heavenly Blue (morning glory)	T40.991	T40.992	T40.993	T40.994	—	—
Heavy metal antidote	T45.8X1	T45.8X2	T45.8X3	T45.8X4	T45.8X5	T45.8X6
Hedaquinium	T49.0X1	T49.0X2	T49.0X3	T49.0X4	T49.0X5	T49.0X6
Hedge hyssop	T62.2X1	T62.2X2	T62.2X3	T62.2X4	—	—
Heet	T49.8X1	T49.8X2	T49.8X3	T49.8X4	T49.8X5	T49.8X6
Helium	T48.991	T48.992	T48.993	T48.994	T48.995	T48.996
Helenin	T37.4X1	T37.4X2	T37.4X3	T37.4X4	T37.4X5	T37.4X6
Hellebore (black) (green) (white)	T62.2X1	T62.2X2	T62.2X3	T62.2X4	—	—
Helium (nonmedicinal) NEC	T59.891	T59.892	T59.893	T59.894	—	—
medicinal	T48.991	T48.992	T48.993	T48.994	T48.995	T48.996
Hematin	T45.8X1	T45.8X2	T45.8X3	T45.8X4	T45.8X5	T45.8X6
Hematinic preparation	T45.8X1	T45.8X2	T45.8X3	T45.8X4	T45.8X5	T45.8X6
Hemlock	T62.2X1	T62.2X2	T62.2X3	T62.2X4	—	—
Hemostatic	T45.621	T45.622	T45.623	T45.624	T45.625	T45.626
drug, systemic	T45.621	T45.622	T45.623	T45.624	T45.625	T45.626
Hemostyptic	T49.4X1	T49.4X2	T49.4X3	T49.4X4	T49.4X5	T49.4X6
Henbane	T62.2X1	T62.2X2	T62.2X3	T62.2X4	—	—
Heparin (sodium)	T45.511	T45.512	T45.513	T45.514	T45.515	T45.516
action reverser	T45.7X1	T45.7X2	T45.7X3	T45.7X4	T45.7X5	T45.7X6
Heparin-fraction	T45.511	T45.512	T45.513	T45.514	T45.515	T45.516

◀ New   ◀|||| Revised   ~~deleted~~ Deleted

Substance	External Cause (T-Code)					
	Poisoning, Accidental (Unintentional)	Poisoning, Intentional Self-Harm	Poisoning, Assault	Poisoning, Undetermined	Adverse Effect	Underdosing
Heparinoid (systemic)	T45.511	T45.512	T45.513	T45.514	T45.515	T45.516
Hepatic secretion stimulant	T47.8X1	T47.8X2	T47.8X3	T47.8X4	T47.8X5	T47.8X6
Hepatitis B						
immune globulin	T50.Z11	T50.Z12	T50.Z13	T50.Z14	T50.Z15	T50.Z16
vaccine	T50.B91	T50.B92	T50.B93	T50.B94	T50.B95	T50.B96
Hepronicate	T46.7X1	T46.7X2	T46.7X3	T46.7X4	T46.7X5	T46.7X6
Heptabarb	T42.3X1	T42.3X2	T42.3X3	T42.3X4	T42.3X5	T42.3X6
Heptabarbitone	T42.3X1	T42.3X2	T42.3X3	T42.3X4	T42.3X5	T42.3X6
Heptabarbital	T42.3X1	T42.3X2	T42.3X3	T42.3X4	T42.3X5	T42.3X6
Heptachlor	T60.1X1	T60.1X2	T60.1X3	T60.1X4	—	—
Heptalgin	T40.2X1	T40.2X2	T40.2X3	T40.2X4	T40.2X5	T40.2X6
Heptaminol	T46.3X1	T46.3X2	T46.3X3	T46.3X4	T46.3X5	T46.3X6
Herbicide NEC	T60.3X1	T60.3X2	T60.3X3	T60.3X4	—	—
Heroin	T40.1X1	T40.1X2	T40.1X3	T40.1X4	—	—
Herplex	T49.5X1	T49.5X2	T49.5X3	T49.5X4	T49.5X5	T49.5X6
HES	T45.8X1	T45.8X2	T45.8X3	T45.8X4	T45.8X5	T45.8X6
Hesperidin	T46.991	T46.992	T46.993	T46.994	T46.995	T46.996
Hetacillin	T36.0X1	T36.0X2	T36.0X3	T36.0X4	T36.0X5	T36.0X6
Hetastarch	T45.8X1	T45.8X2	T45.8X3	T45.8X4	T45.8X5	T45.8X6
HETP	T60.0X1	T60.0X2	T60.0X3	T60.0X4	—	—
Hexachlorobenzene (vapor)	T60.3X1	T60.3X2	T60.3X3	T60.3X4	—	—
Hexachlorocyclohexane	T53.6X1	T53.6X2	T53.6X3	T53.6X4	—	—
Hexachlorophene	T49.0X1	T49.0X2	T49.0X3	T49.0X4	T49.0X5	T49.0X6
Hexadiline	T46.3X1	T46.3X2	T46.3X3	T46.3X4	T46.3X5	T46.3X6
Hexadimethrine (bromide)	T45.7X1	T45.7X2	T45.7X3	T45.7X4	T45.7X5	T45.7X6
Hexadylamine	T46.3X1	T46.3X2	T46.3X3	T46.3X4	T46.3X5	T46.3X6
Hexaethyl tetraphosphate	T60.0X1	T60.0X2	T60.0X3	T60.0X4	—	—
Hexafluorenium bromide	T48.1X1	T48.1X2	T48.1X3	T48.1X4	T48.1X5	T48.1X6
Hexafluorodiethyl ether	T43.291	T43.292	T43.293	T43.294	T43.295	T43.296
Hexafluronium (bromide)	T48.1X1	T48.1X2	T48.1X3	T48.1X4	T48.1X5	T48.1X6
Hexahydrobenzol	T52.8X1	T52.8X2	T52.8X3	T52.8X4	—	—
Hexahydrocresol(s)	T51.8X1	T51.8X2	T51.8X3	T51.8X4	—	—
arsenide	T57.0X1	T57.0X2	T57.0X3	T57.0X4	—	—
arseniurated	T57.0X1	T57.0X2	T57.0X3	T57.0X4	—	—
cyanide	T57.3X1	T57.3X2	T57.3X3	T57.3X4	—	—
gas	T59.891	T59.892	T59.893	T59.894	—	—
Fluoride (liquid)	T57.8X1	T57.8X2	T57.8X3	T57.8X4	—	—
vapor	T59.891	T59.892	T59.893	T59.894	—	—
phophorated	T60.0X1	T60.0X2	T60.0X3	T60.0X4	—	—
sulfate	T57.8X1	T57.8X2	T57.8X3	T57.8X4	—	—

◄ New   ⬅ Revised   ~~deleted~~ Deleted

TABLE OF DRUGS AND CHEMICALS

Substance	External Cause (T-Code)					
	Poisoning, Accidental (Unintentional)	Poisoning, Intentional Self-Harm	Poisoning, Assault	Poisoning, Undetermined	Adverse Effect	Underdosing
Hexahydrocresol(s) *(Continued)*						
sulfide (gas)	T59.6X1	T59.6X2	T59.6X3	T59.6X4	—	—
arseniurated	T57.0X1	T57.0X2	T57.0X3	T57.0X4	—	—
sulfurated	T57.8X1	T57.8X2	T57.8X3	T57.8X4	—	—
Hexahydrophenol	T51.8X1	T51.8X2	T51.8X3	T51.8X4	—	—
Hexa-germ	T49.2X1	T49.2X2	T49.2X3	T49.2X4	T49.2X5	T49.2X6
Hexalen	T51.8X1	T51.8X2	T51.8X3	T51.8X4	—	—
Hexamethonium bromide	T44.2X1	T44.2X2	T44.2X3	T44.2X4	T44.2X5	T44.2X6
Hexamethylene	T52.8X1	T52.8X2	T52.8X3	T52.8X4	—	—
Hexamethylmelamine	T45.1X1	T45.1X2	T45.1X3	T45.1X4	T45.1X5	T45.1X6
Hexamidine	T49.0X1	T49.0X2	T49.0X3	T49.0X4	T49.0X5	T49.0X6
Hexamine (mandelate)	T37.8X1	T37.8X2	T37.8X3	T37.8X4	T37.8X5	T37.8X6
Hexanone, 2-hexanone	T52.4X1	T52.4X2	T52.4X3	T52.4X4	—	—
Hexanuorenium	T48.1X1	T48.1X2	T48.1X3	T48.1X4	T48.1X5	T48.1X6
Hexapropymate	T42.6X1	T42.6X2	T42.6X3	T42.6X4	T42.6X5	T42.6X6
Hexasonium iodide	T44.3X1	T44.3X2	T44.3X3	T44.3X4	T44.3X5	T44.3X6
Hexcarbacholine bromide	T48.1X1	T48.1X2	T48.1X3	T48.1X4	T48.1X5	T48.1X6
Hexemal	T42.3X1	T42.3X2	T42.3X3	T42.3X4	T42.3X5	T42.3X6
Hexestrol	T38.5X1	T38.5X2	T38.5X3	T38.5X4	T38.5X5	T38.5X6
Hexethal (sodium)	T42.3X1	T42.3X2	T42.3X3	T42.3X4	T42.3X5	T42.3X6
Hexetidine	T37.8X1	T37.8X2	T37.8X3	T37.8X4	T37.8X5	T37.8X6
Hexobarbital	T42.3X1	T42.3X2	T42.3X3	T42.3X4	T42.3X5	T42.3X6
rectal	T41.291	T41.292	T41.293	T41.294	T41.295	T41.296
sodium	T41.1X1	T41.1X2	T41.1X3	T41.1X4	T41.1X5	T41.1X6
Hexobendine	T46.3X1	T46.3X2	T46.3X3	T46.3X4	T46.3X5	T46.3X6
Hexocyclium	T44.3X1	T44.3X2	T44.3X3	T44.3X4	T44.3X5	T44.3X6
metilsulfate	T44.3X1	T44.3X2	T44.3X3	T44.3X4	T44.3X5	T44.3X6
Hexoestrol	T38.5X1	T38.5X2	T38.5X3	T38.5X4	T38.5X5	T38.5X6
Hexone	T52.4X1	T52.4X2	T52.4X3	T52.4X4	—	—
Hexoprenaline	T48.6X1	T48.6X2	T48.6X3	T48.6X4	T48.6X5	T48.6X6
Hexylcaine	T41.3X1	T41.3X2	T41.3X3	T41.3X4	T41.3X5	T41.3X6
Hexylresorcinol	T52.2X1	T52.2X2	T52.2X3	T52.2X4	—	—
HGH (human growth hormone)	T38.811	T38.812	T38.813	T38.814	T38.815	T38.816
Hinkle's pills	T47.2X1	T47.2X2	T47.2X3	T47.2X4	T47.2X5	T47.2X6
Histalog	T50.8X1	T50.8X2	T50.8X3	T50.8X4	T50.8X5	T50.8X6
Histamine (phosphate)	T50.8X1	T50.8X2	T50.8X3	T50.8X4	T50.8X5	T50.8X6
Histoplasmin	T50.8X1	T50.8X2	T50.8X3	T50.8X4	T50.8X5	T50.8X6
Holly berries	T62.2X1	T62.2X2	T62.2X3	T62.2X4	—	—
Homatropine	T44.3X1	T44.3X2	T44.3X3	T44.3X4	T44.3X5	T44.3X6
methylbromide	T44.3X1	T44.3X2	T44.3X3	T44.3X4	T44.3X5	T44.3X6

◀ New ◀‖‖ Revised ~~deleted~~ Deleted

Substance	External Cause (T-Code)					
	Poisoning, Accidental (Unintentional)	Poisoning, Intentional Self-Harm	Poisoning, Assault	Poisoning, Undetermined	Adverse Effect	Underdosing
Homochlorcyclizine	T45.0X1	T45.0X2	T45.0X3	T45.0X4	T45.0X5	T45.0X6
Homosalate	T49.3X1	T49.3X2	T49.3X3	T49.3X4	T49.3X5	T49.3X6
Homo-tet	T50.Z11	T50.Z12	T50.Z13	T50.Z14	T50.Z15	T50.Z16
Hormone	T38.801	T38.802	T38.803	T38.804	T38.805	T38.806
adrenal cortical steroids	T38.0X1	T38.0X2	T38.0X3	T38.0X4	T38.0X5	T38.0X6
androgenic	T38.7X1	T38.7X2	T38.7X3	T38.7X4	T38.7X5	T38.7X6
anterior pituitary NEC	T38.811	T38.812	T38.813	T38.814	T38.815	T38.816
antidiabetic agents	T38.3X1	T38.3X2	T38.3X3	T38.3X4	T38.3X5	T38.3X6
antidiuretic	T38.891	T38.892	T38.893	T38.894	T38.895	T38.896
cancer therapy	T45.1X1	T45.1X2	T45.1X3	T45.1X4	T45.1X5	T45.1X6
follicle stimulating	T38.811	T38.812	T38.813	T38.814	T38.815	T38.816
gonadotropic	T38.891	T38.892	T38.893	T38.894	T38.895	T38.896
pituitary	T38.811	T38.812	T38.813	T38.814	T38.815	T38.816
growth	T38.811	T38.812	T38.813	T38.814	T38.815	T38.816
luteinizing	T38.811	T38.812	T38.813	T38.814	T38.815	T38.816
ovarian	T38.5X1	T38.5X2	T38.5X3	T38.5X4	T38.5X5	T38.5X6
oxytocic	T48.0X1	T48.0X2	T48.0X3	T48.0X4	T48.0X5	T48.0X6
parathyroid (derivatives)	T50.991	T50.992	T50.993	T50.994	T50.995	T50.996
pituitary (posterior) NEC	T38.891	T38.892	T38.893	T38.894	T38.895	T38.896
anterior	T38.811	T38.812	T38.813	T38.814	T38.815	T38.816
specified, NEC	T38.891	T38.892	T38.893	T38.894	T38.895	T38.896
thyroid	T38.1X1	T38.1X2	T38.1X3	T38.1X4	T38.1X5	T38.1X6
Hornet (sting)	T63.451	T63.452	T63.453	T63.454	—	—
Horse anti-human lymphocytic serum	T50.Z11	T50.Z12	T50.Z13	T50.Z14	T50.Z15	T50.Z16
Horticulture agent NEC	T65.91	T65.92	T65.93	T65.94	—	—
with pesticide	T60.91	T60.92	T60.93	T60.94	—	—
Human						
albumin	T45.8X1	T45.8X2	T45.8X3	T45.8X4	T45.8X5	T45.8X6
growth hormone (HGH)	T38.811	T38.812	T38.813	T38.814	T38.815	T38.816
immune serum	T50.Z11	T50.Z12	T50.Z13	T50.Z14	T50.Z15	T50.Z16
Hyaluronidase	T45.3X1	T45.3X2	T45.3X3	T45.3X4	T45.3X5	T45.3X6
Hyazyme	T45.3X1	T45.3X2	T45.3X3	T45.3X4	T45.3X5	T45.3X6
Hycodan	T40.2X1	T40.2X2	T40.2X3	T40.2X4	T40.2X5	T40.2X6
Hydantoin derivative NEC	T42.0X1	T42.0X2	T42.0X3	T42.0X4	T42.0X5	T42.0X6
Hydeltra	T38.0X1	T38.0X2	T38.0X3	T38.0X4	T38.0X5	T38.0X6
Hydergine	T44.6X1	T44.6X2	T44.6X3	T44.6X4	T44.6X5	T44.6X6
Hydrabamine penicillin	T36.0X1	T36.0X2	T36.0X3	T36.0X4	T36.0X5	T36.0X6
Hydralazine	T46.5X1	T46.5X2	T46.5X3	T46.5X4	T46.5X5	T46.5X6
Hydrargaphen	T49.0X1	T49.0X2	T49.0X3	T49.0X4	T49.0X5	T49.0X6

TABLE OF DRUGS AND CHEMICALS

◀ New ◀▥ Revised ~~deleted~~ Deleted

Substance	Poisoning, Accidental (Unintentional)	Poisoning, Intentional Self-Harm	Poisoning, Assault	Poisoning, Undetermined	Adverse Effect	Underdosing
Hydrargyri amino-chloridum	T49.0X1	T49.0X2	T49.0X3	T49.0X4	T49.0X5	T49.0X6
Hydrastine	T48.291	T48.292	T48.293	T48.294	T48.295	T48.296
Hydrazine	T54.1X1	T54.1X2	T54.1X3	T54.1X4	—	—
monoamine oxidase inhibitors	T43.1X1	T43.1X2	T43.1X3	T43.1X4	T43.1X5	T43.1X6
Hydrazoic acid, azides	T54.2X1	T54.2X2	T54.2X3	T54.2X4	—	—
Hydriodic acid	T48.4X1	T48.4X2	T48.4X3	T48.4X4	T48.4X5	T48.4X6
Hydrocarbon gas	T59.891	T59.892	T59.893	T59.894	—	
incomplete combustion of — see Carbon, monoxide, fuel, utility						
liquefied (mobile container)	T59.891	T59.892	T59.893	T59.894	—	—
piped (natural)	T59.891	T59.892	T59.893	T59.894	—	—
Hydrochloric acid (liquid)	T54.2X1	T54.2X2	T54.2X3	T54.2X4	—	—
medicinal (digestant)	T47.5X1	T47.5X2	T47.5X3	T47.5X4	T47.5X5	T47.5X6
vapor	T59.891	T59.892	T59.893	T59.894		
Hydrochlorothiazide	T50.2X1	T50.2X2	T50.2X3	T50.2X4	T50.2X5	T50.2X6
Hydrocodone	T40.2X1	T40.2X2	T40.2X3	T40.2X4	T40.2X5	T40.2X6
Hydrocortisone (derivatives)	T49.0X1	T49.0X2	T49.0X3	T49.0X4	T49.0X5	T49.0X6
aceponate	T49.0X1	T49.0X2	T49.0X3	T49.0X4	T49.0X5	T49.0X6
ENT agent	T49.6X1	T49.6X2	T49.6X3	T49.6X4	T49.6X5	T49.6X6
ophthalmic preparation	T49.5X1	T49.5X2	T49.5X3	T49.5X4	T49.5X5	T49.5X6
topical NEC	T49.0X1	T49.0X2	T49.0X3	T49.0X4	T49.0X5	T49.0X6
Hydrocortone	T38.0X1	T38.0X2	T38.0X3	T38.0X4	T38.0X5	T38.0X6
ENT agent	T49.6X1	T49.6X2	T49.6X3	T49.6X4	T49.6X5	T49.6X6
ophthalmic preparation	T49.5X1	T49.5X2	T49.5X3	T49.5X4	T49.5X5	T49.5X6
topical NEC	T49.0X1	T49.0X2	T49.0X3	T49.0X4	T49.0X5	T49.0X6
Hydrocyanic acid (liquid)	T57.3X1	T57.3X2	T57.3X3	T57.3X4	—	—
gas	T65.0X1	T65.0X2	T65.0X3	T65.0X4	—	—
Hydroflumethiazide	T50.2X1	T50.2X2	T50.2X3	T50.2X4	T50.2X5	T50.2X6
Hydrofluoric acid (liquid)	T54.2X1	T54.2X2	T54.2X3	T54.2X4	—	—
vapor	T59.891	T59.892	T59.893	T59.894	—	—
Hydrogen	T59.891	T59.892	T59.893	T59.894	—	—
arsenide	T57.0X1	T57.0X2	T57.0X3	T57.0X4	—	—
arseniureted	T57.0X1	T57.0X2	T57.0X3	T57.0X4	—	—
chloride	T57.8X1	T57.8X2	T57.8X3	T57.8X4	—	—
cyanide (salts)	T57.3X1	T57.3X2	T57.3X3	T57.3X4	—	—
gas	T57.3X1	T57.3X2	T57.3X3	T57.3X4	—	—
Fluoride	T59.5X1	T59.5X2	T59.5X3	T59.5X4	—	—
vapor	T59.5X1	T59.5X2	T59.5X3	T59.5X4	—	—
peroxide	T49.0X1	T49.0X2	T49.0X3	T49.0X4	T49.0X5	T49.0X6
phosphureted	T57.1X1	T57.1X2	T57.1X3	T57.1X4	—	—

◀ New ◀▥▥ Revised ~~deleted~~ Deleted

Substance	External Cause (T-Code)					
	Poisoning, Accidental (Unintentional)	Poisoning, Intentional Self-Harm	Poisoning, Assault	Poisoning, Undetermined	Adverse Effect	Underdosing
Hydrogen *(Continued)*						
sulfide	T59.6X1	T59.6X2	T59.6X3	T59.6X4	—	—
arseniureted	T57.0X1	T57.0X2	T57.0X3	T57.0X4	—	—
sulfureted	T59.6X1	T59.6X2	T59.6X3	T59.6X4	—	—
Hydromethylpyridine	T46.7X1	T46.7X2	T46.7X3	T46.7X4	T46.7X5	T46.7X6
Hydromorphinol	T40.2X1	T40.2X2	T40.2X3	T40.2X4	—	—
Hydromorphinone	T40.2X1	T40.2X2	T40.2X3	T40.2X4	T40.2X5	T40.2X6
Hydromorphone	T40.2X1	T40.2X2	T40.2X3	T40.2X4	T40.2X5	T40.2X6
Hydromox	T50.2X1	T50.2X2	T50.2X3	T50.2X4	T50.2X5	T50.2X6
Hydrophilic lotion	T49.3X1	T49.3X2	T49.3X3	T49.3X4	T49.3X5	T49.3X6
Hydroquinidine	T46.2X1	T46.2X2	T46.2X3	T46.2X4	T46.2X5	T46.2X6
Hydroquinone	T52.2X1	T52.2X2	T52.2X3	T52.2X4	—	—
vapor	T59.891	T59.892	T59.893	T59.894	—	—
Hydrosulfuric acid (gas)	T59.6X1	T59.6X2	T59.6X3	T59.6X4	—	—
Hydrotalcite	T47.1X1	T47.1X2	T47.1X3	T47.1X4	T47.1X5	T47.1X6
Hydrous wool fat	T49.3X1	T49.3X2	T49.3X3	T49.3X4	T49.3X5	T49.3X6
Hydroxide, caustic	T54.3X1	T54.3X2	T54.3X3	T54.3X4	—	—
Hydroxocobalamin	T45.8X1	T45.8X2	T45.8X3	T45.8X4	T45.8X5	T45.8X6
Hydroxyamphetamine	T49.5X1	T49.5X2	T49.5X3	T49.5X4	T49.5X5	T49.5X6
Hydroxycarbamide	T45.1X1	T45.1X2	T45.1X3	T45.1X4	T45.1X5	T45.1X6
Hydroxychloroquine	T37.8X1	T37.8X2	T37.8X3	T37.8X4	T37.8X5	T37.8X6
Hydroxydihydrocodeinone	T40.2X1	T40.2X2	T40.2X3	T40.2X4	T40.2X5	T40.2X6
Hydroxyestrone	T38.5X1	T38.5X2	T38.5X3	T38.5X4	T38.5X5	T38.5X6
Hydroxyethyl starch	T45.8X1	T45.8X2	T45.8X3	T45.8X4	T45.8X5	T45.8X6
Hydroxymethylpentanone	T52.4X1	T52.4X2	T52.4X3	T52.4X4	—	—
Hydroxyphenamate	T43.591	T43.592	T43.593	T43.594	T43.595	T43.596
Hydroxyphenylbutazone	T39.2X1	T39.2X2	T39.2X3	T39.2X4	T39.2X5	T39.2X6
Hydroxyprogesterone	T38.5X1	T38.5X2	T38.5X3	T38.5X4	T38.5X5	T38.5X6
caproate	T38.5X1	T38.5X2	T38.5X3	T38.5X4	T38.5X5	T38.5X6
Hydroxyquinoline (derivatives) NEC	T37.8X1	T37.8X2	T37.8X3	T37.8X4	T37.8X5	T37.8X6
Hydroxystilbamidine	T37.3X1	T37.3X2	T37.3X3	T37.3X4	T37.3X5	T37.3X6
Hydroxytoluene (nonmedicinal)	T54.0X1	T54.0X2	T54.0X3	T54.0X4	—	—
medicinal	T49.0X1	T49.0X2	T49.0X3	T49.0X4	T49.0X5	T49.0X6
Hydroxyurea	T45.1X1	T45.1X2	T45.1X3	T45.1X4	T45.1X5	T45.1X6
Hydroxyzine	T43.591	T43.592	T43.593	T43.594	T43.595	T43.596
Hyoscine	T44.3X1	T44.3X2	T44.3X3	T44.3X4	T44.3X5	T44.3X6
Hyoscyamine	T44.3X1	T44.3X2	T44.3X3	T44.3X4	T44.3X5	T44.3X6
Hyoscyamus	T44.3X1	T44.3X2	T44.3X3	T44.3X4	T44.3X5	T44.3X6
dry extract	T44.3X1	T44.3X2	T44.3X3	T44.3X4	T44.3X5	T44.3X6

TABLE OF DRUGS AND CHEMICALS

◀ New ◀▥ Revised ~~deleted~~ Deleted

Substance	Poisoning, Accidental (Unintentional)	Poisoning, Intentional Self-Harm	Poisoning, Assault	Poisoning, Undetermined	Adverse Effect	Underdosing
	External Cause (T-Code)					
Hypaque	T50.8X1	T50.8X2	T50.8X3	T50.8X4	T50.8X5	T50.8X6
Hypertussis	T50.Z11	T50.Z12	T50.Z13	T50.Z14	T50.Z15	T50.Z16
Hypnotic	T42.71	T42.72	T42.73	T42.74	T42.75	T42.76
anticonvulsant	T42.71	T42.72	T42.73	T42.74	T42.75	T42.76
specified NEC	T42.6X1	T42.6X2	T42.6X3	T42.6X4	T42.6X5	T42.6X6
Hypochlorite	T49.0X1	T49.0X2	T49.0X3	T49.0X4	T49.0X5	T49.0X6
Hypophysis, posterior	T38.891	T38.892	T38.893	T38.894	T38.895	T38.896
Hypotensive NEC	T46.5X1	T46.5X2	T46.5X3	T46.5X4	T46.5X5	T46.5X6
Hypromellose	T49.5X1	T49.5X2	T49.5X3	T49.5X4	T49.5X5	T49.5X6
	I					
Ibacitabine	T37.5X1	T37.5X2	T37.5X3	T37.5X4	T37.5X5	T37.5X6
Ibopamine	T44.991	T44.992	T44.993	T44.994	T44.995	T44.996
Ibufenac	T39.311	T39.312	T39.313	T39.314	T39.315	T39.316
Ibuprofen	T39.311	T39.312	T39.313	T39.314	T39.315	T39.316
Ibuproxam	T39.311	T39.312	T39.313	T39.314	T39.315	T39.316
Ibuterol	T48.6X1	T48.6X2	T48.6X3	T48.6X4	T48.6X5	T48.6X6
Ichthammol	T49.0X1	T49.0X2	T49.0X3	T49.0X4	T49.0X5	T49.0X6
Ichthyol	T49.4X1	T49.4X2	T49.4X3	T49.4X4	T49.4X5	T49.4X6
Idarubicin	T45.1X1	T45.1X2	T45.1X3	T45.1X4	T45.1X5	T45.1X6
Idrocilamide	T42.8X1	T42.8X2	T42.8X3	T42.8X4	T42.8X5	T42.8X6
Ifenprodil	T46.7X1	T46.7X2	T46.7X3	T46.7X4	T46.7X5	T46.7X6
Ifosfamide	T45.1X1	T45.1X2	T45.1X3	T45.1X4	T45.1X5	T45.1X6
Iletin	T38.3X1	T38.3X2	T38.3X3	T38.3X4	T38.3X5	T38.3X6
Ilex	T62.2X1	T62.2X2	T62.2X3	T62.2X4	—	—
Illuminating gas (after combustion)	T58.11	T58.12	T58.13	T58.14	—	—
prior to combustion	T59.891	T59.892	T59.893	T59.894	—	—
Ilopan	T45.2X1	T45.2X2	T45.2X3	T45.2X4	T45.2X5	T45.2X6
Iloprost	T46.7X1	T46.7X2	T46.7X3	T46.7X4	T46.7X5	T46.7X6
Ilotycin	T36.3X1	T36.3X2	T36.3X3	T36.3X4	T36.3X5	T36.3X6
ophthalmic preparation	T49.5X1	T49.5X2	T49.5X3	T49.5X4	T49.5X5	T49.5X6
topical NEC	T49.0X1	T49.0X2	T49.0X3	T49.0X4	T49.0X5	T49.0X6
Imidazole-4-carboxamide	T45.1X1	T45.1X2	T45.1X3	T45.1X4	T45.1X5	T45.1X6
Imipenem	T36.0X1	T36.0X2	T36.0X3	T36.0X4	T36.0X5	T36.0X6
Imipramine	T43.011	T43.012	T43.013	T43.014	T43.015	T43.016
Iminostilbene	T42.1X1	T42.1X2	T42.1X3	T42.1X4	T42.1X5	T42.1X6
Immu-G	T50.Z11	T50.Z12	T50.Z13	T50.Z14	T50.Z15	T50.Z16
Immuglobin	T50.Z11	T50.Z12	T50.Z13	T50.Z14	T50.Z15	T50.Z16
Immune						
globulin	T50.Z11	T50.Z12	T50.Z13	T50.Z14	T50.Z15	T50.Z16
serum globulin	T50.Z11	T50.Z12	T50.Z13	T50.Z14	T50.Z15	T50.Z16

◀ New ◀||| Revised ~~deleted~~ Deleted

Substance	External Cause (T-Code)					
	Poisoning, Accidental (Unintentional)	Poisoning, Intentional Self-Harm	Poisoning, Assault	Poisoning, Undetermined	Adverse Effect	Underdosing
Immunoglobin human (intravenous) (normal)	T50.Z11	T50.Z12	T50.Z13	T50.Z14	T50.Z15	T50.Z16
unmodified	T50.Z11	T50.Z12	T50.Z13	T50.Z14	T50.Z15	T50.Z16
Immunosuppressive drug	T45.1X1	T45.1X2	T45.1X3	T45.1X4	T45.1X5	T45.1X6
Immu-tetanus	T50.Z11	T50.Z12	T50.Z13	T50.Z14	T50.Z15	T50.Z16
Indalpine	T43.221	T43.222	T43.223	T43.224	T43.225	T43.226
Indanazoline	T48.5X1	T48.5X2	T48.5X3	T48.5X4	T48.5X5	T48.5X6
Indandione (derivatives)	T45.511	T45.512	T45.513	T45.514	T45.515	T45.516
Indapamide	T46.5X1	T46.5X2	T46.5X3	T46.5X4	T46.5X5	T46.5X6
Indendione (derivatives)	T45.511	T45.512	T45.513	T45.514	T45.515	T45.516
Indenolol	T44.7X1	T44.7X2	T44.7X3	T44.7X4	T44.7X5	T44.7X6
Inderal	T44.7X1	T44.7X2	T44.7X3	T44.7X4	T44.7X5	T44.7X6
Indian						
hemp	T40.7X1	T40.7X2	T40.7X3	T40.7X4	T40.7X5	T40.7X6
tobacco	T62.2X1	T62.2X2	T62.2X3	T62.2X4	—	—
Indigo carmine	T50.8X1	T50.8X2	T50.8X3	T50.8X4	T50.8X5	T50.8X6
Indobufen	T45.521	T45.522	T45.523	T45.524	T45.525	T45.526
Indocin	T39.2X1	T39.2X2	T39.2X3	T39.2X4	T39.2X5	T39.2X6
Indocyanine green	T50.8X1	T50.8X2	T50.8X3	T50.8X4	T50.8X5	T50.8X6
Indometacin	T39.391	T39.392	T39.393	T39.394	T39.395	T39.396
Indomethacin	T39.391	T39.392	T39.393	T39.394	T39.395	T39.396
farnesil	T39.4X1	T39.4X2	T39.4X3	T39.4X4	T39.4X5	T39.4X6
Indoramin	T44.6X1	T44.6X2	T44.6X3	T44.6X4	T44.6X5	T44.6X6
Industrial						
alcohol	T51.0X1	T51.0X2	T51.0X3	T51.0X4	—	—
fumes	T59.891	T59.892	T59.893	T59.894	—	—
solvents (fumes) (vapors)	T52.91	T52.92	T52.93	T52.94	—	—
Influenza vaccine	T50.B91	T50.B92	T50.B93	T50.B94	T50.B95	T50.B96
Ingested substance NEC	T65.91	T65.92	T65.93	T65.94	—	—
INH	T37.1X1	T37.1X2	T37.1X3	T37.1X4	T37.1X5	T37.1X6
Inhalation, gas (noxious) — see Gas						
Inhibitor						
angiotensin-converting enzyme	T46.4X1	T46.4X2	T46.4X3	T46.4X4	T46.4X5	T46.4X6
carbonic anhydrase	T50.2X1	T50.2X2	T50.2X3	T50.2X4	T50.2X5	T50.2X6
fibrinolysis	T45.621	T45.622	T45.623	T45.624	T45.625	T45.626
monoamine oxidase NEC	T43.1X1	T43.1X2	T43.1X3	T43.1X4	T43.1X5	T43.1X6
hydrazine	T43.1X1	T43.1X2	T43.1X3	T43.1X4	T43.1X5	T43.1X6
postsynaptic	T43.8X1	T43.8X2	T43.8X3	T43.8X4	T43.8X5	T43.8X6
prothrombin synthesis	T45.511	T45.512	T45.513	T45.514	T45.515	T45.516
Ink	T65.891	T65.892	T65.893	T65.894	—	—
Inorganic substance NEC	T57.91	T57.92	T57.93	T57.94	—	—

◀ New   ◀▥ Revised   ~~deleted~~ Deleted

TABLE OF DRUGS AND CHEMICALS

TABLE OF DRUGS AND CHEMICALS

Substance	External Cause (T-Code)					
	Poisoning, Accidental (Unintentional)	Poisoning, Intentional Self-Harm	Poisoning, Assault	Poisoning, Undetermined	Adverse Effect	Underdosing
Inosine pranobex	T37.5X1	T37.5X2	T37.5X3	T37.5X4	T37.5X5	T37.5X6
Inositol	T50.991	T50.992	T50.993	T50.994	T50.995	T50.996
nicotinate	T46.7X1	T46.7X2	T46.7X3	T46.7X4	T46.7X5	T46.7X6
Inproquone	T45.1X1	T45.1X2	T45.1X3	T45.1X4	T45.1X5	T45.1X6
Insect (sting), venomous	T63.481	T63.482	T63.483	T63.484	—	—
ant	T63.421	T63.422	T63.423	T63.424	—	—
bee	T63.441	T63.442	T63.443	T63.444	—	—
caterpillar	T63.431	T63.432	T63.433	T63.434	—	—
hornet	T63.451	T63.452	T63.453	T63.454	—	—
wasp	T63.461	T63.462	T63.463	T63.464	—	—
Insecticide NEC	T60.91	T60.92	T60.93	T60.94	—	—
carbamate	T60.0X1	T60.0X2	T60.0X3	T60.0X4	—	—
chlorinated	T60.1X1	T60.1X2	T60.1X3	T60.1X4	—	—
mixed	T60.91	T60.92	T60.93	T60.94	—	—
organochlorine	T60.1X1	T60.1X2	T60.1X3	T60.1X4	—	—
organophosphorus	T60.0X1	T60.0X2	T60.0X3	T60.0X4	—	—
Insular tissue extract	T38.3X1	T38.3X2	T38.3X3	T38.3X4	T38.3X5	T38.3X6
Insulin (amorphous) (globin) (isophane) (Lente) (NPH) (Semilente) (Ultralente)	T38.3X1	T38.3X2	T38.3X3	T38.3X4	T38.3X5	T38.3X6
defalan	T38.3X1	T38.3X2	T38.3X3	T38.3X4	T38.3X5	T38.3X6
human	T38.3X1	T38.3X2	T38.3X3	T38.3X4	T38.3X5	T38.3X6
injection, soluble	T38.3X1	T38.3X2	T38.3X3	T38.3X4	T38.3X5	T38.3X6
biphasic	T38.3X1	T38.3X2	T38.3X3	T38.3X4	T38.3X5	T38.3X6
intermediate acting	T38.3X1	T38.3X2	T38.3X3	T38.3X4	T38.3X5	T38.3X6
protamine zinc	T38.3X1	T38.3X2	T38.3X3	T38.3X4	T38.3X5	T38.3X6
slow acting	T38.3X1	T38.3X2	T38.3X3	T38.3X4	T38.3X5	T38.3X6
zinc						
protamine injection	T38.3X1	T38.3X2	T38.3X3	T38.3X4	T38.3X5	T38.3X6
suspension (amorphous) (crystalline)	T38.3X1	T38.3X2	T38.3X3	T38.3X4	T38.3X5	T38.3X6
Interferon (alpha) (beta) (gamma)	T37.5X1	T37.5X2	T37.5X3	T37.5X4	T37.5X5	T37.5X6
Intestinal motility control drug	T47.6X1	T47.6X2	T47.6X3	T47.6X4	T47.6X5	T47.6X6
biological	T47.8X1	T47.8X2	T47.8X3	T47.8X4	T47.8X5	T47.8X6
Intranarcon	T41.1X1	T41.1X2	T41.1X3	T41.1X4	T41.1X5	T41.1X6
Intravenous						
amino acids	T50.991	T50.992	T50.993	T50.994	T50.995	T50.996
fat suspension	T50.991	T50.992	T50.993	T50.994	T50.995	T50.996
Inulin	T50.8X1	T50.8X2	T50.8X3	T50.8X4	T50.8X5	T50.8X6
Invert sugar	T50.3X1	T50.3X2	T50.3X3	T50.3X4	T50.3X5	T50.3X6
Inza — see Naproxen						
Iobenzamic acid	T50.8X1	T50.8X2	T50.8X3	T50.8X4	T50.8X5	T50.8X6
Iocarmic acid	T50.8X1	T50.8X2	T50.8X3	T50.8X4	T50.8X5	T50.8X6

◀ New ◀▥ Revised deleted Deleted

Substance	External Cause (T-Code)					
	Poisoning, Accidental (Unintentional)	Poisoning, Intentional Self-Harm	Poisoning, Assault	Poisoning, Undetermined	Adverse Effect	Underdosing
Iocetamic acid	T50.8X1	T50.8X2	T50.8X3	T50.8X4	T50.8X5	T50.8X6
Iodamide	T50.8X1	T50.8X2	T50.8X3	T50.8X4	T50.8X5	T50.8X6
Iodide NEC — *see also Iodine*	T49.0X1	T49.0X2	T49.0X3	T49.0X4	T49.0X5	T49.0X6
mercury (ointment)	T49.0X1	T49.0X2	T49.0X3	T49.0X4	T49.0X5	T49.0X6
methylate	T49.0X1	T49.0X2	T49.0X3	T49.0X4	T49.0X5	T49.0X6
potassium (expectorant) NEC	T48.4X1	T48.4X2	T48.4X3	T48.4X4	T48.4X5	T48.4X6
Iodinated						
contrast medium	T50.8X1	T50.8X2	T50.8X3	T50.8X4	T50.8X5	T50.8X6
glycerol	T48.4X1	T48.4X2	T48.4X3	T48.4X4	T48.4X5	T48.4X6
human serum albumin (131I)	T50.8X1	T50.8X2	T50.8X3	T50.8X4	T50.8X5	T50.8X6
Iodine (antiseptic, external) (tincture) NEC	T49.0X1	T49.0X2	T49.0X3	T49.0X4	T49.0X5	T49.0X6
125 — *see also Radiation sickness, and Exposure to radioactivce isotopes*	T50.8X1	T50.8X2	T50.8X3	T50.8X4	T50.8X5	T50.8X6
therapeutic	T50.991	T50.992	T50.993	T50.994	T50.995	T50.996
131 — *see also Radiation sickness, and Exposure to radioactivce isotopes*	T50.8X1	T50.8X2	T50.8X3	T50.8X4	T50.8X5	T50.8X6
therapeutic	T38.2X1	T38.2X2	T38.2X3	T38.2X4	T38.2X5	T38.2X6
diagnostic	T50.8X1	T50.8X2	T50.8X3	T50.8X4	T50.8X5	T50.8X6
for thyroid conditions (antithyroid)	T38.2X1	T38.2X2	T38.2X3	T38.2X4	T38.2X5	T38.2X6
solution	T49.0X1	T49.0X2	T49.0X3	T49.0X4	T49.0X5	T49.0X6
vapor	T59.891	T59.892	T59.893	T59.894	—	—
Iodipamide	T50.8X1	T50.8X2	T50.8X3	T50.8X4	T50.8X5	T50.8X6
Iodized (poppy seed) oil	T50.8X1	T50.8X2	T50.8X3	T50.8X4	T50.8X5	T50.8X6
Iodobismitol	T37.8X1	T37.8X2	T37.8X3	T37.8X4	T37.8X5	T37.8X6
Iodochlorhydroxyquin	T37.8X1	T37.8X2	T37.8X3	T37.8X4	T37.8X5	T37.8X6
topical	T49.0X1	T49.0X2	T49.0X3	T49.0X4	T49.0X5	T49.0X6
Iodochlorhydroxyquino-line	T37.8X1	T37.8X2	T37.8X3	T37.8X4	T37.8X5	T37.8X6
Iodocholesterol (131I)	T50.8X1	T50.8X2	T50.8X3	T50.8X4	T50.8X5	T50.8X6
Iodoform	T49.0X1	T49.0X2	T49.0X3	T49.0X4	T49.0X5	T49.0X6
Iodohippuric acid	T50.8X1	T50.8X2	T50.8X3	T50.8X4	T50.8X5	T50.8X6
Iodopanoic acid	T50.8X1	T50.8X2	T50.8X3	T50.8X4	T50.8X5	T50.8X6
Iodophthalein (sodium)	T50.8X1	T50.8X2	T50.8X3	T50.8X4	T50.8X5	T50.8X6
Iodopyracet	T50.8X1	T50.8X2	T50.8X3	T50.8X4	T50.8X5	T50.8X6
Iodoquinol	T37.8X1	T37.8X2	T37.8X3	T37.8X4	T37.8X5	T37.8X6
Iodoxamic acid	T50.8X1	T50.8X2	T50.8X3	T50.8X4	T50.8X5	T50.8X6
Iofendylate	T50.8X1	T50.8X2	T50.8X3	T50.8X4	T50.8X5	T50.8X6
Ioglycamic acid	T50.8X1	T50.8X2	T50.8X3	T50.8X4	T50.8X5	T50.8X6
Iohexol	T50.8X1	T50.8X2	T50.8X3	T50.8X4	T50.8X5	T50.8X6
Ion exchange resin						
anion	T47.8X1	T47.8X2	T47.8X3	T47.8X4	T47.8X5	T47.8X6
cation	T50.3X1	T50.3X2	T50.3X3	T50.3X4	T50.3X5	T50.3X6

◀ New   ◀▥ Revised   ~~deleted~~ Deleted

TABLE OF DRUGS AND CHEMICALS

	External Cause (T-Code)					
Substance	Poisoning, Accidental (Unintentional)	Poisoning, Intentional Self-Harm	Poisoning, Assault	Poisoning, Undetermined	Adverse Effect	Underdosing
Ion exchange resin *(Continued)*						
cholestyramine	T46.6X1	T46.6X2	T46.6X3	T46.6X4	T46.6X5	T46.6X6
intestinal	T47.8X1	T47.8X2	T47.8X3	T47.8X4	T47.8X5	T47.8X6
Iopamidol	T50.8X1	T50.8X2	T50.8X3	T50.8X4	T50.8X5	T50.8X6
Iopanoic acid	T50.8X1	T50.8X2	T50.8X3	T50.8X4	T50.8X5	T50.8X6
Iophenoic acid	T50.8X1	T50.8X2	T50.8X3	T50.8X4	T50.8X5	T50.8X6
Iopodate, sodium	T50.8X1	T50.8X2	T50.8X3	T50.8X4	T50.8X5	T50.8X6
Iopodic acid	T50.8X1	T50.8X2	T50.8X3	T50.8X4	T50.8X5	T50.8X6
Iopromide	T50.8X1	T50.8X2	T50.8X3	T50.8X4	T50.8X5	T50.8X6
Iopydol	T50.8X1	T50.8X2	T50.8X3	T50.8X4	T50.8X5	T50.8X6
Iotalamic acid	T50.8X1	T50.8X2	T50.8X3	T50.8X4	T50.8X5	T50.8X6
Iothalamate	T50.8X1	T50.8X2	T50.8X3	T50.8X4	T50.8X5	T50.8X6
Iothiouracil	T38.2X1	T38.2X2	T38.2X3	T38.2X4	T38.2X5	T38.2X6
Iotrol	T50.8X1	T50.8X2	T50.8X3	T50.8X4	T50.8X5	T50.8X6
Iotrolan	T50.8X1	T50.8X2	T50.8X3	T50.8X4	T50.8X5	T50.8X6
Iotroxate	T50.8X1	T50.8X2	T50.8X3	T50.8X4	T50.8X5	T50.8X6
Iotroxic acid	T50.8X1	T50.8X2	T50.8X3	T50.8X4	T50.8X5	T50.8X6
Ioversol	T50.8X1	T50.8X2	T50.8X3	T50.8X4	T50.8X5	T50.8X6
Ioxaglate	T50.8X1	T50.8X2	T50.8X3	T50.8X4	T50.8X5	T50.8X6
Ioxaglic acid	T50.8X1	T50.8X2	T50.8X3	T50.8X4	T50.8X5	T50.8X6
Ioxitalamic acid	T50.8X1	T50.8X2	T50.8X3	T50.8X4	T50.8X5	T50.8X6
Ipecac	T47.7X1	T47.7X2	T47.7X3	T47.7X4	T47.7X5	T47.7X6
Ipecacuanha	T48.4X1	T48.4X2	T48.4X3	T48.4X4	T48.4X5	T48.4X6
Ipodate, calcium	T50.8X1	T50.8X2	T50.8X3	T50.8X4	T50.8X5	T50.8X6
Ipral	T42.3X1	T42.3X2	T42.3X3	T42.3X4	T42.3X5	T42.3X6
Ipratropium (bromide)	T48.6X1	T48.6X2	T48.6X3	T48.6X4	T48.6X5	T48.6X6
Ipriflavone	T46.3X1	T46.3X2	T46.3X3	T46.3X4	T46.3X5	T46.3X6
Iprindole	T43.011	T43.012	T43.013	T43.014	T43.015	T43.016
Iproclozide	T43.1X1	T43.1X2	T43.1X3	T43.1X4	T43.1X5	T43.1X6
Iprofenin	T50.8X1	T50.8X2	T50.8X3	T50.8X4	T50.8X5	T50.8X6
Iproheptine	T49.2X1	T49.2X2	T49.2X3	T49.2X4	T49.2X5	T49.2X6
Iproniazid	T43.1X1	T43.1X2	T43.1X3	T43.1X4	T43.1X5	T43.1X6
Iproplatin	T45.1X1	T45.1X2	T45.1X3	T45.1X4	T45.1X5	T45.1X6
Iproveratril	T46.1X1	T46.1X2	T46.1X3	T46.1X4	T46.1X5	T46.1X6
Iron (compounds) (medicinal) NEC	T45.4X1	T45.4X2	T45.4X3	T45.4X4	T45.4X5	T45.4X6
ammonium	T45.4X1	T45.4X2	T45.4X3	T45.4X4	T45.4X5	T45.4X6
dextran injection	T45.4X1	T45.4X2	T45.4X3	T45.4X4	T45.4X5	T45.4X6
nonmedicinal	T56.891	T56.892	T56.893	T56.894	—	—

◄ New ◄ Revised ~~deleted~~ Deleted

Substance	External Cause (T-Code)					
	Poisoning, Accidental (Unintentional)	Poisoning, Intentional Self-Harm	Poisoning, Assault	Poisoning, Undetermined	Adverse Effect	Underdosing
Iron NEC *(Continued)*						
salts	T45.4X1	T45.4X2	T45.4X3	T45.4X4	T45.4X5	T45.4X6
sorbitex	T45.4X1	T45.4X2	T45.4X3	T45.4X4	T45.4X5	T45.4X6
sorbitol citric acid complex	T45.4X1	T45.4X2	T45.4X3	T45.4X4	T45.4X5	T45.4X6
Irrigating fluid (vaginal)	T49.8X1	T49.8X2	T49.8X3	T49.8X4	T49.8X5	T49.8X6
eye	T49.5X1	T49.5X2	T49.5X3	T49.5X4	T49.5X5	T49.5X6
Isepamicin	T36.5X1	T36.5X2	T36.5X3	T36.5X4	T36.5X5	T36.5X6
Isoaminile (citrate)	T48.3X1	T48.3X2	T48.3X3	T48.3X4	T48.3X5	T48.3X6
Isoamyl nitrite	T46.3X1	T46.3X2	T46.3X3	T46.3X4	T46.3X5	T46.3X6
Isobenzan	T60.1X1	T60.1X2	T60.1X3	T60.1X4	—	—
Isobutyl acetate	T52.8X1	T52.8X2	T52.8X3	T52.8X4	—	—
Isocarboxazid	T43.1X1	T43.1X2	T43.1X3	T43.1X4	T43.1X5	T43.1X6
Isoconazole	T49.0X1	T49.0X2	T49.0X3	T49.0X4	T49.0X5	T49.0X6
Isocyanate	T65.0X1	T65.0X2	T65.0X3	T65.0X4	—	—
Isoephedrine	T44.991	T44.992	T44.993	T44.994	T44.995	T44.996
Isoetarine	T48.6X1	T48.6X2	T48.6X3	T48.6X4	T48.6X5	T48.6X6
Isoethadione	T42.2X1	T42.2X2	T42.2X3	T42.2X4	T42.2X5	T42.2X6
Isoetharine	T44.5X1	T44.5X2	T44.5X3	T44.5X4	T44.5X5	T44.5X6
Isoflurane	T41.0X1	T41.0X2	T41.0X3	T41.0X4	T41.0X5	T41.0X6
Isoflurophate	T44.0X1	T44.0X2	T44.0X3	T44.0X4	T44.0X5	T44.0X6
Isomaltose, ferric complex	T45.4X1	T45.4X2	T45.4X3	T45.4X4	T45.4X5	T45.4X6
Isometheptene	T44.3X1	T44.3X2	T44.3X3	T44.3X4	T44.3X5	T44.3X6
Isoniazid	T37.1X1	T37.1X2	T37.1X3	T37.1X4	T37.1X5	T37.1X6
with						
rifampicin	T36.6X1	T36.6X2	T36.6X3	T36.6X4	T36.6X5	T36.6X6
thioacetazone	T37.1X1	T37.1X2	T37.1X3	T37.1X4	T37.1X5	T37.1X6
Isonicotinic acid hydrazide	T37.1X1	T37.1X2	T37.1X3	T37.1X4	T37.1X5	T37.1X6
Isonipecaine	T40.4X1	T40.4X2	T40.4X3	T40.4X4	T40.4X5	T40.4X6
Isopentaquine	T37.2X1	T37.2X2	T37.2X3	T37.2X4	T37.2X5	T37.2X6
Isophane insulin	T38.3X1	T38.3X2	T38.3X3	T38.3X4	T38.3X5	T38.3X6
Isophorone	T65.891	T65.892	T65.893	T65.894	—	—
Isophosphamide	T45.1X1	T45.1X2	T45.1X3	T45.1X4	T45.1X5	T45.1X6
Isopregnenone	T38.5X1	T38.5X2	T38.5X3	T38.5X4	T38.5X5	T38.5X6
Isoprenaline	T48.6X1	T48.6X2	T48.6X3	T48.6X4	T48.6X5	T48.6X6
Isopromethazine	T43.3X1	T43.3X2	T43.3X3	T43.3X4	T43.3X5	T43.3X6
Isopropamide	T44.3X1	T44.3X2	T44.3X3	T44.3X4	T44.3X5	T44.3X6
iodide	T44.3X1	T44.3X2	T44.3X3	T44.3X4	T44.3X5	T44.3X6
Isopropanol	T51.2X1	T51.2X2	T51.2X3	T51.2X4	—	—

TABLE OF DRUGS AND CHEMICALS

Substance	Poisoning, Accidental (Unintentional)	Poisoning, Intentional Self-Harm	Poisoning, Assault	Poisoning, Undetermined	Adverse Effect	Underdosing
			External Cause (T-Code)			
Isopropyl						
acetate	T52.8X1	T52.8X2	T52.8X3	T52.8X4	—	—
alcohol	T51.2X1	T51.2X2	T51.2X3	T51.2X4	—	—
medicinal	T49.4X1	T49.4X2	T49.4X3	T49.4X4	T49.4X5	T49.4X6
ether	T52.8X1	T52.8X2	T52.8X3	T52.8X4	—	—
Isopropylaminophena-zone	T39.2X1	T39.2X2	T39.2X3	T39.2X4	T39.2X5	T39.2X6
Isoproterenol	T48.6X1	T48.6X2	T48.6X3	T48.6X4	T48.6X5	T48.6X6
Isosorbide dinitrate	T46.3X1	T46.3X2	T46.3X3	T46.3X4	T46.3X5	T46.3X6
Isothipendyl	T45.0X1	T45.0X2	T45.0X3	T45.0X4	T45.0X5	T45.0X6
Isotretinoin	T50.991	T50.992	T50.993	T50.994	T50.995	T50.996
Isoxazolyl penicillin	T36.0X1	T36.0X2	T36.0X3	T36.0X4	T36.0X5	T36.0X6
Isoxicam	T39.391	T39.392	T39.393	T39.394	T39.395	T39.396
Isoxsuprine	T46.7X1	T46.7X2	T46.7X3	T46.7X4	T46.7X5	T46.7X6
Ispagula	T47.4X1	T47.4X2	T47.4X3	T47.4X4	T47.4X5	T47.4X6
husk	T47.4X1	T47.4X2	T47.4X3	T47.4X4	T47.4X5	T47.4X6
Isradipine	T46.1X1	T46.1X2	T46.1X3	T46.1X4	T46.1X5	T46.1X6
l-thyroxine sodium	T38.1X1	T38.1X2	T38.1X3	T38.1X4	T38.1X5	T38.1X6
Itraconazole	T37.8X1	T37.8X2	T37.8X3	T37.8X4	T37.8X5	T37.8X6
Itramin tosilate	T46.3X1	T46.3X2	T46.3X3	T46.3X4	T46.3X5	T46.3X6
Ivermectin	T37.4X1	T37.4X2	T37.4X3	T37.4X4	T37.4X5	T37.4X6
Izoniazid	T37.1X1	T37.1X2	T37.1X3	T37.1X4	T37.1X5	T37.1X6
with thioacetazone	T37.1X1	T37.1X2	T37.1X3	T37.1X4	T37.1X5	T37.1X6
J						
Jalap	T47.2X1	T47.2X2	T47.2X3	T47.2X4	T47.2X5	T47.2X6
Jamaica						
dogwood (bark)	T39.8X1	T39.8X2	T39.8X3	T39.8X4	T39.8X5	T39.8X6
ginger	T65.891	T65.892	T65.893	T65.894	—	—
root	T62.2X1	T62.2X2	T62.2X3	T62.2X4	—	—
Jatropha	T62.2X1	T62.2X2	T62.2X3	T62.2X4	—	—
curcas	T62.2X1	T62.2X2	T62.2X3	T62.2X4	—	—
Jectofer	T45.4X1	T45.4X2	T45.4X3	T45.4X4	T45.4X5	T45.4X6
Jellyfish (sting)	T63.621	T63.622	T63.623	T63.624	—	—
Jequirity (bean)	T62.2X1	T62.2X2	T62.2X3	T62.2X4	—	—
Jimson weed (stramonium)	T62.2X1	T62.2X2	T62.2X3	T62.2X4	—	—
seeds	T62.2X1	T62.2X2	T62.2X3	T62.2X4	—	—
Josamycin	T36.3X1	T36.3X2	T36.3X3	T36.3X4	T36.3X5	T36.3X6
Juniper tar	T49.1X1	T49.1X2	T49.1X3	T49.1X4	T49.1X5	T49.1X6

◀ New   ◀‖‖ Revised   ~~deleted~~ Deleted

Substance	External Cause (T-Code)					
	Poisoning, Accidental (Unintentional)	Poisoning, Intentional Self-Harm	Poisoning, Assault	Poisoning, Undetermined	Adverse Effect	Underdosing
K						
Kallidinogenase	T46.7X1	T46.7X2	T46.7X3	T46.7X4	T46.7X5	T46.7X6
Kallikrein	T46.7X1	T46.7X2	T46.7X3	T46.7X4	T46.7X5	T46.7X6
Kanamycin	T36.5X1	T36.5X2	T36.5X3	T36.5X4	T36.5X5	T36.5X6
Kantrex	T36.5X1	T36.5X2	T36.5X3	T36.5X4	T36.5X5	T36.5X6
Kaolin	T47.6X1	T47.6X2	T47.6X3	T47.6X4	T47.6X5	T47.6X6
light	T47.6X1	T47.6X2	T47.6X3	T47.6X4	T47.6X5	T47.6X6
Karaya (gum)	T47.4X1	T47.4X2	T47.4X3	T47.4X4	T47.4X5	T47.4X6
Kebuzone	T39.2X1	T39.2X2	T39.2X3	T39.2X4	T39.2X5	T39.2X6
Kelevan	T60.1X1	T60.1X2	T60.1X3	T60.1X4	—	—
Kemithal	T41.1X1	T41.1X2	T41.1X3	T41.1X4	T41.1X5	T41.1X6
Kenacort	T38.0X1	T38.0X2	T38.0X3	T38.0X4	T38.0X5	T38.0X6
Keratolytic drug NEC	T49.4X1	T49.4X2	T49.4X3	T49.4X4	T49.4X5	T49.4X6
anthracene	T49.4X1	T49.4X2	T49.4X3	T49.4X4	T49.4X5	T49.4X6
Keratoplastic NEC	T49.4X1	T49.4X2	T49.4X3	T49.4X4	T49.4X5	T49.4X6
Kerosene, kerosine (fuel) (solvent) NEC	T52.0X1	T52.0X2	T52.0X3	T52.0X4	—	—
insecticide	T52.0X1	T52.0X2	T52.0X3	T52.0X4	—	—
vapor	T52.0X1	T52.0X2	T52.0X3	T52.0X4	—	—
Ketamine	T41.291	T41.292	T41.293	T41.294	T41.295	T41.296
Ketazolam	T42.4X1	T42.4X2	T42.4X3	T42.4X4	T42.4X5	T42.4X6
Ketazon	T39.2X1	T39.2X2	T39.2X3	T39.2X4	T39.2X5	T39.2X6
Ketobemidone	T40.4X1	T40.4X2	T40.4X3	T40.4X4	—	—
Ketoconazole	T49.0X1	T49.0X2	T49.0X3	T49.0X4	T49.0X5	T49.0X6
Ketols	T52.4X1	T52.4X2	T52.4X3	T52.4X4	—	—
Ketone oils	T52.4X1	T52.4X2	T52.4X3	T52.4X4	—	—
Ketoprofen	T39.311	T39.312	T39.313	T39.314	T39.315	T39.316
Ketorolac	T39.8X1	T39.8X2	T39.8X3	T39.8X4	T39.8X5	T39.8X6
Ketotifen	T45.0X1	T45.0X2	T45.0X3	T45.0X4	T45.0X5	T45.0X6
Khat	T43.691	T43.692	T43.693	T43.694	—	—
Khellin	T46.3X1	T46.3X2	T46.3X3	T46.3X4	T46.3X5	T46.3X6
Khelloside	T46.3X1	T46.3X2	T46.3X3	T46.3X4	T46.3X5	T46.3X6
Kiln gas or vapor (carbon monoxide)	T58.8X1	T58.8X2	T58.8X3	T58.8X4	—	—
Kitasamycin	T36.3X1	T36.3X2	T36.3X3	T36.3X4	T36.3X5	T36.3X6
Konsyl	T47.4X1	T47.4X2	T47.4X3	T47.4X4	T47.4X5	T47.4X6
Kosam seed	T62.2X1	T62.2X2	T62.2X3	T62.2X4	—	—
Krait (venom)	T63.091	T63.092	T63.093	T63.094	—	—
Kwell (insecticide)	T60.1X1	T60.1X2	T60.1X3	T60.1X4	—	—
anti-infective (topical)	T49.0X1	T49.0X2	T49.0X3	T49.0X4	T49.0X5	T49.0X6

◀ New   ◀▥ Revised   ~~deleted~~ Deleted

Substance	Poisoning, Accidental (Unintentional)	Poisoning, Intentional Self-Harm	Poisoning, Assault	Poisoning, Undetermined	Adverse Effect	Underdosing
L						
Labetalol	T44.8X1	T44.8X2	T44.8X3	T44.8X4	T44.8X5	T44.8X6
Laburnum (seeds)	T62.2X1	T62.2X2	T62.2X3	T62.2X4	—	—
leaves	T62.2X1	T62.2X2	T62.2X3	T62.2X4	—	—
Lachesine	T49.5X1	T49.5X2	T49.5X3	T49.5X4	T49.5X5	T49.5X6
Lacidipine	T46.5X1	T46.5X2	T46.5X3	T46.5X4	T46.5X5	T46.5X6
Lacquer	T65.6X1	T65.6X2	T65.6X3	T65.6X4	—	—
Lacrimogenic gas	T59.3X1	T59.3X2	T59.3X3	T59.3X4	—	—
Lactated potassic saline	T50.3X1	T50.3X2	T50.3X3	T50.3X4	T50.3X5	T50.3X6
Lactic acid	T49.8X1	T49.8X2	T49.8X3	T49.8X4	T49.8X5	T49.8X6
Lactobacillus						
acidophilus	T47.6X1	T47.6X2	T47.6X3	T47.6X4	T47.6X5	T47.6X6
compound	T47.6X1	T47.6X2	T47.6X3	T47.6X4	T47.6X5	T47.6X6
bifidus, lyophilized	T47.6X1	T47.6X2	T47.6X3	T47.6X4	T47.6X5	T47.6X6
bulgaricus	T47.6X1	T47.6X2	T47.6X3	T47.6X4	T47.6X5	T47.6X6
sporogenes	T47.6X1	T47.6X2	T47.6X3	T47.6X4	T47.6X5	T47.6X6
Lactoflavin	T45.2X1	T45.2X2	T45.2X3	T45.2X4	T45.2X5	T45.2X6
Lactose (as excipient)	T50.901	T50.902	T50.903	T50.904	T50.905	T50.906
Lactuca (virosa) (extract)	T42.6X1	T42.6X2	T42.6X3	T42.6X4	T42.6X5	T42.6X6
Lactucarium	T42.6X1	T42.6X2	T42.6X3	T42.6X4	T42.6X5	T42.6X6
Lactulose	T47.3X1	T47.3X2	T47.3X3	T47.3X4	T47.3X5	T47.3X6
Laevo — see Levo-						
Lanatosides	T46.0X1	T46.0X2	T46.0X3	T46.0X4	T46.0X5	T46.0X6
Lanolin	T49.3X1	T49.3X2	T49.3X3	T49.3X4	T49.3X5	T49.3X6
Largactil	T43.3X1	T43.3X2	T43.3X3	T43.3X4	T43.3X5	T43.3X6
Larkspur	T62.2X1	T62.2X2	T62.2X3	T62.2X4	—	—
Laroxyl	T43.011	T43.012	T43.013	T43.014	T43.015	T43.016
Lassar's paste	T49.4X1	T49.4X2	T49.4X3	T49.4X4	T49.4X5	T49.4X6
Lasix	T50.1X1	T50.1X2	T50.1X3	T50.1X4	T50.1X5	T50.1X6
Latamoxef	T36.1X1	T36.1X2	T36.1X3	T36.1X4	T36.1X5	T36.1X6
Latex	T65.811	T65.812	T65.813	T65.814	—	—
Lathyrus (seed)	T62.2X1	T62.2X2	T62.2X3	T62.2X4	—	—
Laudanum	T40.0X1	T40.0X2	T40.0X3	T40.0X4	T40.0X5	T40.0X6
Laudexium	T48.1X1	T48.1X2	T48.1X3	T48.1X4	T48.1X5	T48.1X6
Laughing gas	T41.0X1	T41.0X2	T41.0X3	T41.0X4	T41.0X5	T41.0X6
Laurel, black or cherry	T62.2X1	T62.2X2	T62.2X3	T62.2X4	—	—
Laurolinium	T49.0X1	T49.0X2	T49.0X3	T49.0X4	T49.0X5	T49.0X6
Lauryl sulfoacetate	T49.2X1	T49.2X2	T49.2X3	T49.2X4	T49.2X5	T49.2X6

608   ◀ New   ◀◀◀ Revised   ~~deleted~~ Deleted

Substance	External Cause (T-Code)					
	Poisoning, Accidental (Unintentional)	Poisoning, Intentional Self-Harm	Poisoning, Assault	Poisoning, Undetermined	Adverse Effect	Underdosing
Laxative NEC	T47.4X1	T47.4X2	T47.4X3	T47.4X4	T47.4X5	T47.4X6
osmotic	T47.3X1	T47.3X2	T47.3X3	T47.3X4	T47.3X5	T47.3X6
saline	T47.3X1	T47.3X2	T47.3X3	T47.3X4	T47.3X5	T47.3X6
stimulant	T47.2X1	T47.2X2	T47.2X3	T47.2X4	T47.2X5	T47.2X6
L-dopa	T42.8X1	T42.8X2	T42.8X3	T42.8X4	T42.8X5	T42.8X6
Lead (dust) (fumes) (vapor) NEC	T56.0X1	T56.0X2	T56.0X3	T56.0X4	—	—
acetate	T49.2X1	T49.2X2	T49.2X3	T49.2X4	T49.2X5	T49.2X6
alkyl (fuel additive)	T56.0X1	T56.0X2	T56.0X3	T56.0X4	—	—
anti-infectives	T37.8X1	T37.8X2	T37.8X3	T37.8X4	T37.8X5	T37.8X6
antiknock compound (tetraethyl)	T56.0X1	T56.0X2	T56.0X3	T56.0X4	—	—
arsenate, arsenite (dust) (herbicide) (insecticide) (vapor)	T57.0X1	T57.0X2	T57.0X3	T57.0X4	—	—
carbonate	T56.0X1	T56.0X2	T56.0X3	T56.0X4	—	—
paint	T56.0X1	T56.0X2	T56.0X3	T56.0X4	—	—
chromate	T56.0X1	T56.0X2	T56.0X3	T56.0X4	—	—
paint	T56.0X1	T56.0X2	T56.0X3	T56.0X4	—	—
dioxide	T56.0X1	T56.0X2	T56.0X3	T56.0X4	—	—
inorganic	T56.0X1	T56.0X2	T56.0X3	T56.0X4	—	—
iodide	T56.0X1	T56.0X2	T56.0X3	T56.0X4	—	—
pigment (paint)	T56.0X1	T56.0X2	T56.0X3	T56.0X4	—	—
monoxide (dust)	T56.0X1	T56.0X2	T56.0X3	T56.0X4	—	—
paint	T56.0X1	T56.0X2	T56.0X3	T56.0X4	—	—
organic	T56.0X1	T56.0X2	T56.0X3	T56.0X4	—	—
oxide	T56.0X1	T56.0X2	T56.0X3	T56.0X4	—	—
paint	T56.0X1	T56.0X2	T56.0X3	T56.0X4	—	—
paint	T56.0X1	T56.0X2	T56.0X3	T56.0X4	—	—
salts	T56.0X1	T56.0X2	T56.0X3	T56.0X4	—	—
specified compound NEC	T56.0X1	T56.0X2	T56.0X3	T56.0X4	—	—
tetra-ethyl	T56.0X1	T56.0X2	T56.0X3	T56.0X4	—	—
Lebanese red	T40.7X1	T40.7X2	T40.7X3	T40.7X4	T40.7X5	T40.7X6
Lefetamine	T39.8X1	T39.8X2	T39.8X3	T39.8X4	T39.8X5	T39.8X6
Lenperone	T43.4X1	T43.4X2	T43.4X3	T43.4X4	T43.4X5	T43.4X6
Lente lietin (insulin)	T38.3X1	T38.3X2	T38.3X3	T38.3X4	T38.3X5	T38.3X6
Leptazol	T50.7X1	T50.7X2	T50.7X3	T50.7X4	T50.7X5	T50.7X6
Leptophos	T60.0X1	T60.0X2	T60.0X3	T60.0X4	—	—
Leritine	T40.2X1	T40.2X2	T40.2X3	T40.2X4	T40.2X5	T40.2X6
Letosteine	T48.4X1	T48.4X2	T48.4X3	T48.4X4	T48.4X5	T48.4X6
Letter	T38.1X1	T38.1X2	T38.1X3	T38.1X4	T38.1X5	T38.1X6
Lettuce opium	T42.6X1	T42.6X2	T42.6X3	T42.6X4	T42.6X5	T42.6X6
Leucinocaine	T41.3X1	T41.3X2	T41.3X3	T41.3X4	T41.3X5	T41.3X6

◀ New   ◀▥ Revised   ~~deleted~~ Deleted

TABLE OF DRUGS AND CHEMICALS

Substance	External Cause (T-Code)					
	Poisoning, Accidental (Unintentional)	Poisoning, Intentional Self-Harm	Poisoning, Assault	Poisoning, Undetermined	Adverse Effect	Underdosing
Leucocianidol	T46.991	T46.992	T46.993	T46.994	T46.995	T46.996
Leucovorin (factor)	T45.8X1	T45.8X2	T45.8X3	T45.8X4	T45.8X5	T45.8X6
Leukeran	T45.1X1	T45.1X2	T45.1X3	T45.1X4	T45.1X5	T45.1X6
Leuprolide	T38.891	T38.892	T38.893	T38.894	T38.895	T38.896
Levalbuterol	T48.6X1	T48.6X2	T48.6X3	T48.6X4	T48.6X5	T48.6X6
Levallorphan	T50.7X1	T50.7X2	T50.7X3	T50.7X4	T50.7X5	T50.7X6
Levamisole	T37.4X1	T37.4X2	T37.4X3	T37.4X4	T37.4X5	T37.4X6
Levanil	T42.6X1	T42.6X2	T42.6X3	T42.6X4	T42.6X5	T42.6X6
Levarterenol	T44.4X1	T44.4X2	T44.4X3	T44.4X4	T44.4X5	T44.4X6
Levdropropizine	T48.3X1	T48.3X2	T48.3X3	T48.3X4	T48.3X5	T48.3X6
Levobunolol	T49.5X1	T49.5X2	T49.5X3	T49.5X4	T49.5X5	T49.5X6
Levocabastine (hydrochloride)	T45.0X1	T45.0X2	T45.0X3	T45.0X4	T45.0X5	T45.0X6
Levocarnitine	T50.991	T50.992	T50.993	T50.994	T50.995	T50.996
Levodopa	T42.8X1	T42.8X2	T42.8X3	T42.8X4	T42.8X5	T42.8X6
with carbidopa	T42.8X1	T42.8X2	T42.8X3	T42.8X4	T42.8X5	T42.8X6
Levo-dromoran	T40.2X1	T40.2X2	T40.2X3	T40.2X4	T40.2X5	T40.2X6
Levoglutamide	T50.991	T50.992	T50.993	T50.994	T50.995	T50.996
Levoid	T38.1X1	T38.1X2	T38.1X3	T38.1X4	T38.1X5	T38.1X6
Levo-iso-methadone	T40.3X1	T40.3X2	T40.3X3	T40.3X4	T40.3X5	T40.3X6
Levomepromazine	T43.3X1	T43.3X2	T43.3X3	T43.3X4	T43.3X5	T43.3X6
Levonordefrin	T49.6X1	T49.6X2	T49.6X3	T49.6X4	T49.6X5	T49.6X6
Levonorgestrel	T38.4X1	T38.4X2	T38.4X3	T38.4X4	T38.4X5	T38.4X6
with ethinylestradiol	T38.5X1	T38.5X2	T38.5X3	T38.5X4	T38.5X5	T38.5X6
Levopromazine	T43.3X1	T43.3X2	T43.3X3	T43.3X4	T43.3X5	T43.3X6
Levoprome	T42.6X1	T42.6X2	T42.6X3	T42.6X4	T42.6X5	T42.6X6
Levopropoxyphene	T40.4X1	T40.4X2	T40.4X3	T40.4X4	T40.4X5	T40.4X6
Levopropylhexedrine	T50.5X1	T50.5X2	T50.5X3	T50.5X4	T50.5X5	T50.5X6
Levoproxyphylline	T48.6X1	T48.6X2	T48.6X3	T48.6X4	T48.6X5	T48.6X6
Levorphanol	T40.4X1	T40.4X2	T40.4X3	T40.4X4	T40.4X5	T40.4X6
Levothyroxine	T38.1X1	T38.1X2	T38.1X3	T38.1X4	T38.1X5	T38.1X6
sodium	T38.1X1	T38.1X2	T38.1X3	T38.1X4	T38.1X5	T38.1X6
Levsin	T44.3X1	T44.3X2	T44.3X3	T44.3X4	T44.3X5	T44.3X6
Levulose	T50.3X1	T50.3X2	T50.3X3	T50.3X4	T50.3X5	T50.3X6
Lewisite (gas), not in war	T57.0X1	T57.0X2	T57.0X3	T57.0X4	—	—
Librium	T42.4X1	T42.4X2	T42.4X3	T42.4X4	T42.4X5	T42.4X6
Lidex	T49.0X1	T49.0X2	T49.0X3	T49.0X4	T49.0X5	T49.0X6
Lidocaine	T41.3X1	T41.3X2	T41.3X3	T41.3X4	T41.3X5	T41.3X6
regional	T41.3X1	T41.3X2	T41.3X3	T41.3X4	T41.3X5	T41.3X6
spinal	T41.3X1	T41.3X2	T41.3X3	T41.3X4	T41.3X5	T41.3X6
Lidofenin	T50.8X1	T50.8X2	T50.8X3	T50.8X4	T50.8X5	T50.8X6

◀ New   ◀ꟼ Revised   d̶e̶l̶e̶t̶e̶d̶ Deleted

Substance	External Cause (T-Code)					
	Poisoning, Accidental (Unintentional)	Poisoning, Intentional Self-Harm	Poisoning, Assault	Poisoning, Undetermined	Adverse Effect	Underdosing
Lidoflazine	T46.1X1	T46.1X2	T46.1X3	T46.1X4	T46.1X5	T46.1X6
Lighter fluid	T52.0X1	T52.0X2	T52.0X3	T52.0X4	—	—
Lignin hemicellulose	T47.6X1	T47.6X2	T47.6X3	T47.6X4	T47.6X5	T47.6X6
Lignocaine	T41.3X1	T41.3X2	T41.3X3	T41.3X4	T41.3X5	T41.3X6
regional	T41.3X1	T41.3X2	T41.3X3	T41.3X4	T41.3X5	T41.3X6
spinal	T41.3X1	T41.3X2	T41.3X3	T41.3X4	T41.3X5	T41.3X6
Ligroin(e) (solvent)	T52.0X1	T52.0X2	T52.0X3	T52.0X4	—	—
vapor	T59.891	T59.892	T59.893	T59.894	—	—
Ligustrum vulgare	T62.2X1	T62.2X2	T62.2X3	T62.2X4	—	—
Lily of the valley	T62.2X1	T62.2X2	T62.2X3	T62.2X4	—	—
Lime (chloride)	T54.3X1	T54.3X2	T54.3X3	T54.3X4	—	—
Limonene	T52.8X1	T52.8X2	T52.8X3	T52.8X4	—	—
Lincomycin	T36.8X1	T36.8X2	T36.8X3	T36.8X4	T36.8X5	T36.8X6
Lindane (insecticide) (nonmedicinal) (vapor)	T53.6X1	T53.6X2	T53.6X3	T53.6X4	—	—
medicinal	T49.0X1	T49.0X2	T49.0X3	T49.0X4	T49.0X5	T49.0X6
Liniments NEC	T49.91	T49.92	T49.93	T49.94	T49.95	T49.96
Linoleic acid	T46.6X1	T46.6X2	T46.6X3	T46.6X4	T46.6X5	T46.6X6
Linolenic acid	T46.6X1	T46.6X2	T46.6X3	T46.6X4	T46.6X5	T46.6X6
Linseed	T47.4X1	T47.4X2	T47.4X3	T47.4X4	T47.4X5	T47.4X6
Liothyronine	T38.1X1	T38.1X2	T38.1X3	T38.1X4	T38.1X5	T38.1X6
Liotrix	T38.1X1	T38.1X2	T38.1X3	T38.1X4	T38.1X5	T38.1X6
Lipancreatin	T47.5X1	T47.5X2	T47.5X3	T47.5X4	T47.5X5	T47.5X6
Lipo-alprostadil	T46.7X1	T46.7X2	T46.7X3	T46.7X4	T46.7X5	T46.7X6
Lipo-Lutin	T38.5X1	T38.5X2	T38.5X3	T38.5X4	T38.5X5	T38.5X6
Lipotropic drug NEC	T50.901	T50.902	T50.903	T50.904	T50.905	T50.906
Liquefied petroleum gases	T59.891	T59.892	T59.893	T59.894	—	—
piped (pure or mixed with air)	T59.891	T59.892	T59.893	T59.894	—	—
Liquid						
paraffin	T47.4X1	T47.4X2	T47.4X3	T47.4X4	T47.4X5	T47.4X6
petrolatum	T47.4X1	T47.4X2	T47.4X3	T47.4X4	T47.4X5	T47.4X6
topical	T49.3X1	T49.3X2	T49.3X3	T49.3X4	T49.3X5	T49.3X6
specified NEC	T65.891	T65.892	T65.893	T65.894	—	—
substance	T65.91	T65.92	T65.93	T65.94	—	—
Liquor creosolis compositus	T65.891	T65.892	T65.893	T65.894	—	—
Liquorice	T48.4X1	T48.4X2	T48.4X3	T48.4X4	T48.4X5	T48.4X6
extract	T47.8X1	T47.8X2	T47.8X3	T47.8X4	T47.8X5	T47.8X6
Lirugen	T50.991	T50.992	T50.993	T50.994	T50.995	T50.996
Lisinopril	T46.4X1	T46.4X2	T46.4X3	T46.4X4	T46.4X5	T46.4X6
Lisuride	T42.8X1	T42.8X2	T42.8X3	T42.8X4	T42.8X5	T42.8X6
Lithane	T43.8X1	T43.8X2	T43.8X3	T43.8X4	T43.8X5	T43.8X6

TABLE OF DRUGS AND CHEMICALS

◄ New   ◄⃫ Revised   ~~deleted~~ Deleted

TABLE OF DRUGS AND CHEMICALS

Substance	External Cause (T-Code)					
	Poisoning, Accidental (Unintentional)	Poisoning, Intentional Self-Harm	Poisoning, Assault	Poisoning, Undetermined	Adverse Effect	Underdosing
Lithium	T56.891	T56.892	T56.893	T56.894	—	—
gluconate	T43.591	T43.592	T43.593	T43.594	T43.595	T43.596
salts (carbonate)	T43.591	T43.592	T43.593	T43.594	T43.595	T43.596
Lithonate	T43.8X1	T43.8X2	T43.8X3	T43.8X4	T43.8X5	T43.8X6
Liver						
extract	T45.8X1	T45.8X2	T45.8X3	T45.8X4	T45.8X5	T45.8X6
for parenteral use	T45.8X1	T45.8X2		T45.8X4	T45.8X5	T45.8X6
fraction 1	T45.8X1	T45.8X2	T45.8X3	T45.8X4	T45.8X5	T45.8X6
hydrolysate	T45.8X1	T45.8X2	T45.8X3	T45.8X4	T45.8X5	T45.8X6
Lizard (bite) (venom)	T63.121	T63.122	T63.123	T63.124	—	—
LMD	T45.8X1	T45.8X2	T45.8X3	T45.8X4	T45.8X5	T45.8X6
Lobelia	T62.2X1	T62.2X2	T62.2X3	T62.2X4	—	—
Lobeline	T50.7X1	T50.7X2	T50.7X3	T50.7X4	T50.7X5	T50.7X6
Local action drug NEC	T49.8X1	T49.8X2	T49.8X3	T49.8X4	T49.8X5	T49.8X6
Locorten	T49.0X1	T49.0X2	T49.0X3	T49.0X4	T49.0X5	T49.0X6
Lofepramine	T43.011	T43.012	T43.013	T43.014	T43.015	T43.016
Lolium temulentum	T62.2X1	T62.2X2	T62.2X3	T62.2X4	—	—
Lomotil	T47.6X1	T47.6X2	T47.6X3	T47.6X4	T47.6X5	T47.6X6
Lomustine	T45.1X1	T45.1X2	T45.1X3	T45.1X4	T45.1X5	T45.1X6
Lonidamine	T45.1X1	T45.1X2	T45.1X3	T45.1X4	T45.1X5	T45.1X6
Loperamide	T47.6X1	T47.6X2	T47.6X3	T47.6X4	T47.6X5	T47.6X6
Loprazolam	T42.4X1	T42.4X2	T42.4X3	T42.4X4	T42.4X5	T42.4X6
Lorajmine	T46.2X1	T46.2X2	T46.2X3	T46.2X4	T46.2X5	T46.2X6
Loratidine	T45.0X1	T45.0X2	T45.0X3	T45.0X4	T45.0X5	T45.0X6
Lorazepam	T42.4X1	T42.4X2	T42.4X3	T42.4X4	T42.4X5	T42.4X6
Lorcainide	T46.2X1	T46.2X2	T46.2X3	T46.2X4	T46.2X5	T46.2X6
Lormetazepam	T42.4X1	T42.4X2	T42.4X3	T42.4X4	T42.4X5	T42.4X6
Lotions NEC	T49.91	T49.92	T49.93	T49.94	T49.95	T49.96
Lotusate	T42.3X1	T42.3X2	T42.3X3	T42.3X4	T42.3X5	T42.3X6
Lovastatin	T46.6X1	T46.6X2	T46.6X3	T46.6X4	T46.6X5	T46.6X6
Loxapine	T43.591	T43.592	T43.593	T43.594	T43.595	T43.596
Lowila	T49.2X1	T49.2X2	T49.2X3	T49.2X4	T49.2X5	T49.2X6
Lozenges (throat)	T49.6X1	T49.6X2	T49.6X3	T49.6X4	T49.6X5	T49.6X6
LSD	T40.8X1	T40.8X2	T40.8X3	T40.8X4	—	—
L-Tryptophan — see amino acid						
Lubricant, eye	T49.5X1	T49.5X2	T49.5X3	T49.5X4	T49.5X5	T49.5X6
Lubricating oil NEC	T52.0X1	T52.0X2	T52.0X3	T52.0X4	—	—
Lucanthone	T37.4X1	T37.4X2	T37.4X3	T37.4X4	T37.4X5	T37.4X6
Luminal	T42.3X1	T42.3X2	T42.3X3	T42.3X4	T42.3X5	T42.3X6
Lung irritant (gas) NEC	T59.91	T59.92	T59.93	T59.94	—	—

◀ New   ◀║║ Revised   ~~deleted~~ Deleted

Substance	External Cause (T-Code)					
	Poisoning, Accidental (Unintentional)	Poisoning, Intentional Self-Harm	Poisoning, Assault	Poisoning, Undetermined	Adverse Effect	Underdosing
Luteinizing hormone	T38.811	T38.812	T38.813	T38.814	T38.815	T38.816
Lutocylol	T38.5X1	T38.5X2	T38.5X3	T38.5X4	T38.5X5	T38.5X6
Lutromone	T38.5X1	T38.5X2	T38.5X3	T38.5X4	T38.5X5	T38.5X6
Lututrin	T48.291	T48.292	T48.293	T48.294	T48.295	T48.296
Lye (Concentrated)	T54.3X1	T54.3X2	T54.3X3	T54.3X4	—	—
Lygranum (skin test)	T50.8X1	T50.8X2	T50.8X3	T50.8X4	T50.8X5	T50.8X6
Lymecycline	T36.4X1	T36.4X2	T36.4X3	T36.4X4	T36.4X5	T36.4X6
Lymphogranuloma venereum antigen	T50.8X1	T50.8X2	T50.8X3	T50.8X4	T50.8X5	T50.8X6
Lynestrenol	T38.4X1	T38.4X2	T38.4X3	T38.4X4	T38.4X5	T38.4X6
Lypressin	T38.891	T38.892	T38.893	T38.894	T38.895	T38.896
Lyovac Sodium Edecrin	T50.1X1	T50.1X2	T50.1X3	T50.1X4	T50.1X5	T50.1X6
Lysergic acid diethylamide	T40.8X1	T40.8X2	T40.8X3	T40.8X4	—	— ◄
Lysergide	T40.8X1	T40.8X2	T40.8X3	T40.8X4	—	— ◄
Lysine vasopressin	T38.891	T38.892	T38.893	T38.894	T38.895	T38.896
Lysol	T54.1X1	T54.1X2	T54.1X3	T54.1X4	—	—
Lysozyme	T49.0X1	T49.0X2	T49.0X3	T49.0X4	T49.0X5	T49.0X6
Lytta (vitatta)	T49.8X1	T49.8X2	T49.8X3	T49.8X4	T49.8X5	T49.8X6
M						
Mace	T59.3X1	T59.3X2	T59.3X3	T59.3X4	—	—
Macrogol	T50.991	T50.992	T50.993	T50.994	T50.995	T50.996
Macrolide						
anabolic drug	T38.7X1	T38.7X2	T38.7X3	T38.7X4	T38.7X5	T38.7X6
antibiotic	T36.3X1	T36.3X2	T36.3X3	T36.3X4	T36.3X5	T36.3X6
Mafenide	T49.0X1	T49.0X2	T49.0X3	T49.0X4	T49.0X5	T49.0X6
Magaldrate	T47.1X1	T47.1X2	T47.1X3	T47.1X4	T47.1X5	T47.1X6
Magic mushroom	T40.991	T40.992	T40.993	T40.994	—	—
Magnamycin	T36.8X1	T36.8X2	T36.8X3	T36.8X4	T36.8X5	T36.8X6
Magnesia magma	T47.1X1	T47.1X2	T47.1X3	T47.1X4	T47.1X5	T47.1X6
Magnesium NEC	T56.891	T56.892	T56.893	T56.894	—	—
carbonate	T47.1X1	T47.1X2	T47.1X3	T47.1X4	T47.1X5	T47.1X6
citrate	T47.4X1	T47.4X2	T47.4X3	T47.4X4	T47.4X5	T47.4X6
hydroxide	T47.1X1	T47.1X2	T47.1X3	T47.1X4	T47.1X5	T47.1X6
oxide	T47.1X1	T47.1X2	T47.1X3	T47.1X4	T47.1X5	T47.1X6
peroxide	T49.0X1	T49.0X2	T49.0X3	T49.0X4	T49.0X5	T49.0X6
salicylate	T39.091	T39.092	T39.093	T39.094	T39.095	T39.096
silicofluoride	T50.3X1	T50.3X2	T50.3X3	T50.3X4	T50.3X5	T50.3X6
sulfate	T47.4X1	T47.4X2	T47.4X3	T47.4X4	T47.4X5	T47.4X6
thiosulfate	T45.0X1	T45.0X2	T45.0X3	T45.0X4	T45.0X5	T45.0X6
trisilicate	T47.1X1	T47.1X2	T47.1X3	T47.1X4	T47.1X5	T47.1X6

◄ New ◄ Revised ~~deleted~~ Deleted

	External Cause (T-Code)					
Substance	Poisoning, Accidental (Unintentional)	Poisoning, Intentional Self-Harm	Poisoning, Assault	Poisoning, Undetermined	Adverse Effect	Underdosing
Malathion (medicinal)	T49.0X1	T49.0X2	T49.0X3	T49.0X4	T49.0X5	T49.0X6
insecticide	T60.0X1	T60.0X2	T60.0X3	T60.0X4	—	—
Male fern extract	T37.4X1	T37.4X2	T37.4X3	T37.4X4	T37.4X5	T37.4X6
M-AMSA	T45.1X1	T45.1X2	T45.1X3	T45.1X4	T45.1X5	T45.1X6
Mandelic acid	T37.8X1	T37.8X2	T37.8X3	T37.8X4	T37.8X5	T37.8X6
Manganese (dioxide) (salts)	T57.2X1	T57.2X2	T57.2X3	T57.2X4	—	—
medicinal	T50.991	T50.992	T50.993	T50.994	T50.995	T50.996
Mannitol	T47.3X1	T47.3X2	T47.3X3	T47.3X4	T47.3X5	T47.3X6
hexanitrate	T46.3X1	T46.3X2	T46.3X3	T46.3X4	T46.3X5	T46.3X6
Mannomustine	T45.1X1	T45.1X2	T45.1X3	T45.1X4	T45.1X5	T45.1X6
MAO inhibitors	T43.1X1	T43.1X2	T43.1X3	T43.1X4	T43.1X5	T43.1X6
Mapharsen	T37.8X1	T37.8X2	T37.8X3	T37.8X4	T37.8X5	T37.8X6
Maphenide	T49.0X1	T49.0X2	T49.0X3	T49.0X4	T49.0X5	T49.0X6
Maprotiline	T43.021	T43.022	T43.023	T43.024	T43.025	T43.026
Marcaine	T41.3X1	T41.3X2	T41.3X3	T41.3X4	T41.3X5	T41.3X6
infiltration (subcutaneous)	T41.3X1	T41.3X2	T41.3X3	T41.3X4	T41.3X5	T41.3X6
nerve block (peripheral) (plexus)	T41.3X1	T41.3X2	T41.3X3	T41.3X4	T41.3X5	T41.3X6
Marezine	T45.0X1	T45.0X2	T45.0X3	T45.0X4	T45.0X5	T45.0X6
Marihuana	T40.7X1	T40.7X2	T40.7X3	T40.7X4	T40.7X5	T40.7X6
Marijuana	T40.7X1	T40.7X2	T40.7X3	T40.7X4	T40.7X5	T40.7X6
Marine (sting)	T63.691	T63.692	T63.693	T63.694	—	—
animals (sting)	T63.691	T63.692	T63.693	T63.694	—	—
plants (sting)	T63.711	T63.712	T63.713	T63.714	—	—
Marplan	T43.1X1	T43.1X2	T43.1X3	T43.1X4	T43.1X5	T43.1X6
Marsh gas	T59.891	T59.892	T59.893	T59.894	—	—
Marsilid	T43.1X1	T43.1X2	T43.1X3	T43.1X4	T43.1X5	T43.1X6
Matulane	T45.1X1	T45.1X2	T45.1X3	T45.1X4	T45.1X5	T45.1X6
Mazindol	T50.5X1	T50.5X2	T50.5X3	T50.5X4	T50.5X5	T50.5X6
MCPA	T60.3X1	T60.3X2	T60.3X3	T60.3X4	—	—
MDMA	T43.621	T43.622	T43.623	T43.624	T43.625	T43.626
Meadow saffron	T62.2X1	T62.2X2	T62.2X3	T62.2X4	—	—
Measles virus vaccine (attenuated)	T50.B91	T50.B92	T50.B93	T50.B94	T50.B95	T50.B96
Meat, noxious	T62.8X1	T62.8X2	T62.8X3	T62.8X4	—	—
Meballymal	T42.3X1	T42.3X2	T42.3X3	T42.3X4	T42.3X5	T42.3X6
Mebanazine	T43.1X1	T43.1X2	T43.1X3	T43.1X4	T43.1X5	T43.1X6
Mebaral	T42.3X1	T42.3X2	T42.3X3	T42.3X4	T42.3X5	T42.3X6
Mebendazole	T37.4X1	T37.4X2	T37.4X3	T37.4X4	T37.4X5	T37.4X6
Mebeverine	T44.3X1	T44.3X2	T44.3X3	T44.3X4	T44.3X5	T44.3X6
Mebhydrolin	T45.0X1	T45.0X2	T45.0X3	T45.0X4	T45.0X5	T45.0X6
Mebumal	T42.3X1	T42.3X2	T42.3X3	T42.3X4	T42.3X5	T42.3X6

◀ New   ◀▥ Revised   ~~deleted~~ Deleted

TABLE OF DRUGS AND CHEMICALS

Substance	Poisoning, Accidental (Unintentional)	Poisoning, Intentional Self-Harm	Poisoning, Assault	Poisoning, Undetermined	Adverse Effect	Underdosing
	External Cause (T-Code)					
Mebutamate	T43.591	T43.592	T43.593	T43.594	T43.595	T43.596
Mecamylamine	T44.2X1	T44.2X2	T44.2X3	T44.2X4	T44.2X5	T44.2X6
Mechlorethamine	T45.1X1	T45.1X2	T45.1X3	T45.1X4	T45.1X5	T45.1X6
Mecillinam	T36.0X1	T36.0X2	T36.0X3	T36.0X4	T36.0X5	T36.0X6
Meclizine (hydrochloride)	T45.0X1	T45.0X2	T45.0X3	T45.0X4	T45.0X5	T45.0X6
Meclocycline	T36.4X1	T36.4X2	T36.4X3	T36.4X4	T36.4X5	T36.4X6
Meclofenamate	T39.391	T39.392	T39.393	T39.394	T39.395	T39.396
Meclofenamic acid	T39.391	T39.392	T39.393	T39.394	T39.395	T39.396
Meclofenoxate	T43.691	T43.692	T43.693	T43.694	T43.695	T43.696
Meclozine	T45.0X1	T45.0X2	T45.0X3	T45.0X4	T45.0X5	T45.0X6
Mecobalamin	T45.8X1	T45.8X2	T45.8X3	T45.8X4	T45.8X5	T45.8X6
Mecoprop	T60.3X1	T60.3X2	T60.3X3	T60.3X4	—	—
Mecrilate	T49.3X1	T49.3X2	T49.3X3	T49.3X4	T49.3X5	T49.3X6
Mecysteine	T48.4X1	T48.4X2	T48.4X3	T48.4X4	T48.4X5	T48.4X6
Medazepam	T42.4X1	T42.4X2	T42.4X3	T42.4X4	T42.4X5	T42.4X6
Medicament NEC	T50.901	T50.902	T50.903	T50.904	T50.905	T50.906
Medinal	T42.3X1	T42.3X2	T42.3X3	T42.3X4	T42.3X5	T42.3X6
Medomin	T42.3X1	T42.3X2	T42.3X3	T42.3X4	T42.3X5	T42.3X6
Medrogestone	T38.5X1	T38.5X2	T38.5X3	T38.5X4	T38.5X5	T38.5X6
Medroxalol	T44.8X1	T44.8X2	T44.8X3	T44.8X4	T44.8X5	T44.8X6
Medroxyprogesterone acetate (depot)	T38.5X1	T38.5X2	T38.5X3	T38.5X4	T38.5X5	T38.5X6
Medrysone	T49.0X1	T49.0X2	T49.0X3	T49.0X4	T49.0X5	T49.0X6
Mefenamic acid	T39.391	T39.392	T39.393	T39.394	T39.395	T39.396
Mefenorex	T50.5X1	T50.5X2	T50.5X3	T50.5X4	T50.5X5	T50.5X6
Mefloquine	T37.2X1	T37.2X2	T37.2X3	T37.2X4	T37.2X5	T37.2X6
Mefruside	T50.2X1	T50.2X2	T50.2X3	T50.2X4	T50.2X5	T50.2X6
Megahallucinogen	T40.901	T40.902	T40.903	T40.904	T40.905	T40.906
Megestrol	T38.5X1	T38.5X2	T38.5X3	T38.5X4	T38.5X5	T38.5X6
Meglumine						
antimoniate	T37.8X1	T37.8X2	T37.8X3	T37.8X4	T37.8X5	T37.8X6
diatrizoate	T50.8X1	T50.8X2	T50.8X3	T50.8X4	T50.8X5	T50.8X6
iodipamide	T50.8X1	T50.8X2	T50.8X3	T50.8X4	T50.8X5	T50.8X6
iotroxate	T50.8X1	T50.8X2	T50.8X3	T50.8X4	T50.8X5	T50.8X6
MEK (methyl ethyl ketone)	T52.4X1	T52.4X2	T52.4X3	T52.4X4	—	—
Meladrazine	T44.3X1	T44.3X2	T44.3X3	T44.3X4	T44.3X5	T44.3X6
Meladinin	T49.3X1	T49.3X2	T49.3X3	T49.3X4	T49.3X5	T49.3X6
Melaleuca alternifolia oil	T49.0X1	T49.0X2	T49.0X3	T49.0X4	T49.0X5	T49.0X6
Melanizing agents	T49.3X1	T49.3X2	T49.3X3	T49.3X4	T49.3X5	T49.3X6
Melanocyte-stimulating hormone	T38.891	T38.892	T38.893	T38.894	T38.895	T38.896
Melarsonyl potassium	T37.3X1	T37.3X2	T37.3X3	T37.3X4	T37.3X5	T37.3X6

◀ New   ◀|||| Revised   ~~deleted~~ Deleted

Substance	External Cause (T-Code)					
	Poisoning, Accidental (Unintentional)	Poisoning, Intentional Self-Harm	Poisoning, Assault	Poisoning, Undetermined	Adverse Effect	Underdosing
Melarsoprol	T37.3X1	T37.3X2	T37.3X3	T37.3X4	T37.3X5	T37.3X6
Melia azedarach	T62.2X1	T62.2X2	T62.2X3	T62.2X4	—	—
Melitracen	T43.011	T43.012	T43.013	T43.014	T43.015	T43.016
Mellaril	T43.3X1	T43.3X2	T43.3X3	T43.3X4	T43.3X5	T43.3X6
Meloxine	T49.3X1	T49.3X2	T49.3X3	T49.3X4	T49.3X5	T49.3X6
Melperone	T43.4X1	T43.4X2	T43.4X3	T43.4X4	T43.4X5	T43.4X6
Melphalan	T45.1X1	T45.1X2	T45.1X3	T45.1X4	T45.1X5	T45.1X6
Memantine	T43.8X1	T43.8X2	T43.8X3	T43.8X4	T43.8X5	T43.8X6
Menadiol	T45.7X1	T45.7X2	T45.7X3	T45.7X4	T45.7X5	T45.7X6
sodium sulfate	T45.7X1	T45.7X2	T45.7X3	T45.7X4	T45.7X5	T45.7X6
Menadione	T45.7X1	T45.7X2	T45.7X3	T45.7X4	T45.7X5	T45.7X6
sodium bisulfite	T45.7X1	T45.7X2	T45.7X3	T45.7X4	T45.7X5	T45.7X6
Menaphthone	T45.7X1	T45.7X2	T45.7X3	T45.7X4	T45.7X5	T45.7X6
Menaquinone	T45.7X1	T45.7X2	T45.7X3	T45.7X4	T45.7X5	T45.7X6
Menatetrenone	T45.7X1	T45.7X2	T45.7X3	T45.7X4	T45.7X5	T45.7X6
Meningococcal vaccine	T50.A91	T50.A92	T50.A93	T50.A94	T50.A95	T50.A96
Menningovax (-AC) (-C)	T50.A91	T50.A92	T50.A93	T50.A94	T50.A95	T50.A96
Menotropins	T38.811	T38.812	T38.813	T38.814	T38.815	T38.816
Menthol	T48.5X1	T48.5X2	T48.5X3	T48.5X4	T48.5X5	T48.5X6
Mepacrine	T37.2X1	T37.2X2	T37.2X3	T37.2X4	T37.2X5	T37.2X6
Meparfynol	T42.6X1	T42.6X2	T42.6X3	T42.6X4	T42.6X5	T42.6X6
Mepartricin	T36.7X1	T36.7X2	T36.7X3	T36.7X4	T36.7X5	T36.7X6
Mepazine	T43.3X1	T43.3X2	T43.3X3	T43.3X4	T43.3X5	T43.3X6
Mepenzolate	T44.3X1	T44.3X2	T44.3X3	T44.3X4	T44.3X5	T44.3X6
bromide	T44.3X1	T44.3X2	T44.3X3	T44.3X4	T44.3X5	T44.3X6
Meperidine	T40.4X1	T40.4X2	T40.4X3	T40.4X4	T40.4X5	T40.4X6
Mephebarbital	T42.3X1	T42.3X2	T42.3X3	T42.3X4	T42.3X5	T42.3X6
Mephenamin(e)	T42.8X1	T42.8X2	T42.8X3	T42.8X4	T42.8X5	T42.8X6
Mephenesin	T42.8X1	T42.8X2	T42.8X3	T42.8X4	T42.8X5	T42.8X6
Mephenhydramine	T45.0X1	T45.0X2	T45.0X3	T45.0X4	T45.0X5	T45.0X6
Mephenoxalone	T42.8X1	T42.8X2	T42.8X3	T42.8X4	T42.8X5	T42.8X6
Mephentermine	T44.991	T44.992	T44.993	T44.994	T44.995	T44.996
Mephenytoin	T42.0X1	T42.0X2	T42.0X3	T42.0X4	T42.0X5	T42.0X6
with phenobarbital	T42.3X1	T42.3X2	T42.3X3	T42.3X4	T42.3X5	T42.3X6
Mephobarbital	T42.3X1	T42.3X2	T42.3X3	T42.3X4	T42.3X5	T42.3X6
Mephosfolan	T60.0X1	T60.0X2	T60.0X3	T60.0X4	—	—
Mepindolol	T44.7X1	T44.7X2	T44.7X3	T44.7X4	T44.7X5	T44.7X6
Mepiperphenidol	T44.3X1	T44.3X2	T44.3X3	T44.3X4	T44.3X5	T44.3X6
Mepitiostane	T38.7X1	T38.7X2	T38.7X3	T38.7X4	T38.7X5	T38.7X6

◀ New ◀▥▥ Revised ~~deleted~~ Deleted

Substance	External Cause (T-Code)					
	Poisoning, Accidental (Unintentional)	Poisoning, Intentional Self-Harm	Poisoning, Assault	Poisoning, Undetermined	Adverse Effect	Underdosing
Mepivacaine	T41.3X1	T41.3X2	T41.3X3	T41.3X4	T41.3X5	T41.3X6
epidural	T41.3X1	T41.3X2	T41.3X3	T41.3X4	T41.3X5	T41.3X6
Meprednisone	T38.0X1	T38.0X2	T38.0X3	T38.0X4	T38.0X5	T38.0X6
Meprobam	T43.591	T43.592	T43.593	T43.594	T43.595	T43.596
Meprobamate	T43.591	T43.592	T43.593	T43.594	T43.595	T43.596
Meproscillarin	T46.0X1	T46.0X2	T46.0X3	T46.0X4	T46.0X5	T46.0X6
Meprylcaine	T41.3X1	T41.3X2	T41.3X3	T41.3X4	T41.3X5	T41.3X6
Meptazinol	T39.8X1	T39.8X2	T39.8X3	T39.8X4	T39.8X5	T39.8X6
Mepyramine	T45.0X1	T45.0X2	T45.0X3	T45.0X4	T45.0X5	T45.0X6
Mequitazine	T43.3X1	T43.3X2	T43.3X3	T43.3X4	T43.3X5	T43.3X6
Meralluride	T50.2X1	T50.2X2	T50.2X3	T50.2X4	T50.2X5	T50.2X6
Merbaphen	T50.2X1	T50.2X2	T50.2X3	T50.2X4	T50.2X5	T50.2X6
Merbromin	T49.0X1	T49.0X2	T49.0X3	T49.0X4	T49.0X5	T49.0X6
Mercaptobenzothiazole salts	T49.0X1	T49.0X2	T49.0X3	T49.0X4	T49.0X5	T49.0X6
Mercaptomerin	T50.2X1	T50.2X2	T50.2X3	T50.2X4	T50.2X5	T50.2X6
Mercaptopurine	T45.1X1	T45.1X2	T45.1X3	T45.1X4	T45.1X5	T45.1X6
Mercumatilin	T50.2X1	T50.2X2	T50.2X3	T50.2X4	T50.2X5	T50.2X6
Mercuramide	T50.2X1	T50.2X2	T50.2X3	T50.2X4	T50.2X5	T50.2X6
Mercurochrome	T49.0X1	T49.0X2	T49.0X3	T49.0X4	T49.0X5	T49.0X6
Mercurophylline	T50.2X1	T50.2X2	T50.2X3	T50.2X4	T50.2X5	T50.2X6
Mercury, mercurial, mercuric, mercurous (compounds) (cyanide) (fumes) (nonmedicinal) (vapor) NEC	T56.1X1	T56.1X2	T56.1X3	T56.1X4	—	—
ammoniated	T49.0X1	T49.0X2	T49.0X3	T49.0X4	T49.0X5	T49.0X6
anti-infective						
local	T49.0X1	T49.0X2	T49.0X3	T49.0X4	T49.0X5	T49.0X6
systemic	T37.8X1	T37.8X2	T37.8X3	T37.8X4	T37.8X5	T37.8X6
topical	T49.0X1	T49.0X2	T49.0X3	T49.0X4	T49.0X5	T49.0X6
chloride (ammoniated)	T49.0X1	T49.0X2	T49.0X3	T49.0X4	T49.0X5	T49.0X6
fungicide	T56.1X1	T56.1X2	T56.1X3	T56.1X4	—	—
diuretic NEC	T50.2X1	T50.2X2	T50.2X3	T50.2X4	T50.2X5	T50.2X6
fungicide	T56.1X1	T56.1X2	T56.1X3	T56.1X4	—	—
organic (fungicide)	T56.1X1	T56.1X2	T56.1X3	T56.1X4	—	—
oxide, yellow	T49.0X1	T49.0X2	T49.0X3	T49.0X4	T49.0X5	T49.0X6
Mersalyl	T50.2X1	T50.2X2	T50.2X3	T50.2X4	T50.2X5	T50.2X6
Merthiolate	T49.0X1	T49.0X2	T49.0X3	T49.0X4	T49.0X5	T49.0X6
ophthalmic preparation	T49.5X1	T49.5X2	T49.5X3	T49.5X4	T49.5X5	T49.5X6
Meruvax	T50.B91	T50.B92	T50.B93	T50.B94	T50.B95	T50.B96
Mesalazine	T47.8X1	T47.8X2	T47.8X3	T47.8X4	T47.8X5	T47.8X6
Mescal buttons	T40.991	T40.992	T40.993	T40.994	—	—

TABLE OF DRUGS AND CHEMICALS

◀ New ◀▦ Revised ~~deleted~~ Deleted

Substance	External Cause (T-Code)					
	Poisoning, Accidental (Unintentional)	Poisoning, Intentional Self-Harm	Poisoning, Assault	Poisoning, Undetermined	Adverse Effect	Underdosing
Mescaline	T40.991	T40.992	T40.993	T40.994	—	—
Mesna	T48.4X1	T48.4X2	T48.4X3	T48.4X4	T48.4X5	T48.4X6
Mesoglycan	T46.6X1	T46.6X2	T46.6X3	T46.6X4	T46.6X5	T46.6X6
Mesoridazine	T43.3X1	T43.3X2	T43.3X3	T43.3X4	T43.3X5	T43.3X6
Mestanolone	T38.7X1	T38.7X2	T38.7X3	T38.7X4	T38.7X5	T38.7X6
Mesterolone	T38.7X1	T38.7X2	T38.7X3	T38.7X4	T38.7X5	T38.7X6
Mestranol	T38.5X1	T38.5X2	T38.5X3	T38.5X4	T38.5X5	T38.5X6
Mesulergine	T42.8X1	T42.8X2	T42.8X3	T42.8X4	T42.8X5	T42.8X6
Mesulfen	T49.0X1	T49.0X2	T49.0X3	T49.0X4	T49.0X5	T49.0X6
Mesuximide	T42.2X1	T42.2X2	T42.2X3	T42.2X4	T42.2X5	T42.2X6
Metabutethamine	T41.3X1	T41.3X2	T41.3X3	T41.3X4	T41.3X5	T41.3X6
Metactesylacetate	T49.0X1	T49.0X2	T49.0X3	T49.0X4	T49.0X5	T49.0X6
Metacycline	T36.4X1	T36.4X2	T36.4X3	T36.4X4	T36.4X5	T36.4X6
Metaldehyde (snail killer) NEC	T60.8X1	T60.8X2	T60.8X3	T60.8X4	—	—
Metals (heavy) (nonmedicinal)	T56.91	T56.92	T56.93	T56.94	—	—
dust, fumes, or vapor NEC	T56.91	T56.92	T56.93	T56.94	—	—
light NEC	T56.91	T56.92	T56.93	T56.94	—	—
dust, fumes, or vapor NEC	T56.91	T56.92	T56.93	T56.94	—	—
specified NEC	T56.891	T56.892	T56.893	T56.894	—	—
thallium	T56.811	T56.812	T56.813	T56.814	—	—
Metamfetamine	T43.621	T43.622	T43.623	T43.624	T43.625	T43.626
Metamizole sodium	T39.2X1	T39.2X2	T39.2X3	T39.2X4	T39.2X5	T39.2X6
Metampicillin	T36.0X1	T36.0X2	T36.0X3	T36.0X4	T36.0X5	T36.0X6
Metamucil	T47.4X1	T47.4X2	T47.4X3	T47.4X4	T47.4X5	T47.4X6
Metaphen	T49.0X1	T49.0X2	T49.0X3	T49.0X4	T49.0X5	T49.0X6
Metandienone	T38.7X1	T38.7X2	T38.7X3	T38.7X4	T38.7X5	T38.7X6
Metandrostenolone	T38.7X1	T38.7X2	T38.7X3	T38.7X4	T38.7X5	T38.7X6
Metaphos	T60.0X1	T60.0X2	T60.0X3	T60.0X4	—	—
Metapramine	T43.011	T43.012	T43.013	T43.014	T43.015	T43.016
Metaproterenol	T48.291	T48.292	T48.293	T48.294	T48.295	T48.296
Metaraminol	T44.4X1	T44.4X2	T44.4X3	T44.4X4	T44.4X5	T44.4X6
Metaxalone	T42.8X1	T42.8X2	T42.8X3	T42.8X4	T42.8X5	T42.8X6
Metenolone	T38.7X1	T38.7X2	T38.7X3	T38.7X4	T38.7X5	T38.7X6
Metergoline	T42.8X1	T42.8X2	T42.8X3	T42.8X4	T42.8X5	T42.8X6
Metescufylline	T46.991	T46.992	T46.993	T46.994	T46.995	T46.996
Metetoin	T42.0X1	T42.0X2	T42.0X3	T42.0X4	T42.0X5	T42.0X6
Metformin	T38.3X1	T38.3X2	T38.3X3	T38.3X4	T38.3X5	T38.3X6
Methacholine	T44.1X1	T44.1X2	T44.1X3	T44.1X4	T44.1X5	T44.1X6
Methacycline	T36.4X1	T36.4X2	T36.4X3	T36.4X4	T36.4X5	T36.4X6
Methadone	T40.3X1	T40.3X2	T40.3X3	T40.3X4	T40.3X5	T40.3X6

◀ New   ◀▥ Revised   ~~deleted~~ Deleted

Substance	External Cause (T-Code)					
	Poisoning, Accidental (Unintentional)	Poisoning, Intentional Self-Harm	Poisoning, Assault	Poisoning, Undetermined	Adverse Effect	Underdosing
Methallenestril	T38.5X1	T38.5X2	T38.5X3	T38.5X4	T38.5X5	T38.5X6
Methallenoestril	T38.5X1	T38.5X2	T38.5X3	T38.5X4	T38.5X5	T38.5X6
Methamphetamine	T43.621	T43.622	T43.623	T43.624	T43.625	T43.626
Methampyrone	T39.2X1	T39.2X2	T39.2X3	T39.2X4	T39.2X5	T39.2X6
Methandienone	T38.7X1	T38.7X2	T38.7X3	T38.7X4	T38.7X5	T38.7X6
Methandriol	T38.7X1	T38.7X2	T38.7X3	T38.7X4	T38.7X5	T38.7X6
Methandrostenolone	T38.7X1	T38.7X2	T38.7X3	T38.7X4	T38.7X5	T38.7X6
Methane	T59.891	T59.892	T59.893	T59.894	—	—
Methanethiol	T59.891	T59.892	T59.893	T59.894	—	—
Methaniazide	T37.1X1	T37.1X2	T37.1X3	T37.1X4	T37.1X5	T37.1X6
Methanol (vapor)	T51.1X1	T51.1X2	T51.1X3	T51.1X4	—	—
Methantheline	T44.3X1	T44.3X2	T44.3X3	T44.3X4	T44.3X5	T44.3X6
Methanthelinium bromide	T44.3X1	T44.3X2	T44.3X3	T44.3X4	T44.3X5	T44.3X6
Methaphenilene	T45.0X1	T45.0X2	T45.0X3	T45.0X4	T45.0X5	T45.0X6
Methapyrilene	T45.0X1	T45.0X2	T45.0X3	T45.0X4	T45.0X5	T45.0X6
Methaqualone (compound)	T42.6X1	T42.6X2	T42.6X3	T42.6X4	T42.6X5	T42.6X6
Metharbital	T42.3X1	T42.3X2	T42.3X3	T42.3X4	T42.3X5	T42.3X6
Methazolamide	T50.2X1	T50.2X2	T50.2X3	T50.2X4	T50.2X5	T50.2X6
Methdilazine	T43.3X1	T43.3X2	T43.3X3	T43.3X4	T43.3X5	T43.3X6
Methedrine	T43.621	T43.622	T43.623	T43.624	T43.625	T43.626
Methenamine (mandelate)	T37.8X1	T37.8X2	T37.8X3	T37.8X4	T37.8X5	T37.8X6
Methenolone	T38.7X1	T38.7X2	T38.7X3	T38.7X4	T38.7X5	T38.7X6
Methergine	T48.0X1	T48.0X2	T48.0X3	T48.0X4	T48.0X5	T48.0X6
Methetoin	T42.0X1	T42.0X2	T42.0X3	T42.0X4	T42.0X5	T42.0X6
Methiacil	T38.2X1	T38.2X2	T38.2X3	T38.2X4	T38.2X5	T38.2X6
Methicillin	T36.0X1	T36.0X2	T36.0X3	T36.0X4	T36.0X5	T36.0X6
Methimazole	T38.2X1	T38.2X2	T38.2X3	T38.2X4	T38.2X5	T38.2X6
Methiodal sodium	T50.8X1	T50.8X2	T50.8X3	T50.8X4	T50.8X5	T50.8X6
Methionine	T50.991	T50.992	T50.993	T50.994	T50.995	T50.996
Methisazone	T37.5X1	T37.5X2	T37.5X3	T37.5X4	T37.5X5	T37.5X6
Methisoprinol	T37.5X1	T37.5X2	T37.5X3	T37.5X4	T37.5X5	T37.5X6
Methitural	T42.3X1	T42.3X2	T42.3X3	T42.3X4	T42.3X5	T42.3X6
Methixene	T44.3X1	T44.3X2	T44.3X3	T44.3X4	T44.3X5	T44.3X6
Methobarbital, methobarbitone	T42.3X1	T42.3X2	T42.3X3	T42.3X4	T42.3X5	T42.3X6
Methocarbamol	T42.8X1	T42.8X2	T42.8X3	T42.8X4	T42.8X5	T42.8X6
skeletal muscle relaxant	T48.1X1	T48.1X2	T48.1X3	T48.1X4	T48.1X5	T48.1X6
Methohexital	T41.1X1	T41.1X2	T41.1X3	T41.1X4	T41.1X5	T41.1X6
Methohexitone	T41.1X1	T41.1X2	T41.1X3	T41.1X4	T41.1X5	T41.1X6
Methoin	T42.0X1	T42.0X2	T42.0X3	T42.0X4	T42.0X5	T42.0X6
Methopholine	T39.8X1	T39.8X2	T39.8X3	T39.8X4	T39.8X5	T39.8X6

◀ New ◀▥ Revised ~~deleted~~ Deleted

TABLE OF DRUGS AND CHEMICALS

Substance	External Cause (T-Code)					
	Poisoning, Accidental (Unintentional)	Poisoning, Intentional Self-Harm	Poisoning, Assault	Poisoning, Undetermined	Adverse Effect	Underdosing
Methopromazine	T43.3X1	T43.3X2	T43.3X3	T43.3X4	T43.3X5	T43.3X6
Methorate	T48.3X1	T48.3X2	T48.3X3	T48.3X4	T48.3X5	T48.3X6
Methoserpidine	T46.5X1	T46.5X2	T46.5X3	T46.5X4	T46.5X5	T46.5X6
Methotrexate	T45.1X1	T45.1X2	T45.1X3	T45.1X4	T45.1X5	T45.1X6
Methotrimeprazine	T43.3X1	T43.3X2	T43.3X3	T43.3X4	T43.3X5	T43.3X6
Methoxa-Dome	T49.3X1	T49.3X2	T49.3X3	T49.3X4	T49.3X5	T49.3X6
Methoxamine	T44.4X1	T44.4X2	T44.4X3	T44.4X4	T44.4X5	T44.4X6
Methoxsalen	T50.991	T50.992	T50.993	T50.994	T50.995	T50.996
Methoxyaniline	T65.3X1	T65.3X2	T65.3X3	T65.3X4	—	—
Methoxybenzyl penicillin	T36.0X1	T36.0X2	T36.0X3	T36.0X4	T36.0X5	T36.0X6
Methoxychlor	T53.7X1	T53.7X2	T53.7X3	T53.7X4	—	—
Methoxy-DDT	T53.7X1	T53.7X2	T53.7X3	T53.7X4	—	—
2-Methoxyethanol	T52.3X1	T52.3X2	T52.3X3	T52.3X4	—	—
Methoxyflurane	T41.0X1	T41.0X2	T41.0X3	T41.0X4	T41.0X5	T41.0X6
Methoxyphenamine	T48.6X1	T48.6X2	T48.6X3	T48.6X4	T48.6X5	T48.6X6
Methoxypromazine	T43.3X1	T43.3X2	T43.3X3	T43.3X4	T43.3X5	T43.3X6
5-Methoxypsoralen (5-MOP)	T50.991	T50.992	T50.993	T50.994	T50.995	T50.996
8-Methoxypsoralen (8-MOP)	T50.991	T50.992	T50.993	T50.994	T50.995	T50.996
Methscopolamine bromide	T44.3X1	T44.3X2	T44.3X3	T44.3X4	T44.3X5	T44.3X6
Methsuximide	T42.2X1	T42.2X2	T42.2X3	T42.2X4	T42.2X5	T42.2X6
Methyclothiazide	T50.2X1	T50.2X2	T50.2X3	T50.2X4	T50.2X5	T50.2X6
Methyl						
acetate	T52.4X1	T52.4X2	T52.4X3	T52.4X4	—	—
acetone	T52.4X1	T52.4X2	T52.4X3	T52.4X4	—	—
acrylate	T65.891	T65.892	T65.893	T65.894	—	—
alcohol	T51.1X1	T51.1X2	T51.1X3	T51.1X4	—	—
aminophenol	T65.3X1	T65.3X2	T65.3X3	T65.3X4	—	—
amphetamine	T43.621	T43.622	T43.623	T43.624	T43.625	T43.626
androstanolone	T38.7X1	T38.7X2	T38.7X3	T38.7X4	T38.7X5	T38.7X6
atropine	T44.3X1	T44.3X2	T44.3X3	T44.3X4	T44.3X5	T44.3X6
benzene	T52.2X1	T52.2X2	T52.2X3	T52.2X4	—	—
benzoate	T52.8X1	T52.8X2	T52.8X3	T52.8X4	—	—
benzol	T52.2X1	T52.2X2	T52.2X3	T52.2X4	—	—
bromide (gas)	T59.891	T59.892	T59.893	T59.894	—	—
fumigant	T60.8X1	T60.8X2	T60.8X3	T60.8X4	—	—
butanol	T51.3X1	T51.3X2	T51.3X3	T51.3X4	—	—
carbinol	T51.1X1	T51.1X2	T51.1X3	T51.1X4	—	—
carbonate	T52.8X1	T52.8X2	T52.8X3	T52.8X4	—	—
CCNU	T45.1X1	T45.1X2	T45.1X3	T45.1X4	T45.1X5	T45.1X6
cellosolve	T52.91	T52.92	T52.93	T52.94	—	—

◀ New   ◀‖‖ Revised   ~~deleted~~ Deleted

Substance	External Cause (T-Code)					
	Poisoning, Accidental (Unintentional)	Poisoning, Intentional Self-Harm	Poisoning, Assault	Poisoning, Undetermined	Adverse Effect	Underdosing
Methyl *(Continued)*						
cellulose	T47.4X1	T47.4X2	T47.4X3	T47.4X4	T47.4X5	T47.4X6
chloride (gas)	T59.891	T59.892	T59.893	T59.894	—	—
chloroformate	T59.3X1	T59.3X2	T59.3X3	T59.3X4	—	—
cyclohexane	T52.8X1	T52.8X2	T52.8X3	T52.8X4	—	—
cyclohexanol	T51.8X1	T51.8X2	T51.8X3	T51.8X4	—	—
cyclohexanone	T52.8X1	T52.8X2	T52.8X3	T52.8X4	—	—
cyclohexyl acetate	T52.8X1	T52.8X2	T52.8X3	T52.8X4	—	—
demeton	T60.0X1	T60.0X2	T60.0X3	T60.0X4	—	—
dihydromorphinone	T40.2X1	T40.2X2	T40.2X3	T40.2X4	T40.2X5	T40.2X6
ergometrine	T48.0X1	T48.0X2	T48.0X3	T48.0X4	T48.0X5	T48.0X6
ergonovine	T48.0X1	T48.0X2	T48.0X3	T48.0X4	T48.0X5	T48.0X6
ethyl ketone	T52.4X1	T52.4X2	T52.4X3	T52.4X4	—	—
glucamine antimonate	T37.8X1	T37.8X2	T37.8X3	T37.8X4	T37.8X5	T37.8X6
hydrazine	T65.891	T65.892	T65.893	T65.894	—	—
iodide	T65.891	T65.892	T65.893	T65.894	—	—
isobutyl ketone	T52.4X1	T52.4X2	T52.4X3	T52.4X4	—	—
isothiocyanate	T60.3X1	T60.3X2	T60.3X3	T60.3X4	—	—
mercaptan	T59.891	T59.892	T59.893	T59.894	—	—
morphine NEC	T40.2X1	T40.2X2	T40.2X3	T40.2X4	T40.2X5	T40.2X6
nicotinate	T49.4X1	T49.4X2	T49.4X3	T49.4X4	T49.4X5	T49.4X6
paraben	T49.0X1	T49.0X2	T49.0X3	T49.0X4	T49.0X5	T49.0X6
parafynol	T42.6X1	T42.6X2	T42.6X3	T42.6X4	T42.6X5	T42.6X6
parathion	T60.0X1	T60.0X2	T60.0X3	T60.0X4	—	—
peridol	T43.4X1	T43.4X2	T43.4X3	T43.4X4	T43.4X5	T43.4X6
phenidate	T43.631	T43.632	T43.633	T43.634	T43.635	T43.636
prednisolone	T38.0X1	T38.0X2	T38.0X3	T38.0X4	T38.0X5	T38.0X6
ENT agent	T49.6X1	T49.6X2	T49.6X3	T49.6X4	T49.6X5	T49.6X6
ophthalmic preparation	T49.5X1	T49.5X2	T49.5X3	T49.5X4	T49.5X5	T49.5X6
topical NEC	T49.0X1	T49.0X2	T49.0X3	T49.0X4	T49.0X5	T49.0X6
propylcarbinol	T51.3X1	T51.3X2	T51.3X3	T51.3X4	—	—
rosaniline NEC	T49.0X1	T49.0X2	T49.0X3	T49.0X4	T49.0X5	T49.0X6
salicylate	T49.2X1	T49.2X2	T49.2X3	T49.2X4	T49.2X5	T49.2X6
sulfate (fumes)	T59.891	T59.892	T59.893	T59.894	—	—
liquid	T52.8X1	T52.8X2	T52.8X3	T52.8X4	—	—
sulfonal	T42.6X1	T42.6X2	T42.6X3	T42.6X4	T42.6X5	T42.6X6
testosterone	T38.7X1	T38.7X2	T38.7X3	T38.7X4	T38.7X5	T38.7X6
thiouracil	T38.2X1	T38.2X2	T38.2X3	T38.2X4	T38.2X5	T38.2X6
Methylamphetamine	T43.621	T43.622	T43.623	T43.624	T43.625	T43.626
Methylated spirit	T51.1X1	T51.1X2	T51.1X3	T51.1X4	—	—

◀ New   ◀▥ Revised   ~~deleted~~ Deleted

TABLE OF DRUGS AND CHEMICALS

TABLE OF DRUGS AND CHEMICALS

Substance	External Cause (T-Code)					
	Poisoning, Accidental (Unintentional)	Poisoning, Intentional Self-Harm	Poisoning, Assault	Poisoning, Undetermined	Adverse Effect	Underdosing
Methylatropine nitrate	T44.3X1	T44.3X2	T44.3X3	T44.3X4	T44.3X5	T44.3X6
Methylbenactyzium bromide	T44.3X1	T44.3X2	T44.3X3	T44.3X4	T44.3X5	T44.3X6
Methylbenzethonium chloride	T49.0X1	T49.0X2	T49.0X3	T49.0X4	T49.0X5	T49.0X6
Methylcellulose	T47.4X1	T47.4X2	T47.4X3	T47.4X4	T47.4X5	T47.4X6
laxative	T47.4X1	T47.4X2	T47.4X3	T47.4X4	T47.4X5	T47.4X6
Methylchlorophenoxy-acetic acid	T60.3X1	T60.3X2	T60.3X3	T60.3X4	—	—
Methyldopa	T46.5X1	T46.5X2	T46.5X3	T46.5X4	T46.5X5	T46.5X6
Methyldopate	T46.5X1	T46.5X2	T46.5X3	T46.5X4	T46.5X5	T46.5X6
Methylene						
blue	T50.6X1	T50.6X2	T50.6X3	T50.6X4	T50.6X5	T50.6X6
chloride or dichloride (solvent) NEC	T53.4X1	T53.4X2	T53.4X3	T53.4X4	—	—
Methylenedioxyamphet-amine	T43.621	T43.622	T43.623	T43.624	T43.625	T43.626
Methylenedioxymethamphetamine	T43.621	T43.622	T43.623	T43.624	T43.625	T43.626
Methylergometrine	T48.0X1	T48.0X2	T48.0X3	T48.0X4	T48.0X5	T48.0X6
Methylergonovine	T48.0X1	T48.0X2	T48.0X3	T48.0X4	T48.0X5	T48.0X6
Methylestrenolone	T38.5X1	T38.5X2	T38.5X3	T38.5X4	T38.5X5	T38.5X6
Methylethyl cellulose	T50.991	T50.992	T50.993	T50.994	T50.995	T50.996
Methylhexabital	T42.3X1	T42.3X2	T42.3X3	T42.3X4	T42.3X5	T42.3X6
Methylmorphine	T40.2X1	T40.2X2	T40.2X3	T40.2X4	T40.2X5	T40.2X6
Methylparaben (ophthalmic)	T49.5X1	T49.5X2	T49.5X3	T49.5X4	T49.5X5	T49.5X6
Methylparafynol	T42.6X1	T42.6X2	T42.6X3	T42.6X4	T42.6X5	T42.6X6
Methylpentynol, methylpenthynol	T42.6X1	T42.6X2	T42.6X3	T42.6X4	T42.6X5	T42.6X6
Methylphenidate	T43.631	T43.632	T43.633	T43.634	T43.635	T43.636
Methylphenobarbital	T42.3X1	T42.3X2	T42.3X3	T42.3X4	T42.3X5	T42.3X6
Methylpolysiloxane	T47.1X1	T47.1X2	T47.1X3	T47.1X4	T47.1X5	T47.1X6
Methylprednisolone — see Methyl, prednisolone						
Methylrosaniline	T49.0X1	T49.0X2	T49.0X3	T49.0X4	T49.0X5	T49.0X6
Methylrosanilinium chloride	T49.0X1	T49.0X2	T49.0X3	T49.0X4	T49.0X5	T49.0X6
Methyltestosterone	T38.7X1	T38.7X2	T38.7X3	T38.7X4	T38.7X5	T38.7X6
Methylthionine chloride	T50.6X1	T50.6X2	T50.6X3	T50.6X4	T50.6X5	T50.6X6
Methylthioninium chloride	T50.6X1	T50.6X2	T50.6X3	T50.6X4	T50.6X5	T50.6X6
Methylthiouracil	T38.2X1	T38.2X2	T38.2X3	T38.2X4	T38.2X5	T38.2X6
Methyprylon	T42.6X1	T42.6X2	T42.6X3	T42.6X4	T42.6X5	T42.6X6
Methysergide	T46.5X1	T46.5X2	T46.5X3	T46.5X4	T46.5X5	T46.5X6
Metiamide	T47.1X1	T47.1X2	T47.1X3	T47.1X4	T47.1X5	T47.1X6
Meticillin	T36.0X1	T36.0X2	T36.0X3	T36.0X4	T36.0X5	T36.0X6
Meticrane	T50.2X1	T50.2X2	T50.2X3	T50.2X4	T50.2X5	T50.2X6
Metildigoxin	T46.0X1	T46.0X2	T46.0X3	T46.0X4	T46.0X5	T46.0X6
Metipranolol	T49.5X1	T49.5X2	T49.5X3	T49.5X4	T49.5X5	T49.5X6

◀ New   ◀▦ Revised   ~~deleted~~ Deleted

Substance	Poisoning, Accidental (Unintentional)	Poisoning, Intentional Self-Harm	Poisoning, Assault	Poisoning, Undetermined	Adverse Effect	Underdosing
Metirosine	T46.5X1	T46.5X2	T46.5X3	T46.5X4	T46.5X5	T46.5X6
Metisazone	T37.5X1	T37.5X2	T37.5X3	T37.5X4	T37.5X5	T37.5X6
Metixene	T44.3X1	T44.3X2	T44.3X3	T44.3X4	T44.3X5	T44.3X6
Metizoline	T48.5X1	T48.5X2	T48.5X3	T48.5X4	T48.5X5	T48.5X6
Metoclopramide	T45.0X1	T45.0X2	T45.0X3	T45.0X4	T45.0X5	T45.0X6
Metofenazate	T43.3X1	T43.3X2	T43.3X3	T43.3X4	T43.3X5	T43.3X6
Metofoline	T39.8X1	T39.8X2	T39.8X3	T39.8X4	T39.8X5	T39.8X6
Metolazone	T50.2X1	T50.2X2	T50.2X3	T50.2X4	T50.2X5	T50.2X6
Metopon	T40.2X1	T40.2X2	T40.2X3	T40.2X4	T40.2X5	T40.2X6
Metoprine	T45.1X1	T45.1X2	T45.1X3	T45.1X4	T45.1X5	T45.1X6
Metoprolol	T44.7X1	T44.7X2	T44.7X3	T44.7X4	T44.7X5	T44.7X6
Metrifonate	T60.0X1	T60.0X2	T60.0X3	T60.0X4	—	—
Metrizamide	T50.8X1	T50.8X2	T50.8X3	T50.8X4	T50.8X5	T50.8X6
Metrizoic acid	T50.8X1	T50.8X2	T50.8X3	T50.8X4	T50.8X5	T50.8X6
Metronidazole	T37.8X1	T37.8X2	T37.8X3	T37.8X4	T37.8X5	T37.8X6
Metycaine	T41.3X1	T41.3X2	T41.3X3	T41.3X4	T41.3X5	T41.3X6
infiltration (subcutaneous)	T41.3X1	T41.3X2	T41.3X3	T41.3X4	T41.3X5	T41.3X6
nerve block (peripheral) (plexus)	T41.3X1	T41.3X2	T41.3X3	T41.3X4	T41.3X5	T41.3X6
topical (surface)	T41.3X1	T41.3X2	T41.3X3	T41.3X4	T41.3X5	T41.3X6
Metyrapone	T50.8X1	T50.8X2	T50.8X3	T50.8X4	T50.8X5	T50.8X6
Mevinphos	T60.0X1	T60.0X2	T60.0X3	T60.0X4	—	—
Mexazolam	T42.4X1	T42.4X2	T42.4X3	T42.4X4	T42.4X5	T42.4X6
Mexenone	T49.3X1	T49.3X2	T49.3X3	T49.3X4	T49.3X5	T49.3X6
Mexiletine	T46.2X1	T46.2X2	T46.2X3	T46.2X4	T46.2X5	T46.2X6
Mezereon	T62.2X1	T62.2X2	T62.2X3	T62.2X4	—	—
berries	T62.1X1	T62.1X2	T62.1X3	T62.1X4	—	—
Mezlocillin	T36.0X1	T36.0X2	T36.0X3	T36.0X4	T36.0X5	T36.0X6
Mianserin	T43.021	T43.022	T43.023	T43.024	T43.025	T43.026
Micatin	T49.0X1	T49.0X2	T49.0X3	T49.0X4	T49.0X5	T49.0X6
Miconazole	T49.0X1	T49.0X2	T49.0X3	T49.0X4	T49.0X5	T49.0X6
Micronomicin	T36.5X1	T36.5X2	T36.5X3	T36.5X4	T36.5X5	T36.5X6
Midazolam	T42.4X1	T42.4X2	T42.4X3	T42.4X4	T42.4X5	T42.4X6
Midecamycin	T36.3X1	T36.3X2	T36.3X3	T36.3X4	T36.3X5	T36.3X6
Mifepristone	T38.6X1	T38.6X2	T38.6X3	T38.6X4	T38.6X5	T38.6X6
Milk of magnesia	T47.1X1	T47.1X2	T47.1X3	T47.1X4	T47.1X5	T47.1X6
Millipede (tropical) (venomous)	T63.411	T63.412	T63.413	T63.414	—	—
Miltown	T43.591	T43.592	T43.593	T43.594	T43.595	T43.596
Milverine	T44.3X1	T44.3X2	T44.3X3	T44.3X4	T44.3X5	T44.3X6
Minaprine	T43.291	T43.292	T43.293	T43.294	T43.295	T43.296

TABLE OF DRUGS AND CHEMICALS

◀ New ◀ Revised ~~deleted~~ Deleted

Substance	External Cause (T-Code)					
	Poisoning, Accidental (Unintentional)	Poisoning, Intentional Self-Harm	Poisoning, Assault	Poisoning, Undetermined	Adverse Effect	Underdosing
Minaxolone	T41.291	T41.292	T41.293	T41.294	T41.295	T41.296
Mineral						
acids	T54.2X1	T54.2X2	T54.2X3	T54.2X4	—	—
oil (laxative) (medicinal)	T47.4X1	T47.4X2	T47.4X3	T47.4X4	T47.4X5	T47.4X6
emulsion	T47.2X1	T47.2X2	T47.2X3	T47.2X4	T47.2X5	T47.2X6
nonmedicinal	T52.0X1	T52.0X2	T52.0X3	T52.0X4	—	—
topical	T49.3X1	T49.3X2	T49.3X3	T49.3X4	T49.3X5	T49.3X6
salt NEC	T50.3X1	T50.3X2	T50.3X3	T50.3X4	T50.3X5	T50.3X6
spirits	T52.0X1	T52.0X2	T52.0X3	T52.0X4	—	—
Mineralocorticosteroid	T50.0X1	T50.0X2	T50.0X3	T50.0X4	T50.0X5	T50.0X6
Minocycline	T36.4X1	T36.4X2	T36.4X3	T36.4X4	T36.4X5	T36.4X6
Minoxidil	T46.7X1	T46.7X2	T46.7X3	T46.7X4	T46.7X5	T46.7X6
Miokamycin	T36.3X1	T36.3X2	T36.3X3	T36.3X4	T36.3X5	T36.3X6
Miotic drug	T49.5X1	T49.5X2	T49.5X3	T49.5X4	T49.5X5	T49.5X6
Mipafox	T60.0X1	T60.0X2	T60.0X3	T60.0X4	—	—
Mirex	T60.1X1	T60.1X2	T60.1X3	T60.1X4	—	—
Mirtazapine	T43.021	T43.022	T43.023	T43.024	T43.025	T43.026
Misonidazole	T37.3X1	T37.3X2	T37.3X3	T37.3X4	T37.3X5	T37.3X6
Misoprostol	T47.1X1	T47.1X2	T47.1X3	T47.1X4	T47.1X5	T47.1X6
Mithramycin	T45.1X1	T45.1X2	T45.1X3	T45.1X4	T45.1X5	T45.1X6
Mitobronitol	T45.1X1	T45.1X2	T45.1X3	T45.1X4	T45.1X5	T45.1X6
Mitoguazone	T45.1X1	T45.1X2	T45.1X3	T45.1X4	T45.1X5	T45.1X6
Mitolactol	T45.1X1	T45.1X2	T45.1X3	T45.1X4	T45.1X5	T45.1X6
Mitomycin	T45.1X1	T45.1X2	T45.1X3	T45.1X4	T45.1X5	T45.1X6
Mitopodozide	T45.1X1	T45.1X2	T45.1X3	T45.1X4	T45.1X5	T45.1X6
Mitotane	T45.1X1	T45.1X2	T45.1X3	T45.1X4	T45.1X5	T45.1X6
Mitoxantrone	T45.1X1	T45.1X2	T45.1X3	T45.1X4	T45.1X5	T45.1X6
Mivacurium chloride	T48.1X1	T48.1X2	T48.1X3	T48.1X4	T48.1X5	T48.1X6
Miyari bacteria	T47.6X1	T47.6X2	T47.6X3	T47.6X4	T47.6X5	T47.6X6
Moclobemide	T43.1X1	T43.1X2	T43.1X3	T43.1X4	T43.1X5	T43.1X6
Moderil	T46.5X1	T46.5X2	T46.5X3	T46.5X4	T46.5X5	T46.5X6
Mofebutazone	T39.2X1	T39.2X2	T39.2X3	T39.2X4	T39.2X5	T39.2X6
Mogadon — see Nitrazepam						
Molindone	T43.591	T43.592	T43.593	T43.594	T43.595	T43.596
Molsidomine	T46.3X1	T46.3X2	T46.3X3	T46.3X4	T46.3X5	T46.3X6
Mometasone	T49.0X1	T49.0X2	T49.0X3	T49.0X4	T49.0X5	T49.0X6
Monistat	T49.0X1	T49.0X2	T49.0X3	T49.0X4	T49.0X5	T49.0X6
Monkshood	T62.2X1	T62.2X2	T62.2X3	T62.2X4	—	—
Monoamine oxidase inhibitor NEC	T43.1X1	T43.1X2	T43.1X3	T43.1X4	T43.1X5	T43.1X6
hydrazine	T43.1X1	T43.1X2	T43.1X3	T43.1X4	T43.1X5	T43.1X6

◀ New   ◀▥ Revised   ~~deleted~~ Deleted

Substance	External Cause (T-Code)					
	Poisoning, Accidental (Unintentional)	Poisoning, Intentional Self-Harm	Poisoning, Assault	Poisoning, Undetermined	Adverse Effect	Underdosing
Monobenzone	T49.4X1	T49.4X2	T49.4X3	T49.4X4	T49.4X5	T49.4X6
Monochloroacetic acid	T60.3X1	T60.3X2	T60.3X3	T60.3X4	—	—
Monochlorobenzene	T53.7X1	T53.7X2	T53.7X3	T53.7X4	—	—
Monoethanolamine	T46.8X1	T46.8X2	T46.8X3	T46.8X4	T46.8X5	T46.8X6
oleate	T46.8X1	T46.8X2	T46.8X3	T46.8X4	T46.8X5	T46.8X6
Monooctanoin	T50.991	T50.992	T50.993	T50.994	T50.995	T50.996
Monophenylbutazone	T39.2X1	T39.2X2	T39.2X3	T39.2X4	T39.2X5	T39.2X6
Monosodium glutamate	T65.891	T65.892	T65.893	T65.894	—	—
Monosulfiram	T49.0X1	T49.0X2	T49.0X3	T49.0X4	T49.0X5	T49.0X6
Monoxide, carbon — see Carbon, monoxide	T57.91	T57.92	T57.93	T57.94	—	—
Monoxidine hydrochloride	T46.1X1	T46.1X2	T46.1X3	T46.1X4	T46.1X5	T46.1X6
Monuron	T60.3X1	T60.3X2	T60.3X3	T60.3X4	—	—
Moperone	T43.4X1	T43.4X2	T43.4X3	T43.4X4	T43.4X5	T43.4X6
Mopidamol	T45.1X1	T45.1X2	T45.1X4	T45.1X4	T45.1X5	T45.1X6
MOPP (mechlorethamine + vincristine + prednisone + procarbazine)	T45.1X1	T45.1X2	T45.1X3	T45.1X4	T45.1X5	T45.1X6
Morfin	T40.2X1	T40.2X2	T40.2X3	T40.2X4	T40.2X5	T40.2X6
Morinamide	T37.1X1	T37.1X2	T37.1X3	T37.1X4	T37.1X5	T37.1X6
Morning glory seeds	T40.991	T40.992	T40.993	T40.994	—	—
Moroxydine	T37.5X1	T37.5X2	T37.5X3	T37.5X4	T37.5X5	T37.5X6
Morphazinamide	T37.1X1	T37.1X2	T37.1X3	T37.1X4	T37.1X5	T37.1X6
Morphine	T40.2X1	T40.2X2	T40.2X3	T40.2X4	T40.2X5	T40.2X6
antagonist	T50.7X1	T50.7X2	T50.7X3	T50.7X4	T50.7X5	T50.7X6
Morpholinylethylmorphine	T40.2X1	T40.2X2	T40.2X3	T40.2X4	—	—
Morsuximide	T42.2X1	T42.2X2	T42.2X3	T42.2X4	T42.2X5	T42.2X6
Mosapramine	T43.591	T43.592	T43.593	T43.594	T43.595	T43.596
Moth balls — see also Pesticides	T60.2X1	T60.2X2	T60.2X3	T60.2X4	—	—
naphthalene	T60.2X1	T60.2X2	T60.2X3	T60.2X4	—	—
paradichlorobenzene	T60.1X1	T60.1X2	T60.1X3	T60.1X4	—	—
Motor exhaust gas	T58.01	T58.02	T58.03	T58.04	—	—
Mouthwash (antiseptic) (zinc chloride)	T49.6X1	T49.6X2	T49.6X3	T49.6X4	T49.6X5	T49.6X6
Moxastine	T45.0X1	T45.0X2	T45.0X3	T45.0X4	T45.0X5	T45.0X6
Moxaverine	T44.3X1	T44.3X2	T44.3X3	T44.3X4	T44.3X5	T44.3X6
Moxifensine	T43.291	T43.292	T43.293	T43.294	T43.295	T43.296
Moxisylyte	T46.7X1	T46.7X2	T46.7X3	T46.7X4	T46.7X5	T46.7X6
Mucilage, plant	T47.4X1	T47.4X2	T47.4X3	T47.4X4	T47.4X5	T47.4X6
Mucolytic drug	T48.4X1	T48.4X2	T48.4X3	T48.4X4	T48.4X5	T48.4X6
Mucomyst	T48.4X1	T48.4X2	T48.4X3	T48.4X4	T48.4X5	T48.4X6
Mucous membrane agents (external)	T49.91	T49.92	T49.93	T49.94	T49.95	T49.96
specified NEC	T49.8X1	T49.8X2	T49.8X3	T49.8X4	T49.8X5	T49.8X6

TABLE OF DRUGS AND CHEMICALS

◀ New ◀||| Revised ~~deleted~~ Deleted

TABLE OF DRUGS AND CHEMICALS

Substance	External Cause (T-Code)					
	Poisoning, Accidental (Unintentional)	Poisoning, Intentional Self-Harm	Poisoning, Assault	Poisoning, Undetermined	Adverse Effect	Underdosing
Mumps						
immune globulin (human)	T50.Z11	T50.Z12	T50.Z13	T50.Z14	T50.Z15	T50.Z16
skin test antigen	T50.8X1	T50.8X2	T50.8X3	T50.8X4	T50.8X5	T50.8X6
vaccine	T50.B91	T50.B92	T50.B93	T50.B94	T50.B95	T50.B96
Mumpsvax	T50.B91	T50.B92	T50.B93	T50.B94	T50.B95	T50.B96
Mupirocin	T49.0X1	T49.0X2	T49.0X3	T49.0X4	T49.0X5	T49.0X6
Muriatic acid — *see Hydrochloric acid*						
Muromonab-CD3	T45.1X1	T45.1X2	T45.1X3	T45.1X4	T45.1X5	T45.1X6
Muscle relaxant — *see Relaxant, muscle*						
Muscle-action drug NEC	T48.201	T48.202	T48.203	T48.204	T48.205	T48.206
Muscle affecting agents NEC	T48.201	T48.202	T48.203	T48.204	T48.205	T48.206
oxytocic	T48.0X1	T48.0X2	T48.0X3	T48.0X4	T48.0X5	T48.0X6
relaxants	T48.201	T48.202	T48.203	T48.204	T48.205	T48.206
central nervous system	T42.8X1	T42.8X2	T42.8X3	T42.8X4	T42.8X5	T42.8X6
skeletal	T48.1X1	T48.1X2	T48.1X3	T48.1X4	T48.1X5	T48.1X6
smooth	T44.3X1	T44.3X2	T44.3X3	T44.3X4	T44.3X5	T44.3X6
Muscle-tone depressant, central NEC	T42.8X1	T42.8X2	T42.8X3	T42.8X4	T42.8X5	T42.8X6
specified NEC	T42.8X1	T42.8X2	T42.8X3	T42.8X4	T42.8X5	T42.8X6
Mushroom, noxious	T62.0X1	T62.0X2	T62.0X3	T62.0X4	—	—
Mussel, noxious	T61.781	T61.782	T61.783	T61.784	—	—
Mustard (emetic)	T47.7X1	T47.7X2	T47.7X3	T47.7X4	T47.7X5	T47.7X6
black	T47.7X1	T47.7X2	T47.7X3	T47.7X4	T47.7X5	T47.7X6
gas, not in war	T59.91	T59.92	T59.93	T59.94	—	—
nitrogen	T45.1X1	T45.1X2	T45.1X3	T45.1X4	T45.1X5	T45.1X6
Mustine	T45.1X1	T45.1X2	T45.1X3	T45.1X4	T45.1X5	T45.1X6
M-vac	T45.1X1	T45.1X2	T45.1X3	T45.1X4	T45.1X5	T45.1X6
Mycifradin	T36.5X1	T36.5X2	T36.5X3	T36.5X4	T36.5X5	T36.5X6
topical	T49.0X1	T49.0X2	T49.0X3	T49.0X4	T49.0X5	T49.0X6
Mycitracin	T36.8X1	T36.8X2	T36.8X3	T36.8X4	T36.8X5	T36.8X6
ophthalmic preparation	T49.5X1	T49.5X2	T49.5X3	T49.5X4	T49.5X5	T49.5X6
Mycostatin	T36.7X1	T36.7X2	T36.7X3	T36.7X4	T36.7X5	T36.7X6
topical	T49.0X1	T49.0X2	T49.0X3	T49.0X4	T49.0X5	T49.0X6
Mycotoxins	T64.81	T64.82	T64.83	T64.84	—	—
aflatoxin	T64.01	T64.02	T64.03	T64.04	—	—
specified NEC	T64.81	T64.82	T64.83	T64.84	—	—
Mydriacyl	T44.3X1	T44.3X2	T44.3X3	T44.3X4	T44.3X5	T44.3X6
Mydriatic drug	T49.5X1	T49.5X2	T49.5X3	T49.5X4	T49.5X5	T49.5X6
Myelobromal	T45.1X1	T45.1X2	T45.1X3	T45.1X4	T45.1X5	T45.1X6
Myleran	T45.1X1	T45.1X2	T45.1X3	T45.1X4	T45.1X5	T45.1X6
Myochrysin(e)	T39.2X1	T39.2X2	T39.2X3	T39.2X4	T39.2X5	T39.2X6

◀ New　◀ Revised　~~deleted~~ Deleted

Substance	External Cause (T-Code)					
	Poisoning, Accidental (Unintentional)	Poisoning, Intentional Self-Harm	Poisoning, Assault	Poisoning, Undetermined	Adverse Effect	Underdosing
Myoneural blocking agents	T48.1X1	T48.1X2	T48.1X3	T48.1X4	T48.1X5	T48.1X6
Myralact	T49.0X1	T49.0X2	T49.0X3	T49.0X4	T49.0X5	T49.0X6
Myristica fragrans	T62.2X1	T62.2X2	T62.2X3	T62.2X4	—	—
Myristicin	T65.891	T65.892	T65.893	T65.894	—	—
Mysoline	T42.3X1	T42.3X2	T42.3X3	T42.3X4	T42.3X5	T42.3X6
N						
Nabilone	T40.7X1	T40.7X2	T40.7X3	T40.7X4	T40.7X5	T40.7X6
Nabumetone	T39.391	T39.392	T39.393	T39.394	T39.395	T39.396
Nadolol	T44.7X1	T44.7X2	T44.7X3	T44.7X4	T44.7X5	T44.7X6
Nafcillin	T36.0X1	T36.0X2	T36.0X3	T36.0X4	T36.0X5	T36.0X6
Nafoxidine	T38.6X1	T38.6X2	T38.6X3	T38.6X4	T38.6X5	T38.6X6
Naftazone	T46.991	T46.992	T46.993	T46.994	T46.995	T46.996
Naftidrofuryl (oxalate)	T46.7X1	T46.7X2	T46.7X3	T46.7X4	T46.7X5	T46.7X6
Naftifine	T49.0X1	T49.0X2	T49.0X3	T49.0X4	T49.0X5	T49.0X6
Nail polish remover	T52.91	T52.92	T52.93	T52.94	—	—
Nalbuphine	T40.4X1	T40.4X2	T40.4X3	T40.4X4	T40.4X5	T40.4X6
Naled	T60.0X1	T60.0X2	T60.0X3	T60.0X4	—	—
Nalidixic acid	T37.8X1	T37.8X2	T37.8X3	T37.8X4	T37.8X5	T37.8X6
Nalorphine	T50.7X1	T50.7X2	T50.7X3	T50.7X4	T50.7X5	T50.7X6
Naloxone	T50.7X1	T50.7X2	T50.7X3	T50.7X4	T50.7X5	T50.7X6
Naltrexone	T50.7X1	T50.7X2	T50.7X3	T50.7X4	T50.7X5	T50.7X6
Namenda	T43.8X1	T43.8X2	T43.8X3	T43.8X4	T43.8X5	T43.8X6
Nandrolone	T38.7X1	T38.7X2	T38.7X3	T38.7X4	T38.7X5	T38.7X6
Naphazoline	T48.5X1	T48.5X2	T48.5X3	T48.5X4	T48.5X5	T48.5X6
Naphtha (painters') (petroleum)	T52.0X1	T52.0X2	T52.0X3	T52.0X4	—	—
solvent	T52.0X1	T52.0X2	T52.0X3	T52.0X4	—	—
vapor	T52.0X1	T52.0X2	T52.0X3	T52.0X4	—	—
Naphthalene (non-chlorinated)	T60.2X1	T60.2X2	T60.2X3	T60.2X4	—	—
chlorinated	T60.1X1	T60.1X2	T60.1X3	T60.1X4	—	—
vapor	T60.1X1	T60.1X2	T60.1X3	T60.1X4	—	—
insecticide or moth repellent	T60.2X1	T60.2X2	T60.2X3	T60.2X4	—	—
chlorinated	T60.1X1	T60.1X2	T60.1X3	T60.1X4	—	—
vapor	T60.2X1	T60.2X2	T60.2X3	T60.2X4	—	—
chlorinated	T60.1X1	T60.1X2	T60.1X3	T60.1X4	—	—
Naphthol	T65.891	T65.892	T65.893	T65.894	—	—
Naphthylamine	T65.891	T65.892	T65.893	T65.894	—	—
Naphthylthiourea (ANTU)	T60.4X1	T60.4X2	T60.4X3	T60.4X4	—	—
Naprosyn — see Naproxen						
Naproxen	T39.311	T39.312	T39.313	T39.314	T39.315	T39.316

◄ New   ◄|||| Revised   ~~deleted~~ Deleted

TABLE OF DRUGS AND CHEMICALS

Substance	External Cause (T-Code)					
	Poisoning, Accidental (Unintentional)	Poisoning, Intentional Self-Harm	Poisoning, Assault	Poisoning, Undetermined	Adverse Effect	Underdosing
Narcotic (drug)	T40.601	T40.602	T40.603	T40.604	T40.605	T40.606
analgesic NEC	T40.601	T40.602	T40.603	T40.604	T40.605	T40.606
antagonist	T50.7X1	T50.7X2	T50.7X3	T50.7X4	T50.7X5	T50.7X6
specified NEC	T40.691	T40.692	T40.693	T40.694	T40.695	T40.696
synthetic	T40.4X1	T40.4X2	T40.4X3	T40.4X4	T40.4X5	T40.4X6
Narcotine	T48.3X1	T48.3X2	T48.3X3	T48.3X4	T48.3X5	T48.3X6
Nardil	T43.1X1	T43.1X2	T43.1X3	T43.1X4	T43.1X5	T43.1X6
Nasal drug NEC	T49.6X1	T49.6X2	T49.6X3	T49.6X4	T49.6X5	T49.6X6
Natamycin	T49.0X1	T49.0X2	T49.0X3	T49.0X4	T49.0X5	T49.0X6
Natrium cyanide — see Cyanide(s)						
Natural gas	T59.891	T59.892	T59.893	T59.894	—	—
incomplete combustion	T57.91	T57.92	T57.93	T57.94	—	—
Natural						
blood (product)	T45.8X1	T45.8X2	T45.8X3	T45.8X4	T45.8X5	T45.8X6
gas (piped)	T59.891	T59.892	T59.893	T59.894	—	—
incomplete combustion	T58.11	T58.12	T58.13	T58.14	—	—
Nealbarbital	T42.3X1	T42.3X2	T42.3X3	T42.3X4	T42.3X5	T42.3X6
Nectadon	T48.3X1	T48.3X2	T48.3X3	T48.3X4	T48.3X5	T48.3X6
Nedocromil	T48.6X1	T48.6X2	T48.6X3	T48.6X4	T48.6X5	T48.6X6
Nefopam	T39.8X1	T39.8X2	T39.8X3	T39.8X4	T39.8X5	T39.8X6
Nematocyst (sting)	T63.691	T63.692	T63.693	T63.694	—	—
Nembutal	T42.3X1	T42.3X2	T42.3X3	T42.3X4	T42.3X5	T42.3X6
Nemonapride	T43.591	T43.592	T43.593	T43.594	T43.595	T43.596
Neoarsphenamine	T37.8X1	T37.8X2	T37.8X3	T37.8X4	T37.8X5	T37.8X6
Neocinchophen	T50.4X1	T50.4X2	T50.4X3	T50.4X4	T50.4X5	T50.4X6
Neomycin (derivatives)	T36.5X1	T36.5X2	T36.5X3	T36.5X4	T36.5X5	T36.5X6
with						
bacitracin	T49.0X1	T49.0X2	T49.0X3	T49.0X4	T49.0X5	T49.0X6
neostigmine	T44.0X1	T44.0X2	T44.0X3	T44.0X4	T44.0X5	T44.0X6
ENT agent	T49.6X1	T49.6X2	T49.6X3	T49.6X4	T49.6X5	T49.6X6
ophthalmic preparation	T49.5X1	T49.5X2	T49.5X3	T49.5X4	T49.5X5	T49.5X6
topical NEC	T49.0X1	T49.0X2	T49.0X3	T49.0X4	T49.0X5	T49.0X6
Neonal	T42.3X1	T42.3X2	T42.3X3	T42.3X4	T42.3X5	T42.3X6
Neoprontosil	T37.0X1	T37.0X2	T37.0X3	T37.0X4	T37.0X5	T37.0X6
Neosalvarsan	T37.8X1	T37.8X2	T37.8X3	T37.8X4	T37.8X5	T37.8X6
Neosilversalvarsan	T37.8X1	T37.8X2	T37.8X3	T37.8X4	T37.8X5	T37.8X6
Neosporin	T36.8X1	T36.8X2	T36.8X3	T36.8X4	T36.8X5	T36.8X6
ENT agent	T49.6X1	T49.6X2	T49.6X3	T49.6X4	T49.6X5	T49.6X6
opthalmic preparation	T49.5X1	T49.5X2	T49.5X3	T49.5X4	T49.5X5	T49.5X6
topical NEC	T49.0X1	T49.0X2	T49.0X3	T49.0X4	T49.0X5	T49.0X6

◀ New   ◀░ Revised   ~~deleted~~ Deleted

Substance	External Cause (T-Code)					
	Poisoning, Accidental (Unintentional)	Poisoning, Intentional Self-Harm	Poisoning, Assault	Poisoning, Undetermined	Adverse Effect	Underdosing
Neostigmine bromide	T44.0X1	T44.0X2	T44.0X3	T44.0X4	T44.0X5	T44.0X6
Neraval	T42.3X1	T42.3X2	T42.3X3	T42.3X4	T42.3X5	T42.3X6
Neravan	T42.3X1	T42.3X2	T42.3X3	T42.3X4	T42.3X5	T42.3X6
Nerium oleander	T62.2X1	T62.2X2	T62.2X3	T62.2X4	—	—
Nerve gas, not in war	T59.91	T59.92	T59.93	T59.94	—	—
Nesacaine	T41.3X1	T41.3X2	T41.3X3	T41.3X4	T41.3X5	T41.3X6
infiltration (subcutaneous)	T41.3X1	T41.3X2	T41.3X3	T41.3X4	T41.3X5	T41.3X6
nerve block (peripheral) (plexus)	T41.3X1	T41.3X2	T41.3X3	T41.3X4	T41.3X5	T41.3X6
Netilmicin	T36.5X1	T36.5X2	T36.5X3	T36.5X4	T36.5X5	T36.5X6
Neurobarb	T42.3X1	T42.3X2	T42.3X3	T42.3X4	T42.3X5	T42.3X6
Neuroleptic drug NEC	T43.501	T43.502	T43.503	T43.504	T43.505	T43.506
Neuromuscular blocking drug	T48.1X1	T48.1X2	T48.1X3	T48.1X4	T48.1X5	T48.1X6
Neutral insulin injection	T38.3X1	T38.3X2	T38.3X3	T38.3X4	T38.3X5	T38.3X6
Neutral spirits	T51.0X1	T51.0X2	T51.0X3	T51.0X4	—	—
beverage	T51.0X1	T51.0X2	T51.0X3	T51.0X4	—	—
Niacin	T46.7X1	T46.7X2	T46.7X3	T46.7X4	T46.7X5	T46.7X6
Niacinamide	T45.2X1	T45.2X2	T45.2X3	T45.2X4	T45.2X5	T45.2X6
Nialamide	T43.1X1	T43.1X2	T43.1X3	T43.1X4	T43.1X5	T43.1X6
Niaprazine	T42.6X1	T42.6X2	T42.6X3	T42.6X4	T42.6X5	T42.6X6
Nicametate	T46.7X1	T46.7X2	T46.7X3	T46.7X4	T46.7X5	T46.7X6
Nicardipine	T46.1X1	T46.1X2	T46.1X3	T46.1X4	T46.1X5	T46.1X6
Nicergoline	T46.7X1	T46.7X2	T46.7X3	T46.7X4	T46.7X5	T46.7X6
Nickel (carbonyl) (tetra-carbonyl) (fumes) (vapor)	T56.891	T56.892	T56.893	T56.894	—	—
Nickelocene	T56.891	T56.892	T56.893	T56.894	—	—
Niclosamide	T37.4X1	T37.4X2	T37.4X3	T37.4X4	T37.4X5	T37.4X6
Nicofuranose	T46.7X1	T46.7X2	T46.7X3	T46.7X4	T46.7X5	T46.7X6
Nicomorphine	T40.2X1	T40.2X2	T40.2X3	T40.2X4	—	—
Nicorandil	T46.3X1	T46.3X2	T46.3X3	T46.3X4	T46.3X5	T46.3X6
Nicotiana (plant)	T62.2X1	T62.2X2	T62.2X3	T62.2X4	—	—
Nicotinamide	T45.2X1	T45.2X2	T45.2X3	T45.2X4	T45.2X5	T45.2X6
Nicotine (insecticide) (spray) (sulfate) NEC	T60.2X1	T60.2X2	T60.2X3	T60.2X4	—	—
from tobacco	T65.291	T65.292	T65.293	T65.294	—	—
cigarettes	T65.221	T65.222	T65.223	T65.224	—	—
not insecticide	T65.291	T65.292	T65.293	T65.294	—	—
Nicotinic acid	T46.7X1	T46.7X2	T46.7X3	T46.7X4	T46.7X5	T46.7X6
Nicotinyl alcohol	T46.7X1	T46.7X2	T46.7X3	T46.7X4	T46.7X5	T46.7X6
Nicoumalone	T45.511	T45.512	T45.513	T45.514	T45.515	T45.516
Nifedipine	T46.1X1	T46.1X2	T46.1X3	T46.1X4	T46.1X5	T46.1X6
Nifenazone	T39.2X1	T39.2X2	T39.2X3	T39.2X4	T39.2X5	T39.2X6
Nifuraldezone	T37.91	T37.92	T37.93	T37.94	T37.95	T37.96

◀ New   ◀▥ Revised   ~~deleted~~ Deleted

Substance	External Cause (T-Code)					
	Poisoning, Accidental (Unintentional)	Poisoning, Intentional Self-Harm	Poisoning, Assault	Poisoning, Undetermined	Adverse Effect	Underdosing
Nifuratel	T37.8X1	T37.8X2	T37.8X3	T37.8X4	T37.8X5	T37.8X6
Nifurtimox	T37.3X1	T37.3X2	T37.3X3	T37.3X4	T37.3X5	T37.3X6
Nifurtoinol	T37.8X1	T37.8X2	T37.8X3	T37.8X4	T37.8X5	T37.8X6
Nightshade, deadly (solanum) — see also Belladonna	T62.2X1	T62.2X2	T62.2X3	T62.2X4	—	—
berry	T62.1X1	T62.1X2	T62.1X3	T62.1X4	—	—
Nikethamide	T50.7X1	T50.7X2	T50.7X3	T50.7X4	T50.7X5	T50.7X6
Nilstat	T36.7X1	T36.7X2	T36.7X3	T36.7X4	T36.7X5	T36.7X6
topical	T49.0X1	T49.0X2	T49.0X3	T49.0X4	T49.0X5	T49.0X6
Nilutamide	T38.6X1	T38.6X2	T38.6X3	T38.6X4	T38.6X5	T38.6X6
Nimesulide	T39.391	T39.392	T39.393	T39.394	T39.395	T39.396
Nimetazepam	T42.4X1	T42.4X2	T42.4X3	T42.4X4	T42.4X5	T42.4X6
Nimodipine	T46.1X1	T46.1X2	T46.1X3	T46.1X4	T46.1X5	T46.1X6
Nimorazole	T37.3X1	T37.3X2	T37.3X3	T37.3X4	T37.3X5	T37.3X6
Nimustine	T45.1X1	T45.1X2	T45.1X3	T45.1X4	T45.1X5	T45.1X6
Niridazole	T37.4X1	T37.4X2	T37.4X3	T37.4X4	T37.4X5	T37.4X6
Nisentil	T40.2X1	T40.2X2	T40.2X3	T40.2X4	T40.2X5	T40.2X6
Nisoldipine	T46.1X1	T46.1X2	T46.1X3	T46.1X4	T46.1X5	T46.1X6
Nitramine	T65.3X1	T65.3X2	T65.3X3	T65.3X4	—	—
Nitrate, organic	T46.3X1	T46.3X2	T46.3X3	T46.3X4	T46.3X5	T46.3X6
Nitrazepam	T42.4X1	T42.4X2	T42.4X3	T42.4X4	T42.4X5	T42.4X6
Nitrefazole	T50.6X1	T50.6X2	T50.6X3	T50.6X4	T50.6X5	T50.6X6
Nitrendipine	T46.1X1	T46.1X2	T46.1X3	T46.1X4	T46.1X5	T46.1X6
Nitric						
acid (liquid)	T54.2X1	T54.2X2	T54.2X3	T54.2X4	—	—
vapor	T59.891	T59.892	T59.893	T59.894	—	—
oxide (gas)	T59.0X1	T59.0X2	T59.0X3	T59.0X4	—	—
Nitrimidazine	T37.3X1	T37.3X2	T37.3X3	T37.3X4	T37.3X5	T37.3X6
Nitrite, amyl (medicinal) (vapor)	T46.3X1	T46.3X2	T46.3X3	T46.3X4	T46.3X5	T46.3X6
Nitroaniline	T65.3X1	T65.3X2	T65.3X3	T65.3X4	—	—
vapor	T59.891	T59.892	T59.893	T59.894	—	—
Nitrobenzene, nitrobenzol	T65.3X1	T65.3X2	T65.3X3	T65.3X4	—	—
vapor	T65.3X1	T65.3X2	T65.3X3	T65.3X4	—	—
Nitrocellulose	T65.891	T65.892	T65.893	T65.894	—	—
lacquer	T65.891	T65.892	T65.893	T65.894	—	—
Nitrodiphenyl	T65.3X1	T65.3X2	T65.3X3	T65.3X4	—	—
Nitrofural	T49.0X1	T49.0X2	T49.0X3	T49.0X4	T49.0X5	T49.0X6
Nitrofurantoin	T37.8X1	T37.8X2	T37.8X3	T37.8X4	T37.8X5	T37.8X6
Nitrofurazone	T49.0X1	T49.0X2	T49.0X3	T49.0X4	T49.0X5	T49.0X6
Nitrogen	T59.0X1	T59.0X2	T59.0X3	T59.0X4	—	—
mustard	T45.1X1	T45.1X2	T45.1X3	T45.1X4	T45.1X5	T45.1X6

◀ New   ◀▯ Revised   ~~deleted~~ Deleted

Substance	External Cause (T-Code)					
	Poisoning, Accidental (Unintentional)	Poisoning, Intentional Self-Harm	Poisoning, Assault	Poisoning, Undetermined	Adverse Effect	Underdosing
Nitroglycerin, nitro-glycerol (medicinal)	T46.3X1	T46.3X2	T46.3X3	T46.3X4	T46.3X5	T46.3X6
nonmedicinal	T65.5X1	T65.5X2	T65.5X3	T65.5X4	—	—
fumes	T65.5X1	T65.5X2	T65.5X3	T65.5X4	—	—
Nitroglycol	T52.3X1	T52.3X2	T52.3X3	T52.3X4	—	—
Nitrohydrochloric acid	T54.2X1	T54.2X2	T54.2X3	T54.2X4	—	—
Nitromersol	T49.0X1	T49.0X2	T49.0X3	T49.0X4	T49.0X5	T49.0X6
Nitronaphthalene	T65.891	T65.892	T65.893	T65.894		
Nitrophenol	T54.0X1	T54.0X2	T54.0X3	T54.0X4	—	—
Nitropropane	T52.8X1	T52.8X2	T52.8X3	T52.8X4	—	—
Nitroprusside	T46.5X1	T46.5X2	T46.5X3	T46.5X4	T46.5X5	T46.5X6
Nitrosodimethylamine	T65.3X1	T65.3X2	T65.3X3	T65.3X4	—	—
Nitrothiazol	T37.4X1	T37.4X2	T37.4X3	T37.4X4	T37.4X5	T37.4X6
Nitrotoluene, nitrotoluol	T65.3X1	T65.3X2	T65.3X3	T65.3X4	—	—
vapor	T65.3X1	T65.3X2	T65.3X3	T65.3X4	—	—
Nitrous						
acid (liquid)	T54.2X1	T54.2X2	T54.2X3	T54.2X4	—	—
fumes	T59.891	T59.892	T59.893	T59.894	—	—
ether spirit	T46.3X1	T46.3X2	T46.3X3	T46.3X4	T46.3X5	T46.3X6
oxide	T41.0X1	T41.0X2	T41.0X3	T41.0X4	T41.0X5	T41.0X6
Nitroxoline	T37.8X1	T37.8X2	T37.8X3	T37.8X4	T37.8X5	T37.8X6
Nitrozone	T49.0X1	T49.0X2	T49.0X3	T49.0X4	T49.0X5	T49.0X6
Nizatidine	T47.0X1	T47.0X2	T47.0X3	T47.0X4	T47.0X5	T47.0X6
Nizofenone	T43.8X1	T43.8X2	T43.8X3	T43.8X4	T43.8X5	T43.8X6
Noctec	T42.6X1	T42.6X2	T42.6X3	T42.6X4	T42.6X5	T42.6X6
Noludar	T42.6X1	T42.6X2	T42.6X3	T42.6X4	T42.6X5	T42.6X6
Noptil	T42.3X1	T42.3X2	T42.3X3	T42.3X4	T42.3X5	T42.3X6
Nomegestrol	T38.5X1	T38.5X2	T38.5X3	T38.5X4	T38.5X5	T38.5X6
Nomifensine	T43.291	T43.292	T43.293	T43.294	T43.295	T43.296
Nonoxinol	T49.8X1	T49.8X2	T49.8X3	T49.8X4	T49.8X5	T49.8X6
Nonylphenoxy (polyethoxy-ethanol)	T49.8X1	T49.8X2	T49.8X3	T49.8X4	T49.8X5	T49.8X6
Noptil	T42.3X1	T42.3X2	T42.3X3	T42.3X4	T42.3X5	T42.3X6
Noradrenaline	T44.4X1	T44.4X2	T44.4X3	T44.4X4	T44.4X5	T44.4X6
Noramidopyrine	T39.2X1	T39.2X2	T39.2X3	T39.2X4	T39.2X5	T39.2X6
methanesulfonate sodium	T39.2X1	T39.2X2	T39.2X3	T39.2X4	T39.2X5	T39.2X6
Norbormide	T60.4X1	T60.4X2	T60.4X3	T60.4X4	—	—
Nordazepam	T42.4X1	T42.4X2	T42.4X3	T42.4X4	T42.4X5	T42.4X6
Norepinephrine	T44.4X1	T44.4X2	T44.4X3	T44.4X4	T44.4X5	T44.4X6
Norethandrolone	T38.7X1	T38.7X2	T38.7X3	T38.7X4	T38.7X5	T38.7X6
Norethindrone	T38.4X1	T38.4X2	T38.4X3	T38.4X4	T38.4X5	T38.4X6

◀ New ◀▦ Revised ~~deleted~~ Deleted

Substance	External Cause (T-Code)					
	Poisoning, Accidental (Unintentional)	Poisoning, Intentional Self-Harm	Poisoning, Assault	Poisoning, Undetermined	Adverse Effect	Underdosing
Norethisterone (acetate) (enantate)	T38.4X1	T38.4X2	T38.4X3	T38.4X4	T38.4X5	T38.4X6
with ethinylestradiol	T38.5X1	T38.5X2	T38.5X3	T38.5X4	T38.5X5	T38.5X6
Noretynodrel	T38.5X1	T38.5X2	T38.5X3	T38.5X4	T38.5X5	T38.5X6
Norfenefrine	T44.4X1	T44.4X2	T44.4X3	T44.4X4	T44.4X5	T44.4X6
Norfloxacin	T36.8X1	T36.8X2	T36.8X3	T36.8X4	T36.8X5	T36.8X6
Norgestrel	T38.4X1	T38.4X2	T38.4X3	T38.4X4	T38.4X5	T38.4X6
Norgestrienone	T38.4X1	T38.4X2	T38.4X3	T38.4X4	T38.4X5	T38.4X6
Norlestrin	T38.4X1	T38.4X2	T38.4X3	T38.4X4	T38.4X5	T38.4X6
Norlutin	T38.4X1	T38.4X2	T38.4X3	T38.4X4	T38.4X5	T38.4X6
Normal serum albumin (human), salt-poor	T45.8X1	T45.8X2	T45.8X3	T45.8X4	T45.8X5	T45.8X6
Normethandrone	T38.5X1	T38.5X2	T38.5X3	T38.5X4	T38.5X5	T38.5X6
Normison — *see Benzodiazepines*						
Normorphine	T40.2X1	T40.2X2	T40.2X3	T40.2X4	—	—
Norpseudoephedrine	T50.5X1	T50.5X2	T50.5X3	T50.5X4	T50.5X5	T50.5X6
Nortestosterone (furanpropionate)	T38.7X1	T38.7X2	T38.7X3	T38.7X4	T38.7X5	T38.7X6
Nortriptyline	T43.011	T43.012	T43.013	T43.014	T43.015	T43.016
Noscapine	T48.3X1	T48.3X2	T48.3X3	T48.3X4	T48.3X5	T48.3X6
Nose preparations	T49.6X1	T49.6X2	T49.6X3	T49.6X4	T49.6X5	T49.6X6
Novobiocin	T36.5X1	T36.5X2	T36.5X3	T36.5X4	T36.5X5	T36.5X6
Novocain (infiltration) (topical)	T41.3X1	T41.3X2	T41.3X3	T41.3X4	T41.3X5	T41.3X6
nerve block (peripheral) (plexus)	T41.3X1	T41.3X2	T41.3X3	T41.3X4	T41.3X5	T41.3X6
spinal	T41.3X1	T41.3X2	T41.3X3	T41.3X4	T41.3X5	T41.3X6
Noxious foodstuff	T62.91	T62.92	T62.93	T62.94	—	—
specified NEC	T62.8X1	T62.8X2	T62.8X3	T62.8X4	—	—
Noxiptiline	T43.011	T43.012	T43.013	T43.014	T43.015	T43.016
Noxytiolin	T49.0X1	T49.0X2	T49.0X3	T49.0X4	T49.0X5	T49.0X6
NPH Iletin (insulin)	T38.3X1	T38.3X2	T38.3X3	T38.3X4	T38.3X5	T38.3X6
Numorphan	T40.2X1	T40.2X2	T40.2X3	T40.2X4	T40.2X5	T40.2X6
Nunol	T42.3X1	T42.3X2	T42.3X3	T42.3X4	T42.3X5	T42.3X6
Nupercaine (spinal anesthetic)	T41.3X1	T41.3X2	T41.3X3	T41.3X4	T41.3X5	T41.3X6
topical (surface)	T41.3X1	T41.3X2	T41.3X3	T41.3X4	T41.3X5	T41.3X6
Nutmeg oil (liniment)	T49.3X1	T49.3X2	T49.3X3	T49.3X4	T49.3X5	T49.3X6
Nutritional supplement	T50.901	T50.902	T50.903	T50.904	T50.905	T50.906
Nux vomica	T65.1X1	T65.1X2	T65.1X3	T65.1X4	—	—
Nydrazid	T37.1X1	T37.1X2	T37.1X3	T37.1X4	T37.1X5	T37.1X6
Nylidrin	T46.7X1	T46.7X2	T46.7X3	T46.7X4	T46.7X5	T46.7X6
Nystatin	T36.7X1	T36.7X2	T36.7X3	T36.7X4	T36.7X5	T36.7X6
topical	T49.0X1	T49.0X2	T49.0X3	T49.0X4	T49.0X5	T49.0X6
Nytol	T45.0X1	T45.0X2	T45.0X3	T45.0X4	T45.0X5	T45.0X6

◀ New ◀▥ Revised ~~deleted~~ Deleted

Substance	External Cause (T-Code)					
	Poisoning, Accidental (Unintentional)	Poisoning, Intentional Self-Harm	Poisoning, Assault	Poisoning, Undetermined	Adverse Effect	Underdosing
O						
Obidoxime chloride	T50.6X1	T50.6X2	T50.6X3	T50.6X4	T50.6X5	T50.6X6
Octafonium (chloride)	T49.3X1	T49.3X2	T49.3X3	T49.3X4	T49.3X5	T49.3X6
Octamethyl pyrophos-phoramide	T60.0X1	T60.0X2	T60.0X3	T60.0X4	—	—
Octanoin	T50.991	T50.992	T50.993	T50.994	T50.995	T50.996
Octatropine methyl-bromide	T44.3X1	T44.3X2	T44.3X3	T44.3X4	T44.3X5	T44.3X6
Octotiamine	T45.2X1	T45.2X2	T45.2X3	T45.2X4	T45.2X5	T45.2X6
Octoxinol (9)	T49.8X1	T49.8X2	T49.8X3	T49.8X4	T49.8X5	T49.8X6
Octreotide	T38.991	T38.992	T38.993	T38.994	T38.995	T38.996
Octyl nitrite	T46.3X1	T46.3X2	T46.3X3	T46.3X4	T46.3X5	T46.3X6
Oestradiol	T38.5X1	T38.5X2	T38.5X3	T38.5X4	T38.5X5	T38.5X6
Oestriol	T38.5X1	T38.5X2	T38.5X3	T38.5X4	T38.5X5	T38.5X6
Oestrogen	T38.5X1	T38.5X2	T38.5X3	T38.5X4	T38.5X5	T38.5X6
Oestrone	T38.5X1	T38.5X2	T38.5X3	T38.5X4	T38.5X5	T38.5X6
Ofloxacin	T36.8X1	T36.8X2	T36.8X3	T36.8X4	T36.8X5	T36.8X6
Oil (of)	T65.891	T65.892	T65.893	T65.894	—	—
bitter almond	T62.8X1	T62.8X2	T62.8X3	T62.8X4	—	—
cloves	T49.7X1	T49.7X2	T49.7X3	T49.7X4	T49.7X5	T49.7X6
colors	T65.6X1	T65.6X2	T65.6X3	T65.6X4	—	—
fumes	T59.891	T59.892	T59.893	T59.894	—	—
lubricating	T52.0X1	T52.0X2	T52.0X3	T52.0X4	—	—
Niobe	T52.8X1	T52.8X2	T52.8X3	T52.8X4	—	—
vitriol (liquid)	T54.2X1	T54.2X2	T54.2X3	T54.2X4	—	—
fumes	T54.2X1	T54.2X2	T54.2X3	T54.2X4	—	—
wintergreen (bitter) NEC	T49.3X1	T49.3X2	T49.3X3	T49.3X4	T49.3X5	T49.3X6
Oily preparation (for skin)	T49.3X1	T49.3X2	T49.3X3	T49.3X4	T49.3X5	T49.3X6
Ointment NEC	T49.3X1	T49.3X2	T49.3X3	T49.3X4	T49.3X5	T49.3X6
Olanzapine	T43.591	T43.592	T43.593	T43.594	T43.595	T43.596
Oleander	T62.2X1	T62.2X2	T62.2X3	T62.2X4	—	—
Oleandomycin	T36.3X1	T36.3X2	T36.3X3	T36.3X4	T36.3X5	T36.3X6
Oleandrin	T46.0X1	T46.0X2	T46.0X3	T46.0X4	T46.0X5	T46.0X6
Oleic acid	T46.6X1	T46.6X2	T46.6X3	T46.6X4	T46.6X5	T46.6X6
Oleovitamin A	T45.2X1	T45.2X2	T45.2X3	T45.2X4	T45.2X5	T45.2X6
Oleum ricini	T47.2X1	T47.2X2	T47.2X3	T47.2X4	T47.2X5	T47.2X6
Olive oil (medicinal) NEC	T47.4X1	T47.4X2	T47.4X3	T47.4X4	T47.4X5	T47.4X6
Olivomycin	T45.1X1	T45.1X2	T45.1X3	T45.1X4	T45.1X5	T45.1X6
Olsalazine	T47.8X1	T47.8X2	T47.8X3	T47.8X4	T47.8X5	T47.8X6
Omeprazole	T47.1X1	T47.1X2	T47.1X3	T47.1X4	T47.1X5	T47.1X6

◄ New ◄▥ Revised ~~deleted~~ Deleted

Substance	External Cause (T-Code)					
	Poisoning, Accidental (Unintentional)	Poisoning, Intentional Self-Harm	Poisoning, Assault	Poisoning, Undetermined	Adverse Effect	Underdosing
OMPA	T60.0X1	T60.0X2	T60.0X3	T60.0X4	—	—
Ondansetron	T45.0X1	T45.0X2	T45.0X3	T45.0X4	T45.0X5	T45.0X6
Oncovin	T45.1X1	T45.1X2	T45.1X3	T45.1X4	T45.1X5	T45.1X6
Ophthaine	T41.3X1	T41.3X2	T41.3X3	T41.3X4	T41.3X5	T41.3X6
Ophthetic	T41.3X1	T41.3X2	T41.3X3	T41.3X4	T41.3X5	T41.3X6
Opiate NEC	T40.601	T40.602	T40.603	T40.604	T40.605	T40.606
antagonists	T50.7X1	T50.7X2	T50.7X3	T50.7X4	T50.7X5	T50.7X6
Opioid NEC	T40.2X1	T40.2X2	T40.2X3	T40.2X4	T40.2X5	T40.2X6
Opipramol	T43.011	T43.012	T43.013	T43.014	T43.015	T43.016
Opium alkaloids (total)	T40.0X1	T40.0X2	T40.0X3	T40.0X4	T40.0X5	T40.0X6
standardized powdered	T40.0X1	T40.0X2	T40.0X3	T40.0X4	T40.0X5	T40.0X6
tincture (camphorated)	T40.0X1	T40.0X2	T40.0X3	T40.0X4	T40.0X5	T40.0X6
Oracon	T38.4X1	T38.4X2	T38.4X3	T38.4X4	T38.4X5	T38.4X6
Oragrafin	T50.8X1	T50.8X2	T50.8X3	T50.8X4	T50.8X5	T50.8X6
Oral contraceptives	T38.4X1	T38.4X2	T38.4X3	T38.4X4	T38.4X5	T38.4X6
Oral rehydration salts	T50.3X1	T50.3X2	T50.3X3	T50.3X4	T50.3X5	T50.3X6
Orazamide	T50.991	T50.992	T50.993	T50.994	T50.995	T50.996
Orciprenaline	T48.291	T48.292	T48.293	T48.294	T48.295	T48.296
Organidin	T48.4X1	T48.4X2	T48.4X3	T48.4X4	T48.4X5	T48.4X6
Organonitrate NEC	T46.3X1	T46.3X2	T46.3X3	T46.3X4	T46.3X5	T46.3X6
Organophosphates	T60.0X1	T60.0X2	T60.0X3	T60.0X4	—	—
Orimune	T50.B91	T50.B92	T50.B93	T50.B94	T50.B95	T50.B96
Orinase	T38.3X1	T38.3X2	T38.3X3	T38.3X4	T38.3X5	T38.3X6
Ormeloxifene	T38.6X1	T38.6X2	T38.6X3	T38.6X4	T38.6X5	T38.6X6
Ornidazole	T37.3X1	T37.3X2	T37.3X3	T37.3X4	T37.3X5	T37.3X6
Ornithine aspartate	T50.991	T50.992	T50.993	T50.994	T50.995	T50.996
Ornoprostil	T47.1X1	T47.1X2	T47.1X3	T47.1X4	T47.1X5	T47.1X6
Orphenadrine (hydrochloride)	T42.8X1	T42.8X2	T42.8X3	T42.8X4	T42.8X5	T42.8X6
Ortal (sodium)	T42.3X1	T42.3X2	T42.3X3	T42.3X4	T42.3X5	T42.3X6
Orthoboric acid	T49.0X1	T49.0X2	T49.0X3	T49.0X4	T49.0X5	T49.0X6
ENT agent	T49.6X1	T49.6X2	T49.6X3	T49.6X4	T49.6X5	T49.6X6
ophthalmic preparation	T49.5X1	T49.5X2	T49.5X3	T49.5X4	T49.5X5	T49.5X6
Orthocaine	T41.3X1	T41.3X2	T41.3X3	T41.3X4	T41.3X5	T41.3X6
Orthodichlorobenzene	T53.7X1	T53.7X2	T53.7X3	T53.7X4	—	—
Ortho-Novum	T38.4X1	T38.4X2	T38.4X3	T38.4X4	T38.4X5	T38.4X6
Orthotolidine (reagent)	T54.2X1	T54.2X2	T54.2X3	T54.2X4	—	—
Osmic acid (liquid)	T54.2X1	T54.2X2	T54.2X3	T54.2X4	—	—
fumes	T54.2X1	T54.2X2	T54.2X3	T54.2X4	—	—
Osmotic diuretics	T50.2X1	T50.2X2	T50.2X3	T50.2X4	T50.2X5	T50.2X6
Otilonium bromide	T44.3X1	T44.3X2	T44.3X3	T44.3X4	T44.3X5	T44.3X6

◀ New ◀ Revised ~~deleted~~ Deleted

Substance	External Cause (T-Code)					
	Poisoning, Accidental (Unintentional)	Poisoning, Intentional Self-Harm	Poisoning, Assault	Poisoning, Undetermined	Adverse Effect	Underdosing
Otorhinolaryngological drug NEC	T49.6X1	T49.6X2	T49.6X3	T49.6X4	T49.6X5	T49.6X6
Ouabain(e)	T46.0X1	T46.0X2	T46.0X3	T46.0X4	T46.0X5	T46.0X6
Ovarian						
hormone	T38.5X1	T38.5X2	T38.5X3	T38.5X4	T38.5X5	T38.5X6
stimulant	T38.5X1	T38.5X2	T38.5X3	T38.5X4	T38.5X5	T38.5X6
Ovral	T38.4X1	T38.4X2	T38.4X3	T38.4X4	T38.4X5	T38.4X6
Ovulen	T38.4X1	T38.4X2	T38.4X3	T38.4X4	T38.4X5	T38.4X6
Oxacillin	T36.0X1	T36.0X2	T36.0X3	T36.0X4	T36.0X5	T36.0X6
Oxalic acid	T54.2X1	T54.2X2	T54.2X3	T54.2X4	—	—
ammonium salt	T50.991	T50.992	T50.993	T50.994	T50.995	T50.996
Oxamniquine	T37.4X1	T37.4X2	T37.4X3	T37.4X4	T37.4X5	T37.4X6
Oxanamide	T43.591	T43.592	T43.593	T43.594	T43.595	T43.596
Oxandrolone	T38.7X1	T38.7X2	T38.7X3	T38.7X4	T38.7X5	T38.7X6
Oxantel	T37.4X1	T37.4X2	T37.4X3	T37.4X4	T37.4X5	T37.4X6
Oxapium iodide	T44.3X1	T44.3X2	T44.3X3	T44.3X4	T44.3X5	T44.3X6
Oxaprotiline	T43.021	T43.022	T43.023	T43.024	T43.025	T43.026
Oxaprozin	T39.311	T39.312	T39.313	T39.314	T39.315	T39.316
Oxatomide	T45.0X1	T45.0X2	T45.0X3	T45.0X4	T45.0X5	T45.0X6
Oxazepam	T42.4X1	T42.4X2	T42.4X3	T42.4X4	T42.4X5	T42.4X6
Oxazimedrine	T50.5X1	T50.5X2	T50.5X3	T50.5X4	T50.5X5	T50.5X6
Oxazolam	T42.4X1	T42.4X2	T42.4X3	T42.4X4	T42.4X5	T42.4X6
Oxazolidine derivatives	T42.2X1	T42.2X2	T42.2X3	T42.2X4	T42.2X5	T42.2X6
Oxazolidinedione (derivative)	T42.2X1	T42.2X2	T42.2X3	T42.2X4	T42.2X5	T42.2X6
Ox bile extract	T47.5X1	T47.5X2	T47.5X3	T47.5X4	T47.5X5	T47.5X6
Oxcarbazepine	T42.1X1	T42.1X2	T42.1X3	T42.1X4	T42.1X5	T42.1X6
Oxedrine	T44.4X1	T44.4X2	T44.4X3	T44.4X4	T44.4X5	T44.4X6
Oxeladin (citrate)	T48.3X1	T48.3X2	T48.3X3	T48.3X4	T48.3X5	T48.3X6
Oxendolone	T38.5X1	T38.5X2	T38.5X3	T38.5X4	T38.5X5	T38.5X6
Oxetacaine	T41.3X1	T41.3X2	T41.3X3	T41.3X4	T41.3X5	T41.3X6
Oxethazine	T41.3X1	T41.3X2	T41.3X3	T41.3X4	T41.3X5	T41.3X6
Oxetorone	T39.8X1	T39.8X2	T39.8X3	T39.8X4	T39.8X5	T39.8X6
Oxiconazole	T49.0X1	T49.0X2	T49.0X3	T49.0X4	T49.0X5	T49.0X6
Oxidizing agent NEC	T54.91	T54.92	T54.93	T54.94	—	—
Oxipurinol	T50.4X1	T50.4X2	T50.4X3	T50.4X4	T50.4X5	T50.4X6
Oxitriptan	T43.291	T43.292	T43.293	T43.294	T43.295	T43.296
Oxitropium bromide	T48.6X1	T48.6X2	T48.6X3	T48.6X4	T48.6X5	T48.6X6
Oxodipine	T46.1X1	T46.1X2	T46.1X3	T46.1X4	T46.1X5	T46.1X6
Oxolamine	T48.3X1	T48.3X2	T48.3X3	T48.3X4	T48.3X5	T48.3X6
Oxolinic acid	T37.8X1	T37.8X2	T37.8X3	T37.8X4	T37.8X5	T37.8X6
Oxomemazine	T43.3X1	T43.3X2	T43.3X3	T43.3X4	T43.3X5	T43.3X6

◀ New   ◀≡ Revised   ~~deleted~~ Deleted

TABLE OF DRUGS AND CHEMICALS

Substance	External Cause (T-Code)					
	Poisoning, Accidental (Unintentional)	Poisoning, Intentional Self-Harm	Poisoning, Assault	Poisoning, Undetermined	Adverse Effect	Underdosing
Oxophenarsine	T37.3X1	T37.3X2	T37.3X3	T37.3X4	T37.3X5	T37.3X6
Oxprenolol	T44.7X1	T44.7X2	T44.7X3	T44.7X4	T44.7X5	T44.7X6
Oxsoralen	T49.3X1	T49.3X2	T49.3X3	T49.3X4	T49.3X5	T49.3X6
Oxtriphylline	T48.6X1	T48.6X2	T48.6X3	T48.6X4	T48.6X5	T48.6X6
Oxybate sodium	T41.291	T41.292	T41.293	T41.294	T41.295	T41.296
Oxybuprocaine	T41.3X1	T41.3X2	T41.3X3	T41.3X4	T41.3X5	T41.3X6
Oxybutynin	T44.3X1	T44.3X2	T44.3X3	T44.3X4	T44.3X5	T44.3X6
Oxychlorosene	T49.0X1	T49.0X2	T49.0X3	T49.0X4	T49.0X5	T49.0X6
Oxycodone	T40.2X1	T40.2X2	T40.2X3	T40.2X4	T40.2X5	T40.2X6
Oxyfedrine	T46.3X1	T46.3X2	T46.3X3	T46.3X4	T46.3X5	T46.3X6
Oxygen	T41.5X1	T41.5X2	T41.5X3	T41.5X4	T41.5X5	T41.5X6
Oxylone	T49.0X1	T49.0X2	T49.0X3	T49.0X4	T49.0X5	T49.0X6
ophthalmic preparation	T49.5X1	T49.5X2	T49.5X3	T49.5X4	T49.5X5	T49.5X6
Oxymesterone	T38.7X1	T38.7X2	T38.7X3	T38.7X4	T38.7X5	T38.7X6
Oxymetazoline	T48.5X1	T48.5X2	T48.5X3	T48.5X4	T48.5X5	T48.5X6
Oxymetholone	T38.7X1	T38.7X2	T38.7X3	T38.7X4	T38.7X5	T38.7X6
Oxymorphone	T40.2X1	T40.2X2	T40.2X3	T40.2X4	T40.2X5	T40.2X6
Oxypertine	T43.591	T43.592	T43.593	T43.594	T43.595	T43.596
Oxyphenbutazone	T39.2X1	T39.2X2	T39.2X3	T39.2X4	T39.2X5	T39.2X6
Oxyphencyclimine	T44.3X1	T44.3X2	T44.3X3	T44.3X4	T44.3X5	T44.3X6
Oxyphenisatine	T47.2X1	T47.2X2	T47.2X3	T47.2X4	T47.2X5	T47.2X6
Oxyphenonium bromide	T44.3X1	T44.3X2	T44.3X3	T44.3X4	T44.3X5	T44.3X6
Oxypolygelatin	T45.8X1	T45.8X2	T45.8X3	T45.8X4	T45.8X5	T45.8X6
Oxyquinoline (derivatives)	T37.8X1	T37.8X2	T37.8X3	T37.8X4	T37.8X5	T37.8X6
Oxytetracycline	T36.4X1	T36.4X2	T36.4X3	T36.4X4	T36.4X5	T36.4X6
Oxytocic drug NEC	T48.0X1	T48.0X2	T48.0X3	T48.0X4	T48.0X5	T48.0X6
Oxytocin (synthetic)	T48.0X1	T48.0X2	T48.0X3	T48.0X4	T48.0X5	T48.0X6
Ozone	T59.891	T59.892	T59.893	T59.894	—	—
P						
PABA	T49.3X1	T49.3X2	T49.3X3	T49.3X4	T49.3X5	T49.3X6
Packed red cells	T45.8X1	T45.8X2	T45.8X3	T45.8X4	T45.8X5	T45.8X6
Padimate	T49.3X1	T49.3X2	T49.3X3	T49.3X4	T49.3X5	T49.3X6
Paint NEC	T65.6X1	T65.6X2	T65.6X3	T65.6X4	—	—
cleaner	T52.91	T52.92	T52.93	T52.94	—	—
fumes NEC	T59.891	T59.892	T59.893	T59.894	—	—
lead (fumes)	T56.0X1	T56.0X2	T56.0X3	T56.0X4	—	—
solvent NEC	T52.8X1	T52.8X2	T52.8X3	T52.8X4	—	—
stripper	T52.8X1	T52.8X2	T52.8X3	T52.8X4	—	—
Palfium	T40.2X1	T40.2X2	T40.2X3	T40.2X4	—	—

◀ New   ◀━ Revised   ~~deleted~~ Deleted

Substance	Poisoning, Accidental (Unintentional)	Poisoning, Intentional Self-Harm	Poisoning, Assault	Poisoning, Undetermined	Adverse Effect	Underdosing
	External Cause (T-Code)					
Palm kernel oil	T50.991	T50.992	T50.993	T50.994	T50.995	T50.996
Paludrine	T37.2X1	T37.2X2	T37.2X3	T37.2X4	T37.2X5	T37.2X6
PAM (pralidoxime)	T50.6X1	T50.6X2	T50.6X3	T50.6X4	T50.6X5	T50.6X6
Pamaquine (naphthoute)	T37.2X1	T37.2X2	T37.2X3	T37.2X4	T37.2X5	T37.2X6
Panadol	T39.1X1	T39.1X2	T39.1X3	T39.1X4	T39.1X5	T39.1X6
Pancreatic						
digestive secretion stimulant	T47.8X1	T47.8X2	T47.8X3	T47.8X4	T47.8X5	T47.8X6
dornase	T45.3X1	T45.3X2	T45.3X3	T45.3X4	T45.3X5	T45.3X6
Pancreatin	T47.5X1	T47.5X2	T47.5X3	T47.5X4	T47.5X5	T47.5X6
Pancrelipase	T47.5X1	T47.5X2	T47.5X3	T47.5X4	T47.5X5	T47.5X6
Pancuronium (bromide)	T48.1X1	T48.1X2	T48.1X3	T48.1X4	T48.1X5	T48.1X6
Pangamic acid	T45.2X1	T45.2X2	T45.2X3	T45.2X4	T45.2X5	T45.2X6
Panthenol	T45.2X1	T45.2X2	T45.2X3	T45.2X4	T45.2X5	T45.2X6
topical	T49.8X1	T49.8X2	T49.8X3	T49.8X4	T49.8X5	T49.8X6
Pantopon	T40.0X1	T40.0X2	T40.0X3	T40.0X4	T40.0X5	T40.0X6
Pantothenic acid	T45.2X1	T45.2X2	T45.2X3	T45.2X4	T45.2X5	T45.2X6
Panwarfin	T45.511	T45.512	T45.513	T45.514	T45.515	T45.516
Papain	T47.5X1	T47.5X2	T47.5X3	T47.5X4	T47.5X5	T47.5X6
digestant	T47.5X1	T47.5X2	T47.5X3	T47.5X4	T47.5X5	T47.5X6
Papaveretum	T40.0X1	T40.0X2	T40.0X3	T40.0X4	T40.0X5	T40.0X6
Papaverine	T44.3X1	T44.3X2	T44.3X3	T44.3X4	T44.3X5	T44.3X6
Para-acetamidophenol	T39.1X1	T39.1X2	T39.1X3	T39.1X4	T39.1X5	T39.1X6
Para-aminobenzoic acid	T49.3X1	T49.3X2	T49.3X3	T49.3X4	T49.3X5	T49.3X6
Para-aminophenol derivatives	T39.1X1	T39.1X2	T39.1X3	T39.1X4	T39.1X5	T39.1X6
Para-aminosalicylic acid	T37.1X1	T37.1X2	T37.1X3	T37.1X4	T37.1X5	T37.1X6
Paracetaldehyde	T42.6X1	T42.6X2	T42.6X3	T42.6X4	T42.6X5	T42.6X6
Paracetamol	T39.1X1	T39.1X2	T39.1X3	T39.1X4	T39.1X5	T39.1X6
Parachlorophenol (camphorated)	T49.0X1	T49.0X2	T49.0X3	T49.0X4	T49.0X5	T49.0X6
Paracodin	T40.2X1	T40.2X2	T40.2X3	T40.2X4	T40.2X5	T40.2X6
Paradione	T42.2X1	T42.2X2	T42.2X3	T42.2X4	T42.2X5	T42.2X6
Paraffin(s) (wax)	T52.0X1	T52.0X2	T52.0X3	T52.0X4	—	—
liquid (medicinal)	T47.4X1	T47.4X2	T47.4X3	T47.4X4	T47.4X5	T47.4X6
nonmedicinal	T52.0X1	T52.0X2	T52.0X3	T52.0X4	—	—
Paraformaldehyde	T60.3X1	T60.3X2	T60.3X3	T60.3X4	—	—
Paraldehyde	T42.6X1	T42.6X2	T42.6X3	T42.6X4	T42.6X5	T42.6X6
Paramethadione	T42.2X1	T42.2X2	T42.2X3	T42.2X4	T42.2X5	T42.2X6
Paramethasone	T38.0X1	T38.0X2	T38.0X3	T38.0X4	T38.0X5	T38.0X6
acetate	T49.0X1	T49.0X2	T49.0X3	T49.0X4	T49.0X5	T49.0X6
Paraoxon	T60.0X1	T60.0X2	T60.0X3	T60.0X4	—	—
Paraquat	T60.3X1	T60.3X2	T60.3X3	T60.3X4	—	—

TABLE OF DRUGS AND CHEMICALS

◀ New   ◀▦ Revised   ~~deleted~~ Deleted

Substance	Poisoning, Accidental (Unintentional)	Poisoning, Intentional Self-Harm	Poisoning, Assault	Poisoning, Undetermined	Adverse Effect	Underdosing
	External Cause (T-Code)					
Parasympatholytic NEC	T44.3X1	T44.3X2	T44.3X3	T44.3X4	T44.3X5	T44.3X6
Parasympathomimetic drug NEC	T44.1X1	T44.1X2	T44.1X3	T44.1X4	T44.1X5	T44.1X6
Parathion	T60.0X1	T60.0X2	T60.0X3	T60.0X4	—	—
Parathormone	T50.991	T50.992	T50.993	T50.994	T50.995	T50.996
Parathyroid extract	T50.991	T50.992	T50.993	T50.994	T50.995	T50.996
Paratyphoid vaccine	T50.A91	T50.A92	T50.A93	T50.A94	T50.A95	T50.A96
Paredrine	T44.4X1	T44.4X2	T44.4X3	T44.4X4	T44.4X5	T44.4X6
Paregoric	T40.0X1	T40.0X2	T40.0X3	T40.0X4	T40.0X5	T40.0X6
Pargyline	T46.5X1	T46.5X2	T46.5X3	T46.5X4	T46.5X5	T46.5X6
Paris green	T57.0X1	T57.0X2	T57.0X3	T57.0X4	—	—
insecticide	T57.0X1	T57.0X2	T57.0X3	T57.0X4	—	—
Parnate	T43.1X1	T43.1X2	T43.1X3	T43.1X4	T43.1X5	T43.1X6
Paromomycin	T36.5X1	T36.5X2	T36.5X3	T36.5X4	T36.5X5	T36.5X6
Paroxypropione	T45.1X1	T45.1X2	T45.1X3	T45.1X4	T45.1X5	T45.1X6
Parzone	T40.2X1	T40.2X2	T40.2X3	T40.2X4	T40.2X5	T40.2X6
PAS	T37.1X1	T37.1X2	T37.1X3	T37.1X4	T37.1X5	T37.1X6
Pasiniazid	T37.1X1	T37.1X2	T37.1X3	T37.1X4	T37.1X5	T37.1X6
PBB (polybrominated biphenyls)	T65.891	T65.892	T65.893	T65.894	—	—
PCB	T65.891	T65.892	T65.893	T65.894	—	—
PCP						
meaning pentachlorophenol	T60.1X1	T60.1X2	T60.1X3	T60.1X4	—	—
fungicide	T60.3X1	T60.3X2	T60.3X3	T60.3X4	—	—
herbicide	T60.3X1	T60.3X2	T60.3X3	T60.3X4	—	—
insecticide	T60.1X1	T60.1X2	T60.1X3	T60.1X4	—	—
meaning phencyclidine	T40.991	T40.992	T40.993	T40.994	—	—
Peach kernel oil (emulsion)	T47.4X1	T47.4X2	T47.4X3	T47.4X4	T47.4X5	T47.4X6
Peanut oil (emulsion) NEC	T47.4X1	T47.4X2	T47.4X3	T47.4X4	T47.4X5	T47.4X6
topical	T49.3X1	T49.3X2	T49.3X3	T49.3X4	T49.3X5	T49.3X6
Pearly Gates (morning glory seeds)	T40.991	T40.992	T40.993	T40.994	—	—
Pecazine	T43.3X1	T43.3X2	T43.3X3	T43.3X4	T43.3X5	T43.3X6
Pectin	T47.6X1	T47.6X2	T47.6X3	T47.6X4	T47.6X5	T47.6X6
Pefloxacin	T37.8X1	T37.8X2	T37.8X3	T37.8X4	T37.8X5	T37.8X6
Pegademase, bovine	T50.Z91	T50.Z92	T50.Z93	T50.Z94	T50.Z95	T50.Z96
Pelletierine tannate	T37.4X1	T37.4X2	T37.4X3	T37.4X4	T37.4X5	T37.4X6
Pemirolast (potassium)	T48.6X1	T48.6X2	T48.6X3	T48.6X4	T48.6X5	T48.6X6
Pemoline	T50.7X1	T50.7X2	T50.7X3	T50.7X4	T50.7X5	T50.7X6
Pempidine	T44.2X1	T44.2X2	T44.2X3	T44.2X4	T44.2X5	T44.2X6
Penamecillin	T36.0X1	T36.0X2	T36.0X3	T36.0X4	T36.0X5	T36.0X6
Penbutolol	T44.7X1	T44.7X2	T44.7X3	T44.7X4	T44.7X5	T44.7X6
Penethamate	T36.0X1	T36.0X2	T36.0X3	T36.0X4	T36.0X5	T36.0X6

◄ New   ◄ Revised   ~~deleted~~ Deleted

Substance	Poisoning, Accidental (Unintentional)	Poisoning, Intentional Self-Harm	Poisoning, Assault	Poisoning, Undetermined	Adverse Effect	Underdosing
Penfluridol	T43.591	T43.592	T43.593	T43.594	T43.595	T43.596
Penflutizide	T50.2X1	T50.2X2	T50.2X3	T50.2X4	T50.2X5	T50.2X6
Pengitoxin	T46.0X1	T46.0X2	T46.0X3	T46.0X4	T46.0X5	T46.0X6
Penicillamine	T50.6X1	T50.6X2	T50.6X3	T50.6X4	T50.6X5	T50.6X6
Penicillin (any)	T36.0X1	T36.0X2	T36.0X3	T36.0X4	T36.0X5	T36.0X6
Penicillinase	T45.3X1	T45.3X2	T45.3X3	T45.3X4	T45.3X5	T45.3X6
Penicilloyl polylysine	T50.8X1	T50.8X2	T50.8X3	T50.8X4	T50.8X5	T50.8X6
Penimepicycline	T36.4X1	T36.4X2	T36.4X3	T36.4X4	T36.4X5	T36.4X6
Pentachloroethane	T53.6X1	T53.6X2	T53.6X3	T53.6X4	—	—
Pentachloronaphthalene	T53.7X1	T53.7X2	T53.7X3	T53.7X4	—	—
Pentachlorophenol (pesticide)	T60.1X1	T60.1X2	T60.1X3	T60.1X4	—	—
fungicide	T60.3X1	T60.3X2	T60.3X3	T60.3X4	—	—
herbicide	T60.3X1	T60.3X2	T60.3X3	T60.3X4	—	—
insecticide	T60.1X1	T60.1X2	T60.1X3	T60.1X4	—	—
Pentaerythritol tetranitrate	T46.3X1	T46.3X2	T46.3X3	T46.3X4	T46.3X5	T46.3X6
Pentaerythritol	T46.3X1	T46.3X2	T46.3X3	T46.3X4	T46.3X5	T46.3X6
chloral	T42.6X1	T42.6X2	T42.6X3	T42.6X4	T42.6X5	T42.6X6
tetranitrate NEC	T46.3X1	T46.3X2	T46.3X3	T46.3X4	T46.3X5	T46.3X6
Pentagastrin	T50.8X1	T50.8X2	T50.8X3	T50.8X4	T50.8X5	T50.8X6
Pentalin	T53.6X1	T53.6X2	T53.6X3	T53.6X4	—	—
Pentamethonium bromide	T44.2X1	T44.2X2	T44.2X3	T44.2X4	T44.2X5	T44.2X6
Pentamidine	T37.3X1	T37.3X2	T37.3X3	T37.3X4	T37.3X5	T37.3X6
Pentanol	T51.3X1	T51.3X2	T51.3X3	T51.3X4	—	—
Pentapyrrolinium (bitartrate)	T44.2X1	T44.2X2	T44.2X3	T44.2X4	T44.2X5	T44.2X6
Pentaquine	T37.2X1	T37.2X2	T37.2X3	T37.2X4	T37.2X5	T37.2X6
Pentazocine	T40.4X1	T40.4X2	T40.4X3	T40.4X4	T40.4X5	T40.4X6
Pentetrazole	T50.7X1	T50.7X2	T50.7X3	T50.7X4	T50.7X5	T50.7X6
Penthienate bromide	T44.3X1	T44.3X2	T44.3X3	T44.3X4	T44.3X5	T44.3X6
Pentifylline	T46.7X1	T46.7X2	T46.7X3	T46.7X4	T46.7X5	T46.7X6
Pentobarbital	T42.3X1	T42.3X2	T42.3X3	T42.3X4	T42.3X5	T42.3X6
sodium	T42.3X1	T42.3X2	T42.3X3	T42.3X4	T42.3X5	T42.3X6
Pentobarbitone	T42.3X1	T42.3X2	T42.3X3	T42.3X4	T42.3X5	T42.3X6
Pentolonium tartrate	T44.2X1	T44.2X2	T44.2X3	T44.2X4	T44.2X5	T44.2X6
Pentosan polysulfate (sodium)	T39.8X1	T39.8X2	T39.8X3	T39.8X4	T39.8X5	T39.8X6
Pentostatin	T45.1X1	T45.1X2	T45.1X3	T45.1X4	T45.1X5	T45.1X6
Pentothal	T41.1X1	T41.1X2	T41.1X3	T41.1X4	T41.1X5	T41.1X6
Pentoxifylline	T46.7X1	T46.7X2	T46.7X3	T46.7X4	T46.7X5	T46.7X6
Pentoxyverine	T48.3X1	T48.3X2	T48.3X3	T48.3X4	T48.3X5	T48.3X6
Pentrinat	T46.3X1	T46.3X2	T46.3X3	T46.3X4	T46.3X5	T46.3X6
Pentylenetetrazole	T50.7X1	T50.7X2	T50.7X3	T50.7X4	T50.7X5	T50.7X6

◀ New ◀▥ Revised ~~deleted~~ Deleted

TABLE OF DRUGS AND CHEMICALS

	External Cause (T-Code)					
Substance	Poisoning, Accidental (Unintentional)	Poisoning, Intentional Self-Harm	Poisoning, Assault	Poisoning, Undetermined	Adverse Effect	Underdosing
Pentylsalicylamide	T37.1X1	T37.1X2	T37.1X3	T37.1X4	T37.1X5	T37.1X6
Pentymal	T42.3X1	T42.3X2	T42.3X3	T42.3X4	T42.3X5	T42.3X6
Peplomycin	T45.1X1	T45.1X2	T45.1X3	T45.1X4	T45.1X5	T45.1X6
Peppermint (oil)	T47.5X1	T47.5X2	T47.5X3	T47.5X4	T47.5X5	T47.5X6
Pepsin	T47.5X1	T47.5X2	T47.5X3	T47.5X4	T47.5X5	T47.5X6
digestant	T47.5X1	T47.5X2	T47.5X3	T47.5X4	T47.5X5	T47.5X6
Pepstatin	T47.1X1	T47.1X2	T47.1X3	T47.1X4	T47.1X5	T47.1X6
Peptavlon	T50.8X1	T50.8X2	T50.8X3	T50.8X4	T50.8X5	T50.8X6
Perazine	T43.3X1	T43.3X2	T43.3X3	T43.3X4	T43.3X5	T43.3X6
Percaine (spinal)	T41.3X1	T41.3X2	T41.3X3	T41.3X4	T41.3X5	T41.3X6
topical (surface)	T41.3X1	T41.3X2	T41.3X3	T41.3X4	T41.3X5	T41.3X6
Perchloroethylene	T53.3X1	T53.3X2	T53.3X3	T53.3X4	—	—
medicinal	T37.4X1	T37.4X2	T37.4X3	T37.4X4	T37.4X5	T37.4X6
vapor	T53.3X1	T53.3X2	T53.3X3	T53.3X4	—	—
Percodan	T40.2X1	T40.2X2	T40.2X3	T40.2X4	T40.2X5	T40.2X6
Percogesic — see also acetaminophen	T45.0X1	T45.0X2	T45.0X3	T45.0X4	T45.0X5	T45.0X6
Percorten	T38.0X1	T38.0X2	T38.0X3	T38.0X4	T38.0X5	T38.0X6
Pergolide	T42.8X1	T42.8X2	T42.8X3	T42.8X4	T42.8X5	T42.8X6
Pergonal	T38.811	T38.812	T38.813	T38.814	T38.815	T38.816
Perhexilene	T46.3X1	T46.3X2	T46.3X3	T46.3X4	T46.3X5	T46.3X6
Perhexiline (maleate)	T46.3X1	T46.3X2	T46.3X3	T46.3X4	T46.3X5	T46.3X6
Periactin	T45.0X1	T45.0X2	T45.0X3	T45.0X4	T45.0X5	T45.0X6
Periciazine	T43.3X1	T43.3X2	T43.3X3	T43.3X4	T43.3X5	T43.3X6
Periclor	T42.6X1	T42.6X2	T42.6X3	T42.6X4	T42.6X5	T42.6X6
Perindopril	T46.4X1	T46.4X2	T46.4X3	T46.4X4	T46.4X5	T46.4X6
Perisoxal	T39.8X1	T39.8X2	T39.8X3	T39.8X4	T39.8X5	T39.8X6
Peritrate	T46.3X1	T46.3X2	T46.3X3	T46.3X4	T46.3X5	T46.3X6
Peritoneal dialysis solution	T50.3X1	T50.3X2	T50.3X3	T50.3X4	T50.3X5	T50.3X6
Perlapine	T42.4X1	T42.4X2	T42.4X3	T42.4X4	T42.4X5	T42.4X6
Permanganate	T65.891	T65.892	T65.893	T65.894	—	—
Permethrin	T60.1X1	T60.1X2	T60.1X3	T60.1X4	—	—
Pernocton	T42.3X1	T42.3X2	T42.3X3	T42.3X4	T42.3X5	T42.3X6
Pernoston	T42.3X1	T42.3X2	T42.3X3	T42.3X4	T42.3X5	T42.3X6
Peronine	T40.2X1	T40.2X2	T40.2X3	T40.2X4	—	—
Perphenazine	T43.3X1	T43.3X2	T43.3X3	T43.3X4	T43.3X5	T43.3X6
Pertofrane	T43.011	T43.012	T43.013	T43.014	T43.015	T43.016
Pertussis						
immune serum (human)	T50.Z11	T50.Z12	T50.Z13	T50.Z14	T50.Z15	T50.Z16
vaccine (with diphtheria toxoid) (with tetanus toxoid)	T50.A11	T50.A12	T50.A13	T50.A14	T50.A15	T50.A16
Peruvian balsam	T49.0X1	T49.0X2	T49.0X3	T49.0X4	T49.0X5	T49.0X6

◀ New ◀▥ Revised ~~deleted~~ Deleted

Substance	Poisoning, Accidental (Unintentional)	Poisoning, Intentional Self-Harm	Poisoning, Assault	Poisoning, Undetermined	Adverse Effect	Underdosing
			External Cause (T-Code)			
Peruvoside	T46.0X1	T46.0X2	T46.0X3	T46.0X4	T46.0X5	T46.0X6
Pesticide (dust) (fumes) (vapor) NEC	T60.91	T60.92	T60.93	T60.94	—	—
arsenic	T57.0X1	T57.0X2	T57.0X3	T57.0X4	—	—
chlorinated	T60.1X1	T60.1X2	T60.1X3	T60.1X4	—	—
cyanide	T65.0X1	T65.0X2	T65.0X3	T65.0X4	—	—
kerosene	T52.0X1	T52.0X2	T52.0X3	T52.0X4	—	—
mixture (of compounds)	T60.91	T60.92	T60.93	T60.94	—	—
naphthalene	T60.2X1	T60.2X2	T60.2X3	T60.2X4	—	—
organochlorine (compounds)	T60.1X1	T60.1X2	T60.1X3	T60.1X4	—	—
petroleum (distillate) (products) NEC	T60.8X1	T60.8X2	T60.8X3	T60.8X4	—	—
specified ingredient NEC	T60.8X1	T60.8X2	T60.8X3	T60.8X4	—	—
strychnine	T65.1X1	T65.1X2	T65.1X3	T65.1X4	—	—
thallium	T60.4X1	T60.4X2	T60.4X3	T60.4X4	—	—
Pethidine	T40.4X1	T40.4X2	T40.4X3	T40.4X4	T40.4X5	T40.4X6
Petrichloral	T42.6X1	T42.6X2	T42.6X3	T42.6X4	T42.6X5	T42.6X6
Petrol	T52.0X1	T52.0X2	T52.0X3	T52.0X4	—	—
vapor	T52.0X1	T52.0X2	T52.0X3	T52.0X4	—	—
Petrolatum	T49.3X1	T49.3X2	T49.3X3	T49.3X4	T49.3X5	T49.3X6
hydrophilic	T49.3X1	T49.3X2	T49.3X3	T49.3X4	T49.3X5	T49.3X6
liquid	T47.4X1	T47.4X2	T47.4X3	T47.4X4	T47.4X5	T47.4X6
topical	T49.3X1	T49.3X2	T49.3X3	T49.3X4	T49.3X5	T49.3X6
nonmedicinal	T52.0X1	T52.0X2	T52.0X3	T52.0X4	—	—
red veterinary	T49.3X1	T49.3X2	T49.3X3	T49.3X4	T49.3X5	T49.3X6
white	T49.3X1	T49.3X2	T49.3X3	T49.3X4	T49.3X5	T49.3X6
Petroleum (products) NEC	T52.0X1	T52.0X2	T52.0X3	T52.0X4	—	—
benzine(s) — *see* Ligroin						
ether — *see* Ligroin						
jelly — *see* Petrolatum						
naphtha — *see* Ligroin						
pesticide	T60.8X1	T60.8X2	T60.8X3	T60.8X4	—	—
solids	T52.0X1	T52.0X2	T52.0X3	T52.0X4	—	—
solvents	T52.0X1	T52.0X2	T52.0X3	T52.0X4	—	—
vapor	T52.0X1	T52.0X2	T52.0X3	T52.0X4	—	—
Peyote	T40.991	T40.992	T40.993	T40.994	—	—
Phanodorm, phanodorn	T42.3X1	T42.3X2	T42.3X3	T42.3X4	T42.3X5	T42.3X6
Phanquinone	T37.3X1	T37.3X2	T37.3X3	T37.3X4	T37.3X5	T37.3X6
Phanquone	T37.3X1	T37.3X2	T37.3X3	T37.3X4	T37.3X5	T37.3X6
Pharmaceutical						
adjunct NEC	T50.901	T50.902	T50.903	T50.904	T50.905	T50.906
excipient NEC	T50.901	T50.902	T50.903	T50.904	T50.905	T50.906

◀ New   ◀▥ Revised   ~~deleted~~ Deleted

Substance	External Cause (T-Code)					
	Poisoning, Accidental (Unintentional)	Poisoning, Intentional Self-Harm	Poisoning, Assault	Poisoning, Undetermined	Adverse Effect	Underdosing
Pharmaceutical *(Continued)*						
sweetener	T50.901	T50.902	T50.903	T50.904	T50.905	T50.906
viscous agent	T50.901	T50.902	T50.903	T50.904	T50.905	T50.906
Phemitone	T42.3X1	T42.3X2	T42.3X3	T42.3X4	T42.3X5	T42.3X6
Phenacaine	T41.3X1	T41.3X2	T41.3X3	T41.3X4	T41.3X5	T41.3X6
Phenacemide	T42.6X1	T42.6X2	T42.6X3	T42.6X4	T42.6X5	T42.6X6
Phenacetin	T39.1X1	T39.1X2	T39.1X3	T39.1X4	T39.1X5	T39.1X6
Phenadoxone	T40.2X1	T40.2X2	T40.2X3	T40.2X4	—	—
Phenaglycodol	T43.591	T43.592	T43.593	T43.594	T43.595	T43.596
Phenantoin	T42.0X1	T42.0X2	T42.0X3	T42.0X4	T42.0X5	T42.0X6
Phenaphthazine reagent	T50.991	T50.992	T50.993	T50.994	T50.995	T50.996
Phenazocine	T40.4X1	T40.4X2	T40.4X3	T40.4X4	T40.4X5	T40.4X6
Phenazone	T39.2X1	T39.2X2	T39.2X3	T39.2X4	T39.2X5	T39.2X6
Phenazopyridine	T39.8X1	T39.8X2	T39.8X3	T39.8X4	T39.8X5	T39.8X6
Phenbenicillin	T36.0X1	T36.0X2	T36.0X3	T36.0X4	T36.0X5	T36.0X6
Phenbutrazate	T50.5X1	T50.5X2	T50.5X3	T50.5X4	T50.5X5	T50.5X6
Phencyclidine	T40.991	T40.992	T40.993	T40.994	T40.995	T40.996
Phendimetrazine	T50.5X1	T50.5X2	T50.5X3	T50.5X4	T50.5X5	T50.5X6
Phenelzine	T43.1X1	T43.1X2	T43.1X3	T43.1X4	T43.1X5	T43.1X6
Phenemal	T42.3X1	T42.3X2	T42.3X3	T42.3X4	T42.3X5	T42.3X6
Phenergan	T42.6X1	T42.6X2	T42.6X3	T42.6X4	T42.6X5	T42.6X6
Pheneticillin	T36.0X1	T36.0X2	T36.0X3	T36.0X4	T36.0X5	T36.0X6
Pheneturide	T42.6X1	T42.6X2	T42.6X3	T42.6X4	T42.6X5	T42.6X6
Phenformin	T38.3X1	T38.3X2	T38.3X3	T38.3X4	T38.3X5	T38.3X6
Phenglutarimide	T44.3X1	T44.3X2	T44.3X3	T44.3X4	T44.3X5	T44.3X6
Phenicarbazide	T39.8X1	T39.8X2	T39.8X3	T39.8X4	T39.8X5	T39.8X6
Phenindamine	T45.0X1	T45.0X2	T45.0X3	T45.0X4	T45.0X5	T45.0X6
Phenindione	T45.511	T45.512	T45.513	T45.514	T45.515	T45.516
Pheniprazine	T43.1X1	T43.1X2	T43.1X3	T43.1X4	T43.1X5	T43.1X6
Pheniramine	T45.0X1	T45.0X2	T45.0X3	T45.0X4	T45.0X5	T45.0X6
Phenisatin	T47.2X1	T47.2X2	T47.2X3	T47.2X4	T47.2X5	T47.2X6
Phenmetrazine	T50.5X1	T50.5X2	T50.5X3	T50.5X4	T50.5X5	T50.5X6
Phenobal	T42.3X1	T42.3X2	T42.3X3	T42.3X4	T42.3X5	T42.3X6
Phenobarbital	T42.3X1	T42.3X2	T42.3X3	T42.3X4	T42.3X5	T42.3X6
with						
mephenytoin	T42.3X1	T42.3X2	T42.3X3	T42.3X4	T42.3X5	T42.3X6
phenytoin	T42.3X1	T42.3X2	T42.3X3	T42.3X4	T42.3X5	T42.3X6
sodium	T42.3X1	T42.3X2	T42.3X3	T42.3X4	T42.3X5	T42.3X6
Phenobarbitone	T42.3X1	T42.3X2	T42.3X3	T42.3X4	T42.3X5	T42.3X6

◀ New   ◀▥ Revised   ~~deleted~~ Deleted

Substance	External Cause (T-Code)					
	Poisoning, Accidental (Unintentional)	Poisoning, Intentional Self-Harm	Poisoning, Assault	Poisoning, Undetermined	Adverse Effect	Underdosing
Phenobutiodil	T50.8X1	T50.8X2	T50.8X3	T50.8X4	T50.8X5	T50.8X6
Phenoctide	T49.0X1	T49.0X2	T49.0X3	T49.0X4	T49.0X5	T49.0X6
Phenol	T49.0X1	T49.0X2	T49.0X3	T49.0X4	T49.0X5	T49.0X6
disinfectant	T54.0X1	T54.0X2	T54.0X3	T54.0X4	—	—
in oil injection	T46.8X1	T46.8X2	T46.8X3	T46.8X4	T46.8X5	T46.8X6
medicinal	T49.1X1	T49.1X2	T49.1X3	T49.1X4	T49.1X5	T49.1X6
nonmedicinal NEC	T54.0X1	T54.0X2	T54.0X3	T54.0X4	—	—
pesticide	T60.8X1	T60.8X2	T60.8X3	T60.8X4	—	—
red	T50.8X1	T50.8X2	T50.8X3	T50.8X4	T50.8X5	T50.8X6
Phenolic preparation	T49.1X1	T49.1X2	T49.1X3	T49.1X4	T49.1X5	T49.1X6
Phenolphthalein	T47.2X1	T47.2X2	T47.2X3	T47.2X4	T47.2X5	T47.2X6
Phenolsulfonphthalein	T50.8X1	T50.8X2	T50.8X3	T50.8X4	T50.8X5	T50.8X6
Phenomorphan	T40.2X1	T40.2X2	T40.2X3	T40.2X4	—	—
Phenonyl	T42.3X1	T42.3X2	T42.3X3	T42.3X4	T42.3X5	T42.3X6
Phenoperidine	T40.4X1	T40.4X2	T40.4X3	T40.4X4	—	—
Phenopyrazone	T46.991	T46.992	T46.993	T46.994	T46.995	T46.996
Phenoquin	T50.4X1	T50.4X2	T50.4X3	T50.4X4	T50.4X5	T50.4X6
Phenothiazine (psychotropic) NEC	T43.3X1	T43.3X2	T43.3X3	T43.3X4	T43.3X5	T43.3X6
insecticide	T60.2X1	T60.2X2	T60.2X3	T60.2X4	—	—
Phenothrin	T49.0X1	T49.0X2	T49.0X3	T49.0X4	T49.0X5	T49.0X6
Phenoxybenzamine	T46.7X1	T46.7X2	T46.7X3	T46.7X4	T46.7X5	T46.7X6
Phenoxyethanol	T49.0X1	T49.0X2	T49.0X3	T49.0X4	T49.0X5	T49.0X6
Phenoxymethyl penicillin	T36.0X1	T36.0X2	T36.0X3	T36.0X4	T36.0X5	T36.0X6
Phenprobamate	T42.8X1	T42.8X2	T42.8X3	T42.8X4	T42.8X5	T42.8X6
Phenprocoumon	T45.511	T45.512	T45.513	T45.514	T45.515	T45.516
Phensuximide	T42.2X1	T42.2X2	T42.2X3	T42.2X4	T42.2X5	T42.2X6
Phentermine	T50.5X1	T50.5X2	T50.5X3	T50.5X4	T50.5X5	T50.5X6
Phenthicillin	T36.0X1	T36.0X2	T36.0X3	T36.0X4	T36.0X5	T36.0X6
Phentolamine	T46.7X1	T46.7X2	T46.7X3	T46.7X4	T46.7X5	T46.7X6
Phenyl						
butazone	T39.2X1	T39.2X2	T39.2X3	T39.2X4	T39.2X5	T39.2X6
enediamine	T65.3X1	T65.3X2	T65.3X3	T65.3X4	—	—
hydrazine	T65.3X1	T65.3X2	T65.3X3	T65.3X4	—	—
antineoplastic	T45.1X1	T45.1X2	T45.1X3	T45.1X4	T45.1X5	T45.1X6
mercuric compounds — *see* Mercury						
salicylate	T49.3X1	T49.3X2	T49.3X3	T49.3X4	T49.3X5	T49.3X6
Phenylalanine mustard	T45.1X1	T45.1X2	T45.1X3	T45.1X4	T45.1X5	T45.1X6
Phenylbutazone	T39.2X1	T39.2X2	T39.2X3	T39.2X4	T39.2X5	T39.2X6
Phenylenediamine	T65.3X1	T65.3X2	T65.3X3	T65.3X4	—	—

TABLE OF DRUGS AND CHEMICALS

TABLE OF DRUGS AND CHEMICALS

Substance	External Cause (T-Code)					
	Poisoning, Accidental (Unintentional)	Poisoning, Intentional Self-Harm	Poisoning, Assault	Poisoning, Undetermined	Adverse Effect	Underdosing
Phenylephrine	T44.4X1	T44.4X2	T44.4X3	T44.4X4	T44.4X5	T44.4X6
Phenylethylbiguanide	T38.3X1	T38.3X2	T38.3X3	T38.3X4	T38.3X5	T38.3X6
Phenylmercuric						
acetate	T49.0X1	T49.0X2	T49.0X3	T49.0X4	T49.0X5	T49.0X6
borate	T49.0X1	T49.0X2	T49.0X3	T49.0X4	T49.0X5	T49.0X6
nitrate	T49.0X1	T49.0X2	T49.0X3	T49.0X4	T49.0X5	T49.0X6
Phenylmethylbarbitone	T42.3X1	T42.3X2	T42.3X3	T42.3X4	T42.3X5	T42.3X6
Phenylpropanol	T47.5X1	T47.5X2	T47.5X3	T47.5X4	T47.5X5	T47.5X6
Phenylpropanolamine	T44.991	T44.992	T44.993	T44.994	T44.995	T44.996
Phenylsulfthion	T60.0X1	T60.0X2	T60.0X3	T60.0X4	—	—
Phenyltoloxamine	T45.0X1	T45.0X2	T45.0X3	T45.0X4	T45.0X5	T45.0X6
Phenyramidol, phenyramidon	T39.8X1	T39.8X2	T39.8X3	T39.8X4	T39.8X5	T39.8X6
Phenytoin	T42.0X1	T42.0X2	T42.0X3	T42.0X4	T42.0X5	T42.0X6
with Phenobarbital	T42.3X1	T42.3X2	T42.3X3	T42.3X4	T42.3X5	T42.3X6
pHisoHex	T49.2X1	T49.2X2	T49.2X3	T49.2X4	T49.2X5	T49.2X6
Pholcodine	T48.3X1	T48.3X2	T48.3X3	T48.3X4	T48.3X5	T48.3X6
Pholedrine	T46.991	T46.992	T46.993	T46.994	T46.995	T46.996
Phorate	T60.0X1	T60.0X2	T60.0X3	T60.0X4	—	—
Phosdrin	T60.0X1	T60.0X2	T60.0X3	T60.0X4	—	—
Phosfolan	T60.0X1	T60.0X2	T60.0X3	T60.0X4	—	—
Phosgene (gas)	T59.891	T59.892	T59.893	T59.894	—	—
Phosphamidon	T60.0X1	T60.0X2	T60.0X3	T60.0X4	—	—
Phosphate	T65.891	T65.892	T65.893	T65.894	—	—
laxative	T47.4X1	T47.4X2	T47.4X3	T47.4X4	T47.4X5	T47.4X6
organic	T60.0X1	T60.0X2	T60.0X3	T60.0X4	—	—
solvent	T52.91	T52.92	T52.93	T52.94	—	—
tricresyl	T65.891	T65.892	T65.893	T65.894	—	—
Phosphine	T57.1X1	T57.1X2	T57.1X3	T57.1X4	—	—
fumigant	T57.1X1	T57.1X2	T57.1X3	T57.1X4	—	—
Phospholine	T49.5X1	T49.5X2	T49.5X3	T49.5X4	T49.5X5	T49.5X6
Phosphoric acid	T54.2X1	T54.2X2	T54.2X3	T54.2X4	—	—
Phosphorus (compound) NEC	T57.1X1	T57.1X2	T57.1X3	T57.1X4	—	—
pesticide	T60.0X1	T60.0X2	T60.0X3	T60.0X4	—	—
Phthalates	T65.891	T65.892	T65.893	T65.894	—	—
Phthalic anhydride	T65.891	T65.892	T65.893	T65.894	—	—
Phthalimidoglutarimide	T42.6X1	T42.6X2	T42.6X3	T42.6X4	T42.6X5	T42.6X6
Phthalylsulfathiazole	T37.0X1	T37.0X2	T37.0X3	T37.0X4	T37.0X5	T37.0X6
Phylloquinone	T45.7X1	T45.7X2	T45.7X3	T45.7X4	T45.7X5	T45.7X6
Physeptone	T40.3X1	T40.3X2	T40.3X3	T40.3X4	T40.3X5	T40.3X6

◀ New ◀▥ Revised ~~deleted~~ Deleted

Substance	External Cause (T-Code)					
	Poisoning, Accidental (Unintentional)	Poisoning, Intentional Self-Harm	Poisoning, Assault	Poisoning, Undetermined	Adverse Effect	Underdosing
Physostigma venenosum	T62.2X1	T62.2X2	T62.2X3	T62.2X4	—	—
Physostigmine	T49.5X1	T49.5X2	T49.5X3	T49.5X4	T49.5X5	T49.5X6
Phytolacca decandra	T62.2X1	T62.2X2	T62.2X3	T62.2X4	—	—
berries	T62.1X1	T62.1X2	T62.1X3	T62.1X4	—	—
Phytomenadione	T45.7X1	T45.7X2	T45.7X3	T45.7X4	T45.7X5	T45.7X6
Phytonadione	T45.7X1	T45.7X2	T45.7X3	T45.7X4	T45.7X5	T45.7X6
Picoperine	T48.3X1	T48.3X2	T48.3X3	T48.3X4	T48.3X5	T48.3X6
Picosulfate (sodium)	T47.2X1	T47.2X2	T47.2X3	T47.2X4	T47.2X5	T47.2X6
Picric (acid)	T54.2X1	T54.2X2	T54.2X3	T54.2X4	—	—
Picrotoxin	T50.7X1	T50.7X2	T50.7X3	T50.7X4	T50.7X5	T50.7X6
Piketoprofen	T49.0X1	T49.0X2	T49.0X3	T49.0X4	T49.0X5	T49.0X6
Pilocarpine	T44.1X1	T44.1X2	T44.1X3	T44.1X4	T44.1X5	T44.1X6
Pilocarpus (jaborandi) extract	T44.1X1	T44.1X2	T44.1X3	T44.1X4	T44.1X5	T44.1X6
Pilsicainide (hydrochloride)	T46.2X1	T46.2X2	T46.2X3	T46.2X4	T46.2X5	T46.2X6
Pimaricin	T36.7X1	T36.7X2	T36.7X3	T36.7X4	T36.7X5	T36.7X6
Pimeclone	T50.7X1	T50.7X2	T50.7X3	T50.7X4	T50.7X5	T50.7X6
Pimelic ketone	T52.8X1	T52.8X2	T52.8X3	T52.8X4	—	—
Pimethixene	T45.0X1	T45.0X2	T45.0X3	T45.0X4	T45.0X5	T45.0X6
Piminodine	T40.2X1	T40.2X2	T40.2X3	T40.2X4	T40.2X5	T40.2X6
Pimozide	T43.591	T43.592	T43.593	T43.594	T43.595	T43.596
Pinacidil	T46.5X1	T46.5X2	T46.5X3	T46.5X4	T46.5X5	T46.5X6
Pinaverium bromide	T44.3X1	T44.3X2	T44.3X3	T44.3X4	T44.3X5	T44.3X6
Pinazepam	T42.4X1	T42.4X2	T42.4X3	T42.4X4	T42.4X5	T42.4X6
Pindolol	T44.7X1	T44.7X2	T44.7X3	T44.7X4	T44.7X5	T44.7X6
Pindone	T60.4X1	T60.4X2	T60.4X3	T60.4X4	—	—
Pine oil (disinfectant)	T65.891	T65.892	T65.893	T65.894	—	—
Pinkroot	T37.4X1	T37.4X2	T37.4X3	T37.4X4	T37.4X5	T37.4X6
Pipadone	T40.2X1	T40.2X2	T40.2X3	T40.2X4	—	—
Pipamazine	T45.0X1	T45.0X2	T45.0X3	T45.0X4	T45.0X5	T45.0X6
Pipamperone	T43.4X1	T43.4X2	T43.4X3	T43.4X4	T43.4X5	T43.4X6
Pipazetate	T48.3X1	T48.3X2	T48.3X3	T48.3X4	T48.3X5	T48.3X6
Pipemidic acid	T37.8X1	T37.8X2	T37.8X3	T37.8X4	T37.8X5	T37.8X6
Pipenzolate bromide	T44.3X1	T44.3X2	T44.3X3	T44.3X4	T44.3X5	T44.3X6
Piperacetazine	T43.3X1	T43.3X2	T43.3X3	T43.3X4	T43.3X5	T43.3X6
Piperacillin	T36.0X1	T36.0X2	T36.0X3	T36.0X4	T36.0X5	T36.0X6
Piperazine	T37.4X1	T37.4X2	T37.4X3	T37.4X4	T37.4X5	T37.4X6
estrone sulfate	T38.5X1	T38.5X2	T38.5X3	T38.5X4	T38.5X5	T38.5X6
Piper cubeba	T62.2X1	T62.2X2	T62.2X3	T62.2X4	—	—
Piperidione	T48.3X1	T48.3X2	T48.3X3	T48.3X4	—	—

TABLE OF DRUGS AND CHEMICALS

Substance	External Cause (T-Code)					
	Poisoning, Accidental (Unintentional)	Poisoning, Intentional Self-Harm	Poisoning, Assault	Poisoning, Undetermined	Adverse Effect	Underdosing
Piperidolate	T44.3X1	T44.3X2	T44.3X3	T44.3X4	T44.3X5	T44.3X6
Piperocaine	T41.3X1	T41.3X2	T41.3X3	T41.3X4	T41.3X5	T41.3X6
infiltration (subcutaneous)	T41.3X1	T41.3X2	T41.3X3	T41.3X4	T41.3X5	T41.3X6
nerve block (peripheral) (plexus)	T41.3X1	T41.3X2	T41.3X3	T41.3X4	T41.3X5	T41.3X6
topical (surface)	T41.3X1	T41.3X2	T41.3X3	T41.3X4	T41.3X5	T41.3X6
Piperonyl butoxide	T60.8X1	T60.8X2	T60.8X3	T60.8X4	—	—
Pipethanate	T44.3X1	T44.3X2	T44.3X3	T44.3X4	T44.3X5	T44.3X6
Pipobroman	T45.1X1	T45.1X2	T45.1X3	T45.1X4	T45.1X5	T45.1X6
Pipofezine	T43.0X1	T43.0X2	T43.0X3	T43.0X4	T43.0X5	T43.0X6
Pipotiazine	T43.3X1	T43.3X2	T43.3X3	T43.3X4	T43.3X5	T43.3X6
Pipoxizine	T45.0X1	T45.0X2	T45.0X3	T45.0X4	T45.0X5	T45.0X6
Pipradrol	T43.691	T43.692	T43.693	T43.694	T43.695	T43.696
Piprinhydrinate	T45.0X1	T45.0X2	T45.0X3	T45.0X4	T45.0X5	T45.0X6
Pirarubicin	T45.1X1	T45.1X2	T45.1X3	T45.1X4	T45.1X5	T45.1X6
Pirazinamide	T37.1X1	T37.1X2	T37.1X3	T37.1X4	T37.1X5	T37.1X6
Pirbuterol	T48.6X1	T48.6X2	T48.6X3	T48.6X4	T48.6X5	T48.6X6
Pirenzepine	T47.1X1	T47.1X2	T47.1X3	T47.1X4	T47.1X5	T47.1X6
Piretanide	T50.1X1	T50.1X2	T50.1X3	T50.1X4	T50.1X5	T50.1X6
Piribedil	T42.8X1	T42.8X2	T42.8X3	T42.8X4	T42.8X5	T42.8X6
Piridoxilate	T46.3X1	T46.3X2	T46.3X3	T46.3X4	T46.3X5	T46.3X6
Piritramide	T40.4X1	T40.4X2	T40.4X3	T40.4X4	—	—
Pirlindole	T43.0X1	T43.0X2	T43.0X3	T43.0X4	T43.0X5	T43.0X6
Piromidic acid	T37.8X1	T37.8X2	T37.8X3	T37.8X4	T37.8X5	T37.8X6
Piroxicam	T39.391	T39.392	T39.393	T39.394	T39.395	T39.396
beta-cyclodextrin complex	T39.8X1	T39.8X2	T39.8X3	T39.8X4	T39.8X5	T39.8X6
Pirozadil	T46.6X1	T46.6X2	T46.6X3	T46.6X4	T46.6X5	T46.6X6
Piscidia (bark) (erythrina)	T39.8X1	T39.8X2	T39.8X3	T39.8X4	T39.8X5	T39.8X6
Pitch	T65.891	T65.892	T65.893	T65.894	—	—
Pitkin's solution	T41.3X1	T41.3X2	T41.3X3	T41.3X4	T41.3X5	T41.3X6
Pitocin	T48.0X1	T48.0X2	T48.0X3	T48.0X4	T48.0X5	T48.0X6
Pitressin (tannate)	T38.891	T38.892	T38.893	T38.894	T38.895	T38.896
Pituitary extracts (posterior)	T38.891	T38.892	T38.893	T38.894	T38.895	T38.896
anterior	T38.811	T38.812	T38.813	T38.814	T38.815	T38.816
Pituitrin	T38.891	T38.892	T38.893	T38.894	T38.895	T38.896
Pivampicillin	T36.0X1	T36.0X2	T36.0X3	T36.0X4	T36.0X5	T36.0X6
Pivmecillinam	T36.0X1	T36.0X2	T36.0X3	T36.0X4	T36.0X5	T36.0X6
Placental hormone	T38.891	T38.892	T38.893	T38.894	T38.895	T38.896
Placidyl	T42.6X1	T42.6X2	T42.6X3	T42.6X4	T42.6X5	T42.6X6
Plague vaccine	T50.A91	T50.A92	T50.A93	T50.A94	T50.A95	T50.A96

◀ New ◀◀◀ Revised ~~deleted~~ Deleted

Substance	External Cause (T-Code)					
	Poisoning, Accidental (Unintentional)	Poisoning, Intentional Self-Harm	Poisoning, Assault	Poisoning, Undetermined	Adverse Effect	Underdosing
Plant						
food or fertilizer NEC	T65.891	T65.892	T65.893	T65.894	—	—
containing herbicide	T60.3X1	T60.3X2	T60.3X3	T60.3X4	—	—
noxious, used as food	T62.2X1	T62.2X2	T62.2X3	T62.2X4	—	—
berries	T62.1X1	T62.1X2	T62.1X3	T62.1X4	—	—
seeds	T62.2X1	T62.2X2	T62.2X3	T62.2X4	—	—
specified type NEC	T62.2X1	T62.2X2	T62.2X3	T62.2X4	—	—
Plasma	T45.8X1	T45.8X2	T45.8X3	T45.8X4	T45.8X5	T45.8X6
expander NEC	T45.8X1	T45.8X2	T45.8X3	T45.8X4	T45.8X5	T45.8X6
protein fraction (human)	T45.8X1	T45.8X2	T45.8X3	T45.8X4	T45.8X5	T45.8X6
Plasmanate	T45.8X1	T45.8X2	T45.8X3	T45.8X4	T45.8X5	T45.8X6
Plasminogen (tissue) activator	T45.611	T45.612	T45.613	T45.614	T45.615	T45.616
Plaster dressing	T49.3X1	T49.3X2	T49.3X3	T49.3X4	T49.3X5	T49.3X6
Plastic dressing	T49.3X1	T49.3X2	T49.3X3	T49.3X4	T49.3X5	T49.3X6
Plegicil	T43.3X1	T43.3X2	T43.3X3	T43.3X4	T43.3X5	T43.3X6
Plicamycin	T45.1X1	T45.1X2	T45.1X3	T45.1X4	T45.1X5	T45.1X6
Podophyllotoxin	T49.8X1	T49.8X2	T49.8X3	T49.8X4	T49.8X5	T49.8X6
Podophyllum (resin)	T49.4X1	T49.4X2	T49.4X3	T49.4X4	T49.4X5	T49.4X6
Poison NEC	T65.91	T65.92	T65.93	T65.94	—	—
Poisonous berries	T62.1X1	T62.1X2	T62.1X3	T62.1X4	—	—
Pokeweed (any part)	T62.2X1	T62.2X2	T62.2X3	T62.2X4	—	—
Poldine metilsulfate	T44.3X1	T44.3X2	T44.3X3	T44.3X4	T44.3X5	T44.3X6
Polidexide (sulfate)	T46.6X1	T46.6X2	T46.6X3	T46.6X4	T46.6X5	T46.6X6
Polidocanol	T46.8X1	T46.8X2	T46.8X3	T46.8X4	T46.8X5	T46.8X6
Poliomyelitis vaccine	T50.B91	T50.B92	T50.B93	T50.B94	T50.B95	T50.B96
Polish (car) (floor) (furniture) (metal) (porcelain) (silver)	T65.891	T65.892	T65.893	T65.894	—	—
abrasive	T65.891	T65.892	T65.893	T65.894	—	—
porcelain	T65.891	T65.892	T65.893	T65.894	—	—
Poloxalkol	T47.4X1	T47.4X2	T47.4X3	T47.4X4	T47.4X5	T47.4X6
Poloxamer	T47.4X1	T47.4X2	T47.4X3	T47.4X4	T47.4X5	T47.4X6
Polyaminostyrene resins	T50.3X1	T50.3X2	T50.3X3	T50.3X4	T50.3X5	T50.3X6
Polycarbophil	T47.4X1	T47.4X2	T47.4X3	T47.4X4	T47.4X5	T47.4X6
Polychlorinated biphenyl	T65.891	T65.892	T65.893	T65.894	—	—
Polycycline	T36.4X1	T36.4X2	T36.4X3	T36.4X4	T36.4X5	T36.4X6
Polyester fumes	T59.891	T59.892	T59.893	T59.894	—	—
Polyester resin hardener	T52.91	T52.92	T52.93	T52.94	—	—
fumes	T59.891	T59.892	T59.893	T59.894	—	—
Polyestradiol phosphate	T38.5X1	T38.5X2	T38.5X3	T38.5X4	T38.5X5	T38.5X6
Polyethanolamine alkyl sulfate	T49.2X1	T49.2X2	T49.2X3	T49.2X4	T49.2X5	T49.2X6

◀ New   ◀▌▌ Revised   ~~deleted~~ Deleted

Substance	External Cause (T-Code)					
	Poisoning, Accidental (Unintentional)	Poisoning, Intentional Self-Harm	Poisoning, Assault	Poisoning, Undetermined	Adverse Effect	Underdosing
Polyethylene adhesive	T49.3X1	T49.3X2	T49.3X3	T49.3X4	T49.3X5	T49.3X6
Polyferose	T45.4X1	T45.4X2	T45.4X3	T45.4X4	T45.4X5	T45.4X6
Polygeline	T45.8X1	T45.8X2	T45.8X3	T45.8X4	T45.8X5	T45.8X6
Polymyxin	T36.8X1	T36.8X2	T36.8X3	T36.8X4	T36.8X5	T36.8X6
B	T36.8X1	T36.8X2	T36.8X3	T36.8X4	T36.8X5	T36.8X6
ENT agent	T49.6X1	T49.6X2	T49.6X3	T49.6X4	T49.6X5	T49.6X6
ophthalmic preparation	T49.5X1	T49.5X2	T49.5X3	T49.5X4	T49.5X5	T49.5X6
topical NEC	T49.0X1	T49.0X2	T49.0X3	T49.0X4	T49.0X5	T49.0X6
E sulfate (eye preparation)	T49.5X1	T49.5X2	T49.5X3	T49.5X4	T49.5X5	T49.5X6
Polynoxylin	T49.0X1	T49.0X2	T49.0X3	T49.0X4	T49.0X5	T49.0X6
Polyoestradiol phosphate	T38.5X1	T38.5X2	T38.5X3	T38.5X4	T38.5X5	T38.5X6
Polyoxymethyleneurea	T49.0X1	T49.0X2	T49.0X3	T49.0X4	T49.0X5	T49.0X6
Polysilane	T47.8X1	T47.8X2	T47.8X3	T47.8X4	T47.8X5	T47.8X6
Polytetrafluoroethylene (inhaled)	T59.891	T59.892	T59.893	T59.894	—	—
Polythiazide	T50.2X1	T50.2X2	T50.2X3	T50.2X4	T50.2X5	T50.2X6
Polyvidone	T45.8X1	T45.8X2	T45.8X3	T45.8X4	T45.8X5	T45.8X6
Polyvinylpyrrolidone	T45.8X1	T45.8X2	T45.8X3	T45.8X4	T45.8X5	T45.8X6
Pontocaine (hydrochloride) (infiltration) (topical)	T41.3X1	T41.3X2	T41.3X3	T41.3X4	T41.3X5	T41.3X6
nerve block (peripheral) (plexus)	T41.3X1	T41.3X2	T41.3X3	T41.3X4	T41.3X5	T41.3X6
spinal	T41.3X1	T41.3X2	T41.3X3	T41.3X4	T41.3X5	T41.3X6
Porfiromycin	T45.1X1	T45.1X2	T45.1X3	T45.1X4	T45.1X5	T45.1X6
Posterior pituitary hormone NEC	T38.891	T38.892	T38.893	T38.894	T38.895	T38.896
Pot	T40.7X1	T40.7X2	T40.7X3	T40.7X4	T40.7X5	T40.7X6
Potash (caustic)	T54.3X1	T54.3X2	T54.3X3	T54.3X4	—	—
Potassic saline injection (lactated)	T50.3X1	T50.3X2	T50.3X3	T50.3X4	T50.3X5	T50.3X6
Potassium (salts) NEC	T50.3X1	T50.3X2	T50.3X3	T50.3X4	T50.3X5	T50.3X6
aminobenzoate	T45.8X1	T45.8X2	T45.8X3	T45.8X4	T45.8X5	T45.8X6
aminosalicylate	T37.1X1	T37.1X2	T37.1X3	T37.1X4	T37.1X5	T37.1X6
antimony 'tartrate'	T37.8X1	T37.8X2	T37.8X3	T37.8X4	T37.8X5	T37.8X6
arsenite (solution)	T57.0X1	T57.0X2	T57.0X3	T57.0X4	—	—
bichromate	T56.2X1	T56.2X2	T56.2X3	T56.2X4	—	—
bisulfate	T47.3X1	T47.3X2	T47.3X3	T47.3X4	T47.3X5	T47.3X6
bromide	T42.6X1	T42.6X2	T42.6X3	T42.6X4	T42.6X5	T42.6X6
canrenoate	T50.0X1	T50.0X2	T50.0X3	T50.0X4	T50.0X5	T50.0X6
carbonate	T54.3X1	T54.3X2	T54.3X3	T54.3X4	—	—
chlorate NEC	T65.891	T65.892	T65.893	T65.894	—	—
chloride	T50.3X1	T50.3X2	T50.3X3	T50.3X4	T50.3X5	T50.3X6
citrate	T50.991	T50.992	T50.993	T50.994	T50.995	T50.996
cyanide	T65.0X1	T65.0X2	T65.0X3	T65.0X4	—	—

◀ New ⬅ Revised ~~deleted~~ Deleted

Substance	Poisoning, Accidental (Unintentional)	Poisoning, Intentional Self-Harm	Poisoning, Assault	Poisoning, Undetermined	Adverse Effect	Underdosing
Potassium NEC *(Continued)*						
ferric hexacyanoferrate (medicinal)	T50.6X1	T50.6X2	T50.6X3	T50.6X4	T50.6X5	T50.6X6
nonmedicinal	T65.891	T65.892	T65.893	T65.894	—	—
Fluoride	T57.8X1	T57.8X2	T57.8X3	T57.8X4	—	—
glucaldrate	T47.1X1	T47.1X2	T47.1X3	T47.1X4	T47.1X5	T47.1X6
hydroxide	T54.3X1	T54.3X2	T54.3X3	T54.3X4	—	—
iodate	T49.0X1	T49.0X2	T49.0X3	T49.0X4	T49.0X5	T49.0X6
iodide	T48.4X1	T48.4X2	T48.4X3	T48.4X4	T48.4X5	T48.4X6
nitrate	T57.8X1	T57.8X2	T57.8X3	T57.8X4	—	—
oxalate	T65.891	T65.892	T65.893	T65.894	—	—
perchlorate (nonmedicinal) NEC	T65.891	T65.892	T65.893	T65.894	—	—
antithyroid	T38.2X1	T38.2X2	T38.2X3	T38.2X4	T38.2X5	T38.2X6
medicinal	T38.2X1	T38.2X2	T38.2X3	T38.2X4	T38.2X5	T38.2X6
Permanganate (nonmedicinal)	T65.891	T65.892	T65.893	T65.894	—	—
medicinal	T49.0X1	T49.0X2	T49.0X3	T49.0X4	T49.0X5	T49.0X6
sulfate	T47.2X1	T47.2X2	T47.2X3	T47.2X4	T47.2X5	T47.2X6
Potassium-removing resin	T50.3X1	T50.3X2	T50.3X3	T50.3X4	T50.3X5	T50.3X6
Potassium-retaining drug	T50.3X1	T50.3X2	T50.3X3	T50.3X4	T50.3X5	T50.3X6
Povidone	T45.8X1	T45.8X2	T45.8X3	T45.8X4	T45.8X5	T45.8X6
iodine	T49.0X1	T49.0X2	T49.0X3	T49.0X4	T49.0X5	T49.0X6
Practolol	T44.7X1	T44.7X2	T44.7X3	T44.7X4	T44.7X5	T44.7X6
Prajmalium bitartrate	T46.2X1	T46.2X2	T46.2X3	T46.2X4	T46.2X5	T46.2X6
Pralidoxime (iodide)	T50.6X1	T50.6X2	T50.6X3	T50.6X4	T50.6X5	T50.6X6
chloride	T50.6X1	T50.6X2	T50.6X3	T50.6X4	T50.6X5	T50.6X6
Pramiverine	T44.3X1	T44.3X2	T44.3X3	T44.3X4	T44.3X5	T44.3X6
Pramocaine	T49.1X1	T49.1X2	T49.1X3	T49.1X4	T49.1X5	T49.1X6
Pramoxine	T49.1X1	T49.1X2	T49.1X3	T49.1X4	T49.1X5	T49.1X6
Prasterone	T38.7X1	T38.7X2	T38.7X3	T38.7X4	T38.7X5	T38.7X6
Pravastatin	T46.6X1	T46.6X2	T46.6X3	T46.6X4	T46.6X5	T46.6X6
Prazepam	T42.4X1	T42.4X2	T42.4X3	T42.4X4	T42.4X5	T42.4X6
Praziquantel	T37.4X1	T37.4X2	T37.4X3	T37.4X4	T37.4X5	T37.4X6
Prazitone	T43.291	T43.292	T43.293	T43.294	T43.295	T43.296
Prazosin	T44.6X1	T44.6X2	T44.6X3	T44.6X4	T44.6X5	T44.6X6
Prednicarbate	T49.0X1	T49.0X2	T49.0X3	T49.0X4	T49.0X5	T49.0X6
Prednimustine	T45.1X1	T45.1X2	T45.1X3	T45.1X4	T45.1X5	T45.1X6
Prednisolone	T38.0X1	T38.0X2	T38.0X3	T38.0X4	T38.0X5	T38.0X6
ENT agent	T49.6X1	T49.6X2	T49.6X3	T49.6X4	T49.6X5	T49.6X6
ophthalmic preparation	T49.5X1	T49.5X2	T49.5X3	T49.5X4	T49.5X5	T49.5X6
steaglate	T49.0X1	T49.0X2	T49.0X3	T49.0X4	T49.0X5	T49.0X6
topical NEC	T49.0X1	T49.0X2	T49.0X3	T49.0X4	T49.0X5	T49.0X6

External Cause (T-Code)

TABLE OF DRUGS AND CHEMICALS

◀ New ◀▦ Revised ~~deleted~~ Deleted

TABLE OF DRUGS AND CHEMICALS

Substance	External Cause (T-Code)					
	Poisoning, Accidental (Unintentional)	Poisoning, Intentional Self-Harm	Poisoning, Assault	Poisoning, Undetermined	Adverse Effect	Underdosing
Prednisone	T38.0X1	T38.0X2	T38.0X3	T38.0X4	T38.0X5	T38.0X6
Prednylidene	T38.0X1	T38.0X2	T38.0X3	T38.0X4	T38.0X5	T38.0X6
Pregnandiol	T38.5X1	T38.5X2	T38.5X3	T38.5X4	T38.5X5	T38.5X6
Pregneninolone	T38.5X1	T38.5X2	T38.5X3	T38.5X4	T38.5X5	T38.5X6
Preludin	T43.691	T43.692	T43.693	T43.694	T43.695	T43.696
Premarin	T38.5X1	T38.5X2	T38.5X3	T38.5X4	T38.5X5	T38.5X6
Premedication anesthetic	T41.201	T41.202	T41.203	T41.204	T41.205	T41.206
Prenalterol	T44.5X1	T44.5X2	T44.5X3	T44.5X4	T44.5X5	T44.5X6
Prenoxdiazine	T48.3X1	T48.3X2	T48.3X3	T48.3X4	T48.3X5	T48.3X6
Prenylamine	T46.3X1	T46.3X2	T46.3X3	T46.3X4	T46.3X5	T46.3X6
Preparation, local	T49.4X1	T49.4X2	T49.4X3	T49.4X4	T49.4X5	T49.4X6
Preparation H	T49.8X1	T49.8X2	T49.8X3	T49.8X4	T49.8X5	T49.8X6
Preservative (nonmedicinal)	T65.891	T65.892	T65.893	T65.894	—	—
medicinal	T50.901	T50.902	T50.903	T50.904	T50.905	T50.906
wood	T60.91	T60.92	T60.93	T60.94	—	—
Prethcamide	T50.7X1	T50.7X2	T50.7X3	T50.7X4	T50.7X5	T50.7X6
Pride of China	T62.2X1	T62.2X2	T62.2X3	T62.2X4	—	—
Pridinol	T44.3X1	T44.3X2	T44.3X3	T44.3X4	T44.3X5	T44.3X6
Prifinium bromide	T44.3X1	T44.3X2	T44.3X3	T44.3X4	T44.3X5	T44.3X6
Prilocaine	T41.3X1	T41.3X2	T41.3X3	T41.3X4	T41.3X5	T41.3X6
infiltration (subcutaneous)	T41.3X1	T41.3X2	T41.3X3	T41.3X4	T41.3X5	T41.3X6
nerve block (peripheral) (plexus)	T41.3X1	T41.3X2	T41.3X3	T41.3X4	T41.3X5	T41.3X6
regional	T41.3X1	T41.3X2	T41.3X3	T41.3X4	T41.3X5	T41.3X6
Primaquine	T37.2X1	T37.2X2	T37.2X3	T37.2X4	T37.2X5	T37.2X6
Primidone	T42.6X1	T42.6X2	T42.6X3	T42.6X4	T42.6X5	T42.6X6
Primula (veris)	T62.2X1	T62.2X2	T62.2X3	T62.2X4	—	—
Prinadol	T40.2X1	T40.2X2	T40.2X3	T40.2X4	T40.2X5	T40.2X6
Priscol, Priscoline	T44.6X1	T44.6X2	T44.6X3	T44.6X4	T44.6X5	T44.6X6
Pristinamycin	T36.3X1	T36.3X2	T36.3X3	T36.3X4	T36.3X5	T36.3X6
Privet	T62.2X1	T62.2X2	T62.2X3	T62.2X4	—	—
berries	T62.1X1	T62.1X2	T62.1X3	T62.1X4	—	—
Privine	T44.4X1	T44.4X2	T44.4X3	T44.4X4	T44.4X5	T44.4X6
Pro-Banthine	T44.3X1	T44.3X2	T44.3X3	T44.3X4	T44.3X5	T44.3X6
Probarbital	T42.3X1	T42.3X2	T42.3X3	T42.3X4	T42.3X5	T42.3X6
Probenecid	T50.4X1	T50.4X2	T50.4X3	T50.4X4	T50.4X5	T50.4X6
Probucol	T46.6X1	T46.6X2	T46.6X3	T46.6X4	T46.6X5	T46.6X6
Procainamide	T46.2X1	T46.2X2	T46.2X3	T46.2X4	T46.2X5	T46.2X6
Procaine	T41.3X1	T41.3X2	T41.3X3	T41.3X4	T41.3X5	T41.3X6
benzylpenicillin	T36.0X1	T36.0X2	T36.0X3	T36.0X4	T36.0X5	T36.0X6
nerve block (periphreal) (plexus)	T41.3X1	T41.3X2	T41.3X3	T41.3X4	T41.3X5	T41.3X6

◀ New   ◀||| Revised   ~~deleted~~ Deleted

Substance	Poisoning, Accidental (Unintentional)	Poisoning, Intentional Self-Harm	Poisoning, Assault	Poisoning, Undetermined	Adverse Effect	Underdosing
Procaine *(Continued)*						
penicillin G	T36.0X1	T36.0X2	T36.0X3	T36.0X4	T36.0X5	T36.0X6
regional	T41.3X1	T41.3X2	T41.3X3	T41.3X4	T41.3X5	T41.3X6
spinal	T41.3X1	T41.3X2	T41.3X3	T41.3X4	T41.3X5	T41.3X6
Procalmidol	T43.591	T43.592	T43.593	T43.594	T43.595	T43.596
Procarbazine	T45.1X1	T45.1X2	T45.1X3	T45.1X4	T45.1X5	T45.1X6
Procaterol	T44.5X1	T44.5X2	T44.5X3	T44.5X4	T44.5X5	T44.5X6
Prochlorperazine	T43.3X1	T43.3X2	T43.3X3	T43.3X4	T43.3X5	T43.3X6
Procyclidine	T44.3X1	T44.3X2	T44.3X3	T44.3X4	T44.3X5	T44.3X6
Producer gas	T58.8X1	T58.8X2	T58.8X3	T58.8X4	—	—
Profadol	T40.4X1	T40.4X2	T40.4X3	T40.4X4	T40.4X5	T40.4X6
Profenamine	T44.3X1	T44.3X2	T44.3X3	T44.3X4	T44.3X5	T44.3X6
Profenil	T44.3X1	T44.3X2	T44.3X3	T44.3X4	T44.3X5	T44.3X6
Proflavine	T49.0X1	T49.0X2	T49.0X3	T49.0X4	T49.0X5	T49.0X6
Progabide	T42.6X1	T42.6X2	T42.6X3	T42.6X4	T42.6X5	T42.6X6
Progestin	T38.5X1	T38.5X2	T38.5X3	T38.5X4	T38.5X5	T38.5X6
oral contraceptive	T38.4X1	T38.4X2	T38.4X3	T38.4X4	T38.4X5	T38.4X6
Progesterone	T38.5X1	T38.5X2	T38.5X3	T38.5X4	T38.5X5	T38.5X6
Progestogen NEC	T38.5X1	T38.5X2	T38.5X3	T38.5X4	T38.5X5	T38.5X6
Progestone	T38.5X1	T38.5X2	T38.5X3	T38.5X4	T38.5X5	T38.5X6
Proglumide	T47.1X1	T47.1X2	T47.1X3	T47.1X4	T47.1X5	T47.1X6
Proguanil	T37.2X1	T37.2X2	T37.2X3	T37.2X4	T37.2X5	T37.2X6
Prolactin	T38.811	T38.812	T38.813	T38.814	T38.815	T38.816
Prolintane	T43.691	T43.692	T43.693	T43.694	T43.695	T43.696
Proloid	T38.1X1	T38.1X2	T38.1X3	T38.1X4	T38.1X5	T38.1X6
Proluton	T38.5X1	T38.5X2	T38.5X3	T38.5X4	T38.5X5	T38.5X6
Promacetin	T37.1X1	T37.1X2	T37.1X3	T37.1X4	T37.1X5	T37.1X6
Promazine	T43.3X1	T43.3X2	T43.3X3	T43.3X4	T43.3X5	T43.3X6
Promedol	T40.2X1	T40.2X2	T40.2X3	T40.2X4	—	—
Promegestone	T38.5X1	T38.5X2	T38.5X3	T38.5X4	T38.5X5	T38.5X6
Promethazine (teoclate)	T43.3X1	T43.3X2	T43.3X3	T43.3X4	T43.3X5	T43.3X6
Promin	T37.1X1	T37.1X2	T37.1X3	T37.1X4	T37.1X5	T37.1X6
Pronase	T45.3X1	T45.3X2	T45.3X3	T45.3X4	T45.3X5	T45.3X6
Pronestyl (hydrochloride)	T46.2X1	T46.2X2	T46.2X3	T46.2X4	T46.2X5	T46.2X6
Pronetalol	T44.7X1	T44.7X2	T44.7X3	T44.7X4	T44.7X5	T44.7X6
Prontosil	T37.0X1	T37.0X2	T37.0X3	T37.0X4	T37.0X5	T37.0X6
Propachlor	T60.3X1	T60.3X2	T60.3X3	T60.3X4	—	—
Propafenone	T46.2X1	T46.2X2	T46.2X3	T46.2X4	T46.2X5	T46.2X6
Propallylonal	T42.3X1	T42.3X2	T42.3X3	T42.3X4	T42.3X5	T42.3X6
Propamidine	T49.0X1	T49.0X2	T49.0X3	T49.0X4	T49.0X5	T49.0X6

Substance	External Cause (T-Code)					
	Poisoning, Accidental (Unintentional)	Poisoning, Intentional Self-Harm	Poisoning, Assault	Poisoning, Undetermined	Adverse Effect	Underdosing
Propane (distributed in mobile container)	T59.891	T59.892	T59.893	T59.894	—	—
distributed through pipes	T59.891	T59.892	T59.893	T59.894	—	—
incomplete combustion	T57.11	T57.12	T57.13	T57.14	—	—
Propanidid	T41.291	T41.292	T41.293	T41.294	T41.295	T41.296
Propanil	T60.3X1	T60.3X2	T60.3X3	T60.3X4	—	—
1-Propanol	T51.3X1	T51.3X2	T51.3X3	T51.3X4	—	—
2-Propanol	T51.2X1	T51.2X2	T51.2X3	T51.2X4	—	—
Propantheline	T44.3X1	T44.3X2	T44.3X3	T44.3X4	T44.3X5	T44.3X6
bromide	T44.3X1	T44.3X2	T44.3X3	T44.3X4	T44.3X5	T44.3X6
Proparacaine	T41.3X1	T41.3X2	T41.3X3	T41.3X4	T41.3X5	T41.3X6
Propatylnitrate	T46.3X1	T46.3X2	T46.3X3	T46.3X4	T46.3X5	T46.3X6
Propicillin	T36.0X1	T36.0X2	T36.0X3	T36.0X4	T36.0X5	T36.0X6
Propiolactone	T49.0X1	T49.0X2	T49.0X3	T49.0X4	T49.0X5	T49.0X6
Propiomazine	T45.0X1	T45.0X2	T45.0X3	T45.0X4	T45.0X5	T45.0X6
Propionaidehyde (medicinal)	T42.6X1	T42.6X2	T42.6X3	T42.6X4	T42.6X5	T42.6X6
Propionate (calcium) (sodium)	T49.0X1	T49.0X2	T49.0X3	T49.0X4	T49.0X5	T49.0X6
Propion gel	T49.0X1	T49.0X2	T49.0X3	T49.0X4	T49.0X5	T49.0X6
Propitocaine	T41.3X1	T41.3X2	T41.3X3	T41.3X4	T41.3X5	T41.3X6
infiltration (subcutaneous)	T41.3X1	T41.3X2	T41.3X3	T41.3X4	T41.3X5	T41.3X6
nerve block (peripheral) (plexus)	T41.3X1	T41.3X2	T41.3X3	T41.3X4	T41.3X5	T41.3X6
Propofol	T41.291	T41.292	T41.293	T41.294	T41.295	T41.296
Propoxur	T60.0X1	T60.0X2	T60.0X3	T60.0X4	—	—
Propoxycaine	T41.3X1	T41.3X2	T41.3X3	T41.3X4	T41.3X5	T41.3X6
infiltration (subcutaneous)	T41.3X1	T41.3X2	T41.3X3	T41.3X4	T41.3X5	T41.3X6
nerve block (peripheral) (plexus)	T41.3X1	T41.3X2	T41.3X3	T41.3X4	T41.3X5	T41.3X6
topical (surface)	T41.3X1	T41.3X2	T41.3X3	T41.3X4	T41.3X5	T41.3X6
Propoxyphene	T40.4X1	T40.4X2	T40.4X3	T40.4X4	T40.4X5	T40.4X6
Propranolol	T44.7X1	T44.7X2	T44.7X3	T44.7X4	T44.7X5	T44.7X6
Propyl						
alcohol	T51.3X1	T51.3X2	T51.3X3	T51.3X4		
carbinol	T51.3X1	T51.3X2	T51.3X3	T51.3X4	—	—
hexadrine	T44.4X1	T44.4X2	T44.4X3	T44.4X4	T44.4X5	T44.4X6
iodone	T50.8X1	T50.8X2	T50.8X3	T50.8X4	T50.8X5	T50.8X6
thiouracil	T38.2X1	T38.2X2	T38.2X3	T38.2X4	T38.2X5	T38.2X6
Propylaminophenothiazine	T43.3X1	T43.3X2	T43.3X3	T43.3X4	T43.3X5	T43.3X6
Propylene	T59.891	T59.892	T59.893	T59.894	—	—
Propylhexedrine	T48.5X1	T48.5X2	T48.5X3	T48.5X4	T48.5X5	T48.5X6
Propyliodone	T50.8X1	T50.8X2	T50.8X3	T50.8X4	T50.8X5	T50.8X6
Propylthiouracil	T38.2X1	T38.2X2	T38.2X3	T38.2X4	T38.2X5	T38.2X6
Propylparaben (ophthalmic)	T49.5X1	T49.5X2	T49.5X3	T49.5X4	T49.5X5	T49.5X6

◀ New ◀═ Revised ~~deleted~~ Deleted

Substance	External Cause (T-Code)					
	Poisoning, Accidental (Unintentional)	Poisoning, Intentional Self-Harm	Poisoning, Assault	Poisoning, Undetermined	Adverse Effect	Underdosing
Propyphenazone	T39.2X1	T39.2X2	T39.2X3	T39.2X4	T39.2X5	T39.2X6
Proquazone	T39.391	T39.392	T39.393	T39.394	T39.395	T39.396
Proscillaridin	T46.0X1	T46.0X2	T46.0X3	T46.0X4	T46.0X5	T46.0X6
Prostacyclin	T45.521	T45.522	T45.523	T45.524	T45.525	T45.526
Prostaglandin (I2)	T45.521	T45.522	T45.523	T45.524	T45.525	T45.526
E1	T46.7X1	T46.7X2	T46.7X3	T46.7X4	T46.7X5	T46.7X6
E2	T48.0X1	T48.0X2	T48.0X3	T48.0X4	T48.0X5	T48.0X6
F2 alpha	T48.0X1	T48.0X2	T48.0X3	T48.0X4	T48.0X5	T48.0X6
Prostigmin	T44.0X1	T44.0X2	T44.0X3	T44.0X4	T44.0X5	T44.0X6
Prosultiamine	T45.2X1	T45.2X2	T45.2X3	T45.2X4	T45.2X5	T45.2X6
Protamine sulfate	T45.7X1	T45.7X2	T45.7X3	T45.7X4	T45.7X5	T45.7X6
zinc insulin	T38.3X1	T38.3X2	T38.3X3	T38.3X4	T38.3X5	T38.3X6
Protease	T47.5X1	T47.5X2	T47.5X3	T47.5X4	T47.5X5	T47.5X6
Protectant, skin NEC	T49.3X1	T49.3X2	T49.3X3	T49.3X4	T49.3X5	T49.3X6
Protein hydrolysate	T50.991	T50.992	T50.993	T50.994	T50.995	T50.996
Prothiaden — see Dothiepin hydrochloride						
Prothionamide	T37.1X1	T37.1X2	T37.1X3	T37.1X4	T37.1X5	T37.1X6
Prothipendyl	T43.591	T43.592	T43.593	T43.594	T43.595	T43.596
Prothoate	T60.0X1	T60.0X2	T60.0X3	T60.0X4	—	—
Prothrombin						
activator	T45.7X1	T45.7X2	T45.7X3	T45.7X4	T45.7X5	T45.7X6
synthesis inhibitor	T45.511	T45.512	T45.513	T45.514	T45.515	T45.516
Protionamide	T37.1X1	T37.1X2	T37.1X3	T37.1X4	T37.1X5	T37.1X6
Protirelin	T38.891	T38.892	T38.893	T38.894	T38.895	T38.896
Protokylol	T48.6X1	T48.6X2	T48.6X3	T48.6X4	T48.6X5	T48.6X6
Protopam	T50.6X1	T50.6X2	T50.6X3	T50.6X4	T50.6X5	T50.6X6
Protoveratrine(s) (A) (B)	T46.5X1	T46.5X2	T46.5X3	T46.5X4	T46.5X5	T46.5X6
Protriptyline	T43.011	T43.012	T43.013	T43.014	T43.015	T43.016
Provera	T38.5X1	T38.5X2	T38.5X3	T38.5X4	T38.5X5	T38.5X6
Provitamin A	T45.2X1	T45.2X2	T45.2X3	T45.2X4	T45.2X5	T45.2X6
Proxibarbal	T42.3X1	T42.3X2	T42.3X3	T42.3X4	T42.3X5	T42.3X6
Proxymetacaine	T41.3X1	T41.3X2	T41.3X3	T41.3X4	T41.3X5	T41.3X6
Proxyphylline	T48.6X1	T48.6X2	T48.6X3	T48.6X4	T48.6X5	T48.6X6
Prozac — see Fluoxetine hydrochloride						
Prunus						
laurocerasus	T62.2X1	T62.2X2	T62.2X3	T62.2X4	—	—
virginiana	T62.2X1	T62.2X2	T62.2X3	T62.2X4	—	—
Prussian blue						
commercial	T65.891	T65.892	T65.893	T65.894	—	—
therapeutic	T50.6X1	T50.6X2	T50.6X3	T50.6X4	T50.6X5	T50.6X6

TABLE OF DRUGS AND CHEMICALS

◄ New ◄▭ Revised ~~deleted~~ Deleted

Substance	External Cause (T-Code)					
	Poisoning, Accidental (Unintentional)	Poisoning, Intentional Self-Harm	Poisoning, Assault	Poisoning, Undetermined	Adverse Effect	Underdosing
Prussic acid	T65.0X1	T65.0X2	T65.0X3	T65.0X4	—	—
vapor	T57.3X1	T57.3X2	T57.3X3	T57.3X4	—	—
Pseudoephedrine	T44.991	T44.992	T44.993	T44.994	T44.995	T44.996
Psilocin	T40.991	T40.992	T40.993	T40.994	—	—
Psilocybin	T40.991	T40.992	T40.993	T40.994	—	—
Psilocybine	T40.991	T40.992	T40.993	T40.994	—	—
Psoralene (nonmedicinal)	T65.891	T65.892	T65.893	T65.894	—	—
Psoralens (medicinal)	T50.991	T50.992	T50.993	T50.994	T50.995	T50.996
PSP (phenolsulfonphthalein)	T50.8X1	T50.8X2	T50.8X3	T50.8X4	T50.8X5	T50.8X6
Psychodysleptic drug NEC	T40.901	T40.902	T40.903	T40.904	T40.905	T40.906
Psychostimulant	T43.601	T43.602	T43.603	T43.604	T43.605	T43.606
amphetamine	T43.621	T43.622	T43.623	T43.624	T43.625	T43.626
caffeine	T43.611	T43.612	T43.613	T43.614	T43.615	T43.616
methylphenidate	T43.631	T43.632	T43.633	T43.634	T43.635	T43.636
specified NEC	T43.691	T43.692	T43.693	T43.694	T43.695	T43.696
Psychotherapeutic drug NEC	T43.91	T43.92	T43.93	T43.94	T43.95	T43.96
antidepressants — see also Antidepressant	T43.201	T43.202	T43.203	T43.204	T43.205	T43.206
specified NEC	T43.8X1	T43.8X2	T43.8X3	T43.8X4	T43.8X5	T43.8X6
tranquilizers NEC	T43.501	T43.502	T43.503	T43.504	T43.505	T43.506
Psychotomimetic agents	T40.901	T40.902	T40.903	T40.904	T40.905	T40.906
Psychotropic drug NEC	T43.91	T43.92	T43.93	T43.94	T43.95	T43.96
specified NEC	T43.8X1	T43.8X2	T43.8X3	T43.8X4	T43.8X5	T43.8X6
Psyllium hydrophilic mucilloid	T47.4X1	T47.4X2	T47.4X3	T47.4X4	T47.4X5	T47.4X6
Pteroylglutamic acid	T45.8X1	T45.8X2	T45.8X3	T45.8X4	T45.8X5	T45.8X6
Pteroyltriglutamate	T45.1X1	T45.1X2	T45.1X3	T45.1X4	T45.1X5	T45.1X6
PTFE — see Polytetrafluoroethylene						
Pulp						
devitalizing paste	T49.7X1	T49.7X2	T49.7X3	T49.7X4	T49.7X5	T49.7X6
dressing	T49.7X1	T49.7X2	T49.7X3	T49.7X4	T49.7X5	T49.7X6
Pulsatilla	T62.2X1	T62.2X2	T62.2X3	T62.2X4	—	—
Pumpkin seed extract	T37.4X1	T37.4X2	T37.4X3	T37.4X4	T37.4X5	T37.4X6
Purex (bleach)	T54.91	T54.92	T54.93	T54.94	—	—
Purgative NEC — see also Cathartic	T47.4X1	T47.4X2	T47.4X3	T47.4X4	T47.4X5	T47.4X6
Purine analogue (antineoplastic)	T45.1X1	T45.1X2	T45.1X3	T45.1X4	T45.1X5	T45.1X6
Purine diuretics	T50.2X1	T50.2X2	T50.2X3	T50.2X4	T50.2X5	T50.2X6
Purinethol	T45.1X1	T45.1X2	T45.1X3	T45.1X4	T45.1X5	T45.1X6
PVP	T45.8X1	T45.8X2	T45.8X3	T45.8X4	T45.8X5	T45.8X6
Pyrabital	T39.8X1	T39.8X2	T39.8X3	T39.8X4	T39.8X5	T39.8X6
Pyramidon	T39.2X1	T39.2X2	T39.2X3	T39.2X4	T39.2X5	T39.2X6
Pyrantel	T37.4X1	T37.4X2	T37.4X3	T37.4X4	T37.4X5	T37.4X6

◀ New   ◀▥ Revised   ~~deleted~~ Deleted

Substance	External Cause (T-Code)					
	Poisoning, Accidental (Unintentional)	Poisoning, Intentional Self-Harm	Poisoning, Assault	Poisoning, Undetermined	Adverse Effect	Underdosing
Pyrathiazine	T45.0X1	T45.0X2	T45.0X3	T45.0X4	T45.0X5	T45.0X6
Pyrazinamide	T37.1X1	T37.1X2	T37.1X3	T37.1X4	T37.1X5	T37.1X6
Pyrazinoic acid (amide)	T37.1X1	T37.1X2	T37.1X3	T37.1X4	T37.1X5	T37.1X6
Pyrazole (derivatives)	T39.2X1	T39.2X2	T39.2X3	T39.2X4	T39.2X5	T39.2X6
Pyrazolone analgesic NEC	T39.2X1	T39.2X2	T39.2X3	T39.2X4	T39.2X5	T39.2X6
Pyrethrin, pyrethrum (nonmedicinal)	T60.2X1	T60.2X2	T60.2X3	T60.2X4	—	—
Pyrethrum extract	T49.0X1	T49.0X2	T49.0X3	T49.0X4	T49.0X5	T49.0X6
Pyribenzamine	T45.0X1	T45.0X2	T45.0X3	T45.0X4	T45.0X5	T45.0X6
Pyridine	T52.8X1	T52.8X2	T52.8X3	T52.8X4	—	—
aldoxime methiodide	T50.6X1	T50.6X2	T50.6X3	T50.6X4	T50.6X5	T50.6X6
aldoxime methyl chloride	T50.6X1	T50.6X2	T50.6X3	T50.6X4	T50.6X5	T50.6X6
vapor	T59.891	T59.892	T59.893	T59.894	—	—
Pyridium	T39.8X1	T39.8X2	T39.8X3	T39.8X4	T39.8X5	T39.8X6
Pyridostigmine bromide	T44.0X1	T44.0X2	T44.0X3	T44.0X4	T44.0X5	T44.0X6
Pyridoxal phosphate	T45.2X1	T45.2X2	T45.2X3	T45.2X4	T45.2X5	T45.2X6
Pyridoxine	T45.2X1	T45.2X2	T45.2X3	T45.2X4	T45.2X5	T45.2X6
Pyrilamine	T45.0X1	T45.0X2	T45.0X3	T45.0X4	T45.0X5	T45.0X6
Pyrimethamine	T37.2X1	T37.2X2	T37.2X3	T37.2X4	T37.2X5	T37.2X6
with sulfadoxine	T37.2X1	T37.2X2	T37.2X3	T37.2X4	T37.2X5	T37.2X6
Pyrimidine antagonist	T45.1X1	T45.1X2	T45.1X3	T45.1X4	T45.1X5	T45.1X6
Pyriminil	T60.4X1	T60.4X2	T60.4X3	T60.4X4	—	—
Pyrithione zinc	T49.4X1	T49.4X2	T49.4X3	T49.4X4	T49.4X5	T49.4X6
Pyrithyldione	T42.6X1	T42.6X2	T42.6X3	T42.6X4	T42.6X5	T42.6X6
Pyrogallic acid	T49.0X1	T49.0X2	T49.0X3	T49.0X4	T49.0X5	T49.0X6
Pyrogallol	T49.0X1	T49.0X2	T49.0X3	T49.0X4	T49.0X5	T49.0X6
Pyroxylin	T49.3X1	T49.3X2	T49.3X3	T49.3X4	T49.3X5	T49.3X6
Pyrrobutamine	T45.0X1	T45.0X2	T45.0X3	T45.0X4	T45.0X5	T45.0X6
Pyrrolizidine alkaloids	T62.8X1	T62.8X2	T62.8X3	T62.8X4	—	—
Pyrvinium chloride	T37.4X1	T37.4X2	T37.4X3	T37.4X4	T37.4X5	T37.4X6
PZI	T38.3X1	T38.3X2	T38.3X3	T38.3X4	T38.3X5	T38.3X6
Q						
Quaalude	T42.6X1	T42.6X2	T42.6X3	T42.6X4	T42.6X5	T42.6X6
Quarternary ammonium						
anti-infective	T49.0X1	T49.0X2	T49.0X3	T49.0X4	T49.0X5	T49.0X6
ganglion blocking	T44.2X1	T44.2X2	T44.2X3	T44.2X4	T44.2X5	T44.2X6
parasympatholytic	T44.3X1	T44.3X2	T44.3X3	T44.3X4	T44.3X5	T44.3X6
Quazepam	T42.4X1	T42.4X2	T42.4X3	T42.4X4	T42.4X5	T42.4X6
Quicklime	T54.3X1	T54.3X2	T54.3X3	T54.3X4	—	—
Quillaja extract	T48.4X1	T48.4X2	T48.4X3	T48.4X4	T48.4X5	T48.4X6

◀ New   ◀▥ Revised   ~~deleted~~ Deleted

TABLE OF DRUGS AND CHEMICALS

Substance	External Cause (T-Code)					
	Poisoning, Accidental (Unintentional)	Poisoning, Intentional Self-Harm	Poisoning, Assault	Poisoning, Undetermined	Adverse Effect	Underdosing
Quinacrine	T37.2X1	T37.2X2	T37.2X3	T37.2X4	T37.2X5	T37.2X6
Quinaglute	T46.2X1	T46.2X2	T46.2X3	T46.2X4	T46.2X5	T46.2X6
Quinalbarbital	T42.3X1	T42.3X2	T42.3X3	T42.3X4	T42.3X5	T42.3X6
Quinalbarbitone sodium	T42.3X1	T42.3X2	T42.3X3	T42.3X4	T42.3X5	T42.3X6
Quinalphos	T60.0X1	T60.0X2	T60.0X3	T60.0X4	—	—
Quinapril	T46.4X1	T46.4X2	T46.4X3	T46.4X4	T46.4X5	T46.4X6
Quinestradiol	T38.5X1	T38.5X2	T38.5X3	T38.5X4	T38.5X5	T38.5X6
Quinestradol	T38.5X1	T38.5X2	T38.5X3	T38.5X4	T38.5X5	T38.5X6
Quinestrol	T38.5X1	T38.5X2	T38.5X3	T38.5X4	T38.5X5	T38.5X6
Quinethazone	T50.2X1	T50.2X2	T50.2X3	T50.2X4	T50.2X5	T50.2X6
Quingestanol	T38.4X1	T38.4X2	T38.4X3	T38.4X4	T38.4X5	T38.4X6
Quinidine	T46.2X1	T46.2X2	T46.2X3	T46.2X4	T46.2X5	T46.2X6
Quinine	T37.2X1	T37.2X2	T37.2X3	T37.2X4	T37.2X5	T37.2X6
Quiniobine	T37.8X1	T37.8X2	T37.8X3	T37.8X4	T37.8X5	T37.8X6
Quinisocaine	T49.1X1	T49.1X2	T49.1X3	T49.1X4	T49.1X5	T49.1X6
Quinocide	T37.2X1	T37.2X2	T37.2X3	T37.2X4	T37.2X5	T37.2X6
Quinoline (derivatives) NEC	T37.8X1	T37.8X2	T37.8X3	T37.8X4	T37.8X5	T37.8X6
Quinupramine	T43.011	T43.012	T43.013	T43.014	T43.015	T43.016
Quotane	T41.3X1	T41.3X2	T41.3X3	T41.3X4	T41.3X5	T41.3X6
R						
Rabies						
immune globulin (human)	T50.Z11	T50.Z12	T50.Z13	T50.Z14	T50.Z15	T50.Z16
vaccine	T50.B91	T50.B92	T50.B93	T50.B94	T50.B95	T50.B96
Racemoramide	T40.2X1	T40.2X2	T40.2X3	T40.2X4	—	—
Racemorphan	T40.2X1	T40.2X2	T40.2X3	T40.2X4	T40.2X5	T40.2X6
Racepinefrin	T44.5X1	T44.5X2	T44.5X3	T44.5X4	T44.5X5	T44.5X6
Raclopride	T43.591	T43.592	T43.593	T43.594	T43.595	T43.596
Radiator alcohol	T51.1X1	T51.1X2	T51.1X3	T51.1X4	—	—
Radioactive drug NEC	T50.8X1	T50.8X2	T50.8X3	T50.8X4	T50.8X5	T50.8X6
Radio-opaque (drugs) (materials)	T50.8X1	T50.8X2	T50.8X3	T50.8X4	T50.8X5	T50.8X6
Ramifenazone	T39.2X1	T39.2X2	T39.2X3	T39.2X4	T39.2X5	T39.2X6
Ramipril	T46.4X1	T46.4X2	T46.4X3	T46.4X4	T46.4X5	T46.4X6
Ranitidine	T47.0X1	T47.0X2	T47.0X3	T47.0X4	T47.0X5	T47.0X6
Ranunculus	T62.2X1	T62.2X2	T62.2X3	T62.2X4	—	—
Rat poison NEC	T60.4X1	T60.4X2	T60.4X3	T60.4X4	—	—
Rattlesnake (venom)	T63.011	T63.012	T63.013	T63.014	—	—
Raubasine	T46.7X1	T46.7X2	T46.7X3	T46.7X4	T46.7X5	T46.7X6
Raudixin	T46.5X1	T46.5X2	T46.5X3	T46.5X4	T46.5X5	T46.5X6
Rautensin	T46.5X1	T46.5X2	T46.5X3	T46.5X4	T46.5X5	T46.5X6

◄ New ◄IIII Revised ~~deleted~~ Deleted

Substance	External Cause (T-Code)					
	Poisoning, Accidental (Unintentional)	Poisoning, Intentional Self-Harm	Poisoning, Assault	Poisoning, Undetermined	Adverse Effect	Underdosing
Rautina	T46.5X1	T46.5X2	T46.5X3	T46.5X4	T46.5X5	T46.5X6
Rautotal	T46.5X1	T46.5X2	T46.5X3	T46.5X4	T46.5X5	T46.5X6
Rauwiloid	T46.5X1	T46.5X2	T46.5X3	T46.5X4	T46.5X5	T46.5X6
Rauwoldin	T46.5X1	T46.5X2	T46.5X3	T46.5X4	T46.5X5	T46.5X6
Rauwolfia (alkaloids)	T46.5X1	T46.5X2	T46.5X3	T46.5X4	T46.5X5	T46.5X6
Razoxane	T45.1X1	T45.1X2	T45.1X3	T45.1X4	T45.1X5	T45.1X6
Realgar	T57.0X1	T57.0X2	T57.0X3	T57.0X4	—	—
Recombinant (R) — *see specific protein*						
Red blood cells, packed	T45.8X1	T45.8X2	T45.8X3	T45.8X4	T45.8X5	T45.8X6
Red squill (scilliroside)	T60.4X1	T60.4X2	T60.4X3	T60.4X4	—	—
Reducing agent, industrial NEC	T65.891	T65.892	T65.893	T65.894	—	—
Refrigerant gas (chlorofluoro-carbon)	T53.5X1	T53.5X2	T53.5X3	T53.5X4	—	—
not chlorofluoro-carbon	T59.891	T59.892	T59.893	T59.894	—	—
Regroton	T50.2X1	T50.2X2	T50.2X3	T50.2X4	T50.2X5	T50.2X6
Rehydration salts (oral)	T50.3X1	T50.3X2	T50.3X3	T50.3X4	T50.3X5	T50.3X6
Rela	T42.8X1	T42.8X2	T42.8X3	T42.8X4	T42.8X5	T42.8X6
Relaxant, muscle						
anesthetic	T48.1X1	T48.1X2	T48.1X3	T48.1X4	T48.1X5	T48.1X6
central nervous system	T42.8X1	T42.8X2	T42.8X3	T42.8X4	T42.8X5	T42.8X6
skeletal NEC	T48.1X1	T48.1X2	T48.1X3	T48.1X4	T48.1X5	T48.1X6
smooth NEC	T44.3X1	T44.3X2	T44.3X3	T44.3X4	T44.3X5	T44.3X6
Remoxipride	T43.591	T43.592	T43.593	T43.594	T43.595	T43.596
Renese	T50.2X1	T50.2X2	T50.2X3	T50.2X4	T50.2X5	T50.2X6
Renografin	T50.8X1	T50.8X2	T50.8X3	T50.8X4	T50.8X5	T50.8X6
Replacement solution	T50.3X1	T50.3X2	T50.3X3	T50.3X4	T50.3X5	T50.3X6
Reproterol	T48.6X1	T48.6X2	T48.6X3	T48.6X4	T48.6X5	T48.6X6
Rescinnamine	T46.5X1	T46.5X2	T46.5X3	T46.5X4	T46.5X5	T46.5X6
Reserpin(e)	T46.5X1	T46.5X2	T46.5X3	T46.5X4	T46.5X5	T46.5X6
Resorcin, resorcinol (nonmedicinal)	T65.891	T65.892	T65.893	T65.894	—	—
medicinal	T49.4X1	T49.4X2	T49.4X3	T49.4X4	T49.4X5	T49.4X6
Respaire	T48.4X1	T48.4X2	T48.4X3	T48.4X4	T48.4X5	T48.4X6
Respiratory drug NEC	T48.901	T48.902	T48.903	T48.904	T48.905	T48.906
antiasthmatic NEC	T48.6X1	T48.6X2	T48.6X3	T48.6X4	T48.6X5	T48.6X6
anti-common-cold NEC	T48.5X1	T48.5X2	T48.5X3	T48.5X4	T48.5X5	T48.5X6
expectorant NEC	T48.4X1	T48.4X2	T48.4X3	T48.4X4	T48.4X5	T48.4X6
stimulant	T48.901	T48.902	T48.903	T48.904	T48.905	T48.906
Retinoic acid	T49.0X1	T49.0X2	T49.0X3	T49.0X4	T49.0X5	T49.0X6
Retinol	T45.2X1	T45.2X2	T45.2X3	T45.2X4	T45.2X5	T45.2X6
Rh (D) immune globulin (human)	T50.Z11	T50.Z12	T50.Z13	T50.Z14	T50.Z15	T50.Z16
Rhodine	T39.011	T39.012	T39.013	T39.014	T39.015	T39.016

◀ New　◀▥ Revised　~~deleted~~ Deleted

TABLE OF DRUGS AND CHEMICALS

Substance	Poisoning, Accidental (Unintentional)	Poisoning, Intentional Self-Harm	Poisoning, Assault	Poisoning, Undetermined	Adverse Effect	Underdosing
	External Cause (T-Code)					
RhoGAM	T50.Z11	T50.Z12	T50.Z13	T50.Z14	T50.Z15	T50.Z16
Rhubarb						
dry extract	T47.2X1	T47.2X2	T47.2X3	T47.2X4	T47.2X5	T47.2X6
tincture, compound	T47.2X1	T47.2X2	T47.2X3	T47.2X4	T47.2X5	T47.2X6
Ribavirin	T37.5X1	T37.5X2	T37.5X3	T37.5X4	T37.5X5	T37.5X6
Riboflavin	T45.2X1	T45.2X2	T45.2X3	T45.2X4	T45.2X5	T45.2X6
Ribostamycin	T36.5X1	T36.5X2	T36.5X3	T36.5X4	T36.5X5	T36.5X6
Ricin	T62.2X1	T62.2X2	T62.2X3	T62.2X4	—	—
Ricinus communis	T62.2X1	T62.2X2	T62.2X3	T62.2X4	—	—
Rickettsial vaccine NEC	T50.A91	T50.A92	T50.A93	T50.A94	T50.A95	T50.A96
Rifabutin	T36.6X1	T36.6X2	T36.6X3	T36.6X4	T36.6X5	T36.6X6
Rifamide	T36.6X1	T36.6X2	T36.6X3	T36.6X4	T36.6X5	T36.6X6
Rifampicin	T36.6X1	T36.6X2	T36.6X3	T36.6X4	T36.6X5	T36.6X6
with isoniazid	T37.1X1	T37.1X2	T37.1X3	T37.1X4	T37.1X5	T37.1X6
Rifampin	T36.6X1	T36.6X2	T36.6X3	T36.6X4	T36.6X5	T36.6X6
Rifamycin	T36.6X1	T36.6X2	T36.6X3	T36.6X4	T36.6X5	T36.6X6
Rifaximin	T36.6X1	T36.6X2	T36.6X3	T36.6X4	T36.6X5	T36.6X6
Rimantadine	T37.5X1	T37.5X2	T37.5X3	T37.5X4	T37.5X5	T37.5X6
Rimazolium metilsulfate	T39.8X1	T39.8X2	T39.8X3	T39.8X4	T39.8X5	T39.8X6
Rimifon	T37.1X1	T37.1X2	T37.1X3	T37.1X4	T37.1X5	T37.1X6
Rimiterol	T48.6X1	T48.6X2	T48.6X3	T48.6X4	T48.6X5	T48.6X6
Ringer (lactate) solution	T50.3X1	T50.3X2	T50.3X3	T50.3X4	T50.3X5	T50.3X6
Ristocetin	T36.8X1	T36.8X2	T36.8X3	T36.8X4	T36.8X5	T36.8X6
Ritalin	T43.631	T43.632	T43.633	T43.634	T43.635	T43.636
Ritodrine	T44.5X1	T44.5X2	T44.5X3	T44.5X4	T44.5X5	T44.5X6
Roach killer — see Insecticide						
Rociverine	T44.3X1	T44.3X2	T44.3X3	T44.3X4	T44.3X5	T44.3X6
Rocky Mountain spotted fever vaccine	T50.A91	T50.A92	T50.A93	T50.A94	T50.A95	T50.A96
Rodenticide NEC	T60.4X1	T60.4X2	T60.4X3	T60.4X4	—	—
Rohypnol	T42.4X1	T42.4X2	T42.4X3	T42.4X4	T42.4X5	T42.4X6
Rokitamycin	T36.3X1	T36.3X2	T36.3X3	T36.3X4	T36.3X5	T36.3X6
Rolaids	T47.1X1	T47.1X2	T47.1X3	T47.1X4	T47.1X5	T47.1X6
Rolitetracycline	T36.4X1	T36.4X2	T36.4X3	T36.4X4	T36.4X5	T36.4X6
Romilar	T48.3X1	T48.3X2	T48.3X3	T48.3X4	T48.3X5	T48.3X6
Ronifibrate	T46.6X1	T46.6X2	T46.6X3	T46.6X4	T46.6X5	T46.6X6
Rosaprostol	T47.1X1	T47.1X2	T47.1X3	T47.1X4	T47.1X5	T47.1X6
Rose bengal sodium (131I)	T50.8X1	T50.8X2	T50.8X3	T50.8X4	T50.8X5	T50.8X6
Rose water ointment	T49.3X1	T49.3X2	T49.3X3	T49.3X4	T49.3X5	T49.3X6
Rosoxacin	T37.8X1	T37.8X2	T37.8X3	T37.8X4	T37.8X5	T37.8X6
Rotenone	T60.2X1	T60.2X2	T60.2X3	T60.2X4		—

◀ New   ◀ Revised   ~~deleted~~ Deleted

Substance	External Cause (T-Code)					
	Poisoning, Accidental (Unintentional)	Poisoning, Intentional Self-Harm	Poisoning, Assault	Poisoning, Undetermined	Adverse Effect	Underdosing
Rotoxamine	T45.0X1	T45.0X2	T45.0X3	T45.0X4	T45.0X5	T45.0X6
Rough-on-rats	T60.4X1	T60.4X2	T60.4X3	T60.4X4	—	—
Roxatidine	T47.0X1	T47.0X2	T47.0X3	T47.0X4	T47.0X5	T47.0X6
Roxithromycin	T36.3X1	T36.3X2	T36.3X3	T36.3X4	T36.3X5	T36.3X6
Rt-PA	T45.611	T45.612	T45.613	T45.614	T45.615	T45.616
Rubbing alcohol	T51.2X1	T51.2X2	T51.2X3	T51.2X4	—	—
Rubefacient	T49.4X1	T49.4X2	T49.4X3	T49.4X4	T49.4X5	T49.4X6
Rubella vaccine	T50.B91	T50.B92	T50.B93	T50.B94	T50.B95	T50.B96
Rubelogen	T50.B91	T50.B92	T50.B93	T50.B94	T50.B95	T50.B96
Rubeovax	T50.991	T50.992	T50.993	T50.994	T50.995	T50.996
Rubidium chloride Rb82	T50.8X1	T50.8X2	T50.8X3	T50.8X4	T50.8X5	T50.8X6
Rubidomycin	T45.1X1	T45.1X2	T45.1X3	T45.1X4	T45.1X5	T45.1X6
Rue	T62.2X1	T62.2X2	T62.2X3	T62.2X4	—	—
Rufocromomycin	T45.1X1	T45.1X2	T45.1X3	T45.1X4	T45.1X5	T45.1X6
Russel's viper venin	T45.7X1	T45.7X2	T45.7X3	T45.7X4	T45.7X5	T45.7X6
Ruta (graveolens)	T62.2X1	T62.2X2	T62.2X3	T62.2X4	—	—
Rutinum	T46.991	T46.992	T46.993	T46.994	T46.995	T46.996
Rutoside	T46.991	T46.992	T46.993	T46.994	T46.995	T46.996
S						
Sabadilla (plant)	T62.2X1	T62.2X2	T62.2X3	T62.2X4	—	—
pesticide	T60.2X1	T60.2X2	T60.2X3	T60.2X4	—	—
Saccharated iron oxide	T45.8X1	T45.8X2	T45.8X3	T45.8X4	T45.8X5	T45.8X6
Saccharin	T50.901	T50.902	T50.903	T50.904	T50.905	T50.906
Saccharomyces boulardii	T47.6X1	T47.6X2	T47.6X3	T47.6X4	T47.6X5	T47.6X6
Safflower oil	T46.6X1	T46.6X2	T46.6X3	T46.6X4	T46.6X5	T46.6X6
Safrazine	T43.1X1	T43.1X2	T43.1X3	T43.1X4	T43.1X5	T43.1X6
Salazosulfapyridine	T37.0X1	T37.0X2	T37.0X3	T37.0X4	T37.0X5	T37.0X6
Salbutamol	T48.6X1	T48.6X2	T48.6X3	T48.6X4	T48.6X5	T48.6X6
Salicylamide	T39.091	T39.092	T39.093	T39.094	T39.095	T39.096
Salicylate NEC	T39.091	T39.092	T39.093	T39.094	T39.095	T39.096
methyl	T49.3X1	T49.3X2	T49.3X3	T49.3X4	T49.3X5	T49.3X6
theobromine calcium	T50.2X1	T50.2X2	T50.2X3	T50.2X4	T50.2X5	T50.2X6
Salicylazosulfapyridine	T37.0X1	T37.0X2	T37.0X3	T37.0X4	T37.0X5	T37.0X6
Salicylhydroxamic acid	T49.0X1	T49.0X2	T49.0X3	T49.0X4	T49.0X5	T49.0X6
Salicylic acid	T49.4X1	T49.4X2	T49.4X3	T49.4X4	T49.4X5	T49.4X6
with benzoic acid	T49.4X1	T49.4X2	T49.4X3	T49.4X4	T49.4X5	T49.4X6
congeners	T39.091	T39.092	T39.093	T39.094	T39.095	T39.096
derivative	T39.091	T39.092	T39.093	T39.094	T39.095	T39.096
salts	T39.091	T39.092	T39.093	T39.094	T39.095	T39.096

◀ New   ◀▥ Revised   ~~deleted~~ Deleted

TABLE OF DRUGS AND CHEMICALS

Substance	External Cause (T-Code)					
	Poisoning, Accidental (Unintentional)	Poisoning, Intentional Self-Harm	Poisoning, Assault	Poisoning, Undetermined	Adverse Effect	Underdosing
Salinazid	T37.1X1	T37.1X2	T37.1X3	T37.1X4	T37.1X5	T37.1X6
Salmeterol	T48.6X1	T48.6X2	T48.6X3	T48.6X4	T48.6X5	T48.6X6
Salol	T49.3X1	T49.3X2	T49.3X3	T49.3X4	T49.3X5	T49.3X6
Salsalate	T39.091	T39.092	T39.093	T39.094	T39.095	T39.096
Salt substitute	T50.901	T50.902	T50.903	T50.904	T50.905	T50.906
Salt-replacing drug	T50.901	T50.902	T50.903	T50.904	T50.905	T50.906
Salt-retaining mineralocorticoid	T50.0X1	T50.0X2	T50.0X3	T50.0X4	T50.0X5	T50.0X6
Saluretic NEC	T50.2X1	T50.2X2	T50.2X3	T50.2X4	T50.2X5	T50.2X6
Saluron	T50.2X1	T50.2X2	T50.2X3	T50.2X4	T50.2X5	T50.2X6
Salvarsan 606 (neosilver) (silver)	T37.8X1	T37.8X2	T37.8X3	T37.8X4	T37.8X5	T37.8X6
Sambucus canadensis	T62.2X1	T62.2X2	T62.2X3	T62.2X4	—	—
berry	T62.1X1	T62.1X2	T62.1X3	T62.1X4	—	—
Sandril	T46.5X1	T46.5X2	T46.5X3	T46.5X4	T46.5X5	T46.5X6
Sanguinaria canadensis	T62.2X1	T62.2X2	T62.2X3	T62.2X4		
Saniflush (cleaner)	T54.2X1	T54.2X2	T54.2X3	T54.2X4	—	—
Santonin	T37.4X1	T37.4X2	T37.4X3	T37.4X4	T37.4X5	T37.4X6
Santyl	T49.8X1	T49.8X2	T49.8X3	T49.8X4	T49.8X5	T49.8X6
Saralasin	T46.5X1	T46.5X2	T46.5X3	T46.5X4	T46.5X5	T46.5X6
Sarcolysin	T45.1X1	T45.1X2	T45.1X3	T45.1X4	T45.1X5	T45.1X6
Sarkomycin	T45.1X1	T45.1X2	T45.1X3	T45.1X4	T45.1X5	T45.1X6
Saroten	T43.011	T43.012	T43.013	T43.014	T43.015	T43.016
Saturnine — see Lead						
Savin (oil)	T49.4X1	T49.4X2	T49.4X3	T49.4X4	T49.4X5	T49.4X6
Scammony	T47.2X1	T47.2X2	T47.2X3	T47.2X4	T47.2X5	T47.2X6
Scarlet red	T49.8X1	T49.8X2	T49.8X3	T49.8X4	T49.8X5	T49.8X6
Scheele's green	T57.0X1	T57.0X2	T57.0X3	T57.0X4	—	—
insecticide	T57.0X1	T57.0X2	T57.0X3	T57.0X4	—	—
Schizontozide (blood) (tissue)	T37.2X1	T37.2X2	T37.2X3	T37.2X4	T37.2X5	T37.2X6
Schradan	T60.0X1	T60.0X2	T60.0X3	T60.0X4		
Schweinfurth green	T57.0X1	T57.0X2	T57.0X3	T57.0X4	—	—
insecticide	T57.0X1	T57.0X2	T57.0X3	T57.0X4	—	—
Scilla, rat poison	T60.4X1	T60.4X2	T60.4X3	T60.4X4	—	—
Scillaren	T60.4X1	T60.4X2	T60.4X3	T60.4X4	—	—
Sclerosing agent	T46.8X1	T46.8X2	T46.8X3	T46.8X4	T46.8X5	T46.8X6
Scombrotoxin	T61.11	T61.12	T61.13	T61.14	—	—
Scopolamine	T44.3X1	T44.3X2	T44.3X3	T44.3X4	T44.3X5	T44.3X6
Scopolia extract	T44.3X1	T44.3X2	T44.3X3	T44.3X4	T44.3X5	T44.3X6
Scouring powder	T65.891	T65.892	T65.893	T65.894	—	—

◀ New ◀‖‖ Revised ~~deleted~~ Deleted

Substance	External Cause (T-Code)					
	Poisoning, Accidental (Unintentional)	Poisoning, Intentional Self-Harm	Poisoning, Assault	Poisoning, Undetermined	Adverse Effect	Underdosing
Sea						
anemone (sting)	T63.631	T63.632	T63.633	T63.634	—	—
cucumber (sting)	T63.691	T63.692	T63.693	T63.694	—	—
snake (bite) (venom)	T63.091	T63.092	T63.093	T63.094	—	—
urchin spine (puncture)	T63.691	T63.692	T63.693	T63.694	—	—
Seafood	T61.91	T61.92	T61.93	T61.94	—	—
specified NEC	T61.8X1	T61.8X2	T61.8X3	T61.8X4	—	—
Secbutabarbital	T42.3X1	T42.3X2	T42.3X3	T42.3X4	T42.3X5	T42.3X6
Secbutabarbitone	T42.3X1	T42.3X2	T42.3X3	T42.3X4	T42.3X5	T42.3X6
Secnidazole	T37.3X1	T37.3X2	T37.3X3	T37.3X4	T37.3X5	T37.3X6
Secobarbital	T42.3X1	T42.3X2	T42.3X3	T42.3X4	T42.3X5	T42.3X6
Seconal	T42.3X1	T42.3X2	T42.3X3	T42.3X4	T42.3X5	T42.3X6
Secretin	T50.8X1	T50.8X2	T50.8X3	T50.8X4	T50.8X5	T50.8X6
Sedative NEC	T42.71	T42.72	T42.73	T42.74	T42.75	T42.76
mixed NEC	T42.6X1	T42.6X2	T42.6X3	T42.6X4	T42.6X5	T42.6X6
Sedormid	T42.6X1	T42.6X2	T42.6X3	T42.6X4	T42.6X5	T42.6X6
Seed disinfectant or dressing	T60.8X1	T60.8X2	T60.8X3	T60.8X4	—	—
Seeds (poisonous)	T62.2X1	T62.2X2	T62.2X3	T62.2X4	—	—
Selegiline	T42.8X1	T42.8X2	T42.8X3	T42.8X4	T42.8X5	T42.8X6
Selenium NEC	T56.891	T56.892	T56.893	T56.894	—	—
disulfide or sulfide	T49.4X1	T49.4X2	T49.4X3	T49.4X4	T49.4X5	T49.4X6
fumes	T59.891	T59.892	T59.893	T59.894	—	—
sulfide	T49.4X1	T49.4X2	T49.4X3	T49.4X4	T49.4X5	T49.4X6
Selenomethionine (75Se)	T50.8X1	T50.8X2	T50.8X3	T50.8X4	T50.8X5	T50.8X6
Selsun	T49.4X1	T49.4X2	T49.4X3	T49.4X4	T49.4X5	T49.4X6
Semustine	T45.1X1	T45.1X2	T45.1X3	T45.1X4	T45.1X5	T45.1X6
Senega syrup	T48.4X1	T48.4X2	T48.4X3	T48.4X4	T48.4X5	T48.4X6
Senna	T47.2X1	T47.2X2	T47.2X3	T47.2X4	T47.2X5	T47.2X6
Sennoside A+B	T47.2X1	T47.2X2	T47.2X3	T47.2X4	T47.2X5	T47.2X6
Septisol	T49.2X1	T49.2X2	T49.2X3	T49.2X4	T49.2X5	T49.2X6
Seractide	T38.811	T38.812	T38.813	T38.814	T38.815	T38.816
Serax	T42.4X1	T42.4X2	T42.4X3	T42.4X4	T42.4X5	T42.4X6
Serenesil	T42.6X1	T42.6X2	T42.6X3	T42.6X4	T42.6X5	T42.6X6
Serenium (hydrochloride)	T37.91	T37.92	T37.93	T37.94	T37.95	T37.96
Serepax — see Oxazepam						
Sermorelin	T38.891	T38.892	T38.893	T38.894	T38.895	T38.896
Sernyl	T41.1X1	T41.1X2	T41.1X3	T41.1X4	T41.1X5	T41.1X6
Serotonin	T50.991	T50.992	T50.993	T50.994	T50.995	T50.996

◀ New ◀▥ Revised ~~deleted~~ Deleted

TABLE OF DRUGS AND CHEMICALS

Substance	Poisoning, Accidental (Unintentional)	Poisoning, Intentional Self-Harm	Poisoning, Assault	Poisoning, Undetermined	Adverse Effect	Underdosing
	External Cause (T-Code)					
Serpasil	T46.5X1	T46.5X2	T46.5X3	T46.5X4	T46.5X5	T46.5X6
Serrapeptase	T45.3X1	T45.3X2	T45.3X3	T45.3X4	T45.3X5	T45.3X6
Serum						
antibotulinus	T50.Z11	T50.Z12	T50.Z13	T50.Z14	T50.Z15	T50.Z16
anticytotoxic	T50.Z11	T50.Z12	T50.Z13	T50.Z14	T50.Z15	T50.Z16
antidiphtheria	T50.Z11	T50.Z12	T50.Z13	T50.Z14	T50.Z15	T50.Z16
antimeningococcus	T50.Z11	T50.Z12	T50.Z13	T50.Z14	T50.Z15	T50.Z16
anti-Rh	T50.Z11	T50.Z12	T50.Z13	T50.Z14	T50.Z15	T50.Z16
anti-snake-bite	T50.Z11	T50.Z12	T50.Z13	T50.Z14	T50.Z15	T50.Z16
antitetanic	T50.Z11	T50.Z12	T50.Z13	T50.Z14	T50.Z15	T50.Z16
antitoxic	T50.Z11	T50.Z12	T50.Z13	T50.Z14	T50.Z15	T50.Z16
complement (inhibitor)	T45.8X1	T45.8X2	T45.8X3	T45.8X4	T45.8X5	T45.8X6
convalescent	T50.Z11	T50.Z12	T50.Z13	T50.Z14	T50.Z15	T50.Z16
hemolytic complement	T45.8X1	T45.8X2	T45.8X3	T45.8X4	T45.8X5	T45.8X6
immune (human)	T50.Z11	T50.Z12	T50.Z13	T50.Z14	T50.Z15	T50.Z16
protective NEC	T50.Z11	T50.Z12	T50.Z13	T50.Z14	T50.Z15	T50.Z16
Setastine	T45.0X1	T45.0X2	T45.0X3	T45.0X4	T45.0X5	T45.0X6
Setoperone	T43.591	T43.592	T43.593	T43.594	T43.595	T43.596
Sewer gas	T59.91	T59.92	T59.93	T59.94	—	—
Shampoo	T55.0X1	T55.0X2	T55.0X3	T55.0X4	—	—
Shellfish, noxious, nonbacterial	T61.781	T61.782	T61.783	T61.784	—	—
Sildenafil	T46.7X1	T46.7X2	T46.7X3	T46.7X4	T46.7X5	T46.7X6
Silibinin	T50.991	T50.992	T50.993	T50.994	T50.995	T50.996
Silicone NEC	T65.891	T65.892	T65.893	T65.894	—	—
medicinal	T49.3X1	T49.3X2	T49.3X3	T49.3X4	T49.3X5	T49.3X6
Silvadene	T49.0X1	T49.0X2	T49.0X3	T49.0X4	T49.0X5	T49.0X6
Silver	T49.0X1	T49.0X2	T49.0X3	T49.0X4	T49.0X5	T49.0X6
anti-infectives	T49.0X1	T49.0X2	T49.0X3	T49.0X4	T49.0X5	T49.0X6
arsphenamine	T37.8X1	T37.8X2	T37.8X3	T37.8X4	T37.8X5	T37.8X6
colloidal	T49.0X1	T49.0X2	T49.0X3	T49.0X4	T49.0X5	T49.0X6
nitrate	T49.0X1	T49.0X2	T49.0X3	T49.0X4	T49.0X5	T49.0X6
ophthalmic preparation	T49.5X1	T49.5X2	T49.5X3	T49.5X4	T49.5X5	T49.5X6
toughened (keratolytic)	T49.4X1	T49.4X2	T49.4X3	T49.4X4	T49.4X5	T49.4X6
nonmedicinal (dust)	T56.891	T56.892	T56.893	T56.894	—	—
protein	T49.5X1	T49.5X2	T49.5X3	T49.5X4	T49.5X5	T49.5X6
salvarsan	T37.8X1	T37.8X2	T37.8X3	T37.8X4	T37.8X5	T37.8X6
sulfadiazine	T49.4X1	T49.4X2	T49.4X3	T49.4X4	T49.4X5	T49.4X6
Silymarin	T50.991	T50.992	T50.993	T50.994	T50.995	T50.996
Simaldrate	T47.1X1	T47.1X2	T47.1X3	T47.1X4	T47.1X5	T47.1X6
Simazine	T60.3X1	T60.3X2	T60.3X3	T60.3X4	—	—

◀ New ◀ Revised ~~deleted~~ Deleted

Substance	External Cause (T-Code)					
	Poisoning, Accidental (Unintentional)	Poisoning, Intentional Self-Harm	Poisoning, Assault	Poisoning, Undetermined	Adverse Effect	Underdosing
Simethicone	T47.1X1	T47.1X2	T47.1X3	T47.1X4	T47.1X5	T47.1X6
Simfibrate	T46.6X1	T46.6X2	T46.6X3	T46.6X4	T46.6X5	T46.6X6
Simvastatin	T46.6X1	T46.6X2	T46.6X3	T46.6X4	T46.6X5	T46.6X6
Sincalide	T50.8X1	T50.8X2	T50.8X3	T50.8X4	T50.8X5	T50.8X6
Sinequan	T43.011	T43.012	T43.013	T43.014	T43.015	T43.016
Singoserp	T46.5X1	T46.5X2	T46.5X3	T46.5X4	T46.5X5	T46.5X6
Sintrom	T45.511	T45.512	T45.513	T45.514	T45.515	T45.516
Sisomicin	T36.5X1	T36.5X2	T36.5X3	T36.5X4	T36.5X5	T36.5X6
Sitosterols	T46.6X1	T46.6X2	T46.6X3	T46.6X4	T46.6X5	T46.6X6
Skeletal muscle relaxants	T48.1X1	T48.1X2	T48.1X3	T48.1X4	T48.1X5	T48.1X6
Skin						
agents (external)	T49.91	T49.92	T49.93	T49.94	T49.95	T49.96
specified NEC	T49.8X1	T49.8X2	T49.8X3	T49.8X4	T49.8X5	T49.8X6
test antigen	T50.8X1	T50.8X2	T50.8X3	T50.8X4	T50.8X5	T50.8X6
Sleep-eze	T45.0X1	T45.0X2	T45.0X3	T45.0X4	T45.0X5	T45.0X6
Sleeping draught, pill	T42.71	T42.72	T42.73	T42.74	T42.75	T42.76
Smallpox vaccine	T50.B11	T50.B12	T50.B13	T50.B14	T50.B15	T50.B16
Smelter fumes NEC	T56.91	T56.92	T56.93	T56.94	—	—
Smog	T59.1X1	T59.1X2	T59.1X3	T59.1X4	—	—
Smoke NEC	T59.811	T59.812	T59.813	T59.814	—	—
Smooth muscle relaxant	T44.3X1	T44.3X2	T44.3X3	T44.3X4	T44.3X5	T44.3X6
Snail killer NEC	T60.8X1	T60.8X2	T60.8X3	T60.8X4	—	—
Snake venom or bite	T63.001	T63.002	T63.003	T63.004	—	—
hemocoagulase	T45.7X1	T45.7X2	T45.7X3	T45.7X4	T45.7X5	T45.7X6
Snuff	T65.211	T65.212	T65.213	T65.214	—	—
Soap (powder) (product)	T55.0X1	T55.0X2	T55.0X3	T55.0X4	—	—
enema	T47.4X1	T47.4X2	T47.4X3	T47.4X4	T47.4X5	T47.4X6
medicinal, soft	T49.2X1	T49.2X2	T49.2X3	T49.2X4	T49.2X5	T49.2X6
superfatted	T49.2X1	T49.2X2	T49.2X3	T49.2X4	T49.2X5	T49.2X6
Sobrerol	T48.4X1	T48.4X2	T48.4X3	T48.4X4	T48.4X5	T48.4X6
Soda (caustic)	T54.3X1	T54.3X2	T54.3X3	T54.3X4	—	—
bicarb	T47.1X1	T47.1X2	T47.1X3	T47.1X4	T47.1X5	T47.1X6
chlorinated — *see Sodium, hypochlorite*						
Sodium						
acetosulfone	T37.1X1	T37.1X2	T37.1X3	T37.1X4	T37.1X5	T37.1X6
acetrizoate	T50.8X1	T50.8X2	T50.8X3	T50.8X4	T50.8X5	T50.8X6
acid phosphate	T50.3X1	T50.3X2	T50.3X3	T50.3X4	T50.3X5	T50.3X6
alginate	T47.8X1	T47.8X2	T47.8X3	T47.8X4	T47.8X5	T47.8X6
amidotrizoate	T50.8X1	T50.8X2	T50.8X3	T50.8X4	T50.8X5	T50.8X6
aminopterin	T45.1X1	T45.1X2	T45.1X3	T45.1X4	T45.1X5	T45.1X6

TABLE OF DRUGS AND CHEMICALS

Substance	Poisoning, Accidental (Unintentional)	Poisoning, Intentional Self-Harm	Poisoning, Assault	Poisoning, Undetermined	Adverse Effect	Underdosing
External Cause (T-Code)						
Sodium *(Continued)*						
amylosulfate	T47.8X1	T47.8X2	T47.8X3	T47.8X4	T47.8X5	T47.8X6
amytal	T42.3X1	T42.3X2	T42.3X3	T42.3X4	T42.3X5	T42.3X6
antimony gluconate	T37.3X1	T37.3X2	T37.3X3	T37.3X4	T37.3X5	T37.3X6
arsenate	T57.0X1	T57.0X2	T57.0X3	T57.0X4	—	—
aurothiomalate	T39.4X1	T39.4X2	T39.4X3	T39.4X4	T39.4X5	T39.4X6
aurothiosulfate	T39.4X1	T39.4X2	T39.4X3	T39.4X4	T39.4X5	T39.4X6
barbiturate	T42.3X1	T42.3X2	T42.3X3	T42.3X4	T42.3X5	T42.3X6
basic phosphate	T47.4X1	T47.4X2	T47.4X3	T47.4X4	T47.4X5	T47.4X6
bicarbonate	T47.1X1	T47.1X2	T47.1X3	T47.1X4	T47.1X5	T47.1X6
bichromate	T57.8X1	T57.8X2	T57.8X3	T57.8X4	—	—
biphosphate	T50.3X1	T50.3X2	T50.3X3	T50.3X4	T50.3X5	T50.3X6
bisulfate	T65.891	T65.892	T65.893	T65.894	—	—
borate						
cleanser	T57.8X1	T57.8X2	T57.8X3	T57.8X4	—	—
eye	T49.5X1	T49.5X2	T49.5X3	T49.5X4	T49.5X5	T49.5X6
therapeutic	T49.8X1	T49.8X2	T49.8X3	T49.8X4	T49.8X5	T49.8X6
bromide	T42.6X1	T42.6X2	T42.6X3	T42.6X4	T42.6X5	T42.6X6
cacodylate (nonmedicinal) NEC	T50.8X1	T50.8X2	T50.8X3	T50.8X4	T50.8X5	T50.8X6
anti-infective	T37.8X1	T37.8X2	T37.8X3	T37.8X4	T37.8X5	T37.8X6
herbicide	T60.3X1	T60.3X2	T60.3X3	T60.3X4	—	—
calcium edetate	T45.8X1	T45.8X2	T45.8X3	T45.8X4	T45.8X5	T45.8X6
carbonate NEC	T54.3X1	T54.3X2	T54.3X3	T54.3X4	—	—
chlorate NEC	T65.891	T65.892	T65.893	T65.894	—	—
herbicide	T54.91	T54.92	T54.93	T54.94	—	—
chloride	T50.3X1	T50.3X2	T50.3X3	T50.3X4	T50.3X5	T50.3X6
with glucose	T50.3X1	T50.3X2	T50.3X3	T50.3X4	T50.3X5	T50.3X6
chromate	T65.891	T65.892	T65.893	T65.894	—	—
citrate	T50.991	T50.992	T50.993	T50.994	T50.995	T50.996
cromoglicate	T48.6X1	T48.6X2	T48.6X3	T48.6X4	T48.6X5	T48.6X6
cyanide	T65.0X1	T65.0X2	T65.0X3	T65.0X4	—	—
cyclamate	T50.3X1	T50.3X2	T50.3X3	T50.3X4	T50.3X5	T50.3X6
dehydrocholate	T45.8X1	T45.8X2	T45.8X3	T45.8X4	T45.8X5	T45.8X6
diatrizoate	T50.8X1	T50.8X2	T50.8X3	T50.8X4	T50.8X5	T50.8X6
dibunate	T48.4X1	T48.4X2	T48.4X3	T48.4X4	T48.4X5	T48.4X6
dioctyl sulfosuccinate	T47.4X1	T47.4X2	T47.4X3	T47.4X4	T47.4X5	T47.4X6
dipantoyl ferrate	T45.8X1	T45.8X2	T45.8X3	T45.8X4	T45.8X5	T45.8X6
edetate	T45.8X1	T45.8X2	T45.8X3	T45.8X4	T45.8X5	T45.8X6
ethacrynate	T50.1X1	T50.1X2	T50.1X3	T50.1X4	T50.1X5	T50.1X6
feredetate	T45.8X1	T45.8X2	T45.8X3	T45.8X4	T45.8X5	T45.8X6

◀ New   ◀||| Revised   ~~deleted~~ Deleted

Substance	External Cause (T-Code)					
	Poisoning, Accidental (Unintentional)	Poisoning, Intentional Self-Harm	Poisoning, Assault	Poisoning, Undetermined	Adverse Effect	Underdosing
Sodium *(Continued)*						
Fluoride — *see Fluoride*						
fluoroacetate (dust) (pesticide)	T60.4X1	T60.4X2	T60.4X3	T60.4X4	—	—
free salt	T50.3X1	T50.3X2	T50.3X3	T50.3X4	T50.3X5	T50.3X6
fusidate	T36.8X1	T36.8X2	T36.8X3	T36.8X4	T36.8X5	T36.8X6
glucaldrate	T47.1X1	T47.1X2	T47.1X3	T47.1X4	T47.1X5	T47.1X6
glucosulfone	T37.1X1	T37.1X2	T37.1X3	T37.1X4	T37.1X5	T37.1X6
glutamate	T45.8X1	T45.8X2	T45.8X3	T45.8X4	T45.8X5	T45.8X6
hydrogen carbonate	T50.3X1	T50.3X2	T50.3X3	T50.3X4	T50.3X5	T50.3X6
hydroxide	T54.3X1	T54.3X2	T54.3X3	T54.3X4	—	—
hypochlorite (bleach) NEC	T54.3X1	T54.3X2	T54.3X3	T54.3X4	—	—
disinfectant	T54.3X1	T54.3X2	T54.3X3	T54.3X4	—	—
medicinal (anti-infective) (external)	T49.0X1	T49.0X2	T49.0X3	T49.0X4	T49.0X5	T49.0X6
vapor	T54.3X1	T54.3X2	T54.3X3	T54.3X4	—	—
hyposulfite	T49.0X1	T49.0X2	T49.0X3	T49.0X4	T49.0X5	T49.0X6
indigotin disulfonate	T50.8X1	T50.8X2	T50.8X3	T50.8X4	T50.8X5	T50.8X6
iodide	T50.991	T50.992	T50.993	T50.994	T50.995	T50.996
I-131	T50.8X1	T50.8X2	T50.8X3	T50.8X4	T50.8X5	T50.8X6
therapeutic	T38.2X1	T38.2X2	T38.2X3	T38.2X4	T38.2X5	T38.2X6
iodohippurate (131I)	T50.8X1	T50.8X2	T50.8X3	T50.8X4	T50.8X5	T50.8X6
iopodate	T50.8X1	T50.8X2	T50.8X3	T50.8X4	T50.8X5	T50.8X6
iothalamate	T50.8X1	T50.8X2	T50.8X3	T50.8X4	T50.8X5	T50.8X6
iron edetate	T45.4X1	T45.4X2	T45.4X3	T45.4X4	T45.4X5	T45.4X6
lactate (compound solution)	T45.8X1	T45.8X2	T45.8X3	T45.8X4	T45.8X5	T45.8X6
lauryl (sulfate)	T49.2X1	T49.2X2	T49.2X3	T49.2X4	T49.2X5	T49.2X6
(L)-triiodothyronine	T38.1X1	T38.1X2	T38.1X3	T38.1X4	T38.1X5	T38.1X6
magnesium citrate	T50.991	T50.992	T50.993	T50.994	T50.995	T50.996
mersalate	T50.2X1	T50.2X2	T50.2X3	T50.2X4	T50.2X5	T50.2X6
metasilicate	T65.891	T65.892	T65.893	T65.894	—	—
metrizoate	T50.8X1	T50.8X2	T50.8X3	T50.8X4	T50.8X5	T50.8X6
monofluoroacetate (pesticide)	T60.1X1	T60.1X2	T60.1X3	T60.1X4	—	—
morrhuate	T46.8X1	T46.8X2	T46.8X3	T46.8X4	T46.8X5	T46.8X6
nafcillin	T36.0X1	T36.0X2	T36.0X3	T36.0X4	T36.0X5	T36.0X6
nitrate (oxidizing agent)	T65.891	T65.892	T65.893	T65.894	—	—
nitrite	T50.6X1	T50.6X2	T50.6X3	T50.6X4	T50.6X5	T50.6X6
nitroferricyanide	T46.5X1	T46.5X2	T46.5X3	T46.5X4	T46.5X5	T46.5X6
nitroprusside	T46.5X1	T46.5X2	T46.5X3	T46.5X4	T46.5X5	T46.5X6
oxalate	T65.891	T65.892	T65.893	T65.894	—	—
oxide/peroxide	T65.891	T65.892	T65.893	T65.894	—	—
oxybate	T41.291	T41.292	T41.293	T41.294	T41.295	T41.296

◀ New   ◀▥ Revised   ~~deleted~~ Deleted

| | External Cause (T-Code) | | | | | |
Substance	Poisoning, Accidental (Unintentional)	Poisoning, Intentional Self-Harm	Poisoning, Assault	Poisoning, Undetermined	Adverse Effect	Underdosing
Sodium *(Continued)*						
para-aminohippurate	T50.8X1	T50.8X2	T50.8X3	T50.8X4	T50.8X5	T50.8X6
perborate (nonmedicinal) NEC	T65.891	T65.892	T65.893	T65.894	—	—
medicinal	T49.0X1	T49.0X2	T49.0X3	T49.0X4	T49.0X5	T49.0X6
soap	T55.0X1	T55.0X2	T55.0X3	T55.0X4	—	—
percarbonate — *see Sodium, perborate*						
pertechnetate Tc99m	T50.8X1	T50.8X2	T50.8X3	T50.8X4	T50.8X5	T50.8X6
phosphate						
cellulose	T45.8X1	T45.8X2	T45.8X3	T45.8X4	T45.8X5	T45.8X6
dibasic	T47.2X1	T47.2X2	T47.2X3	T47.2X4	T47.2X5	T47.2X6
monobasic	T47.2X1	T47.2X2	T47.2X3	T47.2X4	T47.2X5	T47.2X6
phytate	T50.6X1	T50.6X2	T50.6X3	T50.6X4	T50.6X5	T50.6X6
picosulfate	T47.2X1	T47.2X2	T47.2X3	T47.2X4	T47.2X5	T47.2X6
polyhydroxyaluminium monocarbonate	T47.1X1	T47.1X2	T47.1X3	T47.1X4	T47.1X5	T47.1X6
polystyrene sulfonate	T50.3X1	T50.3X2	T50.3X3	T50.3X4	T50.3X5	T50.3X6
propionate	T49.0X1	T49.0X2	T49.0X3	T49.0X4	T49.0X5	T49.0X6
propyl hydroxybenzoate	T50.991	T50.992	T50.993	T50.994	T50.995	T50.996
psylliate	T46.8X1	T46.8X2	T46.8X3	T46.8X4	T46.8X5	T46.8X6
removing resins	T50.3X1	T50.3X2	T50.3X3	T50.3X4	T50.3X5	T50.3X6
salicylate	T39.091	T39.092	T39.093	T39.094	T39.095	T39.096
salt NEC	T50.3X1	T50.3X2	T50.3X3	T50.3X4	T50.3X5	T50.3X6
selenate	T60.2X1	T60.2X2	T60.2X3	T60.2X4	—	—
stibogluconate	T37.3X1	T37.3X2	T37.3X3	T37.3X4	T37.3X5	T37.3X6
sulfate	T47.4X1	T47.4X2	T47.4X3	T47.4X4	T47.4X5	T47.4X6
sulfoxone	T37.1X1	T37.1X2	T37.1X3	T37.1X4	T37.1X5	T37.1X6
tetradecyl sulfate	T46.8X1	T46.8X2	T46.8X3	T46.8X4	T46.8X5	T46.8X6
thiopental	T41.1X1	T41.1X2	T41.1X3	T41.1X4	T41.1X5	T41.1X6
thiosalicylate	T39.091	T39.092	T39.093	T39.094	T39.095	T39.096
thiosulfate	T50.6X1	T50.6X2	T50.6X3	T50.6X4	T50.6X5	T50.6X6
tolbutamide	T38.3X1	T38.3X2	T38.3X3	T38.3X4	T38.3X5	T38.3X6
l-triiodothyronine	T38.1X1	T38.1X2	T38.1X3	T38.1X4	T38.1X5	T38.1X6
tyropanoate	T50.8X1	T50.8X2	T50.8X3	T50.8X4	T50.8X5	T50.8X6
valproate	T42.6X1	T42.6X2	T42.6X3	T42.6X4	T42.6X5	T42.6X6
versenate	T50.6X1	T50.6X2	T50.6X3	T50.6X4	T50.6X5	T50.6X6
Sodium-free salt	T50.901	T50.902	T50.903	T50.904	T50.905	T50.906
Sodium-removing resin	T50.3X1	T50.3X2	T50.3X3	T50.3X4	T50.3X5	T50.3X6
Soft soap	T55.0X1	T55.0X2	T55.0X3	T55.0X4	—	—
Solanine	T62.2X1	T62.2X2	T62.2X3	T62.2X4	—	—
berries	T62.1X1	T62.1X2	T62.1X3	T62.1X4	—	—

◀ New ◀ Revised ~~deleted~~ Deleted

Substance	External Cause (T-Code)					
	Poisoning, Accidental (Unintentional)	Poisoning, Intentional Self-Harm	Poisoning, Assault	Poisoning, Undetermined	Adverse Effect	Underdosing
Solanum dulcamara	T62.2X1	T62.2X2	T62.2X3	T62.2X4	—	—
berries	T62.1X1	T62.1X2	T62.1X3	T62.1X4	—	—
Solapsone	T37.1X1	T37.1X2	T37.1X3	T37.1X4	T37.1X5	T37.1X6
Solar lotion	T49.3X1	T49.3X2	T49.3X3	T49.3X4	T49.3X5	T49.3X6
Solasulfone	T37.1X1	T37.1X2	T37.1X3	T37.1X4	T37.1X5	T37.1X6
Soldering fluid	T65.891	T65.892	T65.893	T65.894	—	—
Solid substance	T65.91	T65.92	T65.93	T65.94	—	—
specified NEC	T65.891	T65.892	T65.893	T65.894	—	—
Solvent, industrial NEC	T52.91	T52.92	T52.93	T52.94	—	—
naphtha	T52.0X1	T52.0X2	T52.0X3	T52.0X4	—	—
petroleum	T52.0X1	T52.0X2	T52.0X3	T52.0X4	—	—
specified NEC	T52.8X1	T52.8X2	T52.8X3	T52.8X4	—	—
Soma	T42.8X1	T42.8X2	T42.8X3	T42.8X4	T42.8X5	T42.8X6
Somatorelin	T38.891	T38.892	T38.893	T38.894	T38.895	T38.896
Somatostatin	T38.991	T38.992	T38.993	T38.994	T38.995	T38.996
Somatotropin	T38.811	T38.812	T38.813	T38.814	T38.815	T38.816
Somatrem	T38.811	T38.812	T38.813	T38.814	T38.815	T38.816
Somatropin	T38.811	T38.812	T38.813	T38.814	T38.815	T38.816
Sominex	T45.0X1	T45.0X2	T45.0X3	T45.0X4	T45.0X5	T45.0X6
Somnos	T42.6X1	T42.6X2	T42.6X3	T42.6X4	T42.6X5	T42.6X6
Somonal	T42.3X1	T42.3X2	T42.3X3	T42.3X4	T42.3X5	T42.3X6
Soneryl	T42.3X1	T42.3X2	T42.3X3	T42.3X4	T42.3X5	T42.3X6
Soothing syrup	T50.901	T50.902	T50.903	T50.904	T50.905	T50.906
Sopor	T42.6X1	T42.6X2	T42.6X3	T42.6X4	T42.6X5	T42.6X6
Soporific	T42.71	T42.72	T42.73	T42.74	T42.75	T42.76
Soporific drug	T42.71	T42.72	T42.73	T42.74	T42.75	T42.76
specified type NEC	T42.6X1	T42.6X2	T42.6X3	T42.6X4	T42.6X5	T42.6X6
Sorbide nitrate	T46.3X1	T46.3X2	T46.3X3	T46.3X4	T46.3X5	T46.3X6
Sorbitol	T47.4X1	T47.4X2	T47.4X3	T47.4X4	T47.4X5	T47.4X6
Sotalol	T44.7X1	T44.7X2	T44.7X3	T44.7X4	T44.7X5	T44.7X6
Sotradecol	T46.8X1	T46.8X2	T46.8X3	T46.8X4	T46.8X5	T46.8X6
Soysterol	T46.6X1	T46.6X2	T46.6X3	T46.6X4	T46.6X5	T46.6X6
Spacoline	T44.3X1	T44.3X2	T44.3X3	T44.3X4	T44.3X5	T44.3X6
Spanish fly	T49.8X1	T49.8X2	T49.8X3	T49.8X4	T49.8X5	T49.8X6
Sparine	T43.3X1	T43.3X2	T43.3X3	T43.3X4	T43.3X5	T43.3X6
Sparteine	T48.0X1	T48.0X2	T48.0X3	T48.0X4	T48.0X5	T48.0X6
Spasmolytic						
anticholinergics	T44.3X1	T44.3X2	T44.3X3	T44.3X4	T44.3X5	T44.3X6
autonomic	T44.3X1	T44.3X2	T44.3X3	T44.3X4	T44.3X5	T44.3X6

◀ New   ◀‖‖ Revised   ~~deleted~~ Deleted

Substance	External Cause (T-Code)					
	Poisoning, Accidental (Unintentional)	Poisoning, Intentional Self-Harm	Poisoning, Assault	Poisoning, Undetermined	Adverse Effect	Underdosing
Spasmolytic *(Continued)*						
bronchial NEC	T48.6X1	T48.6X2	T48.6X3	T48.6X4	T48.6X5	T48.6X6
quaternary ammonium	T44.3X1	T44.3X2	T44.3X3	T44.3X4	T44.3X5	T44.3X6
skeletal muscle NEC	T48.1X1	T48.1X2	T48.1X3	T48.1X4	T48.1X5	T48.1X6
Spectinomycin	T36.5X1	T36.5X2	T36.5X3	T36.5X4	T36.5X5	T36.5X6
Speed	T43.621	T43.622	T43.623	T43.624	T43.625	T43.626
Spermicide	T49.8X1	T49.8X2	T49.8X3	T49.8X4	T49.8X5	T49.8X6
Spider (bite) (venom)	T63.391	T63.392	T63.393	T63.394	—	—
antivenin	T50.Z11	T50.Z12	T50.Z13	T50.Z14	T50.Z15	T50.Z16
Spigelia (root)	T37.4X1	T37.4X2	T37.4X3	T37.4X4	T37.4X5	T37.4X6
Spindle inactivator	T50.4X1	T50.4X2	T50.4X3	T50.4X4	T50.4X5	T50.4X6
Spiperone	T43.4X1	T43.4X2	T43.4X3	T43.4X4	T43.4X5	T43.4X6
Spiramycin	T36.3X1	T36.3X2	T36.3X3	T36.3X4	T36.3X5	T36.3X6
Spirapril	T46.4X1	T46.4X2	T46.4X3	T46.4X4	T46.4X5	T46.4X6
Spirilene	T43.591	T43.592	T43.593	T43.594	T43.595	T43.596
Spirit(s) (neutral) NEC	T51.0X1	T51.0X2	T51.0X3	T51.0X4	—	—
beverage	T51.0X1	T51.0X2	T51.0X3	T51.0X4	—	—
industrial	T51.0X1	T51.0X2	T51.0X3	T51.0X4	—	—
mineral	T52.0X1	T52.0X2	T52.0X3	T52.0X4	—	—
of salt — *see* Hydrochloric acid						
surgical	T51.0X1	T51.0X2	T51.0X3	T51.0X4	—	—
Spironolactone	T50.0X1	T50.0X2	T50.0X3	T50.0X4	T50.0X5	T50.0X6
Spiroperidol	T43.4X1	T43.4X2	T43.4X3	T43.4X4	T43.4X5	T43.4X6
Sponge, absorbable (gelatin)	T45.7X1	T45.7X2	T45.7X3	T45.7X4	T45.7X5	T45.7X6
Sporostacin	T49.0X1	T49.0X2	T49.0X3	T49.0X4	T49.0X5	T49.0X6
Spray (aerosol)	T65.91	T65.92	T65.93	T65.94	—	—
cosmetic	T65.891	T65.892	T65.893	T65.894	—	—
medicinal NEC	T50.901	T50.902	T50.903	T50.904	T50.905	T50.906
pesticides — *see* Pesticides						
specified content — *see* specific substance						
Spurge flax	T62.2X1	T62.2X2	T62.2X3	T62.2X4	—	—
Spurges	T62.2X1	T62.2X2	T62.2X3	T62.2X4	—	—
Sputum viscosity-lowering drug	T48.4X1	T48.4X2	T48.4X3	T48.4X4	T48.4X5	T48.4X6
Squill	T46.0X1	T46.0X2	T46.0X3	T46.0X4	T46.0X5	T46.0X6
rat poison	T60.4X1	T60.4X2	T60.4X3	T60.4X4	—	—
Squirting cucumber (cathartic)	T47.2X1	T47.2X2	T47.2X3	T47.2X4	T47.2X5	T47.2X6
Stains	T65.6X1	T65.6X2	T65.6X3	T65.6X4	—	—
Stannous fluoride	T49.7X1	T49.7X2	T49.7X3	T49.7X4	T49.7X5	T49.7X6
Stanolone	T38.7X1	T38.7X2	T38.7X3	T38.7X4	T38.7X5	T38.7X6
Stanozolol	T38.7X1	T38.7X2	T38.7X3	T38.7X4	T38.7X5	T38.7X6

◀ New   ◀▥ Revised   ~~deleted~~ Deleted

Substance	External Cause (T-Code)					
	Poisoning, Accidental (Unintentional)	Poisoning, Intentional Self-Harm	Poisoning, Assault	Poisoning, Undetermined	Adverse Effect	Underdosing
Staphisagria or stavesacre (pediculicide)	T49.0X1	T49.0X2	T49.0X3	T49.0X4	T49.0X5	T49.0X6
Starch	T50.901	T50.902	T50.903	T50.904	T50.905	T50.906
Stelazine	T43.3X1	T43.3X2	T43.3X3	T43.3X4	T43.3X5	T43.3X6
Stemetil	T43.3X1	T43.3X2	T43.3X3	T43.3X4	T43.3X5	T43.3X6
Stepronin	T48.4X1	T48.4X2	T48.4X3	T48.4X4	T48.4X5	T48.4X6
Sterculia	T47.4X1	T47.4X2	T47.4X3	T47.4X4	T47.4X5	T47.4X6
Sternutator gas	T59.891	T59.892	T59.893	T59.894	—	—
Steroid	T38.0X1	T38.0X2	T38.0X3	T38.0X4	T38.0X5	T38.0X6
anabolic	T38.7X1	T38.7X2	T38.7X3	T38.7X4	T38.7X5	T38.7X6
androgenic	T38.7X1	T38.7X2	T38.7X3	T38.7X4	T38.7X5	T38.7X6
antineoplastic, hormone	T38.7X1	T38.7X2	T38.7X3	T38.7X4	T38.7X5	T38.7X6
estrogen	T38.5X1	T38.5X2	T38.5X3	T38.5X4	T38.5X5	T38.5X6
ENT agent	T49.6X1	T49.6X2	T49.6X3	T49.6X4	T49.6X5	T49.6X6
ophthalmic preparation	T49.5X1	T49.5X2	T49.5X3	T49.5X4	T49.5X5	T49.5X6
topical NEC	T49.0X1	T49.0X2	T49.0X3	T49.0X4	T49.0X5	T49.0X6
Stibine	T56.891	T56.892	T56.893	T56.894	—	—
Stibogluconate	T37.3X1	T37.3X2	T37.3X3	T37.3X4	T37.3X5	T37.3X6
Stibophen	T37.4X1	T37.4X2	T37.4X3	T37.4X4	T37.4X5	T37.4X6
Stilbamidine (isetionate)	T37.3X1	T37.3X2	T37.3X3	T37.3X4	T37.3X5	T37.3X6
Stilbestrol	T38.5X1	T38.5X2	T38.5X3	T38.5X4	T38.5X5	T38.5X6
Stilboestrol	T38.5X1	T38.5X2	T38.5X3	T38.5X4	T38.5X5	T38.5X6
Stimulant						
central nervous system — *see also Psychostimulant*	T43.601	T43.602	T43.603	T43.604	T43.605	T43.606
analeptics	T50.7X1	T50.7X2	T50.7X3	T50.7X4	T50.7X5	T50.7X6
opiate antagonist	T50.7X1	T50.7X2	T50.7X3	T50.7X4	T50.7X5	T50.7X6
psychotherapeutic NEC — *see also Psychotherapeutic drug*	T43.601	T43.602	T43.603	T43.604	T43.605	T43.606
specified NEC	T43.691	T43.692	T43.693	T43.694	T43.695	T43.696
respiratory	T48.901	T48.902	T48.903	T48.904	T48.905	T48.906
Stone-dissolving drug	T50.901	T50.902	T50.903	T50.904	T50.905	T50.906
Storage battery (cells) (acid)	T54.2X1	T54.2X2	T54.2X3	T54.2X4	—	—
Stovaine	T41.3X1	T41.3X2	T41.3X3	T41.3X4	T41.3X5	T41.3X6
infiltration (subcutaneous)	T41.3X1	T41.3X2	T41.3X3	T41.3X4	T41.3X5	T41.3X6
nerve block (peripheral) (plexus)	T41.3X1	T41.3X2	T41.3X3	T41.3X4	T41.3X5	T41.3X6
spinal	T41.3X1	T41.3X2	T41.3X3	T41.3X4	T41.3X5	T41.3X6
topical (surface)	T41.3X1	T41.3X2	T41.3X3	T41.3X4	T41.3X5	T41.3X6
Stovarsal	T37.8X1	T37.8X2	T37.8X3	T37.8X4	T37.8X5	T37.8X6
Stove gas — *see Gas, stove*	T57.91	T57.92	T57.93	T57.94	—	—
Stoxil	T49.5X1	T49.5X2	T49.5X3	T49.5X4	T49.5X5	T49.5X6
Stramonium	T48.6X1	T48.6X2	T48.6X3	T48.6X4	T48.6X5	T48.6X6
natural state	T62.2X1	T62.2X2	T62.2X3	T62.2X4	—	—

◀ New   ◀▥ Revised   ~~deleted~~ Deleted

TABLE OF DRUGS AND CHEMICALS

TABLE OF DRUGS AND CHEMICALS

Substance	External Cause (T-Code)					
	Poisoning, Accidental (Unintentional)	Poisoning, Intentional Self-Harm	Poisoning, Assault	Poisoning, Undetermined	Adverse Effect	Underdosing
Streptodornase	T45.3X1	T45.3X2	T45.3X3	T45.3X4	T45.3X5	T45.3X6
Streptoduocin	T36.5X1	T36.5X2	T36.5X3	T36.5X4	T36.5X5	T36.5X6
Streptokinase	T45.611	T45.612	T45.613	T45.614	T45.615	T45.616
Streptomycin (derivative)	T36.5X1	T36.5X2	T36.5X3	T36.5X4	T36.5X5	T36.5X6
Streptonivicin	T36.5X1	T36.5X2	T36.5X3	T36.5X4	T36.5X5	T36.5X6
Streptovarycin	T36.5X1	T36.5X2	T36.5X3	T36.5X4	T36.5X5	T36.5X6
Streptozocin	T45.1X1	T45.1X2	T45.1X3	T45.1X4	T45.1X5	T45.1X6
Streptozotocin	T45.1X1	T45.1X2	T45.1X3	T45.1X4	T45.1X5	T45.1X6
Stripper (paint) (solvent)	T52.8X1	T52.8X2	T52.8X3	T52.8X4	—	—
Strobane	T60.1X1	T60.1X2	T60.1X3	T60.1X4	—	—
Strofantina	T46.0X1	T46.0X2	T46.0X3	T46.0X4	T46.0X5	T46.0X6
Strophanthin (g) (k)	T46.0X1	T46.0X2	T46.0X3	T46.0X4	T46.0X5	T46.0X6
Strophanthus	T46.0X1	T46.0X2	T46.0X3	T46.0X4	T46.0X5	T46.0X6
Strophantin	T46.0X1	T46.0X2	T46.0X3	T46.0X4	T46.0X5	T46.0X6
Strophantin-g	T46.0X1	T46.0X2	T46.0X3	T46.0X4	T46.0X5	T46.0X6
Strychnine (nonmedicinal) (pesticide) (salts)	T65.1X1	T65.1X2	T65.1X3	T65.1X4	—	—
medicinal	T48.291	T48.292	T48.293	T48.294	T48.295	T48.296
Strychnos (ignatii) — see Strychnine						
Styramate	T42.8X1	T42.8X2	T42.8X3	T42.8X4	T42.8X5	T42.8X6
Styrene	T65.891	T65.892	T65.893	T65.894	—	—
Succinimide, antiepileptic or anticonvulsant	T42.2X1	T42.2X2	T42.2X3	T42.2X4	T42.2X5	T42.2X6
mercuric — see Mercury						
Succinylcholine	T48.1X1	T48.1X2	T48.1X3	T48.1X4	T48.1X5	T48.1X6
Succinylsulfathiazole	T37.0X1	T37.0X2	T37.0X3	T37.0X4	T37.0X5	T37.0X6
Sucralfate	T47.1X1	T47.1X2	T47.1X3	T47.1X4	T47.1X5	T47.1X6
Sucrose	T50.3X1	T50.3X2	T50.3X3	T50.3X4	T50.3X5	T50.3X6
Sufentanil	T40.4X1	T40.4X2	T40.4X3	T40.4X4	T40.4X5	T40.4X6
Sulbactam	T36.0X1	T36.0X2	T36.0X3	T36.0X4	T36.0X5	T36.0X6
Sulbenicillin	T36.0X1	T36.0X2	T36.0X3	T36.0X4	T36.0X5	T36.0X6
Sulbentine	T49.0X1	T49.0X2	T49.0X3	T49.0X4	T49.0X5	T49.0X6
Sulfacetamide	T49.0X1	T49.0X2	T49.0X3	T49.0X4	T49.0X5	T49.0X6
ophthalmic preparation	T49.5X1	T49.5X2	T49.5X3	T49.5X4	T49.5X5	T49.5X6
Sulfachlorpyridazine	T37.0X1	T37.0X2	T37.0X3	T37.0X4	T37.0X5	T37.0X6
Sulfacitine	T37.0X1	T37.0X2	T37.0X3	T37.0X4	T37.0X5	T37.0X6
Sulfadiasulfone sodium	T37.0X1	T37.0X2	T37.0X3	T37.0X4	T37.0X5	T37.0X6
Sulfadiazine	T37.0X1	T37.0X2	T37.0X3	T37.0X4	T37.0X5	T37.0X6
silver (topical)	T49.0X1	T49.0X2	T49.0X3	T49.0X4	T49.0X5	T49.0X6
Sulfadimethoxine	T37.0X1	T37.0X2	T37.0X3	T37.0X4	T37.0X5	T37.0X6
Sulfadimidine	T37.0X1	T37.0X2	T37.0X3	T37.0X4	T37.0X5	T37.0X6

◀ New   ◀█ Revised   ~~deleted~~ Deleted

Substance	External Cause (T-Code)					
	Poisoning, Accidental (Unintentional)	Poisoning, Intentional Self-Harm	Poisoning, Assault	Poisoning, Undetermined	Adverse Effect	Underdosing
Sulfadoxine	T37.0X1	T37.0X2	T37.0X3	T37.0X4	T37.0X5	T37.0X6
with pyrimethamine	T37.2X1	T37.2X2	T37.2X3	T37.2X4	T37.2X5	T37.2X6
Sulfaethidole	T37.0X1	T37.0X2	T37.0X3	T37.0X4	T37.0X5	T37.0X6
Sulfafurazole	T37.0X1	T37.0X2	T37.0X3	T37.0X4	T37.0X5	T37.0X6
Sulfaguanidine	T37.0X1	T37.0X2	T37.0X3	T37.0X4	T37.0X5	T37.0X6
Sulfalene	T37.0X1	T37.0X2	T37.0X3	T37.0X4	T37.0X5	T37.0X6
Sulfaloxate	T37.0X1	T37.0X2	T37.0X3	T37.0X4	T37.0X5	T37.0X6
Sulfaloxic acid	T37.0X1	T37.0X2	T37.0X3	T37.0X4	T37.0X5	T37.0X6
Sulfamazone	T39.2X1	T39.2X2	T39.2X3	T39.2X4	T39.2X5	T39.2X6
Sulfamerazine	T37.0X1	T37.0X2	T37.0X3	T37.0X4	T37.0X5	T37.0X6
Sulfameter	T37.0X1	T37.0X2	T37.0X3	T37.0X4	T37.0X5	T37.0X6
Sulfamethazine	T37.0X1	T37.0X2	T37.0X3	T37.0X4	T37.0X5	T37.0X6
Sulfamethizole	T37.0X1	T37.0X2	T37.0X3	T37.0X4	T37.0X5	T37.0X6
Sulfamethoxazole	T37.0X1	T37.0X2	T37.0X3	T37.0X4	T37.0X5	T37.0X6
with trimethoprim	T36.8X1	T36.8X2	T36.8X3	T36.8X4	T36.8X5	T36.8X6
Sulfamethoxydiazine	T37.0X1	T37.0X2	T37.0X3	T37.0X4	T37.0X5	T37.0X6
Sulfamethoxypyridazine	T37.0X1	T37.0X2	T37.0X3	T37.0X4	T37.0X5	T37.0X6
Sulfamethylthiazole	T37.0X1	T37.0X2	T37.0X3	T37.0X4	T37.0X5	T37.0X6
Sulfametoxydiazine	T37.0X1	T37.0X2	T37.0X3	T37.0X4	T37.0X5	T37.0X6
Sulfamidopyrine	T39.2X1	T39.2X2	T39.2X3	T39.2X4	T39.2X5	T39.2X6
Sulfamonomethoxine	T37.0X1	T37.0X2	T37.0X3	T37.0X4	T37.0X5	T37.0X6
Sulfamoxole	T37.0X1	T37.0X2	T37.0X3	T37.0X4	T37.0X5	T37.0X6
Sulfamylon	T49.0X1	T49.0X2	T49.0X3	T49.0X4	T49.0X5	T49.0X6
Sulfan blue (diagnostic dye)	T50.8X1	T50.8X2	T50.8X3	T50.8X4	T50.8X5	T50.8X6
Sulfanilamide	T37.0X1	T37.0X2	T37.0X3	T37.0X4	T37.0X5	T37.0X6
Sulfanilylguanidine	T37.0X1	T37.0X2	T37.0X3	T37.0X4	T37.0X5	T37.0X6
Sulfaperin	T37.0X1	T37.0X2	T37.0X3	T37.0X4	T37.0X5	T37.0X6
Sulfaphenazole	T37.0X1	T37.0X2	T37.0X3	T37.0X4	T37.0X5	T37.0X6
Sulfaphenylthiazole	T37.0X1	T37.0X2	T37.0X3	T37.0X4	T37.0X5	T37.0X6
Sulfaproxyline	T37.0X1	T37.0X2	T37.0X3	T37.0X4	T37.0X5	T37.0X6
Sulfapyridine	T37.0X1	T37.0X2	T37.0X3	T37.0X4	T37.0X5	T37.0X6
Sulfapyrimidine	T37.0X1	T37.0X2	T37.0X3	T37.0X4	T37.0X5	T37.0X6
Sulfarsphenamine	T37.8X1	T37.8X2	T37.8X3	T37.8X4	T37.8X5	T37.8X6
Sulfasalazine	T37.0X1	T37.0X2	T37.0X3	T37.0X4	T37.0X5	T37.0X6
Sulfasuxidine	T37.0X1	T37.0X2	T37.0X3	T37.0X4	T37.0X5	T37.0X6
Sulfasymazine	T37.0X1	T37.0X2	T37.0X3	T37.0X4	T37.0X5	T37.0X6
Sulfated amylopectin	T47.8X1	T47.8X2	T47.8X3	T47.8X4	T47.8X5	T47.8X6
Sulfathiazole	T37.0X1	T37.0X2	T37.0X3	T37.0X4	T37.0X5	T37.0X6
Sulfatostearate	T49.2X1	T49.2X2	T49.2X3	T49.2X4	T49.2X5	T49.2X6

◀ New ◀ Revised deleted Deleted

Substance	Poisoning, Accidental (Unintentional)	Poisoning, Intentional Self-Harm	Poisoning, Assault	Poisoning, Undetermined	Adverse Effect	Underdosing
Sulfinpyrazone	T50.4X1	T50.4X2	T50.4X3	T50.4X4	T50.4X5	T50.4X6
Sulfiram	T49.0X1	T49.0X2	T49.0X3	T49.0X4	T49.0X5	T49.0X6
Sulfisomidine	T37.0X1	T37.0X2	T37.0X3	T37.0X4	T37.0X5	T37.0X6
Sulfisoxazole	T37.0X1	T37.0X2	T37.0X3	T37.0X4	T37.0X5	T37.0X6
ophthalmic preparation	T49.5X1	T49.5X2	T49.5X3	T49.5X4	T49.5X5	T49.5X6
Sulfobromophthalein (sodium)	T50.8X1	T50.8X2	T50.8X3	T50.8X4	T50.8X5	T50.8X6
Sulfobromphthalein	T50.8X1	T50.8X2	T50.8X3	T50.8X4	T50.8X5	T50.8X6
Sulfogaiacol	T48.4X1	T48.4X2	T48.4X3	T48.4X4	T48.4X5	T48.4X6
Sulfomyxin	T36.8X1	T36.8X2	T36.8X3	T36.8X4	T36.8X5	T36.8X6
Sulfonal	T42.6X1	T42.6X2	T42.6X3	T42.6X4	T42.6X5	T42.6X6
Sulfonamide NEC	T37.0X1	T37.0X2	T37.0X3	T37.0X4	T37.0X5	T37.0X6
eye	T49.5X1	T49.5X2	T49.5X3	T49.5X4	T49.5X5	T49.5X6
Sulfonazide	T37.1X1	T37.1X2	T37.1X3	T37.1X4	T37.1X5	T37.1X6
Sulfones	T37.1X1	T37.1X2	T37.1X3	T37.1X4	T37.1X5	T37.1X6
Sulfonethylmethane	T42.6X1	T42.6X2	T42.6X3	T42.6X4	T42.6X5	T42.6X6
Sulfonmethane	T42.6X1	T42.6X2	T42.6X3	T42.6X4	T42.6X5	T42.6X6
Sulfonphthal, sulfonphthol	T50.8X1	T50.8X2	T50.8X3	T50.8X4	T50.8X5	T50.8X6
Sulfonylurea derivatives, oral	T38.3X1	T38.3X2	T38.3X3	T38.3X4	T38.3X5	T38.3X6
Sulforidazine	T43.3X1	T43.3X2	T43.3X3	T43.3X4	T43.3X5	T43.3X6
Sulfoxone	T37.1X1	T37.1X2	T37.1X3	T37.1X4	T37.1X5	T37.1X6
Sulfur, sulfurated, sulfuric, sulfurous, sulfuryl (compounds NEC) (medicinal)	T49.4X1	T49.4X2	T49.4X3	T49.4X4	T49.4X5	T49.4X6
acid	T54.2X1	T54.2X2	T54.2X3	T54.2X4	—	—
dioxide (gas)	T59.1X1	T59.1X2	T59.1X3	T59.1X4	—	—
ether — see Ether(s)						
hydrogen	T59.6X1	T59.6X2	T59.6X3	T59.6X4	—	—
medicinal (keratolytic) (ointment) NEC	T49.4X1	T49.4X2	T49.4X3	T49.4X4	T49.4X5	T49.4X6
ointment	T49.0X1	T49.0X2	T49.0X3	T49.0X4	T49.0X5	T49.0X6
pesticide (vapor)	T60.91	T60.92	T60.93	T60.94	—	—
vapor NEC	T59.891	T59.892	T59.893	T59.894	—	—
Sulfuric acid	T54.2X1	T54.2X2	T54.2X3	T54.2X4	—	—
Sulglicotide	T47.1X1	T47.1X2	T47.1X3	T47.1X4	T47.1X5	T47.1X6
Sulindac	T39.391	T39.392	T39.393	T39.394	T39.395	T39.396
Sulisatin	T47.2X1	T47.2X2	T47.2X3	T47.2X4	T47.2X5	T47.2X6
Sulisobenzone	T49.3X1	T49.3X2	T49.3X3	T49.3X4	T49.3X5	T49.3X6
Sulkowitch's reagent	T50.8X1	T50.8X2	T50.8X3	T50.8X4	T50.8X5	T50.8X6
Sulmetozine	T44.3X1	T44.3X2	T44.3X3	T44.3X4	T44.3X5	T44.3X6
Suloctidil	T46.7X1	T46.7X2	T46.7X3	T46.7X4	T46.7X5	T46.7X6
Sulph — see also Sulf-						
Sulphadiazine	T37.0X1	T37.0X2	T37.0X3	T37.0X4	T37.0X5	T37.0X6
Sulphadimethoxine	T37.0X1	T37.0X2	T37.0X3	T37.0X4	T37.0X5	T37.0X6

◀ New   ◀‖‖ Revised   ~~deleted~~ Deleted

Substance	Poisoning, Accidental (Unintentional)	Poisoning, Intentional Self-Harm	Poisoning, Assault	Poisoning, Undetermined	Adverse Effect	Underdosing
			External Cause (T-Code)			
Sulphadimidine	T37.0X1	T37.0X2	T37.0X3	T37.0X4	T37.0X5	T37.0X6
Sulphadione	T37.1X1	T37.1X2	T37.1X3	T37.1X4	T37.1X5	T37.1X6
Sulphafurazole	T37.0X1	T37.0X2	T37.0X3	T37.0X4	T37.0X5	T37.0X6
Sulphamethizole	T37.0X1	T37.0X2	T37.0X3	T37.0X4	T37.0X5	T37.0X6
Sulphamethoxazole	T37.0X1	T37.0X2	T37.0X3	T37.0X4	T37.0X5	T37.0X6
Sulphan blue	T50.8X1	T50.8X2	T50.8X3	T50.8X4	T50.8X5	T50.8X6
Sulphaphenazole	T37.0X1	T37.0X2	T37.0X3	T37.0X4	T37.0X5	T37.0X6
Sulphapyridine	T37.0X1	T37.0X2	T37.0X3	T37.0X4	T37.0X5	T37.0X6
Sulphasalazine	T37.0X1	T37.0X2	T37.0X3	T37.0X4	T37.0X5	T37.0X6
Sulphinpyrazone	T50.4X1	T50.4X2	T50.4X3	T50.4X4	T50.4X5	T50.4X6
Sulpiride	T43.591	T43.592	T43.593	T43.594	T43.595	T43.596
Sulprostone	T48.0X1	T48.0X2	T48.0X3	T48.0X4	T48.0X5	T48.0X6
Sulpyrine	T39.2X1	T39.2X2	T39.2X3	T39.2X4	T39.2X5	T39.2X6
Sultamicillin	T36.0X1	T36.0X2	T36.0X3	T36.0X4	T36.0X5	T36.0X6
Sulthiame	T42.6X1	T42.6X2	T42.6X3	T42.6X4	T42.6X5	T42.6X6
Sultiame	T42.6X1	T42.6X2	T42.6X3	T42.6X4	T42.6X5	T42.6X6
Sultopride	T43.591	T43.592	T43.593	T43.594	T43.595	T43.596
Sumatriptan	T39.8X1	T39.8X2	T39.8X3	T39.8X4	T39.8X5	T39.8X6
Sunflower seed oil	T46.6X1	T46.6X2	T46.6X3	T46.6X4	T46.6X5	T46.6X6
Superinone	T48.4X1	T48.4X2	T48.4X3	T48.4X4	T48.4X5	T48.4X6
Suprofen	T39.311	T39.312	T39.313	T39.314	T39.315	T39.316
Suramin (sodium)	T37.4X1	T37.4X2	T37.4X3	T37.4X4	T37.4X5	T37.4X6
Surfacaine	T41.3X1	T41.3X2	T41.3X3	T41.3X4	T41.3X5	T41.3X6
Surital	T41.1X1	T41.1X2	T41.1X3	T41.1X4	T41.1X5	T41.1X6
Sutilains	T45.3X1	T45.3X2	T45.3X3	T45.3X4	T45.3X5	T45.3X6
Suxamethonium (chloride)	T48.1X1	T48.1X2	T48.1X3	T48.1X4	T48.1X5	T48.1X6
Suxethonium (chloride)	T48.1X1	T48.1X2	T48.1X3	T48.1X4	T48.1X5	T48.1X6
Suxibuzone	T39.2X1	T39.2X2	T39.2X3	T39.2X4	T39.2X5	T39.2X6
Sweet oil (birch)	T49.3X1	T49.3X2	T49.3X3	T49.3X4	T49.3X5	T49.3X6
Sweet niter spirit	T46.3X1	T46.3X2	T46.3X3	T46.3X4	T46.3X5	T46.3X6
Sweetener	T50.901	T50.902	T50.903	T50.904	T50.905	T50.906
Sym-dichloroethyl ether	T53.6X1	T53.6X2	T53.6X3	T53.6X4	—	—
Sympatholytic NEC	T44.8X1	T44.8X2	T44.8X3	T44.8X4	T44.8X5	T44.8X6
haloalkylamine	T44.8X1	T44.8X2	T44.8X3	T44.8X4	T44.8X5	T44.8X6
Sympathomimetic NEC	T44.901	T44.902	T44.903	T44.904	T44.905	T44.906
anti-common-cold	T48.5X1	T48.5X2	T48.5X3	T48.5X4	T48.5X5	T48.5X6
bronchodilator	T48.6X1	T48.6X2	T48.6X3	T48.6X4	T48.6X5	T48.6X6
specified NEC	T44.991	T44.992	T44.993	T44.994	T44.995	T44.996
Synagis	T50.B91	T50.B92	T50.B93	T50.B94	T50.B95	T50.B96
Synalar	T49.0X1	T49.0X2	T49.0X3	T49.0X4	T49.0X5	T49.0X6

TABLE OF DRUGS AND CHEMICALS

◀ New   ◀ Revised   ~~deleted~~ Deleted

TABLE OF DRUGS AND CHEMICALS

Substance	Poisoning, Accidental (Unintentional)	Poisoning, Intentional Self-Harm	Poisoning, Assault	Poisoning, Undetermined	Adverse Effect	Underdosing
Synthroid	T38.1X1	T38.1X2	T38.1X3	T38.1X4	T38.1X5	T38.1X6
Syntocinon	T48.0X1	T48.0X2	T48.0X3	T48.0X4	T48.0X5	T48.0X6
Syrosingopine	T46.5X1	T46.5X2	T46.5X3	T46.5X4	T46.5X5	T46.5X6
Systemic drug	T45.91	T45.92	T45.93	T45.94	T45.95	T45.96
specified NEC	T45.8X1	T45.8X2	T45.8X3	T45.8X4	T45.8X5	T45.8X6
2,4,5-T	T60.3X1	T60.3X2	T60.3X3	T60.3X4	—	—
T						
Tablets — *see also specified substance*	T50.901	T50.902	T50.903	T50.904	T50.905	T50.906
Tace	T38.5X1	T38.5X2	T38.5X3	T38.5X4	T38.5X5	T38.5X6
Tacrine	T44.0X1	T44.0X2	T44.0X3	T44.0X4	T44.0X5	T44.0X6
Tadalafil	T46.7X1	T46.7X2	T46.7X3	T46.7X4	T46.7X5	T46.7X6
Talampicillin	T36.0X1	T36.0X2	T36.0X3	T36.0X4	T36.0X5	T36.0X6
Talbutal	T42.3X1	T42.3X2	T42.3X3	T42.3X4	T42.3X5	T42.3X6
Talc powder	T49.3X1	T49.3X2	T49.3X3	T49.3X4	T49.3X5	T49.3X6
Talcum	T49.3X1	T49.3X2	T49.3X3	T49.3X4	T49.3X5	T49.3X6
Taleranol	T38.6X1	T38.6X2	T38.6X3	T38.6X4	T38.6X5	T38.6X6
Tamoxifen	T38.6X1	T38.6X2	T38.6X3	T38.6X4	T38.6X5	T38.6X6
Tamsulosin	T44.6X1	T44.6X2	T44.6X3	T44.6X4	T44.6X5	T44.6X6
Tandearil, tanderil	T39.2X1	T39.2X2	T39.2X3	T39.2X4	T39.2X5	T39.2X6
Tannic acid	T49.2X1	T49.2X2	T49.2X3	T49.2X4	T49.2X5	T49.2X6
medicinal (astringent)	T49.2X1	T49.2X2	T49.2X3	T49.2X4	T49.2X5	T49.2X6
Tannin — *see Tannic acid*						
Tansy	T62.2X1	T62.2X2	T62.2X3	T62.2X4	—	—
TAO	T36.3X1	T36.3X2	T36.3X3	T36.3X4	T36.3X5	T36.3X6
Tapazole	T38.2X1	T38.2X2	T38.2X3	T38.2X4	T38.2X5	T38.2X6
Tar NEC	T52.0X1	T52.0X2	T52.0X3	T52.0X4	—	—
camphor	T60.1X1	T60.1X2	T60.1X3	T60.1X4	—	—
distillate	T49.1X1	T49.1X2	T49.1X3	T49.1X4	T49.1X5	T49.1X6
fumes	T59.891	T59.892	T59.893	T59.894	—	—
medicinal	T49.1X1	T49.1X2	T49.1X3	T49.1X4	T49.1X5	T49.1X6
ointment	T49.1X1	T49.1X2	T49.1X3	T49.1X4	T49.1X5	T49.1X6
Taractan	T43.591	T43.592	T43.593	T43.594	T43.595	T43.596
Tarantula (venomous)	T63.321	T63.322	T63.323	T63.324	—	—
Tartar emetic	T37.8X1	T37.8X2	T37.8X3	T37.8X4	T37.8X5	T37.8X6
Tartaric acid	T65.891	T65.892	T65.893	T65.894	—	—
Tartrated antimony (anti-infective)	T37.8X1	T37.8X2	T37.8X3	T37.8X4	T37.8X5	T37.8X6
Tartrate, laxative	T47.4X1	T47.4X2	T47.4X3	T47.4X4	T47.4X5	T47.4X6
Tauromustine	T45.1X1	T45.1X2	T45.1X3	T45.1X4	T45.1X5	T45.1X6
TCA — *see Trichloroacetic acid*						

◀ New   ◀▦ Revised   ~~deleted~~ Deleted

Substance	External Cause (T-Code)					
	Poisoning, Accidental (Unintentional)	Poisoning, Intentional Self-Harm	Poisoning, Assault	Poisoning, Undetermined	Adverse Effect	Underdosing
TCDD	T53.7X1	T53.7X2	T53.7X3	T53.7X4	—	—
TDI (vapor)	T65.0X1	T65.0X2	T65.0X3	T65.0X4	—	—
Tear						
gas	T59.3X1	T59.3X2	T59.3X3	T59.3X4	—	—
solution	T49.5X1	T49.5X2	T49.5X3	T49.5X4	T49.5X5	T49.5X6
Teclothiazide	T50.2X1	T50.2X2	T50.2X3	T50.2X4	T50.2X5	T50.2X6
Teclozan	T37.3X1	T37.3X2	T37.3X3	T37.3X4	T37.3X5	T37.3X6
Tegafur	T45.1X1	T45.1X2	T45.1X3	T45.1X4	T45.1X5	T45.1X6
Tegretol	T42.1X1	T42.1X2	T42.1X3	T42.1X4	T42.1X5	T42.1X6
Teicoplanin	T36.8X1	T36.8X2	T36.8X3	T36.8X4	T36.8X5	T36.8X6
Telepaque	T50.8X1	T50.8X2	T50.8X3	T50.8X4	T50.8X5	T50.8X6
Tellurium	T56.891	T56.892	T56.893	T56.894	—	—
fumes	T56.891	T56.892	T56.893	T56.894	—	—
TEM	T45.1X1	T45.1X2	T45.1X3	T45.1X4	T45.1X5	T45.1X6
Temazepam	T42.4X1	T42.4X2	T42.4X3	T42.4X4	T42.4X5	T42.4X6
Temocillin	T36.0X1	T36.0X2	T36.0X3	T36.0X4	T36.0X5	T36.0X6
Tenamfetamine	T43.621	T43.622	T43.623	T43.624	T43.625	T43.626
Teniposide	T45.1X1	T45.1X2	T45.1X3	T45.1X4	T45.1X5	T45.1X6
Tenitramine	T46.3X1	T46.3X2	T46.3X3	T46.3X4	T46.3X5	T46.3X6
Tenoglicin	T48.4X1	T48.4X2	T48.4X3	T48.4X4	T48.4X5	T48.4X6
Tenonitrozole	T37.3X1	T37.3X2	T37.3X3	T37.3X4	T37.3X5	T37.3X6
Tenoxicam	T39.391	T39.392	T39.393	T39.394	T39.395	T39.396
TEPA	T45.1X1	T45.1X2	T45.1X3	T45.1X4	T45.1X5	T45.1X6
TEPP	T60.0X1	T60.0X2	T60.0X3	T60.0X4	—	—
Teprotide	T46.5X1	T46.5X2	T46.5X3	T46.5X4	T46.5X5	T46.5X6
Terazosin	T44.6X1	T44.6X2	T44.6X3	T44.6X4	T44.6X5	T44.6X6
Terbufos	T60.0X1	T60.0X2	T60.0X3	T60.0X4	—	—
Terbutaline	T48.6X1	T48.6X2	T48.6X3	T48.6X4	T48.6X5	T48.6X6
Terconazole	T49.0X1	T49.0X2	T49.0X3	T49.0X4	T49.0X5	T49.0X6
Terfenadine	T45.0X1	T45.0X2	T45.0X3	T45.0X4	T45.0X5	T45.0X6
Teriparatide (acetate)	T50.991	T50.992	T50.993	T50.994	T50.995	T50.996
Terizidone	T37.1X1	T37.1X2	T37.1X3	T37.1X4	T37.1X5	T37.1X6
Terlipressin	T38.891	T38.892	T38.893	T38.894	T38.895	T38.896
Terodiline	T46.3X1	T46.3X2	T46.3X3	T46.3X4	T46.3X5	T46.3X6
Teroxalene	T37.4X1	T37.4X2	T37.4X3	T37.4X4	T37.4X5	T37.4X6
Terpin(cis) hydrate	T48.4X1	T48.4X2	T48.4X3	T48.4X4	T48.4X5	T48.4X6
Terramycin	T36.4X1	T36.4X2	T36.4X3	T36.4X4	T36.4X5	T36.4X6
Tertatolol	T44.7X1	T44.7X2	T44.7X3	T44.7X4	T44.7X5	T44.7X6
Tessalon	T48.3X1	T48.3X2	T48.3X3	T48.3X4	T48.3X5	T48.3X6
Testolactone	T38.7X1	T38.7X2	T38.7X3	T38.7X4	T38.7X5	T38.7X6

◀ New   ◀▥ Revised   ~~deleted~~ Deleted

TABLE OF DRUGS AND CHEMICALS

Substance	External Cause (T-Code)					
	Poisoning, Accidental (Unintentional)	Poisoning, Intentional Self-Harm	Poisoning, Assault	Poisoning, Undetermined	Adverse Effect	Underdosing
Testosterone	T38.7X1	T38.7X2	T38.7X3	T38.7X4	T38.7X5	T38.7X6
Tetanus toxoid or vaccine	T50.A91	T50.A92	T50.A93	T50.A94	T50.A95	T50.A96
antitoxin	T50.Z11	T50.Z12	T50.Z13	T50.Z14	T50.Z15	T50.Z16
immune globulin (human)	T50.Z11	T50.Z12	T50.Z13	T50.Z14	T50.Z15	T50.Z16
toxoid	T50.A91	T50.A92	T50.A93	T50.A94	T50.A95	T50.A96
with diphtheria toxoid	T50.A21	T50.A22	T50.A23	T50.A24	T50.A25	T50.A26
with pertussis	T50.A11	T50.A12	T50.A13	T50.A14	T50.A15	T50.A16
Tetrabenazine	T43.591	T43.592	T43.593	T43.594	T43.595	T43.596
Tetracaine	T41.3X1	T41.3X2	T41.3X3	T41.3X4	T41.3X5	T41.3X6
nerve block (peripheral) (plexus)	T41.3X1	T41.3X2	T41.3X3	T41.3X4	T41.3X5	T41.3X6
regional	T41.3X1	T41.3X2	T41.3X3	T41.3X4	T41.3X5	T41.3X6
spinal	T41.3X1	T41.3X2	T41.3X3	T41.3X4	T41.3X5	T41.3X6
Tetrachlorethylene — see Tetrachloroethylene						
Tetrachlormethiazide	T50.2X1	T50.2X2	T50.2X3	T50.2X4	T50.2X5	T50.2X6
2,3,7,8-Tetrachlorodibenzo-p-dioxin	T53.7X1	T53.7X2	T53.7X3	T53.7X4	—	—
Tetrachloroethane	T53.6X1	T53.6X2	T53.6X3	T53.6X4	—	—
vapor	T53.6X1	T53.6X2	T53.6X3	T53.6X4	—	—
paint or varnish	T53.6X1	T53.6X2	T53.6X3	T53.6X4	—	—
Tetrachloroethylene (liquid)	T53.3X1	T53.3X2	T53.3X3	T53.3X4	—	—
medicinal	T37.4X1	T37.4X2	T37.4X3	T37.4X4	T37.4X5	T37.4X6
vapor	T53.3X1	T53.3X2	T53.3X3	T53.3X4	—	—
Tetrachloromethane — see Carbon tetrachloride						
Tetracosactide	T38.811	T38.812	T38.813	T38.814	T38.815	T38.816
Tetracosactrin	T38.811	T38.812	T38.813	T38.814	T38.815	T38.816
Tetracycline	T36.4X1	T36.4X2	T36.4X3	T36.4X4	T36.4X5	T36.4X6
ophthalmic preparation	T49.5X1	T49.5X2	T49.5X3	T49.5X4	T49.5X5	T49.5X6
topical NEC	T49.0X1	T49.0X2	T49.0X3	T49.0X4	T49.0X5	T49.0X6
Tetradifon	T60.8X1	T60.8X2	T60.8X3	T60.8X4	—	—
Tetradotoxin	T61.771	T61.772	T61.773	T61.774	—	—
Tetraethyl						
lead	T56.0X1	T56.0X2	T56.0X3	T56.0X4	—	—
pyrophosphate	T60.0X1	T60.0X2	T60.0X3	T60.0X4	—	—
Tetraethylammonium chloride	T44.2X1	T44.2X2	T44.2X3	T44.2X4	T44.2X5	T44.2X6
Tetraethylthiuram disulfide	T50.6X1	T50.6X2	T50.6X3	T50.6X4	T50.6X5	T50.6X6
Tetrahydroaminoacridine	T44.0X1	T44.0X2	T44.0X3	T44.0X4	T44.0X5	T44.0X6
Tetrahydrocannabinol	T40.7X1	T40.7X2	T40.7X3	T40.7X4	T40.7X5	T40.7X6
Tetrahydrofuran	T52.8X1	T52.8X2	T52.8X3	T52.8X4	—	—
Tetrahydronaphthalene	T52.8X1	T52.8X2	T52.8X3	T52.8X4	—	—
Tetrahydrozoline	T49.5X1	T49.5X2	T49.5X3	T49.5X4	T49.5X5	T49.5X6
Tetralin	T52.8X1	T52.8X2	T52.8X3	T52.8X4	—	—

◀ New   ◀▥ Revised   ~~deleted~~ Deleted

Substance	External Cause (T-Code)					
	Poisoning, Accidental (Unintentional)	Poisoning, Intentional Self-Harm	Poisoning, Assault	Poisoning, Undetermined	Adverse Effect	Underdosing
Tetramethrin	T60.2X1	T60.2X2	T60.2X3	T60.2X4	—	—
Tetramethylthiuram (disulfide) NEC	T60.3X1	T60.3X2	T60.3X3	T60.3X4	—	—
medicinal	T49.0X1	T49.0X2	T49.0X3	T49.0X4	T49.0X5	T49.0X6
Tetramisole	T37.4X1	T37.4X2	T37.4X3	T37.4X4	T37.4X5	T37.4X6
Tetranicotinoyl fructose	T46.7X1	T46.7X2	T46.7X3	T46.7X4	T46.7X5	T46.7X6
Tetronal	T42.6X1	T42.6X2	T42.6X3	T42.6X4	T42.6X5	T42.6X6
Tetrazepam	T42.4X1	T42.4X2	T42.4X3	T42.4X4	T42.4X5	T42.4X6
Tetryl	T65.3X1	T65.3X2	T65.3X3	T65.3X4	—	—
Tetrylammonium chloride	T44.2X1	T44.2X2	T44.2X3	T44.2X4	T44.2X5	T44.2X6
Tetryzoline	T49.5X1	T49.5X2	T49.5X3	T49.5X4	T49.5X5	T49.5X6
Thalidomide	T45.1X1	T45.1X2	T45.1X3	T45.1X4	T45.1X5	T45.1X6
Thallium (compounds) (dust) NEC	T56.811	T56.812	T56.813	T56.814	—	—
pesticide	T60.4X1	T60.4X2	T60.4X3	T60.4X4	—	—
THC	T40.7X1	T40.7X2	T40.7X3	T40.7X4	T40.7X5	T40.7X6
Thebacon	T48.3X1	T48.3X2	T48.3X3	T48.3X4	T48.3X5	T48.3X6
Thebaine	T40.2X1	T40.2X2	T40.2X3	T40.2X4	T40.2X5	T40.2X6
Thenoic acid	T49.6X1	T49.6X2	T49.6X3	T49.6X4	T49.6X5	T49.6X6
Thenyldiamine	T45.0X1	T45.0X2	T45.0X3	T45.0X4	T45.0X5	T45.0X6
Theobromine (calcium salicylate)	T48.6X1	T48.6X2	T48.6X3	T48.6X4	T48.6X5	T48.6X6
sodium salicylate	T48.6X1	T48.6X2	T48.6X3	T48.6X4	T48.6X5	T48.6X6
Theophyllamine	T48.6X1	T48.6X2	T48.6X3	T48.6X4	T48.6X5	T48.6X6
Theophylline	T48.6X1	T48.6X2	T48.6X3	T48.6X4	T48.6X5	T48.6X6
aminobenzoic acid	T48.6X1	T48.6X2	T48.6X3	T48.6X4	T48.6X5	T48.6X6
ethylenediamine	T48.6X1	T48.6X2	T48.6X3	T48.6X4	T48.6X5	T48.6X6
piperazine p-amino-benzoate	T48.6X1	T48.6X2	T48.6X3	T48.6X4	T48.6X5	T48.6X6
Thiabendazole	T37.4X1	T37.4X2	T37.4X3	T37.4X4	T37.4X5	T37.4X6
Thialbarbital	T41.1X1	T41.1X2	T41.1X3	T41.1X4	T41.1X5	T41.1X6
Thiamazole	T38.2X1	T38.2X2	T38.2X3	T38.2X4	T38.2X5	T38.2X6
Thiambutosine	T37.1X1	T37.1X2	T37.1X3	T37.1X4	T37.1X5	T37.1X6
Thiamine	T45.2X1	T45.2X2	T45.2X3	T45.2X4	T45.2X5	T45.2X6
Thiamphenicol	T36.2X1	T36.2X2	T36.2X3	T36.2X4	T36.2X5	T36.2X6
Thiamylal	T41.1X1	T41.1X2	T41.1X3	T41.1X4	T41.1X5	T41.1X6
sodium	T41.1X1	T41.1X2	T41.1X3	T41.1X4	T41.1X5	T41.1X6
Thiazesim	T43.291	T43.292	T43.293	T43.294	T43.295	T43.296
Thiazides (diuretics)	T50.2X1	T50.2X2	T50.2X3	T50.2X4	T50.2X5	T50.2X6
Thiazinamium metilsulfate	T43.3X1	T43.3X2	T43.3X4	T43.3X4	T43.3X5	T43.3X6
Thiethylperazine	T43.3X1	T43.3X2	T43.3X3	T43.3X4	T43.3X5	T43.3X6
Thimerosal	T49.0X1	T49.0X2	T49.0X3	T49.0X4	T49.0X5	T49.0X6
ophthalmic preparation	T49.5X1	T49.5X2	T49.5X3	T49.5X4	T49.5X5	T49.5X6

◀ New   ◀▮▮ Revised   ~~deleted~~ Deleted

Substance	External Cause (T-Code)					
	Poisoning, Accidental (Unintentional)	Poisoning, Intentional Self-Harm	Poisoning, Assault	Poisoning, Undetermined	Adverse Effect	Underdosing
Thioacetazone	T37.1X1	T37.1X2	T37.1X3	T37.1X4	T37.1X5	T37.1X6
with isoniazid	T37.1X1	T37.1X2	T37.1X3	T37.1X4	T37.1X5	T37.1X6
Thiobarbital sodium	T41.1X1	T41.1X2	T41.1X3	T41.1X4	T41.1X5	T41.1X6
Thiobarbiturate anesthetic	T41.1X1	T41.1X2	T41.1X3	T41.1X4	T41.1X5	T41.1X6
Thiobismol	T37.8X1	T37.8X2	T37.8X3	T37.8X4	T37.8X5	T37.8X6
Thiobutabarbital sodium	T41.1X1	T41.1X2	T41.1X3	T41.1X4	T41.1X5	T41.1X6
Thiocarbamate (insecticide)	T60.0X1	T60.0X2	T60.0X3	T60.0X4	—	—
Thiocarbamide	T38.2X1	T38.2X2	T38.2X3	T38.2X4	T38.2X5	T38.2X6
Thiocarbarsone	T37.8X1	T37.8X2	T37.8X3	T37.8X4	T37.8X5	T37.8X6
Thiocarlide	T37.1X1	T37.1X2	T37.1X3	T37.1X4	T37.1X5	T37.1X6
Thioctamide	T50.991	T50.992	T50.993	T50.994	T50.995	T50.996
Thioctic acid	T50.991	T50.992	T50.993	T50.994	T50.995	T50.996
Thiofos	T60.0X1	T60.0X2	T60.0X3	T60.0X4	—	—
Thioglycolate	T49.4X1	T49.4X2	T49.4X3	T49.4X4	T49.4X5	T49.4X6
Thioglycolic acid	T65.891	T65.892	T65.893	T65.894	—	—
Thioguanine	T45.1X1	T45.1X2	T45.1X3	T45.1X4	T45.1X5	T45.1X6
Thiomercaptomerin	T50.2X1	T50.2X2	T50.2X3	T50.2X4	T50.2X5	T50.2X6
Thiomerin	T50.2X1	T50.2X2	T50.2X3	T50.2X4	T50.2X5	T50.2X6
Thiomersal	T49.0X1	T49.0X2	T49.0X3	T49.0X4	T49.0X5	T49.0X6
Thionazin	T60.0X1	T60.0X2	T60.0X3	T60.0X4	—	—
Thiopental (sodium)	T41.1X1	T41.1X2	T41.1X3	T41.1X4	T41.1X5	T41.1X6
Thiopentone (sodium)	T41.1X1	T41.1X2	T41.1X3	T41.1X4	T41.1X5	T41.1X6
Thiopropazate	T43.3X1	T43.3X2	T43.3X3	T43.3X4	T43.3X5	T43.3X6
Thioproperazine	T43.3X1	T43.3X2	T43.3X3	T43.3X4	T43.3X5	T43.3X6
Thioridazine	T43.3X1	T43.3X2	T43.3X3	T43.3X4	T43.3X5	T43.3X6
Thiosinamine	T49.3X1	T49.3X2	T49.3X3	T49.3X4	T49.3X5	T49.3X6
Thiotepa	T45.1X1	T45.1X2	T45.1X3	T45.1X4	T45.1X5	T45.1X6
Thiothixene	T43.4X1	T43.4X2	T43.4X3	T43.4X4	T43.4X5	T43.4X6
Thiouracil (benzyl) (methyl) (propyl)	T38.2X1	T38.2X2	T38.2X3	T38.2X4	T38.2X5	T38.2X6
Thiourea	T38.2X1	T38.2X2	T38.2X3	T38.2X4	T38.2X5	T38.2X6
Thiphenamil	T44.3X1	T44.3X2	T44.3X3	T44.3X4	T44.3X5	T44.3X6
Thiram	T60.3X1	T60.3X2	T60.3X3	T60.3X4	—	—
medicinal	T49.2X1	T49.2X2	T49.2X3	T49.2X4	T49.2X5	T49.2X6
Thonzylamine (systemic)	T45.0X1	T45.0X2	T45.0X3	T45.0X4	T45.0X5	T45.0X6
mucosal decongestant	T48.5X1	T48.5X2	T48.5X3	T48.5X4	T48.5X5	T48.5X6
Thorazine	T43.3X1	T43.3X2	T43.3X3	T43.3X4	T43.3X5	T43.3X6
Thorium dioxide suspension	T50.8X1	T50.8X2	T50.8X3	T50.8X4	T50.8X5	T50.8X6
Thornapple	T62.2X1	T62.2X2	T62.2X3	T62.2X4	—	—
Throat drug NEC	T49.6X1	T49.6X2	T49.6X3	T49.6X4	T49.6X5	T49.6X6
Thrombin	T45.7X1	T45.7X2	T45.7X3	T45.7X4	T45.7X5	T45.7X6

◀ New ◀▥▥ Revised ~~deleted~~ Deleted

Substance	External Cause (T-Code)					
	Poisoning, Accidental (Unintentional)	Poisoning, Intentional Self-Harm	Poisoning, Assault	Poisoning, Undetermined	Adverse Effect	Underdosing
Thrombolysin	T45.611	T45.612	T45.613	T45.614	T45.615	T45.616
Thromboplastin	T45.7X1	T45.7X2	T45.7X3	T45.7X4	T45.7X5	T45.7X6
Thurfyl nicotinate	T46.7X1	T46.7X2	T46.7X3	T46.7X4	T46.7X5	T46.7X6
Thymol	T49.0X1	T49.0X2	T49.0X3	T49.0X4	T49.0X5	T49.0X6
Thymopentin	T37.5X1	T37.5X2	T37.5X3	T37.5X4	T37.5X5	T37.5X6
Thymoxamine	T46.7X1	T46.7X2	T46.7X3	T46.7X4	T46.7X5	T46.7X6
Thymus extract	T38.891	T38.892	T38.893	T38.894	T38.895	T38.896
Thyreotrophic hormone	T38.811	T38.812	T38.813	T38.814	T38.815	T38.816
Thyroglobulin	T38.1X1	T38.1X2	T38.1X3	T38.1X4	T38.1X5	T38.1X6
Thyroid (hormone)	T38.1X1	T38.1X2	T38.1X3	T38.1X4	T38.1X5	T38.1X6
Thyrolar	T38.1X1	T38.1X2	T38.1X3	T38.1X4	T38.1X5	T38.1X6
Thyrotrophin	T38.811	T38.812	T38.813	T38.814	T38.815	T38.816
Thyrotropic hormone	T38.811	T38.812	T38.813	T38.814	T38.815	T38.816
Thyroxine	T38.1X1	T38.1X2	T38.1X3	T38.1X4	T38.1X5	T38.1X6
Tiabendazole	T37.4X1	T37.4X2	T37.4X3	T37.4X4	T37.4X5	T37.4X6
Tiamizide	T50.2X1	T50.2X2	T50.2X3	T50.2X4	T50.2X5	T50.2X6
Tianeptine	T43.291	T43.292	T43.293	T43.294	T43.295	T43.296
Tiapamil	T46.1X1	T46.1X2	T46.1X3	T46.1X4	T46.1X5	T46.1X6
Tiapride	T43.591	T43.592	T43.593	T43.594	T43.595	T43.596
Tiaprofenic acid	T39.311	T39.312	T39.313	T39.314	T39.315	T39.316
Tiaramide	T39.8X1	T39.8X2	T39.8X3	T39.8X4	T39.8X5	T39.8X6
Ticarcillin	T36.0X1	T36.0X2	T36.0X3	T36.0X4	T36.0X5	T36.0X6
Ticlatone	T49.0X1	T49.0X2	T49.0X3	T49.0X4	T49.0X5	T49.0X6
Ticlopidine	T45.521	T45.522	T45.523	T45.524	T45.525	T45.526
Ticrynafen	T50.1X1	T50.1X2	T50.1X3	T50.1X4	T50.1X5	T50.1X6
Tidiacic	T50.991	T50.992	T50.993	T50.994	T50.995	T50.996
Tiemonium	T44.3X1	T44.3X2	T44.3X3	T44.3X4	T44.3X5	T44.3X6
iodide	T44.3X1	T44.3X2	T44.3X3	T44.3X4	T44.3X5	T44.3X6
Tienilic acid	T50.1X1	T50.1X2	T50.1X3	T50.1X4	T50.1X5	T50.1X6
Tifenamil	T44.3X1	T44.3X2	T44.3X3	T44.3X4	T44.3X5	T44.3X6
Tigan	T45.0X1	T45.0X2	T45.0X3	T45.0X4	T45.0X5	T45.0X6
Tigloidine	T44.3X1	T44.3X2	T44.3X3	T44.3X4	T44.3X5	T44.3X6
Tilactase	T47.5X1	T47.5X2	T47.5X3	T47.5X4	T47.5X5	T47.5X6
Tiletamine	T41.291	T41.292	T41.293	T41.294	T41.295	T41.296
Tilidine	T40.4X1	T40.4X2	T40.4X3	T40.4X4	—	—
Timepidium bromide	T44.3X1	T44.3X2	T44.3X3	T44.3X4	T44.3X5	T44.3X6
Timiperone	T43.4X1	T43.4X2	T43.4X3	T43.4X4	T43.4X5	T43.4X6
Timolol	T44.7X1	T44.7X2	T44.7X3	T44.7X4	T44.7X5	T44.7X6
Tin (chloride) (dust) (oxide) NEC	T56.6X1	T56.6X2	T56.6X3	T56.6X4	—	—
anti-infectives	T37.8X1	T37.8X2	T37.8X3	T37.8X4	T37.8X5	T37.8X6

◀ New   ◀▥ Revised   deleted Deleted

Substance	External Cause (T-Code)					
	Poisoning, Accidental (Unintentional)	Poisoning, Intentional Self-Harm	Poisoning, Assault	Poisoning, Undetermined	Adverse Effect	Underdosing
Tincture, iodine — see Iodine						
Tindal	T43.3X1	T43.3X2	T43.3X3	T43.3X4	T43.3X5	T43.3X6
Tinidazole	T37.3X1	T37.3X2	T37.3X3	T37.3X4	T37.3X5	T37.3X6
Tinoridine	T39.8X1	T39.8X2	T39.8X3	T39.8X4	T39.8X5	T39.8X6
Tiocarlide	T37.1X1	T37.1X2	T37.1X3	T37.1X4	T37.1X5	T37.1X6
Tioclomarol	T45.511	T45.512	T45.513	T45.514	T45.515	T45.516
Tioconazole	T49.0X1	T49.0X2	T49.0X3	T49.0X4	T49.0X5	T49.0X6
Tioguanine	T45.1X1	T45.1X2	T45.1X3	T45.1X4	T45.1X5	T45.1X6
Tiopronin	T50.991	T50.992	T50.993	T50.994	T50.995	T50.996
Tiotixene	T43.4X1	T43.4X2	T43.4X3	T43.4X4	T43.4X5	T43.4X6
Tioxolone	T49.4X1	T49.4X2	T49.4X3	T49.4X4	T49.4X5	T49.4X6
Tipepidine	T48.3X1	T48.3X2	T48.3X3	T48.3X4	T48.3X5	T48.3X6
Tiquizium bromide	T44.3X1	T44.3X2	T44.3X3	T44.3X4	T44.3X5	T44.3X6
Tiratricol	T38.1X1	T38.1X2	T38.1X3	T38.1X4	T38.1X5	T38.1X6
Tisopurine	T50.4X1	T50.4X2	T50.4X3	T50.4X4	T50.4X5	T50.4X6
Titanium (compounds) (vapor)	T56.891	T56.892	T56.893	T56.894	—	—
dioxide	T49.3X1	T49.3X2	T49.3X3	T49.3X4	T49.3X5	T49.3X6
ointment	T49.3X1	T49.3X2	T49.3X3	T49.3X4	T49.3X5	T49.3X6
oxide	T49.3X1	T49.3X2	T49.3X3	T49.3X4	T49.3X5	T49.3X6
tetrachloride	T56.891	T56.892	T56.893	T56.894	—	—
Titanocene	T56.891	T56.892	T56.893	T56.894	—	—
Titroid	T38.1X1	T38.1X2	T38.1X3	T38.1X4	T38.1X5	T38.1X6
Tizanidine	T42.8X1	T42.8X2	T42.8X3	T42.8X4	T42.8X5	T42.8X6
TMTD	T60.3X1	T60.3X2	T60.3X3	T60.3X4	—	—
TNT (fumes)	T65.3X1	T65.3X2	T65.3X3	T65.3X4	—	—
Toadstool	T62.0X1	T62.0X2	T62.0X3	T62.0X4	—	—
Tobacco NEC	T65.291	T65.292	T65.293	T65.294	—	—
cigarettes	T65.221	T65.222	T65.223	T65.224	—	—
Indian	T62.2X1	T62.2X2	T62.2X3	T62.2X4	—	—
smoke, second-hand	T65.221	T65.222	T65.223	T65.224	—	—
Tobramycin	T36.5X1	T36.5X2	T36.5X3	T36.5X4	T36.5X5	T36.5X6
Tocainide	T46.2X1	T46.2X2	T46.2X3	T46.2X4	T46.2X5	T46.2X6
Tocoferol	T45.2X1	T45.2X2	T45.2X3	T45.2X4	T45.2X5	T45.2X6
Tocopherol	T45.2X1	T45.2X2	T45.2X3	T45.2X4	T45.2X5	T45.2X6
acetate	T45.2X1	T45.2X2	T45.2X3	T45.2X4	T45.2X5	T45.2X6
Tocosamine	T48.0X1	T48.0X2	T48.0X3	T48.0X4	T48.0X5	T48.0X6
Todralazine	T46.5X1	T46.5X2	T46.5X3	T46.5X4	T46.5X5	T46.5X6
Tofisopam	T42.4X1	T42.4X2	T42.4X3	T42.4X4	T42.4X5	T42.4X6
Tofranil	T43.011	T43.012	T43.013	T43.014	T43.015	T43.016
Toilet deodorizer	T65.891	T65.892	T65.893	T65.894	—	—

◀ New ◀▥ Revised ~~deleted~~ Deleted

TABLE OF DRUGS AND CHEMICALS

Substance	Poisoning, Accidental (Unintentional)	Poisoning, Intentional Self-Harm	Poisoning, Assault	Poisoning, Undetermined	Adverse Effect	Underdosing
Tolamolol	T44.7X1	T44.7X2	T44.7X3	T44.7X4	T44.7X5	T44.7X6
Tolazamide	T38.3X1	T38.3X2	T38.3X3	T38.3X4	T38.3X5	T38.3X6
Tolazoline	T46.7X1	T46.7X2	T46.7X3	T46.7X4	T46.7X5	T46.7X6
Tolbutamide (sodium)	T38.3X1	T38.3X2	T38.3X3	T38.3X4	T38.3X5	T38.3X6
Tolciclate	T49.0X1	T49.0X2	T49.0X3	T49.0X4	T49.0X5	T49.0X6
Tolmetin	T39.391	T39.392	T39.393	T39.394	T39.395	T39.396
Tolnaftate	T49.0X1	T49.0X2	T49.0X3	T49.0X4	T49.0X5	T49.0X6
Tolonidine	T46.5X1	T46.5X2	T46.5X3	T46.5X4	T46.5X5	T46.5X6
Toloxatone	T42.6X1	T42.6X2	T42.6X3	T42.6X4	T42.6X5	T42.6X6
Tolperisone	T44.3X1	T44.3X2	T44.3X3	T44.3X4	T44.3X5	T44.3X6
Tolserol	T42.8X1	T42.8X2	T42.8X3	T42.8X4	T42.8X5	T42.8X6
Toluene (liquid)	T52.2X1	T52.2X2	T52.2X3	T52.2X4	—	—
diisocyanate	T65.0X1	T65.0X2	T65.0X3	T65.0X4	—	—
Toluidine	T65.891	T65.892	T65.893	T65.894	—	—
vapor	T59.891	T59.892	T59.893	T59.894	—	—
Toluol (liquid)	T52.2X1	T52.2X2	T52.2X3	T52.2X4	—	—
vapor	T52.2X1	T52.2X2	T52.2X3	T52.2X4	—	—
Toluylenediamine	T65.3X1	T65.3X2	T65.3X3	T65.3X4	—	—
Tolylene-2,4-diisocyanate	T65.0X1	T65.0X2	T65.0X3	T65.0X4	—	—
Tonic NEC	T50.901	T50.902	T50.903	T50.904	T50.905	T50.906
Topical action drug NEC	T49.91	T49.92	T49.93	T49.94	T49.95	T49.96
ear, nose or throat	T49.6X1	T49.6X2	T49.6X3	T49.6X4	T49.6X5	T49.6X6
eye	T49.5X1	T49.5X2	T49.5X3	T49.5X4	T49.5X5	T49.5X6
skin	T49.91	T49.92	T49.93	T49.94	T49.95	T49.96
specified NEC	T49.8X1	T49.8X2	T49.8X3	T49.8X4	T49.8X5	T49.8X6
Toquizine	T44.3X1	T44.3X2	T44.3X3	T44.3X4	T44.3X5	T44.3X6
Toremifene	T38.6X1	T38.6X2	T38.6X3	T38.6X4	T38.6X5	T38.6X6
Tosylchloramide sodium	T49.8X1	T49.8X2	T49.8X3	T49.8X4	T49.8X5	T49.8X6
Toxaphene (dust) (spray)	T60.1X1	T60.1X2	T60.1X3	T60.1X4	—	—
Toxin, diphtheria (Schick Test)	T50.8X1	T50.8X2	T50.8X3	T50.8X4	T50.8X5	T50.8X6
Toxoid						
combined	T50.A21	T50.A22	T50.A23	T50.A24	T50.A25	T50.A26
diphtheria	T50.A91	T50.A92	T50.A93	T50.A94	T50.A95	T50.A96
tetanus	T50.A91	T50.A92	T50.A93	T50.A94	T50.A95	T50.A96
Trace element NEC	T45.8X1	T45.8X2	T45.8X3	T45.8X4	T45.8X5	T45.8X6
Tractor fuel NEC	T52.0X1	T52.0X2	T52.0X3	T52.0X4	—	—
Tragacanth	T50.991	T50.992	T50.993	T50.994	T50.995	T50.996
Tramadol	T40.4X1	T40.4X2	T40.4X3	T40.4X4	T40.4X5	T40.4X6
Tramazoline	T48.5X1	T48.5X2	T48.5X3	T48.5X4	T48.5X5	T48.5X6
Tranexamic acid	T45.621	T45.622	T45.623	T45.624	T45.625	T45.626

◀ New   ◀▥ Revised   ~~deleted~~ Deleted

Substance	External Cause (T-Code)					
	Poisoning, Accidental (Unintentional)	Poisoning, Intentional Self-Harm	Poisoning, Assault	Poisoning, Undetermined	Adverse Effect	Underdosing
Tranilast	T45.0X1	T45.0X2	T45.0X3	T45.0X4	T45.0X5	T45.0X6
Tranquilizer NEC	T43.501	T43.502	T43.503	T43.504	T43.505	T43.506
with hypnotic or sedative	T42.6X1	T42.6X2	T42.6X3	T42.6X4	T42.6X5	T42.6X6
benzodiazepine NEC	T42.4X1	T42.4X2	T42.4X3	T42.4X4	T42.4X5	T42.4X6
butyrophenone NEC	T43.4X1	T43.4X2	T43.4X3	T43.4X4	T43.4X5	T43.4X6
carbamate	T43.591	T43.592	T43.593	T43.594	T43.595	T43.596
dimethylamine	T43.3X1	T43.3X2	T43.3X3	T43.3X4	T43.3X5	T43.3X6
ethylamine	T43.3X1	T43.3X2	T43.3X3	T43.3X4	T43.3X5	T43.3X6
hydroxyzine	T43.591	T43.592	T43.593	T43.594	T43.595	T43.596
major NEC	T43.501	T43.502	T43.503	T43.504	T43.505	T43.506
penothiazine NEC	T43.3X1	T43.3X2	T43.3X3	T43.3X4	T43.3X5	T43.3X6
phenothiazine-based	T43.3X1	T43.3X2	T43.3X3	T43.3X4	T43.3X5	T43.3X6
piperazine NEC	T43.3X1	T43.3X2	T43.3X3	T43.3X4	T43.3X5	T43.3X6
piperidine	T43.3X1	T43.3X2	T43.3X3	T43.3X4	T43.3X5	T43.3X6
propylamine	T43.3X1	T43.3X2	T43.3X3	T43.3X4	T43.3X5	T43.3X6
specified NEC	T43.591	T43.592	T43.593	T43.594	T43.595	T43.596
thioxanthene NEC	T43.591	T43.592	T43.593	T43.594	T43.595	T43.596
Tranxene	T42.4X1	T42.4X2	T42.4X3	T42.4X4	T42.4X5	T42.4X6
Tranylcypromine	T43.1X1	T43.1X2	T43.1X3	T43.1X4	T43.1X5	T43.1X6
Trapidil	T46.3X1	T46.3X2	T46.3X3	T46.3X4	T46.3X5	T46.3X6
Trasentine	T44.3X1	T44.3X2	T44.3X3	T44.3X4	T44.3X5	T44.3X6
Travert	T50.3X1	T50.3X2	T50.3X3	T50.3X4	T50.3X5	T50.3X6
Trazodone	T43.211	T43.212	T43.213	T43.214	T43.215	T43.216
Trecator	T37.1X1	T37.1X2	T37.1X3	T37.1X4	T37.1X5	T37.1X6
Treosulfan	T45.1X1	T45.1X2	T45.1X3	T45.1X4	T45.1X5	T45.1X6
Tretamine	T45.1X1	T45.1X2	T45.1X3	T45.1X4	T45.1X5	T45.1X6
Tretinoin	T49.0X1	T49.0X2	T49.0X3	T49.0X4	T49.0X5	T49.0X6
Tretoquinol	T48.6X1	T48.6X2	T48.6X3	T48.6X4	T48.6X5	T48.6X6
Triacetin	T49.0X1	T49.0X2	T49.0X3	T49.0X4	T49.0X5	T49.0X6
Triacetoxyanthracene	T49.4X1	T49.4X2	T49.4X3	T49.4X4	T49.4X5	T49.4X6
Triacetyloleandomycin	T36.3X1	T36.3X2	T36.3X3	T36.3X4	T36.3X5	T36.3X6
Triamcinolone	T49.0X1	T49.0X2	T49.0X3	T49.0X4	T49.0X5	T49.0X6
ENT agent	T49.6X1	T49.6X2	T49.6X3	T49.6X4	T49.6X5	T49.6X6
hexacetonide	T49.0X1	T49.0X2	T49.0X3	T49.0X4	T49.0X5	T49.0X6
ophthalmic preparation	T49.5X1	T49.5X2	T49.5X3	T49.5X4	T49.5X5	T49.5X6
topical NEC	T49.0X1	T49.0X2	T49.0X3	T49.0X4	T49.0X5	T49.0X6
Triampyzine	T44.3X1	T44.3X2	T44.3X3	T44.3X4	T44.3X5	T44.3X6
Triamterene	T50.2X1	T50.2X2	T50.2X3	T50.2X4	T50.2X5	T50.2X6
Triazine (herbicide)	T60.3X1	T60.3X2	T60.3X3	T60.3X4	—	—
Triaziquone	T45.1X1	T45.1X2	T45.1X3	T45.1X4	T45.1X5	T45.1X6

◄ New ◄◄ Revised deleted Deleted

Substance	External Cause (T-Code)					
	Poisoning, Accidental (Unintentional)	Poisoning, Intentional Self-Harm	Poisoning, Assault	Poisoning, Undetermined	Adverse Effect	Underdosing
Triazolam	T42.4X1	T42.4X2	T42.4X3	T42.4X4	T42.4X5	T42.4X6
Triazole (herbicide)	T60.3X1	T60.3X2	T60.3X3	T60.3X4	—	—
Tribenoside	T46.991	T46.992	T46.993	T46.994	T46.995	T46.996
Tribromacetaldehyde	T42.6X1	T42.6X2	T42.6X3	T42.6X4	T42.6X5	T42.6X6
Tribromoethanol, rectal	T41.291	T41.292	T41.293	T41.294	T41.295	T41.296
Tribromomethane	T42.6X1	T42.6X2	T42.6X3	T42.6X4	T42.6X5	T42.6X6
Trichlorethane	T53.2X1	T53.2X2	T53.2X3	T53.2X4	—	—
Trichlorethylene	T53.2X1	T53.2X2	T53.2X3	T53.2X4	—	—
Trichlorfon	T60.0X1	T60.0X2	T60.0X3	T60.0X4		
Trichlormethiazide	T50.2X1	T50.2X2	T50.2X3	T50.2X4	T50.2X5	T50.2X6
Trichlormethine	T45.1X1	T45.1X2	T45.1X3	T45.1X4	T45.1X5	T45.1X6
Trichloroacetic acid, Trichloracetic acid	T54.2X1	T54.2X2	T54.2X3	T54.2X4	—	—
medicinal	T49.4X1	T49.4X2	T49.4X3	T49.4X4	T49.4X5	T49.4X6
Trichloroethane	T53.2X1	T53.2X2	T53.2X3	T53.2X4	—	—
Trichloroethanol	T42.6X1	T42.6X2	T42.6X3	T42.6X4	T42.6X5	T42.6X6
Trichloroethylene (liquid) (vapor)	T53.2X1	T53.2X2	T53.2X3	T53.2X4	—	—
anesthetic (gas)	T41.0X1	T41.0X2	T41.0X3	T41.0X4	T41.0X5	T41.0X6
vapor NEC	T53.2X1	T53.2X2	T53.2X3	T53.2X4	—	—
Trichloroethyl phosphate	T42.6X1	T42.6X2	T42.6X3	T42.6X4	T42.6X5	T42.6X6
Trichlorofluoromethane NEC	T53.5X1	T53.5X2	T53.5X3	T53.5X4	—	—
Trichloronate	T60.0X1	T60.0X2	T60.0X3	T60.0X4	—	—
2,4,5-Trichlorophen-oxyacetic acid	T60.3X1	T60.3X2	T60.3X3	T60.3X4	—	—
Trichloropropane	T53.6X1	T53.6X2	T53.6X3	T53.6X4	—	—
Trichlorotriethylamine	T45.1X1	T45.1X2	T45.1X3	T45.1X4	T45.1X5	T45.1X6
Trichomonacides NEC	T37.3X1	T37.3X2	T37.3X3	T37.3X4	T37.3X5	T37.3X6
Trichomycin	T36.7X1	T36.7X2	T36.7X3	T36.7X4	T36.7X5	T36.7X6
Triclobisonium chloride	T49.0X1	T49.0X2	T49.0X3	T49.0X4	T49.0X5	T49.0X6
Triclocarban	T49.0X1	T49.0X2	T49.0X3	T49.0X4	T49.0X5	T49.0X6
Triclofos	T42.6X1	T42.6X2	T42.6X3	T42.6X4	T42.6X5	T42.6X6
Triclosan	T49.0X1	T49.0X2	T49.0X3	T49.0X4	T49.0X5	T49.0X6
Tricresyl phosphate	T65.891	T65.892	T65.893	T65.894	—	—
solvent	T52.91	T52.92	T52.93	T52.94	—	—
Tricyclamol chloride	T44.3X1	T44.3X2	T44.3X3	T44.3X4	T44.3X5	T44.3X6
Tridesilon	T49.0X1	T49.0X2	T49.0X3	T49.0X4	T49.0X5	T49.0X6
Tridihexethyl iodide	T44.3X1	T44.3X2	T44.3X3	T44.3X4	T44.3X5	T44.3X6
Tridione	T42.2X1	T42.2X2	T42.2X3	T42.2X4	T42.2X5	T42.2X6
Trientine	T45.8X1	T45.8X2	T45.8X3	T45.8X4	T45.8X5	T45.8X6
Triethanolamine NEC	T54.3X1	T54.3X2	T54.3X3	T54.3X4	—	—
detergent	T54.3X1	T54.3X2	T54.3X3	T54.3X4	—	—
trinitrate (biphosphate)	T46.3X1	T46.3X2	T46.3X3	T46.3X4	T46.3X5	T46.3X6

◀ New ◀▥ Revised ~~deleted~~ Deleted

TABLE OF DRUGS AND CHEMICALS

Substance	External Cause (T-Code)					
	Poisoning, Accidental (Unintentional)	Poisoning, Intentional Self-Harm	Poisoning, Assault	Poisoning, Undetermined	Adverse Effect	Underdosing
Triethanomelamine	T45.1X1	T45.1X2	T45.1X3	T45.1X4	T45.1X5	T45.1X6
Triethylenemelamine	T45.1X1	T45.1X2	T45.1X3	T45.1X4	T45.1X5	T45.1X6
Triethylenephosphoramide	T45.1X1	T45.1X2	T45.1X3	T45.1X4	T45.1X5	T45.1X6
Triethylenethiophosphoramide	T45.1X1	T45.1X2	T45.1X3	T45.1X4	T45.1X5	T45.1X6
Trifluoperazine	T43.3X1	T43.3X2	T43.3X3	T43.3X4	T43.3X5	T43.3X6
Trifluoroethyl vinyl ether	T41.0X1	T41.0X2	T41.0X3	T41.0X4	T41.0X5	T41.0X6
Trifluperidol	T43.4X1	T43.4X2	T43.4X3	T43.4X4	T43.4X5	T43.4X6
Triflupromazine	T43.3X1	T43.3X2	T43.3X3	T43.3X4	T43.3X5	T43.3X6
Trifluridine	T37.5X1	T37.5X2	T37.5X3	T37.5X4	T37.5X5	T37.5X6
Triflusal	T45.521	T45.522	T45.523	T45.524	T45.525	T45.526
Trihexyphenidyl	T44.3X1	T44.3X2	T44.3X3	T44.3X4	T44.3X5	T44.3X6
Triiodothyronine	T38.1X1	T38.1X2	T38.1X3	T38.1X4	T38.1X5	T38.1X6
Trilene	T41.0X1	T41.0X2	T41.0X3	T41.0X4	T41.0X5	T41.0X6
Trilostane	T38.991	T38.992	T38.993	T38.994	T38.995	T38.996
Trimebutine	T44.3X1	T44.3X2	T44.3X3	T44.3X4	T44.3X5	T44.3X6
Trimecaine	T41.3X1	T41.3X2	T41.3X3	T41.3X4	T41.3X5	T41.3X6
Trimeprazine (tartrate)	T44.3X1	T44.3X2	T44.3X3	T44.3X4	T44.3X5	T44.3X6
Trimetaphan camsilate	T44.2X1	T44.2X2	T44.2X3	T44.2X4	T44.2X5	T44.2X6
Trimetazidine	T46.7X1	T46.7X2	T46.7X3	T46.7X4	T46.7X5	T46.7X6
Trimethadione	T42.2X1	T42.2X2	T42.2X3	T42.2X4	T42.2X5	T42.2X6
Trimethaphan	T44.2X1	T44.2X2	T44.2X3	T44.2X4	T44.2X5	T44.2X6
Trimethidinium	T44.2X1	T44.2X2	T44.2X3	T44.2X4	T44.2X5	T44.2X6
Trimethobenzamide	T45.0X1	T45.0X2	T45.0X3	T45.0X4	T45.0X5	T45.0X6
Trimethoprim	T37.8X1	T37.8X2	T37.8X3	T37.8X4	T37.8X5	T37.8X6
with sulfamethoxazole	T36.8X1	T36.8X2	T36.8X3	T36.8X4	T36.8X5	T36.8X6
Trimethylcarbinol	T51.3X1	T51.3X2	T51.3X3	T51.3X4	—	—
Trimethylpsoralen	T49.3X1	T49.3X2	T49.3X3	T49.3X4	T49.3X5	T49.3X6
Trimeton	T45.0X1	T45.0X2	T45.0X3	T45.0X4	T45.0X5	T45.0X6
Trimetrexate	T45.1X1	T45.1X2	T45.1X3	T45.1X4	T45.1X5	T45.1X6
Trimipramine	T43.011	T43.012	T43.013	T43.014	T43.015	T43.016
Trimustine	T45.1X1	T45.1X2	T45.1X3	T45.1X4	T45.1X5	T45.1X6
Trinitrine	T46.3X1	T46.3X2	T46.3X3	T46.3X4	T46.3X5	T46.3X6
Trinitrobenzol	T65.3X1	T65.3X2	T65.3X3	T65.3X4	—	—
Trinitrophenol	T65.3X1	T65.3X2	T65.3X3	T65.3X4	—	—
Trinitrotoluene (fumes)	T65.3X1	T65.3X2	T65.3X3	T65.3X4	—	—
Trional	T42.6X1	T42.6X2	T42.6X3	T42.6X4	T42.6X5	T42.6X6
Triorthocresyl phosphate	T65.891	T65.892	T65.893	T65.894	—	—
Trioxide of arsenic	T57.0X1	T57.0X2	T57.0X3	T57.0X4	—	—
Trioxysalen	T49.4X1	T49.4X2	T49.4X3	T49.4X4	T49.4X5	T49.4X6
Tripamide	T50.2X1	T50.2X2	T50.2X3	T50.2X4	T50.2X5	T50.2X6

TABLE OF DRUGS AND CHEMICALS

◀ New   ◀ Revised   ~~deleted~~ Deleted

Substance	External Cause (T-Code)					
	Poisoning, Accidental (Unintentional)	Poisoning, Intentional Self-Harm	Poisoning, Assault	Poisoning, Undetermined	Adverse Effect	Underdosing
Triparanol	T46.6X1	T46.6X2	T46.6X3	T46.6X4	T46.6X5	T46.6X6
Tripelennamine	T45.0X1	T45.0X2	T45.0X3	T45.0X4	T45.0X5	T45.0X6
Triperiden	T44.3X1	T44.3X2	T44.3X3	T44.3X4	T44.3X5	T44.3X6
Triperidol	T43.4X1	T43.4X2	T43.4X3	T43.4X4	T43.4X5	T43.4X6
Triphenylphosphate	T65.891	T65.892	T65.893	T65.894	—	—
Triple						
bromides	T42.6X1	T42.6X2	T42.6X3	T42.6X4	T42.6X5	T42.6X6
carbonate	T47.1X1	T47.1X2	T47.1X3	T47.1X4	T47.1X5	T47.1X6
vaccine						
DPT	T50.A11	T50.A12	T50.A13	T50.A14	T50.A15	T50.A16
including pertussis	T50.A11	T50.A12	T50.A13	T50.A14	T50.A15	T50.A16
MMR	T50.B91	T50.B92	—	—	—	—
Triprolidine	T45.0X1	T45.0X2	T45.0X3	T45.0X4	T45.0X5	T45.0X6
Trisodium hydrogen edetate	T50.6X1	T50.6X2	T50.6X3	T50.6X4	T50.6X5	T50.6X6
Trisoralen	T49.3X1	T49.3X2	T49.3X3	T49.3X4	T49.3X5	T49.3X6
Trisulfapyrimidines	T37.0X1	T37.0X2	T37.0X3	T37.0X4	T37.0X5	T37.0X6
Trithiozine	T44.3X1	T44.3X2	T44.3X3	T44.3X4	T44.3X5	T44.3X6
Tritiozine	T44.3X1	T44.3X2	T44.3X3	T44.3X4	T44.3X5	T44.3X6
Tritoqualine	T45.0X1	T45.0X2	T45.0X3	T45.0X4	T45.0X5	T45.0X6
Trofosfamide	T45.1X1	T45.1X2	T45.1X3	T45.1X4	T45.1X5	T45.1X6
Troleandomycin	T36.3X1	T36.3X2	T36.3X3	T36.3X4	T36.3X5	T36.3X6
Trolnitrate (phosphate)	T46.3X1	T46.3X2	T46.3X3	T46.3X4	T46.3X5	T46.3X6
Tromantadine	T37.5X1	T37.5X2	T37.5X3	T37.5X4	T37.5X5	T37.5X6
Trometamol	T50.2X1	T50.2X2	T50.2X3	T50.2X4	T50.2X5	T50.2X6
Tromethamine	T50.2X1	T50.2X2	T50.2X3	T50.2X4	T50.2X5	T50.2X6
Tronothane	T41.3X1	T41.3X2	T41.3X3	T41.3X4	T41.3X5	T41.3X6
Tropacine	T44.3X1	T44.3X2	T44.3X3	T44.3X4	T44.3X5	T44.3X6
Tropatepine	T44.3X1	T44.3X2	T44.3X3	T44.3X4	T44.3X5	T44.3X6
Tropicamide	T44.3X1	T44.3X2	T44.3X3	T44.3X4	T44.3X5	T44.3X6
Trospium chloride	T44.3X1	T44.3X2	T44.3X3	T44.3X4	T44.3X5	T44.3X6
Troxerutin	T46.991	T46.992	T46.993	T46.994	T46.995	T46.996
Troxidone	T42.2X1	T42.2X2	T42.2X3	T42.2X4	T42.2X5	T42.2X6
Tryparsamide	T37.3X1	T37.3X2	T37.3X3	T37.3X4	T37.3X5	T37.3X6
Trypsin	T45.3X1	T45.3X2	T45.3X3	T45.3X4	T45.3X5	T45.3X6
Tryptizol	T43.011	T43.012	T43.013	T43.014	T43.015	T43.016
TSH	T38.811	T38.812	T38.813	T38.814	T38.815	T38.816
Tuaminoheptane	T48.5X1	T48.5X2	T48.5X3	T48.5X4	T48.5X5	T48.5X6
Tuberculin, purified protein derivative (PPD)	T50.8X1	T50.8X2	T50.8X3	T50.8X4	T50.8X5	T50.8X6
Tubocurare	T48.1X1	T48.1X2	T48.1X3	T48.1X4	T48.1X5	T48.1X6
Tubocurarine (chloride)	T48.1X1	T48.1X2	T48.1X3	T48.1X4	T48.1X5	T48.1X6

◄ New   ◄▬ Revised   ~~deleted~~ Deleted

TABLE OF DRUGS AND CHEMICALS

Substance	External Cause (T-Code)					
	Poisoning, Accidental (Unintentional)	Poisoning, Intentional Self-Harm	Poisoning, Assault	Poisoning, Undetermined	Adverse Effect	Underdosing
Tulobuterol	T48.6X1	T48.6X2	T48.6X3	T48.6X4	T48.6X5	T48.6X6
Turpentine (spirits of)	T52.8X1	T52.8X2	T52.8X3	T52.8X4	—	—
vapor	T52.8X1	T52.8X2	T52.8X3	T52.8X4	—	—
Tybamate	T43.591	T43.592	T43.593	T43.594	T43.595	T43.596
Tyloxapol	T48.4X1	T48.4X2	T48.4X3	T48.4X4	T48.4X5	T48.4X6
Tymazoline	T48.5X1	T48.5X2	T48.5X3	T48.5X4	T48.5X5	T48.5X6
Typhoid-paratyphoid vaccine	T50.A91	T50.A92	T50.A93	T50.A94	T50.A95	T50.A96
Typhus vaccine	T50.A91	T50.A92	T50.A93	T50.A94	T50.A95	T50.A96
Tyropanoate	T50.8X1	T50.8X2	T50.8X3	T50.8X4	T50.8X5	T50.8X6
Tyrothricin	T49.6X1	T49.6X2	T49.6X3	T49.6X4	T49.6X5	T49.6X6
ENT agent	T49.6X1	T49.6X2	T49.6X3	T49.6X4	T49.6X5	T49.6X6
ophthalmic preparation	T49.5X1	T49.5X2	T49.5X3	T49.5X4	T49.5X5	T49.5X6
U						
Ufenamate	T39.391	T39.392	T39.393	T39.394	T39.395	T39.396
Ultraviolet light protectant	T49.3X1	T49.3X2	T49.3X3	T49.3X4	T49.3X5	T49.3X6
Undecenoic acid	T49.0X1	T49.0X2	T49.0X3	T49.0X4	T49.0X5	T49.0X6
Undecoylium	T49.0X1	T49.0X2	T49.0X3	T49.0X4	T49.0X5	T49.0X6
Undecylenic acid (derivatives)	T49.0X1	T49.0X2	T49.0X3	T49.0X4	T49.0X5	T49.0X6
Unna's boot	T49.3X1	T49.3X2	T49.3X3	T49.3X4	T49.3X5	T49.3X6
Unsaturated fatty acid	T46.6X1	T46.6X2	T46.6X3	T46.6X4	T46.6X5	T46.6X6
Uracil mustard	T45.1X1	T45.1X2	T45.1X3	T45.1X4	T45.1X5	T45.1X6
Uramustine	T45.1X1	T45.1X2	T45.1X3	T45.1X4	T45.1X5	T45.1X6
Urapidil	T46.5X1	T46.5X2	T46.5X3	T46.5X4	T46.5X5	T46.5X6
Urari	T48.1X1	T48.1X2	T48.1X3	T48.1X4	T48.1X5	T48.1X6
Urate oxidase	T50.4X1	T50.4X2	T50.4X3	T50.4X4	T50.4X5	T50.4X6
Urea	T47.3X1	T47.3X2	T47.3X3	T47.3X4	T47.3X5	T47.3X6
peroxide	T49.0X1	T49.0X2	T49.0X3	T49.0X4	T49.0X5	T49.0X6
stibamine	T37.4X1	T37.4X2	T37.4X3	T37.4X4	T37.4X5	T37.4X6
topical	T49.8X1	T49.8X2	T49.8X3	T49.8X4	T49.8X5	T49.8X6
Urethane	T45.1X1	T45.1X2	T45.1X3	T45.1X4	T45.1X5	T45.1X6
Urginea (maritima) (scilla) — *see Squill*						
Uric acid metabolism drug NEC	T50.4X1	T50.4X2	T50.4X3	T50.4X4	T50.4X5	T50.4X6
Uricosuric agent	T50.4X1	T50.4X2	T50.4X3	T50.4X4	T50.4X5	T50.4X6
Urinary anti-infective	T37.8X1	T37.8X2	T37.8X3	T37.8X4	T37.8X5	T37.8X6
Urofollitropin	T38.811	T38.812	T38.813	T38.814	T38.815	T38.816
Urokinase	T45.611	T45.612	T45.613	T45.614	T45.615	T45.616
Urokon	T50.8X1	T50.8X2	T50.8X3	T50.8X4	T50.8X5	T50.8X6
Ursodeoxycholic acid	T50.991	T50.992	T50.993	T50.994	T50.995	T50.996
Ursodiol	T50.991	T50.992	T50.993	T50.994	T50.995	T50.996

◀ New ◀▦ Revised ~~deleted~~ Deleted

Substance	External Cause (T-Code)					
	Poisoning, Accidental (Unintentional)	Poisoning, Intentional Self-Harm	Poisoning, Assault	Poisoning, Undetermined	Adverse Effect	Underdosing
Urtica	T62.2X1	T62.2X2	T62.2X3	T62.2X4	—	—
Utility gas — *see Gas, utility*						
V						
Vaccine NEC	T50.Z91	T50.Z92	T50.Z93	T50.Z94	T50.Z95	T50.Z96
antineoplastic	T50.Z91	T50.Z92	T50.Z93	T50.Z94	T50.Z95	T50.Z96
bacterial NEC	T50.A91	T50.A92	T50.A93	T50.A94	T50.A95	T50.A96
with						
other bacterial component	T50.A91	T50.A92	T50.A93	T50.A94	T50.A95	T50.A96
pertussis component	T50.A91	T50.A92	T50.A93	T50.A94	T50.A95	T50.A96
viral-rickettsial component	T50.A91	T50.A92	T50.A93	T50.A94	T50.A95	T50.A96
mixed NEC	T50.A91	T50.A92	T50.A93	T50.A94	T50.A95	T50.A96
BCG	T50.A91	T50.A92	T50.A93	T50.A94	T50.A95	T50.A96
cholera	T50.A91	T50.A92	T50.A93	T50.A94	T50.A95	T50.A96
diphtheria	T50.A91	T50.A92	T50.A93	T50.A94	T50.A95	T50.A96
with tetanus	T50.A21	T50.A22	T50.A23	T50.A24	T50.A25	T50.A26
and pertussis	T50.A11	T50.A12	T50.A13	T50.A14	T50.A15	T50.A16
influenza	T50.B91	T50.B92	T50.B93	T50.B94	T50.B95	T50.B96
measles	T50.B91	T50.B92	T50.B93	T50.B94	T50.B95	T50.B96
with mumps and rubella	T50.B91	T50.B92	T50.B93	T50.B94	T50.B95	T50.B96
meningococcal	T50.A91	T50.A92	T50.A93	T50.A94	T50.A95	T50.A96
mumps	T50.B91	T50.B92	T50.B93	T50.B94	T50.B95	T50.B96
paratyphoid	T50.A91	T50.A92	T50.A93	T50.A94	T50.A95	T50.A96
pertussis	T50.A11	T50.A12	T50.A13	T50.A14	T50.A15	T50.A16
with diphtheria	T50.A11	T50.A12	T50.A13	T50.A14	T50.A15	T50.A16
and tetanus	T50.A11	T50.A12	T50.A13	T50.A14	T50.A15	T50.A16
plague	T50.A91	T50.A92	T50.A93	T50.A94	T50.A95	T50.A96
poliomyelitis	T50.B91	T50.B92	T50.B93	T50.B94	T50.B95	T50.B96
poliovirus	T50.B91	T50.B92	T50.B93	T50.B94	T50.B95	T50.B96
rabies	T50.B91	T50.B92	T50.B93	T50.B94	T50.B95	T50.B96
respiratory syncytial virus	T50.B91	T50.B92	T50.B93	T50.B94	T50.B95	T50.B96
rickettsial NEC	T50.A91	T50.A92	T50.A93	T50.A94	T50.A95	T50.A96
with						
bacterial component	T50.A21	T50.A22	T50.A23	T50.A24	T50.A25	T50.A26
Rocky Mountain spotted fever	T50.A91	T50.A92	T50.A93	T50.A94	T50.A95	T50.A96
rubella	T50.B91	T50.B92	T50.B93	T50.B94	T50.B95	T50.B96
sabin oral	T50.B91	T50.B92	T50.B93	T50.B94	T50.B95	T50.B96
smallpox	T50.B11	T50.B12	T50.B13	T50.B14	T50.B15	T50.B16
TAB	T50.A91	T50.A92	T50.A93	T50.A94	T50.A95	T50.A96
tetanus	T50.A91	T50.A92	T50.A93	T50.A94	T50.A95	T50.A96

◄ New ◄▥ Revised ~~deleted~~ Deleted

Substance	External Cause (T-Code)					
	Poisoning, Accidental (Unintentional)	Poisoning, Intentional Self-Harm	Poisoning, Assault	Poisoning, Undetermined	Adverse Effect	Underdosing
Vaccine NEC *(Continued)*						
typhoid	T50.A91	T50.A92	T50.A93	T50.A94	T50.A95	T50.A96
typhus	T50.A91	T50.A92	T50.A93	T50.A94	T50.A95	T50.A96
viral NEC	T50.B91	T50.B92	T50.B93	T50.B94	T50.B95	T50.B96
yellow fever	T50.B91	T50.B92	T50.B93	T50.B94	T50.B95	T50.B96
Vaccinia immune globulin	T50.Z11	T50.Z12	T50.Z13	T50.Z14	T50.Z15	T50.Z16
Vaginal contraceptives	T49.8X1	T49.8X2	T49.8X3	T49.8X4	T49.8X5	T49.8X6
Valerian						
root	T42.6X1	T42.6X2	T42.6X3	T42.6X4	T42.6X5	T42.6X6
tincture	T42.6X1	T42.6X2	T42.6X3	T42.6X4	T42.6X5	T42.6X6
Valethamate bromide	T44.3X1	T44.3X2	T44.3X3	T44.3X4	T44.3X5	T44.3X6
Valisone	T49.0X1	T49.0X2	T49.0X3	T49.0X4	T49.0X5	T49.0X6
Valium	T42.4X1	T42.4X2	T42.4X3	T42.4X4	T42.4X5	T42.4X6
Valmid	T42.6X1	T42.6X2	T42.6X3	T42.6X4	T42.6X5	T42.6X6
Valnoctamide	T42.6X1	T42.6X2	T42.6X3	T42.6X4	T42.6X5	T42.6X6
Valproate (sodium)	T42.6X1	T42.6X2	T42.6X3	T42.6X4	T42.6X5	T42.6X6
Valproic acid	T42.6X1	T42.6X2	T42.6X3	T42.6X4	T42.6X5	T42.6X6
Valpromide	T42.6X1	T42.6X2	T42.6X3	T42.6X4	T42.6X5	T42.6X6
Vanadium	T56.891	T56.892	T56.893	T56.894	—	—
Vancomycin	T36.8X1	T36.8X2	T36.8X3	T36.8X4	T36.8X5	T36.8X6
Vapor — *see also Gas*	T59.91	T59.92	T59.93	T59.94	—	—
kiln (carbon monoxide)	T58.8X1	T58.8X2	T58.8X3	T58.8X4	—	—
lead — *see lead*						
specified source NEC	T59.891	T59.892	T59.893	T59.894	—	—
Vardenafil	T46.7X1	T46.7X2	T46.7X3	T46.7X4	T46.7X5	T46.7X6
Varicose reduction drug	T46.8X1	T46.8X2	T46.8X3	T46.8X4	T46.8X5	T46.8X6
Varnish	T65.4X1	T65.4X2	T65.4X3	T65.4X4	—	—
cleaner	T52.91	T52.92	T52.93	T52.94	—	—
Vaseline	T49.3X1	T49.3X2	T49.3X3	T49.3X4	T49.3X5	T49.3X6
Vasodilan	T46.7X1	T46.7X2	T46.7X3	T46.7X4	T46.7X5	T46.7X6
Vasodilator						
coronary NEC	T46.3X1	T46.3X2	T46.3X3	T46.3X4	T46.3X5	T46.3X6
peripheral NEC	T46.7X1	T46.7X2	T46.7X3	T46.7X4	T46.7X5	T46.7X6
Vasopressin	T38.891	T38.892	T38.893	T38.894	T38.895	T38.896
Vasopressor drugs	T38.891	T38.892	T38.893	T38.894	T38.895	T38.896
Vecuronium bromide	T48.1X1	T48.1X2	T48.1X3	T48.1X4	T48.1X5	T48.1X6
Vegetable extract, astringent	T49.2X1	T49.2X2	T49.2X3	T49.2X4	T49.2X5	T49.2X6
Venlafaxine	T43.211	T43.212	T43.213	T43.214	T43.215	T43.216

◀ New ◀▥ Revised ~~deleted~~ Deleted

Substance	External Cause (T-Code)					
	Poisoning, Accidental (Unintentional)	Poisoning, Intentional Self-Harm	Poisoning, Assault	Poisoning, Undetermined	Adverse Effect	Underdosing
Venom, venomous (bite) (sting)	T63.91	T63.92	T63.93	T63.94	—	—
amphibian NEC	T63.831	T63.832	T63.833	T63.834	—	—
animal NEC	T63.891	T63.892	T63.893	T63.894	—	—
ant	T63.421	T63.422	T63.423	T63.424	—	—
arthropod NEC	T63.481	T63.482	T63.483	T63.484	—	—
bee	T63.441	T63.442	T63.443	T63.444	—	—
centipede	T63.411	T63.412	T63.413	T63.414	—	—
fish	T63.591	T63.592	T63.593	T63.594	—	—
frog	T63.811	T63.812	T63.813	T63.814	—	—
hornet	T63.451	T63.452	T63.453	T63.454	—	—
insect NEC	T63.481	T63.482	T63.483	T63.484	—	—
lizard	T63.121	T63.122	T63.123	T63.124	—	—
marine						
animals	T63.691	T63.692	T63.693	T63.694	—	—
bluebottle	T63.611	T63.612	T63.613	T63.614	—	—
jellyfish NEC	T63.621	T63.622	T63.623	T63.624	—	—
Portugese Man-o-war	T63.611	T63.612	T63.613	T63.614	—	—
sea anemone	T63.631	T63.632	T63.633	T63.634	—	—
specified NEC	T63.691	T63.692	T63.693	T63.694	—	—
fish	T63.591	T63.592	T63.593	T63.594	—	—
plants	T63.711	T63.712	T63.713	T63.714	—	—
sting ray	T63.511	T63.512	T63.513	T63.514	—	—
millipede (tropical)	T63.411	T63.412	T63.413	T63.414	—	—
plant NEC	T63.791	T63.792	T63.793	T63.794	—	—
marine	T63.711	T63.712	T63.713	T63.714	—	—
reptile	T63.191	T63.192	T63.193	T63.194	—	—
gila monster	T63.111	T63.112	T63.113	T63.114	—	—
lizard NEC	T63.121	T63.122	T63.123	T63.124	—	—
scorpion	T63.2X1	T63.2X2	T63.2X3	T63.2X4	—	—
snake	T63.001	T63.002	T63.003	T63.004	—	—
African NEC	T63.081	T63.082	T63.083	T63.084	—	—
American (North) (South) NEC	T63.061	T63.062	T63.063	T63.064	—	—
Asian	T63.081	T63.082	T63.083	T63.084	—	—
Australian	T63.071	T63.072	T63.073	T63.074	—	—
cobra	T63.041	T63.042	T63.043	T63.044	—	—
coral snake	T63.021	T63.022	T63.023	T63.024	—	—
rattlesnake	T63.011	T63.012	T63.013	T63.014	—	—
specified NEC	T63.091	T63.092	T63.093	T63.094	—	—
taipan	T63.031	T63.032	T63.033	T63.034	—	—

◀ New   ◀‖‖ Revised   ~~deleted~~ Deleted

Substance	External Cause (T-Code)					
	Poisoning, Accidental (Unintentional)	Poisoning, Intentional Self-Harm	Poisoning, Assault	Poisoning, Undetermined	Adverse Effect	Underdosing
Venom, venomous *(Continued)*						
specified NEC	T63.891	T63.892	T63.893	T63.894	—	—
spider	T63.301	T63.302	T63.303	T63.304	—	—
black widow	T63.311	T63.312	T63.313	T63.314	—	—
brown recluse	T63.331	T63.332	T63.333	T63.334	—	—
specified NEC	T63.391	T63.392	T63.393	T63.394	—	—
tarantula	T63.321	T63.322	T63.323	T63.324	—	—
sting ray	T63.511	T63.512	T63.513	T63.514	—	—
toad	T63.821	T63.822	T63.823	T63.824	—	—
wasp	T63.461	T63.462	T63.463	T63.464	—	—
Venous sclerosing drug NEC	T46.8X1	T46.8X2	T46.8X3	T46.8X4	T46.8X5	T46.8X6
Ventolin — *see Albuterol*						
Verapamil	T46.1X1	T46.1X2	T46.1X3	T46.1X4	T46.1X5	T46.1X6
Veramon	T42.3X1	T42.3X2	T42.3X3	T42.3X4	T42.3X5	T42.3X6
Veratrine	T46.5X1	T46.5X2	T46.5X3	T46.5X4	T46.5X5	T46.5X6
Veratrum						
album	T62.2X1	T62.2X2	T62.2X3	T62.2X4	—	—
alkaloids	T46.5X1	T46.5X2	T46.5X3	T46.5X4	T46.5X5	T46.5X6
viride	T62.2X1	T62.2X2	T62.2X3	T62.2X4	—	—
Verdigris	T60.3X1	T60.3X2	T60.3X3	T60.3X4	—	—
Veronal	T42.3X1	T42.3X2	T42.3X3	T42.3X4	T42.3X5	T42.3X6
Veroxil	T37.4X1	T37.4X2	T37.4X3	T37.4X4	T37.4X5	T37.4X6
Versenate	T50.6X1	T50.6X2	T50.6X3	T50.6X4	T50.6X5	T50.6X6
Versidyne	T39.8X1	T39.8X2	T39.8X3	T39.8X4	T39.8X5	T39.8X6
Vetrabutine	T48.0X1	T48.0X2	T48.0X3	T48.0X4	T48.0X5	T48.0X6
Vidarabine	T37.5X1	T37.5X2	T37.5X3	T37.5X4	T37.5X5	T37.5X6
Vienna						
green	T57.0X1	T57.0X2	T57.0X3	T57.0X4	—	—
insecticide	T60.2X1	T60.2X2	T60.2X3	T60.2X4	—	—
red	T57.0X1	T57.0X2	T57.0X3	T57.0X4	—	—
pharmaceutical dye	T50.991	T50.992	T50.993	T50.994	T50.995	T50.996
Vigabatrin	T42.6X1	T42.6X2	T42.6X3	T42.6X4	T42.6X5	T42.6X6
Viloxazine	T43.291	T43.292	T43.293	T43.294	T43.295	T43.296
Viminol	T39.8X1	T39.8X2	T39.8X3	T39.8X4	T39.8X5	T39.8X6
Vinbarbital, vinbarbitone	T42.3X1	T42.3X2	T42.3X3	T42.3X4	T42.3X5	T42.3X6
Vinblastine	T45.1X1	T45.1X2	T45.1X3	T45.1X4	T45.1X5	T45.1X6
Vinburnine	T46.7X1	T46.7X2	T46.7X3	T46.7X4	T46.7X5	T46.7X6
Vincamine	T45.1X1	T45.1X2	T45.1X3	T45.1X4	T45.1X5	T45.1X6
Vincristine	T45.1X1	T45.1X2	T45.1X3	T45.1X4	T45.1X5	T45.1X6
Vindesine	T45.1X1	T45.1X2	T45.1X3	T45.1X4	T45.1X5	T45.1X6

◀ New   ◀▦ Revised   ~~deleted~~ Deleted

Substance	External Cause (T-Code)					
	Poisoning, Accidental (Unintentional)	Poisoning, Intentional Self-Harm	Poisoning, Assault	Poisoning, Undetermined	Adverse Effect	Underdosing
Vinesthene, vinethene	T41.0X1	T41.0X2	T41.0X3	T41.0X4	T41.0X5	T41.0X6
Vinorelbine tartrate	T45.1X1	T45.1X2	T45.1X3	T45.1X4	T45.1X5	T45.1X6
Vinpocetine	T46.7X1	T46.7X2	T46.7X3	T46.7X4	T46.7X5	T46.7X6
Vinyl						
acetate	T65.891	T65.892	T65.893	T65.894	—	—
bital	T42.3X1	T42.3X2	T42.3X3	T42.3X4	T42.3X5	T42.3X6
bromide	T65.891	T65.892	T65.893	T65.894	—	—
chloride	T59.891	T59.892	T59.893	T59.894	—	—
ether	T41.0X1	T41.0X2	T41.0X3	T41.0X4	T41.0X5	T41.0X6
Vinylbital	T42.3X1	T42.3X2	T42.3X3	T42.3X4	T42.3X5	T42.3X6
Vinylidene chloride	T65.891	T65.892	T65.893	T65.894	—	—
Vioform	T37.8X1	T37.8X2	T37.8X3	T37.8X4	T37.8X5	T37.8X6
topical	T49.0X1	T49.0X2	T49.0X3	T49.0X4	T49.0X5	T49.0X6
Viomycin	T36.8X1	T36.8X2	T36.8X3	T36.8X4	T36.8X5	T36.8X6
Viosterol	T45.2X1	T45.2X2	T45.2X3	T45.2X4	T45.2X5	T45.2X6
Viper (venom)	T63.091	T63.092	T63.093	T63.094	—	—
Viprynium	T37.4X1	T37.4X2	T37.4X3	T37.4X4	T37.4X5	T37.4X6
Viquidil	T46.7X1	T46.7X2	T46.7X3	T46.7X4	T46.7X5	T46.7X6
Viral vaccine NEC	T50.B91	T50.B92	T50.B93	T50.B94	T50.B95	T50.B96
Virginiamycin	T36.8X1	T36.8X2	T36.8X3	T36.8X4	T36.8X5	T36.8X6
Virugon	T37.5X1	T37.5X2	T37.5X3	T37.5X4	T37.5X5	T37.5X6
Viscous agent	T50.901	T50.902	T50.903	T50.904	T50.905	T50.906
Visine	T49.5X1	T49.5X2	T49.5X3	T49.5X4	T49.5X5	T49.5X6
Visnadine	T46.3X1	T46.3X2	T46.3X3	T46.3X4	T46.3X5	T46.3X6
Vitamin NEC	T45.2X1	T45.2X2	T45.2X3	T45.2X4	T45.2X5	T45.2X6
A	T45.2X1	T45.2X2	T45.2X3	T45.2X4	T45.2X5	T45.2X6
B NEC	T45.2X1	T45.2X2	T45.2X3	T45.2X4	T45.2X5	T45.2X6
nicotinic acid	T46.7X1	T46.7X2	T46.7X3	T46.7X4	T46.7X5	T46.7X6
B1	T45.2X1	T45.2X2	T45.2X3	T45.2X4	T45.2X5	T45.2X6
B2	T45.2X1	T45.2X2	T45.2X3	T45.2X4	T45.2X5	T45.2X6
B6	T45.2X1	T45.2X2	T45.2X3	T45.2X4	T45.2X5	T45.2X6
B12	T45.2X1	T45.2X2	T45.2X3	T45.2X4	T45.2X5	T45.2X6
B15	T45.2X1	T45.2X2	T45.2X3	T45.2X4	T45.2X5	T45.2X6
C	T45.2X1	T45.2X2	T45.2X3	T45.2X4	T45.2X5	T45.2X6
D	T45.2X1	T45.2X2	T45.2X3	T45.2X4	T45.2X5	T45.2X6
D2	T45.2X1	T45.2X2	T45.2X3	T45.2X4	T45.2X5	T45.2X6
D3	T45.2X1	T45.2X2	T45.2X3	T45.2X4	T45.2X5	T45.2X6
E	T45.2X1	T45.2X2	T45.2X3	T45.2X4	T45.2X5	T45.2X6
E acetate	T45.2X1	T45.2X2	T45.2X3	T45.2X4	T45.2X5	T45.2X6
hematopoietic	T45.8X1	T45.8X2	T45.8X3	T45.8X4	T45.8X5	T45.8X6

TABLE OF DRUGS AND CHEMICALS

Substance	External Cause (T-Code)					
	Poisoning, Accidental (Unintentional)	Poisoning, Intentional Self-Harm	Poisoning, Assault	Poisoning, Undetermined	Adverse Effect	Underdosing
Vitamin NEC *(Continued)*						
K NEC	T45.7X1	T45.7X2	T45.7X3	T45.7X4	T45.7X5	T45.7X6
K1	T45.7X1	T45.7X2	T45.7X3	T45.7X4	T45.7X5	T45.7X6
K2	T45.7X1	T45.7X2	T45.7X3	T45.7X4	T45.7X5	T45.7X6
PP	T45.2X1	T45.2X2	T45.2X3	T45.2X4	T45.2X5	T45.2X6
ulceroprotectant	T47.1X1	T47.1X2	T47.1X3	T47.1X4	T47.1X5	T47.1X6
Vleminckx's solution	T49.4X1	T49.4X2	T49.4X3	T49.4X4	T49.4X5	T49.4X6
Voltaren — *see Diclofenac sodium*						
W						
Warfarin	T45.511	T45.512	T45.513	T45.514	T45.515	T45.516
rodenticide	T60.4X1	T60.4X2	T60.4X3	T60.4X4	—	—
sodium	T60.4X1	T60.4X2	T60.4X3	T60.4X4	—	—
Wasp (sting)	T63.461	T63.462	T63.463	T63.464	—	—
Water						
balance drug	T50.3X1	T50.3X2	T50.3X3	T50.3X4	T50.3X5	T50.3X6
distilled	T50.3X1	T50.3X2	T50.3X3	T50.3X4	T50.3X5	T50.3X6
gas — *see Gas, water*						
incomplete combustion of — *see Carbon, monoxide, fuel, utility*						
hemlock	T62.2X1	T62.2X2	T62.2X3	T62.2X4	—	—
moccasin (venom)	T63.061	T63.062	T63.063	T63.064	—	—
purified	T50.3X1	T50.3X2	T50.3X3	T50.3X4	T50.3X5	T50.3X6
Wax (paraffin) (petroleum)	T52.0X1	T52.0X2	T52.0X3	T52.0X4	—	—
automobile	T65.891	T65.892	T65.893	T65.894	—	—
floor	T52.0X1	T52.0X2	T52.0X3	T52.0X4	—	—
Weed killers NEC	T60.3X1	T60.3X2	T60.3X3	T60.3X4	—	—
Welldorm	T42.6X1	T42.6X2	T42.6X3	T42.6X4	T42.6X5	T42.6X6
White						
arsenic	T57.0X1	T57.0X2	T57.0X3	T57.0X4	—	—
hellebore	T62.2X1	T62.2X2	T62.2X3	T62.2X4	—	—
lotion (keratolytic)	T49.4X1	T49.4X2	T49.4X3	T49.4X4	T49.4X5	T49.4X6
spirit	T52.0X1	T52.0X2	T52.0X3	T52.0X4	—	—
Whitewash	T65.891	T65.892	T65.893	T65.894	—	—
Whole blood (human)	T45.8X1	T45.8X2	T45.8X3	T45.8X4	T45.8X5	T45.8X6
Wild						
black cherry	T62.2X1	T62.2X2	T62.2X3	T62.2X4	—	—
poisonous plants NEC	T62.2X1	T62.2X2	T62.2X3	T62.2X4	—	—
Window cleaning fluid	T65.891	T65.892	T65.893	T65.894	—	—
Wintergreen (oil)	T49.3X1	T49.3X2	T49.3X3	T49.3X4	T49.3X5	T49.3X6

◀ New   ⬅ Revised   ~~deleted~~ Deleted

Substance	External Cause (T-Code)					
	Poisoning, Accidental (Unintentional)	Poisoning, Intentional Self-Harm	Poisoning, Assault	Poisoning, Undetermined	Adverse Effect	Underdosing
Wisterine	T62.2X1	T62.2X2	T62.2X3	T62.2X4	—	—
Witch hazel	T49.2X1	T49.2X2	T49.2X3	T49.2X4	T49.2X5	T49.2X6
Wood alcohol or spirit	T51.1X1	T51.1X2	T51.1X3	T51.1X4	—	—
Wool fat (hydrous)	T49.3X1	T49.3X2	T49.3X3	T49.3X4	T49.3X5	T49.3X6
Woorali	T48.1X1	T48.1X2	T48.1X3	T48.1X4	T48.1X5	T48.1X6
Wormseed, American	T37.4X1	T37.4X2	T37.4X3	T37.4X4	T37.4X5	T37.4X6
X						
Xamoterol	T44.5X1	T44.5X2	T44.5X3	T44.5X4	T44.5X5	T44.5X6
Xanthine diuretics	T50.2X1	T50.2X2	T50.2X3	T50.2X4	T50.2X5	T50.2X6
Xanthinol nicotinate	T46.7X1	T46.7X2	T46.7X3	T46.7X4	T46.7X5	T46.7X6
Xanthotoxin	T49.3X1	T49.3X2	T49.3X3	T49.3X4	T49.3X5	T49.3X6
Xantinol nicotinate	T46.7X1	T46.7X2	T46.7X3	T46.7X4	T46.7X5	T46.7X6
Xantocillin	T36.0X1	T36.0X2	T36.0X3	T36.0X4	T36.0X5	T36.0X6
Xenon (127Xe) (133Xe)	T50.8X1	T50.8X2	T50.8X3	T50.8X4	T50.8X5	T50.8X6
Xenysalate	T49.4X1	T49.4X2	T49.4X3	T49.4X4	T49.4X5	T49.4X6
Xibornol	T37.8X1	T37.8X2	T37.8X3	T37.8X4	T37.8X5	T37.8X6
Xigris	T45.511	T45.512	T45.513	T45.514	T45.515	T45.516
Xipamide	T50.2X1	T50.2X2	T50.2X3	T50.2X4	T50.2X5	T50.2X6
Xylene (vapor)	T52.2X1	T52.2X2	T52.2X3	T52.2X4	—	—
Xylocaine (infiltration) (topical)	T41.3X1	T41.3X2	T41.3X3	T41.3X4	T41.3X5	T41.3X6
nerve block (peripheral) (plexus)	T41.3X1	T41.3X2	T41.3X3	T41.3X4	T41.3X5	T41.3X6
spinal	T41.3X1	T41.3X2	T41.3X3	T41.3X4	T41.3X5	T41.3X6
Xylol (vapor)	T52.2X1	T52.2X2	T52.2X3	T52.2X4	—	—
Xylometazoline	T48.5X1	T48.5X2	T48.5X3	T48.5X4	T48.5X5	T48.5X6
Y						
Yeast	T45.2X1	T45.2X2	T45.2X3	T45.2X4	T45.2X5	T45.2X6
dried	T45.2X1	T45.2X2	T45.2X3	T45.2X4	T45.2X5	T45.2X6
Yellow						
fever vaccine	T50.B91	T50.B92	T50.B93	T50.B94	T50.B95	T50.B96
jasmine	T62.2X1	T62.2X2	T62.2X3	T62.2X4	—	—
phenolphthalein	T47.2X1	T47.2X2	T47.2X3	T47.2X4	T47.2X5	T47.2X6
Yew	T62.2X1	T62.2X2	T62.2X3	T62.2X4	—	—
Yohimbic acid	T40.991	T40.992	T40.993	T40.994	T40.995	T40.996
Z						
Zactane	T39.8X1	T39.8X2	T39.8X3	T39.8X4	T39.8X5	T39.8X6
Zalcitabine	T37.5X1	T37.5X2	T37.5X3	T37.5X4	T37.5X5	T37.5X6
Zaroxolyn	T50.2X1	T50.2X2	T50.2X3	T50.2X4	T50.2X5	T50.2X6

TABLE OF DRUGS AND CHEMICALS

◀ New   ◀▥ Revised   ~~deleted~~ Deleted

Substance	External Cause (T-Code)					
	Poisoning, Accidental (Unintentional)	Poisoning, Intentional Self-Harm	Poisoning, Assault	Poisoning, Undetermined	Adverse Effect	Underdosing
Zephiran (topical)	T49.0X1	T49.0X2	T49.0X3	T49.0X4	T49.0X5	T49.0X6
ophthalmic preparation	T49.5X1	T49.5X2	T49.5X3	T49.5X4	T49.5X5	T49.5X6
Zeranol	T38.7X1	T38.7X2	T38.7X3	T38.7X4	T38.7X5	T38.7X6
Zerone	T51.1X1	T51.1X2	T51.1X3	T51.1X4	—	—
Zidovudine	T37.5X1	T37.5X2	T37.5X3	T37.5X4	T37.5X5	T37.5X6
Zimeldine	T43.221	T43.222	T43.223	T43.224	T43.225	T43.226
Zinc (compounds) (fumes) (vapor) NEC	T56.5X1	T56.5X2	T56.5X3	T56.5X4	—	—
anti-infectives	T49.0X1	T49.0X2	T49.0X3	T49.0X4	T49.0X5	T49.0X6
antivaricose	T46.8X1	T46.8X2	T46.8X3	T46.8X4	T46.8X5	T46.8X6
bacitracin	T49.0X1	T49.0X2	T49.0X3	T49.0X4	T49.0X5	T49.0X6
chloride (mouthwash)	T49.6X1	T49.6X2	T49.6X3	T49.6X4	T49.6X5	T49.6X6
chromate	T56.5X1	T56.5X2	T56.5X3	T56.5X4	—	—
gelatin	T49.3X1	T49.3X2	T49.3X3	T49.3X4	T49.3X5	T49.3X6
oxide	T49.3X1	T49.3X2	T49.3X3	T49.3X4	T49.3X5	T49.3X6
plaster	T49.3X1	T49.3X2	T49.3X3	T49.3X4	T49.3X5	T49.3X6
peroxide	T49.0X1	T49.0X2	T49.0X3	T49.0X4	T49.0X5	T49.0X6
pesticides	T56.5X1	T56.5X2	T56.5X3	T56.5X4	—	—
phosphide	T60.4X1	T60.4X2	T60.4X3	T60.4X4	—	—
pyrithionate	T49.4X1	T49.4X2	T49.4X3	T49.4X4	T49.4X5	T49.4X6
stearate	T49.3X1	T49.3X2	T49.3X3	T49.3X4	T49.3X5	T49.3X6
sulfate	T49.5X1	T49.5X2	T49.5X3	T49.5X4	T49.5X5	T49.5X6
ENT agent	T49.6X1	T49.6X2	T49.6X3	T49.6X4	T49.6X5	T49.6X6
ophthalmic solution	T49.5X1	T49.5X2	T49.5X3	T49.5X4	T49.5X5	T49.5X6
topical NEC	T49.0X1	T49.0X2	T49.0X3	T49.0X4	T49.0X5	T49.0X6
undecylenate	T49.0X1	T49.0X2	T49.0X3	T49.0X4	T49.0X5	T49.0X6
Zineb	T60.0X1	T60.0X2	T60.0X3	T60.0X4	—	—
Zinostatin	T45.1X1	T45.1X2	T45.1X3	T45.1X4	T45.1X5	T45.1X6
Zipeprol	T48.3X1	T48.3X2	T48.3X3	T48.3X4	T48.3X5	T48.3X6
Zofenopril	T46.4X1	T46.4X2	T46.4X3	T46.4X4	T46.4X5	T46.4X6
Zolpidem	T42.6X1	T42.6X2	T42.6X3	T42.6X4	T42.6X5	T42.6X6
Zomepirac	T39.391	T39.392	T39.393	T39.394	T39.395	T39.396
Zopiclone	T42.6X1	T42.6X2	T42.6X3	T42.6X4	T42.6X5	T42.6X6
Zorubicin	T45.1X1	T45.1X2	T45.1X3	T45.1X4	T45.1X5	T45.1X6
Zotepine	T43.591	T43.592	T43.593	T43.594	T43.595	T43.596
Zovant	T45.511	T45.512	T45.513	T45.514	T45.515	T45.516
Zoxazolamine	T42.8X1	T42.8X2	T42.8X3	T42.8X4	T42.8X5	T42.8X6
Zuclopenthixol	T43.4X1	T43.4X2	T43.4X3	T43.4X4	T43.4X5	T43.4X6
Zygadenus (venenosus)	T62.2X1	T62.2X2	T62.2X3	T62.2X4	—	—
Zyprexa	T43.591	T43.592	T43.593	T43.594	T43.595	T43.596

◀ New ◀||||| Revised ~~deleted~~ Deleted

A

Abandonment (causing exposure to weather conditions) (with intent to injure or kill) NEC X58

Abuse (adult) (child) (mental) (physical) (sexual) X58

Accident (to) X58
 aircraft (in transit) (powered) —*see also* Accident, transport, aircraft
  due to, caused by cataclysm —*see* Forces of nature, by type
 animal-drawn vehicle —*see* Accident, transport, animal-drawn vehicle occupant
 animal-rider —*see* Accident, transport, animal-rider
 automobile —*see* Accident, transport, car occupant
 bare foot water skiier V94.4
 boat, boating —*see also* Accident, watercraft
  striking swimmer
   powered V94.11
   unpowered V94.12
 bus —*see* Accident, transport, bus occupant
 cable car, not on rails V98.0
  on rails —*see* Accident, transport, streetcar occupant
 car —*see* Accident, transport, car occupant
 caused by, due to
  animal NEC W64
  chain hoist W24.0
  cold (excessive) —*see* Exposure, cold
  corrosive liquid, substance —*see* Table of ►Drugs and ◄Chemicals ◄▥
  cutting or piercing instrument —*see* Contact, with, by type of instrument
  drive belt W24.0
  electric
   current —*see* Exposure, electric current
   motor (*see also* Contact, with, by type of machine) W31.3
    current (of) W86.8
  environmental factor NEC X58
  explosive material —*see* Explosion
  fire, flames —*see* Exposure, fire
  firearm missile —*see* Discharge, firearm by type
  heat (excessive) —*see* Heat
  hot —*see* Contact, with, hot
  ignition —*see* Ignition
  lifting device W24.0
  lightning —*see* subcategory T75.0
   causing fire —*see* Exposure, fire
  machine, machinery —*see* Contact, with, by type of machine
  natural factor NEC X58
  pulley (block) W24.0
  radiation —*see* Radiation
  steam X13.1
   inhalation X13.0
   pipe X16
  thunderbolt —*see* subcategory T75.0
   causing fire —*see* Exposure, fire
  transmission device W24.1
 coach —*see* Accident, transport, bus occupant
 coal car —*see* Accident, transport, industrial vehicle occupant
 diving —*see also* Fall, into, water
  with
   drowning or submersion —*see* Drowning
 forklift —*see* Accident, transport, industrial vehicle occupant
 heavy transport vehicle NOS —*see* Accident, transport, truck occupant
 ice yacht V98.2

Accident (*Continued*)
 in
  medical, surgical procedure
   as, or due to misadventure —*see* Misadventure
   causing an abnormal reaction or later complication without mention of misadventure (*see also* Complication of or following, by type of procedure) Y84.9
 land yacht V98.1
 late effect of —*see* W00-X58 with 7th character S
 logging car —*see* Accident, transport, industrial vehicle occupant
 machine, machinery —*see also* Contact, with, by type of machine
  on board watercraft V93.69
   explosion —*see* Explosion, in, watercraft
   fire —*see* Burn, on board watercraft
   powered craft V93.63
    ferry boat V93.61
    fishing boat V93.62
    jetskis V93.63
    liner V93.61
    merchant ship V93.60
    passenger ship V93.61
    sailboat V93.64
 mine tram —*see* Accident, transport, industrial vehicle occupant
 mobility scooter (motorized) —*see* Accident, transport, pedestrian, conveyance, specified type NEC
 motor scooter —*see* Accident, transport, motorcyclist
 motor vehicle NOS (traffic) (*see also* Accident, transport) V89.2
  nontraffic V89.0
  three-wheeled NOS —*see* Accident, transport, three-wheeled motor vehicle occupant
 motorcycle NOS —*see* Accident, transport, motorcyclist
 nonmotor vehicle NOS (nontraffic) (*see also* Accident, transport) V89.1
  traffic NOS V89.3
 nontraffic (victim's mode of transport NOS) V88.9
  collision (between) V88.7
   bus and truck V88.5
   car and:
    bus V88.3
    pickup V88.2
    three-wheeled motor vehicle V88.0
    train V88.6
    truck V88.4
    two-wheeled motor vehicle V88.0
    van V88.2
   specified vehicle NEC and:
    three-wheeled motor vehicle V88.1
    two-wheeled motor vehicle V88.1
   known mode of transport —*see* Accident, transport, by type of vehicle
  noncollision V88.8
 on board watercraft V93.89
  powered craft V93.83
   ferry boat V93.81
   fishing boat V93.82
   jetskis V93.83
   liner V93.81
   merchant ship V93.80
   passenger ship V93.81
  unpowered craft V93.88
   canoe V93.85
   inflatable V93.86
    in tow
     recreational V94.31
     specified NEC V94.32
   kayak V93.85

Accident (*Continued*)
 on board watercraft (*Continued*)
  unpowered craft (*Continued*)
   sailboat V93.84
   surf-board V93.88
   water skis V93.87
   windsurfer V93.88
 parachutist V97.29
  entangled in object V97.21
  injured on landing V97.22
 pedal cycle —*see* Accident, transport, pedal cyclist
 pedestrian (on foot)
  with
   another pedestrian W51
    with fall W03
     due to ice or snow W00.0
    on pedestrian conveyance NEC V00.09
   roller skater (in-line) V00.01
   skate boarder V00.02
   transport vehicle —*see* Accident, transport
  on pedestrian conveyance —*see* Accident, transport, pedestrian, conveyance
 pick-up truck or van —*see* Accident, transport, pickup truck occupant
 quarry truck —*see* Accident, transport, industrial vehicle occupant
 railway vehicle (any) (in motion) —*see* Accident, transport, railway vehicle occupant
  due to cataclysm —*see* Forces of nature, by type
 scooter (non-motorized) —*see* Accident, transport, pedestrian, conveyance, scooter
 sequelae of —*see* W00-X58 with 7th character S
 skateboard —*see* Accident, transport, pedestrian, conveyance, skateboard
 ski (ing) —*see* Accident, transport, pedestrian, conveyance
  lift V98.3
 specified cause NEC X58
 streetcar —*see* Accident, transport, streetcar occupant
 traffic (victim's mode of transport NOS) V87.9
  collision (between) V87.7
   bus and truck V87.5
   car and:
    bus V87.3
    pickup V87.2
    three-wheeled motor vehicle V87.0
    train V87.6
    truck V87.4
    two-wheeled motor vehicle V87.0
    van V87.2
   specified vehicle NEC and:
    three-wheeled motor vehicle V87.1
    two-wheeled motor vehicle V87.1
  known mode of transport —*see* Accident, transport, by type of vehicle
  noncollision V87.8
 transport (involving injury to) V99
  18 wheeler —*see* Accident, transport, truck occupant
  agricultural vehicle occupant (nontraffic) V84.9
   driver V84.5
   hanger-on V84.7
   passenger V84.6
   traffic V84.3
    driver V84.0
    hanger-on V84.2
    passenger V84.1
    while boarding or alighting V84.4

◀ New   ◀▥ Revised   ~~deleted~~ Deleted

Accident (Continued)
 transport (Continued)
  aircraft NEC V97.89
   military NEC V97.818
    with civilian aircraft V97.810
    civilian injured by V97.811
   occupant injured (in)
    nonpowered craft accident
      V96.9
     balloon V96.00
      collision V96.03
      crash V96.01
      explosion V96.05
      fire V96.04
      forced landing V96.02
      specified type NEC V96.09
     glider V96.20
      collision V96.23
      crash V96.21
      explosion V96.25
      fire V96.24
      forced landing V96.22
      specified type NEC V96.29
     hang glider V96.10
      collision V96.13
      crash V96.11
      explosion V96.15
      fire V96.14
      forced landing V96.12
      specified type NEC V96.19
     specified craft NEC V96.8
    powered craft accident V95.9
     fixed wing NEC
      commercial V95.30
       collision V95.33
       crash V95.31
       explosion V95.35
       fire V95.34
       forced landing V95.32
       specified type NEC
         V95.39
      private V95.20
       collision V95.23
       crash V95.21
       explosion V95.25
       fire V95.24
       forced landing V95.22
       specified type NEC
         V95.29
     glider V95.10
      collision V95.13
      crash V95.11
      explosion V95.15
      fire V95.14
      forced landing V95.12
      specified type NEC V95.19
     helicopter V95.00
      collision V95.03
      crash V95.01
      explosion V95.05
      fire V95.04
      forced landing V95.02
      specified type NEC V95.09
     spacecraft V95.40
      collision V95.43
      crash V95.41
      explosion V95.45
      fire V95.44
      forced landing V95.42
      specified type NEC V95.49
     specified craft NEC V95.8
     ultralight V95.10
      collision V95.13
      crash V95.11
      explosion V95.15
      fire V95.14
      forced landing V95.12
      specified type NEC V95.19
   specified accident NEC V97.0
   while boarding or alighting
     V97.1

Accident (Continued)
 transport (Continued)
  aircraft NEC (Continued)
   person (injured by)
    falling from, in or on aircraft V97.0
    machinery on aircraft V97.89
    on ground with aircraft involvement
      V97.39
    rotating propeller V97.32
    struck by object falling from aircraft
      V97.31
    sucked into aircraft jet V97.33
    while boarding or alighting aircraft
      V97.1
  airport (battery-powered) passenger
    vehicle —see Accident, transport,
    industrial vehicle occupant
  all-terrain vehicle occupant (nontraffic)
    V86.99
   driver V86.59
   dune buggy —see Accident, transport,
     dune buggy occupant
   hanger-on V86.79
   passenger V86.69
   snowmobile —see Accident, transport,
     snowmobile occupant
   traffic V86.39
    driver V86.09
    hanger-on V86.29
    passenger V86.19
   while boarding or alighting V86.49
  ambulance occupant (traffic) V86.31
   driver V86.01
   hanger-on V86.21
   nontraffic V86.91
    driver V86.51
    hanger-on V86.71
    passenger V86.61
   passenger V86.11
   while boarding or alighting V86.41
  animal-drawn vehicle occupant (in)
    V80.929
   collision (with)
    animal V80.12
     being ridden V80.711
    animal-drawn vehicle V80.721
    bus V80.42
    car V80.42
    fixed or stationary object V80.82
    military vehicle V80.920
    nonmotor vehicle V80.791
    pedal cycle V80.22
    pedestrian V80.12
    pickup V80.42
    railway train or vehicle V80.62
    specified motor vehicle NEC V80.52
    streetcar V80.731
    truck V80.42
    two-or three-wheeled motor vehicle
      V80.32
    van V80.42
   noncollision V80.02
   specified circumstance NEC V80. 928
  animal-rider V80.919
   collision (with)
    animal V80.11
     being ridden V80.710
    animal-drawn vehicle V80.720
    bus V80.41
    car V80.41
    fixed or stationary object V80.81
    military vehicle V80.910
    nonmotor vehicle V80.790
    pedal cycle V80.21
    pedestrian V80.11
    pickup V80.41
    railway train or vehicle V80.61
    specified motor vehicle NEC
      V80.51
    streetcar V80.730
    truck V80.41

Accident (Continued)
 transport (Continued)
  animal-rider (Continued)
   collision (Continued)
    two- or three-wheeled motor vehicle
      V80.31
    van V80.41
   noncollision V80.018
    specified as horse rider V80.010
   specified circumstance NEC V80.918
  armored car —see Accident, transport,
    truck occupant
  battery-powered truck (baggage) (mail) —
    see Accident, transport, industrial
    vehicle occupant
  bus occupant V79.9
   collision (with)
    animal (traffic) V70.9
     being ridden (traffic) V76.9
      nontraffic V76.3
      while boarding or alighting V76.4
     nontraffic V70.3
     while boarding or alighting V70.4
    animal-drawn vehicle (traffic) V76.9
     nontraffic V76.3
     while boarding or alighting V76.4
    bus (traffic) V74.9
     nontraffic V74.3
     while boarding or alighting V74.4
    car (traffic) V73.9
     nontraffic V73.3
     while boarding or alighting V73.4
    motor vehicle NOS (traffic) V79.60
     nontraffic V79.20
     specified type NEC (traffic) V79.69
      nontraffic V79.29
    pedal cycle (traffic) V71.9
     nontraffic V71.3
     while boarding or alighting V71.4
    pickup truck (traffic) V73.9
     nontraffic V73.3
     while boarding or alighting V73.4
    railway vehicle (traffic) V75.9
     nontraffic V75.3
     while boarding or alighting V75.4
    specified vehicle NEC (traffic) V76.9
     nontraffic V76.3
     while boarding or alighting V76.4
    stationary object (traffic) V77.9
     nontraffic V77.3
     while boarding or alighting V77.4
    streetcar (traffic) V76.9
     nontraffic V76.3
     while boarding or alighting V76.4
    three wheeled motor vehicle (traffic)
      V72.9
     nontraffic V72.3
     while boarding or alighting V72.4
    truck (traffic) V74.9
     nontraffic V74.3
     while boarding or alighting V74.4
    two wheeled motor vehicle (traffic)
      V72.9
     nontraffic V72.3
     while boarding or alighting V72.4
    van (traffic) V73.9
     nontraffic V73.3
     while boarding or alighting V73.4
   driver
    collision (with)
     animal (traffic) V70.5
      being ridden (traffic) V76.5
       nontraffic V76.0
      nontraffic V70.0
     animal-drawn vehicle (traffic)
       V76.5
      nontraffic V76.0
     bus (traffic) V74.5
      nontraffic V74.0
     car (traffic) V73.5
      nontraffic V73.0

A

◄ New   ◄||| Revised   ~~deleted~~ Deleted

Accident (Continued)
  transport (Continued)
    bus occupant (Continued)
      driver (Continued)
        collision (Continued)
          motor vehicle NOS (traffic) V79.40
            nontraffic V79.00
          specified type NEC (traffic)
            V79.49
            nontraffic V79.09
          pedal cycle (traffic) V71.5
            nontraffic V71.0
          pickup truck (traffic) V73.5
            nontraffic V73.0
          railway vehicle (traffic) V75.5
            nontraffic V75.0
          specified vehicle NEC (traffic)
            V76.5
            nontraffic V76.0
          stationary object (traffic) V77.5
            nontraffic V77.0
          streetcar (traffic) V76.5
            nontraffic V76.0
          three wheeled motor vehicle
            (traffic) V72.5
            nontraffic V72.0
          truck (traffic) V74.5
            nontraffic V74.0
          two wheeled motor vehicle (traffic)
            V72.5
            nontraffic V72.0
          van (traffic) V73.5
            nontraffic V73.0
        noncollision accident (traffic) V78.5
          nontraffic V78.0
      hanger-on
        collision (with)
          animal (traffic) V70.7
            being ridden (traffic) V76.7
              nontraffic V76.2
            nontraffic V70.2
          animal-drawn vehicle (traffic) V76.7
            nontraffic V76.2
          bus (traffic) V74.7
            nontraffic V74.2
          car (traffic) V73.7
            nontraffic V73.2
          pedal cycle (traffic) V71.7
            nontraffic V71.2
          pickup truck (traffic) V73.7
            nontraffic V73.2
          railway vehicle (traffic) V75.7
            nontraffic V75.2
          specified vehicle NEC (traffic) V76.7
            nontraffic V76.2
          stationary object (traffic) V77.7
            nontraffic V77.2
          streetcar (traffic) V76.7
            nontraffic V76.2
          three wheeled motor vehicle
            (traffic) V72.7
            nontraffic V72.2
          truck (traffic) V74.7
            nontraffic V74.2
          two wheeled motor vehicle (traffic)
            V72.7
            nontraffic V72.2
          van (traffic) V73.7
            nontraffic V73.2
        noncollision accident (traffic) V78.7
          nontraffic V78.2
      noncollision accident (traffic) V78.9
        nontraffic V78.3
        while boarding or alighting V78.4
      nontraffic V79.3
      passenger
        collision (with)
          animal (traffic) V70.6
            being ridden (traffic) V76.6
              nontraffic V76.1
            nontraffic V70.1

Accident (Continued)
  transport (Continued)
    bus occupant (Continued)
      passenger (Continued)
        collision (Continued)
          animal-drawn vehicle (traffic) V76.6
            nontraffic V76.1
          bus (traffic) V74.6
            nontraffic V74.1
          car (traffic) V73.6
            nontraffic V73.1
          motor vehicle NOS (traffic) V79.50
            nontraffic V79.10
          specified type NEC (traffic)
            V79.59
            nontraffic V79.19
          pedal cycle (traffic) V71.6
            nontraffic V71.1
          pickup truck (traffic) V73.6
            nontraffic V73.1
          railway vehicle (traffic) V75.6
            nontraffic V75.1
          specified vehicle NEC (traffic) V76.6
            nontraffic V76.1
          stationary object (traffic) V77.6
            nontraffic V77.1
          streetcar (traffic) V76.6
            nontraffic V76.1
          three wheeled motor vehicle
            (traffic) V72.6
            nontraffic V72.1
          truck (traffic) V74.6
            nontraffic V74.1
          two wheeled motor vehicle (traffic)
            V72.6
            nontraffic V72.1
          van (traffic) V73.6
            nontraffic V73.1
        noncollision accident (traffic) V78.6
          nontraffic V78.1
      specified type NEC V79.88
      military vehicle V79.81
  cable car, not on rails V98.0
    on rails —see Accident, transport,
      streetcar occupant
  car occupant V49.9
    ambulance occupant —see Accident,
      transport, ambulance occupant
    collision (with)
      animal (traffic) V40.9
        being ridden (traffic) V46.9
          nontraffic V46.3
          while boarding or alighting
            V46.4
        nontraffic V40.3
        while boarding or alighting V40.4
      animal-drawn vehicle (traffic) V46.9
        nontraffic V46.3
        while boarding or alighting V46.4
      bus (traffic) V44.9
        nontraffic V44.3
        while boarding or alighting V44.4
      car (traffic) V43.92
        nontraffic V43.32
        while boarding or alighting V43.42
      motor vehicle NOS (traffic) V49.60
        nontraffic V49.20
        specified type NEC (traffic) V49.69
          nontraffic V49.29
      pedal cycle (traffic) V41.9
        nontraffic V41.3
        while boarding or alighting V41.4
      pickup truck (traffic) V43.93
        nontraffic V43.33
        while boarding or alighting V43.43
      railway vehicle (traffic) V45.9
        nontraffic V45.3
        while boarding or alighting V45.4
      specified vehicle NEC (traffic) V46.9
        nontraffic V46.3
        while boarding or alighting V46.4

Accident (Continued)
  transport (Continued)
    car occupant (Continued)
      collision (Continued)
        sport utility vehicle (traffic) V43.91
          nontraffic V43.31
          while boarding or alighting V43.41
        stationary object (traffic) V47.92
          nontraffic V47.32
          while boarding or alighting V47.4
        streetcar (traffic) V46.9
          nontraffic V46.3
          while boarding or alighting V46.4
        three wheeled motor vehicle (traffic)
          V42.9
          nontraffic V42.3
          while boarding or alighting V42.4
        truck (traffic) V44.9
          nontraffic V44.3
          while boarding or alighting V44.4
        two wheeled motor vehicle (traffic)
          V42.9
          nontraffic V42.3
          while boarding or alighting V42.4
        van (traffic) V43.94
          nontraffic V43.34
          while boarding or alighting V43.44
      driver
        collision (with)
          animal (traffic) V40.5
            being ridden (traffic) V46.5
              nontraffic V46.0
            nontraffic V40.0
          animal-drawn vehicle (traffic) V46.5
            nontraffic V46.0
          bus (traffic) V44.5
            nontraffic V44.0
          car (traffic) V43.52
            nontraffic V43.02
          motor vehicle NOS (traffic) V49.40
            nontraffic V49.00
            specified type NEC (traffic)
              V49.49
              nontraffic V49.09
          pedal cycle (traffic) V41.5
            nontraffic V41.0
          pickup truck (traffic) V43.53
            nontraffic V43.03
          railway vehicle (traffic) V45.5
            nontraffic V45.0
          specified vehicle NEC (traffic) V46.5
            nontraffic V46.0
          sport utility vehicle (traffic) V43.51
            nontraffic V43.01
          stationary object (traffic) V47.52
            nontraffic V47.02
          streetcar (traffic) V46.5
            nontraffic V46.0
          three wheeled motor vehicle
            (traffic) V42.5
            nontraffic V42.0
          truck (traffic) V44.5
            nontraffic V44.0
          two wheeled motor vehicle (traffic)
            V42.5
            nontraffic V42.0
          van (traffic) V43.54
            nontraffic V43.04
        noncollision accident (traffic) V48.5
          nontraffic V48.0
      hanger-on
        collision (with)
          animal (traffic) V40.7
            being ridden (traffic) V46.7
              nontraffic V46.2
            nontraffic V40.2
          animal-drawn vehicle (traffic)
            V46.7
            nontraffic V46.2
          bus (traffic) V44.7
            nontraffic V44.2

◀ New   ◀▥ Revised   ~~deleted~~ Deleted

Accident (Continued)
  transport (Continued)
    car occupant (Continued)
      hanger-on (Continued)
        collision (Continued)
          car (traffic) V43.72
            nontraffic V43.22
          pedal cycle (traffic) V41.7
            nontraffic V41.2
          pickup truck (traffic) V43.73
            nontraffic V43.23
          railway vehicle (traffic) V45.7
            nontraffic V45.2
          specified vehicle NEC (traffic) V46.7
            nontraffic V46.2
          sport utility vehicle (traffic) V43.71
            nontraffic V43.21
          stationary object (traffic) V47.7
            nontraffic V47.2
          streetcar (traffic) V46.7
            nontraffic V46.2
          three wheeled motor vehicle
            (traffic) V42.7
            nontraffic V42.2
          truck (traffic) V44.7
            nontraffic V44.2
          two wheeled motor vehicle (traffic)
            V42.7
            nontraffic V42.2
          van (traffic) V43.74
            nontraffic V43.24
        noncollision accident (traffic) V48.7
          nontraffic V48.2
      noncollision accident (traffic) V48.9
        nontraffic V48.3
      while boarding or alighting V48.4
      nontraffic V49.3
      passenger
        collision (with)
          animal (traffic) V40.6
            being ridden (traffic) V46.6
              nontraffic V46.1
            nontraffic V40.1
          animal-drawn vehicle (traffic) V46.6
            nontraffic V46.1
          bus (traffic) V44.6
            nontraffic V44.1
          car (traffic) V43.62
            nontraffic V43.12
          motor vehicle NOS (traffic) V49.50
            nontraffic V49.10
            specified type NEC (traffic) V49.59
              nontraffic V49.19
          pedal cycle (traffic) V41.6
            nontraffic V41.1
          pickup truck (traffic) V43.63
            nontraffic V43.13
          railway vehicle (traffic) V45.6
            nontraffic V45.1
          specified vehicle NEC (traffic) V46.6
            nontraffic V46.1
          sport utility vehicle (traffic) V43.61
            nontraffic V43.11
          stationary object (traffic) V47.62
            nontraffic V47.12
          streetcar (traffic) V46.6
            nontraffic V46.1
          three wheeled motor vehicle
            (traffic) V42.6
            nontraffic V42.1
          truck (traffic) V44.6
            nontraffic V44.1
          two wheeled motor vehicle (traffic)
            V42.6
            nontraffic V42.1
          van (traffic) V43.64
            nontraffic V43.14
        noncollision accident (traffic) V48.6
          nontraffic V48.1
      specified type NEC V49.88
      military vehicle V49.81

Accident (Continued)
  transport (Continued)
    coal car —see Accident, transport,
      industrial vehicle occupant
    construction vehicle occupant (nontraffic)
      V85.9
      driver V85.5
      hanger-on V85.7
      passenger V85.6
      traffic V85.3
        driver V85.0
        hanger-on V85.2
        passenger V85.1
      while boarding or alighting V85.4
    dirt bike rider —see Accident, transport,
      all-terrain vehicle occupant
    due to cataclysm —see Forces of nature,
      by type
    dune buggy occupant (nontraffic) V86.93
      driver V86.53
      hanger-on V86.73
      passenger V86.63
      traffic V86.33
        driver V86.03
        hanger-on V86.23
        passenger V86.13
      while boarding or alighting V86.43
    forklift —see Accident, transport, industrial
      vehicle occupant
    go cart —see Accident, transport, all-terrain
      vehicle occupant
    golf cart —see Accident, transport, all-
      terrain vehicle occupant
    heavy transport vehicle occupant —see
      Accident, transport, truck occupant
    ice yacht V98.2
    industrial vehicle occupant (nontraffic)
      V83.9
      driver V83.5
      hanger-on V83.7
      passenger V83.6
      traffic V83.3
        driver V83.0
        hanger-on V83.2
        passenger V83.1
      while boarding or alighting V83.4
    interurban electric car —see Accident,
      transport, streetcar
    land yacht V98.1
    logging car —see Accident, transport,
      industrial vehicle occupant
    military vehicle occupant (traffic) V86.34
      driver V86.04
      hanger-on V86.24
      nontraffic V86.94
        driver V86.54
        hanger-on V86.74
        passenger V86.64
      passenger V86.14
      while boarding or alighting V86.44
    mine tram —see Accident, transport,
      industrial vehicle occupant
    motor vehicle NEC occupant (traffic) V86.39
      driver V86.09
      hanger-on V86.29
      nontraffic V86.99
        driver V86.59
        hanger-on V86.79
        passenger V86.69
      passenger V86.19
      while boarding or alighting V86.49
    motorcoach —see Accident, transport, bus
      occupant
    motorcyclist V29.9
      collision (with)
        animal (traffic) V20.9
          being ridden (traffic) V26.9
            nontraffic V26.2
            while boarding or alighting V26.3
          nontraffic V20.2
          while boarding or alighting V20.3

Accident (Continued)
  transport (Continued)
    motorcyclist (Continued)
      collision (Continued)
        animal-drawn vehicle (traffic) V26.9
          nontraffic V26.2
          while boarding or alighting V26.3
        bus (traffic) V24.9
          nontraffic V24.2
          while boarding or alighting V24.3
        car (traffic) V23.9
          nontraffic V23.2
          while boarding or alighting V23.3
        motor vehicle NOS (traffic) V29.60
          nontraffic V29.20
          specified type NEC (traffic) V29.69
            nontraffic V29.29
        pedal cycle (traffic) V21.9
          nontraffic V21.2
          while boarding or alighting V21.3
        pickup truck (traffic) V23.9
          nontraffic V23.2
          while boarding or alighting V23.3
        railway vehicle (traffic) V25.9
          nontraffic V25.2
          while boarding or alighting V25.3
        specified vehicle NEC (traffic) V26.9
          nontraffic V26.2
          while boarding or alighting V26.3
        stationary object (traffic) V27.9
          nontraffic V27.2
          while boarding or alighting V27.3
        streetcar (traffic) V26.9
          nontraffic V26.2
          while boarding or alighting V26.3
        three wheeled motor vehicle (traffic)
          V22.9
          nontraffic V22.2
          while boarding or alighting V22.3
        truck (traffic) V24.9
          nontraffic V24.2
          while boarding or alighting V24.3
        two wheeled motor vehicle (traffic)
          V22.9
          nontraffic V22.2
          while boarding or alighting V22.3
        van (traffic) V23.9
          nontraffic V23.2
          while boarding or alighting V23.3
      driver
        collision (with)
          animal (traffic) V20.4
            being ridden (traffic) V26.4
              nontraffic V26.0
            nontraffic V20.0
          animal-drawn vehicle (traffic) V26.4
            nontraffic V26.0
          bus (traffic) V24.4
            nontraffic V24.0
          car (traffic) V23.4
            nontraffic V23.0
          motor vehicle NOS (traffic) V29.40
            nontraffic V29.00
            specified type NEC (traffic)
              V29.49
              nontraffic V29.09
          pedal cycle (traffic) V21.4
            nontraffic V21.0
          pickup truck (traffic) V23.4
            nontraffic V23.0
          railway vehicle (traffic) V25.4
            nontraffic V25.0
          specified vehicle NEC (traffic) V26.4
            nontraffic V26.0
          stationary object (traffic) V27.4
            nontraffic V27.0
          streetcar (traffic) V26.4
            nontraffic V26.0
          three wheeled motor vehicle
            (traffic) V22.4
            nontraffic V22.0

Accident *(Continued)*
  transport *(Continued)*
    motorcyclist *(Continued)*
      driver *(Continued)*
        collision *(Continued)*
          truck (traffic) V24.4
            nontraffic V24.0
          two wheeled motor vehicle (traffic)
            V22.4
            nontraffic V22.0
          van (traffic) V23.4
            nontraffic V23.0
        noncollision accident (traffic) V28.4
          nontraffic V28.0
        noncollision accident (traffic) V28.9
          nontraffic V28.2
        while boarding or alighting V28.3
      nontraffic V29.3
      passenger
        collision (with)
          animal (traffic) V20.5
            being ridden (traffic) V26.5
              nontraffic V26.1
            nontraffic V20.1
          animal-drawn vehicle (traffic)
            V26.5
            nontraffic V26.1
          bus (traffic) V24.5
            nontraffic V24.1
          car (traffic) V23.5
            nontraffic V23.1
          motor vehicle NOS (traffic) V29.50
            nontraffic V29.10
            specified type NEC (traffic)
              V29.59
              nontraffic V29.19
          pedal cycle (traffic) V21.5
            nontraffic V21.1
          pickup truck (traffic) V23.5
            nontraffic V23.1
          railway vehicle (traffic) V25.5
            nontraffic V25.1
          specified vehicle NEC (traffic)
            V26.5
            nontraffic V26.1
          stationary object (traffic) V27.5
            nontraffic V27.1
          streetcar (traffic) V26.5
            nontraffic V26.1
          three wheeled motor vehicle
            (traffic) V22.5
            nontraffic V22.1
          truck (traffic) V24.5
            nontraffic V24.1
          two wheeled motor vehicle (traffic)
            V22.5
            nontraffic V22.1
          van (traffic) V23.5
            nontraffic V23.1
        noncollision accident (traffic) V28.5
          nontraffic V28.1
      specified type NEC V29.88
      military vehicle V29.81
    occupant (of)
      aircraft (powered) V95.9
        fixed wing
          commercial —*see* Accident,
            transport, aircraft, occupant,
            powered, fixed wing,
            commercial
          private —*see* Accident, transport,
            aircraft, occupant, powered,
            fixed wing, private
        nonpowered V96.9
        specified NEC V95.8
      airport battery-powered vehicle —*see*
        Accident, transport, industrial
        vehicle occupant
      all-terrain vehicle (ATV) —*see* Accident,
        transport, all-terrain vehicle
        occupant

Accident *(Continued)*
  transport *(Continued)*
    occupant *(Continued)*
      animal-drawn vehicle —*see* Accident,
        transport, animal-drawn vehicle
        occupant
      automobile —*see* Accident, transport, car
        occupant
      balloon V96.00
      battery-powered vehicle —*see* Accident,
        transport, industrial vehicle
        occupant
      bicycle —*see* Accident, transport, pedal
        cyclist
        motorized —*see* Accident, transport,
          motorcycle rider
      boat NEC —*see* Accident, watercraft
      bulldozer —*see* Accident, transport,
        construction vehicle occupant
      bus —*see* Accident, transport, bus
        occupant
      cable car (on rails) —*see also* Accident,
        transport, streetcar occupant
        not on rails V98.0
      car —*see also* Accident, transport, car
        occupant
        cable (on rails) —*see also* Accident,
          transport, streetcar occupant
          not on rails V98.0
      coach —*see* Accident, transport, bus
        occupant
      coal-car —*see* Accident, transport,
        industrial vehicle occupant
      digger —*see* Accident, transport,
        construction vehicle occupant
      dump truck —*see* Accident, transport,
        construction vehicle occupant
      earth-leveler —*see* Accident, transport,
        construction vehicle occupant
      farm machinery (self-propelled) —*see*
        Accident, transport, agricultural
        vehicle occupant
      forklift —*see* Accident, transport,
        industrial vehicle occupant
      glider (unpowered) V96.20
        hang V96.10
        powered (microlight) (ultralight) —*see*
          Accident, transport, aircraft,
          occupant, powered, glider
      glider (unpowered) NEC V96.20
      hang-glider V96.10
      harvester —*see* Accident, transport,
        agricultural vehicle occupant
      heavy (transport) vehicle —*see* Accident,
        transport, truck occupant
      helicopter —*see* Accident, transport,
        aircraft, occupant, helicopter
      ice-yacht V98.2
      kite (carrying person) V96.8
      land-yacht V98.1
      logging car —*see* Accident, transport,
        industrial vehicle occupant
      mechanical shovel —*see* Accident,
        transport, construction vehicle
        occupant
      microlight —*see* Accident, transport,
        aircraft, occupant, powered, glider
      minibus —*see* Accident, transport, car
        occupant
      minivan —*see* Accident, transport, car
        occupant
      moped —*see* Accident, transport,
        motorcycle
      motor scooter —*see* Accident, transport,
        motorcycle
      motorcycle (with sidecar) —*see* Accident,
        transport, motorcycle
      pedal cycle —*see also* Accident,
        transport, pedal cyclist
      pick-up (truck) —*see* Accident, transport,
        pickup truck occupant

Accident *(Continued)*
  transport *(Continued)*
    occupant *(Continued)*
      railway (train) (vehicle) (subterranean)
        (elevated) —*see* Accident, transport,
        railway vehicle occupant
      rickshaw —*see* Accident, transport,
        pedal cycle
      pedal driven —*see* Accident, transport,
        pedal cyclist
      road-roller —*see* Accident, transport,
        construction vehicle occupant
      ship NOS V94.9
      ski-lift (chair) (gondola) V98.3
      snowmobile —*see* Accident, transport,
        snowmobile occupant
      spacecraft, spaceship —*see* Accident,
        transport, aircraft, occupant,
        spacecraft
      sport utility vehicle —*see* Accident,
        transport, car occupant
      streetcar (interurban) (operating on
        public street or highway) —*see*
        Accident, transport, streetcar
        occupant
      SUV —*see* Accident, transport, car
        occupant
      téléférique V98.0
      three-wheeled vehicle (motorized) —*see
        also* Accident, transport, three-
        wheeled motor vehicle occupant
        nonmotorized —*see* Accident,
          transport, pedal cycle
      tractor (farm) (and trailer) —*see*
        Accident, transport, agricultural
        vehicle occupant
      train —*see* Accident, transport, railway
        vehicle occupant
      tram —*see* Accident, transport, streetcar
        occupant
        in mine or quarry —*see* Accident,
          transport, industrial vehicle
          occupant
      tricycle —*see* Accident, transport, pedal
        cycle
        motorized —*see* Accident, transport,
          three-wheeled motor vehicle
      trolley —*see* Accident, transport,
        streetcar occupant
        in mine or quarry —*see* Accident,
          transport, industrial vehicle
          occupant
      tub, in mine or quarry —*see* Accident,
        transport, industrial vehicle
        occupant
      ultralight —*see* Accident, transport,
        aircraft, occupant, powered, glider
      van —*see* Accident, transport, van
        occupant
      vehicle NEC V89.9
        heavy transport —*see* Accident,
          transport, truck occupant
        motor (traffic) NEC V89.2
          nontraffic NEC V89.0
      watercraft NOS V94.9
        causing drowning —*see* Drowning,
          resulting from accident to boat
  parachutist V97.29
    after accident to aircraft —*see* Accident,
      transport, aircraft
    entangled in object V97.21
    injured on landing V97.22
  pedal cyclist V19.9
    collision (with)
      animal (traffic) V10.9
        being ridden (traffic) V16.9
          nontraffic V16.2
          while boarding or alighting
            V16.3
        nontraffic V10.2
        while boarding or alighting V10.3

◀ New   ◀▦ Revised   ~~deleted~~ Deleted

Accident *(Continued)*
  transport *(Continued)*
    pedal cyclist *(Continued)*
      collision *(Continued)*
        animal-drawn vehicle (traffic) V16.9
          nontraffic V16.2
          while boarding or alighting V16.3
        bus (traffic) V14.9
          nontraffic V14.2
          while boarding or alighting V14.3
        car (traffic) V13.9
          nontraffic V13.2
          while boarding or alighting V13.3
        motor vehicle NOS (traffic) V19.60
          nontraffic V19.20
          specified type NEC (traffic) V19.69
            nontraffic V19.29
        pedal cycle (traffic) V11.9
          nontraffic V11.2
          while boarding or alighting V11.3
        pickup truck (traffic) V13.9
          nontraffic V13.2
          while boarding or alighting V13.3
        railway vehicle (traffic) V15.9
          nontraffic V15.2
          while boarding or alighting V15.3
        specified vehicle NEC (traffic) V16.9
          nontraffic V16.2
          while boarding or alighting V16.3
        stationary object (traffic) V17.9
          nontraffic V17.2
          while boarding or alighting V17.3
        streetcar (traffic) V16.9
          nontraffic V16.2
          while boarding or alighting V16.3
        three wheeled motor vehicle (traffic) V12.9
          nontraffic V12.2
          while boarding or alighting V12.3
        truck (traffic) V14.9
          nontraffic V14.2
          while boarding or alighting V14.3
        two wheeled motor vehicle (traffic) V12.9
          nontraffic V12.2
          while boarding or alighting V12.3
        van (traffic) V13.9
          nontraffic V13.2
          while boarding or alighting V13.3
      driver
        collision (with)
          animal (traffic) V10.4
            being ridden (traffic) V16.4
              nontraffic V16.0
            nontraffic V10.0
          animal-drawn vehicle (traffic) V16.4
            nontraffic V16.0
          bus (traffic) V14.4
            nontraffic V14.0
          car (traffic) V13.4
            nontraffic V13.0
          motor vehicle NOS (traffic) V19.40
            nontraffic V19.00
            specified type NEC (traffic) V19.49
              nontraffic V19.09
          pedal cycle (traffic) V11.4
            nontraffic V11.0
          pickup truck (traffic) V13.4
            nontraffic V13.0
          railway vehicle (traffic) V15.4
            nontraffic V15.0
          specified vehicle NEC (traffic) V16.4
            nontraffic V16.0
          stationary object (traffic) V17.4
            nontraffic V17.0
          streetcar (traffic) V16.4
            nontraffic V16.0
          three wheeled motor vehicle (traffic) V12.4
            nontraffic V12.0

Accident *(Continued)*
  transport *(Continued)*
    pedal cyclist *(Continued)*
      driver *(Continued)*
        collision *(Continued)*
          truck (traffic) V14.4
            nontraffic V14.0
          two wheeled motor vehicle (traffic) V12.4
            nontraffic V12.0
          van (traffic) V13.4
            nontraffic V13.0
        noncollision accident (traffic) V18.4
          nontraffic V18.0
        noncollision accident (traffic) V18.9
          nontraffic V18.2
          while boarding or alighting V18.3
        nontraffic V19.3
      passenger
        collision (with)
          animal (traffic) V10.5
            being ridden (traffic) V16.5
              nontraffic V16.1
            nontraffic V10.1
          animal-drawn vehicle (traffic) V16.5
            nontraffic V16.1
          bus (traffic) V14.5
            nontraffic V14.1
          car (traffic) V13.5
            nontraffic V13.1
          motor vehicle NOS (traffic) V19.50
            nontraffic V19.10
            specified type NEC (traffic) V19.59
              nontraffic V19.19
          pedal cycle (traffic) V11.5
            nontraffic V11.1
          pickup truck (traffic) V13.5
            nontraffic V13.1
          railway vehicle (traffic) V15.5
            nontraffic V15.1
          specified vehicle NEC (traffic) V16.5
            nontraffic V16.1
          stationary object (traffic) V17.5
            nontraffic V17.1
          streetcar (traffic) V16.5
            nontraffic V16.1
          three wheeled motor vehicle (traffic) V12.5
            nontraffic V12.1
          truck (traffic) V14.5
            nontraffic V14.1
          two wheeled motor vehicle (traffic) V12.5
            nontraffic V12.1
          van (traffic) V13.5
            nontraffic V13.1
        noncollision accident (traffic) V18.5
          nontraffic V18.1
      specified type NEC V19.88
      military vehicle V19.81
    pedestrian
      conveyance (occupant) V09.9
        babystroller V00.828
          collision (with) V09.9
            animal being ridden or animal drawn vehicle V06.99
              nontraffic V06.09
              traffic V06.19
            bus or heavy transport V04.99
              nontraffic V04.09
              traffic V04.19
            car V03.99
              nontraffic V03.09
              traffic V03.19
            pedal cycle V01.99
              nontraffic V01.09
              traffic V01.19
            pick-up truck or van V03.99
              nontraffic V03.09
              traffic V03.19

Accident *(Continued)*
  transport *(Continued)*
    pedestrian *(Continued)*
      conveyance *(Continued)*
        babystroller *(Continued)*
          collision *(Continued)*
            railway (train) (vehicle) V05.99
              nontraffic V05.09
              traffic V05.19
            stationary object V00.822
            streetcar V06.99
              nontraffic V06.09
              traffic V06.19
            two- or three-wheeled motor vehicle V02.99
              nontraffic V02.09
              traffic V02.19
            vehicle V09.9
              animal-drawn V06.99
                nontraffic V06.09
                traffic V06.19
              motor
                nontraffic V09.00
                traffic V09.20
        fall V00.821
        nontraffic V09.1
          involving motor vehicle NEC V09.00
        traffic V09.3
          involving motor vehicle NEC V09.20
        flat-bottomed NEC V00.388
          collision (with) V09.9
            animal being ridden or animal drawn vehicle V06.99
              nontraffic V06.09
              traffic V06.19
            bus or heavy transport V04.99
              nontraffic V04.09
              traffic V04.19
            car V03.99
              nontraffic V03.09
              traffic V03.19
            pedal cycle V01.99
              nontraffic V01.09
              traffic V01.19
            pick-up truck or van V03.99
              nontraffic V03.09
              traffic V03.19
            railway (train) (vehicle) V05.99
              nontraffic V05.09
              traffic V05.19
            stationary object V00.382
            streetcar V06.99
              nontraffic V06.09
              traffic V06.19
            two-or three-wheeled motor vehicle V02.99
              nontraffic V02.09
              traffic V02.19
            vehicle V09.9
              animal-drawn V06.99
                nontraffic V06.09
                traffic V06.19
              motor
                nontraffic V09.00
                traffic V09.20
        fall V00.381
        nontraffic V09.1
          involving motor vehicle NEC V09.00
        snow
          board —*see* Accident, transport, pedestrian, conveyance, snow board
          ski —*see* Accident, transport, pedestrian, conveyance, skis (snow)
        traffic V09.3
          involving motor vehicle NEC V09.20

Accident *(Continued)*
  transport *(Continued)*
    pedestrian *(Continued)*
      conveyance *(Continued)*
        gliding type NEC V00.288
          collision (with) V09.9
            animal being ridden or animal
              drawn vehicle V06.99
              nontraffic V06.09
              traffic V06.19
            bus or heavy transport
              V04.99
              nontraffic V04.09
              traffic V04.19
            car V03.99
              nontraffic V03.09
              traffic V03.19
            pedal cycle V01.99
              nontraffic V01.09
              traffic V01.19
            pick-up truck or van V03.99
              nontraffic V03.09
              traffic V03.19
            railway (train) (vehicle) V05.99
              nontraffic V05.09
              traffic V05.19
            stationary object V00.282
            streetcar V06.99
              nontraffic V06.09
              traffic V06.19
            two- or three-wheeled motor
              vehicle V02.99
              nontraffic V02.09
              traffic V02.19
            vehicle V09.9
              animal-drawn V06.99
                nontraffic V06.09
                traffic V06.19
              motor
                nontraffic V09.00
                traffic V09.20
        fall V00.281
        heelies —*see* Accident, transport,
          pedestrian, conveyance,
          heelies
        ice skate —*see* Accident, transport,
          pedestrian, conveyance, ice
          skate
        nontraffic V09.1
          involving motor vehicle NEC
            V09.00
        sled —*see* Accident, transport,
          pedestrian, conveyance, sled
        traffic V09.3
          involving motor vehicle NEC
            V09.20
          wheelies —*see* Accident,
           transport, pedestrian,
           conveyance, heelies
      heelies V00.158
        colliding with stationary object
          V00.152
        fall V00.151
      ice skates V00.218
        collision (with) V09.9
          animal being ridden or animal
            drawn vehicle V06.99
            nontraffic V06.09
            traffic V06.19
          bus or heavy transport V04.99
            nontraffic V04.09
            traffic V04.19
          car V03.99
            nontraffic V03.09
            traffic V03.19
          pedal cycle V01.99
            nontraffic V01.09
            traffic V01.19
          pick-up truck or van V03.99
            nontraffic V03.09
            traffic V03.19

Accident *(Continued)*
  transport *(Continued)*
    pedestrian *(Continued)*
      conveyance *(Continued)*
        ice skates *(Continued)*
          collision *(Continued)*
            railway (train) (vehicle)
              V05.99
            nontraffic V05.09
            traffic V05.19
            stationary object V00.212
            streetcar V06.99
             nontraffic V06.09
             traffic V06.19
            two- or three-wheeled motor
              vehicle V02.99
             nontraffic V02.09
             traffic V02.19
            vehicle V09.9
             animal-drawn V06.99
              nontraffic V06.09
              traffic V06.19
             motor
              nontraffic V09.00
              traffic V09.20
          fall V00.211
          nontraffic V09.1
            involving motor vehicle NEC
              V09.00
          traffic V09.3
            involving motor vehicle NEC
              V09.20
        motorized mobility scooter
          V00.838
          collision with stationary object
            V00.832
          fall from V00.831
        nontraffic V09.1
          involving motor vehicle
            V09.00
          military V09.01
          specified type NEC V09.09
        roller skates (non in-line) V00.128
          collision (with) V09.9
            animal being ridden or animal
              drawn vehicle V06.91
              nontraffic V06.01
              traffic V06.11
            bus or heavy transport
              V04.91
             nontraffic V04.01
             traffic V04.11
            car V03.91
             nontraffic V03.01
             traffic V03.11
            pedal cycle V01.91
             nontraffic V01.01
             traffic V01.11
            pick-up truck or van V03.91
             nontraffic V03.01
             traffic V03.11
            railway (train) (vehicle)
              V05.91
             nontraffic V05.01
             traffic V05.11
            stationary object V00.122
            streetcar V06.91
             nontraffic V06.01
             traffic V06.11
            two- or three-wheeled motor
              vehicle V02.91
             nontraffic V02.01
             traffic V02.11
            vehicle V09.9
             animal-drawn V06.91
              nontraffic V06.01
              traffic V06.11
             motor
              nontraffic V09.00
              traffic V09.20
          fall V00.121

Accident *(Continued)*
  transport *(Continued)*
    pedestrian *(Continued)*
      conveyance *(Continued)*
        roller skates *(Continued)*
          in-line V00.118
            collision —*see also* Accident,
              transport, pedestrian,
              conveyance occupant, roller
              skates, collision
              with stationary object
                V00.112
            fall V00.111
          nontraffic V09.1
            involving motor vehicle NEC
              V09.00
          traffic V09.3
            involving motor vehicle NEC
              V09.20
        rolling shoes V00.158
          colliding with stationary object
            V00.152
          fall V00.151
        rolling type NEC V00.188
          collision (with) V09.9
            animal being ridden or animal
              drawn vehicle V06.99
              nontraffic V06.09
              traffic V06.19
            bus or heavy transport V04.99
             nontraffic V04.09
             traffic V04.19
            car V03.99
             nontraffic V03.09
             traffic V03.19
            pedal cycle V01.99
             nontraffic V01.09
             traffic V01.19
            pick-up truck or van V03.99
             nontraffic V03.09
             traffic V03.19
            railway (train) (vehicle)
              V05.99
             nontraffic V05.09
             traffic V05.19
            stationary object V00.182
            streetcar V06.99
             nontraffic V06.09
             traffic V06.19
            two- or three-wheeled motor
              vehicle V02.99
             nontraffic V02.09
             traffic V02.19
            vehicle V09.9
             animal-drawn V06.99
              nontraffic V06.09
              traffic V06.19
             motor
              nontraffic V09.00
              traffic V09.20
        fall V00.181
        in-line roller skate —*see* Accident,
          transport, pedestrian,
          conveyance, roller skate,
          in-line
        nontraffic V09.1
          involving motor vehicle NEC
            V09.00
        roller skate —*see* Accident,
          transport, pedestrian,
          conveyance, roller skate
        scooter (non-motorized) —
          see Accident, transport,
          pedestrian, conveyance,
          scooter
        skateboard —*see* Accident,
          transport, pedestrian,
          conveyance, skateboard
        traffic V09.3
          involving motor vehicle NEC
            V09.20

◀ New   ◀◀◀ Revised   ~~deleted~~ Deleted

Accident *(Continued)*
  transport *(Continued)*
    pedestrian *(Continued)*
      conveyance *(Continued)*
        scooter (non-motorized) V00.148
          collision (with) V09.9
            animal being ridden or animal
              drawn vehicle V06.99
              nontraffic V06.09
              traffic V06.19
            bus or heavy transport
              V04.99
              nontraffic V04.09
              traffic V04.19
            car V03.99
              nontraffic V03.09
              traffic V03.19
            pedal cycle V01.99
              nontraffic V01.09
              traffic V01.19
            pick-up truck or van V03.99
              nontraffic V03.09
              traffic V03.19
            railway (train) (vehicle)
              V05.99
              nontraffic V05.09
              traffic V05.19
            stationary object V00.142
            streetcar V06.99
              nontraffic V06.09
              traffic V06.19
            two- or three-wheeled motor
              vehicle V02.99
              nontraffic V02.09
              traffic V02.19
            vehicle V09.9
              animal-drawn V06.99
                nontraffic V06.09
                traffic V06.19
              motor
                nontraffic V09.00
                traffic V09.20
          fall V00.141
          nontraffic V09.1
            involving motor vehicle NEC
              V09.00
          traffic V09.3
            involving motor vehicle NEC
              V09.20
        skate board V00.138
          collision (with) V09.9
            animal being ridden or
              animal drawn vehicle
              V06.92
              nontraffic V06.02
              traffic V06.12
            bus or heavy transport
              V04.92
              nontraffic V04.02
              traffic V04.12
            car V03.92
              nontraffic V03.02
              traffic V03.12
            pedal cycle V01.92
              nontraffic V01.02
              traffic V01.12
            pick-up truck or van V03.92
              nontraffic V03.02
              traffic V03.12
            railway (train) (vehicle)
              V05.92
              nontraffic V05.02
              traffic V05.12
            stationary object V00.132
            streetcar V06.92
              nontraffic V06.02
              traffic V06.12
            two- or three-wheeled motor
              vehicle V02.92
              nontraffic V02.02
              traffic V02.12

Accident *(Continued)*
  transport *(Continued)*
    pedestrian *(Continued)*
      conveyance *(Continued)*
        skate board *(Continued)*
          collision *(Continued)*
            vehicle V09.9
              animal-drawn V06.92
                nontraffic V06.02
                traffic V06.12
              motor
                nontraffic V09.00
                traffic V09.20
          fall V00.131
          nontraffic V09.1
            involving motor vehicle NEC
              V09.00
          traffic V09.3
            involving motor vehicle NEC
              V09.20
        skis (snow) V00.328
          collision (with) V09.9
            animal being ridden or animal
              drawn vehicle V06.99
              nontraffic V06.09
              traffic V06.19
            bus or heavy transport V04.99
              nontraffic V04.09
              traffic V04.19
            car V03.99
              nontraffic V03.09
              traffic V03.19
            pedal cycle V01.99
              nontraffic V01.09
              traffic V01.19
            pick-up truck or van V03.99
              nontraffic V03.09
              traffic V03.19
            railway (train) (vehicle) V05.99
              nontraffic V05.09
              traffic V05.19
            stationary object V00.322
            streetcar V06.99
              nontraffic V06.09
              traffic V06.19
            two- or three-wheeled motor
              vehicle V02.99
              nontraffic V02.09
              traffic V02.19
            vehicle V09.9
              animal-drawn V06.99
                nontraffic V06.09
                traffic V06.19
              motor
                nontraffic V09.00
                traffic V09.20
          fall V00.321
          nontraffic V09.1
            involving motor vehicle NEC
              V09.00
          traffic V09.3
            involving motor vehicle NEC
              V09.20
        sled V00.228
          collision (with) V09.9
            animal being ridden or animal
              drawn vehicle V06.99
              nontraffic V06.09
              traffic V06.19
            bus or heavy transport V04.99
              nontraffic V04.09
              traffic V04.19
            car V03.99
              nontraffic V03.09
              traffic V03.19
            pedal cycle V01.99
              nontraffic V01.09
              traffic V01.19
            pick-up truck or van V03.99
              nontraffic V03.09
              traffic V03.19

Accident *(Continued)*
  transport *(Continued)*
    pedestrian *(Continued)*
      conveyance *(Continued)*
        sled *(Continued)*
          collision *(Continued)*
            railway (train) (vehicle)
              V05.99
              nontraffic V05.09
              traffic V05.19
            stationary object V00.222
            streetcar V06.99
              nontraffic V06.09
              traffic V06.19
            two- or three-wheeled motor
              vehicle V02.99
              nontraffic V02.09
              traffic V02.19
            vehicle V09.9
              animal-drawn V06.99
                nontraffic V06.09
                traffic V06.19
              motor
                nontraffic V09.00
                traffic V09.20
          fall V00.221
          nontraffic V09.1
            involving motor vehicle NEC
              V09.00
          traffic V09.3
            involving motor vehicle NEC
              V09.20
        snow board V00.318
          collision (with) V09.9
            animal being ridden or animal
              drawn vehicle V06.99
              nontraffic V06.09
              traffic V06.19
            bus or heavy transport V04.99
              nontraffic V04.09
              traffic V04.19
            car V03.99
              nontraffic V03.09
              traffic V03.19
            pedal cycle V01.99
              nontraffic V01.09
              traffic V01.19
            pick-up truck or van V03.99
              nontraffic V03.09
              traffic V03.19
            railway (train) (vehicle) V05.99
              nontraffic V05.09
              traffic V05.19
            stationary object V00.312
            streetcar V06.99
              nontraffic V06.09
              traffic V06.19
            two- or three-wheeled motor
              vehicle V02.99
              nontraffic V02.09
              traffic V02.19
            vehicle V09.9
              animal-drawn V06.99
                nontraffic V06.09
                traffic V06.19
              motor
                nontraffic V09.00
                traffic V09.20
          fall V00.311
          nontraffic V09.1
            involving motor vehicle NEC
              V09.00
          traffic V09.3
            involving motor vehicle NEC
              V09.20
        specified type NEC V00.898
          collision (with) V09.9
            animal being ridden or animal
              drawn vehicle V06.99
              nontraffic V06.09
              traffic V06.19

Accident *(Continued)*
  transport *(Continued)*
   pedestrian *(Continued)*
    conveyance *(Continued)*
     specified type NEC *(Continued)*
      collision *(Continued)*
       bus or heavy transport
         V04.99
        nontraffic V04.09
        traffic V04.19
       car V03.99
        nontraffic V03.09
        traffic V03.19
       pedal cycle V01.99
        nontraffic V01.09
        traffic V01.19
       pick-up truck or van V03.99
        nontraffic V03.09
        traffic V03.19
       railway (train) (vehicle)
         V05.99
        nontraffic V05.09
        traffic V05.19
       stationary object V00.892
       streetcar V06.99
        nontraffic V06.09
        traffic V06.19
       two- or three-wheeled motor
         vehicle V02.99
        nontraffic V02.09
        traffic V02.19
       vehicle V09.9
        animal-drawn V06.99
         nontraffic V06.09
         traffic V06.19
        motor
         nontraffic V09.00
         traffic V09.20
      fall V00.891
      nontraffic V09.1
       involving motor vehicle NEC
         V09.00
      traffic V09.3
       involving motor vehicle NEC
         V09.20
     traffic V09.3
      involving motor vehicle V09.20
      military V09.21
      specified type NEC V09.29
    wheelchair (powered) V00.818
     collision (with) V09.9
      animal being ridden or
        animal drawn vehicle
         V06.99
       nontraffic V06.09
       traffic V06.19
      bus or heavy transport
        V04.99
       nontraffic V04.09
       traffic V04.19
      car V03.99
       nontraffic V03.09
       traffic V03.19
      pedal cycle V01.99
       nontraffic V01.09
       traffic V01.19
      pick-up truck or van V03.99
       nontraffic V03.09
       traffic V03.19
      railway (train) (vehicle)
        V05.99
       nontraffic V05.09
       traffic V05.19
      stationary object V00.812
      streetcar V06.99
       nontraffic V06.09
       traffic V06.19
      two- or three-wheeled motor
        vehicle V02.99
       nontraffic V02.09
       traffic V02.19

Accident *(Continued)*
  transport *(Continued)*
   pedestrian *(Continued)*
    conveyance *(Continued)*
     wheelchair *(Continued)*
      collision *(Continued)*
       vehicle V09.9
        animal-drawn V06.99
         nontraffic V06.09
         traffic V06.19
        motor
         nontraffic V09.00
         traffic V09.20
      fall V00.811
      nontraffic V09.1
       involving motor vehicle NEC
         V09.00
      traffic V09.3
       involving motor vehicle NEC
         V09.20
     wheeled shoe V00.158
      colliding with stationary object
        V00.152
      fall V00.151
    on foot —*see also* Accident, pedestrian
     collision (with)
      animal being ridden or animal
        drawn vehicle V06.90
       nontraffic V06.00
       traffic V06.10
      bus or heavy transport V04.90
       nontraffic V04.00
       traffic V04.10
      car V03.90
       nontraffic V03.00
       traffic V03.10
      pedal cycle V01.90
       nontraffic V01.00
       traffic V01.10
      pick-up truck or van V03.90
       nontraffic V03.00
       traffic V03.10
      railway (train) (vehicle) V05.90
       nontraffic V05.00
       traffic V05.10
      streetcar V06.90
       nontraffic V06.00
       traffic V06.10
      two- or three-wheeled motor
        vehicle V02.90
       nontraffic V02.00
       traffic V02.10
      vehicle V09.9
       animal-drawn V06.90
        nontraffic V06.00
        traffic V06.10
       motor
        nontraffic V09.00
        traffic V09.20
      nontraffic V09.1
       involving motor vehicle V09.00
        military V09.01
        specified type NEC V09.09
      traffic V09.3
       involving motor vehicle V09.20
        military V09.21
        specified type NEC V09.29
    person NEC (unknown way or
      transportation) V99
     collision (between)
      bus (with)
       heavy transport vehicle (traffic)
         V87.5
       nontraffic V88.5
      car (with)
       nontraffic V88.5
       bus (traffic) V87.3
        nontraffic V88.3
       heavy transport vehicle (traffic)
         V87.4
        nontraffic V88.4

Accident *(Continued)*
  transport *(Continued)*
   person NEC *(Continued)*
    collision *(Continued)*
     car *(Continued)*
      pick-up truck or van (traffic) V87.2
       nontraffic V88.2
      train or railway vehicle (traffic)
        V87.6
       nontraffic V88.6
      two- or three-wheeled motor
        vehicle (traffic) V87.0
       nontraffic V88.0
      motor vehicle (traffic) NEC V87.7
       nontraffic V88.7
      two- or three-wheeled vehicle (with)
        (traffic)
       motor vehicle NEC V87.1
        nontraffic V88.1
     nonmotor vehicle (collision)
       (noncollision) (traffic) V87.9
      nontraffic V88.9
    pickup truck occupant V59.9
     collision (with)
      animal (traffic) V50.9
       being ridden (traffic) V56.9
        nontraffic V56.3
        while boarding or alighting V56.4
       nontraffic V50.3
       while boarding or alighting V50.4
      animal-drawn vehicle (traffic) V56.9
       nontraffic V56.3
       while boarding or alighting V56.4
      bus (traffic) V54.9
       nontraffic V54.3
       while boarding or alighting V54.4
      car (traffic) V53.9
       nontraffic V53.3
       while boarding or alighting V53.4
      motor vehicle NOS (traffic) V59.60
       nontraffic V59.20
       specified type NEC (traffic) V59.69
        nontraffic V59.29
      pedal cycle (traffic) V51.9
       nontraffic V51.3
       while boarding or alighting V51.4
      pickup truck (traffic) V53.9
       nontraffic V53.3
       while boarding or alighting V53.4
      railway vehicle (traffic) V55.9
       nontraffic V55.3
       while boarding or alighting V55.4
      specified vehicle NEC (traffic) V56.9
       nontraffic V56.3
       while boarding or alighting V56.4
      stationary object (traffic) V57.9
       nontraffic V57.3
       while boarding or alighting V57.4
      streetcar (traffic) V56.9
       nontraffic V56.3
       while boarding or alighting V56.4
      three wheeled motor vehicle (traffic)
        V52.9
       nontraffic V52.3
       while boarding or alighting V52.4
      truck (traffic) V54.9
       nontraffic V54.3
       while boarding or alighting V54.4
      two wheeled motor vehicle (traffic)
        V52.9
       nontraffic V52.3
       while boarding or alighting V52.4
      van (traffic) V53.9
       nontraffic V53.3
       while boarding or alighting V53.4
     driver
      collision (with)
       animal (traffic) V50.5
        being ridden (traffic) V56.5
         nontraffic V56.0
        nontraffic V50.0

◀ New   ◀▥▥ Revised   ~~deleted~~ Deleted

Accident (Continued)
  transport (Continued)
    pickup truck occupant (Continued)
      driver (Continued)
        collision (Continued)
          animal-drawn vehicle (traffic)
            V56.5
            nontraffic V56.0
          bus (traffic) V54.5
            nontraffic V54.0
          car (traffic) V53.5
            nontraffic V53.0
          motor vehicle NOS (traffic) V59.40
            nontraffic V59.00
            specified type NEC (traffic)
              V59.49
              nontraffic V59.09
          pedal cycle (traffic) V51.5
            nontraffic V51.0
          pickup truck (traffic) V53.5
            nontraffic V53.0
          railway vehicle (traffic) V55.5
            nontraffic V55.0
          specified vehicle NEC (traffic) V56.5
            nontraffic V56.0
          stationary object (traffic) V57.5
            nontraffic V57.0
          streetcar (traffic) V56.5
            nontraffic V56.0
          three wheeled motor vehicle
            (traffic) V52.5
            nontraffic V52.0
          truck (traffic) V54.5
            nontraffic V54.0
          two wheeled motor vehicle (traffic)
            V52.5
            nontraffic V52.0
          van (traffic) V53.5
            nontraffic V53.0
        noncollision accident (traffic) V58.5
          nontraffic V58.0
      hanger-on
        collision (with)
          animal (traffic) V50.7
            being ridden (traffic) V56.7
              nontraffic V56.2
            nontraffic V50.2
          animal-drawn vehicle (traffic) V56.7
            nontraffic V56.2
          bus (traffic) V54.7
            nontraffic V54.2
          car (traffic) V53.7
            nontraffic V53.2
          pedal cycle (traffic) V51.7
            nontraffic V51.2
          pickup truck (traffic) V53.7
            nontraffic V53.2
          railway vehicle (traffic) V55.7
            nontraffic V55.2
          specified vehicle NEC (traffic) V56.7
            nontraffic V56.2
          stationary object (traffic) V57.7
            nontraffic V57.2
          streetcar (traffic) V56.7
            nontraffic V56.2
          three wheeled motor vehicle
            (traffic) V52.7
            nontraffic V52.2
          truck (traffic) V54.7
            nontraffic V54.2
          two wheeled motor vehicle (traffic)
            V52.7
            nontraffic V52.2
          van (traffic) V53.7
            nontraffic V53.2
        noncollision accident (traffic) V58.7
          nontraffic V58.2
        noncollision accident (traffic) V58.9
          nontraffic V58.3
          while boarding or alighting V58.4
        nontraffic V59.3

Accident (Continued)
  transport (Continued)
    pickup truck occupant (Continued)
      passenger
        collision (with)
          animal (traffic) V50.6
            being ridden (traffic) V56.6
              nontraffic V56.1
            nontraffic V50.1
          animal-drawn vehicle (traffic)
            V56.6
            nontraffic V56.1
          bus (traffic) V54.6
            nontraffic V54.1
          car (traffic) V53.6
            nontraffic V53.1
          motor vehicle NOS (traffic) V59.50
            nontraffic V59.10
            specified type NEC (traffic)
              V59.59
              nontraffic V59.19
          pedal cycle (traffic) V51.6
            nontraffic V51.1
          pickup truck (traffic) V53.6
            nontraffic V53.1
          railway vehicle (traffic) V55.6
            nontraffic V55.1
          specified vehicle NEC (traffic)
            V56.6
            nontraffic V56.1
          stationary object (traffic) V57.6
            nontraffic V57.1
          streetcar (traffic) V56.6
            nontraffic V56.1
          three wheeled motor vehicle
            (traffic) V52.6
            nontraffic V52.1
          truck (traffic) V54.6
            nontraffic V54.1
          two wheeled motor vehicle (traffic)
            V52.6
            nontraffic V52.1
          van (traffic) V53.6
            nontraffic V53.1
        noncollision accident (traffic) V58.6
          nontraffic V58.1
      specified type NEC V59.88
        military vehicle V59.81
    quarry truck —see Accident, transport,
      industrial vehicle occupant
    race car —see Accident, transport, motor
      vehicle NEC occupant
    railway vehicle occupant V81.9
      collision (with) V81.3
        motor vehicle (non-military) (traffic)
          V81.1
          military V81.83
          nontraffic V81.0
        rolling stock V81.2
        specified object NEC V81.3
      during derailment V81.7
        with antecedent collision —see
          Accident, transport, railway
          vehicle occupant, collision
      explosion V81.81
      fall (in railway vehicle) V81.5
        during derailment V81.7
          with antecedent collision —see
            Accident, transport, railway
            vehicle occupant, collision
        from railway vehicle V81.6
          during derailment V81.7
            with antecedent collision —see
              Accident, transport, railway
              vehicle occupant, collision
        while boarding or alighting V81.4
      fire V81.81
      object falling onto train V81.82
      specified type NEC V81.89
      while boarding or alighting V81.4
    ski lift V98.3

Accident (Continued)
  transport (Continued)
    snowmobile occupant (nontraffic)
      V86.92
      driver V86.52
      hanger-on V86.72
      passenger V86.62
      traffic V86.32
        driver V86.02
        hanger-on V86.22
        passenger V86.12
      while boarding or alighting V86.42
    specified NEC V98.8
    sport utility vehicle occupant —see also
      Accident, transport, car occupant
      collision (with)
        stationary object (traffic) V47.91
          nontraffic V47.31
      driver
        collision (with)
          stationary object (traffic) V47.51
            nontraffic V47.01
      passenger
        collision (with)
          stationary object (traffic) V47.61
            nontraffic V47.11
    streetcar occupant V82.9
      collision (with) V82.3
        motor vehicle (traffic) V82.1
          nontraffic V82.0
        rolling stock V82.2
      during derailment V82.7
        with antecedent collision —see
          Accident, transport, streetcar
          occupant, collision
      fall (in streetcar) V82.5
        during derailment V82.7
          with antecedent collision —see
            Accident, transport, streetcar
            occupant, collision
        from streetcar V82.6
          during derailment V82.7
            with antecedent collision —see
              Accident, transport, streetcar
              occupant, collision
          while boarding or alighting V82.4
        while boarding or alighting V82.4
      specified type NEC V82.8
      while boarding or alighting V82.4
    three-wheeled motor vehicle occupant
      V39.9
      collision (with)
        animal (traffic) V30.9
          being ridden (traffic) V36.9
            nontraffic V36.3
            while boarding or alighting
              V36.4
          nontraffic V30.3
          while boarding or alighting V30.4
        animal-drawn vehicle (traffic) V36.9
          nontraffic V36.3
          while boarding or alighting V36.4
        bus (traffic) V34.9
          nontraffic V34.3
          while boarding or alighting V34.4
        car (traffic) V33.9
          nontraffic V33.3
          while boarding or alighting V33.4
        motor vehicle NOS (traffic) V39.60
          nontraffic V39.20
          specified type NEC (traffic) V39.69
            nontraffic V39.29
        pedal cycle (traffic) V31.9
          nontraffic V31.3
          while boarding or alighting V31.4
        pickup truck (traffic) V33.9
          nontraffic V33.3
          while boarding or alighting V33.4
        railway vehicle (traffic) V35.9
          nontraffic V35.3
          while boarding or alighting V35.4

Accident (Continued)
  transport (Continued)
    three-wheeled motor vehicle occupant
        (Continued)
      collision (Continued)
        specified vehicle NEC (traffic) V36.9
          nontraffic V36.3
          while boarding or alighting V36.4
        stationary object (traffic) V37.9
          nontraffic V37.3
          while boarding or alighting V37.4
        streetcar (traffic) V36.9
          nontraffic V36.3
          while boarding or alighting V36.4
        three wheeled motor vehicle (traffic)
            V32.9
          nontraffic V32.3
          while boarding or alighting V32.4
        truck (traffic) V34.9
          nontraffic V34.3
          while boarding or alighting V34.4
        two wheeled motor vehicle (traffic)
            V32.9
          nontraffic V32.3
          while boarding or alighting V32.4
        van (traffic) V33.9
          nontraffic V33.3
          while boarding or alighting V33.4
      driver
        collision (with)
          animal (traffic) V30.5
            being ridden (traffic) V36.5
              nontraffic V36.0
            nontraffic V30.0
          animal-drawn vehicle (traffic) V36.5
            nontraffic V36.0
          bus (traffic) V34.5
            nontraffic V34.0
          car (traffic) V33.5
            nontraffic V33.0
          motor vehicle NOS (traffic) V39.40
            nontraffic V39.00
            specified type NEC (traffic)
                V39.49
              nontraffic V39.09
          pedal cycle (traffic) V31.5
            nontraffic V31.0
          pickup truck (traffic) V33.5
            nontraffic V33.0
          railway vehicle (traffic) V35.5
            nontraffic V35.0
          specified vehicle NEC (traffic) V36.5
            nontraffic V36.0
          stationary object (traffic) V37.5
            nontraffic V37.0
          streetcar (traffic) V36.5
            nontraffic V36.0
          three wheeled motor vehicle
              (traffic) V32.5
            nontraffic V32.0
          truck (traffic) V34.5
            nontraffic V34.0
          two wheeled motor vehicle (traffic)
              V32.5
            nontraffic V32.0
          van (traffic) V33.5
            nontraffic V33.0
          noncollision accident (traffic) V38.5
            nontraffic V38.0
      hanger-on
        collision (with)
          animal (traffic) V30.7
            being ridden (traffic) V36.7
              nontraffic V36.2
            nontraffic V30.2
          animal-drawn vehicle (traffic) V36.7
            nontraffic V36.2
          bus (traffic) V34.7
            nontraffic V34.2
          car (traffic) V33.7
            nontraffic V33.2

Accident (Continued)
  transport (Continued)
    three-wheeled motor vehicle occupant
        (Continued)
      hanger-on (Continued)
        collision (Continued)
          pedal cycle (traffic) V31.7
            nontraffic V31.2
          pickup truck (traffic) V33.7
            nontraffic V33.2
          railway vehicle (traffic) V35.7
            nontraffic V35.2
          specified vehicle NEC (traffic) V36.7
            nontraffic V36.2
          stationary object (traffic) V37.7
            nontraffic V37.2
          streetcar (traffic) V36.7
            nontraffic V36.2
          three wheeled motor vehicle
              (traffic) V32.7
            nontraffic V32.2
          truck (traffic) V34.7
            nontraffic V34.2
          two wheeled motor vehicle (traffic)
              V32.7
            nontraffic V32.2
          van (traffic) V33.7
            nontraffic V33.2
        noncollision accident (traffic) V38.7
          nontraffic V38.2
      noncollision accident (traffic) V38.9
        nontraffic V38.3
        while boarding or alighting V38.4
      nontraffic V39.3
      passenger
        collision (with)
          animal (traffic) V30.6
            being ridden (traffic) V36.6
              nontraffic V36.1
            nontraffic V30.1
          animal-drawn vehicle (traffic) V36.6
            nontraffic V36.1
          bus (traffic) V34.6
            nontraffic V34.1
          car (traffic) V33.6
            nontraffic V33.1
          motor vehicle NOS (traffic) V39.50
            nontraffic V39.10
            specified type NEC (traffic)
                V39.59
              nontraffic V39.19
          pedal cycle (traffic) V31.6
            nontraffic V31.1
          pickup truck (traffic) V33.6
            nontraffic V33.1
          railway vehicle (traffic) V35.6
            nontraffic V35.1
          specified vehicle NEC (traffic)
              V36.6
            nontraffic V36.1
          stationary object (traffic) V37.6
            nontraffic V37.1
          streetcar (traffic) V36.6
            nontraffic V36.1
          three wheeled motor vehicle
              (traffic) V32.6
            nontraffic V32.1
          truck (traffic) V34.6
            nontraffic V34.1
          two wheeled motor vehicle (traffic)
              V32.6
            nontraffic V32.1
          van (traffic) V33.6
            nontraffic V33.1
        noncollision accident (traffic) V38.6
          nontraffic V38.1
      specified type NEC V39.89
      military vehicle V39.81
    tractor (farm) (and trailer) —see Accident,
        transport, agricultural vehicle
        occupant

Accident (Continued)
  transport (Continued)
    tram —see Accident, transport, streetcar
      in mine or quarry —see Accident,
          transport, industrial vehicle
          occupant
    trolley —see Accident, transport, streetcar
      in mine or quarry —see Accident,
          transport, industrial vehicle
          occupant
    truck (heavy) occupant V69.9
      collision (with)
        animal (traffic) V60.9
          being ridden (traffic) V66.9
            nontraffic V66.3
            while boarding or alighting V66.4
          nontraffic V60.3
          while boarding or alighting V60.4
        animal-drawn vehicle (traffic) V66.9
          nontraffic V66.3
          while boarding or alighting V66.4
        bus (traffic) V64.9
          nontraffic V64.3
          while boarding or alighting V64.4
        car (traffic) V63.9
          nontraffic V63.3
          while boarding or alighting V63.4
        motor vehicle NOS (traffic) V69.60
          nontraffic V69.20
          specified type NEC (traffic) V69.69
            nontraffic V69.29
        pedal cycle (traffic) V61.9
          nontraffic V61.3
          while boarding or alighting V61.4
        pickup truck (traffic) V63.9
          nontraffic V63.3
          while boarding or alighting V63.4
        railway vehicle (traffic) V65.9
          nontraffic V65.3
          while boarding or alighting V65.4
        specified vehicle NEC (traffic) V66.9
          nontraffic V66.3
          while boarding or alighting V66.4
        stationary object (traffic) V67.9
          nontraffic V67.3
          while boarding or alighting V67.4
        streetcar (traffic) V66.9
          nontraffic V66.3
          while boarding or alighting V66.4
        three wheeled motor vehicle (traffic)
            V62.9
          nontraffic V62.3
          while boarding or alighting V62.4
        truck (traffic) V64.9
          nontraffic V64.3
          while boarding or alighting V64.4
        two wheeled motor vehicle (traffic)
            V62.9
          nontraffic V62.3
          while boarding or alighting V62.4
        van (traffic) V63.9
          nontraffic V63.3
          while boarding or alighting V63.4
      driver
        collision (with)
          animal (traffic) V60.5
            being ridden (traffic) V66.5
              nontraffic V66.0
            nontraffic V60.0
          animal-drawn vehicle (traffic)
              V66.5
            nontraffic V66.0
          bus (traffic) V64.5
            nontraffic V64.0
          car (traffic) V63.5
            nontraffic V63.0
          motor vehicle NOS (traffic) V69.40
            nontraffic V69.00
            specified type NEC (traffic)
                V69.49
              nontraffic V69.09

◀ New ◀▥▥ Revised ~~deleted~~ Deleted

Accident *(Continued)*
  transport *(Continued)*
    truck occupant *(Continued)*
      driver *(Continued)*
        collision *(Continued)*
          pedal cycle (traffic) V61.5
            nontraffic V61.0
          pickup truck (traffic) V63.5
            nontraffic V63.0
          railway vehicle (traffic) V65.5
            nontraffic V65.0
          specified vehicle NEC (traffic) V66.5
            nontraffic V66.0
          stationary object (traffic) V67.5
            nontraffic V67.0
          streetcar (traffic) V66.5
            nontraffic V66.0
          three wheeled motor vehicle (traffic) V62.5
            nontraffic V62.0
          truck (traffic) V64.5
            nontraffic V64.0
          two wheeled motor vehicle (traffic) V62.5
            nontraffic V62.0
          van (traffic) V63.5
            nontraffic V63.0
        noncollision accident (traffic) V68.5
          nontraffic V68.0
      dump —*see* Accident, transport, construction vehicle occupant
      hanger-on
        collision (with)
          animal (traffic) V60.7
            being ridden (traffic) V66.7
              nontraffic V66.2
            nontraffic V60.2
          animal-drawn vehicle (traffic) V66.7
            nontraffic V66.2
          bus (traffic) V64.7
            nontraffic V64.2
          car (traffic) V63.7
            nontraffic V63.2
          pedal cycle (traffic) V61.7
            nontraffic V61.2
          pickup truck (traffic) V63.7
            nontraffic V63.2
          railway vehicle (traffic) V65.7
            nontraffic V65.2
          specified vehicle NEC (traffic) V66.7
            nontraffic V66.2
          stationary object (traffic) V67.7
            nontraffic V67.2
          streetcar (traffic) V66.7
            nontraffic V66.2
          three wheeled motor vehicle (traffic) V62.7
            nontraffic V62.2
          truck (traffic) V64.7
            nontraffic V64.2
          two wheeled motor vehicle (traffic) V62.7
            nontraffic V62.2
          van (traffic) V63.7
            nontraffic V63.2
        noncollision accident (traffic) V68.7
          nontraffic V68.2
        noncollision accident (traffic) V68.9
          nontraffic V68.3
          while boarding or alighting V68.4
        nontraffic V69.3
      passenger
        collision (with)
          animal (traffic) V60.6
            being ridden (traffic) V66.6
              nontraffic V66.1
            nontraffic V60.1
          animal-drawn vehicle (traffic) V66.6
            nontraffic V66.1
          bus (traffic) V64.6
            nontraffic V64.1

Accident *(Continued)*
  transport *(Continued)*
    truck occupant *(Continued)*
      passenger *(Continued)*
        collision *(Continued)*
          car (traffic) V63.6
            nontraffic V63.1
          motor vehicle NOS (traffic) V69.50
            nontraffic V69.10
            specified type NEC (traffic) V69.59
              nontraffic V69.19
          pedal cycle (traffic) V61.6
            nontraffic V61.1
          pickup truck (traffic) V63.6
            nontraffic V63.1
          railway vehicle (traffic) V65.6
            nontraffic V65.1
          specified vehicle NEC (traffic) V66.6
            nontraffic V66.1
          stationary object (traffic) V67.6
            nontraffic V67.1
          streetcar (traffic) V66.6
            nontraffic V66.1
          three wheeled motor vehicle (traffic) V62.6
            nontraffic V62.1
          truck (traffic) V64.6
            nontraffic V64.1
          two wheeled motor vehicle (traffic) V62.6
            nontraffic V62.1
          van (traffic) V63.6
            nontraffic V63.1
        noncollision accident (traffic) V68.6
          nontraffic V68.1
      pickup —*see* Accident, transport, pickup truck occupant
      specified type NEC V69.88
      military vehicle V69.81
    van occupant V59.9
      collision (with)
        animal (traffic) V50.9
          being ridden (traffic) V56.9
           nontraffic V56.3
           while boarding or alighting V56.4
          nontraffic V50.3
          while boarding or alighting V50.4
        animal-drawn vehicle (traffic) V56.9
          nontraffic V56.3
          while boarding or alighting V56.4
        bus (traffic) V54.9
          nontraffic V54.3
          while boarding or alighting V54.4
        car (traffic) V53.9
          nontraffic V53.3
          while boarding or alighting V53.4
        motor vehicle NOS (traffic) V59.60
          nontraffic V59.20
          specified type NEC (traffic) V59.69
           nontraffic V59.29
        pedal cycle (traffic) V51.9
          nontraffic V51.3
          while boarding or alighting V51.4
        pickup truck (traffic) V53.9
          nontraffic V53.3
          while boarding or alighting V53.4
        railway vehicle (traffic) V55.9
          nontraffic V55.3
          while boarding or alighting V55.4
        specified vehicle NEC (traffic) V56.9
          nontraffic V56.3
          while boarding or alighting V56.4
        stationary object (traffic) V57.9
          nontraffic V57.3
          while boarding or alighting V57.4
        streetcar (traffic) V56.9
          nontraffic V56.3
          while boarding or alighting V56.4

Accident *(Continued)*
  transport *(Continued)*
    van occupant *(Continued)*
      collision *(Continued)*
        three wheeled motor vehicle (traffic) V52.9
          nontraffic V52.3
          while boarding or alighting V52.4
        truck (traffic) V54.9
          nontraffic V54.3
          while boarding or alighting V54.4
        two wheeled motor vehicle (traffic) V52.9
          nontraffic V52.3
          while boarding or alighting V52.4
        van (traffic) V53.9
          nontraffic V53.3
          while boarding or alighting V53.4
      driver
        collision (with)
          animal (traffic) V50.5
           being ridden (traffic) V56.5
            nontraffic V56.0
           nontraffic V50.0
          animal-drawn vehicle (traffic) V56.5
           nontraffic V56.0
          bus (traffic) V54.5
           nontraffic V54.0
          car (traffic) V53.5
           nontraffic V53.0
          motor vehicle NOS (traffic) V59.40
           nontraffic V59.00
           specified type NEC (traffic) V59.49
            nontraffic V59.09
          pedal cycle (traffic) V51.5
           nontraffic V51.0
          pickup truck (traffic) V53.5
           nontraffic V53.0
          railway vehicle (traffic) V55.5
           nontraffic V55.0
          specified vehicle NEC (traffic) V56.5
           nontraffic V56.0
          stationary object (traffic) V57.5
           nontraffic V57.0
          streetcar (traffic) V56.5
           nontraffic V56.0
          three wheeled motor vehicle (traffic) V52.5
           nontraffic V52.0
          truck (traffic) V54.5
           nontraffic V54.0
          two wheeled motor vehicle (traffic) V52.5
           nontraffic V52.0
          van (traffic) V53.5
           nontraffic V53.0
        noncollision accident (traffic) V58.5
          nontraffic V58.0
      hanger-on
        collision (with)
          animal (traffic) V50.7
           being ridden (traffic) V56.7
            nontraffic V56.2
           nontraffic V50.2
          animal-drawn vehicle (traffic) V56.7
           nontraffic V56.2
          bus (traffic) V54.7
           nontraffic V54.2
          car (traffic) V53.7
           nontraffic V53.2
          pedal cycle (traffic) V51.7
           nontraffic V51.2
          pickup truck (traffic) V53.7
           nontraffic V53.2
          railway vehicle (traffic) V55.7
           nontraffic V55.2
          specified vehicle NEC (traffic) V56.7
           nontraffic V56.2
          stationary object (traffic) V57.7
           nontraffic V57.2

Accident *(Continued)*
  transport *(Continued)*
    van occupant *(Continued)*
      hanger-on *(Continued)*
        collision *(Continued)*
          streetcar (traffic) V56.7
            nontraffic V56.2
          three wheeled motor vehicle
            (traffic) V52.7
            nontraffic V52.2
          truck (traffic) V54.7
            nontraffic V54.2
          two wheeled motor vehicle (traffic)
            V52.7
            nontraffic V52.2
          van (traffic) V53.7
            nontraffic V53.2
        noncollision accident (traffic) V58.7
          nontraffic V58.2
      noncollision accident (traffic) V58.9
        nontraffic V58.3
        while boarding or alighting V58.4
      nontraffic V59.3
      passenger
        collision (with)
          animal (traffic) V50.6
            being ridden (traffic) V56.6
              nontraffic V56.1
            nontraffic V50.1
          animal-drawn vehicle (traffic) V56.6
            nontraffic V56.1
          bus (traffic) V54.6
            nontraffic V54.1
          car (traffic) V53.6
            nontraffic V53.1
          motor vehicle NOS (traffic) V59.50
            nontraffic V59.10
            specified type NEC (traffic) V59.59
              nontraffic V59.19
          pedal cycle (traffic) V51.6
            nontraffic V51.1
          pickup truck (traffic) V53.6
            nontraffic V53.1
          railway vehicle (traffic) V55.6
            nontraffic V55.1
          specified vehicle NEC (traffic) V56.6
            nontraffic V56.1
          stationary object (traffic) V57.6
            nontraffic V57.1
          streetcar (traffic) V56.6
            nontraffic V56.1
          three wheeled motor vehicle
            (traffic) V52.6
            nontraffic V52.1
          truck (traffic) V54.6
            nontraffic V54.1
          two wheeled motor vehicle (traffic)
            V52.6
            nontraffic V52.1
          van (traffic) V53.6
            nontraffic V53.1
        noncollision accident (traffic) V58.6
          nontraffic V58.1
      specified type NEC V59.88
      military vehicle V59.81
    watercraft occupant —*see* Accident,
      watercraft
    vehicle NEC V89.9
      animal-drawn NEC —*see* Accident,
        transport, animal-drawn vehicle
        occupant
    special
      agricultural —*see* Accident, transport,
        agricultural vehicle occupant
      construction —*see* Accident, transport,
        construction vehicle occupant
      industrial —*see* Accident, transport,
        industrial vehicle occupant
      three-wheeled NEC (motorized) —*see*
        Accident, transport, three-wheeled
        motor vehicle occupant

Accident *(Continued)*
  watercraft V94.9
    causing
      drowning —*see* Drowning, due to,
        accident to, watercraft
      injury NEC V91.89
        crushed between craft and object
          V91.19
        powered craft V91.13
          ferry boat V91.11
          fishing boat V91.12
          jetskis V91.13
          liner V91.11
          merchant ship V91.10
          passenger ship V91.11
        unpowered craft V91.18
          canoe V91.15
          inflatable V91.16
          kayak V91.15
          sailboat V91.14
          surf-board V91.18
          windsurfer V91.18
      fall on board V91.29
        powered craft V91.23
          ferry boat V91.21
          fishing boat V91.22
          jetskis V91.23
          liner V91.21
          merchant ship V91.20
          passenger ship V91.21
        unpowered craft
          canoe V91.25
          inflatable V91.26
          kayak V91.25
          sailboat V91.24
      fire on board causing burn V91.09
        powered craft V91.03
          ferry boat V91.01
          fishing boat V91.02
          jetskis V91.03
          liner V91.01
          merchant ship V91.00
          passenger ship V91.01
        unpowered craft V91.08
          canoe V91.05
          inflatable V91.06
          kayak V91.05
          sailboat V91.04
          surf-board V91.08
          water skis V91.07
          windsurfer V91.08
      hit by falling object V91.39
        powered craft V91.33
          ferry boat V91.31
          fishing boat V91.32
          jetskis V91.33
          liner V91.31
          merchant ship V91.30
          passenger ship V91.31
        unpowered craft V91.38
          canoe V91.35
          inflatable V91.36
          kayak V91.35
          sailboat V91.34
          surf-board V91.38
          water skis V91.37
          windsurfer V91.38
      specified type NEC V91.89
        powered craft V91.83
          ferry boat V91.81
          fishing boat V91.82
          jetskis V91.83
          liner V91.81
          merchant ship V91.80
          passenger ship V91.81
        unpowered craft V91.88
          canoe V91.85
          inflatable V91.86
          kayak V91.85
          sailboat V91.84
          surf-board V91.88

Accident *(Continued)*
  watercraft *(Continued)*
    causing *(Continued)*
      injury NEC *(Continued)*
        specified type NEC *(Continued)*
          unpowered craft *(Continued)*
            water skis V91.87
            windsurfer V91.88
      due to, caused by cataclysm —*see* Forces of
        nature, by type
      military NEC V94.818
        with civilian watercraft V94.810
        civilian in water injured by V94.811
      nonpowered, struck by
        nonpowered vessel V94.22
        powered vessel V94.21
      specified type NEC V94.89
      striking swimmer
        powered V94.11
        unpowered V94.12
Acid throwing (assault) Y08.89
Activity (involving) (of victim at time of event)
  Y93.9
  aerobic and step exercise (class) Y93.A3
  alpine skiing Y93.23
  animal care NEC Y93.K9
  arts and handcrafts NEC Y93.D9
  athletics NEC Y93.79
  athletics played as a team or group NEC
    Y93.69
  athletics played individually NEC Y93.59
  baking Y93.G3
  ballet Y93.41
  barbells Y93.B3
  BASE (Building, Antenna, Span, Earth)
    jumping Y93.33
  baseball Y93.64
  basketball Y93.67
  bathing (personal) Y93.E1
  beach volleyball Y93.68
  bike riding Y93.55
  boogie boarding Y93.18
  bowling Y93.54
  boxing Y93.71
  brass instrument playing Y93.J4
  building construction Y93.H3
  bungee jumping Y93.34
  calisthenics Y93.A2
  canoeing (in calm and turbulent water)
    Y93.16
  capture the flag Y93.6A
  cardiorespiratory exercise NEC Y93.A9
  caregiving (providing) NEC Y93.F9
    bathing Y93.F1
    lifting Y93.F2
  cellular
    communication device Y93.C2
    telephone Y93.C2
  challenge course Y93.A5
  cheerleading Y93.45
  circuit training Y93.A4
  cleaning
    floor Y93.E5
  climbing NEC Y93.39
    mountain Y93.31
    rock Y93.31
    wall Y93.31
  clothing care and maintenance NEC
    Y93.E9
  combatives Y93.75
  computer
    keyboarding Y93.C1
    technology NEC Y93.C9
  confidence course Y93.A5
  construction (building) Y93.H3
  cooking and baking Y93.G3
  cool down exercises Y93.A2
  cricket Y93.69
  crocheting Y93.D1
  cross country skiing Y93.24
  dancing (all types) Y93.41

◀ New   ⬅ Revised   ~~deleted~~ Deleted

Activity (Continued)
  digging
    dirt Y93.H1
  dirt digging Y93.H1
  dishwashing Y93.G1
  diving (platform) (springboard) Y93.12
    underwater Y93.15
  dodge ball Y93.6A
  downhill skiing Y93.23
  drum playing Y93.J2
  dumbbells Y93.B3
  electronic
    devices NEC Y93.C9
      hand held interactive Y93.C2
    game playing (using) (with)
      interactive device Y93.C2
      keyboard or other stationary device
        Y93.C1
  elliptical machine Y93.A1
  exercise (s)
    machines ((primarily) for)
      cardiorespiratory conditioning Y93.A1
      muscle strengthening Y93.B1
    muscle strengthening (non-machine) NEC
      Y93.B9
  external motion NEC Y93.I9
    rollercoaster Y93.I1
  field hockey Y93.65
  figure skating (pairs) (singles) Y93.21
  flag football Y93.62
  floor mopping and cleaning Y93.E5
  food preparation and clean up Y93.G1
  football (American) NOS Y93.61
    flag Y93.62
    tackle Y93.61
    touch Y93.62
  four square Y93.6A
  free weights Y93.B3
  frisbee (ultimate) Y93.74
  furniture
    building Y93.D3
    finishing Y93.D3
    repair Y93.D3
  game playing (electronic)
    using interactive device Y93.C2
    using keyboard or other stationary device
      Y93.C1
  gardening Y93.H2
  golf Y93.53
  grass drills Y93.A6
  grilling and smoking food Y93.G2
  grooming and shearing an animal Y93.K3
  guerilla drills Y93.A6
  gymnastics (rhythmic) Y93.43
  hand held interactive electronic device Y93.
    C2
  handball Y93.73
  handcrafts NEC Y93.D9
  hang gliding Y93.35
  hiking (on level or elevated terrain) Y93.01
  hockey (ice) Y93.22
    field Y93.65
  horseback riding Y93.52
  household (interior) maintenance NEC Y93.
    E9
  ice NEC Y93.29
    dancing Y93.21
    hockey Y93.22
    skating Y93.21
  inline roller skating Y93.51
  ironing Y93.E4
  judo Y93.75
  jumping (off) NEC Y93.39
    BASE (Building, Antenna, Span, Earth)
      Y93.33
    bungee Y93.34
    jacks Y93.A2
    rope Y93.56
  jumping jacks Y93.A2
  jumping rope Y93.56
  karate Y93.75

Activity (Continued)
  kayaking (in calm and turbulent water)
    Y93.16
  keyboarding (computer) Y93.C1
  kickball Y93.6A
  knitting Y93.D1
  lacrosse Y93.65
  land maintenance NEC Y93.H9
  landscaping Y93.H2
  laundry Y93.E2
  machines (exercise)
    primarily for cardiorespiratory
      conditioning Y93.A1
    primarily for muscle strengthening Y93.B1
  maintenance
    exterior building NEC Y93.H9
    household (interior) NEC Y93.E9
    land Y93.H9
    property Y93.H9
  marching (on level or elevated terrain) Y93.01
  martial arts Y93.75
  microwave oven Y93.G3
  milking an animal Y93.K2
  mopping (floor) Y93.E5
  mountain climbing Y93.31
  muscle strengthening
    exercises (non-machine) NEC Y93.B9
    machines Y93.B1
  musical keyboard (electronic) playing Y93.J1
  nordic skiing Y93.24
  obstacle course Y93.A5
  oven (microwave) Y93.G3
  packing up and unpacking in moving to a
    new residence Y93.E6
  parasailing Y93.19
  percussion instrument playing NEC Y93.J2
  personal
    bathing and showering Y93.E1
    hygiene NEC Y93.E8
    showering Y93.E1
  physical games generally associated with
    school recess, summer camp and
    children Y93.6A
  physical training NEC Y93.A9
  piano playing Y93.J1
  pilates Y93.B4
  platform diving Y93.12
  playing musical instrument
    brass instrument Y93.J4
    drum Y93.J2
    musical keyboard (electronic) Y93.J1
    percussion instrument NEC Y93.J2
    piano Y93.J1
    string instrument Y93.J3
    winds instrument Y93.J4
  property maintenance
    exterior NEC Y93.H9
    interior NEC Y93.E9
  pruning (garden and lawn) Y93.H2
  pull-ups Y93.B2
  push-ups Y93.B2
  racquetball Y93.73
  rafting (in calm and turbulent water) Y93.16
  raking (leaves) Y93.H1
  rappelling Y93.32
  refereeing a sports activity Y93.81
  residential relocation Y93.E6
  rhythmic gymnastics Y93.43
  rhythmic movement NEC Y93.49
  riding
    horseback Y93.52
    rollercoaster Y93.I1
  rock climbing Y93.31
  roller skating (inline) Y93.51
  rollercoaster riding Y93.I1
  rough housing and horseplay Y93.83
  rowing (in calm and turbulent water)
    Y93.16
  rugby Y93.63
  SCUBA diving Y93.15
  sewing Y93.D2

Activity (Continued)
  shoveling Y93.H1
    dirt Y93.H1
    snow Y93.H1
  showering (personal) Y93.E1
  sit-ups Y93.B2
  skateboarding Y93.51
  skating (ice) Y93.21
    roller Y93.51
  skiing (alpine) (downhill) Y93.23
    cross country Y93.24
    nordic Y93.24
    water Y93.17
  sledding (snow) Y93.23
  sleeping (sleep) Y93.84
  smoking and grilling food Y93.G2
  snorkeling Y93.15
  snow NEC Y93.29
    boarding Y93.23
    shoveling Y93.H1
    sledding Y93.23
    tubing Y93.23
  soccer Y93.66
  softball Y93.64
  specified NEC Y93.89
  spectator at an event Y93.82
  sports NEC Y93.79
    sports played as a team or group NEC
      Y93.69
    sports played individually NEC Y93.59
  springboard diving Y93.12
  squash Y93.73
  stationary bike Y93.A1
  step (stepping) exercise (class) Y93.A3
  stepper machine Y93.A1
  stove Y93.G3
  string instrument playing Y93.J3
  surfing Y93.18
    wind Y93.18
  swimming Y93.11
  tackle football Y93.61
  tap dancing Y93.41
  tennis Y93.73
  tobogganing Y93.23
  touch football Y93.62
  track and field events (non-running) Y93.57
    running Y93.02
  trampoline Y93.44
  treadmill Y93.A1
  trimming shrubs Y93.H2
  tubing (in calm and turbulent water) Y93.16
    snow Y93.23
  ultimate frisbee Y93.74
  underwater diving Y93.15
  unpacking in moving to a new residence
    Y93.E6
  use of stove, oven and microwave oven Y93.
    G3
  vacuuming Y93.E3
  volleyball (beach) (court) Y93.68
  wake boarding Y93.17
  walking (on level or elevated terrain) Y93.01
    an animal Y93.K1
  walking an animal Y93.K1
  wall climbing Y93.31
  warm up and cool down exercises Y93.A2
  water NEC Y93.19
    aerobics Y93.14
    craft NEC Y93.19
    exercise Y93.14
    polo Y93.13
    skiing Y93.17
    sliding Y93.18
    survival training and testing Y93.19
  weeding (garden and lawn) Y93.H2
  wind instrument playing Y93.J4
  windsurfing Y93.18
  wrestling Y93.72
  yoga Y93.42
Adverse effect of drugs —see Table of Drugs
  and Chemicals

Aerosinusitis —see Air, pressure
After-effect, late —see Sequelae
Air
　blast in war operations —see War operations,
　　air blast
　pressure
　　change, rapid
　　　during
　　　　ascent W94.29
　　　　　while (in) (surfacing from)
　　　　　　aircraft W94.23
　　　　　　deep water diving W94.21
　　　　　　underground W94.22
　　　　descent W94.39
　　　　　in
　　　　　　aircraft W94.31
　　　　　　water W94.32
　　　high, prolonged W94.0
　　　low, prolonged W94.12
　　　　due to residence or long visit at high
　　　　　altitude W94.11
Alpine sickness W94.11
Altitude sickness W94.11
Anaphylactic shock, anaphylaxis —see Table of
　Drugs and Chemicals ◀▦
Andes disease W94.11
Arachnidism, arachnoidism X58
Arson (with intent to injure or kill) X97
Asphyxia, asphyxiation
　by
　　food (bone) (seed) —see categories T17
　　　and T18
　　gas —see also Table of Drugs and
　　　Chemicals ◀▦
　　　legal
　　　　execution —see Legal, intervention,
　　　　　gas
　　　　intervention —see Legal, intervention,
　　　　　gas
　　from
　　　fire —see also Exposure, fire
　　　　in war operations —see War operations,
　　　　　fire
　　　ignition —see Ignition
　　　vomitus T17.81
　　in war operations —see War operations,
　　　restriction of airway
Aspiration
　food (any type) (into respiratory tract) (with
　　asphyxia, obstruction respiratory tract,
　　suffocation) —see categories T17 and T18
　foreign body —see Foreign body, aspiration
　vomitus (with asphyxia, obstruction
　　respiratory tract, suffocation) T17.81
Assassination (attempt) —see Assault
Assault (homicidal) (by) (in) Y09
　arson X97
　bite (of human being) Y04.1
　bodily force Y04.8
　　bite Y04.1
　　bumping into Y04.2
　　sexual —see subcategories T74.0, T76.0
　　unarmed fight Y04.0

Assault (Continued)
　bomb X96.9
　　antipersonnel X96.0
　　fertilizer X96.3
　　gasoline X96.1
　　letter X96.2
　　petrol X96.1
　　pipe X96.3
　　specified NEC X96.8
　brawl (hand) (fists) (foot) (unarmed) Y04.0
　burning, burns (by fire) NEC X97
　　acid Y08.89
　　caustic, corrosive substance Y08.89
　　chemical from swallowing caustic,
　　　corrosive substance —see Table of
　　　Drugs and Chemicals ◀▦
　　cigarette (s) X97
　　hot object X98.9
　　　fluid NEC X98.2
　　　household appliance X98.3
　　　specified NEC X98.8
　　　steam X98.0
　　　tap water X98.1
　　　vapors X98.0
　　scalding —see Assault, burning
　　steam X98.0
　　vitriol Y08.89
　caustic, corrosive substance (gas) Y08.89
　crashing of
　　aircraft Y08.81
　　motor vehicle Y03.8
　　　pushed in front of Y02.0
　　　run over Y03.0
　　　specified NEC Y03.8
　cutting or piercing instrument X99.9
　　dagger X99.2
　　glass X99.0
　　knife X99.1
　　specified NEC X99.8
　　sword X99.2
　dagger X99.2
　drowning (in) X92.9
　　bathtub X92.0
　　natural water X92.3
　　specified NEC X92.8
　　swimming pool X92.1
　　following fall X92.2
　dynamite X96.8
　explosive (s) (material) X96.9
　fight (hand) (fists) (foot) (unarmed) Y04.0
　　with weapon —see Assault, by type of
　　　weapon
　fire X97
　firearm X95.9
　　airgun X95.01
　　handgun X93
　　hunting rifle X94.1
　　larger X94.9
　　　specified NEC X94.8
　　machine gun X94.2
　　shotgun X94.0
　　specified NEC X95.8

Assault (Continued)
　from high place Y01
　gunshot (wound) NEC —see Assault, firearm,
　　by type
　incendiary device X97
　injury Y09
　　to child due to criminal abortion attempt
　　　NEC Y08.89
　knife X99.1
　late effect of —see X92-Y08 with 7th character
　　S
　placing before moving object NEC Y02.8
　　motor vehicle Y02.0
　poisoning —see categories T36-T65 with 7th
　　character S
　puncture, any part of body —see Assault,
　　cutting or piercing instrument
　pushing
　　before moving object NEC Y02.8
　　　motor vehicle Y02.0
　　　subway train Y02.1
　　　train Y02.1
　rape T74.2-
　scalding —see Assault, burning
　sequelae of —see X92-Y08 with 7th character
　　S
　sexual (by bodily force) T74.2-
　shooting —see Assault, firearm
　specified means NEC Y08.89
　stab, any part of body —see Assault, cutting
　　or piercing instrument
　steam X98.0
　striking against
　　other person Y04.2
　　sports equipment Y08.09
　　　baseball bat Y08.02
　　　hockey stick Y08.01
　struck by
　　sports equipment Y08.09
　　　baseball bat Y08.02
　　　hockey stick Y08.01
　submersion —see Assault, drowning
　violence Y09
　weapon Y09
　　blunt Y00
　　cutting or piercing —see Assault, cutting or
　　　piercing instrument
　　firearm —see Assault, firearm
　wound Y09
　　cutting —see Assault, cutting or piercing
　　　instrument
　　gunshot —see Assault, firearm
　　knife X99.1
　　piercing —see Assault, cutting or piercing
　　　instrument
　　puncture —see Assault, cutting or piercing
　　　instrument
　　stab —see Assault, cutting or piercing
　　　instrument
Attack by mammals NEC W55.89
Avalanche —see Landslide
Aviator's disease —see Air, pressure

B

Barotitis, barodontalgia, barosinusitis,
    barotrauma (otitic) (sinus) —see Air,
    pressure
Battered (baby) (child) (person) (syndrome)
    X58
Bayonet wound W26.1
    in
        legal intervention —see Legal,
            intervention, sharp object,
            bayonet
        war operations —see War operations,
            combat
    stated as undetermined whether accidental or
        intentional Y28.8
    suicide (attempt) X78.2
Bean in nose —see categories T17 and T18
Bed set on fire NEC —see Exposure, fire,
    uncontrolled, building, bed
Beheading (by guillotine)
    homicide X99.9
    legal execution —see Legal, intervention
Bending, injury in —see category Y93
Bends —see Air, pressure, change
Bite, bitten by
    alligator W58.01
    arthropod (nonvenomous) NEC W57
    bull W55.21
    cat W55.01
    cow W55.21
    crocodile W58.11
    dog W54.0
    goat W55.31
    hoof stock NEC W55.31
    horse W55.11
    human being (accidentally) W50.3
        with intent to injure or kill Y04.1
        as, or caused by, a crowd or human
            stampede (with fall) W52
        assault Y04.1
        homicide (attempt) Y04.1
        in
            fight Y04.1
    insect (nonvenomous) W57
    lizard (nonvenomous) W59.01
    mammal NEC W55.81
        marine W56.31
    marine animal (nonvenomous) W56.81
    millipede W57
    moray eel W56.51
    mouse W53.01
    person (s) (accidentally) W50.3
        with intent to injure or kill Y04.1
        as, or caused by, a crowd or human
            stampede (with fall) W52
        assault Y04.1
        homicide (attempt) Y04.1
        in
            fight Y04.1
    pig W55.41
    raccoon W55.51
    rat W53.11
    reptile W59.81
        lizard W59.01
        snake W59.11
        turtle W59.21
            terrestrial W59.81
    rodent W53.81
        mouse W53.01
        rat W53.11
        specified NEC W53.81
        squirrel W53.21
    shark W56.41
    sheep W55.31
    snake (nonvenomous) W59.11
    spider (nonvenomous) W57
    squirrel W53.21
Blast (air) in war operations —see War
    operations, blast
Blizzard X37.2

Blood alcohol level Y90.9
    20-39mg/100ml Y90.1
    40-59mg/100ml Y90.2
    60-79mg/100ml Y90.3
    80-99mg/100ml Y90.4
    100-119mg/100ml Y90.5
    120-199mg/100ml Y90.6
    200-239mg/100ml Y90.7
    less than 20mg/100ml Y90.0
    presence in blood, level not specified
        Y90.9
Blow X58
    by law-enforcing agent, police (on duty) —see
        Legal, intervention, manhandling
    blunt object —see Legal, intervention, blunt
        object
Blowing up —see Explosion
Brawl (hand) (fists) (foot) Y04.0
Breakage (accidental) (part of)
    ladder (causing fall) W11
    scaffolding (causing fall) W12
Broken
    glass, contact with —see Contact, with, glass
    power line (causing electric shock) W85
Bumping against, into (accidentally)
    object NEC W22.8
        with fall —see Fall, due to, bumping
            against, object
        caused by crowd or human stampede
            (with fall) W52
        sports equipment W21.9
    person (s) W51
        with fall W03
            due to ice or snow W00.0
        assault Y04.2
        caused by, a crowd or human stampede
            (with fall) W52
        homicide (attempt) Y04.2
    sports equipment W21.9
Burn, burned, burning (accidental) (by) (from)
        (on)
    acid NEC —see Table of ₫Drugs and
        ₵Chemicals ◀⃒⃒⃒
    bed linen —see Exposure, fire, uncontrolled,
        in building, bed
    blowtorch X08.8
        with ignition of clothing NEC X06.2
            nightwear X05
    bonfire, campfire (controlled) —see also
        Exposure, fire, controlled, not in
        building
        uncontrolled —see Exposure, fire,
            uncontrolled, not in building
    candle X08.8
        with ignition of clothing NEC X06.2
            nightwear X05
    caustic liquid, substance (external) (internal)
        NEC —see Table of ₫Drugs and
        ₵Chemicals ◀⃒⃒⃒
    chemical (external) (internal) —see also Table
        of ₫Drugs and ₵Chemicals ◀⃒⃒⃒
        in war operations —see War operations, fire
    cigar (s) or cigarette (s) X08.8
        with ignition of clothing NEC X06.2
            nightwear X05
    clothes, clothing NEC (from controlled fire)
        X06.2
        with conflagration —see Exposure, fire,
            uncontrolled, building
        not in building or structure —see
            Exposure, fire, uncontrolled, not in
            building
    cooker (hot) X15.8
        stated as undetermined whether accidental
            or intentional Y27.3
        suicide (attempt) X77.3
    electric blanket X16
    engine (hot) X17
    fire, flames —see Exposure, fire
    flare, Very pistol —see Discharge, firearm
        NEC

Burn, burned, burning (Continued)
    heat
        from appliance (electrical) (household)
            X15.8
            cooker X15.8
            hotplate X15.2
            kettle X15.8
            light bulb X15.8
            saucepan X15.3
            skillet X15.3
            stated as undetermined whether
                accidental or intentional Y27.3
            stove X15.0
            suicide (attempt) X77.3
            toaster X15.1
        in local application or packing during
            medical or surgical procedure
            Y63.5
    heating
        appliance, radiator or pipe X16
    homicide (attempt) —see Assault, burning
    hot
        air X14.1
        cooker X15.8
        drink X10.0
        engine X17
        fat X10.2
        fluid NEC X12
        food X10.1
        gases X14.1
        heating appliance X16
        household appliance NEC X15.8
        kettle X15.8
        liquid NEC X12
        machinery X17
        metal (molten) (liquid) NEC X18
        object (not producing fire or flames) NEC
            X19
        oil (cooking) X10.2
        pipe (s) X16
        radiator X16
        saucepan (glass) (metal) X15.3
        stove (kitchen) X15.0
        substance NEC X19
            caustic or corrosive NEC —see Table of
                ₫Drugs and ₵Chemicals ◀⃒⃒⃒
        toaster X15.1
        tool X17
        vapor X13.1
        water (tap) —see Contact, with, hot, tap
            water
    hotplate X15.2
        suicide (attempt) X77.3
    ignition —see Ignition
    in war operations —see War operations, fire
    inflicted by other person X97
        by hot objects, hot vapor, and steam —see
            Assault, burning, hot object
    internal, from swallowed caustic, corrosive
        liquid, substance —see Table of ₫Drugs
        and ₵Chemicals ◀⃒⃒⃒
    iron (hot) X15.8
        stated as undetermined whether accidental
            or intentional Y27.3
        suicide (attempt) X77.3
    kettle (hot) X15.8
        stated as undetermined whether accidental
            or intentional Y27.3
        suicide (attempt) X77.3
    lamp (flame) X08.8
        with ignition of clothing NEC X06.2
            nightwear X05
    lighter (cigar) (cigarette) X08.8
        with ignition of clothing NEC X06.2
            nightwear X05
    lightning —see subcategory T75.0
        causing fire —see Exposure, fire
    liquid (boiling) (hot) NEC X12
        stated as undetermined whether accidental
            or intentional Y27.2
        suicide (attempt) X77.2

Burn, burned, burning *(Continued)*
  local application of externally applied
      substance in medical or surgical care
      Y63.5
  machinery (hot) X17
  matches X08.8
    with ignition of clothing NEC X06.2
      nightwear X05
  mattress —*see* Exposure, fire, uncontrolled,
    building, bed
  medicament, externally applied Y63.5
  metal (hot) (liquid) (molten) NEC X18
  nightwear (nightclothes, nightdress, gown,
    pajamas, robe) X05
  object (hot) NEC X19
  on board watercraft
    due to
      accident to watercraft V91.09
        powered craft V91.03
          ferry boat V91.01
          fishing boat V91.02
          jetskis V91.03
          liner V91.01
          merchant ship V91.00
          passenger ship V91.01
        unpowered craft V91.08
          canoe V91.05
          inflatable V91.06
          kayak V91.05
          sailboat V91.04
          surf-board V91.08
          water skis V91.07
          windsurfer V91.08
      fire on board V93.09
        ferry boat V93.01
        fishing boat V93.02
        jetskis V93.03
        liner V93.01
        merchant ship V93.00
        passenger ship V93.01
        powered craft NEC V93.03
        sailboat V93.04

Burn, burned, burning *(Continued)*
  on board watercraft *(Continued)*
    due to *(Continued)*
      specified heat source NEC on board
        V93.19
      ferry boat V93.11
      fishing boat V93.12
      jetskis V93.13
      liner V93.11
      merchant ship V93.10
      passenger ship V93.11
      powered craft NEC V93.13
      sailboat V93.14
  pipe (hot) X16
    smoking X08.8
      with ignition of clothing NEC X06.2
        nightwear X05
  powder —*see* Powder burn
  radiator (hot) X16
  saucepan (hot) (glass) (metal) X15.3
    stated as undetermined whether
      accidental or intentional
      Y27.3
    suicide (attempt) X77.3
  self-inflicted X76
    stated as undetermined whether
      accidental or intentional
      Y26
  stated as undetermined whether
    accidental or intentional Y27.0
  steam X13.1
    pipe X16
      stated as undetermined whether
        accidental or intentional
        Y27.8
    stated as undetermined whether
      accidental or intentional Y27.0
    suicide (attempt) X77.0
  stove (hot) (kitchen) X15.0
    stated as undetermined whether
      accidental or intentional Y27.3
    suicide (attempt) X77.3

Burn, burned, burning *(Continued)*
  substance (hot) NEC X19
    boiling X12
      stated as undetermined whether
        accidental or intentional Y27.2
      suicide (attempt) X77.2
    molten (metal) X18
  suicide (attempt) NEC X76
    hot
      household appliance X77.3
      object X77.9
  stated as undetermined whether accidental or
    intentional Y27.0
  therapeutic misadventure
    heat in local application or packing during
      medical or surgical procedure Y63.5
    overdose of radiation Y63.2
  toaster (hot) X15.1
    stated as undetermined whether accidental
      or intentional Y27.3
    suicide (attempt) X77.3
  tool (hot) X17
  torch, welding X08.8
    with ignition of clothing NEC X06.2
      nightwear X05
  trash fire (controlled) —*see* Exposure, fire,
    controlled, not in building
    uncontrolled —*see* Exposure, fire,
      uncontrolled, not in building
  vapor (hot) X13.1
    stated as undetermined whether accidental
      or intentional Y27.0
    suicide (attempt) X77.0
  Very pistol —*see* Discharge, firearm NEC
Butted by animal W55.82
  bull W55.22
  cow W55.22
  goat W55.32
  horse W55.12
  pig W55.42
  sheep W55.32

C

Caisson disease —*see* Air, pressure, change

Campfire (exposure to) (controlled) —*see also* Exposure, fire, controlled, not in building
   uncontrolled —*see* Exposure, fire, uncontrolled, not in building

Capital punishment (any means) —*see* Legal, intervention

Car sickness T75.3

Casualty (not due to war) NEC X58
   war —*see* War operations

Cat
   bite W55.01
   scratch W55.03

Cataclysm, cataclysmic (any injury) NEC —*see* Forces of nature

Catching fire —*see* Exposure, fire

Caught
   between
      folding object W23.0
      objects (moving) (stationary and moving) W23.0
         and machinery —*see* Contact, with, by type of machine
         stationary W23.1
      sliding door and door frame W23.0
   by, in
      machinery (moving parts of) —*see* Contact, with, by type of machine
      washing-machine wringer W23.0
      under packing crate (due to losing grip) W23.1

Cave-in caused by cataclysmic earth surface movement or eruption —*see* Landslide

Change (s) in air pressure —*see* Air, pressure, change

Choked, choking (on) (any object except food or vomitus)
   food (bone) (seed) —*see* categories T17 and T18
   vomitus T17.81-

Civil insurrection —*see* War operations

Cloudburst (any injury) X37.8

Cold, exposure to (accidental) (excessive) (extreme) (natural) (place) NEC —*see* Exposure, cold

Collapse
   building W20.1
      burning (uncontrolled fire) X00.2
   dam or man-made structure (causing earth movement) X36.0
   machinery —*see* Contact, with, by type of machine
   structure W20.1
      burning (uncontrolled fire) X00.2

Collision (accidental) NEC (*see also* Accident, transport) V89.9
   pedestrian W51
      with fall W03
         due to ice or snow W00.0
         involving pedestrian conveyance —*see* Accident, transport, pedestrian, conveyance
      and
         crowd or human stampede (with fall) W52
         object W22.8
            with fall —*see* Fall, due to, bumping against, object
      person (s) —*see* Collision, pedestrian
   transport vehicle NEC V89.9
      and
         avalanche, fallen or not moving —*see* Accident, transport
            falling or moving —*see* Landslide
         landslide, fallen or not moving —*see* Accident, transport
            falling or moving —*see* Landslide

Collision NEC *(Continued)*
   transport vehicle NEC *(Continued)*
      due to cataclysm —*see* Forces of nature, by type
      intentional, purposeful suicide (attempt) —*see* Suicide, collision

Combustion, spontaneous —*see* Ignition

Complication (delayed) of or following (medical or surgical procedure) Y84.9
   with misadventure —*see* Misadventure
   amputation of limb (s) Y83.5
   anastomosis (arteriovenous) (blood vessel) (gastrojejunal) (tendon) (natural or artificial material) Y83.2
   aspiration (of fluid) Y84.4
      tissue Y84.8
   biopsy Y84.8
   blood
      sampling Y84.7
      transfusion
         procedure Y84.8
   bypass Y83.2
   catheterization (urinary) Y84.6
      cardiac Y84.0
   colostomy Y83.3
   cystostomy Y83.3
   dialysis (kidney) Y84.1
   drug —*see* Table of Drugs and Chemicals ◀▥▥▥
   due to misadventure —*see* Misadventure
   duodenostomy Y83.3
   electroshock therapy Y84.3
   external stoma, creation of Y83.3
   formation of external stoma Y83.3
   gastrostomy Y83.3
   graft Y83.2
   hypothermia (medically-induced) Y84.8
   implant, implantation (of)
      artificial
         internal device (cardiac pacemaker) (electrodes in brain) (heart valve prosthesis) (orthopedic) Y83.1
         material or tissue (for anastomosis or bypass) Y83.2
            with creation of external stoma Y83.3
      natural tissues (for anastomosis or bypass) Y83.2
         with creation of external stoma Y83.3
   infusion
      procedure Y84.8
   injection —*see* Table of Drugs and Chemicals ◀▥▥▥
      procedure Y84.8
   insertion of gastric or duodenal sound Y84.5
   insulin-shock therapy Y84.3
   paracentesis (abdominal) (thoracic) (aspirative) Y84.4
   procedures other than surgical operation —*see* Complication of or following, by type of procedure
   radiological procedure or therapy Y84.2
   removal of organ (partial) (total) NEC Y83.6
   sampling
      blood Y84.7
      fluid NEC Y84.4
      tissue Y84.8
   shock therapy Y84.3
   surgical operation NEC (*see also* Complication of or following, by type of operation) Y83.9
      reconstructive NEC Y83.4
        with
            anastomosis, bypass or graft Y83.2
            formation of external stoma Y83.3
      specified NEC Y83.8
   transfusion —*see also* Table of Drugs and Chemicals ◀▥▥▥
      procedure Y84.8
   transplant, transplantation (heart) (kidney) (liver) (whole organ, any) Y83.0
      partial organ Y83.4
   ureterostomy Y83.3

Complication of or following *(Continued)*
   vaccination —*see also* Table of Drugs and Chemicals ◀▥▥▥
      procedure Y84.8

Compression
   divers' squeeze —*see* Air, pressure, change
   trachea by
      food (lodged in esophagus) —*see* categories T17 and T18
      vomitus (lodged in esophagus) T17.81-

Conflagration —*see* Exposure, fire, uncontrolled

Constriction (external)
   hair W49.01
   jewelry W49.04
   ring W49.04
   rubber band W49.03
   specified item NEC W49.09
   string W49.02
   thread W49.02

Contact (accidental)
   with
      abrasive wheel (metalworking) W31.1
      alligator W58.09
         bite W58.01
         crushing W58.03
         strike W58.02
      amphibian W62.9
         frog W62.0
         toad W62.1
      animal (nonvenomous) NEC W64
         marine W56.89
            bite W56.81
            dolphin —*see* Contact, with, dolphin
            fish NEC —*see* Contact, with, fish
            mammal —*see* Contact, with, mammal, marine
            orca —*see* Contact, with, orca
            sea lion —*see* Contact, with, sea lion
            shark —*see* Contact, with, shark
            strike W56.82
      animate mechanical force NEC W64
      arrow W21.89
         not thrown, projected or falling W45.8
      arthropods (nonvenomous) W57
      axe W27.0
      band-saw (industrial) W31.2
      bayonet —*see* Bayonet wound
      bee (s) X58
      bench-saw (industrial) W31.2
      bird W61.99
         bite W61.91
         chicken —*see* Contact, with, chicken
         duck —*see* Contact, with, duck
         goose —*see* Contact, with, goose
         macaw —*see* Contact, with, macaw
         parrot —*see* Contact, with, parrot
         psittacine —*see* Contact, with, psittacine
         strike W61.92
         turkey —*see* Contact, with, turkey
      blender W29.0
      boiling water X12
         stated as undetermined whether accidental or intentional Y27.2
         suicide (attempt) X77.2
      bore, earth-drilling or mining (land) (seabed) W31.0
      buffalo —*see* Contact, with, hoof stock NEC
      bull W55.29
         bite W55.21
         gored W55.22
         strike W55.22
      bumper cars W31.81
      camel —*see* Contact, with, hoof stock NEC
      can
         lid W45.2
         opener W27.4
            powered W29.0
      cat W55.09
         bite W55.01
         scratch W55.03
      caterpillar (venomous) X58

Contact *(Continued)*
  with *(Continued)*
    centipede (venomous) X58
    chain
      hoist W24.0
        agricultural operations W30.89
      saw W29.3
    chicken W61.39
      peck W61.33
      strike W61.32
    chisel W27.0
    circular saw W31.2
    cobra X58
    combine (harvester) W30.0
    conveyer belt W24.1
    cooker (hot) X15.8
      stated as undetermined whether
        accidental or intentional Y27.3
      suicide (attempt) X77.3
    coral X58
    cotton gin W31.82
    cow W55.29
      bite W55.21
      strike W55.22
    crane W24.0
      agricultural operations W30.89
    crocodile W58.19
      bite W58.11
      crushing W58.13
      strike W58.12
    dagger W26.1
      stated as undetermined whether
        accidental or intentional Y28.2
      suicide (attempt) X78.2
    dairy equipment W31.82
    dart W21.89
      not thrown, projected or falling W45.8
    deer —*see* Contact, with, hoof stock
      NEC
    derrick W24.0
      agricultural operations W30.89
        hay W30.2
    dog W54.8
      bite W54.0
      strike W54.1
    dolphin W56.09
      bite W56.01
      strike W56.02
    donkey —*see* Contact, with, hoof stock
      NEC
    drill (powered) W29.8
      earth (land) (seabed) W31.0
      nonpowered W27.8
    drive belt W24.0
      agricultural operations W30.89
    dry ice —*see* Exposure, cold, man-made
    dryer (clothes) (powered) (spin) W29.2
    duck W61.69
      bite W61.61
      strike W61.62
    earth(-)
      drilling machine (industrial) W31.0
      scraping machine in stationary use
        W31.83
    edge of stiff paper W45.1
    electric
      beater W29.0
      blanket X16
      fan W29.2
        commercial W31.82
      knife W29.1
      mixer W29.0
    elevator (building) W24.0
      agricultural operations W30.89
        grain W30.3
    engine (s), hot NEC X17
    excavating machine W31.0
    farm machine W30.9
    feces —*see* Contact, with, by type of
      animal
    fer de lance X58

Contact *(Continued)*
  with *(Continued)*
    fish W56.59
      bite W56.51
      shark —*see* Contact, with, shark
      strike W56.52
    flying horses W31.81
    forging (metalworking) machine
      W31.1
    fork W27.4
    forklift (truck) W24.0
      agricultural operations W30.89
    frog W62.0
    garden
      cultivator (powered) W29.3
        riding W30.89
      fork W27.1
    gas turbine W31.3
    Gila monster X58
    giraffe —*see* Contact, with, hoof stock
      NEC
    glass (sharp) (broken) W25
      with subsequent fall W18.02
      assault X99.0
      due to fall —*see* Fall, by type
      stated as undetermined whether
        accidental or intentional Y28. 0
      suicide (attempt) X78.0
    goat W55.39
      bite W55.31
      strike W55.32
    goose W61.59
      bite W61.51
      strike W61.52
    hand
      saw W27.0
      tool (not powered) NEC W27.8
        powered W29.8
    harvester W30.0
    hay-derrick W30.2
    heat NEC X19
      from appliance (electrical)
        (household) —*see* Contact, with,
        hot, household appliance
      heating appliance X16
    heating
      appliance (hot) X16
      pad (electric) X16
    hedge-trimmer (powered) W29.3
    hoe W27.1
    hoist (chain) (shaft) NEC W24.0
      agricultural W30.89
    hoof stock NEC W55.39
      bite W55.31
      strike W55.32
    hornet (s) X58
    horse W55.19
      bite W55.11
      strike W55.12
    hot
      air X14.1
        inhalation X14.0
      cooker X15.8
      drinks X10.0
      engine X17
      fats X10.2
      fluids NEC X12
        assault X98.2
        suicide (attempt) X77.2
        undetermined whether accidental or
          intentional Y27.2
      food X10.1
      gases X14.1
        inhalation X14.0
      heating appliance X16
      household appliance X15.8
        assault X98.3
        cooker X15.8
        hotplate X15.2
        kettle X15.8
        light bulb X15.8

Contact *(Continued)*
  with *(Continued)*
    hot *(Continued)*
      household appliance *(Continued)*
        object NEC X19
          assault X98.8
          stated as undetermined whether
            accidental or intentional Y27.9
          suicide (attempt) X77.8
        saucepan X15.3
        skillet X15.3
        stated as undetermined whether
          accidental or intentional Y27.3
        stove X15.0
        suicide (attempt) X77.3
        toaster X15.1
      kettle X15.8
      light bulb X15.8
      liquid NEC (*see also* Burning) X12 ◀▥
        drinks X10.0
        stated as undetermined whether
          accidental or intentional Y27.2
        suicide (attempt) X77.2
        tap water X11.8
          stated as undetermined whether
            accidental or intentional Y27.1
          suicide (attempt) X77.1
      machinery X17
      metal (molten) (liquid) NEC X18
      object (not producing fire or flames)
        NEC X19
      oil (cooking) X10.2
      pipe X16
      plate X15.2
      radiator X16
      saucepan (glass) (metal) X15.3
      skillet X15.3
      stove (kitchen) X15.0
      substance NEC X19
      tap-water X11.8
        assault X98.1
        heated on stove X12
          stated as undetermined whether
            accidental or intentional Y27.2
          suicide (attempt) X77.2
        in bathtub X11.0
        running X11.1
        stated as undetermined whether
          accidental or intentional Y27.1
        suicide (attempt) X77.1
      toaster X15.1
      tool X17
      vapors X13.1
        inhalation X13.0
      water (tap) X11.8
        boiling X12
          stated as undetermined whether
            accidental or intentional Y27.2
          suicide (attempt) X77.2
        heated on stove X12
          stated as undetermined whether
            accidental or intentional Y27.2
          suicide (attempt) X77.2
        in bathtub X11.0
        running X11.1
        stated as undetermined whether
          accidental or intentional Y27.1
        suicide (attempt) X77.1
    hotplate X15.2
    ice-pick W27.4
    insect (nonvenomous) NEC W57
    kettle (hot) X15.8
    knife W26.0
      assault X99.1
      electric W29.1
      stated as undetermined whether
        accidental or intentional Y28.1
      suicide (attempt) X78.1
    lathe (metalworking) W31.1
      turnings W45.8
      woodworking W31.2

Contact *(Continued)*
  with *(Continued)*
    lawnmower (powered) (ridden) W28
      causing electrocution W86.8
        suicide (attempt) X83.1
      unpowered W27.1
    lift, lifting (devices) W24.0
      agricultural operations W30.89
      shaft W24.0
    liquefied gas —*see* Exposure, cold,
      man-made
    liquid air, hydrogen, nitrogen —*see*
      Exposure, cold, man-made
    lizard (nonvenomous) W59.09
      bite W59.01
      strike W59.02
    llama —*see* Contact, with, hoof stock NEC
    macaw W61.19
      bite W61.11
      strike W61.12
    machine, machinery W31.9
      abrasive wheel W31.1
      agricultural including animal-powered
        W30.9
        combine harvester W30.0
        grain storage elevator W30.3
        hay derrick W30.2
        power take-off device W30.1
        reaper W30.0
        specified NEC W30.89
        thresher W30.0
        transport vehicle, stationary W30.81
      band saw W31.2
      bench saw W31.2
      circular saw W31.2
      commercial NEC W31.82
      drilling, metal (industrial) W31.1
      earth-drilling W31.0
      earthmoving or scraping W31.89
      excavating W31.89
      forging machine W31.1
      gas turbine W31.3
      hot X17
      internal combustion engine W31.3
      land drill W31.0
      lathe W31.1
      lifting (devices) W24.0
      metal drill W31.1
      metalworking (industrial) W31.1
      milling, metal W31.1
      mining W31.0
      molding W31.2
      overhead plane W31.2
      power press, metal W31.1
      prime mover W31.3
      printing W31.89
      radial saw W31.2
      recreational W31.81
      roller-coaster W31.81
      rolling mill, metal W31.1
      sander W31.2
      seabed drill W31.0
      shaft
        hoist W31.0
        lift W31.0
      specified NEC W31.89
      spinning W31.89
      steam engine W31.3
      transmission W24.1
      undercutter W31.0
      water driven turbine W31.3
      weaving W31.89
      woodworking or forming (industrial)
        W31.2
    mammal (feces) (urine) W55.89
      bull —*see* Contact, with, bull
      cat —*see* Contact, with, cat
      cow —*see* Contact, with, cow
      goat —*see* Contact, with, goat
      hoof stock —*see* Contact, with, hoof
        stock

Contact *(Continued)*
  with *(Continued)*
    mammal *(Continued)*
      horse —*see* Contact, with, horse
      marine W56.39
        dolphin —*see* Contact, with, dolphin
        orca —*see* Contact, with, orca
        sea lion —*see* Contact, with, sea lion
        specified NEC W56.39
          bite W56.31
          strike W56.32
      pig —*see* Contact, with, pig
      raccoon —*see* Contact, with, raccoon
      rodent —*see* Contact, with, rodent
      sheep —*see* Contact, with, sheep
      specified NEC W55.89
        bite W55.81
        strike W55.82
    marine
      animal W56.89
        bite W56.81
        dolphin —*see* Contact, with, dolphin
        fish NEC —*see* Contact, with, fish
        mammal —*see* Contact, with,
          mammal, marine
        orca —*see* Contact, with, orca
        sea lion —*see* Contact, with, sea lion
        shark —*see* Contact, with, shark
        strike W56.82
    meat
      grinder (domestic) W29.0
        industrial W31.82
        nonpowered W27.4
      slicer (domestic) W29.0
        industrial W31.82
    merry go round W31.81
    metal, (hot) (liquid) (molten) NEC X18
    millipede W57
    nail W45.0
      gun W29.4
    needle (sewing) W27.3
      hypodermic W46.0
        contaminated W46.1
    object (blunt) NEC
      hot NEC X19
      legal intervention —*see* Legal,
        intervention, blunt object
      sharp NEC W45.8
        inflicted by other person NEC W45.8
          stated as
            intentional homicide (attempt) —
              see Assault, cutting or
              piercing instrument
        legal intervention —*see* Legal,
          intervention, sharp object
        self-inflicted X78.9
    orca W56.29
      bite W56.21
      strike W56.22
    overhead plane W31.2
    paper (as sharp object) W45.1
    paper-cutter W27.5
    parrot W61.09
      bite W61.01
      strike W61.02
    pig W55.49
      bite W55.41
      strike W55.42
    pipe, hot X16
    pitchfork W27.1
    plane (metal) (wood) W27.0
      overhead W31.2
    plant thorns, spines, sharp leaves or other
      mechanisms W60
    powered
      garden cultivator W29.3
      household appliance, implement, or
        machine W29.8
      saw (industrial) W31.2
        hand W29.8
    printing machine W31.89

Contact *(Continued)*
  with *(Continued)*
    psittacine bird W61.29
      bite W61.21
      macaw —*see* Contact, with, macaw ◀▥
      parrot —*see* Contact, with, parrot
      strike W61.22
    pulley (block) (transmission) W24.0
      agricultural operations W30.89
    raccoon W55.59
      bite W55.51
      strike W55.52
    radial-saw (industrial) W31.2
    radiator (hot) X16
    rake W27.1
    rattlesnake X58
    reaper W30.0
    reptile W59.89
      lizard —*see* Contact, with, lizard
      snake —*see* Contact, with, snake
      specified NEC W59.89
        bite W59.81
        crushing W59.83
        strike W59.82
      turtle —*see* Contact, with, turtle
    rivet gun (powered) W29.4
    road scraper —*see* Accident, transport,
      construction vehicle
    rodent (feces) (urine) W53.89
      bite W53.81
      mouse W53.09
        bite W53.01
      rat W53.19
        bite W53.11
      specified NEC W53.89
        bite W53.81
      squirrel W53.29
        bite W53.21
    roller coaster W31.81
    rope NEC W24.0
      agricultural operations W30.89
    saliva —*see* Contact, with, by type of
      animal
    sander W29.8
      industrial W31.2
    saucepan (hot) (glass) (metal) X15.3
    saw W27.0
      band (industrial) W31.2
      bench (industrial) W31.2
      chain W29.3
      hand W27.0
    sawing machine, metal W31.1
    scissors W27.2
    scorpion X58
    screwdriver W27.0
      powered W29.8
    sea
      anemone, cucumber or urchin (spine)
        X58
      lion W56.19
        bite W56.11
        strike W56.12
    serpent —*see* Contact, with, snake, by type
    sewing-machine (electric) (powered)
      W29.2
      not powered W27.8
    shaft (hoist) (lift) (transmission) NEC
      W24.0
      agricultural W30.89
    shark W56.49
      bite W56.41
      strike W56.42
    shears (hand) W27.2
      powered (industrial) W31.1
        domestic W29.2
    sheep W55.39
      bite W55.31
      strike W55.32
    shovel W27.8
      steam —*see* Accident, transport,
        construction vehicle

Contact (*Continued*)
  with (*Continued*)
    snake (nonvenomous) W59.19
      bite W59.11
      crushing W59.13
      strike W59.12
    spade W27.1
    spider (venomous) X58
    spin-drier W29.2
    spinning machine W31.89
    splinter W45.8
    sports equipment W21.9
    staple gun (powered) W29.8
    steam X13.1
      engine W31.3
      inhalation X13.0
      pipe X16
      shovel W31.89
    stove (hot) (kitchen) X15.0
    substance, hot NEC X19
      molten (metal) X18
    sword W26.1
      assault X99.2
      stated as undetermined whether
        accidental or intentional
        Y28.2
      suicide (attempt) X78.2
    tarantula X58
    thresher W30.0
    tin can lid W45.2
    toad W62.1
    toaster (hot) X15.1
    tool W27.8
      hand (not powered) W27.8
        auger W27.0
        axe W27.0
        can opener W27.4
        chisel W27.0
        fork W27.4
        garden W27.1
        handsaw W27.0
        hoe W27.1
        ice-pick W27.4
        kitchen utensil W27.4
        manual
          lawn mower W27.1
          sewing machine W27.8
        meat grinder W27.4
        needle (sewing) W27.3
          hypodermic W46.0
            contaminated W46.1
        paper cutter W27.5
        pitchfork W27.1
        rake W27.1
        scissors W27.2
        screwdriver W27.0
        specified NEC W27.8
        workbench W27.0
      hot X17
      powered W29.8
        blender W29.0
          commercial W31.82
        can opener W29.0
          commercial W31.82
        chainsaw W29.3
        clothes dryer W29.2
          commercial W31.82
        dishwasher W29.2
          commercial W31.82
        edger W29.3
        electric fan W29.2
          commercial W31.82
        electric knife W29.1
        food processor W29.0
          commercial W31.82
        garbage disposal W29.0
          commercial W31.82

Contact (*Continued*)
  with (*Continued*)
    tool (*Continued*)
      powered (*Continued*)
        garden tool W29.3
        hedge trimmer W29.3
        ice maker W29.0
          commercial W31.82
        kitchen appliance W29.0
          commercial W31.82
        lawn mower W28
        meat grinder W29.0
          commercial W31.82
        mixer W29.0
          commercial W31.82
        rototiller W29.3
        sewing machine W29.2
          commercial W31.82
        washing machine W29.2
          commercial W31.82
    transmission device (belt, cable, chain,
      gear, pinion, shaft) W24.1
      agricultural operations W30.89
    turbine (gas) (water-driven) W31.3
    turkey W61.49
      peck W61.43
      strike W61.42
    turtle (nonvenomous) W59.29
      bite W59.21
      strike W59.22
      terrestrial W59.89
        bite W59.81
        crushing W59.83
        strike W59.82
    under-cutter W31.0
    urine —*see* Contact, with, by type of
      animal
    vehicle
      agricultural use (transport) —*see*
        Accident, transport, agricultural
        vehicle
        not on public highway W30.81
      industrial use (transport) —*see*
        Accident, transport, industrial
        vehicle
        not on public highway W31.83
      off-road use (transport) —*see* Accident,
        transport, all-terrain or off-road
        vehicle
        not on public highway W31.83
      special construction use (transport) —*see*
        Accident, transport, construction
        vehicle
        not on public highway W31.83
    venomous
      animal X58
      arthropods X58
      lizard X58
      marine animal NEC X58
      marine plant NEC X58
      millipedes (tropical) X58
      plant (s) X58
      snake X58
      spider X58
    viper X58
    washing-machine (powered) W29.2
    wasp X58
    weaving-machine W31.89
    winch W24.0
      agricultural operations W30.89
    wire NEC W24.0
      agricultural operations W30.89
    wood slivers W45.8
    yellow jacket X58
    zebra —*see* Contact, with, hoof stock
      NEC
Coup de soleil X32

Crash
  aircraft (in transit) (powered) V95.9
    balloon V96.01
    fixed wing NEC (private) V95.21
      commercial V95.31
    glider V96.21
      hang V96.11
      powered V95.11
    helicopter V95.01
    in war operations —*see* War operations,
      destruction of aircraft
    microlight V95.11
    nonpowered V96.9
      specified NEC V96.8
    powered NEC V95.8
    stated as
      homicide (attempt) Y08.81
      suicide (attempt) X83.0
    ultralight V95.11
  spacecraft V95.41
  transport vehicle NEC (*see also* Accident,
    transport) V89.9
    homicide (attempt) Y03.8
    motor NEC (traffic) V89.2
      homicide (attempt) Y03.8
    suicide (attempt) —*see* Suicide, collision
Cruelty (mental) (physical) (sexual) X58
Crushed (accidentally) X58
  between objects (moving) (stationary and
    moving) W23.0
    stationary W23.1
  by
    alligator W58.03
    avalanche NEC —*see* Landslide
    cave-in W20.0
      caused by cataclysmic earth surface
        movement —*see* Landslide
    crocodile W58.13
    crowd or human stampede W52
    falling
      aircraft V97.39
        in war operations —*see* War
          operations, destruction of aircraft
      earth, material W20.0
        caused by cataclysmic earth surface
          movement —*see* Landslide
      object NEC W20.8
    landslide NEC —*see* Landslide
    lizard (nonvenomous) W59.09
    machinery —*see* Contact, with, by type of
      machine
    reptile NEC W59.89
    snake (nonvenomous) W59.13
  in
    machinery —*see* Contact, with, by type of
      machine
Cut, cutting (any part of body) (accidental) —
  see also Contact, with, by object or machine
  during medical or surgical treatment as
    misadventure —*see* ~~Misadventure, cut,
    by type of procedure~~Index to Diseases
    and Injuries, Complications ◀▦
  homicide (attempt) —*see* Assault, cutting or
    piercing instrument
  inflicted by other person —*see* Assault,
    cutting or piercing instrument
  legal
    execution —*see* Legal, intervention
    intervention —*see* Legal, intervention,
      sharp object
  machine NEC (*see also* Contact, with, by type
    of machine) W31.9
  self-inflicted —*see* Suicide, cutting or piercing
    instrument
  suicide (attempt) —*see* Suicide, cutting or
    piercing instrument
Cyclone (any injury) X37.1

◀ New   ◀▦ Revised   ~~deleted~~ Deleted

D

Decapitation (accidental circumstances)
NEC X58
homicide X99.9
legal execution —*see* Legal, intervention
Dehydration from lack of water X58
Deprivation X58
Derailment (accidental)
railway (rolling stock) (train) (vehicle)
(without antecedent collision) V81.7
with antecedent collision —*see* Accident,
transport, railway vehicle occupant
streetcar (without antecedent collision)
V82.7
with antecedent collision —*see* Accident,
transport, streetcar occupant
Descent
parachute (voluntary) (without accident to
aircraft) V97.29
due to accident to aircraft —*see* Accident,
transport, aircraft
Desertion X58
Destitution X58
Disability, late effect or sequela of injury —*see*
Sequelae
Discharge (accidental)
airgun W34.010
assault X95.01
homicide (attempt) X95.01
stated as undetermined whether accidental
or intentional Y24.0
suicide (attempt) X74.01
BB gun —*see* Discharge, airgun
firearm (accidental) W34.00
assault X95.9
handgun (pistol) (revolver) W32.0
assault X93
homicide (attempt) X93
legal intervention —*see* Legal,
intervention, firearm, handgun
stated as undetermined whether
accidental or intentional Y22
suicide (attempt) X72
homicide (attempt) X95.9
hunting rifle W33.02
assault X94.1
homicide (attempt) X94.1
legal intervention
injuring
bystander Y35.032
law enforcement personnel
Y35.031
suspect Y35.033
stated as undetermined whether
accidental or intentional Y23.1
suicide (attempt) X73.1
larger W33.00
assault X94.9
homicide (attempt) X94.9
hunting rifle —*see* Discharge, firearm,
hunting rifle
legal intervention —*see* Legal,
intervention, firearm by type of
firearm
machine gun —*see* Discharge, firearm,
machine gun
shotgun —*see* Discharge, firearm,
shotgun
specified NEC W33.09
assault X94.8
homicide (attempt) X94.8
legal intervention
injuring
bystander Y35.092
law enforcement personnel
Y35.091
suspect Y35.093
stated as undetermined whether
accidental or intentional Y23.8
suicide (attempt) X73.8

Discharge (*Continued*)
firearm (*Continued*)
larger (*Continued*)
stated as undetermined whether
accidental or intentional Y23.9
suicide (attempt) X73.9
legal intervention
injuring
bystander Y35.002
law enforcement personnel Y35.001
suspect Y35.03
using rubber bullet
injuring
bystander Y35.042
law enforcement personnel
Y35.041
suspect Y35.043
machine gun W33.03
assault X94.2
homicide (attempt) X94.2
legal intervention —*see* Legal,
intervention, firearm, machine gun
stated as undetermined whether
accidental or intentional Y23.3
suicide (attempt) X73.2
pellet gun —*see* Discharge, airgun
shotgun W33.01
assault X94.0
homicide (attempt) X94.0
legal intervention —*see* Legal,
intervention, firearm, specified NEC
stated as undetermined whether
accidental or intentional Y23.0
suicide (attempt) X73.0
specified NEC W34.09
assault X95.8
homicide (attempt) X95.8
legal intervention —*see* Legal,
intervention, firearm, specified NEC
stated as undetermined whether
accidental or intentional Y24.8
suicide (attempt) X74.8
stated as undetermined whether accidental
or intentional Y24.9
suicide (attempt) X74.9
Very pistol W34.09
assault X95.8
homicide (attempt) X95.8
stated as undetermined whether
accidental or intentional Y24.8
suicide (attempt) X74.8
firework (s) W39
stated as undetermined whether accidental
or intentional Y25
gas-operated gun NEC W34.018
airgun —*see* Discharge, airgun
assault X95.09
homicide (attempt) X95.09
paintball gun —*see* Discharge, paintball
gun
stated as undetermined whether accidental
or intentional Y24.8
suicide (attempt) X74.09
gun NEC —*see also* Discharge, firearm NEC
air —*see* Discharge, airgun
BB —*see* Discharge, airgun
for single hand use —*see* Discharge,
firearm, handgun
hand —*see* Discharge, firearm, handgun
machine —*see* Discharge, firearm, machine
gun
other specified —*see* Discharge, firearm
NEC
paintball —*see* Discharge, paintball gun
pellet —*see* Discharge, airgun
handgun —*see* Discharge, firearm, handgun
machine gun —*see* Discharge, firearm,
machine gun
paintball gun W34.011
assault X95.02
homicide (attempt) X95.02

Discharge (*Continued*)
paintball gun (*Continued*)
stated as undetermined whether accidental
or intentional Y24.8
suicide (attempt) X74.02
pistol —*see* Discharge, firearm, handgun
flare —*see* Discharge, firearm, Very pistol
pellet —*see* Discharge, airgun
Very —*see* Discharge, firearm, Very pistol
revolver —*see* Discharge, firearm, handgun
rifle (hunting) —*see* Discharge, firearm,
hunting rifle
shotgun —*see* Discharge, firearm, shotgun
spring-operated gun NEC W34.018
assault X95.09
homicide (attempt) X95.09
stated as undetermined whether accidental
or intentional Y24.8
suicide (attempt) X74.09
Disease
Andes W94.11
aviator's —*see* Air, pressure
range W94.11
Diver's disease, palsy, paralysis, squeeze —*see*
Air, pressure
Diving (into water) —*see* Accident, diving
Dog bite W54.0
Dragged by transport vehicle NEC (*see also*
Accident, transport) V09.9
Drinking poison (accidental) —*see* Table of
~~d~~Drugs and ~~c~~Chemicals ◀━━
Dropped (accidentally) while being carried or
supported by other person W04
Drowning (accidental) W74
assault X92.9
due to
accident (to)
machinery —*see* Contact, with, by type
of machine
watercraft V90.89
burning V90.29
powered V90.23
fishing boat V90.22
jetskis V90.23
merchant ship V90.20
passenger ship V90.21
unpowered V90.28
canoe V90.25
inflatable V90.26
kayak V90.25
sailboat V90.24
water skis V90.27
crushed V90.39
powered V90.33
fishing boat V90.32
jetskis V90.33
merchant ship V90.30
passenger ship V90.31
unpowered V90.38
canoe V90.35
inflatable V90.36
kayak V90.35
sailboat V90.34
water skis V90.37
overturning V90.09
powered V90.03
fishing boat V90.02
jetskis V90.03
merchant ship V90.00
passenger ship V90.01
unpowered V90.08
canoe V90.05
inflatable V90.06
kayak V90.05
sailboat V90.04
sinking V90.19
powered V90.13
fishing boat V90.12
jetskis V90.13
merchant ship V90.10
passenger ship V90.11

Drowning *(Continued)*
  due to *(Continued)*
    accident *(Continued)*
      watercraft *(Continued)*
        sinking *(Continued)*
          unpowered V90.18
            canoe V90.15
            inflatable V90.16
            kayak V90.15
            sailboat V90.14
        specified type NEC V90.89
          powered V90.83
            fishing boat V90.82
            jetskis V90.83
            merchant ship V90.80
            passenger ship V90.81
          unpowered V90.88
            canoe V90.85
            inflatable V90.86
            kayak V90.85
            sailboat V90.84
            water skis V90.87
    avalanche —*see* Landslide
    cataclysmic
      earth surface movement NEC —*see*
        Forces of nature, earth movement
      storm —*see* Forces of nature, cataclysmic
        storm
    cloudburst X37.8
    cyclone X37.1
    fall overboard (from) V92.09
      powered craft V92.03
        ferry boat V92.01
        fishing boat V92.02
        jetskis V92.03
        liner V92.01
        merchant ship V92.00
        passenger ship V92.01
      resulting from
        accident to watercraft —*see* Drowning,
          due to, accident to, watercraft
        being washed overboard (from)
          V92.29
          powered craft V92.23
            ferry boat V92.21
            fishing boat V92.22
            jetskis V92.23
            liner V92.21
            merchant ship V92.20
            passenger ship V92.21
          unpowered craft V92.28
            canoe V92.25
            inflatable V92.26
            kayak V92.25
            sailboat V92.24
            surf-board V92.28
            water skis V92.27
            windsurfer V92.28
        motion of watercraft V92.19
          powered craft V92.13
            ferry boat V92.11
            fishing boat V92.12
            jetskis V92.13
            liner V92.11
            merchant ship V92.10
            passenger ship V92.11
          unpowered craft
            canoe V92.15
            inflatable V92.16
            kayak V92.15
            sailboat V92.14
      unpowered craft V92.08
        canoe V92.05
        inflatable V92.06
        kayak V92.05

Drowning *(Continued)*
  due to *(Continued)*
    fall overboard *(Continued)*
      unpowered craft *(Continued)*
        sailboat V92.04
        surf-board V92.08
        water skis V92.07
        windsurfer V92.08
    hurricane X37.0
    jumping into water from watercraft
      (involved in accident) —*see also*
      Drowning, due to, accident to,
      watercraft
      without accident to or on watercraft
        W16.711
    tidal wave NEC —*see* Forces of nature,
      tidal wave
    torrential rain X37.8
  following
    fall
      into
        bathtub W16.211
        bucket W16.221
        fountain —*see* Drowning, following,
          fall, into, water, specified NEC
        quarry —*see* Drowning, following,
          fall, into, water, specified NEC
        reservoir —*see* Drowning, following,
          fall, into, water, specified NEC
        swimming-pool W16.011
          stated as undetermined whether
            accidental or intentional
            Y21.3
          striking
            bottom W16.021
            wall W16.031
          suicide (attempt) X71.2
        water NOS W16.41
          natural (lake) (open sea) (river)
           (stream) (pond) W16.111
           striking
            bottom W16.121
            side W16.131
          specified NEC W16.311
           striking
            bottom W16.321
            wall W16.331
      overboard NEC —*see* Drowning, due to,
        fall overboard
    jump or dive
      from boat W16.711
        striking bottom W16.721
      into
        fountain —*see* Drowning, following,
          jump or dive, into, water,
          specified NEC
        quarry —*see* Drowning, following,
          jump or dive, into, water,
          specified NEC
        reservoir —*see* Drowning, following,
          jump or dive, into, water,
          specified NEC
        swimming-pool W16.511
          striking
           bottom W16.521
           wall W16.531
          suicide (attempt) X71.2
        water NOS W16.91
          natural (lake) (open sea) (river)
           (stream) (pond) W16.611
          specified NEC W16.811
           striking
            bottom W16.821
            wall W16.831
          striking bottom W16.621

Drowning *(Continued)*
  homicide (attempt) X92.9
  in
    bathtub (accidental) W65
      assault X92.0
      following fall W16.211
        stated as undetermined whether
          accidental or intentional
          Y21.1
      stated as undetermined whether
        accidental or intentional Y21.0
      suicide (attempt) X71.0
    lake —*see* Drowning, in, natural water
    natural water (lake) (open sea) (river)
      (stream) (pond) W69
      assault X92.3
      following
        dive or jump W16.611
          striking bottom W16.621
        fall W16.111
          striking
           bottom W16.121
           side W16.131
      stated as undetermined whether
        accidental or intentional Y21.4
      suicide (attempt) X71.3
    quarry —*see* Drowning, in, specified place
      NEC
    quenching tank —*see* Drowning, in,
      specified place NEC
    reservoir —*see* Drowning, in, specified
      place NEC
    river —*see* Drowning, in, natural water
    sea —*see* Drowning, in, natural water
    specified place NEC W73
      assault X92.8
      following
        dive or jump W16.811
          striking
           bottom W16.821
           wall W16.831
        fall W16.311
          striking
           bottom W16.321
           wall W16.331
      stated as undetermined whether
        accidental or intentional Y21.8
      suicide (attempt) X71.8
    stream —*see* Drowning, in, natural water
    swimming-pool W67
      assault X92.1
        following fall X92.2
      following
        dive or jump W16.511
          striking
           bottom W16.521
           wall W16.531
        fall W16.011
          striking
           bottom W16.021
           wall W16.031
      stated as undetermined whether
        accidental or intentional Y21.2
        following fall Y21.3
      suicide (attempt) X71.1
        following fall X71.2
    war operations —*see* War operations,
      restriction of airway
  resulting from accident to watercraft —*see*
    Drowning, due to, accident, watercraft
  self-inflicted X71.9
  stated as undetermined whether accidental or
    intentional Y21.9
  suicide (attempt) X71.9

◄ New   ◄▦ Revised   ~~deleted~~ Deleted

E

Earth (surface) movement NEC —*see* Forces of
  nature, earth movement
Earth falling (on) W20.0
  caused by cataclysmic earth surface
    movement or eruption —*see* Landslide
Earthquake (any injury) X34
Effect (s) (adverse) of
  air pressure (any) —*see* Air, pressure
  cold, excessive (exposure to) —*see* Exposure,
    cold
  heat (excessive) —*see* Heat
  hot place (weather) —*see* Heat
  insolation X30
  late —*see* Sequelae
  motion —*see* Motion
  nuclear explosion or weapon in war
    operations —*see* War operations, nuclear
    weapon
  radiation —*see* Radiation
  travel —*see* Travel
Electric shock (accidental) (by) (in) —*see*
  Exposure, electric current
Electrocution (accidental) —*see* Exposure,
  electric current
Endotracheal tube wrongly placed during
  anesthetic procedure Y65.3
Entanglement
  in
    bed linen, causing suffocation —*see*
      category T71
    wheel of pedal cycle V19.88
Entry of foreign body or material —*see* Foreign
  body
Environmental pollution related condition —
  see Z57
Execution, legal (any method) —*see* Legal,
  intervention
Exhaustion
  cold —*see* Exposure, cold
  due to excessive exertion —*see* category Y93
  heat —*see* Heat
Explosion (accidental) (of) (with secondary fire)
  W40.9
  acetylene W40.1
  aerosol can W36.1
  air tank (compressed) (in machinery) W36.2
  aircraft (in transit) (powered) NEC V95.9
    balloon V96.05
    fixed wing NEC (private) V95.25
      commercial V95.35
    glider V96.25
      hang V96.15
      powered V95.15
    helicopter V95.05
    in war operations —*see* War operations,
      destruction of aircraft
    microlight V95.15
    nonpowered V96.9
      specified NEC V96.8
    powered NEC V95.8
    stated as
      homicide (attempt) Y03.8
      suicide (attempt) X83.0
    ultralight V95.15
  anesthetic gas in operating room W40.1
  antipersonnel bomb W40.8
    assault X96.0
    homicide (attempt) X96.0
    suicide (attempt) X75
  assault X96.9
  bicycle tire W37.0
  blasting (cap) (materials) W40.0
  boiler (machinery), not on transport vehicle
    W35
    on watercraft —*see* Explosion, in,
      watercraft
  butane W40.1
  caused by other person X96.9
  coal gas W40.1

Explosion (*Continued*)
  detonator W40.0
  dump (munitions) W40.8
  dynamite W40.0
    in
      assault X96.8
      homicide (attempt) X96.8
      legal intervention
        injuring
          bystander Y35.112
          law enforcement personnel Y35.111
          suspect Y35.113
      suicide (attempt) X75
  explosive (material) W40.9
    gas W40.1
    in blasting operation W40.0
    specified NEC W40.8
      in
        assault X96.8
        homicide (attempt) X96.8
        legal intervention
          injuring
            bystander Y35.192
            law enforcement personnel
              Y35.191
            suspect Y35.193
        suicide (attempt) X75
  factory (munitions) W40.8
  fertilizer bomb W40.8
    assault X96.3
    homicide (attempt) X96.3
    suicide (attempt) X75
  fire-damp W40.1
  firearm (parts) NEC W34.19
    airgun W34.110
    BB gun W34.110
    gas, air or spring-operated gun NEC
      W34.118
    handgun W32.1
    hunting rifle W33.12
    larger firearm W33.10
      specified NEC W33.19
    machine gun W33.13
    paintball gun W34.111
    pellet gun W34.110
    shotgun W33.11
    Very pistol [flare] W34.19
  fireworks W39
  gas (coal) (explosive) W40.1
    cylinder W36.9
      aerosol can W36.1
      air tank W36.2
      pressurized W36.3
      specified NEC W36.8
  gasoline (fumes) (tank) not in moving motor
    vehicle W40.1
    bomb W40.8
      assault X96.1
      homicide (attempt) X96.1
      suicide (attempt) X75
    in motor vehicle —*see* Accident, transport,
      by type of vehicle
  grain store W40.8
  grenade W40.8
    in
      assault X96.8
      homicide (attempt) X96.8
      legal intervention
        injuring
          bystander Y35.192
          law enforcement personnel
            Y35.191
          suspect Y35.193
      suicide (attempt) X75
  handgun (parts) —*see* Explosion, firearm,
    handgun (parts)
  homicide (attempt) X96.9
    antipersonnel bomb —*see* Explosion,
      antipersonnel bomb
    fertilizer bomb —*see* Explosion, fertilizer
      bomb

Explosion (*Continued*)
  homicide (*Continued*)
    gasoline bomb —*see* Explosion, gasoline
      bomb
    letter bomb —*see* Explosion, letter bomb
    pipe bomb —*see* Explosion, pipe bomb
    specified NEC X96.8
  hose, pressurized W37.8
  hot water heater, tank (in machinery) W35
    on watercraft —*see* Explosion, in,
      watercraft
  in, on
    dump W40.8
    factory W40.8
    mine (of explosive gases) NEC W40.1
    watercraft V93.59
      powered craft V93.53
        ferry boat V93.51
        fishing boat V93.52
        jetskis V93.53
        liner V93.51
        merchant ship V93.50
        passenger ship V93.51
        sailboat V93.54
  letter bomb W40.8
    assault X96.2
    homicide (attempt) X96.2
    suicide (attempt) X75
  machinery —*see also* Contact, with, by type
    of machine
    on board watercraft —*see* Explosion, in,
      watercraft
    pressure vessel —*see* Explosion, by type
      of vessel
  methane W40.1
  mine W40.1
  missile NEC W40.8
  mortar bomb W40.8
    in
      assault X96.8
      homicide (attempt) X96.8
      legal intervention
        injuring
          bystander Y35.192
          law enforcement personnel
            Y35.191
          suspect Y35.193
      suicide (attempt) X75
  munitions (dump) (factory) W40.8
  pipe, pressurized W37.8
    bomb W40.8
      assault X96.4
      homicide (attempt) X96.4
      suicide (attempt) X75
  pressure, pressurized
    cooker W38
    gas tank (in machinery) W36.3
    hose W37.8
    pipe W37.8
    specified device NEC W38
    tire W37.8
      bicycle W37.0
    vessel (in machinery) W38
  propane W40.1
  self-inflicted X75
  shell (artillery) NEC W40.8
    during war operations —*see* War
      operations, explosion
    in
      legal intervention
        injuring
          bystander Y35.122
          law enforcement personnel Y35.121
          suspect Y35.123
    war —*see* War operations, explosion
  spacecraft V95.45
  stated as undetermined whether accidental or
    intentional Y25
  steam or water lines (in machinery) W37.8
  stove W40.9
  suicide (attempt) X75

Exposure *(Continued)*
    prolonged in deep-freeze unit or refrigerator W93.2
    radiation —*see* Radiation
    smoke —*see also* Exposure, fire
        tobacco, second hand Z77.22
    specified factors NEC X58
    sunlight X32
        man-made (sun lamp) W89.8
            tanning bed W89.1
    supersonic waves W42.0
    transmission line (s), electric W85
    vibration W49.9

Exposure *(Continued)*
    waves
        infrasound W49.9
        sound W42.9
        supersonic W42.0
    weather NEC —*see* Forces of nature
External cause status Y99.9
    child assisting in compensated work for family Y99.8
    civilian activity done for financial or other compensation Y99.0
    civilian activity done for income or pay Y99.0

External cause status *(Continued)*
    family member assisting in compensated work for other family member Y99.8
    hobby not done for income Y99.8
    leisure activity Y99.8
    military activity Y99.1
    off-duty activity of military personnel Y99.8
    recreation or sport not for income or while a student Y99.8
    specified NEC Y99.8
    student activity Y99.8
    volunteer activity Y99.2

F

Factors, supplemental
- alcohol
  - blood level
    - less than 20mg/100ml Y90.0
    - presence in blood, level not specified Y90.9
    - 20-39mg/100ml Y90.1
    - 40-59mg/100ml Y90.2
    - 60-79mg/100ml Y90.3
    - 80-99mg/100ml Y90.4
    - 100-119mg/100ml Y90.5
    - 120-199mg/100ml Y90.6
    - 200-239mg/100ml Y90.7
    - 240mg/100ml or more Y90.8
    - presence in blood, but level not specified Y90.9
  - environmental-pollution-related condition —see Z57
  - nosocomial condition Y95
  - work-related condition Y99.0

Failure
- in suture or ligature during surgical procedure Y65.2
- mechanical, of instrument or apparatus (any) (during any medical or surgical procedure) Y65.8
- sterile precautions (during medical and surgical care) —see Misadventure, failure, sterile precautions, by type of procedure
- to
  - introduce tube or instrument Y65.4
    - endotracheal tube during anesthesia Y65.3
  - make curve (transport vehicle) NEC —see Accident, transport
  - remove tube or instrument Y65.4

Fall, falling (accidental) W19
- building W20.1
  - burning (uncontrolled fire) X00.3
- down
  - embankment W17.81
  - escalator W10.0
  - hill W17.81
  - ladder W11
  - ramp W10.2
  - stairs, steps W10.9
- due to
  - bumping against
    - object W18.00
      - sharp glass W18.02
      - specified NEC W18.09
      - sports equipment W18.01
    - person W03
      - due to ice or snow W00.0
      - on pedestrian conveyance —see Accident, transport, pedestrian, conveyance
  - collision with another person W03
    - due to ice or snow W00.0
    - involving pedestrian conveyance —see Accident, transport, pedestrian, conveyance
  - grocery cart tipping over W17.82
  - ice or snow W00.9
    - from one level to another W00.2
      - on stairs or steps W00.1
    - involving pedestrian conveyance —see Accident, transport, pedestrian, conveyance
    - on same level W00.0
  - slipping (on moving sidewalk) W01.0
    - with subsequent striking against object W01.10
      - furniture W01.190
      - sharp object W01.119
        - glass W01.110
        - power tool or machine W01.111
        - specified NEC W01.118
      - specified NEC W01.198

Fall, falling (Continued)
- due to (Continued)
  - striking against
    - object W18.00
      - sharp glass W18.02
      - specified NEC W18.09
      - sports equipment W18.01
    - person W03
      - due to ice or snow W00.0
      - on pedestrian conveyance —see Accident, transport, pedestrian, conveyance
- earth (with asphyxia or suffocation (by pressure)) —see Earth, falling
- from, off, out of
  - aircraft NEC (with accident to aircraft NEC) V97.0
    - while boarding or alighting V97.1
  - balcony W13.0
  - bed W06
  - boat, ship, watercraft NEC (with drowning or submersion) —see Drowning, due to, fall overboard
    - with hitting bottom or object V94.0
  - bridge W13.1
  - building W13.9
    - burning (uncontrolled fire) X00.3
  - cavity W17.2
  - chair W07
  - cherry picker W17.89
  - cliff W15
  - dock W17.4
  - embankment W17.81
  - escalator W10.0
  - flagpole W13.8
  - furniture NEC W08
  - grocery cart W17.82
  - haystack W17.89
  - high place NEC W17.89
    - stated as undetermined whether accidental or intentional Y30
  - hole W17.2
  - incline W10.2
  - ladder W11
  - lifting device W17.89
  - machine, machinery —see also Contact, with, by type of machine
    - not in operation W17.89
  - manhole W17.1
  - mobile elevated work platform [MEWP] W17.89
  - motorized mobility scooter W05.2
  - one level to another NEC W17.89
    - intentional, purposeful, suicide (attempt) X80
    - stated as undetermined whether accidental or intentional Y30
  - pit W17.2
  - playground equipment W09.8
    - jungle gym W09.2
    - slide W09.0
    - swing W09.1
  - quarry W17.89
  - railing W13.9
  - ramp W10.2
  - roof W13.2
  - scaffolding W12
  - scooter (nonmotorized) W05.1
    - motorized mobility W05.2
  - sky lift W17.89
  - stairs, steps W10.9
    - curb W10.1
    - due to ice or snow W00.1
    - escalator W10.0
    - incline W10.2
    - ramp W10.2
    - sidewalk curb W10.1
    - specified NEC W10.8
  - stepladder W11
  - storm drain W17.1

Fall, falling (Continued)
- from, off, out of (Continued)
  - streetcar NEC V82.6
    - with antecedent collision —see Accident, transport, streetcar occupant
    - while boarding or alighting V82.4
  - structure NEC W13.8
    - burning (uncontrolled fire) X00.3
  - table W08
  - toilet W18.11
    - with subsequent striking against object W18.12
  - train NEC V81.6
    - during derailment (without antecedent collision) V81.7
      - with antecedent collision —see Accident, transport, railway vehicle occupant
    - while boarding or alighting V81.4
  - transport vehicle after collision —see Accident, transport, by type of vehicle, collision
  - tree W14
  - vehicle (in motion) NEC (see also Accident, transport) V89.9
    - motor NEC (see also Accident, transport, occupant, by type of vehicle) V87.8
    - stationary W17.89
      - while boarding or alighting —see Accident, transport, by type of vehicle, while boarding or alighting
  - viaduct W13.8
  - wall W13.8
  - watercraft —see also Drowning, due to, fall overboard
    - with hitting bottom or object V94.0
  - well W17.0
  - wheelchair, non-moving W05.0
    - powered —see Accident, transport, pedestrian, conveyance occupant, specified type NEC
  - window W13.4
- in, on
  - aircraft NEC V97.0
    - with accident to aircraft V97.0
    - while boarding or alighting V97.1
  - bathtub (empty) W18.2
    - filled W16.212
      - causing drowning W16.211
  - escalator W10.0
  - incline W10.2
  - ladder W11
  - machine, machinery —see Contact, with, by type of machine
  - object, edged, pointed or sharp (with cut) —see Fall, by type
  - playground equipment W09.8
    - jungle gym W09.2
    - slide W09.0
    - swing W09.1
  - ramp W10.2
  - scaffolding W12
  - shower W18.2
    - causing drowning W16.211
  - staircase, stairs, steps W10.9
    - curb W10.1
    - due to ice or snow W00.1
    - escalator W10.0
    - incline W10.2
    - specified NEC W10.8
  - streetcar (without antecedent collision) V82.5
    - with antecedent collision —see Accident, transport, streetcar occupant
    - while boarding or alighting V82.4

Fall, falling (Continued)
  in, on (Continued)
    train (without antecedent collision) V81.5
      with antecedent collision —see Accident,
        transport, railway vehicle occupant
      during derailment (without antecedent
        collision) V81.7
        with antecedent collision —see
          Accident, transport, railway
          vehicle occupant
      while boarding or alighting V81.4
      transport vehicle after collision —see
        Accident, transport, by type of
        vehicle, collision
    watercraft V93.39
      due to
        accident to craft V91.29
          powered craft V91.23
            ferry boat V91.21
            fishing boat V91.22
            jetskis V91.23
            liner V91.21
            merchant ship V91.20
            passenger ship V91.21
          unpowered craft
            canoe V91.25
            inflatable V91.26
            kayak V91.25
            sailboat V91.24
        powered craft V93.33
          ferry boat V93.31
          fishing boat V93.32
          jetskis V93.33
          liner V93.31
          merchant ship V93.30
          passenger ship V93.31
        unpowered craft V93.38
          canoe V93.35
          inflatable V93.36
          kayak V93.35
          sailboat V93.34
          surf-board V93.38
          windsurfer V93.38
  into
    cavity W17.2
    dock W17.4
    fire —see Exposure, fire, by type
    haystack W17.89
    hole W17.2
    lake —see Fall, into, water
    manhole W17.1
    moving part of machinery —see Contact,
      with, by type of machine
    ocean —see Fall, into, water
    opening in surface NEC W17.89
    pit W17.2
    pond —see Fall, into, water
    quarry W17.89
    river —see Fall, into, water
    shaft W17.89
    storm drain W17.1
    stream —see Fall, into, water
    swimming pool —see also Fall, into, water,
      in, swimming pool
      empty W17.3
    tank W17.89
    water W16.42
      causing drowning W16.41
      from watercraft —see Drowning, due to,
        fall overboard
      hitting diving board W21.4
      in
        bathtub W16.212
          causing drowning W16.211
        bucket W16.222
          causing drowning W16.221
        natural body of water W16.112
          causing drowning W16.111
          striking
            bottom W16.122
              causing drowning W16.121

Fall, falling (Continued)
  into (Continued)
    water (Continued)
      in (Continued)
        natural body of water (Continued)
          striking (Continued)
            side W16.132
              causing drowning W16.131
        specified water NEC W16.312
          causing drowning W16.311
          striking
            bottom W16.322
              causing drowning W16.321
            wall W16.332
              causing drowning W16.331
        swimming pool W16.012
          causing drowning W16.011
          striking
            bottom W16.022
              causing drowning W16.021
            wall W16.032
              causing drowning W16.031
        utility bucket W16.222
          causing drowning W16.221
    well W17.0
  involving
    bed W06
    chair W07
    furniture NEC W08
    glass —see Fall, by type
    playground equipment W09.8
      jungle gym W09.2
      slide W09.0
      swing W09.1
    roller blades —see Accident, transport,
      pedestrian, conveyance
    skateboard (s) —see Accident, transport,
      pedestrian, conveyance
    skates (ice) (in line) (roller) —see
      Accident, transport, pedestrian,
      conveyance
    skis —see Accident, transport, pedestrian,
      conveyance
    table W08
    wheelchair, non-moving W05.0
      powered —see Accident, transport,
        pedestrian, conveyance, specified
        type NEC
  object —see Struck by, object, falling
  off
    toilet W18.11
      with subsequent striking against object
        W18.12
  on same level W18.30
    due to
      specified NEC W18.39
      stepping on an object W18.31
  out of
    bed W06
    building NEC W13.8
    chair W07
    furniture NEC W08
    wheelchair, non-moving W05.0
      powered —see Accident, transport,
        pedestrian, conveyance, specified
        type NEC
    window W13.4
  over
    animal W01.0
    cliff W15
    embankment W17.81
    small object W01.0
  rock W20.8
  same level W18.30
    from
      being crushed, pushed, or stepped on
        by a crowd or human stampede
        W52
      collision, pushing, shoving, by or with
        other person W03
      slipping, stumbling, tripping W01.0

Fall, falling (Continued)
  same level (Continued)
    involving ice or snow W00.0
    involving skates (ice) (roller),
      skateboard, skis —see Accident,
      transport, pedestrian, conveyance
  snowslide (avalanche) —see Landslide
  stone W20.8
  structure W20.1
    burning (uncontrolled fire) X00.3
  through
    bridge W13.1
    floor W13.3
    roof W13.2
    wall W13.8
    window W13.4
  timber W20.8
  tree (caused by lightning) W20.8
  while being carried or supported by other
    person (s) W04
Fallen on by
  animal (not being ridden) NEC W55.89
Felo-de-se —see Suicide
Fight (hand) (fists) (foot) —see Assault, fight
Fire (accidental) —see Exposure, fire
Firearm discharge —see Discharge, firearm
Fireball effects from nuclear explosion in war
  operations —see War operations, nuclear
  weapons
Fireworks (explosion) W39
Flash burns from explosion —see Explosion
Flood (any injury) (caused by) X38
  collapse of man-made structure causing earth
    movement X36.0
  tidal wave —see Forces of nature, tidal wave
Food (any type) in
  air passages (with asphyxia, obstruction, or
    suffocation) —see categories T17 and T18
  alimentary tract causing asphyxia (due to
    compression of trachea) —see categories
    T17 and T18
Forces of nature X39.8
  avalanche X36.1
    causing transport accident —see Accident,
      transport, by type of vehicle
  blizzard X37.2
  cataclysmic storm X37.9
    with flood X38
    blizzard X37.2
    cloudburst X37.8
    cyclone X37.1
    dust storm X37.3
    hurricane X37.0
    specified storm NEC X37.8
    storm surge X37.0
    tornado X37.1
    twister X37.1
    typhoon X37.0
  cloudburst X37.8
  cold (natural) X31
  cyclone X37.1
  dam collapse causing earth movement X36.0
  dust storm X37.3
  earth movement X36.1
    caused by dam or structure collapse X36.0
    earthquake X34
  earthquake X34
  flood (caused by) X38
    dam collapse X36.0
    tidal wave —see Forces of nature, tidal
      wave
  heat (natural) X30
  hurricane X37.0
  landslide X36.1
    causing transport accident —see Accident,
      transport, by type of vehicle
  lightning —see subcategory T75.0
    causing fire —see Exposure, fire
  mudslide X36.1
    causing transport accident —see Accident,
      transport, by type of vehicle

Forces of nature *(Continued)*
  radiation (natural) X39.08
    radon X39.01
  radon X39.01
  specified force NEC X39.8
  storm surge X37.0
  structure collapse causing
    earth movement
      X36.0
  sunlight X32
  tidal wave X37.41
    due to
      earthquake X37.41
      landslide X37.43
      storm X37.42
      volcanic eruption X37.41
  tornado X37.1
  tsunami X37.41
  twister X37.1

Forces of nature *(Continued)*
  typhoon X37.0
  volcanic eruption X35
~~Foreign body entering through skin W45.8~~
  ~~can lid W45.2~~
  ~~nail W45.0~~
  ~~paper W45.1~~
  ~~specified NEC W45.8~~
  ~~splinter W45.8~~
Foreign body ◄
  aspiration - *see* Index to Diseases and
    Injuries. Foreign body, respitory
    tract ◄
  entering through skin
    W45.8 ◄
    can lid W45.2 ◄
    nail W45.0 ◄
    paper W45.1 ◄

Foreign body *(Continued)*
  entering through skin *(Continued)*
    specified NEC 45.8 ◄
    splinter W45.8 ◄
Forest fire (exposure to) —*see* Exposure, fire,
  uncontrolled, not in building
Found injured X58
  from exposure (to) —*see* Exposure
  on
    highway, road(way), street V89.9
    railway right of way V81.9
Fracture (circumstances unknown or
  unspecified) X58
  due to specified cause NEC X58
Freezing —*see* Exposure, cold
Frostbite X31
  due to man-made conditions —*see* Exposure,
    cold, man-made
Frozen —*see* Exposure, cold

G

Gored by bull W55.22
Gunshot wound W34.00

H

Hailstones, injured by X39.8
Hanged herself or himself —*see* Hanging,
  self-inflicted
Hanging (accidental) (*see also* category T71)
  legal execution —*see* Legal, intervention,
    specified means NEC
Heat (effects of) (excessive) X30
  due to
    man-made conditions W92
      on board watercraft V93.29
        fishing boat V93.22
        merchant ship V93.20
        passenger ship V93.21
        sailboat V93.24
        specified powered craft NEC V93.23
    weather (conditions) X30

Heat *(Continued)*
  from
    electric heating apparatus causing
      burning X16
    nuclear explosion in war operations —*see*
      War operations, nuclear weapons
    inappropriate in local application or packing
      in medical or surgical procedure Y63.5
Hemorrhage
  delayed following medical or surgical
    treatment without mention of
    misadventure —*see* ~~Complication of or~~
    ~~following, by type of procedure~~Index to
    Diseases and Injuries, Complication(s) ◄▥
  during medical or surgical treatment as
    misadventure —*see* ~~Misadventure, cut,~~
    ~~by type of procedure~~Index to Diseases
    and Injuries, Complication(s) ◄▥

High
  altitude (effects) —*see* Air, pressure, low
  level of radioactivity, effects —*see* Radiation
  pressure (effects) —*see* Air, pressure, high
  temperature, effects —*see* Heat
Hit, hitting (accidental) by —*see* Struck by
Hitting against —*see* Striking against
Homicide (attempt) (justifiable) —*see* Assault
Hot
  place, effects —*see also* Heat
  weather, effects X30
House fire (uncontrolled) —*see* Exposure, fire,
  uncontrolled, building
Humidity, causing problem X39.8
Hunger X58
Hurricane (any injury) X37.0
Hypobarism, hypobaropathy —*see* Air,
  pressure, low

◄ New   ◄▥ Revised   ~~deleted~~ Deleted

I

Ictus
  caloris —*see also* Heat
  solaris X30
Ignition (accidental) (*see also* Exposure, fire)
    X08.8
  anesthetic gas in operating room W40.1
  apparel X06.2
    from highly flammable material X04
    nightwear X05
  bed linen (sheets) (spreads) (pillows)
    (mattress) —*see* Exposure, fire,
    uncontrolled, building, bed
  benzine X04
  clothes, clothing NEC (from controlled fire)
    X06.2
    from
      highly flammable material X04
  ether X04
    in operating room W40.1
  explosive material —*see* Explosion
  gasoline X04
  jewelry (plastic) (any) X06.0
  kerosene X04
  material
    explosive —*see* Explosion
    highly flammable with secondary
      explosion X04
  nightwear X05
  paraffin X04
  petrol X04
Immersion (accidental) —*see also* Drowning
  hand or foot due to cold (excessive) X31
Implantation of quills of porcupine
  W55.89
Inanition (from) (hunger) X58
  thirst X58.8
Inappropriate operation performed
  correct operation on wrong side or body
    part (wrong side) (wrong site)
    Y65.53
  operation intended for another patient done
    on wrong patient Y65.52
  wrong operation performed on correct
    patient Y65.51
Inattention after, at birth (homicidal intent)
  (infanticidal intent) X58
Incident, adverse
  device
    anesthesiology Y70.8
      accessory Y70.2
      diagnostic Y70.0
      miscellaneous Y70.8
      monitoring Y70.0
      prosthetic Y70.2
      rehabilitative Y70.1
      surgical Y70.3
      therapeutic Y70.1
    cardiovascular Y71.8
      accessory Y71.2
      diagnostic Y71.0
      miscellaneous Y71.8
      monitoring Y71.0
      prosthetic Y71.2
      rehabilitative Y71.1
      surgical Y71.3
      therapeutic Y71.1
    gastroenterology Y73.8
      accessory Y73.2
      diagnostic Y73.0
      miscellaneous Y73.8
      monitoring Y73.0
      prosthetic Y73.2
      rehabilitative Y73.1
      surgical Y73.3
      therapeutic Y73.1
    general
      hospital Y74.8
        accessory Y74.2
        diagnostic Y74.0

Incident, adverse (*Continued*)
  device (*Continued*)
    general (*Continued*)
      hospital (*Continued*)
        miscellaneous Y74.8
        monitoring Y74.0
        prosthetic Y74.2
        rehabilitative Y74.1
        surgical Y74.3
        therapeutic Y74.1
      surgical Y81.8
        accessory Y81.2
        diagnostic Y81.0
        miscellaneous Y81.8
        monitoring Y81.0
        prosthetic Y81.2
        rehabilitative Y81.1
        surgical Y81.3
        therapeutic Y81.1
    gynecological Y76.8
      accessory Y76.2
      diagnostic Y76.0
      miscellaneous Y76.8
      monitoring Y76.0
      prosthetic Y76.2
      rehabilitative Y76.1
      surgical Y76.3
      therapeutic Y76.1
    medical Y82.9
      specified type NEC Y82.8
    neurological Y75.8
      accessory Y75.2
      diagnostic Y75.0
      miscellaneous Y75.8
      monitoring Y75.0
      prosthetic Y75.2
      rehabilitative Y75.1
      surgical Y75.3
      therapeutic Y75.1
    obstetrical Y76.8
      accessory Y76.2
      diagnostic Y76.0
      miscellaneous Y76.8
      monitoring Y76.0
      prosthetic Y76.2
      rehabilitative Y76.1
      surgical Y76.3
      therapeutic Y76.1
    ophthalmic Y77.8
      accessory Y77.2
      diagnostic Y77.0
      miscellaneous Y77.8
      monitoring Y77.0
      prosthetic Y77.2
      rehabilitative Y77.1
      surgical Y77.3
      therapeutic Y77.1
    orthopedic Y79.8
      accessory Y79.2
      diagnostic Y79.0
      miscellaneous Y79.8
      monitoring Y79.0
      prosthetic Y79.2
      rehabilitative Y79.1
      surgical Y79.3
      therapeutic Y79.1
    otorhinolaryngological Y72.8
      accessory Y72.2
      diagnostic Y72.0
      miscellaneous Y72.8
      monitoring Y72.0
      prosthetic Y72.2
      rehabilitative Y72.1
      surgical Y72.3
      therapeutic Y72.1
    personal use Y74.8
      accessory Y74.2
      diagnostic Y74.0
      miscellaneous Y74.8
      monitoring Y74.0
      prosthetic Y74.2

Incident, adverse (*Continued*)
  device (*Continued*)
    personal use (*Continued*)
      rehabilitative Y74.1
      surgical Y74.3
      therapeutic Y74.1
    physical medicine Y80.8
      accessory Y80.2
      diagnostic Y80.0
      miscellaneous Y80.8
      monitoring Y80.0
      prosthetic Y80.2
      rehabilitative Y80.1
      surgical Y80.3
      therapeutic Y80.1
    plastic surgical Y81.8
      accessory Y81.2
      diagnostic Y81.0
      miscellaneous Y81.8
      monitoring Y81.0
      prosthetic Y81.2
      rehabilitative Y81.1
      surgical Y81.3
      therapeutic Y81.1
    radiological Y78.8
      accessory Y78.2
      diagnostic Y78.0
      miscellaneous Y78.8
      monitoring Y78.0
      prosthetic Y78.2
      rehabilitative Y78.1
      surgical Y78.3
      therapeutic Y78.1
    urology Y73.8
      accessory Y73.2
      diagnostic Y73.0
      miscellaneous Y73.8
      monitoring Y73.0
      prosthetic Y73.2
      rehabilitative Y73.1
      surgical Y73.3
      therapeutic Y73.1
Incineration (accidental) —*see* Exposure, fire
Infanticide —*see* Assault
Infrasound waves (causing injury) W49.9
Ingestion
  foreign body (causing injury) (with
    obstruction) —*see* Foreign body,
    alimentary canal
  poisonous
    plant (s) X58
    substance NEC —*see* Table of ◁Drugs and
    ◁Chemicals ◀▥
Inhalation
  excessively cold substance, man-made —*see*
    Exposure, cold, man-made
  food (any type) (into respiratory tract) (with
    asphyxia, obstruction respiratory tract,
    suffocation) —*see* categories T17 and T18
  foreign body —*see* Foreign body, aspiration
  gastric contents (with asphyxia, obstruction
    respiratory passage, suffocation) T17.81-
  hot air or gases X14.0
  liquid air, hydrogen, nitrogen W93.12
    suicide (attempt) X83.2
  steam X13.0
    assault X98.0
    stated as undetermined whether accidental
      or intentional Y27.0
    suicide (attempt) X77.0
  toxic gas —*see* Table of ◁Drugs and
    ◁Chemicals ◀▥
  vomitus (with asphyxia, obstruction
    respiratory passage, suffocation) T17.81-
Injury, injured (accidental(ly)) NOS X58
  by, caused by, from
    assault —*see* Assault
    law-enforcing agent, police, in course
      of legal intervention —*see* Legal
      intervention
    suicide (attempt) X83.8

Injury, injured NOS *(Continued)*
  due to, in
    civil insurrection —*see* War
      operations
    fight *(see also* Assault, fight)
      Y04.0
    war operations —*see* War
      operations
  homicide *(see also* Assault) Y09
  inflicted (by)
    in course of arrest (attempted), suppression
      of disturbance, maintenance of order,
      by law-enforcing agents —*see* Legal
      intervention

Injury, injured NOS *(Continued)*
  inflicted *(Continued)*
    other person
      stated as
        accidental X58
        intentional, homicide (attempt) —*see*
          Assault
        undetermined whether accidental or
          intentional Y33
    purposely (inflicted) by other person (s) —*see*
      Assault
    self-inflicted X83.8
      stated as accidental X58
    specified cause NEC X58

Injury, injured NOS *(Continued)*
  undetermined whether accidental or
    intentional Y33
Insolation, effects X30
Insufficient nourishment X58
Interruption of respiration (by)
  food (lodged in esophagus) —*see* categories
    T17 and T18
  vomitus (lodged in esophagus) T17.81-
Intervention, legal —*see* Legal intervention
Intoxication
  drug —*see* Table of Drugs and Chemicals ◀▥▥
  poison —*see* Table of Drugs and
    Chemicals ◀▥▥

J

Jammed (accidentally)
  between objects (moving) (stationary and
    moving) W23.0
  stationary W23.1
Jumped, jumping
  before moving object NEC X81.8
    motor vehicle X81.0
    subway train X81.1
    train X81.1
    undetermined whether accidental or
      intentional Y31
  from
    boat (into water) voluntarily,
      without accident (to or on boat)
      W16.712
      with
        accident to or on boat —*see* Accident,
          watercraft
        drowning or submersion W16.711
          suicide (attempt) X71.3

Jumped, jumping *(Continued)*
  from *(Continued)*
    boat voluntarily, without accident
      (Continued)
      striking bottom W16.722
        causing drowning W16.721
    building *(see also* Jumped, from,
      high place) W13.9
      burning (uncontrolled fire)
        X00.5
    high place NEC W17.89
      suicide (attempt) X80
      undetermined whether accidental or
        intentional Y30
    structure *(see also* Jumped, from, high
      place) W13.9
      burning (uncontrolled fire)
        X00.5
    into water W16.92
      causing drowning W16.91
    from, off watercraft —*see* Jumped, from,
      boat

Jumped, jumping *(Continued)*
  into water *(Continued)*
    in
      natural body W16.612
        causing drowning W16.611
        striking bottom W16.622
          causing drowning W16.621
      specified place NEC W16.812
        causing drowning W16.811
        striking
          bottom W16.822
            causing drowning W16.821
          wall W16.832
            causing drowning W16.831
      swimming pool W16.512
        causing drowning W16.511
        striking
          bottom W16.522
            causing drowning W16.521
          wall W16.532
            causing drowning W16.531
    suicide (attempt) X71.3

K

Kicked by
  animal NEC W55.82
  person (s) (accidentally) W50.1
    with intent to injure or kill Y04.0
    as, or caused by, a crowd or human
      stampede (with fall) W52
    assault Y04.0
    homicide (attempt) Y04.0
    in
      fight Y04.0
      legal intervention
        injuring
          bystander Y35.812
          law enforcement personnel Y35.811
          suspect Y35.813

Kicking against
  object W22.8
    sports equipment W21.9
    stationary W22.09
      sports equipment W21.89
  person —*see* Striking against, person
  sports equipment W21.9
Killed, killing (accidentally) NOS *(see also*
  Injury) X58
  in
    action —*see* War operations
    brawl, fight (hand) (fists) (foot) Y04.0
      by weapon —*see also* Assault
        cutting, piercing —*see* Assault, cutting
          or piercing instrument
        firearm —*see* Discharge, firearm, by
          type, homicide

Killed, killing NOS *(Continued)*
  self
    stated as
      accident NOS X58
      suicide —*see* Suicide
      undetermined whether accidental or
        intentional Y33
Knocked down (accidentally) (by) NOS X58
  animal (not being ridden) NEC —*see also*
    Struck by, by type of animal
  crowd or human stampede W52
  person W51
    in brawl, fight Y04.0
  transport vehicle NEC *(see also* Accident,
    transport) V09.9

◀ New   ◀▥▥ Revised   ~~deleted~~ Deleted

L

Laceration NEC —*see* Injury
Lack of
  care (helpless person) (infant) (newborn) X58
  food except as result of abandonment or
    neglect X58
    due to abandonment or neglect X58
  water except as result of transport accident X58
    due to transport accident —*see* Accident,
      transport, by type
    helpless person, infant, newborn X58
Landslide (falling on transport vehicle) X36.1
  caused by collapse of man-made structure
    X36.0
Late effect —*see* Sequelae
Legal
  execution (any method) —*see* Legal,
    intervention
  intervention (by)
    baton —*see* Legal, intervention, blunt
      object, baton
    bayonet —*see* Legal, intervention, sharp
      object, bayonet
    blow —*see* Legal, intervention,
      manhandling
    blunt object
      baton
        injuring
          bystander Y35.312
          law enforcement personnel Y35.311
          suspect Y35.313
      injuring
        bystander Y35.302
        law enforcement personnel Y35.301
        suspect Y35.303
      specified NEC
        injuring
          bystander Y35.392
          law enforcement personnel Y35.391
          suspect Y35.393
      stave
        injuring
          bystander Y35.392
          law enforcement personnel Y35.391
          suspect Y35.393
    bomb —*see* Legal, intervention, explosive
    cutting or piercing instrument —*see* Legal,
      intervention, sharp object
    dynamite —*see* Legal, intervention,
      explosive, dynamite
    explosive (s)
      dynamite
        injuring
          bystander Y35.112
          law enforcement personnel Y35.111
          suspect Y35.113
      grenade
        injuring
          bystander Y35.192
          law enforcement personnel Y35.191
          suspect Y35.193
      injuring
        bystander Y35.102
        law enforcement personnel Y35.101
        suspect Y35.103

Legal *(Continued)*
  intervention *(Continued)*
    explosive *(Continued)*
      mortar bomb
        injuring
          bystander Y35.192
          law enforcement personnel
            Y35.191
          suspect Y35.193
      shell
        injuring
          bystander Y35.122
          law enforcement personnel Y35.121
          suspect Y35.123
      specified NEC
        injuring
          bystander Y35.192
          law enforcement personnel Y35.191
          suspect Y35.193
    firearm (s) (discharge)
      handgun
        injuring
          bystander Y35.022
          law enforcement personnel Y35.021
          suspect Y35.023
      injuring
        bystander Y35.002
        law enforcement personnel Y35.001
        suspect Y35.003
      machine gun
        injuring
          bystander Y35.012
          law enforcement personnel Y35.011
          suspect Y35.013
      rifle pellet
        injuring
          bystander Y35.032
          law enforcement personnel Y35.031
          suspect Y35.033
      rubber bullet
        injuring
          bystander Y35.042
          law enforcement personnel Y35.041
          suspect Y35.043
      shotgun —*see* Legal, intervention,
        firearm, specified NEC
      specified NEC
        injuring
          bystander Y35.092
          law enforcement personnel Y35.091
          suspect Y35.093
    gas (asphyxiation) (poisoning)
      injuring
        bystander Y35.202
        law enforcement personnel Y35.201
        suspect Y35.203
      specified NEC
        injuring
          bystander Y35.292
          law enforcement personnel Y35.291
          suspect Y35.293
      tear gas
        injuring
          bystander Y35.212
          law enforcement personnel Y35.211
          suspect Y35.213

Legal *(Continued)*
  intervention *(Continued)*
    grenade —*see* Legal, intervention,
      explosive, grenade
    injuring
      bystander Y35.92
      law enforcement personnel Y35.91
      suspect Y35.93
    late effect (of) (*see* with 7th character S)
      Y35
    manhandling
      injuring
        bystander Y35.812
        law enforcement personnel Y35.811
        suspect Y35.813
    sequelae (of) (*see* with 7th character S)
      Y35
    sharp objects
      bayonet
        injuring
          bystander Y35.412
          law enforcement personnel
            Y35.411
          suspect Y35.413
      injuring
        bystander Y35.402
        law enforcement personnel Y35.401
        suspect Y35.403
      specified NEC
        injuring
          bystander Y35.492
          law enforcement personnel
            Y35.491
          suspect Y35.493
    specified means NEC
      injuring
        bystander Y35.892
        law enforcement personnel Y35.891
        suspect Y35.893
    stabbing —*see* Legal, intervention, sharp
      object
    stave —*see* Legal, intervention, blunt
      object, stave
    tear gas —*see* Legal, intervention, gas, tear
      gas
    truncheon —*see* Legal, intervention, blunt
      object, stave
Lightning (shock) (stroke) (struck by) —*see*
  subcategory T75.0
  causing fire —*see* Exposure, fire
Loss of control (transport vehicle) NEC —*see*
  Accident, transport
Lost at sea NOS —*see* Drowning, due to, fall
  overboard
Low
  pressure (effects) —*see* Air, pressure, low
  temperature (effects) —*see* Exposure, cold
Lying before train, vehicle or other moving
  object X81.8
  subway train X81.1
  train X81.1
  undetermined whether accidental or
    intentional Y31
Lynching —*see* Assault

M

Malfunction (mechanism or component) (of)
  firearm
    airgun W34.10
    BB gun W34.110
    gas, air or spring-operated gun NEC
      W34.118
    handgun W32.1
    hunting rifle W33.12
    larger firearm W33.10
      specified NEC W33.19
    machine gun W33.13
    paintball gun W34.111
    pellet gun W34.110
    shotgun W33.11
    specified NEC W34.19
    Very pistol [flare] W34.19
  handgun —*see* Malfunction, firearm,
    handgun
Maltreatment —*see* Perpetrator
Mangled (accidentally) NOS X58
Manhandling (in brawl, fight) Y04.0
  legal intervention —*see* Legal, intervention,
    manhandling
Manslaughter (nonaccidental) —*see* Assault
Mauled by animal NEC W55.89
Medical procedure, complication of
  (delayed or as an abnormal reaction
    without mention of misadventure) —*see*
    Complication of or following, by specified
    type of procedure
  due to or as a result of misadventure —*see*
    Misadventure
Melting (due to fire) —*see also* Exposure, fire
  apparel NEC X06.3
  clothes, clothing NEC X06.3
    nightwear X05
  fittings or furniture (burning building)
    (uncontrolled fire) X00.8
  nightwear X05
  plastic jewelry X06.1
Mental cruelty X58
Military operations (injuries to military and
  civilians occuring during peacetime on
  military property and during routine
  military exercises and operations) (by)
  (from) (involving) Y37.90-
  air blast Y37.20-
  aircraft
    destruction —*see* Military operations,
      destruction of aircraft
    airway restriction —*see* Military operations,
      restriction of airways
    asphyxiation —*see* Military operations,
      restriction of airways
  biological weapons Y37.6X-
  blast Y37.20-
  blast fragments Y37.20-
  blast wave Y37.20-
  blast wind Y37.20-
  bomb Y37.20-
    dirty Y37.50-
    gasoline Y37.31-
    incendiary Y37.31-
    petrol Y37.31-
  bullet Y37.43-
    incendiary Y37.32-
    rubber Y37.41-
  chemical weapons Y37.7X-
  combat
    hand to hand (unarmed) combat
      Y37.44-
    using blunt or piercing object Y37.45-
  conflagration —*see* Military operations, fire
  conventional warfare NEC Y37.49-
  depth-charge Y37.01-
  destruction of aircraft Y37.10-
    due to
      air to air missile Y37.11-
      collision with other aircraft Y37.12-

Military operations (*Continued*)
  destruction of aircraft (*Continued*)
    due to (*Continued*)
      detonation (accidental) of onboard
        munitions and explosives Y37.14-
      enemy fire or explosives Y37.11-
      explosive placed on aircraft Y37.11-
      onboard fire Y37.13-
      rocket propelled grenade [RPG] Y37.11-
      small arms fire Y37.11-
      surface to air missile Y37.11-
      specified NEC Y37.19-
  detonation (accidental) of
    onboard marine weapons Y37.05-
    own munitions or munitions launch device
      Y37.24-
  dirty bomb Y37.50-
  explosion (of) Y37.20-
    aerial bomb Y37.21-
    bomb NOS (*see also* Military operations,
      bomb (s)) Y37.20-
    fragments Y37.20-
    grenade Y37.29-
    guided missile Y37.22-
    improvised explosive device [IED] (person-
      borne) (roadside) (vehicle-borne)
      Y37.23-
    land mine Y37.29-
    marine mine (at sea) (in harbor) Y37.02-
    marine weapon Y37.00-
      specified NEC Y37.09-
    own munitions or munitions launch device
      (accidental) Y37.24-
    sea-based artillery shell Y37.03-
    specified NEC Y37.29-
    torpedo Y37.04-
  fire Y37.30-
    specified NEC Y37.39-
  firearms
    discharge Y37.43-
    pellets Y37.42-
  flamethrower Y37.33-
  fragments (from) (of)
    improvised explosive device [IED] (person-
      borne) (roadside) (vehicle-borne)
      Y37.26-
    munitions Y37.25-
    specified NEC Y37.29-
    weapons Y37.27-
  friendly fire Y37.92-
  hand to hand (unarmed) combat Y37.44-
  hot substances —*see* Military operations, fire
  incendiary bullet Y37.32-
  nuclear weapon (effects of) Y37.50-
    acute radiation exposure Y37.54-
    blast pressure Y37.51-
    direct blast Y37.51-
    direct heat Y37.53-
    fallout exposure Y37.54-
    fireball Y37.53-
    indirect blast (struck or crushed by blast
      debris) (being thrown by blast)
      Y37.52-
    ionizing radiation (immediate exposure)
      Y37.54-
    nuclear radiation Y37.54-
    radiation
      ionizing (immediate exposure) Y37.54-
      nuclear Y37.54-
      thermal Y37.53-
    secondary effects Y37.54-
    specified NEC Y37.59-
    thermal radiation Y37.53-
  restriction of air (airway)
    intentional Y37.46-
    unintentional Y37.47-
  rubber bullets Y37.41-
  shrapnel NOS Y37.29-
  suffocation —*see* Military operations,
    restriction of airways
  unconventional warfare NEC Y37.7X-

Military operations (*Continued*)
  underwater blast NOS Y37.00-
  warfare
    conventional NEC Y37.49-
    unconventional NEC Y37.7X-
  weapon of mass destruction [WMD] Y37.91-
  weapons
    biological weapons Y37.6X-
    chemical Y37.7X-
    nuclear (effects of) Y37.50-
      acute radiation exposure Y37.54-
      blast pressure Y37.51-
      direct blast Y37.51-
      direct heat Y37.53-
      fallout exposure Y37.54-
      fireball Y37.53-
      indirect blast (struck or crushed by blast
        debris) (being thrown by blast)
        Y37.52-
      radiation
        ionizing (immediate exposure) Y37.54-
        nuclear Y37.54-
        thermal Y37.53-
      secondary effects Y37.54-
      specified NEC Y37.59-
    of mass destruction [WMD] Y37.91-
Misadventure (s) to patient (s) during surgical
  or medical care Y69
contaminated medical or biological substance
  (blood, drug, fluid) Y64.9
  administered (by) NEC Y64.9
    immunization Y64.1
    infusion Y64.0
    injection Y64.1
    specified means NEC Y64.8
    transfusion Y64.0
    vaccination Y64.1
excessive amount of blood or other fluid
  during transfusion or infusion Y63.0
failure
  in dosage Y63.9
    electroshock therapy Y63.4
    inappropriate temperature (too hot or
      too cold) in local application and
      packing Y63.5
    infusion
      excessive amount of fluid Y63.0
      incorrect dilution of fluid Y63.1
    insulin-shock therapy Y63.4
    nonadministration of necessary drug or
      biological substance Y63.6
    overdose —*see* Table of ◀Drugs and
      ◀Chemicals ◀▥
    radiation, in therapy Y63.2
    radiation
      overdose Y63.2
    specified procedure NEC Y63.8
    transfusion
      excessive amount of blood Y63.0
mechanical, of instrument or apparatus
  (any) (during any procedure) Y65.8
sterile precautions (during procedure)
  Y62.9
  aspiration of fluid or tissue (by puncture
    or catheterization, except heart)
    Y62.6
  biopsy (except needle aspiration) Y62.8
    needle (aspirating) Y62.6
  blood sampling Y62.6
  catheterization Y62.6
    heart Y62.5
  dialysis (kidney) Y62.2
  endoscopic examination Y62.4
  enema Y62.8
  immunization Y62.3
  infusion Y62.1
  injection Y62.3
  needle biopsy Y62.6
  paracentesis (abdominal) (thoracic)
    Y62.6
  perfusion Y62.2

◀ New   ◀▥ Revised   ~~deleted~~ Deleted

Misadventure (s) to patient (s) during surgical
    or medical care *(Continued)*
  failure *(Continued)*
    sterile precautions *(Continued)*
      puncture (lumbar) Y62.6
      removal of catheter or packing
        Y62.8
      specified procedure NEC Y62.8
      surgical operation Y62.0
      transfusion Y62.1
      vaccination Y62.3
    suture or ligature during surgical
      procedure Y65.2
    to introduce or to remove tube or
      instrument —*see* Failure, to
  hemorrhage —*see* ~~Misadventure, cut, by~~
    ~~type of procedure~~Index to Diseases and
    Injuries, Complication(s) ◀▥
  inadvertent exposure of patient to radiation
    Y63.3
  inappropriate
    operation performed —*see*
      Inappropriate operation
      performed
    temperature (too hot or too cold) in
      local application or packing
      Y63.5

Misadventure (s) to patient (s) during surgical
    or medical care *(Continued)*
  infusion (*see also* Misadventure, by type,
    infusion) Y69
    excessive amount of fluid Y63.0
    incorrect dilution of fluid Y63.1
    wrong fluid Y65.1
  mismatched blood in transfusion Y65.0
  nonadministration of necessary drug or
    biological substance Y63.6
  overdose —*see* Table of ~~d~~Drugs and
    ~~c~~Chemicals ◀▥
    radiation (in therapy) Y63.2
  perforation —*see* ~~Misadventure, cut, by type~~
    ~~of procedure~~Index to Diseases and
    Injuries, Complication(s) ◀▥
  performance of inappropriate operation —*see*
    Inappropriate operation performed
  puncture —*see* ~~Misadventure, cut, by type of~~
    ~~procedure~~Index to Diseases and Injuries,
    Complication(s) ◀▥
  specified type NEC Y65.8
    failure
      suture or ligature during surgical
        operation Y65.2
      to introduce or to remove tube or
        instrument —*see* Failure, to

Misadventure (s) to patient (s) during surgical
    or medical care *(Continued)*
  specified type NEC *(Continued)*
    infusion of wrong fluid Y65.1
    performance of inappropriate operation —
      see Inappropriate operation performed
    transfusion of mismatched blood Y65.0
    wrong
      fluid in infusion Y65.1
      placement of endotracheal tube during
        anesthetic procedure Y65.3
  transfusion —*see* Misadventure, by type,
    transfusion
    excessive amount of blood Y63.0
    mismatched blood Y65.0
  wrong
    drug given in error —*see* Table of ~~d~~Drugs
      and ~~c~~Chemicals ◀▥
    fluid in infusion Y65.1
    placement of endotracheal tube during
      anesthetic procedure Y65.3
Mismatched blood in transfusion Y65.0
Motion sickness T75.3
Mountain sickness W94.11
Mudslide (of cataclysmic nature) —*see*
  Landslide
Murder (attempt) —*see* Assault

N

Nail, contact with W45.0
  gun W29.4
Neglect (criminal) (homicidal intent) X58
Noise (causing injury) (pollution) W42.9
  supersonic W42.0

Nonadministration (of)
  drug or biological substance (necessary)
    Y63.6
  surgical and medical care Y66
Nosocomial condition Y95

O

Object
  falling
    from, in, on, hitting
      machinery —*see* Contact, with, by type
        of machine
  set in motion by
    accidental explosion or rupture of pressure
      vessel W38
    firearm —*see* Discharge, firearm, by
      type
    machine (ry) —*see* Contact, with, by type
      of machine

Overdose (drug) —*see* Table of ~~d~~Drugs and
    ~~c~~Chemicals ◀▥
  radiation Y63.2
Overexertion —*see* category Y93
Overexposure (accidental) (to)
  cold (*see also* Exposure, cold) X31
    due to man-made conditions —*see*
      Exposure, cold, man-made
  heat (*see also* Heat) X30
  radiation —*see* Radiation
  radioactivity W88.0
  sun (sunburn) X32
  weather NEC —*see* Forces of nature
  wind NEC —*see* Forces of nature

Overheated —*see* Heat
Overturning (accidental)
  machinery —*see* Contact, with, by type of
    machine
  transport vehicle NEC (*see also* Accident,
    transport) V89.9
  watercraft (causing drowning,
    submersion) —*see also* Drowning, due to,
    accident to, watercraft, overturning
    causing injury except drowning or
      submersion —*see* Accident, watercraft,
      causing, injury NEC

◀ New   ◀▥ Revised   ~~deleted~~ Deleted

P

Parachute descent (voluntary) (without accident to aircraft) V97.29
  due to accident to aircraft —see Accident, transport, aircraft
Pecked by bird W61.99
Perforation during medical or surgical treatment as misadventure —see Misadventure, cut, by type of procedureIndex to Diseases and Injuries, Complication(s) ◀▥
Perpetrator, perpetration, of assault, maltreatment and neglect (by) Y07.9
  boyfriend Y07.03
  brother Y07.410
    stepbrother Y07.435
  coach Y07.53
  cousin
    female Y07.491
    male Y07.490
  daycare provider Y07.519
    at-home
      adult care Y07.512
      childcare Y07.510
    care center
      adult care Y07.513
      childcare Y07.511
  family member NEC Y07.499
  father Y07.11
    adoptive Y07.13
    foster Y07.420
    stepfather Y07.430
  foster father Y07.420
  foster mother Y07.421
  girl friend Y07.04
  healthcare provider Y07.529
    mental health Y07.521
    specified NEC Y07.528
  husband Y07.01
  instructor Y07.53
  mother Y07.12
    adoptive Y07.14
    foster Y07.421
    stepmother Y07.433
  nonfamily member Y07.50
    specified NEC Y07.59
  nurse Y07.528
  occupational therapist Y07.528
  partner of parent
    female Y07.434
    male Y07.432
  physical therapist Y07.528
  sister Y07.411
  speech therapist Y07.528
  stepbrother Y07.435
  stepfather Y07.430
  stepmother Y07.433
  stepsister Y07.436
  teacher Y07.53
  wife Y07.02
Piercing —see Contact, with, by type of object or machine
Pinched
  between objects (moving) (stationary and moving) W23.0
    stationary W23.1
Pinned under machine (ry) —see Contact, with, by type of machine
Place of occurrence Y92.9
  abandoned house Y92.89
  airplane Y92.813
  airport Y92.520
  ambulatory health services establishment NEC Y92.538
  ambulatory surgery center Y92.530
  amusement park Y92.831
  apartment (co-op) —see Place of occurrence, residence, apartment
  assembly hall Y92.29
  bank Y92.510
  barn Y92.71
  baseball field Y92.320

Place of occurrence (Continued)
  basketball court Y92.310
  beach Y92.832
  boarding house —see Place of occurrence, residence, boarding house
  boat Y92.814
  bowling alley Y92.39
  bridge Y92.89
  building under construction Y92.61
  bus Y92.811
    station Y92.521
  cafe Y92.511
  campsite Y92.833
  campus —see Place of occurrence, school
  canal Y92.89
  car Y92.810
  casino Y92.59
  children's home —see Place of occurrence, residence, institutional, orphanage
  church Y92.22
  cinema Y92.26
  clubhouse Y92.29
  coal pit Y92.64
  college (community) Y92.214
  condominium —see Place of occurrence, residence, apartment
  construction area —see Place of occurrence, industrial and construction area
  convalescent home —see Place of occurrence, residence, institutional, nursing home
  court-house Y92.240
  cricket ground Y92.328
  cultural building Y92.258
    art gallery Y92.250
    museum Y92.251
    music hall Y92.252
    opera house Y92.253
    specified NEC Y92.258
    theater Y92.254
  dancehall Y92.252
  day nursery Y92.210
  dentist office Y92.531
  derelict house Y92.89
  desert Y92.820
  dock NOS Y92.89
  dockyard Y92.62
  doctor's office Y92.531
  dormitory —see Place of occurrence, residence, institutional, school dormitory
  dry dock Y92.62
  factory (building) (premises) Y92.63
  farm (land under cultivation) (outbuildings) Y92.79
    barn Y92.71
    chicken coop Y92.72
    field Y92.73
    hen house Y92.72
    house —see Place of occurrence, residence, house
    orchard Y92.74
    specified NEC Y92.79
  football field Y92.321
  forest Y92.821
  freeway Y92.411
  gallery Y92.250
  garage (commercial) Y92.59
    boarding house Y92.044
    military base Y92.135
    mobile home Y92.025
    nursing home Y92.124
    orphanage Y92.114
    private house Y92.015
    reform school Y92.155
  gas station Y92.524
  gasworks Y92.69
  golf course Y92.39
  gravel pit Y92.64
  grocery Y92.512
  gymnasium Y92.39
  handball court Y92.318
  harbor Y92.89

Place of occurrence (Continued)
  harness racing course Y92.39
  healthcare provider office Y92.531
  highway (interstate) Y92.411
  hill Y92.828
  hockey rink Y92.330
  home —see Place of occurrence, residence
  hospice —see Place of occurrence, residence, institutional, nursing home
  hospital Y92.239
    cafeteria Y92.233
    corridor Y92.232
    operating room Y92.234
    patient
      bathroom Y92.231
      room Y92.230
    specified NEC Y92.238
  hotel Y92.59
  house —see also Place of occurrence, residence
    abandoned Y92.89
    under construction Y92.61
  industrial and construction area (yard) Y92.69
    building under construction Y92.61
    dock Y92.62
    dry dock Y92.62
    factory Y92.63
    gasworks Y92.69
    mine Y92.64
    oil rig Y92.65
    pit Y92.64
    power station Y92.69
    shipyard Y92.62
    specified NEC Y92.69
    tunnel under construction Y92.69
    workshop Y92.69
  kindergarten Y92.211
  lacrosse field Y92.328
  lake Y92.828
  library Y92.241
  mall Y92.59
  market Y92.512
  marsh Y92.828
  military
    base —see Place of occurrence, residence, institutional, military base
    training ground Y92.84
  mine Y92.64
  mosque Y92.22
  motel Y92.59
  motorway (interstate) Y92.411
  mountain Y92.828
  movie-house Y92.26
  museum Y92.251
  music-hall Y92.252
  not applicable Y92.9
  nuclear power station Y92.69
  nursing home —see Place of occurrence, residence, institutional, nursing home
  office building Y92.59
  offshore installation Y92.65
  oil rig Y92.65
  old people's home —see Place of occurrence, residence, institutional, specified NEC
  opera-house Y92.253
  orphanage —see Place of occurrence, residence, institutional, orphanage
  outpatient surgery center Y92.530
  park (public) Y92.830
    amusement Y92.831
  parking garage Y92.89
    lot Y92.481
  pavement Y92.480
  physician office Y92.531
  polo field Y92.328
  pond Y92.828
  post office Y92.242
  power station Y92.69
  prairie Y92.828
  prison —see Place of occurrence, residence, institutional, prison

◀ New   ◀▥ Revised   ~~deleted~~ Deleted

Place of occurrence *(Continued)*
  public
    administration building Y92.248
      city hall Y92.243
      courthouse Y92.240
      library Y92.241
      post office Y92.242
      specified NEC Y92.248
    building NEC Y92.29
    hall Y92.29
    place NOS Y92.89
  race course Y92.39
  radio station Y92.59
  railway line (bridge) Y92.85
  ranch (outbuildings) —*see* Place of
    occurrence, farm
  recreation area Y92.838
    amusement park Y92.831
    beach Y92.832
    campsite Y92.833
    park (public) Y92.830
    seashore Y92.832
    specified NEC Y92.838
  reform school —*see* Place of occurrence,
    residence, institutional, reform school
  religious institution Y92.22
  residence (non-institutional) (private) Y92.009
    apartment Y92.039
      bathroom Y92.031
      bedroom Y92.032
      kitchen Y92.030
      specified NEC Y92.038
    bathroom Y92.002
    bedroom Y92.003
    boarding house Y92.049
      bathroom Y92.041
      bedroom Y92.042
      driveway Y92.043
      garage Y92.044
      garden Y92.046
      kitchen Y92.040
      specified NEC Y92.048
      swimming pool Y92.045
      yard Y92.046
    dining room Y92.001
    garden Y92.007
    home Y92.009
    house, single family Y92.019
      bathroom Y92.012
      bedroom Y92.013
      dining room Y92.011
      driveway Y92.014
      garage Y92.015
      garden Y92.017
      kitchen Y92.010
      specified NEC Y92.018
      swimming pool Y92.016
      yard Y92.017
    institutional Y92.10
      children's home —*see* Place of
        occurrence, residence, institutional,
        orphanage
      hospice —*see* Place of occurrence,
        residence, institutional, nursing
        home
      military base Y92.139
        barracks Y92.133
        garage Y92.135
        garden Y92.137
        kitchen Y92.130
        mess hall Y92.131
        specified NEC Y92.138
        swimming pool Y92.136
        yard Y92.137
      nursing home Y92.129
        bathroom Y92.121
        bedroom Y92.122
        driveway Y92.123
        garage Y92.124
        garden Y92.126
        kitchen Y92.120

Place of occurrence *(Continued)*
  residence *(Continued)*
    institutional *(Continued)*
      nursing home *(Continued)*
        specified NEC Y92.128
        swimming pool Y92.125
        yard Y92.126
      orphanage Y92.119
        bathroom Y92.111
        bedroom Y92.112
        driveway Y92.113
        garage Y92.114
        garden Y92.116
        kitchen Y92.110
        specified NEC Y92.118
        swimming pool Y92.115
        yard Y92.116
      prison Y92.149
        bathroom Y92.142
        cell Y92.143
        courtyard Y92.147
        dining room Y92.141
        kitchen Y92.140
        specified NEC Y92.148
        swimming pool Y92.146
      reform school Y92.159
        bathroom Y92.152
        bedroom Y92.153
        dining room Y92.151
        driveway Y92.154
        garage Y92.155
        garden Y92.157
        kitchen Y92.150
        specified NEC Y92.158
        swimming pool Y92.156
        yard Y92.157
      school dormitory Y92.169
        bathroom Y92.162
        bedroom Y92.163
        dining room Y92.161
        kitchen Y92.160
        specified NEC Y92.168
      specified NEC Y92.199
        bathroom Y92.192
        bedroom Y92.193
        dining room Y92.191
        driveway Y92.194
        garage Y92.195
        garden Y92.197
        kitchen Y92.190
        specified NEC Y92.198
        swimming pool Y92.196
        yard Y92.197
    kitchen Y92.000
    mobile home Y92.029
      bathroom Y92.022
      bedroom Y92.023
      dining room Y92.021
      driveway Y92.024
      garage Y92.025
      garden Y92.027
      kitchen Y92.020
      specified NEC Y92.028
      swimming pool Y92.026
      yard Y92.027
    specified place in residence NEC Y92.008
    specified residence type NEC Y92.099
      bathroom Y92.091
      bedroom Y92.092
      driveway Y92.093
      garage Y92.094
      garden Y92.096
      kitchen Y92.090
      specified NEC Y92.098
      swimming pool Y92.095
      yard Y92.096
    restaurant Y92.511
    riding school Y92.39
    river Y92.828
    road Y92.488
    rodeo ring Y92.39

Place of occurrence *(Continued)*
  rugby field Y92.328
  same day surgery center Y92.530
  sand pit Y92.64
  school (private) (public) (state) Y92.219
    college Y92.214
    daycare center Y92.210
    elementary school Y92.211
    high school Y92.213
    kindergarten Y92.211
    middle school Y92.212
    specified NEC Y92.218
    trace school Y92.215
    university Y92.214
    vocational school Y92.215
  sea (shore) Y92.832
  senior citizen center Y92.29
  service area
    airport Y92.520
    bus station Y92.521
    gas station Y92.524
    highway rest stop Y92.523
    railway station Y92.522
  shipyard Y92.62
  shop(commercial) Y92.513
  sidewalk Y92.480
  silo Y92.79
  skating rink (roller) Y92.331
    ice Y92.330
  slaughter house Y92.86
  soccer field Y92.322
  specified place NEC Y92.89
  sports area Y92.39
    athletic
      court Y92.318
        basketball Y92.310
        specified NEC Y92.318
        squash Y92.311
        tennis Y92.312
      field Y92.328
        baseball Y92.320
        cricket ground Y92.328
        football Y92.321
        hockey Y92.328
        soccer Y92.322
        specified NEC Y92.328
    golf course Y92.39
    gymnasium Y92.39
    riding school Y92.39
    skating rink (roller) Y92.331
      ice Y92.330
    stadium Y92.39
    swimming pool Y92.34
  squash court Y92.311
  stadium Y92.39
  steeplechasing course Y92.39
  store Y92.512
  stream Y92.828
  street and highway Y92.410
    bike path Y92.482
    freeway Y92.411
    highway ramp Y92.415
    interstate highway Y92.411
    local residential or business street
      Y92.414
    motorway Y92.411
    parking lot Y92.481
    parkway Y92.412
    sidewalk Y92.480
    specified NEC Y92.488
    state road Y92.413
  subway car Y92.816
  supermarket Y92.512
  swamp Y92.828
  swimming pool (public) Y92.34
    private (at) Y92.095
      boarding house Y92.045
      military base Y92.136
      mobile home Y92.026
      nursing home Y92.125
      orphanage Y92.115

Place of occurrence (Continued)
swimming pool (Continued)
private (Continued)
prison Y92.146
reform school Y92.156
single family residence
Y92.016
synagogue Y92.22
television station Y92.59
tennis court Y92.312
theater Y92.254
trade area Y92.59
bank Y92.510
cafe Y92.511
casino Y92.59
garage Y92.59
hotel Y92.59
market Y92.512
office building Y92.59
radio station Y92.59
restaurant Y92.511
shop Y92.513
shopping mall Y92.59
store Y92.512
supermarket Y92.512
television station Y92.59
warehouse Y92.59
trailer park, residential —see Place of
occurrence, residence, mobile
home
trailer site NOS Y92.89
train Y92.815
station Y92.522
truck Y92.812
tunnel under construction Y92. 69
university Y92.214
urgent (health) care center Y92.532
vehicle (transport) Y92.818
airplane Y92.813
boat Y92.814
bus Y92.811
car Y92.810
specified NEC Y92.818
subway car Y92.816
train Y92.815
truck Y92.812
warehouse Y92.59
water reservoir Y92.89
wilderness area Y92.828
desert Y92.820
forest Y92.821
marsh Y92.828
mountain Y92.828
prairie Y92.828
specified NEC Y92.828
swamp Y92.828
workshop Y92.69
yard, private Y92.096
boarding house Y92.046
mobile home Y92.027
single family house Y92.017

Place of occurrence (Continued)
youth center Y92.29
zoo (zoological garden) Y92.834
Plumbism —see Table of Drugs and
Chemicals, lead ◄▥
Poisoning (accidental) (by) —see also Table of
Drugs and Chemicals ◄▥
by plant, thorns, spines, sharp leaves or other
mechanisms NEC X58
carbon monoxide
generated by
motor vehicle —see Accident, transport
watercraft (in transit) (not in transit)
V93.89
ferry boat V93.81
fishing boat V93.82
jet skis V93.83
liner V93.81
merchant ship V93.80
passenger ship V93.81
powered craft NEC V93.83
caused by injection of poisons into skin by
plant thorns, spines, sharp leaves X58
marine or sea plants (venomous) X58
exhaust gas
generated by
motor vehicle —see Accident, transport
watercraft (in transit) (not in transit)
V93.89
ferry boat V93.81
fishing boat V93.82
jet skis V93.83
liner V93.81
merchant ship V93.80
passenger ship V93.81
powered craft NEC V93.83
fumes or smoke due to
explosion (see also Explosion) W40.9
fire —see Exposure, fire
ignition —see Ignition
gas
in legal intervention —see Legal,
intervention, gas
legal execution —see Legal, intervention,
gas
in war operations —see War operations
legal
execution —see Legal, intervention, gas
intervention
by gas —see Legal, intervention, gas
other specified means —see Legal,
intervention, specified means
NEC
Powder burn (by) (from)
airgun W34.110
BB gun W34.110
firearm NEC W34.19
gas, air or spring-operated gun NEC
W34.118
handgun W32.1
hunting rifle W33.12

Powder burn (Continued)
larger firearm W33.10
specified NEC W33.19
machine gun W33.13
paintball gun W34.111
pellet gun W34.110
shotgun W33.11
Very pistol [flare] W34.19
Premature cessation (of) surgical and medical
care Y66
Privation (food) (water) X58
Procedure (operation)
correct, on wrong side or body part (wrong
side) (wrong site) Y65.53
intended for another patient done on wrong
patient Y65.52
performed on patient not scheduled for
surgery Y65.52
performed on wrong patient Y65.52
wrong, performed on correct patient Y65.51
Prolonged
sitting in transport vehicle —see Travel, by
type of vehicle
stay in
high altitude as cause of anoxia,
barodontalgia, barotitis or hypoxia
W94.11
weightless environment X52
Pulling, excessive —see category Y93
Puncture, puncturing —see also Contact, with,
by type of object or machine
by
plant thorns, spines, sharp leaves or other
mechanisms NEC W60
during medical or surgical treatment as
misadventure —see Misadventure, cut,
by type of procedureIndex to Diseases
and Injuries, Complication(s) ◄▥
Pushed, pushing (accidental) (injury in)
(overexertion) —see also category Y93
by other person (s) (accidental) W51
with fall W03
due to ice or snow W00.0
as, or caused by, a crowd or human
stampede (with fall) W52
before moving object NEC Y02.8
motor vehicle Y02.0
subway train Y02.1
train Y02.1
from
high place NEC
in accidental circumstances W17.89
stated as
intentional, homicide (attempt) Y01
undetermined whether accidental
or intentional Y30
transport vehicle NEC (see also Accident,
transport) V89.9
stated as
intentional, homicide (attempt)
Y08.89

◄ New   ◄▥ Revised   deleted Deleted

R

Radiation (exposure to)
arc lamps W89.0
atomic power plant (malfunction) NEC W88.1
complication of or abnormal reaction to medical radiotherapy Y84.2
electromagnetic, ionizing W88.0
gamma rays W88.1
in
war operations (from or following nuclear explosion) —*see also* War operations
inadvertent exposure of patient (receiving test or therapy) Y63.3
infrared (heaters and lamps) W90.1
excessive heat from W92
ionized, ionizing (particles, artificially accelerated)
radioisotopes W88.1
specified NEC W88.8
x-rays W88.0
isotopes, radioactive —*see* Radiation, radioactive isotopes
laser (s) W90.2
in war operations —*see* War operations
misadventure in medical care Y63.2
light sources (man-made visible and ultraviolet) W89.9
natural X32
specified NEC W89.8
tanning bed W89.1
welding light W89.0
man-made visible light W89.9
specified NEC W89.8
tanning bed W89.1
welding light W89.0
microwave W90.8
misadventure in medical or surgical procedure Y63.2

Radiation (*Continued*)
natural NEC X39.08
radon X39.01
overdose (in medical or surgical procedure) Y63.2
radar W90.0
radioactive isotopes (any) W88.1
atomic power plant malfunction W88.1
misadventure in medical or surgical treatment Y63.2
radiofrequency W90.0
radium NEC W88.1
sun X32
ultraviolet (light) (man-made) W89.9
natural X32
specified NEC W89.8
tanning bed W89.1
welding light W89.0
welding arc, torch, or light W89.0
excessive heat from W92
x-rays (hard) (soft) W88.0
Range disease W94.11
Rape (attempted) T74.2-
Rat bite W53.11
Reaction, abnormal to medical procedure (*see also* Complication of or following, by type of procedure) Y84.9
with misadventure —*see* Misadventure
biologicals —*see* Table of ◁Drugs and ◁Chemicals◁▥
drugs —*see* Table of ◁Drugs and ◁Chemicals◁▥
vaccine —*see* Table of ◁Drugs and ◁Chemicals◁▥
Recoil
airgun W34.110
BB gun W34.110
firearm NEC W34.19
gas, air or spring-operated gun NEC W34.118

Recoil (*Continued*)
handgun W32.1
hunting rifle W33.12
larger firearm W33.10
specified NEC W33.19
machine gun W33.13
paintball gun W34.111
pellet W34.110
shotgun W33.11
Very pistol [flare] W34.19
Reduction in
atmospheric pressure —*see* Air, pressure, change
Rock falling on or hitting (accidentally) (person) W20.8
in cave-in W20.0
Run over (accidentally) (by)
animal (not being ridden) NEC W55.89
machinery —*see* Contact, with, by specified type of machine
transport vehicle NEC (*see also* Accident, transport) V09.9
intentional homicide (attempt) Y03.0
motor NEC V09.20
intentional homicide (attempt) Y03.0
Running
before moving object X81.8
motor vehicle X81.0
Running off, away
animal (being ridden) (*see also* Accident, transport) V80.918
not being ridden W55.89
animal-drawn vehicle NEC (*see also* Accident, transport) V80.928
highway, road(way), street
transport vehicle NEC (*see also* Accident, transport) V89.9
Rupture pressurized devices —*see* Explosion, by type of device

S

Saturnism —*see* Table of ~~d~~Drugs and ~~c~~Chemicals, lead ◀▥▥
Scald, scalding (accidental) (by) (from) (in) X19
  air (hot) X14.1
  gases (hot) X14.1
  homicide (attempt) —*see* Assault, burning, hot object
  inflicted by other person
    stated as intentional, homicide (attempt) — *see* Assault, burning, hot object
  liquid (boiling) (hot) NEC X12
    stated as undetermined whether accidental or intentional Y27.2
    suicide (attempt) X77.2
  local application of externally applied substance in medical or surgical care Y63.5
  metal (molten) (liquid) (hot) NEC X18
  self-inflicted X77.9
  stated as undetermined whether accidental or intentional Y27.8
  steam X13.1
    assault X98.0
    stated as undetermined whether accidental or intentional Y27.0
    suicide (attempt) X77.0
  suicide (attempt) X77.9
  vapor (hot) X13.1
    assault X98.0
    stated as undetermined whether accidental or intentional Y27.0
    suicide (attempt) X77.0
Scratched by
  cat W55.03
  person (s) (accidentally) W50.4
    with intent to injure or kill Y04.0
    as, or caused by, a crowd or human stampede (with fall) W52
    assault Y04.0
    homicide (attempt) Y04.0
    in
      fight Y04.0
      legal intervention
        injuring
          bystander Y35.892
          law enforcement personnel Y35.891
          suspect Y35.893
Seasickness T75.3
Self-harm NEC —*see also* External cause by type, undetermined whether accidental or intentional
  intentional —*see* Suicide
  poisoning NEC —*see* Table of drugs and biologicals, accident
Self-inflicted (injury) NEC —*see also* External cause by type, undetermined whether accidental or intentional
  intentional —*see* Suicide
  poisoning NEC —*see* Table of drugs and biologicals, accident
Sequelae (of)
  accident NEC —*see* W00-X58 with 7th character S
  assault (homicidal) (any means) —*see* X92-Y08 with 7th character S
  homicide, attempt (any means) —*see* X92-Y08 with 7th character S
  injury undetermined whether accidentally or purposely inflicted —*see* Y21-Y33 with 7th character S
  intentional self-harm (classifiable to X71-X83) —*see* X71-X83 with 7th character S
  legal intervention (*see* with 7th character S Y35)
  motor vehicle accident —*see* V00-V99 with 7th character S
  suicide, attempt (any means) —*see* X71-X83 with 7th character S

Sequelae (*Continued*)
  transport accident —*see* V00-V99 with 7th character S
  war operations —*see* War operations
Shock
  electric —*see* Exposure, electric current
  from electric appliance (any) (faulty) W86.8
    domestic W86.0
    suicide (attempt) X83.1
Shooting, shot (accidental (ly)) —*see also* Discharge, firearm, by type
  herself or himself —*see* Discharge, firearm by type, self-inflicted
  homicide (attempt) —*see* Discharge, firearm by type, homicide
  in war operations —*see* War operations
  inflicted by other person —*see* Discharge, firearm by type, homicide
    accidental —*see* Discharge, firearm, by type of firearm
  legal
    execution —*see* Legal, intervention, firearm
    intervention —*see* Legal, intervention, firearm
  self-inflicted —*see* Discharge, firearm by type, suicide
    accidental —*see* Discharge, firearm, by type of firearm
  suicide (attempt) —*see* Discharge, firearm by type, suicide
Shoving (accidentally) **by other person** —*see* Pushe~~ding~~, by other person ◀▥▥
Sickness
  alpine W94.11
  motion —*see* Motion
  mountain W94.11
Sinking (accidental)
  watercraft (causing drowning, submersion) —*see also* Drowning, due to, accident to, watercraft, sinking
    causing injury except drowning or submersion —*see* Accident, watercraft, causing, injury NEC
Siriasis X32
Slashed wrists —*see* Cut, self-inflicted
Slipping (accidental) (on same level) (with fall) W01.0
  without fall W18.40
    due to
      specified NEC W18.49
      stepping from one level to another W18.43
      stepping into hole or opening W18.42
      stepping on object W18.41
    on
      ice W00.0
        with skates —*see* Accident, transport, pedestrian, conveyance
      mud W01.0
      oil W01.0
      snow W00.0
        with skis —*see* Accident, transport, pedestrian, conveyance
      surface (slippery) (wet) NEC W01.0
Sliver, wood, contact with W45.8
Smoldering (due to fire) —*see* Exposure, fire
Sodomy (attempted) by force T74.2-
Sound waves (causing injury) W42.9
  supersonic W42.0
Splinter, contact with W45.8
Stab, stabbing —*see* Cut
Starvation X58
Status of external cause Y99.9
  child assisting in compensated work for family Y99.8
  civilian activity done for financial or other compensation Y99.0
  civilian activity done for income or pay Y99.0
  family member assisting in compensated work for other family member Y99.8
  hobby not done for income Y99.8

Status of external cause (*Continued*)
  leisure activity Y99.8
  military activity Y99.1
  off-duty activity of military personnel Y99.8
  recreation or sport not for income or while a student Y99.8
  specified NEC Y99.8
  student activity Y99.8
  volunteer activity Y99.2
Stepped on
  by
    animal (not being ridden) NEC W55.89
    crowd or human stampede W52
    person W50.0
Stepping on
  object W22.8
    with fall W18.31
    sports equipment W21.9
    stationary W22.09
      sports equipment W21.89
  person W51
    by crowd or human stampede W52
  sports equipment W21.9
Sting
  arthropod, nonvenomous W57
  insect, nonvenomous W57
Storm (cataclysmic) —*see* Forces of nature, cataclysmic storm
Straining, excessive —*see* category Y93
Strangling —*see* Strangulation
Strangulation (accidental) —*see* category T71
Strenuous movements —*see* category Y93
Striking against
  airbag (automobile) W22.10
    driver side W22.11
    front passenger side W22.12
    specified NEC W22.19
  bottom when
    diving or jumping into water (in) W16.822
      causing drowning W16.821
      from boat W16.722
        causing drowning W16.721
      natural body W16.622
        causing drowning W16.821
      swimming pool W16.522
        causing drowning W16.521
    falling into water (in) W16.322
      causing drowning W16.321
      fountain —*see* Striking against, bottom when, falling into water, specified NEC
      natural body W16.122
        causing drowning W16.121
      reservoir —*see* Striking against, bottom when, falling into water, specified NEC
      specified NEC W16.322
        causing drowning W16.321
      swimming pool W16.022
        causing drowning W16.021
  diving board (swimming-pool) W21.4
  object W22.8
    with
      drowning or submersion —*see* Drowning
      fall —*see* Fall, due to, bumping against, object
      caused by crowd or human stampede (with fall) W52
    furniture W22.03
    lamppost W22.02
    sports equipment W21.9
    stationary W22.09
      sports equipment W21.89
    wall W22.01
  person (s) W51
    with fall W03
      due to ice or snow W00.0
    as, or caused by, a crowd or human stampede (with fall) W52

◀ New   ◀▥▥ Revised   ~~deleted~~ Deleted

Striking against *(Continued)*
  person *(Continued)*
    assault Y04.2
    homicide (attempt) Y04.2
  sports equipment W21.9
  wall (when) W22.01
    diving or jumping into water (in) W16.832
      causing drowning W16.831
      swimming pool W16.532
        causing drowning W16.531
    falling into water (in) W16.332
      causing drowning W16.331
      fountain —*see* Striking against, wall
        when, falling into water, specified
        NEC
      natural body W16.132
        causing drowning W16.131
      reservoir —*see* Striking against, wall
        when, falling into water, specified
        NEC
      specified NEC W16.332
        causing drowning W16.331
      swimming pool W16.032
        causing drowning W16.031
    swimming pool (when) W22.042
      causing drowning W22.041
      diving or jumping into water W16.532
        causing drowning W16.531
      falling into water W16.032
        causing drowning W16.031
Struck (accidentally) by
  airbag (automobile) W22.10
    driver side W22.11
    front passenger side W22.12
    specified NEC W22.19
  alligator W58.02
  animal (not being ridden) NEC W55.89
  avalanche —*see* Landslide
  ball (hit) (thrown) W21.00
    assault Y08.09
    baseball W21.03
    basketball W21.05
    football W21.01
    golf ball W21.04
    football W21.01
    soccer W21.02
    softball W21.07
    specified NEC W21.09
    volleyball W21.06
  bat or racquet
    baseball bat W21.11
      assault Y08.02
    golf club W21.13
      assault Y08.09
    specified NEC W21.19
      assault Y08.09
    tennis racquet W21.12
      assault Y08.09
  bullet —*see also* Discharge, firearm by type
    in war operations —*see* War operations
  crocodile W58.12
  dog W54.1
  flare, Very pistol —*see* Discharge, firearm
    NEC
  hailstones X39.8
  hockey (ice)
    field
      puck W21.221
      stick W21.211
    puck W21.220
    stick W21.210
      assault Y08.01
  landslide —*see* Landslide
  law-enforcement agent (on duty) —*see* Legal,
    intervention, manhandling
    with blunt object —*see* Legal, intervention,
      blunt object
  lightning —*see* subcategory T75.0
    causing fire —*see* Exposure, fire
  machine —*see* Contact, with, by type of
    machine

Struck by *(Continued)*
  mammal NEC W55.89
    marine W56.32
  marine animal W56.82
  missile
    firearm —*see* Discharge, firearm by type
    in war operations —*see* War operations,
      missile
  object W22.8
    blunt W22.8
      assault Y00
      suicide (attempt) X79
      undetermined whether accidental or
        intentional Y29
    falling W20.8
      from, in, on
        building W20.1
          burning (uncontrolled fire) X00.4
        cataclysmic
          earth surface movement NEC —*see*
            Landslide
          storm —*see* Forces of nature,
            cataclysmic storm
        cave-in W20.0
        earthquake X34
        machine (in operation) —*see* Contact,
          with, by type of machine
        structure W20.1
          burning X00.4
        transport vehicle (in motion) —*see*
          Accident, transport, by type of
          vehicle
        watercraft V93.49
          due to
            accident to craft V91.39
              powered craft V91.33
                ferry boat V91.31
                fishing boat V91.32
                jetskis V91.33
                liner V91.31
                merchant ship V91.30
                passenger ship V91.31
             unpowered craft V91.38
                canoe V91.35
                inflatable V91.36
                kayak V91.35
                sailboat V91.34
                surf-board V91.38
                windsurfer V91.38
            powered craft V93.43
              ferry boat V93.41
              fishing boat V93.42
              jetskis V93.43
              liner V93.41
              merchant ship V93.40
              passenger ship V93.41
            unpowered craft V93.48
              sailboat V93.44
              surf-board V93.48
              windsurfer V93.48
    moving NEC W20.8
    projected W20.8
      assault Y00
      in sports W21.9
        assault Y08.09
        ball W21.00
          baseball W21.03
          basketball W21.05
          football W21.01
          golf ball W21.04
          soccer W21.02
          softball W21.07
          specified NEC W21.09
          volleyball W21.06
        bat or racquet
          baseball bat W21.11
            assault Y08.02
          golf club W21.13
            assault Y08.09-
          specified NEC W21.19
            assault Y08.09

Struck by *(Continued)*
  object *(Continued)*
    projected *(Continued)*
      in sports *(Continued)*
        bat or racquet *(Continued)*
          tennis racquet W21.12
            assault Y08.09
        hockey (ice)
          field
            puck W21.221
            stick W21.211
          puck W21.220
          stick W21.210
            assault Y08.01
        specified NEC W21.89
    set in motion by explosion —*see*
      Explosion
    thrown W20.8
      assault Y00
      in sports W21.9
        assault Y08.09
        ball W21.00
          baseball W21.03
          basketball W21.05
          football W21.01
          golf ball W21.04
          soccer W21.02
          soft ball W21.07
          specified NEC W21.09
          volleyball W21.06
        bat or racquet
          baseball bat W21.11
            assault Y08.02
          golf club W21.13
            assault Y08.09
          specified NEC W21.19
            assault Y08.09
          tennis racquet W21.12
            assault Y08.09
        hockey (ice)
          field
            puck W21.221
            stick W21.211
          puck W21.220
          stick W21.210
            assault Y08.01
        specified NEC W21.89
  other person (s) W50.0
    with
      blunt object W22.8
        intentional, homicide (attempt) Y00
        sports equipment W21.9
        undetermined whether accidental or
          intentional Y29
      fall W03
        due to ice or snow W00.0
      as, or caused by, a crowd or human
        stampede (with fall) W52
    assault Y04.2
    homicide (attempt) Y04.2
    in legal intervention
      injuring
        bystander Y35.812
        law enforcement personnel Y35.811
        suspect Y35.813
    sports equipment W21.9
  police (on duty) —*see* Legal, intervention,
    manhandling
    with blunt object —*see* Legal, intervention,
      blunt object
  sports equipment W21.9
    assault Y08.09
    ball W21.00
      baseball W21.03
      basketball W21.05
      football W21.01
      golf ball W21.04
      soccer W21.02
      soft ball W21.07
      specified NEC W21.09
      volleyball W21.06

Struck by *(Continued)*
  sports equipment *(Continued)*
    bat or racquet
      baseball bat W21.11
        assault Y08.02
      golf club W21.13
        assault Y08.09
      specified NEC W21.19
      tennis racquet W21.12
        assault Y08.09
    cleats (shoe) W21.31
    foot wear NEC W21.39
    football helmet W21.81
    hockey (ice)
      field
        puck W21.221
        stick W21.211
      puck W21.220
      stick W21.210
        assault Y08.01
    skate blades W21.32
    specified NEC W21.89
      assault Y08.09
  thunderbolt —*see* subcategory
    T75.0
    causing fire —*see* Exposure, fire
  transport vehicle NEC *(see also* Accident,
    transport) V09.9
    intentional, homicide (attempt) Y03.0
    motor NEC *(see also* Accident, transport)
      V09.20
      homicide Y03.0
  vehicle (transport) NEC —*see* Accident,
    transport, by type of vehicle
    stationary (falling from jack,
      hydraulic lift, ramp)
      W20.8
Stumbling
  without fall W18.40
    due to
      specified NEC W18.49
      stepping from one level to another
        W18.43
      stepping into hole or opening
        W18.42
      stepping on object W18.41
  over
    animal NEC W01.0
      with fall W18.09
    carpet, rug or (small) object
      W22.8
      with fall W18.09
    person W51
      with fall W03
        due to ice or snow W00.0
Submersion (accidental) —*see* Drowning

Suffocation (accidental) (by external means) (by
  pressure) (mechanical) —*see also* category
  T71
  due to, by
    avalanche —*see* Landslide
    explosion —*see* Explosion
    fire —*see* Exposure, fire
    food, any type (aspiration) (ingestion)
      (inhalation) —*see* categories T17 and
      T18
    ignition —*see* Ignition
    landslide —*see* Landslide
    machine (ry) —*see* Contact, with, by type
      of machine
    vomitus (aspiration) (inhalation)
      T17.81-
  in
    burning building X00.8
Suicide, suicidal (attempted) (by) X83.8
  blunt object X79
  burning, burns X76
    hot object X77.9
      fluid NEC X77.2
      household appliance X77.3
      specified NEC X77.8
      steam X77.0
      tap water X77.1
      vapors X77.0
  caustic substance —*see* Table of ᵈDrugs and
    ᶜChemicals ◄▥
  cold, extreme X83.2
  collision of motor vehicle with
    motor vehicle X82.0
    specified NEC X82.8
    train X82.1
    tree X82.2
  crashing of aircraft X83.0
  cut (any part of body) X78.9
  cutting or piercing instrument X78.9
    dagger X78.2
    glass X78.0
    knife X78.1
    specified NEC X78.8
    sword X78.2
  drowning (in) X71.9
    bathtub X71.0
    natural water X71.3
    specified NEC X71.8
    swimming pool X71.1
      following fall X71.2
  electrocution X83.1
  explosive (s) (material) X75
  fire, flames X76
  firearm X74.9
    airgun X74.01
    handgun X72

Suicide, suicidal *(Continued)*
  firearm *(Continued)*
    hunting rifle X73.1
    larger X73.9
      specified NEC X73.8
    machine gun X73.2
    shotgun X73.0
    specified NEC X74.8
  hanging X83.8
  hot object —*see* Suicide, burning, hot object
  jumping
    before moving object X81.8
      motor vehicle X81.0
      subway train X81.1
      train X81.1
    from high place X80
  late effect of attempt —*see* X71-X83 with 7th
    character S
  lying before moving object, train, vehicle X81.8
  poisoning —*see* Table of ᵈDrugs and
    ᶜChemicals ◄▥
  puncture (any part of body) —*see* Suicide,
    cutting or piercing instrument
  scald —*see* Suicide, burning, hot object
  sequelae of attempt —*see* X71-X83 with 7th
    character S
  sharp object (any) —*see* Suicide, cutting or
    piercing instrument
  shooting —*see* Suicide, firearm
  specified means NEC X83.8
  stab (any part of body) —*see* Suicide, cutting
    or piercing instrument
  steam, hot vapors X77.0
  strangulation X83.8
  submersion —*see* Suicide, drowning
  suffocation X83.8
  wound NEC X83.8
Sunstroke X32
Supersonic waves (causing injury) W42.0
Surgical procedure, complication of (delayed
  or as an abnormal reaction without
  mention of misadventure) —*see also*
  Complication of or following, by type of
  procedure
  due to or as a result of misadventure —*see*
    Misadventure
Swallowed, swallowing
  foreign body —*see* Foreign body, alimentary
    canal
  poison —*see* Table of ᵈDrugs and
    ᶜChemicals ◄▥
  substance
    caustic or corrosive —*see* Table of ᵈDrugs
      and ᶜChemicals ◄▥
    poisonous —*see* Table of ᵈDrugs and
      ᶜChemicals ◄▥

◄ New   ◄▥ Revised   ~~deleted~~ Deleted

T

Tackle in sport W03
Terrorism (involving) Y38.80
  biological weapons Y38.6X-
  chemical weapons Y38.7X-
  conflagration Y38.3X-
  drowning and submersion Y38.89-
  explosion Y38.2X-
    destruction of aircraft Y38.1X-
    marine weapons Y38.0X-
  fire Y38.3X-
  firearms Y38.4X-
  hot substances Y38.5X-
  lasers Y38.89-
  nuclear weapons Y38.5X-
  piercing or stabbing instruments
    Y38.89-
  secondary effects Y38.9X-
  specified method NEC Y38.89-
  suicide bomber Y38.81-
Thirst X58
Threat to breathing
  aspiration —*see* Aspiration
  due to cave-in, falling earth or substance
    NEC —*see* category T71
Thrown (accidentally)
  against part (any) of or object in transport
    vehicle (in motion) NEC (*see also*
    Accident, transport)

Thrown (*Continued*)
  from
    high place, homicide (attempt) Y01
    machinery —*see* Contact, with, by type of
      machine
    transport vehicle NEC (*see also* Accident,
      transport) V89.9
  off —*see* Thrown, from
Thunderbolt —*see* subcategory T75.0
  causing fire —*see* Exposure, fire
Tidal wave (any injury) NEC —*see* Forces of
  nature, tidal wave
Took
  overdose (drug) —*see* Table of ◄Drugs and
    ◄Chemicals ◄▥
  poison —*see* Table of ◄Drugs and
    ◄Chemicals ◄▥
Tornado (any injury) X37.1
Torrential rain (any injury) X37.8
Torture X58
Trampled by animal NEC W55.89
Trapped (accidentally)
  between objects (moving) (stationary and
    moving) —*see* Caught
  by part (any) of
    motorcycle V29.88
    pedal cycle V19.88
    transport vehicle NEC (*see also* Accident,
      transport) V89.9
Travel (effects) (sickness) T75.3

Tree falling on or hitting (accidentally)
  (person) W20.8
Tripping
  without fall W18.40
    due to
      specified NEC W18.49
      stepping from one level to another
        W18.43
      stepping into hole or opening
        W18.42
      stepping on object W18.41
    over
      animal W01.0
        with fall W01.0
      carpet, rug or (small) object W22.8
        with fall W18.09
      person W51
        with fall W03
    due to ice or snow W00.0
Twisted by person (s) (accidentally) W50.2
  with intent to injure or kill Y04.0
  as, or caused by, a crowd or human stampede
    (with fall) W52
  assault Y04.0
  homicide (attempt) Y04.0
  in
    fight Y04.0
    legal intervention —*see* Legal, intervention,
      manhandling
Twisting, excessive —*see* category Y93

U

Underdosing of necessary drugs, medicaments
  or biological substances Y63.6
Undetermined intent (contact) (exposure)
  automobile collision Y32
  blunt object Y29
  drowning (submersion) (in) Y21.9
    bathtub Y21.0
      after fall Y21.1
    natural water (lake) (ocean) (pond) (river)
      (stream) Y21.4
    specified place NEC Y21.8
    swimming pool Y21.2
      after fall Y21.3
  explosive material Y25
  fall, jump or push from high place Y30
  falling, lying or running before moving object
    Y31
  fire Y26

Undetermined intent (*Continued*)
  firearm discharge Y24.9
    airgun (BB) (pellet) Y24.0
    handgun (pistol) (revolver) Y22
    hunting rifle Y23.1
    larger Y23.9
      hunting rifle Y23.1
      machine gun Y23.3
      military Y23.2
      shotgun Y23.0
      specified type NEC Y23.8
    machine gun Y23.3
    military Y23.2
    shotgun Y23.0
    specified type NEC Y24.8
    Very pistol Y24.8
  hot object Y27.9
    fluid NEC Y27.2
    household appliance Y27.3
    specified object NEC Y27.8

Undetermined intent (*Continued*)
  hot object (*Continued*)
    steam Y27.0
    tap water Y27.1
    vapor Y27.0
  jump, fall or push from high place Y30
  lying, falling or running before moving object
    Y31
  motor vehicle crash Y32
  push, fall or jump from high place Y30
  running, falling or lying before moving object
    Y31
  sharp object Y28.9
    dagger Y28.2
    glass Y28.0
    knife Y28.1
    specified object NEC Y28.8
    sword Y28.2
  smoke Y26
  specified event NEC Y33

V

Vibration (causing injury) W49.9
Victim (of)
  avalanche —*see* Landslide
  earth movements NEC —*see* Forces of nature,
    earth movement
  earthquake X34

Victim (*Continued*)
  flood —*see* Flood
  landslide —*see* Landslide
  lightning —*see* subcategory T75.0
    causing fire —*see* Exposure, fire
  storm (cataclysmic) NEC —*see* Forces of
    nature, cataclysmic storm
  volcanic eruption X35

Volcanic eruption (any injury) X35
Vomitus, gastric contents in air passages
  (with asphyxia, obstruction or
  suffocation) T17.81-

W

Walked into stationary object (any) W22.09
  furniture W22.03
  lamppost W22.02
  wall W22.01
War operations (injuries to military personnel
    and civilians during war, civil insurrection
    and peacekeeping missions) (by) (from)
    (involving) Y36.90-
  after cessation of hostilities Y36.89-
    explosion (of)
      bomb placed during war operations
        Y36.82-
      mine placed during war operations
        Y36.81-
    specified NEC Y36.88-
  air blast Y36.20-
  aircraft
    destruction —*see* War operations,
      destruction of aircraft
  airway restriction —*see* War operations,
    restriction of airways
  asphyxiation —*see* War operations, restriction
    of airways
  biological weapons Y36.6X-
  blast Y36.20-
  blast fragments Y36.20-
  blast wave Y36.20-
  blast wind Y36.20-
  bomb Y36.20-
    dirty Y36.50-
    gasoline Y36.31-
    incendiary Y36.31-
    petrol Y36.31-
  bullet Y36.43-
    incendiary Y36.32-
    rubber Y36.41-
  chemical weapons Y36.7X-
  combat
    hand to hand (unarmed) combat Y36.44-
    using blunt or piercing object Y36.45-
  conflagration —*see* War operations, fire
  conventional warfare NEC Y36.49-
  depth-charge Y36.01-
  destruction of aircraft Y36.10-
    due to
      air to air missile Y36.11-
      collision with other aircraft Y36.12-
      detonation (accidental) of onboard
        munitions and explosives Y36.14-
      enemy fire or explosives Y36.11-
      explosive placed on aircraft Y36.11-
      onboard fire Y36.13-
      rocket propelled grenade [RPG] Y36.11-
      small arms fire Y36.11-
      surface to air missile Y36.11-
      specified NEC Y36.19-
  detonation (accidental) of
    onboard marine weapons Y36.05-
    own munitions or munitions launch device
      Y36.24-

War operations (*Continued*)
  dirty bomb Y36.50-
  explosion (of) Y36.20-
    aerial bomb Y36.21-
    after cessation of hostilities
      bomb placed during war operations
        Y36.82-
      mine placed during war operations
        Y36.81-
    bomb NOS (*see also* War operations,
      bomb (s)) Y36.20-
    fragments Y36.20-
    grenade Y36.29-
    guided missile Y36.22-
    improvised explosive device [IED]
      (person-borne) (roadside)
      (vehicle-borne) Y36.23-
    land mine Y36.29-
    marine mine (at sea) (in harbor)
      Y36.02-
    marine weapon Y36.00-
      specified NEC Y36.09-
    own munitions or munitions launch
      device (accidental) Y36.24-
    sea-based artillery shell Y36.03-
    specified NEC Y36.29-
    torpedo Y36.04-
  fire Y36.30-
    specified NEC Y36.39-
  firearms
    discharge Y36.43-
    pellets Y36.42-
  flamethrower Y36.33-
  fragments (from) (of)
    improvised explosive device [IED]
      (person-borne) (roadside)
      (vehicle-borne) Y36.26-
    munitions Y36.25-
    specified NEC Y36.29-
    weapons Y36.27-
  friendly fire Y36.92
  hand to hand (unarmed) combat
    Y36.44-
  hot substances —*see* War operations,
    fire
  incendiary bullet Y36.32-
  nuclear weapon (effects of) Y36.50-
    acute radiation exposure Y36.54-
    blast pressure Y36.51-
    direct blast Y36.51-
    direct heat Y36.53-
    fallout exposure Y36.54-
    fireball Y36.53-
    indirect blast (struck or crushed by blast
      debris) (being thrown by blast)
      Y36.52-
    ionizing radiation (immediate exposure)
      Y36.54-
    nuclear radiation Y36.54-
    radiation
      ionizing (immediate exposure)
        Y36.54-

War operations (*Continued*)
  nuclear weapon (*Continued*)
    radiation (*Continued*)
      nuclear Y36.54-
      thermal Y36.53-
    secondary effects Y36.54-
    specified NEC Y36.59-
    thermal radiation Y36.53-
  restriction of air (airway)
    intentional Y36.46-
    unintentional Y36.47-
  rubber bullets Y36.41-
  shrapnel NOS Y36.29-
  suffocation —*see* War operations, restriction
    of airways
  unconventional warfare NEC Y36.7X-
  underwater blast NOS Y36.00-
  warfare
    conventional NEC Y36.49-
    unconventional NEC Y36.7X-
  weapon of mass destruction [WMD] Y36.91
  weapons
    biological weapons Y36.6X-
    chemical Y36.7X-
    nuclear (effects of) Y36.50-
      acute radiation exposure Y36.54-
      blast pressure Y36.51-
      direct blast Y36.51-
      direct heat Y36.53-
      fallout exposure Y36.54-
      fireball Y36.53-
      indirect blast (struck or crushed by blast
        debris) (being thrown by blast)
        Y36.52-
      radiation
        ionizing (immediate exposure) Y36.54-
        nuclear Y36.54-
        thermal Y36.53-
      secondary effects Y36.54-
      specified NEC Y36.59-
  of mass destruction [WMD] Y36.91-
Washed
  away by flood —*see* Flood
  off road by storm (transport vehicle) —*see*
    Forces of nature, cataclysmic storm
Weather exposure NEC —*see* Forces of nature
Weightlessness (causing injury) (effects of) (in
    spacecraft, real or simulated) X52
Work related condition Y99.0
Wound (accidental) NEC (*see also* Injury) X58
  battle (*see also* War operations) Y36.90
  gunshot —*see* Discharge, firearm by type
Wreck transport vehicle NEC (*see also* Accident,
    transport) V89.9
Wrong
  device implanted into correct surgical site
    Y65.51
  fluid in infusion Y65.1
  patient, procedure performed on Y65.52
  procedure (operation) on correct patient
    Y65.51

Instructional Notations

Includes:

The word 'Includes' appears immediately under certain categories to further define, or give examples of, the content of the category.

Excludes Notes

The ICD-10-CM has two types of excludes notes. Each note has a different definition for use but they are both similar in that they indicate that codes excluded from each other are independent of each other.

Excludes1

A type 1 Excludes note is a pure excludes. It means 'NOT CODED HERE!' An Excludes1 note indicates that the code excluded should never be used at the same time as the code above the Excludes1 note. An Excludes1 is used when two conditions cannot occur together, such as a congenital form versus an acquired form of the same condition.

Excludes2

A type 2 excludes note represents 'Not included here.' An excludes2 note indicates that the condition excluded is not part of the condition it is excluded from but a patient may have both conditions at the same time. When an Excludes2 note appears under a code, it is acceptable to use both the code and the excluded code together.

Code First/Use Additional Code notes (etiology/manifestation paired codes)

Certain conditions have both an underlying etiology and multiple body system manifestations due to the underlying etiology. For such conditions the ICD-10-CM has a coding convention that requires the underlying condition be sequenced first followed by the manifestation. Wherever such a combination exists there is a 'use additional code' note at the etiology code, and a 'code first' note at the manifestation code. These instructional notes indicate the proper sequencing order of the codes, etiology followed by manifestation.

In most cases the manifestation codes will have in the code title, 'in diseases classified elsewhere.' Codes with this title are a component of the etiology/ manifestation convention. The code title indicates that it is a manifestation code. 'In diseases classified elsewhere' codes are never permitted to be used as first listed or principal diagnosis codes. They must be used in conjunction with an underlying condition code and they must be listed following the underlying condition.

Code Also

A code also note instructs that 2 codes may be required to fully describe a condition but the sequencing of the two codes is discretionary, depending on the severity of the conditions and the reason for the encounter.

7th characters and placeholder X

For codes less than 6 characters that require a 7th character a placeholder X should be assigned for all characters less than 6. The 7th character must always be the 7th character of a code.

CHAPTER 1

CERTAIN INFECTIOUS AND PARASITIC DISEASES (A00-B99)

| Includes | diseases generally recognized as communicable or transmissible |

Use additional code to identify resistance to antimicrobial drugs (Z16.-) ◀▥

| Excludes1 | certain localized infections - see body system-related chapters |

~~infectious and parasitic diseases complicating pregnancy, childbirth and the puerperium (O98.-)~~

~~influenza and other acute respiratory infections (J00-J22)~~

| Excludes2 | carrier or suspected carrier of infectious disease (Z22.-) |

infectious and parasitic diseases complicating pregnancy, childbirth and the puerperium (O98.-) ◀

infectious and parasitic diseases specific to the perinatal period (P35-P39)

influenza and other acute respiratory infections (J00-J22) ◀

This chapter contains the following blocks:

A00-A09	Intestinal infectious diseases
A15-A19	Tuberculosis
A20-A28	Certain zoonotic bacterial diseases
A30-A49	Other bacterial diseases
A50-A64	Infections with a predominantly sexual mode of transmission
A65-A69	Other spirochetal diseases
A70-A74	Other diseases caused by chlamydiae
A75-A79	Rickettsioses
A80-A89	Viral and prion infections of the central nervous system
A90-A99	Arthropod-borne viral fevers and viral hemorrhagic fevers
B00-B09	Viral infections characterized by skin and mucous membrane lesions
B10	Other human herpesviruses
B15-B19	Viral hepatitis
B20	Human immunodeficiency virus [HIV] disease
B25-B34	Other viral diseases
B35-B49	Mycoses
B50-B64	Protozoal diseases
B65-B83	Helminthiases
B85-B89	Pediculosis, acariasis and other infestations
B90-B94	Sequelae of infectious and parasitic diseases
B95-B97	Bacterial and viral infectious agents
B99	Other infectious diseases

INTESTINAL INFECTIOUS DISEASES (A00-A09)

● **A00 Cholera**
A serious, often deadly, infectious disease of the small intestine
(Ex) For category A00 CC codes: A00.0-A00.9

  A00.0 Cholera due to Vibrio cholerae 01, biovar cholerae 🅦
    Classical cholera

  A00.1 Cholera due to Vibrio cholerae 01, biovar eltor 🅦
    Cholera eltor

  A00.9 Cholera, unspecified 🅦

● **A01 Typhoid and paratyphoid fevers**
Caused by Salmonella typhi and Salmonella paratyphi A, B, and C bacteria
(Ex) For category A01 CC codes: A01.00-A01.4

  ● **A01.0 Typhoid fever**
    Infection due to Salmonella typhi

    A01.00 Typhoid fever, unspecified 🅦

    A01.01 Typhoid meningitis 🅦

    A01.02 Typhoid fever with heart involvement 🅦
      Typhoid endocarditis
      Typhoid myocarditis

    A01.03 Typhoid pneumonia 🅦

    A01.04 Typhoid arthritis 🅦

    A01.05 Typhoid osteomyelitis 🅦

    A01.09 Typhoid fever with other complications 🅦

  A01.1 Paratyphoid fever A 🅦

  A01.2 Paratyphoid fever B 🅦

  A01.3 Paratyphoid fever C 🅦

  A01.4 Paratyphoid fever, unspecified 🅦
    Infection due to Salmonella paratyphi NOS

● **A02 Other salmonella infections**

| Includes | infection or foodborne intoxication due to any Salmonella species other than S. typhi and S. paratyphi |

  A02.0 Salmonella enteritis 🅦
    Salmonellosis
    (Ex) A01.00-A01.09, A01.4-A02.0, A03.9-A05.2, A07.4, A08.0-A09, A48.51-A48.52, K30, K52.1-K52.2, K52.82-K52.9, K58.0-K58.9, K65.0, K65.2, K65.8, K68.12-K68.9, P76.8-P77.9, P78.1, P78.3-P78.89

  A02.1 Salmonella sepsis 🅦
    (Ex) A02.1, A20.7, A22.7, A26.7, A32.7, A39.2-A39.4, A40.0-A40.1, A40.8-A41.9, A42.7, A48.2-A48.4, A48.8-A49.9, A54.86, B00.7, B37.7, B92, B94.2-B96.89, P36.0-P36.9, P39.2, P39.4-P39.9, R65.10-R65.20, Z16.10-Z16.39

◀ New   ◀▥ Revised   ~~deleted~~ Deleted   Excludes 1   Excludes 2   Includes   Use additional   Code first   Code also   Unspecified

OGCR Official Guidelines   ● Unacceptable Principal Diagnosis   X Assign placeholder X   ● Use Additional Character(s)   ▸ Manifestation Code   **Coding Clinic**

Item 1–1 Salmonella is a bacterium that lives in the intestines of fowl and mammals and can spread to humans through improper food preparation and cooking. Salmonellosis is an infection with the bacterium. Symptoms include diarrhea, fever, and abdominal cramps 12 to 72 hours after infection. The illness usually lasts 4 to 7 days, and most persons recover without treatment. The diarrhea may be so severe that the patient needs to be hospitalized. Patients with immunocompromised systems in chronic, ill health are more likely to have the infection invade their bloodstream with life-threatening results. For example, patients with sickle cell disease are more prone to salmonella osteomyelitis than others.

● **A02.2 Localized salmonella infections**

A02.20 Localized salmonella infection, unspecified
Specified in the documentation as localized, but unspecified as to type

A02.21 Salmonella meningitis 🔖
Specified as localized in the meninges
(Ex:) A02.21, A17.0-A17.1, A27.81, A39.0, A50.41, A51.41, A52.13, A54.82, A54.84, A54.89-A54.9, A74.81-A74.9, A87.0-A87.9, A96.2, A98.3-A98.4, B26.1, B33.24, B33.4-B33.8, B34.1-B34.2, B34.4-B34.8, B37.5, B38.4, B45.1, B58.2, B92, B94.2-94.9, B97.10, B97.19, B97.29, B97.5-B97.6, B97.81-B97.89, G00.0-G03.9, G04.2, G32.89, G96.8-G96.9, G98.0-G98.8, G99.8

A02.22 Salmonella pneumonia 🔖
Specified as localized in the lungs
(Ex:) A02.22, A15.0-A15.6, A15.8-A15.9, A17.9, A18.82, A18.84, A18.89, A20.2, A21.1, A22.1, A31.0, A37.01, A37.11, A37.81, A37.91, A42.0, A43.0, A48.1, B25.0, B39.0-B39.2, B44.0, B58.3, B59, B67.1, J09.X1-J09.X2, J10.00-J10.1, J11.00-J11.1, J12.0-J12.3, J12.89-J18.1, J18.8-J18.9, J22, J60, J62.0-J67.7, J68.0-J70.4, J70.8-J70.9, J98.4, J98.8-J99, R91.1

A02.23 Salmonella arthritis 🔖
Specified as localized in the joints
(Ex:) A02.23, A18.02, A18.09, A39.83-A39.84, A54.40, A54.42-A54.43, A54.82, A54.84, A54.89-A54.9, B06.82, M00.00-M02.30, M02.319, M02.329, M02.339, M02.349, M02.359, M02.369, M02.379-M02.9, M05.40-M05.59, M05.70-M06.09, M06.20-M06.39, M06.80-M07.69, M11.00-M11.9, M12.10-M15.0, M15.3-M15.9, M16.2-M16.9, M17.2-M17.9, M18.2-M18.9, M19.111-M19.93, M24.10-M24.176, M25.00, M25.08-M25.18, M25.40-M25.676, M25.80-M25.9, M35.2, M36.1-M36.4, R29.4

A02.24 Salmonella osteomyelitis 🔖
Specified as localized in bone
(Ex:) A02.24, A18.03-A18.09, M46.20-M46.39, M86.00-M86.9

A02.25 Salmonella pyelonephritis 🔖
Salmonella tubulo-interstitial nephropathy
(Ex:) A02.25-A02.29

A02.29 Salmonella with other localized infection 🔖
Specified as localized (because it is still under localized heading) but does not assign into any of the above codes
(Ex:) A02.25-A02.29

A02.8 Other specified salmonella infections 🔖
Any specified salmonella infection which does NOT assign into any of the above codes (not specified as localized)
(Ex:) A02.8

A02.9 Salmonella infection, unspecified 🔖
Unspecified in the documentation as to specific type of salmonella
(Ex:) A02.9

● **A03 Shigellosis**
An infectious disease caused by bacteria (Shigella)

A03.0 Shigellosis due to Shigella dysenteriae 🔖
Group A shigellosis [Shiga-Kruse dysentery]
(Ex:) A00.1, A01.00-A01.09, A01.4-A02.0, A03.0, A03.9, A04.9-A05.2, A06.0-A06.2, A06.9, A07.1-A07.9, A08.4-A09, A18.32-A18.39, A18.83, A48.51-A48.52, B37.82, B82.9, J09.X3-J09.X9, J10.2-J10.89, J11.2-J11.89, K30, K31.84, K50.00-K51.919, K52.1-K52.2, K52.82-K55.1, K55.8-K55.9, K58.0-K58.9, P70.0-P70.4, P70.9-P71.9, P72.1, P72.9-P74.4, P74.9, P76.8-P77.9, P78.1, P78.3-P78.89, P94.0

A03.1 Shigellosis due to Shigella flexneri
Group B shigellosis

A03.2 Shigellosis due to Shigella boydii
Group C shigellosis

A03.3 Shigellosis due to Shigella sonnei
Group D shigellosis

A03.8 Other shigellosis

A03.9 Shigellosis, unspecified
Bacillary dysentery NOS

● **A04 Other bacterial intestinal infections**

Excludes1 bacterial foodborne intoxications, NEC (A05.-)
tuberculous enteritis (A18.32)
(Ex:) **For category A04 CC codes A04.0-A04.4:** A02.0, A03.9-A05.0, A05.2, A07.4, A08.0-A09, J09.X3-J09.X9, J10.2-J10.89, J11.2-J11.89, K30, K31.84, K52.1-K52.2, K52.82-K52.9, K58.0-K58.9, K65.0, K65.2, K65.8, K68.12-K68.9, P76.8-P77.9, P78.1, P78.3-P78.89 **For category A04 CC codes A04.5-A04.8:** A00.1, A01.00-A01.09, A01.4-A02.0, A03.9, A04.0-A04.8, A04.9-A05.2, A06.0-A06.2, A06.9, A07.1-A09, A18.32-A18.39, A18.83, A48.51-A48.52, B37.82, B82.9, J09.X3-J09.X9, J10.2-J10.89, J11.2-J11.89, K30, K31.84, K50.00-K51.919, K52.1-K52.2, K52.82-K55.1, K55.8-K55.9, K58.0-K58.9, P70.0-P70.4, P70.9-P71.9, P72.1, P72.9-P74.4, P74.9, P76.8-P77.9, P78.1, P78.3-P78.89, P94.0

A04.0 Enteropathogenic Escherichia coli infection 🔖
Pertaining to or producing intestinal disease

A04.1 Enterotoxigenic Escherichia coli infection 🔖
Producing or containing intestinal toxin

A04.2 Enteroinvasive Escherichia coli infection 🔖
Capable of penetrating and spreading through intestinal mucosal epithelium

A04.3 Enterohemorrhagic Escherichia coli infection 🔖
Causing bloody diarrhea, resulting from microorganisms

A04.4 Other intestinal Escherichia coli infections 🔖
Escherichia coli enteritis NOS

A04.5 Campylobacter enteritis 🔖
Spiral shaped bacterium

A04.6 Enteritis due to Yersinia enterocolitica 🔖

Excludes1 extraintestinal yersiniosis (A28.2)
Transmitted by infected food /water and person-to-person contact, affecting intestinal tract

A04.7 Enterocolitis due to Clostridium difficile 🔖
Foodborne intoxication by Clostridium difficile
Pseudomembraneous colitis
Marked by fibrinous deposit (false membrane) with enmeshed necrotic cells

A04.8 Other specified bacterial intestinal infections 🔖

A04.9 Bacterial intestinal infection, unspecified 🔖
Bacterial enteritis NOS
(Ex:) A00.1, A01.00-A01.09, A01.4-A02.0, A03.9-A05.0, A05.2, A06.0-A06.2, A06.9, A07.1-A09, A18.32-A18.39, A18.83, B37.82, B82.9, J09.X3-J09.X9, J10.2-J10.89, J11.2-J11.89, K30, K31.84, K52.1-K52.2, K52.82-K52.9, K58.0-K58.9, K65.0, K65.2, K65.8, K68.12-K68.9, P76.8-P77.9, P78.1, P78.3-P78.89

Figure 1-1 Electron micrograph of escherichia coli (E. coli) expressing P fimbriae. (From Mandell, Bennett, & Dolin: Principles and Practice of Infectious Diseases, ed 7, Churchill Livingstone, An Imprint of Elsevier, 2009)

Item 1–2 *Escherichia coli [E. coli]* is a gram-negative bacterium found in the intestinal tracts of humans and animals and is usually nonpathogenic. Pathogenic strains can cause diarrhea or pyogenic (pus-producing) infections. Can be a threat to food safety.

N Newborn Age: 0   P Pediatric Age: 0–17   M Maternity DX: 12–55   A Adult Age: 15–124   ♀ Females Only   ♂ Males Only
🔖 Complication\Comorbidity   🔖 Major C\C   (Ex:) CC/MCC Exclusions   🔖 Present on Admission Requirement   🔖 Hospital-Acquired Condition

CHAPTER 1 (A00-B99)

741

● **A05**   **Other bacterial foodborne intoxications, not elsewhere classified**

     Excludes1   Clostridium difficile foodborne intoxication and infection (A04.7)

           Escherichia coli infection (A04.0-A04.4)

           listeriosis (A32.-)

           salmonella foodborne intoxication and infection (A02.-)

           toxic effect of noxious foodstuffs (T61-T62)

     A05.0   **Foodborne staphylococcal intoxication** 🔖

          (Ex:) A00.0-A09, A48.51-A48.52

     A05.1   **Botulism food poisoning** 🔖

          Botulism NOS

          Classical foodborne intoxication due to Clostridium botulinum

          Excludes1   infant botulism (A48.51)

                     wound botulism (A48.52)

          (Ex:) A04.7, A05.0-A05.2, A48.51-A48.52

     A05.2   **Foodborne Clostridium perfringens [Clostridium welchii] intoxication** 🔖

          Type A causes gas gangrene and necrotizing colitis; major cause of food poisoning in humans

          Enteritis necroticans

          Pig-bel

          (Ex:) A02.0, A03.9-A05.2, A07.4, A08.0-A09, A48.51-A48.52, J09.X3-J09.X9, J10.2-J10.89, J11.2-J11.89, K30, K31.84, K52.1-K52.2, K52.82-K52.9, K58.0-K58.9, K65.0, K65.2, K65.8, K68.12-K68.9, P76.8-P77.9, P78.1, P78.3-P78.89

     A05.3   **Foodborne Vibrio parahaemolyticus intoxication** 🔖

          Organism that survives only in high salt environment (halophilic), major cause of gastroenteritis due to consumption of raw or improperly cooked fish/seafood

          (Ex:) A00.0-A09, A48.51-A48.52

     A05.4   **Foodborne Bacillus cereus intoxication** 🔖

          Spore-forming species commonly found in soil, causes food poisoning from formation of intestinal toxins in contaminated foods

          (Ex:) A00.0-A09, A48.51-A48.52

     A05.5   **Foodborne Vibrio vulnificus intoxication** 🔖

          Species that survives in high salt environment (halophilic) with infection by eating raw seafood causes septicemia and cellulitis

          (Ex:) A00.0-A09, A48.51-A48.52

     A05.8   **Other specified bacterial foodborne intoxications** 🔖

          (Ex:) A00.0-A09, A48.51-A48.52

     A05.9   **Bacterial foodborne intoxication, unspecified**

● **A06**   **Amebiasis**

     An intestinal illness caused by the microscopic parasite Entamoeba histolytica

     Includes   infection due to Entamoeba histolytica

     Excludes1   other protozoal intestinal diseases (A07.-)

     Excludes2   acanthamebiasis (B60.1-)

                Naegleriasis (B60.2)

     A06.0   **Acute amebic dysentery** 🔖

          Acute amebiasis

          Intestinal amebiasis NOS

          (Ex:) A06.0-A06.1, A07.4

     A06.1   **Chronic intestinal amebiasis** 🔖

          (Ex:) A06.0-A06.1, A07.4

     A06.2   **Amebic nondysenteric colitis** 🔖

          Pertaining to single cell microorganism

          (Ex:) A02.0, A03.9-A05.0, A05.2, A06.0-A06.2, A06.9, A07.1-A09, B82.9, J09.X3-J09.X9, J10.2-J10.89, J11.2-J11.89, K30, K31.84, K50.00-K51.919, K52.1-K52.2, K52.82-K55.1, K55.8-K55.9, K58.0-K58.9, P76.8-P77.9, P78.1, P78.3, P78.81-P78.89

     A06.3   **Ameboma of intestine** 🔖

          Tumorlike mass produced by localized inflammation often in intestine

          Ameboma NOS

          (Ex:) A06.0-A06.6, A06.81-A06.89

     A06.4   **Amebic liver abscess** 🔖

          Hepatic amebiasis

          (Ex:) A06.4, K75.0

     A06.5   **Amebic lung abscess** 🔖

          Amebic abscess of lung (and liver)

          (Ex:) A06.5, J85.0-J85.2

     A06.6   **Amebic brain abscess** 🔖

          Amebic abscess of brain (and liver) (and lung)

          (Ex:) A06.6, G06.0

     A06.7   **Cutaneous amebiasis**

●   **A06.8**   **Amebic infection of other sites**

         A06.81   **Amebic cystitis** 🔖

               (Ex:) A06.0-A06.6, A06.81-A06.89

         A06.82   **Other amebic genitourinary infections** 🔖

               Amebic balanitis

               Amebic vesiculitis

               Amebic vulvovaginitis

               (Ex:) A06.0-A06.6, A06.81-A06.89

         A06.89   **Other amebic infections** 🔖

               Amebic appendicitis

               Amebic splenic abscess

               (Ex:) A06.0-A06.6, A06.81-A06.89

     A06.9   **Amebiasis, unspecified**

● **A07**   **Other protozoal intestinal diseases**

     (Ex:) For category A07 CC codes unless otherwise indicated: A02.0, A03.9-A05.0, A05.2, A06.0-A06.2, A06.9, A07.1-A09, B82.9, J09.X3-J09.X9, J10.2-J10.89, J11.2-J11.89, K30, K31.84, K52.1-K52.2, K52.82-K52.9, K58.0-K58.9

     A07.0   **Balantidiasis**

          Balantidial dysentery

          Infection by protozoa that may cause diarrhea and dysentery, with ulceration of colonic mucous membranes

     A07.1   **Giardiasis [lambliasis]** 🔖

          Common infection in small intestine spread by contaminated food, water, or direct person-to-person contact

     A07.2   **Cryptosporidiosis** 🔖

          Human infection with protozoa usually seen as self-limited diarrhea in those who work with cattle

     A07.3   **Isosporiasis** 🔖

          Human intestinal disease caused by protozoa

          Infection due to Isospora belli and Isospora hominis

          Intestinal coccidiosis

          Isosporosis

     A07.4   **Cyclosporiasis** 🔖

          Infection by protozoa with most common species infecting humans being C cayetanensis

          (Ex:) A02.0, A03.9-A05.0, A05.2, A06.0-A06.2, A06.9, A07.1-A09, B82.9, J09.X3-J09.X9, J10.2-J10.89, J11.2-J11.89, K30, K31.84, K52.1-K52.2, K52.82-K52.9, K58.0-K58.9, K65.0, K65.2, K65.8, K68.12-K68.9

     A07.8   **Other specified protozoal intestinal diseases** 🔖

          Intestinal microsporidiosis

          Intestinal trichomoniasis

          Sarcocystosis

          Sarcosporidiosis

     A07.9   **Protozoal intestinal disease, unspecified** 🔖

          Flagellate diarrhea

          Protozoal colitis

          Protozoal diarrhea

          Protozoal dysentery

◀ New   ◀⁝⁝ Revised   ~~deleted~~ Deleted   Excludes 1   Excludes 2   Includes   Use additional   Code first   Code also   Unspecified

OGCR Official Guidelines   ● Unacceptable Principal Diagnosis   X Assign placeholder X   ● Use Additional Character(s)   ▌ Manifestation Code   **Coding Clinic**

● **A08**   **Viral and other specified intestinal infections**

> **Excludes1**   influenza with involvement of gastrointestinal tract (J09.X3, J10.2, J11.2)

> (Ex) **For category A08 CC codes:** A02.0, A03.9-A05.0, A05.2, A06.0-A06.2, A06.9, A07.1-A09, A18.32-A18.39, A18.83, B37.82, B82.9, J09.X3-J09.X9, J10.2-J10.89, J11.2-J11.89, K30, K31.84, K52.1-K52.2, K52.82-K52.9, K58.0-K58.9, K65.0, K65.2, K65.8, K68.12-K68.9, P78.1, P78.3-P78.89

A08.0   **Rotaviral enteritis**

● **A08.1**   **Acute gastroenteropathy due to Norwalk agent and other small round viruses**

> **A08.11**   **Acute gastroenteropathy due to Norwalk agent** 🔹
> > Acute gastroenteropathy due to Norovirus
> > Acute gastroenteropathy due to Norwalk-like agent

> **A08.19**   **Acute gastroenteropathy due to other small round viruses** 🔹
> > Acute gastroenteropathy due to small round virus [SRV] NOS

A08.2   **Adenoviral enteritis** 🔹

● **A08.3**   **Other viral enteritis**

> **A08.31**   **Calicivirus enteritis** 🔹
> **A08.32**   **Astrovirus enteritis** 🔹
> **A08.39**   **Other viral enteritis** 🔹
> > Coxsackie virus enteritis
> > Echovirus enteritis
> > Enterovirus enteritis NEC
> > Torovirus enteritis

A08.4   **Viral intestinal infection, unspecified**
> Viral enteritis NOS
> Viral gastroenteritis NOS
> Viral gastroenteropathy NOS

A08.8   **Other specified intestinal infections**

A09   **Infectious gastroenteritis and colitis, unspecified** 🔹
> Infectious colitis NOS
> Infectious enteritis NOS
> Infectious gastroenteritis NOS

> **Excludes1**   colitis NOS (K52.9)
> > diarrhea NOS (R19.7)
> > enteritis NOS (K52.9)
> > gastroenteritis NOS (K52.9)
> > noninfective gastroenteritis and colitis, unspecified (K52.9)

> (Ex) A00.0-A09, A48.51-A48.52

TUBERCULOSIS (A15-A19)

> **Includes**   infections due to Mycobacterium tuberculosis and Mycobacterium bovis

> **Excludes1**   congenital tuberculosis (P37.0)
> > nonspecific reaction to test for tuberculosis without active tuberculosis (R76.1-)
> > pneumoconiosis associated with tuberculosis, any type in A15 (J65)
> > positive PPD (R76.11)
> > positive tuberculin skin test without active tuberculosis (R76.11)
> > sequelae of tuberculosis (B90.-)
> > silicotuberculosis (J65)

● **A15**   **Respiratory tuberculosis**

> (Ex) **For category A15 CC codes unless otherwise indicated:** A15.0-A15.9, A17.9, A18.82, A18.84, A18.89-A19.9, A22.1, A31.0, A31.2-A31.9, A37.01, A37.11, A37.81, A37.91, A48.1, A49.3-A49.9, B25.0, B44.0, B90.9, B92, B94.2-B94.9, B96.0, B96.6-B96.89, J09.X1-J09.X2, J10.00-J10.1, J11.00-J11.1, J12.0-J12.3, J12.89-J18.1, J18.8-J18.9, J44.9, J47.0-J70.4, J70.8-J70.9, J98.4, R91.1

> **A15.0**   **Tuberculosis of lung** 🔹
> > Tuberculous bronchiectasis
> > *Chronic dilatation of bronchi*
> > Tuberculous fibrosis of lung
> > Tuberculous pneumonia
> > Tuberculous pneumothorax

Figure 1-2   Far advanced bilateral pulmonary tuberculosis before and after 8 months of treatment with streptomycin, PAS, and isoniazid. (From Hinshaw HC, Garland LH: Diseases of the Chest, ed 4, Philadelphia, WB Saunders, 1980)

Item 1–3   **Tuberculosis** is a common and deadly infectious disease caused by the *Mycobacterium tuberculosis* organism. The first tuberculosis infection is called the **primary infection** and most commonly attacks the lungs but can affect the central nervous system, lymphatic system, circulatory system, genitourinary system, bones, joints, and even the skin. A **Ghon** lesion is the **initial lesion.** A **secondary lesion** occurs when the tubercle bacilli are carried to other areas.

Item 1–4   **Although** it primarily affects the lungs, the bacteria *Mycobacterium tuberculosis* can travel from the pulmonary circulation to virtually any organ in the body, much as a cancer metastasizes to a secondary site. If the immune system becomes compromised by age or disease, what would otherwise be a self-limiting primary tuberculosis in the lungs will develop in other organs. These are known as extrapulmonary sites.

> **A15.4**   **Tuberculosis of intrathoracic lymph nodes** 🔹
> > Tuberculosis of hilar lymph nodes
> > Tuberculosis of mediastinal lymph nodes
> > Tuberculosis of tracheobronchial lymph nodes
> > > **Excludes1**   tuberculosis specified as primary (A15.7)

> **A15.5**   **Tuberculosis of larynx, trachea and bronchus** 🔹
> > Tuberculosis of bronchus
> > Tuberculosis of glottis
> > Tuberculosis of larynx
> > Tuberculosis of trachea

> **A15.6**   **Tuberculous pleurisy** 🔹
> > Tuberculosis of pleura
> > Tuberculous empyema
> > > **Excludes1**   primary respiratory tuberculosis (A15.7)

> **A15.7**   **Primary respiratory tuberculosis** 🔹
> > (Ex) A15.0-A17.82, A17.89-A19.9

> **A15.8**   **Other respiratory tuberculosis** 🔹
> > Mediastinal tuberculosis
> > Nasopharyngeal tuberculosis
> > Tuberculosis of nose
> > Tuberculosis of sinus [any nasal]
> > (Ex) A15.0-A17.82, A17.89, A18.31-A18.39, A18.83, A19.0-A19.9

> **A15.9**   **Respiratory tuberculosis unspecified** 🔹
> > (Ex) A15.0-A17.82, A17.89, A18.31-A18.39, A18.83, A19.0-A19.9

● **A17**   **Tuberculosis of nervous system**

> **A17.0**   **Tuberculous meningitis** 🔹
> > Tuberculosis of meninges (cerebral) (spinal)
> > Tuberculous leptomeningitis
> > > **Excludes1**   tuberculous meningoencephalitis (A17.82)
> > (Ex) A02.21, A17.0-A17.1, A17.89-A17.9, A18.82, A18.84, A18.89, A27.81, A31.2-A31.9, A39.0, A49.3-A49.9, A50.41, A51.41, A52.13, A54.82, A54.84, A54.89-A54.9, A87.0-A87.9, B00.3, B02.1, B26.1, B37.5, B38.4, B45.1, B58.2, B90.0, B92, B94.2-B94.9, B96.0, B96.6-B96.89, G00.0-G03.9, G04.2, G32.89, G61.0, G96.8-G96.9, G98.0-G98.8, G99.8

> **A17.1**   **Meningeal tuberculoma** 🔹
> > Tuberculoma of meninges (cerebral) (spinal)
> > > **Excludes2**   tuberculoma of brain and spinal cord (A17.81)
> > (Ex) See A17.0

N   Newborn Age: 0   **P**   Pediatric Age: 0–17   **M**   Maternity DX: 12–55   **A**   Adult Age: 15–124   ♀ Females Only   ♂ Males Only

🔹 Complication\Comorbidity   🔹 Major C\C   (Ex) CC/MCC Exclusions   🔹 Present on Admission Requirement   🔹 Hospital-Acquired Condition

- A17.8 **Other tuberculosis of nervous system**
  - A17.81 **Tuberculoma of brain and spinal cord** 🖉
    Tuberculous abscess of brain and spinal cord
    Ⓔⓧ A17.81-A17.82, A17.89-A17.9, A18.82, A18.84, A18.89,
    A31.2-A31.9, A49.3-A49.9, B90.0, B92, B94.2-B94.9, B96.0,
    B96.6-B96.89
  - A17.82 **Tuberculous meningoencephalitis** 🖉
    *Inflammation of brain and meninges; AKA
    cerebromeningitis and encephalomeningitis*
    Tuberculous myelitis
    Ⓔⓧ See A17.81
  - A17.83 **Tuberculous neuritis** 🖉
    Tuberculous mononeuropathy
  - A17.89 **Other tuberculosis of nervous system** 🖉
    Tuberculous polyneuropathy
    Ⓔⓧ A17.89-A17.9, A18.82, A18.84, A18.89, A31.2-A31.9,
    A49.3-A49.9, B90.0, B92, B94.2-B94.9, B96.0, B96.6-B96.89
- A17.9 **Tuberculosis of nervous system, unspecified** 🖉
  Ⓔⓧ A17.9, A18.82, A18.84, A18.89, A31.2-A31.9, A49.3-A49.9, B92, B94.2-B94.9,
  B96.0, B96.6-B96.89

- A18 **Tuberculosis of other organs**
  - A18.0 **Tuberculosis of bones and joints**
    - A18.01 **Tuberculosis of spine** 🖉
      Pott's disease or curvature of spine
      Tuberculous arthritis
      Tuberculous osteomyelitis of spine
      Tuberculous spondylitis
      Ⓔⓧ A18.01
    - A18.02 **Tuberculous arthritis of other joints** 🖉
      Tuberculosis of hip (joint)
      Tuberculosis of knee (joint)
      Ⓔⓧ A18.02
    - A18.03 **Tuberculosis of other bones** 🖉
      Tuberculous mastoiditis
      Tuberculous osteomyelitis
      Ⓔⓧ A18.01, A18.03
    - A18.09 **Other musculoskeletal tuberculosis** 🖉
      Tuberculous myositis
      Tuberculous synovitis
      Tuberculous tenosynovitis
      Ⓔⓧ A18.01-A18.02, A18.09
  - A18.1 **Tuberculosis of genitourinary system**
    - A18.10 **Tuberculosis of genitourinary system,
      unspecified** 🖉
      Ⓔⓧ A17.9, A18.10, A18.82, A18.84, A18.89, A31.2-A31.9,
      A49.3-A49.9, B90.0, B92, B94.2-B94.9, B96.0, B96.6-B96.89
    - A18.11 **Tuberculosis of kidney and ureter** 🖉
      Ⓔⓧ A17.9, A18.10-A18.13, A18.82, A18.84, A18.89, A31.2-A31.9,
      A49.3-A49.9, B90.1, B92, B94.2-B94.9, B96.0, B96.6-B96.89
    - A18.12 **Tuberculosis of bladder** 🖉
      Ⓔⓧ See A18.11
    - A18.13 **Tuberculosis of other urinary organs** 🖉
      Tuberculous urethritis
      Ⓔⓧ See A18.11
    - A18.14 **Tuberculosis of prostate** ♂ 🖉   A
      Ⓔⓧ A17.9, A18.10, A18.82, A18.84, A18.89, A31.2-A31.9,
      A49.3-A49.9, B90.1, B92, B94.2-B94.9, B96.0, B96.6-B96.89
    - A18.15 **Tuberculosis of other male genital organs** ♂ 🖉
      Ⓔⓧ See A18.14
    - A18.16 **Tuberculosis of cervix** ♀ 🖉
      Ⓔⓧ A17.9, A18.0, A18.16-A18.18, A18.82, A18.84, A18.89,
      A31.2-A31.9, A49.3-A49.9, B90.1, B92, B94.2-B94.9, B96.0,
      B96.6-B96.89

- A18.17 **Tuberculous female pelvic inflammatory
  disease** ♀ 🖉
  Tuberculous endometritis
  Tuberculous oophoritis and salpingitis
  Oophoritis = inflammation of ovary
  Salpingitis = inflammation of fallopian tube
  Ⓔⓧ See A18.16
- A18.18 **Tuberculosis of other female genital
  organs** ♀ 🖉
  Tuberculous ulceration of vulva
  Ⓔⓧ See A18.16
- A18.2 **Tuberculous peripheral lymphadenopathy** 🖉
  Tuberculous adenitis
  Excludes2 tuberculosis of bronchial and mediastinal
  lymph nodes (A15.4)
  tuberculosis of mesenteric and
  retroperitoneal lymph nodes
  (A18.39)
  tuberculous tracheobronchial adenopathy
  (A15.4)
  Ⓔⓧ A17.9, A18.2, A18.82, A18.84, A18.89, A31.2-A31.9, A49.3-A49.9, B92,
  B94.2-B94.9, B96.0, B96.6-B96.89
- A18.3 **Tuberculosis of intestines, peritoneum and mesenteric
  glands**
  Ⓔⓧ For category A18.3 CC codes: A17.9, A18.31-A18.39, A18.82-A18.84,
  A18.89, A31.2-A31.9, A49.3-A49.9, B92, B94.2-B94.9, B96.0, B96.6-B96.89
  - A18.31 **Tuberculous peritonitis** 🖉
    Tuberculous ascites
  - A18.32 **Tuberculous enteritis** 🖉
    Tuberculosis of anus and rectum
    Tuberculosis of intestine (large) (small)
  - A18.39 **Retroperitoneal tuberculosis** 🖉
    Tuberculosis of mesenteric glands
    Tuberculosis of retroperitoneal (lymph glands)
- A18.4 **Tuberculosis of skin and subcutaneous tissue** 🖉
  Erythema induratum, tuberculous
  Lupus excedens
  Lupus vulgaris NOS
  Lupus vulgaris of eyelid
  *Cutaneous tuberculosis characterized by reddish brown
  plaque on skin surrounded by papules and nodules*
  Scrofuloderma
  *Type of cutaneous tuberculosis, with direct extension of
  tuberculosis into skin from underlying structures;
  AKA tuberculosis colliquativa*
  Tuberculosis of external ear
  Excludes2 lupus erythematosus (L93.-)
  lupus NOS (M32.9)
  systemic (M32.-)
  Ⓔⓧ A15.0-A17.82, A17.89-A19.9
- A18.5 **Tuberculosis of eye**
  Excludes2 lupus vulgaris of eyelid (A18.4)
  Ⓔⓧ For category A18.5 CC codes: A17.9, A18.50-A18.59, A18.82, A18.84,
  A18.89, A31.2-A31.9, A49.3-A49.9, B92, B94.2-B94.9, B96.0, B96.6-B96.89
  - A18.50 **Tuberculosis of eye, unspecified** 🖉
  - A18.51 **Tuberculous episcleritis** 🖉
    Inflammation of episclera and adjacent tissues
  - A18.52 **Tuberculous keratitis** 🖉
    Tuberculous interstitial keratitis
    Tuberculous keratoconjunctivitis (interstitial)
    (phlyctenular)
    Inflammation of cornea and conjunctiva
  - A18.53 **Tuberculous chorioretinitis** 🖉
    *Inflammation of choroid and retina;
    retinochoroiditis*
  - A18.54 **Tuberculous iridocyclitis** 🖉
    Inflammation of iris and ciliary body
  - A18.59 **Other tuberculosis of eye** 🖉
    Tuberculous conjunctivitis

◀ New   ◀┅ Revised   deleted Deleted   **Excludes 1**   **Excludes 2**   **Includes**   **Use additional**   **Code first**   **Code also**   **Unspecified**
OGCR Official Guidelines   ● Unacceptable Principal Diagnosis   X Assign placeholder X   ● Use Additional Character(s)   ▶ Manifestation Code   **Coding Clinic**

Item 1–5   **Miliary tuberculosis** can be a life-threatening condition. If a tuberculous lesion enters a blood vessel, immense dissemination of tuberculous organisms can occur if the immune system is weak. High-risk populations—children under 4 years of age, the elderly, or the immunocompromised—are particularly prone to this type of infection. The lesions will have a millet seedlike appearance on chest x-ray. Bronchial washings and biopsy may aid in diagnosis.

A18.6   **Tuberculosis of (inner) (middle) ear** 🔾
     Tuberculous otitis media
     Excludes2   tuberculosis of external ear (A18.4)
                  tuberculous mastoiditis (A18.03)
     (Ex) A17.9, A18.6, A18.82, A18.84, A18.89, A31.2-A31.9, A49.3-A49.9, B92, B94.2-B94.9, B96.0, B96.6-B96.89

A18.7   **Tuberculosis of adrenal glands** 🔾
     Tuberculous Addison's disease
     (Ex) A17.9, A18.7, A18.82, A18.84, A18.89, A31.2-A31.9, A49.3-A49.9, B92, B94.2-B94.9, B96.0, B96.6-B96.89

● **A18.8** **Tuberculosis of other specified organs**
     A18.81   **Tuberculosis of thyroid gland** 🔾
           (Ex) A17.9, A18.81-A18.82, A18.84, A18.89, A31.2-A31.9, A49.3-A49.9, B92, B94.2-B94.9, B96.0, B96.6-B96.89

     A18.82   **Tuberculosis of other endocrine glands** 🔾
           Tuberculosis of pituitary gland
           Tuberculosis of thymus gland
           (Ex) A17.9, A18.82, A18.84, A18.89, A31.2-A31.9, A49.3-A49.9, B92, B94.2-B94.9, B96.0, B96.6-B96.89

     A18.83   **Tuberculosis of digestive tract organs, not elsewhere classified** 🔾
           Excludes1   tuberculosis of intestine (A18.32)
           (Ex) See A18.3

     A18.84   **Tuberculosis of heart** 🔾
           Tuberculous cardiomyopathy
           Tuberculous endocarditis
           Tuberculous myocarditis
           Tuberculous pericarditis
           (Ex) See A18.2

     A18.85   **Tuberculosis of spleen** 🔾
           (Ex) A17.9, A18.82, A18.84-A18.85 A18.89, A31.2-A31.9, A49.3-A49.9, B92, B94.2-B94.9, B96.0, B96.6-B96.89

     A18.89   **Tuberculosis of other sites** 🔾
           Tuberculosis of muscle
           Tuberculous cerebral arteritis
           (Ex) See A18.2

● **A19**   **Miliary tuberculosis**
     Includes   disseminated tuberculosis
                   generalized tuberculosis
                   tuberculous polyserositis
     (Ex) For category A19 CC codes: A17.9, A18.82, A18.84, A18.89, A19.0-A19.9, A31.2-A31.9, A49.3-A49.9, B92, B94.2-B94.9, B96.0, B96.6-B96.89

     A19.0   **Acute miliary tuberculosis of a single specified site** 🔾
     A19.1   **Acute miliary tuberculosis of multiple sites** 🔾
     A19.2   **Acute miliary tuberculosis, unspecified** 🔾
     A19.8   **Other miliary tuberculosis** 🔾
     A19.9   **Miliary tuberculosis, unspecified** 🔾

CERTAIN ZOONOTIC BACTERIAL DISEASES (A20-A28)

● **A20**   **Plague**
     Infectious disease caused by a Yersinia pestis bacterium, transmitted by a rodent flea bite or handling of infected animal
     Includes   infection due to Yersinia pestis

     A20.0   **Bubonic plague** 🔾
           (Ex) A20.0-A20.9

     A20.1   **Cellulocutaneous plague** 🔾
           Skin and subcutaneous tissue plague
           (Ex) A20.0-A20.9

     A20.2   **Pneumonic plague** 🔾
           (Ex) A20.2, J12.81

     A20.3   **Plague meningitis** 🔾
           (Ex) A20.3, A20.8

     A20.7   **Septicemic plague** 🔾
           (Ex) A02.1, A20.0-A20.9, A22.7, A26.7, A32.7, A40.0-A40.1, A40.8-A41.9, A42.7, A54.86, B37.7, P36.0-P36.9, P39.2, P39.4-P39.9, R65.10-R65.20

     A20.8   **Other forms of plague** 🔾
           Abortive plague
           Asymptomatic plague
           Pestis minor
           Systemic bacterial disease
           (Ex) See A20.3

     A20.9   **Plague, unspecified** 🔾
           (Ex) A20.9

● **A21**   **Tularemia**
     Caused by Francisella tularensis bacterium found in rodents, rabbits, and hares and transmitted to humans by contact with infected animal tissues or by ticks, biting flies, or mosquitoes
     Includes   deer-fly fever
                   infection due to Francisella tularensis
                   rabbit fever

     A21.0   **Ulceroglandular tularemia** 🔾
           Most common form of tularemia in humans is painful, swollen, erythematous papule at point of inoculation that ruptures to form shallow ulcer
           (Ex) A21.0

     A21.1   **Oculoglandular tularemia** 🔾
           Primary site of entry is conjunctival sac, results in granulomatous corneal lesions
           Ophthalmic tularemia
           (Ex) A21.1, J12.81

     A21.2   **Pulmonary tularemia** 🔾
           (Ex) A22.1, A37.01, A37.11, A37.81, A37.91, A48.1, B25.0, B44.0, J09.X1-J09.X2, J10.00-J10.1, J11.00-J11.1, J15.29, J15.5-J18.0, J18.8-J18.9, J22, J60-J70.4, J70.8-J70.9, J98.4, J98.8-J99, R91.1

     A21.3   **Gastrointestinal tularemia** 🔾
           Abdominal tularemia
           (Ex) A21.3

     A21.7   **Generalized tularemia** 🔾
           (Ex) A21.0-A21.9

     A21.8   **Other forms of tularemia** 🔾
           (Ex) A21.0-A21.9

     A21.9   **Tularemia, unspecified** 🔾
           (Ex) A21.0-A21.9

● **A22**   **Anthrax**
     An acute infectious disease caused by the spore-forming Bacillus anthracis; occurs in humans exposed to infected animals or tissue from infected animals
     Includes   infection due to Bacillus anthracis

     A22.0   **Cutaneous anthrax** 🔾
           Malignant carbuncle
           Malignant pustule
           (Ex) A22.0

     A22.1   **Pulmonary anthrax** 🔾
           Inhalation anthrax
           Ragpicker's disease
           Woolsorter's disease
           (Ex) A15.0-A15.9, A17.9, A18.82, A18.84, A18.89, A20.2, A21.1-A21.2, A22.1, A31.0, A37.01, A37.11, A37.81, A37.91, A42.0, A43.0, A48.1, B25.0, B39.0-B39.2, B44.0, B58.3, B59, B67.1, J09.X1-J09.X2, J10.00-J10.1, J11.00-J11.1, J12.0-J12.3, J12.81-J18.1, J18.8-J18.9, J22, J44.9, J47.0-J70.4, J70.8-J70.9, J98.4, J98.8-J99, R91.1

     A22.2   **Gastrointestinal anthrax** 🔾
           (Ex) A22.2

     A22.7   **Anthrax sepsis** 🔾
           Infectious bacterial disease
           MCC when PDx is its own MCC
           (Ex) A02.1, A20.7, A22.7, A26.7, A32.7, A39.2-A39.4, A40.0-A40.1, A40.8-A41.9, A42.7, A48.2-A48.4, A48.8-A49.9, A54.86, B00.7, B37.7, B92, B94.2-B96.89, P36.0-P36.9, P39.2, P39.4-P39.9, R65.10-R65.20, Z16.10-Z16.39

     A22.8   **Other forms of anthrax** 🔾
           Anthrax meningitis
           (Ex) A22.8

     A22.9   **Anthrax, unspecified** 🔾
           (Ex) A22.0-A22.9

CHAPTER 1 (A00-B99)

N Newborn Age: 0   **P** Pediatric Age: 0–17   **M** Maternity DX: 12–55   **A** Adult Age: 15–124   ♀ Females Only   ♂ Males Only

🔾 Complication\Comorbidity   🔾 Major C\C   (Ex) CC/MCC Exclusions   🔾 Present on Admission Requirement   🔾 Hospital-Acquired Condition

745

Item 1-6 **Brucellosis:** An infectious disease caused by the bacterium Brucella. Humans are infected by contact with contaminated animals or animal products. In humans brucellosis symptoms that are similar to the flu include fever, sweats, headaches, back pains, and physical weakness. Severe infections of the central nervous system or lining of the heart may occur. Brucellosis can also cause chronic symptoms that include recurrent fevers, joint pain, and fatigue.

● **A23   Brucellosis**

    Includes   Malta fever
                    Mediterranean fever
                    undulant fever

    A23.0   Brucellosis due to Brucella melitensis
            *Resulting in flu-like symptoms that may lead to chronic
            symptoms that include recurrent fevers, joint pain, and
            fatigue*

    A23.1   Brucellosis due to Brucella abortus
            *Most common cause of brucellosis in humans; AKA Bang
            bacillus*

    A23.2   Brucellosis due to Brucella suis
            Species found primarily in pigs, rabbits, and reindeer

    A23.3   Brucellosis due to Brucella canis
            Species that causes respiratory tract infection in humans

    A23.8   Other brucellosis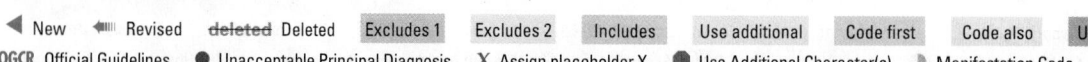
            (Ex) A23.0-A23.9

    A23.9   Brucellosis, unspecified
            (Ex) A23.0-A23.9

● **A24   Glanders and melioidosis**
        *Infection, usually of rodents, which spreads to other animals and
        humans, caused by Burkholderia pseudomallei through break
        in skin contaminated with infested soil or water*
        (Ex) For category A24 CC codes unless otherwise indicated: A24.1-A24.9

    A24.0   Glanders
            Infection due to Pseudomonas mallei
            Malleus
            (Ex) A24.0

    A24.1   Acute and fulminating melioidosis
            Melioidosis pneumonia
            Melioidosis sepsis

    A24.2   Subacute and chronic melioidosis

    A24.3   Other melioidosis

    A24.9   Melioidosis, unspecified
            Infection due to Pseudomonas pseudomallei NOS
            Whitmore's disease

● **A25   Rat-bite fevers**
        *RBF, infectious disease caused by Streptobacillus moniliformis or
        Spirillum minus.*
        (Ex) For category A25 CC codes: A25.0-A25.9

    A25.0   Spirillosis
            Any disease condition caused by spirilla
            Sodoku

    A25.1   Streptobacillosis
            *Acute, febrile human illness caused by bacteria transmitted
            by rats in most cases, passed from rodent to human via
            rodent's urine or mucous secretions; AKA rat fever*
            Epidemic arthritic erythema
            Haverhill fever
            Streptobacillary rat-bite fever

    A25.9   Rat-bite fever, unspecified

● **A26   Erysipeloid**
        *Infection with Erysipelothrix rhusiopathiae, occurring often as
        occupational disease resulting from handling infected fish,
        shellfish, meat, or poultry*

    A26.0   Cutaneous erysipeloid
            Erythema migrans

    A26.7   Erysipelothrix sepsis
            MCC when PDx is its own MCC
            (Ex) A02.1, A20.7, A22.7, A26.7, A32.7, A39.2-A39.4, A40.0-A40.1, A40.8-A41.9,
                A42.7, A48.2-A48.4, A48.8-A49.9, A54.86, B00.7, B3.77, B92,
                B94.2-B96.89, R65.10-R65.20, Z16.10-Z16.39

    A26.8   Other forms of erysipeloid

    A26.9   Erysipeloid, unspecified

● **A27   Leptospirosis**
        Occurs most commonly in the tropics
        (Ex) For category A27 CC codes unless otherwise indicated: A27.0-A27.9

    A27.0   Leptospirosis icterohemorrhagica
            Leptospiral or spirochetal jaundice (hemorrhagic)
            Weil's disease

● **A27.8   Other forms of leptospirosis**

    A27.81   Aseptic meningitis in leptospirosis
            (Ex) A02.21, A17.0-A17.1, A27.0-A27.9, A39.0, A50.41, A51.41,
                A52.13, A54.82, A54.84, A54.89-A54.9, A74.81-A74.9,
                A87.0-A87.9, A96.2, A98.3-A98.4, B26.1, B33.24, B33.4-B33.8,
                B34.1-B34.2, B34.4-B34.8, B37.5, B38.4, B45.1, B58.2, B92,
                B94.2-B94.9, B97.10, B97.19, B97.29, B97.5-B97.6,
                B97.81-B97.89, G00.0-G03.9, G04.2, G32.89, G61.0,
                G96.8-G96.9, G98.0-G98.8, G99.8

    A27.89   Other forms of leptospirosis

    A27.9   Leptospirosis, unspecified

● **A28   Other zoonotic bacterial diseases, not elsewhere classified**
        (Ex) For category A28 CC codes unless otherwise indicated: A26.0, A26.8-A26.9, A28.0,
            A28.2-A28.9, A32.0-A32.12, A32.81-A32.9

    A28.0   Pasteurellosis
            *Infection of humans or other animals by species of
            Pasteurella*

    A28.1   Cat-scratch disease
            Cat-scratch fever
            (Ex) A28.1, B97.21

    A28.2   Extraintestinal yersiniosis
            *Infection from Yersinia enterocolitica; AKA enteric
            yersiniosis, intestinal yersiniosis, Yersinia enteritis*

            Excludes1   enteritis due to Yersinia enterocolitica
                            (A04.6)
                            plague (A20.-)

    **A28.8   Other specified zoonotic bacterial diseases, not
            elsewhere classified**

    A28.9   Zoonotic bacterial disease, unspecified

OTHER BACTERIAL DISEASES (A30-A49)

● **A30   Leprosy [Hansen's disease]**
        *Chronic infectious disease attacking the skin, peripheral nerves, and
        mucous membranes*

        Includes   infection due to Mycobacterium leprae
        Excludes1   sequelae of leprosy (B92)

    A30.0   Indeterminate leprosy
            I leprosy
            (Ex) A30.0

    A30.1   Tuberculoid leprosy
            TT leprosy
            (Ex) A30.1

    A30.2   Borderline tuberculoid leprosy
            BT leprosy
            (Ex) A30.2-A30.4

    A30.3   Borderline leprosy
            BB leprosy
            (Ex) A30.2-A30.4

    A30.4   Borderline lepromatous leprosy
            BL leprosy
            (Ex) A30.2-A30.4

    A30.5   Lepromatous leprosy
            LL leprosy
            (Ex) A30.5

    A30.8   Other forms of leprosy
            (Ex) A30.8

    A30.9   Leprosy, unspecified
            (Ex) A30.9

◄ New   ◄═ Revised   ~~deleted~~ Deleted | Excludes 1 | | Excludes 2 | | Includes | | Use additional | | Code first | | Code also | | Unspecified |

OGCR Official Guidelines   ● Unacceptable Principal Diagnosis   X Assign placeholder X   ● Use Additional Character(s)   ▶ Manifestation Code   **Coding Clinic**

● **A31**   **Infection due to other mycobacteria**
> **Excludes2**   leprosy (A30.-)
>   tuberculosis (A15-A19)
> (Ex) For category A31 CC codes unless otherwise indicated: A31.0-A31.9

     A31.0   **Pulmonary mycobacterial infection**
> Infection due to Mycobacterium avium
> Infection due to Mycobacterium intracellulare [Battey bacillus]
> Infection due to Mycobacterium kansasii
> (Ex) A15.0-A15.9, A17.9, A18.82, A18.84, A18.89, A22.1, A31.0, A31.2-A31.9, A37.01, A37.11, A37.81, A37.91, A48.1, A49.3-A49.9, B25.0, B44.0, B90.0, B92, B94.2-B94.9, B96.0, B96.6-B96.89, J09.X1-J09.X2, J10.00-J10.1, J11.00-J11.1, J12.0-J12.3, J12.89-J18.1, J18.8-J18.9, J44.9, J47.0-J70.4, J70.8-J70.9, J98.4, R91.1

     A31.1   **Cutaneous mycobacterial infection**
> Buruli ulcer
> Infection due to Mycobacterium marinum
> Infection due to Mycobacterium ulcerans

     A31.2   **Disseminated mycobacterium avium-intracellulare complex (DMAC)**
> MAC sepsis

     A31.8   **Other mycobacterial infections**

     A31.9   **Mycobacterial infection, unspecified**
> Atypical mycobacterial infection NOS
> Mycobacteriosis NOS

● **A32**   **Listeriosis**
> *Infection caused by* Listeria monocytogenes
> **Includes**   listerial foodborne infection
> **Excludes1**   neonatal (disseminated) listeriosis (P37.2)
> (Ex) For category A32 CC codes unless otherwise indicated: A26.0, A26.8-A26.9, A28.0, A28.2-A28.9, A32.0-A32.12, A32.81-A32.9

     A32.0   **Cutaneous listeriosis**

●   **A32.1**   **Listerial meningitis and meningoencephalitis**

         A32.11   **Listerial meningitis**

         A32.12   **Listerial meningoencephalitis**

     A32.7   **Listerial sepsis**
> MCC when PDx is its own MCC
> (Ex) A02.1, A20.7, A22.7, A26.7, A32.7, A39.2-A39.4, A40.0-A40.1, A40.8-A41.9, A42.7, A48.2-A48.4, A48.8-A49.9, A54.86, B00.7, B3.77, B92, B94.2-B96.89, R65.10-R65.20, Z16.10-Z16.39

●   **A32.8**   **Other forms of listeriosis**

         A32.81   **Oculoglandular listeriosis**
> *Primary infection site is conjunctival sac, which if untreated may result in perforation of cornea and optic atrophy*

         A32.82   **Listerial endocarditis**
> *Exudative and proliferative inflammatory condition of endocardium caused by listeria bacteria*

         A32.89   **Other forms of listeriosis**
> Listerial cerebral arteritis

     A32.9   **Listeriosis, unspecified**

A33   **Tetanus neonatorum**   **N**
> *Neonate = newborn*
> (Ex) A33, P29.0-P29.2, P29.4, P29.89-P29.9, P94.1-P94.9, P96.0, P96.3-P96.5, P96.82-P96.89

A34   **Obstetrical tetanus** ♀   **M**
> (Ex) A34, 008.0, 008.2-008.9, 020.0-020.9, 025.10-025.3, 026.10-026.13, 026.30-026.43, 026.63-026.819, 026.841-026.86, 026.891-026.93, 029.011-029.93, 035.7XX0-035.7XX9, 044.00-044.13, 045.8X1-045.93, 075.4, 075.81, 075.89-075.9, 080, 090.89, 099.111-099.285, 099.330-099.335, 099.350-099.355, 099.511-099.73, 099.820-099.825, 099.840-09A.53

A35   **Other tetanus**
> Tetanus NOS
> **Excludes1**   tetanus neonatorum (A33)
>   obstetrical tetanus (A34)
> (Ex) A35, B92, B94.2-B94.9

Item 1-7 Diptheria: A highly contagious bacterial disease that results in the formation of an adherent membrane in the throat that may lead to suffocation. In its most poisonous form, it attacks the heart and lungs. It is spread by direct physical contact or breathing the aerosolized secretions of infected individuals. The exact location is specified in the codes.

● **A36**   **Diphtheria**
> (Ex) For category A36 CC codes unless otherwise indicated: A36.0-A36.9

     A36.0   **Pharyngeal diphtheria**
> Diphtheritic membranous angina
> Tonsillar diphtheria

     A36.1   **Nasopharyngeal diphtheria**

     A36.2   **Laryngeal diphtheria**
> Diphtheritic laryngotracheitis

     A36.3   **Cutaneous diphtheria**
> **Excludes2**   erythrasma (L08.1)

●   **A36.8**   **Other diphtheria**

         A36.81   **Diphtheritic cardiomyopathy**
> Diphtheritic myocarditis
> (Ex) A36.81, A52.06, B33.20-B33.22, I00, I01.2-I01.9, I09.0, I09.9, I23.0-I23.3, I23.6-I23.8, I40.0-I41, I51.0, I51.3-I51.4, I87.8, I99.8-I99.9

         A36.82   **Diphtheritic radiculomyelitis**

         A36.83   **Diphtheritic polyneuritis**

         A36.84   **Diphtheritic tubulo-interstitial nephropathy**

         A36.85   **Diphtheritic cystitis**

         A36.86   **Diphtheritic conjunctivitis**

         A36.89   **Other diphtheritic complications**
> Diphtheritic peritonitis

     A36.9   **Diphtheria, unspecified**

● **A37**   **Whooping cough**
> *Pertussis is a highly contagious disease caused by the bacterium Bordetella pertussis and results in a whooping sounding cough.*
> (Ex) For category A37 CC codes A37.00, A37.10, A37.80, A37.90: A37.00-A37.91
> For category A37 CC codes A37.01, A37.11, A37.81, A37.91: A15.0-A15.9, A17.9, A18.82, A18.84, A18.89, A21.2, A22.1, A31.0, A37.00-A37.91, A42.0, A43.0, A48.1, B25.0, B39.0-B39.2, B44.0, B58.3, B59, B67.1, J09.X1-J09.X2, J10.00-J10.1, J11.00-J11.1, J12.0-J12.3, J12.89-J18.1, J18.8-J18.9, J22, J44.9, J47.0-J70.4, J70.8-J70.9, J98.4, J98.8-J98.9, Q33.4, R91.1

●   **A37.0**   **Whooping cough due to Bordetella pertussis**

         A37.00   **Whooping cough due to Bordetella pertussis without pneumonia**

         A37.01   **Whooping cough due to Bordetella pertussis with pneumonia**
> MCC when PDx is its own MCC

●   **A37.1**   **Whooping cough due to Bordetella parapertussis**

         A37.10   **Whooping cough due to Bordetella parapertussis without pneumonia**

         A37.11   **Whooping cough due to Bordetella parapertussis with pneumonia**
> MCC when PDx is its own MCC

●   **A37.8**   **Whooping cough due to other Bordetella species**

         A37.80   **Whooping cough due to other Bordetella species without pneumonia**

         A37.81   **Whooping cough due to other Bordetella species with pneumonia**
> MCC when PDx is its own MCC

●   **A37.9**   **Whooping cough, unspecified species**

         A37.90   **Whooping cough, unspecified species without pneumonia**

         A37.91   **Whooping cough, unspecified species with pneumonia**
> MCC when PDx is its own MCC

N   Newborn Age: 0   **P**   Pediatric Age: 0–17   **M**   Maternity DX: 12–55   **A**   Adult Age: 15–124   ♀   Females Only   ♂   Males Only

 Complication\Comorbidity   Major C\C   (Ex) CC/MCC Exclusions   Present on Admission Requirement   Hospital-Acquired Condition

747

CHAPTER 1 (A00-B99)

● **A38**   **Scarlet fever**
Most commonly caused by the bacteria Streptococcus pneumoniae and Neisseria meningitides
  Includes   scarlatina
  Excludes2   streptococcal sore throat (J02.0)
Ⓔ **For category A38 CC codes:** A38.0-A38.9, A46, J02.0, J03.00-J03.01

A38.0   **Scarlet fever with otitis media** 🔗
A38.1   **Scarlet fever with myocarditis** 🔗
A38.8   **Scarlet fever with other complications** 🔗
A38.9   **Scarlet fever, uncomplicated** 🔗
    Scarlet fever, NOS

● **A39**   **Meningococcal infection**
Most commonly caused by the bacteria Streptococcus pneumoniae and Neisseria meningitides

A39.0   **Meningococcal meningitis** 🔗
    Ⓔ A02.21, A17.0-A17.1, A27.81, A39.0, A39.89-A39.9, A49.3-A49.9, A50.41, A51.41, A52.13, A54.82, A54.84, A54.89-A54.9, A87.0-A87.9, B00.3, B02.1, B26.1, B37.5, B38.4, B45.1, B58.2, B92, B94.2-B94.9, B96.0, B96.6-B96.89, G00.0-G03.9, G04.2, G32.89, G61.0, G96.8-G96.9, G98.0-G98.8, G99.8

A39.1   **Waterhouse-Friderichsen syndrome** 🔗
    Fulminating complication of meningococcemia
    Meningococcal hemorrhagic adrenalitis
    Meningococcic adrenal syndrome
    Ⓔ A39.1, A39.89-A39.9, A49.3-A49.9, B92, B94.2-B94.9, B96.0, B96.6-B96.89

A39.2   **Acute meningococcemia** 🔗
    Ⓔ A02.1, A20.7, A22.7, A26.7, A32.7, A39.2-A39.4, A39.89-A41.9, A42.7, A49.3-A49.9, A54.86, B00.7, B37.7, B92, B94.2-B94.9, B96.0, B96.6-B96.89, R65.10-R65.20

A39.3   **Chronic meningococcemia** 🔗
    Ⓔ See A39.2

A39.4   **Meningococcemia, unspecified** 🔗
    Ⓔ See A39.2

● **A39.5**   **Meningococcal heart disease**
  A39.50   **Meningococcal carditis, unspecified** 🔗
      Ⓔ A39.50, A39.89-A39.9, A49.3-A49.9, B92, B94.2-B94.9, B96.0, B96.6-B96.89
  A39.51   **Meningococcal endocarditis** 🔗
      Ⓔ A39.51, A39.89-A39.9, A49.3-A49.9, B92, B94.2-B94.9, B96.0, B96.6-B96.89
  A39.52   **Meningococcal myocarditis** 🔗
      Ⓔ A39.52, A49.3-A49.9, B92, B94.2-B94.9, B96.0, B96.6-B96.89
  A39.53   **Meningococcal pericarditis** 🔗
      Ⓔ A39.53, A39.89-A39.9, A49.3-A49.9, B92, B94.2-B94.9, B96.0, B96.6-B96.89

● **A39.8**   **Other meningococcal infections**
  A39.81   **Meningococcal encephalitis** 🔗
      Ⓔ A39.81, A39.89-A39.9, A49.3-A49.9, B92, B94.2-B94.9, B96.0, B96.6-B96.89
  A39.82   **Meningococcal retrobulbar neuritis** 🔗
      Optic neuritis in portion of optic nerve posterior to eyeball; AKA postocular optic neuritis
      Ⓔ A39.82, A39.89-A39.9, A49.3-A49.9, B92, B94.2-B94.9, B96.0, B96.6-B96.89
  A39.83   **Meningococcal arthritis** 🔗
      Ⓔ A39.83-A39.9, A49.3-A49.9, B92, B94.2-B94.9, B96.0, B96.6-B96.89
  A39.84   **Postmeningococcal arthritis** 🔗
      Ⓔ See A39.83
  A39.89   **Other meningococcal infections** 🔗
      Meningococcal conjunctivitis
      Ⓔ A39.89-A39.9, A49.3-A49.9, B92, B94.2-B94.9, B96.0, B96.6-B96.89

A39.9   **Meningococcal infection, unspecified** 🔗
    Meningococcal disease NOS
    Ⓔ See A39.89

● **A40**   **Streptococcal sepsis**
Code first
  postprocedural streptococcal sepsis (T81.4)
  streptococcal sepsis during labor (O75.3)
  streptococcal sepsis following abortion or ectopic or molar pregnancy (O03-O07, O08.0)
  streptococcal sepsis following immunization (T88.0)
  streptococcal sepsis following infusion, transfusion or therapeutic injection (T80.2-)
  Excludes1   neonatal (P36.0-P36.1)
          puerperal sepsis (O85)
          sepsis due to Streptococcus, group D (A41.81)
Ⓔ **For category A40 CC codes unless otherwise indicated:** A02.1, A20.7, A22.7, A26.7, A32.7, A39.2-A39.4, A40.0-A40.1, A40.8-A41.9, A42.7, A48.2-A48.4, A48.8-A49.9, A54.86, B00.7, B3.77, B92, B94.2-B96.89, R65.10-R65.20, Z16.10-Z16.39

A40.0   **Sepsis due to streptococcus, group A** 🔗
A40.1   **Sepsis due to streptococcus, group B** 🔗
A40.3   **Sepsis due to Streptococcus pneumoniae** 🔗
    Pneumococcal sepsis
    Ⓔ No exclusions
A40.8   **Other streptococcal sepsis** 🔗
A40.9   **Streptococcal sepsis, unspecified** 🔗

● **A41**   **Other sepsis**
Code first
  postprocedural sepsis (T81.4)
  sepsis during labor (O75.3)
  sepsis following abortion, ectopic or molar pregnancy (O03-O07, O08.0)
  sepsis following immunization (T88.0)
  sepsis following infusion, transfusion or therapeutic injection (T80.2-)
  Excludes1   bacteremia NOS (R78.81)
          neonatal (P36.-)
          puerperal sepsis (O85)
          sepsis NOS (A41.9)
          streptococcal sepsis (A40.-)
  Excludes2   sepsis (due to) (in) actinomycotic (A42.7)
          sepsis (due to) (in) anthrax (A22.7)
          sepsis (due to) (in) candidal (B37.7)
          sepsis (due to) (in) Erysipelothrix (A26.7)
          sepsis (due to) (in) extraintestinal yersiniosis (A28.2)
          sepsis (due to) (in) gonococcal (A54.86)
          sepsis (due to) (in) herpesviral (B00.7)
          sepsis (due to) (in) listerial (A32.7)
          sepsis (due to) (in) melioidosis (A24.1)
          sepsis (due to) (in) meningococcal (A39.2-A39.4)
          sepsis (due to) (in) plague (A20.7)
          sepsis (due to) (in) tularemia (A21.7)
          toxic shock syndrome (A48.3)
Ⓔ **For category A41 CC codes:** A02.1, A20.7, A22.7, A26.7, A32.7, A39.2-A39.4, A40.0-A40.1, A40.8-A41.9, A42.7, A48.2-A48.4, A48.8-A49.9, A54.86, B00.7, B3.77, B92, B94.2-B96.89, R65.10-R65.20, Z16.10-Z16.39

● **A41.0**   **Sepsis due to Staphylococcus aureus**
  A41.01   **Sepsis due to Methicillin susceptible Staphylococcus aureus** 🔗
      MSSA sepsis
      Staphylococcus aureus sepsis NOS
  A41.02   **Sepsis due to Methicillin resistant Staphylococcus aureus** 🔗
A41.1   **Sepsis due to other specified staphylococcus** 🔗
    Coagulase negative staphylococcus sepsis
A41.2   **Sepsis due to unspecified staphylococcus** 🔗
A41.3   **Sepsis due to Hemophilus influenzae** 🔗
A41.4   **Sepsis due to anaerobes** 🔗
  Excludes1   gas gangrene (A48.0)

◀ New   ◀ Revised   ~~deleted~~ Deleted   Excludes 1   Excludes 2   Includes   Use additional   Code first   Code also   Unspecified
OGCR Official Guidelines   ● Unacceptable Principal Diagnosis   X Assign placeholder X   ● Use Additional Character(s)   ▶ Manifestation Code   **Coding Clinic**

● **A41.5**　**Sepsis due to other Gram-negative organisms**
　　A41.50　**Gram-negative sepsis, unspecified** 🔗
　　　　　Gram-negative sepsis NOS
　　A41.51　**Sepsis due to Escherichia coli [E. coli]** 🔗
　　A41.52　**Sepsis due to Pseudomonas** 🔗
　　　　　Pseudomonas aeroginosa
　　A41.53　**Sepsis due to Serratia** 🔗
　　A41.59　**Other Gram-negative sepsis** 🔗
● **A41.8**　**Other specified sepsis**
　　A41.81　**Sepsis due to Enterococcus** 🔗
　　A41.89　**Other specified sepsis** 🔗
　A41.9　**Sepsis, unspecified organism** 🔗
　　　　Septicemia NOS

● **A42**　**Actinomycosis**
　　Excludes1　actinomycetoma (B47.1)
　　A42.0　**Pulmonary actinomycosis** 🔗
　　　　Ⓔ A42.0, A42.81-A43.0, A43.8-A43.9, B47.1, J12.81
　　A42.1　**Abdominal actinomycosis** 🔗
　　　　Ⓔ A42.1, A42.81-A42.9, A43.8-A43.9, B47.1
　　A42.2　**Cervicofacial actinomycosis** 🔗
　　　　Ⓔ A42.2, A42.81-A42.9, A43.8-A43.9, B47.1
　　A42.7　**Actinomycotic sepsis** 🔗
　　　　Ⓔ A02.1, A20.7, A22.7, A26.7, A32.7, A39.2-A39.4, A40.0-A40.1, A40.8-A41.9, A42.7, A48.2-A48.4, A48.8-A49.9, A54.86, B00.7, B3.77, B92, B94.2-B96.89, R65.10-R65.20, Z16.10-Z16.39
　A42.8　**Other forms of actinomycosis**
　　　　Ⓔ **For category A42.8 CC codes:** A42.0-A42.2, A42.81-A43.9, B47.1-B47.9, L08.1
　　A42.81　**Actinomycotic meningitis** 🔗
　　A42.82　**Actinomycotic encephalitis** 🔗
　　A42.89　**Other forms of actinomycosis** 🔗
　A42.9　**Actinomycosis, unspecified** 🔗
　　　　Ⓔ A42.0-A42.2, A42.81-A43.9, B47.1-B47.9, L08.1

● **A43**　**Nocardiosis**
　　A43.0　**Pulmonary nocardiosis** 🔗
　　　　Ⓔ See A42.0
　　A43.1　**Cutaneous nocardiosis** 🔗
　　　　Ⓔ A42.81-A42.9, A43.1-A43.9, B47.1, L08.1
　　A43.8　**Other forms of nocardiosis** 🔗
　　　　Ⓔ See A42.9
　　A43.9　**Nocardiosis, unspecified** 🔗
　　　　Ⓔ See A42.9

● **A44**　**Bartonellosis**
　　Ⓔ **For category A44 CC codes:** A44.0-A44.9, A68.0-A68.9, A69.20-A69.29, A75.0-A79.9, B55.0-B57.5, B60.0
　　A44.0　**Systemic bartonellosis** 🔗
　　　　Oroya fever
　　A44.1　**Cutaneous and mucocutaneous bartonellosis** 🔗
　　　　Verruga peruana
　　A44.8　**Other forms of bartonellosis** 🔗
　　A44.9　**Bartonellosis, unspecified** 🔗

　A46　**Erysipelas**
　　Excludes1　postpartum or puerperal erysipelas (O86.89)

Item 1–8　**Gas gangrene** is a necrotizing subcutaneous infection that will cause tissue death. Patients with poor circulation (e.g., diabetes, peripheral nephropathy) will have low oxygen content in their tissues (hypoxia), which allows the Clostridium bacteria to flourish. Gas gangrene often occurs at the site of a surgical wound or trauma. Onset is sudden and dramatic. Treatment can include debridement, amputation, and/or hyperbaric oxygen treatments.

● **A48**　**Other bacterial diseases, not elsewhere classified**
　　Excludes1　actinomycetoma (B47.1)
　　A48.0　**Gas gangrene** 🔗
　　　　Clostridial cellulitis
　　　　Clostridial myonecrosis
　　　　Ⓔ A48.0, B92, B94.2-B94.9
　　A48.1　**Legionnaires' disease** 🔗
　　　　Ⓔ A15.0-A15.9, A17.9, A18.82, A18.84, A18.89, A21.2, A22.1, A31.0, A37.01, A37.11, A37.81, A37.91, A42.0, A43.0, A48.1, B25.0, B39.0-B39.2, B44.0, B58.3, B59, B67.1, J09.X1-J09.X2, J10.00-J10.1, J11.00-J11.1, J12.0-J12.3, J12.89-J18.1, J18.8-J18.9, J22, J44.9, J47.0-J70.4, J70.8-J70.9, J98.4, J98.8-J98.9, Q33.4, R91.1
　　A48.2　**Nonpneumonic Legionnaires' disease [Pontiac fever]**
　　A48.3　**Toxic shock syndrome** 🔗
　　　　Use additional code to identify the organism (B95, B96)
　　　　Excludes1　endotoxic shock NOS (R57.8)
　　　　　　　　sepsis NOS (A41.9)
　　　　Ⓔ A48.3, G89.0-G89.4, R09.89, R41.0-R41.3, R41.82, R41.9, R44.8-R44.9, R45.83-R45.84, R46.0-R46.89, R52, R57.0-R57.9, R65.21, R68.0-R68.19, R68.81-R68.89, R69
　　A48.4　**Brazilian purpuric fever**
　　　　Systemic Hemophilus aegyptius infection
　● **A48.5**　**Other specified botulism**
　　　　Non-foodborne intoxication due to toxins of Clostridium botulinum [C. botulinum]
　　　　Excludes1　food poisoning due to toxins of Clostridium botulinum (A05.1)
　　A48.51　**Infant botulism**　　　　　　　　　　　　P
　　　　Ⓔ A04.7, A05.0-A05.2, A48.51-A48.52
　　A48.52　**Wound botulism** 🔗
　　　　Non-foodborne botulism NOS
　　　　Use additional code for associated wound
　　　　Ⓔ A04.7, A05.0-A05.2, A48.51-A48.52
　　A48.8　**Other specified bacterial diseases**

● **A49**　**Bacterial infection of unspecified site**
　　Excludes1　bacterial agents as the cause of diseases classified elsewhere (B95-B96)
　　　　　　chlamydial infection NOS (A74.9)
　　　　　　meningococcal infection NOS (A39.9)
　　　　　　rickettsial infection NOS (A79.9)
　　　　　　spirochetal infection NOS (A69.9)
● **A49.0**　**Staphylococcal infection, unspecified site**
　　A49.01　**Methicillin susceptible Staphylococcus aureus infection, unspecified site**
　　　　Methicillin susceptible Staphylococcus aureus (MSSA) infection
　　　　Staphylococcus aureus infection NOS
　　A49.02　**Methicillin resistant Staphylococcus aureus infection, unspecified site**
　　　　Methicillin resistant Staphylococcus aureus (MRSA) infection
　A49.1　**Streptococcal infection, unspecified site**
　A49.2　**Hemophilus influenzae infection, unspecified site**
　　　Any of seven bacterium of genus Haemophilus
　A49.3　**Mycoplasma infection, unspecified site**
　　　Bacterium of class Mollicutes, unusual group of bacteria distinguished by absence of cell wall
　A49.8　**Other bacterial infections of unspecified site**
　A49.9　**Bacterial infection, unspecified**
　　　　Excludes1　bacteremia NOS (R78.81)

CHAPTER 1 (A00-B99)

N　Newborn Age: 0　　**P**　Pediatric Age: 0–17　　**M**　Maternity DX: 12–55　　**A**　Adult Age: 15–124　　♀ Females Only　　♂ Males Only
🔗 Complication\Comorbidity　　🔗 Major C\C　　Ⓔ CC/MCC Exclusions　　🔗 Present on Admission Requirement　　🔗 Hospital-Acquired Condition

749

Figure 1-3 Chancre of primary syphilis. (From Mandell, Bennett, & Dolin: Principles and Practice of Infectious Diseases, ed 7, Churchill Livingstone, An Imprint of Elsevier, 2009)

Item 1–9 Syphilis, also known as lues, is the most serious of the venereal diseases caused by *Treponema pallidum*. The **primary** stage is characterized by an ulceration known as **chancre,** which usually appears on the genitals but can also develop on the anus, lips, tonsils, breasts, or fingers. Syphilis is easy to cure in its early stages. A single intramuscular injection of penicillin will usually cure a person who has had syphilis for less than a year.

The **secondary** stage is characterized by a rash that can affect any area of the body. **Latent** syphilis is divided into **early,** which is diagnosed within two years of infection, and **late,** which is diagnosed two years or more after infection. Additional doses of penicillin or another antibiotic are needed to treat someone who has had syphilis for longer than a year. For those allergic to penicillin, there are other antibiotic treatments. **Congenital** syphilis is also labeled **early** or **late** based on the time of diagnosis.

INFECTIONS WITH A PREDOMINANTLY SEXUAL MODE OF TRANSMISSION (A50-A64)

> **Excludes1** human immunodeficiency virus [HIV] disease (B20)
> nonspecific and nongonococcal urethritis (N34.1)
> Reiter's disease (M02.3-)

● **A50 Congenital syphilis**

● **A50.0 Early congenital syphilis, symptomatic**
Any congenital syphilitic condition specified as early or manifest less than two years after birth
Ex: For category A50.0 CC codes: A50.01-A51.46, A51.5-A53.9

A50.01 Early congenital syphilitic oculopathy

A50.02 Early congenital syphilitic osteochondropathy

A50.03 Early congenital syphilitic pharyngitis
Early congenital syphilitic laryngitis

A50.04 Early congenital syphilitic pneumonia

A50.05 Early congenital syphilitic rhinitis

A50.06 Early cutaneous congenital syphilis

A50.07 Early mucocutaneous congenital syphilis

A50.08 Early visceral congenital syphilis

A50.09 Other early congenital syphilis, symptomatic

A50.1 Early congenital syphilis, latent
Congenital syphilis without clinical manifestations, with positive serological reaction and negative spinal fluid test, less than two years after birth

A50.2 Early congenital syphilis, unspecified
Congenital syphilis NOS less than two years after birth
Ex: A50.01-A51.46, A51.5-A54.85, A54.89-A58, A63.8, A64, B92, B94.2-B94.9, M02.30-M02.39, N34.1

● **A50.3 Late congenital syphilitic oculopathy**
> **Excludes1** Hutchinson's triad (A50.53)
Ex: For category A50.3 CC codes: A50.01-A51.46, A51.5-A53.9

A50.30 Late congenital syphilitic oculopathy, unspecified

A50.31 Late congenital syphilitic interstitial keratitis

A50.32 Late congenital syphilitic chorioretinitis

A50.39 Other late congenital syphilitic oculopathy

● **A50.4 Late congenital neurosyphilis [juvenile neurosyphilis]**
Use additional code to identify any associated mental disorder
> **Excludes1** Hutchinson's triad (A50.53)
Ex: For category A50.4 CC codes unless otherwise indicated: A50.01-A51.46, A51.5-A53.9, A56.00-A56.8, A63.8-A64, B92, B94.2-B94.9, N34.1

A50.40 Late congenital neurosyphilis, unspecified
Juvenile neurosyphilis NOS

A50.41 Late congenital syphilitic meningitis
Ex: A02.21, A17.0-A17.1, A27.81, A39.0, A50.01-A51.46, A51.5-A53.9, A54.82, A54.84, A54.89-A54.9, A56.00-A56.8, A63.8-A64, A87.0-A87.9, B00.3, B02.1, B26.1, B37.5, B38.4, B45.1, B58.2, B92, B94.2-B94.9, G00.0-G03.9, G04.2, G32.89, G61.0, G96.8-G96.9, G98.0-G98.8, G99.8, N34.1

A50.42 Late congenital syphilitic encephalitis

A50.43 Late congenital syphilitic polyneuropathy

A50.44 Late congenital syphilitic optic nerve atrophy
Ex: For category A50.0 CC codes: A50.01-A51.46, A51.5-A53.9

A50.45 Juvenile general paresis
Dementia paralytica juvenilis
Juvenile tabetoparetic neurosyphilis

A50.49 Other late congenital neurosyphilis
Juvenile tabes dorsalis

● **A50.5 Other late congenital syphilis, symptomatic**
Any congenital syphilitic condition specified as late or manifest two years or more after birth
Ex: For category A50.5 CC codes: A50.01-A51.46, A51.5-A53.9

A50.51 Clutton's joints

A50.52 Hutchinson's teeth

A50.53 Hutchinson's triad

A50.54 Late congenital cardiovascular syphilis

A50.55 Late congenital syphilitic arthropathy

A50.56 Late congenital syphilitic osteochondropathy

A50.57 Syphilitic saddle nose

A50.59 Other late congenital syphilis, symptomatic

A50.6 Late congenital syphilis, latent
Congenital syphilis without clinical manifestations, with positive serological reaction and negative spinal fluid test, two years or more after birth.

A50.7 Late congenital syphilis, unspecified
Congenital syphilis NOS two years or more after birth.

A50.9 Congenital syphilis, unspecified

● **A51 Early syphilis**

A51.0 Primary genital syphilis
Syphilitic chancre NOS

A51.1 Primary anal syphilis

A51.2 Primary syphilis of other sites

● **A51.3 Secondary syphilis of skin and mucous membranes**

A51.31 Condyloma latum
Ex: A50.01-A51.46, A51.5-A53.9

A51.32 Syphilitic alopecia
Ex: A50.01-A51.46, A51.5-A54.85, A54.89-A58, A63.8, A64, M02.30-M02.39, N34.1

A51.39 Other secondary syphilis of skin
Syphilitic leukoderma
Syphilitic mucous patch
> **Excludes1** late syphilitic leukoderma (A52.79)
Ex: See A51.31

◄ New ◄ Revised ~~deleted~~ Deleted Excludes 1 Excludes 2 Includes Use additional Code first Code also Unspecified
OGCR Official Guidelines ● Unacceptable Principal Diagnosis X Assign placeholder X ▶ Use Additional Character(s) ▶ Manifestation Code **Coding Clinic**

● **A51.4 Other secondary syphilis**

     A51.41 Secondary syphilitic meningitis 🩺
         Ⓔ A02.21, A17.0-A17.1, A27.81, A39.0, A50.01-A51.46, A51.5-A54.49,
         A54.5-A54.85, A54.89-A58, A63.8-A64, A74.81-A74.9,
         A87.0-A87.9, A96.2, A98.3-A98.4, B26.1, B33.24, B33.4-B33.8,
         B34.1-B34.2, B34.4-B34.8, B37.5, B38.4, B45.1, B58.2, B92,
         B94.2-B94.9, B97.10, B97.19, B97.29, B97.5-B97.6,
         B97.81-B97.89, G00.0-G03.9, G04.2, G32.89, G61.0,
         G96.8-G96.9, G98.0-G98.8, G99.8, M02.30-M02.39, N34.1

     A51.42 Secondary syphilitic female pelvic disease ♀ 🩺
         Ⓔ See A50.2

     A51.43 Secondary syphilitic oculopathy 🩺
         Secondary syphilitic chorioretinitis
         Secondary syphilitic iridocyclitis, iritis
         Secondary syphilitic uveitis
         Ⓔ See A51.31

     A51.44 Secondary syphilitic nephritis 🩺
         Ⓔ See A50.2

     A51.45 Secondary syphilitic hepatitis 🩺
         Ⓔ A50.01-A51.46, A51.5-A54.85, A54.89-A58, A63.8, A64,
         K71.0-K71.9, K73.1-K73.8, K74.0-K74.69, K75.2-K76.0,
         K76.4-K76.5, K76.89-K76.9, M02.30-M02.39, N34.1

     A51.46 Secondary syphilitic osteopathy 🩺
         Ⓔ A18.09, A50.01-A51.46, A51.5-A54.85, A54.89-A58, A63.8, A64,
         A66.6, M02.30-M02.39, M84.80-M84.9, M85.10-M85.19,
         M85.80-M85.89, M86.30-M86.8X9, M89.20-M89.39,
         M89.50-M89.59, M89.8X0-M89.8X9, M94.1,
         M94.351-M94.8X9, N34.1

     A51.49 Other secondary syphilitic conditions 🩺
         Secondary syphilitic lymphadenopathy
         Secondary syphilitic myositis

   A51.5 Early syphilis, latent
         Syphilis (acquired) without clinical manifestations, with
         positive serological reaction and negative spinal
         fluid test, less than two years after infection.

   A51.9 Early syphilis, unspecified

● **A52 Late syphilis**

   ● **A52.0 Cardiovascular and cerebrovascular syphilis**
         Ⓔ For category A52.0 CC codes: A50.01-A51.46, A51.5-A53.9, A56.00-A56.8,
         A63.8-A64, B92, B94.2-B94.9, N34.1

     A52.00 Cardiovascular syphilis, unspecified 🩺

     A52.01 Syphilitic aneurysm of aorta 🩺

     A52.02 Syphilitic aortitis 🩺

     A52.03 Syphilitic endocarditis 🩺
         Syphilitic aortic valve incompetence or stenosis
         Syphilitic mitral valve stenosis
         Syphilitic pulmonary valve regurgitation

     A52.04 Syphilitic cerebral arteritis 🩺

     A52.05 Other cerebrovascular syphilis 🩺
         Syphilitic cerebral aneurysm (ruptured) (non-
         ruptured)
         Syphilitic cerebral thrombosis

     A52.06 Other syphilitic heart involvement 🩺
         Syphilitic coronary artery disease
         Syphilitic myocarditis
         Syphilitic pericarditis

     A52.09 Other cardiovascular syphilis 🩺

   ● **A52.1 Symptomatic neurosyphilis**
         Ⓔ For category A52.1 CC codes unless otherwise indicated: A50.01-A51.46,
         A51.5-A53.9, A56.00-A56.8, A63.8-A64, B92, B94.2-B94.9, N34.1

     A52.10 Symptomatic neurosyphilis, unspecified 🩺

     A52.11 Tabes dorsalis 🩺
         *Cognitive decline with progressive degeneration of
         posterior columns, roots, and ganglia of spinal
         cord, occur 15-20 years after initial infection
         of syphilis; AKA Duchenne disease*
         Locomotor ataxia (progressive)
         Tabetic neurosyphilis

     A52.12 Other cerebrospinal syphilis 🩺

     A52.13 Late syphilitic meningitis 🩺
         Ⓔ A02.21, A17.0-A17.1, A27.81, A39.0, A50.01-A51.46,
         A51.5-A53.9, A54.82, A54.84, A54.89-A54.9, A56.00-A56.8,
         A63.8-A64, A87.0-A87.9, B00.3, B02.1, B26.1, B37.5, B38.4,
         B45.1, B58.2, B92, B94.2-B94.9, G00.0-G03.9, G04.2, G32.89,
         G61.0, G96.8-G96.9, G98.0-G98.8, G99.8, N34.1

     A52.14 Late syphilitic encephalitis 🩺

     A52.15 Late syphilitic neuropathy 🩺
         Late syphilitic acoustic neuritis
         Late syphilitic optic (nerve) atrophy
         Late syphilitic polyneuropathy
         Late syphilitic retrobulbar neuritis

     A52.16 Charcôt's arthropathy (tabetic) 🩺
         *Progressive musculoskeletal condition characterized
         by joint dislocation, fractures, and deformities,
         results in progressive destruction of bone and
         soft tissue of weight-bearing joints*

     A52.17 General paresis 🩺
         *Chronic meningoencephalitis results in loss of
         cortical function, or progressive dementia
         and generalized paralysis, occurring 10-20
         years after initial infection of syphilis; AKA
         Bayle disease, dementia paralytica, paralytic
         dementiaparetic neurosyphilis, syphilitic
         meningoencephalitis*
         Dementia paralytica

     A52.19 Other symptomatic neurosyphilis 🩺
         Syphilitic parkinsonism

   A52.2 Asymptomatic neurosyphilis 🩺
         Ⓔ See A52.10

   A52.3 Neurosyphilis, unspecified 🩺
         Gumma (syphilitic)
         Destructive lesions of syphilis
         Syphilis (late)
         Syphiloma
         Ⓔ See A52.10

● **A52.7 Other symptomatic late syphilis**
         Ⓔ For category A52.7 CC codes unless otherwise indicated: A50.01-A51.46,
         A51.5-A54.85, A54.89-A58, A63.8, A64, M02.30-M02.39, N34.1

     A52.71 Late syphilitic oculopathy 🩺
         Late syphilitic chorioretinitis
         Late syphilitic episcleritis
         Ⓔ A18.50-A18.59, A50.01-A51.46, A51.5-A54.85, A54.89-A58,
         A63.8-A64, H15.001-H15.009, H15.091-H15.129,
         M02.30-M02.39, N34.1

     A52.72 Syphilis of lung and bronchus 🩺

     **A52.73 Symptomatic late syphilis of other respiratory
             organs** 🩺

     A52.74 Syphilis of liver and other viscera 🩺
         Late syphilitic peritonitis

     A52.75 Syphilis of kidney and ureter 🩺
         Syphilitic glomerular disease

     **A52.76 Other genitourinary symptomatic late
             syphilis** 🩺
         Late syphilitic female pelvic inflammatory
         disease

     A52.77 Syphilis of bone and joint 🩺

     A52.78 Syphilis of other musculoskeletal tissue 🩺
         Late syphilitic bursitis
         Syphilis [stage unspecified] of bursa
         Syphilis [stage unspecified] of muscle
         Syphilis [stage unspecified] of synovium
         Syphilis [stage unspecified] of tendon

     A52.79 Other symptomatic late syphilis 🩺
         Late syphilitic leukoderma
         Syphilis of adrenal gland
         Syphilis of pituitary gland
         Syphilis of thyroid gland
         Syphilitic splenomegaly
         Excludes1 syphilitic leukoderma
                 (secondary) (A51.39)

N   Newborn Age: 0   P   Pediatric Age: 0–17   M   Maternity DX: 12–55   A   Adult Age: 15–124   ♀   Females Only   ♂   Males Only

🩺 Complication\Comorbidity   🩺 Major C\C   Ⓔ CC/MCC Exclusions   🩺 Present on Admission Requirement   🩺 Hospital-Acquired Condition

A52.8   Late syphilis, latent
Syphilis (acquired) without clinical manifestations, with positive serological reaction and negative spinal fluid test, two years or more after infection

A52.9   Late syphilis, unspecified

● **A53   Other and unspecified syphilis**

A53.0   Latent syphilis, unspecified as early or late
Latent syphilis NOS
Positive serological reaction for syphilis

A53.9   Syphilis, unspecified
Infection due to Treponema pallidum NOS
Syphilis (acquired) NOS
Excludes1   syphilis NOS under two years of age (A50.2)

● **A54   Gonococcal infection**

● **A54.0   Gonococcal infection of lower genitourinary tract without periurethral or accessory gland abscess**
Excludes1   gonococcal infection with genitourinary gland abscess (A54.1)
gonococcal infection with periurethral abscess (A54.1)
(Ex:) For category A54.0 CC codes: A54.00-A54.29, A54.82, A54.84, A54.89, A54.9, A56.00-A56.8, A63.8-A64, B92, B94.-B94.9, N34.1

A54.00   Gonococcal infection of lower genitourinary tract, unspecified

A54.01   Gonococcal cystitis and urethritis, unspecified

A54.02   Gonococcal vulvovaginitis, unspecified ♀

A54.03   Gonococcal cervicitis, unspecified ♀

A54.09   Other gonococcal infection of lower genitourinary tract

A54.1   Gonococcal infection of lower genitourinary tract with periurethral and accessory gland abscess
Gonococcal Bartholin's gland abscess

● **A54.2   Gonococcal pelviperitonitis and other gonococcal genitourinary infection**
(Ex:) For category A54.2 CC codes: A54.00-A54.29, A54.82, A54.84, A54.89, A54.9, A56.00-A56.8, A63.8-A64, B92, B94.-B94.9, N34.1

A54.21   Gonococcal infection of kidney and ureter

A54.22   Gonococcal prostatitis ♂

A54.23   Gonococcal infection of other male genital organs ♂
Gonococcal epididymitis
Gonococcal orchitis

A54.24   Gonococcal female pelvic inflammatory disease ♀
Gonococcal pelviperitonitis
Excludes1   gonococcal peritonitis (A54.85)

A54.29   Other gonococcal genitourinary infections

● **A54.3   Gonococcal infection of eye**
(Ex:) For category A54.3 CC codes: A50.01-A51.46, A51.5-A54.85, A54.89-A58, A63.8, A64, M02.30-M02.39, N34.1

A54.30   Gonococcal infection of eye, unspecified

A54.31   Gonococcal conjunctivitis
Form of bacterial conjunctivitis contracted by newborns during delivery; AKA neonatal conjunctivitis
Ophthalmia neonatorum due to gonococcus

A54.32   Gonococcal iridocyclitis
Inflammation of iris and of ciliary body due to gonococcal infection

A54.33   Gonococcal keratitis
Inflammation of cornea due to gonococcal infection; AKA keratoconjunctivitis, keratopathy

A54.39   Other gonococcal eye infection
Gonococcal endophthalmia

● **A54.4   Gonococcal infection of musculoskeletal system**
(Ex:) For category A54.4 CC codes: A02.23, A17.9, A18.02, A18.09, A18.82, A18.84, A18.89, A39.83-A39.84, A50.01-A51.9, A52.00-A54.89, A54.9-A58, A63.8, A64, B06.82, M00.00-M02.9, M05.40-M05.59, M05.70-M06.09, M06.20-M06.39, M06.80-M07.69, M11.00-M11.9, M12.10-M15.0, M15.3-M15.9, M16.2-M16.9, M17.2-M17.9, M18.2-M18.9, M19.111-M19.93, M24.10-M24.176, M25.00, M25.08, M25.10-M25.18, M25.40-M25.676, M25.80-M25.9, M35.2, M36.1-M36.4, N34.1, R29.4

A54.40   Gonococcal infection of musculoskeletal system, unspecified

A54.41   Gonococcal spondylopathy
Disorder of vertebrae due to gonococcal infection; AKA rachiopathy

A54.42   Gonococcal arthritis
Excludes2   gonococcal infection of spine (A54.41)

A54.43   Gonococcal osteomyelitis
Excludes2   gonococcal infection of spine (A54.41)

A54.49   Gonococcal infection of other musculoskeletal tissue
Gonococcal bursitis
Gonococcal myositis
Gonococcal synovitis
Gonococcal tenosynovitis

A54.5   Gonococcal pharyngitis

A54.6   Gonococcal infection of anus and rectum

● **A54.8   Other gonococcal infections**

A54.81   Gonococcal meningitis
(Ex:) A02.21, A17.0-A17.1, A27.81, A39.0, A50.01-A51.46, A51.5-A54.49, A54.5-A54.85, A54.89-A58, A63.8-A64, A74.81-A74.9, A87.0-A87.9, A96.2, A98.3-A98.4, B26.1, B33.24, B33.4-B33.8, B34.1-B34.2, B34.4-B34.8, B37.5, B38.4, B45.1, B58.2, B92, B94.2-B94.9, B97.10, B97.19, B97.29, B97.5-B97.6, B97.81-B97.89, G00.0-G03.9, G04.2, G32.89, G61.0, G96.8-G96.9, G98.0-G98.8, G99.8, M02.30-M02.39, N34.1

A54.82   Gonococcal brain abscess
(Ex:) A50.01-A51.46, A51.5-A54.85, A54.89-A58, A63.8, A64, M02.30-M02.39, N25.81-N25.89, N34.1

A54.83   Gonococcal heart infection
Gonococcal endocarditis
Gonococcal myocarditis
Gonococcal pericarditis
(Ex:) A01.00-A01.09, A39.51, A50.01-A58, A63.8-A64, A78, B33.20-B33.22, B37.6, B40.0-B40.9, I00, I01.1-I02.0, I05.0-I05.1, I05.2, I05.8-I08.3, I08.9-I09.1, I09.89-I09.9, I23.0-I23.3, I23.6-I23.8, I33.0-I41, I42.4, I51.0, I51.3-I51.4, I87.8, I99.8-I99.9, M00.00, M00.08-M00.10, M00.18-M00.20, M00.28-M00.80, M00.88-M00.9, M02.30-M02.39, N34.1, Q22.2, Q23.8, Q23.9, Q24.8, T82.6XX[A]

A54.84   Gonococcal pneumonia
(Ex:) See A54.82

A54.85   Gonococcal peritonitis
Excludes1   gonococcal pelviperitonitis (A54.24)

A54.86   Gonococcal sepsis
MCC when PDx is its own MCC
(Ex:) A02.1, A20.7, A22.7, A26.7, A32.7, A39.2-A39.4, A40.0-A40.1, A40.8-A41.9, A42.7, A48.2-A48.4, A48.8-A49.9, A54.86, B00.7, B3.77, B92, B94.2-B96.89, R65.10-R65.20, Z16.10-Z16.39

A54.89   Other gonococcal infections
Gonococcal keratoderma
Gonococcal lymphadenitis
(Ex:) See A54.82

A54.9   Gonococcal infection, unspecified
(Ex:) See A54.82

A55   Chlamydial lymphogranuloma (venereum)
Climatic or tropical bubo
Durand-Nicolas-Favre disease
Esthiomene
Lymphogranuloma inguinale

Item 1-10 An STD (sexually transmitted disease) caused by **Neisseria gonorrhoeae** that flourishes in the warm, moist areas of the reproductive tract. Untreated gonorrhea spreads to other parts of the body, causing inflammation of the testes or prostate or pelvic inflammatory disease (PID).

◄ New   ◄ Revised   ̶d̶e̶l̶e̶t̶e̶d̶ Deleted   Excludes 1   Excludes 2   Includes   Use additional   Code first   Code also   Unspecified
OGCR Official Guidelines   ● Unacceptable Principal Diagnosis   X Assign placeholder X   ● Use Additional Character(s)   ▌ Manifestation Code   **Coding Clinic**

● **A56**   **Other sexually transmitted chlamydial diseases**

> **Includes**   sexually transmitted diseases due to Chlamydia trachomatis

> **Excludes1**   neonatal chlamydial conjunctivitis (P39.1)
> neonatal chlamydial pneumonia (P23.1)

> **Excludes2**   chlamydial lymphogranuloma (A55)
> conditions classified to A74.-

● **A56.0**   **Chlamydial infection of lower genitourinary tract**

     A56.00   **Chlamydial infection of lower genitourinary tract, unspecified**

     A56.01   **Chlamydial cystitis and urethritis**

     A56.02   **Chlamydial vulvovaginitis ♀**

     A56.09   **Other chlamydial infection of lower genitourinary tract**
         Chlamydial cervicitis

● **A56.1**   **Chlamydial infection of pelviperitoneum and other genitourinary organs**

     A56.11   **Chlamydial female pelvic inflammatory disease ♀**

     A56.19   **Other chlamydial genitourinary infection**
         Chlamydial epididymitis
         Chlamydial orchitis

   A56.2   **Chlamydial infection of genitourinary tract, unspecified**

   A56.3   **Chlamydial infection of anus and rectum**

   A56.4   **Chlamydial infection of pharynx**

   A56.8   **Sexually transmitted chlamydial infection of other sites**

A57   **Chancroid**
     Ulcus molle
     Sexually transmitted infection caused by bacteria, Haemophilus ducreyi

A58   **Granuloma inguinale**
     Chronic, progressive, ulcerative granulomatous disease
     Donovanosis

● **A59**   **Trichomoniasis**

> **Excludes2**   intestinal trichomoniasis (A07.8)

     A common STD caused by a parasite, Trichomonas vaginalis

● **A59.0**   **Urogenital trichomoniasis**

     A59.00   **Urogenital trichomoniasis, unspecified**
         Fluor (vaginalis) due to Trichomonas
         Leukorrhea (vaginalis) due to Trichomonas

     A59.01   **Trichomonal vulvovaginitis ♀**

     A59.02   **Trichomonal prostatitis ♂**

     A59.03   **Trichomonal cystitis and urethritis**

     A59.09   **Other urogenital trichomoniasis**
         Common sexually transmitted disease (STD) caused by single-celled protozoan parasite; AKA trich
         Trichomonas cervicitis

   A59.8   **Trichomoniasis of other sites**

   A59.9   **Trichomoniasis, unspecified**

● **A60**   **Anogenital herpesviral [herpes simplex] infections**

● **A60.0**   **Herpesviral infection of genitalia and urogenital tract**

     A60.00   **Herpesviral infection of urogenital system, unspecified**

     A60.01   **Herpesviral infection of penis ♂**

     A60.02   **Herpesviral infection of other male genital organs ♂**

     A60.03   **Herpesviral cervicitis ♀**

     A60.04   **Herpesviral vulvovaginitis ♀**
         Herpesviral [herpes simplex] ulceration
         Herpesviral [herpes simplex] vaginitis
         Herpesviral [herpes simplex] vulvitis

     A60.09   **Herpesviral infection of other urogenital tract**

   A60.1   **Herpesviral infection of perianal skin and rectum**

   A60.9   **Anogenital herpesviral infection, unspecified**

● **A63**   **Other predominantly sexually transmitted diseases, not elsewhere classified**

> **Excludes2**   molluscum contagiosum (B08.1)
> papilloma of cervix (D26.0)

   A63.0   **Anogenital (venereal) warts**
     Anogenital warts due to (human) papillomavirus [HPV]
     Condyloma acuminatum

   A63.8   **Other specified predominantly sexually transmitted diseases**

A64   **Unspecified sexually transmitted disease**

OTHER SPIROCHETAL DISEASES (A65-A69)

> **Excludes2**   leptospirosis (A27.-)
> syphilis (A50-A53)

A65   **Nonvenereal syphilis**
     Bejel
     Endemic syphilis
     Njovera

● **A66**   **Yaws**
     Endemic, infectious, tropical disease caused by spirochete, spread by direct contact; AKA frambesia, framboesia, frambesia tropica

> **Includes**   bouba
> frambesia (tropica)
> pian

   A66.0   **Initial lesions of yaws**
     Chancre of yaws
     Frambesia, initial or primary
     Initial frambesial ulcer
     Mother yaw

   A66.1   **Multiple papillomata and wet crab yaws**
     Frambesioma
     Pianoma
     Plantar or palmar papilloma of yaws

   A66.2   **Other early skin lesions of yaws**
     Cutaneous yaws, less than five years after infection
     Early yaws (cutaneous)(macular)(maculopapular) (micropapular)(papular)
     Frambeside of early yaws

   A66.3   **Hyperkeratosis of yaws**
     Hypertrophy of stratum corneum of skin in which there are small, hard, verrucous scales
     Ghoul hand
     Hyperkeratosis, palmar or plantar (early) (late) due to yaws
     Worm-eaten soles

   A66.4   **Gummata and ulcers of yaws**
     Small, rubbery granuloma with necrotic center and inflamed characteristic of advanced stage of syphilis; AKA syphiloma
     Gummatous frambeside
     Nodular late yaws (ulcerated)

   A66.5   **Gangosa**
     Manifestation of yaws that develops in the soft palate and spreads eroding bone, cartilage, and soft tissue
     Rhinopharyngitis mutilans

   A66.6   **Bone and joint lesions of yaws**
     Yaws ganglion
     Yaws goundou
     Yaws gumma, bone
     Yaws gummatous osteitis or periostitis
     Yaws hydrarthrosis
     Yaws osteitis
     Yaws periostitis (hypertrophic)

   A66.7   **Other manifestations of yaws**
     Juxta-articular nodules of yaws
     Mucosal yaws

   A66.8   **Latent yaws**
     Yaws without clinical manifestations, with positive serology

   A66.9   **Yaws, unspecified**

N   Newborn Age: 0   **P**   Pediatric Age: 0–17   **M**   Maternity DX: 12–55   **A**   Adult Age: 15–124   ♀   Females Only   ♂   Males Only

🔹 Complication\Comorbidity   🔹 Major C\C   (Ex) CC/MCC Exclusions   🔹 Present on Admission Requirement   🔹 Hospital-Acquired Condition

● **A67**   **Pinta [carate]**
     Group of nonvenereal diseases caused by Treponema species

     A67.0   **Primary lesions of pinta**
         Chancre (primary) of pinta
         Papule (primary) of pinta

     A67.1   **Intermediate lesions of pinta**
         Erythematous plaques of pinta
         Hyperchromic lesions of pinta
         Hyperkeratosis of pinta
         Pintids

     A67.2   **Late lesions of pinta**
         Achromic skin lesions of pinta
         Cicatricial skin lesions of pinta
         Dyschromic skin lesions of pinta

     A67.3   **Mixed lesions of pinta**
         Achromic with hyperchromic skin lesions of pinta
         [carate]

     A67.9   **Pinta, unspecified**

● **A68**   **Relapsing fevers**
     Includes   recurrent fever
     Excludes2   Lyme disease (A69.2-)
     (Ex) **For category A68 CC codes:** A44.0-A44.9, A68.0-A68.9, A69.20-A69.29, A75.0-A79.9, B55.0-B57.5, B60.0

     A68.0   **Louse-borne relapsing fever** 🔍
         Relapsing fever due to Borrelia recurrentis

     A68.1   **Tick-borne relapsing fever** 🔍
         Relapsing fever due to any Borrelia species other than
         Borrelia recurrentis

     A68.9   **Relapsing fever, unspecified** 🔍

● **A69**   **Other spirochetal infections**

     A69.0   **Necrotizing ulcerative stomatitis**
         Cancrum oris
         Fusospirochetal gangrene
         Noma
         Stomatitis gangrenosa

     A69.1   **Other Vincent's infections** 🔍
         Fusospirochetal pharyngitis
         Necrotizing ulcerative (acute) gingivitis
         Necrotizing ulcerative (acute) gingivostomatitis
         Spirochetal stomatitis
         Trench mouth
         Vincent's angina
         Vincent's gingivitis
         (Ex) A69.1

●   **A69.2**   **Lyme disease**
         Erythema chronicum migrans due to Borrelia
         burgdorferi
         (Ex) **For category A69.2 CC codes:** A44.0-A44.9, A68.0-A68.9, A69.20-A69.29, A75.0-A79.9, B55.0-B57.5, B60.0

     A69.20   **Lyme disease, unspecified** 🔍

     A69.21   **Meningitis due to Lyme disease** 🔍

     A69.22   **Other neurologic disorders in Lyme disease** 🔍
         Cranial neuritis
         Meningoencephalitis
         Polyneuropathy

     A69.23   **Arthritis due to Lyme disease** 🔍

     A69.29   **Other conditions associated with Lyme disease** 🔍
         Myopericarditis due to Lyme disease

     A69.8   **Other specified spirochetal infections**

     A69.9   **Spirochetal infection, unspecified**

OTHER DISEASES CAUSED BY CHLAMYDIAE (A70-A74)

     Excludes1   sexually transmitted chlamydial diseases
         (A55-A56)

     A70   **Chlamydia psittaci infections** 🔍
         Ornithosis
         Parrot fever
         Psittacosis
         (Ex) A70

● **A71**   **Trachoma**
     Excludes1   sequelae of trachoma (B94.0)

     A71.0   **Initial stage of trachoma**
         Trachoma dubium

     A71.1   **Active stage of trachoma**
         Granular conjunctivitis (trachomatous)
         Trachomatous follicular conjunctivitis
         Trachomatous pannus

     A71.9   **Trachoma, unspecified**

● **A74**   **Other diseases caused by chlamydiae**
     Excludes1   neonatal chlamydial conjunctivitis (P39.1)
         neonatal chlamydial pneumonia (P23.1)
         Reiter's disease (M02.3-)
         sexually transmitted chlamydial diseases
         (A55-A56)

     Excludes2   chlamydial pneumonia (J16.0)

     A74.0   **Chlamydial conjunctivitis** 🔍
         Paratrachoma

●   **A74.8**   **Other chlamydial diseases**

         A74.81   **Chlamydial peritonitis**

         A74.89   **Other chlamydial diseases**

     A74.9   **Chlamydial infection, unspecified**
         Chlamydiosis NOS

RICKETTSIOSES (A75-A79)

● **A75**   **Typhus fever**
     Excludes1   rickettsiosis due to Ehrlichia sennetsu (A79.81) ◀
     (Ex) **For category A75 CC codes unless otherwise indicated:** A44.0-A44.9, A68.0-A68.9, A69.20-A69.29, A75.0-A79.9, B55.0-B57.5, B60.0

     A75.0   **Epidemic louse-borne typhus fever due to Rickettsia prowazekii** 🔍
         Organisms transmitted between humans via louse
         Classical typhus (fever)
         Epidemic (louse-borne) typhus

     A75.1   **Recrudescent typhus [Brill's disease]** 🔍
         Brill-Zinsser disease

     A75.2   **Typhus fever due to Rickettsia typhi** 🔍
         Murine (flea-borne) typhus

     A75.3   **Typhus fever due to Rickettsia tsutsugamushi** 🔍
         Scrub (mite-borne) typhus
         Tsutsugamushi fever

     A75.9   **Typhus fever, unspecified** 🔍
         Typhus (fever) NOS
         (Ex) A17.82, A44.0-A44.9, A50.42, A52.14, A68.0-A68.9, A69.20-A69.29, A75.0-A79.9, A81.1, A81.82-A81.89, A83.0-A85.8, A87.2, A88.0, A88.8, A92.1-A92.8, A93.0, B00.4, B00.82, B01.11-B01.12, B04, B06.01, B08.09, B08.20-B08.22, B08.60-B08.79, B09, B10.01-B10.09, B26.2, B33.1, B45.0, B45.2-B45.9, B50.9, B55.0-B57.5, B58.2, B60.0, B75, B97.10, B97.21, G04.00-G04.01, G04.31, G04.81-G05.4, G37.0, G37.4-G37.5, J09.X3-J09.X9, J10.2-J10.89, J11.2-J11.89, L44.4, M1A.10X0-M1A.19X1, P35.2-P35.9, P37.0-P37.4, P37.8-P37.9, T56.0X1-T56.0X4[A]

Item 1-12   **Rickettsioses** are diseases spread from ticks, lice, fleas, or mites to humans.
     Typhus is spread to humans chiefly by the fleas of rats.
     Endemic identifies a disease as being present in low numbers of humans at all times, whereas **epidemic** identifies a disease as being present in high numbers of humans at a specific time. Morbidity (death) is higher in epidemic diseases.
     Brill's disease, also known as **Brill-Zinsser disease,** is spread from human to human by body lice and also from the lice of flying squirrels. **Scrub typhus** is spread in the same ways as Brill's disease.
     Malaria is spread to humans by mosquitoes.

Item 1-11   **Cancrum oris,** also known as **noma** or **gangrenous stomatitis,** begins as an ulcer of the gingiva and results in a progressive gangrenous process.

◀ New   ◀ Revised   ~~deleted~~ Deleted   Excludes 1   Excludes 2   Includes   Use additional   Code first   Code also   Unspecified

OGCR Official Guidelines   ● Unacceptable Principal Diagnosis   X Assign placeholder X   ● Use Additional Character(s)   ▮ Manifestation Code   **Coding Clinic**

● **A77 Spotted fever [tick-borne rickettsioses]**
(Ex) *For category A77 CC codes: A44.0-A44.9, A68.0-A68.9, A69.20-A69.29, A75.0-A79.9, B55.0-B57.5, B60.0*

A77.0 Spotted fever due to Rickettsia rickettsii 🔖
Rocky Mountain spotted fever
Sao Paulo fever

A77.1 Spotted fever due to Rickettsia conorii 🔖
African tick typhus
Boutonneuse fever
India tick typhus
Kenya tick typhus
Marseilles fever
Mediterranean tick fever

A77.2 Spotted fever due to Rickettsia siberica 🔖
North Asian tick fever
Siberian tick typhus

A77.3 Spotted fever due to Rickettsia australis 🔖
Queensland tick typhus

● **A77.4 Ehrlichiosis**
Type of tick-borne fever caused by bacteria infection
Excludes1 Rickettsiosis due to Ehrlichia sennetsu (A79.81)

A77.40 Ehrlichiosis, unspecified 🔖
A77.41 Ehrlichiosis chafeensis [E. chafeensis] 🔖
A77.49 Other ehrlichiosis 🔖

A77.8 Other spotted fevers 🔖

A77.9 Spotted fever, unspecified 🔖
Tick-borne typhus NOS

A78 Q fever 🔖
Infection due to Coxiella burnetii
Nine Mile fever
Quadrilateral fever
(Ex) See A77.0

● **A79 Other rickettsioses**
(Ex) *For category A79 CC codes unless otherwise indicated: A77.0-A79.9*

A79.0 Trench fever 🔖
Quintan fever
Wolhynian fever
(Ex) See A77.0

A79.1 Rickettsialpox due to Rickettsia akari 🔖
Kew Garden fever
Vesicular rickettsiosis

● **A79.8 Other specified rickettsioses**
A79.81 Rickettsiosis due to Ehrlichia sennetsu 🔖
A79.89 Other specified rickettsioses 🔖

A79.9 Rickettsiosis, unspecified 🔖
Rickettsial infection NOS

VIRAL AND PRION INFECTIONS OF THE CENTRAL NERVOUS SYSTEM (A80-A89)

Excludes1 postpolio syndrome (G14)
sequelae of poliomyelitis (B91)
sequelae of viral encephalitis (B94.1)

● **A80 Acute poliomyelitis**
(Ex) *For category A80 CC codes: A80.0-A80.39*

A80.0 Acute paralytic poliomyelitis, vaccine-associated 🔖
A80.1 Acute paralytic poliomyelitis, wild virus, imported 🔖
A80.2 Acute paralytic poliomyelitis, wild virus, indigenous 🔖
● **A80.3 Acute paralytic poliomyelitis, other and unspecified**
A80.30 Acute paralytic poliomyelitis, unspecified 🔖
A80.39 Other acute paralytic poliomyelitis 🔖
A80.4 Acute nonparalytic poliomyelitis
A80.9 Acute poliomyelitis, unspecified

● **A81 Atypical virus infections of central nervous system**
Includes diseases of the central nervous system caused by prions
Use additional code to identify:
dementia with behavioral disturbance (F02.81)
dementia without behavioral disturbance (F02.80)

● **A81.0 Creutzfeldt-Jakob disease**
(Ex) *For category A81.0 CC codes: A17.82, A50.42, A52.14, A75.9, A79.9, A81.00-A81.9, A83.0-A85.8, A87.2, A88.0, A88.8, A92.1-A92.2, A92.4-A92.8, A93.0, B00.4, B00.82, B01.11-B01.12, B04, B06.01, B08.09, B08.20-B08.22, B08.60-B08.79, B09, B10.01-B10.09, B26.2, B33.1, B45.0, B45.2-B45.9, B58.2, B75, B97.10, G04.00-G04.01, G04.31, G04.81-G05.4, G37.0, G37.4-G37.5, I67.3, J09.X3-J09.X9, J10.2-J10.89, J11.2-J11.89, L44.4, M1A.10X0-M1A.19X1, P35.2-P35.9, P37.0-P37.4, P37.8-P37.9, T56.0X1-T56.0X4[A]*

A81.00 Creutzfeldt-Jakob disease, unspecified 🔖
Jakob-Creutzfeldt disease, unspecified

A81.01 Variant Creutzfeldt-Jakob disease 🔖
vCJD

A81.09 Other Creutzfeldt-Jakob disease 🔖
CJD
Familial Creutzfeldt-Jakob disease
Iatrogenic Creutzfeldt-Jakob disease
Sporadic Creutzfeldt-Jakob disease
Subacute spongiform encephalopathy (with dementia)

A81.1 Subacute sclerosing panencephalitis 🔖
Type of viral encephalitis that causes parenchymatous lesions in gray and white matter of brain
Dawson's inclusion body encephalitis
Van Bogaert's sclerosing leukoencephalopathy
(Ex) A81.1, B92, B94.2-B94.9

A81.2 Progressive multifocal leukoencephalopathy 🔖
Group of diseases affecting white matter of brain
Multifocal leukoencephalopathy NOS
(Ex) A17.82, A50.42, A52.14, A75.9, A79.9, A81.00-A81.9, A83.0-A85.8, A87.2, A88.0, A88.8, A92.1-A92.2, A92.4-A92.8, A93.0, B00.4, B00.82, B01.11-B01.12, B04, B06.01, B08.09, B08.20-B08.22, B08.60-B08.79, B09, B10.01-B10.09, B26.2, B27.00-B27.99, B33.1, B45.0, B45.2-B45.9, B58.2, B75, G04.00-G04.01, G04.31, G04.81-G05.4, G37.0, G37.4-G37.5, I67.3, J09.X3-J09.X9, J10.2-J10.89, J11.2-J11.89, L44.4, M1A.10X0-M1A.19X1, P35.2-P35.9, P37.0-P37.4, P37.8-P37.9, T56.0X1-T56.0X4[A]

● **A81.8 Other atypical virus infections of central nervous system**
(Ex) *For category A81.8 CC codes unless otherwise indicated:*
A81.00-A81.9, A92.30-A92.39, B97.21, I67.3

A81.81 Kuru 🔖
(Ex) A81.00-A81.9, I67.3

A81.82 Gerstmann-Sträussler-Scheinker syndrome 🔖
GSS syndrome

A81.83 Fatal familial insomnia 🔖
FFI

A81.89 Other atypical virus infections of central nervous system 🔖

A81.9 Atypical virus infection of central nervous system, unspecified 🔖
Prion diseases of the central nervous system NOS
(Ex) A81.00-A81.9, I67.3

● **A82 Rabies**
Viral disease affecting the central nervous system and transmitted from infected mammals to man.
(Ex) *For category A82 CC codes: A82.0-A82.9*

A82.0 Sylvatic rabies 🔖
A82.1 Urban rabies 🔖
A82.9 Rabies, unspecified 🔖

Item 1-13 Acute Poliomyelitis: Also called infantile paralysis and is caused by the poliovirus, which enters the body orally and infects the intestinal wall and then enters the blood stream and central nervous system, causing muscle weakness and paralysis. This disease has been nearly eradicated with the polio vaccine.

N Newborn Age: 0 **P** Pediatric Age: 0–17 **M** Maternity DX: 12–55 **A** Adult Age: 15–124 ♀ Females Only ♂ Males Only
🔖 Complication\Comorbidity 🔖 Major C\C (Ex) CC/MCC Exclusions 🔖 Present on Admission Requirement 🔖 Hospital-Acquired Condition

755

CHAPTER 1 (A00-B99)

● **A83**   **Mosquito-borne viral encephalitis**
Inflammation of the brain caused most commonly by Herpes Simplex virus.

Includes	mosquito-borne viral meningoencephalitis
Excludes2	Venezuelan equine encephalitis (A92.2)
	West Nile fever (A92.3-)
	West Nile virus (A92.3-)

(Ex) **For category A83 CC codes:** A17.82, A50.42, A52.14, A75.9, A79.9, A81.1, A81.82-A81.89, A83.0-A85.8, A87.2, A88.0, A88.8, A92.1-A92.8, A93.0, B00.4, B00.82, B01.11-B01.12, B04, B06.01, B08.09, B08.20-B08.22, B08.60-B08.79, B09, B10.01-B10.09, B26.2, B27.00-B27.99, B33.1, B45.0, B45.2-B45.9, B58.2, B75, B97.10-B97.21, G04.00-G04.01, G04.31, G04.81-G04.91, G05.3-G05.4, G37.0, G37.4-G37.5, J09.X3-J09.X9, J10.2-J10.89, J11.2-J11.89, L44.4, M1A.10X0-M1A.19X1, P35.2-P35.9, P37.0-P37.9, T56.0X1-T56.0X4[A]

A83.0   **Japanese encephalitis** 🔊

A83.1   **Western equine encephalitis** 🔊

A83.2   **Eastern equine encephalitis** 🔊

A83.3   **St. Louis encephalitis** 🔊

A83.4   **Australian encephalitis** 🔊
Kunjin virus disease

A83.5   **California encephalitis** 🔊
California meningoencephalitis
La Crosse encephalitis

A83.6   **Rocio virus disease** 🔊
Mosquito-borne virus

A83.8   **Other mosquito-borne viral encephalitis** 🔊

A83.9   **Mosquito-borne viral encephalitis, unspecified** 🔊

● **A84**   **Tick-borne viral encephalitis**

| **Includes** | tick-borne viral meningoencephalitis |

(Ex) **For category A84 CC codes:** A17.82, A50.42, A52.14, A75.9, A79.9, A81.1, A81.82-A81.89, A83.0-A85.8, A87.2, A88.0, A88.8, A92.1-A92.8, A93.0, B00.4, B00.82, B01.11-B01.12, B04, B06.01, B08.09, B08.20-B08.22, B08.60-B08.79, B09, B10.01-B10.09, B26.2, B27.00-B27.99, B33.1, B45.0, B45.2-B45.9, B58.2, B75, B97.10-B97.21, G04.00-G04.01, G04.31, G04.81-G04.91, G05.3-G05.4, G37.0, G37.4-G37.5, J09.X3-J09.X9, J10.2-J10.89, J11.2-J11.89, L44.4, M1A.10X0-M1A.19X1, P35.2-P35.9, P37.0-P37.9, T56.0X1-T56.0X4[A]

A84.0   **Far Eastern tick-borne encephalitis [Russian spring-summer encephalitis]** 🔊

A84.1   **Central European tick-borne encephalitis** 🔊

A84.8   **Other tick-borne viral encephalitis** 🔊
Louping ill
Powassan virus disease

A84.9   **Tick-borne viral encephalitis, unspecified** 🔊

● **A85**   **Other viral encephalitis, not elsewhere classified**

| **Includes** | specified viral encephalomyelitis NEC |
| | specified viral meningoencephalitis NEC |

Excludes1	benign myalgic encephalomyelitis (G93.3)
	encephalitis due to cytomegalovirus (B25.8) ◄▬
	~~cytomegalovirus (B25.8)~~
	encephalitis due to herpesvirus NEC (B10.0-) ◄▬
	encephalitis due to herpesvirus [herpes simplex] (B00.4) ◄▬
	encephalitis due to measles virus (B05.0) ◄▬
	encephalitis due to mumps virus (B26.2) ◄▬
	encephalitis due to poliomyelitis virus (A80.-) ◄▬
	encephalitis due to zoster (B02.0) ◄▬
	lymphocytic choriomeningitis (A87.2)

(Ex) **For category A85 CC codes unless otherwise indicated:** A17.82, A50.42, A52.14, A75.9, A79.9, A81.1, A81.82-A81.89, A83.0-A85.8, A87.2, A88.0, A88.8, A92.1-A92.8, A93.0, B00.4, B00.82, B01.11-B01.12, B04, B06.01, B08.09, B08.20-B08.22, B08.60-B08.79, B09, B10.01-B10.09, B26.2, B27.00-B27.99, B33.1, B45.0, B45.2-B45.9, B58.2, B75, B97.10-B97.21, G04.00-G04.01, G04.31, G04.81-G04.91, G05.3-G05.4, G37.0, G37.4-G37.5, H66.40-H66.43, J09.X3-J09.X9, J10.2-J10.89, J11.2-J11.89, L44.4, M1A.10X0-M1A.19X1, M32.0-M32.9, P35.2-P35.9, P37.0-P37.9, T56.0X1-T56.0X4[A]

A85.0   **Enteroviral encephalitis** 🔊
Enteroviral encephalomyelitis

A85.1   **Adenoviral encephalitis** 🔊
Adenoviral meningoencephalitis

A85.2   **Arthropod-borne viral encephalitis, unspecified** 🔊

| **Excludes1** | West nile virus with encephalitis (A92.31) |

(Ex) See A84.0

A85.8   **Other specified viral encephalitis** 🔊
Encephalitis lethargica
Von Economo-Cruchet disease

Item 1-14   **Encephalitis** is an inflammation of the brain most often caused by a virus but may also be caused by a bacteria and most commonly transmitted by a mosquito. **Myelitis** is an inflammation of the spinal cord that may disrupt CNS function. Untreated myelitis may rapidly lead to permanent damage to the spinal cord. **Encephalomyelitis** is a general term for an inflammation of the brain and spinal cord.

A86   **Unspecified viral encephalitis** 🔊
Viral encephalomyelitis NOS
Viral meningoencephalitis NOS

(Ex) A17.82, A50.42, A52.14, A75.9, A79.9, A81.1, A81.82-A81.89, A83.0-A86, A87.2, A88.0, A88.8-A89, A92.1-A92.2, A92.4-A92.8, A93.0, B00.4, B00.82, B01.11-B01.12, B04, B06.01, B08.09, B08.20-B08.22, B08.60-B08.79, B09, B10.01-B10.09, B26.2, B27.00-B27.99, B33.1, B45.0, B45.2-B45.9, B58.2, B75, B97.10-B97.21, G04.00-G04.01, G04.31, G04.81-G04.91, G05.3-G05.4, G37.0, G37.4-G37.5, H66.40-H66.43, J09.X3-J09.X9, J10.2-J10.89, J11.2-J11.89, L44.4, M1A.10X0-M1A.19X1, M32.0-M32.9, P35.2-P35.9, P37.0-P37.9, T56.0X1-T56.0X4[A]

● **A87**   **Viral meningitis**

Excludes1	meningitis due to herpesvirus [herpes simplex] (B00.3)
	meningitis due to measles virus (B05.1)
	meningitis due to mumps virus (B26.1)
	meningitis due to poliomyelitis virus (A80.-)
	meningitis due to zoster (B02.1)

(Ex) **For category A87 CC codes unless otherwise indicated:** A02.21, A17.0-A17.1, A27.81, A39.0, A50.41, A51.41, A52.13, A54.82-A54.84, A54.89-A54.9, A74.81-A74.9, A87.0-A87.9, A96.2, A98.3-A98.4, B26.1, B33.24, B33.4-B33.8, B34.1-B34.8, B37.5, B38.4, B45.1, B58.2, B92, B94.2-B94.9, B97.10, B97.19, B97.29, B97.5-B97.6, B97.81-B97.89, G00.0-G03.9, G04.2, G32.89, G61.0, G96.8-G96.9, G98.0-G98.8, G99.8

A87.0   **Enteroviral meningitis** 🔊
Group of common viruses responsible for the majority of viral meningitis
Coxsackievirus meningitis
Echovirus meningitis

A87.1   **Adenoviral meningitis** 🔊

A87.2   **Lymphocytic choriomeningitis** 🔊
Lymphocytic meningoencephalitis

(Ex) A02.21, A17.0-A17.1, A27.81, A39.0, A50.41, A51.41, A52.13, A54.82-A54.84, A54.89-A54.9, A74.81-A74.9, A87.0-A87.9, A92-30-A92-39, A96.2, A98.3-A98.4, B26.1, B33.24, B33.4-B33.8, B34.1-B34.8, B37.5, B38.4, B45.1, B58.2, B92, B94.2-B94.9, B97.10, B97.19, B97.21-B97.29, B97.5-B97.6, B97.81-B97.89, G00.0-G03.9, G04.2, G32.89, G61.0, G96.8-G96.9, G98.0-G98.8, G99.8

A87.8   **Other viral meningitis** 🔊

A87.9   **Viral meningitis, unspecified** 🔊

● **A88**   **Other viral infections of central nervous system, not elsewhere classified**

| **Excludes1** | viral encephalitis NOS (A86) |
| | viral meningitis NOS (A87.9) |

A88.0   **Enteroviral exanthematous fever [Boston exanthem]** 🔊
Infectious skin eruption

(Ex) A17.82, A50.42, A52.14, A75.9, A79.9, A81.1, A81.82-A81.89, A83.0-A85.8, A87.2, A88.0, A88.8, A92.1-A92.8, A93.0, B00.4, B00.82, B01.11-B01.12, B04, B06.01, B08.09, B08.20-B08.22, B08.60-B08.79, B09, B10.01-B10.09, B26.2, B27.00-B27.99, B33.1, B45.0, B45.2-B45.9, B58.2, B75, B97.10-B97.21, G04.00-G04.01, G04.31, G04.81-G04.91, G05.3-G05.4, G37.0, G37.4-G37.5, J09.X3-J09.X9, J10.2-J10.89, J11.2-J11.89, L44.4, M1A.10X0-M1A.19X1, P35.2-P35.9, P37.0-P37.9, T56.0X1-T56.0X4[A]

A88.1   **Epidemic vertigo**

A88.8   **Other specified viral infections of central nervous system** 🔊

(Ex) A17.82, A50.42, A52.14, A75.9, A79.9, A81.1, A81.82-A81.89, A83.0-A85.8, A87.2, A88.0, A88.8, A92.1-A92.8, A93.0, B00.4, B00.82, B01.11-B01.12, B04, B06.01, B08.09, B08.20-B08.22, B08.60-B08.79, B09, B10.01-B10.09, B26.2, B27.00-B27.99, B33.1, B45.0, B45.2-B45.9, B58.2, B75, B97.10-B97.21, G04.00-G04.01, G04.31, G04.81-G04.91, G05.3-G05.4, G37.0, G37.4-G37.5, H66.40-H66.43, J09.X3-J09.X9, J10.2-J10.89, J11.2-J11.89, L44.4, M1A.10X0-M1A.19X1, M32.0-M32.9, P35.2-P35.9, P37.0-P37.9, T56.0X1-T56.0X4[A]

A89   **Unspecified viral infection of central nervous system** 🔊

(Ex) A17.82, A50.42, A52.14, A75.9, A79.9, A81.1, A81.82-A81.89, A83.0-A86, A87.2, A88.0, A88.8-A89, A92.1-A92.2, A92.4-A92.8, A93.0, B00.4, B00.82, B01.11-B01.12, B04, B06.01, B08.09, B08.20-B08.22, B08.60-B08.79, B09, B10.01-B10.09, B26.2, B27.00-B27.99, B33.1, B45.0, B45.2-B45.9, B58.2, B75, B97.10, G04.00-G04.01, G04.31, G04.81-G04.91, G05.3-G05.4, G37.0, G37.4-G37.5, H66.40-H66.43, J09.X3-J09.X9, J10.2-J10.89, J11.2-J11.89, L44.4, M1A.10X0-M1A.19X1, M32.0-M32.9, P35.2-P35.9, P37.0-P37.9, T56.0X1-T56.0X4[A]

◄ New   ◄▬ Revised   ~~deleted~~ Deleted   Excludes 1   Excludes 2   Includes   Use additional   Code first   Code also   Unspecified

OGCR Official Guidelines   ● Unacceptable Principal Diagnosis   X Assign placeholder X   ● Use Additional Character(s)   ▌ Manifestation Code   **Coding Clinic**

ARTHROPOD-BORNE VIRAL FEVERS AND VIRAL HEMORRHAGIC FEVERS (A90-A99)

A90   Dengue fever [classical dengue] 🔍
*Acute, self-limited disease, characterized by fever, prostration, severe
muscle pains, headache, rash, lymphadenopathy, and leukopenia,
caused by dengue virus; AKA breakbone, dandy*

Excludes1   dengue hemorrhagic fever (A91)

(Ex:) A90

A91   Dengue hemorrhagic fever 🔍
Serious follow-up to regular dengue, with symptoms of hemorrhage
(Ex:) A91, A92.0-A94, A98.0-A98.2, A98.8-A99, B33.1

⬤ **A92   Other mosquito-borne viral fevers**

Excludes1   Ross River disease (B33.1)

A92.0   Chikungunya virus disease 🔍
Transmitted by mosquitoes
Chikungunya (hemorrhagic) fever
(Ex:) See A91

A92.1   O'nyong-nyong fever 🔍
*Acute, nonfatal febrile disease transmitted by mosquitoes,
which clinically resembles dengue and chikungunya*
(Ex:) A17.82, A50.42, A52.14, A75.9, A79.9, A81.1, A81.82-A81.89, A83.0-A85.8,
A87.2, A88.0, A88.8, A91-A94, A98.0-A98.2, A98.8-A99, B00.4, B00.82,
B01.11-B01.12, B04, B06.01, B08.09, B08.20-B08.22, B08.60-B08.79, B09,
B10.01-B10.09, B26.2, B27.00-B27.99, B33.1, B45.0, B45.2-B45.9, B58.2,
B75, B97.10, B97.21, G04.00-G04.01, G04.31, G04.81-G04.91,
G05.3-G05.4, G37.0, G37.4-G37.5, J09.X3-J09.X9, J10.2-J10.89,
J11.2-J11.89, L44.4, M1A.10X0-M1A.19X1, P35.2-P35.9, P37.0-P37.9,
T56.0X1-T56.0X4[A]

A92.2   Venezuelan equine fever 🔍
Venezuelan equine encephalitis
Venezuelan equine encephalomyelitis virus disease
(Ex:) See A92.1

⬤ **A92.3   West Nile virus infection**
West Nile fever
(Ex:) **For category A92.3 CC codes:** A17.82, A50.42, A52.14, A75.9, A79.9,
A81.1, A81.82-A81.89, A83.0-A85.8, A87.2, A88.0, A88.8, A91,
A92.0-A92.2, A92.4-A94, A98.0-A98.2, A98.8-A99, B00.4, B00.82,
B01.11-B01.12, B04, B06.01, B08.09, B08.20-B08.22, B08.60-B08.79, B09,
B10.01-B10.09, B26.2, B27.00-B27.99, B33.1, B45.0, B45.2-B45.9, B58.2,
B75, B97.10, G04.00-G04.01, G04.31, G04.81-G04.91, G05.3-G05.4, G37.0,
G37.4-G37.5, J09.X3-J09.X9, J10.2-J10.89, J11.2-J11.89, L44.4,
P35.2-P35.9, P37.0-P37.9

A92.30   West Nile virus infection, unspecified 🔍
West Nile fever NOS
West Nile fever without complications
West Nile virus NOS

A92.31   West Nile virus infection with encephalitis 🔍
West Nile encephalitis
West Nile encephalomyelitis

**A92.32   West Nile virus infection with other neurologic
manifestation** 🔍
Use additional code to specify the neurologic
manifestation

**A92.39   West Nile virus infection with other
complications** 🔍
Use additional code to specify the other
conditions

A92.4   Rift Valley fever 🔍
(Ex:) See A92.1

A92.8   Other specified mosquito-borne viral fevers 🔍
(Ex:) See A92.1

A92.9   Mosquito-borne viral fever, unspecified 🔍
(Ex:) See A91

⬤ **A93   Other arthropod-borne viral fevers, not elsewhere classified**

A93.0   Oropouche virus disease 🔍
Tropical viral infection
Oropouche fever
(Ex:) See A92.1

A93.1   Sandfly fever 🔍
Pappataci fever
Phlebotomus fever
(Ex:) See A91

A93.2   Colorado tick fever 🔍
(Ex:) See A91

A93.8   Other specified arthropod-borne viral fevers 🔍
Piry virus disease
Vesicular stomatitis virus disease [Indiana fever]
(Ex:) See A91

A94   Unspecified arthropod-borne viral fever 🔍
Arboviral fever NOS
Arbovirus infection NOS
(Ex:) See A91

⬤ **A95   Yellow fever**
Acute infectious disease transmitted by mosquitoes
(Ex:) **For category A95 CC codes:** A95.0-A95.9

A95.0   Sylvatic yellow fever 🔍
Jungle yellow fever

A95.1   Urban yellow fever 🔍

A95.9   Yellow fever, unspecified 🔍

⬤ **A96   Arenaviral hemorrhagic fever**
Virus that causes various hemorrhagic fevers
(Ex:) **For category A96 CC codes:** A74.81-A74.9, A88.1, A96.0-A96.9, A98.3-A98.5,
B25.8-B25.9, B33.24-B34.2, B34.4-B34.8, B97.0-B97.89

A96.0   Junin hemorrhagic fever 🔍
Argentinian hemorrhagic fever

A96.1   Machupo hemorrhagic fever 🔍
Transmitted by contact with infected rodents
Bolivian hemorrhagic fever

A96.2   Lassa fever 🔍
*Acute type of hemorrhagic fever caused by contact with
disease carrying mouse or person*

A96.8   Other arenaviral hemorrhagic fevers 🔍

A96.9   Arenaviral hemorrhagic fever, unspecified 🔍

⬤ **A98   Other viral hemorrhagic fevers, not elsewhere classified**

Excludes1   chikungunya hemorrhagic fever (A92.0)
dengue hemorrhagic fever (A91)

(Ex:) **For category A98 CC codes unless otherwise indicated:** A91, A92.0-A94,
A98.0-A98.2, A98.8-A99, B33.1

A98.0   Crimean-Congo hemorrhagic fever 🔍
*Virus transmitted by ticks and contact with blood, secretions,
or fluids from infected humans or animals*
Central Asian hemorrhagic fever

A98.1   Omsk hemorrhagic fever 🔍
*Transmitted to humans by bites of infected ticks or contact
with infected muskrats*

A98.2   Kyasanur Forest disease 🔍
Transmitted via infected monkeys, voles, ticks

A98.3   Marburg virus disease 🔍
Rare, acute, often fatal type of hemorrhagic fever

A98.4   Ebola virus disease 🔍

A98.5   Hemorrhagic fever with renal syndrome 🔍
Epidemic hemorrhagic fever
Korean hemorrhagic fever
Russian hemorrhagic fever
Hantaan virus disease
Hantavirus disease with renal manifestations
Nephropathia epidemica
Songo fever

Excludes1   hantavirus (cardio)-pulmonary syndrome
(B33.4)

(Ex:) A17.9, A18.10-A18.11, A18.13, A18.82, A18.84, A18.89, A54.21, A54.29,
A54.82, A54.84, A54.89-A54.9, A59.00, A59.8-A59.9, A98.5,
B37.41-B37.49, B97.21, E08.21-E08.29, E08.618-E08.638, E08.649-E08.8,
E09.21-E09.29, E09.618-E09.638, E09.649-E09.8, E10.21-E10.29,
E10.618-E10.638, E10.649, E10.69-E10.8, E11.21-E11.29, E11.618-E11.638,
E11.649, E11.69-E11.8, E13.21-E13.29, E13.618-E13.638, E13.649-E13.8,
M10.30-M10.39, N00.0-N11.0, N11.8-N13.39, N13.6, N14.0-N17.9, N19,
N25.0-N26.1, N26.9-N27.9, N28.1-N29, N36.41-N36.43, N36.8-N36.9,
N39.8-N39.9, R31.0-R31.9

A98.8   Other specified viral hemorrhagic fevers 🔍

A99   Unspecified viral hemorrhagic fever 🔍
(Ex:) See A98.0

CHAPTER 1 (A00-B99)

N   Newborn Age: 0   P   Pediatric Age: 0–17   M   Maternity DX: 12–55   A   Adult Age: 15–124   ♀   Females Only   ♂   Males Only

🔍 Complication\Comorbidity   Major C\C   (Ex:)   CC/MCC Exclusions   🔍 Present on Admission Requirement   🔍 Hospital-Acquired Condition

757

CHAPTER 1 (A00-B99)

VIRAL INFECTIONS CHARACTERIZED BY SKIN AND MUCOUS MEMBRANE LESIONS (B00-B09)

● **B00**   **Herpesviral [herpes simplex] infections**

Excludes1   congenital herpesviral infections (P35.2)

Excludes2   anogenital herpesviral infection (A60.-)

gammaherpesviral mononucleosis (B27.0-)

herpangina (B08.5)

B00.0   **Eczema herpeticum**

Cutaneous eruption caused by herpes simplex virus (HSV) type 1, HSV-2, coxsackievirus A16, or vaccinia virus

Kaposi's varicelliform eruption

B00.1   **Herpesviral vesicular dermatitis**

Vesicle formation; characteristics include formation of blisters and scabs on feet and legs

Herpes simplex facialis

Herpes simplex labialis

Herpes simplex otitis externa

Vesicular dermatitis of ear

Vesicular dermatitis of lip

B00.2   **Herpesviral gingivostomatitis and pharyngotonsillitis** 🔵

Inflammation involving both gingivae and oral mucosa

Herpesviral pharyngitis

Inflammation of pharynx and tonsils; AKA tonsillopharyngitis

(Ex) B00.2

B00.3   **Herpesviral meningitis** 🔵

(Ex) A02.21, A17.0-A17.1, A27.81, A39.0, A50.41, A51.41, A52.13, A54.82, A54.84, A54.89-A54.9, A87.0-A87.9, B00.3, B00.82-B00.9, B02.1, B10.81-B10.89, B26.1, B37.5, B38.4, B45.1, B58.2, B92, B94.2-B94.9, G00.0-G03.9, G04.2, G32.89, G61.0, G96.8-G96.9, G98.0-G98.8, G99.8

B00.4   **Herpesviral encephalitis** 🔵

Herpesviral meningoencephalitis

Simian B disease

Excludes1   herpesviral encephalitis due to herpesvirus 6 and 7 (B10.01, B10.09)

non-simplex herpesviral encephalitis (B10.0-)

(Ex) B00.4, B00.82-B00.9, B10.01-B10.89, B92, B94.2-B94.9

● **B00.5**   **Herpesviral ocular disease**

(Ex) For category B00.5 CC codes: B00.50-B00.59, B00.89-B00.9, B10.81-B10.89

B00.50   **Herpesviral ocular disease, unspecified** 🔵

B00.51   **Herpesviral iridocyclitis** 🔵

Herpesviral iritis

Herpesviral uveitis, anterior

B00.52   **Herpesviral keratitis** 🔵

Herpesviral keratoconjunctivitis

B00.53   **Herpesviral conjunctivitis** 🔵

B00.59   **Other herpesviral disease of eye** 🔵

Herpesviral dermatitis of eyelid

B00.7   **Disseminated herpesviral disease** 🔵

Herpesviral sepsis

(Ex) A02.1, A20.7, A22.7, A26.7, A32.7, A39.2-A39.4, A40.0-A41.9, A42.7, A54.86, B00.7, B00.82-B00.9, B10.81-B10.89, B37.7, B92, B94.2-B94.9, R65.10-R65.20

● **B00.8**   **Other forms of herpesviral infections**

B00.81   **Herpesviral hepatitis** 🔵

(Ex) B00.3, B00.81-B00.9, B10.81-B10.89, B92, B94.2-B94.9

B00.82   **Herpes simplex myelitis** 🔵

(Ex) A74.81-A74.9, A96.2, A98.3-A98.4, B00.82-B00.9, B01.12, B02.24, B10.81-B10.89, B33.24, B33.4-B33.8, B34.1-B34.2, B34.4-B34.8, B92, B94.2-B94.9, B97.10, B97.19, B97.29, B97.5-B97.6, B97.81-B97.89, G04.00-G04.01, G04.31, G04.81-G04.89, G05.3-G05.4, G37.3

B00.89   **Other herpesviral infection** 🔵

Herpesviral whitlow

(Ex) A74.81-A74.9, A96.2, A98.3-A98.4, B00.82-B00.9, B10.81-B10.89, B33.24, B33.4-B33.8, B34.1-B34.2, B34.4-B34.8, B92, B94.2-B94.9, B97.10, B97.19, B97.29, B97.5-B97.6, B97.81-B97.89

B00.9   **Herpesviral infection, unspecified**

Herpes simplex infection NOS

● **B01**   **Varicella [chickenpox]**

Very contagious disease caused by the varicella zoster virus that results in an itchy outbreak of skin blisters (varicella). The same virus causes shingles (zoster).

B01.0   **Varicella meningitis** 🔵

(Ex) A74.81-A74.9, A96.2, A98.3-A98.4, B01.0, B01.12, B01.81-B01.9, B08.04, B33.24, B33.4-B33.8, B34.1-B34.2, B34.4-B34.8, B92, B94.2-B94.9, B97.10, B97.19, B97.29, B97.5-B97.6, B97.81-B97.89

● **B01.1**   **Varicella encephalitis, myelitis and encephalomyelitis**

Postchickenpox encephalitis, myelitis and encephalomyelitis

B01.11   **Varicella encephalitis and encephalomyelitis** 🔵

Postchickenpox encephalitis and encephalomyelitis

(Ex) A74.81-A74.9, A96.2, A98.3-A98.4, B01.0-B01.12, B01.81-B01.9, B08.04, B33.24, B33.4-B33.8, B34.1-B34.2, B34.4-B34.8, B92, B94.2-B94.9, B97.10, B97.19, B97.29, B97.5-B97.6, B97.81-B97.89

B01.12   **Varicella myelitis** 🔵

Postchickenpox myelitis

(Ex) A74.81-A74.9, A96.2, A98.3-A98.4, B00.82, B01.0, B01.12, B01.81-B01.9, B02.24, B08.04, B33.24, B33.4-B33.8, B34.1-B34.2, B34.4-B34.8, B92, B94.2-B94.9, B97.10, B97.19, B97.29, B97.5-B97.6, B97.81-B97.89, G04.00-G04.01, G04.31, G04.81-G04.89, G05.3-G05.4, G37.3

B01.2   **Varicella pneumonia** 🔵

(Ex) A74.81-A74.9, A96.2, A98.3-A98.4, B01.0, B01.12-B01.9, B08.04, B33.24, B33.4-B33.8, B34.1-B34.2, B34.4-B34.8, B92, B94.2-B94.9, B97.10, B97.19, B97.29, B97.5-B97.6, B97.81-B97.89

● **B01.8**   **Varicella with other complications**

(Ex) For category B01.8 CC codes: A74.81-A74.9, A96.2, A98.3-A98.4, B01.0, B01.12, B01.81-B01.9, B08.04, B33.24, B33.4-B33.8, B34.1-B34.2, B34.4-B34.8, B92, B94.2-B94.9, B97.10, B97.19, B97.29, B97.5-B97.6, B97.81-B97.89

B01.81   **Varicella keratitis** 🔵

B01.89   **Other varicella complications** 🔵

B01.9   **Varicella without complication** 🔵

Varicella NOS

(Ex) See B01.8

● **B02**   **Zoster [herpes zoster]**

Includes   shingles

zona

B02.0   **Zoster encephalitis** 🔵

Zoster meningoencephalitis

(Ex) A74.81-A74.9, A96.2, A98.3-A98.4, B00.3, B00.82-B00.9, B02.0-B02.29, B02.7-B02.9, B10.81-B10.89, B33.24, B33.4-B33.8, B34.1-B34.2, B34.4-B34.8, B92, B94.2-B94.9, B97.10, B97.19, B97.29, B97.5-B97.6, B97.81-B97.89

B02.1   **Zoster meningitis** 🔵

(Ex) A02.21, A17.0-A17.1, A27.81, A39.0, A50.41, A51.41, A52.13, A54.82, A54.84, A54.89-A54.9, A74.81-A74.9, A87.0-A87.9, A96.2, A98.3-A98.4, B00.3, B00.82-B00.9, B02.0-B02.29, B02.7-B02.9, B10.81-B10.89, B26.1, B33.24, B33.4, B33.8, B34.1-B34.2, B34.4-B34.8, B37.5, B38.4, B45.1, B58.2, B92, B94.2-B94.9, B97.10, B97.19, B97.29, B97.5-B97.6, B97.81-B97.89, G00.0-G03.9, G04.2, G32.89, G61.0, G96.8-G96.9, G98.0-G98.8, G99.8

Figure 1-4   Primary herpes simplex in and around the mouth. The infection is usually acquired from siblings or parents and is readily transmitted to other direct contacts. (From Forbes, Jackson: Colour Atlas and Text of Clinical Medicine, International Edition, Mosby, 2002)

Item 1-15   Herpes is a viral disease for which there is no cure. There are two types of the herpes simplex virus: **Type I** causes **cold sores** or **fever blisters,** and **Type II** causes **genital herpes.** The virus can be spread from a sore on the lips to the genitals or from the genitals to the lips.

◀ New   ◀▦ Revised   ~~deleted~~ Deleted   Excludes 1   Excludes 2   Includes   Use additional   Code first   Code also   Unspecified

OGCR Official Guidelines   ● Unacceptable Principal Diagnosis   X Assign placeholder X   ● Use Additional Character(s)   ▶ Manifestation Code   Coding Clinic

Item 1-16 Zoster: Also known as ***shingles*** and is caused by the same virus as chickenpox. After exposure, the virus lies dormant in nerve tissue and is activated by factors including aging, stress, suppression of the immune system, and certain medication. It begins as a unilateral rash that leads to blisters and sores on the skin. It may involve the nerve pathways of the eye, forehead, nose, and eyelids and may be very painful with long term systemic effects.

● **B02.2**   **Zoster with other nervous system involvement**
    (Ex) For category B02.2 CC codes unless otherwise indicated: see B02.0

   B02.21   **Postherpetic geniculate ganglionitis** 🔹

   B02.22   **Postherpetic trigeminal neuralgia** 🔹

   B02.23   **Postherpetic polyneuropathy** 🔹

   B02.24   **Postherpetic myelitis** 🔹
      Herpes zoster myelitis
      (Ex) A74.81-A74.9, A96.2, A98.3-A98.4, B00.3, B00.82-B00.9,
      B01.12, B02.0-B02.29, B02.7-B02.9, B10.81-B10.89, B33.24,
      B33.4-B33.8, B34.1-B34.2, B34.4-B34.8, B92, B94.2-B94.9,
      B97.10, B97.19, B97.29, B97.5-B97.6, B97.81-B97.89,
      G04.00-G04.01, G04.31, G04.81-G04.89, G05.3-G05.4, G37.3

   B02.29   **Other postherpetic nervous system involvement** 🔹
      Postherpetic radiculopathy

● **B02.3**   **Zoster ocular disease**
    (Ex) For category B02.3 CC codes: B02.30-B02.39

   B02.30   **Zoster ocular disease, unspecified** 🔹

   B02.31   **Zoster conjunctivitis** 🔹

   B02.32   **Zoster iridocyclitis** 🔹

   B02.33   **Zoster keratitis** 🔹
      Herpes zoster keratoconjunctivitis

   B02.34   **Zoster scleritis** 🔹

   B02.39   **Other herpes zoster eye disease** 🔹
      Zoster blepharitis

● **B02.7**   **Disseminated zoster** 🔹
    (Ex) A60.00-A60.9, A74.81-A74.9, A96.2, A98.3-A98.4, B00.0-B00.2, B00.4-B00.9,
    B02.0-B02.9, B10.01-B10.89, B33.24, B33.4-B33.8, B34.1-B34.2, B34.4,
    B34.8, B92, B94.2-B94.9, B97.10, B97.19, B97.29, B97.5-B97.6,
    B97.81-B97.89

● **B02.8**   **Zoster with other complications** 🔹
    Herpes zoster otitis externa
    (Ex) See B02.7

● **B02.9**   **Zoster without complications**
    Zoster NOS

B03   **Smallpox** 🔹
    Note: In 1980 the 33rd World Health Assembly declared that smallpox had been eradicated. The classification is maintained for surveillance purposes.
    (Ex) B01.0-B01.9, B03, B08.010-B08.04

B04   **Monkeypox** 🔹
    Disease occurring in captive monkeys and other mammals that may be transmitted to humans, clinically similar to smallpox
    (Ex) B04, B08.010-B08.011, B08.09, B08.3, B08.60-B08.79, B09, L44.4

● **B05**   **Measles**
    Includes   morbilli
    Excludes1   subacute sclerosing panencephalitis (A81.1)

  B05.0   **Measles complicated by encephalitis** 🔹
     Postmeasles encephalitis
     (Ex) A74.81-A74.9, A96.2, A98.3-A98.4, B05.0-B05.1, B05.4, B05.89-B05.9,
     B33.24, B33.4-B33.8, B34.1-B34.2, B34.4-B34.8, B92, B94.2-B94.9, B97.10,
     B97.19, B97.29, B97.5-B97.6, B97.81-B97.89

  B05.1   **Measles complicated by meningitis** 🔹
     Postmeasles meningitis
     (Ex) A74.81-A74.9, A96.2, A98.3-A98.4, B05.1, B05.4, B05.89-B05.9, B33.24,
     B33.4-B33.8, B34.1-B34.2, B34.4-B34.8, B92, B94.2-B94.9, B97.10, B97.19,
     B97.29, B97.5-B97.6, B97.81-B97.89

  B05.2   **Measles complicated by pneumonia** 🔹
     Postmeasles pneumonia
     (Ex) A74.81-A74.9, A96.2, A98.3-A98.4, B05.1-B05.2, B05.4, B05.89-B05.9,
     B33.24, B33.4-B33.8, B34.1-B34.2, B34.4-B34.8, B92, B94.2-B94.9, B97.10,
     B97.19, B97.29, B97.5-B97.6, B97.81-B97.89

  B05.3   **Measles complicated by otitis media**
     Postmeasles otitis media

  B05.4   **Measles with intestinal complications** 🔹
     (Ex) See B05.1

● **B05.8**   **Measles with other complications**

   B05.81   **Measles keratitis and keratoconjunctivitis** 🔹
      (Ex) A74.81-A74.9, A96.2, A98.3-A98.4, B05.1, B05.4, B05.81-B05.9,
      B33.24, B33.4-B33.8, B34.1-B34.2, B34.4-B34.8, B92,
      B94.2-B94.9, B97.10, B97.19, B97.29, B97.5-B97.6,
      B97.81-B97.89

   B05.89   **Other measles complications** 🔹
      (Ex) See B05.1

  B05.9   **Measles without complication**
     Measles NOS

● **B06**   **Rubella [German measles]**
    Excludes1   congenital rubella (P35.0)

● **B06.0**   **Rubella with neurological complications**
    (Ex) For category B06.0 CC codes: A74.81-A74.9, A96.2, A98.3-A98.4, B05.1,
    B05.4, B05.81-B05.9, B06.00-B06.81, B06.89-B06.9, B33.24, B33.4-B33.8,
    B34.1-B34.2, B34.4-B34.8, B92, B94.2-B94.9, B97.10, B97.19, B97.29,
    B97.5-B97.6, B97.81-B97.89

   B06.00   **Rubella with neurological complication, unspecified** 🔹

   B06.01   **Rubella encephalitis** 🔹
      Rubella meningoencephalitis

   B06.02   **Rubella meningitis** 🔹

   B06.09   **Other neurological complications of rubella** 🔹

● **B06.8**   **Rubella with other complications**

   B06.81   **Rubella pneumonia** 🔹
      (Ex) See B06.0

   B06.82   **Rubella arthritis** 🔹
      (Ex) A74.81-A74.9, A96.2, A98.3-A98.4, B05.1, B05.4, B05.81-B05.9,
      B06.81-B06.82, B06.89-B06.9, B33.24, B33.4-B33.8,
      B34.1-B34.2, B34.4-B34.8, B92, B94.2-B94.9, B97.10, B97.19,
      B97.29, B97.5-B97.6, B97.81-B97.89

   B06.89   **Other rubella complications** 🔹
      (Ex) See B06.0

  B06.9   **Rubella without complication**
     Rubella NOS

CHAPTER 1 (A00-B99)

Figure 1-5 Photograph of eyelids with marginal blepharitis. (From Mandell, Bennett, & Dolin: Principles and Practice of Infectious Diseases, ed 7, Churchill Livingstone, An Imprint of Elsevier, 2009)

Item 1-17 Blepharitis is a common condition in which the eyelid is swollen and yellow scaling and conjunctivitis develop. Usually the hair on the scalp and brow is involved.

N Newborn Age: 0   P Pediatric Age: 0–17   M Maternity DX: 12–55   A Adult Age: 15–124   ♀ Females Only   ♂ Males Only

🔹 Complication\Comorbidity   🔹 Major C\C   (Ex) CC/MCC Exclusions   🔹 Present on Admission Requirement   🔹 Hospital-Acquired Condition

CHAPTER 1 (A00–B99)

● **B07   Viral warts**
> **Includes**   verruca simplex
> verruca vulgaris
> viral warts due to human papillomavirus
>
> **Excludes2**   anogenital (venereal) warts (A63.0)
> papilloma of bladder (D41.4)
> papilloma of cervix (D26.0)
> papilloma larynx (D14.1)

   B07.0   Plantar wart
> Verruca plantaris

   B07.8   Other viral warts
> Common wart
> Flat wart
> Verruca plana

   B07.9   Viral wart, unspecified

● **B08   Other viral infections characterized by skin and mucous membrane lesions, not elsewhere classified**
> **Excludes1**   vesicular stomatitis virus disease (A93.8)

● **B08.0   Other orthopoxvirus infections**
> **Excludes2**   monkeypox (B04)

   ● **B08.01   Cowpox and vaccinia not from vaccine**
     B08.010   Cowpox
     B08.011   Vaccinia not from vaccine
> **Excludes1**   vaccinia (from vaccination) (generalized) (T88.1)

   B08.02   Orf virus disease
> Contagious pustular dermatitis
> Ecthyma contagiosum

   B08.03   Pseudocowpox [milker's node]

   B08.04   Paravaccinia, unspecified

   B08.09   Other orthopoxvirus infections
> Orthopoxvirus infection NOS

   B08.1   Molluscum contagiosum
> *Various skin diseases characterized by soft, rounded, cutaneous lesions*

● **B08.2   Exanthema subitum [sixth disease] Roseola infantum**
> *Acute, short-lived high fever in infants and young children followed by a rash mainly on the trunk, caused by human herpesvirus 6*

   B08.20   Exanthema subitum [sixth disease], unspecified Roseola infantum, unspecified   P

   B08.21   Exanthema subitum [sixth disease] due to human herpesvirus 6 Roseola infantum due to human herpesvirus 6   P
> *Virus results in sudden rash; infection results in lifelong persistence*

   B08.22   Exanthema subitum [sixth disease] due to human herpesvirus 7 Roseola infantum due to human herpesvirus 7   P

   B08.3   Erythema infectiosum [fifth disease] 🗨
> *Moderately contagious, epidemic disease in children caused by B19 virus; onset of rash that begins as redness of cheeks, later there is rash on trunk and limbs; when this fades, there may be central clearing that leaves lacelike pattern*
> (Ex) B08.3, B34.3

   B08.4   Enteroviral vesicular stomatitis with exanthem
> Hand, foot and mouth disease
> *Check your documentation—this code is HAND, foot, and mouth disease. Code B08.8 is foot and mouth disease.*

   B08.5   Enteroviral vesicular pharyngitis
> Herpangina

● **B08.6   Parapoxvirus infections**
   B08.60   Parapoxvirus infection, unspecified
   B08.61   Bovine stomatitis
   B08.62   Sealpox
   B08.69   Other parapoxvirus infections

● **B08.7   Yatapoxvirus infections**
   B08.70   Yatapoxvirus infection, unspecified
   B08.71   Tanapox virus disease 🗨
> (Ex) B04, B08.010-B08.011, B08.09, B08.3, B08.60-B08.79, B09, L44.4

   B08.72   Yaba pox virus disease
> Yaba monkey tumor disease

   B08.79   Other yatapoxvirus infections

   B08.8   Other specified viral infections characterized by skin and mucous membrane lesions
> Enteroviral lymphonodular pharyngitis
> Foot-and-mouth disease
> *Check your documentation. Code B08.4 is for HAND, foot, and mouth disease.*
> Poxvirus NEC

B09   Unspecified viral infection characterized by skin and mucous membrane lesions
> Viral enanthema NOS
> Viral exanthema NOS

OTHER HUMAN HERPESVIRUSES (B10)

● **B10   Other human herpesviruses**
> **Excludes2**   cytomegalovirus (B25.9)
> Epstein-Barr virus (B27.0-)
> herpes NOS (B00.9)
> herpes simplex (B00.-)
> herpes zoster (B02.-)
> human herpesvirus NOS (B00.-)
> human herpesvirus 1 and 2 (B00.-)
> human herpesvirus 3 (B01.-, B02.-) ◀
> human herpesvirus 4 (B27.0-)
> human herpesvirus 5 (B25.-)
> varicella (B01.-)
> zoster (B02.-)

● **B10.0   Other human herpesvirus encephalitis**
> **Excludes2**   herpes encephalitis NOS (B00.4)
> herpes simplex encephalitis (B00.4)
> human herpesvirus encephalitis (B00.4)
> simian B herpes virus encephalitis (B00.4)
> (Ex) For category B10.0 CC codes: B00.4, B00.82-B00.9, B10.01-B10.89, B92, B94.2-B94.9

   B10.01   Human herpesvirus 6 encephalitis 🗨
> *Sudden rash or roseola*

   B10.09   Other human herpesvirus encephalitis 🗨
> Human herpesvirus 7 encephalitis
> *Virus closely related to human herpesvirus 6, but not known to cause any disease*

● **B10.8   Other human herpesvirus infection**
   B10.81   Human herpesvirus 6 infection
> *Causative agent of exanthema subitum that results in sudden rash*

   B10.82   Human herpesvirus 7 infection
> *Closely related to human herpesvirus 6, but not known cause any disease*

   B10.89   Other human herpesvirus infection
> Human herpesvirus 8 infection
> *May be the cause of Kaposi sarcoma, a malignant tumor*
> Kaposi's sarcoma-associated herpesvirus infection

◀ New   ◀ Revised   ~~deleted~~ Deleted   Excludes 1   Excludes 2   Includes   Use additional   Code first   Code also   Unspecified

760   OGCR Official Guidelines   ● Unacceptable Principal Diagnosis   X Assign placeholder X   ● Use Additional Character(s)   ▌ Manifestation Code   **Coding Clinic**

Figure 1-6 Hepatitis B viral infection. **A.** Liver parenchyma showing hepatocytes with diffuse granular cytoplasm, so-called ground glass hepatocytes (H&E). **B.** Immunoperoxidase stains from the same case, showing cytoplasmic inclusions of viral particles. (From Kumar: Robbins and Cotran: Pathologic Basis of Disease, ed 8, Saunders, An Imprint of Elsevier, 2009)

Item 1-18 Hepatitis A (HAV) was formerly called epidemic, infectious, short-incubation, or acute catarrhal jaundice hepatitis. The primary transmission mode is the oral–fecal route. **Hepatitis B (HBV)** was formerly called long-incubation period, serum, or homologous serum hepatitis. Transmission modes are through blood from infected persons and from body fluids of infected mother to neonate. **Hepatitis C (HCV),** caused by the hepatitis C virus, is primarily transfusion associated. **Hepatitis D (HDV),** also called delta hepatitis, is caused by the hepatitis D virus in patients formerly or currently infected with hepatitis B. **Hepatitis E (HEV)** is also called enterically transmitted non-A, non-B hepatitis. The primary transmission mode is the oral–fecal route, usually through contaminated water.

VIRAL HEPATITIS (B15-B19)

Excludes1	sequelae of viral hepatitis (B94.2)
Excludes2	cytomegaloviral hepatitis (B25.1)
	herpesviral [herpes simplex] hepatitis (B00.81)

● **B15   Acute hepatitis A**
  Ⓔ **For category B15 CC codes:** A74.81-A74.9, A96.2, A98.3-A98.4, B15.0-B19.9, B33.24, B33.4-B33.8, B34.1-B34.2, B34.4-B34.8, B92, B94.2-B94.9, B97.10, B97.19, B97.29, B97.5-B97.6, B97.81-B97.89

  B15.0   Hepatitis A with hepatic coma 🌑

  B15.9   Hepatitis A without hepatic coma 🌑
      Hepatitis A (acute) (viral) NOS

● **B16   Acute hepatitis B**
  Ⓔ **For category B16 CC codes:** see B15

  B16.0   Acute hepatitis B with delta-agent with hepatic coma 🌑

  B16.1   Acute hepatitis B with delta-agent without hepatic coma 🌑

  B16.2   Acute hepatitis B without delta-agent with hepatic coma 🌑

  B16.9   Acute hepatitis B without delta-agent and without hepatic coma 🌑
      Hepatitis B (acute) (viral) NOS

● **B17   Other acute viral hepatitis**
  Ⓔ **For category B17 CC codes:** see B15

  B17.0   Acute delta-(super) infection of hepatitis B carrier 🌑

● **B17.1   Acute hepatitis C**

      B17.10   Acute hepatitis C without hepatic coma 🌑
          Acute hepatitis C NOS

      B17.11   Acute hepatitis C with hepatic coma 🌑

  B17.2   Acute hepatitis E 🌑

  B17.8   Other specified acute viral hepatitis 🌑
      Hepatitis non-A non-B (acute) (viral) NEC

  B17.9   Acute viral hepatitis, unspecified 🌑
      Acute hepatitis NOS

● **B18   Chronic viral hepatitis**
  Ⓔ **For category B18 CC codes:** see B15

  B18.0   Chronic viral hepatitis B with delta-agent 🌑

  B18.1   Chronic viral hepatitis B without delta-agent 🌑
      Chronic (viral) hepatitis B

  B18.2   Chronic viral hepatitis C 🌑

  B18.8   Other chronic viral hepatitis 🌑

  B18.9   Chronic viral hepatitis, unspecified 🌑

Figure 1-7 Kaposi's sarcoma. There are large confluent hyperpigmented patch-stage lesions with lymphedema. (From Cohen & Powderly: Infectious Diseases, ed 3, Mosby, An Imprint of Elsevier, 2010)

Item 1-19 AIDS (acquired immune deficiency syndrome) is caused by **HIV** (human immunodeficiency virus). HIV affects certain white blood cells (T-4 lymphocytes) and destroys the ability of the cells to fight infections, making patients susceptible to a host of infectious diseases (e.g., ***Pneumocystis carinii pneumonia (PCP), Kaposi's sarcoma,*** and ***lymphoma).*** ***AIDS-related complex (ARC)*** is an early stage of AIDS in which tests for HIV are positive but the symptoms are mild.

● **B19   Unspecified viral hepatitis**
  Ⓔ **For category B19 CC codes:** see B15

  B19.0   Unspecified viral hepatitis with hepatic coma 🌑
● **B19.1   Unspecified viral hepatitis B**

      B19.10   Unspecified viral hepatitis B without hepatic coma 🌑
          Unspecified viral hepatitis B NOS

      B19.11   Unspecified viral hepatitis B with hepatic coma 🌑

● **B19.2   Unspecified viral hepatitis C**

      B19.20   Unspecified viral hepatitis C without hepatic coma 🌑
          Viral hepatitis C NOS

      B19.21   Unspecified viral hepatitis C with hepatic coma 🌑

  B19.9   Unspecified viral hepatitis without hepatic coma 🌑
      Viral hepatitis NOS

  OGCR Section I. C.1.a

  Certain Infectious and Parasitic Diseases (A00-B99)

  a. Human Immunodeficiency Virus (HIV) Infections

      1) Code only confirmed cases

      Code only confirmed cases of HIV infection illness. This is an exception to the hospital inpatient guideline Section II, H.

      In this context, "confirmation" does not require documentation of positive serology or culture for HIV; the provider's diagnostic statement that the patient is HIV positive, or has an HIV-related illness is sufficient.

HUMAN IMMUNODEFICIENCY VIRUS [HIV] DISEASE (B20)

B20   Human immunodeficiency virus [HIV] disease 🌑

Includes	acquired immune deficiency syndrome [AIDS]
	AIDS-related complex [ARC]
	HIV infection, symptomatic

Code first Human immunodeficiency virus [HIV] disease complicating pregnancy, childbirth and the puerperium, if applicable (O98.7-)

Use additional code(s) to identify all manifestations of HIV infection

Excludes1	asymptomatic human immunodeficiency virus [HIV] infection status (Z21)
	exposure to HIV virus (Z20.6)
	inconclusive serologic evidence of HIV (R75)

Ⓔ B20, B92, B94.2-B94.9

N Newborn Age: 0   **P** Pediatric Age: 0–17   **M** Maternity DX: 12–55   **A** Adult Age: 15–124   ♀ Females Only   ♂ Males Only

 Complication\Comorbidity   Major C\C   Ⓔ CC/MCC Exclusions   Present on Admission Requirement   Hospital-Acquired Condition

761

CHAPTER 1 (A00-B99)

OTHER VIRAL DISEASES (B25-B34)

● **B25**   **Cytomegaloviral disease**
AKA: HCMV or Human Herpesvirus 5 (HHV-5)

    Excludes1   congenital cytomegalovirus infection (P35.1)
                 cytomegaloviral mononucleosis (B27.1-)

   B25.0   **Cytomegaloviral pneumonitis** 🔧
MCC when PDx is its own MCC
(Ex:) A15.0-A15.9, A17.9, A18.82, A18.84, A18.89, A21.2, A22.1, A31.0, A37.01,
A37.11, A37.81, A37.91, A42.0, A43.0, A48.1, B25.0, B39.0-B39.2, B44.0,
B58.3, B59, B67.1, J09.X1-J09.X2, J10.00-J10.1, J11.00-J11.1, J12.0-J12.3,
J12.89-J18.1, J18.8-J18.9, J22, J44.9, J47.0-J70.4, J70.8-J70.9, J98.4,
J98.8-J98.9, Q33.4, R91.1

   B25.1   **Cytomegaloviral hepatitis** 🔧
CC when PDx is its own CC
(Ex:) No exclusions

   B25.2   **Cytomegaloviral pancreatitis** 🔧
MCC when PDx is its own MCC
(Ex:) B25.2, K85.0-K86.1, K86.8-K86.9

   B25.8   **Other cytomegaloviral diseases** 🔧
Cytomegaloviral encephalitis
(Ex:) A96.0-A96.9, A98.3-A98.5, B25.8-B25.9, B33.24-B34.2, B34.4-B34.8,
B97.0-B97.32, B97.39, B97.5-B97.89

   B25.9   **Cytomegaloviral disease, unspecified** 🔧
(Ex:) See B25.8

● **B26**   **Mumps**

    Includes   epidemic parotitis
               infectious parotitis
Acute, contagious, viral disease

   B26.0   **Mumps orchitis** ♂ 🔧
(Ex:) A74.81-A74.9, A96.2, A98.3-A98.4, B26.0, B26.82-B26.83, B26.85-B26.9,
B33.24, B33.4-B33.8, B34.1-B34.8, B92, B94.2-B94.9, B97.10, B97.19,
B97.29, B97.5-B97.6, B97.81-B97.89

   B26.1   **Mumps meningitis** 🔧
(Ex:) A02.21, A17.0-A17.1, A27.81, A39.0, A50.41, A51.41, A52.13, A54.82,
A54.84, A54.89-A54.9, A74.81-A74.9, A87.0-A87.9, A96.2, A98.3-A98.4,
B00.3, B02.1, B26.1, B26.82-B26.83, B26.85-B26.9, B33.24, B33.4-B33.8,
B34.1-B34.2, B34.4-B34.8, B37.5, B38.4, B45.1, B58.2, B92, B94.2,
B94.8-B94.9, B97.10, B97.19, B97.29, B97.5-B97.6, B97.81-B97.89,
G00.0-G03.9, G04.2, G32.89, G61.0, G96.8-G96.9, G98.0-G98.8, G99.8

   B26.2   **Mumps encephalitis** 🔧
(Ex:) A74.81-A74.9, A96.2, A98.3-A98.4, B26.2, B26.82-B26.83, B26.85-B26.9,
B33.24, B33.4, B33.8, B34.1-B34.2, B34.4-B34.8, B92, B94.2, B94.8-B94.9,
B97.10, B97.19, B97.29, B97.5-B97.6, B97.81-B97.89

   B26.3   **Mumps pancreatitis** 🔧
(Ex:) A74.81-A74.9, A96.2, A98.3-A98.4, B26.3, B26.82-B26.83, B26.85-B26.9,
B33.24, B33.4, B33.8, B34.1-B34.2, B34.4-B34.8, B92, B94.2, B94.8-B94.9,
B97.10, B97.19, B97.29, B97.5-B97.6, B97.81-B97.89

● **B26.8**   **Mumps with other complications**
(Ex:) For category B26.8 CC codes unless otherwise indicated:
A74.81-A74.9, A96.2, A98.3-A98.4, B26.82-B26.83, B26.85-B26.9, B33.24,
B33.4, B33.8, B34.1-B34.2, B34.4-B34.8, B92, B94.2, B94.8-B94.9, B97.10,
B97.19, B97.29, B97.5-B97.6, B97.81-B97.89

    B26.81   **Mumps hepatitis** 🔧
(Ex:) A74.81-A74.9, A96.2, A98.3-A98.4, B26.81-B26.83,
B26.85-B26.9, B33.24, B33.4, B33.8, B34.1-B34.2,
B34.4-B34.8, B92, B94.2, B94.8-B94.9, B97.10, B97.19,
B97.29, B97.5-B97.6, B97.81-B97.89

    B26.82   **Mumps myocarditis** 🔧

    B26.83   **Mumps nephritis** 🔧

    B26.84   **Mumps polyneuropathy** 🔧
(Ex:) A74.81-A74.9, A96.2, A98.3-A98.4, B26.82-B26.9, B33.24,
B33.4, B33.8, B34.1-B34.2, B34.4-B34.8, B92, B94.2,
B94.8-B94.9, B97.10, B97.19, B97.29, B97.5-B97.6,
B97.81-B97.89

    B26.85   **Mumps arthritis** 🔧

    B26.89   **Other mumps complications** 🔧

   B26.9   **Mumps without complication**
Mumps NOS
Mumps parotitis NOS

● **B27**   **Infectious mononucleosis**

    Includes   glandular fever
               monocytic angina
               Pfeiffer's disease

● **B27.0**   **Gammaherpesviral mononucleosis**
AKA: Pfeiffer's disease, infective mononucleosis
Mononucleosis due to Epstein-Barr virus

    B27.00   **Gammaherpesviral mononucleosis without
complication**
Infective mononucleosis

    B27.01   **Gammaherpesviral mononucleosis with
polyneuropathy**

    B27.02   **Gammaherpesviral mononucleosis with
meningitis**

    B27.09   **Gammaherpesviral mononucleosis with other
complications**
Hepatomegaly in gammaherpesviral
mononucleosis

● **B27.1**   **Cytomegaloviral mononucleosis**
Infectious disease resembling infectious mononucleosis

    B27.10   **Cytomegaloviral mononucleosis without
complications**

    B27.11   **Cytomegaloviral mononucleosis with
polyneuropathy**

    B27.12   **Cytomegaloviral mononucleosis with
meningitis**

    B27.19   **Cytomegaloviral mononucleosis with other
complication**
Hepatomegaly in cytomegaloviral
mononucleosis

● **B27.8**   **Other infectious mononucleosis**

    B27.80   **Other infectious mononucleosis without
complication**

    B27.81   **Other infectious mononucleosis with
polyneuropathy**

    B27.82   **Other infectious mononucleosis with
meningitis**

    B27.89   **Other infectious mononucleosis with other
complication**
Hepatomegaly in other infectious
mononucleosis

● **B27.9**   **Infectious mononucleosis, unspecified**

    B27.90   **Infectious mononucleosis, unspecified without
complication**

    B27.91   **Infectious mononucleosis, unspecified with
polyneuropathy**

    B27.92   **Infectious mononucleosis, unspecified with
meningitis**

    B27.99   **Infectious mononucleosis, unspecified with
other complication**
Hepatomegaly in unspecified infectious
mononucleosis

● **B30**   **Viral conjunctivitis**

    Excludes1   herpesviral [herpes simplex] ocular disease
               (B00.5)
               ocular zoster (B02.3)

   B30.0   **Keratoconjunctivitis due to adenovirus**
Epidemic keratoconjunctivitis
Shipyard eye

   B30.1   **Conjunctivitis due to adenovirus**
Acute adenoviral follicular conjunctivitis
Swimming-pool conjunctivitis

   B30.2   **Viral pharyngoconjunctivitis**

   B30.3   **Acute epidemic hemorrhagic conjunctivitis (enteroviral)**
Conjunctivitis due to coxsackievirus 24
Conjunctivitis due to enterovirus 70
Hemorrhagic conjunctivitis (acute)(epidemic)

   B30.8   **Other viral conjunctivitis**
Newcastle conjunctivitis

   B30.9   **Viral conjunctivitis, unspecified**

◀ New   ◀▥ Revised   ~~deleted~~ Deleted   Excludes 1   Excludes 2   Includes   Use additional   Code first   Code also   Unspecified
OGCR Official Guidelines   ● Unacceptable Principal Diagnosis   X Assign placeholder X   ● Use Additional Character(s)   ▶ Manifestation Code   **Coding Clinic**

● **B33**   **Other viral diseases, not elsewhere classified**

    B33.0   **Epidemic myalgia**
       Acute infectious disease, caused by group A coxsackie viruses
       or other enteroviruses with symptoms that include
       sudden pain in chest or upper abdomen with fever
       Bornholm disease

    B33.1   **Ross River disease** 🔖
       Epidemic polyarthritis and exanthema
       Ross River fever
       (Ex) A17.82, A50.42, A52.14, A75.9, A79.9, A81.1, A81.82-A81.89, A83.0-A85.8,
           A87.2, A88.0, A88.8, A91-A94, A98.0-A98.2, A98.8-A99, B00.4, B00.82,
           B01.11-B01.12, B04, B06.01, B08.09, B08.20-B08.22, B08.60-B08.79, B09,
           B10.01-B10.09, B26.2, B27.00-B27.99, B33.1, B45.0, B45.2-B45.9, B58.2,
           B75, B97.10, B97.21, G04.00-G04.01, G04.31, G04.81-G04.91,
           G05.3-G05.4, G37.0, G37.4-G37.5, J09.X3-J09.X9, J10.2-J10.89,
           J11.2-J11.89, L44.4, M1A.10X0-M1A.19X1, P35.2-P35.9, P37.0-P37.9,
           T56.0X1-T56.0X4[A]

    B33.2   **Viral carditis**
       Coxsackie (virus) carditis

       B33.20   **Viral carditis, unspecified** 🔖
          (Ex) A52.06, B33.20-B33.22, I00, I01.2-I01.9, I09.0, I09.9,
             I23.0-I23.3, I23.6-I23.8, I40.0-I41, I51.0, I51.3-I51.4, I87.8,
             I99.8-I99.9

       B33.21   **Viral endocarditis** 🔖
          (Ex) A01.00-A01.09, A39.51, A52.03, A78, B33.21, B37.6,
             B40.0-B40.9, I00, I01.1, I01.8-I02.0, I05.0-I07.9, I08.1-I08.3,
             I08.9, I09.1, I09.89-I09.9, I33.0-I39, I42.4, I87.8, I99.8-I99.9,
             Q22.2, Q23.8-Q23.9, Q24.8, T82.6XXA

       B33.22   **Viral myocarditis** 🔖
          (Ex) See B33.20

       B33.23   **Viral pericarditis** 🔖
          (Ex) B33.23, I01.0, I09.2, I30.0-I30.9, I31.3-I32, I87.8, I99.8-I99.9

       B33.24   **Viral cardiomyopathy**

    B33.3   **Retrovirus infections, not elsewhere classified**
       Retrovirus infection NOS

    B33.4   **Hantavirus (cardio)-pulmonary syndrome [HPS]**
       [HCPS] 🔖
       Hantavirus disease with pulmonary manifestations
       Sin nombre virus disease
       Use additional code to identify any associated acute
          kidney failure (N17.9)
       Excludes1   hantavirus disease with renal
                manifestations (A98.5)
              hemorrhagic fever with renal
                manifestations (A98.5)
       (Ex) A74.81-A74.9, A88.1, A96.0-A96.9, A98.3-A98.5, B19.20-B19.21,
          B25.8-B25.9, B33.24, B33.3-B34.2, B34.4-B34.8, B97.0-B97.89

    B33.8   **Other specified viral diseases**
       Excludes1   anogenital human papillomavirus
                infection (A63.0)
              viral warts due to human papillomavirus
                infection (B07)

● **B34**   **Viral infection of unspecified site**
    Excludes1   anogenital human papillomavirus infection
             (A63.0)
          cytomegaloviral disease NOS (B25.9)
          herpesvirus [herpes simplex] infection NOS
             (B00.9)
          retrovirus infection NOS (B33.3)
          viral agents as the cause of diseases classified
             elsewhere (B97.-)
          viral warts due to human papillomavirus
             infection (B07)

    B34.0   **Adenovirus infection, unspecified**

    B34.1   **Enterovirus infection, unspecified**
       Intestinal tract infection
       Coxsackievirus infection NOS
       Echovirus infection NOS

    B34.2   **Coronavirus infection, unspecified**
       Excludes1   pneumonia due to SARS-associated
                coronavirus (J12.81)

    B34.3   **Parvovirus infection, unspecified** 🔖
       (Ex) B08.3, B34.3

    B34.4   **Papovavirus infection, unspecified**

    B34.8   **Other viral infections of unspecified site**

    B34.9   **Viral infection, unspecified**
       Viremia NOS

MYCOSES (B35-B49)

    Excludes2   hypersensitivity pneumonitis due to organic dust
             (J67.-)
          mycosis fungoides (C84.0-)

● **B35**   **Dermatophytosis**
       AKA tinea or ringworm
    Includes   favus
          infections due to species of Epidermophyton,
             Micro-sporum and Trichophyton
          tinea, any type except those in B36.-

    B35.0   **Tinea barbae and tinea capitis**
       Beard ringworm
       Kerion
       Scalp ringworm
       Sycosis, mycotic

    B35.1   **Tinea unguium**
       White patches or pits on surface or edges of nails, followed by
          infection under nail plate
       Dermatophytic onychia
       Dermatophytosis of nail
       Onychomycosis
       Ringworm of nails

    B35.2   **Tinea manuum**
       Tinea of hands
       Dermatophytosis of hand
       Hand ringworm

    B35.3   **Tinea pedis**
       Tinea affecting feet
       Athlete's foot
       Dermatophytosis of foot
       Foot ringworm

    B35.4   **Tinea corporis**
       Infecting skin areas other than hands
       Ringworm of the body

    B35.5   **Tinea imbricata**
       Chronic tropical tinea corporis; AKA Oriental ringworm,
          tinea inguinalis, tinea cruris
       Tokelau

    B35.6   **Tinea cruris**
       In groin or perineal area, spreading to adjacent regions; AKA
          jock itch, eczema marginatum, ringworm of groin, or t
          inguinalis
       Dhobi itch
       Groin ringworm
       Jock itch

    B35.8   **Other dermatophytoses**
       Disseminated dermatophytosis
       Granulomatous dermatophytosis

    B35.9   **Dermatophytosis, unspecified**
       Ringworm NOS

CHAPTER 1 (A00-B99)

N   Newborn Age: 0   **P**   Pediatric Age: 0–17   **M**   Maternity DX: 12–55   **A**   Adult Age: 15–124   ♀   Females Only   ♂   Males Only

🔖 Complication\Comorbidity   🔖 Major C\C   (Ex) CC/MCC Exclusions   🔖 Present on Admission Requirement   🔖 Hospital-Acquired Condition

763

● **B36   Other superficial mycoses**

B36.0   Pityriasis versicolor
Common, chronic, symptomless disorder that includes macular patches of various sizes and shapes; AKA liver spots
Tinea flava
Tinea versicolor

B36.1   Tinea nigra
Minor fungal infection, with dark lesions, usually on skin of hands
Keratomycosis nigricans palmaris
Microsporosis nigra
Pityriasis nigra

B36.2   White piedra
White to light brown nodules on hair of beard, axilla, or groin; AKA trichosporosis
Tinea blanca

B36.3   Black piedra
Characterized by small black or brown nodules on shafts of scalp hair

B36.8   Other specified superficial mycoses

B36.9   Superficial mycosis, unspecified

● **B37   Candidiasis**

Includes   candidosis
moniliasis

Excludes1   neonatal candidiasis (P37.5)

B37.0   Candidal stomatitis
Oral thrush
Ex) B37.0-B37.9, B48.3, B49, B92, B94.2-B94.9

B37.1   Pulmonary candidiasis
Candidal bronchitis
Candidal pneumonia
Ex) See B37.0

B37.2   Candidiasis of skin and nail
Candidal onychia
Candidal paronychia
Excludes2   diaper dermatitis (L22)

B37.3   Candidiasis of vulva and vagina ♀
Candidal vulvovaginitis
Monilial vulvovaginitis
Vaginal thrush

● **B37.4   Candidiasis of other urogenital sites**
Ex) For category B37.4 CC codes: B37.1, B37.41-B37.82, B37.84-B37.9, N25.81-N25.89

B37.41   Candidal cystitis and urethritis

B37.42   Candidal balanitis
Male condition only

B37.49   Other urogenital candidiasis
Candidal pyelonephritis

B37.5   Candidal meningitis
Ex) A02.21, A17.0-A17.1, A27.81, A39.0, A50.41, A51.41, A52.13, A54.82, A54.84, A54.89-A54.9, A87.0-A87.9, B00.3, B02.1, B26.1, B37.0-B38.4, B45.1, B48.3, B49, B58.2, B92, B94.2-B94.9, G00.0-G03.9, G04.2, G32.89, G61.0, G96.8-G96.9, G98.0, G98.8-G99.8

B37.6   Candidal endocarditis
Ex) See B37.0

B37.7   Candidal sepsis
Disseminated candidiasis systemic candidiasis
MCC when PDx is its own MCC
Ex) A02.1, A20.7, A22.7, A26.7, A32.7, A39.2-A39.4, A40.0-A40.1, A40.8-A41.9, A42.7, A48.2-A48.4, A48.8-A49.9, A54.86, B00.7, B37.0-B37.9, B48.3, B49, B92, B94.2-B96.89, R65.10-R65.20, Z16.10-Z16.39

● **B37.8   Candidiasis of other sites**
Ex) For category B37.8 CC codes unless otherwise indicated: B37.0-B37.9, B48.3, B49, B92, B94.2-B94.9

B37.81   Candidal esophagitis

B37.82   Candidal enteritis
Candidal proctitis

B37.83   Candidal cheilitis
Inflammation affecting lip

B37.84   Candidal otitis externa
Inflammation of external auditory canal

B37.89   Other sites of candidiasis
Infection manifested by invasive candidiasis
Candidal osteomyelitis
Ex) B37.1, B37.5-B37.82, B37.84-B37.9

B37.9   Candidiasis, unspecified
Thrush NOS

● **B38   Coccidioidomycosis**
Fungal disease; AKA coccidioidosis, coccidioidal granuloma, Posadas, or Posadas-Wernicke disease

B38.0   Acute pulmonary coccidioidomycosis
Ex) B38.0-B38.2, B38.7, B38.89-B39.9, B48.3, B49, B92, B94.2-B94.9

B38.1   Chronic pulmonary coccidioidomycosis
Ex) B38.0-B39.9

B38.2   Pulmonary coccidioidomycosis, unspecified
Ex) See B38.1

B38.3   Cutaneous coccidioidomycosis
Ex) B38.0-B38.9

B38.4   Coccidioidomycosis meningitis
Ex) A02.21, A17.0-A17.1, A27.81, A39.0, A50.41, A51.41, A52.13, A54.82, A54.84, A54.89-A54.9, A87.0-A87.9, B00.3, B02.1, B26.1, B37.5, B38.4-B38.87, B38.89-B39.9, B45.1, B48.3, B49, B58.2, B92, B94.2-B94.9, G00.0-G03.9, G04.2, G32.89, G61.0, G96.8-G96.9, G98.0, G98.8-G99.8

B38.7   Disseminated coccidioidomycosis
Generalized coccidioidomycosis
Ex) B38.7, B38.89-B38.9, B48.3, B49, B92, B94.2-B94.9

● **B38.8   Other forms of coccidioidomycosis**

B38.81   Prostatic coccidioidomycosis ♂
Ex) See B38.3

B38.89   Other forms of coccidioidomycosis
Ex) See B38.7

B38.9   Coccidioidomycosis, unspecified
Ex) See B38.7

● **B39   Histoplasmosis**
Infection resulting from inhalation or ingestion of spores; AKA Darling disease

Code first associated AIDS (B20)

Use additional code for any associated manifestations, such as:
endocarditis (I39)
meningitis (G02)
pericarditis (I32)
retinitits (H32)

B39.0   Acute pulmonary histoplasmosis capsulati
Ex) A22.1, A37.01-A37.11, A37.81, A37.9, A48.1, B25.0, B39.0-B39.4, B39.9-B44.0, B48.3, B49, B92, B94.2-B94.9, J09.X1-J09.X2, J10.00-J10.1, J11.00-J11.1, J12.0-J12.3, J12.89-J18.1, J18.8-J18.9, J44.9, J47.0-J47.9, J60-J70.4, J70.8-J70.9, J98.4, R91.1

B39.1   Chronic pulmonary histoplasmosis capsulati
Ex) See B39.0

B39.2   Pulmonary histoplasmosis capsulati, unspecified
Ex) See B39.0

B39.3   Disseminated histoplasmosis capsulati
Generalized histoplasmosis capsulati
Ex) B38.0-B39.4

Figure 1-8 Oral candidiasis (thrush). *(Courtesy of Stephen Raffanti, MD, MPH.)* (From Mandell, Bennett, & Dolin: Principles and Practice of Infectious Diseases, ed 7, Churchill Livingstone, An Imprint of Elsevier, 2009)

Item 1-20 Candidiasis, also called oidiomycosis or moniliasis, is a fungal infection. It most often appears on moist cutaneous areas of the body but can also be responsible for a variety of systemic infections such as endocarditis, meningitis, arthritis, and myositis. Antifungal medications cure most yeast infections.

◀ New   ◀ Revised   ~~deleted~~ Deleted   Excludes 1   Excludes 2   Includes   Use additional   Code first   Code also   Unspecified
OGCR Official Guidelines   ● Unacceptable Principal Diagnosis   X Assign placeholder X   ● Use Additional Character(s)   ▶ Manifestation Code   **Coding Clinic**

Item 1–21 Bird and bat droppings that fall into the soil give rise to a fungus that can spread airborne spores. When inhaled into the lungs, these spores divide and multiply into lesions. Histoplasmosis capsulatum takes three forms: primary (lodged in the lungs only), chronic (resembles TB), and disseminated (infection has moved to other organs). This is an opportunistic infection in immunosuppressed patients.

B39.4   **Histoplasmosis capsulati, unspecified**
        American histoplasmosis

B39.5   **Histoplasmosis duboisii**
        African histoplasmosis

B39.9   **Histoplasmosis, unspecified**

● **B40**   **Blastomycosis**
     Rare and potentially fatal infection caused by inhaling fungus found in moist soil in temperate climates.

     Excludes1   Brazilian blastomycosis (B41.-)
               keloidal blastomycosis (B48.0)

     (Ex) **For category B40 CC codes:** B40.0-B40.9, B48.3, B49, B92, B94.2-B94.9

B40.0   **Acute pulmonary blastomycosis** 🔒

B40.1   **Chronic pulmonary blastomycosis** 🔒

B40.2   **Pulmonary blastomycosis, unspecified** 🔒

B40.3   **Cutaneous blastomycosis** 🔒

B40.7   **Disseminated blastomycosis** 🔒
        Generalized blastomycosis

● **B40.8**   **Other forms of blastomycosis**

     B40.81   **Blastomycotic meningoencephalitis** 🔒
           Meningomyelitis due to blastomycosis

     B40.89   **Other forms of blastomycosis** 🔒

B40.9   **Blastomycosis, unspecified** 🔒

● **B41**   **Paracoccidioidomycosis**
     Fungal infection usually chronic that begins in lungs, spreads to mucocutaneous areas which may extend to skin, tonsils, gastrointestinal lymphatics, liver, and spleen; AKA Almeida or Lutz-Splendore-Almeida disease, Brazilian or South American blastomycosis, or paracoccidioidal granuloma

     Includes   Brazilian blastomycosis
               Lutz' disease

     (Ex) **For category B41 CC codes:** B41.0-B41.9, B48.3, B49, B92, B94.2-B94.9

B41.0   **Pulmonary paracoccidioidomycosis** 🔒

B41.7   **Disseminated paracoccidioidomycosis** 🔒
        Generalized paracoccidioidomycosis

B41.8   **Other forms of paracoccidioidomycosis** 🔒

B41.9   **Paracoccidioidomycosis, unspecified** 🔒

● **B42**   **Sporotrichosis**
     Chronic fungal infection with nodular lesions

B42.0   **Pulmonary sporotrichosis**

B42.1   **Lymphocutaneous sporotrichosis**

B42.7   **Disseminated sporotrichosis**
        Generalized sporotrichosis

● **B42.8**   **Other forms of sporotrichosis**

     B42.81   **Cerebral sporotrichosis**
           Meningitis due to sporotrichosis

     B42.82   **Sporotrichosis arthritis**

     B42.89   **Other forms of sporotrichosis**

B42.9   **Sporotrichosis, unspecified**

● **B43**   **Chromomycosis and pheomycotic abscess**
     Chronic fungal infection of skin, initiated at site of puncture affecting lower limb or foot (mossy foot)

B43.0   **Cutaneous chromomycosis**
        Dermatitis verrucosa

B43.1   **Pheomycotic brain abscess**
        Cerebral chromomycosis

B43.2   **Subcutaneous pheomycotic abscess and cyst**

B43.8   **Other forms of chromomycosis**

B43.9   **Chromomycosis, unspecified**

● **B44**   **Aspergillosis**
     Infection marked by inflammatory lesions in skin, ear, orbit, nasal sinuses, lungs, and occasionally bones and meninges

     Includes   aspergilloma

     (Ex) **For category B44 CC codes unless otherwise indicated:** B44.1-B44.7, B44.89-B44.9, B48.3-B48.4, B49, B92, B94.2-B94.9

B44.0   **Invasive pulmonary aspergillosis** 🔒
        MCC when PDx is its own MCC
     (Ex) A15.0-A15.9, A17.9, A18.82, A18.84, A18.89, A21.2, A22.1, A31.0, A37.01, A37.11, A37.81, A37.91, A42.0, A43.0, A48.1, B25.0, B39.0-B39.2, B44.0, B58.3, B59, B67.1, J09.X1-J09.X2, J10.00-J10.1, J11.00-J11.1, J12.0-J12.3, J12.89-J18.1, J18.8-J18.9, J22, J44.9, J47.0-J70.4, J70.8-J70.9, J98.4, J98.8-J98.9, Q33.4, R91.1

B44.1   **Other pulmonary aspergillosis** 🔒

B44.2   **Tonsillar aspergillosis** 🔒

B44.7   **Disseminated aspergillosis** 🔒
        Generalized aspergillosis

● **B44.8**   **Other forms of aspergillosis**

     B44.81   **Allergic bronchopulmonary aspergillosis** 🔒
           (Ex) B44.81, J22, J98.8-J98.9

     B44.89   **Other forms of aspergillosis** 🔒

B44.9   **Aspergillosis, unspecified** 🔒

● **B45**   **Cryptococcosis**
     Infection in the immunocompromised and fatal if left untreated; AKA torulosis, Buschke, or Busse-Buschke disease

     (Ex) **For category B45 CC codes unless otherwise indicated:** B45.0, B45.2-B45.9, B48.3, B49, B92, B94.2-B94.9

B45.0   **Pulmonary cryptococcosis** 🔒

B45.1   **Cerebral cryptococcosis** 🔒
        Cryptococcal meningitis
        Cryptococcosis meningocerebralis
        MCC when PDx is its own MCC
     (Ex) A02.21, A17.0-A17.1, A27.81, A39.0, A50.41, A51.41, A52.13, A54.82, A54.84, A54.89-A54.9, A87.0-A87.9, B00.3, B02.1, B26.1, B37.5, B38.4, B45.1, B58.2, E08.40-E08.49, E08.618-E08.638, E08.649-E08.8, E09.40-E09.49, E09.618-E09.638, E09.649-E09.8, E10.40-E10.49, E10.618-E10.638, E10.649, E10.69, E10.8, E11.40-E11.49, E11.618-E11.638, E11.649, E11.69-E11.8, E13.40-E13.49, E13.618-E13.638, E13.649-E13.69, E13.8, G00.0-G03.9, G04.2, G32.89, G61.0, G96.8-G96.9, G98.0-G98.8, G99.8

B45.2   **Cutaneous cryptococcosis** 🔒

B45.3   **Osseous cryptococcosis** 🔒

B45.7   **Disseminated cryptococcosis** 🔒
        Generalized cryptococcosis

B45.8   **Other forms of cryptococcosis** 🔒

B45.9   **Cryptococcosis, unspecified** 🔒

● **B46**   **Zygomycosis**
     Fungal infections including subcutaneous lesions and infection of sinuses, brain, or lungs

     (Ex) **For category B46 CC codes:** B46.0-B46.9, B48.3, B49, B92, B94.2-B94.9

B46.0   **Pulmonary mucormycosis** 🔒
        Fungal infection affecting lung

B46.1   **Rhinocerebral mucormycosis** 🔒

B46.2   **Gastrointestinal mucormycosis** 🔒

B46.3   **Cutaneous mucormycosis** 🔒
        Subcutaneous mucormycosis

B46.4   **Disseminated mucormycosis** 🔒
        Generalized mucormycosis

B46.5   **Mucormycosis, unspecified** 🔒

B46.8   **Other zygomycoses** 🔒
        Entomophthoromycosis

B46.9   **Zygomycosis, unspecified** 🔒
        Phycomycosis NOS

N   Newborn Age: 0   P   Pediatric Age: 0–17   M   Maternity DX: 12–55   A   Adult Age: 15–124   ♀   Females Only   ♂   Males Only

🔒   Complication\Comorbidity   🔒   Major C\C   (Ex)   CC/MCC Exclusions   🔒   Present on Admission Requirement   🔒   Hospital-Acquired Condition

CHAPTER 1 (A00-B99)

● **B47   Mycetoma**
Slow progressive, destructive fungal infection of cutaneous and subcutaneous tissues, fascia, and bone, primarily seen in foot (Madura foot) or leg

B47.0   Eumycetoma 🔧
Madura foot, mycotic Maduromycosis
(Ex) B47.0, B48.3, B49, B92, B94.2-B94.9

B47.1   Actinomycetoma 🔧
(Ex) A42.0-A42.2, A42.81-A43.9, B47.1-B47.9, L08.1

B47.9   Mycetoma, unspecified 🔧
Madura foot NOS
(Ex) A42.81-A42.9, A43.8-A43.9, B47.1-B47.9

● **B48   Other mycoses, not elsewhere classified**

B48.0   Lobomycosis
Infection with symptoms of red, smooth, hard cutaneous nodules resembling keloids
Keloidal blastomycosis
Lobo's disease

B48.1   Rhinosporidiosis
Chronic, localized granulomatous fungal infection, affecting mucocutaneous tissues, usually of nose characterized by polyps, papillomas, and wartlike lesions

B48.2   Allescheriasis 🔧
Fungal infection
Infection due to Pseudallescheria boydii
Excludes1   eumycetoma (B47.0)
(Ex) B48.2-B48.3, B49, B92, B94.2-B94.9

B48.3   Geotrichosis 🔧
Fungal infection usually of bronchi, lungs, mouth, or intestinal tract
Geotrichum stomatitis
(Ex) B48.3, B49

B48.4   Penicillosis 🔧
Fungal infection
(Ex) B44.1-B44.7, B44.89-B44.9, B48.3-B48.4, B49, B92, B94.2-B94.9

B48.8   Other specified mycoses 🔧
Adiaspiromycosis
Infection of tissue and organs by Alternaria
Infection of tissue and organs by Drechslera
Infection of tissue and organs by Fusarium
Infection of tissue and organs by saprophytic fungi NEC
(Ex) B48.3, B48.8-B49, B92, B94.2-B94.9

● **B49   Unspecified mycosis** 🔧
Fungemia NOS
(Ex) B48.3, B49

PROTOZOAL DISEASES (B50-B64)

Excludes1   amebiasis (A06.-)
other protozoal intestinal diseases (A07.-)

● **B50   Plasmodium falciparum malaria**
Severe form of malaria that can be fatal
Includes   mixed infections of Plasmodium falciparum with any other Plasmodium species
(Ex) For category B50 CC codes: B50.0-B57.5

B50.0   Plasmodium falciparum malaria with cerebral complications 🔧
Cerebral malaria NOS

B50.8   Other severe and complicated Plasmodium falciparum malaria 🔧
Severe or complicated Plasmodium falciparum malaria NOS

B50.9   Plasmodium falciparum malaria, unspecified 🔧

● **B51   Plasmodium vivax malaria**
Includes   mixed infections of Plasmodium vivax with other Plasmodium species, except Plasmodium falciparum
Excludes1   plasmodium vivav with Plasmodium falciparum (B50.-)
(Ex) For category B51 CC codes unless otherwise indicated: B50.0-B57.5

B51.0   Plasmodium vivax malaria with rupture of spleen 🔧
B51.8   Plasmodium vivax malaria with other complications 🔧
B51.9   Plasmodium vivax malaria without complication 🔧
Plasmodium vivax malaria NOS
(Ex) A44.0-A44.9, A68.0-A68.9, A69.20-A69.29, B50.0-B57.5, B60.0

● **B52   Plasmodium malariae malaria**
Causes fever that recurs at approximately three-day intervals (quartan fever), longer than two-day (tertian) intervals of other malarial parasites
Includes   mixed infections of Plasmodium malariae with other Plasmodium species, except Plasmodium falciparum and Plasmodium vivax
Excludes1   plasmodium falciparum (B50.-)
plasmodium vivax (B51.-)
(Ex) For category B52 CC codes unless otherwise indicated: B50.0-B57.5

B52.0   Plasmodium malariae malaria with nephropathy 🔧
CC when PDx is its own CC
(Ex) A17.9, A18.10-A18.13, A18.82, A18.84, A18.89, A54.21, A54.29, A54.82, A54.84, A54.89-A54.9, A59.00, A59.8-A59.9, B37.41-B37.49, B50.0-B57.5, E08.21-E08.29, E08.618, E08.620-E08.638, E08.649-E08.8, E09.21-E09.29, E09.618-E09.638, E09.649-E09.8, E10.21-E10.29, E10.618-E10.638, E10.649, E10.69-E10.8, E11.21-E11.29, E11.618-E11.638, E11.649, E11.69-E11.8, E13.21-E13.29, E13.618-E13.638, E13.649-E13.8, E88.3, M10.30-M10.39, N00.0-N11.0, N11.8-N13.39, N13.6, N14.0-N19, N25.0-N26.1, N26.9-N27.9, N28.1-N29, N36.41-N36.43, N36.8-N36.9, N39.8-N39.9, R31.0-R31.9

B52.8   Plasmodium malariae malaria with other complications 🔧

B52.9   Plasmodium malariae malaria without complication 🔧
Plasmodium malariae malaria NOS

● **B53   Other specified malaria**
(Ex) For category B53 CC codes unless otherwise indicated: B50.0-B57.5

B53.0   Plasmodium ovale malaria 🔧
Least diagnosed type of malaria spread by female mosquitoes of rare species
Excludes1   plasmodium ovale with Plasmodium falciparum (B50.-)
plasmodium ovale with Plasmodium malariae (B52.-)
plasmodium ovale with Plasmodium vivax (B51.-)

B53.1   Malaria due to simian plasmodia 🔧
Malaria-like disease (parasite infection)
Excludes1   malaria due to simian plasmodia with Plasmodium falciparum (B50.-)
malaria due to simian plasmodia with Plasmodium malariae (B52.-)
malaria due to simian plasmodia with Plasmodium ovale (B53.0)
malaria due to simian plasmodia with Plasmodium vivax (B51.-)

B53.8   Other malaria, not elsewhere classified 🔧

● **B54   Unspecified malaria** 🔧
(Ex) B50.0-B57.5, B97.21

● **B55   Leishmaniasis**
Protozoal infection
(Ex) For category B55 CC codes: A44.0-A44.9, A68.0-A68.9, A69.20-A69.29, A75.0-A79.9, B50.0-B57.5, B60.0

B55.0   Visceral leishmaniasis 🔧
Kala-azar
Post-kala-azar dermal leishmaniasis

B55.1   Cutaneous leishmaniasis 🔧

B55.2   Mucocutaneous leishmaniasis 🔧

B55.9   Leishmaniasis, unspecified 🔧

◄ New   ◄▬ Revised   ~~deleted~~ Deleted   Excludes 1   Excludes 2   Includes   Use additional   Code first   Code also   Unspecified

OGCR Official Guidelines   ● Unacceptable Principal Diagnosis   X Assign placeholder X   ● Use Additional Character(s)   ▶ Manifestation Code   **Coding Clinic**

● **B56**   **African trypanosomiasis**
Human African trypanosomiasis (HAT) is transmitted by fly bites
(Ex:) For category B56 CC codes: A44.0-A44.9, A68.0-A68.9, A69.20-A69.29, A75.0-A79.9, B50.0-B57.5, B60.0

   B56.0   **Gambiense trypanosomiasis** 🔖
      Infection due to Trypanosoma brucei gambiense
      West African sleeping sickness

   B56.1   **Rhodesiense trypanosomiasis** 🔖
      East African sleeping sickness
      Infection due to Trypanosoma brucei rhodesiense

   B56.9   **African trypanosomiasis, unspecified** 🔖
      Sleeping sickness NOS

● **B57**   **Chagas' disease**
Tropical parasitic disease

   Includes   American trypanosomiasis
            infection due to Trypanosoma cruzi

   B57.0   **Acute Chagas' disease with heart involvement** 🔖
      Acute Chagas' disease with myocarditis
      (Ex:) B57.0, B57.2, B92, B94.2-B94.9

   B57.1   **Acute Chagas' disease without heart involvement** 🔖
      Acute Chagas' disease NOS
      (Ex:) See B56

   B57.2   **Chagas' disease (chronic) with heart involvement** 🔖
      American trypanosomiasis NOS
      Chagas' disease (chronic) NOS
      Chagas' disease (chronic) with myocarditis
      Trypanosomiasis NOS
      (Ex:) See B57.0

●   **B57.3**   **Chagas' disease (chronic) with digestive system involvement**
      (Ex:) For category B57.3 CC codes: A44.0-A44.9, A68.0-A68.9, A69.20-A69.29, A75.0-A79.9, B50.0-B57.5, B60.0

     B57.30   **Chagas' disease with digestive system involvement, unspecified** 🔖

     B57.31   **Megaesophagus in Chagas' disease** 🔖

     B57.32   **Megacolon in Chagas' disease** 🔖

     B57.39   **Other digestive system involvement in Chagas' disease** 🔖

●   **B57.4**   **Chagas' disease (chronic) with nervous system involvement**
      (Ex:) For category B57.4 CC codes: A44.0-A44.9, A68.0-A68.9, A69.20-A69.29, A75.0-A79.9, B50.0-B57.5, B60.0

     B57.40   **Chagas' disease with nervous system involvement, unspecified** 🔖

     B57.41   **Meningitis in Chagas' disease** 🔖

     B57.42   **Meningoencephalitis in Chagas' disease** 🔖

     B57.49   **Other nervous system involvement in Chagas' disease** 🔖

   B57.5   **Chagas' disease (chronic) with other organ involvement** 🔖
      (Ex:) See B57.4

● **B58**   **Toxoplasmosis**
Infection by protozoon transmitted in cysts in feces of cats

   Includes   infection due to Toxoplasma gondii
   Excludes1   congenital toxoplasmosis (P37.1)

●   **B58.0**   **Toxoplasma oculopathy**

     B58.00   **Toxoplasma oculopathy, unspecified** 🔖
        (Ex:) B58.00, B58.82-B58.9, B92, B94.2-B94.9

     B58.01   **Toxoplasma chorioretinitis** 🔖
        (Ex:) B58.00-B58.01, B58.82-B58.9, B92, B94.2-B94.9

     B58.09   **Other toxoplasma oculopathy** 🔖
        Toxoplasma uveitis
        (Ex:) B58.00, B58.09, B58.82-B58.9, B92, B94.2-B94.9

   B58.1   **Toxoplasma hepatitis** 🔖
      (Ex:) B58.00, B58.1, B58.82-B58.9, B92, B94.2-B94.9

   B58.2   **Toxoplasma meningoencephalitis** 🔖
      (Ex:) B58.00, B58.2, B58.82-B58.9, B92, B94.2-B94.9

Item 1–22   **Toxoplasmosis** is caused by the protozoa **Toxoplasma gondii,** of which the house cat can be a host. Human infection occurs when contact is made with materials containing the pathogen, such as feces, contaminated soil, or ingestion of infected lamb, goat, or pork. Of the infected, very few have symptoms because a healthy person's immune system keeps the parasite from causing illness. When the immune system is compromised, symptoms may occur. Clinical symptoms include flu-like symptoms, but the disease progresses to include the eyes and the brain in babies.

   B58.3   **Pulmonary toxoplasmosis** 🔖
      (Ex:) A22.1, A37.01, A37.11, A37.81, A37.91, A48.1, B25.0, B44.0, B58.00, B58.3, B58.82-B58.9, B92, B94.2-B94.9, J09.X1-J09.X2, J10.00-J10.1, J11.00-J11.1, J12.0-J12.3, J12.89-J18.1, J18.8-J18.9, J44.9, J47.0-J70.4, J70.8-J70.9, J98.4, R91.1

●   **B58.8**   **Toxoplasmosis with other organ involvement**
      (Ex:) For category B58.8 CC codes unless otherwise indicated: B58.00, B58.82-B58.9, B92, B94.2-B94.9

     B58.81   **Toxoplasma myocarditis** 🔖
        (Ex:) B58.00, B58.81-B58.9, B92, B94.2-B94.9

     B58.82   **Toxoplasma myositis** 🔖

     B58.83   **Toxoplasma tubulo-interstitial nephropathy** 🔖
        Toxoplasma pyelonephritis

     B58.89   **Toxoplasmosis with other organ involvement** 🔖

   B58.9   **Toxoplasmosis, unspecified** 🔖
      (Ex:) B58.9

   B59   **Pneumocystosis** 🔖
      Caused by fungus
      Pneumonia due to Pneumocystis carinii
      Pneumonia due to Pneumocystis jiroveci
      (Ex:) A22.1, A37.01, A37.11, A37.81, A37.91, A48.1, B25.0, B44.0, B59, B92, B94.2-B94.9, J09.X1-J09.X2, J10.00-J10.1, J11.00-J11.1, J12.0-J12.3, J12.89-J15.20, J15.211-J18.1, J18.8-J18.9, J44.9, J47.0-J70.4, J70.8-J70.9, J98.4, R91.1

● **B60**   **Other protozoal diseases, not elsewhere classified**

   Excludes1   cryptosporidiosis (A07.2)
             intestinal microsporidiosis (A07.8)
             isosporiasis (A07.3)

   B60.0   **Babesiosis** 🔖
      Tickborne disease caused by microscopic organisms
      Piroplasmosis
      (Ex:) A44.0-A44.9, A68.0-A68.9, A69.20-A69.29, A75.0-A79.9, B50.0-B57.5, B60.0

●   **B60.1**   **Acanthamebiasis**
      (Ex:) For category B60.1 CC codes: B59, B60.10-B60.11, B60.19-B64, B89, B99.8-B99.9, L94.6, M35.2

     B60.10   **Acanthamebiasis, unspecified** 🔖

     B60.11   **Meningoencephalitis due to Acanthamoeba (culbertsoni)**

     B60.12   **Conjunctivitis due to Acanthamoeba**

●   **B60.13**   **Keratoconjunctivitis due to Acanthamoeba**

     B60.19   **Other acanthamebic disease** 🔖

   B60.2   **Naegleriasis** 🔖
      Infection with microscopic organisms
      Primary amebic meningoencephalitis
      (Ex:) B59, B60.10-B60.11, B60.19-B64, B89, B99.8-B99.9, L94.6, M35.2

   B60.8   **Other specified protozoal diseases**
      Microsporidiosis

   B64   **Unspecified protozoal disease**

HELMINTHIASES (B65-B83)

Diseases or infestations caused by parasitic worms

● **B65**   **Schistosomiasis [bilharziasis]**
Infection with flukes (flat parasitic worms)

   Includes   snail fever

   (Ex:) For category B64 CC codes: B65.0-B65.9

   B65.0   **Schistosomiasis due to Schistosoma haematobium [urinary schistosomiasis]** 🔖

   B65.1   **Schistosomiasis due to Schistosoma mansoni [intestinal schistosomiasis]** 🔖

CHAPTER 1 (A00-B99)

N   Newborn Age: 0   P   Pediatric Age: 0–17   M   Maternity DX: 12–55   A   Adult Age: 15–124   ♀ Females Only   ♂ Males Only

🔖 Complication\Comorbidity   🔖 Major C\C   (Ex:) CC/MCC Exclusions   🔖 Present on Admission Requirement   🔖 Hospital-Acquired Condition

767

B65.2 **Schistosomiasis due to Schistosoma japonicum** 🔵
Asiatic schistosomiasis

B65.3 **Cercarial dermatitis** 🔵
Swimmer's itch

B65.8 **Other schistosomiasis** 🔵
Infection due to Schistosoma intercalatum
Infection due to Schistosoma mattheei
Infection due to Schistosoma mekongi

B65.9 **Schistosomiasis, unspecified** 🔵

● **B66** **Other fluke infections**
Trematode (parasitic worms)
Ⓔⓧ **For category B66 CC codes: B66.0-B66.9**

B66.0 **Opisthorchiasis** 🔵
Infection due to cat liver fluke
Infection due to Opisthorchis (felineus)(viverrini)

B66.1 **Clonorchiasis** 🔵
Chinese liver fluke disease
Infection due to Clonorchis sinensis
Oriental liver fluke disease

B66.2 **Dicroceliasis** 🔵
Liver fluke
Infection due to Dicrocoelium dendriticum
Lancet fluke infection

B66.3 **Fascioliasis** 🔵
Infection due to Fasciola gigantica
Infection due to Fasciola hepatica
Infection due to Fasciola indica
Sheep liver fluke disease

B66.4 **Paragonimiasis** 🔵
Infection due to Paragonimus species
Lung fluke disease
Pulmonary distomiasis

B66.5 **Fasciolopsiasis** 🔵
Largest intestinal fluke in humans
Infection due to Fasciolopsis buski
Intestinal distomiasis

B66.8 **Other specified fluke infections** 🔵
Echinostomiasis
Heterophyiasis
Metagonimiasis
Nanophyetiasis
Watsoniasis

B66.9 **Fluke infection, unspecified**

● **B67** **Echinococcosis**
Larval forms of tapeworms usually of liver or lungs
  Includes   hydatidosis

B67.0 **Echinococcus granulosus infection of liver** 🔵
Ⓔⓧ B67.0, B67.8-B67.99

B67.1 **Echinococcus granulosus infection of lung** 🔵
Ⓔⓧ B67.1, B67.8-B67.99, J12.81

B67.2 **Echinococcus granulosus infection of bone** 🔵
Ⓔⓧ B67.2, B67.32-B67.39, B67.8-B67.99

● **B67.3** **Echinococcus granulosus infection, other and multiple sites**

B67.31 **Echinococcus granulosus infection, thyroid gland** 🔵
Ⓔⓧ B67.31, B67.8-B67.99

B67.32 **Echinococcus granulosus infection, multiple sites** 🔵
Ⓔⓧ See B67.2

B67.39 **Echinococcus granulosus infection, other sites** 🔵
Ⓔⓧ See B67.2

B67.4 **Echinococcus granulosus infection, unspecified** 🔵
Dog tapeworm (infection)
Ⓔⓧ B67.4, B67.8-B67.99

B67.5 **Echinococcus multilocularis infection of liver** 🔵
Ⓔⓧ B67.5, B67.8-B67.99

Item 1-23 Echinococcosis: Also known as hydatid disease; is caused by Echinococcus granulosus, E. multilocularis, and E. vogeli tapeworms; and is contracted from infected food. Found in southern South America, the Mediterranean, the Middle East, central Asia, and Africa and uncommon in the United States but has been reported in California, New Mexico, Arizona and Utah. The disease is treated with medication over a long course as it is resistive.

● **B67.6** **Echinococcus multilocularis infection, other and multiple sites**
Ⓔⓧ **For category B67.6 CC codes: B67.61-B67.69, B67.8-B67.99**

B67.61 **Echinococcus multilocularis infection, multiple sites** 🔵

B67.69 **Echinococcus multilocularis infection, other sites** 🔵

B67.7 **Echinococcus multilocularis infection, unspecified** 🔵
Ⓔⓧ B67.7-B67.99

B67.8 **Echinococcosis, unspecified, of liver** 🔵
Ⓔⓧ B67.8-B67.99

● **B67.9** **Echinococcosis, other and unspecified**
Ⓔⓧ **For category B67.9 CC codes: B67.8-B67.99**

B67.90 **Echinococcosis, unspecified** 🔵
Echinococcosis NOS

B67.99 **Other echinococcosis** 🔵

● **B68** **Taeniasis**
Intestinal tapeworm (cestode) infection from raw or undercooked meat of infected animal
  Excludes1 cysticercosis (B69.-)

B68.0 **Taenia solium taeniasis** 🔵
Pork tapeworm (infection)
Ⓔⓧ A00.1, A01.00-A01.09, A01.4-A02.0, A03.9-A05.2, A06.0-A06.2, A06.9, A07.1-A09, A18.32-A18.39, A18.83, A48.51-A48.52, B37.82, B68.0-B71.9, B82.9, J09.X3-J09.X9, J10.2-J10.89, J11.2-J11.89, K30, K31.84, K52.1-K52.2, K52.82-K52.9, K58.0-K58.9, P76.8-P77.9, P78.1, P78.3-P78.89

B68.1 **Taenia saginata taeniasis** 🔵
Beef tapeworm (infection)
Infection due to adult tapeworm Taenia saginata
Ⓔⓧ B68.0-B71.9

B68.9 **Taeniasis, unspecified** 🔵
Ⓔⓧ B68.0-B71.9

● **B69** **Cysticercosis**
Systemic illness caused by the larvae of pork tapeworm
  Includes   cysticerciasis infection due to larval form of Taenia solium
Ⓔⓧ **For category B69 CC codes: B68.0-B71.9**

B69.0 **Cysticercosis of central nervous system** 🔵

B69.1 **Cysticercosis of eye** 🔵

● **B69.8** **Cysticercosis of other sites**

B69.81 **Myositis in cysticercosis** 🔵

B69.89 **Cysticercosis of other sites** 🔵

B69.9 **Cysticercosis, unspecified** 🔵

● **B70** **Diphyllobothriasis and sparganosis**
Infection with tapeworms seen most often from inadequately cooked fish
Ⓔⓧ **For category B70 CC codes: B68.0-B71.9**

B70.0 **Diphyllobothriasis** 🔵
Diphyllobothrium (adult) (latum) (pacificum) infection
Fish tapeworm (infection)
  Excludes2 larval diphyllobothriasis (B70.1)

B70.1 **Sparganosis**
Infection with migrating tapeworm larvae, which invade subcutaneous tissues, causing inflammation and fibrosis that resembles cellulitis
Infection due to Sparganum (mansoni) (proliferum)
Infection due to Spirometra larva
Larval diphyllobothriasis
Spirometrosis

◀ New   ⬅ Revised   ~~deleted~~ Deleted   Excludes 1   Excludes 2   Includes   Use additional   Code first   Code also   Unspecified
OGCR Official Guidelines   ● Unacceptable Principal Diagnosis   X Assign placeholder X   ● Use Additional Character(s)   ▸ Manifestation Code   **Coding Clinic**

● **B71**   **Other cestode infections**
    Ex: For category B71 CC codes: B68.0-B71.9

    B71.0   **Hymenolepiasis** 🦠
        Intestinal infestation with tapeworms
        Dwarf tapeworm infection
        Rat tapeworm (infection)

    B71.1   **Dipylidiasis** 🦠
        Infection with tapeworm common to dogs and cats and seen
        in children having close contact with infected pets

    B71.8   **Other specified cestode infections** 🦠
        Infection by the larval stage of a tapeworm, usually through
        fruit or vegetables
        Coenurosis

    B71.9   **Cestode infection, unspecified** 🦠
        Tapeworm (infection) NOS

B72   **Dracunculiasis** 🦠
    Infection with roundworms
    Includes   guinea worm infection
               infection due to Dracunculus medinensis
    Ex: B72-B74.9

● **B73**   **Onchocerciasis**
    Infection with parasitic worm
    Includes   onchocerca volvulus infection
               onchocercosis
               river blindness

  ● **B73.0**   **Onchocerciasis with eye disease**
        Ex: For category B73 CC codes: B72-B74.9

        B73.00   **Onchocerciasis with eye involvement,**
                unspecified 🦠

        B73.01   **Onchocerciasis with endophthalmitis** 🦠

        B73.02   **Onchocerciasis with glaucoma** 🦠

        B73.09   **Onchocerciasis with other eye involvement** 🦠
                Infestation of eyelid due to onchocerciasis

    B73.1   **Onchocerciasis without eye disease** 🦠

● **B74**   **Filariasis**
    Infestation with slender threadlike worms
    Excludes2   onchocerciasis (B73)
                 tropical (pulmonary) eosinophilia NOS (J82)
    Ex: For category B74 CC codes: B72-B74.9

    B74.0   **Filariasis due to Wuchereria bancrofti** 🦠
        Bancroftian elephantiasis
        Bancroftian filariasis

    B74.1   **Filariasis due to Brugia malayi** 🦠

    B74.2   **Filariasis due to Brugia timori** 🦠

    B74.3   **Loiasis** 🦠
        Infection with round worms growing in subcutaneous
                connective tissue
        Calabar swelling
        Eyeworm disease of Africa
        Loa loa infection

    B74.4   **Mansonelliasis** 🦠
        Infection with filarial parasite
        Infection due to Mansonella ozzardi
        Infection due to Mansonella perstans
        Infection due to Mansonella streptocerca

    B74.8   **Other filariases** 🦠
        Dirofilariasis

    B74.9   **Filariasis, unspecified** 🦠

B75   **Trichinellosis** 🦠
    Infestation with parasitic roundworms ingested in undercooked
    contaminated meat
    Includes   infection due to Trichinella species trichiniasis
    Ex: A17.82, A50.42, A52.14, A75.9, A79.9, A81.1, A81.82-A81.89, A83.0-A85.8, A87.2, A88.0, A88.8, A92.1-A92.8, A93.0, B00.4, B00.82, B01.11-B01.12, B04, B06.01, B08.09, B08.20-B08.22, B08.60-B08.79, B09, B10.01-B10.09, B26.2, B33.1, B45.0, B45.2-B45.9, B58.2, B75, B97.10, B97.21, G04.00-G04.01, G04.31, G04.81-G05.4, G37.0, G37.4-G37.5, J09.X3-J09.X9, J10.2-J10.89, J11.2-J11.89, L44.4, M1A.10X0-M1A.10X1, M1A.1110-M1A.19X1, P35.2-P35.9, P37.0-P37.4, P37.8-P37.9, T56.0X1-T56.0X4[A]

● **B76**   **Hookworm diseases**
    Occurs in hot, humid parts of world where larvae are soil borne, enter
    digestive tract through skin of feet/legs or in contaminated food/
    water; AKA ground itch
    Includes   uncinariasis
    Ex: For category B76 CC codes: B76.0-B76.9

    B76.0   **Ancylostomiasis** 🦠
        Infection due to Ancylostoma species

    B76.1   **Necatoriasis** 🦠
        Infection due to Necator americanus

    B76.8   **Other hookworm diseases** 🦠

    B76.9   **Hookworm disease, unspecified** 🦠
        Cutaneous larva migrans NOS

● **B77**   **Ascariasis**
    Infection by roundworm in small intestine
    Includes   ascaridiasis
               roundworm infection

    B77.0   **Ascariasis with intestinal complications** 🦠
        Ex: B77.0-B78.0, B78.7-B82.0

  ● **B77.8**   **Ascariasis with other complications**

        B77.81   **Ascariasis pneumonia** 🦠
                MCC when PDx is its own MCC
            Ex: A15.0-A15.6, A15.8-A15.9, A17.9, A18.82, A18.84, A18.89, A21.2, A22.1, A31.0, A37.01, A37.11, A37.81, A37.91, A42.0, A43.0, A48.1, B25.0, B39.0-B39.2, B44.0, B58.3, B59, B67.1, B77.0-B78.0, B78.7-B82.0, J09.X1-J09.X2, J10.00-J10.1, J11.00-J11.1, J12.0-J12.3, J12.89-J18.1, J18.8-J18.9, J22, J44.9, J47.0-J70.4, J70.8-J70.9, J98.4, J98.8-J99, Q33.4, R91.1

        B77.89   **Ascariasis with other complications** 🦠
                Ex: See B77.0

    B77.9   **Ascariasis, unspecified** 🦠
        Ex: See B77.0

● **B78**   **Strongyloidiasis**
    Infection with adult female roundworms
    Excludes1   trichostrongyliasis (B81.2)
    Ex: For category B78 CC codes: B77.0-B78.0, B78.7-B82.0

    B78.0   **Intestinal strongyloidiasis** 🦠

    B78.1   **Cutaneous strongyloidiasis**

    B78.7   **Disseminated strongyloidiasis** 🦠

    B78.9   **Strongyloidiasis, unspecified** 🦠

B79   **Trichuriasis** 🦠
    Intestinal infection with roundworms
    Includes   trichocephaliasis
               whipworm (disease)(infection)
    Ex: See B78

B80   **Enterobiasis** 🦠
    Intestinal infection with pinworms
    Includes   oxyuriasis
               pinworm infection
               threadworm infection
    Ex: See B78

● **B81**   **Other intestinal helminthiases, not elsewhere classified**
    Diseases or infestations caused by parasitic worms
    Excludes1   angiostrongyliasis due to Parastrongylus
                 cantonensis (B83.2)
    Ex: For category B81 CC codes B81.0-B81.2: B77.0-B78.0, B78.7-B82.0 For category B81 CC codes B81.3-B81.8: B77.0-B78.0, B78.7-B83.3, B83.8-B83.9

    B81.0   **Anisakiasis** 🦠
        Roundworm infection via contaminated undercooked infected
                fish or marine mammals
        Infection due to Anisakis larva

    B81.1   **Intestinal capillariasis** 🦠
        Infestation with of parasites (nematodes)
        Capillariasis NOS
        Infection due to Capillaria philippinensis
        Excludes2   hepatic capillariasis (B83.8)

    B81.2   **Trichostrongyliasis** 🦠

N   Newborn Age: 0   P   Pediatric Age: 0–17   M   Maternity DX: 12–55   A   Adult Age: 15–124   ♀   Females Only   ♂   Males Only

🦠   Complication\Comorbidity   🦠   Major C\C   Ex: CC/MCC Exclusions   🦠   Present on Admission Requirement   🦠   Hospital-Acquired Condition

769

CHAPTER 1 (A00–B99)

CHAPTER 1 (A00-B99)

B81.3 **Intestinal angiostrongyliasis** 🔖
Angiostrongyliasis due to Parastrongylus costaricensis

B81.4 **Mixed intestinal helminthiases** 🔖
Infection due to intestinal helminths classified to more than one of the categories B65.0-B81.3 and B81.8
Mixed helminthiasis NOS

B81.8 **Other specified intestinal helminthiases** 🔖
Infection due to Oesophagostomum species [esophagostomiasis]
Infection due to Ternidens diminutus [ternidensiasis]

● **B82 Unspecified intestinal parasitism**

B82.0 **Intestinal helminthiasis, unspecified** 🔖
Infected with worms
(Ex) See B81.3

B82.9 **Intestinal parasitism, unspecified**

● **B83 Other helminthiases**
Caused by parasitic worms
Excludes1 capillariasis NOS (B81.1)
Excludes2 intestinal capillariasis (B81.1)

B83.0 **Visceral larva migrans**
Prolonged migration of nematode larvae
Toxocariasis

B83.1 **Gnathostomiasis**
Infection with nematode occurring from ingested undercooked fish contaminated with larvae; larvae migrate to subcutaneous tissue or deeper tissues, results are abscesses
Wandering swelling

B83.2 **Angiostrongyliasis due to Parastrongylus cantonensis**
Nematode infection caused by eating contaminated raw snails, slugs, or paratenic hosts such as prawns or crabs; larval worms migrate to central nervous system resulting in eosinophilic meningitis
Eosinophilic meningoencephalitis due to Parastrongylus cantonensis
Excludes2 intestinal angiostrongyliasis (B81.3)

B83.3 **Syngamiasis**
Infestation with gapeworm from turkey, pheasant, guinea fowl, goose, and wild birds
Syngamosis

B83.4 **Internal hirudiniasis**
Infestation by leeches
Excludes2 external hirudiniasis (B88.3)

B83.8 **Other specified helminthiases**
Parasitic worm infestation
Acanthocephaliasis
Gongylonemiasis
Hepatic capillariasis
Metastrongyliasis
Thelaziasis

B83.9 **Helminthiasis, unspecified**
Worms NOS
Excludes1 intestinal helminthiasis NOS (B82.0)

PEDICULOSIS, ACARIASIS AND OTHER INFESTATIONS (B85-B89)
Infestation of lice

● **B85 Pediculosis and phthiriasis**

B85.0 **Pediculosis due to Pediculus humanus capitis**
Head-louse infestation

B85.1 **Pediculosis due to Pediculus humanus corporis**
Body-louse infestation

B85.2 **Pediculosis, unspecified**

B85.3 **Phthiriasis**
Crab or pubic lice
Infestation by crab-louse
Infestation by Phthirus pubis

B85.4 **Mixed pediculosis and phthiriasis**
Infestation classifiable to more than one of the categories B85.0-B85.3 ◀▥▥

● **B86 Scabies**
Sarcoptic itch
Contagious dermatitis caused by mites

● **B87 Myiasis**
Infestation by fly maggots
Includes infestation by larva of flies

B87.0 **Cutaneous myiasis**
Creeping myiasis

B87.1 **Wound myiasis**
Traumatic myiasis

B87.2 **Ocular myiasis**

B87.3 **Nasopharyngeal myiasis**
Laryngeal myiasis

B87.4 **Aural myiasis**

● B87.8 **Myiasis of other sites**
B87.81 **Genitourinary myiasis**
B87.82 **Intestinal myiasis**
B87.89 **Myiasis of other sites**

B87.9 **Myiasis, unspecified**

● **B88 Other infestations**

B88.0 **Other acariasis**
Acarine dermatitis
Dermatitis due to Demodex species
Dermatitis due to Dermanyssus gallinae
Dermatitis due to Liponyssoides sanguineus
Trombiculosis
Excludes2 scabies (B86)

B88.1 **Tungiasis [sandflea infestation]**
Inflammatory skin disease caused by infestation of fleas

B88.2 **Other arthropod infestations**
Scarabiasis

B88.3 **External hirudiniasis**
Leech infestation NOS
Excludes2 internal hirudiniasis (B83.4)

B88.8 **Other specified infestations**
Infection of topical fresh water fish parasite
Ichthyoparasitism due to Vandellia cirrhosa
Linguatulosis
Porocephaliasis

B88.9 **Infestation, unspecified**
Infestation (skin) NOS
Infestation by mites NOS
Skin parasites NOS

B89 **Unspecified parasitic disease**

SEQUELAE OF INFECTIOUS AND PARASITIC DISEASES (B90-B94)

Note: Categories B90-B94 are to be used to indicate conditions in categories A00-B89 as the cause of sequelae, which are themselves classified elsewhere. The 'sequelae' include conditions specified as such; they also include residuals of diseases classifiable to the above categories if there is evidence that the disease itself is no longer present. Codes from these categories are not to be used for chronic infections. Code chronic current infections to active infectious disease as appropriate.

Code first condition resulting from (sequela) the infectious or parasitic disease

● **B90 Sequelae of tuberculosis**
Condition resulting from tuberculosis

B90.0 **Sequelae of central nervous system tuberculosis** 🔖
B90.1 **Sequelae of genitourinary tuberculosis** 🔖
B90.2 **Sequelae of tuberculosis of bones and joints** 🔖
B90.8 **Sequelae of tuberculosis of other organs** 🔖
Excludes2 sequelae of respiratory tuberculosis (B90.9)

B90.9 **Sequelae of respiratory and unspecified tuberculosis** 🔖
Sequelae of tuberculosis NOS

◀ New   ◀▥ Revised   ~~deleted~~ Deleted   Excludes 1   Excludes 2   Includes   Use additional   Code first   Code also   Unspecified
OGCR Official Guidelines   ● Unacceptable Principal Diagnosis   X Assign placeholder X   ● Use Additional Character(s)   ▶ Manifestation Code   **Coding Clinic**

B91   Sequelae of poliomyelitis 🖉

     Excludes1   postpolio syndrome (G14)

B92   Sequelae of leprosy 🖉

● **B94   Sequelae of other and unspecified infectious and parasitic diseases**

     B94.0   Sequelae of trachoma 🖉

     B94.1   Sequelae of viral encephalitis 🖉

     B94.2   Sequelae of viral hepatitis 🖉

     B94.8   Sequelae of other specified infectious and parasitic diseases 🖉

     B94.9   Sequelae of unspecified infectious and parasitic disease 🖉

     OGCR   Section I.C.1.b

     Certain infectious and parasitic diseases

     Infectious agents as the cause of diseases classified to other chapters

     Certain infections are classified in chapters other than Chapter 1 and no organism is identified as part of the infection code. In these instances, it is necessary to use an additional code from Chapter 1 to identify the organism. A code from category B95, Streptococcus, Staphylococcus, and Enterococcus as the cause of diseases classified to other chapters, B96, Other bacterial agents as the cause of diseases classified to other chapters, or B97, Viral agents as the cause of diseases classified to other chapters, is to be used as an additional code to identify the organism. An instructional note will be found at the infection code advising that an additional organism code is required.

BACTERIAL AND VIRAL INFECTIOUS AGENTS (B95-B97)

Note: These categories are provided for use as supplementary or additional codes to identify the infectious agent(s) in diseases classified elsewhere.

Code the disease first, then the bacterium.

● **B95   Streptococcus, Staphylococcus, and Enterococcus as the cause of diseases classified elsewhere**

     B95.0   Streptococcus, group A, as the cause of diseases classified elsewhere

     B95.1   Streptococcus, group B, as the cause of diseases classified elsewhere

     B95.2   Enterococcus as the cause of diseases classified elsewhere

     B95.3   Streptococcus pneumoniae as the cause of diseases classified elsewhere

     B95.4   Other streptococcus as the cause of diseases classified elsewhere

     B95.5   Unspecified streptococcus as the cause of diseases classified elsewhere

     ● **B95.6   Staphylococcus aureus as the cause of diseases classified elsewhere**

         B95.61   Methicillin susceptible Staphylococcus aureus infection as the cause of diseases classified elsewhere

         Methicillin susceptible Staphylococcus aureus (MSSA) infection as the cause of diseases classified elsewhere

         Staphylococcus aureus infection NOS as the cause of diseases classified elsewhere

         B95.62   Methicillin resistant Staphylococcus aureus infection as the cause of diseases classified elsewhere

         Methicillin resistant staphylococcus aureus (MRSA) infection as the cause of diseases classified elsewhere

     B95.7   Other staphylococcus as the cause of diseases classified elsewhere

     B95.8   Unspecified staphylococcus as the cause of diseases classified elsewhere

● **B96   Other bacterial agents as the cause of diseases classified elsewhere**

     B96.0   Mycoplasma pneumoniae [M. pneumoniae] as the cause of diseases classified elsewhere

     Pleuro-pneumonia-like-organism [PPLO]

     B96.1   Klebsiella pneumoniae [K. pneumoniae] as the cause of diseases classified elsewhere

     ● **B96.2   Escherichia coli [E. coli] as the cause of diseases classified elsewhere**

         B96.20   Unspecified Escherichia coli [E. coli] as the cause of diseases classified elsewhere

         Escherichia coli [E. coli] NOS

         B96.21   Shiga toxin-producing Escherichia coli [E. coli] (STEC) O157 as the cause of diseases classified elsewhere

         E. coli O157:H- (nonmotile) with confirmation of Shiga toxin

         E. coli O157 with confirmation of Shiga toxin when H antigen is unknown, or is not H7

         O157:H7 Escherichia coli [E.coli] with or without confirmation of Shiga toxin-production

         Shiga toxin-producing Escherichia coli [E.coli] O157:H7 with or without confirmation of Shiga toxin-production

         STEC O157:H7 with or without confirmation of Shiga toxin-production

         B96.22   Other specified Shiga toxin-producing Escherichia coli [E. coli] (STEC) as the cause of diseases classified elsewhere

         Non-O157 Shiga toxin-producing Escherichia coli [E.coli]

         Non-O157 Shiga toxin-producing Escherichia coli [E.coli] with known O group

         B96.23   Unspecified Shiga toxin-producing Escherichia coli [E. coli] (STEC) as the cause of diseases classified elsewhere

         Shiga toxin-producing Escherichia coli [E. coli] with unspecified O group

         STEC NOS

         B96.29   Other Escherichia coli [E. coli] as the cause of diseases classified elsewhere

         Non-Shiga toxin-producing E. coli

     B96.3   Hemophilus influenzae [H. influenzae] as the cause of diseases classified elsewhere

     B96.4   Proteus (mirabilis) (morganii) as the cause of diseases classified elsewhere

     B96.5   Pseudomonas (aeruginosa) (mallei) (pseudomallei) as the cause of diseases classified elsewhere

     B96.6   Bacteroides fragilis [B. fragilis] as the cause of diseases classified elsewhere

     B96.7   Clostridium perfringens [C. perfringens] as the cause of diseases classified elsewhere

     ● **B96.8   Other specified bacterial agents as the cause of diseases classified elsewhere**

         B96.81   Helicobacter pylori [H. pylori] as the cause of diseases classified elsewhere

         B96.82   Vibrio vulnificus as the cause of diseases classified elsewhere

         B96.89   Other specified bacterial agents as the cause of diseases classified elsewhere

● **B97   Viral agents as the cause of diseases classified elsewhere**

     B97.0   Adenovirus as the cause of diseases classified elsewhere

     ● **B97.1   Enterovirus as the cause of diseases classified elsewhere**

         B97.10   Unspecified enterovirus as the cause of diseases classified elsewhere

         B97.11   Coxsackievirus as the cause of diseases classified elsewhere

         B97.12   Echovirus as the cause of diseases classified elsewhere

         B97.19   Other enterovirus as the cause of diseases classified elsewhere

CHAPTER 1 (A00–B99)

N   Newborn Age: 0   P   Pediatric Age: 0–17   M   Maternity DX: 12–55   A   Adult Age: 15–124   ♀   Females Only   ♂   Males Only

🖉 Complication\Comorbidity   🖉 Major C\C   (Ex) CC/MCC Exclusions   🖉 Present on Admission Requirement   🖉 Hospital-Acquired Condition

● **B97.2** **Coronavirus as the cause of diseases classified elsewhere**

B97.21 SARS-associated coronavirus as the cause of diseases classified elsewhere 🔖

Excludes1 pneumonia due to SARS-associated coronavirus (J12.81)

(Ex:) A15.0-A15.6, A15.8-A15.9, A17.9, A18.82, A18.84, A18.89, A21.2, A22.1, A31.0, A37.01, A37.11, A37.81, A37.91, A42.0, A43.0, A48.1, B25.0, B34.1-B34.2, B34.4-B34.8, B39.0-B39.2, B44.0, B58.3, B59, B67.1, B97.19-B97.29, B97.5-B97.6, B97.81-B97.89, J09.X1-J09.X2, J10.00-J10.1, J11.00-J11.1, J12.0-J12.3, J12.89-J15.20, J15.211-J18.1, J18.8-J18.9, J22, J44.9, J47.0-J70.4, J70.8-J70.9, J98.4, J98.8-J99, Q33.4, R91.1

B97.29 Other coronavirus as the cause of diseases classified elsewhere

● **B97.3** **Retrovirus as the cause of diseases classified elsewhere**

Excludes1 human immunodeficiency virus [HIV] disease (B20)

B97.30 Unspecified retrovirus as the cause of diseases classified elsewhere

B97.31 Lentivirus as the cause of diseases classified elsewhere

B97.32 Oncovirus as the cause of diseases classified elsewhere

B97.33 Human T-cell lymphotrophic virus, type I [HTLV-I] as the cause of diseases classified elsewhere 🔖

(Ex:) A74.81, A74.9, B33.3-B33.4, B34.1-B34.2, B34.4-B34.8, B97.10, B97.19-B97.29, B97.31-B97.39, B97.5-B97.6, B97.81-B97.89

B97.34 Human T-cell lymphotrophic virus, type II [HTLV-II] as the cause of diseases classified elsewhere 🔖

(Ex:) A74.81, A74.9, B33.3-B33.4, B34.1-B34.2, B34.4-B34.8, B97.10, B97.19-B97.39, B97.5-B97.6, B97.81, B97.89

Item 1–24 **Retrovirus** develops by copying its RNA, genetic materials, into the DNA, which then produces new virus particles. It is from the Retroviridae virus family. **Human T-cell lymphotropic virus, Type I (HTLV-I)** is also called human T-cell leukemia virus, Type I, and is a retrovirus thought to cause T-cell leukemia/lymphoma. **Human T-cell lymphotropic virus, Type II (HTLV-II),** is also called human T-cell leukemia virus, Type II, and is a retrovirus associated with hematologic disorders.

HIV-2 is one of the serotypes of HIV and is usually confined to West Africa, whereas HIV-1 is found worldwide.

B97.35 Human immunodeficiency virus, type 2 [HIV 2] as the cause of diseases classified elsewhere 🔖

(Ex:) A74.81, A74.9, B20, B33.3-B33.4, B34.1-B34.2, B34.4, B34.8, B97.10, B97.19-B97.39, B97.5-B97.6, B97.81, B97.89

B97.39 Other retrovirus as the cause of diseases classified elsewhere

B97.4 Respiratory syncytial virus as the cause of diseases classified elsewhere

B97.5 Reovirus as the cause of diseases classified elsewhere

B97.6 Parvovirus as the cause of diseases classified elsewhere

B97.7 Papillomavirus as the cause of diseases classified elsewhere

● **B97.8** Other viral agents as the cause of diseases classified elsewhere

B97.81 Human metapneumovirus as the cause of diseases classified elsewhere

B97.89 Other viral agents as the cause of diseases classified elsewhere

OTHER INFECTIOUS DISEASES (B99)

● **B99** Other and unspecified infectious diseases

B99.8 Other infectious disease

B99.9 Unspecified infectious disease

Item 2–1 Neoplasm: Neo = new, plasm = growth, development, formation. This new growth (mass, tumor) can be malignant or benign, which is confirmed by the pathology report. Do not assign a code to a neoplasm until you review the pathology report. Certain CPT codes will specify benign or malignant lesion, so be certain the diagnosis code supports the procedure code.

OGCR Section I.C.2

General Guidelines

Chapter 2 of the ICD-10-CM contains the codes for the most benign and all malignant neoplasms. Certain benign neoplasms, such as prostatic adenomas, may be found in the specific body system chapters. To properly code a neoplasm, it is necessary to determine from the record if the neoplasm is benign, in-situ, malignant, or, of uncertain histologic behavior. If malignant, any secondary (metastatic) sites should also be determined.

CHAPTER 2

NEOPLASMS (C00-D49)

This chapter contains the following blocks:

C00-C14	Malignant neoplasms of lip, oral cavity and pharynx
C15-C26	Malignant neoplasms of digestive organs
C30-C39	Malignant neoplasms of respiratory and intrathoracic organs
C40-C41	Malignant neoplasms of bone and articular cartilage
C43-C44	Melanoma and other malignant neoplasms of skin
C45-C49	Malignant neoplasms of mesothelial and soft tissue
C50	Malignant neoplasms of breast
C51-C58	Malignant neoplasms of female genital organs
C60-C63	Malignant neoplasms of male genital organs
C64-C68	Malignant neoplasms of urinary tract
C69-C72	Malignant neoplasms of eye, brain and other parts of central nervous system
C73-C75	Malignant neoplasms of thyroid and other endocrine glands
C7A	Malignant neuroendocrine tumors
C7B	Secondary neuroendocrine tumors
C76-C80	Malignant neoplasms of ill-defined, other secondary and unspecified sites
C81-C96	Malignant neoplasms of lymphoid, hematopoietic and related tissue
D00-D09	In situ neoplasms
D10-D36	Benign neoplasms, except benign neuroendocrine tumors
D3A	Benign neuroendocrine tumors
D37-D48	Neoplasms of uncertain behavior, polycythemia vera and myelodysplastic syndromes
D49	Neoplasms of unspecified behavior

Notes: Functional activity

All neoplasms are classified in this chapter, whether they are functionally active or not. An additional code from Chapter 4 may be used, to identify functional activity associated with any neoplasm.

Morphology [Histology]

Chapter 2 classifies neoplasms primarily by site (topography), with broad groupings for behavior, malignant, in situ, benign, etc. The Table of Neoplasms should be used to identify the correct topography code. In a few cases, such as for malignant melanoma and certain neuroendocrine tumors, the morphology (histologic type) is included in the category and codes.

Primary malignant neoplasms overlapping site boundaries

A primary malignant neoplasm that overlaps two or more contiguous (next to each other) sites should be classified to the subcategory/code .8 ('overlapping lesion'), unless the combination is specifically indexed elsewhere. For multiple neoplasms of the same site that are not contiguous, such as tumors in different quadrants of the same breast, codes for each site should be assigned.

Malignant neoplasm of ectopic tissue

Malignant neoplasms of ectopic tissue are to be coded to the site mentioned, e.g., ectopic pancreatic malignant neoplasms are coded to pancreas, unspecified (C25.9).

MALIGNANT NEOPLASMS (C00-C96)

MALIGNANT NEOPLASMS, STATED OR PRESUMED TO BE PRIMARY (OF SPECIFIED SITES), AND CERTAIN SPECIFIED HISTOLOGIES, EXCEPT NEUROENDOCRINE, AND OF LYMPHOID, HEMATOPOIETIC AND RELATED TISSUE (C00-C75)

MALIGNANT NEOPLASMS OF LIP, ORAL CAVITY AND PHARYNX (C00-C14)

● **C00** **Malignant neoplasm of lip**
> Use additional code to identify:
> alcohol abuse and dependence (F10.-)
> history of tobacco use (Z87.891)
> tobacco dependence (F17.-)
> tobacco use (Z72.0)
> **Excludes1**   malignant melanoma of lip (C43.0)
>   Merkel cell carcinoma of lip (C4A.0)
>   other and unspecified malignant neoplasm of skin of lip (C44.0-)

C00.0 **Malignant neoplasm of external upper lip**
> Malignant neoplasm of lipstick area of upper lip
> Malignant neoplasm of upper lip NOS
> Malignant neoplasm of vermilion border of upper lip

C00.1 **Malignant neoplasm of external lower lip**
> Malignant neoplasm of lower lip NOS
> Malignant neoplasm of lipstick area of lower lip
> Malignant neoplasm of vermilion border of lower lip

C00.2 **Malignant neoplasm of external lip, unspecified**
> Malignant neoplasm of vermilion border of lip NOS

C00.3 **Malignant neoplasm of upper lip, inner aspect**
> Malignant neoplasm of buccal aspect of upper lip
> Malignant neoplasm of frenulum of upper lip
> Malignant neoplasm of mucosa of upper lip
> Malignant neoplasm of oral aspect of upper lip

C00.4 **Malignant neoplasm of lower lip, inner aspect**
> Malignant neoplasm of buccal aspect of lower lip
> Malignant neoplasm of frenulum of lower lip
> Malignant neoplasm of mucosa of lower lip
> Malignant neoplasm of oral aspect of lower lip

C00.5 **Malignant neoplasm of lip, unspecified, inner aspect**
> Malignant neoplasm of buccal aspect of lip, unspecified
> Malignant neoplasm of frenulum of lip, unspecified
> Malignant neoplasm of mucosa of lip, unspecified
> Malignant neoplasm of oral aspect of lip, unspecified

C00.6 **Malignant neoplasm of commissure of lip, unspecified**
> *Commissure: Site of union of corresponding parts*

C00.8 **Malignant neoplasm of overlapping sites of lip**

C00.9 **Malignant neoplasm of lip, unspecified**

N Newborn Age: 0   **P** Pediatric Age: 0–17   **M** Maternity DX: 12–55   **A** Adult Age: 15–124   ♀ Females Only   ♂ Males Only

Complication\Comorbidity   Major C\C   (Ex) CC/MCC Exclusions   Present on Admission Requirement   Hospital-Acquired Condition

773

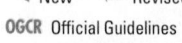

Figure 2-1   Anatomical structures of the mouth and lips. **A.** Transitional or vermilion borders. Lips are connected to the gums by frenulum. **B.** Dorsal surface. **C.** Ventral surface.

C01   **Malignant neoplasm of base of tongue**
     Malignant neoplasm of dorsal surface of base of tongue
     Malignant neoplasm of fixed part of tongue NOS
     Malignant neoplasm of posterior third of tongue
     Use additional code to identify:
         alcohol abuse and dependence (F10.-)
         history of tobacco use (Z87.891)
         tobacco dependence (F17.-)
         tobacco use (Z72.0)

● **C02**   **Malignant neoplasm of other and unspecified parts of tongue**
     Use additional code to identify:
         alcohol abuse and dependence (F10.-)
         history of tobacco use (Z87.891)
         tobacco dependence (F17.-)
         tobacco use (Z72.0)

C02.0   **Malignant neoplasm of dorsal surface of tongue**
     Malignant neoplasm of anterior two-thirds of tongue, dorsal surface

     Excludes2   malignant neoplasm of dorsal surface of base of tongue (C01)

C02.1   **Malignant neoplasm of border of tongue**
     Malignant neoplasm of tip of tongue

C02.2   **Malignant neoplasm of ventral surface of tongue**
     Malignant neoplasm of anterior two-thirds of tongue, ventral surface
     Malignant neoplasm of frenulum linguae

C02.3   **Malignant neoplasm of anterior two-thirds of tongue, part unspecified**
     Malignant neoplasm of middle third of tongue NOS
     Malignant neoplasm of mobile part of tongue NOS

C02.4   **Malignant neoplasm of lingual tonsil**
     Lingual tonsil: Aggregation of lymph follicles at root of tongue

     Excludes2   malignant neoplasm of tonsil NOS (C09.9)

C02.8   **Malignant neoplasm of overlapping sites of tongue**
     Malignant neoplasm of two or more contiguous sites of tongue

C02.9   **Malignant neoplasm of tongue, unspecified**

● **C03**   **Malignant neoplasm of gum**
     Includes   malignant neoplasm of alveolar (ridge) mucosa
                   malignant neoplasm of gingiva
     Use additional code to identify:
         alcohol abuse and dependence (F10.-)
         history of tobacco use (Z87.891)
         tobacco dependence (F17.-)
         tobacco use (Z72.0)

     Excludes2   malignant odontogenic neoplasms (C41.0-C41.1)

C03.0   **Malignant neoplasm of upper gum**

C03.1   **Malignant neoplasm of lower gum**

C03.9   **Malignant neoplasm of gum, unspecified**

● **C04**   **Malignant neoplasm of floor of mouth**
     Use additional code to identify:
         alcohol abuse and dependence (F10.-)
         history of tobacco use (Z87.891)
         tobacco dependence (F17.-)
         tobacco use (Z72.0)

C04.0   **Malignant neoplasm of anterior floor of mouth**
     Malignant neoplasm of anterior to the premolar-canine junction

C04.1   **Malignant neoplasm of lateral floor of mouth**

C04.8   **Malignant neoplasm of overlapping sites of floor of mouth**

C04.9   **Malignant neoplasm of floor of mouth, unspecified**

● **C05**   **Malignant neoplasm of palate**
     Use additional code to identify:
         alcohol abuse and dependence (F10.-)
         history of tobacco use (Z87.891)
         tobacco dependence (F17.-)
         tobacco use (Z72.0)

     Excludes1   Kaposi's sarcoma of palate (C46.2)

C05.0   **Malignant neoplasm of hard palate**

C05.1   **Malignant neoplasm of soft palate**

     Excludes2   malignant neoplasm of nasopharyngeal surface of soft palate (C11.3)

C05.2   **Malignant neoplasm of uvula**

C05.8   **Malignant neoplasm of overlapping sites of palate**

C05.9   **Malignant neoplasm of palate, unspecified**
     Malignant neoplasm of roof of mouth

● **C06**   **Malignant neoplasm of other and unspecified parts of mouth**
     Use additional code to identify:
         alcohol abuse and dependence (F10.-)
         history of tobacco use (Z87.891)
         tobacco dependence (F17.-)
         tobacco use (Z72.0)

C06.0   **Malignant neoplasm of cheek mucosa**
     Malignant neoplasm of buccal mucosa NOS
     Malignant neoplasm of internal cheek

C06.1   **Malignant neoplasm of vestibule of mouth**
     Malignant neoplasm of buccal sulcus (upper) (lower)
     Malignant neoplasm of labial sulcus (upper) (lower)

C06.2   **Malignant neoplasm of retromolar area**

● **C06.8**   **Malignant neoplasm of overlapping sites of other and unspecified parts of mouth**

     C06.80   **Malignant neoplasm of overlapping sites of unspecified parts of mouth**

     C06.89   **Malignant neoplasm of overlapping sites of other parts of mouth 'book leaf' neoplasm [ventral surface of tongue and floor of mouth]**

C06.9   **Malignant neoplasm of mouth, unspecified**
     Malignant neoplasm of minor salivary gland, unspecified site
     Malignant neoplasm of oral cavity NOS

◀ New   ⬅ Revised   ~~deleted~~ Deleted   Excludes 1   Excludes 2   Includes   Use additional   Code first   Code also   Unspecified

774   **OGCR** Official Guidelines   ● Unacceptable Principal Diagnosis   **X** Assign placeholder X   ● Use Additional Character(s)   ▸ Manifestation Code   **Coding Clinic**

CHAPTER 2 (C00-D49)

Figure 2-2 Major salivary glands.

C07 Malignant neoplasm of parotid gland
    Use additional code to identify:
        alcohol abuse and dependence (F10.-)
        exposure to environmental tobacco smoke (Z77.22)
        exposure to tobacco smoke in the perinatal period (P96.81)
        history of tobacco use (Z87.891)
        occupational exposure to environmental tobacco smoke
          (Z57.31)
        tobacco dependence (F17.-)
        tobacco use (Z72.0)

● **C08 Malignant neoplasm of other and unspecified major salivary glands**
    Includes   malignant neoplasm of salivary ducts
    Use additional code to identify:
        alcohol abuse and dependence (F10.-)
        exposure to environmental tobacco smoke (Z77.22)
        exposure to tobacco smoke in the perinatal period (P96.81)
        history of tobacco use (Z87.891)
        occupational exposure to environmental tobacco smoke
          (Z57.31)
        tobacco dependence (F17.-)
        tobacco use (Z72.0)
    Excludes1   malignant neoplasms of specified minor salivary
               glands which are classified according to their
               anatomical location
    Excludes2   malignant neoplasms of minor salivary glands
               NOS (C06.9)
               malignant neoplasm of parotid gland (C07)

C08.0 Malignant neoplasm of submandibular gland
    Malignant neoplasm of submaxillary gland
C08.1 Malignant neoplasm of sublingual gland
C08.9 Malignant neoplasm of major salivary gland, unspecified
    Malignant neoplasm of salivary gland (major) NOS

(See Plate 61 on page 73.)

● **C09 Malignant neoplasm of tonsil**
    Use additional code to identify:
        alcohol abuse and dependence (F10.-)
        exposure to environmental tobacco smoke (Z77.22)
        exposure to tobacco smoke in the perinatal period (P96.81)
        history of tobacco use (Z87.891)
        occupational exposure to environmental tobacco smoke
          (Z57.31)
        tobacco dependence (F17.-)
        tobacco use (Z72.0)
    Excludes2   malignant neoplasm of lingual tonsil (C02.4)
               malignant neoplasm of pharyngeal tonsil (C11.1)

C09.0 Malignant neoplasm of tonsillar fossa
    Surface of palatine (two masses of lymphatic tissue on sides of
    throat) tonsils
C09.1 Malignant neoplasm of tonsillar pillar (anterior) (posterior)
    Extension from palatine (two masses of lymphatic tissue on
    sides of throat) tonsils
C09.8 Malignant neoplasm of overlapping sites of tonsil
C09.9 Malignant neoplasm of tonsil, unspecified
    Malignant neoplasm of tonsil NOS
    Malignant neoplasm of faucial tonsils
    Malignant neoplasm of palatine tonsils

● **C10 Malignant neoplasm of oropharynx**
    Area of throat at back of mouth
    Use additional code to identify:
        alcohol abuse and dependence (F10.-)
        exposure to environmental tobacco smoke (Z77.22)
        exposure to tobacco smoke in the perinatal period (P96.81)
        history of tobacco use (Z87.891)
        occupational exposure to environmental tobacco smoke
          (Z57.31)
        tobacco dependence (F17.-)
        tobacco use (Z72.0)
    Excludes2   malignant neoplasm of tonsil (C09.-)

C10.0 Malignant neoplasm of vallecula
    Vallecula, depression or furrow
C10.1 Malignant neoplasm of anterior surface of epiglottis
    Malignant neoplasm of epiglottis, free border [margin]
    Malignant neoplasm of glossoepiglottic fold(s)
    Excludes2   malignant neoplasm of epiglottis
               (suprahyoid portion) NOS (C32.1)
C10.2 Malignant neoplasm of lateral wall of oropharynx
C10.3 Malignant neoplasm of posterior wall of oropharynx
C10.4 Malignant neoplasm of branchial cleft
    Congenital slitlike openings formed between branchial arches
    pharyngeal groove
    Malignant neoplasm of branchial cyst [site of neoplasm]
C10.8 Malignant neoplasm of overlapping sites of oropharynx
    Malignant neoplasm of junctional region of oropharynx
C10.9 Malignant neoplasm of oropharynx, unspecified

● **C11 Malignant neoplasm of nasopharynx**
    Use additional code to identify:
        exposure to environmental tobacco smoke (Z77.22)
        exposure to tobacco smoke in the perinatal period (P96.81)
        history of tobacco use (Z87.891)
        occupational exposure to environmental tobacco smoke
          (Z57.31)
        tobacco dependence (F17.-)
        tobacco use (Z72.0)

C11.0 Malignant neoplasm of superior wall of nasopharynx
    Part of pharynx that lies above soft palate
    Malignant neoplasm of roof of nasopharynx
C11.1 Malignant neoplasm of posterior wall of nasopharynx
    Malignant neoplasm of adenoid
    Malignant neoplasm of pharyngeal tonsil
C11.2 Malignant neoplasm of lateral wall of nasopharynx
    Malignant neoplasm of fossa of Rosenmüller
    Malignant neoplasm of opening of auditory tube
    Malignant neoplasm of pharyngeal recess
C11.3 Malignant neoplasm of anterior wall of nasopharynx
    Malignant neoplasm of floor of nasopharynx
    Malignant neoplasm of nasopharyngeal (anterior)
      (posterior) surface of soft palate
    Malignant neoplasm of posterior margin of nasal
      choana
    Malignant neoplasm of posterior margin of nasal
      septum
C11.8 Malignant neoplasm of overlapping sites of nasopharynx
C11.9 Malignant neoplasm of nasopharynx, unspecified
    Malignant neoplasm of nasopharyngeal wall NOS

C12 Malignant neoplasm of pyriform sinus
    Malignant neoplasm of pyriform fossa
    Use additional code to identify:
        exposure to environmental tobacco smoke (Z77.22)
        exposure to tobacco smoke in the perinatal period (P96.81)
        history of tobacco use (Z87.891)
        occupational exposure to environmental tobacco smoke
          (Z57.31)
        tobacco dependence (F17.-)
        tobacco use (Z72.0)

CHAPTER 2 (C00-D49)

N Newborn Age: 0   **P** Pediatric Age: 0–17   **M** Maternity DX: 12–55   **A** Adult Age: 15–124   ♀ Females Only   ♂ Males Only

 Complication\Comorbidity   Major C\C   CC/MCC Exclusions   Present on Admission Requirement   Hospital-Acquired Condition   775

CHAPTER 2 (C00-D49)

● C13   **Malignant neoplasm of hypopharynx**
     Use additional code to identify:
        exposure to environmental tobacco smoke (Z77.22)
        exposure to tobacco smoke in the perinatal period (P96.81)
        history of tobacco use (Z87.891)
        occupational exposure to environmental tobacco smoke
          (Z57.31)
        tobacco dependence (F17.-)
        tobacco use (Z72.0)

     Excludes2   malignant neoplasm of pyriform sinus (C12)

   C13.0   **Malignant neoplasm of postcricoid region**
        Behind the cricoid cartilage of neck

   C13.1   **Malignant neoplasm of aryepiglottic fold, hypopharyngeal aspect**
        Arytenoepiglottic fold, triangular opening between side of
          epiglottis and apex of arytenoid cartilage
        Malignant neoplasm of aryepiglottic fold, marginal
          zone ◄
        Malignant neoplasm of aryepiglottic fold NOS
        Malignant neoplasm of interarytenoid fold, marginal
          zone ◄
        Malignant neoplasm of interarytenoid fold NOS
        ~~Malignant neoplasm of aryepiglottic fold marginal zone~~
        ~~Malignant neoplasm of interarytenoid fold marginal zone~~

     Excludes2   malignant neoplasm of aryepiglottic fold
              or interarytenoid fold, laryngeal
              aspect (C32.1)

   C13.2   **Malignant neoplasm of posterior wall of hypopharynx**

   C13.8   **Malignant neoplasm of overlapping sites of hypopharynx**

   C13.9   **Malignant neoplasm of hypopharynx, unspecified**
        Malignant neoplasm of hypopharyngeal wall NOS

● C14   **Malignant neoplasm of other and ill-defined sites in the lip, oral cavity and pharynx**
     Use additional code to identify:
        alcohol abuse and dependence (F10.-)
        exposure to environmental tobacco smoke (Z77.22)
        exposure to tobacco smoke in the perinatal period (P96.81)
        history of tobacco use (Z87.891)
        occupational exposure to environmental tobacco smoke
          (Z57.31)
        tobacco dependence (F17.-)
        tobacco use (Z72.0)

     Excludes1   malignant neoplasm of oral cavity NOS (C06.9)

   C14.0   **Malignant neoplasm of pharynx, unspecified**

   C14.2   **Malignant neoplasm of Waldeyer's ring**

   C14.8   **Malignant neoplasm of overlapping sites of lip, oral cavity and pharynx**
        Primary malignant neoplasm of two or more contiguous
          sites of lip, oral cavity and pharynx

     Excludes1   'book leaf' neoplasm [ventral surface of
              tongue and floor of mouth] (C06.89)

MALIGNANT NEOPLASM OF DIGESTIVE ORGANS (C15-C26)

     Excludes1   Kaposi's sarcoma of gastrointestinal sites (C46.4)

● C15   **Malignant neoplasms of esophagus**
     Use additional code to identify:
        alcohol abuse and dependence (F10.-)
     Ex: **For category C15 CC codes:** C15.3-C15.9, C26.0, C26.9, C45.7-C45.9, C46.4, C76.8,
        C7A.00, C7A.098-C7B.00, C7B.1, C80.0-C80.2, D49.0, D49.81-D49.9

   C15.3   **Malignant neoplasm of upper third of esophagus** 🔲

   C15.4   **Malignant neoplasm of middle third of esophagus** 🔲

   C15.5   **Malignant neoplasm of lower third of esophagus** 🔲

     Excludes1   malignant neoplasm of cardio-esophageal
              junction (C16.0)

   C15.8   **Malignant neoplasm of overlapping sites of esophagus** 🔲

   C15.9   **Malignant neoplasm of esophagus, unspecified** 🔲

● C16   **Malignant neoplasm of stomach**
     Use additional code to identify:
        alcohol abuse and dependence (F10.-)

     Excludes2   malignant carcinoid tumor of the stomach
              (C7A.092)
     Ex: **For category C16 CC codes:** C16.0-C16.9, C26.0, C26.9, C45.7-C45.9, C46.4, C76.8,
        C7A.00, C7A.092, C7A.094-C7B.00, C7B.1, C80.0-C80.2, D49.0, D49.81-D49.9

   C16.0   **Malignant neoplasm of cardia** 🔲
        Malignant neoplasm of cardiac orifice
        Malignant neoplasm of cardio-esophageal junction
        Malignant neoplasm of esophagus and stomach
        Malignant neoplasm of gastro-esophageal junction

   C16.1   **Malignant neoplasm of fundus of stomach** 🔲

   C16.2   **Malignant neoplasm of body of stomach** 🔲

   C16.3   **Malignant neoplasm of pyloric antrum** 🔲
        Malignant neoplasm of gastric antrum

   C16.4   **Malignant neoplasm of pylorus** 🔲
        Malignant neoplasm of prepylorus
        Malignant neoplasm of pyloric canal

   C16.5   **Malignant neoplasm of lesser curvature of stomach, unspecified** 🔲
        Malignant neoplasm of lesser curvature of stomach, not
          classifiable to C16.1-C16.4

   C16.6   **Malignant neoplasm of greater curvature of stomach, unspecified** 🔲
        Malignant neoplasm of greater curvature of stomach,
          not classifiable to C16.0-C16.4

   C16.8   **Malignant neoplasm of overlapping sites of stomach** 🔲

   C16.9   **Malignant neoplasm of stomach, unspecified** 🔲
        Gastric cancer NOS

Figure 2-3   The esophagus is the muscular tube that connects the pharynx and the stomach. The 10 inch (25 cm) long esophagus is divided into three parts: **cervical, thoracic,** and **abdominal.**

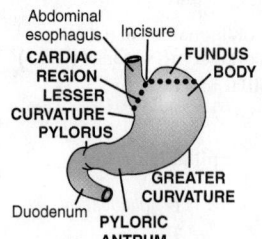

Figure 2-4   Parts of the stomach.

Item 2-2   The esophagus opens into the stomach through the **cardiac orifice,** also called the **cardioesophageal junction.** The **cardia** is adjacent to the cardiac orifice. The stomach widens into the **greater** and **lesser curvatures.** The **pyloric antrum** precedes the **pylorus,** which opens to the duodenum.

◄ New   ◄◄ Revised   ~~deleted~~ Deleted   Excludes 1   Excludes 2   Includes   Use additional   Code first   Code also   Unspecified

   OGCR Official Guidelines   ● Unacceptable Principal Diagnosis   X Assign placeholder X   ● Use Additional Character(s)   ▶ Manifestation Code   **Coding Clinic**

Figure 2-5 Small intestine and colon.

● **C17**   **Malignant neoplasm of small intestine**

> **Excludes1**   malignant carcinoid tumor of the small intestine (C7A.01)

C17.0   **Malignant neoplasm of duodenum**
> *First or proximal portion of small intestine, extending from pylorus to jejunum*
> (Ex:) C17.0, C17.8-C17.9, C26.0, C26.9, C45.7-C45.9, C46.4, C76.8, C7A.00-C7A.010, C7A.019, C7A.098-C7B.00, C7B.1, C80.0-C80.2, D49.0, D49.81-D49.9

C17.1   **Malignant neoplasm of jejunum**
> *Second section of small intestine, extending from duodenum to ileum*
> (Ex:) C17.1, C17.8-C17.9, C26.0, C26.9, C45.7-C45.9, C46.4, C76.8, C7A.00, C7A.011, C7A.019, C7A.098, C7A.1-C7B.00, C7B.1, C80.0-C80.2, D49.0, D49.81-D49.9

C17.2   **Malignant neoplasm of ileum**
> *Distal and longest portion of small intestine, extending from jejunum to cecum*
> > **Excludes1**   malignant neoplasm of ileocecal valve (C18.0)
> (Ex:) C17.2, C17.8-C17.9, C26.0, C26.9, C45.7-C45.9, C46.4, C76.8, C7A.00, C7A.012-C7A.019, C7A.098, C7A.1-C7B.00, C7B.1, C80.0-C80.2, D49.0, D49.81-D49.9

C17.3   **Meckel's diverticulum, malignant**
> *Appendage of ileum*
> > **Excludes1**   Meckel's diverticulum, congenital (Q43.0)
> (Ex:) C17.3-C17.9, C26.0, C26.9, C45.7-C45.9, C46.4, C76.8, C7A.00, C7A.019, C7A.098-C7B.00, C7B.1, C80.0-C80.2, D49.0, D49.81-D49.9

C17.8   **Malignant neoplasm of overlapping sites of small intestine**
> (Ex:) C17.8-C17.9, C26.0, C26.9, C45.7-C45.9, C46.4, C76.8, C7A.00, C7A.019, C7A.098, C7A.1-C7B.00, C7B.1, C80.0-C80.2, D49.0, D49.81-D49.9

C17.9   **Malignant neoplasm of small intestine, unspecified**
> (Ex:) See C17.8

● **C18**   **Malignant neoplasm of colon**

> **Excludes1**   malignant carcinoid tumors of the colon (C7A.02)

C18.0   **Malignant neoplasm of cecum**
> *First section of large intestine*
> Malignant neoplasm of ileocecal valve
> (Ex:) C18.0, C18.8-C18.9, C26.0-C26.9, C45.7-C45.9, C46.4, C76.8, C7A.00, C7A.021, C7A.029, C7A.098-C7B.00, C7B.1, C80.0-C80.2, D49.0, D49.81-D49.9

C18.1   **Malignant neoplasm of appendix**
> *Blind ended tube connected to the cecum; AKA vermiform appendix*
> (Ex:) C18.1, C18.8-C18.9, C26.0, C26.9, C45.7-C45.9, C46.4, C76.8, C7A.00, C7A.020, C7A.029, C7A.098, C7A.1-C7B.00, C7B.1, C80.0-C80.2, D49.0, D49.81-D49.9

C18.2   **Malignant neoplasm of ascending colon**
> *Ascending colon is between cecum and right colic flexure*
> (Ex:) C18.2, C18.8-C18.9, C26.0, C26.9, C45.7-C45.9, C46.4, C76.8, C7A.00, C7A.022, C7A.029, C7A.098, C7A.1-C7B.00, C7B.1, C80.0-C80.2, D49.0, D49.81-D49.9

C18.3   **Malignant neoplasm of hepatic flexure**
> *A flexure is a bending in a structure or organ. Note the three flexures illustrated in Figure 2–5.*
> (Ex:) C18.3, C18.8-C18.9, C26.0, C26.9, C45.7-C45.9, C46.4, C76.8, C7A.00, C7A.029, C7A.098-C7B.00, C7B.1, C80.0-C80.2, D49.0, D49.81-D49.9

C18.4   **Malignant neoplasm of transverse colon**
> *Portion of colon that runs transversely across upper part of abdomen, between right and left colic flexures*
> (Ex:) C18.4, C18.8-C18.9, C26.0, C26.9, C45.7-C45.9, C46.4, C76.8, C7A.00, C7A.023, C7A.029, C7A.098, C7A.1-C7B.00, C7B.1, C80.0-C80.2, D49.0, D49.81-D49.9

C18.5   **Malignant neoplasm of splenic flexure**
> *Bend at junction of transverse and descending colon*
> (Ex:) C18.5, C18.8-C18.9, C26.0, C26.9, C45.7-C45.9, C46.4, C76.8, C7A.00, C7A.029, C7A.098-C7B.00, C7B.1, C80.0-C80.2, D49.0, D49.81-D49.9

C18.6   **Malignant neoplasm of descending colon**
> *Portion between left colic flexure and sigmoid colon at pelvic brim; AKA iliac colon*
> (Ex:) C18.6, C18.8-C18.9, C26.0, C26.9, C45.7-C45.9, C46.4, C76.8, C7A.00, C7A.024, C7A.029, C7A.098-C7B.00, C7B.1, C80.0-C80.2, D49.0, D49.81-D49.9

C18.7   **Malignant neoplasm of sigmoid colon**
> *S-shaped part of colon extending from pelvic brim to third segment of sacrum*
> Malignant neoplasm of sigmoid (flexure)
> > **Excludes1**   malignant neoplasm of rectosigmoid junction (C19)
> (Ex:) C18.7-C18.9, C26.0, C26.9, C45.7-C45.9, C46.4, C76.8, C7A.00, C7A.025, C7A.029, C7A.098, C7A.1-C7B.00, C7B.1, C80.0-C80.2, D49.0, D49.81-D49.9

C18.8   **Malignant neoplasm of overlapping sites of colon**
> (Ex:) C18.8-C18.9, C26.0, C26.9, C45.7-C45.9, C46.4, C76.8, C7A.00, C7A.029, C7A.098, C7A.1-C7B.00, C7B.1, C80.0-C80.2, D49.0, D49.81-D49.9

C18.9   **Malignant neoplasm of colon, unspecified**
> Malignant neoplasm of large intestine NOS
> (Ex:) See C18.8

C19   **Malignant neoplasm of rectosigmoid junction**
> Malignant neoplasm of colon with rectum
> Malignant neoplasm of rectosigmoid (colon)
> > **Excludes1**   malignant carcinoid tumors of the colon (C7A.02-)
> (Ex:) C19, C21.2-C21.8, C26.0, C26.9, C45.7-C45.9, C46.4, C76.8, C7A.00, C7A.098, C7A.1-C7B.00, C7B.1, C80.0-C80.2, D49.0, D49.81-D49.9

C20   **Malignant neoplasm of rectum**
> Malignant neoplasm of rectal ampulla
> > **Excludes1**   malignant carcinoid tumor of the rectum (C7A.026)
> (Ex:) C20, C21.2-C21.8, C26.0, C26.9, C45.7-C45.9, C46.4, C76.8, C7A.00, C7A.026, C7A.098, C7A.1-C7B.00, C7B.1, C80.0-C80.2, D49.0, D49.81-D49.9

● **C21**   **Malignant neoplasm of anus and anal canal**

> **Excludes2**   malignant carcinoid tumors of the colon (C7A.02-)
> malignant melanoma of anal margin (C43.51)
> malignant melanoma of anal skin (C43.51)
> malignant melanoma of perianal skin (C43.51)
> other and unspecified malignant neoplasm of anal margin (C44.500, C44.510, C44.520, C44.590)
> other and unspecified malignant neoplasm of anal skin (C44.500, C44.510, C44.520, C44.590)
> other and unspecified malignant neoplasm of perianal skin (C44.500, C44.510, C44.520, C44.590)
> (Ex:) **For category C21 CC codes C21.0-C21.1:** C21.0-C21.8, C26.0, C26.9, C45.7-C45.9, C46.4, C76.8, C7A.00, C7A.098, C7A.1-C7B.00, C7B.1, C80.0-C80.2, D49.0, D49.81-D49.9 **For category C21 CC codes C21.2-C21.8:** C21.2-C21.8, C26.0, C26.9, C45.7-C45.9, C46.4, C76.8, C7A.00, C7A.098, C7A.1-C7B.00, C7B.1, C80.0-C80.2, D49.0, D49.81-D49.9

C21.0   **Malignant neoplasm of anus, unspecified**

C21.1   **Malignant neoplasm of anal canal**
> *Terminal part of large intestine*
> Malignant neoplasm of anal sphincter

C21.2   **Malignant neoplasm of cloacogenic zone**

CHAPTER 2 (C00-D49)

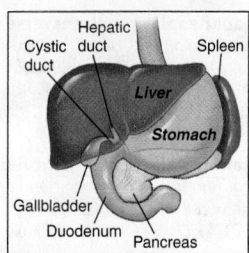

Figure 2-6 Diagram of liver, gallbladder, hepatic duct, pancreas, and spleen. (From Thibodeau and Patton: Anatomy and Physiology, ed 7, Mosby, 2010)

C21.8 **Malignant neoplasm of overlapping sites of rectum, anus and anal canal** 🔞
   Malignant neoplasm of anorectal junction
   Malignant neoplasm of anorectum
   Primary malignant neoplasm of two or more
      contiguous sites of rectum, anus and anal canal

● C22 **Malignant neoplasm of liver and intrahepatic bile ducts**
   Intrahepatic: Within liver
   Use additional code to identify:
      alcohol abuse and dependence (F10.-)
      hepatitis B (B16.-, B18.0-B18.1) hepatitis C (B17.1-, B18.2)
   Excludes1   malignant neoplasm of biliary tract NOS (C24.9)
      secondary malignant neoplasm of liver and
         intrahepatic bile duct (C78.7)
   (Ex:) **For catgory C22 CC codes:** C22.0-C22.9, C26.0, C26.9, C45.7-C45.9, C46.4, C76.8,
   C7A.00, C7A.098, C7A.1-C7B.00, C7B.1, C80.0-C80.2, D49.0, D49.81-D49.9

   C22.0 **Liver cell carcinoma** 🔞
      Hepatocellular carcinoma
      Hepatoma

   C22.1 **Intrahepatic bile duct carcinoma** 🔞
      Cholangiocarcinoma
      Adenocarcinoma (cancer that originates in glandular tissue)
         arising from epithelium of intrahepatic bile ducts
      Excludes1   malignant neoplasm of hepatic duct
         (C24.0)

   C22.2 **Hepatoblastoma** 🔞
      Malignant intrahepatic tumor

   C22.3 **Angiosarcoma of liver** 🔞
      Kupffer cell sarcoma

   C22.4 **Other sarcomas of liver** 🔞

   C22.7 **Other specified carcinomas of liver** 🔞

   C22.8 **Malignant neoplasm of liver, primary, unspecified as to type** 🔞

   C22.9 **Malignant neoplasm of liver, not specified as primary or secondary** 🔞

C23 **Malignant neoplasm of gallbladder** 🔞
   (Ex:) C23, C24.8-C24.9, C26.0, C26.9, C45.7-C45.9, C46.4, C76.8, C7A.00, C7A.098,
   C7A.1-C7B.00, C7B.1, C8.00-C8.02, D49.0, D49.81-D49.9

● C24 **Malignant neoplasm of other and unspecified parts of biliary tract**
   Excludes1   malignant neoplasm of intrahepatic bile duct
      (C22.1)

   C24.0 **Malignant neoplasm of extrahepatic bile duct** 🔞
      Extrahepatic = outside the liver
      Malignant neoplasm of biliary duct or passage NOS
      Malignant neoplasm of common bile duct
      Malignant neoplasm of cystic duct
      Malignant neoplasm of hepatic duct
      (Ex:) C24.0, C24.8-C24.9, C26.0, C26.9, C45.7-C45.9, C46.4, C76.8, C7A.00,
      C7A.098-C7B.00, C7B.1, C80.0-C80.2, D49.0, D49.81-D49.9

   C24.1 **Malignant neoplasm of ampulla of Vater** 🔞
      Union of pancreatic duct and common bile duct
      (Ex:) C24.1, C24.8-C24.9, C26.0, C26.9, C45.7-C45.9, C46.4, C76.8, C7A.00,
      C7A.098, C7A.1, C7A.8, C7B.00, C7B.1, C80.0-C80.2, D49.0, D49.81-D49.9

   C24.8 **Malignant neoplasm of overlapping sites of biliary tract** 🔞
      Malignant neoplasm involving both intrahepatic and
         extrahepatic bile ducts
      Primary malignant neoplasm of two or more
         contiguous sites of biliary tract
      (Ex:) C24.8-C24.9, C26.0, C26.9, C45.7-C45.9, C46.4, C76.8, C7A.00, C7A.098-C7A.8,
      C7B.00, C7B.1, C80.0-C80.2, D49.0, D49.81-D49.9

   C24.9 **Malignant neoplasm of biliary tract, unspecified** 🔞
      (Ex:) See C24.8

● C25 **Malignant neoplasm of pancreas**
   Check documentation for specific site.
   Use additional code to identify:
      alcohol abuse and dependence (F10.-)
   (Ex:) **For catgory C25 CC codes:** C25.0-C26.0, C26.9, C45.7-C45.9, C46.4, C76.8, C7A.00,
   C7A.098, C7A.1-C7B.00, C7B.1, C8.00-C80.2, D49.0, D49.81-D49.9

   C25.0 **Malignant neoplasm of head of pancreas** 🔞
   C25.1 **Malignant neoplasm of body of pancreas** 🔞
   C25.2 **Malignant neoplasm of tail of pancreas** 🔞
   C25.3 **Malignant neoplasm of pancreatic duct** 🔞
   C25.4 **Malignant neoplasm of endocrine pancreas** 🔞
      Malignant neoplasm of islets of Langerhans
      That part of the pancreas that acts as endocrine gland and
         consists of islets of Langerhans
      Use additional code to identify any functional activity.

   C25.7 **Malignant neoplasm of other parts of pancreas** 🔞
      Malignant neoplasm of neck of pancreas

   C25.8 **Malignant neoplasm of overlapping sites of pancreas** 🔞

   C25.9 **Malignant neoplasm of pancreas, unspecified** 🔞

● C26 **Malignant neoplasm of other and ill-defined digestive organs**
   Excludes1   malignant neoplasm of peritoneum and
      retroperitoneum (C48.-)

   C26.0 **Malignant neoplasm of intestinal tract, part unspecified**
      Malignant neoplasm of intestine NOS

   C26.1 **Malignant neoplasm of spleen**
      Excludes1   Hodgkin lymphoma (C81.-)
         non-Hodgkin lymphoma (C82-C85)

   C26.9 **Malignant neoplasm of ill-defined sites within the digestive system**
      Malignant neoplasm of alimentary canal or tract NOS
      Malignant neoplasm of gastrointestinal tract NOS
      Excludes1   malignant neoplasm of abdominal NOS
         (C76.2)
         malignant neoplasm of intra-abdominal
            NOS (C76.2)

Item 2–3 Islets of Langerhans (endocrine producing cells comprising 1% to 2% of the pancreatic mass) make and secrete hormones that regulate the body's production of insulin, glucagon, and stomach acid. Breakdown of the insulin-producing cells can cause diabetes mellitus. Islet cell tumors can be benign or malignant and include glucagonomas, insulinomas, gastrinomas, and neuroendocrine tumor. The neoplasm table must be consulted for the correct neoplasm code.

CHAPTER 2 (C00-D49)

◀ New   ◀ Revised   ~~deleted~~ Deleted   Excludes 1   Excludes 2   Includes   Use additional   Code first   Code also   Unspecified
OGCR Official Guidelines   ● Unacceptable Principal Diagnosis   X Assign placeholder X   ● Use Additional Character(s)   ▶ Manifestation Code   **Coding Clinic**

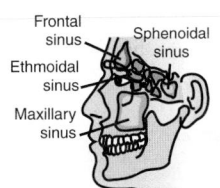

Figure 2-7 Paranasal sinuses. (From Buck CJ: Step-by-Step Medical Coding, ed 2011, Philadelphia, WB Saunders, 2011)

MALIGNANT NEOPLASMS OF RESPIRATORY AND INTRATHORACIC ORGANS (C30-C39)

Includes	malignant neoplasm of middle ear
Excludes1	mesothelioma (C45.-)

● **C30　Malignant neoplasm of nasal cavity and middle ear**

C30.0　Malignant neoplasm of nasal cavity
Malignant neoplasm of cartilage of nose
Malignant neoplasm of nasal concha
Malignant neoplasm of internal nose
Malignant neoplasm of septum of nose
Malignant neoplasm of vestibule of nose
　Anterior part of nasal cavity

Excludes1	malignant neoplasm of nasal bone (C41.0)
	malignant neoplasm of nose NOS (C76.0)
	malignant neoplasm of olfactory bulb (C72.2-)
	malignant neoplasm of posterior margin of nasal septum and choana (C11.3)
	malignant melanoma of skin of nose (C43.31)
	malignant neoplasm of turbinates (C41.0)
	other and unspecified malignant neoplasm of skin of nose C44.301, C44.311, C44.321, C44.391)

C30.1　Malignant neoplasm of middle ear
Malignant neoplasm of antrum tympanicum
　Boney cavity or chamber
Malignant neoplasm of auditory tube
Malignant neoplasm of eustachian tube
Malignant neoplasm of inner ear
Malignant neoplasm of mastoid air cells
Malignant neoplasm of tympanic cavity

Excludes1	malignant neoplasm of auricular canal (external) (C43.2-, C44.2-)
	malignant neoplasm of bone of ear (meatus) (C41.0)
	malignant neoplasm of cartilage of ear (C49.0)
	malignant melanoma of skin of (external) ear (C43.2-)
	other and unspecified malignant neoplasm of skin of (external) ear (C44.2-)

● **C31　Malignant neoplasm of accessory sinuses**
　Paired sinuses in bones of face

C31.0　Malignant neoplasm of maxillary sinus
　Malignant neoplasm of antrum (Highmore) (maxillary)

C31.1　Malignant neoplasm of ethmoidal sinus

C31.2　Malignant neoplasm of frontal sinus

C31.3　Malignant neoplasm of sphenoid sinus

C31.8　Malignant neoplasm of overlapping sites of accessory sinuses

C31.9　Malignant neoplasm of accessory sinus, unspecified

● **C32　Malignant neoplasm of larynx**
Use additional code to identify:
　alcohol abuse and dependence (F10.-)
　exposure to environmental tobacco smoke (Z77.22)
　exposure to tobacco smoke in the perinatal period (P96.81)
　history of tobacco use (Z87.891)
　occupational exposure to environmental tobacco smoke (Z57.31)
　tobacco dependence (F17.-)
　tobacco use (Z72.0)

C32.0　Malignant neoplasm of glottis
　Vocal apparatus of larynx, consisting of true vocal cords (plicae vocales) and opening between them (rima glottidis)
Malignant neoplasm of intrinsic larynx
Malignant neoplasm of laryngeal commissure (anterior) (posterior)
Malignant neoplasm of vocal cord (true) NOS
　True *vocal cords ("lower vocal folds") produce vocalization when air from the lungs passes between them. Check your documentation. Code C32.1 is for malignant neoplasm of the **false** vocal cords.*

C32.1　Malignant neoplasm of supraglottis
　Area of pharynx above glottis
Malignant neoplasm of aryepiglottic fold or interarytenoid fold, laryngeal aspect
Malignant neoplasm of epiglottis (suprahyoid portion) NOS
Malignant neoplasm of extrinsic larynx
Malignant neoplasm of false vocal cord
　False *vocal cords ("upper vocal folds") are not involved in vocalization. Check your documentation. Code C32.0 is for true vocal cords.*
Malignant neoplasm of posterior (laryngeal) surface of epiglottis
Malignant neoplasm of ventricular bands

Excludes2	malignant neoplasm of anterior surface of epiglottis (C10.1)
	malignant neoplasm of aryepiglottic fold or interarytenoid fold, hypopharyngeal aspect (C13.1) ◀
	malignant neoplasm of aryepiglottic fold or interarytenoid fold, marginal zone (C13.1) ◀
	~~hypopharyngeal aspect (C13.1)~~
	malignant neoplasm of aryepiglottic fold or interarytenoid fold NOS (C13.1) ◀

C32.2　Malignant neoplasm of subglottis
　Lowest part of larynx from just below vocal cords down to top of trachea

C32.3　Malignant neoplasm of laryngeal cartilage
　Cartilages of larynx, including cricoid, thyroid, and epiglottic, and two each of arytenoid, corniculate, and cuneiform

C32.8　Malignant neoplasm of overlapping sites of larynx

C32.9　Malignant neoplasm of larynx, unspecified

● **C33　Malignant neoplasm of trachea** 🖋
Use additional code to identify:
　exposure to environmental tobacco smoke (Z77.22)
　exposure to tobacco smoke in the perinatal period (P96.81)
　history of tobacco use (Z87.891)
　occupational exposure to environmental tobacco smoke (Z57.31)
　tobacco dependence (F17.-)
　tobacco use (Z72.0)
　Ⓔⓧ C33, C34.00-C34.92, C39.9, C45.7-C45.9, C46.50-C46.52, C76.1, C76.8, C78.00-C78.1, C78.30-C78.39, C7A.00, C7A.090, C7A.098-C7B.00, C7B.1, C80.0-C80.2, D49.1, D49.81-D49.9

CHAPTER 2 (C00-D49)

N　Newborn Age: 0　　P　Pediatric Age: 0–17　　M　Maternity DX: 12–55　　A　Adult Age: 15–124　　♀　Females Only　　♂　Males Only

🖋 Complication\Comorbidity　　🖋 Major C\C　　Ⓔⓧ CC/MCC Exclusions　　🖋 Present on Admission Requirement　　🖋 Hospital-Acquired Condition

779

● **C34**   **Malignant neoplasm of bronchus and lung**

Use additional code to identify:
exposure to environmental tobacco smoke (Z77.22)
exposure to tobacco smoke in the perinatal period (P96.81)
history of tobacco use (Z87.891)
occupational exposure to environmental tobacco smoke (Z57.31)
tobacco dependence (F17.-)
tobacco use (Z72.0)

Excludes1   Kaposi's sarcoma of lung (C46.5-)
malignant carcinoid tumor of the bronchus and lung (C7A.090)

● **C34.0**   **Malignant neoplasm of main bronchus**
Malignant neoplasm of carina
Ridgelike structure
Malignant neoplasm of hilus (of lung)
Anatomic depression or pit
Ⓔⓧ **For catgory C34.0 CC codes:** C34.00-C34.02, C34.80-C34.92, C39.9, C45.7-C45.9, C46.50-C46.52, C76.8, C7A.00, C7A.090, C7A.098, C7A.1-C7B.00, C7B.1, C80.0-C80.2, D49.1, D49.81-D49.9

C34.00   **Malignant neoplasm of unspecified main bronchus** 🔧

C34.01   **Malignant neoplasm of right main bronchus** 🔧

C34.02   **Malignant neoplasm of left main bronchus** 🔧

● **C34.1**   **Malignant neoplasm of upper lobe, bronchus or lung**
Ⓔⓧ **For catgory C34.1 CC codes:** C34.10-C34.12, C34.80-C34.92, C39.9, C45.7-C45.9, C46.50-C46.52, C76.8, C7A.00, C7A.090, C7A.098-C7B.00, C7B.1, C80.0-C80.2, D49.1, D49.81-D49.9

C34.10   **Malignant neoplasm of unspecified bronchus or lung** 🔧

C34.11   **Malignant neoplasm of upper lobe, right bronchus or lung** 🔧

C34.12   **Malignant neoplasm of upper lobe, left bronchus or lung** 🔧

C34.2   **Malignant neoplasm of middle lobe, bronchus or lung** 🔧
Ⓔⓧ C34.2, C34.80-C34.92, C39.9, C45.7-C45.9, C46.50-C46.52, C76.8, C7A.00, C7A.090, C7A.098-C7B.00, C7B.1, C80.0-C80.2, D49.1, D49.81-D49.9

● **C34.3**   **Malignant neoplasm of lower lobe, bronchus or lung**
Ⓔⓧ **For catgory C34.4 CC codes:** C34.30-C34.92, C39.9, C45.7-C45.9, C46.50-C46.52, C76.8, C7A.00, C7A.090, C7A.098-C7B.00, C7B.1, C80.0-C80.2, D49.1, D49.81-D49.9

C34.30   **Malignant neoplasm of lower lobe, unspecified bronchus or lung** 🔧

C34.31   **Malignant neoplasm of lower lobe, right bronchus or lung** 🔧

C34.32   **Malignant neoplasm of lower lobe, left bronchus or lung** 🔧

● **C34.8**   **Malignant neoplasm of overlapping sites of bronchus and lung**
Ⓔⓧ **For catgory C34.8 CC codes:** C34.80-C34.92, C39.9, C45.7-C45.9, C46.50-C46.52, C76.8, C7A.00, C7A.090, C7A.098-C7B.00, C7B.1, C80.0-C80.2, D49.1, D49.81-D49.9

C34.80   **Malignant neoplasm of overlapping sites of unspecified bronchus and lung** 🔧

C34.81   **Malignant neoplasm of overlapping sites of right bronchus and lung** 🔧

C34.82   **Malignant neoplasm of overlapping sites of left bronchus and lung** 🔧

● **C34.9**   **Malignant neoplasm of unspecified part of bronchus or lung**
Ⓔⓧ **For category C34.9 CC codes:** See C34.8

C34.90   **Malignant neoplasm of unspecified part of unspecified bronchus or lung** 🔧
Lung cancer NOS

C34.91   **Malignant neoplasm of unspecified part of right bronchus or lung** 🔧

C34.92   **Malignant neoplasm of unspecified part of left bronchus or lung** 🔧

● **C37**   **Malignant neoplasm of thymus** 🔧

Excludes1   malignant carcinoid tumor of the thymus (C7A.091)

Ⓔⓧ C37, C7A.091

● **C38**   **Malignant neoplasm of heart, mediastinum and pleura**

Excludes1   mesothelioma (C45.-)

Ⓔⓧ **For catgory C38 CC codes unless otherwise indicated:** C38.1-C38.3, C38.8, C39.9, C45.7-C45.9, C76.8, C7A.00, C7A.098-C7B.00, C7B.1, C80.0-C80.2, D49.1, D49.81-D49.9

C38.0   **Malignant neoplasm of heart** 🔧
Malignant neoplasm of pericardium

Excludes1   malignant neoplasm of great vessels (C49.3)

Ⓔⓧ C38.0, C45.2

C38.1   **Malignant neoplasm of anterior mediastinum** 🔧

C38.2   **Malignant neoplasm of posterior mediastinum** 🔧

C38.3   **Malignant neoplasm of mediastinum, part unspecified** 🔧

C38.4   **Malignant neoplasm of pleura** 🔧
Ⓔⓧ C38.4, C39.9, C45.0, C45.7-C45.9, C76.8, C7A.00, C7A.098, C7A.1-C7B.00, C7B.1, C80.0-C80.2, D49.1, D49.81-D49.9

C38.8   **Malignant neoplasm of overlapping sites of heart, mediastinum and pleura** 🔧
Pleura are comprised of serous membrane that lines the thoracic cavity (parietal) and covers the lungs (visceral).

● **C39**   **Malignant neoplasm of other and ill-defined sites in the respiratory system and intrathoracic organs**
Intrathoracic: within thorax/chest

Use additional code to identify:
exposure to environmental tobacco smoke (Z77.22)
exposure to tobacco smoke in the perinatal period (P96.81)
history of tobacco use (Z87.891)
occupational exposure to environmental tobacco smoke (Z57.31)
tobacco dependence (F17.-)
tobacco use (Z72.0)

Excludes1   intrathoracic malignant neoplasm NOS (C76.1)
thoracic malignant neoplasm NOS (C76.1)

C39.0   **Malignant neoplasm of upper respiratory tract, part unspecified**

C39.9   **Malignant neoplasm of lower respiratory tract, part unspecified**
Malignant neoplasm of respiratory tract NOS

MALIGNANT NEOPLASMS OF BONE AND ARTICULAR CARTILAGE (C40-C41)

Includes   malignant neoplasm of cartilage (articular) (joint)
malignant neoplasm of periosteum

Excludes1   malignant neoplasm of bone marrow NOS (C96.9)
malignant neoplasm of synovia (C49.-)

● **C40**   **Malignant neoplasm of bone and articular cartilage of limbs**

Use additional code to identify major osseous defect, if applicable (M89.7-)

● **C40.0**   **Malignant neoplasm of scapula and long bones of upper limb**
Ⓔⓧ **For catgory C40.0 CC codes:** C40.00-C40.02, C40.80-C40.92, C41.9, Z51.0

C40.00   **Malignant neoplasm of scapula and long bones of unspecified upper limb** 🔧

C40.01   **Malignant neoplasm of scapula and long bones of right upper limb** 🔧

C40.02   **Malignant neoplasm of scapula and long bones of left upper limb** 🔧

● **C40.1**   **Malignant neoplasm of short bones of upper limb**
Ⓔⓧ **For catgory C40.1 CC codes:** C40.10-C40.12, C40.80-C40.92, C41.9, Z51.0

C40.10   **Malignant neoplasm of short bones of unspecified upper limb** 🔧

C40.11   **Malignant neoplasm of short bones of right upper limb** 🔧

C40.12   **Malignant neoplasm of short bones of left upper limb** 🔧

◀ New   ◀┅ Revised   ~~deleted~~ Deleted   Excludes 1   Excludes 2   Includes   Use additional   Code first   Code also   Unspecified

OGCR Official Guidelines   ● Unacceptable Principal Diagnosis   X Assign placeholder X   🔧 Use Additional Character(s)   ▶ Manifestation Code   **Coding Clinic**

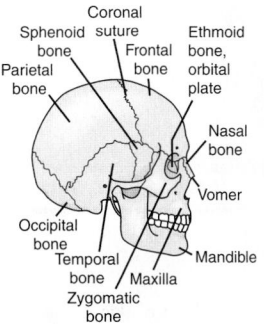

Figure 2-9 Bones of the skull.

Figure 2-8 Diagram of skeleton of trunk and limbs with bones labeled. (From Thibodeau and Patton: Anatomy and Physiology, ed 7, Mosby, 2010)

● **C40.2** Malignant neoplasm of long bones of lower limb
Ⓔⓧ For catgory **C40.2 CC codes:** C40.20-C40.22, C40.80-C40.92, C41.9, Z51.0

    C40.20 Malignant neoplasm of long bones of unspecified lower limb

    C40.21 Malignant neoplasm of long bones of right lower limb

    C40.22 Malignant neoplasm of long bones of left lower limb

● **C40.3** Malignant neoplasm of short bones of lower limb
Ⓔⓧ For catgory **C40.3 CC codes:** C40.30-C40.92, C41.9, Z51.0

    C40.30 Malignant neoplasm of short bones of unspecified lower limb

    C40.31 Malignant neoplasm of short bones of right lower limb

    C40.32 Malignant neoplasm of short bones of left lower limb

● **C40.8** Malignant neoplasm of overlapping sites of bone and articular cartilage of limb
Ⓔⓧ For catgory **C40.8 CC codes:** C40.00-C41.9, Z51.0

    C40.80 Malignant neoplasm of overlapping sites of bone and articular cartilage of unspecified limb

    C40.81 Malignant neoplasm of overlapping sites of bone and articular cartilage of right limb

    C40.82 Malignant neoplasm of overlapping sites of bone and articular cartilage of left limb

● **C40.9** Malignant neoplasm of unspecified bones and articular cartilage of limb
Ⓔⓧ For category **C40.9 CC codes:** See C40.8

    C40.90 Malignant neoplasm of unspecified bones and articular cartilage of unspecified limb

    C40.91 Malignant neoplasm of unspecified bones and articular cartilage of right limb

    C40.92 Malignant neoplasm of unspecified bones and articular cartilage of left limb

● **C41** Malignant neoplasm of bone and articular cartilage of other and unspecified sites
    Excludes1 malignant neoplasm of bones of limbs (C40.-)
        malignant neoplasm of cartilage of ear (C49.0)
        malignant neoplasm of cartilage of eyelid (C49.0)
        ~~eyelid (C49.0)~~
        malignant neoplasm of cartilage of larynx (C32.3)
        malignant neoplasm of cartilage of limbs (C40.-)
        malignant neoplasm of cartilage of nose (C30.0)

C41.0 Malignant neoplasm of bones of skull and face
Malignant neoplasm of maxilla (superior)
Malignant neoplasm of orbital bone
    Excludes2 carcinoma, any type except intraosseous or odontogenic of:
        maxillary sinus (C31.0)
        upper jaw (C03.0)
        malignant neoplasm of jaw bone (lower) (C41.1)
Ⓔⓧ C40.80-C41.0, C41.9, Z51.0

C41.1 Malignant neoplasm of mandible
Malignant neoplasm of inferior maxilla
Malignant neoplasm of lower jaw bone
    Excludes2 carcinoma, any type except intraosseous or odontogenic of:
        jaw NOS (C03.9)
        lower (C03.1)
        malignant neoplasm of upper jaw bone (C41.0)
Ⓔⓧ C40.80-C40.92, C41.1, C41.9, Z51.0

C41.2 Malignant neoplasm of vertebral column
    Excludes1 malignant neoplasm of sacrum and coccyx (C41.4)
Ⓔⓧ C40.80-C40.9, C41.2, C41.9, Z51.0

C41.3 Malignant neoplasm of ribs, sternum and clavicle
Ⓔⓧ C40.80-C40.92, C41.3, C41.9, Z51.0

C41.4 Malignant neoplasm of pelvic bones, sacrum and coccyx
Ⓔⓧ C40.80-C40.92, C41.4-C41.9, Z51.0

C41.9 Malignant neoplasm of bone and articular cartilage, unspecified
Ⓔⓧ See C40.8

MELANOMA AND OTHER MALIGNANT NEOPLASMS OF SKIN (C43-C44)

● **C43** Malignant melanoma of skin
    Excludes1 melanoma in situ (D03.-)
    Excludes2 malignant melanoma of skin of genital organs (C51-C52, C60.-, C63.-)
        Merkel cell carcinoma (C4A.-)
        sites other than skin-code to malignant neoplasm of the site

C43.0 Malignant melanoma of lip
    Excludes1 malignant neoplasm of vermilion border of lip (C00.0-C00.2)

N Newborn Age: 0   **P** Pediatric Age: 0-17   **M** Maternity DX: 12-55   **A** Adult Age: 15-124   ♀ Females Only   ♂ Males Only

Complication\Comorbidity   Major C\C   Ⓔⓧ CC/MCC Exclusions   Present on Admission Requirement   Hospital-Acquired Condition

781

Figure 2-10 Malignant melanoma of skin. (From Goldman: Cecil Textbook of Medicine, ed 22, Saunders, 2004)

Item 2–4 Malignant melanoma is a serious form of skin cancer that affects the melanocytes (pigment-forming cells) and is caused by ultraviolet (UV) rays from the sun that damage skin. It is most commonly seen in the 40- to 60-year-olds with fair skin, blue or green eyes, and red or blond hair who sunburn easily.

Melanoma can spread very rapidly and is the most deadly form of skin cancer. It is less common than other types of skin cancer. The rate of melanoma is increasing and currently is the leading cause of death from skin disease.

● C43.1 **Malignant melanoma of eyelid, including canthus**
  Canthus: Either corner of eye where upper and lower eyelids meet

  C43.10 **Malignant melanoma of unspecified eyelid, including canthus**

  C43.11 **Malignant melanoma of right eyelid, including canthus**

  C43.12 **Malignant melanoma of left eyelid, including canthus**

● C43.2 **Malignant melanoma of ear and external auricular canal**

  C43.20 **Malignant melanoma of unspecified ear and external auricular canal**

  C43.21 **Malignant melanoma of right ear and external auricular canal**

  C43.22 **Malignant melanoma of left ear and external auricular canal**

● C43.3 **Malignant melanoma of other and unspecified parts of face**

  C43.30 **Malignant melanoma of unspecified part of face**

  C43.31 **Malignant melanoma of nose**

  C43.39 **Malignant melanoma of other parts of face**

  C43.4 **Malignant melanoma of scalp and neck**

● C43.5 **Malignant melanoma of trunk**

  Excludes2 malignant neoplasm of anus NOS (C21.0)
  malignant neoplasm of scrotum (C63.2)

  C43.51 **Malignant melanoma of anal skin**
    Malignant melanoma of anal margin
    Malignant melanoma of perianal skin

  C43.52 **Malignant melanoma of skin of breast**

  C43.59 **Malignant melanoma of other part of trunk**

● C43.6 **Malignant melanoma of upper limb, including shoulder**

  C43.60 **Malignant melanoma of upper limb, including shoulder, unspecified side**

  C43.61 **Malignant melanoma of right upper limb, including shoulder**

  C43.62 **Malignant melanoma of left upper limb, including shoulder**

● C43.7 **Malignant melanoma of lower limb, including hip**

  C43.70 **Malignant melanoma of unspecified lower limb, including hip**

  C43.71 **Malignant melanoma of right lower limb, including hip**

  C43.72 **Malignant melanoma of left lower limb, including hip**

  C43.8 **Malignant melanoma of overlapping sites of skin**

  C43.9 **Malignant melanoma of skin, unspecified**
    Malignant melanoma of unspecified site of skin
    Melanoma (malignant) NOS

C4A **Merkel cell carcinoma**
  C4A.0 **Merkel cell carcinoma of lip**

    Excludes1 malignant neoplasm of vermilion border of lip (C00.0-C00.2)

● C4A.1 **Merkel cell carcinoma of eyelid, including canthus**

  C4A.10 **Merkel cell carcinoma of unspecified eyelid, including canthus**

  C4A.11 **Merkel cell carcinoma of right eyelid, including canthus**

  C4A.12 **Merkel cell carcinoma of left eyelid, including canthus**

● C4A.2 **Merkel cell carcinoma of ear and external auricular canal**

  C4A.20 **Merkel cell carcinoma of unspecified ear and external auricular canal**

  C4A.21 **Merkel cell carcinoma of right ear and external auricular canal**

  C4A.22 **Merkel cell carcinoma of left ear and external auricular canal**

● C4A.3 **Merkel cell carcinoma of other and unspecified parts of face**

  C4A.30 **Merkel cell carcinoma of unspecified part of face**

  C4A.31 **Merkel cell carcinoma of nose**

  C4A.39 **Merkel cell carcinoma of other parts of face**

  C4A.4 **Merkel cell carcinoma of scalp and neck**

● C4A.5 **Merkel cell carcinoma of trunk**

    Excludes2 malignant neoplasm of anus NOS (C21.0)
    malignant neoplasm of scrotum (C63.2)

  C4A.51 **Merkel cell carcinoma of anal skin**
    Merkel cell carcinoma of anal margin
    Merkel cell carcinoma of perianal skin

  C4A.52 **Merkel cell carcinoma of skin of breast**

  C4A.59 **Merkel cell carcinoma of other part of trunk**

● C4A.6 **Merkel cell carcinoma of upper limb, including shoulder**

  C4A.60 **Merkel cell carcinoma of unspecified upper limb, including shoulder**

  C4A.61 **Merkel cell carcinoma of right upper limb, including shoulder**

  C4A.62 **Merkel cell carcinoma of left upper limb, including shoulder**

● C4A.7 **Merkel cell carcinoma of lower limb, including hip**

  C4A.70 **Merkel cell carcinoma of unspecified lower limb, including hip**

  C4A.71 **Merkel cell carcinoma of right lower limb, including hip**

  C4A.72 **Merkel cell carcinoma of left lower limb, including hip**

  C4A.8 **Merkel cell carcinoma of overlapping sites**

  C4A.9 **Merkel cell carcinoma, unspecified**
    Merkel cell carcinoma of unspecified site
    Merkel cell carcinoma NOS

● C44 **Other and unspecified malignant neoplasm of skin**

    Includes malignant neoplasm of sebaceous glands
    malignant neoplasm of sweat glands

    Excludes1 Kaposi's sarcoma of skin (C46.0)
    malignant melanoma of skin (C43.-)
    malignant neoplasm of skin of genital organs (C51-C52, C60.-, C63.2)
    Merkel cell carcinoma (C4A.-)

● C44.0 **Other and unspecified malignant neoplasm of skin of lip**

    Excludes1 malignant neoplasm of lip (C00.-)

  C44.00 **Unspecified malignant neoplasm of skin of lip**

  C44.01 **Basal cell carcinoma of skin of lip**

  C44.02 **Squamous cell carcinoma of skin of lip**

  C44.09 **Other specified malignant neoplasm of skin of lip**

◀ New   ◀┅ Revised   d̶e̶l̶e̶t̶e̶d̶ Deleted   Excludes 1   Excludes 2   Includes   Use additional   Code first   Code also   Unspecified

OGCR Official Guidelines   ● Unacceptable Principal Diagnosis   X Assign placeholder X   ● Use Additional Character(s)   ▌ Manifestation Code   **Coding Clinic**

CHAPTER 2 (C00-D49)

● **C44.1**   Other and unspecified malignant neoplasm of skin of eyelid, including canthus

> **Excludes1**   connective tissue of eyelid (C49.0)

● **C44.10**   Unspecified malignant neoplasm of skin of eyelid, including canthus

    C44.101   Unspecified malignant neoplasm of skin of unspecified eyelid, including canthus

    C44.102   Unspecified malignant neoplasm of skin of right eyelid, including canthus

    C44.109   Unspecified malignant neoplasm of skin of left eyelid, including canthus

● **C44.11**   Basal cell carcinoma of skin of eyelid, including canthus

    C44.111   Basal cell carcinoma of skin of unspecified eyelid, including canthus

    C44.112   Basal cell carcinoma of skin of right eyelid, including canthus

    C44.119   Basal cell carcinoma of skin of left eyelid, including canthus

● **C44.12**   Squamous cell carcinoma of skin of eyelid, including canthus

    C44.121   Squamous cell carcinoma of skin of unspecified eyelid, including canthus

    C44.122   Squamous cell carcinoma of skin of right eyelid, including canthus

    C44.129   Squamous cell carcinoma of skin of left eyelid, including canthus

● **C44.19**   Other specified malignant neoplasm of skin of eyelid, including canthus

    C44.191   Other specified malignant neoplasm of skin of unspecified eyelid, including canthus

    C44.192   Other specified malignant neoplasm of skin of right eyelid, including canthus

    C44.199   Other specified malignant neoplasm of skin of left eyelid, including canthus

● **C44.2**   Other and unspecified malignant neoplasm of skin of ear and external auricular canal

> **Excludes1**   connective tissue of ear (C49.0)

● **C44.20**   Unspecified malignant neoplasm of skin of ear and external auricular canal

    C44.201   Unspecified malignant neoplasm of skin of unspecified ear and external auricular canal

    C44.202   Unspecified malignant neoplasm of skin of right ear and external auricular canal

    C44.209   Unspecified malignant neoplasm of skin of left ear and external auricular canal

● **C44.21**   Basal cell carcinoma of skin of ear and external auricular canal

    C44.211   Basal cell carcinoma of skin of unspecified ear and external auricular canal

    C44.212   Basal cell carcinoma of skin of right ear and external auricular canal

    C44.219   Basal cell carcinoma of skin of left ear and external auricular canal

● **C44.22**   Squamous cell carcinoma of skin of ear and external auricular canal

    C44.221   Squamous cell carcinoma of skin of unspecified ear and external auricular canal

    C44.222   Squamous cell carcinoma of skin of right ear and external auricular canal

    C44.229   Squamous cell carcinoma of skin of left ear and external auricular canal

● **C44.29**   Other specified malignant neoplasm of skin of ear and external auricular canal

    C44.291   Other specified malignant neoplasm of skin of unspecified ear and external auricular canal

    C44.292   Other specified malignant neoplasm of skin of right ear and external auricular canal

    C44.299   Other specified malignant neoplasm of skin of left ear and external auricular canal

● **C44.3**   Other and unspecified malignant neoplasm of skin of other and unspecified parts of face

● **C44.30**   Unspecified malignant neoplasm of skin of other and unspecified parts of face

    C44.300   Unspecified malignant neoplasm of skin of unspecified part of face

    C44.301   Unspecified malignant neoplasm of skin of nose

    C44.309   Unspecified malignant neoplasm of skin of other parts of face

● **C44.31**   Basal cell carcinoma of skin of other and unspecified parts of face

    C44.310   Basal cell carcinoma of skin of unspecified parts of face

    C44.311   Basal cell carcinoma of skin of nose

    C44.319   Basal cell carcinoma of skin of other parts of face

● **C44.32**   Squamous cell carcinoma of skin of other and unspecified parts of face

    C44.320   Squamous cell carcinoma of skin of unspecified parts of face

    C44.321   Squamous cell carcinoma of skin of nose

    C44.329   Squamous cell carcinoma of skin of other parts of face

● **C44.39**   Other specified malignant neoplasm of skin of other and unspecified parts of face

    C44.390   Other specified malignant neoplasm of skin of unspecified parts of face

    C44.391   Other specified malignant neoplasm of skin of nose

    C44.399   Other specified malignant neoplasm of skin of other parts of face

● **C44.4**   Other and unspecified malignant neoplasm of skin of scalp and neck

    C44.40   Unspecified malignant neoplasm of skin of scalp and neck

    C44.41   Basal cell carcinoma of skin of scalp and neck

    C44.42   Squamous cell carcinoma of skin of scalp and neck

    C44.49   Other specified malignant neoplasm of skin of scalp and neck

● **C44.5** **Other and unspecified malignant neoplasm of skin of trunk**

> **Excludes1** anus NOS (C21.0)
> scrotum (C63.2)

● **C44.50** **Unspecified malignant neoplasm of skin of trunk**

C44.500 **Unspecified malignant neoplasm of anal skin**
Unspecified malignant neoplasm of anal margin
Unspecified malignant neoplasm of perianal skin

C44.501 **Unspecified malignant neoplasm of skin of breast**

C44.509 **Unspecified malignant neoplasm of skin of other part of trunk**

● **C44.51** **Basal cell carcinoma of skin of trunk**

C44.510 **Basal cell carcinoma of anal skin**
Basal cell carcinoma of anal margin
Basal cell carcinoma of perianal skin

C44.511 **Basal cell carcinoma of skin of breast**

C44.519 **Basal cell carcinoma of skin of other part of trunk**

● **C44.52** **Squamous cell carcinoma of skin of trunk**

C44.520 **Squamous cell carcinoma of anal skin**
Squamous cell carcinoma of anal margin
Squamous cell carcinoma of perianal skin

C44.521 **Squamous cell carcinoma of skin of breast**

C44.529 **Squamous cell carcinoma of skin of other part of trunk**

● **C44.59** **Other specified malignant neoplasm of skin of trunk**

C44.590 **Other specified malignant neoplasm of anal skin**
Other specified malignant neoplasm of anal margin
Other specified malignant neoplasm of perianal skin

C44.591 **Other specified malignant neoplasm of skin of breast**

C44.599 **Other specified malignant neoplasm of skin of other part of trunk**

● **C44.6** **Other and unspecified malignant neoplasm of skin of upper limb, including shoulder**

● **C44.60** **Unspecified malignant neoplasm of skin of upper limb, including shoulder**

C44.601 **Unspecified malignant neoplasm of skin of unspecified upper limb, including shoulder**

C44.602 **Unspecified malignant neoplasm of skin of right upper limb, including shoulder**

C44.609 **Unspecified malignant neoplasm of skin of left upper limb, including shoulder**

● **C44.61** **Basal cell carcinoma of skin of upper limb, including shoulder**

C44.611 **Basal cell carcinoma of skin of unspecified upper limb, including shoulder**

C44.612 **Basal cell carcinoma of skin of right upper limb, including shoulder**

C44.619 **Basal cell carcinoma of skin of left upper limb, including shoulder**

● **C44.62** **Squamous cell carcinoma of skin of upper limb, including shoulder**

C44.621 **Squamous cell carcinoma of skin of unspecified upper limb, including shoulder**

C44.622 **Squamous cell carcinoma of skin of right upper limb, including shoulder**

C44.629 **Squamous cell carcinoma of skin of left upper limb, including shoulder**

● **C44.69** **Other specified malignant neoplasm of skin of upper limb, including shoulder**

C44.691 **Other specified malignant neoplasm of skin of unspecified upper limb, including shoulder**

C44.692 **Other specified malignant neoplasm of skin of right upper limb, including shoulder**

C44.699 **Other specified malignant neoplasm of skin of left upper limb, including shoulder**

● **C44.7** **Other and unspecified malignant neoplasm of skin of lower limb, including hip**

● **C44.70** **Unspecified malignant neoplasm of skin of lower limb, including hip**

C44.701 **Unspecified malignant neoplasm of skin of unspecified lower limb, including hip**

C44.702 **Unspecified malignant neoplasm of skin of right lower limb, including hip**

C44.709 **Unspecified malignant neoplasm of skin of left lower limb, including hip**

● **C44.71** **Basal cell carcinoma of skin of lower limb, including hip**

C44.711 **Basal cell carcinoma of skin of unspecified lower limb, including hip**

C44.712 **Basal cell carcinoma of skin of right lower limb, including hip**

C44.719 **Basal cell carcinoma of skin of left lower limb, including hip**

● **C44.72** **Squamous cell carcinoma of skin of lower limb, including hip**

C44.721 **Squamous cell carcinoma of skin of unspecified lower limb, including hip**

C44.722 **Squamous cell carcinoma of skin of right lower limb, including hip**

C44.729 **Squamous cell carcinoma of skin of left lower limb, including hip**

● **C44.79** **Other specified malignant neoplasm of skin of lower limb, including hip**

C44.791 **Other specified malignant neoplasm of skin of unspecified lower limb, including hip**

C44.792 **Other specified malignant neoplasm of skin of right lower limb, including hip**

C44.799 **Other specified malignant neoplasm of skin of left lower limb, including hip**

● **C44.8**   **Other and unspecified malignant neoplasm of overlapping sites of skin**

     C44.80   Unspecified malignant neoplasm of overlapping sites of skin

     C44.81   Basal cell carcinoma of overlapping sites of skin

     C44.82   Squamous cell carcinoma of overlapping sites of skin

     C44.89   Other specified malignant neoplasm of overlapping sites of skin

● **C44.9**   **Other and unspecified malignant neoplasm of skin, unspecified**

     C44.90   Unspecified malignant neoplasm of skin, unspecified

         Malignant neoplasm of unspecified site of skin

     C44.91   Basal cell carcinoma of skin, unspecified

     C44.92   Squamous cell carcinoma of skin, unspecified

     C44.99   Other specified malignant neoplasm of skin, unspecified

---

MALIGNANT NEOPLASMS OF MESOTHELIAL AND SOFT TISSUE (C45-C49)

● **C45**   **Mesothelioma**

     Malignant cells develop in protective lining that covers internal organs (mesothelium) caused by exposure to asbestos

     C45.0   Mesothelioma of pleura 🦠

         Excludes1   other malignant neoplasm of pleura (C38.4)

         Ex: C38.4, C39.9, C45.0, C45.7-C45.9, C76.8, C7A.00, C7A.098, C7A.1-C7B.00, C7B.1, C80.0-C80.2, D49.1, D49.81-D49.9

     C45.1   Mesothelioma of peritoneum 🦠

         Mesothelioma of cul-de-sac
         Mesothelioma of mesentery
         Mesothelioma of mesocolon
         Mesothelioma of omentum
         Mesothelioma of peritoneum (parietal) (pelvic)

         Excludes1   other malignant neoplasm of soft tissue of peritoneum (C48.-)

         Ex: C45.1, C48.0-C48.8, Z51.0

     C45.2   Mesothelioma of pericardium 🦠

         Excludes1   other malignant neoplasm of pericardium (C38.0)

         Ex: C38.0, C45.2

     C45.7   Mesothelioma of other sites

     C45.9   Mesothelioma, unspecified

● **C46**   **Kaposi's sarcoma**

     Code first any human immunodeficiency virus [HIV] disease (B20)

     C46.0   Kaposi's sarcoma of skin 🦠

         Ex: C46.0, C46.7-C46.9, Z51.0

     C46.1   Kaposi's sarcoma of soft tissue 🦠

         Kaposi's sarcoma of blood vessel
         Kaposi's sarcoma of connective tissue
         Kaposi's sarcoma of fascia
         Kaposi's sarcoma of ligament
         Kaposi's sarcoma of lymphatic(s) NEC
         Kaposi's sarcoma of muscle

         Excludes2   Kaposi's sarcoma of lymph glands and nodes (C46.3)

         Ex: C46.1, C46.7-C46.9, Z51.0

     C46.2   Kaposi's sarcoma of palate 🦠

         Ex: C46.2, C46.7-C46.9, Z51.0

     C46.3   Kaposi's sarcoma of lymph nodes 🦠

         Ex: C45.7-C45.9, C46.3, C76.8-C77.9, C7A.00, C7A.098-C7B.01, C7B.1, C80.0-C80.2, D49.81-D49.9

     C46.4   Kaposi's sarcoma of gastrointestinal sites 🦠

         Ex: C46.4, C46.7-C46.9, Z51.0

Figure 2-11   Kaposi's sarcoma. There are large confluent hyperpigmented patch-stage lesions with lymphedema. (From Cohen & Powderly: Infectious Diseases, ed 3, Mosby, An Imprint of Elsevier, 2010)

Item 2–5   Kaposi's sarcoma is a cancer that causes patches of abnormal tissue to grow under the skin; in the lining of the mouth, nose, and throat; or in other organs, often beginning and spreading to other organs. Patients who have had organ transplants or patients with AIDS are at high risk for this malignancy.

● **C46.5**   **Kaposi's sarcoma of lung**

     Ex: For catgory C46.5 CC codes: C34.80-C34.92, C39.9, C45.7-C45.9, C46.50-C46.52, C76.8, C7A.00, C7A.090, C7A.098-C7B.00, C7B.1, C80.0-C80.2, D49.1, D49.81-D49.9

     C46.50   Kaposi's sarcoma of unspecified lung 🦠

     C46.51   Kaposi's sarcoma of right lung 🦠

     C46.52   Kaposi's sarcoma of left lung 🦠

     C46.7   Kaposi's sarcoma of other sites 🦠

         Ex: C46.0-C46.9, Z51.0

     C46.9   Kaposi's sarcoma, unspecified 🦠

         Kaposi's sarcoma of unspecified site

         Ex: C45.7-C46.9, C51.0-C72.9, C76.0-C79.9, C7A.00, C7A.093, C7A.098-C7B.8, C80.0-C80.2, D00.00-D02.4, D04.0-D09.9, D37.01-D44.9, D48.0-D49.9, Z51.0

● **C47**   **Malignant neoplasm of peripheral nerves and autonomic nervous system**

     Includes   malignant neoplasm of sympathetic and parasympathetic nerves and ganglia

     Excludes1   Kaposi's sarcoma of soft tissue (C46.1)

     Ex: For category C47 CC Codes: Z51.0

     C47.0   Malignant neoplasm of peripheral nerves of head, face and neck 🦠

         Excludes1   malignant neoplasm of peripheral nerves of orbit (C69.6-)

● **C47.1**   **Malignant neoplasm of peripheral nerves of upper limb, including shoulder**

     C47.10   Malignant neoplasm of peripheral nerves of unspecified upper limb, including shoulder 🦠

     C47.11   Malignant neoplasm of peripheral nerves of right upper limb, including shoulder 🦠

     C47.12   Malignant neoplasm of peripheral nerves of left upper limb, including shoulder 🦠

● **C47.2**   **Malignant neoplasm of peripheral nerves of lower limb, including hip**

     C47.20   Malignant neoplasm of peripheral nerves of unspecified lower limb, including hip 🦠

     C47.21   Malignant neoplasm of peripheral nerves of right lower limb, including hip 🦠

     C47.22   Malignant neoplasm of peripheral nerves of left lower limb, including hip 🦠

     C47.3   Malignant neoplasm of peripheral nerves of thorax 🦠

     C47.4   Malignant neoplasm of peripheral nerves of abdomen 🦠

     C47.5   Malignant neoplasm of peripheral nerves of pelvis 🦠

     C47.6   Malignant neoplasm of peripheral nerves of trunk, unspecified 🦠

         Malignant neoplasm of peripheral nerves of unspecified part of trunk

     C47.8   Malignant neoplasm of overlapping sites of peripheral nerves and autonomic nervous system 🦠

     C47.9   Malignant neoplasm of peripheral nerves and autonomic nervous system, unspecified 🦠

         Malignant neoplasm of unspecified site of peripheral nerves and autonomic nervous system

CHAPTER 2 (C00-D49)

N   Newborn Age: 0   P   Pediatric Age: 0–17   M   Maternity DX: 12–55   A   Adult Age: 15–124   ♀   Females Only   ♂   Males Only

🦠   Complication\Comorbidity   🦠   Major C\C   Ex: CC/MCC Exclusions   🦠   Present on Admission Requirement   🦠   Hospital-Acquired Condition

● **C48 Malignant neoplasm of retroperitoneum and peritoneum**

> **Excludes1** Kaposi's sarcoma of connective tissue (C46.1)
> mesothelioma (C45.-)
>
> Ex: For category C48 unless otherwise indicated: C45.1, C48.0-C48.8, Z51.0

C48.0 Malignant neoplasm of retroperitoneum 🔊
Behind/outside of peritoneum
Ex: C48.0, Z51.0

C48.1 Malignant neoplasm of specified parts of peritoneum 🔊
Serous membrane lining abdominopelvic walls and covering viscera
Malignant neoplasm of cul-de-sac
Malignant neoplasm of mesentery
Malignant neoplasm of mesocolon
Malignant neoplasm of omentum
Malignant neoplasm of parietal peritoneum
Malignant neoplasm of pelvic peritoneum

C48.2 Malignant neoplasm of peritoneum, unspecified 🔊

C48.8 Malignant neoplasm of overlapping sites of retroperitoneum and peritoneum 🔊

● **C49 Malignant neoplasm of other connective and soft tissue**

> **Includes** malignant neoplasm of blood vessel
> malignant neoplasm of bursa
> malignant neoplasm of cartilage
> malignant neoplasm of fascia
> malignant neoplasm of fat
> malignant neoplasm of ligament, except uterine
> malignant neoplasm of lymphatic vessel
> malignant neoplasm of muscle
> malignant neoplasm of synovia
> malignant neoplasm of tendon (sheath)
>
> **Excludes1** malignant neoplasm of cartilage (of):
> articular (C40-C41)
> larynx (C32.3)
> nose (C30.0)
> malignant neoplasm of connective tissue of breast (C50.-) ◄
>
> **Excludes2** Kaposi's sarcoma of soft tissue (C46.1)
> malignant neoplasm of heart (C38.0)
> malignant neoplasm of peripheral nerves and autonomic nervous system (C47.-)
> malignant neoplasm of peritoneum (C48.2)
> malignant neoplasm of retroperitoneum (C48.0)
> malignant neoplasm of uterine ligament (C57.3)
> mesothelioma (C45.-)
>
> Ex: For category C49 CC Codes: Z51.0

C49.0 Malignant neoplasm of connective and soft tissue of head, face and neck 🔊
Malignant neoplasm of connective tissue of ear
Malignant neoplasm of connective tissue of eyelid

> **Excludes1** connective tissue of orbit (C69.6-)

C49.1 Malignant neoplasm of connective and soft tissue of upper limb, including shoulder

C49.10 Malignant neoplasm of connective and soft tissue of unspecified upper limb, including shoulder 🔊

C49.11 Malignant neoplasm of connective and soft tissue of right upper limb, including shoulder 🔊

C49.12 Malignant neoplasm of connective and soft tissue of left upper limb, including shoulder 🔊

● **C49.2 Malignant neoplasm of connective and soft tissue of lower limb, including hip**

C49.20 Malignant neoplasm of connective and soft tissue of unspecified lower limb, including hip 🔊

C49.21 Malignant neoplasm of connective and soft tissue of right lower limb, including hip 🔊

C49.22 Malignant neoplasm of connective and soft tissue of left lower limb, including hip 🔊

C49.3 Malignant neoplasm of connective and soft tissue of thorax 🔊
Malignant neoplasm of axilla
Malignant neoplasm of diaphragm
Malignant neoplasm of great vessels

> **Excludes1** malignant neoplasm of breast (C50.-)
> malignant neoplasm of heart (C38.0)
> malignant neoplasm of mediastinum (C38.1-C38.3)
> malignant neoplasm of thymus (C37)

C49.4 Malignant neoplasm of connective and soft tissue of abdomen 🔊
Malignant neoplasm of abdominal wall
Malignant neoplasm of hypochondrium

C49.5 Malignant neoplasm of connective and soft tissue of pelvis 🔊
Malignant neoplasm of buttock
Malignant neoplasm of groin
Malignant neoplasm of perineum

C49.6 Malignant neoplasm of connective and soft tissue of trunk, unspecified 🔊
Malignant neoplasm of back NOS

C49.8 Malignant neoplasm of overlapping sites of connective and soft tissue 🔊
Primary malignant neoplasm of two or more contiguous sites of connective and soft tissue

C49.9 Malignant neoplasm of connective and soft tissue, unspecified 🔊

MALIGNANT NEOPLASMS OF BREAST (C50)

● **C50 Malignant neoplasm of breast**

> **Includes** connective tissue of breast
> Paget's disease of breast
> Paget's disease of nipple
> *Intraductal carcinoma of breast characterized by eczema-like inflammatory skin changes*

Use additional code to identify estrogen receptor status (Z17.0, Z17.1)

> **Excludes1** skin of breast (C44.501, C44.511, C44.521, C44.591)

● **C50.0 Malignant neoplasm of nipple and areola**

● **C50.01 Malignant neoplasm of nipple and areola, female**

C50.011 Malignant neoplasm of nipple and areola, right female breast ♀

C50.012 Malignant neoplasm of nipple and areola, left female breast ♀

C50.019 Malignant neoplasm of nipple and areola, unspecified female breast ♀

● **C50.02 Malignant neoplasm of nipple and areola, male**

C50.021 Malignant neoplasm of nipple and areola, right male breast ♂

C50.022 Malignant neoplasm of nipple and areola, left male breast ♂

C50.029 Malignant neoplasm of nipple and areola, unspecified male breast ♂

Figure 2-12 Female breast quadrants and axillary tail.

◄ New ◄◄ Revised ~~deleted~~ Deleted | Excludes 1 | Excludes 2 | Includes | Use additional | Code first | Code also | Unspecified
OGCR Official Guidelines ● Unacceptable Principal Diagnosis X Assign placeholder X ● Use Additional Character(s) ▸ Manifestation Code **Coding Clinic**

● C50.1 Malignant neoplasm of central portion of breast
  ● C50.11 Malignant neoplasm of central portion of breast, female
    C50.111 Malignant neoplasm of central portion of right female breast ♀
    C50.112 Malignant neoplasm of central portion of left female breast ♀
    C50.119 Malignant neoplasm of central portion of unspecified female breast ♀
  ● C50.12 Malignant neoplasm of central portion of breast, male
    C50.121 Malignant neoplasm of central portion of right male breast ♂
    C50.122 Malignant neoplasm of central portion of left male breast ♂
    C50.129 Malignant neoplasm of central portion of unspecified male breast ♂
● C50.2 Malignant neoplasm of upper-inner quadrant of breast
  ● C50.21 Malignant neoplasm of upper-inner quadrant of breast, female
    C50.211 Malignant neoplasm of upper-inner quadrant of right female breast ♀
    C50.212 Malignant neoplasm of upper-inner quadrant of left female breast ♀
    C50.219 Malignant neoplasm of upper-inner quadrant of unspecified female breast ♀
  ● C50.22 Malignant neoplasm of upper-inner quadrant of breast, male
    C50.221 Malignant neoplasm of upper-inner quadrant of right male breast ♂
    C50.222 Malignant neoplasm of upper-inner quadrant of left male breast ♂
    C50.229 Malignant neoplasm of upper-inner quadrant of unspecified male breast ♂
● C50.3 Malignant neoplasm of lower-inner quadrant of breast
  ● C50.31 Malignant neoplasm of lower-inner quadrant of breast, female
    C50.311 Malignant neoplasm of lower-inner quadrant of right female breast ♀
    C50.312 Malignant neoplasm of lower-inner quadrant of left female breast ♀
    C50.319 Malignant neoplasm of lower-inner quadrant of unspecified female breast ♀
  ● C50.32 Malignant neoplasm of lower-inner quadrant of breast, male
    C50.321 Malignant neoplasm of lower-inner quadrant of right male breast ♂
    C50.322 Malignant neoplasm of lower-inner quadrant of left male breast ♂
    C50.329 Malignant neoplasm of lower-inner quadrant of unspecified male breast ♂
● C50.4 Malignant neoplasm of upper-outer quadrant of breast
  ● C50.41 Malignant neoplasm of upper-outer quadrant of breast, female
    C50.411 Malignant neoplasm of upper-outer quadrant of right female breast ♀
    C50.412 Malignant neoplasm of upper-outer quadrant of left female breast ♀
    C50.419 Malignant neoplasm of upper-outer quadrant of unspecified female breast ♀

● C50.42 Malignant neoplasm of upper-outer quadrant of breast, male
    C50.421 Malignant neoplasm of upper-outer quadrant of right male breast ♂
    C50.422 Malignant neoplasm of upper-outer quadrant of left male breast ♂
    C50.429 Malignant neoplasm of upper-outer quadrant of unspecified male breast ♂
● C50.5 Malignant neoplasm of lower-outer quadrant of breast
  ● C50.51 Malignant neoplasm of lower-outer quadrant of breast, female
    C50.511 Malignant neoplasm of lower-outer quadrant of right female breast ♀
    C50.512 Malignant neoplasm of lower-outer quadrant of left female breast ♀
    C50.519 Malignant neoplasm of lower-outer quadrant of unspecified female breast ♀
  ● C50.52 Malignant neoplasm of lower-outer quadrant of breast, male
    C50.521 Malignant neoplasm of lower-outer quadrant of right male breast ♂
    C50.522 Malignant neoplasm of lower-outer quadrant of left male breast ♂
    C50.529 Malignant neoplasm of lower-outer quadrant of unspecified male breast ♂
● C50.6 Malignant neoplasm of axillary tail of breast
  ● C50.61 Malignant neoplasm of axillary tail of breast, female
    C50.611 Malignant neoplasm of axillary tail of right female breast ♀
    C50.612 Malignant neoplasm of axillary tail of left female breast ♀
    C50.619 Malignant neoplasm of axillary tail of unspecified female breast ♀
  ● C50.62 Malignant neoplasm of axillary tail of breast, male
    C50.621 Malignant neoplasm of axillary tail of right male breast ♂
    C50.622 Malignant neoplasm of axillary tail of left male breast ♂
    C50.629 Malignant neoplasm of axillary tail of unspecified male breast ♂
● C50.8 Malignant neoplasm of overlapping sites of breast
  ● C50.81 Malignant neoplasm of overlapping sites of breast, female
    C50.811 Malignant neoplasm of overlapping sites of right female breast ♀
    C50.812 Malignant neoplasm of overlapping sites of left female breast ♀
    C50.819 Malignant neoplasm of overlapping sites of unspecified female breast ♀
  ● C50.82 Malignant neoplasm of overlapping sites of breast, male
    C50.821 Malignant neoplasm of overlapping sites of right male breast ♂
    C50.822 Malignant neoplasm of overlapping sites of left male breast ♂
    C50.829 Malignant neoplasm of overlapping sites of unspecified male breast ♂
● C50.9 Malignant neoplasm of breast of unspecified site
  ● C50.91 Malignant neoplasm of breast of unspecified site, female
    C50.911 Malignant neoplasm of unspecified site of right female breast ♀
    C50.912 Malignant neoplasm of unspecified site of left female breast ♀
    C50.919 Malignant neoplasm of unspecified site of unspecified female breast ♀

N Newborn Age: 0   P Pediatric Age: 0–17   M Maternity DX: 12–55   A Adult Age: 15–124   ♀ Females Only   ♂ Males Only

◐ Complication\Comorbidity   ◐ Major C\C   (Ex) CC/MCC Exclusions   ◑ Present on Admission Requirement   ◑ Hospital-Acquired Condition

787

● **C50.92**   Malignant neoplasm of breast of unspecified
            site, male
   C50.921   Malignant neoplasm of unspecified
              site of right male breast ♂
   C50.922   Malignant neoplasm of unspecified
              site of left male breast ♂
   C50.929   Malignant neoplasm of unspecified
              site of unspecified male breast ♂

MALIGNANT NEOPLASMS OF FEMALE GENITAL ORGANS (C51-C58)

   Includes   malignant neoplasm of skin of female genital
               organs

● **C51**   Malignant neoplasm of vulva
   Excludes1   carcinoma in situ of vulva (D07.1)
   C51.0   Malignant neoplasm of labium majus ♀
           Outer folds of skin external female genitalia
           Malignant neoplasm of Bartholin's [greater vestibular]
           gland
   C51.1   Malignant neoplasm of labium minus ♀
           Two inner folds surrounding vulva in female genitalia
   C51.2   Malignant neoplasm of clitoris ♀
   C51.8   Malignant neoplasm of overlapping sites of vulva ♀
   C51.9   Malignant neoplasm of vulva, unspecified ♀
           Malignant neoplasm of external female genitalia NOS
           Malignant neoplasm of pudendum

  C52   Malignant neoplasm of vagina ♀
   Excludes1   carcinoma in situ of vagina (D07.2)

● **C53**   Malignant neoplasm of cervix uteri
   Excludes1   carcinoma in situ of cervix uteri (D06.-)
   C53.0   Malignant neoplasm of endocervix ♀
           Inside the cervix
   C53.1   Malignant neoplasm of exocervix ♀
           Outside the cervix
   C53.8   Malignant neoplasm of overlapping sites of cervix
           uteri ♀
   C53.9   Malignant neoplasm of cervix uteri, unspecified ♀

● **C54**   Malignant neoplasm of corpus uteri
   C54.0   Malignant neoplasm of isthmus uteri ♀
           Constricted part of uterus between cervix and body
           Malignant neoplasm of lower uterine segment
   C54.1   Malignant neoplasm of endometrium ♀
           Lining of uterus
   C54.2   Malignant neoplasm of myometrium ♀
           *Middle layer of uterine wall consisting of smooth muscle
           supporting stromal and vascular tissue*
   C54.3   Malignant neoplasm of fundus uteri ♀
           Top rounded portion of uterus
   C54.8   Malignant neoplasm of overlapping sites of corpus
           uteri ♀
           Main body of uterus
   C54.9   Malignant neoplasm of corpus uteri, unspecified ♀

Figure 2-13   Cervix uteri.

  C55   Malignant neoplasm of uterus, part unspecified ♀

● **C56**   Malignant neoplasm of ovary
           Use additional code to identify any functional activity
           Ⓔⓧ **For category C56 CC Codes:** C45.9, C56.1-C57.4, C76.3, C79.60-C79.62, C7A.00,
           C7A.098-C7B.00, C7B.1, C80.0-C80.2
   C56.1   Malignant neoplasm of right ovary ♀ 🔎
   C56.2   Malignant neoplasm of left ovary ♀ 🔎
   C56.9   Malignant neoplasm of unspecified ovary ♀ 🔎

● **C57**   Malignant neoplasm of other and unspecified female genital
         organs
   ● **C57.0**   Malignant neoplasm of fallopian tube
              Malignant neoplasm of oviduct
              Malignant neoplasm of uterine tube
      C57.00   Malignant neoplasm of unspecified fallopian
                tube ♀
      C57.01   Malignant neoplasm of right fallopian tube ♀
      C57.02   Malignant neoplasm of left fallopian tube ♀
   ● **C57.1**   Malignant neoplasm of broad ligament
      C57.10   Malignant neoplasm of unspecified broad
                ligament ♀
      C57.11   Malignant neoplasm of right broad ligament ♀
      C57.12   Malignant neoplasm of left broad ligament ♀
   ● **C57.2**   Malignant neoplasm of round ligament
      C57.20   Malignant neoplasm of unspecified round
                ligament ♀
      C57.21   Malignant neoplasm of right round ligament ♀
      C57.22   Malignant neoplasm of left round ligament ♀
      C57.3   Malignant neoplasm of parametrium ♀
                Malignant neoplasm of uterine ligament NOS
      C57.4   Malignant neoplasm of uterine adnexa, unspecified ♀
      C57.7   Malignant neoplasm of other specified female genital
                organs ♀
                Malignant neoplasm of wolffian body or duct
      C57.8   Malignant neoplasm of overlapping sites of female
                genital organs ♀
                Primary malignant neoplasm of two or more
                   contiguous sites of the female genital organs whose
                   point of origin cannot be determined
                Primary tubo-ovarian malignant neoplasm whose point
                   of origin cannot be determined
                Primary utero-ovarian malignant neoplasm whose
                   point of origin cannot be determined
      C57.9   Malignant neoplasm of female genital
                organ, unspecified ♀
                Malignant neoplasm of female genitourinary tract NOS

  C58   Malignant neoplasm of placenta ♀
   Includes   choriocarcinoma NOS
               chorionepithelioma NOS
   Excludes1   chorioadenoma (destruens) (D39.2)
               hydatidiform mole NOS (O01.9)
               invasive hydatidiform mole (D39.2)
               male choriocarcinoma NOS (C62.9-)
               malignant hydatidiform mole (D39.2)

MALIGNANT NEOPLASMS OF MALE GENITAL ORGANS (C60-C63)

   Includes   malignant neoplasm of skin of male genital
               organs

● **C60**   Malignant neoplasm of penis
   C60.0   Malignant neoplasm of prepuce ♂
           Malignant neoplasm of foreskin
   C60.1   Malignant neoplasm of glans penis ♂
   C60.2   Malignant neoplasm of body of penis ♂
           Malignant neoplasm of corpus cavernosum
   C60.8   Malignant neoplasm of overlapping sites of penis ♂
   C60.9   Malignant neoplasm of penis, unspecified ♂
           Malignant neoplasm of skin of penis NOS

◀ New   ◀▥ Revised   ~~deleted~~ Deleted   Excludes 1   Excludes 2   Includes   Use additional   Code first   Code also   Unspecified

OGCR Official Guidelines   ● Unacceptable Principal Diagnosis   X Assign placeholder X   ● Use Additional Character(s)   ▸ Manifestation Code   **Coding Clinic**

Figure 2-14 Penis and other male genital organs.

C61   Malignant neoplasm of prostate ♂

> **Excludes1**   malignant neoplasm of seminal vesicle (C63.7)

● C62   Malignant neoplasm of testis
Use additional code to identify any functional activity.

● C62.0   Malignant neoplasm of undescended testis
Malignant neoplasm of ectopic testis
Malignant neoplasm of retained testis

C62.00   Malignant neoplasm of unspecified undescended testis ♂

C62.01   Malignant neoplasm of undescended right testis ♂

C62.02   Malignant neoplasm of undescended left testis ♂

● C62.1   Malignant neoplasm of descended testis
Malignant neoplasm of scrotal testis

C62.10   Malignant neoplasm of unspecified descended testis, unspecified side ♂

C62.11   Malignant neoplasm of descended right testis ♂

C62.12   Malignant neoplasm of descended left testis ♂

● C62.9   Malignant neoplasm of testis, unspecified whether descended or undescended

C62.90   Malignant neoplasm of unspecified testis, unspecified whether descended or undescended ♂
Malignant neoplasm of testis NOS

C62.91   Malignant neoplasm of right testis, unspecified whether descended or undescended ♂

C62.92   Malignant neoplasm of left testis, unspecified whether descended or undescended ♂

● C63   Malignant neoplasm of other and unspecified male genital organs

● C63.0   Malignant neoplasm of epididymis

C63.00   Malignant neoplasm of unspecified epididymis ♂

C63.01   Malignant neoplasm of right epididymis ♂

C63.02   Malignant neoplasm of left epididymis ♂

● C63.1   Malignant neoplasm of spermatic cord

C63.10   Malignant neoplasm of unspecified spermatic cord ♂

C63.11   Malignant neoplasm of right spermatic cord ♂

C63.12   Malignant neoplasm of left spermatic cord ♂

C63.2   Malignant neoplasm of scrotum ♂
Malignant neoplasm of skin of scrotum

C63.7   Malignant neoplasm of other specified male genital organs ♂
Malignant neoplasm of seminal vesicle
Malignant neoplasm of tunica vaginalis

C63.8   Malignant neoplasm of overlapping sites of male genital organs ♂
Primary malignant neoplasm of two or more contiguous sites of male genital organs whose point of origin cannot be determined

C63.9   Malignant neoplasm of male genital organ, unspecified ♂
Malignant neoplasm of male genitourinary tract NOS

MALIGNANT NEOPLASMS OF URINARY TRACT (C64-C68)

● C64   Malignant neoplasm of kidney, except renal pelvis

> **Excludes1**   malignant carcinoid tumor of the kidney (C7A.093)
> malignant neoplasm of renal calyces (C65.-)
> malignant neoplasm of renal pelvis (C65.-)

Ex) For category C64 CC Codes: C45.7-C45.9, C64.1-C65.9, C68.8-C68.9, C76.8, C7A.00, C7A.093, C7A.098-C7B.00, C7B.1, C80.0-C80.2, D49.5, D49.81-D49.9

C64.1   Malignant neoplasm of right kidney, except renal pelvis ◐

C64.2   Malignant neoplasm of left kidney, except renal pelvis ◐

C64.9   Malignant neoplasm of unspecified kidney, except renal pelvis ◐

● C65   Malignant neoplasm of renal pelvis

> **Includes**   malignant neoplasm of pelviureteric junction
> malignant neoplasm of renal calyces

Ex) For category C65 CC Codes: See C64

C65.1   Malignant neoplasm of right renal pelvis ◐

C65.2   Malignant neoplasm of left renal pelvis ◐

C65.9   Malignant neoplasm of unspecified renal pelvis ◐

● C66   Malignant neoplasm of ureter

> **Excludes1**   malignant neoplasm of ureteric orifice of bladder (C67.6)

Ex) For category C66 CC Codes: C45.7-C45.9, C66.1-C66.9, C68.8-C68.9, C76.8, C7A.00, C7A.098, C7A.1-C7B.00, C7B.1, C80.0-C80.2, D49.5, D49.81-D49.9

C66.1   Malignant neoplasm of right ureter ◐

C66.2   Malignant neoplasm of left ureter ◐

C66.9   Malignant neoplasm of unspecified ureter ◐

● C67   Malignant neoplasm of bladder

C67.0   Malignant neoplasm of trigone of bladder
Triangular area formed by three openings in the floor of urinary bladder

C67.1   Malignant neoplasm of dome of bladder
Vaulted roof

C67.2   Malignant neoplasm of lateral wall of bladder
Side walls

C67.3   Malignant neoplasm of anterior wall of bladder
Front wall

C67.4   Malignant neoplasm of posterior wall of bladder
Back wall

C67.5   Malignant neoplasm of bladder neck
Joining of bladder and urethra
Malignant neoplasm of internal urethral orifice

C67.6   Malignant neoplasm of ureteric orifice
Opening from bladder to ureters

C67.7   Malignant neoplasm of urachus
Embryonic canal that connects the urinary bladder with the structure that forms the umbilical cord (allantois)

C67.8   Malignant neoplasm of overlapping sites of bladder

C67.9   Malignant neoplasm of bladder, unspecified

● C68   Malignant neoplasm of other and unspecified urinary organs

> **Excludes1**   malignant neoplasm of female genitourinary tract NOS (C57.9)
> malignant neoplasm of male genitourinary tract NOS (C63.9)

Ex) For category C68 CC codes C68.0-C68.1: C68.0-C68.9, C79.82 For category C68 CC codes C68.8-C68.9: C6.41-C66.9, C68.0-C68.9, C76.3, C79.00-C79.19, C7A.093

C68.0   Malignant neoplasm of urethra ◐

> **Excludes1**   malignant neoplasm of urethral orifice of bladder (C67.5)

C68.1   Malignant neoplasm of paraurethral glands ◐
Group of glands of female urethra drained by paraurethral ducts; AKA Skene glands, female prostate

N Newborn Age: 0   P Pediatric Age: 0–17   M Maternity DX: 12–55   A Adult Age: 15–124   ♀ Females Only   ♂ Males Only

◐ Complication\Comorbidity   ◐ Major C\C   Ex) CC/MCC Exclusions   ◐ Present on Admission Requirement   ◐ Hospital-Acquired Condition

CHAPTER 2 (C00–D49)

C68.8   Malignant neoplasm of overlapping sites of urinary organs 🔖

     Primary malignant neoplasm of two or more contiguous sites of urinary organs whose point of origin cannot be determined

C68.9   Malignant neoplasm of urinary organ, unspecified 🔖

     Malignant neoplasm of urinary system NOS

MALIGNANT NEOPLASMS OF EYE, BRAIN AND OTHER PARTS OF CENTRAL NERVOUS SYSTEM (C69-C72)

● **C69**   Malignant neoplasm of eye and adnexa

    Excludes1   malignant neoplasm of connective tissue of eyelid (C49.0)

              malignant neoplasm of eyelid (skin) (C43.1-, C44.1-)

              malignant neoplasm of optic nerve (C72.3-)

● **C69.0**   Malignant neoplasm of conjunctiva

   C69.00   Malignant neoplasm of unspecified conjunctiva

   C69.01   Malignant neoplasm of right conjunctiva

   C69.02   Malignant neoplasm of left conjunctiva

● **C69.1**   Malignant neoplasm of cornea

   C69.10   Malignant neoplasm of unspecified cornea

   C69.11   Malignant neoplasm of right cornea

   C69.12   Malignant neoplasm of left cornea

● **C69.2**   Malignant neoplasm of retina

    Excludes1   dark area on retina (D49.81)

              neoplasm of unspecified behavior of retina and choroid (D49.81)

              retinal freckle (D49.81)

   C69.20   Malignant neoplasm of unspecified retina

   C69.21   Malignant neoplasm of right retina

   C69.22   Malignant neoplasm of left retina

● **C69.3**   Malignant neoplasm of choroid

   C69.30   Malignant neoplasm of unspecified choroid

   C69.31   Malignant neoplasm of right choroid

   C69.32   Malignant neoplasm of left choroid

● **C69.4**   Malignant neoplasm of ciliary body

   C69.40   Malignant neoplasm of unspecified ciliary body

   C69.41   Malignant neoplasm of right ciliary body

   C69.42   Malignant neoplasm of left ciliary body

● **C69.5**   Malignant neoplasm of lacrimal gland and duct

     Malignant neoplasm of lacrimal sac

     Malignant neoplasm of nasolacrimal duct

   C69.50   Malignant neoplasm of unspecified lacrimal gland and duct

   C69.51   Malignant neoplasm of right lacrimal gland and duct

   C69.52   Malignant neoplasm of left lacrimal gland and duct

● **C69.6**   Malignant neoplasm of orbit

     Malignant neoplasm of connective tissue of orbit

     Malignant neoplasm of extraocular muscle

     Malignant neoplasm of peripheral nerves of orbit

     Malignant neoplasm of retrobulbar tissue

     Malignant neoplasm of retro-ocular tissue

    Excludes1   malignant neoplasm of orbital bone (C41.0)

   C69.60   Malignant neoplasm of unspecified orbit

   C69.61   Malignant neoplasm of right orbit

   C69.62   Malignant neoplasm of left orbit

● **C69.8**   Malignant neoplasm of overlapping sites of eye and adnexa

   C69.80   Malignant neoplasm of overlapping sites of unspecified eye and adnexa

   C69.81   Malignant neoplasm of overlapping sites of right eye and adnexa

   C69.82   Malignant neoplasm of overlapping sites of left eye and adnexa

● **C69.9**   Malignant neoplasm of unspecified site of eye

     Malignant neoplasm of eyeball

   C69.90   Malignant neoplasm of unspecified site of unspecified eye

   C69.91   Malignant neoplasm of unspecified site of right eye

   C69.92   Malignant neoplasm of unspecified site of left eye

● **C70**   Malignant neoplasm of meninges

   C70.0   Malignant neoplasm of cerebral meninges 🔖

     Ⓔⓧ C45.7-C45.9, C70.0, C70.9, C72.9, C76.8, C7A.00, C7A.098-C7B.00, C7B.1, C80.0-C80.2, D49.6-D49.9

   C70.1   Malignant neoplasm of spinal meninges 🔖

     Ⓔⓧ C45.7-C45.9, C70.1, C72.9, C76.8, C7A.00, C7A.098-C7B.00, C7B.1, C80.0-C80.2, D49.6-D49.9

   C70.9   Malignant neoplasm of meninges, unspecified 🔖

     Ⓔⓧ See C70.0

● **C71**   Malignant neoplasm of brain

    Excludes1   malignant neoplasm of cranial nerves (C72.2-C72.5)

              retrobulbar malignant neoplasm (C69.6-)

    Ⓔⓧ **For category C71 CC codes:** C45.7-C45.9, C70.0, C70.9-C71.9, C72.20-C72.9, C76.8, C7A.00, C7A.098-C7B.00, C7B.1, C80.0-C80.2, D49.6-D49.9

   C71.0   Malignant neoplasm of cerebrum, except lobes and ventricles 🔖

     Malignant neoplasm of supratentorial NOS

   C71.1   Malignant neoplasm of frontal lobe 🔖

   C71.2   Malignant neoplasm of temporal lobe 🔖

   C71.3   Malignant neoplasm of parietal lobe 🔖

   C71.4   Malignant neoplasm of occipital lobe 🔖

   C71.5   Malignant neoplasm of cerebral ventricle 🔖

      Excludes1   malignant neoplasm of fourth cerebral ventricle (C71.7)

   C71.6   Malignant neoplasm of cerebellum 🔖

   C71.7   Malignant neoplasm of brain stem 🔖

     Malignant neoplasm of fourth cerebral ventricle

     Infratentorial malignant neoplasm NOS

   C71.8   Malignant neoplasm of overlapping sites of brain 🔖

   C71.9   Malignant neoplasm of brain, unspecified 🔖

● **C72**   Malignant neoplasm of spinal cord, cranial nerves and other parts of central nervous system

    Excludes1   malignant neoplasm of meninges (C70.-)

              malignant neoplasm of peripheral nerves and autonomic nervous system (C47.-)

    Ⓔⓧ **For category C72 unless otherwise indicated:** C45.7-C45.9, C72.20-C72.9, C76.8, C7A.00, C7A.098-C7B.00, C7B.1, C80.0-C80.2, D49.6-D49.9

   C72.0   Malignant neoplasm of spinal cord 🔖

     Ⓔⓧ C45.7-C45.9, C72.0-C72.1, C72.9, C76.8, C7A.00, C7A.098, C7A.1-C7B.00, C7B.1, C80.0-C80.2, D49.6-D49.9

FRONTAL LOBE   PARIETAL LOBE

Anterior   Posterior

TEMPORAL LOBE   OCCIPITAL LOBE

CEREBELLUM

Figure 2-15   The brain.

◄ New   ◄ Revised   ~~deleted~~ Deleted   Excludes 1   Excludes 2   Includes   Use additional   Code first   Code also   Unspecified

OGCR Official Guidelines   ● Unacceptable Principal Diagnosis   X Assign placeholder X   ● Use Additional Character(s)   ▶ Manifestation Code   **Coding Clinic**

C72.1   Malignant neoplasm of cauda equina
> *Lower end of spinal column*
> (Ex:) See C72.0

● **C72.2**   Malignant neoplasm of olfactory nerve
Malignant neoplasm of olfactory bulb

    C72.20   Malignant neoplasm of unspecified olfactory nerve

    C72.21   Malignant neoplasm of right olfactory nerve

    C72.22   Malignant neoplasm of left olfactory nerve

● **C72.3**   Malignant neoplasm of optic nerve

    C72.30   Malignant neoplasm of unspecified optic nerve

    C72.31   Malignant neoplasm of right optic nerve

    C72.32   Malignant neoplasm of left optic nerve

● **C72.4**   Malignant neoplasm of acoustic nerve

    C72.40   Malignant neoplasm of unspecified acoustic nerve

    C72.41   Malignant neoplasm of right acoustic nerve

    C72.42   Malignant neoplasm of left acoustic nerve

● **C72.5**   Malignant neoplasm of other and unspecified cranial nerves

    C72.50   Malignant neoplasm of unspecified cranial nerve
       Malignant neoplasm of cranial nerve NOS

    C72.59   Malignant neoplasm of other cranial nerves

C72.9   Malignant neoplasm of central nervous system, unspecified
Malignant neoplasm of unspecified site of central nervous system
Malignant neoplasm of nervous system NOS
> (Ex:) C45.7-C45.9, C70.0-C72.9, C76.8, C79.31-C79.49, C7A.00, C7A.098-C7B.00, C7B.1, C80.0-C80.2, D49.6-D49.9

MALIGNANT NEOPLASMS OF THYROID AND OTHER ENDOCRINE GLANDS (C73-C75)

C73   Malignant neoplasm of thyroid gland
Use additional code to identify any functional activity

● **C74**   Malignant neoplasm of adrenal gland
> (Ex:) For category **C74** CC codes: C45.7-C45.9, C74.00-C74.92, C75.9, C76.2, C76.8, C79.70-C79.72, C7A.00, C7A.098-C7B.00, C7B.1, C80.0-C80.2

  ● **C74.0**   Malignant neoplasm of cortex of adrenal gland

    C74.00   Malignant neoplasm of cortex of unspecified adrenal gland

    C74.01   Malignant neoplasm of cortex of right adrenal gland

    C74.02   Malignant neoplasm of cortex of left adrenal gland

  ● **C74.1**   Malignant neoplasm of medulla of adrenal gland
> *Pair of glands situated on top of or above each kidney ("suprarenal")*

    C74.10   Malignant neoplasm of medulla of unspecified adrenal gland

    C74.11   Malignant neoplasm of medulla of right adrenal gland

    C74.12   Malignant neoplasm of medulla of left adrenal gland

  ● **C74.9**   Malignant neoplasm of unspecified part of adrenal gland

    C74.90   Malignant neoplasm of unspecified part of unspecified adrenal gland

    C74.91   Malignant neoplasm of unspecified part of right adrenal gland

    C74.92   Malignant neoplasm of unspecified part of left adrenal gland

● **C75**   Malignant neoplasm of other endocrine glands and related structures

  Excludes1   malignant carcinoid tumors (C7A.0-)
       malignant neoplasm of adrenal gland (C74.-)
       malignant neoplasm of endocrine pancreas (C25.4)
       malignant neoplasm of islets of Langerhans (C25.4)
       malignant neoplasm of ovary (C56.-) ◂▦
       malignant neoplasm of testis (C62.-)
       malignant neoplasm of thymus (C37)
       malignant neoplasm of thyroid gland (C73)
       malignant neuroendocrine tumors (C7A.-)

  C75.0   Malignant neoplasm of parathyroid gland
> (Ex:) C75.0, C75.8-C75.9

  C75.1   Malignant neoplasm of pituitary gland
> (Ex:) C75.1-C75.2, Z51.0

  C75.2   Malignant neoplasm of craniopharyngeal duct
> (Ex:) See C75.1

  C75.3   Malignant neoplasm of pineal gland
> (Ex:) C75.3, Z51.0

  C75.4   Malignant neoplasm of carotid body
> (Ex:) C75.4, C75.8-C75.9

  C75.5   Malignant neoplasm of aortic body and other paraganglia
> (Ex:) C75.4-C75.9

  C75.8   Malignant neoplasm with pluriglandular involvement, unspecified
> (Ex:) C74.00-C75.9

  C75.9   Malignant neoplasm of endocrine gland, unspecified
> (Ex:) See C75.8

MALIGNANT NEUROENDOCRINE TUMORS (C7A)

● **C7A**   Malignant neuroendocrine tumors
Code also any associated multiple endocrine neoplasia [MEN] syndromes (E31.2-)
Use additional code to identify any associated endocrine syndrome, such as:
carcinoid syndrome (E34.0)

  Excludes2   malignant pancreatic islet cell tumors (C25.4)
       Merkel cell carcinoma (C4A.-)

  ● **C7A.0**   Malignant carcinoid tumors

    C7A.00   Malignant carcinoid tumor of unspecified site
> (Ex:) C45.7-C45.9, C76.8, C79.89-C79.9, C7A.00-C7B.00, C7B.09-C7B.8, C80.0-C80.2, D49.81-D49.9

   ● **C7A.01**   Malignant carcinoid tumors of the small intestine

    C7A.010   Malignant carcinoid tumor of the duodenum
> (Ex:) C17.0, C17.8-C17.9, C26.0, C26.9, C45.7-C45.9, C46.4, C76.8, C7A.00-C7B.00, C7B.1, C80.0-C80.2, D49.0, D49.81-D49.9

    C7A.011   Malignant carcinoid tumor of the jejunum
> (Ex:) C17.1, C17.8-C17.9, C26.0, C26.9, C45.7-C45.9, C46.4, C76.8, C7A.00-C7B.00, C7B.1, C80.0-C80.2, D49.0, D49.81-D49.9

    C7A.012   Malignant carcinoid tumor of the ileum
> (Ex:) C17.2, C17.8-C17.9, C26.0, C26.9, C45.7-C45.9, C46.4, C76.8, C7A.00-C7B.00, C7B.1, C80.0-C80.2, D49.0, D49.81-D49.9

    C7A.019   Malignant carcinoid tumor of the small intestine, unspecified portion
> (Ex:) C17.8-C17.9, C26.0, C26.9, C45.7-C45.9, C46.4, C76.8, C7A.00-C7B.00, C7B.1, C80.0-C80.2, D49.0, D49.81-D49.9

N Newborn Age: 0   **P** Pediatric Age: 0-17   **M** Maternity DX: 12-55   **A** Adult Age: 15-124   ♀ Females Only   ♂ Males Only

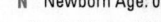 Complication\Comorbidity   Major C\C   (Ex:) CC/MCC Exclusions   Present on Admission Requirement   Hospital-Acquired Condition

791

● **C7A.02   Malignant carcinoid tumors of the appendix, large intestine, and rectum**

    C7A.020   Malignant carcinoid tumor of the appendix 🔍
        (Ex:) C18.1, C18.8-C18.9, C26.0, C26.9, C45.7-C45.9, C46.4, C76.8, C7A.00-C7B.00, C7B.1, C80.0-C80.2, D49.0, D49.81-D49.9

    C7A.021   Malignant carcinoid tumor of the cecum 🔍
        (Ex:) C18.0, C18.8-C18.9, C26.0, C26.9, C45.7-C45.9, C46.4, C76.8, C7A.00-C7B.00, C7B.1, C80.0-C80.2, D49.0, D49.81-D49.9

    C7A.022   Malignant carcinoid tumor of the ascending colon 🔍
        (Ex:) C18.2, C18.8-C18.9, C26.0, C26.9, C45.7-C45.9, C46.4, C76.8, C7A.00-C7B.00, C7B.1, C80.0-C80.2, D49.0, D49.81-D49.9

    C7A.023   Malignant carcinoid tumor of the transverse colon 🔍
        (Ex:) C18.4, C18.8-C18.9, C26.0, C26.9, C45.7-C45.9, C46.4, C76.8, C7A.00-C7B.00, C7B.1, C80.0-C80.2, D49.0, D49.81-D49.9

    C7A.024   Malignant carcinoid tumor of the descending colon 🔍
        (Ex:) C18.6, C18.8-C18.9, C26.0, C26.9, C45.7-C45.9, C46.4, C76.8, C7A.00-C7B.00, C7B.1, C80.0-C80.2, D49.0, D49.81-D49.9

    C7A.025   Malignant carcinoid tumor of the sigmoid colon 🔍
        (Ex:) C18.7-C18.9, C26.0, C26.9, C45.7-C45.9, C46.4, C76.8, C7A.00-C7B.00, C7B.1, C80.0-C80.2, D49.0, D49.81-D49.9

    C7A.026   Malignant carcinoid tumor of the rectum 🔍
        (Ex:) C20, C21.2-C21.8, C26.0, C26.9, C45.7-C45.9, C46.4, C76.8, C7A.00-C7B.00, C7B.1, C80.0-C80.2, D49.0, D49.81-D49.9

    C7A.029   Malignant carcinoid tumor of the large intestine, unspecified portion 🔍
      Malignant carcinoid tumor of the colon NOS
        (Ex:) C18.8-C18.9, C26.0, C26.9, C45.7-C45.9, C46.4, C76.8, C7A.00-C7B.00, C7B.1, C80.0-C80.2, D49.0, D49.81-D49.9

● **C7A.09   Malignant carcinoid tumors of other sites**
    (Ex:) For category C7A.09 CC codes unless otherwise indicated: C16.0-C16.9, C26.0, C26.9, C45.7-C45.9, C46.4, C76.8, C7A.00-C7B.00, C7B.1, C80.0-C80.2, D49.0, D49.81-D49.9

    C7A.090   Malignant carcinoid tumor of the bronchus and lung 🔍
        (Ex:) C34.80-C34.92, C39.9, C45.7-C45.9, C46.50-C46.52, C76.8, C7A.00-C7B.00, C7B.1, C80.0-C80.2, D49.1, D49.81-D49.9

    C7A.091   Malignant carcinoid tumor of the thymus 🔍
        (Ex:) C37, C7A.00-C7A.8

    C7A.092   Malignant carcinoid tumor of the stomach 🔍

    C7A.093   Malignant carcinoid tumor of the kidney 🔍
        (Ex:) C45.7-C45.9, C64.1-C65.9, C68.8-C68.9, C76.8, C7A.00-C7B.00, C7B.1, C80.0-C80.2, D49.5, D49.81-D49.9

    C7A.094   Malignant carcinoid tumor of the foregut NOS 🔍

    C7A.095   Malignant carcinoid tumor of the midgut NOS 🔍

    C7A.096   Malignant carcinoid tumor of the hindgut NOS 🔍

    C7A.098   Malignant carcinoid tumors of other sites 🔍
        (Ex:) C45.7-C45.9, C76.8, C79.89-C79.9, C7A.00-C7B.00, C7B.09-C7B.8, C80.0-C80.2, D49.81-D49.9

C7A.1   Malignant poorly differentiated neuroendocrine tumors 🔍
    Malignant poorly differentiated neuroendocrine tumor NOS
    Malignant poorly differentiated neuroendocrine carcinoma, any site
    High grade neuroendocrine carcinoma, any site
    (Ex:) See C7A.098

C7A.8   Other malignant neuroendocrine tumors 🔍
    Secondary neuroendocrine tumors (C7B)
    (Ex:) See C7A.098

● **C7B   Secondary neuroendocrine tumors**
    Use additional code to identify any functional activity

  ● **C7B.0   Secondary carcinoid tumors**

    C7B.00   Secondary carcinoid tumors, unspecified site

    C7B.01   Secondary carcinoid tumors of distant lymph nodes 🔍
        (Ex:) C45.7-C45.9, C46.3, C76.8-C77.9, C7A.00, C7A.098-C7B.8, C80.0-C80.2, D49.81-D49.9

    C7B.02   Secondary carcinoid tumors of liver 🔍
        (Ex:) C45.7-C45.9, C76.8, C78.7-C78.89, C79.89-C79.9, C7A.00, C7A.098-C7B.8, C80.0-C80.2, D49.81-D49.9

    C7B.03   Secondary carcinoid tumors of bone 🔍
        (Ex:) C45.7-C45.9, C76.8, C79.51-C79.52, C79.89-C79.9, C7A.00, C7A.098-C7B.8, C80.0-C80.2, D49.81-D49.9

    C7B.04   Secondary carcinoid tumors of peritoneum 🔍
      Mesentary metastasis of carcinoid tumor
        (Ex:) C45.7-C45.9, C76.8, C78.6, C78.80-C78.89, C79.89-C79.9, C7A.00, C7A.098-C7B.8, C80.0-C80.2, D49.81-D49.9

    C7B.09   Secondary carcinoid tumors of other sites 🔍
        (Ex:) C45.7-C45.9, C76.8, C79.89-C79.9, C7A.00, C7A.098-C7B.8, C80.0-C80.2, D49.81-D49.9

C7B.1   Secondary Merkel cell carcinoma
    Merkel cell carcinoma nodal presentation
    Merkel cell carcinoma visceral metastatic presentation

C7B.8   Other secondary neuroendocrine tumors 🔍
    (Ex:) See C7B.09

MALIGNANT NEOPLASMS OF ILL-DEFINED, OTHER SECONDARY AND UNSPECIFIED SITES (C76-C80)

● **C76   Malignant neoplasm of other and ill-defined sites**

    Excludes1 malignant neoplasm of female genitourinary tract NOS (C57.9)
        malignant neoplasm of male genitourinary tract NOS (C63.9)
        malignant neoplasm of lymphoid, hematopoietic and related tissue (C81-C96)
        malignant neoplasm of skin (C44.-)
        malignant neoplasm of unspecified site NOS (C80.1)

  C76.0   Malignant neoplasm of head, face and neck
    Malignant neoplasm of cheek NOS
    Malignant neoplasm of nose NOS

  C76.1   Malignant neoplasm of thorax
    Intrathoracic malignant neoplasm NOS
    Malignant neoplasm of axilla NOS
    Thoracic malignant neoplasm NOS

  C76.2   Malignant neoplasm of abdomen

  C76.3   Malignant neoplasm of pelvis
    Malignant neoplasm of groin NOS
    Malignant neoplasm of sites overlapping systems within the pelvis
    Rectovaginal (septum) malignant neoplasm
      Between rectum and vagina
    Rectovesical (septum) malignant neoplasm
      Between rectum and urinary bladder; AKA vesicorectal

● **C76.4   Malignant neoplasm of upper limb**
    C76.40   Malignant neoplasm of unspecified upper limb
    C76.41   Malignant neoplasm of right upper limb
    C76.42   Malignant neoplasm of left upper limb

◄ New   ⬛ Revised   ~~deleted~~ Deleted   Excludes 1   Excludes 2   Includes   Use additional   Code first   Code also   Unspecified

OGCR Official Guidelines   ● Unacceptable Principal Diagnosis   X Assign placeholder X   ● Use Additional Character(s)   ▌ Manifestation Code   **Coding Clinic**

● C76.5   Malignant neoplasm of lower limb
     C76.50   Malignant neoplasm of unspecified lower limb
     C76.51   Malignant neoplasm of right lower limb
     C76.52   Malignant neoplasm of left lower limb
   C76.8   Malignant neoplasm of other specified ill-defined sites
     Malignant neoplasm of overlapping ill-defined sites

● C77   Secondary and unspecified malignant neoplasm of lymph nodes

   Excludes1   malignant neoplasm of lymph nodes, specified as primary (C81-C86, C88, C96.-)
     mesentery metastasis of carcinoid tumor (C7B.04)
     secondary carcinoid tumors of distant lymph nodes (C7B.01)

   Ⓔⓧ **For category C77 CC codes:** C45.7-C45.9, C46.3, C76.8-C77.9, C7A.00, C7A.098-C7B.01, C7B.1, C80.0-C80.2, D49.81-D49.9

   C77.0   Secondary and unspecified malignant neoplasm of lymph nodes of head, face and neck 🔶
     Secondary and unspecified malignant neoplasm of supraclavicular lymph nodes

   C77.1   Secondary and unspecified malignant neoplasm of intrathoracic lymph nodes 🔶

   C77.2   Secondary and unspecified malignant neoplasm of intra-abdominal lymph nodes 🔶

   C77.3   Secondary and unspecified malignant neoplasm of axilla and upper limb lymph nodes 🔶
     Secondary and unspecified malignant neoplasm of pectoral lymph nodes

   C77.4   Secondary and unspecified malignant neoplasm of inguinal and lower limb lymph nodes 🔶

   C77.5   Secondary and unspecified malignant neoplasm of intrapelvic lymph nodes 🔶

   C77.8   Secondary and unspecified malignant neoplasm of lymph nodes of multiple regions 🔶

   C77.9   Secondary and unspecified malignant neoplasm of lymph node, unspecified 🔶

● C78   Secondary malignant neoplasm of respiratory and digestive organs

   Excludes1   lymph node metastases (C77.0)
     secondary carcinoid tumors of liver (C7B.02)
     secondary carcinoid tumors of peritoneum (C7B.04)

● C78.0   Secondary malignant neoplasm of lung
   Ⓔⓧ **For category C78.0 CC Codes:** C45.7-C45.9, C76.8, C78.00-C78.39, C79.89-C79.9, C7A.00, C7A.098-C7B.00, C7B.09-C7B.8, C80.0-C80.2, D49.81-D49.9

     C78.00   Secondary malignant neoplasm of unspecified lung 🔶

     C78.01   Secondary malignant neoplasm of right lung 🔶

     C78.02   Secondary malignant neoplasm of left lung 🔶

   C78.1   Secondary malignant neoplasm of mediastinum 🔶
     Thoracic cavity between pleural cavities
     Ⓔⓧ C45.7-C45.9, C76.8, C78.1, C78.30-C78.39, C79.89-C79.9, C7A.00, C7A.098-C7B.00, C7B.09-C7B.8, C80.0-C80.2, D49.81-D49.9

   C78.2   Secondary malignant neoplasm of pleura 🔶
     Serous membrane covering lungs and lining thoracic cavity
     Ⓔⓧ C45.7-C45.9, C76.8, C78.2-C78.39, C79.89-C79.9, C7A.00, C7A.098-C7B.00, C7B.09-C7B.8, C80.0-C80.2, D49.81-D49.9, J91.0

● C78.3   Secondary malignant neoplasm of other and unspecified respiratory organs
   Ⓔⓧ **For category C78.3 CC Codes:** C45.7-C45.9, C76.8, C78.00-C78.39, C79.89-C79.9, C7A.00, C7A.098-C7B.00, C7B.09-C7B.8, C80.0-C80.2, D49.81-D49.9

     C78.30   Secondary malignant neoplasm of unspecified respiratory organ 🔶

     C78.39   Secondary malignant neoplasm of other respiratory organs 🔶

   C78.4   Secondary malignant neoplasm of small intestine 🔶
     Ⓔⓧ C45.7-C45.9, C76.8, C78.4, C78.80-C78.89, C79.89-C79.9, C7A.00, C7A.098-C7B.00, C7B.09-C7B.8, C80.0-C80.2, D49.81-D49.9

C78.5   Secondary malignant neoplasm of large intestine and rectum 🔶
   Ⓔⓧ C45.7-C45.9, C76.8, C78.5, C78.80-C78.89, C79.89-C79.9, C7A.00, C7A.098-C7B.00, C7B.09-C7B.8, C80.0-C80.2, D49.81-D49.9

C78.6   Secondary malignant neoplasm of retroperitoneum and peritoneum 🔶
   Ⓔⓧ C45.7-C45.9, C76.8, C78.6, C78.80-C78.89, C79.89-C79.9, C7A.00, C7A.098-C7B.00, C7B.04-C7B.8, C80.0-C80.2, D49.81-D49.9

C78.7   Secondary malignant neoplasm of liver and intrahepatic bile duct 🔶
   Ⓔⓧ C45.7-C45.9, C76.8, C78.7-C78.89, C79.89-C79.9, C7A.00, C7A.098-C7A.8, C7B.00, C7B.02, C7B.09-C7B.8, C80.0-C80.2, D49.81-D4.99

● C78.8   Secondary malignant neoplasm of other and unspecified digestive organs
   Ⓔⓧ **For category C78.8 CC Codes:** C45.7-C45.9, C76.8, C78.4-C78.89, C79.89-C79.9, C7A.00, C7A.098-C7B.00, C7B.02, C7B.04-C7B.8, C80.0-C80.2, D49.81-D49.9

     C78.80   Secondary malignant neoplasm of unspecified digestive organ 🔶

     C78.89   Secondary malignant neoplasm of other digestive organs 🔶

● C79   Secondary malignant neoplasm of other and unspecified sites

   Excludes1   lymph node metastases (C77.0)
     secondary carcinoid tumors (C7B.-)
     secondary neuroendocrine tumors (C7B.-)

● C79.0   Secondary malignant neoplasm of kidney and renal pelvis
   Ⓔⓧ **For category C79.0 CC Codes:** C45.7-C45.9, C76.8, C79.00-C79.19, C79.89-C79.9, C7A.00, C7A.098-C7B.00, C7B.09-C7B.8, C80.0-C80.2, D49.81-D49.9

     C79.00   Secondary malignant neoplasm of unspecified kidney and renal pelvis 🔶

     C79.01   Secondary malignant neoplasm of right kidney and renal pelvis 🔶

     C79.02   Secondary malignant neoplasm of left kidney and renal pelvis 🔶

● C79.1   Secondary malignant neoplasm of bladder and other and unspecified urinary organs
   Ⓔⓧ See C79.0

     C79.10   Secondary malignant neoplasm of unspecified urinary organs 🔶

     C79.11   Secondary malignant neoplasm of bladder 🔶

     C79.19   Secondary malignant neoplasm of other urinary organs 🔶

   C79.2   Secondary malignant neoplasm of skin 🔶

     Excludes1   secondary Merkel cell carcinoma (C7B.1)
     Ⓔⓧ C45.7-C45.9, C76.8, C79.2, C79.89-C79.9, C7A.00, C7A.098-C7B.00, C7B.09-C7B.8, C80.0-C80.2, D49.81-D49.9

● C79.3   Secondary malignant neoplasm of brain and cerebral meninges

     C79.31   Secondary malignant neoplasm of brain 🔶
       Ⓔⓧ C45.7-C45.9, C76.8, C79.31, C79.89-C79.9, C7A.00, C7A.098-C7B.00, C7B.09-C7B.8, C80.0-C80.2, D49.81-D49.9

     C79.32   Secondary malignant neoplasm of cerebral meninges 🔶
       Ⓔⓧ C45.7-C45.9, C76.8, C79.32-C79.49, C79.89-C79.9, C7A.00, C7A.098-C7B.00, C7B.09-C7B.8, C80.0-C80.2, D49.81-D49.9

● C79.4   Secondary malignant neoplasm of other and unspecified parts of nervous system
   Ⓔⓧ **For category C79.4 CC codes:** See C79.32

     C79.40   Secondary malignant neoplasm of unspecified part of nervous system 🔶

     C79.49   Secondary malignant neoplasm of other parts of nervous system 🔶

N Newborn Age: 0   **P** Pediatric Age: 0–17   **M** Maternity DX: 12–55   **A** Adult Age: 15–124   ♀ Females Only   ♂ Males Only

🔶 Complication\Comorbidity   🔶 Major C\C   Ⓔⓧ CC/MCC Exclusions   🔶 Present on Admission Requirement   🔶 Hospital-Acquired Condition

793

CHAPTER 2 (C00-D49)

Item 2–6 The adrenal glands are a pair of glands situated on top of or above each kidney ("suprarenal") and chiefly responsible for regulating the stress response through the synthesis of corticosteroids and catecholamines, including cortisol and adrenaline.

● **C79.5 Secondary malignant neoplasm of bone and bone marrow**

> **Excludes1** secondary carcinoid tumors of bone (C7B.03)

> (Ex:) **For category C79.5 CC codes:** C45.7-C45.9, C76.8, C79.51-C79.52, C79.89-C79.9, C7A.00, C7A.098-C7B.00, C7B.03, C7B.09-C7B.8, C80.0-C80.2, D49.81-D49.9

  C79.51 Secondary malignant neoplasm of bone 🗒

  C79.52 Secondary malignant neoplasm of bone marrow 🗒

● **C79.6 Secondary malignant neoplasm of ovary**

> (Ex:) **For category C79.6 CC codes:** C45.7-C45.9, C76.8, C79.60-C79.62, C79.89-C79.9, C7A.00, C7A.098-C7B.00, C7B.09-C7B.8, C80.0-C80.2, D49.81-D49.9

  C79.60 Secondary malignant neoplasm of unspecified ovary ♀ 🗒

  C79.61 Secondary malignant neoplasm of right ovary ♀ 🗒

  C79.62 Secondary malignant neoplasm of left ovary ♀ 🗒

● **C79.7 Secondary malignant neoplasm of adrenal gland**

> (Ex:) **For category C79.7 CC codes:** C45.7-C45.9, C76.8, C79.70-C79.72, C79.89-C79.9, C7A.00, C7A.098-C7B.00, C7B.09-C7B.8, C80.0-C80.2, D49.81-D49.9

  C79.70 Secondary malignant neoplasm of unspecified adrenal gland 🗒

  C79.71 Secondary malignant neoplasm of right adrenal gland 🗒

  C79.72 Secondary malignant neoplasm of left adrenal gland 🗒

● **C79.8 Secondary malignant neoplasm of other specified sites**

  C79.81 Secondary malignant neoplasm of breast 🗒

> (Ex:) C45.7-C45.9, C76.8, C79.81, C79.89-C79.9, C7A.00, C7A.098-C7B.00, C7B.09-C7B.8, C80.0-C80.2, D49.81-D49.9

  C79.82 Secondary malignant neoplasm of genital organs 🗒

> (Ex:) C45.7-C45.9, C76.8, C79.82-C79.9, C7A.00, C7A.098-C7B.00, C7B.09-C7B.8, C80.0-C80.2, D49.81-D49.9

  C79.89 Secondary malignant neoplasm of other specified sites 🗒

> (Ex:) C45.7-C45.9, C76.8, C79.89-C79.9, C7A.00, C7A.098-C7B.00, C7B.09, C7B.1-C7B.8, C80.0-C80.2, D49.81-D49.9

C79.9 Secondary malignant neoplasm of unspecified site 🗒
  Metastatic cancer NOS
  Metastatic disease NOS

> **Excludes1** carcinomatosis NOS (C80.0)
> generalized cancer NOS (C80.0)
> malignant (primary) neoplasm of unspecified site (C80.1)

> (Ex:) See C79.89

OGCR Section I.C.2.j and k

Disseminated malignant neoplasm, unspecified

j. Code C80.0, Disseminated malignant neoplasm, unspecified, is for use only in those cases where the patient has advanced metastatic disease and no known primary or secondary sites are specified. It should not be used in place of assigning codes for the primary site and all known secondary sites.

Malignant neoplasm without specification of site

k. Code C80.1, Malignant (primary) neoplasm, unspecified, equates to Cancer, unspecified. This code should only be used when no determination can be made as to the primary site of a malignancy. This code should rarely be used in the inpatient setting.

● **C80 Malignant neoplasm without specification of site**

> **Excludes1** malignant carcinoid tumor of unspecified site (C7A.00)
> malignant neoplasm of specified multiple sites- code to each site

C80.0 Disseminated malignant neoplasm, unspecified 🗒
  Carcinomatosis NOS
  Generalized cancer, unspecified site (primary) (secondary)
  Generalized malignancy, unspecified site (primary) (secondary)

> (Ex:) C45.7-C45.9, C76.8, C79.89-C79.9, C7A.00, C7A.098-C7B.00, C7B.09, C7B.1-C7B.8, C80.0-C80.2, D49.81-D49.9

C80.1 Malignant (primary) neoplasm, unspecified 🗒
  Cancer NOS
  Cancer unspecified site (primary)
  Carcinoma unspecified site (primary)
  Malignancy unspecified site (primary)

> **Excludes1** secondary malignant neoplasm of unspecified site (C79.9)

● **C80.2 Malignant neoplasm associated with transplanted organ** 🗒

> *Code first complication of transplanted organ (T86.-)*
> Use additional code to identify the specific malignancy

> (Ex:) See C80.0

(See Plate 315 on page 49.)

MALIGNANT NEOPLASMS OF LYMPHOID, HEMATOPOIETIC AND RELATED TISSUE (C81-C96)

> **Excludes2** Kaposi's sarcoma of lymph nodes (C46.3)
> secondary and unspecified neoplasm of lymph nodes (C77.-)
> secondary neoplasm of bone marrow (C79.52)
> secondary neoplasm of spleen (C78.89)

● **C81 Hodgkin lymphoma**

> *Form of malignant lymphoma with four types, nodular sclerosis, mixed cellularity, lymphocyte depleted, and lymphocyte predominant*

> **Excludes1** personal history of Hodgkin lymphoma (Z85.71)

● **C81.0 Nodular lymphocyte predominant Hodgkin lymphoma**
  Least aggressive, least common, typically no symptoms
  Lymphocytic-histiocytic predominance Hodgkin's disease

  C81.00 Nodular lymphocyte predominant Hodgkin lymphoma, unspecified site 🗒

> (Ex:) C81.00-C81.09, C81.40-C81.49, C81.90, C81.98, D49.81-D49.9

  C81.01 Nodular lymphocyte predominant Hodgkin lymphoma, lymph nodes of head, face, and neck 🗒

> (Ex:) C81.00-C81.01, C81.08-C81.09, C81.40-C81.41, C81.48-C81.49, C81.90-C81.91, C81.98, D49.81-D49.9

  C81.02 Nodular lymphocyte predominant Hodgkin lymphoma, intrathoracic lymph nodes 🗒

> (Ex:) C81.00-C81.02, C81.08-C81.09, C81.40-C81.42, C81.48-C81.49, C81.90-C81.92, C81.98, D49.81-D49.9

  C81.03 Nodular lymphocyte predominant Hodgkin lymphoma, intra-abdominal lymph nodes 🗒

> (Ex:) C81.00, C81.03, C81.08-C81.09, C81.40, C81.43, C81.48-C81.49, C81.90, C81.93, C81.98, D49.81-D49.9

  C81.04 Nodular lymphocyte predominant Hodgkin lymphoma, lymph nodes of axilla and upper limb 🗒

> (Ex:) C81.00, C81.04, C81.08-C81.09, C81.40, C81.44, C81.48-C81.49, C81.90, C81.94, C81.98, D49.81-D49.9

  C81.05 Nodular lymphocyte predominant Hodgkin lymphoma, lymph nodes of inguinal region and lower limb 🗒

> (Ex:) C81.00, C81.05, C81.08-C81.09, C81.40, C81.45, C81.48-C81.49, C81.90, C81.95, C81.98, D49.81-D49.9

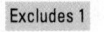

◄ New   ◄||||| Revised   d̶e̶l̶e̶t̶e̶d̶ Deleted   Excludes 1   Excludes 2   Includes   Use additional   Code first   Code also   Unspecified
OGCR Official Guidelines   ● Unacceptable Principal Diagnosis   X Assign placeholder X   ● Use Additional Character(s)   ⟩ Manifestation Code   **Coding Clinic**

C81.06   Nodular lymphocyte predominant Hodgkin lymphoma, intrapelvic lymph nodes 🦠
    (Ex) C81.00, C81.06, C81.08-C81.09, C81.40, C81.46, C81.48-C81.49, C81.90, C81.96, C81.98, D49.81-D49.9

C81.07   Nodular lymphocyte predominant Hodgkin lymphoma, spleen 🦠
    (Ex) C81.00, C81.07-C81.09, C81.40, C81.47-C81.49, C81.90, C81.97-C81.98, D49.81-D49.9

C81.08   Nodular lymphocyte predominant Hodgkin lymphoma, lymph nodes of multiple sites 🦠
    (Ex) See C81.00

C81.09   Nodular lymphocyte predominant Hodgkin lymphoma, extranodal and solid organ sites 🦠
    (Ex) See C81.00

● **C81.1**   **Nodular sclerosis classical Hodgkin lymphoma**
    Moderately aggressive; most common in young adults

C81.10   Nodular sclerosis classical Hodgkin lymphoma, unspecified site 🦠
    (Ex) C81.10-C81.19, C81.90, C81.98, D49.81-D49.9

C81.11   Nodular sclerosis classical Hodgkin lymphoma, lymph nodes of head, face, and neck 🦠
    (Ex) C81.10-C81.11, C81.18-C81.19, C81.90-C81.91, C81.98, D49.81-D49.9

C81.12   Nodular sclerosis classical Hodgkin lymphoma, intrathoracic lymph nodes 🦠
    (Ex) C81.10, C81.12, C81.18-C81.19, C81.90, C81.92, C81.98, D49.81-D49.9

C81.13   Nodular sclerosis classical Hodgkin lymphoma, intra-abdominal lymph nodes 🦠
    (Ex) C81.10, C81.13, C81.18-C81.19, C81.90, C81.93, C81.98, D49.81-D49.9

C81.14   Nodular sclerosis classical Hodgkin lymphoma, lymph nodes of axilla and upper limb 🦠
    (Ex) C81.10, C81.14, C81.18-C81.19, C81.90, C81.94, C81.98, D49.81-D49.9

C81.15   Nodular sclerosis classical Hodgkin lymphoma, lymph nodes of inguinal region and lower limb 🦠
    (Ex) C81.10, C81.15, C81.18-C81.19, C81.90, C81.95, C81.98, D49.81-D49.9

C81.16   Nodular sclerosis classical Hodgkin lymphoma, intrapelvic lymph nodes 🦠
    (Ex) C81.10, C81.16, C81.18-C81.19, C81.90, C81.96, C81.98, D49.81-D49.9

C81.17   Nodular sclerosis classical Hodgkin lymphoma, spleen 🦠
    (Ex) C81.10, C81.17-C81.19, C81.90, C81.97-C81.98, D49.81-D49.9

C81.18   Nodular sclerosis classical Hodgkin lymphoma, lymph nodes of multiple sites 🦠
    (Ex) See C81.10

C81.19   Nodular sclerosis classical Hodgkin lymphoma, extranodal and solid organ sites 🦠
    (Ex) See C81.10

● **C81.2**   **Mixed cellularity classical Hodgkin lymphoma**
    A type of Hodgkin's that is moderately aggressive with mixed cell types

C81.20   Mixed cellularity classical Hodgkin lymphoma, unspecified site 🦠
    (Ex) C81.20-C81.29, C81.90, C81.98, D49.81-D49.9

C81.21   Mixed cellularity classical Hodgkin lymphoma, lymph nodes of head, face, and neck 🦠
    (Ex) C81.20-C81.21, C81.28-C81.29, C81.90-C81.91, C81.98, D49.81-D49.9

C81.22   Mixed cellularity classical Hodgkin lymphoma, intrathoracic lymph nodes 🦠
    (Ex) C81.20, C81.22, C81.28-C81.29, C81.90, C81.92, C81.98, D49.81-D49.9

C81.23   Mixed cellularity classical Hodgkin lymphoma, intra-abdominal lymph nodes 🦠
    (Ex) C81.20, C81.23, C81.28-C81.29, C81.90, C81.93, C81.98, D49.81-D49.9

C81.24   Mixed cellularity classical Hodgkin lymphoma, lymph nodes of axilla and upper limb 🦠
    (Ex) C81.20, C81.24, C81.28-C81.29, C81.90, C81.94, C81.98, D49.81-D49.9

C81.25   Mixed cellularity classical Hodgkin lymphoma, lymph nodes of inguinal region and lower limb 🦠
    (Ex) C81.20, C81.25, C81.28-C81.29, C81.90, C81.95, C81.98, D49.81-D49.9

C81.26   Mixed cellularity classical Hodgkin lymphoma, intrapelvic lymph nodes 🦠
    (Ex) C81.20, C81.26, C81.28-C81.29, C81.90, C81.96, C81.98, D49.81-D49.9

C81.27   Mixed cellularity classical Hodgkin lymphoma, spleen 🦠
    (Ex) C81.20, C81.27, C81.28-C81.29, C81.90, C81.97, C81.98, D49.81-D49.9

C81.28   Mixed cellularity classical Hodgkin lymphoma, lymph nodes of multiple sites 🦠
    (Ex) See C81.20

C81.29   Mixed cellularity classical Hodgkin lymphoma, extranodal and solid organ sites 🦠
    (Ex) See C81.20

● **C81.3**   **Lymphocyte depleted classical Hodgkin lymphoma**
    Most aggressive type with poor prognosis

C81.30   Lymphocyte depleted classical Hodgkin lymphoma, unspecified site 🦠
    (Ex) C81.30-C81.39, C81.90, C81.98, D49.81-D49.9

C81.31   Lymphocyte depleted classical Hodgkin lymphoma, lymph nodes of head, face, and neck 🦠
    (Ex) C81.30-C81.31, C81.38-C81.39, C81.90-C81.91, C81.98, D49.81-D49.9

C81.32   Lymphocyte depleted classical Hodgkin lymphoma, intrathoracic lymph nodes 🦠
    (Ex) C81.30, C81.32, C81.38-C81.39, C81.90, C81.92, C81.98, D49.81-D49.9

C81.33   Lymphocyte depleted classical Hodgkin lymphoma, intra-abdominal lymph nodes 🦠
    (Ex) C81.30, C81.33, C81.38-C81.39, C81.90, C81.93, C81.98, D49.81-D49.9

C81.34   Lymphocyte depleted classical Hodgkin lymphoma, lymph nodes of axilla and upper limb 🦠
    (Ex) C81.30, C81.34, C81.38-C81.39, C81.90, C81.94, C81.98, D49.81-D49.9

C81.35   Lymphocyte depleted classical Hodgkin lymphoma, lymph nodes of inguinal region and lower limb 🦠
    (Ex) C81.30, C81.35, C81.38-C81.39, C81.90, C81.95, C81.98, D49.81-D49.9

C81.36   Lymphocyte depleted classical Hodgkin lymphoma, intrapelvic lymph nodes 🦠
    (Ex) C81.30, C81.36, C81.38-C81.39, C81.90, C81.96, C81.98, D49.81-D49.9

C81.37   Lymphocyte depleted classical Hodgkin lymphoma, spleen 🦠
    (Ex) C81.30, C81.37, C81.38-C81.39, C81.90, C81.97, C81.98, D49.81-D49.9

C81.38   Lymphocyte depleted classical Hodgkin lymphoma, lymph nodes of multiple sites 🦠
    (Ex) C81.30-C81.39, C81.98, D49.81-D49.9

C81.39   Lymphocyte depleted classical Hodgkin lymphoma, extranodal and solid organ sites 🦠
    (Ex) See C81.30

CHAPTER 2 (C00-D49)

N Newborn Age: 0   **P** Pediatric Age: 0–17   **M** Maternity DX: 12–55   **A** Adult Age: 15–124   ♀ Females Only   ♂ Males Only

🦠 Complication\Comorbidity   🦠 Major C\C   (Ex) CC/MCC Exclusions   🦠 Present on Admission Requirement   🦠 Hospital-Acquired Condition

795

● **C81.4**   **Lymphocyte-rich classical Hodgkin lymphoma**

     Excludes1   nodular lymphocyte predominant Hodgkin lymphoma (C81.0-)

     C81.40   **Lymphocyte-rich classical Hodgkin lymphoma, unspecified site** 🅒
         Ex: C81.00-C81.09, C81.40-C81.49, C81.90, C81.98, D49.81-D49.9

     C81.41   **Lymphocyte-rich classical Hodgkin lymphoma, lymph nodes of head, face, and neck** 🅒
         Ex: C81.00-C81.01, C81.08-C81.09, C81.40-C81.41, C81.48-C81.49, C81.90-C81.91, C81.98, D49.81-D49.9

     C81.42   **Lymphocyte-rich classical Hodgkin lymphoma, intrathoracic lymph nodes** 🅒
         Ex: C81.00-C81.02, C81.08-C81.09, C81.40-C81.42, C81.48-C81.49, C81.90-C81.92, C81.98, D49.81-D49.9

     C81.43   **Lymphocyte-rich classical Hodgkin lymphoma, intra-abdominal lymph nodes** 🅒
         Ex: C81.00, C81.03, C81.08-C81.09, C81.40, C81.43, C81.48-C81.49, C81.90, C81.93, C81.98, D49.81-D49.9

     C81.44   **Lymphocyte-rich classical Hodgkin lymphoma, lymph nodes of axilla and upper limb** 🅒
         Ex: C81.00, C81.04, C81.08-C81.09, C81.40, C81.44, C81.48-C81.49, C81.90, C81.94, C81.98, D49.81-D49.9

     C81.45   **Lymphocyte-rich classical Hodgkin lymphoma, lymph nodes of inguinal region and lower limb** 🅒
         Ex: C81.00, C81.05, C81.08-C81.09, C81.40, C81.45, C81.48-C81.49, C81.90, C81.95, C81.98, D49.81-D49.9

     C81.46   **Lymphocyte-rich classical Hodgkin lymphoma, intrapelvic lymph nodes** 🅒
         Ex: C81.00, C81.06, C81.08-C81.09, C81.40, C81.46, C81.48-C81.49, C81.90, C81.96, C81.98, D49.81-D49.9

     C81.47   **Lymphocyte-rich classical Hodgkin lymphoma, spleen** 🅒
         Ex: C81.00, C81.07-C81.09, C81.40, C81.47-C81.49, C81.90, C81.97-C81.98, D49.81-D49.9

     C81.48   **Lymphocyte-rich classical Hodgkin lymphoma, lymph nodes of multiple sites** 🅒
         Ex: See C81.40

     C81.49   **Lymphocyte-rich classical Hodgkin lymphoma, extranodal and solid organ sites** 🅒
         Ex: See C81.40

● **C81.7**   **Other classical Hodgkin lymphoma**
     Classical Hodgkin lymphoma NOS

     C81.70   **Other classical Hodgkin lymphoma, unspecified site** 🅒
         Ex: C81.70-C81.79, C81.90, C81.98, D49.81-D49.9

     C81.71   **Other classical Hodgkin lymphoma, lymph nodes of head, face, and neck** 🅒
         Ex: C81.70-C81.71, C81.78-C81.79, C81.90-C81.91, C81.98, D49.81-D49.9

     C81.72   **Other classical Hodgkin lymphoma, intrathoracic lymph nodes** 🅒
         Ex: C81.70, C81.72, C81.78-C81.79, C81.90, C81.92, C81.98, D49.81-D49.9

     C81.73   **Other classical Hodgkin lymphoma, intra-abdominal lymph nodes** 🅒
         Ex: C81.70, C81.73, C81.78-C81.79, C81.90, C81.93, C81.98, D49.81-D49.9

     C81.74   **Other classical Hodgkin lymphoma, lymph nodes of axilla and upper limb** 🅒
         Ex: C81.70, C81.74, C81.78-C81.79, C81.90, C81.94, C81.98, D49.81-D49.9

     C81.75   **Other classical Hodgkin lymphoma, lymph nodes of inguinal region and lower limb** 🅒
         Ex: C81.70, C81.75, C81.78-C81.79, C81.90, C81.95, C81.98, D49.81-D49.9

     C81.76   **Other classical Hodgkin lymphoma, intrapelvic lymph nodes** 🅒
         Ex: C81.70, C81.76, C81.78-C81.79, C81.90, C81.96, C81.98, D49.81-D49.9

     C81.77   **Other classical Hodgkin lymphoma, spleen** 🅒
         Ex: C81.70, C81.77, C81.78-C81.79, C81.90, C81.97, C81.98, D49.81-D49.9

     C81.78   **Other classical Hodgkin lymphoma, lymph nodes of multiple sites** 🅒
         Ex: See C81.70

     C81.79   **Other classical Hodgkin lymphoma, extranodal and solid organ sites** 🅒
         Ex: See C81.70

● **C81.9**   **Hodgkin lymphoma, unspecified**

     C81.90   **Hodgkin lymphoma, unspecified, unspecified site** 🅒
         Ex: C81.90-C81.98, D49.81-D49.9

     C81.91   **Hodgkin lymphoma, unspecified, lymph nodes of head, face, and neck** 🅒
         Ex: C81.90-C81.91, C81.98, D49.81-D49.9

     C81.92   **Hodgkin lymphoma, unspecified, intrathoracic lymph nodes** 🅒
         Ex: C81.90, C81.92, C81.98, D49.81-D49.9

     C81.93   **Hodgkin lymphoma, unspecified, intra-abdominal lymph nodes** 🅒
         Ex: C81.90, C81.93, C81.98, D49.81-D49.9

     C81.94   **Hodgkin lymphoma, unspecified, lymph nodes of axilla and upper limb** 🅒
         Ex: C81.90, C81.94, C81.98, D49.81-D49.9

     C81.95   **Hodgkin lymphoma, unspecified, lymph nodes of inguinal region and lower limb** 🅒
         Ex: C81.90, C81.95, C81.98, D49.81-D49.9

     C81.96   **Hodgkin lymphoma, unspecified, intrapelvic lymph nodes** 🅒
         Ex: C81.90, C81.96, C81.98, D49.81-D49.9

     C81.97   **Hodgkin lymphoma, unspecified, spleen** 🅒
         Ex: C81.90, C81.97-C81.98, D49.81-D49.9

     C81.98   **Hodgkin lymphoma, unspecified, lymph nodes of multiple sites** 🅒
         Ex: See C81.90

     C81.99   **Hodgkin lymphoma, unspecified, extranodal and solid organ sites** 🅒
         Ex: No exclusions

● **C82**   **Follicular lymphoma**
     Group of malignant lymphomas

     Includes   follicular lymphoma with or without diffuse areas

     Excludes1   mature T/NK-cell lymphomas (C84.-)
                   personal history of non-Hodgkin lymphoma (Z85.72)

● **C82.0**   **Follicular lymphoma grade I**

     C82.00   **Follicular lymphoma grade I, unspecified site** 🅒
         Ex: C82.00-C82.50, C82.59-C82.99, C83.10, C83.19, C84.40, C84.49, C84.60, C84.69-C84.70, C84.79, C84.A0, C84.A9, C84.Z0, C84.Z9, C84.90, C84.99-C85.10, C85.19-C85.20, C85.29-C85.80, C85.89-C85.90, C85.99, C86.4, C88.4, C96.4, C96.9, C96.Z,

     C82.01   **Follicular lymphoma grade I, lymph nodes of head, face, and neck** 🅒
         Ex: C82.00-C82.01, C82.08-C82.11, C82.18-C82.21, C82.28-C82.31, C82.38-C82.41, C82.48-C82.49, C82.51, C82.60-C82.61, C82.68-C82.81, C82.88-C82.91, C82.98-C82.99, C83.11, C84.41, C84.61, C84.71, C84.A1, C84.Z1, C84.91, C85.11, C85.21, C85.81, C85.91, C86.0, D49.81-D49.9

     C82.02   **Follicular lymphoma grade I, intrathoracic lymph nodes** 🅒
         Ex: C82.00, C82.02, C82.08-C82.10, C82.12, C82.18-C82.20, C82.22, C82.28-C82.30, C82.32, C82.38-C82.40, C82.42, C82.48-C82.49, C82.52, C82.60, C82.62, C82.68-C82.80, C82.82, C82.88-C82.90, C82.92, C82.98-C82.99, C83.12, C84.42, C84.62, C84.72, C84.92, C84.A2, C84.Z2, C85.12, C85.22, C85.82, C85.92, D49.81-D49.9

     C82.03   **Follicular lymphoma grade I, intra-abdominal lymph nodes** 🅒
         Ex: C82.00, C82.03, C82.08-C82.10, C82.13, C82.18-C82.20, C12.23, C82.28-C82.30, C82.33, C82.38-C82.40, C82.43, C82.48-C82.49, C82.53, C82.60, C82.63, C82.68-C82.80, C82.83, C82.88-C82.90, C82.93, C82.98-C82.99, C83.13, C84.43, C84.63, C84.73, C84.93, C84.A3, C84.Z3, C85.13, C85.23, C85.83, C85.93, C86.2, C86.3, D49.81-D49.9

◀ New   ◀ Revised   ~~deleted~~ Deleted   Excludes 1   Excludes 2   Includes   Use additional   Code first   Code also   Unspecified

OGCR Official Guidelines   ● Unacceptable Principal Diagnosis   X Assign placeholder X   ● Use Additional Character(s)   ▶ Manifestation Code   **Coding Clinic**

C82.04   Follicular lymphoma grade I, lymph nodes of axilla and upper limb 🦠
     (Ex:) C82.00, C82.04, C82.08-C82.10, C82.14, C82.18-C82.20, C82.24, C82.28-C82.30, C82.34, C82.38-C82.40, C82.44, C82.48-C82.49, C82.54, C82.60, C82.64, C82.68-C82.80, C82.84, C82.88-C82.90, C82.94, C82.98-C82.99, C83.14, C84.44, C84.64, C84.74, C84.94, C84.A4, C84.Z4, C85.14, C85.24, C85.84, C85.94, D49.81-D49.9

C82.05   Follicular lymphoma grade I, lymph nodes of inguinal region and lower limb 🦠
     (Ex:) C82.00, C82.05, C82.08-C82.10, C82.15, C82.18-C82.20, C82.25, C82.28-C82.30, C82.35, C82.38-C82.40, C82.45, C82.48-C82.49, C82.55, C82.60, C82.65, C82.68-C82.80, C82.85, C82.88-C82.90, C82.95, C82.98-C82.99, C83.15, C84.45, C84.65, C84.75, C84.95, C84.A5, C84.Z5, C85.15, C85.25, C85.85, C85.95, D49.81-D49.9

C82.06   Follicular lymphoma grade I, intrapelvic lymph nodes 🦠
     (Ex:) C82.00, C82.06, C82.08-C82.10, C82.16, C82.18-C82.20, C82.26, C82.28-C82.30, C82.36, C82.38-C82.40, C82.46, C82.48-C82.49, C82.56, C82.60, C82.66, C82.68-C82.80, C82.86, C82.88-C82.90, C82.96, C82.98-C82.99, C83.16, C84.46, C84.66, C84.76, C84.96, C84.A6, C84.Z6, C85.16, C85.26, C85.86, C85.96, D49.81-D49.9

C82.07   Follicular lymphoma grade I, spleen 🦠
     (Ex:) C82.00, C82.07, C82.08-C82.10, C82.17-C82.20, C82.27-C82.30, C82.37-C82.40, C82.47-C82.49, C82.57, C82.60, C82.67-C82.80, C82.87-C82.90, C82.97-C82.99, C83.17, C84.47, C84.67, C84.77, C84.97, C84.A7, C84.Z7, C85.17, C85.27, C85.87, C85.97, C86.1, D49.81-D49.9

C82.08   Follicular lymphoma grade I, lymph nodes of multiple sites 🦠
     (Ex:) C82.00-C82.49, C82.58, C82.60-C82.99, C83.18, C84.48, C84.68, C84.78, C84.98, C84.A8, C84.Z8, C85.18, C85.28, C85.88, C85.98, D49.81-D49.9

C82.09   Follicular lymphoma grade I, extranodal and solid organ sites 🦠
     (Ex:) See C82.00

● **C82.1**   Follicular lymphoma grade II

C82.10   Follicular lymphoma grade II, unspecified site 🦠
     (Ex:) See C82.00

C82.11   Follicular lymphoma grade II, lymph nodes of head, face, and neck 🦠
     (Ex:) See C82.01

C82.12   Follicular lymphoma grade II, intrathoracic lymph nodes 🦠
     (Ex:) See C82.02

C82.13   Follicular lymphoma grade II, intra-abdominal lymph nodes 🦠
     (Ex:) See C82.03

C82.14   Follicular lymphoma grade II, lymph nodes of axilla and upper limb 🦠
     (Ex:) See C82.04

C82.15   Follicular lymphoma grade II, lymph nodes of inguinal region and lower limb 🦠
     (Ex:) See C82.05

C82.16   Follicular lymphoma grade II, intrapelvic lymph nodes 🦠
     (Ex:) See C82.06

C82.17   Follicular lymphoma grade II, spleen 🦠
     (Ex:) See C82.07

C82.18   Follicular lymphoma grade II, lymph nodes of multiple sites 🦠
     (Ex:) See C82.08

C82.19   Follicular lymphoma grade II, extranodal and solid organ sites 🦠
     (Ex:) See C82.00

● **C82.2**   Follicular lymphoma grade III, unspecified

C82.20   Follicular lymphoma grade III, unspecified, unspecified site 🦠
     (Ex:) See C82.00

C82.21   Follicular lymphoma grade III, unspecified, lymph nodes of head, face, and neck 🦠
     (Ex:) See C82.01

C82.22   Follicular lymphoma grade III, unspecified, intrathoracic lymph nodes 🦠
     (Ex:) See C82.02

C82.23   Follicular lymphoma grade III, unspecified, intra-abdominal lymph nodes 🦠
     (Ex:) See C82.03

C82.24   Follicular lymphoma grade III, unspecified, lymph nodes of axilla and upper limb 🦠
     (Ex:) See C82.04

C82.25   Follicular lymphoma grade III, unspecified, lymph nodes of inguinal region and lower limb 🦠
     (Ex:) See C82.05

C82.26   Follicular lymphoma grade III, unspecified, intrapelvic lymph nodes 🦠
     (Ex:) See C82.06

C82.27   Follicular lymphoma grade III, unspecified, spleen 🦠
     (Ex:) See C82.07

C82.28   Follicular lymphoma grade III, unspecified, lymph nodes of multiple sites 🦠
     (Ex:) See C82.08

C82.29   Follicular lymphoma grade III, unspecified, extranodal and solid organ sites 🦠
     (Ex:) See C82.00

● **C82.3**   Follicular lymphoma grade IIIa

C82.30   Follicular lymphoma grade IIIa, unspecified site 🦠
     (Ex:) See C82.00

C82.31   Follicular lymphoma grade IIIa, lymph nodes of head, face, and neck 🦠
     (Ex:) See C82.01

C82.32   Follicular lymphoma grade IIIa, intrathoracic lymph nodes 🦠
     (Ex:) See C82.02

C82.33   Follicular lymphoma grade IIIa, intra-abdominal lymph nodes 🦠
     (Ex:) See C82.03

C82.34   Follicular lymphoma grade IIIa, lymph nodes of axilla and upper limb 🦠
     (Ex:) See C82.04

C82.35   Follicular lymphoma grade IIIa, lymph nodes of inguinal region and lower limb 🦠
     (Ex:) See C82.05

C82.36   Follicular lymphoma grade IIIa, intrapelvic lymph nodes 🦠
     (Ex:) See C82.06

C82.37   Follicular lymphoma grade IIIa, spleen 🦠
     (Ex:) See C82.07

C82.38   Follicular lymphoma grade IIIa, lymph nodes of multiple sites 🦠
     (Ex:) See C82.08

C82.39   Follicular lymphoma grade IIIa, extranodal and solid organ sites 🦠
     (Ex:) See C82.00

● **C82.4**   Follicular lymphoma grade IIIb

C82.40   Follicular lymphoma grade IIIb, unspecified site 🦠
     (Ex:) See C82.00

C82.41   Follicular lymphoma grade IIIb, lymph nodes of head, face, and neck 🦠
     (Ex:) See C82.01

C82.42   Follicular lymphoma grade IIIb, intrathoracic lymph nodes 🦠
     (Ex:) See C82.02

CHAPTER 2 (C00-D49)

N   Newborn Age: 0   **P**   Pediatric Age: 0–17   **M**   Maternity DX: 12–55   **A**   Adult Age: 15–124   ♀   Females Only   ♂   Males Only

🦠 Complication\Comorbidity   🦠 Major C\C   (Ex:) CC/MCC Exclusions   🦠 Present on Admission Requirement   🦠 Hospital-Acquired Condition   **797**

C82.43   Follicular lymphoma grade IIIb, intra-abdominal lymph nodes 🖉
Ex: See C82.03

C82.44   Follicular lymphoma grade IIIb, lymph nodes of axilla and upper limb 🖉
Ex: See C82.04

C82.45   Follicular lymphoma grade IIIb, lymph nodes of inguinal region and lower limb 🖉
Ex: See C82.05

C82.46   Follicular lymphoma grade IIIb, intrapelvic lymph nodes 🖉
Ex: See C82.06

C82.47   Follicular lymphoma grade IIIb, spleen 🖉
Ex: See C82.07

C82.48   Follicular lymphoma grade IIIb, lymph nodes of multiple sites 🖉
Ex: See C82.08

C82.49   Follicular lymphoma grade IIIb, extranodal and solid organ sites 🖉
Ex: See C82.00

● **C82.5**   Diffuse follicle center lymphoma

C82.50   Diffuse follicle center lymphoma, unspecified site 🖉
Ex: C82.50-C82.59, C83.10-C83.19, C84.40-C84.49, C84.60-C84.79, C84.90-C84.99, C84.A0-C84.Z9, C85.10-C86.4, C88.4, C96.4, C96.9, C96.Z, D49.81-D49.9

C82.51   Diffuse follicle center lymphoma, lymph nodes of head, face, and neck 🖉
Ex: C82.50-C82.51, C82.58-C82.59, C83.10-C83.11, C83.18-C83.19, C84.40-C84.41, C84.48-C84.61, C84.68-C84.71, C84.78-C84.79, C84.90-C84.91, C84.98-C84.99, C84.A0-C84.A1, C84.A9, C84.Z0-C84.Z1, C84.Z8-C84.Z9, C85.10-C85.11, C85.18-C85.21, C85.28-C85.81, C85.88-C85.91, C85.98-C85.99, C86.0, C86.4, C88.4, D49.81-D49.9

C82.52   Diffuse follicle center lymphoma, intrathoracic lymph nodes 🖉
Ex: C82.50, C82.52, C82.58-C82.59, C83.10, C83.12, C83.18-C83.19, C84.40, C84.42, C84.48-C84.60, C84.62, C84.68-C84.70, C84.72, C84.78-C84.79, C84.90, C84.92, C84.98-C84.99, C84.A0, C84.A2, C84.A8-C84.A9, C84.Z0, C84.Z2, C84.Z8-C84.Z9, C85.10, C85.12, C85.18-C85.20, C85.22, C85.28-C85.80, C85.82, C85.88-C85.90, C85.92, C85.98-C85.99, C86.4, C88.4, D49.81-D49.9

C82.53   Diffuse follicle center lymphoma, intra-abdominal lymph nodes 🖉
Ex: C82.50, C82.53, C82.58-C82.59, C83.10, C83.13, C83.18-C83.19, C84.40, C84.43, C84.48-C84.60, C84.63, C84.68-C84.70, C84.73, C84.78-C84.79, C84.90, C84.93, C84.98-C84.99, C84.A0, C84.A3, C84.A8-C84.A9, C84.Z0, C84.Z3, C84.Z8-C84.Z9, C85.10, C85.13, C85.18-C85.20, C85.22, C85.28-C85.80, C85.83, C85.88-C85.90, C85.93, C85.98-C85.99, C86.2-C86.4, C88.4, D49.81-D49.9

C82.54   Diffuse follicle center lymphoma, lymph nodes of axilla and upper limb 🖉
Ex: C82.50, C82.54, C82.58-C82.59, C83.10, C83.14, C83.18-C83.19, C84.40, C84.44, C84.48-C84.60, C84.64, C84.68-C84.70, C84.74, C84.78-C84.79, C84.90, C84.94, C84.98-C84.99, C84.A0, C84.A4, C84.A8-C84.A9, C84.Z0, C84.Z4, C84.Z8-C84.Z9, C85.10, C85.14, C85.18-C85.20, C85.24, C85.28-C85.80, C85.84, C85.88-C85.90, C85.94, C85.98-C85.99, C86.4, C88.4, D49.81-D49.9

C82.55   Diffuse follicle center lymphoma, lymph nodes of inguinal region and lower limb 🖉
Ex: C82.50, C82.55, C82.58-C82.59, C83.10, C83.15, C83.18-C83.19, C84.40, C84.45, C84.48-C84.60, C84.65, C84.68-C84.70, C84.75, C84.78-C84.79, C84.90, C84.95, C84.98-C84.99, C84.A0, C84.A5, C84.A8-C84.A9, C84.Z0, C84.Z5, C84.Z8-C84.Z9, C85.10, C85.15, C85.18-C85.20, C85.25, C85.28-C85.80, C85.85, C85.88-C85.90, C85.95, C85.98-C85.99, C86.4, C88.4, D49.81-D49.9

C82.56   Diffuse follicle center lymphoma, intrapelvic lymph nodes 🖉
Ex: C82.50, C82.56, C82.58-C82.59, C83.10, C83.16, C83.18-C83.19, C84.40, C84.46, C84.48-C84.60, C84.66, C84.68-C84.70, C84.76, C84.78-C84.79, C84.90, C84.96, C84.98-C84.99, C84.A0, C84.A6, C84.A8-C84.A9, C84.Z0, C84.Z6, C84.Z8-C84.Z9, C85.10, C85.16, C85.18-C85.20, C85.26, C85.28-C85.80, C85.86, C85.88-C85.90, C85.96, C85.98-C85.99, C86.4, C88.4, D49.81-D49.9

C82.57   Diffuse follicle center lymphoma, spleen 🖉
Ex: C82.50, C82.57, C82.58-C82.59, C83.10, C83.17, C83.18-C83.19, C84.40, C84.47-C84.49, C84.60, C84.67, C84.68-C84.69, C84.70, C84.77, C84.78-C84.79, C84.90, C84.97-C84.99, C84.A0, C84.A7-C84.A9, C84.Z0, C84.Z7, C84.Z8-C84.Z9, C85.10, C85.17-C85.20, C85.27-C85.29, C85.80, C85.87-C85.90, C85.97-C85.99, C86.1, C86.4, C88.4, D49.81-D49.9

C82.58   Diffuse follicle center lymphoma, lymph nodes of multiple sites 🖉
Ex: C82.50-C82.59, C83.10-C83.19, C84.40-C84.49, C84.60-C84.79, C84.90-C84.99, C84.A0-C84.Z9, C85.10-C86.4, C88.4, D49.81-D49.9

C82.59   Diffuse follicle center lymphoma, extranodal and solid organ sites 🖉
Ex: See C82.50

● **C82.6**   Cutaneous follicle center lymphoma

C82.60   Cutaneous follicle center lymphoma, unspecified site 🖉
Ex: See C82.00

C82.61   Cutaneous follicle center lymphoma, lymph nodes of head, face, and neck 🖉
Ex: See C82.01

C82.62   Cutaneous follicle center lymphoma, intrathoracic lymph nodes 🖉
Ex: See C82.02

C82.63   Cutaneous follicle center lymphoma, intra-abdominal lymph nodes 🖉
Ex: See C82.03

C82.64   Cutaneous follicle center lymphoma, lymph nodes of axilla and upper limb 🖉
Ex: See C82.04

C82.65   Cutaneous follicle center lymphoma, lymph nodes of inguinal region and lower limb 🖉
Ex: See C82.05

C82.66   Cutaneous follicle center lymphoma, intrapelvic lymph nodes 🖉
Ex: See C82.06

C82.67   Cutaneous follicle center lymphoma, spleen 🖉
Ex: See C82.07

C82.68   Cutaneous follicle center lymphoma, lymph nodes of multiple sites 🖉
Ex: See C82.08

C82.69   Cutaneous follicle center lymphoma, extranodal and solid organ sites 🖉
Ex: See C82.00

● **C82.8**   Other types of follicular lymphoma

C82.80   Other types of follicular lymphoma, unspecified site 🖉
Ex: See C82.00

C82.81   Other types of follicular lymphoma, lymph nodes of head, face, and neck 🖉
Ex: See C82.01

C82.82   Other types of follicular lymphoma, intrathoracic lymph nodes 🖉
Ex: See C82.02

C82.83   Other types of follicular lymphoma, intra-abdominal lymph nodes 🖉
Ex: See C82.03

C82.84   Other types of follicular lymphoma, lymph nodes of axilla and upper limb 🖉
Ex: See C82.04

◄ New   ◄▦ Revised   ~~deleted~~ Deleted   Excludes 1   Excludes 2   Includes   Use additional   Code first   Code also   Unspecified

798   OGCR Official Guidelines   ● Unacceptable Principal Diagnosis   X Assign placeholder X   ● Use Additional Character(s)   ▌ Manifestation Code   **Coding Clinic**

C82.85   Other types of follicular lymphoma, lymph nodes of inguinal region and lower limb 🔧
Ⓔ See C82.05

C82.86   Other types of follicular lymphoma, intrapelvic lymph nodes 🔧
Ⓔ See C82.06

C82.87   Other types of follicular lymphoma, spleen 🔧
Ⓔ See C82.07

C82.88   Other types of follicular lymphoma, lymph nodes of multiple sites 🔧
Ⓔ See C82.08

C82.89   Other types of follicular lymphoma, extranodal and solid organ sites 🔧
Ⓔ See C82.00

● C82.9   Follicular lymphoma, unspecified

C82.90   Follicular lymphoma, unspecified, unspecified site 🔧
Ⓔ See C82.00

C82.91   Follicular lymphoma, unspecified, lymph nodes of head, face, and neck 🔧
Ⓔ See C82.01

C82.92   Follicular lymphoma, unspecified, intrathoracic lymph nodes 🔧
Ⓔ See C82.02

C82.93   Follicular lymphoma, unspecified, intra-abdominal lymph nodes 🔧
Ⓔ See C82.03

C82.94   Follicular lymphoma, unspecified, lymph nodes of axilla and upper limb 🔧
Ⓔ See C82.04

C82.95   Follicular lymphoma, unspecified, lymph nodes of inguinal region and lower limb 🔧
Ⓔ See C82.05

C82.96   Follicular lymphoma, unspecified, intrapelvic lymph nodes 🔧
Ⓔ See C82.06

C82.97   Follicular lymphoma, unspecified, spleen 🔧
Ⓔ See C82.07

C82.98   Follicular lymphoma, unspecified, lymph nodes of multiple sites 🔧
Ⓔ See C82.08

C82.99   Follicular lymphoma, unspecified, extranodal and solid organ sites 🔧
Ⓔ See C82.00

● C83   Non-follicular lymphoma

Excludes1   personal history of non-Hodgkin lymphoma (Z85.72)

● C83.0   Small cell B-cell lymphoma
Lymphoplasmacytic lymphoma
Nodal marginal zone lymphoma
Non-leukemic variant of B-CLL
Splenic marginal zone lymphoma

Excludes1   chronic lymphocytic leukemia (C91.1)
mature T/NK-cell lymphomas (C84.-)
Waldenström macroglobulinemia (C88.0)

C83.00   Small cell B-cell lymphoma, unspecified site 🔧
Ⓔ C83.00-C83.09, C83.80-C83.99, C86.5-C86.6, D49.81-D49.9

C83.01   Small cell B-cell lymphoma, lymph nodes of head, face, and neck 🔧
Ⓔ C83.00-C83.01, C83.08-C83.09, C83.80-C83.81, C83.88-C83.91, C83.98-C83.99, C86.5-C86.6, D49.81-D49.9

C83.02   Small cell B-cell lymphoma, intrathoracic lymph nodes 🔧
Ⓔ C83.00, C83.02, C83.08-C83.09, C83.80, C83.82, C83.88-C83.89, C83.90, C83.92, C83.98-C83.99, C86.5-C86.6, D49.81-D49.9

C83.03   Small cell B-cell lymphoma, intra-abdominal lymph nodes 🔧
Ⓔ C83.00, C83.03, C83.08-C83.09, C83.80, C83.83, C83.88-C83.89, C83.90, C83.93, C83.98-C83.99, C86.5-C86.6, D49.81-D49.9

C83.04   Small cell B-cell lymphoma, lymph nodes of axilla and upper limb 🔧
Ⓔ C83.00, C83.04, C83.08-C83.09, C83.80, C83.84, C83.88-C83.89, C83.90, C83.94, C83.98-C83.99, C86.5-C86.6, D49.81-D49.9

C83.05   Small cell B-cell lymphoma, lymph nodes of inguinal region and lower limb 🔧
Ⓔ C83.00, C83.05, C83.08-C83.09, C83.80, C83.85, C83.88-C83.89, C83.90, C83.95, C83.98-C83.99, C86.5-C86.6, D49.81-D49.9

C83.06   Small cell B-cell lymphoma, intrapelvic lymph nodes 🔧
Ⓔ C83.00, C83.06, C83.08-C83.09, C83.80, C83.86, C83.88-C83.89, C83.90, C83.96, C83.98-C83.99, C86.5-C86.6, D49.81-D49.9

C83.07   Small cell B-cell lymphoma, spleen 🔧
Ⓔ C83.00, C83.07-C83.09, C83.80, C83.87-C83.89, C83.90, C83.97-C83.99, C86.5-C86.6, D49.81-D49.9

C83.08   Small cell B-cell lymphoma, lymph nodes of multiple sites 🔧
Ⓔ See C83.00

C83.09   Small cell B-cell lymphoma, extranodal and solid organ sites 🔧
Ⓔ See C83.00

● C83.1   Mantle cell lymphoma
Centrocytic lymphoma
Malignant lymphomatous polyposis

C83.10   Mantle cell lymphoma, unspecified site 🔧
Ⓔ See C82.50

C83.11   Mantle cell lymphoma, lymph nodes of head, face, and neck 🔧
Ⓔ See C82.51

C83.12   Mantle cell lymphoma, intrathoracic lymph nodes 🔧
Ⓔ See C82.52

C83.13   Mantle cell lymphoma, intra-abdominal lymph nodes 🔧
Ⓔ See C82.53

C83.14   Mantle cell lymphoma, lymph nodes of axilla and upper limb 🔧
Ⓔ See C82.54

C83.15   Mantle cell lymphoma, lymph nodes of inguinal region and lower limb 🔧
Ⓔ See C82.55

C83.16   Mantle cell lymphoma, intrapelvic lymph nodes 🔧
Ⓔ See C82.56

C83.17   Mantle cell lymphoma, spleen 🔧
Ⓔ See C82.57

C83.18   Mantle cell lymphoma, lymph nodes of multiple sites 🔧
Ⓔ See C82.58

C83.19   Mantle cell lymphoma, extranodal and solid organ sites 🔧
Ⓔ See C82.50

● C83.3   Diffuse large B-cell lymphoma
Anaplastic diffuse large B-cell lymphoma
CD30-positive diffuse large B-cell lymphoma
Centroblastic diffuse large B-cell lymphoma
Diffuse large B-cell lymphoma, subtype not specified
Immunoblastic diffuse large B-cell lymphoma
Plasmablastic diffuse large B-cell lymphoma
Diffuse large B-cell lymphoma, subtype not specified
T-cell rich diffuse large B-cell lymphoma

Excludes1   mediastinal (thymic) large B-cell lymphoma (C85.2-)
mature T/NK-cell lymphomas (C84.-)

C83.30   Diffuse large B-cell lymphoma, unspecified site 🔧
Ⓔ C83.30-C83.39, D49.81-D49.9

C83.31   Diffuse large B-cell lymphoma, lymph nodes of head, face, and neck 🔧
Ⓔ C83.30-C83.31, C83.38-C83.39, D49.81-D49.9

CHAPTER 2 (C00-D49)

N   Newborn Age: 0   P   Pediatric Age: 0–17   M   Maternity DX: 12–55   A   Adult Age: 15–124   ♀ Females Only   ♂ Males Only

🔧 Complication\Comorbidity   🔧 Major C\C   Ⓔ CC/MCC Exclusions   🔧 Present on Admission Requirement   🔧 Hospital-Acquired Condition

799

C83.32 Diffuse large B-cell lymphoma, intrathoracic lymph nodes 🔖
(Ex) C83.30, C83.32, C83.38-C83.39, D49.81-D49.9

C83.33 Diffuse large B-cell lymphoma, intra-abdominal lymph nodes 🔖
(Ex) C83.30, C83.33, C83.38-C83.39, D49.81-D49.9

C83.34 Diffuse large B-cell lymphoma, lymph nodes of axilla and upper limb 🔖
(Ex) C83.30, C83.34, C83.38-C83.39, D49.81-D49.9

C83.35 Diffuse large B-cell lymphoma, lymph nodes of inguinal region and lower limb 🔖
(Ex) C83.30, C83.35, C83.38-C83.39, D49.81-D49.9

C83.36 Diffuse large B-cell lymphoma, intrapelvic lymph nodes 🔖
(Ex) C83.30, C83.36, C83.38-C83.39, D49.81-D49.9

C83.37 Diffuse large B-cell lymphoma, spleen 🔖
(Ex) C83.30, C83.37-C83.39, D49.81-D49.9

C83.38 Diffuse large B-cell lymphoma, lymph nodes of multiple sites 🔖
(Ex) See C83.30

C83.39 Diffuse large B-cell lymphoma, extranodal and solid organ sites 🔖
(Ex) See C83.30

● **C83.5** Lymphoblastic (diffuse) lymphoma
Highly malignant type of non-Hodgkin lymphoma with diffuse infiltration
B-precursor lymphoma
Lymphoblastic B-cell lymphoma
Lymphoblastic lymphoma NOS
Lymphoblastic T-cell lymphoma
T-precursor lymphoma

C83.50 Lymphoblastic (diffuse) lymphoma, unspecified site 🔖
(Ex) C83.50-C83.59, D49.81-D49.9

C83.51 Lymphoblastic (diffuse) lymphoma, lymph nodes of head, face, and neck 🔖
(Ex) C83.50-C83.51, C83.58-C83.59, D49.81-D49.9

C83.52 Lymphoblastic (diffuse) lymphoma, intrathoracic lymph nodes 🔖
(Ex) C83.50, C83.52, C83.58-C83.59, D49.81-D49.9

C83.53 Lymphoblastic (diffuse) lymphoma, intra-abdominal lymph nodes 🔖
(Ex) C83.50, C83.53, C83.58-C83.59, D49.81-D49.9

C83.54 Lymphoblastic (diffuse) lymphoma, lymph nodes of axilla and upper limb 🔖
(Ex) C83.50, C83.54, C83.58-C83.59, D49.81-D49.9

C83.55 Lymphoblastic (diffuse) lymphoma, lymph nodes of inguinal region and lower limb 🔖
(Ex) C83.50, C83.55, C83.58-C83.59, D49.81-D49.9

C83.56 Lymphoblastic (diffuse) lymphoma, intrapelvic lymph nodes 🔖
(Ex) C83.50, C83.56, C83.58-C83.59, D49.81-D49.9

C83.57 Lymphoblastic (diffuse) lymphoma, spleen 🔖
(Ex) C83.50, C83.57-C83.59, D49.81-D49.9

C83.58 Lymphoblastic (diffuse) lymphoma, lymph nodes of multiple sites 🔖
(Ex) See C83.50

C83.59 Lymphoblastic (diffuse) lymphoma, extranodal and solid organ sites 🔖
(Ex) See C83.50

● **C83.7** Burkitt lymphoma
Form of small cell lymphoma
Atypical Burkitt lymphoma
Burkitt-like lymphoma
Excludes1   mature B-cell leukemia Burkitt type (C91.A-)

C83.70 Burkitt lymphoma, unspecified site 🔖
(Ex) C83.70-C83.79, D49.81-D49.9

C83.71 Burkitt lymphoma, lymph nodes of head, face, and neck 🔖
(Ex) C83.70-C83.71, C83.78-C83.79, D49.81-D49.9

C83.72 Burkitt lymphoma, intrathoracic lymph nodes 🔖
(Ex) C83.70, C83.72, C83.78-C83.79, D49.81-D49.9

C83.73 Burkitt lymphoma, intra-abdominal lymph nodes 🔖
(Ex) C83.70, C83.73, C83.78-C83.79, D49.81-D49.9

C83.74 Burkitt lymphoma, lymph nodes of axilla and upper limb 🔖
(Ex) C83.70, C83.74, C83.78-C83.79, D49.81-D49.9

C83.75 Burkitt lymphoma, lymph nodes of inguinal region and lower limb 🔖
(Ex) C83.70, C83.75, C83.78-C83.79, D49.81-D49.9

C83.76 Burkitt lymphoma, intrapelvic lymph nodes 🔖
(Ex) C83.70, C83.76, C83.78-C83.79, D49.81-D49.9

C83.77 Burkitt lymphoma, spleen 🔖
(Ex) C83.70, C83.77-C83.79, D49.81-D49.9

C83.78 Burkitt lymphoma, lymph nodes of multiple sites 🔖
(Ex) See C83.70

C83.79 Burkitt lymphoma, extranodal and solid organ sites 🔖
(Ex) See C83.70

● **C83.8** Other non-follicular lymphoma
Intravascular large B-cell lymphoma
Lymphoid granulomatosis
Primary effusion B-cell lymphoma
Excludes1   mediastinal (thymic) large B-cell lymphoma (C85.2-)
T-cell rich B-cell lymphoma (C83.3-)

C83.80 Other non-follicular lymphoma, unspecified site 🔖
(Ex) See C83.00

C83.81 Other non-follicular lymphoma, lymph nodes of head, face, and neck 🔖
(Ex) See C83.01

C83.82 Other non-follicular lymphoma, intrathoracic lymph nodes 🔖
(Ex) See C83.02

C83.83 Other non-follicular lymphoma, intra-abdominal lymph nodes 🔖
(Ex) See C83.03

C83.84 Other non-follicular lymphoma, lymph nodes of axilla and upper limb 🔖
(Ex) See C83.04

C83.85 Other non-follicular lymphoma, lymph nodes of inguinal region and lower limb 🔖
(Ex) See C83.05

C83.86 Other non-follicular lymphoma, intrapelvic lymph nodes 🔖
(Ex) See C83.06

C83.87 Other non-follicular lymphoma, spleen 🔖
(Ex) See C83.07

C83.88 Other non-follicular lymphoma, lymph nodes of multiple sites 🔖
(Ex) See C83.00

C83.89 Other non-follicular lymphoma, extranodal and solid organ sites 🔖
(Ex) See C83.00

● **C83.9** Non-follicular (diffuse) lymphoma, unspecified

C83.90 Non-follicular (diffuse) lymphoma, unspecified, unspecified site 🔖
(Ex) See C83.00

C83.91 Non-follicular (diffuse) lymphoma, unspecified, lymph nodes of head, face, and neck 🔖
(Ex) See C83.01

C83.92 Non-follicular (diffuse) lymphoma, unspecified, intrathoracic lymph nodes 🔖
(Ex) See C83.02

C83.93 Non-follicular (diffuse) lymphoma, unspecified, intra-abdominal lymph nodes 🔖
(Ex) See C83.03

C83.94 Non-follicular (diffuse) lymphoma, unspecified, lymph nodes of axilla and upper limb 🔖
(Ex) See C83.04

◀ New   ◀║║ Revised   ~~deleted~~ Deleted   Excludes 1   Excludes 2   Includes   Use additional   Code first   Code also   Unspecified

OGCR Official Guidelines   ● Unacceptable Principal Diagnosis   X Assign placeholder X   ▶ Use Additional Character(s)   ▶ Manifestation Code   **Coding Clinic**

C83.95   Non-follicular (diffuse) lymphoma, unspecified, lymph nodes of inguinal region and lower limb 🦠
    (Ex:) See C83.05

C83.96   Non-follicular (diffuse) lymphoma, unspecified, intrapelvic lymph nodes 🦠
    (Ex:) See C83.06

C83.97   Non-follicular (diffuse) lymphoma, unspecified, spleen 🦠
    (Ex:) See C83.07

C83.98   Non-follicular (diffuse) lymphoma, unspecified, lymph nodes of multiple sites 🦠
    (Ex:) See C83.00

C83.99   Non-follicular (diffuse) lymphoma, unspecified, extranodal and solid organ sites 🦠
    (Ex:) See C83.00

● **C84**   **Mature T/NK-cell lymphomas**

    Excludes1   personal history of non-Hodgkin lymphoma (Z85.72)

● **C84.0**   **Mycosis fungoides**
    Chronic or rapidly progressive form of cutaneous T-cell lymphoma; AKA granuloma fungoides

    Excludes1   peripheral T-cell lymphoma, not classified (C84.4-)

C84.00   Mycosis fungoides, unspecified site 🦠
    (Ex:) C82.50, C82.59, C83.10, C83.19, C84.00-C84.09, C84.40, C84.49, C84.60, C84.69-C84.70, C84.79, C84.90, C84.99, C84.A0, C84.A9-C84.Z0, C84.Z9, C85.10, C85.19-C85.20, C85.29-C85.80, C85.89-C85.90, C85.99, C86.4, C88.4, C96.4, C96.9, C96.Z, D49.81-D49.9

C84.01   Mycosis fungoides, lymph nodes of head, face, and neck 🦠
    (Ex:) C82.51, C83.11, C84.00-C84.01, C84.08-C84.09, C84.41, C84.61, C84.71, C84.91, C84.A1, C84.Z1, C85.11, C85.21, C85.81, C85.91, C86.0, D49.81-D49.9

C84.02   Mycosis fungoides, intrathoracic lymph nodes 🦠
    (Ex:) C82.52, C83.12, C84.00, C84.02, C84.08-C84.09, C84.42, C84.62, C84.72, C84.92, C84.A2, C84.Z2, C85.12, C85.22, C85.82, C85.92, D49.81-D49.9

C84.03   Mycosis fungoides, intra-abdominal lymph nodes 🦠
    (Ex:) C82.53, C83.13, C84.00, C84.03, C84.08-C84.09, C84.43, C84.63, C84.73, C84.93, C84.A3, C84.Z3, C85.13, C85.23, C85.83, C85.93, C86.2-C86.3, D49.81-D49.9

C84.04   Mycosis fungoides, lymph nodes of axilla and upper limb 🦠
    (Ex:) C82.54, C83.14, C84.00, C84.04, C84.08-C84.09, C84.44, C84.64, C84.74, C84.94, C84.A4, C84.Z4, C85.14, C85.24, C85.84, C85.94, D49.81-D49.9

C84.05   Mycosis fungoides, lymph nodes of inguinal region and lower limb 🦠
    (Ex:) C82.55, C83.15, C84.00, C84.05, C84.08-C84.09, C84.45, C84.65, C84.75, C84.95, C84.A5, C84.Z5, C85.15, C85.25, C85.85, C85.95, D49.81-D49.9

C84.06   Mycosis fungoides, intrapelvic lymph nodes 🦠
    (Ex:) C82.56, C83.16, C84.00, C84.06, C84.08-C84.09, C84.46, C84.66, C84.76, C84.96, C84.A6, C84.Z6, C85.16, C85.26, C85.86, C85.96, D49.81-D49.9

C84.07   Mycosis fungoides, spleen 🦠
    (Ex:) C82.57, C83.17, C84.00, C84.07, C84.08-C84.09, C84.47, C84.67, C84.77, C84.97, C84.A7, C84.Z7, C85.17, C85.27, C85.87, C85.97, D49.81-D49.9

C84.08   Mycosis fungoides, lymph nodes of multiple sites 🦠
    (Ex:) C82.58, C83.18, C84.00-C84.09, C84.48, C84.68, C84.78, C84.98, C84.A8, C84.Z8, C85.18, C85.28, C85.88, C85.98, D49.81-D49.9

C84.09   Mycosis fungoides, extranodal and solid organ sites 🦠
    (Ex:) See C84.00

● **C84.1**   **Sézary disease**
    Type of cutaneous lymphoma affecting T-cells

C84.10   Sézary disease, unspecified site 🦠
    (Ex:) C82.50, C82.59, C83.10, C83.19, C84.10-C84.19, C84.40, C84.49-C84.60, C84.69-C84.70, C84.79, C84.90, C84.99, C84.A0, C84.A9-C84.Z0, C84.Z9, C85.10, C85.19-C85.20, C85.29-C85.80, C85.89-C85.90, C85.99, C86.4, C88.4, C96.4, C96.9, C96.Z, D49.81-D49.9

C84.11   Sézary disease, lymph nodes of head, face, and neck 🦠
    (Ex:) C82.51, C83.11, C84.10-C84.11, C84.18-C84.19, C84.41, C84.61, C84.71, C84.91, C84.A1, C84.Z1, C85.11, C85.21, C85.81, C85.91, C86.0, D49.81-D49.9

C84.12   Sézary disease, intrathoracic lymph nodes 🦠
    (Ex:) C82.52, C83.12, C84.10, C84.12, C84.18-C84.19, C84.42, C84.62, C84.72, C84.92, C84.A2, C84.Z2, C85.12, C85.22, C85.82, C85.92, D49.81-D49.9

C84.13   Sézary disease, intra-abdominal lymph nodes 🦠
    (Ex:) C82.53, C83.13, C84.10, C84.13, C84.18-C84.19, C84.43, C84.63, C84.73, C84.93, C84.A3, C84.Z3, C85.13, C85.23, C85.83, C85.93, C86.2-C86.3, D49.81-D49.9

C84.14   Sézary disease, lymph nodes of axilla and upper limb 🦠
    (Ex:) C82.54, C83.14, C84.10, C84.14, C84.18-C84.19, C84.44, C84.64, C84.74, C84.94, C84.A4, C84.Z4, C85.14, C85.24, C85.84, C85.94, D49.81-D49.9

C84.15   Sézary disease, lymph nodes of inguinal region and lower limb 🦠
    (Ex:) C82.55, C83.15, C84.10, C84.15, C84.18-C84.19, C84.45, C84.65, C84.75, C84.95, C84.A5, C84.Z5, C85.15, C85.25, C85.85, C85.95, D49.81-D49.9

C84.16   Sézary disease, intrapelvic lymph nodes 🦠
    (Ex:) C82.56, C83.16, C84.10, C84.16, C84.18-C84.19, C84.46, C84.66, C84.76, C84.96, C84.A6, C84.Z6, C85.16, C85.26, C85.86, C85.96, D49.81-D49.9

C84.17   Sézary disease, spleen 🦠
    (Ex:) C82.57, C83.17, C84.10, C84.17-C84.19, C84.47, C84.67, C84.77, C84.97, C84.A7, C84.Z7, C85.17, C85.27, C85.87, C85.97, C86.1, D49.81-D49.9

C84.18   Sézary disease, lymph nodes of multiple sites 🦠
    (Ex:) C82.58, C83.18, C84.10-C84.19, C84.48, C84.68, C84.78, C84.98, C84.A8, C84.Z8, C85.18, C85.28, C85.88, C85.98, D49.81-D49.9

C84.19   Sézary disease, extranodal and solid organ sites 🦠
    (Ex:) See C84.10

● **C84.4**   **Peripheral T-cell lymphoma, not classified**
    Diverse group of blood carcinomas originating from T-cells, requiring aggressive chemotherapy
    Lennert's lymphoma
    Lymphoepithelioid lymphoma
    Mature T-cell lymphoma, not elsewhere classified

C84.40   Peripheral T-cell lymphoma, not classified, unspecified site 🦠
    (Ex:) See C82.50

C84.41   Peripheral T-cell lymphoma, not classified, lymph nodes of head, face, and neck 🦠
    (Ex:) See C82.51

C84.42   Peripheral T-cell lymphoma, not classified, intrathoracic lymph nodes 🦠
    (Ex:) See C82.52

C84.43   Peripheral T-cell lymphoma, not classified, intra-abdominal lymph nodes 🦠
    (Ex:) See C82.53

C84.44   Peripheral T-cell lymphoma, not classified, lymph nodes of axilla and upper limb 🦠
    (Ex:) See C82.54

N Newborn Age: 0   **P** Pediatric Age: 0–17   **M** Maternity DX: 12–55   **A** Adult Age: 15–124   ♀ Females Only   ♂ Males Only

🦠 Complication\Comorbidity   🦠 Major C\C   (Ex:) CC/MCC Exclusions   🦠 Present on Admission Requirement   🦠 Hospital-Acquired Condition

801

CHAPTER 2 (C00-D49)

C84.45   Peripheral T-cell lymphoma, not classified, lymph nodes of inguinal region and lower limb

(Ex:) See C82.55

C84.46   Peripheral T-cell lymphoma, not classified, intrapelvic lymph nodes

(Ex:) See C82.56

C84.47   Peripheral T-cell lymphoma, not classified, spleen

(Ex:) See C82.57

C84.48   Peripheral T-cell lymphoma, not classified, lymph nodes of multiple sites

(Ex:) See C82.58

C84.49   Peripheral T-cell lymphoma, not classified, extranodal and solid organ sites

(Ex:) See C82.50

● **C84.6**   Anaplastic large cell lymphoma, ALK-positive

Anaplastic large cell lymphoma, CD30-positive

C84.60   Anaplastic large cell lymphoma, ALK-positive, unspecified site

(Ex:) See C82.50

C84.61   Anaplastic large cell lymphoma, ALK-positive, lymph nodes of head, face, and neck

(Ex:) See C82.51

C84.62   Anaplastic large cell lymphoma, ALK-positive, intrathoracic lymph nodes

(Ex:) See C82.52

C84.63   Anaplastic large cell lymphoma, ALK-positive, intra-abdominal lymph nodes

(Ex:) See C82.53

C84.64   Anaplastic large cell lymphoma, ALK-positive, lymph nodes of axilla and upper limb

(Ex:) See C82.54

C84.65   Anaplastic large cell lymphoma, ALK-positive, lymph nodes of inguinal region and lower limb

(Ex:) See C82.56

C84.66   Anaplastic large cell lymphoma, ALK-positive, intrapelvic lymph nodes

(Ex:) See C82.56

C84.67   Anaplastic large cell lymphoma, ALK-positive, spleen

(Ex:) See C82.57

C84.68   Anaplastic large cell lymphoma, ALK-positive, lymph nodes of multiple sites

(Ex:) See C82.58

C84.69   Anaplastic large cell lymphoma, ALK-positive, extranodal and solid organ sites

(Ex:) See C82.50

● **C84.7**   Anaplastic large cell lymphoma, ALK-negative

Excludes1   primary cutaneous CD30-positive T-cell proliferations (C86.6-)

C84.70   Anaplastic large cell lymphoma, ALK-negative, unspecified site

(Ex:) See C82.50

C84.71   Anaplastic large cell lymphoma, ALK-negative, lymph nodes of head, face, and neck

(Ex:) See C82.51

C84.72   Anaplastic large cell lymphoma, ALK-negative, intrathoracic lymph nodes

(Ex:) See C82.52

C84.73   Anaplastic large cell lymphoma, ALK-negative, intra-abdominal lymph nodes

(Ex:) See C82.53

C84.74   Anaplastic large cell lymphoma, ALK-negative, lymph nodes of axilla and upper limb

(Ex:) See C82.54

C84.75   Anaplastic large cell lymphoma, ALK-negative, lymph nodes of inguinal region and lower limb

(Ex:) See C82.55

Item 2–7 Lymphosarcoma, also known as malignant lymphoma, is a cancer of the lymph system exhibiting abnormal cells encompassing an entire lymph node creating a diffuse pattern without any definite organization. Diffuse pattern lymphoma has a more unfavorable survival outlook than those with a follicular or nodular pattern. Reticulosarcoma is the most common aggressive form of non-Hodgkin's lymphoma.

C84.76   Anaplastic large cell lymphoma, ALK-negative, intrapelvic lymph nodes

(Ex:) See C82.56

C84.77   Anaplastic large cell lymphoma, ALK-negative, spleen

(Ex:) See C82.57

C84.78   Anaplastic large cell lymphoma, ALK-negative, lymph nodes of multiple sites

(Ex:) See C82.58

C84.79   Anaplastic large cell lymphoma, ALK-negative, extranodal and solid organ sites

(Ex:) See C82.50

● **C84.A**   Cutaneous T-cell lymphoma, unspecified

C84.A0   Cutaneous T-cell lymphoma, unspecified, unspecified site

(Ex:) See C82.50

C84.A1   Cutaneous T-cell lymphoma, unspecified lymph nodes of head, face, and neck

(Ex:) See C82.51

C84.A2   Cutaneous T-cell lymphoma, unspecified, intrathoracic lymph nodes

(Ex:) See C82.52

C84.A3   Cutaneous T-cell lymphoma, unspecified, intra-abdominal lymph nodes

(Ex:) See C82.53

C84.A4   Cutaneous T-cell lymphoma, unspecified, lymph nodes of axilla and upper limb

(Ex:) See C82.54

C84.A5   Cutaneous T-cell lymphoma, unspecified, lymph nodes of inguinal region and lower limb

(Ex:) See C82.55

C84.A6   Cutaneous T-cell lymphoma, unspecified, intrapelvic lymph nodes

(Ex:) See C82.56

C84.A7   Cutaneous T-cell lymphoma, unspecified, spleen

(Ex:) See C82.57

C84.A8   Cutaneous T-cell lymphoma, unspecified, lymph nodes of multiple sites

(Ex:) See C82.58

C84.A9   Cutaneous T-cell lymphoma, unspecified, extranodal and solid organ sites

(Ex:) See C82.50

● **C84.Z**   Other mature T/NK-cell lymphomas

Note: If T-cell lineage or involvement is mentioned in conjunction with a specific lymphoma, code to the more specific description.

Excludes1   angioimmunoblastic T-cell lymphoma (C86.5)

blastic NK-cell lymphoma (C86.4)

enteropathy-type T-cell lymphoma (C86.2)

extranodal NK-cell lymphoma, nasal type (C86.0)

hepatosplenic T-cell lymphoma (C86.1)

primary cutaneous CD30-positive T-cell proliferations (C86.6)

subcutaneous panniculitis-like T-cell lymphoma (C86.3)

T-cell leukemia (C91.1-)

C84.Z0   Other mature T/NK-cell lymphomas, unspecified site

(Ex:) See C82.50

C84.Z1   Other mature T/NK-cell lymphomas, lymph nodes of head, face, and neck

(Ex:) See C82.51

C84.Z2 Other mature T/NK-cell lymphomas, intrathoracic lymph nodes 🦠
   (Ex) See C82.52

C84.Z3 Other mature T/NK-cell lymphomas, intra-abdominal lymph nodes 🦠
   (Ex) See C82.53

C84.Z4 Other mature T/NK-cell lymphomas, lymph nodes of axilla and upper limb 🦠
   (Ex) See C82.54

C84.Z5 Other mature T/NK-cell lymphomas, lymph nodes of inguinal region and lower limb 🦠
   (Ex) See C82.55

C84.Z6 Other mature T/NK-cell lymphomas, intrapelvic lymph nodes 🦠
   (Ex) See C82.56

C84.Z7 Other mature T/NK-cell lymphomas, spleen 🦠
   (Ex) See C82.57

C84.Z8 Other mature T/NK-cell lymphomas, lymph nodes of multiple sites 🦠
   (Ex) See C82.58

C84.Z9 Other mature T/NK-cell lymphomas, extranodal and solid organ sites 🦠
   (Ex) See C82.50

● C84.9 **Mature T/NK-cell lymphomas, unspecified**
   NK/T cell lymphoma NOS
   Excludes1   mature T-cell lymphoma, not elsewhere classified (C84.4-)

C84.90 Mature T/NK-cell lymphomas, unspecified, unspecified site 🦠
   (Ex) See C82.50

C84.91 Mature T/NK-cell lymphomas, unspecified, lymph nodes of head, face, and neck 🦠
   (Ex) See C82.51

C84.92 Mature T/NK-cell lymphomas, unspecified, intrathoracic lymph nodes 🦠
   (Ex) See C82.52

C84.93 Mature T/NK-cell lymphomas, unspecified, intra-abdominal lymph nodes 🦠
   (Ex) See C82.53

C84.94 Mature T/NK-cell lymphomas, unspecified, lymph nodes of axilla and upper limb 🦠
   (Ex) See C82.54

C84.95 Mature T/NK-cell lymphomas, unspecified, lymph nodes of inguinal region and lower limb 🦠
   (Ex) See C82.55

C84.96 Mature T/NK-cell lymphomas, unspecified, intrapelvic lymph nodes 🦠
   (Ex) See C82.56

C84.97 Mature T/NK-cell lymphomas, unspecified, spleen 🦠
   (Ex) See C82.57

C84.98 Mature T/NK-cell lymphomas, unspecified, lymph nodes of multiple sites 🦠
   (Ex) See C82.58

C84.99 Mature T/NK-cell lymphomas, unspecified, extranodal and solid organ sites 🦠
   (Ex) See C82.50

● C85 **Other specified and unspecified types of non-Hodgkin lymphoma**
   Excludes1   other specified types of T/NK-cell lymphoma (C86.-)
        personal history of non-Hodgkin lymphoma (Z85.72)

● C85.1 **Unspecified B-cell lymphoma**
   Note: If B-cell lineage or involvement is mentioned in conjunction with a specific lymphoma, code to the more specific description.

C85.10 Unspecified B-cell lymphoma, unspecified site 🦠
   (Ex) See C82.50

C85.11 Unspecified B-cell lymphoma, lymph nodes of head, face, and neck 🦠
   (Ex) See C82.51

C85.12 Unspecified B-cell lymphoma, intrathoracic lymph nodes 🦠
   (Ex) See C82.52

C85.13 Unspecified B-cell lymphoma, intra-abdominal lymph nodes 🦠
   (Ex) See C82.53

C85.14 Unspecified B-cell lymphoma, lymph nodes of axilla and upper limb 🦠
   (Ex) See C82.54

C85.15 Unspecified B-cell lymphoma, lymph nodes of inguinal region and lower limb 🦠
   (Ex) See C82.55

C85.16 Unspecified B-cell lymphoma, intrapelvic lymph nodes 🦠
   (Ex) See C82.56

C85.17 Unspecified B-cell lymphoma, spleen 🦠
   (Ex) See C82.57

C85.18 Unspecified B-cell lymphoma, lymph nodes of multiple sites 🦠
   (Ex) See C82.58

C85.19 Unspecified B-cell lymphoma, extranodal and solid organ sites 🦠
   (Ex) See C82.50

● C85.2 **Mediastinal (thymic) large B-cell lymphoma**

C85.20 Mediastinal (thymic) large B-cell lymphoma, unspecified site 🦠
   (Ex) See C82.50

C85.21 Mediastinal (thymic) large B-cell lymphoma, lymph nodes of head, face, and neck 🦠
   (Ex) See C82.51

C85.22 Mediastinal (thymic) large B-cell lymphoma, intrathoracic lymph nodes 🦠
   (Ex) See C82.52

C85.23 Mediastinal (thymic) large B-cell lymphoma, intra-abdominal lymph nodes 🦠
   (Ex) See C82.53

C85.24 Mediastinal (thymic) large B-cell lymphoma, lymph nodes of axilla and upper limb 🦠
   (Ex) See C82.54

C85.25 Mediastinal (thymic) large B-cell lymphoma, lymph nodes of inguinal region and lower limb 🦠
   (Ex) See C82.55

C85.26 Mediastinal (thymic) large B-cell lymphoma, intrapelvic lymph nodes 🦠
   (Ex) See C82.56

C85.27 Mediastinal (thymic) large B-cell lymphoma, spleen 🦠
   (Ex) See C82.57

C85.28 Mediastinal (thymic) large B-cell lymphoma, lymph nodes of multiple sites 🦠
   (Ex) See C82.58

C85.29 Mediastinal (thymic) large B-cell lymphoma, extranodal and solid organ sites 🦠
   (Ex) See C82.50

● C85.8 **Other specified types of non-Hodgkin lymphoma**

C85.80 Other specified types of non-Hodgkin lymphoma, unspecified site 🦠
   (Ex) See C82.50

C85.81 Other specified types of non-Hodgkin lymphoma, lymph nodes of head, face, and neck 🦠
   (Ex) See C82.51

C85.82 Other specified types of non-Hodgkin lymphoma, intrathoracic lymph nodes 🦠
   (Ex) See C82.52

C85.83 Other specified types of non-Hodgkin lymphoma, intra-abdominal lymph nodes 🦠
   (Ex) See C82.53

N Newborn Age: 0   **P** Pediatric Age: 0–17   **M** Maternity DX: 12–55   **A** Adult Age: 15–124   ♀ Females Only   ♂ Males Only

🦠 Complication\Comorbidity   🦠 Major C\C   (Ex) CC/MCC Exclusions   🦠 Present on Admission Requirement   🦠 Hospital-Acquired Condition

803

C85.84 Other specified types of non-Hodgkin lymphoma, lymph nodes of axilla and upper limb
(Ex:) See C82.54

C85.85 Other specified types of non-Hodgkin lymphoma, lymph nodes of inguinal region and lower limb
(Ex:) See C82.55

C85.86 Other specified types of non-Hodgkin lymphoma, intrapelvic lymph nodes
(Ex:) See C82.56

C85.87 Other specified types of non-Hodgkin lymphoma, spleen
(Ex:) See C82.57

C85.88 Other specified types of non-Hodgkin lymphoma, lymph nodes of multiple sites
(Ex:) See C82.58

C85.89 Other specified types of non-Hodgkin lymphoma, extranodal and solid organ sites
(Ex:) See C82.50

● **C85.9** Non-Hodgkin lymphoma, unspecified
Lymphoma NOS
Malignant lymphoma NOS
Non-Hodgkin lymphoma NOS

C85.90 Non-Hodgkin lymphoma, unspecified, unspecified site
(Ex:) See C82.50

C85.91 Non-Hodgkin lymphoma, unspecified, lymph nodes of head, face, and neck
(Ex:) See C82.51

C85.92 Non-Hodgkin lymphoma, unspecified, intrathoracic lymph nodes
(Ex:) See C82.52

C85.93 Non-Hodgkin lymphoma, unspecified, intra-abdominal lymph nodes
(Ex:) See C82.53

C85.94 Non-Hodgkin lymphoma, unspecified, lymph nodes of axilla and upper limb
(Ex:) See C82.54

C85.95 Non-Hodgkin lymphoma, unspecified, lymph nodes of inguinal region and lower limb
(Ex:) See C82.55

C85.96 Non-Hodgkin lymphoma, unspecified, intrapelvic lymph nodes
(Ex:) See C82.56

C85.97 Non-Hodgkin lymphoma, unspecified, spleen
(Ex:) See C82.57

C85.98 Non-Hodgkin lymphoma, unspecified, lymph nodes of multiple sites
(Ex:) See C82.58

C85.99 Non-Hodgkin lymphoma, unspecified, extranodal and solid organ sites
(Ex:) See C82.50

● **C86** Other specified types of T/NK-cell lymphoma
Excludes1 anaplastic large cell lymphoma, ALK negative (C84.7-)
anaplastic large cell lymphoma, ALK positive (C84.6-)
mature T/NK-cell lymphomas (C84.-)
other specified types of non-Hodgkin lymphoma (C85.8-)

C86.0 Extranodal NK/T-cell lymphoma, nasal type
(Ex:) See C82.51

C86.1 Hepatosplenic T-cell lymphoma
Alpha-beta and gamma delta types
(Ex:) See C82.57

C86.2 Enteropathy-type (intestinal) T-cell lymphoma
Enteropathy associated T-cell lymphoma
(Ex:) See C82.53

C86.3 Subcutaneous panniculitis-like T-cell lymphoma
(Ex:) See C82.53

C86.4 Blastic NK-cell lymphoma
(Ex:) See C82.50

C86.5 Angioimmunoblastic T-cell lymphoma
Angioimmunoblastic lymphadenopathy with dysproteinemia (AILD)
(Ex:) See C83.00

C86.6 Primary cutaneous CD30-positive T-cell proliferations
Lymphomatoid papulosis
Primary cutaneous anaplastic large cell lymphoma
Primary cutaneous CD30-positive large T-cell lymphoma
(Ex:) See C83.00

● **C88** Malignant immunoproliferative diseases and certain other B-cell lymphomas
Diseases involving immune system
Excludes1 B-cell lymphoma, unspecified (C85.1-) ◀▥
personal history of other malignant neoplasms of lymphoid, hematopoietic and related tissues (Z85.79)

C88.0 Waldenström's macroglobulinemia
Lymphoplasmacytic lymphoma with IgM-production
Macroglobulinemia (idiopathic) (primary)
Excludes1 small cell B-cell lymphoma (C83.0)

C88.2 Heavy chain disease
Franklin disease
Gamma heavy chain disease
Mu heavy chain disease
(Ex:) C88.2-C88.3, C88.8-C90.02, C90.10-C90.12, C90.20-C90.22, C90.30-C90.32, C91.00-C91.02, C91.10-C91.12, C91.30-C91.32, C91.50-C91.52, C91.60-C91.62, C91.90-C91.92, C91.A0-C91.A2, C91.Z0-C91.Z2, C92.00-C92.02, C92.10-C92.12, C92.20-C92.22, C92.30-C92.32, C92.40-C92.42, C92.50-C92.52, C92.60-C92.62, C92.90-C92.92, C92.A0-C92.A2, C92.Z0-C92.Z2, C93.00-C93.02, C93.10-C93.12, C93.30-C93.32, C93.90-C93.92, C93.Z0-C93.Z2, C94.00-C94.02, C94.20-C94.22, C94.30-C94.32, C94.80-C94.82, C95.00-C95.02, C95.10-C95.12, C95.90-C95.92, D49.81-D49.9

C88.3 Immunoproliferative small intestinal disease
Alpha heavy chain disease
Mediterranean lymphoma
(Ex:) See C88.2

C88.4 Extranodal marginal zone B-cell lymphoma of mucosa-associated lymphoid tissue [MALT-lymphoma]
Lymphoma of skin-associated lymphoid tissue [SALT-lymphoma]
Lymphoma of bronchial-associated lymphoid tissue [BALT-lymphoma]
Excludes1 high malignant (diffuse large B-cell) lymphoma (C83.3-)
(Ex:) See C82.50

C88.8 Other malignant immunoproliferative diseases
(Ex:) C88.2-C88.3, C88.8-C90.02, C90.10-C90.12, C90.20-C90.22, C90.30-C90.32, C91.00-C91.02, C91.10-C91.12, C91.30-C91.32, C91.40-C91.42, C91.50-C91.52, C91.60-C91.62, C91.90-C91.92, C91.A0-C91.A2, C91.Z0-C91.Z2, C92.00-C92.02, C92.10-C92.12, C92.20-C92.22, C92.30-C92.32, C92.40-C92.42, C92.50-C92.52, C92.60-C92.62, C92.90-C92.92, C92.A0-C92.A2, C92.Z0-C92.Z2, C93.00-C93.02, C93.10-C93.12, C93.30-C93.32, C93.90-C93.92, C93.Z0-C93.Z2, C94.00-C94.02, C94.20-C94.22, C94.30-C94.32, C94.40-C94.42, C94.6, C94.80-C94.82, C95.00-C95.02, C95.10-C95.12, C95.90-C95.92, D45-D46.22, D46.4, D46.9, D46.A-D46.Z, D47.0-D47.1, D47.3, D47.9, D47.Z9, D48.7-D48.9, D49.81-D49.9

C88.9 Malignant immunoproliferative disease, unspecified
Immunoproliferative disease NOS
(Ex:) See C88.2

◀ New   ◀▥ Revised   deleted Deleted   Excludes 1   Excludes 2   Includes   Use additional   Code first   Code also   Unspecified
OGCR Official Guidelines   ● Unacceptable Principal Diagnosis   X Assign placeholder X   ● Use Additional Character(s)   ▶ Manifestation Code   **Coding Clinic**

Item 2–8 Multiple myeloma is a cancer of a plasma cell (a type of white blood cell) and is an incurable but treatable disease. Immunoproliferative neoplasm is a term for diseases (mostly cancers) in which the immune system cells proliferate.

● **C90 Multiple myeloma and malignant plasma cell neoplasms**

 Excludes1 personal history of other malignant neoplasms of lymphoid, hematopoietic and related tissues (Z85.79)

 (Ex) **For category C90 CC codes:** C88.2-C88.3, C88.8-C90.02, C90.10-C90.12, C90.20-C90.22, C90.30-C90.32, C91.00-C91.02, C91.10-C91.12, C91.30-C91.32, C91.50-C91.52, C91.60-C91.62, C91.90-C91.92, C91.A0-C91.A2, C91.Z0-C91.Z2, C92.00-C92.02, C92.10-C92.12, C92.20-C92.22, C92.30-C92.32, C92.40-C92.42, C92.50-C92.52, C92.60-C92.62, C92.90-C92.92, C92.A0-C92.A2, C92.Z0-C92.Z2, C93.00-C93.02, C93.10-C93.12, C93.30-C93.32, C93.90-C93.92, C93.Z0-C93.Z2, C94.00-C94.02, C94.20-C94.22, C94.30-C94.32, C94.80-C94.82, C95.00-C95.02, C95.10-C95.12, C95.90-C95.92, D49.81-D49.9

● **C90.0 Multiple myeloma**
 Kahler's disease
 Medullary plasmacytoma
 Myelomatosis
 Plasma cell myeloma

 Excludes1 solitary myeloma (C90.3-)
 solitary plasmacytoma (C90.3-)

 C90.00 Multiple myeloma not having achieved remission 🔹
  Multiple myeloma with failed remission
  Multiple myeloma NOS

 C90.01 Multiple myeloma in remission 🔹

 C90.02 Multiple myeloma in relapse 🔹

● **C90.1 Plasma cell leukemia**
 Rare type of acute leukemia
 Plasmacytic leukemia

 C90.10 Plasma cell leukemia not having achieved remission 🔹
  Plasma cell leukemia with failed remission
  Plasma cell leukemia NOS

 C90.11 Plasma cell leukemia in remission 🔹

 C90.12 Plasma cell leukemia in relapse 🔹

● **C90.2 Extramedullary plasmacytoma**
 Malignant monoclonal plasma cell tumor growing in soft tissue; AKA plasma cell dyscrasias

 C90.20 Extramedullary plasmacytoma not having achieved remission 🔹
  Extramedullary plasmacytoma with failed remission
  Extramedullary plasmacytoma NOS

 C90.21 Extramedullary plasmacytoma in remission 🔹

 C90.22 Extramedullary plasmacytoma in relapse 🔹

 C90.3 Solitary plasmacytoma
  Localized malignant plasma cell tumor NOS
  Plasmacytoma NOS
  Solitary myeloma

 C90.30 Solitary plasmacytoma not having achieved remission 🔹
  Solitary plasmacytoma with failed remission
  Solitary plasmacytoma NOS

 C90.31 Solitary plasmacytoma in remission 🔹

 C90.32 Solitary plasmacytoma in relapse 🔹

● **C91 Lymphoid leukemia**
 Type of leukemia affecting circulating cells of lymphoid origin

 Excludes1 personal history of leukemia (Z85.6)

 (Ex) **For category C91 CC codes unless otherwise indicated:** C88.2-C88.3, C88.8-C90.02, C90.10-C90.12, C90.20-C90.22, C90.30-C90.32, C91.00-C91.02, C91.10-C91.12, C91.30-C91.32, C91.50-C91.52, C91.60-C91.62, C91.90-C91.92, C91.A0-C91.A2, C91.Z0-C91.Z2, C92.00-C92.02, C92.10-C92.12, C92.20-C92.22, C92.30-C92.32, C92.40-C92.42, C92.50-C92.52, C92.60-C92.62, C92.90-C92.92, C92.A0-C92.A2, C92.Z0-C92.Z2, C93.00-C93.02, C93.10-C93.12, C93.30-C93.32, C93.90-C93.92, C93.Z0-C93.Z2, C94.00-C94.02, C94.20-C94.22, C94.30-C94.32, C94.80-C94.82, C95.00-C95.02, C95.10-C95.12, C95.90-C95.92, D49.81-D49.9

● **C91.0 Acute lymphoblastic leukemia [ALL]**
 Note: Code C91.0 should only be used for T-cell and B-cell precursor leukemia

 C91.00 Acute lymphoblastic leukemia not having achieved remission 🔹
  Acute lymphoblastic leukemia with failed remission
  Acute lymphoblastic leukemia NOS

 C91.01 Acute lymphoblastic leukemia, in remission 🔹

 C91.02 Acute lymphoblastic leukemia, in relapse 🔹

● **C91.1 Chronic lymphocytic leukemia of B-cell type**
 Lymphoplasmacytic leukemia
 Richter syndrome

 Excludes1 lymphoplasmacytic lymphoma (C83.0-)

 C91.10 Chronic lymphocytic leukemia of B-cell type not having achieved remission 🔹
  Chronic lymphocytic leukemia of B-cell type with failed remission
  Chronic lymphocytic leukemia of B-cell type NOS

 C91.11 Chronic lymphocytic leukemia of B-cell type in remission 🔹

 C91.12 Chronic lymphocytic leukemia of B-cell type in relapse 🔹

● **C91.3 Prolymphocytic leukemia of B-cell type**
 Chronic leukemia with symptoms of large number of circulating lymphocytes

 C91.30 Prolymphocytic leukemia of B-cell type not having achieved remission 🔹
  Prolymphocytic leukemia of B-cell type with failed remission
  Prolymphocytic leukemia of B-cell type NOS

 C91.31 Prolymphocytic leukemia of B-cell type, in remission 🔹

 C91.32 Prolymphocytic leukemia of B-cell type, in relapse 🔹

● **C91.4 Hairy cell leukemia**
 Chronic leukemia with splenomegaly and excessive number of abnormal large mononuclear cells covered by hairlike villi
 Leukemic reticuloendotheliosis

 (Ex) **For category C91.4 CC codes:** C82.50, C82.59, C83.10, C83.19, C84.40, C84.49-C84.60, C84.69-C84.70, C84.79, C84.90, C84.99, C84.A0, C84.A9-C84.Z0, C84.Z9, C85.10, C85.19-C85.20, C85.29-C85.80, C85.89-C85.90, C85.99, C86.4, C88.4, C91.40-C91.42, C96.4, C96.9, C96.Z, D49.81-D49.9

 C91.40 Hairy cell leukemia not having achieved remission 🔹
  Hairy cell leukemia with failed remission
  Hairy cell leukemia NOS

 C91.41 Hairy cell leukemia, in remission 🔹

 C91.42 Hairy cell leukemia, in relapse 🔹

Item 2–9 Leukemia is a cancer (acute or chronic) of the blood-forming tissues of the bone marrow. Blood cells all start out as stem cells. They mature and become red cells, white cells, or platelets. There are three main types of leukocytes (white cells that fight infection): monocytes, lymphocytes, and granulocytes. **Acute monocytic leukemia** (AML) affects monocytes. **Acute lymphoid leukemia** (ALL) affects lymphocytes, and **acute myeloid leukemia** (AML) affects cells that typically develop into white blood cells (not lymphocytes), though it may develop in other blood cells.

N Newborn Age: 0 P Pediatric Age: 0–17 M Maternity DX: 12–55 A Adult Age: 15–124 ♀ Females Only ♂ Males Only

🔹 Complication\Comorbidity 🔹 Major C\C (Ex) CC/MCC Exclusions 🔹 Present on Admission Requirement 🔹 Hospital-Acquired Condition

805

● **C91.5 Adult T-cell lymphoma/leukemia (HTLV-1-associated)**
Acute variant of adult T-cell lymphoma/leukemia (HTLV-1-associated)
Chronic variant of adult T-cell lymphoma/leukemia (HTLV-1-associated)
Lymphomatoid variant of adult T-cell lymphoma/leukemia (HTLV-1-associated)
Smouldering variant of adult T-cell lymphoma/leukemia (HTLV-1-associated)

C91.50 Adult T-cell lymphoma/leukemia (HTLV-1-associated) not having achieved remission 🔖 A
Adult T-cell lymphoma/leukemia (HTLV-1-associated) with failed remission
Adult T-cell lymphoma/leukemia (HTLV-1-associated) NOS

C91.51 Adult T-cell lymphoma/leukemia (HTLV-1-associated), in remission 🔖 A

C91.52 Adult T-cell lymphoma/leukemia (HTLV-1-associated), in relapse 🔖 A

● **C91.6 Prolymphocytic leukemia of T-cell type**

C91.60 Prolymphocytic leukemia of T-cell type not having achieved remission 🔖
Prolymphocytic leukemia of T-cell type with failed remission
Prolymphocytic leukemia of T-cell type NOS

C91.61 Prolymphocytic leukemia of T-cell type, in remission 🔖

C91.62 Prolymphocytic leukemia of T-cell type, in relapse 🔖

● **C91.A Mature B-cell leukemia Burkitt-type**
Excludes1 Burkitt lymphoma (C83.7-)

C91.A0 Mature B-cell leukemia Burkitt-type not having achieved remission 🔖
Mature B-cell leukemia Burkitt-type with failed remission
Mature B-cell leukemia Burkitt-type NOS

C91.A1 Mature B-cell leukemia Burkitt-type, in remission 🔖

C91.A2 Mature B-cell leukemia Burkitt-type, in relapse 🔖

● **C91.Z Other lymphoid leukemia**
T-cell large granular lymphocytic leukemia (associated with rheumatoid arthritis)

C91.Z0 Other lymphoid leukemia not having achieved remission 🔖
Other lymphoid leukemia with failed remission
Other lymphoid leukemia NOS

C91.Z1 Other lymphoid leukemia, in remission 🔖

C91.Z2 Other lymphoid leukemia, in relapse 🔖

● **C91.9 Lymphoid leukemia, unspecified**

C91.90 Lymphoid leukemia, unspecified not having achieved remission 🔖
Lymphoid leukemia with failed remission
Lymphoid leukemia NOS

C91.91 Lymphoid leukemia, unspecified, in remission 🔖

C91.92 Lymphoid leukemia, unspecified, in relapse 🔖

● **C92 Myeloid leukemia**
Includes   granulocytic leukemia
myelogenous leukemia

Excludes1   personal history of leukemia (Z85.6)

Ⓔⓧ **For category C92 CC codes:** C88.2-C88.3, C88.8-C90.02, C90.10-C90.12, C90.20-C90.22, C90.30-C90.32, C91.00-C91.02, C91.10-C91.12, C91.30-C91.32, C91.50-C91.52, C91.60-C91.62, C91.90-C91.92, C91.A0-C91.A2, C91.Z0-C91.Z2, C92.00-C92.02, C92.10-C92.12, C92.20-C92.22, C92.30-C92.32, C92.40-C92.42, C92.50-C92.52, C92.60-C92.62, C92.90-C92.92, C92.A0-C92.A2, C92.Z0-C92.Z2, C93.00-C93.02, C93.10-C93.12, C93.30-C93.32, C93.90-C93.92, C93.Z0-C93.Z2, C94.00-C94.02, C94.20-C94.22, C94.30-C94.32, C94.80-C94.82, C95.00-C95.02, C95.10-C95.12, C95.90-C95.92, D49.81-D49.9

● **C92.0 Acute myeloblastic leukemia**
Acute myeloblastic leukemia, minimal differentiation
Acute myeloblastic leukemia (with maturation)
Acute myeloblastic leukemia 1/ETO
Acute myeloblastic leukemia M0
Acute myeloblastic leukemia M1
Acute myeloblastic leukemia M2
Acute myeloblastic leukemia with t(8;21)
Acute myeloblastic leukemia (without a FAB classification) NOS
Refractory anemia with excess blasts in transformation [RAEB T]

Excludes1 acute exacerbation of chronic myeloid leukemia (C92.10)
refractory anemia with excess of blasts not in transformation (D46.2-)

C92.00 Acute myeloblastic leukemia, not having achieved remission 🔖
Acute myeloblastic leukemia with failed remission
Acute myeloblastic leukemia NOS

C92.01 Acute myeloblastic leukemia, in remission 🔖

C92.02 Acute myeloblastic leukemia, in relapse 🔖

● **C92.1 Chronic myeloid leukemia, BCR/ABL-positive**
Chronic myelogenous leukemia, Philadelphia chromosome (Ph1) positive
Chronic myelogenous leukemia, t(9;22) (q34;q11)
Chronic myelogenous leukemia with crisis of blast cells

Excludes1 atypical chronic myeloid leukemia BCR/ABL-negative (C92.2-)
chronic myelomonocytic leukemia (C93.1-)
chronic myeloproliferative disease (D47.1)

C92.10 Chronic myeloid leukemia, BCR/ABL-positive, not having achieved remission 🔖
Chronic myeloid leukemia, BCR/ABL-positive with failed remission
Chronic myeloid leukemia, BCR/ABL-positive NOS

C92.11 Chronic myeloid leukemia, BCR/ABL-positive, in remission 🔖

C92.12 Chronic myeloid leukemia, BCR/ABL-positive, in relapse 🔖

● **C92.2 Atypical chronic myeloid leukemia, BCR/ABL-negative**

C92.20 Atypical chronic myeloid leukemia, BCR/ABL-negative, not having achieved remission 🔖
Atypical chronic myeloid leukemia, BCR/ABL-negative with failed remission
Atypical chronic myeloid leukemia, BCR/ABL-negative NOS

C92.21 Atypical chronic myeloid leukemia, BCR/ABL-negative, in remission 🔖

C92.22 Atypical chronic myeloid leukemia, BCR/ABL-negative, in relapse 🔖

CHAPTER 2 (C00-D49)

● **C92.3**   **Myeloid sarcoma**
A malignant tumor of immature myeloid cells
Chloroma
Granulocytic sarcoma

     C92.30   **Myeloid sarcoma, not having achieved remission** 🔖
Myeloid sarcoma with failed remission
Myeloid sarcoma NOS

     C92.31   **Myeloid sarcoma, in remission** 🔖

     C92.32   **Myeloid sarcoma, in relapse** 🔖

● **C92.4**   **Acute promyelocytic leukemia**
AML M3
AML Me with t(15;17) and variants

     C92.40   **Acute promyelocytic leukemia, not having achieved remission** 🔖
Acute promyelocytic leukemia with failed remission
Acute promyelocytic leukemia NOS

     C92.41   **Acute promyelocytic leukemia, in remission** 🔖

     C92.42   **Acute promyelocytic leukemia, in relapse** 🔖

● **C92.5**   **Acute myelomonocytic leukemia**
AML M4
AML M4 Eo with inv(16) or t(16;16)

     C92.50   **Acute myelomonocytic leukemia, not having achieved remission** 🔖
Acute myelomonocytic leukemia with failed remission
Acute myelomonocytic leukemia NOS

     C92.51   **Acute myelomonocytic leukemia, in remission** 🔖

     C92.52   **Acute myelomonocytic leukemia, in relapse** 🔖

● **C92.6**   **Acute myeloid leukemia with 11q23-abnormality**
Acute myeloid leukemia with variation of MLL-gene

     C92.60   **Acute myeloid leukemia with 11q23-abnormality not having achieved remission** 🔖
Acute myeloid leukemia with 11q23-abnormality with failed remission
Acute myeloid leukemia with 11q23-abnormality NOS

     C92.61   **Acute myeloid leukemia with 11q23-abnormality in remission** 🔖

     C92.62   **Acute myeloid leukemia with 11q23-abnormality in relapse** 🔖

● **C92.A**   **Acute myeloid leukemia with multilineage dysplasia**
Acute myeloid leukemia with dysplasia of remaining hematopoesis and/or myelodysplastic disease in its history

     C92.A0   **Acute myeloid leukemia with multilineage dysplasia, not having achieved remission** 🔖
Acute myeloid leukemia with multilineage dysplasia with failed remission
Acute myeloid leukemia with multilineage dysplasia NOS

     C92.A1   **Acute myeloid leukemia with multilineage dysplasia, in remission** 🔖

     C92.A2   **Acute myeloid leukemia with multilineage dysplasia, in relapse** 🔖

● **C92.Z**   **Other myeloid leukemia**

     C92.Z0   **Other myeloid leukemia not having achieved remission** 🔖
Myeloid leukemia NEC with failed remission
Myeloid leukemia NEC

     C92.Z1   **Other myeloid leukemia, in remission** 🔖

     C92.Z2   **Other myeloid leukemia, in relapse** 🔖

● **C92.9**   **Myeloid leukemia, unspecified**

     C92.90   **Myeloid leukemia, unspecified, not having achieved remission** 🔖
Myeloid leukemia, unspecified with failed remission
Myeloid leukemia, unspecified NOS

     C92.91   **Myeloid leukemia, unspecified in remission** 🔖

     C92.92   **Myeloid leukemia, unspecified in relapse** 🔖

●● **C93**   **Monocytic leukemia**

     Includes   monocytoid leukemia
     Excludes1   personal history of leukemia (Z85.6)
Ⓔₓ **For category C93 CC codes:** C88.2-C88.3, C88.8-C90.02, C90.10-C90.12, C90.20-C90.22, C90.30-C90.32, C91.00-C91.02, C91.10-C91.12, C91.30-C91.32, C91.50-C91.52, C91.60-C91.62, C91.90-C91.92, C91.A0-C91.A2, C91.Z0-C91.Z2, C92.00-C92.02, C92.10-C92.12, C92.20-C92.22, C92.30-C92.32, C92.40-C92.42, C92.50-C92.52, C92.60-C92.62, C92.90-C92.92, C92.A0-C92.A2, C92.Z0-C92.Z2, C93.00-C93.02, C93.10-C93.12, C93.30-C93.32, C93.90-C93.92, C93.Z0-C93.Z2, C94.00-C94.02, C94.20-C94.22, C94.30-C94.32, C94.80-C94.82, C95.00-C95.02, C95.10-C95.12, C95.90-C95.92, D49.81-D49.9

● **C93.0**   **Acute monoblastic/monocytic leukemia**
AML M5
AML M5a
AML M5b

     C93.00   **Acute monoblastic/monocytic leukemia, not having achieved remission** 🔖
Acute monoblastic/monocytic leukemia with failed remission
Acute monoblastic/monocytic leukemia NOS

     C93.01   **Acute monoblastic/monocytic leukemia, in remission** 🔖

     C93.02   **Acute monoblastic/monocytic leukemia, in relapse** 🔖

● **C93.1**   **Chronic myelomonocytic leukemia**
Chronic monocytic leukemia
CMML-1
CMML-2
CMML with eosinophilia

     C93.10   **Chronic myelomonocytic leukemia not having achieved remission** 🔖
Chronic myelomonocytic leukemia with failed remission
Chronic myelomonocytic leukemia NOS

     C93.11   **Chronic myelomonocytic leukemia, in remission** 🔖

     C93.12   **Chronic myelomonocytic leukemia, in relapse** 🔖

● **C93.3**   **Juvenile myelomonocytic leukemia**

     C93.30   **Juvenile myelomonocytic leukemia, not having achieved remission** 🔖   P
Juvenile myelomonocytic leukemia with failed remission
Juvenile myelomonocytic leukemia NOS

     C93.31   **Juvenile myelomonocytic leukemia, in remission** 🔖   P

     C93.32   **Juvenile myelomonocytic leukemia, in relapse** 🔖   P

● **C93.Z**   **Other monocytic leukemia**

     C93.Z0   **Other monocytic leukemia, not having achieved remission** 🔖
Other monocytic leukemia NOS

     C93.Z1   **Other monocytic leukemia, in remission** 🔖

     C93.Z2   **Other monocytic leukemia, in relapse** 🔖

● **C93.9**   **Monocytic leukemia, unspecified**

     C93.90   **Monocytic leukemia, unspecified, not having achieved remission** 🔖
Monocytic leukemia, unspecified with failed remission
Monocytic leukemia, unspecified NOS

     C93.91   **Monocytic leukemia, unspecified in remission** 🔖

     C93.92   **Monocytic leukemia, unspecified in relapse** 🔖

CHAPTER 2 (C00-D49)

N   Newborn Age: 0   P   Pediatric Age: 0–17   M   Maternity DX: 12–55   A   Adult Age: 15–124   ♀   Females Only   ♂   Males Only

🔖   Complication\Comorbidity   🔖   Major C\C   Ⓔₓ   CC/MCC Exclusions   🔖   Present on Admission Requirement   🔖   Hospital-Acquired Condition

807

● **C94**   **Other leukemias of specified cell type**

> **Excludes1**   leukemic reticuloendotheliosis (C91.4-)
> myelodysplastic syndromes (D46.-)
> personal history of leukemia (Z85.6)
> plasma cell leukemia (C90.1-)

(Ex:) **For category C94 CC codes unless otherwise indicated:** C88.2-C88.3, C88.8-C90.02, C90.10-C90.12, C90.20-C90.22, C90.30-C90.32, C91.00-C91.02, C91.10-C91.12, C91.30-C91.32, C91.50-C91.52, C91.60-C91.62, C91.90-C91.92, C91.A0-C91.A2, C91.Z0-C91.Z2, C92.00-C92.02, C92.10-C92.12, C92.20-C92.22, C92.30-C92.32, C92.40-C92.42, C92.50-C92.52, C92.60-C92.62, C92.90-C92.92, C92.A0-C92.A2, C92.Z0-C92.Z2, C93.00-C93.02, C93.10-C93.12, C93.30-C93.32, C93.90-C93.92, C93.Z0-C93.Z2, C94.00-C94.02, C94.20-C94.22, C94.30-C94.32, C94.80-C94.82, C95.00-C95.02, C95.10-C95.12, C95.90-C95.92, D49.81-D49.9

● **C94.0**   **Acute erythroid leukemia**
Acute myeloid leukemia M6(a)(b)
Erythroleukemia

     C94.00   **Acute erythroid leukemia, not having achieved remission** 🔲
Acute erythroid leukemia with failed remission
Acute erythroid leukemia NOS

     C94.01   **Acute erythroid leukemia, in remission** 🔲

     C94.02   **Acute erythroid leukemia, in relapse** 🔲

● **C94.2**   **Acute megakaryoblastic leukemia**
Acute myeloid leukemia M7
Acute megakaryocytic leukemia

     C94.20   **Acute megakaryoblastic leukemia not having achieved remission** 🔲
Acute megakaryoblastic leukemia with failed remission
Acute megakaryoblastic leukemia NOS

     C94.21   **Acute megakaryoblastic leukemia, in remission** 🔲

     C94.22   **Acute megakaryoblastic leukemia, in relapse** 🔲

● **C94.3**   **Mast cell leukemia**

     C94.30   **Mast cell leukemia not having achieved remission** 🔲
Mast cell leukemia with failed remission
Mast cell leukemia NOS

     C94.31   **Mast cell leukemia, in remission** 🔲

     C94.32   **Mast cell leukemia, in relapse** 🔲

● **C94.4**   **Acute panmyelosis with myelofibrosis**
Acute myelofibrosis

> **Excludes1**   myelofibrosis NOS (D75.81)
> secondary myelofibrosis NOS (D75.81)

(Ex:) C88.2-C88.3, C88.8-C88.9, C90.10-C90.11, C90.20-C90.21, C90.30-C90.31, C91.00-C91.02, C91.10-C91.12, C91.30-C91.32, C91.40-C91.42, C91.50-C91.52, C91.60-C91.62, C91.90-C91.92, C91.A0-C91.A2, C91.Z0-C91.Z2, C92.00-C92.02, C92.10-C92.12, C92.20-C92.22, C92.30-C92.32, C92.40-C92.42, C92.50-C92.52, C92.60-C92.62, C92.90-C92.92, C92.A0-C92.A2, C92.Z0-C92.Z2, C93.00-C93.02, C93.10-C93.12, C93.30-C93.32, C93.90-C93.92, C93.Z0-C93.Z2, C94.00-C94.02, C94.20-C94.22, C94.30-C94.32, C94.40-C94.42, C94.6, C94.80-C94.82, C95.00-C95.02, C95.10-C95.12, C95.90-C95.92, D45-D46.22, D46.9, D46.A-D46.Z, D47.0-D47.1, D47.3, D47.9, D47.Z9, D48.7-D48.9

     C94.40   **Acute panmyelosis with myelofibrosis not having achieved remission** 🔲
Acute myelofibrosis NOS
Acute panmyelosis with myelofibrosis with failed remission
Acute panmyelosis NOS

     C94.41   **Acute panmyelosis with myelofibrosis, in remission** 🔲

     C94.42   **Acute panmyelosis with myelofibrosis, in relapse** 🔲

● **C94.6**   **Myelodysplastic disease, not classified** 🔲
Myeloproliferative disease, not classified
(Ex:) See C94.4

● **C94.8**   **Other specified leukemias**
Aggressive NK-cell leukemia
Acute basophilic leukemia

     C94.80   **Other specified leukemias not having achieved remission** 🔲
Other specified leukemia with failed remission
Other specified leukemias NOS

     C94.81   **Other specified leukemias, in remission** 🔲

     C94.82   **Other specified leukemias, in relapse** 🔲

● **C95**   **Leukemia of unspecified cell type**

> **Excludes1**   personal history of leukemia (Z85.6)

(Ex:) **For category C95 CC codes:** C88.2-C88.3, C88.8-C90.02, C90.10-C90.12, C90.20-C90.22, C90.30-C90.32, C91.00-C91.02, C91.10-C91.12, C91.30-C91.32, C91.50-C91.52, C91.60-C91.62, C91.90-C91.92, C91.A0-C91.A2, C91.Z0-C91.Z2, C92.00-C92.02, C92.10-C92.12, C92.20-C92.22, C92.30-C92.32, C92.40-C92.42, C92.50-C92.52, C92.60-C92.62, C92.90-C92.92, C92.A0-C92.A2, C92.Z0-C92.Z2, C93.00-C93.02, C93.10-C93.12, C93.30-C93.32, C93.90-C93.92, C93.Z0-C93.Z2, C94.00-C94.02, C94.20-C94.22, C94.30-C94.32, C94.80-C94.82, C95.00-C95.02, C95.10-C95.12, C95.90-C95.92, D49.81-D49.9

● **C95.0**   **Acute leukemia of unspecified cell type**
Acute bilineal leukemia
Acute mixed lineage leukemia
Biphenotypic acute leukemia
Stem cell leukemia of unclear lineage

> **Excludes1**   acute exacerbation of unspecified chronic leukemia (C95.10)

     C95.00   **Acute leukemia of unspecified cell type not having achieved remission** 🔲
Acute leukemia of unspecified cell type with failed remission
Acute leukemia NOS

     C95.01   **Acute leukemia of unspecified cell type, in remission** 🔲

     C95.02   **Acute leukemia of unspecified cell type, in relapse** 🔲

● **C95.1**   **Chronic leukemia of unspecified cell type**

     C95.10   **Chronic leukemia of unspecified cell type not having achieved remission** 🔲
Chronic leukemia of unspecified cell type with failed remission
Chronic leukemia NOS

     C95.11   **Chronic leukemia of unspecified cell type, in remission** 🔲

     C95.12   **Chronic leukemia of unspecified cell type, in relapse** 🔲

● **C95.9**   **Leukemia, unspecified**

     C95.90   **Leukemia, unspecified not having achieved remission** 🔲
Leukemia, unspecified with failed remission
Leukemia NOS

     C95.91   **Leukemia, unspecified, in remission** 🔲

     C95.92   **Leukemia, unspecified, in relapse** 🔲

◀ New   ◀|||| Revised   ~~deleted~~ Deleted   Excludes 1   Excludes 2   Includes   Use additional   Code first   Code also   Unspecified

OGCR Official Guidelines   ● Unacceptable Principal Diagnosis   X Assign placeholder X   🔲 Use Additional Character(s)   ▌ Manifestation Code   **Coding Clinic**

● **C96　Other and unspecified malignant neoplasms of lymphoid, hematopoietic and related tissue**

　　Excludes1　personal history of other malignant neoplasms of lymphoid, hematopoietic and related tissues (Z85.79)

C96.0　Multifocal and multisystemic (disseminated) Langerhans-cell histiocytosis
　　Histiocytosis X, multisystemic
　　Letterer-Siwe disease

　　Excludes1　adult pulmonary Langerhans cell histiocytosis (J84.82)
　　　　　　　　multifocal and unisystemic Langerhans-cell histiocytosis (C96.5)
　　　　　　　　unifocal Langerhans-cell histiocytosis (C96.6)

　　(Ex:) C82.50, C82.59, C83.10, C83.19, C84.40, C84.49-C84.60, C84.69-C84.70, C84.79, C84.90, C84.99, C84.A0, C84.A9-C84.Z0, C84.Z9, C85.10, C85.19-C85.20, C85.29-C85.80, C85.89-C85.90, C85.99, C86.4, C88.4, C96.0, C96.4, C96.9, C96.Z, D49.81-D49.9

C96.2　Malignant mast cell tumor
　　Aggressive systemic mastocytosis
　　Mast cell sarcoma

　　Excludes1　indolent mastocytosis (D47.0)
　　　　　　　　mast cell leukemia (C94.30)
　　　　　　　　mastocytosis (congenital) (cutaneous) (Q82.2)

　　(Ex:) C82.50, C82.59, C83.10, C83.19, C84.40, C84.49-C84.60, C84.69-C84.70, C84.79, C84.90, C84.99, C84.A0, C84.A9-C84.Z0, C84.Z9, C85.10, C85.19-C85.20, C85.29-C85.80, C85.89-C85.90, C85.99, C86.4, C88.4, C96.2, C96.4, C96.9, C96.Z, D49.81-D49.9

C96.4　Sarcoma of dendritic cells (accessory cells)
　　Follicular dendritic cell sarcoma
　　Interdigitating dendritic cell sarcoma
　　Langerhans cell sarcoma
　　(Ex:) C96.4, C96.9, C96.Z, D49.81-D49.9

C96.5　Multifocal and unisystemic Langerhans-cell histiocytosis
　　Hand-Schüller-Christian disease
　　Histiocytosis X, multifocal

　　Excludes1　multifocal and multisystemic (disseminated) Langerhans-cell histiocytosis (C96.0)
　　　　　　　　unifocal Langerhans-cell histiocytosis (C96.6)

　　(Ex:) E71.310-E71.32, E71.40-E71.548, E80.4-E80.7, E88.40-E88.49, H49.811-H49.819

C96.6　Unifocal Langerhans-cell histiocytosis
　　Eosinophilic granuloma
　　Histiocytosis X, unifocal
　　Histiocytosis X NOS
　　Langerhans-cell histiocytosis NOS

　　Excludes1　multifocal and multisysemic (disseminated) Langerhans-cell histiocytosis (C96.0)
　　　　　　　　multifocal and unisystemic Langerhans-cell histiocytosis (C96.5)

　　(Ex:) See C96.5

C96.A　Histiocytic sarcoma
　　Malignant histiocytosis
　　(Ex:) C82.50, C82.59, C83.10, C83.19, C84.40, C84.49-C84.60, C84.69-C84.70, C84.79, C84.90, C84.99, C84.A0, C84.A9-C84.Z0, C84.Z9, C85.10, C85.19-C85.20, C85.29-C85.80, C85.89-C85.90, C85.99, C86.4, C88.4, C96.4, C96.9, C96.A, C96.Z, D49.81-D49.9

C96.Z　Other specified malignant neoplasms of lymphoid, hematopoietic and related tissue
　　(Ex:) See C96.4

C96.9　Malignant neoplasm of lymphoid, hematopoietic and related tissue, unspecified
　　(Ex:) See C96.4

In situ is carcinoma involving cells in localized tissues that has not spread to nearby tissues

IN SITU NEOPLASMS (D00-D09)

　　Includes　Bowen's disease
　　　　　　　erythroplasia
　　　　　　　grade III intraepithelial neoplasia
　　　　　　　Queyrat's erythroplasia

● **D00　Carcinoma in situ of oral cavity, esophagus and stomach**

　　Excludes1　melanoma in situ (D03.-)

● **D00.0　Carcinoma in situ of lip, oral cavity and pharynx**
　　Use additional code to identify:
　　exposure to environmental tobacco smoke (Z77.22)
　　exposure to tobacco smoke in the perinatal period (P96.81)
　　history of tobacco use (Z87.891)
　　occupational exposure to environmental tobacco smoke (Z57.31)
　　tobacco dependence (F17.-)
　　tobacco use (Z72.0)

　　Excludes1　carcinoma in situ of aryepiglottic fold or interarytenoid fold, laryngeal aspect (D02.0)
　　　　　　　　carcinoma in situ of epiglottis NOS (D02.0)
　　　　　　　　carcinoma in situ of epiglottis suprahyoid portion (D02.0)
　　　　　　　　carcinoma in situ of skin of lip (D03.0, D04.0)

D00.00　Carcinoma in situ of oral cavity, unspecified site

D00.01　Carcinoma in situ of labial mucosa and vermilion border

D00.02　Carcinoma in situ of buccal mucosa

D00.03　Carcinoma in situ of gingiva and edentulous alveolar ridge

D00.04　Carcinoma in situ of soft palate

D00.05　Carcinoma in situ of hard palate

D00.06　Carcinoma in situ of floor of mouth

D00.07　Carcinoma in situ of tongue

D00.08　Carcinoma in situ of pharynx
　　Carcinoma in situ of aryepiglottic fold NOS
　　Carcinoma in situ of hypopharyngeal aspect of aryepiglottic fold
　　Carcinoma in situ of marginal zone of aryepiglottic fold

D00.1　Carcinoma in situ of esophagus

D00.2　Carcinoma in situ of stomach

● **D01　Carcinoma in situ of other and unspecified digestive organs**

　　Excludes1　melanoma in situ (D03.-)

D01.0　Carcinoma in situ of colon

　　Excludes1　carcinoma in situ of rectosigmoid junction (D01.1)

D01.1　Carcinoma in situ of rectosigmoid junction

D01.2　Carcinoma in situ of rectum

D01.3　Carcinoma in situ of anus and anal canal

　　Excludes1　carcinoma in situ of anal margin (D04.5)
　　　　　　　　carcinoma in situ of anal skin (D04.5)
　　　　　　　　carcinoma in situ of perianal skin (D04.5)

● **D01.4　Carcinoma in situ of other and unspecified parts of intestine**

　　Excludes1　carcinoma in situ of ampulla of Vater (D01.5)

D01.40　Carcinoma in situ of unspecified part of intestine

D01.49　Carcinoma in situ of other parts of intestine

D01.5　Carcinoma in situ of liver, gallbladder and bile ducts
　　Carcinoma in situ of ampulla of Vater

D01.7　Carcinoma in situ of other specified digestive organs
　　Carcinoma in situ of pancreas

D01.9　Carcinoma in situ of digestive organ, unspecified

N　Newborn Age: 0　　**P**　Pediatric Age: 0–17　　**M**　Maternity DX: 12–55　　**A**　Adult Age: 15–124　　♀　Females Only　　♂　Males Only

　Complication\Comorbidity　　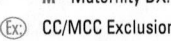　Major C\C　　(Ex:)　CC/MCC Exclusions　　　Present on Admission Requirement　　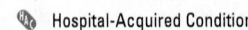　Hospital-Acquired Condition

809

● **D02**   **Carcinoma in situ of middle ear and respiratory system**
Use additional code to identify:
    exposure to environmental tobacco smoke (Z77.22)
    exposure to tobacco smoke in the perinatal period (P96.81)
    history of tobacco use (Z87.891)
    occupational exposure to environmental tobacco smoke
        (Z57.31)
    tobacco dependence (F17.-)
    tobacco use (Z72.0)
> **Excludes1**   melanoma in situ (D03.-)

D02.0   **Carcinoma in situ of larynx**
Carcinoma in situ of aryepiglottic fold or interarytenoid
    fold, laryngeal aspect
Carcinoma in situ of epiglottis (suprahyoid portion)
> **Excludes1**   carcinoma in situ of aryepiglottic fold or
>   interarytenoid fold NOS (D00.08)
> carcinoma in situ of hypopharyngeal
>   aspect (D00.08)
> carcinoma in situ of marginal zone
>   (D00.08)

D02.1   **Carcinoma in situ of trachea**

● **D02.2**   **Carcinoma in situ of bronchus and lung**
     D02.20   Carcinoma in situ of unspecified bronchus and
           lung
     D02.21   Carcinoma in situ of right bronchus and lung
     D02.22   Carcinoma in situ of left bronchus and lung

D02.3   **Carcinoma in situ of other parts of respiratory system**
Carcinoma in situ of accessory sinuses
Carcinoma in situ of middle ear
Carcinoma in situ of nasal cavities
> **Excludes1**   carcinoma in situ of ear (external) (skin)
>   (D04.2-)
> carcinoma in situ of nose NOS (D09.8)
> carcinoma in situ of skin of nose (D04.3)

D02.4   **Carcinoma in situ of respiratory system, unspecified**

● **D03**   **Melanoma in situ**
D03.0   **Melanoma in situ of lip**

● **D03.1**   **Melanoma in situ of eyelid, including canthus**
     D03.10   Melanoma in situ of unspecified eyelid,
           including canthus
     D03.11   Melanoma in situ of right eyelid, including
           canthus
     D03.12   Melanoma in situ of left eyelid, including
           canthus

● **D03.2**   **Melanoma in situ of ear and external auricular canal**
     D03.20   Melanoma in situ of unspecified ear and
           external auricular canal
     D03.21   Melanoma in situ of right ear and external
           auricular canal
     D03.22   Melanoma in situ of left ear and external
           auricular canal

● **D03.3**   **Melanoma in situ of other and unspecified parts of face**
     D03.30   Melanoma in situ of unspecified part of face
     D03.39   Melanoma in situ of other parts of face

D03.4   **Melanoma in situ of scalp and neck**

● **D03.5**   **Melanoma in situ of trunk**
     D03.51   Melanoma in situ of anal skin
            Melanoma in situ of anal margin
            Melanoma in situ of perianal skin
     D03.52   Melanoma in situ of breast (skin) (soft tissue)
     D03.59   Melanoma in situ of other part of trunk

● **D03.6**   **Melanoma in situ of upper limb, including shoulder**
     D03.60   Melanoma in situ of unspecified upper limb,
           including shoulder
     D03.61   Melanoma in situ of right upper limb,
           including shoulder
     D03.62   Melanoma in situ of left upper limb, including
           shoulder

D03.7   **Melanoma in situ of lower limb, including hip**
     D03.70   Melanoma in situ of unspecified lower limb,
           including hip
     D03.71   Melanoma in situ of right lower limb, including
           hip
     D03.72   Melanoma in situ of left lower limb, including
           hip

D03.8   **Melanoma in situ of other sites**
Melanoma in situ of scrotum
> **Excludes1**   carcinoma in situ of scrotum (D07.61)

D03.9   **Melanoma in situ, unspecified**

● **D04**   **Carcinoma in situ of skin**
> **Excludes1**   erythroplasia of Queyrat (penis) NOS (D07.4)
> melanoma in situ (D03.-)

D04.0   **Carcinoma in situ of skin of lip**
> **Excludes1**   carcinoma in situ of vermilion border of lip
>   (D00.01)

● **D04.1**   **Carcinoma in situ of skin of eyelid, including canthus**
     D04.10   Carcinoma in situ of skin of unspecified eyelid,
           including canthus
     D04.11   Carcinoma in situ of skin of right eyelid,
           including canthus
     D04.12   Carcinoma in situ of skin of left eyelid,
           including canthus

● **D04.2**   **Carcinoma in situ of skin of ear and external auricular
canal**
     D04.20   Carcinoma in situ of skin of unspecified ear and
           external auricular canal
     D04.21   Carcinoma in situ of skin of right ear and
           external auricular canal
     D04.22   Carcinoma in situ of skin of left ear and
           external auricular canal

● **D04.3**   **Carcinoma in situ of skin of other and unspecified parts
of face**
     D04.30   Carcinoma in situ of skin of unspecified part of
           face
     D04.39   Carcinoma in situ of skin of other parts of face

D04.4   **Carcinoma in situ of skin of scalp and neck**

D04.5   **Carcinoma in situ of skin of trunk**
Carcinoma in situ of anal margin
Carcinoma in situ of anal skin
Carcinoma in situ of perianal skin
Carcinoma in situ of skin of breast
> **Excludes1**   carcinoma in situ of anus NOS (D01.3)
> carcinoma in situ of scrotum (D07.61)
> carcinoma in situ of skin of genital organs
>   (D07.-)

● **D04.6**   **Carcinoma in situ of skin of upper limb, including
shoulder**
     D04.60   Carcinoma in situ of skin of unspecified upper
           limb, including shoulder
     D04.61   Carcinoma in situ of skin of right upper limb,
           including shoulder
     D04.62   Carcinoma in situ of skin of left upper limb,
           including shoulder

● **D04.7**   **Carcinoma in situ of skin of lower limb, including hip**
     D04.70   Carcinoma in situ of skin of unspecified lower
           limb, including hip
     D04.71   Carcinoma in situ of skin of right lower limb,
           including hip
     D04.72   Carcinoma in situ of skin of left lower limb,
           including hip

D04.8   **Carcinoma in situ of skin of other sites**

D04.9   **Carcinoma in situ of skin, unspecified**

◀ New   ◀ Revised   ~~deleted~~ Deleted   Excludes 1   Excludes 2   Includes   Use additional   Code first   Code also   Unspecified
OGCR Official Guidelines   ● Unacceptable Principal Diagnosis   X Assign placeholder X   ▮ Use Additional Character(s)   ▮ Manifestation Code   **Coding Clinic**

● **D05 Carcinoma in situ of breast**

> **Excludes1** carcinoma in situ of skin of breast (D04.5)
> melanoma in situ of breast (skin) (D03.5)
> Paget's disease of breast or nipple (C50.-)

● **D05.0 Lobular carcinoma in situ of breast**

> **D05.00** Lobular carcinoma in situ of unspecified breast
> **D05.01** Lobular carcinoma in situ of right breast
> **D05.02** Lobular carcinoma in situ of left breast

● **D05.1 Intraductal carcinoma in situ of breast**

> **D05.10** Intraductal carcinoma in situ of unspecified breast
> **D05.11** Intraductal carcinoma in situ of right breast
> **D05.12** Intraductal carcinoma in situ of left breast

● **D05.8 Other specified type of carcinoma in situ of breast**

> **D05.80** Other specified type of carcinoma in situ of unspecified breast
> **D05.81** Other specified type of carcinoma in situ of right breast
> **D05.82** Other specified type of carcinoma in situ of left breast

● **D05.9 Unspecified type of carcinoma in situ of breast**

> **D05.90** Unspecified type of carcinoma in situ of unspecified breast
> **D05.91** Unspecified type of carcinoma in situ of right breast
> **D05.92** Unspecified type of carcinoma in situ of left breast

● **D06 Carcinoma in situ of cervix uteri**

> **Includes** cervical adenocarcinoma in situ
> cervical intraepithelial glandular neoplasia
> cervical intraepithelial neoplasia III [CIN III]
> severe dysplasia of cervix uteri
>
> **Excludes1** cervical intraepithelial neoplasia II [CIN II] (N87.1)
> cytologic evidence of malignancy of cervix without histologic confirmation (R87.614)
> high grade squamous intraepithelial lesion (HGSIL) of cervix (R87.613)
> melanoma in situ of cervix (D03.5)
> moderate cervical dysplasia (N87.1)

D06.0 Carcinoma in situ of endocervix ♀
D06.1 Carcinoma in situ of exocervix ♀
D06.7 Carcinoma in situ of other parts of cervix ♀
D06.9 Carcinoma in situ of cervix, unspecified ♀

● **D07 Carcinoma in situ of other and unspecified genital organs**

> **Excludes1** melanoma in situ of trunk (D03.5)

D07.0 Carcinoma in situ of endometrium ♀
D07.1 Carcinoma in situ of vulva ♀
> Severe dysplasia of vulva
> Vulvar intraepithelial neoplasia III [VIN III]
>
> **Excludes1** moderate dysplasia of vulva (N90.1)
> vulvar intraepithelial neoplasia II [VIN II] (N90.1)

D07.2 Carcinoma in situ of vagina ♀
> Severe dysplasia of vagina
> Vaginal intraepithelial neoplasia III [VIN III]
>
> **Excludes1** moderate dysplasia of vagina (N89.1)
> vaginal intraepithelial neoplasia II [VIN II] (N89.1)

● **D07.3 Carcinoma in situ of other and unspecified female genital organs**

> **D07.30** Carcinoma in situ of unspecified female genital organs ♀
> **D07.39** Carcinoma in situ of other female genital organs ♀

D07.4 Carcinoma in situ of penis ♂
> Erythroplasia of Queyrat NOS

D07.5 Carcinoma in situ of prostate ♂
> Prostatic intraepithelial neoplasia III (PIN III)
> Severe dysplasia of prostate
>
> **Excludes1** dysplasia (mild) (moderate) of prostate (N42.3)

● **D07.6 Carcinoma in situ of other and unspecified male genital organs**

> **D07.60** Carcinoma in situ of unspecified male genital organs ♂
> **D07.61** Carcinoma in situ of scrotum ♂
> **D07.69** Carcinoma in situ of other male genital organs ♂

● **D09 Carcinoma in situ of other and unspecified sites**

> **Excludes1** melanoma in situ (D03.-)

D09.0 Carcinoma in situ of bladder

● **D09.1 Carcinoma in situ of other and unspecified urinary organs**

> **D09.10** Carcinoma in situ of unspecified urinary organ
> **D09.19** Carcinoma in situ of other urinary organs

● **D09.2 Carcinoma in situ of eye**

> **Excludes1** carcinoma in situ of skin of eyelid (D04.1-)
>
> **D09.20** Carcinoma in situ of unspecified eye
> **D09.21** Carcinoma in situ of right eye
> **D09.22** Carcinoma in situ of left eye

D09.3 Carcinoma in situ of thyroid and other endocrine glands

> **Excludes1** carcinoma in situ of endocrine pancreas (D01.7)
> carcinoma in situ of ovary (D07.39)
> carcinoma in situ of testis (D07.69)

D09.8 Carcinoma in situ of other specified sites
D09.9 Carcinoma in situ, unspecified

BENIGN NEOPLASMS, EXCEPT BENIGN NEUROENDOCRINE TUMORS (D10-D36)

● **D10 Benign neoplasm of mouth and pharynx**

D10.0 Benign neoplasm of lip
> Benign neoplasm of lip (frenulum) (inner aspect) (mucosa) (vermilion border)
>
> **Excludes1** benign neoplasm of skin of lip (D22.0, D23.0)

D10.1 Benign neoplasm of tongue
> Benign neoplasm of lingual tonsil

D10.2 Benign neoplasm of floor of mouth

● **D10.3 Other and unspecified parts of mouth**

> **D10.30** Benign neoplasm of unspecified part of mouth
> **D10.39** Benign neoplasm of other parts of mouth
> Benign neoplasm of minor salivary gland NOS
>
> **Excludes1** benign odontogenic neoplasms (D16.4-D16.5)
> benign neoplasm of mucosa of lip (D10.0)
> benign neoplasm of nasopharyngeal surface of soft palate (D10.6)

D10.4 Benign neoplasm of tonsil
> Benign neoplasm of tonsil (faucial) (palatine)
>
> **Excludes1** benign neoplasm of lingual tonsil (D10.1)
> benign neoplasm of pharyngeal tonsil (D10.6)
> benign neoplasm of tonsillar fossa (D10.5)
> benign neoplasm of tonsillar pillars (D10.5)

CHAPTER 2 (C00-D49)

N Newborn Age: 0   **P** Pediatric Age: 0–17   **M** Maternity DX: 12–55   **A** Adult Age: 15–124   ♀ Females Only   ♂ Males Only

 Complication\Comorbidity   Major C\C   (Exc) CC/MCC Exclusions   Present on Admission Requirement   Hospital-Acquired Condition

811

Figure 2-16 The esophagus is the muscular tube that connects the pharynx and the stomach. The 10 inch (25 cm) long esophagus is divided into three parts: **cervical, thoracic,** and **abdominal.**

D10.5   Benign neoplasm of other parts of oropharynx
Division of pharynx lying between soft palate and upper edge of epiglottis
Benign neoplasm of epiglottis, anterior aspect
Benign neoplasm of tonsillar fossa
Benign neoplasm of tonsillar pillars
Benign neoplasm of vallecula
    Excludes1   benign neoplasm of epiglottis NOS (D14.1)
                 benign neoplasm of epiglottis, suprahyoid portion (D14.1)

D10.6   Benign neoplasm of nasopharynx
Segment of pharynx that lies above soft palate
Benign neoplasm of pharyngeal tonsil
Benign neoplasm of posterior margin of septum and choanae

D10.7   Benign neoplasm of hypopharynx
Segment of pharynx that lies below upper edge of epiglottis and opens into larynx and esophagus

D10.9   Benign neoplasm of pharynx, unspecified

● **D11   Benign neoplasm of major salivary glands**
    Excludes1   benign neoplasms of specified minor salivary glands which are classified according to their anatomical location
                 benign neoplasms of minor salivary glands NOS (D10.39)

D11.0   Benign neoplasm of parotid gland

D11.7   Benign neoplasm of other major salivary glands
Benign neoplasm of sublingual salivary gland
Benign neoplasm of submandibular salivary gland

D11.9   Benign neoplasm of major salivary gland, unspecified

● **D12   Benign neoplasm of colon, rectum, anus and anal canal**
    Excludes1   benign carcinoid tumors of the large intestine, and rectum (D3A.02-)

D12.0   Benign neoplasm of cecum
Benign neoplasm of ileocecal valve

D12.1   Benign neoplasm of appendix
    Excludes1   benign carcinoid tumor of the appendix (D3A.020)

D12.2   Benign neoplasm of ascending colon

D12.3   Benign neoplasm of transverse colon
Benign neoplasm of hepatic flexure
Benign neoplasm of splenic flexure
Flexure is a bending in a structure or organ. Note the three flexures illustrated in Figure 2–17. Hepatic = liver, sigmoid = colon, splenic = spleen.

D12.4   Benign neoplasm of descending colon

D12.5   Benign neoplasm of sigmoid colon

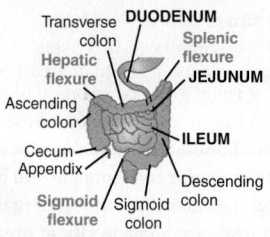

Figure 2-17   Small intestine and colon.

D12.6   Benign neoplasm of colon, unspecified
Adenomatosis of colon
Benign neoplasm of large intestine NOS
Polyposis (hereditary) of colon
    Excludes1   inflammatory polyp of colon (K51.4-)
                 polyp of colon NOS (K63.5)

D12.7   Benign neoplasm of rectosigmoid junction
Angle where sigmoid colon becomes rectum

D12.8   Benign neoplasm of rectum
    Excludes1   benign carcinoid tumor of the rectum (D3A.026)

D12.9   Benign neoplasm of anus and anal canal
Benign neoplasm of anus NOS
    Excludes1   benign neoplasm of anal margin (D22.5, D23.5)
                 benign neoplasm of anal skin (D22.5, D23.5)
                 benign neoplasm of perianal skin (D22.5, D23.5)

● **D13   Benign neoplasm of other and ill-defined parts of digestive system**
    Excludes1   benign stromal tumors of digestive system (D21.4)

D13.0   Benign neoplasm of esophagus

D13.1   Benign neoplasm of stomach
    Excludes1   benign carcinoid tumor of the stomach (D3A.092)

D13.2   Benign neoplasm of duodenum
    Excludes1   benign carcinoid tumor of the duodenum (D3A.010)

● **D13.3   Benign neoplasm of other and unspecified parts of small intestine**
    Excludes1   benign carcinoid tumors of the small intestine (D3A.01-)
                 benign neoplasm of ileocecal valve (D12.0)

D13.30   Benign neoplasm of unspecified part of small intestine

D13.39   Benign neoplasm of other parts of small intestine

D13.4   Benign neoplasm of liver
Benign neoplasm of intrahepatic bile ducts

D13.5   Benign neoplasm of extrahepatic bile ducts
Extensions of common hepatic bile duct (tube that collects bile from liver)

D13.6   Benign neoplasm of pancreas
    Excludes1   benign neoplasm of endocrine pancreas (D13.7)

D13.7   Benign neoplasm of endocrine pancreas
Pancreatic islets: Cells scattered throughout pancreas
Islet cell tumor
Benign neoplasm of islets of Langerhans
Use additional code to identify any functional activity.

D13.9   Benign neoplasm of ill-defined sites within the digestive system
Benign neoplasm of digestive system NOS
Benign neoplasm of intestine NOS
Benign neoplasm of spleen

CHAPTER 2 (C00-D49)

812

◄ New   ◄▦ Revised   ~~deleted~~ Deleted   Excludes 1   Excludes 2   Includes   Use additional   Code first   Code also   Unspecified
OGCR Official Guidelines   ● Unacceptable Principal Diagnosis   X Assign placeholder X   ● Use Additional Character(s)   ▌ Manifestation Code   **Coding Clinic**

● **D14 Benign neoplasm of middle ear and respiratory system**

  D14.0 Benign neoplasm of middle ear, nasal cavity and accessory sinuses
    Benign neoplasm of cartilage of nose

    Excludes1 benign neoplasm of auricular canal (external) (D22.2-, D23.2-)
      benign neoplasm of bone of ear (D16.4)
      benign neoplasm of bone of nose (D16.4)
      benign neoplasm of cartilage of ear (D21.0)
      benign neoplasm of ear (external) (skin) (D22.2-, D23.2-)
      benign neoplasm of nose NOS (D36.7)
      benign neoplasm of skin of nose (D22.39, D23.39)
      benign neoplasm of olfactory bulb (D33.3)
      benign neoplasm of posterior margin of septum and choanae (D10.6)
      polyp of accessory sinus (J33.8)
      polyp of ear (middle) (H74.4)
      polyp of nasal (cavity) (J33.-)

  D14.1 Benign neoplasm of larynx
    Adenomatous polyp of larynx
    Benign neoplasm of epiglottis (suprahyoid portion)
    Horseshoe shaped bone in anterior midline of neck between chin and thyroid cartilage

    Excludes1 benign neoplasm of epiglottis, anterior aspect (D10.5)
      polyp (nonadenomatous) of vocal cord or larynx (J38.1)

  D14.2 Benign neoplasm of trachea

●   **D14.3 Benign neoplasm of bronchus and lung**
    Excludes1 benign carcinoid tumor of the bronchus and lung (D3A.090)

    D14.30 Benign neoplasm of unspecified bronchus and lung

    D14.31 Benign neoplasm of right bronchus and lung

    D14.32 Benign neoplasm of left bronchus and lung

  D14.4 Benign neoplasm of respiratory system, unspecified

● **D15 Benign neoplasm of other and unspecified intrathoracic organs**
  Excludes1 benign neoplasm of mesothelial tissue (D19.-)

  D15.0 Benign neoplasm of thymus
    Excludes1 benign carcinoid tumor of the thymus (D3A.091)

  D15.1 Benign neoplasm of heart
    Excludes1 benign neoplasm of great vessels (D21.3)

  D15.2 Benign neoplasm of mediastinum

  D15.7 Benign neoplasm of other specified intrathoracic organs

  D15.9 Benign neoplasm of intrathoracic organ, unspecified

● **D16 Benign neoplasm of bone and articular cartilage**
  Excludes1 benign neoplasm of connective tissue of ear (D21.0)
    benign neoplasm of connective tissue of eyelid (D21.0)
    benign neoplasm of connective tissue of larynx (D14.1)
    benign neoplasm of connective tissue of nose (D14.0)
    benign neoplasm of synovia (D21.-)

●   **D16.0 Benign neoplasm of scapula and long bones of upper limb**
    D16.00 Benign neoplasm of scapula and long bones of unspecified upper limb

    D16.01 Benign neoplasm of scapula and long bones of right upper limb

    D16.02 Benign neoplasm of scapula and long bones of left upper limb

●   **D16.1 Benign neoplasm of short bones of upper limb**
    D16.10 Benign neoplasm of short bones of unspecified upper limb

    D16.11 Benign neoplasm of short bones of right upper limb

    D16.12 Benign neoplasm of short bones of left upper limb

●   **D16.2 Benign neoplasm of long bones of lower limb**
    D16.20 Benign neoplasm of long bones of unspecified lower limb

    D16.21 Benign neoplasm of long bones of right lower limb

    D16.22 Benign neoplasm of long bones of left lower limb

●   **D16.3 Benign neoplasm of short bones of lower limb**
    D16.30 Benign neoplasm of short bones of unspecified lower limb

    D16.31 Benign neoplasm of short bones of right lower limb

    D16.32 Benign neoplasm of short bones of left lower limb

  D16.4 Benign neoplasm of bones of skull and face
    Benign neoplasm of maxilla (superior)
    Benign neoplasm of orbital bone
    Cavity or socket of skull in which eye and its appendages are located
    Keratocyst of maxilla
    Keratocystic odontogenic tumor of maxilla
    Excludes1 benign neoplasm of lower jaw bone (D16.5)

  D16.5 Benign neoplasm of lower jaw bone
    Keratocyst of mandible
    Keratocystic odontogenic tumor of mandible

  D16.6 Benign neoplasm of vertebral column
    Excludes1 benign neoplasm of sacrum and coccyx (D16.8)

  D16.7 Benign neoplasm of ribs, sternum and clavicle

  D16.8 Benign neoplasm of pelvic bones, sacrum and coccyx

  D16.9 Benign neoplasm of bone and articular cartilage, unspecified

● **D17 Benign lipomatous neoplasm**
  Slow growing benign tumors (rubbery masses) of mature fat cells enclosed in a thin fibrous capsule

  D17.0 Benign lipomatous neoplasm of skin and subcutaneous tissue of head, face and neck

  D17.1 Benign lipomatous neoplasm of skin and subcutaneous tissue of trunk

●   **D17.2 Benign lipomatous neoplasm of skin and subcutaneous tissue of limb**
    D17.20 Benign lipomatous neoplasm of skin and subcutaneous tissue of unspecified limb

    D17.21 Benign lipomatous neoplasm of skin and subcutaneous tissue of right arm

    D17.22 Benign lipomatous neoplasm of skin and subcutaneous tissue of left arm

    D17.23 Benign lipomatous neoplasm of skin and subcutaneous tissue of right leg

    D17.24 Benign lipomatous neoplasm of skin and subcutaneous tissue of left leg

●   **D17.3 Benign lipomatous neoplasm of skin and subcutaneous tissue of other and unspecified sites**
    D17.30 Benign lipomatous neoplasm of skin and subcutaneous tissue of unspecified sites

    D17.39 Benign lipomatous neoplasm of skin and subcutaneous tissue of other sites

  D17.4 Benign lipomatous neoplasm of intrathoracic organs

Figure 2-18 Hemangioma of skin and subcutaneous tissue. (From Yanoff: Ophthalmology, ed 3, Mosby, Inc., 2008)

Item 2–10 Hemangiomas are abnormally dense collections of dilated capillaries that occur on the skin or in internal organs. Hemangiomas are both deep and superficial and undergo a rapid growth phase when the size increases rapidly, followed by a rest phase, in which the tumor changes very little, followed by an involutional phase in which the tumor begins to and can disappear altogether. **Lymphangiomas** or cystic hygroma are benign collections of overgrown lymph vessels and, although rare, may occur anywhere but most commonly on the head and neck of children and infants. Visceral organs, lungs, and gastrointestinal tract may also be involved.

D17.5   **Benign lipomatous neoplasm of intra-abdominal organs**
> **Excludes1**   benign lipomatous neoplasm of peritoneum and retroperitoneum (D17.79)

D17.6   **Benign lipomatous neoplasm of spermatic cord ♂**

● **D17.7**   **Benign lipomatous neoplasm of other sites**
> **D17.71**   **Benign lipomatous neoplasm of kidney**
> **D17.72**   **Benign lipomatous neoplasm of other genitourinary organ**
> **D17.79**   **Benign lipomatous neoplasm of other sites**
> Benign lipomatous neoplasm of peritoneum
> Benign lipomatous neoplasm of retroperitoneum

D17.9   **Benign lipomatous neoplasm, unspecified**
> Lipoma NOS

● **D18**   **Hemangioma and lymphangioma, any site**
> **Excludes1**   benign neoplasm of glomus jugulare (D35.6)
> blue or pigmented nevus (D22.-)
> nevus NOS (D22.-)
> vascular nevus (Q82.5)

● **D18.0**   **Hemangioma**
> *Common type of vascular malformation*
> Angioma NOS
> Cavernous nevus
> **D18.00**   **Hemangioma unspecified site**
> **D18.01**   **Hemangioma of skin and subcutaneous tissue**
> **D18.02**   **Hemangioma of intracranial structures**
> **D18.03**   **Hemangioma of intra-abdominal structures**
> **D18.09**   **Hemangioma of other sites**

D18.1   **Lymphangioma, any site**

● **D19**   **Benign neoplasm of mesothelial tissue**
> *Mesothelial tissue is the membrane lining several body cavities*
> **D19.0**   **Benign neoplasm of mesothelial tissue of pleura**
> **D19.1**   **Benign neoplasm of mesothelial tissue of peritoneum**
> **D19.7**   **Benign neoplasm of mesothelial tissue of other sites**
> **D19.9**   **Benign neoplasm of mesothelial tissue, unspecified**
> Benign mesothelioma NOS

● **D20**   **Benign neoplasm of soft tissue of retroperitoneum and peritoneum**
> **Excludes1**   benign lipomatous neoplasm of peritoneum and retroperitoneum (D17.79)
> benign neoplasm of mesothelial tissue (D19.-)
> **D20.0**   **Benign neoplasm of soft tissue of retroperitoneum**
> **D20.1**   **Benign neoplasm of soft tissue of peritoneum**

● **D21**   **Other benign neoplasms of connective and other soft tissue**
> **Includes**   benign neoplasm of blood vessel
> benign neoplasm of bursa
> benign neoplasm of cartilage
> benign neoplasm of fascia
> benign neoplasm of fat
> benign neoplasm of ligament, except uterine
> benign neoplasm of lymphatic channel
> benign neoplasm of muscle
> benign neoplasm of synovia
> benign neoplasm of tendon (sheath)
> benign stromal tumors

> **Excludes1**   benign neoplasm of articular cartilage (D16.-)
> benign neoplasm of cartilage of larynx (D14.1)
> benign neoplasm of cartilage of nose (D14.0)
> benign neoplasm of connective tissue of breast (D24.-)
> benign neoplasm of peripheral nerves and autonomic nervous system (D36.1-)
> benign neoplasm of peritoneum (D20.1)
> benign neoplasm of retroperitoneum (D20.0)
> benign neoplasm of uterine ligament, any (D28.2)
> benign neoplasm of vascular tissue (D18.-)
> hemangioma (D18.0-)
> lipomatous neoplasm (D17.-)
> lymphangioma (D18.1)
> uterine leiomyoma (D25.-)

D21.0   **Benign neoplasm of connective and other soft tissue of head, face and neck**
> Benign neoplasm of connective tissue of ear
> Benign neoplasm of connective tissue of eyelid
> **Excludes1**   benign neoplasm of connective tissue of orbit (D31.6-)

● **D21.1**   **Benign neoplasm of connective and other soft tissue of upper limb, including shoulder**
> **D21.10**   **Benign neoplasm of connective and other soft tissue of unspecified upper limb, including shoulder**
> **D21.11**   **Benign neoplasm of connective and other soft tissue of right upper limb, including shoulder**
> **D21.12**   **Benign neoplasm of connective and other soft tissue of left upper limb, including shoulder**

● **D21.2**   **Benign neoplasm of connective and other soft tissue of lower limb, including hip**
> **D21.20**   **Benign neoplasm of connective and other soft tissue of unspecified lower limb, including hip**
> **D21.21**   **Benign neoplasm of connective and other soft tissue of right lower limb, including hip**
> **D21.22**   **Benign neoplasm of connective and other soft tissue of left lower limb, including hip**

D21.3   **Benign neoplasm of connective and other soft tissue of thorax**
> Benign neoplasm of axilla
> Benign neoplasm of diaphragm
> Benign neoplasm of great vessels
> **Excludes1**   benign neoplasm of heart (D15.1)
> benign neoplasm of mediastinum (D15.2)
> benign neoplasm of thymus (D15.0)

D21.4   **Benign neoplasm of connective and other soft tissue of abdomen Benign stromal tumors of abdomen**

D21.5   **Benign neoplasm of connective and other soft tissue of pelvis**
> **Excludes1**   benign neoplasm of any uterine ligament (D28.2)
> uterine leiomyoma (D25.-)

D21.6   **Benign neoplasm of connective and other soft tissue of trunk, unspecified**
> Benign neoplasm of back NOS

D21.9   **Benign neoplasm of connective and other soft tissue, unspecified**

◀ New   ◀▬ Revised   ~~deleted~~ Deleted   Excludes 1   Excludes 2   Includes   Use additional   Code first   Code also   Unspecified

814   **OGCR** Official Guidelines   ● Unacceptable Principal Diagnosis   X Assign placeholder X   ● Use Additional Character(s)   ▮ Manifestation Code   **Coding Clinic**

CHAPTER 2 (C00-D49)

● **D22 Melanocytic nevi**

     Includes   atypical nevus
                    blue hairy pigmented nevus
                    nevus NOS

   D22.0   **Melanocytic nevi of lip**

         Skin lesions composed of nests of nevus cells with macules/
         papules

●   D22.1   **Melanocytic nevi of eyelid, including canthus**

     D22.10   Melanocytic nevi of unspecified eyelid,
                including canthus

     D22.11   Melanocytic nevi of right eyelid, including
                canthus

     D22.12   Melanocytic nevi of left eyelid, including
                canthus

●   D22.2   **Melanocytic nevi of ear and external auricular canal**

     D22.20   Melanocytic nevi of unspecified ear and
                external auricular canal

     D22.21   Melanocytic nevi of right ear and external
                auricular canal

     D22.22   Melanocytic nevi of left ear and external
                auricular canal

●   D22.3   **Melanocytic nevi of other and unspecified parts of face**

     D22.30   Melanocytic nevi of unspecified part of face

     D22.39   Melanocytic nevi of other parts of face

   D22.4   **Melanocytic nevi of scalp and neck**

   D22.5   **Melanocytic nevi of trunk**

         Melanocytic nevi of anal margin
         Melanocytic nevi of anal skin
         Melanocytic nevi of perianal skin
         Melanocytic nevi of skin of breast

●   D22.6   **Melanocytic nevi of upper limb, including shoulder**

     D22.60   Melanocytic nevi of unspecified upper limb,
                including shoulder

     D22.61   Melanocytic nevi of right upper limb, including
                shoulder

     D22.62   Melanocytic nevi of left upper limb, including
                shoulder

●   D22.7   **Melanocytic nevi of lower limb, including hip**

     D22.70   Melanocytic nevi of unspecified lower limb,
                including hip

     D22.71   Melanocytic nevi of right lower limb, including
                hip

     D22.72   Melanocytic nevi of left lower limb, including
                hip

   D22.9   **Melanocytic nevi, unspecified**

● **D23 Other benign neoplasms of skin**

     Includes   benign neoplasm of hair follicles
                    benign neoplasm of sebaceous glands
                    benign neoplasm of sweat glands

     Excludes1   benign lipomatous neoplasms of skin
                      (D17.0-D17.3)
                      melanocytic nevi (D22.-)

   D23.0   **Other benign neoplasm of skin of lip**

     Excludes1   benign neoplasm of vermilion border of
                      lip (D10.0)

●   D23.1   **Other benign neoplasm of skin of eyelid, including canthus**

     D23.10   Other benign neoplasm of skin unspecified of
                eyelid, including canthus

     D23.11   Other benign neoplasm of skin of right eyelid,
                including canthus

     D23.12   Other benign neoplasm of skin of left eyelid,
                including canthus

●   D23.2   **Other benign neoplasm of skin of ear and external auricular canal**

     D23.20   Other benign neoplasm of skin of unspecified
                ear and external auricular canal

     D23.21   Other benign neoplasm of skin of right ear and
                external auricular canal

     D23.22   Other benign neoplasm of skin of left ear and
                external auricular canal

●   D23.3   **Other benign neoplasm of skin of other and unspecified parts of face**

     D23.30   Other benign neoplasm of skin of unspecified
                part of face

     D23.39   Other benign neoplasm of skin of other parts of
                face

   D23.4   **Other benign neoplasm of skin of scalp and neck**

   D23.5   **Other benign neoplasm of skin of trunk**

         Other benign neoplasm of anal margin
         Other benign neoplasm of anal skin
         Other benign neoplasm of perianal skin
         Other benign neoplasm of skin of breast

     Excludes1   benign neoplasm of anus NOS (D12.9)

●   D23.6   **Other benign neoplasm of skin of upper limb, including shoulder**

     D23.60   Other benign neoplasm of skin of unspecified
                upper limb, including shoulder

     D23.61   Other benign neoplasm of skin of right upper
                limb, including shoulder

     D23.62   Other benign neoplasm of skin of left upper
                limb, including shoulder

●   D23.7   **Other benign neoplasm of skin of lower limb, including hip**

     D23.70   Other benign neoplasm of skin of unspecified
                lower limb, including hip

     D23.71   Other benign neoplasm of skin of right lower
                limb, including hip

     D23.72   Other benign neoplasm of skin of left lower
                limb, including hip

   D23.9   **Other benign neoplasm of skin, unspecified**

● **D24 Benign neoplasm of breast**

     Includes   benign neoplasm of connective tissue of breast
                    benign neoplasm of soft parts of breast
                    fibroadenoma of breast

     Excludes2   adenofibrosis of breast (N60.2)
                      benign cyst of breast (N60.-)
                      benign mammary dysplasia (N60.-)
                      benign neoplasm of skin of breast (D22.5, D23.5)
                      fibrocystic disease of breast (N60.-)

   D24.1   **Benign neoplasm of right breast**

   D24.2   **Benign neoplasm of left breast**

   D24.9   **Benign neoplasm of unspecified breast**

● **D25 Leiomyoma of uterus**

     Benign tumors or nodules of the uterine wall

     Includes   uterine fibroid
                    uterine fibromyoma
                    uterine myoma

   D25.0   **Submucous leiomyoma of uterus** ♀

   D25.1   **Intramural leiomyoma of uterus** ♀
         Interstitial leiomyoma of uterus

   D25.2   **Subserosal leiomyoma of uterus** ♀
         Subperitoneal leiomyoma of uterus

   D25.9   **Leiomyoma of uterus, unspecified** ♀

● **D26 Other benign neoplasms of uterus**

   D26.0   **Other benign neoplasm of cervix uteri** ♀

   D26.1   **Other benign neoplasm of corpus uteri** ♀

   D26.7   **Other benign neoplasm of other parts of uterus** ♀

   D26.9   **Other benign neoplasm of uterus, unspecified** ♀

CHAPTER 2 (C00-D49)

CHAPTER 2 (C00-D49)

Item 2–11   **Teratoma:** terat = monster, oma = mass, tumor. Alternate terms: dermoid cyst of the ovary, ovarian teratoma. Teratomas are neoplasms and arise from germ cells (ovaries in female and testes in male) and can be benign or malignant. Teratomas have been known to contain hair, nails, and teeth, giving them a bizarre ("monster") appearance.

● **D27**   **Benign neoplasm of ovary**
     Use additional code to identify any functional activity.
     Excludes2   corpus albicans cyst (N83.2)
                 corpus luteum cyst (N83.1)
                 endometrial cyst (N80.1)
                 follicular (atretic) cyst (N83.0)
                 graafian follicle cyst (N83.0)
                 ovarian cyst NEC (N83.2)
                 ovarian retention cyst (N83.2)
    D27.0   **Benign neoplasm of right ovary** ♀
    D27.1   **Benign neoplasm of left ovary** ♀
    D27.9   **Benign neoplasm of unspecified ovary** ♀

● **D28**   **Benign neoplasm of other and unspecified female genital organs**
     Includes   adenomatous polyp
                 benign neoplasm of skin of female genital organs
                 benign teratoma
     Excludes1   epoophoron cyst (Q50.5)
                 fimbrial cyst (Q50.4)
                 Gartner's duct cyst (Q52.4)
                 parovarian cyst (Q50.5)
    D28.0   **Benign neoplasm of vulva** ♀
    D28.1   **Benign neoplasm of vagina** ♀
    D28.2   **Benign neoplasm of uterine tubes and ligaments** ♀
        Benign neoplasm of fallopian tube
        Benign neoplasm of uterine ligament (broad) (round)
    D28.7   **Benign neoplasm of other specified female genital organs** ♀
    D28.9   **Benign neoplasm of female genital organ, unspecified** ♀

● **D29**   **Benign neoplasm of male genital organs**
     Includes   benign neoplasm of skin of male genital organs
    D29.0   **Benign neoplasm of penis** ♂
    D29.1   **Benign neoplasm of prostate** ♂
        Excludes1   enlarged prostate (N40.-)
   ● D29.2   **Benign neoplasm of testis**
        Use additional code to identify any functional activity.
        D29.20   **Benign neoplasm of unspecified testis** ♂
        D29.21   **Benign neoplasm of right testis** ♂
        D29.22   **Benign neoplasm of left testis** ♂
   ● D29.3   **Benign neoplasm of epididymis**
        D29.30   **Benign neoplasm of unspecified epididymis** ♂
        D29.31   **Benign neoplasm of right epididymis** ♂
        D29.32   **Benign neoplasm of left epididymis** ♂
    D29.4   **Benign neoplasm of scrotum** ♂
        Benign neoplasm of skin of scrotum
    D29.8   **Benign neoplasm of other specified male genital organs** ♂
        Benign neoplasm of seminal vesicle
        Benign neoplasm of spermatic cord
        Benign neoplasm of tunica vaginalis
    D29.9   **Benign neoplasm of male genital organ, unspecified** ♂

● **D30**   **Benign neoplasm of urinary organs**
   ● D30.0   **Benign neoplasm of kidney**
        Excludes1   benign carcinoid tumor of the kidney (D3A.093)
                 benign neoplasm of renal calyces (D30.1-)
                 benign neoplasm of renal pelvis (D30.1-)
        D30.00   **Benign neoplasm of unspecified kidney**
        D30.01   **Benign neoplasm of right kidney**
        D30.02   **Benign neoplasm of left kidney**
   ● D30.1   **Benign neoplasm of renal pelvis**
        D30.10   **Benign neoplasm of unspecified renal pelvis**
        D30.11   **Benign neoplasm of right renal pelvis**
        D30.12   **Benign neoplasm of left renal pelvis**
   ● D30.2   **Benign neoplasm of ureter**
        Excludes1   benign neoplasm of ureteric orifice of bladder (D30.3)
        D30.20   **Benign neoplasm of unspecified ureter**
        D30.21   **Benign neoplasm of right ureter**
        D30.22   **Benign neoplasm of left ureter**
    D30.3   **Benign neoplasm of bladder**
        Benign neoplasm of ureteric orifice of bladder
        Benign neoplasm of urethral orifice of bladder
    D30.4   **Benign neoplasm of urethra**
        Excludes1   benign neoplasm of urethral orifice of bladder (D30.3)
    D30.8   **Benign neoplasm of other specified urinary organs**
        Benign neoplasm of paraurethral glands
    D30.9   **Benign neoplasm of urinary organ, unspecified**
        Benign neoplasm of urinary system NOS

● **D31**   **Benign neoplasm of eye and adnexa**
     Excludes1   benign neoplasm of connective tissue of eyelid (D21.0)
                 benign neoplasm of optic nerve (D33.3)
                 benign neoplasm of skin of eyelid (D22.1-, D23.1-)
   ● D31.0   **Benign neoplasm of conjunctiva**
        D31.00   **Benign neoplasm of unspecified conjunctiva**
        D31.01   **Benign neoplasm of right conjunctiva**
        D31.02   **Benign neoplasm of left conjunctiva**
   ● D31.1   **Benign neoplasm of cornea**
        D31.10   **Benign neoplasm of unspecified cornea**
        D31.11   **Benign neoplasm of right cornea**
        D31.12   **Benign neoplasm of left cornea**
   ● D31.2   **Benign neoplasm of retina**
        Excludes1   dark area on retina (D49.81)
                 hemangioma of retina (D49.81)
                 neoplasm of unspecified behavior of retina and choroid (D49.81)
                 retinal freckle (D49.81)
        D31.20   **Benign neoplasm of unspecified retina**
        D31.21   **Benign neoplasm of right retina**
        D31.22   **Benign neoplasm of left retina**
   ● D31.3   **Benign neoplasm of choroid**
        D31.30   **Benign neoplasm of unspecified choroid**
        D31.31   **Benign neoplasm of right choroid**
        D31.32   **Benign neoplasm of left choroid**
   ● D31.4   **Benign neoplasm of ciliary body**
        D31.40   **Benign neoplasm of unspecified ciliary body**
        D31.41   **Benign neoplasm of right ciliary body**
        D31.42   **Benign neoplasm of left ciliary body**

◀ New   ◀━ Revised   ~~deleted~~ Deleted   Excludes 1   Excludes 2   Includes   Use additional   Code first   Code also   Unspecified

OGCR Official Guidelines   ● Unacceptable Principal Diagnosis   X Assign placeholder X   ● Use Additional Character(s)   ▶ Manifestation Code   **Coding Clinic**

● **D31.5 Benign neoplasm of lacrimal gland and duct**
  Benign neoplasm of lacrimal sac
  Benign neoplasm of nasolacrimal duct
    D31.50 Benign neoplasm of unspecified lacrimal gland and duct
    D31.51 Benign neoplasm of right lacrimal gland and duct
    D31.52 Benign neoplasm of left lacrimal gland and duct
● **D31.6 Benign neoplasm of unspecified site of orbit**
  Benign neoplasm of connective tissue of orbit
  Benign neoplasm of extraocular muscle
  Benign neoplasm of peripheral nerves of orbit
  Benign neoplasm of retrobulbar tissue
  Benign neoplasm of retro-ocular tissue
    Excludes1 benign neoplasm of orbital bone (D16.4)
    D31.60 Benign neoplasm of unspecified site of unspecified orbit
    D31.61 Benign neoplasm of unspecified site of right orbit
    D31.62 Benign neoplasm of unspecified site of left orbit
● **D31.9 Benign neoplasm of unspecified part of eye**
  Benign neoplasm of eyeball
    D31.90 Benign neoplasm of unspecified part of unspecified eye
    D31.91 Benign neoplasm of unspecified part of right eye
    D31.92 Benign neoplasm of unspecified part of left eye
● **D32 Benign neoplasm of meninges**
  D32.0 Benign neoplasm of cerebral meninges
  D32.1 Benign neoplasm of spinal meninges
  D32.9 Benign neoplasm of meninges, unspecified
    Meningioma NOS
● **D33 Benign neoplasm of brain and other parts of central nervous system**
    Excludes1 angioma (D18.0-)
      benign neoplasm of meninges (D32.-)
      benign neoplasm of peripheral nerves and
        autonomic nervous system (D36.1-)
      hemangioma (D18.0-)
      neurofibromatosis (Q85.0-)
      retro-ocular benign neoplasm (D31.6-)
  D33.0 Benign neoplasm of brain, supratentorial
    Benign neoplasm of cerebral ventricle
    Benign neoplasm of cerebrum
    Benign neoplasm of frontal lobe
    Benign neoplasm of occipital lobe
    Benign neoplasm of parietal lobe
    Benign neoplasm of temporal lobe
      Excludes1 benign neoplasm of fourth ventricle
        (D33.1)
  D33.1 Benign neoplasm of brain, infratentorial
    Benign neoplasm of brain stem
    Benign neoplasm of cerebellum
    Benign neoplasm of fourth ventricle
  D33.2 Benign neoplasm of brain, unspecified
  D33.3 Benign neoplasm of cranial nerves
    Benign neoplasm of olfactory bulb
  D33.4 Benign neoplasm of spinal cord
  D33.7 Benign neoplasm of other specified parts of central nervous system
  D33.9 Benign neoplasm of central nervous system, unspecified
    Benign neoplasm of nervous system (central) NOS
D34 Benign neoplasm of thyroid gland
  Use additional code to identify any functional activity.

● **D35 Benign neoplasm of other and unspecified endocrine glands**
  Use additional code to identify any functional activity.
    Excludes1 benign neoplasm of endocrine pancreas (D13.7)
      benign neoplasm of ovary (D27.-)
      benign neoplasm of testis (D29.2.-)
      benign neoplasm of thymus (D15.0)
  ● **D35.0 Benign neoplasm of adrenal gland**
    D35.00 Benign neoplasm of unspecified adrenal gland
    D35.01 Benign neoplasm of right adrenal gland
    D35.02 Benign neoplasm of left adrenal gland
  D35.1 Benign neoplasm of parathyroid gland
  D35.2 Benign neoplasm of pituitary gland
  D35.3 Benign neoplasm of craniopharyngeal duct
  D35.4 Benign neoplasm of pineal gland
  D35.5 Benign neoplasm of carotid body
  D35.6 Benign neoplasm of aortic body and other paraganglia
    Benign tumor of glomus jugulare
  D35.7 Benign neoplasm of other specified endocrine glands
  D35.9 Benign neoplasm of endocrine gland, unspecified
    Benign neoplasm of unspecified endocrine gland
● **D36 Benign neoplasm of other and unspecified sites**
  D36.0 Benign neoplasm of lymph nodes
    Excludes1 lymphangioma (D18.1)
  ● **D36.1 Benign neoplasm of peripheral nerves and autonomic nervous system**
    Excludes1 benign neoplasm of peripheral nerves of
      orbit (D31.6-)
      neurofibromatosis (Q85.0-)
    D36.10 Benign neoplasm of peripheral nerves and autonomic nervous system, unspecified
    D36.11 Benign neoplasm of peripheral nerves and autonomic nervous system of face, head, and neck
    D36.12 Benign neoplasm of peripheral nerves and autonomic nervous system, upper limb, including shoulder
    D36.13 Benign neoplasm of peripheral nerves and autonomic nervous system of lower limb, including hip
    D36.14 Benign neoplasm of peripheral nerves and autonomic nervous system of thorax
    D36.15 Benign neoplasm of peripheral nerves and autonomic nervous system of abdomen
    D36.16 Benign neoplasm of peripheral nerves and autonomic nervous system of pelvis
    D36.17 Benign neoplasm of peripheral nerves and autonomic nervous system of trunk, unspecified
  D36.7 Benign neoplasm of other specified sites
    Benign neoplasm of nose NOS
  D36.9 Benign neoplasm, unspecified site

BENIGN NEUROENDOCRINE TUMORS (D3A)

● **D3A Benign neuroendocrine tumors**
  Code also any associated multiple endocrine neoplasia [MEN] syndromes (E31.2-)
  Use additional code to identify any associated endocrine syndrome, such as:
    carcinoid syndrome (E34.0)
    Excludes2 benign pancreatic islet cell tumors (D13.7)
  ● **D3A.0 Benign carcinoid tumors**
    D3A.00 Benign carcinoid tumor of unspecified site
      Carcinoid tumor NOS

N Newborn Age: 0   P Pediatric Age: 0–17   M Maternity DX: 12–55   A Adult Age: 15–124   ♀ Females Only   ♂ Males Only
Complication\Comorbidity   Major C\C   (Ex) CC/MCC Exclusions   Present on Admission Requirement   Hospital-Acquired Condition

817

- D3A.01 **Benign carcinoid tumors of the small intestine**
  - D3A.010 **Benign carcinoid tumor of the duodenum**
  - D3A.011 **Benign carcinoid tumor of the jejunum**
  - D3A.012 **Benign carcinoid tumor of the ileum**
  - D3A.019 **Benign carcinoid tumor of the small intestine, unspecified portion**
- D3A.02 **Benign carcinoid tumors of the appendix, large intestine, and rectum**
  - D3A.020 **Benign carcinoid tumor of the appendix**
  - D3A.021 **Benign carcinoid tumor of the cecum**
  - D3A.022 **Benign carcinoid tumor of the ascending colon**
  - D3A.023 **Benign carcinoid tumor of the transverse colon**
  - D3A.024 **Benign carcinoid tumor of the descending colon**
  - D3A.025 **Benign carcinoid tumor of the sigmoid colon**
  - D3A.026 **Benign carcinoid tumor of the rectum**
  - D3A.029 **Benign carcinoid tumor of the large intestine, unspecified portion**
    Benign carcinoid tumor of the colon NOS
- D3A.09 **Benign carcinoid tumors of other sites**
  - D3A.090 **Benign carcinoid tumor of the bronchus and lung**
  - D3A.091 **Benign carcinoid tumor of the thymus**
  - D3A.092 **Benign carcinoid tumor of the stomach**
  - D3A.093 **Benign carcinoid tumor of the kidney**
  - D3A.094 **Benign carcinoid tumor of the foregut NOS**
  - D3A.095 **Benign carcinoid tumor of the midgut NOS**
  - D3A.096 **Benign carcinoid tumor of the hindgut NOS**
  - D3A.098 **Benign carcinoid tumors of other sites**
- D3A.8 **Other benign neuroendocrine tumors**
  Neuroendocrine tumor NOS

NEOPLASMS OF UNCERTAIN BEHAVIOR, POLYCYTHEMIA VERA AND MYELODYSPLASTIC SYNDROMES (D37-D48)

Note: Categories D37-D44, and D48 classify by site neoplasms of uncertain behavior, i.e., histologic confirmation whether the neoplasm is malignant or benign cannot be made.

Excludes1   neoplasms of unspecified behavior (D49.-) ◄

- D37 **Neoplasm of uncertain behavior of oral cavity and digestive organs**
  Excludes1   stromal tumors of uncertain behavior of digestive system (D48.1)
  - D37.0 **Neoplasm of uncertain behavior of lip, oral cavity and pharynx**
    Excludes1   neoplasm of uncertain behavior of aryepiglottic fold or interarytenoid fold, laryngeal aspect (D38.0)
    neoplasm of uncertain behavior of epiglottis NOS (D38.0)
    neoplasm of uncertain behavior of skin of lip (D48.5)
    neoplasm of uncertain behavior of suprahyoid portion of epiglottis (D38.0)
    - D37.01 **Neoplasm of uncertain behavior of lip**
      Neoplasm of uncertain behavior of vermilion border of lip
    - D37.02 **Neoplasm of uncertain behavior of tongue**

Figure 2-19 Major salivary glands.

Parotid gland
Sublingual gland
Submandibular gland

- D37.03 **Neoplasm of uncertain behavior of the major salivary glands**
  - D37.030 **Neoplasm of uncertain behavior of the parotid salivary glands**
  - D37.031 **Neoplasm of uncertain behavior of the sublingual salivary glands**
  - D37.032 **Neoplasm of uncertain behavior of the submandibular salivary glands**
  - D37.039 **Neoplasm of uncertain behavior of the major salivary glands, unspecified**
- D37.04 **Neoplasm of uncertain behavior of the minor salivary glands**
  Neoplasm of uncertain behavior of submucosal salivary glands of lip
  Neoplasm of uncertain behavior of submucosal salivary glands of cheek
  Neoplasm of uncertain behavior of submucosal salivary glands of hard palate
  Neoplasm of uncertain behavior of submucosal salivary glands of soft palate
- D37.05 **Neoplasm of uncertain behavior of pharynx**
  Neoplasm of uncertain behavior of aryepiglottic fold of pharynx NOS
  Neoplasm of uncertain behavior of hypopharyngeal aspect of aryepiglottic fold of pharynx
  Neoplasm of uncertain behavior of marginal zone of aryepiglottic fold of pharynx
- D37.09 **Neoplasm of uncertain behavior of other specified sites of the oral cavity**
- D37.1 **Neoplasm of uncertain behavior of stomach**
- D37.2 **Neoplasm of uncertain behavior of small intestine**
- D37.3 **Neoplasm of uncertain behavior of appendix**
- D37.4 **Neoplasm of uncertain behavior of colon**
- D37.5 **Neoplasm of uncertain behavior of rectum**
  Neoplasm of uncertain behavior of rectosigmoid junction
  Rectosigmoid junction: Angle where sigmoid colon becomes rectum
- D37.6 **Neoplasm of uncertain behavior of liver, gallbladder and bile ducts**
  Neoplasm of uncertain behavior of ampulla of Vater
  Ampulla of Vater: Enlarged segment of ducts from liver and pancreas at entry point to small intestine
- D37.8 **Neoplasm of uncertain behavior of other specified digestive organs**
  Neoplasm of uncertain behavior of anal canal
  Neoplasm of uncertain behavior of anal sphincter
  Neoplasm of uncertain behavior of anus NOS
  Neoplasm of uncertain behavior of esophagus
  Neoplasm of uncertain behavior of intestine NOS
  Neoplasm of uncertain behavior of pancreas
  Excludes1   neoplasm of uncertain behavior of anal margin (D48.5)
  neoplasm of uncertain behavior of anal skin (D48.5)
  neoplasm of uncertain behavior of perianal skin (D48.5)
- D37.9 **Neoplasm of uncertain behavior of digestive organ, unspecified**

◄ New   ◄ⅢⅢ Revised   ~~deleted~~ Deleted   Excludes 1   Excludes 2   Includes   Use additional   Code first   Code also   Unspecified

818   OGCR Official Guidelines   ● Unacceptable Principal Diagnosis   X Assign placeholder X   ● Use Additional Character(s)   ▶ Manifestation Code   **Coding Clinic**

● **D38 Neoplasm of uncertain behavior of middle ear and respiratory and intrathoracic organs**

> **Excludes1** neoplasm of uncertain behavior of heart (D48.7)

D38.0 **Neoplasm of uncertain behavior of larynx**
Neoplasm of uncertain behavior of aryepiglottic fold or interarytenoid fold, laryngeal aspect
Neoplasm of uncertain behavior of epiglottis (suprahyoid portion)

> **Excludes1** neoplasm of uncertain behavior of aryepiglottic fold or interarytenoid fold NOS (D37.05)
> neoplasm of uncertain behavior of hypopharyngeal aspect of aryepiglottic fold (D37.05)
> neoplasm of uncertain behavior of marginal zone of aryepiglottic fold (D37.05)

D38.1 **Neoplasm of uncertain behavior of trachea, bronchus and lung**

D38.2 **Neoplasm of uncertain behavior of pleura**

D38.3 **Neoplasm of uncertain behavior of mediastinum**

D38.4 **Neoplasm of uncertain behavior of thymus**

D38.5 **Neoplasm of uncertain behavior of other respiratory organs**
Neoplasm of uncertain behavior of accessory sinuses
Neoplasm of uncertain behavior of cartilage of nose
Neoplasm of uncertain behavior of middle ear
Neoplasm of uncertain behavior of nasal cavities

> **Excludes1** neoplasm of uncertain behavior of ear (external) (skin) (D48.5)
> neoplasm of uncertain behavior of nose NOS (D48.7)
> neoplasm of uncertain behavior of skin of nose (D48.5)

D38.6 **Neoplasm of uncertain behavior of respiratory organ, unspecified**

● **D39 Neoplasm of uncertain behavior of female genital organs**

D39.0 **Neoplasm of uncertain behavior of uterus** ♀

● D39.1 **Neoplasm of uncertain behavior of ovary**
Use additional code to identify any functional activity.

D39.10 **Neoplasm of uncertain behavior of unspecified ovary** ♀

D39.11 **Neoplasm of uncertain behavior of right ovary** ♀

D39.12 **Neoplasm of uncertain behavior of left ovary** ♀

D39.2 **Neoplasm of uncertain behavior of placenta** ♀
Chorioadenoma destruens
Invasive hydatidiform mole
Malignant hydatidiform mole

> **Excludes1** hydatidiform mole NOS (O01.9)

D39.8 **Neoplasm of uncertain behavior of other specified female genital organs** ♀
Neoplasm of uncertain behavior of skin of female genital organs

D39.9 **Neoplasm of uncertain behavior of female genital organ, unspecified** ♀

● **D40 Neoplasm of uncertain behavior of male genital organs**

D40.0 **Neoplasm of uncertain behavior of prostate** ♂

● D40.1 **Neoplasm of uncertain behavior of testis**

D40.10 **Neoplasm of uncertain behavior of unspecified testis** ♂

D40.11 **Neoplasm of uncertain behavior of right testis** ♂

D40.12 **Neoplasm of uncertain behavior of left testis** ♂

D40.8 **Neoplasm of uncertain behavior of other specified male genital organs** ♂
Neoplasm of uncertain behavior of skin of male genital organs

D40.9 **Neoplasm of uncertain behavior of male genital organ, unspecified** ♂

● **D41 Neoplasm of uncertain behavior of urinary organs**

● D41.0 **Neoplasm of uncertain behavior of kidney**

> **Excludes1** neoplasm of uncertain behavior of renal pelvis (D41.1-)

D41.00 **Neoplasm of uncertain behavior of unspecified kidney**

D41.01 **Neoplasm of uncertain behavior of right kidney**

D41.02 **Neoplasm of uncertain behavior of left kidney**

● D41.1 **Neoplasm of uncertain behavior of renal pelvis**

D41.10 **Neoplasm of uncertain behavior of unspecified renal pelvis**

D41.11 **Neoplasm of uncertain behavior of right renal pelvis**

D41.12 **Neoplasm of uncertain behavior of left renal pelvis**

● D41.2 **Neoplasm of uncertain behavior of ureter**

D41.20 **Neoplasm of uncertain behavior of unspecified ureter**

D41.21 **Neoplasm of uncertain behavior of right ureter**

D41.22 **Neoplasm of uncertain behavior of left ureter**

D41.3 **Neoplasm of uncertain behavior of urethra**

D41.4 **Neoplasm of uncertain behavior of bladder**

D41.8 **Neoplasm of uncertain behavior of other specified urinary organs**

D41.9 **Neoplasm of uncertain behavior of unspecified urinary organ**

● **D42 Neoplasm of uncertain behavior of meninges**

D42.0 **Neoplasm of uncertain behavior of cerebral meninges**

D42.1 **Neoplasm of uncertain behavior of spinal meninges**

D42.9 **Neoplasm of uncertain behavior of meninges, unspecified**

● **D43 Neoplasm of uncertain behavior of brain and central nervous system**

> **Excludes1** neoplasm of uncertain behavior of peripheral nerves and autonomic nervous system (D48.2)

D43.0 **Neoplasm of uncertain behavior of brain, supratentorial**
Superior to tentorium of cerebellum
Neoplasm of uncertain behavior of cerebral ventricle
Neoplasm of uncertain behavior of cerebrum
Neoplasm of uncertain behavior of frontal lobe
Neoplasm of uncertain behavior of occipital lobe
Neoplasm of uncertain behavior of parietal lobe
Neoplasm of uncertain behavior of temporal lobe

> **Excludes1** neoplasm of uncertain behavior of fourth ventricle (D43.1)

D43.1 **Neoplasm of uncertain behavior of brain, infratentorial**
Beneath the tentorium of cerebellum
Neoplasm of uncertain behavior of brain stem
Neoplasm of uncertain behavior of cerebellum
Neoplasm of uncertain behavior of fourth ventricle

D43.2 **Neoplasm of uncertain behavior of brain, unspecified**

D43.3 **Neoplasm of uncertain behavior of cranial nerves**

D43.4 **Neoplasm of uncertain behavior of spinal cord**

D43.8 **Neoplasm of uncertain behavior of other specified parts of central nervous system**

D43.9 **Neoplasm of uncertain behavior of central nervous system, unspecified**
Neoplasm of uncertain behavior of nervous system (central) NOS

CHAPTER 2 (C00-D49)

CHAPTER 2 (C00-D49)

● **D44 Neoplasm of uncertain behavior of endocrine glands**

    Excludes1   multiple endocrine adenomatosis (E31.2-)
                   multiple endocrine neoplasia (E31.2-)
                   neoplasm of uncertain behavior of endocrine pancreas (D37.8)
                   neoplasm of uncertain behavior of ovary (D39.1-)
                   neoplasm of uncertain behavior of testis (D40.1-)
                   neoplasm of uncertain behavior of thymus (D38.4)

    D44.0 Neoplasm of uncertain behavior of thyroid gland

●   **D44.1 Neoplasm of uncertain behavior of adrenal gland**

      Use additional code to identify any functional activity.

      D44.10 Neoplasm of uncertain behavior of unspecified adrenal gland

      D44.11 Neoplasm of uncertain behavior of right adrenal gland

      D44.12 Neoplasm of uncertain behavior of left adrenal gland

    D44.2 Neoplasm of uncertain behavior of parathyroid gland

    D44.3 Neoplasm of uncertain behavior of pituitary gland

      Use additional code to identify any functional activity.

    D44.4 Neoplasm of uncertain behavior of craniopharyngeal duct

    D44.5 Neoplasm of uncertain behavior of pineal gland

    D44.6 Neoplasm of uncertain behavior of carotid body

    D44.7 Neoplasm of uncertain behavior of aortic body and other paraganglia

    D44.9 Neoplasm of uncertain behavior of unspecified endocrine gland

D45 Polycythemia vera

    Excludes1   familial polycythemia (D75.0)
                   secondary polycythemia (D75.1)

    Primary polycythemia. Secondary polycythemia is D75.1. Check your documentation. Polycythemia is caused by too many red blood cells, which increase the thickness of blood (viscosity). This can cause engorgement of the spleen (splenomegaly) with extra RBCs and potential clot formation.

● **D46 Myelodysplastic syndromes**

    Use additional code for adverse effect, if applicable, to identify drug (T36-T50 with fifth or sixth character 5)

    Excludes2   drug-induced aplastic anemia (D61.1)

    D46.0 Refractory anemia without ring sideroblasts, so stated
      Refractory anemia without sideroblasts, without excess of blasts

    D46.1 Refractory anemia with ring sideroblasts RARS

●   **D46.2 Refractory anemia with excess of blasts**
      Form of myelodysplasia with increased immature white blood cells (blasts) in bone marrow

      D46.20 Refractory anemia with excess of blasts, unspecified RAEB NOS

      D46.21 Refractory anemia with excess of blasts 1 RAEB 1
        Bone marrow disease which results in insufficient RBCs (anemia) in which level of blasts is less than 10%

      D46.22 Refractory anemia with excess of blasts 2 RAEB 2 🔗
        Bone marrow disease manifested by insufficient numbers of RBCs (anemia) with level of blasts 10-20%
        (Ex:) C88.2-C88.3, C88.8-C88.9, C90.10-C90.11, C90.20-C90.21, C90.30-C90.31, C91.00-C91.02, C91.10-C91.12, C91.30-C91.32, C91.40-C91.42, C91.50-C91.52, C91.60-C91.62, C91.90-C91.92, C91.A0-C91.A2, C92.10-C92.22, C92.00-C92.02, C92.10-C92.12, C92.20-C92.22, C92.30-C92.32, C92.40-C92.42, C92.50-C92.52, C92.60-C92.62, C92.90-C92.92, C92.A0-C92.A2, C92.Z0-C92.Z2, C93.00-C93.02, C93.10-C93.12, C93.30-C93.32, C93.90-C93.92, C93.Z0-C93.Z2, C94.00-C94.02, C94.20-C94.22, C94.30-C94.32, C94.40-C94.42, C94.6, C94.80-C94.82, C95.00-C95.02, C95.10-C95.12, C95.90-C95.92, D45-D46.22, D46.9, D46.A-D46.Z, D47.0-D47.1, D47.3, D47.9, D47.Z9, D48.7-D48.9

D46.A Refractory cytopenia with multilineage dysplasia

D46.B Refractory cytopenia with multilineage dysplasia and ring sideroblasts
    RCMD RS

D46.C Myelodysplastic syndrome with isolated del(5q) chromosomal abnormality 🔗
    Myelodysplastic syndrome with 5q deletion
    5q minus syndrome NOS
    (Ex:) See D46.22

D46.4 Refractory anemia, unspecified

D46.Z Other myelodysplastic syndromes
    Excludes1   chronic myelomonocytic leukemia (C93.1-)

D46.9 Myelodysplastic syndrome, unspecified
    Myelodysplasia NOS

● **D47 Other neoplasms of uncertain behavior of lymphoid, hematopoietic and related tissue**

    D47.0 Histiocytic and mast cell tumors of uncertain behavior 🔗
      Indolent systemic mastocytosis
      Mast cell tumor NOS
      Mastocytoma NOS
      Excludes1   malignant mast cell tumor (C96.2)
                  mastocytosis (congenital) (cutaneous) (Q82.2)
      (Ex:) C88.8, C94.40-C94.42, C94.6, D45-D46.22, D46.4, D46.9, D46.A-D46.C, D46.Z, D47.0-D47.1, D47.3, D47.9, D47.Z9, D75.81, Z51.0

    D47.1 Chronic myeloproliferative disease 🔗
      Chronic neutrophilic leukemia
      Myeloproliferative disease, unspecified
      Excludes1   atypical chronic myeloid leukemia BCR/ABL-negative (C92.2-)
                  chronic myeloid leukemia BCR/ABL-positive (C92.1-)
                  myelofibrosis NOS (D75.81)
                  myelophthisic anemia (D61.82)
                  myelophthisis (D61.82)
                  secondary myelofibrosis NOS (D75.81)
      (Ex:) See D46.22

    D47.2 Monoclonal gammopathy
      Monoclonal gammopathy of undetermined significance [MGUS]

    D47.3 Essential (hemorrhagic) thrombocythemia
      Essential thrombocytosis
      Idiopathic hemorrhagic thrombocythemia

    D47.4 Osteomyelofibrosis
      Chronic idiopathic myelofibrosis
      Myelofibrosis (idiopathic) (with myeloid metaplasia)
      Myelosclerosis (megakaryocytic) with myeloid metaplasia
      Secondary myelofibrosis in myeloproliferative disease
      Excludes1   acute myelofibrosis (C94.4-)

● **D47.Z Other specified neoplasms of uncertain behavior of lymphoid, hematopoietic and related tissue**

    ● **D47.Z1 Post-transplant lymphoproliferative disorder (PTLD)** 🔗
      Code first complications of transplanted organs and tissue (T86.-)
      (Ex:) D47.Z1, D78.81-D78.89, E89.810-E89.89, H59.011-H59.019, H59.031-H59.099, H59.811-H59.89, H95.811-H95.89, I97.3, M96.89, N98.1-N98.9, T86.850-T86.99

    D47.Z9 Other specified neoplasms of uncertain behavior of lymphoid, hematopoietic and related tissue 🔗
      Histiocytic tumors of uncertain behavior
      (Ex:) See D46.22

    D47.9 Neoplasm of uncertain behavior of lymphoid, hematopoietic and related tissue, unspecified 🔗
      Lymphoproliferative disease NOS
      (Ex:) See D46.22

◀ New   ◀⁞⁞ Revised   ~~deleted~~ Deleted   Excludes 1   Excludes 2   Includes   Use additional   Code first   Code also   Unspecified
OGCR Official Guidelines   ● Unacceptable Principal Diagnosis   X Assign placeholder X   ● Use Additional Character(s)   ▶ Manifestation Code   **Coding Clinic**

● **D48**   **Neoplasm of uncertain behavior of other and unspecified sites**

     Excludes1   neurofibromatosis (nonmalignant) (Q85.0-)

   D48.0   **Neoplasm of uncertain behavior of bone and articular cartilage**

       Excludes1   neoplasm of uncertain behavior of cartilage of ear (D48.1)

                   neoplasm of uncertain behavior of cartilage of larynx (D38.0)

                   neoplasm of uncertain behavior of cartilage of nose (D38.5)

                   neoplasm of uncertain behavior of connective tissue of eyelid (D48.1)

                   neoplasm of uncertain behavior of synovia (D48.1)

   D48.1   **Neoplasm of uncertain behavior of connective and other soft tissue**

       Neoplasm of uncertain behavior of connective tissue of ear

       Neoplasm of uncertain behavior of connective tissue of eyelid

       Stromal tumors of uncertain behavior of digestive system

       Excludes1   neoplasm of uncertain behavior of articular cartilage (D48.0)

                   neoplasm of uncertain behavior of cartilage of larynx (D38.0)

                   neoplasm of uncertain behavior of cartilage of nose (D38.5)

                   neoplasm of uncertain behavior of connective tissue of breast (D48.6-)

   D48.2   **Neoplasm of uncertain behavior of peripheral nerves and autonomic nervous system**

       Excludes1   neoplasm of uncertain behavior of peripheral nerves of orbit (D48.7)

   D48.3   **Neoplasm of uncertain behavior of retroperitoneum**

   D48.4   **Neoplasm of uncertain behavior of peritoneum**

   D48.5   **Neoplasm of uncertain behavior of skin**

       Neoplasm of uncertain behavior of anal margin

       Neoplasm of uncertain behavior of anal skin

       Neoplasm of uncertain behavior of perianal skin

       Neoplasm of uncertain behavior of skin of breast

       Excludes1   neoplasm of uncertain behavior of anus NOS (D37.8)

                   neoplasm of uncertain behavior of skin of genital organs (D39.8, D40.8) ◀▥

                   neoplasm of uncertain behavior of vermilion border of lip (D37.0)

● **D48.6**   **Neoplasm of uncertain behavior of breast**

       Neoplasm of uncertain behavior of connective tissue of breast

       Cystosarcoma phyllodes

       Excludes1   neoplasm of uncertain behavior of skin of breast (D48.5)

     D48.60   **Neoplasm of uncertain behavior of unspecified breast**

     D48.61   **Neoplasm of uncertain behavior of right breast**

     D48.62   **Neoplasm of uncertain behavior of left breast**

   D48.7   **Neoplasm of uncertain behavior of other specified sites**

       Neoplasm of uncertain behavior of eye

       Neoplasm of uncertain behavior of heart

       Neoplasm of uncertain behavior of peripheral nerves of orbit

       Excludes1   neoplasm of uncertain behavior of connective tissue (D48.1)

                   neoplasm of uncertain behavior of skin of eyelid (D48.5)

   D48.9   **Neoplasm of uncertain behavior, unspecified**

● **D49**   **Neoplasms of unspecified behavior**

     Note: Category D49 classifies by site neoplasms of unspecified morphology and behavior. The term 'mass,' unless otherwise stated, is not to be regarded as a neoplastic growth.

     Includes   'growth' NOS

               neoplasm NOS

               new growth NOS

               tumor NOS

     Excludes1   neoplasms of uncertain behavior (D37-D44, D48)

   D49.0   **Neoplasm of unspecified behavior of digestive system**

       Excludes1   neoplasm of unspecified behavior of margin of anus (D49.2)

                   neoplasm of unspecified behavior of perianal skin (D49.2)

                   neoplasm of unspecified behavior of skin of anus (D49.2)

   D49.1   **Neoplasm of unspecified behavior of respiratory system**

   D49.2   **Neoplasm of unspecified behavior of bone, soft tissue, and skin**

       Excludes1   neoplasm of unspecified behavior of anal canal (D49.0)

                   neoplasm of unspecified behavior of anus NOS (D49.0)

                   neoplasm of unspecified behavior of bone marrow (D49.89) ◀▥

                   neoplasm of unspecified behavior of cartilage of larynx (D49.1)

                   neoplasm of unspecified behavior of cartilage of nose (D49.1)

                   neoplasm of unspecified behavior of connective tissue of breast (D49.3)

                   neoplasm of unspecified behavior of skin of genital organs (D49.5)

                   neoplasm of unspecified behavior of vermilion border of lip (D49.0)

   D49.3   **Neoplasm of unspecified behavior of breast**

       Excludes1   neoplasm of unspecified behavior of skin of breast (D49.2)

   D49.4   **Neoplasm of unspecified behavior of bladder**

   D49.5   **Neoplasm of unspecified behavior of other genitourinary organs**

   D49.6   **Neoplasm of unspecified behavior of brain**

       Excludes1   neoplasm of unspecified behavior of cerebral meninges (D49.7)

                   neoplasm of unspecified behavior of cranial nerves (D49.7)

● **D49.7**   **Neoplasm of unspecified behavior of endocrine glands and other parts of nervous system**

       Excludes1   neoplasm of unspecified behavior of peripheral, sympathetic, and parasympathetic nerves and ganglia (D49.2)

● **D49.8**   **Neoplasm of unspecified behavior of other specified sites**

       Excludes1   neoplasm of unspecified behavior of eyelid (skin) (D49.2)

                   neoplasm of unspecified behavior of eyelid cartilage (D49.2)

                   neoplasm of unspecified behavior of great vessels (D49.2)

                   neoplasm of unspecified behavior of optic nerve (D49.7)

     D49.81   **Neoplasm of unspecified behavior of retina and choroid**

         Dark area on retina

         Retinal freckle

     D49.89   **Neoplasm of unspecified behavior of other specified sites**

   D49.9   **Neoplasm of unspecified behavior of unspecified site**

N Newborn Age: 0   **P** Pediatric Age: 0–17   **M** Maternity DX: 12–55   **A** Adult Age: 15–124   ♀ Females Only   ♂ Males Only

Complication\Comorbidity   Major C\C   (Ex) CC/MCC Exclusions   Present on Admission Requirement   Hospital-Acquired Condition   **821**

CHAPTER 3

DISEASES OF THE BLOOD AND BLOOD-FORMING ORGANS AND CERTAIN DISORDERS INVOLVING THE IMMUNE MECHANISM (D50-D89)

Excludes2   autoimmune disease (systemic) NOS (M35.9)
certain conditions originating in the perinatal period (P00-P96)
complications of pregnancy, childbirth and the puerperium (O00-O9A)
congenital malformations, deformations and chromosomal abnormalities (Q00-Q99)
endocrine, nutritional and metabolic diseases (E00-E88)
human immunodeficiency virus [HIV] disease (B20)
injury, poisoning and certain other consequences of external causes (S00-T88)
neoplasms (C00-D49)
symptoms, signs and abnormal clinical and laboratory findings, not elsewhere classified (R00-R94)

This chapter contains the following blocks:

D50-D53	Nutritional anemias
D55-D59	Hemolytic anemias
D60-D64	Aplastic and other anemias and other bone marrow failure syndromes
D65-D69	Coagulation defects, purpura and other hemorrhagic conditions
D70-D77	Other disorders of blood and blood-forming organs
D78	Intraoperative and postprocedural complications of the spleen
D80-D89	Certain disorders involving the immune mechanism

NUTRITIONAL ANEMIAS (D50-D53)

● **D50   Iron deficiency anemia**
A disease characterized by a decrease in the number of red cells (hemoglobin) in the blood.

Includes   asiderotic anemia
hypochromic anemia

D50.0   Iron deficiency anemia secondary to blood loss (chronic)
Posthemorrhagic anemia (chronic)

Excludes1   acute posthemorrhagic anemia (D62)
congenital anemia from fetal blood loss (P61.3)

D50.1   Sideropenic dysphagia
Web-like growth of membranes in throat that makes swallowing difficult
Kelly-Paterson syndrome
Plummer-Vinson syndrome

D50.8   Other iron deficiency anemias
Iron deficiency anemia due to inadequate dietary iron intake

D50.9   Iron deficiency anemia, unspecified

● **D51   Vitamin B12 deficiency anemia**

Excludes1   vitamin B12 deficiency (E53.8)

D51.0   Vitamin B12 deficiency anemia due to intrinsic factor deficiency
Addison anemia
Biermer anemia
Pernicious (congenital) anemia
Congenital intrinsic factor deficiency

D51.1   Vitamin B12 deficiency anemia due to selective vitamin B12 malabsorption with proteinuria
Imerslund (Gräsbeck) syndrome
Megaloblastic hereditary anemia

D51.2   Transcobalamin II deficiency

D51.3   Other dietary vitamin B12 deficiency anemia
Vegan anemia

D51.8   Other vitamin B12 deficiency anemias

D51.9   Vitamin B12 deficiency anemia, unspecified

● **D52   Folate deficiency anemia**

Excludes1   folate deficiency without anemia (E53.8)

D52.0   Dietary folate deficiency anemia
Nutritional megaloblastic anemia

D52.1   Drug-induced folate deficiency anemia
Use additional code for adverse effect, if applicable, to identify drug (T36-T50 with fifth or sixth character 5)

D52.8   Other folate deficiency anemias

D52.9   Folate deficiency anemia, unspecified
Folic acid deficiency anemia NOS

● **D53   Other nutritional anemias**

Includes   megaloblastic anemia unresponsive to vitamin B12 or folate therapy

D53.0   Protein deficiency anemia
Amino-acid deficiency anemia
Orotaciduric anemia

Excludes1   Lesch-Nyhan syndrome (E79.1)

D53.1   Other megaloblastic anemias, not elsewhere classified
Megaloblastic anemia NOS

Excludes1   Di Guglielmo's disease (C94.0)

D53.2   Scorbutic anemia
Anemia resulting from deficiency of ascorbic acid (vitamin C)

Excludes1   scurvy (E54)

D53.8   Other specified nutritional anemias
Anemia associated with deficiency of copper
Anemia associated with deficiency of molybdenum
Anemia associated with deficiency of zinc

Excludes1   nutritional deficiencies without anemia, such as:
copper deficiency NOS (E61.0)
molybdenum deficiency NOS (E61.5)
zinc deficiency NOS (E60)

D53.9   Nutritional anemia, unspecified
Simple chronic anemia

Excludes1   anemia NOS (D64.9)

HEMOLYTIC ANEMIAS (D55-D59)

● **D55   Anemia due to enzyme disorders**

Excludes1   drug-induced enzyme deficiency anemia (D59.2)

D55.0   Anemia due to glucose-6-phosphate dehydrogenase [G6PD] deficiency
Favism
G6PD deficiency anemia

D55.1   Anemia due to other disorders of glutathione metabolism
Anemia (due to) enzyme deficiencies, except G6PD, related to the hexose monophosphate [HMP] shunt pathway
Anemia (due to) hemolytic nonspherocytic (hereditary), type I

D55.2   Anemia due to disorders of glycolytic enzymes
Hemolytic nonspherocytic (hereditary) anemia, type II
Hexokinase deficiency anemia
Pyruvate kinase [PK] deficiency anemia
Triose-phosphate isomerase deficiency anemia

Excludes1   disorders of glycolysis not associated with anemia (E74.8)

D55.3   Anemia due to disorders of nucleotide metabolism

D55.8   Other anemias due to enzyme disorders

D55.9   Anemia due to enzyme disorder, unspecified

◀ New   ◀▥ Revised   ~~deleted~~ Deleted   Excludes 1   Excludes 2   Includes   Use additional   Code first   Code also   Unspecified
OGCR Official Guidelines   ● Unacceptable Principal Diagnosis   X Assign placeholder X   ● Use Additional Character(s)   ▶ Manifestation Code   **Coding Clinic**

● **D56   Thalassemia**
Hereditary disorders characterized by low production of hemoglobin or excessive destruction of red blood cells

> **Excludes1**   sickle-cell thalassemia (D57.4-)

D56.0   Alpha thalassemia
Alpha thalassemia major
Hemoglobin H Constant Spring
Hemoglobin H disease
Hydrops fetalis due to alpha thalassemia
Severe alpha thalassemia
Triple gene defect alpha thalassemia

Use additional code, if applicable, for hydrops fetalis due to alpha thalassemia (P56.99)

> **Excludes1**   alpha thalassemia trait or minor (D56.3)
> asymptomatic alpha thalassemia (D56.3)
> hydrops fetalis due to isoimmunization (P56.0)
> hydrops fetalis not due to immune hemolysis (P83.2)

D56.1   Beta thalassemia
Beta thalassemia major
Cooley's anemia
Homozygous beta thalassemia
Severe beta thalassemia
Thalassemia intermedia
Thalassemia major

> **Excludes1**   beta thalassemia minor (D56.3)
> beta thalassemia trait (D56.3)
> delta-beta thalassemia (D56.2)
> hemoglobin E-beta thalassemia (D56.5)
> sickle-cell beta thalassemia (D57.4-)

D56.2   Delta-beta thalassemia
Homozygous delta-beta thalassemia

> **Excludes1**   delta-beta thalassemia minor (D56.3)
> delta-beta thalassemia trait (D56.3)

D56.3   Thalassemia minor
Genetic disorders that have in common defective production of hemoglobin
Alpha thalassemia minor
Alpha thalassemia silent carrier
Alpha thalassemia trait
Beta thalassemia minor
Beta thalassemia trait
Delta-beta thalassemia minor
Delta-beta thalassemia trait
Thalassemia trait NOS

> **Excludes1**   alpha thalassemia (D56.0)
> beta thalassemia (D56.1)
> delta-beta thalassemia (D56.2)
> hemoglobin E-beta thalassemia (D56.5)
> sickle-cell trait (D57.3)

D56.4   Hereditary persistence of fetal hemoglobin [HPFH]
Persistent production of hemoglobin

D56.5   Hemoglobin E-beta thalassemia

> **Excludes1**   beta thalassemia (D56.1)
> beta thalassemia minor (D56.3)
> beta thalassemia trait (D56.3)
> delta-beta thalassemia (D56.2)
> delta-beta thalassemia trait (D56.3)
> hemoglobin E disease (D58.2)
> other hemoglobinopathies (D58.2)
> sickle-cell beta thalassemia (D57.4-)

D56.8   Other thalassemias
Dominant thalassemia
Hemoglobin C thalassemia
Mixed thalassemia
Thalassemia with other hemoglobinopathy

> **Excludes1**   hemoglobin C disease (D58.2)
> hemoglobin E disease (D58.2)
> other hemoglobinopathies (D58.2)
> sickle cell anemia (D57.-)
> sickle-cell thalassemia (D57.4)

D56.9   Thalassemia, unspecified
Mediterranean anemia (with other hemoglobinopathy)

● **D57   Sickle-cell disorders**
Inherited disease in which red blood cells, normally disc-shaped, become crescent shaped.

Use additional code for any associated fever (R50.81)

> **Excludes1**   other hemoglobinopathies (D58.-)

Ⓔ **For category D57 CC codes:** D47.4, D50.0-D64.9, D68.312, D68.51-D68.69, D75.81, D75.89-D75.9, D77, D89.2

● **D57.0   Hb-SS disease with crisis**
Sickle-cell disease NOS with crisis
Hb-SS disease with vasoocclusive pain

D57.00   Hb-SS disease with crisis, unspecified 🔹

D57.01   Hb-SS disease with acute chest syndrome 🔹

D57.02   Hb-SS disease with splenic sequestration 🔹

D57.1   Sickle-cell disease without crisis Hb-SS disease without crisis
Sickle-cell anemia NOS
Sickle-cell disease NOS
Sickle-cell disorder NOS

● **D57.2   Sickle-cell/Hb-C disease**
Hb-SC disease
Hb-S/Hb-C disease

D57.20   Sickle-cell/Hb-C disease without crisis

● **D57.21   Sickle-cell/Hb-C disease with crisis**

D57.211   Sickle-cell/Hb-C disease with acute chest syndrome 🔹🔹
CC when PDX is its own CC

D57.212   Sickle-cell/Hb-C disease with splenic sequestration 🔹

D57.219   Sickle-cell/Hb-C disease with crisis, unspecified 🔹
Sickle-cell/Hb-C disease with crisis NOS

D57.3   Sickle-cell trait
Hb-S trait
Heterozygous hemoglobin S

● **D57.4   Sickle-cell thalassemia**
Sickle-cell beta thalassemia
Thalassemia Hb-S disease

D57.40   Sickle-cell thalassemia without crisis
Microdrepanocytosis
Sickle-cell thalassemia NOS

● **D57.41   Sickle-cell thalassemia with crisis**
Sickle-cell "crisis" is precipitated when abnormally crescent-shaped red blood cells form clots and interrupt blood flow to major organs, causing severe pain and organ damage.
Sickle-cell thalassemia with vasoocclusive pain

D57.411   Sickle-cell thalassemia with acute chest syndrome 🔹🔹
CC when PDX is its own CC

D57.412   Sickle-cell thalassemia with splenic sequestration 🔹

D57.419   Sickle-cell thalassemia with crisis, unspecified 🔹
Sickle-cell thalassemia with crisis NOS

● **D57.8   Other sickle-cell disorders**
Hb-SD disease
Hb-SE disease

D57.80   Other sickle-cell disorders without crisis

● **D57.81   Other sickle-cell disorders with crisis**

D57.811   Other sickle-cell disorders with acute chest syndrome 🔹

D57.812   Other sickle-cell disorders with splenic sequestration 🔹

D57.819   Other sickle-cell disorders with crisis, unspecified 🔹
Other sickle-cell disorders with crisis NOS

N Newborn Age: 0   **P** Pediatric Age: 0–17   **M** Maternity DX: 12–55   **A** Adult Age: 15–124   ♀ Females Only   ♂ Males Only

🔹 Complication\Comorbidity   🔹 Major C\C   Ⓔ CC/MCC Exclusions   🔹 Present on Admission Requirement   🔹 Hospital-Acquired Condition

823

CHAPTER 3 (D50–D89)

● **D58**   **Other hereditary hemolytic anemias**
Genetic condition in which bone marrow is unable to compensate for premature destruction of red blood cells

> **Excludes1**   hemolytic anemia of the newborn (P55.-)

D58.0   **Hereditary spherocytosis**
Presence of spherocytes (spherically shaped red blood cells)
Acholuric (familial) jaundice
Congenital (spherocytic) hemolytic icterus
Minkowski-Chauffard syndrome

D58.1   **Hereditary elliptocytosis**
Presence of large numbers of elliptocytes in blood
Elliptocytosis (congenital)
Ovalocytosis (congenital) (hereditary)

D58.2   **Other hemoglobinopathies**
Abnormal hemoglobin NOS
Congenital Heinz body anemia
Hb-C disease
Hb-D disease
Hb-E disease
Hemoglobinopathy NOS
Unstable hemoglobin hemolytic disease

> **Excludes1**   familial polycythemia (D75.0)
> Hb-M disease (D74.0)
> hemoglobin E-beta thalassemia (D56.5)
> hereditary persistence of fetal hemoglobin [HPFH] (D56.4)
> high-altitude polycythemia (D75.1)
> methemoglobinemia (D74.-)
> other hemoglobinopathies with thalassemia (D56.8)

D58.8   **Other specified hereditary hemolytic anemias**
Stomatocytosis
(Ex:) D50.0-D64.9, D75.9, P61.2-P61.4

D58.9   **Hereditary hemolytic anemia, unspecified**
(Ex:) See D58.8

● **D59**   **Acquired hemolytic anemia**
(Ex:) For category D59 CC codes: D47.4, D50.0-D64.9, D68.312, D68.51-D68.69, D75.81, D75.89-D75.9, D77, D89.2

D59.0   **Drug-induced autoimmune hemolytic anemia**
Use additional code for adverse effect, if applicable, to identify drug (T36-T50 with fifth or sixth character 5)

D59.1   **Other autoimmune hemolytic anemias**
Autoimmune hemolytic disease (cold type) (warm type)
Chronic cold hemagglutinin disease
Cold agglutinin disease
Cold agglutinin hemoglobinuria
Cold type (secondary) (symptomatic) hemolytic anemia
Warm type (secondary) (symptomatic) hemolytic anemia

> **Excludes1**   Evans syndrome (D69.41)
> hemolytic disease of newborn (P55.-)
> paroxysmal cold hemoglobinuria (D59.6)

D59.2   **Drug-induced nonautoimmune hemolytic anemia**
Drug-induced enzyme deficiency anemia
Use additional code for adverse effect, if applicable, to identify drug (T36-T50 with fifth or sixth character 5)

D59.3   **Hemolytic-uremic syndrome**
Use additional code to identify associated:
E. coli infection (B96.2-)
Pneumococcal pneumonia (J13)
Shigella dysenteriae (A03.9)

D59.4   **Other nonautoimmune hemolytic anemias**
Mechanical hemolytic anemia
Microangiopathic hemolytic anemia
Toxic hemolytic anemia

D59.5   **Paroxysmal nocturnal hemoglobinuria [Marchiafava-Micheli]**

> **Excludes1**   hemoglobinuria NOS (R82.3)

D59.6   **Hemoglobinuria due to hemolysis from other external causes**
Hemoglobinuria from exertion
March hemoglobinuria
Paroxysmal cold hemoglobinuria
Use additional code (Chapter 20) to identify external cause

> **Excludes1**   hemoglobinuria NOS (R82.3)

D59.8   **Other acquired hemolytic anemias**

D59.9   **Acquired hemolytic anemia, unspecified**
Idiopathic hemolytic anemia, chronic

APLASTIC AND OTHER ANEMIAS AND OTHER BONE MARROW FAILURE SYNDROMES (D60-D64)

● **D60**   **Acquired pure red cell aplasia [erythroblastopenia]**
Deficiency of erythroblasts

> **Includes**   red cell aplasia (acquired) (adult) (with thymoma)
> **Excludes1**   congenital red cell aplasia (D61.01)

(Ex:) For category D60 CC codes: D47.4, D50.0-D64.9, D68.312, D68.51-D68.69, D75.81, D75.89-D75.9, D77, D89.2

D60.0   **Chronic acquired pure red cell aplasia**
Lack of development of blood cell

D60.1   **Transient acquired pure red cell aplasia**

D60.8   **Other acquired pure red cell aplasias**

D60.9   **Acquired pure red cell aplasia, unspecified**

● **D61**   **Other aplastic anemias and other bone marrow failure syndromes**

> **Excludes1**   neutropenia (D70.-)

● **D61.0**   **Constitutional aplastic anemia**
Condition where bone marrow is unable to produce blood cells

D61.01   **Constitutional (pure) red blood cell aplasia**
Blackfan-Diamond syndrome
Congenital (pure) red cell aplasia
Familial hypoplastic anemia
Primary (pure) red cell aplasia
Red cell (pure) aplasia of infants

> **Excludes1**   acquired red cell aplasia (D60.9)

(Ex:) D50.0-D64.9, D75.9, P61.2-P61.4

D61.09   **Other constitutional aplastic anemia**
Fanconi's anemia
Pancytopenia with malformations
(Ex:) D50.0-D64.9, D69.3-D69.49, D75.9, P61.2-P61.4

D61.1   **Drug-induced aplastic anemia**
Use additional code for adverse effect, if applicable, to identify drug (T36-T50 with fifth or sixth character 5)
(Ex:) See D60

D61.2   **Aplastic anemia due to other external agents**
Code first , if applicable, toxic effects of substances chiefly nonmedicinal as to source (T51-T65)
(Ex:) See D60

D61.3   **Idiopathic aplastic anemia**
(Ex:) See D60

● **D61.8   Other specified aplastic anemias and other bone marrow failure syndromes**

(Ex) **For category D61.8 CC codes unless otherwise indicated:** D60.0-D60.9, D61.1-D64.9, D70.0-D70.9, D72.810-D72.820, D72.823, D72.825-D72.829, D75.9-D76.3, P61.2

● **D61.81   Pancytopenia**

Marked deficiency of all the blood elements: Red blood cells (erythrocytes), white blood cells (leukocytes), and platelets (thrombocytes). Check laboratory results.

Excludes1   pancytopenia (due to) (with) aplastic anemia (D61.9)

pancytopenia (due to) (with) bone marrow infiltration (D61.82)

pancytopenia (due to) (with) congenital (pure) red cell aplasia (D61.01)

pancytopenia (due to) (with) hairy cell leukemia (C91.4-)

pancytopenia (due to) (with) human immunodeficiency virus disease (B20.-)

pancytopenia (due to) (with) leukoerythroblastic anemia (D61.82)

pancytopenia (due to) (with) myelodysplastic syndromes (D46.-)

pancytopenia (due to) (with) myeloproliferative disease (D47.1)

D61.810   Antineoplastic chemotherapy induced pancytopenia 🔹

Excludes2   aplastic anemia due to antineoplastic chemotherapy (D61.1)

D61.811   Other drug-induced pancytopenia 🔹

Excludes2   aplastic anemia due to drugs (D61.1)

D61.818   Other pancytopenia 🔹

D61.82   Myelophthisis 🔹🔹

Leukoerythroblastic anemia
Myelophthisic anemia
Panmyelophthisis

Code also the underlying disorder, such as:
malignant neoplasm of breast (C50.-)
tuberculosis (A15.-)

Excludes1   idiopathic myelofibrosis (D47.1)

myelofibrosis NOS (D75.81)

myelofibrosis with myeloid metaplasia (D47.4)

primary myelofibrosis (D47.1)

secondary myelofibrosis (D75.81)

D61.89   Other specified aplastic anemias and other bone marrow failure syndromes 🔹

(Ex) See D60

D61.9   Aplastic anemia, unspecified 🔹

Hypoplastic anemia NOS
Medullary hypoplasia

(Ex) See D60

D62   Acute posthemorrhagic anemia 🔹

Excludes1   anemia due to chronic blood loss (D50.0)
blood loss anemia NOS (D50.0)
congenital anemia from fetal blood loss (P61.3)

(Ex) D47.4, D50.0-D64.9, D68.312, D68.51-D68.69, D75.81, D75.89-D75.9, D77, D89.2, T79.2XX[A]

▷ **D63   Anemia in chronic diseases classified elsewhere**

▷ **D63.0   Anemia in neoplastic disease**

Code first neoplasm (C00-D49)

Excludes1   anemia due to antineoplastic chemotherapy (D64.81)

aplastic anemia due to antineoplastic chemotherapy (D61.1)

OGCR   Section I.C.2.e.2.

2) Anemia associated with chemotherapy, immunotherapy and radiation therapy

When the admission/encounter is for management of an anemia associated with an adverse effect of the administration of chemotherapy or immunotherapy and the only treatment is for the anemia, the anemia code is sequenced first followed by the appropriate codes for the neoplasm and the adverse effect (T45.1X5, Adverse effect of antineoplastic and immunosuppressive drugs).

▷ **D63.1   Anemia in chronic kidney disease**

Erythropoietin resistant anemia (EPO resistant anemia)

Code first underlying chronic kidney disease (CKD) (N18.-)

▷ **D63.8   Anemia in other chronic diseases classified elsewhere**

Code first underlying disease, such as:
diphyllobothriasis (B70.0)
hookworm disease (B76.0-B76.9)
hypothyroidism (E00.0-E03.9)
malaria (B50.0-B54)
symptomatic late syphilis (A52.79)
tuberculosis (A18.89)

● **D64   Other anemias**

Excludes1   refractory anemia (D46.-)

refractory anemia with excess blasts in transformation [RAEB T] (C92.0-)

D64.0   Hereditary sideroblastic anemia

Abnormal production RBCs (erythrocytes)
Sex-linked hypochromic sideroblastic anemia

▷ **D64.1   Secondary sideroblastic anemia due to disease**

Code first underlying disease

D64.2   Secondary sideroblastic anemia due to drugs and toxins

Code first poisoning due to drug or toxin, if applicable (T36-T65 with fifth or sixth character 1-4 or 6)

Use additional code for adverse effect, if applicable, to identify drug (T36-T50 with fifth or sixth character 5)

D64.3   Other sideroblastic anemias

Sideroblastic anemia NOS
Pyridoxine-responsive sideroblastic anemia NEC

D64.4   Congenital dyserythropoietic anemia

Any of several rare hereditary anemias, mostly types of macrocytic anemia

Dyshematopoietic anemia (congenital)

Excludes1   Blackfan-Diamond syndrome (D61.01)
Di Guglielmo's disease (C94.0)

● **D64.8   Other specified anemias**

D64.81   Anemia due to antineoplastic chemotherapy

Antineoplastic chemotherapy induced anemia

Excludes1   anemia in neoplastic disease (D63.0)

aplastic anemia due to antineoplastic chemotherapy (D61.1)

D64.89   Other specified anemias

Infantile pseudoleukemia

D64.9   Anemia, unspecified

N Newborn Age: 0   **P** Pediatric Age: 0–17   **M** Maternity DX: 12–55   **A** Adult Age: 15–124   ♀ Females Only   ♂ Males Only

🔹 Complication\Comorbidity   🔹 Major C\C   (Ex) CC/MCC Exclusions   🔹 Present on Admission Requirement   🔹 Hospital-Acquired Condition

825

CHAPTER 3 (D50-D89)

CHAPTER 3 (D50-D89)

COAGULATION DEFECTS, PURPURA AND OTHER HEMORRHAGIC CONDITIONS (D65-D69)

D65   Disseminated intravascular coagulation [defibrination syndrome]

Blood clots form and consume all coagulation proteins and platelets and disrupt normal coagulation, resulting in abnormal bleeding

Afibrinogenemia, acquired
Consumption coagulopathy
Diffuse or disseminated intravascular coagulation [DIC]
Fibrinolytic hemorrhage, acquired
Fibrinolytic purpura
Purpura fulminans

> **Excludes1**   disseminated intravascular coagulation (complicating):
> abortion or ectopic or molar pregnancy (O00-O07, O08.1)
> in newborn (P60)
> pregnancy, childbirth and the puerperium (O45.0, O46.0, O67.0, O72.3)

(Ex:) D47.4, D65-D69.9, D75.81-D75.9, D77, D89.2

D66   Hereditary factor VIII deficiency

Inherited coagulation disorder carried by females but most often affecting males

Classical hemophilia
Deficiency factor VIII (with functional defect)
Hemophilia NOS
Hemophilia A

> **Excludes1**   factor VIII deficiency with vascular defect (D68.0)

(Ex:) See D65

D67   Hereditary factor IX deficiency

Christmas disease
Factor IX deficiency (with functional defect)
Hemophilia B
Plasma thromboplastin component [PTC] deficiency

(Ex:) See D65

● D68   Other coagulation defects

> **Excludes1**   abnormal coagulation profile (R79.1)
> coagulation defects complicating abortion or ectopic or molar pregnancy (O00-O07, O08.1) ◄
> ~~abortion or ectopic or molar pregnancy (O00-O07, O08.1)~~
> coagulation defects complicating pregnancy, childbirth and the puerperium (O45.0, O46.0, O67.0, O72.3) ◄

D68.0   Von Willebrand's disease

Congenital bleeding disorder

Angiohemophilia
Factor VIII deficiency with vascular defect
Vascular hemophilia

> **Excludes1**   capillary fragility (hereditary) (D69.8)
> factor VIII deficiency NOS (D66)
> factor VIII deficiency with functional defect (D66)

D68.1   Hereditary factor XI deficiency

Deficiency of blood coagulation resulting in systemic blood-clotting defect

Hemophilia C
Plasma thromboplastin antecedent [PTA] deficiency
Rosenthal's disease

D68.2   Hereditary deficiency of other clotting factors

Blood clotting disorders caused by hereditary deficiencies of one or more clotting factors

AC globulin deficiency
Congenital afibrinogenemia
Deficiency of factor I [fibrinogen]
Deficiency of factor II [prothrombin]
Deficiency of factor V [labile]
Deficiency of factor VII [stable]
Deficiency of factor X [Stuart-Prower]
Deficiency of factor XII [Hageman]
Deficiency of factor XIII [fibrin stabilizing]
Dysfibrinogenemia (congenital)
Hypoproconvertinemia
Owren's disease
Proaccelerin deficiency

● D68.3   Hemorrhagic disorder due to circulating anticoagulants

Blood clotting disorders caused by anticoagulants (warfarin and heparin)

● D68.31   Hemorrhagic disorder due to intrinsic circulating anticoagulants, antibodies, or inhibitors

D68.311   Acquired hemophilia

Autoimmune hemophilia
Autoimmune inhibitors to clotting factors
Secondary hemophilia

(Ex:) D47.4, D65-D69.9, D75.82-D75.9, D77, D89.2

D68.312   Antiphospholipid antibody with hemorrhagic disorder

Lupus anticoagulant (LAC) with hemorrhagic disorder
Systemic lupus erythematosus [SLE] inhibitor with hemorrhagic disorder

> **Excludes1**   antiphospholipid antibody, finding without diagnosis (R76.0)
> antiphospholipid antibody syndrome (D68.61)
> antiphospholipid antibody with hypercoagulable state (D68.61)
> lupus anticoagulant (LAC) finding without diagnosis (R76.0)
> lupus anticoagulant (LAC) with hypercoagulable state (D68.62)
> systemic lupus erythematosus [SLE] inhibitor finding without diagnosis (R76.0)
> systemic lupus erythematosus [SLE] inhibitor with hypercoagulable state (D68.62)

(Ex:) D47.4, D68.311-D68.318, D68.51-D68.69, D70.0-D72.9, D73.81, D75.81, D75.89-D77, D89.2

D68.318   Other hemorrhagic disorder due to intrinsic circulating anticoagulants, antibodies, or inhibitors

Antithromboplastinemia
Antithromboplastinogenemia
Hemorrhagic disorder due to intrinsic increase in antithrombin
Hemorrhagic disorder due to intrinsic increase in anti-VIIIa
Hemorrhagic disorder due to intrinsic increase in anti-IXa
Hemorrhagic disorder due to intrinsic increase in anti-XIa

(Ex:) See 68.31

◄ New   ◄ⅿ Revised   ~~deleted~~ Deleted   Excludes 1   Excludes 2   Includes   Use additional   Code first   Code also   Unspecified

OGCR Official Guidelines   ● Unacceptable Principal Diagnosis   X Assign placeholder X   ● Use Additional Character(s)   ▸ Manifestation Code   **Coding Clinic**

D68.32   **Hemorrhagic disorder due to extrinsic circulating anticoagulants** 🔹
Drug-induced hemorrhagic disorder
Hemorrhagic disorder due to increase in anti-IIa
Hemorrhagic disorder due to increase in anti-Xa
Hyperheparinemia
Use additional code for adverse effect, if applicable, to identify drug (T45.515, T45.525)
(Ex:) D47.4, D65-D69.9, D75.81-D75.9, D77, D89.2

D68.4   **Acquired coagulation factor deficiency** 🔹
Deficiency of coagulation factor due to liver disease
Deficiency of coagulation factor due to vitamin K deficiency
Excludes1   vitamin K deficiency of newborn (P53)
(Ex:) See D68.32

● D68.5   **Primary thrombophilia**
AKA idiopathic thrombocytopenia, may be acquired or congenital and is a common cause of coagulation disorders.
Primary hypercoagulable states
Excludes1   antiphospholipid syndrome (D68.61)
lupus anticoagulant (D68.62)
secondary activated protein C resistance (D68.69)
secondary antiphospholipid antibody syndrome (D68.69)
secondary lupus anticoagulant with hypercoagulable state (D68.69)
secondary systemic lupus erythematosus [SLE] inhibitor with hypercoagulable state (D68.69)
systemic lupus erythematosus [SLE] inhibitor finding without diagnosis (R76.0)
systemic lupus erythematosus [SLE] inhibitor with hemorrhagic disorder (D68.312)
thrombotic thrombocytopenic purpura (M31.1)
(Ex:) **For category D68.5 CC codes:** D47.4, D68.312, D68.51-D68.69, D70.0-D72.9, D73.81, D75.81, D75.89-D77, D89.2

D68.51   **Activated protein C resistance** 🔹
Factor V Leiden mutation

D68.52   **Prothrombin gene mutation** 🔹

D68.59   **Other primary thrombophilia** 🔹
Antithrombin III deficiency
Hypercoagulable state NOS
Primary hypercoagulable state NEC
Primary thrombophilia NEC
Protein C deficiency
Protein S deficiency
Thrombophilia NOS

● D68.6   **Other thrombophilia**
Other hypercoagulable states
Excludes1   diffuse or disseminated intravascular coagulation [DIC] (D65)
heparin induced thrombocytopenia (HIT) (D75.82)
hyperhomocysteinemia (E72.11)
(Ex:) **For category D68.6 CC codes:** D47.4, D68.312, D68.51-D68.69, D70.0-D72.9, D73.81, D75.81, D75.89-D77, D89.2

D68.61   **Antiphospholipid syndrome** 🔹
Anticardiolipin syndrome
Antiphospholipid antibody syndrome
Excludes1   anti-phospholipid antibody, finding without diagnosis (R76.0)
anti-phospholipid antibody with hemorrhagic disorder (D68.312)
lupus anticoagulant syndrome (D68.62)

D68.62   **Lupus anticoagulant syndrome** 🔹
Lupus anticoagulant
Presence of systemic lupus erythematosus [SLE] inhibitor
Excludes1   anticardiolipin syndrome (D68.61)
antiphospholipid syndrome (D68.61)
lupus anticoagulant (LAC) finding without diagnosis (R79.0)
lupus anticoagulant (LAC) with hemorrhagic disorder (D68.312)

D68.69   **Other thrombophilia** 🔹
Hypercoagulable states NEC
Secondary hypercoagulable state NOS

D68.8   **Other specified coagulation defects** 🔹
Excludes1   hemorrhagic disease of newborn (P53)
(Ex:) See D68.32

D68.9   **Coagulation defect, unspecified** 🔹
(Ex:) See D68.32

● D69   **Purpura and other hemorrhagic conditions**
Group of conditions characterized by small hemorrhages in skin, mucous membranes, or serosal surfaces
Excludes1   benign hypergammaglobulinemic purpura (D89.0)
cryoglobulinemic purpura (D89.1)
essential (hemorrhagic) thrombocythemia (D47.3)
hemorrhagic thrombocythemia (D47.3)
purpura fulminans (D65)
thrombotic thrombocytopenic purpura (M31.1)
Waldenström hypergammaglobulinemic purpura (D89.0)

D69.0   **Allergic purpura** 🔹
Allergic vasculitis
Nonthrombocytopenic hemorrhagic purpura
Nonthrombocytopenic idiopathic purpura
Purpura anaphylactoid
Purpura Henoch(-Schönlein)
Purpura rheumatica
Vascular purpura
Excludes1   thrombocytopenic hemorrhagic purpura (D69.3)
(Ex:) See D68.32

N Newborn Age: 0   **P** Pediatric Age: 0–17   **M** Maternity DX: 12–55   **A** Adult Age: 15–124   ♀ Females Only   ♂ Males Only
🔹 Complication\Comorbidity   Major C\C   (Ex:) CC/MCC Exclusions   Present on Admission Requirement   Hospital-Acquired Condition

827

CHAPTER 3 (D50-D89)

CHAPTER 3 (D50-D89)

D69.1 Qualitative platelet defects
Bernard-Soulier [giant platelet] syndrome
Glanzmann's disease
Grey platelet syndrome
Thromboasthenia (hemorrhagic) (hereditary)
Thrombocytopathy
> **Excludes1** von Willebrand's disease (D68.0)

D69.2 Other nonthrombocytopenic purpura
Purpura NOS
Purpura simplex
Senile purpura

D69.3 Immune thrombocytopenic purpura
Hemorrhagic (thrombocytopenic) purpura
Idiopathic thrombocytopenic purpura
Tidal platelet dysgenesis
Ex) See D68.32

● **D69.4 Other primary thrombocytopenia**
> **Excludes1** transient neonatal thrombocytopenia (P61.0)
> Wiskott-Aldrich syndrome (D82.0)

D69.41 Evans syndrome
Acquired hemolytic anemia and thrombocytopenia
Ex) See D68.32

D69.42 Congenital and hereditary thrombocytopenia purpura
Congenital thrombocytopenia
Hereditary thrombocytopenia
> *Code first* congenital or hereditary disorder, such as:
> thrombocytopenia with absent radius (TAR syndrome) (Q87.2)
Ex) See D68.32

D69.49 Other primary thrombocytopenia
Megakaryocytic hypoplasia
Primary thrombocytopenia NOS

● **D69.5 Secondary thrombocytopenia**
Acquired reduction of number of platelets required for blood clotting
> **Excludes1** heparin induced thrombocytopenia (HIT) (D75.82)
> transient thrombocytopenia of newborn (P61.0)

D69.51 Posttransfusion purpura
Posttransfusion purpura from whole blood (fresh) or blood products PTP

D69.59 Other secondary thrombocytopenia

D69.6 Thrombocytopenia, unspecified

D69.8 Other specified hemorrhagic conditions
Capillary fragility (hereditary)
Vascular pseudohemophilia

D69.9 Hemorrhagic condition, unspecified

OTHER DISORDERS OF BLOOD AND BLOOD-FORMING ORGANS (D70-D77)

● **D70 Neutropenia**
Decrease in number of neutrophils (type of white blood cell)
> **Includes** agranulocytosis
> decreased absolute neurophile count (ANC)
Use additional code for any associated:
fever (R50.81)
mucositis (J34.81, K12.3-, K92.81, N76.81)
> **Excludes1** neutropenic splenomegaly (D73.81)
> transient neonatal neutropenia (P61.5)

D70.0 Congenital agranulocytosis
Reduced numbers of neutrophils (type of white blood cell)
Congenital neutropenia
Infantile genetic agranulocytosis
Kostmann's disease

D70.1 Agranulocytosis secondary to cancer chemotherapy
Decreased numbers of granulocytes (type of white blood cell)
> *Code also* underlying neoplasm
Use additional code for adverse effect, if applicable, to identify drug (T45.1X5)

D70.2 Other drug-induced agranulocytosis
Use additional code for adverse effect, if applicable, to identify drug (T36-T50 with fifth or sixth character 5)

D70.3 Neutropenia due to infection

D70.4 Cyclic neutropenia
Chronic neutropenia (low number of type of white blood cell)
Cyclic hematopoiesis
Periodic neutropenia

D70.8 Other neutropenia

D70.9 Neutropenia, unspecified

D71 Functional disorders of polymorphonuclear neutrophils
Polymorphonuclear: varying shapes of nucleus; AKA PMNs
Cell membrane receptor complex [CR3] defect
Chronic (childhood) granulomatous disease
Congenital dysphagocytosis
Progressive septic granulomatosis

● **D72 Other disorders of white blood cells**
> **Excludes1** basophilia (D72.824)
> immunity disorders (D80-D89)
> neutropenia (D70)
> preleukemia (syndrome) (D46.9)

D72.0 Genetic anomalies of leukocytes
Alder (granulation) (granulocyte) anomaly
Alder syndrome
Hereditary leukocytic hypersegmentation
Hereditary leukocytic hyposegmentation
Hereditary leukomelanopathy
May-Hegglin (granulation) (granulocyte) anomaly
May-Hegglin syndrome
Pelger-Huët (granulation) (granulocyte) anomaly
Pelger-Huët syndrome
> **Excludes1** Chédiak (-Steinbrinck)-Higashi syndrome (E70.330)

D72.1 Eosinophilia
Formation and accumulation of high number of white cells in blood/tissue
Allergic eosinophilia
Hereditary eosinophilia
> **Excludes1** Löffler's syndrome (J82)
> pulmonary eosinophilia (J82)

● **D72.8 Other specified disorders of white blood cells**
> **Excludes1** leukemia (C91-C95)

● **D72.81 Decreased white blood cell count**
> **Excludes1** neutropenia (D70.-)

D72.810 Lymphocytopenia
Decreased lymphocytes
Reduction in number of lympho cytes in blood

D72.818 Other decreased white blood cell count
Basophilic leukopenia
Eosinophilic leukopenia
Monocytopenia
Other decreased leukocytes
Plasmacytopenia

D72.819 Decreased white blood cell count, unspecified
Decreased leukocytes, unspecified
Leukocytopenia, unspecified
Leukopenia
> **Excludes1** malignant leukopenia (D70.9)

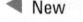

◀ New   ◀ Revised   ~~deleted~~ Deleted   Excludes 1   Excludes 2   Includes   Use additional   Code first   Code also   Unspecified
OGCR Official Guidelines   ● Unacceptable Principal Diagnosis   X Assign placeholder X   ● Use Additional Character(s)   ▶ Manifestation Code   **Coding Clinic**

● **D72.82**   **Elevated white blood cell count**
> **Excludes1**   eosinophilia (D72.1)

   D72.820   **Lymphocytosis (symptomatic)**
> Elevated lymphocytes
> *Excess of normal lymphocytes*

   D72.821   **Monocytosis (symptomatic)**
> **Excludes1**   infectious mononucleosis (B27.-)

   D72.822   **Plasmacytosis**
> *Presence of excess plasma cells*

   D72.823   **Leukemoid reaction**
> Basophilic leukemoid reaction
> Leukemoid reaction NOS
> Lymphocytic leukemoid reaction
> Monocytic leukemoid reaction
> Myelocytic leukemoid reaction
> Neutrophilic leukemoid reaction

   D72.824   **Basophilia**
> *Increase of basophils in blood*

   D72.825   **Bandemia**
> Bandemia without diagnosis of specific infection
> *Excess number of band cells (immature white blood cells) released by bone marrow*
> **Excludes1**   confirmed infection -code to infection
> leukemia (C91.-, C92.-, C93.-, C94.-, C95.-)

   D72.828   **Other elevated white blood cell count**

   D72.829   **Elevated white blood cell count, unspecified**
> Elevated leukocytes, unspecified
> Leukocytosis, unspecified

   D72.89   **Other specified disorders of white blood cells**
> Abnormality of white blood cells NEC

● **D72.9**   **Disorder of white blood cells, unspecified**
> Abnormal leukocyte differential NOS

● **D73**   **Diseases of spleen**

   D73.0   **Hyposplenism**
> *Diminished functioning of spleen*
> Atrophy of spleen
> **Excludes1**   asplenia (congenital) (Q89.01)
> postsurgical absence of spleen (Z90.81)

   D73.1   **Hypersplenism**
> *Accelerated function of spleen*
> **Excludes1**   neutropenic splenomegaly (D73.81)
> primary splenic neutropenia (D73.81)
> splenitis, splenomegaly in late syphilis (A52.79)
> splenitis, splenomegaly in tuberculosis (A18.85)
> splenomegaly NOS (R16.1)
> splenomegaly congenital (Q89.0)

   D73.2   **Chronic congestive splenomegaly**
> *Enlargement of spleen*

   D73.3   **Abscess of spleen**

   D73.4   **Cyst of spleen**

   D73.5   **Infarction of spleen**
> Splenic rupture, nontraumatic
> Torsion of spleen
> **Excludes1**   rupture of spleen due to Plasmodium vivax malaria (B51.0)
> traumatic rupture of spleen (S36.03-)

● **D73.8**   **Other diseases of spleen**

   D73.81   **Neutropenic splenomegaly**
> Werner-Schultz disease
> *Enlarged spleen responding to inadequate number of neutrophils*

   D73.89   **Other diseases of spleen**
> Fibrosis of spleen NOS
> Perisplenitis
> Splenitis NOS

● **D73.9**   **Disease of spleen, unspecified**

● **D74**   **Methemoglobinemia**
> *Excessive methemoglobin (form of hemoglobin)*
> Ⓔ **For category D74 CC codes:** D56.4, D58.2-D59.2, D59.4-D59.9, D64.4-D64.9, D74.0-D74.9, D75.9

   D74.0   **Congenital methemoglobinemia** 🔖
> Congenital NADH-methemoglobin reductase deficiency
> Hemoglobin-M [Hb-M] disease
> Methemoglobinemia, hereditary

   D74.8   **Other methemoglobinemias** 🔖
> Acquired methemoglobinemia (with sulfhemoglobinemia)
> Toxic methemoglobinemia

● **D74.9**   **Methemoglobinemia, unspecified** 🔖

● **D75**   **Other and unspecified diseases of blood and blood-forming organs**
> **Excludes2**   acute lymphadenitis (L04.-)
> chronic lymphadenitis (I88.1)
> enlarged lymph nodes (R59.-)
> hypergammaglobulinemia NOS (D89.2)
> lymphadenitis NOS (I88.9)
> mesenteric lymphadenitis (acute) (chronic) (I88.0)

   D75.0   **Familial erythrocytosis**
> *Genetic mutation of gene that results in increased circulating RBCs*
> Benign polycythemia
> Familial polycythemia
> **Excludes1**   hereditary ovalocytosis (D58.1)

   D75.1   **Secondary polycythemia**
> *Increase in total red cell mass*
> Acquired polycythemia
> Emotional polycythemia
> Erythrocytosis NOS
> Hypoxemic polycythemia
> Nephrogenous polycythemia
> Polycythemia due to erythropoietin
> Polycythemia due to fall in plasma volume
> Polycythemia due to high altitude
> Polycythemia due to stress
> Polycythemia NOS
> Relative polycythemia
> **Excludes1**   polycythemia neonatorum (P61.1)
> polycythemia vera (D45)

CHAPTER 3 (D50-D89)

N Newborn Age: 0   **P** Pediatric Age: 0–17   **M** Maternity DX: 12–55   **A** Adult Age: 15–124   ♀ Females Only   ♂ Males Only

● Complication\Comorbidity   🔖 Major C\C   Ⓔ CC/MCC Exclusions   🔖 Present on Admission Requirement   🔖 Hospital-Acquired Condition

829

● **D75.8   Other specified diseases of blood and blood-forming organs**

D75.81   Myelofibrosis 🔾

Replacing bone marrow by fibrous tissue
Myelofibrosis NOS
Secondary myelofibrosis NOS

Code first the underlying disorder, such as:
malignant neoplasm of breast (C50.-)

Use additional code, if applicable,
for associated therapy-related
myelodysplastic syndrome (D46.-)

Use additional code for adverse effect, if
applicable, to identify drug (T45.1X5)

Excludes1   acute myelofibrosis (C94.4-)
idiopathic myelofibrosis (D47.1)
leukoerythroblastic anemia
(D61.82)
myelofibrosis with myeloid
metaplasia (D47.4)
myelophthisic anemia (D61.82)
myelophthisis (D61.82)
primary myelofibrosis (D47.1)

Ex) C88.2-C88.3, C88.8-C88.9, C90.10-C90.11, C90.20-C90.21,
C90.30-C90.31, C91.00-C91.02, C91.10-C91.12, C91.30-C91.32,
C91.40-C91.42, C91.50-C91.52, C91.60-C91.62, C91.90-C91.92,
C91.A0-C91.A2, C91.Z0-C91.Z2, C92.00-C92.02, C92.10-C92.12,
C92.20-C92.22, C92.30-C92.32, C92.40-C92.42, C92.50-C92.52,
C92.60-C92.62, C92.90-C92.92, C92.A0-C92.A2, C92.Z0-C92.Z2,
C93.00-C93.02, C93.10-C93.12, C93.30-C93.32, C93.90-C93.92,
C93.Z0-C93.Z2, C94.00-C94.02, C94.20-C94.22, C94.30-C94.32,
C94.40-C94.42, C94.6, C94.80-C94.82, C95.00-C95.02,
C95.10-C95.12, C95.90-C95.92, D45-D46.22, D46.4, D46.9,
D46.A-D46.Z, D47.0-D47.1, D47.3, D47.9, D47.Z9,
D48.7-D48.9

D75.82   Heparin induced thrombocytopenia (HIT)

D75.89   Other specified diseases of blood and blood-forming organs

D75.9   Disease of blood and blood-forming organs, unspecified

● **D76   Other specified diseases with participation of lymphoreticular and reticulohistiocytic tissue**

Excludes1   (Abt-) Letterer-Siwe disease (C96.0)
eosinophilic granuloma (C96.6)
Hand-Schüller-Christian disease (C96.5)
histiocytic sarcoma (C96.A)
histiocytosis X, multifocal (C96.5)
histiocytosis X, unifocal (C96.6)
malignant histiocytosis (C96.A)
Langerhans-cell histiocytosis, multifocal (C96.5)
Langerhans-cell histiocytosis NOS (C96.6)
Langerhans-cell histiocytosis, unifocal (C96.6)

Excludes1   leukemic reticuloendotheliosis or reticulosis
(C91.4-)
lipomelanotic reticuloendotheliosis or reticulosis
(I89.8)

Ex) For category D76 CC codes: D60.0-D60.9, D61.1-D61.9, D65, D69.3-D70.9,
D72.818-D72.819, D75.82, D75.9

D76.1   Hemophagocytic lymphohistiocytosis 🔾
Familial hemophagocytic reticulosis
Histiocytoses of mononuclear phagocytes

D76.2   Hemophagocytic syndrome, infection-associated 🔾
Use additional code to identify infectious agent or
disease.

D76.3   Other histiocytosis syndromes 🔾
Reticulohistiocytoma (giant-cell)
Sinus histiocytosis with massive lymphadenopathy
Xanthogranuloma

▷ **D77   Other disorders of blood and blood-forming organs in diseases classified elsewhere**

Code first underlying disease, such as:
amyloidosis (E85.-) ◀▦
congenital early syphilis (A50.0)
echinococcosis (B67.0-B67.9)
malaria (B50.0-B54)
schistosomiasis [bilharziasis] (B65.0-B65.9)
vitamin C deficiency (E54)

Excludes1   rupture of spleen due to Plasmodium vivax
malaria (B51.0)
splenitis, splenomegaly in late syphilis
(A52.79) ◀▦
late syphilis (A52.79)
splenitis, splenomegaly in tuberculosis
(A18.85) ◀▦

INTRAOPERATIVE AND POSTPROCEDURAL COMPLICATIONS OF THE SPLEEN (D78)

● **D78   Intraoperative and postprocedural complications of the spleen**

● **D78.0   Intraoperative hemorrhage and hematoma of the spleen complicating a procedure**

Excludes1   intraoperative hemorrhage and
hematoma of the spleen due to
accidental puncture or laceration
during a procedure (D78.1-)

Ex) For category D78.0 CC codes: D78.01-D78.02, D78.21-D78.89,
H95.811-H95.89, I85.01, I85.11, I97.3, K21.9, K22.8, K23-K25.0, K25.2,
K25.4, K25.6, K26.0, K26.2, K26.4, K26.6, K27.0, K27.2, K27.4, K27.6,
K28.0, K28.2, K28.4, K28.6, K29.01, K29.21, K29.31, K29.41, K29.51,
K29.61, K29.71, K29.81, K29.91, K31.811, K55.21, K57.01, K57.11,
K57.13, K57.21, K57.31, K57.33, K57.41, K57.51, K57.53, K57.81, K57.91,
K57.93, K62.5, K92.0-K92.2, M96.89, N98.1-N98.9, P54.1-P54.3,
T81.10X-T81.19X[A], T81.82X[A], T81.89X-T81.9XX[A]

**D78.01   Intraoperative hemorrhage and hematoma of
the spleen complicating a procedure on the
spleen** 🔾

**D78.02   Intraoperative hemorrhage and hematoma of
the spleen complicating other procedure** 🔾

● **D78.1   Accidental puncture and laceration of the spleen during
a procedure**

Ex) For category D78.1 CC codes: D78.11-D78.12, D78.81-D78.89,
E36.11-E36.8, E89.810-E89.89, G96.11, G97.41-G97.49, H59.011-H59.019,
H59.031-H59.099, H59.211-H59.229, H59.811-H59.89, H95.31-H95.32,
H95.811-H95.89, I97.3, I97.51-I97.52, J95.71-J95.72, K91.71-K91.72,
L76.11-L76.12, L76.81-L76.82, M96.820-M96.821, M96.89, N98.1-N98.9,
N99.71-N99.72, T81.82X[A], T81.89X-T81.9XX[A]

**D78.11   Accidental puncture and laceration of the
spleen during a procedure on the spleen** 🔾

**D78.12   Accidental puncture and laceration of the
spleen during other procedure** 🔾

● **D78.2   Postprocedural hemorrhage and hematoma of the spleen
following a procedure**

Ex) For category D78.2 CC codes: See D78.0

**D78.21   Postprocedural hemorrhage and hematoma of
the spleen following a procedure on the
spleen** 🔾

**D78.22   Postprocedural hemorrhage and hematoma of
the spleen following other procedure** 🔾

● **D78.8   Other intraoperative and postprocedural complications
of the spleen**

Use additional code, if applicable, to further specify
disorder

Ex) For category D78.8 CC codes: D78.81-D78.89, H95.811-H95.89, I97.3,
M96.89, N98.1-N98.9, T81.82X[A], T81.89X-T81.9XX[A]

**D78.81   Other intraoperative complications of the
spleen** 🔾

**D78.89   Other postprocedural complications of the
spleen** 🔾

◀ New   ◀▦ Revised   deleted Deleted   Excludes 1   Excludes 2   Includes   Use additional   Code first   Code also   Unspecified

OGCR Official Guidelines   ● Unacceptable Principal Diagnosis   X Assign placeholder X   ● Use Additional Character(s)   ▷ Manifestation Code   **Coding Clinic**

CERTAIN DISORDERS INVOLVING THE IMMUNE MECHANISM (D80-D89)

Includes	defects in the complement system
	immunodeficiency disorders, except human immunodeficiency virus [HIV] disease
	sarcoidosis

Excludes1	autoimmune disease (systemic) NOS (M35.9)
	functional disorders of polymorphonuclear neutrophils (D71)
	human immunodeficiency virus [HIV] disease (B20)

● **D80   Immunodeficiency with predominantly antibody defects**
  (Ex:) For category D80 CC codes unless otherwise indicated: D80.0, D80.3-D81.4, D81.6-D81.7, D81.89-D84.0, D84.8-D84.9, D89.3-D89.9

  D80.0   Hereditary hypogammaglobulinemia 🔾
      Autosomal recessive agammaglobulinemia (Swiss type)
      X-linked agammaglobulinemia [Bruton] (with growth hormone deficiency)

  D80.1   Nonfamilial hypogammaglobulinemia 🔾
      Abnormally low levels of all classes of immunoglobulins
      Agammaglobulinemia with immunoglobulin-bearing B-lymphocytes
      Common variable agammaglobulinemia [CVAgamma]
      Hypogammaglobulinemia NOS
      (Ex:) D80.0-D81.2, D81.4, D81.6-D81.7, D81.89-D84.0, D84.8-D84.9, D89.3-D89.9

  D80.2   Selective deficiency of immunoglobulin A [IgA] 🔾
      (Ex:) See D80.1

  D80.3   Selective deficiency of immunoglobulin G [IgG] subclasses 🔾

  D80.4   Selective deficiency of immunoglobulin M [IgM] 🔾

  D80.5   Immunodeficiency with increased immunoglobulin M [IgM] 🔾

  D80.6   Antibody deficiency with near-normal immunoglobulins or with hyperimmunoglobulinemia 🔾
      Abnormally high levels of immunoglobulins in serum

  D80.7   Transient hypogammaglobulinemia of infancy 🔾   **N**

  D80.8   Other immunodeficiencies with predominantly antibody defects
      Kappa light chain deficiency

  D80.9   Immunodeficiency with predominantly antibody defects, unspecified 🔾

● **D81   Combined immunodeficiencies**
Excludes1	autosomal recessive agammaglobulinemia (Swiss type) (D80.0)
  (Ex:) For category D81 CC codes unless otherwise indicated: D80.0, D80.3-D81.4, D81.6-D81.7, D81.89-D84.0, D84.8-D84.9, D89.3-D89.9

  D81.0   Severe combined immunodeficiency [SCID] with reticular dysgenesis 🔾

  D81.1   Severe combined immunodeficiency [SCID] with low T- and B-cell numbers 🔾

  D81.2   Severe combined immunodeficiency [SCID] with low or normal B-cell numbers 🔾

  D81.3   Adenosine deaminase [ADA] deficiency 🔾
      (Ex:) D81.3, D81.5, D81.810, D84.1, E76.01-E76.9, E79.1-E80.29, E80.4-E80.7, E88.81

  D81.4   Nezelof's syndrome 🔾

  D81.5   Purine nucleoside phosphorylase [PNP] deficiency 🔾
      (Ex:) See D81.3

  D81.6   Major histocompatibility complex class I deficiency 🔾
      Bare lymphocyte syndrome

  D81.7   Major histocompatibility complex class II deficiency 🔾

● **D81.8   Other combined immunodeficiencies**

● **D81.81   Biotin-dependent carboxylase deficiency**
      Multiple carboxylase deficiency
Excludes1	biotin-dependent carboxylase deficiency due to dietary deficiency of biotin (E53.8)

  D81.810   Biotinidase deficiency

  D81.818   Other biotin-dependent carboxylase deficiency
      Holocarboxylase synthetase deficiency
      Other multiple carboxylase deficiency

  D81.819   Biotin-dependent carboxylase deficiency, unspecified
      Multiple carboxylase deficiency, unspecified

  D81.89   Other combined immunodeficiencies 🔾

  D81.9   Combined immunodeficiency, unspecified 🔾
      Severe combined immunodeficiency disorder [SCID] NOS

● **D82   Immunodeficiency associated with other major defects**
Excludes1	ataxia telangiectasia [Louis-Bar] (G11.3)

  D82.0   Wiskott-Aldrich syndrome 🔾
      X-linked immunodeficiency
      Immunodeficiency with thrombocytopenia and eczema
      (Ex:) See D81

  D82.1   Di George's syndrome 🔾
      Congenital disorder with defective development of third and fourth pharyngeal pouches
      Pharyngeal pouch syndrome
      Thymic alymphoplasia
      Thymic aplasia or hypoplasia with immunodeficiency
      (Ex:) See D81

  D82.2   Immunodeficiency with short-limbed stature

  D82.3   Immunodeficiency following hereditary defective response to Epstein-Barr virus
      X-linked lymphoproliferative disease

  D82.4   Hyperimmunoglobulin E [IgE] syndrome
      Suspected genetic defect that produces high levels of antibody immunoglobulin (IgE) that causes skin and lung infections and eczema

  D82.8   Immunodeficiency associated with other specified major defects

  D82.9   Immunodeficiency associated with major defect, unspecified

● **D83   Common variable immunodeficiency**
  (Ex:) For category D83 CC codes: D80.0, D80.3-D81.4, D81.6-D81.7, D81.89-D84.0, D84.8-D84.9, D89.3-D89.9

  D83.0   Common variable immunodeficiency with predominant abnormalities of B-cell numbers and function 🔾

  D83.1   Common variable immunodeficiency with predominant immunoregulatory T-cell disorders 🔾

  D83.2   Common variable immunodeficiency with autoantibodies to B- or T-cells 🔾

  D83.8   Other common variable immunodeficiencies 🔾

  D83.9   Common variable immunodeficiency, unspecified 🔾

● **D84   Other immunodeficiencies**

  D84.0   Lymphocyte function antigen-1 [LFA-1] defect

  D84.1   Defects in the complement system
      C1 esterase inhibitor [C1-INH] deficiency

  D84.8   Other specified immunodeficiencies 🔾
      (Ex:) See D83

  D84.9   Immunodeficiency, unspecified 🔾
      (Ex:) See D83

CHAPTER 3 (D50-D89)

Item 3-1 Sarcoidosis: A symptom of an inflammation producing tiny lumps of cells (granulomas) in various organs, most commonly the lungs and lymph nodes, that affect organ function. Cause is unknown occurring primarily in 20- to 40-year-olds, African-American, especially women, and those of Asian, German, Irish, Scandinavian, and Puerto Rican heritage.

● **D86**   **Sarcoidosis**

     D86.0   **Sarcoidosis of lung**

     D86.1   **Sarcoidosis of lymph nodes**

     D86.2   **Sarcoidosis of lung with sarcoidosis of lymph nodes**

     D86.3   **Sarcoidosis of skin**

     ● **D86.8**   **Sarcoidosis of other sites**

         D86.81   **Sarcoid meningitis**

         D86.82   **Multiple cranial nerve palsies in sarcoidosis**

         D86.83   **Sarcoid iridocyclitis**
                 Rare large tumor with irregular surface of iris

         D86.84   **Sarcoid pyelonephritis**
                 Systemic disease of unknown etiology characterized by chronic granulomatous inflammation with tissue destruction of pelvis kidney
                 Tubulo-interstitial nephropathy in sarcoidosis

         D86.85   **Sarcoid myocarditis**

         D86.86   **Sarcoid arthropathy**
                 Polyarthritis in sarcoidosis

         D86.87   **Sarcoid myositis**
                 Granumloma of muscle

         D86.89   **Sarcoidosis of other sites**
                 Hepatic granuloma
                 Uveoparotid fever [Heerfordt]

     D86.9   **Sarcoidosis, unspecified**

● **D89**   **Other disorders involving the immune mechanism, not elsewhere classified**

     Excludes1   hyperglobulinemia NOS (R77.1)
                 monoclonal gammopathy (of undetermined significance) (D47.2)

     Excludes2   transplant failure and rejection (T86.-)

     D89.0   **Polyclonal hypergammaglobulinemia**
         Benign hypergammaglobulinemic purpura
         Polyclonal gammopathy NOS

     D89.1   **Cryoglobulinemia**
         Cryoglobulin (proteins) in blood that precipitate temperatures below 98.6° F; usually symptomatic of underlying disease
         Cryoglobulinemic purpura
         Cryoglobulinemic vasculitis
         Essential cryoglobulinemia
         Idiopathic cryoglobulinemia
         Mixed cryoglobulinemia
         Primary cryoglobulinemia
         Secondary cryoglobulinemia

     D89.2   **Hypergammaglobulinemia, unspecified**

     D89.3   **Immune reconstitution syndrome**
         Immune reconstitution inflammatory syndrome [IRIS]
         Use additional code for adverse effect, if applicable, to identify drug (T36-T50 with fifth or sixth character 5)

●   **D89.8**   **Other specified disorders involving the immune mechanism, not elsewhere classified**

     ● **D89.81**   **Graft-versus-host disease**
         Code first underlying cause, such as:
             complications of transplanted organs and tissue (T86.-)
             complications of blood transfusion (T80.89)
         Use additional code to identify associated manifestations, such as:
         desquamative dermatitis (L30.8)
         diarrhea (R19.7)
         elevated bilirubin (R17)
         hair loss (L65.9)
         ⒺⓍ **For category D89.81 CC codes:** D78.81-D78.89, D89.810-D89.813, E89.810-E89.89, H59.011-H59.019, H59.031-H59.099, H59.811-H59.89, H95.811-H95.89, I97.3, M96.89, N98.1-N98.9, T86.00-T86.09

         ● **D89.810**   **Acute graft-versus-host disease** 🔖

         ● **D89.811**   **Chronic graft-versus-host disease** 🔖

         ● **D89.812**   **Acute on chronic graft-versus-host disease** 🔖

         ● **D89.813**   **Graft-versus-host disease, unspecified** 🔖

     D89.82   **Autoimmune lymphoproliferative syndrome [ALPS]**

     D89.89   **Other specified disorders involving the immune mechanism, not elsewhere classified**

         Excludes1   human immunodeficiency virus disease (B20)

     D89.9   **Disorder involving the immune mechanism, unspecified**
         Immune disease NOS

◀ New   ◀▥ Revised   ~~deleted~~ Deleted   Excludes 1   Excludes 2   Includes   Use additional   Code first   Code also   Unspecified

OGCR Official Guidelines   ● Unacceptable Principal Diagnosis   X Assign placeholder X   ● Use Additional Character(s)   ▶ Manifestation Code   **Coding Clinic**

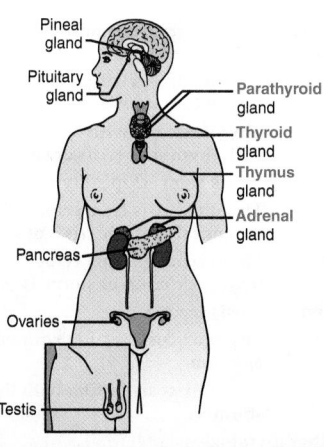

Figure 4-1 The endocrine system. (From Buck CJ: Step-by-Step Medical Coding, ed 2011, Philadelphia, WB Saunders, 2011)

CHAPTER 4

ENDOCRINE, NUTRITIONAL AND METABOLIC DISEASES (E00-E89)

All neoplasms, whether functionally active or not, are classified in Chapter 2. Appropriate codes in this chapter (i.e., E05.8, E07.0, E16-E31, E34.-) may be used as additional codes to indicate either functional activity by neoplasms and ectopic endocrine tissue or hyperfunction and hypofunction of endocrine glands associated with neoplasms and other conditions classified elsewhere.

Excludes1   transitory endocrine and metabolic disorders specific to newborn (P70-P74)

This chapter contains the following blocks:

E00-E07	Disorders of thyroid gland
E08-E13	Diabetes mellitus
E15-E16	Other disorders of glucose regulation and pancreatic internal secretion
E20-E35	Disorders of other endocrine glands
E36	Intraoperative complications of endocrine system
E40-E46	Malnutrition
E50-E64	Other nutritional deficiencies
E65-E68	Overweight, obesity and other hyperalimentation
E70-E88	Metabolic disorders
E89	Postprocedural endocrine and metabolic complications and disorders, not elsewhere classified

DISORDERS OF THYROID GLAND (E00-E07)

● **E00   Congenital iodine-deficiency syndrome**

Use additional code (F70-F79) to identify associated intellectual disabilities.

Excludes1   subclinical iodine-deficiency hypothyroidism (E02)

E00.0   Congenital iodine-deficiency syndrome, neurological type
Endemic cretinism, neurological type

E00.1   Congenital iodine-deficiency syndrome, myxedematous type
Dry, waxy type of swelling (nonpitting edema) with abnormal deposits of mucin in skin (mucinosis) and other tissues
Endemic hypothyroid cretinism
Endemic cretinism, myxedematous type

E00.2   Congenital iodine-deficiency syndrome, mixed type
Endemic cretinism, mixed type

E00.9   Congenital iodine-deficiency syndrome, unspecified
Congenital iodine-deficiency hypothyroidism NOS
Endemic cretinism NOS

Figure 4-2   Goiter is an enlargement of the thyroid gland.

Item 4–1   Simple goiter indicates no nodules are present. The most common type of goiter is a **diffuse colloidal**, also called a **nontoxic** or **endemic** goiter.

● **E01   Iodine-deficiency related thyroid disorders and allied conditions**

Excludes1   congenital iodine-deficiency syndrome (E00.-)
subclinical iodine-deficiency hypothyroidism (E02)

E01.0   Iodine-deficiency related diffuse (endemic) goiter
Thyroid gland is enlarged

E01.1   Iodine-deficiency related multinodular (endemic) goiter
Iodine-deficiency related nodular goiter

E01.2   Iodine-deficiency related (endemic) goiter, unspecified
Endemic goiter NOS

E01.8   Other iodine-deficiency related thyroid disorders and allied conditions
Acquired iodine-deficiency hypothyroidism NOS

E02   Subclinical iodine-deficiency hypothyroidism

● **E03   Other hypothyroidism**

Excludes1   iodine-deficiency related hypothyroidism (E00-E02)
postprocedural hypothyroidism (E89.0)

E03.0   Congenital hypothyroidism with diffuse goiter
Congenital parenchymatous goiter (nontoxic)
Congenital goiter (nontoxic) NOS

Excludes1   transitory congenital goiter with normal function (P72.0)

E03.1   Congenital hypothyroidism without goiter
Aplasia of thyroid (with myxedema)
Congenital atrophy of thyroid
Congenital hypothyroidism NOS

E03.2   Hypothyroidism due to medicaments and other exogenous substances
Code first poisoning due to drug or toxin, if applicable (T36-T65 with fifth or sixth character 1-4 or 6)
Use additional code for adverse effect, if applicable, to identify drug (T36-T50 with fifth or sixth character 5)

E03.3   Postinfectious hypothyroidism

E03.4   Atrophy of thyroid (acquired)
Excludes1   congenital atrophy of thyroid (E03.1)

Item 4–2   Hypothyroidism is a condition in which there are insufficient levels of thyroxine. **Cretinism** is congenital hypothyroidism, which can result in mental and physical retardation.

Figure 4-3 Typical appearance of patients with moderately severe primary hypothyroidism or myxedema. (From Larsen: Williams Textbook of Endocrinology, ed 10, Saunders, An Imprint of Elsevier, 2003)

N Newborn Age: 0   **P** Pediatric Age: 0–17   **M** Maternity DX: 12–55   **A** Adult Age: 15–124   ♀ Females Only   ♂ Males Only

🏷 Complication\Comorbidity   🏷 Major C\C   (Ex) CC/MCC Exclusions   🏷 Present on Admission Requirement   🏷 Hospital-Acquired Condition

833

CHAPTER 4 (E00-E90)

CHAPTER 4 (E00-E90)

E03.5   Myxedema coma
Often fatal complication of long-term hypothyroidism
(Ex) B15.0-B19.9, E03.5, E08.00-E08.59, E08.618-E09.59, E09.618-E10.59, E10.618-E10.649, E10.69-E11.59, E11.618-E11.649, E11.69-E13.59, E13.618-E16.2, E89.1, G32.89, G89.0-G89.4, G93.81-G93.9, G96.8-G96.9, G98.0-G98.8, G99.8, I60.00-I62.9, K72.91, R40.0-R40.2124, R40.2210-R40.2224, R40.2310-R40.2324, R40.2340-R40.2344, R40.3-R41.3, R41.82, R41.9-R42, R44.8-R44.9, R45.83-R45.84, R46.0-R46.89, R52, R55, R68.0-R68.83, R68.89-R69, S02.0XX-S02.19X[A,B], S02.91X[A,B], S06.0X0-S06.9X9[A]

E03.8   Other specified hypothyroidism

E03.9   Hypothyroidism, unspecified
Myxedema NOS

● **E04   Other nontoxic goiter**
     Excludes1   congenital goiter (NOS) (diffuse)
                     (parenchymatous) (E03.0)
                     iodine-deficiency related goiter (E00-E02)

E04.0   Nontoxic diffuse goiter
Thyroid gland is enlarged
Diffuse (colloid) nontoxic goiter
Simple nontoxic goiter

E04.1   Nontoxic single thyroid nodule
Colloid nodule (cystic) (thyroid)
Nontoxic uninodular goiter
Thyroid (cystic) nodule NOS

E04.2   Nontoxic multinodular goiter
Enlarged thyroid gland with multiple nodules
Cystic goiter NOS
Multinodular (cystic) goiter NOS

E04.8   Other specified nontoxic goiter

E04.9   Nontoxic goiter, unspecified
Goiter NOS
Nodular goiter (nontoxic) NOS

● **E05   Thyrotoxicosis [hyperthyroidism]**
Enlarged thyroid gland with multiple nodules
     Excludes1   chronic thyroiditis with transient thyrotoxicosis
                     (E06.2)
                     neonatal thyrotoxicosis (P72.1)
     (Ex) **For category E05 CC codes:** A17.9, A18.81-A18.82, A18.84, A18.89, E00.0-E03.4, E03.8-E07.1, E07.89-E07.9, E30.9, E34.1, E34.50-E35, E89.0

● **E05.0   Thyrotoxicosis with diffuse goiter**
Exophthalmic or toxic goiter NOS
Graves' disease
Toxic diffuse goiter

E05.00   Thyrotoxicosis with diffuse goiter without thyrotoxic crisis or storm

E05.01   Thyrotoxicosis with diffuse goiter with thyrotoxic crisis or storm

● **E05.1   Thyrotoxicosis with toxic single thyroid nodule**
Thyrotoxicosis with toxic uninodular goiter

E05.10   Thyrotoxicosis with toxic single thyroid nodule without thyrotoxic crisis or storm

E05.11   Thyrotoxicosis with toxic single thyroid nodule with thyrotoxic crisis or storm

● **E05.2   Thyrotoxicosis with toxic multinodular goiter**
Toxic nodular goiter NOS

E05.20   Thyrotoxicosis with toxic multinodular goiter without thyrotoxic crisis or storm

E05.21   Thyrotoxicosis with toxic multinodular goiter with thyrotoxic crisis or storm

● **E05.3   Thyrotoxicosis from ectopic thyroid tissue**

E05.30   Thyrotoxicosis from ectopic thyroid tissue without thyrotoxic crisis or storm

E05.31   Thyrotoxicosis from ectopic thyroid tissue with thyrotoxic crisis or storm

● **E05.4   Thyrotoxicosis factitia**

E05.40   Thyrotoxicosis factitia without thyrotoxic crisis or storm

E05.41   Thyrotoxicosis factitia with thyrotoxic crisis or storm

● **E05.8   Other thyrotoxicosis**
Overproduction of thyroid-stimulating hormone

E05.80   Other thyrotoxicosis without thyrotoxic crisis or storm

E05.81   Other thyrotoxicosis with thyrotoxic crisis or storm

● **E05.9   Thyrotoxicosis, unspecified**
Hyperthyroidism NOS

E05.90   Thyrotoxicosis, unspecified without thyrotoxic crisis or storm

E05.91   Thyrotoxicosis, unspecified with thyrotoxic crisis or storm

● **E06   Thyroiditis**
An inflammation of the thyroid gland which results in an inability to convert iodine into thyroid hormone
     Excludes1   postpartum thyroiditis (O90.5)

E06.0   Acute thyroiditis
Abscess of thyroid
Pyogenic thyroiditis
Suppurative thyroiditis
Use additional code (B95-B97) to identify infectious agent.
     (Ex) E06.0-E06.9

E06.1   Subacute thyroiditis
Inflammation of thyroid gland following viral upper respiratory infection
de Quervain thyroiditis
Giant-cell thyroiditis
Granulomatous thyroiditis
Nonsuppurative thyroiditis
Viral thyroiditis
     Excludes1   autoimmune thyroiditis (E06.3)

E06.2   Chronic thyroiditis with transient thyrotoxicosis
Chronic inflammation of thyroid gland with intermittent overproduction of thyroid hormone
     Excludes1   autoimmune thyroiditis (E06.3)

E06.3   Autoimmune thyroiditis
Hashimoto's thyroiditis
Hashitoxicosis (transient)
Lymphadenoid goiter
Lymphocytic thyroiditis
Struma lymphomatosa

E06.4   Drug-induced thyroiditis
Use additional code for adverse effect, if applicable, to identify drug (T36-T50 with fifth or sixth character 5)

E06.5   Other chronic thyroiditis
Chronic fibrous thyroiditis
Chronic thyroiditis NOS
Ligneous thyroiditis
Riedel thyroiditis

E06.9   Thyroiditis, unspecified

Figure 4-4   Graves' disease. In Graves' disease, exophthalmos often looks more pronounced than it actually is because of the extreme lid retraction that may occur. This patient, for instance, had minimal proptosis of the left eye but marked lid retraction.
(Courtesy Dr. HG Scheie. From Yanoff M, Fine BS: Ocular Pathology, ed 6, St. Louis, Mosby, 2008)

Item 4–3   Thyrotoxicosis is a condition caused by excessive amounts of the thyroid hormone thyroxine production or hyperthyroidism. **Graves' disease is associated with hyperthyroidism** (known as **Basedow's disease** in Europe).

◀ New   ⬅ Revised   ~~deleted~~ Deleted   Excludes 1   Excludes 2   Includes   Use additional   Code first   Code also   Unspecified
OGCR Official Guidelines   ● Unacceptable Principal Diagnosis   X Assign placeholder X   ● Use Additional Character(s)   〽 Manifestation Code   **Coding Clinic**

- **E07   Other disorders of thyroid**
  - **E07.0   Hypersecretion of calcitonin**
    - C-cell hyperplasia of thyroid
    - Hypersecretion of thyrocalcitonin
  - **E07.1   Dyshormogenetic goiter**
    - *Group of several types of goiter resulting from enzyme defects in hormone synthesis*
    - Familial dyshormogenetic goiter
    - Pendred's syndrome
    - **Excludes1**   transitory congenital goiter with normal function (P72.0)
  - **E07.8   Other specified disorders of thyroid**
    - **E07.81   Sick-euthyroid syndrome**
      - Euthyroid sick-syndrome
    - **E07.89   Other specified disorders of thyroid**
      - Abnormality of thyroid-binding globulin
      - Hemorrhage of thyroid
      - Infarction of thyroid
  - **E07.9   Disorder of thyroid, unspecified**

  OGCR   Section I.C.4.a

  4.1 Diabetes mellitus

  The diabetes mellitus codes are combination codes that include the type of diabetes mellitus, body system affected, and the complications affecting that body system. As many codes within a particular category as are necessary to describe all of the complications of the disease may be used. They should be sequenced based on the reason for a particular visit. Assign as many codes from categories E08–E13 as needed to identify all of the associated conditions that the patient has.

  ### DIABETES MELLITUS (E08-E13)

  A metabolic disease that results in persistent hyperglycemia.

- **E08   Diabetes mellitus due to underlying condition**
  - *Code first the underlying condition, such as:*
    - congenital rubella (P35.0)
    - Cushing's syndrome (E24.-)
    - cystic fibrosis (E84.-)
    - malignant neoplasm (C00-C96)
    - malnutrition (E40-E46)
    - pancreatitis and other diseases of the pancreas (K85-K86.-)
  - Use additional code to identify any insulin use (Z79.4)
  - **Excludes1**   drug or chemical induced diabetes mellitus (E09.-)
    - gestational diabetes (O24.4-)
    - neonatal diabetes mellitus (P70.2)
    - postpancreatectomy diabetes mellitus (E13.-)
    - postprocedural diabetes mellitus (E13.-)
    - secondary diabetes mellitus NEC (E13.-)
    - type 1 diabetes mellitus (E10.-)
    - type 2 diabetes mellitus (E11.-)
  - **E08.0   Diabetes mellitus due to underlying condition with hyperosmolarity**
    - Ex: **For category E08.0 CC codes:** E08.00-E08.59, E08.618-E09.59, E09.618-E10.52, E10.59, E10.618-E10.649, E10.69-E11.59, E11.618-E11.649, E11.69-E13.59, E13.618-E16.2, E30.9, E34.1, E34.8-E35, E89.1
    - **E08.00   Diabetes mellitus due to underlying condition with hyperosmolarity without nonketotic hyperglycemic-hyperosmolar coma (NKHHC)** 🔹🔹
    - **E08.01   Diabetes mellitus due to underlying condition with hyperosmolarity with coma** 🔹🔹
  - **E08.1   Diabetes mellitus due to underlying condition with ketoacidosis**
    - Ex: **For category E08.1 CC codes:** See E08.0
    - **E08.10   Diabetes mellitus due to underlying condition with ketoacidosis without coma** 🔹🔹
    - **E08.11   Diabetes mellitus due to underlying condition with ketoacidosis with coma** 🔹

- **E08.2   Diabetes mellitus due to underlying condition with kidney complications**
  - **E08.21   Diabetes mellitus due to underlying condition with diabetic nephropathy**
    - Diabetes mellitus due to underlying condition with intercapillary glomerulosclerosis
    - Diabetes mellitus due to underlying condition with intracapillary glomerulonephrosis
    - Diabetes mellitus due to underlying condition with Kimmelstiel-Wilson disease
  - **E08.22   Diabetes mellitus due to underlying condition with diabetic chronic kidney disease**
    - ~~Diabetes mellitus due to underlying condition with chronic kidney disease due to conditions classified to .21 and .22~~
    - Use additional code to identify stage of chronic kidney disease (N18.1-N18.6)
  - **E08.29   Diabetes mellitus due to underlying condition with other diabetic kidney complication**
    - Renal tubular degeneration in diabetes mellitus due to underlying condition
- **E08.3   Diabetes mellitus due to underlying condition with ophthalmic complications**
  - *Changes in blood vessels of retina in which blood vessels swell and leak fluid into retinal surface.*
  - **E08.31   Diabetes mellitus due to underlying condition with unspecified diabetic retinopathy**
    - **E08.311   Diabetes mellitus due to underlying condition with unspecified diabetic retinopathy with macular edema**
    - **E08.319   Diabetes mellitus due to underlying condition with unspecified diabetic retinopathy without macular edema**
  - **E08.32   Diabetes mellitus due to underlying condition with mild nonproliferative diabetic retinopathy**
    - Diabetes mellitus due to underlying condition with nonproliferative diabetic retinopathy NOS
    - **E08.321   Diabetes mellitus due to underlying condition with mild nonproliferative diabetic retinopathy with macular edema**
    - **E08.329   Diabetes mellitus due to underlying condition with mild nonproliferative diabetic retinopathy without macular edema**
  - **E08.33   Diabetes mellitus due to underlying condition with moderate nonproliferative diabetic retinopathy**
    - **E08.331   Diabetes mellitus due to underlying condition with moderate nonproliferative diabetic retinopathy with macular edema**
    - **E08.339   Diabetes mellitus due to underlying condition with moderate nonproliferative diabetic retinopathy without macular edema**
  - **E08.34   Diabetes mellitus due to underlying condition with severe nonproliferative diabetic retinopathy**
    - **E08.341   Diabetes mellitus due to underlying condition with severe nonproliferative diabetic retinopathy with macular edema**
    - **E08.349   Diabetes mellitus due to underlying condition with severe nonproliferative diabetic retinopathy without macular edema**

N Newborn Age: 0   P   Pediatric Age: 0–17   M   Maternity DX: 12–55   A   Adult Age: 15–124   ♀ Females Only   ♂ Males Only

🔹 Complication\Comorbidity   🔹 Major C\C   Ex CC/MCC Exclusions   🔹 Present on Admission Requirement   🔹 Hospital-Acquired Condition

835

CHAPTER 4 (E00-E90)

● E08.35   Diabetes mellitus due to underlying condition with proliferative diabetic retinopathy

    E08.351   Diabetes mellitus due to underlying condition with proliferative diabetic retinopathy with macular edema

    E08.359   Diabetes mellitus due to underlying condition with proliferative diabetic retinopathy without macular edema

  E08.36   Diabetes mellitus due to underlying condition with diabetic cataract

  E08.39   Diabetes mellitus due to underlying condition with other diabetic ophthalmic complication

    Use additional code to identify manifestation, such as: ◀
      diabetic glaucoma (H40-H42) ◀

● E08.4   Diabetes mellitus due to underlying condition with neurological complications

  E08.40   Diabetes mellitus due to underlying condition with diabetic neuropathy, unspecified

  E08.41   Diabetes mellitus due to underlying condition with diabetic mononeuropathy

  E08.42   Diabetes mellitus due to underlying condition with diabetic polyneuropathy
    Diabetes mellitus due to underlying condition with diabetic neuralgia

  E08.43   Diabetes mellitus due to underlying condition with diabetic autonomic (poly)neuropathy
    Diabetes mellitus due to underlying condition with diabetic gastroparesis

  E08.44   Diabetes mellitus due to underlying condition with diabetic amyotrophy

  E08.49   Diabetes mellitus due to underlying condition with other diabetic neurological complication

● E08.5   Diabetes mellitus due to underlying condition with circulatory complications

  E08.51   Diabetes mellitus due to underlying condition with diabetic peripheral angiopathy without gangrene

  E08.52   Diabetes mellitus due to underlying condition with diabetic peripheral angiopathy with gangrene 🖋
    Diabetes mellitus due to underlying condition with diabetic gangrene
    CC when PDx is its own CC
    (Ex) G89.0-G89.4, I70.261-I70.269, I96, R41.0-R41.3, R41.82, R41.9, R44.8-R44.9, R45.83-R45.84, R46.0-R46.89, R52, R68.0-R68.19, R68.81-R68.83, R68.89-R69

  E08.59   Diabetes mellitus due to underlying condition with other circulatory complications

● E08.6   Diabetes mellitus due to underlying condition with other specified complications

 ● E08.61   Diabetes mellitus due to underlying condition with diabetic arthropathy

    E08.610   Diabetes mellitus due to underlying condition with diabetic neuropathic arthropathy
      Diabetes mellitus due to underlying condition with Charcôt's joints

    E08.618   Diabetes mellitus due to underlying condition with other diabetic arthropathy

 ● E08.62   Diabetes mellitus due to underlying condition with skin complications

    E08.620   Diabetes mellitus due to underlying condition with diabetic dermatitis
      Diabetes mellitus due to underlying condition with diabetic necrobiosis lipoidica

    E08.621   Diabetes mellitus due to underlying condition with foot ulcer
      Use additional code to identify site of ulcer (L97.4-, L97.5-)

    E08.622   Diabetes mellitus due to underlying condition with other skin ulcer
      Use additional code to identify site of ulcer (L97.1-L97.9, L98.41-L98.49)

    E08.628   Diabetes mellitus due to underlying condition with other skin complications

 ● E08.63   Diabetes mellitus due to underlying condition with oral complications

    E08.630   Diabetes mellitus due to underlying condition with periodontal disease

    E08.638   Diabetes mellitus due to underlying condition with other oral complications

 ● E08.64   Diabetes mellitus due to underlying condition with hypoglycemia

    E08.641   Diabetes mellitus due to underlying condition with hypoglycemia with coma 🖋
      (Ex) E08.00-E08.59, E08.618-E09.59, E09.618-E10.52, E10.59, E10.618-E10.649, E10.69-E11.59, E11.618-E11.649, E11.69-E13.59, E13.618-E16.2, E30.9, E34.1, E34.8-E35, E89.1

    E08.649   Diabetes mellitus due to underlying condition with hypoglycemia without coma

  E08.65   Diabetes mellitus due to underlying condition with hyperglycemia

  E08.69   Diabetes mellitus due to underlying condition with other specified complication
    Use additional code to identify complication

 E08.8   Diabetes mellitus due to underlying condition with unspecified complications

 E08.9   Diabetes mellitus due to underlying condition without complications

● E09   Drug or chemical induced diabetes mellitus
  Code first poisoning due to drug or toxin, if applicable (T36-T65 with fifth or sixth character 1-4 or 6)

  Use additional code for adverse effect, if applicable, to identify drug (T36-T50 with fifth or sixth character 5)

  Use additional code to identify any insulin use (Z79.4)

  Excludes1   diabetes mellitus due to underlying condition (E08.-)
    gestational diabetes (O24.4-)
    neonatal diabetes mellitus (P70.2)
    postpancreatectomy diabetes mellitus (E13.-)
    postprocedural diabetes mellitus (E13.-)
    secondary diabetes mellitus NEC (E13.-)
    type 1 diabetes mellitus (E10.-)
    type 2 diabetes mellitus (E11.-)

● E09.0   Drug or chemical induced diabetes mellitus with hyperosmolarity
  (Ex) For category E09.0 CC codes: See E08.641

  E09.00   Drug or chemical induced diabetes mellitus with hyperosmolarity without nonketotic hyperglycemic-hyperosmolar coma (NKHHC) 🖋 🖋

  E09.01   Drug or chemical induced diabetes mellitus with hyperosmolarity with coma 🖋 🖋

● E09.1   Drug or chemical induced diabetes mellitus with ketoacidosis
  (Ex) For category E09.1 CC codes: See E08.641

  E09.10   Drug or chemical induced diabetes mellitus with ketoacidosis without coma 🖋 🖋

  E09.11   Drug or chemical induced diabetes mellitus with ketoacidosis with coma 🖋

◀ New   ◀▥ Revised   ~~deleted~~ Deleted   Excludes 1   Excludes 2   Includes   Use additional   Code first   Code also   Unspecified
OGCR Official Guidelines   ● Unacceptable Principal Diagnosis   X Assign placeholder X   ● Use Additional Character(s)   ▌ Manifestation Code   **Coding Clinic**

● **E09.2 Drug or chemical induced diabetes mellitus with kidney complications**

E09.21 Drug or chemical induced diabetes mellitus with diabetic nephropathy
Drug or chemical induced diabetes mellitus with intercapillary glomerulosclerosis
Drug or chemical induced diabetes mellitus with intracapillary glomerulonephrosis
Drug or chemical induced diabetes mellitus with Kimmelstiel-Wilson disease

E09.22 Drug or chemical induced diabetes mellitus with diabetic chronic kidney disease
~~Drug or chemical induced diabetes mellitus with chronic kidney disease due to conditions classified to .21 and .22~~
Use additional code to identify stage of chronic kidney disease (N18.1-N18.6)

E09.29 Drug or chemical induced diabetes mellitus with other diabetic kidney complication
Drug or chemical induced diabetes mellitus with renal tubular degeneration

● **E09.3 Drug or chemical induced diabetes mellitus with ophthalmic complications**

● **E09.31 Drug or chemical induced diabetes mellitus with unspecified diabetic retinopathy**

E09.311 Drug or chemical induced diabetes mellitus with unspecified diabetic retinopathy with macular edema

E09.319 Drug or chemical induced diabetes mellitus with unspecified diabetic retinopathy without macular edema

● **E09.32 Drug or chemical induced diabetes mellitus with mild nonproliferative diabetic retinopathy**
Drug or chemical induced diabetes mellitus with nonproliferative diabetic retinopathy NOS

E09.321 Drug or chemical induced diabetes mellitus with mild nonproliferative diabetic retinopathy with macular edema

E09.329 Drug or chemical induced diabetes mellitus with mild nonproliferative diabetic retinopathy without macular edema

● **E09.33 Drug or chemical induced diabetes mellitus with moderate nonproliferative diabetic retinopathy**

E09.331 Drug or chemical induced diabetes mellitus with moderate nonproliferative diabetic retinopathy with macular edema

E09.339 Drug or chemical induced diabetes mellitus with moderate nonproliferative diabetic retinopathy without macular edema

● **E09.34 Drug or chemical induced diabetes mellitus with severe nonproliferative diabetic retinopathy**

E09.341 Drug or chemical induced diabetes mellitus with severe nonproliferative diabetic retinopathy with macular edema

E09.349 Drug or chemical induced diabetes mellitus with severe nonproliferative diabetic retinopathy without macular edema

● **E09.35 Drug or chemical induced diabetes mellitus with proliferative diabetic retinopathy**

E09.351 Drug or chemical induced diabetes mellitus with proliferative diabetic retinopathy with macular edema

E09.359 Drug or chemical induced diabetes mellitus with proliferative diabetic retinopathy without macular edema

E09.36 Drug or chemical induced diabetes mellitus with diabetic cataract

E09.39 Drug or chemical induced diabetes mellitus with other diabetic ophthalmic complication
Use additional code to identify manifestation, such as: ◄
diabetic glaucoma (H40-H42) ◄

● **E09.4 Drug or chemical induced diabetes mellitus with neurological complications**

E09.40 Drug or chemical induced diabetes mellitus with neurological complications with diabetic neuropathy, unspecified

E09.41 Drug or chemical induced diabetes mellitus with neurological complications with diabetic mononeuropathy

E09.42 Drug or chemical induced diabetes mellitus with neurological complications with diabetic polyneuropathy
Drug or chemical induced diabetes mellitus with diabetic neuralgia

E09.43 Drug or chemical induced diabetes mellitus with neurological complications with diabetic autonomic (poly)neuropathy
Drug or chemical induced diabetes mellitus with diabetic gastroparesis

E09.44 Drug or chemical induced diabetes mellitus with neurological complications with diabetic amyotrophy

E09.49 Drug or chemical induced diabetes mellitus with neurological complications with other diabetic neurological complication

● **E09.5 Drug or chemical induced diabetes mellitus with circulatory complications**

E09.51 Drug or chemical induced diabetes mellitus with diabetic peripheral angiopathy without gangrene

E09.52 Drug or chemical induced diabetes mellitus with diabetic peripheral angiopathy with gangrene 🔖
Drug or chemical induced diabetes mellitus with diabetic gangrene
CC when PDx is its own CC
(Ex) G89.0-G89.4, I70.261-I70.269, I96, R41.0-R41.3, R41.82, R41.9, R44.8-R44.9, R45.83-R45.84, R46.0-R46.89, R52, R68.0-R68.19, R68.81-R68.83, R68.89-R69

E09.59 Drug or chemical induced diabetes mellitus with other circulatory complications

● **E09.6 Drug or chemical induced diabetes mellitus with other specified complications**

● **E09.61 Drug or chemical induced diabetes mellitus with diabetic arthropathy**

E09.610 Drug or chemical induced diabetes mellitus with diabetic neuropathic arthropathy
Drug or chemical induced diabetes mellitus with Charcôt's joints
Progressive degeneration of weight bearing joint

E09.618 Drug or chemical induced diabetes mellitus with other diabetic arthropathy

CHAPTER 4 (E00-E90)

N Newborn Age: 0   P Pediatric Age: 0–17   M Maternity DX: 12–55   A Adult Age: 15–124   ♀ Females Only   ♂ Males Only

🔖 Complication\Comorbidity   📘 Major C\C   (Ex) CC/MCC Exclusions   🔖 Present on Admission Requirement   🔖 Hospital-Acquired Condition

837

● E09.62   Drug or chemical induced diabetes mellitus
           with skin complications

    E09.620   Drug or chemical induced diabetes
              mellitus with diabetic dermatitis
                 Drug or chemical induced diabetes
                 mellitus with diabetic
                 necrobiosis lipoidica
                 Necrotizing skin condition

    E09.621   Drug or chemical induced diabetes
              mellitus with foot ulcer
                 Use additional code to identify site
                    of ulcer (L97.4-, L97.5-)

    E09.622   Drug or chemical induced diabetes
              mellitus with other skin ulcer 🐾
                 Use additional code to identify
                    site of ulcer (L97.1-L97.9,
                    L98.41-L98.49)

    E09.628   Drug or chemical induced
              diabetes mellitus with other skin
              complications

● E09.63   Drug or chemical induced diabetes mellitus
           with oral complications

    E09.630   Drug or chemical induced diabetes
              mellitus with periodontal disease

    E09.638   Drug or chemical induced diabetes
              mellitus with other oral complications

● E09.64   Drug or chemical induced diabetes mellitus
           with hypoglycemia

    E09.641   Drug or chemical induced diabetes
              mellitus with hypoglycemia with
              coma 🐾
                 Ⓔ⒳ E08.00-E08.59, E08.618-E09.59, E09.618-E10.52,
                    E10.59, E10.618-E10.649, E10.69-E11.59,
                    E11.618-E11.649, E11.69-E13.59,
                    E13.618-E16.2, E30.9, E34.1, E34.8-E35, E89.1

    E09.649   Drug or chemical induced diabetes
              mellitus with hypoglycemia without
              coma

    E09.65   Drug or chemical induced diabetes mellitus
             with hyperglycemia

    E09.69   Drug or chemical induced diabetes mellitus
             with other specified complication
                 Use additional code to identify complication

E09.8   Drug or chemical induced diabetes mellitus
        with unspecified complications

E09.9   Drug or chemical induced diabetes mellitus without
        complications

● E10   Type 1 diabetes mellitus

    Includes   brittle diabetes (mellitus)
                   diabetes (mellitus) due to autoimmune process
                   diabetes (mellitus) due to immune mediated
                       pancreatic islet beta-cell destruction
                   idiopathic diabetes (mellitus)
                   juvenile onset diabetes (mellitus)
                   ketosis-prone diabetes (mellitus)

    Excludes1 diabetes mellitus due to underlying condition
                       (E08.-)
                   drug or chemical induced diabetes mellitus
                       (E09.-)
                   gestational diabetes (O24.4-)
                   hyperglycemia NOS (R73.9)
                   neonatal diabetes mellitus (P70.2)
                   postpancreatectomy diabetes mellitus (E13.-)
                   postprocedural diabetes mellitus (E13.-)
                   secondary diabetes mellitus NEC (E13.-)
                   type 2 diabetes mellitus (E11.-)

● E10.1   Type 1 diabetes mellitus with ketoacidosis
             *Acidosis accompanied by accumulation of ketone bodies
             (ketosis) in body tissues and fluids*
             Ⓔ⒳ **For category E.10.1 CC codes:** E08.00-E08.59,
                E09.618-E10.59, E10.618-E10.649, E10.69-E11.59, E11.618-E11.649,
                E11.69-E13.59, E13.618-E16.2, E30.9, E34.1, E34.50-E35, E89.1

    E10.10   Type 1 diabetes mellitus with ketoacidosis
             without coma 🐾 🐾

    E10.11   Type 1 diabetes mellitus with ketoacidosis with
             coma 🐾

● E10.2   Type 1 diabetes mellitus with kidney complications

    E10.21   Type 1 diabetes mellitus with diabetic
             nephropathy
                 Type 1 diabetes mellitus with intercapillary
                    glomerulosclerosis
                 Type 1 diabetes mellitus with intracapillary
                    glomerulonephrosis
                 Type 1 diabetes mellitus with Kimmelstiel-
                    Wilson disease

    E10.22   Type 1 diabetes mellitus with diabetic chronic
             kidney disease
                 ~~Type 1 diabetes mellitus with chronic kidney
                    disease due to conditions classified to .21
                    and .22~~
                 Use additional code to identify stage of chronic
                    kidney disease (N18.1-N18.6)

    E10.29   Type 1 diabetes mellitus with other diabetic
             kidney complication
                 Type 1 diabetes mellitus with renal tubular
                    degeneration

● E10.3   Type 1 diabetes mellitus with ophthalmic complications

    ● E10.31   Type 1 diabetes mellitus with unspecified
               diabetic retinopathy

        E10.311   Type 1 diabetes mellitus
                  with unspecified diabetic retinopathy
                  with macular edema

        E10.319   Type 1 diabetes mellitus
                  with unspecified diabetic retinopathy
                  without macular edema

    ● E10.32   Type 1 diabetes mellitus with mild
               nonproliferative diabetic retinopathy
                   Type 1 diabetes mellitus with nonproliferative
                      diabetic retinopathy NOS

        E10.321   Type 1 diabetes mellitus with mild
                  nonproliferative diabetic retinopathy
                  with macular edema

        E10.329   Type 1 diabetes mellitus with mild
                  nonproliferative diabetic retinopathy
                  without macular edema

    ● E10.33   Type 1 diabetes mellitus with moderate
               nonproliferative diabetic retinopathy

        E10.331   Type 1 diabetes mellitus with
                  moderate nonproliferative diabetic
                  retinopathy with macular edema

        E10.339   Type 1 diabetes mellitus with
                  moderate nonproliferative diabetic
                  retinopathy without macular edema

    ● E10.34   Type 1 diabetes mellitus with severe
               nonproliferative diabetic retinopathy

        E10.341   Type 1 diabetes mellitus with severe
                  nonproliferative diabetic retinopathy
                  with macular edema

        E10.349   Type 1 diabetes mellitus with severe
                  nonproliferative diabetic retinopathy
                  without macular edema

CHAPTER 4 (E00-E90)

● E10.35   Type 1 diabetes mellitus with proliferative
             diabetic retinopathy
   E10.351   Type 1 diabetes mellitus with
             proliferative diabetic retinopathy
             with macular edema
   E10.359   Type 1 diabetes mellitus with
             proliferative diabetic retinopathy
             without macular edema
   E10.36   Type 1 diabetes mellitus with diabetic cataract
   E10.39   Type 1 diabetes mellitus with other diabetic
             ophthalmic complication
             ◄ Use additional code to identify manifestation,
                such as: ◄
                diabetic glaucoma (H40-H42) ◄

● E10.4   Type 1 diabetes mellitus with neurological
          complications
   E10.40   Type 1 diabetes mellitus with diabetic
             neuropathy, unspecified
   E10.41   Type 1 diabetes mellitus with diabetic
             mononeuropathy
   E10.42   Type 1 diabetes mellitus with diabetic
             polyneuropathy
                Type 1 diabetes mellitus with diabetic
                   neuralgia
   E10.43   Type 1 diabetes mellitus with diabetic
             autonomic (poly)neuropathy
                Type 1 diabetes mellitus with diabetic
                   gastroparesis
   E10.44   Type 1 diabetes mellitus with diabetic
             amyotrophy
   E10.49   Type 1 diabetes mellitus with other diabetic
             neurological complication

● E10.5   Type 1 diabetes mellitus with circulatory complications
   E10.51   Type 1 diabetes mellitus with diabetic
             peripheral angiopathy without gangrene
   E10.52   Type 1 diabetes mellitus with diabetic
             peripheral angiopathy with gangrene
                Type 1 diabetes mellitus with diabetic
                   gangrene 🖎
                CC when PDx is its own CC
                (Ex:) See E09.52
   E10.59   Type 1 diabetes mellitus with other circulatory
             complications

● E10.6   Type 1 diabetes mellitus with other specified
          complications
● E10.61   Type 1 diabetes mellitus with diabetic
            arthropathy
   E10.610   Type 1 diabetes mellitus with diabetic
             neuropathic arthropathy
                Type 1 diabetes mellitus with
                   Charcôt's joints
   E10.618   Type 1 diabetes mellitus with other
             diabetic arthropathy
● E10.62   Type 1 diabetes mellitus with skin
            complications
   E10.620   Type 1 diabetes mellitus with diabetic
             dermatitis
                Type 1 diabetes mellitus with
                   diabetic necrobiosis lipoidica
   E10.621   Type 1 diabetes mellitus with foot
             ulcer
                Use additional code to identify site
                   of ulcer (L97.4-, L97.5-)
   E10.622   Type 1 diabetes mellitus with other
             skin ulcer
                Use additional code to identify
                   site of ulcer (L97.1-L97.9,
                   L98.41-L98.49)
   E10.628   Type 1 diabetes mellitus with other
             skin complications

● E10.63   Type 1 diabetes mellitus with oral
             complications
   E10.630   Type 1 diabetes mellitus with
             periodontal disease
   E10.638   Type 1 diabetes mellitus with other
             oral complications
● E10.64   Type 1 diabetes mellitus with hypoglycemia
   E10.641   Type 1 diabetes mellitus with
             hypoglycemia with coma 🖎
                (Ex:) See E10.1
   E10.649   Type 1 diabetes mellitus with
             hypoglycemia without coma
   E10.65   Type 1 diabetes mellitus with hyperglycemia
   E10.69   Type 1 diabetes mellitus with other specified
             complication
                Use additional code to identify complication

   E10.8   Type 1 diabetes mellitus with unspecified complications
   E10.9   Type 1 diabetes mellitus without complications

● E11   Type 2 diabetes mellitus
   Includes   diabetes (mellitus) due to insulin secretory defect
                   diabetes NOS
                   insulin resistant diabetes (mellitus)
   Use additional code to identify any insulin use (Z79.4)
   Excludes1   diabetes mellitus due to underlying condition
                      (E08.-)
                   drug or chemical induced diabetes mellitus
                      (E09.-)
                   gestational diabetes (O24.4-)
                   neonatal diabetes mellitus (P70.2)
                   postpancreatectomy diabetes mellitus (E13.-)
                   postprocedural diabetes mellitus (E13.-)
                   secondary diabetes mellitus NEC (E13.-)
                   type 1 diabetes mellitus (E10.-)

● E11.0   Type 2 diabetes mellitus with hyperosmolarity
   (Ex:) For category E11.0 CC codes: E08.00-E08.59, E08.618-E09.59,
         E09.618-E10.52, E10.59, E10.618-E10.649, E10.69-E11.59,
         E11.618-E11.649, E11.69-E13.59, E13.618-E16.2, E30.9, E34.1,
         E34.8-E35, E89.1

   E11.00   Type 2 diabetes mellitus with hyperosmolarity
             without nonketotic hyperglycemic-
             hyperosmolar coma (NKHHC) 🖎 🖎
   E11.01   Type 2 diabetes mellitus with hyperosmolarity
             with coma 🖎 🖎

● E11.2   Type 2 diabetes mellitus with kidney complications
   E11.21   Type 2 diabetes mellitus with diabetic
             nephropathy
                Type 2 diabetes mellitus with intercapillary
                   glomerulosclerosis
                Type 2 diabetes mellitus with intracapillary
                   glomerulonephrosis
                Type 2 diabetes mellitus with Kimmelstiel-
                   Wilson disease
   E11.22   Type 2 diabetes mellitus with diabetic chronic
             kidney disease
                ~~Type 2 diabetes mellitus with chronic kidney~~
                   ~~disease due to conditions classified to .21~~
                   ~~and .22~~
                Use additional code to identify stage of chronic
                   kidney disease (N18.1-N18.6)
   E11.29   Type 2 diabetes mellitus with other diabetic
             kidney complication
                Type 2 diabetes mellitus with renal tubular
                   degeneration

N Newborn Age: 0   P Pediatric Age: 0–17   M Maternity DX: 12–55   A Adult Age: 15–124   ♀ Females Only   ♂ Males Only

🖎 Complication\Comorbidity   🖎 Major C\C   (Ex:) CC/MCC Exclusions   🖎 Present on Admission Requirement   🖎 Hospital-Acquired Condition

CHAPTER 4 (E00-E90)

839

● **E11.3** Type 2 diabetes mellitus with ophthalmic complications

  ● **E11.31** Type 2 diabetes mellitus with unspecified diabetic retinopathy

    E11.311 Type 2 diabetes mellitus with unspecified diabetic retinopathy with macular edema

    E11.319 Type 2 diabetes mellitus with unspecified diabetic retinopathy without macular edema

  ● **E11.32** Type 2 diabetes mellitus with mild nonproliferative diabetic retinopathy
    Type 2 diabetes mellitus with nonproliferative diabetic retinopathy NOS

    E11.321 Type 2 diabetes mellitus with mild nonproliferative diabetic retinopathy with macular edema

    E11.329 Type 2 diabetes mellitus with mild nonproliferative diabetic retinopathy without macular edema

  ● **E11.33** Type 2 diabetes mellitus with moderate nonproliferative diabetic retinopathy

    E11.331 Type 2 diabetes mellitus with moderate nonproliferative diabetic retinopathy with macular edema

    E11.339 Type 2 diabetes mellitus with moderate nonproliferative diabetic retinopathy without macular edema

  ● **E11.34** Type 2 diabetes mellitus with severe nonproliferative diabetic retinopathy

    E11.341 Type 2 diabetes mellitus with severe nonproliferative diabetic retinopathy with macular edema

    E11.349 Type 2 diabetes mellitus with severe nonproliferative diabetic retinopathy without macular edema

  ● **E11.35** Type 2 diabetes mellitus with proliferative diabetic retinopathy

    E11.351 Type 2 diabetes mellitus with proliferative diabetic retinopathy with macular edema

    E11.359 Type 2 diabetes mellitus with proliferative diabetic retinopathy without macular edema

    E11.36 Type 2 diabetes mellitus with diabetic cataract

    E11.39 Type 2 diabetes mellitus with other diabetic ophthalmic complication
      Use additional code to identify manifestation, such as: ◄
        diabetic glaucoma (H40-H42) ◄

● **E11.4** Type 2 diabetes mellitus with neurological complications

    E11.40 Type 2 diabetes mellitus with diabetic neuropathy, unspecified

    E11.41 Type 2 diabetes mellitus with diabetic mononeuropathy

    E11.42 Type 2 diabetes mellitus with diabetic polyneuropathy
      Type 2 diabetes mellitus with diabetic neuralgia

    E11.43 Type 2 diabetes mellitus with diabetic autonomic (poly)neuropathy
      Type 2 diabetes mellitus with diabetic gastroparesis

    E11.44 Type 2 diabetes mellitus with diabetic amyotrophy

    E11.49 Type 2 diabetes mellitus with other diabetic neurological complication

● **E11.5** Type 2 diabetes mellitus with circulatory complications

    E11.51 Type 2 diabetes mellitus with diabetic peripheral angiopathy without gangrene

    E11.52 Type 2 diabetes mellitus with diabetic peripheral angiopathy with gangrene
      Type 2 diabetes mellitus with diabetic gangrene 🅒
      CC when PDx is its own CC
      (Ex:) See E09.52

    E11.59 Type 2 diabetes mellitus with other circulatory complications

● **E11.6** Type 2 diabetes mellitus with other specified complications

  ● **E11.61** Type 2 diabetes mellitus with diabetic arthropathy

    E11.610 Type 2 diabetes mellitus with diabetic neuropathic arthropathy
      Type 2 diabetes mellitus with Charcôt's joints

    E11.618 Type 2 diabetes mellitus with other diabetic arthropathy

  ● **E11.62** Type 2 diabetes mellitus with skin complications

    E11.620 Type 2 diabetes mellitus with diabetic dermatitis
      Type 2 diabetes mellitus with diabetic necrobiosis lipoidica

    E11.621 Type 2 diabetes mellitus with foot ulcer
      Use additional code to identify site of ulcer (L97.4-, L97.5-)

    E11.622 Type 2 diabetes mellitus with other skin ulcer
      Use additional code to identify site of ulcer (L97.1-L97.9, L98.41-L98.49)

    E11.628 Type 2 diabetes mellitus with other skin complications

  ● **E11.63** Type 2 diabetes mellitus with oral complications

    E11.630 Type 2 diabetes mellitus with periodontal disease

    E11.638 Type 2 diabetes mellitus with other oral complications

  ● **E11.64** Type 2 diabetes mellitus with hypoglycemia

    E11.641 Type 2 diabetes mellitus with hypoglycemia with coma 🅒
      (Ex:) See E11.0

    E11.649 Type 2 diabetes mellitus with hypoglycemia without coma

    E11.65 Type 2 diabetes mellitus with hyperglycemia

    E11.69 Type 2 diabetes mellitus with other specified complication
      Use additional code to identify complication

  E11.8 Type 2 diabetes mellitus with unspecified complications

  E11.9 Type 2 diabetes mellitus without complications
    MCE: Questionable admission when principal dx

◄ New   ◄‖‖ Revised   ~~deleted~~ Deleted   Excludes 1   Excludes 2   Includes   Use additional   Code first   Code also   Unspecified

OGCR Official Guidelines   ● Unacceptable Principal Diagnosis   X Assign placeholder X   ● Use Additional Character(s)   ▮ Manifestation Code   **Coding Clinic**

● **E13   Other specified diabetes mellitus**

Includes   diabetes mellitus due to genetic defects of beta-cell function

diabetes mellitus due to genetic defects in insulin action

postpancreatectomy diabetes mellitus

postprocedural diabetes mellitus

secondary diabetes mellitus NEC

Use additional code to identify any insulin use (Z79.4)

Excludes 1   diabetes (mellitus) due to autoimmune process (E10.-)

diabetes (mellitus) due to immune mediated pancreatic islet beta-cell destruction (E10.-)

diabetes mellitus due to underlying condition (E08.-)

drug or chemical induced diabetes mellitus (E09.-)

gestational diabetes (O24.4-)

neonatal diabetes mellitus (P70.2)

type 2 diabetes mellitus (E11.-)

● **E13.0   Other specified diabetes mellitus with hyperosmolarity**
(Ex) For category E13.0 CC codes: See E11.0

E13.00   Other specified diabetes mellitus with hyperosmolarity without nonketotic hyperglycemic-hyperosmolar coma (NKHHC) 🔾 🔾

E13.01   Other specified diabetes mellitus with hyperosmolarity with coma 🔾 🔾

● **E13.1   Other specified diabetes mellitus with ketoacidosis**
(Ex) For category E13.1 CC codes: See E11.0

E13.10   Other specified diabetes mellitus with ketoacidosis without coma 🔾 🔾

E13.11   Other specified diabetes mellitus with ketoacidosis with coma 🔾

● **E13.2   Other specified diabetes mellitus with kidney complications**

E13.21   Other specified diabetes mellitus with diabetic nephropathy

Other specified diabetes mellitus with intercapillary glomerulosclerosis

Other specified diabetes mellitus with intracapillary glomerulonephrosis

Other specified diabetes mellitus with Kimmelstiel-Wilson disease

E13.22   Other specified diabetes mellitus with diabetic chronic kidney disease

~~Other specified diabetes mellitus with chronic kidney disease due to conditions classified to .21 and .22~~

Use additional code to identify stage of chronic kidney disease (N18.1-N18.6)

E13.29   Other specified diabetes mellitus with other diabetic kidney complication

Other specified diabetes mellitus with renal tubular degeneration

● **E13.3   Other specified diabetes mellitus with ophthalmic complications**

● **E13.31   Other specified diabetes mellitus with unspecified diabetic retinopathy**

E13.311   Other specified diabetes mellitus with unspecified diabetic retinopathy with macular edema

E13.319   Other specified diabetes mellitus with unspecified diabetic retinopathy without macular edema

● **E13.32   Other specified diabetes mellitus with mild nonproliferative diabetic retinopathy**

Other specified diabetes mellitus with nonproliferative diabetic retinopathy NOS

E13.321   Other specified diabetes mellitus with mild nonproliferative diabetic retinopathy with macular edema

E13.329   Other specified diabetes mellitus with mild nonproliferative diabetic retinopathy without macular edema

● **E13.33   Other specified diabetes mellitus with moderate nonproliferative diabetic retinopathy**

E13.331   Other specified diabetes mellitus with moderate nonproliferative diabetic retinopathy with macular edema

E13.339   Other specified diabetes mellitus with moderate nonproliferative diabetic retinopathy without macular edema

● **E13.34   Other specified diabetes mellitus with severe nonproliferative diabetic retinopathy**

E13.341   Other specified diabetes mellitus with severe nonproliferative diabetic retinopathy with macular edema

E13.349   Other specified diabetes mellitus with severe nonproliferative diabetic retinopathy without macular edema

● **E13.35   Other specified diabetes mellitus with proliferative diabetic retinopathy**

E13.351   Other specified diabetes mellitus with proliferative diabetic retinopathy with macular edema

E13.359   Other specified diabetes mellitus with proliferative diabetic retinopathy without macular edema

E13.36   Other specified diabetes mellitus with diabetic cataract

E13.39   Other specified diabetes mellitus with other diabetic ophthalmic complication

Use additional code to identify manifestation, such as: ◄

diabetic glaucoma (H40-H42) ◄

● **E13.4   Other specified diabetes mellitus with neurological complications**

E13.40   Other specified diabetes mellitus with diabetic neuropathy, unspecified

E13.41   Other specified diabetes mellitus with diabetic mononeuropathy

E13.42   Other specified diabetes mellitus with diabetic polyneuropathy

Other specified diabetes mellitus with diabetic neuralgia

E13.43   Other specified diabetes mellitus with diabetic autonomic (poly)neuropathy

Other specified diabetes mellitus with diabetic gastroparesis

E13.44   Other specified diabetes mellitus with diabetic amyotrophy

E13.49   Other specified diabetes mellitus with other diabetic neurological complication

● **E13.5   Other specified diabetes mellitus with circulatory complications**

E13.51   Other specified diabetes mellitus with diabetic peripheral angiopathy without gangrene

E13.52   Other specified diabetes mellitus with diabetic peripheral angiopathy with gangrene

Other specified diabetes mellitus with diabetic gangrene 🔾

CC when PDx is its own CC

(Ex) See E09.52

E13.59   Other specified diabetes mellitus with other circulatory complications

N Newborn Age: 0   **P** Pediatric Age: 0–17   **M** Maternity DX: 12–55   **A** Adult Age: 15–124   ♀ Females Only   ♂ Males Only

🔾 Complication\Comorbidity   🔾 Major C\C   (Ex) CC/MCC Exclusions   🔾 Present on Admission Requirement   🔾 Hospital-Acquired Condition

841

CHAPTER 4 (E00-E90)

CHAPTER 4 (E00-E90)

● E13.6   Other specified diabetes mellitus with other specified complications

  ● E13.61   Other specified diabetes mellitus with diabetic arthropathy

     E13.610   Other specified diabetes mellitus with diabetic neuropathic arthropathy
        Other specified diabetes mellitus with Charcôt's joints

     E13.618   Other specified diabetes mellitus with other diabetic arthropathy

  ● E13.62   Other specified diabetes mellitus with skin complications

     E13.620   Other specified diabetes mellitus with diabetic dermatitis
        Other specified diabetes mellitus with diabetic necrobiosis lipoidica

     E13.621   Other specified diabetes mellitus with foot ulcer
        Use additional code to identify site of ulcer (L97.4-, L97.5-)

     E13.622   Other specified diabetes mellitus with other skin ulcer
        Use additional code to identify site of ulcer (L97.1-L97.9, L98.41-L98.49)

     E13.628   Other specified diabetes mellitus with other skin complications

  ● E13.63   Other specified diabetes mellitus with oral complications

     E13.630   Other specified diabetes mellitus with periodontal disease

     E13.638   Other specified diabetes mellitus with other oral complications

  ● E13.64   Other specified diabetes mellitus with hypoglycemia

     E13.641   Other specified diabetes mellitus with hypoglycemia with coma 🔲
        Ex: See E11.0

     E13.649   Other specified diabetes mellitus with hypoglycemia without coma

     E13.65   Other specified diabetes mellitus with hyperglycemia

     E13.69   Other specified diabetes mellitus with other specified complication
        Use additional code to identify complication

   E13.8   Other specified diabetes mellitus with unspecified complications

   E13.9   Other specified diabetes mellitus without complications
     MCE: Questionable admission when principal dx

OTHER DISORDERS OF GLUCOSE REGULATION AND PANCREATIC INTERNAL SECRETION (E15-E16)

E15   Nondiabetic hypoglycemic coma 🔲 🔲
   Includes   drug-induced insulin coma in nondiabetic
     hyperinsulinism with hypoglycemic coma
     hypoglycemic coma NOS
   Ex: A74.81, A74.9, B33.3-B33.4, B34.1-B34.2, B34.4-B34.8, B97.10, B97.19-B97.29, B97.31-B97.39, B97.5-B97.6, B97.81-B97.89

● E16   Other disorders of pancreatic internal secretion

   E16.0   Drug-induced hypoglycemia without coma
     Use additional code for adverse effect, if applicable, to identify drug (T36-T50 with fifth or sixth character 5)

   E16.1   Other hypoglycemia
     Functional hyperinsulinism
     Functional nonhyperinsulinemic hypoglycemia
     Hyperinsulinism NOS
     Hyperplasia of pancreatic islet beta cells NOS
     Excludes1   hypoglycemia in infant of diabetic mother (P70.1)
        neonatal hypoglycemia (P70.4)

E16.2   Hypoglycemia, unspecified

E16.3   Increased secretion of glucagon
   Hyperplasia of pancreatic endocrine cells with glucagon excess

E16.4   Increased secretion of gastrin
   Hypergastrinemia
   Hyperplasia of pancreatic endocrine cells with gastrin excess
   Zollinger-Ellison syndrome

E16.8   Other specified disorders of pancreatic internal secretion
   Increased secretion from endocrine pancreas of growth hormone-releasing hormone
   Increased secretion from endocrine pancreas of pancreatic polypeptide
   Increased secretion from endocrine pancreas of somatostatin
   Increased secretion from endocrine pancreas of vasoactive-intestinal polypeptide

E16.9   Disorder of pancreatic internal secretion, unspecified
   Islet-cell hyperplasia NOS
   Pancreatic endocrine cell hyperplasia NOS

DISORDERS OF OTHER ENDOCRINE GLANDS (E20-E35)

   Excludes1   galactorrhea (N64.3)
     gynecomastia (N62)

● E20   Hypoparathyroidism
   Greatly reduced function of parathyroid glands; AKA parathyroid insufficiency
   Excludes1   Di George's syndrome (D82.1)
     postprocedural hypoparathyroidism (E89.2)
     tetany NOS (R29.0)
     transitory neonatal hypoparathyroidism (P71.4)

   E20.0   Idiopathic hypoparathyroidism
     Rare condition, unknown cause; short dwarf-like with round face

   E20.1   Pseudohypoparathyroidism
     Hereditary condition resembling hypoparathyroidism, but caused by inability to respond to parathyroid hormone

   E20.8   Other hypoparathyroidism

   E20.9   Hypoparathyroidism, unspecified
     Parathyroid tetany

● E21   Hyperparathyroidism and other disorders of parathyroid gland
   Excludes1   adult osteomalacia (M83.-)
     ectopic hyperparathyroidism (E34.2)
     familial hypocalciuric hypercalcemia (E83.52)
     hungry bone syndrome (E83.81)
     infantile and juvenile osteomalacia (E55.0)

   E21.0   Primary hyperparathyroidism
     Hyperplasia of parathyroid
     Osteitis fibrosa cystica generalisata [von Recklinghausen's disease of bone]

   E21.1   Secondary hyperparathyroidism, not elsewhere classified
     Excludes1   secondary hyperparathyroidism of renal origin (N25.81)

Item 4–4 Hyperparathyroidism is an overactive parathyroid gland that secretes excessive parathormone, causing increased levels of circulating calcium. This results in a loss of calcium in the bone (osteoporosis).

Hypoparathyroidism is an underactive parathyroid gland that results in decreased levels of circulating calcium. The primary manifestation is **tetany,** a continuous muscle spasm.

Figure 4-5 Tetany caused by hypoparathyroidism.

◄ New   ◄ Revised   ~~deleted~~ Deleted   Excludes 1   Excludes 2   Includes   Use additional   Code first   Code also   Unspecified

OGCR Official Guidelines   ● Unacceptable Principal Diagnosis   X Assign placeholder X   ● Use Additional Character(s)   ▌ Manifestation Code   **Coding Clinic**

Item 4–5 Hyperadrenalism is overactivity of the adrenal cortex, which secretes corticosteroid hormones. Excessive glucocorticoid hormone results in hyperglycemia **(Cushing's syndrome)**, and excessive aldosterone results in **Conn's syndrome. Adrenogenital syndrome** is the result of excessive secretion of androgens, male hormones, which stimulates premature sexual development. **Hypoadrenalism, Addison's disease,** is a condition in which the adrenal glands atrophy.

Figure 4-6 Centripetal and generalized obesity and dorsal kyphosis in a 30-year-old woman with Cushing's disease. (From Larsen: Williams Textbook of Endocrinology, ed 10, Saunders, An Imprint of Elsevier, 2003)

E21.2   **Other hyperparathyroidism**
        Tertiary hyperparathyroidism
        Excludes1 familial hypocalciuric hypercalcemia (E83.52)

E21.3   **Hyperparathyroidism, unspecified**
E21.4   **Other specified disorders of parathyroid gland**
E21.5   **Disorder of parathyroid gland, unspecified**

● E22   **Hyperfunction of pituitary gland**
        Excludes1 Cushing's syndrome (E24.-)
                Nelson's syndrome (E24.1)
                overproduction of ACTH not associated with Cushing's disease (E27.0)
                overproduction of pituitary ACTH (E24.0)
                overproduction of thyroid-stimulating hormone (E05.8-)
        (Ex) **For category E.22 CC codes unless otherwise indicated:** E22.1-E22.9

E22.0   **Acromegaly and pituitary gigantism**
        Chronic disease caused by hypersecretion of growth hormone
        Overproduction of growth hormone
        Excludes1 constitutional gigantism (E34.4)
                constitutional tall stature (E34.4)
                increased secretion from endocrine pancreas of growth hormone-releasing hormone (E16.8)

E22.1   **Hyperprolactinemia** 🔍
        Increased levels of prolactin
        Use additional code for adverse effect, if applicable, to identify drug (T36-T50 with fifth or sixth character 5)

E22.2   **Syndrome of inappropriate secretion of antidiuretic hormone** 🔍
        (Ex) E22.0-E23.7, E24.1, E30.9, E34.1, E34.8-E35, E89.3

E22.8   **Other hyperfunction of pituitary gland** 🔍
        Central precocious puberty

E22.9   **Hyperfunction of pituitary gland, unspecified** 🔍

● E23   **Hypofunction and other disorders of the pituitary gland**
        Includes the listed conditions whether the disorder is in the pituitary or the hypothalamus
        Excludes1 postprocedural hypopituitarism (E89.3)

E23.0   **Hypopituitarism** 🔍
        Fertile eunuch syndrome
        Hypogonadotropic hypogonadism
        Idiopathic growth hormone deficiency
        Isolated deficiency of gonadotropin
        Isolated deficiency of growth hormone
        Isolated deficiency of pituitary hormone
        Kallmann's syndrome
        Lorain-Levi short stature
        Necrosis of pituitary gland (postpartum)
        Panhypopituitarism
        Pituitary cachexia
        Pituitary insufficiency NOS
        Pituitary short stature
        Sheehan's syndrome
        Simmonds' disease
        (Ex) E22.0-E23.7, E24.1, E30.9, E34.1, E34.4-E35, E89.3

E23.1   **Drug-induced hypopituitarism**
        Use additional code for adverse effect, if applicable, to identify drug (T36-T50 with fifth or sixth character 5)

E23.2   **Diabetes insipidus** 🔍
        Excludes1 nephrogenic diabetes insipidus (N25.1)
        (Ex) E22.1-E23.7, E24.1, E30.9, E34.1, E34.50-E35, E89.3

E23.3   **Hypothalamic dysfunction, not elsewhere classified**
        Excludes1 Prader-Willi syndrome (Q87.1)
                Russell-Silver syndrome (Q87.1)

E23.6   **Other disorders of pituitary gland**
        Abscess of pituitary
        Adiposogenital dystrophy

E23.7   **Disorder of pituitary gland, unspecified**

● E24   **Cushing's syndrome**
        Excludes1 congenital adrenal hyperplasia (E25.0)
        (Ex) **For category E24 CC codes:** E24.0, E24.2-E26.9, E30.9, E34.1, E34.50-E35

E24.0   **Pituitary-dependent Cushing's disease** 🔍
        Overproduction of pituitary ACTH
        Pituitary-dependent hypercorticalism

E24.1   **Nelson's syndrome**

E24.2   **Drug-induced Cushing's syndrome** 🔍
        Use additional code for adverse effect, if applicable, to identify drug (T36-T50 with fifth or sixth character 5)

E24.3   **Ectopic ACTH syndrome** 🔍
E24.4   **Alcohol-induced pseudo-Cushing's syndrome** 🔍
E24.8   **Other Cushing's syndrome** 🔍
E24.9   **Cushing's syndrome, unspecified** 🔍

● E25   **Adrenogenital disorders**
        Disorder of production of steroid hormone in adrenal gland
        Includes adrenogenital syndromes, virilizing or feminizing, whether acquired or due to adrenal hyperplasia consequent on inborn enzyme defects in hormone synthesis
                female adrenal pseudohermaphroditism
                female heterosexual precocious pseudopuberty
                male isosexual precocious pseudopuberty
                male macrogenitosomia praecox
                male sexual precocity with adrenal hyperplasia
                male virilization (female)
        Excludes1 indeterminate sex and pseudohermaphroditism (Q56)
                chromosomal abnormalities (Q90-Q99)

E25.0   **Congenital adrenogenital disorders associated with enzyme deficiency**
        Congenital adrenal hyperplasia
        21-Hydroxylase deficiency
        Salt-losing congenital adrenal hyperplasia

E25.8   **Other adrenogenital disorders**
        Idiopathic adrenogenital disorder
        Use additional code for adverse effect, if applicable, to identify drug (T36-T50 with fifth or sixth character 5)

E25.9   **Adrenogenital disorder, unspecified**
        Adrenogenital syndrome NOS

CHAPTER 4 (E00-E90)

N Newborn Age: 0   **P** Pediatric Age: 0–17   **M** Maternity DX: 12–55   **A** Adult Age: 15–124   ♀ Females Only   ♂ Males Only

🔍 Complication\Comorbidity   🔍 Major C\C   (Ex) CC/MCC Exclusions   🔍 Present on Admission Requirement   🔍 Hospital-Acquired Condition

843

CHAPTER 4 (E00-E90)

● **E26** **Hyperaldosteronism**
Abnormality of electrolyte metabolism caused by excessive secretion of aldosterone

  ● **E26.0** **Primary hyperaldosteronism**

    E26.01 **Conn's syndrome**
      Code also adrenal adenoma (D35.0-)

    E26.02 **Glucocorticoid-remediable aldosteronism**
      Familial aldosteronism type I

    E26.09 **Other primary hyperaldosteronism**
      Primary aldosteronism due to adrenal hyperplasia (bilateral)

  E26.1 **Secondary hyperaldosteronism**

  ● **E26.8** **Other hyperaldosteronism**

    E26.81 **Bartter's syndrome**

    E26.89 **Other hyperaldosteronism**

  E26.9 **Hyperaldosteronism, unspecified**
    Aldosteronism NOS
    Hyperaldosteronism NOS

● **E27** **Other disorders of adrenal gland**
  Ⓔⓧ **For category E27 CC codes:** A17.9, A18.7, A18.82, A18.84, A18.89, E27.0-E27.9, E30.9, E34.1, E34.50-E35, E89.6

  E27.0 **Other adrenocortical overactivity** 🔖
    Overproduction of ACTH, not associated with Cushing's disease
    Premature adrenarche

    Excludes1   Cushing's syndrome (E24.-)

  E27.1 **Primary adrenocortical insufficiency** 🔖
    Addison's disease
    Autoimmune adrenalitis

    Excludes1   Addison only phenotype adrenoleukodystrophy (E71.528)
      amyloidosis (E85.-) ◀▥
      tuberculous Addison's disease (A18.7)
      Waterhouse-Friderichsen syndrome (A39.1)

  E27.2 **Addisonian crisis** 🔖
    Acute onset of adrenocortical insufficiency
    Adrenal crisis
    Adrenocortical crisis

  E27.3 **Drug-induced adrenocortical insufficiency** 🔖
    Use additional code for adverse effect, if applicable, to identify drug (T36-T50 with fifth or sixth character 5)

  ● **E27.4** **Other and unspecified adrenocortical insufficiency**

    Excludes1   adrenoleukodystrophy [Addison-Schilder] (E71.528)
      Waterhouse-Friderichsen syndrome (A39.1)

    E27.40 **Unspecified adrenocortical insufficiency** 🔖
      Adrenocortical insufficiency NOS
      Hypoaldosteronism

    E27.49 **Other adrenocortical insufficiency** 🔖
      Adrenal hemorrhage
      Adrenal infarction

  E27.5 **Adrenomedullary hyperfunction** 🔖
    Adrenomedullary hyperplasia
    Catecholamine hypersecretion

  E27.8 **Other specified disorders of adrenal gland**
    Abnormality of cortisol-binding globulin

  E27.9 **Disorder of adrenal gland, unspecified**

● **E28** **Ovarian dysfunction**

  Excludes1   isolated gonadotropin deficiency (E23.0)
    postprocedural ovarian failure (E89.4-)

  E28.0 **Estrogen excess** ♀
    Use additional code for adverse effect, if applicable, to identify drug (T36-T50 with fifth or sixth character 5)

  E28.1 **Androgen excess** ♀
    Hypersecretion of ovarian androgens
    Use additional code for adverse effect, if applicable, to identify drug (T36-T50 with fifth or sixth character 5)

  E28.2 **Polycystic ovarian syndrome** ♀
    Sclerocystic ovary syndrome
    Stein-Leventhal syndrome

  ● **E28.3** **Primary ovarian failure**

    Excludes1   pure gonadal dysgenesis (Q99.1)
      Turner's syndrome (Q96.-)

    ● **E28.31** **Premature menopause**

      E28.310 **Symptomatic premature menopause** ♀   A
        Symptoms such as flushing, sleeplessness, headache, lack of concentration, associated with premature menopause

      E28.319 **Asymptomatic premature menopause** ♀   A
        Premature menopause NOS

    E28.39 **Other primary ovarian failure** ♀
      Decreased estrogen
      Resistant ovary syndrome

  E28.8 **Other ovarian dysfunction** ♀
    Ovarian hyperfunction NOS

    Excludes1   postprocedural ovarian failure (E89.4-)

  E28.9 **Ovarian dysfunction, unspecified** ♀

● **E29** **Testicular dysfunction**

  Excludes1   androgen insensitivity syndrome (E34.5-)
    azoospermia or oligospermia NOS (N46.0-N46.1)
    isolated gonadotropin deficiency (E23.0)
    Klinefelter's syndrome (Q98.0-Q98.2, Q98.4)

  E29.0 **Testicular hyperfunction** ♂
    Hypersecretion of testicular hormones

  E29.1 **Testicular hypofunction** ♂
    Defective biosynthesis of testicular androgen NOS
    5-delta-Reductase deficiency (with male pseudohermaphroditism)
    Testicular hypogonadism NOS
    Use additional code for adverse effect, if applicable, to identify drug (T36-T50 with fifth or sixth character 5)

    Excludes1   postprocedural testicular hypofunction (E89.5)

  E29.8 **Other testicular dysfunction** ♂

  E29.9 **Testicular dysfunction, unspecified** ♂

● **E30** **Disorders of puberty, not elsewhere classified**

  E30.0 **Delayed puberty**
    Constitutional delay of puberty
    Delayed sexual development

  E30.1 **Precocious puberty**   P
    Sexual maturation at earlier age than normal, or before age 8 in girls and 9 in boys, usually hormonal; AKA sexual precocity or pubertas praecox
    Precocious menstruation

    Excludes1   Albright (-McCune) (-Sternberg) syndrome (Q78.1)
      central precocious puberty (E22.8)
      congenital adrenal hyperplasia (E25.0)
      female heterosexual precocious pseudopuberty (E25.-)
      male isosexual precocious pseudopuberty (E25.-)

  E30.8 **Other disorders of puberty**   P
    Premature thelarche

  E30.9 **Disorder of puberty, unspecified**

◀ New   ◀▥ Revised   ~~deleted~~ Deleted   Excludes 1   Excludes 2   Includes   Use additional   Code first   Code also   Unspecified
OGCR Official Guidelines   ● Unacceptable Principal Diagnosis   X Assign placeholder X   ● Use Additional Character(s)   ▶ Manifestation Code   **Coding Clinic**

● **E31   Polyglandular dysfunction**

　　Excludes1　ataxia telangiectasia [Louis-Bar] (G11.3)
　　　　　　dystrophia myotonica [Steinert] (G71.11)
　　　　　　pseudohypoparathyroidism (E20.1)

E31.0   Autoimmune polyglandular failure
　　Schmidt's syndrome

E31.1   Polyglandular hyperfunction
　　Excludes1　multiple endocrine adenomatosis (E31.2-)
　　　　　　multiple endocrine neoplasia (E31.2-)

● **E31.2   Multiple endocrine neoplasia [MEN] syndromes**
　　*Adenomatous hyperplasia and malignant tumors in
　　　endocrine glands*
　　Multiple endocrine adenomatosis
　　Code also any associated malignancies and other
　　　conditions associated with the syndromes

　　**E31.20   Multiple endocrine neoplasia [MEN]
　　　　　syndrome, unspecified**
　　　　Multiple endocrine adenomatosis NOS
　　　　Multiple endocrine neoplasia [MEN]
　　　　　syndrome NOS

　　E31.21   Multiple endocrine neoplasia [MEN] type I
　　　　Wermer's syndrome

　　E31.22   Multiple endocrine neoplasia [MEN] type IIA
　　　　Sipple's syndrome

　　E31.23   Multiple endocrine neoplasia [MEN] type IIB

E31.8   Other polyglandular dysfunction

E31.9   Polyglandular dysfunction, unspecified

● **E32   Diseases of thymus**

　　Excludes1　aplasia or hypoplasia of thymus with
　　　　　　immunodeficiency (D82.1)
　　　　　　myasthenia gravis (G70.0)

E32.0   Persistent hyperplasia of thymus
　　Hypertrophy of thymus

E32.1   Abscess of thymus 🦠
　　(Ex) E30.9, E32.0-E32.9, E34.1, E34.50-E35

E32.8   Other diseases of thymus
　　Excludes1　aplasia or hypoplasia with
　　　　　　immunodeficiency (D82.1)
　　　　　　thymoma (D15.0)

E32.9   Disease of thymus, unspecified

● **E34   Other endocrine disorders**

　　Excludes1　pseudohypoparathyroidism (E20.1)

E34.0   Carcinoid syndrome 🦠
　　Note: May be used as an additional code to identify
　　　functional activity associated with a carcinoid
　　　tumor.
　　(Ex) E30.9, E34.0-E34.2, E34.50-E35

E34.1   Other hypersecretion of intestinal hormones

E34.2   Ectopic hormone secretion, not elsewhere classified
　　Excludes1　ectopic ACTH syndrome (E24.3)

E34.3   Short stature due to endocrine disorder
　　Constitutional short stature
　　Laron-type short stature
　　Excludes1　achondroplastic short stature (Q77.4)
　　　　　　hypochondroplastic short stature (Q77.4)
　　　　　　nutritional short stature (E45)
　　　　　　pituitary short stature (E23.0)
　　　　　　progeria (E34.8)
　　　　　　renal short stature (N25.0)
　　　　　　Russell-Silver syndrome (Q87.1)
　　　　　　short-limbed stature with
　　　　　　　immunodeficiency (D82.2)
　　　　　　short stature in specific dysmorphic
　　　　　　　syndromes - code to syndrome - see
　　　　　　　Alphabetical Index
　　　　　　short stature NOS (R62.52)

E34.4   Constitutional tall stature
　　Constitutional gigantism

E34.5   Androgen insensitivity syndrome

　　E34.50   Androgen insensitivity syndrome, unspecified
　　　　Androgen insensitivity NOS

　　E34.51   Complete androgen insensitivity syndrome
　　　　Complete androgen insensitivity
　　　　de Quervain syndrome
　　　　Goldberg-Maxwell syndrome

　　E34.52   Partial androgen insensitivity syndrome
　　　　Partial androgen insensitivity
　　　　Reifenstein syndrome

E34.8   Other specified endocrine disorders
　　Pineal gland dysfunction
　　Progeria
　　Excludes2　pseudohypoparathyroidism (E20.1)

E34.9   Endocrine disorder, unspecified
　　Endocrine disturbance NOS
　　Hormone disturbance NOS

▶ **E35   Disorders of endocrine glands in diseases classified elsewhere**
　　Code first underlying disease, such as:
　　　late congenital syphilis of thymus gland [Dubois disease]
　　　　(A50.5)
　　　~~tuberculous calcification of adrenal gland (B90.8)~~
　　Use additional code, if applicable, to identify: ◀
　　　sequelae of tuberculosis of other organs (B90.8) ◀
　　Excludes1　Echinococcus granulosus infection of thyroid
　　　　　　gland (B67.3)
　　　　　　meningococcal hemorrhagic adrenalitis (A39.1)
　　　　　　syphilis of endocrine gland (A52.79)
　　　　　　tuberculosis of adrenal gland, except calcification
　　　　　　　(A18.7)
　　　　　　tuberculosis of endocrine gland NEC (A18.82)
　　　　　　tuberculosis of thyroid gland (A18.81)
　　　　　　Waterhouse-Friderichsen syndrome (A39.1)

INTRAOPERATIVE COMPLICATIONS OF ENDOCRINE SYSTEM (E36)

● **E36   Intraoperative complications of endocrine system**
　　Excludes2　postprocedural endocrine and metabolic
　　　　　　complications and disorders, not elsewhere
　　　　　　classified (E89.-)

● **E36.0   Intraoperative hemorrhage and hematoma of an
　　endocrine system organ or structure complicating a
　　procedure**
　　Excludes1　intraoperative hemorrhage and
　　　　　　hematoma of an endocrine system
　　　　　　organ or structure due to accidental
　　　　　　puncture or laceration during a
　　　　　　procedure (E36.1-)
　　(Ex) For category E36.0 CC codes: E36.01-E36.02, E36.8, E89.810-E89.89,
　　　H95.811-H95.89, I85.01, I85.11, I97.3, K21.9, K22.8, K23-K25.0, K25.2,
　　　K25.4, K25.6, K26.0, K26.2, K26.4, K26.6, K27.0, K27.2, K27.4, K27.6,
　　　K28.0, K28.2, K28.4, K28.6, K29.01, K29.21, K29.31, K29.41, K29.51,
　　　K29.61, K29.71, K29.81, K29.91, K31.811, K55.21, K57.01, K57.11,
　　　K57.13, K57.21, K57.31, K57.33, K57.41, K57.51, K57.53, K57.81, K57.91,
　　　K57.93, K62.5, K92.0-K92.2, M96.89, N98.1-N98.9, P54.1-P54.3,
　　　T81.10X-T81.19X[A], T81.82X[A], T81.89X-T81.9XX[A]

　　**E36.01   Intraoperative hemorrhage and hematoma of an
　　　　　endocrine system organ or structure
　　　　　complicating an endocrine system procedure** 🦠

　　**E36.02   Intraoperative hemorrhage and hematoma of an
　　　　　endocrine system organ or structure
　　　　　complicating other procedure** 🦠

● **E36.1   Accidental puncture and laceration of an endocrine
　　system organ or structure during a procedure**
　　(Ex) For category E36.1 CC codes: D78.11-D78.12, D78.81-D78.89,
　　　E36.11-E36.8, E89.810-E89.89, G96.11, G97.41-G97.49, H59.011-H59.019,
　　　H59.031-H59.099, H59.211-H59.229, H59.811-H59.89, H95.31-H95.32,
　　　H95.811-H95.89, I97.3, I97.51-I97.52, J95.71-J95.72, K91.71-K91.72,
　　　L76.11-L76.12, L76.81-L76.82, M96.820-M96.821, M96.89, N98.1-N98.9,
　　　N99.71-N99.72, T81.82X[A], T81.89X-T81.9XX[A]

　　**E36.11   Accidental puncture and laceration of an
　　　　　endocrine system organ or structure during an
　　　　　endocrine system procedure** 🦠

N Newborn Age: 0　　**P** Pediatric Age: 0–17　　**M** Maternity DX: 12–55　　**A** Adult Age: 15–124　　♀ Females Only　　♂ Males Only

🦠 Complication\Comorbidity　　🦠 Major C\C　　(Ex) CC/MCC Exclusions　　🦠 Present on Admission Requirement　　🦠 Hospital-Acquired Condition

845

CHAPTER 4 (E00-E90)

E36.12   Accidental puncture and laceration of an endocrine system organ or structure during other procedure 🖉

E36.8   Other intraoperative complications of endocrine system

 Use additional code, if applicable, to further specify disorder

---

MALNUTRITION (E40-E46)

Excludes1   intestinal malabsorption (K90.-)
     sequelae of protein-calorie malnutrition (E64.0)

Excludes2   nutritional anemias (D50-D53)
     starvation (T73.0)

E40   Kwashiorkor 🖉
Malnutrition produced by severe protein deficiency
Severe malnutrition with nutritional edema with dyspigmentation of skin and hair

 Excludes1   marasmic kwashiorkor (E42)

 (Ex) E40-E46, E64.0

E41   Nutritional marasmus 🖉
Severe malnutrition with marasmus

 Excludes1   marasmic kwashiorkor (E42)

 (Ex) E40-E46, E64.0

E42   Marasmic kwashiorkor 🖉
Severe protein malnutrition
Intermediate form severe protein-calorie malnutrition
Severe protein-calorie malnutrition with signs of both kwashiorkor and marasmus

 (Ex) E40-E46, E64.0

E43   Unspecified severe protein-calorie malnutrition 🖉
Starvation edema

 (Ex) E40-E46, E64.0

● E44   Protein-calorie malnutrition of moderate and mild degree
 (Ex) For category E44 CC codes: E40-E46, E64.0

E44.0   Moderate protein-calorie malnutrition 🖉

E44.1   Mild protein-calorie malnutrition 🖉

E45   Retarded development following protein-calorie malnutrition 🖉
Nutritional short stature
Nutritional stunting
Physical retardation due to malnutrition

 (Ex) E40-E46, E64.0

E46   Unspecified protein-calorie malnutrition 🖉
Malnutrition NOS
Protein-calorie imbalance NOS

 Excludes1   nutritional deficiency NOS (E63.9)

 (Ex) E40-E46, E64.0

OTHER NUTRITIONAL DEFICIENCIES (E50-E64)

Excludes2   nutritional anemias (D50-D53)

● E50   Vitamin A deficiency

 Excludes1   sequelae of vitamin A deficiency (E64.1)

E50.0   Vitamin A deficiency with conjunctival xerosis

E50.1   Vitamin A deficiency with Bitot's spot and conjunctival xerosis
 Bitot's spot in the young child

E50.2   Vitamin A deficiency with corneal xerosis

E50.3   Vitamin A deficiency with corneal ulceration and xerosis

E50.4   Vitamin A deficiency with keratomalacia
 Eye disorder that results in dry cornea caused by vitamin A deficiency

E50.5   Vitamin A deficiency with night blindness

E50.6   Vitamin A deficiency with xerophthalmic scars of cornea
 Abnormal dryness and thickening of conjunctiva and cornea due to vitamin A deficiency

E50.7   Other ocular manifestations of vitamin A deficiency
 Xerophthalmia NOS

E50.8   Other manifestations of vitamin A deficiency
 Follicular keratosis
 Xeroderma

E50.9   Vitamin A deficiency, unspecified
 Hypovitaminosis A NOS

● E51   Thiamine deficiency

 Excludes1   sequelae of thiamine deficiency (E64.8)

● E51.1   Beriberi
 (Ex) For category E51.1 CC codes: D81.818-D81.819, E51.11-E53.9, E56.0, E56.8-E63.9, E64.8-E64.9

 E51.11   Dry beriberi 🖉
  Thiamine deficiency with nervous system manifestation most often caused by excessive alcohol consumption
  Beriberi NOS
  Beriberi with polyneuropathy

 E51.12   Wet beriberi 🖉
  Thiamine deficiency with cardiovascular manifestation most often caused by excessive alcohol consumption
  Beriberi with cardiovascular manifestations
  Cardiovascular beriberi
  Shoshin disease

E51.2   Wernicke's encephalopathy 🖉
 Acute disease of brain due to thiamine deficiency most often associated with excessive alcohol consumption
 (Ex) See E51.1

E51.8   Other manifestations of thiamine deficiency 🖉
 (Ex) See E51.1

E51.9   Thiamine deficiency, unspecified 🖉
 (Ex) See E51.1

Item 4–6   Bitot's spots are the result of a buildup of keratin debris found on the superficial surface the conjunctiva; oval, triangular, or irregular in shape; and a sign of vitamin A deficiency and associated with night blindness. The disease may progress to **keratomalacia,** which can result in eventual prolapse of the iris and loss of the lens.

    Figure 4-7   Bitot's spot on the conjunctiva.

Figure 4-8   The sharply demarcated, characteristic scaling dermatitis of pellagra. (From Kumar: Robbins and Cotran: Pathologic Basis of Disease, ed 8, Saunders, An Imprint of Elsevier, 2009)

Item 4–7   Pellagra is associated with a deficiency of niacin and its precursor, **tryptophan.** Characteristics of the condition include diarrhea, dermatitis on exposed skin surfaces, dementia, and death. It is prevalent in developing countries where nutrition is inadequate. **Beriberi** is associated with thiamine deficiency.

◀ New   ◀ Revised   ~~deleted~~ Deleted   Excludes 1   Excludes 2   Includes   Use additional   Code first   Code also   Unspecified

OGCR Official Guidelines   ● Unacceptable Principal Diagnosis   X Assign placeholder X   ● Use Additional Character(s)   ▶ Manifestation Code   **Coding Clinic**

E52   **Niacin deficiency [pellagra]**
      Niacin (-tryptophan) deficiency
      Nicotinamide deficiency
      Pellagra (alcoholic)
      Excludes1   sequelae of niacin deficiency (E64.8)

● **E53**   **Deficiency of other B group vitamins**
      Excludes1   sequelae of vitamin B deficiency (E64.8)
      E53.0   **Riboflavin deficiency** 🔧
           Ariboflavinosis
           Vitamin B2 deficiency
           (Ex:) See E51.1
      E53.1   **Pyridoxine deficiency**
           Vitamin B6 deficiency
           Excludes1   pyridoxine-responsive sideroblastic
                  anemia (D64.3)
      E53.8   **Deficiency of other specified B group vitamins**
           Biotin deficiency
           Cyanocobalamin deficiency
           Folate deficiency
           Folic acid deficiency
           Pantothenic acid deficiency
           Vitamin B12 deficiency
           Excludes1   folate deficiency anemia (D52.-)
                  vitamin B12 deficiency anemia (D51.-)
      E53.9   **Vitamin B deficiency, unspecified**

E54   **Ascorbic acid deficiency**
      Deficiency of vitamin C
      Scurvy
      Excludes1   scorbutic anemia (D53.2)
                  sequelae of vitamin C deficiency (E64.2)

● **E55**   **Vitamin D deficiency**
      Excludes1   adult osteomalacia (M83.-)
                  osteoporosis (M80.-) ◄▥
                  sequelae of rickets (E64.3)
      E55.0   **Rickets, active** 🔧
           Infantile ⊖osteomalacia ◄▥
           Juvenile ⊖osteomalacia ◄▥
           Softening of bone
           Excludes1   celiac rickets (K90.0)
                  Crohn's rickets (K50.-)
                  hereditary vitamin D-dependent rickets
                     (E83.32)
                  inactive rickets (E64.3)
                  renal rickets (N25.0)
                  sequelae of rickets (E64.3)
                  vitamin D-resistant rickets (E83.31)
           (Ex:) E55.0-E63.9, E64.3-E64.9, M83.0-M83.9
      E55.9   **Vitamin D deficiency, unspecified**
           Avitaminosis D

● **E56**   **Other vitamin deficiencies**
      Excludes1   sequelae of other vitamin deficiencies (E64.8)
      E56.0   **Deficiency of vitamin E**
      E56.1   **Deficiency of vitamin K**
           Excludes1   deficiency of coagulation factor due to
                  vitamin K deficiency (D68.4)
                  vitamin K deficiency of newborn (P53)
      E56.8   **Deficiency of other vitamins**
      E56.9   **Vitamin deficiency, unspecified**

E58   **Dietary calcium deficiency**
      Excludes1   disorders of calcium metabolism (E83.5-)
                  sequelae of calcium deficiency (E64.8)

E59   **Dietary selenium deficiency**
      Keshan disease
      Excludes1   sequelae of selenium deficiency (E64.8)

E60   **Dietary zinc deficiency**

● **E61**   **Deficiency of other nutrient elements**
      Use additional code for adverse effect, if applicable, to identify
      drug (T36-T50 with fifth or sixth character 5)
      Excludes1   disorders of mineral metabolism (E83.-)
                  iodine deficiency related thyroid disorders
                     (E00-E02)
                  sequelae of malnutrition and other nutritional
                     deficiencies (E64.-)
      E61.0   **Copper deficiency**
      E61.1   **Iron deficiency**
           Excludes1   iron deficiency anemia (D50.-)
      E61.2   **Magnesium deficiency**
      E61.3   **Manganese deficiency**
      E61.4   **Chromium deficiency**
      E61.5   **Molybdenum deficiency**
      E61.6   **Vanadium deficiency**
      E61.7   **Deficiency of multiple nutrient elements**
      E61.8   **Deficiency of other specified nutrient elements**
      E61.9   **Deficiency of nutrient element, unspecified**

● **E63**   **Other nutritional deficiencies**
      Excludes1   dehydration (E86.0)
                  failure to thrive, adult (R62.7)
                  failure to thrive, child (R62.51)
                  feeding problems in newborn (P92.-)
                  sequelae of malnutrition and other nutritional
                     deficiencies (E64.-)
      E63.0   **Essential fatty acid [EFA] deficiency**
      E63.1   **Imbalance of constituents of food intake**
      E63.8   **Other specified nutritional deficiencies**
      E63.9   **Nutritional deficiency, unspecified**

● **E64**   **Sequelae of malnutrition and other nutritional deficiencies**
      Pathological condition resulting from disease, injury, or other trauma
      Note: This category is to be used to indicate conditions in
      categories E43, E44, E46, E50-E63 as the cause of sequelae,
      which are themselves classified elsewhere. The 'sequelae'
      include conditions specified as such; they also include the
      late effects of diseases classifiable to the above categories if
      the disease itself is no longer present
      Code first condition resulting from (sequela) of malnutrition and
      other nutritional deficiencies
      E64.0   **Sequelae of protein-calorie malnutrition** 🔧🔧
           Excludes2   retarded development following
                  protein-calorie malnutrition (E45)
           (Ex:) E40-E46, E64.0
      E64.1   **Sequelae of vitamin A deficiency** 🔧
      E64.2   **Sequelae of vitamin C deficiency** 🔧
      E64.3   **Sequelae of rickets** 🔧
      E64.8   **Sequelae of other nutritional deficiencies** 🔧
      E64.9   **Sequelae of unspecified nutritional deficiency** 🔧

CHAPTER 4 (E00-E90)

N Newborn Age: 0   **P** Pediatric Age: 0–17   **M** Maternity DX: 12–55   **A** Adult Age: 15–124   ♀ Females Only   ♂ Males Only

🔧 Complication\Comorbidity   🔧 Major C\C   (Ex:) CC/MCC Exclusions   🔧 Present on Admission Requirement   🔧 Hospital-Acquired Condition

847

CHAPTER 4 (E00-E90)

OVERWEIGHT, OBESITY AND OTHER HYPERALIMENTATION (E65-E68)

E65   **Localized adiposity**
Fat pad

● **E66**   **Overweight and obesity**
Code first obesity complicating pregnancy, childbirth and the puerperium, if applicable (O99.21-)
Use additional code to identify body mass index (BMI), if known (Z68.-)
Excludes1   adiposogenital dystrophy (E23.6)
lipomatosis NOS (E88.2)
lipomatosis dolorosa [Dercum] (E88.2)
Prader-Willi syndrome (Q87.1)

● **E66.0**   **Obesity due to excess calories**

     E66.01   **Morbid (severe) obesity due to excess calories** 🔖
         Excludes1   morbid (severe) obesity with alveolar hypoventilation (E66.2)

     E66.09   **Other obesity due to excess calories**
         MCE: Questionable admission when principal dx

   E66.1   **Drug-induced obesity**
     MCE: Questionable admission when principal dx
     Use additional code for adverse effect, if applicable, to identify drug (T36-T50 with fifth or sixth character 5)

   E66.2   **Morbid (severe) obesity with alveolar hypoventilation** 🔖
     Uncommon condition of unknown cause leading to inadequate ventilation in lungs, even though lungs and airways are normal
     Pickwickian syndrome
     (Ex) E66.2, I27.0-I27.81, I27.89-I27.9

   E66.3   **Overweight**

   E66.8   **Other obesity**
     MCE: Questionable admission when principal dx

   E66.9   **Obesity, unspecified**
     Obesity NOS
     MCE: Questionable admission when principal dx

● **E67**   **Other hyperalimentation**
Ingestion of more than optimal amount of nutrients
Excludes1   hyperalimentation NOS (R63.2)
sequelae of hyperalimentation (E68)

   E67.0   **Hypervitaminosis A**

   E67.1   **Hypercarotinemia**

   E67.2   **Megavitamin-B6 syndrome**

   E67.3   **Hypervitaminosis D**

   E67.8   **Other specified hyperalimentation**

E68   **Sequelae of hyperalimentation**
Code first condition resulting from (sequela) of hyperalimentation

METABOLIC DISORDERS (E70-E88)

Excludes1   androgen insensitivity syndrome (E34.5-)
congenital adrenal hyperplasia (E25.0)
Ehlers-Danlos syndrome (Q79.6)
hemolytic anemias attributable to enzyme disorders (D55.-)
Marfan's syndrome (Q87.4)
5-alpha-reductase deficiency (E29.1)

● **E70**   **Disorders of aromatic amino-acid metabolism**
(Ex) **For category E70 CC codes:** C88.0, D47.2, D89.0-D89.1, E70.0-E71.30, E72.00-E72.02, E72.04-E74.9, E75.21-E75.249, E75.3, E75.5-E75.6, E77.0-E78.70, E78.79-E78.9, E88.09-E88.2, E88.89

   E70.0   **Classical phenylketonuria** 🔖
     Inherited disorder that increases to harmful levels amino acid phenylalanine

   E70.1   **Other hyperphenylalaninemias** 🔖

● **E70.2**   **Disorders of tyrosine metabolism**
Excludes1   transitory tyrosinemia of newborn (P74.5)

   E70.20   **Disorder of tyrosine metabolism, unspecified** 🔖
     Tyrosine: Nonessential amino acid occurring in most proteins

   E70.21   **Tyrosinemia** 🔖
     Congenital amino acid metabolism
     Hypertyrosinemia

   E70.29   **Other disorders of tyrosine metabolism** 🔖
     Alkaptonuria
     Ochronosis

● **E70.3**   **Albinism**
Congenital condition of reduced or absent pigment in eyes, skin, and hair

   E70.30   **Albinism, unspecified** 🔖

● **E70.31**   **Ocular albinism**

     E70.310   **X-linked ocular albinism** 🔖

     E70.311   **Autosomal recessive ocular albinism** 🔖

     E70.318   **Other ocular albinism** 🔖

     E70.319   **Ocular albinism, unspecified** 🔖

● **E70.32**   **Oculocutaneous albinism**
Partial or total lack of melanin pigment in eyes
Excludes1   Chediak-Higashi syndrome (E70.330)
Hermansky-Pudlak syndrome (E70.331)

     E70.320   **Tyrosinase negative oculocutaneous albinism** 🔖
       Albinism I
       Oculocutaneous albinism ty-neg

     E70.321   **Tyrosinase positive oculocutaneous albinism** 🔖
       Albinism II
       Oculocutaneous albinism ty-pos

     E70.328   **Other oculocutaneous albinism** 🔖
       Cross syndrome

     E70.329   **Oculocutaneous albinism, unspecified** 🔖

● **E70.33**   **Albinism with hematologic abnormality**

     E70.330   **Chediak-Higashi syndrome** 🔖

     E70.331   **Hermansky-Pudlak syndrome** 🔖

     E70.338   **Other albinism with hematologic abnormality** 🔖

     E70.339   **Albinism with hematologic abnormality, unspecified** 🔖

   E70.39   **Other specified albinism** 🔖
     Piebaldism

● **E70.4**   **Disorders of histidine metabolism**

   E70.40   **Disorders of histidine metabolism, unspecified** 🔖

   E70.41   **Histidinemia** 🔖

   E70.49   **Other disorders of histidine metabolism** 🔖

   E70.5   **Disorders of tryptophan metabolism** 🔖

   E70.8   **Other disorders of aromatic amino-acid metabolism** 🔖

   E70.9   **Disorder of aromatic amino-acid metabolism, unspecified** 🔖

◄ New   ◄ Revised   ~~deleted~~ Deleted   Excludes 1   Excludes 2   Includes   Use additional   Code first   Code also   Unspecified
OGCR Official Guidelines   ● Unacceptable Principal Diagnosis   X Assign placeholder X   🔖 Use Additional Character(s)   ▶ Manifestation Code   **Coding Clinic**

● **E71**   **Disorders of branched-chain amino-acid metabolism and fatty-acid metabolism**

   E71.0   **Maple-syrup-urine disease** 🕮
       Due to defect in amino acid catabolism, causing severe
       ketoacidosis with smell of maple syrup in urine and on
       body

● **E71.1**   **Other disorders of branched-chain amino-acid metabolism**
      (Ex) **For category E71.1 CC codes:** C88.0, D47.2, D89.0-D89.1, E70.0-E71.30,
      E72.00-E72.02, E72.04-E74.9, E75.21-E75.249, E75.3, E75.5-E75.6,
      E77.0-E78.70, E78.79-E78.9, E88.09-E88.2, E88.89

     ● **E71.11**   **Branched-chain organic acidurias**
        E71.110   **Isovaleric acidemia** 🕮
        E71.111   **3-methylglutaconic aciduria** 🕮
        E71.118   **Other branched-chain organic acidurias** 🕮

     ● **E71.12**   **Disorders of propionate metabolism**
        E71.120   **Methylmalonic acidemia** 🕮
        E71.121   **Propionic acidemia** 🕮
        E71.128   **Other disorders of propionate metabolism** 🕮

     E71.19   **Other disorders of branched-chain amino-acid metabolism** 🕮
       Hyperleucine-isoleucinemia
       Hypervalinemia

   E71.2   **Disorder of branched-chain amino-acid metabolism, unspecified** 🕮
      (Ex) See E71.1

● **E71.3**   **Disorders of fatty-acid metabolism**
     Excludes1   peroxisomal disorders (E71.5)
           Refsum's disease (G60.1)
           Schilder's disease (G37.0)
     Excludes2   carnitine deficiency due to inborn error of
           metabolism (E71.42)

     E71.30   **Disorder of fatty-acid metabolism, unspecified**

     ● **E71.31**   **Disorders of fatty-acid oxidation**
       (Ex) **For category E71.31 CC codes:** C96.5-C96.6, E71.39-E71.548,
       E80.3, E88.40-E88.49, E88.89, H49.811-H49.819

        E71.310   **Long chain/very long chain acyl CoA dehydrogenase deficiency** 🕮
           LCAD
           VLCAD
        E71.311   **Medium chain acyl CoA dehydrogenase deficiency** 🕮
           MCAD
        E71.312   **Short chain acyl CoA dehydrogenase deficiency** 🕮
           SCAD
        E71.313   **Glutaric aciduria type II** 🕮
           Glutaric aciduria type II A
           Glutaric aciduria type II B
           Glutaric aciduria type II C
           Excludes1   glutaric aciduria (type 1) NOS (E72.3)
        E71.314   **Muscle carnitine palmitoyltransferase deficiency** 🕮
        E71.318   **Other disorders of fatty-acid oxidation** 🕮

     E71.32   **Disorders of ketone metabolism** 🕮
       (Ex) See E71.31

     E71.39   **Other disorders of fatty-acid metabolism** 🕮
       (Ex) E71.310-E71.32, E71.40-E71.548, E80.4-E80.7, E88.40-E88.49,
       H49.811-H49.819

● **E71.4**   **Disorders of carnitine metabolism**
     Excludes1   muscle carnitine palmitoyltransferase
           deficiency (E71.314)

     E71.40   **Disorder of carnitine metabolism, unspecified**
     E71.41   **Primary carnitine deficiency**
     E71.42   **Carnitine deficiency due to inborn errors of metabolism**
       Code also associated inborn error or
       metabolism
     E71.43   **Iatrogenic carnitine deficiency**
       Iatrogenic: Outcomes from activity of physicians
       Carnitine deficiency due to hemodialysis ◀▥
       ~~hemodialysis~~
       Carnitine deficiency due to Valproic acid
       therapy ◀▥

     ● **E71.44**   **Other secondary carnitine deficiency**
        E71.440   **Ruvalcaba-Myhre-Smith syndrome**
        E71.448   **Other secondary carnitine deficiency**

● **E71.5**   **Peroxisomal disorders**
     Class of conditions which lead to disorders of lipid
     metabolism
     Excludes1   Schilder's disease (G37.0)
       (Ex) **For category E71.5 CC codes:** C96.5-C96.6, E71.310-E71.448, E80.3-E80.7,
       E88.40-E88.49, E88.89, H49.811-H49.819

     E71.50   **Peroxisomal disorder, unspecified** 🕮

     ● **E71.51**   **Disorders of peroxisome biogenesis**
       Group 1 peroxisomal disorders
       Excludes1   Refsum's disease (G60.1)
        E71.510   **Zellweger syndrome** 🕮
        E71.511   **Neonatal adrenoleukodystrophy** 🕮   N
           Excludes1   X-linked adrenoleuko-
             dystrophy
             (E71.42-)
        E71.518   **Other disorders of peroxisome biogenesis** 🕮

     ● **E71.52**   **X-linked adrenoleukodystrophy**
        E71.520   **Childhood cerebral X-linked adrenoleukodystrophy** 🕮
        E71.521   **Adolescent X-linked adrenoleukodystrophy** 🕮
        E71.522   **Adrenomyeloneuropathy** 🕮
        E71.528   **Other X-linked adrenoleukodystrophy** 🕮
           Addison only phenotype
           adrenoleukodystrophy
           Addison-Schilder
           adrenoleukodystrophy
        E71.529   **X-linked adrenoleukodystrophy, unspecified type** 🕮

     E71.53   **Other group 2 peroxisomal disorders** 🕮

     ● **E71.54**   **Other peroxisomal disorders**
        E71.540   **Rhizomelic chondrodysplasia punctata** 🕮
           Rare, severe, inherited disorder with
           limb shortening, bone and
           cartilage abnormalities, abnormal
           facial appearance, severe mental
           retardation, psychomotor
           retardation, and cataracts
           Excludes1   chondrodysplasia
             punctata NOS
             (Q77.3)
        E71.541   **Zellweger-like syndrome** 🕮
        E71.542   **Other group 3 peroxisomal disorders** 🕮
        E71.548   **Other peroxisomal disorders** 🕮

CHAPTER 4 (E00-E90)

N   Newborn Age: 0   P   Pediatric Age: 0–17   M   Maternity DX: 12–55   A   Adult Age: 15–124   ♀   Females Only   ♂   Males Only

🕮   Complication\Comorbidity   🕮   Major C\C   (Ex)   CC/MCC Exclusions   🕮   Present on Admission Requirement   🕮   Hospital-Acquired Condition

● **E72   Other disorders of amino-acid metabolism**

    Excludes1   disorders of:
        aromatic amino-acid metabolism (E70.-)
        branched-chain amino-acid metabolism
          (E71.0-E71.2)
        fatty-acid metabolism (E71.3)
        purine and pyrimidine metabolism (E79.-)
        gout (M1A.-, M10.-) ◀▥

    (Ex) **For category E72 CC codes unless otherwise noted:** C88.0, D47.2, D89.0-D89.1, E70.0-E71.30, E72.00-E72.02, E72.04-E74.9, E75.21-E75.249, E75.3, E75.5-E75.6, E77.0-E78.70, E78.79-E78.9, E88.09-E88.2, E88.89

● **E72.0   Disorders of amino-acid transport**

    Excludes1   disorders of tryptophan metabolism
        (E70.5)

    E72.00   Disorders of amino-acid transport, unspecified 🔗

    E72.01   Cystinuria 🔗
        Hereditary aminoaciduria due to impairment of renal transport with predominant symptom of urinary cystine calculi

    E72.02   Hartnup's disease 🔗
        Inborn error of metabolism

    E72.03   Lowe's syndrome 🔗
        X-linked disorder with rickets, hydrophthalmia, congenital glaucoma, cataracts, mental retardation, and renal tubule dysfunction

        Use additional code for associated glaucoma (H42)

        (Ex) No exclusion

    E72.04   Cystinosis 🔗
        Genetic disease with excessive depostits of amino acid cystine in cells
        Fanconi (-de Toni) (-Debré) syndrome with cystinosis

        Excludes1   Fanconi (-de Toni) (-Debré) syndrome without cystinosis (E72.09)

    E72.09   Other disorders of amino-acid transport 🔗
        Fanconi (-de Toni) (-Debré) syndrome, unspecified

● **E72.1   Disorders of sulfur-bearing amino-acid metabolism**

    Excludes1   cystinosis (E72.04)
        cystinuria (E72.01)
        transcobalamin II deficiency (D51.2)

    E72.10   Disorders of sulfur-bearing amino-acid metabolism, unspecified 🔗

    E72.11   Homocystinuria 🔗
        Cystathionine synthase deficiency

    E72.12   Methylenetetrahydrofolate reductase deficiency 🔗

    E72.19   Other disorders of sulfur-bearing amino-acid metabolism 🔗
        Cystathioninuria
        Methioninemia
        Sulfite oxidase deficiency

● **E72.2   Disorders of urea cycle metabolism**

    Excludes1   disorders of ornithine metabolism (E72.4)

    E72.20   Disorder of urea cycle metabolism, unspecified 🔗
        Hyperammonemia
        Elevated levels of ammonia

        Excludes1   hyperammonemia-hyperornithinemia-homocitrullinemia syndrome E72.4
          transient hyperammonemia of newborn (P74.6)

    E72.21   Argininemia 🔗
        Disorder in which deficiency of enzyme arginase causes build up of arginine and ammonia in blood

    E72.22   Arginosuccinic aciduria 🔗
        Gene disorder of urea cycle resulting accumulation of ammonia

    E72.23   Citrullinemia 🔗
        Urea cycle disorder that causes ammonia and other toxic substances to accumulate in blood

    E72.29   Other disorders of urea cycle metabolism 🔗

● **E72.3   Disorders of lysine and hydroxylysine metabolism** 🔗
    Glutaric aciduria NOS
    Glutaric aciduria (type I)
    Hydroxylysinemia
    Hyperlysinemia

    Excludes1   glutaric aciduria type II (E71.313)
        Refsum's disease (G60.1)
        Zellweger syndrome (E71.510)

● **E72.4   Disorders of ornithine metabolism** 🔗
    Hyperammonemia-Hyperornithinemia-Homocitrullinemia syndrome
    Ornithinemia (types I, II)
    Ornithine transcarbamylase deficiency

    Excludes1   hereditary choroidal dystrophy (H31.2-)

● **E72.5   Disorders of glycine metabolism**

    E72.50   Disorder of glycine metabolism, unspecified 🔗

    E72.51   Non-ketotic hyperglycinemia

    E72.52   Trimethylaminuria 🔗

    E72.53   Hyperoxaluria 🔗
        Oxalosis
        Oxaluria

    E72.59   Other disorders of glycine metabolism 🔗
        D-glycericacidemia
        Hyperhydroxyprolinemia
        Hyperprolinemia (types I, II)
        Sarcosinemia

E72.8   Other specified disorders of amino-acid metabolism 🔗
    Disorders of beta-amino-acid metabolism
    Disorders of gamma-glutamyl cycle

E72.9   Disorder of amino-acid metabolism, unspecified 🔗

● **E73   Lactose intolerance**
    Intolerance for lactose, due to inherited deficiency of lactase activity in intestinal mucosa

    E73.0   Congenital lactase deficiency

    E73.1   Secondary lactase deficiency

    E73.8   Other lactose intolerance

    E73.9   Lactose intolerance, unspecified

● **E74   Other disorders of carbohydrate metabolism**

    Excludes1   diabetes mellitus (E08-E13)
        hypoglycemia NOS (E16.2)
        increased secretion of glucagon (E16.3)
        mucopolysaccharidosis (E76.0-E76.3)

    (Ex) **For category E74 CC codes:** C88.0, D47.2, D89.0-D89.1, E70.0-E71.30, E72.00-E72.02, E72.04-E74.9, E75.21-E75.249, E75.3, E75.5-E75.6, E77.0-E78.70, E78.79-E78.9, E88.09-E88.2, E88.89

● **E74.0   Glycogen storage disease**

    E74.00   Glycogen storage disease, unspecified 🔗

    E74.01   von Gierke's disease 🔗
        Type I glycogen storage disease

    E74.02   Pompe disease 🔗
        Cardiac glycogenosis
        Type II glycogen storage disease

    E74.03   Cori disease 🔗
        Forbes' disease
        Type III glycogen storage disease

    E74.04   McArdle disease 🔗
        Type V glycogen storage disease

    E74.09   Other glycogen storage disease 🔗
        Andersen disease
        Hers disease
        Tauri disease
        Glycogen storage disease, types 0, IV, VI-XI
        Liver phosphorylase deficiency
        Muscle phosphofructokinase deficiency

◀ New   ◀▥ Revised   ~~deleted~~ Deleted   Excludes 1   Excludes 2   Includes   Use additional   Code first   Code also   Unspecified

OGCR Official Guidelines   ● Unacceptable Principal Diagnosis   X Assign placeholder X   ● Use Additional Character(s)   ▶ Manifestation Code   **Coding Clinic**

● **E74.1** **Disorders of fructose metabolism**

> **Excludes1** muscle phosphofructokinase deficiency (E74.09)

E74.10 **Disorder of fructose metabolism, unspecified**

E74.11 **Essential fructosuria**
Fructokinase deficiency

E74.12 **Hereditary fructose intolerance**
Fructosemia

E74.19 **Other disorders of fructose metabolism**
Fructose-1, 6-diphosphatase deficiency

● **E74.2** **Disorders of galactose metabolism**

E74.20 **Disorders of galactose metabolism, unspecified** 🦠

E74.21 **Galactosemia** 🦠
Genetic disorders resulting from defective simple sugar (galactose) metabolism

E74.29 **Other disorders of galactose metabolism** 🦠
Galactokinase deficiency

● **E74.3** **Other disorders of intestinal carbohydrate absorption**

> **Excludes2** lactose intolerance (E73.-)

E74.31 **Sucrase-isomaltase deficiency**
Deficiency in metabolism in intestinal mucosa results in malabsorption of sucrose and starch

E74.39 **Other disorders of intestinal carbohydrate absorption**
Disorder of intestinal carbohydrate absorption NOS
Glucose-galactose malabsorption
Sucrase deficiency

● **E74.4** **Disorders of pyruvate metabolism and gluconeogenesis** 🦠
Deficiency of phosphoenolpyruvate carboxykinase
Deficiency of pyruvate carboxylase
Deficiency of pyruvate dehydrogenase

> **Excludes1** disorders of pyruvate metabolism and gluconeogenesis with anemia (D55.-)
> Leigh's syndrome (G31.82)

● **E74.8** **Other specified disorders of carbohydrate metabolism** 🦠
Essential pentosuria
Renal glycosuria

● **E74.9** **Disorder of carbohydrate metabolism, unspecified**

● **E75** **Disorders of sphingolipid metabolism and other lipid storage disorders**

> **Excludes1** mucolipidosis, types I-III (E77.0-E77.1)
> Refsum's disease (G60.1)

● **E75.0** **GM2 gangliosidosis**
Rare metabolic disorder that causes destruction of nerve cells of brain and spinal cord
(Ex) **For category E75.0 CC codes:** E75.00-E75.19, E75.4, F84.2, G13.2-G13.8, G30.0-G31.82, G31.84-G31.9, G91.4, G94

E75.00 **GM2 gangliosidosis, unspecified** 🦠

E75.01 **Sandhoff disease** 🦠

E75.02 **Tay-Sachs disease** 🦠

E75.09 **Other GM2 gangliosidosis** 🦠
Adult GM2 gangliosidosis
Juvenile GM2 gangliosidosis

● **E75.1** **Other and unspecified gangliosidosis**
(Ex) **For category E75.1 CC codes:** See E75.0

E75.10 **Unspecified gangliosidosis**
Gangliosidosis NOS

E75.11 **Mucolipidosis IV** 🦠
Disorder with symptoms of psychomotor retardation and severe visual impairment

E75.19 **Other gangliosidosis** 🦠
GM1 gangliosidosis
GM3 gangliosidosis

Item 4–8 **Leukodystrophy** is characterized by degeneration and/or failure of the myelin formation of the central nervous system and sometimes of the peripheral nervous system. The disease is inherited and progressive.

● **E75.2** **Other sphingolipidosis**
Lysosomal (a particle in a cytoplasm cell that contains digestive enzymes) storage diseases with symptoms of abnormal storage of amino acids

> **Excludes1** adrenoleukodystrophy [Addison-Schilder] (E71.528)

E75.21 **Fabry (-Anderson) disease**

E75.22 **Gaucher disease**

E75.23 **Krabbe disease** 🦠
(Ex) E75.00-E75.19, E75.23, E75.25-E75.29, E75.4, F84.2, G13.2-G13.8, G31.2-G31.82, G32.89, G91.4, G93.81, G93.89-G94, G96.8-G96.9, G98.0-G98.8, G99.8

● **E75.24** **Niemann-Pick disease**

E75.240 **Niemann-Pick disease type A**

E75.241 **Niemann-Pick disease type B**

E75.242 **Niemann-Pick disease type C**

E75.243 **Niemann-Pick disease type D**

E75.248 **Other Niemann-Pick disease**

E75.249 **Niemann-Pick disease, unspecified**

E75.25 **Metachromatic leukodystrophy** 🦠
(Ex) See E75.23

E75.29 **Other sphingolipidosis** 🦠
Farber's syndrome
Sulfatase deficiency
Sulfatide lipidosis
(Ex) See E75.23

● **E75.3** **Sphingolipidosis, unspecified**

● **E75.4** **Neuronal ceroid lipofuscinosis** 🦠
Batten disease
Bielschowsky-Jansky disease
Kufs disease
Spielmeyer-Vogt disease
(Ex) See E75.0

● **E75.5** **Other lipid storage disorders**
Cerebrotendinous cholesterosis [van Bogaert-Scherer-Epstein]
Wolman's disease

● **E75.6** **Lipid storage disorder, unspecified**

● **E76** **Disorders of glycosaminoglycan metabolism**
(Ex) **For category E76 CC codes:** D81.3, D81.5, D81.810, D84.1, E76.01-E76.9, E79.1-E80.29, E80.4-E80.7, E85.0, E85.9, E88.81

● **E76.0** **Mucopolysaccharidosis, type I**
Inborn metabolic disorder of enzymes that break down carbohydrates

E76.01 **Hurler's syndrome** 🦠

E76.02 **Hurler-Scheie syndrome** 🦠

E76.03 **Scheie's syndrome** 🦠

● **E76.1** **Mucopolysaccharidosis, type II** 🦠
Inborn metabolic disorder of enzymes that break down carbohydrates occurs in 2-4 year old males
Hunter's syndrome

● **E76.2** **Other mucopolysaccharidoses**

● **E76.21** **Morquio mucopolysaccharidoses**

E76.210 **Morquio A mucopolysaccharidoses** 🦠
Classic Morquio syndrome
Morquio syndrome A
Mucopolysaccharidosis, type IVA

E76.211 **Morquio B mucopolysaccharidoses** 🦠
Morquio-like mucopolysaccharidoses
Morquio-like syndrome
Morquio syndrome B
Mucopolysaccharidosis, type IVB

E76.219 **Morquio mucopolysaccharidoses, unspecified**
Morquio syndrome
Mucopolysaccharidosis, type IV

N Newborn Age: 0   P Pediatric Age: 0–17   M Maternity DX: 12–55   A Adult Age: 15–124   ♀ Females Only   ♂ Males Only

🦠 Complication\Comorbidity   🦠 Major C\C   (Ex) CC/MCC Exclusions   ⊙ Present on Admission Requirement   🦠 Hospital-Acquired Condition

851

E76.22   **Sanfilippo mucopolysaccharidoses** 🔹
      Mucopolysaccharidosis, type III (A) (B) (C) (D)
      Sanfilippo A syndrome
      Sanfilippo B syndrome
      Sanfilippo C syndrome
      Sanfilippo D syndrome

E76.29   **Other mucopolysaccharidoses** 🔹
      beta-Glucuronidase deficiency
      Maroteaux-Lamy (mild) (severe) syndrome
      Mucopolysaccharidosis, types VI, VII

E76.3   **Mucopolysaccharidosis, unspecified** 🔹

E76.8   **Other disorders of glucosaminoglycan metabolism** 🔹

E76.9   **Glucosaminoglycan metabolism disorder, unspecified** 🔹

● **E77**   **Disorders of glycoprotein metabolism**

E77.0   **Defects in post-translational modification of lysosomal enzymes**
      Mucolipidosis II [I-cell disease]
      Mucolipidosis III [pseudo-Hurler polydystrophy]

E77.1   **Defects in glycoprotein degradation**
      Aspartylglucosaminuria
      Fucosidosis
      Mannosidosis
      Sialidosis [mucolipidosis I]

E77.8   **Other disorders of glycoprotein metabolism**

E77.9   **Disorder of glycoprotein metabolism, unspecified**

● **E78**   **Disorders of lipoprotein metabolism and other lipidemias**
    Excludes1   sphingolipidosis (E75.0-E75.3)

E78.0   **Pure hypercholesterolemia**
      Familial hypercholesterolemia
      Fredrickson's hyperlipoproteinemia, type IIa
      Hyperbetalipoproteinemia
      Hyperlipidemia, Group A
      Low-density-lipoprotein-type [LDL]
        hyperlipoproteinemia

E78.1   **Pure hyperglyceridemia**
      Elevated fasting triglycerides
      Endogenous hyperglyceridemia
      Fredrickson's hyperlipoproteinemia, type IV
      Hyperlipidemia, group B
      Hyperprebetalipoproteinemia
      Very-low-density-lipoprotein-type [VLDL]
        hyperlipoproteinemia

E78.2   **Mixed hyperlipidemia**
      Broad- or floating-betalipoproteinemia
      Combined hyperlipidemia NOS
      Elevated cholesterol with elevated triglycerides NEC
      Fredrickson's hyperlipoproteinemia, type IIb or III
      Hyperbetalipoproteinemia with prebetalipoproteinemia
      Hypercholesteremia with endogenous
        hyperglyceridemia
      Hyperlipidemia, group C
      Tubo-eruptive xanthoma
      Xanthoma tuberosum
    Excludes1   cerebrotendinous cholesterosis [van Bogaert-Scherer-Epstein] (E75.5)
         familial combined hyperlipidemia (E78.4)

E78.3   **Hyperchylomicronemia**
      Chylomicron retention disease
      Fredrickson's hyperlipoproteinemia, type I or V
      Hyperlipidemia, group D
      Mixed hyperglyceridemia

E78.4   **Other hyperlipidemia**
      Familial combined hyperlipidemia

E78.5   **Hyperlipidemia, unspecified**

E78.6   **Lipoprotein deficiency**
      Abetalipoproteinemia
      Depressed HDL cholesterol
      High-density lipoprotein deficiency
      Hypoalphalipoproteinemia
      Hypobetalipoproteinemia (familial)
      Lecithin cholesterol acyltransferase deficiency
      Tangier disease

● **E78.7**   **Disorders of bile acid and cholesterol metabolism**
    Excludes1   Niemann-Pick disease type C (E75.242)
    (Ex) **For category E78.7 CC codes:** E78.71-E78.72, Q87.1-Q87.89, Q89.8, Q99.2

E78.70   **Disorder of bile acid and cholesterol metabolism, unspecified**

E78.71   **Barth syndrome** 🔹🔹

E78.72   **Smith-Lemli-Opitz syndrome** 🔹🔹

E78.79   **Other disorders of bile acid and cholesterol metabolism**

● **E78.8**   **Other disorders of lipoprotein metabolism**

E78.81   **Lipoid dermatoarthritis**

E78.89   **Other lipoprotein metabolism disorders**

E78.9   **Disorder of lipoprotein metabolism, unspecified**

● **E79**   **Disorders of purine and pyrimidine metabolism**
   Purines, along with pyrimidines, signal RNA and DNA production
    Excludes1   Ataxia-telangiectasia (Q87.1)
         Bloom's syndrome (Q82.8)
         Cockayne's syndrome (Q87.1)
         calculus of kidney (N20.0)
         combined immunodeficiency disorders (D81.-)
         Fanconi's anemia (D61.09)
         gout (M1A.-, M10.-) ◀◀◀
         orotaciduric anemia (D53.0)
         progeria (E34.8)
         Werner's syndrome (E34.8)
         xeroderma pigmentosum (Q82.1)
    (Ex) **For category E79 CC codes:** D81.3, D81.5, D81.810, D84.1, E76.01-E76.9, E79.1-E80.29, E80.4-E80.7, E88.81

E79.0   **Hyperuricemia without signs of inflammatory arthritis and tophaceous disease**
      Asymptomatic hyperuricemia

E79.1   **Lesch-Nyhan syndrome** 🔹
      HGPRT deficiency

E79.2   **Myoadenylate deaminase deficiency** 🔹

E79.8   **Other disorders of purine and pyrimidine metabolism** 🔹
      Hereditary xanthinuria

E79.9   **Disorder of purine and pyrimidine metabolism, unspecified** 🔹

● **E80**   **Disorders of porphyrin and bilirubin metabolism**
   Group of chemical compounds in RBC's that combine with iron to form heme
    Includes   defects of catalase and peroxidase
    (Ex) **For category E80 CC codes unless otherwise indicated:** D81.3, D81.5, D81.810, D84.1, E76.01-E76.9, E79.1-E80.29, E80.4-E80.7, E88.81

E80.0   **Hereditary erythropoietic porphyria** 🔹
      Congenital erythropoietic porphyria
      Erythropoietic protoporphyria

E80.1   **Porphyria cutanea tarda** 🔹

● **E80.2**   **Other and unspecified porphyria**

E80.20   **Unspecified porphyria** 🔹
      Porphyria NOS

E80.21   **Acute intermittent (hepatic) porphyria** 🔹

E80.29   **Other porphyria** 🔹
      Hereditary coproporphyria

E80.3   **Defects of catalase and peroxidase** 🔹
      Acatalasia [Takahara]
    (Ex) E71.310-E71.32, E71.40-E71.548, E80.4-E80.7, E88.40-E88.49, H49.811-H49.819

E80.4   **Gilbert syndrome**

E80.5   **Crigler-Najjar syndrome**

E80.6   **Other disorders of bilirubin metabolism**
      Dubin-Johnson syndrome
      Rotor's syndrome

E80.7   **Disorder of bilirubin metabolism, unspecified**

◀ New   ◀◀◀ Revised   ~~deleted~~ Deleted   Excludes 1   Excludes 2   Includes   Use additional   Code first   Code also   Unspecified

OGCR Official Guidelines   ● Unacceptable Principal Diagnosis   X Assign placeholder X   🔹 Use Additional Character(s)   ▶ Manifestation Code   **Coding Clinic**

● **E83**   **Disorders of mineral metabolism**
    Excludes1   dietary mineral deficiency (E58-E61)
                  parathyroid disorders (E20-E21)
                  vitamin D deficiency (E55.-)

● **E83.0**   **Disorders of copper metabolism**
     E83.00   **Disorder of copper metabolism, unspecified**
     E83.01   **Wilson's disease**
             Code also associated Kayser Fleischer ring
               (H18.04-)
     E83.09   **Other disorders of copper metabolism**
             Menkes' (kinky hair) (steely hair) disease

● **E83.1**   **Disorders of iron metabolism**
     Excludes1   iron deficiency anemia (D50.-)
                    sideroblastic anemia (D64.0-D64.3)
     E83.10   **Disorder of iron metabolism, unspecified**
     ● **E83.11**   **Hemochromatosis**
         E83.110   **Hereditary hemochromatosis**
               Bronzed diabetes
               Pigmentary cirrhosis (of liver)
               Primary (hereditary)
                 hemochromatosis
         E83.111   **Hemochromatosis due to repeated red blood cell transfusions**
               Iron overload due to repeated red
                 blood cell transfusions
               Transfusion (red blood cell)
                 associated hemochromatosis
         E83.118   **Other hemochromatosis**
         E83.119   **Hemochromatosis, unspecified**
     E83.19   **Other disorders of iron metabolism**
             Use additional code, if applicable, for
               idiopathic pulmonary hemosiderosis
               (J84.03)

● **E83.2**   **Disorders of zinc metabolism**
      Acrodermatitis enteropathica

● **E83.3**   **Disorders of phosphorus metabolism and phosphatases**
     Excludes1   adult osteomalacia (M83.-)
                  osteoporosis (M80.-) ◄▥
     E83.30   **Disorder of phosphorus metabolism, unspecified**
     E83.31   **Familial hypophosphatemia**
             Vitamin D-resistant osteomalacia
             Vitamin D-resistant rickets
         Excludes1   vitamin D-deficiency rickets
                      (E55.0)
     E83.32   **Hereditary vitamin D-dependent rickets (type 1) (type 2)**
             25-hydroxyvitamin D 1-alpha-hydroxylase
               deficiency
             Pseudovitamin D deficiency
             Vitamin D receptor defect
     E83.39   **Other disorders of phosphorus metabolism**
             Acid phosphatase deficiency
             Hypophosphatasia

● **E83.4**   **Disorders of magnesium metabolism**
     E83.40   **Disorders of magnesium metabolism, unspecified**
     E83.41   **Hypermagnesemia**
     E83.42   **Hypomagnesemia**
     E83.49   **Other disorders of magnesium metabolism**

● **E83.5**   **Disorders of calcium metabolism**
     Excludes1   chondrocalcinosis (M11.1-M11.2)
                  hungry bone syndrome (E83.81)
                  hyperparathyroidism (E21.0-E21.3)
     E83.50   **Unspecified disorder of calcium metabolism**
     E83.51   **Hypocalcemia**
     E83.52   **Hypercalcemia**
             Familial hypocalciuric hypercalcemia
     E83.59   **Other disorders of calcium metabolism**
             Idiopathic hypercalciuria

● **E83.8**   **Other disorders of mineral metabolism**
     E83.81   **Hungry bone syndrome**
     E83.89   **Other disorders of mineral metabolism**
● **E83.9**   **Disorder of mineral metabolism, unspecified**

● **E84**   **Cystic fibrosis**
     Includes   mucoviscidosis
     (Ex) **For category E84 CC codes: E84.0-E84.9**
     E84.0   **Cystic fibrosis with pulmonary manifestations** 🔧
            Use additional code to identify any infectious organism
               present, such as:
               Pseudomonas (B96.5)
● **E84.1**   **Cystic fibrosis with intestinal manifestations**
     E84.11   **Meconium ileus in cystic fibrosis** 🔧   N
         Excludes1   meconium ileus not due to cystic
                    fibrosis (P76.0)
     E84.19   **Cystic fibrosis with other intestinal manifestations** 🔧
             Distal intestinal obstruction syndrome
  E84.8   **Cystic fibrosis with other manifestations** 🔧
  E84.9   **Cystic fibrosis, unspecified** 🔧

● **E85**   **Amyloidosis**
     A disorder resulting from the abnormal deposition of a particular
     protein (amyloid) into tissues of the body.
     Excludes1   Alzheimer's disease (G30.0-)
     (Ex) **For category E85 CC codes: E85.0-E85.9, E88.81**
     E85.0   **Non-neuropathic heredofamilial amyloidosis** 🔧
            Familial Mediterranean fever
            Hereditary amyloid nephropathy
     E85.1   **Neuropathic heredofamilial amyloidosis** 🔧
            Amyloid polyneuropathy (Portuguese)
            Coding Clinic: 2012, Q4, P100
     E85.2   **Heredofamilial amyloidosis, unspecified** 🔧
     E85.3   **Secondary systemic amyloidosis** 🔧
            Hemodialysis-associated amyloidosis
     E85.4   **Organ-limited amyloidosis** 🔧
            Localized amyloidosis
     E85.8   **Other amyloidosis** 🔧
     E85.9   **Amyloidosis, unspecified** 🔧

● **E86**   **Volume depletion**
     Excludes1   dehydration of newborn (P74.1)
                  hypovolemic shock NOS (R57.1)
                  postprocedural hypovolemic shock (T81.19) ◄▥
                  traumatic hypovolemic shock (T79.4)
     E86.0   **Dehydration**
            Excessive loss of body water
     E86.1   **Hypovolemia**
            Diminished volume of circulating blood
            Depletion of volume of plasma
     E86.9   **Volume depletion, unspecified**

Item 4–9   Circulating fluid volume is regulated by the amount of water and sodium ingested, excreted by the kidneys into the urine, and lost through the gastrointestinal tract, lungs, and skin. To maintain blood volume within a normal range, the kidneys regulate the amount of water and sodium lost into the urine. Too much **(fluid overload)** or too little fluid volume **(volume depletion)** will affect blood pressure. Severe cases of vomiting, diarrhea, bleeding, and burns (fluid loss through exposed burn surface area) can contribute to fluid loss. Internal body environment must maintain a precise balance (homeostasis) between too much fluid and too little fluid. This complex balancing mechanism is critical to good health.

N Newborn Age: 0   **P** Pediatric Age: 0–17   **M** Maternity DX: 12–55   **A** Adult Age: 15–124   ♀ Females Only   ♂ Males Only

🔧 Complication\Comorbidity   🔧 Major C\C   (Ex) CC/MCC Exclusions   🔧 Present on Admission Requirement   🔧 Hospital-Acquired Condition   853

CHAPTER 4 (E00-E90)

CHAPTER 4 (E00-E90)

● **E87   Other disorders of fluid, electrolyte and acid-base balance**

Excludes1   diabetes insipidus (E23.2)
electrolyte imbalance associated with
hyperemesis gravidarum (O21.1)
electrolyte imbalance following ectopic or molar
pregnancy (O08.5)
familial periodic paralysis (G72.3)

(Ex) For category E87 CC codes: E86.0-E87.8

E87.0   Hyperosmolality and hypernatremia 🔖
Sodium [Na] excess
Sodium [Na] overload

E87.1   Hypo-osmolality and hyponatremia 🔖
Sodium [Na] deficiency

Excludes1   syndrome of inappropriate secretion of
antidiuretic hormone (E22.2)

E87.2   Acidosis 🔖
Acidosis NOS
Lactic acidosis
Metabolic acidosis
Respiratory acidosis

Excludes1   diabetic acidosis - see categories E08-E10,
E13 with ketoacidosis ◄▥

E87.3   Alkalosis 🔖
Alkalosis NOS
Metabolic alkalosis
Respiratory alkalosis

E87.4   Mixed disorder of acid-base balance 🔖

E87.5   Hyperkalemia
Potassium [K] excess
Potassium [K] overload

E87.6   Hypokalemia
Potassium [K] deficiency

● **E87.7   Fluid overload**

Excludes1   edema NOS (R60.9)
fluid retention (R60.9)

E87.70   Fluid overload, unspecified

E87.71   Transfusion associated circulatory overload
Fluid overload due to transfusion (blood)
(blood components) TACO

E87.79   Other fluid overload

E87.8   Other disorders of electrolyte and fluid balance, not elsewhere classified
Electrolyte imbalance NOS
Hyperchloremia
Hypochloremia

● **E88   Other and unspecified metabolic disorders**

Use additional codes for associated conditions

Excludes1   histiocytosis X (chronic) (C96.6)

● **E88.0   Disorders of plasma-protein metabolism, not elsewhere classified**

Excludes1   disorder of lipoprotein metabolism (E78.-)
monoclonal gammopathy (of
undetermined significance) (D47.2)
polyclonal hypergammaglobulinemia
(D89.0)
Waldenström macroglobulinemia (C88.0)

E88.01   Alpha-1-antitrypsin deficiency AAT deficiency

E88.09   Other disorders of plasma-protein metabolism, not elsewhere classified
Bisalbuminemia

E88.1   Lipodystrophy, not elsewhere classified
*Defective fat metabolism resulting in absence of subcutaneous
fat*
Lipodystrophy NOS

Excludes1   Whipple's disease (K90.81)

E88.2   Lipomatosis, not elsewhere classified
Abnormal tumorlike accumulations of fat in tissue
Lipomatosis NOS
Lipomatosis (Check) dolorosa [Dercum]

E88.3   Tumor lysis syndrome 🔖
Tumor lysis syndrome (spontaneous)
Tumor lysis syndrome following antineoplastic drug
chemotherapy

Use additional code for adverse effect, if applicable, to
identify drug (T45.1X5)

(Ex) E08.21-E08.29, E09.21-E09.29, E88.3, N00.0-N01.9, N02.8-N02.9,
N04.7-N05.1, N05.6-N06.1, N06.6-N07.1, N07.6-N08, N14.0-N15.0,
N15.8-N17.9

● **E88.4   Mitochondrial metabolism disorders**
Congenital disorder of metabolism

Excludes1   disorders of pyruvate metabolism (E74.4)
Kearns-Sayre syndrome (H49.81)
Leber's disease (H47.22)
Leigh's encephalopathy (G31.82)
Mitochondrial myopathy, NEC (G71.3)
Reye's syndrome (G93.7)

(Ex) For category E88.4 CC codes: C96.5-C96.6, E71.310-E71.548, E80.3-E80.7,
E88.89

E88.40   Mitochondrial metabolism disorder, unspecified 🔖

E88.41   MELAS syndrome 🔖
Mitochondrial myopathy, encephalopathy,
lactic acidosis and stroke-like episodes

E88.42   MERRF syndrome 🔖
Myoclonic epilepsy associated with ragged-red
fibers

Code also myoclonic epilepsy (G40.3-)

E88.49   Other mitochondrial metabolism disorders 🔖

● **E88.8   Other specified metabolic disorders**

E88.81   Metabolic syndrome
Dysmetabolic syndrome X

Use additional codes for associated
manifestations, such as:
obesity (E66.-)

E88.89   Other specified metabolic disorders 🔖
Launois-Bensaude adenolipomatosis

Excludes1   adult pulmonary Langerhans cell
histiocytosis (J84.82)

E88.9   Metabolic disorder, unspecified

**POSTPROCEDURAL ENDOCRINE AND METABOLIC COMPLICATIONS
AND DISORDERS, NOT ELSEWHERE CLASSIFIED (E89)**

● **E89   Postprocedural endocrine and metabolic complications and
disorders, not elsewhere classified**

Excludes2   intraoperative complications of endocrine system
organ or structure (E36.0-, E36.1-, E36.8)

E89.0   Postprocedural hypothyroidism
Postirradiation hypothyroidism
Postsurgical hypothyroidism

E89.1   Postprocedural hypoinsulinemia 🔖
Postpancreatectomy hyperglycemia
Postsurgical hypoinsulinemia

Use additional code, if applicable, to identify:
acquired absence of pancreas (Z90.41-)
diabetes mellitus (postpancreatectomy)
(postprocedural) (E13.-)
insulin use (Z79.4)

Excludes1   transient postprocedural hyperglycemia
(R73.9)
transient postprocedural hypoglycemia
(E16.2)

(Ex) E08.00-E08.59, E08.618-E09.59, E09.618-E10.59, E10.618-E10.649,
E10.69-E11.59, E11.618-E11.649, E11.69-E13.59, E13.618-E16.2, E30.9,
E34.1, E34.50-E35, E89.1

E89.2   Postprocedural hypoparathyroidism
Parathyroprival tetany

E89.3   Postprocedural hypopituitarism
Postirradiation hypopituitarism

◄ New   ◄▥ Revised   ~~deleted~~ Deleted   Excludes 1   Excludes 2   Includes   Use additional   Code first   Code also   Unspecified

OGCR Official Guidelines   ● Unacceptable Principal Diagnosis   X Assign placeholder X   🔖 Use Additional Character(s)   ▶ Manifestation Code   **Coding Clinic**

● E89.4   **Postprocedural ovarian failure**

    E89.40   **Asymptomatic postprocedural ovarian failure** ♀
        Postprocedural ovarian failure NOS

    E89.41   **Symptomatic postprocedural ovarian failure** ♀
        Symptoms such as flushing, sleeplessness,
        headache, lack of concentration,
        associated with postprocedural
        menopause

E89.5   **Postprocedural testicular hypofunction** ♂

E89.6   **Postprocedural adrenocortical (-medullary) hypofunction** 🔖
    (Ex) A17.9, A18.7, A18.82, A18.84, A18.89, E27.0-E27.9, E30.9, E34.1,
    E34.50-E35, E89.6

● E89.8   **Other postprocedural endocrine and metabolic complications and disorders**
    (Ex) **For category E89.8 CC codes:** E36.8, E89.810-E89.89, H95.811-H95.89,
    I97.3, M96.89, N98.1-N98.9, T81.82X[A], T81.89X-T81.9XX[A]

● E89.81   **Postprocedural hemorrhage and hematoma of an endocrine system organ or structure following a procedure**

    E89.810   **Postprocedural hemorrhage and hematoma of an endocrine system organ or structure following an endocrine system procedure** 🔖

    E89.811   **Postprocedural hemorrhage and hematoma of an endocrine system organ or structure following other procedure** 🔖

    E89.89   **Other postprocedural endocrine and metabolic complications and disorders** 🔖
        Use additional code, if applicable, to further
        specify disorder

N Newborn Age: 0   **P** Pediatric Age: 0–17   **M** Maternity DX: 12–55   **A** Adult Age: 15–124   ♀ Females Only   ♂ Males Only

🔖 Complication\Comorbidity   🔖 Major C\C   (Ex) CC/MCC Exclusions   🔖 Present on Admission Requirement   🔖 Hospital-Acquired Condition   855

CHAPTER 5

MENTAL, BEHAVIORAL AND NEURODEVELOPMENTAL DISORDERS (F01-F99)

Includes disorders of psychological development

Excludes2 symptoms, signs and abnormal clinical laboratory findings, not elsewhere classified (R00-R99)

This chapter contains the following blocks:

F01-F09	Mental disorders due to known physiological conditions
F10-F19	Mental and behavioral disorders due to psychoactive substance use
F20-F29	Schizophrenia, schizotypal, delusional, and other non-mood psychotic disorders
F30-F39	Mood [affective] disorders
F40-F48	Anxiety, dissociative, stress-related, somatoform and other nonpsychotic mental disorders
F50-F59	Behavioral syndromes associated with physiological disturbances and physical factors
F60-F69	Disorders of adult personality and behavior
F70-F79	Intellectual disabilities
F80-F89	Pervasive and specific developmental disorders
F90-F98	Behavioral and emotional disorders with onset usually occurring in childhood and adolescence
F99	Unspecified mental disorder

MENTAL DISORDERS DUE TO KNOWN PHYSIOLOGICAL CONDITIONS (F01-F09)

This block comprises a range of mental disorders grouped together on the basis of their having in common a demonstrable etiology in cerebral disease, brain injury, or other insult leading to cerebral dysfunction. The dysfunction may be primary, as in diseases, injuries, and insults that affect the brain directly and selectively; or secondary, as in systemic diseases and disorders that attack the brain only as one of the multiple organs or systems of the body that are involved.

● **F01　Vascular dementia**

Vascular dementia as a result of infarction of the brain due to vascular disease, including hypertensive cerebrovascular disease.

Includes arteriosclerotic dementia

Code first the underlying physiological condition or sequelae of cerebrovascular disease.

● **F01.5　Vascular dementia**

F01.50　Vascular dementia without behavioral disturbance　　　　A

F01.51　Vascular dementia with behavioral disturbance 🔖　　　　A

Vascular dementia with aggressive behavior
Vascular dementia with combative behavior
Vascular dementia with violent behavior

Use additional code, if applicable, to identify wandering in vascular dementia (Z91.83)

(Ex) F01.51

● **F02　Dementia in other diseases classified elsewhere**

Code first the underlying physiological condition, such as:
Alzheimer's (G30.-)
cerebral lipidosis (E75.4)
Creutzfeldt-Jakob disease (A81.0-)
dementia with Lewy bodies (G31.83)
epilepsy and recurrent seizures (G40.-)
frontotemporal dementia (G31.09)
hepatolenticular degeneration (E83.0)
human immunodeficiency virus [HIV] disease (B20)
hypercalcemia (E83.52)
hypothyroidism, acquired (E00-E03.-)
intoxications (T36-T65)
Jakob-Creutzfeldt disease (A81.0-)
multiple sclerosis (G35)
neurosyphilis (A52.17)
niacin deficiency [pellagra] (E52)
Parkinson's disease (G20)
Pick's disease (G31.01)
polyarteritis nodosa (M30.0)
systemic lupus erythematosus (M32.-)
trypanosomiasis (B56.-, B57.-)
vitamin B deficiency (E53.8)

Excludes1 dementia with Parkinsonism (G31.83)

Excludes2 dementia in alcohol and psychoactive substance disorders (F10-F19, with .17, .27, .97)
vascular dementia (F01.5-)

● **F02.8　Dementia in other diseases classified elsewhere**

▸ **F02.80　Dementia in other diseases classified elsewhere without behavioral disturbance**

Dementia in other diseases classified elsewhere NOS

▸ **F02.81　Dementia in other diseases classified elsewhere with behavioral disturbance** 🔖

Dementia in other diseases classified elsewhere with aggressive behavior
Dementia in other diseases classified elsewhere with combative behavior
Dementia in other diseases classified elsewhere with violent behavior

Use additional code, if applicable, to identify wandering in dementia in conditions classified elsewhere (Z91.83)

(Ex) F02.81, F03.91

● **F03　Unspecified dementia**

Presenile dementia NOS
Presenile psychosis NOS
Primary degenerative dementia NOS
Senile dementia NOS
Senile dementia depressed or paranoid type
Senile psychosis NOS

Excludes1 senility NOS (R41.81)

Excludes2 mild memory disturbance due to known physiological condition (F06.8)
senile dementia with delirium or acute confusional state (F05)

● **F03.9　Unspecified dementia**

F03.90　Unspecified dementia without behavioral disturbance　　　　A

Dementia NOS
Coding Clinic: 2012, Q4, P92

F03.91　Unspecified dementia with behavioral disturbance 🔖　　　　A

Unspecified dementia with aggressive behavior
Unspecified dementia with combative behavior
Unspecified dementia with violent behavior

Use additional code, if applicable, to identify wandering in unspecified dementia (Z91.83)

(Ex) F02.81, F03.91

Item 5-1 Psychosis was a term formerly applied to any mental disorder but is now restricted to disturbances of a great magnitude in which there is a personality disintegration and loss of contact with reality.

◀ New　◀ Revised　~~deleted~~ Deleted　Excludes 1　Excludes 2　Includes　Use additional　Code first　Code also　Unspecified

OGCR Official Guidelines　● Unacceptable Principal Diagnosis　X Assign placeholder X　● Use Additional Character(s)　▸ Manifestation Code　Coding Clinic

CHAPTER 5 (F01-F99)

F04   Amnestic disorder due to known physiological condition

Korsakov's psychosis or syndrome, nonalcoholic

Code first the underlying physiological condition

Excludes1   amnesia NOS (R41.3)
anterograde amnesia (R41.1)
dissociative amnesia (F44.0)
retrograde amnesia (R41.2)

Excludes2   alcohol-induced or unspecified Korsakov's syndrome (F10.26, F10.96)
Korsakov's syndrome induced by other psychoactive substances (F13.26, F13.96, F19.16, F19.26, F19.96)

F05   Delirium due to known physiological condition 🔹

Acute or subacute brain syndrome
Acute or subacute confusional state (nonalcoholic)
Acute or subacute infective psychosis
Acute or subacute organic reaction
Acute or subacute psycho-organic syndrome
Delirium of mixed etiology
Delirium superimposed on dementia
Sundowning

Code first the underlying physiological condition

Excludes1   delirium NOS (R41.0)

Excludes2   delirium tremens alcohol-induced or unspecified (F10.231, F10.921)

(Ex:) F05, R45.851

● F06   Other mental disorders due to known physiological condition

Includes   mental disorders due to endocrine disorder
mental disorders due to exogenous hormone
mental disorders due to exogenous toxic substance
mental disorders due to primary cerebral disease
mental disorders due to somatic illness
mental disorders due to systemic disease affecting the brain

Code first the underlying physiological condition

Excludes1   unspecified dementia (F03)

Excludes2   delirium due to known physiological condition (F05)
dementia as classified in F01-F02
other mental disorders associated with alcohol and other psychoactive substances (F10-F19)

(Ex:) For category F06 CC codes: F02.80-F02.81, F04-F06.8, F10.10-F11.19, F11.21-F13.19, F13.21-F14.19, F14.21-F15.19, F15.21-F16.19, F16.21-F17.209, F17.213-F17.219, F17.223-F17.229, F17.293-F18.19, F18.21-F19.19, F19.21-F19.99, F53-F55.8, R78

F06.0   Psychotic disorder with hallucinations due to known physiological condition 🔹

Organic hallucinatory state (nonalcoholic)

Excludes2   hallucinations and perceptual disturbance induced by alcohol and other psychoactive substances (F10-F19 with .151, .251, .951)
schizophrenia (F20.-)

F06.1   Catatonic disorder due to known physiological condition

Excludes1   catatonic stupor (R40.1)
stupor NOS (R40.1)

Excludes2   catatonic schizophrenia (F20.2)
dissociative stupor (F44.2)

F06.2   Psychotic disorder with delusions due to known physiological condition 🔹

Paranoid and paranoid-hallucinatory organic states
Schizophrenia-like psychosis in epilepsy

Excludes2   alcohol and drug-induced psychotic disorder (F10-F19 with .150, .250, .950)
brief psychotic disorder (F23)
delusional disorder (F22)
schizophrenia (F20.-)

F06.3   Mood disorder due to known physiological condition

Excludes2   mood disorders due to alcohol and other psychoactive substances (F10-F19 with .14, .24, .94)
mood disorders, not due to known physiological condition or unspecified (F30-F39)

F06.30   Mood disorder due to known physiological condition, unspecified

F06.31   Mood disorder due to known physiological condition with depressive features

F06.32   Mood disorder due to known physiological condition with major depressive-like episode

F06.33   Mood disorder due to known physiological condition with manic features

F06.34   Mood disorder due to known physiological condition with mixed features

F06.4   Anxiety disorder due to known physiological condition

Excludes2   anxiety disorders due to alcohol and other psychoactive substances (F10-F19 with .180, .280, .980)
anxiety disorders, not due to known physiological condition or unspecified (F40.-, F41.-)

F06.8   Other specified mental disorders due to known physiological condition

Epileptic psychosis NOS
Organic dissociative disorder
Organic emotionally labile [asthenic] disorder

● F07   Personality and behavioral disorders due to known physiological condition

Code first the underlying physiological condition

F07.0   Personality change due to known physiological condition

Frontal lobe syndrome
Limbic epilepsy personality syndrome
Lobotomy syndrome
Organic personality disorder
Organic pseudopsychopathic personality
Organic pseudoretarded personality
Postleucotomy syndrome

Code first underlying physiological condition

Excludes1   mild cognitive impairment (G31.84)
postconcussional syndrome (F07.81)
postencephalitic syndrome (F07.89)
signs and symptoms involving emotional state (R45.-)

Excludes2   specific personality disorder (F60.-)

● F07.8   Other personality and behavioral disorders due to known physiological condition

F07.81   Postconcussional syndrome

Postcontusional syndrome (encephalopathy)
Post-traumatic brain syndrome, nonpsychotic

Use additional code to identify associated post-traumatic headache, if applicable (G44.3-)

Excludes1   current concussion (brain) (S06.0-)
postencephalitic syndrome (F07.89)

F07.89   Other personality and behavioral disorders due to known physiological condition

Postencephalitic syndrome
Damage to temporal brain lobes with memory loss and abnormal behavior
Right hemispheric organic affective disorder

F07.9   Unspecified personality and behavioral disorder due to known physiological condition

Organic psychosyndrome
Due to exposure to organic solvents

| N | Newborn Age: 0 | P | Pediatric Age: 0–17 | M | Maternity DX: 12–55 | A | Adult Age: 15–124 | ♀ | Females Only | ♂ | Males Only |

🔹 Complication\Comorbidity   🔹 Major C\C   (Ex:) CC/MCC Exclusions   🔹 Present on Admission Requirement   🔹 Hospital-Acquired Condition

857

CHAPTER 5 (F01-F99)

F09   Unspecified mental disorder due to known physiological condition
Mental disorder NOS due to known physiological condition
Organic brain syndrome NOS
Organic mental disorder NOS
Organic psychosis NOS
Symptomatic psychosis NOS
Code first the underlying physiological condition
Excludes1   psychosis NOS (F29)

**MENTAL AND BEHAVIORAL DISORDERS DUE TO
PSYCHOACTIVE SUBSTANCE USE (F10-F19)**

● **F10   Alcohol related disorders**
Use additional code for blood alcohol level, if applicable (Y90.-)
(Ex) For category F10 CC codes: F02.80-F02.81, F04-F06.8, F10.10-F11.19, F11.21-F13.19, F13.21-F14.19, F14.21-F15.19, F15.21-F16.19, F16.21-F17.209, F17.213-F17.219, F17.223-F17.229, F17.293-F18.19, F18.21-F19.19, F19.21-F19.99, F53-F55.8, R78

● **F10.1   Alcohol abuse**
     Excludes1   alcohol dependence (F10.2-)
                 alcohol use, unspecified (F10.9-)
     F10.10   Alcohol abuse, uncomplicated
     ● **F10.12   Alcohol abuse with intoxication**
         F10.120   Alcohol abuse with intoxication, uncomplicated
         F10.121   Alcohol abuse with intoxication, delirium ⚕
         F10.129   Alcohol abuse with intoxication, unspecified
     F10.14   Alcohol abuse with alcohol-induced mood disorder ⚕
     ● **F10.15   Alcohol abuse with alcohol-induced psychotic disorder**
         F10.150   Alcohol abuse with alcohol-induced psychotic disorder with delusions
         F10.151   Alcohol abuse with alcohol-induced psychotic disorder with hallucinations ⚕
         F10.159   Alcohol abuse with alcohol-induced psychotic disorder, unspecified ⚕
     ● **F10.18   Alcohol abuse with other alcohol-induced disorders**
         F10.180   Alcohol abuse with alcohol-induced anxiety disorder ⚕
         F10.181   Alcohol abuse with alcohol-induced sexual dysfunction ⚕
         F10.182   Alcohol abuse with alcohol-induced sleep disorder
         F10.188   Alcohol abuse with other alcohol-induced disorder ⚕
     F10.19   Alcohol abuse with unspecified alcohol-induced disorder ⚕
● **F10.2   Alcohol dependence**
     Excludes1   alcohol abuse (F10.1-)
                 alcohol use, unspecified (F10.9-)
     Excludes2   toxic effect of alcohol (T51.0-)
     F10.20   Alcohol dependence, uncomplicated
     F10.21   Alcohol dependence, in remission
     ● **F10.22   Alcohol dependence with intoxication**
         Acute drunkenness (in alcoholism)
         Excludes1   alcohol dependence with withdrawal (F10.23-)
         F10.220   Alcohol dependence with intoxication, uncomplicated
         F10.221   Alcohol dependence with intoxication delirium ⚕
         F10.229   Alcohol dependence with intoxication, unspecified

● **F10.23   Alcohol dependence with withdrawal**
     Excludes1   alcohol dependence with intoxication (F10.22-)
     F10.230   Alcohol dependence with withdrawal, uncomplicated ⚕
     F10.231   Alcohol dependence with withdrawal delirium ⚕
     F10.232   Alcohol dependence with withdrawal with perceptual disturbance ⚕
     F10.239   Alcohol dependence with withdrawal, unspecified ⚕
F10.24   Alcohol dependence with alcohol-induced mood disorder ⚕
● **F10.25   Alcohol dependence with alcohol-induced psychotic disorder**
     F10.250   Alcohol dependence with alcohol-induced psychotic disorder with delusions
     F10.251   Alcohol dependence with alcohol-induced psychotic disorder with hallucinations ⚕
     F10.259   Alcohol dependence with alcohol-induced psychotic disorder, unspecified ⚕
F10.26   Alcohol dependence with alcohol-induced persisting amnestic disorder
F10.27   Alcohol dependence with alcohol-induced persisting dementia ⚕
● **F10.28   Alcohol dependence with other alcohol-induced disorders**
     F10.280   Alcohol dependence with alcohol-induced anxiety disorder ⚕
     F10.281   Alcohol dependence with alcohol-induced sexual dysfunction ⚕
     F10.282   Alcohol dependence with alcohol-induced sleep disorder
     F10.288   Alcohol dependence with other alcohol-induced disorder ⚕
F10.29   Alcohol dependence with unspecified alcohol-induced disorder ⚕
● **F10.9   Alcohol use, unspecified**
     Excludes1   alcohol abuse (F10.1-)
                 alcohol dependence (F10.2-)
     ● **F10.92   Alcohol use, unspecified with intoxication**
         F10.920   Alcohol use, unspecified with intoxication, uncomplicated
         F10.921   Alcohol use, unspecified with intoxication delirium ⚕
         F10.929   Alcohol use, unspecified with intoxication, unspecified
     F10.94   Alcohol use, unspecified with alcohol-induced mood disorder ⚕
     ● **F10.95   Alcohol use, unspecified with alcohol-induced psychotic disorder**
         F10.950   Alcohol use, unspecified with alcohol-induced psychotic disorder with delusions
         F10.951   Alcohol use, unspecified with alcohol-induced psychotic disorder with hallucinations ⚕
         F10.959   Alcohol use, unspecified with alcohol-induced psychotic disorder, unspecified ⚕
     F10.96   Alcohol use, unspecified with alcohol-induced persisting amnestic disorder
     F10.97   Alcohol use, unspecified with alcohol-induced persisting dementia

● F10.98   Alcohol use, unspecified with other alcohol-induced disorders

     F10.980   Alcohol use, unspecified with alcohol-induced anxiety disorder 🗝

     F10.981   Alcohol use, unspecified with alcohol-induced sexual dysfunction 🗝

     F10.982   Alcohol use, unspecified with alcohol-induced sleep disorder 🗝

     F10.988   Alcohol use, unspecified with other alcohol-induced disorder 🗝

   F10.99   Alcohol use, unspecified with unspecified alcohol-induced disorder 🗝

● **F11**   **Opioid related disorders**

   (Ex) **For category F11 CC codes unless otherwise indicated:** F02.80-F02.81, F04-F06.8, F10.10-F11.19, F11.21-F13.19, F13.21-F14.19, F14.21-F15.19, F15.21-F16.19, F16.21-F17.209, F17.213-F17.219, F17.223-F17.229, F17.293-F18.19, F18.21-F19.19, F19.21-F19.99, F53-F55.8, R78

   ● F11.1   **Opioid abuse**

     Excludes1   opioid dependence (F11.2-)
                opioid use, unspecified (F11.9-)

     F11.10   Opioid abuse, uncomplicated

   ● F11.12   Opioid abuse with intoxication

     F11.120   Opioid abuse with intoxication, uncomplicated

     F11.121   Opioid abuse with intoxication delirium 🗝

     F11.122   Opioid abuse with intoxication with perceptual disturbance 🗝

     F11.129   Opioid abuse with intoxication, unspecified

     F11.14   Opioid abuse with opioid-induced mood disorder

   ● F11.15   Opioid abuse with opioid-induced psychotic disorder

     F11.150   Opioid abuse with opioid-induced psychotic disorder with delusions 🗝

     F11.151   Opioid abuse with opioid-induced psychotic disorder with hallucinations 🗝

     F11.159   Opioid abuse with opioid-induced psychotic disorder, unspecified

   ● F11.18   Opioid abuse with other opioid-induced disorder

     F11.181   Opioid abuse with opioid-induced sexual dysfunction

     F11.182   Opioid abuse with opioid-induced sleep disorder

     F11.188   Opioid abuse with other opioid-induced disorder

     F11.19   Opioid abuse with unspecified opioid-induced disorder

   ● F11.2   **Opioid dependence**

     Excludes1   opioid abuse (F11.1-)
                opioid use, unspecified (F11.9-)

     Excludes2   opioid poisoning (T40.0--T40.2-)

     F11.20   Opioid dependence, uncomplicated 🗝
         (Ex) No exclusions

     F11.21   Opioid dependence, in remission

   ● F11.22   Opioid dependence with intoxication

     Excludes1   opioid dependence with withdrawal (F11.23)

     F11.220   Opioid dependence with intoxication, uncomplicated

     F11.221   Opioid dependence with intoxication delirium 🗝

     F11.222   Opioid dependence with intoxication with perceptual disturbance 🗝
         (Ex) No exclusions

     F11.229   Opioid dependence with intoxication, unspecified

     F11.23   Opioid dependence with withdrawal 🗝

     Excludes1   opioid dependence with intoxication (F11.22-)

     F11.24   Opioid dependence with opioid-induced mood disorder

   ● F11.25   Opioid dependence with opioid-induced psychotic disorder

     F11.250   Opioid dependence with opioid-induced psychotic disorder with delusions 🗝

     F11.251   Opioid dependence with opioid-induced psychotic disorder with hallucinations 🗝

     F11.259   Opioid dependence with opioid-induced psychotic disorder, unspecified 🗝
         (Ex) No exclusions

   ● F11.28   Opioid dependence with other opioid-induced disorder
         (Ex) **For category F11.28 CC codes:** No exclusions

     F11.281   Opioid dependence with opioid-induced sexual dysfunction 🗝

     F11.282   Opioid dependence with opioid-induced sleep disorder 🗝

     F11.288   Opioid dependence with other opioid-induced disorder 🗝

     F11.29   Opioid dependence with unspecified opioid-induced disorder

   ● F11.9   **Opioid use, unspecified**

     Excludes1   opioid abuse (F11.1-)
                opioid dependence (F11.2-)

     F11.90   Opioid use, unspecified, uncomplicated

   ● F11.92   Opioid use, unspecified with intoxication

     Excludes1   opioid use, unspecified with withdrawal (F11.93)

     F11.920   Opioid use, unspecified with intoxication, uncomplicated

     F11.921   Opioid use, unspecified with intoxication delirium 🗝

     F11.922   Opioid use, unspecified with intoxication with perceptual disturbance

     F11.929   Opioid use, unspecified with intoxication, unspecified

     F11.93   Opioid use, unspecified with withdrawal 🗝

     Excludes1   opioid use, unspecified with intoxication (F11.92-)

     F11.94   Opioid use, unspecified with opioid-induced mood disorder

   ● F11.95   Opioid use, unspecified with opioid-induced psychotic disorder

     F11.950   Opioid use, unspecified with opioid-induced psychotic disorder with delusions 🗝

     F11.951   Opioid use, unspecified with opioid-induced psychotic disorder with hallucinations 🗝

     F11.959   Opioid use, unspecified with opioid-induced psychotic disorder, unspecified

   ● F11.98   Opioid use, unspecified with other specified opioid-induced disorder

     F11.981   Opioid use, unspecified with opioid-induced sexual dysfunction

     F11.982   Opioid use, unspecified with opioid-induced sleep disorder

     F11.988   Opioid use, unspecified with other opioid-induced disorder

     F11.99   Opioid use, unspecified with unspecified opioid-induced disorder

CHAPTER 5 (F01-F99)

N   Newborn Age: 0   **P**   Pediatric Age: 0–17   **M**   Maternity DX: 12–55   **A**   Adult Age: 15–124   ♀   Females Only   ♂   Males Only

🗝   Complication\Comorbidity   🗝   Major C\C   (Ex)   CC/MCC Exclusions   🗝   Present on Admission Requirement   Hospital-Acquired Condition

859

● F12   **Cannabis related disorders**
     Includes   marijuana
     (Ex) **For category F12 CC codes:** F02.80-F02.81, F04-F06.8, F10.10-F11.19, F11.21-F13.19, F13.21-F14.19, F14.21-F15.19, F15.21-F16.19, F16.21-F17.209, F17.213-F17.219, F17.223-F17.229, F17.293-F18.19, F18.21-F19.19, F19.21-F19.99, F53-F55.8, R78

   ● F12.1   **Cannabis abuse**
       Excludes1   cannabis dependence (F12.2-)
                   cannabis use, unspecified (F12.9-)

     F12.10   Cannabis abuse, uncomplicated
   ● F12.12   Cannabis abuse with intoxication
       F12.120   Cannabis abuse with intoxication, uncomplicated
       F12.121   Cannabis abuse with intoxication delirium 🔗
       F12.122   Cannabis abuse with intoxication with perceptual disturbance
       F12.129   Cannabis abuse with intoxication, unspecified

   ● F12.15   Cannabis abuse with psychotic disorder
       F12.150   Cannabis abuse with psychotic disorder with delusions 🔗
       F12.151   Cannabis abuse with psychotic disorder with hallucinations 🔗
       F12.159   Cannabis abuse with psychotic disorder, unspecified

   ● F12.18   Cannabis abuse with other cannabis-induced disorder
       F12.180   Cannabis abuse with cannabis-induced anxiety disorder
       F12.188   Cannabis abuse with other cannabis-induced disorder

     F12.19   Cannabis abuse with unspecified cannabis-induced disorder

   ● F12.2   **Cannabis dependence**
       Excludes1   cannabis abuse (F12.1-)
                   cannabis use, unspecified (F12.9-)
       Excludes2   cannabis poisoning (T40.7-)

     F12.20   Cannabis dependence, uncomplicated
     F12.21   Cannabis dependence, in remission
   ● F12.22   Cannabis dependence with intoxication
       F12.220   Cannabis dependence with intoxication, uncomplicated
       F12.221   Cannabis dependence with intoxication delirium 🔗
       F12.222   Cannabis dependence with intoxication with perceptual disturbance
       F12.229   Cannabis dependence with intoxication, unspecified

   ● F12.25   Cannabis dependence with psychotic disorder
       F12.250   Cannabis dependence with psychotic disorder with delusions 🔗
       F12.251   Cannabis dependence with psychotic disorder with hallucinations 🔗
       F12.259   Cannabis dependence with psychotic disorder, unspecified

   ● F12.28   Cannabis dependence with other cannabis-induced disorder
       F12.280   Cannabis dependence with cannabis-induced anxiety disorder
       F12.288   Cannabis dependence with other cannabis-induced disorder

     F12.29   Cannabis dependence with unspecified cannabis-induced disorder

   ● F12.9   **Cannabis use, unspecified**
       Excludes1   cannabis abuse (F12.1-)
                   cannabis dependence (F12.2-)

     F12.90   Cannabis use, unspecified, uncomplicated
   ● F12.92   Cannabis use, unspecified with intoxication
       F12.920   Cannabis use, unspecified with intoxication, uncomplicated
       F12.921   Cannabis use, unspecified with intoxication delirium 🔗
       F12.922   Cannabis use, unspecified with intoxication with perceptual disturbance
       F12.929   Cannabis use, unspecified with intoxication, unspecified

   ● F12.95   Cannabis use, unspecified with psychotic disorder
       F12.950   Cannabis use, unspecified with psychotic disorder with delusions 🔗
       F12.951   Cannabis use, unspecified with psychotic disorder with hallucinations 🔗
       F12.959   Cannabis use, unspecified with psychotic disorder, unspecified

   ● F12.98   Cannabis use, unspecified with other cannabis-induced disorder
       F12.980   Cannabis use, unspecified with anxiety disorder
       F12.988   Cannabis use, unspecified with other cannabis-induced disorder

     F12.99   Cannabis use, unspecified with unspecified cannabis-induced disorder

● F13   **Sedative, hypnotic, or anxiolytic related disorders**
     (Ex) **For category F13 CC codes unless otherwise indicated:** F02.80-F02.81, F04-F06.8, F10.10-F11.19, F11.21-F13.19, F13.21-F14.19, F14.21-F15.19, F15.21-F16.19, F16.21-F17.209, F17.213-F17.219, F17.223-F17.229, F17.293-F18.19, F18.21-F19.19, F19.21-F19.99, F53-F55.8, R78

   ● F13.1   **Sedative, hypnotic or anxiolytic-related abuse**
       Excludes1   sedative, hypnotic or anxiolytic-related dependence (F13.2-)
                   sedative, hypnotic, or anxiolytic use, unspecified (F13.9-)

     F13.10   Sedative, hypnotic or anxiolytic abuse, uncomplicated
   ● F13.12   Sedative, hypnotic or anxiolytic abuse with intoxication
       F13.120   Sedative, hypnotic or anxiolytic abuse with intoxication, uncomplicated
       F13.121   Sedative, hypnotic or anxiolytic abuse with intoxication delirium 🔗
       F13.129   Sedative, hypnotic or anxiolytic abuse with intoxication, unspecified

     F13.14   Sedative, hypnotic or anxiolytic abuse with sedative, hypnotic or anxiolytic-induced mood disorder
   ● F13.15   Sedative, hypnotic or anxiolytic abuse with sedative, hypnotic or anxiolyticinduced psychotic disorder
       F13.150   Sedative, hypnotic or anxiolytic abuse with sedative, hypnotic or anxiolytic-induced psychotic disorder with delusions 🔗
       F13.151   Sedative, hypnotic or anxiolytic abuse with sedative, hypnotic or anxiolytic-induced psychotic disorder with hallucinations 🔗
       F13.159   Sedative, hypnotic or anxiolytic abuse with sedative, hypnotic or anxiolytic-induced psychotic disorder, unspecified

CHAPTER 5 (F01-F99)

◀ New   ◀ Revised   ~~deleted~~ Deleted   Excludes 1   Excludes 2   Includes   Use additional   Code first   Code also   Unspecified
OGCR Official Guidelines   ● Unacceptable Principal Diagnosis   X Assign placeholder X   ● Use Additional Character(s)   🔗 Manifestation Code   **Coding Clinic**

● **F13.18**   Sedative, hypnotic or anxiolytic abuse with other sedative, hypnotic or anxiolytic-induced disorders

    F13.180   Sedative, hypnotic or anxiolytic abuse with sedative, hypnotic or anxiolytic-induced anxiety disorder

    F13.181   Sedative, hypnotic or anxiolytic abuse with sedative, hypnotic or anxiolytic-induced sexual dysfunction

    F13.182   Sedative, hypnotic or anxiolytic abuse with sedative, hypnotic or anxiolytic-induced sleep disorder

    F13.188   Sedative, hypnotic or anxiolytic abuse with other sedative, hypnotic or anxiolytic-induced disorder

  F13.19   Sedative, hypnotic or anxiolytic abuse with unspecified sedative, hypnotic or anxiolytic-induced disorder

● **F13.2**   Sedative, hypnotic or anxiolytic-related dependence

    Excludes1   sedative, hypnotic or anxiolytic-related abuse (F13.1-)
         sedative, hypnotic, or anxiolytic use, unspecified (F13.9-)

    Excludes2   sedative, hypnotic, or anxiolytic poisoning (T42.-)

  F13.20   Sedative, hypnotic or anxiolytic dependence, uncomplicated
      (Ex:) No exclusions

  F13.21   Sedative, hypnotic or anxiolytic dependence, in remission

● **F13.22**   Sedative, hypnotic or anxiolytic dependence with intoxication

    Excludes1   sedative, hypnotic or anxiolytic dependence with withdrawal (F13.23-)

    F13.220   Sedative, hypnotic or anxiolytic dependence with intoxication, uncomplicated

    F13.221   Sedative, hypnotic or anxiolytic dependence with intoxication delirium

    F13.229   Sedative, hypnotic or anxiolytic dependence with intoxication, unspecified

● **F13.23**   Sedative, hypnotic or anxiolytic dependence with withdrawal

    Excludes1   sedative, hypnotic or anxiolytic dependence with intoxication (F13.22-)

    F13.230   Sedative, hypnotic or anxiolytic dependence with withdrawal, uncomplicated

    F13.231   Sedative, hypnotic or anxiolytic dependence with withdrawal delirium

    F13.232   Sedative, hypnotic or anxiolytic dependence with withdrawal with perceptual disturbance

    F13.239   Sedative, hypnotic or anxiolytic dependence with withdrawal, unspecified

  F13.24   Sedative, hypnotic or anxiolytic dependence with sedative, hypnotic or anxiolytic-induced mood disorder

● **F13.25**   Sedative, hypnotic or anxiolytic dependence with sedative, hypnotic or anxiolytic-induced psychotic disorder

    F13.250   Sedative, hypnotic or anxiolytic dependence with sedative, hypnotic or anxiolytic-induced psychotic disorder with delusions

    F13.251   Sedative, hypnotic or anxiolytic dependence with sedative, hypnotic or anxiolytic-induced psychotic disorder with hallucinations

    F13.259   Sedative, hypnotic or anxiolytic dependence with sedative, hypnotic or anxiolytic-induced psychotic disorder, unspecified
      (Ex:) No exclusions

  F13.26   Sedative, hypnotic or anxiolytic dependence with sedative, hypnotic or anxiolytic-induced persisting amnestic disorder
      (Ex:) No exclusions

  F13.27   Sedative, hypnotic or anxiolytic dependence with sedative, hypnotic or anxiolytic-induced persisting dementia

● **F13.28**   Sedative, hypnotic or anxiolytic dependence with other sedative, hypnotic or anxiolytic-induced disorders
      (Ex:) For category F13.28 CC codes: No exclusions

    F13.280   Sedative, hypnotic or anxiolytic dependence with sedative, hypnotic or anxiolytic-induced anxiety disorder

    F13.281   Sedative, hypnotic or anxiolytic dependence with sedative, hypnotic or anxiolytic-induced sexual dysfunction

    F13.282   Sedative, hypnotic or anxiolytic dependence with sedative, hypnotic or anxiolytic-induced sleep disorder

    F13.288   Sedative, hypnotic or anxiolytic dependence with other sedative, hypnotic or anxiolytic-induced disorder

  F13.29   Sedative, hypnotic or anxiolytic dependence with unspecified sedative, hypnotic or anxiolytic-induced disorder

● **F13.9**   Sedative, hypnotic or anxiolytic-related use, unspecified

    Excludes1   sedative, hypnotic or anxiolytic-related abuse (F13.1-)
         sedative, hypnotic or anxiolytic-related dependence (F13.2-)

  F13.90   Sedative, hypnotic, or anxiolytic use, unspecified, uncomplicated

● **F13.92**   Sedative, hypnotic or anxiolytic use, unspecified with intoxication

    Excludes1   sedative, hypnotic or anxiolytic use, unspecified with withdrawal (F13.93-)

    F13.920   Sedative, hypnotic or anxiolytic use, unspecified with intoxication, uncomplicated

    F13.921   Sedative, hypnotic or anxiolytic use, unspecified with intoxication delirium

    F13.929   Sedative, hypnotic or anxiolytic use, unspecified with intoxication, unspecified

CHAPTER 5 (F01-F99)

N Newborn Age: 0   **P** Pediatric Age: 0–17   **M** Maternity DX: 12–55   **A** Adult Age: 15–124   ♀ Females Only   ♂ Males Only

🍷 Complication\Comorbidity   🍷 Major C\C   (Ex:) CC/MCC Exclusions   🍷 Present on Admission Requirement   🍷 Hospital-Acquired Condition

861

● **F13.93** Sedative, hypnotic or anxiolytic use, unspecified with withdrawal

    Excludes1 sedative, hypnotic or anxiolytic use, unspecified with intoxication (F13.92-)

    F13.930 Sedative, hypnotic or anxiolytic use, unspecified with withdrawal, uncomplicated

    F13.931 Sedative, hypnotic or anxiolytic use, unspecified with withdrawal delirium

    F13.932 Sedative, hypnotic or anxiolytic use, unspecified with withdrawal with perceptual disturbances

    F13.939 Sedative, hypnotic or anxiolytic use, unspecified with withdrawal, unspecified

F13.94 Sedative, hypnotic or anxiolytic use, unspecified with sedative, hypnotic or anxiolytic-induced mood disorder

● **F13.95** Sedative, hypnotic or anxiolytic use, unspecified with sedative, hypnotic or anxiolytic-induced psychotic disorder

    F13.950 Sedative, hypnotic or anxiolytic use, unspecified with sedative, hypnotic or anxiolytic-induced psychotic disorder with delusions

    F13.951 Sedative, hypnotic or anxiolytic use, unspecified with sedative, hypnotic or anxiolytic-induced psychotic disorder with hallucinations

    F13.959 Sedative, hypnotic or anxiolytic use, unspecified with sedative, hypnotic or anxiolytic-induced psychotic disorder, unspecified

F13.96 Sedative, hypnotic or anxiolytic use, unspecified with sedative, hypnotic or anxiolytic-induced persisting amnestic disorder

F13.97 Sedative, hypnotic or anxiolytic use, unspecified with sedative, hypnotic or anxiolytic-induced persisting dementia

● **F13.98** Sedative, hypnotic or anxiolytic use, unspecified with other sedative, hypnotic or anxiolytic-induced disorders

    F13.980 Sedative, hypnotic or anxiolytic use, unspecified with sedative, hypnotic or anxiolytic-induced anxiety disorder

    F13.981 Sedative, hypnotic or anxiolytic use, unspecified with sedative, hypnotic or anxiolytic-induced sexual dysfunction

    F13.982 Sedative, hypnotic or anxiolytic use, unspecified with sedative, hypnotic or anxiolytic-induced sleep disorder

    F13.988 Sedative, hypnotic or anxiolytic use, unspecified with other sedative, hypnotic or anxiolytic-induced disorder

F13.99 Sedative, hypnotic or anxiolytic use, unspecified with unspecified sedative, hypnotic or anxiolytic-induced disorder

● **F14** Cocaine related disorders

    Excludes2 other stimulant-related disorders (F15.-)

    (Ex) For category F14 CC codes unless otherwise indicated: F02.80-F02.81, F04-F06.8, F10.10-F11.19, F11.21-F13.19, F13.21-F14.19, F14.21-F15.19, F15.21-F16.19, F16.21-F17.209, F17.213-F17.219, F17.223-F17.229, F17.293-F18.19, F18.21-F19.19, F19.21-F19.99, F53-F55.8, R78

● **F14.1** Cocaine abuse

    Excludes1 cocaine dependence (F14.2-)
                    cocaine use, unspecified (F14.9-)

    F14.10 Cocaine abuse, uncomplicated

●   **F14.12** Cocaine abuse with intoxication

    F14.120 Cocaine abuse with intoxication, uncomplicated

    F14.121 Cocaine abuse with intoxication with delirium

    F14.122 Cocaine abuse with intoxication with perceptual disturbance

    F14.129 Cocaine abuse with intoxication, unspecified

    F14.14 Cocaine abuse with cocaine-induced mood disorder

●   **F14.15** Cocaine abuse with cocaine-induced psychotic disorder

    F14.150 Cocaine abuse with cocaine-induced psychotic disorder with delusions

    F14.151 Cocaine abuse with cocaine-induced psychotic disorder with hallucinations

    F14.159 Cocaine abuse with cocaine-induced psychotic disorder, unspecified

●   **F14.18** Cocaine abuse with other cocaine-induced disorder

    F14.180 Cocaine abuse with cocaine-induced anxiety disorder

    F14.181 Cocaine abuse with cocaine-induced sexual dysfunction

    F14.182 Cocaine abuse with cocaine-induced sleep disorder

    F14.188 Cocaine abuse with other cocaine-induced disorder

    F14.19 Cocaine abuse with unspecified cocaine-induced disorder

● **F14.2** Cocaine dependence

    Excludes1 cocaine abuse (F14.1-)
                    cocaine use, unspecified (F14.9-)

    Excludes2 cocaine poisoning (T40.5-)

    F14.20 Cocaine dependence, uncomplicated
        (Ex) No exclusions

    F14.21 Cocaine dependence, in remission

●   **F14.22** Cocaine dependence with intoxication

    Excludes1 cocaine dependence with withdrawal (F14.23)

    F14.220 Cocaine dependence with intoxication, uncomplicated

    F14.221 Cocaine dependence with intoxication delirium

    F14.222 Cocaine dependence with intoxication with perceptual disturbance
        (Ex) No exclusions

    F14.229 Cocaine dependence with intoxication, unspecified
        (Ex) No exclusions

    F14.23 Cocaine dependence with withdrawal

    Excludes1 cocaine dependence with intoxication (F14.22-)

    F14.24 Cocaine dependence with cocaine-induced mood disorder

◀ New   ◀ Revised   ~~deleted~~ Deleted   Excludes 1   Excludes 2   Includes   Use additional   Code first   Code also   **Unspecified**

OGCR Official Guidelines   ● Unacceptable Principal Diagnosis   X Assign placeholder X   ● Use Additional Character(s)   ▶ Manifestation Code   **Coding Clinic**

● F14.25   Cocaine dependence with cocaine-induced
           psychotic disorder
    F14.250   Cocaine dependence with cocaine-
               induced psychotic disorder with
               delusions 🦠
    F14.251   Cocaine dependence with cocaine-
               induced psychotic disorder with
               hallucinations 🦠
    F14.259   Cocaine dependence with cocaine-
               induced psychotic disorder,
               unspecified 🦠
               Ⓔ No exclusions
● F14.28   Cocaine dependence with other cocaine-
           induced disorder
           Ⓔ For category F14.28 CC codes: No exclusions
    F14.280   Cocaine dependence with cocaine-
               induced anxiety disorder 🦠
    F14.281   Cocaine dependence with cocaine-
               induced sexual dysfunction 🦠
    F14.282   Cocaine dependence with cocaine-
               induced sleep disorder 🦠
    F14.288   Cocaine dependence with other
               cocaine-induced disorder 🦠
    F14.29   Cocaine dependence with unspecified
             cocaine-induced disorder
● F14.9   Cocaine use, unspecified
           Excludes1   cocaine abuse (F14.1-)
                          cocaine dependence (F14.2-)
    F14.90   Cocaine use, unspecified, uncomplicated
● F14.92   Cocaine use, unspecified with intoxication
    F14.920   Cocaine use, unspecified with
               intoxication, uncomplicated
    F14.921   Cocaine use, unspecified with
               intoxication delirium 🦠
    F14.922   Cocaine use, unspecified with
               intoxication with perceptual
               disturbance
    F14.929   Cocaine use, unspecified with
               intoxication, unspecified
    F14.94   Cocaine use, unspecified with cocaine-induced
             mood disorder
● F14.95   Cocaine use, unspecified with cocaine-induced
           psychotic disorder
    F14.950   Cocaine use, unspecified with
               cocaine-induced psychotic disorder
               with delusions 🦠
    F14.951   Cocaine use, unspecified with
               cocaine-induced psychotic disorder
               with hallucinations 🦠
    F14.959   Cocaine use, unspecified with
               cocaine-induced psychotic disorder,
               unspecified
● F14.98   Cocaine use, unspecified with other specified
           cocaine-induced disorder
    F14.980   Cocaine use, unspecified with
               cocaine-induced anxiety disorder
    F14.981   Cocaine use, unspecified with
               cocaine-induced sexual dysfunction
    F14.982   Cocaine use, unspecified with
               cocaine-induced sleep disorder
    F14.988   Cocaine use, unspecified with other
               cocaine-induced disorder
    F14.99   Cocaine use, unspecified with unspecified
             cocaine-induced disorder

● F15   Other stimulant related disorders
    Includes   amphetamine-related disorders
                   ∈caffeine ◀▥▥
    Excludes2   cocaine-related disorders (F14.-)
    Ⓔ **For category F15 CC codes unless otherwise indicated:** F02.80-F02.81, F04-F06.8,
      F10.10-F11.19, F11.21-F13.19, F13.21-F14.19, F14.21-F15.19, F15.21-F16.19,
      F16.21-F17.209, F17.213-F17.219, F17.223-F17.229, F17.293-F18.19, F18.21-F19.19,
      F19.21-F19.99, F53-F55.8, R78
● F15.1   Other stimulant abuse
           Excludes1   other stimulant dependence (F15.2-)
                          other stimulant use, unspecified (F15.9-)
    F15.10   Other stimulant abuse, uncomplicated
● F15.12   Other stimulant abuse with intoxication
    F15.120   Other stimulant abuse with
               intoxication, uncomplicated
    F15.121   Other stimulant abuse with
               intoxication delirium 🦠
    F15.122   Other stimulant abuse with
               intoxication with perceptual
               disturbance
    F15.129   Other stimulant abuse with
               intoxication, unspecified
    F15.14   Other stimulant abuse with stimulant-induced
             mood disorder
● F15.15   Other stimulant abuse with stimulant-induced
           psychotic disorder
    F15.150   Other stimulant abuse with
               stimulant-induced psychotic disorder
               with delusions 🦠
    F15.151   Other stimulant abuse with
               stimulant-induced psychotic disorder
               with hallucinations 🦠
    F15.159   Other stimulant abuse with
               stimulant-induced psychotic
               disorder, unspecified
● F15.18   Other stimulant abuse with other stimulant-
           induced disorder
    F15.180   Other stimulant abuse with
               stimulant-induced anxiety disorder
    F15.181   Other stimulant abuse with
               stimulant-induced sexual dysfunction
    F15.182   Other stimulant abuse with
               stimulant-induced sleep disorder
    F15.188   Other stimulant abuse with other
               stimulant-induced disorder
    F15.19   Other stimulant abuse with unspecified
             stimulant-induced disorder
● F15.2   Other stimulant dependence
           Excludes1   other stimulant abuse (F15.1-)
                          other stimulant use, unspecified (F15.9-)
    F15.20   Other stimulant dependence, uncomplicated 🦠
             Ⓔ No exclusions
    F15.21   Other stimulant dependence, in remission
● F15.22   Other stimulant dependence with intoxication
           Excludes1   other stimulant dependence with
                          withdrawal (F15.23)
    F15.220   Other stimulant dependence with
               intoxication, uncomplicated
    F15.221   Other stimulant dependence with
               intoxication delirium 🦠
    F15.222   Other stimulant dependence with
               intoxication with perceptual
               disturbance 🦠
               Ⓔ No exclusions
    F15.229   Other stimulant dependence with
               intoxication, unspecified

CHAPTER 5 (F01-F99)

F15.23 Other stimulant dependence with withdrawal 🔾

    Excludes1 other stimulant dependence with intoxication (F15.22-)

F15.24 Other stimulant dependence with stimulant-induced mood disorder

● **F15.25** Other stimulant dependence with stimulant-induced psychotic disorder

    F15.250 Other stimulant dependence with stimulant-induced psychotic disorder with delusions 🔾

    F15.251 Other stimulant dependence with stimulant-induced psychotic disorder with hallucinations 🔾

    F15.259 Other stimulant dependence with stimulant-induced psychotic disorder, unspecified 🔾
        (Ex:) No exclusions

● **F15.28** Other stimulant dependence with other stimulant-induced disorder
        (Ex:) For category F15.28 CC codes: No exclusions

    F15.280 Other stimulant dependence with stimulant-induced anxiety disorder 🔾

    F15.281 Other stimulant dependence with stimulant-induced sexual dysfunction 🔾

    F15.282 Other stimulant dependence with stimulant-induced sleep disorder 🔾

    F15.288 Other stimulant dependence with other stimulant-induced disorder 🔾

F15.29 Other stimulant dependence with unspecified stimulant-induced disorder

● **F15.9** Other stimulant use, unspecified

    Excludes1 other stimulant abuse (F15.1-)
           other stimulant dependence (F15.2-)

F15.90 Other stimulant use, unspecified, uncomplicated

● **F15.92** Other stimulant use, unspecified with intoxication

    Excludes1 other stimulant use, unspecified with withdrawal (F15.93)

    F15.920 Other stimulant use, unspecified with intoxication, uncomplicated

    F15.921 Other stimulant use, unspecified with intoxication delirium 🔾

    F15.922 Other stimulant use, unspecified with intoxication with perceptual disturbance

    F15.929 Other stimulant use, unspecified with intoxication, unspecified

F15.93 Other stimulant use, unspecified with withdrawal 🔾

    Excludes1 other stimulant use, unspecified with intoxication (F15.92-)

F15.94 Other stimulant use, unspecified with stimulant-induced mood disorder

● **F15.95** Other stimulant use, unspecified with stimulant-induced psychotic disorder

    F15.950 Other stimulant use, unspecified with stimulant-induced psychotic disorder with delusions 🔾

    F15.951 Other stimulant use, unspecified with stimulant-induced psychotic disorder with hallucinations 🔾

    F15.959 Other stimulant use, unspecified with stimulant-induced psychotic disorder, unspecified

● **F15.98** Other stimulant use, unspecified with other stimulant-induced disorder

    F15.980 Other stimulant use, unspecified with stimulant-induced anxiety disorder

    F15.981 Other stimulant use, unspecified with stimulant-induced sexual dysfunction

    F15.982 Other stimulant use, unspecified with stimulant-induced sleep disorder

    F15.988 Other stimulant use, unspecified with other stimulant-induced disorder

F15.99 Other stimulant use, unspecified with unspecified stimulant-induced disorder

● **F16** Hallucinogen related disorders

    Includes ecstasy
               PCP
               phencyclidine

    (Ex:) **For category F16 CC codes unless otherwise indicated:** F02.80-F02.81, F04-F06.8, F10.10-F11.19, F11.21-F13.19, F13.21-F14.19, F14.21-F15.19, F15.21-F16.19, F16.21-F17.209, F17.213-F17.219, F17.223-F17.229, F17.293-F18.19, F18.21-F19.19, F19.21-F19.99, F53-F55.8, R78

● **F16.1** Hallucinogen abuse

    Excludes1 hallucinogen dependence (F16.2-)
           hallucinogen use, unspecified (F16.9-)

F16.10 Hallucinogen abuse, uncomplicated

● **F16.12** Hallucinogen abuse with intoxication

    F16.120 Hallucinogen abuse with intoxication, uncomplicated

    F16.121 Hallucinogen abuse with intoxication with delirium 🔾

    F16.122 Hallucinogen abuse with intoxication with perceptual disturbance

    F16.129 Hallucinogen abuse with intoxication, unspecified

F16.14 Hallucinogen abuse with hallucinogen-induced mood disorder

● **F16.15** Hallucinogen abuse with hallucinogen-induced psychotic disorder

    F16.150 Hallucinogen abuse with hallucinogen-induced psychotic disorder with delusions 🔾

    F16.151 Hallucinogen abuse with hallucinogen-induced psychotic disorder with hallucinations 🔾

    F16.159 Hallucinogen abuse with hallucinogen-induced psychotic disorder, unspecified

● **F16.18** Hallucinogen abuse with other hallucinogen-induced disorder

    F16.180 Hallucinogen abuse with hallucinogen-induced anxiety disorder

    F16.183 Hallucinogen abuse with hallucinogen persisting perception disorder (flashbacks)

    F16.188 Hallucinogen abuse with other hallucinogen-induced disorder

F16.19 Hallucinogen abuse with unspecified hallucinogen-induced disorder

● **F16.2** Hallucinogen dependence

    Excludes1 hallucinogen abuse (F16.1-)
           hallucinogen use, unspecified (F16.9-)

F16.20 Hallucinogen dependence, uncomplicated 🔾
        (Ex:) No exclusions

F16.21 Hallucinogen dependence, in remission

◀ New   ◀⁞⁞⁞ Revised   ~~deleted~~ Deleted   Excludes 1   Excludes 2   Includes   Use additional   Code first   Code also   Unspecified

OGCR Official Guidelines   ● Unacceptable Principal Diagnosis   X Assign placeholder X   🔾 Use Additional Character(s)   ▌ Manifestation Code   **Coding Clinic**

● F16.22   Hallucinogen dependence with intoxication
    F16.220   Hallucinogen dependence with intoxication, uncomplicated
    F16.221   Hallucinogen dependence with intoxication with delirium 🕭
    F16.229   Hallucinogen dependence with intoxication, unspecified

F16.24   Hallucinogen dependence with hallucinogen-induced mood disorder

● F16.25   Hallucinogen dependence with hallucinogen-induced psychotic disorder
    F16.250   Hallucinogen dependence with hallucinogen-induced psychotic disorder with delusions 🕭
    F16.251   Hallucinogen dependence with hallucinogen-induced psychotic disorder with hallucinations 🕭
    F16.259   Hallucinogen dependence with hallucinogen-induced psychotic disorder, unspecified 🕭
        Ex: No exclusions

● F16.28   Hallucinogen dependence with other hallucinogen-induced disorder
    Ex: **For category F16.28 CC codes:** No exclusions
    F16.280   Hallucinogen dependence with hallucinogen-induced anxiety disorder 🕭
    F16.283   Hallucinogen dependence with hallucinogen persisting perception disorder (flashbacks) 🕭
    F16.288   Hallucinogen dependence with other hallucinogen-induced disorder 🕭

F16.29   Hallucinogen dependence with unspecified hallucinogen-induced disorder

● F16.9   Hallucinogen use, unspecified
    Excludes1   hallucinogen abuse (F16.1-)
              hallucinogen dependence (F16.2-)

F16.90   Hallucinogen use, unspecified, uncomplicated

● F16.92   Hallucinogen use, unspecified with intoxication
    F16.920   Hallucinogen use, unspecified with intoxication, uncomplicated
    F16.921   Hallucinogen use, unspecified with intoxication with delirium 🕭
    F16.929   Hallucinogen use, unspecified with intoxication, unspecified

F16.94   Hallucinogen use, unspecified with hallucinogen-induced mood disorder

● F16.95   Hallucinogen use, unspecified with hallucinogen-induced psychotic disorder
    F16.950   Hallucinogen use, unspecified with hallucinogen-induced psychotic disorder with delusions 🕭
    F16.951   Hallucinogen use, unspecified with hallucinogen-induced psychotic disorder with hallucinations 🕭
    F16.959   Hallucinogen use, unspecified with hallucinogen-induced psychotic disorder, unspecified

● F16.98   Hallucinogen use, unspecified with other specified hallucinogen-induced disorder
    F16.980   Hallucinogen use, unspecified with hallucinogen-induced anxiety disorder
    F16.983   Hallucinogen use, unspecified with hallucinogen persisting perception disorder (flashbacks)
    F16.988   Hallucinogen use, unspecified with other hallucinogen-induced disorder

F16.99   Hallucinogen use, unspecified with unspecified hallucinogen-induced disorder

● F17   Nicotine dependence
    Excludes1   history of tobacco dependence (Z87.891)
              tobacco use NOS (Z72.0)
    Excludes2   tobacco use (smoking) during pregnancy, childbirth and the puerperium (O99.33-)
              toxic effect of nicotine (T65.2-)
    Ex: **For category F17 CC codes:** F02.80-F02.81, F04-F06.8, F10.10-F11.19, F11.21-F13.19, F13.21-F14.19, F14.21-F15.19, F15.21-F16.19, F16.21-F17.209, F17.213-F17.219, F17.223-F17.229, F17.293-F18.19, F18.21-F19.19, F19.21-F19.99, F53-F55.8, R78

● F17.2   Nicotine dependence
  ● F17.20   Nicotine dependence, unspecified
    ● F17.200   Nicotine dependence, unspecified, uncomplicated
    ● F17.201   Nicotine dependence, unspecified, in remission
    F17.203   Nicotine dependence unspecified, with withdrawal 🕭
    F17.208   Nicotine dependence, unspecified, with other nicotine-induced disorders
    F17.209   Nicotine dependence, unspecified, with unspecified nicotine-induced disorders

  ● F17.21   Nicotine dependence, cigarettes
    ● F17.210   Nicotine dependence, cigarettes, uncomplicated
    ● F17.211   Nicotine dependence, cigarettes, in remission
    F17.213   Nicotine dependence, cigarettes, with withdrawal 🕭
    F17.218   Nicotine dependence, cigarettes, with other nicotine-induced disorders
    F17.219   Nicotine dependence, cigarettes, with unspecified nicotine-induced disorders

  ● F17.22   Nicotine dependence, chewing tobacco
    ● F17.220   Nicotine dependence, chewing tobacco, uncomplicated
    ● F17.221   Nicotine dependence, chewing tobacco, in remission
    F17.223   Nicotine dependence, chewing tobacco, with withdrawal 🕭
    F17.228   Nicotine dependence, chewing tobacco, with other nicotine-induced disorders
    F17.229   Nicotine dependence, chewing tobacco, with unspecified nicotine-induced disorders

  ● F17.29   Nicotine dependence, other tobacco product
    ● F17.290   Nicotine dependence, other tobacco product, uncomplicated
    ● F17.291   Nicotine dependence, other tobacco product, in remission
    F17.293   Nicotine dependence, other tobacco product, with withdrawal 🕭
    F17.298   Nicotine dependence, other tobacco product, with other nicotine-induced disorders
    F17.299   Nicotine dependence, other tobacco product, with unspecified nicotine-induced disorders

N   Newborn Age: 0   P   Pediatric Age: 0–17   M   Maternity DX: 12–55   A   Adult Age: 15–124   ♀   Females Only   ♂   Males Only
🕭   Complication\Comorbidity   🕭   Major C\C   Ex: CC/MCC Exclusions   🕭   Present on Admission Requirement   🕭   Hospital-Acquired Condition

- **F18**   **Inhalant related disorders**
  - **Includes**   volatile solvents
  - (Ex) **For category F18 CC codes unless otherwise indicated:** F02.80-F02.81, F04-F06.8, F10.10-F11.19, F11.21-F13.19, F13.21-F14.19, F14.21-F15.19, F15.21-F16.19, F16.21-F17.209, F17.213-F17.219, F17.223-F17.229, F17.293-F18.19, F18.21-F19.19, F19.21-F19.99, F53-F55.8, R78
  - **F18.1**   **Inhalant abuse**
    - **Excludes1**   inhalant dependence (F18.2-)
      - inhalant use, unspecified (F18.9-)
    - F18.10   Inhalant abuse, uncomplicated
    - **F18.12**   **Inhalant abuse with intoxication**
      - F18.120   Inhalant abuse with intoxication, uncomplicated
      - F18.121   Inhalant abuse with intoxication delirium
      - F18.129   Inhalant abuse with intoxication, unspecified
    - F18.14   Inhalant abuse with inhalant-induced mood disorder
    - **F18.15**   **Inhalant abuse with inhalant-induced psychotic disorder**
      - F18.150   Inhalant abuse with inhalant-induced psychotic disorder with delusions
      - F18.151   Inhalant abuse with inhalant-induced psychotic disorder with hallucinations
      - F18.159   Inhalant abuse with inhalant-induced psychotic disorder, unspecified
    - F18.17   Inhalant abuse with inhalant-induced dementia
    - **F18.18**   **Inhalant abuse with other inhalant-induced disorders**
      - F18.180   Inhalant abuse with inhalant-induced anxiety disorder
      - F18.188   Inhalant abuse with other inhalant-induced disorder
    - F18.19   Inhalant abuse with unspecified inhalant-induced disorder
  - **F18.2**   **Inhalant dependence**
    - **Excludes1**   inhalant abuse (F18.1-)
      - inhalant use, unspecified (F18.9-)
    - F18.20   Inhalant dependence, uncomplicated
      - (Ex) No exclusions
    - F18.21   Inhalant dependence, in remission
    - **F18.22**   **Inhalant dependence with intoxication**
      - F18.220   Inhalant dependence with intoxication, uncomplicated
      - F18.221   Inhalant dependence with intoxication delirium
      - F18.229   Inhalant dependence with intoxication, unspecified
    - F18.24   Inhalant dependence with inhalant-induced mood disorder
    - **F18.25**   **Inhalant dependence with inhalant-induced psychotic disorder**
      - F18.250   Inhalant dependence with inhalant-induced psychotic disorder with delusions
      - F18.251   Inhalant dependence with inhalant-induced psychotic disorder with hallucinations
      - F18.259   Inhalant dependence with inhalant-induced psychotic disorder, unspecified
        - (Ex) No exclusions
    - F18.27   Inhalant dependence with inhalant-induced dementia

-    **F18.28**   **Inhalant dependence with other inhalant-induced disorders**
  - (Ex) **For category F18.28 CC codes:** No exclusions
  - F18.280   Inhalant dependence with inhalant-induced anxiety disorder
  - F18.288   Inhalant dependence with other inhalant-induced disorder
-    F18.29   Inhalant dependence with unspecified inhalant-induced disorder
- **F18.9**   **Inhalant use, unspecified**
  - **Excludes1**   inhalant abuse (F18.1-)
    - inhalant dependence (F18.2-)
  - F18.90   Inhalant use, unspecified, uncomplicated
  - **F18.92**   **Inhalant use, unspecified with intoxication**
    - F18.920   Inhalant use, unspecified with intoxication, uncomplicated
    - F18.921   Inhalant use, unspecified with intoxication with delirium
    - F18.929   Inhalant use, unspecified with intoxication, unspecified
  - F18.94   Inhalant use, unspecified with inhalant-induced mood disorder
  - **F18.95**   **Inhalant use, unspecified with inhalant-induced psychotic disorder**
    - F18.950   Inhalant use, unspecified with inhalant-induced psychotic disorder with delusions
    - F18.951   Inhalant use, unspecified with inhalant-induced psychotic disorder with hallucinations
    - F18.959   Inhalant use, unspecified with inhalant-induced psychotic disorder, unspecified
  - F18.97   Inhalant use, unspecified with inhalant-induced persisting dementia
  - **F18.98**   **Inhalant use, unspecified with other inhalant-induced disorders**
    - F18.980   Inhalant use, unspecified with inhalant-induced anxiety disorder
    - F18.988   Inhalant use, unspecified with other inhalant-induced disorder
  - F18.99   Inhalant use, unspecified with unspecified inhalant-induced disorder

- **F19**   **Other psychoactive substance related disorders**
  - **Includes**   polysubstance drug use (indiscriminate drug use)
  - (Ex) **For category F19 CC codes unless otherwise indicated:** F02.80-F02.81, F04-F06.8, F10.10-F11.19, F11.21-F13.19, F13.21-F14.19, F14.21-F15.19, F15.21-F16.19, F16.21-F17.209, F17.213-F17.219, F17.223-F17.229, F17.293-F18.19, F18.21-F19.19, F19.21-F19.99, F53-F55.8, R78
  - **F19.1**   **Other psychoactive substance abuse**
    - **Excludes1**   other psychoactive substance dependence (F19.2-)
      - other psychoactive substance use, unspecified (F19.9-)
    - F19.10   Other psychoactive substance abuse, uncomplicated
    - **F19.12**   **Other psychoactive substance abuse with intoxication**
      - F19.120   Other psychoactive substance abuse with intoxication, uncomplicated
      - F19.121   Other psychoactive substance abuse with intoxication delirium
      - F19.122   Other psychoactive substance abuse with intoxication with perceptual disturbances
      - F19.129   Other psychoactive substance abuse with intoxication, unspecified

◀ New   ◀ Revised   ~~deleted~~ Deleted   Excludes 1   Excludes 2   Includes   Use additional   Code first   Code also   Unspecified

OGCR Official Guidelines   ● Unacceptable Principal Diagnosis   X Assign placeholder X   ● Use Additional Character(s)   ▶ Manifestation Code   **Coding Clinic**

F19.14   Other psychoactive substance abuse with psychoactive substance-induced mood disorder

● F19.15   Other psychoactive substance abuse with psychoactive substance-induced psychotic disorder

    F19.150   Other psychoactive substance abuse with psychoactive substance-induced psychotic disorder with delusions 🔗

    F19.151   Other psychoactive substance abuse with psychoactive substance-induced psychotic disorder with hallucinations 🔗

    F19.159   Other psychoactive substance abuse with psychoactive substance-induced psychotic disorder, unspecified

F19.16   Other psychoactive substance abuse with psychoactive substance-induced persisting amnestic disorder

F19.17   Other psychoactive substance abuse with psychoactive substance-induced persisting dementia 🔗

● F19.18   Other psychoactive substance abuse with other psychoactive substance-induced disorders

    F19.180   Other psychoactive substance abuse with psychoactive substance-induced anxiety disorder

    F19.181   Other psychoactive substance abuse with psychoactive substance-induced sexual dysfunction

    F19.182   Other psychoactive substance abuse with psychoactive substance-induced sleep disorder

    F19.188   Other psychoactive substance abuse with other psychoactive substance-induced disorder

F19.19   Other psychoactive substance abuse with unspecified psychoactive substance-induced disorder

● F19.2   Other psychoactive substance dependence

    Excludes1   other psychoactive substance abuse (F19.1-)
                other psychoactive substance use, unspecified (F19.9-)

F19.20   Other psychoactive substance dependence, uncomplicated 🔗
      (Ex:) No exclusions

F19.21   Other psychoactive substance dependence, in remission

● F19.22   Other psychoactive substance dependence with intoxication

    Excludes1   other psychoactive substance dependence with withdrawal (F19.23-)

    F19.220   Other psychoactive substance dependence with intoxication, uncomplicated

    F19.221   Other psychoactive substance dependence with intoxication delirium 🔗

    F19.222   Other psychoactive substance dependence with intoxication with perceptual disturbance 🔗
      (Ex:) No exclusions

    F19.229   Other psychoactive substance dependence with intoxication, unspecified

● F19.23   Other psychoactive substance dependence with withdrawal

    Excludes1   other psychoactive substance dependence with intoxication (F19.22-)

    F19.230   Other psychoactive substance dependence with withdrawal, uncomplicated 🔗

    F19.231   Other psychoactive substance dependence with withdrawal delirium 🔗

    F19.232   Other psychoactive substance dependence with withdrawal with perceptual disturbance 🔗

    F19.239   Other psychoactive substance dependence with withdrawal, unspecified 🔗

F19.24   Other psychoactive substance dependence with psychoactive substance-induced mood disorder

● F19.25   Other psychoactive substance dependence with psychoactive substance-induced psychotic disorder

    F19.250   Other psychoactive substance dependence with psychoactive substance-induced psychotic disorder with delusions 🔗

    F19.251   Other psychoactive substance dependence with psychoactive substance-induced psychotic disorder with hallucinations 🔗

    F19.259   Other psychoactive substance dependence with psychoactive substance-induced psychotic disorder, unspecified 🔗
      (Ex:) No exclusions

F19.26   Other psychoactive substance dependence with psychoactive substance-induced persisting amnestic disorder 🔗
    (Ex:) No exclusions

F19.27   Other psychoactive substance dependence with psychoactive substance-induced persisting dementia 🔗

● F19.28   Other psychoactive substance dependence with other psychoactive substance-induced disorders
    (Ex:) For category F19.28 CC codes: No exclusions

    F19.280   Other psychoactive substance dependence with psychoactive substance-induced anxiety disorder 🔗

    F19.281   Other psychoactive substance dependence with psychoactive substance-induced sexual dysfunction 🔗

    F19.282   Other psychoactive substance dependence with psychoactive substance-induced sleep disorder 🔗

    F19.288   Other psychoactive substance dependence with other psychoactive substance-induced disorder 🔗

F19.29   Other psychoactive substance dependence with unspecified psychoactive substance-induced disorder

N Newborn Age: 0   P Pediatric Age: 0–17   M Maternity DX: 12–55   A Adult Age: 15–124   ♀ Females Only   ♂ Males Only

🔗 Complication\Comorbidity   🔗 Major C\C   (Ex:) CC/MCC Exclusions   🔗 Present on Admission Requirement   🔗 Hospital-Acquired Condition

867

● **F19.9**   Other psychoactive substance use, unspecified

       Excludes1   other psychoactive substance abuse (F19.1-)

                        other psychoactive substance dependence (F19.2-)

    F19.90   Other psychoactive substance use, unspecified, uncomplicated

● **F19.92**   Other psychoactive substance use, unspecified with intoxication

       Excludes1   other psychoactive substance use, unspecified with withdrawal (F19.93)

       F19.920   Other psychoactive substance use, unspecified with intoxication, uncomplicated

       F19.921   Other psychoactive substance use, unspecified with intoxication with delirium

       F19.922   Other psychoactive substance use, unspecified with intoxication with perceptual disturbance

       F19.929   Other psychoactive substance use, unspecified with intoxication, unspecified

● **F19.93**   Other psychoactive substance use, unspecified with withdrawal

       Excludes1   other psychoactive substance use, unspecified with intoxication (F19.92-)

       F19.930   Other psychoactive substance use, unspecified with withdrawal, uncomplicated

       F19.931   Other psychoactive substance use, unspecified with withdrawal delirium

       F19.932   Other psychoactive substance use, unspecified with withdrawal with perceptual disturbance

       F19.939   Other psychoactive substance use, unspecified with withdrawal, unspecified

    F19.94   Other psychoactive substance use, unspecified with psychoactive substance-induced mood disorder

● **F19.95**   Other psychoactive substance use, unspecified with psychoactive substance-induced psychotic disorder

       F19.950   Other psychoactive substance use, unspecified with psychoactive substance-induced psychotic disorder with delusions

       F19.951   Other psychoactive substance use, unspecified with psychoactive substance-induced psychotic disorder with hallucinations

       F19.959   Other psychoactive substance use, unspecified with psychoactive substance-induced psychotic disorder, unspecified

    F19.96   Other psychoactive substance use, unspecified with psychoactive substance-induced persisting amnestic disorder

    F19.97   Other psychoactive substance use, unspecified with psychoactive substance-induced persisting dementia

    F19.98   Other psychoactive substance use, unspecified with other psychoactive substance-induced disorders

       F19.980   Other psychoactive substance use, unspecified with psychoactive substance-induced anxiety disorder

       F19.981   Other psychoactive substance use, unspecified with psychoactive substance-induced sexual dysfunction

       F19.982   Other psychoactive substance use, unspecified with psychoactive substance-induced sleep disorder

       F19.988   Other psychoactive substance use, unspecified with other psychoactive substance-induced disorder

    F19.99   Other psychoactive substance use, unspecified with unspecified psychoactive substance-induced disorder

SCHIZOPHRENIA, SCHIZOTYPAL, DELUSIONAL, AND OTHER NON-MOOD PSYCHOTIC DISORDERS (F20-F29)

● **F20**   Schizophrenia

Personality disorders characterized by multiple mental and behavioral irregularities (may exhibit disorganized thinking, delusions, and auditory hallucinations).

   Excludes1   brief psychotic disorder (F23)

                    cyclic schizophrenia (F25.0)

                    mood [affective] disorders with psychotic symptoms (F30.2, F31.2, F31.5, F31.64, F32.3, F33.3)

                    schizoaffective disorder (F25.-)

                    schizophrenic reaction NOS (F23)

   Excludes2   schizophrenic reaction in:

                    alcoholism (F10.15-, F10.25-, F10.95-)

                    brain disease (F06.2)

                    epilepsy (F06.2)

                    psychoactive drug use (F11-F19 with .15, .25, .95)

                    schizotypal disorder (F21)

(Ex:) **For category F20 CC codes:** F07.0-F07.81, F07.9-F09, F20.0-F51.03, F51.12, F51.3-F51.9, F52.5, F54, F59-F63.2, F63.81-F63.9, F68.10-F80.4, F80.89-F84.0, F84.3-F99, G44.201-G44.229, H93.25, R45.1-R45.2, R45.5-R45.82, R45.86-R45.87

   F20.0   Paranoid schizophrenia

       Paraphrenic schizophrenia

       Excludes1   involutional paranoid state (F22)

                     paranoia (F22)

   F20.1   Disorganized schizophrenia

       Hebephrenic schizophrenia

       Hebephrenia

   F20.2   Catatonic schizophrenia

       Schizophrenic catalepsy

       Schizophrenic catatonia

       Schizophrenic flexibilitas cerea

       Excludes1   catatonic stupor (R40.1)

   F20.3   Undifferentiated schizophrenia

       Atypical schizophrenia

       Excludes1   acute schizophrenia-like psychotic disorder (F23)

       Excludes2   post-schizophrenic depression (F32.8)

   F20.5   Residual schizophrenia

       Restzustand (schizophrenic)

       Schizophrenic residual state

● **F20.8**   Other schizophrenia

      F20.81   Schizophreniform disorder

            Schizophreniform psychosis NOS

      F20.89   Other schizophrenia

            Cenesthopathic schizophrenia

            Simple schizophrenia

   F20.9   Schizophrenia, unspecified

F21   Schizotypal disorder
Personality disorder characterized by need for social isolation, odd behavior and thinking, and often unconventional beliefs
Borderline schizophrenia
Latent schizophrenia
Latent schizophrenic reaction
Prepsychotic schizophrenia
Prodromal schizophrenia
Pseudoneurotic schizophrenia
Pseudopsychopathic schizophrenia
Schizotypal personality disorder

> **Excludes2**   Asperger's syndrome (F84.5)
> schizoid personality disorder (F60.1)

F22   Delusional disorders
Delusional dysmorphophobia
Involutional paranoid state
Paranoia
Paranoia querulans
Paranoid psychosis
Paranoid state
Paraphrenia (late)
Sensitiver Beziehungswahn

> **Excludes1**   mood [affective] disorders with psychotic symptoms (F30.2, F31.2, F31.5, F31.64, F32.3, F33.3)
> paranoid schizophrenia (F20.0)

> **Excludes2**   paranoid personality disorder (F60.0)
> paranoid psychosis, psychogenic (F23)
> paranoid reaction (F23)

F23   Brief psychotic disorder 🔹
Paranoid reaction
Psychogenic paranoid psychosis

> **Excludes2**   mood [affective] disorders with psychotic symptoms (F30.2, F31.2, F31.5, F31.64, F32.3, F33.3)

> (Ex) No exclusions

F24   Shared psychotic disorder
Folie à deux
Induced paranoid disorder
Induced psychotic disorder

● **F25   Schizoaffective disorders**
Mental disorder exhibiting major depressive episode, manic episode, or mixed episode occurs with symptoms of schizophrenia, and mood disorder

> **Excludes1**   mood [affective] disorders with psychotic symptoms (F30.2, F31.2, F31.5, F31.64, F32.3, F33.3)
> schizophrenia (F20.-)

F25.0   Schizoaffective disorder, bipolar type
Cyclic schizophrenia
Schizoaffective disorder, manic type
Schizoaffective disorder, mixed type
Schizoaffective psychosis, bipolar type
Schizophreniform psychosis, manic type

F25.1   Schizoaffective disorder, depressive type
Schizoaffective psychosis, depressive type
Schizophreniform psychosis, depressive type

F25.8   Other schizoaffective disorders

F25.9   Schizoaffective disorder, unspecified
Schizoaffective psychosis NOS

F28   Other psychotic disorder not due to a substance or known physiological condition
Chronic hallucinatory psychosis

F29   Unspecified psychosis not due to a substance or known physiological condition
Psychosis NOS

> **Excludes1**   mental disorder NOS (F99)
> unspecified mental disorder due to known physiological condition (F09)

MOOD [AFFECTIVE] DISORDERS (F30-F39)

● **F30   Manic episode**
Elevated, expansive, or irritable mood

> **Includes**   bipolar disorder, single manic episode
> mixed affective episode

> **Excludes1**   bipolar disorder (F31.-)
> major depressive disorder, single episode (F32.-)
> major depressive disorder, recurrent (F33.-)

> (Ex) For category F30 CC codes unless otherwise indicated: F07.0-F07.81, F07.9-F09, F20.0-F51.03, F51.12, F51.3-F51.9, F52.5, F54, F59-F63.2, F63.81-F63.9, F68.10-F80.4, F80.89-F84.0, F84.3-F99, G44.201-G44.229, H93.25, R45.1-R45.2, R45.5-R45.82, R45.86-R45.87

● **F30.1   Manic episode without psychotic symptoms**

F30.10   Manic episode without psychotic symptoms, unspecified 🔹

F30.11   Manic episode without psychotic symptoms, mild 🔹

F30.12   Manic episode without psychotic symptoms, moderate 🔹

F30.13   Manic episode, severe, without psychotic symptoms 🔹
> (Ex) F30.13, F30.2, F31.13-F31.2, F31.4-F31.5, F31.63-F31.64

F30.2   Manic episode, severe with psychotic symptoms 🔹
Manic stupor
Mania with mood-congruent psychotic symptoms
Mania with mood-incongruent psychotic symptoms

F30.3   Manic episode in partial remission

F30.4   Manic episode in full remission

F30.8   Other manic episodes
Abnormality of mood resembling mania but less intense
Hypomania

F30.9   Manic episode, unspecified 🔹
Mania NOS

● **F31   Bipolar disorder**
Mood disorders with history of manic, mixed, or hypomanic episodes

> **Includes**   manic-depressive illness
> manic-depressive psychosis
> manic-depressive reaction

> **Excludes1**   bipolar disorder, single manic episode (F30.-)
> major depressive disorder, single episode (F32.-)
> major depressive disorder, recurrent (F33.-)

> **Excludes2**   cyclothymia (F34.0)

> (Ex) For category F31 CC codes unless otherwise indicated: F07.0-F07.81, F07.9-F09, F20.0-F51.03, F51.12, F51.3-F51.9, F52.5, F54, F59-F63.2, F63.81-F63.9, F68.10-F80.4, F80.89-F84.0, F84.3-F99, G44.201-G44.229, H93.25, R45.1-R45.2, R45.5-R45.82, R45.86-R45.87

F31.0   Bipolar disorder, current episode hypomanic 🔹

● **F31.1   Bipolar disorder, current episode manic without psychotic features**

F31.10   Bipolar disorder, current episode manic without psychotic features, unspecified 🔹

F31.11   Bipolar disorder, current episode manic without psychotic features, mild 🔹

F31.12   Bipolar disorder, current episode manic without psychotic features, moderate 🔹

F31.13   Bipolar disorder, current episode manic without psychotic features, severe 🔹
> (Ex) F31.13-F31.2, F31.63-F31.64

F31.2   Bipolar disorder, current episode manic severe with psychotic features 🔹
Bipolar disorder, current episode manic with mood-congruent psychotic symptoms
Bipolar disorder, current episode manic with mood-incongruent psychotic symptoms

---

N Newborn Age: 0   P Pediatric Age: 0–17   M Maternity DX: 12–55   A Adult Age: 15–124   ♀ Females Only   ♂ Males Only

🔹 Complication\Comorbidity   🔹 Major C\C   (Ex) CC/MCC Exclusions   🔹 Present on Admission Requirement   🔹 Hospital-Acquired Condition

CHAPTER 5 (F01-F99)

● **F31.3**   **Bipolar disorder, current episode depressed, mild or moderate severity**

     F31.30   Bipolar disorder, current episode depressed, mild or moderate severity, unspecified 🔧

     F31.31   Bipolar disorder, current episode depressed, mild 🔧

     F31.32   Bipolar disorder, current episode depressed, moderate

F31.4   **Bipolar disorder, current episode depressed, severe, without psychotic features** 🔧
     (Ex:) F31.13-F31.2, F31.4-F31.5, F31.63-F31.64

F31.5   **Bipolar disorder, current episode depressed, severe, with psychotic features** 🔧
     Bipolar disorder, current episode depressed with mood-incongruent psychotic symptoms
     Bipolar disorder, current episode depressed with mood-congruent psychotic symptoms

● **F31.6**   **Bipolar disorder, current episode mixed**

     F31.60   Bipolar disorder, current episode mixed, unspecified 🔧

     F31.61   Bipolar disorder, current episode mixed, mild 🔧

     F31.62   Bipolar disorder, current episode mixed, moderate 🔧

     F31.63   Bipolar disorder, current episode mixed, severe, without psychotic features 🔧

     F31.64   Bipolar disorder, current episode mixed, severe, with psychotic features 🔧
         Bipolar disorder, current episode mixed with mood-congruent psychotic symptoms
         Bipolar disorder, current episode mixed with mood-incongruent psychotic symptoms

● **F31.7**   **Bipolar disorder, currently in remission**

     F31.70   Bipolar disorder, currently in remission, most recent episode unspecified

     F31.71   Bipolar disorder, in partial remission, most recent episode hypomanic

     F31.72   Bipolar disorder, in full remission, most recent episode hypomanic

     F31.73   Bipolar disorder, in partial remission, most recent episode manic

     F31.74   Bipolar disorder, in full remission, most recent episode manic

     F31.75   Bipolar disorder, in partial remission, most recent episode depressed

     F31.76   Bipolar disorder, in full remission, most recent episode depressed

     F31.77   Bipolar disorder, in partial remission, most recent episode mixed

     F31.78   Bipolar disorder, in full remission, most recent episode mixed

● **F31.8**   **Other bipolar disorders**

     F31.81   Bipolar II disorder 🔧

     F31.89   Other bipolar disorder 🔧
         Recurrent manic episodes NOS

F31.9   **Bipolar disorder, unspecified**

● **F32**   **Major depressive disorder, single episode**

     Includes   single episode of agitated depression
         single episode of depressive reaction
         single episode of major depression
         single episode of psychogenic depression
         single episode of reactive depression
         single episode of vital depression

     Excludes1   bipolar disorder (F31.-) ◀▥
         manic episode (F30.-) ◀▥
         recurrent depressive disorder (F33.-)

     Excludes2   adjustment disorder (F43.2)

F32.0   **Major depressive disorder, single episode, mild** 🔧
     (Ex:) F32.0-F32.3, F33.0-F33.40, F33.9

F32.1   **Major depressive disorder, single episode, moderate** 🔧
     (Ex:) F32.0-F32.3, F33.0-F33.40, F33.9

F32.2   **Major depressive disorder, single episode, severe without psychotic features** 🔧
     (Ex:) F32.0-F32.3, F33.0-F33.40, F33.9

F32.3   **Major depressive disorder, single episode, severe with psychotic features** 🔧
     Single episode of major depression with mood-congruent psychotic symptoms
     Single episode of major depression with mood-incongruent psychotic symptoms
     Single episode of major depression with psychotic symptoms
     Single episode of psychogenic depressive psychosis
     Single episode of psychotic depression
     Single episode of reactive depressive psychosis
     (Ex:) F32.0-F32.3, F33.0-F33.40, F33.9

F32.4   **Major depressive disorder, single episode, in partial remission**

F32.5   **Major depressive disorder, single episode, in full remission**

F32.8   **Other depressive episodes**
     Atypical depression
     Post-schizophrenic depression
     Single episode of 'masked' depression NOS

F32.9   **Major depressive disorder, single episode, unspecified**
     Depression NOS
     Depressive disorder NOS
     Major depression NOS

● **F33**   **Major depressive disorder, recurrent**

     Includes   recurrent episodes of depressive reaction
         recurrent episodes of endogenous depression
         recurrent episodes of major depression
         recurrent episodes of psychogenic depression
         recurrent episodes of reactive depression
         recurrent episodes of seasonal depressive disorder
         recurrent episodes of vital depression

     Excludes1   bipolar disorder (F31.-)
         manic episode (F30.-)

     (Ex:) **For category F33 CC codes unless otherwise indicated:** F32.0-F32.3, F33.0-F33.40, F33.9

F33.0   **Major depressive disorder, recurrent, mild** 🔧

F33.1   **Major depressive disorder, recurrent, moderate** 🔧

F33.2   **Major depressive disorder, recurrent severe without psychotic features** 🔧

F33.3   **Major depressive disorder, recurrent, severe with psychotic symptoms** 🔧
     Endogenous depression with psychotic symptoms
     Recurrent severe episodes of major depression with mood-congruent psychotic symptoms
     Recurrent severe episodes of major depression with mood-incongruent psychotic symptoms
     Recurrent severe episodes of major depression with psychotic symptoms
     Recurrent severe episodes of psychogenic depressive psychosis
     Recurrent severe episodes of psychotic depression
     Recurrent severe episodes of reactive depressive psychosis
     (Ex:) See F31

● **F33.4**   **Major depressive disorder, recurrent, in remission**

     F33.40   Major depressive disorder, recurrent, in remission, unspecified 🔧

     F33.41   Major depressive disorder, recurrent, in partial remission

     F33.42   Major depressive disorder, recurrent, in full remission

F33.8   **Other recurrent depressive disorders** 🔧
     Recurrent brief depressive episodes
     (Ex:) See F31

F33.9   **Major depressive disorder, recurrent, unspecified** 🔧
     Monopolar depression NOS

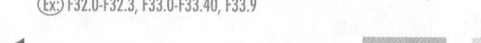 ◀ New   ◀▥ Revised   ~~deleted~~ Deleted   Excludes 1   Excludes 2   Includes   Use additional   Code first   Code also   Unspecified

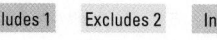 **OGCR** Official Guidelines   ● Unacceptable Principal Diagnosis   X Assign placeholder X   ● Use Additional Character(s)   ▶ Manifestation Code   **Coding Clinic**

● **F34   Persistent mood [affective] disorders**
   (Ex) **For category F34 CC codes:** F07.0-F07.81, F07.9-F09, F20.0-F51.03, F51.12,
      F51.3-F51.9, F52.5, F54, F59-F63.2, F63.81-F63.9, F68.10-F80.4, F80.89-F84.0,
      F84.3-F99, G44.201-G44.229, H93.25, R45.1-R45.2, R45.5-R45.82, R45.86-R45.87

  F34.0   Cyclothymic disorder
     Affective personality disorder
     Cycloid personality
     Cyclothymia
     Cyclothymic personality

  F34.1   Dysthymic disorder
     Depressive neurosis
     Depressive personality disorder
     Dysthymia
     Neurotic depression
     Persistent anxiety depression
       Excludes2   anxiety depression (mild or not
               persistent) (F41.8)

  F34.8   Other persistent mood [affective] disorders ⍟

  F34.9   Persistent mood [affective] disorder, unspecified ⍟

● **F39   Unspecified mood [affective] disorder**
     Affective psychosis NOS

ANXIETY, DISSOCIATIVE, STRESS-RELATED, SOMATOFORM AND OTHER NONPSYCHOTIC MENTAL DISORDERS (F40-F48)

● **F40   Phobic anxiety disorders**
   Irrational fear with avoidance of the feared subject, activity, or
   situation even though the individual knows that the reaction is
   excessive.

 ● **F40.0   Agoraphobia**
     Intense, irrational fear of open spaces

   F40.00   Agoraphobia, unspecified

   F40.01   Agoraphobia with panic disorder
      Panic disorder with agoraphobia
       Excludes1   panic disorder without
              agoraphobia (F41.0)

   F40.02   Agoraphobia without panic disorder

 ● **F40.1   Social phobias**
     Anthropophobia
     Social anxiety disorder of childhood
     Social neurosis

   F40.10   Social phobia, unspecified

   F40.11   Social phobia, generalized

 ● **F40.2   Specific (isolated) phobias**
      Excludes2   dysmorphophobia (nondelusional)
             (F45.22)
             nosophobia (F45.22)

  ● **F40.21   Animal type phobia**
     F40.210   Arachnophobia
       Fear of spiders
     F40.218   Other animal type phobia

  ● **F40.22   Natural environment type phobia**
     F40.220   Fear of thunderstorms
     F40.228   Other natural environment type
            phobia

  ● **F40.23   Blood, injection, injury type phobia**
     F40.230   Fear of blood
     F40.231   Fear of injections and transfusions
     F40.232   Fear of other medical care
     F40.233   Fear of injury

  ● **F40.24   Situational type phobia**
     F40.240   Claustrophobia
       Fear of closed spaces
     F40.241   Acrophobia
       Fear of heights
     F40.242   Fear of bridges
     F40.243   Fear of flying
     F40.248   Other situational type phobia

● **F40.29   Other specified phobia**
   F40.290   Androphobia
      Fear of men
   F40.291   Gynephobia
      Fear of women
   F40.298   Other specified phobia

  F40.8   Other phobic anxiety disorders
     Phobic anxiety disorder of childhood

  F40.9   Phobic anxiety disorder, unspecified
     Phobia NOS
     Phobic state NOS

● **F41   Other anxiety disorders**
     Excludes2   anxiety in:
        acute stress reaction (F43.0)
        transient adjustment reaction (F43.2)
        neurasthenia (F48.8)
        psychophysiologic disorders (F45.-)
        separation anxiety (F93.0)

  F41.0   Panic disorder [episodic paroxysmal anxiety] without
     agoraphobia
     Panic attack
     Panic state
       Excludes1   panic disorder with agoraphobia (F40.01)

  F41.1   Generalized anxiety disorder
     Anxiety neurosis
     Anxiety reaction
     Anxiety state
     Overanxious disorder
       Excludes2   neurasthenia (F48.8)

  F41.3   Other mixed anxiety disorders

  F41.8   Other specified anxiety disorders
     Anxiety depression (mild or not persistent)
     Anxiety hysteria
     Mixed anxiety and depressive disorder

  F41.9   Anxiety disorder, unspecified
     Anxiety NOS

  F42   Obsessive-compulsive disorder
   Anxiety disorder with recurrent obsessions or compulsions
     Anancastic neurosis
     Obsessive-compulsive neurosis
       Excludes2   obsessive-compulsive personality (disorder)
             (F60.5)
            obsessive-compulsive symptoms occurring in
             depression (F32-F33) ◀‖
            ~~depression (F32-F33)~~
            obsessive-compulsive symptoms occurring in
             schizophrenia (F20.-) ◀‖

● **F43   Reaction to severe stress and adjustment disorders**
  F43.0   Acute stress reaction
     Acute crisis reaction
     Acute reaction to stress
     Combat and operational stress reaction
     Combat fatigue
     Crisis state
     Psychic shock

 ● **F43.1   Post-traumatic stress disorder (PTSD)**
     Traumatic neurosis
     F43.10   Post-traumatic stress disorder, unspecified
     F43.11   Post-traumatic stress disorder, acute
     F43.12   Post-traumatic stress disorder, chronic

 ● **F43.2   Adjustment disorders**
     Culture shock
     Grief reaction
     Hospitalism in children
       Excludes2   separation anxiety disorder of childhood
             (F93.0)
     F43.20   Adjustment disorder, unspecified
     F43.21   Adjustment disorder with depressed mood
     F43.22   Adjustment disorder with anxiety
     F43.23   Adjustment disorder with mixed anxiety and
            depressed mood

CHAPTER 5 (F01-F99)

N Newborn Age: 0   **P** Pediatric Age: 0–17   **M** Maternity DX: 12–55   **A** Adult Age: 15–124   ♀ Females Only   ♂ Males Only

 Complication\Comorbidity   ⍟ Major C\C   (Ex) CC/MCC Exclusions   ⍟ Present on Admission Requirement   ⍟ Hospital-Acquired Condition   **871**

CHAPTER 5 (F01-F99)

F43.24 **Adjustment disorder with disturbance of conduct**

F43.25 **Adjustment disorder with mixed disturbance of emotions and conduct**

F43.29 **Adjustment disorder with other symptoms**

F43.8 **Other reactions to severe stress**

F43.9 **Reaction to severe stress, unspecified**

● F44 **Dissociative and conversion disorders**

Includes   conversion hysteria
            conversion reaction
            hysteria
            hysterical psychosis

Excludes2   malingering [conscious simulation] (Z76.5)

F44.0 **Dissociative amnesia**
Sudden loss of memory for personal information

Excludes1   amnesia NOS (R41.3)
            anterograde amnesia (R41.1)
            retrograde amnesia (R41.2)

Excludes2   alcohol-or other psychoactive substance-induced amnestic disorder (F10, F13, F19 with .26, .96)
            amnestic disorder due to known physiological condition (F04)
            postictal amnesia in epilepsy (G40.-)

F44.1 **Dissociative fugue**
Characterized by episode of sudden, unexpected travel with amnesia for past and partial to total confusion about identity or assumption of new identity

Excludes2   postictal fugue in epilepsy (G40.-)

F44.2 **Dissociative stupor**
Profound diminution or absence of voluntary movement and responsiveness to external stimuli

Excludes1   catatonic stupor (R40.1)
            stupor NOS (R40.1)

Excludes2   catatonic disorder due to known physiological condition (F06.1)
            depressive stupor (F32, F33)
            manic stupor (F30, F31)

F44.4 **Conversion disorder with motor symptom or deficit**
Dissociative motor disorders
Psychogenic aphonia
Psychogenic dysphonia

F44.5 **Conversion disorder with seizures or convulsions**
Dissociative convulsions

F44.6 **Conversion disorder with sensory symptom or deficit**
Dissociative anesthesia and sensory loss
Psychogenic deafness

F44.7 **Conversion disorder with mixed symptom presentation**

● F44.8 **Other dissociative and conversion disorders**

F44.81 **Dissociative identity disorder**
Multiple personality disorder

F44.89 **Other dissociative and conversion disorders**
Ganser's syndrome
Psychogenic confusion
Psychogenic twilight state
Trance and possession disorders

F44.9 **Dissociative and conversion disorder, unspecified**
Dissociative disorder NOS

OGCR **Section I.C.5.a**

Pain disorders related to psychological factors

Assign code F45.41, for pain that is exclusively psychological. Code F45.41, Pain disorder exclusively related to psychological factors, should be used following the appropriate code from category G89, Pain, not elsewhere classified, if there is documentation of a psychological component for a patient with acute or chronic pain.
See Section I.C.6. Pain

● F45 **Somatoform disorders**
Mental disorders characterized by symptoms suggesting general medical condition

Excludes2   dissociative and conversion disorders (F44.-)
            factitious disorders (F68.1-)
            hair-plucking (F63.3)
            lalling (F80.0)
            lisping (F80.0)
            malingering [conscious simulation] (Z76.5)
            nail-biting (F98.8)
            psychological or behavioral factors associated with disorders or diseases classified elsewhere (F54)
            sexual dysfunction, not due to a substance or known physiological condition (F52.-)
            thumb-sucking (F98.8)
            tic disorders (in childhood and adolescence) (F95.-)
            Tourette's syndrome (F95.2)
            trichotillomania (F63.3)

F45.0 **Somatization disorder**
Briquet's disorder
Multiple psychosomatic disorder

F45.1 **Undifferentiated somatoform disorder**
Undifferentiated psychosomatic disorder

● F45.2 **Hypochondriacal disorders**
Persistent, unrealistic preoccupation with possibility of having serious disease

Excludes2   delusional dysmorphophobia (F22)
            fixed delusions about bodily functions or shape (F22)

F45.20 **Hypochondriacal disorder, unspecified**

F45.21 **Hypochondriasis**
Hypochondriacal neurosis

F45.22 **Body dysmorphic disorder**
Dysmorphophobia (nondelusional)
Nosophobia

F45.29 **Other hypochondriacal disorders**

● F45.4 **Pain disorders related to psychological factors**

Excludes1   pain NOS (R52)

F45.41 **Pain disorder exclusively related to psychological factors**
Somatoform pain disorder (persistent)

F45.42 **Pain disorder with related psychological factors**
Code also associated acute or chronic pain (G89.-)

F45.8 **Other somatoform disorders**
Psychogenic dysmenorrhea
Psychogenic dysphagia, including 'globus hystericus'
Psychogenic pruritus
Psychogenic torticollis
Somatoform autonomic dysfunction
Teeth grinding

Excludes1   sleep related teeth grinding (G47.63)

F45.9 **Somatoform disorder, unspecified**
Psychosomatic disorder NOS

● F48 **Other nonpsychotic mental disorders**

F48.1 **Depersonalization-derealization syndrome**

F48.2 **Pseudobulbar affect**
Involuntary emotional expression disorder

Code first underlying cause, if known, such as:
amyotrophic lateral sclerosis (G12.21)
multiple sclerosis (G35)
sequelae of cerebrovascular disease (I69.-)
sequelae of traumatic intracranial injury (S06.-)

F48.8 **Other specified nonpsychotic mental disorders**
Dhat syndrome
Neurasthenia
Occupational neurosis, including writer's cramp
Psychasthenia
Psychasthenic neurosis
Psychogenic syncope

F48.9 **Nonpsychotic mental disorder, unspecified**
Neurosis NOS

◀ New   ◀▬ Revised   ~~deleted~~ Deleted   Excludes 1   Excludes 2   Includes   Use additional   Code first   Code also   Unspecified

OGCR Official Guidelines   ● Unacceptable Principal Diagnosis   X Assign placeholder X   ▶ Use Additional Character(s)   ▶ Manifestation Code   **Coding Clinic**

BEHAVIORAL SYNDROMES ASSOCIATED WITH PHYSIOLOGICAL DISTURBANCES AND PHYSICAL FACTORS (F50-F59)

● **F50　Eating disorders**

　　Excludes1　anorexia NOS (R63.0)
　　　　　　　　　feeding difficulties (R63.3)
　　　　　　　　　polyphagia (R63.2)

　　Excludes2　feeding disorder in infancy or childhood (F98.2-)

● **F50.0　Anorexia nervosa**

　　Excludes1　loss of appetite (R63.0)
　　　　　　　　　psychogenic loss of appetite (F50.8)

　　(Ex) For category F50.0 CC codes: F45.9, F50.00-F50.9, F59, F98.21-F98.3

　　F50.00　Anorexia nervosa, unspecified 🔖

　　F50.01　Anorexia nervosa, restricting type 🔖

　　F50.02　Anorexia nervosa, binge eating/purging type 🔖

　　　　Excludes1　bulimia nervosa (F50.2)

　F50.2　Bulimia nervosa 🔖
　　　Bulimia NOS
　　　Hyperorexia nervosa

　　　Excludes1　anorexia nervosa, binge eating/purging type (F50.02)

　　　(Ex) F50.00-F50.9, F98.21-F98.29

　F50.8　Other eating disorders
　　　Pica in adults
　　　Psychogenic loss of appetite

　　　Excludes2　pica of infancy and childhood (F98.3)

　F50.9　Eating disorder, unspecified
　　　Atypical anorexia nervosa
　　　Atypical bulimia nervosa

● **F51　Sleep disorders not due to a substance or known physiological condition**

　　Excludes2　organic sleep disorders (G47.-)

● **F51.0　Insomnia not due to a substance or known physiological condition**

　　Excludes2　alcohol related insomnia (F10.182,
　　　　　　　　　F10.282, F10.982)
　　　　　　　　drug-related insomnia (F11.182, F11.282,
　　　　　　　　　F11.982, F13.182, F13.282, F13.982,
　　　　　　　　　F14.182, F14.282, F14.982, F15.182,
　　　　　　　　　F15.282, F15.982, F19.182, F19.282,
　　　　　　　　　F19.982) ◄▦
　　　　　　　　insomnia NOS (G47.0-)
　　　　　　　　insomnia due to known physiological
　　　　　　　　　condition (G47.0-)
　　　　　　　　organic insomnia (G47.0-)
　　　　　　　　sleep deprivation (Z72.820)

　　F51.01　Primary insomnia
　　　　　Idiopathic insomnia

　　F51.02　Adjustment insomnia

　　F51.03　Paradoxical insomnia

　　F51.04　Psychophysiologic insomnia

　　F51.05　Insomnia due to other mental disorder
　　　　　Code also associated mental disorder

　　F51.09　Other insomnia not due to a substance or known physiological condition

● **F51.1　Hypersomnia not due to a substance or known physiological condition**
　　　Hypersomnia: Excessive sleeping/sleepiness

　　Excludes2　alcohol related hypersomnia (F10.182,
　　　　　　　　　F10.282, F10.982)
　　　　　　　　drug-related hypersomnia (F11.182,
　　　　　　　　　F11.282, F11.982, F13.182, F13.282,
　　　　　　　　　F13.982, F14.182, F14.282, F14.982,
　　　　　　　　　F15.182, F15.282, F15.982, F19.182,
　　　　　　　　　F19.282, F19.982) ◄▦
　　　　　　　　hypersomnia NOS (G47.10)
　　　　　　　　hypersomnia due to known physiological
　　　　　　　　　condition (G47.10)
　　　　　　　　idiopathic hypersomnia (G47.11, G47.12)
　　　　　　　　narcolepsy (G47.4-)

　　F51.11　Primary hypersomnia

　　F51.12　Insufficient sleep syndrome

　　　　Excludes1　sleep deprivation (Z72.820)

　　F51.13　Hypersomnia due to other mental disorder
　　　　　Code also associated mental disorder

　　F51.19　Other hypersomnia not due to a substance or known physiological condition

　F51.3　Sleepwalking [somnambulism]

　F51.4　Sleep terrors [night terrors]

　F51.5　Nightmare disorder
　　　Dream anxiety disorder

　F51.8　Other sleep disorders not due to a substance or known physiological condition

　F51.9　Sleep disorder not due to a substance or known physiological condition, unspecified
　　　Emotional sleep disorder NOS

● **F52　Sexual dysfunction not due to a substance or known physiological condition**

　　Excludes2　Dhat syndrome (F48.8)

　F52.0　Hypoactive sexual desire disorder
　　　Anhedonia (sexual)
　　　　Total loss of feeling of sexual pleasure
　　　Lack or loss of sexual desire

　　　Excludes1　decreased libido (R68.82)

　F52.1　Sexual aversion disorder
　　　Sexual aversion and lack of sexual enjoyment

● **F52.2　Sexual arousal disorders**
　　　Failure of genital response

　　F52.21　Male erectile disorder ♂
　　　　　Psychogenic impotence

　　　　Excludes1　impotence of organic origin
　　　　　　　　　　　(N52.-)
　　　　　　　　　　impotence NOS (N52.-)

　　F52.22　Female sexual arousal disorder ♀
　　　　　Frigidity

● **F52.3　Orgasmic disorder**
　　　Inhibited orgasm
　　　Psychogenic anorgasmy

　　F52.31　Female orgasmic disorder ♀

　　F52.32　Male orgasmic disorder ♂

　F52.4　Premature ejaculation ♂

　F52.5　Vaginismus not due to a substance or known physiological condition ♀
　　　Psychogenic vaginismus

　　　Excludes2　vaginismus (due to a known
　　　　　　　　　　physiological condition) (N94.2)

　F52.6　Dyspareunia not due to a substance or known physiological condition ♀
　　　Dyspareunia: Difficult or painful sexual intercourse
　　　Psychogenic dyspareunia

　　　Excludes2　dyspareunia (due to a known
　　　　　　　　　　physiological condition) (N94.1)

N Newborn Age: 0　**P** Pediatric Age: 0–17　**M** Maternity DX: 12–55　**A** Adult Age: 15–124　♀ Females Only　♂ Males Only

🔖 Complication\Comorbidity　🔖 Major C\C　(Ex) CC/MCC Exclusions　🔖 Present on Admission Requirement　🔖 Hospital-Acquired Condition

CHAPTER 5 (F01-F99)

873

F52.8   **Other sexual dysfunction not due to a substance or known physiological condition**
Excessive sexual drive
Nymphomania
Satyriasis

● **F52.9**   Unspecified **sexual dysfunction not due to a substance or known physiological condition**
Sexual dysfunction NOS

F53   **Puerperal psychosis ♀**
Postpartum depression
Acute mental illness with sudden onset following childbirth with symptoms of affective psychosis, disorientation, and confusion are prevalent

    Excludes1   mood disorders with psychotic features (F30.2, F31.2, F31.5, F31.64, F32.3, F33.3)
postpartum dysphoria (O90.6)
psychosis in schizophrenia, schizotypal, delusional, and other psychotic disorders (F20-F29)

▶ **F54**   *Psychological and behavioral factors associated with disorders or diseases classified elsewhere*
Psychological factors affecting physical conditions

   Code first the associated physical disorder, such as:
asthma (J45.-)
dermatitis (L23-L25)
gastric ulcer (K25.-)
mucous colitis (K58.-)
ulcerative colitis (K51.-)
urticaria (L50.-)

    Excludes2   tension-type headache (G44.2)

● **F55**   **Abuse of non-psychoactive substances**

    Excludes2   abuse of psychoactive substances (F10-F19)

    F55.0   **Abuse of antacids**

    F55.1   **Abuse of herbal or folk remedies**

    F55.2   **Abuse of laxatives**

    F55.3   **Abuse of steroids or hormones**

    F55.4   **Abuse of vitamins**

    F55.8   **Abuse of other non-psychoactive substances**

F59   Unspecified **behavioral syndromes associated with physiological disturbances and physical factors**
Psychogenic physiological dysfunction NOS

DISORDERS OF ADULT PERSONALITY AND BEHAVIOR (F60-F69)

● **F60**   **Specific personality disorders**
Long-term patterns of thoughts and behaviors causing serious problems with relationships and work.

    F60.0   **Paranoid personality disorder**
Hostile, devious, and combative response to disappointments
Expansive paranoid personality (disorder)
Fanatic personality (disorder)
Querulant personality (disorder)
Paranoid personality (disorder)
Sensitive paranoid personality (disorder)

      Excludes2   paranoia (F22)
paranoia querulans (F22)
paranoid psychosis (F22)
paranoid schizophrenia (F20.0)
paranoid state (F22)

    F60.1   **Schizoid personality disorder**
Detachment from social relationships with minimal emotional experiences and expressions

      Excludes2   Asperger's syndrome (F84.5)
delusional disorder (F22)
schizoid disorder of childhood (F84.5)
schizophrenia (F20.-)
schizotypal disorder (F21)

    F60.2   **Antisocial personality disorder**
Continuous and chronic antisocial behavior
Amoral personality (disorder)
Asocial personality (disorder)
Dissocial personality disorder
Psychopathic personality (disorder)
Sociopathic personality (disorder)

      Excludes1   conduct disorders (F91.-)

      Excludes2   borderline personality disorder (F60.3)

    F60.3   **Borderline personality disorder**
Instability of mood, self-image or sense of self, and interpersonal relationships
Aggressive personality (disorder)
Emotionally unstable personality disorder
Explosive personality (disorder)

      Excludes2   antisocial personality disorder (F60.2)

    F60.4   **Histrionic personality disorder**
Personality disorder with excessive emotional and attention-seeking behavior
Hysterical personality (disorder)
Psychoinfantile personality (disorder)

    F60.5   **Obsessive-compulsive personality disorder**
Anankastic personality (disorder)
Compulsive personality (disorder)
Obsessional personality (disorder)

      Excludes2   obsessive-compulsive disorder (F42)

    F60.6   **Avoidant personality disorder**
Anxious personality disorder

    F60.7   **Dependent personality disorder**
Asthenic personality (disorder)
Inadequate personality (disorder)
Passive personality (disorder)

●   **F60.8**   **Other specific personality disorders**

      F60.81   **Narcissistic personality disorder**
Vanity, conceit, egotism or indifference to plight of others

      F60.89   **Other specific personality disorders**
Eccentric personality disorder
'Haltlose' type personality disorder
Immature personality disorder
Passive-aggressive personality disorder
Psychoneurotic personality disorder
Self-defeating personality disorder

    F60.9   **Personality disorder,** unspecified
Character disorder NOS
Character neurosis NOS
Pathological personality NOS

● **F63**   **Impulse disorders**

    Excludes2   habitual excessive use of alcohol or psychoactive substances (F10-F19)
impulse disorders involving sexual behavior (F65.-)

    F63.0   **Pathological gambling**
Compulsive gambling

      Excludes1   gambling and betting NOS (Z72.6)

      Excludes2   excessive gambling by manic patients (F30, F31)
gambling in antisocial personality disorder (F60.2)

    F63.1   **Pyromania**
Pathological fire-setting

      Excludes2   fire-setting (by) (in):
adult with antisocial personality disorder (F60.2)
alcohol or psychoactive substance intoxication (F10-F19)
conduct disorders (F91.-)
mental disorders due to known physiological condition (F01-F09)
schizophrenia (F20.-)

CHAPTER 5 (F01-F99)

◀ New   ◀▦ Revised   ~~deleted~~ Deleted   Excludes 1   Excludes 2   Includes   Use additional   Code first   Code also   Unspecified

OGCR Official Guidelines   ● Unacceptable Principal Diagnosis   X Assign placeholder X   ● Use Additional Character(s)   ▶ Manifestation Code   **Coding Clinic**

F63.2   **Kleptomania**
Pathological stealing

> **Excludes1**   shoplifting as the reason for observation for suspected mental disorder (Z03.8)

> **Excludes2**   depressive disorder with stealing (F31-F33)
> stealing due to underlying mental condition-code to mental condition
> stealing in mental disorders due to known physiological condition (F01-F09)

F63.3   **Trichotillomania**
Hair plucking

> **Excludes2**   other stereotyped movement disorder (F98.4)

● **F63.8**   **Other impulse disorders**

     F63.81   **Intermittent explosive disorder**

     F63.89   **Other impulse disorders**

F63.9   **Impulse disorder, unspecified**
Impulse control disorder NOS

● **F64 Gender identity disorders**

   F64.1   **Gender identity disorder in adolescence and adulthood**
Dual role transvestism
Transsexualism

> Use additional code to identify sex reassignment status (Z87.890)

> **Excludes1**   gender identity disorder in childhood (F64.2)

> **Excludes2**   fetishistic transvestism (F65.1)

   F64.2   **Gender identity disorder of childhood**   P

> **Excludes1**   gender identity disorder in adolescence and adulthood (F64.1)

> **Excludes2**   sexual maturation disorder (F66)

   F64.8   **Other gender identity disorders**

   F64.9   **Gender identity disorder, unspecified**
Gender-role disorder NOS

● **F65**   **Paraphilias**

   F65.0   **Fetishism**
Intense sexual urges and arousing fantasies using inanimate objects

   F65.1   **Transvestic fetishism**
Intense sexual urges, arousal, or orgasm associated with fantasized/actual cross-dressing
Fetishistic transvestism

   F65.2   **Exhibitionism**

   F65.3   **Voyeurism**
Sexual urges or arousal involving real or fantasized observation of unsuspecting people who are naked, disrobing, or engaging in sexual activity

   F65.4   **Pedophilia**

● **F65.5**   **Sadomasochism**

     F65.50   **Sadomasochism, unspecified**

     F65.51   **Sexual masochism**

     F65.52   **Sexual sadism**

● **F65.8**   **Other paraphilias**

     F65.81   **Frotteurism**
Sexual arousal or orgasm is achieved by rubbing up against another person (or fantasies of), in crowded place with unsuspecting victim

     F65.89   **Other paraphilias**
Necrophilia

F65.9   **Paraphilia, unspecified**
Sexual deviation NOS

F66   **Other sexual disorders**
Sexual maturation disorder
Sexual relationship disorder

● **F68**   **Other disorders of adult personality and behavior**

   ● **F68.1**   **Factitious disorder**
Compensation neurosis
Elaboration of physical symptoms for psychological reasons
Hospital hopper syndrome
Münchhausen's syndrome
Peregrinating patient

> **Excludes2**   factitial dermatitis (L98.1)
> person feigning illness (with obvious motivation) (Z76.5)

> (Ex) **For category F68.1 CC codes:** F07.0-F07.81, F07.9-F09, F20.0-F51.03, F51.12, F51.3-F51.9, F52.5, F54, F59-F63.2, F63.81-F63.9, F68.10-F80.4, F80.89-F84.0, F84.3-F99, G44.201-G44.229, H93.25, R45.1-R45.2, R45.5-R45.82, R45.86-R45.87

     F68.10   **Factitious disorder, unspecified** 🔹

     F68.11   **Factitious disorder with predominantly psychological signs and symptoms**

     F68.12   **Factitious disorder with predominantly physical signs and symptoms** 🔹

     F68.13   **Factitious disorder with combined psychological and physical signs and symptoms**

   F68.8   **Other specified disorders of adult personality and behavior**

F69   **Unspecified disorder of adult personality and behavior**   A

INTELLECTUAL DISABILITIES (F70-F79)

Code first any associated physical or developmental disorders

> **Excludes1**   borderline intellectual functioning, IQ above 70 to 84 (R41.83)

F70   **Mild intellectual disabilities**
IQ level 50-55 to approximately 70
Mild mental subnormality

F71   **Moderate intellectual disabilities**
IQ level 35-40 to 50-55
Moderate mental subnormality

F72   **Severe intellectual disabilities** 🔹
IQ 20-25 to 35-40
Severe mental subnormality
(Ex) F72-F73

F73   **Profound intellectual disabilities** 🔹
IQ level below 20-25
Profound mental subnormality
(Ex) F72-F73

F78   **Other intellectual disabilities**

F79   **Unspecified intellectual disabilities**
Mental deficiency NOS
Mental subnormality NOS

CHAPTER 5 (F01-F99)

N Newborn Age: 0   **P** Pediatric Age: 0–17   **M** Maternity DX: 12–55   **A** Adult Age: 15–124   ♀ Females Only   ♂ Males Only

🔹 Complication\Comorbidity   🔹 Major C\C   (Ex) CC/MCC Exclusions   🔹 Present on Admission Requirement   🔹 Hospital-Acquired Condition

875

PERVASIVE AND SPECIFIC DEVELOPMENTAL DISORDERS (F80-F89)

● **F80**   **Specific developmental disorders of speech and language**

     F80.0   **Phonological disorder**

         Communication disorder of unknown cause, characterized by
         failure to use age-appropriate sounds

         Dyslalia

         Functional speech articulation disorder

         Lalling

         Lisping

         Phonological developmental disorder

         Speech articulation developmental disorder

         Excludes1   speech articulation impairment due to
                 aphasia NOS (R47.01)
               speech articulation impairment due to
                 apraxia (R48.2)

         Excludes2   speech articulation impairment due to
                 hearing loss (F80.4)
               speech articulation impairment due to
                 intellectual disabilities (F70-F79)
               speech articulation impairment with
                 expressive language developmental
                 disorder (F80.1)
               speech articulation impairment with
                 mixed receptive expressive language
                 developmental disorder (F80.2)

     F80.1   **Expressive language disorder**

         Developmental dysphasia or aphasia, expressive type

         Excludes1   mixed receptive-expressive language
                 disorder (F80.2)
               dysphasia and aphasia NOS (R47.-)

         Excludes2   acquired aphasia with epilepsy [Landau-
                 Kleffner] (G40.80-)
               intellectual disabilities (F70-F79)
               pervasive developmental disorders
                 (F84.-)
               selective mutism (F94.0)

     F80.2   **Mixed receptive-expressive language disorder**

         Developmental dysphasia or aphasia, receptive type

         Developmental Wernicke's aphasia

         Excludes1   central auditory processing disorder
                 (H93.25)
               dysphasia or aphasia NOS (R47.-)
               expressive language disorder (F80.1)
               expressive type dysphasia or aphasia
                 (F80.1)
               word deafness (H93.25)

         Excludes2   acquired aphasia with epilepsy [Landau-
                 Kleffner] (G40.80-)
               intellectual disabilities (F70-F79)
               pervasive developmental disorders
                 (F84.-)
               selective mutism (F94.0)

     F80.4   **Speech and language development delay due to hearing**
           loss

         Code also type of hearing loss (H90.-, H91.-)

●   **F80.8**   **Other developmental disorders of speech or language**

         F80.81   **Childhood onset fluency disorder**

            Cluttering NOS

            Stuttering NOS

            Excludes1   adult onset fluency disorder
                 (F98.5)
               fluency disorder in conditions
                 classified elsewhere (R47.82)
               fluency disorder (stuttering)
                 following cerebrovascular
                 disease (I69. with final
                 characters -23)

         F80.89   **Other developmental disorders of speech and**
                language

     F80.9   **Developmental disorder of speech and**
           language, unspecified

         Communication disorder NOS

         Language disorder NOS

●   **F81**   **Specific developmental disorders of scholastic skills**

     F81.0   **Specific reading disorder**

         'Backward reading'

         Developmental dyslexia

         Specific reading retardation

         Excludes1   alexia NOS (R48.0)
               dyslexia NOS (R48.0)

     F81.2   **Mathematics disorder**

         Developmental acalculia

         Developmental arithmetical disorder

         Developmental Gerstmann's syndrome

         Excludes1   acalculia NOS (R48.8)

         Excludes2   arithmetical difficulties associated with a
                 reading disorder (F81.0)
               arithmetical difficulties associated with a
                 spelling disorder (F81.81)
               arithmetical difficulties due to inadequate
                 teaching (Z55.8)

●   **F81.8**   **Other developmental disorders of scholastic skills**

         F81.81   **Disorder of written expression**

            Specific spelling disorder

         F81.89   **Other developmental disorders of scholastic**
                skills

●   **F81.9**   **Developmental disorder of scholastic skills, unspecified**

         Knowledge acquisition disability NOS

         Learning disability NOS

         Learning disorder NOS

  F82   **Specific developmental disorder of motor function**

         Clumsy child syndrome

         Developmental coordination disorder

         Developmental dyspraxia

         Excludes1   abnormalities of gait and mobility (R26.-)
               lack of coordination (R27.-)

         Excludes2   lack of coordination secondary to intellectual
                 disabilities (F70-F79)

●   **F84**   **Pervasive developmental disorders**

         Use additional code to identify any associated medical
         condition and intellectual disabilities.

         (Ex) For category F84 CC codes unless otherwise indicated: F07.0-F07.81, F07.9-F09,
         F20.0-F51.03, F51.12, F51.3-F51.9, F52.5, F54, F59-F63.2, F63.81-F63.9, F68.10-F80.4,
         F80.89-F84.0, F84.3-F99, G44.201-G44.229, H93.25, R45.1-R45.2, R45.5-R45.82,
         R45.86-R45.87

     F84.0   **Autistic disorder**

         Infantile autism

         Infantile psychosis

         Kanner's syndrome

         Excludes1   Asperger's syndrome (F84.5)

     F84.2   **Rett's syndrome**

         Neurodevelopmental disorder

         Excludes1   Asperger's syndrome (F84.5)
               Autistic disorder (F84.0)
               other childhood disintegrative disorder
                 (F84.3)

         (Ex) E75.00-E75.19, E75.4, F84.2, G13.2-G13.8, G30.0-G31.82, G31.84-G31.9,
         G91.4, G94

     F84.3   **Other childhood disintegrative disorder**   P

         Dementia infantilis

         At least two years of normal development followed by
         significant loss of language abilities, social skills,
         bowel/bladder control, motor skills

         Disintegrative psychosis

         Heller's syndrome

         At least two years of normal development followed by
         significant loss of language abilities, social skills,
         bowel/bladder control, motor skills

         Symbiotic psychosis

         Abnormal relationship to mothering figure, characterized
         by intense separation anxiety, severe regression,
         giving up of useful speech, and autism

         Use additional code to identify any associated
         neurological condition.

         Excludes1   Asperger's syndrome (F84.5)
               Autistic disorder (F84.0)
               Rett's syndrome (F84.2)

◀ New   ◀▥ Revised   ~~deleted~~ Deleted   Excludes 1   Excludes 2   Includes   Use additional   Code first   Code also   Unspecified

OGCR Official Guidelines   ● Unacceptable Principal Diagnosis   X Assign placeholder X   ● Use Additional Character(s)   ▌ Manifestation Code   **Coding Clinic**

F84.5   Asperger's syndrome 🔗
Developmental disorder
Asperger's disorder
Autistic psychopathy
Schizoid disorder of childhood

F84.8   Other pervasive developmental disorders 🔗
Overactive disorder associated with intellectual disabilities and stereotyped movements

F84.9   Pervasive developmental disorder, unspecified 🔗
Atypical autism

F88   Other disorders of psychological development
Developmental agnosia

F89   Unspecified disorder of psychological development
Developmental disorder NOS

BEHAVIORAL AND EMOTIONAL DISORDERS WITH ONSET USUALLY OCCURRING IN CHILDHOOD AND ADOLESCENCE (F90-F98)

Note: Codes within categories F90-F98 may be used regardless of the age of a patient. These disorders generally have onset within the childhood or adolescent years, but may continue throughout life or not be diagnosed until adulthood.

● F90   Attention-deficit hyperactivity disorders
> **Includes**   attention deficit disorder with hyperactivity
> attention deficit syndrome with hyperactivity
>
> **Excludes2**   anxiety disorders (F40.-, F41.-)
> mood [affective] disorders (F30-F39)
> pervasive developmental disorders (F84.-)
> schizophrenia (F20.-)

Attention deficit disorder with hyperactivity=ADHD

F90.0   Attention-deficit hyperactivity disorder, predominantly inattentive type

F90.1   Attention-deficit hyperactivity disorder, predominantly hyperactive type

F90.2   Attention-deficit hyperactivity disorder, combined type

F90.8   Attention-deficit hyperactivity disorder, other type

F90.9   Attention-deficit hyperactivity disorder, unspecified type
Attention-deficit hyperactivity disorder of childhood or adolescence NOS
Attention-deficit hyperactivity disorder NOS

● F91   Conduct disorders
Childhood/adolescence disruptive behavior disorder
> **Excludes1**   antisocial behavior (Z72.81-)
> antisocial personality disorder (F60.2)
>
> **Excludes2**   conduct problems associated with attention-deficit hyperactivity disorder (F90.-)
> mood [affective] disorders (F30-F39)
> pervasive developmental disorders (F84.-)
> schizophrenia (F20.-)

F91.0   Conduct disorder confined to family context

F91.1   Conduct disorder, childhood-onset type
Unsocialized conduct disorder
Conduct disorder, solitary aggressive type
Unsocialized aggressive disorder

F91.2   Conduct disorder, adolescent-onset type
Socialized conduct disorder
Conduct disorder, group type

F91.3   Oppositional defiant disorder

F91.8   Other conduct disorders

F91.9   Conduct disorder, unspecified
Behavioral disorder NOS
Conduct disorder NOS
Disruptive behavior disorder NOS

● F93   Emotional disorders with onset specific to childhood

F93.0   Separation anxiety disorder of childhood   P
> **Excludes2**   mood [affective] disorders (F30-F39)
> nonpsychotic mental disorders (F40-F48)
> phobic anxiety disorder of childhood (F40.8)
> social phobia (F40.1)

F93.8   Other childhood emotional disorders   P
Identity disorder
> **Excludes2**   gender identity disorder of childhood (F64.2)

F93.9   Childhood emotional disorder, unspecified   P

● F94   Disorders of social functioning with onset specific to childhood and adolescence

F94.0   Selective mutism
Elective mutism
> **Excludes2**   pervasive developmental disorders (F84.-)
> schizophrenia (F20.-)
> specific developmental disorders of speech and language (F80.-)
> transient mutism as part of separation anxiety in young children (F93.0)

F94.1   Reactive attachment disorder of childhood   P
Use additional code to identify any associated failure to thrive or growth retardation
> **Excludes1**   disinhibited attachment disorder of childhood (F94.2)
> normal variation in pattern of selective attachment
>
> **Excludes2**   Asperger's syndrome (F84.5)
> maltreatment syndromes (T74.-)
> sexual or physical abuse in childhood, resulting in psychosocial problems (Z62.81-)

F94.2   Disinhibited attachment disorder of childhood   P
Affectionless psychopathy
Institutional syndrome
> **Excludes1**   reactive attachment disorder of childhood (F94.1) ◀▥
>
> **Excludes2**   Asperger's syndrome (F84.5)
> attention-deficit hyperactivity disorders (F90.-)
> hospitalism in children (F43.2-)

F94.8   Other childhood disorders of social functioning   P

F94.9   Childhood disorder of social functioning, unspecified   P

● F95   Tic disorder
Involuntary twitch

F95.0   Transient tic disorder

F95.1   Chronic motor or vocal tic disorder

F95.2   Tourette's disorder
Combined vocal and multiple motor tic disorder [de la Tourette]
Tourette's syndrome

F95.8   Other tic disorders

F95.9   Tic disorder, unspecified
Tic NOS

N Newborn Age: 0   **P** Pediatric Age: 0–17   **M** Maternity DX: 12–55   **A** Adult Age: 15–124   ♀ Females Only   ♂ Males Only

🔗 Complication\Comorbidity   🔗 Major C\C   (Ex) CC/MCC Exclusions   🔗 Present on Admission Requirement   🔗 Hospital-Acquired Condition

877

CHAPTER 5 (F01-F99)

Item 5–2 Enuresis: Bed wetting by children at night. Causes can be either psychological or medical (diabetes, urinary tract infections, or abnormalities). **Encopresis:** Overflow incontinence of bowels sometimes resulting from chronic constipation or fecal impaction. Check the documentation for additional diagnoses.

● **F98**   **Other behavioral and emotional disorders with onset usually occurring in childhood and adolescence**

    Excludes2   breath-holding spells (R06.89)
               gender identity disorder of childhood (F64.2)
               Kleine-Levin syndrome (G47.13)
               obsessive-compulsive disorder (F42)
               sleep disorders not due to a substance or known physiological condition (F51.-)

    F98.0   **Enuresis not due to a substance or known physiological condition**
          Enuresis: Urinary incontinence
          Enuresis (primary) (secondary) of nonorganic origin
          Functional enuresis
          Psychogenic enuresis
          Urinary incontinence of nonorganic origin
          Excludes1   enuresis NOS (R32)

    F98.1   **Encopresis not due to a substance or known physiological condition**
          Encopresis: Fecal incontinence
          Functional encopresis
          Incontinence of feces of nonorganic origin
          Psychogenic encopresis
          Use additional code to identify the cause of any coexisting constipation.
          Excludes1   encopresis NOS (R15.-) ◀▥

● **F98.2**   **Other feeding disorders of infancy and childhood**
          Excludes1   feeding difficulties (R63.3)
          Excludes2   anorexia nervosa and other eating disorders (F50.-)
                   feeding problems of newborn (P92.-)
                   pica of infancy or childhood (F98.3)

      F98.21   **Rumination disorder of infancy**   P

      F98.29   **Other feeding disorders of infancy and early childhood**   P

    F98.3   **Pica of infancy and childhood**   P
          Craving and eating substances such as paint, clay, or dirt to replace a nutritional deficit in the body.

    F98.4   **Stereotyped movement disorders**
          Stereotype/habit disorder
          Excludes1   abnormal involuntary movements (R25.-)
          Excludes2   compulsions in obsessive-compulsive disorder (F42)
                   hair plucking (F63.3)
                   movement disorders of organic origin (G20-G25)
                   nail-biting (F98.8)
                   nose-picking (F98.8)
                   stereotypies that are part of a broader psychiatric condition (F01-F95)
                   thumb-sucking (F98.8)
                   tic disorders (F95.-)
                   trichotillomania (F63.3)

    F98.5   **Adult onset fluency disorder**
          Excludes1   childhood onset fluency disorder (F80.81)
                   dysphasia (R47.02)
                   fluency disorder in conditions classified elsewhere (R47.82)
                   fluency disorder (stuttering) following cerebrovascular disease (I69. with final characters -23)
                   tic disorders (F95.-)

    F98.8   **Other specified behavioral and emotional disorders with onset usually occurring in childhood and adolescence**   P
          Excessive masturbation
          Nail-biting
          Nose-picking
          Thumb-sucking

    F98.9   **Unspecified behavioral and emotional disorders with onset usually occurring in childhood and adolescence**   P

UNSPECIFIED MENTAL DISORDER (F99)

F99   **Mental disorder, not otherwise specified**
      Mental illness NOS
      Excludes1   unspecified mental disorder due to known physiological condition (F09)

◀ New   ◀▥ Revised   ~~deleted~~ Deleted   Excludes 1   Excludes 2   Includes   Use additional   Code first   Code also   Unspecified

OGCR Official Guidelines   ● Unacceptable Principal Diagnosis   X Assign placeholder X   ● Use Additional Character(s)   ▶ Manifestation Code   **Coding Clinic**

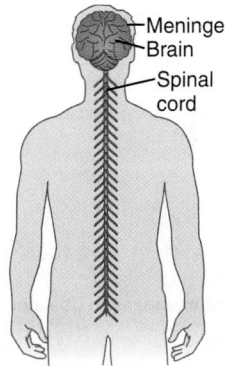

—Meninges
—Brain
—Spinal cord

Figure 6-1 The brain and spinal cord make up the central nervous system.

Item 6-1 The two major classifications of the nervous system are the peripheral nervous system and the central nervous system (CNS). The central nervous system is comprised of the brain and the spinal cord. The peripheral nervous system is comprised of the parasympathetic and sympathetic systems. **Encephalitis** is the swelling of the brain. **Meningitis** is swelling of the covering of the brain, the meninges. Types and causes of brain infections are:

Type	Cause
purulent	bacterial
aseptic/abacterial	viral
chronic meningitis	mycobacterial and fungal

CHAPTER 6

DISEASES OF THE NERVOUS SYSTEM
(G00-G99)

Excludes2　certain conditions originating in the perinatal period (P04-P96)
certain infectious and parasitic diseases (A00-B99)
complications of pregnancy, childbirth and the puerperium (O00-O9A)
congenital malformations, deformations, and chromosomal abnormalities (Q00-Q99)
endocrine, nutritional and metabolic diseases (E00-E88)
injury, poisoning and certain other consequences of external causes (S00-T88)
neoplasms (C00-D49)
symptoms, signs and abnormal clinical and laboratory findings, not elsewhere classified (R00-R94)

This chapter contains the following blocks:

G00-G09	Inflammatory diseases of the central nervous system
G10-G14	Systemic atrophies primarily affecting the central nervous system
G20-G26	Extrapyramidal and movement disorders
G30-G32	Other degenerative diseases of the nervous system
G35-G37	Demyelinating diseases of the central nervous system
G40-G47	Episodic and paroxysmal disorders
G50-G59	Nerve, nerve root and plexus disorders
G60-G65	Polyneuropathies and other disorders of the peripheral nervous system
G70-G73	Diseases of myoneural junction and muscle
G80-G83	Cerebral palsy and other paralytic syndromes
G89-G99	Other disorders of the nervous system

INFLAMMATORY DISEASES OF THE CENTRAL NERVOUS SYSTEM (G00-G09)

● **G00**　**Bacterial meningitis, not elsewhere classified**
An infection of the cerebrospinal fluid surrounding the spinal cord and brain.

Includes　bacterial arachnoiditis
bacterial leptomeningitis
bacterial meningitis
bacterial pachymeningitis

Excludes1　bacterial:
meningoencephalitis (G04.2)
meningomyelitis (G04.2)

(Ex) **For category G00 CC codes:** 02.21, A17.0-A17.1, A27.81, A39.0, A50.41, A51.41, A52.13, A54.82, A54.84, A54.89-A54.9, A87.0-A87.9, B00.3, B02.1, B26.1, B37.5, B38.4, B45.1, B58.2, E08.40-E08.49, E08.618-E08.638, E08.649-E08.8, E09.40-E09.49, E09.618-E09.638, E09.649-E09.8, E10.40-E10.49, E10.618-E10.638, E10.649, E10.69, E10.8, E11.40-E11.49, E11.618-E11.638, E11.649, E11.69-E11.8, E13.40-E13.49, E13.618-E13.638, E13.649-E13.69, E13.8, G00.0-G03.9, G04.2, G32.89, G61.0, G96.8-G96.9, G98.0-G98.8, G99.9

G00.0　**Hemophilus meningitis** 🔹
Meningitis due to Hemophilus influenzae

G00.1　**Pneumococcal meningitis** 🔹

G00.2　**Streptococcal meningitis** 🔹
Use additional code to further identify organism (B95.0-B95.5)

G00.3　**Staphylococcal meningitis** 🔹
Use additional code to further identify organism (B95.61-B95.8)

G00.8　**Other bacterial meningitis** 🔹
Meningitis due to Escherichia coli
Meningitis due to Friedländer bacillus
Meningitis due to Klebsiella
Use additional code to further identify organism (B96.-)

G00.9　**Bacterial meningitis, unspecified** 🔹
Meningitis due to gram-negative bacteria, unspecified
Purulent meningitis NOS
Pyogenic meningitis NOS
Suppurative meningitis NOS

▶ **G01**　*Meningitis in bacterial diseases classified elsewhere* 🔹
Code first underlying disease
Excludes1　meningitis (in):
gonococcal (A54.81)
leptospirosis (A27.81)
listeriosis (A32.11)
Lyme disease (A69.21)
meningococcal (A39.0)
neurosyphilis (A52.13)
tuberculosis (A17.0)
meningoencephalitis and meningomyelitis in bacterial diseases classified elsewhere (G05)

(Ex) See G00

▶ **G02**　*Meningitis in other infectious and parasitic diseases classified elsewhere* 🔹
Code first underlying disease, such as:
African trypanosomiasis (B56.-)
poliovirus infection (A80.-)
Excludes1　candidal meningitis (B37.5)
coccidioidomycosis meningitis (B38.4)
cryptococcal meningitis (B45.1)
herpesviral [herpes simplex] meningitis (B00.3)
infectious mononucleosis complicated by meningitis (B27.- with fourth character 2)
measles complicated by meningitis (B05.1)
meningoencephalitis and meningomyelitis in other infectious and parasitic diseases classified elsewhere (G05)
mumps meningitis (B26.1)
rubella meningitis (B06.02)
varicella [chickenpox] meningitis (B01.0)
zoster meningitis (B02.1)

(Ex) A02.21, A17.0-A17.1, A27.81, A39.0, A50.41, A51.41, A52.13, A54.82, A54.84, A54.89-A54.9, A87.0-A87.9, B00.3, B02.1, B26.1, B37.5, B38.4, B45.1, B58.2, G00.0-G03.9, G04.2, G32.89, G61.0, G96.8-G96.9, G98.0-G98.8, G99.8

N Newborn Age: 0　　**P** Pediatric Age: 0–17　　**M** Maternity DX: 12–55　　**A** Adult Age: 15–124　　♀ Females Only　　♂ Males Only
🔹 Complication\Comorbidity　　🔹 Major C\C　　(Ex) CC/MCC Exclusions　　🔹 Present on Admission Requirement　　🔹 Hospital-Acquired Condition

879

CHAPTER 6 (G00–G99)

● **G03**   **Meningitis due to other and unspecified causes**

     Includes   arachnoiditis NOS
                  leptomeningitis NOS
                  meningitis NOS
                  pachymeningitis NOS

     Excludes1   meningoencephalitis (G04.-)
                     meningomyelitis (G04.-)

     (Ex:) For category G03 CC codes unless otherwise indicated: See G00

   G03.0   **Nonpyogenic meningitis** 🔖
          Aseptic meningitis
          Nonbacterial meningitis

   G03.1   **Chronic meningitis** 🔖

   G03.2   **Benign recurrent meningitis [Mollaret]** 🔖
          (Ex:) A02.21, A17.0-A17.1, A27.81, A39.0, A50.41, A51.41, A52.13,
          A54.82-A54.84, A54.89-A54.9, A74.81-A74.9, A87.0-A87.9, A96.2,
          A98.3-A98.4, B26.1, B33.24, B33.4-B33.8, B34.1-B34.8, B37.5, B38.4,
          B45.1, B58.2, B92, B94.2-B94.9, B97.10, B97.19, B97.29, B97.5-B97.6,
          B97.81-B97.89, G00.0-G03.9, G04.2, G32.89, G61.0, G96.8-G96.9,
          G98.0-G98.8, G99.8

   G03.8   **Meningitis due to other specified causes** 🔖

   G03.9   **Meningitis, unspecified** 🔖
          Arachnoiditis (spinal) NOS

● **G04**   Encephalitis, myelitis and encephalomyelitis

     Includes   acute ascending myelitis
                  meningoencephalitis
                  meningomyelitis

     Excludes1   encephalopathy NOS (G93.40)
                     other noninfectious acute disseminated
                        encephalomyelitis (noninfectious ADEM)
                        (G04.81)

     Excludes2   acute transverse myelitis (G37.3-)
                     alcoholic encephalopathy (G31.2)
                     benign myalgic encephalomyelitis (G93.3)
                     multiple sclerosis (G35)
                     subacute necrotizing myelitis (G37.4)
                     toxic encephalitis (G92)
                     toxic encephalopathy (G92)

● **G04.0**   **Acute disseminated encephalitis and encephalomyelitis (ADEM)**

     Excludes1   acute necrotizing hemorrhagic
                     encephalopathy (G04.3-)

     (Ex:) For category G04.0 CC codes unless otherwise indicated: A02.21,
     A17.0-A17.1, A17.82, A27.81, A39.0, A50.41-A50.42, A51.41,
     A52.13-A52.14, A54.82, A54.84, A54.89-A54.9, A81.1, A81.82-A81.89,
     A83.0-A85.8, A87.0-A88.0, A88.8, A92.1-A92.8, A93.0, A96.2, A98.3-A98.4,
     B00.3-B00.4, B00.89-B01.11, B01.81-B02.23, B02.29, B02.7-B02.9, B04,
     B06.01, B08.04-B08.09, B08.20-B08.22, B08.60-B08.79, B09-B10.89,
     B26.1-B26.2, B27.00-B27.99, B33.1, B33.24, B33.4-B33.8, B34.1-B34.2,
     B34.4, B34.8, B37.5, B38.4, B45.1-B58.2, B92, B94.2, B94.8-B94.9, B97.10,
     B97.19-B97.29, B97.5-B97.6, B97.81-B97.89, G00.0-G04.01, G04.2,
     G04.31, G04.81-G05.4, G32.89, G37.0, G37.4-G37.5, G61.0, G96.8-G96.9,
     G98.0-G98.8, G99.8, J09.X3-J09.X9, J10.2-J10.89, J11.2-J11.89, L44.4,
     P35.2-P35.9, P37.0-P37.4, P37.8-P37.9

   G04.00   **Acute disseminated encephalitis and encephalomyelitis, unspecified** 🔖

▌   *G04.01*   *Postinfectious acute disseminated encephalitis and encephalomyelitis (postinfectious ADEM)* 🔖

       Excludes1   post chickenpox encephalitis
                        (B01.1)
                        post measles encephalitis (B05.0)
                        post measles myelitis (B05.1)

   G04.02   **Postimmunization acute disseminated encephalitis, myelitis and encephalomyelitis** 🔖
          Encephalitis, post immunization
          Encephalomyelitis, post immunization
          Use additional code to identify the vaccine
              (T50.A-, T50.B-, T50.Z-)
          (Ex:) No exclusions

   G04.1   **Tropical spastic paraplegia** 🔖
          (Ex:) G04.1, G11.0-G12.9, G32.0-G37.3, G37.5-G37.9, G80.0-G80.2, G80.4-G80.9,
          G81.00-G83.9, G90.01-G90.09, G90.2, G90.4, G90.50-G90.9, G92,
          G93.40-G93.49, G93.81, G93.89-G95.9, G96.8-G96.9, G98.0-G99.8, I67.83,
          R53.2

   G04.2   **Bacterial meningoencephalitis and meningomyelitis, not elsewhere classified** 🔖
          (Ex:) See G00

● **G04.3**   **Acute necrotizing hemorrhagic encephalopathy**
          Sudden and severe CNS disease with pathology of hemorrhages and necrosis of white matter

     Excludes1   acute disseminated encephalitis and
                     encephalomyelitis (G04.0-)

   G04.30   **Acute necrotizing hemorrhagic encephalopathy, unspecified** 🔖
          (Ex:) No exclusions

▌   *G04.31*   *Postinfectious acute necrotizing hemorrhagic encephalopathy* 🔖
          (Ex:) See G04.0

   G04.32   **Postimmunization acute necrotizing hemorrhagic encephalopathy** 🔖
          Use additional code to identify vaccine
              (T50.A-, T50.B-, T50.Z-)
          (Ex:) No exclusions

▌   *G04.39*   *Other acute necrotizing hemorrhagic encephalopathy* 🔖
          Code also underlying etiology, if applicable
          (Ex:) No exclusions

● **G04.8**   **Other encephalitis, myelitis and encephalomyelitis**
          Code also any associated seizure (G40.-, R56.9)
          (Ex:) For category G04.8 CC codes: See G04.0

   G04.81   **Other encephalitis and encephalomyelitis** 🔖
          Noninfectious acute disseminated
              encephalomyelitis (noninfectious ADEM)

   G04.89   **Other myelitis** 🔖

● **G04.9**   **Encephalitis, myelitis and encephalomyelitis, unspecified**
          (Ex:) For category G04.9 CC codes: A17.82, A28.1, A50.42, A52.14, A75.9,
          A79.9, A81.1, A81.82-A81.89, A83.0-A85.8, A87.2, A88.0, A88.8,
          A92.1-A92.8, A93.0, B00.4, B00.82, B01.11-B01.12, B04, B06.01, B08.09,
          B08.20-B08.22, B08.60-B08.79, B09, B10.01-B10.09, B26.2,
          B27.00-B27.99, B33.1, B45.0, B45.2-B45.9, B54, B58.2, B75, B97.10,
          B97.21, G04.00-G04.01, G04.31, G04.81-G05.4, G37.0, G37.4-G37.5,
          H66.40-H66.43, J09.X3-J09.X9, J10.2-J10.89, J11.2-J11.89, L44.4,
          M1A.10X0-M1A.19X1, M32.0-M32.9, P35.2-P35.9, P37.0-P37.9,
          T56.0X1-T56.0X4[A]

   G04.90   **Encephalitis and encephalomyelitis, unspecified** 🔖
          Ventriculitis (cerebral) NOS

   G04.91   **Myelitis, unspecified** 🔖

◀ New   ◀▥ Revised   ~~deleted~~ Deleted   Excludes 1   Excludes 2   Includes   Use additional   Code first   Code also   Unspecified

OGCR Official Guidelines   ● Unacceptable Principal Diagnosis   X Assign placeholder X   ● Use Additional Character(s)   ▌ Manifestation Code   **Coding Clinic**

● **G05**   **Encephalitis, myelitis and encephalomyelitis in diseases classified elsewhere**

     Code first underlying disease, such as:
       human immunodeficiency virus [HIV] disease (B20)
       poliovirus (A80.-)
       suppurative otitis media (H66.01-H66.4)
       trichinellosis (B75)

     Excludes1   adenoviral encephalitis, myelitis and encephalomyelitis (A85.1)
       congenital toxoplasmosis encephalitis, myelitis and encephalomyelitis (P37.1)
       cytomegaloviral encephalitis, myelitis and encephalomyelitis (B25.8)
       encephalitis, myelitis and encephalomyelitis (in) measles (B05.0)
       encephalitis, myelitis and encephalomyelitis (in) systemic lupus erythematosus (M32.19)
       enteroviral encephalitis, myelitis and encephalomyelitis (A85.0)
       herpesviral [herpes simplex] encephalitis, myelitis and encephalomyelitis (B00.4)
       listerial encephalitis, myelitis and encephalomyelitis (A32.12)
       meningococcal encephalitis, myelitis and encephalomyelitis (A39.81)
       mumps encephalitis, myelitis and encephalomyelitis (B26.2)
       postchickenpox encephalitis, myelitis and encephalomyelitis (B01.1-)
       rubella encephalitis, myelitis and encephalomyelitis (B06.01)
       toxoplasmosis encephalitis, myelitis and encephalomyelitis (B58.2)
       zoster encephalitis, myelitis and encephalomyelitis (B02.0)

     (Ex:) **For category G05 CC codes: See G04.0**

▷ **G05.3**   *Encephalitis and encephalomyelitis in diseases classified elsewhere* 🔖
       Meningoencephalitis in diseases classified elsewhere

▷ **G05.4**   *Myelitis in diseases classified elsewhere* 🔖
       Meningomyelitis in diseases classified elsewhere

● **G06**   **Intracranial and intraspinal abscess and granuloma**
     An accumulation of pus in either the brain or spinal cord

     Use additional code (B95-B97) to identify infectious agent.

     G06.0   **Intracranial abscess and granuloma** 🔖
       Brain [any part] abscess (embolic)
       Cerebellar abscess (embolic)
       Cerebral abscess (embolic)
       Intracranial epidural abscess or granuloma
       Intracranial extradural abscess or granuloma
       Intracranial subdural abscess or granuloma
       Otogenic abscess (embolic)

       Excludes1   tuberculous intracranial abscess and granuloma (A17.81)

       (Ex:) A06.6, A17.81, E08.40-E08.49, E08.618-E08.638, E08.649-E08.8,
       E09.40-E09.49, E09.618-E09.638, E09.649-E09.8, E10.40-E10.49,
       E10.618-E10.638, E10.649, E10.69-E10.8, E11.40-E11.49, E11.618-E11.638,
       E11.649, E11.69-E11.8, E13.40-E13.49, E13.618-E13.638, E13.649-E13.8,
       G06.0-G08, G93.81, G93.89-G93.9

     G06.1   **Intraspinal abscess and granuloma** 🔖
       Abscess (embolic) of spinal cord [any part]
       Intraspinal epidural abscess or granuloma
       Intraspinal extradural abscess or granuloma
       Intraspinal subdural abscess or granuloma

       Excludes1   tuberculous intraspinal abscess and granuloma (A17.81)

       (Ex:) A06.6, A17.81, E08.40-A08.49, E08.618-E08.638, E08.649-E08.8,
       E09.40-E09.49, E09.618-E09.638, E09.649-E09.8, E10.40-E10.49,
       E10.618-E10.638, E10.649, E10.69-E10.8, E11.40-E11.49, E11.618-E11.638,
       E11.649, E11.69-E11.8, E13.40-E13.49, E13.618-E13.638, E13.649-E13.8,
       G06.1

     G06.2   **Extradural and subdural abscess, unspecified** 🔖
       (Ex:) A06.6, A17.81, E08.40-E08.49, E08.618-E08.638, E08.649-E08.8,
       E09.40-E09.49, E09.618-E09.638, E09.649-E09.8, E10.40-E10.49,
       E10.618-E10.638, E10.649, E10.69-E10.8, E11.40-E11.49, E11.618-E11.638,
       E11.649, E11.69-E11.8, E13.40-E13.49, E13.618-E13.638, E13.649-E13.8,
       G06.0-G06.2, G07-G08

▷ **G07**   *Intracranial and intraspinal abscess and granuloma in diseases classified elsewhere* 🔖

     Code first underlying disease, such as: ◀▥
       schistosomiasis granuloma of brain (B65.-)

     Excludes1   abscess of brain:
       amebic (A06.6)
       chromomycotic (B43.1)
       gonococcal (A54.82)
       tuberculous (A17.81)
       tuberculoma of meninges (A17.1)

     (Ex:) See G06.2

● **G08**   **Intracranial and intraspinal phlebitis and thrombophlebitis** 🔖
     Septic embolism of intracranial or intraspinal venous sinuses and veins
     Septic endophlebitis of intracranial or intraspinal venous sinuses and veins
     Septic phlebitis of intracranial or intraspinal venous sinuses and veins
     Septic thrombophlebitis of intracranial or intraspinal venous sinuses and veins
     Septic thrombosis of intracranial or intraspinal venous sinuses and veins

     Excludes1   intracranial phlebitis and thrombophlebitis complicating:
       abortion, ectopic or molar pregnancy (O00-O07, O08.7)
       pregnancy, childbirth and the puerperium (O22.5, O87.3)
       nonpyogenic intracranial phlebitis and thrombophlebitis (I67.6)
       ~~nonpyogenic intraspinal phlebitis and thrombophlebitis (G95.1)~~

     Excludes2   intracranial phlebitis and thrombophlebitis complicating nonpyogenic intraspinal phlebitis and thrombophlebitis (G95.1) ◀

     (Ex:) See G06.2

● **G09**   **Sequelae of inflammatory diseases of central nervous system** 🔖
     Note: Category G09 is to be used to indicate conditions whose primary classification is to G00-G08 as the cause of sequelae, themselves classifiable elsewhere. The 'sequelae' include conditions specified as residuals.

     Code first condition resulting from (sequela) of inflammatory diseases of central nervous system

---

**SYSTEMIC ATROPHIES PRIMARILY AFFECTING
THE CENTRAL NERVOUS SYSTEM (G10-G14)**

● **G10**   **Huntington's disease** 🔖
     Genetic disease with degeneration of cells of the nervous system, including brain
     Huntington's chorea
     Huntington's dementia
     (Ex:) G04.1, G20, G21.11-G21.9, G32.89-G37.9, G80.0-G80.2, G80.4-G80.9, G82.20-G83.0,
     G92, G93.1, G93.40-G93.6, G93.81, G93.89-G93.9, G96.8-G96.9, G98.0-G98.8, G99.8,
     I67.83, R53.2

Item 6–2 Huntington's chorea is an inherited degenerative disorder of the central nervous system and is characterized by ceaseless, jerky movements and progressive cognitive and behavioral deterioration.

CHAPTER 6 (G00-G99)

N   Newborn Age: 0   **P**   Pediatric Age: 0–17   **M**   Maternity DX: 12–55   **A**   Adult Age: 15–124   ♀   Females Only   ♂   Males Only

 Complication\Comorbidity   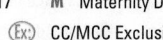 Major C\C   (Ex:) CC/MCC Exclusions   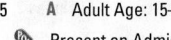 Present on Admission Requirement   🔖 Hospital-Acquired Condition

881

● **G11 Hereditary ataxia**
   Genetic neurological disorder affecting coordination
   Excludes2   cerebral palsy (G80.-)
                  hereditary and idiopathic neuropathy (G60.-)
                  metabolic disorders (E70-E88)
   (Ex) **For category G11 CC codes unless otherwise indicated:** G04.1, G10-G12.9, G21.0,
   G23.0-G25.79, G25.82-G26, G32.0-G37.9, G80.0-G83.9, G90.01-G90.09, G90.2-G90.9,
   G92-G93.1, G93.40-G93.49, G93.81, G93.89-G95.9, G96.8-G96.9, G98.0-G99.8, I67.83,
   R53.2

   G11.0 Congenital nonprogressive ataxia %

   G11.1 Early-onset cerebellar ataxia %
            Early-onset cerebellar ataxia with essential tremor
            Early-onset cerebellar ataxia with myoclonus [Hunt's
               ataxia]
            Early-onset cerebellar ataxia with retained tendon
               reflexes
            Friedreich's ataxia (autosomal recessive)
            X-linked recessive spinocerebellar ataxia

   G11.2 Late-onset cerebellar ataxia   A

   G11.3 Cerebellar ataxia with defective DNA repair %
            Ataxia telangiectasia [Louis-Bar]
            Excludes2   Cockayne's syndrome (Q87.1)
                           other disorders of purine and pyrimidine
                              metabolism (E79.-)
                           xeroderma pigmentosum (Q82.1)

   G11.4 Hereditary spastic paraplegia %
            (Ex) G04.1, G10-G12.9, G21.0, G23.0-G25.79, G25.82-G26, G32.0-G37.3,
            G37.5-G37.9, G80.0-G83.9, G90.01-G90.09, G90.2-G90.9, G92, G93.1,
            G93.40-G93.49, G93.81, G93.89-G93.9, G95.0-G95.9, G96.12-G96.9, G97.1,
            G98.0-G99.8, I67.83, R53.2

   G11.8 Other hereditary ataxias %

   G11.9 Hereditary ataxia, unspecified %
            Hereditary cerebellar ataxia NOS
            Hereditary cerebellar degeneration
            Hereditary cerebellar disease
            Hereditary cerebellar syndrome
            (Ex) G11.0-G11.9, G32.81

● **G12 Spinal muscular atrophy and related syndromes**
   (Ex) **For category G12 CC codes:** E08.40-E08.49, E08.618-E08.638, E08.649-E08.8,
   E09.40-E09.49, E09.618-E09.638, E09.649-E09.8, E10.40-E10.49, E10.618-E10.638,
   E10.649, E10.69-E10.8, E11.40-E11.49, E11.618-E11.638, E11.649, E11.69-E11.8,
   E13.40-E13.49, E13.618-E13.638, E13.649-E13.8, G11.3, G11.8-G12.9, G32.0, G32.89,
   G90.01-G90.09, G90.2, G90.4, G90.50-G90.9, G95.0-G95.9, G96.8-G96.9, G98.0-G99.8

   **G12.0 Infantile spinal muscular atrophy, type I
            [Werdnig-Hoffman]** %

   G12.1 Other inherited spinal muscular atrophy %
            Adult form spinal muscular atrophy
            Childhood form, type II spinal muscular atrophy
            Distal spinal muscular atrophy
            Juvenile form, type III spinal muscular atrophy
               [Kugelberg-Welander]
            Progressive bulbar palsy of childhood [Fazio-Londe]
            Scapuloperoneal form spinal muscular atrophy

   ● **G12.2 Motor neuron disease**
            *Progressive disease of motor neurons that carry impulses to
               muscles to move*

            G12.20 Motor neuron disease, unspecified %

            G12.21 Amyotrophic lateral sclerosis %   A
                      Lou Gehrig's disease (ALS)
                      Progressive spinal muscle atrophy

            G12.22 Progressive bulbar palsy %

            G12.29 Other motor neuron disease %
                      Familial motor neuron disease
                      Primary lateral sclerosis

   **G12.8 Other spinal muscular atrophies and related
            syndromes** %

   G12.9 Spinal muscular atrophy, unspecified %

▶ **G13 Systemic atrophies primarily affecting central nervous system
         in diseases classified elsewhere**

   ▶ **G13.0 *Paraneoplastic neuromyopathy and neuropathy***
            Carcinomatous neuromyopathy
            Sensorial paraneoplastic neuropathy [Denny Brown]
            Code first underlying neoplasm (C00-D49)

   ▶ **G13.1 *Other systemic atrophy primarily affecting central
            nervous system in neoplastic disease***
            Paraneoplastic limbic encephalopathy
            Code first underlying neoplasm (C00-D49)

   ▶ **G13.2 *Systemic atrophy primarily affecting the central nervous
            system in myxedema***
            Code first underlying disease, such as:
               hypothyroidism (E03.-)
               myxedematous congenital iodine deficiency (E00.1)

   ▶ **G13.8 *Systemic atrophy primarily affecting central nervous
            system in other diseases classified elsewhere***
            Code first underlying disease

   G14 Postpolio syndrome %
         Includes   Postpolio myelitic syndrome
         Excludes1   sequelae of poliomyelitis (B91)

   _____
   EXTRAPYRAMIDAL AND MOVEMENT DISORDERS (G20-G26)
   _____

   G20 Parkinson's disease
         *Progressive disease of the nervous system that affects muscle
            coordination*
         Hemiparkinsonism
         Idiopathic Parkinsonism or Parkinson's disease
         Paralysis agitans
         Parkinsonism or Parkinson's disease NOS
         Primary Parkinsonism or Parkinson's disease
         Excludes1   dementia with Parkinsonism (G31.83)

● **G21 Secondary parkinsonism**
         *Symptoms of Parkinson's caused by medicines, illness, or other
            nervous system disorder*
         Excludes1   dementia with Parkinsonism (G31.83)
                        Huntington's disease (G10)
                        Shy-Drager syndrome (G90.3)
                        syphilitic Parkinsonism (A52.19)

   G21.0 Malignant neuroleptic syndrome %
            Use additional code for adverse effect, if applicable, to
               identify drug (T43.3X5, T43.4X5, T43.505, T43.595)
            Excludes1   neuroleptic induced parkinsonism
                           (G21.11)
            (Ex) G10, G21.0, G23.0-G25.79, G25.82-G26, G80.3, G81.00-G81.94, G90.3,
            G93.2, G93.40-G93.49, I67.83

   ● **G21.1 Other drug-induced secondary parkinsonism**
            (Ex) **For category G21.1 CC codes:** G20, G21.11-G21.9

            G21.11 Neuroleptic induced parkinsonism %
                      Use additional code for adverse effect, if
                         applicable, to identify drug (T43.3X5,
                         T43.4X5, T43.505, T43.595)
                      Excludes1   malignant neuroleptic syndrome
                                     (G21.0)

            G21.19 Other drug induced secondary parkinsonism %
                      Use additional code for adverse effect, if
                         applicable, to identify drug (T36-T50 with
                         fifth or sixth character 5)

   G21.2 Secondary parkinsonism due to other external agents %
            Code first (T51-T65) to identify external agent

   G21.3 Postencephalitic parkinsonism

   G21.4 Vascular parkinsonism

   G21.8 Other secondary parkinsonism %

   G21.9 Secondary parkinsonism, unspecified %

◀ New   ◀▥ Revised   ~~deleted~~ Deleted   Excludes 1   Excludes 2   Includes   Use additional   Code first   Code also   Unspecified

882   OGCR Official Guidelines   ● Unacceptable Principal Diagnosis   X Assign placeholder X   % Use Additional Character(s)   ▶ Manifestation Code   Coding Clinic

CHAPTER 6 (G00-G99)

● G23   Other degenerative diseases of basal ganglia

> **Excludes2**   multi-system degeneration of the autonomic nervous system (G90.3)
>
> (Ex) **For category G23 CC codes:** G20, G21.11-G21.9, G90.01-G90.09, G93.40-G93.49, I67.83

   G23.0   Hallervorden-Spatz disease 🔖
       Pigmentary pallidal degeneration

   G23.1   Progressive supranuclear ophthalmoplegia [Steele-Richardson-Olszewski] 🔖
       Progressive supranuclear palsy

   G23.2   Striatonigral degeneration 🔖

   G23.8   Other specified degenerative diseases of basal ganglia 🔖
       Calcification of basal ganglia

   G23.9   Degenerative disease of basal ganglia, unspecified 🔖

● G24   Dystonia

> *Involuntary movements*
>
> **Includes**   dyskinesia
>
> **Excludes2**   athetoid cerebral palsy (G80.3)

 ● G24.0   Drug induced dystonia

> Use additional code for adverse effect, if applicable, to identify drug (T36-T50 with fifth or sixth character 5)

   G24.01   Drug induced subacute dyskinesia
       Drug induced blepharospasm
       Drug induced orofacial dyskinesia
       Neuroleptic induced tardive dyskinesia
       Tardive dyskinesia

   G24.02   Drug induced acute dystonia 🔖
       Acute dystonic reaction to drugs
       Neuroleptic induced acute dystonia
       (Ex) G20, G21.11-G21.9, G25.70-G25.79, G25.89-G26, G80.3, G93.40, G93.41-G93.49, I67.83

   G24.09   Other drug induced dystonia 🔖
       (Ex) See G24.02

   G24.1   Genetic torsion dystonia
       Dystonia deformans progressiva
       Dystonia musculorum deformans
       Familial torsion dystonia
       Idiopathic familial dystonia
       Idiopathic (torsion) dystonia NOS
       (Schwalbe-) Ziehen-Oppenheim disease

   G24.2   Idiopathic nonfamilial dystonia 🔖
       (Ex) See G24.02

   G24.3   Spasmodic torticollis

> *Head tilts toward one side and chin is elevated and turned toward opposite side (wry neck)*
>
> **Excludes1**   congenital torticollis (Q68.0)
>   hysterical torticollis (F44.4)
>   ocular torticollis (R29.891)
>   psychogenic torticollis (F45.8)
>   torticollis NOS (M43.6)
>   traumatic recurrent torticollis (S13.4)

   G24.4   Idiopathic orofacial dystonia
       Orofacial dyskinesia

> **Excludes1**   drug induced orofacial dyskinesia (G24.01)

   G24.5   Blepharospasm

> *Tonic spasm of orbicularis oculi muscle, producing closure of eyelids*
>
> **Excludes1**   drug induced blepharospasm (G24.01)

   G24.8   Other dystonia 🔖
       Acquired torsion dystonia NOS
       (Ex) See G24.02

   G24.9   Dystonia, unspecified 🔖
       Dyskinesia NOS

● G25   Other extrapyramidal and movement disorders

> *Extrapyramidal: Other than pyramidal tracts*
>
> **Excludes2**   sleep related movement disorders (G47.6-)

   G25.0   Essential tremor
       Familial tremor

> **Excludes1**   tremor NOS (R25.1)

   G25.1   Drug-induced tremor

> Use additional code for adverse effect, if applicable, to identify drug (T36-T50 with fifth or sixth character 5)

   G25.2   Other specified forms of tremor
       Intention tremor

   G25.3   Myoclonus

> *Shocklike contractions muscle(s)*
>
> Drug-induced myoclonus
> Palatal myoclonus

> Use additional code for adverse effect, if applicable, to identify drug (T36-T50 with fifth or sixth character 5)
>
> **Excludes1**   facial myokymia (G51.4)
>   myoclonic epilepsy (G40.-)

   G25.4   Drug-induced chorea

> Use additional code for adverse effect, if applicable, to identify drug (T36-T50 with fifth or sixth character 5)

   G25.5   Other chorea

> *Continual, involuntary, jerky, movements*
>
> Chorea NOS
>
> **Excludes1**   chorea NOS with heart involvement (I02.0)
>   Huntington's chorea (G10)
>   rheumatic chorea (I02.-)
>   Sydenham's chorea (I02.-)

 ● G25.6   Drug induced tics and other tics of organic origin

   G25.61   Drug induced tics

> Use additional code for adverse effect, if applicable, to identify drug (T36-T50 with fifth or sixth character 5)

   G25.69   Other tics of organic origin

> **Excludes1**   habit spasm (F95.9)
>   tic NOS (F95.9)
>   Tourette's syndrome (F95.2)

 ● G25.7   Other and unspecified drug induced movement disorders

> Use additional code for adverse effect, if applicable, to identify drug (T36-T50 with fifth or sixth character 5)

   G25.70   Drug induced movement disorder, unspecified

   G25.71   Drug induced akathisia
       Drug induced acathisia
       Neuroleptic induced acute akathisia

   G25.79   Other drug induced movement disorders

 ● G25.8   Other specified extrapyramidal and movement disorders

   G25.81   Restless legs syndrome

   G25.82   Stiff-man syndrome 🔖
       (Ex) G04.1, G10, G12.22, G20-G21.9, G24.01-G25.79, G25.82-G26, G32.89-G37.2, G37.5-G37.9, G80.0-G80.9, G82.20-G83.0, G92, G93.1, G93.40-G93.6, G93.81, G93.89-G93.9, G96.8-G96.9, G98.0-G98.8, G99.8, I67.83, R53.2

   G25.83   Benign shuddering attacks

   G25.89   Other specified extrapyramidal and movement disorders

   G25.9   Extrapyramidal and movement disorder, unspecified 🔖
       (Ex) See G25.82

▷ G26   Extrapyramidal and movement disorders in diseases classified elsewhere

> Code first underlying disease

N   Newborn Age: 0   P   Pediatric Age: 0–17   M   Maternity DX: 12–55   A   Adult Age: 15–124   ♀   Females Only   ♂   Males Only

🔖 Complication\Comorbidity   🔖 Major C\C   (Ex) CC/MCC Exclusions   Present on Admission Requirement   🔖 Hospital-Acquired Condition

883

CHAPTER 6 (G00-G99)

CHAPTER 6 (G00-G99)

OTHER DEGENERATIVE DISEASES OF THE NERVOUS SYSTEM (G30-G32)

● **G30**   **Alzheimer's disease**
      Progressive central neurodegenerative disorder

    Includes   Alzheimer's dementia senile and presenile forms

    Use additional code to identify:
      delirium, if applicable (F05)
      dementia with behavioral disturbance (F02.81)
      dementia without behavioral disturbance (F02.80)

    Excludes1   senile degeneration of brain NEC (G31.1)
                  senile dementia NOS (F03)
                  senility NOS (R41.81)

  G30.0   **Alzheimer's disease with early onset**

  G30.1   **Alzheimer's disease with late onset**   A

  G30.8   **Other Alzheimer's disease**

  G30.9   **Alzheimer's disease, unspecified**
        Coding Clinic: 2012, Q4, P95

● **G31**   **Other degenerative diseases of nervous system, not elsewhere classified**

    Use additional code to identify:
      dementia with behavioral disturbance (F02.81)
      dementia without behavioral disturbance (F02.80)

    Excludes2   Reye's syndrome (G93.7)

● **G31.0**   **Frontotemporal dementia**

    G31.01   **Pick's disease**
          Primary progressive aphasia
          Progressive isolated aphasia

    G31.09   **Other frontotemporal dementia**
          Frontal dementia

  G31.1   **Senile degeneration of brain, not elsewhere classified**

    Excludes1   Alzheimer's disease (G30.-)
                  senility NOS (R41.81)

  G31.2   **Degeneration of nervous system due to alcohol**
      Alcoholic cerebellar ataxia
      Alcoholic cerebellar degeneration
      Alcoholic cerebral degeneration
      Alcoholic encephalopathy
      Dysfunction of the autonomic nervous system due to alcohol
      Code also associated alcoholism (F10.-)

● **G31.8**   **Other specified degenerative diseases of nervous system**

    G31.81   **Alpers' disease** 🔒
          Rare neuronal degeneration of cerebral cortex disease of young children
          Grey-matter degeneration
          Ⓔ E75.00-E75.19, E75.4, F84.2, G13.2-G13.8, G30.0-G31.82, G31.84-G31.9, G91.4, G94

    G31.82   **Leigh's disease** 🔒
          Rare neurometabolic disorder that affects central nervous system
          Subacute necrotizing encephalopathy
          Ⓔ See G31.81

    G31.83   **Dementia with Lewy bodies**
          Closely allied to Parkinson's Disease
          Dementia with Parkinsonism
          Lewy body dementia
          Lewy body disease

    G31.84   **Mild cognitive impairment, so stated**

      Excludes1   age related cognitive decline (R41.81)
                    altered mental status (R41.82)
                    cerebral degeneration (G31.9)
                    change in mental status (R41.82)
                    cognitive deficits following (sequelae of) cerebral hemorrhage or infarction (I69.01, I69.11, I69.21, I69.31, I69.81, I69.91)
                    cognitive impairment due to intracranial or head injury (S06.-)
                    dementia (F01.-, F02.-, F03)
                    mild memory disturbance (F06.8)
                    neurologic neglect syndrome (R41.4)
                    personality change, nonpsychotic (F68.8)

    G31.85   **Corticobasal degeneration**

    G31.89   **Other specified degenerative diseases of nervous system**

  G31.9   **Degenerative disease of nervous system, unspecified**

● **G32**   **Other degenerative disorders of nervous system in diseases classified elsewhere**

▶ **G32.0**   *Subacute combined degeneration of spinal cord in diseases classified elsewhere* 🔒
      Dana-Putnam syndrome
      Sclerosis of spinal cord (combined) (dorsolateral) (posterolateral)

    Code first underlying disease, such as:
      anemia (D51.9)
      dietary (D51.3)
      pernicious (D51.0)
      vitamin B12 deficiency (E53.8)

    Excludes1   syphilitic combined degeneration of spinal cord (A52.11)
    Ⓔ G04.1, G11.3, G11.8-G12.9, G32.0, G32.89-G37.3, G37.5-G37.9, G80.0-G83.9, G90.01-G90.09, G90.2, G90.4-G90.9, G93.1, G93.40-G93.49, G95.0-G96.9, G97.1, G98.0-G99.8, I67.83, R53.2

● **G32.8**   **Other specified degenerative disorders of nervous system in diseases classified elsewhere**

    Code first underlying disease, such as:
      amyloidosis cerebral degeneration (E85.-) ◀▬
      cerebral degeneration (due to) hypothyroidism (E00.0-E03.9)
      cerebral degeneration (due to) neoplasm (C00-D49)
      cerebral degeneration (due to) vitamin B deficiency, except thiamine (E52-E53.-)

    Excludes1   superior hemorrhagic polioencephalitis [Wernicke's encephalopathy] (E51.2)

▶ **G32.81**   *Cerebellar ataxia in diseases classified elsewhere* 🔒

      Code first underlying disease, such as:
        celiac disease (with gluten ataxia) (K90.0) ◀
        cerebellar ataxia (in) neoplastic disease (paraneoplastic cerebellar degeneration) (C00-D49)
        non-celiac gluten ataxia (M35.9) ◀

      Excludes1   systemic atrophy primarily affecting the central nervous system in alcoholic cerebellar ataxia (G31.2)
                      systemic atrophy primarily affecting the central nervous system in myxedema (G13.2)
      Ⓔ G04.1, G10-G12.9, G21.0, G23.0-G25.79, G25.82-G26, G32.0-G37.9, G80.0-G83.9, G90.01-G90.09, G90.2-G90.9, G92-G93.1, G93.40-G93.49, G93.81, G93.89-G95.9, G96.8-G96.9, G98.0-G99.8, I67.83, R53.2

▶ **G32.89**   *Other specified degenerative disorders of nervous system in diseases classified elsewhere*
      Degenerative encephalopathy in diseases classified elsewhere

---

◀ New   ◀▬ Revised   ~~deleted~~ Deleted   Excludes 1   Excludes 2   Includes   Use additional   Code first   Code also   Unspecified

OGCR Official Guidelines   ● Unacceptable Principal Diagnosis   X Assign placeholder X   ● Use Additional Character(s)   ▶ Manifestation Code   **Coding Clinic**

DEMYELINATING DISEASES OF THE CENTRAL NERVOUS SYSTEM (G35-G37)

G35   **Multiple sclerosis**
Destruction of central nervous system; four types: relapsing remitting, secondary progressive, primary progressive, and progressive relapsing
Disseminated multiple sclerosis
Generalized multiple sclerosis
Multiple sclerosis NOS
Multiple sclerosis of brain stem
Multiple sclerosis of cord

● **G36**   **Other acute disseminated demyelination**
> **Excludes1**   postinfectious encephalitis and encephalomyelitis NOS (G04.01)

Ⓔ **For category G36 CC codes unless otherwise indicated:** G04.1, G10-G12.9, G21.0, G24.01-G25.79, G25.82-G26, G32.0-G37.3, G37.5, G37.8-G37.9, G80.0-G83.9, G90.01-G90.09, G90.2, G90.4-G90.9, G92, G93.40-G93.49, G93.81, G93.89-G95.9, G96.8-G96.9, G98.0-G99.8, I67.83, R53.2

G36.0   **Neuromyelitis optica [Devic]** Ⓜ
Inflammatory disorder in which immune system attacks optic nerves and spinal cord producing inflammation of optic nerve (optic neuritis) and spinal cord (myelitis)
Demyelination in optic neuritis
> **Excludes1**   optic neuritis NOS (H46)

Ⓔ G36.0, G93.40-G93.49, I67.83

G36.1   **Acute and subacute hemorrhagic leukoencephalitis [Hurst]** Ⓜ

G36.8   **Other specified acute disseminated demyelination** Ⓜ

G36.9   **Acute disseminated demyelination, unspecified** Ⓜ

● **G37**   **Other demyelinating diseases of central nervous system**
Destruction of central nervous system

G37.0   **Diffuse sclerosis of central nervous system** Ⓜ
Periaxial encephalitis
Schilder's disease
> **Excludes1**   X linked adrenoleukodystrophy (E71.52-)

Ⓔ A92.30-A92.39, B97.21, G93.40-G93.49, I67.83

G37.1   **Central demyelination of corpus callosum** Ⓜ
Ⓔ See G36

G37.2   **Central pontine myelinolysis** Ⓜ
Ⓔ See G36

G37.3   **Acute transverse myelitis in demyelinating disease of central nervous system** Ⓜ
Acute transverse myelitis NOS
Acute transverse myelopathy
> **Excludes1**   multiple sclerosis (G35)
> neuromyelitis optica [Devic] (G36.0)

Ⓔ A02.21, A17.0-A27.81, A39.0, A50.41, A51.41, A52.13, A54.82, A54.84, A54.89-A54.9, A87.0-A87.9, A96.2, A98.3-A98.4, B00.3, B00.89-B00.9, B02.0-B02.29, B02.7-B02.9, B10.81-B10.89, B26.1, B33.24-B33.8, B34.1-B34.2, B34.4-B34.8, B37.5, B38.4, B45.1, B58.2, B92, B94.2-B94.9, B97.10, B97.19, B97.29, B97.5-B97.6, B97.81-B97.89, E08.40-E08.49, E09.40-E09.49, E10.40-E10.49, E11.40-E11.49, E13.40-E13.49, G00.0-G03.9, G04.1-G04.2, G11.3, G11.8-G12.9, G32.0, G32.89-G37.2, G37.5-G37.9, G61.0, G80.0-G80.2, G80.4-G83.9, G90.01-G90.09, G90.2, G90.4-G90.9, G93.1, G93.40-G93.49, G95.0-G95.9, G96.12-G96.9, G97.1, G98.0-G99.8, I67.83, R53.2

G37.4   **Subacute necrotizing myelitis of central nervous system** Ⓜ
Ⓔ A17.82, A28.1, A50.42, A52.14, A75.9, A79.9, A81.1, A81.82-A81.89, A83.0-A85.8, A87.2, A88.0, A88.8, A92.1-A92.8, A93.0, B00.4, B00.82, B01.11-B01.12, B04, B06.01, B08.09, B08.20-B08.22, B08.60-B08.79, B09, B10.01-B10.09, B26.2, B27.00-B27.99, B33.1, B45.0, B45.2-B45.9, B54, B58.2, B75, B97.10, B97.21, G04.00-G04.01, G04.31, G04.81-G05.4, G37.0, G37.4-G37.5, H66.40-H66.43, J09.X3-J09.X9, J10.2-J10.89, J11.2-J11.89, L44.4, M1A.10X0-M1A.19X1, M32.0-M32.9, P35.2-P35.9, P37.0-P37.9, T56.0X1-T56.0X4[A]

Item 6–3   **Multiple sclerosis** (MS) is a nervous system disease affecting the brain and spinal cord by damaging the myelin sheath surrounding and protecting nerve cells. The damage slows down/blocks messages between the brain and body. Symptoms are: visual disturbances, muscle weakness, coordination and balance issues, numbness, prickling, thinking and memory problems. The cause is unknown, though it is thought that it may be an autoimmune disease. It affects women more than men, between 20 and 40 years of age. MS can be mild, but it may cause the loss of ability to write, walk, and speak. There is no cure, but medication may slow or control symptoms.

G37.5   **Concentric sclerosis [Baló] of central nervous system** Ⓜ
Ⓔ See G37.0

G37.8   **Other specified demyelinating diseases of central nervous system** Ⓜ
Ⓔ See G36

G37.9   **Demyelinating disease of central nervous system, unspecified** Ⓜ
Ⓔ See G36

EPISODIC AND PAROXYSMAL DISORDERS (G40-G47)

● **G40**   **Epilepsy and recurrent seizures**
> **Note:** The following terms are to be considered equivalent to intractable: pharmacoresistant (pharmacologically resistant), treatment resistant, refractory (medically) and poorly controlled
> **Excludes1**   conversion disorder with seizures (F44.5)
> convulsions NOS (R56.9)
> hippocampal sclerosis (G93.81)
> mesial temporal sclerosis (G93.81)
> post traumatic seizures (R56.1)
> seizure (convulsive) NOS (R56.9)
> seizure of newborn (P90)
> temporal sclerosis (G93.81)
> Todd's paralysis (G83.8)

● **G40.0**   **Localization-related (focal) (partial) idiopathic epilepsy and epileptic syndromes with seizures of localized onset**
Benign childhood epilepsy with centrotemporal EEG spikes
Childhood epilepsy with occipital EEG paroxysms
> **Excludes1**   adult onset localization-related epilepsy (G40.1-, G40.2-)

● **G40.00**   **Localization-related (focal) (partial) idiopathic epilepsy and epileptic syndromes with seizures of localized onset, not intractable**
Localization-related (focal) (partial) idiopathic epilepsy and epileptic syndromes with seizures of localized onset without intractability

G40.001   **Localization-related (focal) (partial) idiopathic epilepsy and epileptic syndromes with seizures of localized onset, not intractable, with status epilepticus** Ⓜ
Ⓔ G32.89, G40.001-G40.319, G40.401-G40.919, G40.A01-G40.B19, G93.40-G93.49, G93.9, G96.8-G96.9, G98.0-G98.8, G99.8. I67.83, R56.1

G40.009   **Localization-related (focal) (partial) idiopathic epilepsy and epileptic syndromes with seizures of localized onset, not intractable, without status epilepticus** Ⓜ
Localization-related (focal) (partial) idiopathic epilepsy and epileptic syndromes with seizures of localized onset NOS
Ⓔ See G40.001

N Newborn Age: 0   **P** Pediatric Age: 0–17   **M** Maternity DX: 12–55   **A** Adult Age: 15–124   ♀ Females Only   ♂ Males Only
Ⓜ Complication\Comorbidity   Ⓜ Major C\C   Ⓔ CC/MCC Exclusions   Ⓜ Present on Admission Requirement   Ⓜ Hospital-Acquired Condition

885

● G40.01 Localization-related (focal) (partial) idiopathic epilepsy and epileptic syndromes with seizures of localized onset, intractable

 G40.011 Localization-related (focal) (partial) idiopathic epilepsy and epileptic syndromes with seizures of localized onset, intractable, with status epilepticus 🔖
  (Ex:) E08.40-E08.49, E09.40-E09.49, E10.40-E10.49, E11.40-E11.49, E13.40-E13.49, G32.89, G40.001-G40.319, G40.401-G40.919, G40.A01-G40.A19, G40.B01-G40.B19, G93.81, G93.89-G93.9, G96.8-G96.9, G98.0-G98.8, G99.8, R56.1

 G40.019 Localization-related (focal) (partial) idiopathic epilepsy and epileptic syndromes with seizures of localized onset, intractable, without status epilepticus 🔖
  (Ex:) See G40.011

● G40.1 Localization-related (focal) (partial) symptomatic epilepsy and epileptic syndromes with simple partial seizures
 Attacks without alteration of consciousness
 Epilepsia partialis continua [Kozhevnikof]
 Simple partial seizures developing into secondarily generalized seizures

 ● G40.10 Localization-related (focal) (partial) symptomatic epilepsy and epileptic syndromes with simple partial seizures, not intractable
  Localization-related (focal) (partial) symptomatic epilepsy and epileptic syndromes with simple partial seizures without intractability

  G40.101 Localization-related (focal) (partial) symptomatic epilepsy and epileptic syndromes with simple partial seizures, not intractable, with status epilepticus 🔖
   (Ex:) See G40.001

  G40.109 Localization-related (focal) (partial) symptomatic epilepsy and epileptic syndromes with simple partial seizures, not intractable, without status epilepticus 🔖
   Localization-related (focal) (partial) symptomatic epilepsy and epileptic syndromes with simple partial seizures NOS
   (Ex:) See G40.001

 ● G40.11 Localization-related (focal) (partial) symptomatic epilepsy and epileptic syndromes with simple partial seizures, intractable

  G40.111 Localization-related (focal) (partial) symptomatic epilepsy and epileptic syndromes with simple partial seizures, intractable, with status epilepticus 🔖
   (Ex:) See G40.011

  G40.119 Localization-related (focal) (partial) symptomatic epilepsy and epileptic syndromes with simple partial seizures, intractable, without status epilepticus 🔖
   (Ex:) See G40.011

● G40.2 Localization-related (focal) (partial) symptomatic epilepsy and epileptic syndromes with complex partial seizures
 Attacks with alteration of consciousness, often with automatisms
 Complex partial seizures developing into secondarily generalized seizures

 ● G40.20 Localization-related (focal) (partial) symptomatic epilepsy and epileptic syndromes with complex partial seizures, not intractable
  Localization-related (focal) (partial) symptomatic epilepsy and epileptic syndromes with complex partial seizures without intractability

  G40.201 Localization-related (focal) (partial) symptomatic epilepsy and epileptic syndromes with complex partial seizures, not intractable, with status epilepticus 🔖
   (Ex:) See G40.001

  G40.209 Localization-related (focal) (partial) symptomatic epilepsy and epileptic syndromes with complex partial seizures, not intractable, without status epilepticus 🔖
   Localization-related (focal) (partial) symptomatic epilepsy and epileptic syndromes with complex partial seizures NOS
   (Ex:) See G40.001

 ● G40.21 Localization-related (focal) (partial) symptomatic epilepsy and epileptic syndromes with complex partial seizures, intractable

  G40.211 Localization-related (focal) (partial) symptomatic epilepsy and epileptic syndromes with complex partial seizures, intractable, with status epilepticus 🔖
   (Ex:) See G40.011

  G40.219 Localization-related (focal) (partial) symptomatic epilepsy and epileptic syndromes with complex partial seizures, intractable, without status epilepticus 🔖
   (Ex:) See G40.011

● G40.3 Generalized idiopathic epilepsy and epileptic syndromes
 Code also MERRF syndrome, if applicable (E88.42)

 ● G40.30 Generalized idiopathic epilepsy and epileptic syndromes, not intractable
  Generalized idiopathic epilepsy and epileptic syndromes without intractability

  G40.301 Generalized idiopathic epilepsy and epileptic syndromes, not intractable, with status epilepticus 🔖
   (Ex:) E08.40-E08.49, E08.618-E08.638, E08.649-E08.8, E09.40-E09.49, E09.618-E09.638, E09.649-E09.8, E10.40-E10.49, E10.618-E10.638, E10.649, E10.69-E10.8, E11.40-E11.49, E11.618-E11.638, E11.649, E11.69-E11.8, E13.40-E13.49, E13.618-E13.638, E13.649-E13.8, G32.89, G40.001-G40.319, G40.401-G40.419, G40.501-G40.919, G40.A01-G40.B19, G93.81, G93.89-G93.9, G96.8-G96.9, G98.0-G98.8, G99.8, R56.1

  G40.309 Generalized idiopathic epilepsy and epileptic syndromes, not intractable, without status epilepticus
   Generalized idiopathic epilepsy and epileptic syndromes NOS

● **G40.31　Generalized idiopathic epilepsy and epileptic syndromes, intractable**

　　G40.311　Generalized idiopathic epilepsy and epileptic syndromes, intractable, with status epilepticus 🔖
　　　　Ⓔ See G40.301

　　G40.319　Generalized idiopathic epilepsy and epileptic syndromes, intractable, without status epilepticus 🔖
　　　　Ⓔ See G40.301

● **G40.A　Absence epileptic syndrome**
　　Childhood absence epilepsy [pyknolepsy]
　　Juvenile absence epilepsy
　　Absence epileptic syndrome, NOS
　　Ⓔ **For category G40.A CC codes:** See G40.011

● **G40.A0　Absence epileptic syndrome, not intractable**

　　G40.A01　Absence epileptic syndrome, not intractable, with status epilepticus 🔖

　　G40.A09　Absence epileptic syndrome, not intractable, without status epilepticus 🔖

● **G40.A1　Absence epileptic syndrome, intractable**

　　G40.A11　Absence epileptic syndrome, intractable, with status epilepticus 🔖

　　G40.A19　Absence epileptic syndrome, intractable, without status epilepticus 🔖

● **G40.B　Juvenile myoclonic epilepsy [impulsive petit mal]**
　　Ⓔ **For category G40.B CC codes:** See G40.011

● **G40.B0　Juvenile myoclonic epilepsy, not intractable**

　　G40.B01　Juvenile myoclonic epilepsy, not intractable, with status epilepticus 🔖

　　G40.B09　Juvenile myoclonic epilepsy, not intractable, without status epilepticus 🔖

● **G40.B1　Juvenile myoclonic epilepsy, intractable**

　　G40.B11　Juvenile myoclonic epilepsy, intractable, with status epilepticus 🔖

　　G40.B19　Juvenile myoclonic epilepsy, intractable, without status epilepticus 🔖

● **G40.4　Other generalized epilepsy and epileptic syndromes**
　　Epilepsy with grand mal seizures on awakening
　　Epilepsy with myoclonic absences
　　Epilepsy with myoclonic-astatic seizures
　　Grand mal seizure NOS
　　Nonspecific atonic epileptic seizures
　　Nonspecific clonic epileptic seizures
　　Nonspecific myoclonic epileptic seizures
　　Nonspecific tonic epileptic seizures
　　Nonspecific tonic-clonic epileptic seizures
　　Symptomatic early myoclonic encephalopathy

● **G40.40　Other generalized epilepsy and epileptic syndromes, not intractable**
　　Other generalized epilepsy and epileptic syndromes without intractability
　　Other generalized epilepsy and epileptic syndromes NOS

　　G40.401　Other generalized epilepsy and epileptic syndromes, not intractable, with status epilepticus 🔖
　　　　Ⓔ See G40.001

　　G40.409　Other generalized epilepsy and epileptic syndromes, not intractable, without status epilepticus 🔖
　　　　Ⓔ See G40.001

● **G40.41　Other generalized epilepsy and epileptic syndromes, intractable**

　　G40.411　Other generalized epilepsy and epileptic syndromes, intractable, with status epilepticus 🔖
　　　　Ⓔ See G40.011

　　G40.419　Other generalized epilepsy and epileptic syndromes, intractable, without status epilepticus 🔖
　　　　Ⓔ See G40.011

● **G40.5　Epileptic seizures related to external causes**
　　Epileptic seizures related to alcohol
　　Epileptic seizures related to drugs
　　Epileptic seizures related to hormonal changes
　　Epileptic seizures related to sleep deprivation
　　Epileptic seizures related to stress
　　Code also, if applicable, associated epilepsy and recurrent seizures (G40.-)
　　Use additional code for adverse effect, if applicable, to identify drug (T36-T50 with fifth or sixth character 5)
　　Ⓔ **For category G40.5 CC codes:** See G40.011

● **G40.50　Epileptic seizures related to external causes, not intractable**

　　G40.501　Epileptic seizures related to external causes, not intractable, with status epilepticus 🔖

　　G40.509　Epileptic seizures related to external causes, not intractable, without status epilepticus 🔖
　　　　Epileptic seizures related to external causes, NOS

● **G40.8　Other epilepsy and recurrent seizures**
　　Epilepsies and epileptic syndromes undetermined as to whether they are focal or generalized
　　Landau-Kleffner syndrome
　　Ⓔ **For category G40.8 CC codes:** See G40.011

● **G40.80　Other epilepsy**

　　G40.801　Other epilepsy, not intractable, with status epilepticus 🔖
　　　　Other epilepsy without intractability with status epilepticus

　　G40.802　Other epilepsy, not intractable, without status epilepticus 🔖
　　　　Other epilepsy NOS
　　　　Other epilepsy without intractability without status epilepticus

　　G40.803　Other epilepsy, intractable, with status epilepticus 🔖

　　G40.804　Other epilepsy, intractable, without status epilepticus 🔖

● **G40.81　Lennox-Gastaut syndrome**

　　G40.811　Lennox-Gastaut syndrome, not intractable, with status epilepticus 🔖

　　G40.812　Lennox-Gastaut syndrome, not intractable, without status epilepticus 🔖

　　G40.813　Lennox-Gastaut syndrome, intractable, with status epilepticus 🔖

　　G40.814　Lennox-Gastaut syndrome, intractable, without status epilepticus 🔖

● **G40.82　Epileptic spasms**
　　Infantile spasms
　　Salaam attacks
　　West's syndrome

　　G40.821　Epileptic spasms, not intractable, with status epilepticus 🔖

　　G40.822　Epileptic spasms, not intractable, without status epilepticus 🔖

CHAPTER 6 (G00-G99)

N Newborn Age: 0　　**P** Pediatric Age: 0–17　　**M** Maternity DX: 12–55　　**A** Adult Age: 15–124　　♀ Females Only　　♂ Males Only

🔖 Complication\Comorbidity　　🔖 Major C\C　　Ⓔ CC/MCC Exclusions　　🔖 Present on Admission Requirement　　🔖 Hospital-Acquired Condition

887

G40.823 Epileptic spasms, intractable, with status epilepticus 🔵

G40.824 Epileptic spasms, intractable, without status epilepticus 🔵

G40.89 Other seizures 🔵

> **Excludes1** post traumatic seizures (R56.1)
> recurrent seizures NOS (G40.909)
> seizure NOS (R56.9)

G40.9 Epilepsy, unspecified

G40.90 Epilepsy, unspecified, not intractable
Epilepsy, unspecified, without intractability

G40.901 Epilepsy, unspecified, not intractable, with status epilepticus

G40.909 Epilepsy, unspecified, not intractable, without status epilepticus
Epilepsy NOS
Epileptic convulsions NOS
Epileptic fits NOS
Epileptic seizures NOS
Recurrent seizures NOS
Seizure disorder NOS

G40.91 Epilepsy, unspecified, intractable
Intractable seizure disorder NOS
🅔🅧 For category G40.91 CC codes: See G40.011

G40.911 Epilepsy, unspecified, intractable, with status epilepticus 🔵

G40.919 Epilepsy, unspecified, intractable, without status epilepticus 🔵

G43 **Migraine**

Note: The following terms are to be considered equivalent to intractable: pharmacoresistant (pharmacologically resistant), treatment resistant, refractory (medically) and poorly controlled

Use additional code for adverse effect, if applicable, to identify drug (T36-T50 with fifth or sixth character 5)

> **Excludes1** headache NOS (R51)
> ~~headache syndromes (G44.-)~~
> lower half migraine (G44.00)

> **Excludes2** headache syndromes (G44.-) ◄

G43.0 Migraine without aura
Neurological disorder, generally recurring headaches without early symptom (aura)
Common migraine

> **Excludes1** chronic migraine without aura (G43.7-)

G43.00 Migraine without aura, not intractable
Migraine without aura without mention of refractory migraine
Neurological disorder, generally recurring headaches without early symptom (aura); resistant to cure, relief, or control

G43.001 Migraine without aura, not intractable, with status migrainosus

G43.009 Migraine without aura, not intractable, without status migrainosus
Migraine without aura NOS

G43.01 Migraine without aura, intractable
Migraine without aura with refractory migraine
Intractable migraine: Not easily cured or managed; relentless pain from a migraine

G43.011 Migraine without aura, intractable, with status migrainosus

G43.019 Migraine without aura, intractable, without status migrainosus

Item 6-4 Migraine headache is described as an intense pulsing or throbbing pain in one area of the head. It can be accompanied by extreme sensitivity to light (photophobic) and sound and is three times more common in women than in men. Symptoms include nausea and vomiting. Research indicates migraine headaches are caused by inherited abnormalities in genes that control the activities of certain cell populations in the brain.

G43.1 Migraine with aura
Basilar migraine
Classical migraine
Migraine equivalents
Migraine preceded or accompanied by transient focal neurological phenomena
Migraine triggered seizures
Migraine with acute-onset aura
Migraine with aura without headache (migraine equivalents)
Migraine with prolonged aura
Migraine with typical aura
Retinal migraine
Code also any associated seizure (G40.-, R56.9)

> **Excludes1** persistent migraine aura (G43.5-, G43.6-)

G43.10 Migraine with aura, not intractable
Migraine with aura without mention of refractory migraine

G43.101 Migraine with aura, not intractable, with status migrainosus

G43.109 Migraine with aura, not intractable, without status migrainosus
Migraine with aura NOS

G43.11 Migraine with aura, intractable
Migraine with aura with refractory migraine

G43.111 Migraine with aura, intractable, with status migrainosus

G43.119 Migraine with aura, intractable, without status migrainosus

G43.4 Hemiplegic migraine
Familial migraine
Sporadic migraine
Inherited migraine disorder causing temporary paralysis of one side of body followed by severe headache and nausea

G43.40 Hemiplegic migraine, not intractable
Hemiplegic migraine without refractory migraine

G43.401 Hemiplegic migraine, not intractable, with status migrainosus

G43.409 Hemiplegic migraine, not intractable, without status migrainosus
Hemiplegic migraine NOS

G43.41 Hemiplegic migraine, intractable
Hemiplegic migraine with refractory migraine

G43.411 Hemiplegic migraine, intractable, with status migrainosus

G43.419 Hemiplegic migraine, intractable, without status migrainosus

G43.5 Persistent migraine aura without cerebral infarction

G43.50 Persistent migraine aura without cerebral infarction, not intractable
Persistent migraine aura without cerebral infarction, without refractory migraine

G43.501 Persistent migraine aura without cerebral infarction, not intractable, with status migrainosus

G43.509 Persistent migraine aura without cerebral infarction, not intractable, without status migrainosus
Persistent migraine aura NOS

● **G43.51** **Persistent migraine aura without cerebral infarction, intractable**
> Persistent migraine aura without cerebral infarction, with refractory migraine

    G43.511 **Persistent migraine aura without cerebral infarction, intractable, with status migrainosus**

    G43.519 **Persistent migraine aura without cerebral infarction, intractable, without status migrainosus**

● **G43.6** **Persistent migraine aura with cerebral infarction**
> *Visual, motor, or psychic disturbances, paresthesias, and related neurologic abnormalities accompanying migraine*

> Code also the type of cerebral infarction (I63.-)

● **G43.60** **Persistent migraine aura with cerebral infarction, not intractable**
> Persistent migraine aura with cerebral infarction, without refractory migraine
>
> (Ex) For category G43.6 CC codes: G43.601-G43.619, I63.00-I66.9

    G43.601 **Persistent migraine aura with cerebral infarction, not intractable, with status migrainosus** ℅

    G43.609 **Persistent migraine aura with cerebral infarction, not intractable, without status migrainosus** ℅

● **G43.61** **Persistent migraine aura with cerebral infarction, intractable**
> Persistent migraine aura with cerebral infarction, with refractory migraine

    G43.611 **Persistent migraine aura with cerebral infarction, intractable, with status migrainosus** ℅

    G43.619 **Persistent migraine aura with cerebral infarction, intractable, without status migrainosus** ℅

● **G43.7** **Chronic migraine without aura**
> Transformed migraine
>
> **Excludes1**   migraine without aura (G43.0-)

● **G43.70** **Chronic migraine without aura, not intractable**
> Chronic migraine without aura, without refractory migraine

    G43.701 **Chronic migraine without aura, not intractable, with status migrainosus**

    G43.709 **Chronic migraine without aura, not intractable, without status migrainosus**
> > Chronic migraine without aura NOS

● **G43.71** **Chronic migraine without aura, intractable**
> Chronic migraine without aura, with refractory migraine

    G43.711 **Chronic migraine without aura, intractable, with status migrainosus**

    G43.719 **Chronic migraine without aura, intractable, without status migrainosus**

● **G43.A** **Cyclical vomiting**

    G43.A0 **Cyclical vomiting, not intractable**
> > Cyclical vomiting, without refractory migraine

    G43.A1 **Cyclical vomiting, intractable**
> > Cyclical vomiting, with refractory migraine

● **G43.B** **Ophthalmoplegic migraine**

    G43.B0 **Ophthalmoplegic migraine, not intractable**
> > Ophthalmoplegic migraine, without refractory migraine

    G43.B1 **Ophthalmoplegic migraine, intractable**
> > Ophthalmoplegic migraine, with refractory migraine

● **G43.C** **Periodic headache syndromes in child or adult**

    G43.C0 **Periodic headache syndromes in child or adult, not intractable**
> > Periodic headache syndromes in child or adult, without refractory migraine

    G43.C1 **Periodic headache syndromes in child or adult, intractable**
> > Periodic headache syndromes in child or adult, with refractory migraine

● **G43.D** **Abdominal migraine**

    G43.D0 **Abdominal migraine, not intractable**
> > Abdominal migraine, without refractory migraine

    G43.D1 **Abdominal migraine, intractable**
> > Abdominal migraine, with refractory migraine

● **G43.8** **Other migraine**

● **G43.80** **Other migraine, not intractable**
> Other migraine, without refractory migraine

    G43.801 **Other migraine, not intractable, with status migrainosus**

    G43.809 **Other migraine, not intractable, without status migrainosus**

● **G43.81** **Other migraine, intractable**
> Other migraine, with refractory migraine

    G43.811 **Other migraine, intractable, with status migrainosus**

    G43.819 **Other migraine, intractable, without status migrainosus**

● **G43.82** **Menstrual migraine, not intractable**
> Menstrual headache, not intractable
> Menstrual migraine, without refractory migraine
> Menstrually related migraine, not intractable
> Pre-menstrual headache, not intractable
> Pre-menstrual migraine, not intractable
> Pure menstrual migraine, not intractable
>
> Code also associated premenstrual tension syndrome (N94.3)

    G43.821 **Menstrual migraine, not intractable, with status migrainosus** ♀

    G43.829 **Menstrual migraine, not intractable, without status migrainosus** ♀
> > Menstrual migraine NOS

● **G43.83** **Menstrual migraine, intractable**
> Menstrual headache, intractable
> Menstrual migraine, with refractory migraine
> Menstrually related migraine, intractable
> Pre-menstrual headache, intractable
> Pre-menstrual migraine, intractable
> Pure menstrual migraine, intractable
>
> Code also associated premenstrual tension syndrome (N94.3)

    G43.831 **Menstrual migraine, intractable, with status migrainosus** ♀

    G43.839 **Menstrual migraine, intractable, without status migrainosus** ♀

● **G43.9** **Migraine, unspecified**

● **G43.90** **Migraine, unspecified, not intractable**
> Migraine, unspecified, without refractory migraine

    G43.901 **Migraine, unspecified, not intractable, with status migrainosus**
> > Status migrainosus NOS

    G43.909 **Migraine, unspecified, not intractable, without status migrainosus**
> > Migraine NOS

N Newborn Age: 0   **P** Pediatric Age: 0–17   **M** Maternity DX: 12–55   **A** Adult Age: 15–124   ♀ Females Only   ♂ Males Only

℅ Complication\Comorbidity   Major C\C   (Ex) CC/MCC Exclusions   Present on Admission Requirement   Hospital-Acquired Condition

889

CHAPTER 6 (G00-G99)

● **G43.91**   **Migraine, unspecified, intractable**
Migraine, unspecified, with refractory
migraine

G43.911   **Migraine, unspecified, intractable, with status migrainosus**

G43.919   **Migraine, unspecified, intractable, without status migrainosus**

● **G44**   **Other headache syndromes**

Excludes1   headache NOS (R51)

Excludes2   atypical facial pain (G50.1)
headache due to lumbar puncture (G97.1)
migraines (G43.-)
trigeminal neuralgia (G50.0)

● **G44.0**   **Cluster headaches and other trigeminal autonomic cephalgias (TAC)**

● **G44.00**   **Cluster headache syndrome, unspecified**
Ciliary neuralgia
Cluster headache NOS
Histamine cephalgia
Lower half migraine
Migrainous neuralgia

G44.001   **Cluster headache syndrome, unspecified, intractable**

G44.009   **Cluster headache syndrome, unspecified, not intractable**
Cluster headache syndrome NOS

● **G44.01**   **Episodic cluster headache**

G44.011   **Episodic cluster headache, intractable**

G44.019   **Episodic cluster headache, not intractable**
Episodic cluster headache NOS

● **G44.02**   **Chronic cluster headache**

G44.021   **Chronic cluster headache, intractable**

G44.029   **Chronic cluster headache, not intractable**
Chronic cluster headache NOS

● **G44.03**   **Episodic paroxysmal hemicrania**
Paroxysmal hemicrania NOS

G44.031   **Episodic paroxysmal hemicrania, intractable**

G44.039   **Episodic paroxysmal hemicrania, not intractable**
Episodic paroxysmal hemicrania NOS

● **G44.04**   **Chronic paroxysmal hemicrania**
Unilateral headache

G44.041   **Chronic paroxysmal hemicrania, intractable**

G44.049   **Chronic paroxysmal hemicrania, not intractable**
Chronic paroxysmal hemicrania NOS

● **G44.05**   **Short lasting unilateral neuralgiform headache with conjunctival injection and tearing (SUNCT)**

G44.051   **Short lasting unilateral neuralgiform headache with conjunctival injection and tearing (SUNCT), intractable**

G44.059   **Short lasting unilateral neuralgiform headache with conjunctival injection and tearing (SUNCT), not intractable**
Short lasting unilateral neuralgiform headache with conjunctival injection and tearing (SUNCT) NOS

● **G44.09**   **Other trigeminal autonomic cephalgias (TAC)**
Cluster headaches

G44.091   **Other trigeminal autonomic cephalgias (TAC), intractable**

G44.099   **Other trigeminal autonomic cephalgias (TAC), not intractable**

● **G44.1**   **Vascular headache, not elsewhere classified**

Excludes2   cluster headache (G44.0)
complicated headache syndromes (G44.5-)
drug-induced headache (G44.4-)
migraine (G43.-)
other specified headache syndromes (G44.8-)
post-traumatic headache (G44.3-)
tension-type headache (G44.2-)

● **G44.2**   **Tension-type headache**

● **G44.20**   **Tension-type headache, unspecified**

G44.201   **Tension-type headache, unspecified, intractable**

G44.209   **Tension-type headache, unspecified, not intractable**
Tension headache NOS

● **G44.21**   **Episodic tension-type headache**

G44.211   **Episodic tension-type headache, intractable**

G44.219   **Episodic tension-type headache, not intractable**
Episodic tension-type headache NOS

● **G44.22**   **Chronic tension-type headache**

G44.221   **Chronic tension-type headache, intractable**

G44.229   **Chronic tension-type headache, not intractable**
Chronic tension-type headache NOS

● **G44.3**   **Post-traumatic headache**

● **G44.30**   **Post-traumatic headache, unspecified**

G44.301   **Post-traumatic headache, unspecified, intractable**

G44.309   **Post-traumatic headache, unspecified, not intractable**
Post-traumatic headache NOS

● **G44.31**   **Acute post-traumatic headache**

G44.311   **Acute post-traumatic headache, intractable**

G44.319   **Acute post-traumatic headache, not intractable**
Acute post-traumatic headache NOS

● **G44.32**   **Chronic post-traumatic headache**

G44.321   **Chronic post-traumatic headache, intractable**

G44.329   **Chronic post-traumatic headache, not intractable**
Chronic post-traumatic headache NOS

● **G44.4**   **Drug-induced headache, not elsewhere classified**
Medication overuse headache

Use additional code for adverse effect, if applicable, to identify drug (T36-T50 with fifth or sixth character 5)

G44.40   **Drug-induced headache, not elsewhere classified, not intractable**

G44.41   **Drug-induced headache, not elsewhere classified, intractable**

● **G44.5**   **Complicated headache syndromes**

G44.51   **Hemicrania continua**
Persistent unilateral headache

G44.52   **New daily persistent headache (NDPH)**

G44.53   **Primary thunderclap headache**

G44.59   **Other complicated headache syndrome**

● **G44.8   Other specified headache syndromes**

     G44.81   Hypnic headache
         Benign primary headaches

     G44.82   Headache associated with sexual activity
         Orgasmic headache
         Preorgasmic headache

     G44.83   Primary cough headache

     G44.84   Primary exertional headache

     G44.85   Primary stabbing headache

     G44.89   Other headache syndrome

● **G45   Transient cerebral ischemic attacks and related syndromes**

     Excludes1   neonatal cerebral ischemia (P91.0)
                 transient retinal artery occlusion (H34.0-)

     (Ex) **For category G45 CC codes:** E08.51-E08.59, E08.618-E08.638, E08.649-E08.8, E09.51-E09.59, E09.618-E09.638, E09.649-E09.8, E10.51-E10.59, E10.618-E10.638, E10.649, E10.69-E10.8, E11.51-E11.59, E11.618-E11.638, E11.649, E11.69, E11.8, E13.51-E13.59, E13.618-E13.638, E13.649-E13.8, G45.0-G45.2, G45.8-G46.2, I63.00-I63.02, I63.29, I65.01-I65.9, I67.841-I67.848, I87.8, I99.8-I99.9

     G45.0   Vertebro-basilar artery syndrome 🔗

     G45.1   Carotid artery syndrome (hemispheric) 🔗

     G45.2   Multiple and bilateral precerebral artery syndromes 🔗

     G45.3   Amaurosis fugax 🔗
         Transient visual loss in one eye

     G45.4   Transient global amnesia
         Episode of short-term memory loss, nonrecurrent, lasting few hours

         Excludes1   amnesia NOS (R41.3)

     G45.8   Other transient cerebral ischemic attacks and related syndromes 🔗

     G45.9   Transient cerebral ischemic attack, unspecified 🔗
         Spasm of cerebral artery
         TIA
         Transient cerebral ischemia NOS

● **G46   Vascular syndromes of brain in cerebrovascular diseases**

     Code first underlying cerebrovascular disease (I60-I69)

     G46.0   Middle cerebral artery syndrome 🔗
         (Ex) See G45

     G46.1   Anterior cerebral artery syndrome 🔗
         (Ex) See G45

     G46.2   Posterior cerebral artery syndrome 🔗
         (Ex) See G45

     G46.3   Brain stem stroke syndrome
         Benedikt syndrome
         Claude syndrome
         Foville syndrome
         Millard-Gubler syndrome
         Wallenberg syndrome
         Weber syndrome

     G46.4   Cerebellar stroke syndrome

     G46.5   Pure motor lacunar syndrome
         Occlusion of single deep penetrating artery

     G46.6   Pure sensory lacunar syndrome

     G46.7   Other lacunar syndromes

     G46.8   Other vascular syndromes of brain in cerebrovascular diseases

● **G47   Sleep disorders**

     Excludes2   nightmares (F51.5)
                 nonorganic sleep disorders (F51.-)
                 sleep terrors (F51.4)
                 sleepwalking (F51.3)

● **G47.0   Insomnia**

     Excludes2   alcohol related insomnia (F10.182, F10.282, F10.982)
                 ~~drug related insomnia F11.182, F11.282, F11.982, F13.182, F13.282, F13.982, F14.182, F14.282, F14.982, F15.182, F15.282, F15.982, F19.182, F19.282, F19.982~~
                 drug-related insomnia (F11.182, F11.282, F11.982, F13.182, F13.282, F13.982, F14.182, F14.282, F14.982, F15.182, F15.282, F15.982, F19.182, F19.282, F19.982) ◄
                 idiopathic insomnia (F51.01)
                 insomnia due to a mental disorder (F51.05)
                 insomnia not due to a substance or known physiological condition (F51.0-)
                 nonorganic insomnia (F51.0-)
                 primary insomnia (F51.01)
                 sleep apnea (G47.3-)

     G47.00   Insomnia, unspecified
         Insomnia NOS

     G47.01   Insomnia due to medical condition
         Code also associated medical condition

     G47.09   Other insomnia

● **G47.1   Hypersomnia**

     Excludes2   alcohol-related hypersomnia (F10.182, F10.282, F10.982)
                 ~~drug-related hypersomnia F11.182, F11.282, F11.982, F13.182, F13.282, F13.982, F14.182, F14.282, F14.982, F15.182, F15.282, F15.982, F19.182, F19.282, F19.982~~
                 drug-related hypersomnia (F11.182, F11.282, F11.982, F13.182, F13.282, F13.982, F14.182, F14.282, F14.982, F15.182, F15.282, F15.982, F19.182, F19.282, F19.982) ◄
                 hypersomnia due to a mental disorder (F51.13)
                 hypersomnia not due to a substance or known physiological condition (F51.1-)
                 primary hypersomnia (F51.11)
                 sleep apnea (G47.3-)

     G47.10   Hypersomnia, unspecified
         Hypersomnia NOS

     G47.11   Idiopathic hypersomnia with long sleep time
         Idiopathic hypersomnia NOS

     G47.12   Idiopathic hypersomnia without long sleep time

     G47.13   Recurrent hypersomnia
         Kleine-Levin syndrome
         Menstrual related hypersomnia

     G47.14   Hypersomnia due to medical condition
         Code also associated medical condition

     G47.19   Other hypersomnia

● **G47.2   Circadian rhythm sleep disorders**
     Disorders of the sleep wake schedule
     Inversion of nyctohemeral rhythm
     Inversion of sleep rhythm

     G47.20   Circadian rhythm sleep disorder, unspecified type
         Sleep wake schedule disorder NOS

     G47.21   Circadian rhythm sleep disorder, delayed sleep phase type
         Delayed sleep phase syndrome

     G47.22   Circadian rhythm sleep disorder, advanced sleep phase type

     G47.23   Circadian rhythm sleep disorder, irregular sleep wake type
         Irregular sleep-wake pattern

CHAPTER 6 (G00-G99)

N   Newborn Age: 0   **P**   Pediatric Age: 0–17   **M**   Maternity DX: 12–55   **A**   Adult Age: 15–124   ♀   Females Only   ♂   Males Only

🔗   Complication\Comorbidity   🔗   Major C\C   (Ex)   CC/MCC Exclusions   🔗   Present on Admission Requirement   🔗   Hospital-Acquired Condition

891

G47.24   Circadian rhythm sleep disorder, free running type

G47.25   Circadian rhythm sleep disorder, jet lag type

G47.26   Circadian rhythm sleep disorder, shift work type

▷ *G47.27   Circadian rhythm sleep disorder in conditions classified elsewhere*
        Code first underlying condition

G47.29   Other circadian rhythm sleep disorder

● G47.3   Sleep apnea
        Characterized by episodes in which breathing stops during sleep
        Code also any associated underlying condition

        Excludes1   apnea NOS (R06.81) ◀▥
                Cheyne-Stokes breathing (R06.3)
                pickwickian syndrome (E66.2)
                sleep apnea of newborn (P28.3)

    G47.30   Sleep apnea, unspecified
            Sleep apnea NOS

    G47.31   Primary central sleep apnea

    G47.32   High altitude periodic breathing

    G47.33   Obstructive sleep apnea (adult) (pediatric)
            Excludes1   obstructive sleep apnea of newborn (P28.3)

    G47.34   Idiopathic sleep related nonobstructive alveolar hypoventilation
            Sleep related hypoxia

    G47.35   Congenital central alveolar hypoventilation syndrome

▷ *G47.36   Sleep related hypoventilation in conditions classified elsewhere*
            Sleep related hypoxemia in conditions classified elsewhere
            Code first underlying condition

▷ *G47.37   Central sleep apnea in conditions classified elsewhere*
            Code first underlying condition

    G47.39   Other sleep apnea

● G47.4   Narcolepsy and cataplexy
        *Cataplexy is a disorder evidenced by seizures including minor slacking of the facial muscles to complete collapse and often affects people who have **narcolepsy**, a disorder in which there is great difficulty remaining awake during the daytime.*

    ● G47.41   Narcolepsy
            G47.411   Narcolepsy with cataplexy
            G47.419   Narcolepsy without cataplexy
                    Narcolepsy NOS

    ● G47.42   Narcolepsy in conditions classified elsewhere
            Code first underlying condition ◀
        ▷ *G47.421   Narcolepsy in conditions classified elsewhere with cataplexy*
        ▷ *G47.429   Narcolepsy in conditions classified elsewhere without cataplexy*

● G47.5   Parasomnia
        Excludes1   alcohol induced parasomnia (F10.182, F10.282, F10.982)
                drug induced parasomnia (F11.182, F11.282, F11.982, F13.182, F13.282, F13.982, F14.182, F14.282, F14.982, F15.182, F15.282, F15.982, F19.182, F19.282, F19.982)
                parasomnia not due to a substance or known physiological condition (F51.8)

    G47.50   Parasomnia, unspecified
            Parasomnia NOS

    G47.51   Confusional arousals

    G47.52   REM sleep behavior disorder

    G47.53   Recurrent isolated sleep paralysis

▷ *G47.54   Parasomnia in conditions classified elsewhere*
            Code first underlying condition

    G47.59   Other parasomnia

● G47.6   Sleep related movement disorders
        Excludes2   restless legs syndrome (G25.81)

    G47.61   Periodic limb movement disorder
            Periodic limb movement disorder

    G47.62   Sleep related leg cramps

    G47.63   Sleep related bruxism
            Excludes1   psychogenic bruxism (F45.8)

    G47.69   Other sleep related movement disorders

G47.8   Other sleep disorders

G47.9   Sleep disorder, unspecified
        Sleep disorder NOS

(See Plate 118 on page 54.)

NERVE, NERVE ROOT AND PLEXUS DISORDERS (G50-G59)

Excludes1   current traumatic nerve, nerve root and plexus disorders - see Injury, nerve by body region
        neuralgia NOS (M79.2)
        neuritis NOS (M79.2)
        peripheral neuritis in pregnancy (O26.82-)
        radiculitis NOS (M54.1-)

● G50   Disorders of trigeminal nerve
        Includes   disorders of 5th cranial nerve

    G50.0   Trigeminal neuralgia
            Syndrome of paroxysmal facial pain
            Tic douloureux

    G50.1   Atypical facial pain

    G50.8   Other disorders of trigeminal nerve

    G50.9   Disorder of trigeminal nerve, unspecified

● G51   Facial nerve disorders
        Includes   disorders of 7th cranial nerve

    G51.0   Bell's palsy
            Facial palsy

    G51.1   Geniculate ganglionitis
            Rare disorder with symptoms of severe pain deep in ear, spreading to ear canal, outer ear, mastoid or eye regions
            Excludes1   postherpetic geniculate ganglionitis (B02.21)

    G51.2   Melkersson's syndrome
            Melkersson-Rosenthal syndrome

    G51.3   Clonic hemifacial spasm

    G51.4   Facial myokymia
            Involuntary facial muscle movement

    G51.8   Other disorders of facial nerve

    G51.9   Disorder of facial nerve, unspecified

● G52   Disorders of other cranial nerves
        Excludes2   disorders of acoustic [8th] nerve (H93.3)
                disorders of optic [2nd] nerve (H46, H47.0)
                paralytic strabismus due to nerve palsy (H49.0-H49.2)

    G52.0   Disorders of olfactory nerve
            Disorders of 1st cranial nerve

    G52.1   Disorders of glossopharyngeal nerve
            Disorder of 9th cranial nerve
            Glossopharyngeal neuralgia

    G52.2   Disorders of vagus nerve
            Disorders of pneumogastric [10th] nerve

Item 6-5   Trigeminal neuralgia, tic douloureux, is a pain syndrome diagnosed from the patient's history alone. The condition is characterized by pain and a brief facial spasm or tic. Pain is unilateral and follows the sensory distribution of cranial nerve V, typically radiating to the maxillary (V2) or mandibular (V3) area.

Item 6-6   The most common facial nerve disorder is **Bell's Palsy,** which occurs suddenly and results in facial drooping unilaterally. This disorder is the result of a reaction to a virus that causes the facial nerve in the ear to swell resulting in pressure in the bony canal.

◀ New   ◀▥ Revised   ~~deleted~~ Deleted   Excludes 1   Excludes 2   Includes   Use additional   Code first   Code also   Unspecified

OGCR Official Guidelines   ● Unacceptable Principal Diagnosis   X Assign placeholder X   ● Use Additional Character(s)   ▷ Manifestation Code   **Coding Clinic**

G52.3   **Disorders of hypoglossal nerve**
Disorders of 12th cranial nerve

G52.7   **Disorders of multiple cranial nerves**
Polyneuritis cranialis

G52.8   **Disorders of other specified cranial nerves**

G52.9   **Cranial nerve disorder, unspecified**

▶ *G53*   *Cranial nerve disorders in diseases classified elsewhere*
Code first underlying disease, such as:
neoplasm (C00-D49)

> **Excludes1**   multiple cranial nerve palsy in sarcoidosis
> (D86.82)
> multiple cranial nerve palsy in syphilis (A52.15)
> postherpetic geniculate ganglionitis (B02.21)
> postherpetic trigeminal neuralgia (B02.22)

● **G54**   **Nerve root and plexus disorders**
Raiculopathy (nerve root disorder) caused by pressure on nerve root,
most common cause is herniation of intervertebral disk. Plexus
disorders (plexopathies) are due to compression or injury.

> **Excludes1**   current traumatic nerve root and plexus disorders
> - see nerve injury by body region
> intervertebral disc disorders (M50-M51)
> neuralgia or neuritis NOS (M79.2)
> neuritis or radiculitis brachial NOS (M54.13) ◀▥
> ~~brachial NOS (M54.13)~~
> neuritis or radiculitis lumbar NOS (M54.16) ◀▥
> neuritis or radiculitis lumbosacral NOS
> (M54.17) ◀▥
> neuritis or radiculitis thoracic NOS (M54.14) ◀▥
> radiculitis NOS (M54.10) ◀▥
> radiculopathy NOS (M54.10) ◀▥
> spondylosis (M47.-) ◀▥

G54.0   **Brachial plexus disorders**
Thoracic outlet syndrome

G54.1   **Lumbosacral plexus disorders**

G54.2   **Cervical root disorders, not elsewhere classified**

● **G54.3**   **Thoracic root disorders, not elsewhere classified**

G54.4   **Lumbosacral root disorders, not elsewhere classified**

G54.5   **Neuralgic amyotrophy**
Parsonage-Aldren-Turner syndrome
Shoulder-girdle neuritis

> **Excludes1**   neuralgic amyotrophy in diabetes
> mellitus (E08-E13 with .44)

G54.6   **Phantom limb syndrome with pain**
Sensations (cramping, itching) in a limb that no longer
exists.

G54.7   **Phantom limb syndrome without pain**
Phantom limb syndrome NOS

G54.8   **Other nerve root and plexus disorders**

G54.9   **Nerve root and plexus disorder, unspecified**

▶ *G55*   *Nerve root and plexus compressions in diseases classified*
elsewhere
Code first underlying disease, such as:
neoplasm (C00-D49)

> **Excludes1**   nerve root compression (due to) (in) ankylosing
> spondylitis (M45.-)
> nerve root compression (due to) (in)dorsopathies
> (M53.-, M54.-)
> nerve root compression (due to) (in)intervertebral
> disc disorders (M50.1.-, M51.1.-)
> nerve root compression (due to) (in)
> spondylopathies (M46.-, M48.-)
> ~~nerve root compression (due to) (in)spondylosis~~
> ~~(M47.0-M47.2.-)~~

(See Plates 472 and 473 on pages 56 and 57.)

● **G56**   **Mononeuropathies of upper limb**

> **Excludes1**   current traumatic nerve disorder - see nerve
> injury by body region

● **G56.0**   **Carpal tunnel syndrome**

   G56.00   Carpal tunnel syndrome, unspecified upper
limb

   G56.01   Carpal tunnel syndrome, right upper limb

   G56.02   Carpal tunnel syndrome, left upper limb

● **G56.1**   **Other lesions of median nerve**

   G56.10   Other lesions of median nerve, unspecified side

   G56.11   Other lesions of median nerve, right upper
limb

   G56.12   Other lesions of median nerve, left upper limb

● **G56.2**   **Lesion of ulnar nerve**
Tardy ulnar nerve palsy

   G56.20   Lesion of ulnar nerve, unspecified upper limb

   G56.21   Lesion of ulnar nerve, right upper limb

   G56.22   Lesion of ulnar nerve, left upper limb

● **G56.3**   **Lesion of radial nerve**

   G56.30   Lesion of radial nerve, unspecified upper limb

   G56.31   Lesion of radial nerve, right upper limb

   G56.32   Lesion of radial nerve, left upper limb

● **G56.4**   **Causalgia of upper limb**
Intense burning pain and sensitivity to slight touch
Complex regional pain syndrome II of upper limb

> **Excludes1**   complex regional pain syndrome I of
> lower limb (G90.52-)
> complex regional pain syndrome I of
> upper limb (G90.51-)
> complex regional pain syndrome II of
> lower limb (G57.7-)
> reflex sympathetic dystrophy of lower
> limb (G90.52-)
> reflex sympathetic dystrophy (G90.51-)

   G56.40   Causalgia of unspecified upper limb

   G56.41   Causalgia of right upper limb

   G56.42   Causalgia of left upper limb

● **G56.8**   **Other specified mononeuropathies of upper limb**
Disease of a single nerve
Interdigital neuroma of upper limb

   G56.80   Other specified mononeuropathies
of unspecified upper limb

   G56.81   Other specified mononeuropathies of right
upper limb

   G56.82   Other specified mononeuropathies of left upper
limb

● **G56.9**   **Unspecified mononeuropathy of upper limb**
Disease of a single nerve

   G56.90   Unspecified mononeuropathy of unspecified
upper limb

   G56.91   Unspecified mononeuropathy of right upper
limb

   G56.92   Unspecified mononeuropathy of left upper
limb

● **G57**   **Mononeuropathies of lower limb**

> **Excludes1**   current traumatic nerve disorder - see nerve
> injury by body region

(See Plates 544 and 545 on pages 58 and 59.)

● **G57.0**   **Lesion of sciatic nerve**

> **Excludes1**   sciatica NOS (M54.3-)
> **Excludes2**   sciatica attributed to intervertebral disc
> disorder (M51.1.-)

   G57.00   Lesion of sciatic nerve, unspecified lower limb

   G57.01   Lesion of sciatic nerve, right lower limb

   G57.02   Lesion of sciatic nerve, left lower limb

CHAPTER 6 (G00-G99)

N   Newborn Age: 0   P   Pediatric Age: 0–17   M   Maternity DX: 12–55   A   Adult Age: 15–124   ♀   Females Only   ♂   Males Only

🝢 Complication\Comorbidity   🝢 Major C\C   (Ex) CC/MCC Exclusions   ◉ Present on Admission Requirement   🝢 Hospital-Acquired Condition

● **G57.1   Meralgia paresthetica**
Numbness or pain in outer thigh caused by injury to nerve
Lateral cutaneous nerve of thigh syndrome

    G57.10   Meralgia paresthetica, unspecified lower limb

    G57.11   Meralgia paresthetica, right lower limb

    G57.12   Meralgia paresthetica, left lower limb

● **G57.2   Lesion of femoral nerve**

    G57.20   Lesion of femoral nerve, unspecified lower limb

    G57.21   Lesion of femoral nerve, right lower limb

    G57.22   Lesion of femoral nerve, left lower limb

● **G57.3   Lesion of lateral popliteal nerve**
Peroneal nerve palsy

    G57.30   Lesion of lateral popliteal nerve, unspecified lower limb

    G57.31   Lesion of lateral popliteal nerve, right lower limb

    G57.32   Lesion of lateral popliteal nerve, left lower limb

● **G57.4   Lesion of medial popliteal nerve**

    G57.40   Lesion of medial popliteal nerve, unspecified lower limb

    G57.41   Lesion of medial popliteal nerve, right lower limb

    G57.42   Lesion of medial popliteal nerve, left lower limb

● **G57.5   Tarsal tunnel syndrome**

    G57.50   Tarsal tunnel syndrome, unspecified lower limb

    G57.51   Tarsal tunnel syndrome, right lower limb

    G57.52   Tarsal tunnel syndrome, left lower limb

● **G57.6   Lesion of plantar nerve**
Morton's metatarsalgia

    G57.60   Lesion of plantar nerve, unspecified lower limb

    G57.61   Lesion of plantar nerve, right lower limb

    G57.62   Lesion of plantar nerve, left lower limb

● **G57.7   Causalgia of lower limb**
Complex regional pain syndrome II of lower limb

    Excludes1   complex regional pain syndrome I of lower limb (G90.52-)
               complex regional pain syndrome I of upper limb (G90.51-)
               complex regional pain syndrome II of upper limb (G56.4-)
               reflex sympathetic dystrophy of lower limb (G90.52-)
               reflex sympathetic dystrophy of upper limb (G90.51-)

    G57.70   Causalgia of unspecified lower limb

    G57.71   Causalgia of right lower limb

    G57.72   Causalgia of left lower limb

● **G57.8   Other specified mononeuropathies of lower limb**
Interdigital neuroma of lower limb

    G57.80   Other specified mononeuropathies of unspecified lower limb

    G57.81   Other specified mononeuropathies of right lower limb

    G57.82   Other specified mononeuropathies of left lower limb

● **G57.9   Unspecified mononeuropathy of lower limb**

    G57.90   Unspecified mononeuropathy of unspecified lower limb

    G57.91   Unspecified mononeuropathy of right lower limb

    G57.92   Unspecified mononeuropathy of left lower limb

● **G58   Other mononeuropathies**

    G58.0   Intercostal neuropathy

    G58.7   Mononeuritis multiplex

    G58.8   Other specified mononeuropathies

    G58.9   Mononeuropathy, unspecified

▌ *G59   Mononeuropathy in diseases classified elsewhere*
    Code first underlying disease

    Excludes1   diabetic mononeuropathy (E08-E13 with .41) ◄▥
               syphilitic nerve paralysis (A52.19)
               syphilitic neuritis (A52.15)
               tuberculous mononeuropathy (A17.83)

POLYNEUROPATHIES AND OTHER DISORDERS OF THE PERIPHERAL NERVOUS SYSTEM (G60-G65)

    Excludes1   neuralgia NOS (M79.2)
               neuritis NOS (M79.2)
               peripheral neuritis in pregnancy (O26.82-)
               radiculitis NOS (M54.10)

● **G60   Hereditary and idiopathic neuropathy**

    G60.0   **Hereditary motor and sensory neuropathy**
       Charcot-Marie-Tooth disease
       Déjerine-Sottas disease
       Hereditary motor and sensory neuropathy, types I-IV
       Hypertrophic neuropathy of infancy
       Peroneal muscular atrophy (axonal type) (hypertrophic type)
       Roussy-Lévy syndrome

    G60.1   **Refsum's disease** ✿
       Genetic disorder affecting fatty acid metabolism
       Infantile Refsum disease
       (Ex:) E11.42, G13.0, G13.1, G50.0-G65.2, M34.83

    G60.2   **Neuropathy in association with hereditary ataxia**

    G60.3   **Idiopathic progressive neuropathy**

    G60.8   **Other hereditary and idiopathic neuropathies**
       Dominantly inherited sensory neuropathy
       Morvan's disease
       Nelaton's syndrome
       Recessively inherited sensory neuropathy

    G60.9   **Hereditary and idiopathic neuropathy, unspecified**

● **G61   Inflammatory polyneuropathy**

    G61.0   **Guillain-Barré syndrome** ✿
       Autoimmune disease affecting peripheral nervous system
       Acute (post-)infective polyneuritis
       Miller Fisher Syndrome
       (Ex:) A02.21, A17.0-A17.1, A27.81, A39.0, A39.89-A39.9, A49.3-A49.9, A50.41, A51.41, A52.13, A54.82, A54.84, A54.89-A54.9, A87.0-A87.9, B00.3, B02.1, B26.1, B37.5, B38.4, B45.1, B58.2, B92, B94.2-B94.9, B96.0, B96.6-B96.89, G00.0-G03.9, G04.2, G32.89, G61.0, G96.8-G96.9, G98.0-G98.8, G99.8

    G61.1   **Serum neuropathy**
       Use additional code for adverse effect, if applicable, to identify serum (T50.-)

● **G61.8   Other inflammatory polyneuropathies**

    G61.81   **Chronic inflammatory demyelinating polyneuritis** ✿
       (Ex:) G51.0-G54.5, G54.8-G60.9, G61.81-G61.89, G62.81-G62.89, G64

    G61.89   Other inflammatory polyneuropathies

    G61.9   Inflammatory polyneuropathy, unspecified

Item 6–7 The **peripheral nervous system** consists of 31 pairs of spinal nerves, 12 pairs of cranial nerves, and the autonomic nerves, which are divided into the parasympathetic and sympathetic nerves. The cranial nerves are: olfactory (I), optic (II), oculomotor (III), trochlear (IV), trigeminal (V), abducens (VI), facial (VII), vestibulocochlear (VIII), glossopharyngeal (IX), vagus (X), accessory (XI), and hypoglossal (XII).

◄ New   ◄▥ Revised   ~~deleted~~ Deleted   Excludes 1   Excludes 2   Includes   Use additional   Code first   Code also   Unspecified

OGCR Official Guidelines   ● Unacceptable Principal Diagnosis   X Assign placeholder X   ● Use Additional Character(s)   ▌ Manifestation Code   **Coding Clinic**

● **G62   Other and unspecified polyneuropathies**
    G62.0   Drug-induced polyneuropathy
        Use additional code for adverse effect, if applicable, to identify drug (T36-T50 with fifth or sixth character 5)
    G62.1   Alcoholic polyneuropathy
        Malfunction of many peripheral nerves throughout the body
    G62.2   Polyneuropathy due to other toxic agents
        Code first (T51-T65) to identify toxic agent
●   **G62.8   Other specified polyneuropathies**
        G62.81   Critical illness polyneuropathy 🅒
            Acute motor neuropathy
            (Ex) G51.0-G54.5, G54.8-G60.9, G61.81-G61.9, G62.81, G62.89-G62.9, G64
        G62.82   Radiation-induced polyneuropathy
            Use additional external cause code (W88-W90, X39.0-) to identify cause
        G62.89   Other specified polyneuropathies
    G62.9   Polyneuropathy, unspecified
        Neuropathy NOS

▸ *G63   Polyneuropathy in diseases classified elsewhere*
    Code first underlying disease, such as:
      amyloidosis (E85.-) ◂▪▪▪
      endocrine disease, except diabetes (E00-E07, E15-E16, E20-E34)
      metabolic diseases (E70-E88)
      neoplasm (C00-D49)
      nutritional deficiency (E40-E64)
    Excludes1 polyneuropathy (in):
          diabetes mellitus (E08-E13 with .42)
          diphtheria (A36.83)
          infectious mononucleosis (B27.0-B27.9 with 1)
          Lyme disease (A69.22)
          mumps (B26.84)
          postherpetic (B02.23)
          rheumatoid arthritis (M05.33)
          scleroderma (M34.83)
          systemic lupus erythematosus (M32.19)
  Coding Clinic: 2012, Q4, P100

G64   Other disorders of peripheral nervous system
    Disorder of peripheral nervous system NOS

● **G65   Sequelae of inflammatory and toxic polyneuropathies**
    Code first condition resulting from (sequela) of inflammatory and toxic polyneuropathies
    G65.0   Sequelae of Guillain-Barré syndrome
    G65.1   Sequelae of other inflammatory polyneuropathy
    G65.2   Sequelae of toxic polyneuropathy

DISEASES OF MYONEURAL JUNCTION AND MUSCLE (G70-G73)

● **G70   Myasthenia gravis and other myoneural disorders**
    Excludes1 botulism (A05.1, A48.51-A48.52)
              transient neonatal myasthenia gravis (P94.0)
●   **G70.0   Myasthenia gravis**
        Acquired and results in fatigable muscle weakness exacerbated by activity and improved with rest.
    G70.00   Myasthenia gravis without (acute) exacerbation
        Myasthenia gravis NOS
    G70.01   Myasthenia gravis with (acute) exacerbation 🅒
        Myasthenia gravis in crisis
        (Ex) E08.40-E08.49, E08.618-E08.638, E08.649-E08.8, E09.40-E09.49, E09.618-E09.638, E09.649-E09.8, E10.40-E10.49, E10.618-E10.638, E10.649, E10.69-E10.8, E11.40-E11.49, E11.618-E11.638, E11.649, E11.69-E11.8, E13.40-E13.49, E13.618-E13.638, E13.649-E13.8, G32.89, G70.00-G70.01, G70.80-G70.81, G73.1-G73.3, G96.8-G96.9, G98.0-G98.8, G99.8
    G70.1   Toxic myoneural disorders
        Dysfunction at junction of muscle and motor nerve (myoneural junction)
        Code first (T51-T65) to identify toxic agent
    G70.2   Congenital and developmental myasthenia
●   **G70.8   Other specified myoneural disorders**
    G70.80   Lambert-Eaton syndrome, unspecified 🅒
        Lambert-Eaton syndrome NOS
        (Ex) See G70.01
    ▸ *G70.81   Lambert-Eaton syndrome in disease classified elsewhere* 🅒
        Code first underlying disease
        Excludes1 Lambert-Eaton syndrome in neoplastic disease (G73.1)
        (Ex) See G70.01
    G70.89   Other specified myoneural disorders
    G70.9   Myoneural disorder, unspecified

CHAPTER 6 (G00-G99)

Figure 6-2   A. Parasympathetic nervous system. **B.** Sympathetic nervous system. (From Buck CJ: Step-by-Step Medical Coding, Philadelphia, WB Saunders, 1998)

N   Newborn Age: 0   P   Pediatric Age: 0–17   M   Maternity DX: 12–55   A   Adult Age: 15–124   ♀   Females Only   ♂   Males Only

🅒   Complication\Comorbidity   🅜   Major C\C   (Ex)   CC/MCC Exclusions   🄿   Present on Admission Requirement   🄷   Hospital-Acquired Condition

Item 6–8 Muscular dystrophies (MD) are a group of rare inherited muscle diseases. Voluntary muscles become progressively weaker. In the late stages of MD, fat and connective tissue replace muscle fibers. In some types of muscular dystrophy, heart muscles, other involuntary muscles, and other organs are affected. **Myopathies** is a general term for neuromuscular diseases in which the muscle fibers dysfunction for any one of many reasons, resulting in muscular weakness.

● **G71**   **Primary disorders of muscles**
>   **Excludes2**   arthrogryposis multiplex congenita (Q74.3)
>   metabolic disorders (E70-E88)
>   myositis (M60.-)

  G71.0   **Muscular dystrophy** 🔓
> Autosomal recessive, childhood type, muscular dystrophy resembling Duchenne or Becker muscular dystrophy
> Benign [Becker] muscular dystrophy
> Benign scapuloperoneal muscular dystrophy with early contractures [Emery-Dreifuss]
> Congenital muscular dystrophy NOS
> Congenital muscular dystrophy with specific morphological abnormalities of the muscle fiber
> Distal muscular dystrophy
> Facioscapulohumeral muscular dystrophy
> Limb-girdle muscular dystrophy
> Ocular muscular dystrophy
> Oculopharyngeal muscular dystrophy
> Scapuloperoneal muscular dystrophy
> Severe [Duchenne] muscular dystrophy
>   (Ex:) E08.40-E08.49, E08.618-E08.638, E08.649-E08.8, E09.40-E09.49,
>   E09.618-E09.638, E09.649-E09.8, E10.40-E10.49, E10.618-E10.638,
>   E10.649, E10.69-E10.8, E11.40-E11.49, E11.618-E11.638, E11.649,
>   E11.69-E11.8, E13.40-E13.49, E13.618-E13.638, E13.649-E13.8, G32.89,
>   G71.0, G71.2, G96.8-G96.9, G98.0-G98.8, G99.8

● **G71.1**   **Myotonic disorders**
> *Inherited disorder that affects muscles tone*

    G71.11   **Myotonic muscular dystrophy**
> Dystrophia myotonica [Steinert]
> Myotonia atrophica
> Myotonic dystrophy
> Proximal myotonic myopathy (PROMM)
> Steinert disease

    G71.12   **Myotonia congenita**
> Acetazolamide responsive myotonia congenita
> Dominant myotonia congenita [Thomsen disease]
> Myotonia levior
> Recessive myotonia congenita [Becker disease]

    G71.13   **Myotonic chondrodystrophy**
> Chondrodystrophic myotonia
> Congenital myotonic chondrodystrophy
> Schwartz-Jampel disease

    G71.14   **Drug induced myotonia**
> Use additional code for adverse effect, if applicable, to identify drug (T36-T50 with fifth or sixth character 5)

    G71.19   **Other specified myotonic disorders**
> Myotonia fluctuans
> Myotonia permanens
> Neuromyotonia [Isaacs]
> Paramyotonia congenita (of von Eulenburg)
> Pseudomyotonia
> Symptomatic myotonia

  G71.2   **Congenital myopathies** 🔓
> Central core disease
> Fiber-type disproportion
> Minicore disease
> Multicore disease
> Myotubular (centronuclear) myopathy
> Nemaline myopathy
>   **Excludes1**   arthrogryposis multiplex congenita (Q74.3)
>   (Ex:) See G71.0

  G71.3   **Mitochondrial myopathy, not elsewhere classified**
> *Myopathies associated with increased number of enlarged, often abnormal, mitochondria in muscle fibers*
>   **Excludes1**   Kearns-Sayre syndrome (H49.81)
>   Leber's disease (H47.21)
>   Leigh's encephalopathy (G31.82)
>   mitochondrial metabolism disorders (E88.4.-)
>   Reye's syndrome (G93.7)

  G71.8   **Other primary disorders of muscles**
  G71.9   **Primary disorder of muscle, unspecified**
> Hereditary myopathy NOS

● **G72**   **Other and unspecified myopathies**
>   **Excludes1**   arthrogryposis multiplex congenita (Q74.3)
>   dermatopolymyositis (M33.-)
>   ischemic infarction of muscle (M62.2-)
>   myositis (M60.-)
>   polymyositis (M33.2.-)

  G72.0   **Drug-induced myopathy** 🔓
> Use additional code for adverse effect, if applicable, to identify drug (T36-T50 with fifth or sixth character 5)
>   (Ex:) G32.89, G70.00-G71.0, G71.11-G72.3, G72.81-G73.7, G96.8-G96.9,
>   G98.0-G98.8, G99.8

  G72.1   **Alcoholic myopathy** 🔓
> Use additional code to identify alcoholism (F10.-)
>   (Ex:) See G72.0

  G72.2   **Myopathy due to other toxic agents** 🔓
> *Code first (T51-T65) to identify toxic agent*
>   (Ex:) See G72.0

  G72.3   **Periodic paralysis**
> Familial periodic paralysis
> Hyperkalemic periodic paralysis (familial)
> Hypokalemic periodic paralysis (familial)
> Myotonic periodic paralysis (familial)
> Normokalemic paralysis (familial)
> Potassium sensitive periodic paralysis
>   **Excludes1**   paramyotonia congenita (of von Eulenburg) (G71.19)

● **G72.4**   **Inflammatory and immune myopathies, not elsewhere classified**
    G72.41   **Inclusion body myositis [IBM]**
    G72.49   **Other inflammatory and immune myopathies, not elsewhere classified**
> Inflammatory myopathy NOS

● **G72.8**   **Other specified myopathies**
    G72.81   **Critical illness myopathy** 🔓
> Acute necrotizing myopathy
> Acute quadriplegic myopathy
> Intensive care (ICU) myopathy
> Myopathy of critical illness
>   (Ex:) G70.1-G72.3, G72.81-G73.7

    G72.89   **Other specified myopathies**
  G72.9   **Myopathy, unspecified**

● **G73**   **Disorders of myoneural junction and muscle in diseases classified elsewhere**
>   (Ex:) **For category G73 CC codes:** See G70.01

● ▶ **G73.1**   *Lambert-Eaton syndrome in neoplastic disease* 🔓
> *Rare autoimmune disorder affecting calcium channels of nerve-muscle (neuromuscular) junction*
> *Code first underlying neoplasm (C00-D49)*
>   **Excludes1**   Lambert-Eaton syndrome not associated with neoplasm (G70.80-G70.81)

▶ **G73.3**   *Myasthenic syndromes in other diseases classified elsewhere* 🔓
> *Code first underlying disease, such as:*
> neoplasm (C00-D49)
> thyrotoxicosis (E05.-)

◀ New   ◀ Revised   deleted Deleted   Excludes 1   Excludes 2   Includes   Use additional   Code first   Code also   Unspecified

896

OGCR Official Guidelines   ● Unacceptable Principal Diagnosis   X Assign placeholder X   ● Use Additional Character(s)   ▶ Manifestation Code   **Coding Clinic**

▶ *G73.7* *Myopathy in diseases classified elsewhere*
    Code first underlying disease, such as:
      hyperparathyroidism (E21.0, E21.3)
      hypoparathyroidism (E20.-)
      glycogen storage disease (E74.0)
      lipid storage disorders (E75.-)
    Excludes1 myopathy in:
      rheumatoid arthritis (M05.32)
      sarcoidosis (D86.87)
      scleroderma (M34.82)
      sicca syndrome [Sjögren] (M35.03)
      systemic lupus erythematosus (M32.19)

CEREBRAL PALSY AND OTHER PARALYTIC SYNDROMES (G80-G83)

● **G80** **Cerebral palsy**
    Excludes1 hereditary spastic paraplegia (G11.4)
  G80.0 **Spastic quadriplegic cerebral palsy** 🔧
    Congenital spastic paralysis (cerebral)
    (Ex) E08.40-E08.49, E08.618-E08.638, E08.649-E08.8, E09.40-E09.49,
      E09.618-E09.638, E09.649-E09.8, E10.40-E10.49, E10.618-E10.638,
      E10.649, E10.69-E10.8, E11.40-E11.49, E11.618-E11.638, E11.649,
      E11.69-E11.8, E13.40-E13.49, E13.618-E13.638, E13.649-E13.8, G04.1,
      G32.89, G80.0-G80.2, G80.4-G83.9, G90.1, G93.81, G93.89-G93.9,
      G96.8-G96.9, G98.0-G98.8, G99.8, Q06.0-Q06.1, Q06.3, Q06.8-Q06.9,
      Q07.8-Q07.9, R53.2
  G80.1 **Spastic diplegic cerebral palsy** 🔧
    Spastic cerebral palsy NOS
    (Ex) G80.1, G93.40-G93.49, I67.83
  G80.2 **Spastic hemiplegic cerebral palsy** 🔧
    (Ex) G80.2, G93.40-G93.49, I67.83
  G80.3 **Athetoid cerebral palsy** 🔧
    Result of damage to cerebellum or basal ganglia responsible
    for processing neuromuscular signals
    Double athetosis (syndrome)
    Dyskinetic cerebral palsy
    Dystonic cerebral palsy
    Vogt disease
    (Ex) G20, G21.11-G21.9, G25.70-G25.79, G25.89-G26, G80.0-G80.9,
      G93.40-G93.49, I67.83
  G80.4 **Ataxic cerebral palsy**
    Poor muscle tone and coordination
  G80.8 **Other cerebral palsy**
    Mixed cerebral palsy syndromes
  G80.9 **Cerebral palsy, unspecified**
    Cerebral palsy NOS

OGCR Section I.C.6.a.

Dominant/nondominant side
Codes from category G81, Hemiplegia and hemiparesis, and
subcategories, G83.1, Monoplegia of lower limb, G83.2, Monoplegia of
upper limb, and G83.3, Monoplegia, unspecified, identify whether the
dominant and nondominant side is affected. Should the affected side
be documented, but not specified as dominant or nondominant, and
the classification system does not indicate a default, code selection is
as follows:
- For ambidextrous patients, the default should be dominant.
- If the left side is affected, the default is non-dominant.
- If the right side is affected, the default is dominant.

Item 6-9 **Hemiplegia** is complete paralysis of one side of the body—
arm, leg, and trunk. **Hemiparesis** is a generalized weakness or incomplete
paralysis of one side of the body. If most activities (eating, writing) are
performed with the right hand, the right is the dominant side, and the left is
the nondominant side. **Quadriplegia,** also called tetraplegia, is the complete
paralysis of all four limbs. **Quadriparesis** is the incomplete paralysis of all
four limbs. Nerve damage in C1–C4 is associated with lower limb paralysis,
and C5–C7 damage is associated with upper limb paralysis. **Diplegia** is the
paralysis of the upper limbs. **Monoplegia** is the complete paralysis of one
limb.

● **G81** **Hemiplegia and hemiparesis**
    Note: This category is to be used only when hemiplegia
    (complete)(incomplete) is reported without further
    specification, or is stated to be old or longstanding but of
    unspecified cause. The category is also for use in multiple
    coding to identify these types of hemiplegia resulting
    from any cause.
    Excludes1 congenital cerebral palsy (G80.-)
      hemiplegia and hemiparesis due to sequela of
      cerebrovascular disease (I69.05-, I69.15-,
      I69.25-, I69.35-, I69.85-, I69.95-)
    (Ex) For category G81 CC codes: G04.1, G11.0-G12.9, G32.0-G37.3, G37.5-G37.9,
      G80.0-G80.2, G80.4-G83.9, G81.0-G83.9, G90.01-G90.09, G90.2, G90.4,
      G90.50-G90.9, G92, G93.40-G93.49, G93.81, G93.89-G95.9, G96.8-G96.9,
      G98.0-G99.8, I67.83, R53.2
    Coding Clinic: 2012, Q4, P106
  ● **G81.0** **Flaccid hemiplegia**
    Paralysis of half of body with loss of tone of muscles of
    paralyzed part and absence of tendon reflexes
    G81.00 **Flaccid hemiplegia affecting unspecified side** 🔧
    G81.01 **Flaccid hemiplegia affecting right dominant side** 🔧
    G81.02 **Flaccid hemiplegia affecting left dominant side** 🔧
    G81.03 **Flaccid hemiplegia affecting right nondominant side** 🔧
    G81.04 **Flaccid hemiplegia affecting left nondominant side** 🔧
  ● **G81.1** **Spastic hemiplegia**
    Paralysis of half of body with spasticity of muscles of
    paralyzed part and increased tendon reflexes
    G81.10 **Spastic hemiplegia affecting unspecified side** 🔧
    G81.11 **Spastic hemiplegia affecting right dominant side** 🔧
    G81.12 **Spastic hemiplegia affecting left dominant side** 🔧
    G81.13 **Spastic hemiplegia affecting right nondominant side** 🔧
    G81.14 **Spastic hemiplegia affecting left nondominant side** 🔧
  ● **G81.9** **Hemiplegia, unspecified**
    G81.90 **Hemiplegia, unspecified affecting unspecified side** 🔧
    G81.91 **Hemiplegia, unspecified affecting right dominant side** 🔧
    G81.92 **Hemiplegia, unspecified affecting left dominant side** 🔧
    G81.93 **Hemiplegia, unspecified affecting right nondominant side** 🔧
    G81.94 **Hemiplegia, unspecified affecting left nondominant side** 🔧

● **G82** **Paraplegia (paraparesis) and quadriplegia (quadriparesis)**
    Note: This category is to be used only when the listed
    conditions are reported without further specification, or
    are stated to be old or longstanding but of unspecified
    cause. The category is also for use in multiple coding to
    identify these conditions resulting from any cause.
    Excludes1 congenital cerebral palsy (G80.-)
      functional quadriplegia (R53.2)
      hysterical paralysis (F44.4)
  ● **G82.2** **Paraplegia**
    Paralysis of both lower limbs NOS
    Paraparesis (lower) NOS
    Paraplegia (lower) NOS
    (Ex) For category G82.2 CC codes: G04.1, G11.0-G12.9, G32.0-G37.3,
      G37.5-G37.9, G80.0-G80.2, G80.4-G80.9, G81.0-G83.9, G90.01-G90.09,
      G90.2, G90.4, G90.50-G90.9, G92, G93.40-G93.49, G93.81, G93.89-G95.9,
      G96.8-G96.9, G98.0-G99.8, I67.83, R53.2
    G82.20 **Paraplegia, unspecified**
    G82.21 **Paraplegia, complete** 🔧
    G82.22 **Paraplegia, incomplete** 🔧

CHAPTER 6 (G00-G99)

N Newborn Age: 0   **P** Pediatric Age: 0–17   **M** Maternity DX: 12–55   **A** Adult Age: 15–124   ♀ Females Only   ♂ Males Only

🔧 Complication\Comorbidity   🔧 Major C\C   (Ex) CC/MCC Exclusions   🔧 Present on Admission Requirement   🔧 Hospital-Acquired Condition

897

● **G82.5 Quadriplegia**
Paralysis of all limbs; AKA tetraplegia
Ⓔ See G80.0

     G82.50 Quadriplegia, unspecified 🔖

     G82.51 Quadriplegia, C1-C4 complete 🔖

     G82.52 Quadriplegia, C1-C4 incomplete 🔖

     G82.53 Quadriplegia, C5-C7 complete 🔖

     G82.54 Quadriplegia, C5-C7 incomplete 🔖

● **G83 Other paralytic syndromes**

     Note: This category is to be used only when the listed conditions are reported without further specification, or are stated to be old or longstanding but of unspecified cause. The category is also for use in multiple coding to identify these conditions resulting from any cause.

     Includes paralysis (complete) (incomplete), except as in G80-G82

   G83.0 Diplegia of upper limbs 🔖
Paralysis affecting limbs on both sides; AKA bilateral paralysis
Diplegia (upper)
Paralysis of both upper limbs
Ⓔ G32.89, G82.50-G83.0, G83.5-G83.9, G96.8-G96.9, G98.0-G98.8, G99.8, R53.2

   G83.1 Monoplegia of lower limb
Paralysis of limb on one side
Paralysis of lower limb

     Excludes1 monoplegia of lower limbs due to sequela of cerebrovascular disease (I69.04-, I69.14-, I69.24-, I69.34-, I69.84-, I69.94-)

     Coding Clinic: 2012, Q4, P106

     G83.10 Monoplegia of lower limb affecting unspecified side

     G83.11 Monoplegia of lower limb affecting right dominant side

     G83.12 Monoplegia of lower limb affecting left dominant side

     G83.13 Monoplegia of lower limb affecting right nondominant side

     G83.14 Monoplegia of lower limb affecting left nondominant side

● **G83.2 Monoplegia of upper limb**
Paralysis of upper limb

     Excludes1 monoplegia of upper limbs due to sequela of cerebrovascular disease (I69.03-, I69.13-, I69.23-, I69.33-, I69.83-, I69.93-)

     Coding Clinic: 2012, Q4, P106

     G83.20 Monoplegia of upper limb affecting unspecified side

     G83.21 Monoplegia of upper limb affecting right dominant side

     G83.22 Monoplegia of upper limb affecting left dominant side

     G83.23 Monoplegia of upper limb affecting right nondominant side

     G83.24 Monoplegia of upper limb affecting left nondominant side

● **G83.3 Monoplegia, unspecified**
     Coding Clinic: 2012, Q4, P106

     G83.30 Monoplegia, unspecified affecting unspecified side

     G83.31 Monoplegia, unspecified affecting right dominant side

     G83.32 Monoplegia, unspecified affecting left dominant side

     G83.33 Monoplegia, unspecified affecting right nondominant side

     G83.34 Monoplegia, unspecified affecting left nondominant side

   G83.4 Cauda equina syndrome 🔖
Aching pain due to compression of spinal nerve roots
Neurogenic bladder due to cauda equina syndrome

     Excludes1 cord bladder NOS (G95.89)
                neurogenic bladder NOS (N31.9)
     Ⓔ G04.1, G32.89, G82.20-G82.54, G83.10-G83.14, G83.4-G83.9, G96.8-G96.9, G98.0-G98.8, G99.8, R53.2

   G83.5 Locked-in state
     Ⓔ G04.1, G32.89, G80.0-G83.9, G92, G93.40-G93.49, G93.81, G93.89-G93.9, G96.8-G96.9, G98.0-G98.8, G99.8, I67.83, R53.2

● **G83.8 Other specified paralytic syndromes**

     Excludes1 paralytic syndromes due to current spinal cord injury-code to spinal cord injury (S14, S24, S34)

   G83.81 Brown-Séquard syndrome

   G83.82 Anterior cord syndrome

   G83.83 Posterior cord syndrome

   G83.84 Todd's paralysis (postepileptic)

   G83.89 Other specified paralytic syndromes

   G83.9 Paralytic syndrome, unspecified

OTHER DISORDERS OF THE NERVOUS SYSTEM (G89-G99)

● **G89 Pain, not elsewhere classified**
Code also related psychological factors associated with pain (F45.42)

     Excludes1 generalized pain NOS (R52)
                pain disorders exclusively related to psychological factors (F45.41)
                pain NOS (R52)

     Excludes2 atypical face pain (G50.1)
                headache syndromes (G44.-)
                localized pain, unspecified type - code to pain by site, such as:
                   abdomen pain (R10.-)
                   back pain (M54.9)
                   breast pain (N64.4)
                   chest pain (R07.1-R07.9)
                   ear pain (H92.0-)
                   eye pain (H57.1)
                   headache (R51)
                   joint pain (M25.5-)
                   limb pain (M79.6-)
                   lumbar region pain (M54.5)
                   painful urination (R30.9)
                   pelvic and perineal pain (R10.2)
                   shoulder pain (M25.51-)
                   spine pain (M54.-)
                   throat pain (R07.0)
                   tongue pain (K14.6)
                   tooth pain (K08.8)
                 renal colic (N23)
                 migraines (G43.-)
                 myalgia (M79.1)
                 pain from prosthetic devices, implants, and grafts (T82.84, T83.84, T84.84, T85.84)
                 phantom limb syndrome with pain (G54.6)
                 vulvar vestibulitis (N94.810)
                 vulvodynia (N94.81-)

   G89.0 Central pain syndrome
Neurological condition causing intractable pain resulting from damage to CNS
Déjérine-Roussy syndrome
Myelopathic pain syndrome
Thalamic pain syndrome (hyperesthetic)

● **G89.1 Acute pain, not elsewhere classified**

   G89.11 Acute pain due to trauma

   G89.12 Acute post-thoracotomy pain
Post-thoracotomy pain NOS

   G89.18 Other acute postprocedural pain
Postoperative pain NOS
Postprocedural pain NOS

CHAPTER 6 (G00-G99)

◀ New   ◀▦ Revised   ~~deleted~~ Deleted   Excludes 1   Excludes 2   Includes   Use additional   Code first   Code also   Unspecified

OGCR Official Guidelines   ● Unacceptable Principal Diagnosis   X Assign placeholder X   🔖 Use Additional Character(s)   ▶ Manifestation Code   **Coding Clinic**

● **G89.2** **Chronic pain, not elsewhere classified**

     Excludes1   causalgia, lower limb (G57.7-)
          causalgia, upper limb (G56.4-)
          central pain syndrome (G89.0)
          chronic pain syndrome (G89.4)
          complex regional pain syndrome II, lower limb (G57.7-)
          complex regional pain syndrome II, upper limb (G56.4-)
          neoplasm related chronic pain (G89.3)
          reflex sympathetic dystrophy (G90.5-)

    G89.21   **Chronic pain due to trauma**

    G89.22   **Chronic post-thoracotomy pain**

    G89.28   **Other chronic postprocedural pain**
          Other chronic postoperative pain

    G89.29   **Other chronic pain**

G89.3   **Neoplasm related pain (acute) (chronic)**
      Cancer associated pain
      Pain due to malignancy (primary) (secondary)
      Tumor associated pain

G89.4   **Chronic pain syndrome**
      Chronic pain associated with significant psychosocial dysfunction

● **G90**   **Disorders of autonomic nervous system**

     Excludes1   dysfunction of the autonomic nervous system due to alcohol (G31.2)

● **G90.0**   **Idiopathic peripheral autonomic neuropathy**

    G90.01   **Carotid sinus syncope**
          Carotid sinus syndrome

    G90.09   **Other idiopathic peripheral autonomic neuropathy**
          Idiopathic peripheral autonomic neuropathy NOS

G90.1   **Familial dysautonomia [Riley-Day]** 🔧
      Inherited disorder that affects nerve function

G90.2   **Horner's syndrome**
      Due to damage of the sympathetic nervous system
      Bernard(-Horner) syndrome
      Cervical sympathetic dystrophy or paralysis

G90.3   **Multi-system degeneration of the autonomic nervous system** 🔧
      Neurogenic orthostatic hypotension [Shy-Drager]
     Excludes1   orthostatic hypotension NOS (I95.1)
     (Ex:) G20, G21.11-G21.9, G90.01-G90.09, G93.40-G93.49, I67.83

G90.4   **Autonomic dysreflexia**
      Syndrome resulting from lesions of spinal cord
      Use additional code to identify the cause, such as:
        fecal impaction (K56.41)
        pressure ulcer (pressure area) (L89.-)
        urinary tract infection (N39.0)

● **G90.5**   **Complex regional pain syndrome I (CRPS I)**
      Reflex sympathetic dystrophy
     Excludes1   causalgia of lower limb (G57.7-)
          causalgia of upper limb (G56.4-)
          complex regional pain syndrome II of lower limb (G57.7-)
          complex regional pain syndrome II of upper limb (G56.4-)

     (Ex:) **For category G90.5 CC codes unless otherwise indicated:**
      E08.40-E08.49, E09.40-E09.49, E10.40-E10.49, E11.40-E11.49,
      E13.40-E13.49, G04.1, G11.3, G11.8-G12.9, G32.0, G32.89-G37.3,
      G37.5-G37.9, G80.0-G80.2, G80.4-G83.9, G90.01-G90.09, G90.2,
      G90.4-G90.9, G93.1, G93.40-G93.49, G95.0-G95.9, G96.12-G96.9, G97.1,
      G98.0-G99.8, I67.83, R53.2

    G90.50   **Complex regional pain syndrome I, unspecified** 🔧
        (Ex:) G90.50-G90.59

    ● **G90.51**   **Complex regional pain syndrome I of upper limb**

        G90.511   **Complex regional pain syndrome I of right upper limb** 🔧

        G90.512   **Complex regional pain syndrome I of left upper limb** 🔧

        G90.513   **Complex regional pain syndrome I of upper limb, bilateral** 🔧

        G90.519   **Complex regional pain syndrome I of unspecified upper limb** 🔧

    ● **G90.52**   **Complex regional pain syndrome I of lower limb**

        G90.521   **Complex regional pain syndrome I of right lower limb** 🔧

        G90.522   **Complex regional pain syndrome I of left lower limb** 🔧

        G90.523   **Complex regional pain syndrome I of lower limb, bilateral** 🔧

        G90.529   **Complex regional pain syndrome I of unspecified lower limb** 🔧

    G90.59   **Complex regional pain syndrome I of other specified site** 🔧

   G90.8   **Other disorders of autonomic nervous system**

   G90.9   **Disorder of the autonomic nervous system, unspecified**

● **G91**   **Hydrocephalus**
      Dilatation of cerebral ventricles, accompanied by accumulation of cerebrospinal fluid
     Includes   acquired hydrocephalus
     Excludes1   Arnold-Chiari syndrome with hydrocephalus (Q07.-)
          congenital hydrocephalus (Q03.-)
          spina bifida with hydrocephalus (Q05.-)
     (Ex:) **For category G91 CC codes unless otherwise indicated:** E08.40-E08.49,
      E08.618-E08.638, E08.649-E08.8, E09.40-E09.49, E09.618-E09.638, E09.649-E09.8,
      E10.40-E10.49, E10.618-E10.638, E10.649, E10.69-E10.8, E11.40-E11.49,
      E11.618-E11.638, E11.649, E11.69-E11.8, E13.40-E13.49, E13.618-E13.638,
      E13.649-E13.8, G13.2-G13.8, G31.2, G31.83-G31.9, G90.1, G91.0-G91.9, G93.81,
      G93.89-G94, Q03.0-Q03.9, Q04.4-Q04.8, Q05.0-Q05.4, Q05.9-Q06.1, Q06.3,
      Q06.8-Q06.9, Q07.01-Q07.9

   G91.0   **Communicating hydrocephalus** 🔧
      Secondary normal pressure hydrocephalus
       (Ex:) G91.0-G91.3, G91.8-G91.9

   G91.1   **Obstructive hydrocephalus** 🔧

   G91.2   **(Idiopathic) normal pressure hydrocephalus** 🔧
      Normal pressure hydrocephalus NOS
       (Ex:) G91.0-G91.3, G91.8-G91.9

   G91.3   **Post-traumatic hydrocephalus, unspecified** 🔧

▌ **G91.4**   *Hydrocephalus in diseases classified elsewhere*
      Code first underlying condition, such as:
        congenital syphilis (A50.4-)
        neoplasm (C00-D49)
     Excludes1   hydrocephalus due to congenital toxoplasmosis (P37.1)

   G91.8   **Other hydrocephalus** 🔧

   G91.9   **Hydrocephalus, unspecified** 🔧

G92   **Toxic encephalopathy** 🔧
      Disorder or disease of brain caused by chemicals
      Toxic encephalitis
      Toxic metabolic encephalopathy
      Code first (T51-T65) to identify toxic agent
     (Ex:) A17.82, A17.9, A18.82, A18.84, A18.89, A39.81, A50.42, A52.14, A83.0-A85.1,
      A85.8-A86, A88.8-A89, B00.4, B01.11, B10.01-B10.09, B26.2, B58.2, E08.40-E08.49,
      E08.618-E08.638, E08.649-E08.8, E09.40-E09.49, E09.618-E09.638, E09.649-E09.8,
      E10.40-E10.49, E10.618-E10.638, E10.649, E10.69-E10.8, E11.40-E11.49,
      E11.618-E11.638, E11.649, E11.69-E11.8, E13.40-E13.49, E13.618-E13.638,
      E13.649-E13.8, G04.00-G04.01, G04.31, G04.81-G05.4, G32.89, G37.3-G37.4, G92,
      G93.40-G93.49, G93.81, G93.89-G93.9, G96.8-G96.9, G98.0-G98.8, G99.8, I67.83

CHAPTER 6 (G00-G99)

N   Newborn Age: 0   P   Pediatric Age: 0–17   M   Maternity DX: 12–55   A   Adult Age: 15–124   ♀   Females Only   ♂   Males Only

🔧 Complication\Comorbidity   🔧 Major C\C   (Ex:) CC/MCC Exclusions   🔧 Present on Admission Requirement   🔧 Hospital-Acquired Condition

899

● **G93   Other disorders of brain**

G93.0   Cerebral cysts
Arachnoid cyst
Porencephalic cyst, acquired

> **Excludes1**   acquired periventricular cysts of newborn (P91.1)
> congenital cerebral cysts (Q04.6)

G93.1   Anoxic brain damage, not elsewhere classified 🔖
Permanent brain damage by lack of oxygen perfusion through brain tissues.

> **Excludes1**   cerebral anoxia due to anesthesia during labor and delivery (O74.3)
> cerebral anoxia due to anesthesia during the puerperium (O89.2)
> neonatal anoxia (P84)

(Ex:) E08.40-E08.49, E08.618-E08.638, E08.649-E08.8, E09.40-E09.49, E09.618-E09.638, E09.649-E09.8, E10.40-E10.49, E10.618-E10.638, E10.649, E10.69-E10.8, E11.40-E11.49, E11.618-E11.638, E11.649, E11.69-E11.8, E13.40-E13.49, E13.618-E13.638, E13.649-E13.8, G32.89, G93.1-G93.2, G96.8-G96.9, G98.0-G98.8, G99.8

G93.2   Benign intracranial hypertension

> **Excludes1**   hypertensive encephalopathy (I67.4)

G93.3   Postviral fatigue syndrome
Benign myalgic encephalomyelitis

> **Excludes1**   chronic fatigue syndrome NOS (R53.82)

● **G93.4   Other and unspecified encephalopathy**

> **Excludes1**   alcoholic encephalopathy (G31.2)
> encephalopathy in diseases classified elsewhere (G94)
> hypertensive encephalopathy (I67.4)
> toxic (metabolic) encephalopathy (G92)

G93.40   Encephalopathy, unspecified 🔖
(Ex:) G21.0, G83.5, G93.41-G93.49, I67.83

G93.41   Metabolic encephalopathy 🔖
Septic encephalopathy
(Ex:) G21.0, G83.5, G93.40-G93.49, I67.83

G93.49   Other encephalopathy 🔖
Encephalopathy NEC
(Ex:) G21.0, G83.5, G93.40-G93.41

G93.5   Compression of brain 🔖
Arnold-Chiari type 1 compression of brain
Compression of brain (stem)
Herniation of brain (stem)

> **Excludes1**   diffuse traumatic compression of brain (S06.2-)
> focal traumatic compression of brain (S06.3-)

(Ex:) G81.90, G93.82

G93.6   Cerebral edema 🔖

> **Excludes1**   cerebral edema due to birth injury (P11.0)
> traumatic cerebral edema (S06.1-)

(Ex:) G93.6, G93.82

G93.7   Reye's syndrome 🔖   P
Life-threatening neurological condition, usually follows viral illness

Code first (T39.0-), *if salicylates-induced*

(Ex:) G93.7

● **G93.8   Other specified disorders of brain**

G93.81   Temporal sclerosis
Hippocampal sclerosis
Mesial temporal sclerosis

G93.82   Brain death 🔖
(Ex:) B15.0-B19.9, E03.5, E08.00-E08.59, E08.618-E09.59, E09.618-E10.59, E10.618-E10.649, E10.69-E11.59, E11.618-E11.649, E11.69-E13.59, E13.618-E16.2, E89.1, G32.89, G89.0-G89.4, G93.81-G93.9, G96.8-G96.9, G98.0-G98.8, G99.8, I60.00-I62.9, K72.91, R40.0-R40.2124, R40.2210-R40.2224, R40.2310-R40.2324, R40.2340-R40.2344, R40.3-R41.3, R41.82, R41.9-R42, R44.8-R44.9, R45.83-R45.84, R46.0-R46.89, R52, R55, R68.0-R68.83, R68.89-R69, S02.0XX-S02.19X[A,B], S02.91X[A,B], S06.0X0-S06.9X9[A]

G93.89   Other specified disorders of brain
Postradiation encephalopathy

G93.9   Disorder of brain, unspecified

▷ **G94   Other disorders of brain in diseases classified elsewhere**
Code first underlying disease

> **Excludes1**   encephalopathy in congenital syphilis (A50.49)
> encephalopathy in influenza (J09.X9, J10.81, J11.81)
> encephalopathy in syphilis (A52.19)
> hydrocephalus in diseases classified elsewhere (G91.4)

● **G95   Other and unspecified diseases of spinal cord**

> **Excludes2**   myelitis (G04.-)

G95.0   Syringomyelia and syringobulbia 🔖
(Ex:) G04.1, G11.3, G11.8-G12.9, G32.0, G32.89-G37.3, G37.5-G37.9, G80.0-G80.2, G80.4-G83.9, G90.01-G90.09, G90.2, G90.4-G90.9, G93.40-G93.49, G93.81, G93.89-G93.9, G95.0-G95.9, G96.12-G96.9, G97.1, G98.0-G99.8, I67.83, R53.2

● **G95.1   Vascular myelopathies**

> **Excludes2**   intraspinal phlebitis and thrombophlebitis, except non-pyogenic (G08)

(Ex:) For category G95.1 CC codes: See G90.5

G95.11   Acute infarction of spinal cord (embolic) (nonembolic) 🔖
Anoxia of spinal cord
Arterial thrombosis of spinal cord

G95.19   Other vascular myelopathies 🔖
Edema of spinal cord
Hematomyelia
Nonpyogenic intraspinal phlebitis and thrombophlebitis
Subacute necrotic myelopathy

● **G95.2   Other and unspecified cord compression**
(Ex:) For category G95.2 CC codes: E08.40-E08.49, E09.40-E09.49, E10.40-E10.49, E11.40-E11.49, E13.40-E13.49, G04.1, G11.3-G12.9, G32.0, G32.89-G37.9, G80.0-G80.2, G80.4-G83.9, G90.01-G90.09, G90.2, G90.4-G90.9, G93.1, G93.40-G93.49, G95.0-G95.9, G96.12-G96.9, G97.1, G98.0-G99.8, I67.83, R53.2

G95.20   Unspecified cord compression 🔖

G95.29   Other cord compression 🔖

● **G95.8   Other specified diseases of spinal cord**

> **Excludes1**   neurogenic bladder NOS (N31.9)
> neurogenic bladder due to cauda equina syndrome (G83.4)
> neuromuscular dysfunction of bladder without spinal cord lesion (N31.-)

(Ex:) For category G95.8 CC codes: See G90.5

G95.81   Conus medullaris syndrome 🔖
Damage to gray matter and/or nerve roots in lower end of spinal cord

G95.89   Other specified diseases of spinal cord 🔖
Cord bladder NOS
Drug-induced myelopathy
Radiation-induced myelopathy

> **Excludes1**   myelopathy NOS (G95.9)

G95.9   Disease of spinal cord, unspecified 🔖
Myelopathy NOS
(Ex:) See G95.2

● **G96   Other disorders of central nervous system**

G96.0   Cerebrospinal fluid leak 🔖

> **Excludes1**   cerebrospinal fluid leak from spinal puncture (G97.0)

(Ex:) E08.40-E08.49, E08.618-E08.638, E08.649-E08.8, E09.40-E09.49, E09.618-E09.638, E09.649-E09.8, E10.40-E10.49, E10.618-E10.638, E10.649, E10.69-E10.8, E11.40-E11.49, E11.618-E11.638, E11.649, E11.69-E11.8, E13.40-E13.49, E13.618-E13.638, E13.649-E13.8, G32.89, G96.0, G96.8-G96.9, G98.0-G98.8, G99.8

◀ New   ◀ Revised   ~~deleted~~ Deleted   Excludes 1   Excludes 2   Includes   Use additional   Code first   Code also   Unspecified

OGCR Official Guidelines   ● Unacceptable Principal Diagnosis   X Assign placeholder X   ● Use Additional Character(s)   ▶ Manifestation Code   **Coding Clinic**

● G96.1   **Disorders of meninges, not elsewhere classified**

　　　G96.11   **Dural tear** 🅒

　　　　　Excludes1   accidental puncture or laceration
　　　　　　　　　　of dura during a procedure
　　　　　　　　　　(G97.41)

　　　　　Ⓔⓧ D78.11-D78.12, D78.81-D78.89, E36.11-E36.8, E89.810-E89.89,
　　　　　　　G96.11, G97.41-G97.49, H59.011-H59.019, H59.031-H59.099,
　　　　　　　H59.211-H59.229, H59.811-H59.89, H95.31-H95.32,
　　　　　　　H95.811-H95.89, I97.3, I97.51-I97.52, J95.71-J95.72,
　　　　　　　K91.71-K91.72, L76.11-L76.12, L76.81-L76.82,
　　　　　　　M96.820-M96.821, M96.89, N98.1-N98.9, N99.71-N99.72,
　　　　　　　T81.82X[A], T81.89X-T81.9XX[A]

　　　G96.12   **Meningeal adhesions (cerebral) (spinal)**

　　　G96.19   **Other disorders of meninges, not elsewhere
　　　　　　　classified**

　　G96.8   **Other specified disorders of central nervous system**

　　G96.9   **Disorder of central nervous system, unspecified**

● G97   **Intraoperative and postprocedural complications and disorders
　　　of nervous system, not elsewhere classified**

　　　　Excludes2   intraoperative and postprocedural
　　　　　　　　cerebrovascular infarction (I97.81-, I97.82-)

　　G97.0   **Cerebrospinal fluid leak from spinal puncture** 🅒

　　　　　Ⓔⓧ D78.81-D78.89, E36.8, E89.810-E89.89, G97.0, G97.2-G97.32,
　　　　　　　G97.81-G97.82, H59.011-H59.019, H59.031-H59.099, H59.811-H59.89,
　　　　　　　H95.811-H95.89, I97.3, I97.810-I97.821, L76.81-L76.82, M96.89,
　　　　　　　N98.1-N98.9, T81.82X[A], T81.89X-T81.9XX[A]

　　G97.1   **Other reaction to spinal and lumbar puncture**
　　　　　Headache due to lumbar puncture

　　G97.2   **Intracranial hypotension following ventricular
　　　　　shunting** 🅒
　　　　　Ⓔⓧ See G97.0

● G97.3   **Intraoperative hemorrhage and hematoma of a nervous
　　　system organ or structure complicating a procedure**

　　　　　Excludes1   intraoperative hemorrhage and
　　　　　　　　hematoma of a nervous system
　　　　　　　　organ or structure due to accidental
　　　　　　　　puncture and laceration during a
　　　　　　　　procedure (G97.4-)

　　　　Ⓔⓧ **For category G97.3 CC codes:** G97.0, G97.2-G97.32, G97.81-G97.82,
　　　　　　　H95.811-H95.89, I97.3, I97.810-I97.821, M96.89, N98.1-N98.9,
　　　　　　　T81.82X[A], T81.89X-T81.9XX[A]

　　　G97.31   **Intraoperative hemorrhage and hematoma of a
　　　　　　　nervous system organ or structure complicating
　　　　　　　a nervous system procedure** 🅒

　　　G97.32   **Intraoperative hemorrhage and hematoma of a
　　　　　　　nervous system organ or structure complicating
　　　　　　　other procedure** 🅒

● G97.4   **Accidental puncture and laceration of a nervous system
　　　organ or structure during a procedure**
　　　　Ⓔⓧ **For category G97.4 CC codes:** See G96.11

　　　G97.41   **Accidental puncture or laceration of dura
　　　　　　　during a procedure** 🅒
　　　　　　　Incidental (inadvertent) durotomy

　　　G97.48   **Accidental puncture and laceration of other
　　　　　　　nervous system organ or structure during a
　　　　　　　nervous system procedure** 🅒

　　　G97.49   **Accidental puncture and laceration of other
　　　　　　　nervous system organ or structure during other
　　　　　　　procedure** 🅒

● G97.5   **Postprocedural hemorrhage and hematoma of a nervous
　　　system organ or structure following a procedure**
　　　　Ⓔⓧ **For category G97.5 CC codes:** G97.51-G97.52, H95.811-H95.89, I85.01,
　　　　　　　I85.11, I97.3, K21.9, K22.8, K23-K25.0, K25.2, K25.4, K25.6, K26.0, K26.2,
　　　　　　　K26.4, K26.6, K27.0, K27.2, K27.4, K27.6, K28.0, K28.2, K28.4, K28.6,
　　　　　　　K29.01, K29.21, K29.31, K29.41, K29.51, K29.61, K29.71, K29.81, K29.91,
　　　　　　　K31.811, K55.21, K57.01, K57.11, K57.13, K57.21, K57.31, K57.33,
　　　　　　　K57.41, K57.51, K57.53, K57.81, K57.91, K57.93, K62.5, K92.0-K92.2,
　　　　　　　M96.89, N98.1-N98.9, P54.1-P54.3, T81.10X-T81.19X[A],
　　　　　　　T81.82X-T81.9XX[A]

　　　G97.51   **Postprocedural hemorrhage and hematoma of a
　　　　　　　nervous system organ or structure following a
　　　　　　　nervous system procedure** 🅒

　　　G97.52   **Postprocedural hemorrhage and hematoma of a
　　　　　　　nervous system organ or structure following
　　　　　　　other procedure** 🅒

● G97.8   **Other intraoperative and postprocedural complications
　　　and disorders of nervous system**
　　　　Use additional code to further specify disorder
　　　　Ⓔⓧ **For category G97.8 CC codes:** See G97.0

　　　G97.81   **Other intraoperative complications of nervous
　　　　　　　system** 🅒

　　　G97.82   **Other postprocedural complications and
　　　　　　　disorders of nervous system** 🅒

● G98   **Other disorders of nervous system not elsewhere classified**
　　　　Includes   nervous system disorder NOS

　　G98.0   **Neurogenic arthritis, not elsewhere classified**
　　　　　Nonsyphilitic neurogenic arthropathy NEC
　　　　　Nonsyphilitic neurogenic spondylopathy NEC
　　　　　Excludes1   spondylopathy (in):
　　　　　　　　　syringomyelia and syringobulbia
　　　　　　　　　　(G95.0)
　　　　　　　　tabes dorsalis (A52.11)

　　G98.8   **Other disorders of nervous system**
　　　　　Nervous system disorder NOS

● G99   **Other disorders of nervous system in diseases classified
　　　elsewhere**

　▸ G99.0   *Autonomic neuropathy in diseases classified elsewhere* 🅒
　　　　　Code first underlying disease, such as:
　　　　　　amyloidosis (E85.-) ◀▥
　　　　　　gout (M1A.-, M10.-) ◀▥
　　　　　　hyperthyroidism (E05.-)
　　　　　Excludes1   diabetic autonomic neuropathy
　　　　　　　　(E08-E13 with .43) ◀▥
　　　　　Ⓔⓧ G90.50-G90.59

　▸ G99.2   *Myelopathy in diseases classified elsewhere* 🅒
　　　　　Code first underlying disease, such as:
　　　　　　neoplasm (C00-D49)
　　　　　Excludes1   myelopathy in:
　　　　　　　　intervertebral disease (M50.0-, M51.0-)
　　　　　　　　spondylosis (M47.0-, M47.1-)
　　　　　Ⓔⓧ See G90.5

　▸ G99.8   *Other specified disorders of nervous system in diseases
　　　　　classified elsewhere*
　　　　　Code first underlying disorder, such as:
　　　　　　amyloidosis (E85.-) ◀▥
　　　　　　avitaminosis (E56.9)
　　　　　Excludes1   nervous system involvement in:
　　　　　　　　cysticercosis (B69.0)
　　　　　　　　rubella (B06.0-)
　　　　　　　　syphilis (A52.1-)

N   Newborn Age: 0   P   Pediatric Age: 0–17   M   Maternity DX: 12–55   A   Adult Age: 15–124   ♀   Females Only   ♂   Males Only

🅒   Complication\Comorbidity   🅜   Major C\C   Ⓔⓧ   CC/MCC Exclusions   🅟   Present on Admission Requirement   ▥   Hospital-Acquired Condition

901

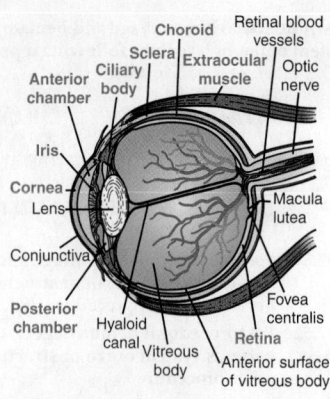

Anterior chamber, Ciliary body, Iris, Cornea, Lens, Conjunctiva, Posterior chamber, Hyaloid canal, Vitreous body, Anterior surface of vitreous body, Choroid, Sclera, Extraocular muscle, Retinal blood vessels, Optic nerve, Macula lutea, Fovea centralis, Retina

Figure 7–1 Eye and ocular adnexa. (From Buck CJ: Step-by-Step Medical Coding, ed 2011, Philadelphia, WB Saunders, 2011)

(See Plate 87 on page 63.)

CHAPTER 7

DISEASES OF THE EYE AND ADNEXA (H00-H59)

Note: Use an external cause code following the code for the eye condition, if applicable, to identify the cause of the eye condition

Excludes2 certain conditions originating in the perinatal period (P04-P96)
certain infectious and parasitic diseases (A00-B99)
complications of pregnancy, childbirth and the puerperium (O00-O9A)
congenital malformations, deformations, and chromosomal abnormalities (Q00-Q99)
diabetes mellitus related eye conditions (E09.3-, E10.3-, E11.3-, E13.3-)
endocrine, nutritional and metabolic diseases (E00-E88)
injury (trauma) of eye and orbit (S05.-)
injury, poisoning and certain other consequences of external causes (S00-T88)
neoplasms (C00-D49)
symptoms, signs and abnormal clinical and laboratory findings, not elsewhere classified (R00-R94)
syphilis related eye disorders (A50.01, A50.3-, A51.43, A52.71)

This chapter contains the following blocks:

H00-H05	Disorders of eyelid, lacrimal system and orbit
H10-H11	Disorders of conjunctiva
H15-H22	Disorders of sclera, cornea, iris and ciliary body
H25-H28	Disorders of lens
H30-H36	Disorders of choroid and retina
H40-H42	Glaucoma
H43-H44	Disorders of vitreous body and globe
H46-H47	Disorders of optic nerve and visual pathways
H49-H52	Disorders of ocular muscles, binocular movement, accommodation and refraction
H53-H54	Visual disturbances and blindness
H55-H57	Other disorders of eye and adnexa
H59	Intraoperative and postprocedural complications and disorders of eye and adnexa, not elsewhere classified

DISORDERS OF EYELID, LACRIMAL SYSTEM AND ORBIT (H00-H05)

Excludes2 open wound of eyelid (S01.1-)
superficial injury of eyelid (S00.1-, S00.2-)

● **H00   Hordeolum and chalazion**
Hordeolum: inflammatory staphylococcal infection of sebaceous glands of eyelids; AKA stye. Chalazion: eyelid mass

● **H00.0   Hordeolum (externum) (internum) of eyelid**
Bacterial infection (staphylococcus) of the sebaceous gland of the eyelid (stye)

● **H00.01   Hordeolum externum**
Hordeolum NOS
Stye

   H00.011   Hordeolum externum right upper eyelid
   H00.012   Hordeolum externum right lower eyelid
   H00.013   Hordeolum externum right eye, unspecified eyelid
   H00.014   Hordeolum externum left upper eyelid
   H00.015   Hordeolum externum left lower eyelid
   H00.016   Hordeolum externum left eye, unspecified eyelid
   H00.019   Hordeolum externum unspecified eye, unspecified eyelid

● **H00.02   Hordeolum internum**
Infection of meibomian gland

   H00.021   Hordeolum internum right upper eyelid
   H00.022   Hordeolum internum right lower eyelid
   H00.023   Hordeolum internum right eye, unspecified eyelid
   H00.024   Hordeolum internum left upper eyelid
   H00.025   Hordeolum internum left lower eyelid
   H00.026   Hordeolum internum left eye, unspecified eyelid
   H00.029   Hordeolum internum unspecified eye, unspecified eyelid

● **H00.03   Abscess of eyelid**
Furuncle of eyelid

   H00.031   Abscess of right upper eyelid
   H00.032   Abscess of right lower eyelid
   H00.033   Abscess of eyelid right eye, unspecified eyelid
   H00.034   Abscess of left upper eyelid
   H00.035   Abscess of left lower eyelid
   H00.036   Abscess of eyelid left eye, unspecified eyelid
   H00.039   Abscess of eyelid unspecified eye, unspecified eyelid

● **H00.1   Chalazion**
Often caused by accumulation of meibomian gland secretions resulting from a blockage of duct.
Meibomian (gland) cyst

   Excludes2   infected meibomian gland (H00.02-)

   H00.11   Chalazion right upper eyelid
   H00.12   Chalazion right lower eyelid
   H00.13   Chalazion right eye, unspecified eyelid
   H00.14   Chalazion left upper eyelid
   H00.15   Chalazion left lower eyelid
   H00.16   Chalazion left eye, unspecified eyelid
   H00.19   Chalazion unspecified eye, unspecified eyelid

◀ New   ◀ Revised   ~~deleted~~ Deleted   Excludes 1   Excludes 2   Includes   Use additional   Code first   Code also   Unspecified
OGCR Official Guidelines   ● Unacceptable Principal Diagnosis   X Assign placeholder X   ▸ Use Additional Character(s)   ▸ Manifestation Code   **Coding Clinic**

● H01   Other inflammation of eyelid
  ● H01.0   **Blepharitis**
    Inflammation of eyelids
      Excludes1   blepharoconjunctivitis (H10.5-)
    ● H01.00   Unspecified blepharitis
      H01.001   Unspecified blepharitis right upper eyelid
      H01.002   Unspecified blepharitis right lower eyelid
      H01.003   Unspecified blepharitis right eye, unspecified eyelid
      H01.004   Unspecified blepharitis left upper eyelid
      H01.005   Unspecified blepharitis left lower eyelid
      H01.006   Unspecified blepharitis left eye, unspecified eyelid
      H01.009   Unspecified blepharitis unspecified eye, unspecified eyelid
    ● H01.01   Ulcerative blepharitis
      H01.011   Ulcerative blepharitis right upper eyelid
      H01.012   Ulcerative blepharitis right lower eyelid
      H01.013   Ulcerative blepharitis right eye, unspecified eyelid
      H01.014   Ulcerative blepharitis left upper eyelid
      H01.015   Ulcerative blepharitis left lower eyelid
      H01.016   Ulcerative blepharitis left eye, unspecified eyelid
      H01.019   Ulcerative blepharitis unspecified eye, unspecified eyelid
    ● H01.02   Squamous blepharitis
      H01.021   Squamous blepharitis right upper eyelid
      H01.022   Squamous blepharitis right lower eyelid
      H01.023   Squamous blepharitis right eye, unspecified eyelid
      H01.024   Squamous blepharitis left upper eyelid
      H01.025   Squamous blepharitis left lower eyelid
      H01.026   Squamous blepharitis left eye, unspecified eyelid
      H01.029   Squamous blepharitis unspecified eye, unspecified eyelid
  ● H01.1   Noninfectious dermatoses of eyelid
    ● H01.11   Allergic dermatitis of eyelid
      Contact dermatitis of eyelid
      H01.111   Allergic dermatitis of right upper eyelid
      H01.112   Allergic dermatitis of right lower eyelid
      H01.113   Allergic dermatitis of right eye, unspecified eyelid
      H01.114   Allergic dermatitis of left upper eyelid
      H01.115   Allergic dermatitis of left lower eyelid
      H01.116   Allergic dermatitis of left eye, unspecified eyelid
      H01.119   Allergic dermatitis of unspecified eye, unspecified eyelid

    ● H01.12   Discoid lupus erythematosus of eyelid
      H01.121   Discoid lupus erythematosus of right upper eyelid
      H01.122   Discoid lupus erythematosus of right lower eyelid
      H01.123   Discoid lupus erythematosus of right eye, unspecified eyelid
      H01.124   Discoid lupus erythematosus of left upper eyelid
      H01.125   Discoid lupus erythematosus of left lower eyelid
      H01.126   Discoid lupus erythematosus of left eye, unspecified eyelid
      H01.129   Discoid lupus erythematosus of unspecified eye, unspecified eyelid
    ● H01.13   Eczematous dermatitis of eyelid
      H01.131   Eczematous dermatitis of right upper eyelid
      H01.132   Eczematous dermatitis of right lower eyelid
      H01.133   Eczematous dermatitis of right eye, unspecified eyelid
      H01.134   Eczematous dermatitis of left upper eyelid
      H01.135   Eczematous dermatitis of left lower eyelid
      H01.136   Eczematous dermatitis of left eye, unspecified eyelid
      H01.139   Eczematous dermatitis of unspecified eye, unspecified eyelid
    ● H01.14   Xeroderma of eyelid
      Abnormally dry
      H01.141   Xeroderma of right upper eyelid
      H01.142   Xeroderma of right lower eyelid
      H01.143   Xeroderma of right eye, unspecified eyelid
      H01.144   Xeroderma of left upper eyelid
      H01.145   Xeroderma of left lower eyelid
      H01.146   Xeroderma of left eye, unspecified eyelid
      H01.149   Xeroderma of unspecified eye, unspecified eyelid
  H01.8   Other specified inflammations of eyelid
  H01.9   Unspecified inflammation of eyelid
    Inflammation of eyelid NOS

● H02   Other disorders of eyelid
  Turning inward (inversion) of eyelid margin and ingrowing eyelashes
    Excludes1   congenital malformations of eyelid (Q10.0-Q10.3)
  ● H02.0   Entropion and trichiasis of eyelid
    ● H02.00   Unspecified entropion of eyelid
      H02.001   Unspecified entropion of right upper eyelid
      H02.002   Unspecified entropion of right lower eyelid
      H02.003   Unspecified entropion of right eye, unspecified eyelid
      H02.004   Unspecified entropion of left upper eyelid

Figure 7-2 Right lower eyelid entropion. Note the inward rotation of the tarsal plate about the horizontal axis and the resultant contact between the mucocutaneous junction and ocular surface. (From Yanoff: Ophthalmology, ed 3, Mosby, Inc., 2008)

CHAPTER 7 (H00-H59)

CHAPTER 7 (H00-H59)

H02.005 Unspecified entropion of left lower eyelid

H02.006 Unspecified entropion of left eye, unspecified eyelid

H02.009 Unspecified entropion of unspecified eye, unspecified eyelid

● H02.01 Cicatricial entropion of eyelid
Scar

H02.011 Cicatricial entropion of right upper eyelid

H02.012 Cicatricial entropion of right lower eyelid

H02.013 Cicatricial entropion of right eye, unspecified eyelid

H02.014 Cicatricial entropion of left upper eyelid

H02.015 Cicatricial entropion of left lower eyelid

H02.016 Cicatricial entropion of left eye, unspecified eyelid

H02.019 Cicatricial entropion of unspecified eye, unspecified eyelid

● H02.02 Mechanical entropion of eyelid
Turning inward (inversion) of eyelid margin due to lack of support

H02.021 Mechanical entropion of right upper eyelid

H02.022 Mechanical entropion of right lower eyelid

H02.023 Mechanical entropion of right eye, unspecified eyelid

H02.024 Mechanical entropion of left upper eyelid

H02.025 Mechanical entropion of left lower eyelid

H02.026 Mechanical entropion of left eye, unspecified eyelid

H02.029 Mechanical entropion of unspecified eye, unspecified eyelid

● H02.03 Senile entropion of eyelid
Turning inward (inversion) of eyelid margin due to aging

H02.031 Senile entropion of right upper eyelid   A

H02.032 Senile entropion of right lower eyelid   A

H02.033 Senile entropion of right eye, unspecified eyelid   A

H02.034 Senile entropion of left upper eyelid A

H02.035 Senile entropion of left lower eyelid A

H02.036 Senile entropion of left eye, unspecified eyelid   A

H02.039 Senile entropion of unspecified eye, unspecified eyelid   A

● H02.04 Spastic entropion of eyelid
Turning inward (inversion) of eyelid margin caused by spasm of muscle

H02.041 Spastic entropion of right upper eyelid

H02.042 Spastic entropion of right lower eyelid

H02.043 Spastic entropion of right eye, unspecified eyelid

H02.044 Spastic entropion of left upper eyelid

H02.045 Spastic entropion of left lower eyelid

H02.046 Spastic entropion of left eye, unspecified eyelid

H02.049 Spastic entropion of unspecified eye, unspecified eyelid

● H02.05 Trichiasis without entropian
Ingrowing hairs of eyelashes

H02.051 Trichiasis without entropian right upper eyelid

H02.052 Trichiasis without entropian right lower eyelid

H02.053 Trichiasis without entropian right eye, unspecified eyelid

H02.054 Trichiasis without entropian left upper eyelid

H02.055 Trichiasis without entropian left lower eyelid

H02.056 Trichiasis without entropian left eye, unspecified eyelid

H02.059 Trichiasis without entropian unspecified eye, unspecified eyelid

● H02.1 Ectropion of eyelid
Eversion (pulling away) of eyelid

● H02.10 Unspecified ectropion of eyelid

H02.101 Unspecified ectropion of right upper eyelid

H02.102 Unspecified ectropion of right lower eyelid

H02.103 Unspecified ectropion of right eye, unspecified eyelid

H02.104 Unspecified ectropion of left upper eyelid

H02.105 Unspecified ectropion of left lower eyelid

H02.106 Unspecified ectropion of left eye, unspecified eyelid

H02.109 Unspecified ectropion of unspecified eye, unspecified eyelid

● H02.11 Cicatricial ectropion of eyelid
Pulling of eyelid down and away from eye due to scar or tightening

H02.111 Cicatricial ectropion of right upper eyelid

H02.112 Cicatricial ectropion of right lower eyelid

H02.113 Cicatricial ectropion of right eye, unspecified eyelid

H02.114 Cicatricial ectropion of left upper eyelid

H02.115 Cicatricial ectropion of left lower eyelid

H02.116 Cicatricial ectropion of left eye, unspecified eyelid

H02.119 Cicatricial ectropion of unspecified eye, unspecified eyelid

● H02.12 Mechanical ectropion of eyelid
Eversion (pulling away) of eyelid due to lack of support

H02.121 Mechanical ectropion of right upper eyelid

H02.122 Mechanical ectropion of right lower eyelid

H02.123 Mechanical ectropion of right eye, unspecified eyelid

H02.124 Mechanical ectropion of left upper eyelid

H02.125 Mechanical ectropion of left lower eyelid

H02.126 Mechanical ectropion of left eye, unspecified eyelid

H02.129 Mechanical ectropion of unspecified eye, unspecified eyelid

◀ New   ◀ Revised   deleted Deleted   Excludes 1   Excludes 2   Includes   Use additional   Code first   Code also   Unspecified

OGCR Official Guidelines   ● Unacceptable Principal Diagnosis   X Assign placeholder X   ● Use Additional Character(s)   ▶ Manifestation Code   **Coding Clinic**

● **H02.13   Senile ectropion of eyelid**
    Eversion (pulling away) of eyelid due to age

  H02.131 Senile ectropion of right upper
      eyelid   A

  H02.132 Senile ectropion of right lower
      eyelid   A

  H02.133 Senile ectropion of right eye,
      unspecified eyelid   A

  H02.134 Senile ectropion of left upper eyelid A

  H02.135 Senile ectropion of left lower eyelid A

  H02.136 Senile ectropion of left eye,
      unspecified eyelid   A

  H02.139 Senile ectropion of unspecified eye,
      unspecified eyelid   A

● **H02.14   Spastic ectropion of eyelid**
    Eversion (pulling away) of eyelid due to tonic
      muscle spasm

  H02.141 Spastic ectropion of right upper
      eyelid

  H02.142 Spastic ectropion of right lower
      eyelid

  H02.143 Spastic ectropion of right eye,
      unspecified eyelid

  H02.144 Spastic ectropion of left upper eyelid

  H02.145 Spastic ectropion of left lower eyelid

  H02.146 Spastic ectropion of left eye,
      unspecified eyelid

  H02.149 Spastic ectropion of unspecified eye,
      unspecified eyelid

● **H02.2   Lagophthalmos**
    Condition in which eye cannot completely close

● **H02.20   Unspecified lagophthalmos**

  H02.201 Unspecified lagophthalmos right
      upper eyelid

  H02.202 Unspecified lagophthalmos right
      lower eyelid

  H02.203 Unspecified lagophthalmos right eye,
      unspecified eyelid

  H02.204 Unspecified lagophthalmos left upper
      eyelid

  H02.205 Unspecified lagophthalmos left lower
      eyelid

  H02.206 Unspecified lagophthalmos left eye,
      unspecified eyelid

  H02.209 Unspecified lagophthalmos
      unspecified eye, unspecified eyelid

● **H02.21   Cicatricial lagophthalmos**
    Upper or lower eyelid does not close due to scar or
      tightening

  H02.211 Cicatricial lagophthalmos right upper
      eyelid

  H02.212 Cicatricial lagophthalmos right lower
      eyelid

  H02.213 Cicatricial lagophthalmos right eye,
      unspecified eyelid

  H02.214 Cicatricial lagophthalmos left upper
      eyelid

  H02.215 Cicatricial lagophthalmos left lower
      eyelid

  H02.216 Cicatricial lagophthalmos left eye,
      unspecified eyelid

  H02.219 Cicatricial lagophthalmos unspecified
      eye, unspecified eyelid

● **H02.22   Mechanical lagophthalmos**
    Inability to close lids due to structural disorder

  H02.221 Mechanical lagophthalmos right
      upper eyelid

  H02.222 Mechanical lagophthalmos right
      lower eyelid

  H02.223 Mechanical lagophthalmos right eye,
      unspecified eyelid

  H02.224 Mechanical lagophthalmos left upper
      eyelid

  H02.225 Mechanical lagophthalmos left lower
      eyelid

  H02.226 Mechanical lagophthalmos left eye,
      unspecified eyelid

  H02.229 Mechanical lagophthalmos
      unspecified eye, unspecified eyelid

● **H02.23   Paralytic lagophthalmos**
    Eyelids do not close due to paralysis

  H02.231 Paralytic lagophthalmos right upper
      eyelid

  H02.232 Paralytic lagophthalmos right lower
      eyelid

  H02.233 Paralytic lagophthalmos right eye,
      unspecified eyelid

  H02.234 Paralytic lagophthalmos left upper
      eyelid

  H02.235 Paralytic lagophthalmos left lower
      eyelid

  H02.236 Paralytic lagophthalmos left eye,
      unspecified eyelid

  H02.239 Paralytic lagophthalmos unspecified
      eye, unspecified eyelid

(See Plate 81, middle, on page 65.)

● **H02.3   Blepharochalasis**
    Relaxation of skin of eyelid, due to atrophy of intercellular
    tissue
    Pseudoptosis

  H02.30 Blepharochalasis unspecified eye, unspecified
      eyelid

  H02.31 Blepharochalasis right upper eyelid

  H02.32 Blepharochalasis right lower eyelid

  H02.33 Blepharochalasis right eye, unspecified eyelid

  H02.34 Blepharochalasis left upper eyelid

  H02.35 Blepharochalasis left lower eyelid

  H02.36 Blepharochalasis left eye, unspecified eyelid

● **H02.4   Ptosis of eyelid**
    Falling forward, drooping, sagging of eyelid

● **H02.40   Unspecified ptosis of eyelid**

  H02.401 Unspecified ptosis of right eyelid

  H02.402 Unspecified ptosis of left eyelid

  H02.403 Unspecified ptosis of bilateral eyelids

  H02.409 Unspecified ptosis of unspecified
      eyelid

● **H02.41   Mechanical ptosis of eyelid**

  H02.411 Mechanical ptosis of right eyelid

  H02.412 Mechanical ptosis of left eyelid

  H02.413 Mechanical ptosis of bilateral eyelids

  H02.419 Mechanical ptosis of unspecified
      eyelid

Figure 7-3 Ptosis of eyelid. (From Yanoff:
Ophthalmology, ed 3, Mosby, Inc., 2008)

Item 7-1 Ptosis of eyelid is drooping of the upper eyelid over the pupil when
the eyes are fully opened resulting from nerve or muscle damage, which may
require surgical correction.

N Newborn Age: 0 **P** Pediatric Age: 0–17 **M** Maternity DX: 12–55 **A** Adult Age: 15–124 ♀ Females Only ♂ Males Only

Complication\Comorbidity Major C\C (Ex) CC/MCC Exclusions Present on Admission Requirement Hospital-Acquired Condition   **905**

- H02.42   Myogenic ptosis of eyelid
  - H02.421   Myogenic ptosis of right eyelid
  - H02.422   Myogenic ptosis of left eyelid
  - H02.423   Myogenic ptosis of bilateral eyelids
  - H02.429   Myogenic ptosis of unspecified eyelid
- H02.43   Paralytic ptosis of eyelid
  - Neurogenic ptosis of eyelid
  - H02.431   Paralytic ptosis of right eyelid
  - H02.432   Paralytic ptosis of left eyelid
  - H02.433   Paralytic ptosis of bilateral eyelids
  - H02.439   Paralytic ptosis unspecified eyelid
- H02.5   Other disorders affecting eyelid function

  Excludes2   blepharospasm (G24.5)

  organic tic (G25.69)

  psychogenic tic (F95.-)

  - H02.51   Abnormal innervation syndrome
    - H02.511   Abnormal innervation syndrome right upper eyelid
    - H02.512   Abnormal innervation syndrome right lower eyelid
    - H02.513   Abnormal innervation syndrome right eye, unspecified eyelid
    - H02.514   Abnormal innervation syndrome left upper eyelid
    - H02.515   Abnormal innervation syndrome left lower eyelid
    - H02.516   Abnormal innervation syndrome left eye, unspecified eyelid
    - H02.519   Abnormal innervation syndrome unspecified eye, unspecified eyelid
  - H02.52   Blepharophimosis
    - *Drooping of eyelid with reduced lid size*
    - Ankyloblepharon
    - H02.521   Blepharophimosis right upper eyelid
    - H02.522   Blepharophimosis right lower eyelid
    - H02.523   Blepharophimosis right eye, unspecified eyelid
    - H02.524   Blepharophimosis left upper eyelid
    - H02.525   Blepharophimosis left lower eyelid
    - H02.526   Blepharophimosis left eye, unspecified eyelid
    - H02.529   Blepharophimosis unspecified eye, unspecified lid
  - H02.53   Eyelid retraction
    - Eyelid lag
    - H02.531   Eyelid retraction right upper eyelid
    - H02.532   Eyelid retraction right lower eyelid
    - H02.533   Eyelid retraction right eye, unspecified eyelid
    - H02.534   Eyelid retraction left upper eyelid
    - H02.535   Eyelid retraction left lower eyelid
    - H02.536   Eyelid retraction left eye, unspecified eyelid
    - H02.539   Eyelid retraction unspecified eye, unspecified lid
  - H02.59   Other disorders affecting eyelid function
    - Deficient blink reflex
    - Sensory disorders

- H02.6   Xanthelasma of eyelid
  - *Yellow-to-orange patches or pimples clustered together on eyelid*
  - H02.60   Xanthelasma of unspecified eye, unspecified eyelid
  - H02.61   Xanthelasma of right upper eyelid
  - H02.62   Xanthelasma of right lower eyelid
  - H02.63   Xanthelasma of right eye, unspecified eyelid
  - H02.64   Xanthelasma of left upper eyelid
  - H02.65   Xanthelasma of left lower eyelid
  - H02.66   Xanthelasma of left eye, unspecified eyelid
- H02.7   Other and unspecified degenerative disorders of eyelid and periocular area
  - H02.70   Unspecified degenerative disorders of eyelid and periocular area
  - H02.71   Chloasma of eyelid and periocular area
    - Dyspigmentation of eyelid
    - Hyperpigmentation of eyelid
    - H02.711   Chloasma of right upper eyelid and periocular area
    - H02.712   Chloasma of right lower eyelid and periocular area
    - H02.713   Chloasma of right eye, unspecified eyelid and periocular area
    - H02.714   Chloasma of left upper eyelid and periocular area
    - H02.715   Chloasma of left lower eyelid and periocular area
    - H02.716   Chloasma of left eye, unspecified eyelid and periocular area
    - H02.719   Chloasma of unspecified eye, unspecified eyelid and periocular area
  - H02.72   Madarosis of eyelid and periocular area
    - *Loss of eyelashes and/or eyebrows*
    - Hypotrichosis of eyelid
    - H02.721   Madarosis of right upper eyelid and periocular area
    - H02.722   Madarosis of right lower eyelid and periocular area
    - H02.723   Madarosis of right eye, unspecified eyelid and periocular area
    - H02.724   Madarosis of left upper eyelid and periocular area
    - H02.725   Madarosis of left lower eyelid and periocular area
    - H02.726   Madarosis of left eye, unspecified eyelid and periocular area
    - H02.729   Madarosis of unspecified eye, unspecified eyelid and periocular area
  - H02.73   Vitiligo of eyelid and periocular area
    - *Skin pigmentation disease characterized by white patches*
    - Hypopigmentation of eyelid
    - H02.731   Vitiligo of right upper eyelid and periocular area
    - H02.732   Vitiligo of right lower eyelid and periocular area
    - H02.733   Vitiligo of right eye, unspecified eyelid and periocular area
    - H02.734   Vitiligo of left upper eyelid and periocular area
    - H02.735   Vitiligo of left lower eyelid and periocular area
    - H02.736   Vitiligo of left eye, unspecified eyelid and periocular area
    - H02.739   Vitiligo of unspecified eye, unspecified eyelid and periocular area
  - H02.79   Other degenerative disorders of eyelid and periocular area

● **H02.8   Other specified disorders of eyelid**

   ● **H02.81   Retained foreign body in eyelid**

       Use additional code to identify the type of retained foreign body (Z18.-)

       Excludes1   laceration of eyelid with foreign body (S01.12-)
          retained intraocular foreign body (H44.6-, H44.7-)
          superficial foreign body of eyelid and periocular area (S00.25-)

       H02.811   Retained foreign body in right upper eyelid
       H02.812   Retained foreign body in right lower eyelid
       H02.813   Retained foreign body in right eye, unspecified eyelid
       H02.814   Retained foreign body in left upper eyelid
       H02.815   Retained foreign body in left lower eyelid
       H02.816   Retained foreign body in left eye, unspecified eyelid
       H02.819   Retained foreign body in unspecified eye, unspecified eyelid

   ● **H02.82   Cysts of eyelid**
       Sebaceous cyst of eyelid
       H02.821   Cysts of right upper eyelid
       H02.822   Cysts of right lower eyelid
       H02.823   Cysts of right eye, unspecified eyelid
       H02.824   Cysts of left upper eyelid
       H02.825   Cysts of left lower eyelid
       H02.826   Cysts of left eye, unspecified eyelid
       H02.829   Cysts of unspecified eye, unspecified eyelid

   ● **H02.83   Dermatochalasis of eyelid**
       Skin is inelastic and hangs loosely in folds
       H02.831   Dermatochalasis of right upper eyelid
       H02.832   Dermatochalasis of right lower eyelid
       H02.833   Dermatochalasis of right eye, unspecified eyelid
       H02.834   Dermatochalasis of left upper eyelid
       H02.835   Dermatochalasis of left lower eyelid
       H02.836   Dermatochalasis of left eye, unspecified eyelid
       H02.839   Dermatochalasis of unspecified eye, unspecified eyelid

   ● **H02.84   Edema of eyelid**
       Hyperemia of eyelid
       H02.841   Edema of right upper eyelid
       H02.842   Edema of right lower eyelid
       H02.843   Edema of right eye, unspecified eyelid
       H02.844   Edema of left upper eyelid
       H02.845   Edema of left lower eyelid
       H02.846   Edema of left eye, unspecified eyelid
       H02.849   Edema of unspecified eye, unspecified eyelid

   ● **H02.85   Elephantiasis of eyelid**
       Massive secondary lymphedema with hypertrophy of skin and subcutaneous tissues (pachyderma)
       H02.851   Elephantiasis of right upper eyelid
       H02.852   Elephantiasis of right lower eyelid
       H02.853   Elephantiasis of right eye, unspecified eyelid
       H02.854   Elephantiasis of left upper eyelid
       H02.855   Elephantiasis of left lower eyelid

       H02.856   Elephantiasis of left eye, unspecified eyelid
       H02.859   Elephantiasis of unspecified eye, unspecified eyelid

   ● **H02.86   Hypertrichosis of eyelid**
       Excessive growth of hair
       H02.861   Hypertrichosis of right upper eyelid
       H02.862   Hypertrichosis of right lower eyelid
       H02.863   Hypertrichosis of right eye, unspecified eyelid
       H02.864   Hypertrichosis of left upper eyelid
       H02.865   Hypertrichosis of left lower eyelid
       H02.866   Hypertrichosis of left eye, unspecified eyelid
       H02.869   Hypertrichosis of unspecified eye, unspecified eyelid

   ● **H02.87   Vascular anomalies of eyelid**
       H02.871   Vascular anomalies of right upper eyelid
       H02.872   Vascular anomalies of right lower eyelid
       H02.873   Vascular anomalies of right eye, unspecified eyelid
       H02.874   Vascular anomalies of left upper eyelid
       H02.875   Vascular anomalies of left lower eyelid
       H02.876   Vascular anomalies of left eye, unspecified eyelid
       H02.879   Vascular anomalies of unspecified eye, unspecified eyelid

     H02.89   Other specified disorders of eyelid
       Hemorrhage of eyelid

   H02.9   Unspecified disorder of eyelid
       Disorder of eyelid NOS

● **H04   Disorders of lacrimal system**

       Excludes1   congenital malformations of lacrimal system (Q10.4-Q10.6)

   ● **H04.0   Dacryoadenitis**
       Inflammation of lacrimal gland

     ● **H04.00   Unspecified dacryoadenitis**
       H04.001   Unspecified dacryoadenitis, right lacrimal gland
       H04.002   Unspecified dacryoadenitis, left lacrimal gland
       H04.003   Unspecified dacryoadenitis, bilateral lacrimal glands
       H04.009   Unspecified dacryoadenitis, unspecified lacrimal gland

     ● **H04.01   Acute dacryoadenitis**
       H04.011   Acute dacryoadenitis, right lacrimal gland
       H04.012   Acute dacryoadenitis, left lacrimal gland
       H04.013   Acute dacryoadenitis, bilateral lacrimal glands
       H04.019   Acute dacryoadenitis, unspecified lacrimal gland

Figure 7-4   Lacrimal apparatus. (From Buck CJ: Step-by-Step Medical Coding, Philadelphia, WB Saunders, 2006, p 302)

(See Plate 82 on page 67.)

N Newborn Age: 0   **P** Pediatric Age: 0–17   **M** Maternity DX: 12–55   **A** Adult Age: 15–124   ♀ Females Only   ♂ Males Only

Complication\Comorbidity   Major C\C   (Ex) CC/MCC Exclusions   Present on Admission Requirement   Hospital-Acquired Condition

907

● **H04.02**   Chronic dacryoadenitis

    H04.021   Chronic dacryoadenitis, right lacrimal gland

    H04.022   Chronic dacryoadenitis, left lacrimal gland

    H04.023   Chronic dacryoadenitis, bilateral lacrimal gland

    H04.029   Chronic dacryoadenitis, `unspecified` lacrimal gland

● **H04.03**   Chronic enlargement of lacrimal gland

    H04.031   Chronic enlargement of right lacrimal gland

    H04.032   Chronic enlargement of left lacrimal gland

    H04.033   Chronic enlargement of bilateral lacrimal glands

    H04.039   Chronic enlargement of `unspecified` lacrimal gland

● **H04.1**   Other disorders of lacrimal gland

● **H04.11**   Dacryops

    Watery eye or distention of lacrimal duct due to fluid

    H04.111   Dacryops of right lacrimal gland

    H04.112   Dacryops of left lacrimal gland

    H04.113   Dacryops of bilateral lacrimal glands

    H04.119   Dacryops of `unspecified` lacrimal gland

● **H04.12**   Dry eye syndrome

    Tear film insufficiency, NOS

    H04.121   Dry eye syndrome of right lacrimal gland

    H04.122   Dry eye syndrome of left lacrimal gland

    H04.123   Dry eye syndrome of bilateral lacrimal glands

    H04.129   Dry eye syndrome of `unspecified` lacrimal gland

● **H04.13**   Lacrimal cyst

    Lacrimal cystic degeneration

    H04.131   Lacrimal cyst right lacrimal gland

    H04.132   Lacrimal cyst left lacrimal gland

    H04.133   Lacrimal cyst bilateral lacrimal glands

    H04.139   Lacrimal cyst `unspecified` lacrimal gland

● **H04.14**   Primary lacrimal gland atrophy

    H04.141   Primary lacrimal gland atrophy, right lacrimal gland

    H04.142   Primary lacrimal gland atrophy, left lacrimal gland

    H04.143   Primary lacrimal gland atrophy, bilateral lacrimal glands

    H04.149   Primary lacrimal gland atrophy, `unspecified` lacrimal gland

● **H04.15**   Secondary lacrimal gland atrophy

    H04.151   Secondary lacrimal gland atrophy, right lacrimal gland

    H04.152   Secondary lacrimal gland atrophy, left lacrimal gland

    H04.153   Secondary lacrimal gland atrophy, bilateral lacrimal glands

    H04.159   Secondary lacrimal gland atrophy, `unspecified` lacrimal gland

● **H04.16**   Lacrimal gland dislocation

    H04.161   Lacrimal gland dislocation, right lacrimal gland

    H04.162   Lacrimal gland dislocation, left lacrimal gland

    H04.163   Lacrimal gland dislocation, bilateral lacrimal glands

    H04.169   Lacrimal gland dislocation, `unspecified` lacrimal gland

    H04.19   Other specified disorders of lacrimal gland

● **H04.2**   Epiphora

    Overflow of tears due to stricture of lacrimal passages; AKA lacrimation

● **H04.20**   Unspecified epiphora

    H04.201   `Unspecified` epiphora, right lacrimal gland

    H04.202   `Unspecified` epiphora, left lacrimal gland

    H04.203   `Unspecified` epiphora, bilateral lacrimal glands

    H04.209   `Unspecified` epiphora, unspecified lacrimal gland

● **H04.21**   Epiphora due to excess lacrimation

    H04.211   Epiphora due to excess lacrimation, right lacrimal gland

    H04.212   Epiphora due to excess lacrimation, left lacrimal gland

    H04.213   Epiphora due to excess lacrimation, bilateral lacrimal glands

    H04.219   Epiphora due to excess lacrimation, `unspecified` lacrimal gland

● **H04.22**   Epiphora due to insufficient drainage

    H04.221   Epiphora due to insufficient drainage, right lacrimal gland

    H04.222   Epiphora due to insufficient drainage, left lacrimal gland

    H04.223   Epiphora due to insufficient drainage, bilateral lacrimal glands

    H04.229   Epiphora due to insufficient drainage, `unspecified` lacrimal gland

● **H04.3**   Acute and unspecified inflammation of lacrimal passages

    Excludes1   neonatal dacryocystitis (P39.1)

● **H04.30**   Unspecified dacryocystitis

    H04.301   `Unspecified` dacryocystitis of right lacrimal passage

    H04.302   `Unspecified` dacryocystitis of left lacrimal passage

    H04.303   `Unspecified` dacryocystitis of bilateral lacrimal passages

    H04.309   `Unspecified` dacryocystitis of unspecified lacrimal passage

● **H04.31**   Phlegmonous dacryocystitis

    Cellulitis of lacrimal sac

    H04.311   Phlegmonous dacryocystitis of right lacrimal passage

    H04.312   Phlegmonous dacryocystitis of left lacrimal passage

    H04.313   Phlegmonous dacryocystitis of bilateral lacrimal passages

    H04.319   Phlegmonous dacryocystitis of `unspecified` lacrimal passage

● **H04.32**   Acute dacryocystitis

    Acute dacryopericystitis

    H04.321   Acute dacryocystitis of right lacrimal passage

    H04.322   Acute dacryocystitis of left lacrimal passage

    H04.323   Acute dacryocystitis of bilateral lacrimal passages

    H04.329   Acute dacryocystitis of `unspecified` lacrimal passage

● H04.33   Acute lacrimal canaliculitis
    H04.331   Acute lacrimal canaliculitis of right lacrimal passage
    H04.332   Acute lacrimal canaliculitis of left lacrimal passage
    H04.333   Acute lacrimal canaliculitis of bilateral lacrimal passages
    H04.339   Acute lacrimal canaliculitis of unspecified lacrimal passage

● H04.4   Chronic inflammation of lacrimal passages

 ● H04.41   Chronic dacryocystitis
    Inflammation of lacrimal sac
    H04.411   Chronic dacryocystitis of right lacrimal passage
    H04.412   Chronic dacryocystitis of left lacrimal passage
    H04.413   Chronic dacryocystitis of bilateral lacrimal passages
    H04.419   Chronic dacryocystitis of unspecified lacrimal passage

 ● H04.42   Chronic lacrimal canaliculitis
    Inflammation of lacrimal ducts
    H04.421   Chronic lacrimal canaliculitis of right lacrimal passage
    H04.422   Chronic lacrimal canaliculitis of left lacrimal passage
    H04.423   Chronic lacrimal canaliculitis of bilateral lacrimal passages
    H04.429   Chronic lacrimal canaliculitis of unspecified lacrimal passage

 ● H04.43   Chronic lacrimal mucocele
    Accumulation of mucous secretion
    H04.431   Chronic lacrimal mucocele of right lacrimal passage
    H04.432   Chronic lacrimal mucocele of left lacrimal passage
    H04.433   Chronic lacrimal mucocele of bilateral lacrimal passages
    H04.439   Chronic lacrimal mucocele of unspecified lacrimal passage

● H04.5   Stenosis and insufficiency of lacrimal passages

 ● H04.51   Dacryolith
    Concretion in lacrimal sac/duct; AKA lacrimal calculus
    H04.511   Dacryolith of right lacrimal passage
    H04.512   Dacryolith of left lacrimal passage
    H04.513   Dacryolith of bilateral lacrimal passages
    H04.519   Dacryolith of unspecified lacrimal passage

 ● H04.52   Eversion of lacrimal punctum
    Turning out of lacrimal drainage opening
    H04.521   Eversion of right lacrimal punctum
    H04.522   Eversion of left lacrimal punctum
    H04.523   Eversion of bilateral lacrimal punctum
    H04.529   Eversion of unspecified lacrimal punctum

 ● H04.53   Neonatal obstruction of nasolacrimal duct
    Excludes1   congenital stenosis and stricture of lacrimal duct (Q10.5)
    H04.531   Neonatal obstruction of right nasolacrimal duct   N
    H04.532   Neonatal obstruction of left nasolacrimal duct   N
    H04.533   Neonatal obstruction of bilateral nasolacrimal duct   N
    H04.539   Neonatal obstruction of unspecified nasolacrimal duct   N

 ● H04.54   Stenosis of lacrimal canaliculi
    H04.541   Stenosis of right lacrimal canaliculi
    H04.542   Stenosis of left lacrimal canaliculi
    H04.543   Stenosis of bilateral lacrimal canaliculi
    H04.549   Stenosis of unspecified lacrimal canaliculi

 ● H04.55   Acquired stenosis of nasolacrimal duct
    H04.551   Acquired stenosis of right nasolacrimal duct
    H04.552   Acquired stenosis of left nasolacrimal duct
    H04.553   Acquired stenosis of bilateral nasolacrimal duct
    H04.559   Acquired stenosis of unspecified nasolacrimal duct

 ● H04.56   Stenosis of lacrimal punctum
    H04.561   Stenosis of right lacrimal punctum
    H04.562   Stenosis of left lacrimal punctum
    H04.563   Stenosis of bilateral lacrimal punctum
    H04.569   Stenosis of unspecified lacrimal punctum

 ● H04.57   Stenosis of lacrimal sac
    H04.571   Stenosis of right lacrimal sac
    H04.572   Stenosis of left lacrimal sac
    H04.573   Stenosis of bilateral lacrimal sac
    H04.579   Stenosis of unspecified lacrimal sac

● H04.6   Other changes of lacrimal passages

 ● H04.61   Lacrimal fistula
    H04.611   Lacrimal fistula right lacrimal passage
    H04.612   Lacrimal fistula left lacrimal passage
    H04.613   Lacrimal fistula bilateral lacrimal passages
    H04.619   Lacrimal fistula unspecified lacrimal passage
    H04.69   Other changes of lacrimal passages

● H04.8   Other disorders of lacrimal system

 ● H04.81   Granuloma of lacrimal passages
    Inflammatory response due to infectious or noninfectious agents
    H04.811   Granuloma of right lacrimal passage
    H04.812   Granuloma of left lacrimal passage
    H04.813   Granuloma of bilateral lacrimal passages
    H04.819   Granuloma of unspecified lacrimal passage
    H04.89   Other disorders of lacrimal system

    H04.9   Disorder of lacrimal system, unspecified

● H05   Disorders of orbit
    Excludes1   congenital malformation of orbit (Q10.7)

● H05.0   Acute inflammation of orbit
    H05.00   Unspecified acute inflammation of orbit
 ● H05.01   Cellulitis of orbit
    Infection of soft tissue of orbit
    Abscess of orbit
    (Ex) **For category H05.01 CC codes:** H05.00-H05.049
    H05.011   Cellulitis of right orbit 🔊
    H05.012   Cellulitis of left orbit 🔊
    H05.013   Cellulitis of bilateral orbits 🔊
    H05.019   Cellulitis of unspecified orbit 🔊

N   Newborn Age: 0   **P**   Pediatric Age: 0–17   **M**   Maternity DX: 12–55   **A**   Adult Age: 15–124   ♀   Females Only   ♂   Males Only

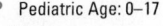   Complication\Comorbidity   🔊   Major C\C   (Ex)   CC/MCC Exclusions   🔊   Present on Admission Requirement   🔊   Hospital-Acquired Condition   **909**

CHAPTER 7 (H00-H59)

● **H05.02   Osteomyelitis of orbit**
  Infection of boney orbit of eye
  (Ex) **For category H05.02 CC codes:** A02.24, A17.9,
  A18.03-A18.09, A18.82, A18.84, A18.89, H05.021-H05.029,
  M46.20-M46.39, M86.00-M86.9

  H05.021   Osteomyelitis of right orbit 🖉
  H05.022   Osteomyelitis of left orbit 🖉
  H05.023   Osteomyelitis of bilateral orbits 🖉
  H05.029   Osteomyelitis of unspecified orbit 🖉

● **H05.03   Periostitis of orbit**
  *Inflammation of periosteum (membrane covering
  bone surface)*
  (Ex) **For category H05.03 CC codes:** A02.24, A17.9,
  A18.03-A18.09, A18.82, A18.84, A18.89, H05.031-H05.039,
  M46.20-M46.39, M86.00-M86.9

  H05.031   Periostitis of right orbit 🖉
  H05.032   Periostitis of left orbit 🖉
  H05.033   Periostitis of bilateral orbits 🖉
  H05.039   Periostitis of unspecified orbit 🖉

● **H05.04   Tenonitis of orbit**
  *Inflammation of tenon capsule (space enclosing
  fascia of Tenon between eyeball and fat of
  orbit)*

  H05.041   Tenonitis of right orbit
  H05.042   Tenonitis of left orbit
  H05.043   Tenonitis of bilateral orbits
  H05.049   Tenonitis of unspecified orbit

● **H05.1   Chronic inflammatory disorders of orbit**

  **H05.10   Unspecified chronic inflammatory disorders of
  orbit**

● **H05.11   Granuloma of orbit**
  Pseudotumor (inflammatory) of orbit

  H05.111   Granuloma of right orbit
  H05.112   Granuloma of left orbit
  H05.113   Granuloma of bilateral orbits
  H05.119   Granuloma of unspecified orbit

● **H05.12   Orbital myositis**
  Inflammation of extraocular muscles of orbit

  H05.121   Orbital myositis, right orbit
  H05.122   Orbital myositis, left orbit
  H05.123   Orbital myositis, bilateral
  H05.129   Orbital myositis, unspecified orbit

● **H05.2   Exophthalmic conditions**
  Bulging eyes

  H05.20   Unspecified exophthalmos

● **H05.21   Displacement (lateral) of globe**

  H05.211   Displacement (lateral) of globe, right
            eye
  H05.212   Displacement (lateral) of globe, left
            eye
  H05.213   Displacement (lateral) of globe,
            bilateral
  H05.219   Displacement (lateral) of globe,
            unspecified eye

● **H05.22   Edema of orbit**
  Orbital congestion

  H05.221   Edema of right orbit
  H05.222   Edema of left orbit
  H05.223   Edema of bilateral orbit
  H05.229   Edema of unspecified orbit

● **H05.23   Hemorrhage of orbit**

  H05.231   Hemorrhage of right orbit
  H05.232   Hemorrhage of left orbit
  H05.233   Hemorrhage of bilateral orbit
  H05.239   Hemorrhage of unspecified orbit

● **H05.24   Constant exophthalmos**
  *Constant bulging eyes, often symptom of Graves
  disease*

  H05.241   Constant exophthalmos, right eye
  H05.242   Constant exophthalmos, left eye
  H05.243   Constant exophthalmos, bilateral
  H05.249   Constant exophthalmos, unspecified
            eye

● **H05.25   Intermittent exophthalmos**
  *Intermittent bulging eye occurring with bending
  forward or sharp turning of head*

  H05.251   Intermittent exophthalmos, right eye
  H05.252   Intermittent exophthalmos, left eye
  H05.253   Intermittent exophthalmos, bilateral
  H05.259   Intermittent exophthalmos,
            unspecified eye

● **H05.26   Pulsating exophthalmos**
  *Bulging eyes with pulsation and bruit, often due to
  aneurysm pushing eye forward*

  H05.261   Pulsating exophthalmos, right eye
  H05.262   Pulsating exophthalmos, left eye
  H05.263   Pulsating exophthalmos, bilateral
  H05.269   Pulsating exophthalmos, unspecified
            eye

● **H05.3   Deformity of orbit**

  Excludes1   congenital deformity of orbit (Q10.7)
                  hypertelorism (Q75.2)

  H05.30   Unspecified deformity of orbit

● **H05.31   Atrophy of orbit**

  H05.311   Atrophy of right orbit
  H05.312   Atrophy of left orbit
  H05.313   Atrophy of bilateral orbit
  H05.319   Atrophy of unspecified orbit

● **H05.32   Deformity of orbit due to bone disease**
  Code also associated bone disease

  H05.321   Deformity of right orbit due to bone
            disease
  H05.322   Deformity of left orbit due to bone
            disease
  H05.323   Deformity of bilateral orbits due to
            bone disease
  H05.329   Deformity of unspecified orbit due to
            bone disease

● **H05.33   Deformity of orbit due to trauma or surgery**

  H05.331   Deformity of right orbit due to
            trauma or surgery
  H05.332   Deformity of left orbit due to trauma
            or surgery
  H05.333   Deformity of bilateral orbits due to
            trauma or surgery
  H05.339   Deformity of unspecified orbit due to
            trauma or surgery

● **H05.34   Enlargement of orbit**

  H05.341   Enlargement of right orbit
  H05.342   Enlargement of left orbit
  H05.343   Enlargement of bilateral orbits
  H05.349   Enlargement of unspecified orbit

● **H05.35   Exostosis of orbit**

  H05.351   Exostosis of right orbit
  H05.352   Exostosis of left orbit
  H05.353   Exostosis of bilateral orbits
  H05.359   Exostosis of unspecified orbit

◄ New   ◄┅ Revised   deleted Deleted   Excludes 1   Excludes 2   Includes   Use additional   Code first   Code also   Unspecified

910   **OGCR** Official Guidelines   ● Unacceptable Principal Diagnosis   X Assign placeholder X   ● Use Additional Character(s)   ▶ Manifestation Code   **Coding Clinic**

● H05.4   Enophthalmos
     Recessed eyeball into orbit
     ● H05.40   Unspecified enophthalmos
         H05.401   Unspecified enophthalmos, right eye
         H05.402   Unspecified enophthalmos, left eye
         H05.403   Unspecified enophthalmos, bilateral
         H05.409   Unspecified enophthalmos, unspecified eye
     ● H05.41   Enophthalmos due to atrophy of orbital tissue
         H05.411   Enophthalmos due to atrophy of orbital tissue, right eye
         H05.412   Enophthalmos due to atrophy of orbital tissue, left eye
         H05.413   Enophthalmos due to atrophy of orbital tissue, bilateral
         H05.419   Enophthalmos due to atrophy of orbital tissue, unspecified eye
     ● H05.42   Enophthalmos due to trauma or surgery
         H05.421   Enophthalmos due to trauma or surgery, right eye
         H05.422   Enophthalmos due to trauma or surgery, left eye
         H05.423   Enophthalmos due to trauma or surgery, bilateral
         H05.429   Enophthalmos due to trauma or surgery, unspecified eye
● H05.5   Retained (old) foreign body following penetrating wound of orbit
     Retrobulbar foreign body
     Use additional code to identify the type of retained foreign body (Z18.-)
     Excludes1   current penetrating wound of orbit (S05.4-)
     Excludes2   retained foreign body of eyelid (H02.81-)
                      retained intraocular foreign body (H44.6-, H44.7-)
     H05.50   Retained (old) foreign body following penetrating wound of unspecified orbit
     H05.51   Retained (old) foreign body following penetrating wound of right orbit
     H05.52   Retained (old) foreign body following penetrating wound of left orbit
     H05.53   Retained (old) foreign body following penetrating wound of bilateral orbits
● H05.8   Other disorders of orbit
     ● H05.81   Cyst of orbit
         Encephalocele of orbit
         H05.811   Cyst of right orbit
         H05.812   Cyst of left orbit
         H05.813   Cyst of bilateral orbits
         H05.819   Cyst of unspecified orbit
     ● H05.82   Myopathy of extraocular muscles
         Weakness of muscles of eye
         H05.821   Myopathy of extraocular muscles, right orbit
         H05.822   Myopathy of extraocular muscles, left orbit
         H05.823   Myopathy of extraocular muscles, bilateral
         H05.829   Myopathy of extraocular muscles, unspecified orbit
     H05.89   Other disorders of orbit
● H05.9   Unspecified disorder of orbit

DISORDERS OF CONJUNCTIVA (H10-H11)

(See Plate 81, upper, on page 66.)

● H10   Conjunctivitis
     Inflammation of membrane of the inside of the eyelid or on surface of eye (conjunctiva)
     Excludes1   keratoconjunctivitis (H16.2-)
     ● H10.0   Mucopurulent conjunctivitis
         ● H10.01   Acute follicular conjunctivitis
             H10.011   Acute follicular conjunctivitis, right eye
             H10.012   Acute follicular conjunctivitis, left eye
             H10.013   Acute follicular conjunctivitis, bilateral
             H10.019   Acute follicular conjunctivitis, unspecified eye
         ● H10.02   Other mucopurulent conjunctivitis
             H10.021   Other mucopurulent conjunctivitis, right eye
             H10.022   Other mucopurulent conjunctivitis, left eye
             H10.023   Other mucopurulent conjunctivitis, bilateral
             H10.029   Other mucopurulent conjunctivitis, unspecified eye
     ● H10.1   Acute atopic conjunctivitis
         Acute papillary conjunctivitis
         H10.10   Acute atopic conjunctivitis, unspecified eye
         H10.11   Acute atopic conjunctivitis, right eye
         H10.12   Acute atopic conjunctivitis, left eye
         H10.13   Acute atopic conjunctivitis, bilateral
     ● H10.2   Other acute conjunctivitis
         ● H10.21   Acute toxic conjunctivitis
             Acute chemical conjunctivitis
             Code first (T51-T65) to identify chemical and intent
             Excludes1   burn and corrosion of eye and adnexa (T26.-)
             H10.211   Acute toxic conjunctivitis, right eye
             H10.212   Acute toxic conjunctivitis, left eye
             H10.213   Acute toxic conjunctivitis, bilateral
             H10.219   Acute toxic conjunctivitis, unspecified eye
         ● H10.22   Pseudomembranous conjunctivitis
             H10.221   Pseudomembranous conjunctivitis, right eye
             H10.222   Pseudomembranous conjunctivitis, left eye
             H10.223   Pseudomembranous conjunctivitis, bilateral
             H10.229   Pseudomembranous conjunctivitis, unspecified eye
         ● H10.23   Serous conjunctivitis, except viral
             Excludes1   viral conjunctivitis (B30.-)
             H10.231   Serous conjunctivitis, except viral, right eye
             H10.232   Serous conjunctivitis, except viral, left eye
             H10.233   Serous conjunctivitis, except viral, bilateral
             H10.239   Serous conjunctivitis, except viral, unspecified eye

CHAPTER 7 (H00-H59)

N   Newborn Age: 0   P   Pediatric Age: 0-17   M   Maternity DX: 12-55   A   Adult Age: 15-124   ♀   Females Only   ♂   Males Only

●   Complication\Comorbidity   ●   Major C\C   Ⓔⓧ   CC/MCC Exclusions   ●   Present on Admission Requirement   ●   Hospital-Acquired Condition

911

● **H10.3 Unspecified acute conjunctivitis**
     Excludes1   ophthalmia neonatorum NOS (P39.1)
     H10.30   Unspecified acute conjunctivitis, unspecified eye
     H10.31   Unspecified acute conjunctivitis, right eye
     H10.32   Unspecified acute conjunctivitis, left eye
     H10.33   Unspecified acute conjunctivitis, bilateral

● **H10.4 Chronic conjunctivitis**
     ● **H10.40 Unspecified chronic conjunctivitis**
         H10.401   Unspecified chronic conjunctivitis, right eye
         H10.402   Unspecified chronic conjunctivitis, left eye
         H10.403   Unspecified chronic conjunctivitis, bilateral
         H10.409   Unspecified chronic conjunctivitis, unspecified eye
     ● **H10.41 Chronic giant papillary conjunctivitis**
         Inflammation of membrane of the inside of the eyelid or on surface of eye often associated with contact lens wear
         H10.411   Chronic giant papillary conjunctivitis, right eye
         H10.412   Chronic giant papillary conjunctivitis, left eye
         H10.413   Chronic giant papillary conjunctivitis, bilateral
         H10.419   Chronic giant papillary conjunctivitis, unspecified eye
     ● **H10.42 Simple chronic conjunctivitis**
         H10.421   Simple chronic conjunctivitis, right eye
         H10.422   Simple chronic conjunctivitis, left eye
         H10.423   Simple chronic conjunctivitis, bilateral
         H10.429   Simple chronic conjunctivitis, unspecified eye
     ● **H10.43 Chronic follicular conjunctivitis**
         Inflammation of membrane of the inside of the eyelid or on surface of eye due to topical medications or infection
         H10.431   Chronic follicular conjunctivitis, right eye
         H10.432   Chronic follicular conjunctivitis, left eye
         H10.433   Chronic follicular conjunctivitis, bilateral
         H10.439   Chronic follicular conjunctivitis, unspecified eye
     H10.44   Vernal conjunctivitis
         Affecting children, especially boys in which there are flattened papules with thick, gelatinous exudate on conjunctivae on inside of upper lid
         Excludes1   vernal keratoconjunctivitis with limbar and corneal involvement (H16.26-)
     H10.45   Other chronic allergic conjunctivitis

● **H10.5 Blepharoconjunctivitis**
     Inflammation of eyelids and conjunctiva
     ● **H10.50 Unspecified blepharoconjunctivitis**
         H10.501   Unspecified blepharoconjunctivitis, right eye
         H10.502   Unspecified blepharoconjunctivitis, left eye
         H10.503   Unspecified blepharoconjunctivitis, bilateral
         H10.509   Unspecified blepharoconjunctivitis, unspecified eye

● **H10.51 Ligneous conjunctivitis**
     H10.511   Ligneous conjunctivitis, right eye
     H10.512   Ligneous conjunctivitis, left eye
     H10.513   Ligneous conjunctivitis, bilateral
     H10.519   Ligneous conjunctivitis, unspecified eye
● **H10.52 Angular blepharoconjunctivitis**
     H10.521   Angular blepharoconjunctivitis, right eye
     H10.522   Angular blepharoconjunctivitis, left eye
     H10.523   Angular blepharoconjunctivitis, bilateral
     H10.529   Angular blepharoconjunctivitis, unspecified eye
● **H10.53 Contact blepharoconjunctivitis**
     H10.531   Contact blepharoconjunctivitis, right eye
     H10.532   Contact blepharoconjunctivitis, left eye
     H10.533   Contact blepharoconjunctivitis, bilateral
     H10.539   Contact blepharoconjunctivitis, unspecified eye
● **H10.8 Other conjunctivitis**
     ● **H10.81 Pingueculitis**
         Inflammation of a yellow, raised thickening on the white of the eye associated with chronic dry eyes
         Excludes1   pinguecula (H11.15-)
         H10.811   Pingueculitis, right eye
         H10.812   Pingueculitis, left eye
         H10.813   Pingueculitis, bilateral
         H10.819   Pingueculitis, unspecified eye
     H10.89   Other conjunctivitis
● **H10.9 Unspecified conjunctivitis**

● **H11 Other disorders of conjunctiva**
     Excludes1   keratoconjunctivitis (H16.2-)
     ● **H11.0 Pterygium of eye**
         Excludes1   pseudopterygium (H11.81-)
     ● **H11.00 Unspecified pterygium of eye**
         H11.001   Unspecified pterygium of right eye
         H11.002   Unspecified pterygium of left eye
         H11.003   Unspecified pterygium of eye, bilateral
         H11.009   Unspecified pterygium of unspecified eye
     ● **H11.01 Amyloid pterygium**
         H11.011   Amyloid pterygium of right eye
         H11.012   Amyloid pterygium of left eye
         H11.013   Amyloid pterygium of eye, bilateral
         H11.019   Amyloid pterygium of unspecified eye

Figure 7-5   Double pterygium. Note both nasal and temporal pterygia in a 57-year-old farmer. (From Yanoff: Ophthalmology, ed 3, Mosby, Inc., 2008)

Item 7-2   Pterygium is Greek for batlike. The condition is characterized by a membrane that extends from the limbus to the center of the cornea and resembles a wing.

◀ New   ◀ꞁꞁꞁ Revised   ~~deleted~~ Deleted   Excludes 1   Excludes 2   Includes   Use additional   Code first   Code also   Unspecified
OGCR Official Guidelines   ● Unacceptable Principal Diagnosis   X Assign placeholder X   ▶ Use Additional Character(s)   ▶ Manifestation Code   **Coding Clinic**

● H11.02   Central pterygium of eye
    H11.021   Central pterygium of right eye
    H11.022   Central pterygium of left eye
    H11.023   Central pterygium of eye, bilateral
    H11.029   Central pterygium of unspecified eye
● H11.03   Double pterygium of eye
    H11.031   Double pterygium of right eye
    H11.032   Double pterygium of left eye
    H11.033   Double pterygium of eye, bilateral
    H11.039   Double pterygium of unspecified eye
● H11.04   Peripheral pterygium of eye, stationary
    H11.041   Peripheral pterygium, stationary, right eye
    H11.042   Peripheral pterygium, stationary, left eye
    H11.043   Peripheral pterygium, stationary, bilateral
    H11.049   Peripheral pterygium, stationary, unspecified eye
● H11.05   Peripheral pterygium of eye, progressive
    H11.051   Peripheral pterygium, progressive, right eye
    H11.052   Peripheral pterygium, progressive, left eye
    H11.053   Peripheral pterygium, progressive, bilateral
    H11.059   Peripheral pterygium, progressive, unspecified eye
● H11.06   Recurrent pterygium of eye
    H11.061   Recurrent pterygium of right eye
    H11.062   Recurrent pterygium of left eye
    H11.063   Recurrent pterygium of eye, bilateral
    H11.069   Recurrent pterygium of unspecified eye
● H11.1   Conjunctival degenerations and deposits
    Excludes2   pseudopterygium (H11.81)
    H11.10   Unspecified conjunctival degenerations
● H11.11   Conjunctival deposits
    H11.111   Conjunctival deposits, right eye
    H11.112   Conjunctival deposits, left eye
    H11.113   Conjunctival deposits, bilateral
    H11.119   Conjunctival deposits, unspecified eye
● H11.12   Conjunctival concretions
    White to yellow nodules within or beneath conjunctiva
    H11.121   Conjunctival concretions, right eye
    H11.122   Conjunctival concretions, left eye
    H11.123   Conjunctival concretions, bilateral
    H11.129   Conjunctival concretions, unspecified eye
● H11.13   Conjunctival pigmentations
    Conjunctival argyrosis [argyria]
    H11.131   Conjunctival pigmentations, right eye
    H11.132   Conjunctival pigmentations, left eye
    H11.133   Conjunctival pigmentations, bilateral
    H11.139   Conjunctival pigmentations, unspecified eye

● H11.14   Conjunctival xerosis, unspecified
    Excludes1   xerosis of conjunctiva due to vitamin A deficiency (E50.0, E50.1)
    H11.141   Conjunctival xerosis, unspecified, right eye
    H11.142   Conjunctival xerosis, unspecified, left eye
    H11.143   Conjunctival xerosis, unspecified, bilateral
    H11.149   Conjunctival xerosis, unspecified, unspecified eye
● H11.15   Pinguecula
    Yellowish spot near sclerocorneal junction, usually on nasal side; associated with aging
    Excludes1   pingueculitis (H10.81-)
    H11.151   Pinguecula, right eye
    H11.152   Pinguecula, left eye
    H11.153   Pinguecula, bilateral
    H11.159   Pinguecula, unspecified eye
● H11.2   Conjunctival scars
  ● H11.21   Conjunctival adhesions and strands (localized)
    H11.211   Conjunctival adhesions and strands (localized), right eye
    H11.212   Conjunctival adhesions and strands (localized), left eye
    H11.213   Conjunctival adhesions and strands (localized), bilateral
    H11.219   Conjunctival adhesions and strands (localized), unspecified eye
  ● H11.22   Conjunctival granuloma
    H11.221   Conjunctival granuloma, right eye
    H11.222   Conjunctival granuloma, left eye
    H11.223   Conjunctival granuloma, bilateral
    H11.229   Conjunctival granuloma, unspecified
  ● H11.23   Symblepharon
    Adhesion between tarsal conjunctiva and bulbar conjunctiva
    H11.231   Symblepharon, right eye
    H11.232   Symblepharon, left eye
    H11.233   Symblepharon, bilateral
    H11.239   Symblepharon, unspecified eye
  ● H11.24   Scarring of conjunctiva
    H11.241   Scarring of conjunctiva, right eye
    H11.242   Scarring of conjunctiva, left eye
    H11.243   Scarring of conjunctiva, bilateral
    H11.249   Scarring of conjunctiva, unspecified eye
● H11.3   Conjunctival hemorrhage
    Subconjunctival hemorrhage
    H11.30   Conjunctival hemorrhage, unspecified eye
    H11.31   Conjunctival hemorrhage, right eye
    H11.32   Conjunctival hemorrhage, left eye
    H11.33   Conjunctival hemorrhage, bilateral
● H11.4   Other conjunctival vascular disorders and cysts
  ● H11.41   Vascular abnormalities of conjunctiva
    Conjunctival aneurysm
    H11.411   Vascular abnormalities of conjunctiva, right eye
    H11.412   Vascular abnormalities of conjunctiva, left eye
    H11.413   Vascular abnormalities of conjunctiva, bilateral
    H11.419   Vascular abnormalities of conjunctiva, unspecified eye

N   Newborn Age: 0   P   Pediatric Age: 0–17   M   Maternity DX: 12–55   A   Adult Age: 15–124   ♀   Females Only   ♂   Males Only
Complication\Comorbidity   Major C\C   (Ex)   CC/MCC Exclusions   Present on Admission Requirement   Hospital-Acquired Condition
913

CHAPTER 7 (H00-H59)

- ● H11.42   Conjunctival edema
  - H11.421   Conjunctival edema, right eye
  - H11.422   Conjunctival edema, left eye
  - H11.423   Conjunctival edema, bilateral
  - H11.429   Conjunctival edema, unspecified eye
- ● H11.43   Conjunctival hyperemia
  - H11.431   Conjunctival hyperemia, right eye
  - H11.432   Conjunctival hyperemia, left eye
  - H11.433   Conjunctival hyperemia, bilateral
  - H11.439   Conjunctival hyperemia, unspecified eye
- ● H11.44   Conjunctival cysts
  - H11.441   Conjunctival cysts, right eye
  - H11.442   Conjunctival cysts, left eye
  - H11.443   Conjunctival cysts, bilateral
  - H11.449   Conjunctival cysts, unspecified eye
- ● H11.8   Other specified disorders of conjunctiva
  - ● H11.81   Pseudopterygium of conjunctiva
    - *Conjunctival scar attached to cornea*
    - H11.811   Pseudopterygium of conjunctiva, right eye
    - H11.812   Pseudopterygium of conjunctiva, left eye
    - H11.813   Pseudopterygium of conjunctiva, bilateral
    - H11.819   Pseudopterygium of conjunctiva, unspecified eye
  - ● H11.82   Conjunctivochalasis
    - *Conjunctiva bulges over eyelid margin or covers lower punctum*
    - H11.821   Conjunctivochalasis, right eye
    - H11.822   Conjunctivochalasis, left eye
    - H11.823   Conjunctivochalasis, bilateral
    - H11.829   Conjunctivochalasis, unspecified eye
  - H11.89   Other specified disorders of conjunctiva
- H11.9   Unspecified disorder of conjunctiva

DISORDERS OF SCLERA, CORNEA, IRIS AND CILIARY BODY (H15-H22)

- ● H15   Disorders of sclera
  - ● H15.0   Scleritis
    - *Inflammation of the white (sclera and episclera) of the eye.*
    - ● H15.00   Unspecified scleritis
      - H15.001   Unspecified scleritis, right eye
      - H15.002   Unspecified scleritis, left eye
      - H15.003   Unspecified scleritis, bilateral
      - H15.009   Unspecified scleritis, unspecified eye
    - ● H15.01   Anterior scleritis
      - H15.011   Anterior scleritis, right eye
      - H15.012   Anterior scleritis, left eye
      - H15.013   Anterior scleritis, bilateral
      - H15.019   Anterior scleritis, unspecified eye
    - ● H15.02   Brawny scleritis
      - *Swelling around the cornea that is gelantinous in appearance*
      - H15.021   Brawny scleritis, right eye
      - H15.022   Brawny scleritis, left eye
      - H15.023   Brawny scleritis, bilateral
      - H15.029   Brawny scleritis, unspecified eye
    - ● H15.03   Posterior scleritis
      - Sclerotenonitis
      - H15.031   Posterior scleritis, right eye
      - H15.032   Posterior scleritis, left eye
      - H15.033   Posterior scleritis, bilateral
      - H15.039   Posterior scleritis, unspecified eye
    - ● H15.04   Scleritis with corneal involvement
      - H15.041   Scleritis with corneal involvement, right eye
      - H15.042   Scleritis with corneal involvement, left eye
      - H15.043   Scleritis with corneal involvement, bilateral
      - H15.049   Scleritis with corneal involvement, unspecified eye
    - ● H15.05   Scleromalacia perforans
      - *Necrotic without inflammation; usually associated with rheumatoid arthritis*
      - H15.051   Scleromalacia perforans, right eye
      - H15.052   Scleromalacia perforans, left eye
      - H15.053   Scleromalacia perforans, bilateral
      - H15.059   Scleromalacia perforans, unspecified eye
    - ● H15.09   Other scleritis
      - Scleral abscess
      - H15.091   Other scleritis, right eye
      - H15.092   Other scleritis, left eye
      - H15.093   Other scleritis, bilateral
      - H15.099   Other scleritis, unspecified eye
  - ● H15.1   Episcleritis
    - *Inflammation of the white (sclera and episclera) of the eye.*
    - ● H15.10   Unspecified episcleritis
      - H15.101   Unspecified episcleritis, right eye
      - H15.102   Unspecified episcleritis, left eye
      - H15.103   Unspecified episcleritis, bilateral
      - H15.109   Unspecified episcleritis, unspecified eye
    - ● H15.11   Episcleritis periodica fugax
      - *Transient, recurrent inflammation of portion of episclera (connective tissue on the surface of the sclera)*
      - H15.111   Episcleritis periodica fugax, right eye
      - H15.112   Episcleritis periodica fugax, left eye
      - H15.113   Episcleritis periodica fugax, bilateral
      - H15.119   Episcleritis periodica fugax, unspecified eye
    - ● H15.12   Nodular episcleritis
      - *Characterized by tender, localized, moveable nodule within inflamed area*
      - H15.121   Nodular episcleritis, right eye
      - H15.122   Nodular episcleritis, left eye
      - H15.123   Nodular episcleritis, bilateral
      - H15.129   Nodular episcleritis, unspecified eye
  - ● H15.8   Other disorders of sclera
    - **Excludes2**   blue sclera (Q13.5)
      - degenerative myopia (H44.2-)
    - ● H15.81   Equatorial staphyloma
      - H15.811   Equatorial staphyloma, right eye
      - H15.812   Equatorial staphyloma, left eye
      - H15.813   Equatorial staphyloma, bilateral
      - H15.819   Equatorial staphyloma, unspecified eye
    - ● H15.82   Localized anterior staphyloma
      - H15.821   Localized anterior staphyloma, right eye
      - H15.822   Localized anterior staphyloma, left eye
      - H15.823   Localized anterior staphyloma, bilateral
      - H15.829   Localized anterior staphyloma, unspecified eye

◀ New   ◀◀ Revised   ~~deleted~~ Deleted   Excludes 1   Excludes 2   Includes   Use additional   Code first   Code also   Unspecified

OGCR Official Guidelines   ● Unacceptable Principal Diagnosis   X Assign placeholder X   ● Use Additional Character(s)   ▶ Manifestation Code   **Coding Clinic**

H15.83 Staphyloma posticum
    H15.831 Staphyloma posticum, right eye
    H15.832 Staphyloma posticum, left eye
    H15.833 Staphyloma posticum, bilateral
    H15.839 Staphyloma posticum, unspecified eye
H15.84 Scleral ectasia
    H15.841 Scleral ectasia, right eye
    H15.842 Scleral ectasia, left eye
    H15.843 Scleral ectasia, bilateral
    H15.849 Scleral ectasia, unspecified eye
H15.85 Ring staphyloma
    H15.851 Ring staphyloma, right eye
    H15.852 Ring staphyloma, left eye
    H15.853 Ring staphyloma, bilateral
    H15.859 Ring staphyloma, unspecified eye
H15.89 Other disorders of sclera
H15.9 Unspecified disorder of sclera

● H16 Keratitis
  ● H16.0 Corneal ulcer
    ● H16.00 Unspecified corneal ulcer
      H16.001 Unspecified corneal ulcer, right eye
      H16.002 Unspecified corneal ulcer, left eye
      H16.003 Unspecified corneal ulcer, bilateral
      H16.009 Unspecified corneal ulcer, unspecified eye
    ● H16.01 Central corneal ulcer
      H16.011 Central corneal ulcer, right eye
      H16.012 Central corneal ulcer, left eye
      H16.013 Central corneal ulcer, bilateral
      H16.019 Central corneal ulcer, unspecified eye
    ● H16.02 Ring corneal ulcer
      H16.021 Ring corneal ulcer, right eye
      H16.022 Ring corneal ulcer, left eye
      H16.023 Ring corneal ulcer, bilateral
      H16.029 Ring corneal ulcer, unspecified eye
    ● H16.03 Corneal ulcer with hypopyon
      H16.031 Corneal ulcer with hypopyon, right eye
      H16.032 Corneal ulcer with hypopyon, left eye
      H16.033 Corneal ulcer with hypopyon, bilateral
      H16.039 Corneal ulcer with hypopyon, unspecified eye

| Marginal (catarrhal) ulcer | Ring ulcer | Central corneal ulcer | Rosacea ulcer | Mooren's (rodent) ulcer |

Figure 7-6 Corneal ulcers: marginal, ring, central corneal, rosacea, and Mooren's.

Item 7-3 An infected ulcer is usually called a **serpiginous** or **hypopyon** ulcer which is a pus sac in the anterior chamber of the eye. **Marginal** ulcers are usually asymptomatic, not primary, and are often superficial and simple. More severe marginal ulcers spread to form a ring ulcer. **Ring** ulcers can extend around the entire corneal periphery. **Central corneal** ulcers develop when there is an abrasion to the epithelium and an infection develops in the eroded area. The **pyocyaneal** ulcer is the most serious corneal infection, which, if left untreated, can lead to loss of the eye.

● H16.04 Marginal corneal ulcer
    H16.041 Marginal corneal ulcer, right eye
    H16.042 Marginal corneal ulcer, left eye
    H16.043 Marginal corneal ulcer, bilateral
    H16.049 Marginal corneal ulcer, unspecified eye
● H16.05 Mooren's corneal ulcer
    H16.051 Mooren's corneal ulcer, right eye
    H16.052 Mooren's corneal ulcer, left eye
    H16.053 Mooren's corneal ulcer, bilateral
    H16.059 Mooren's corneal ulcer, unspecified eye
● H16.06 Mycotic corneal ulcer
    H16.061 Mycotic corneal ulcer, right eye
    H16.062 Mycotic corneal ulcer, left eye
    H16.063 Mycotic corneal ulcer, bilateral
    H16.069 Mycotic corneal ulcer, unspecified eye
● H16.07 Perforated corneal ulcer
    H16.071 Perforated corneal ulcer, right eye
    H16.072 Perforated corneal ulcer, left eye
    H16.073 Perforated corneal ulcer, bilateral
    H16.079 Perforated corneal ulcer, unspecified eye
● H16.1 Other and unspecified superficial keratitis without conjunctivitis
  ● H16.10 Unspecified superficial keratitis
    H16.101 Unspecified superficial keratitis, right eye
    H16.102 Unspecified superficial keratitis, left eye
    H16.103 Unspecified superficial keratitis, bilateral
    H16.109 Unspecified superficial keratitis, unspecified eye
  ● H16.11 Macular keratitis
    Areolar keratitis
    Nummular keratitis
    Stellate keratitis
    Striate keratitis
    H16.111 Macular keratitis, right eye
    H16.112 Macular keratitis, left eye
    H16.113 Macular keratitis, bilateral
    H16.119 Macular keratitis, unspecified eye
  ● H16.12 Filamentary keratitis
    H16.121 Filamentary keratitis, right eye
    H16.122 Filamentary keratitis, left eye
    H16.123 Filamentary keratitis, bilateral
    H16.129 Filamentary keratitis, unspecified eye
  ● H16.13 Photokeratitis
    Snow blindness
    Welders' keratitis
    H16.131 Photokeratitis, right eye
    H16.132 Photokeratitis, left eye
    H16.133 Photokeratitis, bilateral
    H16.139 Photokeratitis, unspecified eye
  ● H16.14 Punctate keratitis
    H16.141 Punctate keratitis, right eye
    H16.142 Punctate keratitis, left eye
    H16.143 Punctate keratitis, bilateral
    H16.149 Punctate keratitis, unspecified eye

CHAPTER 7 (H00-H59)

- ● H16.2 Keratoconjunctivitis
  - ● H16.20 Unspecified keratoconjunctivitis
    Superficial keratitis with conjunctivitis NOS
    - H16.201 Unspecified keratoconjunctivitis, right eye
    - H16.202 Unspecified keratoconjunctivitis, left eye
    - H16.203 Unspecified keratoconjunctivitis, bilateral
    - H16.209 Unspecified keratoconjunctivitis, unspecified eye
  - ● H16.21 Exposure keratoconjunctivitis
    - H16.211 Exposure keratoconjunctivitis, right eye
    - H16.212 Exposure keratoconjunctivitis, left eye
    - H16.213 Exposure keratoconjunctivitis, bilateral
    - H16.219 Exposure keratoconjunctivitis, unspecified eye
  - ● H16.22 Keratoconjunctivitis sicca, not specified as Sjögren's
    - **Excludes1** Sjogren's syndrome (M35.01)
    - H16.221 Keratoconjunctivitis sicca, not specified as Sjögren's, right eye
    - H16.222 Keratoconjunctivitis sicca, not specified as Sjögren's, left eye
    - H16.223 Keratoconjunctivitis sicca, not specified as Sjögren's, bilateral
    - H16.229 Keratoconjunctivitis sicca, not specified as Sjögren's, unspecified eye
  - ● H16.23 Neurotrophic keratoconjunctivitis
    - H16.231 Neurotrophic keratoconjunctivitis, right eye
    - H16.232 Neurotrophic keratoconjunctivitis, left eye
    - H16.233 Neurotrophic keratoconjunctivitis, bilateral
    - H16.239 Neurotrophic keratoconjunctivitis, unspecified eye
  - ● H16.24 Ophthalmia nodosa
    - H16.241 Ophthalmia nodosa, right eye
    - H16.242 Ophthalmia nodosa, left eye
    - H16.243 Ophthalmia nodosa, bilateral
    - H16.249 Ophthalmia nodosa, unspecified eye
  - ● H16.25 Phlyctenular keratoconjunctivitis
    - H16.251 Phlyctenular keratoconjunctivitis, right eye
    - H16.252 Phlyctenular keratoconjunctivitis, left eye
    - H16.253 Phlyctenular keratoconjunctivitis, bilateral
    - H16.259 Phlyctenular keratoconjunctivitis, unspecified eye
  - ● H16.26 Vernal keratoconjunctivitis, with limbar and corneal involvement
    - **Excludes1** vernal conjunctivitis without limbar and corneal involvement (H10.44)
    - H16.261 Vernal keratoconjunctivitis, with limbar and corneal involvement, right eye
    - H16.262 Vernal keratoconjunctivitis, with limbar and corneal involvement, left eye
    - H16.263 Vernal keratoconjunctivitis, with limbar and corneal involvement, bilateral
    - H16.269 Vernal keratoconjunctivitis, with limbar and corneal involvement, unspecified eye
  - ● H16.29 Other keratoconjunctivitis
    - H16.291 Other keratoconjunctivitis, right eye
    - H16.292 Other keratoconjunctivitis, left eye
    - H16.293 Other keratoconjunctivitis, bilateral
    - H16.299 Other keratoconjunctivitis, unspecified eye
- ● H16.3 Interstitial and deep keratitis
  - ● H16.30 Unspecified interstitial keratitis
    - H16.301 Unspecified interstitial keratitis, right eye
    - H16.302 Unspecified interstitial keratitis, left eye
    - H16.303 Unspecified interstitial keratitis, bilateral
    - H16.309 Unspecified interstitial keratitis, unspecified eye
  - ● H16.31 Corneal abscess
    - H16.311 Corneal abscess, right eye
    - H16.312 Corneal abscess, left eye
    - H16.313 Corneal abscess, bilateral
    - H16.319 Corneal abscess, unspecified eye
  - ● H16.32 Diffuse interstitial keratitis
    Cogan's syndrome
    - H16.321 Diffuse interstitial keratitis, right eye
    - H16.322 Diffuse interstitial keratitis, left eye
    - H16.323 Diffuse interstitial keratitis, bilateral
    - H16.329 Diffuse interstitial keratitis, unspecified eye
  - ● H16.33 Sclerosing keratitis
    - H16.331 Sclerosing keratitis, right eye
    - H16.332 Sclerosing keratitis, left eye
    - H16.333 Sclerosing keratitis, bilateral
    - H16.339 Sclerosing keratitis, unspecified eye
  - ● H16.39 Other interstitial and deep keratitis
    - H16.391 Other interstitial and deep keratitis, right eye
    - H16.392 Other interstitial and deep keratitis, left eye
    - H16.393 Other interstitial and deep keratitis, bilateral
    - H16.399 Other interstitial and deep keratitis, unspecified eye
- ● H16.4 Corneal neovascularization
  - ● H16.40 Unspecified corneal neovascularization
    - H16.401 Unspecified corneal neovascularization, right eye
    - H16.402 Unspecified corneal neovascularization, left eye
    - H16.403 Unspecified corneal neovascularization, bilateral
    - H16.409 Unspecified corneal neovascularization, unspecified eye
  - ● H16.41 Ghost vessels (corneal)
    - H16.411 Ghost vessels (corneal), right eye
    - H16.412 Ghost vessels (corneal), left eye
    - H16.413 Ghost vessels (corneal), bilateral
    - H16.419 Ghost vessels (corneal), unspecified eye

- H16.42   Pannus (corneal)
  - H16.421   Pannus (corneal), right eye
  - H16.422   Pannus (corneal), left eye
  - H16.423   Pannus (corneal), bilateral
  - H16.429   Pannus (corneal), unspecified eye
- H16.43   Localized vascularization of cornea
  - H16.431   Localized vascularization of cornea, right eye
  - H16.432   Localized vascularization of cornea, left eye
  - H16.433   Localized vascularization of cornea, bilateral
  - H16.439   Localized vascularization of cornea, unspecified eye
- H16.44   Deep vascularization of cornea
  - H16.441   Deep vascularization of cornea, right eye
  - H16.442   Deep vascularization of cornea, left eye
  - H16.443   Deep vascularization of cornea, bilateral
  - H16.449   Deep vascularization of cornea, unspecified eye
- H16.8   Other keratitis
- H16.9   Unspecified keratitis

- H17   **Corneal scars and opacities**
  - H17.0   Adherent leukoma
    - H17.00   Adherent leukoma, unspecified eye
    - H17.01   Adherent leukoma, right eye
    - H17.02   Adherent leukoma, left eye
    - H17.03   Adherent leukoma, bilateral
  - H17.1   Central corneal opacity
    - H17.10   Central corneal opacity, unspecified eye
    - H17.11   Central corneal opacity, right eye
    - H17.12   Central corneal opacity, left eye
    - H17.13   Central corneal opacity, bilateral
  - H17.8   Other corneal scars and opacities
    - H17.81   Minor opacity of cornea
      Corneal nebula
      - H17.811   Minor opacity of cornea, right eye
      - H17.812   Minor opacity of cornea, left eye
      - H17.813   Minor opacity of cornea, bilateral
      - H17.819   Minor opacity of cornea, unspecified eye
    - H17.82   Peripheral opacity of cornea
      - H17.821   Peripheral opacity of cornea, right eye
      - H17.822   Peripheral opacity of cornea, left eye
      - H17.823   Peripheral opacity of cornea, bilateral
      - H17.829   Peripheral opacity of cornea, unspecified eye
    - H17.89   Other corneal scars and opacities
  - H17.9   Unspecified corneal scar and opacity

- H18   **Other disorders of cornea**
  - H18.0   Corneal pigmentations and deposits
    - H18.00   Unspecified corneal deposit
      - H18.001   Unspecified corneal deposit, right eye
      - H18.002   Unspecified corneal deposit, left eye
      - H18.003   Unspecified corneal deposit, bilateral
      - H18.009   Unspecified corneal deposit, unspecified eye
    - H18.01   Anterior corneal pigmentations
      Staehli's line
      - H18.011   Anterior corneal pigmentations, right eye
      - H18.012   Anterior corneal pigmentations, left eye
      - H18.013   Anterior corneal pigmentations, bilateral
      - H18.019   Anterior corneal pigmentations, unspecified eye
    - H18.02   Argentous corneal deposits
      - H18.021   Argentous corneal deposits, right eye
      - H18.022   Argentous corneal deposits, left eye
      - H18.023   Argentous corneal deposits, bilateral
      - H18.029   Argentous corneal deposits, unspecified eye
    - H18.03   Corneal deposits in metabolic disorders
      Code also associated metabolic disorder
      - H18.031   Corneal deposits in metabolic disorders, right eye
      - H18.032   Corneal deposits in metabolic disorders, left eye
      - H18.033   Corneal deposits in metabolic disorders, bilateral
      - H18.039   Corneal deposits in metabolic disorders, unspecified eye
    - H18.04   Kayser-Fleischer ring
      Code also associated Wilson's disease (E83.01)
      - H18.041   Kayser-Fleischer ring, right eye
      - H18.042   Kayser-Fleischer ring, left eye
      - H18.043   Kayser-Fleischer ring, bilateral
      - H18.049   Kayser-Fleischer ring, unspecified eye
    - H18.05   Posterior corneal pigmentations
      Krukenberg's spindle
      - H18.051   Posterior corneal pigmentations, right eye
      - H18.052   Posterior corneal pigmentations, left eye
      - H18.053   Posterior corneal pigmentations, bilateral
      - H18.059   Posterior corneal pigmentations, unspecified eye
    - H18.06   Stromal corneal pigmentations
      Hematocornea
      - H18.061   Stromal corneal pigmentations, right eye
      - H18.062   Stromal corneal pigmentations, left eye
      - H18.063   Stromal corneal pigmentations, bilateral
      - H18.069   Stromal corneal pigmentations, unspecified eye
  - H18.1   Bullous keratopathy
    - H18.10   Bullous keratopathy, unspecified eye
    - H18.11   Bullous keratopathy, right eye
    - H18.12   Bullous keratopathy, left eye
    - H18.13   Bullous keratopathy, bilateral
  - H18.2   Other and unspecified corneal edema
    - H18.20   Unspecified corneal edema
    - H18.21   Corneal edema secondary to contact lens

      Excludes2   other corneal disorders due to contact lens (H18.82-)
      - H18.211   Corneal edema secondary to contact lens, right eye
      - H18.212   Corneal edema secondary to contact lens, left eye
      - H18.213   Corneal edema secondary to contact lens, bilateral
      - H18.219   Corneal edema secondary to contact lens, unspecified eye

CHAPTER 7 (H00-H59)

 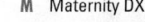

● H18.22 Idiopathic corneal edema
 H18.221 Idiopathic corneal edema, right eye
 H18.222 Idiopathic corneal edema, left eye
 H18.223 Idiopathic corneal edema, bilateral
 H18.229 Idiopathic corneal edema, unspecified eye

● H18.23 Secondary corneal edema
 H18.231 Secondary corneal edema, right eye
 H18.232 Secondary corneal edema, left eye
 H18.233 Secondary corneal edema, bilateral
 H18.239 Secondary corneal edema, unspecified eye

● H18.3 Changes of corneal membranes
 H18.30 Unspecified corneal membrane change

● H18.31 Folds and rupture in Bowman's membrane
 H18.311 Folds and rupture in Bowman's membrane, right eye
 H18.312 Folds and rupture in Bowman's membrane, left eye
 H18.313 Folds and rupture in Bowman's membrane, bilateral
 H18.319 Folds and rupture in Bowman's membrane, unspecified eye

● H18.32 Folds in Descemet's membrane
 H18.321 Folds in Descemet's membrane, right eye
 H18.322 Folds in Descemet's membrane, left eye
 H18.323 Folds in Descemet's membrane, bilateral
 H18.329 Folds in Descemet's membrane, unspecified eye

● H18.33 Rupture in Descemet's membrane
 H18.331 Rupture in Descemet's membrane, right eye
 H18.332 Rupture in Descemet's membrane, left eye
 H18.333 Rupture in Descemet's membrane, bilateral
 H18.339 Rupture in Descemet's membrane, unspecified eye

● H18.4 Corneal degeneration
 Excludes1 Mooren's ulcer (H16.0-)
  recurrent erosion of cornea (H18.83-)

 H18.40 Unspecified corneal degeneration

● H18.41 Arcus senilis
 Senile corneal changes
 H18.411 Arcus senilis, right eye
 H18.412 Arcus senilis, left eye
 H18.413 Arcus senilis, bilateral
 H18.419 Arcus senilis, unspecified eye

● H18.42 Band keratopathy
 H18.421 Band keratopathy, right eye
 H18.422 Band keratopathy, left eye
 H18.423 Band keratopathy, bilateral
 H18.429 Band keratopathy, unspecified eye

 H18.43 Other calcerous corneal degeneration

● H18.44 Keratomalacia
 Excludes1 keratomalacia due to vitamin A deficiency (E50.4)
 H18.441 Keratomalacia, right eye
 H18.442 Keratomalacia, left eye
 H18.443 Keratomalacia, bilateral
 H18.449 Keratomalacia, unspecified eye

● H18.45 Nodular corneal degeneration
 H18.451 Nodular corneal degeneration, right eye
 H18.452 Nodular corneal degeneration, left eye
 H18.453 Nodular corneal degeneration, bilateral
 H18.459 Nodular corneal degeneration, unspecified eye

● H18.46 Peripheral corneal degeneration
 H18.461 Peripheral corneal degeneration, right eye
 H18.462 Peripheral corneal degeneration, left eye
 H18.463 Peripheral corneal degeneration, bilateral
 H18.469 Peripheral corneal degeneration, unspecified eye

 H18.49 Other corneal degeneration

● H18.5 Hereditary corneal dystrophies
 H18.50 Unspecified hereditary corneal dystrophies
 H18.51 Endothelial corneal dystrophy
  Fuchs' dystrophy
 H18.52 Epithelial (juvenile) corneal dystrophy
 H18.53 Granular corneal dystrophy
 H18.54 Lattice corneal dystrophy
 H18.55 Macular corneal dystrophy
 H18.59 Other hereditary corneal dystrophies

● H18.6 Keratoconus
● H18.60 Keratoconus, unspecified
 H18.601 Keratoconus, unspecified, right eye
 H18.602 Keratoconus, unspecified, left eye
 H18.603 Keratoconus, unspecified, bilateral
 H18.609 Keratoconus, unspecified, unspecified eye

● H18.61 Keratoconus, stable
 H18.611 Keratoconus, stable, right eye
 H18.612 Keratoconus, stable, left eye
 H18.613 Keratoconus, stable, bilateral
 H18.619 Keratoconus, stable, unspecified eye

● H18.62 Keratoconus, unstable
 Acute hydrops
 H18.621 Keratoconus, unstable, right eye
 H18.622 Keratoconus, unstable, left eye
 H18.623 Keratoconus, unstable, bilateral
 H18.629 Keratoconus, unstable, unspecified eye

Figure 7-7 Lateral view of the displacement of the cone apex in keratoconus. (From Yanoff: Ophthalmology, ed 3, Mosby, Inc., 2008)

Item 7–4 Keratoconus results in corneal degeneration that begins in childhood, gradually changes the cornea from a round to cone shape, decreasing visual acuity. Treatment includes contact lenses. In severe cases the need for corneal transplant may be the treatment of choice; however, newer technologies may use high frequency radio energy to shrink the edges of the cornea, pulling the central area back to a more normal shape. It can help delay or avoid the need for a corneal transplantation.

◄ New   ◄≡ Revised   ~~deleted~~ Deleted   Excludes 1   Excludes 2   Includes   Use additional   Code first   Code also   Unspecified

OGCR Official Guidelines   ● Unacceptable Principal Diagnosis   X Assign placeholder X   ● Use Additional Character(s)   ▶ Manifestation Code   **Coding Clinic**

● **H18.7   Other and unspecified corneal deformities**
  Excludes1 congenital malformations of cornea
      (Q13.3-Q13.4)
 H18.70 Unspecified corneal deformity
 ● H18.71 Corneal ectasia
  H18.711 Corneal ectasia, right eye
  H18.712 Corneal ectasia, left eye
  H18.713 Corneal ectasia, bilateral
  H18.719 Corneal ectasia, unspecified eye
 ● H18.72 Corneal staphyloma
  H18.721 Corneal staphyloma, right eye
  H18.722 Corneal staphyloma, left eye
  H18.723 Corneal staphyloma, bilateral
  H18.729 Corneal staphyloma, unspecified eye
 ● H18.73 Descemetocele
  H18.731 Descemetocele, right eye
  H18.732 Descemetocele, left eye
  H18.733 Descemetocele, bilateral
  H18.739 Descemetocele, unspecified eye
 ● H18.79 Other corneal deformities
  H18.791 Other corneal deformities, right eye
  H18.792 Other corneal deformities, left eye
  H18.793 Other corneal deformities, bilateral
  H18.799 Other corneal deformities, unspecified eye

● **H18.8   Other specified disorders of cornea**
 ● H18.81 Anesthesia and hypoesthesia of cornea
  H18.811 Anesthesia and hypoesthesia of cornea, right eye
  H18.812 Anesthesia and hypoesthesia of cornea, left eye
  H18.813 Anesthesia and hypoesthesia of cornea, bilateral
  H18.819 Anesthesia and hypoesthesia of cornea, unspecified eye
 ● H18.82 Corneal disorder due to contact lens
  Excludes2 corneal edema due to contact lens (H18.21-)
  H18.821 Corneal disorder due to contact lens, right eye
  H18.822 Corneal disorder due to contact lens, left eye
  H18.823 Corneal disorder due to contact lens, bilateral
  H18.829 Corneal disorder due to contact lens, unspecified eye
 ● H18.83 Recurrent erosion of cornea
  H18.831 Recurrent erosion of cornea, right eye
  H18.832 Recurrent erosion of cornea, left eye
  H18.833 Recurrent erosion of cornea, bilateral
  H18.839 Recurrent erosion of cornea, unspecified eye
 ● H18.89 Other specified disorders of cornea
  H18.891 Other specified disorders of cornea, right eye
  H18.892 Other specified disorders of cornea, left eye
  H18.893 Other specified disorders of cornea, bilateral
  H18.899 Other specified disorders of cornea, unspecified eye
 H18.9 Unspecified disorder of cornea

● **H20   Iridocyclitis**
 ● **H20.0   Acute and subacute iridocyclitis**
  Acute anterior uveitis
  Acute cyclitis
  Acute iritis
  Subacute anterior uveitis
  Subacute cyclitis
  Subacute iritis
  Excludes1 iridocyclitis, iritis, uveitis (due to) (in) diabetes mellitus (E08-E13 with .39)
    iridocyclitis, iritis, uveitis (due to) (in) diphtheria (A36.89)
    iridocyclitis, iritis, uveitis (due to) (in) gonococcal (A54.32)
    iridocyclitis, iritis, uveitis (due to) (in) herpes (simplex) (B00.51)
    iridocyclitis, iritis, uveitis (due to) (in) herpes zoster (B02.32)
    iridocyclitis, iritis, uveitis (due to) (in) late congenital syphilis (A50.39)
    iridocyclitis, iritis, uveitis (due to) (in) late syphilis (A52.71)
    iridocyclitis, iritis, uveitis (due to) (in) sarcoidosis (D86.83)
    iridocyclitis, iritis, uveitis (due to) (in) syphilis (A51.43)
    iridocyclitis, iritis, uveitis (due to) (in) toxoplasmosis (B58.09)
    iridocyclitis, iritis, uveitis (due to) (in) tuberculosis (A18.54)
  (Ex:) For category H20 CC codes: A18.54, H20.00-H20.9
  H20.00 Unspecified acute and subacute iridocyclitis
 ● H20.01 Primary iridocyclitis
  H20.011 Primary iridocyclitis, right eye
  H20.012 Primary iridocyclitis, left eye
  H20.013 Primary iridocyclitis, bilateral
  H20.019 Primary iridocyclitis, unspecified eye
 ● H20.02 Recurrent acute iridocyclitis
  H20.021 Recurrent acute iridocyclitis, right eye
  H20.022 Recurrent acute iridocyclitis, left eye
  H20.023 Recurrent acute iridocyclitis, bilateral
  H20.029 Recurrent acute iridocyclitis, unspecified eye
 ● H20.03 Secondary infectious iridocyclitis
  H20.031 Secondary infectious iridocyclitis, right eye
  H20.032 Secondary infectious iridocyclitis, left eye
  H20.033 Secondary infectious iridocyclitis, bilateral
  H20.039 Secondary infectious iridocyclitis, unspecified eye
 ● H20.04 Secondary noninfectious iridocyclitis
  H20.041 Secondary noninfectious iridocyclitis, right eye
  H20.042 Secondary noninfectious iridocyclitis, left eye
  H20.043 Secondary noninfectious iridocyclitis, bilateral
  H20.049 Secondary noninfectious iridocyclitis, unspecified eye
 ● H20.05 Hypopyon
  H20.051 Hypopyon, right eye
  H20.052 Hypopyon, left eye
  H20.053 Hypopyon, bilateral
  H20.059 Hypopyon, unspecified eye

CHAPTER 7 (H00-H59)

N Newborn Age: 0 P Pediatric Age: 0–17 M Maternity DX: 12–55 A Adult Age: 15–124 ♀ Females Only ♂ Males Only

 Complication\Comorbidity Major C\C (Ex:) CC/MCC Exclusions Present on Admission Requirement Hospital-Acquired Condition

919

● H20.1   Chronic iridocyclitis
          Use additional code for any associated cataract
          (H26.21-)
          Excludes2   posterior cyclitis (H30.2-)
    H20.10   Chronic iridocyclitis, unspecified eye
    H20.11   Chronic iridocyclitis, right eye
    H20.12   Chronic iridocyclitis, left eye
    H20.13   Chronic iridocyclitis, bilateral
● H20.2   Lens-induced iridocyclitis
    H20.20   Lens-induced iridocyclitis, unspecified eye
    H20.21   Lens-induced iridocyclitis, right eye
    H20.22   Lens-induced iridocyclitis, left eye
    H20.23   Lens-induced iridocyclitis, bilateral
● H20.8   Other iridocyclitis
          Excludes2   glaucomatocyclitis crises (H40.4-)
                          posterior cyclitis (H30.2-)
                          sympathetic uveitis (H44.13-)
    ● H20.81   Fuchs' heterochromic cyclitis
          H20.811   Fuchs' heterochromic cyclitis, right
                    eye
          H20.812   Fuchs' heterochromic cyclitis, left eye
          H20.813   Fuchs' heterochromic cyclitis,
                    bilateral
          H20.819   Fuchs' heterochromic cyclitis,
                    unspecified eye
    ● H20.82   Vogt-Koyanagi syndrome
          H20.821   Vogt-Koyanagi syndrome, right eye
          H20.822   Vogt-Koyanagi syndrome, left eye
          H20.823   Vogt-Koyanagi syndrome, bilateral
          H20.829   Vogt-Koyanagi syndrome, unspecified
                    eye
● H20.9   Unspecified iridocyclitis
          Uveitis NOS

●H21   Other disorders of iris and ciliary body
          Excludes2   sympathetic uveitis (H44.1-)
● H21.0   Hyphema
          Excludes1   traumatic hyphema (S05.1-)
    H21.00   Hyphema, unspecified eye
    H21.01   Hyphema, right eye
    H21.02   Hyphema, left eye
    H21.03   Hyphema, bilateral
● H21.1   Other vascular disorders of iris and ciliary body
          Neovascularization of iris or ciliary body
          Rubeosis iridis
          Rubeosis of iris
    ● H21.1X   Other vascular disorders of iris and ciliary body
          H21.1X1   Other vascular disorders of iris and
                    ciliary body, right eye
          H21.1X2   Other vascular disorders of iris and
                    ciliary body, left eye
          H21.1X3   Other vascular disorders of iris and
                    ciliary body, bilateral
          H21.1X9   Other vascular disorders of iris and
                    ciliary body, unspecified eye
● H21.2   Degeneration of iris and ciliary body
    ● H21.21   Degeneration of chamber angle
          H21.211   Degeneration of chamber angle, right
                    eye
          H21.212   Degeneration of chamber angle, left
                    eye
          H21.213   Degeneration of chamber angle,
                    bilateral
          H21.219   Degeneration of chamber angle,
                    unspecified eye

● H21.22   Degeneration of ciliary body
    H21.221   Degeneration of ciliary body, right
              eye
    H21.222   Degeneration of ciliary body, left eye
    H21.223   Degeneration of ciliary body, bilateral
    H21.229   Degeneration of ciliary body,
              unspecified eye
● H21.23   Degeneration of iris (pigmentary)
          Translucency of iris
    H21.231   Degeneration of iris (pigmentary),
              right eye
    H21.232   Degeneration of iris (pigmentary), left
              eye
    H21.233   Degeneration of iris (pigmentary),
              bilateral
    H21.239   Degeneration of iris (pigmentary),
              unspecified eye
● H21.24   Degeneration of pupillary margin
    H21.241   Degeneration of pupillary margin,
              right eye
    H21.242   Degeneration of pupillary margin,
              left eye
    H21.243   Degeneration of pupillary margin,
              bilateral
    H21.249   Degeneration of pupillary margin,
              unspecified eye
● H21.25   Iridoschisis
    H21.251   Iridoschisis, right eye
    H21.252   Iridoschisis, left eye
    H21.253   Iridoschisis, bilateral
    H21.259   Iridoschisis, unspecified eye
● H21.26   Iris atrophy (essential) (progressive)
    H21.261   Iris atrophy (essential) (progressive),
              right eye
    H21.262   Iris atrophy (essential) (progressive),
              left eye
    H21.263   Iris atrophy (essential) (progressive),
              bilateral
    H21.269   Iris atrophy (essential) (progressive),
              unspecified eye
● H21.27   Miotic pupillary cyst
    H21.271   Miotic pupillary cyst, right eye
    H21.272   Miotic pupillary cyst, left eye
    H21.273   Miotic pupillary cyst, bilateral
    H21.279   Miotic pupillary cyst, unspecified eye
  H21.29   Other iris atrophy
● H21.3   Cyst of iris, ciliary body and anterior chamber
          Excludes2   miotic pupillary cyst (H21.27-)
● H21.30   Idiopathic cysts of iris, ciliary body or anterior
          chamber
          Cyst of iris, ciliary body or anterior chamber
          NOS
    H21.301   Idiopathic cysts of iris, ciliary body or
              anterior chamber, right eye
    H21.302   Idiopathic cysts of iris, ciliary body or
              anterior chamber, left eye
    H21.303   Idiopathic cysts of iris, ciliary body or
              anterior chamber, bilateral
    H21.309   Idiopathic cysts of iris, ciliary body or
              anterior chamber, unspecified eye
● H21.31   Exudative cysts of iris or anterior chamber
    H21.311   Exudative cysts of iris or anterior
              chamber, right eye
    H21.312   Exudative cysts of iris or anterior
              chamber, left eye
    H21.313   Exudative cysts of iris or anterior
              chamber, bilateral
    H21.319   Exudative cysts of iris or anterior
              chamber, unspecified eye

◀ New   ◀▦ Revised   ~~deleted~~ Deleted   Excludes 1   Excludes 2   Includes   Use additional   Code first   Code also   Unspecified

OGCR Official Guidelines   ● Unacceptable Principal Diagnosis   X Assign placeholder X   ▶ Use Additional Character(s)   ▶ Manifestation Code   **Coding Clinic**

● H21.32   Implantation cysts of iris, ciliary body or anterior chamber

     H21.321   Implantation cysts of iris, ciliary body or anterior chamber, right eye

     H21.322   Implantation cysts of iris, ciliary body or anterior chamber, left eye

     H21.323   Implantation cysts of iris, ciliary body or anterior chamber, bilateral

     H21.329   Implantation cysts of iris, ciliary body or anterior chamber, unspecified eye

● H21.33   Parasitic cyst of iris, ciliary body or anterior chamber

     (Ex) **For category H21.33 CC codes:** H20.051-H20.059, H21.331-H21.339, H33.121-H33.129, H44.001-H44.029, H44.121-H44.129, H44.19

     H21.331   Parasitic cyst of iris, ciliary body or anterior chamber, right eye 🖐

     H21.332   Parasitic cyst of iris, ciliary body or anterior chamber, left eye 🖐

     H21.333   Parasitic cyst of iris, ciliary body or anterior chamber, bilateral 🖐

     H21.339   Parasitic cyst of iris, ciliary body or anterior chamber, unspecified eye 🖐

● H21.34   Primary cyst of pars plana

     H21.341   Primary cyst of pars plana, right eye

     H21.342   Primary cyst of pars plana, left eye

     H21.343   Primary cyst of pars plana, bilateral

     H21.349   Primary cyst of pars plana, unspecified eye

● H21.35   Exudative cyst of pars plana

     H21.351   Exudative cyst of pars plana, right eye

     H21.352   Exudative cyst of pars plana, left eye

     H21.353   Exudative cyst of pars plana, bilateral

     H21.359   Exudative cyst of pars plana, unspecified eye

● H21.4   Pupillary membranes

     Iris bombé
     Pupillary occlusion
     Pupillary seclusion

     Excludes1   congenital pupillary membranes (Q13.8)

     H21.40   Pupillary membranes, unspecified eye

     H21.41   Pupillary membranes, right eye

     H21.42   Pupillary membranes, left eye

     H21.43   Pupillary membranes, bilateral

● H21.5   Other and unspecified adhesions and disruptions of iris and ciliary body

     Excludes1   corectopia (Q13.2)

● H21.50   Unspecified adhesions of iris

     Synechia (iris) NOS

     H21.501   Unspecified adhesions of iris, right eye

     H21.502   Unspecified adhesions of iris, left eye

     H21.503   Unspecified adhesions of iris, bilateral

     H21.509   Unspecified adhesions of iris and ciliary body, unspecified eye

● H21.51   Anterior synechiae (iris)

     H21.511   Anterior synechiae (iris), right eye

     H21.512   Anterior synechiae (iris), left eye

     H21.513   Anterior synechiae (iris), bilateral

     H21.519   Anterior synechiae (iris), unspecified eye

● H21.52   Goniosynechiae

     H21.521   Goniosynechiae, right eye

     H21.522   Goniosynechiae, left eye

     H21.523   Goniosynechiae, bilateral

     H21.529   Goniosynechiae, unspecified eye

● H21.53   Iridodialysis

     H21.531   Iridodialysis, right eye

     H21.532   Iridodialysis, left eye

     H21.533   Iridodialysis, bilateral

     H21.539   Iridodialysis, unspecified eye

● H21.54   Posterior synechiae (iris)

     H21.541   Posterior synechiae (iris), right eye

     H21.542   Posterior synechiae (iris), left eye

     H21.543   Posterior synechiae (iris), bilateral

     H21.549   Posterior synechiae (iris), unspecified eye

● H21.55   Recession of chamber angle

     H21.551   Recession of chamber angle, right eye

     H21.552   Recession of chamber angle, left eye

     H21.553   Recession of chamber angle, bilateral

     H21.559   Recession of chamber angle, unspecified eye

● H21.56   Pupillary abnormalities

     Deformed pupil
     Ectopic pupil
     Rupture of sphincter, pupil

     Excludes1   congenital deformity of pupil (Q13.2-)

     H21.561   Pupillary abnormality, right eye

     H21.562   Pupillary abnormality, left eye

     H21.563   Pupillary abnormality, bilateral

     H21.569   Pupillary abnormality, unspecified eye

● H21.8   Other specified disorders of iris and ciliary body

     H21.81   Floppy iris syndrome

         Intraoperative floppy iris syndrome (IFIS)

         Use additional code for adverse effect, if applicable, to identify drug (T36-T50 with fifth or sixth character 5)

     H21.82   Plateau iris syndrome (post-iridectomy) (postprocedural)

     H21.89   Other specified disorders of iris and ciliary body

   H21.9   Unspecified disorder of iris and ciliary body

▶ *H22*   *Disorders of iris and ciliary body in diseases classified elsewhere*

     Code first underlying disease, such as:
     gout (M1A.-, M10.-) ◀▥
     leprosy (A30.-) ◀
     parasitic disease (B89) ◀

DISORDERS OF LENS (H25-H28)

● H25   Age-related cataract

     Senile cataract

     Excludes2   capsular glaucoma with pseudoexfoliation of lens (H40.1-)

● H25.0   Age-related incipient cataract

   ● H25.01   Cortical age-related cataract

     H25.011   Cortical age-related cataract, right eye   A

     H25.012   Cortical age-related cataract, left eye   A

     H25.013   Cortical age-related cataract, bilateral   A

     H25.019   Cortical age-related cataract, unspecified eye   A

   ● H25.03   Anterior subcapsular polar age-related cataract

     H25.031   Anterior subcapsular polar age-related cataract, right eye   A

     H25.032   Anterior subcapsular polar age-related cataract, left eye   A

     H25.033   Anterior subcapsular polar age-related cataract, bilateral   A

     H25.039   Anterior subcapsular polar age-related cataract, unspecified eye   A

N Newborn Age: 0   **P** Pediatric Age: 0–17   **M** Maternity DX: 12–55   **A** Adult Age: 15–124   ♀ Females Only   ♂ Males Only

🖐 Complication\Comorbidity   🖐 Major C\C   (Ex) CC/MCC Exclusions   🖐 Present on Admission Requirement   🖐 Hospital-Acquired Condition

921

CHAPTER 7 (H00-H59)

Figure 7-8   Age-related cataract.
Nuclear sclerosis and cortical lens opacities are present. (From Yanoff: Ophthalmology, ed 3, Mosby, Inc., 2008)

Item 7–5 Senile cataracts are linked to the aging process. The most common area for the formation of a cataract is the cortical area of the lens. **Polar cataracts** can be either anterior or posterior. **Anterior polar cataracts** are more common and are small, white, capsular cataracts located on the anterior portion of the lens. **Total cataracts,** also called **complete** or **mature,** cause an opacity of all fibers of the lens. **Hypermature** describes a mature cataract with a swollen, milky cortex that covers the entire lens. **Immature,** also called **incipient,** cataracts have a clear cortex and are only slightly opaque. Treatment for all cataracts is the removal of the lens.

● H25.04   Posterior subcapsular polar age-related cataract

     H25.041   Posterior subcapsular polar age-related cataract, right eye   A

     H25.042   Posterior subcapsular polar age-related cataract, left eye   A

     H25.043   Posterior subcapsular polar age-related cataract, bilateral   A

     H25.049   Posterior subcapsular polar age-related cataract, unspecified eye   A

● H25.09   Other age-related incipient cataract
     Coronary age-related cataract
     Punctate age-related cataract
     Water clefts

     H25.091   Other age-related incipient cataract, right eye   A

     H25.092   Other age-related incipient cataract, left eye   A

     H25.093   Other age-related incipient cataract, bilateral   A

     H25.099   Other age-related incipient cataract, unspecified eye   A

● H25.1   Age-related nuclear cataract
     Cataracta brunescens
     Nuclear sclerosis cataract

     H25.10   Age-related nuclear cataract, unspecified eye   A

     H25.11   Age-related nuclear cataract, right eye   A

     H25.12   Age-related nuclear cataract, left eye   A

     H25.13   Age-related nuclear cataract, bilateral   A

● H25.2   Age-related cataract, morgagnian type
     Age-related hypermature cataract

     H25.20   Age-related cataract, morgagnian type, unspecified eye   A

     H25.21   Age-related cataract, morgagnian type, right eye   A

     H25.22   Age-related cataract, morgagnian type, left eye   A

     H25.23   Age-related cataract, morgagnian type, bilateral   A

● H25.8   Other age-related cataract

   ● H25.81   Combined forms of age-related cataract

     H25.811   Combined forms of age-related cataract, right eye   A

     H25.812   Combined forms of age-related cataract, left eye   A

     H25.813   Combined forms of age-related cataract, bilateral   A

     H25.819   Combined forms of age-related cataract, unspecified eye   A

     H25.89   Other age-related cataract   A

H25.9   Unspecified age-related cataract   A

● H26   Other cataract
    Excludes1   congenital cataract (Q12.0)

  ● H26.0   Infantile and juvenile cataract

    ● H26.00   Unspecified infantile and juvenile cataract

       H26.001   Unspecified infantile and juvenile cataract, right eye   P

       H26.002   Unspecified infantile and juvenile cataract, left eye   P

       H26.003   Unspecified infantile and juvenile cataract, bilateral   P

       H26.009   Unspecified infantile and juvenile cataract, unspecified eye   P

    ● H26.01   Infantile and juvenile cortical, lamellar, or zonular cataract

       H26.011   Infantile and juvenile cortical, lamellar, or zonular cataract, right eye   P

       H26.012   Infantile and juvenile cortical, lamellar, or zonular cataract, left eye   P

       H26.013   Infantile and juvenile cortical, lamellar, or zonular cataract, bilateral   P

       H26.019   Infantile and juvenile cortical, lamellar, or zonular cataract, unspecified eye   P

    ● H26.03   Infantile and juvenile nuclear cataract

       H26.031   Infantile and juvenile nuclear cataract, right eye   P

       H26.032   Infantile and juvenile nuclear cataract, left eye   P

       H26.033   Infantile and juvenile nuclear cataract, bilateral   P

       H26.039   Infantile and juvenile nuclear cataract, unspecified eye   P

    ● H26.04   Anterior subcapsular polar infantile and juvenile cataract

       H26.041   Anterior subcapsular polar infantile and juvenile cataract, right eye   P

       H26.042   Anterior subcapsular polar infantile and juvenile cataract, left eye   P

       H26.043   Anterior subcapsular polar infantile and juvenile cataract, bilateral   P

       H26.049   Anterior subcapsular polar infantile and juvenile cataract, unspecified eye   P

    ● H26.05   Posterior subcapsular polar infantile and juvenile cataract

       H26.051   Posterior subcapsular polar infantile and juvenile cataract, right eye   P

       H26.052   Posterior subcapsular polar infantile and juvenile cataract, left eye   P

       H26.053   Posterior subcapsular polar infantile and juvenile cataract, bilateral   P

       H26.059   Posterior subcapsular polar infantile and juvenile cataract, unspecified eye   P

    ● H26.06   Combined forms of infantile and juvenile cataract

       H26.061   Combined forms of infantile and juvenile cataract, right eye   P

       H26.062   Combined forms of infantile and juvenile cataract, left eye   P

       H26.063   Combined forms of infantile and juvenile cataract bilateral   P

       H26.069   Combined forms of infantile and juvenile cataract, unspecified eye   P

     H26.09   Other infantile and juvenile cataract   P

◀ New   ◀▥ Revised   ~~deleted~~ Deleted   Excludes 1   Excludes 2   Includes   Use additional   Code first   Code also   Unspecified

OGCR Official Guidelines   ● Unacceptable Principal Diagnosis   X Assign placeholder X   ● Use Additional Character(s)   ▶ Manifestation Code   **Coding Clinic**

● H26.1   Traumatic cataract
   Use additional code (Chapter 20) to identify external cause
   ● H26.10   Unspecified traumatic cataract
     H26.101   Unspecified traumatic cataract, right eye
     H26.102   Unspecified traumatic cataract, left eye
     H26.103   Unspecified traumatic cataract, bilateral
     H26.109   Unspecified traumatic cataract, unspecified eye
   ● H26.11   Localized traumatic opacities
     H26.111   Localized traumatic opacities, right eye
     H26.112   Localized traumatic opacities, left eye
     H26.113   Localized traumatic opacities, bilateral
     H26.119   Localized traumatic opacities, unspecified eye
   ● H26.12   Partially resolved traumatic cataract
     H26.121   Partially resolved traumatic cataract, right eye
     H26.122   Partially resolved traumatic cataract, left eye
     H26.123   Partially resolved traumatic cataract, bilateral
     H26.129   Partially resolved traumatic cataract, unspecified eye
   ● H26.13   Total traumatic cataract
     H26.131   Total traumatic cataract, right eye
     H26.132   Total traumatic cataract, left eye
     H26.133   Total traumatic cataract, bilateral
     H26.139   Total traumatic cataract, unspecified eye

● H26.2   Complicated cataract
     H26.20   Unspecified complicated cataract
       Cataracta complicata NOS
   ● H26.21   Cataract with neovascularization
     Code also associated condition, such as: chronic iridocyclitis (H20.1-)
     H26.211   Cataract with neovascularization, right eye
     H26.212   Cataract with neovascularization, left eye
     H26.213   Cataract with neovascularization, bilateral
     H26.219   Cataract with neovascularization, unspecified eye
   ● H26.22   Cataract secondary to ocular disorders (degenerative) (inflammatory)
     Code also associated ocular disorder
     H26.221   Cataract secondary to ocular disorders (degenerative) (inflammatory), right eye
     H26.222   Cataract secondary to ocular disorders (degenerative) (inflammatory), left eye
     H26.223   Cataract secondary to ocular disorders (degenerative) (inflammatory), bilateral
     H26.229   Cataract secondary to ocular disorders (degenerative) (inflammatory), unspecified eye
   ● H26.23   Glaucomatous flecks (subcapsular)
     Code first underlying glaucoma (H40-H42)
     H26.231   Glaucomatous flecks (subcapsular), right eye
     H26.232   Glaucomatous flecks (subcapsular), left eye

     H26.233   Glaucomatous flecks (subcapsular), bilateral
     H26.239   Glaucomatous flecks (subcapsular), unspecified eye
● H26.3   Drug-induced cataract
     Toxic cataract
     Use additional code for adverse effect, if applicable, to identify drug (T36-T50 with fifth or sixth character 5)
     H26.30   Drug-induced cataract, unspecified eye
     H26.31   Drug-induced cataract, right eye
     H26.32   Drug-induced cataract, left eye
     H26.33   Drug-induced cataract, bilateral
● H26.4   Secondary cataract
     H26.40   Unspecified secondary cataract
   ● H26.41   Soemmering's ring
     H26.411   Soemmering's ring, right eye
     H26.412   Soemmering's ring, left eye
     H26.413   Soemmering's ring, bilateral
     H26.419   Soemmering's ring, unspecified eye
   ● H26.49   Other secondary cataract
     H26.491   Other secondary cataract, right eye
     H26.492   Other secondary cataract, left eye
     H26.493   Other secondary cataract, bilateral
     H26.499   Other secondary cataract, unspecified eye
   H26.8   Other specified cataract
   H26.9   Unspecified cataract

● H27   Other disorders of lens
   Excludes1   congenital lens malformations (Q12.-)
     mechanical complications of intraocular lens implant (T85.2)
     pseudophakia (Z96.1)
   ● H27.0   Aphakia
     Acquired absence of lens
     Acquired aphakia
     Aphakia due to trauma
     Excludes1   cataract extraction status (Z98.4-)
       congenital absence of lens (Q12.3)
       congenital aphakia (Q12.3)
     H27.00   Aphakia, unspecified eye
     H27.01   Aphakia, right eye
     H27.02   Aphakia, left eye
     H27.03   Aphakia, bilateral
   ● H27.1   Dislocation of lens
     H27.10   Unspecified dislocation of lens
   ● H27.11   Subluxation of lens
     H27.111   Subluxation of lens, right eye
     H27.112   Subluxation of lens, left eye
     H27.113   Subluxation of lens, bilateral
     H27.119   Subluxation of lens, unspecified eye
   ● H27.12   Anterior dislocation of lens
     H27.121   Anterior dislocation of lens, right eye
     H27.122   Anterior dislocation of lens, left eye
     H27.123   Anterior dislocation of lens, bilateral
     H27.129   Anterior dislocation of lens, unspecified eye
   ● H27.13   Posterior dislocation of lens
     H27.131   Posterior dislocation of lens, right eye
     H27.132   Posterior dislocation of lens, left eye
     H27.133   Posterior dislocation of lens, bilateral
     H27.139   Posterior dislocation of lens, unspecified eye
   H27.8   Other specified disorders of lens
   H27.9   Unspecified disorder of lens

N   Newborn Age: 0   P   Pediatric Age: 0–17   M   Maternity DX: 12–55   A   Adult Age: 15–124   ♀   Females Only   ♂   Males Only
  Complication\Comorbidity   Major C\C   (Ex:)   CC/MCC Exclusions   Present on Admission Requirement   Hospital-Acquired Condition

◗ **H28** *Cataract in diseases classified elsewhere*
    Code first underlying disease, such as:
        hypoparathyroidism (E20.-)
        myotonia (G71.1-)
        myxedema (E03.-)
        protein-calorie malnutrition (E40-E46)
    Excludes1 cataract in diabetes mellitus (E08.36, E09.36,
                E10.36, E11.36, E13.36) ◀▥

DISORDERS OF CHOROID AND RETINA (H30-H36)

(See Plate 90 on page 64.)

● H30 Chorioretinal inflammation
    ● H30.0 Focal chorioretinal inflammation
            Focal chorioretinitis
            Focal choroiditis
            Focal retinitis
            Focal retinochoroiditis
        ● H30.00 Unspecified focal chorioretinal inflammation
                Focal chorioretinitis NOS
                Focal choroiditis NOS
                Focal retinitis NOS
                Focal retinochoroiditis NOS
            H30.001 Unspecified focal chorioretinal
                    inflammation, right eye
            H30.002 Unspecified focal chorioretinal
                    inflammation, left eye
            H30.003 Unspecified focal chorioretinal
                    inflammation, bilateral
            H30.009 Unspecified focal chorioretinal
                    inflammation, unspecified eye
        ● H30.01 Focal chorioretinal inflammation, juxtapapillary
            H30.011 Focal chorioretinal inflammation,
                    juxtapapillary, right eye
            H30.012 Focal chorioretinal inflammation,
                    juxtapapillary, left eye
            H30.013 Focal chorioretinal inflammation,
                    juxtapapillary, bilateral
            H30.019 Focal chorioretinal inflammation,
                    juxtapapillary, unspecified eye
        ● H30.02 Focal chorioretinal inflammation of posterior
                pole
            H30.021 Focal chorioretinal inflammation of
                    posterior pole, right eye
            H30.022 Focal chorioretinal inflammation of
                    posterior pole, left eye
            H30.023 Focal chorioretinal inflammation of
                    posterior pole, bilateral
            H30.029 Focal chorioretinal inflammation of
                    posterior pole, unspecified eye
        ● H30.03 Focal chorioretinal inflammation, peripheral
            H30.031 Focal chorioretinal inflammation,
                    peripheral, right eye
            H30.032 Focal chorioretinal inflammation,
                    peripheral, left eye
            H30.033 Focal chorioretinal inflammation,
                    peripheral, bilateral
            H30.039 Focal chorioretinal inflammation,
                    peripheral, unspecified eye
        ● H30.04 Focal chorioretinal inflammation, macular or
                paramacular
            H30.041 Focal chorioretinal inflammation,
                    macular or paramacular, right eye
            H30.042 Focal chorioretinal inflammation,
                    macular or paramacular, left eye
            H30.043 Focal chorioretinal inflammation,
                    macular or paramacular, bilateral
            H30.049 Focal chorioretinal inflammation,
                    macular or paramacular, unspecified
                    eye

● H30.1 Disseminated chorioretinal inflammation
        Disseminated chorioretinitis
        Disseminated choroiditis
        Disseminated retinitis
        Disseminated retinochoroiditis
    Excludes2 exudative retinopathy (H35.02-)
    Ⓔ **For category H30.1 CC codes:** H30.001-H30.93
    ● H30.10 Unspecified disseminated chorioretinal
            inflammation
            Disseminated chorioretinitis NOS
            Disseminated choroiditis NOS
            Disseminated retinitis NOS
            Disseminated retinochoroiditis NOS
        H30.101 Unspecified disseminated
                chorioretinal inflammation, right
                eye
        H30.102 Unspecified disseminated
                chorioretinal inflammation, left eye
        H30.103 Unspecified disseminated
                chorioretinal inflammation,
                bilateral
        H30.109 Unspecified disseminated
                chorioretinal inflammation,
                unspecified eye
    ● H30.11 Disseminated chorioretinal inflammation of
            posterior pole
        H30.111 Disseminated chorioretinal
                inflammation of posterior pole, right
                eye
        H30.112 Disseminated chorioretinal
                inflammation of posterior pole, left
                eye
        H30.113 Disseminated chorioretinal
                inflammation of posterior pole,
                bilateral
        H30.119 Disseminated chorioretinal
                inflammation of posterior pole,
                unspecified eye
    ● H30.12 Disseminated chorioretinal inflammation,
            peripheral
        H30.121 Disseminated chorioretinal
                inflammation, peripheral right eye
        H30.122 Disseminated chorioretinal
                inflammation, peripheral, left eye
        H30.123 Disseminated chorioretinal
                inflammation, peripheral, bilateral
        H30.129 Disseminated chorioretinal
                inflammation, peripheral, unspecified
                eye
    ● H30.13 Disseminated chorioretinal inflammation,
            generalized
        H30.131 Disseminated chorioretinal
                inflammation, generalized, right
                eye
        H30.132 Disseminated chorioretinal
                inflammation, generalized, left eye
        H30.133 Disseminated chorioretinal
                inflammation, generalized,
                bilateral
        H30.139 Disseminated chorioretinal
                inflammation, generalized,
                unspecified eye
    ● H30.14 Acute posterior multifocal placoid pigment
            epitheliopathy
        H30.141 Acute posterior multifocal placoid
                pigment epitheliopathy, right eye
        H30.142 Acute posterior multifocal placoid
                pigment epitheliopathy, left eye

◀ New   ◀▥ Revised   ~~deleted~~ Deleted   Excludes 1   Excludes 2   Includes   Use additional   Code first   Code also   Unspecified

OGCR Official Guidelines   ● Unacceptable Principal Diagnosis   X Assign placeholder X   ● Use Additional Character(s)   ◗ Manifestation Code   **Coding Clinic**

H30.143   Acute posterior multifocal placoid pigment epitheliopathy, bilateral

H30.149   Acute posterior multifocal placoid pigment epitheliopathy, unspecified eye

● H30.2   **Posterior cyclitis**
     Pars planitis

    H30.20   Posterior cyclitis, unspecified eye

    H30.21   Posterior cyclitis, right eye

    H30.22   Posterior cyclitis, left eye

    H30.23   Posterior cyclitis, bilateral

● H30.8   **Other chorioretinal inflammations**

   ● H30.81   Harada's disease

      H30.811   Harada's disease, right eye

      H30.812   Harada's disease, left eye

      H30.813   Harada's disease, bilateral

      H30.819   Harada's disease, unspecified eye

   ● H30.89   Other chorioretinal inflammations
      (Ex) **For category H30.89 CC codes:** H30.001-H30.93

      H30.891   Other chorioretinal inflammations, right eye

      H30.892   Other chorioretinal inflammations, left eye

      H30.893   Other chorioretinal inflammations, bilateral

      H30.899   Other chorioretinal inflammations, unspecified eye

● H30.9   **Unspecified chorioretinal inflammation**
     Chorioretinitis NOS
     Choroiditis NOS
     Neuroretinitis NOS
     Retinitis NOS
     Retinochoroiditis NOS
     (Ex) **For category H30.9 CC codes:** H30.001-H30.93

    H30.90   Unspecified chorioretinal inflammation, unspecified eye

    H30.91   Unspecified chorioretinal inflammation, right eye

    H30.92   Unspecified chorioretinal inflammation, left eye

    H30.93   Unspecified chorioretinal inflammation, bilateral

● **H31   Other disorders of choroid**

   ● H31.0   **Chorioretinal scars**

     Excludes2   postsurgical chorioretinal scars (H59.81-)

   ● H31.00   Unspecified chorioretinal scars

      H31.001   Unspecified chorioretinal scars, right eye

      H31.002   Unspecified chorioretinal scars, left eye

      H31.003   Unspecified chorioretinal scars, bilateral

      H31.009   Unspecified chorioretinal scars, unspecified eye

   ● H31.01   Macula scars of posterior pole (postinflammatory) (post-traumatic)

     Excludes1   postprocedural choriorentinal scar (H59.81-)

      H31.011   Macula scars of posterior pole (postinflammatory) (post-traumatic), right eye

      H31.012   Macula scars of posterior pole (postinflammatory) (post-traumatic), left eye

      H31.013   Macula scars of posterior pole (postinflammatory) (post-traumatic), bilateral

      H31.019   Macula scars of posterior pole (postinflammatory) (post-traumatic), unspecified eye

   ● H31.02   Solar retinopathy

      H31.021   Solar retinopathy, right eye

      H31.022   Solar retinopathy, left eye

      H31.023   Solar retinopathy, bilateral

      H31.029   Solar retinopathy, unspecified eye

   ● H31.09   Other chorioretinal scars

      H31.091   Other chorioretinal scars, right eye

      H31.092   Other chorioretinal scars, left eye

      H31.093   Other chorioretinal scars, bilateral

      H31.099   Other chorioretinal scars, unspecified eye

● H31.1   **Choroidal degeneration**

     Excludes2   angioid streaks of macula (H35.33)

   ● H31.10   Unspecified choroidal degeneration
     Choroidal sclerosis NOS

      H31.101   Choroidal degeneration, unspecified, right eye

      H31.102   Choroidal degeneration, unspecified, left eye

      H31.103   Choroidal degeneration, unspecified, bilateral

      H31.109   Choroidal degeneration, unspecified, unspecified eye

   ● H31.11   Age-related choroidal atrophy

      H31.111   Age-related choroidal atrophy, right eye   A

      H31.112   Age-related choroidal atrophy, left eye   A

      H31.113   Age-related choroidal atrophy, bilateral   A

      H31.119   Age-related choroidal atrophy, unspecified eye   A

   ● H31.12   Diffuse secondary atrophy of choroid

      H31.121   Diffuse secondary atrophy of choroid, right eye

      H31.122   Diffuse secondary atrophy of choroid, left eye

      H31.123   Diffuse secondary atrophy of choroid, bilateral

      H31.129   Diffuse secondary atrophy of choroid, unspecified eye

● H31.2   **Hereditary choroidal dystrophy**

     Excludes2   hyperornithinemia (E72.4)
                ornithinemia (E72.4)

    H31.20   Hereditary choroidal dystrophy, unspecified

    H31.21   Choroideremia

    H31.22   Choroidal dystrophy (central areolar) (generalized) (peripapillary)

    H31.23   Gyrate atrophy, choroid

    H31.29   Other hereditary choroidal dystrophy

● H31.3   **Choroidal hemorrhage and rupture**

   ● H31.30   Unspecified choroidal hemorrhage

      H31.301   Unspecified choroidal hemorrhage, right eye

      H31.302   Unspecified choroidal hemorrhage, left eye

      H31.303   Unspecified choroidal hemorrhage, bilateral

      H31.309   Unspecified choroidal hemorrhage, unspecified eye

CHAPTER 7 (H00-H59)

● H31.31   Expulsive choroidal hemorrhage

     H31.311   Expulsive choroidal hemorrhage, right eye

     H31.312   Expulsive choroidal hemorrhage, left eye

     H31.313   Expulsive choroidal hemorrhage, bilateral

     H31.319   Expulsive choroidal hemorrhage, unspecified eye

● H31.32   Choroidal rupture

     Ⓔⓧ For category H31.32 CC codes: H31.301-H32

     H31.321   Choroidal rupture, right eye 🅒

     H31.322   Choroidal rupture, left eye 🅒

     H31.323   Choroidal rupture, bilateral 🅒

     H31.329   Choroidal rupture, unspecified eye 🅒

● H31.4   Choroidal detachment

     Ⓔⓧ For category H31.4 CC codes: H31.301-H32

  ● H31.40   Unspecified choroidal detachment

     H31.401   Unspecified choroidal detachment, right eye 🅒

     H31.402   Unspecified choroidal detachment, left eye 🅒

     H31.403   Unspecified choroidal detachment, bilateral 🅒

     H31.409   Unspecified choroidal detachment, unspecified eye 🅒

  ● H31.41   Hemorrhagic choroidal detachment

     H31.411   Hemorrhagic choroidal detachment, right eye 🅒

     H31.412   Hemorrhagic choroidal detachment, left eye 🅒

     H31.413   Hemorrhagic choroidal detachment, bilateral 🅒

     H31.419   Hemorrhagic choroidal detachment, unspecified eye 🅒

  ● H31.42   Serous choroidal detachment

     H31.421   Serous choroidal detachment, right eye 🅒

     H31.422   Serous choroidal detachment, left eye 🅒

     H31.423   Serous choroidal detachment, bilateral 🅒

     H31.429   Serous choroidal detachment, unspecified eye 🅒

H31.8   Other specified disorders of choroid

H31.9   Unspecified disorder of choroid

▷ H32   *Chorioretinal disorders in diseases classified elsewhere*

     Code first underlying disease, such as:
     congenital toxoplasmosis (P37.1)
     histoplasmosis (B39.-)
     leprosy (A30.-)

     Excludes1   chorioretinitis (in):
           toxoplasmosis (acquired) (B58.01)
           tuberculosis (A18.53)

● H33   Retinal detachments and breaks

     Excludes1   detachment of retinal pigment epithelium (H35.72-, H35.73-)

  ● H33.0   Retinal detachment with retinal break
     Rhegmatogenous retinal detachment

     Excludes1   serous retinal detachment (without retinal break) (H33.2-)

    ● H33.00   Unspecified retinal detachment with retinal break

     H33.001   Unspecified retinal detachment with retinal break, right eye

     H33.002   Unspecified retinal detachment with retinal break, left eye

---

Figure 7-9   Retinal detachment. (From Kumar: Robbins and Cotran: Pathologic Basis of Disease, ed 7, Saunders, 2005)

Item 7–6   Retinal detachments and defects are conditions of the eye in which the retina separates from the underlying tissue. Initial detachment may be localized, requiring rapid treatment (medical emergency) to avoid the entire retina from detaching which leads to vision loss and blindness.

     H33.003   Unspecified retinal detachment with retinal break, bilateral

     H33.009   Unspecified retinal detachment with retinal break, unspecified eye

  ● H33.01   Retinal detachment with single break

     H33.011   Retinal detachment with single break, right eye

     H33.012   Retinal detachment with single break, left eye

     H33.013   Retinal detachment with single break, bilateral

     H33.019   Retinal detachment with single break, unspecified eye

  ● H33.02   Retinal detachment with multiple breaks

     H33.021   Retinal detachment with multiple breaks, right eye

     H33.022   Retinal detachment with multiple breaks, left eye

     H33.023   Retinal detachment with multiple breaks, bilateral

     H33.029   Retinal detachment with multiple breaks, unspecified eye

  ● H33.03   Retinal detachment with giant retinal tear

     H33.031   Retinal detachment with giant retinal tear, right eye

     H33.032   Retinal detachment with giant retinal tear, left eye

     H33.033   Retinal detachment with giant retinal tear, bilateral

     H33.039   Retinal detachment with giant retinal tear, unspecified eye

---

◀ New   ◀▦ Revised   ~~deleted~~ Deleted   Excludes 1   Excludes 2   Includes   Use additional   Code first   Code also   Unspecified

OGCR Official Guidelines   ● Unacceptable Principal Diagnosis   X Assign placeholder X   ● Use Additional Character(s)   ▷ Manifestation Code   **Coding Clinic**

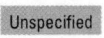

● H33.04 Retinal detachment with retinal dialysis
  H33.041 Retinal detachment with retinal dialysis, right eye
  H33.042 Retinal detachment with retinal dialysis, left eye
  H33.043 Retinal detachment with retinal dialysis, bilateral
  H33.049 Retinal detachment with retinal dialysis, unspecified eye
● H33.05 Total retinal detachment
  H33.051 Total retinal detachment, right eye
  H33.052 Total retinal detachment, left eye
  H33.053 Total retinal detachment, bilateral
  H33.059 Total retinal detachment, unspecified eye
● H33.1 Retinoschisis and retinal cysts
  Excludes1 congenital retinoschisis (Q14.1)
    microcystoid degeneration of retina (H35.42-)
● H33.10 Unspecified retinoschisis
  H33.101 Unspecified retinoschisis, right eye
  H33.102 Unspecified retinoschisis, left eye
  H33.103 Unspecified retinoschisis, bilateral
  H33.109 Unspecified retinoschisis, unspecified eye
● H33.11 Cyst of ora serrata
  H33.111 Cyst of ora serrata, right eye
  H33.112 Cyst of ora serrata, left eye
  H33.113 Cyst of ora serrata, bilateral
  H33.119 Cyst of ora serrata, unspecified eye
● H33.12 Parasitic cyst of retina
  (Ex:) For category H33.12 CC codes: H20.051-H20.059, H21.331-H21.339, H33.121-H33.129, H44.001-H44.029, H44.121-H44.129, H44.19
  H33.121 Parasitic cyst of retina, right eye ⚙
  H33.122 Parasitic cyst of retina, left eye ⚙
  H33.123 Parasitic cyst of retina, bilateral ⚙
  H33.129 Parasitic cyst of retina, unspecified eye ⚙
● H33.19 Other retinoschisis and retinal cysts
  Pseudocyst of retina
  H33.191 Other retinoschisis and retinal cysts, right eye
  H33.192 Other retinoschisis and retinal cysts, left eye
  H33.193 Other retinoschisis and retinal cysts, bilateral
  H33.199 Other retinoschisis and retinal cysts, unspecified eye
● H33.2 Serous retinal detachment
  Retinal detachment NOS
  Retinal detachment without retinal break
  Excludes1 central serous chorioretinopathy (H35.71-)
  (Ex:) For category H33.2 CC codes: H33.001-H33.119, H33.191-H33.8, H35.70-H35.739
  H33.20 Serous retinal detachment, unspecified eye ⚙
  H33.21 Serous retinal detachment, right eye ⚙
  H33.22 Serous retinal detachment, left eye ⚙
  H33.23 Serous retinal detachment, bilateral ⚙

● H33.3 Retinal breaks without detachment
  Excludes1 chorioretinal scars after surgery for detachment (H59.81-)
    peripheral retinal degeneration without break (H35.4-)
● H33.30 Unspecified retinal break
  H33.301 Unspecified retinal break, right eye
  H33.302 Unspecified retinal break, left eye
  H33.303 Unspecified retinal break, bilateral
  H33.309 Unspecified retinal break, unspecified eye
● H33.31 Horseshoe tear of retina without detachment
  Operculum of retina without detachment
  H33.311 Horseshoe tear of retina without detachment, right eye
  H33.312 Horseshoe tear of retina without detachment, left eye
  H33.313 Horseshoe tear of retina without detachment, bilateral
  H33.319 Horseshoe tear of retina without detachment, unspecified eye
● H33.32 Round hole of retina without detachment
  H33.321 Round hole, right eye
  H33.322 Round hole, left eye
  H33.323 Round hole, bilateral
  H33.329 Round hole, unspecified eye
● H33.33 Multiple defects of retina without detachment
  H33.331 Multiple defects of retina without detachment, right eye
  H33.332 Multiple defects of retina without detachment, left eye
  H33.333 Multiple defects of retina without detachment, bilateral
  H33.339 Multiple defects of retina without detachment, unspecified eye
● H33.4 Traction detachment of retina
  Proliferative vitreo-retinopathy with retinal detachment
  (Ex:) For category H33.4 CC codes: See H33.2
  H33.40 Traction detachment of retina, unspecified eye ⚙
  H33.41 Traction detachment of retina, right eye ⚙
  H33.42 Traction detachment of retina, left eye ⚙
  H33.43 Traction detachment of retina, bilateral ⚙
H33.8 Other retinal detachments ⚙
  (Ex:) See H33.2

● H34 Retinal vascular occlusions
  Blockage in vessel of the retina
  Excludes1 amaurosis fugax (G45.3)
  (Ex:) For category H34 CC codes: G45.3, H34.00-H34.9
● H34.0 Transient retinal artery occlusion
  H34.00 Transient retinal artery occlusion, unspecified eye ⚙
  H34.01 Transient retinal artery occlusion, right eye ⚙
  H34.02 Transient retinal artery occlusion, left eye ⚙
  H34.03 Transient retinal artery occlusion, bilateral ⚙
● H34.1 Central retinal artery occlusion
  H34.10 Central retinal artery occlusion, unspecified eye ⚙
  H34.11 Central retinal artery occlusion, right eye ⚙
  H34.12 Central retinal artery occlusion, left eye ⚙
  H34.13 Central retinal artery occlusion, bilateral ⚙

CHAPTER 7 (H00–H59)

● H34.2   Other retinal artery occlusions
   ● H34.21   Partial retinal artery occlusion
        Hollenhorst's plaque
        Retinal microembolism
        H34.211   Partial retinal artery occlusion, right eye
        H34.212   Partial retinal artery occlusion, left eye
        H34.213   Partial retinal artery occlusion, bilateral
        H34.219   Partial retinal artery occlusion, unspecified eye
   ● H34.23   Retinal artery branch occlusion
        H34.231   Retinal artery branch occlusion, right eye
        H34.232   Retinal artery branch occlusion, left eye
        H34.233   Retinal artery branch occlusion, bilateral
        H34.239   Retinal artery branch occlusion, unspecified eye

● H34.8   Other retinal vascular occlusions
   ● H34.81   Central retinal vein occlusion
        H34.811   Central retinal vein occlusion, right eye
        H34.812   Central retinal vein occlusion, left eye
        H34.813   Central retinal vein occlusion, bilateral
        H34.819   Central retinal vein occlusion, unspecified eye
   ● H34.82   Venous engorgement
        Incipient retinal vein occlusion
        Partial retinal vein occlusion
        H34.821   Venous engorgement, right eye
        H34.822   Venous engorgement, left eye
        H34.823   Venous engorgement, bilateral
        H34.829   Venous engorgement, unspecified eye
   ● H34.83   Tributary (branch) retinal vein occlusion
        H34.831   Tributary (branch) retinal vein occlusion, right eye
        H34.832   Tributary (branch) retinal vein occlusion, left eye
        H34.833   Tributary (branch) retinal vein occlusion, bilateral
        H34.839   Tributary (branch) retinal vein occlusion, unspecified eye

  H34.9   Unspecified retinal vascular occlusion
    OGCR   Section I. C.9.a.5.

    Hypertensive Retinopathy
    Subcategory H35.0, Background retinopathy and retinal vascular changes, should be used with a code from category I10–I15, Hypertensive disease to include the systemic hypertension. The sequencing is based on the reason for the encounter.

● H35   Other retinal disorders
    Excludes2   diabetic retinal disorders (E08.311-E08.359, E09.311-E09.359, E10.311-E10.359, E11.311-E11.359, E13.311-E13.359) ◄▥

● H35.0   Background retinopathy and retinal vascular changes
    Code also any associated hypertension (I10.-) ◄▥
    H35.00   Unspecified background retinopathy
   ● H35.01   Changes in retinal vascular appearance
        Retinal vascular sheathing
        H35.011   Changes in retinal vascular appearance, right eye
        H35.012   Changes in retinal vascular appearance, left eye

        H35.013   Changes in retinal vascular appearance, bilateral
        H35.019   Changes in retinal vascular appearance, unspecified eye
   ● H35.02   Exudative retinopathy
        Coats retinopathy
        H35.021   Exudative retinopathy, right eye
        H35.022   Exudative retinopathy, left eye
        H35.023   Exudative retinopathy, bilateral
        H35.029   Exudative retinopathy, unspecified eye
   ● H35.03   Hypertensive retinopathy
        H35.031   Hypertensive retinopathy, right eye
        H35.032   Hypertensive retinopathy, left eye
        H35.033   Hypertensive retinopathy, bilateral
        H35.039   Hypertensive retinopathy, unspecified eye
   ● H35.04   Retinal micro-aneurysms, unspecified
        H35.041   Retinal micro-aneurysms, unspecified, right eye
        H35.042   Retinal micro-aneurysms, unspecified, left eye
        H35.043   Retinal micro-aneurysms, unspecified, bilateral
        H35.049   Retinal micro-aneurysms, unspecified, unspecified eye
   ● H35.05   Retinal neovascularization, unspecified
        H35.051   Retinal neovascularization, unspecified, right eye
        H35.052   Retinal neovascularization, unspecified, left eye
        H35.053   Retinal neovascularization, unspecified, bilateral
        H35.059   Retinal neovascularization, unspecified, unspecified eye
   ● H35.06   Retinal vasculitis
        Eales disease
        Retinal perivasculitis
        H35.061   Retinal vasculitis, right eye
        H35.062   Retinal vasculitis, left eye
        H35.063   Retinal vasculitis, bilateral
        H35.069   Retinal vasculitis, unspecified eye
   ● H35.07   Retinal telangiectasis
        H35.071   Retinal telangiectasis, right eye
        H35.072   Retinal telangiectasis, left eye
        H35.073   Retinal telangiectasis, bilateral
        H35.079   Retinal telangiectasis, unspecified eye
    H35.09   Other intraretinal microvascular abnormalities
        Retinal varices

  H35.1   Retinopathy of prematurity
   ● H35.10   Retinopathy of prematurity, unspecified
        Retinopathy of prematurity NOS
        H35.101   Retinopathy of prematurity, unspecified, right eye
        H35.102   Retinopathy of prematurity, unspecified, left eye
        H35.103   Retinopathy of prematurity, unspecified, bilateral
        H35.109   Retinopathy of prematurity, unspecified, unspecified eye
   ● H35.11   Retinopathy of prematurity, stage 0
        H35.111   Retinopathy of prematurity, stage 0, right eye
        H35.112   Retinopathy of prematurity, stage 0, left eye
        H35.113   Retinopathy of prematurity, stage 0, bilateral
        H35.119   Retinopathy of prematurity, stage 0, unspecified eye

◄ New   ◄▥ Revised   ~~deleted~~ Deleted   Excludes 1   Excludes 2   Includes   Use additional   Code first   Code also   Unspecified
OGCR Official Guidelines   ● Unacceptable Principal Diagnosis   X Assign placeholder X   ● Use Additional Character(s)   ▶ Manifestation Code   **Coding Clinic**

● **H35.12**   **Retinopathy of prematurity, stage 1**
    H35.121   Retinopathy of prematurity, stage 1, right eye
    H35.122   Retinopathy of prematurity, stage 1, left eye
    H35.123   Retinopathy of prematurity, stage 1, bilateral
    H35.129   Retinopathy of prematurity, stage 1, unspecified eye

● **H35.13**   **Retinopathy of prematurity, stage 2**
    H35.131   Retinopathy of prematurity, stage 2, right eye
    H35.132   Retinopathy of prematurity, stage 2, left eye
    H35.133   Retinopathy of prematurity, stage 2, bilateral
    H35.139   Retinopathy of prematurity, stage 2, unspecified eye

● **H35.14**   **Retinopathy of prematurity, stage 3**
    H35.141   Retinopathy of prematurity, stage 3, right eye
    H35.142   Retinopathy of prematurity, stage 3, left eye
    H35.143   Retinopathy of prematurity, stage 3, bilateral
    H35.149   Retinopathy of prematurity, stage 3, unspecified eye

● **H35.15**   **Retinopathy of prematurity, stage 4**
    H35.151   Retinopathy of prematurity, stage 4, right eye
    H35.152   Retinopathy of prematurity, stage 4, left eye
    H35.153   Retinopathy of prematurity, stage 4, bilateral
    H35.159   Retinopathy of prematurity, stage 4, unspecified eye

● **H35.16**   **Retinopathy of prematurity, stage 5**
    H35.161   Retinopathy of prematurity, stage 5, right eye
    H35.162   Retinopathy of prematurity, stage 5, left eye
    H35.163   Retinopathy of prematurity, stage 5, bilateral
    H35.169   Retinopathy of prematurity, stage 5, unspecified eye

● **H35.17**   **Retrolental fibroplasia**
    H35.171   Retrolental fibroplasia, right eye
    H35.172   Retrolental fibroplasia, left eye
    H35.173   Retrolental fibroplasia, bilateral
    H35.179   Retrolental fibroplasia, unspecified eye

● **H35.2**   **Other non-diabetic proliferative retinopathy**
    Proliferative vitreo-retinopathy
    Excludes1   proliferative vitreo-retinopathy with retinal detachment (H33.4-)
    H35.20   Other non-diabetic proliferative retinopathy, unspecified eye
    H35.21   Other non-diabetic proliferative retinopathy, right eye
    H35.22   Other non-diabetic proliferative retinopathy, left eye
    H35.23   Other non-diabetic proliferative retinopathy, bilateral

Item 7–7   Macular degeneration is typically age-related, chronic, and is evidenced by deterioration of the macula (the part of the retina that provides for central field vision), resulting in blurred vision or a blind spot in the center of visual field while not affecting peripheral vision.

● **H35.3**   **Degeneration of macula and posterior pole**
    H35.30   Unspecified macular degeneration   A
       Age-related macular degeneration
    H35.31   Nonexudative age-related macular degeneration   A
       Atrophic age-related macular degeneration
    H35.32   Exudative age-related macular degeneration   A
    H35.33   Angioid streaks of macula
● **H35.34**   **Macular cyst, hole, or pseudohole**
    H35.341   Macular cyst, hole, or pseudohole, right eye
    H35.342   Macular cyst, hole, or pseudohole, left eye
    H35.343   Macular cyst, hole, or pseudohole, bilateral
    H35.349   Macular cyst, hole, or pseudohole, unspecified eye
● **H35.35**   **Cystoid macular degeneration**
    Excludes1   cystoid macular edema following cataract surgery (H59.03-)
    H35.351   Cystoid macular degeneration, right eye
    H35.352   Cystoid macular degeneration, left eye
    H35.353   Cystoid macular degeneration, bilateral
    H35.359   Cystoid macular degeneration, unspecified eye
● **H35.36**   **Drusen (degenerative) of macula**
    H35.361   Drusen (degenerative) of macula, right eye
    H35.362   Drusen (degenerative) of macula, left eye
    H35.363   Drusen (degenerative) of macula, bilateral
    H35.369   Drusen (degenerative) of macula, unspecified eye
● **H35.37**   **Puckering of macula**
    H35.371   Puckering of macula, right eye
    H35.372   Puckering of macula, left eye
    H35.373   Puckering of macula, bilateral
    H35.379   Puckering of macula, unspecified eye
● **H35.38**   **Toxic maculopathy**
    Code first poisoning due to drug or toxin, if applicable (T36-T65 with fifth or sixth character 1-4 or 6)
    Use additional code for adverse effect, if applicable, to identify drug (T36-T50 with fifth or sixth character 5)
    H35.381   Toxic maculopathy, right eye
    H35.382   Toxic maculopathy, left eye
    H35.383   Toxic maculopathy, bilateral
    H35.389   Toxic maculopathy, unspecified eye

CHAPTER 7 (H00-H59)

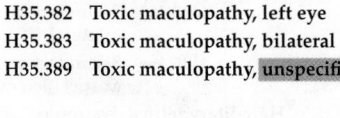

CHAPTER 7 (H00–H59)

- **H35.4   Peripheral retinal degeneration**
  - **Excludes1**   hereditary retinal degeneration (dystrophy) (H35.5-)
  - peripheral retinal degeneration with retinal break (H33.3-)
  - H35.40   Unspecified peripheral retinal degeneration
  - • H35.41   Lattice degeneration of retina
    - Palisade degeneration of retina
    - H35.411   Lattice degeneration of retina, right eye
    - H35.412   Lattice degeneration of retina, left eye
    - H35.413   Lattice degeneration of retina, bilateral
    - H35.419   Lattice degeneration of retina, unspecified eye
  - • H35.42   Microcystoid degeneration of retina
    - H35.421   Microcystoid degeneration of retina, right eye
    - H35.422   Microcystoid degeneration of retina, left eye
    - H35.423   Microcystoid degeneration of retina, bilateral
    - H35.429   Microcystoid degeneration of retina, unspecified eye
  - • H35.43   Paving stone degeneration of retina
    - H35.431   Paving stone degeneration of retina, right eye
    - H35.432   Paving stone degeneration of retina, left eye
    - H35.433   Paving stone degeneration of retina, bilateral
    - H35.439   Paving stone degeneration of retina, unspecified eye
  - • H35.44   Age-related reticular degeneration of retina
    - H35.441   Age-related reticular degeneration of retina, right eye   A
    - H35.442   Age-related reticular degeneration of retina, left eye   A
    - H35.443   Age-related reticular degeneration of retina, bilateral   A
    - H35.449   Age-related reticular degeneration of retina, unspecified eye   A
  - • H35.45   Secondary pigmentary degeneration
    - H35.451   Secondary pigmentary degeneration, right eye
    - H35.452   Secondary pigmentary degeneration, left eye
    - H35.453   Secondary pigmentary degeneration, bilateral
    - H35.459   Secondary pigmentary degeneration, unspecified eye
  - • H35.46   Secondary vitreoretinal degeneration
    - H35.461   Secondary vitreoretinal degeneration, right eye
    - H35.462   Secondary vitreoretinal degeneration, left eye
    - H35.463   Secondary vitreoretinal degeneration, bilateral
    - H35.469   Secondary vitreoretinal degeneration, unspecified eye
- • **H35.5   Hereditary retinal dystrophy**
  - **Excludes1**   dystrophies primarily involving Bruch's membrane (H31.1-)
  - H35.50   Unspecified hereditary retinal dystrophy
  - H35.51   Vitreoretinal dystrophy
  - H35.52   Pigmentary retinal dystrophy
    - Albipunctate retinal dystrophy
    - Retinitis pigmentosa
    - Tapetoretinal dystrophy

- H35.53   Other dystrophies primarily involving the sensory retina
  - Stargardt's disease
- H35.54   Dystrophies primarily involving the retinal pigment epithelium
  - Vitelliform retinal dystrophy
- • **H35.6   Retinal hemorrhage**
  - H35.60   Retinal hemorrhage, unspecified eye
  - H35.61   Retinal hemorrhage, right eye
  - H35.62   Retinal hemorrhage, left eye
  - H35.63   Retinal hemorrhage, bilateral
- • **H35.7   Separation of retinal layers**
  - **Excludes1**   retinal detachment (serous) (H33.2-)
  - rhegmatogenous retinal detachment (H33.0-)
  - (Ex) **For category H35.7 CC codes:** H33.001-H33.119, H33.191-H33.8, H35.70-H35.739
  - H35.70   Unspecified separation of retinal layers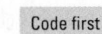
  - • H35.71   Central serous chorioretinopathy
    - H35.711   Central serous chorioretinopathy, right eye
    - H35.712   Central serous chorioretinopathy, left eye
    - H35.713   Central serous chorioretinopathy, bilateral
    - H35.719   Central serous chorioretinopathy, unspecified eye
  - • H35.72   Serous detachment of retinal pigment epithelium
    - H35.721   Serous detachment of retinal pigment epithelium, right eye
    - H35.722   Serous detachment of retinal pigment epithelium, left eye
    - H35.723   Serous detachment of retinal pigment epithelium, bilateral
    - H35.729   Serous detachment of retinal pigment epithelium, unspecified eye
  - • H35.73   Hemorrhagic detachment of retinal pigment epithelium
    - H35.731   Hemorrhagic detachment of retinal pigment epithelium, right eye
    - H35.732   Hemorrhagic detachment of retinal pigment epithelium, left eye
    - H35.733   Hemorrhagic detachment of retinal pigment epithelium, bilateral
    - H35.739   Hemorrhagic detachment of retinal pigment epithelium, unspecified eye
- • **H35.8   Other specified retinal disorders**
  - **Excludes2**   retinal hemorrhage (H35.6-)
  - H35.81   Retinal edema
    - Retinal cotton wool spots
  - H35.82   Retinal ischemia
    - (Ex) H35.60-H35.63, H35.81-H35.89
  - H35.89   Other specified retinal disorders
- H35.9   Unspecified retinal disorder

- ▌ **H36   _Retinal disorders in diseases classified elsewhere_**
  - _Code first_ underlying disease, such as:
    - lipid storage disorders (E75.-)
    - sickle-cell disorders (D57.-)
  - **Excludes1**   arteriosclerotic retinopathy (H35.0-)
    - diabetic retinopathy (E08.3-, E09.3-, E10.3-, E11.3-, E13.3-)

GLAUCOMA (H40-H42)

● **H40   Glaucoma**

Intraocular pressure (IOP) that is too high results from too much aqueous humor and because of excess production or inadequate drainage, optic nerve damage and vision loss may occur.

Excludes 1   absolute glaucoma (H44.51-)
congenital glaucoma (Q15.0)
traumatic glaucoma due to birth injury (P15.3)

● **H40.0   Glaucoma suspect**

● **H40.00   Preglaucoma, unspecified**

H40.001   Preglaucoma, unspecified, right eye

H40.002   Preglaucoma, unspecified, left eye

H40.003   Preglaucoma, unspecified, bilateral

H40.009   Preglaucoma, unspecified, unspecified eye

● **H40.01   Open angle with borderline findings, low risk**
Open angle, low risk

H40.011   Open angle with borderline findings, low risk, right eye

H40.012   Open angle with borderline findings, low risk, left eye

H40.013   Open angle with borderline findings, low risk, bilateral

H40.019   Open angle with borderline findings, low risk, unspecified eye

● **H40.02   Open angle with borderline findings, high risk**
Open angle, high risk

H40.021   Open angle with borderline findings, high risk, right eye

H40.022   Open angle with borderline findings, high risk, left eye

H40.023   Open angle with borderline findings, high risk, bilateral

H40.029   Open angle with borderline findings, high risk, unspecified eye

● **H40.03   Anatomical narrow angle**
Primary angle closure suspect

H40.031   Anatomical narrow angle, right eye

H40.032   Anatomical narrow angle, left eye

H40.033   Anatomical narrow angle, bilateral

H40.039   Anatomical narrow angle, unspecified eye

● **H40.04   Steroid responder**

H40.041   Steroid responder, right eye

H40.042   Steroid responder, left eye

H40.043   Steroid responder, bilateral

H40.049   Steroid responder, unspecified eye

● **H40.05   Ocular hypertension**

H40.051   Ocular hypertension, right eye

H40.052   Ocular hypertension, left eye

H40.053   Ocular hypertension, bilateral

H40.059   Ocular hypertension, unspecified eye

● **H40.06   Primary angle closure without glaucoma damage**

H40.061   Primary angle closure without glaucoma damage, right eye

H40.062   Primary angle closure without glaucoma damage, left eye

H40.063   Primary angle closure without glaucoma damage, bilateral

H40.069   Primary angle closure without glaucoma damage, unspecified eye

● **H40.1   Open-angle glaucoma**

X ● **H40.10   Unspecified open-angle glaucoma**

One of the following 7th characters is to be assigned to code H40.10 to designate the stage of glaucoma

0	stage unspecified
1	mild stage
2	moderate stage
3	severe stage
4	indeterminate stage

X ● **H40.11   Primary open-angle glaucoma**
Chronic simple glaucoma

One of the following 7th characters is to be assigned to code H40.11 to designate the stage of glaucoma

0	stage unspecified
1	mild stage
2	moderate stage
3	severe stage
4	indeterminate stage

● **H40.12   Low-tension glaucoma**

One of the following 7th characters is to be assigned to each code in subcategory H40.12 to designate the stage of glaucoma

0	stage unspecified
1	mild stage
2	moderate stage
3	severe stage
4	indeterminate stage

●● H40.121   Low-tension glaucoma, right eye

●● H40.122   Low-tension glaucoma, left eye

●● H40.123   Low-tension glaucoma, bilateral

●● H40.129   Low-tension glaucoma, unspecified eye

● **H40.13   Pigmentary glaucoma**

One of the following 7th characters is to be assigned to each code in subcategory H40.13 to designate the stage of glaucoma

0	stage unspecified
1	mild stage
2	moderate stage
3	severe stage
4	indeterminate stage

●● H40.131   Pigmentary glaucoma, right eye

●● H40.132   Pigmentary glaucoma, left eye

●● H40.133   Pigmentary glaucoma, bilateral

●● H40.139   Pigmentary glaucoma, unspecified eye

● **H40.14   Capsular glaucoma with pseudoexfoliation of lens**

One of the following 7th characters is to be assigned to each code in subcategory H40.14 to designate the stage of glaucoma

0	stage unspecified
1	mild stage
2	moderate stage
3	severe stage
4	indeterminate stage

● H40.141   Capsular glaucoma with pseudoexfoliation of lens, right eye

● H40.142   Capsular glaucoma with pseudoexfoliation of lens, left eye

CHAPTER 7 (H00-H59)

● H40.143　Capsular glaucoma with pseudoexfoliation of lens, bilateral

● H40.149　Capsular glaucoma with pseudoexfoliation of lens, unspecified eye

● H40.15　Residual stage of open-angle glaucoma

  ● H40.151　Residual stage of open-angle glaucoma, right eye

  ● H40.152　Residual stage of open-angle glaucoma, left eye

  ● H40.153　Residual stage of open-angle glaucoma, bilateral

  ● H40.159　Residual stage of open-angle glaucoma, unspecified eye

● H40.2　Primary angle-closure glaucoma

  Excludes1　aqueous misdirection (H40.83-)
             malignant glaucoma (H40.83-)

● H40.20　Unspecified primary angle-closure glaucoma

  One of the following 7th characters is to be assigned to code H40.20 to designate the stage of glaucoma

0	stage unspecified
1	mild stage
2	moderate stage
3	severe stage
4	indeterminate stage

● H40.21　Acute angle-closure glaucoma

  Acute angle-closure glaucoma attack
  Acute angle-closure glaucoma crisis
  (Ex) For category H40.21 CC codes: H40.211-H40.219

  H40.211　Acute angle-closure glaucoma, right eye

  H40.212　Acute angle-closure glaucoma, left eye

  H40.213　Acute angle-closure glaucoma, bilateral

  H40.219　Acute angle-closure glaucoma, unspecified eye

● H40.22　Chronic angle-closure glaucoma

  Chronic primary angle closure glaucoma

  One of the following 7th characters is to be assigned to each code in subcategory H40.22 to designate the stage of glaucoma

0	stage unspecified
1	mild stage
2	moderate stage
3	severe stage
4	indeterminate stage

  ● H40.221　Chronic angle-closure glaucoma, right eye

  ● H40.222　Chronic angle-closure glaucoma, left eye

  ● H40.223　Chronic angle-closure glaucoma, bilateral

  ● H40.229　Chronic angle-closure glaucoma, unspecified eye

● H40.23　Intermittent angle-closure glaucoma

  H40.231　Intermittent angle-closure glaucoma, right eye

  H40.232　Intermittent angle-closure glaucoma, left eye

  H40.233　Intermittent angle-closure glaucoma, bilateral

  H40.239　Intermittent angle-closure glaucoma, unspecified eye

● H40.24　Residual stage of angle-closure glaucoma

  H40.241　Residual stage of angle-closure glaucoma, right eye

  H40.242　Residual stage of angle-closure glaucoma, left eye

  H40.243　Residual stage of angle-closure glaucoma, bilateral

  H40.249　Residual stage of angle-closure glaucoma, unspecified eye

● H40.3　Glaucoma secondary to eye trauma

  Code also underlying condition

  One of the following 7th characters is to be assigned to each code in subcategory H40.3 to designate the stage of glaucoma

0	stage unspecified
1	mild stage
2	moderate stage
3	severe stage
4	indeterminate stage

X ● H40.30　Glaucoma secondary to eye trauma, unspecified eye

X ● H40.31　Glaucoma secondary to eye trauma, right eye

X ● H40.32　Glaucoma secondary to eye trauma, left eye

X ● H40.33　Glaucoma secondary to eye trauma, bilateral

● H40.4　Glaucoma secondary to eye inflammation

  Code also underlying condition

  One of the following 7th characters is to be assigned to each code in subcategory H40.4 to designate the stage of glaucoma

0	stage unspecified
1	mild stage
2	moderate stage
3	severe stage
4	indeterminate stage

X ● H40.40　Glaucoma secondary to eye inflammation, unspecified eye

X ● H40.41　Glaucoma secondary to eye inflammation, right eye

X ● H40.42　Glaucoma secondary to eye inflammation, left eye

X ● H40.43　Glaucoma secondary to eye inflammation, bilateral

● H40.5　Glaucoma secondary to other eye disorders

  Code also underlying eye disorder

  One of the following 7th characters is to be assigned to each code in subcategory H40.5 to designate the stage of glaucoma

0	stage unspecified
1	mild stage
2	moderate stage
3	severe stage
4	indeterminate stage

X ● H40.50　Glaucoma secondary to other eye disorders, unspecified eye

X ● H40.51　Glaucoma secondary to other eye disorders, right eye

X ● H40.52　Glaucoma secondary to other eye disorders, left eye

X ● H40.53　Glaucoma secondary to other eye disorders, bilateral

◀ New　◀■ Revised　deleted Deleted　Excludes 1　Excludes 2　Includes　Use additional　Code first　Code also　Unspecified

OGCR Official Guidelines　● Unacceptable Principal Diagnosis　X Assign placeholder X　▶ Use Additional Character(s)　▶ Manifestation Code　**Coding Clinic**

● **H40.6 Glaucoma secondary to drugs**

Use additional code for adverse effect, if applicable, to identify drug (T36-T50 with fifth or sixth character 5)

One of the following 7th characters is to be assigned to each code in subcategory H40.6 to designate the stage of glaucoma

0	stage unspecified
1	mild stage
2	moderate stage
3	severe stage
4	indeterminate stage

X● **H40.60 Glaucoma secondary to drugs, unspecified eye**
X● **H40.61 Glaucoma secondary to drugs, right eye**
X● **H40.62 Glaucoma secondary to drugs, left eye**
X● **H40.63 Glaucoma secondary to drugs, bilateral**

● **H40.8 Other glaucoma**

  ● **H40.81 Glaucoma with increased episcleral venous pressure**

    H40.811 Glaucoma with increased episcleral venous pressure, right eye

    H40.812 Glaucoma with increased episcleral venous pressure, left eye

    H40.813 Glaucoma with increased episcleral venous pressure, bilateral

    H40.819 Glaucoma with increased episcleral venous pressure, unspecified eye

  ● **H40.82 Hypersecretion glaucoma**

    H40.821 Hypersecretion glaucoma, right eye

    H40.822 Hypersecretion glaucoma, left eye

    H40.823 Hypersecretion glaucoma, bilateral

    H40.829 Hypersecretion glaucoma, unspecified eye

  ● **H40.83 Aqueous misdirection**

Malignant glaucoma

    H40.831 Aqueous misdirection, right eye

    H40.832 Aqueous misdirection, left eye

    H40.833 Aqueous misdirection, bilateral

    H40.839 Aqueous misdirection, unspecified eye

  H40.89 Other specified glaucoma

H40.9 Unspecified glaucoma

▷ *H42 Glaucoma in diseases classified elsewhere*

Code first underlying condition, such as:
amyloidosis (E85.-) ◀▥
aniridia (Q13.1)
Lowe's syndrome (E72.03)
Reiger's anomaly (Q13.81)
specified metabolic disorder (E70-E88)

Excludes1 glaucoma (in):
diabetes mellitus (E08.39, E09.39, E10.39, E11.39, E13.39)
onchocerciasis (B73.02)
syphilis (A52.71)
tuberculous (A18.59)

DISORDERS OF VITREOUS BODY AND GLOBE (H43-H44)

● **H43 Disorders of vitreous body**

  ● **H43.0 Vitreous prolapse**

    Excludes1 vitreous syndrome following cataract surgery (H59.0-)
traumatic vitreous prolapse (S05.2-)

  H43.00 Vitreous prolapse, unspecified eye

  H43.01 Vitreous prolapse, right eye

  H43.02 Vitreous prolapse, left eye

  H43.03 Vitreous prolapse, bilateral

● **H43.1 Vitreous hemorrhage**

  H43.10 Vitreous hemorrhage, unspecified eye

  H43.11 Vitreous hemorrhage, right eye

  H43.12 Vitreous hemorrhage, left eye

  H43.13 Vitreous hemorrhage, bilateral

● **H43.2 Crystalline deposits in vitreous body**

  H43.20 Crystalline deposits in vitreous body, unspecified eye

  H43.21 Crystalline deposits in vitreous body, right eye

  H43.22 Crystalline deposits in vitreous body, left eye

  H43.23 Crystalline deposits in vitreous body, bilateral

● **H43.3 Other vitreous opacities**

  ● **H43.31 Vitreous membranes and strands**

    H43.311 Vitreous membranes and strands, right eye

    H43.312 Vitreous membranes and strands, left eye

    H43.313 Vitreous membranes and strands, bilateral

    H43.319 Vitreous membranes and strands, unspecified eye

  ● **H43.39 Other vitreous opacities**

Vitreous floaters
Small clumps of cells that float in the vitreous of the eye, appearing as black specks or dots in the field of vision and common in the aging eye.

    H43.391 Other vitreous opacities, right eye

    H43.392 Other vitreous opacities, left eye

    H43.393 Other vitreous opacities, bilateral

    H43.399 Other vitreous opacities, unspecified eye

● **H43.8 Other disorders of vitreous body**

  Excludes1 proliferative vitreo-retinopathy with retinal detachment (H33.4)

  Excludes2 vitreous abscess (H44.02-)

  ● **H43.81 Vitreous degeneration**

Vitreous detachment

    H43.811 Vitreous degeneration, right eye

    H43.812 Vitreous degeneration, left eye

    H43.813 Vitreous degeneration, bilateral

    H43.819 Vitreous degeneration, unspecified eye

  ● **H43.82 Vitreomacular adhesion**

Vitreomacular traction

    H43.821 Vitreomacular adhesion, right eye   A

    H43.822 Vitreomacular adhesion, left eye   A

    H43.823 Vitreomacular adhesion, bilateral   A

    H43.829 Vitreomacular adhesion, unspecified eye   A

  H43.89 Other disorders of vitreous body

H43.9 Unspecified disorder of vitreous body

● **H44 Disorders of globe**

  Includes disorders affecting multiple structures of eye

  ● **H44.0 Purulent endophthalmitis**

Use additional code to identify organism

    Excludes1 bleb associated endophthalmitis (H59.4-)

  ● **H44.00 Unspecified purulent endophthalmitis**

    (Ex) **For category H44.00 CC codes:** H20.051-H20.059, H21.331-H21.339, H33.121-H33.129, H44.001-H44.029, H44.121-H44.129, H44.19

    H44.001 Unspecified purulent endophthalmitis, right eye 🔖

    H44.002 Unspecified purulent endophthalmitis, left eye 🔖

    H44.003 Unspecified purulent endophthalmitis, bilateral 🔖

    H44.009 Unspecified purulent endophthalmitis, unspecified eye 🔖

N   Newborn Age: 0   P   Pediatric Age: 0–17   M   Maternity DX: 12–55   A   Adult Age: 15–124   ♀ Females Only   ♂ Males Only

 Complication\Comorbidity   🔖 Major C\C   (Ex) CC/MCC Exclusions   🔖 Present on Admission Requirement   🔖 Hospital-Acquired Condition

933

CHAPTER 7 (H00-H59)

● H44.01 Panophthalmitis (acute)
     (Ex) For category H44.01 CC codes: See H44.00
     H44.011 Panophthalmitis (acute), right eye
     H44.012 Panophthalmitis (acute), left eye
     H44.013 Panophthalmitis (acute), bilateral
     H44.019 Panophthalmitis (acute), unspecified eye

● H44.02 Vitreous abscess (chronic)
     (Ex) For category H44.02 CC codes: H16.241-H16.249,
         H21.331-H21.339, H33.121-H33.129, H44.001-H44.19
     H44.021 Vitreous abscess (chronic), right eye
     H44.022 Vitreous abscess (chronic), left eye
     H44.023 Vitreous abscess (chronic), bilateral
     H44.029 Vitreous abscess (chronic), unspecified eye

● H44.1 Other endophthalmitis
     Excludes1 bleb associated endophthalmitis (H59.4-)
     Excludes2 ophthalmia nodosa (H16.2-)
● H44.11 Panuveitis
     (Ex) For category H44.11 CC codes: H44.111-H44.119,
         H44.131-H44.139
     H44.111 Panuveitis, right eye
     H44.112 Panuveitis, left eye
     H44.113 Panuveitis, bilateral
     H44.119 Panuveitis, unspecified eye

● H44.12 Parasitic endophthalmitis, unspecified
     (Ex) For category H44.12 CC codes: See H44.00
     H44.121 Parasitic endophthalmitis, unspecified, right eye
     H44.122 Parasitic endophthalmitis, unspecified, left eye
     H44.123 Parasitic endophthalmitis, unspecified, bilateral
     H44.129 Parasitic endophthalmitis, unspecified, unspecified eye

● H44.13 Sympathetic uveitis
     (Ex) For category H44.13 CC codes: See H44.11
     H44.131 Sympathetic uveitis, right eye
     H44.132 Sympathetic uveitis, left eye
     H44.133 Sympathetic uveitis, bilateral
     H44.139 Sympathetic uveitis, unspecified eye

H44.19 Other endophthalmitis
     (Ex) See H44.00

● H44.2 Degenerative myopia
     Malignant myopia
     H44.20 Degenerative myopia, unspecified eye
     H44.21 Degenerative myopia, right eye
     H44.22 Degenerative myopia, left eye
     H44.23 Degenerative myopia, bilateral
● H44.3 Other and unspecified degenerative disorders of globe
     H44.30 Unspecified degenerative disorder of globe
● H44.31 Chalcosis
     H44.311 Chalcosis, right eye
     H44.312 Chalcosis, left eye
     H44.313 Chalcosis, bilateral
     H44.319 Chalcosis, unspecified eye
● H44.32 Siderosis of eye
     H44.321 Siderosis of eye, right eye
     H44.322 Siderosis of eye, left eye
     H44.323 Siderosis of eye, bilateral
     H44.329 Siderosis of eye, unspecified eye

● H44.39 Other degenerative disorders of globe
     H44.391 Other degenerative disorders of globe, right eye
     H44.392 Other degenerative disorders of globe, left eye
     H44.393 Other degenerative disorders of globe, bilateral
     H44.399 Other degenerative disorders of globe, unspecified eye
● H44.4 Hypotony of eye
     H44.40 Unspecified hypotony of eye
● H44.41 Flat anterior chamber hypotony of eye
     H44.411 Flat anterior chamber hypotony of right eye
     H44.412 Flat anterior chamber hypotony of left eye
     H44.413 Flat anterior chamber hypotony of eye, bilateral
     H44.419 Flat anterior chamber hypotony of unspecified eye
● H44.42 Hypotony of eye due to ocular fistula
     H44.421 Hypotony of right eye due to ocular fistula
     H44.422 Hypotony of left eye due to ocular fistula
     H44.423 Hypotony of eye due to ocular fistula, bilateral
     H44.429 Hypotony of unspecified eye due to ocular fistula
● H44.43 Hypotony of eye due to other ocular disorders
     H44.431 Hypotony of eye due to other ocular disorders, right eye
     H44.432 Hypotony of eye due to other ocular disorders, left eye
     H44.433 Hypotony of eye due to other ocular disorders, bilateral
     H44.439 Hypotony of eye due to other ocular disorders, unspecified eye
● H44.44 Primary hypotony of eye
     H44.441 Primary hypotony of right eye
     H44.442 Primary hypotony of left eye
     H44.443 Primary hypotony of eye, bilateral
     H44.449 Primary hypotony of unspecified eye
● H44.5 Degenerated conditions of globe
     H44.50 Unspecified degenerated conditions of globe
● H44.51 Absolute glaucoma
     H44.511 Absolute glaucoma, right eye
     H44.512 Absolute glaucoma, left eye
     H44.513 Absolute glaucoma, bilateral
     H44.519 Absolute glaucoma, unspecified eye
● H44.52 Atrophy of globe
     Phthisis bulbi
     H44.521 Atrophy of globe, right eye
     H44.522 Atrophy of globe, left eye
     H44.523 Atrophy of globe, bilateral
     H44.529 Atrophy of globe, unspecified eye
● H44.53 Leucocoria
     H44.531 Leucocoria, right eye
     H44.532 Leucocoria, left eye
     H44.533 Leucocoria, bilateral
     H44.539 Leucocoria, unspecified eye

◄ New   ◄ Revised   ~~deleted~~ Deleted   Excludes 1   Excludes 2   Includes   Use additional   Code first   Code also   Unspecified
OGCR Official Guidelines   ● Unacceptable Principal Diagnosis   X Assign placeholder X   ● Use Additional Character(s)   ▶ Manifestation Code   **Coding Clinic**

● H44.6   Retained (old) intraocular foreign body, magnetic

    Use additional code to identify magnetic foreign body (Z18.11)

    Excludes1   current intraocular foreign body (S05.-)

    Excludes2   retained foreign body in eyelid (H02.81-)

        retained (old) foreign body following penetrating wound of orbit (H05.5-)

        retained (old) intraocular foreign body, nonmagnetic (H44.7-)

● H44.60   Unspecified retained (old) intraocular foreign body, magnetic

    H44.601   Unspecified retained (old) intraocular foreign body, magnetic, right eye

    H44.602   Unspecified retained (old) intraocular foreign body, magnetic, left eye

    H44.603   Unspecified retained (old) intraocular foreign body, magnetic, bilateral

    H44.609   Unspecified retained (old) intraocular foreign body, magnetic, unspecified eye

● H44.61   Retained (old) magnetic foreign body in anterior chamber

    H44.611   Retained (old) magnetic foreign body in anterior chamber, right eye

    H44.612   Retained (old) magnetic foreign body in anterior chamber, left eye

    H44.613   Retained (old) magnetic foreign body in anterior chamber, bilateral

    H44.619   Retained (old) magnetic foreign body in anterior chamber, unspecified eye

● H44.62   Retained (old) magnetic foreign body in iris or ciliary body

    H44.621   Retained (old) magnetic foreign body in iris or ciliary body, right eye

    H44.622   Retained (old) magnetic foreign body in iris or ciliary body, left eye

    H44.623   Retained (old) magnetic foreign body in iris or ciliary body, bilateral

    H44.629   Retained (old) magnetic foreign body in iris or ciliary body, unspecified eye

● H44.63   Retained (old) magnetic foreign body in lens

    H44.631   Retained (old) magnetic foreign body in lens, right eye

    H44.632   Retained (old) magnetic foreign body in lens, left eye

    H44.633   Retained (old) magnetic foreign body in lens, bilateral

    H44.639   Retained (old) magnetic foreign body in lens, unspecified eye

● H44.64   Retained (old) magnetic foreign body in posterior wall of globe

    H44.641   Retained (old) magnetic foreign body in posterior wall of globe, right eye

    H44.642   Retained (old) magnetic foreign body in posterior wall of globe, left eye

    H44.643   Retained (old) magnetic foreign body in posterior wall of globe, bilateral

    H44.649   Retained (old) magnetic foreign body in posterior wall of globe, unspecified eye

● H44.65   Retained (old) magnetic foreign body in vitreous body

    H44.651   Retained (old) magnetic foreign body in vitreous body, right eye

    H44.652   Retained (old) magnetic foreign body in vitreous body, left eye

    H44.653   Retained (old) magnetic foreign body in vitreous body, bilateral

    H44.659   Retained (old) magnetic foreign body in vitreous body, unspecified eye

● H44.69   Retained (old) intraocular foreign body, magnetic, in other or multiple sites

    H44.691   Retained (old) intraocular foreign body, magnetic, in other or multiple sites, right eye

    H44.692   Retained (old) intraocular foreign body, magnetic, in other or multiple sites, left eye

    H44.693   Retained (old) intraocular foreign body, magnetic, in other or multiple sites, bilateral

    H44.699   Retained (old) intraocular foreign body, magnetic, in other or multiple sites, unspecified eye

● H44.7   Retained (old) intraocular foreign body, nonmagnetic

    Use additional code to identify nonmagnetic foreign body (Z18.01-Z18.10, Z18.12, Z18.2-Z18.9)

    Excludes1   current intraocular foreign body (S05.-)

    Excludes2   retained foreign body in eyelid (H02.81-)

        retained (old) foreign body following penetrating wound of orbit (H05.5-)

        retained (old) intraocular foreign body, magnetic (H44.6-)

● H44.70   Unspecified retained (old) intraocular foreign body, nonmagnetic

    H44.701   Unspecified retained (old) intraocular foreign body, nonmagnetic, right eye

    H44.702   Unspecified retained (old) intraocular foreign body, nonmagnetic, left eye

    H44.703   Unspecified retained (old) intraocular foreign body, nonmagnetic, bilateral

    H44.709   Unspecified retained (old) intraocular foreign body, nonmagnetic, unspecified eye

        Retained (old) intraocular foreign body NOS

● H44.71   Retained (nonmagnetic) (old) foreign body in anterior chamber

    H44.711   Retained (nonmagnetic) (old) foreign body in anterior chamber, right eye

    H44.712   Retained (nonmagnetic) (old) foreign body in anterior chamber, left eye

    H44.713   Retained (nonmagnetic) (old) foreign body in anterior chamber, bilateral

    H44.719   Retained (nonmagnetic) (old) foreign body in anterior chamber, unspecified eye

● H44.72   Retained (nonmagnetic) (old) foreign body in iris or ciliary body

    H44.721   Retained (nonmagnetic) (old) foreign body in iris or ciliary body, right eye

    H44.722   Retained (nonmagnetic) (old) foreign body in iris or ciliary body, left eye

    H44.723   Retained (nonmagnetic) (old) foreign body in iris or ciliary body, bilateral

    H44.729   Retained (nonmagnetic) (old) foreign body in iris or ciliary body, unspecified eye

● H44.73   Retained (nonmagnetic) (old) foreign body in lens

    H44.731   Retained (nonmagnetic) (old) foreign body in lens, right eye

    H44.732   Retained (nonmagnetic) (old) foreign body in lens, left eye

    H44.733   Retained (nonmagnetic) (old) foreign body in lens, bilateral

    H44.739   Retained (nonmagnetic) (old) foreign body in lens, unspecified eye

N Newborn Age: 0   **P** Pediatric Age: 0–17   **M** Maternity DX: 12–55   **A** Adult Age: 15–124   ♀ Females Only   ♂ Males Only

Complication\Comorbidity   Major C\C   (Ex) CC/MCC Exclusions   Present on Admission Requirement   Hospital-Acquired Condition

935

CHAPTER 7 (H00-H59)

CHAPTER 7 (H00-H59)

● H44.74   Retained (nonmagnetic) (old) foreign body in posterior wall of globe

     H44.741   Retained (nonmagnetic) (old) foreign body in posterior wall of globe, right eye

     H44.742   Retained (nonmagnetic) (old) foreign body in posterior wall of globe, left eye

     H44.743   Retained (nonmagnetic) (old) foreign body in posterior wall of globe, bilateral

     H44.749   Retained (nonmagnetic) (old) foreign body in posterior wall of globe, unspecified eye

● H44.75   Retained (nonmagnetic) (old) foreign body in vitreous body

     H44.751   Retained (nonmagnetic) (old) foreign body in vitreous body, right eye

     H44.752   Retained (nonmagnetic) (old) foreign body in vitreous body, left eye

     H44.753   Retained (nonmagnetic) (old) foreign body in vitreous body, bilateral

     H44.759   Retained (nonmagnetic) (old) foreign body in vitreous body, unspecified eye

● H44.79   Retained (old) intraocular foreign body, nonmagnetic, in other or multiple sites

     H44.791   Retained (old) intraocular foreign body, nonmagnetic, in other or multiple sites, right eye

     H44.792   Retained (old) intraocular foreign body, nonmagnetic, in other or multiple sites, left eye

     H44.793   Retained (old) intraocular foreign body, nonmagnetic, in other or multiple sites, bilateral

     H44.799   Retained (old) intraocular foreign body, nonmagnetic, in other or multiple sites, unspecified eye

● H44.8   Other disorders of globe

   ● H44.81   Hemophthalmos

     H44.811   Hemophthalmos, right eye

     H44.812   Hemophthalmos, left eye

     H44.813   Hemophthalmos, bilateral

     H44.819   Hemophthalmos, unspecified eye

   ● H44.82   Luxation of globe

     H44.821   Luxation of globe, right eye

     H44.822   Luxation of globe, left eye

     H44.823   Luxation of globe, bilateral

     H44.829   Luxation of globe, unspecified eye

   H44.89   Other disorders of globe

   H44.9   Unspecified disorder of globe

(See Plate 86 on page 55.)

DISORDERS OF OPTIC NERVE AND VISUAL PATHWAYS (H46-H47)

● H46   Optic neuritis

   Excludes2   ischemic optic neuropathy (H47.01-)
               neuromyelitis optica [Devic] (G36.0)

   Ex: For category H46 CC codes: H46.00-H46.9

   ● H46.0   Optic papillitis

     H46.00   Optic papillitis, unspecified eye

     H46.01   Optic papillitis, right eye

     H46.02   Optic papillitis, left eye

     H46.03   Optic papillitis, bilateral

● H46.1   Retrobulbar neuritis

   Retrobulbar neuritis NOS

   Excludes1   syphilitic retrobulbar neuritis (A52.15)

   H46.10   Retrobulbar neuritis, unspecified eye

   H46.11   Retrobulbar neuritis, right eye

   H46.12   Retrobulbar neuritis, left eye

   H46.13   Retrobulbar neuritis, bilateral

H46.2   Nutritional optic neuropathy

H46.3   Toxic optic neuropathy

   Code first (T51-T65) to identify cause

H46.8   Other optic neuritis

H46.9   Unspecified optic neuritis

● H47   Other disorders of optic [2nd] nerve and visual pathways

   ● H47.0   Disorders of optic nerve, not elsewhere classified

     ● H47.01   Ischemic optic neuropathy

       H47.011   Ischemic optic neuropathy, right eye

       H47.012   Ischemic optic neuropathy, left eye

       H47.013   Ischemic optic neuropathy, bilateral

       H47.019   Ischemic optic neuropathy, unspecified eye

     ● H47.02   Hemorrhage in optic nerve sheath

       H47.021   Hemorrhage in optic nerve sheath, right eye

       H47.022   Hemorrhage in optic nerve sheath, left eye

       H47.023   Hemorrhage in optic nerve sheath, bilateral

       H47.029   Hemorrhage in optic nerve sheath, unspecified eye

     ● H47.03   Optic nerve hypoplasia

       H47.031   Optic nerve hypoplasia, right eye

       H47.032   Optic nerve hypoplasia, left eye

       H47.033   Optic nerve hypoplasia, bilateral

       H47.039   Optic nerve hypoplasia, unspecified eye

     ● H47.09   Other disorders of optic nerve, not elsewhere classified

       Compression of optic nerve

       H47.091   Other disorders of optic nerve, not elsewhere classified, right eye

       H47.092   Other disorders of optic nerve, not elsewhere classified, left eye

       H47.093   Other disorders of optic nerve, not elsewhere classified, bilateral

       H47.099   Other disorders of optic nerve, not elsewhere classified, unspecified eye

   ● H47.1   Papilledema

     H47.10   Unspecified papilledema

       Ex: A17.9, A18.50-A18.59, A18.82, A18.84, A18.89, A39.82, E08.311-E08.39, E08.618-E08.638, E08.649-E08.8, E09.311-E09.39, E09.618-E09.638, E09.649-E09.8, E10.311-E10.39, E10.618-E10.638, E10.649, E10.69-E10.8, E11.311-E11.39, E11.618-E11.638, E11.649, E11.69-E11.8, E13.311-E13.39, E13.618-E13.638, E13.649-E13.8, H47.10-H47.13, H47.231-H47.239, H47.331-H47.339, H57.8-H57.9, H59.40-H59.43, Q11.3, Q15.8-Q15.9

     H47.11   Papilledema associated with increased intracranial pressure

       Ex: See H47.10

     H47.12   Papilledema associated with decreased ocular pressure

     H47.13   Papilledema associated with retinal disorder

     ● H47.14   Foster-Kennedy syndrome

       H47.141   Foster-Kennedy syndrome, right eye

       H47.142   Foster-Kennedy syndrome, left eye

       H47.143   Foster-Kennedy syndrome, bilateral

       H47.149   Foster-Kennedy syndrome, unspecified eye

◀ New   ◀ Revised   ~~deleted~~ Deleted   Excludes 1   Excludes 2   Includes   Use additional   Code first   Code also   Unspecified

OGCR Official Guidelines   ● Unacceptable Principal Diagnosis   X Assign placeholder X   ● Use Additional Character(s)   ▸ Manifestation Code   **Coding Clinic**

Figure 7-10   Papilledema. (From Behrma: Nelson Textbook of Pediatrics, ed 17, Saunders, 2004)

Item 7-8   Papilledema is swelling of the optic disc caused by increased intracranial pressure. It is most often bilateral and occurs quickly (hours) or over weeks of time. It is a common symptom of a brain tumor. The term should not be used to describe optic disc swelling with underlying infectious, infiltrative, or inflammatory etiologies.

● **H47.2**   **Optic atrophy**
     H47.20   Unspecified optic atrophy
   ● H47.21   Primary optic atrophy
       H47.211   Primary optic atrophy, right eye
       H47.212   Primary optic atrophy, left eye
       H47.213   Primary optic atrophy, bilateral
       H47.219   Primary optic atrophy, unspecified eye
     H47.22   Hereditary optic atrophy
       Leber's optic atrophy
   ● H47.23   Glaucomatous optic atrophy
       H47.231   Glaucomatous optic atrophy, right eye
       H47.232   Glaucomatous optic atrophy, left eye
       H47.233   Glaucomatous optic atrophy, bilateral
       H47.239   Glaucomatous optic atrophy, unspecified eye
   ● H47.29   Other optic atrophy
       Temporal pallor of optic disc
       H47.291   Other optic atrophy, right eye
       H47.292   Other optic atrophy, left eye
       H47.293   Other optic atrophy, bilateral
       H47.299   Other optic atrophy, unspecified eye
● **H47.3**   **Other disorders of optic disc**
   ● H47.31   Coloboma of optic disc
       H47.311   Coloboma of optic disc, right eye
       H47.312   Coloboma of optic disc, left eye
       H47.313   Coloboma of optic disc, bilateral
       H47.319   Coloboma of optic disc, unspecified eye
   ● H47.32   Drusen of optic disc
       H47.321   Drusen of optic disc, right eye
       H47.322   Drusen of optic disc, left eye
       H47.323   Drusen of optic disc, bilateral
       H47.329   Drusen of optic disc, unspecified eye

   ● H47.33   Pseudopapilledema of optic disc
       H47.331   Pseudopapilledema of optic disc, right eye
       H47.332   Pseudopapilledema of optic disc, left eye
       H47.333   Pseudopapilledema of optic disc, bilateral
       H47.339   Pseudopapilledema of optic disc, unspecified eye
   ● H47.39   Other disorders of optic disc
       H47.391   Other disorders of optic disc, right eye
       H47.392   Other disorders of optic disc, left eye
       H47.393   Other disorders of optic disc, bilateral
       H47.399   Other disorders of optic disc, unspecified eye
● **H47.4**   **Disorders of optic chiasm**
     Code also underlying condition
     (Ex) **For category H47.4 CC codes:** H47.41-H47.539
     H47.41   Disorders of optic chiasm in (due to) inflammatory disorders 🅒
     H47.42   Disorders of optic chiasm in (due to) neoplasm 🅒
     H47.43   Disorders of optic chiasm in (due to) vascular disorders 🅒
     H47.49   Disorders of optic chiasm in (due to) other disorders 🅒
● **H47.5**   **Disorders of other visual pathways**
     Disorders of optic tracts, geniculate nuclei and optic radiations
     Code also underlying condition
     (Ex) **For category H47.5 CC codes:** H47.41-H47.539
   ● H47.51   Disorders of visual pathways in (due to) inflammatory disorders
       H47.511   Disorders of visual pathways in (due to) inflammatory disorders, right side 🅒
       H47.512   Disorders of visual pathways in (due to) inflammatory disorders, left side 🅒
       H47.519   Disorders of visual pathways in (due to) inflammatory disorders, unspecified side 🅒
   ● H47.52   Disorders of visual pathways in (due to) neoplasm
       H47.521   Disorders of visual pathways in (due to) neoplasm, right side 🅒
       H47.522   Disorders of visual pathways in (due to) neoplasm, left side 🅒
       H47.529   Disorders of visual pathways in (due to) neoplasm, unspecified side 🅒
   ● H47.53   Disorders of visual pathways in (due to) vascular disorders
       H47.531   Disorders of visual pathways in (due to) vascular disorders, right side 🅒
       H47.532   Disorders of visual pathways in (due to) vascular disorders, left side 🅒
       H47.539   Disorders of visual pathways in (due to) vascular disorders, unspecified side 🅒
● **H47.6**   **Disorders of visual cortex**
     Code also underlying condition
     Excludes1   injury to visual cortex S04.04
     (Ex) **For category H47.6 CC codes:** H47.611-H47.9
   ● H47.61   Cortical blindness
       H47.611   Cortical blindness, right side of brain
       H47.612   Cortical blindness, left side of brain
       H47.619   Cortical blindness, unspecified side of brain

CHAPTER 7 (H00-H59)

N   Newborn Age: 0   **P**   Pediatric Age: 0–17   **M**   Maternity DX: 12–55   **A**   Adult Age: 15–124   ♀ Females Only   ♂ Males Only

🅒 Complication\Comorbidity   🅜 Major C\C   (Ex) CC/MCC Exclusions   🅟 Present on Admission Requirement   🅗 Hospital-Acquired Condition

H47.62 Disorders of visual cortex in (due to) inflammatory disorders

H47.621 Disorders of visual cortex in (due to) inflammatory disorders, right side of brain

H47.622 Disorders of visual cortex in (due to) inflammatory disorders, left side of brain

H47.629 Disorders of visual cortex in (due to) inflammatory disorders, unspecified side of brain

H47.63 Disorders of visual cortex in (due to) neoplasm

H47.631 Disorders of visual cortex in (due to) neoplasm, right side of brain

H47.632 Disorders of visual cortex in (due to) neoplasm, left side of brain

H47.639 Disorders of visual cortex in (due to) neoplasm, unspecified side of brain

H47.64 Disorders of visual cortex in (due to) vascular disorders

H47.641 Disorders of visual cortex in (due to) vascular disorders, right side of brain

H47.642 Disorders of visual cortex in (due to) vascular disorders, left side of brain

H47.649 Disorders of visual cortex in (due to) vascular disorders, unspecified side of brain

H47.9 Unspecified disorder of visual pathways

DISORDERS OF OCULAR MUSCLES, BINOCULAR MOVEMENT, ACCOMMODATION AND REFRACTION (H49-H52)

Excludes2 nystagmus and other irregular eye movements (H55)

H49 Paralytic strabismus

Excludes2 internal ophthalmoplegia (H52.51-)
internuclear ophthalmoplegia (H51.2-)
progressive supranuclear ophthalmoplegia (G23.1)

H49.0 Third [oculomotor] nerve palsy

H49.00 Third [oculomotor] nerve palsy, unspecified eye

H49.01 Third [oculomotor] nerve palsy, right eye

H49.02 Third [oculomotor] nerve palsy, left eye

H49.03 Third [oculomotor] nerve palsy, bilateral

H49.1 Fourth [trochlear] nerve palsy

H49.10 Fourth [trochlear] nerve palsy, unspecified eye

H49.11 Fourth [trochlear] nerve palsy, right eye

H49.12 Fourth [trochlear] nerve palsy, left eye

H49.13 Fourth [trochlear] nerve palsy, bilateral

Item 7-9 Strabismus or esotropia (crossed eyes) is a condition of the extraocular eye muscles, resulting in an inability of the eyes to focus and also affects depth perception.

Figure 7-11 **A.** Image of strabismus. **B.** Exotropia. (**A** from Yanoff: Ophthalmology, ed 3, Mosby, Inc., 2008. **B** from Rakel: Textbook of Family Practice, ed 7, Saunders, 2007)

H49.2 Sixth [abducent] nerve palsy

H49.20 Sixth [abducent] nerve palsy, unspecified eye

H49.21 Sixth [abducent] nerve palsy, right eye

H49.22 Sixth [abducent] nerve palsy, left eye

H49.23 Sixth [abducent] nerve palsy, bilateral

H49.3 Total (external) ophthalmoplegia

H49.30 Total (external) ophthalmoplegia, unspecified eye

H49.31 Total (external) ophthalmoplegia, right eye

H49.32 Total (external) ophthalmoplegia, left eye

H49.33 Total (external) ophthalmoplegia, bilateral

H49.4 Progressive external ophthalmoplegia

Excludes1 Kearns-Sayre syndrome (H49.81-)

H49.40 Progressive external ophthalmoplegia, unspecified eye

H49.41 Progressive external ophthalmoplegia, right eye

H49.42 Progressive external ophthalmoplegia, left eye

H49.43 Progressive external ophthalmoplegia, bilateral

H49.8 Other paralytic strabismus

H49.81 Kearns-Sayre syndrome

Progressive external ophthalmoplegia with pigmentary retinopathy

Use additional code for other manifestation, such as:
heart block (I45.9)

(Ex) For category H49.81 CC codes: C96.5-C96.6, E71.310-E71.548, E80.3-E80.7, E88.89

H49.811 Kearns-Sayre syndrome, right eye

H49.812 Kearns-Sayre syndrome, left eye

H49.813 Kearns-Sayre syndrome, bilateral

H49.819 Kearns-Sayre syndrome, unspecified eye

H49.88 Other paralytic strabismus

External ophthalmoplegia NOS

H49.881 Other paralytic strabismus, right eye

H49.882 Other paralytic strabismus, left eye

H49.883 Other paralytic strabismus, bilateral

H49.889 Other paralytic strabismus, unspecified eye

H49.9 Unspecified paralytic strabismus

H50 Other strabismus

H50.0 Esotropia

Convergent concomitant strabismus

Excludes1 intermittent esotropia (H50.31-, H50.32)

H50.00 Unspecified esotropia

H50.01 Monocular esotropia

H50.011 Monocular esotropia, right eye

H50.012 Monocular esotropia, left eye

H50.02 Monocular esotropia with A pattern

H50.021 Monocular esotropia with A pattern, right eye

H50.022 Monocular esotropia with A pattern, left eye

H50.03 Monocular esotropia with V pattern

H50.031 Monocular esotropia with V pattern, right eye

H50.032 Monocular esotropia with V pattern, left eye

◀ New   ◀▥ Revised   ~~deleted~~ Deleted   Excludes 1   Excludes 2   Includes   Use additional   Code first   Code also   Unspecified

OGCR Official Guidelines   ● Unacceptable Principal Diagnosis   X Assign placeholder X   ● Use Additional Character(s)   ▸ Manifestation Code   **Coding Clinic**

● H50.04   Monocular esotropia with other noncomitancies
    H50.041   Monocular esotropia with other noncomitancies, right eye
    H50.042   Monocular esotropia with other noncomitancies, left eye
  H50.05   Alternating esotropia
  H50.06   Alternating esotropia with A pattern
  H50.07   Alternating esotropia with V pattern
  H50.08   Alternating esotropia with other noncomitancies

● H50.1   Exotropia
    Misalignment in which one eye deviates outward (away from nose) while the other fixates normally
    Divergent concomitant strabismus
    Excludes1   intermittent exotropia (H50.33-, H50.34)
  H50.10   Unspecified exotropia
● H50.11   Monocular exotropia
    H50.111   Monocular exotropia, right eye
    H50.112   Monocular exotropia, left eye
● H50.12   Monocular exotropia with A pattern
    H50.121   Monocular exotropia with A pattern, right eye
    H50.122   Monocular exotropia with A pattern, left eye
● H50.13   Monocular exotropia with V pattern
    H50.131   Monocular exotropia with V pattern, right eye
    H50.132   Monocular exotropia with V pattern, left eye
● H50.14   Monocular exotropia with other noncomitancies
    H50.141   Monocular exotropia with other noncomitancies, right eye
    H50.142   Monocular exotropia with other noncomitancies, left eye
  H50.15   Alternating exotropia
  H50.16   Alternating exotropia with A pattern
  H50.17   Alternating exotropia with V pattern
  H50.18   Alternating exotropia with other noncomitancies

● H50.2   Vertical strabismus
    Hypertropia
  H50.21   Vertical strabismus, right eye
  H50.22   Vertical strabismus, left eye
● H50.3   Intermittent heterotropia
    Displacement of an organ or part of an organ from its normal position
  H50.30   Unspecified intermittent heterotropia
● H50.31   Intermittent monocular esotropia
    H50.311   Intermittent monocular esotropia, right eye
    H50.312   Intermittent monocular esotropia, left eye
  H50.32   Intermittent alternating esotropia
● H50.33   Intermittent monocular exotropia
    H50.331   Intermittent monocular exotropia, right eye
    H50.332   Intermittent monocular exotropia, left eye
  H50.34   Intermittent alternating exotropia
● H50.4   Other and unspecified heterotropia
  H50.40   Unspecified heterotropia
● H50.41   Cyclotropia
    H50.411   Cyclotropia, right eye
    H50.412   Cyclotropia, left eye
  H50.42   Monofixation syndrome
  H50.43   Accommodative component in esotropia

● H50.5   Heterophoria
    One or both eyes wander away from the position where both eyes are looking together in the same direction
  H50.50   Unspecified heterophoria
  H50.51   Esophoria
    Eye deviates inward (toward the nose)
  H50.52   Exophoria
    Eye deviates outward (toward the ear)
  H50.53   Vertical heterophoria
  H50.54   Cyclophoria
  H50.55   Alternating heterophoria
● H50.6   Mechanical strabismus
  H50.60   Mechanical strabismus, unspecified
● H50.61   Brown's sheath syndrome
    H50.611   Brown's sheath syndrome, right eye
    H50.612   Brown's sheath syndrome, left eye
  H50.69   Other mechanical strabismus
    Strabismus due to adhesions
    Traumatic limitation of duction of eye muscle
● H50.8   Other specified strabismus
● H50.81   Duane's syndrome
    H50.811   Duane's syndrome, right eye
    H50.812   Duane's syndrome, left eye
  H50.89   Other specified strabismus
  H50.9   Unspecified strabismus

● H51   Other disorders of binocular movement
  H51.0   Palsy (spasm) of conjugate gaze
● H51.1   Convergence insufficiency and excess
  H51.11   Convergence insufficiency
  H51.12   Convergence excess
● H51.2   Internuclear ophthalmoplegia
  H51.20   Internuclear ophthalmoplegia, unspecified eye
  H51.21   Internuclear ophthalmoplegia, right eye
  H51.22   Internuclear ophthalmoplegia, left eye
  H51.23   Internuclear ophthalmoplegia, bilateral
  H51.8   Other specified disorders of binocular movement
  H51.9   Unspecified disorder of binocular movement

● H52   Disorders of refraction and accommodation
● H52.0   Hypermetropia
  H52.00   Hypermetropia, unspecified eye
  H52.01   Hypermetropia, right eye
  H52.02   Hypermetropia, left eye
  H52.03   Hypermetropia, bilateral
● H52.1   Myopia
    Excludes1   degenerative myopia (H44.2-)
  H52.10   Myopia, unspecified eye
  H52.11   Myopia, right eye
  H52.12   Myopia, left eye
  H52.13   Myopia, bilateral

Item 7–10 Disorders of refraction: **Hypermetropia,** or farsightedness, means focus at a distance is adequate but not on close objects. **Myopia** is near-sightedness or short-sightedness and means the focus on nearby objects is clear but distant objects appear blurred. **Astigmatism** is warping of the curvature of the cornea so light rays entering do not meet a single focal point, resulting in a distorted image. **Anisometropia** is unequal refractive power in which one eye may be myopic (near-sighted) and the other hyperopic (far-sighted). **Presbyopia** is the loss of focus on near objects, which occurs with age because the lens loses elasticity.

CHAPTER 7 (H00–H59)

● H52.2 **Astigmatism**
  ● H52.20 **Unspecified astigmatism**
      H52.201 Unspecified astigmatism, right eye
      H52.202 Unspecified astigmatism, left eye
      H52.203 Unspecified astigmatism, bilateral
      H52.209 Unspecified astigmatism, unspecified eye
  ● H52.21 **Irregular astigmatism**
      H52.211 Irregular astigmatism, right eye
      H52.212 Irregular astigmatism, left eye
      H52.213 Irregular astigmatism, bilateral
      H52.219 Irregular astigmatism, unspecified eye
  ● H52.22 **Regular astigmatism**
      H52.221 Regular astigmatism, right eye
      H52.222 Regular astigmatism, left eye
      H52.223 Regular astigmatism, bilateral
      H52.229 Regular astigmatism, unspecified eye
● H52.3 **Anisometropia and aniseikonia**
    H52.31 **Anisometropia**
    H52.32 **Aniseikonia**
  H52.4 **Presbyopia**
● H52.5 **Disorders of accommodation**
  ● H52.51 **Internal ophthalmoplegia (complete) (total)**
      H52.511 Internal ophthalmoplegia (complete) (total), right eye
      H52.512 Internal ophthalmoplegia (complete) (total), left eye
      H52.513 Internal ophthalmoplegia (complete) (total), bilateral
      H52.519 Internal ophthalmoplegia (complete) (total), unspecified eye
  ● H52.52 **Paresis of accommodation**
      H52.521 Paresis of accommodation, right eye
      H52.522 Paresis of accommodation, left eye
      H52.523 Paresis of accommodation, bilateral
      H52.529 Paresis of accommodation, unspecified eye
  ● H52.53 **Spasm of accommodation**
      H52.531 Spasm of accommodation, right eye
      H52.532 Spasm of accommodation, left eye
      H52.533 Spasm of accommodation, bilateral
      H52.539 Spasm of accommodation, unspecified eye

  H52.6 **Other disorders of refraction**
  H52.7 **Unspecified disorder of refraction**

VISUAL DISTURBANCES AND BLINDNESS (H53-H54)

● H53 **Visual disturbances**
  ● H53.0 **Amblyopia ex anopsia**
        Excludes1 amblyopia due to vitamin A deficiency (E50.5)
    ● H53.00 **Unspecified amblyopia**
        H53.001 Unspecified amblyopia, right eye
        H53.002 Unspecified amblyopia, left eye
        H53.003 Unspecified amblyopia, bilateral
        H53.009 Unspecified amblyopia, unspecified eye
    ● H53.01 **Deprivation amblyopia**
        H53.011 Deprivation amblyopia, right eye
        H53.012 Deprivation amblyopia, left eye
        H53.013 Deprivation amblyopia, bilateral
        H53.019 Deprivation amblyopia, unspecified eye
    ● H53.02 **Refractive amblyopia**
        H53.021 Refractive amblyopia, right eye
        H53.022 Refractive amblyopia, left eye
        H53.023 Refractive amblyopia, bilateral
        H53.029 Refractive amblyopia, unspecified eye
    ● H53.03 **Strabismic amblyopia**
          Excludes1 strabismus (H50.-)
        H53.031 Strabismic amblyopia, right eye
        H53.032 Strabismic amblyopia, left eye
        H53.033 Strabismic amblyopia, bilateral
        H53.039 Strabismic amblyopia, unspecified eye
  ● H53.1 **Subjective visual disturbances**
        Excludes1 subjective visual disturbances due to vitamin A deficiency (E50.5)
                     visual hallucinations (R44.1)
      H53.10 **Unspecified subjective visual disturbances**
      H53.11 **Day blindness**
              Hemeralopia
    ● H53.12 **Transient visual loss**
              Scintillating scotoma
          Excludes1 amaurosis fugax (G45.3-)
                       transient retinal artery occlusion (H34.0-)
          (Ex) For category H53.12 CC codes: H53.10-H53.139, H53.16, R44.1, R48.3
        H53.121 Transient visual loss, right eye
        H53.122 Transient visual loss, left eye
        H53.123 Transient visual loss, bilateral
        H53.129 Transient visual loss, unspecified eye
    ● H53.13 **Sudden visual loss**
          (Ex) For category H53.13 CC codes: See H53.12
        H53.131 Sudden visual loss, right eye
        H53.132 Sudden visual loss, left eye
        H53.133 Sudden visual loss, bilateral
        H53.139 Sudden visual loss, unspecified eye
    ● H53.14 **Visual discomfort**
              Asthenopia
              Photophobia
        H53.141 Visual discomfort, right eye
        H53.142 Visual discomfort, left eye
        H53.143 Visual discomfort, bilateral
        H53.149 Visual discomfort, unspecified
      H53.15 **Visual distortions of shape and size**
              Metamorphopsia
      H53.16 **Psychophysical visual disturbances**
      H53.19 **Other subjective visual disturbances**
              Visual halos
  H53.2 **Diplopia**
          Double vision
● H53.3 **Other and unspecified disorders of binocular vision**
      H53.30 **Unspecified disorder of binocular vision**
      H53.31 **Abnormal retinal correspondence**
      H53.32 **Fusion with defective stereopsis**
      H53.33 **Simultaneous visual perception without fusion**
      H53.34 **Suppression of binocular vision**

◀ New   ◀ Revised   ~~deleted~~ Deleted   Excludes 1   Excludes 2   Includes   Use additional   Code first   Code also   Unspecified
OGCR Official Guidelines   ● Unacceptable Principal Diagnosis   X Assign placeholder X   ● Use Additional Character(s)   ▌Manifestation Code   Coding Clinic

- H53.4   **Visual field defects**
    - H53.40   **Unspecified** visual field defects
  - H53.41   **Scotoma involving central area**
    Central scotoma
    - H53.411   **Scotoma involving central area, right eye**
    - H53.412   **Scotoma involving central area, left eye**
    - H53.413   **Scotoma involving central area, bilateral**
    - H53.419   **Scotoma involving central area, unspecified eye**
  - H53.42   **Scotoma of blind spot area**
    Enlarged blind spot
    - H53.421   **Scotoma of blind spot area, right eye**
    - H53.422   **Scotoma of blind spot area, left eye**
    - H53.423   **Scotoma of blind spot area, bilateral**
    - H53.429   **Scotoma of blind spot area, unspecified eye**
  - H53.43   **Sector or arcuate defects**
    Arcuate scotoma
    Bjerrum scotoma
    - H53.431   **Sector or arcuate defects, right eye**
    - H53.432   **Sector or arcuate defects, left eye**
    - H53.433   **Sector or arcuate defects, bilateral**
    - H53.439   **Sector or arcuate defects, unspecified eye**
  - H53.45   **Other localized visual field defect**
    Peripheral visual field defect
    Ring scotoma NOS
    Scotoma NOS
    - H53.451   **Other localized visual field defect, right eye**
    - H53.452   **Other localized visual field defect, left eye**
    - H53.453   **Other localized visual field defect, bilateral**
    - H53.459   **Other localized visual field defect, unspecified eye**
  - H53.46   **Homonymous bilateral field defects**
    Homonymous hemianopia ◄▥
    ~~Quadrant anop(s)ia~~
    Homonymous hemianopsia ◄
    Quadrant anopia ◄
    Quadrant anopsia ◄
    - H53.461   **Homonymous bilateral field defects, right side**
    - H53.462   **Homonymous bilateral field defects, left side**
    - H53.469   **Homonymous bilateral field defects, unspecified side**
      Homonymous bilateral field defects NOS
  - H53.47   **Heteronymous bilateral field defects**
    Heteronymous hemianop(s)ia
  - H53.48   **Generalized contraction of visual field**
    - H53.481   **Generalized contraction of visual field, right eye**
    - H53.482   **Generalized contraction of visual field, left eye**
    - H53.483   **Generalized contraction of visual field, bilateral**
    - H53.489   **Generalized contraction of visual field, unspecified eye**

- H53.5   **Color vision deficiencies**
  Color blindness
  Excludes2   day blindness (H53.11)
    - H53.50   **Unspecified** color vision deficiencies
      Color blindness NOS
    - H53.51   **Achromatopsia**
    - H53.52   **Acquired color vision deficiency**
    - H53.53   **Deuteranomaly**
      Deuteranopia
    - H53.54   **Protanomaly**
      Protanopia
    - H53.55   **Tritanomaly**
      Tritanopia
    - H53.59   **Other color vision deficiencies**
- H53.6   **Night blindness**
  Excludes1   night blindness due to vitamin A deficiency (E50.5)
    - H53.60   **Unspecified** night blindness
    - H53.61   **Abnormal dark adaptation curve**
    - H53.62   **Acquired night blindness**
    - H53.63   **Congenital night blindness**
    - H53.69   **Other night blindness**
  - H53.7   **Vision sensitivity deficiencies**
    - H53.71   **Glare sensitivity**
    - H53.72   **Impaired contrast sensitivity**
  - H53.8   **Other visual disturbances**
  - H53.9   **Unspecified** visual disturbance

- H54   **Blindness and low vision**
  Note: For definition of visual impairment categories see table below.
  Code first any associated underlying cause of the blindness
  Excludes1   amaurosis fugax (G45.3)
  - H54.0   **Blindness, both eyes**
    Visual impairment categories 3, 4, 5 in both eyes.
  - H54.1   **Blindness, one eye, low vision other eye**
    Visual impairment categories 3, 4, 5 in one eye, with categories 1 or 2 in the other eye.
    - H54.10   **Blindness, one eye, low vision other eye, unspecified eyes**
    - H54.11   **Blindness, right eye, low vision left eye**
    - H54.12   **Blindness, left eye, low vision right eye**
  - H54.2   **Low vision, both eyes**
    Visual impairment categories 1 or 2 in both eyes.
  - H54.3   **Unqualified visual loss, both eyes**
    Visual impairment category 9 in both eyes.
  - H54.4   **Blindness, one eye**
    Visual impairment categories 3, 4, 5 in one eye [normal vision in other eye]
    - H54.40   **Blindness, one eye, unspecified eye**
    - H54.41   **Blindness, right eye, normal vision left eye**
    - H54.42   **Blindness, left eye, normal vision right eye**
  - H54.5   **Low vision, one eye**
    Visual impairment categories 1 or 2 in one eye [normal vision in other eye].
    - H54.50   **Low vision, one eye, unspecified eye**
    - H54.51   **Low vision, right eye, normal vision left eye**
    - H54.52   **Low vision, left eye, normal vision right eye**
  - H54.6   **Unqualified visual loss, one eye**
    Visual impairment category 9 in one eye [normal vision in other eye].
    - H54.60   **Unqualified visual loss, one eye, unspecified**
    - H54.61   **Unqualified visual loss, right eye, normal vision left eye**
    - H54.62   **Unqualified visual loss, left eye, normal vision right eye**

CHAPTER 7 (H00–H59)

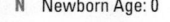

● **H54.7** **Unspecified** visual loss
     Visual impairment category 9 NOS

H54.8 **Legal blindness, as defined in USA**
     Blindness NOS according to USA definition
     Excludes1   legal blindness with specification of impairment level (H54.0-H54.7)

Note: The table below gives a classification of severity of visual impairment recommended by a WHO Study Group on the Prevention of Blindness, Geneva, 6-10 November 1972.

The term 'low vision' in category H54 comprises categories 1 and 2 of the table, the term 'blindness' categories 3, 4 and 5, and the term 'unqualified visual loss' category 9.

If the extent of the visual field is taken into account, patients with a field no greater than 10 but greater than 5 around central fixation should be placed in category 3 and patients with a field no greater than 5 around central fixation should be placed in category 4, even if the central acuity is not impaired.

Category of visual impairment	Visual acuity with best possible correction	
	Maximum less than:	**Minimum equal to or better than:**
	6/18	6/60
3/10 (0.3)	1/10 (0.1)	
20/70	20/200	
	6/60	3/60
1/10 (0.1)	1/20 (0.05)	
20/200	20/400	
	3/60	1/60 (finger counting at one meter)
1/20 (0.05)	1/50 (0.02)	
20/400	5/300 (20/1200)	
	1/60 (finger counting at one meter)	Light perception
1/50 (0.02)		
5/300		
	No light perception	
	Undetermined or unspecified	

OTHER DISORDERS OF EYE AND ADNEXA (H55-H57)

● **H55** **Nystagmus and other irregular eye movements**
   ● **H55.0** **Nystagmus**
     Rapid, involuntary movements of the eyes in the horizontal or vertical direction.
     H55.00 **Unspecified** nystagmus
     H55.01 **Congenital nystagmus**
     H55.02 **Latent nystagmus**
     H55.03 **Visual deprivation nystagmus**
     H55.04 **Dissociated nystagmus**
     H55.09 **Other forms of nystagmus**
   ● **H55.8** **Other irregular eye movements**
     H55.81 **Saccadic eye movements**
     H55.89 **Other irregular eye movements**

● **H57** **Other disorders of eye and adnexa**
   ● **H57.0** **Anomalies of pupillary function**
     H57.00 **Unspecified** anomaly of pupillary function
     H57.01 **Argyll Robertson pupil, atypical**
     Excludes1   syphilitic Argyll Robertson pupil (A52.19)
     H57.02 **Anisocoria**
     H57.03 **Miosis**
     H57.04 **Mydriasis**
   ● **H57.05** **Tonic pupil**
     H57.051 **Tonic pupil, right eye**
     H57.052 **Tonic pupil, left eye**
     H57.053 **Tonic pupil, bilateral**
     H57.059 **Tonic pupil, unspecified eye**
     H57.09 **Other anomalies of pupillary function**
   ● **H57.1** **Ocular pain**
     H57.10 **Ocular pain, unspecified eye**
     H57.11 **Ocular pain, right eye**
     H57.12 **Ocular pain, left eye**
     H57.13 **Ocular pain, bilateral**
   H57.8 **Other specified disorders of eye and adnexa**
   ● **H57.9** **Unspecified** disorder of eye and adnexa

INTRAOPERATIVE AND POSTPROCEDURAL COMPLICATIONS AND DISORDERS OF EYE AND ADNEXA, NOT ELSEWHERE CLASSIFIED (H59)

● **H59** **Intraoperative and postprocedural complications and disorders of eye and adnexa, not elsewhere classified**
     Excludes1   mechanical complication of intraocular lens (T85.2)
       mechanical complication of other ocular prosthetic devices, implants and grafts (T85.3)
       pseudophakia (Z96.1)
       secondary cataracts (H26.4-)
   ● **H59.0** **Disorders of the eye following cataract surgery**
     (Ex) **For category H59.0 CC codes:** H59.011-H59.019, H59.031-H59.099, H59.811-H59.89, H95.811-H95.89, I97.3, M96.89, N98.1-N98.9, T81.82X[A], T81.89X-T81.9XX[A]
   ● **H59.01** **Keratopathy (bullous aphakic) following cataract surgery**
     Vitreal corneal syndrome
     Vitreous (touch) syndrome
     H59.011 **Keratopathy (bullous aphakic) following cataract surgery, right eye**
     H59.012 **Keratopathy (bullous aphakic) following cataract surgery, left eye**
     H59.013 **Keratopathy (bullous aphakic) following cataract surgery, bilateral**
     H59.019 **Keratopathy (bullous aphakic) following cataract surgery, unspecified eye**
   ● **H59.02** **Cataract (lens) fragments in eye following cataract surgery**
     H59.021 **Cataract (lens) fragments in eye following cataract surgery, right eye**
     H59.022 **Cataract (lens) fragments in eye following cataract surgery, left eye**
     H59.023 **Cataract (lens) fragments in eye following cataract surgery, bilateral**
     H59.029 **Cataract (lens) fragments in eye following cataract surgery, unspecified eye**

◄ New   ◄ Revised   ~~deleted~~ Deleted   Excludes 1   Excludes 2   Includes   Use additional   Code first   Code also   Unspecified
OGCR Official Guidelines   ● Unacceptable Principal Diagnosis   X Assign placeholder X   ● Use Additional Character(s)   ▌ Manifestation Code   **Coding Clinic**

● **H59.03**   Cystoid macular edema following cataract surgery

     H59.031   Cystoid macular edema following cataract surgery, right eye

     H59.032   Cystoid macular edema following cataract surgery, left eye

     H59.033   Cystoid macular edema following cataract surgery, bilateral

     H59.039   Cystoid macular edema following cataract surgery, unspecified eye

● **H59.09**   Other disorders of the eye following cataract surgery

     H59.091   Other disorders of the right eye following cataract surgery

     H59.092   Other disorders of the left eye following cataract surgery

     H59.093   Other disorders of the eye following cataract surgery, bilateral

     H59.099   Other disorders of unspecified eye following cataract surgery

● **H59.1**   Intraoperative hemorrhage and hematoma of eye and adnexa complicating a procedure

     Excludes1   intraoperative hemorrhage and hematoma of eye and adnexa due to accidental puncture or laceration during a procedure (H59.2-)

     (Ex) **For category H59.1 CC codes:** H59.011-H59.019, H59.031-H59.129, H59.311-H59.329, H59.811-H59.89, H95.811-H95.89, I85.01, I85.11, I97.3, K21.9, K22.8, K23-K25.0, K25.2, K25.4, K25.6, K26.0, K26.2, K26.4, K26.6, K27.0, K27.2, K27.4, K27.6, K28.0, K28.2, K28.4, K28.6, K29.01, K29.21, K29.31, K29.41, K29.51, K29.61, K29.71, K29.81, K29.91, K31.811, K55.21, K57.01, K57.11, K57.13, K57.21, K57.31, K57.33, K57.41, K57.51, K57.53, K57.81, K57.91, K57.93, K62.5, K92.0-K92.2, M96.89, N98.1-N98.9, P54.1-P54.3, T81.10X-T81.19X[A], T81.82X[A], T81.89X-T81.9XX[A]

● **H59.11**   Intraoperative hemorrhage and hematoma of eye and adnexa complicating an ophthalmic procedure

     (Ex) **For category H59.3 CC codes:** See H59.1

     H59.111   Intraoperative hemorrhage and hematoma of right eye and adnexa complicating an ophthalmic procedure

     H59.112   Intraoperative hemorrhage and hematoma of left eye and adnexa complicating an ophthalmic procedure

     H59.113   Intraoperative hemorrhage and hematoma of eye and adnexa complicating an ophthalmic procedure, bilateral

     H59.119   Intraoperative hemorrhage and hematoma of unspecified eye and adnexa complicating an ophthalmic procedure

● **H59.12**   Intraoperative hemorrhage and hematoma of eye and adnexa complicating other procedure

     H59.121   Intraoperative hemorrhage and hematoma of right eye and adnexa complicating other procedure

     H59.122   Intraoperative hemorrhage and hematoma of left eye and adnexa complicating other procedure

     H59.123   Intraoperative hemorrhage and hematoma of eye and adnexa complicating other procedure, bilateral

     H59.129   Intraoperative hemorrhage and hematoma of unspecified eye and adnexa complicating other procedure

● **H59.2**   Accidental puncture and laceration of eye and adnexa during a procedure

     (Ex) **For category H59.2 CC codes:** D78.11-D78.12, D78.81-D78.89, E36.11-E36.8, E89.810-E89.89, G96.11, G97.41-G97.49, H59.011-H59.019, H59.031-H59.099, H59.211-H59.229, H59.811-H59.89, H95.31-H95.32, H95.811-H95.89, I97.3, I97.51-I97.52, J95.71-J95.72, K91.71-K91.72, L76.11-L76.12, L76.81-L76.82, M96.820-M96.821, M96.89, N98.1-N98.9, N99.71-N99.72, T81.82X[A], T81.89X-T81.9XX[A]

● **H59.21**   Accidental puncture and laceration of eye and adnexa during an ophthalmic procedure

     H59.211   Accidental puncture and laceration of right eye and adnexa during an ophthalmic procedure

     H59.212   Accidental puncture and laceration of left eye and adnexa during an ophthalmic procedure

     H59.213   Accidental puncture and laceration of eye and adnexa during an ophthalmic procedure, bilateral

     H59.219   Accidental puncture and laceration of unspecified eye and adnexa during an ophthalmic procedure

● **H59.22**   Accidental puncture and laceration of eye and adnexa during other procedure

     H59.221   Accidental puncture and laceration of right eye and adnexa during other procedure

     H59.222   Accidental puncture and laceration of left eye and adnexa during other procedure

     H59.223   Accidental puncture and laceration of eye and adnexa during other procedure, bilateral

     H59.229   Accidental puncture and laceration of unspecified eye and adnexa during other procedure

● **H59.3**   Postprocedural hemorrhage and hematoma of eye and adnexa following a procedure

     (Ex) **For category H59.3 CC codes:** See H59.1

● **H59.31**   Postprocedural hemorrhage and hematoma of eye and adnexa following an ophthalmic procedure

     H59.311   Postprocedural hemorrhage and hematoma of right eye and avdnexa following an ophthalmic procedure

     H59.312   Postprocedural hemorrhage and hematoma of left eye and adnexa following an ophthalmic procedure

     H59.313   Postprocedural hemorrhage and hematoma of eye and adnexa following an ophthalmic procedure, bilateral

     H59.319   Postprocedural hemorrhage and hematoma of unspecified eye and adnexa following an ophthalmic procedure

● **H59.32**   Postprocedural hemorrhage and hematoma of eye and adnexa following other procedure

     H59.321   Postprocedural hemorrhage and hematoma of right eye and adnexa following other procedure

     H59.322   Postprocedural hemorrhage and hematoma of left eye and adnexa following other procedure

     H59.323   Postprocedural hemorrhage and hematoma of eye and adnexa following other procedure, bilateral

     H59.329   Postprocedural hemorrhage and hematoma of unspecified eye and adnexa following other procedure

N Newborn Age: 0   **P** Pediatric Age: 0–17   **M** Maternity DX: 12–55   **A** Adult Age: 15–124   ♀ Females Only   ♂ Males Only

Complication\Comorbidity   Major C\C   (Ex) CC/MCC Exclusions   Present on Admission Requirement   Hospital-Acquired Condition

943

● **H59.4** **Inflammation (infection) of postprocedural bleb**
       Postprocedural blebitis

      Excludes1   filtering (vitreous) bleb after glaucoma
                   surgery status (Z98.83)

    H59.40 **Inflammation (infection) of postprocedural
            bleb, unspecified**

    H59.41 **Inflammation (infection) of postprocedural
            bleb, stage 1**

    H59.42 **Inflammation (infection) of postprocedural
            bleb, stage 2**

    H59.43 **Inflammation (infection) of postprocedural
            bleb, stage 3**

          Bleb endophthalmitis

● **H59.8** **Other intraoperative and postprocedural complications
and disorders of eye and adnexa, not elsewhere
classified**

    (Ex) **For category H59.8 CC codes:** See H59.0

● **H59.81** **Chorioretinal scars after surgery for detachment**

    H59.811 **Chorioretinal scars after surgery for
              detachment, right eye** 🔍

    H59.812 **Chorioretinal scars after surgery for
              detachment, left eye** 🔍

    H59.813 **Chorioretinal scars after surgery for
              detachment, bilateral** 🔍

    H59.819 **Chorioretinal scars after surgery for
              detachment, unspecified eye** 🔍

    H59.88 **Other intraoperative complications of eye and
           adnexa, not elsewhere classified** 🔍

    H59.89 **Other postprocedural complications and
           disorders of eye and adnexa, not elsewhere
           classified** 🔍

◀ New   ◀ Revised   deleted Deleted   Excludes 1   Excludes 2   Includes   Use additional   Code first   Code also   Unspecified

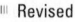 OGCR Official Guidelines   ● Unacceptable Principal Diagnosis   X Assign placeholder X   ● Use Additional Character(s)   ▶ Manifestation Code   **Coding Clinic**

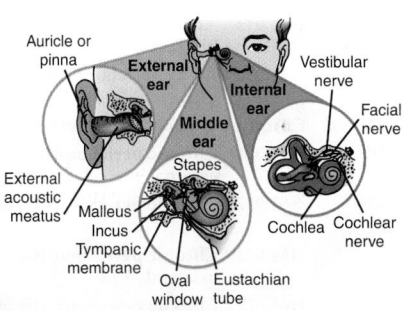

Figure 8-1 Auditory system. (From Buck CJ: Step-by-Step Medical Coding, ed 2010, Philadelphia, WB Saunders, 2010)

(See Plate 92 on page 68.)

CHAPTER 8

DISEASES OF THE EAR AND MASTOID PROCESS (H60-H95)

Note: Use an external cause code following the code for the ear condition, if applicable, to identify the cause of the ear condition

Excludes2   certain conditions originating in the perinatal period (P04-P96)

certain infectious and parasitic diseases (A00-B99)

complications of pregnancy, childbirth and the puerperium (O00-O9A)

congenital malformations, deformations and chromosomal abnormalities (Q00-Q99)

endocrine, nutritional and metabolic diseases (E00-E88)

injury, poisoning and certain other consequences of external causes (S00-T88)

neoplasms (C00-D49)

symptoms, signs and abnormal clinical and laboratory findings, not elsewhere classified (R00-R94)

This chapter contains the following blocks:

H60-H62	Diseases of external ear
H65-H75	Diseases of middle ear and mastoid
H80-H83	Diseases of inner ear
H90-H94	Other disorders of ear
H95	Intraoperative and postprocedural complications and disorders of ear and mastoid process, not elsewhere classified

DISEASES OF EXTERNAL EAR (H60-H62)

● **H60 Otitis externa**

  ● **H60.0 Abscess of external ear**
      Boil of external ear
      Carbuncle of auricle or external auditory canal
      Furuncle of external ear

    H60.00   Abscess of external ear, unspecified ear
    H60.01   Abscess of right external ear
    H60.02   Abscess of left external ear
    H60.03   Abscess of external ear, bilateral

  ● **H60.1 Cellulitis of external ear**
      Cellulitis of auricle
      Cellulitis of external auditory canal

    H60.10   Cellulitis of external ear, unspecified ear
    H60.11   Cellulitis of right external ear
    H60.12   Cellulitis of left external ear
    H60.13   Cellulitis of external ear, bilateral

● **H60.2 Malignant otitis externa**
    ⊕ For category H60.2 CC codes: H60.20-H60.23, H70.001-H70.13

    H60.20   Malignant otitis externa, unspecified ear ⊚
    H60.21   Malignant otitis externa, right ear ⊚
    H60.22   Malignant otitis externa, left ear ⊚
    H60.23   Malignant otitis externa, bilateral ⊚

● **H60.3 Other infective otitis externa**

  ● **H60.31 Diffuse otitis externa**
    H60.311   Diffuse otitis externa, right ear
    H60.312   Diffuse otitis externa, left ear
    H60.313   Diffuse otitis externa, bilateral
    H60.319   Diffuse otitis externa, unspecified ear

  ● **H60.32 Hemorrhagic otitis externa**
    H60.321   Hemorrhagic otitis externa, right ear
    H60.322   Hemorrhagic otitis externa, left ear
    H60.323   Hemorrhagic otitis externa, bilateral
    H60.329   Hemorrhagic otitis externa, unspecified ear

  ● **H60.33 Swimmer's ear**
    H60.331   Swimmer's ear, right ear
    H60.332   Swimmer's ear, left ear
    H60.333   Swimmer's ear, bilateral
    H60.339   Swimmer's ear, unspecified ear

  ● **H60.39 Other infective otitis externa**
    H60.391   Other infective otitis externa, right ear
    H60.392   Other infective otitis externa, left ear
    H60.393   Other infective otitis externa, bilateral
    H60.399   Other infective otitis externa, unspecified ear

● **H60.4 Cholesteatoma of external ear**
    Keratosis obturans of external ear (canal)

    Excludes2   cholesteatoma of middle ear (H71.-)
         recurrent cholesteatoma of postmastoidectomy cavity (H95.0-)

    H60.40   Cholesteatoma of external ear, unspecified ear
    H60.41   Cholesteatoma of right external ear
    H60.42   Cholesteatoma of left external ear
    H60.43   Cholesteatoma of external ear, bilateral

● **H60.5 Acute noninfective otitis externa**

  ● **H60.50 Unspecified acute noninfective otitis externa**
      Acute otitis externa NOS

    H60.501   Unspecified acute noninfective otitis externa, right ear
    H60.502   Unspecified acute noninfective otitis externa, left ear
    H60.503   Unspecified acute noninfective otitis externa, bilateral
    H60.509   Unspecified acute noninfective otitis externa, unspecified ear

  ● **H60.51 Acute actinic otitis externa**
    H60.511   Acute actinic otitis externa, right ear
    H60.512   Acute actinic otitis externa, left ear
    H60.513   Acute actinic otitis externa, bilateral
    H60.519   Acute actinic otitis externa, unspecified ear

  ● **H60.52 Acute chemical otitis externa**
    H60.521   Acute chemical otitis externa, right ear
    H60.522   Acute chemical otitis externa, left ear
    H60.523   Acute chemical otitis externa, bilateral
    H60.529   Acute chemical otitis externa, unspecified ear

N Newborn Age: 0   **P** Pediatric Age: 0–17   **M** Maternity DX: 12–55   **A** Adult Age: 15–124   ♀ Females Only   ♂ Males Only

⊚ Complication\Comorbidity   ◆ Major C\C   ⊕ CC/MCC Exclusions   ⊛ Present on Admission Requirement   ⊚ Hospital-Acquired Condition

945

● H60.53   Acute contact otitis externa
     H60.531   Acute contact otitis externa, right ear
     H60.532   Acute contact otitis externa, left ear
     H60.533   Acute contact otitis externa, bilateral
     H60.539   Acute contact otitis externa, unspecified ear

● H60.54   Acute eczematoid otitis externa
     H60.541   Acute eczematoid otitis externa, right ear
     H60.542   Acute eczematoid otitis externa, left ear
     H60.543   Acute eczematoid otitis externa, bilateral
     H60.549   Acute eczematoid otitis externa, unspecified ear

● H60.55   Acute reactive otitis externa
     H60.551   Acute reactive otitis externa, right ear
     H60.552   Acute reactive otitis externa, left ear
     H60.553   Acute reactive otitis externa, bilateral
     H60.559   Acute reactive otitis externa, unspecified ear

● H60.59   Other noninfective acute otitis externa
     H60.591   Other noninfective acute otitis externa, right ear
     H60.592   Other noninfective acute otitis externa, left ear
     H60.593   Other noninfective acute otitis externa, bilateral
     H60.599   Other noninfective acute otitis externa, unspecified ear

● H60.6   Unspecified chronic otitis externa
     H60.60   Unspecified chronic otitis externa, unspecified ear
     H60.61   Unspecified chronic otitis externa, right ear
     H60.62   Unspecified chronic otitis externa, left ear
     H60.63   Unspecified chronic otitis externa, bilateral

● H60.8   Other otitis externa
   ● H60.8X   Other otitis externa
     H60.8X1   Other otitis externa, right ear
     H60.8X2   Other otitis externa, left ear
     H60.8X3   Other otitis externa, bilateral
     H60.8X9   Other otitis externa, unspecified ear

● H60.9   Unspecified otitis externa
     H60.90   Unspecified otitis externa, unspecified ear
     H60.91   Unspecified otitis externa, right ear
     H60.92   Unspecified otitis externa, left ear
     H60.93   Unspecified otitis externa, bilateral

● H61   Other disorders of external ear
   ● H61.0   Chondritis and perichondritis of external ear
     Chondrodermatitis nodularis chronica helicis
     Perichondritis of auricle
     Perichondritis of pinna
   ● H61.00   Unspecified perichondritis of external ear
     H61.001   Unspecified perichondritis of right external ear
     H61.002   Unspecified perichondritis of left external ear
     H61.003   Unspecified perichondritis of external ear, bilateral
     H61.009   Unspecified perichondritis of external ear, unspecified ear
   ● H61.01   Acute perichondritis of external ear
     H61.011   Acute perichondritis of right external ear
     H61.012   Acute perichondritis of left external ear

     H61.013   Acute perichondritis of external ear, bilateral
     H61.019   Acute perichondritis of external ear, unspecified ear
   ● H61.02   Chronic perichondritis of external ear
     H61.021   Chronic perichondritis of right external ear
     H61.022   Chronic perichondritis of left external ear
     H61.023   Chronic perichondritis of external ear, bilateral
     H61.029   Chronic perichondritis of external ear, unspecified ear
   ● H61.03   Chondritis of external ear
     Chondritis of auricle
     Chondritis of pinna
     H61.031   Chondritis of right external ear
     H61.032   Chondritis of left external ear
     H61.033   Chondritis of external ear, bilateral
     H61.039   Chondritis of external ear, unspecified ear

● H61.1   Noninfective disorders of pinna
     Excludes2   cauliflower ear (M95.1-)
                   gouty tophi of ear (M1A.-) ◀
   ● H61.10   Unspecified noninfective disorders of pinna
     Disorder of pinna NOS
     H61.101   Unspecified noninfective disorders of pinna, right ear
     H61.102   Unspecified noninfective disorders of pinna, left ear
     H61.103   Unspecified noninfective disorders of pinna, bilateral
     H61.109   Unspecified noninfective disorders of pinna, unspecified ear
   ● H61.11   Acquired deformity of pinna
     Acquired deformity of auricle
     Excludes2   cauliflower ear (M95.1-)
     H61.111   Acquired deformity of pinna, right ear
     H61.112   Acquired deformity of pinna, left ear
     H61.113   Acquired deformity of pinna, bilateral
     H61.119   Acquired deformity of pinna, unspecified ear
   ● H61.12   Hematoma of pinna
     Hematoma of auricle
     H61.121   Hematoma of pinna, right ear
     H61.122   Hematoma of pinna, left ear
     H61.123   Hematoma of pinna, bilateral
     H61.129   Hematoma of pinna, unspecified ear
   ● H61.19   Other noninfective disorders of pinna
     H61.191   Noninfective disorders of pinna, right ear
     H61.192   Noninfective disorders of pinna, left ear
     H61.193   Noninfective disorders of pinna, bilateral
     H61.199   Noninfective disorders of pinna, unspecified ear

● H61.2   Impacted cerumen
     Wax in ear
     H61.20   Impacted cerumen, unspecified ear
        MCE: Questionable admission when principal dx
     H61.21   Impacted cerumen, right ear
        MCE: Questionable admission when principal dx
     H61.22   Impacted cerumen, left ear
        MCE: Questionable admission when principal dx
     H61.23   Impacted cerumen, bilateral
        MCE: Questionable admission when principal dx

● **H61.3** **Acquired stenosis of external ear canal**
Collapse of external ear canal

> **Excludes1** postprocedural stenosis of external ear canal (H95.81-)

● **H61.30** Acquired stenosis of external ear canal, unspecified

  H61.301 Acquired stenosis of right external ear canal, unspecified

  H61.302 Acquired stenosis of left external ear canal, unspecified

  H61.303 Acquired stenosis of external ear canal, unspecified, bilateral

  H61.309 Acquired stenosis of external ear canal, unspecified, unspecified ear

● **H61.31** Acquired stenosis of external ear canal secondary to trauma

  H61.311 Acquired stenosis of right external ear canal secondary to trauma

  H61.312 Acquired stenosis of left external ear canal secondary to trauma

  H61.313 Acquired stenosis of external ear canal secondary to trauma, bilateral

  H61.319 Acquired stenosis of external ear canal secondary to trauma, unspecified ear

● **H61.32** Acquired stenosis of external ear canal secondary to inflammation and infection

  H61.321 Acquired stenosis of right external ear canal secondary to inflammation and infection

  H61.322 Acquired stenosis of left external ear canal secondary to inflammation and infection

  H61.323 Acquired stenosis of external ear canal secondary to inflammation and infection, bilateral

  H61.329 Acquired stenosis of external ear canal secondary to inflammation and infection, unspecified ear

● **H61.39** Other acquired stenosis of external ear canal

  H61.391 Other acquired stenosis of right external ear canal

  H61.392 Other acquired stenosis of left external ear canal

  H61.393 Other acquired stenosis of external ear canal, bilateral

  H61.399 Other acquired stenosis of external ear canal, unspecified ear

● **H61.8** **Other specified disorders of external ear**

● **H61.81** Exostosis of external canal

  H61.811 Exostosis of right external canal

  H61.812 Exostosis of left external canal

  H61.813 Exostosis of external canal, bilateral

  H61.819 Exostosis of external canal, unspecified ear

● **H61.89** Other specified disorders of external ear

  H61.891 Other specified disorders of right external ear

  H61.892 Other specified disorders of left external ear

  H61.893 Other specified disorders of external ear, bilateral

  H61.899 Other specified disorders of external ear, unspecified ear

● **H61.9** **Disorder of external ear, unspecified**

  H61.90 Disorder of external ear, unspecified, unspecified ear

  H61.91 Disorder of right external ear, unspecified

  H61.92 Disorder of left external ear, unspecified

  H61.93 Disorder of external ear, unspecified, bilateral

● **H62** **Disorders of external ear in diseases classified elsewhere**

● **H62.4** **Otitis externa in other diseases classified elsewhere**

Code first underlying disease, such as:
erysipelas (A46)
impetigo (L01.0)

> **Excludes1** otitis externa (in):
> candidiasis (B37.84)
> herpes viral [herpes simplex] (B00.1)
> herpes zoster (B02.8)

  ▷ *H62.40* *Otitis externa in other diseases classified elsewhere, unspecified ear*

  ▷ *H62.41* *Otitis externa in other diseases classified elsewhere, right ear*

  ▷ *H62.42* *Otitis externa in other diseases classified elsewhere, left ear*

  ▷ *H62.43* *Otitis externa in other diseases classified elsewhere, bilateral*

● **H62.8** **Other disorders of external ear in diseases classified elsewhere**

Code first underlying disease, such as:
gout (M1A.-, M10.-) ◀▥

● **H62.8X** Other disorders of external ear in diseases classified elsewhere

  ▷ *H62.8X1* *Other disorders of right external ear in diseases classified elsewhere*

  ▷ *H62.8X2* *Other disorders of left external ear in diseases classified elsewhere*

  ▷ *H62.8X3* *Other disorders of external ear in diseases classified elsewhere, bilateral*

  ▷ *H62.8X9* *Other disorders of external ear in diseases classified elsewhere, unspecified ear*

DISEASES OF MIDDLE EAR AND MASTOID (H65-H75)

(See Plate 94 on page 69.)

● **H65** **Nonsuppurative otitis media**

Bacterial or viral infection or inflammation of the middle ear; may result in fluid accumulation with pain and temporary hearing loss.

> **Includes** nonsuppurative otitis media with myringitis

Use additional code for any associated perforated tympanic membrane (H72.-)

Use additional code to identify:
exposure to environmental tobacco smoke (Z77.22)
exposure to tobacco smoke in the perinatal period (P96.81)
history of tobacco use (Z87.891)
occupational exposure to environmental tobacco smoke (Z57.31)
tobacco dependence (F17.-)
tobacco use (Z72.0)

● **H65.0** **Acute serous otitis media**
Acute and subacute secretory otitis

  H65.00 Acute serous otitis media, unspecified ear

  H65.01 Acute serous otitis media, right ear

  H65.02 Acute serous otitis media, left ear

  H65.03 Acute serous otitis media, bilateral

  H65.04 Acute serous otitis media, recurrent, right ear

  H65.05 Acute serous otitis media, recurrent, left ear

  H65.06 Acute serous otitis media, recurrent, bilateral

  H65.07 Acute serous otitis media, recurrent, unspecified ear

N Newborn Age: 0   **P** Pediatric Age: 0–17   **M** Maternity DX: 12–55   **A** Adult Age: 15–124   ♀ Females Only   ♂ Males Only

🗲 Complication\Comorbidity   🗲 Major C\C   (Ex) CC/MCC Exclusions   🗲 Present on Admission Requirement   🗲 Hospital-Acquired Condition

947

● **H65.1** **Other acute nonsuppurative otitis media**

 Excludes1 otitic barotrauma (T70.0)
otitis media (acute) NOS (H66.9)

 ● **H65.11** **Acute and subacute allergic otitis media (mucoid) (sanguinous) (serous)**

  H65.111 Acute and subacute allergic otitis media (mucoid) (sanguinous) (serous), right ear

  H65.112 Acute and subacute allergic otitis media (mucoid) (sanguinous) (serous), left ear

  H65.113 Acute and subacute allergic otitis media (mucoid) (sanguinous) (serous), bilateral

  H65.114 Acute and subacute allergic otitis media (mucoid) (sanguinous) (serous), recurrent, right ear

  H65.115 Acute and subacute allergic otitis media (mucoid) (sanguinous) (serous), recurrent, left ear

  H65.116 Acute and subacute allergic otitis media (mucoid) (sanguinous) (serous), recurrent, bilateral

  H65.117 Acute and subacute allergic otitis media (mucoid) (sanguinous) (serous), recurrent, unspecified ear

  H65.119 Acute and subacute allergic otitis media (mucoid) (sanguinous) (serous), unspecified ear

 ● **H65.19** **Other acute nonsuppurative otitis media**
Acute and subacute mucoid otitis media
Acute and subacute nonsuppurative otitis media NOS
Acute and subacute sanguinous otitis media
Acute and subacute seromucinous otitis media

  H65.191 Other acute nonsuppurative otitis media, right ear

  H65.192 Other acute nonsuppurative otitis media, left ear

  H65.193 Other acute nonsuppurative otitis media, bilateral

  H65.194 Other acute nonsuppurative otitis media, recurrent, right ear

  H65.195 Other acute nonsuppurative otitis media, recurrent, left ear

  H65.196 Other acute nonsuppurative otitis media, recurrent, bilateral

  H65.197 Other acute nonsuppurative otitis media recurrent, unspecified ear

  H65.199 Other acute nonsuppurative otitis media, unspecified ear

● **H65.2** **Chronic serous otitis media**
Chronic tubotympanal catarrh

 H65.20 Chronic serous otitis media, unspecified ear

 H65.21 Chronic serous otitis media, right ear

 H65.22 Chronic serous otitis media, left ear

 H65.23 Chronic serous otitis media, bilateral

● **H65.3** **Chronic mucoid otitis media**
Chronic mucinous otitis media
Chronic secretory otitis media
Chronic transudative otitis media
Glue ear

 Excludes1 adhesive middle ear disease (H74.1)

 H65.30 Chronic mucoid otitis media, unspecified ear

 H65.31 Chronic mucoid otitis media, right ear

 H65.32 Chronic mucoid otitis media, left ear

 H65.33 Chronic mucoid otitis media, bilateral

● **H65.4** **Other chronic nonsuppurative otitis media**

 ● **H65.41** **Chronic allergic otitis media**

  H65.411 Chronic allergic otitis media, right ear

  H65.412 Chronic allergic otitis media, left ear

  H65.413 Chronic allergic otitis media, bilateral

  H65.419 Chronic allergic otitis media, unspecified ear

 ● **H65.49** **Other chronic nonsuppurative otitis media**
Chronic exudative otitis media
Chronic nonsuppurative otitis media NOS
Chronic otitis media with effusion (nonpurulent)
Chronic seromucinous otitis media

  H65.491 Other chronic nonsuppurative otitis media, right ear

  H65.492 Other chronic nonsuppurative otitis media, left ear

  H65.493 Other chronic nonsuppurative otitis media, bilateral

  H65.499 Other chronic nonsuppurative otitis media, unspecified ear

● **H65.9** **Unspecified nonsuppurative otitis media**
Allergic otitis media NOS
Catarrhal otitis media NOS
Exudative otitis media NOS
Mucoid otitis media NOS
Otitis media with effusion (nonpurulent) NOS
Secretory otitis media NOS
Seromucinous otitis media NOS
Serous otitis media NOS
Transudative otitis media NOS

 H65.90 Unspecified nonsuppurative otitis media, unspecified ear

 H65.91 Unspecified nonsuppurative otitis media, right ear

 H65.92 Unspecified nonsuppurative otitis media, left ear

 H65.93 Unspecified nonsuppurative otitis media, bilateral

● **H66** **Suppurative and unspecified otitis media**
 Suppurative: Discharging pus

 Includes suppurative and unspecified otitis media with myringitis

 ~~Use additional code for any associated perforated tympanic membrane (H72.-)~~

 Use additional code to identify:
exposure to environmental tobacco smoke (Z77.22)
exposure to tobacco smoke in the perinatal period (P96.81)
history of tobacco use (Z87.891)
occupational exposure to environmental tobacco smoke (Z57.31)
tobacco dependence (F17.-)
tobacco use (Z72.0)

 ● **H66.0** **Acute suppurative otitis media**

  ● **H66.00** **Acute suppurative otitis media without spontaneous rupture of ear drum**

   H66.001 Acute suppurative otitis media without spontaneous rupture of ear drum, right ear

   H66.002 Acute suppurative otitis media without spontaneous rupture of ear drum, left ear

   H66.003 Acute suppurative otitis media without spontaneous rupture of ear drum, bilateral

   H66.004 Acute suppurative otitis media without spontaneous rupture of ear drum, recurrent, right ear

   H66.005 Acute suppurative otitis media without spontaneous rupture of ear drum, recurrent, left ear

   H66.006 Acute suppurative otitis media without spontaneous rupture of ear drum, recurrent, bilateral

   H66.007 Acute suppurative otitis media without spontaneous rupture of ear drum, recurrent, unspecified ear

   H66.009 Acute suppurative otitis media without spontaneous rupture of ear drum, unspecified ear

● H66.01   Acute suppurative otitis media with spontaneous rupture of ear drum

    H66.011   Acute suppurative otitis media with spontaneous rupture of ear drum, right ear

    H66.012   Acute suppurative otitis media with spontaneous rupture of ear drum, left ear

    H66.013   Acute suppurative otitis media with spontaneous rupture of ear drum, bilateral

    H66.014   Acute suppurative otitis media with spontaneous rupture of ear drum, recurrent, right ear

    H66.015   Acute suppurative otitis media with spontaneous rupture of ear drum, recurrent, left ear

    H66.016   Acute suppurative otitis media with spontaneous rupture of ear drum, recurrent, bilateral

    H66.017   Acute suppurative otitis media with spontaneous rupture of ear drum, recurrent, unspecified ear

    H66.019   Acute suppurative otitis media with spontaneous rupture of ear drum, unspecified ear

● H66.1   Chronic tubotympanic suppurative otitis media

    Benign chronic suppurative otitis media
    Chronic tubotympanic disease

    Use additional code for any associated perforated tympanic membrane (H72.-) ◀

    H66.10   Chronic tubotympanic suppurative otitis media, unspecified

    H66.11   Chronic tubotympanic suppurative otitis media, right ear

    H66.12   Chronic tubotympanic suppurative otitis media, left ear

    H66.13   Chronic tubotympanic suppurative otitis media, bilateral

● H66.2   Chronic atticoantral suppurative otitis media

    Chronic atticoantral disease

    Use additional code for any associated perforated tympanic membrane (H72.-) ◀

    H66.20   Chronic atticoantral suppurative otitis media, unspecified ear

    H66.21   Chronic atticoantral suppurative otitis media, right ear

    H66.22   Chronic atticoantral suppurative otitis media, left ear

    H66.23   Chronic atticoantral suppurative otitis media, bilateral

● H66.3   Other chronic suppurative otitis media

    Chronic suppurative otitis media NOS

    Use additional code for any associated perforated tympanic membrane (H72.-) ◀

    Excludes1   tuberculous otitis media (A18.6)

● H66.3X   Other chronic suppurative otitis media

    H66.3X1   Other chronic suppurative otitis media, right ear

    H66.3X2   Other chronic suppurative otitis media, left ear

    H66.3X3   Other chronic suppurative otitis media, bilateral

    H66.3X9   Other chronic suppurative otitis media, unspecified ear

● H66.4   Suppurative otitis media, unspecified

    Purulent otitis media NOS

    Use additional code for any associated perforated tympanic membrane (H72.-) ◀

    H66.40   Suppurative otitis media, unspecified, unspecified ear

    H66.41   Suppurative otitis media, unspecified, right ear

    H66.42   Suppurative otitis media, unspecified, left ear

    H66.43   Suppurative otitis media, unspecified, bilateral

● H66.9   Otitis media, unspecified

    Otitis media NOS
    Acute otitis media NOS
    Chronic otitis media NOS

    Use additional code for any associated perforated tympanic membrane (H72.-) ◀

    H66.90   Otitis media, unspecified, unspecified ear

    H66.91   Otitis media, unspecified, right ear

    H66.92   Otitis media, unspecified, left ear

    H66.93   Otitis media, unspecified, bilateral

● H67   Otitis media in diseases classified elsewhere

    Code first underlying disease, such as:
    viral disease NEC (B00-B34)

    Use additional code for any associated perforated tympanic membrane (H72.-)

    Excludes1   otitis media in:
         influenza (J09.X9, J10.83, J11.83)
         measles (B05.3)
         scarlet fever (A38.0)
         tuberculosis (A18.6)

▌ *H67.1*   *Otitis media in diseases classified elsewhere, right ear*

▌ *H67.2*   *Otitis media in diseases classified elsewhere, left ear*

▌ *H67.3*   *Otitis media in diseases classified elsewhere, bilateral*

▌ *H67.9*   *Otitis media in diseases classified elsewhere, unspecified ear*

● H68   Eustachian salpingitis and obstruction

   ● H68.0   Eustachian salpingitis

     ● H68.00   Unspecified Eustachian salpingitis

       H68.001   Unspecified Eustachian salpingitis, right ear

       H68.002   Unspecified Eustachian salpingitis, left ear

       H68.003   Unspecified Eustachian salpingitis, bilateral

       H68.009   Unspecified Eustachian salpingitis, unspecified ear

     ● H68.01   Acute Eustachian salpingitis

       H68.011   Acute Eustachian salpingitis, right ear

       H68.012   Acute Eustachian salpingitis, left ear

       H68.013   Acute Eustachian salpingitis, bilateral

       H68.019   Acute Eustachian salpingitis, unspecified ear

     ● H68.02   Chronic Eustachian salpingitis

       H68.021   Chronic Eustachian salpingitis, right ear

       H68.022   Chronic Eustachian salpingitis, left ear

       H68.023   Chronic Eustachian salpingitis, bilateral

       H68.029   Chronic Eustachian salpingitis, unspecified ear

   ● H68.1   Obstruction of Eustachian tube

     Stenosis of Eustachian tube
     Stricture of Eustachian tube

     ● H68.10   Unspecified obstruction of Eustachian tube

       H68.101   Unspecified obstruction of Eustachian tube, right ear

       H68.102   Unspecified obstruction of Eustachian tube, left ear

       H68.103   Unspecified obstruction of Eustachian tube, bilateral

       H68.109   Unspecified obstruction of Eustachian tube, unspecified ear

CHAPTER 8 (H60-H95)

N   Newborn Age: 0   P   Pediatric Age: 0–17   M   Maternity DX: 12–55   A   Adult Age: 15–124   ♀   Females Only   ♂   Males Only

🔖 Complication\Comorbidity   🔖 Major C\C   (Ex) CC/MCC Exclusions   🔖 Present on Admission Requirement   🔖 Hospital-Acquired Condition

949

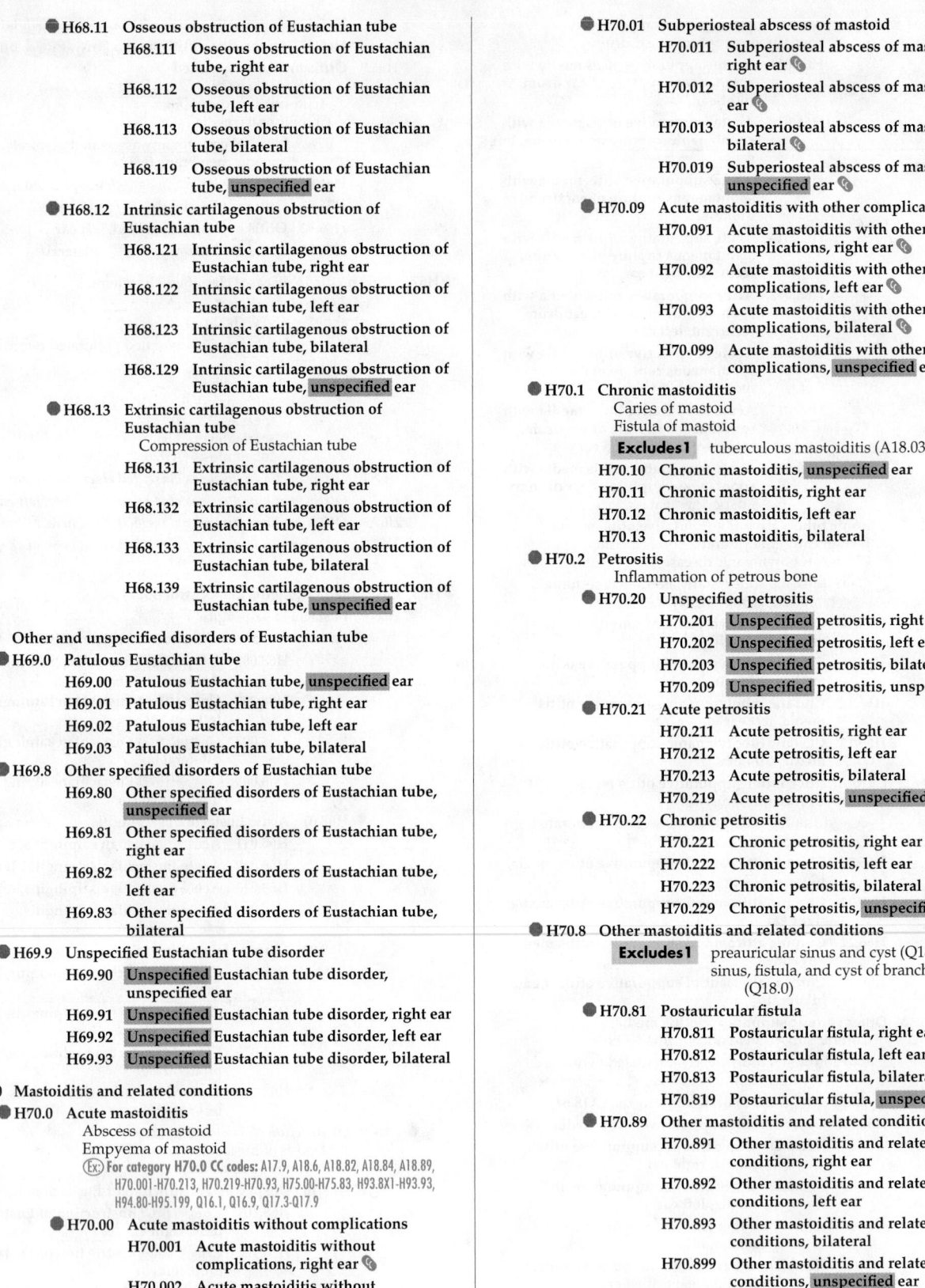

CHAPTER 8 (H60-H95)

● H68.11 Osseous obstruction of Eustachian tube
    H68.111 Osseous obstruction of Eustachian tube, right ear
    H68.112 Osseous obstruction of Eustachian tube, left ear
    H68.113 Osseous obstruction of Eustachian tube, bilateral
    H68.119 Osseous obstruction of Eustachian tube, unspecified ear

● H68.12 Intrinsic cartilagenous obstruction of Eustachian tube
    H68.121 Intrinsic cartilagenous obstruction of Eustachian tube, right ear
    H68.122 Intrinsic cartilagenous obstruction of Eustachian tube, left ear
    H68.123 Intrinsic cartilagenous obstruction of Eustachian tube, bilateral
    H68.129 Intrinsic cartilagenous obstruction of Eustachian tube, unspecified ear

● H68.13 Extrinsic cartilagenous obstruction of Eustachian tube
    Compression of Eustachian tube
    H68.131 Extrinsic cartilagenous obstruction of Eustachian tube, right ear
    H68.132 Extrinsic cartilagenous obstruction of Eustachian tube, left ear
    H68.133 Extrinsic cartilagenous obstruction of Eustachian tube, bilateral
    H68.139 Extrinsic cartilagenous obstruction of Eustachian tube, unspecified ear

● H69 Other and unspecified disorders of Eustachian tube
● H69.0 Patulous Eustachian tube
    H69.00 Patulous Eustachian tube, unspecified ear
    H69.01 Patulous Eustachian tube, right ear
    H69.02 Patulous Eustachian tube, left ear
    H69.03 Patulous Eustachian tube, bilateral
● H69.8 Other specified disorders of Eustachian tube
    H69.80 Other specified disorders of Eustachian tube, unspecified ear
    H69.81 Other specified disorders of Eustachian tube, right ear
    H69.82 Other specified disorders of Eustachian tube, left ear
    H69.83 Other specified disorders of Eustachian tube, bilateral

● H69.9 Unspecified Eustachian tube disorder
    H69.90 Unspecified Eustachian tube disorder, unspecified ear
    H69.91 Unspecified Eustachian tube disorder, right ear
    H69.92 Unspecified Eustachian tube disorder, left ear
    H69.93 Unspecified Eustachian tube disorder, bilateral

● H70 Mastoiditis and related conditions
● H70.0 Acute mastoiditis
    Abscess of mastoid
    Empyema of mastoid
    (Ex) For category H70.0 CC codes: A17.9, A18.6, A18.82, A18.84, A18.89, H70.001-H70.213, H70.219-H70.93, H75.00-H75.83, H93.8X1-H93.93, H94.80-H95.199, Q16.1, Q16.9, Q17.3-Q17.9
    ● H70.00 Acute mastoiditis without complications
        H70.001 Acute mastoiditis without complications, right ear
        H70.002 Acute mastoiditis without complications, left ear
        H70.003 Acute mastoiditis without complications, bilateral
        H70.009 Acute mastoiditis without complications, unspecified ear

● H70.01 Subperiosteal abscess of mastoid
    H70.011 Subperiosteal abscess of mastoid, right ear
    H70.012 Subperiosteal abscess of mastoid, left ear
    H70.013 Subperiosteal abscess of mastoid, bilateral
    H70.019 Subperiosteal abscess of mastoid, unspecified ear
● H70.09 Acute mastoiditis with other complications
    H70.091 Acute mastoiditis with other complications, right ear
    H70.092 Acute mastoiditis with other complications, left ear
    H70.093 Acute mastoiditis with other complications, bilateral
    H70.099 Acute mastoiditis with other complications, unspecified ear

● H70.1 Chronic mastoiditis
    Caries of mastoid
    Fistula of mastoid
    Excludes1 tuberculous mastoiditis (A18.03)
    H70.10 Chronic mastoiditis, unspecified ear
    H70.11 Chronic mastoiditis, right ear
    H70.12 Chronic mastoiditis, left ear
    H70.13 Chronic mastoiditis, bilateral
● H70.2 Petrositis
    Inflammation of petrous bone
    ● H70.20 Unspecified petrositis
        H70.201 Unspecified petrositis, right ear
        H70.202 Unspecified petrositis, left ear
        H70.203 Unspecified petrositis, bilateral
        H70.209 Unspecified petrositis, unspecified ear
    ● H70.21 Acute petrositis
        H70.211 Acute petrositis, right ear
        H70.212 Acute petrositis, left ear
        H70.213 Acute petrositis, bilateral
        H70.219 Acute petrositis, unspecified ear
    ● H70.22 Chronic petrositis
        H70.221 Chronic petrositis, right ear
        H70.222 Chronic petrositis, left ear
        H70.223 Chronic petrositis, bilateral
        H70.229 Chronic petrositis, unspecified ear
● H70.8 Other mastoiditis and related conditions
    Excludes1 preauricular sinus and cyst (Q18.1)
        sinus, fistula, and cyst of branchial cleft (Q18.0)
    ● H70.81 Postauricular fistula
        H70.811 Postauricular fistula, right ear
        H70.812 Postauricular fistula, left ear
        H70.813 Postauricular fistula, bilateral
        H70.819 Postauricular fistula, unspecified ear
    ● H70.89 Other mastoiditis and related conditions
        H70.891 Other mastoiditis and related conditions, right ear
        H70.892 Other mastoiditis and related conditions, left ear
        H70.893 Other mastoiditis and related conditions, bilateral
        H70.899 Other mastoiditis and related conditions, unspecified ear

Item 8-1 Mastoiditis is an infection of the portion of the temporal bone of the skull that is behind the ear (mastoid process) caused by an untreated otitis media, leading to an infection of the surrounding structures which may include the brain.

◀ New   ⬅ Revised   ~~deleted~~ Deleted   Excludes 1   Excludes 2   Includes   Use additional   Code first   Code also   Unspecified

OGCR Official Guidelines   ● Unacceptable Principal Diagnosis   X Assign placeholder X   ● Use Additional Character(s)   ▷ Manifestation Code   **Coding Clinic**

- H70.9   Unspecified mastoiditis
  - H70.90   Unspecified mastoiditis, unspecified ear
  - H70.91   Unspecified mastoiditis, right ear
  - H70.92   Unspecified mastoiditis, left ear
  - H70.93   Unspecified mastoiditis, bilateral
- H71   Cholesteatoma of middle ear
  - **Excludes2**   cholesteatoma of external ear (H60.4-)
    recurrent cholesteatoma of postmastoidectomy cavity (H95.0-)
  - H71.0   Cholesteatoma of attic
    - H71.00   Cholesteatoma of attic, unspecified ear
    - H71.01   Cholesteatoma of attic, right ear
    - H71.02   Cholesteatoma of attic, left ear
    - H71.03   Cholesteatoma of attic, bilateral
  - H71.1   Cholesteatoma of tympanum
    - H71.10   Cholesteatoma of tympanum, unspecified ear
    - H71.11   Cholesteatoma of tympanum, right ear
    - H71.12   Cholesteatoma of tympanum, left ear
    - H71.13   Cholesteatoma of tympanum, bilateral
  - H71.2   Cholesteatoma of mastoid
    - H71.20   Cholesteatoma of mastoid, unspecified ear
    - H71.21   Cholesteatoma of mastoid, right ear
    - H71.22   Cholesteatoma of mastoid, left ear
    - H71.23   Cholesteatoma of mastoid, bilateral
  - H71.3   Diffuse cholesteatosis
    - H71.30   Diffuse cholesteatosis, unspecified ear
    - H71.31   Diffuse cholesteatosis, right ear
    - H71.32   Diffuse cholesteatosis, left ear
    - H71.33   Diffuse cholesteatosis, bilateral
  - H71.9   Unspecified cholesteatoma
    - H71.90   Unspecified cholesteatoma, unspecified ear
    - H71.91   Unspecified cholesteatoma, right ear
    - H71.92   Unspecified cholesteatoma, left ear
    - H71.93   Unspecified cholesteatoma, bilateral

(See Plate 93 on page 69.)

- H72   Perforation of tympanic membrane
  Hole or rupture in ear drum
  - **Includes**   persistent post-traumatic perforation of ear drum
    postinflammatory perforation of ear drum
  - *Code first any associated otitis media (H65.-, H66.1-, H66.2-, H66.3-, H66.4-, H66.9-, H67.-)*
  - **Excludes1**   acute suppurative otitis media with rupture of the tympanic membrane (H66.01-)
    traumatic rupture of ear drum (S09.2-)
  - H72.0   Central perforation of tympanic membrane
    - H72.00   Central perforation of tympanic membrane, unspecified ear
    - H72.01   Central perforation of tympanic membrane, right ear
    - H72.02   Central perforation of tympanic membrane, left ear
    - H72.03   Central perforation of tympanic membrane, bilateral
  - H72.1   Attic perforation of tympanic membrane
    Perforation of pars flaccida
    - H72.10   Attic perforation of tympanic membrane, unspecified ear
    - H72.11   Attic perforation of tympanic membrane, right ear
    - H72.12   Attic perforation of tympanic membrane, left ear
    - H72.13   Attic perforation of tympanic membrane, bilateral

- H72.2   Other marginal perforations of tympanic membrane
  - H72.2X   Other marginal perforations of tympanic membrane
    - H72.2X1   Other marginal perforations of tympanic membrane, right ear
    - H72.2X2   Other marginal perforations of tympanic membrane, left ear
    - H72.2X3   Other marginal perforations of tympanic membrane, bilateral
    - H72.2X9   Other marginal perforations of tympanic membrane, unspecified ear
- H72.8   Other perforations of tympanic membrane
  - H72.81   Multiple perforations of tympanic membrane
    - H72.811   Multiple perforations of tympanic membrane, right ear
    - H72.812   Multiple perforations of tympanic membrane, left ear
    - H72.813   Multiple perforations of tympanic membrane, bilateral
    - H72.819   Multiple perforations of tympanic membrane, unspecified ear
  - H72.82   Total perforations of tympanic membrane
    - H72.821   Total perforations of tympanic membrane, right ear
    - H72.822   Total perforations of tympanic membrane, left ear
    - H72.823   Total perforations of tympanic membrane, bilateral
    - H72.829   Total perforations of tympanic membrane, unspecified ear
- H72.9   Unspecified perforation of tympanic membrane
  - H72.90   Unspecified perforation of tympanic membrane, unspecified ear
  - H72.91   Unspecified perforation of tympanic membrane, right ear
  - H72.92   Unspecified perforation of tympanic membrane, left ear
  - H72.93   Unspecified perforation of tympanic membrane, bilateral

- H73   Other disorders of tympanic membrane
  - H73.0   Acute myringitis
    - **Excludes1**   acute myringitis with otitis media (H65, H66)
    - H73.00   Unspecified acute myringitis
      Acute tympanitis NOS
      - H73.001   Acute myringitis, right ear
      - H73.002   Acute myringitis, left ear
      - H73.003   Acute myringitis, bilateral
      - H73.009   Acute myringitis, unspecified ear
    - H73.01   Bullous myringitis
      - H73.011   Bullous myringitis, right ear
      - H73.012   Bullous myringitis, left ear
      - H73.013   Bullous myringitis, bilateral
      - H73.019   Bullous myringitis, unspecified ear
    - H73.09   Other acute myringitis
      - H73.091   Other acute myringitis, right ear
      - H73.092   Other acute myringitis, left ear
      - H73.093   Other acute myringitis, bilateral
      - H73.099   Other acute myringitis, unspecified ear
  - H73.1   Chronic myringitis
    Chronic tympanitis
    - **Excludes1**   chronic myringitis with otitis media (H65, H66)
    - H73.10   Chronic myringitis, unspecified ear
    - H73.11   Chronic myringitis, right ear
    - H73.12   Chronic myringitis, left ear
    - H73.13   Chronic myringitis, bilateral

CHAPTER 8 (H60–H95)

- **H73.2**   Unspecified myringitis
  - H73.20   Unspecified myringitis, unspecified ear
  - H73.21   Unspecified myringitis, right ear
  - H73.22   Unspecified myringitis, left ear
  - H73.23   Unspecified myringitis, bilateral
- **H73.8**   Other specified disorders of tympanic membrane
  - **H73.81**   Atrophic flaccid tympanic membrane
    - H73.811   Atrophic flaccid tympanic membrane, right ear
    - H73.812   Atrophic flaccid tympanic membrane, left ear
    - H73.813   Atrophic flaccid tympanic membrane, bilateral
    - H73.819   Atrophic flaccid tympanic membrane, unspecified ear
  - **H73.82**   Atrophic nonflaccid tympanic membrane
    - H73.821   Atrophic nonflaccid tympanic membrane, right ear
    - H73.822   Atrophic nonflaccid tympanic membrane, left ear
    - H73.823   Atrophic nonflaccid tympanic membrane, bilateral
    - H73.829   Atrophic nonflaccid tympanic membrane, unspecified ear
  - **H73.89**   Other specified disorders of tympanic membrane
    - H73.891   Other specified disorders of tympanic membrane, right ear
    - H73.892   Other specified disorders of tympanic membrane, left ear
    - H73.893   Other specified disorders of tympanic membrane, bilateral
    - H73.899   Other specified disorders of tympanic membrane, unspecified ear
- **H73.9**   Unspecified disorder of tympanic membrane
  - H73.90   Unspecified disorder of tympanic membrane, unspecified ear
  - H73.91   Unspecified disorder of tympanic membrane, right ear
  - H73.92   Unspecified disorder of tympanic membrane, left ear
  - H73.93   Unspecified disorder of tympanic membrane, bilateral
- **H74**   Other disorders of middle ear mastoid

  Excludes2   mastoiditis (H70.-)
- **H74.0**   Tympanosclerosis
  - H74.01   Tympanosclerosis, right ear
  - H74.02   Tympanosclerosis, left ear
  - H74.03   Tympanosclerosis, bilateral
  - H74.09   Tympanosclerosis, unspecified ear
- **H74.1**   Adhesive middle ear disease

      Adhesive otitis

      Excludes1   glue ear (H65.3-)
  - H74.11   Adhesive right middle ear disease
  - H74.12   Adhesive left middle ear disease
  - H74.13   Adhesive middle ear disease, bilateral
  - H74.19   Adhesive middle ear disease, unspecified ear
- **H74.2**   Discontinuity and dislocation of ear ossicles
  - H74.20   Discontinuity and dislocation of ear ossicles, unspecified ear
  - H74.21   Discontinuity and dislocation of right ear ossicles
  - H74.22   Discontinuity and dislocation of left ear ossicles
  - H74.23   Discontinuity and dislocation of ear ossicles, bilateral

- **H74.3**   Other acquired abnormalities of ear ossicles
  - **H74.31**   Ankylosis of ear ossicles
    - H74.311   Ankylosis of ear ossicles, right ear
    - H74.312   Ankylosis of ear ossicles, left ear
    - H74.313   Ankylosis of ear ossicles, bilateral
    - H74.319   Ankylosis of ear ossicles, unspecified ear
  - **H74.32**   Partial loss of ear ossicles
    - H74.321   Partial loss of ear ossicles, right ear
    - H74.322   Partial loss of ear ossicles, left ear
    - H74.323   Partial loss of ear ossicles, bilateral
    - H74.329   Partial loss of ear ossicles, unspecified ear
  - **H74.39**   Other acquired abnormalities of ear ossicles
    - H74.391   Other acquired abnormalities of right ear ossicles
    - H74.392   Other acquired abnormalities of left ear ossicles
    - H74.393   Other acquired abnormalities of ear ossicles, bilateral
    - H74.399   Other acquired abnormalities of ear ossicles, unspecified ear
- **H74.4**   Polyp of middle ear
  - H74.40   Polyp of middle ear, unspecified ear
  - H74.41   Polyp of right middle ear
  - H74.42   Polyp of left middle ear
  - H74.43   Polyp of middle ear, bilateral
- **H74.8**   Other specified disorders of middle ear and mastoid
  - **H74.8X**   Other specified disorders of middle ear and mastoid
    - H74.8X1   Other specified disorders of right middle ear and mastoid
    - H74.8X2   Other specified disorders of left middle ear and mastoid
    - H74.8X3   Other specified disorders of middle ear and mastoid, bilateral
    - H74.8X9   Other specified disorders of middle ear and mastoid, unspecified ear
- **H74.9**   Unspecified disorder of middle ear and mastoid
  - H74.90   Unspecified disorder of middle ear and mastoid, unspecified ear
  - H74.91   Unspecified disorder of right middle ear and mastoid
  - H74.92   Unspecified disorder of left middle ear and mastoid
  - H74.93   Unspecified disorder of middle ear and mastoid, bilateral
- **H75**   Other disorders of middle ear and mastoid in diseases classified elsewhere

  Code first underlying disease
  - **H75.0**   Mastoiditis in infectious and parasitic diseases classified elsewhere

        Excludes1   mastoiditis (in):

                   syphilis (A52.77)

                   tuberculosis (A18.03)
    - *H75.00*   *Mastoiditis in infectious and parasitic diseases classified elsewhere, unspecified ear*
    - *H75.01*   *Mastoiditis in infectious and parasitic diseases classified elsewhere, right ear*
    - *H75.02*   *Mastoiditis in infectious and parasitic diseases classified elsewhere, left ear*
    - *H75.03*   *Mastoiditis in infectious and parasitic diseases classified elsewhere, bilateral*

◀ New   ◀▥ Revised   ~~deleted~~ Deleted   Excludes 1   Excludes 2   Includes   Use additional   Code first   Code also   Unspecified

OGCR Official Guidelines   ● Unacceptable Principal Diagnosis   X Assign placeholder X   ● Use Additional Character(s)   ▌ Manifestation Code   **Coding Clinic**

CHAPTER 8 (H60-H95)

● H75.8   Other specified disorders of middle ear and mastoid in diseases classified elsewhere

   ▸ *H75.80*   *Other specified disorders of middle ear and mastoid in diseases classified elsewhere, unspecified ear*

   ▸ *H75.81*   *Other specified disorders of right middle ear and mastoid in diseases classified elsewhere*

   ▸ *H75.82*   *Other specified disorders of left middle ear and mastoid in diseases classified elsewhere*

   ▸ *H75.83*   *Other specified disorders of middle ear and mastoid in diseases classified elsewhere, bilateral*

DISEASES OF INNER EAR (H80-H83)

(See Plate 95 on page 69.)

● H80   Otosclerosis

   Inherited middle ear spongelike bone growth causing hearing loss

   Includes   Otospongiosis

● H80.0   Otosclerosis involving oval window, nonobliterative

    H80.00   Otosclerosis involving oval window, nonobliterative, unspecified ear

    H80.01   Otosclerosis involving oval window, nonobliterative, right ear

    H80.02   Otosclerosis involving oval window, nonobliterative, left ear

    H80.03   Otosclerosis involving oval window, nonobliterative, bilateral

● H80.1   Otosclerosis involving oval window, obliterative

    H80.10   Otosclerosis involving oval window, obliterative, unspecified ear

    H80.11   Otosclerosis involving oval window, obliterative, right ear

    H80.12   Otosclerosis involving oval window, obliterative, left ear

    H80.13   Otosclerosis involving oval window, obliterative, bilateral

● H80.2   Cochlear otosclerosis

   Otosclerosis involving otic capsule
   Otosclerosis involving round window

    H80.20   Cochlear otosclerosis, unspecified ear

    H80.21   Cochlear otosclerosis, right ear

    H80.22   Cochlear otosclerosis, left ear

    H80.23   Cochlear otosclerosis, bilateral

● H80.8   Other otosclerosis

    H80.80   Other otosclerosis, unspecified ear

    H80.81   Other otosclerosis, right ear

    H80.82   Other otosclerosis, left ear

    H80.83   Other otosclerosis, bilateral

● H80.9   Unspecified otosclerosis

    H80.90   Unspecified otosclerosis, unspecified ear

    H80.91   Unspecified otosclerosis, right ear

    H80.92   Unspecified otosclerosis, left ear

    H80.93   Unspecified otosclerosis, bilateral

● H81   Disorders of vestibular function

   Excludes 1   epidemic vertigo (A88.1)
                  vertigo NOS (R42)

● H81.0   Ménière's disease

   Vestibular disorder that produces recurring symptoms including severe and intermittent hearing loss including the feeling of ear pressure or pain.

   Labyrinthine hydrops
   Ménière's syndrome or vertigo

    H81.01   Ménière's disease, right ear

    H81.02   Ménière's disease, left ear

    H81.03   Ménière's disease, bilateral

    H81.09   Ménière's disease, unspecified ear

● H81.1   Benign paroxysmal vertigo

    H81.10   Benign paroxysmal vertigo, unspecified ear

    H81.11   Benign paroxysmal vertigo, right ear

    H81.12   Benign paroxysmal vertigo, left ear

    H81.13   Benign paroxysmal vertigo, bilateral

● H81.2   Vestibular neuronitis

    H81.20   Vestibular neuronitis, unspecified ear

    H81.21   Vestibular neuronitis, right ear

    H81.22   Vestibular neuronitis, left ear

    H81.23   Vestibular neuronitis, bilateral

● H81.3   Other peripheral vertigo

  ● H81.31   Aural vertigo

      H81.311   Aural vertigo, right ear

      H81.312   Aural vertigo, left ear

      H81.313   Aural vertigo, bilateral

      H81.319   Aural vertigo, unspecified ear

  ● H81.39   Other peripheral vertigo

     Lermoyez' syndrome
     Otogenic vertigo
     Peripheral vertigo NOS

      H81.391   Other peripheral vertigo, right ear

      H81.392   Other peripheral vertigo, left ear

      H81.393   Other peripheral vertigo, bilateral

      H81.399   Other peripheral vertigo, unspecified ear

● H81.4   Vertigo of central origin

   Central positional nystagmus

    H81.41   Vertigo of central origin, right ear

    H81.42   Vertigo of central origin, left ear

    H81.43   Vertigo of central origin, bilateral

    H81.49   Vertigo of central origin, unspecified ear

● H81.8   Other disorders of vestibular function

  ● H81.8X   Other disorders of vestibular function

      H81.8X1   Other disorders of vestibular function, right ear

      H81.8X2   Other disorders of vestibular function, left ear

      H81.8X3   Other disorders of vestibular function, bilateral

      H81.8X9   Other disorders of vestibular function, unspecified ear

● H81.9   Unspecified disorder of vestibular function

   Vertiginous syndrome NOS

    H81.90   Unspecified disorder of vestibular function, unspecified ear

    H81.91   Unspecified disorder of vestibular function, right ear

    H81.92   Unspecified disorder of vestibular function, left ear

    H81.93   Unspecified disorder of vestibular function, bilateral

● H82   Vertiginous syndromes in diseases classified elsewhere

   Code first underlying disease

   Excludes 1   epidemic vertigo (A88.1)

   ▸ *H82.1*   *Vertiginous syndromes in diseases classified elsewhere, right ear*

   ▸ *H82.2*   *Vertiginous syndromes in diseases classified elsewhere, left ear*

   ▸ *H82.3*   *Vertiginous syndromes in diseases classified elsewhere, bilateral*

   ▸ *H82.9*   *Vertiginous syndromes in diseases classified elsewhere, unspecified ear*

● **H83   Other diseases of inner ear**
  ● **H83.0   Labyrinthitis**
     Balance disorder that follows URI or head injury.
    H83.01   Labyrinthitis, right ear
    H83.02   Labyrinthitis, left ear
    H83.03   Labyrinthitis, bilateral
    H83.09   Labyrinthitis, unspecified ear
  ● **H83.1   Labyrinthine fistula**
    H83.11   Labyrinthine fistula, right ear
    H83.12   Labyrinthine fistula, left ear
    H83.13   Labyrinthine fistula, bilateral
    H83.19   Labyrinthine fistula, unspecified ear
  ● **H83.2   Labyrinthine dysfunction**
     Labyrinthine hypersensitivity
     Labyrinthine hypofunction
     Labyrinthine loss of function
    ● **H83.2X   Labyrinthine dysfunction**
      H83.2X1   Labyrinthine dysfunction, right ear
      H83.2X2   Labyrinthine dysfunction, left ear
      H83.2X3   Labyrinthine dysfunction, bilateral
      H83.2X9   Labyrinthine dysfunction, unspecified ear
  ● **H83.3   Noise effects on inner ear**
     Acoustic trauma of inner ear
     Noise-induced hearing loss of inner ear
    ● **H83.3X   Noise effects on inner ear**
      H83.3X1   Noise effects on right inner ear
      H83.3X2   Noise effects on left inner ear
      H83.3X3   Noise effects on inner ear, bilateral
      H83.3X9   Noise effects on inner ear, unspecified ear
  ● **H83.8   Other specified diseases of inner ear**
    ● **H83.8X   Other specified diseases of inner ear**
      H83.8X1   Other specified diseases of right inner ear
      H83.8X2   Other specified diseases of left inner ear
      H83.8X3   Other specified diseases of inner ear, bilateral
      H83.8X9   Other specified diseases of inner ear, unspecified ear
  ● **H83.9   Unspecified disease of inner ear**
    H83.90   Unspecified disease of inner ear, unspecified ear
    H83.91   Unspecified disease of right inner ear
    H83.92   Unspecified disease of left inner ear
    H83.93   Unspecified disease of inner ear, bilateral

OTHER DISORDERS OF EAR (H90-H94)

● **H90   Conductive and sensorineural hearing loss**
    Excludes1   deaf nonspeaking NEC (H91.3)
               deafness NOS (H91.9-)
               hearing loss NOS (H91.9-)
               noise-induced hearing loss (H83.3-)
               ototoxic hearing loss (H91.0-)
               sudden (idiopathic) hearing loss (H91.2-)
  H90.0   Conductive hearing loss, bilateral
  ● **H90.1   Conductive hearing loss, unilateral with unrestricted hearing on the contralateral side**
    H90.11   Conductive hearing loss, unilateral, right ear, with unrestricted hearing on the contralateral side
    H90.12   Conductive hearing loss, unilateral, left ear, with unrestricted hearing on the contralateral side
  H90.2   Conductive hearing loss, unspecified
     Conductive deafness NOS
  H90.3   Sensorineural hearing loss, bilateral

● **H90.4   Sensorineural hearing loss, unilateral with unrestricted hearing on the contralateral side**
    H90.41   Sensorineural hearing loss, unilateral, right ear, with unrestricted hearing on the contralateral side
    H90.42   Sensorineural hearing loss, unilateral, left ear, with unrestricted hearing on the contralateral side
  H90.5   Unspecified sensorineural hearing loss
     Central hearing loss NOS
     Congenital deafness NOS
     Neural hearing loss NOS
     Perceptive hearing loss NOS
     Sensorineural deafness NOS
     Sensory hearing loss NOS
    Excludes1   abnormal auditory perception (H93.2-)
               psychogenic deafness (F44.6)
  H90.6   Mixed conductive and sensorineural hearing loss, bilateral
  ● **H90.7   Mixed conductive and sensorineural hearing loss, unilateral with unrestricted hearing on the contralateral side**
    H90.71   Mixed conductive and sensorineural hearing loss, unilateral, right ear, with unrestricted hearing on the contralateral side
    H90.72   Mixed conductive and sensorineural hearing loss, unilateral, left ear, with unrestricted hearing on the contralateral side
  H90.8   Mixed conductive and sensorineural hearing loss, unspecified

● **H91   Other and unspecified hearing loss**
    Excludes1   abnormal auditory perception (H93.2-)
               hearing loss as classified in H90.-
               impacted cerumen (H61.2-)
               noise-induced hearing loss (H83.3-)
               psychogenic deafness (F44.6)
               transient ischemic deafness (H93.01-)
  ● **H91.0   Ototoxic hearing loss**
     Code first poisoning due to drug or toxin, if applicable (T36-T65 with fifth or sixth character 1-4 or 6)
     Use additional code for adverse effect, if applicable, to identify drug (T36-T50 with fifth or sixth character 5)
    H91.01   Ototoxic hearing loss, right ear
    H91.02   Ototoxic hearing loss, left ear
    H91.03   Ototoxic hearing loss, bilateral
    H91.09   Ototoxic hearing loss, unspecified ear
  ● **H91.1   Presbycusis**
     Presbyacusia
    H91.10   Presbycusis, unspecified ear
    H91.11   Presbycusis, right ear
    H91.12   Presbycusis, left ear
    H91.13   Presbycusis, bilateral
  ● **H91.2   Sudden idiopathic hearing loss**
     Sudden hearing loss NOS
    H91.20   Sudden idiopathic hearing loss, unspecified ear
    H91.21   Sudden idiopathic hearing loss, right ear
    H91.22   Sudden idiopathic hearing loss, left ear
    H91.23   Sudden idiopathic hearing loss, bilateral
  H91.3   Deaf nonspeaking, not elsewhere classified
  ● **H91.8   Other specified hearing loss**
    ● **H91.8X   Other specified hearing loss**
      H91.8X1   Other specified hearing loss, right ear
      H91.8X2   Other specified hearing loss, left ear
      H91.8X3   Other specified hearing loss, bilateral
      H91.8X9   Other specified hearing loss, unspecified ear

◀ New   ◀|||| Revised   ~~deleted~~ Deleted   Excludes 1   Excludes 2   Includes   Use additional   Code first   Code also   Unspecified

OGCR Official Guidelines   ● Unacceptable Principal Diagnosis   X Assign placeholder X   ● Use Additional Character(s)   ▶ Manifestation Code   **Coding Clinic**

● H91.9   **Unspecified hearing loss**
     Deafness NOS
     High frequency deafness
     Low frequency deafness
   H91.90   Unspecified hearing loss, unspecified ear
   H91.91   Unspecified hearing loss, right ear
   H91.92   Unspecified hearing loss, left ear
   H91.93   Unspecified hearing loss, bilateral

● H92   **Otalgia and effusion of ear**
  ● H92.0   **Otalgia**
   H92.01   Otalgia, right ear
   H92.02   Otalgia, left ear
   H92.03   Otalgia, bilateral
   H92.09   Otalgia, unspecified ear
  ● H92.1   **Otorrhea**
    Excludes1   leakage of cerebrospinal fluid through ear
           (G96.0)
   H92.10   Otorrhea, unspecified ear
   H92.11   Otorrhea, right ear
   H92.12   Otorrhea, left ear
   H92.13   Otorrhea, bilateral
  ● H92.2   **Otorrhagia**
    Excludes1   traumatic otorrhagia - code to injury
   H92.20   Otorrhagia, unspecified ear
   H92.21   Otorrhagia, right ear
   H92.22   Otorrhagia, left ear
   H92.23   Otorrhagia, bilateral

● H93   **Other disorders of ear, not elsewhere classified**
  ● H93.0   **Degenerative and vascular disorders of ear**
    Excludes1   presbycusis (H91.1)
   ● H93.01   **Transient ischemic deafness**
    H93.011   Transient ischemic deafness, right ear
    H93.012   Transient ischemic deafness, left ear
    H93.013   Transient ischemic deafness, bilateral
    H93.019   Transient ischemic deafness, unspecified ear
   ● H93.09   **Unspecified degenerative and vascular disorders of ear**
    H93.091   Unspecified degenerative and vascular disorders of right ear
    H93.092   Unspecified degenerative and vascular disorders of left ear
    H93.093   Unspecified degenerative and vascular disorders of ear, bilateral
    H93.099   Unspecified degenerative and vascular disorders of unspecified ear
  ● H93.1   **Tinnitus**
     Perception of sound (ringing, buzzing, humming, whistling tunes, or singing)
   H93.11   Tinnitus, right ear
   H93.12   Tinnitus, left ear
   H93.13   Tinnitus, bilateral
   H93.19   Tinnitus, unspecified ear
  ● H93.2   **Other abnormal auditory perceptions**
    Excludes2   auditory hallucinations (R44.0)
   ● H93.21   **Auditory recruitment**
    H93.211   Auditory recruitment, right ear
    H93.212   Auditory recruitment, left ear
    H93.213   Auditory recruitment, bilateral
    H93.219   Auditory recruitment, unspecified ear
   ● H93.22   **Diplacusis**
    H93.221   Diplacusis, right ear
    H93.222   Diplacusis, left ear
    H93.223   Diplacusis, bilateral
    H93.229   Diplacusis, unspecified ear

   ● H93.23   **Hyperacusis**
    H93.231   Hyperacusis, right ear
    H93.232   Hyperacusis, left ear
    H93.233   Hyperacusis, bilateral
    H93.239   Hyperacusis, unspecified ear
   ● H93.24   **Temporary auditory threshold shift**
    H93.241   Temporary auditory threshold shift, right ear
    H93.242   Temporary auditory threshold shift, left ear
    H93.243   Temporary auditory threshold shift, bilateral
    H93.249   Temporary auditory threshold shift, unspecified ear
   H93.25   **Central auditory processing disorder**
     Congenital auditory imperception
     Word deafness
    Excludes1   mixed receptive-expressive language disorder (F80.2)
   ● H93.29   **Other abnormal auditory perceptions**
    H93.291   Other abnormal auditory perceptions, right ear
    H93.292   Other abnormal auditory perceptions, left ear
    H93.293   Other abnormal auditory perceptions, bilateral
    H93.299   Other abnormal auditory perceptions, unspecified ear
  ● H93.3   **Disorders of acoustic nerve**
     Disorder of 8th cranial nerve
    Excludes1   acoustic neuroma (D33.3)
             syphilitic acoustic neuritis (A52.15)
   ● H93.3X   **Disorders of acoustic nerve**
    H93.3X1   Disorders of right acoustic nerve
    H93.3X2   Disorders of left acoustic nerve
    H93.3X3   Disorders of bilateral acoustic nerves
    H93.3X9   Disorders of unspecified acoustic nerve
  ● H93.8   **Other specified disorders of ear**
   ● H93.8X   **Other specified disorders of ear**
    H93.8X1   Other specified disorders of right ear
    H93.8X2   Other specified disorders of left ear
    H93.8X3   Other specified disorders of ear, bilateral
    H93.8X9   Other specified disorders of ear, unspecified ear
  ● H93.9   **Unspecified disorder of ear**
   ● H93.90   Unspecified disorder of ear, unspecified ear
   ● H93.91   Unspecified disorder of right ear
   ● H93.92   Unspecified disorder of left ear
   ● H93.93   Unspecified disorder of ear, bilateral

● H94   **Other disorders of ear in diseases classified elsewhere**
  ● H94.0   **Acoustic neuritis in infectious and parasitic diseases classified elsewhere**
     Code first underlying disease, such as:
     parasitic disease (B65-B89)
    Excludes1   acoustic neuritis (in):
             herpes zoster (B02.29)
             syphilis (A52.15)
   ▸ H94.00   *Acoustic neuritis in infectious and parasitic diseases classified elsewhere, unspecified ear*
   ▸ H94.01   *Acoustic neuritis in infectious and parasitic diseases classified elsewhere, right ear*
   ▸ H94.02   *Acoustic neuritis in infectious and parasitic diseases classified elsewhere, left ear*
   ▸ H94.03   *Acoustic neuritis in infectious and parasitic diseases classified elsewhere, bilateral*

CHAPTER 8 (H60-H95)

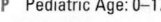

H94.8   **Other specified disorders of ear in diseases classified elsewhere**

Code first underlying disease, such as:
congenital syphilis (A50.0)

Excludes1   aural myiasis (B87.4)
syphilitic labyrinthitis (A52.79)

▸ *H94.80*   *Other specified disorders of ear in diseases classified elsewhere, unspecified ear*

▸ *H94.81*   *Other specified disorders of right ear in diseases classified elsewhere*

▸ *H94.82*   *Other specified disorders of left ear in diseases classified elsewhere*

▸ *H94.83*   *Other specified disorders of ear in diseases classified elsewhere, bilateral*

● **H95**   **Intraoperative and postprocedural complications and disorders of ear and mastoid process, not elsewhere classified**

● **H95.0**   **Recurrent cholesteatoma of postmastoidectomy cavity**

   H95.00   Recurrent cholesteatoma of postmastoidectomy cavity, unspecified ear

   H95.01   Recurrent cholesteatoma of postmastoidectomy cavity, right ear

   H95.02   Recurrent cholesteatoma of postmastoidectomy cavity, left ear

   H95.03   Recurrent cholesteatoma of postmastoidectomy cavity, bilateral ears

● **H95.1**   **Other disorders of ear and mastoid process following mastoidectomy**

   ● **H95.11**   Chronic inflammation of postmastoidectomy cavity

     H95.111   Chronic inflammation of postmastoidectomy cavity, right ear

     H95.112   Chronic inflammation of postmastoidectomy cavity, left ear

     H95.113   Chronic inflammation of postmastoidectomy cavity, bilateral ears

     H95.119   Chronic inflammation of postmastoidectomy cavity, unspecified ear

   ● **H95.12**   Granulation of postmastoidectomy cavity

     H95.121   Granulation of postmastoidectomy cavity, right ear

     H95.122   Granulation of postmastoidectomy cavity, left ear

     H95.123   Granulation of postmastoidectomy cavity, bilateral ears

     H95.129   Granulation of postmastoidectomy cavity, unspecified ear

   ● **H95.13**   Mucosal cyst of postmastoidectomy cavity

     H95.131   Mucosal cyst of postmastoidectomy cavity, right ear

     H95.132   Mucosal cyst of postmastoidectomy cavity, left ear

     H95.133   Mucosal cyst of postmastoidectomy cavity, bilateral ears

     H95.139   Mucosal cyst of postmastoidectomy cavity, unspecified ear

   ● **H95.19**   Other disorders following mastoidectomy

     H95.191   Other disorders following mastoidectomy, right ear

     H95.192   Other disorders following mastoidectomy, left ear

     H95.193   Other disorders following mastoidectomy, bilateral ears

     H95.199   Other disorders following mastoidectomy, unspecified ear

● **H95.2**   **Intraoperative hemorrhage and hematoma of ear and mastoid process complicating a procedure**

Excludes1   intraoperative hemorrhage and hematoma of ear and mastoid process due to accidental puncture or laceration during a procedure (H95.3-)

(Ex) **For category H95.2 CC codes:** H95.21-H95.22, H95.41-H95.89, I85.01, I85.11, I97.3, K21.9, K22.8, K23-K25.2, K25.4, K25.6, K26.0, K26.2, K26.4, K26.6, K27.0, K27.2, K27.4, K27.6, K28.0, K28.2, K28.4, K28.6, K29.01, K29.21, K29.31, K29.41, K29.51, K29.61, K29.71, K29.81, K29.91, K31.811, K55.21, K57.01, K57.11, K57.13, K57.21, K57.31, K57.33, K57.41, K57.51, K57.53, K57.81, K57.91, K57.93, K62.5, K92.0-K92.2, M96.89, N98.1-N98.9, P54.1-P54.3, T81.10X-T81.19X[A], T81.82X[A], T81.89X-T81.9XX[A]

   H95.21   Intraoperative hemorrhage and hematoma of ear and mastoid process complicating a procedure on the ear and mastoid process 🔖

   H95.22   Intraoperative hemorrhage and hematoma of ear and mastoid process complicating other procedure 🔖

● **H95.3**   **Accidental puncture and laceration of ear and mastoid process during a procedure**

(Ex) **For category H95.3 CC codes:** D78.11-D78.12, D78.81-D78.89, E36.11-E36.8, E89.810-E89.89, G96.11, G97.41-G97.49, H59.011-H59.019, H59.031-H59.099, H59.211-H59.229, H59.811-H59.89, H95.31-H95.32, H95.811-H95.89, I97.3, I97.51-I97.52, J95.71-J95.72, K91.71-K91.72, L76.11-L76.12, L76.81-L76.82, M96.820-M96.821, M96.89, N98.1-N98.9, N99.71-N99.72, T81.82X[A], T81.89X-T81.9XX[A]

   H95.31   Accidental puncture and laceration of the ear and mastoid process during a procedure on the ear and mastoid process 🔖

   H95.32   Accidental puncture and laceration of the ear and mastoid process during other procedure 🔖

● **H95.4**   **Postprocedural hemorrhage and hematoma of ear and mastoid process following a procedure**

(Ex) **For category H95.4 CC codes:** See H95.2

   H95.41   Postprocedural hemorrhage and hematoma of ear and mastoid process following a procedure on the ear and mastoid process 🔖

   H95.42   Postprocedural hemorrhage and hematoma of ear and mastoid process following other procedure 🔖

● **H95.8**   **Other intraoperative and postprocedural complications and disorders of the ear and mastoid process, not elsewhere classified**

Excludes2   postprocedural complications and disorders following mastoidectomy (H95.0-, H95.1-)

(Ex) **For category H95.8 CC codes:** D78.81-D78.89, E36.8, E89.810-E89.89, H59.011-H59.019, H59.031-H59.099, H59.811-H59.89, H95.811-H95.89, I97.3, L76.81-L76.82, M96.89, N98.1-N98.9, T81.82X[A], T81.89X-T81.9XX[A]

   ● **H95.81**   Postprocedural stenosis of external ear canal

     H95.811   Postprocedural stenosis of right external ear canal 🔖

     H95.812   Postprocedural stenosis of left external ear canal 🔖

     H95.813   Postprocedural stenosis of external ear canal, bilateral 🔖

     H95.819   Postprocedural stenosis of unspecified external ear canal 🔖

   H95.88   Other intraoperative complications and disorders of the ear and mastoid process, not elsewhere classified 🔖

     Use additional code, if applicable, to further specify disorder

   H95.89   Other postprocedural complications and disorders of the ear and mastoid process, not elsewhere classified 🔖

     Use additional code, if applicable, to further specify disorder

◀ New   ◀ Revised   ~~deleted~~ Deleted   Excludes 1   Excludes 2   Includes   Use additional   Code first   Code also   Unspecified

OGCR Official Guidelines   ● Unacceptable Principal Diagnosis   X Assign placeholder X   ● Use Additional Character(s)   ▸ Manifestation Code   **Coding Clinic**

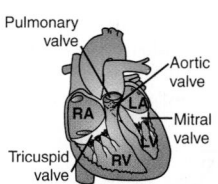

Figure 9-1 Cardiovascular valves.

Item 9-1 Rheumatic fever is the inflammation of the valve(s) of the heart, usually the mitral or aortic, which leads to valve damage. Rheumatic heart inflammations are usually **pericarditis** (sac surrounding heart), **endocarditis** (heart cavity), or **myocarditis** (heart muscle).

CHAPTER 9   DISEASES OF THE CIRCULATORY SYSTEM (I00-I99)

Excludes2   certain conditions originating in the perinatal period (P04-P96)
certain infectious and parasitic diseases (A00-B99)
complications of pregnancy, childbirth and the puerperium (O00-O9A)
congenital malformations, deformations, and chromosomal abnormalities (Q00-Q99)
endocrine, nutritional and metabolic diseases (E00-E88)
injury, poisoning and certain other consequences of external causes (S00-T88)
neoplasms (C00-D49)
symptoms, signs and abnormal clinical and laboratory findings, not elsewhere classified (R00-R94)
systemic connective tissue disorders (M30-M36)
transient cerebral ischemic attacks and related syndromes (G45.-)

This chapter contains the following blocks:

I00-I02	Acute rheumatic fever
I05-I09	Chronic rheumatic heart diseases
I10-I15	Hypertensive diseases
I20-I25	Ischemic heart diseases
I26-I28	Pulmonary heart disease and diseases of pulmonary circulation
I30-I52	Other forms of heart disease
I60-I69	Cerebrovascular diseases
I70-I79	Diseases of arteries, arterioles and capillaries
I80-I89	Diseases of veins, lymphatic vessels and lymph nodes, not elsewhere classified
I95-I99	Other and unspecified disorders of the circulatory system

ACUTE RHEUMATIC FEVER (I00-I02)

I00   **Rheumatic fever without heart involvement**
     Includes   arthritis, rheumatic, acute or subacute
     Excludes1   rheumatic fever with heart involvement (I01.0-I01.9) ◀▥

● **I01**   **Rheumatic fever with heart involvement**
     Excludes1   chronic diseases of rheumatic origin (I05-I09) unless rheumatic fever is also present or there is evidence of reactivation or activity of the rheumatic process.

   I01.0   **Acute rheumatic pericarditis** 🔖
     Any condition in I00 with pericarditis
     Rheumatic pericarditis (acute)
       Excludes1   acute pericarditis not specified as rheumatic (I30.-)
       (Ex) B33.23, I01.0, I09.2, I30.0-I30.9, I31.3-I32, I87.8, I99.8-I99.9

   I01.1   **Acute rheumatic endocarditis** 🔖
     Any condition in I00 with endocarditis or valvulitis
     Acute rheumatic valvulitis
       (Ex) A01.00-A01.09, A39.51, A52.03, A78, B33.21, B37.6, I00, I01.1, I01.8-I02.0, I05.0-I07.9, I08.1-I08.3, I08.9, I09.1, I09.89-I09.9, I33.0-I39, I42.4, I87.8, I99.8-I99.9, Q22.2, Q23.8-Q23.9, Q24.8, T82.6XX[A]

Item 9-2 Rheumatic chorea, also called Sydenham's, juvenile, minor, simple, or St. Vitus' dance, is a major symptom of rheumatic fever and is characterized by ceaseless, involuntary, jerky, purposeless movements.

   I01.2   **Acute rheumatic myocarditis** 🔖
     Any condition in I00 with myocarditis
       (Ex) A52.06, B33.20-B33.22, I00, I01.2-I01.9, I09.0, I09.9, I23.0-I23.3, I23.6-I23.8, I40.0-I41, I51.0, I51.3-I51.4, I87.8, I99.8-I99.9

   I01.8   **Other acute rheumatic heart disease** 🔖
     Any condition in I00 with other or multiple types of heart involvement
     Acute rheumatic pancarditis
       (Ex) I01.0-I09.9, I50.20-I50.43

   I01.9   **Acute rheumatic heart disease, unspecified** 🔖
     Any condition in I00 with unspecified type of heart involvement
     Rheumatic carditis, acute
     Rheumatic heart disease, active or acute
       (Ex) I01.0-I09.9

● **I02**   **Rheumatic chorea**
     Includes   Sydenham's chorea
     Excludes1   chorea NOS (G25.5)
               Huntington's chorea (G10)

   I02.0   **Rheumatic chorea with heart involvement** 🔖
     Chorea NOS with heart involvement
     Rheumatic chorea with heart involvement of any type classifiable under I01.-
       (Ex) See I01.8

   I02.9   **Rheumatic chorea without heart involvement** 🔖
     Rheumatic chorea NOS
       (Ex) See I01.9

CHRONIC RHEUMATIC HEART DISEASES (I05-I09)

● **I05**   **Rheumatic mitral valve diseases**
     Includes   conditions classifiable to both I05.0 and I05.2-I05.9, whether specified as rheumatic or not
     Excludes1   mitral valve disease specified as nonrheumatic (I34.-)
               mitral valve disease with aortic and/or tricuspid valve involvement (I08.-)

   I05.0   **Rheumatic mitral stenosis**
     Mitral (valve) obstruction (rheumatic)

   I05.1   **Rheumatic mitral insufficiency**
     Rheumatic mitral incompetence
     Rheumatic mitral regurgitation
       Excludes1   mitral insufficiency not specified as rheumatic (I34.0)

   I05.2   **Rheumatic mitral stenosis with insufficiency**
     Rheumatic mitral stenosis with incompetence or regurgitation

   I05.8   **Other rheumatic mitral valve diseases**
     Rheumatic mitral (valve) failure

   I05.9   **Rheumatic mitral valve disease, unspecified**
     Rheumatic mitral (valve) disorder (chronic) NOS

● **I06**   **Rheumatic aortic valve diseases**
     Excludes1   aortic valve disease not specified as rheumatic (I35.-)
               aortic valve disease with mitral and/or tricuspid valve involvement (I08.-)

   I06.0   **Rheumatic aortic stenosis**
     Rheumatic aortic (valve) obstruction

   I06.1   **Rheumatic aortic insufficiency**
     Rheumatic aortic incompetence
     Rheumatic aortic regurgitation

(See Plate 244 on page 78.)

Item 9-3 Mitral stenosis is the narrowing of the mitral valve separating the left atrium from the left ventricle. **Mitral insufficiency** is the improper closure of the mitral valve which may lead to enlargement (hypertrophy) of the left atrium.

N Newborn Age: 0   **P** Pediatric Age: 0–17   **M** Maternity DX: 12–55   **A** Adult Age: 15–124   ♀ Females Only   ♂ Males Only
🔖 Complication\Comorbidity   🔖 Major C\C   (Ex) CC/MCC Exclusions   🔖 Present on Admission Requirement   🔖 Hospital-Acquired Condition
957

Item 9–4 Aortic stenosis is the narrowing of the aortic valve located between the left ventricle and the aorta. **Aortic insufficiency** is the improper closure of the aortic valve which may lead to enlargement (hypertrophy) of the left ventricle.

I06.2   **Rheumatic aortic stenosis with insufficiency**
Rheumatic aortic stenosis with incompetence or regurgitation

I06.8   **Other rheumatic aortic valve diseases**

I06.9   **Rheumatic aortic valve disease, unspecified**
Rheumatic aortic (valve) disease NOS

● **I07**   **Rheumatic tricuspid valve diseases**

   Includes   rheumatic tricuspid valve diseases specified as rheumatic or unspecified

   Excludes1   tricuspid valve disease specified as nonrheumatic (I36.-)
tricuspid valve disease with aortic and/or mitral valve involvement (I08.-)

I07.0   **Rheumatic tricuspid stenosis**
Tricuspid (valve) stenosis (rheumatic)

I07.1   **Rheumatic tricuspid insufficiency**
Tricuspid (valve) insufficiency (rheumatic)

I07.2   **Rheumatic tricuspid stenosis and insufficiency**

I07.8   **Other rheumatic tricuspid valve diseases**

I07.9   **Rheumatic tricuspid valve disease, unspecified**
Rheumatic tricuspid valve disorder NOS

● **I08**   **Multiple valve diseases**

   Includes   multiple valve diseases specified as rheumatic or unspecified

   Excludes1   endocarditis, valve unspecified (I38)
multiple valve disease specified a nonrheumatic (I34.-, I35.-, I36.-, I37.-, I38.-, Q22.-, Q23.-, Q24.8-)
rheumatic valve disease NOS (I09.1)

I08.0   **Rheumatic disorders of both mitral and aortic valves**
Involvement of both mitral and aortic valves specified as rheumatic or unspecified

I08.1   **Rheumatic disorders of both mitral and tricuspid valves**

I08.2   **Rheumatic disorders of both aortic and tricuspid valves**

I08.3   **Combined rheumatic disorders of mitral, aortic and tricuspid valves**

I08.8   **Other rheumatic multiple valve diseases**

I08.9   **Rheumatic multiple valve disease, unspecified**

● **I09**   **Other rheumatic heart diseases**

I09.0   **Rheumatic myocarditis** 🔊

   Excludes1   myocarditis not specified as rheumatic (I51.4)
Ⓔⓧ I00, I01.2-I01.9, I09.0, I09.9, I23.0-I23.3, I23.6-I23.8, I40.0-I41, I51.0, I51.3-I51.4, I87.8, I99.8-I99.9

I09.1   **Rheumatic diseases of endocardium, valve unspecified**
Rheumatic endocarditis (chronic)
Rheumatic valvulitis (chronic)

   Excludes1   endocarditis, valve unspecified (I38)

I09.2   **Chronic rheumatic pericarditis** 🔊
Adherent pericardium, rheumatic
Chronic rheumatic mediastinopericarditis
Chronic rheumatic myopericarditis

   Excludes1   chronic pericarditis not specified as rheumatic (I31.-)
Ⓔⓧ See I01.0

● **I09.8**   **Other specified rheumatic heart diseases**

I09.81   **Rheumatic heart failure** 🔊
Use additional code to identify type of heart failure (I50.-)
Ⓔⓧ I09.81, I09.9, I11.0, I50.1-I50.9, I87.8, I99.8-I99.9

I09.89   **Other specified rheumatic heart diseases**
Rheumatic disease of pulmonary valve

I09.9   **Rheumatic heart disease, unspecified**
Rheumatic carditis

   Excludes1   rheumatoid carditis (M05.31)

Item 9–5 Hypertension is caused by high arterial blood pressure in the arteries. **Essential, primary,** or **idiopathic** hypertension occurs without identifiable organic cause. **Secondary** hypertension is that which has an organic cause. **Malignant** hypertension is severely elevated blood pressure. **Benign** hypertension is mildly elevated blood pressure.

HYPERTENSIVE DISEASES (I10-I15)

Use additional code to identify:
exposure to environmental tobacco smoke (Z77.22)
history of tobacco use (Z87.891)
occupational exposure to environmental tobacco smoke (Z57.31)
tobacco dependence (F17.-)
tobacco use (Z72.0)

   Excludes1   hypertensive disease complicating pregnancy, childbirth and the puerperium (O10-O11, O13-O16)
neonatal hypertension (P29.2)
primary pulmonary hypertension (I27.0)

I10   **Essential (primary) hypertension**

   Includes   high blood pressure
hypertension (arterial) (benign) (essential) (malignant) (primary) (systemic)

   Excludes1   hypertensive disease complicating pregnancy, childbirth and the puerperium (O10-O11, O13-O16)

   Excludes2   essential (primary) hypertension involving vessels of brain (I60-I69)
essential (primary) hypertension involving vessels of eye (H35.0-)

MCE: Questionable admission when principal dx

● **I11**   **Hypertensive heart disease**

   Includes   any condition in I51.4-I51.9 due to hypertension

I11.0   **Hypertensive heart disease with heart failure**
Hypertensive heart failure
Use additional code to identify type of heart failure (I50.-)

I11.9   **Hypertensive heart disease without heart failure**
Hypertensive heart disease NOS

OGCR Section I.C.9.a.2

Hypertensive Chronic Kidney Disease

Assign codes from category I12, Hypertensive chronic kidney disease, when both hypertension and a condition classifiable to category N18, Chronic kidney disease (CKD), are present. Unlike hypertension with heart disease, ICD-10-CM presumes a cause-and-effect relationship and classifies chronic kidney disease with hypertension as hypertensive chronic kidney disease.

The appropriate code from category N18 should be used as a secondary code with a code from category I12 to identify the stage of chronic kidney disease.

See Section I.C.14. Chronic kidney disease.

If a patient has hypertensive chronic kidney disease and acute renal failure, an additional code for the acute renal failure is required.

● **I12**   **Hypertensive chronic kidney disease**

   Includes   any condition in N18 and N26 - due to hypertension
arteriosclerosis of kidney
arteriosclerotic nephritis (chronic) (interstitial)
hypertensive nephropathy
nephrosclerosis

   Excludes1   hypertension due to kidney disease (I15.0, I15.1)
renovascular hypertension (I15.0)
secondary hypertension (I15.-)

   Excludes2   acute kidney failure (N17.-)

I12.0   **Hypertensive chronic kidney disease with stage 5 chronic kidney disease or end stage renal disease** 🔊
Use additional code to identify the stage of chronic kidney disease (N18.5, N18.6)
Ⓔⓧ I10-I15.9, I87.8, I99.8-I99.9, N18.6, N26.2

I12.9   **Hypertensive chronic kidney disease with stage 1 through stage 4 chronic kidney disease, or unspecified chronic kidney disease**

      Hypertensive chronic kidney disease NOS

      Hypertensive renal disease NOS

      Use additional code to identify the stage of chronic kidney disease (N18.1-N18.4, N18.9)

OGCR   Section I.c.9.a.6

Hypertensive Heart and Chronic Kidney Disease

Assign codes from combination category I13, Hypertensive heart and chronic kidney disease, when both hypertensive kidney disease and hypertensive heart disease are stated in the diagnosis. Assume a relationship between the hypertension and the chronic kidney disease, whether or not the condition is so designated. If heart failure is present, assign an additional code from category I50 to identify the type of heart failure.

The appropriate code from category N18, Chronic kidney disease, should be used as a secondary code with a code from category I13 to identify the stage of chronic kidney disease. *See Section I.C.14. Chronic kidney disease.*

The codes in category I13, Hypertensive heart and chronic kidney disease, are combination codes that include hypertension, heart disease and chronic kidney disease. The Includes note at I13 specifies that the conditions included at I11 and I12 are included together in I13. If a patient has hypertension, heart disease and chronic kidney disease then a code from I13 should be used, not individual codes for hypertension, heart disease and chronic kidney disease, or codes from I11 or I12.

For patients with both acute renal failure and chronic kidney disease an additional code for acute renal failure is required.

●I13   **Hypertensive heart and chronic kidney disease**

     Includes   any condition in I11.- with any condition in I12.-

          cardiorenal disease

          cardiovascular renal disease

     (Ex) **For category I13 CC codes:** I10-I15.9, I87.8, I99.8-I99.9, N26.2

I13.0   **Hypertensive heart and chronic kidney disease with heart failure and stage 1 through stage 4 chronic kidney disease, or unspecified chronic kidney disease** 🅒

      Use additional code to identify type of heart failure (I50.-)

      Use additional code to identify stage of chronic kidney disease (N18.1-N18.4, N18.9)

●I13.1   **Hypertensive heart and chronic kidney disease without heart failure**

     I13.10   **Hypertensive heart and chronic kidney disease without heart failure, with stage 1 through stage 4 chronic kidney disease, or unspecified chronic kidney disease**

         Hypertensive heart disease and hypertensive chronic kidney disease NOS

         Use additional code to identify the stage of chronic kidney disease (N18.1-N18.4, N18.9)

     I13.11   **Hypertensive heart and chronic kidney disease without heart failure, with stage 5 chronic kidney disease, or end stage renal disease** 🅒

         Use additional code to identify the stage of chronic kidney disease (N18.5, N18.6)

I13.2   **Hypertensive heart and chronic kidney disease with heart failure and with stage 5 chronic kidney disease, or end stage renal disease** 🅒

      Use additional code to identify type of heart failure (I50.-)

      Use additional code to identify the stage of chronic kidney disease (N18.5, N18.6)

OGCR   Section I.9.a.6

Hypertension, Secondary

Secondary hypertension is due to an underlying condition. Two codes are required: one to identify the underlying etiology and one from category I15 to identify the hypertension. Sequencing of codes is determined by the reason for admission/encounter.

●I15   **Secondary hypertension**

     Code also underlying condition

     Excludes1   postprocedural hypertension (I97.3)

     Excludes2   secondary hypertension involving vessels of brain (I60-I69)

               secondary hypertension involving vessels of eye (H35.0-)

I15.0   **Renovascular hypertension**

I15.1   **Hypertension secondary to other renal disorders**

I15.2   **Hypertension secondary to endocrine disorders**

I15.8   **Other secondary hypertension**

I15.9   **Secondary hypertension, unspecified**

ISCHEMIC HEART DISEASES (I20-I25)

Use additional code to identify presence of hypertension (I10-I15)

●I20   **Angina pectoris**

Chest pain/discomfort due to lack of oxygen to the heart muscle. Principal symptom of myocardial infarction.

     Use additional code to identify:

      exposure to environmental tobacco smoke (Z77.22)

      history of tobacco use (Z87.891)

      occupational exposure to environmental tobacco smoke (Z57.31)

      tobacco dependence (F17.-)

      tobacco use (Z72.0)

     Excludes1   angina pectoris with atherosclerotic heart disease of native coronary arteries (I25.1-)

               atherosclerosis of coronary artery bypass graft(s) and coronary artery of transplanted heart with angina pectoris (I25.7-)

               postinfarction angina (I23.7)

I20.0   **Unstable angina** 🅒

      Accelerated angina

      Crescendo angina

      De novo effort angina

      Intermediate coronary syndrome

      Preinfarction syndrome

      Worsening effort angina

     (Ex) I09.81, I11.0, I13.0, I13.2, I20.0-I22.9, I24.0, I24.8-I24.9, I25.5-I25.6, I25.82-I25.83, I25.89-I25.9, I50.1, I50.9, I87.8, I99.8-I99.9, R57.0, R57.9

I20.1   **Angina pectoris with documented spasm** 🅒

      Angiospastic angina

      Prinzmetal angina

      Spasm-induced angina

      Variant angina

     (Ex) I20.0-I22.9, I24.0, I24.8-I24.9, I25.5-I25.6, I25.89-I25.9, I87.8, I99.8-I99.9

I20.8   **Other forms of angina pectoris**

      Angina equivalent

      Angina of effort

      Coronary slow flow syndrome

      Stenocardia

      Use additional code(s) for symptoms associated with angina equivalent

I20.9   **Angina pectoris, unspecified**

      Angina NOS

      Anginal syndrome

      Cardiac angina

      Ischemic chest pain

CHAPTER 9 (I00-I99)

OGCR See Section I.c.9.e.3

Acute myocardial infarction, unspecified
Code I21.3, ST elevation (STEMI) myocardial infarction of unspecified site, is the default for unspecified acute myocardial infarction. If only STEMI or transmural MI without the site is documented, assign I21.3.

I21   **ST elevation (STEMI) and non-ST elevation (NSTEMI) myocardial infarction**

     Includes   cardiac infarction
                coronary (artery) embolism
                coronary (artery) occlusion
                coronary (artery) rupture
                coronary (artery) thrombosis
                infarction of heart, myocardium, or ventricle
                myocardial infarction specified as acute or with a stated duration of 4 weeks (28 days) or less from onset

Use additional code, if applicable, to identify:
     exposure to environmental tobacco smoke (Z77.22)
     history of tobacco use (Z87.891)
     occupational exposure to environmental tobacco smoke (Z57.31)
     status post administration of tPA (rtPA) in a different facility within the last 24 hours prior to admission to current facility (Z92.82)
     tobacco dependence (F17.-)
     tobacco use (Z72.0)

     Excludes2   old myocardial infarction (I25.2)
                 postmyocardial infarction syndrome (I24.1)
                 subsequent myocardial infarction (I22.-)

Ⓔ⒳ For category I21 CC codes: I21.01-I22.9, I87.8, I99.8-I99.9

Coding Clinic: 2012, Q4, P103

● **I21.0**   **ST elevation (STEMI) myocardial infarction of anterior wall**

     I21.01   **ST elevation (STEMI) myocardial infarction involving left main coronary artery** 🔖

     I21.02   **ST elevation (STEMI) myocardial infarction involving left anterior descending coronary artery** 🔖
              ST elevation (STEMI) myocardial infarction involving diagonal coronary artery

     I21.09   **ST elevation (STEMI) myocardial infarction involving other coronary artery of anterior wall** 🔖
              Acute transmural myocardial infarction of anterior wall
              Anteroapical transmural (Q wave) infarction (acute)
              Anterolateral transmural (Q wave) infarction (acute)
              Anteroseptal transmural (Q wave) infarction (acute)
              Transmural (Q wave) infarction (acute) (of) anterior (wall) NOS

              Coding Clinic: 2012, Q4, P102, 104

● **I21.1**   **ST elevation (STEMI) myocardial infarction of inferior wall**

     I21.11   **ST elevation (STEMI) myocardial infarction involving right coronary artery** 🔖
              Inferoposterior transmural (Q wave) infarction (acute)

     I21.19   **ST elevation (STEMI) myocardial infarction involving other coronary artery of inferior wall** 🔖
              Acute transmural myocardial infarction of inferior wall
              Inferolateral transmural (Q wave) infarction (acute)
              Transmural (Q wave) infarction (acute) (of) diaphragmatic wall
              Transmural (Q wave) infarction (acute) (of) inferior (wall) NOS

          Excludes2   ST elevation (STEMI) myocardial infarction involving left circumflex coronary artery (I21.21)

         Coding Clinic: 2012, Q4, P97

● **I21.2**   **ST elevation (STEMI) myocardial infarction of other sites**
       Ⓔ⒳ For category I21.2 CC codes: I21.01-I22.9, I87.8, I99.8-I99.9

     I21.21   **ST elevation (STEMI) myocardial infarction involving left circumflex coronary artery** 🔖
              ST elevation (STEMI) myocardial infarction involving oblique marginal coronary artery

     I21.29   **ST elevation (STEMI) myocardial infarction involving other sites** 🔖
              Acute transmural myocardial infarction of other sites
              Apical-lateral transmural (Q wave) infarction (acute)
              Basal-lateral transmural (Q wave) infarction (acute)
              High lateral transmural (Q wave) infarction (acute)
              Lateral (wall) NOS transmural (Q wave) infarction (acute)
              Posterior (true) transmural (Q wave) infarction (acute)
              Posterobasal transmural (Q wave) infarction (acute)
              Posterolateral transmural (Q wave) infarction (acute)
              Posteroseptal transmural (Q wave) infarction (acute)
              Septal transmural (Q wave) infarction (acute) NOS

     I21.3   **ST elevation (STEMI) myocardial infarction of unspecified site** 🔖
              Acute transmural myocardial infarction of unspecified site
              Myocardial infarction (acute) NOS
              Transmural (Q wave) myocardial infarction NOS

     I21.4   **Non-ST elevation (NSTEMI) myocardial infarction** 🔖
              Acute subendocardial myocardial infarction
              Non-Q wave myocardial infarction NOS
              Nontransmural myocardial infarction NOS

◀ New   ◀▥ Revised   ~~deleted~~ Deleted   Excludes 1   Excludes 2   Includes   Use additional   Code first   Code also   Unspecified

OGCR Official Guidelines   ● Unacceptable Principal Diagnosis   X Assign placeholder X   ● Use Additional Character(s)   ▌ Manifestation Code   **Coding Clinic**

● **I22**   **Subsequent ST elevation (STEMI) and non-ST elevation (NSTEMI) myocardial infarction**

   Includes   acute myocardial infarction occurring within four weeks (28 days) of a previous acute myocardial infarction, regardless of site
   cardiac infarction
   coronary (artery) embolism
   coronary (artery) occlusion
   coronary (artery) rupture
   coronary (artery) thrombosis
   infarction of heart, myocardium, or ventricle
   recurrent myocardial infarction
   reinfarction of myocardium
   rupture of heart, myocardium, or ventricle

   Use additional code, if applicable, to identify:
   exposure to environmental tobacco smoke (Z77.22)
   history of tobacco use (Z87.891)
   occupational exposure to environmental tobacco smoke (Z57.31)
   status post administration of tPA (rtPA) in a different facility within the last 24 hours prior to admission to current facility (Z92.82)
   tobacco dependence (F17.-)
   tobacco use (Z72.0)

   Ⓔ **For category I22 CC codes:** I21.01-I22.9, I87.8, I99.8-I99.9

   Coding Clinic: 2012, Q4, P103

   I22.0   **Subsequent ST elevation (STEMI) myocardial infarction of anterior wall** 🅒
      Subsequent acute transmural myocardial infarction of anterior wall
      Subsequent transmural (Q wave) infarction (acute)(of) anterior (wall) NOS
      Subsequent anteroapical transmural (Q wave) infarction (acute)
      Subsequent anterolateral transmural (Q wave) infarction (acute)
      Subsequent anteroseptal transmural (Q wave) infarction (acute)

   I22.1   **Subsequent ST elevation (STEMI) myocardial infarction of inferior wall** 🅒
      Subsequent acute transmural myocardial infarction of inferior wall
      Subsequent transmural (Q wave) infarction (acute)(of) diaphragmatic wall
      Subsequent transmural (Q wave) infarction (acute)(of) inferior (wall) NOS
      Subsequent inferolateral transmural (Q wave) infarction (acute)
      Subsequent inferoposterior transmural (Q wave) infarction (acute)

      Coding Clinic: 2012, Q4, P97, 102, 104

   I22.2   **Subsequent non-ST elevation (NSTEMI) myocardial infarction** 🅒
      Subsequent acute subendocardial myocardial infarction
      Subsequent non-Q wave myocardial infarction NOS
      Subsequent nontransmural myocardial infarction NOS

   I22.8   **Subsequent ST elevation (STEMI) myocardial infarction of other sites** 🅒
      Subsequent acute transmural myocardial infarction of other sites
      Subsequent apical-lateral transmural (Q wave) myocardial infarction (acute)
      Subsequent basal-lateral transmural (Q wave) myocardial infarction (acute)
      Subsequent high lateral transmural (Q wave) myocardial infarction (acute)
      Subsequent transmural (Q wave) myocardial infarction (acute)(of) lateral (wall) NOS
      Subsequent posterior (true) transmural (Q wave) myocardial infarction (acute)
      Subsequent posterobasal transmural (Q wave) myocardial infarction (acute)
      Subsequent posterolateral transmural (Q wave) myocardial infarction (acute)
      Subsequent posteroseptal transmural (Q wave) myocardial infarction (acute)
      Subsequent septal NOS transmural (Q wave) myocardial infarction (acute)

   I22.9   **Subsequent ST elevation (STEMI) myocardial infarction of unspecified site** 🅒
      Subsequent acute myocardial infarction of unspecified site
      Subsequent myocardial infarction (acute) NOS

● **I23**   **Certain current complications following ST elevation (STEMI) and non-ST elevation (NSTEMI) myocardial infarction (within the 28 day period)**

   ~~Note: A code from category I23 must be used in conjunction with a code from category I21 or category I22. The I23 code should be sequenced first, if it is the reason for encounter, or, it should be sequenced after the I21 or I22 code if the complication of the MI occurs during the encounter for the MI.~~

   Ⓔ **For category I23 CC codes unless otherwise indicated:** E78.71-E78.72, I23.0-I23.8, I40.0-I41, I51.0-I51.4, I87.8, I97.0-I97.191, I99.8-I99.9, P29.3, Q20.0-Q21.9, Q23.8-Q23.9, Q24.8-Q24.9, Q27.30, Q27.4, Q28.0-Q28.1, Q28.8-Q28.9, Q87.1-Q87.89, Q89.7-Q89.8, Q99.2

   I23.0   **Hemopericardium as current complication following acute myocardial infarction** 🅒   A
      Excludes1   hemopericardium not specified as current complication following acute myocardial infarction (I31.2)

   I23.1   **Atrial septal defect as current complication following acute myocardial infarction** 🅒   A
      Excludes1   acquired atrial septal defect not specified as current complication following acute myocardial infarction (I51.0)

   I23.2   **Ventricular septal defect as current complication following acute myocardial infarction** 🅒   A
      Excludes1   acquired ventricular septal defect not specified as current complication following acute myocardial infarction (I51.0)

   I23.3   **Rupture of cardiac wall without hemopericardium as current complication following acute myocardial infarction** 🅒   A

N Newborn Age: 0   P Pediatric Age: 0–17   M Maternity DX: 12–55   A Adult Age: 15–124   ♀ Females Only   ♂ Males Only

🅒 Complication\Comorbidity   🅜 Major C\C   Ⓔ CC/MCC Exclusions   🅟 Present on Admission Requirement   🅗 Hospital-Acquired Condition

961

I23.4   **Rupture of chordae tendineae as current complication following acute myocardial infarction** 🔹

> **Excludes1**   rupture of chordae tendineae not specified as current complication following acute myocardial infarction (I51.1)
>
> (Ex) I23.0-I23.4, I23.6-I23.8, I51.0-I51.1, I51.3, I87.8, I99.8-I99.9

I23.5   **Rupture of papillary muscle as current complication following acute myocardial infarction** 🔹

> **Excludes1**   rupture of papillary muscle not specified as current complication following acute myocardial infarction (I51.2)
>
> (Ex) I23.0-I23.3, I23.5-I23.8, I51.0, I51.2-I51.3, I87.8, I99.8-I99.9

I23.6   **Thrombosis of atrium, auricular appendage, and ventricle as current complications following acute myocardial infarction** 🔹   A

> **Excludes1**   thrombosis of atrium, auricular appendage, and ventricle not specified as current complication following acute myocardial infarction (I51.3)

I23.7   **Postinfarction angina** 🔹   A

I23.8   **Other current complications following acute myocardial infarction** 🔹   A

● **I24**   **Other acute ischemic heart diseases**

> **Excludes1**   angina pectoris (I20.-)
> transient myocardial ischemia in newborn (P29.4)
>
> (Ex) **For category I24 CC codes unless otherwise indicated:** I20.0-I22.9, I24.0-I24.9, I25.5-I25.6, I25.89-I25.9, I87.8, I99.8-I99.9

I24.0   **Acute coronary thrombosis not resulting in myocardial infarction** 🔹

> Acute coronary (artery) (vein) embolism not resulting in myocardial infarction
> Acute coronary (artery) (vein) occlusion not resulting in myocardial infarction
> Acute coronary (artery) (vein) thromboembolism not resulting in myocardial infarction
>
> > **Excludes1**   atherosclerotic heart disease (I25.1-)

I24.1   **Dressler's syndrome** 🔹

> Postmyocardial infarction syndrome
>
> **Excludes1**   postinfarction angina (I23.7)
>
> (Ex) I24.0-I24.9, I87.8, I99.8-I99.9

I24.8   **Other forms of acute ischemic heart disease** 🔹

I24.9   **Acute ischemic heart disease, unspecified** 🔹

> **Excludes1**   ischemic heart disease (chronic) NOS (I25.9)

● **I25**   **Chronic ischemic heart disease**

> Use additional code to identify:
> chronic total occlusion of coronary artery (I25.82)
> exposure to environmental tobacco smoke (Z77.22)
> history of tobacco use (Z87.891)
> occupational exposure to environmental tobacco smoke (Z57.31)
> tobacco dependence (F17.-)
> tobacco use (Z72.0)

OGCR   See Section I.9.b.

Atherosclerotic Coronary Artery Disease and Angina

ICD-10-CM has combination codes for atherosclerotic heart disease with angina pectoris. The subcategories for these codes are I25.11, Atherosclerotic heart disease of native coronary artery with angina pectoris and I25.7, Atherosclerosis of coronary artery bypass graft(s) and coronary artery of transplanted heart with angina pectoris.

When using one of these combination codes it is not necessary to use an additional code for angina pectoris. A causal relationship can be assumed in a patient with both atherosclerosis and angina pectoris, unless the documentation indicates the angina is due to something other than the atherosclerosis.

If a patient with coronary artery disease is admitted due to an acute myocardial infarction (AMI), the AMI should be sequenced before the coronary artery disease.

See Section I.C.9. Acute myocardial infarction (AMI)

(See Plates 218 and 219 on pages 74 and 75.)

● **I25.1**   **Atherosclerotic heart disease of native coronary artery**

> *Disease in which fatty deposits form on the walls of arteries*
> Atherosclerotic cardiovascular disease
> Coronary (artery) atheroma
> Coronary (artery) atherosclerosis
> Coronary (artery) disease
> Coronary (artery) sclerosis
>
> Use additional code, if applicable, to identify:
> coronary atherosclerosis due to calcified coronary lesion (I25.84)
> coronary atherosclerosis due to lipid rich plaque (I25.83)
>
> **Excludes2**   atheroembolism (I75.-)
> atherosclerosis of coronary artery bypass graft(s) and transplanted heart (I25.7-)

I25.10   **Atherosclerotic heart disease of native coronary artery without angina pectoris**   A

> Atherosclerotic heart disease NOS
>
> **Coding Clinic: 2012, Q4, P92**

● **I25.11**   **Atherosclerotic heart disease of native coronary artery with angina pectoris**

> **I25.110**   **Atherosclerotic heart disease of native coronary artery with unstable angina pectoris** 🔹   A
>
> > **Excludes1**   unstable angina without atherosclerotic heart disease (I20.0)
>
> > CC when PDx is its own CC
> > (Ex) I09.81, I11.0, I13.0, I13.2, I20.0-I22.9, I24.0, I24.8-I24.9, I25.5-I25.6, I25.82-I25.83, I25.89-I25.9, I50.1, I50.9, I87.8, I99.8-I99.9, R57.0, R57.9
>
> **I25.111**   **Atherosclerotic heart disease of native coronary artery with angina pectoris with documented spasm**   A
>
> > **Excludes1**   angina pectoris with documented spasm without atherosclerotic heart disease (I20.1)

Item 9–6   **Classification** is based on the location of the atherosclerosis. **"Of native coronary artery"** indicates the atherosclerosis is within an original heart artery. **"Of autologous vein bypass graft"** indicates that the atherosclerosis is within a vein graft that was taken from within the patient. **"Of nonautologous biological bypass graft"** indicates the atherosclerosis is within a vessel grafted from other than the patient. **"Of artery bypass graft"** indicates the atherosclerosis is within an artery that was grafted from within the patient.

Atherosclerotic plaque (atheromas)

Figure 9-2   Atherosclerotic plaque.

◀ New   ◀ Revised   ~~deleted~~ Deleted   Excludes 1   Excludes 2   Includes   Use additional   Code first   Code also   Unspecified

OGCR Official Guidelines   ● Unacceptable Principal Diagnosis   X Assign placeholder X   🔹 Use Additional Character(s)   ▶ Manifestation Code   **Coding Clinic**

I25.118   Atherosclerotic heart disease of native coronary artery with other forms of angina pectoris   A

> **Excludes1**   other forms of angina pectoris without atherosclerotic heart disease (I20.8)

I25.119   Atherosclerotic heart disease of native coronary artery with unspecified angina pectoris   A

Atherosclerotic heart disease with angina NOS
Atherosclerotic heart disease with ischemic chest pain

> **Excludes1**   unspecified angina pectoris without atherosclerotic heart disease (I20.9)

I25.2   Old myocardial infarction 🔖
Healed myocardial infarction
Past myocardial infarction diagnosed by ECG or other investigation, but currently presenting no symptoms

I25.3   Aneurysm of heart 🔖
Mural aneurysm
Ventricular aneurysm
(Ex) I25.3-I25.41

● **I25.4   Coronary artery aneurysm and dissection**

I25.41   Coronary artery aneurysm
Coronary arteriovenous fistula, acquired

> **Excludes1**   congenital coronary (artery) aneurysm (Q24.5)

I25.42   Coronary artery dissection 🔖
(Ex) I25.42, I67.0, I77.2-I77.3, I77.5-I77.6, I77.79, I77.89-I77.9, M31.8-M31.9

I25.5   Ischemic cardiomyopathy

> **Excludes2**   coronary atherosclerosis (I25.1-, I25.7-)

I25.6   Silent myocardial ischemia

● **I25.7   Atherosclerosis of coronary artery bypass graft(s) and coronary artery of transplanted heart with angina pectoris**

Use additional code, if applicable, to identify:
coronary atherosclerosis due to calcified coronary lesion (I25.84)
coronary atherosclerosis due to lipid rich plaque (I25.83)

> **Excludes1**   atherosclerosis of bypass graft(s) of transplanted heart without angina pectoris (I25.812)
> atherosclerosis of coronary artery bypass graft(s) without angina pectoris (I25.810)
> atherosclerosis of native coronary artery of transplanted heart without angina pectoris (I25.811)
> embolism or thrombus of coronary artery bypass graft(s) (T82.8-)

● **I25.70   Atherosclerosis of coronary artery bypass graft(s), unspecified, with angina pectoris**

I25.700   Atherosclerosis of coronary artery bypass graft(s), unspecified, with unstable angina pectoris 🔖   A

> **Excludes1**   unstable angina pectoris without atherosclerosis of coronary artery bypass graft (I20.0)

CC when PDx is its own CC
(Ex) See I25.11

I25.701   Atherosclerosis of coronary artery bypass graft(s), unspecified, with angina pectoris with documented spasm   A

> **Excludes1**   angina pectoris with documented spasm without atherosclerosis of coronary artery bypass graft (I20.1)

I25.708   Atherosclerosis of coronary artery bypass graft(s), unspecified, with other forms of angina pectoris   A

> **Excludes1**   other forms of angina pectoris without atherosclerosis of coronary artery bypass graft (I20.8)

I25.709   Atherosclerosis of coronary artery bypass graft(s), unspecified, with unspecified angina pectoris   A

> **Excludes1**   unspecified angina pectoris without atherosclerosis of coronary artery bypass graft (I20.9)

● **I25.71   Atherosclerosis of autologous vein coronary artery bypass graft(s) with angina pectoris**
(Ex) For category I25.71 CC codes unless otherwise indicated: I25.10-I25.119, I25.700-I25.739, I25.760-I25.799, I25.812-I25.84

I25.710   Atherosclerosis of autologous vein coronary artery bypass graft(s) with unstable angina pectoris 🔖   A

> **Excludes1**   unstable angina without atherosclerosis of autologous vein coronary artery bypass graft(s) (I20.0)

CC when PDx is its own CC
(Ex) I09.81, I11.0, I13.0, I13.2, I20.0-I22.9, I24.0, I24.8-I25.119, I25.5-I25.739, I25.760-I25.799, I25.812-I25.9, I50.1, I50.9, I87.8, I99.8-I99.9, R57.0, R57.9

I25.711   Atherosclerosis of autologous vein coronary artery bypass graft(s) with angina pectoris with documented spasm 🔖   A

> **Excludes1**   angina pectoris with documented spasm without atherosclerosis of autologous vein coronary artery bypass graft(s) (I20.1)

CHAPTER 9 (I00-I99)

I25.718 **Atherosclerosis of autologous vein coronary artery bypass graft(s) with other forms of angina pectoris** 🕭 A

Excludes1 other forms of angina pectoris without atherosclerosis of autologous vein coronary artery bypass graft(s) (I20.8) ◄▥

I25.719 **Atherosclerosis of autologous vein coronary artery bypass graft(s) with unspecified angina pectoris** 🕭 A

Excludes1 unspecified angina pectoris without atherosclerosis of autologous vein coronary artery bypass graft(s) (I20.9)

● **I25.72** **Atherosclerosis of autologous artery coronary artery bypass graft(s) with angina pectoris**
Atherosclerosis of internal mammary artery graft with angina pectoris
Ex For category I25.72 CC codes unless otherwise indicated: See I25.71

I25.720 **Atherosclerosis of autologous artery coronary artery bypass graft(s) with unstable angina pectoris** 🕭 A

Excludes1 unstable angina without atherosclerosis of autologous artery coronary artery bypass graft(s) (I20.0)
CC when PDx is its own CC
Ex See I25.710

I25.721 **Atherosclerosis of autologous artery coronary artery bypass graft(s) with angina pectoris with documented spasm** 🕭 A

Excludes1 angina pectoris with documented spasm without atherosclerosis of autologous artery coronary artery bypass graft(s) (I20.1)

I25.728 **Atherosclerosis of autologous artery coronary artery bypass graft(s) with other forms of angina pectoris** 🕭 A

Excludes1 other forms of angina pectoris without atherosclerosis of autologous artery coronary artery bypass graft(s) (I20.8)

I25.729 **Atherosclerosis of autologous artery coronary artery bypass graft(s) with unspecified angina pectoris** 🕭 A

Excludes1 unspecified angina pectoris without atherosclerosis of autologous artery coronary artery bypass graft(s) (I20.9)

● **I25.73** **Atherosclerosis of nonautologous biological coronary artery bypass graft(s) with angina pectoris**
Ex For category I25.73 CC codes unless otherwise indicated: See I25.71

I25.730 **Atherosclerosis of nonautologous biological coronary artery bypass graft(s) with unstable angina pectoris** 🕭 A

Excludes1 unstable angina without atherosclerosis of nonautologous biological coronary artery bypass graft(s) (I20.0)
CC when PDx is its own CC
Ex See I25.710

I25.731 **Atherosclerosis of nonautologous biological coronary artery bypass graft(s) with angina pectoris with documented spasm** 🕭 A

Excludes1 angina pectoris with documented spasm without atherosclerosis of nonautologous biological coronary artery bypass graft(s) (I20.1)

I25.738 **Atherosclerosis of nonautologous biological coronary artery bypass graft(s) with other forms of angina pectoris** 🕭 A

Excludes1 other forms of angina pectoris without atherosclerosis of nonautologous biological coronary artery bypass graft(s) (I20.8)

I25.739 **Atherosclerosis of nonautologous biological coronary artery bypass graft(s) with unspecified angina pectoris** 🕭 A

Excludes1 unspecified angina pectoris without atherosclerosis of nonautologous biological coronary artery bypass graft(s) (I20.9)

● **I25.75** **Atherosclerosis of native coronary artery of transplanted heart with angina pectoris**

Excludes1 atherosclerosis of native coronary artery of transplanted heart without angina pectoris (I25.811)
Ex For category I25.75 CC codes unless otherwise indicated: I25.10-I25.119, I25.700-I25.799, I25.811-I25.84

I25.750 **Atherosclerosis of native coronary artery of transplanted heart with unstable angina** 🕭
CC when PDx is its own CC
Ex I09.81, I11.0, I13.0, I13.2, I20.0-I22.9, I24.0, I24.8-I25.119, I25.5-I25.799, I25.811-I25.9, I50.1, I50.9, I87.8, I99.8-I99.9, R57.0, R57.9

I25.751 **Atherosclerosis of native coronary artery of transplanted heart with angina pectoris with documented spasm** 🕭

◄ New   ◄▥ Revised   ~~deleted~~ Deleted   Excludes 1   Excludes 2   Includes   Use additional   Code first   Code also   Unspecified
OGCR Official Guidelines   ● Unacceptable Principal Diagnosis   X Assign placeholder X   ● Use Additional Character(s)   ▶ Manifestation Code   **Coding Clinic**

CHAPTER 9 (I00-I99)

I25.758   Atherosclerosis of native coronary artery of transplanted heart with other forms of angina pectoris 🔹

I25.759   Atherosclerosis of native coronary artery of transplanted heart with unspecified angina pectoris 🔹

● I25.76   Atherosclerosis of bypass graft of coronary artery of transplanted heart with angina pectoris

     Excludes1   atherosclerosis of bypass graft of coronary artery of transplanted heart without angina pectoris (I25.812)

     (Ex) For category I25.76 CC codes unless otherwise indicated: I25.10-I25.119, I25.700-I25.759, I25.790-I25.799, I25.811, I25.82-I25.84

I25.760   Atherosclerosis of bypass graft of coronary artery of transplanted heart with unstable angina 🔹   A
     CC when PDx is its own CC
     (Ex) I09.81, I11.0, I13.0, I13.2, I20.0-I22.9, I24.0, I24.8-I25.119, I25.5-I25.759, I25.790-I25.799, I25.811, I25.82-I25.9, I50.1, I50.9, I87.8, I99.8-I99.9, R57.0, R57.9

I25.761   Atherosclerosis of bypass graft of coronary artery of transplanted heart with angina pectoris with documented spasm 🔹   A

I25.768   Atherosclerosis of bypass graft of coronary artery of transplanted heart with other forms of angina pectoris 🔹   A

I25.769   Atherosclerosis of bypass graft of coronary artery of transplanted heart with unspecified angina pectoris 🔹   A

● I25.79   Atherosclerosis of other coronary artery bypass graft(s) with angina pectoris   A

     (Ex) For category I25.79 CC codes unless otherwise indicated: No exclusions

I25.790   Atherosclerosis of other coronary artery bypass graft(s) with unstable angina pectoris 🔹

     Excludes1   unstable angina without atherosclerosis of other coronary artery bypass graft(s) (I20.0)
     CC when PDx is its own CC
     (Ex) See I25.11

I25.791   Atherosclerosis of other coronary artery bypass graft(s) with angina pectoris with documented spasm 🔹   A

     Excludes1   angina pectoris with documented spasm without atherosclerosis of other coronary artery bypass graft(s) (I20.1)

I25.798   Atherosclerosis of other coronary artery bypass graft(s) with other forms of angina pectoris 🔹   A

     Excludes1   other forms of angina pectoris without atherosclerosis of other coronary artery bypass graft(s) (I20.8) ◄━━

I25.799   Atherosclerosis of other coronary artery bypass graft(s) with unspecified angina pectoris 🔹   A

     Excludes1   unspecified angina pectoris without atherosclerosis of other coronary artery bypass graft(s) (I20.9)

● I25.8   Other forms of chronic ischemic heart disease

   ● I25.81   Atherosclerosis of other coronary vessels without angina pectoris

     Use additional code, if applicable, to identify:
     coronary atherosclerosis due to calcified coronary lesion (I25.84)
     coronary atherosclerosis due to lipid rich plaque (I25.83)

     Excludes1   atherosclerotic heart disease of native coronary artery without angina pectoris (I25.10)

I25.810   Atherosclerosis of coronary artery bypass graft(s) without angina pectoris 🔹   A
     Atherosclerosis of coronary artery bypass graft NOS

     Excludes1   atherosclerosis of coronary bypass graft(s) with angina pectoris (I25.70- -I25.73-, I25.79-)

     (Ex) No exclusions

I25.811   Atherosclerosis of native coronary artery of transplanted heart without angina pectoris 🔹
     Atherosclerosis of native coronary artery of transplanted heart NOS

     Excludes1   atherosclerosis of native coronary artery of transplanted heart with angina pectoris (I25.75-)

     (Ex) See I25.75

I25.812   Atherosclerosis of bypass graft of coronary artery of transplanted heart without angina pectoris 🔹   A
     Atherosclerosis of bypass graft of transplanted heart NOS

     Excludes1   atherosclerosis of bypass graft of transplanted heart with angina pectoris (I25.76)

   ● I25.82   Chronic total occlusion of coronary artery
     Complete occlusion of coronary artery
     Total occlusion of coronary artery
     Code first coronary atherosclerosis (I25.1-, I25.7-, I25.81-)

     Excludes1   acute coronary occlusion with myocardial infarction (I21.-, I22.-)
     acute coronary occlusion without myocardial infarction (I24.0)

     (Ex) See I25.76

   ● I25.83   Coronary atherosclerosis due to lipid rich plaque   A

     Code first coronary atherosclerosis (I25.1-, I25.7-, I25.81-)

N   Newborn Age: 0   P   Pediatric Age: 0–17   M   Maternity DX: 12–55   A   Adult Age: 15–124   ♀   Females Only   ♂   Males Only

🔹 Complication\Comorbidity   🔹 Major C\C   (Ex) CC/MCC Exclusions   🔹 Present on Admission Requirement   🔹 Hospital-Acquired Condition

965

CHAPTER 9 (I00–I99)

Item 9–7 Pulmonary heart disease or **cor pulmonale** is right ventricle hypertrophy or RVH as a result of a respiratory disorder increasing back flow pressure to the right ventricle. Left untreated, cor pulmonale leads to right-heart failure and death.

●● I25.84   **Coronary atherosclerosis due to calcified coronary lesion**
         Coronary atherosclerosis due to severely calcified coronary lesion
         Code first coronary atherosclerosis (I25.1-, I25.7-, I25.81-)

   I25.89   **Other forms of chronic ischemic heart disease**

   I25.9   **Chronic ischemic heart disease, unspecified**
         Ischemic heart disease (chronic) NOS

PULMONARY HEART DISEASE AND DISEASES OF PULMONARY CIRCULATION (I26-I28)

● I26   **Pulmonary embolism**

   Includes   pulmonary (acute)(artery)(vein) infarction
           pulmonary (acute)(artery)(vein) thromboembolism
           pulmonary (acute)(artery)(vein) thrombosis

   Excludes2   chronic pulmonary embolism (I27.82)
           personal history of pulmonary embolism (Z86.711)
           pulmonary embolism due to trauma (T79.0, T79.1)
           pulmonary embolism due to complications of surgical and medical care (T80.0, T81.7-, T82.8-)
           pulmonary embolism complicating abortion, ectopic or molar pregnancy (O00-O07, O08.2) ◀
           pulmonary embolism complicating pregnancy, childbirth and the puerperium (O88.-) ◀
           ~~pulmonary embolism complicating:~~
             ~~abortion, ectopic or molar pregnancy (O00-O07, O08.2)~~
             ~~pregnancy, childbirth and the puerperium (O88.-)~~
           septic (non-pulmonary) arterial embolism (I76)

● I26.0   **Pulmonary embolism with acute cor pulmonale**
      (Ex:) For category I26.0 CC codes: I26.01-I26.99, I27.2-I27.9, I74.01-I74.10, I74.19, I87.8, I99.8-I99.9

     ● I26.01   **Septic pulmonary embolism with acute cor pulmonale** 🔒
         Code first underlying infection
         MCC when PDx is its own MCC

     I26.02   **Saddle embolus of pulmonary artery with acute cor pulmonale** 🔒🔒
         MCC when PDx is its own MCC

     I26.09   **Other pulmonary embolism with acute cor pulmonale** 🔒🔒
         Acute cor pulmonale NOS
         MCC when PDx is its own MCC

● I26.9   **Pulmonary embolism without acute cor pulmonale**

     ● I26.90   **Septic pulmonary embolism without acute cor pulmonale** 🔒
         Code first underlying infection
         (Ex:) I26.01-I26.99, I27.82, I74.01-I74.10, I74.19, I87.8, I99.8-I99.9, T80.0XX[A], T81.718[A], T81.72X[A,] T82.817-T82.818[A]

     I26.92   **Saddle embolus of pulmonary artery without acute cor pulmonale** 🔒 🔒
         (Ex:) I26.01-I26.99, I27.82, I74.01-I74.10, I74.19, I87.8, I99.8-I99.9

     I26.99   **Other pulmonary embolism without acute cor pulmonale** 🔒 🔒
         Acute pulmonary embolism NOS
         Pulmonary embolism NOS
         (Ex:) I26.01-I26.99, I27.82, I74.01-I74.10, I74.19, I87.8, I99.8-I99.9, T80.0XX[A], T81.718[A], T81.72X[A], T82.817-T82.818[A]

● I27   **Other pulmonary heart diseases**

   I27.0   **Primary pulmonary hypertension** 🔒
     Excludes1   pulmonary hypertension NOS (I27.2)
           secondary pulmonary hypertension (I27.2)
     (Ex:) E66.2, I27.0, I27.2-I27.81, I27.89-I27.9, I28.8-I28.9, I87.8, I99.8-I99.9

   I27.1   **Kyphoscoliotic heart disease** 🔒
     (Ex:) E66.2, I27.0-I27.81, I27.89-I27.9

   I27.2   **Other secondary pulmonary hypertension**
         Pulmonary hypertension NOS
         Code also associated underlying condition

● I27.8   **Other specified pulmonary heart diseases**

     I27.81   **Cor pulmonale (chronic)**
         Cor pulmonale NOS
       Excludes1   acute cor pulmonale (I26.0-)

     I27.82   **Chronic pulmonary embolism** 🔒
         Use additional code, if applicable, for associated long-term (current) use of anticoagulants (Z79.01)
       Excludes1   personal history of pulmonary embolism (Z86.711)
       (Ex:) See I26.92

     I27.89   **Other specified pulmonary heart diseases**
         Eisenmenger's complex
         Eisenmenger's syndrome
       Excludes1   Eisenmenger's defect (Q21.8)

   I27.9   **Pulmonary heart disease, unspecified**
         Chronic cardiopulmonary disease

● I28   **Other diseases of pulmonary vessels**
   (Ex:) For category I28 CC codes: I28.0-I28.9

   I28.0   **Arteriovenous fistula of pulmonary vessels** 🔒
     Excludes1   congenital arteriovenous fistula (Q25.72)

   I28.1   **Aneurysm of pulmonary artery** 🔒
     Excludes1   congenital aneurysm (Q25.79)
           congenital arteriovenous aneurysm (Q25.72)

   I28.8   **Other diseases of pulmonary vessels**
         Pulmonary arteritis
         Pulmonary endarteritis
         Rupture of pulmonary vessels
         Stenosis of pulmonary vessels
         Stricture of pulmonary vessels

   I28.9   **Disease of pulmonary vessels, unspecified**

OTHER FORMS OF HEART DISEASE (I30-I52)

● I30   **Acute pericarditis**
     Inflammation of pericardium (sac surrounding the heart) caused by an infection.

   Includes   acute mediastinopericarditis
           acute myopericarditis
           acute pericardial effusion
           acute pleuropericarditis
           acute pneumopericarditis

   Excludes1   Dressler's syndrome (I24.1)
           rheumatic pericarditis (acute) (I01.0)
   (Ex:) For category I30 CC codes: I01.0, I09.2, I30.0-I30.9, I31.3-I32, I87.8, I99.8-I99.9

   I30.0   **Acute nonspecific idiopathic pericarditis** 🔒

   I30.1   **Infective pericarditis** 🔒
         Pneumococcal pericarditis
         Pneumopyopericardium
         Purulent pericarditis
         Pyopericarditis
         Pyopericardium
         Pyopneumopericardium
         Staphylococcal pericarditis
         Streptococcal pericarditis
         Suppurative pericarditis
         Viral pericarditis
         Use additional code (B95-B97) to identify infectious agent

   I30.8   **Other forms of acute pericarditis** 🔒

   I30.9   **Acute pericarditis, unspecified** 🔒

◀ New   ◀▦ Revised   ~~deleted~~ Deleted   Excludes 1   Excludes 2   Includes   Use additional   Code first   Code also   Unspecified

OGCR Official Guidelines   ● Unacceptable Principal Diagnosis   X Assign placeholder X   ● Use Additional Character(s)   ▶ Manifestation Code   **Coding Clinic**

● **I31**   **Other diseases of pericardium**

> **Excludes1**   diseases of pericardium specified as rheumatic (I09.2)
> postcardiotomy syndrome (I97.0)
> traumatic injury to pericardium (S26.-)

> (Ex) For category I31 CC codes unless otherwise indicated: B33.23, I01.0, I09.2, I30.0-I30.9, I31.3-I32, I87.8, I99.8-I99.9

I31.0   **Chronic adhesive pericarditis** 🔖
> Accretio cordis
> Adherent pericardium
> Adhesive mediastinopericarditis
> (Ex) I31.0-I31.9, I87.8, I99.8-I99.9

I31.1   **Chronic constrictive pericarditis** 🔖
> Concretio cordis
> Pericardial calcification
> (Ex) I31.0-I31.9, I87.8, I99.8-I99.9

I31.2   **Hemopericardium, not elsewhere classified** 🔖
> **Excludes1**   hemopericardium as current complication following acute myocardial infarction (I23.0)
> (Ex) I31.0-I31.9, I87.8, I99.8-I99.9

I31.3   **Pericardial effusion (noninflammatory)** 🔖
> Chylopericardium
> **Excludes1**   acute pericardial effusion (I30.9)

● **I31.4**   **Cardiac tamponade** 🔖
> *Code first* underlying cause

I31.8   **Other specified diseases of pericardium** 🔖
> Epicardial plaques
> Focal pericardial adhesions

I31.9   **Disease of pericardium, unspecified** 🔖
> Pericarditis (chronic) NOS

▷ *I32*   *Pericarditis in diseases classified elsewhere* 🔖
> *Code first* underlying disease
> **Excludes1**   pericarditis (in):
> coxsackie (virus) (B33.23)
> gonococcal (A54.83)
> meningococcal (A39.53)
> rheumatoid (arthritis) (M05.31)
> syphilitic (A52.06)
> systemic lupus erythematosus (M32.12)
> tuberculosis (A18.84)

> (Ex) See I30

● **I33**   **Acute and subacute endocarditis**

> *Inflammation/infection of lining of heart, affecting heart valves including replacement valves and is usually caused by a bacterial infection*

> **Excludes1**   acute rheumatic endocarditis (I01.1)
> endocarditis NOS (I38)

> (Ex) For category I33 CC codes: I01.1, I08.1-I08.3, I09.1, I33.0-I33.9, I38-I39, I87.8, I99.8-I99.9

I33.0   **Acute and subacute infective endocarditis** 🔖
> Bacterial endocarditis (acute) (subacute)
> Infective endocarditis (acute) (subacute) NOS
> Endocarditis lenta (acute) (subacute)
> Malignant endocarditis (acute) (subacute)
> Purulent endocarditis (acute) (subacute)
> Septic endocarditis (acute) (subacute)
> Ulcerative endocarditis (acute) (subacute)
> Vegetative endocarditis (acute) (subacute)
> Use additional code (B95-B97) to identify infectious agent

I33.9   **Acute and subacute endocarditis, unspecified** 🔖
> Acute endocarditis NOS
> Acute myoendocarditis NOS
> Acute periendocarditis NOS
> Subacute endocarditis NOS
> Subacute myoendocarditis NOS
> Subacute periendocarditis NOS

● **I34**   **Nonrheumatic mitral valve disorders**

> **Excludes1**   mitral valve disease (I05.9)
> mitral valve failure (I05.8)
> mitral valve stenosis (I05.0)
> mitral valve disorder of unspecified cause with diseases of aortic and/or tricuspid valve(s) (I08.-)
> mitral valve disorder of unspecified cause with mitral stenosis or obstruction (I05.0)
> mitral valve disorder specified as congenital (Q23.2, Q23.3)
> mitral valve disorder specified as rheumatic (I05.-)

I34.0   **Nonrheumatic mitral (valve) insufficiency**
> Nonrheumatic mitral (valve) incompetence NOS
> Nonrheumatic mitral (valve) regurgitation NOS

I34.1   **Nonrheumatic mitral (valve) prolapse**
> Floppy nonrheumatic mitral valve syndrome
> **Excludes1**   Marfan's syndrome (Q87.4-)

I34.2   **Nonrheumatic mitral (valve) stenosis**

I34.8   **Other nonrheumatic mitral valve disorders**

I34.9   **Nonrheumatic mitral valve disorder, unspecified**

● **I35**   **Nonrheumatic aortic valve disorders**

> **Excludes1**   aortic valve disorder of unspecified cause but with diseases of mitral and/or tricuspid valve(s) (I08.-)
> aortic valve disorder specified as congenital (Q23.0, Q23.1)
> aortic valve disorder specified as rheumatic (I06.-)
> hypertrophic subaortic stenosis (I42.1)

I35.0   **Nonrheumatic aortic (valve) stenosis**

I35.1   **Nonrheumatic aortic (valve) insufficiency**
> Nonrheumatic aortic (valve) incompetence NOS
> Nonrheumatic aortic (valve) regurgitation NOS

I35.2   **Nonrheumatic aortic (valve) stenosis with insufficiency**

I35.8   **Other nonrheumatic aortic valve disorders**

I35.9   **Nonrheumatic aortic valve disorder, unspecified**

● **I36**   **Nonrheumatic tricuspid valve disorders**

> **Excludes1**   tricuspid valve disorders of unspecified cause (I07.-)
> tricuspid valve disorders specified as congenital (Q22.4, Q22.8, Q22.9)
> tricuspid valve disorders specified as rheumatic (I07.-)
> tricuspid valve disorders with aortic and/or mitral valve involvement (I08.-)

I36.0   **Nonrheumatic tricuspid (valve) stenosis**

I36.1   **Nonrheumatic tricuspid (valve) insufficiency**
> Nonrheumatic tricuspid (valve) incompetence
> Nonrheumatic tricuspid (valve) regurgitation

I36.2   **Nonrheumatic tricuspid (valve) stenosis with insufficiency**

I36.8   **Other nonrheumatic tricuspid valve disorders**

I36.9   **Nonrheumatic tricuspid valve disorder, unspecified**

● **I37**   **Nonrheumatic pulmonary valve disorders**

> **Excludes1**   pulmonary valve disorder specified as congenital (Q22.1, Q22.2, Q22.3)
> pulmonary valve disorder specified as rheumatic (I09.89)

I37.0   **Nonrheumatic pulmonary valve stenosis**

I37.1   **Nonrheumatic pulmonary valve insufficiency**
> Nonrheumatic pulmonary valve incompetence
> Nonrheumatic pulmonary valve regurgitation

I37.2   **Nonrheumatic pulmonary valve stenosis with insufficiency**

I37.8   **Other nonrheumatic pulmonary valve disorders**

I37.9   **Nonrheumatic pulmonary valve disorder, unspecified**

N Newborn Age: 0   **P** Pediatric Age: 0–17   **M** Maternity DX: 12–55   **A** Adult Age: 15–124   ♀ Females Only   ♂ Males Only

🔖 Complication\Comorbidity   🔖 Major C\C   (Ex) CC/MCC Exclusions   🔖 Present on Admission Requirement   🔖 Hospital-Acquired Condition

967

I38   Endocarditis, valve unspecified 🔍

    Includes   endocarditis (chronic) NOS
               valvular incompetence NOS
               valvular insufficiency NOS
               valvular regurgitation NOS
               valvular stenosis NOS
               valvulitis (chronic) NOS

    Excludes1   congenital insufficiency of cardiac valve NOS
                 (Q24.8)
               congenital stenosis of cardiac valve NOS (Q24.8)
               endocardial fibroelastosis (I42.4)
               endocarditis specified as rheumatic (I09.1)
    (Ex:) I38-I39, I87.8, I99.8-I99.9

I39   Endocarditis and heart valve disorders in diseases classified elsewhere 🔍

    Code first underlying disease, such as:
       Q fever (A78)

    Excludes1   endocardial involvement in:
               candidiasis (B37.6)
               gonococcal infection (A54.83)
               Libman-Sacks disease (M32.11)
               listerosis (A32.82)
               meningococcal infection (A39.51)
               rheumatoid arthritis (M05.31)
               syphilis (A52.03)
               tuberculosis (A18.84)
               typhoid fever (A01.02)
    (Ex:) I38-I39, I87.8, I99.8-I99.9

● I40   Acute myocarditis

    Inflammation of heart muscle due to infection (viral/bacterial).

    Includes   subacute myocarditis

    Excludes1   acute rheumatic myocarditis (I01.2)
    (Ex:) For category I40 CC codes: I01.2, I09.0, I23.0-I23.3, I23.6-I23.8, I40.0-I41, I51.0, I51.3-I51.4, I87.8, I99.8-I99.9

    I40.0   **Infective myocarditis** 🔍
           Septic myocarditis

           Use additional code (B95-B97) to identify infectious
                 agent

    I40.1   **Isolated myocarditis** 🔍
           Fiedler's myocarditis
           Giant cell myocarditis
           Idiopathic myocarditis

    I40.8   **Other acute myocarditis** 🔍

    I40.9   **Acute myocarditis, unspecified** 🔍

I41   Myocarditis in diseases classified elsewhere 🔍

    Code first underlying disease, such as:
       typhus (A75.0-A75.9)

    Excludes1   myocarditis (in):
               Chagas' disease (chronic) (B57.2)
               acute (B57.0)
               coxsackie (virus) infection (B33.22)
               diphtheritic (A36.81)
               gonococcal (A54.83)
               influenzal (J09.X9, J10.82, J11.82)
               meningococcal (A39.52)
               mumps (B26.82)
               rheumatoid arthritis (M05.31)
               sarcoid (D86.85)
               syphilis (A52.06)
               toxoplasmosis (B58.81)
               tuberculous (A18.84)
    (Ex:) See I40

● I42   Cardiomyopathy

    Disease of the heart muscle resulting in an abnormally enlarged, weakened, thickened, and/or stiffened muscles

    Includes   myocardiopathy

    Code first pre-existing cardiomyopathy complicating pregnancy and puerperium (O99.4) ◀

    Excludes1   ischemic cardiomyopathy (I25.5)
               peripartum cardiomyopathy (O90.3)

    Excludes2   ventricular hypertrophy (I51.7)
    (Ex:) For category I42 CC codes: I09.81, I11.0, I13.0, I13.2, I25.10-I25.119, I25.5-I25.799, I25.811-I25.9, I42.0-I44.1, I44.30-I44.39, I45.2-I45.4, I45.81-I45.89, I48.0-I49.1, I49.3-I49.8, I50.1, I50.9, I87.8, I99.8-I99.9, Q24.6, R00.0-R00.2, R57.0, R57.9

    I42.0   **Dilated cardiomyopathy** 🔍
           Congestive cardiomyopathy

    I42.1   **Obstructive hypertrophic cardiomyopathy** 🔍
           Hypertrophic subaortic stenosis (idiopathic)

    I42.2   **Other hypertrophic cardiomyopathy** 🔍
           Nonobstructive hypertrophic cardiomyopathy

    I42.3   **Endomyocardial (eosinophilic) disease** 🔍
           Endomyocardial (tropical) fibrosis
           Löffler's endocarditis

    I42.4   **Endocardial fibroelastosis** 🔍
           Congenital cardiomyopathy
           Elastomyofibrosis

    I42.5   **Other restrictive cardiomyopathy** 🔍
           Constrictive cardiomyopathy NOS

    I42.6   **Alcoholic cardiomyopathy** 🔍
           Code also presence of alcoholism (F10.-)

    I42.7   **Cardiomyopathy due to drug and external agent** 🔍
           Code first poisoning due to drug or toxin, if applicable (T36-T65 with fifth or sixth character 1-4 or 6)
           Use additional code for adverse effect, if applicable, to identify drug (T36-T50 with fifth or sixth character 5)

    I42.8   **Other cardiomyopathies** 🔍

    I42.9   **Cardiomyopathy, unspecified** 🔍
           Cardiomyopathy (primary) (secondary) NOS

I43   Cardiomyopathy in diseases classified elsewhere 🔍

    Code first underlying disease, such as:
       amyloidosis (E85.-) ◀
       glycogen storage disease (E74.0)
       gout (M10.0-)
       thyrotoxicosis (E05.0-E05.9-)

    Excludes1   cardiomyopathy (in):
               coxsackie (virus) (B33.24)
               diphtheria (A36.81)
               sarcoidosis (D86.85)
               tuberculosis (A18.84)
    (Ex:) See I42

● I44   Atrioventricular and left bundle-branch block

    Conduction problem resulting in arrhythmias/dysrhythmias due to a lack of electrical impulses being transmitted normally through the heart.

    I44.0   **Atrioventricular block, first degree**

    I44.1   **Atrioventricular block, second degree**
           Atrioventricular block, type I and II
           Möbitz block, type I and II
           Second degree block, type I and II
           Wenckebach's block

    I44.2   **Atrioventricular block, complete** 🔍
           Complete heart block NOS
           Third degree block
           (Ex:) I44.0-I49.02, I49.2, I49.8, I87.8, I99.8-I99.9, R00.1

    ● I44.3   **Other and unspecified atrioventricular block**
           Atrioventricular block NOS

        I44.30   **Unspecified atrioventricular block**

        I44.39   **Other atrioventricular block**

◀ New   ◀⋯ Revised   ~~deleted~~ Deleted   Excludes 1   Excludes 2   Includes   Use additional   Code first   Code also   Unspecified

OGCR Official Guidelines   ● Unacceptable Principal Diagnosis   X Assign placeholder X   ● Use Additional Character(s)   ▌ Manifestation Code   **Coding Clinic**

CHAPTER 9 (I00-I99)

I44.4   **Left anterior fascicular block**
       MCE: Questionable admission when principal dx

I44.5   **Left posterior fascicular block**
       MCE: Questionable admission when principal dx

● **I44.6**   **Other and unspecified fascicular block**

     I44.60   `Unspecified` **fascicular block**
           Left bundle-branch hemiblock NOS
           MCE: Questionable admission when principal dx

     I44.69   **Other fascicular block**
           MCE: Questionable admission when principal dx

I44.7   **Left bundle-branch block,** `unspecified`
       MCE: Questionable admission when principal dx

● **I45**   **Other conduction disorders**

   I45.0   **Right fascicular block**
       MCE: Questionable admission when principal dx

● **I45.1**   **Other and unspecified right bundle-branch block**

     I45.10   `Unspecified` **right bundle-branch block**
           Right bundle-branch block NOS
           MCE: Questionable admission when principal dx

     I45.19   **Other right bundle-branch block**
           MCE: Questionable admission when principal dx

   I45.2   **Bifascicular block** 🔖
       (Ex) See I44.2

   I45.3   **Trifascicular block** 🔖
       (Ex) See I44.2

   I45.4   **Nonspecific intraventricular block**
       Bundle-branch block NOS

   I45.5   **Other specified heart block**
       Sinoatrial block
       Sinoauricular block

     Excludes1   heart block NOS (I45.9)

   I45.6   **Pre-excitation syndrome**
       Accelerated atrioventricular conduction
       Accessory atrioventricular conduction
       Anomalous atrioventricular excitation
       Lown-Ganong-Levine syndrome
       Pre-excitation atrioventricular conduction
       Wolff-Parkinson-White syndrome

● **I45.8**   **Other specified conduction disorders**

     I45.81   **Long QT syndrome**

     I45.89   **Other specified conduction disorders** 🔖
           Atrioventricular [AV] dissociation
           Interference dissociation
           Isorhythmic dissociation
           Nonparoxysmal AV nodal tachycardia
           (Ex) See I44.2

   I45.9   **Conduction disorder,** `unspecified`
       Heart block NOS
       Stokes-Adams syndrome

● **I46**   **Cardiac arrest**

     Excludes1   cardiogenic shock (R57.0)

     (Ex) **For category I46 CC codes:** I46.2-I49.02, I49.2, I87.8, I99.8-I99.9

   I46.2   **Cardiac arrest due to underlying cardiac condition** 🔖
       Code first underlying cardiac condition
       MCC: If patient discharged alive

   I46.8   **Cardiac arrest due to other underlying condition** 🔖
       Code first underlying condition
       MCC: If patient discharged alive

   I46.9   **Cardiac arrest, cause** `unspecified` 🔖
       MCC: If patient discharged alive

● **I47**   **Paroxysmal tachycardia**
       Code first tachycardia complicating:
           abortion or ectopic or molar pregnancy (O00-O07, O08.8)
           obstetric surgery and procedures (O75.4)

     Excludes1   tachycardia NOS (R00.0) ⬅
           sinoauricular tachycardia NOS (R00.0) ⬅
           sinus [sinusal] tachycardia NOS (R00.0) ⬅
           ~~sinus [sinusal] NOS (R00.0)~~

     (Ex) **For category I47 CC codes:** See I44.2

   I47.0   **Re-entry ventricular arrhythmia** 🔖

   I47.1   **Supraventricular tachycardia** 🔖
       Atrial (paroxysmal) tachycardia
       Atrioventricular [AV] (paroxysmal) tachycardia
       Atrioventricular re-entrant (nodal) tachycardia
           [AVNRT] [AVRT]
       Junctional (paroxysmal) tachycardia
       Nodal (paroxysmal) tachycardia

   I47.2   **Ventricular tachycardia** 🔖

   I47.9   **Paroxysmal tachycardia,** `unspecified`
       Bouveret (-Hoffman) syndrome

● **I48**   **Atrial fibrillation and flutter**
       Most common abnormal heart rhythm (arrhythmia) presenting
       as irregular, rapid beating (tachycardia) of the heart's upper
       chamber.
     (Ex) **For category I48 CC codes:** See I44.2

   I48.0   **Paroxysmal atrial fibrillation**

   I48.1   **Persistent atrial fibrillation** 🔖
       Rapid contractions of the upper heart chamber

   I48.2   **Chronic atrial fibrillation**
       Permanent atrial fibrillation

   I48.3   **Typical atrial flutter** 🔖
       Type I atrial flutter

   I48.4   **Atypical atrial flutter** 🔖
       Type II atrial flutter

● **I48.9**   **Unspecified atrial fibrillation and atrial flutter**

     I48.91   `Unspecified` **atrial fibrillation**

     I48.92   `Unspecified` **atrial flutter** 🔖

● **I49**   **Other cardiac arrhythmias**
       Code first cardiac arrhythmia complicating:
           abortion or ectopic or molar pregnancy (O00-O07, O08.8)
           obstetric surgery and procedures (O75.4)

     Excludes1   bradycardia NOS (R00.1) ⬅
           ~~NOS (R00.1)~~
           ~~sinoatrial (R00.1)~~
           ~~sinus (R00.1)~~
           ~~vagal (R00.1)~~
           neonatal dysrhythmia (P29.1-)
           sinoatrial bradycardia (R00.1) ◀
           sinus bradycardia (R00.1) ◀
           vagal bradycardia (R00.1) ◀

● **I49.0**   **Ventricular fibrillation and flutter**

     I49.01   **Ventricular fibrillation** 🔖
           MCC: If patient discharged alive
           (Ex) See I44.2

     I49.02   **Ventricular flutter** 🔖
           (Ex) See I44.2

   I49.1   **Atrial premature depolarization**
       Atrial premature beats

   I49.2   **Junctional premature depolarization** 🔖
       (Ex) See I44.2

   I49.3   **Ventricular premature depolarization**

● **I49.4**   **Other and unspecified premature depolarization**

     I49.40   `Unspecified` **premature depolarization**
           Premature beats NOS

     I49.49   **Other premature depolarization**
           Ectopic beats
           Extrasystoles
           Extrasystolic arrhythmias
           Premature contractions

N Newborn Age: 0   **P** Pediatric Age: 0–17   **M** Maternity DX: 12–55   **A** Adult Age: 15–124   ♀ Females Only   ♂ Males Only

🔖 Complication\Comorbidity   🔖 Major C\C   (Ex) CC/MCC Exclusions   🔖 Present on Admission Requirement   🔖 Hospital-Acquired Condition

969

CHAPTER 9 (I00-I99)

I49.5   **Sick sinus syndrome**
       Tachycardia-bradycardia syndrome

I49.8   **Other specified cardiac arrhythmias**
       Coronary sinus rhythm disorder
       Ectopic rhythm disorder
       Nodal rhythm disorder

I49.9   **Cardiac arrhythmia, unspecified**
       Arrhythmia (cardiac) NOS

● **I50**   **Heart failure**
       Code first heart failure complicating abortion or ectopic or molar
          pregnancy (O00-O07, O08.8)
       heart failure due to hypertension (I11.0)
       heart failure due to hypertension with chronic kidney disease
          (I13.-)
       heart failure following surgery (I97.13-)
       obstetric surgery and procedures (O75.4)
       rheumatic heart failure (I09.81)
      Excludes1   cardiac arrest (I46.-)
                   neonatal cardiac failure (P29.0)

I50.1   **Left ventricular failure**
       Cardiac asthma
       Edema of lung with heart disease NOS
       Edema of lung with heart failure
       Left heart failure
       Pulmonary edema with heart disease NOS
       Pulmonary edema with heart failure
      Excludes1   edema of lung without heart disease or
                   heart failure (J81.-)
                pulmonary edema without heart disease
                   or failure (J81.-)
      (Ex) I09.81, I11.0, I50.1-I50.9, I87.8, I99.8-I99.9

● **I50.2**   **Systolic (congestive) heart failure**
      Excludes1   combined systolic (congestive) and
                   diastolic (congestive) heart failure
                   (I50.4-)
      (Ex) **For category I50.2 CC codes:** I09.81, I11.0, I50.1-I50.9, I87.8, I99.8-I99.9,
           J81.0

    I50.20   **Unspecified systolic (congestive) heart**
              failure

    I50.21   **Acute systolic (congestive) heart failure**
              Presenting a short and relatively severe episode

    I50.22   **Chronic systolic (congestive) heart failure**
              Long-lasting, presenting over time

    I50.23   **Acute on chronic systolic (congestive) heart**
              failure
              Combination code. What was a chronic condition
                 now has an acute exacerbation (to make more
                 severe).

● **I50.3**   **Diastolic (congestive) heart failure**
      Excludes1   combined systolic (congestive) and
                   diastolic (congestive) heart failure
                   (I50.4-)
      (Ex) **For category I50.3 CC codes:** See I50.2

    I50.30   **Unspecified diastolic (congestive) heart**
              failure

    I50.31   **Acute diastolic (congestive) heart failure**

    I50.32   **Chronic diastolic (congestive) heart failure**

    I50.33   **Acute on chronic diastolic (congestive) heart**
              failure

● **I50.4**   **Combined systolic (congestive) and diastolic**
       (congestive) heart failure
         (Ex) **For category I50.4 CC codes:** See I50.2

    I50.40   **Unspecified combined systolic (congestive) and**
              diastolic (congestive) heart failure

    I50.41   **Acute combined systolic (congestive) and**
              diastolic (congestive) heart failure

    I50.42   **Chronic combined systolic (congestive) and**
              diastolic (congestive) heart failure

    I50.43   **Acute on chronic combined systolic**
              (congestive) and diastolic (congestive) heart
              failure

Item 9-8 Congestive heart failure (CHF) is a condition in which the left ventricle of the heart cannot pump enough blood to the body. The blood flow from the heart slows or returns to the heart from the venous system back flow resulting in congestion (fluid accumulation) particularly in the abdomen. Most commonly, fluid collects in the lungs and results in shortness of breath, especially when in a reclining position.

I50.9   **Heart failure, unspecified**
       Biventricular (heart) failure NOS
       Cardiac, heart or myocardial failure NOS
       Congestive heart disease
       Congestive heart failure NOS
       Right ventricular failure (secondary to left heart failure)
      Excludes1   fluid overload (E87.70)
      Coding Clinic: 2012, Q4, P92

● **I51**   **Complications and ill-defined descriptions of heart disease**
      Excludes1   any condition in I51.4-I51.9 due to hypertension
                   (I11.-)
                any condition in I51.4-I51.9 due to hypertension
                   and chronic kidney disease (I13.-)
                heart disease specified as rheumatic (I00-I09)

I51.0   **Cardiac septal defect, acquired**   A
       Acquired septal atrial defect (old)
       Acquired septal auricular defect (old)
       Acquired septal ventricular defect (old)
      Excludes1   cardiac septal defect as current
                   complication following acute
                   myocardial infarction (I23.1, I23.2)
      (Ex) E78.71-E78.72, I23.0-I23.8, I40.0-I41, I51.0-I51.4, I87.8, I97.0-I97.191,
           I99.8-I99.9, P29.3, Q20.0-Q21.9, Q23.8-Q23.9, Q24.8-Q24.9, Q27.30,
           Q27.4, Q28.0-Q28.1, Q28.8-Q28.9, Q87.1-Q87.89, Q89.7-Q89.8, Q99.2

I51.1   **Rupture of chordae tendineae, not elsewhere classified**
      Excludes1   rupture of chordae tendineae as current
                   complication following acute
                   myocardial infarction (I23.4)
      (Ex) I23.0-I23.4, I23.6-I23.8, I51.0-I51.1, I51.3, I87.8, I99.8-I99.9

I51.2   **Rupture of papillary muscle, not elsewhere classified**
      Excludes1   rupture of papillary muscle as current
                   complication following acute
                   myocardial infarction (I23.5)
      (Ex) I23.0-I23.3, I23.5-I23.8, I51.0, I51.2-I51.3, I87.8, I99.8-I99.9

I51.3   **Intracardiac thrombosis, not elsewhere classified**   A
       Apical thrombosis (old)
       Atrial thrombosis (old)
       Auricular thrombosis (old)
       Mural thrombosis (old)
       Ventricular thrombosis (old)
      Excludes1   intracardiac thrombosis as current
                   complication following acute
                   myocardial infarction (I23.6)
      (Ex) See I51.0

I51.4   **Myocarditis, unspecified**
       Chronic (interstitial) myocarditis
       Myocardial fibrosis
       Myocarditis NOS
      Excludes1   acute or subacute myocarditis (I40.-)

I51.5   **Myocardial degeneration**
       Fatty degeneration of heart or myocardium
       Myocardial disease
       Senile degeneration of heart or myocardium

I51.7   **Cardiomegaly**
       Cardiac dilatation
       Cardiac hypertrophy
       Ventricular dilatation

◄ New   ◄▬ Revised   ~~deleted~~ Deleted   Excludes 1   Excludes 2   Includes   Use additional   Code first   Code also   Unspecified

OGCR Official Guidelines   ● Unacceptable Principal Diagnosis   X Assign placeholder X   ● Use Additional Character(s)   ▸ Manifestation Code   **Coding Clinic**

● **I51.8** **Other ill-defined heart diseases**

    I51.81 **Takotsubo syndrome** 🖐

        Reversible left ventricular dysfunction following sudden emotional stress

        Stress induced cardiomyopathy

        Takotsubo cardiomyopathy

        Transient left ventricular apical ballooning syndrome

        🔵Ex I09.81, I11.0, I50.1-I50.9, I51.81, I51.9-I52, I87.8, I99.8-I99.9

    I51.89 **Other ill-defined heart diseases**

        Carditis (acute)(chronic)

        Pancarditis (acute)(chronic)

  I51.9 **Heart disease, unspecified**

▷ **I52** *Other heart disorders in diseases classified elsewhere*

    Code first underlying disease, such as:

      congenital syphilis (A50.5)

      mucopolysaccharidosis (E76.3)

      schistosomiasis (B65.0-B65.9)

    Excludes1 heart disease (in):

        gonococcal infection (A54.83)

        meningococcal infection (A39.50)

        rheumatoid arthritis (M05.31)

        syphilis (A52.06)

CEREBROVASCULAR DISEASES (I60-I69)

Use additional code to identify presence of:

  alcohol abuse and dependence (F10.-)

  exposure to environmental tobacco smoke (Z77.22)

  history of tobacco use (Z87.891)

  hypertension (I10-I15)

  occupational exposure to environmental tobacco smoke (Z57.31)

  tobacco dependence (F17.-)

  tobacco use (Z72.0)

    Excludes1 transient cerebral ischemic attacks and related syndromes (G45.-)

        traumatic intracranial hemorrhage (S06.-)

● **I60** **Nontraumatic subarachnoid hemorrhage**

    Includes ruptured cerebral aneurysm

    Excludes1 sequelae of subarachnoid hemorrhage (I69.0-)

        syphilitic ruptured cerebral aneurysm (A52.05)

    🔵Ex **For category I60 CC codes:** E03.5, G93.82, I60.00-I62.9, I87.8, I99.8-I99.9, R40.0-R40.2224, R40.2310-R40.2324, R40.2340-R40.2344, R40.3-R40.4, S02.0XX-S02.19X[A,B], S02.91X[A,B], S06.0X0-S06.9X9[A]

  ● **I60.0** **Nontraumatic subarachnoid hemorrhage from carotid siphon and bifurcation**

    I60.00 **Nontraumatic subarachnoid hemorrhage from unspecified carotid siphon and bifurcation** 🖐

    I60.01 **Nontraumatic subarachnoid hemorrhage from right carotid siphon and bifurcation** 🖐

    I60.02 **Nontraumatic subarachnoid hemorrhage from left carotid siphon and bifurcation** 🖐

  ● **I60.1** **Nontraumatic subarachnoid hemorrhage from middle cerebral artery**

    I60.10 **Nontraumatic subarachnoid hemorrhage from unspecified middle cerebral artery** 🖐

    I60.11 **Nontraumatic subarachnoid hemorrhage from right middle cerebral artery** 🖐

    I60.12 **Nontraumatic subarachnoid hemorrhage from left middle cerebral artery** 🖐

  ● **I60.2** **Nontraumatic subarachnoid hemorrhage from anterior communicating artery**

    I60.20 **Nontraumatic subarachnoid hemorrhage from unspecified anterior communicating artery** 🖐

    I60.21 **Nontraumatic subarachnoid hemorrhage from right anterior communicating artery** 🖐

    I60.22 **Nontraumatic subarachnoid hemorrhage from left anterior communicating artery** 🖐

● **I60.3** **Nontraumatic subarachnoid hemorrhage from posterior communicating artery**

    I60.30 **Nontraumatic subarachnoid hemorrhage from unspecified posterior communicating artery** 🖐

    I60.31 **Nontraumatic subarachnoid hemorrhage from right posterior communicating artery** 🖐

    I60.32 **Nontraumatic subarachnoid hemorrhage from left posterior communicating artery** 🖐

  I60.4 **Nontraumatic subarachnoid hemorrhage from basilar artery** 🖐

● **I60.5** **Nontraumatic subarachnoid hemorrhage from vertebral artery**

    I60.50 **Nontraumatic subarachnoid hemorrhage from unspecified vertebral artery** 🖐

    I60.51 **Nontraumatic subarachnoid hemorrhage from right vertebral artery** 🖐

    I60.52 **Nontraumatic subarachnoid hemorrhage from left vertebral artery** 🖐

  I60.6 **Nontraumatic subarachnoid hemorrhage from other intracranial arteries** 🖐

  I60.7 **Nontraumatic subarachnoid hemorrhage from unspecified intracranial artery** 🖐

    Ruptured (congenital) berry aneurysm

    Ruptured (congenital) cerebral aneurysm

    Subarachnoid hemorrhage (nontraumatic) from cerebral artery NOS

    Subarachnoid hemorrhage (nontraumatic) from communicating artery NOS

    Excludes1 berry aneurysm, nonruptured (I67.1)

  I60.8 **Other nontraumatic subarachnoid hemorrhage** 🖐

    Meningeal hemorrhage

    Rupture of cerebral arteriovenous malformation

  I60.9 **Nontraumatic subarachnoid hemorrhage, unspecified** 🖐

● **I61** **Nontraumatic intracerebral hemorrhage**

    Excludes1 sequelae of intracerebral hemorrhage (I69.1-)

    🔵Ex **For category I61 CC codes:** See I60

  I61.0 **Nontraumatic intracerebral hemorrhage in hemisphere, subcortical** 🖐

    Deep intracerebral hemorrhage (nontraumatic)

  I61.1 **Nontraumatic intracerebral hemorrhage in hemisphere, cortical** 🖐

    Cerebral lobe hemorrhage (nontraumatic)

    Superficial intracerebral hemorrhage (nontraumatic)

  I61.2 **Nontraumatic intracerebral hemorrhage in hemisphere, unspecified** 🖐

  I61.3 **Nontraumatic intracerebral hemorrhage in brain stem** 🖐

  I61.4 **Nontraumatic intracerebral hemorrhage in cerebellum** 🖐

  I61.5 **Nontraumatic intracerebral hemorrhage, intraventricular** 🖐

  I61.6 **Nontraumatic intracerebral hemorrhage, multiple localized** 🖐

  I61.8 **Other nontraumatic intracerebral hemorrhage** 🖐

  I61.9 **Nontraumatic intracerebral hemorrhage, unspecified** 🖐

● **I62** **Other and unspecified nontraumatic intracranial hemorrhage**

    Excludes1 sequelae of intracranial hemorrhage (I69.2)

    🔵Ex **For category I62 CC codes:** See I60

  ● **I62.0** **Nontraumatic subdural hemorrhage**

    I62.00 **Nontraumatic subdural hemorrhage, unspecified** 🖐

    I62.01 **Nontraumatic acute subdural hemorrhage** 🖐

    I62.02 **Nontraumatic subacute subdural hemorrhage** 🖐

    I62.03 **Nontraumatic chronic subdural hemorrhage** 🖐

  I62.1 **Nontraumatic extradural hemorrhage** 🖐

    Nontraumatic epidural hemorrhage

  I62.9 **Nontraumatic intracranial hemorrhage, unspecified** 🖐

N Newborn Age: 0   P Pediatric Age: 0–17   M Maternity DX: 12–55   A Adult Age: 15–124   ♀ Females Only   ♂ Males Only

🖐 Complication\Comorbidity   🖐 Major C\C   Ex CC/MCC Exclusions   🖐 Present on Admission Requirement   🖐 Hospital-Acquired Condition   **971**

(See Plate 141 on page 76.)

● **I63**   **Cerebral infarction**

> **Includes**   occlusion and stenosis of cerebral and precerebral arteries, resulting in cerebral infarction
>
> Use additional code, if applicable, to identify status post administration of tPA (rtPA) in a different facility within the last 24 hours prior to admission to current facility (Z92.82)
>
> **Excludes1**   sequelae of cerebral infarction (I69.3-)

● **I63.0**   **Cerebral infarction due to thrombosis of precerebral arteries**

     I63.00   **Cerebral infarction due to thrombosis of unspecified precerebral artery** 🔍

> (Ex:) E08.51-E08.59, E08.618-E08.638, E08.649-E08.8, E09.51-E09.59, E09.618-E09.638, E09.649-E09.8, E10.51-E10.59, E10.618-E10.638, E10.649, E10.69-E10.8, E11.51-E11.59, E11.618-E11.638, E11.649, E11.69-E11.8, E13.51-E13.59, E13.618-E13.638, E13.649-E13.8, G43.601-G43.619, I63.00-I63.29, I65.01-I65.9, I87.8, I99.8, I99.9

     ● **I63.01**   **Cerebral infarction due to thrombosis of vertebral artery**

> (Ex:) For category I63.01 CC codes: E08.51-E08.59, E08.618-E08.638, E08.649-E08.8, E09.51-E09.59, E09.618-E09.638, E09.649-E09.8, E10.51-E10.59, E10.618-E10.638, E10.649, E10.69-E10.8, E11.51-E11.59, E11.618-E11.638, E11.649, E11.69-E11.8, E13.51-E13.59, E13.618-E13.638, E13.649-E13.8, G43.601-G43.619, I63.00-I63.29, I65.01-I65.9, I87.8, I99.8-I99.9

         I63.011   **Cerebral infarction due to thrombosis of right vertebral artery** 🔍

         I63.012   **Cerebral infarction due to thrombosis of left vertebral artery** 🔍

         I63.019   **Cerebral infarction due to thrombosis of unspecified vertebral artery** 🔍

     I63.02   **Cerebral infarction due to thrombosis of basilar artery** 🔍

> (Ex:) See I63.00

     ● **I63.03**   **Cerebral infarction due to thrombosis of carotid artery**

> (Ex:) For category I63.03 CC codes: E08.51-E08.59, E08.618-E08.638, E08.649-E08.8, E09.51-E09.59, E09.618-E09.638, E09.649-E09.8, E10.51-E10.59, E10.618-E10.638, E10.649, E10.69-E10.8, E11.51-E11.59, E11.618-E11.638, E11.649, E11.69-E11.8, E13.51-E13.59, E13.618-E13.638, E13.649-E13.8, G43.601-G43.619, I63.00-I63.29, I65.01-I65.9, I87.8, I99.8-I99.9

         I63.031   **Cerebral infarction due to thrombosis of right carotid artery** 🔍

         I63.032   **Cerebral infarction due to thrombosis of left carotid artery** 🔍

         I63.039   **Cerebral infarction due to thrombosis of unspecified carotid artery** 🔍

     I63.09   **Cerebral infarction due to thrombosis of other precerebral artery** 🔍

> (Ex:) See I63.00

● **I63.1**   **Cerebral infarction due to embolism of precerebral arteries**

     I63.10   **Cerebral infarction due to embolism of unspecified precerebral artery** 🔍

> (Ex:) See I63.00

     ● **I63.11**   **Cerebral infarction due to embolism of vertebral artery**

> (Ex:) For category I63.11 CC codes: See I63.01

         I63.111   **Cerebral infarction due to embolism of right vertebral artery** 🔍

         I63.112   **Cerebral infarction due to embolism of left vertebral artery** 🔍

         I63.119   **Cerebral infarction due to embolism of unspecified vertebral artery** 🔍

     I63.12   **Cerebral infarction due to embolism of basilar artery** 🔍

> (Ex:) See I63.00

     ● **I63.13**   **Cerebral infarction due to embolism of carotid artery**

> (Ex:) For category I63.13 CC codes: See I63.03

         I63.131   **Cerebral infarction due to embolism of right carotid artery** 🔍

         I63.132   **Cerebral infarction due to embolism of left carotid artery** 🔍

         I63.139   **Cerebral infarction due to embolism of unspecified carotid artery** 🔍

     I63.19   **Cerebral infarction due to embolism of other precerebral artery** 🔍

> (Ex:) See I63.00

● **I63.2**   **Cerebral infarction due to unspecified occlusion or stenosis of precerebral arteries**

     I63.20   **Cerebral infarction due to unspecified occlusion or stenosis of unspecified precerebral arteries** 🔍

> (Ex:) See I63.00

     ● **I63.21**   **Cerebral infarction due to unspecified occlusion or stenosis of vertebral arteries**

> (Ex:) For category I63.21 CC codes: See I63.01

         I63.211   **Cerebral infarction due to unspecified occlusion or stenosis of right vertebral arteries** 🔍

         I63.212   **Cerebral infarction due to unspecified occlusion or stenosis of left vertebral arteries** 🔍

         I63.219   **Cerebral infarction due to unspecified occlusion or stenosis of unspecified vertebral arteries** 🔍

     I63.22   **Cerebral infarction due to unspecified occlusion or stenosis of basilar arteries** 🔍

> (Ex:) See I63.00

     ● **I63.23**   **Cerebral infarction due to unspecified occlusion or stenosis of carotid arteries**

> (Ex:) For category I63.23 CC codes: See I63.03

         I63.231   **Cerebral infarction due to unspecified occlusion or stenosis of right carotid arteries** 🔍

         I63.232   **Cerebral infarction due to unspecified occlusion or stenosis of left carotid arteries** 🔍

         I63.239   **Cerebral infarction due to unspecified occlusion or stenosis of unspecified carotid arteries** 🔍

     I63.29   **Cerebral infarction due to unspecified occlusion or stenosis of other precerebral arteries** 🔍

> (Ex:) See I63.00

● **I63.3**   **Cerebral infarction due to thrombosis of cerebral arteries**

> (Ex:) For category I63.3 CC codes: E08.51-E08.59, E08.618-E08.638, E08.649-E08.8, E09.51-E09.59, E09.618-E09.638, E09.649-E09.8, E10.51-E10.59, E10.618-E10.638, E10.649, E10.69-E10.8, E11.51-E11.59, E11.618-E11.638, E11.649, E11.69-E11.8, E13.51-E13.59, E13.618-E13.638, E13.649-E13.8, G43.601-G43.619, I63.30-I63.9, I66.01-I66.9, I87.8, I99.8-I99.9

     I63.30   **Cerebral infarction due to thrombosis of unspecified cerebral artery** 🔍

     ● **I63.31**   **Cerebral infarction due to thrombosis of middle cerebral artery**

         I63.311   **Cerebral infarction due to thrombosis of right middle cerebral artery** 🔍

         I63.312   **Cerebral infarction due to thrombosis of left middle cerebral artery** 🔍

         I63.319   **Cerebral infarction due to thrombosis of unspecified middle cerebral artery** 🔍

● **I63.32**   Cerebral infarction due to thrombosis of anterior cerebral artery

     I63.321   Cerebral infarction due to thrombosis of right anterior cerebral artery 🔖

     I63.322   Cerebral infarction due to thrombosis of left anterior cerebral artery 🔖

     I63.329   Cerebral infarction due to thrombosis of unspecified anterior cerebral artery 🔖

● **I63.33**   Cerebral infarction due to thrombosis of posterior cerebral artery

     I63.331   Cerebral infarction due to thrombosis of right posterior cerebral artery 🔖

     I63.332   Cerebral infarction due to thrombosis of left posterior cerebral artery 🔖

     I63.339   Cerebral infarction due to thrombosis of unspecified posterior cerebral artery 🔖

● **I63.34**   Cerebral infarction due to thrombosis of cerebellar artery

     I63.341   Cerebral infarction due to thrombosis of right cerebellar artery 🔖

     I63.342   Cerebral infarction due to thrombosis of left cerebellar artery 🔖

     I63.349   Cerebral infarction due to thrombosis of unspecified cerebellar artery 🔖

   I63.39   Cerebral infarction due to thrombosis of other cerebral artery 🔖

● **I63.4**   Cerebral infarction due to embolism of cerebral arteries

     (Ex) For category I63.4 CC codes: See I63.3

   I63.40   Cerebral infarction due to embolism of unspecified cerebral artery 🔖

● **I63.41**   Cerebral infarction due to embolism of middle cerebral artery

     I63.411   Cerebral infarction due to embolism of right middle cerebral artery 🔖

     I63.412   Cerebral infarction due to embolism of left middle cerebral artery 🔖

     I63.419   Cerebral infarction due to embolism of unspecified middle cerebral artery 🔖

● **I63.42**   Cerebral infarction due to embolism of anterior cerebral artery

     I63.421   Cerebral infarction due to embolism of right anterior cerebral artery 🔖

     I63.422   Cerebral infarction due to embolism of left anterior cerebral artery 🔖

     I63.429   Cerebral infarction due to embolism of unspecified anterior cerebral artery 🔖

● **I63.43**   Cerebral infarction due to embolism of posterior cerebral artery

     I63.431   Cerebral infarction due to embolism of right posterior cerebral artery 🔖

     I63.432   Cerebral infarction due to embolism of left posterior cerebral artery 🔖

     I63.439   Cerebral infarction due to embolism of unspecified posterior cerebral artery 🔖

● **I63.44**   Cerebral infarction due to embolism of cerebellar artery

     I63.441   Cerebral infarction due to embolism of right cerebellar artery 🔖

     I63.442   Cerebral infarction due to embolism of left cerebellar artery 🔖

     I63.449   Cerebral infarction due to embolism of unspecified cerebellar artery 🔖

   I63.49   Cerebral infarction due to embolism of other cerebral artery 🔖

● **I63.5**   Cerebral infarction due to unspecified occlusion or stenosis of cerebral arteries

     (Ex) For category I63.5 CC codes: See I63.3

   I63.50   Cerebral infarction due to unspecified occlusion or stenosis of unspecified cerebral artery 🔖

● **I63.51**   Cerebral infarction due to unspecified occlusion or stenosis of middle cerebral artery

     I63.511   Cerebral infarction due to unspecified occlusion or stenosis of right middle cerebral artery 🔖

     I63.512   Cerebral infarction due to unspecified occlusion or stenosis of left middle cerebral artery 🔖

     I63.519   Cerebral infarction due to unspecified occlusion or stenosis of unspecified middle cerebral artery 🔖

● **I63.52**   Cerebral infarction due to unspecified occlusion or stenosis of anterior cerebral artery

     I63.521   Cerebral infarction due to unspecified occlusion or stenosis of right anterior cerebral artery 🔖

     I63.522   Cerebral infarction due to unspecified occlusion or stenosis of left anterior cerebral artery 🔖

     I63.529   Cerebral infarction due to unspecified occlusion or stenosis of unspecified anterior cerebral artery 🔖

● **I63.53**   Cerebral infarction due to unspecified occlusion or stenosis of posterior cerebral artery

     I63.531   Cerebral infarction due to unspecified occlusion or stenosis of right posterior cerebral artery 🔖

     I63.532   Cerebral infarction due to unspecified occlusion or stenosis of left posterior cerebral artery 🔖

     I63.539   Cerebral infarction due to unspecified occlusion or stenosis of unspecified posterior cerebral artery 🔖

● **I63.54**   Cerebral infarction due to unspecified occlusion or stenosis of cerebellar artery

     I63.541   Cerebral infarction due to unspecified occlusion or stenosis of right cerebellar artery 🔖

     I63.542   Cerebral infarction due to unspecified occlusion or stenosis of left cerebellar artery 🔖

     I63.549   Cerebral infarction due to unspecified occlusion or stenosis of unspecified cerebellar artery 🔖

   I63.59   Cerebral infarction due to unspecified occlusion or stenosis of other cerebral artery 🔖

I63.6   Cerebral infarction due to cerebral venous thrombosis, nonpyogenic 🔖

     (Ex) See I63.3

I63.8   Other cerebral infarction 🔖

     (Ex) See I63.3

I63.9   Cerebral infarction, unspecified 🔖

     Stroke NOS

     (Ex) See I63.3

CHAPTER 9 (I00-I99)

N   Newborn Age: 0   **P**   Pediatric Age: 0–17   **M**   Maternity DX: 12–55   **A**   Adult Age: 15–124   ♀   Females Only   ♂   Males Only

🔖   Complication\Comorbidity   🔖   Major C\C   (Ex)   CC/MCC Exclusions   🔖   Present on Admission Requirement   Hospital-Acquired Condition

973

● I65   **Occlusion and stenosis of precerebral arteries, not resulting in cerebral infarction**

     Includes   embolism of precerebral artery
                   narrowing of precerebral artery
                   obstruction (complete) (partial) of precerebral artery
                   thrombosis of precerebral artery

     Excludes1   insufficiency, NOS, of precerebral artery (G45.-)
                   insufficiency of precerebral arteries causing cerebral infarction (I63.0-I63.2)

   ● **I65.0**   Occlusion and stenosis of vertebral artery

     I65.01   Occlusion and stenosis of right vertebral artery

     I65.02   Occlusion and stenosis of left vertebral artery

     I65.03   Occlusion and stenosis of bilateral vertebral arteries

     I65.09   Occlusion and stenosis of unspecified vertebral artery

   I65.1   Occlusion and stenosis of basilar artery

   ● **I65.2**   Occlusion and stenosis of carotid artery

     I65.21   Occlusion and stenosis of right carotid artery

     I65.22   Occlusion and stenosis of left carotid artery

     I65.23   Occlusion and stenosis of bilateral carotid arteries

     I65.29   Occlusion and stenosis of unspecified carotid artery

   I65.8   Occlusion and stenosis of other precerebral arteries

   I65.9   Occlusion and stenosis of unspecified precerebral artery
           Occlusion and stenosis of precerebral artery NOS

● I66   **Occlusion and stenosis of cerebral arteries, not resulting in cerebral infarction**

     Includes   embolism of cerebral artery
                   narrowing of cerebral artery
                   obstruction (complete) (partial) of cerebral artery
                   thrombosis of cerebral artery

     Excludes1   occlusion and stenosis of cerebral artery causing cerebral infarction (I63.3-I63.5)

   ● **I66.0**   Occlusion and stenosis of middle cerebral artery

     I66.01   Occlusion and stenosis of right middle cerebral artery

     I66.02   Occlusion and stenosis of left middle cerebral artery

     I66.03   Occlusion and stenosis of bilateral middle cerebral arteries

     I66.09   Occlusion and stenosis of unspecified middle cerebral artery

   ● **I66.1**   Occlusion and stenosis of anterior cerebral artery

     I66.11   Occlusion and stenosis of right anterior cerebral artery

     I66.12   Occlusion and stenosis of left anterior cerebral artery

     I66.13   Occlusion and stenosis of bilateral anterior cerebral arteries

     I66.19   Occlusion and stenosis of unspecified anterior cerebral artery

   ● **I66.2**   Occlusion and stenosis of posterior cerebral artery

     I66.21   Occlusion and stenosis of right posterior cerebral artery

     I66.22   Occlusion and stenosis of left posterior cerebral artery

     I66.23   Occlusion and stenosis of bilateral posterior cerebral arteries

     I66.29   Occlusion and stenosis of unspecified posterior cerebral artery

   I66.3   Occlusion and stenosis of cerebellar arteries

   I66.8   Occlusion and stenosis of other cerebral arteries
           Occlusion and stenosis of perforating arteries

   I66.9   Occlusion and stenosis of unspecified cerebral artery

● I67   **Other cerebrovascular diseases**

     Excludes1   sequelae of the listed conditions (I69.8)

   I67.0   **Dissection of cerebral arteries, nonruptured** ✎

     Excludes1   ruptured cerebral arteries (I60.7)

     (Ex:) I77.2-I77.3, I77.5-I77.6, I77.89-I77.9, M31.8-M31.9

   I67.1   **Cerebral aneurysm, nonruptured**
           Cerebral aneurysm NOS
           Cerebral arteriovenous fistula, acquired
           Internal carotid artery aneurysm, intracranial portion
           Internal carotid artery aneurysm, NOS

     Excludes1   congenital cerebral aneurysm, nonruptured (Q28.-)
                   ruptured cerebral aneurysm (I60.7)

   I67.2   **Cerebral atherosclerosis**   A
           Atheroma of cerebral and precerebral arteries

   I67.3   **Progressive vascular leukoencephalopathy** ✎
           Binswanger's disease
     (Ex:) A17.82, A50.42, A52.14, A75.9, A79.9, A81.00-A81.9, A83.0-A85.8, A87.2, A88.0, A88.8, A92.1-A92.2, A92.4-A92.8, A93.0, B00.4, B00.82, B01.11-B01.12, B04, B06.01, B08.09, B08.20-B08.22, B08.60-B08.79, B09, B10.01-B10.09, B26.2, B27.00-B27.99, B33.1, B45.0, B45.2-B45.9, B58.2, B75, G04.00-G04.01, G04.31, G04.81-G05.4, G37.0, G37.4-G37.5, I67.3, J09.X3-J09.X9, J10.2-J10.89, J11.2-J11.89, L44.4, M1A.10X0-M1A.19X1, P35.2-P35.9, P37.0-P37.4, P37.8-P37.9, T56.0X1-T56.0X4[A]

   I67.4   **Hypertensive encephalopathy** ✎
     (Ex:) E08.51-E08.59, E08.618-E08.638, E08.649-E08.8, E09.51-E09.59, E09.618-E09.638, E09.649-E09.8, E10.51-E10.59, E10.618-E10.638, E10.649, E10.69-E10.8, E11.51-E11.59, E11.618-E11.638, E11.649, E11.69-E11.8, E13.51-E13.59, E13.618-E13.638, E13.649-E13.8, I67.4, I87.8, I99.8-I99.9

   I67.5   **Moyamoya disease** ✎
     (Ex:) E08.51-E08.59, E08.618-E08.638, E08.649-E08.8, E09.51-E09.59, E09.618-E09.638, E09.649-E09.8, E10.51-E10.59, E10.618-E10.638, E10.649, E10.69-E10.8, E11.51-E11.59, E11.618-E11.638, E11.649, E11.69-E11.8, E13.51-E13.59, E13.618-E13.638, E13.649-E13.8, I67.5, I87.8, I99.8-I99.9

   I67.6   **Nonpyogenic thrombosis of intracranial venous system** ✎
           Nonpyogenic thrombosis of cerebral vein
           Nonpyogenic thrombosis of intracranial venous sinus

     Excludes1   nonpyogenic thrombosis of intracranial venous system causing infarction (I63.6)

     (Ex:) E08.51-E08.59, E08.618-E08.638, E08.649-E08.8, E09.51-E09.59, E09.618-E09.638, E09.649-E09.8, E10.51-E10.59, E10.618-E10.638, E10.649, E10.69-E10.8, E11.51-E11.59, E11.618-E11.638, E11.649, E11.69-E11.8, E13.51-E13.59, E13.618-E13.638, E13.649-E13.8, I67.6, I87.8, I99.8-I99.9

   I67.7   **Cerebral arteritis, not elsewhere classified** ✎
           Granulomatous angiitis of the nervous system

     Excludes1   allergic granulomatous angiitis (M30.1)

     (Ex:) E08.51-E08.59, E08.618-E08.638, E08.649-E08.8, E09.51-E09.59, E09.618-E09.638, E09.649-E09.8, E10.51-E10.59, E10.618-E10.638, E10.649, E10.69-E10.8, E11.51-E11.59, E11.618-E11.638, E11.649, E11.69-E11.8, E13.51-E13.59, E13.618-E13.638, E13.649-E13.8, I67.7, I68.2, I87.8, I99.8-I99.9

   ● **I67.8**   **Other specified cerebrovascular diseases**

     I67.81   **Acute cerebrovascular insufficiency** ✎
           Acute cerebrovascular insufficiency unspecified as to location or reversibility
       (Ex:) E08.51-E08.59, E08.618-E08.638, E08.649-E08.8, E09.51-E09.59, E09.618-E09.638, E09.649-E09.8, E10.51-E10.59, E10.618-E10.638, E10.649, E10.69-E10.8, E11.51-E11.59, E11.618-E11.638, E11.649, E11.69-E11.8, E13.51-E13.59, E13.618-E13.638, E13.649-E13.8, G45.0-G45.2, G45.8-G46.2, I60.00-I62.9, I63.30-I63.9, I66.01-I66.9, I67.81-I67.82, I67.841-I67.89, I87.8, I99.8-I99.9

     I67.82   **Cerebral ischemia** ✎
           Chronic cerebral ischemia
       (Ex:) See I67.81

     I67.83   **Posterior reversible encephalopathy syndrome** ✎
           PRES
       (Ex:) G21.0, G83.5, G93.40-G93.41

◀ New   ◀ Revised   ~~deleted~~ Deleted   Excludes 1   Excludes 2   Includes   Use additional   Code first   Code also   Unspecified

OGCR Official Guidelines   ● Unacceptable Principal Diagnosis   X Assign placeholder X   ● Use Additional Character(s)   ✎ Manifestation Code   **Coding Clinic**

● **I67.84**   **Cerebral vasospasm and vasoconstriction**

     (Ex) For category I67.84 CC codes: E08.51-E08.59,
     E08.618-E08.638, E08.649-E08.8, E09.51-E09.59,
     E09.618-E09.638, E09.649-E09.8, E10.51-E10.59,
     E10.618-E10.638, E10.649-E10.8, E11.51-E11.59,
     E11.618-E11.638, E11.649, E11.69, E11.8, E13.51-E13.59,
     E13.618-E13.638, E13.649-E13.8, G45.0-G45.2, G45.8-G46.2,
     I63.00-I63.02, I63.29, I65.01-I65.9, I67.841-I67.848, I87.8,
     I99.8-I99.9

     I67.841   **Reversible cerebrovascular vasoconstriction syndrome** 🔍
          Call-Fleming syndrome

          Code first underlying condition, if applicable, such as eclampsia (O15.00-O15.9)

     I67.848   **Other cerebrovascular vasospasm and vasoconstriction** 🔍

   I67.89   **Other cerebrovascular disease** 🔍
       (Ex) See I67.81

   I67.9   **Cerebrovascular disease, unspecified**

● **I68**   **Cerebrovascular disorders in diseases classified elsewhere**

▌ **I68.0**   *Cerebral amyloid angiopathy*
     Code first underlying amyloidosis (E85.-) ◀▥

▌ **I68.2**   *Cerebral arteritis in other diseases classified elsewhere* 🔍
     Code first underlying disease

     Excludes1   cerebral arteritis (in):
          listerosis (A32.89)
          systemic lupus erythematosus (M32.19)
          syphilis (A52.04)
          tuberculosis (A18.89)

     (Ex) See I67.7

▌ **I68.8**   *Other cerebrovascular disorders in diseases classified elsewhere*
     Code first underlying disease

     Excludes1   syphilitic cerebral aneurysm (A52.05)

OGCR   Section I.c.9.d.

Sequelae of Cerebrovascular Disease

1) Category I69, Sequelae of Cerebrovascular disease
Category I69 is used to indicate conditions classifiable to categories I60-I67 as the causes of sequela (neurologic deficits), themselves classified elsewhere. These "late effects" include neurologic deficits that persist after initial onset of conditions classifiable to categories I60-I67. The neurologic deficits caused by cerebrovascular disease may be present from the onset of may arise at any time after the onset of the condition classifiable to categories I60-I67.

2) Codes from category I69 with codes from I60-I67
Codes from category I69 may be assigned on a health care record with codes from I60-I67, if the patient has a current cerebrovascular disease and deficits from an old cerebrovascular disease.

● **I69**   **Sequelae of cerebrovascular disease**

   Note: Category I69 is to be used to indicate conditions in I60-I67 as the cause of sequelae. The 'sequelae' include conditions specified as such or as residuals which may occur at any time after the onset of the causal condition.

   Excludes1   personal history of cerebral infarction without residual deficit (Z86.73)
       personal history of prolonged reversible ischemic neurologic deficit (PRIND) (Z86.73)
       personal history of reversible ischemic neurolgcial deficit (RIND) (Z86.73)
       sequelae of traumatic intracranial injury (S06.-)
       transient ischemic attack (TIA) (G45.9)

Coding Clinic: 2012, Q4, P107

● **I69.0**   **Sequelae of nontraumatic subarachnoid hemorrhage**

   I69.00   **Unspecified sequelae of nontraumatic subarachnoid hemorrhage** 🔍

   I69.01   **Cognitive deficits following nontraumatic subarachnoid hemorrhage** 🔍

● **I69.02**   **Speech and language deficits following nontraumatic subarachnoid hemorrhage**

     I69.020   **Aphasia following nontraumatic subarachnoid hemorrhage** 🔍

     I69.021   **Dysphasia following nontraumatic subarachnoid hemorrhage** 🔍

     I69.022   **Dysarthria following nontraumatic subarachnoid hemorrhage** 🔍

     I69.023   **Fluency disorder following nontraumatic subarachnoid hemorrhage** 🔍
          Stuttering following nontraumatic subarachnoid hemorrhage

     I69.028   **Other speech and language deficits following nontraumatic subarachnoid hemorrhage** 🔍

● **I69.03**   **Monoplegia of upper limb following nontraumatic subarachnoid hemorrhage**

     I69.031   **Monoplegia of upper limb following nontraumatic subarachnoid hemorrhage affecting right dominant side** 🔍

     I69.032   **Monoplegia of upper limb following nontraumatic subarachnoid hemorrhage affecting left dominant side** 🔍

     I69.033   **Monoplegia of upper limb following nontraumatic subarachnoid hemorrhage affecting right non-dominant side** 🔍

     I69.034   **Monoplegia of upper limb following nontraumatic subarachnoid hemorrhage affecting left non-dominant side** 🔍

     I69.039   **Monoplegia of upper limb following nontraumatic subarachnoid hemorrhage affecting unspecified side** 🔍

● **I69.04**   **Monoplegia of lower limb following nontraumatic subarachnoid hemorrhage**

     I69.041   **Monoplegia of lower limb following nontraumatic subarachnoid hemorrhage affecting right dominant side** 🔍

     I69.042   **Monoplegia of lower limb following nontraumatic subarachnoid hemorrhage affecting left dominant side** 🔍

     I69.043   **Monoplegia of lower limb following nontraumatic subarachnoid hemorrhage affecting right non-dominant side** 🔍

     I69.044   **Monoplegia of lower limb following nontraumatic subarachnoid hemorrhage affecting left non-dominant side** 🔍

     I69.049   **Monoplegia of lower limb following nontraumatic subarachnoid hemorrhage affecting unspecified side** 🔍

CHAPTER 9 (I00-I99)

N   Newborn Age: 0   **P**   Pediatric Age: 0–17   **M**   Maternity DX: 12–55   **A**   Adult Age: 15–124   ♀   Females Only   ♂   Males Only

 Complication\Comorbidity   Major C\C   (Ex) CC/MCC Exclusions   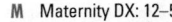 Present on Admission Requirement   🔍 Hospital-Acquired Condition

975

● **I69.05**   **Hemiplegia and hemiparesis following nontraumatic subarachnoid hemorrhage**

I69.051   Hemiplegia and hemiparesis following nontraumatic subarachnoid hemorrhage affecting right dominant side 🖐🖐
Ex: I69.051-I69.052, I69.151-I69.152, I69.251-I69.252, I69.351-I69.352, I69.851-I69.852, I69.951-I69.952

I69.052   Hemiplegia and hemiparesis following nontraumatic subarachnoid hemorrhage affecting left dominant side 🖐🖐
Ex: See I69.051

I69.053   Hemiplegia and hemiparesis following nontraumatic subarachnoid hemorrhage affecting right non-dominant side 🖐🖐
Ex: I69.053-I69.054, I69.153-I69.154, I69.253-I69.254, I69.353-I69.354, I69.853-I69.854, I69.953-I69.954

I69.054   Hemiplegia and hemiparesis following nontraumatic subarachnoid hemorrhage affecting left non-dominant side 🖐🖐
Ex: See I69.053

I69.059   Hemiplegia and hemiparesis following nontraumatic subarachnoid hemorrhage affecting unspecified side 🖐🖐
Ex: I69.059, I69.159, I69.259, I69.359, I69.859, I69.959

● **I69.06**   **Other paralytic syndrome following nontraumatic subarachnoid hemorrhage**
Use additional code to identify type of paralytic syndrome, such as:
locked-in state (G83.5)
quadriplegia (G82.5-)
Excludes1   hemiplegia/hemiparesis following nontraumatic subarachnoid hemorrhage (I69.05-)
monoplegia of lower limb following nontraumatic subarachnoid hemorrhage (I69.04-)
monoplegia of upper limb following nontraumatic subarachnoid hemorrhage (I69.03-)

I69.061   Other paralytic syndrome following nontraumatic subarachnoid hemorrhage affecting right dominant side 🖐

I69.062   Other paralytic syndrome following nontraumatic subarachnoid hemorrhage affecting left dominant side 🖐

I69.063   Other paralytic syndrome following nontraumatic subarachnoid hemorrhage affecting right non-dominant side 🖐

I69.064   Other paralytic syndrome following nontraumatic subarachnoid hemorrhage affecting left non-dominant side 🖐

I69.065   Other paralytic syndrome following nontraumatic subarachnoid hemorrhage, bilateral 🖐

I69.069   Other paralytic syndrome following nontraumatic subarachnoid hemorrhage affecting unspecified side 🖐

● **I69.09**   **Other sequelae of nontraumatic subarachnoid hemorrhage**

I69.090   Apraxia following nontraumatic subarachnoid hemorrhage 🖐

I69.091   Dysphagia following nontraumatic subarachnoid hemorrhage 🖐
Use additional code to identify the type of dysphagia, if known (R13.1-)

I69.092   Facial weakness following nontraumatic subarachnoid hemorrhage 🖐
Facial droop following nontraumatic subarachnoid hemorrhage

I69.093   Ataxia following nontraumatic subarachnoid hemorrhage 🖐

I69.098   Other sequelae following nontraumatic subarachnoid hemorrhage 🖐
Alterations of sensation following nontraumatic subarachnoid hemorrhage
Disturbance of vision following nontraumatic subarachnoid hemorrhage
Use additional code to identify the sequelae

● **I69.1**   **Sequelae of nontraumatic intracerebral hemorrhage**

I69.10   Unspecified sequelae of nontraumatic intracerebral hemorrhage 🖐

I69.11   Cognitive deficits following nontraumatic intracerebral hemorrhage 🖐

● **I69.12**   **Speech and language deficits following nontraumatic intracerebral hemorrhage**

I69.120   Aphasia following nontraumatic intracerebral hemorrhage 🖐

I69.121   Dysphasia following nontraumatic intracerebral hemorrhage 🖐

I69.122   Dysarthria following nontraumatic intracerebral hemorrhage 🖐

I69.123   Fluency disorder following nontraumatic intracerebral hemorrhage 🖐
Stuttering following nontraumatic subarachnoid hemorrhage

I69.128   Other speech and language deficits following nontraumatic intracerebral hemorrhage 🖐

● **I69.13**   **Monoplegia of upper limb following nontraumatic intracerebral hemorrhage**

I69.131   Monoplegia of upper limb following nontraumatic intracerebral hemorrhage affecting right dominant side 🖐

I69.132   Monoplegia of upper limb following nontraumatic intracerebral hemorrhage affecting left dominant side 🖐

I69.133   Monoplegia of upper limb following nontraumatic intracerebral hemorrhage affecting right non-dominant side 🖐

I69.134   Monoplegia of upper limb following nontraumatic intracerebral hemorrhage affecting left non-dominant side 🖐

I69.139   Monoplegia of upper limb following nontraumatic intracerebral hemorrhage affecting unspecified side 🖐

◄ New   ◄ Revised   ~~deleted~~ Deleted   Excludes 1   Excludes 2   Includes   Use additional   Code first   Code also   Unspecified
OGCR Official Guidelines   ● Unacceptable Principal Diagnosis   X Assign placeholder X   ● Use Additional Character(s)   ▶ Manifestation Code   **Coding Clinic**

● **I69.14** Monoplegia of lower limb following nontraumatic intracerebral hemorrhage

  I69.141 Monoplegia of lower limb following nontraumatic intracerebral hemorrhage affecting right dominant side 🖫

  I69.142 Monoplegia of lower limb following nontraumatic intracerebral hemorrhage affecting left dominant side 🖫

  I69.143 Monoplegia of lower limb following nontraumatic intracerebral hemorrhage affecting right non-dominant side 🖫

  I69.144 Monoplegia of lower limb following nontraumatic intracerebral hemorrhage affecting left non-dominant side 🖫

  I69.149 Monoplegia of lower limb following nontraumatic intracerebral hemorrhage affecting unspecified side 🖫

● **I69.15** Hemiplegia and hemiparesis following nontraumatic intracerebral hemorrhage

  I69.151 Hemiplegia and hemiparesis following nontraumatic intracerebral hemorrhage affecting right dominant side 🖫 🖫
    (Ex:) See I69.051

  I69.152 Hemiplegia and hemiparesis following nontraumatic intracerebral hemorrhage affecting left dominant side 🖫 🖫
    (Ex:) See I69.051

  I69.153 Hemiplegia and hemiparesis following nontraumatic intracerebral hemorrhage affecting right non-dominant side 🖫 🖫
    (Ex:) See I69.053

  I69.154 Hemiplegia and hemiparesis following nontraumatic intracerebral hemorrhage affecting left non-dominant side 🖫 🖫
    (Ex:) See I69.053

  I69.159 Hemiplegia and hemiparesis following nontraumatic intracerebral hemorrhage affecting unspecified side 🖫 🖫
    (Ex:) See I69.059

● **I69.16** Other paralytic syndrome following nontraumatic intracerebral hemorrhage

  Use additional code to identify type of paralytic syndrome, such as:
    locked-in state (G83.5)
    quadriplegia (G82.5-)

  Excludes1 hemiplegia/hemiparesis following nontraumatic intracerebral hemorrhage (I69.15-)
    monoplegia of lower limb following nontraumatic intracerebral hemorrhage (I69.14-)
    monoplegia of upper limb following nontraumatic intracerebral hemorrhage (I69.13-)

  I69.161 Other paralytic syndrome following nontraumatic intracerebral hemorrhage affecting right dominant side 🖫

  I69.162 Other paralytic syndrome following nontraumatic intracerebral hemorrhage affecting left dominant side 🖫

  I69.163 Other paralytic syndrome following nontraumatic intracerebral hemorrhage affecting right non-dominant side 🖫

  I69.164 Other paralytic syndrome following nontraumatic intracerebral hemorrhage affecting left non-dominant side 🖫

  I69.165 Other paralytic syndrome following nontraumatic intracerebral hemorrhage, bilateral 🖫

  I69.169 Other paralytic syndrome following nontraumatic intracerebral hemorrhage affecting unspecified side 🖫

● **I69.19** Other sequelae of nontraumatic intracerebral hemorrhage

  I69.190 Apraxia following nontraumatic intracerebral hemorrhage 🖫

  I69.191 Dysphagia following nontraumatic intracerebral hemorrhage 🖫

    Use additional code to identify the type of dysphagia, if known (R13.1-)

  I69.192 Facial weakness following nontraumatic intracerebral hemorrhage 🖫

    Facial droop following nontraumatic intracerebral hemorrhage

  I69.193 Ataxia following nontraumatic intracerebral hemorrhage 🖫

  I69.198 Other sequelae of nontraumatic intracerebral hemorrhage 🖫

    Alteration of sensations following nontraumatic intracerebral hemorrhage
    Disturbance of vision following nontraumatic intracerebral hemorrhage

    Use additional code to identify the sequelae

● **I69.2** Sequelae of other nontraumatic intracranial hemorrhage

  I69.20 Unspecified sequelae of other nontraumatic intracranial hemorrhage 🖫

  I69.21 Cognitive deficits following other nontraumatic intracranial hemorrhage 🖫

● **I69.22** Speech and language deficits following other nontraumatic intracranial hemorrhage

  I69.220 Aphasia following other nontraumatic intracranial hemorrhage 🖫

  I69.221 Dysphasia following other nontraumatic intracranial hemorrhage 🖫

  I69.222 Dysarthria following other nontraumatic intracranial hemorrhage 🖫

  I69.223 Fluency disorder following other nontraumatic intracranial hemorrhage 🖫

    Stuttering following nontraumatic subarachnoid hemorrhage

  I69.228 Other speech and language deficits following other nontraumatic intracranial hemorrhage 🖫

CHAPTER 9 (I00-I99)

N Newborn Age: 0   P Pediatric Age: 0–17   M Maternity DX: 12–55   A Adult Age: 15–124   ♀ Females Only   ♂ Males Only

🖫 Complication\Comorbidity   🖫 Major C\C   (Ex:) CC/MCC Exclusions   🖫 Present on Admission Requirement   🖫 Hospital-Acquired Condition

977

I69.23 Monoplegia of upper limb following other nontraumatic intracranial hemorrhage

    I69.231 Monoplegia of upper limb following other nontraumatic intracranial hemorrhage affecting right dominant side

    I69.232 Monoplegia of upper limb following other nontraumatic intracranial hemorrhage affecting left dominant side

    I69.233 Monoplegia of upper limb following other nontraumatic intracranial hemorrhage affecting right non-dominant side

    I69.234 Monoplegia of upper limb following other nontraumatic intracranial hemorrhage affecting left non-dominant side

    I69.239 Monoplegia of upper limb following other nontraumatic intracranial hemorrhage affecting unspecified side

I69.24 Monoplegia of lower limb following other nontraumatic intracranial hemorrhage

    I69.241 Monoplegia of lower limb following other nontraumatic intracranial hemorrhage affecting right dominant side

    I69.242 Monoplegia of lower limb following other nontraumatic intracranial hemorrhage affecting left dominant side

    I69.243 Monoplegia of lower limb following other nontraumatic intracranial hemorrhage affecting right non-dominant side

    I69.244 Monoplegia of lower limb following other nontraumatic intracranial hemorrhage affecting left non-dominant side

    I69.249 Monoplegia of lower limb following other nontraumatic intracranial hemorrhage affecting unspecified side

I69.25 Hemiplegia and hemiparesis following other nontraumatic intracranial hemorrhage

    I69.251 Hemiplegia and hemiparesis following other nontraumatic intracranial hemorrhage affecting right dominant side
        (Ex) See I69.051

    I69.252 Hemiplegia and hemiparesis following other nontraumatic intracranial hemorrhage affecting left dominant side
        (Ex) See I69.051

    I69.253 Hemiplegia and hemiparesis following other nontraumatic intracranial hemorrhage affecting right non-dominant side
        (Ex) See I69.053

    I69.254 Hemiplegia and hemiparesis following other nontraumatic intracranial hemorrhage affecting left non-dominant side
        (Ex) See I69.053

    I69.259 Hemiplegia and hemiparesis following other nontraumatic intracranial hemorrhage affecting unspecified side
        (Ex) See I69.059

I69.26 Other paralytic syndrome following other nontraumatic intracranial hemorrhage

    Use additional code to identify type of paralytic syndrome, such as:
    locked-in state (G83.5)
    quadriplegia (G82.5-)

    Excludes1 hemiplegia/hemiparesis following other nontraumatic intracranial hemorrhage (I69.25-)
        monoplegia of lower limb following other nontraumatic intracranial hemorrhage (I69.24-)
        monoplegia of upper limb following other nontraumatic intracranial hemorrhage (I69.23-)

    I69.261 Other paralytic syndrome following other nontraumatic intracranial hemorrhage affecting right dominant side

    I69.262 Other paralytic syndrome following other nontraumatic intracranial hemorrhage affecting left dominant side

    I69.263 Other paralytic syndrome following other nontraumatic intracranial hemorrhage affecting right non-dominant side

    I69.264 Other paralytic syndrome following other nontraumatic intracranial hemorrhage affecting left non-dominant side

    I69.265 Other paralytic syndrome following other nontraumatic intracranial hemorrhage, bilateral

    I69.269 Other paralytic syndrome following other nontraumatic intracranial hemorrhage affecting unspecified side

I69.29 Other sequelae of other nontraumatic intracranial hemorrhage

    I69.290 Apraxia following other nontraumatic intracranial hemorrhage

    I69.291 Dysphagia following other nontraumatic intracranial hemorrhage

        Use additional code to identify the type of dysphagia, if known (R13.1-)

    I69.292 Facial weakness following other nontraumatic intracranial hemorrhage

        Facial droop following other nontraumatic intracranial hemorrhage

    I69.293 Ataxia following other nontraumatic intracranial hemorrhage

    I69.298 Other sequelae of other nontraumatic intracranial hemorrhage

        Alteration of sensation following other nontraumatic intracranial hemorrhage
        Disturbance of vision following other nontraumatic intracranial hemorrhage

        Use additional code to identify the sequelae

CHAPTER 9 (I00-I99)

◄ New ◄▥ Revised ~~deleted~~ Deleted | Excludes 1 | Excludes 2 | Includes | Use additional | Code first | Code also | Unspecified
OGCR Official Guidelines ● Unacceptable Principal Diagnosis X Assign placeholder X ● Use Additional Character(s) ▸ Manifestation Code **Coding Clinic**

● **I69.3** **Sequelae of cerebral infarction**
Sequelae of stroke NOS
Coding Clinic: 2012, Q4, P92, 95

     I69.30   Unspecified sequelae of cerebral infarction

     I69.31   Cognitive deficits following cerebral infarction

●   I69.32   Speech and language deficits following cerebral infarction

         I69.320   Aphasia following cerebral infarction

         I69.321   Dysphasia following cerebral infarction
                 Coding Clinic: 2012, Q4, P91

         I69.322   Dysarthria following cerebral infarction

         I69.323   Fluency disorder following cerebral infarction
                 Stuttering following nontraumatic subarachnoid hemorrhage

         I69.328   Other speech and language deficits following cerebral infarction

●   I69.33   Monoplegia of upper limb following cerebral infarction

         I69.331   Monoplegia of upper limb following cerebral infarction affecting right dominant side

         I69.332   Monoplegia of upper limb following cerebral infarction affecting left dominant side

         I69.333   Monoplegia of upper limb following cerebral infarction affecting right non-dominant side

         I69.334   Monoplegia of upper limb following cerebral infarction affecting left non-dominant side

         I69.339   Monoplegia of upper limb following cerebral infarction affecting unspecified side

●   I69.34   Monoplegia of lower limb following cerebral infarction

         I69.341   Monoplegia of lower limb following cerebral infarction affecting right dominant side

         I69.342   Monoplegia of lower limb following cerebral infarction affecting left dominant side

         I69.343   Monoplegia of lower limb following cerebral infarction affecting right non-dominant side

         I69.344   Monoplegia of lower limb following cerebral infarction affecting left non-dominant side

         I69.349   Monoplegia of lower limb following cerebral infarction affecting unspecified side

●   I69.35   Hemiplegia and hemiparesis following cerebral infarction

         I69.351   Hemiplegia and hemiparesis following cerebral infarction affecting right dominant side
                 Ex: See I69.051

         I69.352   Hemiplegia and hemiparesis following cerebral infarction affecting left dominant side
                 Ex: See I69.051

         I69.353   Hemiplegia and hemiparesis following cerebral infarction affecting right non-dominant side
                 Ex: See I69.053

         I69.354   Hemiplegia and hemiparesis following cerebral infarction affecting left non-dominant side
                 Ex: See I69.053
                 Coding Clinic: 2012, Q4, P91

         I69.359   Hemiplegia and hemiparesis following cerebral infarction affecting unspecified side
                 Ex: See I69.059

● I69.36 **Other paralytic syndrome following cerebral infarction**
       Use additional code to identify type of paralytic syndrome, such as:
         locked-in state (G83.5)
         quadriplegia (G82.5-)

       Excludes1   hemiplegia/hemiparesis following cerebral infarction (I69.35-)
                 monoplegia of lower limb following cerebral infarction (I69.34-)
                 monoplegia of upper limb following cerebral infarction (I69.33-)

         I69.361   Other paralytic syndrome following cerebral infarction affecting right dominant side

         I69.362   Other paralytic syndrome following cerebral infarction affecting left dominant side

         I69.363   Other paralytic syndrome following cerebral infarction affecting right non-dominant side

         I69.364   Other paralytic syndrome following cerebral infarction affecting left non-dominant side

         I69.365   Other paralytic syndrome following cerebral infarction, bilateral

         I69.369   Other paralytic syndrome following cerebral infarction affecting unspecified side

●   I69.39   Other sequelae of cerebral infarction

         I69.390   Apraxia following cerebral infarction

         I69.391   Dysphagia following cerebral infarction
                 Use additional code to identify the type of dysphagia, if known (R13.1-)

         I69.392   Facial weakness following cerebral infarction
                 Facial droop following cerebral infarction

         I69.393   Ataxia following cerebral infarction

         I69.398   Other sequelae of cerebral infarction
                 Alteration of sensation following cerebral infarction
                 Disturbance of vision following cerebral infarction
                 Use additional code to identify the sequelae

CHAPTER 9 (I00-I99)

N   Newborn Age: 0   **P**   Pediatric Age: 0–17   **M**   Maternity DX: 12–55   **A**   Adult Age: 15–124   ♀   Females Only   ♂   Males Only

 Complication\Comorbidity   Major C\C   Ex: CC/MCC Exclusions   Present on Admission Requirement   Hospital-Acquired Condition

979

● **I69.8 Sequelae of other cerebrovascular diseases**

> **Excludes1**   sequelae of traumatic intracranial injury (S06.-)

I69.80   Unspecified sequelae of other cerebrovascular disease ✎

I69.81   Cognitive deficits following other cerebrovascular disease ✎

● **I69.82**   Speech and language deficits following other cerebrovascular disease

     I69.820   Aphasia following other cerebrovascular disease ✎

     I69.821   Dysphasia following other cerebrovascular disease ✎

     I69.822   Dysarthria following other cerebrovascular disease ✎

     I69.823   Fluency disorder following other cerebrovascular disease ✎
              Stuttering following nontraumatic subarachnoid hemorrhage

     I69.828   Other speech and language deficits following other cerebrovascular disease ✎

● **I69.83**   Monoplegia of upper limb following other cerebrovascular disease

     I69.831   Monoplegia of upper limb following other cerebrovascular disease affecting right dominant side ✎

     I69.832   Monoplegia of upper limb following other cerebrovascular disease affecting left dominant side ✎

     I69.833   Monoplegia of upper limb following other cerebrovascular disease affecting right non-dominant side ✎

     I69.834   Monoplegia of upper limb following other cerebrovascular disease affecting left non-dominant side ✎

     I69.839   Monoplegia of upper limb following other cerebrovascular disease affecting unspecified side ✎

● **I69.84**   Monoplegia of lower limb following other cerebrovascular disease

     I69.841   Monoplegia of lower limb following other cerebrovascular disease affecting right dominant side ✎

     I69.842   Monoplegia of lower limb following other cerebrovascular disease affecting left dominant side ✎

     I69.843   Monoplegia of lower limb following other cerebrovascular disease affecting right non-dominant side ✎

     I69.844   Monoplegia of lower limb following other cerebrovascular disease affecting left non-dominant side ✎

     I69.849   Monoplegia of lower limb following other cerebrovascular disease affecting unspecified side ✎

● **I69.85**   Hemiplegia and hemiparesis following other cerebrovascular disease

     I69.851   Hemiplegia and hemiparesis following other cerebrovascular disease affecting right dominant side ✎ ✎
              (Ex:) See I69.051

     I69.852   Hemiplegia and hemiparesis following other cerebrovascular disease affecting left dominant side ✎ ✎
              (Ex:) See I69.051

     I69.853   Hemiplegia and hemiparesis following other cerebrovascular disease affecting right non-dominant side ✎
              (Ex:) See I69.053

     I69.854   Hemiplegia and hemiparesis following other cerebrovascular disease affecting left non-dominant side ✎
              (Ex:) See I69.053

     I69.859   Hemiplegia and hemiparesis following other cerebrovascular disease affecting unspecified side ✎
              (Ex:) See I69.059

● **I69.86**   Other paralytic syndrome following other cerebrovascular disease

> Use additional code to identify type of paralytic syndrome, such as:
> locked-in state (G83.5)
> quadriplegia (G82.5-)

> **Excludes1**   hemiplegia/hemiparesis following other cerebrovascular disease (I69.85-)
> monoplegia of lower limb following other cerebrovascular disease (I69.84-)
> monoplegia of upper limb following other cerebrovascular disease (I69.83-)

     I69.861   Other paralytic syndrome following other cerebrovascular disease affecting right dominant side ✎

     I69.862   Other paralytic syndrome following other cerebrovascular disease affecting left dominant side ✎

     I69.863   Other paralytic syndrome following other cerebrovascular disease affecting right non-dominant side ✎

     I69.864   Other paralytic syndrome following other cerebrovascular disease affecting left non-dominant side ✎

     I69.865   Other paralytic syndrome following other cerebrovascular disease, bilateral ✎

     I69.869   Other paralytic syndrome following other cerebrovascular disease affecting unspecified side ✎

● **I69.89**   Other sequelae of other cerebrovascular disease

     I69.890   Apraxia following other cerebrovascular disease ✎

     I69.891   Dysphagia following other cerebrovascular disease ✎

> Use additional code to identify the type of dysphagia, if known (R13.1-)

     I69.892   Facial weakness following other cerebrovascular disease ✎
              Facial droop following other cerebrovascular disease

     I69.893   Ataxia following other cerebrovascular disease ✎

     I69.898   Other sequelae of other cerebrovascular disease ✎
              Alteration of sensation following other cerebrovascular disease
              Disturbance of vision following other cerebrovascular disease

> Use additional code to identify the sequelae

◀ New   ◀ Revised   ~~deleted~~ Deleted   Excludes 1   Excludes 2   Includes   Use additional   Code first   Code also   Unspecified

OGCR Official Guidelines   ● Unacceptable Principal Diagnosis   X Assign placeholder X   ● Use Additional Character(s)   ▶ Manifestation Code   **Coding Clinic**

● **I69.9**   **Sequelae of unspecified cerebrovascular diseases**

     Excludes1   sequelae of stroke (I69.3)
                 sequelae of traumatic intracranial injury
                   (S06.-)

I69.90   Unspecified sequelae of unspecified cerebrovascular disease 🖉

I69.91   Cognitive deficits following unspecified cerebrovascular disease 🖉

● **I69.92**   Speech and language deficits following unspecified cerebrovascular disease

    I69.920   Aphasia following unspecified cerebrovascular disease 🖉

    I69.921   Dysphasia following unspecified cerebrovascular disease 🖉

    I69.922   Dysarthria following unspecified cerebrovascular disease 🖉

    I69.923   Fluency disorder following unspecified cerebrovascular disease 🖉

           Stuttering following nontraumatic subarachnoid hemorrhage

    I69.928   Other speech and language deficits following unspecified cerebrovascular disease 🖉

● **I69.93**   Monoplegia of upper limb following unspecified cerebrovascular disease

    I69.931   Monoplegia of upper limb following unspecified cerebrovascular disease affecting right dominant side 🖉

    I69.932   Monoplegia of upper limb following unspecified cerebrovascular disease affecting left dominant side 🖉

    I69.933   Monoplegia of upper limb following unspecified cerebrovascular disease affecting right non-dominant side 🖉

    I69.934   Monoplegia of upper limb following unspecified cerebrovascular disease affecting left non-dominant side 🖉

    I69.939   Monoplegia of upper limb following unspecified cerebrovascular disease affecting unspecified side 🖉

● **I69.94**   Monoplegia of lower limb following unspecified cerebrovascular disease

    I69.941   Monoplegia of lower limb following unspecified cerebrovascular disease affecting right dominant side 🖉

    I69.942   Monoplegia of lower limb following unspecified cerebrovascular disease affecting left dominant side 🖉

    I69.943   Monoplegia of lower limb following unspecified cerebrovascular disease affecting right non-dominant side 🖉

    I69.944   Monoplegia of lower limb following unspecified cerebrovascular disease affecting left non-dominant side 🖉

    I69.949   Monoplegia of lower limb following unspecified cerebrovascular disease affecting unspecified side 🖉

● **I69.95**   Hemiplegia and hemiparesis following unspecified cerebrovascular disease

    I69.951   Hemiplegia and hemiparesis following unspecified cerebrovascular disease affecting right dominant side 🖉 🖉
           Ⓔ See I69.051

    I69.952   Hemiplegia and hemiparesis following unspecified cerebrovascular disease affecting left dominant side 🖉 🖉
           Ⓔ See I69.051

    I69.953   Hemiplegia and hemiparesis following unspecified cerebrovascular disease affecting right non-dominant side 🖉 🖉
           Ⓔ See I69.053

    I69.954   Hemiplegia and hemiparesis following unspecified cerebrovascular disease affecting left non-dominant side 🖉 🖉
           Ⓔ See I69.053

    I69.959   Hemiplegia and hemiparesis following unspecified cerebrovascular disease affecting unspecified side 🖉 🖉
           Ⓔ See I69.059

● **I69.96**   Other paralytic syndrome following unspecified cerebrovascular disease

    Use additional code to identify type of paralytic syndrome, such as:
      locked-in state (G83.5)
      quadriplegia (G82.5-)

    Excludes1   hemiplegia/hemiparesis following unspecified cerebrovascular disease (I69.95-)
           monoplegia of lower limb following unspecified cerebrovascular disease (I69.94-)
           monoplegia of upper limb following unspecified cerebrovascular disease (I69.93-)

    I69.961   Other paralytic syndrome following unspecified cerebrovascular disease affecting right dominant side 🖉

    I69.962   Other paralytic syndrome following unspecified cerebrovascular disease affecting left dominant side 🖉

    I69.963   Other paralytic syndrome following unspecified cerebrovascular disease affecting right non-dominant side 🖉

    I69.964   Other paralytic syndrome following unspecified cerebrovascular disease affecting left non-dominant side 🖉

    I69.965   Other paralytic syndrome following unspecified cerebrovascular disease, bilateral 🖉

    I69.969   Other paralytic syndrome following unspecified cerebrovascular disease affecting unspecified side 🖉

● **I69.99**   Other sequelae of unspecified cerebrovascular disease

    I69.990   Apraxia following unspecified cerebrovascular disease 🖉

    I69.991   Dysphagia following unspecified cerebrovascular disease 🖉

           Use additional code to identify the type of dysphagia, if known (R13.1-)

    I69.992   Facial weakness following unspecified cerebrovascular disease 🖉

           Facial droop following unspecified cerebrovascular disease

    I69.993   Ataxia following unspecified cerebrovascular disease 🖉

    I69.998   Other sequelae following unspecified cerebrovascular disease 🖉

           Alteration in sensation following unspecified cerebrovascular disease

           Disturbance of vision following unspecified cerebrovascular disease

           Use additional code to identify the sequelae

CHAPTER 9 (I00-I99)

N Newborn Age: 0   P Pediatric Age: 0–17   M Maternity DX: 12–55   A Adult Age: 15–124   ♀ Females Only   ♂ Males Only

🖉 Complication\Comorbidity   🖉 Major C\C   Ⓔ CC/MCC Exclusions   🖉 Present on Admission Requirement   🖉 Hospital-Acquired Condition

981

DISEASES OF ARTERIES, ARTERIOLES AND CAPILLARIES (I70-I79)

- I70   **Atherosclerosis**

  Includes   arteriolosclerosis
  arterial degeneration
  arteriosclerosis
  arteriosclerotic vascular disease
  arteriovascular degeneration
  atheroma
  endarteritis deformans or obliterans
  senile arteritis
  senile endarteritis
  vascular degeneration

  Use additional code to identify:
  exposure to environmental tobacco smoke (Z77.22)
  history of tobacco use (Z87.891)
  occupational exposure to environmental tobacco smoke
  (Z57.31)
  tobacco dependence (F17.-)
  tobacco use (Z72.0)

  Excludes2   arteriosclerotic cardiovascular disease (I25.1-)
  arteriosclerotic heart disease (I25.1-)
  atheroembolism (I75.-)
  cerebral atherosclerosis (I67.2)
  coronary atherosclerosis (I25.1-)
  mesenteric atherosclerosis (K55.1)
  precerebral atherosclerosis (I67.2)
  primary pulmonary atherosclerosis (I27.0)

  I70.0   **Atherosclerosis of aorta**   A
  I70.1   **Atherosclerosis of renal artery**   A
           Goldblatt's kidney

           Excludes2   atherosclerosis of renal arterioles (I12.-)

(See Plates 500, 501, and 502 on pages 60 – 62.)

- I70.2   **Atherosclerosis of native arteries of the extremities**
           Mönckeberg's (medial) sclerosis
           Use additional code, if applicable, to identify chronic
           total occlusion of artery of extremity (I70.92)

           Excludes2   atherosclerosis of bypass graft of
           extremities (I70.30-I70.79)

  - I70.20   **Unspecified atherosclerosis of native arteries of
              extremities**

    I70.201   **Unspecified atherosclerosis of native
               arteries of extremities, right leg**   A
    I70.202   **Unspecified atherosclerosis of native
               arteries of extremities, left leg**   A
    I70.203   **Unspecified atherosclerosis of native
               arteries of extremities, bilateral legs**   A
    I70.208   **Unspecified atherosclerosis of native
               arteries of extremities, other extremity**
                                                             A
    I70.209   **Unspecified atherosclerosis of native
               arteries of extremities, unspecified
               extremity**   A

  - I70.21   **Atherosclerosis of native arteries of extremities
              with intermittent claudication**
    I70.211   **Atherosclerosis of native arteries
               of extremities with intermittent
               claudication, right leg**   A
    I70.212   **Atherosclerosis of native arteries
               of extremities with intermittent
               claudication, left leg**   A
    I70.213   **Atherosclerosis of native arteries
               of extremities with intermittent
               claudication, bilateral legs**   A
    I70.218   **Atherosclerosis of native arteries
               of extremities with intermittent
               claudication, other extremity**   A
    I70.219   **Atherosclerosis of native arteries
               of extremities with intermittent
               claudication, unspecified extremity**   A

- I70.22   **Atherosclerosis of native arteries of extremities
            with rest pain**

    Includes   any condition classifiable to
                    I70.21-
    I70.221   **Atherosclerosis of native arteries of
               extremities with rest pain, right leg**   A
    I70.222   **Atherosclerosis of native arteries of
               extremities with rest pain, left leg**   A
    I70.223   **Atherosclerosis of native arteries of
               extremities with rest pain, bilateral
               legs**   A
    I70.228   **Atherosclerosis of native arteries
               of extremities with rest pain, other
               extremity**   A
    I70.229   **Atherosclerosis of native arteries of
               extremities with rest pain, unspecified
               extremity**   A

- I70.23   **Atherosclerosis of native arteries of right leg
            with ulceration**

    Includes   any condition classifiable to
                    I70.211 and I70.221

    Use additional code to identify severity of
    ulcer (L97.-) ◀▥
    I70.231   **Atherosclerosis of native arteries of
               right leg with ulceration of thigh**   A
    I70.232   **Atherosclerosis of native arteries of
               right leg with ulceration of calf**   A
    I70.233   **Atherosclerosis of native arteries of
               right leg with ulceration of ankle**   A
    I70.234   **Atherosclerosis of native arteries of
               right leg with ulceration of heel and
               midfoot**   A
               Atherosclerosis of native arteries
               of right leg with ulceration of
               plantar surface of midfoot
    I70.235   **Atherosclerosis of native arteries of
               right leg with ulceration of other part
               of foot**   A
               Atherosclerosis of native arteries
               of right leg extremities with
               ulceration of toe
    I70.238   **Atherosclerosis of native arteries of
               right leg with ulceration of other part
               of lower right leg**   A
    I70.239   **Atherosclerosis of native arteries
               of right leg with ulceration of
               unspecified site**   A

- I70.24   **Atherosclerosis of native arteries of left leg
            with ulceration**

    Includes   any condition classifiable to
                    I70.212 and I70.222

    Use additional code to identify severity of
    ulcer (L97.-) ◀▥
    I70.241   **Atherosclerosis of native arteries of
               left leg with ulceration of thigh**   A
    I70.242   **Atherosclerosis of native arteries of
               left leg with ulceration of calf**   A
    I70.243   **Atherosclerosis of native arteries of
               left leg with ulceration of ankle**   A
    I70.244   **Atherosclerosis of native arteries of
               left leg with ulceration of heel and
               midfoot**   A
               Atherosclerosis of native arteries
               of left leg with ulceration of
               plantar surface of midfoot
    I70.245   **Atherosclerosis of native arteries of
               left leg with ulceration of other part
               of foot**   A
               Atherosclerosis of native arteries
               of left leg extremities with
               ulceration of toe

◀ New   ◀▥ Revised   ~~deleted~~ Deleted   Excludes 1   Excludes 2   Includes   Use additional   Code first   Code also   Unspecified

OGCR Official Guidelines   ● Unacceptable Principal Diagnosis   X Assign placeholder X   ● Use Additional Character(s)   ▌ Manifestation Code   **Coding Clinic**

I70.248　Atherosclerosis of native arteries of left leg with ulceration of other part of lower left leg　A

I70.249　Atherosclerosis of native arteries of left leg with ulceration of unspecified site　A

I70.25　Atherosclerosis of native arteries of other extremities with ulceration　A

> **Includes**　any condition classifiable to I70.218 and I70.228
>
> Use additional code to identify the severity of the ulcer (L98.49-)

● **I70.26**　Atherosclerosis of native arteries of extremities with gangrene

> **Includes**　any condition classifiable to I70.21-, I70.22-, I70.23-, I70.24-, and I70.25-
>
> Use additional code to identify the severity of any ulcer (L97.-, L98.49-), if applicable ◄▥
>
> (Ex) For category I70.26 CC codes: G89.0-G89.4, I70.261-I70.269, I96, R41.0-R41.3, R41.82, R41.9, R44.8-R44.9, R45.83-R45.84, R46.0-R46.89, R52, R68.0-R68.19, R68.81-R68.83, R68.89-R69

I70.261　Atherosclerosis of native arteries of extremities with gangrene, right leg 🅒　A

I70.262　Atherosclerosis of native arteries of extremities with gangrene, left leg 🅒A

I70.263　Atherosclerosis of native arteries of extremities with gangrene, bilateral legs 🅒　A

I70.268　Atherosclerosis of native arteries of extremities with gangrene, other extremity 🅒　A

I70.269　Atherosclerosis of native arteries of extremities with gangrene, unspecified extremity 🅒　A

● **I70.29**　Other atherosclerosis of native arteries of extremities

I70.291　Other atherosclerosis of native arteries of extremities, right leg　A

I70.292　Other atherosclerosis of native arteries of extremities, left leg　A

I70.293　Other atherosclerosis of native arteries of extremities, bilateral legs　A

I70.298　Other atherosclerosis of native arteries of extremities, other extremity

I70.299　Other atherosclerosis of native arteries of extremities, unspecified extremity　A

● **I70.3**　Atherosclerosis of unspecified type of bypass graft(s) of the extremities

> Use additional code, if applicable, to identify chronic total occlusion of artery of extremity (I70.92)
>
> **Excludes1**　embolism or thrombus of bypass graft(s) of extremities (T82.8-)

● **I70.30**　Unspecified atherosclerosis of unspecified type of bypass graft(s) of the extremities

70.301　Unspecified atherosclerosis of unspecified type of bypass graft(s) of the extremities, right leg　A

I70.302　Unspecified atherosclerosis of unspecified type of bypass graft(s) of the extremities, left leg　A

I70.303　Unspecified atherosclerosis of unspecified type of bypass graft(s) of the extremities, bilateral legs　A

I70.308　Unspecified atherosclerosis of unspecified type of bypass graft(s) of the extremities, other extremity　A

I70.309　Unspecified atherosclerosis of unspecified type of bypass graft(s) of the extremities, unspecified extremity

● **I70.31**　Atherosclerosis of unspecified type of bypass graft(s) of the extremities with intermittent claudication

I70.311　Atherosclerosis of unspecified type of bypass graft(s) of the extremities with intermittent claudication, right leg　A

I70.312　Atherosclerosis of unspecified type of bypass graft(s) of the extremities with intermittent claudication, left leg　A

I70.313　Atherosclerosis of unspecified type of bypass graft(s) of the extremities with intermittent claudication, bilateral legs　A

I70.318　Atherosclerosis of unspecified type of bypass graft(s) of the extremities with intermittent claudication, other extremity　A

I70.319　Atherosclerosis of unspecified type of bypass graft(s) of the extremities with intermittent claudication, unspecified extremity　A

● **I70.32**　Atherosclerosis of unspecified type of bypass graft(s) of the extremities with rest pain

> **Includes**　any condition classifiable to I70.31-

I70.321　Atherosclerosis of unspecified type of bypass graft(s) of the extremities with rest pain, right leg　A

I70.322　Atherosclerosis of unspecified type of bypass graft(s) of the extremities with rest pain, left leg　A

I70.323　Atherosclerosis of unspecified type of bypass graft(s) of the extremities with rest pain, bilateral legs　A

I70.328　Atherosclerosis of unspecified type of bypass graft(s) of the extremities with rest pain, other extremity　A

I70.329　Atherosclerosis of unspecified type of bypass graft(s) of the extremities with rest pain, unspecified extremity　A

● **I70.33**　Atherosclerosis of unspecified type of bypass graft(s) of the right leg with ulceration

> **Includes**　any condition classifiable to I70.311 and I70.321
>
> Use additional code to identify severity of ulcer (L97.-) ◄▥
>
> (Ex) For category I70.33 CC codes: I70.231-I70.25, L44.8-L45, L94.2, L94.4, L97.101-L97.929, L98.411-L98.499, L98.8-L99

I70.331　Atherosclerosis of unspecified type of bypass graft(s) of the right leg with ulceration of thigh 🅒　A
　　　　CC when PDx is its own CC

I70.332　Atherosclerosis of unspecified type of bypass graft(s) of the right leg with ulceration of calf 🅒　A
　　　　CC when PDx is its own CC

I70.333　Atherosclerosis of unspecified type of bypass graft(s) of the right leg with ulceration of ankle 🅒　A
　　　　CC when PDx is its own CC

CHAPTER 9 (I00-I99)

N　Newborn Age: 0　　P　Pediatric Age: 0–17　　M　Maternity DX: 12–55　　A　Adult Age: 15–124　　♀　Females Only　　♂　Males Only

🅒　Complication\Comorbidity　　🅜　Major C\C　　(Ex)　CC/MCC Exclusions　　🅟　Present on Admission Requirement　　🅗　Hospital-Acquired Condition

983

I70.334   Atherosclerosis of unspecified type of bypass graft(s) of the right leg with ulceration of heel and midfoot 🔎   A
Atherosclerosis of unspecified type of bypass graft(s) of right leg with ulceration of plantar surface of midfoot
CC when PDx is its own CC

I70.335   Atherosclerosis of unspecified type of bypass graft(s) of the right leg with ulceration of other part of foot
Atherosclerosis of unspecified type of bypass graft(s) of the right leg with ulceration of toe

I70.338   Atherosclerosis of unspecified type of bypass graft(s) of the right leg with ulceration of other part of lower leg 🔎   A
CC when PDx is its own CC

I70.339   Atherosclerosis of unspecified type of bypass graft(s) of the right leg with ulceration of unspecified site 🔎   A
CC when PDx is its own CC

● I70.34   Atherosclerosis of unspecified type of bypass graft(s) of the left leg with ulceration
Includes   any condition classifiable to I70.312 and I70.322
Use additional code to identify severity of ulcer (L97.-) ◀▥
(Ex) For category I70.34 CC codes: See I70.33

I70.341   Atherosclerosis of unspecified type of bypass graft(s) of the left leg with ulceration of thigh 🔎   A
CC when PDx is its own CC

I70.342   Atherosclerosis of unspecified type of bypass graft(s) of the left leg with ulceration of calf 🔎   A
CC when PDx is its own CC

I70.343   Atherosclerosis of unspecified type of bypass graft(s) of the left leg with ulceration of ankle 🔎   A
CC when PDx is its own CC

I70.344   Atherosclerosis of unspecified type of bypass graft(s) of the left leg with ulceration of heel and midfoot 🔎   A
Atherosclerosis of unspecified type of bypass graft(s) of left leg with ulceration of plantar surface of midfoot
CC when PDx is its own CC

I70.345   Atherosclerosis of unspecified type of bypass graft(s) of the left leg with ulceration of other part of foot   A
Atherosclerosis of unspecified type of bypass graft(s) of the left leg with ulceration of toe

I70.348   Atherosclerosis of unspecified type of bypass graft(s) of the left leg with ulceration of other part of lower leg 🔎   A
CC when PDx is its own CC

I70.349   Atherosclerosis of unspecified type of bypass graft(s) of the left leg with ulceration of unspecified site 🔎   A
CC when PDx is its own CC

I70.35   Atherosclerosis of unspecified type of bypass graft(s) of other extremity with ulceration   A
Includes   any condition classifiable to I70.318 and I70.328
Use additional code to identify severity of ulcer (L98.49-)

● I70.36   Atherosclerosis of unspecified type of bypass graft(s) of the extremities with gangrene
Includes   any condition classifiable to I70.31-, I70.32-, I70.33-, I70.34-, I70.35
Use additional code to identify the severity of any ulcer (L97.-, L98.49-), if applicable ◀▥
(Ex) For category I70.36 CC codes: See I70.26

I70.361   Atherosclerosis of unspecified type of bypass graft(s) of the extremities with gangrene, right leg 🔎   A
CC when PDx is its own CC

I70.362   Atherosclerosis of unspecified type of bypass graft(s) of the extremities with gangrene, left leg 🔎   A
CC when PDx is its own CC

I70.363   Atherosclerosis of unspecified type of bypass graft(s) of the extremities with gangrene, bilateral legs 🔎   A
CC when PDx is its own CC

I70.368   Atherosclerosis of unspecified type of bypass graft(s) of the extremities with gangrene, other extremity 🔎   A
CC when PDx is its own CC

I70.369   Atherosclerosis of unspecified type of bypass graft(s) of the extremities with gangrene, unspecified extremity 🔎   A
CC when PDx is its own CC

● I70.39   Other atherosclerosis of unspecified type of bypass graft(s) of the extremities

I70.391   Other atherosclerosis of unspecified type of bypass graft(s) of the extremities, right leg   A

I70.392   Other atherosclerosis of unspecified type of bypass graft(s) of the extremities, left leg   A

I70.393   Other atherosclerosis of unspecified type of bypass graft(s) of the extremities, bilateral legs   A

I70.398   Other atherosclerosis of unspecified type of bypass graft(s) of the extremities, other extremity   A

I70.399   Other atherosclerosis of unspecified type of bypass graft(s) of the extremities, unspecified extremity   A

● I70.4   Atherosclerosis of autologous vein bypass graft(s) of the extremities
Use additional code, if applicable, to identify chronic total occlusion of artery of extremity (I70.92)

● I70.40   Unspecified atherosclerosis of autologous vein bypass graft(s) of the extremities

I70.401   Unspecified atherosclerosis of autologous vein bypass graft(s) of the extremities, right leg   A

I70.402   Unspecified atherosclerosis of autologous vein bypass graft(s) of the extremities, left leg   A

I70.403   Unspecified atherosclerosis of autologous vein bypass graft(s) of the extremities, bilateral legs   A

I70.408   Unspecified atherosclerosis of autologous vein bypass graft(s) of the extremities, other extremity   A

I70.409   Unspecified atherosclerosis of autologous vein bypass graft(s) of the extremities, unspecified extremity   A

◀ New   ◀▥ Revised   ~~deleted~~ Deleted   Excludes 1   Excludes 2   Includes   Use additional   Code first   Code also   Unspecified
OGCR Official Guidelines   ● Unacceptable Principal Diagnosis   X Assign placeholder X   ● Use Additional Character(s)   ▌ Manifestation Code   Coding Clinic

● **I70.41 Atherosclerosis of autologous vein bypass graft(s) of the extremities with intermittent claudication**

    I70.411   Atherosclerosis of autologous vein bypass graft(s) of the extremities with intermittent claudication, right leg   A

    I70.412   Atherosclerosis of autologous vein bypass graft(s) of the extremities with intermittent claudication, left leg   A

    I70.413   Atherosclerosis of autologous vein bypass graft(s) of the extremities with intermittent claudication, bilateral legs   A

    I70.418   Atherosclerosis of autologous vein bypass graft(s) of the extremities with intermittent claudication, other extremity   A

    I70.419   Atherosclerosis of autologous vein bypass graft(s) of the extremities with intermittent claudication, unspecified extremity

● **I70.42 Atherosclerosis of autologous vein bypass graft(s) of the extremities with rest pain**

    Includes   any condition classifiable to I70.41-

    I70.421   Atherosclerosis of autologous vein bypass graft(s) of the extremities with rest pain, right leg   A

    I70.422   Atherosclerosis of autologous vein bypass graft(s) of the extremities with rest pain, left leg   A

    I70.423   Atherosclerosis of autologous vein bypass graft(s) of the extremities with rest pain, bilateral legs   A

    I70.428   Atherosclerosis of autologous vein bypass graft(s) of the extremities with rest pain, other extremity

    I70.429   Atherosclerosis of autologous vein bypass graft(s) of the extremities with rest pain, unspecified extremity   A

● **I70.43 Atherosclerosis of autologous vein bypass graft(s) of the right leg with ulceration**

    Includes   any condition classifiable to I70.411 and I70.421

    Use additional code to identify severity of ulcer (L97.-) ◄▬

    (Ex) **For category I70.43 CC codes:** See I70.33

    I70.431   Atherosclerosis of autologous vein bypass graft(s) of the right leg with ulceration of thigh 🜂   A
         CC when PDx is its own CC

    I70.432   Atherosclerosis of autologous vein bypass graft(s) of the right leg with ulceration of calf 🜂   A
         CC when PDx is its own CC

    I70.433   Atherosclerosis of autologous vein bypass graft(s) of the right leg with ulceration of ankle 🜂   A
         CC when PDx is its own CC

    I70.434   Atherosclerosis of autologous vein bypass graft(s) of the right leg with ulceration of heel and midfoot 🜂   A
         Atherosclerosis of autologous vein bypass graft(s) of right leg with ulceration of plantar surface of midfoot
         CC when PDx is its own CC

    I70.435   Atherosclerosis of autologous vein bypass graft(s) of the right leg with ulceration of other part of foot   A
         Atherosclerosis of autologous vein bypass graft(s) of right leg with ulceration of toe

    I70.438   Atherosclerosis of autologous vein bypass graft(s) of the right leg with ulceration of other part of lower leg 🜂   A
         CC when PDx is its own CC

    I70.439   Atherosclerosis of autologous vein bypass graft(s) of the right leg with ulceration of unspecified site 🜂   A
         CC when PDx is its own CC

● **I70.44 Atherosclerosis of autologous vein bypass graft(s) of the left leg with ulceration**

    Includes   any condition classifiable to I70.412 and I70.422

    Use additional code to identify severity of ulcer (L97.-) ◄▬

    (Ex) **For category I70.44 CC codes:** See I70.33

    I70.441   Atherosclerosis of autologous vein bypass graft(s) of the left leg with ulceration of thigh 🜂   A
         CC when PDx is its own CC

    I70.442   Atherosclerosis of autologous vein bypass graft(s) of the left leg with ulceration of calf 🜂   A
         CC when PDx is its own CC

    I70.443   Atherosclerosis of autologous vein bypass graft(s) of the left leg with ulceration of ankle 🜂   A
         CC when PDx is its own CC

    I70.444   Atherosclerosis of autologous vein bypass graft(s) of the left leg with ulceration of heel and midfoot 🜂   A
         Atherosclerosis of autologous vein bypass graft(s) of left leg with ulceration of plantar surface of midfoot
         CC when PDx is its own CC

    I70.445   Atherosclerosis of autologous vein bypass graft(s) of the left leg with ulceration of other part of foot   A
         Atherosclerosis of autologous vein bypass graft(s) of left leg with ulceration of toe

    I70.448   Atherosclerosis of autologous vein bypass graft(s) of the left leg with ulceration of other part of lower leg 🜂   A
         CC when PDx is its own CC

    I70.449   Atherosclerosis of autologous vein bypass graft(s) of the left leg with ulceration of unspecified site 🜂   A
         CC when PDx is its own CC

I70.45 Atherosclerosis of autologous vein bypass graft(s) of other extremity with ulceration   A

    Includes   any condition classifiable to I70.418, I70.428, and I70.438

    Use additional code to identify severity of ulcer (L98.49-)

● **I70.46 Atherosclerosis of autologous vein bypass graft(s) of the extremities with gangrene**

    Includes   any condition classifiable to I70.41-, I70.42-, and I70.43-, I70.44-, I70.45

    Use additional code to identify the severity of any ulcer (L97.-, L98.49-), if applicable ◄▬

    (Ex) **For category I70.46 CC codes:** See I70.26

    I70.461   Atherosclerosis of autologous vein bypass graft(s) of the extremities with gangrene, right leg 🜂   A
         CC when PDx is its own CC

    I70.462   Atherosclerosis of autologous vein bypass graft(s) of the extremities with gangrene, left leg 🜂   A
         CC when PDx is its own CC

N   Newborn Age: 0   P   Pediatric Age: 0–17   M   Maternity DX: 12–55   A   Adult Age: 15–124   ♀   Females Only   ♂   Males Only

🜂   Complication\Comorbidity   🜂   Major C\C   (Ex)   CC/MCC Exclusions   🜂   Present on Admission Requirement   🜂   Hospital-Acquired Condition

I70.463   **Atherosclerosis of autologous vein bypass graft(s) of the extremities with gangrene, bilateral legs** 🔖   A
     CC when PDx is its own CC

I70.468   **Atherosclerosis of autologous vein bypass graft(s) of the extremities with gangrene, other extremity** 🔖   A
     CC when PDx is its own CC

I70.469   **Atherosclerosis of autologous vein bypass graft(s) of the extremities with gangrene, unspecified extremity** 🔖   A
     CC when PDx is its own CC

● **I70.49**   **Other atherosclerosis of autologous vein bypass graft(s) of the extremities**

I70.491   **Other atherosclerosis of autologous vein bypass graft(s) of the extremities, right leg**   A

I70.492   **Other atherosclerosis of autologous vein bypass graft(s) of the extremities, left leg**   A

I70.493   **Other atherosclerosis of autologous vein bypass graft(s) of the extremities, bilateral legs**   A

I70.498   **Other atherosclerosis of autologous vein bypass graft(s) of the extremities, other extremity**   A

I70.499   **Other atherosclerosis of autologous vein bypass graft(s) of the extremities, unspecified extremity**   A

● **I70.5**   **Atherosclerosis of nonautologous biological bypass graft(s) of the extremities**
     Use additional code, if applicable, to identify chronic total occlusion of artery of extremity (I70.92)

● **I70.50**   **Unspecified atherosclerosis of nonautologous biological bypass graft(s) of the extremities**

I70.501   **Unspecified atherosclerosis of nonautologous biological bypass graft(s) of the extremities, right leg**   A

I70.502   **Unspecified atherosclerosis of nonautologous biological bypass graft(s) of the extremities, left leg**   A

I70.503   **Unspecified atherosclerosis of nonautologous biological bypass graft(s) of the extremities, bilateral legs**   A

I70.508   **Unspecified atherosclerosis of nonautologous biological bypass graft(s) of the extremities, other extremity**   A

I70.509   **Unspecified atherosclerosis of nonautologous biological bypass graft(s) of the extremities, unspecified extremity**   A

● **I70.51**   **Atherosclerosis of nonautologous biological bypass graft(s) of the extremities intermittent claudication**

I70.511   **Atherosclerosis of nonautologous biological bypass graft(s) of the extremities with intermittent claudication, right leg**   A

I70.512   **Atherosclerosis of nonautologous biological bypass graft(s) of the extremities with intermittent claudication, left leg**   A

I70.513   **Atherosclerosis of nonautologous biological bypass graft(s) of the extremities with intermittent claudication, bilateral legs**   A

I70.518   **Atherosclerosis of nonautologous biological bypass graft(s) of the extremities with intermittent claudication, other extremity**   A

I70.519   **Atherosclerosis of nonautologous biological bypass graft(s) of the extremities with intermittent claudication, unspecified extremity**   A

● **I70.52**   **Atherosclerosis of nonautologous biological bypass graft(s) of the extremities with rest pain**
     Includes   any condition classifiable to I70.51-

I70.521   **Atherosclerosis of nonautologous biological bypass graft(s) of the extremities with rest pain, right leg**   A

I70.522   **Atherosclerosis of nonautologous biological bypass graft(s) of the extremities with rest pain, left leg**   A

I70.523   **Atherosclerosis of nonautologous biological bypass graft(s) of the extremities with rest pain, bilateral legs**   A

I70.528   **Atherosclerosis of nonautologous biological bypass graft(s) of the extremities with rest pain, other extremity**   A

I70.529   **Atherosclerosis of nonautologous biological bypass graft(s) of the extremities with rest pain, unspecified extremity**   A

● **I70.53**   **Atherosclerosis of nonautologous biological bypass graft(s) of the right leg with ulceration**
     Includes   any condition classifiable to I70.511 and I70.521
     Use additional code to identify severity of ulcer (L97.-) ◀▥
     (Ex) For category I70.53 CC codes: See I70.33

I70.531   **Atherosclerosis of nonautologous biological bypass graft(s) of the right leg with ulceration of thigh** 🔖   A
     CC when PDx is its own CC

I70.532   **Atherosclerosis of nonautologous biological bypass graft(s) of the right leg with ulceration of calf** 🔖   A
     CC when PDx is its own CC

I70.533   **Atherosclerosis of nonautologous biological bypass graft(s) of the right leg with ulceration of ankle** 🔖   A
     CC when PDx is its own CC

I70.534   **Atherosclerosis of nonautologous biological bypass graft(s) of the right leg with ulceration of heel and midfoot** 🔖   A
     Atherosclerosis of nonautologous biological bypass graft(s) of right leg with ulceration of plantar surface of midfoot
     CC when PDx is its own CC

I70.535   **Atherosclerosis of nonautologous biological bypass graft(s) of the right leg with ulceration of other part of foot**   A
     Atherosclerosis of nonautologous biological bypass graft(s) of the right leg with ulceration of toe

I70.538   **Atherosclerosis of nonautologous biological bypass graft(s) of the right leg with ulceration of other part of lower leg** 🔖   A
     CC when PDx is its own CC

I70.539   **Atherosclerosis of nonautologous biological bypass graft(s) of the right leg with ulceration of unspecified site** 🔖   A
     CC when PDx is its own CC

◀ New   ◀▥ Revised   ~~deleted~~ Deleted   Excludes 1   Excludes 2   Includes   Use additional   Code first   Code also   Unspecified

OGCR Official Guidelines   ● Unacceptable Principal Diagnosis   X Assign placeholder X   ● Use Additional Character(s)   ▌ Manifestation Code   **Coding Clinic**

● **I70.54**   Atherosclerosis of nonautologous biological bypass graft(s) of the left leg with ulceration

    Includes   any condition classifiable to I70.512 and I70.522

    Use additional code to identify severity of ulcer (L97.-) ◀▥

    (Ex) **For category I70.54 CC codes:** See I70.33

    I70.541   Atherosclerosis of nonautologous biological bypass graft(s) of the left leg with ulceration of thigh 🔵   A
        CC when PDx is its own CC

    I70.542   Atherosclerosis of nonautologous biological bypass graft(s) of the left leg with ulceration of calf 🔵   A
        CC when PDx is its own CC

    I70.543   Atherosclerosis of nonautologous biological bypass graft(s) of the left leg with ulceration of ankle 🔵   A
        CC when PDx is its own CC

    I70.544   Atherosclerosis of nonautologous biological bypass graft(s) of the left leg with ulceration of heel and midfoot 🔵   A
        Atherosclerosis of nonautologous biological bypass graft(s) of left leg with ulceration of plantar surface of midfoot
        CC when PDx is its own CC

    I70.545   Atherosclerosis of nonautologous biological bypass graft(s) of the left leg with ulceration of other part of foot   A
        Atherosclerosis of nonautologous biological bypass graft(s) of the left leg with ulceration of toe

    I70.548   Atherosclerosis of nonautologous biological bypass graft(s) of the left leg with ulceration of other part of lower leg 🔵   A
        CC when PDx is its own CC

    I70.549   Atherosclerosis of nonautologous biological bypass graft(s) of the left leg with ulceration of unspecified site 🔵   A
        CC when PDx is its own CC

I70.55   Atherosclerosis of nonautologous biological bypass graft(s) of other extremity with ulceration   A

    Includes   any condition classifiable to I70.518, I70.528, and I70.538

    Use additional code to identify severity of ulcer (L98.49)

● **I70.56**   Atherosclerosis of nonautologous biological bypass graft(s) of the extremities with gangrene

    Includes   any condition classifiable to I70.51-, I70.52-, and I70.53-, I70.54-, I70.55

    Use additional code to identify the severity of any ulcer (L97.-, L98.49-), if applicable ◀▥

    (Ex) **For category I70.56 CC codes:** See I70.26

    I70.561   Atherosclerosis of nonautologous biological bypass graft(s) of the extremities with gangrene, right leg 🔵   A
        CC when PDx is its own CC

    I70.562   Atherosclerosis of nonautologous biological bypass graft(s) of the extremities with gangrene, left leg 🔵A
        CC when PDx is its own CC

    I70.563   Atherosclerosis of nonautologous biological bypass graft(s) of the extremities with gangrene, bilateral legs 🔵   A
        CC when PDx is its own CC

    I70.568   Atherosclerosis of nonautologous biological bypass graft(s) of the extremities with gangrene, other extremity 🔵   A
        CC when PDx is its own CC

    I70.569   Atherosclerosis of nonautologous biological bypass graft(s) of the extremities with gangrene, unspecified extremity 🔵   A
        CC when PDx is its own CC

● **I70.59**   Other atherosclerosis of nonautologous biological bypass graft(s) of the extremities

    I70.591   Other atherosclerosis of nonautologous biological bypass graft(s) of the extremities, right leg   A

    I70.592   Other atherosclerosis of nonautologous biological bypass graft(s) of the extremities, left leg   A

    I70.593   Other atherosclerosis of nonautologous biological bypass graft(s) of the extremities, bilateral legs   A

    I70.598   Other atherosclerosis of nonautologous biological bypass graft(s) of the extremities, other extremity   A

    I70.599   Other atherosclerosis of nonautologous biological bypass graft(s) of the extremities, unspecified extremity   A

● **I70.6**   Atherosclerosis of nonbiological bypass graft(s) of the extremities

    Use additional code, if applicable, to identify chronic total occlusion of artery of extremity (I70.92)

● **I70.60**   Unspecified atherosclerosis of nonbiological bypass graft(s) of the extremities

    I70.601   Unspecified atherosclerosis of nonbiological bypass graft(s) of the extremities, right leg   A

    I70.602   Unspecified atherosclerosis of nonbiological bypass graft(s) of the extremities, left leg   A

    I70.603   Unspecified atherosclerosis of nonbiological bypass graft(s) of the extremities, bilateral legs   A

    I70.608   Unspecified atherosclerosis of nonbiological bypass graft(s) of the extremities, other extremity   A

    I70.609   Unspecified atherosclerosis of nonbiological bypass graft(s) of the extremities, unspecified extremity   A

● **I70.61**   Atherosclerosis of nonbiological bypass graft(s) of the extremities with intermittent claudication

    I70.611   Atherosclerosis of nonbiological bypass graft(s) of the extremities with intermittent claudication, right leg   A

    I70.612   Atherosclerosis of nonbiological bypass graft(s) of the extremities with intermittent claudication, left leg   A

    I70.613   Atherosclerosis of nonbiological bypass graft(s) of the extremities with intermittent claudication, bilateral legs   A

    I70.618   Atherosclerosis of nonbiological bypass graft(s) of the extremities with intermittent claudication, other extremity   A

    I70.619   Atherosclerosis of nonbiological bypass graft(s) of the extremities with intermittent claudication, unspecified extremity   A

CHAPTER 9 (I00–I99)

N Newborn Age: 0   P Pediatric Age: 0–17   M Maternity DX: 12–55   A Adult Age: 15–124   ♀ Females Only   ♂ Males Only

🔵 Complication\Comorbidity   Major C\C   (Ex) CC/MCC Exclusions   Present on Admission Requirement   🔵 Hospital-Acquired Condition

987

● **I70.62 Atherosclerosis of nonbiological bypass graft(s) of the extremities with rest pain**

> **Includes** any condition classifiable to I70.61-

I70.621 Atherosclerosis of nonbiological bypass graft(s) of the extremities with rest pain, right leg A

I70.622 Atherosclerosis of nonbiological bypass graft(s) of the extremities with rest pain, left leg A

I70.623 Atherosclerosis of nonbiological bypass graft(s) of the extremities with rest pain, bilateral legs A

I70.628 Atherosclerosis of nonbiological bypass graft(s) of the extremities with rest pain, other extremity A

I70.629 Atherosclerosis of nonbiological bypass graft(s) of the extremities with rest pain, unspecified extremity A

● **I70.63 Atherosclerosis of nonbiological bypass graft(s) of the right leg with ulceration**

> **Includes** any condition classifiable to I70.611 and I70.621

Use additional code to identify severity of ulcer (L97.-) ◀

(Ex) **For category I70.63 CC codes:** See I70.33

I70.631 Atherosclerosis of nonbiological bypass graft(s) of the right leg with ulceration of thigh A
> CC when PDx is its own CC

I70.632 Atherosclerosis of nonbiological bypass graft(s) of the right leg with ulceration of calf A
> CC when PDx is its own CC

I70.633 Atherosclerosis of nonbiological bypass graft(s) of the right leg with ulceration of ankle A
> CC when PDx is its own CC

I70.634 Atherosclerosis of nonbiological bypass graft(s) of the right leg with ulceration of heel and midfoot A
> Atherosclerosis of nonbiological bypass graft(s) of right leg with ulceration of plantar surface of midfoot
> CC when PDx is its own CC

I70.635 Atherosclerosis of nonbiological bypass graft(s) of the right leg with ulceration of other part of foot A
> Atherosclerosis of nonbiological bypass graft(s) of the right leg with ulceration of toe

I70.638 Atherosclerosis of nonbiological bypass graft(s) of the right leg with ulceration of other part of lower leg A
> CC when PDx is its own CC

I70.639 Atherosclerosis of nonbiological bypass graft(s) of the right leg with ulceration of unspecified site A
> CC when PDx is its own CC

● **I70.64 Atherosclerosis of nonbiological bypass graft(s) of the left leg with ulceration**

> **Includes** any condition classifiable to I70.612 and I70.622

Use additional code to identify severity of ulcer (L97.-) ◀

(Ex) **For category I70.64 CC codes:** See I70.33

I70.641 Atherosclerosis of nonbiological bypass graft(s) of the left leg with ulceration of thigh A
> CC when PDx is its own CC

I70.642 Atherosclerosis of nonbiological bypass graft(s) of the left leg with ulceration of calf A
> CC when PDx is its own CC

I70.643 Atherosclerosis of nonbiological bypass graft(s) of the left leg with ulceration of ankle A
> CC when PDx is its own CC

I70.644 Atherosclerosis of nonbiological bypass graft(s) of the left leg with ulceration of heel and midfoot A
> Atherosclerosis of nonbiological bypass graft(s) of left leg with ulceration of plantar surface of midfoot
> CC when PDx is its own CC

I70.645 Atherosclerosis of nonbiological bypass graft(s) of the left leg with ulceration of other part of foot A
> Atherosclerosis of nonbiological bypass graft(s) of the left leg with ulceration of toe

I70.648 Atherosclerosis of nonbiological bypass graft(s) of the left leg with ulceration of other part of lower leg A
> CC when PDx is its own CC

I70.649 Atherosclerosis of nonbiological bypass graft(s) of the left leg with ulceration of unspecified site A
> CC when PDx is its own CC

I70.65 Atherosclerosis of nonbiological bypass graft(s) of other extremity with ulceration A

> **Includes** any condition classifiable to I70.618 and I70.628

Use additional code to identify severity of ulcer (L98.49-)

● **I70.66 Atherosclerosis of nonbiological bypass graft(s) of the extremities with gangrene**

> **Includes** any condition classifiable to I70.61-, I70.62-, I70.63-, I70.64-, I70.65

Use additional code to identify the severity of any ulcer (L97.-, L98.49-), if applicable ◀

(Ex) **For category I70.66 CC codes:** See I70.26

I70.661 Atherosclerosis of nonbiological bypass graft(s) of the extremities with gangrene, right leg A
> CC when PDx is its own CC

I70.662 Atherosclerosis of nonbiological bypass graft(s) of the extremities with gangrene, left leg A
> CC when PDx is its own CC

I70.663 Atherosclerosis of nonbiological bypass graft(s) of the extremities with gangrene, bilateral legs A
> CC when PDx is its own CC

I70.668   Atherosclerosis of nonbiological bypass graft(s) of the extremities with gangrene, other extremity 🅟   A
       CC when PDx is its own CC

I70.669   Atherosclerosis of nonbiological bypass graft(s) of the extremities with gangrene, unspecified extremity 🅟   A
       CC when PDx is its own CC

● **I70.69**   Other atherosclerosis of nonbiological bypass graft(s) of the extremities

I70.691   Other atherosclerosis of nonbiological bypass graft(s) of the extremities, right leg   A

I70.692   Other atherosclerosis of nonbiological bypass graft(s) of the extremities, left leg   A

I70.693   Other atherosclerosis of nonbiological bypass graft(s) of the extremities, bilateral legs   A

I70.698   Other atherosclerosis of nonbiological bypass graft(s) of the extremities, other extremity   A

I70.699   Other atherosclerosis of nonbiological bypass graft(s) of the extremities, unspecified extremity   A

● **I70.7**   Atherosclerosis of other type of bypass graft(s) of the extremities

     Use additional code, if applicable, to identify chronic total occlusion of artery of extremity (I70.92)

● **I70.70**   Unspecified atherosclerosis of other type of bypass graft(s) of the extremities

I70.701   Unspecified atherosclerosis of other type of bypass graft(s) of the extremities, right leg   A

I70.702   Unspecified atherosclerosis of other type of bypass graft(s) of the extremities, left leg   A

I70.703   Unspecified atherosclerosis of other type of bypass graft(s) of the extremities, bilateral legs   A

I70.708   Unspecified atherosclerosis of other type of bypass graft(s) of the extremities, other extremity   A

I70.709   Unspecified atherosclerosis of other type of bypass graft(s) of the extremities, unspecified extremity   A

● **I70.71**   Atherosclerosis of other type of bypass graft(s) of the extremities with intermittent claudication

I70.711   Atherosclerosis of other type of bypass graft(s) of the extremities with intermittent claudication, right leg   A

I70.712   Atherosclerosis of other type of bypass graft(s) of the extremities with intermittent claudication, left leg   A

I70.713   Atherosclerosis of other type of bypass graft(s) of the extremities with intermittent claudication, bilateral legs   A

I70.718   Atherosclerosis of other type of bypass graft(s) of the extremities with intermittent claudication, other extremity   A

I70.719   Atherosclerosis of other type of bypass graft(s) of the extremities with intermittent claudication, unspecified extremity   A

● **I70.72**   Atherosclerosis of other type of bypass graft(s) of the extremities with rest pain

     Includes   any condition classifiable to I70.71-

I70.721   Atherosclerosis of other type of bypass graft(s) of the extremities with rest pain, right leg   A

I70.722   Atherosclerosis of other type of bypass graft(s) of the extremities with rest pain, left leg   A

I70.723   Atherosclerosis of other type of bypass graft(s) of the extremities with rest pain, bilateral legs   A

I70.728   Atherosclerosis of other type of bypass graft(s) of the extremities with rest pain, other extremity   A

I70.729   Atherosclerosis of other type of bypass graft(s) of the extremities with rest pain, unspecified extremity   A

● **I70.73**   Atherosclerosis of other type of bypass graft(s) of the right leg with ulceration

     Includes   any condition classifiable to I70.711 and I70.721

     Use additional code to identify severity of ulcer (L97.-) ◄▥

     (Ex) **For category I70.73 CC codes:** See I70.33

I70.731   Atherosclerosis of other type of bypass graft(s) of the right leg with ulceration of thigh 🅟   A
       CC when PDx is its own CC

I70.732   Atherosclerosis of other type of bypass graft(s) of the right leg with ulceration of calf 🅟   A
       CC when PDx is its own CC

I70.733   Atherosclerosis of other type of bypass graft(s) of the right leg with ulceration of ankle 🅟   A
       CC when PDx is its own CC

I70.734   Atherosclerosis of other type of bypass graft(s) of the right leg with ulceration of heel and midfoot 🅟   A
       Atherosclerosis of other type of bypass graft(s) of right leg with ulceration of plantar surface of midfoot
       CC when PDx is its own CC

I70.735   Atherosclerosis of other type of bypass graft(s) of the right leg with ulceration of other part of foot   A
       Atherosclerosis of other type of bypass graft(s) of right leg with ulceration of toe

I70.738   Atherosclerosis of other type of bypass graft(s) of the right leg with ulceration of other part of lower leg 🅟   A
       CC when PDx is its own CC

I70.739   Atherosclerosis of other type of bypass graft(s) of the right leg with ulceration of unspecified site 🅟   A
       CC when PDx is its own CC

CHAPTER 9 (I00–I99)

N   Newborn Age: 0   **P**   Pediatric Age: 0–17   **M**   Maternity DX: 12–55   **A**   Adult Age: 15–124   ♀   Females Only   ♂   Males Only

🅒   Complication\Comorbidity   🅜   Major C\C   (Ex)   CC/MCC Exclusions   🅟   Present on Admission Requirement   🅗   Hospital-Acquired Condition

989

● **I70.74** **Atherosclerosis of other type of bypass graft(s) of the left leg with ulceration**

> **Includes**   any condition classifiable to I70.712 and I70.722

Use additional code to identify severity of ulcer (L97.-) ◀▥

Ⓔ **For category I70.74 CC codes:** See I70.33

I70.741 **Atherosclerosis of other type of bypass graft(s) of the left leg with ulceration of thigh** 🏵   A
CC when PDx is its own CC

I70.742 **Atherosclerosis of other type of bypass graft(s) of the left leg with ulceration of calf** 🏵   A
CC when PDx is its own CC

I70.743 **Atherosclerosis of other type of bypass graft(s) of the left leg with ulceration of ankle** 🏵   A
CC when PDx is its own CC

I70.744 **Atherosclerosis of other type of bypass graft(s) of the left leg with ulceration of heel and midfoot** 🏵   A
Atherosclerosis of other type of bypass graft(s) of left leg with ulceration of plantar surface of midfoot
CC when PDx is its own CC

I70.745 **Atherosclerosis of other type of bypass graft(s) of the left leg with ulceration of other part of foot**   A
Atherosclerosis of other type of bypass graft(s) of left leg with ulceration of toe

I70.748 **Atherosclerosis of other type of bypass graft(s) of the left leg with ulceration of other part of lower leg** 🏵   A
CC when PDx is its own CC

I70.749 **Atherosclerosis of other type of bypass graft(s) of the left leg with ulceration of unspecified site** 🏵   A
CC when PDx is its own CC

I70.75 **Atherosclerosis of other type of bypass graft(s) of other extremity with ulceration**   A

> **Includes**   any condition classifiable to I70.718 and I70.728

Use additional code to identify severity of ulcer (L98.49)

● **I70.76** **Atherosclerosis of other type of bypass graft(s) of the extremities with gangrene**

> **Includes**   any condition classifiable to I70.71-, I70.72-, I70.73-, I70.74-, I70.75

Use additional code to identify the severity of any ulcer (L97.-, L98.49-), if applicable ◀▥
Ⓔ **For category I70.76 CC codes:** See I70.26

I70.761 **Atherosclerosis of other type of bypass graft(s) of the extremities with gangrene, right leg** 🏵   A
CC when PDx is its own CC

I70.762 **Atherosclerosis of other type of bypass graft(s) of the extremities with gangrene, left leg** 🏵   A
CC when PDx is its own CC

I70.763 **Atherosclerosis of other type of bypass graft(s) of the extremities with gangrene, bilateral legs** 🏵   A
CC when PDx is its own CC

I70.768 **Atherosclerosis of other type of bypass graft(s) of the extremities with gangrene, other extremity** 🏵   A
CC when PDx is its own CC

I70.769 **Atherosclerosis of other type of bypass graft(s) of the extremities with gangrene, unspecified extremity** 🏵   A
CC when PDx is its own CC

● **I70.79** **Other atherosclerosis of other type of bypass graft(s) of the extremities**

I70.791 **Other atherosclerosis of other type of bypass graft(s) of the extremities, right leg**   A

I70.792 **Other atherosclerosis of other type of bypass graft(s) of the extremities, left leg**   A

I70.793 **Other atherosclerosis of other type of bypass graft(s) of the extremities, bilateral legs**   A

I70.798 **Other atherosclerosis of other type of bypass graft(s) of the extremities, other extremity**   A

I70.799 **Other atherosclerosis of other type of bypass graft(s) of the extremities, unspecified extremity**   A

I70.8 **Atherosclerosis of other arteries**   A

● **I70.9** **Other and unspecified atherosclerosis**

I70.90 **Unspecified atherosclerosis**   A

I70.91 **Generalized atherosclerosis**   A

● **I70.92** **Chronic total occlusion of artery of the extremities** 🏵   A
Complete occlusion of artery of the extremities
Total occlusion of artery of the extremities

> *Code first* atherosclerosis of arteries of the extremities (I70.2-, I70.3-, I70.4-, I70.5-, I70.6-, I70.7-)

> ~~Excludes1~~ ~~acute occlusion of artery of the extremity (I70.2-, I70.3-, I70.4-)~~

Ⓔ 167.0, I70.201-I70.799, I70.92-I71.9, I72.1, I72.3-I72.4, I72.9, I73.81-I74.19, .I74.2-I77.2, I77.5-I77.6, I77.72, I77.79-I77.819, I79.0-I79.8, M31.8-M31.9

● **I71** **Aortic aneurysm and dissection**

> **Excludes1**   aortic ectasia (I77.81-)
> syphilitic aortic aneurysm (A52.01)
> traumatic aortic aneurysm (S25.09, S35.09)

Ⓔ **For category I71 CC codes:** E08.51-E08.59, E08.618-E08.638, E08.649-E08.8, E09.51-E09.59, E09.618-E09.638, E09.649, E09.65-E09.8, E10.51-E10.59, E10.618-E10.638, E10.649, E10.69-E10.8, E11.51-E11.59, E11.618-E11.638, E11.649, E11.69-E11.8, E13.51-E13.59, E13.618-E13.638, E13.649-E13.8, I71.00-I71.9, I77.810-I77.819, I79.0, I87.8, I99.8-I99.9

● **I71.0** **Dissection of aorta**

I71.00 **Dissection of unspecified site of aorta** 🏵

I71.01 **Dissection of thoracic aorta** 🏵

I71.02 **Dissection of abdominal aorta** 🏵

I71.03 **Dissection of thoracoabdominal aorta** 🏵

I71.1 **Thoracic aortic aneurysm, ruptured** 🏵

I71.2 **Thoracic aortic aneurysm, without rupture**

I71.3 **Abdominal aortic aneurysm, ruptured** 🏵

I71.4 **Abdominal aortic aneurysm, without rupture**

I71.5 **Thoracoabdominal aortic aneurysm, ruptured** 🏵

I71.6 **Thoracoabdominal aortic aneurysm, without rupture**

I71.8 **Aortic aneurysm of unspecified site, ruptured** 🏵
Rupture of aorta NOS

I71.9 **Aortic aneurysm of unspecified site, without rupture**
Aneurysm of aorta
Dilatation of aorta
Hyaline necrosis of aorta

◀ New   ◀▥ Revised   ~~deleted~~ Deleted   Excludes 1   Excludes 2   Includes   Use additional   Code first   Code also   Unspecified

OGCR Official Guidelines   ● Unacceptable Principal Diagnosis   X Assign placeholder X   🏵 Use Additional Character(s)   ▶ Manifestation Code   **Coding Clinic**

● **I72**   **Other aneurysm**

> **Includes**   aneurysm (cirsoid) (false) (ruptured)
>
> **Excludes2**   acquired aneurysm (I77.0)
> aneurysm (of) aorta (I71.-)
> aneurysm (of) arteriovenous NOS (Q27.3-)
> carotid artery dissection (I77.71)
> cerebral (nonruptured) aneurysm (I67.1)
> coronary aneurysm (I25.4)
> coronary artery dissection (I25.42)
> dissection of artery NEC (I77.79)
> heart aneurysm (I25.3)
> iliac artery dissection (I77.72)
> pulmonary artery aneurysm (I28.1)
> renal artery dissection (I77.73)
> retinal aneurysm (H35.0)
> ruptured cerebral aneurysm (I60.7)
> varicose aneurysm (I77.0)
> vertebral artery dissection (I77.74)

I72.0   **Aneurysm of carotid artery**
Aneurysm of common carotid artery
Aneurysm of external carotid artery
Aneurysm of internal carotid artery, extracranial portion

> **Excludes1**   aneurysm of internal carotid artery, intracranial portion (I67.1)
> aneurysm of internal carotid artery NOS (I67.1)

I72.1   **Aneurysm of artery of upper extremity**

I72.2   **Aneurysm of renal artery**

I72.3   **Aneurysm of iliac artery**

I72.4   **Aneurysm of artery of lower extremity**

I72.8   **Aneurysm of other specified arteries**

I72.9   **Aneurysm of unspecified site**

● **I73**   **Other peripheral vascular diseases**

> **Excludes2**   chilblains (T69.1)
> frostbite (T33-T34) ◀
> immersion hand or foot (T69.0-)
> spasm of cerebral artery (G45.9)

● **I73.0**   **Raynaud's syndrome**
Diminishing oxygen supply to fingers, toes, nose, and ears when exposed to temperature changes or stress
Raynaud's disease
Raynaud's phenomenon (secondary)

I73.00   **Raynaud's syndrome without gangrene**

I73.01   **Raynaud's syndrome with gangrene** 🔿
CC when PDx is its own CC
(Ex) G89.0-G89.4, I70.261-I70.269, I96, R41.0-R41.3, R41.82, R41.9, R44.8-R44.9, R45.83-R45.84, R46.0-R46.89, R52, R68.0-R68.19, R68.81-R68.83, R68.89-R69

I73.1   **Thromboangiitis obliterans [Buerger's disease]**
Inflammatory occlusive disease resulting in poor circulation to the legs, feet, and sometimes the hands due to progressive inflammatory narrowing and eventually obliteration of the small arteries

● **I73.8**   **Other specified peripheral vascular diseases**

> **Excludes1**   diabetic (peripheral) angiopathy (E08-E13 with .51-.52)

I73.81   **Erythromelalgia**

I73.89   **Other specified peripheral vascular diseases**
Acrocyanosis
Erythrocyanosis
Simple acroparesthesia [Schultze's type]
Vasomotor acroparesthesia [Nothnagel's type]

I73.9   **Peripheral vascular disease, unspecified**
Intermittent claudication
Peripheral angiopathy NOS
Spasm of artery

> **Excludes1**   atherosclerosis of the extremities (I70.2--I70.7-)

Item 9–9   An **embolus** is a mass of undissolved matter present in the blood that is transported by the blood current. A **thrombus** is a blood clot that occludes or shuts off a vessel. When a thrombus is dislodged, it becomes an embolus.

Embolus

Figure 9-3   An arterial embolus.

● **I74**   **Arterial embolism and thrombosis**

> **Includes**   embolic infarction
> embolic occlusion
> thrombotic infarction
> thrombotic occlusion

Code first embolism and thrombosis complicating abortion or ectopic or molar pregnancy (O00-O07, O08.2)
embolism and thrombosis complicating pregnancy, childbirth and the puerperium (O88.-)

> **Excludes2**   atheroembolism (I75.-)
> basilar embolism and thrombosis (I63.0-I63.2, I65.1)
> carotid embolism and thrombosis (I63.0-I63.2, I65.2)
> cerebral embolism and thrombosis (I63.3-I63.5, I66.-)
> coronary embolism and thrombosis (I21-I25)
> mesenteric embolism and thrombosis (K55.0)
> ophthalmic embolism and thrombosis (H34.-)
> precerebral embolism and thrombosis NOS (I63.0-I63.2, I65.9)
> pulmonary embolism and thrombosis (I26.-)
> renal embolism and thrombosis (N28.0)
> retinal embolism and thrombosis (H34.-)
> septic embolism and thrombosis (I76)
> vertebral embolism and thrombosis (I63.0-I63.2, I65.0)

● **I74.0**   **Embolism and thrombosis of abdominal aorta**
(Ex) For category I74.0 CC codes: I26.01-I26.99, I27.82, I74.01-I74.10, I74.19, I87.8, I99.8-I99.9

I74.01   **Saddle embolus of abdominal aorta** 🔿

I74.09   **Other arterial embolism and thrombosis of abdominal aorta** 🔿
Aortic bifurcation syndrome
Aortoiliac obstruction
Leriche's syndrome

● **I74.1**   **Embolism and thrombosis of other and unspecified parts of aorta**
(Ex) For category I74.1 CC codes unless otherwise indicated: See I74.0

I74.10   **Embolism and thrombosis of unspecified parts of aorta** 🔿

I74.11   **Embolism and thrombosis of thoracic aorta** 🔿
(Ex) E08.51-E08.59, E08.618-E08.638, E08.649-E08.8, E09.51-E09.59, E09.618-E09.638, E09.649, E09.65-E09.8, E10.51-E10.59, E10.618-E10.638, E10.649, E10.69-E10.8, E11.51-E11.59, E11.618-E11.638, E11.649, E11.69-E11.8, E13.51-E13.59, E13.618-E13.638, E13.649-E13.8, I74.11, I74.8-I74.9, I76, I87.8, I99.8-I99.9

I74.19   **Embolism and thrombosis of other parts of aorta** 🔿

I74.2   **Embolism and thrombosis of arteries of the upper extremities** 🔿
(Ex) E08.51-E08.59, E08.618-E08.638, E08.649-E08.8, E09.51-E09.59, E09.618-E09.638, E09.649, E09.65-E09.8, E10.51-E10.59, E10.618-E10.638, E10.649, E10.69-E10.8, E11.51-E11.59, E11.618-E11.638, E11.649, E11.69-E11.8, E13.51-E13.59, E13.618-E13.638, E13.649-E13.8, I74.2, I74.8-I74.9, I76, I87.8, I99.8-I99.9

CHAPTER 9 (I00–I99)

N Newborn Age: 0   **P** Pediatric Age: 0–17   **M** Maternity DX: 12–55   **A** Adult Age: 15–124   ♀ Females Only   ♂ Males Only
🔿 Complication\Comorbidity   🔿 Major C\C   (Ex) CC/MCC Exclusions   🔿 Present on Admission Requirement   🔿 Hospital-Acquired Condition

991

CHAPTER 9 (I00-I99)

I74.3   **Embolism and thrombosis of arteries of the lower extremity** 🔧
> Ex: E08.51-E08.59, E08.618-E08.638, E08.649-E08.8, E09.51-E09.59, E09.618-E09.638, E09.649, E09.65-E09.8, E10.51-E10.59, E10.618-E10.638, E10.649, E10.69-E10.8, E11.51-E11.59, E11.618-E11.638, E11.649, E11.69-E11.8, E13.51-E13.59, E13.618-E13.638, E13.649-E13.8, I74.3-I74.4, I74.8-I74.9, I76, I87.8, I99.8-I99.9

I74.4   **Embolism and thrombosis of arteries of extremities, unspecified** 🔧
> Peripheral arterial embolism NOS
> Ex: See I74.3

I74.5   **Embolism and thrombosis of iliac artery** 🔧
> Ex: E08.51-E08.59, E08.618-E08.638, E08.649-E08.8, E09.51-E09.59, E09.618-E09.638, E09.649, E09.65-E09.8, E10.51-E10.59, E10.618-E10.638, E10.649, E10.69-E10.8, E11.51-E11.59, E11.618-E11.638, E11.649, E11.69-E11.8, E13.51-E13.59, E13.618-E13.638, E13.649-E13.8, I74.5-I74.9, I76, I87.8, I99.8-I99.9

I74.8   **Embolism and thrombosis of other arteries** 🔧
> Ex: E08.51-E08.59, E08.618-E08.638, E08.649-E08.8, E09.51-E09.59, E09.618-E09.638, E09.649, E09.65-E09.8, E10.51-E10.59, E10.618-E10.638, E10.649, E10.69-E10.8, E11.51-E11.59, E11.618-E11.638, E11.649, E11.69-E11.8, E13.51-E13.59, E13.618-E13.638, E13.649-E13.8, I74.8-I74.9, I76, I87.8, I99.8-I99.9

I74.9   **Embolism and thrombosis of unspecified artery** 🔧
> Ex: See I74.8

● **I75**   **Atheroembolism**
> **Includes**   atherothrombotic microembolism
>   cholesterol embolism

● **I75.0**   **Atheroembolism of extremities**

● **I75.01**   **Atheroembolism of upper extremity**
> Ex: For category I75.01 CC codes: E08.51-E08.59, E08.618-E08.638, E08.649-E08.8, E09.51-E09.59, E09.618-E09.638, E09.649, E09.65-E09.8, E10.51-E10.59, E10.618-E10.638, E10.649, E10.69-E10.8, E11.51-E11.59, E11.618-E11.638, E11.649, E11.69-E11.8, E13.51-E13.59, E13.618-E13.638, E13.649-E13.8, I74.8-I75.019, I76, I87.8, I99.8-I99.9

I75.011   **Atheroembolism of right upper extremity** 🔧

I75.012   **Atheroembolism of left upper extremity** 🔧

I75.013   **Atheroembolism of bilateral upper extremities** 🔧

I75.019   **Atheroembolism of unspecified upper extremity** 🔧

● **I75.02**   **Atheroembolism of lower extremity**
> Ex: For category I75.02 CC codes: E08.51-E08.59, E08.618-E08.638, E08.649-E08.8, E09.51-E09.59, E09.618-E09.638, E09.649, E09.65-E09.8, E10.51-E10.59, E10.618-E10.638, E10.649, E10.69-E10.8, E11.51-E11.59, E11.618-E11.638, E11.649, E11.69-E11.8, E13.51-E13.59, E13.618-E13.638, E13.649-E13.8, I74.8-I74.9, I75.021-I75.029, I76, I87.8, I99.8-I99.9

I75.021   **Atheroembolism of right lower extremity** 🔧

I75.022   **Atheroembolism of left lower extremity** 🔧

I75.023   **Atheroembolism of bilateral lower extremities** 🔧

I75.029   **Atheroembolism of unspecified lower extremity** 🔧

● **I75.8**   **Atheroembolism of other sites**

I75.81   **Atheroembolism of kidney** 🔧
> Use additional code for any associated acute kidney failure and chronic kidney disease (N17.-, N18.-)
> Ex: E08.51-E08.59, E08.618-E08.638, E08.649-E08.8, E09.51-E09.59, E09.618-E09.638, E09.649, E09.65-E09.8, E10.51-E10.59, E10.618-E10.638, E10.649, E10.69-E10.8, E11.51-E11.59, E11.618-E11.638, E11.649, E11.69-E11.8, E13.51-E13.59, E13.618-E13.638, E13.649-E13.8, I74.8-I74.9, I75.81, I76, I87.8, I99.8-I99.9

I75.89   **Atheroembolism of other site** 🔧
> Ex: E08.51-E08.59, E08.618-E08.638, E08.649-E08.8, E09.51-E09.59, E09.618-E09.638, E09.649, E09.65-E09.8, E10.51-E10.59, E10.618-E10.638, E10.649, E10.69-E10.8, E11.51-E11.59, E11.618-E11.638, E11.649, E11.69-E11.8, E13.51-E13.59, E13.618-E13.638, E13.649-E13.8, I74.8-I74.9, I75.89, I76, I87.8, I99.8-I99.9

● **I76**   **Septic arterial embolism** 🔧
> *Code first* underlying infection, such as:
>   infective endocarditis (I33.0)
>   lung abscess (J85.-)
> Use additional code to identify the site of the embolism (I74.-)
> **Excludes2**   septic pulmonary embolism (I26.01, I26.90)
> Ex: See I74.8

● **I77**   **Other disorders of arteries and arterioles**
> **Excludes2**   collagen (vascular) diseases (M30-M36)
>   hypersensitivity angiitis (M31.0)
>   pulmonary artery (I28.-)

I77.0   **Arteriovenous fistula, acquired**
> Aneurysmal varix
> Arteriovenous aneurysm, acquired
> **Excludes1**   arteriovenous aneurysm NOS (Q27.3-)
>   presence of arteriovenous shunt (fistula) for dialysis (Z99.2)
>   traumatic - see injury of blood vessel by body region
> **Excludes2**   cerebral (I67.1)
>   coronary (I25.4)

I77.1   **Stricture of artery**
> Narrowing of artery

I77.2   **Rupture of artery** 🔧
> Erosion of artery
> Fistula of artery
> Ulcer of artery
> **Excludes1**   traumatic rupture of artery - see injury of blood vessel by body region
> Ex: I25.42, I67.0, I77.2, I77.72-I77.79

I77.3   **Arterial fibromuscular dysplasia**
> Fibromuscular hyperplasia (of) carotid artery
> Fibromuscular hyperplasia (of) renal artery

I77.4   **Celiac artery compression syndrome** 🔧
> Ex: I77.4

I77.5   **Necrosis of artery** 🔧
> Ex: I77.5, M31.8-M31.9

I77.6   **Arteritis, unspecified**
> Aortitis NOS
> Endarteritis NOS
> **Excludes1**   arteritis or endarteritis:
>   aortic arch (M31.4)
>   cerebral NEC (I67.7)
>   coronary (I25.89)
>   deformans (I70.-)
>   giant cell (M31.5., M31.6)
>   obliterans (I70.-)
>   senile (I70.-)

◀ New   ◀ Revised   ~~deleted~~ Deleted   Excludes 1   Excludes 2   Includes   Use additional   Code first   Code also   Unspecified

992   OGCR Official Guidelines   ● Unacceptable Principal Diagnosis   X Assign placeholder X   ● Use Additional Character(s)   ▶ Manifestation Code   **Coding Clinic**

● **I77.7**   **Other arterial dissection**

> **Excludes2**   dissection of aorta (I71.0-)
> dissection of coronary artery (I25.42)
>
> (Ex) For category **I77.7 CC codes:** I77.2-I77.3, I77.5-I77.6, I77.89-I77.9, M31.8-M31.9

    I77.71   Dissection of carotid artery 🔗

    I77.72   Dissection of iliac artery 🔗

    I77.73   Dissection of renal artery 🔗

    I77.74   Dissection of vertebral artery 🔗

    I77.79   Dissection of other artery 🔗

● **I77.8**   **Other specified disorders of arteries and arterioles**

    I77.81   **Aortic ectasia**

> Ectasis aorta
>
> > **Excludes1**   aortic aneurysm and dissection (I71.0-)

      I77.810   Thoracic aortic ectasia

      I77.811   Abdominal aortic ectasia

      I77.812   Thoracoabdominal aortic ectasia

      I77.819   Aortic ectasia, unspecified site

    I77.89   Other specified disorders of arteries and arterioles

● **I77.9**   Disorder of arteries and arterioles, unspecified

● **I78**   **Diseases of capillaries**

    I78.0   **Hereditary hemorrhagic telangiectasia**

> Rendu-Osler-Weber disease

    I78.1   **Nevus, non-neoplastic**

> Araneus nevus   Spider nevus
> Senile nevus   Stellar nevus
>
> > **Excludes1**   nevus NOS (D22.-)
> > vascular NOS (Q82.5)
> >
> > **Excludes2**   blue nevus (D22.-)
> > flammeus nevus (Q82.5)
> > hairy nevus (D22.-)
> > melanocytic nevus (D22.-)
> > pigmented nevus (D22.-)
> > portwine nevus (Q82.5)
> > sanguineous nevus (Q82.5)
> > strawberry nevus (Q82.5)
> > verrucous nevus (Q82.5)

    I78.8   Other diseases of capillaries

    I78.9   Disease of capillaries, unspecified

● **I79**   **Disorders of arteries, arterioles and capillaries in diseases classified elsewhere**

   ▹ *I79.0*   *Aneurysm of aorta in diseases classified elsewhere*

> *Code first* underlying disease
>
> > **Excludes1**   syphilitic aneurysm (A52.01)

   ▹ *I79.1*   *Aortitis in diseases classified elsewhere*

> *Code first* underlying disease
>
> > **Excludes1**   syphilitic aortitis (A52.02)

   ▹ *I79.8*   *Other disorders of arteries, arterioles and capillaries in diseases classified elsewhere*

> *Code first* underlying disease, such as:
> amyloidosis (E85.-) ◀▥
>
> > **Excludes1**   diabetic (peripheral) angiopathy (E08-E13 with .51-.52)
> > ~~endarteritis:~~ ◀▥
> > syphilitic endarteritis (A52.09) ◀▥
> > tuberculous endarteritis (A18.89) ◀▥

DISEASES OF VEINS, LYMPHATIC VESSELS AND LYMPH NODES, NOT ELSEWHERE CLASSIFIED (I80-I89)

● **I80**   **Phlebitis and thrombophlebitis**

> *Inflammation of a vein with infiltration of walls (phlebitis).*
>
> **Includes**   endophlebitis
> inflammation, vein
> periphlebitis
> suppurative phlebitis
>
> *Code first* phlebitis and thrombophlebitis complicating abortion, ectopic or molar pregnancy (O00-O07, O08.7)
> phlebitis and thrombophlebitis complicating pregnancy, childbirth and the puerperium (O22.-, O87.-)
>
> **Excludes1**   venous embolism and thrombosis of lower extremities (I82.4-, I82.5-, I82.81-)

● **I80.0**   **Phlebitis and thrombophlebitis of superficial vessels of lower extremities**

> Phlebitis and thrombophlebitis of femoropopliteal vein

    I80.00   Phlebitis and thrombophlebitis of superficial vessels of unspecified lower extremity

    I80.01   Phlebitis and thrombophlebitis of superficial vessels of right lower extremity

    I80.02   Phlebitis and thrombophlebitis of superficial vessels of left lower extremity

    I80.03   Phlebitis and thrombophlebitis of superficial vessels of lower extremities, bilateral

● **I80.1**   **Phlebitis and thrombophlebitis of femoral vein**

> (Ex) For category **I80.1 CC codes:** E08.51-E08.59, E08.618-E08.638, E08.649-E08.8, E09.51-E09.59, E09.618-E09.638, E09.649, E09.65-E09.8, E10.51-E10.59, E10.618-E10.638, E10.649, E10.69-E10.8, E11.51-E11.59, E11.618-E11.638, E11.649, E11.69-E11.8, E13.51-E13.59, E13.618-E13.638, E13.649-E13.8, I80.00-I80.9, I87.8, I99.8-I99.9

    I80.10   Phlebitis and thrombophlebitis of unspecified femoral vein 🔗

    I80.11   Phlebitis and thrombophlebitis of right femoral vein 🔗

    I80.12   Phlebitis and thrombophlebitis of left femoral vein 🔗

    I80.13   Phlebitis and thrombophlebitis of femoral vein, bilateral 🔗

● **I80.2**   **Phlebitis and thrombophlebitis of other and unspecified deep vessels of lower extremities**

> (Ex) For category **I80.2 CC codes:** See I80.1

 ● **I80.20**   Phlebitis and thrombophlebitis of unspecified deep vessels of lower extremities

      I80.201   Phlebitis and thrombophlebitis of unspecified deep vessels of right lower extremity 🔗

      I80.202   Phlebitis and thrombophlebitis of unspecified deep vessels of left lower extremity 🔗

      I80.203   Phlebitis and thrombophlebitis of unspecified deep vessels of lower extremities, bilateral 🔗

      I80.209   Phlebitis and thrombophlebitis of unspecified deep vessels of unspecified lower extremity 🔗

 ● **I80.21**   Phlebitis and thrombophlebitis of iliac vein

      I80.211   Phlebitis and thrombophlebitis of right iliac vein 🔗

      I80.212   Phlebitis and thrombophlebitis of left iliac vein 🔗

      I80.213   Phlebitis and thrombophlebitis of iliac vein, bilateral 🔗

      I80.219   Phlebitis and thrombophlebitis of unspecified iliac vein 🔗

N Newborn Age: 0   **P** Pediatric Age: 0–17   **M** Maternity DX: 12–55   **A** Adult Age: 15–124   ♀ Females Only   ♂ Males Only

🔗 Complication\Comorbidity   🔗 Major C\C   (Ex) CC/MCC Exclusions   🔗 Present on Admission Requirement   🔗 Hospital-Acquired Condition

993

CHAPTER 9 (I00-I99)

● I80.22 Phlebitis and thrombophlebitis of popliteal vein
  I80.221 Phlebitis and thrombophlebitis of right popliteal vein 🔍
  I80.222 Phlebitis and thrombophlebitis of left popliteal vein 🔍
  I80.223 Phlebitis and thrombophlebitis of popliteal vein, bilateral 🔍
  I80.229 Phlebitis and thrombophlebitis of unspecified popliteal vein 🔍

● I80.23 Phlebitis and thrombophlebitis of tibial vein
  I80.231 Phlebitis and thrombophlebitis of right tibial vein 🔍
  I80.232 Phlebitis and thrombophlebitis of left tibial vein 🔍
  I80.233 Phlebitis and thrombophlebitis of tibial vein, bilateral 🔍
  I80.239 Phlebitis and thrombophlebitis of unspecified tibial vein 🔍

● I80.29 Phlebitis and thrombophlebitis of other deep vessels of lower extremities
  I80.291 Phlebitis and thrombophlebitis of other deep vessels of right lower extremity 🔍
  I80.292 Phlebitis and thrombophlebitis of other deep vessels of left lower extremity 🔍
  I80.293 Phlebitis and thrombophlebitis of other deep vessels of lower extremity, bilateral 🔍
  I80.299 Phlebitis and thrombophlebitis of other deep vessels of unspecified lower extremity 🔍

I80.3 Phlebitis and thrombophlebitis of lower extremities, unspecified

I80.8 Phlebitis and thrombophlebitis of other sites

I80.9 Phlebitis and thrombophlebitis of unspecified site

I81 Portal vein thrombosis 🔍
 Portal (vein) obstruction
  Excludes2 hepatic vein thrombosis (I82.0)
       phlebitis of portal vein (K75.1)
 (Ex) E08.51-E08.59, E08.618-E08.638, E08.649-E08.8, E09.51-E09.59, E09.618-E09.638, E09.649, E09.65-E09.8, E10.51-E10.59, E10.618-E10.638, E10.649, E10.69-E10.8, E11.51-E11.59, E11.618-E11.638, E11.649, E11.69-E11.8, E13.51-E13.59, E13.618-E13.638, E13.649-E13.8, I81, I82.210-I82.291, I82.401-I82.729, I82.811-I82.91, I82.A11-I82.C29, I87.8, I99.8-I99.9

● I82 Other venous embolism and thrombosis
 Code first venous embolism and thrombosis complicating:
  abortion, ectopic or molar pregnancy (O00-O07, O08.7)
  pregnancy, childbirth and the puerperium (O22.-, O87.-)
 Excludes2 venous embolism and thrombosis (of):
     cerebral (I63.6, I67.6)
     coronary (I21-I25)
     intracranial and intraspinal, septic or NOS (G08)
     intracranial, nonpyogenic (I67.6)
     intraspinal, nonpyogenic (G95.1)
     mesenteric (K55.0)
     portal (I81)
     pulmonary (I26.-)

I82.0 **Budd-Chiari syndrome** 🔍
 Hepatic vein thrombosis
 (Ex) E08.51-E08.59, E08.618-E08.638, E08.649-E08.8, E09.51-E09.59, E09.618-E09.638, E09.649, E09.65-E09.8, E10.51-E10.59, E10.618-E10.638, E10.649, E10.69-E10.8, E11.51-E11.59, E11.618-E11.638, E11.649, E11.69-E11.8, E13.51-E13.59, E13.618-E13.638, E13.649-E13.8, I82.0, I82.210-I82.291, I82.401-I82.729, I82.811-I82.91, I82.A11-I82.C29, I87.8, I99.8-I99.9

I82.1 Thrombophlebitis migrans 🔍
 "White leg" is the other term to describe a migrating thrombus.
 (Ex) E08.51-E08.59, E08.618-E08.638, E08.649-E08.8, E09.51-E09.59, E09.618-E09.638, E09.649, E09.65-E09.8, E10.51-E10.59, E10.618-E10.638, E10.649, E10.69-E10.8, E11.51-E11.59, E11.618-E11.638, E11.649, E11.69-E11.8, E13.51-E13.59, E13.618-E13.638, E13.649-E13.8, I82.1, I82.210-I82.291, I82.401-I82.729, I82.811-I82.91, I82.A11-I82.C29, I87.8, I99.8-I99.9

● I82.2 Embolism and thrombosis of vena cava and other thoracic veins
 (Ex) For category I82.2 CC codes unless otherwise indicated: E08.51-E08.59, E08.618-E08.638, E08.649-E08.8, E09.51-E09.59, E09.618-E09.638, E09.649, E09.65-E09.8, E10.51-E10.59, E10.618-E10.638, E10.649, E10.69-E10.8, E11.51-E11.59, E11.618-E11.638, E11.649, E11.69-E11.8, E13.51-E13.59, E13.618-E13.638, E13.649-E13.8, I82.210-I82.291, I82.401-I82.729, I82.811-I82.91, I82.A11-I82.C29, I87.8, I99.8-I99.9

 ● I82.21 Embolism and thrombosis of superior vena cava
  I82.210 Acute embolism and thrombosis of superior vena cava 🔍
    Embolism and thrombosis of superior vena cava NOS
  I82.211 Chronic embolism and thrombosis of superior vena cava 🔍

 ● I82.22 Embolism and thrombosis of inferior vena cava
  (Ex) For category I82.22 CC codes: E08.51-E08.59, E08.618-E08.638, E08.649-E08.8, E09.51-E09.59, E09.618-E09.638, E09.649, E09.65-E09.8, E10.51-E10.59, E10.618-E10.638, E10.649, E10.69-E10.8, E11.51-E11.59, E11.618-E11.638, E11.649, E11.69-E11.8, E13.51-E13.59, E13.618-E13.638, E13.649-E13.8, I82.210-I82.291, I82.401-I82.729, I82.811-I82.91, I82.A11-I82.C29, I87.8, I99.8-I99.9

  I82.220 Acute embolism and thrombosis of inferior vena cava 🔍
    Embolism and thrombosis of inferior vena cava NOS
  I82.221 Chronic embolism and thrombosis of inferior vena cava 🔍

 ● I82.29 Embolism and thrombosis of other thoracic veins
  Embolism and thrombosis of brachiocephalic (innominate) vein
  I82.290 Acute embolism and thrombosis of other thoracic veins 🔍
  I82.291 Chronic embolism and thrombosis of other thoracic veins 🔍

I82.3 Embolism and thrombosis of renal vein 🔍
 (Ex) E08.51-E08.59, E08.618-E08.638, E08.649-E08.8, E09.51-E09.59, E09.618-E09.638, E09.649, E09.65-E09.8, E10.51-E10.59, E10.618-E10.638, E10.649, E10.69-E10.8, E11.51-E11.59, E11.618-E11.638, E11.649, E11.69-E11.8, E13.51-E13.59, E13.618-E13.638, E13.649-E13.8, I82.210-I82.291, I82.3, I82.401-I82.729, I82.811-I82.91, I82.A11-I82.C29, I87.8, I99.8-I99.9

● I82.4 Acute embolism and thrombosis of deep veins of lower extremity
 (Ex) For category I82.4 CC codes unless otherwise indicated: See I82.2

 I82.40 Acute embolism and thrombosis of unspecified deep veins of lower extremity
  Deep vein thrombosis NOS
  DVT NOS
  Excludes1 acute embolism and thrombosis of unspecified deep veins of distal lower extremity (I82.4Z-) ◄▥
     acute embolism and thrombosis of unspecified deep veins of proximal lower extremity (I82.4Y-) ◄▥

 I82.401 Acute embolism and thrombosis of unspecified deep veins of right lower extremity 🔍 🔍

◄ New ◄▥ Revised ~~deleted~~ Deleted Excludes 1 Excludes 2 Includes Use additional Code first Code also Unspecified

OGCR Official Guidelines ● Unacceptable Principal Diagnosis X Assign placeholder X ● Use Additional Character(s) ▶ Manifestation Code **Coding Clinic**

I82.402   Acute embolism and thrombosis of **unspecified** deep veins of left lower extremity 🐾🐾

I82.403   Acute embolism and thrombosis of **unspecified** deep veins of lower extremity, bilateral 🐾🐾

I82.409   Acute embolism and thrombosis of **unspecified** deep veins of unspecified lower extremity 🐾🐾

● **I82.41**   Acute embolism and thrombosis of femoral vein

     I82.411   Acute embolism and thrombosis of right femoral vein 🐾🐾

     I82.412   Acute embolism and thrombosis of left femoral vein 🐾🐾

     I82.413   Acute embolism and thrombosis of femoral vein, bilateral 🐾🐾

     I82.419   Acute embolism and thrombosis of **unspecified** femoral vein 🐾🐾

● **I82.42**   Acute embolism and thrombosis of iliac vein

     I82.421   Acute embolism and thrombosis of right iliac vein 🐾🐾

     I82.422   Acute embolism and thrombosis of left iliac vein 🐾🐾

     I82.423   Acute embolism and thrombosis of iliac vein, bilateral 🐾🐾

     I82.429   Acute embolism and thrombosis of **unspecified** iliac vein 🐾🐾

● **I82.43**   Acute embolism and thrombosis of popliteal vein

     I82.431   Acute embolism and thrombosis of right popliteal vein 🐾🐾

     I82.432   Acute embolism and thrombosis of left popliteal vein 🐾🐾

     I82.433   Acute embolism and thrombosis of popliteal vein, bilateral 🐾🐾

     I82.439   Acute embolism and thrombosis of **unspecified** popliteal vein 🐾🐾

● **I82.44**   Acute embolism and thrombosis of tibial vein

     I82.441   Acute embolism and thrombosis of right tibial vein 🐾🐾

     I82.442   Acute embolism and thrombosis of left tibial vein 🐾🐾

     I82.443   Acute embolism and thrombosis of tibial vein, bilateral 🐾🐾

     I82.449   Acute embolism and thrombosis of **unspecified** tibial vein 🐾🐾

● **I82.49**   Acute embolism and thrombosis of other specified deep vein of lower extremity

     I82.491   Acute embolism and thrombosis of other specified deep vein of right lower extremity 🐾🐾

     I82.492   Acute embolism and thrombosis of other specified deep vein of left lower extremity 🐾🐾

     I82.493   Acute embolism and thrombosis of other specified deep vein of lower extremity, bilateral 🐾🐾

     I82.499   Acute embolism and thrombosis of other specified deep vein of **unspecified** lower extremity 🐾🐾

● **I82.4Y**   Acute embolism and thrombosis of unspecified deep veins of proximal lower extremity

     Acute embolism and thrombosis of deep vein of thigh NOS

     Acute embolism and thrombosis of deep vein of upper leg NOS

     I82.4Y1   Acute embolism and thrombosis of **unspecified** deep veins of right proximal lower extremity 🐾🐾

I82.4Y2   Acute embolism and thrombosis of **unspecified** deep veins of left proximal lower extremity 🐾🐾

I82.4Y3   Acute embolism and thrombosis of **unspecified** deep veins of proximal lower extremity, bilateral 🐾🐾

I82.4Y9   Acute embolism and thrombosis of **unspecified** deep veins of unspecified proximal lower extremity 🐾🐾

● **I82.4Z**   Acute embolism and thrombosis of unspecified deep veins of distal lower extremity

     Acute embolism and thrombosis of deep vein of calf NOS

     Acute embolism and thrombosis of deep vein of lower leg NOS

     I82.4Z1   Acute embolism and thrombosis of **unspecified** deep veins of right distal lower extremity 🐾🐾

     I82.4Z2   Acute embolism and thrombosis of **unspecified** deep veins of left distal lower extremity 🐾🐾

     I82.4Z3   Acute embolism and thrombosis of **unspecified** deep veins of distal lower extremity, bilateral 🐾🐾

     I82.4Z9   Acute embolism and thrombosis of **unspecified** deep veins of unspecified distal lower extremity 🐾🐾

● **I82.5**   Chronic embolism and thrombosis of deep veins of lower extremity

     Use additional code, if applicable, for associated long-term (current) use of anticoagulants (Z79.01)

     Excludes1   personal history of venous embolism and thrombosis (Z86.718)

     (Ex) For category I82.5 CC codes unless otherwise indicated: See I82.2

● **I82.50**   Chronic embolism and thrombosis of unspecified deep veins of lower extremity

     Excludes1   chronic embolism and thrombosis of unspecified deep veins of distal lower extremity (I82.5Z-) ◄▭
                  chronic embolism and thrombosis of unspecified deep veins of proximal lower extremity (I82.5Y-) ◄▭

     I82.501   Chronic embolism and thrombosis of **unspecified** deep veins of right lower extremity 🐾

     I82.502   Chronic embolism and thrombosis of **unspecified** deep veins of left lower extremity 🐾

     I82.503   Chronic embolism and thrombosis of **unspecified** deep veins of lower extremity, bilateral 🐾

     I82.509   Chronic embolism and thrombosis of **unspecified** deep veins of unspecified lower extremity 🐾

● **I82.51**   Chronic embolism and thrombosis of femoral vein

     I82.511   Chronic embolism and thrombosis of right femoral vein 🐾

     I82.512   Chronic embolism and thrombosis of left femoral vein 🐾

     I82.513   Chronic embolism and thrombosis of femoral vein, bilateral 🐾

     I82.519   Chronic embolism and thrombosis of **unspecified** femoral vein 🐾

N   Newborn Age: 0   P   Pediatric Age: 0–17   M   Maternity DX: 12–55   A   Adult Age: 15–124   ♀   Females Only   ♂   Males Only

🐾   Complication\Comorbidity   🐾   Major C\C   (Ex)   CC/MCC Exclusions   🐾   Present on Admission Requirement   🐾   Hospital-Acquired Condition

995

Item 9–10 Varicose/Varicosities (varix = singular, varices = plural): Enlarged, engorged, tortuous, twisted vascular vessels (veins, arteries, lymphatics). As such, the condition can present in various parts of the body, although the most familiar locations are the lower extremities. A common complication of varices is thrombophlebitis. Varicosities of the anus and rectum are called hemorrhoids.

Figure 9-4 Varicose veins of the legs. (From Goldman: Cecil Medicine, ed 23, Saunders, 2008)

● **I82.52** Chronic embolism and thrombosis of iliac vein

    I82.521 Chronic embolism and thrombosis of right iliac vein 🔊

    I82.522 Chronic embolism and thrombosis of left iliac vein 🔊

    I82.523 Chronic embolism and thrombosis of iliac vein, bilateral 🔊

    I82.529 Chronic embolism and thrombosis of unspecified iliac vein 🔊

● **I82.53** Chronic embolism and thrombosis of popliteal vein

    I82.531 Chronic embolism and thrombosis of right popliteal vein 🔊

    I82.532 Chronic embolism and thrombosis of left popliteal vein 🔊

    I82.533 Chronic embolism and thrombosis of popliteal vein, bilateral 🔊

    I82.539 Chronic embolism and thrombosis of unspecified popliteal vein 🔊

● **I82.54** Chronic embolism and thrombosis of tibial vein

    I82.541 Chronic embolism and thrombosis of right tibial vein 🔊

    I82.542 Chronic embolism and thrombosis of left tibial vein 🔊

    I82.543 Chronic embolism and thrombosis of tibial vein, bilateral 🔊

    I82.549 Chronic embolism and thrombosis of unspecified tibial vein 🔊

● **I82.59** Chronic embolism and thrombosis of other specified deep vein of lower extremity

    I82.591 Chronic embolism and thrombosis of other specified deep vein of right lower extremity 🔊

    I82.592 Chronic embolism and thrombosis of other specified deep vein of left lower extremity 🔊

    I82.593 Chronic embolism and thrombosis of other specified deep vein of lower extremity, bilateral 🔊

    I82.599 Chronic embolism and thrombosis of other specified deep vein of unspecified lower extremity 🔊

● **I82.5Y** Chronic embolism and thrombosis of unspecified deep veins of proximal lower extremity

    Chronic embolism and thrombosis of deep veins of thigh NOS

    Chronic embolism and thrombosis of deep veins of upper leg NOS

    I82.5Y1 Chronic embolism and thrombosis of unspecified deep veins of right proximal lower extremity 🔊

    I82.5Y2 Chronic embolism and thrombosis of unspecified deep veins of left proximal lower extremity 🔊

    I82.5Y3 Chronic embolism and thrombosis of unspecified deep veins of proximal lower extremity, bilateral 🔊

    I82.5Y9 Chronic embolism and thrombosis of unspecified deep veins of unspecified proximal lower extremity 🔊

● **I82.5Z** Chronic embolism and thrombosis of unspecified deep veins of distal lower extremity

    Chronic embolism and thrombosis of deep veins of calf NOS

    Chronic embolism and thrombosis of deep veins of lower leg NOS

    I82.5Z1 Chronic embolism and thrombosis of unspecified deep veins of right distal lower extremity 🔊

    I82.5Z2 Chronic embolism and thrombosis of unspecified deep veins of left distal lower extremity 🔊

    I82.5Z3 Chronic embolism and thrombosis of unspecified deep veins of distal lower extremity, bilateral 🔊

    I82.5Z9 Chronic embolism and thrombosis of unspecified deep veins of unspecified distal lower extremity 🔊

● **I82.6** Acute embolism and thrombosis of veins of upper extremity

    Ⓔⓧ **For category I82.6 CC codes unless otherwise indicated:** See I82.2

● **I82.60** Acute embolism and thrombosis of unspecified veins of upper extremity

    I82.601 Acute embolism and thrombosis of unspecified veins of right upper extremity 🔊

    I82.602 Acute embolism and thrombosis of unspecified veins of left upper extremity 🔊

    I82.603 Acute embolism and thrombosis of unspecified veins of upper extremity, bilateral 🔊

    I82.609 Acute embolism and thrombosis of unspecified veins of unspecified upper extremity 🔊

● **I82.61** Acute embolism and thrombosis of superficial veins of upper extremity

    Acute embolism and thrombosis of antecubital vein

    Acute embolism and thrombosis of basilic vein

    Acute embolism and thrombosis of cephalic vein

    I82.611 Acute embolism and thrombosis of superficial veins of right upper extremity 🔊

    I82.612 Acute embolism and thrombosis of superficial veins of left upper extremity 🔊

    I82.613 Acute embolism and thrombosis of superficial veins of upper extremity, bilateral 🔊

    I82.619 Acute embolism and thrombosis of superficial veins of unspecified upper extremity 🔊

◀ New   ◀ⁱⁱⁱ Revised   ~~deleted~~ Deleted   Excludes 1   Excludes 2   Includes   Use additional   Code first   Code also   Unspecified

OGCR Official Guidelines   ● Unacceptable Principal Diagnosis   X Assign placeholder X   ● Use Additional Character(s)   ▶ Manifestation Code   **Coding Clinic**

CHAPTER 9 (I00-I99)

● **I82.62   Acute embolism and thrombosis of deep veins of upper extremity**
Acute embolism and thrombosis of brachial vein
Acute embolism and thrombosis of radial vein
Acute embolism and thrombosis of ulnar vein

    I82.621   Acute embolism and thrombosis of deep veins of right upper extremity

    I82.622   Acute embolism and thrombosis of deep veins of left upper extremity

    I82.623   Acute embolism and thrombosis of deep veins of upper extremity, bilateral

    I82.629   Acute embolism and thrombosis of deep veins of unspecified upper extremity

● **I82.7   Chronic embolism and thrombosis of veins of upper extremity**
Use additional code, if applicable, for associated long-term (current) use of anticoagulants (Z79.01)

  Excludes1   personal history of venous embolism and thrombosis (Z86.718)

  (Ex) For category I82.7 CC codes unless otherwise indicated: See I82.2

● **I82.70   Chronic embolism and thrombosis of unspecified veins of upper extremity**

    I82.701   Chronic embolism and thrombosis of unspecified veins of right upper extremity

    I82.702   Chronic embolism and thrombosis of unspecified veins of left upper extremity

    I82.703   Chronic embolism and thrombosis of unspecified veins of upper extremity, bilateral

    I82.709   Chronic embolism and thrombosis of unspecified veins of unspecified upper extremity

● **I82.71   Chronic embolism and thrombosis of superficial veins of upper extremity**
Chronic embolism and thrombosis of antecubital vein
Chronic embolism and thrombosis of basilic vein
Chronic embolism and thrombosis of cephalic vein

    I82.711   Chronic embolism and thrombosis of superficial veins of right upper extremity

    I82.712   Chronic embolism and thrombosis of superficial veins of left upper extremity

    I82.713   Chronic embolism and thrombosis of superficial veins of upper extremity, bilateral

    I82.719   Chronic embolism and thrombosis of superficial veins of unspecified upper extremity

● **I82.72   Chronic embolism and thrombosis of deep veins of upper extremity**
Chronic embolism and thrombosis of brachial vein
Chronic embolism and thrombosis of radial vein
Chronic embolism and thrombosis of ulnar vein

    I82.721   Chronic embolism and thrombosis of deep veins of right upper extremity

    I82.722   Chronic embolism and thrombosis of deep veins of left upper extremity

    I82.723   Chronic embolism and thrombosis of deep veins of upper extremity, bilateral

    I82.729   Chronic embolism and thrombosis of deep veins of unspecified upper extremity

● **I82.A   Embolism and thrombosis of axillary vein**
(Ex) For category I82.A CC codes unless otherwise indicated: See I82.2

● **I82.A1   Acute embolism and thrombosis of axillary vein**

    I82.A11   Acute embolism and thrombosis of right axillary vein

    I82.A12   Acute embolism and thrombosis of left axillary vein

    I82.A13   Acute embolism and thrombosis of axillary vein, bilateral

    I82.A19   Acute embolism and thrombosis of unspecified axillary vein

● **I82.A2   Chronic embolism and thrombosis of axillary vein**

    I82.A21   Chronic embolism and thrombosis of right axillary vein

    I82.A22   Chronic embolism and thrombosis of left axillary vein

    I82.A23   Chronic embolism and thrombosis of axillary vein, bilateral

    I82.A29   Chronic embolism and thrombosis of unspecified axillary vein

● **I82.B   Embolism and thrombosis of subclavian vein**
(Ex) For category I82.B CC codes unless otherwise indicated: See I82.2

● **I82.B1   Acute embolism and thrombosis of subclavian vein**

    I82.B11   Acute embolism and thrombosis of right subclavian vein

    I82.B12   Acute embolism and thrombosis of left subclavian vein

    I82.B13   Acute embolism and thrombosis of subclavian vein, bilateral

    I82.B19   Acute embolism and thrombosis of unspecified subclavian vein

● **I82.B2   Chronic embolism and thrombosis of subclavian vein**

    I82.B21   Chronic embolism and thrombosis of right subclavian vein

    I82.B22   Chronic embolism and thrombosis of left subclavian vein

    I82.B23   Chronic embolism and thrombosis of subclavian vein, bilateral

    I82.B29   Chronic embolism and thrombosis of unspecified subclavian vein

● **I82.C   Embolism and thrombosis of internal jugular vein**
(Ex) For category I82.C CC codes unless otherwise indicated: See I82.2

● **I82.C1   Acute embolism and thrombosis of internal jugular vein**

    I82.C11   Acute embolism and thrombosis of right internal jugular vein

    I82.C12   Acute embolism and thrombosis of left internal jugular vein

    I82.C13   Acute embolism and thrombosis of internal jugular vein, bilateral

    I82.C19   Acute embolism and thrombosis of unspecified internal jugular vein

● **I82.C2   Chronic embolism and thrombosis of internal jugular vein**

    I82.C21   Chronic embolism and thrombosis of right internal jugular vein

    I82.C22   Chronic embolism and thrombosis of left internal jugular vein

    I82.C23   Chronic embolism and thrombosis of internal jugular vein, bilateral

    I82.C29   Chronic embolism and thrombosis of unspecified internal jugular vein

CHAPTER 9 (I00-I99)

CHAPTER 9 (I00-I99)

● **I82.8**   **Embolism and thrombosis of other specified veins**
　　Use additional code, if applicable, for associated
　　long-term (current) use of anticoagulants (Z79.01)
　　Ⓔⓧ For category I82.8 CC codes unless otherwise indicated: See I82.2

● **I82.81**   **Embolism and thrombosis of superficial veins of lower extremities**
　　Embolism and thrombosis of saphenous vein (greater) (lesser)

     I82.811   **Embolism and thrombosis of superficial veins of right lower extremities** 🔗

     I82.812   **Embolism and thrombosis of superficial veins of left lower extremities** 🔗

     I82.813   **Embolism and thrombosis of superficial veins of lower extremities, bilateral** 🔗

     I82.819   **Embolism and thrombosis of superficial veins of unspecified lower extremities** 🔗

● **I82.89**   **Embolism and thrombosis of other specified veins**

     I82.890   **Acute embolism and thrombosis of other specified veins** 🔗

     I82.891   **Chronic embolism and thrombosis of other specified veins** 🔗

● **I82.9**   **Embolism and thrombosis of unspecified vein**
　　Ⓔⓧ For category I82.9 CC codes unless otherwise indicated: See I82.2

     I82.90   **Acute embolism and thrombosis of unspecified vein** 🔗
　　Embolism of vein NOS
　　Thrombosis (vein) NOS

     I82.91   **Chronic embolism and thrombosis of unspecified vein** 🔗

● **I83**   **Varicose veins of lower extremities**
　　Excludes 1   varicose veins complicating pregnancy (O22.0-)
　　　　varicose veins complicating the puerperium (O87.4)

● **I83.0**   **Varicose veins of lower extremities with ulcer**
　　Use additional code to identify severity of ulcer (L97.-)

● **I83.00**   **Varicose veins of unspecified lower extremity with ulcer**

     I83.001   **Varicose veins of unspecified lower extremity with ulcer of thigh**   A

     I83.002   **Varicose veins of unspecified lower extremity with ulcer of calf**   A

     I83.003   **Varicose veins of unspecified lower extremity with ulcer of ankle**   A

     I83.004   **Varicose veins of unspecified lower extremity with ulcer of heel and midfoot**   A
　　Varicose veins of unspecified lower extremity with ulcer of plantar surface of midfoot

     I83.005   **Varicose veins of unspecified lower extremity with ulcer other part of foot**   A
　　Varicose veins of unspecified lower extremity with ulcer of toe

     I83.008   **Varicose veins of unspecified lower extremity with ulcer other part of lower leg**   A

     I83.009   **Varicose veins of unspecified lower extremity with ulcer of unspecified site**   A

● **I83.01**   **Varicose veins of right lower extremity with ulcer**

     I83.011   **Varicose veins of right lower extremity with ulcer of thigh**   A

     I83.012   **Varicose veins of right lower extremity with ulcer of calf**   A

     I83.013   **Varicose veins of right lower extremity with ulcer of ankle**   A

     I83.014   **Varicose veins of right lower extremity with ulcer of heel and midfoot**   A
　　Varicose veins of right lower extremity with ulcer of plantar surface of midfoot

     I83.015   **Varicose veins of right lower extremity with ulcer other part of foot**   A
　　Varicose veins of right lower extremity with ulcer of toe

     I83.018   **Varicose veins of right lower extremity with ulcer other part of lower leg**   A

     I83.019   **Varicose veins of right lower extremity with ulcer of unspecified site**   A

● **I83.02**   **Varicose veins of left lower extremity with ulcer**

     I83.021   **Varicose veins of left lower extremity with ulcer of thigh**   A

     I83.022   **Varicose veins of left lower extremity with ulcer of calf**   A

     I83.023   **Varicose veins of left lower extremity with ulcer of ankle**   A

     I83.024   **Varicose veins of left lower extremity with ulcer of heel and midfoot**   A
　　Varicose veins of left lower extremity with ulcer of plantar surface of midfoot

     I83.025   **Varicose veins of left lower extremity with ulcer other part of foot**   A
　　Varicose veins of left lower extremity with ulcer of toe

     I83.028   **Varicose veins of left lower extremity with ulcer other part of lower leg**   A

     I83.029   **Varicose veins of left lower extremity with ulcer of unspecified site**   A

● **I83.1**   **Varicose veins of lower extremities with inflammation**
　　Stasis dermatitis

     I83.10   **Varicose veins of unspecified lower extremity with inflammation**   A

     I83.11   **Varicose veins of right lower extremity with inflammation**   A

     I83.12   **Varicose veins of left lower extremity with inflammation**   A

● **I83.2**   **Varicose veins of lower extremities with both ulcer and inflammation**
　　Use additional code to identify severity of ulcer (L97.-)
　　Ⓔⓧ For category I83.2 CC codes: I83.001-I83.229, I83.90-I83.93

● **I83.20**   **Varicose veins of unspecified lower extremity with both ulcer and inflammation**

     I83.201   **Varicose veins of unspecified lower extremity with both ulcer of thigh and inflammation** 🔗   A

     I83.202   **Varicose veins of unspecified lower extremity with both ulcer of calf and inflammation** 🔗   A

     I83.203   **Varicose veins of unspecified lower extremity with both ulcer of ankle and inflammation** 🔗   A

◀ New   ◀▥ Revised   ~~deleted~~ Deleted   Excludes 1   Excludes 2   Includes   Use additional   Code first   Code also   Unspecified

OGCR Official Guidelines   ● Unacceptable Principal Diagnosis   X Assign placeholder X   ● Use Additional Character(s)   ▶ Manifestation Code   **Coding Clinic**

I83.204   Varicose veins of unspecified lower extremity with both ulcer of heel and midfoot and inflammation 🦠   A
     Varicose veins of unspecified lower extremity with both ulcer of plantar surface of midfoot and inflammation

I83.205   Varicose veins of unspecified lower extremity with both ulcer other part of foot and inflammation 🦠   A
     Varicose veins of unspecified lower extremity with both ulcer of toe and inflammation

I83.208   Varicose veins of unspecified lower extremity with both ulcer of other part of lower extremity and inflammation 🦠   A

I83.209   Varicose veins of unspecified lower extremity with both ulcer of unspecified site and inflammation 🦠 A

● I83.21   Varicose veins of right lower extremity with both ulcer and inflammation

I83.211   Varicose veins of right lower extremity with both ulcer of thigh and inflammation 🦠   A

I83.212   Varicose veins of right lower extremity with both ulcer of calf and inflammation 🦠   A

I83.213   Varicose veins of right lower extremity with both ulcer of ankle and inflammation 🦠   A

I83.214   Varicose veins of right lower extremity with both ulcer of heel and midfoot and inflammation 🦠   A
     Varicose veins of right lower extremity with both ulcer of plantar surface of midfoot and inflammation

I83.215   Varicose veins of right lower extremity with both ulcer other part of foot and inflammation 🦠   A
     Varicose veins of right lower extremity with both ulcer of toe and inflammation

I83.218   Varicose veins of right lower extremity with both ulcer of other part of lower extremity and inflammation 🦠   A

I83.219   Varicose veins of right lower extremity with both ulcer of unspecified site and inflammation 🦠 A

● I83.22   Varicose veins of left lower extremity with both ulcer and inflammation

I83.221   Varicose veins of left lower extremity with both ulcer of thigh and inflammation 🦠   A

I83.222   Varicose veins of left lower extremity with both ulcer of calf and inflammation 🦠   A

I83.223   Varicose veins of left lower extremity with both ulcer of ankle and inflammation 🦠   A

I83.224   Varicose veins of left lower extremity with both ulcer of heel and midfoot and inflammation 🦠   A
     Varicose veins of left lower extremity with both ulcer of plantar surface of midfoot and inflammation

I83.225   Varicose veins of left lower extremity with both ulcer other part of foot and inflammation 🦠   A
     Varicose veins of left lower extremity with both ulcer of toe and inflammation

I83.228   Varicose veins of left lower extremity with both ulcer of other part of lower extremity and inflammation 🦠   A

I83.229   Varicose veins of left lower extremity with both ulcer of unspecified site and inflammation 🦠   A

● I83.8   Varicose veins of lower extremities with other complications

● I83.81   Varicose veins of lower extremities with pain

I83.811   Varicose veins of right lower extremities with pain   A

I83.812   Varicose veins of left lower extremities with pain   A

I83.813   Varicose veins of bilateral lower extremities with pain   A

I83.819   Varicose veins of unspecified lower extremities with pain   A

● I83.89   Varicose veins of lower extremities with other complications
     Varicose veins of lower extremities with edema
     Varicose veins of lower extremities with swelling

I83.891   Varicose veins of right lower extremities with other complications A

I83.892   Varicose veins of left lower extremities with other complications A

I83.893   Varicose veins of bilateral lower extremities with other complications A

I83.899   Varicose veins of unspecified lower extremities with other complications A

● I83.9   Asymptomatic varicose veins of lower extremities
     Phlebectasia of lower extremities
     Varicose veins of lower extremities
     Varix of lower extremities

I83.90   Asymptomatic varicose veins of unspecified lower extremity   A
     Varicose veins NOS

I83.91   Asymptomatic varicose veins of right lower extremity   A

I83.92   Asymptomatic varicose veins of left lower extremity   A

I83.93   Asymptomatic varicose veins of bilateral lower extremities   A

● I85   **Esophageal varices**
     Use additional code to identify:
     alcohol abuse and dependence (F10.-)

● I85.0   **Esophageal varices**
     Idiopathic esophageal varices
     Primary esophageal varices

I85.00   **Esophageal varices without bleeding** 🦠
     Esophageal varices NOS
     (Ex) E16.4, I85.00-I85.01, I85.11, I87.8, I99.8-I99.9, K22.6, K25.0-K28.9, K29.01, K29.21, K29.31, K29.41, K29.51, K29.61, K29.71, K29.81, K29.91, K31.811, K92.0-K92.2

I85.01   **Esophageal varices with bleeding** 🦠
     (Ex) E16.4, I85.01, I85.11, I87.8, I99.8-I99.9, K22.10-K22.11, K22.6-K22.70, K22.710-K22.719, K25.0-K28.9, K29.01, K29.21, K29.31, K29.41, K29.51, K29.61, K29.71, K29.81, K29.91, K31.811, K55.21, K57.01, K57.11, K57.13, K57.21, K57.31, K57.33, K57.41, K57.51, K57.53, K57.81, K57.91, K57.93, K62.5, K92.0-K92.2

N Newborn Age: 0   **P** Pediatric Age: 0–17   **M** Maternity DX: 12–55   **A** Adult Age: 15–124   ♀ Females Only   ♂ Males Only

🦠 Complication\Comorbidity   🦠 Major C\C   (Ex) CC/MCC Exclusions   🦠 Present on Admission Requirement   🦠 Hospital-Acquired Condition

999

● **I85.1**   **Secondary esophageal varices**
       Esophageal varices secondary to alcoholic liver disease
       Esophageal varices secondary to cirrhosis of liver
       Esophageal varices secondary to schistosomiasis
       Esophageal varices secondary to toxic liver disease
       Code first underlying disease

     I85.10   **Secondary esophageal varices without bleeding** 🔖
         (Ex:) E16.4, I85.01, I85.10-I85.11, I87.8, I99.8-I99.9, K22.6,
            K25.0-K28.9, K29.01, K29.21, K29.31, K29.41, K29.51,
            K29.61, K29.71, K29.81, K29.91, K31.811, K92.0-K92.2

     I85.11   **Secondary esophageal varices with bleeding** 🔖
         (Ex:) I85.01, I85.11, I87.8, I99.8-I99.9

● **I86**   **Varicose veins of other sites**
     Excludes1   varicose veins of unspecified site (I83.9-)
     Excludes2   retinal varices (H35.0-)

   I86.0   **Sublingual varices**

   I86.1   **Scrotal varices** ♂
       Varicocele

   I86.2   **Pelvic varices**

   I86.3   **Vulval varices** ♀
     Excludes1   vulval varices complicating childbirth
               and the puerperium (O87.8)
            vulval varices complicating pregnancy
               (O22.1-)

   I86.4   **Gastric varices**

   I86.8   **Varicose veins of other specified sites**   A
       Varicose ulcer of nasal septum

● **I87**   **Other disorders of veins**

   ● **I87.0**   **Postthrombotic syndrome**
       Chronic venous hypertension due to deep vein
           thrombosis
       Postphlebitic syndrome
     Excludes1   chronic venous hypertension without
               deep vein thrombosis (I87.3-)

    ● **I87.00**   **Postthrombotic syndrome without complications**
         Asymptomatic Postthrombotic syndrome

     I87.001   **Postthrombotic syndrome without complications of right lower extremity**

     I87.002   **Postthrombotic syndrome without complications of left lower extremity**

     I87.003   **Postthrombotic syndrome without complications of bilateral lower extremity**

     I87.009   **Postthrombotic syndrome without complications of unspecified extremity**
         Postthrombotic syndrome NOS

    ● **I87.01**   **Postthrombotic syndrome with ulcer**
       Use additional code to specify site and severity
          of ulcer (L97.-)
       (Ex:) **For category I87.01 CC codes:** I80.00-I80.9

     I87.011   **Postthrombotic syndrome with ulcer of right lower extremity** 🔖

     I87.012   **Postthrombotic syndrome with ulcer of left lower extremity** 🔖

     I87.013   **Postthrombotic syndrome with ulcer of bilateral lower extremity** 🔖

     I87.019   **Postthrombotic syndrome with ulcer of unspecified lower extremity** 🔖

    ● **I87.02**   **Postthrombotic syndrome with inflammation**

     I87.021   **Postthrombotic syndrome with inflammation of right lower extremity**

     I87.022   **Postthrombotic syndrome with inflammation of left lower extremity**

     I87.023   **Postthrombotic syndrome with inflammation of bilateral lower extremity**

     I87.029   **Postthrombotic syndrome with inflammation of unspecified lower extremity**

    ● **I87.03**   **Postthrombotic syndrome with ulcer and inflammation**
       Use additional code to specify site and severity
          of ulcer (L97.-)
       (Ex:) **For category I87.03 CC codes:** I80.00-I80.9

     I87.031   **Postthrombotic syndrome with ulcer and inflammation of right lower extremity** 🔖

     I87.032   **Postthrombotic syndrome with ulcer and inflammation of left lower extremity** 🔖

     I87.033   **Postthrombotic syndrome with ulcer and inflammation of bilateral lower extremity** 🔖

     I87.039   **Postthrombotic syndrome with ulcer and inflammation of unspecified lower extremity** 🔖

    ● **I87.09**   **Postthrombotic syndrome with other complications**

     I87.091   **Postthrombotic syndrome with other complications of right lower extremity**

     I87.092   **Postthrombotic syndrome with other complications of left lower extremity**

     I87.093   **Postthrombotic syndrome with other complications of bilateral lower extremity**

     I87.099   **Postthrombotic syndrome with other complications of unspecified lower extremity**

   I87.1   **Compression of vein** 🔖
       Stricture of vein
       Vena cava syndrome (inferior) (superior)
     Excludes2   compression of pulmonary vein (I28.8)
       (Ex:) I87.1

   I87.2   **Venous insufficiency (chronic) (peripheral)**

   ● **I87.3**   **Chronic venous hypertension (idiopathic)**
       Stasis edema
     Excludes1   chronic venous hypertension due to deep
               vein thrombosis (I87.0-)
            varicose veins of lower extremities (I83.-)

    ● **I87.30**   **Chronic venous hypertension (idiopathic) without complications**
         Asymptomatic chronic venous hypertension
            (idiopathic)

     I87.301   **Chronic venous hypertension (idiopathic) without complications of right lower extremity**

     I87.302   **Chronic venous hypertension (idiopathic) without complications of left lower extremity**

     I87.303   **Chronic venous hypertension (idiopathic) without complications of bilateral lower extremity**

     I87.309   **Chronic venous hypertension (idiopathic) without complications of unspecified lower extremity**
         Chronic venous hypertension NOS

CHAPTER 9 (I00-I99)

◄ New   ◄■ Revised   ~~deleted~~ Deleted   Excludes 1   Excludes 2   Includes   Use additional   Code first   Code also   Unspecified

OGCR Official Guidelines   ● Unacceptable Principal Diagnosis   X Assign placeholder X   ● Use Additional Character(s)   ▶ Manifestation Code   **Coding Clinic**

● **I87.31** Chronic venous hypertension (idiopathic) with ulcer

Use additional code to specify site and severity of ulcer (L97.-)

(Ex) **For category I87.31 CC codes:** I83.001-I83.229, I83.90-I83.93, I87.2, I87.8-I87.9, I99.8-I99.9

I87.311 Chronic venous hypertension (idiopathic) with ulcer of right lower extremity

I87.312 Chronic venous hypertension (idiopathic) with ulcer of left lower extremity

I87.313 Chronic venous hypertension (idiopathic) with ulcer of bilateral lower extremity

I87.319 Chronic venous hypertension (idiopathic) with ulcer of unspecified lower extremity

● **I87.32** Chronic venous hypertension (idiopathic) with inflammation

I87.321 Chronic venous hypertension (idiopathic) with inflammation of right lower extremity

I87.322 Chronic venous hypertension (idiopathic) with inflammation of left lower extremity

I87.323 Chronic venous hypertension (idiopathic) with inflammation of bilateral lower extremity

I87.329 Chronic venous hypertension (idiopathic) with inflammation of unspecified lower extremity

● **I87.33** Chronic venous hypertension (idiopathic) with ulcer and inflammation

Use additional code to specify site and severity of ulcer (L97.-)

(Ex) **For category I87.33 CC codes:** See I87.31

I87.331 Chronic venous hypertension (idiopathic) with ulcer and inflammation of right lower extremity

I87.332 Chronic venous hypertension (idiopathic) with ulcer and inflammation of left lower extremity

I87.333 Chronic venous hypertension (idiopathic) with ulcer and inflammation of bilateral lower extremity

I87.339 Chronic venous hypertension (idiopathic) with ulcer and inflammation of unspecified lower extremity

● **I87.39** Chronic venous hypertension (idiopathic) with other complications

I87.391 Chronic venous hypertension (idiopathic) with other complications of right lower extremity

I87.392 Chronic venous hypertension (idiopathic) with other complications of left lower extremity

I87.393 Chronic venous hypertension (idiopathic) with other complications of bilateral lower extremity

I87.399 Chronic venous hypertension (idiopathic) with other complications of unspecified lower extremity

I87.8 Other specified disorders of veins
Phlebosclerosis
Venofibrosis

I87.9 Disorder of vein, unspecified

● **I88** Nonspecific lymphadenitis

Excludes1 acute lymphadenitis, except mesenteric (L04.-)
enlarged lymph nodes NOS (R59.-)
human immunodeficiency virus [HIV] disease resulting in generalized lymphadenopathy (B20)

I88.0 Nonspecific mesenteric lymphadenitis
Mesenteric lymphadenitis (acute)(chronic)

I88.1 Chronic lymphadenitis, except mesenteric
Adenitis
Lymphadenitis

I88.8 Other nonspecific lymphadenitis

I88.9 Nonspecific lymphadenitis, unspecified
Lymphadenitis NOS

● **I89** Other noninfective disorders of lymphatic vessels and lymph nodes

Excludes1 chylocele, tunica vaginalis (nonfilarial) NOS (N50.8)
enlarged lymph nodes NOS (R59.-)
filarial chylocele (B74.-)
hereditary lymphedema (Q82.0)

I89.0 Lymphedema, not elsewhere classified
Elephantiasis (nonfilarial) NOS
Lymphangiectasis
Obliteration, lymphatic vessel
Praecox lymphedema
Secondary lymphedema

Excludes1 postmastectomy lymphedema (I97.2)

I89.1 Lymphangitis
Chronic lymphangitis
Lymphangitis NOS
Subacute lymphangitis

Excludes1 acute lymphangitis (L03.-)

I89.8 Other specified noninfective disorders of lymphatic vessels and lymph nodes
Chylocele (nonfilarial)
Chylous ascites
Chylous cyst
Lipomelanotic reticulosis
Lymph node or vessel fistula
Lymph node or vessel infarction
Lymph node or vessel rupture

I89.9 Noninfective disorder of lymphatic vessels and lymph nodes, unspecified
Disease of lymphatic vessels NOS

OTHER AND UNSPECIFIED DISORDERS OF THE CIRCULATORY SYSTEM (I95-I99)

● **I95** Hypotension
Subnormal arterial blood pressure

Excludes1 cardiovascular collapse (R57.9)
maternal hypotension syndrome (O26.5-)
nonspecific low blood pressure reading NOS (R03.1)

I95.0 Idiopathic hypotension

I95.1 Orthostatic hypotension
Hypotension, postural
Moving from a sitting or reclining position to a standing position precipitates a sudden drop in blood pressure (hypotension).

Excludes1 neurogenic orthostatic hypotension [Shy-Drager] (G90.3)
orthostatic hypotension due to drugs (I95.2)

I95.2 Hypotension due to drugs
Orthostatic hypotension due to drugs

Use additional code for adverse effect, if applicable, to identify drug (T36-T50 with fifth or sixth character 5)

I95.3 Hypotension of hemodialysis
Intra-dialytic hypotension

N Newborn Age: 0   **P** Pediatric Age: 0–17   **M** Maternity DX: 12–55   **A** Adult Age: 15–124   ♀ Females Only   ♂ Males Only

 Complication\Comorbidity   Major C\C   (Ex) CC/MCC Exclusions   Present on Admission Requirement   Hospital-Acquired Condition

1001

CHAPTER 9 (I00-I99)

CHAPTER 9 (I00-I99)

● I95.8   **Other hypotension**
       I95.81   **Postprocedural hypotension**
       I95.89   **Other hypotension**
              Chronic hypotension
    I95.9   **Hypotension, unspecified**

I96   **Gangrene, not elsewhere classified**
      Gangrenous cellulitis
      Excludes1   gangrene in atherosclerosis of native arteries of
                 the extremities (I70.26)
               gangrene of certain specified sites - *see*
                 Alphabetical Index
               gangrene in diabetes mellitus (E08-E13)
               gangrene in hernia (K40.1, K40.4, K41.1, K41.4,
                 K42.1, K43.1-, K44.1, K45.1, K46.1)
               gangrene in other peripheral vascular diseases
                 (I73.-)
               gas gangrene (A48.0)
               pyoderma gangrenosum (L88)
     (Ex) G89.0-G89.4, I70.261-I70.269, I96, R41.0-R41.3, R41.82, R41.9, R44.8-R44.9,
       R45.83-R45.84, R46.0-R46.89, R52, R68.0-R68.19, R68.81-R68.83, R68.89-R69

● I97   **Intraoperative and postprocedural complications and disorders**
      of circulatory system, not elsewhere classified
      Excludes2   postprocedural shock (T81.1-)
    I97.0   **Postcardiotomy syndrome**
● I97.1   **Other postprocedural cardiac functional disturbances**
      Excludes2   acute pulmonary insufficiency following
                 thoracic surgery (J95.1)
               intraoperative cardiac functional
                 disturbances (I97.7-)
     (Ex) **For category I97.1 CC codes:** D78.81-D78.89, E36.8, E89.810-E89.89,
       H59.011-H59.019, H59.031-H59.099, H59.811-H95.89, H95.811-H95.89,
       I97.110-I97.191, I97.3, I97.710-I97.791, I97.88-I97.89, L76.81-L76.82,
       M96.89, N98.1-N98.9, T81.82X[A], T81.89X-T81.9XX[A]
   ● I97.11   **Postprocedural cardiac insufficiency**
       I97.110   **Postprocedural cardiac insufficiency**
               following cardiac surgery 🔎
       I97.111   **Postprocedural cardiac insufficiency**
               following other surgery 🔎
   ● I97.12   **Postprocedural cardiac arrest**
       I97.120   **Postprocedural cardiac arrest**
               following cardiac surgery 🔎
       I97.121   **Postprocedural cardiac arrest**
               following other surgery 🔎
   ● I97.13   **Postprocedural heart failure**
       Use additional code to identify the heart
          failure (I50.-)
       I97.130   **Postprocedural heart failure**
               following cardiac surgery 🔎
       I97.131   **Postprocedural heart failure**
               following other surgery 🔎
   ● I97.19   **Other postprocedural cardiac functional**
       disturbances
       Use additional code, if applicable, to further
          specify disorder
       I97.190   **Other postprocedural cardiac**
               functional disturbances following
               cardiac surgery 🔎
       I97.191   **Other postprocedural cardiac**
               functional disturbances following
               other surgery 🔎

I97.2   **Postmastectomy lymphedema syndrome**   A
      Elephantiasis due to mastectomy
      Obliteration of lymphatic vessels
I97.3   **Postprocedural hypertension**
● I97.4   **Intraoperative hemorrhage and hematoma of a**
      circulatory system organ or structure complicating a
      procedure
      Excludes1   intraoperative hemorrhage and
               hematoma of a circulatory system
               organ or structure due to accidental
               puncture and laceration during a
               procedure (I97.5-)
      Excludes2   intraoperative cerebrovascular
               hemorrhage complicating a
               procedure (G97.3-)
     (Ex) **For category I97.4 CC codes:** H95.811-H95.89, I85.01, I85.11,
       I97.3-I97.42, I97.610-I97.62, K21.9, K22.8, K23-K25.0, K25.2, K25.4,
       K25.6, K26.0, K26.2, K26.4, K26.6, K27.0, K27.2, K27.4, K27.6, K28.0,
       K28.2, K28.4, K28.6, K29.01, K29.21, K29.31, K29.41, K29.51, K29.61,
       K29.71, K29.81, K29.91, K31.811, K55.21, K57.01, K57.11, K57.13,
       K57.21, K57.31, K57.33, K57.41, K57.51, K57.53, K57.81, K57.91, K57.93,
       K62.5, K92.0-K92.2, M96.89, N98.1-N98.9, P54.1-P54.3,
       T81.10X-T81.19X[A], T81.82X[A], T81.89X-T81.9XX[A]
   ● I97.41   **Intraoperative hemorrhage and hematoma**
       of a circulatory system organ or structure
       complicating a circulatory system procedure
       I97.410   **Intraoperative hemorrhage and**
               hematoma of a circulatory system
               organ or structure complicating a
               cardiac catheterization 🔎
       I97.411   **Intraoperative hemorrhage and**
               hematoma of a circulatory system
               organ or structure complicating a
               cardiac bypass 🔎
       I97.418   **Intraoperative hemorrhage and**
               hematoma of a circulatory system
               organ or structure complicating other
               circulatory system procedure 🔎
     I97.42   **Intraoperative hemorrhage and hematoma of a**
       circulatory system organ or structure
       complicating other procedure 🔎
● I97.5   **Accidental puncture and laceration of a circulatory**
      system organ or structure during a procedure
      Excludes2   accidental puncture and laceration of
               brain during a procedure (G97.4-)
     (Ex) **For category I97.5 CC codes:** D78.11-D78.12, D78.81-D78.89,
       E36.11-E36.8, E89.810-E89.89, G96.11, G97.41-G97.49, H59.011-H59.019,
       H59.031-H59.099, H59.211-H59.229, H59.811-H59.89, H95.31-H95.32,
       H95.811-H95.89, I97.3, I97.51-I97.52, J95.71-J95.72, K91.71-K91.72,
       L76.11-L76.12, L76.81-L76.82, M96.820-M96.821, M96.89, N98.1-N98.9,
       N99.71-N99.72, T81.82X[A], T81.89X-T81.9XX[A]
     I97.51   **Accidental puncture and laceration of a**
       circulatory system organ or structure during a
       circulatory system procedure 🔎
     I97.52   **Accidental puncture and laceration of a**
       circulatory system organ or structure during
       other procedure 🔎

◄ New   ◄ Revised   ~~deleted~~ Deleted   Excludes 1   Excludes 2   Includes   Use additional   Code first   Code also   Unspecified
OGCR Official Guidelines   ● Unacceptable Principal Diagnosis   X Assign placeholder X   ● Use Additional Character(s)   ▶ Manifestation Code   **Coding Clinic**

● **I97.6**   **Postprocedural hemorrhage and hematoma of a circulatory system organ or structure following a procedure**

> **Excludes2**   postprocedural cerebrovascular hemorrhage complicating a procedure (G97.5-)
>
> (Ex) **For category I97.6 CC codes:** See I97.4

   ● **I97.61**   **Postprocedural hemorrhage and hematoma of a circulatory system organ or structure following a circulatory system procedure**

       I97.610   Postprocedural hemorrhage and hematoma of a circulatory system organ or structure following a cardiac catheterization 🗅

       I97.611   Postprocedural hemorrhage and hematoma of a circulatory system organ or structure following cardiac bypass 🗅

       I97.618   Postprocedural hemorrhage and hematoma of a circulatory system organ or structure following other circulatory system procedure 🗅

   I97.62   Postprocedural hemorrhage and hematoma of a circulatory system organ or structure following other procedure 🗅

● **I97.7**   **Intraoperative cardiac functional disturbances**

> **Excludes2**   acute pulmonary insufficiency following thoracic surgery (J95.1)
> postprocedural cardiac functional disturbances (I97.1-)
>
> (Ex) **For category I97.7 CC codes:** See I97.1

   ● **I97.71**   **Intraoperative cardiac arrest**

       I97.710   Intraoperative cardiac arrest during cardiac surgery 🗅

       I97.711   Intraoperative cardiac arrest during other surgery 🗅

   ● **I97.79**   **Other intraoperative cardiac functional disturbances**

> Use additional code, if applicable, to further specify disorder

       I97.790   Other intraoperative cardiac functional disturbances during cardiac surgery 🗅

       I97.791   Other intraoperative cardiac functional disturbances during other surgery 🗅

● **I97.8**   **Other intraoperative and postprocedural complications and disorders of the circulatory system, not elsewhere classified**

> Use additional code, if applicable, to further specify disorder
>
> (Ex) **For category I97.8 CC codes unless otherwise indicated:** D78.81-D78.89, E36.8, E89.810-E89.89, G97.0, G97.2-G97.32, G97.81-G97.82, H59.011-H59.019, H59.031-H59.099, H59.811-H59.89, H95.811-H95.89, I97.3, I97.810-I97.821, L76.81-L76.82, M96.89, N98.1-N98.9, T81.82X[A], T81.89X-T81.9XX[A]

   ● **I97.81**   **Intraoperative cerebrovascular infarction**

       I97.810   Intraoperative cerebrovascular infarction during cardiac surgery 🗅

       I97.811   Intraoperative cerebrovascular infarction during other surgery 🗅

   ● **I97.82**   **Postprocedural cerebrovascular infarction**

       I97.820   Postprocedural cerebrovascular infarction during cardiac surgery 🗅

       I97.821   Postprocedural cerebrovascular infarction during other surgery 🗅

       I97.88   Other intraoperative complications of the circulatory system, not elsewhere classified 🗅

>   (Ex) See I97.1

       I97.89   Other postprocedural complications and disorders of the circulatory system, not elsewhere classified 🗅

>   (Ex) See I97.1

● **I99**   **Other and unspecified disorders of circulatory system**

   I99.8   Other disorder of circulatory system

   I99.9   Unspecified disorder of circulatory system

N Newborn Age: 0   **P** Pediatric Age: 0–17   **M** Maternity DX: 12–55   **A** Adult Age: 15–124   ♀ Females Only   ♂ Males Only

🗅 Complication\Comorbidity   🗅 Major C\C   (Ex) CC/MCC Exclusions   🗅 Present on Admission Requirement   🗅 Hospital-Acquired Condition   **1003**

CHAPTER 9 (I00-I99)

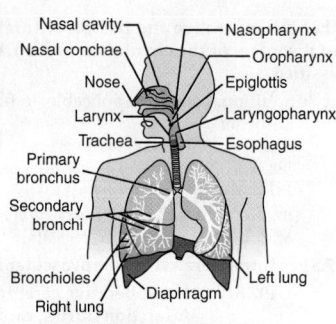

Figure 10-1 Respiratory system. (From Buck CJ: Step-by-Step Medical Coding, ed 2011, Philadelphia, WB Saunders, 2011)

Figure 10-2 Paranasal sinuses. (From Buck CJ: Step-by-Step Medical Coding, ed 2011, Philadelphia, WB Saunders, 2011)

Item 10-1 Pharyngitis is painful inflammation of the pharynx (sore throat). Ninety percent of the infections are caused by a virus with the remaining being bacterial and rarely a fungus (candidiasis). Other irritants such as pollutants, chemicals, or smoke may cause similar symptoms.

OGCR Section I.C.10.a.1

10.1 Chronic Obstructive Pulmonary Disease (COPD) and Asthma

CHAPTER 10

DISEASES OF THE RESPIRATORY SYSTEM (J00-J99)

Note: When a respiratory condition is described as occurring in more than one site and is not specifically indexed, it should be classified to the lower anatomic site (e.g., tracheobronchitis to bronchitis in J40).

Use additional code, where applicable, to identify:
exposure to environmental tobacco smoke (Z77.22)
exposure to tobacco smoke in the perinatal period (P96.81)
history of tobacco use (Z87.891)
occupational exposure to environmental tobacco smoke (Z57.31)
tobacco dependence (F17.-)
tobacco use (Z72.0)

Excludes2 certain conditions originating in the perinatal period (P04-P96)
certain infectious and parasitic diseases (A00-B99)
complications of pregnancy, childbirth and the puerperium (O00-O99A)
congenital malformations, deformations and chromosomal abnormalities (Q00-Q99)
endocrine, nutritional and metabolic diseases (E00-E88)
injury, poisoning and certain other consequences of external causes (S00-T88)
neoplasms (C00-D49)
smoke inhalation (T59.81-)
symptoms, signs and abnormal clinical and laboratory findings, not elsewhere classified (R00-R94)

This chapter contains the following blocks:

J00-J06	Acute upper respiratory infections
J09-J18	Influenza and pneumonia
J20-J22	Other acute lower respiratory infections
J30-J39	Other diseases of upper respiratory tract
J40-J47	Chronic lower respiratory diseases
J60-J70	Lung diseases due to external agents
J80-J84	Other respiratory diseases principally affecting the interstitium
J85-J86	Suppurative and necrotic conditions of the lower respiratory tract
J90-J94	Other diseases of the pleura
J95	Intraoperative and postprocedural complications and disorders of respiratory system, not elsewhere classified
J96-J99	Other diseases of the respiratory system

ACUTE UPPER RESPIRATORY INFECTIONS (J00-J06)

Excludes1 chronic obstructive pulmonary disease with acute lower respiratory infection (J44.0)
influenza virus with other respiratory manifestations (J09.X2, J10.1, J11.1)

J00   Acute nasopharyngitis [common cold]
Acute rhinitis
Coryza (acute)
Infective nasopharyngitis NOS
Infective rhinitis
Nasal catarrh, acute
Nasopharyngitis NOS

Excludes1 acute pharyngitis (J02.-)
acute sore throat NOS (J02.9)
pharyngitis NOS (J02.9)
rhinitis NOS (J31.0)
sore throat NOS (J02.9)

Excludes2 allergic rhinitis (J30.1-J30.9)
chronic pharyngitis (J31.2)
chronic rhinitis (J31.0)
chronic sore throat (J31.2)
nasopharyngitis, chronic (J31.1)
vasomotor rhinitis (J30.0)

(See Plate 49 on page 72.)

● **J01   Acute sinusitis**
Includes acute abscess of sinus
acute empyema of sinus
acute infection of sinus
acute inflammation of sinus
acute suppuration of sinus

Use additional code (B95-B97) to identify infectious agent.

Excludes1 sinusitis NOS (J32.9)
Excludes2 chronic sinusitis (J32.0-J32.8)

● **J01.0   Acute maxillary sinusitis**
Acute antritis
    J01.00   Acute maxillary sinusitis, unspecified
    J01.01   Acute recurrent maxillary sinusitis

● **J01.1   Acute frontal sinusitis**
    J01.10   Acute frontal sinusitis, unspecified
    J01.11   Acute recurrent frontal sinusitis

● **J01.2   Acute ethmoidal sinusitis**
    J01.20   Acute ethmoidal sinusitis, unspecified
    J01.21   Acute recurrent ethmoidal sinusitis

● **J01.3   Acute sphenoidal sinusitis**
    J01.30   Acute sphenoidal sinusitis, unspecified
    J01.31   Acute recurrent sphenoidal sinusitis

● **J01.4   Acute pansinusitis**
    J01.40   Acute pansinusitis, unspecified
    J01.41   Acute recurrent pansinusitis

◄ New   ⬅ Revised   ~~deleted~~ Deleted   Excludes 1   Excludes 2   Includes   Use additional   Code first   Code also   Unspecified

OGCR Official Guidelines   ● Unacceptable Principal Diagnosis   X Assign placeholder X   ● Use Additional Character(s)   ▷ Manifestation Code   **Coding Clinic**

- **J01.8**   **Other acute sinusitis**
  - **J01.80**   **Other acute sinusitis**
    Acute sinusitis involving more than one sinus but not pansinusitis
  - **J01.81**   **Other acute recurrent sinusitis**
    Acute recurrent sinusitis involving more than one sinus but not pansinusitis
- **J01.9**   **Acute sinusitis, unspecified**
  - **J01.90**   **Acute sinusitis, unspecified**
  - **J01.91**   **Acute recurrent sinusitis, unspecified**
- **J02**   **Acute pharyngitis**
  - **Includes**   acute sore throat
  - **Excludes1**   acute laryngopharyngitis (J06.0)
    peritonsillar abscess (J36)
    pharyngeal abscess (J39.1)
    retropharyngeal abscess (J39.0)
  - **Excludes2**   chronic pharyngitis (J31.2)
  - **J02.0**   **Streptococcal pharyngitis**
    Septic pharyngitis
    Streptococcal sore throat
    - **Excludes2**   scarlet fever (A38.-)
  - **J02.8**   **Acute pharyngitis due to other specified organisms**
    Use additional code (B95-B97) to identify infectious agent
    - **Excludes1**   pharyngitis due to coxsackie virus (B08.5)
      pharyngitis due to gonococcus (A54.5)
      acute pharyngitis due to herpes [simplex] virus (B00.2)
      acute pharyngitis due to infectious mononucleosis (B27.-)
      enteroviral vesicular pharyngitis (B08.5)
  - **J02.9**   **Acute pharyngitis, unspecified**
    Gangrenous pharyngitis (acute)
    Infective pharyngitis (acute) NOS
    Pharyngitis (acute) NOS
    Sore throat (acute) NOS
    Suppurative pharyngitis (acute)
    Ulcerative pharyngitis (acute)
- **J03**   **Acute tonsillitis**
  Inflammation of pharyngeal tonsils caused by virus or bacteria
  - **Excludes1**   acute sore throat (J02.-)
    hypertrophy of tonsils (J35.1)
    peritonsillar abscess (J36)
    sore throat NOS (J02.9)
    streptococcal sore throat (J02.0)
  - **Excludes2**   chronic tonsillitis (J35.0)
  - **J03.0**   **Streptococcal tonsillitis**
    - **J03.00**   **Acute streptococcal tonsillitis, unspecified**
    - **J03.01**   **Acute recurrent streptococcal tonsillitis**
  - **J03.8**   **Acute tonsillitis due to other specified organisms**
    Use additional code (B95-B97) to identify infectious agent.
    - **Excludes1**   diphtheritic tonsillitis (A36.0)
      herpesviral pharyngotonsillitis (B00.2)
      streptococcal tonsillitis (J03.0)
      tuberculous tonsillitis (A15.8)
      Vincent's tonsillitis (A69.1)
    - **J03.80**   **Acute tonsillitis due to other specified organisms**
    - **J03.81**   **Acute recurrent tonsillitis due to other specified organisms**
  - **J03.9**   **Acute tonsillitis, unspecified**
    Follicular tonsillitis (acute)
    Gangrenous tonsillitis (acute)
    Infective tonsillitis (acute)
    Tonsillitis (acute) NOS
    Ulcerative tonsillitis (acute)
    - **J03.90**   **Acute tonsillitis, unspecified**
    - **J03.91**   **Acute recurrent tonsillitis, unspecified**

Item 10–2   **Laryngitis** is an inflammation of the larynx (voice box) resulting in hoarse voice or the complete loss of the voice. **Tracheitis** is an inflammation of the trachea (often following a URI) commonly caused by *staphylococcus aureus* resulting in inspiratory stridor (crowing sound on inspiration) and a croup like cough.

- **J04**   **Acute laryngitis and tracheitis**
  Use additional code (B95-B97) to identify infectious agent.
  - **Excludes1**   acute obstructive laryngitis [croup] and epiglottitis (J05.-)
  - **Excludes2**   laryngismus (stridulus) (J38.5)
  - **J04.0**   **Acute laryngitis**
    Edematous laryngitis (acute)
    Laryngitis (acute) NOS
    Subglottic laryngitis (acute)
    Suppurative laryngitis (acute)
    Ulcerative laryngitis (acute)
    - **Excludes1**   acute obstructive laryngitis (J05.0)
    - **Excludes2**   chronic laryngitis (J37.0)
  - **J04.1**   **Acute tracheitis**
    Acute viral tracheitis
    Catarrhal tracheitis (acute)
    Tracheitis (acute) NOS
    - **Excludes2**   chronic tracheitis (J42)
    - **J04.10**   **Acute tracheitis without obstruction**
    - **J04.11**   **Acute tracheitis with obstruction**
      (Ex) A15.8-A15.9, A17.9, A18.82, A18.84, A18.89, J04.10-J04.2, J05.10-J05.11, J22, J98.8-J98.9
  - **J04.2**   **Acute laryngotracheitis**
    Laryngotracheitis NOS
    Tracheitis (acute) with laryngitis (acute)
    - **Excludes1**   acute obstructive laryngotracheitis (J05.0)
    - **Excludes2**   chronic laryngotracheitis (J37.1)
  - **J04.3**   **Supraglottitis, unspecified**
    - **J04.30**   **Supraglottitis, unspecified, without obstruction**
    - **J04.31**   **Supraglottitis, unspecified, with obstruction**
      (Ex) A15.8-A15.9, A17.9, A18.82, A18.84, A18.89, J04.0-J04.2, J05.10-J05.11, J22, J98.8-J98.9
- **J05**   **Acute obstructive laryngitis [croup] and epiglottitis**
  Use additional code (B95-B97) to identify infectious agent.
  - **J05.0**   **Acute obstructive laryngitis [croup]**
    Obstructive laryngitis (acute) NOS
    Obstructive laryngotracheitis NOS
  - **J05.1**   **Acute epiglottitis**
    - **Excludes2**   epiglottitis, chronic (J37.0)
    - **J05.10**   **Acute epiglottitis without obstruction**
      Epiglottitis NOS
      (Ex) J04.31, J05.10-J05.11
    - **J05.11**   **Acute epiglottitis with obstruction**
      (Ex) See J04.10
- **J06**   **Acute upper respiratory infections of multiple and unspecified sites**
  - **Excludes1**   acute respiratory infection NOS (J22)
    streptococcal pharyngitis (J02.0)
  - **J06.0**   **Acute laryngopharyngitis**
  - **J06.9**   **Acute upper respiratory infection, unspecified**
    Upper respiratory disease, acute
    Upper respiratory infection NOS

CHAPTER 10 (J00–J99)

INFLUENZA AND PNEUMONIA (J09-J18)

Excludes2   allergic or eosinophilic pneumonia (J82)
aspiration pneumonia NOS (J69.0)
meconium pneumonia (P24.01)
neonatal aspiration pneumonia (P24.-)
pneumonia due to solids and liquids (J69.-) ◄▦
congenital pneumonia (P23.9)
lipid pneumonia (J69.1)
rheumatic pneumonia (I00)
ventilator associated pneumonia (J95.851)

● **J09**   **Influenza due to certain identified influenza viruses**

Excludes1   influenza due to other influenza viruses (J10.-)
influenza due to unidentified influenza virus (J11.-)
seasonal influenza due to other identified influenza virus (J10.-)
seasonal influenza due to unidentified influenza virus (J11.-)

● **J09.X**   **Influenza due to identified novel influenza A virus**
Avian influenza
Bird influenza
Influenza A/H5N1
Influenza of other animal origin, not bird or swine
Swine influenza virus (viruses that normally cause infections in pigs)

J09.X1   **Influenza due to identified novel influenza A virus with pneumonia** 🔖

Code also , if applicable, associated:
lung abscess (J85.1)
other specified type of pneumonia
Ⓔⓧ A15.0-A15.9, A17.9, A18.82, A18.84, A18.89, A21.2, A22.1, A31.0, A37.01, A37.11, A37.81, A37.91, A42.0, A43.0, A48.1, B25.0, B39.0-B39.2, B44.0, B58.3, B59, B67.1, J09.X1-J09.X2, J10.00-J10.1, J11.00-J11.1, J12.0-J12.3, J12.89-J18.1, J18.8-J18.9, J22, J44.9, J47.0-J70.4, J70.8-J70.9, J98.4, J98.8-J98.9, Q33.4, R91.1

J09.X2   **Influenza due to identified novel influenza A virus with other respiratory manifestations**
Influenza due to identified novel influenza A virus NOS
Influenza due to identified novel influenza A virus with laryngitis
Influenza due to identified novel influenza A virus with pharyngitis
Influenza due to identified novel influenza A virus with upper respiratory symptoms

Use additional code, if applicable, for associated:
pleural effusion (J91.8)
sinusitis (J01.-)

J09.X3   **Influenza due to identified novel influenza A virus with gastrointestinal manifestations**
Influenza due to identified novel influenza A virus gastroenteritis

Excludes1   'intestinal flu' [viral gastroenteritis] (A08.-)

J09.X9   **Influenza due to identified novel influenza A virus with other manifestations**
Influenza due to identified novel influenza A virus with encephalopathy
Influenza due to identified novel influenza A virus with myocarditis
Influenza due to identified novel influenza A virus with otitis media

Use additional code to identify manifestation

● **J10**   **Influenza due to other identified influenza virus**
~~Use additional code to identify the virus (B97.-)~~

Excludes1   influenza due to avian influenza virus (J09.X-)
influenza due to swine flu (J09.X-)
influenza due to unidentified influenza virus (J11.-)

● **J10.0**   **Influenza due to other identified influenza virus with pneumonia**

Code also associated lung abscess, if applicable (J85.1)

J10.00   **Influenza due to other identified influenza virus with unspecified type of pneumonia** 🔖
Ⓔⓧ See J09.X1

J10.01   **Influenza due to other identified influenza virus with the same other identified influenza virus pneumonia**

J10.08   **Influenza due to other identified influenza virus with other specified pneumonia** 🔖

Code also other specified type of pneumonia
Ⓔⓧ A15.0-A15.6, A15.8-A15.9, A17.9, A18.82, A18.84, A18.89, A21.2, A22.1, A31.0, A37.01, A37.11, A37.81, A37.91, A42.0, A43.0, A48.1, B25.0, B39.0-B39.2, B44.0, B58.3, B59, B67.1, J09.X1-J09.X2, J10.00-J10.1, J11.00-J11.1, J12.0-J12.3, J12.89-J18.1, J18.8-J18.9, J22, J44.0-J44.9, J45.21-J45.22, J45.31-J45.32, J45.41-J45.42, J45.51-J45.902, J47.0-J70.4, J70.8-J70.9, J98.4, J98.8-J99, Q33.4, R91.1

J10.1   **Influenza due to other identified influenza virus with other respiratory manifestations**
Influenza due to other identified influenza virus NOS
Influenza due to other identified influenza virus with laryngitis
Influenza due to other identified influenza virus with pharyngitis
Influenza due to other identified influenza virus with upper respiratory symptoms

Use additional code for associated pleural effusion, if applicable (J91.8)
Use additional code for associated sinusitis, if applicable (J01.-)

J10.2   **Influenza due to other identified influenza virus with gastrointestinal manifestations**
Influenza due to other identified influenza virus gastroenteritis

Excludes1   'intestinal flu' [viral gastroenteritis] (A08.-)

● **J10.8**   **Influenza due to other identified influenza virus with other manifestations**

J10.81   **Influenza due to other identified influenza virus with encephalopathy**

J10.82   **Influenza due to other identified influenza virus with myocarditis**

J10.83   **Influenza due to other identified influenza virus with otitis media**

Use additional code for any associated perforated tympanic membrane (H72.-)

J10.89   **Influenza due to other identified influenza virus with other manifestations**

Use additional codes to identify the manifestations

● **J11**   **Influenza due to unidentified influenza virus**

● **J11.0**   **Influenza due to unidentified influenza virus with pneumonia**

Code also associated lung abscess, if applicable (J85.1)
Ⓔⓧ **For category J11.0 CC codes:** See J09.X1

J11.00   **Influenza due to unidentified influenza virus with unspecified type of pneumonia** 🔖
Influenza with pneumonia NOS

J11.08   **Influenza due to unidentified influenza virus with specified pneumonia** 🔖

Code also other specified type of pneumonia

◄ New   ◄▦ Revised   ~~deleted~~ Deleted   Excludes 1   Excludes 2   Includes   Use additional   Code first   Code also   Unspecified
OGCR Official Guidelines   ● Unacceptable Principal Diagnosis   X Assign placeholder X   ▶ Use Additional Character(s)   ▌ Manifestation Code   **Coding Clinic**

J11.1 Influenza due to unidentified influenza virus with other respiratory manifestations
Influenza NOS
Influenzal laryngitis NOS
Influenzal pharyngitis NOS
Influenza with upper respiratory symptoms NOS

> Use additional code for associated pleural effusion, if applicable (J91.8)

> Use additional code for associated sinusitis, if applicable (J01.-)

J11.2 Influenza due to unidentified influenza virus with gastrointestinal manifestations
Influenza gastroenteritis NOS

> **Excludes1** 'intestinal flu' [viral gastroenteritis] (A08.-)

● **J11.8 Influenza due to unidentified influenza virus with other manifestations**

J11.81 Influenza due to unidentified influenza virus with encephalopathy
Influenzal encephalopathy NOS

J11.82 Influenza due to unidentified influenza virus with myocarditis
Influenzal myocarditis NOS

J11.83 Influenza due to unidentified influenza virus with otitis media
Influenzal otitis media NOS

> Use additional code for any associated perforated tympanic membrane (H72.-)

J11.89 Influenza due to unidentified influenza virus with other manifestations

> Use additional codes to identify the manifestations

● **J12 Viral pneumonia, not elsewhere classified**

> **Includes** bronchopneumonia due to viruses other than influenza viruses

Code first associated influenza, if applicable (J09.X1, J10.0-, J11.0-)

Code also associated abscess, if applicable (J85.1)

> **Excludes1** aspiration pneumonia due to anesthesia during labor and delivery (O74.0)
> aspiration pneumonia due to anesthesia during pregnancy (O29)
> aspiration pneumonia due to anesthesia during puerperium (O89.0)
> aspiration pneumonia due to solids and liquids (J69.-)
> aspiration pneumonia NOS (J69.0)
> congenital pneumonia (P23.0)
> congenital rubella pneumonitis (P35.0)
> interstitial pneumonia NOS (J84.9)
> lipid pneumonia (J69.1)
> neonatal aspiration pneumonia (P24.-)

(Ex) **For category J12 CC codes unless otherwise indicated:** A15.0-A15.6, A15.8-A15.9, A17.9, A18.82, A18.84, A18.89, A20.2, A21.1, A22.1, A31.0, A37.01, A37.11, A37.81, A37.91, A42.0, A43.0, A48.1, B25.0, B39.0-B39.2, B44.0, B58.3, B59, B67.1, J09.X1-J09.X2, J10.00-J10.1, J11.00-J11.1, J12.0-J12.3, J12.81-J18.1, J18.8-J18.9, J22, J60-J70.4, J70.8-J70.9, J98.4, J98.8-J99, R91.1

J12.0 Adenoviral pneumonia 🗞

J12.1 Respiratory syncytial virus pneumonia 🗞

J12.2 Parainfluenza virus pneumonia 🗞

J12.3 Human metapneumovirus pneumonia 🗞

● **J12.8 Other viral pneumonia**

J12.81 Pneumonia due to SARS-associated coronavirus 🗞
Severe acute respiratory syndrome NOS

(Ex) A15.0-A15.6, A15.8-A15.9, A17.9, A18.82, A18.84, A18.89, A21.2, A22.1, A31.0, A37.01, A37.11, A37.81, A37.91, A42.0, A43.0, A48.1, B25.0, B39.0-B39.2, B44.0, B58.3, B59, B67.1, J09.X1-J09.X2, J10.00-J10.1, J11.00-J11.1, J12.0-J12.3, J12.81-J18.1, J18.8-J18.9, J22, J44.9, J47.0-J70.4, J70.8-J70.9, J98.4, J98.8-J99, Q33.4, R91.1

J12.89 Other viral pneumonia

J12.9 Viral pneumonia, unspecified 🗞

Item 10–3 Pneumonia is an infection of the lungs, caused by a variety of microorganisms, including viruses, most commonly the Streptococcus pneumoniae (pneumococcus) bacteria, fungi, and parasites. Pneumonia occurs when the immune system is weakened, often by a URI or influenza.

J13 Pneumonia due to Streptococcus pneumoniae 🗞
Bronchopneumonia due to S. pneumoniae

Code first associated influenza, if applicable (J09.X1, J10.0-, J11.0-) ◄▥

Code also associated abscess, if applicable (J85.1)

> **Excludes1** congenital pneumonia due to S. pneumoniae (P23.6)
> lobar pneumonia, unspecified organism (J18.1)
> pneumonia due to other streptococci (J15.3-J15.4)

(Ex) See J09.X1

J14 Pneumonia due to Hemophilus influenzae 🗞
Bronchopneumonia due to H. influenzae

Code first associated influenza, if applicable (J09.X1, J10.0-, J11.0-) ◄▥

Code also associated abscess, if applicable (J85.1)

> **Excludes1** congenital pneumonia due to H. influenzae (P23.6)

(Ex) See J09.X1

● **J15 Bacterial pneumonia, not elsewhere classified**

> **Includes** bronchopneumonia due to bacteria other than S. pneumoniae and H. influenzae

Code first associated influenza, if applicable (J09.X1, J10.0-, J11.0-) ◄▥

Code also associated abscess, if applicable (J85.1)

> **Excludes1** chlamydial pneumonia (J16.0)
> congenital pneumonia (P23.-)
> Legionnaires' disease (A48.1)
> spirochetal pneumonia (A69.8)

(Ex) **For category J15 CC codes: See** J09.X1

J15.0 Pneumonia due to Klebsiella pneumoniae 🗞

J15.1 Pneumonia due to Pseudomonas 🗞

● **J15.2 Pneumonia due to staphylococcus**

J15.20 Pneumonia due to staphylococcus, unspecified 🗞

● **J15.21 Pneumonia due to staphylococcus aureus**

J15.211 Pneumonia due to Methicillin susceptible Staphylococcus aureus 🗞
MSSA pneumonia
Pneumonia due to Staphylococcus aureus NOS

J15.212 Pneumonia due to Methicillin resistant Staphylococcus aureus 🗞

J15.29 Pneumonia due to other staphylococcus 🗞

J15.3 Pneumonia due to streptococcus, group B 🗞

J15.4 Pneumonia due to other streptococci 🗞

> **Excludes1** pneumonia due to streptococcus, group B (J15.3)
> pneumonia due to Streptococcus pneumoniae (J13)

J15.5 Pneumonia due to Escherichia coli 🗞

J15.6 Pneumonia due to other aerobic Gram-negative bacteria 🗞
Pneumonia due to Serratia marcescens

J15.7 Pneumonia due to Mycoplasma pneumoniae 🗞

J15.8 Pneumonia due to other specified bacteria 🗞

J15.9 Unspecified bacterial pneumonia 🗞
Pneumonia due to gram-positive bacteria

CHAPTER 10 (J00-J99)

N Newborn Age: 0   P Pediatric Age: 0–17   M Maternity DX: 12–55   A Adult Age: 15–124   ♀ Females Only   ♂ Males Only
🗞 Complication\Comorbidity   🗞 Major C\C   (Ex) CC/MCC Exclusions   🗞 Present on Admission Requirement   🗞 Hospital-Acquired Condition
1007

J16   Pneumonia due to other infectious organisms, not elsewhere classified

Code first associated influenza, if applicable (J09.X1, J10.0-, J11.0-) ◄▥

Code also associated abscess, if applicable (J85.1)

> **Excludes1**   congenital pneumonia (P23.-)
> ornithosis (A70)
> pneumocystosis (B59)
> pneumonia NOS (J18.9)

(Ex) For category J16 CC codes: See J09.X1

J16.0   Chlamydial pneumonia 🐾

J16.8   Pneumonia due to other specified infectious organisms 🐾

J17   Pneumonia in diseases classified elsewhere 🐾

Code first underlying disease, such as:
> Q fever (A78)
> rheumatic fever (I00)
> schistosomiasis (B65.0-B65.9)

> **Excludes1**   candidial pneumonia (B37.1)
> chlamydial pneumonia (J16.0)
> gonorrheal pneumonia (A54.84)
> histoplasmosis pneumonia (B39.0-B39.2)
> measles pneumonia (B05.2)
> nocardiosis pneumonia (A43.0)
> pneumocystosis (B59)
> pneumonia due to Pneumocystis carinii (B59)
> pneumonia due to Pneumocystis jiroveci (B59)
> pneumonia in actinomycosis (A42.0)
> pneumonia in anthrax (A22.1)
> pneumonia in ascariasis (B77.81)
> pneumonia in aspergillosis (B44.0-B44.1)
> pneumonia in coccidioidomycosis (B38.0-B38.2)
> pneumonia in cytomegalovirus disease (B25.0)
> pneumonia in toxoplasmosis (B58.3)
> rubella pneumonia (B06.81)
> salmonella pneumonia (A02.22)
> spirochetal infection NEC with pneumonia (A69.8)
> tularemia pneumonia (A21.2)
> typhoid fever with pneumonia (A01.03)
> varicella pneumonia (B01.2)
> whooping cough with pneumonia (A37 with fifth-character 1)

(Ex) See J09.X1

J18   Pneumonia, unspecified organism

Code first associated influenza, if applicable (J09.X1, J10.0-, J11.0-) ◄▥

> **Excludes1**   abscess of lung with pneumonia (J85.1)
> aspiration pneumonia due to anesthesia during labor and delivery (O74.0)
> aspiration pneumonia due to anesthesia during pregnancy (O29)
> aspiration pneumonia due to anesthesia during puerperium (O89.0)
> aspiration pneumonia due to solids and liquids (J69.-)
> aspiration pneumonia NOS (J69.0)
> congenital pneumonia (P23.0)
> drug-induced interstitial lung disorder (J70.2-J70.4)
> interstitial pneumonia NOS (J84.9)
> lipid pneumonia (J69.1)
> neonatal aspiration pneumonia (P24.-)
> pneumonitis due to external agents (J67-J70)
> pneumonitis due to fumes and vapors (J68.0)
> usual interstitial pneumonia (J84.17)

(Ex) For category J18 CC code unless otherwise indicated: See J09.X1

J18.0   Bronchopneumonia, unspecified organism 🐾

> **Excludes1**   hypostatic bronchopneumonia (J18.2)
> lipid pneumonia (J69.1)

> **Excludes2**   acute bronchiolitis (J21.-)
> chronic bronchiolitis (J44.9)

J18.1   Lobar pneumonia, unspecified organism 🐾

J18.2   Hypostatic pneumonia, unspecified organism 🐾
Hypostatic bronchopneumonia
Passive pneumonia
> (Ex) J18.2, J22, J81.1, J98.4, J98.8-J99, R91.1

J18.8   Other pneumonia, unspecified organism 🐾

J18.9   Pneumonia, unspecified organism 🐾
Coding Clinic: 2012, Q4, P94

OTHER ACUTE LOWER RESPIRATORY INFECTIONS (J20-J22)

> **Excludes2**   chronic obstructive pulmonary disease with acute lower respiratory infection (J44.0)

J20   Acute bronchitis
Inflammation/irritation of the bronchial tubes lasting 2-3 weeks, most commonly caused by a virus.

> **Includes**   acute and subacute bronchitis (with) bronchospasm
> acute and subacute bronchitis (with) tracheitis
> acute and subacute bronchitis (with) tracheobronchitis, acute
> acute and subacute fibrinous bronchitis
> acute and subacute membranous bronchitis
> acute and subacute purulent bronchitis
> acute and subacute septic bronchitis

> **Excludes1**   bronchitis NOS (J40) ◄
> tracheobronchitis NOS (J40) ◄

> **Excludes2**   acute bronchitis with bronchiectasis (J47.0)
> acute bronchitis with chronic obstructive asthma (J44.0)
> acute bronchitis with chronic obstructive pulmonary disease (J44.0)
> allergic bronchitis NOS (J45.909-)
> bronchitis due to chemicals, fumes and vapors (J68.0)
> ~~bronchitis NOS (J40)~~
> chronic bronchitis NOS (J42)
> chronic mucopurulent bronchitis (J41.1)
> chronic obstructive bronchitis (J44.-)
> chronic obstructive tracheobronchitis (J44.-)
> chronic simple bronchitis (J41.0)
> chronic tracheobronchitis (J42)
> ~~tracheobronchitis NOS (J40)~~

J20.0   Acute bronchitis due to Mycoplasma pneumoniae

J20.1   Acute bronchitis due to Hemophilus influenzae

J20.2   Acute bronchitis due to streptococcus

J20.3   Acute bronchitis due to coxsackievirus

J20.4   Acute bronchitis due to parainfluenza virus

J20.5   Acute bronchitis due to respiratory syncytial virus

J20.6   Acute bronchitis due to rhinovirus

J20.7   Acute bronchitis due to echovirus

J20.8   Acute bronchitis due to other specified organisms

J20.9   Acute bronchitis, unspecified

J21   Acute bronchiolitis
Bronchiolitis obliterans with organizing pneumonia (BOOP) inflammation of bronchioles and surrounding tissue in lung.

> **Includes**   acute bronchiolitis with bronchospasm
> **Excludes2**   respiratory bronchiolitis interstitial lung disease (J84.115)

(Ex) For category J21 CC codes unless otherwise indicated: J20.0-J21.9

J21.0   Acute bronchiolitis due to respiratory syncytial virus 🐾
(Ex) J21.0

J21.1   Acute bronchiolitis due to human metapneumovirus 🐾

J21.8   Acute bronchiolitis due to other specified organisms 🐾

J21.9   Acute bronchiolitis, unspecified 🐾
Bronchiolitis (acute)

> **Excludes1**   chronic bronchiolitis (J44.-)

J22   Unspecified acute lower respiratory infection
Acute (lower) respiratory (tract) infection NOS

> **Excludes1**   upper respiratory infection (acute) (J06.9)

◄ New   ◄▥ Revised   ~~deleted~~ Deleted   Excludes 1   Excludes 2   Includes   Use additional   Code first   Code also   Unspecified
OGCR Official Guidelines   ● Unacceptable Principal Diagnosis   X Assign placeholder X   ● Use Additional Character(s)   ▌ Manifestation Code   **Coding Clinic**

CHAPTER 10 (J00-J99)

OTHER DISEASES OF UPPER RESPIRATORY TRACT (J30-J39)

● **J30   Vasomotor and allergic rhinitis**

> **Includes** spasmodic rhinorrhea
> **Excludes1** allergic rhinitis with asthma (bronchial) (J45.909)
> rhinitis NOS (J31.0)

J30.0   Vasomotor rhinitis

J30.1   Allergic rhinitis due to pollen
> Allergy NOS due to pollen
> Hay fever
> Pollinosis

J30.2   Other seasonal allergic rhinitis

J30.5   Allergic rhinitis due to food

J30.8   Other allergic rhinitis
> **J30.81   Allergic rhinitis due to animal (cat) (dog) hair and dander**
> **J30.89   Other allergic rhinitis**
> > Perennial allergic rhinitis

J30.9   Allergic rhinitis, unspecified

● **J31   Chronic rhinitis, nasopharyngitis and pharyngitis**

> Use additional code to identify:
> exposure to environmental tobacco smoke (Z77.22)
> exposure to tobacco smoke in the perinatal period (P96.81)
> history of tobacco use (Z87.891)
> occupational exposure to environmental tobacco smoke (Z57.31)
> tobacco dependence (F17.-)
> tobacco use (Z72.0)

J31.0   Chronic rhinitis
> Atrophic rhinitis (chronic)
> Granulomatous rhinitis (chronic)
> Hypertrophic rhinitis (chronic)
> Obstructive rhinitis (chronic)
> Ozena
> Purulent rhinitis (chronic)
> Rhinitis (chronic) NOS
> Ulcerative rhinitis (chronic)
>
> > **Excludes1** allergic rhinitis (J30.1-J30.9)
> > vasomotor rhinitis (J30.0)

J31.1   Chronic nasopharyngitis
> **Excludes2** acute nasopharyngitis (J00)

J31.2   Chronic pharyngitis
> Chronic sore throat
> Atrophic pharyngitis (chronic)
> Granular pharyngitis (chronic)
> Hypertrophic pharyngitis (chronic)
>
> > **Excludes2** acute pharyngitis (J02.9)

● **J32   Chronic sinusitis**

> **Includes** sinus abscess
> sinus empyema
> sinus infection
> sinus suppuration
>
> Use additional code to identify:
> exposure to environmental tobacco smoke (Z77.22)
> exposure to tobacco smoke in the perinatal period (P96.81)
> history of tobacco use (Z87.891)
> infectious agent (B95-B97)
> occupational exposure to environmental tobacco smoke (Z57.31)
> tobacco dependence (F17.-)
> tobacco use (Z72.0)
>
> **Excludes2** acute sinusitis (J01.-)

J32.0   Chronic maxillary sinusitis
> Antritis (chronic)
> Maxillary sinusitis NOS

J32.1   Chronic frontal sinusitis
> Frontal sinusitis NOS

Item 10–4 Nasal polyps are an abnormal growth of tissue (tumor) projecting from a mucous membrane and attached to the surface by a narrow elongated stalk (pedunculated). Nasal polyps usually originate in the ethmoid sinus but also may occur in the maxillary sinus. Symptoms are nasal block, sinusitis, anosmia, and secondary infections.

J32.2   Chronic ethmoidal sinusitis
> Ethmoidal sinusitis NOS
>
> > **Excludes1** Woakes' ethmoiditis (J33.1)

J32.3   Chronic sphenoidal sinusitis
> Sphenoidal sinusitis NOS

J32.4   Chronic pansinusitis
> Pansinusitis NOS

J32.8   Other chronic sinusitis
> Sinusitis (chronic) involving more than one sinus but not pansinusitis

J32.9   Chronic sinusitis, unspecified
> Sinusitis (chronic) NOS

● **J33   Nasal polyp**

> Use additional code to identify:
> exposure to environmental tobacco smoke (Z77.22)
> exposure to tobacco smoke in the perinatal period (P96.81)
> history of tobacco use (Z87.891)
> occupational exposure to environmental tobacco smoke (Z57.31)
> tobacco dependence (F17.-)
> tobacco use (Z72.0)
>
> **Excludes1** adenomatous polyps (D14.0)

J33.0   Polyp of nasal cavity
> Choanal polyp
> Nasopharyngeal polyp

J33.1   Polypoid sinus degeneration
> Woakes' syndrome or ethmoiditis

J33.8   Other polyp of sinus
> Accessory polyp of sinus
> Ethmoidal polyp of sinus
> Maxillary polyp of sinus
> Sphenoidal polyp of sinus

J33.9   Nasal polyp, unspecified

● **J34   Other and unspecified disorders of nose and nasal sinuses**

> **Excludes2** varicose ulcer of nasal septum (I86.8)

J34.0   Abscess, furuncle and carbuncle of nose
> Cellulitis of nose
> Necrosis of nose
> Ulceration of nose

J34.1   Cyst and mucocele of nose and nasal sinus

J34.2   Deviated nasal septum
> Deflection or deviation of septum (nasal) (acquired)
>
> > **Excludes1** congenital deviated nasal septum (Q67.4)

J34.3   Hypertrophy of nasal turbinates

Deviated septal cartilage

Figure 10-3 Deviated nasal septum.

Item 10–5 A **deviated nasal septum** is the displacement of the septal cartilage that separates the nares. This displacement causes obstructed air flow through the nasal passages. A child can be born with this displacement (congenital), or the condition may be acquired through trauma, such as a sports injury. Symptoms include nasal block, sinusitis, and related secondary infections. Septoplasty is surgical repair of this condition.

CHAPTER 10 (J00-J99)

● **J34.8**   **Other specified disorders of nose and nasal sinuses**

     J34.81   **Nasal mucositis (ulcerative)**

         Code also type of associated therapy, such as:
           antineoplastic and immunosuppressive
           drugs (T45.1X-) ◀▦
           radiological procedure and radiotherapy
           (Y84.2)

         Excludes2   gastrointestinal mucositis
           (ulcerative) (K92.81)
           mucositis (ulcerative) of vagina
           and vulva (N76.81)
           oral mucositis (ulcerative)
           (K12.3-)

     J34.89   **Other specified disorders of nose and nasal sinuses**
         Perforation of nasal septum NOS
         Rhinolith

J34.9   **Unspecified disorder of nose and nasal sinuses**

● **J35**   **Chronic diseases of tonsils and adenoids**

     Use additional code to identify:
       exposure to environmental tobacco smoke (Z77.22)
       exposure to tobacco smoke in the perinatal period (P96.81)
       history of tobacco use (Z87.891)
       occupational exposure to environmental tobacco smoke
         (Z57.31)
       tobacco dependence (F17.-)
       tobacco use (Z72.0)

● **J35.0**   **Chronic tonsillitis and adenoiditis**

     Excludes2   acute tonsillitis (J03.-)

     J35.01   **Chronic tonsillitis**

     J35.02   **Chronic adenoiditis**

     J35.03   **Chronic tonsillitis and adenoiditis**

J35.1   **Hypertrophy of tonsils**
     Enlargement of tonsils

     Excludes1   hypertrophy of tonsils with tonsillitis
         (J35.0-)

J35.2   **Hypertrophy of adenoids**
     Enlargement of adenoids

     Excludes1   hypertrophy of adenoids with adenoiditis
         (J35.0-)

J35.3   **Hypertrophy of tonsils with hypertrophy of adenoids**

     Excludes1   hypertrophy of tonsils and adenoids with
         tonsillitis and adenoiditis (J35.03)

J35.8   **Other chronic diseases of tonsils and adenoids**
     Adenoid vegetations
     Amygdalolith
     Calculus, tonsil
     Cicatrix of tonsil (and adenoid)
     Tonsillar tag
     Ulcer of tonsil

J35.9   **Chronic disease of tonsils and adenoids, unspecified**
     Disease (chronic) of tonsils and adenoids NOS

J36   **Peritonsillar abscess** ⊛

     Includes   abscess of tonsil
          peritonsillar cellulitis
          quinsy

     Use additional code (B95-B97) to identify infectious agent.

     Excludes1   acute tonsillitis (J03.-)
         chronic tonsillitis (J35.0)
         retropharyngeal abscess (J39.0)
         tonsillitis NOS (J03.9-)

     (Ex) J22, J36, J98.8-J98.9

● **J37**   **Chronic laryngitis and laryngotracheitis**

     Use additional code to identify:
       exposure to environmental tobacco smoke (Z77.22)
       exposure to tobacco smoke in the perinatal period (P96.81)
       history of tobacco use (Z87.891)
       infectious agent (B95-B97)
       occupational exposure to environmental tobacco smoke
         (Z57.31)
       tobacco dependence (F17.-)
       tobacco use (Z72.0)

J37.0   **Chronic laryngitis**
     Catarrhal laryngitis
     Hypertrophic laryngitis
     Sicca laryngitis

     Excludes2   acute laryngitis (J04.0)
         obstructive (acute) laryngitis (J05.0)

J37.1   **Chronic laryngotracheitis**
     Laryngitis, chronic, with tracheitis (chronic)
     Tracheitis, chronic, with laryngitis

     Excludes1   chronic tracheitis (J42)

     Excludes2   acute laryngotracheitis (J04.2)
         acute tracheitis (J04.1)

● **J38**   **Diseases of vocal cords and larynx, not elsewhere classified**

     Use additional code to identify:
       exposure to environmental tobacco smoke (Z77.22)
       exposure to tobacco smoke in the perinatal period (P96.81)
       history of tobacco use (Z87.891)
       occupational exposure to environmental tobacco smoke
         (Z57.31)
       tobacco dependence (F17.-)
       tobacco use (Z72.0)

     Excludes1   congenital laryngeal stridor (P28.89)
         obstructive laryngitis (acute) (J05.0)
         postprocedural subglottic stenosis (J95.5)
         stridor (R06.1)
         ulcerative laryngitis (J04.0)

● **J38.0**   **Paralysis of vocal cords and larynx**
     Laryngoplegia
     Paralysis of glottis

     J38.00   **Paralysis of vocal cords and larynx, unspecified**

     J38.01   **Paralysis of vocal cords and larynx, unilateral**

     J38.02   **Paralysis of vocal cords and larynx, bilateral**

J38.1   **Polyp of vocal cord and larynx**

     Excludes1   adenomatous polyps (D14.1)

J38.2   **Nodules of vocal cords**
     Chorditis (fibrinous)(nodosa)(tuberosa)
     Singer's nodes
     Teacher's nodes

Figure 10-4   Coronal section of the larynx.

Item 10–6 The **larynx** extends from the tongue to the trachea and is divided into an upper and lower portion separated by folds. The framework of the larynx is cartilage composed of the single cricoid, thyroid, and epiglottic cartilages, and the paired arytenoid, cuneiform, and corniculate cartilages.

◀ New   ◀▦ Revised   ~~deleted~~ Deleted   Excludes 1   Excludes 2   Includes   Use additional   Code first   Code also   Unspecified

OGCR Official Guidelines   ● Unacceptable Principal Diagnosis   X Assign placeholder X   ⊛ Use Additional Character(s)   ▌ Manifestation Code   **Coding Clinic**

J38.3   **Other diseases of vocal cords**
Abscess of vocal cords
Cellulitis of vocal cords
Granuloma of vocal cords
Leukokeratosis of vocal cords
Leukoplakia of vocal cords

J38.4   **Edema of larynx**
Edema (of) glottis
Subglottic edema
Supraglottic edema

> **Excludes1**   acute obstructive laryngitis [croup] (J05.0)
> edematous laryngitis (J04.0)

J38.5   **Laryngeal spasm**
Laryngismus (stridulus)

J38.6   **Stenosis of larynx**

J38.7   **Other diseases of larynx**
Abscess of larynx
Cellulitis of larynx
Disease of larynx NOS
Necrosis of larynx
Pachyderma of larynx
Perichondritis of larynx
Ulcer of larynx

● **J39**   **Other diseases of upper respiratory tract**

> **Excludes1**   acute respiratory infection NOS (J22)
> acute upper respiratory infection (J06.9)
> upper respiratory inflammation due to chemicals, gases, fumes or vapors (J68.2)

J39.0   **Retropharyngeal and parapharyngeal abscess** 🔖
Peripharyngeal abscess

> **Excludes1**   peritonsillar abscess (J36)
> (Ex) J22, J39.0-J39.1, J98.8-J98.9

J39.1   **Other abscess of pharynx** 🔖
Cellulitis of pharynx
Nasopharyngeal abscess
(Ex) J22, J39.0-J39.1, J98.8-J98.9

J39.2   **Other diseases of pharynx**
Cyst of pharynx
Edema of pharynx

> **Excludes2**   chronic pharyngitis (J31.2)
> ulcerative pharyngitis (J02.9)

J39.3   **Upper respiratory tract hypersensitivity reaction, site unspecified**

> **Excludes1**   hypersensitivity reaction of upper respiratory tract, such as:
> extrinsic allergic alveolitis (J67.9)
> pneumoconiosis (J60-J67.9)

J39.8   **Other specified diseases of upper respiratory tract**

J39.9   **Disease of upper respiratory tract, unspecified**

Item 10-8   **Chronic bronchitis** is usually defined as being present in any patient who has persistent cough with sputum production for at least three months in at least two consecutive years. **Simple chronic bronchitis** is marked by a productive cough but no pathological airflow obstruction. **Chronic obstructive pulmonary disease (COPD)** is a group of conditions—bronchitis, emphysema, asthma, bronchiectasis, allergic alveolitis—marked by dyspnea. **Catarrhal** bronchitis is an acute form of bronchitis marked by profuse mucus and pus production (**mucopurulent** discharge). **Croupous** bronchitis, also known as pseudomembranous, fibrinous, plastic, exudative, or membranous, is marked by a violent cough and dyspnea.

CHRONIC LOWER RESPIRATORY DISEASES (J40-J47)

> **Excludes1**   bronchitis due to chemicals, gases, fumes and vapors (J68.0)
>
> **Excludes2**   cystic fibrosis (E84.-)

J40   **Bronchitis, not specified as acute or chronic**
Bronchitis NOS
Catarrhal bronchitis
Bronchitis with tracheitis NOS
Tracheobronchitis NOS

Use additional code to identify:
exposure to environmental tobacco smoke (Z77.22)
exposure to tobacco smoke in the perinatal period (P96.81)
history of tobacco use (Z87.891)
occupational exposure to environmental tobacco smoke (Z57.31)
tobacco dependence (F17.-)
tobacco use (Z72.0)

> **Excludes1**   acute bronchitis (J20.-) ◄
> allergic bronchitis NOS (J45.909-)
> asthmatic bronchitis NOS (J45.9-)
> bronchitis due to chemicals, gases, fumes and vapors (J68.0)

● **J41**   **Simple and mucopurulent chronic bronchitis**
Use additional code to identify:
exposure to environmental tobacco smoke (Z77.22)
exposure to tobacco smoke in the perinatal period (P96.81)
history of tobacco use (Z87.891)
occupational exposure to environmental tobacco smoke (Z57.31)
tobacco dependence (F17.-)
tobacco use (Z72.0)

> **Excludes1**   chronic bronchitis NOS (J42)
> chronic obstructive bronchitis (J44.-)

J41.0   **Simple chronic bronchitis**

J41.1   **Mucopurulent chronic bronchitis**

J41.8   **Mixed simple and mucopurulent chronic bronchitis**

J42   **Unspecified chronic bronchitis**
Chronic bronchitis NOS
Chronic tracheitis
Chronic tracheobronchitis

Use additional code to identify:
exposure to environmental tobacco smoke (Z77.22)
exposure to tobacco smoke in the perinatal period (P96.81)
history of tobacco use (Z87.891)
occupational exposure to environmental tobacco smoke (Z57.31)
tobacco dependence (F17.-)
tobacco use (Z72.0)

> **Excludes1**   chronic asthmatic bronchitis (J44.-)
> chronic bronchitis with airways obstruction (J44.-)
> chronic emphysematous bronchitis (J44.-)
> chronic obstructive pulmonary disease NOS (J44.9)
> simple and mucopurulent chronic bronchitis (J41.-)

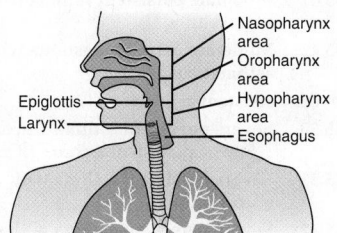

Figure 10-5   The pharynx.

Item 10-7   The **pharynx** is the passage for both food and air between the mouth and the esophagus and is divided into three areas: nasopharynx, oropharynx, and hypopharynx. The hypopharynx branches into the esophagus and the voice box.

N Newborn Age: 0   **P** Pediatric Age: 0–17   **M** Maternity DX: 12–55   **A** Adult Age: 15–124   ♀ Females Only   ♂ Males Only

🔖 Complication\Comorbidity   🔖 Major C\C   (Ex) CC/MCC Exclusions   🔖 Present on Admission Requirement   🔖 Hospital-Acquired Condition

1011

● J43   Emphysema

Use additional code to identify:
exposure to environmental tobacco smoke (Z77.22)
history of tobacco use (Z87.891)
occupational exposure to environmental tobacco smoke
(Z57.31)
tobacco dependence (F17.-)
tobacco use (Z72.0)

> **Excludes1**   compensatory emphysema (J98.3)
> emphysema due to inhalation of chemicals, gases,
> fumes or vapors (J68.4)
> emphysema with chronic (obstructive) bronchitis
> (J44.-)
> emphysematous (obstructive) bronchitis (J44.-)
> interstitial emphysema (J98.2)
> mediastinal emphysema (J98.2)
> neonatal interstitial emphysema (P25.0)
> surgical (subcutaneous) emphysema (T81.82)
> traumatic subcutaneous emphysema (T79.7)

J43.0   Unilateral pulmonary emphysema [MacLeod's syndrome]
Swyer-James syndrome
Unilateral emphysema
Unilateral hyperlucent lung
Unilateral pulmonary artery functional hypoplasia
Unilateral transparency of lung

J43.1   Panlobular emphysema
Panacinar emphysema

J43.2   Centrilobular emphysema

J43.8   Other emphysema

J43.9   Emphysema, unspecified
Bullous emphysema (lung)(pulmonary)
Emphysema (lung)(pulmonary) NOS
Emphysematous bleb
Vesicular emphysema (lung)(pulmonary)

● J44   Other chronic obstructive pulmonary disease

> **Includes**   asthma with chronic obstructive pulmonary
> disease
> chronic asthmatic (obstructive) bronchitis
> chronic bronchitis with airways obstruction
> chronic bronchitis with emphysema
> chronic emphysematous bronchitis
> chronic obstructive asthma
> chronic obstructive bronchitis
> chronic obstructive tracheobronchitis

Code also type of asthma, if applicable (J45.-): ◀▥
Use additional code to identify:
exposure to environmental tobacco smoke (Z77.22)
history of tobacco use (Z87.891)
occupational exposure to environmental tobacco smoke
(Z57.31)
tobacco dependence (F17.-)
tobacco use (Z72.0)

> **Excludes1**   bronchiectasis (J47.-)
> chronic bronchitis NOS (J42)
> chronic simple and mucopurulent bronchitis (J41.-)
> chronic tracheitis (J42)
> chronic tracheobronchitis (J42)
> emphysema without chronic bronchitis (J43.-)
> lung diseases due to external agents (J60-J70)

J44.0   Chronic obstructive pulmonary disease with acute lower respiratory infection ✥
Use additional code to identify the infection
Ⓔⓧ J10.08, J41.1-J42, J44.0-J44.1

J44.1   Chronic obstructive pulmonary disease with (acute) exacerbation ✥
Decompensated COPD
Decompensated COPD with (acute) exacerbation

> **Excludes2**   chronic obstructive pulmonary disease
> [COPD] with acute bronchitis (J44.0)
> Ⓔⓧ J10.08, J41.1-J42, J44.0-J44.1

J44.9   Chronic obstructive pulmonary disease, unspecified
Chronic obstructive airway disease NOS
Chronic obstructive lung disease NOS

Item 10–9   Asthma is a bronchial condition marked by airway obstruction, hyper-responsiveness, and inflammation. **Extrinsic** asthma, also known as allergic asthma, is characterized by the same symptoms that occur with exposure to allergens and is divided into the following types: **atopic, occupational, and allergic bronchopulmonary aspergillosis. Intrinsic** asthma occurs in patients who have no history of allergy or sensitivities to allergens and is divided into the following types: **nonreaginic and pharmacologic. Status asthmaticus** is the most severe form of asthma attack and can last for days or weeks.

● J45   Asthma
Allergic (predominantly) asthma
Allergic bronchitis NOS
Allergic rhinitis with asthma
Atopic asthma
Extrinsic allergic asthma
Hay fever with asthma
Idiosyncratic asthma
Intrinsic nonallergic asthma
Nonallergic asthma

Use additional code to identify:
exposure to environmental tobacco smoke (Z77.22)
exposure to tobacco smoke in the perinatal period (P96.81)
history of tobacco use (Z87.891)
occupational exposure to environmental tobacco smoke
(Z57.31)
tobacco dependence (F17.-)
tobacco use (Z72.0)

> **Excludes1**   detergent asthma (J69.8)
> eosinophilic asthma (J82)
> lung diseases due to external agents (J60-J70)
> miner's asthma (J60)
> wheezing NOS (R06.2)
> wood asthma (J67.8)

> **Excludes2**   asthma with chronic obstructive pulmonary
> disease (J44.9)
> chronic asthmatic (obstructive) bronchitis (J44.9)
> chronic obstructive asthma (J44.9)

Ⓔⓧ For category J45 CC codes: J10.08, J22, J45.20-J45.998, J98.4, J98.8-J99, R91.1

● J45.2   Mild intermittent asthma

J45.20   Mild intermittent asthma, uncomplicated
Mild intermittent asthma NOS

J45.21   Mild intermittent asthma with (acute) exacerbation ✥

J45.22   Mild intermittent asthma with status asthmaticus ✥

● J45.3   Mild persistent asthma

J45.30   Mild persistent asthma, uncomplicated
Mild persistent asthma NOS

J45.31   Mild persistent asthma with (acute) exacerbation ✥

J45.32   Mild persistent asthma with status asthmaticus ✥

● J45.4   Moderate persistent asthma

J45.40   Moderate persistent asthma, uncomplicated
Moderate persistent asthma NOS

J45.41   Moderate persistent asthma with (acute) exacerbation ✥

J45.42   Moderate persistent asthma with status asthmaticus ✥

● J45.5   Severe persistent asthma

J45.50   Severe persistent asthma, uncomplicated
Severe persistent asthma NOS

J45.51   Severe persistent asthma with (acute) exacerbation ✥

J45.52   Severe persistent asthma with status asthmaticus ✥

◀ New   ◀▥ Revised   ~~deleted~~ Deleted   Excludes 1   Excludes 2   Includes   Use additional   Code first   Code also   Unspecified

OGCR Official Guidelines   ● Unacceptable Principal Diagnosis   X Assign placeholder X   ✥ Use Additional Character(s)   ▶ Manifestation Code   **Coding Clinic**

- **J45.9   Other and unspecified asthma**
  - **J45.90   Unspecified asthma**
    Asthmatic bronchitis NOS
    Childhood asthma NOS
    Late onset asthma
    - J45.901   Unspecified asthma with (acute) exacerbation 🔗
    - J45.902   Unspecified asthma with status asthmaticus 🔗
    - J45.909   Unspecified asthma, uncomplicated
      Asthma NOS
  - **J45.99   Other asthma**
    - J45.990   **Exercise induced bronchospasm**
    - J45.991   **Cough variant asthma**
    - J45.998   **Other asthma**

- **J47   Bronchiectasis**
  - **Includes**   bronchiolectasis
  Use additional code to identify:
    exposure to environmental tobacco smoke (Z77.22)
    exposure to tobacco smoke in the perinatal period (P96.81)
    history of tobacco use (Z87.891)
    occupational exposure to environmental tobacco smoke (Z57.31)
    tobacco dependence (F17.-)
    tobacco use (Z72.0)
  - **Excludes1**   congenital bronchiectasis (Q33.4)
    tuberculous bronchiectasis (current disease) (A15.0)
  - (Ex) **For category J47 CC codes:** A17.9, A18.82, A18.84, A18.89, J09.X2, J10.01-J10.1, J11.1, J44.9, J47.0-J47.1, J68.1, J68.4-J68.9, Q33.4
  - **J47.0   Bronchiectasis with acute lower respiratory infection** 🔗
    Bronchiectasis with acute bronchitis
  - **J47.1   Bronchiectasis with (acute) exacerbation** 🔗
  - **J47.9   Bronchiectasis, uncomplicated**
    Bronchiectasis NOS

LUNG DISEASES DUE TO EXTERNAL AGENTS (J60-J70)

- **Excludes2**   asthma (J45.-)
  malignant neoplasm of bronchus and lung (C34.-)

- **J60   Coalworker's pneumoconiosis**   A
  Anthracosilicosis
  Anthracosis
  Black lung disease
  Coalworker's lung
  - **Excludes1**   coalworker pneumoconiosis with tuberculosis, any type in A15 (J65)

- **J61   Pneumoconiosis due to asbestos and other mineral fibers**   A
  Asbestosis
  - **Excludes1**   pleural plaque with asbestosis (J92.0)
    pneumoconiosis with tuberculosis, any type in A15 (J65)

- **J62   Pneumoconiosis due to dust containing silica**
  - **Includes**   silicotic fibrosis (massive) of lung
  - **Excludes1**   pneumoconiosis with tuberculosis, any type in A15 (J65)
  - **J62.0   Pneumoconiosis due to talc dust**
  - **J62.8   Pneumoconiosis due to other dust containing silica**
    Silicosis NOS

Figure 10-6   Progressive massive fibrosis superimposed on coal workers' pneumoconiosis. The large, blackened scars are located principally in the upper lobe. (From Cotran R, Kumar V, Collins T: Robbins Pathologic Basis of Disease, ed 8, Philadelphia, WB Saunders, 2009. Courtesy of Dr. Warner Laquer, Dr. Jerome Kleinerman, and the National Institute of Occupational Safety and Health, Morgantown, WV)

Item 10-10   **Pneumoconiosis** refers to a lung condition resulting from exposure to inorganic or organic airborne particles, such as coal dust or moldy hay, as well as chemical fumes and vapors, such as insecticides. In this condition, the lungs retain the airborne particles.

- **J63   Pneumoconiosis due to other inorganic dusts**
  - **Excludes1**   pneumoconiosis with tuberculosis, any type in A15 (J65)
  - **J63.0   Aluminosis (of lung)**
  - **J63.1   Bauxite fibrosis (of lung)**
  - **J63.2   Berylliosis**
  - **J63.3   Graphite fibrosis (of lung)**
  - **J63.4   Siderosis**
  - **J63.5   Stannosis**
  - **J63.6   Pneumoconiosis due to other specified inorganic dusts**

- **J64   Unspecified pneumoconiosis**
  - **Excludes1**   pneumonoconiosis with tuberculosis, any type in A15 (J65)

- **J65   Pneumoconiosis associated with tuberculosis**
  Any condition in J60-J64 with tuberculosis, any type in A15
  Silicotuberculosis

- **J66   Airway disease due to specific organic dust**
  - **Excludes2**   allergic alveolitis (J67.-)
    asbestosis (J61)
    bagassosis (J67.1)
    farmer's lung (J67.0)
    hypersensitivity pneumonitis due to organic dust (J67.-)
    reactive airways dysfunction syndrome (J68.3)
  - **J66.0   Byssinosis**
    Airway disease due to cotton dust
  - **J66.1   Flax-dressers' disease**
  - **J66.2   Cannabinosis**
  - **J66.8   Airway disease due to other specific organic dusts**

- **J67   Hypersensitivity pneumonitis due to organic dust**
  - **Includes**   allergic alveolitis and pneumonitis due to inhaled organic dust and particles of fungal, actinomycetic or other origin
  - **Excludes1**   pneumonitis due to inhalation of chemicals, gases, fumes or vapors (J68.0)
  - **J67.0   Farmer's lung**
    Harvester's lung
    Haymaker's lung
    Moldy hay disease
  - **J67.1   Bagassosis**
    Bagasse disease
    Bagasse pneumonitis
  - **J67.2   Bird fancier's lung**
    Budgerigar fancier's disease or lung
    Pigeon fancier's disease or lung

CHAPTER 10 (J00-J99)

N   Newborn Age: 0   P   Pediatric Age: 0–17   M   Maternity DX: 12–55   A   Adult Age: 15–124   ♀   Females Only   ♂   Males Only

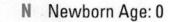   Complication\Comorbidity   🔗   Major C\C   (Ex)   CC/MCC Exclusions   🔗   Present on Admission Requirement   🔗   Hospital-Acquired Condition

1013

CHAPTER 10 (J00-J99)

J67.3   **Suberosis**
Corkhandler's disease or lung
Corkworker's disease or lung

J67.4   **Maltworker's lung**
Alveolitis due to Aspergillus clavatus

J67.5   **Mushroom-worker's lung**

J67.6   **Maple-bark-stripper's lung**
Alveolitis due to Cryptostroma corticale
Cryptostromosis

J67.7   **Air conditioner and humidifier lung** 🔖
Allergic alveolitis due to fungal, thermophilic
actinomycetes and other organisms growing in
ventilation [air conditioning] systems
(Ex:) A15.0-A15.9, A17.9, A18.82, A18.84, A18.89, A21.2, A22.1, A31.0, A37.01,
A37.11, A37.81, A37.91, A42.0, A43.0, A48.1, B25.0, B39.0-B39.2, B44.0,
B58.3, B59, B67.1, J09.X1-J09.X2, J10.00-J10.1, J11.00-J11.1, J12.0-J12.3,
J12.89-J18.1, J18.8-J18.9, J22, J44.9, J47.0-J70.4, J70.8-J70.9, J98.4,
J98.8-J98.9, Q33.4, R91.1

J67.8   **Hypersensitivity pneumonitis due to other organic dusts** 🔖
Cheese-washer's lung
Coffee-worker's lung
Fish-meal worker's lung
Furrier's lung
Sequoiosis
(Ex:) See J67.7

J67.9   **Hypersensitivity pneumonitis due to unspecified organic dust** 🔖
Allergic alveolitis (extrinsic) NOS
Hypersensitivity pneumonitis NOS
(Ex:) See J67.7

● **J68**   **Respiratory conditions due to inhalation of chemicals, gases, fumes and vapors**
Code first (T51-T65) to identify cause
Use additional code to identify associated respiratory
conditions, such as:
acute respiratory failure (J96.0-)

J68.0   **Bronchitis and pneumonitis due to chemicals, gases, fumes and vapors** 🔖
Chemical bronchitis (acute)
(Ex:) See J67.7

J68.1   **Pulmonary edema due to chemicals, gases, fumes and vapors** 🔖
Chemical pulmonary edema (acute) (chronic)
  Excludes1   pulmonary edema (acute) (chronic) NOS
(J81.-)
(Ex:) See J67.7

J68.2   **Upper respiratory inflammation due to chemicals, gases, fumes and vapors, not elsewhere classified**

J68.3   **Other acute and subacute respiratory conditions due to chemicals, gases, fumes and vapors**
Reactive airways dysfunction syndrome

J68.4   **Chronic respiratory conditions due to chemicals, gases, fumes and vapors**
Emphysema (diffuse) (chronic) due to inhalation of
chemicals, gases, fumes and vapors
Obliterative bronchiolitis (chronic) (subacute) due to
inhalation of chemicals, gases, fumes and vapors
Pulmonary fibrosis (chronic) due to inhalation of
chemicals, gases, fumes and vapors
  Excludes1   chronic pulmonary edema due to
chemicals, gases, fumes and vapors
(J68.1)

J68.8   **Other respiratory conditions due to chemicals, gases, fumes and vapors**

J68.9   **Unspecified respiratory condition due to chemicals, gases, fumes and vapors**

● **J69**   **Pneumonitis due to solids and liquids**
  Excludes1   neonatal aspiration syndromes (P24.-)
postprocedural pneumonitis (J95.4)
(Ex:) For category J69 CC codes: See J67.7

J69.0   **Pneumonitis due to inhalation of food and vomit** 🔖
Aspiration pneumonia NOS
Aspiration pneumonia (due to) food (regurgitated)
Aspiration pneumonia (due to) gastric secretions
Aspiration pneumonia (due to) milk
Aspiration pneumonia (due to) vomit
Code also any associated foreign body in respiratory
tract (T17.-)
  Excludes1   chemical pneumonitis due to anesthesia
(J95.4)
obstetric aspiration pneumonia (O74.0)

J69.1   **Pneumonitis due to inhalation of oils and essences** 🔖
Exogenous lipoid pneumonia
Lipid pneumonia NOS
Code first (T51-T65) to identify substance
  Excludes1   endogenous lipoid pneumonia (J84.89)

J69.8   **Pneumonitis due to inhalation of other solids and liquids** 🔖
Pneumonitis due to aspiration of blood
Pneumonitis due to aspiration of detergent
Code first (T51-T65) to identify substance

● **J70**   **Respiratory conditions due to other external agents**

J70.0   **Acute pulmonary manifestations due to radiation** 🔖
Radiation pneumonitis
Use additional code (W88-W90, X39.0-) to identify the
external cause
(Ex:) See J67.7

J70.1   **Chronic and other pulmonary manifestations due to radiation** 🔖
Fibrosis of lung following radiation
Use additional code (W88-W90, X39.0-) to identify the
external cause
(Ex:) See J67.7

J70.2   **Acute drug-induced interstitial lung disorders**
Use additional code for adverse effect, if applicable,
to identify drug (T36-T50 with fifth or sixth
character 5)
  Excludes1   interstitial pneumonia NOS (J84.9)
lymphoid interstitial pneumonia (J84.2)

J70.3   **Chronic drug-induced interstitial lung disorders**
Use additional code for adverse effect, if applicable,
to identify drug (T36-T50 with fifth or sixth
character 5)
  Excludes1   interstitial pneumonia NOS (J84.9)
lymphoid interstitial pneumonia (J84.2)

J70.4   **Drug-induced interstitial lung disorders, unspecified**
Use additional code for adverse effect, if applicable,
to identify drug (T36-T50 with fifth or sixth
character 5)
  Excludes1   interstitial pneumonia NOS (J84.9)
lymphoid interstitial pneumonia (J84.2)

J70.5   **Respiratory conditions due to smoke inhalation**
Smoke inhalation NOS
  Excludes1   smoke inhalation due to chemicals, gases,
fumes and vapors (J68.9)

J70.8   **Respiratory conditions due to other specified external agents**
Code first (T51-T65) to identify the external agent

J70.9   **Respiratory conditions due to unspecified external agent**
Code first (T51-T65) to identify the external agent

◀ New   ◀ Revised   ~~deleted~~ Deleted   Excludes 1   Excludes 2   Includes   Use additional   Code first   Code also   Unspecified
OGCR Official Guidelines   ● Unacceptable Principal Diagnosis   X Assign placeholder X   ● Use Additional Character(s)   ▌ Manifestation Code   **Coding Clinic**

OTHER RESPIRATORY DISEASES PRINCIPALLY AFFECTING THE INTERSTITIUM (J80-J84)

J80   **Acute respiratory distress syndrome**
Acute respiratory distress syndrome in adult or child
Adult hyaline membrane disease

> **Excludes1**   respiratory distress syndrome in newborn (perinatal) (P22.0)

Ex: J22, J80, J96.00-J96.92, J98.8-J98.9, R09.2

● **J81**   **Pulmonary edema**
Use additional code to identify:
exposure to environmental tobacco smoke (Z77.22)
history of tobacco use (Z87.891)
occupational exposure to environmental tobacco smoke (Z57.31)
tobacco dependence (F17.-)
tobacco use (Z72.0)

> **Excludes1**   chemical (acute) pulmonary edema (J68.1)
> hypostatic pneumonia (J18.2)
> passive pneumonia (J18.2)
> pulmonary edema due to external agents (J60-J70)
> pulmonary edema with heart disease NOS (I50.1)
> pulmonary edema with heart failure (I50.1)

J81.0   **Acute pulmonary edema**
Acute edema of lung
Ex: I09.81, I50.1-I50.9, J22, J81.0, J98.8-J98.9

J81.1   **Chronic pulmonary edema**
Pulmonary congestion (chronic) (passive)
Pulmonary edema NOS
Ex: J18.2, J22, J81.1, J98.4, J98.8-J99, R91.1

J82   **Pulmonary eosinophilia, not elsewhere classified**
Allergic pneumonia
Eosinophilic asthma
Eosinophilic pneumonia
Löffler's pneumonia
Tropical (pulmonary) eosinophilia NOS

> **Excludes1**   pulmonary eosinophilia due to aspergillosis (B44.-)
> pulmonary eosinophilia due to drugs (J70.2-J70.4)
> pulmonary eosinophilia due to specified parasitic infection (B50-B83)
> pulmonary eosinophilia due to systemic connective tissue disorders (M30-M36)
> pulmonary infiltrate NOS (R91.8)

Ex: A15.0-A15.6, A15.8-A15.9, A17.9, A18.82, A18.84, A18.89, A20.2, A21.1, A22.1, A31.0, A37.01, A37.11, A37.81, A37.91, A42.0, A43.0, A48.1, B25.0, B39.0-B39.2, B44.0, B58.3, B59, B67.1, J09.X1-J09.X2, J10.00-J10.1, J11.00-J11.1, J12.0-J12.3, J12.89-J18.1, J18.8-J18.9, J22, J47.0-J70.4, J70.8-J70.9, J82, J98.4, J98.8-J99, Q33.4, R91.1

● **J84**   **Other interstitial pulmonary diseases**

> **Excludes1**   drug-induced interstitial lung disorders (J70.2-J70.4)
> interstitial emphysema (J98.2)
> lung diseases due to external agents (J60-J70)

Ex: **For category J84 CC codes unless otherwise indicated:** A15.0-A15.6, A15.8-A15.9, A17.9, A18.82, A18.84, A18.89, J22, J44.9, J47.0-J70.4, J70.8-J70.9, J84.01-J84.82, J84.89-J84.9, J98.4, J98.8-J99, Q33.4, R91.1

● **J84.0**   **Alveolar and parieto-alveolar conditions**

J84.01   **Alveolar proteinosis**

J84.02   **Pulmonary alveolar microlithiasis**

J84.03   *Idiopathic pulmonary hemosiderosis*
Essential brown induration of lung

> *Code first* underlying disease, such as:
> disorders of iron metabolism (E83.1-)

> **Excludes1**   acute idiopathic pulmonary hemorrhage in infants [AIPHI] (R04.81)

J84.09   **Other alveolar and parieto-alveolar conditions**

Figure 10-7   Bullous emphysema with large subpleural bullae *(upper left)*. (From Kumar: Robbins and Cotran: Pathologic Basis of Disease, ed 8, Saunders, An Imprint of Elsevier, 2009)

● **J84.1**   **Other interstitial pulmonary diseases with fibrosis**

> **Excludes1**   pulmonary fibrosis (chronic) due to inhalation of chemicals, gases, fumes or vapors (J68.4)
> pulmonary fibrosis (chronic) following radiation (J70.1)

J84.10   **Pulmonary fibrosis, unspecified**
Capillary fibrosis of lung
Cirrhosis of lung (chronic) NOS
Fibrosis of lung (atrophic) (chronic) (confluent) (massive) (perialveolar) (peribronchial) NOS
Induration of lung (chronic) NOS
Postinflammatory pulmonary fibrosis

● **J84.11**   **Idiopathic interstitial pneumonia**

> **Excludes1**   lymphoid interstitial pneumonia (J84.2)
> pneumocystis pneumonia (B59)

J84.111   **Idiopathic interstitial pneumonia, not otherwise specified**

J84.112   **Idiopathic pulmonary fibrosis**
Cryptogenic fibrosing alveolitis
Idiopathic fibrosing alveolitis

J84.113   **Idiopathic non-specific interstitial pneumonitis**

> **Excludes1**   non-specific interstitial pneumonia NOS, or due to known underlying cause (J84.89)

J84.114   **Acute interstitial pneumonitis**
Hamman-Rich syndrome

> **Excludes1**   pneumocystis pneumonia (B59)

J84.115   **Respiratory bronchiolitis interstitial lung disease**

J84.116   **Cryptogenic organizing pneumonia**

> **Excludes1**   organizing pneumonia NOS, or due to known underlying cause (J84.89)

J84.117   **Desquamative interstitial pneumonia**

J84.17   *Other interstitial pulmonary diseases with fibrosis in diseases classified elsewhere*
Interstitial pneumonia (nonspecific) (usual) due to collagen vascular disease
Interstitial pneumonia (nonspecific) (usual) in diseases classified elsewhere
Organizing pneumonia due to collagen vascular disease
Organizing pneumonia in diseases classified elsewhere

> *Code first* underlying disease, such as:
> progressive systemic sclerosis (M34.0)
> rheumatoid arthritis (M05.00-M06.9)
> systemic lupus erythematosis (M32.0-M32.9)

CHAPTER 10 (J00-J99)

N   Newborn Age: 0   P   Pediatric Age: 0–17   M   Maternity DX: 12–55   A   Adult Age: 15–124   ♀   Females Only   ♂   Males Only

Complication\Comorbidity   Major C\C   Ex: CC/MCC Exclusions   Present on Admission Requirement   Hospital-Acquired Condition   **1015**

J84.2 **Lymphoid interstitial pneumonia** 🔿
       Lymphoid interstitial pneumonitis

● J84.8 **Other specified interstitial pulmonary diseases**
       Excludes1 exogenous lipoid pneumonia (J69.1)
                    unspecified lipoid pneumonia (J69.1)

J84.81 **Lymphangioleiomyomatosis** ♀ 🔿
        Lymphangiomyomatosis

J84.82 **Adult pulmonary Langerhans cell
        histiocytosis** 🔿   A
        Adult PLCH

J84.83 **Surfactant mutations of the lung** 🔿
        (Ex:) J84.83-J84.848, P22.0-P28.5, P28.89-P29.2, P29.4,
              P29.89-P29.9, P84, P94.1-P96.0, P96.3-P96.5, P96.82-P96.89

● J84.84 **Other interstitial lung diseases of childhood**
        (Ex:) For category J84.84 CC codes: See J84.83

J84.841 **Neuroendocrine cell hyperplasia of
         infancy** 🔿

J84.842 **Pulmonary interstitial glycogenosis** 🔿

J84.843 **Alveolar capillary dysplasia with vein
         misalignment** 🔿

J84.848 **Other interstitial lung diseases of
         childhood** 🔿

J84.89 **Other specified interstitial pulmonary diseases**
        Endogenous lipoid pneumonia
        Interstitial pneumonitis
        Non-specific interstitial pneumonitis NOS
        Organizing pneumonia due to known
            underlying cause
        Organizing pneumonia NOS

        Code first, if applicable:
            poisoning due to drug or toxin (T51-T65
                with fifth or sixth character to indicate
                intent), for toxic pneumonopathy
            underlying cause of pneumonopathy, if
                known
        Use additional code, for adverse effect, to
            identify drug (T36-T50 with fifth or sixth
            character 5), if drug-induced
        Excludes1 cryptogenic organizing
                     pneumonia (J84.116)
                     idiopathic non-specific
                         interstitial pneumonitis
                         (J84.113) ⬅
                     lipoid pneumonia, exogenous or
                         unspecified (J69.1)
                     lymphoid interstitial pneumonia
                         (J84.2)

J84.9 **Interstitial pulmonary disease, unspecified** 🔿
       Interstitial pneumonia NOS

SUPPURATIVE AND NECROTIC CONDITIONS OF THE LOWER RESPIRATORY TRACT (J85-J86)

● J85 **Abscess of lung and mediastinum**
       Use additional code (B95-B97) to identify infectious agent.
       (Ex:) **For category J85 CC codes unless otherwise indicated:** A06.5, A15.0-A15.6,
             A15.8-A15.9, A17.9, A18.82, A18.84, A18.89, J22, J85.0-J85.2, J98.8-J98.9

J85.0 **Gangrene and necrosis of lung** 🔿

J85.1 **Abscess of lung with pneumonia** 🔿
       Code also the type of pneumonia

J85.2 **Abscess of lung without pneumonia** 🔿
       Abscess of lung NOS

J85.3 **Abscess of mediastinum** 🔿
       (Ex:) J22, J85.3, J98.8-J98.9

Item 10-11 Empyema is a condition in which pus accumulates in a body cavity. Empyema **with fistula** occurs when the pus passes from one cavity to another organ or structure.

● J86 **Pyothorax**
       Use additional code (B95-B97) to identify infectious agent.
       Excludes1 abscess of lung (J85.-)
                    pyothorax due to tuberculosis (A15.6)
       (Ex:) **For category J86 CC codes:** J22, J86.0-J86.9, J98.4, J98.8-J99, R91.1

J86.0 **Pyothorax with fistula** 🔿
       Bronchocutaneous fistula
       Bronchopleural fistula
       Hepatopleural fistula
       Mediastinal fistula
       Pleural fistula
       Thoracic fistula
       Any condition classifiable to J86.9 with fistula

J86.9 **Pyothorax without fistula** 🔿
       Abscess of pleura
       Abscess of thorax
       Empyema (chest) (lung) (pleura)
       Fibrinopurulent pleurisy
       Purulent pleurisy
       Pyopneumothorax
       Septic pleurisy
       Seropurulent pleurisy
       Suppurative pleurisy

OTHER DISEASES OF THE PLEURA (J90-J94)

J90 **Pleural effusion, not elsewhere classified** 🔿
     Encysted pleurisy
     Pleural effusion NOS
     Pleurisy with effusion (exudative) (serous)
     Excludes1 chylous (pleural) effusion (J94.0)
                  malignant pleural effusion (J91.0))
                  pleurisy NOS (R09.1)
                  tuberculous pleural effusion (A15.6)
     (Ex:) A15.0-A15.6, A15.8-A15.9, A17.9, A18.82, A18.84, A18.89, J22, J90-J92.9, J94.0-J94.9,
           J98.4, J98.8-J99, R09.1, R91.1

● J91 **Pleural effusion in conditions classified elsewhere**
       Excludes2 pleural effusion in heart failure (I50.-)
                    pleural effusion in systemic lupus erythematosus
                        (M32.13)

▷ J91.0 *Malignant pleural effusion* 🔿
       Code first underlying neoplasm
       (Ex:) C45.7-C45.9, C76.8, C78.2-C78.39, C79.89-C79.9, C7A.00, C7A.098,
             C7A.1-C7B.00, C7B.09-C7B.8, C80.0-C80.2, D49.81-D49.9, J90-J91.0, J94.0,
             J94.2

▷ J91.8 *Pleural effusion in other conditions classified
       elsewhere* 🔿
       Code first underlying disease, such as:
           filariasis (B74.0-B74.9)
           influenza (J09.X2, J10.1, J11.1)
       (Ex:) See J90

● J92 **Pleural plaque**
       Includes pleural thickening

J92.0 **Pleural plaque with presence of asbestos**

J92.9 **Pleural plaque without asbestos**
       Pleural plaque NOS

◀ New   ⬅ Revised   ~~deleted~~ Deleted   Excludes 1   Excludes 2   Includes   Use additional   Code first   Code also   Unspecified
OGCR Official Guidelines   ● Unacceptable Principal Diagnosis   X Assign placeholder X   🔿 Use Additional Character(s)   ▷ Manifestation Code   **Coding Clinic**

● **J93**   **Pneumothorax and air leak**
        Collapsed lung

        Excludes1   congenital or perinatal pneumothorax (P25.1)
                    postprocedural air leak (J95.812)
                    postprocedural pneumothorax (J95.811)
                    traumatic pneumothorax (S27.0)
                    tuberculous (current disease) pneumothorax
                        (A15.-)
                    pyopneumothorax (J86.-)

     (Ex) **For category J93 CC codes:** J22, J93.0-J93.9, J95.811-J95.812, J98.4, J98.8-J99, R91.1

     J93.0   **Spontaneous tension pneumothorax** 🔹
           Tension pneumothorax (most serious type) occurs when air
             (positive pressure) collects in the pleural space

●   **J93.1**   **Other spontaneous pneumothorax**

          J93.11   **Primary spontaneous pneumothorax** 🔹

   ●   **J93.12**   **Secondary spontaneous pneumothorax** 🔹

               Code first underlying condition, such as:
                  catamenial pneumothorax due to
                      endometriosis (N80.8)
                  cystic fibrosis (E84.-)
                  eosinophilic pneumonia (J82)
                  lymphangioleiomyomatosis (J84.81)
                  malignant neoplasm of bronchus and lung
                      (C34.-)
                  Marfan's syndrome (Q87.4)
                  pneumonia due to Pneumocystis carinii
                      (B59)
                  secondary malignant neoplasm of lung
                      (C78.0-)
                  spontaneous rupture of the esophagus
                      (K22.3)

●   **J93.8**   **Other pneumothorax and air leak**

          J93.81   **Chronic pneumothorax** 🔹

          J93.82   **Other air leak** 🔹
                  Persistent air leak

          J93.83   **Other pneumothorax** 🔹
                  Acute pneumothorax
                  Spontaneous pneumothorax NOS

     J93.9   Pneumothorax, **unspecified** 🔹
           Pneumothorax NOS

● **J94**   **Other pleural conditions**

        Excludes1   pleurisy NOS (R09.1)
                    traumatic hemopneumothorax (S27.2)
                    traumatic hemothorax (S27.1)
                    tuberculous pleural conditions (current disease)
                        (A15.-)

     (Ex) **For category J94 CC codes unless otherwise indicated:** See J90

     J94.0   **Chylous effusion** 🔹
          Chyliform effusion

     J94.1   **Fibrothorax**

     J94.2   **Hemothorax** 🔹
          Hemopneumothorax

     J94.8   **Other specified pleural conditions** 🔹
          Hydropneumothorax
          Hydrothorax
          (Ex) No exclusions

     J94.9   Pleural condition, **unspecified**

INTRAOPERATIVE AND POSTPROCEDURAL COMPLICATIONS AND DISORDERS OF RESPIRATORY SYSTEM, NOT ELSEWHERE CLASSIFIED (J95)

● **J95**   **Intraoperative and postprocedural complications and disorders of respiratory system, not elsewhere classified**

        Excludes2   aspiration pneumonia (J69.-)
                    emphysema (subcutaneous) resulting from a
                      procedure (T81.82)
                    hypostatic pneumonia (J18.2)
                    pulmonary manifestations due to radiation
                      (J70.0- J70.1) ◀▥▥

● **J95.0**   **Tracheostomy complications**
        (Ex) **For category J95.0 CC codes:** J22, J39.8, J95.00-J95.09, J98.01-J98.09,
           J98.8-J98.9

     J95.00   **Unspecified** tracheostomy complication 🔹

     J95.01   **Hemorrhage from tracheostomy stoma** 🔹

     J95.02   **Infection of tracheostomy stoma** 🔹

          Use additional code to identify type of
             infection, such as:
                cellulitis of neck (L03.8)
                sepsis (A40, A41.-)

     J95.03   **Malfunction of tracheostomy stoma** 🔹
          Mechanical complication of tracheostomy
             stoma
          Obstruction of tracheostomy airway
          Tracheal stenosis due to tracheostomy

     J95.04   **Tracheo-esophageal fistula following
                 tracheostomy** ◀

     J95.09   **Other tracheostomy complication** 🔹

     J95.1   **Acute pulmonary insufficiency following thoracic
            surgery** 🔹

        Excludes2   functional disturbances following cardiac
                    surgery (I97.0, I97.1-)
        (Ex) J22, J95.1-J95.3, J95.821-J95.822, J98.8-J98.9

     J95.2   **Acute pulmonary insufficiency following nonthoracic
            surgery** 🔹

        Excludes2   functional disturbances following cardiac
                    surgery (I97.0, I97.1-)
        (Ex) See J95.1

     J95.3   **Chronic pulmonary insufficiency following surgery** 🔹

        Excludes2   functional disturbances following cardiac
                    surgery (I97.0, I97.1-)
        (Ex) See J95.1

     J95.4   **Chemical pneumonitis due to anesthesia** 🔹
          Mendelson's syndrome
          Postprocedural aspiration pneumonia

          Use additional code for adverse effect, if applicable, to
             identify drug (T41.- with fifth or sixth character 5)

        Excludes1   aspiration pneumonitis due to anesthesia
                    complicating labor and delivery
                      (O74.0)
                    aspiration pneumonitis due to anesthesia
                      complicating pregnancy (O29)
                    aspiration pneumonitis due to anesthesia
                      complicating the puerperium
                      (O89.01)
        (Ex) D78.81-D78.89, E36.8, E89.810-E89.89, H59.011-H59.019,
           H59.031-H59.099, H59.811-H59.89, H95.811-H95.89, I97.3, J95.4-J95.5,
           J95.84, J95.851-J95.89, L76.81-L76.82, M96.89, N98.1-N98.9, T81.82X[A],
           T81.89X-T81.9XX[A]

     J95.5   **Postprocedural subglottic stenosis** 🔹
          (Ex) See J95.4

N   Newborn Age: 0   P   Pediatric Age: 0–17   M   Maternity DX: 12–55   A   Adult Age: 15–124   ♀   Females Only   ♂   Males Only

🔹 Complication\Comorbidity   🔹 Major C\C   (Ex) CC/MCC Exclusions   🔹 Present on Admission Requirement   🔹 Hospital-Acquired Condition

● **J95.6** **Intraoperative hemorrhage and hematoma of a respiratory system organ or structure complicating a procedure**

> **Excludes1** intraoperative hemorrhage and hematoma of a respiratory system organ or structure due to accidental puncture and laceration during procedure (J95.7-)

> Ex: **For category J95.6 CC codes:** H95.811-H95.89, I85.01, I85.11, I97.3, J95.61-J95.62, J95.830-J95.831, K21.9, K22.8, K23-K25.0, K25.2, K25.4, K25.6, K26.0, K26.2, K26.4, K26.6, K27.0, K27.2, K27.4, K27.6, K28.0, K28.2, K28.4, K28.6, K29.01, K29.21, K29.31, K29.41, K29.51, K29.61, K29.71, K29.81, K29.91, K31.811, K55.21, K57.01, K57.11, K57.13, K57.21, K57.31, K57.33, K57.41, K57.51, K57.53, K57.81, K57.91, K57.93, K62.5, K92.0-K92.2, M96.89, N98.1-N98.9, P54.1-P54.3, T81.10X-T81.19X[A], T81.82X[A], T81.89X-T81.9XX[A]

J95.61 Intraoperative hemorrhage and hematoma of a respiratory system organ or structure complicating a respiratory system procedure 🔍

J95.62 Intraoperative hemorrhage and hematoma of a respiratory system organ or structure complicating other procedure 🔍

● **J95.7** **Accidental puncture and laceration of a respiratory system organ or structure during a procedure**

> **Excludes2** postprocedural pneumothorax (J95.811) ◀━

> Ex: **For category J95.7 CC codes:** D78.11-D78.12, D78.81-D78.89, E36.11-E36.8, E89.810-E89.89, G96.11, G97.41-G97.49, H59.011-H59.019, H59.031-H59.099, H59.211-H59.229, H59.811-H59.89, H95.31-H95.32, H95.811-H95.89, I97.3, I97.51-I97.52, J95.71-J95.72, K91.71-K91.72, L76.11-L76.12, L76.81-L76.82, M96.820-M96.821, M96.89, N98.1-N98.9, N99.71-N99.72, T81.82X[A], T81.89X-T81.9XX[A]

J95.71 Accidental puncture and laceration of a respiratory system organ or structure during a respiratory system procedure 🔍

J95.72 Accidental puncture and laceration of a respiratory system organ or structure during other procedure 🔍

● **J95.8** **Other intraoperative and postprocedural complications and disorders of respiratory system, not elsewhere classified**

● **J95.81** **Postprocedural pneumothorax and air leak**

> Ex: **For category J95.81 CC codes:** J22, J93.0-J93.9, J95.811-J95.812, J98.4, J98.8-J99, R91.1

J95.811 Postprocedural pneumothorax 🔍🔍

J95.812 Postprocedural air leak 🔍

● **J95.82** **Postprocedural respiratory failure**

> **Excludes1** Respiratory failure in other conditions (J96.-)

> Ex: **For category J95.82 CC codes:** See J95.1

J95.821 Acute postprocedural respiratory failure 🔍

Postprocedural respiratory failure NOS

J95.822 Acute and chronic postprocedural respiratory failure 🔍

● **J95.83** **Postprocedural hemorrhage and hematoma of a respiratory system organ or structure following a procedure**

> Ex: **For category J95.83 CC codes:** See J95.6

J95.830 Postprocedural hemorrhage and hematoma of a respiratory system organ or structure following a respiratory system procedure 🔍

J95.831 Postprocedural hemorrhage and hematoma of a respiratory system organ or structure following other procedure 🔍

J95.84 Transfusion-related acute lung injury (TRALI) 🔍

> Ex: See J95.4

● **J95.85** **Complication of respirator [ventilator]**

J95.850 Mechanical complication of respirator 🔍🔍

> **Excludes1** encounter for respirator [ventilator] dependence during power failure (Z99.12)

> Ex: J95.850, Z99.0-Z99.12, Z99.81-Z99.89

J95.851 Ventilator associated pneumonia 🔍

Ventilator associated pneumonitis

Use additional code to identify the organism, if known (B95.-, B96.-, B97.-)

> **Excludes1** ventilator lung in newborn (P27.8)

> Ex: See J95.4

J95.859 Other complication of respirator [ventilator] 🔍

> Ex: See J95.4

J95.88 Other intraoperative complications of respiratory system, not elsewhere classified 🔍

> Ex: See J95.4

J95.89 Other postprocedural complications and disorders of respiratory system, not elsewhere classified 🔍

Use additional code to identify disorder, such as:
aspiration pneumonia (J69.-)
bacterial or viral pneumonia (J12-J18)

> **Excludes2** acute pulmonary insufficiency following thoracic surgery (J95.1)
> postprocedural subglottic stenosis (J95.5)

> Ex: See J95.4

OTHER DISEASES OF THE RESPIRATORY SYSTEM (J96-J99)

● **J96** **Respiratory failure, not elsewhere classified**

> **Excludes1** acute respiratory distress syndrome (J80)
> cardiorespiratory failure (R09.2)
> newborn respiratory distress syndrome (P22.0)
> postprocedural respiratory failure (J95.82-)
> respiratory arrest (R09.2)
> respiratory arrest of newborn (P28.81)
> respiratory failure of newborn (P28.5)

> Ex: **For category J96 CC codes:** J22, J80, J96.00-J96.92, J98.8-J98.9, R09.2

● **J96.0** **Acute respiratory failure**

J96.00 Acute respiratory failure, unspecified whether with hypoxia or hypercapnia

J96.01 Acute respiratory failure with hypoxia 🔍

J96.02 Acute respiratory failure with hypercapnia 🔍

● **J96.1** **Chronic respiratory failure**

J96.10 Chronic respiratory failure, unspecified whether with hypoxia or hypercapnia 🔍

J96.11 Chronic respiratory failure with hypoxia 🔍

J96.12 Chronic respiratory failure with hypercapnia 🔍

● **J96.2** **Acute and chronic respiratory failure**

Acute on chronic respiratory failure

J96.20 Acute and chronic respiratory failure, unspecified whether with hypoxia or hypercapnia 🔍

J96.21 Acute and chronic respiratory failure with hypoxia 🔍

J96.22 Acute and chronic respiratory failure with hypercapnia 🔍

◀ New   ◀━ Revised   ~~deleted~~ Deleted   Excludes 1   Excludes 2   Includes   Use additional   Code first   Code also   Unspecified

OGCR Official Guidelines   ● Unacceptable Principal Diagnosis   X Assign placeholder X   ● Use Additional Character(s)   ▶ Manifestation Code   **Coding Clinic**

● **J96.9   Respiratory failure, unspecified**
    J96.90   Respiratory failure, unspecified, unspecified whether with hypoxia or hypercapnia 🦠
    J96.91   Respiratory failure, unspecified with hypoxia 🦠
    J96.92   Respiratory failure, unspecified with hypercapnia 🦠

● **J98   Other respiratory disorders**
    Use additional code to identify:
        exposure to environmental tobacco smoke (Z77.22)
        exposure to tobacco smoke in the perinatal period (P96.81)
        history of tobacco use (Z87.891)
        occupational exposure to environmental tobacco smoke (Z57.31)
        tobacco dependence (F17.-)
        tobacco use (Z72.0)
    Excludes1   newborn apnea (P28.4)
                newborn sleep apnea (P28.3)
    Excludes2   apnea NOS (R06.81)
                sleep apnea (G47.3-)

● **J98.0   Diseases of bronchus, not elsewhere classified**
    J98.01   Acute bronchospasm
        Excludes1   acute bronchiolitis with bronchospasm (J21.-)
                  acute bronchitis with bronchospasm (J20.-)
                  asthma (J45.-)
                  exercise induced bronchospasm (J45.990)
    J98.09   Other diseases of bronchus, not elsewhere classified
        Broncholithiasis
        Calcification of bronchus
        Stenosis of bronchus
        Tracheobronchial collapse
        Tracheobronchial dyskinesia
        Ulcer of bronchus

● **J98.1   Pulmonary collapse**
    Excludes1   therapeutic collapse of lung status (Z98.3)
    (Ex:) **For category J98.1 CC codes: J22, J98.11-J98.19, J98.8-J98.9**
    J98.11   Atelectasis 🦠
        Excludes1   newborn atelectasis
                  tuberculous atelectasis (current disease) (A15)
    J98.19   Other pulmonary collapse 🦠

● **J98.2   Interstitial emphysema**
    Mediastinal emphysema
    Excludes1   emphysema NOS (J43.9)
                emphysema in newborn (P25.0)
                surgical emphysema (subcutaneous) (T81.82)
                traumatic subcutaneous emphysema (T79.7)

J98.3   Compensatory emphysema

J98.4   Other disorders of lung
    Calcification of lung
    Cystic lung disease (acquired)
    Lung disease NOS
    Pulmolithiasis
    Excludes1   acute interstitial pneumonitis (J84.114)
                pulmonary insufficiency following surgery (J95.1-J95.2)

J98.5   Diseases of mediastinum, not elsewhere classified 🦠🦠
    Fibrosis of mediastinum
    Hernia of mediastinum
    Retraction of mediastinum
    Mediastinitis
    Excludes2   abscess of mediastinum (J85.3)
    (Ex:) No exclusions

J98.6   Disorders of diaphragm
    Diaphragmatitis
    Paralysis of diaphragm
    Relaxation of diaphragm
    Excludes1   congenital malformation of diaphragm NEC (Q79.1)
                congenital diaphragmatic hernia (Q79.0)
    Excludes2   diaphragmatic hernia (K44.-)

J98.8   Other specified respiratory disorders

J98.9   Respiratory disorder, unspecified
    Respiratory disease (chronic) NOS

◗ *J99   Respiratory disorders in diseases classified elsewhere*
    Code first underlying disease, such as:
        amyloidosis (E85.-) ◀||||
        ankylosing spondylitis (M45)
        congenital syphilis (A50.5)
        cryoglobulinemia (D89.1)
        early congenital syphilis (A50.0)
        schistosomiasis (B65.0-B65.9)
    Excludes1   respiratory disorders in:
            amebiasis (A06.5)
            blastomycosis (B40.0-B40.2)
            candidiasis (B37.1)
            coccidioidomycosis (B38.0-B38.2)
            cystic fibrosis with pulmonary manifestations (E84.0)
            dermatomyositis (M33.01, M33.11)
            histoplasmosis (B39.0-B39.2)
            late syphilis (A52.72, A52.73)
            polymyositis (M33.21)
            sicca syndrome (M35.02)
            systemic lupus erythematosus (M32.13)
            systemic sclerosis (M34.81)
            Wegener's granulomatosis (M31.30-M31.31)

CHAPTER 10 (J00-J99)

N Newborn Age: 0   **P** Pediatric Age: 0–17   **M** Maternity DX: 12–55   **A** Adult Age: 15–124   ♀ Females Only   ♂ Males Only

🦠 Complication\Comorbidity   🦠 Major C\C   (Ex:) CC/MCC Exclusions   🦠 Present on Admission Requirement   🦠 Hospital-Acquired Condition

1019

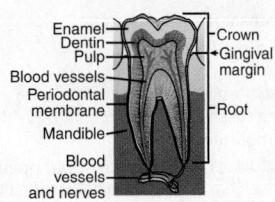

Figure 11-1 Anatomy of a tooth.

Item 11-1 Anodontia is the congenital absence of teeth. **Hypodontia** is partial anodontia. **Oligodontia** is the congenital absence of some teeth, whereas **supernumerary** is having more teeth than the normal number. **Mesiodens** are small extra teeth that often appear in pairs, although single small teeth are not uncommon.

CHAPTER 11

DISEASES OF THE DIGESTIVE SYSTEM (K00-K95)

Excludes2 certain conditions originating in the perinatal period (P04-P96)
certain infectious and parasitic diseases (A00-B99)
complications of pregnancy, childbirth and the puerperium (O00-O9A)
congenital malformations, deformations and chromosomal abnormalities (Q00-Q99)
endocrine, nutritional and metabolic diseases (E00-E88)
injury, poisoning and certain other consequences of external causes (S00-T88)
neoplasms (C00-D49)
symptoms, signs and abnormal clinical and laboratory findings, not elsewhere classified (R00-R94)

This chapter contains the following blocks:

K00-K14	Diseases of oral cavity and salivary glands
K20-K31	Diseases of esophagus, stomach and duodenum
K35-K38	Diseases of appendix
K40-K46	Hernia
K50-K52	Noninfective enteritis and colitis
K55-K64	Other diseases of intestines
K65-K68	Diseases of peritoneum and retroperitoneum
K70-K77	Diseases of liver
K80-K87	Disorders of gallbladder, biliary tract and pancreas
K90-K95	Other diseases of the digestive system

DISEASES OF ORAL CAVITY AND SALIVARY GLANDS (K00-K14)

● **K00 Disorders of tooth development and eruption**
Excludes2 embedded and impacted teeth (K01.-)

K00.0 Anodontia
Hypodontia
Oligodontia
Excludes1 acquired absence of teeth (K08.1-)

K00.1 Supernumerary teeth
Distomolar
Fourth molar
Mesiodens
Paramolar
Supplementary teeth
Excludes2 supernumerary roots (K00.2)

K00.2 Abnormalities of size and form of teeth
Concrescence of teeth
Fusion of teeth
Gemination of teeth
Dens evaginatus
Dens in dente
Dens invaginatus
Enamel pearls
Macrodontia
Microdontia
Peg-shaped [conical] teeth
Supernumerary roots
Taurodontism
Tuberculum paramolare
Excludes1 abnormalities of teeth due to congenital syphilis (A50.5)
tuberculum Carabelli, which is regarded as a normal variation and should not be coded

K00.3 Mottled teeth
Dental fluorosis
Mottling of enamel
Nonfluoride enamel opacities
Excludes2 deposits [accretions] on teeth (K03.6)

K00.4 Disturbances in tooth formation
Aplasia and hypoplasia of cementum
Dilaceration of tooth
Enamel hypoplasia (neonatal) (postnatal) (prenatal)
Regional odontodysplasia
Turner's tooth
Excludes1 Hutchinson's teeth and mulberry molars in congenital syphilis (A50.5)
Excludes2 mottled teeth (K00.3)

K00.5 Hereditary disturbances in tooth structure, not elsewhere classified
Amelogenesis imperfecta
Dentinogenesis imperfecta
Odontogenesis imperfecta
Dentinal dysplasia
Shell teeth

K00.6 Disturbances in tooth eruption
Dentia praecox
Natal tooth
Neonatal tooth
Premature eruption of tooth
Premature shedding of primary [deciduous] tooth
Prenatal teeth
Retained [persistent] primary tooth
Excludes2 embedded and impacted teeth (K01.-)

K00.7 Teething syndrome

K00.8 Other disorders of tooth development
Color changes during tooth formation
Intrinsic staining of teeth NOS
Excludes2 posteruptive color changes (K03.7)

K00.9 Disorder of tooth development, unspecified
Disorder of odontogenesis NOS

● **K01 Embedded and impacted teeth**
Excludes1 abnormal position of fully erupted teeth (M26.3-)

K01.0 Embedded teeth

K01.1 Impacted teeth

1020

◄ New ◄ Revised deleted Deleted Excludes 1 Excludes 2 Includes Use additional Code first Code also Unspecified

OGCR Official Guidelines ● Unacceptable Principal Diagnosis X Assign placeholder X ● Use Additional Character(s) ▌ Manifestation Code Coding Clinic

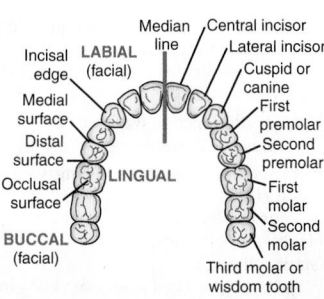

Figure 11-2   The permanent teeth within the dental arch.

Item 11–2   Each dental arch (jaw) normally contains 16 teeth. Tooth decay or **dental caries** is a disease of the enamel, dentin, and cementum of the tooth and can result in a cavity.

● **K02**   **Dental caries**
     Includes   dental cavities
                     tooth decay

    K02.3   **Arrested dental caries**
            Arrested coronal and root caries

●   **K02.5**   **Dental caries on pit and fissure surface**
            Dental caries on chewing surface of tooth

       K02.51   **Dental caries on pit and fissure surface limited to enamel**
               White spot lesions [initial caries] on pit and fissure surface of tooth

       K02.52   **Dental caries on pit and fissure surface penetrating into dentin**

       K02.53   **Dental caries on pit and fissure surface penetrating into pulp**

●   **K02.6**   **Dental caries on smooth surface**

       K02.61   **Dental caries on smooth surface limited to enamel**
               White spot lesions [initial caries] on smooth surface of tooth

       K02.62   **Dental caries on smooth surface penetrating into dentin**

       K02.63   **Dental caries on smooth surface penetrating into pulp**

    K02.7   **Dental root caries**

    K02.9   **Dental caries, unspecified**

● **K03**   **Other diseases of hard tissues of teeth**
     Excludes2   bruxism (F45.8)
                     dental caries (K02.-)
                     teeth-grinding NOS (F45.8)

    K03.0   **Excessive attrition of teeth**
            Approximal wear of teeth
            Occlusal wear of teeth

    K03.1   **Abrasion of teeth**
            Dentifrice abrasion of teeth
            Habitual abrasion of teeth
            Occupational abrasion of teeth
            Ritual abrasion of teeth
            Traditional abrasion of teeth
            Wedge defect NOS

    K03.2   **Erosion of teeth**
            Erosion of teeth due to diet
            Erosion of teeth due to drugs and medicaments
            Erosion of teeth due to persistent vomiting
            Erosion of teeth NOS
            Idiopathic erosion of teeth
            Occupational erosion of teeth

    K03.3   **Pathological resorption of teeth**
            Internal granuloma of pulp
            Resorption of teeth (external)

    K03.4   **Hypercementosis**
            Cementation hyperplasia

    K03.5   **Ankylosis of teeth**

    K03.6   **Deposits [accretions] on teeth**
            Betel deposits [accretions] on teeth
            Black deposits [accretions] on teeth
            Extrinsic staining of teeth NOS
            Green deposits [accretions] on teeth
            Materia alba deposits [accretions] on teeth
            Orange deposits [accretions] on teeth
            Staining of teeth NOS
            Subgingival dental calculus
            Supragingival dental calculus
            Tobacco deposits [accretions] on teeth

    K03.7   **Posteruptive color changes of dental hard tissues**
            Excludes2   deposits [accretions] on teeth (K03.6)

●   **K03.8**   **Other specified diseases of hard tissues of teeth**

       K03.81   **Cracked tooth**
               Excludes1   asymptomatic craze lines in enamel - omit code
                                   broken or fractured tooth due to trauma (S02.5)

       K03.89   **Other specified diseases of hard tissues of teeth**

    K03.9   **Disease of hard tissues of teeth, unspecified**

   K04   **Diseases of pulp and periapical tissues**

    K04.0   **Pulpitis**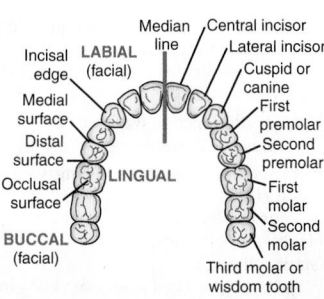
            Acute pulpitis
            Chronic (hyperplastic) (ulcerative) pulpitis
            Irreversible pulpitis
            Reversible pulpitis
            (Ex) K00.0-K08.9, M26.00-M26.9, M27.61-M27.69

    K04.1   **Necrosis of pulp**
            Pulpal gangrene

    K04.2   **Pulp degeneration**
            Denticles
            Pulpal calcifications
            Pulpal stones

    K04.3   **Abnormal hard tissue formation in pulp**
            Secondary or irregular dentine

    K04.4   **Acute apical periodontitis of pulpal origin**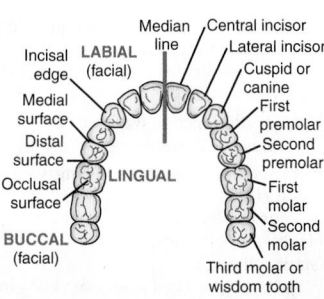
            Acute apical periodontitis NOS
            Excludes1   acute periodontitis (K05.2-)
            (Ex) See K04.0

    K04.5   **Chronic apical periodontitis**
            Apical or periapical granuloma
            Apical periodontitis NOS
            Excludes1   chronic periodontitis (K05.3-)

    K04.6   **Periapical abscess with sinus**
            Dental abscess with sinus
            Dentoalveolar abscess with sinus

    K04.7   **Periapical abscess without sinus**
            Dental abscess without sinus
            Dentoalveolar abscess without sinus
            Periapical abscess without sinus

    K04.8   **Radicular cyst**
            Apical (periodontal) cyst
            Periapical cyst
            Residual radicular cyst
            Excludes2   lateral periodontal cyst (K09.0)

●   **K04.9**   **Other and unspecified diseases of pulp and periapical tissues**

       K04.90   **Unspecified diseases of pulp and periapical tissues**

       K04.99   **Other diseases of pulp and periapical tissues**

N   Newborn Age: 0   **P**   Pediatric Age: 0–17   **M**   Maternity DX: 12–55   **A**   Adult Age: 15–124   ♀   Females Only   ♂   Males Only

Complication\Comorbidity   Major C\C   (Ex) CC/MCC Exclusions   Present on Admission Requirement   Hospital-Acquired Condition   **1021**

Item 11–3 Acute gingivitis, also known as orilitis or ulitis, is the short-term, severe inflammation of the gums (gingiva) caused by bacteria. **Chronic gingivitis** is persistent inflammation of the gums. When the gingivitis moves into the periodontium it is called periodontitis, also known as paradentitis.

● **K05   Gingivitis and periodontal diseases**
　　　Use additional code to identify:
　　　　alcohol abuse and dependence (F10.-)
　　　　exposure to environmental tobacco smoke (Z77.22)
　　　　exposure to tobacco smoke in the perinatal period (P96.81)
　　　　history of tobacco use (Z87.891)
　　　　occupational exposure to environmental tobacco smoke
　　　　　(Z57.31)
　　　　tobacco dependence (F17.-)
　　　　tobacco use (Z72.0)

● **K05.0   Acute gingivitis**
　　　Excludes1   acute necrotizing ulcerative gingivitis
　　　　　　　　　　(A69.1)
　　　　　　　　　　herpesviral [herpes simplex]
　　　　　　　　　　gingivostomatitis (B00.2)
　　　K05.00   Acute gingivitis, plaque induced
　　　　　　Acute gingivitis NOS
　　　K05.01   Acute gingivitis, non-plaque induced

● **K05.1   Chronic gingivitis**
　　　Desquamative gingivitis (chronic)
　　　Gingivitis (chronic) NOS
　　　Hyperplastic gingivitis (chronic)
　　　Simple marginal gingivitis (chronic)
　　　Ulcerative gingivitis (chronic)
　　　K05.10   Chronic gingivitis, plaque induced
　　　　　　Chronic gingivitis NOS
　　　　　　Gingivitis NOS
　　　K05.11   Chronic gingivitis, non-plaque induced

● **K05.2   Aggressive periodontitis**
　　　Acute pericoronitis
　　　Excludes1   acute apical periodontitis (K04.4)
　　　　　　　　　　periapical abscess (K04.7)
　　　　　　　　　　periapical abscess with sinus (K04.6)
　　　K05.20   Aggressive periodontitis, unspecified
　　　K05.21   Aggressive periodontitis, localized
　　　　　　Periodontal abscess
　　　K05.22   Aggressive periodontitis, generalized

● **K05.3   Chronic periodontitis**
　　　Chronic pericoronitis
　　　Complex periodontitis
　　　Periodontitis NOS
　　　Simplex periodontitis
　　　Excludes1   chronic apical periodontitis (K04.5)
　　　K05.30   Chronic periodontitis, unspecified
　　　K05.31   Chronic periodontitis, localized
　　　K05.32   Chronic periodontitis, generalized

K05.4   Periodontosis
　　　Juvenile periodontosis

K05.5   Other periodontal diseases
　　　Excludes2   leukoplakia of gingiva (K13.21)

K05.6   Periodontal disease, unspecified

● **K06   Other disorders of gingiva and edentulous alveolar ridge**
　　　Excludes2   acute gingivitis (K05.0)
　　　　　　　　　　atrophy of edentulous alveolar ridge (K08.2)
　　　　　　　　　　chronic gingivitis (K05.1)
　　　　　　　　　　gingivitis NOS (K05.1)

K06.0   Gingival recession
　　　Gingival recession (generalized) (localized)
　　　　(postinfective) (postprocedural)

K06.1   Gingival enlargement
　　　Gingival fibromatosis

**K06.2   Gingival and edentulous alveolar ridge lesions
　　　associated with trauma**
　　　Irritative hyperplasia of edentulous ridge [denture
　　　　hyperplasia]
　　　Use additional code (Chapter 20) to identify external
　　　　cause or denture status (Z97.2)

**K06.8   Other specified disorders of gingiva and edentulous
　　　alveolar ridge**
　　　Fibrous epulis
　　　Flabby alveolar ridge
　　　Giant cell epulis
　　　Peripheral giant cell granuloma of gingiva
　　　Pyogenic granuloma of gingiva
　　　Excludes2   gingival cyst (K09.0)

**K06.9   Disorder of gingiva and edentulous alveolar ridge,
　　　unspecified**

● **K08   Other disorders of teeth and supporting structures**
　　　Excludes2   dentofacial anomalies [including malocclusion]
　　　　　　　　　　(M26.-)
　　　　　　　　　　disorders of jaw (M27.-)

K08.0   Exfoliation of teeth due to systemic causes
　　　Code also underlying systemic condition

● **K08.1   Complete loss of teeth**
　　　Acquired loss of teeth, complete
　　　Excludes1   congenital absence of teeth (K00.0)
　　　　　　　　　　exfoliation of teeth due to systemic causes
　　　　　　　　　　(K08.0)
　　　　　　　　　　partial loss of teeth (K08.4-)

● **K08.10   Complete loss of teeth, unspecified cause**
　　　**K08.101   Complete loss of teeth, unspecified
　　　　　　cause, class I**
　　　**K08.102   Complete loss of teeth, unspecified
　　　　　　cause, class II**
　　　**K08.103   Complete loss of teeth, unspecified
　　　　　　cause, class III**
　　　**K08.104   Complete loss of teeth, unspecified
　　　　　　cause, class IV**
　　　**K08.109   Complete loss of teeth, unspecified
　　　　　　cause, unspecified class**
　　　　　　Edentulism NOS

● **K08.11   Complete loss of teeth due to trauma**
　　　**K08.111   Complete loss of teeth due to trauma,
　　　　　　class I**
　　　**K08.112   Complete loss of teeth due to trauma,
　　　　　　class II**
　　　**K08.113   Complete loss of teeth due to trauma,
　　　　　　class III**
　　　**K08.114   Complete loss of teeth due to trauma,
　　　　　　class IV**
　　　**K08.119   Complete loss of teeth due to trauma,
　　　　　　unspecified class**

● **K08.12   Complete loss of teeth due to periodontal
　　　diseases**
　　　**K08.121   Complete loss of teeth due to
　　　　　　periodontal diseases, class I**
　　　**K08.122   Complete loss of teeth due to
　　　　　　periodontal diseases, class II**
　　　**K08.123   Complete loss of teeth due to
　　　　　　periodontal diseases, class III**
　　　**K08.124   Complete loss of teeth due to
　　　　　　periodontal diseases, class IV**
　　　**K08.129   Complete loss of teeth due to
　　　　　　periodontal diseases, unspecified
　　　　　　class**

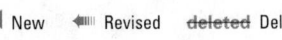

◄ New   ◄▮ Revised   ~~deleted~~ Deleted   Excludes 1   Excludes 2   Includes   Use additional   Code first   Code also   Unspecified
OGCR Official Guidelines   ● Unacceptable Principal Diagnosis   X Assign placeholder X   ● Use Additional Character(s)   ▶ Manifestation Code   **Coding Clinic**

● **K08.13**   **Complete loss of teeth due to caries**

     K08.131   Complete loss of teeth due to caries, class I

     K08.132   Complete loss of teeth due to caries, class II

     K08.133   Complete loss of teeth due to caries, class III

     K08.134   Complete loss of teeth due to caries, class IV

     K08.139   Complete loss of teeth due to caries, unspecified class

● **K08.19**   **Complete loss of teeth due to other specified cause**

     K08.191   Complete loss of teeth due to other specified cause, class I

     K08.192   Complete loss of teeth due to other specified cause, class II

     K08.193   Complete loss of teeth due to other specified cause, class III

     K08.194   Complete loss of teeth due to other specified cause, class IV

     K08.199   Complete loss of teeth due to other specified cause, unspecified class

● **K08.2**   **Atrophy of edentulous alveolar ridge**

     K08.20   Unspecified atrophy of edentulous alveolar ridge
         Atrophy of the mandible NOS
         Atrophy of the maxilla NOS

     K08.21   Minimal atrophy of the mandible
         Minimal atrophy of the edentulous mandible

     K08.22   Moderate atrophy of the mandible
         Moderate atrophy of the edentulous mandible

     K08.23   Severe atrophy of the mandible
         Severe atrophy of the edentulous mandible

     K08.24   Minimal atrophy of maxilla
         Minimal atrophy of the edentulous maxilla

     K08.25   Moderate atrophy of the maxilla
         Moderate atrophy of the edentulous maxilla

     K08.26   Severe atrophy of the maxilla
         Severe atrophy of the edentulous maxilla

   K08.3   **Retained dental root**

● **K08.4**   **Partial loss of teeth**
     Acquired loss of teeth, partial

     Excludes1   complete loss of teeth (K08.1-)
                 congenital absence of teeth (K00.0)

     Excludes2   exfoliation of teeth due to systemic causes (K08.0)

● **K08.40**   **Partial loss of teeth, unspecified cause**

     K08.401   Partial loss of teeth, unspecified cause, class I

     K08.402   Partial loss of teeth, unspecified cause, class II

     K08.403   Partial loss of teeth, unspecified cause, class III

     K08.404   Partial loss of teeth, unspecified cause, class IV

     K08.409   Partial loss of teeth, unspecified cause, unspecified class
         Tooth extraction status NOS

● **K08.41**   **Partial loss of teeth due to trauma**

     K08.411   Partial loss of teeth due to trauma, class I

     K08.412   Partial loss of teeth due to trauma, class II

     K08.413   Partial loss of teeth due to trauma, class III

     K08.414   Partial loss of teeth due to trauma, class IV

     K08.419   Partial loss of teeth due to trauma, unspecified class

● **K08.42**   **Partial loss of teeth due to periodontal diseases**

     K08.421   Partial loss of teeth due to periodontal diseases, class I

     K08.422   Partial loss of teeth due to periodontal diseases, class II

     K08.423   Partial loss of teeth due to periodontal diseases, class III

     K08.424   Partial loss of teeth due to periodontal diseases, class IV

     K08.429   Partial loss of teeth due to periodontal diseases, unspecified class

● **K08.43**   **Partial loss of teeth due to caries**

     K08.431   Partial loss of teeth due to caries, class I

     K08.432   Partial loss of teeth due to caries, class II

     K08.433   Partial loss of teeth due to caries, class III

     K08.434   Partial loss of teeth due to caries, class IV

     K08.439   Partial loss of teeth due to caries, unspecified class

● **K08.49**   **Partial loss of teeth due to other specified cause**

     K08.491   Partial loss of teeth due to other specified cause, class I

     K08.492   Partial loss of teeth due to other specified cause, class II

     K08.493   Partial loss of teeth due to other specified cause, class III

     K08.494   Partial loss of teeth due to other specified cause, class IV

     K08.499   Partial loss of teeth due to other specified cause, unspecified class

● **K08.5**   **Unsatisfactory restoration of tooth**
     Defective bridge, crown, filling
     Defective dental restoration

     Excludes1   dental restoration status (Z98.811)
     Excludes2   endosseous dental implant failure (M27.6-)
                 unsatisfactory endodontic treatment (M27.5-)

     K08.50   Unsatisfactory restoration of tooth, unspecified
         Defective dental restoration NOS

     K08.51   Open restoration margins of tooth
         Dental restoration failure of marginal integrity
         Open margin on tooth restoration
         Poor gingival margin to tooth restoration

     K08.52   Unrepairable overhanging of dental restorative materials
         Overhanging of tooth restoration

CHAPTER 11 (K00–K95)

N Newborn Age: 0   **P** Pediatric Age: 0–17   **M** Maternity DX: 12–55   **A** Adult Age: 15–124   ♀ Females Only   ♂ Males Only

Complication\Comorbidity   Major C\C   CC/MCC Exclusions   Present on Admission Requirement   Hospital-Acquired Condition   **1023**

● **K08.53　Fractured dental restorative material**
　　Excludes1　cracked tooth (K03.81)
　　　　　　　　　traumatic fracture of tooth
　　　　　　　　　(S02.5)

　　K08.530　Fractured dental restorative material without loss of material

　　K08.531　Fractured dental restorative material with loss of material

　　K08.539　Fractured dental restorative material, unspecified

K08.54　Contour of existing restoration of tooth biologically incompatible with oral health
　　Dental restoration failure of periodontal anatomical integrity
　　Unacceptable contours of existing restoration of tooth
　　Unacceptable morphology of existing restoration of tooth

K08.55　Allergy to existing dental restorative material
　　Use additional code to identify the specific type of allergy

K08.56　Poor aesthetic of existing restoration of tooth
　　Dental restoration aesthetically inadequate or displeasing

K08.59　Other unsatisfactory restoration of tooth
　　Other defective dental restoration

K08.8　Other specified disorders of teeth and supporting structures
　　Enlargement of alveolar ridge NOS
　　Irregular alveolar process
　　Toothache NOS

K08.9　Disorder of teeth and supporting structures, unspecified

● **K09　Cysts of oral region, not elsewhere classified**
　　Includes　lesions showing histological features both of aneurysmal cyst and of another fibro-osseous lesion
　　Excludes2　cysts of jaw (M27.0-, M27.4-)
　　　　　　　　　radicular cyst (K04.8)

K09.0　Developmental odontogenic cysts
　　Dentigerous cyst
　　Eruption cyst
　　Follicular cyst
　　Gingival cyst
　　Lateral periodontal cyst
　　Primordial cyst
　　Excludes2　keratocysts (D16.4, D16.5) ◀▥
　　　　　　　　　odontogenic keratocystic tumors (D16.4, D16.5) ◀▥

K09.1　Developmental (nonodontogenic) cysts of oral region
　　Cyst (of) incisive canal
　　Cyst (of) palatine of papilla
　　Globulomaxillary cyst
　　Median palatal cyst
　　Nasoalveolar cyst
　　Nasolabial cyst
　　Nasopalatine duct cyst

K09.8　Other cysts of oral region, not elsewhere classified
　　Dermoid cyst
　　Epidermoid cyst
　　Lymphoepithelial cyst
　　Epstein's pearl

K09.9　Cyst of oral region, unspecified

Item 11–4　Atrophy is wasting away of a tissue or organ, whereas **hypertrophy** is overdevelopment or enlargement of a tissue or organ. **Sialoadenitis** is salivary gland inflammation. **Parotitis** is the inflammation of the parotid gland. In the epidemic form, parotitis is also known as mumps. **Sialolithiasis** is the formation of calculus within a salivary gland. **Mucocele** is a polyp composed of mucus.

Figure 11-3　Major salivary glands.

Parotid gland
Sublingual gland
Submandibular gland

(See Plate 61 on page 73.)

● **K11　Diseases of salivary glands**
　　Use additional code to identify:
　　alcohol abuse and dependence (F10.-)
　　exposure to environmental tobacco smoke (Z77.22)
　　exposure to tobacco smoke in the perinatal period (P96.81)
　　history of tobacco use (Z87.891)
　　occupational exposure to environmental tobacco smoke (Z57.31)
　　tobacco dependence (F17.-)
　　tobacco use (Z72.0)

K11.0　Atrophy of salivary gland

K11.1　Hypertrophy of salivary gland

● **K11.2　Sialoadenitis**
　　Parotitis
　　Excludes1　epidemic parotitis (B26.-)
　　　　　　　　　mumps (B26.-)
　　　　　　　　　uveoparotid fever [Heerfordt] (D86.89)

　　K11.20　Sialoadenitis, unspecified

　　K11.21　Acute sialoadenitis
　　　　Excludes1　acute recurrent sialoadenitis (K11.22)

　　K11.22　Acute recurrent sialoadenitis

　　K11.23　Chronic sialoadenitis

K11.3　Abscess of salivary gland 🔊
　　(Ex) K11.0-K11.9, K31.89-K31.9, K92.81, R68.2

K11.4　Fistula of salivary gland 🔊
　　Excludes1　congenital fistula of salivary gland (Q38.4)
　　(Ex) See K11.3

K11.5　Sialolithiasis
　　Calculus of salivary gland or duct
　　Stone of salivary gland or duct

K11.6　Mucocele of salivary gland
　　Mucous extravasation cyst of salivary gland
　　Mucous retention cyst of salivary gland
　　Ranula

K11.7　Disturbances of salivary secretion
　　Hypoptyalism
　　Ptyalism
　　Xerostomia
　　Excludes2　dry mouth NOS (R68.2)

K11.8　Other diseases of salivary glands
　　Benign lymphoepithelial lesion of salivary gland
　　Mikulicz' disease
　　Necrotizing sialometaplasia
　　Sialectasia
　　Stenosis of salivary duct
　　Stricture of salivary duct
　　Excludes1　sicca syndrome [Sjögren] (M35.0-)

K11.9　Disease of salivary gland, unspecified
　　Sialoadenopathy NOS

CHAPTER 11 (K00-K95)

Item 11–5 **Stomatitis** is the inflammation of the oral mucosa. **Mucositis** is the inflammation of the mucous membranes lining the digestive tract from the mouth to the anus. It is a common side effect of chemotherapy and of radiotherapy that involves any part of the digestive tract.

● **K12 Stomatitis and related lesions**
    Use additional code to identify:
      alcohol abuse and dependence (F10.-)
      exposure to environmental tobacco smoke (Z77.22)
      exposure to tobacco smoke in the perinatal period (P96.81)
      history of tobacco use (Z87.891)
      occupational exposure to environmental tobacco smoke
        (Z57.31)
      tobacco dependence (F17.-)
      tobacco use (Z72.0)

    Excludes1   cancrum oris (A69.0)
              cheilitis (K13.0)
              gangrenous stomatitis (A69.0)
              herpesviral [herpes simplex] gingivostomatitis
                (B00.2)
              noma (A69.0)

K12.0 Recurrent oral aphthae
    Aphthous stomatitis (major) (minor)
    Bednar's aphthae
    Periadenitis mucosa necrotica recurrens
    Recurrent aphthous ulcer
    Stomatitis herpetiformis

K12.1 Other forms of stomatitis
    Stomatitis NOS
    Denture stomatitis
    Ulcerative stomatitis
    Vesicular stomatitis

    Excludes1   acute necrotizing ulcerative stomatitis
                (A69.1)
              Vincent's stomatitis (A69.1)

K12.2 Cellulitis and abscess of mouth 🔖
    Cellulitis of mouth (floor)
    Submandibular abscess

    Excludes2   abscess of salivary gland (K11.3)
              abscess of tongue (K14.0)
              periapical abscess (K04.6-K04.7)
              periodontal abscess (K05.21)
              peritonsillar abscess (J36)
       (Ex) K12.1-K12.39, K14.0, K14.2

● **K12.3 Oral mucositis (ulcerative)**
    Mucositis (oral) (oropharyneal)

    Excludes2   gastrointestinal mucositis (ulcerative)
              (K92.81)
              mucositis (ulcerative) of vagina and vulva
                (N76.81)
              nasal mucositis (ulcerative) (J34.81)

K12.30 Oral mucositis (ulcerative), unspecified

K12.31 Oral mucositis (ulcerative) due to antineoplastic therapy
    Use additional code for adverse effect, if
      applicable, to identify antineoplastic and
      immunosuppressive drugs (T45.1X5) ◀▥
    Use additional code for other antineoplastic
      therapy, such as:
      radiological procedure and radiotherapy
        (Y84.2)

K12.32 Oral mucositis (ulcerative) due to other drugs
    Use additional code for adverse effect, if
      applicable, to identify drug (T36-T50 with
      fifth or sixth character 5)

K12.33 Oral mucositis (ulcerative) due to radiation
    Use additional external cause code (W88-W90,
      X39.0-) to identify cause

K12.39 Other oral mucositis (ulcerative)
    Viral oral mucositis (ulcerative)

● **K13 Other diseases of lip and oral mucosa**
    Includes   epithelial disturbances of tongue
    Use additional code to identify:
      alcohol abuse and dependence (F10.-)
      exposure to environmental tobacco smoke (Z77.22)
      exposure to tobacco smoke in the perinatal period (P96.81)
      history of tobacco use (Z87.891)
      occupational exposure to environmental tobacco smoke
        (Z57.31)
      tobacco dependence (F17.-)
      tobacco use (Z72.0)

    Excludes2   certain disorders of gingiva and edentulous
              alveolar ridge (K05-K06)
              cysts of oral region (K09.-)
              diseases of tongue (K14.-)
              stomatitis and related lesions (K12.-)

K13.0 Diseases of lips
    Abscess of lips   Exfoliative cheilitis
    Angular cheilitis   Fistula of lips
    Cellulitis of lips   Glandular cheilitis
    Cheilitis NOS   Hypertrophy of lips
    Cheilodynia   Perlèche NEC
    Cheilosis

    Excludes1   ariboflavinosis (E53.0)
              cheilitis due to radiation-related disorders
                (L55-L59)
              congenital fistula of lips (Q38.0)
              congenital hypertrophy of lips (Q18.6)
              Perlèche due to candidiasis (B37.83)
              Perlèche due to riboflavin deficiency
                (E53.0)

K13.1 Cheek and lip biting

● **K13.2 Leukoplakia and other disturbances of oral epithelium, including tongue**
    Excludes1   carcinoma in situ of oral epithelium
              (D00.0-)
              hairy leukoplakia (K13.3)

K13.21 Leukoplakia of oral mucosa, including tongue
    *Considered precancerous and evidenced by
      thickened white patches of epithelium on
      mucous membranes*
    Leukokeratosis of oral mucosa
    Leukoplakia of gingiva, lips, tongue

    Excludes1   hairy leukoplakia (K13.3)
              leukokeratosis nicotina palati
                (K13.24)

K13.22 Minimal keratinized residual ridge mucosa
    Minimal keratinization of alveolar ridge
      mucosa

K13.23 Excessive keratinized residual ridge mucosa
    Excessive keratinization of alveolar ridge
      mucosa

K13.24 Leukokeratosis nicotina palati
    Smoker's palate

K13.29 Other disturbances of oral epithelium, including tongue
    Erythroplakia of mouth or tongue
    Focal epithelial hyperplasia of mouth or
      tongue
    Leukoedema of mouth or tongue
    Other oral epithelium disturbances

K13.3 Hairy leukoplakia

Figure 11-4 Oral leukoplakia and associated squamous carcinoma. (From Feldman: Sleisenger & Fordtran's Gastrointestinal and Liver Disease, ed 8, Saunders, An Imprint of Elsevier, 2006)

N Newborn Age: 0   P Pediatric Age: 0–17   M Maternity DX: 12–55   A Adult Age: 15–124   ♀ Females Only   ♂ Males Only

🔖 Complication\Comorbidity   🔖 Major C\C   (Ex) CC/MCC Exclusions   🔖 Present on Admission Requirement   🔖 Hospital-Acquired Condition   **1025**

CHAPTER 11 (K00-K95)

K13.4   **Granuloma and granuloma-like lesions of oral mucosa**
     Eosinophilic granuloma
     Granuloma pyogenicum
     Verrucous xanthoma

K13.5   **Oral submucous fibrosis**
     Submucous fibrosis of tongue

K13.6   **Irritative hyperplasia of oral mucosa**
     Excludes2   irritative hyperplasia of edentulous ridge [denture hyperplasia] (K06.2)

● **K13.7**   **Other and unspecified lesions of oral mucosa**

(See Plate 58 on page 71.)

     K13.70   **Unspecified lesions of oral mucosa**

     K13.79   **Other lesions of oral mucosa**
         Focal oral mucinosis

● **K14**   **Diseases of tongue**
     Use additional code to identify:
       alcohol abuse and dependence (F10.-)
       exposure to environmental tobacco smoke (Z77.22)
       history of tobacco use (Z87.891)
       occupational exposure to environmental tobacco smoke (Z57.31)
       tobacco dependence (F17.-)
       tobacco use (Z72.0)
     Excludes2   erythroplakia (K13.29)
         focal epithelial hyperplasia (K13.29)
         leukedema of tongue (K13.29)
         leukoplakia of tongue (K13.21)
         hairy leukoplakia (K13.3)
         macroglossia (congenital) (Q38.2)
         submucous fibrosis of tongue (K13.5)

K14.0   **Glossitis**
     Abscess of tongue
     Ulceration (traumatic) of tongue
     Excludes1   atrophic glossitis (K14.4)

K14.1   **Geographic tongue**
     Benign migratory glossitis
     Glossitis areata exfoliativa

K14.2   **Median rhomboid glossitis**

K14.3   **Hypertrophy of tongue papillae**
     Black hairy tongue
     Coated tongue
     Hypertrophy of foliate papillae
     Lingua villosa nigra

K14.4   **Atrophy of tongue papillae**
     Atrophic glossitis

K14.5   **Plicated tongue**
     Fissured tongue   Scrotal tongue
     Furrowed tongue
     Excludes1   fissured tongue, congenital (Q38.3)

K14.6   **Glossodynia**
     Glossopyrosis   Painful tongue

K14.8   **Other diseases of tongue**
     Atrophy of tongue   Glossocele
     Crenated tongue   Glossoptosis
     Enlargement of tongue   Hypertrophy of tongue

K14.9   **Disease of tongue, unspecified**
     Glossopathy NOS

DISEASES OF ESOPHAGUS, STOMACH AND DUODENUM (K20-K31)

     Excludes2   hiatus hernia (K44.-)

● **K20**   **Esophagitis**
     Use additional code to identify:
       alcohol abuse and dependence (F10.-)
     Excludes1   erosion of esophagus (K22.1-)
         esophagitis with gastro-esophageal reflux disease (K21.0)
         reflux esophagitis (K21.0)
         ulcerative esophagitis (K22.1-)
     Excludes2   eosinophilic gastritis or gastroenteritis (K52.81)

K20.0   **Eosinophilic esophagitis**

K20.8   **Other esophagitis**
     Abscess of esophagus

K20.9   **Esophagitis, unspecified**
     Esophagitis NOS

● **K21**   **Gastro-esophageal reflux disease**
     Excludes1   newborn esophageal reflux (P78.83)

K21.0   **Gastro-esophageal reflux disease with esophagitis**
     Reflux esophagitis

K21.9   **Gastro-esophageal reflux disease without esophagitis**
     Esophageal reflux NOS

● **K22**   **Other diseases of esophagus**
     Excludes2   esophageal varices (I85.-)

K22.0   **Achalasia of cardia**
     Achalasia NOS
     Cardiospasm
     Excludes1   congenital cardiospasm (Q39.5)

● **K22.1**   **Ulcer of esophagus**
     Barrett's ulcer
     Erosion of esophagus
     Fungal ulcer of esophagus
     Peptic ulcer of esophagus
     Ulcer of esophagus due to ingestion of chemicals
     Ulcer of esophagus due to ingestion of drugs and medicaments
     Ulcerative esophagitis

     Code first poisoning due to drug or toxin, if applicable (T36-T65 with fifth or sixth character 1-4 or 6)

     Use additional code for adverse effect, if applicable, to identify drug (T36-T50 with fifth or sixth character 5)

     Excludes1   Barrett's esophagus (K22.87-)

K22.10   **Ulcer of esophagus without bleeding** 🔖
     Ulcer of esophagus NOS
     Ex: K22.11, K22.8-K23, K31.82

K22.11   **Ulcer of esophagus with bleeding** 🔖
     Excludes2   bleeding esophageal varices (I85.01, I85.11)
     Ex: E16.4, I85.01, K22.10-K22.11, K22.6-K22.719, K25.0-K28.9, K29.01, K29.21, K29.31, K29.41, K29.51, K29.61, K29.71, K29.81, K29.91, K31.811, K31.89-K31.9, K55.21, K57.01, K57.11, K57.13, K57.21, K57.31, K57.33, K57.41, K57.51, K57.53, K57.81, K57.91, K57.93, K62.5, K92.0-K92.81

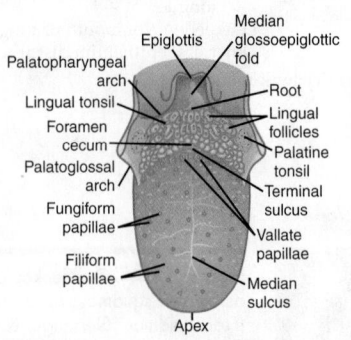

Figure 11-5   Structure of the tongue.

    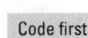
CHAPTER 11 (K00-K95)

Item 11-6 Esophageal reflux is the return flow of the contents of the stomach to the esophagus and is referred to as GERD and/or "heartburn." **Gastroesophageal reflux** is the return flow of the contents of the stomach and duodenum to the esophagus. **Esophageal leukoplakia** are white areas on the mucous membrane of the esophagus for which no specific cause can be identified.

CERVICAL ESOPHAGUS
Left subclavian artery
First rib
Arch of aorta
THORACIC ESOPHAGUS
Diaphragm
ABDOMINAL ESOPHAGUS
Stomach

Figure 11-6 The esophagus is the muscular tube that connects the pharynx and the stomach. The 10 inch (25 cm) long esophagus is divided into three parts: **cervical, thoracic,** and **abdominal.**

K22.2 Esophageal obstruction
Compression of esophagus
Constriction of esophagus
Stenosis of esophagus
Stricture of esophagus
> **Excludes1** congenital stenosis or stricture of esophagus (Q39.3)

K22.3 Perforation of esophagus 🔧
Rupture of esophagus
> **Excludes1** traumatic perforation of (thoracic) esophagus (S27.8-)

Ex: K21.9, K22.3, K22.6, K22.8-K23

K22.4 Dyskinesia of esophagus
Difficulty in moving
Corkscrew esophagus
Diffuse esophageal spasm
Spasm of esophagus
> **Excludes1** cardiospasm (K22.0)

K22.5 Diverticulum of esophagus, acquired
Esophageal pouch, acquired
> **Excludes1** diverticulum of esophagus (congenital) (Q39.6)

K22.6 Gastro-esophageal laceration-hemorrhage syndrome 🔧
Mallory-Weiss syndrome
Ex: E16.4, I85.01, K21.9, K22.10-K22.11, K22.3, K22.6-K28.9, K29.01, K29.21, K29.31, K29.41, K29.51, K29.61, K29.71, K29.81, K29.91, K31.811, K55.21, K57.01, K57.11, K57.13, K57.21, K57.31, K57.33, K57.41, K57.51, K57.53, K57.81, K57.91, K57.93, K62.5, K92.0-K92.2

● **K22.7 Barrett's esophagus**
Barrett's disease
Barrett's syndrome
> **Excludes1** Barrett's ulcer (K22.1)
> malignant neoplasm of esophagus (C15.-)

K22.70 Barrett's esophagus without dysplasia
Barrett's esophagus NOS

● **K22.71 Barrett's esophagus with dysplasia**
K22.710 Barrett's esophagus with low grade dysplasia
K22.711 Barrett's esophagus with high grade dysplasia
K22.719 Barrett's esophagus with dysplasia, unspecified

K22.8 Other specified diseases of esophagus
Hemorrhage of esophagus NOS
> **Excludes2** esophageal varices (I85.-)
> Paterson-Kelly syndrome (D50.1)

K22.9 Disease of esophagus, unspecified

▶ **K23 Disorders of esophagus in diseases classified elsewhere**
Code first underlying disease, such as:
congenital syphilis (A50.5)
> **Excludes1** late syphilis (A52.79)
> megaesophagus due to Chagas' disease (B57.31)
> tuberculosis (A18.83)

● **K25 Gastric ulcer**
Includes erosion (acute) of stomach
pylorus ulcer (peptic)
stomach ulcer (peptic)
Use additional code to identify:
alcohol abuse and dependence (F10.-)
> **Excludes1** acute gastritis (K29.0-)
> peptic ulcer NOS (K27.-)

Ex: **For category K25 CC codes:** E16.4, I85.01, K22.10-K22.11, K22.6-K22.719, K25.0-K28.9, K29.01, K29.21, K29.31, K29.41, K29.51, K29.61, K29.71, K29.81, K29.91, K31.811, K31.89-K31.9, K55.21, K57.01, K57.11, K57.13, K57.21, K57.31, K57.33, K57.41, K57.51, K57.53, K57.81, K57.91, K57.93, K62.5, K92.0-K92.81

K25.0 Acute gastric ulcer with hemorrhage 🔧
K25.1 Acute gastric ulcer with perforation 🔧
K25.2 Acute gastric ulcer with both hemorrhage and perforation 🔧
K25.3 Acute gastric ulcer without hemorrhage or perforation 🔧
K25.4 Chronic or unspecified gastric ulcer with hemorrhage 🔧
K25.5 Chronic or unspecified gastric ulcer with perforation 🔧
K25.6 Chronic or unspecified gastric ulcer with both hemorrhage and perforation 🔧
K25.7 Chronic gastric ulcer without hemorrhage or perforation 🔧
K25.9 Gastric ulcer, unspecified as acute or chronic, without hemorrhage or perforation

● **K26 Duodenal ulcer**
Includes erosion (acute) of duodenum
duodenum ulcer (peptic)
postpyloric ulcer (peptic)
Use additional code to identify:
alcohol abuse and dependence (F10.-)
> **Excludes1** peptic ulcer NOS (K27.-)

Ex: **For category K26 CC codes unless otherwise indicated:** E16.4, I85.01, K22.10-K22.11, K22.6-K22.719, K25.0-K28.9, K29.01, K29.21, K29.31, K29.41, K29.51, K29.61, K29.71, K29.81, K29.91, K31.5, K31.811, K31.89-K31.9, K55.21, K57.01, K57.11, K57.13, K57.21, K57.31, K57.33, K57.41, K57.51, K57.53, K57.81, K57.91, K57.93, K62.5, K92.0-K92.81

K26.0 Acute duodenal ulcer with hemorrhage 🔧
K26.1 Acute duodenal ulcer with perforation 🔧
K26.2 Acute duodenal ulcer with both hemorrhage and perforation 🔧
K26.3 Acute duodenal ulcer without hemorrhage or perforation 🔧
Ex: E16.4, I85.01, K22.6, K25.0-K28.9, K29.01, K29.21, K29.31, K29.41, K29.51, K29.61, K29.71, K29.81, K29.91, K31.5, K31.811, K31.82, K31.89-K31.9, K55.21, K57.01, K57.11, K57.13, K57.21, K57.31, K57.33, K57.41, K57.51, K57.53, K57.81, K57.91, K57.93, K62.5, K92.0-K92.81

K26.4 Chronic or unspecified duodenal ulcer with hemorrhage 🔧
K26.5 Chronic or unspecified duodenal ulcer with perforation 🔧

Item 11-7 Achalasia is a condition in which the smooth muscle fibers of the esophagus do not relax. Most frequently, this condition occurs at the esophagogastric sphincter. **Cardiospasm,** also known as **megaesophagus,** is achalasia of the thoracic esophagus.

A   B   C

Figure 11-7 A. Ulcer. **B.** Perforated ulcer. **C.** Laparoscopic view of a perforated duodenal ulcer *(arrow)* with fibrinous exudate on the adjacent peritoneum. (**C** from Feldman: Sleisenger & Fordtran's Gastrointestinal and Liver Disease, ed 8, Saunders, An Imprint of Elsevier, 2006)

Item 11–8 Gastric ulcers are lesions of the stomach that result in the death of the tissue and a defect of the surface. **Perforated ulcers** are those in which the lesion penetrates the gastric wall, leaving a hole. **Peptic ulcers** are lesions of the stomach or the duodenum. **Peptic** refers to the gastric juice, pepsin.

K26.6   Chronic or unspecified duodenal ulcer with both hemorrhage and perforation 🔖

K26.7   Chronic duodenal ulcer without hemorrhage or perforation

K26.9   Duodenal ulcer, unspecified as acute or chronic, without hemorrhage or perforation

● **K27**   Peptic ulcer, site unspecified

    Includes   gastroduodenal ulcer NOS
               peptic ulcer NOS

    Use additional code to identify:
      alcohol abuse and dependence (F10.-)

    Excludes1   peptic ulcer of newborn (P78.82)

    (Ex) **For category K27 CC codes:** See K26

K27.0   Acute peptic ulcer, site unspecified, with hemorrhage 🔖

K27.1   Acute peptic ulcer, site unspecified, with perforation 🔖

K27.2   Acute peptic ulcer, site unspecified, with both hemorrhage and perforation 🔖

K27.3   Acute peptic ulcer, site unspecified, without hemorrhage or perforation 🔖

K27.4   Chronic or unspecified peptic ulcer, site unspecified, with hemorrhage 🔖

K27.5   Chronic or unspecified peptic ulcer, site unspecified, with perforation 🔖

K27.6   Chronic or unspecified peptic ulcer, site unspecified, with both hemorrhage and perforation 🔖

K27.7   Chronic peptic ulcer, site unspecified, without hemorrhage or perforation

K27.9   Peptic ulcer, site unspecified, unspecified as acute or chronic, without hemorrhage or perforation

● **K28**   Gastrojejunal ulcer

    Includes   anastomotic ulcer (peptic) or erosion
               gastrocolic ulcer (peptic) or erosion
               gastrointestinal ulcer (peptic) or erosion
               gastrojejunal ulcer (peptic) or erosion
               jejunal ulcer (peptic) or erosion
               marginal ulcer (peptic) or erosion
               stomal ulcer (peptic) or erosion

    Use additional code to identify:
      alcohol abuse and dependence (F10.-)

    Excludes1   primary ulcer of small intestine (K63.3)

    (Ex) **For category K28 CC codes:** See K25

K28.0   Acute gastrojejunal ulcer with hemorrhage 🔖

K28.1   Acute gastrojejunal ulcer with perforation 🔖

K28.2   Acute gastrojejunal ulcer with both hemorrhage and perforation 🔖

K28.3   Acute gastrojejunal ulcer without hemorrhage or perforation 🔖

K28.4   Chronic or unspecified gastrojejunal ulcer with hemorrhage 🔖

K28.5   Chronic or unspecified gastrojejunal ulcer with perforation 🔖

K28.6   Chronic or unspecified gastrojejunal ulcer with both hemorrhage and perforation 🔖

K28.7   Chronic gastrojejunal ulcer without hemorrhage or perforation

K28.9   Gastrojejunal ulcer, unspecified as acute or chronic, without hemorrhage or perforation

● **K29**   Gastritis and duodenitis

    Excludes1   eosinophilic gastritis or gastroenteritis (K52.81)
                    Zollinger-Ellison syndrome (E16.4)

    (Ex) **For category K29 CC codes:** E16.4, I85.01, K22.10-K22.11, K22.6-K22.719, K25.0-K28.9, K29.01, K29.21, K29.31, K29.41, K29.51, K29.61, K29.71, K29.81, K29.91, K31.811, K55.21, K57.01, K57.11, K57.13, K57.21, K57.31, K57.33, K57.41, K57.51, K57.53, K57.81, K57.91, K57.93, K62.5, K92.0-K92.2

● **K29.0**   Acute gastritis

    Use additional code to identify:
      alcohol abuse and dependence (F10.-)

    Excludes1   erosion (acute) of stomach (K25.-)

K29.00   Acute gastritis without bleeding

K29.01   Acute gastritis with bleeding 🔖

● **K29.2**   Alcoholic gastritis

    Use additional code to identify:
      alcohol abuse and dependence (F10.-)

K29.20   Alcoholic gastritis without bleeding

K29.21   Alcoholic gastritis with bleeding 🔖

● **K29.3**   Chronic superficial gastritis

K29.30   Chronic superficial gastritis without bleeding

K29.31   Chronic superficial gastritis with bleeding 🔖

● **K29.4**   Chronic atrophic gastritis

    Gastric atrophy

K29.40   Chronic atrophic gastritis without bleeding

K29.41   Chronic atrophic gastritis with bleeding 🔖

● **K29.5**   Unspecified chronic gastritis

    Chronic antral gastritis
    Chronic fundal gastritis

K29.50   Unspecified chronic gastritis without bleeding

K29.51   Unspecified chronic gastritis with bleeding 🔖

● **K29.6**   Other gastritis

    Giant hypertrophic gastritis
    Granulomatous gastritis
    Ménétrier's disease

K29.60   Other gastritis without bleeding

K29.61   Other gastritis with bleeding 🔖

● **K29.7**   Gastritis, unspecified

K29.70   Gastritis, unspecified, without bleeding

K29.71   Gastritis, unspecified, with bleeding 🔖

● **K29.8**   Duodenitis

K29.80   Duodenitis without bleeding

K29.81   Duodenitis with bleeding 🔖

● **K29.9**   Gastroduodenitis, unspecified

K29.90   Gastroduodenitis, unspecified, without bleeding

K29.91   Gastroduodenitis, unspecified, with bleeding 🔖

Item 11–9 Gastritis is a severe inflammation of the stomach. **Atrophic gastritis** is a chronic inflammation of the stomach that results in destruction of the cells of the mucosa of the stomach. Duodenitis is an inflammation of the duodenum, the first section of the small intestine.

◀ New   ◀▦ Revised   ~~deleted~~ Deleted   Excludes 1   Excludes 2   Includes   Use additional   Code first   Code also   Unspecified

OGCR Official Guidelines   ● Unacceptable Principal Diagnosis   X Assign placeholder X   ● Use Additional Character(s)   ▌ Manifestation Code   **Coding Clinic**

K30 Functional dyspepsia
    Indigestion
    Excludes1 dyspepsia NOS (R10.13)
                heartburn (R12)
                nervous dyspepsia (F45.8)
                neurotic dyspepsia (F45.8)
                psychogenic dyspepsia (F45.8)

● **K31 Other diseases of stomach and duodenum**
    Includes   functional disorders of stomach
    Excludes2 diabetic gastroparesis (E08.43, E09.43,
                E11.43, E13.43)
                diverticulum of duodenum (K57.00-K57.13)

  K31.0 Acute dilatation of stomach 🔖
      Acute distention of stomach
      (Ex:) K31.0

  K31.1 Adult hypertrophic pyloric stenosis 🔖   A
      Pyloric stenosis NOS
      Excludes1 congenital or infantile pyloric stenosis
                (Q40.0)
      (Ex:) K30-K31.1, K31.5, K31.84, Q38.5, Q40.0, Q40.8-Q41.9, Q43.4-Q43.9

  K31.2 Hourglass stricture and stenosis of stomach
      Excludes1 congenital hourglass stomach (Q40.2)
                hourglass contraction of stomach (K31.89)

  K31.3 Pylorospasm, not elsewhere classified
      Excludes1 congenital or infantile pylorospasm
                (Q40.0)
                neurotic pylorospasm (F45.8)
                psychogenic pylorospasm (F45.8)

  K31.4 Gastric diverticulum
      Excludes1 congenital diverticulum of stomach
                (Q40.2)

  K31.5 Obstruction of duodenum 🔖
      Constriction of duodenum
      Duodenal ileus (chronic)
      Stenosis of duodenum
        Narrowing
      Stricture of duodenum
        Narrowing
      Volvulus of duodenum
        Twisting/knotting
      Excludes1 congenital stenosis of duodenum (Q41.0)
      (Ex:) K31.5, Q38.5, Q40.8-Q41.9, Q43.4-Q43.9

  K31.6 Fistula of stomach and duodenum 🔖
      Gastrocolic fistula
      Gastrojejunocolic fistula
      (Ex:) K31.6, Q38.5, Q40.8-Q40.9, Q43.4-Q43.9

  K31.7 Polyp of stomach and duodenum
      Excludes1 adenomatous polyp of stomach (D13.1)

● **K31.8 Other specified diseases of stomach and duodenum**
    ● **K31.81 Angiodysplasia of stomach and duodenum**
        K31.811 Angiodysplasia of stomach and
                duodenum with bleeding 🔖
                (Ex:) See K29

        K31.819 Angiodysplasia of stomach and
                duodenum without bleeding
                Angiodysplasia of stomach and
                duodenum NOS

    K31.82 Dieulafoy lesion (hemorrhagic) of stomach and duodenum 🔖
        Excludes2 Dieulafoy lesion of intestine
                  (K63.81)
        (Ex:) E16.4, I85.01, K22.10-K22.11, K22.6-K22.719, K25.0-K28.9, K29.01, K29.21, K29.31, K29.41, K29.51, K29.61, K29.71, K29.81, K29.91, K31.811, K31.82, K55.21, K57.01, K57.11, K57.13, K57.21, K57.31, K57.33, K57.41, K57.51, K57.53, K57.81, K57.91, K57.93, K62.5, K92.0-K92.2

Item 11–10 Achlorhydria, also known as gastric anacidity, is the absence of gastric acid.

  K31.83 Achlorhydria
  K31.84 Gastroparesis
      Gastroparalysis
      Code first underlying disease, if known, such as:
        anorexia nervosa (F50.0-)
        diabetes mellitus (E08.43, E09.43, E10.43,
          E11.43, E13.43)
        scleroderma (M34.-)
  K31.89 Other diseases of stomach and duodenum
  K31.9 Disease of stomach and duodenum, unspecified

DISEASES OF APPENDIX (K35-K38)

● **K35 Acute appendicitis**
    (Ex:) For category K35 CC codes: K31.89-K38.9, K92.81
  K35.2 Acute appendicitis with generalized peritonitis 🔖
      Appendicitis (acute) with generalized (diffuse)
        peritonitis following rupture or perforation of
        appendix
      ~~Appendicitis with peritonitis NOS~~
      Perforated appendix NOS
      Ruptured appendix NOS
  K35.3 Acute appendicitis with localized peritonitis 🔖
      Acute appendicitis with or without perforation or
        rupture NOS ◀▦
      Acute appendicitis with or without perforation or
        rupture with localized peritonitis ◀
      Acute appendicitis with peritoneal abscess
● **K35.8 Other and unspecified acute appendicitis**
    K35.80 Unspecified acute appendicitis 🔖
        Acute appendicitis NOS
        Acute appendicitis without (localized)
          (generalized) peritonitis
    K35.89 Other acute appendicitis 🔖

  K36 Other appendicitis
    Chronic appendicitis
    Recurrent appendicitis

  K37 Unspecified appendicitis
    Excludes1 -unspecified appendicitis with peritonitis
             (K35.2-K35.3)

● **K38 Other diseases of appendix**
  K38.0 Hyperplasia of appendix
  K38.1 Appendicular concretions
      Fecalith of appendix
      Stercolith of appendix
  K38.2 Diverticulum of appendix
  K38.3 Fistula of appendix
  K38.8 Other specified diseases of appendix
      Intussusception of appendix
  K38.9 Disease of appendix, unspecified

Hepatic flexure Transverse colon Ascending colon Cecum Appendix

Figure 11-8 Acute appendicitis is the inflammation of the appendix, usually associated with obstruction. Most often this is a disease of adolescents and young adults.

N Newborn Age: 0   P Pediatric Age: 0–17   M Maternity DX: 12–55   A Adult Age: 15–124   ♀ Females Only   ♂ Males Only

🔖 Complication\Comorbidity   🔖 Major C\C   (Ex:) CC/MCC Exclusions   🔖 Present on Admission Requirement   🔖 Hospital-Acquired Condition

1029

CHAPTER 11 (K00-K95)

CHAPTER 11 (K00-K95)

Item 11-11 Hernias of the groin are the most common type, accounting for 80 percent of all hernias. There are two major types of inguinal hernias: indirect (oblique) affecting men only and direct. **Indirect inguinal hernias** result when the intestines emerge through the abdominal wall in an indirect fashion through the inguinal canal. **Direct inguinal hernias** penetrate through the abdominal wall in a direct fashion. **Femoral hernias** occur at the femoral ring where the femoral vessels enter the thigh and is most common in women. An abdominal wall hernia is also called a ventral or epigastric hernia and occurs in both sexes. Classification is based on location of the hernia and whether there is obstruction or gangrene.

Ventral, epigastric, or incisional hernia occurs on the abdominal surface caused by musculature weakness or a tear at a previous surgical site and is evidenced by a bulge that changes in size, becoming larger with exertion. An **incarcerated** hernia is one in which the intestines become trapped in the hernia. A **strangulated** hernia is one in which the blood supply to the intestines is lost. Hiatal hernia occurs when a loop of the stomach protrudes upward through the small opening in the diaphragm through which the esophagus passes, leaving the abdominal cavity and entering the chest. It occurs in both sexes.

HERNIA (K40-K46)

Note: Hernia with both gangrene and obstruction is classified to hernia with gangrene.

Includes acquired hernia
congenital [except diaphragmatic or hiatus] hernia
recurrent hernia

● **K40 Inguinal hernia**
Includes bubonocele
direct inguinal hernia
double inguinal hernia
indirect inguinal hernia
inguinal hernia NOS
oblique inguinal hernia
scrotal hernia
(Ex:) **For category K40 CC codes:** K31.89-K31.9, K40.00-K40.91, K45.0, K45.8-K46.0, K92.81

● **K40.0 Bilateral inguinal hernia, with obstruction, without gangrene**
Inguinal hernia (bilateral) causing obstruction without gangrene
Incarcerated inguinal hernia (bilateral) without gangrene
Irreducible inguinal hernia (bilateral) without gangrene
Strangulated inguinal hernia (bilateral) without gangrene

   K40.00 Bilateral inguinal hernia, with obstruction, without gangrene, not specified as recurrent
   Bilateral inguinal hernia, with obstruction, without gangrene NOS

   K40.01 Bilateral inguinal hernia, with obstruction, without gangrene, recurrent

● **K40.1 Bilateral inguinal hernia, with gangrene**
   K40.10 Bilateral inguinal hernia, with gangrene, not specified as recurrent
   Bilateral inguinal hernia, with gangrene NOS

   K40.11 Bilateral inguinal hernia, with gangrene, recurrent

● **K40.2 Bilateral inguinal hernia, without obstruction or gangrene**
   K40.20 Bilateral inguinal hernia, without obstruction or gangrene, not specified as recurrent
   Bilateral inguinal hernia NOS

   K40.21 Bilateral inguinal hernia, without obstruction or gangrene, recurrent

Figure 11-9 Inguinal hernias are those that are located in the inguinal or iliac areas of the abdomen.

● **K40.3 Unilateral inguinal hernia, with obstruction, without gangrene**
Inguinal hernia (unilateral) causing obstruction without gangrene
Incarcerated inguinal hernia (unilateral) without gangrene
Irreducible inguinal hernia (unilateral) without gangrene
Strangulated inguinal hernia (unilateral) without gangrene

   K40.30 Unilateral inguinal hernia, with obstruction, without gangrene, not specified as recurrent
   Inguinal hernia, with obstruction NOS
   Unilateral inguinal hernia, with obstruction, without gangrene NOS

   K40.31 Unilateral inguinal hernia, with obstruction, without gangrene, recurrent

● **K40.4 Unilateral inguinal hernia, with gangrene**
   K40.40 Unilateral inguinal hernia, with gangrene, not specified as recurrent
   Inguinal hernia with gangrene NOS
   Unilateral inguinal hernia with gangrene NOS

   K40.41 Unilateral inguinal hernia, with gangrene, recurrent

● **K40.9 Unilateral inguinal hernia, without obstruction or gangrene**
   K40.90 Unilateral inguinal hernia, without obstruction or gangrene, not specified as recurrent
   Inguinal hernia NOS
   Unilateral inguinal hernia NOS

   K40.91 Unilateral inguinal hernia, without obstruction or gangrene, recurrent

● **K41 Femoral hernia**
● **K41.0 Bilateral femoral hernia, with obstruction, without gangrene**
Femoral hernia (bilateral) causing obstruction, without gangrene
Incarcerated femoral hernia (bilateral), without gangrene
Irreducible femoral hernia (bilateral), without gangrene
Strangulated femoral hernia (bilateral), without gangrene
(Ex:) **For category K41.0 CC codes:** K31.89-K31.9, K41.00-K41.91, K45.0, K45.8-K46.0, K92.81

   K41.00 Bilateral femoral hernia, with obstruction, without gangrene, not specified as recurrent
   Bilateral femoral hernia, with obstruction, without gangrene NOS

   K41.01 Bilateral femoral hernia, with obstruction, without gangrene, recurrent

◀ New   ◀▥ Revised   ~~deleted~~ Deleted   Excludes 1   Excludes 2   Includes   Use additional   Code first   Code also   Unspecified

OGCR Official Guidelines   ● Unacceptable Principal Diagnosis   X Assign placeholder X   Use Additional Character(s)   Manifestation Code   **Coding Clinic**

● **K41.1** **Bilateral femoral hernia, with gangrene**
   (Ex) For category K41.1 CC codes: K31.89-K31.9, K41.10-K41.21, K41.40-K41.91, K45.0, K45.8-K46.0, K92.81

   K41.10 **Bilateral femoral hernia, with gangrene, not specified as recurrent** 🏥
      Bilateral femoral hernia, with gangrene NOS

   K41.11 **Bilateral femoral hernia, with gangrene, recurrent**

● **K41.2** **Bilateral femoral hernia, without obstruction or gangrene**

   K41.20 **Bilateral femoral hernia, without obstruction or gangrene, not specified as recurrent**
      Bilateral femoral hernia NOS

   K41.21 **Bilateral femoral hernia, without obstruction or gangrene, recurrent**

● **K41.3** **Unilateral femoral hernia, with obstruction, without gangrene**
   Femoral hernia (unilateral) causing obstruction, without gangrene
   Incarcerated femoral hernia (unilateral), without gangrene
   Irreducible femoral hernia (unilateral), without gangrene
   Strangulated femoral hernia (unilateral), without gangrene
   (Ex) For category K41.3 CC codes: See K41.0

   K41.30 **Unilateral femoral hernia, with obstruction, without gangrene, not specified as recurrent** 🏥
      Femoral hernia, with obstruction NOS
      Unilateral femoral hernia, with obstruction NOS

   K41.31 **Unilateral femoral hernia, with obstruction, without gangrene, recurrent** 🏥

● **K41.4** **Unilateral femoral hernia, with gangrene**
   (Ex) For category K41.4 CC codes: K41.1

   K41.40 **Unilateral femoral hernia, with gangrene, not specified as recurrent** 🏥
      Femoral hernia, with gangrene NOS
      Unilateral femoral hernia, with gangrene NOS

   K41.41 **Unilateral femoral hernia, with gangrene, recurrent** 🏥

● **K41.9** **Unilateral femoral hernia, without obstruction or gangrene**

   K41.90 **Unilateral femoral hernia, without obstruction or gangrene, not specified as recurrent**
      Femoral hernia NOS
      Unilateral femoral hernia NOS

   K41.91 **Unilateral femoral hernia, without obstruction or gangrene, recurrent**

● **K42** **Umbilical hernia**
   Includes paraumbilical hernia
   Excludes1 omphalocele (Q79.2)

   K42.0 **Umbilical hernia with obstruction, without gangrene** 🏥
      Umbilical hernia causing obstruction, without gangrene
      Incarcerated umbilical hernia, without gangrene
      Irreducible umbilical hernia, without gangrene
      Strangulated umbilical hernia, without gangrene
      (Ex) K42.0-K42.1, K43.0-K43.1, K43.3-K43.4, K43.6-K43.7, K45.0, K45.8-K46.0

   K42.1 **Umbilical hernia with gangrene** 🏥
      Gangrenous umbilical hernia
      (Ex) K31.89-K31.9, K42.0-K43.9, K45.0, K45.8-K46.0, K46.9, K92.81

   K42.9 **Umbilical hernia without obstruction or gangrene**
      Umbilical hernia NOS

● **K43** **Ventral hernia**

   K43.0 **Incisional hernia with obstruction, without gangrene** 🏥
      Incisional hernia causing obstruction, without gangrene
      Incarcerated incisional hernia, without gangrene
      Irreducible incisional hernia, without gangrene
      Strangulated incisional hernia, without gangrene
      (Ex) See K42.0

   K43.1 **Incisional hernia with gangrene** 🏥
      Gangrenous incisional hernia
      (Ex) See K42.1

   K43.2 **Incisional hernia without obstruction or gangrene**
      Incisional hernia NOS

   K43.3 **Parastomal hernia with obstruction, without gangrene** 🏥
      Incarcerated parastomal hernia, without gangrene
      Irreducible parastomal hernia, without gangrene
      Parastomal hernia causing obstruction, without gangrene
      Strangulated parastomal hernia, without gangrene
      (Ex) See K42.0

   K43.4 **Parastomal hernia with gangrene** 🏥
      Gangrenous parastomal hernia
      (Ex) See K42.1

   K43.5 **Parastomal hernia without obstruction or gangrene**
      Parastomal hernia NOS

   K43.6 **Other and unspecified ventral hernia with obstruction, without gangrene** 🏥
      Epigastric hernia causing obstruction, without gangrene
      Hypogastric hernia causing obstruction, without gangrene
      Incarcerated epigastric hernia without gangrene
      Incarcerated hypogastric hernia without gangrene
      Incarcerated midline hernia without gangrene
      Incarcerated spigelian hernia without gangrene
      Incarcerated subxiphoid hernia without gangrene
      Irreducible epigastric hernia without gangrene
      Irreducible hypogastric hernia without gangrene
      Irreducible midline hernia without gangrene
      Irreducible spigelian hernia without gangrene
      Irreducible subxiphoid hernia without gangrene
      Midline hernia causing obstruction, without gangrene
      Spigelian hernia causing obstruction, without gangrene
      Strangulated epigastric hernia without gangrene
      Strangulated hypogastric hernia without gangrene
      Strangulated midline hernia without gangrene
      Strangulated spigelian hernia without gangrene
      Strangulated subxiphoid hernia without gangrene
      Subxiphoid hernia causing obstruction, without gangrene
      (Ex) See K42.0

   K43.7 **Other and unspecified ventral hernia with gangrene** 🏥
      Any condition listed under K43.6 specified as gangrenous
      (Ex) See K42.1

   K43.9 **Ventral hernia without obstruction or gangrene**
      Epigastric hernia
      Ventral hernia NOS

● **K44** **Diaphragmatic hernia**
   Includes hiatus hernia (esophageal) (sliding)
      paraesophageal hernia
   Excludes1 congenital diaphragmatic hernia (Q79.0)
      congenital hiatus hernia (Q40.1)
   (Ex) For category K44 CC codes: K44.0-K46.0

   K44.0 **Diaphragmatic hernia with obstruction, without gangrene** 🏥
      Diaphragmatic hernia causing obstruction
      Incarcerated diaphragmatic hernia
      Irreducible diaphragmatic hernia
      Strangulated diaphragmatic hernia

   K44.1 **Diaphragmatic hernia with gangrene** 🏥
      Gangrenous diaphragmatic hernia

   K44.9 **Diaphragmatic hernia without obstruction or gangrene**
      Diaphragmatic hernia NOS

N Newborn Age: 0   **P** Pediatric Age: 0–17   **M** Maternity DX: 12–55   **A** Adult Age: 15–124   ♀ Females Only   ♂ Males Only

🏥 Complication\Comorbidity   🏥 Major C\C   (Ex) CC/MCC Exclusions   🏥 Present on Admission Requirement   🏥 Hospital-Acquired Condition   1031

K45 Other abdominal hernia

> **Includes**   abdominal hernia, specified site NEC
> lumbar hernia
> obturator hernia
> pudendal hernia
> retroperitoneal hernia
> sciatic hernia

K45.0 **Other specified abdominal hernia with obstruction, without gangrene** 🔍
> Other specified abdominal hernia causing obstruction
> Other specified incarcerated abdominal hernia
> Other specified irreducible abdominal hernia
> Other specified strangulated abdominal hernia
> (Ex) K40.00-K46.9

K45.1 **Other specified abdominal hernia with gangrene** 🔍
> Any condition listed under K45 specified as gangrenous
> (Ex) K31.89-K31.9, K40.00-K46.9, K92.81

K45.8 **Other specified abdominal hernia without obstruction or gangrene**

K46 Unspecified abdominal hernia

> **Includes**   enterocele
> epiplocele
> hernia NOS
> interstitial hernia
> intestinal hernia
> intra-abdominal hernia

> **Excludes1** vaginal enterocele (N81.5)

K46.0 **Unspecified abdominal hernia with obstruction, without gangrene** 🔍
> Unspecified abdominal hernia causing obstruction
> Unspecified incarcerated abdominal hernia
> Unspecified irreducible abdominal hernia
> Unspecified strangulated abdominal hernia
> (Ex) K40.00-K46.9

K46.1 **Unspecified abdominal hernia with gangrene** 🔍
> Any condition listed under K46 specified as gangrenous
> (Ex) K31.89-K31.9, K40.00-K46.9, K92.81

K46.9 **Unspecified abdominal hernia without obstruction or gangrene**
> Abdominal hernia NOS

(See Plate 284 on page 77.)

NONINFECTIVE ENTERITIS AND COLITIS (K50-K52)

> **Includes**   noninfective inflammatory bowel disease
> **Excludes1** irritable bowel syndrome (K58.-)
> megacolon (K59.3)

K50 Crohn's disease [regional enteritis]

> **Includes**   granulomatous enteritis
> Use additional code to identify manifestations, such as:
> pyoderma gangrenosum (L88)
> **Excludes1** ulcerative colitis (K51.-)
> (Ex) For category K50 CC codes unless otherwise indicated: K50.00-K51.919

K50.0 **Crohn's disease of small intestine**
> Crohn's disease [regional enteritis] of duodenum
> Crohn's disease [regional enteritis] of ileum
> Crohn's disease [regional enteritis] of jejunum
> Regional ileitis
> Terminal ileitis
> **Excludes1** Crohn's disease of both small and large intestine (K50.8-)

K50.00 **Crohn's disease of small intestine without complications** 🔍

K50.01 **Crohn's disease of small intestine with complications**

K50.011 **Crohn's disease of small intestine with rectal bleeding** 🔍

K50.012 **Crohn's disease of small intestine with intestinal obstruction** 🔍
> CC when PDx is its own CC

K50.013 **Crohn's disease of small intestine with fistula** 🔍
> CC when PDx is its own CC

K50.014 **Crohn's disease of small intestine with abscess** 🔍
> CC when PDx is its own CC
> **Coding Clinic: 2012, Q4, P104**

K50.018 **Crohn's disease of small intestine with other complication** 🔍

K50.019 **Crohn's disease of small intestine with unspecified complications** 🔍

K50.1 **Crohn's disease of large intestine**
> Crohn's disease [regional enteritis] of colon
> Crohn's disease [regional enteritis] of large bowel
> Crohn's disease [regional enteritis] of rectum
> Granulomatous colitis
> Regional colitis
> **Excludes1** Crohn's disease of both small and large intestine (K50.8)

K50.10 **Crohn's disease of large intestine without complications** 🔍

K50.11 **Crohn's disease of large intestine with complications**

K50.111 **Crohn's disease of large intestine with rectal bleeding** 🔍

K50.112 **Crohn's disease of large intestine with intestinal obstruction** 🔍
> CC when PDx is its own CC

K50.113 **Crohn's disease of large intestine with fistula** 🔍
> CC when PDx is its own CC

K50.114 **Crohn's disease of large intestine with abscess** 🔍
> CC when PDx is its own CC
> **Coding Clinic: 2012, Q4, P104**

K50.118 **Crohn's disease of large intestine with other complication** 🔍

K50.119 **Crohn's disease of large intestine with unspecified complications** 🔍

K50.8 **Crohn's disease of both small and large intestine**

K50.80 **Crohn's disease of both small and large intestine without complications** 🔍

K50.81 **Crohn's disease of both small and large intestine with complications**

K50.811 **Crohn's disease of both small and large intestine with rectal bleeding** 🔍

K50.812 **Crohn's disease of both small and large intestine with intestinal obstruction** 🔍
> CC when PDx is its own CC

K50.813 **Crohn's disease of both small and large intestine with fistula** 🔍
> CC when PDx is its own CC

K50.814 **Crohn's disease of both small and large intestine with abscess** 🔍
> CC when PDx is its own CC
> **Coding Clinic: 2012, Q4, P104**

K50.818 **Crohn's disease of both small and large intestine with other complication** 🔍

K50.819 **Crohn's disease of both small and large intestine with unspecified complications** 🔍

Item 11-12 Crohn's disease, also known as **regional enteritis,** is a chronic inflammatory disease of the intestines. Classification is based on location in the small (duodenum, ileum, jejunum) or large (cecum, colon, rectum, anal canal) intestine.

◀ New   ◀▥ Revised   ~~deleted~~ Deleted   Excludes 1   Excludes 2   Includes   Use additional   Code first   Code also   Unspecified

OGCR Official Guidelines   ● Unacceptable Principal Diagnosis   X Assign placeholder X   ● Use Additional Character(s)   ▶ Manifestation Code   **Coding Clinic**

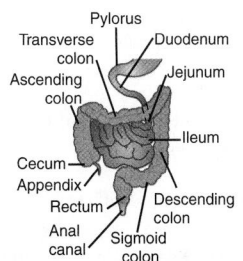

Figure 11-10   Small and large intestines.

(Labels: Pylorus, Transverse colon, Duodenum, Ascending colon, Jejunum, Ileum, Cecum, Appendix, Rectum, Descending colon, Anal canal, Sigmoid colon*)*

● **K50.9**   **Crohn's disease, unspecified**
  (Ex) **For category K50.9 CC codes:** K50.00-K50.919
  K50.90   Crohn's disease, unspecified, without complications 🦠
      Crohn's disease NOS
      Regional enteritis NOS
  ● **K50.91**   Crohn's disease, unspecified, with complications
     K50.911   Crohn's disease, unspecified, with rectal bleeding 🦠
     K50.912   Crohn's disease, unspecified, with intestinal obstruction 🦠
       CC when PDx is its own CC
     K50.913   Crohn's disease, unspecified, with fistula 🦠
       CC when PDx is its own CC
     K50.914   Crohn's disease, unspecified, with abscess 🦠
       CC when PDx is its own CC
       Coding Clinic: 2012, Q4, P104
     K50.918   Crohn's disease, unspecified, with other complication 🦠
     K50.919   Crohn's disease, unspecified, with unspecified complications 🦠

● **K51**   **Ulcerative colitis**
  Use additional code to identify manifestations, such as:
  pyoderma gangrenosum (L88)
  Excludes1   Crohn's disease [regional enteritis] (K50.-)
  (Ex) **For category K51 CC codes unless otherwise indicated:** K50.00-K51.919
  ● **K51.0**   Ulcerative (chronic) pancolitis
     Backwash ileitis
     K51.00   Ulcerative (chronic) pancolitis without complications 🦠
       Ulcerative (chronic) pancolitis NOS
  ● **K51.01**   Ulcerative (chronic) pancolitis with complications
     K51.011   Ulcerative (chronic) pancolitis with rectal bleeding 🦠
     K51.012   Ulcerative (chronic) pancolitis with intestinal obstruction 🦠
       CC when PDx is its own CC
     K51.013   Ulcerative (chronic) pancolitis with fistula 🦠
       CC when PDx is its own CC
     K51.014   Ulcerative (chronic) pancolitis with abscess 🦠
       CC when PDx is its own CC
     K51.018   Ulcerative (chronic) pancolitis with other complication 🦠
     K51.019   Ulcerative (chronic) pancolitis with unspecified complications 🦠

● **K51.2**   Ulcerative (chronic) proctitis
     K51.20   Ulcerative (chronic) proctitis without complications 🦠
       Ulcerative (chronic) proctitis NOS
  ● **K51.21**   Ulcerative (chronic) proctitis with complications
     K51.211   Ulcerative (chronic) proctitis with rectal bleeding 🦠
     K51.212   Ulcerative (chronic) proctitis with intestinal obstruction 🦠
       CC when PDx is its own CC
     K51.213   Ulcerative (chronic) proctitis with fistula 🦠
       CC when PDx is its own CC
     K51.214   Ulcerative (chronic) proctitis with abscess 🦠
       CC when PDx is its own CC
     K51.218   Ulcerative (chronic) proctitis with other complication 🦠
     K51.219   Ulcerative (chronic) proctitis with unspecified complications 🦠
● **K51.3**   Ulcerative (chronic) rectosigmoiditis
     K51.30   Ulcerative (chronic) rectosigmoiditis without complications 🦠
       Ulcerative (chronic) rectosigmoiditis NOS
  ● **K51.31**   Ulcerative (chronic) rectosigmoiditis with complications
     K51.311   Ulcerative (chronic) rectosigmoiditis with rectal bleeding 🦠
     K51.312   Ulcerative (chronic) rectosigmoiditis with intestinal obstruction 🦠
       CC when PDx is its own CC
     K51.313   Ulcerative (chronic) rectosigmoiditis with fistula 🦠
       CC when PDx is its own CC
     K51.314   Ulcerative (chronic) rectosigmoiditis with abscess 🦠
       CC when PDx is its own CC
     K51.318   Ulcerative (chronic) rectosigmoiditis with other complication 🦠
     K51.319   Ulcerative (chronic) rectosigmoiditis with unspecified complications 🦠
● **K51.4**   Inflammatory polyps of colon
     Excludes1   adenomatous polyp of colon (D12.6)
       polyposis of colon (D12.6)
       polyps of colon NOS (K63.5)
     K51.40   Inflammatory polyps of colon without complications 🦠
       Inflammatory polyps of colon NOS
  ● **K51.41**   Inflammatory polyps of colon with complications
     K51.411   Inflammatory polyps of colon with rectal bleeding 🦠
     K51.412   Inflammatory polyps of colon with intestinal obstruction 🦠
       CC when PDx is its own CC
     K51.413   Inflammatory polyps of colon with fistula 🦠
       CC when PDx is its own CC
     K51.414   Inflammatory polyps of colon with abscess 🦠
       CC when PDx is its own CC
     K51.418   Inflammatory polyps of colon with other complication 🦠
     K51.419   Inflammatory polyps of colon with unspecified complications 🦠

Item 11-13   Ulcerative colitis attacks the colonic mucosa and forms abscesses. The disease involves the intestines. Classification is based on the location:
- Enterocolitis: large and small intestine
- Ileocolitis: ileum and colon
- Proctitis: rectum
- Proctosigmoiditis: sigmoid colon and rectum

N Newborn Age: 0   **P** Pediatric Age: 0–17   **M** Maternity DX: 12–55   **A** Adult Age: 15–124   ♀ Females Only   ♂ Males Only

🦠 Complication\Comorbidity   Major C\C   (Ex) CC/MCC Exclusions   Present on Admission Requirement   Hospital-Acquired Condition

1033

(Side tab: **CHAPTER 11 (K00-K95)** *)*

● **K51.5** **Left sided colitis**
  Left hemicolitis
  K51.50 **Left sided colitis without complications** 🔎
  Left sided colitis NOS
● **K51.51** **Left sided colitis with complications**
  K51.511 **Left sided colitis with rectal bleeding** 🔎
  K51.512 **Left sided colitis with intestinal obstruction** 🔎
  CC when PDx is its own CC
  K51.513 **Left sided colitis with fistula** 🔎
  CC when PDx is its own CC
  K51.514 **Left sided colitis with abscess** 🔎
  CC when PDx is its own CC
  K51.518 **Left sided colitis with other complication** 🔎
  K51.519 **Left sided colitis with unspecified complications** 🔎
● **K51.8** **Other ulcerative colitis**
  K51.80 **Other ulcerative colitis without complications** 🔎
● **K51.81** **Other ulcerative colitis with complications**
  K51.811 **Other ulcerative colitis with rectal bleeding** 🔎
  K51.812 **Other ulcerative colitis with intestinal obstruction** 🔎
  CC when PDx is its own CC
  K51.813 **Other ulcerative colitis with fistula** 🔎
  CC when PDx is its own CC
  K51.814 **Other ulcerative colitis with abscess** 🔎
  CC when PDx is its own CC
  K51.818 **Other ulcerative colitis with other complication** 🔎
  K51.819 **Other ulcerative colitis with unspecified complications** 🔎
● **K51.9** **Ulcerative colitis, unspecified**
  (Ex:) For category K51.9 CC codes: K51.00-K51.919
  K51.90 **Ulcerative colitis, unspecified, without complications** 🔎
● **K51.91** **Ulcerative colitis, unspecified, with complications**
  K51.911 **Ulcerative colitis, unspecified with rectal bleeding** 🔎
  K51.912 **Ulcerative colitis, unspecified with intestinal obstruction** 🔎
  CC when PDx is its own CC
  K51.913 **Ulcerative colitis, unspecified with fistula** 🔎
  CC when PDx is its own CC
  K51.914 **Ulcerative colitis, unspecified with abscess** 🔎
  CC when PDx is its own CC
  K51.918 **Ulcerative colitis, unspecified with other complication** 🔎
  K51.919 **Ulcerative colitis, unspecified with unspecified complications** 🔎
● **K52** **Other and unspecified noninfective gastroenteritis and colitis**
  K52.0 **Gastroenteritis and colitis due to radiation** 🔎
  (Ex:) K52.0
  K52.1 **Toxic gastroenteritis and colitis** 🔎
  Drug-induced gastroenteritis and colitis
  Code first (T51-T65) to identify toxic agent
  Use additional code for adverse effect, if applicable, to identify drug (T36-T50 with fifth or sixth character 5)
  (Ex:) K52.1

K52.2 **Allergic and dietetic gastroenteritis and colitis**
  Food hypersensitivity gastroenteritis or colitis
  Use additional code to identify type of food allergy (Z91.01-, Z91.02-)
● **K52.8** **Other specified noninfective gastroenteritis and colitis**
  K52.81 **Eosinophilic gastritis or gastroenteritis**
  Eosinophilic enteritis
  Excludes1 eosinophilic esophagitis (K20.0)
  K52.82 **Eosinophilic colitis**
  K52.89 **Other specified noninfective gastroenteritis and colitis**
  Collagenous colitis
  Lymphocytic colitis
  Microscopic colitis (collagenous or lymphocytic)
● **K52.9** **Noninfective gastroenteritis and colitis, unspecified**
  Colitis NOS   Ileitis NOS
  Enteritis NOS   Jejunitis NOS
  Gastroenteritis NOS Sigmoiditis NOS
  Excludes1 diarrhea NOS (R19.7)
  functional diarrhea (K59.1)
  infectious gastroenteritis and colitis NOS (A09)
  neonatal diarrhea (noninfective) (P78.3)
  psychogenic diarrhea (F45.8)

OTHER DISEASES OF INTESTINES (K55-K64)

● **K55** **Vascular disorders of intestine**
  Excludes1 necrotizing enterocolitis of newborn (P77.-)
  (Ex:) For category K55 CC codes unless otherwise indicated: K55.0-K55.1, K55.8-K55.9
  K55.0 **Acute vascular disorders of intestine** 🔎
  Acute fulminant ischemic colitis
  Acute intestinal infarction
  Acute small intestine ischemia
  Infarction of appendices epiploicae
  Mesenteric (artery) (vein) embolism
  Mesenteric (artery) (vein) infarction
  Mesenteric (artery) (vein) thrombosis
  Necrosis of intestine
  Subacute ischemic colitis
  (Ex:) K55.0-K55.1
  K55.1 **Chronic vascular disorders of intestine** 🔎
  Chronic ischemic colitis
  Chronic ischemic enteritis
  Chronic ischemic enterocolitis
  Ischemic stricture of intestine
  Mesenteric atherosclerosis
  Mesenteric vascular insufficiency
● **K55.2** **Angiodysplasia of colon**
  K55.20 **Angiodysplasia of colon without hemorrhage**
  K55.21 **Angiodysplasia of colon with hemorrhage** 🔎
  (Ex:) E16.4, I85.01, K22.10-K22.11, K22.6-K22.719, K25.0-K28.9, K29.01, K29.21, K29.31, K29.41, K29.51, K29.61, K29.71, K29.81, K29.91, K31.811, K55.21, K57.01, K57.11, K57.13, K57.21, K57.31, K57.33, K57.41, K57.51, K57.53, K57.81, K57.91, K57.93, K62.5, K92.0-K92.2
  K55.8 **Other vascular disorders of intestine** 🔎
  K55.9 **Vascular disorder of intestine, unspecified** 🔎
  Ischemic colitis
  Ischemic enteritis
  Ischemic enterocolitis

◀ New   ◀▥▥ Revised   ~~deleted~~ Deleted   Excludes 1   Excludes 2   Includes   Use additional   Code first   Code also   Unspecified
OGCR Official Guidelines   ● Unacceptable Principal Diagnosis   X Assign placeholder X   ● Use Additional Character(s)   ▶ Manifestation Code   **Coding Clinic**

SIMPLE TYPES   DOUBLE TYPES

Cecum and appendix

Ileum
Ileocecal valve   Ileum   Ileocecal valve

ILEOCOLIC

ILEOCECAL

Figure 11-11   Types of intussusception.

Item 11-14   Intussusception is the prolapse (telescoping) of a part of the intestine into another adjacent part of the intestine. Intussusception may be enteric (ileoileal, jejunoileal, jejunojejunal), colic (colocolic), or intracolic (ileocecal, ileocolic).

Item 11-15   Volvulus is the twisting of a segment of the intestine, resulting in obstruction. Paralytic ileus is paralysis of the intestine. It need not be a complete paralysis, but it must prohibit the passage of food through the intestine and lead to intestinal blockage. It is a common aftermath of some types of surgery.

● **K56   Paralytic ileus and intestinal obstruction without hernia**

    Excludes1   congenital stricture or stenosis of intestine (Q41-Q42)
        cystic fibrosis with meconium ileus (E84.11)
        ischemic stricture of intestine (K55.1)
        meconium ileus NOS (P76.0)
        neonatal intestinal obstructions classifiable to P76.-
        obstruction of duodenum (K31.5)
        postprocedural intestinal obstruction (K91.3)
        stenosis of anus or rectum (K62.4)
        intestinal obstruction with hernia (K40-K46)

    Ⓔⓧ **For category K56 CC codes:** K56.0-K56.3, K56.49-K56.7, K63.4, K63.89-K63.9, K92.89-K92.9, R11.13

    K56.0   Paralytic ileus 🅒
       Paralysis of bowel
       Paralysis of colon
       Paralysis of intestine
       Excludes1   gallstone ileus (K56.3)
              ileus NOS (K56.7)
              obstructive ileus NOS (K56.69)

    K56.1   Intussusception 🅒
       Intussusception or invagination of bowel
       Intussusception or invagination of colon
       Intussusception or invagination of intestine
       Intussusception or invagination of rectum
       Excludes2   intussusception of appendix (K38.8)

    K56.2   Volvulus 🅒
       Strangulation of colon or intestine
       Torsion of colon or intestine
       Twist of colon or intestine
       Excludes2   volvulus of duodenum (K31.5)

    K56.3   Gallstone ileus 🅒
       Obstruction of intestine by gallstone

●   **K56.4   Other impaction of intestine**
      K56.41   Fecal impaction
         Excludes1   constipation (K59.0-)
                incomplete defecation (R15.0)
      K56.49   Other impaction of intestine 🅒

    K56.5   Intestinal adhesions [bands] with obstruction (postprocedural) (postinfection) 🅒
       Abdominal hernia due to adhesions with obstruction
       Peritoneal adhesions [bands] with intestinal obstruction (postprocedural) (postinfection)

●   **K56.6   Other and unspecified intestinal obstruction**
      K56.60   Unspecified intestinal obstruction Intestinal obstruction NOS 🅒
         Excludes1   intestinal obstruction due to specified condition-code to condition

      K56.69   Other intestinal obstruction 🅒
        Enterostenosis NOS
        Obstructive ileus NOS
        Occlusion of colon or intestine NOS
        Stenosis of colon or intestine NOS
        Stricture of colon or intestine NOS
        Excludes1   intestinal obstruction due to specified condition-code to condition

    K56.7   Ileus, unspecified 🅒
       Excludes1   obstructive ileus (K56.69)

● **K57   Diverticular disease of intestine**
    Excludes1   congenital diverticulum of intestine (Q43.8)
              Meckel's diverticulum (Q43.0)
    Excludes2   diverticulum of appendix (K38.2)

    Ⓔⓧ **For category K57 CC codes unless otherwise indicated:** E16.4, I85.01, K22.10-K22.11, K22.6-K22.719, K25.0-K28.9, K29.01, K29.21, K29.31, K29.41, K29.51, K29.61, K29.71, K29.81, K29.91, K31.811, K55.21, K57.01, K57.11, K57.13, K57.21, K57.31, K57.33, K57.41, K57.51, K57.53, K57.81, K57.91, K57.93, K62.5, K92.0-K92.2

● **K57.0   Diverticulitis of small intestine with perforation and abscess**
       Diverticulitis of small intestine with peritonitis
    Excludes1   diverticulitis of both small and large intestine with perforation and abscess (K57.4-)

    K57.00   Diverticulitis of small intestine with perforation and abscess without bleeding 🅒
       CC when PDx is its own CC
       Ⓔⓧ K57.00-K57.13

    K57.01   Diverticulitis of small intestine with perforation and abscess with bleeding 🅒 🅒
       CC when PDx is its own CC

● **K57.1   Diverticular disease of small intestine without perforation or abscess**
    Excludes1   diverticular disease of both small and large intestine without perforation or abscess (K57.5-)

    K57.10   Diverticulosis of small intestine without perforation or abscess without bleeding
       Diverticular disease of small intestine NOS

    K57.11   Diverticulosis of small intestine without perforation or abscess with bleeding 🅒

    K57.12   Diverticulitis of small intestine without perforation or abscess without bleeding 🅒
       Ⓔⓧ K57.00-K57.13

    K57.13   Diverticulitis of small intestine without perforation or abscess with bleeding 🅒

● **K57.2   Diverticulitis of large intestine with perforation and abscess**
       Diverticulitis of colon with peritonitis
    Excludes1   diverticulitis of both small and large intestine with perforation and abscess (K57.4-)

    K57.20   Diverticulitis of large intestine with perforation and abscess without bleeding 🅒
       CC when PDx is its own CC
       Ⓔⓧ K57.20-K57.93

    K57.21   Diverticulitis of large intestine with perforation and abscess with bleeding 🅒
       CC when PDx is its own CC

N Newborn Age: 0   **P** Pediatric Age: 0-17   **M** Maternity DX: 12-55   **A** Adult Age: 15-124   ♀ Females Only   ♂ Males Only

🅒 Complication\Comorbidity   🅜 Major C\C   Ⓔⓧ CC/MCC Exclusions   🅟 Present on Admission Requirement   🅗 Hospital-Acquired Condition

1035

CHAPTER 11 (K00-K95)

Item 11-16 **Diverticula** of the intestines are acquired herniations of the mucosa. Diverticulum (singular): Pocket or pouch that bulges outward through a weak spot (herniation) in the colon. Diverticula (plural). **Diverticulosis** is the condition of having diverticula. **Diverticulitis** is inflammation of these pouches or herniations. Classification is based on location (small intestine or colon) and whether it occurs with or without hemorrhage.

● **K57.3** **Diverticular disease of large intestine without perforation or abscess**

    Excludes1   diverticular disease of both small and large intestine without perforation or abscess (K57.5-)

   K57.30 **Diverticulosis of large intestine without perforation or abscess without bleeding**
      Diverticular disease of colon NOS

   K57.31 **Diverticulosis of large intestine without perforation or abscess with bleeding** 🔹

   K57.32 **Diverticulitis of large intestine without perforation or abscess without bleeding** 🔹
      (Ex:) K57.20-K57.93

   K57.33 **Diverticulitis of large intestine without perforation or abscess with bleeding** 🔹

● **K57.4** **Diverticulitis of both small and large intestine with perforation and abscess**
     Diverticulitis of both small and large intestine with peritonitis

   K57.40 **Diverticulitis of both small and large intestine with perforation and abscess without bleeding** 🔹
      CC when PDx is its own CC
      (Ex:) K57.20-K57.93

   K57.41 **Diverticulitis of both small and large intestine with perforation and abscess with bleeding** 🔹 🔹
      CC when PDx is its own CC

● **K57.5** **Diverticular disease of both small and large intestine without perforation or abscess**

   K57.50 **Diverticulosis of both small and large intestine without perforation or abscess without bleeding**
      Diverticular disease of both small and large intestine NOS

   K57.51 **Diverticulosis of both small and large intestine without perforation or abscess with bleeding** 🔹

   K57.52 **Diverticulitis of both small and large intestine without perforation or abscess without bleeding** 🔹
      CC when PDx is its own CC
      (Ex:) K57.20-K57.93

   K57.53 **Diverticulitis of both small and large intestine without perforation or abscess with bleeding** 🔹

● **K57.8** **Diverticulitis of intestine, part unspecified, with perforation and abscess**
     Diverticulitis of intestine NOS with peritonitis

   K57.80 **Diverticulitis of intestine, part unspecified, with perforation and abscess without bleeding** 🔹
      CC when PDx is its own CC
      (Ex:) K57.20-K57.93

   K57.81 **Diverticulitis of intestine, part unspecified, with perforation and abscess with bleeding** 🔹 🔹
      CC when PDx is its own CC

● **K57.9** **Diverticular disease of intestine, part unspecified, without perforation or abscess**

   K57.90 **Diverticulosis of intestine, part unspecified, without perforation or abscess without bleeding**
      Diverticular disease of intestine NOS

   K57.91 **Diverticulosis of intestine, part unspecified, without perforation or abscess with bleeding** 🔹

   K57.92 **Diverticulitis of intestine, part unspecified, without perforation or abscess without bleeding** 🔹
      (Ex:) K57.20-K57.93

   K57.93 **Diverticulitis of intestine, part unspecified, without perforation or abscess with bleeding** 🔹

● **K58** **Irritable bowel syndrome**

    Includes   irritable colon
              spastic colon

   K58.0 **Irritable bowel syndrome with diarrhea**

   K58.9 **Irritable bowel syndrome without diarrhea**
      Irritable bowel syndrome NOS

● **K59** **Other functional intestinal disorders**

    Excludes1   change in bowel habit NOS (R19.4)
                intestinal malabsorption (K90.-)
                psychogenic intestinal disorders (F45.8)

    Excludes2   functional disorders of stomach (K31.-)

● **K59.0** **Constipation**

    Excludes1   fecal impaction (K56.41)
                incomplete defecation (R15.0)

   K59.00 **Constipation, unspecified**

   K59.01 **Slow transit constipation**

   K59.02 **Outlet dysfunction constipation**

   K59.09 **Other constipation**

   K59.1 **Functional diarrhea**

    Excludes1   diarrhea NOS (R19.7)
                irritable bowel syndrome with diarrhea (K58.0)

   K59.2 **Neurogenic bowel, not elsewhere classified** 🔹
      (Ex:) K58.0-K58.9, K59.1-K59.9, K91.0-K91.1

   K59.3 **Megacolon, not elsewhere classified** 🔹
      Dilatation of colon
      Toxic megacolon
      Code first (T51-T65) *to identify toxic agent*

    Excludes1   congenital megacolon (aganglionic) (Q43.1)
                megacolon (due to) (in) Chagas' disease (B57.32)
                megacolon (due to) (in) Clostridium difficile (A04.7)
                megacolon (due to) (in) Hirschsprung's disease (Q43.1)
      (Ex:) K58.0-K58.9, K59.1-K59.9, K91.0-K91.1

   K59.4 **Anal spasm**
      Proctalgia fugax

   K59.8 **Other specified functional intestinal disorders**
      Atony of colon Pseudo-obstruction (acute) (chronic) of intestine

   K59.9 **Functional intestinal disorder, unspecified**

● **K60** **Fissure and fistula of anal and rectal regions**

    Excludes1   fissure and fistula of anal and rectal regions with abscess or cellulitis (K61.-)

    Excludes2   anal sphincter tear (healed) (nontraumatic) (old) (K62.81)

   K60.0 **Acute anal fissure**

   K60.1 **Chronic anal fissure**

   K60.2 **Anal fissure, unspecified**

   K60.3 **Anal fistula**

   K60.4 **Rectal fistula**
      Fistula of rectum to skin

    Excludes1   rectovaginal fistula (N82.3)
                vesicorectal fistula (N32.1)

   K60.5 **Anorectal fistula**

Item 11-17 A **fissure** is a groove in the surface, whereas a **fistula** is an abnormal passage. An **abscess** is an accumulation of pus in a tissue cavity resulting from a bacterial or parasitic infection.

◄ New   ◄▥ Revised   ~~deleted~~ Deleted   Excludes 1   Excludes 2   Includes   Use additional   Code first   Code also   Unspecified

OGCR Official Guidelines   ● Unacceptable Principal Diagnosis   X Assign placeholder X   ● Use Additional Character(s)   ▮ Manifestation Code   **Coding Clinic**

● **K61**   **Abscess of anal and rectal regions**

     Includes   abscess of anal and rectal regions
                      cellulitis of anal and rectal regions

     (Ex) **For category K61 CC codes: K61.0-K61.4**

   K61.0   **Anal abscess** 🔖
          Perianal abscess

         Excludes1   intrasphincteric abscess (K61.4)

   K61.1   **Rectal abscess** 🔖
          Perirectal abscess

         Excludes1   ischiorectal abscess (K61.3)

         Coding Clinic: 2012, Q4, P104

   K61.2   **Anorectal abscess** 🔖

   K61.3   **Ischiorectal abscess** 🔖
          Abscess of ischiorectal fossa

   K61.4   **Intrasphincteric abscess** 🔖

● **K62**   **Other diseases of anus and rectum**

     Includes   anal canal

     Excludes2   colostomy and enterostomy malfunction (K94.0-, K91.4-)
                       fecal incontinence (R15.-) ◀▥
                       hemorrhoids (K64.-)

   K62.0   **Anal polyp**

   K62.1   **Rectal polyp**

         Excludes1   adenomatous polyp (D12.8)

   K62.2   **Anal prolapse**
          Prolapse of anal canal

   K62.3   **Rectal prolapse**
          Prolapse of rectal mucosa

   K62.4   **Stenosis of anus and rectum**
          Stricture of anus (sphincter)

   K62.5   **Hemorrhage of anus and rectum** 🔖

         Excludes1   gastrointestinal bleeding NOS (K92.2)
                         melena (K92.1)
                         neonatal rectal hemorrhage (P54.2)

     (Ex) **See K57**

   K62.6   **Ulcer of anus and rectum** 🔖
          Solitary ulcer of anus and rectum
          Stercoral ulcer of anus and rectum

         Excludes1   fissure and fistula of anus and rectum (K60.-)
                         ulcerative colitis (K51.-)

     (Ex) **K62.6**

   K62.7   **Radiation proctitis**

         Use additional code to identify the type of radiation (W90.-)

● **K62.8**   **Other specified diseases of anus and rectum**

         Excludes2   ulcerative proctitis (K51.2)

   K62.81   **Anal sphincter tear (healed) (nontraumatic) (old)**
          Tear of anus, nontraumatic

         Use additional code for any associated fecal incontinence (R15.-) ◀▥

         Excludes2   anal fissure (K60.-)
                         anal sphincter tear (healed) (old) complicating delivery (O34.7-)
                         traumatic tear of anal sphincter (S31.831)

   K62.82   **Dysplasia of anus**
          Anal intraepithelial neoplasia I and II (AIN I and II) (histologically confirmed)
          Dysplasia of anus NOS
          Mild and moderate dysplasia of anus (histologically confirmed)

         Excludes1   abnormal results from anal cytologic examination without histologic confirmation (R85.61-)
                         anal intraepithelial neoplasia III (D01.3)
                         carcinoma in situ of anus (D01.3)
                         HGSIL of anus (R85.613)
                         severe dysplasia of anus (D01.3)

   K62.89   **Other specified diseases of anus and rectum**
          Proctitis NOS

         Use additional code for any associated fecal incontinence (R15.-) ◀▥

   K62.9   **Disease of anus and rectum, unspecified**

● **K63**   **Other diseases of intestine**

   K63.0   **Abscess of intestine** 🔖

         Excludes1   abscess of intestine with Crohn's disease (K50.014, K50.114, K50.814, K50.914)
                         abscess of intestine with diverticular disease (K57.0, K57.2, K57.4, K57.8)
                         abscess of intestine with ulcerative colitis (K51.014, K51.214, K51.314, K51.414, K51.514, K51.814, K51.914) ◀▥

         Excludes2   abscess of anal and rectal regions (K61.-)
                         abscess of appendix (K35.3)

     (Ex) **K63.0**

   K63.1   **Perforation of intestine (nontraumatic)** 🔖
          Perforation (nontraumatic) of rectum

         Excludes1   perforation (nontraumatic) of duodenum (K26.-)
                         perforation (nontraumatic) of intestine with diverticular disease (K57.0, K57.2, K57.4, K57.8)

         Excludes2   perforation (nontraumatic) of appendix (K35.2, K35.3)

     (Ex) **K63.1**

   K63.2   **Fistula of intestine** 🔖

         Excludes1   fistula of duodenum (K31.6)
                         fistula of intestine with Crohn's disease (K50.013, K50.113, K50.813, K50.913)
                         fistula of intestine with ulcerative colitis (K51.013, K51.213, K51.313, K51.413, K51.513, K51.813, K51.913) ◀▥

         Excludes2   fistula of anal and rectal regions (K60.-)
                         fistula of appendix (K38.3)
                         intestinal-genital fistula, female (N82.2-N82.4)
                         vesicointestinal fistula (N32.1)

     (Ex) **K63.2**

N   Newborn Age: 0   **P**   Pediatric Age: 0–17   **M**   Maternity DX: 12–55   **A**   Adult Age: 15–124   ♀   Females Only   ♂   Males Only

🔖   Complication\Comorbidity   🔖   Major C\C   (Ex)   CC/MCC Exclusions   🔖   Present on Admission Requirement   🔖   Hospital-Acquired Condition

1037

K63.3 Ulcer of intestine 🔖
  Primary ulcer of small intestine
  Excludes1 duodenal ulcer (K26.-)
         gastrointestinal ulcer (K28.-)
         gastrojejunal ulcer (K28.-)
         jejunal ulcer (K28.-)
         peptic ulcer, site unspecified (K27.-)
         ulcer of intestine with perforation (K63.1)
         ulcer of anus or rectum (K62.6)
         ulcerative colitis (K51.-)
  (Ex) K63.3

K63.4 Enteroptosis

K63.5 Polyp of colon
  Excludes1 adenomatous polyp of colon (D12.6)
         inflammatory polyp of colon (K51.4-)
         polyposis of colon (D12.6)

● **K63.8 Other specified diseases of intestine**
  K63.81 Dieulafoy lesion of intestine 🔖
       Excludes2 Dieulafoy lesion of stomach and
                   duodenum (K31.82)
       (Ex) E16.4, I85.01, K22.10-K22.11, K22.6-K22.719, K25.0-K28.9,
             K29.01, K29.21, K29.31, K29.41, K29.51, K29.61, K29.71,
             K29.81, K29.91, K31.811, K55.21, K57.01, K57.11, K57.13,
             K57.21, K57.31, K57.33, K57.41, K57.51, K57.53, K57.81,
             K57.91, K57.93, K62.5, K63.81, K92.0-K92.2

  K63.89 Other specified diseases of intestine

K63.9 Disease of intestine, unspecified

● **K64 Hemorrhoids and perianal venous thrombosis**
  Includes piles
  Excludes1 hemorrhoids complicating childbirth and the
               puerperium (O87.2)
         hemorrhoids complicating pregnancy (O22.4)

K64.0 First degree hemorrhoids
  Grade/stage I hemorrhoids
  Hemorrhoids (bleeding) without prolapse outside of
    anal canal

K64.1 Second degree hemorrhoids
  Grade/stage II hemorrhoids
  Hemorrhoids (bleeding) that prolapse with straining,
    but retract spontaneously

K64.2 Third degree hemorrhoids
  Grade/stage III hemorrhoids
  Hemorrhoids (bleeding) that prolapse with straining
    and require manual replacement back inside anal
    canal

K64.3 Fourth degree hemorrhoids
  Grade/stage IV hemorrhoids
  Hemorrhoids (bleeding) with prolapsed tissue that
    cannot be manually replaced

K64.4 Residual hemorrhoidal skin tags
  External hemorrhoids, NOS
  Skin tags of anus

K64.5 Perianal venous thrombosis
  External hemorrhoids with thrombosis
  Perianal hematoma
  Thrombosed hemorrhoids NOS

K64.8 Other hemorrhoids
  Internal hemorrhoids, without mention of degree
  Prolapsed hemorrhoids, degree not specified

K64.9 Unspecified hemorrhoids
  Hemorrhoids (bleeding) NOS
  Hemorrhoids (bleeding) without mention of degree

Item 11–18 Peritonitis is an inflammation of the lining (peritoneum) of
the abdominal cavity and surface of the intestines.

Item 11–19 Retroperitoneal infections occur between the posterior
parietal peritoneum and posterior abdominal wall where the kidneys, adrenal
glands, ureters, duodenum, ascending colon, descending colon, pancreas, and
the large vessels and nerves are located.

DISEASES OF PERITONEUM AND RETROPERITONEUM (K65-K68)

● **K65 Peritonitis**
  Use additional code (B95-B97), to identify infectious agent
  Excludes1 acute appendicitis with generalized peritonitis
               (K35.2)
         aseptic peritonitis (T81.6)
         benign paroxysmal peritonitis (E85.0)
         chemical peritonitis (T81.6)
         diverticulitis of both small and large intestine
             with peritonitis (K57.4-)
         diverticulitis of colon with peritonitis (K57.2-)
         diverticulitis of intestine, NOS, with peritonitis
             (K57.8-)
         diverticulitis of small intestine with peritonitis
             (K57.0-)
         gonococcal peritonitis (A54.85)
         neonatal peritonitis (P78.0-P78.1)
         pelvic peritonitis, female (N73.3-N73.5)
         periodic familial peritonitis (E85.0)
         peritonitis due to talc or other foreign substance
             (T81.6)
         peritonitis in chlamydia (A74.81)
         peritonitis in diphtheria (A36.89)
         peritonitis in syphilis (late) (A52.74)
         peritonitis in tuberculosis (A18.31)
         peritonitis with or following abortion or ectopic
             or molar pregnancy (O00-O07, O08.0)
         peritonitis with or following appendicitis (K35.-)
         peritonitis with or following diverticular disease
             of intestine (K57.-)
         puerperal peritonitis (O85)
         retroperitoneal infections (K68.-)
  (Ex) **For category K65 CC codes:** K63.4, K63.89-K63.9, K65.0-K65.9, K67, K68.19-K68.9,
       K92.89-K92.9, R11.13

K65.0 Generalized (acute) peritonitis 🔖
  Pelvic peritonitis (acute), male
  Subphrenic peritonitis (acute)
  Suppurative peritonitis (acute)

K65.1 Peritoneal abscess 🔖
  Abdominopelvic abscess
  Abscess (of) omentum
  Abscess (of) peritoneum
  Mesenteric abscess
  Retrocecal abscess
  Subdiaphragmatic abscess
  Subhepatic abscess
  Subphrenic abscess

K65.2 Spontaneous bacterial peritonitis 🔖
  Excludes1 bacterial peritonitis NOS (K65.9) ◀

K65.3 Choleperitonitis 🔖
  Peritonitis due to bile

K65.4 Sclerosing mesenteritis 🔖
  Fat necrosis of peritoneum
  (Idiopathic) sclerosing mesenteric fibrosis
  Mesenteric lipodystrophy
  Mesenteric panniculitis
  Retractile mesenteritis

K65.8 Other peritonitis 🔖
  Chronic proliferative peritonitis
  Peritonitis due to urine

K65.9 Peritonitis, unspecified 🔖
  Bacterial peritonitis NOS

◀ New   ◀‖ Revised   ~~deleted~~ Deleted   Excludes 1   Excludes 2   Includes   Use additional   Code first   Code also   Unspecified
OGCR Official Guidelines   ● Unacceptable Principal Diagnosis   X Assign placeholder X   ‖ Use Additional Character(s)   ‖ Manifestation Code   **Coding Clinic**

● **K66**   **Other disorders of peritoneum**
     Excludes2   ascites (R18.-)
                peritoneal effusion (chronic) (R18.8)

     K66.0   **Peritoneal adhesions (postprocedural) (postinfection)**
          Adhesions (of) abdominal (wall)
          Adhesions (of) diaphragm
          Adhesions (of) intestine
          Adhesions (of) male pelvis
          Adhesions (of) omentum
          Adhesions (of) stomach
          Adhesive bands
          Mesenteric adhesions
          Excludes1   female pelvic adhesions [bands] (N73.6)
                   peritoneal adhesions with intestinal
                       obstruction (K56.5)

     K66.1   **Hemoperitoneum** 🔷
          Excludes1   traumatic hemoperitoneum (S36.8-)
          (Ex:) K66.1

     K66.8   **Other specified disorders of peritoneum**

     K66.9   **Disorder of peritoneum, unspecified**

▶ *K67*   *Disorders of peritoneum in infectious diseases classified elsewhere* 🔷
     Code first underlying disease, such as:
          congenital syphilis (A50.0)
          helminthiasis (B65.0-B83.9) ◄▥
     Excludes1   peritonitis in chlamydia (A74.81)
                 peritonitis in diphtheria (A36.89)
                 peritonitis in gonococcal (A54.85)
                 peritonitis in syphilis (late) (A52.74)
                 peritonitis in tuberculosis (A18.31)
     (Ex:) See K65

● **K68**   **Disorders of retroperitoneum**
     ● **K68.1**   **Retroperitoneal abscess**
          K68.11   **Postprocedural retroperitoneal abscess** 🔷 🔷
                     (Ex:) D78.81-D78.89, E36.8, E89.810-E89.89, H59.011-H59.019,
                         H59.031-H59.099, H59.811-H59.89, H95.811-H95.89, I97.3,
                         K68.11, L76.81-L76.82, M96.89, N98.1-N98.9, T81.4XX[A],
                         T81.82X[A], T81.89X-T81.9XX[A]

          K68.12   **Psoas muscle abscess** 🔷
                     (Ex:) K68.12, M60.00-M60.19, M61.00-M61.19, M61.30-M61.59,
                         M62.3, M62.50-M62.59, M62.89, M72.6

          K68.19   **Other retroperitoneal abscess** 🔷
                     (Ex:) See K65

     K68.9   **Other disorders of retroperitoneum** 🔷
          (Ex:) See K65

DISEASES OF LIVER (K70-K77)

     Excludes1   jaundice NOS (R17)
     Excludes2   hemochromatosis (E83.11-)
                  Reye's syndrome (G93.7)
                  viral hepatitis (B15-B19)
                  Wilson's disease (E83.0)

● **K70**   **Alcoholic liver disease**
     Use additional code to identify:
          alcohol abuse and dependence (F10.-)

     K70.0   **Alcoholic fatty liver**   A

     ● **K70.1**   **Alcoholic hepatitis**
          K70.10   **Alcoholic hepatitis without ascites**   A
          K70.11   **Alcoholic hepatitis with ascites**   A

     K70.2   **Alcoholic fibrosis and sclerosis of liver**   A

     ● **K70.3**   **Alcoholic cirrhosis of liver**
          Alcoholic cirrhosis NOS
          K70.30   **Alcoholic cirrhosis of liver without ascites**   A
          K70.31   **Alcoholic cirrhosis of liver with ascites**   A

Item 11-20 Cirrhosis is the progressive fibrosis of the liver resulting in loss of liver function. The main causes of cirrhosis of the liver are alcohol abuse, chronic hepatitis (inflammation of the liver), biliary disease, and excessive amounts of iron. **Alcoholic cirrhosis of the liver** is also called portal, Laënnec's, or fatty nutritional cirrhosis.

     ● **K70.4**   **Alcoholic hepatic failure**
          Acute alcoholic hepatic failure
          Alcoholic hepatic failure NOS
          Chronic alcoholic hepatic failure
          Subacute alcoholic hepatic failure
          K70.40   **Alcoholic hepatic failure without coma**   A
          K70.41   **Alcoholic hepatic failure with coma** 🔷   A
                   MCC when PDx is its own MCC
                   (Ex:) K72.91, K76.5, K76.89-K76.9

     K70.9   **Alcoholic liver disease, unspecified**   A

● **K71**   **Toxic liver disease**
     Includes   drug-induced idiosyncratic (unpredictable) liver
                     disease
               drug-induced toxic (predictable) liver disease
     Code first poisoning due to drug or toxin, if applicable (T36-T65 with
          fifth or sixth character 1-4 or 6)
     Use additional code for adverse effect, if applicable, to identify
          drug (T36-T50 with fifth or sixth character 5)
     Excludes2   alcoholic liver disease (K70.-)
                  Budd-Chiari syndrome (I82.0)

     K71.0   **Toxic liver disease with cholestasis**
          Cholestasis with hepatocyte injury
          'Pure' cholestasis

     ● **K71.1**   **Toxic liver disease with hepatic necrosis**
          Hepatic failure (acute) (chronic) due to drugs
          K71.10   **Toxic liver disease with hepatic necrosis,**
                     without coma
          K71.11   **Toxic liver disease with hepatic necrosis, with**
                     coma 🔷
                     MCC when PDx is its own MCC
                     (Ex:) K72.91, K76.5, K76.89-K76.9

     K71.2   **Toxic liver disease with acute hepatitis**

     K71.3   **Toxic liver disease with chronic persistent hepatitis**

     K71.4   **Toxic liver disease with chronic lobular hepatitis**

     ● **K71.5**   **Toxic liver disease with chronic active hepatitis**
          Toxic liver disease with lupoid hepatitis
          K71.50   **Toxic liver disease with chronic active hepatitis**
                     without ascites
          K71.51   **Toxic liver disease with chronic active hepatitis**
                     with ascites

     K71.6   **Toxic liver disease with hepatitis, not elsewhere classified**

     K71.7   **Toxic liver disease with fibrosis and cirrhosis of liver**

     K71.8   **Toxic liver disease with other disorders of liver**
          Toxic liver disease with focal nodular hyperplasia
          Toxic liver disease with hepatic granulomas
          Toxic liver disease with peliosis hepatis
          Toxic liver disease with veno-occlusive disease of liver

     K71.9   **Toxic liver disease, unspecified**

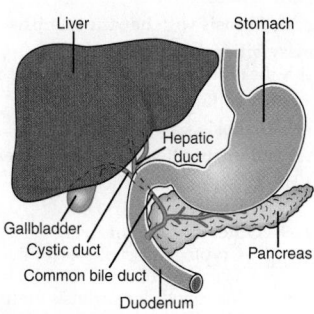

Figure 11-12   Liver and bile ducts.

N Newborn Age: 0   **P** Pediatric Age: 0–17   **M** Maternity DX: 12–55   **A** Adult Age: 15–124   ♀ Females Only   ♂ Males Only

🔷 Complication\Comorbidity   🔷 Major C\C   (Ex:) CC/MCC Exclusions   🔷 Present on Admission Requirement   🔷 Hospital-Acquired Condition

1039

CHAPTER 11 (K00-K95)

● **K72** **Hepatic failure, not elsewhere classified**

   Includes　acute hepatitis NEC, with hepatic failure
        fulminant hepatitis NEC, with hepatic failure
        hepatic encephalopathy NOS
        liver (cell) necrosis with hepatic failure
        malignant hepatitis NEC, with hepatic failure
        yellow liver atrophy or dystrophy

   Excludes1　alcoholic hepatic failure (K70.4)
       ~~hepatic failure complicating abortion or ectopic~~
         ~~or molar pregnancy (O00-O07, O08.8)~~
       ~~hepatic failure complicating pregnancy, childbirth~~
         ~~and the puerperium (O26.6-)~~
       hepatic failure with toxic liver disease (K71.1-)
       icterus of newborn (P55-P59)
       postprocedural hepatic failure (K91.82)
       viral hepatitis with hepatic coma (B15-B19)

   Excludes2　hepatic failure complicating abortion or ectopic
        or molar pregnancy (O00-O07, O08.8) ◄
       hepatic failure complicating pregnancy, childbirth
        and the puerperium (O26.6-) ◄

● **K72.0** **Acute and subacute hepatic failure**
    Ex For category **K72.0** CC codes: K72.00-K72.01, K76.2-K76.3, K76.5,
      K76.89-K76.9

   K72.00　**Acute and subacute hepatic failure without coma** 🐾

   K72.01　**Acute and subacute hepatic failure with coma** 🐾
      MCC when PDx is its own MCC

● **K72.1** **Chronic hepatic failure**
   K72.10　**Chronic hepatic failure without coma**
   K72.11　**Chronic hepatic failure with coma** 🐾
      MCC when PDx is its own MCC
      Ex K72.91, K76.5, K76.89-K76.9

● **K72.9** **Hepatic failure, unspecified**
   K72.90　**Hepatic failure, unspecified without coma**
   K72.91　**Hepatic failure, unspecified with coma** 🐾
      Hepatic coma NOS
      Ex K72.91, K76.5, K76.89-K76.9

● **K73** **Chronic hepatitis, not elsewhere classified**

   Excludes1　alcoholic hepatitis (chronic) (K70.1-)
       drug-induced hepatitis (chronic) (K71.-)
       granulomatous hepatitis (chronic) NEC (K75.3)
       reactive, nonspecific hepatitis (chronic) (K75.2)
       viral hepatitis (chronic) (B15-B19)

  K73.0 **Chronic persistent hepatitis, not elsewhere classified**
  K73.1 **Chronic lobular hepatitis, not elsewhere classified**
  K73.2 **Chronic active hepatitis, not elsewhere classified**
  K73.8 **Other chronic hepatitis, not elsewhere classified**
  K73.9 **Chronic hepatitis, unspecified**

● **K74** **Fibrosis and cirrhosis of liver**
   Code also, if applicable, viral hepatitis (acute) (chronic) (B15-B19)
   Excludes1　alcoholic cirrhosis (of liver) (K70.3)
       alcoholic fibrosis of liver (K70.2)
       cardiac sclerosis of liver (K76.1)
       cirrhosis (of liver) with toxic liver disease (K71.7)
       congenital cirrhosis (of liver) (P78.81)
       pigmentary cirrhosis (of liver) (E83.110)

  K74.0 **Hepatic fibrosis**
  K74.1 **Hepatic sclerosis**
  K74.2 **Hepatic fibrosis with hepatic sclerosis**
  K74.3 **Primary biliary cirrhosis**
     Chronic nonsuppurative destructive cholangitis
  K74.4 **Secondary biliary cirrhosis**
  K74.5 **Biliary cirrhosis, unspecified**
● **K74.6** **Other and unspecified cirrhosis of liver**
   K74.60　**Unspecified cirrhosis of liver**
      Cirrhosis (of liver) NOS

   K74.69　**Other cirrhosis of liver**
      Cryptogenic cirrhosis (of liver)
      Macronodular cirrhosis (of liver)
      Micronodular cirrhosis (of liver)
      Mixed type cirrhosis (of liver)
      Portal cirrhosis (of liver)
      Postnecrotic cirrhosis (of liver)

● **K75** **Other inflammatory liver diseases**
   Excludes2　toxic liver disease (K71.-)
  K75.0 **Abscess of liver** 🐾
     Cholangitic hepatic abscess
     Hematogenic hepatic abscess
     Hepatic abscess NOS
     Lymphogenic hepatic abscess
     Pylephlebitic hepatic abscess
   Excludes1　amebic liver abscess (A06.4)
       cholangitis without liver abscess (K83.0)
       pylephlebitis without liver abscess
        (K75.1)
    Ex A06.4, K75.0-K75.1, K76.5, K76.89-K76.9

  K75.1 **Phlebitis of portal vein** 🐾
     Pylephlebitis
   Excludes1　pylephlebitic liver abscess (K75.0)
    Ex A06.4, K75.0-K75.1, K76.5, K76.89-K76.9

  K75.2 **Nonspecific reactive hepatitis**
   Excludes1　acute or subacute hepatitis (K72.0-)
       chronic hepatitis NEC (K73.-)
       viral hepatitis (B15-B19)

  K75.3 **Granulomatous hepatitis, not elsewhere classified**
   Excludes1　acute or subacute hepatitis (K72.0-)
       chronic hepatitis NEC (K73.-)
       viral hepatitis (B15-B19)

  K75.4 **Autoimmune hepatitis**
     Lupoid hepatitis NEC

● **K75.8** **Other specified inflammatory liver diseases**
   K75.81　**Nonalcoholic steatohepatitis (NASH)**
   K75.89　**Other specified inflammatory liver diseases**

  K75.9 **Inflammatory liver disease, unspecified**
     Hepatitis NOS
   Excludes1　acute or subacute hepatitis (K72.0-)
       chronic hepatitis NEC (K73.-)
       viral hepatitis (B15-B19)

● **K76** **Other diseases of liver**
   Excludes2　alcoholic liver disease (K70.-)
       amyloid degeneration of liver (E85.-) ◄▥
       cystic disease of liver (congenital) (Q44.6)
       hepatic vein thrombosis (I82.0)
       hepatomegaly NOS (R16.0)
       pigmentary cirrhosis (of liver) (E83.110)
       portal vein thrombosis (I81)
       toxic liver disease (K71.-)

  K76.0 **Fatty (change of) liver, not elsewhere classified**
     Nonalcoholic fatty liver disease (NAFLD)
   Excludes1　nonalcoholic steatohepatitis (NASH)
       (K75.81)

  K76.1 **Chronic passive congestion of liver**
     Cardiac cirrhosis
     Cardiac sclerosis

  K76.2 **Central hemorrhagic necrosis of liver** 🐾
   Excludes1　liver necrosis with hepatic failure (K72.-)
    Ex K72.00-K72.01, K76.2-K76.3, K76.5, K76.89-K76.9

  K76.3 **Infarction of liver** 🐾
    Ex See K76.2

  K76.4 **Peliosis hepatis**
     Hepatic angiomatosis

  K76.5 **Hepatic veno-occlusive disease**
   Excludes1　Budd-Chiari syndrome (I82.0)

  K76.6 **Portal hypertension** 🐾
    Use additional code for any associated complications,
      such as:
      portal hypertensive gastropathy (K31.89)
    Ex K72.91, K76.5-K76.6, K76.89-K76.9

  K76.7 **Hepatorenal syndrome** 🐾
   Excludes1　hepatorenal syndrome following labor
       and delivery (O90.4)
       postprocedural hepatorenal syndrome
        (K91.82)
    Ex K76.5, K76.7, K76.89-K76.9

◄ New　◄▥ Revised　~~deleted~~ Deleted　Excludes 1　Excludes 2　Includes　Use additional　Code first　Code also　Unspecified

OGCR Official Guidelines　● Unacceptable Principal Diagnosis　X Assign placeholder X　🐾 Use Additional Character(s)　▶ Manifestation Code　**Coding Clinic**

● **K76.8 Other specified diseases of liver**

  ● **K76.81 Hepatopulmonary syndrome**
      Code first underlying liver disease, such as:
        alcoholic cirrhosis of liver (K70.3-)
        cirrhosis of liver without mention of alcohol
          (K74.6-)

  K76.89 Other specified diseases of liver
      Cyst (simple) of liver
      Focal nodular hyperplasia of liver
      Hepatoptosis

K76.9 Liver disease, unspecified

▌*K77 Liver disorders in diseases classified elsewhere* 🦠

  Code first underlying disease, such as:
    amyloidosis (E85.-) ◀▯▯
    congenital syphilis (A50.0, A50.5)
    congenital toxoplasmosis (P37.1)
    schistosomiasis (B65.0-B65.9)

   Excludes1   alcoholic hepatitis (K70.1-)
           alcoholic liver disease (K70.-)
           cytomegaloviral hepatitis (B25.1)
           herpesviral [herpes simplex] hepatitis (B00.81)
           infectious mononucleosis with liver disease
             (B27.0-B27.9 with .9)
           mumps hepatitis (B26.81)
           sarcoidosis with liver disease (D86.89)
           secondary syphilis with liver disease (A51.45)
           syphilis (late) with liver disease (A52.74)
           toxoplasmosis (acquired) hepatitis (B58.1)
           tuberculosis with liver disease (A18.83)

  Ⓔⓧ No exclusions

DISORDERS OF GALLBLADDER, BILIARY TRACT AND PANCREAS (K80–K87)

● **K80 Cholelithiasis**
  Presence or formation of gallstones

   Excludes1   retained cholelithiasis following cholecystectomy
           (K91.86)

  ● **K80.0 Calculus of gallbladder with acute cholecystitis**
    Any condition listed in K80.2 with acute cholecystitis
    Check documentation for acute/chronic gallbladder/common
     bile duct either with or without obstruction.

    K80.00 Calculus of gallbladder with acute cholecystitis
       without obstruction 🦠
       Ⓔⓧ K80.00-K80.21, K80.40, K80.44, K80.62-K80.63,
          K80.66-K80.67, K80.80, K81.0-K81.9, K82.9, K83.5-K83.9,
          K87

    K80.01 Calculus of gallbladder with acute cholecystitis
       with obstruction 🦠
       Ⓔⓧ K80.00-K80.21, K80.62-K80.63, K80.66-K80.67, K80.80,
          K81.0-K81.9, K82.9, K83.5-K83.9, K87

  ● **K80.1 Calculus of gallbladder with other cholecystitis**
    Ⓔⓧ **For category K80.1 CC codes unless otherwise indicated:** See K80.01

    K80.10 Calculus of gallbladder with chronic
       cholecystitis without obstruction 🦠
       Cholelithiasis with cholecystitis NOS

    K80.11 Calculus of gallbladder with chronic
       cholecystitis with obstruction 🦠

    K80.12 Calculus of gallbladder with acute and chronic
       cholecystitis without obstruction 🦠
       Ⓔⓧ See K80.00

    K80.13 Calculus of gallbladder with acute and chronic
       cholecystitis with obstruction 🦠

    K80.18 Calculus of gallbladder with other cholecystitis
       without obstruction 🦠

    K80.19 Calculus of gallbladder with other cholecystitis
       with obstruction 🦠

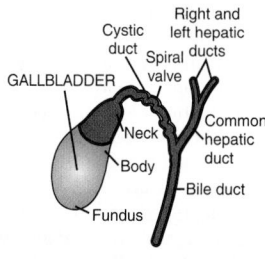

Figure 11-13   Gallbladder and bile ducts.

  ● **K80.2 Calculus of gallbladder without cholecystitis**
    Cholecystolithiasis without cholecystitis
    Cholelithiasis (without cholecystitis)
    Colic (recurrent) of gallbladder (without cholecystitis)
    Gallstone (impacted) of cystic duct (without
      cholecystitis)
    Gallstone (impacted) of gallbladder (without
      cholecystitis)

    K80.20 Calculus of gallbladder without cholecystitis
       without obstruction

    K80.21 Calculus of gallbladder without cholecystitis
       with obstruction 🦠
       Ⓔⓧ See K80.01

  ● **K80.3 Calculus of bile duct with cholangitis**
    Any condition listed in K80.5 with cholangitis

    K80.30 Calculus of bile duct with cholangitis,
       unspecified, without obstruction 🦠
       CC when PDx is its own CC
       Ⓔⓧ K83.0, K83.5-K83.9, K87

    K80.31 Calculus of bile duct with cholangitis,
       unspecified, with obstruction 🦠
       CC when PDx is its own CC
       Ⓔⓧ K80.30-K80.71, K80.81-K81.9, K83.5-K83.9, K87

    K80.32 Calculus of bile duct with acute cholangitis
       without obstruction 🦠
       CC when PDx is its own CC
       Ⓔⓧ See K80.30

    K80.33 Calculus of bile duct with acute cholangitis
       with obstruction 🦠
       CC when PDx is its own CC
       Ⓔⓧ See K80.31

    K80.34 Calculus of bile duct with chronic cholangitis
       without obstruction 🦠
       CC when PDx is its own CC
       Ⓔⓧ See K80.30

    K80.35 Calculus of bile duct with chronic cholangitis
       with obstruction 🦠
       CC when PDx is its own CC
       Ⓔⓧ See K80.31

    K80.36 Calculus of bile duct with acute and chronic
       cholangitis without obstruction 🦠
       CC when PDx is its own CC
       Ⓔⓧ See K80.30

    K80.37 Calculus of bile duct with acute and chronic
       cholangitis with obstruction 🦠
       CC when PDx is its own CC
       Ⓔⓧ See K80.31

  ● **K80.4 Calculus of bile duct with cholecystitis**
    Any condition listed in K80.5 with cholecystitis (with
     cholangitis)
    Ⓔⓧ **For category K80.4 CC codes:** K80.30-K80.71, K80.81-K81.9,
      K83.5-K83.9, K87

    K80.40 Calculus of bile duct with cholecystitis,
       unspecified, without obstruction 🦠

    K80.41 Calculus of bile duct with cholecystitis,
       unspecified, with obstruction 🦠

N Newborn Age: 0   **P** Pediatric Age: 0–17   **M** Maternity DX: 12–55   **A** Adult Age: 15–124   ♀ Females Only   ♂ Males Only

🦠 Complication\Comorbidity   🦠 Major C\C   Ⓔⓧ CC/MCC Exclusions   🦠 Present on Admission Requirement   🦠 Hospital-Acquired Condition

1041

K80.42　Calculus of bile duct with acute cholecystitis without obstruction 🔍

K80.43　Calculus of bile duct with acute cholecystitis with obstruction 🔍

K80.44　Calculus of bile duct with chronic cholecystitis without obstruction 🔍

K80.45　Calculus of bile duct with chronic cholecystitis with obstruction 🔍

K80.46　Calculus of bile duct with acute and chronic cholecystitis without obstruction 🔍

K80.47　Calculus of bile duct with acute and chronic cholecystitis with obstruction 🔍

● K80.5　Calculus of bile duct without cholangitis or cholecystitis
　　Choledocholithiasis (without cholangitis or cholecystitis)
　　Gallstone (impacted) of bile duct NOS (without cholangitis or cholecystitis)
　　Gallstone (impacted) of common duct (without cholangitis or cholecystitis)
　　Gallstone (impacted) of hepatic duct (without cholangitis or cholecystitis)
　　Hepatic cholelithiasis (without cholangitis or cholecystitis)
　　Hepatic colic (recurrent) (without cholangitis or cholecystitis)

K80.50　Calculus of bile duct without cholangitis or cholecystitis without obstruction

K80.51　Calculus of bile duct without cholangitis or cholecystitis with obstruction 🔍
　　　　Ex: See K80.4

● K80.6　Calculus of gallbladder and bile duct with cholecystitis

K80.60　Calculus of gallbladder and bile duct with cholecystitis, unspecified, without obstruction 🔍
　　　　Ex: See K80.4

K80.61　Calculus of gallbladder and bile duct with cholecystitis, unspecified, with obstruction 🔍
　　　　Ex: See K80.4

K80.62　Calculus of gallbladder and bile duct with acute cholecystitis without obstruction 🔍
　　　　Ex: K80.62-K80.63, K81.0-K81.9, K82.9, K83.5-K83.9, K87

K80.63　Calculus of gallbladder and bile duct with acute cholecystitis with obstruction 🔍
　　　　Ex: See K80.62

K80.64　Calculus of gallbladder and bile duct with chronic cholecystitis without obstruction 🔍
　　　　Ex: See K80.4

K80.65　Calculus of gallbladder and bile duct with chronic cholecystitis with obstruction 🔍
　　　　Ex: See K80.4

K80.66　Calculus of gallbladder and bile duct with acute and chronic cholecystitis without obstruction 🔍
　　　　Ex: K80.66-K80.67, K81.0-K81.9, K82.9, K83.5-K83.9, K87

K80.67　Calculus of gallbladder and bile duct with acute and chronic cholecystitis with obstruction 🔍
　　　　Ex: See K80.66

● K80.7　Calculus of gallbladder and bile duct without cholecystitis

K80.70　Calculus of gallbladder and bile duct without cholecystitis without obstruction

K80.71　Calculus of gallbladder and bile duct without cholecystitis with obstruction 🔍
　　　　Ex: See K80.4

● K80.8　Other cholelithiasis

K80.80　Other cholelithiasis without obstruction

K80.81　Other cholelithiasis with obstruction 🔍
　　　　Ex: See K80.4

● K81　Cholecystitis
　　Chronic or acute inflammation of the gallbladder.
　　Excludes1　cholecystitis with cholelithiasis (K80.-)

K81.0　Acute cholecystitis 🔍
　　Abscess of gallbladder
　　Angiocholecystitis
　　Emphysematous (acute) cholecystitis
　　Empyema of gallbladder
　　Gangrene of gallbladder
　　Gangrenous cholecystitis
　　Suppurative cholecystitis
　　Ex: K80.62-K80.63, K80.66-K80.67, K81.0-K81.9, K82.9, K83.5-K83.9, K87

K81.1　Chronic cholecystitis

K81.2　Acute cholecystitis with chronic cholecystitis 🔍
　　Ex: K81.0-K81.9, K82.9, K83.5-K83.9, K87

K81.9　Cholecystitis, unspecified

● K82　Other diseases of gallbladder
　　Excludes1　nonvisualization of gallbladder (R93.2)
　　　　　　　　postcholecystectomy syndrome (K91.5)
　　Ex: For category K82 CC codes: K82.0-K82.9, K83.5-K83.9, K87

K82.0　Obstruction of gallbladder 🔍
　　Occlusion of cystic duct or gallbladder without cholelithiasis
　　Stenosis of cystic duct or gallbladder without cholelithiasis
　　Stricture of cystic duct or gallbladder without cholelithiasis
　　Excludes1　obstruction of gallbladder with cholelithiasis (K80.-)

K82.1　Hydrops of gallbladder 🔍
　　Mucocele of gallbladder

K82.2　Perforation of gallbladder 🔍
　　Rupture of cystic duct or gallbladder

K82.3　Fistula of gallbladder 🔍
　　Cholecystocolic fistula
　　Cholecystoduodenal fistula

K82.4　Cholesterolosis of gallbladder
　　Strawberry gallbladder
　　Excludes1　cholesterolosis of gallbladder with cholecystitis (K81.-)
　　　　　　　　cholesterolosis of gallbladder with cholelithiasis (K80.-)

K82.8　Other specified diseases of gallbladder
　　Adhesions of cystic duct or gallbladder
　　Atrophy of cystic duct or gallbladder
　　Cyst of cystic duct or gallbladder
　　Dyskinesia of cystic duct or gallbladder
　　Hypertrophy of cystic duct or gallbladder
　　Nonfunctioning of cystic duct or gallbladder
　　Ulcer of cystic duct or gallbladder

K82.9　Disease of gallbladder, unspecified

● K83　Other diseases of biliary tract
　　Excludes1　postcholecystectomy syndrome (K91.5)
　　Excludes2　conditions involving the gallbladder (K81-K82)
　　　　　　　　conditions involving the cystic duct (K81-K82)

K83.0　Cholangitis 🔍
　　Ascending cholangitis　　Sclerosing cholangitis
　　Cholangitis NOS　　　　Secondary cholangitis
　　Primary cholangitis　　 Stenosing cholangitis
　　Recurrent cholangitis　 Suppurative cholangitis
　　Excludes1　cholangitic liver abscess (K75.0)
　　　　　　　　cholangitis with choledocholithiasis (K80.3-, K80.4-)
　　　　　　　　chronic nonsuppurative destructive cholangitis (K74.3)
　　Ex: K83.0, K83.5-K83.9, K87

◀ New　◀ⁱⁱⁱ Revised　d̶e̶l̶e̶t̶e̶d̶ Deleted　Excludes 1　Excludes 2　Includes　Use additional　Code first　Code also　Unspecified
OGCR Official Guidelines　● Unacceptable Principal Diagnosis　✗ Assign placeholder X　● Use Additional Character(s)　▶ Manifestation Code　**Coding Clinic**

CHAPTER 11 (K00-K95)

K83.1   **Obstruction of bile duct**
Occlusion of bile duct without cholelithiasis
Stenosis of bile duct without cholelithiasis
Stricture of bile duct without cholelithiasis
> **Excludes1**   congenital obstruction of bile duct (Q44.3)
> obstruction of bile duct with cholelithiasis
> (K80.-)
(Ex) K80.31, K80.33, K80.35, K80.37, K80.41, K80.43, K80.45, K80.47, K80.51,
K80.81, K83.1, K83.5-K83.9, K87, Q44.2-Q44.3

K83.2   **Perforation of bile duct**
Rupture of bile duct
(Ex) K83.2-K83.3, K83.5-K83.9, K87

K83.3   **Fistula of bile duct**
Choledochoduodenal fistula
(Ex) K83.2-K83.3, K83.5-K83.9, K87

K83.4   **Spasm of sphincter of Oddi**

K83.5   **Biliary cyst**

K83.8   **Other specified diseases of biliary tract**
Adhesions of biliary tract
Atrophy of biliary tract
Hypertrophy of biliary tract
Ulcer of biliary tract

K83.9   **Disease of biliary tract, unspecified**

● **K85**   **Acute pancreatitis**
Inflammatory process in which pancreatic enzymes autodigest the gland.
> **Includes**   abscess of pancreas
> acute necrosis of pancreas
> acute (recurrent) pancreatitis
> gangrene of (gangrenous) pancreas
> hemorrhagic pancreatitis
> infective necrosis of pancreas
> subacute pancreatitis
> suppurative pancreatitis
(Ex) For category K85 CC codes: B25.2, K85.0-K86.1, K86.8-K86.9

K85.0   **Idiopathic acute pancreatitis**

K85.1   **Biliary acute pancreatitis**
Gallstone pancreatitis

K85.2   **Alcohol induced acute pancreatitis**
> **Excludes2**   alcohol induced chronic pancreatitis (K86.0)

K85.3   **Drug induced acute pancreatitis**
> Use additional code for adverse effect, if applicable, to identify drug (T36-T50 with fifth or sixth character 5)
> Use additional code to identify drug abuse and dependence (F11.-F17.-) ◄

K85.8   **Other acute pancreatitis**

K85.9   **Acute pancreatitis, unspecified**
Pancreatitis NOS

● **K86**   **Other diseases of pancreas**
> **Excludes2**   fibrocystic disease of pancreas (E84.-)
> islet cell tumor (of pancreas) (D13.7)
> pancreatic steatorrhea (K90.3)

K86.0   **Alcohol-induced chronic pancreatitis**
> Use additional code to identify:
> alcohol abuse and dependence (F10.-)
> **Excludes2**   alcohol induced acute pancreatitis (K85.2)
(Ex) B25.2, E16.8, K85.0-K86.9

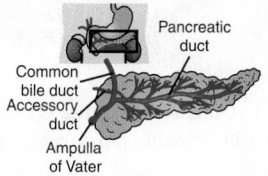

Figure 11-14   Pancreatic ductal system.

K86.1   **Other chronic pancreatitis**
Chronic pancreatitis NOS
Infectious chronic pancreatitis
Recurrent chronic pancreatitis
Relapsing chronic pancreatitis
(Ex) B25.2, E16.8, K85.0-K86.9

K86.2   **Cyst of pancreas**
(Ex) K86.2-K86.9

K86.3   **Pseudocyst of pancreas**
(Ex) K86.2-K86.9

K86.8   **Other specified diseases of pancreas**
Aseptic pancreatic necrosis
Atrophy of pancreas
Calculus of pancreas
Cirrhosis of pancreas
Fibrosis of pancreas
Pancreatic fat necrosis
Pancreatic infantilism
Pancreatic necrosis NOS

K86.9   **Disease of pancreas, unspecified**

▌ **K87**   *Disorders of gallbladder, biliary tract and pancreas in diseases classified elsewhere*
> *Code first* underlying disease
> **Excludes1**   cytomegaloviral pancreatitis (B25.2)
> mumps pancreatitis (B26.3)
> syphilitic gallbladder (A52.74)
> syphilitic pancreas (A52.74)
> tuberculosis of gallbladder (A18.83)
> tuberculosis of pancreas (A18.83)

OTHER DISEASES OF THE DIGESTIVE SYSTEM (K90-K95)

● **K90**   **Intestinal malabsorption**
> **Excludes1**   intestinal malabsorption following gastrointestinal surgery (K91.2)
(Ex) For category K90 cc does unless otherwise indicated: E84.19, K90.0-K90.4,
K90.89-K90.9, K91.2

K90.0   **Celiac disease**
Gluten-sensitive enteropathy
Idiopathic steatorrhea
Nontropical sprue
> Use additional code for associated disorders including: ◄
> dermatitis herpetiformis (L13.0) ◄
> gluten ataxia (G32.81) ◄

K90.1   **Tropical sprue**
Sprue NOS
Tropical steatorrhea

K90.2   **Blind loop syndrome, not elsewhere classified**
Blind loop syndrome NOS
> **Excludes1**   congenital blind loop syndrome (Q43.8)
> postsurgical blind loop syndrome (K91.2)

K90.3   **Pancreatic steatorrhea**

K90.4   **Malabsorption due to intolerance, not elsewhere classified**
Malabsorption due to intolerance to carbohydrate
Malabsorption due to intolerance to fat
Malabsorption due to intolerance to protein
Malabsorption due to intolerance to starch
> **Excludes2**   gluten-sensitive enteropathy (K90.0)
> lactose intolerance (E73.-)

● **K90.8**   **Other intestinal malabsorption**
     K90.81   **Whipple's disease**
         (Ex) K90.81
     K90.89   **Other intestinal malabsorption**

K90.9   **Intestinal malabsorption, unspecified**

CHAPTER 11 (K00-K95)

N   Newborn Age: 0   P   Pediatric Age: 0–17   M   Maternity DX: 12–55   A   Adult Age: 15–124   ♀   Females Only   ♂   Males Only
Complication\Comorbidity   Major C\C   (Ex)   CC/MCC Exclusions   Present on Admission Requirement   Hospital-Acquired Condition

● K91   Intraoperative and postprocedural complications and disorders of digestive system, not elsewhere classified

Excludes2   complications of artificial opening of digestive system (K94.-)
complications of bariatric procedures (K95.-)
gastrojejunal ulcer (K28.-)
postprocedural (radiation) retroperitoneal abscess (K68.11)
radiation colitis (K52.0)
radiation gastroenteritis (K52.0)
radiation proctitis (K62.7)

K91.0   Vomiting following gastrointestinal surgery

K91.1   Postgastric surgery syndromes
Dumping syndrome
Postgastrectomy syndrome
Postvagotomy syndrome

K91.2   Postsurgical malabsorption, not elsewhere classified 🔖
Postsurgical blind loop syndrome
Excludes1   malabsorption osteomalacia in adults (M83.2)
malabsorption osteoporosis, postsurgical (M80.8-, M81.8)
(Ex:) K90.3-K90.4, K90.89-K90.9, K91.2

K91.3   Postprocedural intestinal obstruction 🔖
(Ex:) D78.81-D78.89, E36.8, E89.810-E89.89, H59.011-H59.019, H59.031-H59.099, H59.811-H59.89, H95.811-H95.89, I97.3, K91.3, K91.81-K91.83, K91.850-K91.89, K94.20-K95.89, L76.81-L76.82, M96.89, N98.1-N98.9, T81.710[A], T81.82X[A], T81.89X-T81.9XX[A]

K91.5   Postcholecystectomy syndrome

● K91.6   Intraoperative hemorrhage and hematoma of a digestive system organ or structure complicating a procedure
Excludes1   intraoperative hemorrhage and hematoma of a digestive system organ or structure due to accidental puncture and laceration during a procedure (K91.7-)
(Ex:) For category K91.6 CC codes: H95.811-H95.89, I85.01, I85.11, I97.3, K21.9, K22.8, K23-K25.0, K25.2, K25.4, K25.6, K26.0, K26.2, K26.4, K26.6, K27.0, K27.2, K27.4, K27.6, K28.0, K28.2, K28.4, K28.6, K29.01, K29.21, K29.31, K29.41, K29.51, K29.61, K29.71, K29.81, K29.91, K31.811, K55.21, K57.01, K57.11, K57.13, K57.21, K57.31, K57.33, K57.41, K57.51, K57.53, K57.81, K57.91, K57.93, K62.5, K91.61-K91.62, K91.840-K91.841, K92.0-K92.2, M96.89, N98.1-N98.9, P54.1-P54.3, T81.10X-T81.19X[A], T81.82X[A], T81.89X-T81.9XX[A]

K91.61   Intraoperative hemorrhage and hematoma of a digestive system organ or structure complicating a digestive sytem procedure 🔖

K91.62   Intraoperative hemorrhage and hematoma of a digestive system organ or structure complicating other procedure 🔖

● K91.7   Accidental puncture and laceration of a digestive system organ or structure during a procedure
(Ex:) For category K91.7 CC codes: D78.11-D78.12, D78.81-D78.89, E36.11-E36.8, E89.810-E89.89, G96.11, G97.41-G97.49, H59.011-H59.019, H59.031-H59.099, H59.211-H59.229, H59.811-H59.89, H95.31-H95.32, H95.811-H95.89, I97.3, I97.51-I97.52, J95.71-J95.72, K91.71-K91.72, L76.11-L76.12, L76.81-L76.82, M96.820-M96.821, M96.89, N98.1-N98.9, N99.71-N99.72, T81.82X[A], T81.89X-T81.9XX[A]

K91.71   Accidental puncture and laceration of a digestive system organ or structure during a digestive system procedure 🔖

K91.72   Accidental puncture and laceration of a digestive system organ or structure during other procedure 🔖

● K91.8   Other intraoperative and postprocedural complications and disorders of digestive system
(Ex:) For category K91.8 CC codes unless otherwise indicated: See K91.3

K91.81   Other intraoperative complications of digestive system 🔖

K91.82   Postprocedural hepatic failure 🔖

K91.83   Postprocedural hepatorenal syndrome 🔖

● K91.84   Postprocedural hemorrhage and hematoma of a digestive system organ or structure following a procedure
(Ex:) For category K91.84 CC codes: K96.1

K91.840   Postprocedural hemorrhage and hematoma of a digestive system organ or structure following a digestive system procedure 🔖

K91.841   Postprocedural hemorrhage and hematoma of a digestive system organ or structure following other procedure 🔖

● K91.85   Complications of intestinal pouch

K91.850   Pouchitis 🔖
Inflammation of internal ileoanal pouch

K91.858   Other complications of intestinal pouch 🔖

K91.86   Retained cholelithiasis following cholecystectomy 🔖

K91.89   Other postprocedural complications and disorders of digestive system 🔖
Use additional code, if applicable, to further specify disorder
Excludes2   postprocedural retroperitoneal abscess (K68.11)

● K92   Other diseases of digestive system
Excludes1   neonatal gastrointestinal hemorrhage (P54.0-P54.3)
(Ex:) For category K92 CC codes unless otherwise indicated: E16.4, I85.01, K22.10-K22.11, K22.6-K22.719, K25.0-K28.9, K29.01, K29.21, K29.31, K29.41, K29.51, K29.61, K29.71, K29.81, K29.91, K31.811, K55.21, K57.01, K57.11, K57.13, K57.21, K57.31, K57.33, K57.41, K57.51, K57.53, K57.81, K57.91, K57.93, K62.5, K92.0-K92.2

K92.0   Hematemesis 🔖

K92.1   Melena 🔖
Excludes1   occult blood in feces (R19.5)

K92.2   Gastrointestinal hemorrhage, unspecified 🔖
Gastric hemorrhage NOS
Intestinal hemorrhage NOS
Excludes1   acute hemorrhagic gastritis (K29.01)
hemorrhage of anus and rectum (K62.5)
angiodysplasia of stomach with hemorrhage (K31.811)
diverticular disease with hemorrhage (K57.-)
gastritis and duodenitis with hemorrhage (K29.-)
peptic ulcer with hemorrhage (K25-K28)

● K92.8   Other specified diseases of the digestive system

K92.81   Gastrointestinal mucositis (ulcerative) 🔖
Code also type of associated therapy, such as: antineoplastic and immunosuppressive drugs (T45.1X-) ◀▥
radiological procedure and radiotherapy (Y84.2)
Excludes2   mucositis (ulcerative) of vagina and vulva (N76.81)
nasal mucositis (ulcerative) (J34.81)
oral mucositis (ulcerative) (K12.3-)
(Ex:) E16.4, I85.01, K22.10-K22.11, K22.6-K22.719, K25.0-K28.9, K29.01, K29.21, K29.31, K29.41, K29.51, K29.61, K29.71, K29.81, K29.91, K31.811, K31.89-K31.9, K55.21, K57.01, K57.11, K57.13, K57.21, K57.31, K57.33, K57.41, K57.51, K57.53, K57.81, K57.91, K57.93, K62.5, K92.0-K92.81

K92.89   Other specified diseases of the digestive system

K92.9   Disease of digestive system, unspecified

◀ New   ◀▥ Revised   ̶d̶e̶l̶e̶t̶e̶d̶ Deleted   Excludes 1   Excludes 2   Includes   Use additional   Code first   Code also   Unspecified

OGCR Official Guidelines   ● Unacceptable Principal Diagnosis   X Assign placeholder X   ● Use Additional Character(s)   ▌ Manifestation Code   Coding Clinic

● **K94   Complications of artificial openings of the digestive system**
  ● **K94.0   Colostomy complications**
    (Ex) **For category K94.0 CC does unless otherwise indicated:**
         K94.00-K94.19
    K94.00   Colostomy complication, unspecified
    K94.01   Colostomy hemorrhage 🔗
    K94.02   Colostomy infection 🔗
         Use additional code to specify type of
            infection, such as:
              cellulitis of abdominal wall (L03.311)
              sepsis (A40.-, A41.-)
    K94.03   Colostomy malfunction 🔗
         Mechanical complication of colostomy
        (Ex) D78.81-D78.89, E36.8, E89.810-E89.89, H59.011-H59.019,
              H59.031-H59.099, H59.811-H59.89, H95.811-H95.89, I97.3,
              K91.3, K91.81-K91.83, K91.850-K91.89, K94.00-K95.89,
              L76.81-L76.82, M96.89, N98.1-N98.9, T81.710[A], T81.82X[A],
              T81.89X-T81.9XX[A]
    K94.09   Other complications of colostomy 🔗
  ● **K94.1   Enterostomy complications**
    (Ex) **For category K94.1 CC does unless otherwise indicated:**
         K94.00-K94.19
    K94.10   Enterostomy complication, unspecified
    K94.11   Enterostomy hemorrhage 🔗
    K94.12   Enterostomy infection 🔗
         Use additional code to specify type of
            infection, such as:
             cellulitis of abdominal wall (L03.311)
             sepsis (A40.-, A41.-)
    K94.13   Enterostomy malfunction 🔗
         Mechanical complication of enterostomy
        (Ex) See K94.03
    K94.19   Other complications of enterostomy 🔗
  ● **K94.2   Gastrostomy complications**
    K94.20   Gastrostomy complication, unspecified
    K94.21   Gastrostomy hemorrhage
    K94.22   Gastrostomy infection 🔗
         Use additional code to specify type of
            infection, such as:
             cellulitis of abdominal wall (L03.311)
             sepsis (A40.-, A41.-)
        (Ex) See K91.3
    K94.23   Gastrostomy malfunction 🔗
         Mechanical complication of gastrostomy
        (Ex) See K91.3
    K94.29   Other complications of gastrostomy

  ● **K94.3   Esophagostomy complications**
    (Ex) **For category K94.3 CC codes:** See K91.3
    K94.30   Esophagostomy complications, unspecified 🔗
    K94.31   Esophagostomy hemorrhage 🔗
    K94.32   Esophagostomy infection 🔗
         Use additional code to identify the infection
    K94.33   Esophagostomy malfunction 🔗
         Mechanical complication of esophagostomy
    K94.39   Other complications of esophagostomy 🔗
● **K95   Complications of bariatric procedures**
    (Ex) **For category K95 CC codes:** See K91.3
  ● **K95.0   Complications of gastric band procedure**
    K95.01   Infection due to gastric band procedure 🔗 🔗
         Use additional code to specify type of infection
            or organism, such as:
            bacterial and viral infectious agents
              (B95.-, B96.-) ◀▥
            cellulitis of abdominal wall (L03.311)
            sepsis (A40.-, A41.-)
    **K95.09   Other complications of gastric band
         procedure** 🔗
         Use additional code, if applicable, to further
            specify complication
  ● **K95.8   Complications of other bariatric procedure**
    Excludes1   complications of gastric band surgery
                 (K95.0-)
    K95.81   Infection due to other bariatric procedure 🔗 🔗
         Use additional code to specify type of infection
            or organism, such as:
            bacterial and viral infectious agents
              (B95.-, B96.-) ◀▥
            cellulitis of abdominal wall (L03.311)
            sepsis (A40.-, A41.-)
    **K95.89   Other complications of other bariatric
         procedure** 🔗
         Use additional code, if applicable, to further
            specify complication

CHAPTER 11 (K00-K95)

N   Newborn Age: 0   P   Pediatric Age: 0–17   M   Maternity DX: 12–55   A   Adult Age: 15–124   ♀   Females Only   ♂   Males Only

🔗 Complication\Comorbidity   🔗 Major C\C   (Ex) CC/MCC Exclusions   🔗 Present on Admission Requirement   🔗 Hospital-Acquired Condition

1045

Carbuncle   Furuncle   Deep folliculitis   Superficial folliculitis

A   B

Figure 12-1   Furuncle, also known as a boil, is a staphylococcal infection. The organism enters the body through a hair follicle and so furuncles usually appear in hairy areas of the body. A cluster of furuncles is known as a carbuncle and involves infection into the deep subcutaneous fascia. These usually appear on the back and neck. (**B** from Habif: Clinical Dermatology, ed 5, Mosby, 2009)

CHAPTER 12

DISEASES OF THE SKIN AND SUBCUTANEOUS TISSUE (L00-L99)

Excludes2   certain conditions originating in the perinatal period (P04-P96)
certain infectious and parasitic diseases (A00-B99)
complications of pregnancy, childbirth and the puerperium (O00-O9A)
congenital malformations, deformations, and chromosomal abnormalities (Q00-Q99)
endocrine, nutritional and metabolic diseases (E00-E88)
lipomelanotic reticulosis (I89.8)
neoplasms (C00-D49)
symptoms, signs and abnormal clinical and laboratory findings, not elsewhere classified (R00-R94)
systemic connective tissue disorders (M30-M36)
viral warts (B07.-)

This chapter contains the following blocks:

L00-L08	Infections of the skin and subcutaneous tissue
L10-L14	Bullous disorders
L20-L30	Dermatitis and eczema
L40-L45	Papulosquamous disorders
L49-L54	Urticaria and erythema
L55-L59	Radiation-related disorders of the skin and subcutaneous tissue
L60-L75	Disorders of skin appendages
L76	Intraoperative and postprocedural complications of skin and subcutaneous tissue
L80-L99	Other disorders of the skin and subcutaneous tissue

INFECTIONS OF THE SKIN AND SUBCUTANEOUS TISSUE (L00-L08)

Use additional code (B95-B97) to identify infectious agent.

Excludes2   hordeolum (H00.0)
infective dermatitis (L30.3)
local infections of skin classified in Chapter 1
lupus panniculitis (L93.2)
panniculitis NOS (M79.3)
panniculitis of neck and back (M54.0-)
Perlèche NOS (K13.0)
Perlèche due to candidiasis (B37.0)
Perlèche due to riboflavin deficiency (E53.0)
pyogenic granuloma (L98.0)
relapsing panniculitis [Weber-Christian] (M35.6)
viral warts (B07.-)
zoster (B02.-)

L00   **Staphylococcal scalded skin syndrome**
Ritter's disease
Use additional code to identify percentage of skin exfoliation (L49.-) ◀▥

     Excludes1   bullous impetigo (L01.03)
pemphigus neonatorum (L01.03)
toxic epidermal necrolysis [Lyell] (L51.2)

● **L01**   **Impetigo**
Contagious skin infection caused by a streptococcus or staphylococcus aureus, common skin infections among children.

     Excludes1   impetigo herpetiformis (L40.1)

● **L01.0**   **Impetigo**
Impetigo contagiosa
Impetigo vulgaris

     L01.00   **Impetigo, unspecified**
Impetigo NOS

     L01.01   **Non-bullous impetigo**

     L01.02   **Bockhart's impetigo**
Impetigo follicularis
Perifolliculitis NOS
Superficial pustular perifolliculitis

     L01.03   **Bullous impetigo**
Impetigo neonatorum
Pemphigus neonatorum
Neonate = newborn

     L01.09   **Other impetigo**
Ulcerative impetigo

    L01.1   **Impetiginization of other dermatoses**

● **L02**   **Cutaneous abscess, furuncle and carbuncle**
Use additional code to identify organism (B95-B96)

     Excludes2   abscess of anus and rectal regions (K61.-)
abscess of female genital organs (external) (N76.4)
abscess of male genital organs (external) (N48.2, N49.-)

● **L02.0**   **Cutaneous abscess, furuncle and carbuncle of face**

     Excludes2   abscess of ear, external (H60.0)
abscess of eyelid (H00.0)
abscess of head [any part, except face] (L02.8)
abscess of lacrimal gland (H04.0)
abscess of lacrimal passages (H04.3)
abscess of mouth (K12.2)
abscess of nose (J34.0)
abscess of orbit (H05.0)
submandibular abscess (K12.2)

     L02.01   **Cutaneous abscess of face** ✎
       Ⓔⓧ No exclusions

     L02.02   **Furuncle of face**
Boil of face
Folliculitis of face

     L02.03   **Carbuncle of face**

◀ New   ◀▥ Revised   ~~deleted~~ Deleted   Excludes 1   Excludes 2   Includes   Use additional   Code first   Code also   Unspecified
OGCR Official Guidelines   ● Unacceptable Principal Diagnosis   X Assign placeholder X   ● Use Additional Character(s)   ▶ Manifestation Code   **Coding Clinic**

● **L02.1** **Cutaneous abscess, furuncle and carbuncle of neck**

L02.11 **Cutaneous abscess of neck** 🖲
(Ex) A17.9, A18.4, A18.82, A18.84, A18.89, A48.2-A48.4, A48.8-A49.9, B78.1, B95.0-B96.89, E83.2, L02.11, L02.811-L02.818, L02.91, L03.221-L03.222, L03.811-L03.91, L08.0-L08.9, L44.8-L45, L73.2, L88, L92.8, L94.2, L94.4, L98.0, L98.3, L98.8, L99, Z16.10-Z16.39

L02.12 **Furuncle of neck**
Boil of neck
Folliculitis of neck

L02.13 **Carbuncle of neck**

● **L02.2** **Cutaneous abscess, furuncle and carbuncle of trunk**

Excludes1   non-newborn omphalitis (L08.82)
omphalitis of newborn (P38.-)

Excludes2   abscess of breast (N61)
abscess of buttocks (L02.3)
abscess of female external genital organs (N76.4)
abscess of male external genital organs (N48.2, N49.-)
abscess of hip (L02.4)

● **L02.21** **Cutaneous abscess of trunk**
(Ex) For category **L02.21** CC codes: A17.9, A18.4, A18.82, A18.84, A18.89, A48.2-A48.4, A48.8-A49.9, B78.1, B95.0-B96.89, E83.2, L02.211-L02.219, L02.811-L02.818, L02.91, L03.311-L03.316, L03.319-L03.326, L03.329-L03.91, L08.0, L08.81-L08.9, L44.8-L45, L73.2, L88, L92.8, L94.2, L94.4, L98.0, L98.3, L98.8, L99, Z16.10-Z16.39

L02.211 **Cutaneous abscess of abdominal wall** 🖲

L02.212 **Cutaneous abscess of back [any part, except buttock]** 🖲

L02.213 **Cutaneous abscess of chest wall** 🖲

L02.214 **Cutaneous abscess of groin** 🖲

L02.215 **Cutaneous abscess of perineum** 🖲

L02.216 **Cutaneous abscess of umbilicus** 🖲

L02.219 **Cutaneous abscess of trunk, unspecified** 🖲

● **L02.22** **Furuncle of trunk**
Boil of trunk
Folliculitis of trunk

L02.221 **Furuncle of abdominal wall**

L02.222 **Furuncle of back [any part, except buttock]**

L02.223 **Furuncle of chest wall**

L02.224 **Furuncle of groin**

L02.225 **Furuncle of perineum**

L02.226 **Furuncle of umbilicus**

L02.229 **Furuncle of trunk, unspecified**

● **L02.23** **Carbuncle of trunk**

L02.231 **Carbuncle of abdominal wall**

L02.232 **Carbuncle of back [any part, except buttock]**

L02.233 **Carbuncle of chest wall**

L02.234 **Carbuncle of groin**

L02.235 **Carbuncle of perineum**

L02.236 **Carbuncle of umbilicus**

L02.239 **Carbuncle of trunk, unspecified**

● **L02.3** **Cutaneous abscess, furuncle and carbuncle of buttock**

Excludes1   pilonidal cyst with abscess (L05.01)

L02.31 **Cutaneous abscess of buttock** 🖲
Cutaneous abscess of gluteal region
(Ex) A17.9, A18.4, A18.82, A18.84, A18.89, A48.2-A48.4, A48.8-A49.9, B78.1, B95.0-B96.89, E83.2, L02.31, L02.811-L02.818, L02.91, L03.317, L03.327, L03.811-L03.91, L08.0, L08.81-L08.9, L44.8-L45, L73.2, L88, L92.8, L94.2, L94.4, L98.0, L98.3, L98.8, L99, Z16.10-Z16.39

L02.32 **Furuncle of buttock**
Boil of buttock
Folliculitis of buttock
Furuncle of gluteal region

L02.33 **Carbuncle of buttock**
Carbuncle of gluteal region

● **L02.4** **Cutaneous abscess, furuncle and carbuncle of limb**

Excludes2   Cutaneous abscess, furuncle and carbuncle of groin (L02.214, L02.224, L02.234)
Cutaneous abscess, furuncle and carbuncle of hand (L02.5-)
Cutaneous abscess, furuncle and carbuncle of foot (L02.6-)

● **L02.41** **Cutaneous abscess of limb**

L02.411 **Cutaneous abscess of right axilla** 🖲
(Ex) A17.9, A18.4, A18.82, A18.84, A18.89, A48.2-A48.4, A48.8-A49.9, B78.1, B95.0-B96.89, E83.2, L02.411-L02.414, L02.811-L02.818, L02.91, L03.111-L03.114, L03.121-L03.124, L03.811-L03.91, L08.0, L08.81-L08.9, L44.8-L45, L73.2, L88, L92.8, L94.2, L94.4, L98.0, L98.3, L98.8, L99, Z16.10-Z16.39

L02.412 **Cutaneous abscess of left axilla** 🖲
(Ex) See L02.411

L02.413 **Cutaneous abscess of right upper limb** 🖲
(Ex) See L02.411

L02.414 **Cutaneous abscess of left upper limb** 🖲
(Ex) See L02.411

L02.415 **Cutaneous abscess of right lower limb** 🖲
(Ex) A17.9, A18.4, A18.82, A18.84, A18.89, A48.2-A48.4, A48.8-A49.9, B78.1, B95.0-B96.89, E83.2, L02.415-L02.419, L02.811-L02.818, L02.91, L03.115-L03.119, L03.125-L03.129, L03.811-L03.91, L08.0, L08.81-L08.9, L44.8-L45, L73.2, L88, L92.8, L94.2, L94.4, L98.0, L98.3, L98.8, L99, Z16.10-Z16.39

L02.416 **Cutaneous abscess of left lower limb** 🖲
(Ex) See L02.415

L02.419 **Cutaneous abscess of limb, unspecified** 🖲
(Ex) See L02.415

● **L02.42** **Furuncle of limb**
Boil of limb
Folliculitis of limb

L02.421 **Furuncle of right axilla**

L02.422 **Furuncle of left axilla**

L02.423 **Furuncle of right upper limb**

L02.424 **Furuncle of left upper limb**

L02.425 **Furuncle of right lower limb**

L02.426 **Furuncle of left lower limb**

L02.429 **Furuncle of limb, unspecified**

● **L02.43** **Carbuncle of limb**

L02.431 **Carbuncle of right axilla**

L02.432 **Carbuncle of left axilla**

L02.433 **Carbuncle of right upper limb**

L02.434 **Carbuncle of left upper limb**

L02.435 **Carbuncle of right lower limb**

L02.436 **Carbuncle of left lower limb**

L02.439 **Carbuncle of limb, unspecified**

CHAPTER 12 (L00-L99)

N   Newborn Age: 0   P   Pediatric Age: 0–17   M   Maternity DX: 12–55   A   Adult Age: 15–124   ♀ Females Only   ♂ Males Only

🖲 Complication\Comorbidity   Major C\C   (Ex) CC/MCC Exclusions   Present on Admission Requirement   Hospital-Acquired Condition

1047

CHAPTER 12 (L00-L99)

- **L02.5 Cutaneous abscess, furuncle and carbuncle of hand**
  - **L02.51 Cutaneous abscess of hand**
    - (Ex) For category L02.51 CC codes: A17.9, A18.4, A18.82, A18.84, A18.89, A48.2-A48.4, A48.8-A49.9, B78.1, B95.0-B96.89, E83.2, L02.511-L02.519, L02.811-L02.818, L02.91, L03.811-L03.91, L08.0, L08.81-L08.9, L44.8-L45, L73.2, L88, L92.8, L94.2, L94.4, L98.0, L98.3, L98.8, L99, Z16.10-Z16.39
    - L02.511 Cutaneous abscess of right hand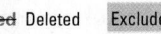
    - L02.512 Cutaneous abscess of left hand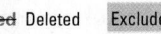
    - L02.519 Cutaneous abscess of unspecified hand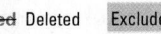
  - **L02.52 Furuncle hand**
    - Boil of hand
    - Folliculitis of hand
    - L02.521 Furuncle right hand
    - L02.522 Furuncle left hand
    - L02.529 Furuncle unspecified hand
  - **L02.53 Carbuncle of hand**
    - L02.531 Carbuncle of right hand
    - L02.532 Carbuncle of left hand
    - L02.539 Carbuncle of unspecified hand
- **L02.6 Cutaneous abscess, furuncle and carbuncle of foot**
  - **L02.61 Cutaneous abscess of foot**
    - (Ex) For category L02.61 CC codes: A17.9, A18.4, A18.82, A18.84, A18.89, A48.2-A48.4, A48.8-A49.9, B78.1, B95.0-B96.89, E83.2, L02.611-L02.619, L02.811-L02.818, L02.91, L03.811-L03.91, L08.0, L08.81-L08.9, L44.8-L45, L73.2, L88, L92.8, L94.2, L94.4, L98.0, L98.3, L98.8, L99, Z16.10-Z16.39
    - L02.611 Cutaneous abscess of right foot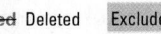
    - L02.612 Cutaneous abscess of left foot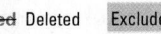
    - L02.619 Cutaneous abscess of unspecified foot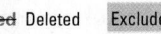
  - **L02.62 Furuncle of foot**
    - Boil of foot
    - Folliculitis of foot
    - L02.621 Furuncle of right foot
    - L02.622 Furuncle of left foot
    - L02.629 Furuncle of unspecified foot
  - **L02.63 Carbuncle of foot**
    - L02.631 Carbuncle of right foot
    - L02.632 Carbuncle of left foot
    - L02.639 Carbuncle of unspecified foot
- **L02.8 Cutaneous abscess, furuncle and carbuncle of other sites**
  - **L02.81 Cutaneous abscess of other sites**
    - (Ex) For category L02.81 CC codes: A17.9, A18.4, A18.82, A18.84, A18.89, A48.2-A48.4, A48.8-A49.9, B78.1, B95.0-B96.89, E83.2, L02.811-L02.818, L02.91, L03.811-L03.91, L08.0, L08.81-L08.9, L44.8-L45, L73.2, L88, L92.8, L94.2, L94.4, L98.0, L98.3, L98.8, L99, Z16.10-Z16.39
    - L02.811 Cutaneous abscess of head [any part, except face]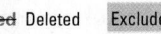
    - L02.818 Cutaneous abscess of other sites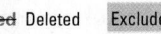
  - **L02.82 Furuncle of other sites**
    - Boil of other sites
    - Folliculitis of other sites
    - L02.821 Furuncle of head [any part, except face]
    - L02.828 Furuncle of other sites
  - **L02.83 Carbuncle of other sites**
    - L02.831 Carbuncle of head [any part, except face]
    - L02.838 Carbuncle of other sites
- **L02.9 Cutaneous abscess, furuncle and carbuncle, unspecified**
  - L02.91 Cutaneous abscess, unspecified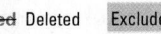
    - (Ex) See L02.81
  - L02.92 Furuncle, unspecified
    - Boil NOS
    - Furunculosis NOS
  - L02.93 Carbuncle, unspecified

Item 12-1 Onychia is an inflammation of the tissue surrounding the nail with pus accumulation and loss of the nail, resulting from microscopic pathogens entering through small wounds. **Paronychia** is a nail disease also known as felon or whitlow and is a bacterial or fungal infection.

- **L03 Cellulitis and acute lymphangitis**
  - Excludes2 cellulitis of anal and rectal region (K61.-)
    - cellulitis of external auditory canal (H60.1)
    - cellulitis of eyelid (H00.0)
    - cellulitis of female external genital organs (N76.4)
    - cellulitis of lacrimal apparatus (H04.3)
    - cellulitis of male external genital organs (N48.2, N49.-)
    - cellulitis of mouth (K12.2)
    - cellulitis of nose (J34.0)
    - eosinophilic cellulitis [Wells] (L98.3)
    - febrile neutrophilic dermatosis [Sweet] (L98.2)
    - lymphangitis (chronic) (subacute) (I89.1)
  - **L03.0 Cellulitis and acute lymphangitis of finger and toe**
    - Infection of nail
    - Onychia
    - Paronychia
    - Perionychia
    - **L03.01 Cellulitis of finger**
      - Felon
      - Whitlow
      - Excludes1 herpetic whitlow (B00.89)
      - L03.011 Cellulitis of right finger
      - L03.012 Cellulitis of left finger
      - L03.019 Cellulitis of unspecified finger
    - **L03.02 Acute lymphangitis of finger**
      - Hangnail with lymphangitis of finger
      - L03.021 Acute lymphangitis of right finger
      - L03.022 Acute lymphangitis of left finger
      - L03.029 Acute lymphangitis of unspecified finger
    - **L03.03 Cellulitis of toe**
      - L03.031 Cellulitis of right toe
      - L03.032 Cellulitis of left toe
      - L03.039 Cellulitis of unspecified toe
    - **L03.04 Acute lymphangitis of toe**
      - Hangnail with lymphangitis of toe
      - L03.041 Acute lymphangitis of right toe
      - L03.042 Acute lymphangitis of left toe
      - L03.049 Acute lymphangitis of unspecified toe
  - **L03.1 Cellulitis and acute lymphangitis of other parts of limb**
    - **L03.11 Cellulitis of other parts of limb**
      - Excludes2 cellulitis of fingers (L03.01-)
        - cellulitis of toes (L03.03-)
        - groin (L03.314)
      - L03.111 Cellulitis of right axilla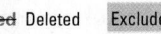
        - (Ex) See L02.411
      - L03.112 Cellulitis of left axilla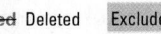
        - (Ex) See L02.411
      - L03.113 Cellulitis of right upper limb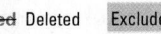
        - (Ex) See L02.411
      - L03.114 Cellulitis of left upper limb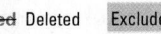
        - (Ex) See L02.411
      - L03.115 Cellulitis of right lower limb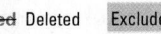
        - (Ex) See L02.415
      - L03.116 Cellulitis of left lower limb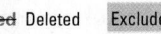
        - (Ex) See L02.415
      - L03.119 Cellulitis of unspecified part of limb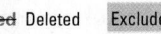
        - (Ex) See L02.415

◀ New   ◀ Revised   ~~deleted~~ Deleted   Excludes 1   Excludes 2   Includes   Use additional   Code first   Code also   Unspecified

OGCR Official Guidelines   ● Unacceptable Principal Diagnosis   X Assign placeholder X   ● Use Additional Character(s)   ▶ Manifestation Code   **Coding Clinic**

● **L03.12   Acute lymphangitis of other parts of limb**
    Excludes2   acute lymphangitis of fingers
       (L03.2-)
       acute lymphangitis of toes
       (L03.04-) ◄▮▮▮
       acute lymphangitis of groin
       (L03.324)

    L03.121   Acute lymphangitis of right axilla 🗞
        (Ex:) See L02.411

    L03.122   Acute lymphangitis of left axilla 🗞
        (Ex:) See L02.411

    L03.123   Acute lymphangitis of right upper limb 🗞
        (Ex:) See L02.411

    L03.124   Acute lymphangitis of left upper limb 🗞
        (Ex:) See L02.411

    L03.125   Acute lymphangitis of right lower limb 🗞
        (Ex:) See L02.415

    L03.126   Acute lymphangitis of left lower limb 🗞
        (Ex:) See L02.415

    L03.129   Acute lymphangitis of unspecified part of limb 🗞
        (Ex:) See L02.415

● **L03.2   Cellulitis and acute lymphangitis of face and neck**
 ● **L03.21   Cellulitis and acute lymphangitis of face**
    L03.211   **Cellulitis of face** 🗞
       Excludes2   cellulitis of ear
         (H60.1-)
         cellulitis of eyelid
         (H00.0-)
         cellulitis of head
         (L03.81)
         cellulitis of lacrimal
         apparatus (H04.3)
         cellulitis of lip (K13.0)
         cellulitis of mouth
         (K12.2)
         cellulitis of nose
         (internal) (J34.0)
         cellulitis of orbit
         (H05.0)
         cellulitis of scalp
         (L03.81)
        (Ex:) A17.9, A18.4, A18.82, A18.84, A18.89,
        A48.2-A48.4, A48.8-A49.9, B78.1,
        B95.0-B96.89, E83.2, L02.811-L02.818, L02.91,
        L03.211, L03.811-L03.91, L08.0, L08.81-L08.9,
        L44.8-L45, L73.2, L88, L92.8, L94.2, L94.4,
        L98.0, L98.3, L98.8, L99, Z16.10-Z16.39

    L03.212   **Acute lymphangitis of face** 🗞
        (Ex:) No exclusions

 ● **L03.22   Cellulitis and acute lymphangitis of neck**
     (Ex:) For category L03.22 CC codes: See L02.11
    L03.221   **Cellulitis of neck** 🗞
    L03.222   **Acute lymphangitis of neck** 🗞

Item 12–2   Cellulitis is an acute spreading bacterial infection below the surface of the skin characterized by redness (erythema), warmth, swelling, pain, fever, chills, and enlarged lymph nodes ("swollen glands").

● **L03.3   Cellulitis and acute lymphangitis of trunk**
 ● **L03.31   Cellulitis of trunk**
      Excludes2   cellulitis of anal and rectal
        regions (K61.-)
        cellulitis of breast NOS (N61)
        cellulitis of female external
        genital organs (N76.4)
        cellulitis of male external genital
        organs (N48.2, N49.-)
        omphalitis of newborn (P38.-)
        puerperal cellulitis of breast
        (O91.2)
     (Ex:) For category L03.31 CC codes unless otherwise indicated:
       See L02.21

    L03.311   **Cellulitis of abdominal wall** 🗞
       Excludes2   cellulitis of umbilicus
         (L03.316)
         cellulitis of groin
         (L03.314)

    L03.312   **Cellulitis of back [any part except buttock]** 🗞
    L03.313   **Cellulitis of chest wall** 🗞
    L03.314   **Cellulitis of groin** 🗞
    L03.315   **Cellulitis of perineum** 🗞
    L03.316   **Cellulitis of umbilicus** 🗞
    L03.317   **Cellulitis of buttock** 🗞
        (Ex:) See L02.31
    L03.319   **Cellulitis of trunk, unspecified** 🗞

 ● **L03.32   Acute lymphangitis of trunk**
     (Ex:) For category L03.32 CC codes unless otherwise indicated:
       See L02.21
    L03.321   **Acute lymphangitis of abdominal wall** 🗞
    L03.322   **Acute lymphangitis of back [any part except buttock]** 🗞
    L03.323   **Acute lymphangitis of chest wall** 🗞
    L03.324   **Acute lymphangitis of groin** 🗞
    L03.325   **Acute lymphangitis of perineum** 🗞
    L03.326   **Acute lymphangitis of umbilicus** 🗞
    L03.327   **Acute lymphangitis of buttock** 🗞
        (Ex:) See L02.31
    L03.329   **Acute lymphangitis of trunk, unspecified** 🗞

● **L03.8   Cellulitis and acute lymphangitis of other sites**
   (Ex:) A17.9, A18.4, A18.82, A18.84, A18.89, A48.2-A48.4, A48.8-A49.9, B78.1,
    B95.0-B96.89, E83.2, L02.811-L02.818, L02.91, L03.811-L03.91, L08.0,
    L08.81-L08.9, L44.8-L45, L73.2, L88, L92.8, L94.2, L94.4, L98.0, L98.3,
    L98.8, L99, Z16.10-Z16.39

 ● **L03.81   Cellulitis of other sites**
    L03.811   **Cellulitis of head [any part, except face]** 🗞
       Cellulitis of scalp
       Excludes2   cellulitis of face
         (L03.211)
    L03.818   **Cellulitis of other sites** 🗞

 ● **L03.89   Acute lymphangitis of other sites**
    L03.891   **Acute lymphangitis of head [any part, except face]** 🗞
    L03.898   **Acute lymphangitis of other sites** 🗞

● **L03.9   Cellulitis and acute lymphangitis, unspecified**
   (Ex:) For category L03.9 CC codes: See L02.81
    L03.90   **Cellulitis, unspecified** 🗞
    L03.91   **Acute lymphangitis, unspecified** 🗞
       Excludes1   lymphangitis NOS (I89.1)

N   Newborn Age: 0   P   Pediatric Age: 0–17   M   Maternity DX: 12–55   A   Adult Age: 15–124   ♀   Females Only   ♂   Males Only
🗞 Complication\Comorbidity   🗞 Major C\C   (Ex:) CC/MCC Exclusions   🗞 Present on Admission Requirement   🗞 Hospital-Acquired Condition

● **L04** **Acute lymphadenitis**
Short-term inflammation of lymph nodes which can be regionalized to involve a given area of the lymph system or systemic involving much of the body

Includes abscess (acute) of lymph nodes, except mesenteric
acute lymphadenitis, except mesenteric

Excludes1 chronic or subacute lymphadenitis, except mesenteric (I88.1)
enlarged lymph nodes (R59.-)
human immunodeficiency virus [HIV] disease resulting in generalized lymphadenopathy (B20)
lymphadenitis NOS (I88.9)
nonspecific mesenteric lymphadenitis (I88.0)

L04.0 **Acute lymphadenitis of face, head and neck**

L04.1 **Acute lymphadenitis of trunk**

L04.2 **Acute lymphadenitis of upper limb**
Acute lymphadenitis of axilla
Acute lymphadenitis of shoulder

L04.3 **Acute lymphadenitis of lower limb**
Acute lymphadenitis of hip
Excludes2 acute lymphadenitis of groin (L04.1)

L04.8 **Acute lymphadenitis of other sites**

L04.9 **Acute lymphadenitis, unspecified**

● **L05** **Pilonidal cyst and sinus**

● **L05.0** **Pilonidal cyst and sinus with abscess**
(Ex) For category L05.0 CC codes: L05.01-L05.92, L44.8-L45, L94.2, L94.4, L98.8, L99

L05.01 **Pilonidal cyst with abscess** 🖐
Parasacral dimple with abscess
Pilonidal abscess
Pilonidal dimple with abscess
Postanal dimple with abscess

L05.02 **Pilonidal sinus with abscess** 🖐
Coccygeal fistula with abscess
Coccygeal sinus with abscess
Pilonidal fistula with abscess

● **L05.9** **Pilonidal cyst and sinus without abscess**

L05.91 **Pilonidal cyst without abscess**
Parasacral dimple
Pilonidal dimple
Postanal dimple
Pilonidal cyst NOS

L05.92 **Pilonidal sinus without abscess**
Coccygeal fistula
Coccygeal sinus without abscess
Pilonidal fistula

● **L08** **Other local infections of skin and subcutaneous tissue**

L08.0 **Pyoderma**
Dermatitis gangrenosa
Purulent dermatitis
Septic dermatitis
Suppurative dermatitis
Excludes1 pyoderma gangrenosum (L88)
pyoderma vegetans (L08.81)

L08.1 **Erythrasma** 🖐
(Ex) A42.81-A42.9, A43.1-A43.9, B47.1, L08.

Figure 12-2 Impetigo. A thick, honey-yellow adherent crust covers the entire eroded surface. (From Habif: Clinical Dermatology, ed 4, Mosby, Inc., 2004)

Item 12–3 **Abscess** is a localized collection of pus in tissues or organs and is a sign of infection resulting in swelling and inflammation.

Item 12–4 **Pilonidal cyst,** also called a coccygeal cyst, is the result of a disorder called pilonidal disease. The cyst usually contains hair and pus.

● **L08.8** **Other specified local infections of the skin and subcutaneous tissue**

L08.81 **Pyoderma vegetans**
Excludes1 pyoderma gangrenosum (L88)
pyoderma NOS (L08.0)

L08.82 **Omphalitis not of newborn**
Excludes1 omphalitis of newborn (P38.-)

L08.89 **Other specified local infections of the skin and subcutaneous tissue**

L08.9 **Local infection of the skin and subcutaneous tissue, unspecified**

BULLOUS DISORDERS (L10-L14)

Excludes1 benign familial pemphigus [Hailey-Hailey] (Q82.8)
staphylococcal scalded skin syndrome (L00)
toxic epidermal necrolysis [Lyell] (L51.2)

● **L10** **Pemphigus**
Excludes1 pemphigus neonatorum (L01.03)
(Ex) For category L10 CC codes: L10.0-L10.9, L12.0-L12.1, L12.8-L12.9, L13.8-L14, L44.8-L45, L94.2, L94.4, L98.8, L99

L10.0 **Pemphigus vulgaris** 🖐

L10.1 **Pemphigus vegetans** 🖐

L10.2 **Pemphigus foliaceous** 🖐

L10.3 **Brazilian pemphigus [fogo selvagem]** 🖐

L10.4 **Pemphigus erythematosus** 🖐
Senear-Usher syndrome

L10.5 **Drug-induced pemphigus** 🖐
Use additional code for adverse effect, if applicable, to identify drug (T36-T50 with fifth or sixth character 5)

● **L10.8** **Other pemphigus**
L10.81 **Paraneoplastic pemphigus** 🖐
L10.89 **Other pemphigus** 🖐

L10.9 **Pemphigus, unspecified** 🖐

● **L11** **Other acantholytic disorders**

L11.0 **Acquired keratosis follicularis**
Excludes1 keratosis follicularis (congenital) [Darier-White] (Q82.8)

L11.1 **Transient acantholytic dermatosis [Grover]**

L11.8 **Other specified acantholytic disorders**

L11.9 **Acantholytic disorder, unspecified**

● **L12** **Pemphigoid**
Excludes1 herpes gestationis (O26.4-)
impetigo herpetiformis (L40.1)

L12.0 **Bullous pemphigoid** 🖐
(Ex) See L10

L12.1 **Cicatricial pemphigoid**
Benign mucous membrane pemphigoid

L12.2 **Chronic bullous disease of childhood**   P
Juvenile dermatitis herpetiformis

● **L12.3** **Acquired epidermolysis bullosa**
Excludes1 epidermolysis bullosa (congenital) (Q81.-)
(Ex) For category L12.3 CC codes: L00, L12.30-L12.35, L26, L30.4, L44.8-L45, L51.0-L54, L71.0-L71.9, L92.0, L93.0-L93.2, L94.2, L94.4, L95.1, L98.2, L98.8, L99

L12.30 **Acquired epidermolysis bullosa, unspecified** 🖐

L12.31 **Epidermolysis bullosa due to drug** 🖐
Use additional code for adverse effect, if applicable, to identify drug (T36-T50 with fifth or sixth character 5)

L12.35 **Other acquired epidermolysis bullosa** 🖐

L12.8 **Other pemphigoid** 🖐
(Ex) See L10

L12.9 **Pemphigoid, unspecified** 🖐
(Ex) See L10

◀ New   ◀▥▥ Revised   ~~deleted~~ Deleted   Excludes 1   Excludes 2   Includes   Use additional   Code first   Code also   Unspecified

OGCR Official Guidelines   ● Unacceptable Principal Diagnosis   X Assign placeholder X   ● Use Additional Character(s)   ▶ Manifestation Code   **Coding Clinic**

● **L13 Other bullous disorders**
    L13.0 Dermatitis herpetiformis
        Duhring's disease
        Hydroa herpetiformis
        Excludes1 juvenile dermatitis herpetiformis (L12.2)
                    senile dermatitis herpetiformis (L12.0)
    L13.1 Subcorneal pustular dermatitis
        Sneddon-Wilkinson disease
    L13.8 Other specified bullous disorders
    L13.9 Bullous disorder, unspecified

▶ *L14 Bullous disorders in diseases classified elsewhere*
    Code first underlying disease

DERMATITIS AND ECZEMA (L20-L30)

    Note: In this block the terms dermatitis and eczema are used synonymously and interchangeably.
    Excludes2 chronic (childhood) granulomatous disease (D71)
                dermatitis gangrenosa (L08.0)
                dermatitis herpetiformis (L13.0)
                dry skin dermatitis (L85.3)
                factitial dermatitis (L98.1)
                perioral dermatitis (L71.0)
                radiation-related disorders of the skin and subcutaneous tissue (L55-L59)
                stasis dermatitis (I83.1-I83.2)

● **L20 Atopic dermatitis**
    L20.0 Besnier's prurigo
  ● **L20.8 Other atopic dermatitis**
        Excludes2 circumscribed neurodermatitis (L28.0)
        L20.81 Atopic neurodermatitis
            Diffuse neurodermatitis
        L20.82 Flexural eczema
        L20.83 Infantile (acute) (chronic) eczema   **P**
        L20.84 Intrinsic (allergic) eczema
        L20.89 Other atopic dermatitis
    L20.9 Atopic dermatitis, unspecified

● **L21 Seborrheic dermatitis**
    Excludes2 infective dermatitis (L30.3)
                seborrheic keratosis (L82.-)
    L21.0 Seborrhea capitis   **P**
        Cradle cap
    L21.1 Seborrheic infantile dermatitis   **P**
    L21.8 Other seborrheic dermatitis
    L21.9 Seborrheic dermatitis, unspecified
        Seborrhea NOS

Item 12–5 Dermatitis herpetiformis, also known as Duhring's disease, is a systemic disease characterized by small blisters (3 to 5 mm) and occasionally large bullae (> 5 mm).

Figure 12-3 Dermatitis herpetiformis. (From Arnold HL, Odom RB, James WD: Andrews' Diseases of the Skin, Clinical Dermatology, ed 8, Philadelphia, WB Saunders, 1990)

Item 12–6 Seborrheic dermatitis is characterized by greasy, scaly, red patches and is associated with oily skin and scalp.

Figure 12-4 Seborrheic dermatitis. (From Cohen BA: Atlas of Pediatric Dermatology, St. Louis, Mosby, 1993)

Item 12–7 Atopic dermatitis, also known as atopic eczema, infantile eczema, disseminated neuro dermatitis, flexural eczema, and *prurigo diathesique* (Besnier), is characterized by intense itching and is often hereditary.

Figure 12-5 Atopic dermatitis. (From Moschella SL, Hurley HJ: Dermatology, ed 3, Philadelphia, WB Saunders, 1993)

    L22 Diaper dermatitis
        Diaper erythema
        Diaper rash
        Psoriasiform diaper rash

● **L23 Allergic contact dermatitis**
    Excludes1 allergy NOS (T78.40)
                contact dermatitis NOS (L25.9)
                dermatitis NOS (L30.9)
    Excludes2 dermatitis due to substances taken internally (L27.-)
                dermatitis of eyelid (H01.1-)
                diaper dermatitis (L22)
                eczema of external ear (H60.5-)
                irritant contact dermatitis (L24.-)
                perioral dermatitis (L71.0)
                radiation-related disorders of the skin and subcutaneous tissue (L55-L59)
    L23.0 Allergic contact dermatitis due to metals
        Allergic contact dermatitis due to chromium
        Allergic contact dermatitis due to nickel
    L23.1 Allergic contact dermatitis due to adhesives
    L23.2 Allergic contact dermatitis due to cosmetics
    L23.3 Allergic contact dermatitis due to drugs in contact with skin
        Use additional code for adverse effect, if applicable, to identify drug (T36-T50 with fifth or sixth character 5)
        Excludes2 dermatitis due to ingested drugs and medicaments (L27.0-L27.1)
    L23.4 Allergic contact dermatitis due to dyes
    L23.5 Allergic contact dermatitis due to other chemical products
        Allergic contact dermatitis due to cement
        Allergic contact dermatitis due to insecticide
        Allergic contact dermatitis due to plastic
        Allergic contact dermatitis due to rubber
    L23.6 Allergic contact dermatitis due to food in contact with the skin
        Excludes2 dermatitis due to ingested food (L27.2)
    L23.7 Allergic contact dermatitis due to plants, except food
        Excludes2 allergy NOS due to pollen (J30.1)

N Newborn Age: 0   **P** Pediatric Age: 0–17   **M** Maternity DX: 12–55   **A** Adult Age: 15–124   ♀ Females Only   ♂ Males Only
🔵 Complication\Comorbidity   🔷 Major C\C   (Ex:) CC/MCC Exclusions   🔶 Present on Admission Requirement   🔷 Hospital-Acquired Condition

● **L23.8   Allergic contact dermatitis due to other agents**

L23.81   Allergic contact dermatitis due to animal (cat) (dog) dander

Allergic contact dermatitis due to animal (cat) (dog) hair

L23.89   Allergic contact dermatitis due to other agents

L23.9   Allergic contact dermatitis, unspecified cause

Allergic contact eczema NOS

● **L24   Irritant contact dermatitis**

Excludes1   allergy NOS (T78.40)
contact dermatitis NOS (L25.9)
dermatitis NOS (L30.9)

Excludes2   allergic contact dermatitis (L23.-)
dermatitis due to substances taken internally (L27.-)
dermatitis of eyelid (H01.1-)
diaper dermatitis (L22)
eczema of external ear (H60.5-)
perioral dermatitis (L71.0)
radiation-related disorders of the skin and subcutaneous tissue (L55-L59)

L24.0   Irritant contact dermatitis due to detergents

L24.1   Irritant contact dermatitis due to oils and greases

L24.2   Irritant contact dermatitis due to solvents

Irritant contact dermatitis due to chlorocompound
Irritant contact dermatitis due to cyclohexane
Irritant contact dermatitis due to ester
Irritant contact dermatitis due to glycol
Irritant contact dermatitis due to hydrocarbon
Irritant contact dermatitis due to ketone

L24.3   Irritant contact dermatitis due to cosmetics

L24.4   Irritant contact dermatitis due to drugs in contact with skin

Use additional code for adverse effect, if applicable, to identify drug (T36-T50 with fifth or sixth character 5)

L24.5   Irritant contact dermatitis due to other chemical products

Irritant contact dermatitis due to cement
Irritant contact dermatitis due to insecticide
Irritant contact dermatitis due to plastic
Irritant contact dermatitis due to rubber

L24.6   Irritant contact dermatitis due to food in contact with skin

Excludes2   dermatitis due to ingested food (L27.2)

L24.7   Irritant contact dermatitis due to plants, except food

Excludes2   allergy NOS to pollen (J30.1)

● **L24.8   Irritant contact dermatitis due to other agents**

L24.81   Irritant contact dermatitis due to metals

Irritant contact dermatitis due to chromium
Irritant contact dermatitis due to nickel

L24.89   Irritant contact dermatitis due to other agents

Irritant contact dermatitis due to dyes

L24.9   Irritant contact dermatitis, unspecified cause

Irritant contact eczema NOS

● **L25   Unspecified contact dermatitis**

Excludes1   allergic contact dermatitis (L23.-)
allergy NOS (T78.40)
dermatitis NOS (L30.9)
irritant contact dermatitis (L24.-)

Excludes2   dermatitis due to ingested substances (L27.-)
dermatitis of eyelid (H01.1-)
eczema of external ear (H60.5-)
perioral dermatitis (L71.0)
radiation-related disorders of the skin and subcutaneous tissue (L55-L59)

L25.0   Unspecified contact dermatitis due to cosmetics

L25.1   Unspecified contact dermatitis due to drugs in contact with skin

Use additional code for adverse effect, if applicable, to identify drug (T36-T50 with fifth or sixth character 5)

Excludes2   dermatitis due to ingested drugs and medicaments (L27.0-L27.1)

L25.2   Unspecified contact dermatitis due to dyes

L25.3   Unspecified contact dermatitis due to other chemical products

Unspecified contact dermatitis due to cement
Unspecified contact dermatitis due to insecticide

L25.4   Unspecified contact dermatitis due to food in contact with skin

Excludes2   dermatitis due to ingested food (L27.2)

L25.5   Unspecified contact dermatitis due to plants, except food

Excludes1   nettle rash (L50.9)

Excludes2   allergy NOS due to pollen (J30.1)

L25.8   Unspecified contact dermatitis due to other agents

L25.9   Unspecified contact dermatitis, unspecified cause

Contact dermatitis (occupational) NOS
Contact eczema (occupational) NOS

L26   Exfoliative dermatitis

Hebra's pityriasis

Excludes1   Ritter's disease (L00)

● **L27   Dermatitis due to substances taken internally**

Excludes1   allergy NOS (T78.40)

Excludes2   adverse food reaction, except dermatitis (T78.0-T78.1)
contact dermatitis (L23-L25)
drug photoallergic response (L56.1)
drug phototoxic response (L56.0)
urticaria (L50.-)

L27.0   Generalized skin eruption due to drugs and medicaments taken internally

Use additional code for adverse effect, if applicable, to identify drug (T36-T50 with fifth or sixth character 5)

L27.1   Localized skin eruption due to drugs and medicaments taken internally

Use additional code for adverse effect, if applicable, to identify drug (T36-T50 with fifth or sixth character 5)

L27.2   Dermatitis due to ingested food

Excludes2   dermatitis due to food in contact with skin (L23.6, L24.6, L25.4)

L27.8   Dermatitis due to other substances taken internally

L27.9   Dermatitis due to unspecified substance taken internally

◀ New   ◀▦ Revised   ~~deleted~~ Deleted   Excludes 1   Excludes 2   Includes   Use additional   Code first   Code also   Unspecified

OGCR Official Guidelines   ● Unacceptable Principal Diagnosis   X Assign placeholder X   ● Use Additional Character(s)   ▶ Manifestation Code   **Coding Clinic**

● **L28   Lichen simplex chronicus and prurigo**

    L28.0   **Lichen simplex chronicus**
          Circumscribed neurodermatitis
          Lichen NOS

    L28.1   **Prurigo nodularis**

    L28.2   **Other prurigo**
          Prurigo NOS   Prurigo mitis
          Prurigo Hebra   Urticaria papulosa

● **L29   Pruritus**

    Excludes1   neurotic excoriation (L98.1)
                 psychogenic pruritus (F45.8)

    L29.0   **Pruritus ani**

    L29.1   **Pruritus scroti** ♂

    L29.2   **Pruritus vulvae** ♀

    L29.3   **Anogenital pruritus, unspecified**

    L29.8   **Other pruritus**

    L29.9   **Pruritus, unspecified**
          Itch NOS

● **L30   Other and unspecified dermatitis**

    Excludes2   contact dermatitis (L23-L25)
                 dry skin dermatitis (L85.3)
                 small plaque parapsoriasis (L41.3)
                 stasis dermatitis (I83.1-.2)

    L30.0   **Nummular dermatitis**

    L30.1   **Dyshidrosis [pompholyx]**

    L30.2   **Cutaneous autosensitization**
          Candidid [levurid]   Eczematid
          Dermatophytid

    L30.3   **Infective dermatitis**
          Infectious eczematoid dermatitis

    L30.4   **Erythema intertrigo**

    L30.5   **Pityriasis alba**

    L30.8   **Other specified dermatitis**

    L30.9   **Dermatitis, unspecified**
          Eczema NOS

PAPULOSQUAMOUS DISORDERS (L40-L45)

● **L40   Psoriasis**

    L40.0   **Psoriasis vulgaris**
          Nummular psoriasis   Plaque psoriasis

    L40.1   **Generalized pustular psoriasis**
          Impetigo herpetiformis
          Von Zumbusch's disease

    L40.2   **Acrodermatitis continua**

    L40.3   **Pustulosis palmaris et plantaris**

    L40.4   **Guttate psoriasis**

 ● L40.5   **Arthropathic psoriasis**

       L40.50   **Arthropathic psoriasis, unspecified**

       L40.51   **Distal interphalangeal psoriatic arthropathy**

       L40.52   **Psoriatic arthritis mutilans**

       L40.53   **Psoriatic spondylitis**

       L40.54   **Psoriatic juvenile arthropathy**

       L40.59   **Other psoriatic arthropathy**

    L40.8   **Other psoriasis**
          Flexural psoriasis

    L40.9   **Psoriasis, unspecified**

● **L41   Parapsoriasis**

    Excludes1   poikiloderma vasculare atrophicans (L94.5)

    L41.0   **Pityriasis lichenoides et varioliformis acuta**
          Mucha-Habermann disease

    L41.1   **Pityriasis lichenoides chronica**

    L41.3   **Small plaque parapsoriasis**

    L41.4   **Large plaque parapsoriasis**

    L41.5   **Retiform parapsoriasis**

    L41.8   **Other parapsoriasis**

    L41.9   **Parapsoriasis, unspecified**

    L42   **Pityriasis rosea**

● **L43   Lichen planus**

    Excludes1   lichen planopilaris (L66.1)

    L43.0   **Hypertrophic lichen planus**

    L43.1   **Bullous lichen planus**

    L43.2   **Lichenoid drug reaction**

         Use additional code for adverse effect, if applicable, to identify drug (T36-T50 with fifth or sixth character 5)

    L43.3   **Subacute (active) lichen planus**
          Lichen planus tropicus

    L43.8   **Other lichen planus**

    L43.9   **Lichen planus, unspecified**

● **L44   Other papulosquamous disorders**

    L44.0   **Pityriasis rubra pilaris**

    L44.1   **Lichen nitidus**

    L44.2   **Lichen striatus**

    L44.3   **Lichen ruber moniliformis**

    L44.4   **Infantile papular acrodermatitis [Gianotti-Crosti]**   P

    L44.8   **Other specified papulosquamous disorders**

    L44.9   **Papulosquamous disorder, unspecified**

▌ *L45*   *Papulosquamous disorders in diseases classified elsewhere*
       Code first underlying disease

URTICARIA AND ERYTHEMA (L49-L54)

    Excludes1   Lyme disease (A69.2-)
                 rosacea (L71.-)

● **L49   Exfoliation due to erythematous conditions according to extent of body surface involved**

       Code first erythematous condition causing exfoliation, such as:
          Ritter's disease (L00)
          (Staphylococcal) scalded skin syndrome (L00)
          Stevens-Johnson syndrome (L51.1)
          Stevens-Johnson syndrome-toxic epidermal necrolysis overlap syndrome (L51.3)
          Toxic epidermal necrolysis (L51.2)

 ● **L49.0**   **Exfoliation due to erythematous condition involving less than 10 percent of body surface**
          Exfoliation due to erythematous condition NOS

 ● **L49.1**   **Exfoliation due to erythematous condition involving 10-19 percent of body surface**

 ● **L49.2**   **Exfoliation due to erythematous condition involving 20-29 percent of body surface**

 ● **L49.3**   **Exfoliation due to erythematous condition involving 30-39 percent of body surface**
         (Ex) L49.3

 ● **L49.4**   **Exfoliation due to erythematous condition involving 40-49 percent of body surface**
         (Ex) L49.4

 ● **L49.5**   **Exfoliation due to erythematous condition involving 50-59 percent of body surface**
         (Ex) L49.5

CHAPTER 12 (L00-L99)

Item 12–8 Psoriasis is a chronic, recurrent inflammatory skin disease characterized by small patches covered with thick silvery scales. **Parapsoriasis** is a treatment-resistant erythroderma. **Pityriasis rosea** is characterized by a herald patch that is a single large lesion and that usually appears on the trunk and is followed by scattered, smaller lesions.

Figure 12-6 Erythematous plaques with silvery scales in a patient with psoriasis. (From Goldman: Cecil Textbook of Medicine, ed 22, Saunders, 2004)

● **L49.6** **Exfoliation due to erythematous condition involving 60-69 percent of body surface** 🅱
  (Ex:) L49.6

● **L49.7** **Exfoliation due to erythematous condition involving 70-79 percent of body surface** 🅱
  (Ex:) L49.7

● **L49.8** **Exfoliation due to erythematous condition involving 80-89 percent of body surface** 🅱
  (Ex:) L49.8

● **L49.9** **Exfoliation due to erythematous condition involving 90 or more percent of body surface** 🅱
  (Ex:) L49.9

● **L50** **Urticaria**

  Excludes1   allergic contact dermatitis (L23.-)
  angioneurotic edema (T78.3)
  giant urticaria (T78.3)
  hereditary angio-edema (D84.1)
  Quincke's edema (T78.3)
  serum urticaria (T80.6-)
  solar urticaria (L56.3)
  urticaria neonatorum (P83.8)
  urticaria papulosa (L28.2)
  urticaria pigmentosa (Q82.2)

  L50.0 **Allergic urticaria**

  L50.1 **Idiopathic urticaria**

  L50.2 **Urticaria due to cold and heat**

  L50.3 **Dermatographic urticaria**

  L50.4 **Vibratory urticaria**

  L50.5 **Cholinergic urticaria**

  L50.6 **Contact urticaria**

  L50.8 **Other urticaria**
    Chronic urticaria
    Recurrent periodic urticaria

  L50.9 **Urticaria, unspecified**

Figure 12-7 Urticaria (hives). *(Courtesy of David Effron, MD.)* (From Marx: Rosen's Emergency Medicine: Concepts and Clinical Practice, ed 6, Mosby, Inc., 2006)

Item 12–9 Urticaria is a vascular reaction in which wheals surrounded by a red halo appear and cause severe itching. The causes of urticaria or hives are extensive and varied (e.g., food, heat, cold, drugs, stress, infections).

● **L51** **Erythema multiforme**

  Use additional code for adverse effect, if applicable, to identify drug (T36-T50 with fifth or sixth character 5)

  Use additional code to identify associated manifestations, such as:
    arthropathy associated with dermatological disorders (M14.8-)
    conjunctival edema (H11.42)
    conjunctivitis (H10.22-)
    corneal scars and opacities (H17.-)
    corneal ulcer (H16.0-)
    edema of eyelid (H02.84)
    inflammation of eyelid (H01.8)
    keratoconjunctivitis sicca (H16.22-)
    mechanical lagophthalmos (H02.22-)
    stomatitis (K12.-)
    symblepharon (H11.23-)

  Use additional code to identify percentage of skin exfoliation (L49.-) ◄━━

  Excludes1   staphylococcal scalded skin syndrome (L00)
    Ritter's disease (L00)
  (Ex:) For category L51 CC codes: L00, L12.30-L12.35, L26, L30.4, L44.8-L45, L51.0-L54, L71.0-L71.9, L92.0, L93.0-L93.2, L94.2, L94.4, L95.1, L98.2, L98.8, L99

  L51.0 **Nonbullous erythema multiforme**

  L51.1 **Stevens-Johnson syndrome** 🅱

  L51.2 **Toxic epidermal necrolysis [Lyell]** 🅱

  L51.3 **Stevens-Johnson syndrome-toxic epidermal necrolysis overlap syndrome** 🅱
    SJS-TEN overlap syndrome

  L51.8 **Other erythema multiforme**

  L51.9 **Erythema multiforme, unspecified**
    Erythema iris
    Erythema multiforme major NOS
    Erythema multiforme minor NOS
    Herpes iris

● **L52** **Erythema nodosum**

  Excludes1   tuberculous erythema nodosum (A18.4)

● **L53** **Other erythematous conditions**

  Excludes1   erythema ab igne (L59.0)
    erythema due to external agents in contact with skin (L23-L25)
    erythema intertrigo (L30.4)
  (Ex:) For category L53 CC codes: L12.30-L12.35, L44.8-L45, L51.0-L53.3, L71.0-L71.9, L93.0-L93.2, L94.2, L94.4, L98.8, L99

  L53.0 **Toxic erythema** 🅱
    Code first poisoning due to drug or toxin, if applicable (T36-T65 with fifth or sixth character 1-4 or 6)

    Use additional code for adverse effect, if applicable, to identify drug (T36-T50 with fifth or sixth character 5)
    Excludes1   neonatal erythema toxicum (P83.1)

  L53.1 **Erythema annulare centrifugum** 🅱

  L53.2 **Erythema marginatum** 🅱

  L53.3 **Other chronic figurate erythema** 🅱

  L53.8 **Other specified erythematous conditions**

  L53.9 **Erythematous condition, unspecified**
    Erythema NOS
    Erythroderma NOS

▸ *L54* *Erythema in diseases classified elsewhere*
    Code first underlying disease

RADIATION-RELATED DISORDERS OF THE SKIN AND SUBCUTANEOUS TISSUE (L55-L59)

● **L55** **Sunburn**

  L55.0 **Sunburn of first degree**

  L55.1 **Sunburn of second degree**

  L55.2 **Sunburn of third degree**

  L55.9 **Sunburn, unspecified**

●**L56**   **Other acute skin changes due to ultraviolet radiation**
          Use additional code to identify the source of the ultraviolet radiation (W89, X32)
   L56.0   **Drug phototoxic response**
          Use additional code for adverse effect, if applicable, to identify drug (T36-T50 with fifth or sixth character 5)
   L56.1   **Drug photoallergic response**
          Use additional code for adverse effect, if applicable, to identify drug (T36-T50 with fifth or sixth character 5)
   L56.2   **Photocontact dermatitis [berloque dermatitis]**
   L56.3   **Solar urticaria**
   L56.4   **Polymorphous light eruption**
   L56.5   **Disseminated superficial actinic porokeratosis (DSAP)**
   L56.8   **Other specified acute skin changes due to ultraviolet radiation**
   L56.9   **Acute skin change due to ultraviolet radiation, unspecified**

●**L57**   **Skin changes due to chronic exposure to nonionizing radiation**
          Use additional code to identify the source of the ultraviolet radiation (W89, X32)
   L57.0   **Actinic keratosis**
          Keratosis NOS   Solar keratosis
          Senile keratosis
   L57.1   **Actinic reticuloid**
   L57.2   **Cutis rhomboidalis nuchae**
   L57.3   **Poikiloderma of Civatte**
   L57.4   **Cutis laxa senilis**
          Elastosis senilis
   L57.5   **Actinic granuloma**
   L57.8   **Other skin changes due to chronic exposure to nonionizing radiation**
          Farmer's skin   Solar dermatitis
          Sailor's skin
   L57.9   **Skin changes due to chronic exposure to nonionizing radiation, unspecified**

●**L58**   **Radiodermatitis**
          Use additional code to identify the source of the radiation (W88, W90)
   L58.0   **Acute radiodermatitis**
   L58.1   **Chronic radiodermatitis**
   L58.9   **Radiodermatitis, unspecified**

●**L59**   **Other disorders of skin and subcutaneous tissue related to radiation**
   L59.0   **Erythema ab igne [dermatitis ab igne]**
   L59.8   **Other specified disorders of the skin and subcutaneous tissue related to radiation**
   L59.9   **Disorder of the skin and subcutaneous tissue related to radiation, unspecified**

DISORDERS OF SKIN APPENDAGES (L60-L75)

   Excludes1   congenital malformations of integument (Q84.-)

●**L60**   **Nail disorders**
   Excludes2   clubbing of nails (R68.3)
                  onychia and paronychia (L03.0-)
   L60.0   **Ingrowing nail**
   L60.1   **Onycholysis**
   L60.2   **Onychogryphosis**
   L60.3   **Nail dystrophy**
   L60.4   **Beau's lines**
   L60.5   **Yellow nail syndrome**
   L60.8   **Other nail disorders**
   L60.9   **Nail disorder, unspecified**

Item 12-10   **Alopecia** is lack of hair and takes many forms. The most common is male pattern alopecia, also known as **androgenetic alopecia.** **Telogen effluvium** is early and excessive loss of hair resulting from a trauma to the hair follicle (fever, drugs, surgery, etc.).

Figure 12-8   Male pattern alopecia.

▸**L62**   *Nail disorders in diseases classified elsewhere*
          Code first underlying disease, such as:
          pachydermoperiostosis (M89.4-)

●**L63**   **Alopecia areata**
   L63.0   **Alopecia (capitis) totalis**
   L63.1   **Alopecia universalis**
   L63.2   **Ophiasis**
   L63.8   **Other alopecia areata**
   L63.9   **Alopecia areata, unspecified**

●**L64**   **Androgenic alopecia**
   Includes   male-pattern baldness
   L64.0   **Drug-induced androgenic alopecia**
          Use additional code for adverse effect, if applicable, to identify drug (T36-T50 with fifth or sixth character 5)
   L64.8   **Other androgenic alopecia**
   L64.9   **Androgenic alopecia, unspecified**

●**L65**   **Other nonscarring hair loss**
          Use additional code for adverse effect, if applicable, to identify drug (T36-T50 with fifth or sixth character 5)
   Excludes1   trichotillomania (F63.3)
   L65.0   **Telogen effluvium**
   L65.1   **Anagen effluvium**
   L65.2   **Alopecia mucinosa**
   L65.8   **Other specified nonscarring hair loss**
   L65.9   **Nonscarring hair loss, unspecified**
          Alopecia NOS

●**L66**   **Cicatricial alopecia [scarring hair loss]**
   L66.0   **Pseudopelade**
   L66.1   **Lichen planopilaris**
          Follicular lichen planus
   L66.2   **Folliculitis decalvans**
   L66.3   **Perifolliculitis capitis abscedens**
   L66.4   **Folliculitis ulerythematosa reticulata**
   L66.8   **Other cicatricial alopecia**
   L66.9   **Cicatricial alopecia, unspecified**

N Newborn Age: 0   **P** Pediatric Age: 0–17   **M** Maternity DX: 12–55   **A** Adult Age: 15–124   ♀ Females Only   ♂ Males Only

🔶 Complication\Comorbidity   🔶 Major C\C   ⒺⓍ CC/MCC Exclusions   🔶 Present on Admission Requirement   🔶 Hospital-Acquired Condition

● **L67**   **Hair color and hair shaft abnormalities**
     Excludes1   monilethrix (Q84.1)
                    pili annulati (Q84.1)
                    telogen effluvium (L65.0)

     L67.0   Trichorrhexis nodosa

     L67.1   **Variations in hair color**
           Canities
           Greyness, hair (premature)
           Heterochromia of hair
           Poliosis circumscripta, acquired
           Poliosis NOS

     L67.8   **Other hair color and hair shaft abnormalities**
           Fragilitas crinium

     L67.9   **Hair color and hair shaft abnormality, unspecified**

● **L68**   **Hypertrichosis**
     Includes   excess hair
     Excludes1   congenital hypertrichosis (Q84.2)
                    persistent lanugo (Q84.2)

     L68.0   **Hirsutism**
           Excessive growth of hair

     L68.1   Acquired hypertrichosis lanuginosa

     L68.2   Localized hypertrichosis

     L68.3   Polytrichia

     L68.8   Other hypertrichosis

     L68.9   **Hypertrichosis, unspecified**

● **L70**   **Acne**
     Excludes2   acne keloid (L73.0)

     L70.0   Acne vulgaris

     L70.1   Acne conglobata

     L70.2   **Acne varioliformis**
           Acne necrotica miliaris

     L70.3   Acne tropica

     L70.4   Infantile acne   P

     L70.5   **Acné excoriée des jeunes filles**
           Picker's acne

     L70.8   Other acne

     L70.9   **Acne, unspecified**

● **L71**   **Rosacea**
     Use additional code for adverse effect, if applicable, to identify drug (T36-T50 with fifth or sixth character 5)

     L71.0   Perioral dermatitis

     L71.1   Rhinophyma

     L71.8   Other rosacea

     L71.9   **Rosacea, unspecified**

● **L72**   **Follicular cysts of skin and subcutaneous tissue**

     L72.0   Epidermal cyst

   ● **L72.1**   **Pilar and trichodermal cyst**

         L72.11   Pilar cyst

         L72.12   **Trichodermal cyst**
                Trichilemmal (proliferating) cyst

     L72.3   **Sebaceous cyst**
         Excludes2   pilar cyst (L72.11)
                       trichilemmal (proliferating) cyst (L72.12)

     L72.2   Steatocystoma multiplex

     L72.8   Other follicular cysts of the skin and subcutaneous tissue

     L72.9   **Follicular cyst of the skin and subcutaneous tissue, unspecified**

● **L73**   **Other follicular disorders**

     L73.0   Acne keloid

     L73.1   Pseudofolliculitis barbae

     L73.2   Hidradenitis suppurativa

     L73.8   **Other specified follicular disorders**
           Sycosis barbae

     L73.9   **Follicular disorder, unspecified**

● **L74**   **Eccrine sweat disorders**
     Excludes2   generalized hyperhidrosis (R61)

     L74.0   Miliaria rubra

     L74.1   Miliaria crystallina

     L74.2   **Miliaria profunda**
           Miliaria tropicalis

     L74.3   **Miliaria, unspecified**

     L74.4   **Anhidrosis**
           Hypohidrosis

   ● **L74.5**   **Focal hyperhidrosis**

      ● **L74.51**   **Primary focal hyperhidrosis**

         L74.510   Primary focal hyperhidrosis, axilla

         L74.511   Primary focal hyperhidrosis, face

         L74.512   Primary focal hyperhidrosis, palms

         L74.513   Primary focal hyperhidrosis, soles

         L74.519   **Primary focal hyperhidrosis, unspecified**

      L74.52   **Secondary focal hyperhidrosis**
              Frey's syndrome

     L74.8   Other eccrine sweat disorders

     L74.9   **Eccrine sweat disorder, unspecified**
           Sweat gland disorder NOS

● **L75**   **Apocrine sweat disorders**
     Excludes1   dyshidrosis (L30.1)
                    hidradenitis suppurativa (L73.2)

     L75.0   Bromhidrosis

     L75.1   Chromhidrosis

     L75.2   **Apocrine miliaria**
           Fox-Fordyce disease

     L75.8   Other apocrine sweat disorders

     L75.9   **Apocrine sweat disorder, unspecified**
           Intraoperative and postprocedural complications of skin and subcutaneous tissue (L76)

INTRAOPERATIVE AND POSTPROCEDURAL COMPLICATIONS OF SKIN AND SUBCUTANEOUS TISSUE (L76)

● **L76**   **Intraoperative and postprocedural complications of skin and subcutaneous tissue**
     (Ex) **For category L76 CC codes unless otherwise indicated:** H95.811-H95.89, I85.01, I85.11, I97.3, K21.9, K22.8, K23, K25.0, K25.2, K25.4, K25.6, K26.0, K26.2, K26.4, K26.6, K27.0, K27.2, K27.4, K27.6, K28.0, K28.2, K28.4, K28.6, K29.01, K29.21, K29.31, K29.41, K29.51, K29.61, K29.71, K29.81, K29.91, K31.811, K55.21, K57.01, K57.11, K57.13, K57.21, K57.31, K57.33, K57.41, K57.51, K57.53, K57.81, K57.91, K57.93, K62.5, K92.0-K92.2, L76.01-L76.02, L76.21-L76.82, M96.89, N98.1-N98.9, P54.1-P54.3, T81.10X-T81.19X[A], T81.82X[A], T81.89X-T81.9XX[A]

   ● **L76.0**   **Intraoperative hemorrhage and hematoma of skin and subcutaneous tissue complicating a procedure**
         Excludes1   intraoperative hemorrhage and hematoma of skin and subcutaneous tissue due to accidental puncture and laceration during a procedure (L76.1-)

      L76.01   Intraoperative hemorrhage and hematoma of skin and subcutaneous tissue complicating a dermatologic procedure 🔗

      L76.02   Intraoperative hemorrhage and hematoma of skin and subcutaneous tissue complicating other procedure 🔗

● **L76.1** **Accidental puncture and laceration of skin and subcutaneous tissue during a procedure**
    (Ex) For category **L76.1** CC codes: D78.11-D78.12, D78.81-D78.89, E36.11-E36.8, E89.810-E89.89, G96.11, G97.41-G97.49, H59.011-H59.019, H59.031-H59.099, H59.211-H59.229, H59.811-H59.89, H95.31-H95.32, H95.811-H95.89, I97.3, I97.51-I97.52, J95.71-J95.72, K91.71-K91.72, L76.11-L76.12, L76.81-L76.82, M96.820-M96.821, M96.89, N98.1-N98.9, N99.71-N99.72, T81.82X[A], T81.89X-T81.9XX[A]

    L76.11 **Accidental puncture and laceration of skin and subcutaneous tissue during a dermatologic procedure** 🔖

    L76.12 **Accidental puncture and laceration of skin and subcutaneous tissue during other procedure** 🔖

● **L76.2** **Postprocedural hemorrhage and hematoma of skin and subcutaneous tissue following a procedure**

    L76.21 **Postprocedural hemorrhage and hematoma of skin and subcutaneous tissue following a dermatologic procedure** 🔖

    L76.22 **Postprocedural hemorrhage and hematoma of skin and subcutaneous tissue following other procedure** 🔖

● **L76.8** **Other intraoperative and postprocedural complications of skin and subcutaneous tissue**
    Use additional code, if applicable, to further specify disorder

    L76.81 **Other intraoperative complications of skin and subcutaneous tissue**

    L76.82 **Other postprocedural complications of skin and subcutaneous tissue**

OTHER DISORDERS OF THE SKIN AND SUBCUTANEOUS TISSUE (L80-L99)

L80 **Vitiligo**
    Excludes2   vitiligo of eyelids (H02.73-)
               vitiligo of vulva (N90.89)

● **L81** **Other disorders of pigmentation**
    Excludes1   birthmark NOS (Q82.5)
               Peutz-Jeghers syndrome (Q85.8)
    Excludes2   nevus - see Alphabetical Index

    L81.0 **Postinflammatory hyperpigmentation**
    L81.1 **Chloasma**
    L81.2 **Freckles**
    L81.3 **Café au lait spots**
    L81.4 **Other melanin hyperpigmentation**
         Lentigo
    L81.5 **Leukoderma, not elsewhere classified**
    L81.6 **Other disorders of diminished melanin formation**
    L81.7 **Pigmented purpuric dermatosis**
         Angioma serpiginosum
    L81.8 **Other specified disorders of pigmentation**
         Iron pigmentation
         Tattoo pigmentation
    L81.9 **Disorder of pigmentation, unspecified**

● **L82** **Seborrheic keratosis**
    Includes   dermatosis papulosa nigra
             Leser-Trélat disease
    Excludes2   seborrheic dermatitis (L21.-)
    L82.0 **Inflamed seborrheic keratosis**
    L82.1 **Other seborrheic keratosis**
         Seborrheic keratosis NOS

L83 **Acanthosis nigricans**
    Confluent and reticulated papillomatosis

L84 **Corns and callosities**
    Callus
    Clavus

● **L85** **Other epidermal thickening**
    Excludes2   hypertrophic disorders of the skin (L91.-)

    L85.0 **Acquired ichthyosis**
        Excludes1   congenital ichthyosis (Q80.-)

    L85.1 **Acquired keratosis [keratoderma] palmaris et plantaris**
        Excludes1   inherited keratosis palmaris et plantaris (Q82.8)

    L85.2 **Keratosis punctata (palmaris et plantaris) L85.3**
        Xerosis cutis
        Dry skin dermatitis

    L85.8 **Other specified epidermal thickening**
        Cutaneous horn

    L85.9 **Epidermal thickening, unspecified**

▷ **L86** *Keratoderma in diseases classified elsewhere*
    Firm horny papules that have a cobblestone appearance.
    Code first underlying disease, such as:
        Reiter's disease (M02.3-)
    Excludes1   gonococcal keratoderma (A54.89)
               gonococcal keratosis (A54.89)
               keratoderma due to vitamin A deficiency (E50.8)
               keratosis due to vitamin A deficiency (E50.8)
               xeroderma due to vitamin A deficiency (E50.8)

● **L87** **Transepidermal elimination disorders**
    Excludes1   granuloma annulare (perforating) (L92.0)

    L87.0 **Keratosis follicularis et parafollicularis in cutem penetrans**
        Kyrle disease
        Hyperkeratosis follicularis penetrans

    L87.1 **Reactive perforating collagenosis**
    L87.2 **Elastosis perforans serpiginosa**
    L87.8 **Other transepidermal elimination disorders**
    L87.9 **Transepidermal elimination disorder, unspecified**

● **L88** **Pyoderma gangrenosum** 🔖
    Phagedenic pyoderma
    Excludes1   dermatitis gangrenosa (L08.0)
    (Ex) L08.0, L08.81, L88

● **L89** **Pressure ulcer**
    Includes   bed sore   pressure area
             decubitus ulcer   pressure sore
             plaster ulcer
    Code first any associated gangrene (I96)
    Excludes2   decubitus (trophic) ulcer of cervix (uteri) (N86)
               diabetic ulcers (E08.621, E08.622, E09.621, E09.622, E10.621, E10.622, E11.621, E11.622, E13.621, E13.622)
               non-pressure chronic ulcer of skin (L97.-)
               skin infections (L00-L08)
               varicose ulcer (I83.0, I83.2)
    (Ex) For category **L89** CC codes: L89.000-L89.95, L97.101-L97.929, L98.411-L98.499

    ● **L89.0** **Pressure ulcer of elbow**
       ● **L89.00** **Pressure ulcer of unspecified elbow**

          L89.000 **Pressure ulcer of unspecified elbow, unstageable**

          L89.001 **Pressure ulcer of unspecified elbow, stage 1**
              Healing pressure ulcer of unspecified elbow, stage 1
              Pressure pre-ulcer skin changes limited to persistent focal edema, unspecified elbow

          L89.002 **Pressure ulcer of unspecified elbow, stage 2**
              Healing pressure ulcer of unspecified elbow, stage 2
              Pressure ulcer with abrasion, blister, partial thickness skin loss involving epidermis and/or dermis, unspecified elbow

N Newborn Age: 0   P Pediatric Age: 0–17   M Maternity DX: 12–55   A Adult Age: 15–124   ♀ Females Only   ♂ Males Only

🔖 Complication\Comorbidity   🔖 Major C\C   (Ex) CC/MCC Exclusions   🔖 Present on Admission Requirement   🔖 Hospital-Acquired Condition

1057

CHAPTER 12 (L00-L99)

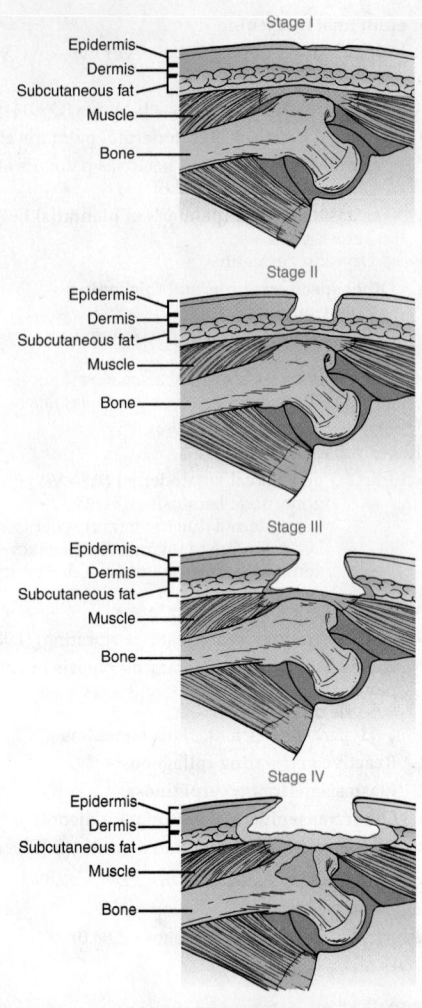

Stage I

Epidermis
Dermis
Subcutaneous fat
Muscle
Bone

Stage II

Epidermis
Dermis
Subcutaneous fat
Muscle
Bone

Stage III

Epidermis
Dermis
Subcutaneous fat
Muscle
Bone

Stage IV

Epidermis
Dermis
Subcutaneous fat
Muscle
Bone

Figure 12-9   Stage I, II, III, and IV of pressure ulcers.

L89.003   **Pressure ulcer of unspecified elbow, stage 3** 🦠 🦠
Healing pressure ulcer of unspecified elbow, stage 3
Pressure ulcer with full thickness skin loss involving damage or necrosis of subcutaneous tissue, unspecified elbow
MCC when PDx is its own MCC

L89.004   **Pressure ulcer of unspecified elbow, stage 4** 🦠 🦠
Healing pressure ulcer of unspecified elbow, stage 4
Pressure ulcer with necrosis of soft tissues through to underlying muscle, tendon, or bone, unspecified elbow
MCC when PDx is its own MCC

L89.009   **Pressure ulcer of unspecified elbow, unspecified stage**
Healing pressure ulcer of elbow NOS
Healing pressure ulcer of unspecified elbow, unspecified stage

● L89.01   **Pressure ulcer of right elbow**

L89.010   **Pressure ulcer of right elbow, unstageable**

L89.011   **Pressure ulcer of right elbow, stage 1**
Healing pressure ulcer of right elbow, stage 1
Pressure pre-ulcer skin changes limited to persistent focal edema, right elbow

L89.012   **Pressure ulcer of right elbow, stage 2**
Healing pressure ulcer of right elbow, stage 2
Pressure ulcer with abrasion, blister, partial thickness skin loss involving epidermis and/or dermis, right elbow

L89.013   **Pressure ulcer of right elbow, stage 3** 🦠 🦠
Healing pressure ulcer of right elbow, stage 3
Pressure ulcer with full thickness skin loss involving damage or necrosis of subcutaneous tissue, right elbow
MCC when PDx is its own MCC

L89.014   **Pressure ulcer of right elbow, stage 4** 🦠 🦠
Healing pressure ulcer of right elbow, stage 4
Pressure ulcer with necrosis of soft tissues through to underlying muscle, tendon, or bone, right elbow
MCC when PDx is its own MCC

L89.019   **Pressure ulcer of right elbow, unspecified stage**
Healing pressure right of elbow NOS
Healing pressure ulcer of unspecified elbow, unspecified stage

● L89.02   **Pressure ulcer of left elbow**

L89.020   **Pressure ulcer of left elbow, unstageable**

L89.021   **Pressure ulcer of left elbow, stage 1**
Healing pressure ulcer of left elbow, stage 1
Pressure pre-ulcer skin changes limited to persistent focal edema, left elbow

L89.022   **Pressure ulcer of left elbow, stage 2**
Healing pressure ulcer of left elbow, stage 2
Pressure ulcer with abrasion, blister, partial thickness skin loss involving epidermis and/or dermis, left elbow

L89.023   **Pressure ulcer of left elbow, stage 3** 🦠 🦠
Healing pressure ulcer of left elbow, stage 3
Pressure ulcer with full thickness skin loss involving damage or necrosis of subcutaneous tissue, left elbow
MCC when PDx is its own MCC

◀ New   ◀▥ Revised   ~~deleted~~ Deleted | Excludes 1 | | Excludes 2 | | Includes | | Use additional | | Code first | | Code also | | Unspecified |
OGCR Official Guidelines   ● Unacceptable Principal Diagnosis   X Assign placeholder X   ▸ Use Additional Character(s)   ▸ Manifestation Code   **Coding Clinic**

L89.024   **Pressure ulcer of left elbow, stage 4** 🔲 🔲
    Healing pressure ulcer of left elbow, stage 4
    Pressure ulcer with necrosis of soft tissues through to underlying muscle, tendon, or bone, left elbow
    MCC when PDx is its own MCC

L89.029   **Pressure ulcer of left elbow, unspecified stage**
    Healing pressure ulcer of left of elbow NOS
    Healing pressure ulcer of unspecified elbow, unspecified stage

● **L89.1   Pressure ulcer of back**

  ● **L89.10   Pressure ulcer of unspecified part of back**

L89.100   **Pressure ulcer of unspecified part of back, unstageable**

L89.101   **Pressure ulcer of unspecified part of back, stage 1**
    Healing pressure ulcer of unspecified part of back, stage 1
    Pressure pre-ulcer skin changes limited to persistent focal edema, unspecified part of back

L89.102   **Pressure ulcer of unspecified part of back, stage 2**
    Healing pressure ulcer of unspecified part of back, stage 2
    Pressure ulcer with abrasion, blister, partial thickness skin loss involving epidermis and/or dermis, unspecified part of back

L89.103   **Pressure ulcer of unspecified part of back, stage 3** 🔲 🔲
    Healing pressure ulcer of unspecified part of back, stage 3
    Pressure ulcer with full thickness skin loss involving damage or necrosis of subcutaneous tissue, unspecified part of back
    MCC when PDx is its own MCC

L89.104   **Pressure ulcer of unspecified part of back, stage 4** 🔲 🔲
    Healing pressure ulcer of unspecified part of back, stage 4
    Pressure ulcer with necrosis of soft tissues through to underlying muscle, tendon, or bone, unspecified part of back
    MCC when PDx is its own MCC

L89.109   **Pressure ulcer of unspecified part of back, unspecified stage**
    Healing pressure ulcer of unspecified part of back NOS
    Healing pressure ulcer of unspecified part of back, unspecified stage

  ● **L89.11   Pressure ulcer of right upper back**
    Pressure ulcer of right shoulder blade

L89.110   **Pressure ulcer of right upper back, unstageable**

L89.111   **Pressure ulcer of right upper back, stage 1**
    Healing pressure ulcer of right upper back, stage 1
    Pressure pre-ulcer skin changes limited to persistent focal edema, right upper back

L89.112   **Pressure ulcer of right upper back, stage 2**
    Healing pressure ulcer of right upper back, stage 2
    Pressure ulcer with abrasion, blister, partial thickness skin loss involving epidermis and/or dermis, right upper back

L89.113   **Pressure ulcer of right upper back, stage 3** 🔲 🔲
    Healing pressure ulcer of right upper back, stage 3
    Pressure ulcer with full thickness skin loss involving damage or necrosis of subcutaneous tissue, right upper back
    MCC when PDx is its own MCC

L89.114   **Pressure ulcer of right upper back, stage 4** 🔲 🔲
    Healing pressure ulcer of right upper back, stage 4
    Pressure ulcer with necrosis of soft tissues through to underlying muscle, tendon, or bone, right upper back
    MCC when PDx is its own MCC

L89.119   **Pressure ulcer of right upper back, unspecified stage**
    Healing pressure ulcer of right upper back NOS
    Healing pressure ulcer of right upper back, unspecified stage

  ● **L89.12   Pressure ulcer of left upper back**
    Pressure ulcer of left shoulder blade

L89.120   **Pressure ulcer of left upper back, unstageable**

L89.121   **Pressure ulcer of left upper back, stage 1**
    Healing pressure ulcer of left upper back, stage 1
    Pressure pre-ulcer skin changes limited to persistent focal edema, left upper back

L89.122   **Pressure ulcer of left upper back, stage 2**
    Healing pressure ulcer of left upper back, stage 2
    Pressure ulcer with abrasion, blister, partial thickness skin loss involving epidermis and/or dermis, left upper back

L89.123   **Pressure ulcer of left upper back, stage 3** 🔲 🔲
    Healing pressure ulcer of left upper back, stage 3
    Pressure ulcer with full thickness skin loss involving damage or necrosis of subcutaneous tissue, left upper back
    MCC when PDx is its own MCC

L89.124   **Pressure ulcer of left upper back, stage 4** 🔲 🔲
    Healing pressure ulcer of left upper back, stage 4
    Pressure ulcer with necrosis of soft tissues through to underlying muscle, tendon, or bone, left upper back
    MCC when PDx is its own MCC

L89.129   **Pressure ulcer of left upper back, unspecified stage**
    Healing pressure ulcer of left upper back NOS
    Healing pressure ulcer of left upper back, unspecified stage

N Newborn Age: 0   P Pediatric Age: 0–17   M Maternity DX: 12–55   A Adult Age: 15–124   ♀ Females Only   ♂ Males Only

🔲 Complication\Comorbidity   🔲 Major C\C   (Ex) CC/MCC Exclusions   🔲 Present on Admission Requirement   🔲 Hospital-Acquired Condition

1059

● **L89.13** **Pressure ulcer of right lower back**

L89.130 **Pressure ulcer of right lower back, unstageable**

L89.131 **Pressure ulcer of right lower back, stage 1**
　　Healing pressure ulcer of right lower back, stage 1
　　Pressure pre-ulcer skin changes limited to persistent focal edema, right lower back

L89.132 **Pressure ulcer of right lower back, stage 2**
　　Healing pressure ulcer of right lower back, stage 2
　　Pressure ulcer with abrasion, blister, partial thickness skin loss involving epidermis and/or dermis, right lower back

L89.133 **Pressure ulcer of right lower back, stage 3** 🔖🔖
　　Healing pressure ulcer of right lower back, stage 3
　　Pressure ulcer with full thickness skin loss involving damage or necrosis of subcutaneous tissue, right lower back
　　MCC when PDx is its own MCC

L89.134 **Pressure ulcer of right lower back, stage 4** 🔖🔖
　　Healing pressure ulcer of right lower back, stage 4
　　Pressure ulcer with necrosis of soft tissues through to underlying muscle, tendon, or bone, right lower back
　　MCC when PDx is its own MCC

L89.139 **Pressure ulcer of right lower back, unspecified stage**
　　Healing pressure ulcer of right lower back NOS
　　Healing pressure ulcer of right lower back, unspecified stage

● **L89.14** **Pressure ulcer of left lower back**

L89.140 **Pressure ulcer of left lower back, unstageable**

L89.141 **Pressure ulcer of left lower back, stage 1**
　　Healing pressure ulcer of left lower back, stage 1
　　Pressure pre-ulcer skin changes limited to persistent focal edema, left lower back

L89.142 **Pressure ulcer of left lower back, stage 2**
　　Healing pressure ulcer of left lower back, stage 2
　　Pressure ulcer with abrasion, blister, partial thickness skin loss involving epidermis and/or dermis, left lower back

L89.143 **Pressure ulcer of left lower back, stage 3** 🔖🔖
　　Healing pressure ulcer of left lower back, stage 3
　　Pressure ulcer with full thickness skin loss involving damage or necrosis of subcutaneous tissue, left lower back
　　MCC when PDx is its own MCC

L89.144 **Pressure ulcer of left lower back, stage 4** 🔖🔖
　　Healing pressure ulcer of left lower back, stage 4
　　Pressure ulcer with necrosis of soft tissues through to underlying muscle, tendon, or bone, left lower back
　　MCC when PDx is its own MCC

L89.149 **Pressure ulcer of left lower back, unspecified stage**
　　Healing pressure ulcer of left lower back NOS
　　Healing pressure ulcer of left lower back, unspecified stage

● **L89.15** **Pressure ulcer of sacral region**
　Pressure ulcer of coccyx
　Pressure ulcer of tailbone

L89.150 **Pressure ulcer of sacral region, unstageable**

L89.151 **Pressure ulcer of sacral region, stage 1**
　　Healing pressure ulcer of sacral region, stage 1
　　Pressure pre-ulcer skin changes limited to persistent focal edema, sacral region

L89.152 **Pressure ulcer of sacral region, stage 2**
　　Healing pressure ulcer of sacral region, stage 2
　　Pressure ulcer with abrasion, blister, partial thickness skin loss involving epidermis and/or dermis, sacral region

L89.153 **Pressure ulcer of sacral region, stage 3** 🔖🔖
　　Healing pressure ulcer of sacral region, stage 3
　　Pressure ulcer with full thickness skin loss involving damage or necrosis of subcutaneous tissue, sacral region
　　MCC when PDx is its own MCC

L89.154 **Pressure ulcer of sacral region, stage 4** 🔖🔖
　　Healing pressure ulcer of sacral region, stage 4
　　Pressure ulcer with necrosis of soft tissues through to underlying muscle, tendon, or bone, sacral region
　　MCC when PDx is its own MCC

L89.159 **Pressure ulcer of sacral region, unspecified stage**
　　Healing pressure ulcer of sacral region NOS
　　Healing pressure ulcer of sacral region, unspecified stage

● **L89.2** **Pressure ulcer of hip**

● **L89.20** **Pressure ulcer of unspecified hip**

L89.200 **Pressure ulcer of unspecified hip, unstageable**

L89.201 **Pressure ulcer of unspecified hip, stage 1**
　　Healing pressure ulcer of unspecified hip back, stage 1
　　Pressure pre-ulcer skin changes limited to persistent focal edema, unspecified hip

L89.202 **Pressure ulcer of unspecified hip, stage 2**
　　Healing pressure ulcer of unspecified hip, stage 2
　　Pressure ulcer with abrasion, blister, partial thickness skin loss involving epidermis and/or dermis, unspecified hip

◀ New　◀▥ Revised　d̶e̶l̶e̶t̶e̶d̶ Deleted　Excludes 1　Excludes 2　Includes　Use additional　Code first　Code also　Unspecified
OGCR Official Guidelines　● Unacceptable Principal Diagnosis　X Assign placeholder X　● Use Additional Character(s)　▌ Manifestation Code　**Coding Clinic**

L89.203 **Pressure ulcer of** unspecified **hip, stage 3** 🐾 🐾
> Healing pressure ulcer of unspecified hip, stage 3
> Pressure ulcer with full thickness skin loss involving damage or necrosis of subcutaneous tissue, unspecified hip
> MCC when PDx is its own MCC

L89.204 **Pressure ulcer of** unspecified **hip, stage 4** 🐾 🐾
> Healing pressure ulcer of unspecified hip, stage 4
> Pressure ulcer with necrosis of soft tissues through to underlying muscle, tendon, or bone, unspecified hip
> MCC when PDx is its own MCC

L89.209 **Pressure ulcer of** unspecified **hip, unspecified stage**
> Healing pressure ulcer of unspecified hip NOS
> Healing pressure ulcer of unspecified hip, unspecified stage

● L89.21 **Pressure ulcer of right hip**

L89.210 **Pressure ulcer of right hip, unstageable**

L89.211 **Pressure ulcer of right hip, stage 1**
> Healing pressure ulcer of right hip back, stage 1
> Pressure pre-ulcer skin changes limited to persistent focal edema, right hip

L89.212 **Pressure ulcer of right hip, stage 2**
> Healing pressure ulcer of right hip, stage 2
> Pressure ulcer with abrasion, blister, partial thickness skin loss involving epidermis and/or dermis, right hip

L89.213 **Pressure ulcer of right hip, stage 3** 🐾 🐾
> Healing pressure ulcer of right hip, stage 3
> Pressure ulcer with full thickness skin loss involving damage or necrosis of subcutaneous tissue, right hip
> MCC when PDx is its own MCC

L89.214 **Pressure ulcer of right hip, stage 4** 🐾 🐾
> Healing pressure ulcer of right hip, stage 4
> Pressure ulcer with necrosis of soft tissues through to underlying muscle, tendon, or bone, right hip
> MCC when PDx is its own MCC

L89.219 **Pressure ulcer of right hip,** unspecified **stage**
> Healing pressure ulcer of right hip NOS
> Healing pressure ulcer of right hip, unspecified stage

● L89.22 **Pressure ulcer of left hip**

L89.220 **Pressure ulcer of left hip, unstageable**

L89.221 **Pressure ulcer of left hip, stage 1**
> Healing pressure ulcer of left hip back, stage 1
> Pressure pre-ulcer skin changes limited to persistent focal edema, left hip

L89.222 **Pressure ulcer of left hip, stage 2**
> Healing pressure ulcer of left hip, stage 2
> Pressure ulcer with abrasion, blister, partial thickness skin loss involving epidermis and/or dermis, left hip

L89.223 **Pressure ulcer of left hip, stage 3** 🐾 🐾
> Healing pressure ulcer of left hip, stage 3
> Pressure ulcer with full thickness skin loss involving damage or necrosis of subcutaneous tissue, left hip
> MCC when PDx is its own MCC

L89.224 **Pressure ulcer of left hip, stage 4** 🐾 🐾
> Healing pressure ulcer of left hip, stage 4
> Pressure ulcer with necrosis of soft tissues through to underlying muscle, tendon, or bone, left hip
> MCC when PDx is its own MCC

L89.229 **Pressure ulcer of left hip,** unspecified **stage**
> Healing pressure ulcer of left hip NOS
> Healing pressure ulcer of left hip, unspecified stage

● L89.3 **Pressure ulcer of buttock**

● L89.30 **Pressure ulcer of unspecified buttock**

L89.300 **Pressure ulcer of** unspecified **buttock, unstageable**

L89.301 **Pressure ulcer of** unspecified **buttock, stage 1**
> Healing pressure ulcer of unspecified buttock, stage 1
> Pressure pre-ulcer skin changes limited to persistent focal edema, unspecified buttock

L89.302 **Pressure ulcer of** unspecified **buttock, stage 2**
> Healing pressure ulcer of unspecified buttock, stage 2
> Pressure ulcer with abrasion, blister, partial thickness skin loss involving epidermis and/or dermis, unspecified buttock

L89.303 **Pressure ulcer of** unspecified **buttock, stage 3** 🐾 🐾
> Healing pressure ulcer of unspecified buttock, stage 3
> Pressure ulcer with full thickness skin loss involving damage or necrosis of subcutaneous tissue, unspecified buttock
> MCC when PDx is its own MCC

N Newborn Age: 0 P Pediatric Age: 0–17 M Maternity DX: 12–55 A Adult Age: 15–124 ♀ Females Only ♂ Males Only

🐾 Complication\Comorbidity 🐾 Major C\C (Ex) CC/MCC Exclusions 🐾 Present on Admission Requirement 🐾 Hospital-Acquired Condition

1061

L89.304 **Pressure ulcer of** unspecified **buttock, stage 4** 🖐🖐
  Healing pressure ulcer of unspecified buttock, stage 4
  Pressure ulcer with necrosis of soft tissues through to underlying muscle, tendon, or bone, unspecified buttock
  MCC when PDx is its own MCC

L89.309 **Pressure ulcer of** unspecified **buttock, unspecified stage**
  Healing pressure ulcer of unspecified buttock NOS
  Healing pressure ulcer of unspecified buttock, unspecified stage

● **L89.31** **Pressure ulcer of right buttock**

L89.310 **Pressure ulcer of right buttock, unstageable**

L89.311 **Pressure ulcer of right buttock, stage 1**
  Healing pressure ulcer of right buttock, stage 1
  Pressure pre-ulcer skin changes limited to persistent focal edema, right buttock

L89.312 **Pressure ulcer of right buttock, stage 2**
  Healing pressure ulcer of right buttock, stage 2
  Pressure ulcer with abrasion, blister, partial thickness skin loss involving epidermis and/or dermis, right buttock

L89.313 **Pressure ulcer of right buttock, stage 3** 🖐🖐
  Healing pressure ulcer of right buttock, stage 3
  Pressure ulcer with full thickness skin loss involving damage or necrosis of subcutaneous tissue, right buttock
  MCC when PDx is its own MCC

L89.314 **Pressure ulcer of right buttock, stage 4** 🖐🖐
  Healing pressure ulcer of right buttock, stage 4
  Pressure ulcer with necrosis of soft tissues through to underlying muscle, tendon, or bone, right buttock
  MCC when PDx is its own MCC

L89.319 **Pressure ulcer of right buttock,** unspecified **stage**
  Healing pressure ulcer of right buttock NOS
  Healing pressure ulcer of right buttock, unspecified stage

● **L89.32** **Pressure ulcer of left buttock**

L89.320 **Pressure ulcer of left buttock, unstageable**

L89.321 **Pressure ulcer of left buttock, stage 1**
  Healing pressure ulcer of left buttock, stage 1
  Pressure pre-ulcer skin changes limited to persistent focal edema, left buttock

L89.322 **Pressure ulcer of left buttock, stage 2**
  Healing pressure ulcer of left buttock, stage 2
  Pressure ulcer with abrasion, blister, partial thickness skin loss involving epidermis and/or dermis, left buttock

L89.323 **Pressure ulcer of left buttock, stage 3** 🖐🖐
  Healing pressure ulcer of left buttock, stage 3
  Pressure ulcer with full thickness skin loss involving damage or necrosis of subcutaneous tissue, left buttock
  MCC when PDx is its own MCC

L89.324 **Pressure ulcer of left buttock, stage 4** 🖐🖐
  Healing pressure ulcer of left buttock, stage 4
  Pressure ulcer with necrosis of soft tissues through to underlying muscle, tendon, or bone, left buttock
  MCC when PDx is its own MCC

L89.329 **Pressure ulcer of left buttock,** unspecified **stage**
  Healing pressure ulcer of left buttock NOS
  Healing pressure ulcer of left buttock, unspecified stage

● **L89.4** **Pressure ulcer of contiguous site of back, buttock and hip**

L89.40 **Pressure ulcer of contiguous site of back, buttock and hip,** unspecified **stage**
  Healing pressure ulcer of contiguous site of back, buttock and hip NOS
  Healing pressure ulcer of contiguous site of back, buttock and hip, unspecified stage

L89.41 **Pressure ulcer of contiguous site of back, buttock and hip, stage 1**
  Healing pressure ulcer of contiguous site of back, buttock and hip, stage 1
  Pressure pre-ulcer skin changes limited to persistent focal edema, contiguous site of back, buttock and hip

L89.42 **Pressure ulcer of contiguous site of back, buttock and hip, stage 2**
  Healing pressure ulcer of contiguous site of back, buttock and hip, stage 2
  Pressure ulcer with abrasion, blister, partial thickness skin loss involving epidermis and/or dermis, contiguous site of back, buttock and hip

L89.43 **Pressure ulcer of contiguous site of back, buttock and hip, stage 3** 🖐🖐
  Healing pressure ulcer of contiguous site of back, buttock and hip, stage 3
  Pressure ulcer with full thickness skin loss involving damage or necrosis of subcutaneous tissue, contiguous site of back, buttock and hip
  MCC when PDx is its own MCC

L89.44 **Pressure ulcer of contiguous site of back, buttock and hip, stage 4** 🖐🖐
  Healing pressure ulcer of contiguous site of back, buttock and hip, stage 4
  Pressure ulcer with necrosis of soft tissues through to underlying muscle, tendon, or bone, contiguous site of back, buttock and hip
  MCC when PDx is its own MCC

L89.45 **Pressure ulcer of contiguous site of back, buttock and hip, unstageable**

◀ New   ◀▦ Revised   ~~deleted~~ Deleted   Excludes 1   Excludes 2   Includes   Use additional   Code first   Code also   Unspecified
OGCR Official Guidelines   ● Unacceptable Principal Diagnosis   X Assign placeholder X   ● Use Additional Character(s)   ▶ Manifestation Code   **Coding Clinic**

● **L89.5**   **Pressure ulcer of ankle**

   ● **L89.50**   **Pressure ulcer of unspecified ankle**

     L89.500   **Pressure ulcer of unspecified ankle, unstageable**

     L89.501   **Pressure ulcer of unspecified ankle, stage 1**
         Healing pressure ulcer of unspecified ankle, stage 1
         Pressure pre-ulcer skin changes limited to persistent focal edema, unspecified ankle

     L89.502   **Pressure ulcer of unspecified ankle, stage 2**
         Healing pressure ulcer of unspecified ankle, stage 2
         Pressure ulcer with abrasion, blister, partial thickness skin loss involving epidermis and/or dermis, unspecified ankle

     L89.503   **Pressure ulcer of unspecified ankle, stage 3** 🖐🖐
         Healing pressure ulcer of unspecified ankle, stage 3
         Pressure ulcer with full thickness skin loss involving damage or necrosis of subcutaneous tissue, unspecified ankle
         MCC when PDx is its own MCC

     L89.504   **Pressure ulcer of unspecified ankle, stage 4** 🖐🖐
         Healing pressure ulcer of unspecified ankle, stage 4
         Pressure ulcer with necrosis of soft tissues through to underlying muscle, tendon, or bone, unspecified ankle
         MCC when PDx is its own MCC

     L89.509   **Pressure ulcer of unspecified ankle, unspecified stage**
         Healing pressure ulcer of unspecified ankle NOS
         Healing pressure ulcer of unspecified ankle, unspecified stage

   ● **L89.51**   **Pressure ulcer of right ankle**

     L89.510   **Pressure ulcer of right ankle, unstageable**

     L89.511   **Pressure ulcer of right ankle, stage 1**
         Healing pressure ulcer of right ankle, stage 1
         Pressure pre-ulcer skin changes limited to persistent focal edema, right ankle

     L89.512   **Pressure ulcer of right ankle, stage 2**
         Healing pressure ulcer of right ankle, stage 2
         Pressure ulcer with abrasion, blister, partial thickness skin loss involving epidermis and/or dermis, right ankle

     L89.513   **Pressure ulcer of right ankle, stage 3** 🖐🖐
         Healing pressure ulcer of right ankle, stage 3
         Pressure ulcer with full thickness skin loss involving damage or necrosis of subcutaneous tissue, right ankle
         MCC when PDx is its own MCC

     L89.514   **Pressure ulcer of right ankle, stage 4** 🖐🖐
         Healing pressure ulcer of right ankle, stage 4
         Pressure ulcer with necrosis of soft tissues through to underlying muscle, tendon, or bone, right ankle
         MCC when PDx is its own MCC

     L89.519   **Pressure ulcer of right ankle, unspecified stage**
         Healing pressure ulcer of right ankle NOS
         Healing pressure ulcer of right ankle, unspecified stage

   ● **L89.52**   **Pressure ulcer of left ankle**

     L89.520   **Pressure ulcer of left ankle, unstageable**

     L89.521   **Pressure ulcer of left ankle, stage 1**
         Healing pressure ulcer of left ankle, stage 1
         Pressure pre-ulcer skin changes limited to persistent focal edema, left ankle

     L89.522   **Pressure ulcer of left ankle, stage 2**
         Healing pressure ulcer of left ankle, stage 2
         Pressure ulcer with abrasion, blister, partial thickness skin loss involving epidermis and/or dermis, left ankle

     L89.523   **Pressure ulcer of left ankle, stage 3** 🖐🖐
         Healing pressure ulcer of left ankle, stage 3
         Pressure ulcer with full thickness skin loss involving damage or necrosis of subcutaneous tissue, left ankle
         MCC when PDx is its own MCC

     L89.524   **Pressure ulcer of left ankle, stage 4** 🖐🖐
         Healing pressure ulcer of left ankle, stage 4
         Pressure ulcer with necrosis of soft tissues through to underlying muscle, tendon, or bone, left ankle
         MCC when PDx is its own MCC

     L89.529   **Pressure ulcer of left ankle, unspecified stage**
         Healing pressure ulcer of left ankle NOS
         Healing pressure ulcer of left ankle, unspecified stage

● **L89.6**   **Pressure ulcer of heel**

   ● **L89.60**   **Pressure ulcer of unspecified heel**

     L89.600   **Pressure ulcer of unspecified heel, unstageable**

     L89.601   **Pressure ulcer of unspecified heel, stage 1**
         Healing pressure ulcer of unspecified heel, stage 1
         Pressure pre-ulcer skin changes limited to persistent focal edema, unspecified heel

     L89.602   **Pressure ulcer of unspecified heel, stage 2**
         Healing pressure ulcer of unspecified heel, stage 2
         Pressure ulcer with abrasion, blister, partial thickness skin loss involving epidermis and/or dermis, unspecified heel

N   Newborn Age: 0   **P**   Pediatric Age: 0–17   **M**   Maternity DX: 12–55   **A**   Adult Age: 15–124   ♀   Females Only   ♂   Males Only

🖐   Complication\Comorbidity   🖐🖐   Major C\C   Ⓧ   CC/MCC Exclusions   🖐   Present on Admission Requirement   🖐   Hospital-Acquired Condition

1063

L89.603   **Pressure ulcer of unspecified heel, stage 3**
     Healing pressure ulcer of unspecified heel, stage 3
     Pressure ulcer with full thickness skin loss involving damage or necrosis of subcutaneous tissue, unspecified heel
     MCC when PDx is its own MCC

L89.604   **Pressure ulcer of unspecified heel, stage 4**
     Healing pressure ulcer of unspecified heel, stage 4
     Pressure ulcer with necrosis of soft tissues through to underlying muscle, tendon, or bone, unspecified heel
     MCC when PDx is its own MCC

L89.609   **Pressure ulcer of unspecified heel, unspecified stage**
     Healing pressure ulcer of unspecified heel NOS
     Healing pressure ulcer of unspecified heel, unspecified stage

● **L89.61**   **Pressure ulcer of right heel**

L89.610   **Pressure ulcer of right heel, unstageable**

L89.611   **Pressure ulcer of right heel, stage 1**
     Healing pressure ulcer of right heel, stage 1
     Pressure pre-ulcer skin changes limited to persistent focal edema, right heel

L89.612   **Pressure ulcer of right heel, stage 2**
     Healing pressure ulcer of right heel, stage 2
     Pressure ulcer with abrasion, blister, partial thickness skin loss involving epidermis and/or dermis, right heel

L89.613   **Pressure ulcer of right heel, stage 3**
     Healing pressure ulcer of right heel, stage 3
     Pressure ulcer with full thickness skin loss involving damage or necrosis of subcutaneous tissue, right heel
     MCC when PDx is its own MCC

L89.614   **Pressure ulcer of right heel, stage 4**
     Healing pressure ulcer of right heel, stage 4
     Pressure ulcer with necrosis of soft tissues through to underlying muscle, tendon, or bone, right heel
     MCC when PDx is its own MCC

L89.619   **Pressure ulcer of right heel, unspecified stage**
     Healing pressure ulcer of right heel NOS
     Healing pressure ulcer of unspecified heel, right stage

● **L89.62**   **Pressure ulcer of left heel**

L89.620   **Pressure ulcer of left heel, unstageable**

L89.621   **Pressure ulcer of left heel, stage 1**
     Healing pressure ulcer of left heel, stage 1
     Pressure pre-ulcer skin changes limited to persistent focal edema, left heel

L89.622   **Pressure ulcer of left heel, stage 2**
     Healing pressure ulcer of left heel, stage 2
     Pressure ulcer with abrasion, blister, partial thickness skin loss involving epidermis and/or dermis, left heel

L89.623   **Pressure ulcer of left heel, stage 3**
     Healing pressure ulcer of left heel, stage 3
     Pressure ulcer with full thickness skin loss involving damage or necrosis of subcutaneous tissue, left heel
     MCC when PDx is its own MCC

L89.624   **Pressure ulcer of left heel, stage 4**
     Healing pressure ulcer of left heel, stage 4
     Pressure ulcer with necrosis of soft tissues through to underlying muscle, tendon, or bone, left heel
     MCC when PDx is its own MCC

L89.629   **Pressure ulcer of left heel, unspecified stage**
     Healing pressure ulcer of left heel NOS
     Healing pressure ulcer of left heel, unspecified stage

● **L89.8**   **Pressure ulcer of other site**

● **L89.81**   **Pressure ulcer of head**
     Pressure ulcer of face

L89.810   **Pressure ulcer of head, unstageable**

L89.811   **Pressure ulcer of head, stage 1**
     Healing pressure ulcer of head, stage 1
     Pressure pre-ulcer skin changes limited to persistent focal edema, head

L89.812   **Pressure ulcer of head, stage 2**
     Healing pressure ulcer of head, stage 2
     Pressure ulcer with abrasion, blister, partial thickness skin loss involving epidermis and/or dermis, head

L89.813   **Pressure ulcer of head, stage 3**
     Healing pressure ulcer of head, stage 3
     Pressure ulcer with full thickness skin loss involving damage or necrosis of subcutaneous tissue, head
     MCC when PDx is its own MCC

L89.814   **Pressure ulcer of head, stage 4**
     Healing pressure ulcer of head, stage 4
     Pressure ulcer with necrosis of soft tissues through to underlying muscle, tendon, or bone, head
     MCC when PDx is its own MCC

L89.819   **Pressure ulcer of head, unspecified stage**
     Healing pressure ulcer of head NOS
     Healing pressure ulcer of head, unspecified stage

CHAPTER 12 (L00-L99)

◄ New   ⬅ Revised   ~~deleted~~ Deleted   Excludes 1   Excludes 2   Includes   Use additional   Code first   Code also   Unspecified

 OGCR Official Guidelines   ● Unacceptable Principal Diagnosis   X Assign placeholder X   ● Use Additional Character(s)   Manifestation Code   **Coding Clinic**

● **L89.89   Pressure ulcer of other site**

     L89.890   Pressure ulcer of other site, unstageable

     L89.891   Pressure ulcer of other site, stage 1
        Healing pressure ulcer of other site, stage 1
        Pressure pre-ulcer skin changes limited to persistent focal edema, other site

     L89.892   Pressure ulcer of other site, stage 2
        Healing pressure ulcer of other site, stage 2
        Pressure ulcer with abrasion, blister, partial thickness skin loss involving epidermis and/or dermis, other site

     L89.893   Pressure ulcer of other site, stage 3 🝆 🝆
        Healing pressure ulcer of other site, stage 3
        Pressure ulcer with full thickness skin loss involving damage or necrosis of subcutaneous tissue, other site
        MCC when PDx is its own MCC

     L89.894   Pressure ulcer of other site, stage 4 🝆 🝆
        Healing pressure ulcer of other site, stage 4
        Pressure ulcer with necrosis of soft tissues through to underlying muscle, tendon, or bone, other site
        MCC when PDx is its own MCC

     L89.899   Pressure ulcer of other site, unspecified stage
        Healing pressure ulcer of other site NOS
        Healing pressure ulcer of other site, unspecified stage

● **L89.9   Pressure ulcer of unspecified site**

     L89.90   Pressure ulcer of unspecified site, unspecified stage
        Healing pressure ulcer of unspecified site NOS
        Healing pressure ulcer of unspecified site, unspecified stage

     L89.91   Pressure ulcer of unspecified site, stage 1
        Healing pressure ulcer of unspecified site, stage 1
        Pressure pre-ulcer skin changes limited to persistent focal edema, unspecified site

     L89.92   Pressure ulcer of unspecified site, stage 2
        Healing pressure ulcer of unspecified site, stage 2
        Pressure ulcer with abrasion, blister, partial thickness skin loss involving epidermis and/or dermis, unspecified site

     L89.93   Pressure ulcer of unspecified site, stage 3 🝆 🝆
        Healing pressure ulcer of unspecified site, stage 3
        Pressure ulcer with full thickness skin loss involving damage or necrosis of subcutaneous tissue, unspecified site
        MCC when PDx is its own MCC

     L89.94   Pressure ulcer of unspecified site, stage 4 🝆 🝆
        Healing pressure ulcer of unspecified site, stage 4
        Pressure ulcer with necrosis of soft tissues through to underlying muscle, tendon, or bone, unspecified site
        MCC when PDx is its own MCC

     L89.95   Pressure ulcer of unspecified site, unstageable

---

● **L90   Atrophic disorders of skin**

   L90.0   **Lichen sclerosus et atrophicus**
        Excludes2   lichen sclerosus of external female genital organs (N90.4)
                  lichen sclerosus of external male genital organs (N48.0)

   L90.1   **Anetoderma of Schweninger-Buzzi**

   L90.2   **Anetoderma of Jadassohn-Pellizzari**

   L90.3   **Atrophoderma of Pasini and Pierini**

   L90.4   **Acrodermatitis chronica atrophicans**

   L90.5   **Scar conditions and fibrosis of skin**
        Adherent scar (skin)
        Cicatrix
        Disfigurement of skin due to scar
        Fibrosis of skin NOS
        Scar NOS
        Excludes2   hypertrophic scar (L91.0)
                  keloid scar (L91.0)

   L90.6   **Striae atrophicae**

   L90.8   **Other atrophic disorders of skin**

   L90.9   **Atrophic disorder of skin, unspecified**

● **L91   Hypertrophic disorders of skin**

   L91.0   **Keloid scar**
        Hypertrophic scar
        Keloid
        Excludes2   acne keloid (L73.0)
                  scar NOS (L90.5)

   L91.8   **Other hypertrophic disorders of the skin**

   L91.9   **Hypertrophic disorder of the skin, unspecified**

● **L92   Granulomatous disorders of skin and subcutaneous tissue**
     Excludes2   actinic granuloma (L57.5)

   L92.0   **Granuloma annulare**
        Perforating granuloma annulare

   L92.1   **Necrobiosis lipoidica, not elsewhere classified**
        Excludes1   necrobiosis lipoidica associated with diabetes mellitus (E08-E13 with .620)

   L92.2   **Granuloma faciale [eosinophilic granuloma of skin]**

   L92.3   **Foreign body granuloma of the skin and subcutaneous tissue**
        Use additional code to identify the type of retained foreign body (Z18.-)

   L92.8   **Other granulomatous disorders of the skin and subcutaneous tissue**

   L92.9   **Granulomatous disorder of the skin and subcutaneous tissue, unspecified**

● **L93   Lupus erythematosus**
     Use additional code for adverse effect, if applicable, to identify drug (T36-T50 with fifth or sixth character 5)
     Excludes1   lupus exedens (A18.4)
                 lupus vulgaris (A18.4)
                 scleroderma (M34.-)
                 systemic lupus erythematosus (M32.-)

   L93.0   **Discoid lupus erythematosus**
        Lupus erythematosus NOS

   L93.1   **Subacute cutaneous lupus erythematosus**

   L93.2   **Other local lupus erythematosus**
        Lupus erythematosus profundus
        Lupus panniculitis

Item 12-11   Scleroderma means hard skin. It is a group of diseases that causes abnormal growth of connective tissues that support the skin and organs. There are two types: localized scleroderma affecting the skin and systemic scleroderma affecting blood vessels and internal organs and the skin.

CHAPTER 12 (L00-L99)

N Newborn Age: 0   **P** Pediatric Age: 0-17   **M** Maternity DX: 12-55   **A** Adult Age: 15-124   ♀ Females Only   ♂ Males Only

🝆 Complication\Comorbidity   🝆 Major C\C   (Ex) CC/MCC Exclusions   🝆 Present on Admission Requirement   🝆 Hospital-Acquired Condition

1065

● **L94**   **Other localized connective tissue disorders**
> **Excludes1**   systemic connective tissue disorders (M30-M36)

L94.0   **Localized scleroderma [morphea]**
> Circumscribed scleroderma

L94.1   **Linear scleroderma**
> En coup de sabre lesion

L94.2   **Calcinosis cutis**

L94.3   **Sclerodactyly**

L94.4   **Gottron's papules**

L94.5   **Poikiloderma vasculare atrophicans**

L94.6   **Ainhum**

L94.8   **Other specified localized connective tissue disorders**

L94.9   **Localized connective tissue disorder, unspecified**

● **L95**   **Vasculitis limited to skin, not elsewhere classified**
> **Excludes1**   angioma serpiginosum (L81.7)
> Henoch(-Schönlein) purpura (D69.0)
> hypersensitivity angiitis (M31.0)
> lupus panniculitis (L93.2)
> panniculitis NOS (M79.3)
> panniculitis of neck and back (M54.0-)
> polyarteritis nodosa (M30.0)
> relapsing panniculitis (M35.6)
> rheumatoid vasculitis (M05.2)
> serum sickness (T80.6-)
> urticaria (L50.-)
> Wegener's granulomatosis (M31.3-)

L95.0   **Livedoid vasculitis**
> Atrophie blanche (en plaque)

L95.1   **Erythema elevatum diutinum**

L95.8   **Other vasculitis limited to the skin**

L95.9   **Vasculitis limited to the skin, unspecified**

● **L97**   **Non-pressure chronic ulcer of lower limb, not elsewhere classified**
> **Includes**   chronic ulcer of skin of lower limb NOS
> non-healing ulcer of skin
> non-infected sinus of skin
> trophic ulcer NOS
> tropical ulcer NOS
> ulcer of skin of lower limb NOS

> *Code first* any associated underlying condition, such as:
> any associated gangrene (I96)
> atherosclerosis of the lower extremities (I70.23-, I70.24-,
> I70.33-, I70.34-, I70.43-, I70.44-, I70.53-, I70.54-, I70.63-,
> I70.64-, I70.73-, I70.74-)
> chronic venous hypertension (I87.31-, I87.33-)
> diabetic ulcers (E08.621, E08.622, E09.621, E09.622, E10.621,
> E10.622, E11.621, E11.622, E13.621, E13.622)
> postphlebitic syndrome (I87.01-, I87.03-)
> postthrombotic syndrome (I87.01-, I87.03-)
> varicose ulcer (I83.0-, I83.2-)

> **Excludes2**   pressure ulcer (pressure area) (L89.-)
> skin infections (L00-L08)
> specific infections classified to A00-B99
> (Ex) **For category L97 CC codes:** I70.231-I70.25, L44.8-L45, L94.2, L94.4,
> L97.101-L97.929, L98.411-L98.499, L98.8-L99

● **L97.1**   **Non-pressure chronic ulcer of thigh**
> ● **L97.10**   **Non-pressure chronic ulcer of unspecified thigh**
> > **L97.101**   Non-pressure chronic ulcer of unspecified thigh limited to breakdown of skin
> > **L97.102**   Non-pressure chronic ulcer of unspecified thigh with fat layer exposed
> > **L97.103**   Non-pressure chronic ulcer of unspecified thigh with necrosis of muscle

L97.104   Non-pressure chronic ulcer of unspecified thigh with necrosis of bone

L97.109   Non-pressure chronic ulcer of unspecified thigh with unspecified severity

● **L97.11**   **Non-pressure chronic ulcer of right thigh**
> **L97.111**   Non-pressure chronic ulcer of right thigh limited to breakdown of skin
> **L97.112**   Non-pressure chronic ulcer of right thigh with fat layer exposed
> **L97.113**   Non-pressure chronic ulcer of right thigh with necrosis of muscle
> **L97.114**   Non-pressure chronic ulcer of right thigh with necrosis of bone
> **L97.119**   Non-pressure chronic ulcer of right thigh with unspecified severity

● **L97.12**   **Non-pressure chronic ulcer of left thigh**
> **L97.121**   Non-pressure chronic ulcer of left thigh limited to breakdown of skin
> **L97.122**   Non-pressure chronic ulcer of left thigh with fat layer exposed
> **L97.123**   Non-pressure chronic ulcer of left thigh with necrosis of muscle
> **L97.124**   Non-pressure chronic ulcer of left thigh with necrosis of bone
> **L97.129**   Non-pressure chronic ulcer of left thigh with unspecified severity

● **L97.2**   **Non-pressure chronic ulcer of calf**
> ● **L97.20**   **Non-pressure chronic ulcer of unspecified calf**
> > **L97.201**   Non-pressure chronic ulcer of unspecified calf limited to breakdown of skin
> > **L97.202**   Non-pressure chronic ulcer of unspecified calf with fat layer exposed
> > **L97.203**   Non-pressure chronic ulcer of unspecified calf with necrosis of muscle
> > **L97.204**   Non-pressure chronic ulcer of unspecified calf with necrosis of bone
> > **L97.209**   Non-pressure chronic ulcer of unspecified calf with unspecified severity

● **L97.21**   **Non-pressure chronic ulcer of right calf**
> **L97.211**   Non-pressure chronic ulcer of right calf limited to breakdown of skin
> **L97.212**   Non-pressure chronic ulcer of right calf with fat layer exposed
> **L97.213**   Non-pressure chronic ulcer of right calf with necrosis of muscle
> **L97.214**   Non-pressure chronic ulcer of right calf with necrosis of bone
> **L97.219**   Non-pressure chronic ulcer of right calf with unspecified severity

● **L97.22**   **Non-pressure chronic ulcer of left calf**
> **L97.221**   Non-pressure chronic ulcer of left calf limited to breakdown of skin
> **L97.222**   Non-pressure chronic ulcer of left calf with fat layer exposed
> **L97.223**   Non-pressure chronic ulcer of left calf with necrosis of muscle
> **L97.224**   Non-pressure chronic ulcer of left calf with necrosis of bone
> **L97.229**   Non-pressure chronic ulcer of left calf with unspecified severity

◀ New   ◀‖ Revised   ~~deleted~~ Deleted   Excludes 1   Excludes 2   Includes   Use additional   Code first   Code also   Unspecified

OGCR Official Guidelines   ● Unacceptable Principal Diagnosis   X Assign placeholder X   ▌ Use Additional Character(s)   ▐ Manifestation Code   **Coding Clinic**

● **L97.3**   Non-pressure chronic ulcer of ankle
  ● **L97.30**   Non-pressure chronic ulcer of unspecified ankle
     L97.301   Non-pressure chronic ulcer of unspecified ankle limited to breakdown of skin 🅰
     L97.302   Non-pressure chronic ulcer of unspecified ankle with fat layer exposed 🅰
     L97.303   Non-pressure chronic ulcer of unspecified ankle with necrosis of muscle 🅰
     L97.304   Non-pressure chronic ulcer of unspecified ankle with necrosis of bone 🅰
     L97.309   Non-pressure chronic ulcer of unspecified ankle with unspecified severity 🅰
  ● **L97.31**   Non-pressure chronic ulcer of right ankle
     L97.311   Non-pressure chronic ulcer of right ankle limited to breakdown of skin 🅰
     L97.312   Non-pressure chronic ulcer of right ankle with fat layer exposed 🅰
     L97.313   Non-pressure chronic ulcer of right ankle with necrosis of muscle 🅰
     L97.314   Non-pressure chronic ulcer of right ankle with necrosis of bone 🅰
     L97.319   Non-pressure chronic ulcer of right ankle with unspecified severity 🅰
  ● **L97.32**   Non-pressure chronic ulcer of left ankle
     L97.321   Non-pressure chronic ulcer of left ankle limited to breakdown of skin 🅰
     L97.322   Non-pressure chronic ulcer of left ankle with fat layer exposed 🅰
     L97.323   Non-pressure chronic ulcer of left ankle with necrosis of muscle 🅰
     L97.324   Non-pressure chronic ulcer of left ankle with necrosis of bone 🅰
     L97.329   Non-pressure chronic ulcer of left ankle with unspecified severity 🅰
● **L97.4**   Non-pressure chronic ulcer of heel and midfoot
     Non-pressure chronic ulcer of plantar surface of midfoot
  ● **L97.40**   Non-pressure chronic ulcer of unspecified heel and midfoot
     L97.401   Non-pressure chronic ulcer of unspecified heel and midfoot limited to breakdown of skin 🅰
     L97.402   Non-pressure chronic ulcer of unspecified heel and midfoot with fat layer exposed 🅰
     L97.403   Non-pressure chronic ulcer of unspecified heel and midfoot with necrosis of muscle 🅰
     L97.404   Non-pressure chronic ulcer of unspecified heel and midfoot with necrosis of bone 🅰
     L97.409   Non-pressure chronic ulcer of unspecified heel and midfoot with unspecified severity 🅰
  ● **L97.41**   Non-pressure chronic ulcer of right heel and midfoot
     L97.411   Non-pressure chronic ulcer of right heel and midfoot limited to breakdown of skin 🅰
     L97.412   Non-pressure chronic ulcer of right heel and midfoot with fat layer exposed 🅰
     L97.413   Non-pressure chronic ulcer of right heel and midfoot with necrosis of muscle 🅰

     L97.414   Non-pressure chronic ulcer of right heel and midfoot with necrosis of bone 🅰
     L97.419   Non-pressure chronic ulcer of right heel and midfoot with unspecified severity 🅰
  ● **L97.42**   Non-pressure chronic ulcer of left heel and midfoot
     L97.421   Non-pressure chronic ulcer of left heel and midfoot limited to breakdown of skin 🅰
     L97.422   Non-pressure chronic ulcer of left heel and midfoot with fat layer exposed 🅰
     L97.423   Non-pressure chronic ulcer of left heel and midfoot with necrosis of muscle 🅰
     L97.424   Non-pressure chronic ulcer of left heel and midfoot with necrosis of bone 🅰
     L97.429   Non-pressure chronic ulcer of left heel and midfoot with unspecified severity 🅰
● **L97.5**   Non-pressure chronic ulcer of other part of foot
     Non-pressure chronic ulcer of toe
  ● **L97.50**   Non-pressure chronic ulcer of other part of unspecified foot
     L97.501   Non-pressure chronic ulcer of other part of unspecified foot limited to breakdown of skin
     L97.502   Non-pressure chronic ulcer of other part of unspecified foot with fat layer exposed
     L97.503   Non-pressure chronic ulcer of other part of unspecified foot with necrosis of muscle
     L97.504   Non-pressure chronic ulcer of other part of unspecified foot with necrosis of bone
     L97.509   Non-pressure chronic ulcer of other part of unspecified foot with unspecified severity
  ● **L97.51**   Non-pressure chronic ulcer of other part of right foot
     L97.511   Non-pressure chronic ulcer of other part of right foot limited to breakdown of skin
     L97.512   Non-pressure chronic ulcer of other part of right foot with fat layer exposed
     L97.513   Non-pressure chronic ulcer of other part of right foot with necrosis of muscle
     L97.514   Non-pressure chronic ulcer of other part of right foot with necrosis of bone
     L97.519   Non-pressure chronic ulcer of other part of right foot with unspecified severity
  ● **L97.52**   Non-pressure chronic ulcer of other part of left foot
     L97.521   Non-pressure chronic ulcer of other part of left foot limited to breakdown of skin
     L97.522   Non-pressure chronic ulcer of other part of left foot with fat layer exposed
     L97.523   Non-pressure chronic ulcer of other part of left foot with necrosis of muscle

N Newborn Age: 0   **P** Pediatric Age: 0–17   **M** Maternity DX: 12–55   **A** Adult Age: 15–124   ♀ Females Only   ♂ Males Only

🅰 Complication\Comorbidity   🅰 Major C\C   (Ex) CC/MCC Exclusions   🅰 Present on Admission Requirement   🅰 Hospital-Acquired Condition

1067

CHAPTER 12 (L00-L99)

L97.524 Non-pressure chronic ulcer of other part of left foot with necrosis of bone

L97.529 Non-pressure chronic ulcer of other part of left foot with unspecified severity

● **L97.8** Non-pressure chronic ulcer of other part of lower leg

● **L97.80** Non-pressure chronic ulcer of other part of unspecified lower leg

L97.801 Non-pressure chronic ulcer of other part of unspecified lower leg limited to breakdown of skin ⌖

L97.802 Non-pressure chronic ulcer of other part of unspecified lower leg with fat layer exposed ⌖

L97.803 Non-pressure chronic ulcer of other part of unspecified lower leg with necrosis of muscle ⌖

L97.804 Non-pressure chronic ulcer of other part of unspecified lower leg with necrosis of bone ⌖

L97.809 Non-pressure chronic ulcer of other part of unspecified lower leg with unspecified severity ⌖

● **L97.81** Non-pressure chronic ulcer of other part of right lower leg

L97.811 Non-pressure chronic ulcer of other part of right lower leg limited to breakdown of skin ⌖

L97.812 Non-pressure chronic ulcer of other part of right lower leg with fat layer exposed ⌖

L97.813 Non-pressure chronic ulcer of other part of right lower leg with necrosis of muscle ⌖

L97.814 Non-pressure chronic ulcer of other part of right lower leg with necrosis of bone ⌖

L97.819 Non-pressure chronic ulcer of other part of right lower leg with unspecified severity ⌖

● **L97.82** Non-pressure chronic ulcer of other part of left lower leg

L97.821 Non-pressure chronic ulcer of other part of left lower leg limited to breakdown of skin ⌖

L97.822 Non-pressure chronic ulcer of other part of left lower leg with fat layer exposed ⌖

L97.823 Non-pressure chronic ulcer of other part of left lower leg with necrosis of muscle ⌖

L97.824 Non-pressure chronic ulcer of other part of left lower leg with necrosis of bone ⌖

L97.829 Non-pressure chronic ulcer of other part of left lower leg with unspecified severity ⌖

● **L97.9** Non-pressure chronic ulcer of unspecified part of lower leg

● **L97.90** Non-pressure chronic ulcer of unspecified part of unspecified lower leg

L97.901 Non-pressure chronic ulcer of unspecified part of unspecified lower leg limited to breakdown of skin ⌖

L97.902 Non-pressure chronic ulcer of unspecified part of unspecified lower leg with fat layer exposed ⌖

L97.903 Non-pressure chronic ulcer of unspecified part of unspecified lower leg with necrosis of muscle ⌖

L97.904 Non-pressure chronic ulcer of unspecified part of unspecified lower leg with necrosis of bone ⌖

L97.909 Non-pressure chronic ulcer of unspecified part of unspecified lower leg with unspecified severity ⌖

● **L97.91** Non-pressure chronic ulcer of unspecified part of right lower leg

L97.911 Non-pressure chronic ulcer of unspecified part of right lower leg limited to breakdown of skin ⌖

L97.912 Non-pressure chronic ulcer of unspecified part of right lower leg with fat layer exposed ⌖

L97.913 Non-pressure chronic ulcer of unspecified part of right lower leg with necrosis of muscle ⌖

L97.914 Non-pressure chronic ulcer of unspecified part of right lower leg with necrosis of bone ⌖

L97.919 Non-pressure chronic ulcer of unspecified part of right lower leg with unspecified severity ⌖

● **L97.92** Non-pressure chronic ulcer of unspecified part of left lower leg

L97.921 Non-pressure chronic ulcer of unspecified part of left lower leg limited to breakdown of skin ⌖

L97.922 Non-pressure chronic ulcer of unspecified part of left lower leg with fat layer exposed ⌖

L97.923 Non-pressure chronic ulcer of unspecified part of left lower leg with necrosis of muscle ⌖

L97.924 Non-pressure chronic ulcer of unspecified part of left lower leg with necrosis of bone ⌖

L97.929 Non-pressure chronic ulcer of unspecified part of left lower leg with unspecified severity ⌖

● **L98** Other disorders of skin and subcutaneous tissue, not elsewhere classified

L98.0 Pyogenic granuloma

> **Excludes2** pyogenic granuloma of gingiva (K06.8)
> pyogenic granuloma of maxillary alveolar ridge (K04.5)
> pyogenic granuloma of oral mucosa (K13.4)

L98.1 Factitial dermatitis
Neurotic excoriation

L98.2 Febrile neutrophilic dermatosis [Sweet]

L98.3 Eosinophilic cellulitis [Wells] ⌖
(Ex) A17.9, A18.4, A18.82, A18.84, A18.89, A48.2-A48.4, A48.8-A49.9, B78.1, B95.0-B96.89, E83.2, L02.811-L02.818, L02.91, L03.811-L03.91, L08.0, L08.81-L08.9, L44.8-L45, L73.2, L88, L92.8, L94.2, L94.4, L98.0, L98.3, L98.8, L99, Z16.10-Z16.39

● **L98.4** Non-pressure chronic ulcer of skin, not elsewhere classified
Chronic ulcer of skin NOS
Tropical ulcer NOS
Ulcer of skin NOS

> **Excludes2** pressure ulcer (pressure area) (L89.-)
> gangrene (I96)
> skin infections (L00-L08)
> specific infections classified to A00-B99
> ulcer of lower limb NEC (L97.-)
> varicose ulcer (I83.0-I82.2)

● **L98.41** Non-pressure chronic ulcer of buttock

L98.411 Non-pressure chronic ulcer of buttock limited to breakdown of skin

L98.412 Non-pressure chronic ulcer of buttock with fat layer exposed

◄ New   ◄⊪ Revised   ~~deleted~~ Deleted   Excludes 1   Excludes 2   Includes   Use additional   Code first   Code also   Unspecified
OGCR Official Guidelines   ● Unacceptable Principal Diagnosis   X Assign placeholder X   ● Use Additional Character(s)   ▸ Manifestation Code   **Coding Clinic**

L98.413 Non-pressure chronic ulcer of buttock with necrosis of muscle

L98.414 Non-pressure chronic ulcer of buttock with necrosis of bone

L98.419 Non-pressure chronic ulcer of buttock with unspecified severity

● L98.42 Non-pressure chronic ulcer of back

L98.421 Non-pressure chronic ulcer of back limited to breakdown of skin

L98.422 Non-pressure chronic ulcer of back with fat layer exposed

L98.423 Non-pressure chronic ulcer of back with necrosis of muscle

L98.424 Non-pressure chronic ulcer of back with necrosis of bone

L98.429 Non-pressure chronic ulcer of back with unspecified severity

● L98.49 Non-pressure chronic ulcer of skin of other sites
Non-pressure chronic ulcer of skin NOS

L98.491 Non-pressure chronic ulcer of skin of other sites limited to breakdown of skin

L98.492 Non-pressure chronic ulcer of skin of other sites with fat layer exposed

L98.493 Non-pressure chronic ulcer of skin of other sites with necrosis of muscle

L98.494 Non-pressure chronic ulcer of skin of other sites with necrosis of bone

L98.499 Non-pressure chronic ulcer of skin of other sites with unspecified severity

L98.5 **Mucinosis of the skin**
Focal mucinosis
Lichen myxedematosus
Reticular erythematous mucinosis

Excludes1 focal oral mucinosis (K13.79)
myxedema (E03.9)

L98.6 **Other infiltrative disorders of the skin and subcutaneous tissue**

Excludes1 hyalinosis cutis et mucosae (E78.89)

L98.8 **Other specified disorders of the skin and subcutaneous tissue**

L98.9 **Disorder of the skin and subcutaneous tissue, unspecified**

▸ *L99* *Other disorders of skin and subcutaneous tissue in diseases classified elsewhere*

Code first underlying disease, such as:
amyloidosis (E85.-) ◂▥

Excludes1 skin disorders in diabetes (E08-E13 with .62)
skin disorders in gonorrhea (A54.89)
skin disorders in syphilis (A51.31, A52.79)

N Newborn Age: 0 **P** Pediatric Age: 0–17 **M** Maternity DX: 12–55 **A** Adult Age: 15–124 ♀ Females Only ♂ Males Only

Complication\Comorbidity Major C\C (Ex) CC/MCC Exclusions Present on Admission Requirement Hospital-Acquired Condition

1069

OGCR Section I.C.a.-c.

a. Site and laterality

Most of the codes within Chapter 13 have site and laterality designations. The site represents the bone, joint or the muscle involved. For some conditions where more than one bone, joint or muscle is usually involved, such as osteoarthritis, there is a "multiple sites" code available. For categories where no multiple site code is provided and more than one bone, joint or muscle is involved, multiple codes should be used to indicate the different sites involved.

1) Bone versus joint

For certain conditions, the bone may be affected at the upper or lower end, (e.g., avascular necrosis of bone, M87, Osteoporosis, M80, M81). Though the portion of the bone affected may be at the joint, the site designation will be the bone, not the joint.

b. Acute traumatic versus chronic or recurrent musculoskeletal conditions

Many musculoskeletal conditions are a result of previous injury or trauma to a site, or are recurrent conditions. Bone, joint or muscle conditions that are the result of a healed injury are usually found in chapter 13. Recurrent bone, joint or muscle conditions are also usually found in chapter 13. Any current, acute injury should be coded to the appropriate injury code from chapter 19. Chronic or recurrent conditions should generally be coded with a code from chapter 13. If it is difficult to determine from the documentation in the record which code is best to describe a condition, query the provider.

c. Coding of Pathologic Fractures

7th character A is for use as long as the patient is receiving active treatment for the fracture. Examples of active treatment are: surgical treatment, emergency department encounter, evaluation and treatment by a new physician. 7th character, D is to be used for encounters after the patient has completed active treatment. The other 7th characters, listed under each subcategory in the Tabular List, are to be used for subsequent encounters for treatment of problems associated with the healing, such as malunions and nonunions, and sequelae. Care for complications of surgical treatment for fracture repairs during the healing or recovery phase should be coded with the appropriate complication codes.

See Section I.C.19. Coding of traumatic fractures.

CHAPTER 13

DISEASES OF THE MUSCULOSKELETAL SYSTEM AND CONNECTIVE TISSUE (M00-M99)

Note: Use an external cause code following the code for the musculoskeletal condition, if applicable, to identify the cause of the musculoskeletal condition

Excludes2   arthropathic psoriasis (L40.5-)
certain conditions originating in the perinatal period (P04-P96)
certain infectious and parasitic diseases (A00-B99)
compartment syndrome (traumatic) (T79.A-)
complications of pregnancy, childbirth and the puerperium (O00-O9A)
congenital malformations, deformations, and chromosomal abnormalities (Q00-Q99)
endocrine, nutritional and metabolic diseases (E00-E88)
injury, poisoning and certain other consequences of external causes (S00-T88)
neoplasms (C00-D49)
symptoms, signs and abnormal clinical and laboratory findings, not elsewhere classified (R00-R94)

This chapter contains the following blocks:

M00-M02	Infectious arthropathies
M05-M14	Inflammatory polyarthropathies
M15-M19	Osteoarthritis
M20-M25	Other joint disorders
M26-M27	Dentofacial anomalies [including malocclusion] and other disorders of jaw
M30-M36	Systemic connective tissue disorders
M40-M43	Deforming dorsopathies
M45-M49	Spondylopathies
M50-M54	Other dorsopathies
M60-M63	Disorders of muscles
M65-M67	Disorders of synovium and tendon
M70-M79	Other soft tissue disorders
M80-M85	Disorders of bone density and structure
M86-M90	Other osteopathies
M91-M94	Chondropathies
M95	Other disorders of the musculoskeletal system and connective tissue
M96	Intraoperative and postprocedural complications and disorders of musculoskeletal system, not elsewhere classified
M99	Biomechanical lesions, not elsewhere classified

ARTHROPATHIES (M00-M25)

Includes   Disorders affecting predominantly peripheral (limb) joints

INFECTIOUS ARTHROPATHIES (M00-M02)

Note: This block comprises arthropathies due to microbiological agents.

Distinction is made between the following types of etiological relationship:

a) direct infection of joint, where organisms invade synovial tissue and microbial antigen is present in the joint;

b) indirect infection, which may be of two types: a reactive arthropathy, where microbial infection of the body is established but neither organisms nor antigens can be identified in the joint, and a postinfective arthropathy, where microbial antigen is present but recovery of an organism is inconstant and evidence of local multiplication is lacking.

● **M00   Pyogenic arthritis**

   ● **M00.0   Staphylococcal arthritis and polyarthritis**

     Use additional code (B95.61-B95.8) to identify bacterial agent

     Excludes2   infection and inflammatory reaction due to internal joint prosthesis (T84.5-)

     M00.00   Staphylococcal arthritis, unspecified joint 🔗

       (Ex) A17.9, A18.02, A18.09, A18.82, A18.84, A18.89, A39.83-A39.84, A54.40, A54.42-A54.43, A54.82, A54.84, A54.89-A54.9, B06.82, M00.00-M02.30, M02.319, M02.329, M02.339, M02.349, M02.359, M02.369, M02.379-M02.9, M05.40-M05.59, M05.70-M06.09, M06.20-M07.69, M11.00-M11.9, M12.10-M15.0, M15.3-M15.9, M16.2-M16.9, M17.2-M17.9, M18.2-M19.93, M24.10-M24.176, M25.00, M25.08-M25.18, M25.40-M25.676, M25.80-M25.9, M35.2, M36.1-M36.4, R26.2, R29.4

◀ New   ◀|||| Revised   ~~deleted~~ Deleted   Excludes 1   Excludes 2   Includes   Use additional   Code first   Code also   Unspecified
OGCR Official Guidelines   ● Unacceptable Principal Diagnosis   X Assign placeholder X   ▶ Use Additional Character(s)   ▶ Manifestation Code   **Coding Clinic**

● M00.01 Staphylococcal arthritis, shoulder
    (Ex:) **For category M00.01 CC codes:** A17.9, A18.02, A18.09,
      A18.82, A18.84, A18.89, A39.83-A39.84, A54.40,
      A54.42-A54.43, A54.82, A54.84, A54.89-A54.9, B06.82,
      M00.00-M02.30, M02.319, M02.38-M02.819, M02.88-M02.9,
      M05.40-M05.59, M05.70-M06.09, M06.20-M07.69,
      M11.00-M11.9, M11.20-M11.219, M11.28-M11.819,
      M11.88-M11.9, M12.10-M15.0, M15.3-M15.9,
      M19.011-M19.019, M19.111-M19.119, M19.211-M19.219,
      M19.90-M19.93, M24.10-M24.119, M25.00,
      M25.011-M25.019, M25.08-M25.119, M25.18,
      M25.40-M25.419, M25.48-M25.519, M25.60-M25.619,
      M25.80-M25.819, M25.9, M35.2, M36.1-M36.4, R26.2

   M00.011   Staphylococcal arthritis, right
           shoulder 🦠

   M00.012   Staphylococcal arthritis, left
           shoulder 🦠

   M00.019   Staphylococcal arthritis, unspecified
           shoulder 🦠

● M00.02 Staphylococcal arthritis, elbow
    (Ex:) **For category M00.02 CC codes:** A17.9, A18.02, A18.09,
      A18.82, A18.84, A18.89, A39.83-A39.84, A54.40,
      A54.42-A54.43, A54.82, A54.84, A54.89-A54.9, B06.82,
      M00.00-M02.30, M02.329, M02.38-M02.80,
      M02.821-M02.829, M02.88-M02.9, M05.40-M05.59,
      M05.70-M07.60, M07.621-M07.629, M07.68-M07.69, M11.00,
      M11.021-M11.029, M11.08-M11.10, M11.121-M11.129,
      M11.18-M11.20, M11.221-M11.229, M11.28-M11.80,
      M11.821-M11.829, M11.88-M11.9, M12.10,
      M12.121-M12.129, M12.18-M12.20, M12.221-M12.229,
      M12.28-M12.30, M12.321-M12.329, M12.38-M12.40,
      M12.421-M12.429, M12.48-M12.50, M12.521-M12.529,
      M12.58-M12.80, M12.821-M12.829, M12.88-M12.9,
      M13.0-M13.10, M13.121-M13.129, M13.80,
      M13.821-M13.829, M13.88-M13.9, M14.60-M15.9,
      M19.021-M19.029, M19.121-M19.129, M19.221-M19.229,
      M19.90-M19.93, M24.10, M24.121-M24.129, M25.00,
      M25.021-M25.029, M25.08-M25.10, M25.121-M25.129,
      M25.18, M25.40, M25.421-M25.429, M25.48-M25.50,
      M25.521-M25.529, M25.60, M25.621-M25.629, M25.80,
      M25.821-M25.829, M25.9, M35.2, M36.1-M36.4, R26.2

   M00.021   Staphylococcal arthritis, right
           elbow 🦠

   M00.022   Staphylococcal arthritis, left elbow 🦠

   M00.029   Staphylococcal arthritis, unspecified
           elbow 🦠

● M00.03 Staphylococcal arthritis, wrist
    Staphylococcal arthritis of carpal bones
    (Ex:) **For category M00.03 CC codes:** A17.9, A18.02, A18.09,
      A18.82, A18.84, A18.89, A39.83-A39.84, A54.40,
      A54.42-A54.43, A54.82, A54.84, A54.89-A54.9, B06.82,
      M00.00-M02.30, M02.339, M02.38-M02.80,
      M02.831-M02.839, M02.88-M02.9, M05.40-M05.59,
      M05.70-M07.60, M07.631-M07.639, M07.68-M07.69, M11.00,
      M11.031-M11.039, M11.08-M11.10, M11.131-M11.139,
      M11.18-M11.20, M11.231-M11.239, M11.28-M11.80,
      M11.831-M11.839, M11.88-M11.9, M12.10,
      M12.131-M12.139, M12.18-M12.20, M12.231-M12.239,
      M12.28-M12.30, M12.331-M12.339, M12.38-M12.40,
      M12.431-M12.439, M12.48-M12.50, M12.531-M12.539,
      M12.58-M12.80, M12.831-M12.839, M12.88-M12.9,
      M13.0-M13.10, M13.131-M13.139, M13.80,
      M13.831-M13.839, M13.88-M15.9, M19.031-M19.039,
      M19.131-M19.139, M19.231-M19.239, M19.90-M19.93,
      M24.10, M24.131-M24.139, M25.00, M25.031-M25.039,
      M25.08-M25.10, M25.131-M25.139, M25.18, M25.40,
      M25.431-M25.439, M25.48-M25.50, M25.531-M25.539,
      M25.60, M25.631-M25.639, M25.80, M25.831-M25.839,
      M25.9, M35.2, M36.1-M36.4, R26.2

   M00.031   Staphylococcal arthritis, right wrist 🦠

   M00.032   Staphylococcal arthritis, left wrist 🦠

   M00.039   Staphylococcal arthritis, unspecified
           wrist 🦠

● M00.04 Staphylococcal arthritis, hand
    Staphylococcal arthritis of metacarpus and
    phalanges
    (Ex:) **For category M00.04 CC codes:** A17.9, A18.02, A18.09,
      A18.82, A18.84, A18.89, A39.83-A39.84, A54.40,
      A54.42-A54.43, A54.82, A54.84, A54.89-A54.9, B06.82,
      M00.00, M00.041-M00.049, M00.08-M00.10,
      M00.141-M00.149, M00.18-M00.20, M00.241-M00.249,
      M00.28-M00.80, M00.841-M00.849, M00.88-M01.X0, M01.
      X41-M01.X49, M01.X8-M02.10, M02.141-M02.149,
      M02.18-M02.30, M02.349, M02.38-M02.80,
      M02.841-M02.849, M02.88-M02.9, M05.40-M05.59,
      M05.70-M06.09, M06.20-M07.60, M07.641-M07.649,
      M07.68-M07.69, M11.00, M11.041-M11.049, M11.08-M11.10,
      M11.141-M11.149, M11.18-M11.20, M11.241-M11.249,
      M11.28-M11.80, M11.841-M11.849, M11.88-M11.9, M12.10,
      M12.141-M12.149, M12.18-M12.20, M12.241-M12.249,
      M12.28-M12.30, M12.341-M12.349, M12.38-M12.40,
      M12.441-M12.449, M12.48-M12.50, M12.541-M12.549,
      M12.58-M12.80, M12.841-M12.849, M12.88-M13.10,
      M13.141-M13.149, M13.80, M13.841-M13.849,
      M13.88-M15.9, M18.0-M18.9, M19.041-M19.049,
      M19.141-M19.149, M19.241-M19.249, M19.90-M19.93,
      M24.10, M24.141-M24.149, M25.00, M25.041-M25.049,
      M25.08-M25.10, M25.141-M25.149, M25.18, M25.40,
      M25.441-M25.449, M25.48-M25.50, M25.60,
      M25.641-M25.649, M25.80, M25.841-M25.849, M25.9, M35.2,
      M36.1-M36.4, R26.2

   M00.041   Staphylococcal arthritis, right hand 🦠

   M00.042   Staphylococcal arthritis, left hand 🦠

   M00.049   Staphylococcal arthritis, unspecified
           hand 🦠

● M00.05 Staphylococcal arthritis, hip
    (Ex:) **For category M00.05 CC codes:** A17.9, A18.02, A18.09,
      A18.82, A18.84, A18.89, A39.83-A39.84, A54.40,
      A54.42-A54.43, A54.82, A54.84, A54.89-A54.9, B06.82,
      M00.00, M00.051-M00.059, M00.08-M00.10,
      M00.151-M00.159, M00.18-M00.20, M00.251-M00.259,
      M00.28-M00.29, M00.80, M00.851-M00.859, M00.88-M00.9,
      M01.X0, M01.X51-M01.X59 , M01.X8-M02.10,
      M02.151-M02.159, M02.18-M02.30, M02.359,
      M02.38-M02.80, M02.851-M02.9, M05.40-M05.59,
      M05.70-M06.09, M06.20-M06.39, M06.80-M07.60,
      M07.651-M07.659, M07.68-M07.69, M11.00,
      M11.051-M11.059, M11.08-M11.10, M11.151-M11.159,
      M11.18-M11.20, M11.251-M11.259, M11.28-M11.80,
      M11.851-M11.859, M11.88-M12.10, M12.151-M12.159,
      M12.18-M12.20, M12.251-M12.259, M12.28-M12.30,
      M12.351-M12.359, M12.38-M12.40, M12.451-M12.459,
      M12.48-M12.50, M12.551-M12.559, M12.58-M12.80,
      M12.851-M12.859, M12.88-M13.10, M13.151-M13.159,
      M13.80, M13.851-M13.859, M13.88-M15.0, M15.3-M16.9,
      M19.90-M19.93, M24.10, M24.151-M24.159, M25.00,
      M25.051-M25.059, M25.08-M25.10, M25.151-M25.159,
      M25.18, M25.40, M25.451-M25.459, M25.48-M25.559,
      M25.60, M25.651-M25.659, M25.80, M25.851-M25.859,
      M25.9, M35.2, M36.1-M36.4, R26.2, R29.4

   M00.051   Staphylococcal arthritis, right hip 🦠

   M00.052   Staphylococcal arthritis, left hip 🦠

   M00.059   Staphylococcal arthritis, unspecified
           hip 🦠

CHAPTER 13 (M00-M99)

N   Newborn Age: 0   P   Pediatric Age: 0–17   M   Maternity DX: 12–55   A   Adult Age: 15–124   ♀   Females Only   ♂   Males Only

🦠   Complication\Comorbidity   🦠   Major C\C   (Ex:)   CC/MCC Exclusions   🦠   Present on Admission Requirement   🦠   Hospital-Acquired Condition

1071

● **M00.06 Staphylococcal arthritis, knee**
Ex For category M00.06 CC codes: A17.9, A18.02, A18.09,
A18.82, A18.84, A18.89, A39.83-A39.84, A54.40,
A54.42-A54.43, A54.82, A54.84, A54.89-A54.9, B06.82,
M00.00, M00.061-M00.069, M00.08-M00.10,
M00.161-M00.169, M00.18-M00.20, M00.261-M00.269,
M00.28-M00.29, M00.80, M00.861-M00.869, M00.88-M00.9,
M01.X0, M01.X61-M01.X69 , M01.X8-M02.10,
M02.161-M02.169, M02.18-M02.30, M02.369,
M02.38-M02.80, M02.861-M02.869, M02.88-M02.9,
M05.40-M05.59, M05.70-M06.09, M06.20-M06.39,
M06.80-M07.60, M07.661-M07.669, M07.68-M07.69, M11.00,
M11.061-M11.069, M11.08-M11.10, M11.161-M11.169,
M11.18-M11.20, M11.261-M11.269, M11.28-M11.80,
M11.861-M11.869, M11.88-M12.10, M12.161-M12.169,
M12.18-M12.20, M12.261-M12.269, M12.28-M12.30,
M12.361-M12.369, M12.38-M12.40, M12.461-M12.469,
M12.48-M12.50, M12.561-M12.569, M12.58-M12.80,
M12.861-M12.869, M12.88-M13.10, M13.161-M13.169,
M13.80, M13.861-M13.869, M13.88-M15.0, M15.3-M15.9,
M17.0-M17.9, M19.90-M19.93, M24.10, M25.00,
M25.061-M25.069, M25.08-M25.10, M25.161-M25.169,
M25.18, M25.40, M25.461-M25.469, M25.48-M25.50,
M25.561-M25.569, M25.60, M25.661-M25.669, M25.80,
M25.861-M25.869, M25.9, M35.2, M36.1-M36.4, R26.2

M00.061 Staphylococcal arthritis, right knee ◐
M00.062 Staphylococcal arthritis, left knee ◐
M00.069 Staphylococcal arthritis, unspecified
knee ◐

● **M00.07 Staphylococcal arthritis, ankle and foot**
Staphylococcal arthritis, tarsus, metatarsus and
phalanges
Ex For category M00.07 CC codes: A17.9, A18.02, A18.09,
A18.82, A18.84, A18.89, A39.83-A39.84, A54.40,
A54.42-A54.43, A54.82, A54.84, A54.89-A54.9, B06.82,
M00.00, M00.071-M00.079, M00.08-M00.10,
M00.171-M00.179, M00.18-M00.20, M00.271-M00.279,
M00.28-M00.29, M00.80, M00.871-M00.879, M00.88-M00.9,
M01.X0, M01.X71-M01.X79 , M01.X8-M02.10,
M02.171-M02.179, M02.18-M02.9, M05.40-M05.59,
M05.70-M06.09, M06.20-M06.39, M06.80-M07.60,
M07.671-M07.679, M07.68-M07.69, M11.00,
M11.071-M11.079, M11.08-M11.10, M11.171-M11.179,
M11.18-M11.20, M11.271-M11.279, M11.28-M11.80,
M11.871-M11.879, M11.88-M11.9, M12.10,
M12.171-M12.179, M12.18-M12.20, M12.271-M12.279,
M12.28-M12.30, M12.371-M12.379, M12.38-M12.40,
M12.471-M12.479, M12.48-M12.50, M12.571-M12.579,
M12.58-M12.80, M12.871-M12.879, M12.88-M13.10,
M13.171-M13.179, M13.80, M13.871-M13.879,
M13.88-M15.0, M15.3-M15.9, M19.071-M19.079,
M19.171-M19.179, M19.271-M19.279, M19.90-M19.93,
M24.10, M24.171-M24.176, M25.00, M25.071-M25.10,
M25.171-M25.18, M25.40, M25.471-M25.50,
M25.571-M25.60, M25.671-M25.676, M25.80,
M25.871-M25.9, M35.2, M36.1-M36.4, R26.2

M00.071 Staphylococcal arthritis, right ankle
and foot ◐
M00.072 Staphylococcal arthritis, left ankle
and foot ◐
M00.079 Staphylococcal arthritis, unspecified
ankle and foot ◐

M00.08 Staphylococcal arthritis, vertebrae ◐
Ex See M00.00

M00.09 Staphylococcal polyarthritis ◐
Ex See M00.00

● **M00.1 Pneumococcal arthritis and polyarthritis**
M00.10 Pneumococcal arthritis, unspecified joint ◐
Ex See M00.00

● M00.11 Pneumococcal arthritis, shoulder
Ex For category M00.11 CC codes: See M00.01
M00.111 Pneumococcal arthritis, right
shoulder ◐
M00.112 Pneumococcal arthritis, left
shoulder ◐
M00.119 Pneumococcal arthritis, unspecified
shoulder ◐

● M00.12 Pneumococcal arthritis, elbow
Ex For category M00.12 CC codes: See M00.02
M00.121 Pneumococcal arthritis, right elbow ◐
M00.122 Pneumococcal arthritis, left elbow ◐
M00.129 Pneumococcal arthritis, unspecified
elbow ◐

● M00.13 Pneumococcal arthritis, wrist
Pneumococcal arthritis of carpal bones
Ex For category M00.13 CC codes: See M00.03
M00.131 Pneumococcal arthritis, right wrist ◐
M00.132 Pneumococcal arthritis, left wrist ◐
M00.139 Pneumococcal arthritis, unspecified
wrist ◐

● M00.14 Pneumococcal arthritis, hand
Pneumococcal arthritis of metacarpus and
phalanges
Ex For category M00.14 CC codes: See M00.04
M00.141 Pneumococcal arthritis, right hand ◐
M00.142 Pneumococcal arthritis, left hand ◐
M00.149 Pneumococcal arthritis, unspecified
hand ◐

● M00.15 Pneumococcal arthritis, hip
Ex For category M00.15 CC codes: See M00.05
M00.151 Pneumococcal arthritis, right hip ◐
M00.152 Pneumococcal arthritis, left hip ◐
M00.159 Pneumococcal arthritis, unspecified
hip ◐

● M00.16 Pneumococcal arthritis, knee
Ex For category M00.16 CC codes: See M00.06
M00.161 Pneumococcal arthritis, right knee ◐
M00.162 Pneumococcal arthritis, left knee ◐
M00.169 Pneumococcal arthritis, unspecified
knee ◐

● M00.17 Pneumococcal arthritis, ankle and foot
Pneumococcal arthritis, tarsus, metatarsus and
phalanges
Ex For category M00.17 CC codes: See M00.07
M00.171 Pneumococcal arthritis, right ankle
and foot ◐
M00.172 Pneumococcal arthritis, left ankle and
foot ◐
M00.179 Pneumococcal arthritis, unspecified
ankle and foot ◐

M00.18 Pneumococcal arthritis, vertebrae ◐
Ex See M00.00

M00.19 Pneumococcal polyarthritis ◐
Ex See M00.00

◀ New   ◀ Revised   deleted Deleted   Excludes 1   Excludes 2   Includes   Use additional   Code first   Code also   Unspecified
OGCR Official Guidelines   ● Unacceptable Principal Diagnosis   X Assign placeholder X   ● Use Additional Character(s)   ▶ Manifestation Code   Coding Clinic

● **M00.2**   **Other streptococcal arthritis and polyarthritis**
     Use additional code (B95.0-B95.2, B95.4-B95.5) to identify bacterial agent

   M00.20   **Other streptococcal arthritis, unspecified joint** 🦴
       Ⓔ See M00.00

●   **M00.21**   **Other streptococcal arthritis, shoulder**
       Ⓔ For category M00.21 CC codes: See M00.01

      M00.211   Other streptococcal arthritis, right shoulder 🦴

      M00.212   Other streptococcal arthritis, left shoulder 🦴

      M00.219   Other streptococcal arthritis, unspecified shoulder 🦴

●   **M00.22**   **Other streptococcal arthritis, elbow**
       Ⓔ For category M00.22 CC codes: See M00.02

      M00.221   Other streptococcal arthritis, right elbow 🦴

      M00.222   Other streptococcal arthritis, left elbow 🦴

      M00.229   Other streptococcal arthritis, unspecified elbow 🦴

●   **M00.23**   **Other streptococcal arthritis, wrist**
       Other streptococcal arthritis of carpal bones
       Ⓔ For category M00.23 CC codes: See M00.03

      M00.231   Other streptococcal arthritis, right wrist 🦴

      M00.232   Other streptococcal arthritis, left wrist 🦴

      M00.239   Other streptococcal arthritis, unspecified wrist 🦴

●   **M00.24**   **Other streptococcal arthritis, hand**
       Other streptococcal arthritis metacarpus and phalanges
       Ⓔ For category M00.24 CC codes: See M00.04

      M00.241   Other streptococcal arthritis, right hand 🦴

      M00.242   Other streptococcal arthritis, left hand 🦴

      M00.249   Other streptococcal arthritis, unspecified hand 🦴

●   **M00.25**   **Other streptococcal arthritis, hip**
       Ⓔ For category M00.25 CC codes: See M00.05

      M00.251   Other streptococcal arthritis, right hip 🦴

      M00.252   Other streptococcal arthritis, left hip 🦴

      M00.259   Other streptococcal arthritis, unspecified hip 🦴

●   **M00.26**   **Other streptococcal arthritis, knee**
       Ⓔ For category M00.26 CC codes: See M00.06

      M00.261   Other streptococcal arthritis, right knee 🦴

      M00.262   Other streptococcal arthritis, left knee 🦴

      M00.269   Other streptococcal arthritis, unspecified knee 🦴

●   **M00.27**   **Other streptococcal arthritis, ankle and foot**
       Other streptococcal arthritis, tarsus, metatarsus and phalanges
       Ⓔ For category M00.27 CC codes: See M00.07

      M00.271   Other streptococcal arthritis, right ankle and foot 🦴

      M00.272   Other streptococcal arthritis, left ankle and foot 🦴

      M00.279   Other streptococcal arthritis, unspecified ankle and foot 🦴

   M00.28   **Other streptococcal arthritis, vertebrae** 🦴
       Ⓔ See M00.00

   M00.29   **Other streptococcal polyarthritis** 🦴
       Ⓔ See M00.00

● **M00.8**   **Arthritis and polyarthritis due to other bacteria**
     Use additional code (B96) to identify bacteria

   M00.80   **Arthritis due to other bacteria, unspecified joint** 🦴
       Ⓔ See M00.00

●   **M00.81**   **Arthritis due to other bacteria, shoulder**
       Ⓔ For category M00.81 CC codes: See M00.01

      M00.811   Arthritis due to other bacteria, right shoulder 🦴

      M00.812   Arthritis due to other bacteria, left shoulder 🦴

      M00.819   Arthritis due to other bacteria, unspecified shoulder 🦴

●   **M00.82**   **Arthritis due to other bacteria, elbow**
       Ⓔ For category M00.82 CC codes: See M00.02

      M00.821   Arthritis due to other bacteria, right elbow 🦴

      M00.822   Arthritis due to other bacteria, left elbow 🦴

      M00.829   Arthritis due to other bacteria, unspecified elbow 🦴

●   **M00.83**   **Arthritis due to other bacteria, wrist**
       Arthritis due to other bacteria, carpal bones
       Ⓔ For category M00.83 CC codes: See M00.03

      M00.831   Arthritis due to other bacteria, right wrist 🦴

      M00.832   Arthritis due to other bacteria, left wrist 🦴

      M00.839   Arthritis due to other bacteria, unspecified wrist 🦴

●   **M00.84**   **Arthritis due to other bacteria, hand**
       Arthritis due to other bacteria, metacarpus and phalanges
       Ⓔ For category M00.84 CC codes: See M00.04

      M00.841   Arthritis due to other bacteria, right hand 🦴

      M00.842   Arthritis due to other bacteria, left hand 🦴

      M00.849   Arthritis due to other bacteria, unspecified hand 🦴

●   **M00.85**   **Arthritis due to other bacteria, hip**
       Ⓔ For category M00.85 CC codes: See M00.05

      M00.851   Arthritis due to other bacteria, right hip 🦴

      M00.852   Arthritis due to other bacteria, left hip 🦴

      M00.859   Arthritis due to other bacteria, unspecified hip 🦴

●   **M00.86**   **Arthritis due to other bacteria, knee**
       Ⓔ For category M00.86 CC codes: See M00.06

      M00.861   Arthritis due to other bacteria, right knee 🦴

      M00.862   Arthritis due to other bacteria, left knee 🦴

      M00.869   Arthritis due to other bacteria, unspecified knee 🦴

●   **M00.87**   **Arthritis due to other bacteria, ankle and foot**
       Arthritis due to other bacteria, tarsus, metatarsus, and phalanges
       Ⓔ For category M00.87 CC codes: See M00.07

      M00.871   Arthritis due to other bacteria, right ankle and foot 🦴

      M00.872   Arthritis due to other bacteria, left ankle and foot 🦴

      M00.879   Arthritis due to other bacteria, unspecified ankle and foot 🦴

   M00.88   **Arthritis due to other bacteria, vertebrae** 🦴
       Ⓔ See M00.00

   M00.89   **Polyarthritis due to other bacteria** 🦴
       Ⓔ See M00.00

M00.9   **Pyogenic arthritis, unspecified** 🦴
     Infective arthritis NOS
     Ⓔ See M00.00

N Newborn Age: 0   **P** Pediatric Age: 0–17   **M** Maternity DX: 12–55   **A** Adult Age: 15–124   ♀ Females Only   ♂ Males Only

🦴 Complication\Comorbidity   🦴 Major C\C   Ⓔ CC/MCC Exclusions   🦴 Present on Admission Requirement   🦴 Hospital-Acquired Condition

1073

CHAPTER 13 (M00-M99)

● **M01** **Direct infections of joint in infectious and parasitic diseases classified elsewhere**

Code first underlying disease, such as:
leprosy [Hansen's disease] (A30.-)
mycoses (B35-B49)
O'nyong-nyong fever (A92.1)
paratyphoid fever (A01.1-A01.4)

Excludes1 arthritis, arthropathy (in):
~~gonococcal (A54.42)~~
arthropathy in Lyme disease (A69.23) ◄▥
~~meningococcal (A39.83)~~
~~postmeningococcal (A39.84)~~
~~mumps (B26.85)~~
~~postinfective (M02.-)~~
~~reactive (M04.0-)~~
~~rubella (B06.82)~~
~~sarcoidosis (D86.86)~~
~~typhoid fever (A01.04)~~
~~tuberculosis (A18.02)~~
~~spine (A18.01)~~
gonococcal arthritis (A54.42) ◄
meningococcal arthritis (A39.83) ◄
mumps arthritis (B26.85) ◄
postinfective arthropathy (M02.-) ◄
postmeningococcal arthritis (A39.84) ◄
reactive arthritis (M02.3) ◄
rubella arthritis (B06.82) ◄
sarcoidosis arthritis (D86.86) ◄
typhoid fever arthritis (A01.04) ◄
tuberculosis arthritis (A18.01-A18.02) ◄

● **M01.X** **Direct infection of joint in infectious and parasitic diseases classified elsewhere**

Ⓔ: **For category M01.X CC codes unless otherwise indicated:** A02.23, A17.9, A18.02, A18.09, A18.82, A18.84, A18.89, A39.83-A39.84, A54.40, A54.42-A54.43, A54.82, A54.84, A54.89-A54.9, B06.82, M00.00, M00.011-M02.30, M02.319, M02.329, M02.339, M02.349, M02.359, M02.369, M02.379, M02.38-M02.9, M05.40-M05.59, M05.70-M07.69, M11.00-M15.0, M15.3-M15.9, M16.2-M16.9, M17.2-M17.9, M18.2-M18.9, M19.111-M19.93, M24.10-M24.176, M25.00, M25.08-M25.18, M25.40-M25.676, M25.80-M25.9, M35.2, M36.1-M36.4, R29.4

▷ *M01.X0* *Direct infection of* unspecified *joint in infectious and parasitic diseases classified elsewhere* ✎

● *M01.X1* **Direct infection of shoulder joint in infectious and parasitic diseases classified elsewhere**

Ⓔ: **For category M01.X1 CC codes:** A02.23, A17.9, A18.02, A18.09, A18.82, A18.84, A18.89, A39.83-A39.84, A54.40, A54.42-A54.43, A54.82, A54.84, A54.89-A54.9, B06.82, M00.00, M00.011-M02.30, M02.319, M02.329, M02.339, M02.349, M02.359, M02.369, M02.379, M02.38-M02.9, M05.40-M05.59, M05.70-M07.69, M11.00-M15.0, M15.3-M15.9, M16.2-M16.9, M17.2-M17.9, M18.2-M18.9, M19.111-M19.93, M24.10-M24.176, M25.00, M25.08-M25.18, M25.40-M25.676, M25.80-M25.9, M35.2, M36.1-M36.4, R29.4

▷ *M01.X11* *Direct infection of right shoulder in infectious and parasitic diseases classified elsewhere* ✎

▷ *M01.X12* *Direct infection of left shoulder in infectious and parasitic diseases classified elsewhere* ✎

▷ *M01.X19* *Direct infection of* unspecified *shoulder in infectious and parasitic diseases classified elsewhere* ✎

● *M01.X2* **Direct infection of elbow in infectious and parasitic diseases classified elsewhere**

▷ *M01.X21* *Direct infection of right elbow in infectious and parasitic diseases classified elsewhere* ✎

▷ *M01.X22* *Direct infection of left elbow in infectious and parasitic diseases classified elsewhere* ✎

▷ *M01.X29* *Direct infection of* unspecified *elbow in infectious and parasitic diseases classified elsewhere* ✎

● *M01.X3* **Direct infection of wrist in infectious and parasitic diseases classified elsewhere**
Direct infection of carpal bones in infectious and parasitic diseases classified elsewhere

▷ *M01.X31* *Direct infection of right wrist in infectious and parasitic diseases classified elsewhere* ✎

▷ *M01.X32* *Direct infection of left wrist in infectious and parasitic diseases classified elsewhere* ✎

▷ *M01.X39* *Direct infection of* unspecified *wrist in infectious and parasitic diseases classified elsewhere* ✎

● *M01.X4* **Direct infection of hand in infectious and parasitic diseases classified elsewhere**
Direct infection of metacarpus and phalanges in infectious and parasitic diseases classified elsewhere

▷ *M01.X41* *Direct infection of right hand in infectious and parasitic diseases classified elsewhere* ✎

▷ *M01.X42* *Direct infection of left hand in infectious and parasitic diseases classified elsewhere* ✎

▷ *M01.X49* *Direct infection of* unspecified *hand in infectious and parasitic diseases classified elsewhere* ✎

● *M01.X5* **Direct infection of hip in infectious and parasitic diseases classified elsewhere**

▷ *M01.X51* *Direct infection of right hip in infectious and parasitic diseases classified elsewhere* ✎

▷ *M01.X52* *Direct infection of left hip in infectious and parasitic diseases classified elsewhere* ✎

▷ *M01.X59* *Direct infection of* unspecified *hip in infectious and parasitic diseases classified elsewhere* ✎

● *M01.X6* **Direct infection of knee in infectious and parasitic diseases classified elsewhere**

▷ *M01.X61* *Direct infection of right knee in infectious and parasitic diseases classified elsewhere* ✎

▷ *M01.X62* *Direct infection of left knee in infectious and parasitic diseases classified elsewhere* ✎

▷ *M01.X69* *Direct infection of* unspecified *knee in infectious and parasitic diseases classified elsewhere* ✎

● *M01.X7* **Direct infection of ankle and foot in infectious and parasitic diseases classified elsewhere**
Direct infection of tarsus, metatarsus and phalanges in infectious and parasitic diseases classified elsewhere

▷ *M01.X71* *Direct infection of right ankle and foot in infectious and parasitic diseases classified elsewhere* ✎

▷ *M01.X72* *Direct infection of left ankle and foot in infectious and parasitic diseases classified elsewhere* ✎

▷ *M01.X79* *Direct infection of* unspecified *ankle and foot in infectious and parasitic diseases classified elsewhere* ✎

▷ *M01.X8* *Direct infection of vertebrae in infectious and parasitic diseases classified elsewhere* ✎

▷ *M01.X9* *Direct infection of multiple joints in infectious and parasitic diseases classified elsewhere* ✎

◄ New   ◄▥ Revised   ~~deleted~~ Deleted   Excludes 1   Excludes 2   Includes   Use additional   Code first   Code also   Unspecified
OGCR Official Guidelines   ● Unacceptable Principal Diagnosis   X Assign placeholder X   ● Use Additional Character(s)   ▷ Manifestation Code   **Coding Clinic**

● **M02   Postinfective and reactive arthropathies**

     Code first underlying disease, such as:
        congenital syphilis [Clutton's joints] (A50.5)
        enteritis due to Yersinia enterocolitica (A04.6)
        infective endocarditis (I33.0)
        viral hepatitis (B15-B19)

     Excludes1   Behçet's disease (M35.2)
                  direct infections of joint in infectious and parasitic
                      diseases classified elsewhere (M01.-)
                  ~~postinfectious arthritis (in):~~
                      ~~meningococcal~~ postmeningococcal arthritis
                      (A39.84) ◀▥
                  mumps arthritis (B26.85) ◀▥
                  rubella arthritis (B06.82) ◀▥
                  syphilis arthritis (late) (A52.77) ◀▥
                  rheumatic fever (I00)
                  tabetic arthropathy [Charcôt's] (A52.16)

    Ⓔⓧ For category M02 CC codes unless otherwise indicated: See M01.X

● **M02.0   Arthropathy following intestinal bypass**

    M02.00   Arthropathy following intestinal bypass, **unspecified** site

    ● **M02.01**   Arthropathy following intestinal bypass, shoulder

       M02.011   Arthropathy following intestinal bypass, right shoulder

       M02.012   Arthropathy following intestinal bypass, left shoulder

       M02.019   Arthropathy following intestinal bypass, **unspecified** shoulder

    ● **M02.02**   Arthropathy following intestinal bypass, elbow

       M02.021   Arthropathy following intestinal bypass, right elbow

       M02.022   Arthropathy following intestinal bypass, left elbow

       M02.029   Arthropathy following intestinal bypass, **unspecified** elbow

    ● **M02.03**   Arthropathy following intestinal bypass, wrist
               Arthropathy following intestinal bypass, carpal bones

       M02.031   Arthropathy following intestinal bypass, right wrist

       M02.032   Arthropathy following intestinal bypass, left wrist

       M02.039   Arthropathy following intestinal bypass, **unspecified** wrist

    ● **M02.04**   Arthropathy following intestinal bypass, hand
               Arthropathy following intestinal bypass, metacarpals and phalanges

       M02.041   Arthropathy following intestinal bypass, right hand

       M02.042   Arthropathy following intestinal bypass, left hand

       M02.049   Arthropathy following intestinal bypass, **unspecified** hand

    ● **M02.05**   Arthropathy following intestinal bypass, hip

       M02.051   Arthropathy following intestinal bypass, right hip

       M02.052   Arthropathy following intestinal bypass, left hip

       M02.059   Arthropathy following intestinal bypass, **unspecified** hip

    ● **M02.06**   Arthropathy following intestinal bypass, knee

       M02.061   Arthropathy following intestinal bypass, right knee

       M02.062   Arthropathy following intestinal bypass, left knee

       M02.069   Arthropathy following intestinal bypass, **unspecified** knee

● **M02.07**   Arthropathy following intestinal bypass, ankle and foot
             Arthropathy following intestinal bypass, tarsus, metatarsus and phalanges

       M02.071   Arthropathy following intestinal bypass, right ankle and foot

       M02.072   Arthropathy following intestinal bypass, left ankle and foot

       M02.079   Arthropathy following intestinal bypass, **unspecified** ankle and foot

    M02.08   Arthropathy following intestinal bypass, vertebrae

    M02.09   Arthropathy following intestinal bypass, multiple sites

● **M02.1   Postdysenteric arthropathy**

    M02.10   Postdysenteric arthropathy, **unspecified** site 🦠

    ● **M02.11**   Postdysenteric arthropathy, shoulder

       M02.111   Postdysenteric arthropathy, right shoulder 🦠

       M02.112   Postdysenteric arthropathy, left shoulder 🦠

       M02.119   Postdysenteric arthropathy, **unspecified** shoulder 🦠

    ● **M02.12**   Postdysenteric arthropathy, elbow

       M02.121   Postdysenteric arthropathy, right elbow 🦠

       M02.122   Postdysenteric arthropathy, left elbow 🦠

       M02.129   Postdysenteric arthropathy, **unspecified** elbow 🦠

    ● **M02.13**   Postdysenteric arthropathy, wrist
               Postdysenteric arthropathy, carpal bones

       M02.131   Postdysenteric arthropathy, right wrist 🦠

       M02.132   Postdysenteric arthropathy, left wrist 🦠

       M02.139   Postdysenteric arthropathy, **unspecified** wrist 🦠

    ● **M02.14**   Postdysenteric arthropathy, hand
               Postdysenteric arthropathy, metacarpus and phalanges

       M02.141   Postdysenteric arthropathy, right hand 🦠

       M02.142   Postdysenteric arthropathy, left hand 🦠

       M02.149   Postdysenteric arthropathy, **unspecified** hand 🦠

    ● **M02.15**   Postdysenteric arthropathy, hip

       M02.151   Postdysenteric arthropathy, right hip 🦠

       M02.152   Postdysenteric arthropathy, left hip 🦠

       M02.159   Postdysenteric arthropathy, **unspecified** hip 🦠

    ● **M02.16**   Postdysenteric arthropathy, knee

       Ⓔⓧ For category M02.16 CC codes: A02.23, A17.9, A18.02, A18.09, A18.82, A18.84, A18.89, A39.83-A39.84, A54.40, A54.42-A54.43, A54.82, A54.84, A54.89-A54.9, B06.82, M00.00, M00.011-M02.30, M02.319, M02.329, M02.339, M02.349, M02.359, M02.369, M02.379, M02.38-M02.9, M05.40-M05.59, M05.70-M07.69, M11.00-M15.0, M15.3-M15.9, M16.2-M16.9, M17.2-M17.9, M18.2-M18.9, M19.111-M19.93, M24.10-M24.176, M25.00, M25.08-M25.18, M25.40-M25.676, M25.80-M25.9, M35.2, M36.1-M36.4, R29.4

       M02.161   Postdysenteric arthropathy, right knee 🦠

       M02.162   Postdysenteric arthropathy, left knee 🦠

       M02.169   Postdysenteric arthropathy, **unspecified** knee 🦠

N Newborn Age: 0   **P** Pediatric Age: 0–17   **M** Maternity DX: 12–55   **A** Adult Age: 15–124   ♀ Females Only   ♂ Males Only

🦠 Complication\Comorbidity   🦠 Major C\C   Ⓔⓧ CC/MCC Exclusions   🦠 Present on Admission Requirement   🦠 Hospital-Acquired Condition

1075

● **M02.17 Postdysenteric arthropathy, ankle and foot**
Postdysenteric arthropathy, tarsus, metatarsus and phalanges

    M02.171 Postdysenteric arthropathy, right ankle and foot 🗘

    M02.172 Postdysenteric arthropathy, left ankle and foot 🗘

    M02.179 Postdysenteric arthropathy, unspecified ankle and foot 🗘

M02.18 Postdysenteric arthropathy, vertebrae 🗘
(Ex:) A02.23, A17.9, A18.02, A18.09, A18.82, A18.84, A18.89, A39.83-A39.84, A54.40, A54.42-A54.43, A54.82, A54.84, A54.89-A54.9, B06.82, M00.00, M00.011-M02.30, M02.319, M02.329, M02.339, M02.349, M02.359, M02.369, M02.379, M02.38-M02.9, M05.40-M05.59, M05.70-M07.69, M11.00-M15.0, M15.3-M15.9, M16.2-M16.9, M17.2-M17.9, M18.2-M18.9, M19.111-M19.93, M24.10-M24.176, M25.00, M25.08-M25.18, M25.40-M25.676, M25.80-M25.9, M35.2, M36.1-M36.4, R29.4

M02.19 Postdysenteric arthropathy, multiple sites 🗘

● **M02.2 Postimmunization arthropathy**

    M02.20 Postimmunization arthropathy, unspecified site

● **M02.21 Postimmunization arthropathy, shoulder**

    M02.211 Postimmunization arthropathy, right shoulder

    M02.212 Postimmunization arthropathy, left shoulder

    M02.219 Postimmunization arthropathy, unspecified shoulder

● **M02.22 Postimmunization arthropathy, elbow**

    M02.221 Postimmunization arthropathy, right elbow

    M02.222 Postimmunization arthropathy, left elbow

    M02.229 Postimmunization arthropathy, unspecified elbow

● **M02.23 Postimmunization arthropathy, wrist**
Postimmunization arthropathy, carpal bones

    M02.231 Postimmunization arthropathy, right wrist

    M02.232 Postimmunization arthropathy, left wrist

    M02.239 Postimmunization arthropathy, unspecified wrist

● **M02.24 Postimmunization arthropathy, hand**
Postimmunization arthropathy, metacarpus and phalanges

    M02.241 Postimmunization arthropathy, right hand

    M02.242 Postimmunization arthropathy, left hand

    M02.249 Postimmunization arthropathy, unspecified hand

● **M02.25 Postimmunization arthropathy, hip**

    M02.251 Postimmunization arthropathy, right hip

    M02.252 Postimmunization arthropathy, left hip

    M02.259 Postimmunization arthropathy, unspecified hip

● **M02.26 Postimmunization arthropathy, knee**

    M02.261 Postimmunization arthropathy, right knee

    M02.262 Postimmunization arthropathy, left knee

    M02.269 Postimmunization arthropathy, unspecified knee

● **M02.27 Postimmunization arthropathy, ankle and foot**
Postimmunization arthropathy, tarsus, metatarsus and phalanges

    M02.271 Postimmunization arthropathy, right ankle and foot

    M02.272 Postimmunization arthropathy, left ankle and foot

    M02.279 Postimmunization arthropathy, unspecified ankle and foot

M02.28 Postimmunization arthropathy, vertebrae

M02.29 Postimmunization arthropathy, multiple sites

● **M02.3 Reiter's disease**
Reactive arthritis

    M02.30 Reiter's disease, unspecified site 🗘
CC when PDx is its own CC

● **M02.31 Reiter's disease, shoulder**

    M02.311 Reiter's disease, right shoulder 🗘
CC when PDx is its own CC

    M02.312 Reiter's disease, left shoulder 🗘
CC when PDx is its own CC

    M02.319 Reiter's disease, unspecified shoulder 🗘
CC when PDx is its own CC

● **M02.32 Reiter's disease, elbow**

    M02.321 Reiter's disease, right elbow 🗘
CC when PDx is its own CC

    M02.322 Reiter's disease, left elbow 🗘
CC when PDx is its own CC

    M02.329 Reiter's disease, unspecified elbow 🗘
CC when PDx is its own CC

● **M02.33 Reiter's disease, wrist**
Reiter's disease, carpal bones

    M02.331 Reiter's disease, right wrist 🗘
CC when PDx is its own CC

    M02.332 Reiter's disease, left wrist 🗘
CC when PDx is its own CC

    M02.339 Reiter's disease, unspecified wrist 🗘
CC when PDx is its own CC

● **M02.34 Reiter's disease, hand**
Reiter's disease, metacarpus and phalanges

    M02.341 Reiter's disease, right hand 🗘
CC when PDx is its own CC

    M02.342 Reiter's disease, left hand 🗘
CC when PDx is its own CC

    M02.349 Reiter's disease, unspecified hand 🗘
CC when PDx is its own CC

● **M02.35 Reiter's disease, hip**

    M02.351 Reiter's disease, right hip 🗘
CC when PDx is its own CC

    M02.352 Reiter's disease, left hip 🗘
CC when PDx is its own CC

    M02.359 Reiter's disease, unspecified hip 🗘
CC when PDx is its own CC

● **M02.36 Reiter's disease, knee**

    M02.361 Reiter's disease, right knee 🗘
CC when PDx is its own CC

    M02.362 Reiter's disease, left knee 🗘
CC when PDx is its own CC

    M02.369 Reiter's disease, unspecified knee 🗘
CC when PDx is its own CC

● **M02.37 Reiter's disease, ankle and foot**
Reiter's disease, tarsus, metatarsus and phalanges

    M02.371 Reiter's disease, right ankle and foot 🗘
CC when PDx is its own CC

    M02.372 Reiter's disease, left ankle and foot 🗘
CC when PDx is its own CC

    M02.379 Reiter's disease, unspecified ankle and foot 🗘
CC when PDx is its own CC

◀ New ◀⋯ Revised ~~deleted~~ Deleted | Excludes 1 | Excludes 2 | Includes | Use additional | Code first | Code also | Unspecified
OGCR Official Guidelines ● Unacceptable Principal Diagnosis X Assign placeholder X ● Use Additional Character(s) ▶ Manifestation Code **Coding Clinic**

M02.38 Reiter's disease, vertebrae 🔖
    CC when PDx is its own CC

M02.39 Reiter's disease, multiple sites 🔖
    CC when PDx is its own CC

● M02.8 Other reactive arthropathies

M02.80 Other reactive arthropathies, unspecified site 🔖

● M02.81 Other reactive arthropathies, shoulder
    (Ex) For category M02.81 CC codes: See M01.X1

    M02.811 Other reactive arthropathies, right shoulder 🔖

    M02.812 Other reactive arthropathies, left shoulder 🔖

    M02.819 Other reactive arthropathies, unspecified shoulder 🔖

● M02.82 Other reactive arthropathies, elbow

    M02.821 Other reactive arthropathies, right elbow 🔖

    M02.822 Other reactive arthropathies, left elbow 🔖

    M02.829 Other reactive arthropathies, unspecified elbow 🔖

● M02.83 Other reactive arthropathies, wrist
    Other reactive arthropathies, carpal bones

    M02.831 Other reactive arthropathies, right wrist 🔖

    M02.832 Other reactive arthropathies, left wrist 🔖

    M02.839 Other reactive arthropathies, unspecified wrist 🔖

● M02.84 Other reactive arthropathies, hand
    Other reactive arthropathies, metacarpus and phalanges

    M02.841 Other reactive arthropathies, right hand 🔖

    M02.842 Other reactive arthropathies, left hand 🔖

    M02.849 Other reactive arthropathies, unspecified hand 🔖

● M02.85 Other reactive arthropathies, hip

    M02.851 Other reactive arthropathies, right hip 🔖

    M02.852 Other reactive arthropathies, left hip 🔖

    M02.859 Other reactive arthropathies, unspecified hip 🔖

● M02.86 Other reactive arthropathies, knee

    M02.861 Other reactive arthropathies, right knee 🔖

    M02.862 Other reactive arthropathies, left knee 🔖

    M02.869 Other reactive arthropathies, unspecified knee 🔖

● M02.87 Other reactive arthropathies, ankle and foot
    Other reactive arthropathies, tarsus, metatarsus and phalanges

    M02.871 Other reactive arthropathies, right ankle and foot 🔖

    M02.872 Other reactive arthropathies, left ankle and foot 🔖

    M02.879 Other reactive arthropathies, unspecified ankle and foot 🔖

▷ M02.88 Other reactive arthropathies, vertebrae 🔖

▷ M02.89 Other reactive arthropathies, multiple sites 🔖

▷ M02.9 Reactive arthropathy, unspecified

Item 13–1 Rheumatoid arthritis (RA) is a chronic systemic inflammatory disease of undetermined etiology involving primarily the synovial membranes and articular structures of multiple joints. The disease is often progressive and results in pain, stiffness, and swelling of joints. In late stages, deformity, ankylosis, and other **inflammatory polyarthropathies** develop.

INFLAMMATORY POLYARTHROPATHIES (M05-M14)

● M05 Rheumatoid arthritis with rheumatoid factor
    Excludes1 rheumatic fever (I00)
              juvenile rheumatoid arthritis (M08.-)
              rheumatoid arthritis of spine (M45.-)

● M05.0 Felty's syndrome
    Rheumatoid arthritis with splenoadenomegaly and leukopenia

    M05.00 Felty's syndrome, unspecified site

● M05.01 Felty's syndrome, shoulder

    M05.011 Felty's syndrome, right shoulder

    M05.012 Felty's syndrome, left shoulder

    M05.019 Felty's syndrome, unspecified shoulder

● M05.02 Felty's syndrome, elbow

    M05.021 Felty's syndrome, right elbow

    M05.022 Felty's syndrome, left elbow

    M05.029 Felty's syndrome, unspecified elbow

● M05.03 Felty's syndrome, wrist
    Felty's syndrome, carpal bones

    M05.031 Felty's syndrome, right wrist

    M05.032 Felty's syndrome, left wrist

    M05.039 Felty's syndrome, unspecified wrist

● M05.04 Felty's syndrome, hand
    Felty's syndrome, metacarpus and phalanges

    M05.041 Felty's syndrome, right hand

    M05.042 Felty's syndrome, left hand

    M05.049 Felty's syndrome, unspecified hand

● M05.05 Felty's syndrome, hip

    M05.051 Felty's syndrome, right hip

    M05.052 Felty's syndrome, left hip

    M05.059 Felty's syndrome, unspecified hip

● M05.06 Felty's syndrome, knee

    M05.061 Felty's syndrome, right knee

    M05.062 Felty's syndrome, left knee

    M05.069 Felty's syndrome, unspecified knee

● M05.07 Felty's syndrome, ankle and foot
    Felty's syndrome, tarsus, metatarsus and phalanges

    M05.071 Felty's syndrome, right ankle and foot

    M05.072 Felty's syndrome, left ankle and foot

    M05.079 Felty's syndrome, unspecified ankle and foot

    M05.09 Felty's syndrome, multiple sites

● M05.1 Rheumatoid lung disease with rheumatoid arthritis

    M05.10 Rheumatoid lung disease with rheumatoid arthritis of unspecified site

● M05.11 Rheumatoid lung disease with rheumatoid arthritis of shoulder

    M05.111 Rheumatoid lung disease with rheumatoid arthritis of right shoulder

    M05.112 Rheumatoid lung disease with rheumatoid arthritis of left shoulder

    M05.119 Rheumatoid lung disease with rheumatoid arthritis of unspecified shoulder

CHAPTER 13 (M00-M99)

N Newborn Age: 0   P Pediatric Age: 0–17   M Maternity DX: 12–55   A Adult Age: 15–124   ♀ Females Only   ♂ Males Only

🔖 Complication\Comorbidity   🔖 Major C\C   (Ex) CC/MCC Exclusions   🔖 Present on Admission Requirement   🔖 Hospital-Acquired Condition

1077

● M05.12　Rheumatoid lung disease with rheumatoid arthritis of elbow

　　　M05.121　Rheumatoid lung disease with rheumatoid arthritis of right elbow

　　　M05.122　Rheumatoid lung disease with rheumatoid arthritis of left elbow

　　　M05.129　Rheumatoid lung disease with rheumatoid arthritis of unspecified elbow

● M05.13　Rheumatoid lung disease with rheumatoid arthritis of wrist
　　　　　　Rheumatoid lung disease with rheumatoid arthritis, carpal bones

　　　M05.131　Rheumatoid lung disease with rheumatoid arthritis of right wrist

　　　M05.132　Rheumatoid lung disease with rheumatoid arthritis of left wrist

　　　M05.139　Rheumatoid lung disease with rheumatoid arthritis of unspecified wrist

● M05.14　Rheumatoid lung disease with rheumatoid arthritis of hand
　　　　　　Rheumatoid lung disease with rheumatoid arthritis, metacarpus and phalanges

　　　M05.141　Rheumatoid lung disease with rheumatoid arthritis of right hand

　　　M05.142　Rheumatoid lung disease with rheumatoid arthritis of left hand

　　　M05.149　Rheumatoid lung disease with rheumatoid arthritis of unspecified hand

● M05.15　Rheumatoid lung disease with rheumatoid arthritis of hip

　　　M05.151　Rheumatoid lung disease with rheumatoid arthritis of right hip

　　　M05.152　Rheumatoid lung disease with rheumatoid arthritis of left hip

　　　M05.159　Rheumatoid lung disease with rheumatoid arthritis of unspecified hip

● M05.16　Rheumatoid lung disease with rheumatoid arthritis of knee

　　　M05.161　Rheumatoid lung disease with rheumatoid arthritis of right knee

　　　M05.162　Rheumatoid lung disease with rheumatoid arthritis of left knee

　　　M05.169　Rheumatoid lung disease with rheumatoid arthritis of unspecified knee

● M05.17　Rheumatoid lung disease with rheumatoid arthritis of ankle and foot
　　　　　　Rheumatoid lung disease with rheumatoid arthritis, tarsus, metatarsus and phalanges

　　　M05.171　Rheumatoid lung disease with rheumatoid arthritis of right ankle and foot

　　　M05.172　Rheumatoid lung disease with rheumatoid arthritis of left ankle and foot

　　　M05.179　Rheumatoid lung disease with rheumatoid arthritis of unspecified ankle and foot

　 M05.19　Rheumatoid lung disease with rheumatoid arthritis of multiple sites

● M05.2　Rheumatoid vasculitis with rheumatoid arthritis

　　　M05.20　Rheumatoid vasculitis with rheumatoid arthritis of unspecified site

● M05.21　Rheumatoid vasculitis with rheumatoid arthritis of shoulder

　　　M05.211　Rheumatoid vasculitis with rheumatoid arthritis of right shoulder

　　　M05.212　Rheumatoid vasculitis with rheumatoid arthritis of left shoulder

　　　M05.219　Rheumatoid vasculitis with rheumatoid arthritis of unspecified shoulder

● M05.22　Rheumatoid vasculitis with rheumatoid arthritis of elbow

　　　M05.221　Rheumatoid vasculitis with rheumatoid arthritis of right elbow

　　　M05.222　Rheumatoid vasculitis with rheumatoid arthritis of left elbow

　　　M05.229　Rheumatoid vasculitis with rheumatoid arthritis of unspecified elbow

● M05.23　Rheumatoid vasculitis with rheumatoid arthritis of wrist
　　　　　　Rheumatoid vasculitis with rheumatoid arthritis, carpal bones

　　　M05.231　Rheumatoid vasculitis with rheumatoid arthritis of right wrist

　　　M05.232　Rheumatoid vasculitis with rheumatoid arthritis of left wrist

　　　M05.239　Rheumatoid vasculitis with rheumatoid arthritis of unspecified wrist

● M05.24　Rheumatoid vasculitis with rheumatoid arthritis of hand
　　　　　　Rheumatoid vasculitis with rheumatoid arthritis, metacarpus and phalanges

　　　M05.241　Rheumatoid vasculitis with rheumatoid arthritis of right hand

　　　M05.242　Rheumatoid vasculitis with rheumatoid arthritis of left hand

　　　M05.249　Rheumatoid vasculitis with rheumatoid arthritis of unspecified hand

● M05.25　Rheumatoid vasculitis with rheumatoid arthritis of hip

　　　M05.251　Rheumatoid vasculitis with rheumatoid arthritis of right hip

　　　M05.252　Rheumatoid vasculitis with rheumatoid arthritis of left hip

　　　M05.259　Rheumatoid vasculitis with rheumatoid arthritis of unspecified hip

● M05.26　Rheumatoid vasculitis with rheumatoid arthritis of knee

　　　M05.261　Rheumatoid vasculitis with rheumatoid arthritis of right knee

　　　M05.262　Rheumatoid vasculitis with rheumatoid arthritis of left knee

　　　M05.269　Rheumatoid vasculitis with rheumatoid arthritis of unspecified knee

◄ New　◄ Revised　deleted Deleted　Excludes 1　Excludes 2　Includes　Use additional　Code first　Code also　Unspecified
OGCR Official Guidelines　● Unacceptable Principal Diagnosis　X Assign placeholder X　● Use Additional Character(s)　▌Manifestation Code　Coding Clinic

● **M05.27**   **Rheumatoid vasculitis with rheumatoid arthritis of ankle and foot**
    Rheumatoid vasculitis with rheumatoid arthritis, tarsus, metatarsus and phalanges

    M05.271   **Rheumatoid vasculitis with rheumatoid arthritis of right ankle and foot**

    M05.272   **Rheumatoid vasculitis with rheumatoid arthritis of left ankle and foot**

    M05.279   **Rheumatoid vasculitis with rheumatoid arthritis of unspecified ankle and foot**

   M05.29   **Rheumatoid vasculitis with rheumatoid arthritis of multiple sites**

● **M05.3**   **Rheumatoid heart disease with rheumatoid arthritis**
    Rheumatoid carditis
    Rheumatoid endocarditis
    Rheumatoid myocarditis
    Rheumatoid pericarditis

   M05.30   **Rheumatoid heart disease with rheumatoid arthritis of unspecified site**

● **M05.31**   **Rheumatoid heart disease with rheumatoid arthritis of shoulder**

    M05.311   **Rheumatoid heart disease with rheumatoid arthritis of right shoulder**

    M05.312   **Rheumatoid heart disease with rheumatoid arthritis of left shoulder**

    M05.319   **Rheumatoid heart disease with rheumatoid arthritis of unspecified shoulder**

● **M05.32**   **Rheumatoid heart disease with rheumatoid arthritis of elbow**

    M05.321   **Rheumatoid heart disease with rheumatoid arthritis of right elbow**

    M05.322   **Rheumatoid heart disease with rheumatoid arthritis of left elbow**

    M05.329   **Rheumatoid heart disease with rheumatoid arthritis of unspecified elbow**

● **M05.33**   **Rheumatoid heart disease with rheumatoid arthritis of wrist**
    Rheumatoid heart disease with rheumatoid arthritis, carpal bones

    M05.331   **Rheumatoid heart disease with rheumatoid arthritis of right wrist**

    M05.332   **Rheumatoid heart disease with rheumatoid arthritis of left wrist**

    M05.339   **Rheumatoid heart disease with rheumatoid arthritis of unspecified wrist**

● **M05.34**   **Rheumatoid heart disease with rheumatoid arthritis of hand**
    Rheumatoid heart disease with rheumatoid arthritis, metacarpus and phalanges

    M05.341   **Rheumatoid heart disease with rheumatoid arthritis of right hand**

    M05.342   **Rheumatoid heart disease with rheumatoid arthritis of left hand**

    M05.349   **Rheumatoid heart disease with rheumatoid arthritis of unspecified hand**

● **M05.35**   **Rheumatoid heart disease with rheumatoid arthritis of hip**

    M05.351   **Rheumatoid heart disease with rheumatoid arthritis of right hip**

    M05.352   **Rheumatoid heart disease with rheumatoid arthritis of left hip**

    M05.359   **Rheumatoid heart disease with rheumatoid arthritis of unspecified hip**

● **M05.36**   **Rheumatoid heart disease with rheumatoid arthritis of knee**

    M05.361   **Rheumatoid heart disease with rheumatoid arthritis of right knee**

    M05.362   **Rheumatoid heart disease with rheumatoid arthritis of left knee**

    M05.369   **Rheumatoid heart disease with rheumatoid arthritis of unspecified knee**

● **M05.37**   **Rheumatoid heart disease with rheumatoid arthritis of ankle and foot**
    Rheumatoid heart disease with rheumatoid arthritis, tarsus, metatarsus and phalanges

    M05.371   **Rheumatoid heart disease with rheumatoid arthritis of right ankle and foot**

    M05.372   **Rheumatoid heart disease with rheumatoid arthritis of left ankle and foot**

    M05.379   **Rheumatoid heart disease with rheumatoid arthritis of unspecified ankle and foot**

   M05.39   **Rheumatoid heart disease with rheumatoid arthritis of multiple sites**

● **M05.4**   **Rheumatoid myopathy with rheumatoid arthritis**
    (Ex): **For category M05.4 CC codes:** E08.40-E08.49, E08.618-E08.638, E08.649-E08.8, E09.40-E09.49, E09.618-E09.638, E09.649-E09.8, E10.40-E10.49, E10.618-E10.638, E10.649, E10.69-E10.8, E11.40-E11.49, E11.618-E11.638, E11.649, E11.69-E11.8, E13.40-E13.49, E13.618-E13.638, E13.649-E13.8, G32.89, G70.00-G72.3, G72.81-G73.7, G96.8-G96.9, G98.0-G98.8, G99.8

   M05.40   **Rheumatoid myopathy with rheumatoid arthritis of unspecified site** 🖥
     CC when PDx is its own CC

● **M05.41**   **Rheumatoid myopathy with rheumatoid arthritis of shoulder**

    M05.411   **Rheumatoid myopathy with rheumatoid arthritis of right shoulder** 🖥
     CC when PDx is its own CC

    M05.412   **Rheumatoid myopathy with rheumatoid arthritis of left shoulder** 🖥
     CC when PDx is its own CC

    M05.419   **Rheumatoid myopathy with rheumatoid arthritis of unspecified shoulder** 🖥
     CC when PDx is its own CC

● **M05.42**   **Rheumatoid myopathy with rheumatoid arthritis of elbow**

    M05.421   **Rheumatoid myopathy with rheumatoid arthritis of right elbow** 🖥
     CC when PDx is its own CC

    M05.422   **Rheumatoid myopathy with rheumatoid arthritis of left elbow** 🖥
     CC when PDx is its own CC

    M05.429   **Rheumatoid myopathy with rheumatoid arthritis of unspecified elbow** 🖥
     CC when PDx is its own CC

● **M05.43**   **Rheumatoid myopathy with rheumatoid arthritis of wrist**
    Rheumatoid myopathy with rheumatoid arthritis, carpal bones

    M05.431   **Rheumatoid myopathy with rheumatoid arthritis of right wrist** 🖥
     CC when PDx is its own CC

    M05.432   **Rheumatoid myopathy with rheumatoid arthritis of left wrist** 🖥
     CC when PDx is its own CC

    M05.439   **Rheumatoid myopathy with rheumatoid arthritis of unspecified wrist** 🖥
     CC when PDx is its own CC

N Newborn Age: 0   **P** Pediatric Age: 0–17   **M** Maternity DX: 12–55   **A** Adult Age: 15–124   ♀ Females Only   ♂ Males Only

Complication\Comorbidity   Major C\C   (Ex) CC/MCC Exclusions   Present on Admission Requirement   Hospital-Acquired Condition

1079

CHAPTER 13 (M00-M99)

● M05.44   **Rheumatoid myopathy with rheumatoid arthritis of hand**
           Rheumatoid myopathy with rheumatoid arthritis, metacarpus and phalanges

   M05.441   **Rheumatoid myopathy with rheumatoid arthritis of right hand** 🔵
             CC when PDx is its own CC

   M05.442   **Rheumatoid myopathy with rheumatoid arthritis of left hand** 🔵
             CC when PDx is its own CC

   M05.449   **Rheumatoid myopathy with rheumatoid arthritis of** unspecified **hand** 🔵
             CC when PDx is its own CC

● M05.45   **Rheumatoid myopathy with rheumatoid arthritis of hip**

   M05.451   **Rheumatoid myopathy with rheumatoid arthritis of right hip** 🔵
             CC when PDx is its own CC

   M05.452   **Rheumatoid myopathy with rheumatoid arthritis of left hip** 🔵
             CC when PDx is its own CC

   M05.459   **Rheumatoid myopathy with rheumatoid arthritis of** unspecified **hip** 🔵
             CC when PDx is its own CC

● M05.46   **Rheumatoid myopathy with rheumatoid arthritis of knee**

   M05.461   **Rheumatoid myopathy with rheumatoid arthritis of right knee** 🔵
             CC when PDx is its own CC

   M05.462   **Rheumatoid myopathy with rheumatoid arthritis of left knee** 🔵
             CC when PDx is its own CC

   M05.469   **Rheumatoid myopathy with rheumatoid arthritis of** unspecified **knee** 🔵
             CC when PDx is its own CC

● M05.47   **Rheumatoid myopathy with rheumatoid arthritis of ankle and foot**
           Rheumatoid myopathy with rheumatoid arthritis, tarsus, metatarsus and phalanges

   M05.471   **Rheumatoid myopathy with rheumatoid arthritis of right ankle and foot** 🔵
             CC when PDx is its own CC

   M05.472   **Rheumatoid myopathy with rheumatoid arthritis of left ankle and foot** 🔵
             CC when PDx is its own CC

   M05.479   **Rheumatoid myopathy with rheumatoid arthritis of** unspecified **ankle and foot** 🔵
             CC when PDx is its own CC

   M05.49   **Rheumatoid myopathy with rheumatoid arthritis of multiple sites** 🔵
             CC when PDx is its own CC

● M05.5   **Rheumatoid polyneuropathy with rheumatoid arthritis**

   M05.50   **Rheumatoid polyneuropathy with rheumatoid arthritis of** unspecified **site**

● M05.51   **Rheumatoid polyneuropathy with rheumatoid arthritis of shoulder**

   M05.511   **Rheumatoid polyneuropathy with rheumatoid arthritis of right shoulder**

   M05.512   **Rheumatoid polyneuropathy with rheumatoid arthritis of left shoulder**

   M05.519   **Rheumatoid polyneuropathy with rheumatoid arthritis of** unspecified **shoulder**

● M05.52   **Rheumatoid polyneuropathy with rheumatoid arthritis of elbow**

   M05.521   **Rheumatoid polyneuropathy with rheumatoid arthritis of right elbow**

   M05.522   **Rheumatoid polyneuropathy with rheumatoid arthritis of left elbow**

   M05.529   **Rheumatoid polyneuropathy with rheumatoid arthritis of** unspecified **elbow**

● M05.53   **Rheumatoid polyneuropathy with rheumatoid arthritis of wrist**
           Rheumatoid polyneuropathy with rheumatoid arthritis, carpal bones

   M05.531   **Rheumatoid polyneuropathy with rheumatoid arthritis of right wrist**

   M05.532   **Rheumatoid polyneuropathy with rheumatoid arthritis of left wrist**

   M05.539   **Rheumatoid polyneuropathy with rheumatoid arthritis of** unspecified **wrist**

● M05.54   **Rheumatoid polyneuropathy with rheumatoid arthritis of hand**
           Rheumatoid polyneuropathy with rheumatoid arthritis, metacarpus and phalanges

   M05.541   **Rheumatoid polyneuropathy with rheumatoid arthritis of right hand**

   M05.542   **Rheumatoid polyneuropathy with rheumatoid arthritis of left hand**

   M05.549   **Rheumatoid polyneuropathy with rheumatoid arthritis of** unspecified **hand**

● M05.55   **Rheumatoid polyneuropathy with rheumatoid arthritis of hip**

   M05.551   **Rheumatoid polyneuropathy with rheumatoid arthritis of right hip**

   M05.552   **Rheumatoid polyneuropathy with rheumatoid arthritis of left hip**

   M05.559   **Rheumatoid polyneuropathy with rheumatoid arthritis of** unspecified **hip**

● M05.56   **Rheumatoid polyneuropathy with rheumatoid arthritis of knee**

   M05.561   **Rheumatoid polyneuropathy with rheumatoid arthritis of right knee**

   M05.562   **Rheumatoid polyneuropathy with rheumatoid arthritis of left knee**

   M05.569   **Rheumatoid polyneuropathy with rheumatoid arthritis of** unspecified **knee**

● M05.57   **Rheumatoid polyneuropathy with rheumatoid arthritis of ankle and foot**
           Rheumatoid polyneuropathy with rheumatoid arthritis, tarsus, metatarsus and phalanges

   M05.571   **Rheumatoid polyneuropathy with rheumatoid arthritis of right ankle and foot**

   M05.572   **Rheumatoid polyneuropathy with rheumatoid arthritis of left ankle and foot**

   M05.579   **Rheumatoid polyneuropathy with rheumatoid arthritis of** unspecified **ankle and foot**

   M05.59   **Rheumatoid polyneuropathy with rheumatoid arthritis of multiple sites**

◄ New   ◄ Revised   ~~deleted~~ Deleted   Excludes 1   Excludes 2   Includes   Use additional   Code first   Code also   Unspecified

OGCR Official Guidelines   ● Unacceptable Principal Diagnosis   X Assign placeholder X   ● Use Additional Character(s)   ▌ Manifestation Code   **Coding Clinic**

● **M05.6**   Rheumatoid arthritis with involvement of other organs and systems

     M05.60   Rheumatoid arthritis of unspecified site with involvement of other organs and systems

● **M05.61**   Rheumatoid arthritis of shoulder with involvement of other organs and systems

       M05.611   Rheumatoid arthritis of right shoulder with involvement of other organs and systems

       M05.612   Rheumatoid arthritis of left shoulder with involvement of other organs and systems

       M05.619   Rheumatoid arthritis of unspecified shoulder with involvement of other organs and systems

● **M05.62**   Rheumatoid arthritis of elbow with involvement of other organs and systems

       M05.621   Rheumatoid arthritis of right elbow with involvement of other organs and systems

       M05.622   Rheumatoid arthritis of left elbow with involvement of other organs and systems

       M05.629   Rheumatoid arthritis of unspecified elbow with involvement of other organs and systems

● **M05.63**   Rheumatoid arthritis of wrist with involvement of other organs and systems

       Rheumatoid arthritis of carpal bones with involvement of other organs and systems

       M05.631   Rheumatoid arthritis of right wrist with involvement of other organs and systems

       M05.632   Rheumatoid arthritis of left wrist with involvement of other organs and systems

       M05.639   Rheumatoid arthritis of unspecified wrist with involvement of other organs and systems

● **M05.64**   Rheumatoid arthritis of hand with involvement of other organs and systems

       Rheumatoid arthritis of metacarpus and phalanges with involvement of other organs and systems

       M05.641   Rheumatoid arthritis of right hand with involvement of other organs and systems

       M05.642   Rheumatoid arthritis of left hand with involvement of other organs and systems

       M05.649   Rheumatoid arthritis of unspecified hand with involvement of other organs and systems

● **M05.65**   Rheumatoid arthritis of hip with involvement of other organs and systems

       M05.651   Rheumatoid arthritis of right hip with involvement of other organs and systems

       M05.652   Rheumatoid arthritis of left hip with involvement of other organs and systems

       M05.659   Rheumatoid arthritis of unspecified hip with involvement of other organs and systems

● **M05.66**   Rheumatoid arthritis of knee with involvement of other organs and systems

       M05.661   Rheumatoid arthritis of right knee with involvement of other organs and systems

       M05.662   Rheumatoid arthritis of left knee with involvement of other organs and systems

       M05.669   Rheumatoid arthritis of unspecified knee with involvement of other organs and systems

● **M05.67**   Rheumatoid arthritis of ankle and foot with involvement of other organs and systems

       Rheumatoid arthritis of tarsus, metatarsus and phalanges with involvement of other organs and systems

       M05.671   Rheumatoid arthritis of right ankle and foot with involvement of other organs and systems

       M05.672   Rheumatoid arthritis of left ankle and foot with involvement of other organs and systems

       M05.679   Rheumatoid arthritis of unspecified ankle and foot with involvement of other organs and systems

     M05.69   Rheumatoid arthritis of multiple sites with involvement of other organs and systems

● **M05.7**   Rheumatoid arthritis with rheumatoid factor without organ or systems involvement

     M05.70   Rheumatoid arthritis with rheumatoid factor of unspecified site without organ or systems involvement

● **M05.71**   Rheumatoid arthritis with rheumatoid factor of shoulder without organ or systems involvement

       M05.711   Rheumatoid arthritis with rheumatoid factor of right shoulder without organ or systems involvement

       M05.712   Rheumatoid arthritis with rheumatoid factor of left shoulder without organ or systems involvement

       M05.719   Rheumatoid arthritis with rheumatoid factor of unspecified shoulder without organ or systems involvement

● **M05.72**   Rheumatoid arthritis with rheumatoid factor of elbow without organ or systems involvement

       M05.721   Rheumatoid arthritis with rheumatoid factor of right elbow without organ or systems involvement

       M05.722   Rheumatoid arthritis with rheumatoid factor of left elbow without organ or systems involvement

       M05.729   Rheumatoid arthritis with rheumatoid factor of unspecified elbow without organ or systems involvement

● **M05.73**   Rheumatoid arthritis with rheumatoid factor of wrist without organ or systems involvement

       M05.731   Rheumatoid arthritis with rheumatoid factor of right wrist without organ or systems involvement

       M05.732   Rheumatoid arthritis with rheumatoid factor of left wrist without organ or systems involvement

       M05.739   Rheumatoid arthritis with rheumatoid factor of unspecified wrist without organ or systems involvement

N   Newborn Age: 0   **P**   Pediatric Age: 0–17   **M**   Maternity DX: 12–55   **A**   Adult Age: 15–124   ♀   Females Only   ♂   Males Only

  Complication\Comorbidity   Major C\C   (Ex)   CC/MCC Exclusions   Present on Admission Requirement   Hospital-Acquired Condition

1081

CHAPTER 13 (M00-M99)

● M05.74   Rheumatoid arthritis with rheumatoid factor of hand without organ or systems involvement

    M05.741   Rheumatoid arthritis with rheumatoid factor of right hand without organ or systems involvement

    M05.742   Rheumatoid arthritis with rheumatoid factor of left hand without organ or systems involvement

    M05.749   Rheumatoid arthritis with rheumatoid factor of unspecified hand without organ or systems involvement

● M05.75   Rheumatoid arthritis with rheumatoid factor of hip without organ or systems involvement

    M05.751   Rheumatoid arthritis with rheumatoid factor of right hip without organ or systems involvement

    M05.752   Rheumatoid arthritis with rheumatoid factor of left hip without organ or systems involvement

    M05.759   Rheumatoid arthritis with rheumatoid factor of unspecified hip without organ or systems involvement

● M05.76   Rheumatoid arthritis with rheumatoid factor of knee without organ or systems involvement

    M05.761   Rheumatoid arthritis with rheumatoid factor of right knee without organ or systems involvement

    M05.762   Rheumatoid arthritis with rheumatoid factor of left knee without organ or systems involvement

    M05.769   Rheumatoid arthritis with rheumatoid factor of unspecified knee without organ or systems involvement

● M05.77   Rheumatoid arthritis with rheumatoid factor of ankle and foot without organ or systems involvement

    M05.771   Rheumatoid arthritis with rheumatoid factor of right ankle and foot without organ or systems involvement

    M05.772   Rheumatoid arthritis with rheumatoid factor of left ankle and foot without organ or systems involvement

    M05.779   Rheumatoid arthritis with rheumatoid factor of unspecified ankle and foot without organ or systems involvement

   M05.79   Rheumatoid arthritis with rheumatoid factor of multiple sites without organ or systems involvement

● M05.8   Other rheumatoid arthritis with rheumatoid factor

   M05.80   Other rheumatoid arthritis with rheumatoid factor of unspecified site

● M05.81   Other rheumatoid arthritis with rheumatoid factor of shoulder

    M05.811   Other rheumatoid arthritis with rheumatoid factor of right shoulder

    M05.812   Other rheumatoid arthritis with rheumatoid factor of left shoulder

    M05.819   Other rheumatoid arthritis with rheumatoid factor of unspecified shoulder

● M05.82   Other rheumatoid arthritis with rheumatoid factor of elbow

    M05.821   Other rheumatoid arthritis with rheumatoid factor of right elbow

    M05.822   Other rheumatoid arthritis with rheumatoid factor of left elbow

    M05.829   Other rheumatoid arthritis with rheumatoid factor of unspecified elbow

● M05.83   Other rheumatoid arthritis with rheumatoid factor of wrist

    M05.831   Other rheumatoid arthritis with rheumatoid factor of right wrist

    M05.832   Other rheumatoid arthritis with rheumatoid factor of left wrist

    M05.839   Other rheumatoid arthritis with rheumatoid factor of unspecified wrist

● M05.84   Other rheumatoid arthritis with rheumatoid factor of hand

    M05.841   Other rheumatoid arthritis with rheumatoid factor of right hand

    M05.842   Other rheumatoid arthritis with rheumatoid factor of left hand

    M05.849   Other rheumatoid arthritis with rheumatoid factor of unspecified hand

● M05.85   Other rheumatoid arthritis with rheumatoid factor of hip

    M05.851   Other rheumatoid arthritis with rheumatoid factor of right hip

    M05.852   Other rheumatoid arthritis with rheumatoid factor of left hip

    M05.859   Other rheumatoid arthritis with rheumatoid factor of unspecified hip

● M05.86   Other rheumatoid arthritis with rheumatoid factor of knee

    M05.861   Other rheumatoid arthritis with rheumatoid factor of right knee

    M05.862   Other rheumatoid arthritis with rheumatoid factor of left knee

    M05.869   Other rheumatoid arthritis with rheumatoid factor of unspecified knee

● M05.87   Other rheumatoid arthritis with rheumatoid factor of ankle and foot

    M05.871   Other rheumatoid arthritis with rheumatoid factor of right ankle and foot

    M05.872   Other rheumatoid arthritis with rheumatoid factor of left ankle and foot

    M05.879   Other rheumatoid arthritis with rheumatoid factor of unspecified ankle and foot

   M05.89   Other rheumatoid arthritis with rheumatoid factor of multiple sites

  M05.9   Rheumatoid arthritis with rheumatoid factor, unspecified

◀ New   ◀▥ Revised   ~~deleted~~ Deleted   Excludes 1   Excludes 2   Includes   Use additional   Code first   Code also   Unspecified

OGCR Official Guidelines   ● Unacceptable Principal Diagnosis   X Assign placeholder X   ● Use Additional Character(s)   ▶ Manifestation Code   **Coding Clinic**

● **M06   Other rheumatoid arthritis**
  ● **M06.0   Rheumatoid arthritis without rheumatoid factor**
     M06.00   Rheumatoid arthritis without rheumatoid factor, unspecified site
    ● M06.01   Rheumatoid arthritis without rheumatoid factor, shoulder
       M06.011   Rheumatoid arthritis without rheumatoid factor, right shoulder
       M06.012   Rheumatoid arthritis without rheumatoid factor, left shoulder
       M06.019   Rheumatoid arthritis without rheumatoid factor, unspecified shoulder
    ● M06.02   Rheumatoid arthritis without rheumatoid factor, elbow
       M06.021   Rheumatoid arthritis without rheumatoid factor, right elbow
       M06.022   Rheumatoid arthritis without rheumatoid factor, left elbow
       M06.029   Rheumatoid arthritis without rheumatoid factor, unspecified elbow
    ● M06.03   Rheumatoid arthritis without rheumatoid factor, wrist
       M06.031   Rheumatoid arthritis without rheumatoid factor, right wrist
       M06.032   Rheumatoid arthritis without rheumatoid factor, left wrist
       M06.039   Rheumatoid arthritis without rheumatoid factor, unspecified wrist
    ● M06.04   Rheumatoid arthritis without rheumatoid factor, hand
       M06.041   Rheumatoid arthritis without rheumatoid factor, right hand
       M06.042   Rheumatoid arthritis without rheumatoid factor, left hand
       M06.049   Rheumatoid arthritis without rheumatoid factor, unspecified hand
    ● M06.05   Rheumatoid arthritis without rheumatoid factor, hip
       M06.051   Rheumatoid arthritis without rheumatoid factor, right hip
       M06.052   Rheumatoid arthritis without rheumatoid factor, left hip
       M06.059   Rheumatoid arthritis without rheumatoid factor, unspecified hip
    ● M06.06   Rheumatoid arthritis without rheumatoid factor, knee
       M06.061   Rheumatoid arthritis without rheumatoid factor, right knee
       M06.062   Rheumatoid arthritis without rheumatoid factor, left knee
       M06.069   Rheumatoid arthritis without rheumatoid factor, unspecified knee
    ● M06.07   Rheumatoid arthritis without rheumatoid factor, ankle and foot
       M06.071   Rheumatoid arthritis without rheumatoid factor, right ankle and foot
       M06.072   Rheumatoid arthritis without rheumatoid factor, left ankle and foot
       M06.079   Rheumatoid arthritis without rheumatoid factor, unspecified ankle and foot
     M06.08   Rheumatoid arthritis without rheumatoid factor, vertebrae
     M06.09   Rheumatoid arthritis without rheumatoid factor, multiple sites
   M06.1   Adult-onset Still's disease   A
     Excludes1   Still's disease NOS (M08.2-)

  ● **M06.2   Rheumatoid bursitis**
     M06.20   Rheumatoid bursitis, unspecified site
    ● M06.21   Rheumatoid bursitis, shoulder
       M06.211   Rheumatoid bursitis, right shoulder
       M06.212   Rheumatoid bursitis, left shoulder
       M06.219   Rheumatoid bursitis, unspecified shoulder
    ● M06.22   Rheumatoid bursitis, elbow
       M06.221   Rheumatoid bursitis, right elbow
       M06.222   Rheumatoid bursitis, left elbow
       M06.229   Rheumatoid bursitis, unspecified elbow
    ● M06.23   Rheumatoid bursitis, wrist
       M06.231   Rheumatoid bursitis, right wrist
       M06.232   Rheumatoid bursitis, left wrist
       M06.239   Rheumatoid bursitis, unspecified wrist
    ● M06.24   Rheumatoid bursitis, hand
       M06.241   Rheumatoid bursitis, right hand
       M06.242   Rheumatoid bursitis, left hand
       M06.249   Rheumatoid bursitis, unspecified hand
    ● M06.25   Rheumatoid bursitis, hip
       M06.251   Rheumatoid bursitis, right hip
       M06.252   Rheumatoid bursitis, left hip
       M06.259   Rheumatoid bursitis, unspecified hip
    ● M06.26   Rheumatoid bursitis, knee
       M06.261   Rheumatoid bursitis, right knee
       M06.262   Rheumatoid bursitis, left knee
       M06.269   Rheumatoid bursitis, unspecified knee
    ● M06.27   Rheumatoid bursitis, ankle and foot
       M06.271   Rheumatoid bursitis, right ankle and foot
       M06.272   Rheumatoid bursitis, left ankle and foot
       M06.279   Rheumatoid bursitis, unspecified ankle and foot
     M06.28   Rheumatoid bursitis, vertebrae
     M06.29   Rheumatoid bursitis, multiple sites
  ● **M06.3   Rheumatoid nodule**
     M06.30   Rheumatoid nodule, unspecified site
    ● M06.31   Rheumatoid nodule, shoulder
       M06.311   Rheumatoid nodule, right shoulder
       M06.312   Rheumatoid nodule, left shoulder
       M06.319   Rheumatoid nodule, unspecified shoulder
    ● M06.32   Rheumatoid nodule, elbow
       M06.321   Rheumatoid nodule, right elbow
       M06.322   Rheumatoid nodule, left elbow
       M06.329   Rheumatoid nodule, unspecified elbow
    ● M06.33   Rheumatoid nodule, wrist
       M06.331   Rheumatoid nodule, right wrist
       M06.332   Rheumatoid nodule, left wrist
       M06.339   Rheumatoid nodule, unspecified wrist
    ● M06.34   Rheumatoid nodule, hand
       M06.341   Rheumatoid nodule, right hand
       M06.342   Rheumatoid nodule, left hand
       M06.349   Rheumatoid nodule, unspecified hand

CHAPTER 13 (M00-M99)

N   Newborn Age: 0   P   Pediatric Age: 0–17   M   Maternity DX: 12–55   A   Adult Age: 15–124   ♀   Females Only   ♂   Males Only

● Complication\Comorbidity   ● Major C\C   ℰ℥   CC/MCC Exclusions   ● Present on Admission Requirement   ● Hospital-Acquired Condition

1083

CHAPTER 13 (M00-M99)

● M06.35   Rheumatoid nodule, hip
    M06.351   Rheumatoid nodule, right hip
    M06.352   Rheumatoid nodule, left hip
    M06.359   Rheumatoid nodule, unspecified hip
● M06.36   Rheumatoid nodule, knee
    M06.361   Rheumatoid nodule, right knee
    M06.362   Rheumatoid nodule, left knee
    M06.369   Rheumatoid nodule, unspecified knee
● M06.37   Rheumatoid nodule, ankle and foot
    M06.371   Rheumatoid nodule, right ankle and foot
    M06.372   Rheumatoid nodule, left ankle and foot
    M06.379   Rheumatoid nodule, unspecified ankle and foot
   M06.38   Rheumatoid nodule, vertebrae
   M06.39   Rheumatoid nodule, multiple sites
  M06.4   Inflammatory polyarthropathy
    Excludes1   polyarthritis NOS (M13.0)
● M06.8   Other specified rheumatoid arthritis
   M06.80   Other specified rheumatoid arthritis, unspecified site
● M06.81   Other specified rheumatoid arthritis, shoulder
    M06.811   Other specified rheumatoid arthritis, right shoulder
    M06.812   Other specified rheumatoid arthritis, left shoulder
    M06.819   Other specified rheumatoid arthritis, unspecified shoulder
● M06.82   Other specified rheumatoid arthritis, elbow
    M06.821   Other specified rheumatoid arthritis, right elbow
    M06.822   Other specified rheumatoid arthritis, left elbow
    M06.829   Other specified rheumatoid arthritis, unspecified elbow
● M06.83   Other specified rheumatoid arthritis, wrist
    M06.831   Other specified rheumatoid arthritis, right wrist
    M06.832   Other specified rheumatoid arthritis, left wrist
    M06.839   Other specified rheumatoid arthritis, unspecified wrist
● M06.84   Other specified rheumatoid arthritis, hand
    M06.841   Other specified rheumatoid arthritis, right hand
    M06.842   Other specified rheumatoid arthritis, left hand
    M06.849   Other specified rheumatoid arthritis, unspecified hand
● M06.85   Other specified rheumatoid arthritis, hip
    M06.851   Other specified rheumatoid arthritis, right hip
    M06.852   Other specified rheumatoid arthritis, left hip
    M06.859   Other specified rheumatoid arthritis, unspecified hip
● M06.86   Other specified rheumatoid arthritis, knee
    M06.861   Other specified rheumatoid arthritis, right knee
    M06.862   Other specified rheumatoid arthritis, left knee
    M06.869   Other specified rheumatoid arthritis, unspecified knee

● M06.87   Other specified rheumatoid arthritis, ankle and foot
    M06.871   Other specified rheumatoid arthritis, right ankle and foot
    M06.872   Other specified rheumatoid arthritis, left ankle and foot
    M06.879   Other specified rheumatoid arthritis, unspecified ankle and foot
   M06.88   Other specified rheumatoid arthritis, vertebrae
   M06.89   Other specified rheumatoid arthritis, multiple sites
  M06.9   Rheumatoid arthritis, unspecified
● M07   Enteropathic arthropathies
   Code also associated enteropathy, such as:
    regional enteritis [Crohn's disease] (K50.-)
    ulcerative colitis (K51.-)
   Excludes1   psoriatic arthropathies (L40.5-)
● M07.6   Enteropathic arthropathies
   M07.60   Enteropathic arthropathies, unspecified site
● M07.61   Enteropathic arthropathies, shoulder
    M07.611   Enteropathic arthropathies, right shoulder
    M07.612   Enteropathic arthropathies, left shoulder
    M07.619   Enteropathic arthropathies, unspecified shoulder
● M07.62   Enteropathic arthropathies, elbow
    M07.621   Enteropathic arthropathies, right elbow
    M07.622   Enteropathic arthropathies, left elbow
    M07.629   Enteropathic arthropathies, unspecified elbow
● M07.63   Enteropathic arthropathies, wrist
    M07.631   Enteropathic arthropathies, right wrist
    M07.632   Enteropathic arthropathies, left wrist
    M07.639   Enteropathic arthropathies, unspecified wrist
● M07.64   Enteropathic arthropathies, hand
    M07.641   Enteropathic arthropathies, right hand
    M07.642   Enteropathic arthropathies, left hand
    M07.649   Enteropathic arthropathies, unspecified hand
● M07.65   Enteropathic arthropathies, hip
    M07.651   Enteropathic arthropathies, right hip
    M07.652   Enteropathic arthropathies, left hip
    M07.659   Enteropathic arthropathies, unspecified hip
● M07.66   Enteropathic arthropathies, knee
    M07.661   Enteropathic arthropathies, right knee
    M07.662   Enteropathic arthropathies, left knee
    M07.669   Enteropathic arthropathies, unspecified knee
● M07.67   Enteropathic arthropathies, ankle and foot
    M07.671   Enteropathic arthropathies, right ankle and foot
    M07.672   Enteropathic arthropathies, left ankle and foot
    M07.679   Enteropathic arthropathies, unspecified ankle and foot
   M07.68   Enteropathic arthropathies, vertebrae
   M07.69   Enteropathic arthropathies, multiple sites

◄ New   ◄ Revised   deleted Deleted   Excludes 1   Excludes 2   Includes   Use additional   Code first   Code also   Unspecified
OGCR Official Guidelines   ● Unacceptable Principal Diagnosis   X Assign placeholder X   ● Use Additional Character(s)   ▌ Manifestation Code   **Coding Clinic**

● **M08   Juvenile arthritis**

     Code also any associated underlying condition, such as:
       regional enteritis [Crohn's disease] (K50.-)
       ulcerative colitis (K51.-)

     Excludes1   arthropathy in Whipple's disease (M14.8)
       Felty's syndrome (M05.0)
       juvenile dermatomyositis (M33.0-)
       psoriatic juvenile arthropathy (L40.54)

● **M08.0   Unspecified juvenile rheumatoid arthritis**
     Juvenile rheumatoid arthritis with or without rheumatoid factor

     M08.00   Unspecified juvenile rheumatoid arthritis of unspecified site

●   **M08.01**   Unspecified juvenile rheumatoid arthritis, shoulder

       M08.011   Unspecified juvenile rheumatoid arthritis, right shoulder

       M08.012   Unspecified juvenile rheumatoid arthritis, left shoulder

       M08.019   Unspecified juvenile rheumatoid arthritis, unspecified shoulder

●   **M08.02**   Unspecified juvenile rheumatoid arthritis of elbow

       M08.021   Unspecified juvenile rheumatoid arthritis, right elbow

       M08.022   Unspecified juvenile rheumatoid arthritis, left elbow

       M08.029   Unspecified juvenile rheumatoid arthritis, unspecified elbow

●   **M08.03**   Unspecified juvenile rheumatoid arthritis, wrist

       M08.031   Unspecified juvenile rheumatoid arthritis, right wrist

       M08.032   Unspecified juvenile rheumatoid arthritis, left wrist

       M08.039   Unspecified juvenile rheumatoid arthritis, unspecified wrist

●   **M08.04**   Unspecified juvenile rheumatoid arthritis, hand

       M08.041   Unspecified juvenile rheumatoid arthritis, right hand

       M08.042   Unspecified juvenile rheumatoid arthritis, left hand

       M08.049   Unspecified juvenile rheumatoid arthritis, unspecified hand

●   **M08.05**   Unspecified juvenile rheumatoid arthritis, hip

       M08.051   Unspecified juvenile rheumatoid arthritis, right hip

       M08.052   Unspecified juvenile rheumatoid arthritis, left hip

       M08.059   Unspecified juvenile rheumatoid arthritis, unspecified hip

●   **M08.06**   Unspecified juvenile rheumatoid arthritis, knee

       M08.061   Unspecified juvenile rheumatoid arthritis, right knee

       M08.062   Unspecified juvenile rheumatoid arthritis, left knee

       M08.069   Unspecified juvenile rheumatoid arthritis, unspecified knee

●   **M08.07**   Unspecified juvenile rheumatoid arthritis, ankle and foot

       M08.071   Unspecified juvenile rheumatoid arthritis, right ankle and foot

       M08.072   Unspecified juvenile rheumatoid arthritis, left ankle and foot

       M08.079   Unspecified juvenile rheumatoid arthritis, unspecified ankle and foot

     M08.08   Unspecified juvenile rheumatoid arthritis, vertebrae

     M08.09   Unspecified juvenile rheumatoid arthritis, multiple sites

M08.1   Juvenile ankylosing spondylitis

     Excludes1   ankylosing spondylitis in adults (M45.0-)

● **M08.2   Juvenile rheumatoid arthritis with systemic onset**
     Still's disease NOS

     Excludes1   adult-onset Still's disease (M06.1-)

     M08.20   Juvenile rheumatoid arthritis with systemic onset, unspecified site

●   **M08.21**   Juvenile rheumatoid arthritis with systemic onset, shoulder

       M08.211   Juvenile rheumatoid arthritis with systemic onset, right shoulder

       M08.212   Juvenile rheumatoid arthritis with systemic onset, left shoulder

       M08.219   Juvenile rheumatoid arthritis with systemic onset, unspecified shoulder

●   **M08.22**   Juvenile rheumatoid arthritis with systemic onset, elbow

       M08.221   Juvenile rheumatoid arthritis with systemic onset, right elbow

       M08.222   Juvenile rheumatoid arthritis with systemic onset, left elbow

       M08.229   Juvenile rheumatoid arthritis with systemic onset, unspecified elbow

●   **M08.23**   Juvenile rheumatoid arthritis with systemic onset, wrist

       M08.231   Juvenile rheumatoid arthritis with systemic onset, right wrist

       M08.232   Juvenile rheumatoid arthritis with systemic onset, left wrist

       M08.239   Juvenile rheumatoid arthritis with systemic onset, unspecified wrist

●   **M08.24**   Juvenile rheumatoid arthritis with systemic onset, hand

       M08.241   Juvenile rheumatoid arthritis with systemic onset, right hand

       M08.242   Juvenile rheumatoid arthritis with systemic onset, left hand

       M08.249   Juvenile rheumatoid arthritis with systemic onset, unspecified hand

●   **M08.25**   Juvenile rheumatoid arthritis with systemic onset, hip

       M08.251   Juvenile rheumatoid arthritis with systemic onset, right hip

       M08.252   Juvenile rheumatoid arthritis with systemic onset, left hip

       M08.259   Juvenile rheumatoid arthritis with systemic onset, unspecified hip

●   **M08.26**   Juvenile rheumatoid arthritis with systemic onset, knee

       M08.261   Juvenile rheumatoid arthritis with systemic onset, right knee

       M08.262   Juvenile rheumatoid arthritis with systemic onset, left knee

       M08.269   Juvenile rheumatoid arthritis with systemic onset, unspecified knee

●   **M08.27**   Juvenile rheumatoid arthritis with systemic onset, ankle and foot

       M08.271   Juvenile rheumatoid arthritis with systemic onset, right ankle and foot

       M08.272   Juvenile rheumatoid arthritis with systemic onset, left ankle and foot

       M08.279   Juvenile rheumatoid arthritis with systemic onset, unspecified ankle and foot

     M08.28   Juvenile rheumatoid arthritis with systemic onset, vertebrae

     M08.29   Juvenile rheumatoid arthritis with systemic onset, multiple sites

N   Newborn Age: 0   **P**   Pediatric Age: 0–17   **M**   Maternity DX: 12–55   **A**   Adult Age: 15–124   ♀   Females Only   ♂   Males Only

Complication\Comorbidity   Major C\C   (Ex)   CC/MCC Exclusions   Present on Admission Requirement   Hospital-Acquired Condition   **1085**

CHAPTER 13 (M00-M99)

M08.3   Juvenile rheumatoid polyarthritis (seronegative)
● M08.4   Pauciarticular juvenile rheumatoid arthritis
    M08.40   Pauciarticular juvenile rheumatoid arthritis, unspecified site
    ● M08.41   Pauciarticular juvenile rheumatoid arthritis, shoulder
        M08.411   Pauciarticular juvenile rheumatoid arthritis, right shoulder
        M08.412   Pauciarticular juvenile rheumatoid arthritis, left shoulder
        M08.419   Pauciarticular juvenile rheumatoid arthritis, unspecified shoulder
    ● M08.42   Pauciarticular juvenile rheumatoid arthritis, elbow
        M08.421   Pauciarticular juvenile rheumatoid arthritis, right elbow
        M08.422   Pauciarticular juvenile rheumatoid arthritis, left elbow
        M08.429   Pauciarticular juvenile rheumatoid arthritis, unspecified elbow
    ● M08.43   Pauciarticular juvenile rheumatoid arthritis, wrist
        M08.431   Pauciarticular juvenile rheumatoid arthritis, right wrist
        M08.432   Pauciarticular juvenile rheumatoid arthritis, left wrist
        M08.439   Pauciarticular juvenile rheumatoid arthritis, unspecified wrist
    ● M08.44   Pauciarticular juvenile rheumatoid arthritis, hand
        M08.441   Pauciarticular juvenile rheumatoid arthritis, right hand
        M08.442   Pauciarticular juvenile rheumatoid arthritis, left hand
        M08.449   Pauciarticular juvenile rheumatoid arthritis, unspecified hand
    ● M08.45   Pauciarticular juvenile rheumatoid arthritis, hip
        M08.451   Pauciarticular juvenile rheumatoid arthritis, right hip
        M08.452   Pauciarticular juvenile rheumatoid arthritis, left hip
        M08.459   Pauciarticular juvenile rheumatoid arthritis, unspecified hip
    ● M08.46   Pauciarticular juvenile rheumatoid arthritis, knee
        M08.461   Pauciarticular juvenile rheumatoid arthritis, right knee
        M08.462   Pauciarticular juvenile rheumatoid arthritis, left knee
        M08.469   Pauciarticular juvenile rheumatoid arthritis, unspecified knee
    ● M08.47   Pauciarticular juvenile rheumatoid arthritis, ankle and foot
        M08.471   Pauciarticular juvenile rheumatoid arthritis, right ankle and foot
        M08.472   Pauciarticular juvenile rheumatoid arthritis, left ankle and foot
        M08.479   Pauciarticular juvenile rheumatoid arthritis, unspecified ankle and foot
    M08.48   Pauciarticular juvenile rheumatoid arthritis, vertebrae
● M08.8   Other juvenile arthritis
    M08.80   Other juvenile arthritis, unspecified site
    ● M08.81   Other juvenile arthritis, shoulder
        M08.811   Other juvenile arthritis, right shoulder
        M08.812   Other juvenile arthritis, left shoulder
        M08.819   Other juvenile arthritis, unspecified shoulder

    ● M08.82   Other juvenile arthritis, elbow
        M08.821   Other juvenile arthritis, right elbow
        M08.822   Other juvenile arthritis, left elbow
        M08.829   Other juvenile arthritis, unspecified elbow
    ● M08.83   Other juvenile arthritis, wrist
        M08.831   Other juvenile arthritis, right wrist
        M08.832   Other juvenile arthritis, left wrist
        M08.839   Other juvenile arthritis, unspecified wrist
    ● M08.84   Other juvenile arthritis, hand
        M08.841   Other juvenile arthritis, right hand
        M08.842   Other juvenile arthritis, left hand
        M08.849   Other juvenile arthritis, unspecified hand
    ● M08.85   Other juvenile arthritis, hip
        M08.851   Other juvenile arthritis, right hip
        M08.852   Other juvenile arthritis, left hip
        M08.859   Other juvenile arthritis, unspecified hip
    ● M08.86   Other juvenile arthritis, knee
        M08.861   Other juvenile arthritis, right knee
        M08.862   Other juvenile arthritis, left knee
        M08.869   Other juvenile arthritis, unspecified knee
    ● M08.87   Other juvenile arthritis, ankle and foot
        M08.871   Other juvenile arthritis, right ankle and foot
        M08.872   Other juvenile arthritis, left ankle and foot
        M08.879   Other juvenile arthritis, unspecified ankle and foot
    M08.88   Other juvenile arthritis, other specified site ◄▥
        Other juvenile arthritis, vertebrae ◄
    M08.89   Other juvenile arthritis, multiple sites
● M08.9   Juvenile arthritis, unspecified
    Excludes1   juvenile rheumatoid arthritis, unspecified (M08.0-)
    M08.90   Juvenile arthritis, unspecified, unspecified site
    ● M08.91   Juvenile arthritis, unspecified, shoulder
        M08.911   Juvenile arthritis, unspecified, right shoulder
        M08.912   Juvenile arthritis, unspecified, left shoulder
        M08.919   Juvenile arthritis, unspecified, unspecified shoulder
    ● M08.92   Juvenile arthritis, unspecified, elbow
        M08.921   Juvenile arthritis, unspecified, right elbow
        M08.922   Juvenile arthritis, unspecified, left elbow
        M08.929   Juvenile arthritis, unspecified, unspecified elbow
    ● M08.93   Juvenile arthritis, unspecified, wrist
        M08.931   Juvenile arthritis, unspecified, right wrist
        M08.932   Juvenile arthritis, unspecified, left wrist
        M08.939   Juvenile arthritis, unspecified, unspecified wrist
    ● M08.94   Juvenile arthritis, unspecified, hand
        M08.941   Juvenile arthritis, unspecified, right hand
        M08.942   Juvenile arthritis, unspecified, left hand
        M08.949   Juvenile arthritis, unspecified, unspecified hand

◄ New   ◄▥ Revised   ~~deleted~~ Deleted   Excludes 1   Excludes 2   Includes   Use additional   Code first   Code also   Unspecified
OGCR Official Guidelines   ● Unacceptable Principal Diagnosis   X Assign placeholder X   ● Use Additional Character(s)   ▸ Manifestation Code   **Coding Clinic**

● M08.95   Juvenile arthritis, unspecified, hip

    M08.951   Juvenile arthritis, unspecified, right hip

    M08.952   Juvenile arthritis, unspecified, left hip

    M08.959   Juvenile arthritis, unspecified, unspecified hip

● M08.96   Juvenile arthritis, unspecified, knee

    M08.961   Juvenile arthritis, unspecified, right knee

    M08.962   Juvenile arthritis, unspecified, left knee

    M08.969   Juvenile arthritis, unspecified, unspecified knee

● M08.97   Juvenile arthritis, unspecified, ankle and foot

    M08.971   Juvenile arthritis, unspecified, right ankle and foot

    M08.972   Juvenile arthritis, unspecified, left ankle and foot

    M08.979   Juvenile arthritis, unspecified, unspecified ankle and foot

    M08.98   Juvenile arthritis, unspecified, vertebrae

    M08.99   Juvenile arthritis, unspecified, multiple sites

● **M1A   Chronic gout**

    Use additional code to identify:

      Autonomic neuropathy in diseases classified elsewhere (G99.0)

      Calculus of urinary tract in diseases classified elsewhere (N22)

      Cardiomyopathy in diseases classified elsewhere (I43)

      Disorders of external ear in diseases classified elsewhere (H61.1-, H62.8-)

      Disorders of iris and ciliary body in diseases classified elsewhere (H22)

      Glomerular disorders in diseases classified elsewhere (N08)

    Excludes1   acute gout (M10.-) ◄▥

            gout NOS (M10.-)

    The appropriate 7th character is to be added to each code from category M1A

| 0 | without tophus (tophi) |
| 1 | with tophus (tophi) |

● **M1A.0   Idiopathic chronic gout**

    Chronic gouty bursitis

    Primary chronic gout

X ● **M1A.00**   Idiopathic chronic gout, unspecified site

● **M1A.01**   Idiopathic chronic gout, shoulder

    ● M1A.011   Idiopathic chronic gout, right shoulder

    ● M1A.012   Idiopathic chronic gout, left shoulder

    ● M1A.019   Idiopathic chronic gout, unspecified shoulder

● **M1A.02**   Idiopathic chronic gout, elbow

    ● M1A.021   Idiopathic chronic gout, right elbow

    ● M1A.022   Idiopathic chronic gout, left elbow

    ● M1A.029   Idiopathic chronic gout, unspecified elbow

● **M1A.03**   Idiopathic chronic gout, wrist

    ● M1A.031   Idiopathic chronic gout, right wrist

    ● M1A.032   Idiopathic chronic gout, left wrist

    ● M1A.039   Idiopathic chronic gout, unspecified wrist

● **M1A.04**   Idiopathic chronic gout, hand

    ● M1A.041   Idiopathic chronic gout, right hand

    ● M1A.042   Idiopathic chronic gout, left hand

    ● M1A.049   Idiopathic chronic gout, unspecified hand

● **M1A.05**   Idiopathic chronic gout, hip

    ● M1A.051   Idiopathic chronic gout, right hip

    ● M1A.052   Idiopathic chronic gout, left hip

    ● M1A.059   Idiopathic chronic gout, unspecified hip

● **M1A.06**   Idiopathic chronic gout, knee

    ● M1A.061   Idiopathic chronic gout, right knee

    ● M1A.062   Idiopathic chronic gout, left knee

    ● M1A.069   Idiopathic chronic gout, unspecified knee

● **M1A.07**   Idiopathic chronic gout, ankle and foot

    ● M1A.071   Idiopathic chronic gout, right ankle and foot

    ● M1A.072   Idiopathic chronic gout, left ankle and foot

    ● M1A.079   Idiopathic chronic gout, unspecified ankle and foot

X ● **M1A.08**   Idiopathic chronic gout, vertebrae

X ● **M1A.09**   Idiopathic chronic gout, multiple sites

● **M1A.1   Lead-induced chronic gout**

    Code first toxic effects of lead and its compounds (T56.0-)

X ● **M1A.10**   Lead-induced chronic gout, unspecified site

● **M1A.11**   Lead-induced chronic gout, shoulder

    ● M1A.111   Lead-induced chronic gout, right shoulder

    ● M1A.112   Lead-induced chronic gout, left shoulder

    ● M1A.119   Lead-induced chronic gout, unspecified shoulder

● **M1A.12**   Lead-induced chronic gout, elbow

    ● M1A.121   Lead-induced chronic gout, right elbow

    ● M1A.122   Lead-induced chronic gout, left elbow

    ● M1A.129   Lead-induced chronic gout, unspecified elbow

● **M1A.13**   Lead-induced chronic gout, wrist

    ● M1A.131   Lead-induced chronic gout, right wrist

    ● M1A.132   Lead-induced chronic gout, left wrist

    ● M1A.139   Lead-induced chronic gout, unspecified wrist

● **M1A.14**   Lead-induced chronic gout, hand

    ● M1A.141   Lead-induced chronic gout, right hand

    ● M1A.142   Lead-induced chronic gout, left hand

    ● M1A.149   Lead-induced chronic gout, unspecified hand

● **M1A.15**   Lead-induced chronic gout, hip

    ● M1A.151   Lead-induced chronic gout, right hip

    ● M1A.152   Lead-induced chronic gout, left hip

    ● M1A.159   Lead-induced chronic gout, unspecified hip

● **M1A.16**   Lead-induced chronic gout, knee

    ● M1A.161   Lead-induced chronic gout, right knee

    ● M1A.162   Lead-induced chronic gout, left knee

    ● M1A.169   Lead-induced chronic gout, unspecified knee

● **M1A.17**   Lead-induced chronic gout, ankle and foot

    ● M1A.171   Lead-induced chronic gout, right ankle and foot

    ● M1A.172   Lead-induced chronic gout, left ankle and foot

    ● M1A.179   Lead-induced chronic gout, unspecified ankle and foot

X ● **M1A.18**   Lead-induced chronic gout, vertebrae

X ● **M1A.19**   Lead-induced chronic gout, multiple sites

N   Newborn Age: 0   **P**   Pediatric Age: 0–17   **M**   Maternity DX: 12–55   **A**   Adult Age: 15–124   ♀   Females Only   ♂   Males Only

 Complication\Comorbidity   Major C\C   (Ex) CC/MCC Exclusions   Present on Admission Requirement   ● Hospital-Acquired Condition

1087

CHAPTER 13 (M00-M99)

● M1A.2 Drug-induced chronic gout
    Use additional code for adverse effect, if applicable, to identify drug (T36-T50 with fifth or sixth character 5)

X● M1A.20 Drug-induced chronic gout, unspecified site

● M1A.21 Drug-induced chronic gout, shoulder
  ● M1A.211 Drug-induced chronic gout, right shoulder
  ● M1A.212 Drug-induced chronic gout, left shoulder
  ● M1A.219 Drug-induced chronic gout, unspecified shoulder

● M1A.22 Drug-induced chronic gout, elbow
  ● M1A.221 Drug-induced chronic gout, right elbow
  ● M1A.222 Drug-induced chronic gout, left elbow
  ● M1A.229 Drug-induced chronic gout, unspecified elbow

● M1A.23 Drug-induced chronic gout, wrist
  ● M1A.231 Drug-induced chronic gout, right wrist
  ● M1A.232 Drug-induced chronic gout, left wrist
  ● M1A.239 Drug-induced chronic gout, unspecified wrist

● M1A.24 Drug-induced chronic gout, hand
  ● M1A.241 Drug-induced chronic gout, right hand
  ● M1A.242 Drug-induced chronic gout, left hand
  ● M1A.249 Drug-induced chronic gout, unspecified hand

● M1A.25 Drug-induced chronic gout, hip
  ● M1A.251 Drug-induced chronic gout, right hip
  ● M1A.252 Drug-induced chronic gout, left hip
  ● M1A.259 Drug-induced chronic gout, unspecified hip

● M1A.26 Drug-induced chronic gout, knee
  ● M1A.261 Drug-induced chronic gout, right knee
  ● M1A.262 Drug-induced chronic gout, left knee
  ● M1A.269 Drug-induced chronic gout, unspecified knee

● M1A.27 Drug-induced chronic gout, ankle and foot
  ● M1A.271 Drug-induced chronic gout, right ankle and foot
  ● M1A.272 Drug-induced chronic gout, left ankle and foot
  ● M1A.279 Drug-induced chronic gout, unspecified ankle and foot

X● M1A.28 Drug-induced chronic gout, vertebrae

X● M1A.29 Drug-induced chronic gout, multiple sites

● M1A.3 Chronic gout due to renal impairment
    Code first associated renal disease

X● M1A.30 Chronic gout due to renal impairment, unspecified site

● M1A.31 Chronic gout due to renal impairment, shoulder
  ● M1A.311 Chronic gout due to renal impairment, right shoulder
  ● M1A.312 Chronic gout due to renal impairment, left shoulder
  ● M1A.319 Chronic gout due to renal impairment, unspecified shoulder

● M1A.32 Chronic gout due to renal impairment, elbow
  ● M1A.321 Chronic gout due to renal impairment, right elbow
  ● M1A.322 Chronic gout due to renal impairment, left elbow
  ● M1A.329 Chronic gout due to renal impairment, unspecified elbow

● M1A.33 Chronic gout due to renal impairment, wrist
  ● M1A.331 Chronic gout due to renal impairment, right wrist
  ● M1A.332 Chronic gout due to renal impairment, left wrist
  ● M1A.339 Chronic gout due to renal impairment, unspecified wrist

● M1A.34 Chronic gout due to renal impairment, hand
  ● M1A.341 Chronic gout due to renal impairment, right hand
  ● M1A.342 Chronic gout due to renal impairment, left hand
  ● M1A.349 Chronic gout due to renal impairment, unspecified hand

● M1A.35 Chronic gout due to renal impairment, hip
  ● M1A.351 Chronic gout due to renal impairment, right hip
  ● M1A.352 Chronic gout due to renal impairment, left hip
  ● M1A.359 Chronic gout due to renal impairment, unspecified hip

● M1A.36 Chronic gout due to renal impairment, knee
  ● M1A.361 Chronic gout due to renal impairment, right knee
  ● M1A.362 Chronic gout due to renal impairment, left knee
  ● M1A.369 Chronic gout due to renal impairment, unspecified knee

● M1A.37 Chronic gout due to renal impairment, ankle and foot
  ● M1A.371 Chronic gout due to renal impairment, right ankle and foot
  ● M1A.372 Chronic gout due to renal impairment, left ankle and foot
  ● M1A.379 Chronic gout due to renal impairment, unspecified ankle and foot

X● M1A.38 Chronic gout due to renal impairment, vertebrae

X● M1A.39 Chronic gout due to renal impairment, multiple sites

X● M1A.4 Other secondary chronic gout
    Code first associated condition

● M1A.40 Other secondary chronic gout, unspecified site

● M1A.41 Other secondary chronic gout, shoulder
  ● M1A.411 Other secondary chronic gout, right shoulder
  ● M1A.412 Other secondary chronic gout, left shoulder
  ● M1A.419 Other secondary chronic gout, unspecified shoulder

● M1A.42 Other secondary chronic gout, elbow
  ● M1A.421 Other secondary chronic gout, right elbow
  ● M1A.422 Other secondary chronic gout, left elbow
  ● M1A.429 Other secondary chronic gout, unspecified elbow

◀ New   ◀ Revised   ~~deleted~~ Deleted   Excludes 1   Excludes 2   Includes   Use additional   Code first   Code also   Unspecified
OGCR Official Guidelines   ● Unacceptable Principal Diagnosis   X Assign placeholder X   ● Use Additional Character(s)   ▌ Manifestation Code   **Coding Clinic**

● M1A.43   Other secondary chronic gout, wrist
   ● M1A.431   Other secondary chronic gout, right wrist
   ● M1A.432   Other secondary chronic gout, left wrist
   ● M1A.439   Other secondary chronic gout, unspecified wrist

● M1A.44   Other secondary chronic gout, hand
   ● M1A.441   Other secondary chronic gout, right hand
   ● M1A.442   Other secondary chronic gout, left hand
   ● M1A.449   Other secondary chronic gout, unspecified hand

● M1A.45   Other secondary chronic gout, hip
   ● M1A.451   Other secondary chronic gout, right hip
   ● M1A.452   Other secondary chronic gout, left hip
   ● M1A.459   Other secondary chronic gout, unspecified hip

● M1A.46   Other secondary chronic gout, knee
   ● M1A.461   Other secondary chronic gout, right knee
   ● M1A.462   Other secondary chronic gout, left knee
   ● M1A.469   Other secondary chronic gout, unspecified knee

● M1A.47   Other secondary chronic gout, ankle and foot
   ● M1A.471   Other secondary chronic gout, right ankle and foot
   ● M1A.472   Other secondary chronic gout, left ankle and foot
   ● M1A.479   Other secondary chronic gout, unspecified ankle and foot

X ● M1A.48   Other secondary chronic gout, vertebrae
X ● M1A.49   Other secondary chronic gout, multiple sites

X ● M1A.9   Chronic gout, unspecified

● **M10   Gout**
   Accumulation of uric acid that results in swollen, red, hot, painful, stiff joints.
   Acute gout
   Gout attack
   Gout flare
   Gout NOS
   Podagra
   Use additional code to identify:
     Autonomic neuropathy in diseases classified elsewhere (G99.0)
     Calculus of urinary tract in diseases classified elsewhere (N22)
     Cardiomyopathy in diseases classified elsewhere (I43)
     Disorders of external ear in diseases classified elsewhere (H61.1-, H62.8-)
     Disorders of iris and ciliary body in diseases classified elsewhere (H22)
     Glomerular disorders in diseases classified elsewhere (N08)
   Excludes1   chronic gout (M1A.-) ◀

● M10.0   Idiopathic gout
   Gouty bursitis
   Primary gout
   M10.00   Idiopathic gout, unspecified site
   ● M10.01   Idiopathic gout, shoulder
     M10.011   Idiopathic gout, right shoulder
     M10.012   Idiopathic gout, left shoulder
     M10.019   Idiopathic gout, unspecified shoulder
   ● M10.02   Idiopathic gout, elbow
     M10.021   Idiopathic gout, right elbow
     M10.022   Idiopathic gout, left elbow
     M10.029   Idiopathic gout, unspecified elbow

● M10.03   Idiopathic gout, wrist
   M10.031   Idiopathic gout, right wrist
   M10.032   Idiopathic gout, left wrist
   M10.039   Idiopathic gout, unspecified wrist

● M10.04   Idiopathic gout, hand
   M10.041   Idiopathic gout, right hand
   M10.042   Idiopathic gout, left hand
   M10.049   Idiopathic gout, unspecified hand

● M10.05   Idiopathic gout, hip
   M10.051   Idiopathic gout, right hip
   M10.052   Idiopathic gout, left hip
   M10.059   Idiopathic gout, unspecified hip

● M10.06   Idiopathic gout, knee
   M10.061   Idiopathic gout, right knee
   M10.062   Idiopathic gout, left knee
   M10.069   Idiopathic gout, unspecified knee

● M10.07   Idiopathic gout, ankle and foot
   M10.071   Idiopathic gout, right ankle and foot
   M10.072   Idiopathic gout, left ankle and foot
   M10.079   Idiopathic gout, unspecified ankle and foot

M10.08   Idiopathic gout, vertebrae
M10.09   Idiopathic gout, multiple sites

● M10.1   Lead-induced gout
   Code first toxic effects of lead and its compounds (T56.0-)
   M10.10   Lead-induced gout, unspecified site
   ● M10.11   Lead-induced gout, shoulder
     M10.111   Lead-induced gout, right shoulder
     M10.112   Lead-induced gout, left shoulder
     M10.119   Lead-induced gout, unspecified shoulder
   ● M10.12   Lead-induced gout, elbow
     M10.121   Lead-induced gout, right elbow
     M10.122   Lead-induced gout, left elbow
     M10.129   Lead-induced gout, unspecified elbow
   ● M10.13   Lead-induced gout, wrist
     M10.131   Lead-induced gout, right wrist
     M10.132   Lead-induced gout, left wrist
     M10.139   Lead-induced gout, unspecified wrist
   ● M10.14   Lead-induced gout, hand
     M10.141   Lead-induced gout, right hand
     M10.142   Lead-induced gout, left hand
     M10.149   Lead-induced gout, unspecified hand
   ● M10.15   Lead-induced gout, hip
     M10.151   Lead-induced gout, right hip
     M10.152   Lead-induced gout, left hip
     M10.159   Lead-induced gout, unspecified hip
   ● M10.16   Lead-induced gout, knee
     M10.161   Lead-induced gout, right knee
     M10.162   Lead-induced gout, left knee
     M10.169   Lead-induced gout, unspecified knee
   ● M10.17   Lead-induced gout, ankle and foot
     M10.171   Lead-induced gout, right ankle and foot
     M10.172   Lead-induced gout, left ankle and foot
     M10.179   Lead-induced gout, unspecified ankle and foot
   M10.18   Lead-induced gout, vertebrae
   M10.19   Lead-induced gout, multiple sites

CHAPTER 13 (M00-M99)

N Newborn Age: 0   P Pediatric Age: 0–17   M Maternity DX: 12–55   A Adult Age: 15–124   ♀ Females Only   ♂ Males Only

Complication\Comorbidity   Major C\C   (Ex) CC/MCC Exclusions   Present on Admission Requirement   Hospital-Acquired Condition   **1089**

● **M10.2 Drug-induced gout**
    Use additional code for adverse effect, if applicable, to identify drug (T36-T50 with fifth or sixth character 5)

    M10.20   Drug-induced gout, unspecified site

● M10.21   Drug-induced gout, shoulder
      M10.211   Drug-induced gout, right shoulder
      M10.212   Drug-induced gout, left shoulder
      M10.219   Drug-induced gout, unspecified shoulder

● M10.22   Drug-induced gout, elbow
      M10.221   Drug-induced gout, right elbow
      M10.222   Drug-induced gout, left elbow
      M10.229   Drug-induced gout, unspecified elbow

● M10.23   Drug-induced gout, wrist
      M10.231   Drug-induced gout, right wrist
      M10.232   Drug-induced gout, left wrist
      M10.239   Drug-induced gout, unspecified wrist

● M10.24   Drug-induced gout, hand
      M10.241   Drug-induced gout, right hand
      M10.242   Drug-induced gout, left hand
      M10.249   Drug-induced gout, unspecified hand

● M10.25   Drug-induced gout, hip
      M10.251   Drug-induced gout, right hip
      M10.252   Drug-induced gout, left hip
      M10.259   Drug-induced gout, unspecified hip

● M10.26   Drug-induced gout, knee
      M10.261   Drug-induced gout, right knee
      M10.262   Drug-induced gout, left knee
      M10.269   Drug-induced gout, unspecified knee

● M10.27   Drug-induced gout, ankle and foot
      M10.271   Drug-induced gout, right ankle and foot
      M10.272   Drug-induced gout, left ankle and foot
      M10.279   Drug-induced gout, unspecified ankle and foot

    M10.28   Drug-induced gout, vertebrae
    M10.29   Drug-induced gout, multiple sites

● **M10.3 Gout due to renal impairment**
    Code also associated renal disease

    M10.30   Gout due to renal impairment, unspecified site

● M10.31   Gout due to renal impairment, shoulder
      M10.311   Gout due to renal impairment, right shoulder
      M10.312   Gout due to renal impairment, left shoulder
      M10.319   Gout due to renal impairment, unspecified shoulder

● M10.32   Gout due to renal impairment, elbow
      M10.321   Gout due to renal impairment, right elbow
      M10.322   Gout due to renal impairment, left elbow
      M10.329   Gout due to renal impairment, unspecified elbow

● M10.33   Gout due to renal impairment, wrist
      M10.331   Gout due to renal impairment, right wrist
      M10.332   Gout due to renal impairment, left wrist
      M10.339   Gout due to renal impairment, unspecified wrist

● M10.34   Gout due to renal impairment, hand
      M10.341   Gout due to renal impairment, right hand
      M10.342   Gout due to renal impairment, left hand
      M10.349   Gout due to renal impairment, unspecified hand

● M10.35   Gout due to renal impairment, hip
      M10.351   Gout due to renal impairment, right hip
      M10.352   Gout due to renal impairment, left hip
      M10.359   Gout due to renal impairment, unspecified hip

● M10.36   Gout due to renal impairment, knee
      M10.361   Gout due to renal impairment, right knee
      M10.362   Gout due to renal impairment, left knee
      M10.369   Gout due to renal impairment, unspecified knee

● M10.37   Gout due to renal impairment, ankle and foot
      M10.371   Gout due to renal impairment, right ankle and foot
      M10.372   Gout due to renal impairment, left ankle and foot
      M10.379   Gout due to renal impairment, unspecified ankle and foot

    M10.38   Gout due to renal impairment, vertebrae
    M10.39   Gout due to renal impairment, multiple sites

● **M10.4 Other secondary gout**
    Code first associated condition

    M10.40   Other secondary gout, unspecified site

● M10.41   Other secondary gout, shoulder
      M10.411   Other secondary gout, right shoulder
      M10.412   Other secondary gout, left shoulder
      M10.419   Other secondary gout, unspecified shoulder

● M10.42   Other secondary gout, elbow
      M10.421   Other secondary gout, right elbow
      M10.422   Other secondary gout, left elbow
      M10.429   Other secondary gout, unspecified elbow

● M10.43   Other secondary gout, wrist
      M10.431   Other secondary gout, right wrist
      M10.432   Other secondary gout, left wrist
      M10.439   Other secondary gout, unspecified wrist

● M10.44   Other secondary gout, hand
      M10.441   Other secondary gout, right hand
      M10.442   Other secondary gout, left hand
      M10.449   Other secondary gout, unspecified hand

● M10.45   Other secondary gout, hip
      M10.451   Other secondary gout, right hip
      M10.452   Other secondary gout, left hip
      M10.459   Other secondary gout, unspecified hip

● M10.46   Other secondary gout, knee
      M10.461   Other secondary gout, right knee
      M10.462   Other secondary gout, left knee
      M10.469   Other secondary gout, unspecified knee

● M10.47   Other secondary gout, ankle and foot

     M10.471   Other secondary gout, right ankle and foot

     M10.472   Other secondary gout, left ankle and foot

     M10.479   Other secondary gout, unspecified ankle and foot

   M10.48   Other secondary gout, vertebrae

   M10.49   Other secondary gout, multiple sites

M10.9   Gout, unspecified

     Gout NOS

● M11   Other crystal arthropathies

   ● M11.0   Hydroxyapatite deposition disease

     M11.00   Hydroxyapatite deposition disease, unspecified site

     ● M11.01   Hydroxyapatite deposition disease, shoulder

       M11.011   Hydroxyapatite deposition disease, right shoulder

       M11.012   Hydroxyapatite deposition disease, left shoulder

       M11.019   Hydroxyapatite deposition disease, unspecified shoulder

     ● M11.02   Hydroxyapatite deposition disease, elbow

       M11.021   Hydroxyapatite deposition disease, right elbow

       M11.022   Hydroxyapatite deposition disease, left elbow

       M11.029   Hydroxyapatite deposition disease, unspecified elbow

     ● M11.03   Hydroxyapatite deposition disease, wrist

       M11.031   Hydroxyapatite deposition disease, right wrist

       M11.032   Hydroxyapatite deposition disease, left wrist

       M11.039   Hydroxyapatite deposition disease, unspecified wrist

     ● M11.04   Hydroxyapatite deposition disease, hand

       M11.041   Hydroxyapatite deposition disease, right hand

       M11.042   Hydroxyapatite deposition disease, left hand

       M11.049   Hydroxyapatite deposition disease, unspecified hand

     ● M11.05   Hydroxyapatite deposition disease, hip

       M11.051   Hydroxyapatite deposition disease, right hip

       M11.052   Hydroxyapatite deposition disease, left hip

       M11.059   Hydroxyapatite deposition disease, unspecified hip

     ● M11.06   Hydroxyapatite deposition disease, knee

       M11.061   Hydroxyapatite deposition disease, right knee

       M11.062   Hydroxyapatite deposition disease, left knee

       M11.069   Hydroxyapatite deposition disease, unspecified knee

     ● M11.07   Hydroxyapatite deposition disease, ankle and foot

       M11.071   Hydroxyapatite deposition disease, right ankle and foot

       M11.072   Hydroxyapatite deposition disease, left ankle and foot

       M11.079   Hydroxyapatite deposition disease, unspecified ankle and foot

     M11.08   Hydroxyapatite deposition disease, vertebrae

     M11.09   Hydroxyapatite deposition disease, multiple sites

● M11.1   Familial chondrocalcinosis

     M11.10   Familial chondrocalcinosis, unspecified site

   ● M11.11   Familial chondrocalcinosis, shoulder

     M11.111   Familial chondrocalcinosis, right shoulder

     M11.112   Familial chondrocalcinosis, left shoulder

     M11.119   Familial chondrocalcinosis, unspecified shoulder

   ● M11.12   Familial chondrocalcinosis, elbow

     M11.121   Familial chondrocalcinosis, right elbow

     M11.122   Familial chondrocalcinosis, left elbow

     M11.129   Familial chondrocalcinosis, unspecified elbow

   ● M11.13   Familial chondrocalcinosis, wrist

     M11.131   Familial chondrocalcinosis, right wrist

     M11.132   Familial chondrocalcinosis, left wrist

     M11.139   Familial chondrocalcinosis, unspecified wrist

   ● M11.14   Familial chondrocalcinosis, hand

     M11.141   Familial chondrocalcinosis, right hand

     M11.142   Familial chondrocalcinosis, left hand

     M11.149   Familial chondrocalcinosis, unspecified hand

   ● M11.15   Familial chondrocalcinosis, hip

     M11.151   Familial chondrocalcinosis, right hip

     M11.152   Familial chondrocalcinosis, left hip

     M11.159   Familial chondrocalcinosis, unspecified hip

   ● M11.16   Familial chondrocalcinosis, knee

     M11.161   Familial chondrocalcinosis, right knee

     M11.162   Familial chondrocalcinosis, left knee

     M11.169   Familial chondrocalcinosis, unspecified knee

   ● M11.17   Familial chondrocalcinosis, ankle and foot

     M11.171   Familial chondrocalcinosis, right ankle and foot

     M11.172   Familial chondrocalcinosis, left ankle and foot

     M11.179   Familial chondrocalcinosis, unspecified ankle and foot

     M11.18   Familial chondrocalcinosis, vertebrae

     M11.19   Familial chondrocalcinosis, multiple sites

● M11.2   Other chondrocalcinosis

     Chondrocalcinosis NOS

     M11.20   Other chondrocalcinosis, unspecified site

   ● M11.21   Other chondrocalcinosis, shoulder

     M11.211   Other chondrocalcinosis, right shoulder

     M11.212   Other chondrocalcinosis, left shoulder

     M11.219   Other chondrocalcinosis, unspecified shoulder

   ● M11.22   Other chondrocalcinosis, elbow

     M11.221   Other chondrocalcinosis, right elbow

     M11.222   Other chondrocalcinosis, left elbow

     M11.229   Other chondrocalcinosis, unspecified elbow

   ● M11.23   Other chondrocalcinosis, wrist

     M11.231   Other chondrocalcinosis, right wrist

     M11.232   Other chondrocalcinosis, left wrist

     M11.239   Other chondrocalcinosis, unspecified wrist

CHAPTER 13 (M00-M99)

- **M11.24** Other chondrocalcinosis, hand
  - M11.241 Other chondrocalcinosis, right hand
  - M11.242 Other chondrocalcinosis, left hand
  - M11.249 Other chondrocalcinosis, unspecified hand
- **M11.25** Other chondrocalcinosis, hip
  - M11.251 Other chondrocalcinosis, right hip
  - M11.252 Other chondrocalcinosis, left hip
  - M11.259 Other chondrocalcinosis, unspecified hip
- **M11.26** Other chondrocalcinosis, knee
  - M11.261 Other chondrocalcinosis, right knee
  - M11.262 Other chondrocalcinosis, left knee
  - M11.269 Other chondrocalcinosis, unspecified knee
- **M11.27** Other chondrocalcinosis, ankle and foot
  - M11.271 Other chondrocalcinosis, right ankle and foot
  - M11.272 Other chondrocalcinosis, left ankle and foot
  - M11.279 Other chondrocalcinosis, unspecified ankle and foot
- **M11.28** Other chondrocalcinosis, vertebrae
- **M11.29** Other chondrocalcinosis, multiple sites
- **M11.8** Other specified crystal arthropathies
  - M11.80 Other specified crystal arthropathies, unspecified site
- **M11.81** Other specified crystal arthropathies, shoulder
  - M11.811 Other specified crystal arthropathies, right shoulder
  - M11.812 Other specified crystal arthropathies, left shoulder
  - M11.819 Other specified crystal arthropathies, unspecified shoulder
- **M11.82** Other specified crystal arthropathies, elbow
  - M11.821 Other specified crystal arthropathies, right elbow
  - M11.822 Other specified crystal arthropathies, left elbow
  - M11.829 Other specified crystal arthropathies, unspecified elbow
- **M11.83** Other specified crystal arthropathies, wrist
  - M11.831 Other specified crystal arthropathies, right wrist
  - M11.832 Other specified crystal arthropathies, left wrist
  - M11.839 Other specified crystal arthropathies, unspecified wrist
- **M11.84** Other specified crystal arthropathies, hand
  - M11.841 Other specified crystal arthropathies, right hand
  - M11.842 Other specified crystal arthropathies, left hand
  - M11.849 Other specified crystal arthropathies, unspecified hand
- **M11.85** Other specified crystal arthropathies, hip
  - M11.851 Other specified crystal arthropathies, right hip
  - M11.852 Other specified crystal arthropathies, left hip
  - M11.859 Other specified crystal arthropathies, unspecified hip
- **M11.86** Other specified crystal arthropathies, knee
  - M11.861 Other specified crystal arthropathies, right knee
  - M11.862 Other specified crystal arthropathies, left knee
  - M11.869 Other specified crystal arthropathies, unspecified knee

- **M11.87** Other specified crystal arthropathies, ankle and foot
  - M11.871 Other specified crystal arthropathies, right ankle and foot
  - M11.872 Other specified crystal arthropathies, left ankle and foot
  - M11.879 Other specified crystal arthropathies, unspecified ankle and foot
- **M11.88** Other specified crystal arthropathies, vertebrae
- **M11.89** Other specified crystal arthropathies, multiple sites
- **M11.9** Crystal arthropathy, unspecified

- **M12** Other and unspecified arthropathy
  - **Excludes1**   arthrosis (M15-M19)
  -            cricoarytenoid arthropathy (J38.7)
- **M12.0** Chronic postrheumatic arthropathy [Jaccoud]
  - M12.00 Chronic postrheumatic arthropathy [Jaccoud], unspecified site
- **M12.01** Chronic postrheumatic arthropathy [Jaccoud], shoulder
  - M12.011 Chronic postrheumatic arthropathy [Jaccoud], right shoulder
  - M12.012 Chronic postrheumatic arthropathy [Jaccoud], left shoulder
  - M12.019 Chronic postrheumatic arthropathy [Jaccoud], unspecified shoulder
- **M12.02** Chronic postrheumatic arthropathy [Jaccoud], elbow
  - M12.021 Chronic postrheumatic arthropathy [Jaccoud], right elbow
  - M12.022 Chronic postrheumatic arthropathy [Jaccoud], left elbow
  - M12.029 Chronic postrheumatic arthropathy [Jaccoud], unspecified elbow
- **M12.03** Chronic postrheumatic arthropathy [Jaccoud], wrist
  - M12.031 Chronic postrheumatic arthropathy [Jaccoud], right wrist
  - M12.032 Chronic postrheumatic arthropathy [Jaccoud], left wrist
  - M12.039 Chronic postrheumatic arthropathy [Jaccoud], unspecified wrist
- **M12.04** Chronic postrheumatic arthropathy [Jaccoud], hand
  - M12.041 Chronic postrheumatic arthropathy [Jaccoud], right hand
  - M12.042 Chronic postrheumatic arthropathy [Jaccoud], left hand
  - M12.049 Chronic postrheumatic arthropathy [Jaccoud], unspecified hand
- **M12.05** Chronic postrheumatic arthropathy [Jaccoud], hip
  - M12.051 Chronic postrheumatic arthropathy [Jaccoud], right hip
  - M12.052 Chronic postrheumatic arthropathy [Jaccoud], left hip
  - M12.059 Chronic postrheumatic arthropathy [Jaccoud], unspecified hip
- **M12.06** Chronic postrheumatic arthropathy [Jaccoud], knee
  - M12.061 Chronic postrheumatic arthropathy [Jaccoud], right knee
  - M12.062 Chronic postrheumatic arthropathy [Jaccoud], left knee
  - M12.069 Chronic postrheumatic arthropathy [Jaccoud], unspecified knee

◄ New   ◄ Revised   ~~deleted~~ Deleted   Excludes 1   Excludes 2   Includes   Use additional   Code first   Code also   Unspecified

OGCR Official Guidelines   ● Unacceptable Principal Diagnosis   X Assign placeholder X   ● Use Additional Character(s)   ▶ Manifestation Code   **Coding Clinic**

● M12.07 Chronic postrheumatic arthropathy [Jaccoud], ankle and foot
    M12.071 Chronic postrheumatic arthropathy [Jaccoud], right ankle and foot
    M12.072 Chronic postrheumatic arthropathy [Jaccoud], left ankle and foot
    M12.079 Chronic postrheumatic arthropathy [Jaccoud], unspecified ankle and foot
  M12.08 Chronic postrheumatic arthropathy [Jaccoud], other specified site ◀⊪
     Chronic postrheumatic arthropathy [Jaccoud], vertebrae ◀
  M12.09 Chronic postrheumatic arthropathy [Jaccoud], multiple sites

● M12.1 Kaschin-Beck disease
   Osteochondroarthrosis deformans endemica
  M12.10 Kaschin-Beck disease, unspecified site
● M12.11 Kaschin-Beck disease, shoulder
    M12.111 Kaschin-Beck disease, right shoulder
    M12.112 Kaschin-Beck disease, left shoulder
    M12.119 Kaschin-Beck disease, unspecified shoulder
● M12.12 Kaschin-Beck disease, elbow
    M12.121 Kaschin-Beck disease, right elbow
    M12.122 Kaschin-Beck disease, left elbow
    M12.129 Kaschin-Beck disease, unspecified elbow
● M12.13 Kaschin-Beck disease, wrist
    M12.131 Kaschin-Beck disease, right wrist
    M12.132 Kaschin-Beck disease, left wrist
    M12.139 Kaschin-Beck disease, unspecified wrist
● M12.14 Kaschin-Beck disease, hand
    M12.141 Kaschin-Beck disease, right hand
    M12.142 Kaschin-Beck disease, left hand
    M12.149 Kaschin-Beck disease, unspecified hand
● M12.15 Kaschin-Beck disease, hip
    M12.151 Kaschin-Beck disease, right hip
    M12.152 Kaschin-Beck disease, left hip
    M12.159 Kaschin-Beck disease, unspecified hip
● M12.16 Kaschin-Beck disease, knee
    M12.161 Kaschin-Beck disease, right knee
    M12.162 Kaschin-Beck disease, left knee
    M12.169 Kaschin-Beck disease, unspecified knee
● M12.17 Kaschin-Beck disease, ankle and foot
    M12.171 Kaschin-Beck disease, right ankle and foot
    M12.172 Kaschin-Beck disease, left ankle and foot
    M12.179 Kaschin-Beck disease, unspecified ankle and foot
  M12.18 Kaschin-Beck disease, vertebrae
  M12.19 Kaschin-Beck disease, multiple sites
● M12.2 Villonodular synovitis (pigmented)
  M12.20 Villonodular synovitis (pigmented), unspecified site
● M12.21 Villonodular synovitis (pigmented), shoulder
    M12.211 Villonodular synovitis (pigmented), right shoulder
    M12.212 Villonodular synovitis (pigmented), left shoulder
    M12.219 Villonodular synovitis (pigmented), unspecified shoulder

● M12.22 Villonodular synovitis (pigmented), elbow
    M12.221 Villonodular synovitis (pigmented), right elbow
    M12.222 Villonodular synovitis (pigmented), left elbow
    M12.229 Villonodular synovitis (pigmented), unspecified elbow
● M12.23 Villonodular synovitis (pigmented), wrist
    M12.231 Villonodular synovitis (pigmented), right wrist
    M12.232 Villonodular synovitis (pigmented), left wrist
    M12.239 Villonodular synovitis (pigmented), unspecified wrist
● M12.24 Villonodular synovitis (pigmented), hand
    M12.241 Villonodular synovitis (pigmented), right hand
    M12.242 Villonodular synovitis (pigmented), left hand
    M12.249 Villonodular synovitis (pigmented), unspecified hand
● M12.25 Villonodular synovitis (pigmented), hip
    M12.251 Villonodular synovitis (pigmented), right hip
    M12.252 Villonodular synovitis (pigmented), left hip
    M12.259 Villonodular synovitis (pigmented), unspecified hip
● M12.26 Villonodular synovitis (pigmented), knee
    M12.261 Villonodular synovitis (pigmented), right knee
    M12.262 Villonodular synovitis (pigmented), left knee
    M12.269 Villonodular synovitis (pigmented), unspecified knee
● M12.27 Villonodular synovitis (pigmented), ankle and foot
    M12.271 Villonodular synovitis (pigmented), right ankle and foot
    M12.272 Villonodular synovitis (pigmented), left ankle and foot
    M12.279 Villonodular synovitis (pigmented), unspecified ankle and foot
  M12.28 Villonodular synovitis (pigmented), other specified site ◀⊪
     Villonodular synovitis (pigmented), vertebrae ◀
  M12.29 Villonodular synovitis (pigmented), multiple sites
● M12.3 Palindromic rheumatism
  M12.30 Palindromic rheumatism, unspecified site
● M12.31 Palindromic rheumatism, shoulder
    M12.311 Palindromic rheumatism, right shoulder
    M12.312 Palindromic rheumatism, left shoulder
    M12.319 Palindromic rheumatism, unspecified shoulder
● M12.32 Palindromic rheumatism, elbow
    M12.321 Palindromic rheumatism, right elbow
    M12.322 Palindromic rheumatism, left elbow
    M12.329 Palindromic rheumatism, unspecified elbow
● M12.33 Palindromic rheumatism, wrist
    M12.331 Palindromic rheumatism, right wrist
    M12.332 Palindromic rheumatism, left wrist
    M12.339 Palindromic rheumatism, unspecified wrist

N   Newborn Age: 0   P   Pediatric Age: 0–17   M   Maternity DX: 12–55   A   Adult Age: 15–124   ♀   Females Only   ♂   Males Only

🐾 Complication\Comorbidity   🐾 Major C\C   (Ex) CC/MCC Exclusions   🗅 Present on Admission Requirement   🐾 Hospital-Acquired Condition

1093

● M12.34 Palindromic rheumatism, hand
    M12.341 Palindromic rheumatism, right hand
    M12.342 Palindromic rheumatism, left hand
    M12.349 Palindromic rheumatism, `unspecified` hand
● M12.35 Palindromic rheumatism, hip
    M12.351 Palindromic rheumatism, right hip
    M12.352 Palindromic rheumatism, left hip
    M12.359 Palindromic rheumatism, `unspecified` hip
● M12.36 Palindromic rheumatism, knee
    M12.361 Palindromic rheumatism, right knee
    M12.362 Palindromic rheumatism, left knee
    M12.369 Palindromic rheumatism, `unspecified` knee
● M12.37 Palindromic rheumatism, ankle and foot
    M12.371 Palindromic rheumatism, right ankle and foot
    M12.372 Palindromic rheumatism, left ankle and foot
    M12.379 Palindromic rheumatism, `unspecified` ankle and foot
  M12.38 Palindromic rheumatism, other specified site ◀▦
    Palindromic rheumatism, vertebrae ◀
  M12.39 Palindromic rheumatism, multiple sites
● M12.4 Intermittent hydrarthrosis
  M12.40 Intermittent hydrarthrosis, `unspecified` site
● M12.41 Intermittent hydrarthrosis, shoulder
    M12.411 Intermittent hydrarthrosis, right shoulder
    M12.412 Intermittent hydrarthrosis, left shoulder
    M12.419 Intermittent hydrarthrosis, `unspecified` shoulder
● M12.42 Intermittent hydrarthrosis, elbow
    M12.421 Intermittent hydrarthrosis, right elbow
    M12.422 Intermittent hydrarthrosis, left elbow
    M12.429 Intermittent hydrarthrosis, `unspecified` elbow
● M12.43 Intermittent hydrarthrosis, wrist
    M12.431 Intermittent hydrarthrosis, right wrist
    M12.432 Intermittent hydrarthrosis, left wrist
    M12.439 Intermittent hydrarthrosis, `unspecified` wrist
● M12.44 Intermittent hydrarthrosis, hand
    M12.441 Intermittent hydrarthrosis, right hand
    M12.442 Intermittent hydrarthrosis, left hand
    M12.449 Intermittent hydrarthrosis, `unspecified` hand
● M12.45 Intermittent hydrarthrosis, hip
    M12.451 Intermittent hydrarthrosis, right hip
    M12.452 Intermittent hydrarthrosis, left hip
    M12.459 Intermittent hydrarthrosis, `unspecified` hip
● M12.46 Intermittent hydrarthrosis, knee
    M12.461 Intermittent hydrarthrosis, right knee
    M12.462 Intermittent hydrarthrosis, left knee
    M12.469 Intermittent hydrarthrosis, `unspecified` knee

● M12.47 Intermittent hydrarthrosis, ankle and foot
    M12.471 Intermittent hydrarthrosis, right ankle and foot
    M12.472 Intermittent hydrarthrosis, left ankle and foot
    M12.479 Intermittent hydrarthrosis, `unspecified` ankle and foot
  M12.48 Intermittent hydrarthrosis, other site
  M12.49 Intermittent hydrarthrosis, multiple sites
● M12.5 Traumatic arthropathy
    `Excludes1`   current injury-see Alphabetic Index
        post-traumatic osteoarthritis of first carpometacarpal joint (M18.2-M18.3) ◀▦
        ~~NOS (M19.1-)~~
        ~~first carpometacarpal joint (M18.2-M18.3)~~
        post-traumatic osteoarthritis of hip (M16.4-M16.5) ◀▦
        post-traumatic osteoarthritis of knee (M17.2-M17.3) ◀▦
        post-traumatic osteoarthritis NOS (M19.1-) ◀▦
        post-traumatic osteoarthritis of other single joints (M19.1-) ◀
  M12.50 Traumatic arthropathy, `unspecified` site
● M12.51 Traumatic arthropathy, shoulder
    M12.511 Traumatic arthropathy, right shoulder
    M12.512 Traumatic arthropathy, left shoulder
    M12.519 Traumatic arthropathy, `unspecified` shoulder
● M12.52 Traumatic arthropathy, elbow
    M12.521 Traumatic arthropathy, right elbow
    M12.522 Traumatic arthropathy, left elbow
    M12.529 Traumatic arthropathy, `unspecified` elbow
● M12.53 Traumatic arthropathy, wrist
    M12.531 Traumatic arthropathy, right wrist
    M12.532 Traumatic arthropathy, left wrist
    M12.539 Traumatic arthropathy, `unspecified` wrist
● M12.54 Traumatic arthropathy, hand
    M12.541 Traumatic arthropathy, right hand
    M12.542 Traumatic arthropathy, left hand
    M12.549 Traumatic arthropathy, `unspecified` hand
● M12.55 Traumatic arthropathy, hip
    M12.551 Traumatic arthropathy, right hip
    M12.552 Traumatic arthropathy, left hip
    M12.559 Traumatic arthropathy, `unspecified` hip
● M12.56 Traumatic arthropathy, knee
    M12.561 Traumatic arthropathy, right knee
    M12.562 Traumatic arthropathy, left knee
    M12.569 Traumatic arthropathy, `unspecified` knee
● M12.57 Traumatic arthropathy, ankle and foot
    M12.571 Traumatic arthropathy, right ankle and foot
    M12.572 Traumatic arthropathy, left ankle and foot
    M12.579 Traumatic arthropathy, `unspecified` ankle and foot
  M12.58 Traumatic arthropathy, other specified site ◀▦
    Traumatic arthropathy, vertebrae ◀
  M12.59 Traumatic arthropathy, multiple sites

◀ New   ◀▦ Revised   ~~deleted~~ Deleted   `Excludes 1`   `Excludes 2`   `Includes`   `Use additional`   `Code first`   `Code also`   `Unspecified`

   OGCR Official Guidelines   ● Unacceptable Principal Diagnosis   X Assign placeholder X   ● Use Additional Character(s)   ▌ Manifestation Code   **Coding Clinic**

● **M12.8 Other specific arthropathies, not elsewhere classified**
  Transient arthropathy
  M12.80 Other specific arthropathies, not elsewhere classified, unspecified site
● **M12.81** Other specific arthropathies, not elsewhere classified, shoulder
  M12.811 Other specific arthropathies, not elsewhere classified, right shoulder
  M12.812 Other specific arthropathies, not elsewhere classified, left shoulder
  M12.819 Other specific arthropathies, not elsewhere classified, unspecified shoulder
● **M12.82** Other specific arthropathies, not elsewhere classified, elbow
  M12.821 Other specific arthropathies, not elsewhere classified, right elbow
  M12.822 Other specific arthropathies, not elsewhere classified, left elbow
  M12.829 Other specific arthropathies, not elsewhere classified, unspecified elbow
● **M12.83** Other specific arthropathies, not elsewhere classified, wrist
  M12.831 Other specific arthropathies, not elsewhere classified, right wrist
  M12.832 Other specific arthropathies, not elsewhere classified, left wrist
  M12.839 Other specific arthropathies, not elsewhere classified, unspecified wrist
● **M12.84** Other specific arthropathies, not elsewhere classified, hand
  M12.841 Other specific arthropathies, not elsewhere classified, right hand
  M12.842 Other specific arthropathies, not elsewhere classified, left hand
  M12.849 Other specific arthropathies, not elsewhere classified, unspecified hand
● **M12.85** Other specific arthropathies, not elsewhere classified, hip
  M12.851 Other specific arthropathies, not elsewhere classified, right hip
  M12.852 Other specific arthropathies, not elsewhere classified, left hip
  M12.859 Other specific arthropathies, not elsewhere classified, unspecified hip
● **M12.86** Other specific arthropathies, not elsewhere classified, knee
  M12.861 Other specific arthropathies, not elsewhere classified, right knee
  M12.862 Other specific arthropathies, not elsewhere classified, left knee
  M12.869 Other specific arthropathies, not elsewhere classified, unspecified knee
● **M12.87** Other specific arthropathies, not elsewhere classified, ankle and foot
  M12.871 Other specific arthropathies, not elsewhere classified, right ankle and foot
  M12.872 Other specific arthropathies, not elsewhere classified, left ankle and foot
  M12.879 Other specific arthropathies, not elsewhere classified, unspecified ankle and foot
  M12.88 Other specific arthropathies, not elsewhere classified, other specified site ◀‖‖
    Other specific arthropathies, not elsewhere classified, vertebrae ◀
  M12.89 Other specific arthropathies, not elsewhere classified, multiple sites
M12.9 Arthropathy, unspecified

● **M13 Other arthritis**
  Excludes1 arthrosis (M15-M19)
    osteoarthritis (M15-M19)
  M13.0 Polyarthritis, unspecified
● **M13.1 Monoarthritis, not elsewhere classified**
  M13.10 Monoarthritis, not elsewhere classified, unspecified site
● **M13.11** Monoarthritis, not elsewhere classified, shoulder
  M13.111 Monoarthritis, not elsewhere classified, right shoulder
  M13.112 Monoarthritis, not elsewhere classified, left shoulder
  M13.119 Monoarthritis, not elsewhere classified, unspecified shoulder
● **M13.12** Monoarthritis, not elsewhere classified, elbow
  M13.121 Monoarthritis, not elsewhere classified, right elbow
  M13.122 Monoarthritis, not elsewhere classified, left elbow
  M13.129 Monoarthritis, not elsewhere classified, unspecified elbow
● **M13.13** Monoarthritis, not elsewhere classified, wrist
  M13.131 Monoarthritis, not elsewhere classified, right wrist
  M13.132 Monoarthritis, not elsewhere classified, left wrist
  M13.139 Monoarthritis, not elsewhere classified, unspecified wrist
● **M13.14** Monoarthritis, not elsewhere classified, hand
  M13.141 Monoarthritis, not elsewhere classified, right hand
  M13.142 Monoarthritis, not elsewhere classified, left hand
  M13.149 Monoarthritis, not elsewhere classified, unspecified hand
● **M13.15** Monoarthritis, not elsewhere classified, hip
  M13.151 Monoarthritis, not elsewhere classified, right hip
  M13.152 Monoarthritis, not elsewhere classified, left hip
  M13.159 Monoarthritis, not elsewhere classified, unspecified hip
● **M13.16** Monoarthritis, not elsewhere classified, knee
  M13.161 Monoarthritis, not elsewhere classified, right knee
  M13.162 Monoarthritis, not elsewhere classified, left knee
  M13.169 Monoarthritis, not elsewhere classified, unspecified knee
● **M13.17** Monoarthritis, not elsewhere classified, ankle and foot
  M13.171 Monoarthritis, not elsewhere classified, right ankle and foot
  M13.172 Monoarthritis, not elsewhere classified, left ankle and foot
  M13.179 Monoarthritis, not elsewhere classified, unspecified ankle and foot
● **M13.8 Other specified arthritis**
  Allergic arthritis
  Excludes1 osteoarthritis (M15-M19)
  M13.80 Other specified arthritis, unspecified site
● **M13.81** Other specified arthritis, shoulder
  M13.811 Other specified arthritis, right shoulder
  M13.812 Other specified arthritis, left shoulder
  M13.819 Other specified arthritis, unspecified shoulder

N Newborn Age: 0   **P** Pediatric Age: 0–17   **M** Maternity DX: 12–55   **A** Adult Age: 15–124   ♀ Females Only   ♂ Males Only

Complication\Comorbidity   Major C\C   (Ex) CC/MCC Exclusions   Present on Admission Requirement   Hospital-Acquired Condition

1095

CHAPTER 13 (M00-M99)

● M13.82   Other specified arthritis, elbow
    M13.821   Other specified arthritis, right elbow
    M13.822   Other specified arthritis, left elbow
    M13.829   Other specified arthritis, unspecified elbow

● M13.83   Other specified arthritis, wrist
    M13.831   Other specified arthritis, right wrist
    M13.832   Other specified arthritis, left wrist
    M13.839   Other specified arthritis, unspecified wrist

● M13.84   Other specified arthritis, hand
    M13.841   Other specified arthritis, right hand
    M13.842   Other specified arthritis, left hand
    M13.849   Other specified arthritis, unspecified hand

● M13.85   Other specified arthritis, hip
    M13.851   Other specified arthritis, right hip
    M13.852   Other specified arthritis, left hip
    M13.859   Other specified arthritis, unspecified hip

● M13.86   Other specified arthritis, knee
    M13.861   Other specified arthritis, right knee
    M13.862   Other specified arthritis, left knee
    M13.869   Other specified arthritis, unspecified knee

● M13.87   Other specified arthritis, ankle and foot
    M13.871   Other specified arthritis, right ankle and foot
    M13.872   Other specified arthritis, left ankle and foot
    M13.879   Other specified arthritis, unspecified ankle and foot

    M13.88   Other specified arthritis, other site
    M13.89   Other specified arthritis, multiple sites

● M14   **Arthropathies in other diseases classified elsewhere**
    Excludes1   arthropathy in:
      diabetes mellitus (E08-E13 with .61-) ◀▥
      hematological disorders (M36.2-M36.3)
      hypersensitivity reactions (M36.4)
      neoplastic disease (M36.1)
      neurosyphillis (A52.16)
      sarcoidosis (D86.86)
     enteropathic arthropathies (M07.0-)
     juvenile psoriatic arthropathy (L40.54)
     lipoid dermatoarthritis (E78.81)

● M14.6   **Charcôt's joint**
    Neuropathic arthropathy
    Excludes1   Charcôt's joint in diabetes mellitus (E08-E13 with .610) ◀▥
       Charcôt's joint in tabes dorsalis (A52.16)

    M14.60   Charcôt's joint, unspecified site
● M14.61   Charcôt's joint, shoulder
    M14.611   Charcôt's joint, right shoulder
    M14.612   Charcôt's joint, left shoulder
    M14.619   Charcôt's joint, unspecified shoulder

● M14.62   Charcôt's joint, elbow
    M14.621   Charcôt's joint, right elbow
    M14.622   Charcôt's joint, left elbow
    M14.629   Charcôt's joint, unspecified elbow

● M14.63   Charcôt's joint, wrist
    M14.631   Charcôt's joint, right wrist
    M14.632   Charcôt's joint, left wrist
    M14.639   Charcôt's joint, unspecified wrist

● M14.64   Charcôt's joint, hand
    M14.641   Charcôt's joint, right hand
    M14.642   Charcôt's joint, left hand
    M14.649   Charcôt's joint, unspecified hand

● M14.65   Charcôt's joint, hip
    M14.651   Charcôt's joint, right hip
    M14.652   Charcôt's joint, left hip
    M14.659   Charcôt's joint, unspecified hip

● M14.66   Charcôt's joint, knee
    M14.661   Charcôt's joint, right knee
    M14.662   Charcôt's joint, left knee
    M14.669   Charcôt's joint, unspecified knee

● M14.67   Charcôt's joint, ankle and foot
    M14.671   Charcôt's joint, right ankle and foot
    M14.672   Charcôt's joint, left ankle and foot
    M14.679   Charcôt's joint, unspecified ankle and foot

    M14.68   Charcôt's joint, vertebrae
    M14.69   Charcôt's joint, multiple sites

● M14.8   **Arthropathies in other specified diseases classified elsewhere**
    Code first underlying disease, such as:
     amyloidosis (E85.-) ◀▥
     erythema multiforme (L51.-)
     erythema nodosum (L52)
     hemochromatosis (E83.11-)
     hyperparathyroidism (E21.-)
     hypothyroidism (E00-E03)
     sickle-cell disorders (D57.-)
     thyrotoxicosis [hyperthyroidism] (E05.-)
     Whipple's disease (K90.81)

▷ *M14.80   Arthropathies in other specified diseases classified elsewhere, unspecified site*

● M14.81   Arthropathies in other specified diseases classified elsewhere, shoulder
    ▷ *M14.811   Arthropathies in other specified diseases classified elsewhere, right shoulder*
    ▷ *M14.812   Arthropathies in other specified diseases classified elsewhere, left shoulder*
    ▷ *M14.819   Arthropathies in other specified diseases classified elsewhere, unspecified shoulder*

● M14.82   Arthropathies in other specified diseases classified elsewhere, elbow
    ▷ *M14.821   Arthropathies in other specified diseases classified elsewhere, right elbow*
    ▷ *M14.822   Arthropathies in other specified diseases classified elsewhere, left elbow*
    ▷ *M14.829   Arthropathies in other specified diseases classified elsewhere, unspecified elbow*

● M14.83   Arthropathies in other specified diseases classified elsewhere, wrist
    ▷ *M14.831   Arthropathies in other specified diseases classified elsewhere, right wrist*
    ▷ *M14.832   Arthropathies in other specified diseases classified elsewhere, left wrist*
    ▷ *M14.839   Arthropathies in other specified diseases classified elsewhere, unspecified wrist*

◀ New   ◀▥ Revised   ~~deleted~~ Deleted   Excludes 1   Excludes 2   Includes   Use additional   Code first   Code also   Unspecified
OGCR Official Guidelines   ● Unacceptable Principal Diagnosis   X Assign placeholder X   ● Use Additional Character(s)   ▷ Manifestation Code   **Coding Clinic**

● **M14.84** Arthropathies in other specified diseases classified elsewhere, hand

▶ *M14.841* *Arthropathies in other specified diseases classified elsewhere, right hand*

▶ *M14.842* *Arthropathies in other specified diseases classified elsewhere, left hand*

▶ *M14.849* *Arthropathies in other specified diseases classified elsewhere, unspecified hand*

● **M14.85** Arthropathies in other specified diseases classified elsewhere, hip

▶ *M14.851* *Arthropathies in other specified diseases classified elsewhere, right hip*

▶ *M14.852* *Arthropathies in other specified diseases classified elsewhere, left hip*

▶ *M14.859* *Arthropathies in other specified diseases classified elsewhere, unspecified hip*

● **M14.86** Arthropathies in other specified diseases classified elsewhere, knee

▶ *M14.861* *Arthropathies in other specified diseases classified elsewhere, right knee*

▶ *M14.862* *Arthropathies in other specified diseases classified elsewhere, left knee*

▶ *M14.869* *Arthropathies in other specified diseases classified elsewhere, unspecified knee*

● **M14.87** Arthropathies in other specified diseases classified elsewhere, ankle and foot

▶ *M14.871* *Arthropathies in other specified diseases classified elsewhere, right ankle and foot*

▶ *M14.872* *Arthropathies in other specified diseases classified elsewhere, left ankle and foot*

▶ *M14.879* *Arthropathies in other specified diseases classified elsewhere, unspecified ankle and foot*

▶ *M14.88* *Arthropathies in other specified diseases classified elsewhere, vertebrae*

▶ *M14.89* *Arthropathies in other specified diseases classified elsewhere, multiple sites*

OSTEOARTHRITIS (M15-M19)

Osteoarthritis is the most common degenerative joint disease and form of arthritis that breaks down the cartilage causing pain, swelling, and reduced motion in the joints.

> **Excludes2**　osteoarthritis of spine (M47.-)

● **M15** Polyosteoarthritis

> **Includes**　arthritis of multiple sites
>
> **Excludes1**　bilateral involvement of single joint (M16-M19)

M15.0 Primary generalized (osteo)arthritis

M15.1 Heberden's nodes (with arthropathy)
Interphalangeal distal osteoarthritis

M15.2 Bouchard's nodes (with arthropathy)
Juxtaphalangeal distal osteoarthritis

M15.3 Secondary multiple arthritis
Post-traumatic polyosteoarthritis

M15.4 Erosive (osteo)arthritis

M15.8 Other polyosteoarthritis

M15.9 Polyosteoarthritis, unspecified
Generalized osteoarthritis NOS

● **M16** Osteoarthritis of hip

M16.0 Bilateral primary osteoarthritis of hip

● **M16.1** Unilateral primary osteoarthritis of hip
Primary osteoarthritis of hip NOS

M16.10 Unilateral primary osteoarthritis, unspecified hip

M16.11 Unilateral primary osteoarthritis, right hip

M16.12 Unilateral primary osteoarthritis, left hip

M16.2 Bilateral osteoarthritis resulting from hip dysplasia

● **M16.3** Unilateral osteoarthritis resulting from hip dysplasia
Dysplastic osteoarthritis of hip NOS

M16.30 Unilateral osteoarthritis resulting from hip dysplasia, unspecified hip

M16.31 Unilateral osteoarthritis resulting from hip dysplasia, right hip

M16.32 Unilateral osteoarthritis resulting from hip dysplasia, left hip

M16.4 Bilateral post-traumatic osteoarthritis of hip

● **M16.5** Unilateral post-traumatic osteoarthritis of hip
Post-traumatic osteoarthritis of hip NOS

M16.50 Unilateral post-traumatic osteoarthritis, unspecified hip

M16.51 Unilateral post-traumatic osteoarthritis, right hip

M16.52 Unilateral post-traumatic osteoarthritis, left hip

M16.6 Other bilateral secondary osteoarthritis of hip

M16.7 Other unilateral secondary osteoarthritis of hip
Secondary osteoarthritis of hip NOS

M16.9 Osteoarthritis of hip, unspecified

● **M17** Osteoarthritis of knee

M17.0 Bilateral primary osteoarthritis of knee

● **M17.1** Unilateral primary osteoarthritis of knee
Primary osteoarthritis of knee NOS

M17.10 Unilateral primary osteoarthritis, unspecified knee

M17.11 Unilateral primary osteoarthritis, right knee

M17.12 Unilateral primary osteoarthritis, left knee

M17.2 Bilateral post-traumatic osteoarthritis of knee

● **M17.3** Unilateral post-traumatic osteoarthritis of knee
Post-traumatic osteoarthritis of knee NOS

M17.30 Unilateral post-traumatic osteoarthritis, unspecified knee

M17.31 Unilateral post-traumatic osteoarthritis, right knee

M17.32 Unilateral post-traumatic osteoarthritis, left knee

M17.4 Other bilateral secondary osteoarthritis of knee

M17.5 Other unilateral secondary osteoarthritis of knee
Secondary osteoarthritis of knee NOS

M17.9 Osteoarthritis of knee, unspecified

● **M18** Osteoarthritis of first carpometacarpal joint

M18.0 Bilateral primary osteoarthritis of first carpometacarpal joints

● **M18.1** Unilateral primary osteoarthritis of first carpometacarpal joint
Primary osteoarthritis of first carpometacarpal joint NOS

M18.10 Unilateral primary osteoarthritis of first carpometacarpal joint, unspecified hand

M18.11 Unilateral primary osteoarthritis of first carpometacarpal joint, right hand

M18.12 Unilateral primary osteoarthritis of first carpometacarpal joint, left hand

M18.2 Bilateral post-traumatic osteoarthritis of first carpometacarpal joints

CHAPTER 13 (M00-M99)

N Newborn Age: 0　　**P** Pediatric Age: 0–17　　**M** Maternity DX: 12–55　　**A** Adult Age: 15–124　　♀ Females Only　　♂ Males Only

Complication\Comorbidity　　Major C\C　　(Ex) CC/MCC Exclusions　　Present on Admission Requirement　　Hospital-Acquired Condition

1097

● M18.3   Unilateral post-traumatic osteoarthritis of first carpometacarpal joint
     Post-traumatic osteoarthritis of first carpometacarpal joint NOS

   M18.30   Unilateral post-traumatic osteoarthritis of first carpometacarpal joint, unspecified hand

   M18.31   Unilateral post-traumatic osteoarthritis of first carpometacarpal joint, right hand

   M18.32   Unilateral post-traumatic osteoarthritis of first carpometacarpal joint, left hand

  M18.4   Other bilateral secondary osteoarthritis of first carpometacarpal joints

● M18.5   Other unilateral secondary osteoarthritis of first carpometacarpal joint
     Secondary osteoarthritis of first carpometacarpal joint NOS

   M18.50   Other unilateral secondary osteoarthritis of first carpometacarpal joint, unspecified hand

   M18.51   Other unilateral secondary osteoarthritis of first carpometacarpal joint, right hand

   M18.52   Other unilateral secondary osteoarthritis of first carpometacarpal joint, left hand

  M18.9   Osteoarthritis of first carpometacarpal joint, unspecified

● M19   Other and unspecified osteoarthritis

   Excludes1   polyarthritis (M15.-)

   Excludes2   arthrosis of spine (M47.-)
           hallux rigidus (M20.2)
           osteoarthritis of spine (M47.-)

● M19.0   Primary osteoarthritis of other joints

   ● M19.01   Primary osteoarthritis, shoulder

     M19.011   Primary osteoarthritis, right shoulder
     M19.012   Primary osteoarthritis, left shoulder
     M19.019   Primary osteoarthritis, unspecified shoulder

   ● M19.02   Primary osteoarthritis, elbow

     M19.021   Primary osteoarthritis, right elbow
     M19.022   Primary osteoarthritis, left elbow
     M19.029   Primary osteoarthritis, unspecified elbow

   ● M19.03   Primary osteoarthritis, wrist

     M19.031   Primary osteoarthritis, right wrist
     M19.032   Primary osteoarthritis, left wrist
     M19.039   Primary osteoarthritis, unspecified wrist

   ● M19.04   Primary osteoarthritis, hand

     Excludes2   primary osteoarthritis of first carpometacarpal joint (M18.0-, M18.1-)

     M19.041   Primary osteoarthritis, right hand
     M19.042   Primary osteoarthritis, left hand
     M19.049   Primary osteoarthritis, unspecified hand

   ● M19.07   Primary osteoarthritis ankle and foot

     M19.071   Primary osteoarthritis, right ankle and foot
     M19.072   Primary osteoarthritis, left ankle and foot
     M19.079   Primary osteoarthritis, unspecified ankle and foot

● M19.1   Post-traumatic osteoarthritis of other joints

   ● M19.11   Post-traumatic osteoarthritis, shoulder

     M19.111   Post-traumatic osteoarthritis, right shoulder
     M19.112   Post-traumatic osteoarthritis, left shoulder
     M19.119   Post-traumatic osteoarthritis, unspecified shoulder

   ● M19.12   Post-traumatic osteoarthritis, elbow

     M19.121   Post-traumatic osteoarthritis, right elbow
     M19.122   Post-traumatic osteoarthritis, left elbow
     M19.129   Post-traumatic osteoarthritis, unspecified elbow

   ● M19.13   Post-traumatic osteoarthritis, wrist

     M19.131   Post-traumatic osteoarthritis, right wrist
     M19.132   Post-traumatic osteoarthritis, left wrist
     M19.139   Post-traumatic osteoarthritis, unspecified wrist

   ● M19.14   Post-traumatic osteoarthritis, hand

     Excludes2   post-traumatic osteoarthritis of first carpometacarpal joint (M18.2-, M18.3-)

     M19.141   Post-traumatic osteoarthritis, right hand
     M19.142   Post-traumatic osteoarthritis, left hand
     M19.149   Post-traumatic osteoarthritis, unspecified hand

   ● M19.17   Post-traumatic osteoarthritis, ankle and foot

     M19.171   Post-traumatic osteoarthritis, right ankle and foot
     M19.172   Post-traumatic osteoarthritis, left ankle and foot
     M19.179   Post-traumatic osteoarthritis, unspecified ankle and foot

● M19.2   Secondary osteoarthritis of other joints

   ● M19.21   Secondary osteoarthritis, shoulder

     M19.211   Secondary osteoarthritis, right shoulder
     M19.212   Secondary osteoarthritis, left shoulder
     M19.219   Secondary osteoarthritis, unspecified shoulder

   ● M19.22   Secondary osteoarthritis, elbow

     M19.221   Secondary osteoarthritis, right elbow
     M19.222   Secondary osteoarthritis, left elbow
     M19.229   Secondary osteoarthritis, unspecified elbow

   ● M19.23   Secondary osteoarthritis, wrist

     M19.231   Secondary osteoarthritis, right wrist
     M19.232   Secondary osteoarthritis, left wrist
     M19.239   Secondary osteoarthritis, unspecified wrist

   ● M19.24   Secondary osteoarthritis, hand

     M19.241   Secondary osteoarthritis, right hand
     M19.242   Secondary osteoarthritis, left hand
     M19.249   Secondary osteoarthritis, unspecified hand

   ● M19.27   Secondary osteoarthritis, ankle and foot

     M19.271   Secondary osteoarthritis, right ankle and foot
     M19.272   Secondary osteoarthritis, left ankle and foot
     M19.279   Secondary osteoarthritis, unspecified ankle and foot

◀ New   ◀ Revised   ~~deleted~~ Deleted   Excludes 1   Excludes 2   Includes   Use additional   Code first   Code also   Unspecified

OGCR Official Guidelines   ● Unacceptable Principal Diagnosis   X Assign placeholder X   ● Use Additional Character(s)   ▶ Manifestation Code   **Coding Clinic**

● M19.9 **Osteoarthritis, unspecified site**
     M19.90   **Unspecified osteoarthritis, unspecified site**
           Arthrosis NOS
           Arthritis NOS
           Osteoarthritis NOS
     M19.91   **Primary osteoarthritis, unspecified site**
           Primary osteoarthritis NOS
     M19.92   **Post-traumatic osteoarthritis, unspecified site**
           Post-traumatic osteoarthritis NOS
     M19.93   **Secondary osteoarthritis, unspecified site**
           Secondary osteoarthritis NOS

OTHER JOINT DISORDERS (M20-M25)

     Excludes2   joints of the spine (M40-M54)

● M20   **Acquired deformities of fingers and toes**
     Excludes1   acquired absence of fingers and toes (Z89.-)
           congenital absence of fingers and toes (Q71.3-,
             Q72.3-)
           congenital deformities and malformations of
             fingers and toes (Q66.-, Q68-Q70, Q74.-)
   ● M20.0   **Deformity of finger(s)**
         Excludes1   clubbing of fingers (R68.3)
                palmar fascial fibromatosis [Dupuytren]
                  (M72.0)
                trigger finger (M65.3)
     ● M20.00   **Unspecified deformity of finger(s)**
         M20.001   **Unspecified deformity of right
                 finger(s)**
         M20.002   **Unspecified deformity of left finger(s)**
         M20.009   **Unspecified deformity of unspecified
                 finger(s)**
     ● M20.01   **Mallet finger**
         M20.011   **Mallet finger of right finger(s)**
         M20.012   **Mallet finger of left finger(s)**
         M20.019   **Mallet finger of unspecified finger(s)**
     ● M20.02   **Boutonnière deformity**
         M20.021   **Boutonnière deformity of right
                 finger(s)**
         M20.022   **Boutonnière deformity of left
                 finger(s)**
         M20.029   **Boutonnière deformity of unspecified
                 finger(s)**
     ● M20.03   **Swan-neck deformity**
         M20.031   **Swan-neck deformity of right
                 finger(s)**
         M20.032   **Swan-neck deformity of left finger(s)**
         M20.039   **Swan-neck deformity of unspecified
                 finger(s)**
     ● M20.09   **Other deformity of finger(s)**
         M20.091   **Other deformity of right finger(s)**
         M20.092   **Other deformity of left finger(s)**
         M20.099   **Other deformity of finger(s),
                 unspecified finger(s)**
   ● M20.1   **Hallux valgus (acquired)**
         Bunion
     M20.10   **Hallux valgus (acquired), unspecified foot**
     M20.11   **Hallux valgus (acquired), right foot**
     M20.12   **Hallux valgus (acquired), left foot**
   ● M20.2   **Hallux rigidus**
     M20.20   **Hallux rigidus, unspecified foot**
     M20.21   **Hallux rigidus, right foot**
     M20.22   **Hallux rigidus, left foot**
   ● M20.3   **Hallux varus (acquired)**
     M20.30   **Hallux varus (acquired), unspecified foot**
     M20.31   **Hallux varus (acquired), right foot**
     M20.32   **Hallux varus (acquired), left foot**

Figure 13-1   Hallux valgus or bunion.

Item 13-2   Hallux valgus or bunion is a sometimes painful structural deformity caused by an inflammation of the bursal sac at the base of the metatarsophalangeal joint (big toe). **Hallus varus** is a deviation of the great toe to the inner side of the foot or away from the next toe.

Item 13-3   Cubitus valgus is a deformity of the elbow resulting in an increased carrying angle in which the arm extends at the side and the palm faces forward, which results in the forearm and hand extended at a greater than 15 degrees.

   ● M20.4   **Other hammer toe(s) (acquired)**
     M20.40   **Other hammer toe(s) (acquired), unspecified
                foot**
     M20.41   **Other hammer toe(s) (acquired), right foot**
     M20.42   **Other hammer toe(s) (acquired), left foot**
   ● M20.5   **Other deformities of toe(s) (acquired)**
     ● M20.5X   **Other deformities of toe(s) (acquired)**
         M20.5X1   **Other deformities of toe(s) (acquired),
                 right foot**
         M20.5X2   **Other deformities of toe(s) (acquired),
                 left foot**
         M20.5X9   **Other deformities of toe(s) (acquired),
                 unspecified foot**
   ● M20.6   **Acquired deformities of toe(s), unspecified**
     M20.60   **Acquired deformities of toe(s), unspecified,
                unspecified foot**
     M20.61   **Acquired deformities of toe(s), unspecified,
                right foot**
     M20.62   **Acquired deformities of toe(s), unspecified, left
                foot**

● M21   **Other acquired deformities of limbs**
     Excludes1   acquired absence of limb (Z89.-)
           congenital absence of limbs (Q71-Q73)
           congenital deformities and malformations of
             limbs (Q65-Q66, Q68-Q74)
     Excludes2   acquired deformities of fingers or toes (M20.-)
           coxa plana (M91.2)
   ● M21.0   **Valgus deformity, not elsewhere classified**
         Excludes1   metatarsus valgus (Q66.6)
                talipes calcaneovalgus (Q66.4)
     M21.00   **Valgus deformity, not elsewhere classified,
                unspecified site**
     ● M21.02   **Valgus deformity, not elsewhere classified,
                elbow**
           Cubitus valgus
         M21.021   **Valgus deformity, not elsewhere
                 classified, right elbow**
         M21.022   **Valgus deformity, not elsewhere
                 classified, left elbow**
         M21.029   **Valgus deformity, not elsewhere
                 classified, unspecified elbow**

CHAPTER 13 (M00-M99)

Item 13–4 Cubitus varus is a deformity of the elbow resulting in the arm extended at the side and the palm facing forward so that the forearm and hand are held at less than 5 degrees, decreasing the carrying angle.

● M21.05 Valgus deformity, not elsewhere classified, hip
    M21.051 Valgus deformity, not elsewhere classified, right hip
    M21.052 Valgus deformity, not elsewhere classified, left hip
    M21.059 Valgus deformity, not elsewhere classified, unspecified hip

● M21.06 Valgus deformity, not elsewhere classified, knee
    Genu valgum
    Knock knee
    M21.061 Valgus deformity, not elsewhere classified, right knee
    M21.062 Valgus deformity, not elsewhere classified, left knee
    M21.069 Valgus deformity, not elsewhere classified, unspecified knee

● M21.07 Valgus deformity, not elsewhere classified, ankle
    M21.071 Valgus deformity, not elsewhere classified, right ankle
    M21.072 Valgus deformity, not elsewhere classified, left ankle
    M21.079 Valgus deformity, not elsewhere classified, unspecified ankle

● M21.1 Varus deformity, not elsewhere classified
    Excludes1 metatarsus varus (Q66.2)
             tibia vara (M92.5)

    M21.10 Varus deformity, not elsewhere classified, unspecified site

● M21.12 Varus deformity, not elsewhere classified, elbow
    Cubitus varus, elbow
    M21.121 Varus deformity, not elsewhere classified, right elbow
    M21.122 Varus deformity, not elsewhere classified, left elbow
    M21.129 Varus deformity, not elsewhere classified, unspecified elbow

● M21.15 Varus deformity, not elsewhere classified, hip
    M21.151 Varus deformity, not elsewhere classified, right hip
    M21.152 Varus deformity, not elsewhere classified, left hip
    M21.159 Varus deformity, not elsewhere classified, unspecified

● M21.16 Varus deformity, not elsewhere classified, knee
    Bow leg
    Genu varum
    M21.161 Varus deformity, not elsewhere classified, right knee
    M21.162 Varus deformity, not elsewhere classified, left knee
    M21.169 Varus deformity, not elsewhere classified, unspecified knee

● M21.17 Varus deformity, not elsewhere classified, ankle
    M21.171 Varus deformity, not elsewhere classified, right ankle
    M21.172 Varus deformity, not elsewhere classified, left ankle
    M21.179 Varus deformity, not elsewhere classified, unspecified ankle

● M21.2 Flexion deformity
    M21.20 Flexion deformity, unspecified site

● M21.21 Flexion deformity, shoulder
    M21.211 Flexion deformity, right shoulder
    M21.212 Flexion deformity, left shoulder
    M21.219 Flexion deformity, unspecified shoulder

● M21.22 Flexion deformity, elbow
    M21.221 Flexion deformity, right elbow
    M21.222 Flexion deformity, left elbow
    M21.229 Flexion deformity, unspecified elbow

● M21.23 Flexion deformity, wrist
    M21.231 Flexion deformity, right wrist
    M21.232 Flexion deformity, left wrist
    M21.239 Flexion deformity, unspecified wrist

● M21.24 Flexion deformity, finger joints
    M21.241 Flexion deformity, right finger joints
    M21.242 Flexion deformity, left finger joints
    M21.249 Flexion deformity, unspecified finger joints

● M21.25 Flexion deformity, hip
    M21.251 Flexion deformity, right hip
    M21.252 Flexion deformity, left hip
    M21.259 Flexion deformity, unspecified hip

● M21.26 Flexion deformity, knee
    M21.261 Flexion deformity, right knee
    M21.262 Flexion deformity, left knee
    M21.269 Flexion deformity, unspecified knee

● M21.27 Flexion deformity, ankle and toes
    M21.271 Flexion deformity, right ankle and toes
    M21.272 Flexion deformity, left ankle and toes
    M21.279 Flexion deformity, unspecified ankle and toes

● M21.3 Wrist or foot drop (acquired)
● M21.33 Wrist drop (acquired)
    M21.331 Wrist drop, right wrist
    M21.332 Wrist drop, left wrist
    M21.339 Wrist drop, unspecified wrist

● M21.37 Foot drop (acquired)
    M21.371 Foot drop, right foot
    M21.372 Foot drop, left foot
    M21.379 Foot drop, unspecified foot

● M21.4 Flat foot [pes planus] (acquired)
    Excludes1 congenital pes planus (Q66.5-)
    M21.40 Flat foot [pes planus] (acquired), unspecified foot
    M21.41 Flat foot [pes planus] (acquired), right foot
    M21.42 Flat foot [pes planus] (acquired), left foot

● M21.5 Acquired clawhand, clubhand, clawfoot and clubfoot
    Excludes1 clubfoot, not specified as acquired (Q66.89)

● M21.51 Acquired clawhand
    M21.511 Acquired clawhand, right hand
    M21.512 Acquired clawhand, left hand
    M21.519 Acquired clawhand, unspecified hand

● M21.52 Acquired clubhand
    M21.521 Acquired clubhand, right hand
    M21.522 Acquired clubhand, left hand
    M21.529 Acquired clubhand, unspecified hand

● M21.53 Acquired clawfoot
    M21.531 Acquired clawfoot, right foot
    M21.532 Acquired clawfoot, left foot
    M21.539 Acquired clawfoot, unspecified foot

◀ New   ◀ⁿⁿⁿ Revised   ~~deleted~~ Deleted   Excludes 1   Excludes 2   Includes   Use additional   Code first   Code also   Unspecified

OGCR Official Guidelines   ● Unacceptable Principal Diagnosis   X Assign placeholder X   ● Use Additional Character(s)   ▌ Manifestation Code   **Coding Clinic**

● M21.54　Acquired clubfoot
　　　　M21.541　Acquired clubfoot, right foot
　　　　M21.542　Acquired clubfoot, left foot
　　　　M21.549　Acquired clubfoot, unspecified foot
● M21.6　Other acquired deformities of foot
　　　Excludes2　deformities of toe (acquired)
　　　　　　　　(M20.1-M20.6) ◄
　　● M21.6X　Other acquired deformities of foot
　　　　M21.6X1　Other acquired deformities of right foot
　　　　M21.6X2　Other acquired deformities of left foot
　　　　M21.6X9　Other acquired deformities of unspecified foot
● M21.7　Unequal limb length (acquired)
　　　Note: The site used should correspond to the shorter limb.
　　　M21.70　Unequal limb length (acquired), unspecified site
　　● M21.72　Unequal limb length (acquired), humerus
　　　　M21.721　Unequal limb length (acquired), right humerus
　　　　M21.722　Unequal limb length (acquired), left humerus
　　　　M21.729　Unequal limb length (acquired), unspecified humerus
　　● M21.73　Unequal limb length (acquired), ulna and radius
　　　　M21.731　Unequal limb length (acquired), right ulna
　　　　M21.732　Unequal limb length (acquired), left ulna
　　　　M21.733　Unequal limb length (acquired), right radius
　　　　M21.734　Unequal limb length (acquired), left radius
　　　　M21.739　Unequal limb length (acquired), unspecified ulna and radius
　　● M21.75　Unequal limb length (acquired), femur
　　　　M21.751　Unequal limb length (acquired), right femur
　　　　M21.752　Unequal limb length (acquired), left femur
　　　　M21.759　Unequal limb length (acquired), unspecified femur
　　● M21.76　Unequal limb length (acquired), tibia and fibula
　　　　M21.761　Unequal limb length (acquired), right tibia
　　　　M21.762　Unequal limb length (acquired), left tibia
　　　　M21.763　Unequal limb length (acquired), right fibula
　　　　M21.764　Unequal limb length (acquired), left fibula
　　　　M21.769　Unequal limb length (acquired), unspecified tibia and fibula
● M21.8　Other specified acquired deformities of limbs
　　　Excludes2　coxa plana (M91.2)
　　　M21.80　Other specified acquired deformities of unspecified limb
　　● M21.82　Other specified acquired deformities of upper arm
　　　　M21.821　Other specified acquired deformities of right upper arm
　　　　M21.822　Other specified acquired deformities of left upper arm
　　　　M21.829　Other specified acquired deformities of unspecified upper arm

● M21.83　Other specified acquired deformities of forearm
　　　　M21.831　Other specified acquired deformities of right forearm
　　　　M21.832　Other specified acquired deformities of left forearm
　　　　M21.839　Other specified acquired deformities of unspecified forearm
● M21.85　Other specified acquired deformities of thigh
　　　　M21.851　Other specified acquired deformities of right thigh
　　　　M21.852　Other specified acquired deformities of left thigh
　　　　M21.859　Other specified acquired deformities of unspecified thigh
● M21.86　Other specified acquired deformities of lower leg
　　　　M21.861　Other specified acquired deformities of right lower leg
　　　　M21.862　Other specified acquired deformities of left lower leg
　　　　M21.869　Other specified acquired deformities of unspecified lower leg
● M21.9　Unspecified acquired deformity of limb and hand
　　　M21.90　Unspecified acquired deformity of unspecified limb
　　● M21.92　Unspecified acquired deformity of upper arm
　　　　M21.921　Unspecified acquired deformity of right upper arm
　　　　M21.922　Unspecified acquired deformity of left upper arm
　　　　M21.929　Unspecified acquired deformity of unspecified upper arm
　　● M21.93　Unspecified acquired deformity of forearm
　　　　M21.931　Unspecified acquired deformity of right forearm
　　　　M21.932　Unspecified acquired deformity of left forearm
　　　　M21.939　Unspecified acquired deformity of unspecified forearm
　　● M21.94　Unspecified acquired deformity of hand
　　　　M21.941　Unspecified acquired deformity of hand, right hand
　　　　M21.942　Unspecified acquired deformity of hand, left hand
　　　　M21.949　Unspecified acquired deformity of hand, unspecified hand
　　● M21.95　Unspecified acquired deformity of thigh
　　　　M21.951　Unspecified acquired deformity of right thigh
　　　　M21.952　Unspecified acquired deformity of left thigh
　　　　M21.959　Unspecified acquired deformity of unspecified thigh
　　● M21.96　Unspecified acquired deformity of lower leg
　　　　M21.961　Unspecified acquired deformity of right lower leg
　　　　M21.962　Unspecified acquired deformity of left lower leg
　　　　M21.969　Unspecified acquired deformity of unspecified lower leg

● M22　Disorder of patella
　　　Excludes1　traumatic dislocation of patella (S83.0-)
　　● M22.0　Recurrent dislocation of patella
　　　　M22.00　Recurrent dislocation of patella, unspecified knee
　　　　M22.01　Recurrent dislocation of patella, right knee
　　　　M22.02　Recurrent dislocation of patella, left knee

CHAPTER 13 (M00-M99)

N Newborn Age: 0　　**P** Pediatric Age: 0–17　　**M** Maternity DX: 12–55　　**A** Adult Age: 15–124　　♀ Females Only　　♂ Males Only

Complication\Comorbidity　　Major C\C　　(Ex) CC/MCC Exclusions　　Present on Admission Requirement　　Hospital-Acquired Condition　　**1101**

CHAPTER 13 (M00-M99)

● M22.1 **Recurrent subluxation of patella**
  Incomplete dislocation of patella
  M22.10   Recurrent subluxation of patella, unspecified knee
  M22.11   Recurrent subluxation of patella, right knee
  M22.12   Recurrent subluxation of patella, left knee
● M22.2 **Patellofemoral disorders**
  ● M22.2X **Patellofemoral disorders**
    M22.2X1   Patellofemoral disorders, right knee
    M22.2X2   Patellofemoral disorders, left knee
    M22.2X9   Patellofemoral disorders, unspecified knee
● M22.3 **Other derangements of patella**
  ● M22.3X **Other derangements of patella**
    M22.3X1   Other derangements of patella, right knee
    M22.3X2   Other derangements of patella, left knee
    M22.3X9   Other derangements of patella, unspecified knee
● M22.4 **Chondromalacia patellae**
    M22.40   Chondromalacia patellae, unspecified knee
    M22.41   Chondromalacia patellae, right knee
    M22.42   Chondromalacia patellae, left knee
● M22.8 **Other disorders of patella**
  ● M22.8X **Other disorders of patella**
    M22.8X1   Other disorders of patella, right knee
    M22.8X2   Other disorders of patella, left knee
    M22.8X9   Other disorders of patella, unspecified knee
● M22.9 **Unspecified disorder of patella**
    M22.90   Unspecified disorder of patella, unspecified knee
    M22.91   Unspecified disorder of patella, right knee
    M22.92   Unspecified disorder of patella, left knee

● M23 **Internal derangement of knee**
  Excludes1   ankylosis (M24.66)
                current injury - see injury of knee and lower leg (S80-S89)
                deformity of knee (M21.-)
                osteochondritis dissecans (M93.2)
                recurrent dislocation or subluxation of joints (M24.4)
                recurrent dislocation or subluxation of patella (M22.0-M22.1)

● M23.0 **Cystic meniscus**
  ● M23.00 **Cystic meniscus, unspecified meniscus**
    Cystic meniscus, unspecified lateral meniscus
    Cystic meniscus, unspecified medial meniscus
    M23.000   Cystic meniscus, unspecified lateral meniscus, right knee
    M23.001   Cystic meniscus, unspecified lateral meniscus, left knee
    M23.002   Cystic meniscus, unspecified lateral meniscus, unspecified knee
    M23.003   Cystic meniscus, unspecified medial meniscus, right knee
    M23.004   Cystic meniscus, unspecified medial meniscus, left knee
    M23.005   Cystic meniscus, unspecified medial meniscus, unspecified knee
    M23.006   Cystic meniscus, unspecified meniscus, right knee
    M23.007   Cystic meniscus, unspecified meniscus, left knee
    M23.009   Cystic meniscus, unspecified meniscus, unspecified knee

● M23.01 **Cystic meniscus, anterior horn of medial meniscus**
    M23.011   Cystic meniscus, anterior horn of medial meniscus, right knee
    M23.012   Cystic meniscus, anterior horn of medial meniscus, left knee
    M23.019   Cystic meniscus, anterior horn of medial meniscus, unspecified knee
● M23.02 **Cystic meniscus, posterior horn of medial meniscus**
    M23.021   Cystic meniscus, posterior horn of medial meniscus, right knee
    M23.022   Cystic meniscus, posterior horn of medial meniscus, left knee
    M23.029   Cystic meniscus, posterior horn of medial meniscus, unspecified knee
● M23.03 **Cystic meniscus, other medial meniscus**
    M23.031   Cystic meniscus, other medial meniscus, right knee
    M23.032   Cystic meniscus, other medial meniscus, left knee
    M23.039   Cystic meniscus, other medial meniscus, unspecified knee
● M23.04 **Cystic meniscus, anterior horn of lateral meniscus**
    M23.041   Cystic meniscus, anterior horn of lateral meniscus, right knee
    M23.042   Cystic meniscus, anterior horn of lateral meniscus, left knee
    M23.049   Cystic meniscus, anterior horn of lateral meniscus, unspecified knee
● M23.05 **Cystic meniscus, posterior horn of lateral meniscus**
    M23.051   Cystic meniscus, posterior horn of lateral meniscus, right knee
    M23.052   Cystic meniscus, posterior horn of lateral meniscus, left knee
    M23.059   Cystic meniscus, posterior horn of lateral meniscus, unspecified knee
● M23.06 **Cystic meniscus, other lateral meniscus**
    M23.061   Cystic meniscus, other lateral meniscus, right knee
    M23.062   Cystic meniscus, other lateral meniscus, left knee
    M23.069   Cystic meniscus, other lateral meniscus, unspecified knee

(See Plate 509 on page 79.)

● M23.2 **Derangement of meniscus due to old tear or injury**
  Old bucket-handle tear
  ● M23.20 **Derangement of unspecified meniscus due to old tear or injury**
    Derangement of unspecified lateral meniscus due to old tear or injury
    Derangement of unspecified medial meniscus due to old tear or injury
    M23.200   Derangement of unspecified lateral meniscus due to old tear or injury, right knee
    M23.201   Derangement of unspecified lateral meniscus due to old tear or injury, left knee
    M23.202   Derangement of unspecified lateral meniscus due to old tear or injury, unspecified knee
    M23.203   Derangement of unspecified medial meniscus due to old tear or injury, right knee

◀ New   ◀▥ Revised   ~~deleted~~ Deleted   Excludes 1   Excludes 2   Includes   Use additional   Code first   Code also   Unspecified
OGCR Official Guidelines   ● Unacceptable Principal Diagnosis   X Assign placeholder X   ● Use Additional Character(s)   ▌ Manifestation Code   **Coding Clinic**

M23.204　Derangement of unspecified medial meniscus due to old tear or injury, left knee

M23.205　Derangement of unspecified medial meniscus due to old tear or injury, unspecified knee

M23.206　Derangement of unspecified meniscus due to old tear or injury, right knee

M23.207　Derangement of unspecified meniscus due to old tear or injury, left knee

M23.209　Derangement of unspecified meniscus due to old tear or injury, unspecified knee

● M23.21　Derangement of anterior horn of medial meniscus due to old tear or injury

　　M23.211　Derangement of anterior horn of medial meniscus due to old tear or injury, right knee

　　M23.212　Derangement of anterior horn of medial meniscus due to old tear or injury, left knee

　　M23.219　Derangement of anterior horn of medial meniscus due to old tear or injury, unspecified knee

● M23.22　Derangement of posterior horn of medial meniscus due to old tear or injury

　　M23.221　Derangement of posterior horn of medial meniscus due to old tear or injury, right knee

　　M23.222　Derangement of posterior horn of medial meniscus due to old tear or injury, left knee

　　M23.229　Derangement of posterior horn of medial meniscus due to old tear or injury, unspecified knee

● M23.23　Derangement of other medial meniscus due to old tear or injury

　　M23.231　Derangement of other medial meniscus due to old tear or injury, right knee

　　M23.232　Derangement of other medial meniscus due to old tear or injury, left knee

　　M23.239　Derangement of other medial meniscus due to old tear or injury, unspecified knee

● M23.24　Derangement of anterior horn of lateral meniscus due to old tear or injury

　　M23.241　Derangement of anterior horn of lateral meniscus due to old tear or injury, right knee

　　M23.242　Derangement of anterior horn of lateral meniscus due to old tear or injury, left knee

　　M23.249　Derangement of anterior horn of lateral meniscus due to old tear or injury, unspecified knee

● M23.25　Derangement of posterior horn of lateral meniscus due to old tear or injury

　　M23.251　Derangement of posterior horn of lateral meniscus due to old tear or injury, right knee

　　M23.252　Derangement of posterior horn of lateral meniscus due to old tear or injury, left knee

　　M23.259　Derangement of posterior horn of lateral meniscus due to old tear or injury, unspecified knee

● M23.26　Derangement of other lateral meniscus due to old tear or injury

　　M23.261　Derangement of other lateral meniscus due to old tear or injury, right knee

　　M23.262　Derangement of other lateral meniscus due to old tear or injury, left knee

　　M23.269　Derangement of other lateral meniscus due to old tear or injury, unspecified knee

● M23.3　Other meniscus derangements
　　Degenerate meniscus
　　Detached meniscus
　　Retained meniscus

● M23.30　Other meniscus derangements, unspecified meniscus
　　Other meniscus derangements, unspecified lateral meniscus
　　Other meniscus derangements, unspecified medial meniscus

　　M23.300　Other meniscus derangements, unspecified lateral meniscus, right knee

　　M23.301　Other meniscus derangements, unspecified lateral meniscus, left knee

　　M23.302　Other meniscus derangements, unspecified lateral meniscus, unspecified knee

　　M23.303　Other meniscus derangements, unspecified medial meniscus, right knee

　　M23.304　Other meniscus derangements, unspecified medial meniscus, left knee

　　M23.305　Other meniscus derangements, unspecified medial meniscus, unspecified knee

　　M23.306　Other meniscus derangements, unspecified meniscus, right knee

　　M23.307　Other meniscus derangements, unspecified meniscus, left knee

　　M23.309　Other meniscus derangements, unspecified meniscus, unspecified knee

● M23.31　Other meniscus derangements, anterior horn of medial meniscus

　　M23.311　Other meniscus derangements, anterior horn of medial meniscus, right knee

　　M23.312　Other meniscus derangements, anterior horn of medial meniscus, left knee

　　M23.319　Other meniscus derangements, anterior horn of medial meniscus, unspecified knee

● M23.32　Other meniscus derangements, posterior horn of medial meniscus

　　M23.321　Other meniscus derangements, posterior horn of medial meniscus, right knee

　　M23.322　Other meniscus derangements, posterior horn of medial meniscus, left knee

　　M23.329　Other meniscus derangements, posterior horn of medial meniscus, unspecified knee

N Newborn Age: 0　　**P** Pediatric Age: 0–17　　**M** Maternity DX: 12–55　　**A** Adult Age: 15–124　　♀ Females Only　　♂ Males Only

🔗 Complication\Comorbidity　　🔗 Major C\C　　(Ex) CC/MCC Exclusions　　🔗 Present on Admission Requirement　　🔗 Hospital-Acquired Condition

1103

CHAPTER 13 (M00-M99)

● M23.33 Other meniscus derangements, other medial meniscus
   M23.331 Other meniscus derangements, other medial meniscus, right knee
   M23.332 Other meniscus derangements, other medial meniscus, left knee
   M23.339 Other meniscus derangements, other medial meniscus, unspecified knee
● M23.34 Other meniscus derangements, anterior horn of lateral meniscus
   M23.341 Other meniscus derangements, anterior horn of lateral meniscus, right knee
   M23.342 Other meniscus derangements, anterior horn of lateral meniscus, left knee
   M23.349 Other meniscus derangements, anterior horn of lateral meniscus, unspecified knee
● M23.35 Other meniscus derangements, posterior horn of lateral meniscus
   M23.351 Other meniscus derangements, posterior horn of lateral meniscus, right knee
   M23.352 Other meniscus derangements, posterior horn of lateral meniscus, left knee
   M23.359 Other meniscus derangements, posterior horn of lateral meniscus, unspecified knee
● M23.36 Other meniscus derangements, other lateral meniscus
   M23.361 Other meniscus derangements, other lateral meniscus, right knee
   M23.362 Other meniscus derangements, other lateral meniscus, left knee
   M23.369 Other meniscus derangements, other lateral meniscus, unspecified knee
● M23.4 Loose body in knee
   M23.40 Loose body in knee, unspecified knee
   M23.41 Loose body in knee, right knee
   M23.42 Loose body in knee, left knee
● M23.5 Chronic instability of knee
   M23.50 Chronic instability of knee, unspecified knee
   M23.51 Chronic instability of knee, right knee
   M23.52 Chronic instability of knee, left knee
● M23.6 Other spontaneous disruption of ligament(s) of knee
● M23.60 Other spontaneous disruption of unspecified ligament of knee
   M23.601 Other spontaneous disruption of unspecified ligament of right knee
   M23.602 Other spontaneous disruption of unspecified ligament of left knee
   M23.609 Other spontaneous disruption of unspecified ligament of unspecified knee
● M23.61 Other spontaneous disruption of anterior cruciate ligament of knee
   M23.611 Other spontaneous disruption of anterior cruciate ligament of right knee
   M23.612 Other spontaneous disruption of anterior cruciate ligament of left knee
   M23.619 Other spontaneous disruption of anterior cruciate ligament of unspecified knee

Figure 13-2 Collateral and cruciate ligament of knee. (From DeLee: DeLee and Drez's Orthopaedic Sports Medicine, ed 3, Saunders, 2009)

● M23.62 Other spontaneous disruption of posterior cruciate ligament of knee
   M23.621 Other spontaneous disruption of posterior cruciate ligament of right knee
   M23.622 Other spontaneous disruption of posterior cruciate ligament of left knee
   M23.629 Other spontaneous disruption of posterior cruciate ligament of unspecified knee
● M23.63 Other spontaneous disruption of medial collateral ligament of knee
   M23.631 Other spontaneous disruption of medial collateral ligament of right knee
   M23.632 Other spontaneous disruption of medial collateral ligament of left knee
   M23.639 Other spontaneous disruption of medial collateral ligament of unspecified knee
● M23.64 Other spontaneous disruption of lateral collateral ligament of knee
   M23.641 Other spontaneous disruption of lateral collateral ligament of right knee
   M23.642 Other spontaneous disruption of lateral collateral ligament of left knee
   M23.649 Other spontaneous disruption of lateral collateral ligament of unspecified knee
● M23.67 Other spontaneous disruption of capsular ligament of knee
   M23.671 Other spontaneous disruption of capsular ligament of right knee
   M23.672 Other spontaneous disruption of capsular ligament of left knee
   M23.679 Other spontaneous disruption of capsular ligament of unspecified knee
● M23.8 Other internal derangements of knee
   Laxity of ligament of knee
   Snapping knee
● M23.8X Other internal derangements of knee
   M23.8X1 Other internal derangements of right knee
   M23.8X2 Other internal derangements of left knee
   M23.8X9 Other internal derangements of unspecified knee
● M23.9 Unspecified internal derangement of knee
   M23.90 Unspecified internal derangement of unspecified knee
   M23.91 Unspecified internal derangement of right knee
   M23.92 Unspecified internal derangement of left knee

◀ New   ◀▥ Revised   ~~deleted~~ Deleted   Excludes 1   Excludes 2   Includes   Use additional   Code first   Code also   Unspecified
OGCR Official Guidelines   ● Unacceptable Principal Diagnosis   X Assign placeholder X   ● Use Additional Character(s)   ▶ Manifestation Code   **Coding Clinic**

● **M24 Other specific joint derangements**
    Excludes1   current injury - see injury of joint by body region
    Excludes2   ganglion (M67.4)
                  snapping knee (M23.8-)
                  temporomandibular joint disorders (M26.6-)

● **M24.0 Loose body in joint**
    Excludes2   loose body in knee (M23.4)
   M24.00   Loose body in unspecified joint
● M24.01   Loose body in shoulder
     M24.011   Loose body in right shoulder
     M24.012   Loose body in left shoulder
     M24.019   Loose body in unspecified shoulder
● M24.02   Loose body in elbow
     M24.021   Loose body in right elbow
     M24.022   Loose body in left elbow
     M24.029   Loose body in unspecified elbow
● M24.03   Loose body in wrist
     M24.031   Loose body in right wrist
     M24.032   Loose body in left wrist
     M24.039   Loose body in unspecified wrist
● M24.04   Loose body in finger joints
     M24.041   Loose body in right finger joint(s)
     M24.042   Loose body in left finger joint(s)
     M24.049   Loose body in unspecified finger joint(s)
● M24.05   Loose body in hip
     M24.051   Loose body in right hip
     M24.052   Loose body in left hip
     M24.059   Loose body in unspecified hip
● M24.07   Loose body in ankle and toe joints
     M24.071   Loose body in right ankle
     M24.072   Loose body in left ankle
     M24.073   Loose body in unspecified ankle
     M24.074   Loose body in right toe joint(s)
     M24.075   Loose body in left toe joint(s)
     M24.076   Loose body in unspecified toe joints
   M24.08   Loose body, other site
● **M24.1 Other articular cartilage disorders**
    Excludes2   chondrocalcinosis (M11.1, M11.2-)
                  internal derangement of knee (M23.-)
                  metastatic calcification (E83.5)
                  ochronosis (E70.2)
   M24.10   Other articular cartilage disorders, unspecified site
● M24.11   Other articular cartilage disorders, shoulder
     M24.111   Other articular cartilage disorders, right shoulder
     M24.112   Other articular cartilage disorders, left shoulder
     M24.119   Other articular cartilage disorders, unspecified shoulder
● M24.12   Other articular cartilage disorders, elbow
     M24.121   Other articular cartilage disorders, right elbow
     M24.122   Other articular cartilage disorders, left elbow
     M24.129   Other articular cartilage disorders, unspecified elbow
● M24.13   Other articular cartilage disorders, wrist
     M24.131   Other articular cartilage disorders, right wrist
     M24.132   Other articular cartilage disorders, left wrist
     M24.139   Other articular cartilage disorders, unspecified wrist

● M24.14   Other articular cartilage disorders, hand
     M24.141   Other articular cartilage disorders, right hand
     M24.142   Other articular cartilage disorders, left hand
     M24.149   Other articular cartilage disorders, unspecified hand
● M24.15   Other articular cartilage disorders, hip
     M24.151   Other articular cartilage disorders, right hip
     M24.152   Other articular cartilage disorders, left hip
     M24.159   Other articular cartilage disorders, unspecified hip
● M24.17   Other articular cartilage disorders, ankle and foot
     M24.171   Other articular cartilage disorders, right ankle
     M24.172   Other articular cartilage disorders, left ankle
     M24.173   Other articular cartilage disorders, unspecified ankle
     M24.174   Other articular cartilage disorders, right foot
     M24.175   Other articular cartilage disorders, left foot
     M24.176   Other articular cartilage disorders, unspecified foot

● **M24.2 Disorder of ligament**
    Instability secondary to old ligament injury
    Ligamentous laxity NOS
    Excludes1   familial ligamentous laxity (M35.7)
    Excludes2   internal derangement of knee (M23.5-M23.89)
   M24.20   Disorder of ligament, unspecified site
● M24.21   Disorder of ligament, shoulder
     M24.211   Disorder of ligament, right shoulder
     M24.212   Disorder of ligament, left shoulder
     M24.219   Disorder of ligament, unspecified shoulder
● M24.22   Disorder of ligament, elbow
     M24.221   Disorder of ligament, right elbow
     M24.222   Disorder of ligament, left elbow
     M24.229   Disorder of ligament, unspecified elbow
● M24.23   Disorder of ligament, wrist
     M24.231   Disorder of ligament, right wrist
     M24.232   Disorder of ligament, left wrist
     M24.239   Disorder of ligament, unspecified wrist
● M24.24   Disorder of ligament, hand
     M24.241   Disorder of ligament, right hand
     M24.242   Disorder of ligament, left hand
     M24.249   Disorder of ligament, unspecified hand
● M24.25   Disorder of ligament, hip
     M24.251   Disorder of ligament, right hip
     M24.252   Disorder of ligament, left hip
     M24.259   Disorder of ligament, unspecified hip
● M24.27   Disorder of ligament, ankle and foot
     M24.271   Disorder of ligament, right ankle
     M24.272   Disorder of ligament, left ankle
     M24.273   Disorder of ligament, unspecified ankle
     M24.274   Disorder of ligament, right foot
     M24.275   Disorder of ligament, left foot
     M24.276   Disorder of ligament, unspecified foot
   M24.28   Disorder of ligament, vertebrae

N   Newborn Age: 0   **P**   Pediatric Age: 0–17   **M**   Maternity DX: 12–55   **A**   Adult Age: 15–124   ♀   Females Only   ♂   Males Only

   Complication\Comorbidity   Major C\C   (Ex)   CC/MCC Exclusions   Present on Admission Requirement   Hospital-Acquired Condition

1105

● M24.3 Pathological dislocation of joint, not elsewhere classified
   Excludes1   congenital dislocation or displacement of
                  joint - see congenital malformations
                  and deformations of the
                  musculoskeletal system (Q65-Q79)
                  current injury - see injury of joints and
                  ligaments by body region
                  recurrent dislocation of joint (M24.4-)
   M24.30 Pathological dislocation of unspecified joint,
           not elsewhere classified
● M24.31 Pathological dislocation of shoulder, not
           elsewhere classified
   M24.311 Pathological dislocation of right
            shoulder, not elsewhere classified
   M24.312 Pathological dislocation of left
            shoulder, not elsewhere classified
   M24.319 Pathological dislocation of
            unspecified shoulder, not elsewhere
            classified
● M24.32 Pathological dislocation of elbow, not
           elsewhere classified
   M24.321 Pathological dislocation of right
            elbow, not elsewhere classified
   M24.322 Pathological dislocation of left elbow,
            not elsewhere classified
   M24.329 Pathological dislocation of
            unspecified elbow, not elsewhere
            classified
● M24.33 Pathological dislocation of wrist, not elsewhere
           classified
   M24.331 Pathological dislocation of right
            wrist, not elsewhere classified
   M24.332 Pathological dislocation of left wrist,
            not elsewhere classified
   M24.339 Pathological dislocation of
            unspecified wrist, not elsewhere
            classified
● M24.34 Pathological dislocation of hand, not elsewhere
           classified
   M24.341 Pathological dislocation of right
            hand, not elsewhere classified
   M24.342 Pathological dislocation of left hand,
            not elsewhere classified
   M24.349 Pathological dislocation of
            unspecified hand, not elsewhere
            classified
● M24.35 Pathological dislocation of hip, not elsewhere
           classified
   M24.351 Pathological dislocation of right hip,
            not elsewhere classified
   M24.352 Pathological dislocation of left hip,
            not elsewhere classified
   M24.359 Pathological dislocation of
            unspecified hip, not elsewhere
            classified
● M24.36 Pathological dislocation of knee, not elsewhere
           classified
   M24.361 Pathological dislocation of right knee,
            not elsewhere classified
   M24.362 Pathological dislocation of left knee,
            not elsewhere classified
   M24.369 Pathological dislocation of
            unspecified knee, not elsewhere
            classified
● M24.37 Pathological dislocation of ankle and foot, not
           elsewhere classified
   M24.371 Pathological dislocation of right
            ankle, not elsewhere classified
   M24.372 Pathological dislocation of left ankle,
            not elsewhere classified

   M24.373 Pathological dislocation of
            unspecified ankle, not elsewhere
            classified
   M24.374 Pathological dislocation of right foot,
            not elsewhere classified
   M24.375 Pathological dislocation of left foot,
            not elsewhere classified
   M24.376 Pathological dislocation of
            unspecified foot, not elsewhere
            classified
● M24.4 Recurrent dislocation of joint
   Recurrent subluxation of joint
   Excludes2   recurrent dislocation of patella
                  (M22.0-M22.1)
                  recurrent vertebral dislocation (M43.3-,
                  M43.4, M43.5-)
   M24.40 Recurrent dislocation, unspecified joint
● M24.41 Recurrent dislocation, shoulder
   M24.411 Recurrent dislocation, right shoulder
   M24.412 Recurrent dislocation, left shoulder
   M24.419 Recurrent dislocation, unspecified
            shoulder
● M24.42 Recurrent dislocation, elbow
   M24.421 Recurrent dislocation, right elbow
   M24.422 Recurrent dislocation, left elbow
   M24.429 Recurrent dislocation, unspecified
            elbow
● M24.43 Recurrent dislocation, wrist
   M24.431 Recurrent dislocation, right wrist
   M24.432 Recurrent dislocation, left wrist
   M24.439 Recurrent dislocation, unspecified
            wrist
● M24.44 Recurrent dislocation, hand and finger(s)
   M24.441 Recurrent dislocation, right hand
   M24.442 Recurrent dislocation, left hand
   M24.443 Recurrent dislocation, unspecified
            hand
   M24.444 Recurrent dislocation, right finger
   M24.445 Recurrent dislocation, left finger
   M24.446 Recurrent dislocation, unspecified
            finger
● M24.45 Recurrent dislocation, hip
   M24.451 Recurrent dislocation, right hip
   M24.452 Recurrent dislocation, left hip
   M24.459 Recurrent dislocation, unspecified hip
● M24.46 Recurrent dislocation, knee
   M24.461 Recurrent dislocation, right knee
   M24.462 Recurrent dislocation, left knee
   M24.469 Recurrent dislocation, unspecified
            knee
● M24.47 Recurrent dislocation, ankle, foot and toes
   M24.471 Recurrent dislocation, right ankle
   M24.472 Recurrent dislocation, left ankle
   M24.473 Recurrent dislocation, unspecified
            ankle
   M24.474 Recurrent dislocation, right foot
   M24.475 Recurrent dislocation, left foot
   M24.476 Recurrent dislocation, unspecified
            foot
   M24.477 Recurrent dislocation, right toe(s)
   M24.478 Recurrent dislocation, left toe(s)
   M24.479 Recurrent dislocation, unspecified
            toe(s)

CHAPTER 13 (M00-M99)

◀ New   ◀▥ Revised   ~~deleted~~ Deleted   Excludes 1   Excludes 2   Includes   Use additional   Code first   Code also   Unspecified
OGCR Official Guidelines   ● Unacceptable Principal Diagnosis   X Assign placeholder X   ● Use Additional Character(s)   ▶ Manifestation Code   **Coding Clinic**

● M24.5   **Contracture of joint**

    Excludes1   contracture of muscle without contracture of joint (M62.4-)
                     contracture of tendon (sheath) without contracture of joint (M62.4-)
                     Dupuytren's contracture (M72.0)

    Excludes2   acquired deformities of limbs (M20-M21)

   M24.50   Contracture, unspecified joint

● M24.51   Contracture, shoulder
     M24.511   Contracture, right shoulder
     M24.512   Contracture, left shoulder
     M24.519   Contracture, unspecified shoulder

● M24.52   Contracture, elbow
     M24.521   Contracture, right elbow
     M24.522   Contracture, left elbow
     M24.529   Contracture, unspecified elbow

● M24.53   Contracture, wrist
     M24.531   Contracture, right wrist
     M24.532   Contracture, left wrist
     M24.539   Contracture, unspecified wrist

● M24.54   Contracture, hand
     M24.541   Contracture, right hand
     M24.542   Contracture, left hand
     M24.549   Contracture, unspecified hand

● M24.55   Contracture, hip
     M24.551   Contracture, right hip
     M24.552   Contracture, left hip
     M24.559   Contracture, unspecified hip

● M24.56   Contracture, knee
     M24.561   Contracture, right knee
     M24.562   Contracture, left knee
     M24.569   Contracture, unspecified knee

● M24.57   Contracture, ankle and foot
     M24.571   Contracture, right ankle
     M24.572   Contracture, left ankle
     M24.573   Contracture, unspecified ankle
     M24.574   Contracture, right foot
     M24.575   Contracture, left foot
     M24.576   Contracture, unspecified foot

● M24.6   **Ankylosis of joint**

    Excludes1   stiffness of joint without ankylosis (M25.6-)

    Excludes2   spine (M43.2-)

   M24.60   Ankylosis, unspecified joint

● M24.61   Ankylosis, shoulder
     M24.611   Ankylosis, right shoulder
     M24.612   Ankylosis, left shoulder
     M24.619   Ankylosis, unspecified shoulder

● M24.62   Ankylosis, elbow
     M24.621   Ankylosis, right elbow
     M24.622   Ankylosis, left elbow
     M24.629   Ankylosis, unspecified elbow

● M24.63   Ankylosis, wrist
     M24.631   Ankylosis, right wrist
     M24.632   Ankylosis, left wrist
     M24.639   Ankylosis, unspecified wrist

● M24.64   Ankylosis, hand
     M24.641   Ankylosis, right hand
     M24.642   Ankylosis, left hand
     M24.649   Ankylosis, unspecified hand

● M24.65   Ankylosis, hip
     M24.651   Ankylosis, right hip
     M24.652   Ankylosis, left hip
     M24.659   Ankylosis, unspecified hip

Item 13–5   Ankylosis or arthrokleisis is a consolidation of a joint due to disease, injury, or surgical procedure. Spondylosis is the degeneration of the vertebral processes and formation of osteophytes and commonly occurs with age. **Spondylitis** or ankylosing spondylitis is a type of arthritis that affects the spine or backbone causing back pain and stiffness.

● M24.66   Ankylosis, knee
     M24.661   Ankylosis, right knee
     M24.662   Ankylosis, left knee
     M24.669   Ankylosis, unspecified knee

● M24.67   Ankylosis, ankle and foot
     M24.671   Ankylosis, right ankle
     M24.672   Ankylosis, left ankle
     M24.673   Ankylosis, unspecified ankle
     M24.674   Ankylosis, right foot
     M24.675   Ankylosis, left foot
     M24.676   Ankylosis, unspecified foot

   M24.7   Protrusio acetabuli

● M24.8   Other specific joint derangements, not elsewhere classified

    Excludes2   iliotibial band syndrome (M76.3)

   M24.80   Other specific joint derangements of unspecified joint, not elsewhere classified

● M24.81   Other specific joint derangements of shoulder, not elsewhere classified
     M24.811   Other specific joint derangements of right shoulder, not elsewhere classified
     M24.812   Other specific joint derangements of left shoulder, not elsewhere classified
     M24.819   Other specific joint derangements of unspecified shoulder, not elsewhere classified

● M24.82   Other specific joint derangements of elbow, not elsewhere classified
     M24.821   Other specific joint derangements of right elbow, not elsewhere classified
     M24.822   Other specific joint derangements of left elbow, not elsewhere classified
     M24.829   Other specific joint derangements of unspecified elbow, not elsewhere classified

● M24.83   Other specific joint derangements of wrist, not elsewhere classified
     M24.831   Other specific joint derangements of right wrist, not elsewhere classified
     M24.832   Other specific joint derangements of left wrist, not elsewhere classified
     M24.839   Other specific joint derangements of unspecified wrist, not elsewhere classified

● M24.84   Other specific joint derangements of hand, not elsewhere classified
     M24.841   Other specific joint derangements of right hand, not elsewhere classified
     M24.842   Other specific joint derangements of left hand, not elsewhere classified
     M24.849   Other specific joint derangements of unspecified hand, not elsewhere classified

● M24.85   Other specific joint derangements of hip, not elsewhere classified
     Irritable hip
     M24.851   Other specific joint derangements of right hip, not elsewhere classified
     M24.852   Other specific joint derangements of left hip, not elsewhere classified
     M24.859   Other specific joint derangements of unspecified hip, not elsewhere classified

---

N   Newborn Age: 0   P   Pediatric Age: 0–17   M   Maternity DX: 12–55   A   Adult Age: 15–124   ♀   Females Only   ♂   Males Only

Complication\Comorbidity   Major C\C   (Ex)   CC/MCC Exclusions   Present on Admission Requirement   Hospital-Acquired Condition

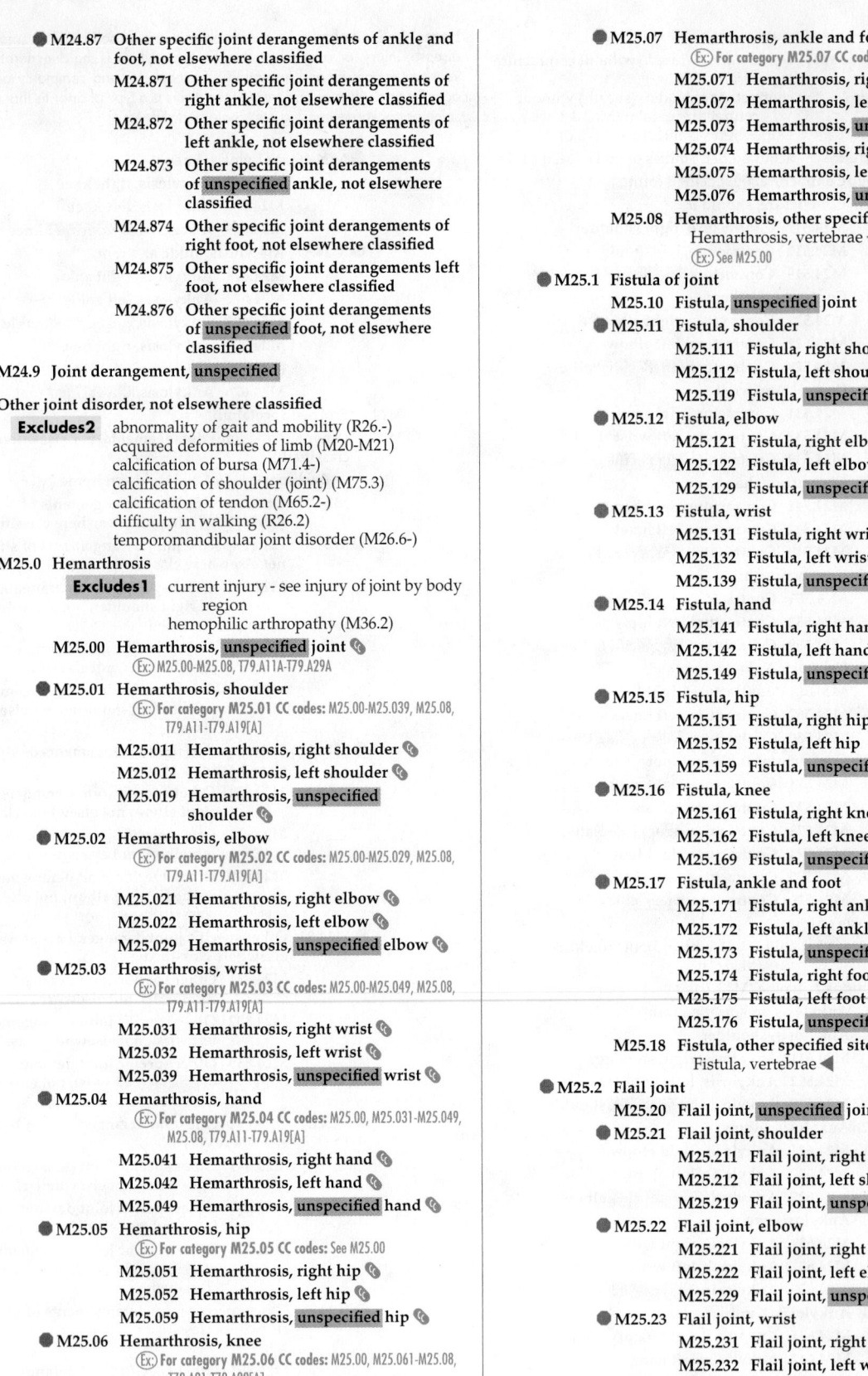

● M24.87 Other specific joint derangements of ankle and foot, not elsewhere classified

     M24.871 Other specific joint derangements of right ankle, not elsewhere classified

     M24.872 Other specific joint derangements of left ankle, not elsewhere classified

     M24.873 Other specific joint derangements of unspecified ankle, not elsewhere classified

     M24.874 Other specific joint derangements of right foot, not elsewhere classified

     M24.875 Other specific joint derangements left foot, not elsewhere classified

     M24.876 Other specific joint derangements of unspecified foot, not elsewhere classified

    M24.9 Joint derangement, unspecified

● M25 Other joint disorder, not elsewhere classified

    Excludes2   abnormality of gait and mobility (R26.-)
                   acquired deformities of limb (M20-M21)
                   calcification of bursa (M71.4-)
                   calcification of shoulder (joint) (M75.3)
                   calcification of tendon (M65.2-)
                   difficulty in walking (R26.2)
                   temporomandibular joint disorder (M26.6-)

● M25.0 Hemarthrosis

    Excludes1   current injury - see injury of joint by body region
                   hemophilic arthropathy (M36.2)

    M25.00 Hemarthrosis, unspecified joint
           (Ex:) M25.00-M25.08, T79.A11A-T79.A29A

   ● M25.01 Hemarthrosis, shoulder
           (Ex:) **For category M25.01 CC codes:** M25.00-M25.039, M25.08, T79.A11-T79.A19[A]

     M25.011 Hemarthrosis, right shoulder
     M25.012 Hemarthrosis, left shoulder
     M25.019 Hemarthrosis, unspecified shoulder

   ● M25.02 Hemarthrosis, elbow
           (Ex:) **For category M25.02 CC codes:** M25.00-M25.029, M25.08, T79.A11-T79.A19[A]

     M25.021 Hemarthrosis, right elbow
     M25.022 Hemarthrosis, left elbow
     M25.029 Hemarthrosis, unspecified elbow

   ● M25.03 Hemarthrosis, wrist
           (Ex:) **For category M25.03 CC codes:** M25.00-M25.049, M25.08, T79.A11-T79.A19[A]

     M25.031 Hemarthrosis, right wrist
     M25.032 Hemarthrosis, left wrist
     M25.039 Hemarthrosis, unspecified wrist

   ● M25.04 Hemarthrosis, hand
           (Ex:) **For category M25.04 CC codes:** M25.00, M25.031-M25.049, M25.08, T79.A11-T79.A19[A]

     M25.041 Hemarthrosis, right hand
     M25.042 Hemarthrosis, left hand
     M25.049 Hemarthrosis, unspecified hand

   ● M25.05 Hemarthrosis, hip
           (Ex:) **For category M25.05 CC codes:** See M25.00

     M25.051 Hemarthrosis, right hip
     M25.052 Hemarthrosis, left hip
     M25.059 Hemarthrosis, unspecified hip

   ● M25.06 Hemarthrosis, knee
           (Ex:) **For category M25.06 CC codes:** M25.00, M25.061-M25.08, T79.A21-T79.A29[A]

     M25.061 Hemarthrosis, right knee
     M25.062 Hemarthrosis, left knee
     M25.069 Hemarthrosis, unspecified knee

   ● M25.07 Hemarthrosis, ankle and foot
           (Ex:) **For category M25.07 CC codes:** See M25.06

     M25.071 Hemarthrosis, right ankle
     M25.072 Hemarthrosis, left ankle
     M25.073 Hemarthrosis, unspecified ankle
     M25.074 Hemarthrosis, right foot
     M25.075 Hemarthrosis, left foot
     M25.076 Hemarthrosis, unspecified foot

    M25.08 Hemarthrosis, other specified site ◀▥▥▥
         Hemarthrosis, vertebrae ◀
         (Ex:) See M25.00

● M25.1 Fistula of joint

    M25.10 Fistula, unspecified joint

   ● M25.11 Fistula, shoulder
     M25.111 Fistula, right shoulder
     M25.112 Fistula, left shoulder
     M25.119 Fistula, unspecified shoulder

   ● M25.12 Fistula, elbow
     M25.121 Fistula, right elbow
     M25.122 Fistula, left elbow
     M25.129 Fistula, unspecified elbow

   ● M25.13 Fistula, wrist
     M25.131 Fistula, right wrist
     M25.132 Fistula, left wrist
     M25.139 Fistula, unspecified wrist

   ● M25.14 Fistula, hand
     M25.141 Fistula, right hand
     M25.142 Fistula, left hand
     M25.149 Fistula, unspecified hand

   ● M25.15 Fistula, hip
     M25.151 Fistula, right hip
     M25.152 Fistula, left hip
     M25.159 Fistula, unspecified hip

   ● M25.16 Fistula, knee
     M25.161 Fistula, right knee
     M25.162 Fistula, left knee
     M25.169 Fistula, unspecified knee

   ● M25.17 Fistula, ankle and foot
     M25.171 Fistula, right ankle
     M25.172 Fistula, left ankle
     M25.173 Fistula, unspecified ankle
     M25.174 Fistula, right foot
     M25.175 Fistula, left foot
     M25.176 Fistula, unspecified foot

    M25.18 Fistula, other specified site ◀▥▥▥
         Fistula, vertebrae ◀

● M25.2 Flail joint

    M25.20 Flail joint, unspecified joint

   ● M25.21 Flail joint, shoulder
     M25.211 Flail joint, right shoulder
     M25.212 Flail joint, left shoulder
     M25.219 Flail joint, unspecified shoulder

   ● M25.22 Flail joint, elbow
     M25.221 Flail joint, right elbow
     M25.222 Flail joint, left elbow
     M25.229 Flail joint, unspecified elbow

   ● M25.23 Flail joint, wrist
     M25.231 Flail joint, right wrist
     M25.232 Flail joint, left wrist
     M25.239 Flail joint, unspecified wrist

   ● M25.24 Flail joint, hand
     M25.241 Flail joint, right hand
     M25.242 Flail joint, left hand
     M25.249 Flail joint, unspecified hand

◀ New   ◀▥▥▥ Revised   ~~deleted~~ Deleted   Excludes 1   Excludes 2   Includes   Use additional   Code first   Code also   Unspecified
OGCR Official Guidelines   ● Unacceptable Principal Diagnosis   X Assign placeholder X   ● Use Additional Character(s)   ▶ Manifestation Code   **Coding Clinic**

● M25.25   Flail joint, hip
     M25.251   Flail joint, right hip
     M25.252   Flail joint, left hip
     M25.259   Flail joint, unspecified hip
● M25.26   Flail joint, knee
     M25.261   Flail joint, right knee
     M25.262   Flail joint, left knee
     M25.269   Flail joint, unspecified knee
● M25.27   Flail joint, ankle and foot
     M25.271   Flail joint, right ankle and foot
     M25.272   Flail joint, left ankle and foot
     M25.279   Flail joint, unspecified ankle and foot
     M25.28   Flail joint, other site
● M25.3   Other instability of joint

> **Excludes1**   instability of joint secondary to old ligament injury (M24.2-)
> instability of joint secondary to removal of joint prosthesis (M96.8-)

> **Excludes2**   spinal instabilities (M53.2-)

     M25.30   Other instability, unspecified joint
● M25.31   Other instability, shoulder
     M25.311   Other instability, right shoulder
     M25.312   Other instability, left shoulder
     M25.319   Other instability, unspecified shoulder
● M25.32   Other instability, elbow
     M25.321   Other instability, right elbow
     M25.322   Other instability, left elbow
     M25.329   Other instability, unspecified elbow
● M25.33   Other instability, wrist
     M25.331   Other instability, right wrist
     M25.332   Other instability, left wrist
     M25.339   Other instability, unspecified wrist
● M25.34   Other instability, hand
     M25.341   Other instability, right hand
     M25.342   Other instability, left hand
     M25.349   Other instability, unspecified hand
● M25.35   Other instability, hip
     M25.351   Other instability, right hip
     M25.352   Other instability, left hip
     M25.359   Other instability, unspecified hip
● M25.36   Other instability, knee
     M25.361   Other instability, right knee
     M25.362   Other instability, left knee
     M25.369   Other instability, unspecified knee
● M25.37   Other instability, ankle and foot
     M25.371   Other instability, right ankle
     M25.372   Other instability, left ankle
     M25.373   Other instability, unspecified ankle
     M25.374   Other instability, right foot
     M25.375   Other instability, left foot
     M25.376   Other instability, unspecified foot
● M25.4   Effusion of joint

> **Excludes1**   hydrarthrosis in yaws (A66.6)
> intermittent hydrarthrosis (M12.4-)
> other infective (teno)synovitis (M65.1-)

     M25.40   Effusion, unspecified joint
● M25.41   Effusion, shoulder
     M25.411   Effusion, right shoulder
     M25.412   Effusion, left shoulder
     M25.419   Effusion, unspecified shoulder

● M25.42   Effusion, elbow
     M25.421   Effusion, right elbow
     M25.422   Effusion, left elbow
     M25.429   Effusion, unspecified elbow
● M25.43   Effusion, wrist
     M25.431   Effusion, right wrist
     M25.432   Effusion, left wrist
     M25.439   Effusion, unspecified wrist
● M25.44   Effusion, hand
     M25.441   Effusion, right hand
     M25.442   Effusion, left hand
     M25.449   Effusion, unspecified hand
● M25.45   Effusion, hip
     M25.451   Effusion, right hip
     M25.452   Effusion, left hip
     M25.459   Effusion, unspecified hip
● M25.46   Effusion, knee
     M25.461   Effusion, right knee
     M25.462   Effusion, left knee
     M25.469   Effusion, unspecified knee
● M25.47   Effusion, ankle and foot
     M25.471   Effusion, right ankle
     M25.472   Effusion, left ankle
     M25.473   Effusion, unspecified ankle
     M25.474   Effusion, right foot
     M25.475   Effusion, left foot
     M25.476   Effusion, unspecified foot
     M25.48   Effusion, other site
● M25.5   Pain in joint

> **Excludes2**   pain in hand (M79.64-)
> pain in fingers (M79.64-)
> pain in foot (M79.67-)
> pain in limb (M79.6-)
> pain in toes (M79.67-)

     M25.50   Pain in unspecified joint
● M25.51   Pain in shoulder
     M25.511   Pain in right shoulder
     M25.512   Pain in left shoulder
     M25.519   Pain in unspecified shoulder
● M25.52   Pain in elbow
     M25.521   Pain in right elbow
     M25.522   Pain in left elbow
     M25.529   Pain in unspecified elbow
● M25.53   Pain in wrist
     M25.531   Pain in right wrist
     M25.532   Pain in left wrist
     M25.539   Pain in unspecified wrist
● M25.55   Pain in hip
     M25.551   Pain in right hip
     M25.552   Pain in left hip
     M25.559   Pain in unspecified hip
● M25.56   Pain in knee
     M25.561   Pain in right knee
     M25.562   Pain in left knee
     M25.569   Pain in unspecified knee
● M25.57   Pain in ankle and joints of foot
     M25.571   Pain in right ankle and joints of right foot
     M25.572   Pain in left ankle and joints of left foot
     M25.579   Pain in unspecified ankle and joints of unspecified foot

CHAPTER 13 (M00–M99)

N Newborn Age: 0   **P** Pediatric Age: 0–17   **M** Maternity DX: 12–55   **A** Adult Age: 15–124   ♀ Females Only   ♂ Males Only

℀ Complication\Comorbidity   ℀ Major C\C   (Ex) CC/MCC Exclusions   ℀ Present on Admission Requirement   ℀ Hospital-Acquired Condition

1109

● **M25.6** **Stiffness of joint, not elsewhere classified**

     Excludes1   ankylosis of joint (M24.6-)
                       contracture of joint (M24.5-)

   M25.60   Stiffness of unspecified joint, not elsewhere classified

● M25.61   Stiffness of shoulder, not elsewhere classified

     M25.611   Stiffness of right shoulder, not elsewhere classified

     M25.612   Stiffness of left shoulder, not elsewhere classified

     M25.619   Stiffness of unspecified shoulder, not elsewhere classified

● M25.62   Stiffness of elbow, not elsewhere classified

     M25.621   Stiffness of right elbow, not elsewhere classified

     M25.622   Stiffness of left elbow, not elsewhere classified

     M25.629   Stiffness of unspecified elbow, not elsewhere classified

● M25.63   Stiffness of wrist, not elsewhere classified

     M25.631   Stiffness of right wrist, not elsewhere classified

     M25.632   Stiffness of left wrist, not elsewhere classified

     M25.639   Stiffness of unspecified wrist, not elsewhere classified

● M25.64   Stiffness of hand, not elsewhere classified

     M25.641   Stiffness of right hand, not elsewhere classified

     M25.642   Stiffness of left hand, not elsewhere classified

     M25.649   Stiffness of unspecified hand, not elsewhere classified

● M25.65   Stiffness of hip, not elsewhere classified

     M25.651   Stiffness of right hip, not elsewhere classified

     M25.652   Stiffness of left hip, not elsewhere classified

     M25.659   Stiffness of unspecified hip, not elsewhere classified

● M25.66   Stiffness of knee, not elsewhere classified

     M25.661   Stiffness of right knee, not elsewhere classified

     M25.662   Stiffness of left knee, not elsewhere classified

     M25.669   Stiffness of unspecified knee, not elsewhere classified

● M25.67   Stiffness of ankle and foot, not elsewhere classified

     M25.671   Stiffness of right ankle, not elsewhere classified

     M25.672   Stiffness of left ankle, not elsewhere classified

     M25.673   Stiffness of unspecified ankle, not elsewhere classified

     M25.674   Stiffness of right foot, not elsewhere classified

     M25.675   Stiffness of left foot, not elsewhere classified

     M25.676   Stiffness of unspecified foot, not elsewhere classified

● **M25.7** **Osteophyte**

   M25.70   Osteophyte, unspecified joint

● M25.71   Osteophyte, shoulder

     M25.711   Osteophyte, right shoulder

     M25.712   Osteophyte, left shoulder

     M25.719   Osteophyte, unspecified shoulder

● M25.72   Osteophyte, elbow

     M25.721   Osteophyte, right elbow

     M25.722   Osteophyte, left elbow

     M25.729   Osteophyte, unspecified elbow

● M25.73   Osteophyte, wrist

     M25.731   Osteophyte, right wrist

     M25.732   Osteophyte, left wrist

     M25.739   Osteophyte, unspecified wrist

● M25.74   Osteophyte, hand

     M25.741   Osteophyte, right hand

     M25.742   Osteophyte, left hand

     M25.749   Osteophyte, unspecified hand

● M25.75   Osteophyte, hip

     M25.751   Osteophyte, right hip

     M25.752   Osteophyte, left hip

     M25.759   Osteophyte, unspecified hip

● M25.76   Osteophyte, knee

     M25.761   Osteophyte, right knee

     M25.762   Osteophyte, left knee

     M25.769   Osteophyte, unspecified knee

● M25.77   Osteophyte, ankle and foot

     M25.771   Osteophyte, right ankle

     M25.772   Osteophyte, left ankle

     M25.773   Osteophyte, unspecified ankle

     M25.774   Osteophyte, right foot

     M25.775   Osteophyte, left foot

     M25.776   Osteophyte, unspecified foot

   M25.78   Osteophyte, vertebrae

● **M25.8** **Other specified joint disorders**

   M25.80   Other specified joint disorders, unspecified joint

● M25.81   Other specified joint disorders, shoulder

     M25.811   Other specified joint disorders, right shoulder

     M25.812   Other specified joint disorders, left shoulder

     M25.819   Other specified joint disorders, unspecified shoulder

● M25.82   Other specified joint disorders, elbow

     M25.821   Other specified joint disorders, right elbow

     M25.822   Other specified joint disorders, left elbow

     M25.829   Other specified joint disorders, unspecified elbow

● M25.83   Other specified joint disorders, wrist

     M25.831   Other specified joint disorders, right wrist

     M25.832   Other specified joint disorders, left wrist

     M25.839   Other specified joint disorders, unspecified wrist

● M25.84 Other specified joint disorders, hand

M25.841 Other specified joint disorders, right hand

M25.842 Other specified joint disorders, left hand

M25.849 Other specified joint disorders, unspecified hand

● M25.85 Other specified joint disorders, hip

M25.851 Other specified joint disorders, right hip

M25.852 Other specified joint disorders, left hip

M25.859 Other specified joint disorders, unspecified hip

● M25.86 Other specified joint disorders, knee

M25.861 Other specified joint disorders, right knee

M25.862 Other specified joint disorders, left knee

M25.869 Other specified joint disorders, unspecified knee

● M25.87 Other specified joint disorders, ankle and foot

M25.871 Other specified joint disorders, right ankle and foot

M25.872 Other specified joint disorders, left ankle and foot

M25.879 Other specified joint disorders, unspecified ankle and foot

M25.9 Joint disorder, unspecified

DENTOFACIAL ANOMALIES [INCLUDING MALOCCLUSION] AND OTHER DISORDERS OF JAW (M26-M27)

Excludes 1 hemifacial atrophy or hypertrophy (Q67.4)
unilateral condylar hyperplasia or hypoplasia (M27.8)

● M26 Dentofacial anomalies [including malocclusion]

● M26.0 Major anomalies of jaw size

Excludes 1 acromegaly (E22.0)
Robin's syndrome (Q87.0)

M26.00 Unspecified anomaly of jaw size

M26.01 Maxillary hyperplasia

M26.02 Maxillary hypoplasia

M26.03 Mandibular hyperplasia

M26.04 Mandibular hypoplasia

M26.05 Macrogenia

M26.06 Microgenia

M26.07 Excessive tuberosity of jaw
Entire maxillary tuberosity

M26.09 Other specified anomalies of jaw size

● M26.1 Anomalies of jaw-cranial base relationship

M26.10 Unspecified anomaly of jaw-cranial base relationship

M26.11 Maxillary asymmetry

M26.12 Other jaw asymmetry

M26.19 Other specified anomalies of jaw-cranial base relationship

Figure 13-3 Dentofacial malocclusion.

Item 13–6 Hyperplasia is a condition of overdevelopment, whereas **hypoplasia** is a condition of underdevelopment. **Macrogenia** is overdevelopment of the chin, whereas **microgenia** is underdevelopment of the chin.

● M26.2 Anomalies of dental arch relationship

M26.20 Unspecified anomaly of dental arch relationship

● M26.21 Malocclusion, Angle's class

M26.211 Malocclusion, Angle's class I
Neutro-occlusion

M26.212 Malocclusion, Angle's class II
Disto-occlusion Division I
Disto-occlusion Division II

M26.213 Malocclusion, Angle's class III
Mesio-occlusion

M26.219 Malocclusion, Angle's class, unspecified

● M26.22 Open occlusal relationship

M26.220 Open anterior occlusal relationship
Anterior openbite

M26.221 Open posterior occlusal relationship
Posterior openbite

M26.23 Excessive horizontal overlap
Excessive horizontal overjet

M26.24 Reverse articulation
Crossbite (anterior) (posterior)

M26.25 Anomalies of interarch distance

M26.29 Other anomalies of dental arch relationship
Midline deviation of dental arch
Overbite (excessive) deep
Overbite (excessive) horizontal
Overbite (excessive) vertical
Posterior lingual occlusion of mandibular teeth

● M26.3 Anomalies of tooth position of fully erupted tooth or teeth

Excludes 2 embedded and impacted teeth (K01.-)

M26.30 Unspecified anomaly of tooth position of fully erupted tooth or teeth
Abnormal spacing of fully erupted tooth or teeth NOS
Displacement of fully erupted tooth or teeth NOS
Transposition of fully erupted tooth or teeth NOS

M26.31 Crowding of fully erupted teeth

M26.32 Excessive spacing of fully erupted teeth
Diastema of fully erupted tooth or teeth NOS

M26.33 Horizontal displacement of fully erupted tooth or teeth
Tipped tooth or teeth
Tipping of fully erupted tooth

M26.34 Vertical displacement of fully erupted tooth or teeth
Extruded tooth
Infraeruption of tooth or teeth
Supraeruption of tooth or teeth

M26.35 Rotation of fully erupted tooth or teeth

N Newborn Age: 0   P Pediatric Age: 0–17   M Maternity DX: 12–55   A Adult Age: 15–124   ♀ Females Only   ♂ Males Only

🔗 Complication\Comorbidity   🔗 Major C\C   (Ex) CC/MCC Exclusions   🔗 Present on Admission Requirement   🔗 Hospital-Acquired Condition

1111

M26.36 Insufficient interocclusal distance of fully erupted teeth (ridge)
Lack of adequate intermaxillary vertical dimension of fully erupted teeth

M26.37 Excessive interocclusal distance of fully erupted teeth
Excessive intermaxillary vertical dimension of fully erupted teeth
Loss of occlusal vertical dimension of fully erupted teeth

M26.39 Other anomalies of tooth position of fully erupted tooth or teeth

M26.4 Malocclusion, unspecified

● **M26.5 Dentofacial functional abnormalities**
   Excludes1   bruxism (F45.8)
              teeth-grinding NOS (F45.8)

M26.50 Dentofacial functional abnormalities, unspecified

M26.51 Abnormal jaw closure

M26.52 Limited mandibular range of motion

M26.53 Deviation in opening and closing of the mandible

M26.54 Insufficient anterior guidance
Insufficient anterior occlusal guidance

M26.55 Centric occlusion maximum intercuspation discrepancy
   Excludes1   centric occlusion NOS (M26.59)

M26.56 Non-working side interference
Balancing side interference

M26.57 Lack of posterior occlusal support

M26.59 Other dentofacial functional abnormalities
Centric occlusion (of teeth) NOS
Malocclusion due to abnormal swallowing
Malocclusion due to mouth breathing
Malocclusion due to tongue, lip or finger habits

● **M26.6 Temporomandibular joint disorders**
   Excludes2   current temporomandibular joint dislocation (S03.0)
              current temporomandibular joint sprain (S03.4)

M26.60 Temporomandibular joint disorder, unspecified

M26.61 Adhesions and ankylosis of temporomandibular joint

M26.62 Arthralgia of temporomandibular joint

M26.63 Articular disc disorder of temporomandibular joint

M26.69 Other specified disorders of temporomandibular joint

● **M26.7 Dental alveolar anomalies**

M26.70 Unspecified alveolar anomaly

M26.71 Alveolar maxillary hyperplasia

M26.72 Alveolar mandibular hyperplasia

M26.73 Alveolar maxillary hypoplasia

M26.74 Alveolar mandibular hypoplasia

M26.79 Other specified alveolar anomalies

● **M26.8 Other dentofacial anomalies**

M26.81 Anterior soft tissue impingement
Anterior soft tissue impingement on teeth

M26.82 Posterior soft tissue impingement
Posterior soft tissue impingement on teeth

M26.89 Other dentofacial anomalies

M26.9 Dentofacial anomaly, unspecified

● **M27 Other diseases of jaws**

M27.0 Developmental disorders of jaws
Latent bone cyst of jaw
Stafne's cyst
Torus mandibularis
Torus palatinus

M27.1 Giant cell granuloma, central
Giant cell granuloma NOS
   Excludes1   peripheral giant cell granuloma (K06.8)

M27.2 Inflammatory conditions of jaws
Osteitis of jaw(s)
Osteomyelitis (neonatal) jaw(s)
Osteoradionecrosis jaw(s)
Periostitis jaw(s)
Sequestrum of jaw bone
Use additional code (W88-W90, X39.0) to identify radiation, if radiation-induced
   Excludes2   osteonecrosis of jaw due to drug (M87.180)

M27.3 Alveolitis of jaws
Alveolar osteitis
Dry socket

● **M27.4 Other and unspecified cysts of jaw**
   Excludes1   cysts of oral region (K09.-)
             latent bone cyst of jaw (M27.0)
             Stafne's cyst (M27.0)

M27.40 Unspecified cyst of jaw
Cyst of jaw NOS

M27.49 Other cysts of jaw
Aneurysmal cyst of jaw
Hemorrhagic cyst of jaw
Traumatic cyst of jaw

● **M27.5 Periradicular pathology associated with previous endodontic treatment**

M27.51 Perforation of root canal space due to endodontic treatment

M27.52 Endodontic overfill

M27.53 Endodontic underfill

M27.59 Other periradicular pathology associated with previous endodontic treatment

● **M27.6 Endosseous dental implant failure**

M27.61 Osseointegration failure of dental implant
Hemorrhagic complications of dental implant placement
Iatrogenic osseointegration failure of dental implant
Osseointegration failure of dental implant due to complications of systemic disease
Osseointegration failure of dental implant due to poor bone quality
Pre-integration failure of dental implant NOS
Pre-osseointegration failure of dental implant

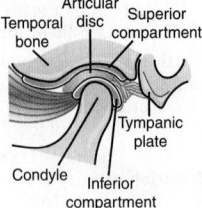

Figure 13-4   Temporomandibular joint.

Item 13-7 Dysfunction of the temporomandibular joint is termed **temporomandibular joint (TMJ) syndrome** and is characterized by pain and tenderness/spasm of the muscles of mastication, joint noise, and in the later stages, limited mandibular movement.

◀ New   ◀ Revised   ~~deleted~~ Deleted   Excludes 1   Excludes 2   Includes   Use additional   Code first   Code also   Unspecified
OGCR Official Guidelines   ● Unacceptable Principal Diagnosis   X Assign placeholder X   ● Use Additional Character(s)   ▶ Manifestation Code   **Coding Clinic**

M27.62 Post-osseointegration biological failure of dental implant
   Failure of dental implant due to lack of attached gingiva
   Failure of dental implant due to occlusal trauma (caused by poor prosthetic design)
   Failure of dental implant due to parafunctional habits
   Failure of dental implant due to periodontal infection (peri–implantitis)
   Failure of dental implant due to poor oral hygiene
   Iatrogenic post-osseointegration failure of dental implant
   Post-osseointegration failure of dental implant due to complications of systemic disease

M27.63 Post-osseointegration mechanical failure of dental implant
   Failure of dental prosthesis causing loss of dental implant
   Fracture of dental implant
   Excludes2 cracked tooth (K03.81)
            fractured dental restorative material with loss of material (K08.531)
            fractured dental restorative material without loss of material (K08.530)
            fractured tooth (S02.5)

M27.69 Other endosseous dental implant failure
   Dental implant failure NOS

M27.8 Other specified diseases of jaws
   Cherubism
   Exostosis
   Fibrous dysplasia
   Unilateral condylar hyperplasia
   Unilateral condylar hypoplasia
   Excludes1 jaw pain (R68.84)

M27.9 Disease of jaws, unspecified

SYSTEMIC CONNECTIVE TISSUE DISORDERS (M30-M36)

   Includes   autoimmune disease NOS
            collagen (vascular) disease NOS
            systemic autoimmune disease
            systemic collagen (vascular) disease
   Excludes1   autoimmune disease, single organ or single cell-type - code to relevant condition category

● **M30 Polyarteritis nodosa and related conditions**
   Excludes1   microscopic polyarteritis (M31.7)
   (Ex) **For category M30 CC codes unless otherwise indicated:** E08.51-E08.59, E08.618-E08.638, E08.649-E08.8, E09.51-E09.59, E09.618-E09.638, E09.649-E09.8, E10.51-E10.59, E10.618-E10.638, E10.649, E10.69-E10.8, E11.51-E11.59, E11.618-E11.638, E11.649, E11.69-E11.8, E13.51-E13.59, E13.618-E13.638, E13.649-E13.8, I87.8, I99.8-I99.9, M30.0-M31.7

M30.0 Polyarteritis nodosa ⬥

M30.1 Polyarteritis with lung involvement [Churg-Strauss] ⬥
   Allergic granulomatous angiitis

M30.2 Juvenile polyarteritis ⬥

M30.3 Mucocutaneous lymph node syndrome [Kawasaki] ⬥
   (Ex) I87.8, I99.8-I99.9, M30.0-M31.7

M30.8 Other conditions related to polyarteritis nodosa ⬥
   Polyangiitis overlap syndrome

● **M31 Other necrotizing vasculopathies**
   (Ex) **For category M31 CC codes unless otherwise indicated:** See M30

M31.0 Hypersensitivity angiitis ⬥
   Goodpasture's syndrome

M31.1 Thrombotic microangiopathy ⬥
   Thrombotic thrombocytopenic purpura

M31.2 Lethal midline granuloma ⬥

M31.3 Wegener's granulomatosis
   Necrotizing respiratory granulomatosis

   M31.30 Wegener's granulomatosis without renal involvement ⬥
      Wegener's granulomatosis NOS

   M31.31 Wegener's granulomatosis with renal involvement ⬥

M31.4 Aortic arch syndrome [Takayasu] ⬥

M31.5 Giant cell arteritis with polymyalgia rheumatica

M31.6 Other giant cell arteritis

M31.7 Microscopic polyangiitis ⬥
   Microscopic polyarteritis
   Excludes1   polyarteritis nodosa (M30.0)

M31.8 Other specified necrotizing vasculopathies ⬥
   Hypocomplementemic vasculitis
   Septic vasculitis
   (Ex) I77.5, M31.8-M31.9

M31.9 Necrotizing vasculopathy, unspecified ⬥
   (Ex) I77.5, M31.8-M31.9

● **M32 Systemic lupus erythematosus (SLE)**
   Autoimmune inflammatory connective tissue disease of unknown cause that occurs most often in women.
   Excludes1   lupus erythematosus (discoid) (NOS) (L93.0)

M32.0 Drug-induced systemic lupus erythematosus
   Use additional code for adverse effect, if applicable, to identify drug (T36-T50 with fifth or sixth character 5)

● **M32.1 Systemic lupus erythematosus with organ or system involvement**

   M32.10 Systemic lupus erythematosus, organ or system involvement unspecified

   M32.11 Endocarditis in systemic lupus erythematosus ⬥
      Libman-Sacks disease
      CC when PDx is its own CC
      (Ex) I38-I39, I87.8, I99.8-I99.9

   M32.12 Pericarditis in systemic lupus erythematosus ⬥
      Lupus pericarditis
      CC when PDx is its own CC
      (Ex) I01.0, I09.2, I30.0-I30.9, I31.3-I32, I87.8, I99.8-I99.9

   M32.13 Lung involvement in systemic lupus erythematosus
      Pleural effusion due to systemic lupus erythematosus

   M32.14 Glomerular disease in systemic lupus erythematosus
      Lupus renal disease NOS

   M32.15 Tubulo-interstitial nephropathy in systemic lupus erythematosus

   M32.19 Other organ or system involvement in systemic lupus erythematosus

M32.8 Other forms of systemic lupus erythematosus

M32.9 Systemic lupus erythematosus, unspecified
   SLE NOS
   Systemic lupus erythematosus NOS
   Systemic lupus erythematosus without organ involvement

CHAPTER 13 (M00-M99)

N Newborn Age: 0   **P** Pediatric Age: 0–17   **M** Maternity DX: 12–55   **A** Adult Age: 15–124   ♀ Females Only   ♂ Males Only

⬥ Complication\Comorbidity   Major C\C   (Ex) CC/MCC Exclusions   Present on Admission Requirement   Hospital-Acquired Condition

1113

CHAPTER 13 (M00-M99)

● **M33 Dermatopolymyositis**

Ex: For category M33 CC codes unless otherwise indicated: M33.00-M33.19, M33.90-M33.99, M36.0

● **M33.0 Juvenile dermatopolymyositis**

M33.00 Juvenile dermatopolymyositis, organ involvement unspecified 🗝

M33.01 Juvenile dermatopolymyositis with respiratory involvement 🗝

M33.02 Juvenile dermatopolymyositis with myopathy 🗝
CC when PDx is its own CC
Ex: E08.40-E08.49, E08.618-E08.638, E08.649-E08.8, E09.40-E09.49, E09.618-E09.638, E09.649-E09.8, E10.40-E10.49, E10.618-E10.638, E10.649, E10.69-E10.8, E11.40-E11.49, E11.618-E11.638, E11.649, E11.69-E11.8, E13.40-E13.49, E13.618-E13.638, E13.649-E13.8, G32.89, G70.00-G72.3, G72.81-G73.7, G96.8-G96.9, G98.0-G98.8, G99.8, M33.00-M33.19, M33.90-M33.99, M36.0

M33.09 Juvenile dermatopolymyositis with other organ involvement 🗝

● **M33.1 Other dermatopolymyositis**

M33.10 Other dermatopolymyositis, organ involvement unspecified 🗝

M33.11 Other dermatopolymyositis with respiratory involvement 🗝

M33.12 Other dermatopolymyositis with myopathy 🗝
CC when PDx is its own CC
Ex: See M33.02

M33.19 Other dermatopolymyositis with other organ involvement 🗝

● **M33.2 Polymyositis**

M33.20 Polymyositis, organ involvement unspecified 🗝
Ex: M33.20-M33.29

M33.21 Polymyositis with respiratory involvement 🗝
Ex: M33.20-M33.29

M33.22 Polymyositis with myopathy 🗝
CC when PDx is its own CC
Ex: E08.40-E08.49, E08.618-E08.638, E08.649-E08.8, E09.40-E09.49, E09.618-E09.638, E09.649-E09.8, E10.40-E10.49, E10.618-E10.638, E10.649, E10.69-E10.8, E11.40-E11.49, E11.618-E11.638, E11.649, E11.69-E11.8, E13.40-E13.49, E13.618-E13.638, E13.649-E13.8, G32.89, G70.00-G72.3, G72.81-G73.7, G96.8-G96.9, G98.0-G98.8, G99.8, M33.20-M33.29

M33.29 Polymyositis with other organ involvement 🗝
Ex: M33.20-M33.29

● **M33.9 Dermatopolymyositis, unspecified**

M33.90 Dermatopolymyositis, unspecified, organ involvement unspecified 🗝

M33.91 Dermatopolymyositis, unspecified with respiratory involvement 🗝

M33.92 Dermatopolymyositis, unspecified with myopathy 🗝
CC when PDx is its own CC
Ex: See M33.02

M33.99 Dermatopolymyositis, unspecified with other organ involvement 🗝

● **M34 Systemic sclerosis [scleroderma]**

Excludes1   circumscribed scleroderma (L94.0)
neonatal scleroderma (P83.8)

M34.0 Progressive systemic sclerosis

M34.1 CR(E)ST syndrome
Combination of calcinosis, Raynaud's phenomenon, esophageal dysfunction, sclerodactyly, telangiectasia

M34.2 Systemic sclerosis induced by drug and chemical

Code first poisoning due to drug or toxin, if applicable (T36-T65 with fifth or sixth character 1-4 or 6)

Use additional code for adverse effect, if applicable, to identify drug (T36-T50 with fifth or sixth character 5)

Item 13-8 Polymyalgia rheumatica is a syndrome characterized by aching and morning stiffness and is related to aging and hereditary predisposition.

● **M34.8 Other forms of systemic sclerosis**

M34.81 Systemic sclerosis with lung involvement 🗝
CC when PDx is its own CC
Ex: No exclusions

M34.82 Systemic sclerosis with myopathy 🗝
CC when PDx is its own CC
Ex: E08.40-E08.49, E08.618-E08.638, E08.649-E08.8, E09.40-E09.49, E09.618-E09.638, E09.649-E09.8, E10.40-E10.49, E10.618-E10.638, E10.649, E10.69-E10.8, E11.40-E11.49, E11.618-E11.638, E11.649, E11.69-E11.8, E13.40-E13.49, E13.618-E13.638, E13.649-E13.8, G32.89, G70.00-G72.3, G72.81-G73.7, G96.8-G96.9, G98.0-G98.8, G99.8

M34.83 Systemic sclerosis with polyneuropathy

M34.89 Other systemic sclerosis

M34.9 Systemic sclerosis, unspecified

● **M35 Other systemic involvement of connective tissue**

Excludes1   reactive perforating collagenosis (L87.1)

● **M35.0 Sicca syndrome [Sjögren]**

M35.00 Sicca syndrome, unspecified

M35.01 Sicca syndrome with keratoconjunctivitis

M35.02 Sicca syndrome with lung involvement

M35.03 Sicca syndrome with myopathy 🗝
CC when PDx is its own CC
Ex: See M34.82

M35.04 Sicca syndrome with tubulo-interstitial nephropathy
Renal tubular acidosis in sicca syndrome

M35.09 Sicca syndrome with other organ involvement

M35.1 Other overlap syndromes
Mixed connective tissue disease

Excludes1   polyangiitis overlap syndrome (M30.8)

Ex: G72.41-G72.49, M35.1, M35.5, M35.8

M35.2 Behçet's disease 🗝
Ex: A02.23, A17.9, A18.02, A18.09, A18.82, A18.84, A18.89, A39.83-A39.84, A54.40, A54.42-A54.43, A54.82, A54.84, A54.89-A54.9, B06.82, M00.00, M00.011-M02.30, M02.319, M02.329, M02.339, M02.349, M02.359, M02.369, M02.379, M02.38-M02.9, M05.40-M05.59, M05.70-M07.69, M11.00-M15.0, M15.3-M15.9, M16.2-M16.9, M17.2-M17.9, M18.2-M18.9, M19.111-M19.93, M24.10-M24.176, M25.00, M25.08-M25.18, M25.40-M25.676, M25.80-M25.9, M35.2, M36.1-M36.4, R29.4

M35.3 Polymyalgia rheumatica

Excludes1   polymyalgia rheumatica with giant cell arteritis (M31.5)

M35.4 Diffuse (eosinophilic) fasciitis

M35.5 Multifocal fibrosclerosis 🗝
Ex: G72.41-G72.49, M35.1, M35.5, M35.8

M35.6 Relapsing panniculitis [Weber-Christian]

Excludes1   lupus panniculitis (L93.2)
panniculitis NOS (M79.3-)

M35.7 Hypermobility syndrome
Familial ligamentous laxity

Excludes1   Ehlers-Danlos syndrome (Q79.6)
ligamentous laxity, NOS (M24.2-)

M35.8 Other specified systemic involvement of connective tissue 🗝
Ex: G72.41-G72.49, M35.1, M35.5, M35.8

M35.9 Systemic involvement of connective tissue, unspecified
Autoimmune disease (systemic) NOS
Collagen (vascular) disease NOS

◀ New   ◀ Revised   ~~deleted~~ Deleted   Excludes 1   Excludes 2   Includes   Use additional   Code first   Code also   Unspecified

OGCR Official Guidelines   ● Unacceptable Principal Diagnosis   X Assign placeholder X   🗝 Use Additional Character(s)   ▸ Manifestation Code   **Coding Clinic**

● **M36** **Systemic disorders of connective tissue in diseases classified elsewhere**

　　Excludes2　arthropathies in diseases classified elsewhere (M14.-)

▶ *M36.0*　*Dermato(poly)myositis in neoplastic disease* 🅖

　　　　Code first underlying neoplasm (C00-D49)

　　　　Ⓔ🅧 M33.00-M33.19, M33.90-M33.99, M36.0

▶ *M36.1*　*Arthropathy in neoplastic disease*

　　　　Code first underlying neoplasm, such as:
　　　　　leukemia (C91-C95)
　　　　　malignant histiocytosis (C96.A)
　　　　　multiple myeloma (C90.0)

▶ *M36.2*　*Hemophilic arthropathy*

　　　　Hemarthrosis in hemophilic arthropathy

　　　　Code first underlying disease, such as:
　　　　　factor VIII deficiency (D66)
　　　　　　with vascular defect (D68.0)
　　　　　factor IX deficiency (D67)
　　　　　hemophilia (classical) (D66)
　　　　　hemophilia B (D67)
　　　　　hemophilia C (D68.1)

▶ *M36.3*　*Arthropathy in other blood disorders*

▶ *M36.4*　*Arthropathy in hypersensitivity reactions classified elsewhere*

　　　　Code first underlying disease, such as:
　　　　　Henoch (-Schönlein) purpura (D69.0)
　　　　　serum sickness (T80.6-)

▶ *M36.8*　*Systemic disorders of connective tissue in other diseases classified elsewhere*

　　　　Code first underlying disease, such as:
　　　　　alkaptonuria (E70.2)
　　　　　hypogammaglobulinemia (D80.-)
　　　　　ochronosis (E70.2)

DORSOPATHIES (M40-M54)

DEFORMING DORSOPATHIES (M40-M43)

● **M40**　**Kyphosis and lordosis**

　　Excludes1　congenital kyphosis and lordosis (Q76.4)
　　　　　　kyphoscoliosis (M41.-)
　　　　　　postprocedural kyphosis and lordosis (M96.-)

● **M40.0**　Postural kyphosis

　　Excludes1　osteochondrosis of spine (M42.-)

　　M40.00　**Postural kyphosis, site unspecified**

　　M40.03　**Postural kyphosis, cervicothoracic region**

　　M40.04　**Postural kyphosis, thoracic region**

　　M40.05　**Postural kyphosis, thoracolumbar region**

● **M40.1**　Other secondary kyphosis

　　M40.10　**Other secondary kyphosis, site unspecified**

　　M40.12　**Other secondary kyphosis, cervical region**

　　M40.13　**Other secondary kyphosis, cervicothoracic region**

　　M40.14　**Other secondary kyphosis, thoracic region**

　　M40.15　**Other secondary kyphosis, thoracolumbar region**

● **M40.2**　Other and unspecified kyphosis

● **M40.20**　Unspecified kyphosis

　　M40.202　Unspecified kyphosis, cervical region

　　M40.203　Unspecified kyphosis, cervicothoracic region

　　M40.204　Unspecified kyphosis, thoracic region

　　M40.205　Unspecified kyphosis, thoracolumbar region

　　M40.209　Unspecified kyphosis, site unspecified

● **M40.29**　Other kyphosis

　　M40.292　Other kyphosis, cervical region

　　M40.293　Other kyphosis, cervicothoracic region

　　M40.294　Other kyphosis, thoracic region

　　M40.295　Other kyphosis, thoracolumbar region

　　M40.299　Other kyphosis, site unspecified

● **M40.3**　Flatback syndrome

　　M40.30　Flatback syndrome, site unspecified

　　M40.35　Flatback syndrome, thoracolumbar region

　　M40.36　Flatback syndrome, lumbar region

　　M40.37　Flatback syndrome, lumbosacral region

● **M40.4**　Postural lordosis

　　Abnormal increase in the normal curvature of the lumbar spine (sway back)

　　　Acquired lordosis

　　M40.40　Postural lordosis, site unspecified

　　M40.45　Postural lordosis, thoracolumbar region

　　M40.46　Postural lordosis, lumbar region

　　M40.47　Postural lordosis, lumbosacral region

● **M40.5**　Lordosis, unspecified

　　M40.50　Lordosis, unspecified, site unspecified

　　M40.55　Lordosis, unspecified, thoracolumbar region

　　M40.56　Lordosis, unspecified, lumbar region

　　M40.57　Lordosis, unspecified, lumbosacral region

● **M41**　**Scoliosis**

　　Includes　kyphoscoliosis

　　Excludes1　congenital scoliosis NOS (Q67.5)
　　　　　　congenital scoliosis due to bony malformation (Q76.3)
　　　　　　postural congenital scoliosis (Q67.5)
　　　　　　kyphoscoliotic heart disease (I27.1)
　　　　　　postprocedural scoliosis (M96.-)

● **M41.0**　Infantile idiopathic scoliosis

　　M41.00　Infantile idiopathic scoliosis, site unspecified

　　M41.02　Infantile idiopathic scoliosis, cervical region

　　M41.03　Infantile idiopathic scoliosis, cervicothoracic region

　　M41.04　Infantile idiopathic scoliosis, thoracic region

　　M41.05　Infantile idiopathic scoliosis, thoracolumbar region

　　M41.06　Infantile idiopathic scoliosis, lumbar region

　　M41.07　Infantile idiopathic scoliosis, lumbosacral region

　　M41.08　Infantile idiopathic scoliosis, sacral and sacrococcygeal region

● **M41.1**　Juvenile and adolescent idiopathic scoliosis

● **M41.11**　Juvenile idiopathic scoliosis

　　M41.112　Juvenile idiopathic scoliosis, cervical region

　　M41.113　Juvenile idiopathic scoliosis, cervicothoracic region

　　M41.114　Juvenile idiopathic scoliosis, thoracic region

　　M41.115　Juvenile idiopathic scoliosis, thoracolumbar region

Item 13-9 Kyphosis is an abnormal curvature of the spine. **Senile kyphosis** is a result of disc degeneration causing ossification (turning to bone). **Adolescent** or **juvenile** kyphosis is also known as **Scheuermann's disease,** a condition in which the discs of the lower thoracic spine herniate, causing the disc space to narrow and the spine to tilt forward. This condition is attributed to poor posture. Lordosis or swayback is an abnormal curvature of the spine resulting in an inward curve of the lumbar spine just above the buttocks. Scoliosis causes a sideways curve to the spine. The curves are S- or C-shaped, and it is most commonly acquired in late childhood and early teen years, when growth is fast.

N Newborn Age: 0　　**P** Pediatric Age: 0–17　　**M** Maternity DX: 12–55　　**A** Adult Age: 15–124　　♀ Females Only　　♂ Males Only

🅖 Complication\Comorbidity　　🅖 Major C\C　　Ⓔ🅧 CC/MCC Exclusions　　🅟 Present on Admission Requirement　　🅗 Hospital-Acquired Condition

1115

CHAPTER 13 (M00-M99)

      M41.116   Juvenile idiopathic scoliosis, lumbar region

      M41.117   Juvenile idiopathic scoliosis, lumbosacral region

      M41.119   Juvenile idiopathic scoliosis, site unspecified

● M41.12   Adolescent scoliosis

      M41.122   Adolescent idiopathic scoliosis, cervical region

      M41.123   Adolescent idiopathic scoliosis, cervicothoracic region

      M41.124   Adolescent idiopathic scoliosis, thoracic region

      M41.125   Adolescent idiopathic scoliosis, thoracolumbar region

      M41.126   Adolescent idiopathic scoliosis, lumbar region

      M41.127   Adolescent idiopathic scoliosis, lumbosacral region

      M41.129   Adolescent idiopathic scoliosis, site unspecified

● M41.2   Other idiopathic scoliosis

    M41.20   Other idiopathic scoliosis, site unspecified

    M41.22   Other idiopathic scoliosis, cervical region

    M41.23   Other idiopathic scoliosis, cervicothoracic region

    M41.24   Other idiopathic scoliosis, thoracic region

    M41.25   Other idiopathic scoliosis, thoracolumbar region

    M41.26   Other idiopathic scoliosis, lumbar region

    M41.27   Other idiopathic scoliosis, lumbosacral region

● M41.3   Thoracogenic scoliosis

    M41.30   Thoracogenic scoliosis, site unspecified

    M41.34   Thoracogenic scoliosis, thoracic region

    M41.35   Thoracogenic scoliosis, thoracolumbar region

● M41.4   Neuromuscular scoliosis

    Scoliosis secondary to cerebral palsy, Friedreich's ataxia, poliomyelitis and other neuromuscular disorders

    Code also underlying condition

    M41.40   Neuromuscular scoliosis, site unspecified

    M41.41   Neuromuscular scoliosis, occipito-atlanto-axial region

    M41.42   Neuromuscular scoliosis, cervical region

    M41.43   Neuromuscular scoliosis, cervicothoracic region

    M41.44   Neuromuscular scoliosis, thoracic region

    M41.45   Neuromuscular scoliosis, thoracolumbar region

    M41.46   Neuromuscular scoliosis, lumbar region

    M41.47   Neuromuscular scoliosis, lumbosacral region

● M41.5   Other secondary scoliosis

    M41.50   Other secondary scoliosis, site unspecified

    M41.52   Other secondary scoliosis, cervical region

    M41.53   Other secondary scoliosis, cervicothoracic region

    M41.54   Other secondary scoliosis, thoracic region

    M41.55   Other secondary scoliosis, thoracolumbar region

    M41.56   Other secondary scoliosis, lumbar region

    M41.57   Other secondary scoliosis, lumbosacral region

● M41.8   Other forms of scoliosis

    M41.80   Other forms of scoliosis, site unspecified

    M41.82   Other forms of scoliosis, cervical region

    M41.83   Other forms of scoliosis, cervicothoracic region

    M41.84   Other forms of scoliosis, thoracic region

    M41.85   Other forms of scoliosis, thoracolumbar region

    M41.86   Other forms of scoliosis, lumbar region

    M41.87   Other forms of scoliosis, lumbosacral region

  M41.9   Scoliosis, unspecified

● M42   Spinal osteochondrosis

● M42.0   Juvenile osteochondrosis of spine

    Calvé's disease

    Scheuermann's disease

    Excludes1   postural kyphosis (M40.0)

    M42.00   Juvenile osteochondrosis of spine, site unspecified

    M42.01   Juvenile osteochondrosis of spine, occipito-atlanto-axial region

    M42.02   Juvenile osteochondrosis of spine, cervical region

    M42.03   Juvenile osteochondrosis of spine, cervicothoracic region

    M42.04   Juvenile osteochondrosis of spine, thoracic region

    M42.05   Juvenile osteochondrosis of spine, thoracolumbar region

    M42.06   Juvenile osteochondrosis of spine, lumbar region

    M42.07   Juvenile osteochondrosis of spine, lumbosacral region

    M42.08   Juvenile osteochondrosis of spine, sacral and sacrococcygeal region

    M42.09   Juvenile osteochondrosis of spine, multiple sites in spine

● M42.1   Adult osteochondrosis of spine

    M42.10   Adult osteochondrosis of spine, site unspecified   A

    M42.11   Adult osteochondrosis of spine, occipitoatlanto-axial region   A

    M42.12   Adult osteochondrosis of spine, cervical region   A

    M42.13   Adult osteochondrosis of spine, cervicothoracic region   A

    M42.14   Adult osteochondrosis of spine, thoracic region   A

    M42.15   Adult osteochondrosis of spine, thoracolumbar region   A

    M42.16   Adult osteochondrosis of spine, lumbar region   A

    M42.17   Adult osteochondrosis of spine, lumbosacral region   A

    M42.18   Adult osteochondrosis of spine, sacral and sacrococcygeal region   A

    M42.19   Adult osteochondrosis of spine, multiple sites in spine   A

  M42.9   Spinal osteochondrosis, unspecified

● M43   Other deforming dorsopathies

    Excludes1   congenital spondylolysis and spondylolisthesis (Q76.2)

        hemivertebra (Q76.3-Q76.4)

        Klippel-Feil syndrome (Q76.1)

        lumbarization and sacralization (Q76.4)

        platyspondylisis (Q76.4)

        spina bifida occulta (Q76.0)

        spinal curvature in osteoporosis (M80.-) ◄|||

        spinal curvature in Paget's disease of bone [osteitis deformans] (M88.-)

● M43.0   Spondylolysis

    Excludes1   congenital spondylolysis (Q76.2)

        spondylolisthesis (M43.1)

    M43.00   Spondylolysis, site unspecified

    M43.01   Spondylolysis, occipito-atlanto-axial region

    M43.02   Spondylolysis, cervical region

    M43.03   Spondylolysis, cervicothoracic region

    M43.04   Spondylolysis, thoracic region

    M43.05   Spondylolysis, thoracolumbar region

    M43.06   Spondylolysis, lumbar region

    M43.07   Spondylolysis, lumbosacral region

    M43.08   Spondylolysis, sacral and sacrococcygeal region

    M43.09   Spondylolysis, multiple sites in spine

◄ New   ◄||| Revised   ~~deleted~~ Deleted   Excludes 1   Excludes 2   Includes   Use additional   Code first   Code also   Unspecified

OGCR Official Guidelines   ● Unacceptable Principal Diagnosis   X Assign placeholder X   ● Use Additional Character(s)   ▌ Manifestation Code   **Coding Clinic**

Item 13–10 **Spondylolisthesis** is a condition caused by the slipping forward of one disc over another.

- M43.1 Spondylolisthesis
  - **Excludes1** acute traumatic of lumbosacral region (S33.1)
    acute traumatic of sites other than lumbosacral - code to Fracture, vertebra, by region
    congenital spondylolisthesis (Q76.2)
  - M43.10 Spondylolisthesis, site unspecified
  - M43.11 Spondylolisthesis, occipito-atlanto-axial region
  - M43.12 Spondylolisthesis, cervical region
  - M43.13 Spondylolisthesis, cervicothoracic region
  - M43.14 Spondylolisthesis, thoracic region
  - M43.15 Spondylolisthesis, thoracolumbar region
  - M43.16 Spondylolisthesis, lumbar region
  - M43.17 Spondylolisthesis, lumbosacral region
  - M43.18 Spondylolisthesis, sacral and sacrococcygeal region
  - M43.19 Spondylolisthesis, multiple sites in spine
- M43.2 Fusion of spine
  Ankylosis of spinal joint
  - **Excludes1** ankylosing spondylitis (M45.0-)
    congenital fusion of spine (Q76.4)
  - **Excludes2** arthrodesis status (Z98.1)
    pseudoarthrosis after fusion or arthrodesis (M96.0)
  - M43.20 Fusion of spine, site unspecified
  - M43.21 Fusion of spine, occipito-atlanto-axial region
  - M43.22 Fusion of spine, cervical region
  - M43.23 Fusion of spine, cervicothoracic region
  - M43.24 Fusion of spine, thoracic region
  - M43.25 Fusion of spine, thoracolumbar region
  - M43.26 Fusion of spine, lumbar region
  - M43.27 Fusion of spine, lumbosacral region
  - M43.28 Fusion of spine, sacral and sacrococcygeal region
- M43.3 Recurrent atlantoaxial dislocation with myelopathy
- M43.4 Other recurrent atlantoaxial dislocation
- M43.5 Other recurrent vertebral dislocation
  - **Excludes1** biomechanical lesions NEC (M99.-)
  - M43.5X Other recurrent vertebral dislocation
    - M43.5X2 Other recurrent vertebral dislocation, cervical region
    - M43.5X3 Other recurrent vertebral dislocation, cervicothoracic region
    - M43.5X4 Other recurrent vertebral dislocation, thoracic region
    - M43.5X5 Other recurrent vertebral dislocation, thoracolumbar region
    - M43.5X6 Other recurrent vertebral dislocation, lumbar region
    - M43.5X7 Other recurrent vertebral dislocation, lumbosacral region
    - M43.5X8 Other recurrent vertebral dislocation, sacral and sacrococcygeal region
    - M43.5X9 Other recurrent vertebral dislocation, site unspecified
- M43.6 Torticollis
  - **Excludes1** congenital (sternomastoid) torticollis (Q68.0)
    current injury - see Injury, of spine, by body region ocular torticollis (R29.891)
    psychogenic torticollis (F45.8)
    spasmodic torticollis (G24.3)
    torticollis due to birth injury (P15.2)

- M43.8 Other specified deforming dorsopathies
  - **Excludes2** kyphosis and lordosis (M40.-)
    scoliosis (M41.-)
  - M43.8X Other specified deforming dorsopathies
    - M43.8X1 Other specified deforming dorsopathies, occipito-atlanto-axial region
    - M43.8X2 Other specified deforming dorsopathies, cervical region
    - M43.8X3 Other specified deforming dorsopathies, cervicothoracic region
    - M43.8X4 Other specified deforming dorsopathies, thoracic region
    - M43.8X5 Other specified deforming dorsopathies, thoracolumbar region
    - M43.8X6 Other specified deforming dorsopathies, lumbar region
    - M43.8X7 Other specified deforming dorsopathies, lumbosacral region
    - M43.8X8 Other specified deforming dorsopathies, sacral and sacrococcygeal region
    - M43.8X9 Other specified deforming dorsopathies, site unspecified
  - M43.9 Deforming dorsopathy, unspecified
    Curvature of spine NOS

SPONDYLOPATHIES (M45-M49)

- M45 Ankylosing spondylitis
  Rheumatoid arthritis of spine
  - **Excludes1** arthropathy in Reiter's disease (M02.3-)
    juvenile (ankylosing) spondylitis (M08.1)
  - **Excludes2** Behçet's disease (M35.2)
  - M45.0 Ankylosing spondylitis of multiple sites in spine
  - M45.1 Ankylosing spondylitis of occipito-atlanto-axial region
  - M45.2 Ankylosing spondylitis of cervical region
  - M45.3 Ankylosing spondylitis of cervicothoracic region
  - M45.4 Ankylosing spondylitis of thoracic region
  - M45.5 Ankylosing spondylitis of thoracolumbar region
  - M45.6 Ankylosing spondylitis lumbar region
  - M45.7 Ankylosing spondylitis of lumbosacral region
  - M45.8 Ankylosing spondylitis sacral and sacrococcygeal region
  - M45.9 Ankylosing spondylitis of unspecified sites in spine
- M46 Other inflammatory spondylopathies
  - M46.0 Spinal enthesopathy
    Disorder of ligamentous or muscular attachments of spine
    - M46.00 Spinal enthesopathy, site unspecified
    - M46.01 Spinal enthesopathy, occipito-atlanto-axial region
    - M46.02 Spinal enthesopathy, cervical region
    - M46.03 Spinal enthesopathy, cervicothoracic region
    - M46.04 Spinal enthesopathy, thoracic region
    - M46.05 Spinal enthesopathy, thoracolumbar region
    - M46.06 Spinal enthesopathy, lumbar region
    - M46.07 Spinal enthesopathy, lumbosacral region
    - M46.08 Spinal enthesopathy, sacral and sacrococcygeal region
    - M46.09 Spinal enthesopathy, multiple sites in spine
  - M46.1 Sacroiliitis, not elsewhere classified

CHAPTER 13 (M00-M99)

● **M46.2 Osteomyelitis of vertebra**
Ex: For category M46.2 CC codes: A02.24, A17.9, A18.03, A18.09, A18.82, A18.84, A18.89, M46.20-M46.39, M86.00-M86.9

    M46.20   Osteomyelitis of vertebra, site unspecified 🔖

    M46.21   Osteomyelitis of vertebra, occipito-atlanto-axial region 🔖

    M46.22   Osteomyelitis of vertebra, cervical region 🔖

    M46.23   Osteomyelitis of vertebra, cervicothoracic region 🔖

    M46.24   Osteomyelitis of vertebra, thoracic region 🔖

    M46.25   Osteomyelitis of vertebra, thoracolumbar region 🔖

    M46.26   Osteomyelitis of vertebra, lumbar region 🔖

    M46.27   Osteomyelitis of vertebra, lumbosacral region 🔖

    M46.28   Osteomyelitis of vertebra, sacral and sacrococcygeal region 🔖

● **M46.3 Infection of intervertebral disc (pyogenic)**
Use additional code (B95-B97) to identify infectious agent
Ex: For category M46.3 CC codes: A17.9, A18.01, A18.03, A18.09, A18.82, A18.84, A18.89, M46.20-M46.39, M86.00-M86.9

    M46.30   Infection of intervertebral disc (pyogenic), site unspecified 🔖

    M46.31   Infection of intervertebral disc (pyogenic), occipito-atlanto-axial region 🔖

    M46.32   Infection of intervertebral disc (pyogenic), cervical region 🔖

    M46.33   Infection of intervertebral disc (pyogenic), cervicothoracic region 🔖

    M46.34   Infection of intervertebral disc (pyogenic), thoracic region 🔖

    M46.35   Infection of intervertebral disc (pyogenic), thoracolumbar region 🔖

    M46.36   Infection of intervertebral disc (pyogenic), lumbar region 🔖

    M46.37   Infection of intervertebral disc (pyogenic), lumbosacral region 🔖

    M46.38   Infection of intervertebral disc (pyogenic), sacral and sacrococcygeal region 🔖

    M46.39   Infection of intervertebral disc (pyogenic), multiple sites in spine 🔖

● **M46.4 Discitis, unspecified**

    M46.40   Discitis, unspecified, site unspecified

    M46.41   Discitis, unspecified, occipito-atlanto-axial region

    M46.42   Discitis, unspecified, cervical region

    M46.43   Discitis, unspecified, cervicothoracic region

    M46.44   Discitis, unspecified, thoracic region

    M46.45   Discitis, unspecified, thoracolumbar region

    M46.46   Discitis, unspecified, lumbar region

    M46.47   Discitis, unspecified, lumbosacral region

    M46.48   Discitis, unspecified, sacral and sacrococcygeal region

    M46.49   Discitis, unspecified, multiple sites in spine

● **M46.5 Other infective spondylopathies**

    M46.50   Other infective spondylopathies, site unspecified

    M46.51   Other infective spondylopathies, occipitoatlanto-axial region

    M46.52   Other infective spondylopathies, cervical region

    M46.53   Other infective spondylopathies, cervicothoracic region

    M46.54   Other infective spondylopathies, thoracic region

    M46.55   Other infective spondylopathies, thoracolumbar region

    M46.56   Other infective spondylopathies, lumbar region

    M46.57   Other infective spondylopathies, lumbosacral region

    M46.58   Other infective spondylopathies, sacral and sacrococcygeal region

    M46.59   Other infective spondylopathies, multiple sites in spine

● **M46.8 Other specified inflammatory spondylopathies**

    M46.80   Other specified inflammatory spondylopathies, site unspecified

    M46.81   Other specified inflammatory spondylopathies, occipito-atlanto-axial region

    M46.82   Other specified inflammatory spondylopathies, cervical region

    M46.83   Other specified inflammatory spondylopathies, cervicothoracic region

    M46.84   Other specified inflammatory spondylopathies, thoracic region

    M46.85   Other specified inflammatory spondylopathies, thoracolumbar region

    M46.86   Other specified inflammatory spondylopathies, lumbar region

    M46.87   Other specified inflammatory spondylopathies, lumbosacral region

    M46.88   Other specified inflammatory spondylopathies, sacral and sacrococcygeal region

    M46.89   Other specified inflammatory spondylopathies, multiple sites in spine

● **M46.9 Unspecified inflammatory spondylopathy**

    M46.90   Unspecified inflammatory spondylopathy, site unspecified

    M46.91   Unspecified inflammatory spondylopathy, occipito-atlanto-axial region

    M46.92   Unspecified inflammatory spondylopathy, cervical region

    M46.93   Unspecified inflammatory spondylopathy, cervicothoracic region

    M46.94   Unspecified inflammatory spondylopathy, thoracic region

    M46.95   Unspecified inflammatory spondylopathy, thoracolumbar region

    M46.96   Unspecified inflammatory spondylopathy, lumbar region

    M46.97   Unspecified inflammatory spondylopathy, lumbosacral region

    M46.98   Unspecified inflammatory spondylopathy, sacral and sacrococcygeal region

    M46.99   Unspecified inflammatory spondylopathy, multiple sites in spine

● **M47 Spondylosis**
Includes   arthrosis or osteoarthritis of spine
degeneration of facet joints

● **M47.0 Anterior spinal and vertebral artery compression syndromes**
Ex: For category M47.0 CC codes: M47.011-M47.029, M47.11-M47.13, M47.21-M47.23, M47.811-M47.813, M47.891-M47.893

● **M47.01 Anterior spinal artery compression syndromes**

    M47.011   Anterior spinal artery compression syndromes, occipito-atlanto-axial region 🔖

    M47.012   Anterior spinal artery compression syndromes, cervical region 🔖

    M47.013   Anterior spinal artery compression syndromes, cervicothoracic region 🔖

◀ New   ◀ Revised   ~~deleted~~ Deleted   Excludes 1   Excludes 2   Includes   Use additional   Code first   Code also   Unspecified
OGCR Official Guidelines   ● Unacceptable Principal Diagnosis   X Assign placeholder X   ● Use Additional Character(s)   ▶ Manifestation Code   **Coding Clinic**

M47.014   Anterior spinal artery compression syndromes, thoracic region 🔹

M47.015   Anterior spinal artery compression syndromes, thoracolumbar region 🔹

M47.016   Anterior spinal artery compression syndromes, lumbar region 🔹

M47.019   Anterior spinal artery compression syndromes, site unspecified 🔹

● M47.02   Vertebral artery compression syndromes

M47.021   Vertebral artery compression syndromes, occipito-atlanto-axial region 🔹

M47.022   Vertebral artery compression syndromes, cervical region 🔹

M47.029   Vertebral artery compression syndromes, site unspecified 🔹

● M47.1   Other spondylosis with myelopathy
Spondylogenic compression of spinal cord

Excludes1   vertebral subluxation (M43.3-M43.59)

M47.10   Other spondylosis with myelopathy, site unspecified 🔹
Ⓔ M25.78, M47.011-M47.9, M48.10-M48.38, M48.9

M47.11   Other spondylosis with myelopathy, occipito-atlanto-axial region 🔹
Ⓔ See M47.0

M47.12   Other spondylosis with myelopathy, cervical region 🔹
Ⓔ See M47.0

M47.13   Other spondylosis with myelopathy, cervicothoracic region 🔹
Ⓔ See M47.0

M47.14   Other spondylosis with myelopathy, thoracic region 🔹
Ⓔ M47.14-M47.15

M47.15   Other spondylosis with myelopathy, thoracolumbar region 🔹
Ⓔ M47.14-M47.15

M47.16   Other spondylosis with myelopathy, lumbar region 🔹
Ⓔ M46.40, M46.46-M46.49, M47.16-M47.18, M47.26-M47.28, M47.816-M47.818, M47.896-M47.898, M51.06-M51.07, M51.26-M51.27, M51.36-M51.37, M51.46-M51.47, M51.86-M51.9

~~M47.17   Other spondylosis with myelopathy, lumbosacral region~~

~~M47.18   Other spondylosis with myelopathy, sacral and sacrococcygeal region~~

● M47.2   Other spondylosis with radiculopathy

M47.20   Other spondylosis with radiculopathy, site unspecified

M47.21   Other spondylosis with radiculopathy, occipito-atlanto-axial region

M47.22   Other spondylosis with radiculopathy, cervical region

M47.23   Other spondylosis with radiculopathy, cervicothoracic region

M47.24   Other spondylosis with radiculopathy, thoracic region

M47.25   Other spondylosis with radiculopathy, thoracolumbar region

M47.26   Other spondylosis with radiculopathy, lumbar region

M47.27   Other spondylosis with radiculopathy, lumbosacral region

M47.28   Other spondylosis with radiculopathy, sacral and sacrococcygeal region

● M47.8   Other spondylosis

● M47.81   Spondylosis without myelopathy or radiculopathy

M47.811   Spondylosis without myelopathy or radiculopathy, occipito-atlanto-axial region

M47.812   Spondylosis without myelopathy or radiculopathy, cervical region

M47.813   Spondylosis without myelopathy or radiculopathy, cervicothoracic region

M47.814   Spondylosis without myelopathy or radiculopathy, thoracic region

M47.815   Spondylosis without myelopathy or radiculopathy, thoracolumbar region

M47.816   Spondylosis without myelopathy or radiculopathy, lumbar region

M47.817   Spondylosis without myelopathy or radiculopathy, lumbosacral region

M47.818   Spondylosis without myelopathy or radiculopathy, sacral and sacrococcygeal region

M47.819   Spondylosis without myelopathy or radiculopathy, site unspecified

● M47.89   Other spondylosis

M47.891   Other spondylosis, occipito-atlanto-axial region

M47.892   Other spondylosis, cervical region

M47.893   Other spondylosis, cervicothoracic region

M47.894   Other spondylosis, thoracic region

M47.895   Other spondylosis, thoracolumbar region

M47.896   Other spondylosis, lumbar region

M47.897   Other spondylosis, lumbosacral region

M47.898   Other spondylosis, sacral and sacrococcygeal region

M47.899   Other spondylosis, site unspecified

M47.9   Spondylosis, unspecified

● M48   Other spondylopathies

● M48.0   Spinal stenosis
Caudal stenosis

M48.00   Spinal stenosis, site unspecified

M48.01   Spinal stenosis, occipito-atlanto-axial region

M48.02   Spinal stenosis, cervical region

M48.03   Spinal stenosis, cervicothoracic region

M48.04   Spinal stenosis, thoracic region

M48.05   Spinal stenosis, thoracolumbar region

M48.06   Spinal stenosis, lumbar region

M48.07   Spinal stenosis, lumbosacral region

M48.08   Spinal stenosis, sacral and sacrococcygeal region

● M48.1   Ankylosing hyperostosis [Forestier]
Diffuse idiopathic skeletal hyperostosis [DISH]

M48.10   Ankylosing hyperostosis [Forestier], site unspecified

M48.11   Ankylosing hyperostosis [Forestier], occipito-atlanto-axial region

M48.12   Ankylosing hyperostosis [Forestier], cervical region

M48.13   Ankylosing hyperostosis [Forestier], cervicothoracic region

M48.14   Ankylosing hyperostosis [Forestier], thoracic region

M48.15   Ankylosing hyperostosis [Forestier], thoracolumbar region

N   Newborn Age: 0   P   Pediatric Age: 0–17   M   Maternity DX: 12–55   A   Adult Age: 15–124   ♀   Females Only   ♂   Males Only

🔹 Complication\Comorbidity   🔹 Major C\C   Ⓔ CC/MCC Exclusions   🔹 Present on Admission Requirement   🔹 Hospital-Acquired Condition

1119

M48.16   Ankylosing hyperostosis [Forestier], lumbar region

M48.17   Ankylosing hyperostosis [Forestier], lumbosacral region

M48.18   Ankylosing hyperostosis [Forestier], sacral and sacrococcygeal region

M48.19   Ankylosing hyperostosis [Forestier], multiple sites in spine

● M48.2   Kissing spine

M48.20   Kissing spine, site unspecified

M48.21   Kissing spine, occipito-atlanto-axial region

M48.22   Kissing spine, cervical region

M48.23   Kissing spine, cervicothoracic region

M48.24   Kissing spine, thoracic region

M48.25   Kissing spine, thoracolumbar region

M48.26   Kissing spine, lumbar region

M48.27   Kissing spine, lumbosacral region

● M48.3   Traumatic spondylopathy

    Ⓔⓧ For category M48.3 CC codes: M48.30-M48.38

M48.30   Traumatic spondylopathy, site unspecified ✎

M48.31   Traumatic spondylopathy, occipito-atlanto-axial region ✎

M48.32   Traumatic spondylopathy, cervical region ✎

M48.33   Traumatic spondylopathy, cervicothoracic region ✎

M48.34   Traumatic spondylopathy, thoracic region ✎

M48.35   Traumatic spondylopathy, thoracolumbar region ✎

M48.36   Traumatic spondylopathy, lumbar region ✎

M48.37   Traumatic spondylopathy, lumbosacral region ✎

M48.38   Traumatic spondylopathy, sacral and sacrococcygeal region ✎

● M48.4   Fatigue fracture of vertebra

    Stress fracture of vertebra

    Excludes1   pathological fracture NOS (M84.4-)

              pathological fracture of vertebra due to neoplasm (M84.58)

              pathological fracture of vertebra due to other diagnosis (M84.68)

              pathological fracture of vertebra due to osteoporosis (M80.-)

              traumatic fracture of vertebrae (S12.0-S12.3-, S22.0-, S32.0-)

The appropriate 7th character is to be added to each code from subcategory M48.4:

A	initial encounter for fracture
D	subsequent encounter for fracture with routine healing
G	subsequent encounter for fracture with delayed healing
S	sequela of fracture

X ● M48.40   Fatigue fracture of vertebra, site unspecified

X ● M48.41   Fatigue fracture of vertebra, occipitoatlanto-axial region

X ● M48.42   Fatigue fracture of vertebra, cervical region

X ● M48.43   Fatigue fracture of vertebra, cervicothoracic region

X ● M48.44   Fatigue fracture of vertebra, thoracic region

X ● M48.45   Fatigue fracture of vertebra, thoracolumbar region

X ● M48.46   Fatigue fracture of vertebra, lumbar region

X ● M48.47   Fatigue fracture of vertebra, lumbosacral region

X ● M48.48   Fatigue fracture of vertebra, sacral and sacrococcygeal region

● M48.5   Collapsed vertebra, not elsewhere classified

    Collapsed vertebra NOS

    Wedging of vertebra NOS

    Excludes1   current injury - see Injury of spine, by body region

              fatigue fracture of vertebra (M48.4)

              pathological fracture of vertebra due to neoplasm (M84.58)

              pathological fracture of vertebra due to other diagnosis (M84.68)

              pathological fracture of vertebra due to osteoporosis (M80.-)

              pathological fracture NOS (M84.4-)

              stress fracture of vertebra (M48.4-)

              traumatic fracture of vertebra (S12.-, S22.-, S32.-)

The appropriate 7th character is to be added to each code from subcategory M48.5:

A	initial encounter for fracture
D	subsequent encounter for fracture with routine healing
G	subsequent encounter for fracture with delayed healing
S	sequela of fracture

    Ⓔⓧ For category M48.5 CC codes: M48.40X-M48.58X[A], M80.00X-M80.88X[A], M84.30X-M84.68X[A]

X ● M48.50   Collapsed vertebra, not elsewhere classified, site unspecified A ✎

X ● M48.51   Collapsed vertebra, not elsewhere classified, occipito-atlanto-axial region A ✎

X ● M48.52   Collapsed vertebra, not elsewhere classified, cervical region A ✎

X ● M48.53   Collapsed vertebra, not elsewhere classified, cervicothoracic region A ✎

X ● M48.54   Collapsed vertebra, not elsewhere classified, thoracic region A ✎

X ● M48.55   Collapsed vertebra, not elsewhere classified, thoracolumbar region A ✎

X ● M48.56   Collapsed vertebra, not elsewhere classified, lumbar region A ✎

X ● M48.57   Collapsed vertebra, not elsewhere classified, lumbosacral region A ✎

X ● M48.58   Collapsed vertebra, not elsewhere classified, sacral and sacrococcygeal region A ✎

● M48.8   Other specified spondylopathies

    Ossification of posterior longitudinal ligament

● M48.8X   Other specified spondylopathies

M48.8X1   Other specified spondylopathies, occipito-atlanto-axial region

M48.8X2   Other specified spondylopathies, cervical region

M48.8X3   Other specified spondylopathies, cervicothoracic region

M48.8X4   Other specified spondylopathies, thoracic region

M48.8X5   Other specified spondylopathies, thoracolumbar region

M48.8X6   Other specified spondylopathies, lumbar region

M48.8X7   Other specified spondylopathies, lumbosacral region

M48.8X8   Other specified spondylopathies, sacral and sacrococcygeal region

M48.8X9   Other specified spondylopathies, site unspecified

M48.9   Spondylopathy, unspecified

◀ New   ◀ Revised   deleted Deleted   Excludes 1   Excludes 2   Includes   Use additional   Code first   Code also   Unspecified

OGCR Official Guidelines   ● Unacceptable Principal Diagnosis   X Assign placeholder X   ● Use Additional Character(s)   ▶ Manifestation Code   Coding Clinic

● **M49 Spondylopathies in diseases classified elsewhere**

Includes   curvature of spine in diseases classified elsewhere
deformity of spine in diseases classified elsewhere
kyphosis in diseases classified elsewhere
scoliosis in diseases classified elsewhere
spondylopathy in diseases classified elsewhere

Code first underlying disease, such as:
brucellosis (A23.-)
Charcot-Marie-Tooth disease (G60.0)
enterobacterial infections (A01-A04)
osteitis fibrosa cystica (E21.0)

Excludes1   curvature of spine in tuberculosis [Pott's] (A18.01)
enteropathic arthropathies (M07.-)
~~neuropathic spondylopathy (in):~~
~~nonsyphilitic NEC (G98.0)~~
~~syringomyelia (G95.0)~~
~~tabes dorsalis (A52.11)~~
~~spondylitis (in):~~
gonococcal spondylitis (A54.41) ◀▥
~~syphilis (acquired) (A52.77)~~
neuropathic [tabes dorsalis] spondylitis (A52.11) ◀▥
~~tuberculosis (A18.01)~~
~~typhoid fever (A01.05)~~
neuropathic spondylopathy in syringomyelia (G95.0) ◀
neuropathic spondylopathy in tabes dorsalis (A52.11) ◀
nonsyphilitic neuropathic spondylopathy NEC (G98.0) ◀
spondylitis in syphilis (acquired) (A52.77) ◀
tuberculous spondylitis (A18.01) ◀
typhoid fever spondylitis (A01.05) ◀

● **M49.8 Spondylopathy in diseases classified elsewhere**

▹ *M49.80*   *Spondylopathy in diseases classified elsewhere, site unspecified*

▹ *M49.81*   *Spondylopathy in diseases classified elsewhere, occipito-atlanto-axial region*

▹ *M49.82*   *Spondylopathy in diseases classified elsewhere, cervical region*

▹ *M49.83*   *Spondylopathy in diseases classified elsewhere, cervicothoracic region*

▹ *M49.84*   *Spondylopathy in diseases classified elsewhere, thoracic region*

▹ *M49.85*   *Spondylopathy in diseases classified elsewhere, thoracolumbar region*

▹ *M49.86*   *Spondylopathy in diseases classified elsewhere, lumbar region*

▹ *M49.87*   *Spondylopathy in diseases classified elsewhere, lumbosacral region*

▹ *M49.88*   *Spondylopathy in diseases classified elsewhere, sacral and sacrococcygeal region*

▹ *M49.89*   *Spondylopathy in diseases classified elsewhere, multiple sites in spine*

OTHER DORSOPATHIES (M50-M54)

Excludes1   current injury - see injury of spine by body region
discitis NOS (M46.4-)

● **M50 Cervical disc disorders**

Note: Code to the most superior level of disorder.

Includes   cervicothoracic disc disorders with cervicalgia
cervicothoracic disc disorders

● **M50.0 Cervical disc disorder with myelopathy**

(Ex) **For category M50.0 CC codes:** M50.00-M50.03, M50.20-M50.23

M50.00 Cervical disc disorder with myelopathy, unspecified cervical region 🏥

M50.01 Cervical disc disorder with myelopathy, high cervical region 🏥 ◀▥
C2-C3 disc disorder with myelopathy ◀
C3-C4 disc disorder with myelopathy ◀

M50.02 Cervical disc disorder with myelopathy, mid-cervical region 🏥
C4-C5 disc disorder with myelopathy ◀
C5-C6 disc disorder with myelopathy ◀
C6-C7 disc disorder with myelopathy ◀

M50.03 Cervical disc disorder with myelopathy, cervicothoracic region 🏥
C7-T1 disc disorder with myelopathy ◀

● **M50.1 Cervical disc disorder with radiculopathy**

Excludes2   brachial radiculitis NOS (M54.13)

M50.10 Cervical disc disorder with radiculopathy, unspecified cervical region

M50.11 Cervical disc disorder with radiculopathy, high cervical region ◀▥
C2-C3 disc disorder with radiculopathy ◀
C3 radiculopathy due to disc disorder ◀
C3-C4 disc disorder with radiculopathy ◀
C4 radiculopathy due to disc disorder ◀

M50.12 Cervical disc disorder with radiculopathy, mid-cervical region
C4-C5 disc disorder with radiculopathy ◀
C5 radiculopathy due to disc disorder ◀
C5-C6 disc disorder with radiculopathy ◀
C6 radiculopathy due to disc disorder ◀
C6-C7 disc disorder with radiculopathy ◀
C7 radiculopathy due to disc disorder ◀

M50.13 Cervical disc disorder with radiculopathy, cervicothoracic region
C7-T1 disc disorder with radiculopathy ◀
C8 radiculopathy due to disc disorder ◀

● **M50.2 Other cervical disc displacement**

M50.20 Other cervical disc displacement, unspecified cervical region

M50.21 Other cervical disc displacement, high cervical region ◀▥
Other C2-C3 cervical disc displacement ◀
Other C3-C4 cervical disc displacement ◀

M50.22 Other cervical disc displacement, mid-cervical region
Other C4-C5 cervical disc displacement ◀
Other C5-C6 cervical disc displacement ◀
Other C6-C7 cervical disc displacement ◀

M50.23 Other cervical disc displacement, cervicothoracic region
Other C7-T1 cervical disc displacement ◀

● **M50.3 Other cervical disc degeneration**

M50.30 Other cervical disc degeneration, unspecified cervical region

M50.31 Other cervical disc degeneration, high cervical region ◀▥
Other C2-C3 cervical disc degeneration ◀
Other C3-C4 cervical disc degeneration ◀

M50.32 Other cervical disc degeneration, mid-cervical region
Other C4-C5 cervical disc degeneration ◀
Other C5-C6 cervical disc degeneration ◀
Other C6-C7 cervical disc degeneration ◀

M50.33 Other cervical disc degeneration, cervicothoracic region
Other C7-T1 cervical disc degeneration ◀

● **M50.8 Other cervical disc disorders**

M50.80 Other cervical disc disorders, unspecified cervical region

M50.81 Other cervical disc disorders, high cervical region ◀▥
Other C2-C3 cervical disc disorders ◀
Other C3-C4 cervical disc disorders ◀

M50.82 Other cervical disc disorders, mid-cervical region
Other C4-C5 cervical disc disorders ◀
Other C5-C6 cervical disc disorders ◀
Other C6-C7 cervical disc disorders ◀

M50.83 Other cervical disc disorders, cervicothoracic region
Other C7-T1 cervical disc disorders ◀

CHAPTER 13 (M00-M99)

● M50.9   Cervical disc disorder, unspecified

     M50.90   Cervical disc disorder, unspecified, unspecified cervical region

     M50.91   Cervical disc disorder, unspecified, high cervical region ◀▦
          C2-C3 cervical disc disorder, unspecified ◀
          C3-C4 cervical disc disorder, unspecified ◀

     M50.92   Cervical disc disorder, unspecified, mid-cervical region
          C4-C5 cervical disc disorder, unspecified ◀
          C5-C6 cervical disc disorder, unspecified ◀
          C6-C7 cervical disc disorder, unspecified ◀

     M50.93   Cervical disc disorder, unspecified, cervicothoracic region
          C7-T1 cervical disc disorder, unspecified ◀

● M51   Thoracic, thoracolumbar, and lumbosacral intervertebral disc disorders

     Excludes2   cervical and cervicothoracic disc disorders (M50.-)
                  sacral and sacrococcygeal disorders (M53.3)

● M51.0   Thoracic, thoracolumbar and lumbosacral intervertebral disc disorders with myelopathy
     Ⓔ⊼ For category M51.0 CC codes M51.04-M51.05: M51.04-M51.05, M51.24-M51.25 For category M51.0 CC codes M51.06-M51.07: M51.06-M51.07, M51.24-M51.25

     M51.04   Intervertebral disc disorders with myelopathy, thoracic region ◔

     M51.05   Intervertebral disc disorders with myelopathy, thoracolumbar region ◔

     M51.06   Intervertebral disc disorders with myelopathy, lumbar region ◔

     ~~M51.07~~   ~~Intervertebral disc disorders with myelopathy, lumbosacral region~~

● M51.1   Thoracic, thoracolumbar and lumbosacral intervertebral disc disorders with radiculopathy
     Sciatica due to intervertebral disc disorder

     Excludes1   lumbar radiculitis NOS (M54.16)
                  sciatica NOS (M54.3)

     M51.14   Intervertebral disc disorders with radiculopathy, thoracic region

     M51.15   Intervertebral disc disorders with radiculopathy, thoracolumbar region

     M51.16   Intervertebral disc disorders with radiculopathy, lumbar region

     M51.17   Intervertebral disc disorders with radiculopathy, lumbosacral region

● M51.2   Other thoracic, thoracolumbar and lumbosacral intervertebral disc displacement
     Lumbago due to displacement of intervertebral disc

     M51.24   Other intervertebral disc displacement, thoracic region

     M51.25   Other intervertebral disc displacement, thoracolumbar region

     M51.26   Other intervertebral disc displacement, lumbar region

     M51.27   Other intervertebral disc displacement, lumbosacral region

● M51.3   Other thoracic, thoracolumbar and lumbosacral intervertebral disc degeneration

     M51.34   Other intervertebral disc degeneration, thoracic region

     M51.35   Other intervertebral disc degeneration, thoracolumbar region

     M51.36   Other intervertebral disc degeneration, lumbar region

     M51.37   Other intervertebral disc degeneration, lumbosacral region

● M51.4   Schmorl's nodes

     M51.44   Schmorl's nodes, thoracic region

     M51.45   Schmorl's nodes, thoracolumbar region

     M51.46   Schmorl's nodes, lumbar region

     M51.47   Schmorl's nodes, lumbosacral region

● M51.8   Other thoracic, thoracolumbar and lumbosacral intervertebral disc disorders

     M51.84   Other intervertebral disc disorders, thoracic region

     M51.85   Other intervertebral disc disorders, thoracolumbar region

     M51.86   Other intervertebral disc disorders, lumbar region

     M51.87   Other intervertebral disc disorders, lumbosacral region

     M51.9   Unspecified thoracic, thoracolumbar and lumbosacral intervertebral disc disorder

● M53   Other and unspecified dorsopathies, not elsewhere classified

     M53.0   Cervicocranial syndrome
          Posterior cervical sympathetic syndrome

     M53.1   Cervicobrachial syndrome

          Excludes2   cervical disc disorder (M50.-)
                        thoracic outlet syndrome (G54.0)

● M53.2   Spinal instabilities

     ● M53.2X   Spinal instabilities

          M53.2X1   Spinal instabilities, occipito-atlanto-axial region

          M53.2X2   Spinal instabilities, cervical region

          M53.2X3   Spinal instabilities, cervicothoracic region

          M53.2X4   Spinal instabilities, thoracic region

          M53.2X5   Spinal instabilities, thoracolumbar region

          M53.2X6   Spinal instabilities, lumbar region

          M53.2X7   Spinal instabilities, lumbosacral region

          M53.2X8   Spinal instabilities, sacral and sacrococcygeal region

          M53.2X9   Spinal instabilities, site unspecified

     M53.3   Sacrococcygeal disorders, not elsewhere classified
          Coccygodynia

● M53.8   Other specified dorsopathies

     M53.80   Other specified dorsopathies, site unspecified

     M53.81   Other specified dorsopathies, occipito-atlanto-axial region

     M53.82   Other specified dorsopathies, cervical region

     M53.83   Other specified dorsopathies, cervicothoracic region

     M53.84   Other specified dorsopathies, thoracic region

     M53.85   Other specified dorsopathies, thoracolumbar region

     M53.86   Other specified dorsopathies, lumbar region

     M53.87   Other specified dorsopathies, lumbosacral region

     M53.88   Other specified dorsopathies, sacral and sacrococcygeal region

     M53.9   Dorsopathy, unspecified

● M54   Dorsalgia

     Excludes1   psychogenic dorsalgia (F45.41)

● M54.0   Panniculitis affecting regions of neck and back

     Excludes1   lupus panniculitis (L93.2)
                  panniculitis NOS (M79.3)
                  relapsing [Weber-Christian] panniculitis (M35.6)

     M54.00   Panniculitis affecting regions of neck and back, site unspecified

     M54.01   Panniculitis affecting regions of neck and back, occipito-atlanto-axial region

     M54.02   Panniculitis affecting regions of neck and back, cervical region

     M54.03   Panniculitis affecting regions of neck and back, cervicothoracic region

---

◀ New   ◀▦ Revised   ~~deleted~~ Deleted   Excludes 1   Excludes 2   Includes   Use additional   Code first   Code also   Unspecified

1122   OGCR Official Guidelines   ● Unacceptable Principal Diagnosis   X Assign placeholder X   ● Use Additional Character(s)   ▌ Manifestation Code   **Coding Clinic**

M54.04   Panniculitis affecting regions of neck and back, thoracic region

M54.05   Panniculitis affecting regions of neck and back, thoracolumbar region

M54.06   Panniculitis affecting regions of neck and back, lumbar region

M54.07   Panniculitis affecting regions of neck and back, lumbosacral region

M54.08   Panniculitis affecting regions of neck and back, sacral and sacrococcygeal region

M54.09   Panniculitis affecting regions, neck and back, multiple sites in spine

● **M54.1   Radiculopathy**
    Brachial neuritis or radiculitis NOS
    Lumbar neuritis or radiculitis NOS
    Lumbosacral neuritis or radiculitis NOS
    Thoracic neuritis or radiculitis NOS
    Radiculitis NOS

    Excludes1   neuralgia and neuritis NOS (M79.2)
        radiculopathy with cervical disc disorder (M50.1)
        radiculopathy with lumbar and other intervertebral disc disorder (M51.1-)
        radiculopathy with spondylosis (M47.2-)

M54.10   Radiculopathy, site unspecified

M54.11   Radiculopathy, occipito-atlanto-axial region

M54.12   Radiculopathy, cervical region

M54.13   Radiculopathy, cervicothoracic region

M54.14   Radiculopathy, thoracic region

M54.15   Radiculopathy, thoracolumbar region

M54.16   Radiculopathy, lumbar region

M54.17   Radiculopathy, lumbosacral region

M54.18   Radiculopathy, sacral and sacrococcygeal region

M54.2   Cervicalgia
    Excludes1   cervicalgia due to intervertebral cervical disc disorder (M50.-)

● **M54.3   Sciatica**
    Excludes1   lesion of sciatic nerve (G57.0)
        sciatica due to intervertebral disc disorder (M51.1-)
        sciatica with lumbago (M54.4-)

M54.30   Sciatica, unspecified side

M54.31   Sciatica, right side

M54.32   Sciatica, left side

● **M54.4   Lumbago with sciatica**
    Excludes1   lumbago with sciatica due to intervertebral disc disorder (M51.1-)

M54.40   Lumbago with sciatica, unspecified side

M54.41   Lumbago with sciatica, right side

M54.42   Lumbago with sciatica, left side

M54.5   Low back pain
    Loin pain
    Lumbago NOS

    Excludes1   low back strain (S39.012) ◄
        lumbago due to intervertebral disc displacement (M51.2-)
        lumbago with sciatica (M54.4-)

M54.6   Pain in thoracic spine
    Excludes1   pain in thoracic spine due to intervertebral disc disorder (M51.)

● **M54.8   Other dorsalgia**
    Excludes1   dorsalgia in thoracic region (M54.6)
        low back pain (M54.5)

M54.81   Occipital neuralgia

M54.89   Other dorsalgia

M54.9   Dorsalgia, unspecified
    Backache NOS
    Back pain NOS

SOFT TISSUE DISORDERS (M60-M79)

DISORDERS OF MUSCLES (M60-M63)

Excludes1   dermatopolymyositis (M33.-)
    muscular dystrophies and myopathies (G71-G72)
    myopathy in amyloidosis (E85.-)
    ~~amyloidosis (E85-)~~ ◄
    myopathy in polyarteritis nodosa (M30.0) ◄
    myopathy in rheumatoid arthritis (M05.32) ◄
    myopathy in scleroderma (M34.-) ◄
    myopathy in Sjögren's syndrome (M35.03) ◄
    myopathy in systemic lupus erythematosus (M32.-) ◄

● **M60   Myositis**
    Excludes2   inclusion body myositis [IBM] (G72.41)

● **M60.0   Infective myositis**
    Tropical pyomyositis
    Use additional code (B95-B97) to identify infectious agent

    Ⓔⓧ **For category M60.0 CC codes:** K68.12, M60.000-M60.19, M61.00-M61.19, M61.30-M61.59, M62.3, M62.50-M62.59, M62.89, M72.6

    ● **M60.00   Infective myositis, unspecified site**

      M60.000   Infective myositis, unspecified right arm 🔖
          Infective myositis, right upper limb NOS

      M60.001   Infective myositis, unspecified left arm 🔖
          Infective myositis, left upper limb NOS

      M60.002   Infective myositis, unspecified arm 🔖
          Infective myositis, upper limb NOS

      M60.003   Infective myositis, unspecified right leg 🔖
          Infective myositis, right lower limb NOS

      M60.004   Infective myositis, unspecified leg 🔖
          Infective myositis, left lower limb NOS

      M60.005   Infective myositis, unspecified leg 🔖
          Infective myositis, lower limb NOS

      M60.009   Infective myositis, unspecified site 🔖

    ● **M60.01   Infective myositis, shoulder**

      M60.011   Infective myositis, right shoulder 🔖

      M60.012   Infective myositis, left shoulder 🔖

      M60.019   Infective myositis, unspecified shoulder 🔖

    ● **M60.02   Infective myositis, upper arm**

      M60.021   Infective myositis, right upper arm 🔖

      M60.022   Infective myositis, left upper arm 🔖

      M60.029   Infective myositis, unspecified upper arm 🔖

    ● **M60.03   Infective myositis, forearm**

      M60.031   Infective myositis, right forearm 🔖

      M60.032   Infective myositis, left forearm 🔖

      M60.039   Infective myositis, unspecified forearm 🔖

    ● **M60.04   Infective myositis, hand and fingers**

      M60.041   Infective myositis, right hand 🔖

      M60.042   Infective myositis, left hand 🔖

      M60.043   Infective myositis, unspecified hand 🔖

      M60.044   Infective myositis, right finger(s) 🔖

      M60.045   Infective myositis, left finger(s) 🔖

      M60.046   Infective myositis, unspecified finger(s) 🔖

N   Newborn Age: 0   **P**   Pediatric Age: 0–17   **M**   Maternity DX: 12–55   **A**   Adult Age: 15–124   ♀   Females Only   ♂   Males Only

🔖 Complication\Comorbidity   🔖 Major C\C   Ⓔⓧ CC/MCC Exclusions   🔖 Present on Admission Requirement   🔖 Hospital-Acquired Condition

1123

● M60.05 Infective myositis, thigh
   M60.051 Infective myositis, right thigh 🔊
   M60.052 Infective myositis, left thigh 🔊
   M60.059 Infective myositis, unspecified
            thigh 🔊
● M60.06 Infective myositis, lower leg
   M60.061 Infective myositis, right lower leg 🔊
   M60.062 Infective myositis, left lower leg 🔊
   M60.069 Infective myositis, unspecified lower
            leg 🔊
● M60.07 Infective myositis, ankle, foot and toes
   M60.070 Infective myositis, right ankle 🔊
   M60.071 Infective myositis, left ankle 🔊
   M60.072 Infective myositis, unspecified
            ankle 🔊
   M60.073 Infective myositis, right foot 🔊
   M60.074 Infective myositis, left foot 🔊
   M60.075 Infective myositis, unspecified foot 🔊
   M60.076 Infective myositis, right toe(s) 🔊
   M60.077 Infective myositis, left toe(s) 🔊
   M60.078 Infective myositis, unspecified
            toe(s) 🔊
   M60.08 Infective myositis, other site 🔊
   M60.09 Infective myositis, multiple sites 🔊
● M60.1 Interstitial myositis
   M60.10 Interstitial myositis of unspecified site
● M60.11 Interstitial myositis, shoulder
   M60.111 Interstitial myositis, right shoulder
   M60.112 Interstitial myositis, left shoulder
   M60.119 Interstitial myositis, unspecified
            shoulder
● M60.12 Interstitial myositis, upper arm
   M60.121 Interstitial myositis, right upper arm
   M60.122 Interstitial myositis, left upper arm
   M60.129 Interstitial myositis, unspecified
            upper arm
● M60.13 Interstitial myositis, forearm
   M60.131 Interstitial myositis, right forearm
   M60.132 Interstitial myositis, left forearm
   M60.139 Interstitial myositis, unspecified
            forearm
● M60.14 Interstitial myositis, hand
   M60.141 Interstitial myositis, right hand
   M60.142 Interstitial myositis, left hand
   M60.149 Interstitial myositis, unspecified hand
● M60.15 Interstitial myositis, thigh
   M60.151 Interstitial myositis, right thigh
   M60.152 Interstitial myositis, left thigh
   M60.159 Interstitial myositis, unspecified thigh
● M60.16 Interstitial myositis, lower leg
   M60.161 Interstitial myositis, right lower leg
   M60.162 Interstitial myositis, left lower leg
   M60.169 Interstitial myositis, unspecified
            lower leg
● M60.17 Interstitial myositis, ankle and foot
   M60.171 Interstitial myositis, right ankle and
            foot
   M60.172 Interstitial myositis, left ankle and
            foot
   M60.179 Interstitial myositis, unspecified
            ankle and foot
   M60.18 Interstitial myositis, other site
   M60.19 Interstitial myositis, multiple sites

● M60.2 Foreign body granuloma of soft tissue, not elsewhere
         classified
   Use additional code to identify the type of retained
   foreign body (Z18.-)
   Excludes1 foreign body granuloma of skin and
                  subcutaneous tissue (L92.3)
   M60.20 Foreign body granuloma of soft tissue, not
           elsewhere classified, unspecified site
● M60.21 Foreign body granuloma of soft tissue, not
          elsewhere classified, shoulder
   M60.211 Foreign body granuloma of soft
            tissue, not elsewhere classified, right
            shoulder
   M60.212 Foreign body granuloma of soft
            tissue, not elsewhere classified, left
            shoulder
   M60.219 Foreign body granuloma of soft
            tissue, not elsewhere classified,
            unspecified shoulder
● M60.22 Foreign body granuloma of soft tissue, not
          elsewhere classified, upper arm
   M60.221 Foreign body granuloma of soft
            tissue, not elsewhere classified, right
            upper arm
   M60.222 Foreign body granuloma of soft
            tissue, not elsewhere classified, left
            upper arm
   M60.229 Foreign body granuloma of soft
            tissue, not elsewhere classified,
            unspecified upper arm
● M60.23 Foreign body granuloma of soft tissue, not
          elsewhere classified, forearm
   M60.231 Foreign body granuloma of soft
            tissue, not elsewhere classified, right
            forearm
   M60.232 Foreign body granuloma of soft
            tissue, not elsewhere classified, left
            forearm
   M60.239 Foreign body granuloma of soft
            tissue, not elsewhere classified,
            unspecified forearm
● M60.24 Foreign body granuloma of soft tissue, not
          elsewhere classified, hand
   M60.241 Foreign body granuloma of soft tissue,
            not elsewhere classified, right hand
   M60.242 Foreign body granuloma of soft
            tissue, not elsewhere classified, left
            hand
   M60.249 Foreign body granuloma of soft
            tissue, not elsewhere classified,
            unspecified hand
● M60.25 Foreign body granuloma of soft tissue, not
          elsewhere classified, thigh
   M60.251 Foreign body granuloma of soft
            tissue, not elsewhere classified, right
            thigh
   M60.252 Foreign body granuloma of soft
            tissue, not elsewhere classified, left
            thigh
   M60.259 Foreign body granuloma of soft
            tissue, not elsewhere classified,
            unspecified thigh
● M60.26 Foreign body granuloma of soft tissue, not
          elsewhere classified, lower leg
   M60.261 Foreign body granuloma of soft
            tissue, not elsewhere classified, right
            lower leg
   M60.262 Foreign body granuloma of soft
            tissue, not elsewhere classified, left
            lower leg
   M60.269 Foreign body granuloma of soft
            tissue, not elsewhere classified,
            unspecified lower leg

◀ New   ◀◀ Revised   ~~deleted~~ Deleted   Excludes 1   Excludes 2   Includes   Use additional   Code first   Code also   Unspecified
OGCR Official Guidelines   ● Unacceptable Principal Diagnosis   X Assign placeholder X   ● Use Additional Character(s)   ▶ Manifestation Code   **Coding Clinic**

● M60.27　Foreign body granuloma of soft tissue, not elsewhere classified, ankle and foot
　　M60.271　Foreign body granuloma of soft tissue, not elsewhere classified, right ankle and foot
　　M60.272　Foreign body granuloma of soft tissue, not elsewhere classified, left ankle and foot
　　M60.279　Foreign body granuloma of soft tissue, not elsewhere classified, unspecified ankle and foot
　M60.28　Foreign body granuloma of soft tissue, not elsewhere classified, other site
● M60.8　Other myositis
　M60.80　Other myositis, unspecified site
● M60.81　Other myositis shoulder
　　M60.811　Other myositis, right shoulder
　　M60.812　Other myositis, left shoulder
　　M60.819　Other myositis, unspecified shoulder
● M60.82　Other myositis, upper arm
　　M60.821　Other myositis, right upper arm
　　M60.822　Other myositis, left upper arm
　　M60.829　Other myositis, unspecified upper arm
● M60.83　Other myositis, forearm
　　M60.831　Other myositis, right forearm
　　M60.832　Other myositis, left forearm
　　M60.839　Other myositis, unspecified forearm
● M60.84　Other myositis, hand
　　M60.841　Other myositis, right hand
　　M60.842　Other myositis, left hand
　　M60.849　Other myositis, unspecified hand
● M60.85　Other myositis, thigh
　　M60.851　Other myositis, right thigh
　　M60.852　Other myositis, left thigh
　　M60.859　Other myositis, unspecified thigh
● M60.86　Other myositis, lower leg
　　M60.861　Other myositis, right lower leg
　　M60.862　Other myositis, left lower leg
　　M60.869　Other myositis, unspecified lower leg
● M60.87　Other myositis, ankle and foot
　　M60.871　Other myositis, right ankle and foot
　　M60.872　Other myositis, left ankle and foot
　　M60.879　Other myositis, unspecified ankle and foot
　M60.88　Other myositis, other site
　M60.89　Other myositis, multiple sites
　M60.9　Myositis, unspecified

● M61　Calcification and ossification of muscle
● M61.0　Myositis ossificans traumatica
　M61.00　Myositis ossificans traumatica, unspecified site
● M61.01　Myositis ossificans traumatica, shoulder
　　M61.011　Myositis ossificans traumatica, right shoulder
　　M61.012　Myositis ossificans traumatica, left shoulder
　　M61.019　Myositis ossificans traumatica, unspecified shoulder
● M61.02　Myositis ossificans traumatica, upper arm
　　M61.021　Myositis ossificans traumatica, right upper arm
　　M61.022　Myositis ossificans traumatica, left upper arm
　　M61.029　Myositis ossificans traumatica, unspecified upper arm

● M61.03　Myositis ossificans traumatica, forearm
　　M61.031　Myositis ossificans traumatica, right forearm
　　M61.032　Myositis ossificans traumatica, left forearm
　　M61.039　Myositis ossificans traumatica, unspecified forearm
● M61.04　Myositis ossificans traumatica, hand
　　M61.041　Myositis ossificans traumatica, right hand
　　M61.042　Myositis ossificans traumatica, left hand
　　M61.049　Myositis ossificans traumatica, unspecified hand
● M61.05　Myositis ossificans traumatica, thigh
　　M61.051　Myositis ossificans traumatica, right thigh
　　M61.052　Myositis ossificans traumatica, left thigh
　　M61.059　Myositis ossificans traumatica, unspecified thigh
● M61.06　Myositis ossificans traumatica, lower leg
　　M61.061　Myositis ossificans traumatica, right lower leg
　　M61.062　Myositis ossificans traumatica, left lower leg
　　M61.069　Myositis ossificans traumatica, unspecified lower leg
● M61.07　Myositis ossificans traumatica, ankle and foot
　　M61.071　Myositis ossificans traumatica, right ankle and foot
　　M61.072　Myositis ossificans traumatica, left ankle and foot
　　M61.079　Myositis ossificans traumatica, unspecified ankle and foot
　M61.08　Myositis ossificans traumatica, other site
　M61.09　Myositis ossificans traumatica, multiple sites
● M61.1　Myositis ossificans progressiva
　　　Fibrodysplasia ossificans progressiva
　M61.10　Myositis ossificans progressiva, unspecified site
● M61.11　Myositis ossificans progressiva, shoulder
　　M61.111　Myositis ossificans progressiva, right shoulder
　　M61.112　Myositis ossificans progressiva, left shoulder
　　M61.119　Myositis ossificans progressiva, unspecified shoulder
● M61.12　Myositis ossificans progressiva, upper arm
　　M61.121　Myositis ossificans progressiva, right upper arm
　　M61.122　Myositis ossificans progressiva, left upper arm
　　M61.129　Myositis ossificans progressiva, unspecified arm
● M61.13　Myositis ossificans progressiva, forearm
　　M61.131　Myositis ossificans progressiva, right forearm
　　M61.132　Myositis ossificans progressiva, left forearm
　　M61.139　Myositis ossificans progressiva, unspecified forearm
● M61.14　Myositis ossificans progressiva, hand and finger(s)
　　M61.141　Myositis ossificans progressiva, right hand
　　M61.142　Myositis ossificans progressiva, left hand
　　M61.143　Myositis ossificans progressiva, unspecified hand

N Newborn Age: 0　　**P** Pediatric Age: 0–17　　**M** Maternity DX: 12–55　　**A** Adult Age: 15–124　　♀ Females Only　　♂ Males Only

 Complication\Comorbidity　　 Major C\C　　(Ex) CC/MCC Exclusions　　Present on Admission Requirement　　Hospital-Acquired Condition

1125

M61.144 Myositis ossificans progressiva, right finger(s)

M61.145 Myositis ossificans progressiva, left finger(s)

M61.146 Myositis ossificans progressiva, unspecified finger(s)

● M61.15 Myositis ossificans progressiva, thigh

M61.151 Myositis ossificans progressiva, right thigh

M61.152 Myositis ossificans progressiva, left thigh

M61.159 Myositis ossificans progressiva, unspecified thigh

● M61.16 Myositis ossificans progressiva, lower leg

M61.161 Myositis ossificans progressiva, right lower leg

M61.162 Myositis ossificans progressiva, left lower leg

M61.169 Myositis ossificans progressiva, unspecified lower leg

● M61.17 Myositis ossificans progressiva, ankle, foot and toe(s)

M61.171 Myositis ossificans progressiva, right ankle

M61.172 Myositis ossificans progressiva, left ankle

M61.173 Myositis ossificans progressiva, unspecified ankle

M61.174 Myositis ossificans progressiva, right foot

M61.175 Myositis ossificans progressiva, left foot

M61.176 Myositis ossificans progressiva, unspecified foot

M61.177 Myositis ossificans progressiva, right toe(s)

M61.178 Myositis ossificans progressiva, left toe(s)

M61.179 Myositis ossificans progressiva, unspecified toe(s)

M61.18 Myositis ossificans progressiva, other site

M61.19 Myositis ossificans progressiva, multiple sites

● M61.2 Paralytic calcification and ossification of muscle

Myositis ossificans associated with quadriplegia or paraplegia

M61.20 Paralytic calcification and ossification of muscle, unspecified site

● M61.21 Paralytic calcification and ossification of muscle, shoulder

M61.211 Paralytic calcification and ossification of muscle, right shoulder

M61.212 Paralytic calcification and ossification of muscle, left shoulder

M61.219 Paralytic calcification and ossification of muscle, unspecified shoulder

● M61.22 Paralytic calcification and ossification of muscle, upper arm

M61.221 Paralytic calcification and ossification of muscle, right upper arm

M61.222 Paralytic calcification and ossification of muscle, left upper arm

M61.229 Paralytic calcification and ossification of muscle, unspecified upper arm

● M61.23 Paralytic calcification and ossification of muscle, forearm

M61.231 Paralytic calcification and ossification of muscle, right forearm

M61.232 Paralytic calcification and ossification of muscle, left forearm

M61.239 Paralytic calcification and ossification of muscle, unspecified forearm

● M61.24 Paralytic calcification and ossification of muscle, hand

M61.241 Paralytic calcification and ossification of muscle, right hand

M61.242 Paralytic calcification and ossification of muscle, left hand

M61.249 Paralytic calcification and ossification of muscle, unspecified hand

● M61.25 Paralytic calcification and ossification of muscle, thigh

M61.251 Paralytic calcification and ossification of muscle, right thigh

M61.252 Paralytic calcification and ossification of muscle, left thigh

M61.259 Paralytic calcification and ossification of muscle, unspecified thigh

● M61.26 Paralytic calcification and ossification of muscle, lower leg

M61.261 Paralytic calcification and ossification of muscle, right lower leg

M61.262 Paralytic calcification and ossification of muscle, left lower leg

M61.269 Paralytic calcification and ossification of muscle, unspecified lower leg

● M61.27 Paralytic calcification and ossification of muscle, ankle and foot

M61.271 Paralytic calcification and ossification of muscle, right ankle and foot

M61.272 Paralytic calcification and ossification of muscle, left ankle and foot

M61.279 Paralytic calcification and ossification of muscle, unspecified ankle and foot

M61.28 Paralytic calcification and ossification of muscle, other site

M61.29 Paralytic calcification and ossification of muscle, multiple sites

● M61.3 Calcification and ossification of muscles associated with burns

Myositis ossificans associated with burns

M61.30 Calcification and ossification of muscles associated with burns, unspecified site

● M61.31 Calcification and ossification of muscles associated with burns, shoulder

M61.311 Calcification and ossification of muscles associated with burns, right shoulder

M61.312 Calcification and ossification of muscles associated with burns, left shoulder

M61.319 Calcification and ossification of muscles associated with burns, unspecified shoulder

● M61.32 Calcification and ossification of muscles associated with burns, upper arm

M61.321 Calcification and ossification of muscles associated with burns, right upper arm

M61.322 Calcification and ossification of muscles associated with burns, left upper arm

M61.329 Calcification and ossification of muscles associated with burns, unspecified upper arm

◄ New   ◄▦ Revised   d̶e̶l̶e̶t̶e̶d̶ Deleted   Excludes 1   Excludes 2   Includes   Use additional   Code first   Code also   Unspecified

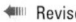 OGCR Official Guidelines   ● Unacceptable Principal Diagnosis   X Assign placeholder X   ● Use Additional Character(s)   ▶ Manifestation Code   Coding Clinic

● M61.33　Calcification and ossification of muscles associated with burns, forearm
　　M61.331　Calcification and ossification of muscles associated with burns, right forearm
　　M61.332　Calcification and ossification of muscles associated with burns, left forearm
　　M61.339　Calcification and ossification of muscles associated with burns, unspecified forearm

● M61.34　Calcification and ossification of muscles associated with burns, hand
　　M61.341　Calcification and ossification of muscles associated with burns, right hand
　　M61.342　Calcification and ossification of muscles associated with burns, left hand
　　M61.349　Calcification and ossification of muscles associated with burns, unspecified hand

● M61.35　Calcification and ossification of muscles associated with burns, thigh
　　M61.351　Calcification and ossification of muscles associated with burns, right thigh
　　M61.352　Calcification and ossification of muscles associated with burns, left thigh
　　M61.359　Calcification and ossification of muscles associated with burns, unspecified thigh

● M61.36　Calcification and ossification of muscles associated with burns, lower leg
　　M61.361　Calcification and ossification of muscles associated with burns, right lower leg
　　M61.362　Calcification and ossification of muscles associated with burns, left lower leg
　　M61.369　Calcification and ossification of muscles associated with burns, unspecified lower leg

● M61.37　Calcification and ossification of muscles associated with burns, ankle and foot
　　M61.371　Calcification and ossification of muscles associated with burns, right ankle and foot
　　M61.372　Calcification and ossification of muscles associated with burns, left ankle and foot
　　M61.379　Calcification and ossification of muscles associated with burns, unspecified ankle and foot
　　M61.38　Calcification and ossification of muscles associated with burns, other site
　　M61.39　Calcification and ossification of muscles associated with burns, multiple sites

● M61.4　Other calcification of muscle
　　Excludes1　calcific tendinitis NOS (M65.2-)
　　　　　　　　calcific tendinitis of shoulder (M75.3)
　　M61.40　Other calcification of muscle, unspecified site
● M61.41　Other calcification of muscle, shoulder
　　M61.411　Other calcification of muscle, right shoulder
　　M61.412　Other calcification of muscle, left shoulder
　　M61.419　Other calcification of muscle, unspecified shoulder

● M61.42　Other calcification of muscle, upper arm
　　M61.421　Other calcification of muscle, right upper arm
　　M61.422　Other calcification of muscle, left upper arm
　　M61.429　Other calcification of muscle, unspecified upper arm
● M61.43　Other calcification of muscle, forearm
　　M61.431　Other calcification of muscle, right forearm
　　M61.432　Other calcification of muscle, left forearm
　　M61.439　Other calcification of muscle, unspecified forearm
● M61.44　Other calcification of muscle, hand
　　M61.441　Other calcification of muscle, right hand
　　M61.442　Other calcification of muscle, left hand
　　M61.449　Other calcification of muscle, unspecified hand
● M61.45　Other calcification of muscle, thigh
　　M61.451　Other calcification of muscle, right thigh
　　M61.452　Other calcification of muscle, left thigh
　　M61.459　Other calcification of muscle, unspecified thigh
● M61.46　Other calcification of muscle, lower leg
　　M61.461　Other calcification of muscle, right lower leg
　　M61.462　Other calcification of muscle, left lower leg
　　M61.469　Other calcification of muscle, unspecified lower leg
● M61.47　Other calcification of muscle, ankle and foot
　　M61.471　Other calcification of muscle, right ankle and foot
　　M61.472　Other calcification of muscle, left ankle and foot
　　M61.479　Other calcification of muscle, unspecified ankle and foot
　　M61.48　Other calcification of muscle, other site
　　M61.49　Other calcification of muscle, multiple sites
● M61.5　Other ossification of muscle
　　M61.50　Other ossification of muscle, unspecified site
● M61.51　Other ossification of muscle, shoulder
　　M61.511　Other ossification of muscle, right shoulder
　　M61.512　Other ossification of muscle, left shoulder
　　M61.519　Other ossification of muscle, unspecified shoulder
● M61.52　Other ossification of muscle, upper arm
　　M61.521　Other ossification of muscle, right upper arm
　　M61.522　Other ossification of muscle, left upper arm
　　M61.529　Other ossification of muscle, unspecified upper arm
● M61.53　Other ossification of muscle, forearm
　　M61.531　Other ossification of muscle, right forearm
　　M61.532　Other ossification of muscle, left forearm
　　M61.539　Other ossification of muscle, unspecified forearm

N Newborn Age: 0　　**P** Pediatric Age: 0–17　　**M** Maternity DX: 12–55　　**A** Adult Age: 15–124　　♀ Females Only　　♂ Males Only

🅒 Complication\Comorbidity　　🅜 Major C\C　　(Ex) CC/MCC Exclusions　　🅟 Present on Admission Requirement　　🅗 Hospital-Acquired Condition

1127

● M61.54   Other ossification of muscle, hand

     M61.541   Other ossification of muscle, right hand

     M61.542   Other ossification of muscle, left hand

     M61.549   Other ossification of muscle, unspecified hand

● M61.55   Other ossification of muscle, thigh

     M61.551   Other ossification of muscle, right thigh

     M61.552   Other ossification of muscle, left thigh

     M61.559   Other ossification of muscle, unspecified thigh

● M61.56   Other ossification of muscle, lower leg

     M61.561   Other ossification of muscle, right lower leg

     M61.562   Other ossification of muscle, left lower leg

     M61.569   Other ossification of muscle, unspecified lower leg

● M61.57   Other ossification of muscle, ankle and foot

     M61.571   Other ossification of muscle, right ankle and foot

     M61.572   Other ossification of muscle, left ankle and foot

     M61.579   Other ossification of muscle, unspecified ankle and foot

   M61.58   Other ossification of muscle, other site

   M61.59   Other ossification of muscle, multiple sites

M61.9   Calcification and ossification of muscle, unspecified

● M62   **Other disorders of muscle**

     Excludes1   alcoholic myopathy (G72.1)
                cramp and spasm (R25.2)
                drug-induced myopathy (G72.0)
                myalgia (M79.1)
                stiff-man syndrome (G25.82)

     Excludes2   nontraumatic hematoma of muscle (M79.81)

● M62.0   Separation of muscle (nontraumatic)

     Diastasis of muscle

     Excludes1   diastasis recti complicating pregnancy, labor and delivery (O71.8)
                traumatic separation of muscle - see strain of muscle by body region

   M62.00   Separation of muscle (nontraumatic), unspecified site

● M62.01   Separation of muscle (nontraumatic), shoulder

     M62.011   Separation of muscle (nontraumatic), right shoulder

     M62.012   Separation of muscle (nontraumatic), left shoulder

     M62.019   Separation of muscle (nontraumatic), unspecified shoulder

● M62.02   Separation of muscle (nontraumatic), upper arm

     M62.021   Separation of muscle (nontraumatic), right upper arm

     M62.022   Separation of muscle (nontraumatic), left upper arm

     M62.029   Separation of muscle (nontraumatic), unspecified upper arm

● M62.03   Separation of muscle (nontraumatic), forearm

     M62.031   Separation of muscle (nontraumatic), right forearm

     M62.032   Separation of muscle (nontraumatic), left forearm

     M62.039   Separation of muscle (nontraumatic), unspecified forearm

● M62.04   Separation of muscle (nontraumatic), hand

     M62.041   Separation of muscle (nontraumatic), right hand

     M62.042   Separation of muscle (nontraumatic), left hand

     M62.049   Separation of muscle (nontraumatic), unspecified hand

● M62.05   Separation of muscle (nontraumatic), thigh

     M62.051   Separation of muscle (nontraumatic), right thigh

     M62.052   Separation of muscle (nontraumatic), left thigh

     M62.059   Separation of muscle (nontraumatic), unspecified thigh

● M62.06   Separation of muscle (nontraumatic), lower leg

     M62.061   Separation of muscle (nontraumatic), right lower leg

     M62.062   Separation of muscle (nontraumatic), left lower leg

     M62.069   Separation of muscle (nontraumatic), unspecified lower leg

● M62.07   Separation of muscle (nontraumatic), ankle and foot

     M62.071   Separation of muscle (nontraumatic), right ankle and foot

     M62.072   Separation of muscle (nontraumatic), left ankle and foot

     M62.079   Separation of muscle (nontraumatic), unspecified ankle and foot

   M62.08   Separation of muscle (nontraumatic), other site

● M62.1   Other rupture of muscle (nontraumatic)

     Excludes1   traumatic rupture of muscle - see strain of muscle by body region

     Excludes2   rupture of tendon (M66.-)

   M62.10   Other rupture of muscle (nontraumatic), unspecified site

● M62.11   Other rupture of muscle (nontraumatic), shoulder

     M62.111   Other rupture of muscle (nontraumatic), right shoulder

     M62.112   Other rupture of muscle (nontraumatic), left shoulder

     M62.119   Other rupture of muscle (nontraumatic), unspecified shoulder

● M62.12   Other rupture of muscle (nontraumatic), upper arm

     M62.121   Other rupture of muscle (nontraumatic), right upper arm

     M62.122   Other rupture of muscle (nontraumatic), left upper arm

     M62.129   Other rupture of muscle (nontraumatic), unspecified upper arm

● M62.13   Other rupture of muscle (nontraumatic), forearm

     M62.131   Other rupture of muscle (nontraumatic), right forearm

     M62.132   Other rupture of muscle (nontraumatic), left forearm

     M62.139   Other rupture of muscle (nontraumatic), unspecified forearm

● M62.14   Other rupture of muscle (nontraumatic), hand

     M62.141   Other rupture of muscle (nontraumatic), right hand

     M62.142   Other rupture of muscle (nontraumatic), left hand

     M62.149   Other rupture of muscle (nontraumatic), unspecified hand

◀ New   ◀▥ Revised   ~~deleted~~ Deleted   Excludes 1   Excludes 2   Includes   Use additional   Code first   Code also   Unspecified

OGCR Official Guidelines   ● Unacceptable Principal Diagnosis   X Assign placeholder X   ● Use Additional Character(s)   ▶ Manifestation Code   **Coding Clinic**

● M62.15 Other rupture of muscle (nontraumatic), thigh
    M62.151 Other rupture of muscle (nontraumatic), right thigh
    M62.152 Other rupture of muscle (nontraumatic), left thigh
    M62.159 Other rupture of muscle (nontraumatic), unspecified thigh
● M62.16 Other rupture of muscle (nontraumatic), lower leg
    M62.161 Other rupture of muscle (nontraumatic), right lower leg
    M62.162 Other rupture of muscle (nontraumatic), left lower leg
    M62.169 Other rupture of muscle (nontraumatic), unspecified lower leg
● M62.17 Other rupture of muscle (nontraumatic), ankle and foot
    M62.171 Other rupture of muscle (nontraumatic), right ankle and foot
    M62.172 Other rupture of muscle (nontraumatic), left ankle and foot
    M62.179 Other rupture of muscle (nontraumatic), unspecified ankle and foot
  M62.18 Other rupture of muscle (nontraumatic), other site
● M62.2 Nontraumatic ischemic infarction of muscle

    Excludes1 compartment syndrome (traumatic) (T79.A-)
        nontraumatic compartment syndrome (M79.A-)
        traumatic ischemia of muscle (T79.6)
        rhabdomyolysis (M62.82)
        Volkmann's ischemic contracture (T79.6)

  M62.20 Nontraumatic ischemic infarction of muscle, unspecified site
● M62.21 Nontraumatic ischemic infarction of muscle, shoulder
    M62.211 Nontraumatic ischemic infarction of muscle, right shoulder
    M62.212 Nontraumatic ischemic infarction of muscle, left shoulder
    M62.219 Nontraumatic ischemic infarction of muscle, unspecified shoulder
● M62.22 Nontraumatic ischemic infarction of muscle, upper arm
    M62.221 Nontraumatic ischemic infarction of muscle, right upper arm
    M62.222 Nontraumatic ischemic infarction of muscle, left upper arm
    M62.229 Nontraumatic ischemic infarction of muscle, unspecified upper arm
● M62.23 Nontraumatic ischemic infarction of muscle, forearm
    M62.231 Nontraumatic ischemic infarction of muscle, right forearm
    M62.232 Nontraumatic ischemic infarction of muscle, left forearm
    M62.239 Nontraumatic ischemic infarction of muscle, unspecified forearm
● M62.24 Nontraumatic ischemic infarction of muscle, hand
    M62.241 Nontraumatic ischemic infarction of muscle, right hand
    M62.242 Nontraumatic ischemic infarction of muscle, left hand
    M62.249 Nontraumatic ischemic infarction of muscle, unspecified hand

● M62.25 Nontraumatic ischemic infarction of muscle, thigh
    M62.251 Nontraumatic ischemic infarction of muscle, right thigh
    M62.252 Nontraumatic ischemic infarction of muscle, left thigh
    M62.259 Nontraumatic ischemic infarction of muscle, unspecified thigh
● M62.26 Nontraumatic ischemic infarction of muscle, lower leg
    M62.261 Nontraumatic ischemic infarction of muscle, right lower leg
    M62.262 Nontraumatic ischemic infarction of muscle, left lower leg
    M62.269 Nontraumatic ischemic infarction of muscle, unspecified lower leg
● M62.27 Nontraumatic ischemic infarction of muscle, ankle and foot
    M62.271 Nontraumatic ischemic infarction of muscle, right ankle and foot
    M62.272 Nontraumatic ischemic infarction of muscle, left ankle and foot
    M62.279 Nontraumatic ischemic infarction of muscle, unspecified ankle and foot
  M62.28 Nontraumatic ischemic infarction of muscle, other site
M62.3 Immobility syndrome (paraplegic)
M62.4 Contracture of muscle

CONTRACTURE OF TENDON (SHEATH)

Excludes1 contracture of joint (M24.5-)
  M62.40 Contracture of muscle, unspecified site
● M62.41 Contracture of muscle, shoulder
    M62.411 Contracture of muscle, right shoulder
    M62.412 Contracture of muscle, left shoulder
    M62.419 Contracture of muscle, unspecified shoulder
● M62.42 Contracture of muscle, upper arm
    M62.421 Contracture of muscle, right upper arm
    M62.422 Contracture of muscle, left upper arm
    M62.429 Contracture of muscle, unspecified upper arm
● M62.43 Contracture of muscle, forearm
    M62.431 Contracture of muscle, right forearm
    M62.432 Contracture of muscle, left forearm
    M62.439 Contracture of muscle, unspecified forearm
● M62.44 Contracture of muscle, hand
    M62.441 Contracture of muscle, right hand
    M62.442 Contracture of muscle, left hand
    M62.449 Contracture of muscle, unspecified hand
● M62.45 Contracture of muscle, thigh
    M62.451 Contracture of muscle, right thigh
    M62.452 Contracture of muscle, left thigh
    M62.459 Contracture of muscle, unspecified thigh
● M62.46 Contracture of muscle, lower leg
    M62.461 Contracture of muscle, right lower leg
    M62.462 Contracture of muscle, left lower leg
    M62.469 Contracture of muscle, unspecified lower leg

N Newborn Age: 0   P Pediatric Age: 0–17   M Maternity DX: 12–55   A Adult Age: 15–124   ♀ Females Only   ♂ Males Only
Complication\Comorbidity   Major C\C   (Ex:) CC/MCC Exclusions   Present on Admission Requirement   Hospital-Acquired Condition

1129

CHAPTER 13 (M00-M99)

● M62.47   **Contracture of muscle, ankle and foot**
     M62.471   Contracture of muscle, right ankle and foot
     M62.472   Contracture of muscle, left ankle and foot
     M62.479   Contracture of muscle, unspecified ankle and foot
   M62.48   **Contracture of muscle, other site**
   M62.49   **Contracture of muscle, multiple sites**

● M62.5   **Muscle wasting and atrophy, not elsewhere classified**
     Disuse atrophy NEC
     Excludes1   neuralgic amyotrophy (G54.5)
                     progressive muscular atrophy (G12.29)
     Excludes2   pelvic muscle wasting (N81.84)
   M62.50   **Muscle wasting and atrophy, not elsewhere classified, unspecified site**
● M62.51   **Muscle wasting and atrophy, not elsewhere classified, shoulder**
     M62.511   Muscle wasting and atrophy, not elsewhere classified, right shoulder
     M62.512   Muscle wasting and atrophy, not elsewhere classified, left shoulder
     M62.519   Muscle wasting and atrophy, not elsewhere classified, unspecified shoulder
● M62.52   **Muscle wasting and atrophy, not elsewhere classified, upper arm**
     M62.521   Muscle wasting and atrophy, not elsewhere classified, right upper arm
     M62.522   Muscle wasting and atrophy, not elsewhere classified, left upper arm
     M62.529   Muscle wasting and atrophy, not elsewhere classified, unspecified upper arm
● M62.53   **Muscle wasting and atrophy, not elsewhere classified, forearm**
     M62.531   Muscle wasting and atrophy, not elsewhere classified, right forearm
     M62.532   Muscle wasting and atrophy, not elsewhere classified, left forearm
     M62.539   Muscle wasting and atrophy, not elsewhere classified, unspecified forearm
● M62.54   **Muscle wasting and atrophy, not elsewhere classified, hand**
     M62.541   Muscle wasting and atrophy, not elsewhere classified, right hand
     M62.542   Muscle wasting and atrophy, not elsewhere classified, left hand
     M62.549   Muscle wasting and atrophy, not elsewhere classified, unspecified hand
● M62.55   **Muscle wasting and atrophy, not elsewhere classified, thigh**
     M62.551   Muscle wasting and atrophy, not elsewhere classified, right thigh
     M62.552   Muscle wasting and atrophy, not elsewhere classified, left thigh
     M62.559   Muscle wasting and atrophy, not elsewhere classified, unspecified thigh
● M62.56   **Muscle wasting and atrophy, not elsewhere classified, lower leg**
     M62.561   Muscle wasting and atrophy, not elsewhere classified, right lower leg
     M62.562   Muscle wasting and atrophy, not elsewhere classified, left lower leg
     M62.569   Muscle wasting and atrophy, not elsewhere classified, unspecified lower leg

● M62.57   **Muscle wasting and atrophy, not elsewhere classified, ankle and foot**
     M62.571   Muscle wasting and atrophy, not elsewhere classified, right ankle and foot
     M62.572   Muscle wasting and atrophy, not elsewhere classified, left ankle and foot
     M62.579   Muscle wasting and atrophy, not elsewhere classified, unspecified ankle and foot
   M62.58   **Muscle wasting and atrophy, not elsewhere classified, other site**
   M62.59   **Muscle wasting and atrophy, not elsewhere classified, multiple sites**

● M62.8   **Other specified disorders of muscle**
     Excludes2   nontraumatic hematoma of muscle (M79.81)
   M62.81   **Muscle weakness (generalized)**
   M62.82   **Rhabdomyolysis** 🔖
     Excludes1   traumatic rhabdomyolysis (T79.6)
     (Ex) K68.12, M60.000-M60.19, M61.00-M61.19, M61.30-M61.59, M62.3, M62.50-M62.59, M62.82, M62.89, M72.6
● M62.83   **Muscle spasm**
     M62.830   Muscle spasm of back
     M62.831   Muscle spasm of calf
                  Charley-horse
     M62.838   Other muscle spasm
   M62.89   **Other specified disorders of muscle**
     Muscle (sheath) hernia
   M62.9   **Disorder of muscle, unspecified**

● M63   **Disorders of muscle in diseases classified elsewhere**
     Code first underlying disease, such as:
     leprosy (A30.-)
     neoplasm (C49.-, C79.89, D21., D48.1)
     schistosomiasis (B65.-)
     trichinellosis (B75)
     Excludes1   myopathy in cysticercosis (B69.81)
                     myopathy in endocrine diseases (G73.7)
                     myopathy in metabolic diseases (G73.7)
                     myopathy in sarcoidosis (D86.87)
                     myopathy in secondary syphilis (A51.49)
                     myopathy in syphilis (late) (A52.78)
                     myopathy in toxoplasmosis (B58.82)
                     myopathy in tuberculosis (A18.09)
● M63.8   **Disorders of muscle in diseases classified elsewhere**
   ▸ *M63.80*   *Disorders of muscle in diseases classified elsewhere, unspecified site*
● M63.81   **Disorders of muscle in diseases classified elsewhere, shoulder**
   ▸ *M63.811*   *Disorders of muscle in diseases classified elsewhere, right shoulder*
   ▸ *M63.812*   *Disorders of muscle in diseases classified elsewhere, left shoulder*
   ▸ *M63.819*   *Disorders of muscle in diseases classified elsewhere, unspecified shoulder*
● M63.82   **Disorders of muscle in diseases classified elsewhere, upper arm**
   ▸ *M63.821*   *Disorders of muscle in diseases classified elsewhere, right upper arm*
   ▸ *M63.822*   *Disorders of muscle in diseases classified elsewhere, left upper arm*
   ▸ *M63.829*   *Disorders of muscle in diseases classified elsewhere, unspecified upper arm*

◀ New   ◀▥ Revised   ~~deleted~~ Deleted   Excludes 1   Excludes 2   Includes   Use additional   Code first   Code also   Unspecified
OGCR Official Guidelines   ● Unacceptable Principal Diagnosis   X Assign placeholder X   ● Use Additional Character(s)   ▸ Manifestation Code   **Coding Clinic**

● M63.83　Disorders of muscle in diseases classified elsewhere, forearm

> *M63.831　Disorders of muscle in diseases classified elsewhere, right forearm*

> *M63.832　Disorders of muscle in diseases classified elsewhere, left forearm*

> *M63.839　Disorders of muscle in diseases classified elsewhere, unspecified forearm*

● M63.84　Disorders of muscle in diseases classified elsewhere, hand

> *M63.841　Disorders of muscle in diseases classified elsewhere, right hand*

> *M63.842　Disorders of muscle in diseases classified elsewhere, left hand*

> *M63.849　Disorders of muscle in diseases classified elsewhere, unspecified hand*

● M63.85　Disorders of muscle in diseases classified elsewhere, thigh

> *M63.851　Disorders of muscle in diseases classified elsewhere, right thigh*

> *M63.852　Disorders of muscle in diseases classified elsewhere, left thigh*

> *M63.859　Disorders of muscle in diseases classified elsewhere, unspecified thigh*

● M63.86　Disorders of muscle in diseases classified elsewhere, lower leg

> *M63.861　Disorders of muscle in diseases classified elsewhere, right lower leg*

> *M63.862　Disorders of muscle in diseases classified elsewhere, left lower leg*

> *M63.869　Disorders of muscle in diseases classified elsewhere, unspecified lower leg*

● M63.87　Disorders of muscle in diseases classified elsewhere, ankle and foot

> *M63.871　Disorders of muscle in diseases classified elsewhere, right ankle and foot*

> *M63.872　Disorders of muscle in diseases classified elsewhere, left ankle and foot*

> *M63.879　Disorders of muscle in diseases classified elsewhere, unspecified ankle and foot*

> *M63.88　Disorders of muscle in diseases classified elsewhere, other site*

> *M63.89　Disorders of muscle in diseases classified elsewhere, multiple sites*

DISORDERS OF SYNOVIUM AND TENDON (M65-M67)

● M65　Synovitis and tenosynovitis

> **Excludes1**　chronic crepitant synovitis of hand and wrist (M70.0-)
> current injury - see injury of ligament or tendon by body region
> soft tissue disorders related to use, overuse and pressure (M70.-)

● M65.0　Abscess of tendon sheath

> Use additional code (B95-B96) to identify bacterial agent

　M65.00　Abscess of tendon sheath, unspecified site

● M65.01　Abscess of tendon sheath, shoulder

　　M65.011　Abscess of tendon sheath, right shoulder

　　M65.012　Abscess of tendon sheath, left shoulder

　　M65.019　Abscess of tendon sheath, unspecified shoulder

Item 13–11　Synovitis is an inflammation of a synovial membrane resulting in pain on motion and is characterized by fluctuating swelling due to effusion in a synovial sac. **Tenosynovitis** is an inflammation of a tendon sheath and occurs most commonly in the wrists, hands, and feet. Bursitis is inflammation of a bursa (fluid filled sac) caused by repetitive use, trauma, infection, or systemic inflammatory disease. Bursae act as protectors and facilitate movement between bones and overlapping muscles (deep bursae) or between bones and tendons/skin (superficial bursae).

● M65.02　Abscess of tendon sheath, upper arm

　　M65.021　Abscess of tendon sheath, right upper arm

　　M65.022　Abscess of tendon sheath, left upper arm

　　M65.029　Abscess of tendon sheath, unspecified upper arm

● M65.03　Abscess of tendon sheath, forearm

　　M65.031　Abscess of tendon sheath, right forearm

　　M65.032　Abscess of tendon sheath, left forearm

　　M65.039　Abscess of tendon sheath, unspecified forearm

● M65.04　Abscess of tendon sheath, hand

　　M65.041　Abscess of tendon sheath, right hand

　　M65.042　Abscess of tendon sheath, left hand

　　M65.049　Abscess of tendon sheath, unspecified hand

● M65.05　Abscess of tendon sheath, thigh

　　M65.051　Abscess of tendon sheath, right thigh

　　M65.052　Abscess of tendon sheath, left thigh

　　M65.059　Abscess of tendon sheath, unspecified thigh

● M65.06　Abscess of tendon sheath, lower leg

　　M65.061　Abscess of tendon sheath, right lower leg

　　M65.062　Abscess of tendon sheath, left lower leg

　　M65.069　Abscess of tendon sheath, unspecified lower leg

● M65.07　Abscess of tendon sheath, ankle and foot

　　M65.071　Abscess of tendon sheath, right ankle and foot

　　M65.072　Abscess of tendon sheath, left ankle and foot

　　M65.079　Abscess of tendon sheath, unspecified ankle and foot

　　M65.08　Abscess of tendon sheath, other site

● M65.1　Other infective (teno)synovitis

　　M65.10　Other infective (teno)synovitis, unspecified site

● M65.11　Other infective (teno)synovitis, shoulder

　　M65.111　Other infective (teno)synovitis, right shoulder

　　M65.112　Other infective (teno)synovitis, left shoulder

　　M65.119　Other infective (teno)synovitis, unspecified shoulder

● M65.12　Other infective (teno)synovitis, elbow

　　M65.121　Other infective (teno)synovitis, right elbow

　　M65.122　Other infective (teno)synovitis, left elbow

　　M65.129　Other infective (teno)synovitis, unspecified elbow

CHAPTER 13 (M00-M99)

N Newborn Age: 0　　**P** Pediatric Age: 0–17　　**M** Maternity DX: 12–55　　**A** Adult Age: 15–124　　♀ Females Only　　♂ Males Only

🏥 Complication\Comorbidity　　🏥 Major C\C　　(Ex:) CC/MCC Exclusions　　🏥 Present on Admission Requirement　　🏥 Hospital-Acquired Condition　　　　1131

● M65.13　Other infective (teno)synovitis, wrist
　　　M65.131　Other infective (teno)synovitis, right wrist
　　　M65.132　Other infective (teno)synovitis, left wrist
　　　M65.139　Other infective (teno)synovitis, unspecified wrist
● M65.14　Other infective (teno)synovitis, hand
　　　M65.141　Other infective (teno)synovitis, right hand
　　　M65.142　Other infective (teno)synovitis, left hand
　　　M65.149　Other infective (teno)synovitis, unspecified hand
● M65.15　Other infective (teno)synovitis, hip
　　　M65.151　Other infective (teno)synovitis, right hip
　　　M65.152　Other infective (teno)synovitis, left hip
　　　M65.159　Other infective (teno)synovitis, unspecified hip
● M65.16　Other infective (teno)synovitis, knee
　　　M65.161　Other infective (teno)synovitis, right knee
　　　M65.162　Other infective (teno)synovitis, left knee
　　　M65.169　Other infective (teno)synovitis, unspecified knee
● M65.17　Other infective (teno)synovitis, ankle and foot
　　　M65.171　Other infective (teno)synovitis, right ankle and foot
　　　M65.172　Other infective (teno)synovitis, left ankle and foot
　　　M65.179　Other infective (teno)synovitis, unspecified ankle and foot
　　M65.18　Other infective (teno)synovitis, other site
　　M65.19　Other infective (teno)synovitis, multiple sites
● M65.2　Calcific tendinitis
　　Excludes1　tendinitis as classified in M75-M77
　　　　　　　　calcified tendinitis of shoulder (M75.3)
　　M65.20　Calcific tendinitis, unspecified site
● M65.22　Calcific tendinitis, upper arm
　　　M65.221　Calcific tendinitis, right upper arm
　　　M65.222　Calcific tendinitis, left upper arm
　　　M65.229　Calcific tendinitis, unspecified upper arm
● M65.23　Calcific tendinitis, forearm
　　　M65.231　Calcific tendinitis, right forearm
　　　M65.232　Calcific tendinitis, left forearm
　　　M65.239　Calcific tendinitis, unspecified forearm
● M65.24　Calcific tendinitis, hand
　　　M65.241　Calcific tendinitis, right hand
　　　M65.242　Calcific tendinitis, left hand
　　　M65.249　Calcific tendinitis, unspecified hand
● M65.25　Calcific tendinitis, thigh
　　　M65.251　Calcific tendinitis, right thigh
　　　M65.252　Calcific tendinitis, left thigh
　　　M65.259　Calcific tendinitis, unspecified thigh
● M65.26　Calcific tendinitis, lower leg
　　　M65.261　Calcific tendinitis, right lower leg
　　　M65.262　Calcific tendinitis, left lower leg
　　　M65.269　Calcific tendinitis, unspecified lower leg

● M65.27　Calcific tendinitis, ankle and foot
　　　M65.271　Calcific tendinitis, right ankle and foot
　　　M65.272　Calcific tendinitis, left ankle and foot
　　　M65.279　Calcific tendinitis, unspecified ankle and foot
　　M65.28　Calcific tendinitis, other site
　　M65.29　Calcific tendinitis, multiple sites
● M65.3　Trigger finger
　　　Nodular tendinous disease
　　M65.30　Trigger finger, unspecified finger
● M65.31　Trigger thumb
　　　M65.311　Trigger thumb, right thumb
　　　M65.312　Trigger thumb, left thumb
　　　M65.319　Trigger thumb, unspecified thumb
● M65.32　Trigger finger, index finger
　　　M65.321　Trigger finger, right index finger
　　　M65.322　Trigger finger, left index finger
　　　M65.329　Trigger finger, unspecified index finger
● M65.33　Trigger finger, middle finger
　　　M65.331　Trigger finger, right middle finger
　　　M65.332　Trigger finger, left middle finger
　　　M65.339　Trigger finger, unspecified middle finger
● M65.34　Trigger finger, ring finger
　　　M65.341　Trigger finger, right ring finger
　　　M65.342　Trigger finger, left ring finger
　　　M65.349　Trigger finger, unspecified ring finger
● M65.35　Trigger finger, little finger
　　　M65.351　Trigger finger, right little finger
　　　M65.352　Trigger finger, left little finger
　　　M65.359　Trigger finger, unspecified little finger
　　M65.4　Radial styloid tenosynovitis [de Quervain]
● M65.8　Other synovitis and tenosynovitis
　　M65.80　Other synovitis and tenosynovitis, unspecified site
● M65.81　Other synovitis and tenosynovitis, shoulder
　　　M65.811　Other synovitis and tenosynovitis, right shoulder
　　　M65.812　Other synovitis and tenosynovitis, left shoulder
　　　M65.819　Other synovitis and tenosynovitis, unspecified shoulder
● M65.82　Other synovitis and tenosynovitis, upper arm
　　　M65.821　Other synovitis and tenosynovitis, right upper arm
　　　M65.822　Other synovitis and tenosynovitis, left upper arm
　　　M65.829　Other synovitis and tenosynovitis, unspecified upper arm
● M65.83　Other synovitis and tenosynovitis, forearm
　　　M65.831　Other synovitis and tenosynovitis, right forearm
　　　M65.832　Other synovitis and tenosynovitis, left forearm
　　　M65.839　Other synovitis and tenosynovitis, unspecified forearm
● M65.84　Other synovitis and tenosynovitis, hand
　　　M65.841　Other synovitis and tenosynovitis, right hand
　　　M65.842　Other synovitis and tenosynovitis, left hand
　　　M65.849　Other synovitis and tenosynovitis, unspecified hand

◀ New　　◀ Revised　　deleted Deleted　　Excludes 1　　Excludes 2　　Includes　　Use additional　　Code first　　Code also　　Unspecified
OGCR Official Guidelines　　● Unacceptable Principal Diagnosis　　X Assign placeholder X　　● Use Additional Character(s)　　▶ Manifestation Code　　**Coding Clinic**

● **M65.85** Other synovitis and tenosynovitis, thigh

    M65.851 Other synovitis and tenosynovitis, right thigh

    M65.852 Other synovitis and tenosynovitis, left thigh

    M65.859 Other synovitis and tenosynovitis, unspecified thigh

● **M65.86** Other synovitis and tenosynovitis, lower leg

    M65.861 Other synovitis and tenosynovitis, right lower leg

    M65.862 Other synovitis and tenosynovitis, left lower leg

    M65.869 Other synovitis and tenosynovitis, unspecified lower leg

● **M65.87** Other synovitis and tenosynovitis, ankle and foot

    M65.871 Other synovitis and tenosynovitis, right ankle and foot

    M65.872 Other synovitis and tenosynovitis, left ankle and foot

    M65.879 Other synovitis and tenosynovitis, unspecified ankle and foot

  M65.88 Other synovitis and tenosynovitis, other site

  M65.89 Other synovitis and tenosynovitis, multiple sites

  M65.9 Synovitis and tenosynovitis, unspecified

● **M66** Spontaneous rupture of synovium and tendon

    Includes   rupture that occurs when a normal force is applied to tissues that are inferred to have less than normal strength

    Excludes2   rotator cuff syndrome (M75.1-)

                 rupture where an abnormal force is applied to normal tissue - see injury of tendon by body region

  M66.0 Rupture of popliteal cyst

● **M66.1** Rupture of synovium

    Rupture of synovial cyst

    Excludes2   rupture of popliteal cyst (M66.0)

  M66.10 Rupture of synovium, unspecified joint

● **M66.11** Rupture of synovium, shoulder

    M66.111 Rupture of synovium, right shoulder

    M66.112 Rupture of synovium, left shoulder

    M66.119 Rupture of synovium, unspecified shoulder

● **M66.12** Rupture of synovium, elbow

    M66.121 Rupture of synovium, right elbow

    M66.122 Rupture of synovium, left elbow

    M66.129 Rupture of synovium, unspecified elbow

● **M66.13** Rupture of synovium, wrist

    M66.131 Rupture of synovium, right wrist

    M66.132 Rupture of synovium, left wrist

    M66.139 Rupture of synovium, unspecified wrist

● **M66.14** Rupture of synovium, hand and fingers

    M66.141 Rupture of synovium, right hand

    M66.142 Rupture of synovium, left hand

    M66.143 Rupture of synovium, unspecified hand

    M66.144 Rupture of synovium, right finger(s)

    M66.145 Rupture of synovium, left finger(s)

    M66.146 Rupture of synovium, unspecified finger(s)

● **M66.15** Rupture of synovium, hip

    M66.151 Rupture of synovium, right hip

    M66.152 Rupture of synovium, left hip

    M66.159 Rupture of synovium, unspecified hip

● **M66.17** Rupture of synovium, ankle, foot and toes

    M66.171 Rupture of synovium, right ankle

    M66.172 Rupture of synovium, left ankle

    M66.173 Rupture of synovium, unspecified ankle

    M66.174 Rupture of synovium, right foot

    M66.175 Rupture of synovium, left foot

    M66.176 Rupture of synovium, unspecified foot

    M66.177 Rupture of synovium, right toe(s)

    M66.178 Rupture of synovium, left toe(s)

    M66.179 Rupture of synovium, unspecified toe(s)

  M66.18 Rupture of synovium, other site

● **M66.2** Spontaneous rupture of extensor tendons

  M66.20 Spontaneous rupture of extensor tendons, unspecified site

● **M66.21** Spontaneous rupture of extensor tendons, shoulder

    M66.211 Spontaneous rupture of extensor tendons, right shoulder

    M66.212 Spontaneous rupture of extensor tendons, left shoulder

    M66.219 Spontaneous rupture of extensor tendons, unspecified shoulder

● **M66.22** Spontaneous rupture of extensor tendons, upper arm

    M66.221 Spontaneous rupture of extensor tendons, right upper arm

    M66.222 Spontaneous rupture of extensor tendons, left upper arm

    M66.229 Spontaneous rupture of extensor tendons, unspecified upper arm

● **M66.23** Spontaneous rupture of extensor tendons, forearm

    M66.231 Spontaneous rupture of extensor tendons, right forearm

    M66.232 Spontaneous rupture of extensor tendons, left forearm

    M66.239 Spontaneous rupture of extensor tendons, unspecified forearm

● **M66.24** Spontaneous rupture of extensor tendons, hand

    M66.241 Spontaneous rupture of extensor tendons, right hand

    M66.242 Spontaneous rupture of extensor tendons, left hand

    M66.249 Spontaneous rupture of extensor tendons, unspecified hand

● **M66.25** Spontaneous rupture of extensor tendons, thigh

    M66.251 Spontaneous rupture of extensor tendons, right thigh

    M66.252 Spontaneous rupture of extensor tendons, left thigh

    M66.259 Spontaneous rupture of extensor tendons, unspecified thigh

● **M66.26** Spontaneous rupture of extensor tendons, lower leg

    M66.261 Spontaneous rupture of extensor tendons, right lower leg

    M66.262 Spontaneous rupture of extensor tendons, left lower leg

    M66.269 Spontaneous rupture of extensor tendons, unspecified lower leg

CHAPTER 13 (M00-M99)

● M66.27   Spontaneous rupture of extensor tendons, ankle and foot

     M66.271   Spontaneous rupture of extensor tendons, right ankle and foot

     M66.272   Spontaneous rupture of extensor tendons, left ankle and foot

     M66.279   Spontaneous rupture of extensor tendons, unspecified ankle and foot

   M66.28   Spontaneous rupture of extensor tendons, other site

   M66.29   Spontaneous rupture of extensor tendons, multiple sites

● M66.3   Spontaneous rupture of flexor tendons

   M66.30   Spontaneous rupture of flexor tendons, unspecified site

● M66.31   Spontaneous rupture of flexor tendons, shoulder

     M66.311   Spontaneous rupture of flexor tendons, right shoulder

     M66.312   Spontaneous rupture of flexor tendons, left shoulder

     M66.319   Spontaneous rupture of flexor tendons, unspecified shoulder

● M66.32   Spontaneous rupture of flexor tendons, upper arm

     M66.321   Spontaneous rupture of flexor tendons, right upper arm

     M66.322   Spontaneous rupture of flexor tendons, left upper arm

     M66.329   Spontaneous rupture of flexor tendons, unspecified upper arm

● M66.33   Spontaneous rupture of flexor tendons, forearm

     M66.331   Spontaneous rupture of flexor tendons, right forearm

     M66.332   Spontaneous rupture of flexor tendons, left forearm

     M66.339   Spontaneous rupture of flexor tendons, unspecified forearm

● M66.34   Spontaneous rupture of flexor tendons, hand

     M66.341   Spontaneous rupture of flexor tendons, right hand

     M66.342   Spontaneous rupture of flexor tendons, left hand

     M66.349   Spontaneous rupture of flexor tendons, unspecified hand

● M66.35   Spontaneous rupture of flexor tendons, thigh

     M66.351   Spontaneous rupture of flexor tendons, right thigh

     M66.352   Spontaneous rupture of flexor tendons, left thigh

     M66.359   Spontaneous rupture of flexor tendons, unspecified thigh

● M66.36   Spontaneous rupture of flexor tendons, lower leg

     M66.361   Spontaneous rupture of flexor tendons, right lower leg

     M66.362   Spontaneous rupture of flexor tendons, left lower leg

     M66.369   Spontaneous rupture of flexor tendons, unspecified lower leg

● M66.37   Spontaneous rupture of flexor tendons, ankle and foot

     M66.371   Spontaneous rupture of flexor tendons, right ankle and foot

     M66.372   Spontaneous rupture of flexor tendons, left ankle and foot

     M66.379   Spontaneous rupture of flexor tendons, unspecified ankle and foot

   M66.38   Spontaneous rupture of flexor tendons, other site

   M66.39   Spontaneous rupture of flexor tendons, multiple sites

● M66.8   Spontaneous rupture of other tendons

   M66.80   Spontaneous rupture of other tendons, unspecified site

● M66.81   Spontaneous rupture of other tendons, shoulder

     M66.811   Spontaneous rupture of other tendons, right shoulder

     M66.812   Spontaneous rupture of other tendons, left shoulder

     M66.819   Spontaneous rupture of other tendons, unspecified shoulder

● M66.82   Spontaneous rupture of other tendons, upper arm

     M66.821   Spontaneous rupture of other tendons, right upper arm

     M66.822   Spontaneous rupture of other tendons, left upper arm

     M66.829   Spontaneous rupture of other tendons, unspecified upper arm

● M66.83   Spontaneous rupture of other tendons, forearm

     M66.831   Spontaneous rupture of other tendons, right forearm

     M66.832   Spontaneous rupture of other tendons, left forearm

     M66.839   Spontaneous rupture of other tendons, unspecified forearm

● M66.84   Spontaneous rupture of other tendons, hand

     M66.841   Spontaneous rupture of other tendons, right hand

     M66.842   Spontaneous rupture of other tendons, left hand

     M66.849   Spontaneous rupture of other tendons, unspecified hand

● M66.85   Spontaneous rupture of other tendons, thigh

     M66.851   Spontaneous rupture of other tendons, right thigh

     M66.852   Spontaneous rupture of other tendons, left thigh

     M66.859   Spontaneous rupture of other tendons, unspecified thigh

● M66.86   Spontaneous rupture of other tendons, lower leg

     M66.861   Spontaneous rupture of other tendons, right lower leg

     M66.862   Spontaneous rupture of other tendons, left lower leg

     M66.869   Spontaneous rupture of other tendons, unspecified lower leg

● M66.87   Spontaneous rupture of other tendons, ankle and foot

     M66.871   Spontaneous rupture of other tendons, right ankle and foot

     M66.872   Spontaneous rupture of other tendons, left ankle and foot

     M66.879   Spontaneous rupture of other tendons, unspecified ankle and foot

   M66.88   Spontaneous rupture of other tendons, other

   M66.89   Spontaneous rupture of other tendons, multiple sites

M66.9   Spontaneous rupture of unspecified tendon

     Rupture at musculotendinous junction, nontraumatic

● **M67   Other disorders of synovium and tendon**

     Excludes1   palmar fascial fibromatosis [Dupuytren] (M72.0)

                  tendinitis NOS (M77.9-)

                  xanthomatosis localized to tendons (E78.2)

● **M67.0   Short Achilles tendon (acquired)**

     M67.00   Short Achilles tendon (acquired), unspecified ankle

     M67.01   Short Achilles tendon (acquired), right ankle

     M67.02   Short Achilles tendon (acquired), left ankle

● **M67.2   Synovial hypertrophy, not elsewhere classified**

     Excludes1   villonodular synovitis (pigmented) (M12.2-)

     M67.20   Synovial hypertrophy, not elsewhere classified, unspecified site

   ● **M67.21**   Synovial hypertrophy, not elsewhere classified, shoulder

       M67.211   Synovial hypertrophy, not elsewhere classified, right shoulder

       M67.212   Synovial hypertrophy, not elsewhere classified, left shoulder

       M67.219   Synovial hypertrophy, not elsewhere classified, unspecified shoulder

   ● **M67.22**   Synovial hypertrophy, not elsewhere classified, upper arm

       M67.221   Synovial hypertrophy, not elsewhere classified, right upper arm

       M67.222   Synovial hypertrophy, not elsewhere classified, left upper arm

       M67.229   Synovial hypertrophy, not elsewhere classified, unspecified upper arm

   ● **M67.23**   Synovial hypertrophy, not elsewhere classified, forearm

       M67.231   Synovial hypertrophy, not elsewhere classified, right forearm

       M67.232   Synovial hypertrophy, not elsewhere classified, left forearm

       M67.239   Synovial hypertrophy, not elsewhere classified, unspecified forearm

   ● **M67.24**   Synovial hypertrophy, not elsewhere classified, hand

       M67.241   Synovial hypertrophy, not elsewhere classified, right hand

       M67.242   Synovial hypertrophy, not elsewhere classified, left hand

       M67.249   Synovial hypertrophy, not elsewhere classified, unspecified hand

   ● **M67.25**   Synovial hypertrophy, not elsewhere classified, thigh

       M67.251   Synovial hypertrophy, not elsewhere classified, right thigh

       M67.252   Synovial hypertrophy, not elsewhere classified, left thigh

       M67.259   Synovial hypertrophy, not elsewhere classified, unspecified thigh

   ● **M67.26**   Synovial hypertrophy, not elsewhere classified, lower leg

       M67.261   Synovial hypertrophy, not elsewhere classified, right lower leg

       M67.262   Synovial hypertrophy, not elsewhere classified, left lower leg

       M67.269   Synovial hypertrophy, not elsewhere classified, unspecified lower leg

   ● **M67.27**   Synovial hypertrophy, not elsewhere classified, ankle and foot

       M67.271   Synovial hypertrophy, not elsewhere classified, right ankle and foot

       M67.272   Synovial hypertrophy, not elsewhere classified, left ankle and foot

       M67.279   Synovial hypertrophy, not elsewhere classified, unspecified ankle and foot

     M67.28   Synovial hypertrophy, not elsewhere classified, other site

     M67.29   Synovial hypertrophy, not elsewhere classified, multiple sites

● **M67.3   Transient synovitis**

     Toxic synovitis

     Excludes1   palindromic rheumatism (M12.3-)

     M67.30   Transient synovitis, unspecified site

   ● **M67.31**   Transient synovitis, shoulder

       M67.311   Transient synovitis, right shoulder

       M67.312   Transient synovitis, left shoulder

       M67.319   Transient synovitis, unspecified shoulder

   ● **M67.32**   Transient synovitis, elbow

       M67.321   Transient synovitis, right elbow

       M67.322   Transient synovitis, left elbow

       M67.329   Transient synovitis, unspecified elbow

   ● **M67.33**   Transient synovitis, wrist

       M67.331   Transient synovitis, right wrist

       M67.332   Transient synovitis, left wrist

       M67.339   Transient synovitis, unspecified wrist

   ● **M67.34**   Transient synovitis, hand

       M67.341   Transient synovitis, right hand

       M67.342   Transient synovitis, left hand

       M67.349   Transient synovitis, unspecified hand

   ● **M67.35**   Transient synovitis, hip

       M67.351   Transient synovitis, right hip

       M67.352   Transient synovitis, left hip

       M67.359   Transient synovitis, unspecified hip

   ● **M67.36**   Transient synovitis, knee

       M67.361   Transient synovitis, right knee

       M67.362   Transient synovitis, left knee

       M67.369   Transient synovitis, unspecified knee

   ● **M67.37**   Transient synovitis, ankle and foot

       M67.371   Transient synovitis, right ankle and foot

       M67.372   Transient synovitis, left ankle and foot

       M67.379   Transient synovitis, unspecified ankle and foot

     M67.38   Transient synovitis, other site

     M67.39   Transient synovitis, multiple sites

● **M67.4   Ganglion**

     Ganglion of joint or tendon (sheath)

     Excludes1   ganglion in yaws (A66.6)

     Excludes2   cyst of bursa (M71.2-M71.3)

                  cyst of synovium (M71.2-M71.3)

     M67.40   Ganglion, unspecified site

   ● **M67.41**   Ganglion, shoulder

       M67.411   Ganglion, right shoulder

       M67.412   Ganglion, left shoulder

       M67.419   Ganglion, unspecified shoulder

   ● **M67.42**   Ganglion, elbow

       M67.421   Ganglion, right elbow

       M67.422   Ganglion, left elbow

       M67.429   Ganglion, unspecified elbow

CHAPTER 13 (M00-M99)

N Newborn Age: 0   **P** Pediatric Age: 0–17   **M** Maternity DX: 12–55   **A** Adult Age: 15–124   ♀ Females Only   ♂ Males Only

Complication\Comorbidity   Major C\C   (Ex) CC/MCC Exclusions   Present on Admission Requirement   Hospital-Acquired Condition

1135

● M67.43 Ganglion, wrist
     M67.431 Ganglion, right wrist
     M67.432 Ganglion, left wrist
     M67.439 Ganglion, unspecified wrist
● M67.44 Ganglion, hand
     M67.441 Ganglion, right hand
     M67.442 Ganglion, left hand
     M67.449 Ganglion, unspecified hand
● M67.45 Ganglion, hip
     M67.451 Ganglion, right hip
     M67.452 Ganglion, left hip
     M67.459 Ganglion, unspecified hip
● M67.46 Ganglion, knee
     M67.461 Ganglion, right knee
     M67.462 Ganglion, left knee
     M67.469 Ganglion, unspecified knee
● M67.47 Ganglion, ankle and foot
     M67.471 Ganglion, right ankle and foot
     M67.472 Ganglion, left ankle and foot
     M67.479 Ganglion, unspecified ankle and foot
   M67.48 Ganglion, other site
   M67.49 Ganglion, multiple sites
● M67.5 Plica syndrome
          Plica knee
   M67.50 Plica syndrome, unspecified knee
   M67.51 Plica syndrome, right knee
   M67.52 Plica syndrome, left knee
● M67.8 Other specified disorders of synovium and tendon
   M67.80 Other specified disorders of synovium and tendon, unspecified site
● M67.81 Other specified disorders of synovium and tendon, shoulder
     M67.811 Other specified disorders of synovium, right shoulder
     M67.812 Other specified disorders of synovium, left shoulder
     M67.813 Other specified disorders of tendon, right shoulder
     M67.814 Other specified disorders of tendon, left shoulder
     M67.819 Other specified disorders of synovium and tendon, unspecified shoulder
● M67.82 Other specified disorders of synovium and tendon, elbow
     M67.821 Other specified disorders of synovium, right elbow
     M67.822 Other specified disorders of synovium, left elbow
     M67.823 Other specified disorders of tendon, right elbow
     M67.824 Other specified disorders of tendon, left elbow
     M67.829 Other specified disorders of synovium and tendon, unspecified elbow
● M67.83 Other specified disorders of synovium and tendon, wrist
     M67.831 Other specified disorders of synovium, right wrist
     M67.832 Other specified disorders of synovium, left wrist

     M67.833 Other specified disorders of tendon, right wrist
     M67.834 Other specified disorders of tendon, left wrist
     M67.839 Other specified disorders of synovium and tendon, unspecified forearm
● M67.84 Other specified disorders of synovium and tendon, hand
     M67.841 Other specified disorders of synovium, right hand
     M67.842 Other specified disorders of synovium, left hand
     M67.843 Other specified disorders of tendon, right hand
     M67.844 Other specified disorders of tendon, left hand
     M67.849 Other specified disorders of synovium and tendon, unspecified hand
● M67.85 Other specified disorders of synovium and tendon, hip
     M67.851 Other specified disorders of synovium, right hip
     M67.852 Other specified disorders of synovium, left hip
     M67.853 Other specified disorders of tendon, right hip
     M67.854 Other specified disorders of tendon, left hip
     M67.859 Other specified disorders of synovium and tendon, unspecified hip
● M67.86 Other specified disorders of synovium and tendon, knee
     M67.861 Other specified disorders of synovium, right knee
     M67.862 Other specified disorders of synovium, left knee
     M67.863 Other specified disorders of tendon, right knee
     M67.864 Other specified disorders of tendon, left knee
     M67.869 Other specified disorders of synovium and tendon, unspecified knee
● M67.87 Other specified disorders of synovium and tendon, ankle and foot
     M67.871 Other specified disorders of synovium, right ankle and foot
     M67.872 Other specified disorders of synovium, left ankle and foot
     M67.873 Other specified disorders of tendon, right ankle and foot
     M67.874 Other specified disorders of tendon, left ankle and foot
     M67.879 Other specified disorders of synovium and tendon, unspecified ankle and foot
   M67.88 Other specified disorders of synovium and tendon, other site
   M67.89 Other specified disorders of synovium and tendon, multiple sites

◀ New   ◀▥ Revised   ~~deleted~~ Deleted   Excludes 1   Excludes 2   Includes   Use additional   Code first   Code also   Unspecified

OGCR Official Guidelines   ● Unacceptable Principal Diagnosis   X Assign placeholder X   ● Use Additional Character(s)   ▷ Manifestation Code   Coding Clinic

● M67.9 Unspecified disorder of synovium and tendon

    M67.90 Unspecified disorder of synovium and tendon, unspecified site

● M67.91 Unspecified disorder of synovium and tendon, shoulder

    M67.911 Unspecified disorder of synovium and tendon, right shoulder

    M67.912 Unspecified disorder of synovium and tendon, left shoulder

    M67.919 Unspecified disorder of synovium and tendon, unspecified shoulder

● M67.92 Unspecified disorder of synovium and tendon, upper arm

    M67.921 Unspecified disorder of synovium and tendon, right upper arm

    M67.922 Unspecified disorder of synovium and tendon, left upper arm

    M67.929 Unspecified disorder of synovium and tendon, unspecified upper arm

● M67.93 Unspecified disorder of synovium and tendon, forearm

    M67.931 Unspecified disorder of synovium and tendon, right forearm

    M67.932 Unspecified disorder of synovium and tendon, left forearm

    M67.939 Unspecified disorder of synovium and tendon, unspecified forearm

● M67.94 Unspecified disorder of synovium and tendon, hand

    M67.941 Unspecified disorder of synovium and tendon, right hand

    M67.942 Unspecified disorder of synovium and tendon, left hand

    M67.949 Unspecified disorder of synovium and tendon, unspecified hand

● M67.95 Unspecified disorder of synovium and tendon, thigh

    M67.951 Unspecified disorder of synovium and tendon, right thigh

    M67.952 Unspecified disorder of synovium and tendon, left thigh

    M67.959 Unspecified disorder of synovium and tendon, unspecified thigh

● M67.96 Unspecified disorder of synovium and tendon, lower leg

    M67.961 Unspecified disorder of synovium and tendon, right lower leg

    M67.962 Unspecified disorder of synovium and tendon, left lower leg

    M67.969 Unspecified disorder of synovium and tendon, unspecified lower leg

● M67.97 Unspecified disorder of synovium and tendon, ankle and foot

    M67.971 Unspecified disorder of synovium and tendon, right ankle and foot

    M67.972 Unspecified disorder of synovium and tendon, left ankle and foot

    M67.979 Unspecified disorder of synovium and tendon, unspecified ankle and foot

  M67.98 Unspecified disorder of synovium and tendon, other site

  M67.99 Unspecified disorder of synovium and tendon, multiple sites

---

OTHER SOFT TISSUE DISORDERS (M70-M79)

● M70 Soft tissue disorders related to use, overuse and pressure

    Includes   soft tissue disorders of occupational origin

    Use additional external cause code to identify activity causing disorder (Y93.-)

    Excludes1   bursitis NOS (M71.9-)

    Excludes2   bursitis of shoulder (M75.5)
                enthesopathies (M76-M77)
                pressure ulcer (pressure area) (L89.-)

● M70.0 Crepitant synovitis (acute) (chronic) of hand and wrist

  ● M70.03 Crepitant synovitis (acute) (chronic), wrist

    M70.031 Crepitant synovitis (acute) (chronic), right wrist

    M70.032 Crepitant synovitis (acute) (chronic), left wrist

    M70.039 Crepitant synovitis (acute) (chronic), unspecified wrist

  ● M70.04 Crepitant synovitis (acute) (chronic), hand

    M70.041 Crepitant synovitis (acute) (chronic), right hand

    M70.042 Crepitant synovitis (acute) (chronic), left hand

    M70.049 Crepitant synovitis (acute) (chronic), unspecified hand

● M70.1 Bursitis of hand

    M70.10 Bursitis, unspecified hand

    M70.11 Bursitis, right hand

    M70.12 Bursitis, left hand

● M70.2 Olecranon bursitis

    M70.20 Olecranon bursitis, unspecified elbow

    M70.21 Olecranon bursitis, right elbow

    M70.22 Olecranon bursitis, left elbow

● M70.3 Other bursitis of elbow

    M70.30 Other bursitis of elbow, unspecified elbow

    M70.31 Other bursitis of elbow, right elbow

    M70.32 Other bursitis of elbow, left elbow

● M70.4 Prepatellar bursitis

    M70.40 Prepatellar bursitis, unspecified knee

    M70.41 Prepatellar bursitis, right knee

    M70.42 Prepatellar bursitis, left knee

● M70.5 Other bursitis of knee

    M70.50 Other bursitis of knee, unspecified knee

    M70.51 Other bursitis of knee, right knee

    M70.52 Other bursitis of knee, left knee

● M70.6 Trochanteric bursitis
    Trochanteric tendinitis

    M70.60 Trochanteric bursitis, unspecified hip

    M70.61 Trochanteric bursitis, right hip

    M70.62 Trochanteric bursitis, left hip

● M70.7 Other bursitis of hip
    Ischial bursitis

    M70.70 Other bursitis of hip, unspecified hip

    M70.71 Other bursitis of hip, right hip

    M70.72 Other bursitis of hip, left hip

CHAPTER 13 (M00-M99)

CHAPTER 13 (M00-M99)

● M70.8   Other soft tissue disorders related to use, overuse and pressure

    M70.80   Other soft tissue disorders related to use, overuse and pressure of unspecified site

● M70.81   Other soft tissue disorders related to use, overuse and pressure of shoulder

    M70.811   Other soft tissue disorders related to use, overuse and pressure, right shoulder

    M70.812   Other soft tissue disorders related to use, overuse and pressure, left shoulder

    M70.819   Other soft tissue disorders related to use, overuse and pressure, unspecified shoulder

● M70.82   Other soft tissue disorders related to use, overuse and pressure of upper arm

    M70.821   Other soft tissue disorders related to use, overuse and pressure, right upper arm

    M70.822   Other soft tissue disorders related to use, overuse and pressure, left upper arm

    M70.829   Other soft tissue disorders related to use, overuse and pressure, unspecified upper arms

● M70.83   Other soft tissue disorders related to use, overuse and pressure of forearm

    M70.831   Other soft tissue disorders related to use, overuse and pressure, right forearm

    M70.832   Other soft tissue disorders related to use, overuse and pressure, left forearm

    M70.839   Other soft tissue disorders related to use, overuse and pressure, unspecified forearm

● M70.84   Other soft tissue disorders related to use, overuse and pressure of hand

    M70.841   Other soft tissue disorders related to use, overuse and pressure, right hand

    M70.842   Other soft tissue disorders related to use, overuse and pressure, left hand

    M70.849   Other soft tissue disorders related to use, overuse and pressure, unspecified hand

● M70.85   Other soft tissue disorders related to use, overuse and pressure of thigh

    M70.851   Other soft tissue disorders related to use, overuse and pressure, right thigh

    M70.852   Other soft tissue disorders related to use, overuse and pressure, left thigh

    M70.859   Other soft tissue disorders related to use, overuse and pressure, unspecified thigh

● M70.86   Other soft tissue disorders related to use, overuse and pressure lower leg

    M70.861   Other soft tissue disorders related to use, overuse and pressure, right lower leg

    M70.862   Other soft tissue disorders related to use, overuse and pressure, left lower leg

    M70.869   Other soft tissue disorders related to use, overuse and pressure, unspecified leg

● M70.87   Other soft tissue disorders related to use, overuse and pressure of ankle and foot

    M70.871   Other soft tissue disorders related to use, overuse and pressure, right ankle and foot

    M70.872   Other soft tissue disorders related to use, overuse and pressure, left ankle and foot

    M70.879   Other soft tissue disorders related to use, overuse and pressure, unspecified ankle and foot

    M70.88   Other soft tissue disorders related to use, overuse and pressure other site

    M70.89   Other soft tissue disorders related to use, overuse and pressure multiple sites

● M70.9   Unspecified soft tissue disorder related to use, overuse and pressure

    M70.90   Unspecified soft tissue disorder related to use, overuse and pressure of unspecified site

● M70.91   Unspecified soft tissue disorder related to use, overuse and pressure of shoulder

    M70.911   Unspecified soft tissue disorder related to use, overuse and pressure, right shoulder

    M70.912   Unspecified soft tissue disorder related to use, overuse and pressure, left shoulder

    M70.919   Unspecified soft tissue disorder related to use, overuse and pressure, unspecified shoulder

● M70.92   Unspecified soft tissue disorder related to use, overuse and pressure of upper arm

    M70.921   Unspecified soft tissue disorder related to use, overuse and pressure, right upper arm

    M70.922   Unspecified soft tissue disorder related to use, overuse and pressure, left upper arm

    M70.929   Unspecified soft tissue disorder related to use, overuse and pressure, unspecified upper arm

● M70.93   Unspecified soft tissue disorder related to use, overuse and pressure of forearm

    M70.931   Unspecified soft tissue disorder related to use, overuse and pressure, right forearm

    M70.932   Unspecified soft tissue disorder related to use, overuse and pressure, left forearm

    M70.939   Unspecified soft tissue disorder related to use, overuse and pressure, unspecified forearm

● M70.94   Unspecified soft tissue disorder related to use, overuse and pressure of hand

    M70.941   Unspecified soft tissue disorder related to use, overuse and pressure, right hand

    M70.942   Unspecified soft tissue disorder related to use, overuse and pressure, left hand

    M70.949   Unspecified soft tissue disorder related to use, overuse and pressure, unspecified hand

◀ New   ◀|||| Revised   ~~deleted~~ Deleted   Excludes 1   Excludes 2   Includes   Use additional   Code first   Code also   Unspecified

OGCR Official Guidelines   ● Unacceptable Principal Diagnosis   X Assign placeholder X   ● Use Additional Character(s)   ▶ Manifestation Code   **Coding Clinic**

● M70.95 Unspecified soft tissue disorder related to use, overuse and pressure of thigh

M70.951 Unspecified soft tissue disorder related to use, overuse and pressure, right thigh

M70.952 Unspecified soft tissue disorder related to use, overuse and pressure, left thigh

M70.959 Unspecified soft tissue disorder related to use, overuse and pressure, unspecified thigh

● M70.96 Unspecified soft tissue disorder related to use, overuse and pressure lower leg

M70.961 Unspecified soft tissue disorder related to use, overuse and pressure, right lower leg

M70.962 Unspecified soft tissue disorder related to use, overuse and pressure, left lower leg

M70.969 Unspecified soft tissue disorder related to use, overuse and pressure, unspecified lower leg

● M70.97 Unspecified soft tissue disorder related to use, overuse and pressure of ankle and foot

M70.971 Unspecified soft tissue disorder related to use, overuse and pressure, right ankle and foot

M70.972 Unspecified soft tissue disorder related to use, overuse and pressure, left ankle and foot

M70.979 Unspecified soft tissue disorder related to use, overuse and pressure, unspecified ankle and foot

M70.98 Unspecified soft tissue disorder related to use, overuse and pressure other

M70.99 Unspecified soft tissue disorder related to use, overuse and pressure multiple sites

● M71 Other bursopathies

Excludes1 bunion (M20.1)
bursitis related to use, overuse or pressure (M70.-)
enthesopathies (M76-M77)

● M71.0 Abscess of bursa

Use additional code (B95.-, B96.-) to identify causative organism

M71.00 Abscess of bursa, unspecified site

● M71.01 Abscess of bursa, shoulder

M71.011 Abscess of bursa, right shoulder

M71.012 Abscess of bursa, left shoulder

M71.019 Abscess of bursa, unspecified shoulder

● M71.02 Abscess of bursa, elbow

M71.021 Abscess of bursa, right elbow

M71.022 Abscess of bursa, left elbow

M71.029 Abscess of bursa, unspecified elbow

● M71.03 Abscess of bursa, wrist

M71.031 Abscess of bursa, right wrist

M71.032 Abscess of bursa, left wrist

M71.039 Abscess of bursa, unspecified wrist

● M71.04 Abscess of bursa, hand

M71.041 Abscess of bursa, right hand

M71.042 Abscess of bursa, left hand

M71.049 Abscess of bursa, unspecified hand

● M71.05 Abscess of bursa, hip

M71.051 Abscess of bursa, right hip

M71.052 Abscess of bursa, left hip

M71.059 Abscess of bursa, unspecified hip

● M71.06 Abscess of bursa, knee

M71.061 Abscess of bursa, right knee

M71.062 Abscess of bursa, left knee

M71.069 Abscess of bursa, unspecified knee

● M71.07 Abscess of bursa, ankle and foot

M71.071 Abscess of bursa, right ankle and foot

M71.072 Abscess of bursa, left ankle and foot

M71.079 Abscess of bursa, unspecified ankle and foot

M71.08 Abscess of bursa, other site

M71.09 Abscess of bursa, multiple sites

● M71.1 Other infective bursitis

Use additional code (B95.-, B96.-) to identify causative organism

M71.10 Other infective bursitis, unspecified site

● M71.11 Other infective bursitis, shoulder

M71.111 Other infective bursitis, right shoulder

M71.112 Other infective bursitis, left shoulder

M71.119 Other infective bursitis, unspecified shoulder

● M71.12 Other infective bursitis, elbow

M71.121 Other infective bursitis, right elbow

M71.122 Other infective bursitis, left elbow

M71.129 Other infective bursitis, unspecified elbow

● M71.13 Other infective bursitis, wrist

M71.131 Other infective bursitis, right wrist

M71.132 Other infective bursitis, left wrist

M71.139 Other infective bursitis, unspecified wrist

● M71.14 Other infective bursitis, hand

M71.141 Other infective bursitis, right hand

M71.142 Other infective bursitis, left hand

M71.149 Other infective bursitis, unspecified hand

● M71.15 Other infective bursitis, hip

M71.151 Other infective bursitis, right hip

M71.152 Other infective bursitis, left hip

M71.159 Other infective bursitis, unspecified hip

● M71.16 Other infective bursitis, knee

M71.161 Other infective bursitis, right knee

M71.162 Other infective bursitis, left knee

M71.169 Other infective bursitis, unspecified knee

● M71.17 Other infective bursitis, ankle and foot

M71.171 Other infective bursitis, right ankle and foot

M71.172 Other infective bursitis, left ankle and foot

M71.179 Other infective bursitis, unspecified ankle and foot

M71.18 Other infective bursitis, other site

M71.19 Other infective bursitis, multiple sites

● **M71.2 Synovial cyst of popliteal space [Baker]**
Popliteal space = popliteal cavity, popliteal fossa. Depression in the posterior aspect of the knee (behind the knee).

> **Excludes1** synovial cyst of popliteal space with rupture (M66.0)

M71.20 Synovial cyst of popliteal space [Baker], unspecified knee

M71.21 Synovial cyst of popliteal space [Baker], right knee

M71.22 Synovial cyst of popliteal space [Baker], left knee

● **M71.3 Other bursal cyst**
Synovial cyst NOS

> **Excludes1** synovial cyst with rupture (M66.1-)

M71.30 Other bursal cyst, unspecified site

● M71.31 Other bursal cyst, shoulder
  M71.311 Other bursal cyst, right shoulder
  M71.312 Other bursal cyst, left shoulder
  M71.319 Other bursal cyst, unspecified shoulder

● M71.32 Other bursal cyst, elbow
  M71.321 Other bursal cyst, right elbow
  M71.322 Other bursal cyst, left elbow
  M71.329 Other bursal cyst, unspecified elbow

● M71.33 Other bursal cyst, wrist
  M71.331 Other bursal cyst, right wrist
  M71.332 Other bursal cyst, left wrist
  M71.339 Other bursal cyst, unspecified wrist

● M71.34 Other bursal cyst, hand
  M71.341 Other bursal cyst, right hand
  M71.342 Other bursal cyst, left hand
  M71.349 Other bursal cyst, unspecified hand

● M71.35 Other bursal cyst, hip
  M71.351 Other bursal cyst, right hip
  M71.352 Other bursal cyst, left hip
  M71.359 Other bursal cyst, unspecified hip

● M71.37 Other bursal cyst, ankle and foot
  M71.371 Other bursal cyst, right ankle and foot
  M71.372 Other bursal cyst, left ankle and foot
  M71.379 Other bursal cyst, unspecified ankle and foot

M71.38 Other bursal cyst, other site

M71.39 Other bursal cyst, multiple sites

● **M71.4 Calcium deposit in bursa**

> **Excludes2** calcium deposit in bursa of shoulder (M75.3)

M71.40 Calcium deposit in bursa, unspecified site

● M71.42 Calcium deposit in bursa, elbow
  M71.421 Calcium deposit in bursa, right elbow
  M71.422 Calcium deposit in bursa, left elbow
  M71.429 Calcium deposit in bursa, unspecified elbow

● M71.43 Calcium deposit in bursa, wrist
  M71.431 Calcium deposit in bursa, right wrist
  M71.432 Calcium deposit in bursa, left wrist
  M71.439 Calcium deposit in bursa, unspecified wrist

● M71.44 Calcium deposit in bursa, hand
  M71.441 Calcium deposit in bursa, right hand
  M71.442 Calcium deposit in bursa, left hand
  M71.449 Calcium deposit in bursa, unspecified hand

● M71.45 Calcium deposit in bursa, hip
  M71.451 Calcium deposit in bursa, right hip
  M71.452 Calcium deposit in bursa, left hip
  M71.459 Calcium deposit in bursa, unspecified hip

● M71.46 Calcium deposit in bursa, knee
  M71.461 Calcium deposit in bursa, right knee
  M71.462 Calcium deposit in bursa, left knee
  M71.469 Calcium deposit in bursa, unspecified knee

● M71.47 Calcium deposit in bursa, ankle and foot
  M71.471 Calcium deposit in bursa, right ankle and foot
  M71.472 Calcium deposit in bursa, left ankle and foot
  M71.479 Calcium deposit in bursa, unspecified ankle and foot

M71.48 Calcium deposit in bursa, other site

M71.49 Calcium deposit in bursa, multiple sites

● **M71.5 Other bursitis, not elsewhere classified**

> **Excludes1** bursitis NOS (M71.9-)
> **Excludes2** bursitis of shoulder (M75.5)
> bursitis of tibial collateral [Pellegrini-Stieda] (M76.4)

M71.50 Other bursitis, not elsewhere classified, unspecified site

● M71.52 Other bursitis, not elsewhere classified, elbow
  M71.521 Other bursitis, not elsewhere classified, right elbow
  M71.522 Other bursitis, not elsewhere classified, left elbow
  M71.529 Other bursitis, not elsewhere classified, unspecified elbow

● M71.53 Other bursitis, not elsewhere classified, wrist
  M71.531 Other bursitis, not elsewhere classified, right wrist
  M71.532 Other bursitis, not elsewhere classified, left wrist
  M71.539 Other bursitis, not elsewhere classified, unspecified wrist

● M71.54 Other bursitis, not elsewhere classified, hand
  M71.541 Other bursitis, not elsewhere classified, right hand
  M71.542 Other bursitis, not elsewhere classified, left hand
  M71.549 Other bursitis, not elsewhere classified, unspecified hand

● M71.55 Other bursitis, not elsewhere classified, hip
  M71.551 Other bursitis, not elsewhere classified, right hip
  M71.552 Other bursitis, not elsewhere classified, left hip
  M71.559 Other bursitis, not elsewhere classified, unspecified hip

● M71.56 Other bursitis, not elsewhere classified, knee
  M71.561 Other bursitis, not elsewhere classified, right knee
  M71.562 Other bursitis, not elsewhere classified, left knee
  M71.569 Other bursitis, not elsewhere classified, unspecified knee

● M71.57 Other bursitis, not elsewhere classified, ankle and foot
  M71.571 Other bursitis, not elsewhere classified, right ankle and foot
  M71.572 Other bursitis, not elsewhere classified, left ankle and foot
  M71.579 Other bursitis, not elsewhere classified, unspecified ankle and foot

M71.58 Other bursitis, not elsewhere classified, other site

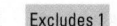

◄ New   ◄ Revised   ~~deleted~~ Deleted   Excludes 1   Excludes 2   Includes   Use additional   Code first   Code also   Unspecified

OGCR Official Guidelines   ● Unacceptable Principal Diagnosis   X Assign placeholder X   ● Use Additional Character(s)   ▷ Manifestation Code   **Coding Clinic**

● **M71.8   Other specified bursopathies**
  M71.80   Other specified bursopathies, unspecified site
● **M71.81**   Other specified bursopathies, shoulder
  M71.811   Other specified bursopathies, right shoulder
  M71.812   Other specified bursopathies, left shoulder
  M71.819   Other specified bursopathies, unspecified shoulder
● **M71.82**   Other specified bursopathies, elbow
  M71.821   Other specified bursopathies, right elbow
  M71.822   Other specified bursopathies, left elbow
  M71.829   Other specified bursopathies, unspecified elbow
● **M71.83**   Other specified bursopathies, wrist
  M71.831   Other specified bursopathies, right wrist
  M71.832   Other specified bursopathies, left wrist
  M71.839   Other specified bursopathies, unspecified wrist
● **M71.84**   Other specified bursopathies, hand
  M71.841   Other specified bursopathies, right hand
  M71.842   Other specified bursopathies, left hand
  M71.849   Other specified bursopathies, unspecified hand
● **M71.85**   Other specified bursopathies, hip
  M71.851   Other specified bursopathies, right hip
  M71.852   Other specified bursopathies, left hip
  M71.859   Other specified bursopathies, unspecified hip
● **M71.86**   Other specified bursopathies, knee
  M71.861   Other specified bursopathies, right knee
  M71.862   Other specified bursopathies, left knee
  M71.869   Other specified bursopathies, unspecified knee
● **M71.87**   Other specified bursopathies, ankle and foot
  M71.871   Other specified bursopathies, right ankle and foot
  M71.872   Other specified bursopathies, left ankle and foot
  M71.879   Other specified bursopathies, unspecified ankle and foot
  M71.88   Other specified bursopathies, other site
  M71.89   Other specified bursopathies, multiple sites
M71.9   Bursopathy, unspecified
  Bursitis NOS

● **M72   Fibroblastic disorders**
  Excludes2   retroperitoneal fibromatosis (D48.3)
  M72.0   Palmar fascial fibromatosis [Dupuytren]   A
  M72.1   Knuckle pads
  M72.2   Plantar fascial fibromatosis
     Plantar fasciitis
  M72.4   Pseudosarcomatous fibromatosis
     Nodular fasciitis

M72.6   Necrotizing fasciitis 🔖
  Use additional code (B95.-, B96.-) to identify causative organism
  (Ex:) K68.12, M60.000-M60.19, M61.00-M61.19, M61.30-M61.59, M62.3, M62.50-M62.59, M62.89, M72.6
M72.8   Other fibroblastic disorders
  Abscess of fascia
  Fasciitis NEC
  Other infective fasciitis
  Use additional code to (B95.-, B96.-) identify causative organism
  Excludes1   diffuse (eosinophilic) fasciitis (M35.4)
            necrotizing fasciitis (M72.6)
            nodular fasciitis (M72.4)
            perirenal fasciitis NOS (N13.5)
            perirenal fasciitis with infection (N13.6)
            plantar fasciitis (M72.2)
M72.9   Fibroblastic disorder, unspecified
  Fasciitis NOS
  Fibromatosis NOS

● **M75   Shoulder lesions**
  Excludes2   shoulder-hand syndrome (M89.0-)
● **M75.0   Adhesive capsulitis of shoulder**
  Frozen shoulder
  Periarthritis of shoulder
  M75.00   Adhesive capsulitis of unspecified shoulder
  M75.01   Adhesive capsulitis of right shoulder
  M75.02   Adhesive capsulitis of left shoulder
● **M75.1   Rotator cuff tear or rupture, not specified as traumatic**
  Rotator cuff syndrome
  Supraspinatus syndrome
  Supraspinatus tear or rupture, not specified as traumatic
  Excludes1   tear of rotator cuff, traumatic (S46.01-)
● **M75.10**   Unspecified rotator cuff tear or rupture, not specified as traumatic
  M75.100   Unspecified rotator cuff tear or rupture of unspecified shoulder, not specified as traumatic
  M75.101   Unspecified rotator cuff tear or rupture of right shoulder, not specified as traumatic
  M75.102   Unspecified rotator cuff tear or rupture of left shoulder, not specified as traumatic
● **M75.11**   Incomplete rotator cuff tear or rupture not specified as traumatic
  M75.110   Incomplete rotator cuff tear or rupture of unspecified shoulder, not specified as traumatic
  M75.111   Incomplete rotator cuff tear or rupture of right shoulder, not specified as traumatic
  M75.112   Incomplete rotator cuff tear or rupture of left shoulder, not specified as traumatic
● **M75.12**   Complete rotator cuff tear or rupture not specified as traumatic
  M75.120   Complete rotator cuff tear or rupture of unspecified shoulder, not specified as traumatic
  M75.121   Complete rotator cuff tear or rupture of right shoulder, not specified as traumatic
  M75.122   Complete rotator cuff tear or rupture of left shoulder, not specified as traumatic

N Newborn Age: 0   **P** Pediatric Age: 0–17   **M** Maternity DX: 12–55   **A** Adult Age: 15–124   ♀ Females Only   ♂ Males Only
🔖 Complication\Comorbidity   🔖 Major C\C   (Ex:) CC/MCC Exclusions   Present on Admission Requirement   🔖 Hospital-Acquired Condition
1141

CHAPTER 13 (M00-M99)

● M75.2 Bicipital tendinitis
　　　M75.20 Bicipital tendinitis, unspecified shoulder
　　　M75.21 Bicipital tendinitis, right shoulder
　　　M75.22 Bicipital tendinitis, left shoulder
● M75.3 Calcific tendinitis of shoulder
　　　　　Calcified bursa of shoulder
　　　M75.30 Calcific tendinitis of unspecified shoulder
　　　M75.31 Calcific tendinitis of right shoulder
　　　M75.32 Calcific tendinitis of left shoulder
● M75.4 Impingement syndrome of shoulder
　　　M75.40 Impingement syndrome of unspecified shoulder
　　　M75.41 Impingement syndrome of right shoulder
　　　M75.42 Impingement syndrome of left shoulder
● M75.5 Bursitis of shoulder
　　　M75.50 Bursitis of unspecified shoulder
　　　M75.51 Bursitis of right shoulder
　　　M75.52 Bursitis of left shoulder
● M75.8 Other shoulder lesions
　　　M75.80 Other shoulder lesions, unspecified shoulder
　　　M75.81 Other shoulder lesions, right shoulder
　　　M75.82 Other shoulder lesions, left shoulder
● M75.9 Shoulder lesion, unspecified
　　　M75.90 Shoulder lesion, unspecified, unspecified shoulder
　　　M75.91 Shoulder lesion, unspecified, right shoulder
　　　M75.92 Shoulder lesion, unspecified, left shoulder
● M76 Enthesopathies, lower limb, excluding foot
　　　Excludes2 bursitis due to use, overuse and pressure (M70.-)
　　　　　　　　enthesopathies of ankle and foot (M77.5-)
● M76.0 Gluteal tendinitis
　　　M76.00 Gluteal tendinitis, unspecified hip
　　　M76.01 Gluteal tendinitis, right hip
　　　M76.02 Gluteal tendinitis, left hip
● M76.1 Psoas tendinitis
　　　M76.10 Psoas tendinitis, unspecified hip
　　　M76.11 Psoas tendinitis, right hip
　　　M76.12 Psoas tendinitis, left hip
● M76.2 Iliac crest spur
　　　M76.20 Iliac crest spur, unspecified hip
　　　M76.21 Iliac crest spur, right hip
　　　M76.22 Iliac crest spur, left hip
● M76.3 Iliotibial band syndrome
　　　M76.30 Iliotibial band syndrome, unspecified leg
　　　M76.31 Iliotibial band syndrome, right leg
　　　M76.32 Iliotibial band syndrome, left leg
● M76.4 Tibial collateral bursitis [Pellegrini-Stieda]
　　　M76.40 Tibial collateral bursitis [Pellegrini-Stieda], unspecified leg
　　　M76.41 Tibial collateral bursitis [Pellegrini-Stieda], right leg
　　　M76.42 Tibial collateral bursitis [Pellegrini-Stieda], left leg
● M76.5 Patellar tendinitis
　　　M76.50 Patellar tendinitis, unspecified knee
　　　M76.51 Patellar tendinitis, right knee
　　　M76.52 Patellar tendinitis, left knee
● M76.6 Achilles tendinitis
　　　　　Achilles bursitis
　　　M76.60 Achilles tendinitis, unspecified leg
　　　M76.61 Achilles tendinitis, right leg
　　　M76.62 Achilles tendinitis, left leg

● M76.7 Peroneal tendinitis
　　　M76.70 Peroneal tendinitis, unspecified leg
　　　M76.71 Peroneal tendinitis, right leg
　　　M76.72 Peroneal tendinitis, left leg
● M76.8 Other specified enthesopathies of lower limb, excluding foot
　　● M76.81 Anterior tibial syndrome
　　　　　M76.811 Anterior tibial syndrome, right leg
　　　　　M76.812 Anterior tibial syndrome, left leg
　　　　　M76.819 Anterior tibial syndrome, unspecified leg
　　● M76.82 Posterior tibial tendinitis
　　　　　M76.821 Posterior tibial tendinitis, right leg
　　　　　M76.822 Posterior tibial tendinitis, left leg
　　　　　M76.829 Posterior tibial tendinitis, unspecified leg
　　● M76.89 Other specified enthesopathies of lower limb, excluding foot
　　　　　M76.891 Other specified enthesopathies of right lower limb, excluding foot
　　　　　M76.892 Other specified enthesopathies of left lower limb, excluding foot
　　　　　M76.899 Other specified enthesopathies of unspecified lower limb, excluding foot
　　M76.9 Unspecified enthesopathy, lower limb, excluding foot
● M77 Other enthesopathies
　　　Excludes1 bursitis NOS (M71.9-)
　　　Excludes2 bursitis due to use, overuse and pressure (M70.-)
　　　　　　　　osteophyte (M25.7)
　　　　　　　　spinal enthesopathy (M46.0-)
● M77.0 Medial epicondylitis
　　　M77.00 Medial epicondylitis, unspecified elbow
　　　M77.01 Medial epicondylitis, right elbow
　　　M77.02 Medial epicondylitis, left elbow
● M77.1 Lateral epicondylitis
　　　　　Tennis elbow
　　　M77.10 Lateral epicondylitis, unspecified elbow
　　　M77.11 Lateral epicondylitis, right elbow
　　　M77.12 Lateral epicondylitis, left elbow
● M77.2 Periarthritis of wrist
　　　M77.20 Periarthritis, unspecified wrist
　　　M77.21 Periarthritis, right wrist
　　　M77.22 Periarthritis, left wrist
● M77.3 Calcaneal spur
　　　M77.30 Calcaneal spur, unspecified foot
　　　M77.31 Calcaneal spur, right foot
　　　M77.32 Calcaneal spur, left foot
● M77.4 Metatarsalgia
　　　Excludes1 Morton's metatarsalgia (G57.6)
　　　M77.40 Metatarsalgia, unspecified foot
　　　M77.41 Metatarsalgia, right foot
　　　M77.42 Metatarsalgia, left foot
● M77.5 Other enthesopathy of foot
　　　M77.50 Other enthesopathy of unspecified foot
　　　M77.51 Other enthesopathy of right foot
　　　M77.52 Other enthesopathy of left foot
　　M77.8 Other enthesopathies, not elsewhere classified
　　M77.9 Enthesopathy, unspecified
　　　　　Bone spur NOS
　　　　　Capsulitis NOS
　　　　　Periarthritis NOS
　　　　　Tendinitis NOS

CHAPTER 13 (M00-M99)

◀ New　　◀▥ Revised　　d̶e̶l̶e̶t̶e̶d̶ Deleted　　Excludes 1　　Excludes 2　　Includes　　Use additional　　Code first　　Code also　　Unspecified

OGCR Official Guidelines　　● Unacceptable Principal Diagnosis　　X Assign placeholder X　　● Use Additional Character(s)　　▌ Manifestation Code　　**Coding Clinic**

● **M79**   **Other and unspecified soft tissue disorders, not elsewhere classified**

     Excludes1   psychogenic rheumatism (F45.8)
                      soft tissue pain, psychogenic (F45.41)

   M79.0   **Rheumatism, unspecified**

     Excludes1   fibromyalgia (M79.7)
                      palindromic rheumatism (M12.3-)

   M79.1   **Myalgia**

      Myofascial pain syndrome

     Excludes1   fibromyalgia (M79.7)
                      myositis (M60.-)

   M79.2   **Neuralgia and neuritis, unspecified**

     Excludes1   brachial radiculitis NOS (M54.1)
                      lumbosacral radiculitis NOS (M54.1)
                      mononeuropathies (G56-G58)
                      radiculitis NOS (M54.1)
                      sciatica (M54.3-M54.4)

   M79.3   **Panniculitis, unspecified**

     Excludes1   lupus panniculitis (L93.2)
                      neck and back panniculitis (M54.0-)
                      relapsing [Weber-Christian] panniculitis (M35.6)

   M79.4   **Hypertrophy of (infrapatellar) fat pad**

   M79.5   **Residual foreign body in soft tissue**

     Excludes1   foreign body granuloma of skin and subcutaneous tissue (L92.3)
                      foreign body granuloma of soft tissue (M60.2-)

● **M79.6**   **Pain in limb, hand, foot, fingers and toes**

     Excludes2   pain in joint (M25.5-)

   ● **M79.60**   **Pain in limb, unspecified**

      M79.601   **Pain in right arm**
            Pain in right upper limb NOS

      M79.602   **Pain in left arm**
            Pain in left upper limb NOS

      M79.603   **Pain in arm, unspecified**
            Pain in upper limb NOS

      M79.604   **Pain in right leg**
            Pain in right lower limb NOS

      M79.605   **Pain in left leg**
            Pain in left lower limb NOS

      M79.606   **Pain in leg, unspecified**
            Pain in lower limb NOS

      M79.609   **Pain in unspecified limb**
            Pain in limb NOS

   ● **M79.62**   **Pain in upper arm**
       Pain in axillary region

      M79.621   **Pain in right upper arm**

      M79.622   **Pain in left upper arm**

      M79.629   **Pain in unspecified upper arm**

   ● **M79.63**   **Pain in forearm**

      M79.631   **Pain in right forearm**

      M79.632   **Pain in left forearm**

      M79.639   **Pain in unspecified forearm**

   ● **M79.64**   **Pain in hand and fingers**

      M79.641   **Pain in right hand**

      M79.642   **Pain in left hand**

      M79.643   **Pain in unspecified hand**

      M79.644   **Pain in right finger(s)**

      M79.645   **Pain in left finger(s)**

      M79.646   **Pain in unspecified finger(s)**

   ● **M79.65**   **Pain in thigh**

      M79.651   **Pain in right thigh**

      M79.652   **Pain in left thigh**

      M79.659   **Pain in unspecified thigh**

   ● **M79.66**   **Pain in lower leg**

      M79.661   **Pain in right lower leg**

      M79.662   **Pain in left lower leg**

      M79.669   **Pain in unspecified lower leg**

   ● **M79.67**   **Pain in foot and toes**

      M79.671   **Pain in right foot**

      M79.672   **Pain in left foot**

      M79.673   **Pain in unspecified foot**

      M79.674   **Pain in right toe(s)**

      M79.675   **Pain in left toe(s)**

      M79.676   **Pain in unspecified toe(s)**

   M79.7   **Fibromyalgia**

      Fibromyositis
      Fibrositis
      Myofibrositis

● **M79.A**   **Nontraumatic compartment syndrome**

     Code first, if applicable, associated postprocedural complication

     Excludes1   compartment syndrome NOS (T79.A-)
                      fibromyalgia (M79.7) nontraumatic ischemic infarction of muscle (M62.2-)
                      traumatic compartment syndrome (T79.A-)

   ● **M79.A1**   **Nontraumatic compartment syndrome of upper extremity**

      Nontraumatic compartment syndrome of shoulder, arm, forearm, wrist, hand, and fingers

      Ⓔⓧ For category M79.A1 CC codes: M70.80-M70.99, M79.81-M79.9, R29.898, S45.301-S45.899[A], S55.201-S55.899[A], S65.801-S65.899[A]

      M79.A11   **Nontraumatic compartment syndrome of right upper extremity** 🦠

      M79.A12   **Nontraumatic compartment syndrome of left upper extremity** 🦠

      M79.A19   **Nontraumatic compartment syndrome of unspecified upper extremity** 🦠

   ● **M79.A2**   **Nontraumatic compartment syndrome of lower extremity**

      Nontraumatic compartment syndrome of hip, buttock, thigh, leg, foot, and toes

      Ⓔⓧ For category M79.A2 CC codes: M70.80-M70.99, M79.81-M79.9, R29.898, S75.801-S75.899[A], S85.201-S85.899[A], S95.001-S95.099[A], S95.201-S95.899[A]

      M79.A21   **Nontraumatic compartment syndrome of right lower extremity** 🦠

      M79.A22   **Nontraumatic compartment syndrome of left lower extremity** 🦠

      M79.A29   **Nontraumatic compartment syndrome of unspecified lower extremity** 🦠

   M79.A3   **Nontraumatic compartment syndrome of abdomen** 🦠

      Ⓔⓧ S31.001[A], S31.011[A], S31.021[A], S31.031[A], S31.041[A], S31.051-S31.159[A], S31.600-S31.659[A], S31.831-S31.839[A], S36.00X-S37.599[A], S37.812-S37.99X[A], S38.3XX[A], S39.021-S39.023[A], T14.8-T14.91, T79.8XX-T79.9XX[A]

   M79.A9   **Nontraumatic compartment syndrome of other sites** 🦠

      Ⓔⓧ S31.001[A], S31.011[A], S31.021[A], S31.031[A], S31.041[A], S31.051[A], S31.600-S31.659[A], S36.81X-S36.899[A]

● **M79.8**   **Other specified soft tissue disorders**

      M79.81   **Nontraumatic hematoma of soft tissue**
            Nontraumatic hematoma of muscle
            Nontraumatic seroma of muscle and soft tissue

      M79.89   **Other specified soft tissue disorders**
            Polyalgia

   M79.9   **Soft tissue disorder, unspecified**

N Newborn Age: 0   **P** Pediatric Age: 0–17   **M** Maternity DX: 12–55   **A** Adult Age: 15–124   ♀ Females Only   ♂ Males Only

🦠 Complication\Comorbidity   🦠 Major C\C   Ⓔⓧ CC/MCC Exclusions   🦠 Present on Admission Requirement   🦠 Hospital-Acquired Condition

1143

CHAPTER 13 (M00-M99)

CHAPTER 13 (M00-M99)

OGCR See Section I.C., Chapter 13.d.

Osteoporosis

OSTEOPATHIES AND CHONDROPATHIES (M80-M94)

DISORDERS OF BONE DENSITY AND STRUCTURE (M80-M85)

M80 Osteoporosis with current pathological fracture
Excessive skeletal fragility (porous bone) resulting in bone fractures

Includes osteoporosis with current fragility fracture

Use additional code to identify major osseous defect, if applicable (M89.7-)

Excludes1 collapsed vertebra NOS (M48.5)
pathological fracture NOS (M84.4)
wedging of vertebra NOS (M48.5)

Excludes2 personal history of (healed) osteoporosis fracture (Z87.310)

The appropriate 7th character is to be added to each code from category M80:

A	initial encounter for fracture
D	subsequent encounter for fracture with routine healing
G	subsequent encounter for fracture with delayed healing
K	subsequent encounter for fracture with nonunion
	Total failure of fracture healing
P	subsequent encounter for fracture with malunion
	Fracture ends do not heal together correctly.
S	sequela

(Ex) **For category M80[A] CC codes:** M48.40X-M48.58X[A], M80.00X-M80.88X[A], M84.30X-M84.68X[A] **For category M80[K,P] CC codes:** M80.00X-M80.88X[K,P], M84.30X-M84.68X[K,P], S02.0XX-S02.92X[K], S12.000-S12.691[K], S22.000-S22.9XX[K], S32.000-S32.9XX[K], S42.001-S42.92X[K,P], S49.001-S49.199[K,P], S52.001-S52.92X[K,M,N,P,Q,R], S59.001-S59.299[K,P], S62.001-S62.92X[K,P], S72.001-S72.92X[K,M,N,P,Q,R], S79.001-S79.199[K,P], S82.001-S82.92X[K,M,N,P,Q,R], S89.001-S89.399[K,P], S92.001-S92.919[K,P]

● **M80.0 Age-related osteoporosis with current pathological fracture**
Involutional osteoporosis with current pathological fracture
Osteoporosis NOS with current pathological fracture
Postmenopausal osteoporosis with current pathological fracture
Senile osteoporosis with current pathological fracture

X● **M80.00 Age-related osteoporosis with current pathological fracture, unspecified site** A, K, P   A

● **M80.01 Age-related osteoporosis with current pathological fracture, shoulder**

   ● **M80.011 Age-related osteoporosis with current pathological fracture, right shoulder** A, K, P   A

   ● **M80.012 Age-related osteoporosis with current pathological fracture, left shoulder** A, K, P   A

   ● **M80.019 Age-related osteoporosis with current pathological fracture, unspecified shoulder** A, K, P   A

● **M80.02 Age-related osteoporosis with current pathological fracture, humerus**

   ● **M80.021 Age-related osteoporosis with current pathological fracture, right humerus** A, K, P   A

   ● **M80.022 Age-related osteoporosis with current pathological fracture, left humerus** A, K, P   A

   ● **M80.029 Age-related osteoporosis with current pathological fracture, unspecified humerus** A, K, P   A

● **M80.03 Age-related osteoporosis with current pathological fracture, forearm**
Age-related osteoporosis with current pathological fracture of wrist

   ● **M80.031 Age-related osteoporosis with current pathological fracture, right forearm** A, K, P   A

   ● **M80.032 Age-related osteoporosis with current pathological fracture, left forearm** A, K, P   A

   ● **M80.039 Age-related osteoporosis with current pathological fracture, unspecified forearm** A, K, P   A

● **M80.04 Age-related osteoporosis with current pathological fracture, hand**

   ● **M80.041 Age-related osteoporosis with current pathological fracture, right hand** A, K, P   A

   ● **M80.042 Age-related osteoporosis with current pathological fracture, left hand** A, K, P   A

   ● **M80.049 Age-related osteoporosis with current pathological fracture, unspecified hand** A, K, P   A

● **M80.05 Age-related osteoporosis with current pathological fracture, femur**
Age-related osteoporosis with current pathological fracture of hip

   ● **M80.051 Age-related osteoporosis with current pathological fracture, right femur** A, K, P   A

   ● **M80.052 Age-related osteoporosis with current pathological fracture, left femur** A, K, P   A

   ● **M80.059 Age-related osteoporosis with current pathological fracture, unspecified femur** A, K, P   A

● **M80.06 Age-related osteoporosis with current pathological fracture, lower leg**

   ● **M80.061 Age-related osteoporosis with current pathological fracture, right lower leg** A, K, P   A

   ● **M80.062 Age-related osteoporosis with current pathological fracture, left lower leg** A, K, P   A

   ● **M80.069 Age-related osteoporosis with current pathological fracture, unspecified lower leg** A, K, P   A

● **M80.07 Age-related osteoporosis with current pathological fracture, ankle and foot**

   ● **M80.071 Age-related osteoporosis with current pathological fracture, right ankle and foot** A, K, P   A

   ● **M80.072 Age-related osteoporosis with current pathological fracture, left ankle and foot** A, K, P   A

   ● **M80.079 Age-related osteoporosis with current pathological fracture, unspecified ankle and foot** A, K, P   A

X● **M80.08 Age-related osteoporosis with current pathological fracture, vertebra(e)** A, K, P   A

◀ New   ◀ Revised   ~~deleted~~ Deleted   Excludes 1   Excludes 2   Includes   Use additional   Code first   Code also   Unspecified

OGCR Official Guidelines   ● Unacceptable Principal Diagnosis   X Assign placeholder X   ● Use Additional Character(s)   ▶ Manifestation Code   **Coding Clinic**

● **M80.8   Other osteoporosis with current pathological fracture**
     Drug-induced osteoporosis with current pathological fracture
     Idiopathic osteoporosis with current pathological fracture
     Osteoporosis of disuse with current pathological fracture
     Postoophorectomy osteoporosis with current pathological fracture
     Postsurgical malabsorption osteoporosis with current pathological fracture
     Post-traumatic osteoporosis with current pathological fracture
     Use additional code for adverse effect, if applicable, to identify drug (T36-T50 with fifth or sixth character 5)

X ● **M80.80   Other osteoporosis with current pathological fracture, unspecified site** A, K, P 🐾   A

● **M80.81   Other osteoporosis with pathological fracture, shoulder**

    ● **M80.811   Other osteoporosis with current pathological fracture, right shoulder** A, K, P 🐾

    ● **M80.812   Other osteoporosis with current pathological fracture, left shoulder** A, K, P 🐾

    ● **M80.819   Other osteoporosis with current pathological fracture, unspecified shoulder** A, K, P 🐾

● **M80.82   Other osteoporosis with current pathological fracture, humerus**

    ● **M80.821   Other osteoporosis with current pathological fracture, right humerus** A, K, P 🐾

    ● **M80.822   Other osteoporosis with current pathological fracture, left humerus** A, K, P 🐾

    ● **M80.829   Other osteoporosis with current pathological fracture, unspecified humerus** A, K, P 🐾

● **M80.83   Other osteoporosis with current pathological fracture, forearm**
     Other osteoporosis with current pathological fracture of wrist

    ● **M80.831   Other osteoporosis with current pathological fracture, right forearm** A, K, P 🐾

    ● **M80.832   Other osteoporosis with current pathological fracture, left forearm** A, K, P 🐾

    ● **M80.839   Other osteoporosis with current pathological fracture, unspecified forearm** A, K, P 🐾

● **M80.84   Other osteoporosis with current pathological fracture, hand**

    ● **M80.841   Other osteoporosis with current pathological fracture, right hand** A, K, P 🐾

    ● **M80.842   Other osteoporosis with current pathological fracture, left hand** A, K, P 🐾

    ● **M80.849   Other osteoporosis with current pathological fracture, unspecified hand** A, K, P 🐾

● **M80.85   Other osteoporosis with current pathological fracture, femur**
     Other osteoporosis with current pathological fracture of hip

    ● **M80.851   Other osteoporosis with current pathological fracture, right femur** A, K, P 🐾

    ● **M80.852   Other osteoporosis with current pathological fracture, left femur** A, K, P 🐾

    ● **M80.859   Other osteoporosis with current pathological fracture, unspecified femur** A, K, P 🐾

● **M80.86   Other osteoporosis with current pathological fracture, lower leg**

    ● **M80.861   Other osteoporosis with current pathological fracture, right lower leg** A, K, P 🐾

    ● **M80.862   Other osteoporosis with current pathological fracture, left lower leg** A, K, P 🐾

    ● **M80.869   Other osteoporosis with current pathological fracture, unspecified lower leg** A, K, P 🐾

● **M80.87   Other osteoporosis with current pathological fracture, ankle and foot**

    ● **M80.871   Other osteoporosis with current pathological fracture, right ankle and foot** A, K, P 🐾

    ● **M80.872   Other osteoporosis with current pathological fracture, left ankle and foot** A, K, P 🐾

    ● **M80.879   Other osteoporosis with current pathological fracture, unspecified ankle and foot** A, K, P 🐾

X ● **M80.88   Other osteoporosis with current pathological fracture, vertebra(e)** A, K, P 🐾

● **M81   Osteoporosis without current pathological fracture**
     Use additional code to identify:
      major osseous defect, if applicable (M89.7-)
      personal history of (healed) osteoporosis fracture, if applicable (Z87.310)
     Excludes1   osteoporosis with current pathological fracture (M80.-)
      Sudeck's atrophy (M89.0)

M81.0   Age-related osteoporosis without current pathological fracture   A
     Involutional osteoporosis without current pathological fracture
     Osteoporosis NOS
     Postmenopausal osteoporosis without current pathological fracture
     Senile osteoporosis without current pathological fracture

M81.6   Localized osteoporosis [Lequesne]
     Excludes1   Sudeck's atrophy (M89.0)

M81.8   Other osteoporosis without current pathological fracture
     Drug-induced osteoporosis without current pathological fracture
     Idiopathic osteoporosis without current pathological fracture
     Osteoporosis of disuse without current pathological fracture
     Postoophorectomy osteoporosis without current pathological fracture
     Postsurgical malabsorption osteoporosis without current pathological fracture
     Post-traumatic osteoporosis without current pathological fracture
     Use additional code for adverse effect, if applicable, to identify drug (T36-T50 with fifth or sixth character 5)

● M83 **Adult osteomalacia**

　　Excludes1 infantile and juvenile osteomalacia (E55.0)
　　　　　　　　renal osteodystrophy (N25.0)
　　　　　　　　rickets (active) (E55.0)
　　　　　　　　rickets (active) sequelae (E64.3)
　　　　　　　　vitamin D-resistant osteomalacia (E83.3)
　　　　　　　　vitamin D-resistant rickets (active) (E83.3)

　　M83.0 **Puerperal osteomalacia** ♀　　　　　　　　M

　　M83.1 **Senile osteomalacia**　　　　　　　　　　A

　　M83.2 **Adult osteomalacia due to malabsorption**　　A
　　　　　Postsurgical malabsorption osteomalacia in adults

　　M83.3 **Adult osteomalacia due to malnutrition**　　A

　　M83.4 **Aluminum bone disease**

　　M83.5 **Other drug-induced osteomalacia in adults**　　A
　　　　　Use additional code for adverse effect, if applicable,
　　　　　　to identify drug (T36-T50 with fifth or sixth
　　　　　　character 5)

　　M83.8 **Other adult osteomalacia**　　　　　　　　A

　　M83.9 **Adult osteomalacia, unspecified**　　　　　A

● M84 **Disorder of continuity of bone**

　　Excludes2 traumatic fracture of bone-see fracture, by site

　　Ex: For category **M84[A]** CC codes: M48.40X-M48.58X[A], M80.00X-M80.88X[A],
　　M84.30X-M84.68X[A] For category **M84[K,P]** CC codes: M80.00X-M80.88X[K,P],
　　M84.30X-M84.68X[K,P], S02.0XX-S02.92X[K], S12.000-S12.691[K],
　　S22.000-S22.9XX[K], S32.000-S32.9XX[K], S42.001-S42.92X[K,P],
　　S49.001-S49.199[K,P], S52.001-S52.92X[K,M,N,P,Q,R], S59.001-S59.299[K,P],
　　S62.001-S62.92X[K,P], S72.001-S72.92X[K,M,N,P,Q,R], S79.001-S79.199[K,P],
　　S82.001-S82.92X[K,M,N,P,Q,R], S89.001-S89.399[K,P], S92.001-S92.919[K,P]

　● M84.3 **Stress fracture**
　　　　Fatigue fracture
　　　　March fracture
　　　　Stress fracture NOS
　　　　Stress reaction
　　　　Use additional external cause code(s) to identify the
　　　　　cause of the stress fracture

　　　　Excludes1 pathological fracture NOS (M84.4.-)
　　　　　　　　　pathological fracture due to osteoporosis
　　　　　　　　　　(M80.-)
　　　　　　　　　traumatic fracture (S12.-, S22.-, S32.-,
　　　　　　　　　　S42.-, S52.-, S62.-, S72.-, S82.-, S92.-)

　　　　Excludes2 personal history of (healed) stress
　　　　　　　　　(fatigue) fracture (Z87.312)
　　　　　　　　　stress fracture of vertebra (M48.4-)

　　　　The appropriate 7th character is to be added to each
　　　　　code from subcategory M84.3:

　　　　| A | initial encounter for fracture |
　　　　| D | subsequent encounter for fracture with routine healing |
　　　　| G | subsequent encounter for fracture with delayed healing |
　　　　| K | subsequent encounter for fracture with nonunion |
　　　　| P | subsequent encounter for fracture with malunion |
　　　　| S | sequela |

　　　　Ex: See M84

X ● M84.30 **Stress fracture, unspecified** site K, P 🦴

　● M84.31 **Stress fracture, shoulder**
　　　　● M84.311 **Stress fracture, right shoulder** K, P 🦴
　　　　● M84.312 **Stress fracture, left shoulder** K, P 🦴
　　　　● M84.319 **Stress fracture, unspecified shoulder** K, P 🦴

　● M84.32 **Stress fracture, humerus**
　　　　● M84.321 **Stress fracture, right humerus** K, P 🦴
　　　　● M84.322 **Stress fracture, left humerus** K, P 🦴
　　　　● M84.329 **Stress fracture, unspecified humerus** K, P 🦴

　● M84.33 **Stress fracture, ulna and radius**
　　　　● M84.331 **Stress fracture, right ulna** K, P 🦴
　　　　● M84.332 **Stress fracture, left ulna** K, P 🦴
　　　　● M84.333 **Stress fracture, right radius** K, P 🦴
　　　　● M84.334 **Stress fracture, left radius** K, P 🦴
　　　　● M84.339 **Stress fracture, unspecified ulna and radius** K, P 🦴

　● M84.34 **Stress fracture, hand and fingers**
　　　　● M84.341 **Stress fracture, right hand** K, P 🦴
　　　　● M84.342 **Stress fracture, left hand** K, P 🦴
　　　　● M84.343 **Stress fracture, unspecified hand** K, P 🦴
　　　　● M84.344 **Stress fracture, right finger(s)** K, P 🦴
　　　　● M84.345 **Stress fracture, left finger(s)** K, P 🦴
　　　　● M84.346 **Stress fracture, unspecified finger(s)** K, P 🦴

　● M84.35 **Stress fracture, pelvis and femur**
　　　　Stress fracture, hip
　　　　● M84.350 **Stress fracture, pelvis** K, P 🦴
　　　　● M84.351 **Stress fracture, right femur** K, P 🦴
　　　　● M84.352 **Stress fracture, left femur** K, P 🦴
　　　　● M84.353 **Stress fracture, unspecified femur** K, P 🦴
　　　　● M84.359 **Stress fracture, hip, unspecified** K, P 🦴

　● M84.36 **Stress fracture, tibia and fibula**
　　　　● M84.361 **Stress fracture, right tibia** K, P 🦴
　　　　● M84.362 **Stress fracture, left tibia** K, P 🦴
　　　　● M84.363 **Stress fracture, right fibula** K, P 🦴
　　　　● M84.364 **Stress fracture, left fibula** K, P 🦴
　　　　● M84.369 **Stress fracture, unspecified tibia and fibula** K, P 🦴

　● M84.37 **Stress fracture, ankle, foot and toes**
　　　　● M84.371 **Stress fracture, right ankle** K, P 🦴
　　　　● M84.372 **Stress fracture, left ankle** K, P 🦴
　　　　● M84.373 **Stress fracture, unspecified ankle** K, P 🦴
　　　　● M84.374 **Stress fracture, right foot** K, P 🦴
　　　　● M84.375 **Stress fracture, left foot** K, P 🦴
　　　　● M84.376 **Stress fracture, unspecified foot** K, P 🦴
　　　　● M84.377 **Stress fracture, right toe(s)** K, P 🦴
　　　　● M84.378 **Stress fracture, left toe(s)** K, P 🦴
　　　　● M84.379 **Stress fracture, unspecified toe(s)** K, P 🦴

X ● M84.38 **Stress fracture, other site** K, P 🦴
　　　　Excludes2 stress fracture of vertebra (M48.4-)

◄ New　◄ Revised　~~deleted~~ Deleted　Excludes 1　Excludes 2　Includes　Use additional　Code first　Code also　Unspecified
OGCR Official Guidelines　● Unacceptable Principal Diagnosis　X Assign placeholder X　● Use Additional Character(s)　▶ Manifestation Code　**Coding Clinic**

● **M84.4**   Pathological fracture, not elsewhere classified
      Chronic fracture
      Pathological fracture NOS

      Excludes1   collapsed vertebra NEC (M48.5)
                     pathological fracture in neoplastic disease
                        (M84.5-)
                     pathological fracture in osteoporosis
                        (M80.-)
                     pathological fracture in other disease
                        (M84.6-)
                     stress fracture (M84.3-)
                     traumatic fracture (S12.-, S22.-, S32.-,
                        S42.-, S52.-, S62.-, S72.-, S82.-, S92.-)

      Excludes2   personal history of (healed) pathological
                        fracture (Z87.311)

      The appropriate 7th character is to be added to each
        code from subcategory M84.4:

> A   initial encounter for fracture
> D   subsequent encounter for fracture with routine
>   healing
> G   subsequent encounter for fracture with
>   delayed healing
> K   subsequent encounter for fracture with
>   nonunion
> P   subsequent encounter for fracture with
>   malunion
> S   sequela

      (Ex) See M84

X ● **M84.40**   Pathological fracture, unspecified site A, K, P
● **M84.41**   Pathological fracture, shoulder
      ● **M84.411**   Pathological fracture, right shoulder
                   A, K, P
      ● **M84.412**   Pathological fracture, left shoulder
                   A, K, P
      ● **M84.419**   Pathological fracture, unspecified
                   shoulder A, K, P
● **M84.42**   Pathological fracture, humerus
      ● **M84.421**   Pathological fracture, right humerus
                   A, K, P
      ● **M84.422**   Pathological fracture, left humerus
                   A, K, P
      ● **M84.429**   Pathological fracture, unspecified
                   humerus A, K, P
● **M84.43**   Pathological fracture, ulna and radius
      ● **M84.431**   Pathological fracture, right ulna
                   A, K, P
      ● **M84.432**   Pathological fracture, left ulna
                   A, K, P
      ● **M84.433**   Pathological fracture, right radius
                   A, K, P
      ● **M84.434**   Pathological fracture, left radius
                   A, K, P
      ● **M84.439**   Pathological fracture, unspecified
                   ulna and radius A, K, P

● **M84.44**   Pathological fracture, hand and fingers
      ● **M84.441**   Pathological fracture, right hand
                   A, K, P
      ● **M84.442**   Pathological fracture, left hand
                   A, K, P
      ● **M84.443**   Pathological fracture, unspecified
                   hand A, K, P
      ● **M84.444**   Pathological fracture, right finger(s)
                   A, K, P
      ● **M84.445**   Pathological fracture, left finger(s)
                   A, K, P
      ● **M84.446**   Pathological fracture, unspecified
                   finger(s) A, K, P
● **M84.45**   Pathological fracture, femur and pelvis
      ● **M84.451**   Pathological fracture, right femur
                   A, K, P
      ● **M84.452**   Pathological fracture, left femur
                   A, K, P
      ● **M84.453**   Pathological fracture, unspecified
                   femur A, K, P
      ● **M84.454**   Pathological fracture, pelvis A, K, P
      ● **M84.459**   Pathological fracture, hip, unspecified
                   A, K, P
● **M84.46**   Pathological fracture, tibia and fibula
      ● **M84.461**   Pathological fracture, right tibia
                   A, K, P
      ● **M84.462**   Pathological fracture, left tibia
                   A, K, P
      ● **M84.463**   Pathological fracture, right fibula
                   A, K, P
      ● **M84.464**   Pathological fracture, left fibula
                   A, K, P
      ● **M84.469**   Pathological fracture, unspecified
                   tibia and fibula A, K, P
● **M84.47**   Pathological fracture, ankle, foot and toes
      ● **M84.471**   Pathological fracture, right ankle
                   A, K, P
      ● **M84.472**   Pathological fracture, left ankle
                   A, K, P
      ● **M84.473**   Pathological fracture, unspecified
                   ankle A, K, P
      ● **M84.474**   Pathological fracture, right foot
                   A, K, P
      ● **M84.475**   Pathological fracture, left foot
                   A, K, P
      ● **M84.476**   Pathological fracture, unspecified foot
                   A, K, P
      ● **M84.477**   Pathological fracture, right toe(s)
                   A, K, P
      ● **M84.478**   Pathological fracture, left toe(s)
                   A, K, P
      ● **M84.479**   Pathological fracture, unspecified
                   toe(s) A, K, P
X ● **M84.48**   Pathological fracture, other site A, K, P

N Newborn Age: 0   **P** Pediatric Age: 0–17   **M** Maternity DX: 12–55   **A** Adult Age: 15–124   ♀ Females Only   ♂ Males Only
Complication\Comorbidity   Major C\C   (Ex) CC/MCC Exclusions   Present on Admission Requirement   Hospital-Acquired Condition

1147

CHAPTER 13 (M00-M99)

CHAPTER 13 (M00-M99)

Coding of Pathologic Fractures

7th character A is for use as long as the patient is receiving active treatment for the fracture. Examples of active treatment are: surgical treatment, emergency department encounter, evaluation and treatment by a new physician. 7th character, D is to be used for encounters after the patient has completed active treatment. The other 7th characters, listed under each subcategory in the Tabular List, are to be used for subsequent encounters for treatment of problems associated with the healing, such as malunions, nonunions, and sequelae.

Care for complications of surgical treatment for fracture repairs during the healing or recovery phase should be coded with the appropriate complication codes.

See Section I.C.19. Coding of traumatic fractures.

● M84.5　Pathological fracture in neoplastic disease
　　Code also underlying neoplasm
　　The appropriate 7th character is to be added to each
　　　code from subcategory M84.5:

A	initial encounter for fracture
D	subsequent encounter for fracture with routine healing
G	subsequent encounter for fracture with delayed healing
K	subsequent encounter for fracture with nonunion
P	subsequent encounter for fracture with malunion
S	sequela

　　(Ex:) See M84

X ● M84.50　Pathological fracture in neoplastic disease,
　　　unspecified site A, K, P &

● M84.51　Pathological fracture in neoplastic disease,
　　　shoulder
　　● M84.511　Pathological fracture in neoplastic
　　　　disease, right shoulder A, K, P &
　　● M84.512　Pathological fracture in neoplastic
　　　　disease, left shoulder A, K, P &
　　● M84.519　Pathological fracture in neoplastic
　　　　disease, unspecified shoulder
　　　　A, K, P &

● M84.52　Pathological fracture in neoplastic disease,
　　　humerus
　　● M84.521　Pathological fracture in neoplastic
　　　　disease, right humerus A, K, P &
　　● M84.522　Pathological fracture in neoplastic
　　　　disease, left humerus A, K, P &
　　● M84.529　Pathological fracture in neoplastic
　　　　disease, unspecified humerus
　　　　A, K, P &

● M84.53　Pathological fracture in neoplastic disease, ulna
　　　and radius
　　● M84.531　Pathological fracture in neoplastic
　　　　disease, right ulna A, K, P &
　　● M84.532　Pathological fracture in neoplastic
　　　　disease, left ulna A, K, P &
　　● M84.533　Pathological fracture in neoplastic
　　　　disease, right radius A, K, P &
　　● M84.534　Pathological fracture in neoplastic
　　　　disease, left radius A, K, P &
　　● M84.539　Pathological fracture in neoplastic
　　　　disease, unspecified ulna and radius
　　　　A, K, P &

● M84.54　Pathological fracture in neoplastic disease,
　　　hand
　　● M84.541　Pathological fracture in neoplastic
　　　　disease, right hand A, K, P &
　　● M84.542　Pathological fracture in neoplastic
　　　　disease, left hand A, K, P &
　　● M84.549　Pathological fracture in neoplastic
　　　　disease, unspecified hand A, K, P &

● M84.55　Pathological fracture in neoplastic disease,
　　　pelvis and femur
　　● M84.550　Pathological fracture in neoplastic
　　　　disease, pelvis A, K, P &
　　● M84.551　Pathological fracture in neoplastic
　　　　disease, right femur A, K, P &
　　● M84.552　Pathological fracture in neoplastic
　　　　disease, left femur A, K, P &
　　● M84.553　Pathological fracture in neoplastic
　　　　disease, unspecified femur A, K, P &
　　● M84.559　Pathological fracture in neoplastic
　　　　disease, hip, unspecified A, K, P &

● M84.56　Pathological fracture in neoplastic disease, tibia
　　　and fibula
　　● M84.561　Pathological fracture in neoplastic
　　　　disease, right tibia A, K, P &
　　● M84.562　Pathological fracture in neoplastic
　　　　disease, left tibia A, K, P &
　　● M84.563　Pathological fracture in neoplastic
　　　　disease, right fibula A, K, P &
　　● M84.564　Pathological fracture in neoplastic
　　　　disease, left fibula A, K, P &
　　● M84.569　Pathological fracture in neoplastic
　　　　disease, unspecified tibia and fibula
　　　　A, K, P &

● M84.57　Pathological fracture in neoplastic disease,
　　　ankle and foot
　　● M84.571　Pathological fracture in neoplastic
　　　　disease, right ankle A, K, P &
　　● M84.572　Pathological fracture in neoplastic
　　　　disease, left ankle A, K, P &
　　● M84.573　Pathological fracture in neoplastic
　　　　disease, unspecified ankle A, K, P &
　　● M84.574　Pathological fracture in neoplastic
　　　　disease, right foot A, K, P &
　　● M84.575　Pathological fracture in neoplastic
　　　　disease, left foot A, K, P &
　　● M84.576　Pathological fracture in neoplastic
　　　　disease, unspecified foot A, K, P &

X ● M84.58　Pathological fracture in neoplastic disease,
　　　other specified site A, K, P & ◀▬
　　　Pathological fracture in neoplastic disease,
　　　　vertebrae ◀

● M84.6　Pathological fracture in other disease
　　Code also underlying condition
　　Excludes1　pathological fracture in osteoporosis
　　　　(M80.-)

　　The appropriate 7th character is to be added to each
　　　code from subcategory M84.6:

A	initial encounter for fracture
D	subsequent encounter for fracture with routine healing
G	subsequent encounter for fracture with delayed healing
K	subsequent encounter for fracture with nonunion
P	subsequent encounter for fracture with malunion
S	sequela

　　(Ex:) See M84

X ● M84.60　Pathological fracture in other disease,
　　　unspecified site A, K, P &

● M84.61　Pathological fracture in other disease, shoulder
　　● M84.611　Pathological fracture in other disease,
　　　　right shoulder A, K, P &
　　● M84.612　Pathological fracture in other disease,
　　　　left shoulder A, K, P &
　　● M84.619　Pathological fracture in other disease,
　　　　unspecified shoulder A, K, P &

◀ New　◀▬ Revised　d̶e̶l̶e̶t̶e̶d̶ Deleted　Excludes 1　Excludes 2　Includes　Use additional　Code first　Code also　Unspecified

OGCR Official Guidelines　● Unacceptable Principal Diagnosis　X Assign placeholder X　● Use Additional Character(s)　▌ Manifestation Code　**Coding Clinic**

● M84.62　Pathological fracture in other disease, humerus
　　● M84.621　Pathological fracture in other disease, right humerus A, K, P 🔒
　　● M84.622　Pathological fracture in other disease, left humerus A, K, P 🔒
　　● M84.629　Pathological fracture in other disease, unspecified humerus A, K, P 🔒
● M84.63　Pathological fracture in other disease, ulna and radius
　　● M84.631　Pathological fracture in other disease, right ulna A, K, P 🔒
　　● M84.632　Pathological fracture in other disease, left ulna A, K, P 🔒
　　● M84.633　Pathological fracture in other disease, right radius A, K, P 🔒
　　● M84.634　Pathological fracture in other disease, left radius A, K, P 🔒
　　● M84.639　Pathological fracture in other disease, unspecified ulna and radius A, K, P 🔒
● M84.64　Pathological fracture in other disease, hand
　　● M84.641　Pathological fracture in other disease, right hand A, K, P 🔒
　　● M84.642　Pathological fracture in other disease, left hand A, K, P 🔒
　　● M84.649　Pathological fracture in other disease, unspecified hand A, K, P 🔒
● M84.65　Pathological fracture in other disease, pelvis and femur
　　● M84.650　Pathological fracture in other disease, pelvis A, K, P 🔒
　　● M84.651　Pathological fracture in other disease, right femur A, K, P 🔒
　　● M84.652　Pathological fracture in other disease, left femur A, K, P 🔒
　　● M84.653　Pathological fracture in other disease, unspecified femur A, K, P 🔒
　　● M84.659　Pathological fracture in other disease, hip, unspecified A, K, P 🔒
● M84.66　Pathological fracture in other disease, tibia and fibula
　　● M84.661　Pathological fracture in other disease, right tibia A, K, P 🔒
　　● M84.662　Pathological fracture in other disease, left tibia A, K, P 🔒
　　● M84.663　Pathological fracture in other disease, right fibula A, K, P 🔒
　　● M84.664　Pathological fracture in other disease, left fibula A, K, P 🔒
　　● M84.669　Pathological fracture in other disease, unspecified tibia and fibula A, K, P 🔒
● M84.67　Pathological fracture in other disease, ankle and foot
　　● M84.671　Pathological fracture in other disease, right ankle A, K, P 🔒
　　● M84.672　Pathological fracture in other disease, left ankle A, K, P 🔒
　　● M84.673　Pathological fracture in other disease, unspecified ankle A, K, P 🔒
　　● M84.674　Pathological fracture in other disease, right foot A, K, P 🔒
　　● M84.675　Pathological fracture in other disease, left foot A, K, P 🔒
　　● M84.676　Pathological fracture in other disease, unspecified foot A, K, P 🔒
X ● M84.68　Pathological fracture in other disease, other site A, K, P 🔒

● M84.8　Other disorders of continuity of bone
　　M84.80　Other disorders of continuity of bone, unspecified site
　● M84.81　Other disorders of continuity of bone, shoulder
　　　M84.811　Other disorders of continuity of bone, right shoulder
　　　M84.812　Other disorders of continuity of bone, left shoulder
　　　M84.819　Other disorders of continuity of bone, unspecified shoulder
　● M84.82　Other disorders of continuity of bone, humerus
　　　M84.821　Other disorders of continuity of bone, right humerus
　　　M84.822　Other disorders of continuity of bone, left humerus
　　　M84.829　Other disorders of continuity of bone, unspecified humerus
　● M84.83　Other disorders of continuity of bone, ulna and radius
　　　M84.831　Other disorders of continuity of bone, right ulna
　　　M84.832　Other disorders of continuity of bone, left ulna
　　　M84.833　Other disorders of continuity of bone, right radius
　　　M84.834　Other disorders of continuity of bone, left radius
　　　M84.839　Other disorders of continuity of bone, unspecified ulna and radius
　● M84.84　Other disorders of continuity of bone, hand
　　　M84.841　Other disorders of continuity of bone, right hand
　　　M84.842　Other disorders of continuity of bone, left hand
　　　M84.849　Other disorders of continuity of bone, unspecified hand
　● M84.85　Other disorders of continuity of bone, pelvic region and thigh
　　　M84.851　Other disorders of continuity of bone, right pelvic region and thigh
　　　M84.852　Other disorders of continuity of bone, left pelvic region and thigh
　　　M84.859　Other disorders of continuity of bone, unspecified pelvic region and thigh
　● M84.86　Other disorders of continuity of bone, tibia and fibula
　　　M84.861　Other disorders of continuity of bone, right tibia
　　　M84.862　Other disorders of continuity of bone, left tibia
　　　M84.863　Other disorders of continuity of bone, right fibula
　　　M84.864　Other disorders of continuity of bone, left fibula
　　　M84.869　Other disorders of continuity of bone, unspecified tibia and fibula
　● M84.87　Other disorders of continuity of bone, ankle and foot
　　　M84.871　Other disorders of continuity of bone, right ankle and foot
　　　M84.872　Other disorders of continuity of bone, left ankle and foot
　　　M84.879　Other disorders of continuity of bone, unspecified ankle and foot
　　M84.88　Other disorders of continuity of bone, other site
M84.9　Disorder of continuity of bone, unspecified

N　Newborn Age: 0　　　P　Pediatric Age: 0–17　　　M　Maternity DX: 12–55　　　A　Adult Age: 15–124　　　♀　Females Only　　　♂　Males Only

🔒 Complication\Comorbidity　　　🔒 Major C\C　　　(Ex) CC/MCC Exclusions　　　🔒 Present on Admission Requirement　　　🔒 Hospital-Acquired Condition

1149

CHAPTER 13 (M00-M99)

● M85   **Other disorders of bone density and structure**

     Excludes1   osteogenesis imperfecta (Q78.0)
                  osteopetrosis (Q78.2)
                  osteopoikilosis (Q78.8)
                  polyostotic fibrous dysplasia (Q78.1)

● M85.0   **Fibrous dysplasia (monostotic)**

     Excludes2   fibrous dysplasia of jaw (M27.8)

    M85.00   Fibrous dysplasia (monostotic), unspecified site

● M85.01   Fibrous dysplasia (monostotic), shoulder

      M85.011   Fibrous dysplasia (monostotic), right shoulder

      M85.012   Fibrous dysplasia (monostotic), left shoulder

      M85.019   Fibrous dysplasia (monostotic), unspecified shoulder

● M85.02   Fibrous dysplasia (monostotic), upper arm

      M85.021   Fibrous dysplasia (monostotic), right upper arm

      M85.022   Fibrous dysplasia (monostotic), left upper arm

      M85.029   Fibrous dysplasia (monostotic), unspecified upper arm

● M85.03   Fibrous dysplasia (monostotic), forearm

      M85.031   Fibrous dysplasia (monostotic), right forearm

      M85.032   Fibrous dysplasia (monostotic), left forearm

      M85.039   Fibrous dysplasia (monostotic), unspecified forearm

● M85.04   Fibrous dysplasia (monostotic), hand

      M85.041   Fibrous dysplasia (monostotic), right hand

      M85.042   Fibrous dysplasia (monostotic), left hand

      M85.049   Fibrous dysplasia (monostotic), unspecified hand

● M85.05   Fibrous dysplasia (monostotic), thigh

      M85.051   Fibrous dysplasia (monostotic), right thigh

      M85.052   Fibrous dysplasia (monostotic), left thigh

      M85.059   Fibrous dysplasia (monostotic), unspecified thigh

● M85.06   Fibrous dysplasia (monostotic), lower leg

      M85.061   Fibrous dysplasia (monostotic), right lower leg

      M85.062   Fibrous dysplasia (monostotic), left lower leg

      M85.069   Fibrous dysplasia (monostotic), unspecified lower leg

● M85.07   Fibrous dysplasia (monostotic), ankle and foot

      M85.071   Fibrous dysplasia (monostotic), right ankle and foot

      M85.072   Fibrous dysplasia (monostotic), left ankle and foot

      M85.079   Fibrous dysplasia (monostotic), unspecified ankle and foot

    M85.08   Fibrous dysplasia (monostotic), other site

    M85.09   Fibrous dysplasia (monostotic), multiple sites

● M85.1   **Skeletal fluorosis**

    M85.10   Skeletal fluorosis, unspecified site

● M85.11   Skeletal fluorosis, shoulder

      M85.111   Skeletal fluorosis, right shoulder

      M85.112   Skeletal fluorosis, left shoulder

      M85.119   Skeletal fluorosis, unspecified shoulder

● M85.12   Skeletal fluorosis, upper arm

      M85.121   Skeletal fluorosis, right upper arm

      M85.122   Skeletal fluorosis, left upper arm

      M85.129   Skeletal fluorosis, unspecified upper arm

● M85.13   Skeletal fluorosis, forearm

      M85.131   Skeletal fluorosis, right forearm

      M85.132   Skeletal fluorosis, left forearm

      M85.139   Skeletal fluorosis, unspecified forearm

● M85.14   Skeletal fluorosis, hand

      M85.141   Skeletal fluorosis, right hand

      M85.142   Skeletal fluorosis, left hand

      M85.149   Skeletal fluorosis, unspecified hand

● M85.15   Skeletal fluorosis, thigh

      M85.151   Skeletal fluorosis, right thigh

      M85.152   Skeletal fluorosis, left thigh

      M85.159   Skeletal fluorosis, unspecified thigh

● M85.16   Skeletal fluorosis, lower leg

      M85.161   Skeletal fluorosis, right lower leg

      M85.162   Skeletal fluorosis, left lower leg

      M85.169   Skeletal fluorosis, unspecified lower leg

● M85.17   Skeletal fluorosis, ankle and foot

      M85.171   Skeletal fluorosis, right ankle and foot

      M85.172   Skeletal fluorosis, left ankle and foot

      M85.179   Skeletal fluorosis, unspecified ankle and foot

    M85.18   Skeletal fluorosis, other site

    M85.19   Skeletal fluorosis, multiple sites

   M85.2   **Hyperostosis of skull**

● M85.3   **Osteitis condensans**

    M85.30   Osteitis condensans, unspecified site

● M85.31   Osteitis condensans, shoulder

      M85.311   Osteitis condensans, right shoulder

      M85.312   Osteitis condensans, left shoulder

      M85.319   Osteitis condensans, unspecified shoulder

● M85.32   Osteitis condensans, upper arm

      M85.321   Osteitis condensans, right upper arm

      M85.322   Osteitis condensans, left upper arm

      M85.329   Osteitis condensans, unspecified upper arm

● M85.33   Osteitis condensans, forearm

      M85.331   Osteitis condensans, right forearm

      M85.332   Osteitis condensans, left forearm

      M85.339   Osteitis condensans, unspecified forearm

● M85.34   Osteitis condensans, hand

      M85.341   Osteitis condensans, right hand

      M85.342   Osteitis condensans, left hand

      M85.349   Osteitis condensans, unspecified hand

● M85.35   Osteitis condensans, thigh

      M85.351   Osteitis condensans, right thigh

      M85.352   Osteitis condensans, left thigh

      M85.359   Osteitis condensans, unspecified thigh

● M85.36   Osteitis condensans, lower leg

      M85.361   Osteitis condensans, right lower leg

      M85.362   Osteitis condensans, left lower leg

      M85.369   Osteitis condensans, unspecified lower leg

◀ New   ◀▥ Revised   ~~deleted~~ Deleted   Excludes 1   Excludes 2   Includes   Use additional   Code first   Code also   Unspecified

OGCR Official Guidelines   ● Unacceptable Principal Diagnosis   X Assign placeholder X   ● Use Additional Character(s)   ▶ Manifestation Code   **Coding Clinic**

● M85.37　Osteitis condensans, ankle and foot
　　　M85.371　Osteitis condensans, right ankle and foot
　　　M85.372　Osteitis condensans, left ankle and foot
　　　M85.379　Osteitis condensans, unspecified ankle and foot
　　M85.38　Osteitis condensans, other site
　　M85.39　Osteitis condensans, multiple sites
● M85.4　Solitary bone cyst
　　　Excludes2　solitary cyst of jaw (M27.4)
　　M85.40　Solitary bone cyst, unspecified site
● M85.41　Solitary bone cyst, shoulder
　　　M85.411　Solitary bone cyst, right shoulder
　　　M85.412　Solitary bone cyst, left shoulder
　　　M85.419　Solitary bone cyst, unspecified shoulder
● M85.42　Solitary bone cyst, humerus
　　　M85.421　Solitary bone cyst, right humerus
　　　M85.422　Solitary bone cyst, left humerus
　　　M85.429　Solitary bone cyst, unspecified humerus
● M85.43　Solitary bone cyst, ulna and radius
　　　M85.431　Solitary bone cyst, right ulna and radius
　　　M85.432　Solitary bone cyst, left ulna and radius
　　　M85.439　Solitary bone cyst, unspecified ulna and radius
● M85.44　Solitary bone cyst, hand
　　　M85.441　Solitary bone cyst, right hand
　　　M85.442　Solitary bone cyst, left hand
　　　M85.449　Solitary bone cyst, unspecified hand
● M85.45　Solitary bone cyst, pelvis
　　　M85.451　Solitary bone cyst, right pelvis
　　　M85.452　Solitary bone cyst, left pelvis
　　　M85.459　Solitary bone cyst, unspecified pelvis
● M85.46　Solitary bone cyst, tibia and fibula
　　　M85.461　Solitary bone cyst, right tibia and fibula
　　　M85.462　Solitary bone cyst, left tibia and fibula
　　　M85.469　Solitary bone cyst, unspecified tibia and fibula
● M85.47　Solitary bone cyst, ankle and foot
　　　M85.471　Solitary bone cyst, right ankle and foot
　　　M85.472　Solitary bone cyst, left ankle and foot
　　　M85.479　Solitary bone cyst, unspecified ankle and foot
　　M85.48　Solitary bone cyst, other site
● M85.5　Aneurysmal bone cyst
　　　Excludes2　aneurysmal cyst of jaw (M27.4)
　　M85.50　Aneurysmal bone cyst, unspecified site
● M85.51　Aneurysmal bone cyst, shoulder
　　　M85.511　Aneurysmal bone cyst, right shoulder
　　　M85.512　Aneurysmal bone cyst, left shoulder
　　　M85.519　Aneurysmal bone cyst, unspecified shoulder
● M85.52　Aneurysmal bone cyst, upper arm
　　　M85.521　Aneurysmal bone cyst, right upper arm
　　　M85.522　Aneurysmal bone cyst, left upper arm
　　　M85.529　Aneurysmal bone cyst, unspecified upper arm

● M85.53　Aneurysmal bone cyst, forearm
　　　M85.531　Aneurysmal bone cyst, right forearm
　　　M85.532　Aneurysmal bone cyst, left forearm
　　　M85.539　Aneurysmal bone cyst, unspecified forearm
● M85.54　Aneurysmal bone cyst, hand
　　　M85.541　Aneurysmal bone cyst, right hand
　　　M85.542　Aneurysmal bone cyst, left hand
　　　M85.549　Aneurysmal bone cyst, unspecified hand
● M85.55　Aneurysmal bone cyst, thigh
　　　M85.551　Aneurysmal bone cyst, right thigh
　　　M85.552　Aneurysmal bone cyst, left thigh
　　　M85.559　Aneurysmal bone cyst, unspecified thigh
● M85.56　Aneurysmal bone cyst, lower leg
　　　M85.561　Aneurysmal bone cyst, right lower leg
　　　M85.562　Aneurysmal bone cyst, left lower leg
　　　M85.569　Aneurysmal bone cyst, unspecified lower leg
● M85.57　Aneurysmal bone cyst, ankle and foot
　　　M85.571　Aneurysmal bone cyst, right ankle and foot
　　　M85.572　Aneurysmal bone cyst, left ankle and foot
　　　M85.579　Aneurysmal bone cyst, unspecified ankle and foot
　　M85.58　Aneurysmal bone cyst, other site
　　M85.59　Aneurysmal bone cyst, multiple sites
● M85.6　Other cyst of bone
　　　Excludes1　cyst of jaw NEC (M27.4)
　　　　　　osteitis fibrosa cystica generalisata [von Recklinghausen's disease of bone] (E21.0)
　　M85.60　Other cyst of bone, unspecified site
● M85.61　Other cyst of bone, shoulder
　　　M85.611　Other cyst of bone, right shoulder
　　　M85.612　Other cyst of bone, left shoulder
　　　M85.619　Other cyst of bone, unspecified shoulder
● M85.62　Other cyst of bone, upper arm
　　　M85.621　Other cyst of bone, right upper arm
　　　M85.622　Other cyst of bone, left upper arm
　　　M85.629　Other cyst of bone, unspecified upper arm
● M85.63　Other cyst of bone, forearm
　　　M85.631　Other cyst of bone, right forearm
　　　M85.632　Other cyst of bone, left forearm
　　　M85.639　Other cyst of bone, unspecified forearm
● M85.64　Other cyst of bone, hand
　　　M85.641　Other cyst of bone, right hand
　　　M85.642　Other cyst of bone, left hand
　　　M85.649　Other cyst of bone, unspecified hand
● M85.65　Other cyst of bone, thigh
　　　M85.651　Other cyst of bone, right thigh
　　　M85.652　Other cyst of bone, left thigh
　　　M85.659　Other cyst of bone, unspecified thigh
● M85.66　Other cyst of bone, lower leg
　　　M85.661　Other cyst of bone, right lower leg
　　　M85.662　Other cyst of bone, left lower leg
　　　M85.669　Other cyst of bone, unspecified lower leg

CHAPTER 13 (M00-M99)

N Newborn Age: 0　　**P** Pediatric Age: 0–17　　**M** Maternity DX: 12–55　　**A** Adult Age: 15–124　　♀ Females Only　　♂ Males Only

🐾 Complication\Comorbidity　　🐾 Major C\C　　Ⓔⓧ CC/MCC Exclusions　　🐾 Present on Admission Requirement　　🐾 Hospital-Acquired Condition

1151

● M85.67 Other cyst of bone, ankle and foot
  M85.671 Other cyst of bone, right ankle and foot
  M85.672 Other cyst of bone, left ankle and foot
  M85.679 Other cyst of bone, unspecified ankle and foot
 M85.68 Other cyst of bone, other site
 M85.69 Other cyst of bone, multiple sites
● M85.8 Other specified disorders of bone density and structure
  Hyperostosis of bones, except skull
  Osteosclerosis, acquired
  Excludes1 diffuse idiopathic skeletal hyperostosis [DISH] (M48.1)
           osteosclerosis congenita (Q77.4)
           osteosclerosis fragilitas (generalista) (Q78.2)
           osteosclerosis myelofibrosis (D75.81)
 M85.80 Other specified disorders of bone density and structure, unspecified site
● M85.81 Other specified disorders of bone density and structure, shoulder
  M85.811 Other specified disorders of bone density and structure, right shoulder
  M85.812 Other specified disorders of bone density and structure, left shoulder
  M85.819 Other specified disorders of bone density and structure, unspecified shoulder
● M85.82 Other specified disorders of bone density and structure, upper arm
  M85.821 Other specified disorders of bone density and structure, right upper arm
  M85.822 Other specified disorders of bone density and structure, left upper arm
  M85.829 Other specified disorders of bone density and structure, unspecified upper arm
● M85.83 Other specified disorders of bone density and structure, forearm
  M85.831 Other specified disorders of bone density and structure, right forearm
  M85.832 Other specified disorders of bone density and structure, left forearm
  M85.839 Other specified disorders of bone density and structure, unspecified forearm
● M85.84 Other specified disorders of bone density and structure, hand
  M85.841 Other specified disorders of bone density and structure, right hand
  M85.842 Other specified disorders of bone density and structure, left hand
  M85.849 Other specified disorders of bone density and structure, unspecified hand
● M85.85 Other specified disorders of bone density and structure, thigh
  M85.851 Other specified disorders of bone density and structure, right thigh
  M85.852 Other specified disorders of bone density and structure, left thigh
  M85.859 Other specified disorders of bone density and structure, unspecified thigh

● M85.86 Other specified disorders of bone density and structure, lower leg
  M85.861 Other specified disorders of bone density and structure, right lower leg
  M85.862 Other specified disorders of bone density and structure, left lower leg
  M85.869 Other specified disorders of bone density and structure, unspecified lower leg
● M85.87 Other specified disorders of bone density and structure, ankle and foot
  M85.871 Other specified disorders of bone density and structure, right ankle and foot
  M85.872 Other specified disorders of bone density and structure, left ankle and foot
  M85.879 Other specified disorders of bone density and structure, unspecified ankle and foot
 M85.88 Other specified disorders of bone density and structure, other site
 M85.89 Other specified disorders of bone density and structure, multiple sites
 M85.9 Disorder of bone density and structure, unspecified

OTHER OSTEOPATHIES (M86-M90)

Excludes1 postprocedural osteopathies (M96.-)

● M86 Osteomyelitis
  Use additional code (B95-B97) to identify infectious agent
  Use additional code to identify major osseous defect, if applicable (M89.7-)
  Excludes1 osteomyelitis due to:
           echinococcus (B67.2)
           gonococcus (A54.43)
           salmonella (A02.24)
  Excludes2 ostemyelitis of:
           orbit (H05.0-)
           petrous bone (H70.2-)
           vertebra (M46.2-)
● M86.0 Acute hematogenous osteomyelitis
  M86.00 Acute hematogenous osteomyelitis, unspecified site 🔖
         Ex: A17.9, A18.03-A18.09, A18.82, A18.84, A18.89, M46.20-M46.39, M86.00-M86.9
● M86.01 Acute hematogenous osteomyelitis, shoulder
         Ex: For category M86.01 CC codes: A17.9, A18.03-A18.09, A18.82, A18.84, A18.89, M46.20-M46.39, M86.00, M86.08-M86.10, M86.18-M86.20, M86.28-M86.319, M86.38-M86.419, M86.48-M86.519, M86.58-M86.619, M86.68-M86.8X1, M86.8X8-M86.9
  M86.011 Acute hematogenous osteomyelitis, right shoulder 🔖
  M86.012 Acute hematogenous osteomyelitis, left shoulder 🔖
  M86.019 Acute hematogenous osteomyelitis, unspecified shoulder 🔖
● M86.02 Acute hematogenous osteomyelitis, humerus
         Ex: For category M86.02 CC codes: A17.9, A18.03-A18.09, A18.82, A18.84, A18.89, M46.20-M46.39, M86.00, M86.08-M86.10, M86.18-M86.20, M86.28-M86.30, M86.321-M86.329, M86.38-M86.40, M86.421-M86.429, M86.48-M86.50, M86.521-M86.529, M86.58-M86.60, M86.621-M86.629, M86.68-M86.69, M86.8X0, M86.8X2, M86.8X8-M86.9
  M86.021 Acute hematogenous osteomyelitis, right humerus 🔖
  M86.022 Acute hematogenous osteomyelitis, left humerus 🔖
  M86.029 Acute hematogenous osteomyelitis, unspecified humerus 🔖

◀ New   ◀▥ Revised   deleted Deleted   Excludes 1   Excludes 2   Includes   Use additional   Code first   Code also   Unspecified
OGCR Official Guidelines   ● Unacceptable Principal Diagnosis   X Assign placeholder X   ● Use Additional Character(s)   ▌ Manifestation Code   **Coding Clinic**

Figure 13-5 Osteomyelitis of the spine. A lateral view of the lower thoracic spine demonstrates destruction of the disk space *(arrow)* as well as destruction of the adjoining vertebral bodies. (From Mettler: Essentials of Radiology, ed 2, Saunders, An Imprint of Elsevier, 2005)

Item 13–12 Osteomyelitis is an inflammation of the bone. **Acute osteomyelitis** is a rapidly destructive, pus-producing infection capable of causing severe bone destruction. **Chronic osteomyelitis** can remain long after the initial acute episode has passed and may lead to a recurrence of the acute phase. **Brodie's abscess** is an encapsulated focal abscess that must be surgically drained. Periostitis is an inflammation of the periosteum, a dense membrane composed of fibrous connective tissue that closely wraps all bone, except those with articulating surfaces in joints, which are covered by synovial membranes.

● **M86.03** Acute hematogenous osteomyelitis, radius and ulna
   (Ex) **For category M86.03 CC codes:** A17.9, A18.03-A18.09, A18.82, A18.84, A18.89, M46.20-M46.39, M86.00, M86.08-M86.10, M86.18-M86.20, M86.28-M86.30, M86.331-M86.339, M86.38-M86.40, M86.431-M86.439, M86.48-M86.50, M86.531-M86.539, M86.58-M86.60, M86.631-M86.639, M86.68-M86.8X0, M86.8X3, M86.8X8-M86.9

   M86.031   Acute hematogenous osteomyelitis, right radius and ulna 🔹

   M86.032   Acute hematogenous osteomyelitis, left radius and ulna 🔹

   M86.039   Acute hematogenous osteomyelitis, unspecified radius and ulna 🔹

● **M86.04** Acute hematogenous osteomyelitis, hand
   (Ex) **For category M86.04 CC codes:** A17.9, A18.03-A18.09, A18.82, A18.84, A18.89, M46.20-M46.39, M86.00, M86.08-M86.10, M86.18-M86.20, M86.28-M86.30, M86.341-M86.349, M86.38-M86.40, M86.441-M86.449, M86.48-M86.50, M86.541-M86.549, M86.58-M86.60, M86.41-M86.649, M86.68-M86.69, M86.8X0, M86.8X4, M86.8X8-M86.9

   M86.041   Acute hematogenous osteomyelitis, right hand 🔹

   M86.042   Acute hematogenous osteomyelitis, left hand 🔹

   M86.049   Acute hematogenous osteomyelitis, unspecified hand 🔹

● **M86.05** Acute hematogenous osteomyelitis, femur
   (Ex) **For category M86.05 CC codes:** A17.9, A18.03-A18.09, A18.82, A18.84, A18.89, M46.20-M46.39, M86.00, M86.08-M86.10, M86.18-M86.20, M86.28-M86.30, M86.351-M86.359, M86.38-M86.40, M86.451-M86.459, M86.48-M86.50, M86.551-M86.559, M86.58-M86.60, M86.651-M86.659, M86.68-M86.8X0, M86.8X5, M86.8X8-M86.9

   M86.051   Acute hematogenous osteomyelitis, right femur 🔹

   M86.052   Acute hematogenous osteomyelitis, left femur 🔹

   M86.059   Acute hematogenous osteomyelitis, unspecified femur 🔹

● **M86.06** Acute hematogenous osteomyelitis, tibia and fibula
   (Ex) **For category M86.06 CC codes:** A17.9, A18.03-A18.09, A18.82, A18.84, A18.89, M46.20-M46.39, M86.00, M86.08-M86.10, M86.18-M86.20, M86.28-M86.30, M86.361-M86.369, M86.38-M86.40, M86.461-M86.469, M86.48-M86.50, M86.561-M86.569, M86.58-M86.60, M86.661-M86.669, M86.68-M86.8X0, M86.8X6, M86.8X8-M86.9

   M86.061   Acute hematogenous osteomyelitis, right tibia and fibula 🔹

   M86.062   Acute hematogenous osteomyelitis, left tibia and fibula 🔹

   M86.069   Acute hematogenous osteomyelitis, unspecified tibia and fibula 🔹

● **M86.07** Acute hematogenous osteomyelitis, ankle and foot
   (Ex) **For category M86.07 CC codes:** A17.9, A18.03-A18.09, A18.82, A18.84, A18.89, M46.20-M46.39, M86.00, M86.08-M86.10, M86.18-M86.20, M86.28-M86.30, M86.371-M86.379, M86.38-M86.40, M86.471-M86.479, M86.48-M86.50, M86.571-M86.579, M86.58-M86.60, M86.671-M86.679, M86.68-M86.8X0, M86.8X7-M86.9

   M86.071   Acute hematogenous osteomyelitis, right ankle and foot 🔹

   M86.072   Acute hematogenous osteomyelitis, left ankle and foot 🔹

   M86.079   Acute hematogenous osteomyelitis, unspecified ankle and foot 🔹

   M86.08 Acute hematogenous osteomyelitis, other sites 🔹
   (Ex) A17.9, A18.01, A18.03, A18.09, A18.82, A18.84, A18.89, M46.20-M46.39, M86.00-M86.9

   M86.09 Acute hematogenous osteomyelitis, multiple sites 🔹
   (Ex) See M86.00

● **M86.1** Other acute osteomyelitis

   M86.10 Other acute osteomyelitis, unspecified site 🔹
   (Ex) See M86.00

● **M86.11** Other acute osteomyelitis, shoulder
   (Ex) **For category M86.11 CC codes:** See M86.01

   M86.111   Other acute osteomyelitis, right shoulder 🔹

   M86.112   Other acute osteomyelitis, left shoulder 🔹

   M86.119   Other acute osteomyelitis, unspecified shoulder 🔹

● **M86.12** Other acute osteomyelitis, humerus
   (Ex) **For category M86.12 CC codes:** See M86.02

   M86.121   Other acute osteomyelitis, right humerus 🔹

   M86.122   Other acute osteomyelitis, left humerus 🔹

   M86.129   Other acute osteomyelitis, unspecified humerus 🔹

● **M86.13** Other acute osteomyelitis, radius and ulna
   (Ex) **For category M86.13 CC codes:** See M86.03

   M86.131   Other acute osteomyelitis, right radius and ulna 🔹

   M86.132   Other acute osteomyelitis, left radius and ulna 🔹

   M86.139   Other acute osteomyelitis, unspecified radius and ulna 🔹

● **M86.14** Other acute osteomyelitis, hand
   (Ex) **For category M86.14 CC codes:** See M86.04

   M86.141   Other acute osteomyelitis, right hand 🔹

   M86.142   Other acute osteomyelitis, left hand 🔹

   M86.149   Other acute osteomyelitis, unspecified hand 🔹

N Newborn Age: 0   **P** Pediatric Age: 0–17   **M** Maternity DX: 12–55   **A** Adult Age: 15–124   ♀ Females Only   ♂ Males Only
🔹 Complication\Comorbidity   🔹 Major C\C   (Ex) CC/MCC Exclusions   🔹 Present on Admission Requirement   🔹 Hospital-Acquired Condition

1153

CHAPTER 13 (M00-M99)

● **M86.15   Other acute osteomyelitis, femur**
    (Ex:) For category M86.15 CC codes: See M86.05

    M86.151   Other acute osteomyelitis, right femur

    M86.152   Other acute osteomyelitis, left femur

    M86.159   Other acute osteomyelitis, unspecified femur

● **M86.16   Other acute osteomyelitis, tibia and fibula**
    (Ex:) For category M86.16 CC codes: See M86.06

    M86.161   Other acute osteomyelitis, right tibia and fibula

    M86.162   Other acute osteomyelitis, left tibia and fibula

    M86.169   Other acute osteomyelitis, unspecified tibia and fibula

● **M86.17   Other acute osteomyelitis, ankle and foot**
    (Ex:) For category M86.17 CC codes: See M86.07

    M86.171   Other acute osteomyelitis, right ankle and foot

    M86.172   Other acute osteomyelitis, left ankle and foot

    M86.179   Other acute osteomyelitis, unspecified ankle and foot

    M86.18   Other acute osteomyelitis, other site
        (Ex:) See M86.08

    M86.19   Other acute osteomyelitis, multiple sites
        (Ex:) See M86.00

● **M86.2   Subacute osteomyelitis**

    M86.20   Subacute osteomyelitis, unspecified site
        (Ex:) See M86.00

● **M86.21   Subacute osteomyelitis, shoulder**
    (Ex:) For category M86.21 CC codes: See M86.01

    M86.211   Subacute osteomyelitis, right shoulder

    M86.212   Subacute osteomyelitis, left shoulder

    M86.219   Subacute osteomyelitis, unspecified shoulder

● **M86.22   Subacute osteomyelitis, humerus**
    (Ex:) For category M86.22 CC codes: See M86.02

    M86.221   Subacute osteomyelitis, right humerus

    M86.222   Subacute osteomyelitis, left humerus

    M86.229   Subacute osteomyelitis, unspecified humerus

● **M86.23   Subacute osteomyelitis, radius and ulna**
    (Ex:) For category M86.23 CC codes: See M86.03

    M86.231   Subacute osteomyelitis, right radius and ulna

    M86.232   Subacute osteomyelitis, left radius and ulna

    M86.239   Subacute osteomyelitis, unspecified radius and ulna

● **M86.24   Subacute osteomyelitis, hand**
    (Ex:) For category M86.24 CC codes: See M86.04

    M86.241   Subacute osteomyelitis, right hand
    M86.242   Subacute osteomyelitis, left hand
    M86.249   Subacute osteomyelitis, unspecified hand

● **M86.25   Subacute osteomyelitis, femur**
    (Ex:) For category M86.25 CC codes: See M86.05

    M86.251   Subacute osteomyelitis, right femur

    M86.252   Subacute osteomyelitis, left femur

    M86.259   Subacute osteomyelitis, unspecified femur

● **M86.26   Subacute osteomyelitis, tibia and fibula**
    (Ex:) For category M86.26 CC codes: See M86.06

    M86.261   Subacute osteomyelitis, right tibia and fibula

    M86.262   Subacute osteomyelitis, left tibia and fibula

    M86.269   Subacute osteomyelitis, unspecified tibia and fibula

● **M86.27   Subacute osteomyelitis, ankle and foot**
    (Ex:) For category M86.27 CC codes: See M86.07

    M86.271   Subacute osteomyelitis, right ankle and foot

    M86.272   Subacute osteomyelitis, left ankle and foot

    M86.279   Subacute osteomyelitis, unspecified ankle and foot

    M86.28   Subacute osteomyelitis, other site
        (Ex:) See M86.08

    M86.29   Subacute osteomyelitis, multiple sites
        (Ex:) See M86.00

● **M86.3   Chronic multifocal osteomyelitis**
    (Ex:) For category M86.3 CC codes unless otherwise indicated: A02.24, A17.9, A18.03, A18.09, A18.82, A18.84, A18.89, M46.20-M46.39, M86.00-M86.9

    M86.30   Chronic multifocal osteomyelitis, unspecified site
        (Ex:) M46.20-M46.39, M86.30-M86.9, M88.0-M88.9, M90.60-M90.69

● **M86.31   Chronic multifocal osteomyelitis, shoulder**

    M86.311   Chronic multifocal osteomyelitis, right shoulder

    M86.312   Chronic multifocal osteomyelitis, left shoulder

    M86.319   Chronic multifocal osteomyelitis, unspecified shoulder

● **M86.32   Chronic multifocal osteomyelitis, humerus**

    M86.321   Chronic multifocal osteomyelitis, right humerus

    M86.322   Chronic multifocal osteomyelitis, left humerus

    M86.329   Chronic multifocal osteomyelitis, unspecified humerus

● **M86.33   Chronic multifocal osteomyelitis, radius and ulna**

    M86.331   Chronic multifocal osteomyelitis, right radius and ulna

    M86.332   Chronic multifocal osteomyelitis, left radius and ulna

    M86.339   Chronic multifocal osteomyelitis, unspecified radius and ulna

● **M86.34   Chronic multifocal osteomyelitis, hand**

    M86.341   Chronic multifocal osteomyelitis, right hand

    M86.342   Chronic multifocal osteomyelitis, left hand

    M86.349   Chronic multifocal osteomyelitis, unspecified hand

● **M86.35   Chronic multifocal osteomyelitis, femur**

    M86.351   Chronic multifocal osteomyelitis, right femur

    M86.352   Chronic multifocal osteomyelitis, left femur

    M86.359   Chronic multifocal osteomyelitis, unspecified femur

◀ New   ◀▥ Revised   ~~deleted~~ Deleted   Excludes 1   Excludes 2   Includes   Use additional   Code first   Code also   Unspecified

OGCR Official Guidelines   ● Unacceptable Principal Diagnosis   X Assign placeholder X   ● Use Additional Character(s)   ▶ Manifestation Code   **Coding Clinic**

● M86.36   Chronic multifocal osteomyelitis, tibia and fibula

    M86.361   Chronic multifocal osteomyelitis, right tibia and fibula 🦠

    M86.362   Chronic multifocal osteomyelitis, left tibia and fibula 🦠

    M86.369   Chronic multifocal osteomyelitis, unspecified tibia and fibula 🦠

● M86.37   Chronic multifocal osteomyelitis, ankle and foot

    M86.371   Chronic multifocal osteomyelitis, right ankle and foot 🦠

    M86.372   Chronic multifocal osteomyelitis, left ankle and foot 🦠

    M86.379   Chronic multifocal osteomyelitis, unspecified ankle and foot 🦠

   M86.38   Chronic multifocal osteomyelitis, other site 🦠

   M86.39   Chronic multifocal osteomyelitis, multiple sites 🦠

● M86.4   Chronic osteomyelitis with draining sinus

    (Ex:) For category M86.4 CC codes unless otherwise indicated: See M86.3

   M86.40   Chronic osteomyelitis with draining sinus, unspecified site 🦠

     (Ex:) See M86.30

● M86.41   Chronic osteomyelitis with draining sinus, shoulder

    M86.411   Chronic osteomyelitis with draining sinus, right shoulder 🦠

    M86.412   Chronic osteomyelitis with draining sinus, left shoulder 🦠

    M86.419   Chronic osteomyelitis with draining sinus, unspecified shoulder 🦠

● M86.42   Chronic osteomyelitis with draining sinus, humerus

    M86.421   Chronic osteomyelitis with draining sinus, right humerus 🦠

    M86.422   Chronic osteomyelitis with draining sinus, left humerus 🦠

    M86.429   Chronic osteomyelitis with draining sinus, unspecified humerus 🦠

● M86.43   Chronic osteomyelitis with draining sinus, radius and ulna

    M86.431   Chronic osteomyelitis with draining sinus, right radius and ulna 🦠

    M86.432   Chronic osteomyelitis with draining sinus, left radius and ulna 🦠

    M86.439   Chronic osteomyelitis with draining sinus, unspecified radius and ulna 🦠

● M86.44   Chronic osteomyelitis with draining sinus, hand

    M86.441   Chronic osteomyelitis with draining sinus, right hand 🦠

    M86.442   Chronic osteomyelitis with draining sinus, left hand 🦠

    M86.449   Chronic osteomyelitis with draining sinus, unspecified hand 🦠

● M86.45   Chronic osteomyelitis with draining sinus, femur

    M86.451   Chronic osteomyelitis with draining sinus, right femur 🦠

    M86.452   Chronic osteomyelitis with draining sinus, left femur 🦠

    M86.459   Chronic osteomyelitis with draining sinus, unspecified femur 🦠

● M86.46   Chronic osteomyelitis with draining sinus, tibia and fibula

    M86.461   Chronic osteomyelitis with draining sinus, right tibia and fibula 🦠

    M86.462   Chronic osteomyelitis with draining sinus, left tibia and fibula 🦠

    M86.469   Chronic osteomyelitis with draining sinus, unspecified tibia and fibula 🦠

● M86.47   Chronic osteomyelitis with draining sinus, ankle and foot

    M86.471   Chronic osteomyelitis with draining sinus, right ankle and foot 🦠

    M86.472   Chronic osteomyelitis with draining sinus, left ankle and foot 🦠

    M86.479   Chronic osteomyelitis with draining sinus, unspecified ankle and foot 🦠

   M86.48   Chronic osteomyelitis with draining sinus, other site 🦠

   M86.49   Chronic osteomyelitis with draining sinus, multiple sites 🦠

● M86.5   Other chronic hematogenous osteomyelitis

    (Ex:) For category M86.5 CC codes unless otherwise indicated: See M86.3

   M86.50   Other chronic hematogenous osteomyelitis, unspecified site 🦠

     (Ex:) See M86.30

● M86.51   Other chronic hematogenous osteomyelitis, shoulder

    M86.511   Other chronic hematogenous osteomyelitis, right shoulder 🦠

    M86.512   Other chronic hematogenous osteomyelitis, left shoulder 🦠

    M86.519   Other chronic hematogenous osteomyelitis, unspecified shoulder 🦠

● M86.52   Other chronic hematogenous osteomyelitis, humerus

    M86.521   Other chronic hematogenous osteomyelitis, right humerus 🦠

    M86.522   Other chronic hematogenous osteomyelitis, left humerus 🦠

    M86.529   Other chronic hematogenous osteomyelitis, unspecified humerus 🦠

● M86.53   Other chronic hematogenous osteomyelitis, radius and ulna

    M86.531   Other chronic hematogenous osteomyelitis, right radius and ulna 🦠

    M86.532   Other chronic hematogenous osteomyelitis, left radius and ulna 🦠

    M86.539   Other chronic hematogenous osteomyelitis, unspecified radius and ulna 🦠

● M86.54   Other chronic hematogenous osteomyelitis, hand

    M86.541   Other chronic hematogenous osteomyelitis, right hand 🦠

    M86.542   Other chronic hematogenous osteomyelitis, left hand 🦠

    M86.549   Other chronic hematogenous osteomyelitis, unspecified hand 🦠

● M86.55   Other chronic hematogenous osteomyelitis, femur

    M86.551   Other chronic hematogenous osteomyelitis, right femur 🦠

    M86.552   Other chronic hematogenous osteomyelitis, left femur 🦠

    M86.559   Other chronic hematogenous osteomyelitis, unspecified femur 🦠

N   Newborn Age: 0   **P**   Pediatric Age: 0–17   **M**   Maternity DX: 12–55   **A**   Adult Age: 15–124   ♀   Females Only   ♂   Males Only

🦠   Complication\Comorbidity   🦠   Major C\C   (Ex:)   CC/MCC Exclusions   🦠   Present on Admission Requirement   🦠   Hospital-Acquired Condition

1155

CHAPTER 13 (M00-M99)

CHAPTER 13 (M00-M99)

● M86.56 Other chronic hematogenous osteomyelitis, tibia and fibula

    M86.561 Other chronic hematogenous osteomyelitis, right tibia and fibula 🔗

    M86.562 Other chronic hematogenous osteomyelitis, left tibia and fibula 🔗

    M86.569 Other chronic hematogenous osteomyelitis, unspecified tibia and fibula 🔗

● M86.57 Other chronic hematogenous osteomyelitis, ankle and foot

    M86.571 Other chronic hematogenous osteomyelitis, right ankle and foot 🔗

    M86.572 Other chronic hematogenous osteomyelitis, left ankle and foot 🔗

    M86.579 Other chronic hematogenous osteomyelitis, unspecified ankle and foot 🔗

  M86.58 Other chronic hematogenous osteomyelitis, other site 🔗

  M86.59 Other chronic hematogenous osteomyelitis, multiple sites 🔗

● M86.6 Other chronic osteomyelitis

    Ⓔⓧ For category M86.6 CC codes unless otherwise indicated: See M86.3

  M86.60 Other chronic osteomyelitis, unspecified site 🔗

    Ⓔⓧ See M86.30

● M86.61 Other chronic osteomyelitis, shoulder

    M86.611 Other chronic osteomyelitis, right shoulder 🔗

    M86.612 Other chronic osteomyelitis, left shoulder 🔗

    M86.619 Other chronic osteomyelitis, unspecified shoulder 🔗

● M86.62 Other chronic osteomyelitis, humerus

    M86.621 Other chronic osteomyelitis, right humerus 🔗

    M86.622 Other chronic osteomyelitis, left humerus 🔗

    M86.629 Other chronic osteomyelitis, unspecified humerus 🔗

● M86.63 Other chronic osteomyelitis, radius and ulna

    M86.631 Other chronic osteomyelitis, right radius and ulna 🔗

    M86.632 Other chronic osteomyelitis, left radius and ulna 🔗

    M86.639 Other chronic osteomyelitis, unspecified radius and ulna 🔗

● M86.64 Other chronic osteomyelitis, hand

    M86.641 Other chronic osteomyelitis, right hand 🔗

    M86.642 Other chronic osteomyelitis, left hand 🔗

    M86.649 Other chronic osteomyelitis, unspecified hand 🔗

● M86.65 Other chronic osteomyelitis, thigh

    M86.651 Other chronic osteomyelitis, right thigh 🔗

    M86.652 Other chronic osteomyelitis, left thigh 🔗

    M86.659 Other chronic osteomyelitis, unspecified thigh 🔗

● M86.66 Other chronic osteomyelitis, tibia and fibula

    M86.661 Other chronic osteomyelitis, right tibia and fibula 🔗

    M86.662 Other chronic osteomyelitis, left tibia and fibula 🔗

    M86.669 Other chronic osteomyelitis, unspecified tibia and fibula 🔗

● M86.67 Other chronic osteomyelitis, ankle and foot

    M86.671 Other chronic osteomyelitis, right ankle and foot 🔗

    M86.672 Other chronic osteomyelitis, left ankle and foot 🔗

    M86.679 Other chronic osteomyelitis, unspecified ankle and foot 🔗

  M86.68 Other chronic osteomyelitis, other site 🔗

  M86.69 Other chronic osteomyelitis, multiple sites 🔗

● M86.8 Other osteomyelitis

    Brodie's abscess

    Ⓔⓧ For category M86.8 CC codes unless otherwise indicated: See M86.3

● M86.8X Other osteomyelitis

    M86.8X0 Other osteomyelitis, multiple sites 🔗

    M86.8X1 Other osteomyelitis, shoulder 🔗

    M86.8X2 Other osteomyelitis, upper arm 🔗

    M86.8X3 Other osteomyelitis, forearm 🔗

    M86.8X4 Other osteomyelitis, hand 🔗

    M86.8X5 Other osteomyelitis, thigh 🔗

    M86.8X6 Other osteomyelitis, lower leg 🔗

    M86.8X7 Other osteomyelitis, ankle and foot 🔗

    M86.8X8 Other osteomyelitis, other site 🔗

    M86.8X9 Other osteomyelitis, unspecified sites 🔗

    Ⓔⓧ See M86.30

  M86.9 Osteomyelitis, unspecified 🔗

    Infection of bone NOS

    Periostitis without osteomyelitis

    Ⓔⓧ See M86.30

● M87 Osteonecrosis

    Includes avascular necrosis of bone

    Use additional code to identify major osseous defect, if applicable (M89.7-)

    Excludes 1 juvenile osteonecrosis (M91-M92) osteochondropathies (M90-M93)

    Ⓔⓧ For category M87 CC codes unless otherwise indicated: M87.00-M87.9, M90.50-M90.59

● M87.0 Idiopathic aseptic necrosis of bone

  M87.00 Idiopathic aseptic necrosis of unspecified bone 🔗

● M87.01 Idiopathic aseptic necrosis of shoulder

    Idiopathic aseptic necrosis of clavicle and scapula

    Ⓔⓧ For category M87.01 CC codes: M87.00-M87.9, M90.50-M90.59

    M87.011 Idiopathic aseptic necrosis of right shoulder 🔗

    M87.012 Idiopathic aseptic necrosis of left shoulder 🔗

    M87.019 Idiopathic aseptic necrosis of unspecified shoulder 🔗

  M87.02 Idiopathic aseptic necrosis of humerus

    Ⓔⓧ For category M87.02 CC codes: See M87.01

    M87.021 Idiopathic aseptic necrosis of right humerus 🔗

    M87.022 Idiopathic aseptic necrosis of left humerus 🔗

    M87.029 Idiopathic aseptic necrosis of unspecified humerus 🔗

● M87.03 Idiopathic aseptic necrosis of radius, ulna and carpus

    M87.031 Idiopathic aseptic necrosis of right radius 🔗

    M87.032 Idiopathic aseptic necrosis of left radius 🔗

    M87.033 Idiopathic aseptic necrosis of unspecified radius 🔗

◀ New   ◀ Revised   ~~deleted~~ Deleted   Excludes 1   Excludes 2   Includes   Use additional   Code first   Code also   Unspecified

OGCR Official Guidelines   ● Unacceptable Principal Diagnosis   X Assign placeholder X   🔗 Use Additional Character(s)   ▶ Manifestation Code   **Coding Clinic**

M87.034   Idiopathic aseptic necrosis of right ulna 🦠

M87.035   Idiopathic aseptic necrosis of left ulna 🦠

M87.036   Idiopathic aseptic necrosis of unspecified ulna 🦠

M87.037   Idiopathic aseptic necrosis of right carpus 🦠

M87.038   Idiopathic aseptic necrosis of left carpus 🦠

M87.039   Idiopathic aseptic necrosis of unspecified carpus 🦠

● **M87.04**   **Idiopathic aseptic necrosis of hand and fingers**
     Idiopathic aseptic necrosis of metacarpals and phalanges of hands

M87.041   Idiopathic aseptic necrosis of right hand 🦠

M87.042   Idiopathic aseptic necrosis of left hand 🦠

M87.043   Idiopathic aseptic necrosis of unspecified hand 🦠

M87.044   Idiopathic aseptic necrosis of right finger(s) 🦠

M87.045   Idiopathic aseptic necrosis of left finger(s) 🦠

M87.046   Idiopathic aseptic necrosis of unspecified finger(s) 🦠

● **M87.05**   **Idiopathic aseptic necrosis of pelvis and femur**

M87.050   Idiopathic aseptic necrosis of pelvis 🦠

M87.051   Idiopathic aseptic necrosis of right femur 🦠
     (Ex) M87.00-M87.9, M90.50-M90.59

M87.052   Idiopathic aseptic necrosis of left femur 🦠
     (Ex) See M87.501

M87.059   Idiopathic aseptic necrosis of unspecified femur 🦠
     Idiopathic aseptic necrosis of hip NOS
     (Ex) See M87.501

● **M87.06**   **Idiopathic aseptic necrosis of tibia and fibula**

M87.061   Idiopathic aseptic necrosis of right tibia 🦠

M87.062   Idiopathic aseptic necrosis of left tibia 🦠

M87.063   Idiopathic aseptic necrosis of unspecified tibia 🦠

M87.064   Idiopathic aseptic necrosis of right fibula 🦠

M87.065   Idiopathic aseptic necrosis of left fibula 🦠

M87.066   Idiopathic aseptic necrosis of unspecified fibula 🦠

● **M87.07**   **Idiopathic aseptic necrosis of ankle, foot and toes**
     Idiopathic aseptic necrosis of metatarsus, tarsus, and phalanges of toes

M87.071   Idiopathic aseptic necrosis of right ankle 🦠

M87.072   Idiopathic aseptic necrosis of left ankle 🦠

M87.073   Idiopathic aseptic necrosis of unspecified ankle 🦠

M87.074   Idiopathic aseptic necrosis of right foot 🦠
     (Ex) M87.00, M87.031-M87.819, M87.831-M87.849, M87.861-M87.9, M90.50, M90.521-M90.549, M90.561-M90.59

M87.075   Idiopathic aseptic necrosis of left foot 🦠
     (Ex) See M87.074

M87.076   Idiopathic aseptic necrosis of unspecified foot 🦠
     (Ex) See M87.074

M87.077   Idiopathic aseptic necrosis of right toe(s) 🦠

M87.078   Idiopathic aseptic necrosis of left toe(s) 🦠

M87.079   Idiopathic aseptic necrosis of unspecified toe(s) 🦠

M87.08   Idiopathic aseptic necrosis of bone, other site 🦠

M87.09   Idiopathic aseptic necrosis of bone, multiple sites 🦠

● **M87.1**   **Osteonecrosis due to drugs**
     Use additional code for adverse effect, if applicable, to identify drug (T36-T50 with fifth or sixth character 5)
     (Ex) See M87

M87.10   Osteonecrosis due to drugs, unspecified bone 🦠

● **M87.11**   **Osteonecrosis due to drugs, shoulder**

M87.111   Osteonecrosis due to drugs, right shoulder 🦠

M87.112   Osteonecrosis due to drugs, left shoulder 🦠

M87.119   Osteonecrosis due to drugs, unspecified shoulder 🦠

● **M87.12**   **Osteonecrosis due to drugs, humerus**
     (Ex) For category M87.12 CC codes: See M87.01

M87.121   Osteonecrosis due to drugs, right humerus 🦠

M87.122   Osteonecrosis due to drugs, left humerus 🦠

M87.129   Osteonecrosis due to drugs, unspecified humerus 🦠

● **M87.13**   **Osteonecrosis due to drugs of radius, ulna and carpus**

M87.131   Osteonecrosis due to drugs of right radius 🦠

M87.132   Osteonecrosis due to drugs of left radius 🦠

M87.133   Osteonecrosis due to drugs of unspecified radius 🦠

M87.134   Osteonecrosis due to drugs of right ulna 🦠

M87.135   Osteonecrosis due to drugs of left ulna 🦠

M87.136   Osteonecrosis due to drugs of unspecified ulna 🦠

M87.137   Osteonecrosis due to drugs of right carpus 🦠

M87.138   Osteonecrosis due to drugs of left carpus 🦠

M87.139   Osteonecrosis due to drugs of unspecified carpus 🦠

● **M87.14**   **Osteonecrosis due to drugs, hand and fingers**

M87.141   Osteonecrosis due to drugs, right hand 🦠

M87.142   Osteonecrosis due to drugs, left hand 🦠

M87.143   Osteonecrosis due to drugs, unspecified hand 🦠

M87.144   Osteonecrosis due to drugs, right finger(s) 🦠

M87.145   Osteonecrosis due to drugs, left finger(s) 🦠

M87.146   Osteonecrosis due to drugs, unspecified finger(s) 🦠

N   Newborn Age: 0   P   Pediatric Age: 0–17   M   Maternity DX: 12–55   A   Adult Age: 15–124   ♀   Females Only   ♂   Males Only

🦠 Complication\Comorbidity   🦠 Major C\C   (Ex) CC/MCC Exclusions   🦠 Present on Admission Requirement   🦠 Hospital-Acquired Condition

1157

CHAPTER 13 (M00-M99)

● **M87.15**   Osteonecrosis due to drugs, pelvis and femur
     (Ex:) **For category M87.15 CC codes:** See M87.051

     M87.150   Osteonecrosis due to drugs, pelvis 🦴

     M87.151   Osteonecrosis due to drugs, right femur 🦴

     M87.152   Osteonecrosis due to drugs, left femur 🦴

     M87.159   Osteonecrosis due to drugs, unspecified femur 🦴

● **M87.16**   Osteonecrosis due to drugs, tibia and fibula

     M87.161   Osteonecrosis due to drugs, right tibia 🦴

     M87.162   Osteonecrosis due to drugs, left tibia 🦴

     M87.163   Osteonecrosis due to drugs, unspecified tibia 🦴

     M87.164   Osteonecrosis due to drugs, right fibula 🦴

     M87.165   Osteonecrosis due to drugs, left fibula 🦴

     M87.166   Osteonecrosis due to drugs, unspecified fibula 🦴

● **M87.17**   Osteonecrosis due to drugs, ankle, foot and toes

     M87.171   Osteonecrosis due to drugs, right ankle 🦴

     M87.172   Osteonecrosis due to drugs, left ankle 🦴

     M87.173   Osteonecrosis due to drugs, unspecified ankle 🦴

     M87.174   Osteonecrosis due to drugs, right foot 🦴
         (Ex:) See M87.074

     M87.175   Osteonecrosis due to drugs, left foot 🦴
         (Ex:) See M87.074

     M87.176   Osteonecrosis due to drugs, unspecified foot 🦴
         (Ex:) See M87.074

     M87.177   Osteonecrosis due to drugs, right toe(s) 🦴

     M87.178   Osteonecrosis due to drugs, left toe(s) 🦴

     M87.179   Osteonecrosis due to drugs, unspecified toe(s) 🦴

● **M87.18**   Osteonecrosis due to drugs, other site

     M87.180   Osteonecrosis due to drugs, jaw 🦴

     M87.188   Osteonecrosis due to drugs, other site 🦴

     M87.19   Osteonecrosis due to drugs, multiple sites 🦴

● **M87.2**   Osteonecrosis due to previous trauma
     (Ex:) See M87

     M87.20   Osteonecrosis due to previous trauma, unspecified bone 🦴

● **M87.21**   Osteonecrosis due to previous trauma, shoulder

     M87.211   Osteonecrosis due to previous trauma, right shoulder 🦴

     M87.212   Osteonecrosis due to previous trauma, left shoulder 🦴

     M87.219   Osteonecrosis due to previous trauma, unspecified shoulder 🦴

● **M87.22**   Osteonecrosis due to previous trauma, humerus
     (Ex:) **For category M87.22 CC codes:** See M87.01

     M87.221   Osteonecrosis due to previous trauma, right humerus 🦴

     M87.222   Osteonecrosis due to previous trauma, left humerus 🦴

     M87.229   Osteonecrosis due to previous trauma, unspecified humerus 🦴

● **M87.23**   Osteonecrosis due to previous trauma of radius, ulna and carpus

     M87.231   Osteonecrosis due to previous trauma of right radius 🦴

     M87.232   Osteonecrosis due to previous trauma of left radius 🦴

     M87.233   Osteonecrosis due to previous trauma of unspecified radius 🦴

     M87.234   Osteonecrosis due to previous trauma of right ulna 🦴

     M87.235   Osteonecrosis due to previous trauma of left ulna 🦴

     M87.236   Osteonecrosis due to previous trauma of unspecified ulna 🦴

     M87.237   Osteonecrosis due to previous trauma of right carpus 🦴

     M87.238   Osteonecrosis due to previous trauma of left carpus 🦴

     M87.239   Osteonecrosis due to previous trauma of unspecified carpus 🦴

● **M87.24**   Osteonecrosis due to previous trauma, hand and fingers

     M87.241   Osteonecrosis due to previous trauma, right hand 🦴

     M87.242   Osteonecrosis due to previous trauma, left hand 🦴

     M87.243   Osteonecrosis due to previous trauma, unspecified hand 🦴

     M87.244   Osteonecrosis due to previous trauma, right finger(s) 🦴

     M87.245   Osteonecrosis due to previous trauma, left finger(s) 🦴

     M87.246   Osteonecrosis due to previous trauma, unspecified finger(s) 🦴

● **M87.25**   Osteonecrosis due to previous trauma, pelvis and femur

     M87.250   Osteonecrosis due to previous trauma, pelvis 🦴

     M87.251   Osteonecrosis due to previous trauma, right femur 🦴
         (Ex:) See M87.051

     M87.252   Osteonecrosis due to previous trauma, left femur 🦴
         (Ex:) See M87.051

     M87.256   Osteonecrosis due to previous trauma, unspecified femur 🦴
         (Ex:) See M87.051

● **M87.26**   Osteonecrosis due to previous trauma, tibia and fibula

     M87.261   Osteonecrosis due to previous trauma, right tibia 🦴

     M87.262   Osteonecrosis due to previous trauma, left tibia 🦴

     M87.263   Osteonecrosis due to previous trauma, unspecified tibia 🦴

     M87.264   Osteonecrosis due to previous trauma, right fibula 🦴

     M87.265   Osteonecrosis due to previous trauma, left fibula 🦴

     M87.266   Osteonecrosis due to previous trauma, unspecified fibula 🦴

● **M87.27**   Osteonecrosis due to previous trauma, ankle, foot and toes

     M87.271   Osteonecrosis due to previous trauma, right ankle 🦴

     M87.272   Osteonecrosis due to previous trauma, left ankle 🦴

     M87.273   Osteonecrosis due to previous trauma, unspecified ankle 🦴

◀ New   ◀▥ Revised   ~~deleted~~ Deleted   Excludes 1   Excludes 2   Includes   Use additional   Code first   Code also   Unspecified

OGCR Official Guidelines   ● Unacceptable Principal Diagnosis   X Assign placeholder X   ● Use Additional Character(s)   ▷ Manifestation Code   **Coding Clinic**

M87.274 Osteonecrosis due to previous trauma, right foot 🦠
(Ex) See M87.074

M87.275 Osteonecrosis due to previous trauma, left foot 🦠
(Ex) See M87.074

M87.276 Osteonecrosis due to previous trauma, unspecified foot 🦠
(Ex) See M87.074

M87.277 Osteonecrosis due to previous trauma, right toe(s) 🦠

M87.278 Osteonecrosis due to previous trauma, left toe(s) 🦠

M87.279 Osteonecrosis due to previous trauma, unspecified toe(s) 🦠

M87.28 Osteonecrosis due to previous trauma, other site 🦠

M87.29 Osteonecrosis due to previous trauma, multiple sites 🦠

● M87.3 Other secondary osteonecrosis
(Ex) See M87

M87.30 Other secondary osteonecrosis, unspecified bone 🦠

● M87.31 Other secondary osteonecrosis, shoulder

M87.311 Other secondary osteonecrosis, right shoulder 🦠

M87.312 Other secondary osteonecrosis, left shoulder 🦠

M87.319 Other secondary osteonecrosis, unspecified shoulder 🦠

● M87.32 Other secondary osteonecrosis, humerus
(Ex) For category M87.32 CC codes: See M87.01

M87.321 Other secondary osteonecrosis, right humerus 🦠

M87.322 Other secondary osteonecrosis, left humerus 🦠

M87.329 Other secondary osteonecrosis, unspecified humerus 🦠

● M87.33 Other secondary osteonecrosis of radius, ulna and carpus

M87.331 Other secondary osteonecrosis of right radius 🦠

M87.332 Other secondary osteonecrosis of left radius 🦠

M87.333 Other secondary osteonecrosis of unspecified radius 🦠

M87.334 Other secondary osteonecrosis of right ulna 🦠

M87.335 Other secondary osteonecrosis of left ulna 🦠

M87.336 Other secondary osteonecrosis of unspecified ulna 🦠

M87.337 Other secondary osteonecrosis of right carpus 🦠

M87.338 Other secondary osteonecrosis of left carpus 🦠

M87.339 Other secondary osteonecrosis of unspecified carpus 🦠

● M87.34 Other secondary osteonecrosis, hand and fingers

M87.341 Other secondary osteonecrosis, right hand 🦠

M87.342 Other secondary osteonecrosis, left hand 🦠

M87.343 Other secondary osteonecrosis, unspecified hand 🦠

M87.344 Other secondary osteonecrosis, right finger(s) 🦠

M87.345 Other secondary osteonecrosis, left finger(s) 🦠

M87.346 Other secondary osteonecrosis, unspecified finger(s) 🦠

● M87.35 Other secondary osteonecrosis, pelvis and femur
(Ex) For category M87.35 CC codes: See M87.051

M87.350 Other secondary osteonecrosis, pelvis 🦠

M87.351 Other secondary osteonecrosis, right femur 🦠

M87.352 Other secondary osteonecrosis, left femur 🦠

M87.353 Other secondary osteonecrosis, unspecified femur 🦠

● M87.36 Other secondary osteonecrosis, tibia and fibula

M87.361 Other secondary osteonecrosis, right tibia 🦠

M87.362 Other secondary osteonecrosis, left tibia 🦠

M87.363 Other secondary osteonecrosis, unspecified tibia 🦠

M87.364 Other secondary osteonecrosis, right fibula 🦠

M87.365 Other secondary osteonecrosis, left fibula 🦠

M87.366 Other secondary osteonecrosis, unspecified fibula 🦠

● M87.37 Other secondary osteonecrosis, ankle and foot

M87.371 Other secondary osteonecrosis, right ankle 🦠

M87.372 Other secondary osteonecrosis, left ankle 🦠

M87.373 Other secondary osteonecrosis, unspecified ankle 🦠

M87.374 Other secondary osteonecrosis, right foot 🦠
(Ex) See M87.074

M87.375 Other secondary osteonecrosis, left foot 🦠
(Ex) See M87.074

M87.376 Other secondary osteonecrosis, unspecified foot 🦠
(Ex) See M87.074

M87.377 Other secondary osteonecrosis, right toe(s) 🦠

M87.378 Other secondary osteonecrosis, left toe(s) 🦠

M87.379 Other secondary osteonecrosis, unspecified toe(s) 🦠

M87.38 Other secondary osteonecrosis, other site 🦠

M87.39 Other secondary osteonecrosis, multiple sites 🦠

● M87.8 Other osteonecrosis
(Ex) See M87

M87.80 Other osteonecrosis, unspecified bone 🦠

● M87.81 Other osteonecrosis, shoulder

M87.811 Other osteonecrosis, right shoulder 🦠

M87.812 Other osteonecrosis, left shoulder 🦠

M87.819 Other osteonecrosis, unspecified shoulder 🦠

● M87.82 Other osteonecrosis, humerus
(Ex) For category M87.82 CC codes: See M87.01

M87.821 Other osteonecrosis, right humerus 🦠

M87.822 Other osteonecrosis, left humerus 🦠

M87.829 Other osteonecrosis, unspecified humerus 🦠

N Newborn Age: 0   P Pediatric Age: 0–17   M Maternity DX: 12–55   A Adult Age: 15–124   ♀ Females Only   ♂ Males Only

🦠 Complication\Comorbidity   🦠 Major C\C   (Ex) CC/MCC Exclusions   🦠 Present on Admission Requirement   🦠 Hospital-Acquired Condition

1159

CHAPTER 13 (M00–M99)

CHAPTER 13 (M00-M99)

● M87.83   Other osteonecrosis of radius, ulna and carpus
     M87.831   Other osteonecrosis of right radius
     M87.832   Other osteonecrosis of left radius
     M87.833   Other osteonecrosis of unspecified radius
     M87.834   Other osteonecrosis of right ulna
     M87.835   Other osteonecrosis of left ulna
     M87.836   Other osteonecrosis of unspecified ulna
     M87.837   Other osteonecrosis of right carpus
     M87.838   Other osteonecrosis of left carpus
     M87.839   Other osteonecrosis of unspecified carpus

● M87.84   Other osteonecrosis, hand and fingers
     M87.841   Other osteonecrosis, right hand
     M87.842   Other osteonecrosis, left hand
     M87.843   Other osteonecrosis, unspecified hand
     M87.844   Other osteonecrosis, right finger(s)
     M87.845   Other osteonecrosis, left finger(s)
     M87.849   Other osteonecrosis, unspecified finger(s)

● M87.85   Other osteonecrosis, pelvis and femur
     (Ex:) **For category M87.85 CC codes: See M87.051**
     M87.850   Other osteonecrosis, pelvis
     M87.851   Other osteonecrosis, right femur
     M87.852   Other osteonecrosis, left femur
     M87.859   Other osteonecrosis, unspecified femur

● M87.86   Other osteonecrosis, tibia and fibula
     M87.861   Other osteonecrosis, right tibia
     M87.862   Other osteonecrosis, left tibia
     M87.863   Other osteonecrosis, unspecified tibia
     M87.864   Other osteonecrosis, right fibula
     M87.865   Other osteonecrosis, left fibula
     M87.869   Other osteonecrosis, unspecified fibula

● M87.87   Other osteonecrosis, ankle, foot and toes
     M87.871   Other osteonecrosis, right ankle
     M87.872   Other osteonecrosis, left ankle
     M87.873   Other osteonecrosis, unspecified ankle
     M87.874   Other osteonecrosis, right foot
         (Ex:) See M87.074
     M87.875   Other osteonecrosis, left foot
         (Ex:) See M87.074
     M87.876   Other osteonecrosis, unspecified foot
         (Ex:) See M87.074
     M87.877   Other osteonecrosis, right toe(s)
     M87.878   Other osteonecrosis, left toe(s)
     M87.879   Other osteonecrosis, unspecified toe(s)

   M87.88   Other osteonecrosis, other site
   M87.89   Other osteonecrosis, multiple sites

M87.9   Osteonecrosis, unspecified
     Necrosis of bone NOS
     (Ex:) See M87

● M88   Osteitis deformans [Paget's disease of bone]
     Chronic disorder that results in enlarged and deformed bones. The excessive breakdown and formation of bone tissue causes bones to weaken and results in bone pain, arthritis, deformities, and fractures.
     Excludes1   osteitis deformans in neoplastic disease (M90.6)

   M88.0   Osteitis deformans of skull
   M88.1   Osteitis deformans of vertebrae
● M88.8   Osteitis deformans of other bones
   ● M88.81   Osteitis deformans of shoulder
     M88.811   Osteitis deformans of right shoulder
     M88.812   Osteitis deformans of left shoulder
     M88.819   Osteitis deformans of unspecified shoulder
   ● M88.82   Osteitis deformans of upper arm
     M88.821   Osteitis deformans of right upper arm
     M88.822   Osteitis deformans of left upper arm
     M88.829   Osteitis deformans of unspecified upper arm
   ● M88.83   Osteitis deformans of forearm
     M88.831   Osteitis deformans of right forearm
     M88.832   Osteitis deformans of left forearm
     M88.839   Osteitis deformans of unspecified forearm
   ● M88.84   Osteitis deformans of hand
     M88.841   Osteitis deformans of right hand
     M88.842   Osteitis deformans of left hand
     M88.849   Osteitis deformans of unspecified hand
   ● M88.85   Osteitis deformans of thigh
     M88.851   Osteitis deformans of right thigh
     M88.852   Osteitis deformans of left thigh
     M88.859   Osteitis deformans of unspecified thigh
   ● M88.86   Osteitis deformans of lower leg
     M88.861   Osteitis deformans of right lower leg
     M88.862   Osteitis deformans of left lower leg
     M88.869   Osteitis deformans of unspecified lower leg
   ● M88.87   Osteitis deformans of ankle and foot
     M88.871   Osteitis deformans of right ankle and foot
     M88.872   Osteitis deformans of left ankle and foot
     M88.879   Osteitis deformans of unspecified ankle and foot
     M88.88   Osteitis deformans of other bones
         Excludes2   osteitis deformans of skull (M88.0)
                   osteitis deformans of vertebrae (M88.1)
     M88.89   Osteitis deformans of multiple sites
   M88.9   Osteitis deformans of unspecified bone

● **M89** **Other disorders of bone**
  ● **M89.0** **Algoneurodystrophy**
    Shoulder-hand syndrome
    Sudeck's atrophy
    Excludes1 causalgia, lower limb (G57.7-)
                causalgia, upper limb (G56.4-)
                complex regional pain syndrome II, lower limb (G57.7-)
                complex regional pain syndrome II, upper limb (G56.4-)
                reflex sympathetic dystrophy (G90.5-)

    M89.00 Algoneurodystrophy, unspecified site
    ● **M89.01** Algoneurodystrophy, shoulder
      M89.011 Algoneurodystrophy, right shoulder
      M89.012 Algoneurodystrophy, left shoulder
      M89.019 Algoneurodystrophy, unspecified shoulder
    ● **M89.02** Algoneurodystrophy, upper arm
      M89.021 Algoneurodystrophy, right upper arm
      M89.022 Algoneurodystrophy, left upper arm
      M89.029 Algoneurodystrophy, unspecified upper arm
    ● **M89.03** Algoneurodystrophy, forearm
      M89.031 Algoneurodystrophy, right forearm
      M89.032 Algoneurodystrophy, left forearm
      M89.039 Algoneurodystrophy, unspecified forearm
    ● **M89.04** Algoneurodystrophy, hand
      M89.041 Algoneurodystrophy, right hand
      M89.042 Algoneurodystrophy, left hand
      M89.049 Algoneurodystrophy, unspecified hand
    ● **M89.05** Algoneurodystrophy, thigh
      M89.051 Algoneurodystrophy, right thigh
      M89.052 Algoneurodystrophy, left thigh
      M89.059 Algoneurodystrophy, unspecified thigh
    ● **M89.06** Algoneurodystrophy, lower leg
      M89.061 Algoneurodystrophy, right lower leg
      M89.062 Algoneurodystrophy, left lower leg
      M89.069 Algoneurodystrophy, unspecified lower leg
    ● **M89.07** Algoneurodystrophy, ankle and foot
      M89.071 Algoneurodystrophy, right ankle and foot
      M89.072 Algoneurodystrophy, left ankle and foot
      M89.079 Algoneurodystrophy, unspecified ankle and foot
    M89.08 Algoneurodystrophy, other site
    M89.09 Algoneurodystrophy, multiple sites
  ● **M89.1** **Physeal arrest**
    Arrest of growth plate
    Epiphyseal arrest
    Growth plate arrest
    ● **M89.12** Physeal arrest, humerus
      M89.121 Complete physeal arrest, right proximal humerus
      M89.122 Complete physeal arrest, left proximal humerus
      M89.123 Partial physeal arrest, right proximal humerus
      M89.124 Partial physeal arrest, left proximal humerus
      M89.125 Complete physeal arrest, right distal humerus

      M89.126 Complete physeal arrest, left distal humerus
      M89.127 Partial physeal arrest, right distal humerus
      M89.128 Partial physeal arrest, left distal humerus
      M89.129 Physeal arrest, humerus, unspecified
    ● **M89.13** Physeal arrest, forearm
      M89.131 Complete physeal arrest, right distal radius
      M89.132 Complete physeal arrest, left distal radius
      M89.133 Partial physeal arrest, right distal radius
      M89.134 Partial physeal arrest, left distal radius
      M89.138 Other physeal arrest of forearm
      M89.139 Physeal arrest, forearm, unspecified
    ● **M89.15** Physeal arrest, femur
      M89.151 Complete physeal arrest, right proximal femur
      M89.152 Complete physeal arrest, left proximal femur
      M89.153 Partial physeal arrest, right proximal femur
      M89.154 Partial physeal arrest, left proximal femur
      M89.155 Complete physeal arrest, right distal femur
      M89.156 Complete physeal arrest, left distal femur
      M89.157 Partial physeal arrest, right distal femur
      M89.158 Partial physeal arrest, left distal femur
      M89.159 Physeal arrest, femur, unspecified
    ● **M89.16** Physeal arrest, lower leg
      M89.160 Complete physeal arrest, right proximal tibia
      M89.161 Complete physeal arrest, left proximal tibia
      M89.162 Partial physeal arrest, right proximal tibia
      M89.163 Partial physeal arrest, left proximal tibia
      M89.164 Complete physeal arrest, right distal tibia
      M89.165 Complete physeal arrest, left distal tibia
      M89.166 Partial physeal arrest, right distal tibia
      M89.167 Partial physeal arrest, left distal tibia
      M89.168 Other physeal arrest of lower leg
      M89.169 Physeal arrest, lower leg, unspecified
    M89.18 Physeal arrest, other site
  ● **M89.2** **Other disorders of bone development and growth**
    M89.20 Other disorders of bone development and growth, unspecified site
    ● **M89.21** Other disorders of bone development and growth, shoulder
      M89.211 Other disorders of bone development and growth, right shoulder
      M89.212 Other disorders of bone development and growth, left shoulder
      M89.219 Other disorders of bone development and growth, unspecified shoulder

---

N Newborn Age: 0   **P** Pediatric Age: 0–17   **M** Maternity DX: 12–55   **A** Adult Age: 15–124   ♀ Females Only   ♂ Males Only

Complication\Comorbidity   Major C\C   (Ex) CC/MCC Exclusions   Present on Admission Requirement   Hospital-Acquired Condition

● M89.22 Other disorders of bone development and growth, humerus

     M89.221 Other disorders of bone development and growth, right humerus

     M89.222 Other disorders of bone development and growth, left humerus

     M89.229 Other disorders of bone development and growth, unspecified humerus

● M89.23 Other disorders of bone development and growth, ulna and radius

     M89.231 Other disorders of bone development and growth, right ulna

     M89.232 Other disorders of bone development and growth, left ulna

     M89.233 Other disorders of bone development and growth, right radius

     M89.234 Other disorders of bone development and growth, left radius

     M89.239 Other disorders of bone development and growth, unspecified ulna and radius

● M89.24 Other disorders of bone development and growth, hand

     M89.241 Other disorders of bone development and growth, right hand

     M89.242 Other disorders of bone development and growth, left hand

     M89.249 Other disorders of bone development and growth, unspecified hand

● M89.25 Other disorders of bone development and growth, femur

     M89.251 Other disorders of bone development and growth, right femur

     M89.252 Other disorders of bone development and growth, left femur

     M89.259 Other disorders of bone development and growth, unspecified femur

● M89.26 Other disorders of bone development and growth, tibia and fibula

     M89.261 Other disorders of bone development and growth, right tibia

     M89.262 Other disorders of bone development and growth, left tibia

     M89.263 Other disorders of bone development and growth, right fibula

     M89.264 Other disorders of bone development and growth, left fibula

     M89.269 Other disorders of bone development and growth, unspecified lower leg

● M89.27 Other disorders of bone development and growth, ankle and foot

     M89.271 Other disorders of bone development and growth, right ankle and foot

     M89.272 Other disorders of bone development and growth, left ankle and foot

     M89.279 Other disorders of bone development and growth, unspecified ankle and foot

M89.28 Other disorders of bone development and growth, other site

M89.29 Other disorders of bone development and growth, multiple sites

● M89.3 Hypertrophy of bone

     M89.30 Hypertrophy of bone, unspecified site

● M89.31 Hypertrophy of bone, shoulder

     M89.311 Hypertrophy of bone, right shoulder

     M89.312 Hypertrophy of bone, left shoulder

     M89.319 Hypertrophy of bone, unspecified shoulder

● M89.32 Hypertrophy of bone, humerus

     M89.321 Hypertrophy of bone, right humerus

     M89.322 Hypertrophy of bone, left humerus

     M89.329 Hypertrophy of bone, unspecified humerus

● M89.33 Hypertrophy of bone, ulna and radius

     M89.331 Hypertrophy of bone, right ulna

     M89.332 Hypertrophy of bone, left ulna

     M89.333 Hypertrophy of bone, right radius

     M89.334 Hypertrophy of bone, left radius

     M89.339 Hypertrophy of bone, unspecified ulna and radius

● M89.34 Hypertrophy of bone, hand

     M89.341 Hypertrophy of bone, right hand

     M89.342 Hypertrophy of bone, left hand

     M89.349 Hypertrophy of bone, unspecified hand

● M89.35 Hypertrophy of bone, femur

     M89.351 Hypertrophy of bone, right femur

     M89.352 Hypertrophy of bone, left femur

     M89.359 Hypertrophy of bone, unspecified femur

● M89.36 Hypertrophy of bone, tibia and fibula

     M89.361 Hypertrophy of bone, right tibia

     M89.362 Hypertrophy of bone, left tibia

     M89.363 Hypertrophy of bone, right fibula

     M89.364 Hypertrophy of bone, left fibula

     M89.369 Hypertrophy of bone, unspecified tibia and fibula

● M89.37 Hypertrophy of bone, ankle and foot

     M89.371 Hypertrophy of bone, right ankle and foot

     M89.372 Hypertrophy of bone, left ankle and foot

     M89.379 Hypertrophy of bone, unspecified ankle and foot

M89.38 Hypertrophy of bone, other site

M89.39 Hypertrophy of bone, multiple sites

● M89.4 Other hypertrophic osteoarthropathy

     Marie-Bamberger disease
     Pachydermoperiostosis

     M89.40 Other hypertrophic osteoarthropathy, unspecified site

● M89.41 Other hypertrophic osteoarthropathy, shoulder

     M89.411 Other hypertrophic osteoarthropathy, right shoulder

     M89.412 Other hypertrophic osteoarthropathy, left shoulder

     M89.419 Other hypertrophic osteoarthropathy, unspecified shoulder

● M89.42 Other hypertrophic osteoarthropathy, upper arm

     M89.421 Other hypertrophic osteoarthropathy, right upper arm

     M89.422 Other hypertrophic osteoarthropathy, left upper arm

     M89.429 Other hypertrophic osteoarthropathy, unspecified upper arm

● **M89.43**   Other hypertrophic osteoarthropathy, forearm
    M89.431   Other hypertrophic osteoarthropathy, right forearm
    M89.432   Other hypertrophic osteoarthropathy, left forearm
    M89.439   Other hypertrophic osteoarthropathy, unspecified forearm
● **M89.44**   Other hypertrophic osteoarthropathy, hand
    M89.441   Other hypertrophic osteoarthropathy, right hand
    M89.442   Other hypertrophic osteoarthropathy, left hand
    M89.449   Other hypertrophic osteoarthropathy, unspecified hand
● **M89.45**   Other hypertrophic osteoarthropathy, thigh
    M89.451   Other hypertrophic osteoarthropathy, right thigh
    M89.452   Other hypertrophic osteoarthropathy, left thigh
    M89.459   Other hypertrophic osteoarthropathy, unspecified thigh
● **M89.46**   Other hypertrophic osteoarthropathy, lower leg
    M89.461   Other hypertrophic osteoarthropathy, right lower leg
    M89.462   Other hypertrophic osteoarthropathy, left lower leg
    M89.469   Other hypertrophic osteoarthropathy, unspecified lower leg
● **M89.47**   Other hypertrophic osteoarthropathy, ankle and foot
    M89.471   Other hypertrophic osteoarthropathy, right ankle and foot
    M89.472   Other hypertrophic osteoarthropathy, left ankle and foot
    M89.479   Other hypertrophic osteoarthropathy, unspecified ankle and foot
    M89.48   Other hypertrophic osteoarthropathy, other site
    M89.49   Other hypertrophic osteoarthropathy, multiple sites
● **M89.5**   **Osteolysis**
    Use additional code to identify major osseous defect, if applicable (M89.7-)
    Excludes2   periprosthetic osteolysis of internal prosthetic joint (T84.05-)
    M89.50   Osteolysis, unspecified site
● **M89.51**   Osteolysis, shoulder
    M89.511   Osteolysis, right shoulder
    M89.512   Osteolysis, left shoulder
    M89.519   Osteolysis, unspecified shoulder
● **M89.52**   Osteolysis, upper arm
    M89.521   Osteolysis, right upper arm
    M89.522   Osteolysis, left upper arm
    M89.529   Osteolysis, unspecified upper arm
● **M89.53**   Osteolysis, forearm
    M89.531   Osteolysis, right forearm
    M89.532   Osteolysis, left forearm
    M89.539   Osteolysis, unspecified forearm
● **M89.54**   Osteolysis, hand
    M89.541   Osteolysis, right hand
    M89.542   Osteolysis, left hand
    M89.549   Osteolysis, unspecified hand
● **M89.55**   Osteolysis, thigh
    M89.551   Osteolysis, right thigh
    M89.552   Osteolysis, left thigh
    M89.559   Osteolysis, unspecified thigh

● **M89.56**   Osteolysis, lower leg
    M89.561   Osteolysis, right lower leg
    M89.562   Osteolysis, left lower leg
    M89.569   Osteolysis, unspecified lower leg
● **M89.57**   Osteolysis, ankle and foot
    M89.571   Osteolysis, right ankle and foot
    M89.572   Osteolysis, left ankle and foot
    M89.579   Osteolysis, unspecified ankle and foot
    M89.58   Osteolysis, other site
    M89.59   Osteolysis, multiple sites
● **M89.6**   **Osteopathy after poliomyelitis**
    Use additional code (B91) to identify previous poliomyelitis
    Excludes1   postpolio syndrome (G14)
    M89.60   Osteopathy after poliomyelitis, unspecified site
● **M89.61**   Osteopathy after poliomyelitis, shoulder
    M89.611   Osteopathy after poliomyelitis, right shoulder
    M89.612   Osteopathy after poliomyelitis, left shoulder
    M89.619   Osteopathy after poliomyelitis, unspecified shoulder
● **M89.62**   Osteopathy after poliomyelitis, upper arm
    M89.621   Osteopathy after poliomyelitis, right upper arm
    M89.622   Osteopathy after poliomyelitis, left upper arm
    M89.629   Osteopathy after poliomyelitis, unspecified upper arm
● **M89.63**   Osteopathy after poliomyelitis, forearm
    M89.631   Osteopathy after poliomyelitis, right forearm
    M89.632   Osteopathy after poliomyelitis, left forearm
    M89.639   Osteopathy after poliomyelitis, unspecified forearm
● **M89.64**   Osteopathy after poliomyelitis, hand
    M89.641   Osteopathy after poliomyelitis, right hand
    M89.642   Osteopathy after poliomyelitis, left hand
    M89.649   Osteopathy after poliomyelitis, unspecified hand
● **M89.65**   Osteopathy after poliomyelitis, thigh
    M89.651   Osteopathy after poliomyelitis, right thigh
    M89.652   Osteopathy after poliomyelitis, left thigh
    M89.659   Osteopathy after poliomyelitis, unspecified thigh
● **M89.66**   Osteopathy after poliomyelitis, lower leg
    M89.661   Osteopathy after poliomyelitis, right lower leg
    M89.662   Osteopathy after poliomyelitis, left lower leg
    M89.669   Osteopathy after poliomyelitis, unspecified lower leg
● **M89.67**   Osteopathy after poliomyelitis, ankle and foot
    M89.671   Osteopathy after poliomyelitis, right ankle and foot
    M89.672   Osteopathy after poliomyelitis, left ankle and foot
    M89.679   Osteopathy after poliomyelitis, unspecified ankle and foot
    M89.68   Osteopathy after poliomyelitis, other site
    M89.69   Osteopathy after poliomyelitis, multiple sites

CHAPTER 13 (M00-M99)

N   Newborn Age: 0   P   Pediatric Age: 0–17   M   Maternity DX: 12–55   A   Adult Age: 15–124   ♀ Females Only   ♂ Males Only

Complication\Comorbidity   Major C\C   (Exc) CC/MCC Exclusions   Present on Admission Requirement   Hospital-Acquired Condition   **1163**

● **M89.7   Major osseous defect**
  Code first underlying disease, if known, such as:
    aseptic necrosis of bone (M87.-)
    malignant neoplasm of bone (C40.-)
    osteolysis (M89.5)
    osteomyelitis (M86.-)
    osteonecrosis (M87.-)
    osteoporosis (M80.-, M81.-)
    periprosthetic osteolysis (T84.05-)

  M89.70   Major osseous defect, unspecified site

● **M89.71   Major osseous defect, shoulder region**
    Major osseous defect clavicle or scapula
    M89.711   Major osseous defect, right shoulder region
    M89.712   Major osseous defect, left shoulder region
    M89.719   Major osseous defect, unspecified shoulder region

● **M89.72   Major osseous defect, humerus**
    M89.721   Major osseous defect, right humerus
    M89.722   Major osseous defect, left humerus
    M89.729   Major osseous defect, unspecified humerus

● **M89.73   Major osseous defect, forearm**
    Major osseous defect of radius and ulna
    M89.731   Major osseous defect, right forearm
    M89.732   Major osseous defect, left forearm
    M89.739   Major osseous defect, unspecified forearm

● **M89.74   Major osseous defect, hand**
    Major osseous defect of carpus, fingers, metacarpus
    M89.741   Major osseous defect, right hand
    M89.742   Major osseous defect, left hand
    M89.749   Major osseous defect, unspecified hand

● **M89.75   Major osseous defect, pelvic region and thigh**
    Major osseous defect of femur and pelvis
    M89.751   Major osseous defect, right pelvic region and thigh
    M89.752   Major osseous defect, left pelvic region and thigh
    M89.759   Major osseous defect, unspecified pelvic region and thigh

● **M89.76   Major osseous defect, lower leg**
    Major osseous defect of fibula and tibia
    M89.761   Major osseous defect, right lower leg
    M89.762   Major osseous defect, left lower leg
    M89.769   Major osseous defect, unspecified lower leg

● **M89.77   Major osseous defect, ankle and foot**
    Major osseous defect of metatarsus, tarsus, toes
    M89.771   Major osseous defect, right ankle and foot
    M89.772   Major osseous defect, left ankle and foot
    M89.779   Major osseous defect, unspecified ankle and foot

  M89.78   Major osseous defect, other site

  M89.79   Major osseous defect, multiple sites

● **M89.8   Other specified disorders of bone**
    Infantile cortical hyperostoses
    Post-traumatic subperiosteal ossification

● **M89.8X   Other specified disorders of bone**
    M89.8X0   Other specified disorders of bone, multiple sites
    M89.8X1   Other specified disorders of bone, shoulder
    M89.8X2   Other specified disorders of bone, upper arm
    M89.8X3   Other specified disorders of bone, forearm
    M89.8X4   Other specified disorders of bone, hand
    M89.8X5   Other specified disorders of bone, thigh
    M89.8X6   Other specified disorders of bone, lower leg
    M89.8X7   Other specified disorders of bone, ankle and foot
    M89.8X8   Other specified disorders of bone, other site
    M89.8X9   Other specified disorders of bone, unspecified site

  M89.9   Disorder of bone, unspecified

● **M90   Osteopathies in diseases classified elsewhere**
    Excludes1   osteochondritis, osteomyelitis, and osteopathy (in):
        cryptococcosis (B45.3)
        diabetes mellitus (E08-E13 with .61-) ◄▥
        gonococcal (A54.43)
        neurogenic syphilis (A52.11)
        renal osteodystrophy (N25.0)
        salmonellosis (A02.24)
        secondary syphilis (A51.46)
        syphilis (late) (A52.77)

● **M90.5   Osteonecrosis in diseases classified elsewhere**
    Code first underlying disease, such as:
      caisson disease (T70.3)
      hemoglobinopathy (D50-D64)
    (Ex:) **For category M90.5 CC codes unless otherwise indicated:** M87.00-M87.9, M90.50-M90.59

  ▌ *M90.50   Osteonecrosis in diseases classified elsewhere, unspecified site* 🕭
        CC when PDx is its own CC

● **M90.51   Osteonecrosis in diseases classified elsewhere, shoulder**
    (Ex:) **For category M90.51 CC codes:** M87.00-M87.9, M90.50-M90.59

  ▌ *M90.511   Osteonecrosis in diseases classified elsewhere, right shoulder* 🕭
        CC when PDx is its own CC

  ▌ *M90.512   Osteonecrosis in diseases classified elsewhere, left shoulder* 🕭
        CC when PDx is its own CC

  ▌ *M90.519   Osteonecrosis in diseases classified elsewhere, unspecified shoulder* 🕭
        CC when PDx is its own CC

● **M90.52   Osteonecrosis in diseases classified elsewhere, upper arm**

  ▌ *M90.521   Osteonecrosis in diseases classified elsewhere, right upper arm* 🕭
        CC when PDx is its own CC

  ▌ *M90.522   Osteonecrosis in diseases classified elsewhere, left upper arm* 🕭
        CC when PDx is its own CC

  ▌ *M90.529   Osteonecrosis in diseases classified elsewhere, unspecified upper arm* 🕭
        CC when PDx is its own CC

◄ New   ◀▥ Revised   ~~deleted~~ Deleted   Excludes 1   Excludes 2   Includes   Use additional   Code first   Code also   Unspecified
OGCR Official Guidelines   ● Unacceptable Principal Diagnosis   X Assign placeholder X   ● Use Additional Character(s)   ▌ Manifestation Code   **Coding Clinic**

● **M90.53** Osteonecrosis in diseases classified elsewhere, forearm

⟩ *M90.531 Osteonecrosis in diseases classified elsewhere, right forearm* 🦴
    CC when PDx is its own CC

⟩ *M90.532 Osteonecrosis in diseases classified elsewhere, left forearm* 🦴
    CC when PDx is its own CC

⟩ *M90.539 Osteonecrosis in diseases classified elsewhere, unspecified forearm* 🦴
    CC when PDx is its own CC

● **M90.54** Osteonecrosis in diseases classified elsewhere, hand

⟩ *M90.541 Osteonecrosis in diseases classified elsewhere, right hand* 🦴
    CC when PDx is its own CC

⟩ *M90.542 Osteonecrosis in diseases classified elsewhere, left hand* 🦴
    CC when PDx is its own CC

⟩ *M90.549 Osteonecrosis in diseases classified elsewhere, unspecified hand* 🦴
    CC when PDx is its own CC

● **M90.55** Osteonecrosis in diseases classified elsewhere, thigh
    Ⓔ **For category M90.55 CC codes:** M87.00-M87.9, M90.50-M90.59, M87.9

⟩ *M90.551 Osteonecrosis in diseases classified elsewhere, right thigh* 🦴
    CC when PDx is its own CC

⟩ *M90.552 Osteonecrosis in diseases classified elsewhere, left thigh* 🦴
    CC when PDx is its own CC

⟩ *M90.559 Osteonecrosis in diseases classified elsewhere, unspecified thigh* 🦴
    CC when PDx is its own CC

● **M90.56** Osteonecrosis in diseases classified elsewhere, lower leg

⟩ *M90.561 Osteonecrosis in diseases classified elsewhere, right lower leg* 🦴
    CC when PDx is its own CC

⟩ *M90.562 Osteonecrosis in diseases classified elsewhere, left lower leg* 🦴
    CC when PDx is its own CC

⟩ *M90.569 Osteonecrosis in diseases classified elsewhere, unspecified lower leg* 🦴
    CC when PDx is its own CC

● **M90.57** Osteonecrosis in diseases classified elsewhere, ankle and foot

⟩ *M90.571 Osteonecrosis in diseases classified elsewhere, right ankle and foot* 🦴
    CC when PDx is its own CC

⟩ *M90.572 Osteonecrosis in diseases classified elsewhere, left ankle and foot* 🦴
    CC when PDx is its own CC

⟩ *M90.579 Osteonecrosis in diseases classified elsewhere, unspecified ankle and foot* 🦴
    CC when PDx is its own CC

⟩ *M90.58 Osteonecrosis in diseases classified elsewhere, other site* 🦴
    CC when PDx is its own CC

⟩ *M90.59 Osteonecrosis in diseases classified elsewhere, multiple sites* 🦴
    CC when PDx is its own CC

● **M90.6** Osteitis deformans in neoplastic diseases
    Osteitis deformans in malignant neoplasm of bone
    Code first the neoplasm (C40.-, C41.-)
    Excludes1 osteitis deformans [Paget's disease of bone] (M88.-)

⟩ *M90.60 Osteitis deformans in neoplastic diseases, unspecified site*

● **M90.61** Osteitis deformans in neoplastic diseases, shoulder

⟩ *M90.611 Osteitis deformans in neoplastic diseases, right shoulder*

⟩ *M90.612 Osteitis deformans in neoplastic diseases, left shoulder*

⟩ *M90.619 Osteitis deformans in neoplastic diseases, unspecified shoulder*

● **M90.62** Osteitis deformans in neoplastic diseases, upper arm

⟩ *M90.621 Osteitis deformans in neoplastic diseases, right upper arm*

⟩ *M90.622 Osteitis deformans in neoplastic diseases, left upper arm*

⟩ *M90.629 Osteitis deformans in neoplastic diseases, unspecified upper arm*

● **M90.63** Osteitis deformans in neoplastic diseases, forearm

⟩ *M90.631 Osteitis deformans in neoplastic diseases, right forearm*

⟩ *M90.632 Osteitis deformans in neoplastic diseases, left forearm*

⟩ *M90.639 Osteitis deformans in neoplastic diseases, unspecified forearm*

● **M90.64** Osteitis deformans in neoplastic diseases, hand

⟩ *M90.641 Osteitis deformans in neoplastic diseases, right hand*

⟩ *M90.642 Osteitis deformans in neoplastic diseases, left hand*

⟩ *M90.649 Osteitis deformans in neoplastic diseases, unspecified hand*

● **M90.65** Osteitis deformans in neoplastic diseases, thigh

⟩ *M90.651 Osteitis deformans in neoplastic diseases, right thigh*

⟩ *M90.652 Osteitis deformans in neoplastic diseases, left thigh*

⟩ *M90.659 Osteitis deformans in neoplastic diseases, unspecified thigh*

● **M90.66** Osteitis deformans in neoplastic diseases, lower leg

⟩ *M90.661 Osteitis deformans in neoplastic diseases, right lower leg*

⟩ *M90.662 Osteitis deformans in neoplastic diseases, left lower leg*

⟩ *M90.669 Osteitis deformans in neoplastic diseases, unspecified lower leg*

● **M90.67** Osteitis deformans in neoplastic diseases, ankle and foot

⟩ *M90.671 Osteitis deformans in neoplastic diseases, right ankle and foot*

⟩ *M90.672 Osteitis deformans in neoplastic diseases, left ankle and foot*

⟩ *M90.679 Osteitis deformans in neoplastic diseases, unspecified ankle and foot*

⟩ *M90.68 Osteitis deformans in neoplastic diseases, other site*

⟩ *M90.69 Osteitis deformans in neoplastic diseases, multiple sites*

CHAPTER 13 (M00-M99)

N Newborn Age: 0   **P** Pediatric Age: 0–17   **M** Maternity DX: 12–55   **A** Adult Age: 15–124   ♀ Females Only   ♂ Males Only

🦴 Complication\Comorbidity   🦴 Major C\C   Ⓔ CC/MCC Exclusions   🦴 Present on Admission Requirement   🦴 Hospital-Acquired Condition

CHAPTER 13 (M00-M99)

● **M90.8 Osteopathy in diseases classified elsewhere**

Code first underlying disease, such as:
rickets (E55.0)
vitamin-D-resistant rickets (E83.3)

▷ *M90.80 Osteopathy in diseases classified elsewhere, unspecified site*

● **M90.81 Osteopathy in diseases classified elsewhere, shoulder**

▷ *M90.811 Osteopathy in diseases classified elsewhere, right shoulder*

▷ *M90.812 Osteopathy in diseases classified elsewhere, left shoulder*

▷ *M90.819 Osteopathy in diseases classified elsewhere, unspecified shoulder*

● **M90.82 Osteopathy in diseases classified elsewhere, upper arm**

▷ *M90.821 Osteopathy in diseases classified elsewhere, right upper arm*

▷ *M90.822 Osteopathy in diseases classified elsewhere, left upper arm*

▷ *M90.829 Osteopathy in diseases classified elsewhere, unspecified upper arm*

● **M90.83 Osteopathy in diseases classified elsewhere, forearm**

▷ *M90.831 Osteopathy in diseases classified elsewhere, right forearm*

▷ *M90.832 Osteopathy in diseases classified elsewhere, left forearm*

▷ *M90.839 Osteopathy in diseases classified elsewhere, unspecified forearm*

● **M90.84 Osteopathy in diseases classified elsewhere, hand**

▷ *M90.841 Osteopathy in diseases classified elsewhere, right hand*

▷ *M90.842 Osteopathy in diseases classified elsewhere, left hand*

▷ *M90.849 Osteopathy in diseases classified elsewhere, unspecified hand*

● **M90.85 Osteopathy in diseases classified elsewhere, thigh**

▷ *M90.851 Osteopathy in diseases classified elsewhere, right thigh*

▷ *M90.852 Osteopathy in diseases classified elsewhere, left thigh*

▷ *M90.859 Osteopathy in diseases classified elsewhere, unspecified thigh*

● **M90.86 Osteopathy in diseases classified elsewhere, lower leg**

▷ *M90.861 Osteopathy in diseases classified elsewhere, right lower leg*

▷ *M90.862 Osteopathy in diseases classified elsewhere, left lower leg*

▷ *M90.869 Osteopathy in diseases classified elsewhere, unspecified lower leg*

● **M90.87 Osteopathy in diseases classified elsewhere, ankle and foot**

▷ *M90.871 Osteopathy in diseases classified elsewhere, right ankle and foot*

▷ *M90.872 Osteopathy in diseases classified elsewhere, left ankle and foot*

▷ *M90.879 Osteopathy in diseases classified elsewhere, unspecified ankle and foot*

▷ *M90.88 Osteopathy in diseases classified elsewhere, other site*

▷ *M90.89 Osteopathy in diseases classified elsewhere, multiple sites*

CHONDROPATHIES (M91-M94)

Excludes1 postprocedural chondropathies (M96.-)

● **M91 Juvenile osteochondrosis of hip and pelvis**

Excludes1 slipped upper femoral epiphysis (nontraumatic) (M93.0)

M91.0 Juvenile osteochondrosis of pelvis
Osteochondrosis (juvenile) of acetabulum ◀▥
~~acetabulum~~
Osteochondrosis (juvenile) of iliac crest [Buchanan] ◀▥
Osteochondrosis (juvenile) of ischiopubic synchondrosis [van Neck] ◀▥
Osteochondrosis (juvenile) of symphysis pubis [Pierson] ◀▥

● **M91.1 Juvenile osteochondrosis of head of femur [Legg-Calvé-Perthes]**

M91.10 Juvenile osteochondrosis of head of femur [Legg-Calvé-Perthes], unspecified leg

M91.11 Juvenile osteochondrosis of head of femur [Legg-Calvé-Perthes], right leg

M91.12 Juvenile osteochondrosis of head of femur [Legg-Calvé-Perthes], left leg

● **M91.2 Coxa plana**
Hip deformity due to previous juvenile osteochondrosis

M91.20 Coxa plana, unspecified hip

M91.21 Coxa plana, right hip

M91.22 Coxa plana, left hip

● **M91.3 Pseudocoxalgia**

M91.30 Pseudocoxalgia, unspecified hip

M91.31 Pseudocoxalgia, right hip

M91.32 Pseudocoxalgia, left hip

● **M91.4 Coxa magna**

M91.40 Coxa magna, unspecified hip

M91.41 Coxa magna, right hip

M91.42 Coxa magna, left hip

● **M91.8 Other juvenile osteochondrosis of hip and pelvis**
Juvenile osteochondrosis after reduction of congenital dislocation of hip

M91.80 Other juvenile osteochondrosis of hip and pelvis, unspecified leg

M91.81 Other juvenile osteochondrosis of hip and pelvis, right leg

M91.82 Other juvenile osteochondrosis of hip and pelvis, left leg

● **M91.9 Juvenile osteochondrosis of hip and pelvis, unspecified**

M91.90 Juvenile osteochondrosis of hip and pelvis, unspecified, unspecified leg

M91.91 Juvenile osteochondrosis of hip and pelvis, unspecified, right leg

M91.92 Juvenile osteochondrosis of hip and pelvis, unspecified, left leg

● **M92 Other juvenile osteochondrosis**

● **M92.0 Juvenile osteochondrosis of humerus**
Osteochondrosis (juvenile) of capitulum of humerus [Panner]
Osteochondrosis (juvenile) of head of humerus [Haas]

M92.00 Juvenile osteochondrosis of humerus, unspecified arm

M92.01 Juvenile osteochondrosis of humerus, right arm

M92.02 Juvenile osteochondrosis of humerus, left arm

● **M92.1 Juvenile osteochondrosis of radius and ulna**
Osteochondrosis (juvenile) of lower ulna [Burns]
Osteochondrosis (juvenile) of radial head [Brailsford]

M92.10 Juvenile osteochondrosis of radius and ulna, unspecified arm

M92.11 Juvenile osteochondrosis of radius and ulna, right arm

M92.12 Juvenile osteochondrosis of radius and ulna, left arm

◀ New   ◀▥ Revised   ~~deleted~~ Deleted   Excludes 1   Excludes 2   Includes   Use additional   Code first   Code also   Unspecified

OGCR Official Guidelines   ● Unacceptable Principal Diagnosis   X Assign placeholder X   ● Use Additional Character(s)   ▷ Manifestation Code   **Coding Clinic**

● **M92.2 Juvenile osteochondrosis, hand**
   ● **M92.20 Unspecified juvenile osteochondrosis, hand**
     M92.201 Unspecified juvenile osteochondrosis, right hand
     M92.202 Unspecified juvenile osteochondrosis, left hand
     M92.209 Unspecified juvenile osteochondrosis, unspecified hand
   ● **M92.21 Osteochondrosis (juvenile) of carpal lunate [Kienböck]**
     M92.211 Osteochondrosis (juvenile) of carpal lunate [Kienböck], right hand
     M92.212 Osteochondrosis (juvenile) of carpal lunate [Kienböck], left hand
     M92.219 Osteochondrosis (juvenile) of carpal lunate [Kienböck], unspecified hand
   ● **M92.22 Osteochondrosis (juvenile) of metacarpal heads [Mauclaire]**
     M92.221 Osteochondrosis (juvenile) of metacarpal heads [Mauclaire], right hand
     M92.222 Osteochondrosis (juvenile) of metacarpal heads [Mauclaire], left hand
     M92.229 Osteochondrosis (juvenile) of metacarpal heads [Mauclaire], unspecified hand
   ● **M92.29 Other juvenile osteochondrosis, hand**
     M92.291 Other juvenile osteochondrosis, right hand
     M92.292 Other juvenile osteochondrosis, left hand
     M92.299 Other juvenile osteochondrosis, unspecified hand
● **M92.3 Other juvenile osteochondrosis, upper limb**
     M92.30 Other juvenile osteochondrosis, unspecified upper limb
     M92.31 Other juvenile osteochondrosis, right upper limb
     M92.32 Other juvenile osteochondrosis, left upper limb
● **M92.4 Juvenile osteochondrosis of patella**
   Osteochondrosis (juvenile) of primary patellar center [Köhler]
   Osteochondrosis (juvenile) of secondary patellar center [Sinding Larsen]
     M92.40 Juvenile osteochondrosis of patella, unspecified knee
     M92.41 Juvenile osteochondrosis of patella, right knee
     M92.42 Juvenile osteochondrosis of patella, left knee
● **M92.5 Juvenile osteochondrosis of tibia and fibula**
   Osteochondrosis (juvenile) of proximal tibia [Blount]
   Osteochondrosis (juvenile) of tibial tubercle [Osgood-Schlatter]
   Tibia vara
     M92.50 Juvenile osteochondrosis of tibia and fibula, unspecified leg
     M92.51 Juvenile osteochondrosis of tibia and fibula, right leg
     M92.52 Juvenile osteochondrosis of tibia and fibula, left leg
● **M92.6 Juvenile osteochondrosis of tarsus**
   Osteochondrosis (juvenile) of calcaneum [Sever]
   Osteochondrosis (juvenile) of os tibiale externum [Haglund]
   Osteochondrosis (juvenile) of talus [Diaz]
   Osteochondrosis (juvenile) of tarsal navicular [Köhler]
     M92.60 Juvenile osteochondrosis of tarsus, unspecified ankle
     M92.61 Juvenile osteochondrosis of tarsus, right ankle
     M92.62 Juvenile osteochondrosis of tarsus, left ankle

● **M92.7 Juvenile osteochondrosis of metatarsus**
   Osteochondrosis (juvenile) of fifth metatarsus [Iselin]
   Osteochondrosis (juvenile) of second metatarsus [Freiberg]
     M92.70 Juvenile osteochondrosis of metatarsus, unspecified foot
     M92.71 Juvenile osteochondrosis of metatarsus, right foot
     M92.72 Juvenile osteochondrosis of metatarsus, left foot
   M92.8 Other specified juvenile osteochondrosis
     Calcaneal apophysitis
   M92.9 Juvenile osteochondrosis, unspecified
     Juvenile apophysitis NOS
     Juvenile epiphysitis NOS
     Juvenile osteochondritis NOS
     Juvenile osteochondrosis NOS

● **M93 Other osteochondropathies**
   Excludes2   osteochondrosis of spine (M42.-)
   ● **M93.0 Slipped upper femoral epiphysis (nontraumatic)**
     Use additional code for associated chondrolysis (M94.3)
     ● **M93.00 Unspecified slipped upper femoral epiphysis (nontraumatic)**
       M93.001 Unspecified slipped upper femoral epiphysis (nontraumatic), right hip
       M93.002 Unspecified slipped upper femoral epiphysis (nontraumatic), left hip
       M93.003 Unspecified slipped upper femoral epiphysis (nontraumatic), unspecified hip
     ● **M93.01 Acute slipped upper femoral epiphysis (nontraumatic)**
       M93.011 Acute slipped upper femoral epiphysis (nontraumatic), right hip
       M93.012 Acute slipped upper femoral epiphysis (nontraumatic), left hip
       M93.013 Acute slipped upper femoral epiphysis (nontraumatic), unspecified hip
     ● **M93.02 Chronic slipped upper femoral epiphysis (nontraumatic)**
       M93.021 Chronic slipped upper femoral epiphysis (nontraumatic), right hip
       M93.022 Chronic slipped upper femoral epiphysis (nontraumatic), left hip
       M93.023 Chronic slipped upper femoral epiphysis (nontraumatic), unspecified hip
     ● **M93.03 Acute on chronic slipped upper femoral epiphysis (nontraumatic)**
       M93.031 Acute on chronic slipped upper femoral epiphysis (nontraumatic), right hip
       M93.032 Acute on chronic slipped upper femoral epiphysis (nontraumatic), left hip
       M93.033 Acute on chronic slipped upper femoral epiphysis (nontraumatic), unspecified hip
   M93.1 Kienböck's disease of adults   A
     Adult osteochondrosis of carpal lunates
   ● **M93.2 Osteochondritis dissecans**
     M93.20 Osteochondritis dissecans of unspecified site
     ● **M93.21 Osteochondritis dissecans of shoulder**
       M93.211 Osteochondritis dissecans, right shoulder
       M93.212 Osteochondritis dissecans, left shoulder
       M93.219 Osteochondritis dissecans, unspecified shoulder

CHAPTER 13 (M00-M99)

CHAPTER 13 (M00-M99)

● M93.22 Osteochondritis dissecans of elbow
   M93.221 Osteochondritis dissecans, right elbow
   M93.222 Osteochondritis dissecans, left elbow
   M93.229 Osteochondritis dissecans, unspecified elbow
● M93.23 Osteochondritis dissecans of wrist
   M93.231 Osteochondritis dissecans, right wrist
   M93.232 Osteochondritis dissecans, left wrist
   M93.239 Osteochondritis dissecans, unspecified wrist
● M93.24 Osteochondritis dissecans of joints of hand
   M93.241 Osteochondritis dissecans, joints of right hand
   M93.242 Osteochondritis dissecans, joints of left hand
   M93.249 Osteochondritis dissecans, joints of unspecified hand
● M93.25 Osteochondritis dissecans of hip
   M93.251 Osteochondritis dissecans, right hip
   M93.252 Osteochondritis dissecans, left hip
   M93.259 Osteochondritis dissecans, unspecified hip
● M93.26 Osteochondritis dissecans knee
   M93.261 Osteochondritis dissecans, right knee
   M93.262 Osteochondritis dissecans, left knee
   M93.269 Osteochondritis dissecans, unspecified knee
● M93.27 Osteochondritis dissecans of ankle and joints of foot
   M93.271 Osteochondritis dissecans, right ankle and joints of right foot
   M93.272 Osteochondritis dissecans, left ankle and joints of left foot
   M93.279 Osteochondritis dissecans, unspecified ankle and joints of foot
   M93.28 Osteochondritis dissecans other site
   M93.29 Osteochondritis dissecans multiple sites
● M93.8 Other specified osteochondropathies
   M93.80 Other specified osteochondropathies of unspecified site
● M93.81 Other specified osteochondropathies of shoulder
   M93.811 Other specified osteochondropathies, right shoulder
   M93.812 Other specified osteochondropathies, left shoulder
   M93.819 Other specified osteochondropathies, unspecified shoulder
● M93.82 Other specified osteochondropathies of upper arm
   M93.821 Other specified osteochondropathies, right upper arm
   M93.822 Other specified osteochondropathies, left upper arm
   M93.829 Other specified osteochondropathies, unspecified upper arm
● M93.83 Other specified osteochondropathies of forearm
   M93.831 Other specified osteochondropathies, right forearm
   M93.832 Other specified osteochondropathies, left forearm
   M93.839 Other specified osteochondropathies, unspecified forearm

● M93.84 Other specified osteochondropathies of hand
   M93.841 Other specified osteochondropathies, right hand
   M93.842 Other specified osteochondropathies, left hand
   M93.849 Other specified osteochondropathies, unspecified hand
● M93.85 Other specified osteochondropathies of thigh
   M93.851 Other specified osteochondropathies, right thigh
   M93.852 Other specified osteochondropathies, left thigh
   M93.859 Other specified osteochondropathies, unspecified thigh
● M93.86 Other specified osteochondropathies lower leg
   M93.861 Other specified osteochondropathies, right lower leg
   M93.862 Other specified osteochondropathies, left lower leg
   M93.869 Other specified osteochondropathies, unspecified lower leg
● M93.87 Other specified osteochondropathies of ankle and foot
   M93.871 Other specified osteochondropathies, right ankle and foot
   M93.872 Other specified osteochondropathies, left ankle and foot
   M93.879 Other specified osteochondropathies, unspecified ankle and foot
   M93.88 Other specified osteochondropathies other
   M93.89 Other specified osteochondropathies multiple sites
M93.9 Osteochondropathy, unspecified
   Apophysitis NOS
   Epiphysitis NOS
   Osteochondritis NOS
   Osteochondrosis NOS
   M93.90 Osteochondropathy, unspecified of unspecified site
● M93.91 Osteochondropathy, unspecified of shoulder
   M93.911 Osteochondropathy, unspecified, right shoulder
   M93.912 Osteochondropathy, unspecified, left shoulder
   M93.919 Osteochondropathy, unspecified, unspecified shoulder
● M93.92 Osteochondropathy, unspecified of upper arm
   M93.921 Osteochondropathy, unspecified, right upper arm
   M93.922 Osteochondropathy, unspecified, left upper arm
   M93.929 Osteochondropathy, unspecified, unspecified upper arm
● M93.93 Osteochondropathy, unspecified of forearm
   M93.931 Osteochondropathy, unspecified, right forearm
   M93.932 Osteochondropathy, unspecified, left forearm
   M93.939 Osteochondropathy, unspecified, unspecified forearm
● M93.94 Osteochondropathy, unspecified of hand
   M93.941 Osteochondropathy, unspecified, right hand
   M93.942 Osteochondropathy, unspecified, left hand
   M93.949 Osteochondropathy, unspecified, unspecified hand

◀ New   ◀▥ Revised   deleted Deleted   Excludes 1   Excludes 2   Includes   Use additional   Code first   Code also   Unspecified

OGCR Official Guidelines   ● Unacceptable Principal Diagnosis   X Assign placeholder X   ● Use Additional Character(s)   ▶ Manifestation Code   Coding Clinic

● M93.95   Osteochondropathy, unspecified of thigh

     M93.951   Osteochondropathy, unspecified, right thigh

     M93.952   Osteochondropathy, unspecified, left thigh

     M93.959   Osteochondropathy, unspecified, unspecified thigh

● M93.96   Osteochondropathy, unspecified lower leg

     M93.961   Osteochondropathy, unspecified, right lower leg

     M93.962   Osteochondropathy, unspecified, left lower leg

     M93.969   Osteochondropathy, unspecified, unspecified lower leg

● M93.97   Osteochondropathy, unspecified of ankle and foot

     M93.971   Osteochondropathy, unspecified, right ankle and foot

     M93.972   Osteochondropathy, unspecified, left ankle and foot

     M93.979   Osteochondropathy, unspecified, unspecified ankle and foot

   M93.98   Osteochondropathy, unspecified other

   M93.99   Osteochondropathy, unspecified multiple sites

● M94   Other disorders of cartilage

   M94.0   Chondrocostal junction syndrome [Tietze]
             Costochondritis

   M94.1   Relapsing polychondritis

● M94.2   Chondromalacia

     Excludes1   chondromalacia patellae (M22.4)

   M94.20   Chondromalacia, unspecified site

● M94.21   Chondromalacia, shoulder

     M94.211   Chondromalacia, right shoulder

     M94.212   Chondromalacia, left shoulder

     M94.219   Chondromalacia, unspecified shoulder

● M94.22   Chondromalacia, elbow

     M94.221   Chondromalacia, right elbow

     M94.222   Chondromalacia, left elbow

     M94.229   Chondromalacia, unspecified elbow

● M94.23   Chondromalacia, wrist

     M94.231   Chondromalacia, right wrist

     M94.232   Chondromalacia, left wrist

     M94.239   Chondromalacia, unspecified wrist

● M94.24   Chondromalacia, joints of hand

     M94.241   Chondromalacia, joints of right hand

     M94.242   Chondromalacia, joints of left hand

     M94.249   Chondromalacia, joints of unspecified hand

● M94.25   Chondromalacia, hip

     M94.251   Chondromalacia, right hip

     M94.252   Chondromalacia, left hip

     M94.259   Chondromalacia, unspecified hip

● M94.26   Chondromalacia, knee

     M94.261   Chondromalacia, right knee

     M94.262   Chondromalacia, left knee

     M94.269   Chondromalacia, unspecified knee

● M94.27   Chondromalacia, ankle and joints of foot

     M94.271   Chondromalacia, right ankle and joints of right foot

     M94.272   Chondromalacia, left ankle and joints of left foot

     M94.279   Chondromalacia, unspecified ankle and joints of foot

   M94.28   Chondromalacia, other site

   M94.29   Chondromalacia, multiple sites

● M94.3   Chondrolysis

     Code first any associated slipped upper femoral epiphysis (nontraumatic) (M93.0-)

● M94.35   Chondrolysis, hip

     M94.351   Chondrolysis, right hip

     M94.352   Chondrolysis, left hip

     M94.359   Chondrolysis, unspecified hip

● M94.8   Other specified disorders of cartilage

● M94.8X   Other specified disorders of cartilage

     M94.8X0   Other specified disorders of cartilage, multiple sites

     M94.8X1   Other specified disorders of cartilage, shoulder

     M94.8X2   Other specified disorders of cartilage, upper arm

     M94.8X3   Other specified disorders of cartilage, forearm

     M94.8X4   Other specified disorders of cartilage, hand

     M94.8X5   Other specified disorders of cartilage, thigh

     M94.8X6   Other specified disorders of cartilage, lower leg

     M94.8X7   Other specified disorders of cartilage, ankle and foot

     M94.8X8   Other specified disorders of cartilage, other site

     M94.8X9   Other specified disorders of cartilage, unspecified sites

   M94.9   Disorder of cartilage, unspecified

OTHER DISORDERS OF THE MUSCULOSKELETAL SYSTEM AND CONNECTIVE TISSUE (M95)

● M95   Other acquired deformities of musculoskeletal system and connective tissue

     Excludes2   acquired absence of limbs and organs (Z89-Z90)
                   acquired deformities of limbs (M20-M21)
                   congenital malformations and deformations of the musculoskeletal system (Q65-Q79)
                   deforming dorsopathies (M40-M43)
                   dentofacial anomalies [including malocclusion] (M26.-)
                   postprocedural musculoskeletal disorders (M96.-)

   M95.0   Acquired deformity of nose

     Excludes2   deviated nasal septum (J34.2)

● M95.1   Cauliflower ear

     Excludes2   other acquired deformities of ear (H61.1)

   M95.10   Cauliflower ear, unspecified ear

   M95.11   Cauliflower ear, right ear

   M95.12   Cauliflower ear, left ear

   M95.2   Other acquired deformity of head

   M95.3   Acquired deformity of neck

   M95.4   Acquired deformity of chest and rib

   M95.5   Acquired deformity of pelvis

     Excludes1   maternal care for known or suspected disproportion (O33.-)

   M95.8   Other specified acquired deformities of musculoskeletal system

   M95.9   Acquired deformity of musculoskeletal system, unspecified

CHAPTER 13 (M00-M99)

INTRAOPERATIVE AND POSTPROCEDURAL COMPLICATIONS AND DISORDERS OF MUSCULOSKELETAL SYSTEM, NOT ELSEWHERE CLASSIFIED (M96)

● **M96**   **Intraoperative and postprocedural complications and disorders of musculoskeletal system, not elsewhere classified**

> **Excludes2**   arthropathy following intestinal bypass (M02.0-)
> complications of internal orthopedic prosthetic devices, implants and grafts (T84.-)
> disorders associated with osteoporosis (M80)
> presence of functional implants and other devices (Z96-Z97)

● **M96.0**   Pseudarthrosis after fusion or arthrodesis

M96.1   Postlaminectomy syndrome, not elsewhere classified

M96.2   Postradiation kyphosis

M96.3   Postlaminectomy kyphosis

M96.4   Postsurgical lordosis

M96.5   Postradiation scoliosis

● **M96.6**   Fracture of bone following insertion of orthopedic implant, joint prosthesis, or bone plate
Intraoperative fracture of bone during insertion of orthopedic implant, joint prosthesis, or bone plate

> **Excludes2**   complication of internal orthopedic devices, implants or grafts (T84.-)

> (Ex) **For category M96.6 CC codes:** D78.81, D78.89, E36.8, E89.810-E89.89, H59.011-H59.019, H59.031-H59.819, H59.88-H59.89, H95.811-H95.89, I97.3, L76.81-L76.82, M96.621-M96.69, M96.89, N98.1-N98.9, T81.82X[A], T81.89X-T81.9XX[A], T84.010-T84.9XX[A]

   ● **M96.62**   Fracture of humerus following insertion of orthopedic implant, joint prosthesis, or bone plate

       M96.621   Fracture of humerus following insertion of orthopedic implant, joint prosthesis, or bone plate, right arm

       M96.622   Fracture of humerus following insertion of orthopedic implant, joint prosthesis, or bone plate, left arm

       M96.629   Fracture of humerus following insertion of orthopedic implant, joint prosthesis, or bone plate, unspecified arm

   ● **M96.63**   Fracture of radius or ulna following insertion of orthopedic implant, joint prosthesis, or bone plate

       M96.631   Fracture of radius or ulna following insertion of orthopedic implant, joint prosthesis, or bone plate, right arm

       M96.632   Fracture of radius or ulna following insertion of orthopedic implant, joint prosthesis, or bone plate, left arm

       M96.639   Fracture of radius or ulna following insertion of orthopedic implant, joint prosthesis, or bone plate, unspecified arm

    M96.65   Fracture of pelvis following insertion of orthopedic implant, joint prosthesis, or bone plate

   ● **M96.66**   Fracture of femur following insertion of orthopedic implant, joint prosthesis, or bone plate

       M96.661   Fracture of femur following insertion of orthopedic implant, joint prosthesis, or bone plate, right leg

       M96.662   Fracture of femur following insertion of orthopedic implant, joint prosthesis, or bone plate, left leg

       M96.669   Fracture of femur following insertion of orthopedic implant, joint prosthesis, or bone plate, unspecified leg

   ● **M96.67**   Fracture of tibia or fibula following insertion of orthopedic implant, joint prosthesis, or bone plate

       M96.671   Fracture of tibia or fibula following insertion of orthopedic implant, joint prosthesis, or bone plate, right leg

       M96.672   Fracture of tibia or fibula following insertion of orthopedic implant, joint prosthesis, or bone plate, left leg

       M96.679   Fracture of tibia or fibula following insertion of orthopedic implant, joint prosthesis, or bone plate, unspecified leg

    M96.69   Fracture of other bone following insertion of orthopedic implant, joint prosthesis, or bone plate

● **M96.8**   Other intraoperative and postprocedural complications and disorders of musculoskeletal system, not elsewhere classified

● **M96.81**   Intraoperative hemorrhage and hematoma of a musculoskeletal structure complicating a procedure

> **Excludes1**   intraoperative hemorrhage and hematoma of a musculoskeletal structure due to accidental puncture and laceration during a procedure (M96.82-) ◀━

> (Ex) **For category M96.81 CC codes:** H95.811-H95.89, I85.01, I85.11, I97.3, K21.9, K22.8, K23-K25.2, K25.4, K25.6, K26.0, K26.2, K26.4, K26.6, K27.0, K27.2, K27.4, K27.6, K28.0, K28.2, K28.4, K28.6, K29.01, K29.21, K29.31, K29.41, K29.51, K29.61, K29.71, K29.81, K29.91, K31.811, K55.21, K57.01, K57.11, K57.13, K57.21, K57.31, K57.33, K57.41, K57.51, K57.53, K57.81, K57.91, K57.93, K62.5, K92.0-K92.2, M96.810-M96.811, M96.830-M96.89, N98.1-N98.9, P54.1-P54.3, T81.10X-T81.19X[A], T81.82X[A], T81.89X-T81.9XX[A]

       M96.810   Intraoperative hemorrhage and hematoma of a musculoskeletal structure complicating a musculoskeletal system procedure

       M96.811   Intraoperative hemorrhage and hematoma of a musculoskeletal structure complicating other procedure

● **M96.82**   Accidental puncture and laceration of a musculoskeletal structure during a procedure

> (Ex) **For category M96.82 CC codes:** D78.11-D78.12, D78.81-D78.89, E36.11-E36.8, E89.810-E89.89, G96.11, G97.41-G97.49, H59.011-H59.019, H59.031-H59.099, H59.211-H59.229, H59.811-H59.89, H95.31-H95.32, H95.811-H95.89, I97.3, I97.51-I97.52, J95.71-J95.72, K91.71-K91.72, L76.11-L76.12, L76.81-L76.82, M96.820-M96.821, M96.89, N98.1-N98.9, N99.71-N99.72, T81.82X[A], T81.89X-T81.9XX[A]

       M96.820   Accidental puncture and laceration of a musculoskeletal structure during a musculoskeletal system procedure

       M96.821   Accidental puncture and laceration of a musculoskeletal structure during other procedure

● **M96.83**   Postprocedural hemorrhage and hematoma of a musculoskeletal structure following a procedure

> (Ex) **For category M96.83 CC codes:** See M96.81

       M96.830   Postprocedural hemorrhage and hematoma of a musculoskeletal structure following a musculoskeletal system procedure

       M96.831   Postprocedural hemorrhage and hematoma of a musculoskeletal structure following other procedure

◀ New   ◀━ Revised   ~~deleted~~ Deleted   Excludes 1   Excludes 2   Includes   Use additional   Code first   Code also   Unspecified
OGCR Official Guidelines   ● Unacceptable Principal Diagnosis   X Assign placeholder X   ● Use Additional Character(s)   ▶ Manifestation Code   **Coding Clinic**

M96.89   Other intraoperative and postprocedural complications and disorders of the musculoskeletal system 🔗

     Instability of joint secondary to removal of joint prosthesis

     Use additional code, if applicable, to further specify disorder

     (Ex) D78.81-D78.89, E36.8, E89.810-E89.89, H59.011-H59.019, H59.031-H59.099, H59.811-H59.89, H95.811-H95.89, I97.3, L76.81-L76.82, M96.89, N98.1-N98.9, T81.82X[A], T81.89X-T81.9XX[A]

BIOMECHANICAL LESIONS, NOT ELSEWHERE CLASSIFIED (M99)

● **M99**   Biomechanical lesions, not elsewhere classified

     Note: This category should not be used if the condition can be classified elsewhere.

● **M99.0**   Segmental and somatic dysfunction

   M99.00   Segmental and somatic dysfunction of head region

   M99.01   Segmental and somatic dysfunction of cervical region

   M99.02   Segmental and somatic dysfunction of thoracic region

   M99.03   Segmental and somatic dysfunction of lumbar region

   M99.04   Segmental and somatic dysfunction of sacral region

   M99.05   Segmental and somatic dysfunction of pelvic region

   M99.06   Segmental and somatic dysfunction of lower extremity

   M99.07   Segmental and somatic dysfunction of upper extremity

   M99.08   Segmental and somatic dysfunction of rib cage

   M99.09   Segmental and somatic dysfunction of abdomen and other regions

● **M99.1**   Subluxation complex (vertebral)

   M99.10   Subluxation complex (vertebral) of head region 🔗 🔗

     (Ex) M99.10-M99.11, S03.8XX-S03.9XX[A], S12.000-S12.691[A,B], S12.9XX-S13.4XX[A], S13.8XX[A], S14.0XX-S14.108[A], S14.111-S14.118[A], S14.121-S14.128[A], S14.131-S14.138[A], S14.141-S14.148[A], S14.151-S14.158[A], S16.1XX[A], S29.011-S29.019[A], S38.3XX[A], S39.011-S39.013[A], T14.8-T14.91, T79.A0X-T79.9XX[A]

   M99.11   Subluxation complex (vertebral) of cervical region 🔗 🔗

     (Ex) See M99.10

   M99.12   Subluxation complex (vertebral) of thoracic region

   M99.13   Subluxation complex (vertebral) of lumbar region

   M99.14   Subluxation complex (vertebral) of sacral region

   M99.15   Subluxation complex (vertebral) of pelvic region

   M99.16   Subluxation complex (vertebral) of lower extremity

   M99.17   Subluxation complex (vertebral) of upper extremity

   M99.18   Subluxation complex (vertebral) of rib cage 🔗 🔗

     (Ex) M99.18, S43.201A-S43.226[A]

   M99.19   Subluxation complex (vertebral) of abdomen and other regions

● **M99.2**   Subluxation stenosis of neural canal

   M99.20   Subluxation stenosis of neural canal of head region

   M99.21   Subluxation stenosis of neural canal of cervical region

   M99.22   Subluxation stenosis of neural canal of thoracic region

   M99.23   Subluxation stenosis of neural canal of lumbar region

   M99.24   Subluxation stenosis of neural canal of sacral region

   M99.25   Subluxation stenosis of neural canal of pelvic region

   M99.26   Subluxation stenosis of neural canal of lower extremity

   M99.27   Subluxation stenosis of neural canal of upper extremity

   M99.28   Subluxation stenosis of neural canal of rib cage

   M99.29   Subluxation stenosis of neural canal of abdomen and other regions

● **M99.3**   Osseous stenosis of neural canal

   M99.30   Osseous stenosis of neural canal of head region

   M99.31   Osseous stenosis of neural canal of cervical region

   M99.32   Osseous stenosis of neural canal of thoracic region

   M99.33   Osseous stenosis of neural canal of lumbar region

   M99.34   Osseous stenosis of neural canal of sacral region

   M99.35   Osseous stenosis of neural canal of pelvic region

   M99.36   Osseous stenosis of neural canal of lower extremity

   M99.37   Osseous stenosis of neural canal of upper extremity

   M99.38   Osseous stenosis of neural canal of rib cage

   M99.39   Osseous stenosis of neural canal of abdomen and other regions

● **M99.4**   Connective tissue stenosis of neural canal

   M99.40   Connective tissue stenosis of neural canal of head region

   M99.41   Connective tissue stenosis of neural canal of cervical region

   M99.42   Connective tissue stenosis of neural canal of thoracic region

   M99.43   Connective tissue stenosis of neural canal of lumbar region

   M99.44   Connective tissue stenosis of neural canal of sacral region

   M99.45   Connective tissue stenosis of neural canal of pelvic region

   M99.46   Connective tissue stenosis of neural canal of lower extremity

   M99.47   Connective tissue stenosis of neural canal of upper extremity

   M99.48   Connective tissue stenosis of neural canal of rib cage

   M99.49   Connective tissue stenosis of neural canal of abdomen and other regions

CHAPTER 13 (M00–M99)

N   Newborn Age: 0   P   Pediatric Age: 0–17   M   Maternity DX: 12–55   A   Adult Age: 15–124   ♀   Females Only   ♂   Males Only

🔗 Complication\Comorbidity   🔗 Major C\C   (Ex) CC/MCC Exclusions   🔗 Present on Admission Requirement   🔗 Hospital-Acquired Condition

1171

● M99.5 Intervertebral disc stenosis of neural canal

M99.50 Intervertebral disc stenosis of neural canal of head region

M99.51 Intervertebral disc stenosis of neural canal of cervical region

M99.52 Intervertebral disc stenosis of neural canal of thoracic region

M99.53 Intervertebral disc stenosis of neural canal of lumbar region

M99.54 Intervertebral disc stenosis of neural canal of sacral region

M99.55 Intervertebral disc stenosis of neural canal of pelvic region

M99.56 Intervertebral disc stenosis of neural canal of lower extremity

M99.57 Intervertebral disc stenosis of neural canal of upper extremity

M99.58 Intervertebral disc stenosis of neural canal of rib cage

M99.59 Intervertebral disc stenosis of neural canal of abdomen and other regions

● M99.6 Osseous and subluxation stenosis of intervertebral foramina

M99.60 Osseous and subluxation stenosis of intervertebral foramina of head region

M99.61 Osseous and subluxation stenosis of intervertebral foramina of cervical region

M99.62 Osseous and subluxation stenosis of intervertebral foramina of thoracic region

M99.63 Osseous and subluxation stenosis of intervertebral foramina of lumbar region

M99.64 Osseous and subluxation stenosis of intervertebral foramina of sacral region

M99.65 Osseous and subluxation stenosis of intervertebral foramina of pelvic region

M99.66 Osseous and subluxation stenosis of intervertebral foramina of lower extremity

M99.67 Osseous and subluxation stenosis of intervertebral foramina of upper extremity

M99.68 Osseous and subluxation stenosis of intervertebral foramina of rib cage

M99.69 Osseous and subluxation stenosis of intervertebral foramina of abdomen and other regions

● M99.7 Connective tissue and disc stenosis of intervertebral foramina

M99.70 Connective tissue and disc stenosis of intervertebral foramina of head region

M99.71 Connective tissue and disc stenosis of intervertebral foramina of cervical region

M99.72 Connective tissue and disc stenosis of intervertebral foramina of thoracic region

M99.73 Connective tissue and disc stenosis of intervertebral foramina of lumbar region

M99.74 Connective tissue and disc stenosis of intervertebral foramina of sacral region

M99.75 Connective tissue and disc stenosis of intervertebral foramina of pelvic region

M99.76 Connective tissue and disc stenosis of intervertebral foramina of lower extremity

M99.77 Connective tissue and disc stenosis of intervertebral foramina of upper extremity

M99.78 Connective tissue and disc stenosis of intervertebral foramina of rib cage

M99.79 Connective tissue and disc stenosis of intervertebral foramina of abdomen and other regions

● M99.8 Other biomechanical lesions

M99.80 Other biomechanical lesions of head region

M99.81 Other biomechanical lesions of cervical region

M99.82 Other biomechanical lesions of thoracic region

M99.83 Other biomechanical lesions of lumbar region

M99.84 Other biomechanical lesions of sacral region

M99.85 Other biomechanical lesions of pelvic region

M99.86 Other biomechanical lesions of lower extremity

M99.87 Other biomechanical lesions of upper extremity

M99.88 Other biomechanical lesions of rib cage

M99.89 Other biomechanical lesions of abdomen and other regions

M99.9 Biomechanical lesion, unspecified

◀ New   ◀⫶⫶⫶ Revised   ~~deleted~~ Deleted   Excludes 1   Excludes 2   Includes   Use additional   Code first   Code also   Unspecified

1172   OGCR Official Guidelines   ● Unacceptable Principal Diagnosis   X Assign placeholder X   ● Use Additional Character(s)   ▌ Manifestation Code   Coding Clinic

Item 14–1 Nephritis (inflammation) or **nephropathy** (disease) **with lesion of proliferative glomerulonephritis** results from a streptococcal infection.

   Nephritis (inflammation) or **nephropathy** (disease) **with lesion of membranous glomerulonephritis** is characterized by deposits along the epithelial side of the basement membrane.

   Nephritis (inflammation) or **nephropathy** (disease) **with lesion of membranoproliferative glomerulonephritis** is characterized by alterations in the basement membranes of the kidney and the glomerular cells.

   Nephritis (inflammation) or **nephropathy** (disease) **with lesion of rapidly progressive glomerulonephritis** is characterized by rapid and progressive decline in renal function.

   Nephritis (inflammation) or **nephropathy** (disease) **with lesion of renal cortical necrosis** is characterized by death of the cortical tissues.

   Nephritis (inflammation) or **nephropathy** (disease) **with lesion of renal medullary necrosis** is characterized by death of the tissues that collect urine.

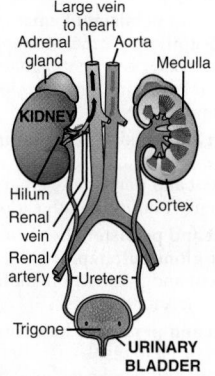

Figure 14-1   Kidneys within the urinary system.

Item 14–2 Glomerulonephritis is nephritis accompanied by inflammation of the glomeruli of the kidney, resulting in the degeneration of the glomeruli and the nephrons.

   Acute glomerulonephritis primarily affects children and young adults and is usually a result of a streptococcal infection.

   Proliferative glomerulonephritis is the acute form of the disease resulting from a streptococcal infection.

   Rapidly progressive glomerulonephritis, also known as **crescentic** or **malignant glomerulonephritis**, is the acute form of the disease, which leads quickly to rapid and progressive decline in renal function.

CHAPTER 14

DISEASES OF THE GENITOURINARY SYSTEM (N00-N99)

Excludes2   certain conditions originating in the perinatal period (P04-P96)

certain infectious and parasitic diseases (A00-B99)

complications of pregnancy, childbirth and the puerperium (O00-O9A)

congenital malformations, deformations and chromosomal abnormalities (Q00-Q99)

endocrine, nutritional and metabolic diseases (E00-E88)

injury, poisoning and certain other consequences of external causes (S00-T88)

neoplasms (C00-D49)

symptoms, signs and abnormal clinical and laboratory findings, not elsewhere classified (R00-R94)

This chapter contains the following blocks:

N00-N08	Glomerular diseases
N10-N16	Renal tubulo-interstitial diseases
N17-N19	Acute kidney failure and chronic kidney disease
N20-N23	Urolithiasis
N25-N29	Other disorders of kidney and ureter
N30-N39	Other diseases of the urinary system
N40-N53	Diseases of male genital organs
N60-N65	Disorders of breast
N70-N77	Inflammatory diseases of female pelvic organs
N80-N98	Noninflammatory disorders of female genital tract
N99	Intraoperative and postprocedural complications and disorders of genitourinary system, not elsewhere classified

GLOMERULAR DISEASES (N00-N08)

Code also any associated kidney failure (N17-N19)

   Excludes1   hypertensive chronic kidney disease (I12.-)

● **N00**   **Acute nephritic syndrome**

   Includes   acute glomerular disease
acute glomerulonephritis
acute nephritis

   Excludes1   acute tubulo-interstitial nephritis (N10)
nephritic syndrome NOS (N05.-)

   (Ex) For category N00 CC codes unless otherwise indicated: A17.9, A18.10-A18.11, A18.13, A18.82, A18.84, A18.89, A54.21, A54.29, A54.82, A54.84, A54.89-A54.9, A59.00, A59.8-A59.9, B37.41-B37.49, E08.21-E08.29, E08.618-E08.638, E08.649, E08.65-E08.8, E09.21-E09.29, E09.618-E09.638, E09.649-E09.8, E10.21-E10.29, E10.618-E10.638, E10.649, E10.69-E10.8, E11.21-E11.29, E11.618-E11.638, E11.649, E11.69-E11.8, E13.21-E13.29, E13.618-E13.638, E13.649-E13.69, E13.8, E88.3, M10.30-M10.39, N00.0-N13.39, N13.6, N14.0-N19, N25.0-N27.9, N28.1-N29, N36.41-N36.43, N36.8-N36.9, N39.8-N39.9, R31.0-R31.9

N00.0   **Acute nephritic syndrome with minor glomerular abnormality** 🔖
Acute nephritic syndrome with minimal change lesion

N00.1   **Acute nephritic syndrome with focal and segmental glomerular lesions** 🔖
Acute nephritic syndrome with focal and segmental hyalinosis
Acute nephritic syndrome with focal and segmental sclerosis
Acute nephritic syndrome with focal glomerulonephritis

N00.2   **Acute nephritic syndrome with diffuse membranous glomerulonephritis** 🔖

N00.3   **Acute nephritic syndrome with diffuse mesangial proliferative glomerulonephritis** 🔖

N00.4   **Acute nephritic syndrome with diffuse endocapillary proliferative glomerulonephritis** 🔖

N00.5   **Acute nephritic syndrome with diffuse mesangiocapillary glomerulonephritis** 🔖
Acute nephritic syndrome with membranoproliferative glomerulonephritis, types 1 and 3, or NOS

N00.6   **Acute nephritic syndrome with dense deposit disease** 🔖
Acute nephritic syndrome with membranoproliferative glomerulonephritis, type 2

N00.7   **Acute nephritic syndrome with diffuse crescentic glomerulonephritis** 🔖
Acute nephritic syndrome with extracapillary glomerulonephritis

N00.8   **Acute nephritic syndrome with other morphologic changes** 🔖
Acute nephritic syndrome with proliferative glomerulonephritis NOS
   (Ex) A17.9, A18.10-A18.11, A18.13, A18.82, A18.84, A18.89, A54.21, A54.29, A54.82, A54.84, A54.89-A54.9, A59.00, A59.8-A59.9, B37.41-B37.49, E08.21-E08.29, E09.21-E09.29, E88.3, M10.30-M10.39, N00.0-N13.39, N13.6, N14.0-N19, N25.0-N27.9, N28.1-N29, N36.41-N36.43, N36.8-N36.9, N39.8-N39.9, R31.0-R31.9

N00.9   **Acute nephritic syndrome with** `unspecified` **morphologic changes** 🔖

N   Newborn Age: 0   **P**   Pediatric Age: 0–17   **M**   Maternity DX: 12–55   **A**   Adult Age: 15–124   ♀   Females Only   ♂   Males Only

🔖 Complication\Comorbidity   🔖 Major C\C   (Ex) CC/MCC Exclusions   🔖 Present on Admission Requirement   🔖 Hospital-Acquired Condition

1173

● **N01   Rapidly progressive nephritic syndrome**

> **Includes**   rapidly progressive glomerular disease
> rapidly progressive glomerulonephritis
> rapidly progressive nephritis

> **Excludes1**   nephritic syndrome NOS (N05.-)

Ex: **For category N01 CC codes: See N00**

N01.0   Rapidly progressive nephritic syndrome with minor glomerular abnormality 🖊
> Rapidly progressive nephritic syndrome with minimal change lesion

N01.1   Rapidly progressive nephritic syndrome with focal and segmental glomerular lesions 🖊
> Rapidly progressive nephritic syndrome with focal and segmental hyalinosis
> Rapidly progressive nephritic syndrome with focal and segmental sclerosis
> Rapidly progressive nephritic syndrome with focal glomerulonephritis

N01.2   Rapidly progressive nephritic syndrome with diffuse membranous glomerulonephritis 🖊

N01.3   Rapidly progressive nephritic syndrome with diffuse mesangial proliferative glomerulonephritis 🖊

N01.4   Rapidly progressive nephritic syndrome with diffuse endocapillary proliferative glomerulonephritis 🖊

N01.5   Rapidly progressive nephritic syndrome with diffuse mesangiocapillary glomerulonephritis 🖊
> Rapidly progressive nephritic syndrome with membranoproliferative glomerulonephritis, types 1 and 3, or NOS

N01.6   Rapidly progressive nephritic syndrome with dense deposit disease 🖊
> Rapidly progressive nephritic syndrome with membranoproliferative glomerulonephritis, type 2

N01.7   Rapidly progressive nephritic syndrome with diffuse crescentic glomerulonephritis 🖊
> Rapidly progressive nephritic syndrome with extracapillary glomerulonephritis

N01.8   Rapidly progressive nephritic syndrome with other morphologic changes 🖊
> Rapidly progressive nephritic syndrome with proliferative glomerulonephritis NOS

N01.9   Rapidly progressive nephritic syndrome with unspecified morphologic changes 🖊

● **N02   Recurrent and persistent hematuria**

> **Excludes1**   acute cystitis with hematuria (N30.01)
> ~~acute prostatitis with hematuria (N41.01)~~
> ~~chronic prostatitis with hematuria (N41.11)~~
> hematuria NOS (R31.9)
> hematuria not associated with specified morphologic lesions (R31.-)

Ex: **For category N02 CC codes unless otherwise indicated:** A17.9, A18.10-A18.11, A18.13, A18.82, A18.84, A18.89, A54.21, A54.29, A54.82, A54.84, A54.89-A54.9, A59.00, A59.8-A59.9, B37.41-B37.49, E08.21-E08.29, E08.618-E08.638, E08.649, E08.65-E08.8, E09.21-E09.29, E09.618-E09.638, E09.649-E09.8, E10.21-E10.29, E10.618-E10.638, E10.649, E10.69-E10.8, E11.21-E11.29, E11.618-E11.638, E11.649, E11.69-E11.8, E13.21-E13.29, E13.618-E13.638, E13.649-E13.69, E13.8, M10.30-M10.39, N00.0-N13.39, N13.6, N14.0-N19, N25.0-N27.9, N28.1-N29, N36.41-N36.43, N36.8-N36.9, N39.8-N39.9, R31.0-R31.9

N02.0   Recurrent and persistent hematuria with minor glomerular abnormality 🖊
> Recurrent and persistent hematuria with minimal change lesion

N02.1   Recurrent and persistent hematuria with focal and segmental glomerular lesions 🖊
> Recurrent and persistent hematuria with focal and segmental hyalinosis
> Recurrent and persistent hematuria with focal and segmental sclerosis
> Recurrent and persistent hematuria with focal glomerulonephritis

N02.2   Recurrent and persistent hematuria with diffuse membranous glomerulonephritis 🖊

Item 14–3 Chronic glomerulonephritis (GN) persists over a period of years, with remissions and exacerbation.

Chronic GN with lesion of proliferative glomerulonephritis results from a streptococcal infection.

Chronic GN with lesion of membranous glomerulonephritis, also known as membranous nephropathy, is characterized by deposits along the epithelial side of the basement membrane.

Chronic GN with lesion of membrano-proliferative glomerulonephritis (MPGN) is a group of disorders characterized by alterations in the basement membranes of the kidney and the glomerular cells.

Chronic GN with lesion of rapidly progressive glomerulonephritis is characterized by necrosis, endothelial proliferation, and mesangial proliferation. The condition is marked by rapid and progressive decline in renal function.

N02.3   Recurrent and persistent hematuria with diffuse mesangial proliferative glomerulonephritis 🖊

N02.4   Recurrent and persistent hematuria with diffuse endocapillary proliferative glomerulonephritis 🖊

N02.5   Recurrent and persistent hematuria with diffuse mesangiocapillary glomerulonephritis 🖊
> Recurrent and persistent hematuria with membranoproliferative glomerulonephritis, types 1 and 3, or NOS

N02.6   Recurrent and persistent hematuria with dense deposit disease 🖊
> Recurrent and persistent hematuria with membranoproliferative glomerulonephritis, type 2

N02.7   Recurrent and persistent hematuria with diffuse crescentic glomerulonephritis 🖊
> Recurrent and persistent hematuria with extracapillary glomerulonephritis

N02.8   Recurrent and persistent hematuria with other morphologic changes 🖊
> Recurrent and persistent hematuria with proliferative glomerulonephritis NOS
> Ex: See N00

N02.9   Recurrent and persistent hematuria with unspecified morphologic changes 🖊
> Ex: See N00

● **N03   Chronic nephritic syndrome**

> **Includes**   chronic glomerular disease
> chronic glomerulonephritis
> chronic nephritis

> **Excludes1**   chronic tubulo-interstitial nephritis (N11.-)
> diffuse sclerosing glomerulonephritis (N05.8-)
> nephritic syndrome NOS (N05.-)

Ex: **For category N03 CC codes:** A17.9, A18.10-A18.11, A18.13, A18.82, A18.84, A18.89, A54.21, A54.29, A54.82, A54.84, A54.89-A54.9, A59.00, A59.8-A59.9, A98.5, B37.41-B37.49, E08.21-E08.29, E08.618-E08.638, E08.649, E08.65-E08.8, E09.21-E09.29, E09.618-E09.638, E09.649-E09.8, E10.21-E10.29, E10.618-E10.638, E10.649, E10.69-E10.8, E11.21-E11.29, E11.618-E11.638, E11.649, E11.69-E11.8, E13.21-E13.29, E13.618-E13.638, E13.649-E13.69, E13.8, M10.30-M10.39, N00.0-N13.39, N13.6, N14.0-N19, N25.0-N27.9, N28.1-N29, N36.41-N36.43, N36.8-N36.9, N39.8-N39.9, R31.0-R31.9

N03.0   Chronic nephritic syndrome with minor glomerular abnormality 🖊
> Chronic nephritic syndrome with minimal change lesion

N03.1   Chronic nephritic syndrome with focal and segmental glomerular lesions 🖊
> Chronic nephritic syndrome with focal and segmental hyalinosis
> Chronic nephritic syndrome with focal and segmental sclerosis
> Chronic nephritic syndrome with focal glomerulonephritis

N03.2   Chronic nephritic syndrome with diffuse membranous glomerulonephritis 🖊

N03.3   Chronic nephritic syndrome with diffuse mesangial proliferative glomerulonephritis 🖊

N03.4   Chronic nephritic syndrome with diffuse endocapillary proliferative glomerulonephritis 🖊

◀ New   ◀ Revised   ~~deleted~~ Deleted   Excludes 1   Excludes 2   Includes   Use additional   Code first   Code also   Unspecified

OGCR Official Guidelines   ● Unacceptable Principal Diagnosis   X Assign placeholder X   ● Use Additional Character(s)   ▶ Manifestation Code   **Coding Clinic**

N03.5 **Chronic nephritic syndrome with diffuse mesangiocapillary glomerulonephritis** 🔵
> Chronic nephritic syndrome with membranoproliferative glomerulonephritis, types 1 and 3, or NOS

N03.6 **Chronic nephritic syndrome with dense deposit disease** 🔵
> Chronic nephritic syndrome with membranoproliferative glomerulonephritis, type 2

N03.7 **Chronic nephritic syndrome with diffuse crescentic glomerulonephritis** 🔵
> Chronic nephritic syndrome with extracapillary glomerulonephritis

N03.8 **Chronic nephritic syndrome with other morphologic changes** 🔵
> Chronic nephritic syndrome with proliferative glomerulonephritis NOS

N03.9 **Chronic nephritic syndrome with unspecified morphologic changes** 🔵

● **N04** **Nephrotic syndrome**
> **Includes**   congenital nephrotic syndrome
>   lipoid nephrosis
>
> (Ex:) For category N04 CC codes unless otherwise indicated: See N02

N04.0 **Nephrotic syndrome with minor glomerular abnormality** 🔵
> Nephrotic syndrome with minimal change lesion

N04.1 **Nephrotic syndrome with focal and segmental glomerular lesions** 🔵
> Nephrotic syndrome with focal and segmental hyalinosis
> Nephrotic syndrome with focal and segmental sclerosis
> Nephrotic syndrome with focal glomerulonephritis

N04.2 **Nephrotic syndrome with diffuse membranous glomerulonephritis** 🔵

N04.3 **Nephrotic syndrome with diffuse mesangial proliferative glomerulonephritis** 🔵

N04.4 **Nephrotic syndrome with diffuse endocapillary proliferative glomerulonephritis** 🔵

N04.5 **Nephrotic syndrome with diffuse mesangiocapillary glomerulonephritis** 🔵
> Nephrotic syndrome with membranoproliferative glomerulonephritis, types 1 and 3, or NOS

N04.6 **Nephrotic syndrome with dense deposit disease** 🔵
> Nephrotic syndrome with membranoproliferative glomerulonephritis, type 2

N04.7 **Nephrotic syndrome with diffuse crescentic glomerulonephritis** 🔵
> Nephrotic syndrome with extracapillary glomerulonephritis
> (Ex:) See N00

N04.8 **Nephrotic syndrome with other morphologic changes** 🔵
> Nephrotic syndrome with proliferative glomerulonephritis NOS
> (Ex:) See N00

N04.9 **Nephrotic syndrome with unspecified morphologic changes** 🔵
> (Ex:) See N00

● **N05** **Unspecified nephritic syndrome**
> **Includes**   glomerular disease NOS
>   glomerulonephritis NOS
>   nephritis NOS
>   nephropathy NOS and renal disease NOS with morphological lesion specified in .0-.8
>
> **Excludes1**   nephropathy NOS with no stated morphological lesion (N28.9)
>   renal disease NOS with no stated morphological lesion (N28.9)
>   tubulo-interstitial nephritis NOS (N12)

N05.0 **Unspecified nephritic syndrome with minor glomerular abnormality**
> Unspecified nephritic syndrome with minimal change lesion

N05.1 **Unspecified nephritic syndrome with focal and segmental glomerular lesions**
> Unspecified nephritic syndrome with focal and segmental hyalinosis
> Unspecified nephritic syndrome with focal and segmental sclerosis
> Unspecified nephritic syndrome with focal glomerulonephritis

N05.2 **Unspecified nephritic syndrome with diffuse membranous glomerulonephritis** 🔵
> (Ex:) See N03

N05.3 **Unspecified nephritic syndrome with diffuse mesangial proliferative glomerulonephritis** 🔵
> (Ex:) See N03

N05.4 **Unspecified nephritic syndrome with diffuse endocapillary proliferative glomerulonephritis** 🔵
> (Ex:) See N03

N05.5 **Unspecified nephritic syndrome with diffuse mesangiocapillary glomerulonephritis** 🔵
> Unspecified nephritic syndrome with membranoproliferative glomerulonephritis, types 1 and 3, or NOS
> (Ex:) See N03

N05.6 **Unspecified nephritic syndrome with dense deposit disease**
> Unspecified nephritic syndrome with membranoproliferative glomerulonephritis, type 2

N05.7 **Unspecified nephritic syndrome with diffuse crescentic glomerulonephritis**
> Unspecified nephritic syndrome with extracapillary glomerulonephritis

N05.8 **Unspecified nephritic syndrome with other morphologic changes**
> Unspecified nephritic syndrome with proliferative glomerulonephritis NOS

N05.9 **Unspecified nephritic syndrome with unspecified morphologic changes**

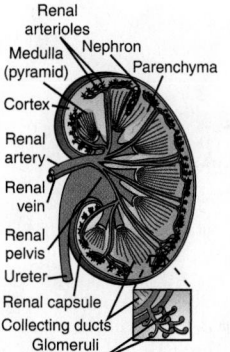

Renal arterioles
Nephron
Medulla (pyramid)
Parenchyma
Cortex
Renal artery
Renal vein
Renal pelvis
Ureter
Renal capsule
Collecting ducts
Glomeruli (microscopic)

Figure 14-2 Kidney cross section.

Item 14-4 Nephrotic syndrome (NS) is marked by massive proteinuria (protein in the urine) and water retention. Patients with NS are particularly vulnerable to staphylococcal and pneumococcal infections. NS with lesion of proliferative glomerulonephritis results from a streptococcal infection. NS with lesion of membranous glomerulonephritis results in thickening of the capillary walls. NS with lesion of minimal change glomerulonephritis is usually a benign disorder that occurs mostly in children and requires electron microscopy (biopsy) to verify changes in the glomeruli.

CHAPTER 14 (N00-N99)

N Newborn Age: 0   P Pediatric Age: 0-17   M Maternity DX: 12-55   A Adult Age: 15-124   ♀ Females Only   ♂ Males Only

🔵 Complication\Comorbidity   🔵 Major C\C   (Ex:) CC/MCC Exclusions   🔵 Present on Admission Requirement   Hospital-Acquired Condition

CHAPTER 14 (N00–N99)

● **N06**   **Isolated proteinuria with specified morphological lesion**

     Excludes1   proteinuria not associated with specific morphologic lesions (R80.0)

N06.0   **Isolated proteinuria with minor glomerular abnormality**
     Isolated proteinuria with minimal change lesion

N06.1   **Isolated proteinuria with focal and segmental glomerular lesions**
     Isolated proteinuria with focal and segmental hyalinosis
     Isolated proteinuria with focal and segmental sclerosis
     Isolated proteinuria with focal glomerulonephritis

N06.2   **Isolated proteinuria with diffuse membranous glomerulonephritis** 🔗
     (Ex:) See N03

N06.3   **Isolated proteinuria with diffuse mesangial proliferative glomerulonephritis** 🔗
     (Ex:) See N03

N06.4   **Isolated proteinuria with diffuse endocapillary proliferative glomerulonephritis** 🔗
     (Ex:) See N03

N06.5   **Isolated proteinuria with diffuse mesangiocapillary glomerulonephritis** 🔗
     Isolated proteinuria with membranoproliferative glomerulonephritis, types 1 and 3, or NOS
     (Ex:) See N03

N06.6   **Isolated proteinuria with dense deposit disease**
     Isolated proteinuria with membranoproliferative glomerulonephritis, type 2

N06.7   **Isolated proteinuria with diffuse crescentic glomerulonephritis**
     Isolated proteinuria with extracapillary glomerulonephritis

N06.8   **Isolated proteinuria with other morphologic lesion**
     Isolated proteinuria with proliferative glomerulonephritis NOS

N06.9   **Isolated proteinuria with unspecified morphologic lesion**

● **N07**   **Hereditary nephropathy, not elsewhere classified**

     Excludes2   Alport's syndrome (Q87.81-)
         hereditary amyloid nephropathy (E85.-) ◀▦
         nail patella syndrome (Q87.2)
         non-neuropathic heredofamilial amyloidosis (E85.-) ◀▦

N07.0   **Hereditary nephropathy, not elsewhere classified with minor glomerular abnormality**
     Hereditary nephropathy, not elsewhere classified with minimal change lesion

N07.1   **Hereditary nephropathy, not elsewhere classified with focal and segmental glomerular lesions**
     Hereditary nephropathy, not elsewhere classified with focal and segmental hyalinosis
     Hereditary nephropathy, not elsewhere classified with focal and segmental sclerosis
     Hereditary nephropathy, not elsewhere classified with focal glomerulonephritis

N07.2   **Hereditary nephropathy, not elsewhere classified with diffuse membranous glomerulonephritis** 🔗
     (Ex:) See N03

N07.3   **Hereditary nephropathy, not elsewhere classified with diffuse mesangial proliferative glomerulonephritis** 🔗
     (Ex:) See N03

N07.4   **Hereditary nephropathy, not elsewhere classified with diffuse endocapillary proliferative glomerulonephritis** 🔗
     (Ex:) See N03

N07.5   **Hereditary nephropathy, not elsewhere classified with diffuse mesangiocapillary glomerulonephritis** 🔗
     Hereditary nephropathy, not elsewhere classified with membranoproliferative glomerulonephritis, types 1 and 3, or NOS
     (Ex:) See N03

N07.6   **Hereditary nephropathy, not elsewhere classified with dense deposit disease**
     Hereditary nephropathy, not elsewhere classified with membranoproliferative glomerulonephritis, type 2

N07.7   **Hereditary nephropathy, not elsewhere classified with diffuse crescentic glomerulonephritis**
     Hereditary nephropathy, not elsewhere classified with extracapillary glomerulonephritis

N07.8   **Hereditary nephropathy, not elsewhere classified with other morphologic lesions**
     Hereditary nephropathy, not elsewhere classified with proliferative glomerulonephritis NOS

N07.9   **Hereditary nephropathy, not elsewhere classified with unspecified morphologic lesions**

▌ *N08*   *Glomerular disorders in diseases classified elsewhere*
     Glomerulonephritis
     Nephritis
     Nephropathy

     Code first underlying disease, such as:
         amyloidosis (E85.-) ◀▦
         congenital syphilis (A50.5)
         cryoglobulinemia (D89.1)
         disseminated intravascular coagulation (D65)
         gout (M1A.-, M10.-) ◀▦
         microscopic polyangiitis (M31.7)
         multiple myeloma (C90.0-)
         sepsis (A40.0-A41.9)
         sickle-cell disease (D57.0-D57.8)

     Excludes1   glomerulonephritis, nephritis and nephropathy (in):
         antiglomerular basement membrane disease (M31.0)
         diabetes (E08-E13 with .21)
         gonococcal (A54.21)
         Goodpasture's syndrome (M31.0)
         hemolytic-uremic syndrome (D59.3)
         lupus (M32.14)
         mumps (B26.83)
         syphilis (A52.75)
         systemic lupus erythematosus (M32.14)
         Wegener's granulomatosis (M31.31)
     pyelonephritis in diseases classified elsewhere (N16)
     renal tubulo-interstitial disorders classified elsewhere (N16)

RENAL TUBULO-INTERSTITIAL DISEASES (N10-N16)

     Includes   pyelonephritis
     Excludes1   pyeloureteritis cystica (N28.85)

N10   **Acute tubulo-interstitial nephritis** 🔗 🔗
     Acute infectious interstitial nephritis
     Acute pyelitis
     Acute pyelonephritis
     Hemoglobin nephrosis
     Myoglobin nephrosis
     Use additional code (B95-B97), to identify infectious agent
     (Ex:) A17.9, A18.10-A18.11, A18.13, A18.82, A18.84, A18.89, A54.21, A54.29, A54.82,
         A54.84, A54.89-A54.9, A59.00, A59.8-A59.9, B37.41-B37.49, E08.21-E08.29,
         E08.618-E08.638, E08.649, E08.65-E08.8, E09.21-E09.29, E09.618-E09.638,
         E09.649-E09.8, E10.21-E10.29, E10.618-E10.638, E10.649, E10.69-E10.8,
         E11.21-E11.29, E11.618-E11.638, E11.649, E11.69-E11.8, E13.21-E13.29,
         E13.618-E13.638, E13.649-E13.69, E13.8, M10.30-M10.39, N00.0-N13.39, N13.6,
         N14.0-N19, N25.0-N27.9, N28.1-N29, N36.41-N36.43, N36.8-N36.9, N39.0,
         N39.8-N39.9, R31.0-R31.9

● **N11**   **Chronic tubulo-interstitial nephritis**
     Includes   chronic infectious interstitial nephritis
         chronic pyelitis
         chronic pyelonephritis
     Use additional code (B95-B97), to identify infectious agent

N11.0   **Nonobstructive reflux-associated chronic pyelonephritis**
     Pyelonephritis (chronic) associated with (vesicoureteral) reflux
     Excludes1   vesicoureteral reflux NOS (N13.70)

◀ New   ◀▦ Revised   ~~deleted~~ Deleted   Excludes 1   Excludes 2   Includes   Use additional   Code first   Code also   Unspecified

OGCR Official Guidelines   ● Unacceptable Principal Diagnosis   X Assign placeholder X   ● Use Additional Character(s)   ▌ Manifestation Code   **Coding Clinic**

Figure 14-3 Acute pyelonephritis. Cortical surface exhibits grayish white areas of inflammation and abscess formation. (From Kumar: Robbins and Cotran: Pathologic Basis of Disease, ed 8, Saunders, An Imprint of Elsevier, 2009)

Figure 14-4 Hydronephrosis of the kidney, with marked dilatation of pelvis and calyces and thinning of renal parenchyma. (From Kumar: Robbins and Cotran: Pathologic Basis of Disease, ed 8, Saunders, An Imprint of Elsevier, 2009)

Item 14–5 Pyelonephritis is an infection of the kidneys and ureters and may be chronic or acute in one or both kidneys.

N11.1   Chronic obstructive pyelonephritis 🔲
Pyelonephritis (chronic) associated with anomaly of pelviureteric junction
Pyelonephritis (chronic) associated with anomaly of pyelouretic junction
Pyelonephritis (chronic) associated with crossing of vessel
Pyelonephritis (chronic) associated with kinking of ureter
Pyelonephritis (chronic) associated with obstruction of ureter
Pyelonephritis (chronic) associated with stricture of pelviureteric junction
Pyelonephritis (chronic) associated with stricture of ureter

   Excludes1   calculous pyelonephritis (N20.9)
           obstructive uropathy (N13.-)
CC when PDx is its own CC
(Ex) N11.1, N13.4-N13.5, N13.8-N13.9, N28.82, N28.89-N30.91, N32.89-N33, N36.41-N36.43, N36.8-N36.9, N39.0, N39.8-N39.9, Q62.4-Q62.8, Q64.10-Q64.19, Q64.8-Q64.9, R31.0-R31.9, Z90.6

N11.8   Other chronic tubulo-interstitial nephritis 🔲
Nonobstructive chronic pyelonephritis NOS
(Ex) A17.9, A18.10-A18.11, A18.13, A18.82, A18.84, A18.89, A54.21, A54.29, A54.82, A54.84, A54.89-A54.9, A59.00, A59.8-A59.9, A98.5, B37.41-B37.49, E08.21-E08.29, E08.618-E08.638, E08.649, E08.65-E08.8, E09.21-E09.29, E09.618-E09.638, E09.649-E09.8, E10.21-E10.29, E10.618-E10.638, E10.649, E10.69-E10.8, E11.21-E11.29, E11.618-E11.638, E11.649, E11.69-E11.8, E13.21-E13.29, E13.618-E13.638, E13.649-E13.69, E13.8, M10.30-M10.39, N00.0-N13.39, N13.6, N14.0-N19, N25.0-N27.9, N28.1-N29, N36.41-N36.43, N36.8-N36.9, N39.8-N39.9, O23.01-O23.03, O23.11-O23.13, O23.21-O23.23, O23.31-O23.33, O23.41-O23.43, O23.511-O23.513, O23.521-O23.523, O23.591-O23.593, O23.91-O23.93, O86.11, O86.13-O86.29, R31.0-R31.9

N11.9   Chronic tubulo-interstitial nephritis, unspecified 🔲 🔲
Chronic interstitial nephritis NOS
Chronic pyelitis NOS
Chronic pyelonephritis NOS
(Ex) A17.9, A18.10-A18.11, A18.13, A18.82, A18.84, A18.89, A54.21, A54.29, A54.82, A54.84, A54.89-A54.9, A59.00, A59.8-A59.9, B37.41-B37.49, E08.21-E08.29, E09.21-E09.29, M10.30-M10.39, N00.0-N13.39, N13.6, N14.0-N19, N25.0-N27.9, N28.1-N29, N36.41-N36.43, N36.8-N36.9, N39.0, N39.8-N39.9, R31.0-R31.9

N12   Tubulo-interstitial nephritis, not specified as acute or chronic 🔲 🔲
Interstitial nephritis NOS
Pyelitis NOS
Pyelonephritis NOS

   Excludes1   calculous pyelonephritis (N20.9)
     (Ex) See N11.9

● **N13   Obstructive and reflux uropathy**

   Excludes2   calculus of kidney and ureter without hydronephrosis (N20.-)
          congenital obstructive defects of renal pelvis and ureter (Q62.0-Q62.3)
          hydronephrosis with ureteropelvic junction obstruction (Q62.1)
          obstructive pyelonephritis (N11.1)
   (Ex) For category N13 CC codes unless otherwise indicated: See N11.9

N13.1   Hydronephrosis with ureteral stricture, not elsewhere classified 🔲
   Excludes1   hydronephrosis with ureteral stricture with infection (N13.6)

N13.2   Hydronephrosis with renal and ureteral calculous obstruction 🔲
   Excludes1   hydronephrosis with renal and ureteral calculous obstruction with infection (N13.6)

● **N13.3   Other and unspecified hydronephrosis**
   Excludes1   hydronephrosis with infection (N13.6)
   N13.30   Unspecified hydronephrosis 🔲
   N13.39   Other hydronephrosis 🔲

N13.4   Hydroureter 🔲
   Excludes1   congenital hydroureter (Q62.3-)
          hydroureter with infection (N13.6)
          vesicoureteral-reflux with hydroureter (N13.73-)
     (Ex) N11.1, N13.4-N13.5, N13.8-N13.9, N28.82, N28.89-N30.91, N32.89-N33, N36.41-N36.43, N36.8-N36.9, N39.0, N39.8-N39.9, Q62.4-Q62.8, Q64.10-Q64.19, Q64.8-Q64.9, R31.0-R31.9

N13.5   Crossing vessel and stricture of ureter without hydronephrosis
Kinking and stricture of ureter without hydronephrosis
   Excludes1   crossing vessel and stricture of ureter without hydronephrosis with infection (N13.6)

N13.6   Pyonephrosis 🔲 🔲
Conditions in N13.1-N13.5 with infection
Obstructive uropathy with infection
   Use additional code (B95-B97), to identify infectious agent

● **N13.7   Vesicoureteral-reflux**
   Excludes1   reflux-associated pyelonephritis (N11.0)
   N13.70   Vesicoureteral-reflux, unspecified
     Occurs when urine flows from bladder back into ureters
     Vesicoureteral-reflux NOS
   N13.71   Vesicoureteral-reflux without reflux nephropathy
● **N13.72   Vesicoureteral-reflux with reflux nephropathy without hydroureter**
     N13.721   Vesicoureteral-reflux with reflux nephropathy without hydroureter, unilateral
     N13.722   Vesicoureteral-reflux with reflux nephropathy without hydroureter, bilateral
     N13.729   Vesicoureteral-reflux with reflux nephropathy without hydroureter, unspecified

N Newborn Age: 0   **P** Pediatric Age: 0–17   **M** Maternity DX: 12–55   **A** Adult Age: 15–124   ♀ Females Only   ♂ Males Only
🔲 Complication\Comorbidity   Major C\C   (Ex) CC/MCC Exclusions   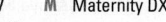 Present on Admission Requirement   🔲 Hospital-Acquired Condition

1177

● N13.73   **Vesicoureteral-reflux with reflux nephropathy with hydroureter**

     N13.731   **Vesicoureteral-reflux with reflux nephropathy with hydroureter, unilateral**

     N13.732   **Vesicoureteral-reflux with reflux nephropathy with hydroureter, bilateral**

     N13.739   **Vesicoureteral-reflux with reflux nephropathy with hydroureter, unspecified**

N13.8   **Other obstructive and reflux uropathy** 🐾
     Urinary tract obstruction due to specified cause
     Code first, if applicable, any causal condition first, such as:
     enlarged prostate (N40.1)
     Ex: See N11.1

N13.9   **Obstructive and reflux uropathy, unspecified**
     Urinary tract obstruction NOS

● N14   **Drug- and heavy-metal-induced tubulo-interstitial and tubular conditions**
     Code first poisoning due to drug or toxin, if applicable (T36-T65 with fifth or sixth character 1-4 or 6)
     Use additional code for adverse effect, if applicable, to identify drug (T36-T50 with fifth or sixth character 5)

   N14.0   **Analgesic nephropathy**

   N14.1   **Nephropathy induced by other drugs, medicaments and biological substances**

   N14.2   **Nephropathy induced by unspecified drug, medicament or biological substance**

   N14.3   **Nephropathy induced by heavy metals**

   N14.4   **Toxic nephropathy, not elsewhere classified**

● N15   **Other renal tubulo-interstitial diseases**

   N15.0   **Balkan nephropathy**
     Balkan endemic nephropathy

   N15.1   **Renal and perinephric abscess** 🐾 🐾
     Ex: See N10

   N15.8   **Other specified renal tubulo-interstitial diseases**

   N15.9   **Renal tubulo-interstitial disease, unspecified**
     Infection of kidney NOS
     Excludes1   urinary tract infection NOS (N39.0)

▷ N16   *Renal tubulo-interstitial disorders in diseases classified elsewhere*
     Pyelonephritis
     Tubulo-interstitial nephritis
     Code first underlying disease, such as:
       brucellosis (A23.0-A23.9)
       cryoglobulinemia (D89.1)
       glycogen storage disease (E74.0)
       leukemia (C91-C95)
       lymphoma (C81.0-C85.9, C96.0-C96.9)
       multiple myeloma (C90.0-)
       sepsis (A40.0-A41.9)
       Wilson's disease (E83.0)

     Excludes1   diphtheritic pyelonephritis and tubulo-interstitial nephritis (A36.84)
       pyelonephritis and tubulo-interstitial nephritis in candidiasis (B37.49)
       pyelonephritis and tubulo-interstitial nephritis in cystinosis (E72.04)
       pyelonephritis and tubulo-interstitial nephritis in salmonella infection (A02.25)
       pyelonephritis and tubulo-interstitial nephritis in sarcoidosis (D86.84)
       pyelonephritis and tubulo-interstitial nephritis in sicca syndrome [Sjogren's] (M35.04)
       pyelonephritis and tubulo-interstitial nephritis in systemic lupus erythematosus (M32.15)
       pyelonephritis and tubulo-interstitial nephritis in toxoplasmosis (B58.83)
       renal tubular degeneration in diabetes (E08-E13 with .29)
       syphilitic pyelonephritis and tubulo-interstitial nephritis (A52.75)

Item 14–6 Decreased blood flow is the usual cause of **acute renal failure** that offers a good prognosis for recovery.
   Chronic renal failure is usually the result of long-standing kidney disease and is a very serious condition that generally results in death.

ACUTE KIDNEY FAILURE AND CHRONIC KIDNEY DISEASE (N17-N19)

   Excludes2   congenital renal failure (P96.0)
     drug- and heavy-metal-induced tubulo-interstitial and tubular conditions (N14.-)
     extrarenal uremia (R39.2)
     hemolytic-uremic syndrome (D59.3)
     hepatorenal syndrome (K76.7)
     postpartum hepatorenal syndrome (O90.4)
     posttraumatic renal failure (T79.5)
     prerenal uremia (R39.2)
     renal failure complicating abortion or ectopic or molar pregnancy (O00-O07, O08.4) ◀▥
     ~~complicating abortion or ectopic or molar pregnancy (O00-O07, O08.4)~~
     renal failure following labor and delivery (O90.4) ◀▥
     renal failure postprocedural (N99.0) ◀▥

● N17   **Acute kidney failure**
     Code also associated underlying condition
     Excludes1   posttraumatic renal failure (T79.5)
     Ex: For category N17 CC codes unless otherwise indicated: E08.21-E08.29, E08.618-E08.638, E08.649-E08.8, E09.21-E09.29, E09.618-E09.638, E09.649-E09.8, E10.21-E10.29, E10.618-E10.638, E10.649, E10.69-E10.8, E11.21-E11.29, E11.618-E11.638, E11.649, E11.69-E11.8, E13.21-E13.29, E13.618-E13.638, E13.649-E13.8, E88.3, M10.30-M10.39, N00.0-N13.39, N13.6, N14.0-N19, N25.0-N27.9, N28.1-N29, N36.41-N36.43, N36.8-N36.9, N39.8-N39.9, Q60.0-Q62.39, Q63.0-Q63.9, Q64.8-Q64.9, R31.0-R31.9

   N17.0   **Acute kidney failure with tubular necrosis** 🐾
     Acute tubular necrosis
     Renal tubular necrosis
     Tubular necrosis NOS

   N17.1   **Acute kidney failure with acute cortical necrosis** 🐾
     Acute cortical necrosis
     Cortical necrosis NOS
     Renal cortical necrosis

   N17.2   **Acute kidney failure with medullary necrosis** 🐾
     Medullary [papillary] necrosis NOS
     Acute medullary [papillary] necrosis
     Renal medullary [papillary] necrosis

   N17.8   **Other acute kidney failure** 🐾
     Ex: E08.21-E08.29, E08.618-E08.638, E08.649-E08.8, E09.21-E09.29, E09.618-E09.638, E09.649-E09.8, E10.21-E10.29, E10.618-E10.638, E10.649, E10.69-E10.8, E11.21-E11.29, E11.618-E11.638, E11.649, E11.69-E11.8, E13.21-E13.29, E13.618-E13.638, E13.649-E13.8, E88.3, M10.30-M10.39, N00.0-N13.39, N13.6, N14.0-N19, N25.0-N27.9, N28.1-N29, N36.41-N36.43, N36.8-N36.9, N39.8-N39.9, R31.0-R31.9

   N17.9   **Acute kidney failure, unspecified** 🐾
     Acute kidney injury (nontraumatic)
     Excludes2   traumatic kidney injury (S37.0-)

● N18   **Chronic kidney disease (CKD)**
     Code first any associated:
     diabetic chronic kidney disease (E08.22, E09.22, E10.22, E11.22, E13.22)
     hypertensive chronic kidney disease (I12.-, I13.-)
     Use additional code to identify kidney transplant status, if applicable, (Z94.0)

   N18.1   **Chronic kidney disease, stage 1**

   N18.2   **Chronic kidney disease, stage 2 (mild)**

   N18.3   **Chronic kidney disease, stage 3 (moderate)**

   N18.4   **Chronic kidney disease, stage 4 (severe)** 🐾
     Ex: E08.21-E08.29, E08.618-E08.638, E08.649-E08.8, E09.21-E09.29, E09.618-E09.638, E09.649-E09.8, E10.21-E10.29, E10.618-E10.638, E10.649, E10.69-E10.8, E11.21-E11.29, E11.618-E11.638, E11.649, E11.69-E11.8, E13.21-E13.29, E13.618-E13.638, E13.649-E13.8, M10.30-M10.39, N00.0-N13.39, N13.6, N14.0-N19, N25.0-N27.9, N28.1-N29, N36.41-N36.43, N36.8-N36.9, N39.8-N39.9, Q60.0-Q62.39, Q63.0-Q63.9, Q64.8-Q64.9, R31.0-R31.9

◀ New   ◀▥ Revised   ~~deleted~~ Deleted   Excludes 1   Excludes 2   Includes   Use additional   Code first   Code also   Unspecified

OGCR Official Guidelines   ● Unacceptable Principal Diagnosis   X Assign placeholder X   ● Use Additional Character(s)   ▷ Manifestation Code   **Coding Clinic**

N18.5   **Chronic kidney disease, stage 5** 🦠
> **Excludes1**   chronic kidney disease, stage 5 requiring chronic dialysis (N18.6)
>
> (Ex) See N18.4

N18.6   **End stage renal disease** ♀
> Chronic kidney disease requiring chronic dialysis
>
> Use additional code to identify dialysis status (Z99.2)
>
> (Ex) E08.21-E08.29, E08.618-E08.638, E08.649-E08.8, E09.21-E09.29, E09.618-E09.638, E09.649-E09.8, E10.21-E10.29, E10.618-E10.638, E10.649, E10.69-E10.8, E11.21-E11.29, E11.618-E11.638, E11.649, E11.69-E11.8, E13.21-E13.29, E13.618-E13.638, E13.649-E13.8, I12.9, M10.30-M10.39, N00.0-N13.39, N13.6, N14.0-N19, N25.0-N27.9, N28.1-N29, N36.41-N36.43, N36.8-N36.9, N39.8-N39.9, Q60.0-Q62.39, Q63.0-Q63.9, Q64.8-Q64.9, R31.0-R31.9

N18.9   **Chronic kidney disease, unspecified**
> Chronic renal disease
> Chronic renal failure NOS
> Chronic renal insufficiency
> Chronic uremia
> ~~Renal disease NOS~~

N19   **Unspecified kidney failure**
> Uremia NOS
> **Excludes1**   acute kidney failure (N17.-)
>   chronic kidney disease (N18.-)
>   chronic uremia (N18.9)
>   extrarenal uremia (R39.2)
>   prerenal uremia (R39.2)
>   renal insufficiency (acute) (N28.9)
>   uremia of newborn (P96.0)

UROLITHIASIS (N20-N23)

🔴 **N20**   **Calculus of kidney and ureter**
> Calculous pyelonephritis
> **Excludes1**   nephrocalcinosis (E83.5)
>   that with hydronephrosis (N13.2)

N20.0   **Calculus of kidney**
> Nephrolithiasis NOS   Staghorn calculus
> Renal calculus   Stone in kidney
> Renal stone

N20.1   **Calculus of ureter** 🦠
> Ureteric stone
> (Ex) N11.1, N13.4-N13.5, N13.8-N13.9, N20.0-N22, N28.82, N28.89-N29, N36.41-N36.43, N36.8-N36.9, N39.8-N39.9, R31.0-R31.9

N20.2   **Calculus of kidney with calculus of ureter**

N20.9   **Urinary calculus, unspecified**

🔴 **N21**   **Calculus of lower urinary tract**
> **Includes**   calculus of lower urinary tract with cystitis and urethritis

N21.0   **Calculus in bladder**
> Calculus in diverticulum of bladder
> Urinary bladder stone
> **Excludes2**   staghorn calculus (N20.0)

N21.1   **Calculus in urethra**
> **Excludes2**   calculus of prostate (N42.0)

N21.8   **Other lower urinary tract calculus**

N21.9   **Calculus of lower urinary tract, unspecified**
> **Excludes1**   calculus of urinary tract NOS (N20.9)

▷ **N22**   *Calculus of urinary tract in diseases classified elsewhere*
> *Code first* underlying disease, such as:
>   gout (M1A.-, M10.-) ◀▥
>   schistosomiasis (B65.0-B65.9)

N23   **Unspecified renal colic**

Figure 14-5   Multiple urinary calculi.

Multiple calculi

OTHER DISORDERS OF KIDNEY AND URETER (N25-N29)

> **Excludes2**   disorders of kidney and ureter with urolithiasis (N20-N23)

🔴 **N25**   **Disorders resulting from impaired renal tubular function**
> **Excludes1**   metabolic disorders classifiable to E70-E88

N25.0   **Renal osteodystrophy**
> Azotemic osteodystrophy
> Phosphate-losing tubular disorders
> Renal rickets
> Renal short stature

N25.1   **Nephrogenic diabetes insipidus** 🦠
> **Excludes1**   diabetes insipidus NOS (E23.2)
> (Ex) A17.9, A18.10-A18.11, A18.13, A18.82, A18.84, A18.89, A54.21, A54.29, A54.82, A54.84, A54.89-A54.9, A59.00, A59.8-A59.9, A98.5, B37.41-B37.49, E08.21-E08.29, E08.618-E08.638, E08.649, E08.65-E08.8, E09.21-E09.29, E09.618-E09.638, E09.649-E09.8, E10.21-E10.29, E10.618-E10.638, E10.649, E10.69-E10.8, E11.21-E11.29, E11.618-E11.638, E11.649, E11.69-E11.8, E13.21-E13.29, E13.618-E13.638, E13.649-E13.69, E13.8, M10.30-M10.39, N00.0-N13.39, N13.6, N14.0-N19, N25.0-N27.9, N28.1-N29, N36.41-N36.43, N36.8-N36.9, N39.8-N39.9, R31.0-R31.9

🔴 **N25.8**   **Other disorders resulting from impaired renal tubular function**

N25.81   **Secondary hyperparathyroidism of renal origin** 🦠
> **Excludes1**   secondary hyperparathyroidism, non-renal (E21.1)
> (Ex) A17.9, A18.10-A18.11, A18.13, A18.82, A18.84, A18.89, A54.21, A54.29, A54.82, A54.84, A54.89-A54.9, A59.00, A59.8-A59.9, A98.5, B37.41-B37.49, E08.21-E08.29, E08.618-E08.638, E08.649, E08.65-E08.8, E09.21-E09.29, E09.618-E09.638, E09.649-E09.8, E10.21-E10.29, E10.618-E10.638, E10.649, E10.69-E10.8, E11.21-E11.29, E11.618-E11.638, E11.649, E11.69-E11.8, E13.21-E13.29, E13.618-E13.638, E13.649-E13.69, E13.8, M10.30-M10.39, N00.0-N13.39, N13.6, N14.0-N19, N25.0-N27.9, N28.1-N29, N36.41-N36.43, N36.8-N36.9, N39.8-N39.9, R31.0-R31.9

N25.89   **Other disorders resulting from impaired renal tubular function**
> Hypokalemic nephropathy
> Lightwood-Albright syndrome
> Renal tubular acidosis NOS

N25.9   **Disorder resulting from impaired renal tubular function, unspecified**

🔴 **N26**   **Unspecified contracted kidney**
> **Excludes1**   contracted kidney due to hypertension (I12.-)
>   diffuse sclerosing glomerulonephritis (N05.8.-)
>   hypertensive nephrosclerosis (arteriolar) (arteriosclerotic) (I12.-)
>   small kidney of unknown cause (N27.-)

N26.1   **Atrophy of kidney (terminal)**

N26.2   **Page kidney**

N26.9   **Renal sclerosis, unspecified**

🔴 **N27**   **Small kidney of unknown cause**
> **Includes**   oligonephronia

N27.0   **Small kidney, unilateral**

N27.1   **Small kidney, bilateral**

N27.9   **Small kidney, unspecified**

N   Newborn Age: 0   **P**   Pediatric Age: 0–17   **M**   Maternity DX: 12–55   **A**   Adult Age: 15–124   ♀   Females Only   ♂   Males Only

🦠   Complication\Comorbidity   🦠   Major C\C   (Ex)   CC/MCC Exclusions   ●   Present on Admission Requirement   🦠   Hospital-Acquired Condition

1179

CHAPTER 14 (N00-N99)

● **N28   Other disorders of kidney and ureter, not elsewhere classified**

     N28.0   Ischemia and infarction of kidney 🔖
         Renal artery embolism
         Renal artery obstruction
         Renal artery occlusion
         Renal artery thrombosis
         Renal infarct

         Excludes1   atherosclerosis of renal artery (extrarenal part) (I70.1)
                     congenital stenosis of renal artery (Q27.1)
                     Goldblatt's kidney (I70.1)
         (Ex) N13.70-N13.739, N28.0, N28.9-N29

     N28.1   Cyst of kidney, acquired
         Cyst (multiple)(solitary) of kidney, acquired

         Excludes1   cystic kidney disease (congenital) (Q61.-)

     ● **N28.8   Other specified disorders of kidney and ureter**

         Excludes1   hydroureter (N13.4)
                     ureteric stricture with hydronephrosis (N13.1)
                     ureteric stricture without hydronephrosis (N13.5)

         N28.81   Hypertrophy of kidney

         N28.82   Megaloureter

         N28.83   Nephroptosis

         N28.84   Pyelitis cystica 🔖 🔖
             (Ex) See N11.9

         N28.85   Pyeloureteritis cystica 🔖 🔖
             (Ex) See N11.9

         N28.86   Ureteritis cystica 🔖 🔖
             (Ex) See N11.9

         N28.89   Other specified disorders of kidney and ureter

     N28.9   Disorder of kidney and ureter, unspecified
         Nephropathy NOS
         Renal disease (acute) NOS
         Renal insufficiency (acute)

         Excludes1   chronic renal insufficiency (N18.9)
                     unspecified nephritic syndrome (N05.-) ◀▥

▶ **N29   *Other disorders of kidney and ureter in diseases classified elsewhere***

     Code first underlying disease, such as:
         amyloidosis (E85.-) ◀▥
         nephrocalcinosis (E83.5)
         schistosomiasis (B65.0-B65.9)

     Excludes1   disorders of kidney and ureter in:
                 cystinosis (E72.0)
                 gonorrhea (A54.21)
                 syphilis (A52.75)
                 tuberculosis (A18.11)

OTHER DISEASES OF THE URINARY SYSTEM (N30-N39)

     Excludes1   urinary infection (complicating):
                 abortion or ectopic or molar pregnancy (O00-O07, O08.8)
                 pregnancy, childbirth and the puerperium (O23.-, O75.3, O86.2-)

● **N30   Cystitis**
     Infection of bladder and irritation in lower urinary tract
     Use additional code to identify infectious agent (B95-B97)

     Excludes1   prostatocystitis (N41.3)

     ● **N30.0   Acute cystitis**

         Excludes1   irradiation cystitis (N30.4-)
                     trigonitis (N30.3-)
         (Ex) **For category N30.0 CC codes:** A17.9, A18.10, A18.12-A18.13, A18.82, A18.84, A18.89, A54.00-A54.02, A54.09-A54.1, A54.82, A54.84, A54.89-A54.9, A59.00, A59.8-A59.9, B37.41-B37.49, N11.1, N13.4-N13.5, N13.8-N13.9, N28.82, N28.89-N30.91, N32.89-N33, N36.41-N36.43, N36.8-N36.9, N39.0, N39.8-N39.9, R31.0-R31.9

         N30.00   Acute cystitis without hematuria 🔖 🔖

         N30.01   Acute cystitis with hematuria 🔖 🔖

     ● **N30.1   Interstitial cystitis (chronic)**
         Ongoing infection of kidney glomeruli and tubules

         N30.10   Interstitial cystitis (chronic) without hematuria

         N30.11   Interstitial cystitis (chronic) with hematuria

     ● **N30.2   Other chronic cystitis**

         N30.20   Other chronic cystitis without hematuria

         N30.21   Other chronic cystitis with hematuria

     ● **N30.3   Trigonitis**
         Inflammation of triangular area of bladder (where the ureters and urethra come together)
         Urethrotrigonitis

         N30.30   Trigonitis without hematuria

         N30.31   Trigonitis with hematuria

     ● **N30.4   Irradiation cystitis**
         (Ex) **For category N30.4 CC codes:** See N30.0

         N30.40   Irradiation cystitis without hematuria 🔖

         N30.41   Irradiation cystitis with hematuria 🔖

     ● **N30.8   Other cystitis**
         Abscess of bladder

         N30.80   Other cystitis without hematuria

         N30.81   Other cystitis with hematuria

     ● **N30.9   Cystitis, unspecified**

         N30.90   Cystitis, unspecified without hematuria

         N30.91   Cystitis, unspecified with hematuria

● **N31   Neuromuscular dysfunction of bladder, not elsewhere classified**
     Use additional code to identify any associated urinary incontinence (N39.3-N39.4-)

     Excludes1   cord bladder NOS (G95.89)
                 neurogenic bladder due to cauda equina syndrome (G83.4)
                 neuromuscular dysfunction due to spinal cord lesion (G95.89)

     N31.0   Uninhibited neuropathic bladder, not elsewhere classified

     N31.1   Reflex neuropathic bladder, not elsewhere classified

     N31.2   Flaccid neuropathic bladder, not elsewhere classified
         Atonic (motor) (sensory) neuropathic bladder
         Diminished tone of bladder muscle
         Autonomous neuropathic bladder
         Nonreflex neuropathic bladder

     N31.8   Other neuromuscular dysfunction of bladder

     N31.9   Neuromuscular dysfunction of bladder, unspecified
         Neurogenic bladder dysfunction NOS

● **N32   Other disorders of bladder**

     Excludes2   calculus of bladder (N21.0)
                 cystocele (N81.1-)
                 hernia or prolapse of bladder, female (N81.1-)

     N32.0   Bladder-neck obstruction
         Bladder-neck stenosis (acquired)

         Excludes1   congenital bladder-neck obstruction (Q64.3-)

     N32.1   Vesicointestinal fistula 🔖
         Vesicorectal fistula
         (Ex) A54.00-A54.02, A54.09-A54.1, A54.82, A54.84, A54.89-A54.9, N32.1-N32.2, N32.89-N33, N36.41-N36.43, N36.8-N36.9, N39.8-N39.9, R30.0, R30.9, R31.0-R31.9

     N32.2   Vesical fistula, not elsewhere classified 🔖

         Excludes1   fistula between bladder and female genital tract (N82.0-N82.1)
         (Ex) See N32.1

     N32.3   Diverticulum of bladder
         Formation of sac from a herniation of wall of bladder

         Excludes1   congenital diverticulum of bladder (Q64.6)
                 diverticulitis of bladder (N30.8-)

◀ New   ◀▥ Revised   ~~deleted~~ Deleted   Excludes 1   Excludes 2   Includes   Use additional   Code first   Code also   Unspecified

OGCR Official Guidelines   ● Unacceptable Principal Diagnosis   X Assign placeholder X   ● Use Additional Character(s)   ▶ Manifestation Code   **Coding Clinic**

● **N32.8   Other specified disorders of bladder**

    N32.81   Overactive bladder

       Detrusor muscle hyperactivity

       Excludes1   frequent urination due to specified bladder condition-code to condition

    N32.89   Other specified disorders of bladder

       Bladder hemorrhage

       Bladder hypertrophy

       Calcified bladder

       Contracted bladder

N32.9   Bladder disorder, unspecified

▷ **N33   Bladder disorders in diseases classified elsewhere**

    Code first underlying disease, such as:

       schistosomiasis (B65.0-B65.9)

    Excludes1   bladder disorder in syphilis (A52.76) ◀▥

       ~~syphilis (A52.76)~~

       bladder disorder in tuberculosis (A18.12) ◀▥

       ~~cystitis (in):~~

       candidal cystitis (B37.41) ◀▥

       chlamydial cystitis (A56.01) ◀▥

       ~~diphtheritic (A36.85)~~

       cystitis in gonorrhea (A54.01) ◀▥

       ~~syphilitic (A52.76)~~

       ~~trichomonal infection (A59.03)~~ ◀▥

       cystitis in neurogenic bladder (N31.-) ◀▥

       diphtheritic cystitis (A36.85) ◀

       syphilitic cystitis (A52.76) ◀

       trichomonal cystitis (A59.03) ◀

● **N34   Urethritis and urethral syndrome**

    Use additional code (B95-B97), to identify infectious agent

    Excludes2   Reiter's disease (M02.3-)

       urethritis in diseases with a predominantly sexual mode of transmission (A50-A64)

       urethrotrigonitis (N30.3-)

    N34.0   Urethral abscess 🅒 🅒

       Abscess (of) Cowper's gland

       Abscess (of) Littré's gland

       Abscess (of) urethral (gland)

       Periurethral abscess

       Excludes1   urethral caruncle (N36.2)

       (Ex) A54.00-A54.02, A54.09-A54.1, A54.82, A54.84, A54.89-A54.9, A59.00, A59.03, A59.8-A59.9, B37.41-B37.49, N13.9, N34.0-N34.3, N35.111-N35.9, N36.41-N36.43, N36.8-N39.0, N39.8-N39.9, N44.1-N44.8, N47.6, N48.1-N48.9, N49.1-N49.9, N50.3-N50.8, N51, N53.11-N53.9, Q54.0-Q55.9, Q64.0, Q64.2-Q64.9, R30.0, R30.9-R31.9

    N34.1   Nonspecific urethritis

       Nongonococcal urethritis

       Nonvenereal urethritis

    N34.2   Other urethritis

       Inflammation of urethra

       Meatitis, urethral

       Postmenopausal urethritis

       Ulcer of urethra (meatus)

       Urethritis NOS

    N34.3   Urethral syndrome, unspecified

● **N35   Urethral stricture**

    Narrowing of lumen of urethra caused by scarring due to infection or injury

    Excludes1   congenital urethral stricture (Q64.3-)

       postprocedural urethral stricture (N99.1-)

   ● **N35.0   Post-traumatic urethral stricture**

       Urethral stricture due to injury

       Excludes1   postprocedural urethral stricture (N99.1-)

    ● **N35.01   Post-traumatic urethral stricture, male**

       N35.010   Post-traumatic urethral stricture, male, meatal ♂

       N35.011   Post-traumatic bulbous urethral stricture

       N35.012   Post-traumatic membranous urethral stricture

       N35.013   Post-traumatic anterior urethral stricture

       N35.014   Post-traumatic urethral stricture, male, unspecified ♂

   ● **N35.02   Post-traumatic urethral stricture, female**

       N35.021   Urethral stricture due to childbirth ♀

       N35.028   Other post-traumatic urethral stricture, female ♀

● **N35.1   Postinfective urethral stricture, not elsewhere classified**

    Excludes1   urethral stricture associated with schistosomiasis (B65.-, N29)

       gonococcal urethral stricture (A54.01)

       syphilitic urethral stricture (A52.76)

   ● **N35.11   Postinfective urethral stricture, not elsewhere classified, male**

       N35.111   Postinfective urethral stricture, not elsewhere classified, male, meatal ♂

       N35.112   Postinfective bulbous urethral stricture, not elsewhere classified

       N35.113   Postinfective membranous urethral stricture, not elsewhere classified

       N35.114   Postinfective anterior urethral stricture, not elsewhere classified

       N35.119   Postinfective urethral stricture, not elsewhere classified, male, unspecified ♂

    N35.12   Postinfective urethral stricture, not elsewhere classified, female ♀

N35.8   Other urethral stricture

    Excludes1   postprocedural urethral stricture (N99.1-)

N35.9   Urethral stricture, unspecified

● **N36   Other disorders of urethra**

    N36.0   Urethral fistula 🅒

       Urethroperineal fistula

       Urethrorectal fistula

       Urinary fistula NOS

       Excludes1   urethroscrotal fistula (N50.8)

       urethrovaginal fistula (N82.1)

       urethrovesicovaginal fistula (N82.1)

       (Ex) N13.9, N34.0, N34.2-N36.43, N36.5-N37, N39.8-N39.9, N44.1-N44.8, N47.6, N48.1-N48.9, N49.1-N49.9, N50.3-N50.8, N51, N53.11-N53.9, N99.110-N99.12, Q54.0-Q55.21, Q55.23-Q55.9, Q64.0, Q64.8-Q64.9, R30.0, R30.9-R31.9

    N36.1   Urethral diverticulum

    N36.2   Urethral caruncle

   ● **N36.4   Urethral functional and muscular disorders**

       Use additional code to identify associated urinary stress incontinence (N39.3)

       N36.41   Hypermobility of urethra

       N36.42   Intrinsic sphincter deficiency (ISD)

       N36.43   Combined hypermobility of urethra and intrinsic sphincter deficiency

       N36.44   Muscular disorders of urethra

          Bladder sphincter dyssynergy

    N36.5   Urethral false passage

    N36.8   Other specified disorders of urethra

    N36.9   Urethral disorder, unspecified

▷ **N37   Urethral disorders in diseases classified elsewhere**

    Code first underlying disease

    Excludes1   urethritis (in):

       candidal infection (B37.41)

       chlamydial (A56.01)

       gonorrhea (A54.01)

       syphilis (A52.76)

       trichomonal infection (A59.03)

       tuberculosis (A18.13)

N Newborn Age: 0   **P** Pediatric Age: 0–17   **M** Maternity DX: 12–55   **A** Adult Age: 15–124   ♀ Females Only   ♂ Males Only

🅒 Complication\Comorbidity   🅒 Major C\C   (Ex) CC/MCC Exclusions   🅟 Present on Admission Requirement   🅗 Hospital-Acquired Condition

1181

● N39　Other disorders of urinary system

Excludes2　hematuria NOS (R31.-) ◀▦
recurrent or persistent hematuria (N02.-)
recurrent or persistent hematuria with specified
morphological lesion (N02.-)
proteinuria NOS (R80.-)

N39.0　Urinary tract infection, site not specified 🦠 🦠

Use additional code (B95-B97), to identify infectious
agent

Excludes1　candidiasis of urinary tract (B37.4-)
neonatal urinary tract infection (P39.3)
urinary tract infection of specified site,
such as:
cystitis (N30.-)
urethritis (N34.-)

Ⓔⓧ A54.82, A54.84, A54.89-A54.9, A59.00, A59.8-A59.9, B37.41-B37.49, N10,
N11.9-N13.39, N13.6, N13.9, N15.1, N28.82, N28.84-N30.91, N34.1,
N36.41-N36.43, N36.8-N36.9, N39.0, N39.8-N39.9, N99.511, R30.0,
R30.9-R31.9, T83.51X[A]

Coding Clinic: 2012, Q4, P94

N39.3　Stress incontinence (female) (male)

Code also any associated overactive bladder (N32.81)

Excludes1　mixed incontinence (N39.46)

● N39.4　Other specified urinary incontinence

Code also any associated overactive bladder (N32.81)

Excludes1　enuresis NOS (R32)
functional urinary incontinence (R39.81)
urinary incontinence associated with
cognitive impairment (R39.81)
urinary incontinence NOS (R32)
urinary incontinence of nonorganic origin
(F98.0)

N39.41　Urge incontinence

Excludes1　mixed incontinence (N39.46)

N39.42　Incontinence without sensory awareness

N39.43　Post-void dribbling

N39.44　Nocturnal enuresis

N39.45　Continuous leakage

N39.46　Mixed incontinence
Urge and stress incontinence

● N39.49　Other specified urinary incontinence

N39.490　Overflow incontinence

N39.498　Other specified urinary incontinence
Reflex incontinence
Total incontinence

N39.8　Other specified disorders of urinary system

N39.9　Disorder of urinary system, unspecified

DISEASES OF MALE GENITAL ORGANS (N40-N53)

(See Plate 387 on page 53.)

● N40　Enlarged prostate

Includes　adenofibromatous hypertrophy of prostate
benign hypertrophy of the prostate
*Enlargement of prostate gland usually occurring
with age and causing obstructed urine flow*
benign prostatic hyperplasia
benign prostatic hypertrophy
BPH
nodular prostate
polyp of prostate

Excludes1　benign neoplasms of prostate (adenoma, benign)
(fibroadenoma) (fibroma) (myoma) (D29.1)
malignant neoplasm of prostate (C61)

N40.0　Enlarged prostate without lower urinary tract
symptoms ♂　　　　　　　　　　　　　　　A
Enlarged prostate without LUTS
Enlarged prostate NOS

N40.1　Enlarged prostate with lower urinary tract symptoms
(LUTS) ♂　　　　　　　　　　　　　　　A
Enlarged prostate with LUTS
Use additional code for associated symptoms, when
specified:
incomplete bladder emptying (R39.14)
nocturia (R35.1)
straining on urination (R39.16)
urinary frequency (R35.0)
urinary hesitancy (R39.11)
urinary incontinence (N39.4-)
urinary obstruction (N13.8)
urinary retention (R33.8)
urinary urgency (R39.15)
weak urinary stream (R39.12)

N40.2　Nodular prostate without lower urinary tract
symptoms ♂　　　　　　　　　　　　　　　A
Nodular prostate without LUTS

N40.3　Nodular prostate with lower urinary tract symptoms ♂　A
Use additional code for associated symptoms, when
specified:
incomplete bladder emptying (R39.14)
nocturia (R35.1)
straining on urination (R39.16)
urinary frequency (R35.0)
urinary hesitancy (R39.11)
urinary incontinence (N39.4-)
urinary obstruction (N13.8)
urinary retention (R33.8)
urinary urgency (R39.15)
weak urinary stream (R39.12)

● N41　Inflammatory diseases of prostate

Use additional code (B95-B97), to identify infectious agent

N41.0　Acute prostatitis ♂ 🦠　　　　　　　　　　　A
Ⓔⓧ A18.14, A54.22, A54.82, A54.84, A54.89-A54.9, A59.00, A59.02,
A59.8-A59.9, B37.41-B37.49, N40.0-N42.9

N41.1　Chronic prostatitis ♂　　　　　　　　　　　　　A

N41.2　Abscess of prostate ♂ 🦠　　　　　　　　　　　A
Ⓔⓧ See N41.0

N41.3　Prostatocystitis ♂　　　　　　　　　　　　　　A

N41.4　Granulomatous prostatitis ♂　　　　　　　　　　A

N41.8　Other inflammatory diseases of prostate ♂　　　　A

N41.9　Inflammatory disease of prostate, unspecified ♂　A
Prostatitis NOS

● N42　Other and unspecified disorders of prostate

N42.0　Calculus of prostate ♂　　　　　　　　　　　　A
Prostatic stone

N42.1　Congestion and hemorrhage of prostate ♂　　　　A
Excludes1　enlarged prostate (N40.-)
hematuria (R31.-)
hyperplasia of prostate (N40.-)
inflammatory diseases of prostate (N41.-)

N42.3　Dysplasia of prostate ♂
Prostatic intraepithelial neoplasia I (PIN I)
Prostatic intraepithelial neoplasia II (PIN II)
Excludes1　prostatic intraepithelial neoplasia III (PIN
III) (D07.5)

● N42.8　Other specified disorders of prostate

N42.81　Prostatodynia syndrome ♂　　　　　　　A
Painful prostate syndrome

N42.82　Prostatosis syndrome ♂　　　　　　　　A

N42.83　Cyst of prostate ♂　　　　　　　　　　A

N42.89　Other specified disorders of prostate ♂　A

N42.9　Disorder of prostate, unspecified ♂　　　　　　A

◀ New　◀▦ Revised　~~deleted~~ Deleted　Excludes 1　Excludes 2　Includes　Use additional　Code first　Code also　Unspecified

OGCR Official Guidelines　● Unacceptable Principal Diagnosis　X Assign placeholder X　● Use Additional Character(s)　▶ Manifestation Code　**Coding Clinic**

Item 14–7 **Hydrocele** is a sac of fluid accumulating in the testes membrane.

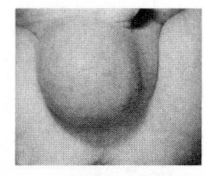

Blood
vessels
Vas
deferens
Epididymis
Testis
A
Hydrocele
B

Figure 14-6　A. Hydrocele. **B.** Newborn with large right hydrocele. (**B** from Behrman: Nelson Textbook of Pediatrics, ed 18, Saunders, An Imprint of Elsevier, 2007)

● **N43　Hydrocele and spermatocele**

　　Includes　hydrocele of spermatic cord, testis or tunica vaginalis

　　Excludes1　congenital hydrocele (P83.5)

　　N43.0　Encysted hydrocele ♂

　　N43.1　Infected hydrocele♂ 🔵

　　　　　　Use additional code (B95-B97), to identify infectious agent
　　　　　　Ⓔⓧ A59.00, A59.8-A59.9, B37.41-B37.49, N43.0-N43.3

　　N43.2　Other hydrocele ♂

　　N43.3　Hydrocele, unspecified ♂

　● N43.4　Spermatocele of epididymis
　　　　　　Spermatic cyst

　　　　　N43.40　Spermatocele of epididymis, unspecified ♂

　　　　　N43.41　Spermatocele of epididymis, single ♂

　　　　　N43.42　Spermatocele of epididymis, multiple ♂

● **N44　Noninflammatory disorders of testis**

　● N44.0　Torsion of testis
　　　　　　Ⓔⓧ For category N44.0 CC codes: N44.00-N44.04

　　　　　N44.00　Torsion of testis, unspecified ♂ 🔵

　　　　　N44.01　Extravaginal torsion of spermatic cord ♂ 🔵

　　　　　N44.02　Intravaginal torsion of spermatic cord ♂ 🔵
　　　　　　　　　Torsion of spermatic cord NOS

　　　　　N44.03　Torsion of appendix testis ♂ 🔵

　　　　　N44.04　Torsion of appendix epididymis ♂ 🔵

　　N44.1　Cyst of tunica albuginea testis ♂

　　N44.2　Benign cyst of testis ♂

　　N44.8　Other noninflammatory disorders of the testis ♂

● **N45　Orchitis and epididymitis**

　　Orchitis is inflammation of one or both of the testes as a result of mumps or other infection, trauma, or metastasis. Epididymitis is inflammation of the tubular structure that connects the testicle with the vas deferens.

　　　　Use additional code (B95-B97), to identify infectious agent

　　N45.1　Epididymitis ♂

　　N45.2　Orchitis ♂

　　N45.3　Epididymo-orchitis ♂

　　N45.4　Abscess of epididymis or testis ♂ 🔵
　　　　　　Ⓔⓧ A54.23, A54.82, A54.84, A54.89-A54.9, A59.00, A59.8-A59.9, B26.0, B37.41-B37.49, N45.1-N45.4

Item 14-8 Male infertility is the inability of the female sex partner to conceive after one year of unprotected intercourse.

　　Azoospermia is no sperm ejaculated and **oligospermia** is few sperm ejaculated—both resulting in infertility. Extratesticular causes such as injury, infections, radiation, and chemotherapy may also cause male infertility.

● **N46　Male infertility**

　　Excludes1　vasectomy status (Z98.52)

　● N46.0　Azoospermia
　　　　　　Absolute male infertility
　　　　　　Male infertility due to germinal (cell) aplasia
　　　　　　Male infertility due to spermatogenic arrest (complete)

　　　　　N46.01　Organic azoospermia ♂　　　　　　　A
　　　　　　　　　Azoospermia NOS

　● N46.02　Azoospermia due to extratesticular causes
　　　　　　Code also associated cause

　　　　　N46.021　Azoospermia due to drug therapy ♂ A

　　　　　N46.022　Azoospermia due to infection ♂　　A

　　　　　N46.023　Azoospermia due to obstruction of efferent ducts ♂　　　　　　　　　　A

　　　　　N46.024　Azoospermia due to radiation ♂　A

　　　　　N46.025　Azoospermia due to systemic disease ♂　　　　　　　　　　　　　A

　　　　　N46.029　Azoospermia due to other extratesticular causes ♂　　　　A

　● N46.1　Oligospermia
　　　　　　Male infertility due to germinal cell desquamation
　　　　　　Male infertility due to hypospermatogenesis
　　　　　　Male infertility due to incomplete spermatogenic arrest

　　　　　N46.11　Organic oligospermia ♂　　　　　　　A
　　　　　　　　　Oligospermia NOS

　● N46.12　Oligospermia due to extratesticular causes
　　　　　　Code also associated cause

　　　　　N46.121　Oligospermia due to drug therapy ♂ A

　　　　　N46.122　Oligospermia due to infection ♂　A

　　　　　N46.123　Oligospermia due to obstruction of efferent ducts ♂　　　　　　　A

　　　　　N46.124　Oligospermia due to radiation ♂　A

　　　　　N46.125　Oligospermia due to systemic disease ♂　　　　　　　　　　　A

　　　　　N46.129　Oligospermia due to other extratesticular causes ♂　　　A

　　N46.8　Other male infertility ♂　　　　　　　　A

　　N46.9　Male infertility, unspecified ♂　　　　　A

● **N47　Disorders of prepuce**

　　N47.0　Adherent prepuce, newborn ♂　　　　　　N

　　N47.1　Phimosis ♂

　　N47.2　Paraphimosis ♂

　　N47.3　Deficient foreskin ♂

　　N47.4　Benign cyst of prepuce ♂

　　N47.5　Adhesions of prepuce and glans penis ♂

　　N47.6　Balanoposthitis ♂
　　　　　　Use additional code (B95-B97), to identify infectious agent

　　　　　Excludes1　balanitis (N48.1)

　　N47.7　Other inflammatory diseases of prepuce ♂
　　　　　　Use additional code (B95-B97), to identify infectious agent

　　N47.8　Other disorders of prepuce ♂

CHAPTER 14 (N00-N99)

N　Newborn Age: 0　　　P　Pediatric Age: 0–17　　　M　Maternity DX: 12–55　　　A　Adult Age: 15–124　　　♀　Females Only　　　♂　Males Only

🔵 Complication\Comorbidity　　🔵 Major C\C　　Ⓔⓧ CC/MCC Exclusions　　🔵 Present on Admission Requirement　　🔵 Hospital-Acquired Condition

1183

CHAPTER 14 (N00-N99)

● **N48 Other disorders of penis**

N48.0 Leukoplakia of penis ♂
Balanitis xerotica obliterans
Kraurosis of penis
Lichen sclerosus of external male genital organs
> **Excludes1** carcinoma in situ of penis (D07.4)

N48.1 Balanitis ♂
Use additional code (B95-B97), to identify infectious agent
> **Excludes1** amebic balanitis (A06.8)
> balanitis xerotica obliterans (N48.0)
> candidal balanitis (B37.42)
> gonococcal balanitis (A54.23)
> herpesviral [herpes simplex] balanitis (A60.01)

● **N48.2 Other inflammatory disorders of penis**
Use additional code (B95-B97), to identify infectious agent
> **Excludes1** balanitis (N48.1)
> balanitis xerotica obliterans (N48.0)
> balanoposthitis (N47.6)

N48.21 Abscess of corpus cavernosum and penis ♂

N48.22 Cellulitis of corpus cavernosum and penis ♂

N48.29 Other inflammatory disorders of penis ♂

● **N48.3 Priapism**
Painful erection
Code first underlying cause
> (Ex) **For category N48.3 CC codes:** N47.6, N48.0-N48.9, N52.01-N52.9

N48.30 Priapism, unspecified ♂ 🔒

N48.31 Priapism due to trauma ♂ 🔒

▷ **N48.32 Priapism due to disease classified elsewhere** ♂ 🔒

N48.33 Priapism, drug-induced ♂ 🔒

N48.39 Other priapism ♂ 🔒

N48.5 Ulcer of penis ♂

N48.6 Induration penis plastica ♂
Peyronie's disease
Plastic induration of penis

● **N48.8 Other specified disorders of penis**

N48.81 Thrombosis of superficial vein of penis ♂

N48.82 Acquired torsion of penis ♂
Acquired torsion of penis NOS
> **Excludes1** congenital torsion of penis (Q55.63)

N48.83 Acquired buried penis ♂
> **Excludes1** congenital hidden penis (Q55.64)

N48.89 Other specified disorders of penis ♂

N48.9 Disorder of penis, unspecified ♂

● **N49 Inflammatory disorders of male genital organs, not elsewhere classified**
Use additional code (B95-B97), to identify infectious agent
> **Excludes1** inflammation of penis (N48.1, N48.2-)
> orchitis and epididymitis (N45.-)

N49.0 Inflammatory disorders of seminal vesicle ♂
Vesiculitis NOS

N49.1 Inflammatory disorders of spermatic cord, tunica vaginalis and vas deferens ♂
Vasitis

N49.2 Inflammatory disorders of scrotum ♂

N49.3 Fournier gangrene ♂

N49.8 Inflammatory disorders of other specified male genital organs ♂
Inflammation of multiple sites in male genital organs

N49.9 Inflammatory disorder of unspecified male genital organ ♂
Abscess of unspecified male genital organ
Boil of unspecified male genital organ
Carbuncle of unspecified male genital organ
Cellulitis of unspecified male genital organ

Item 14-9 Seminal vesiculitis is an inflammation of the seminal vesicle. Spermatocele is a benign cystic accumulation of sperm arising from the head of the epididymis. Torsion of the testis is a medical emergency occurring most commonly in boys 7 to 12 years of age and results from a congenital abnormality of the covering of the testis allowing the testis to twist within its sac and cutting off the blood supply to the testis.

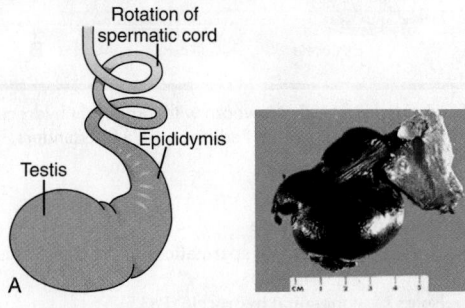

Figure 14-7 A. Torsion of testis. **B.** Torsion of the testis. (**B** from Kumar: Robbins and Cotran: Pathologic Basis of Disease, ed 8, Saunders, An Imprint of Elsevier, 2009)

● **N50 Other and unspecified disorders of male genital organs**
> **Excludes2** torsion of testis (N44.0-)

N50.0 Atrophy of testis ♂

N50.1 Vascular disorders of male genital organs ♂
Hematocele, NOS, of male genital organs
Hemorrhage of male genital organs
Thrombosis of male genital organs

N50.3 Cyst of epididymis ♂

N50.8 Other specified disorders of male genital organs ♂
Atrophy of scrotum, seminal vesicle, spermatic cord, tunica vaginalis and vas deferens
Edema of scrotum, seminal vesicle, spermatic cord, testis, tunica vaginalis and vas deferens
Hypertrophy of scrotum, seminal vesicle, spermatic cord, testis, tunica vaginalis and vas deferens
Ulcer of scrotum, seminal vesicle, spermatic cord, testis, tunica vaginalis and vas deferens
Chylocele, tunica vaginalis (nonfilarial) NOS
Urethroscrotal fistula
Stricture of spermatic cord, tunica vaginalis, and vas deferens

N50.9 Disorder of male genital organs, unspecified ♂

▷ **N51 Disorders of male genital organs in diseases classified elsewhere** ♂
Code first underlying disease, such as:
filariasis (B74.0-B74.9)
> **Excludes1** amebic balanitis (A06.8)
> candidal balanitis (B37.42)
> gonococcal balanitis (A54.23)
> gonococcal prostatitis (A54.22)
> herpesviral [herpes simplex] balanitis (A60.01)
> trichomonal prostatitis (A59.02)
> tuberculous prostatitis (A18.14)

● **N52 Male erectile dysfunction**
> **Excludes1** psychogenic impotence (F52.21)

● **N52.0 Vasculogenic erectile dysfunction**

N52.01 Erectile dysfunction due to arterial insufficiency ♂   A

N52.02 Corporo-venous occlusive erectile dysfunction ♂   A

N52.03 Combined arterial insufficiency and corporo-venous occlusive erectile dysfunction ♂   A

▷ **N52.1 Erectile dysfunction due to diseases classified elsewhere** ♂   A
Code first underlying disease

N52.2 Drug-induced erectile dysfunction ♂   A

◀ New   ◀ Revised   ~~deleted~~ Deleted   Excludes 1   Excludes 2   Includes   Use additional   Code first   Code also   Unspecified
OGCR Official Guidelines   ● Unacceptable Principal Diagnosis   X Assign placeholder X   ● Use Additional Character(s)   ▷ Manifestation Code   **Coding Clinic**

● N52.3   Post-surgical erectile dysfunction

    N52.31   Erectile dysfunction following radical prostatectomy ♂   A

    N52.32   Erectile dysfunction following radical cystectomy ♂   A

    N52.33   Erectile dysfunction following urethral surgery ♂   A

    N52.34   Erectile dysfunction following simple prostatectomy ♂   A

    N52.39   Other post-surgical erectile dysfunction ♂   A

  N52.8   Other male erectile dysfunction ♂   A

  N52.9   Male erectile dysfunction, unspecified ♂   A
       Impotence NOS

● N53   Other male sexual dysfunction

    Excludes1   psychogenic sexual dysfunction (F52.-)

  ● N53.1   Ejaculatory dysfunction

       Excludes1   premature ejaculation (F52.4)

    N53.11   Retarded ejaculation ♂

    N53.12   Painful ejaculation ♂

    N53.13   Anejaculatory orgasm ♂

    N53.14   Retrograde ejaculation ♂

    N53.19   Other ejaculatory dysfunction ♂
       Ejaculatory dysfunction NOS

  N53.8   Other male sexual dysfunction ♂

  N53.9   Unspecified male sexual dysfunction ♂

DISORDERS OF BREAST (N60-N65)

    Excludes1   disorders of breast associated with childbirth (O91-O92)

● N60   Benign mammary dysplasia
    Benign lumpiness of breast

    Includes   fibrocystic mastopathy

  ● N60.0   Solitary cyst of breast
    Cyst of breast

    N60.01   Solitary cyst of right breast

    N60.02   Solitary cyst of left breast

    N60.09   Solitary cyst of unspecified breast

  ● N60.1   Diffuse cystic mastopathy
    Cystic breast
    Fibrocystic disease of breast

       Excludes1   diffuse cystic mastopathy with epithelial proliferation (N60.3-)

    N60.11   Diffuse cystic mastopathy of right breast   A

    N60.12   Diffuse cystic mastopathy of left breast   A

    N60.19   Diffuse cystic mastopathy of unspecified breast   A

  ● N60.2   Fibroadenosis of breast
    Adenofibrosis of breast

       Excludes2   fibroadenoma of breast (D24.-)

    N60.21   Fibroadenosis of right breast

    N60.22   Fibroadenosis of left breast

    N60.29   Fibroadenosis of unspecified breast

  ● N60.3   Fibrosclerosis of breast
    Cystic mastopathy with epithelial proliferation

    N60.31   Fibrosclerosis of right breast

    N60.32   Fibrosclerosis of left breast

    N60.39   Fibrosclerosis of unspecified breast

  ● N60.4   Mammary duct ectasia

    N60.41   Mammary duct ectasia of right breast

    N60.42   Mammary duct ectasia of left breast

    N60.49   Mammary duct ectasia of unspecified breast

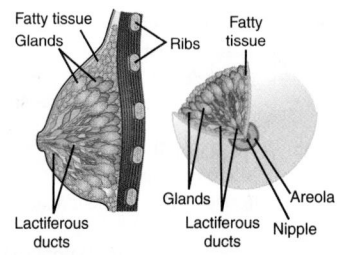

Figure 14-8   Breast.

  ● N60.8   Other benign mammary dysplasias

    N60.81   Other benign mammary dysplasias of right breast

    N60.82   Other benign mammary dysplasias of left breast

    N60.89   Other benign mammary dysplasias of unspecified breast

  ● N60.9   Unspecified benign mammary dysplasia

    N60.91   Unspecified benign mammary dysplasia of right breast

    N60.92   Unspecified benign mammary dysplasia of left breast

    N60.99   Unspecified benign mammary dysplasia of unspecified breast

N61   Inflammatory disorders of breast
    Abscess (acute) (chronic) (nonpuerperal) of areola
    Abscess (acute) (chronic) (nonpuerperal) of breast
    Carbuncle of breast
    Infective mastitis (acute) (subacute) (nonpuerperal)
    Mastitis (acute) (subacute) (nonpuerperal) NOS

    Excludes1   inflammatory carcinoma of breast (C50.9)
       inflammatory disorder of breast associated with childbirth (O91.-)
       neonatal infective mastitis (P39.0)
       thrombophlebitis of breast [Mondor's disease] (I80.8)

N62   Hypertrophy of breast
    Gynecomastia
    Hypertrophy of breast NOS
    Massive pubertal hypertrophy of breast

    Excludes1   breast engorgement of newborn (P83.4)
       disproportion of reconstructed breast (N65.1)

N63   Unspecified lump in breast
    Nodule(s) NOS in breast

● N64   Other disorders of breast

    Excludes2   mechanical complication of breast prosthesis and implant (T85.4-)

  N64.0   Fissure and fistula of nipple

  ● N64.1   Fat necrosis of breast
    Fat necrosis (segmental) of breast
    Code first breast necrosis due to breast graft (T85.89)

  N64.2   Atrophy of breast

  N64.3   Galactorrhea not associated with childbirth
    Excessive or spontaneous flow of milk

  N64.4   Mastodynia

  ● N64.5   Other signs and symptoms in breast

       Excludes2   abnormal findings on diagnostic imaging of breast (R92.-)

    N64.51   Induration of breast

    N64.52   Nipple discharge

       Excludes1   abnormal findings in nipple discharge (R89.-)

    N64.53   Retraction of nipple

    N64.59   Other signs and symptoms in breast

N Newborn Age: 0   **P** Pediatric Age: 0–17   **M** Maternity DX: 12–55   **A** Adult Age: 15–124   ♀ Females Only   ♂ Males Only

Complication\Comorbidity   Major C\C   (Ex) CC/MCC Exclusions   Present on Admission Requirement   Hospital-Acquired Condition

1185

CHAPTER 14 (N00-N99)

CHAPTER 14 (N00-N99)

● **N64.8   Other specified disorders of breast**

     N64.81   Ptosis of breast   A

         Excludes1   ptosis of native breast in relation to reconstructed breast (N65.1)

     N64.82   Hypoplasia of breast   A

         Micromastia

         Excludes1   congenital absence of breast (Q83.0)

                   hypoplasia of native breast in relation to reconstructed breast (N65.1)

     N64.89   Other specified disorders of breast

         Galactocele

         Subinvolution of breast (postlactational)

     N64.9   Disorder of breast, unspecified

● **N65   Deformity and disproportion of reconstructed breast**

     N65.0   Deformity of reconstructed breast   A

         Contour irregularity in reconstructed breast

         Excess tissue in reconstructed breast

         Misshapen reconstructed breast

     N65.1   Disproportion of reconstructed breast   A

         Breast asymmetry between native breast and reconstructed breast

         Disproportion between native and reconstructed breast

---

INFLAMMATORY DISEASES OF FEMALE PELVIC ORGANS (N70-N77)

     Excludes1   inflammatory diseases of female pelvic organs complicating:

                 abortion or ectopic or molar pregnancy (O00-O07, O08.0)

                 pregnancy, childbirth and the puerperium (O23.-, O75.3, O85, O86.-)

(See Plate 360 on page 80.)

● **N70   Salpingitis and oophoritis**

     Oophoritis = inflammation of ovary

     Salpingitis = inflammation of falloplan tube

     Includes   abscess (of) fallopian tube

             abscess (of) ovary

             pyosalpinx

             salpingo-oophoritis

             tubo-ovarian abscess

             tubo-ovarian inflammatory disease

     Use additional code (B95-B97), to identify infectious agent

     Excludes1   gonococcal infection (A54.24)

                 tuberculous infection (A18.17)

● **N70.0   Acute salpingitis and oophoritis**

     Ex: **For category N70.0 CC codes:** A17.9, A18.10, A18.16-A18.18, A18.82, A18.84, A18.89, A54.03, A54.24, A54.82, A54.84, A54.89-A54.9, A59.00, A59.8-A59.9, B37.41-B37.49, N70.01-N71.9, N72, N73.0-N74, N75.9, N76.5, N76.81-N76.89, N90.810-N90.818, N94.818-N94.9, N96, Q55.0-Q55.4, Q55.7-Q55.9

     N70.01   Acute salpingitis ♀ 🔩

     N70.02   Acute oophoritis ♀ 🔩

     N70.03   Acute salpingitis and oophoritis ♀ 🔩

● **N70.1   Chronic salpingitis and oophoritis**

     Hydrosalpinx

     N70.11   Chronic salpingitis ♀

     N70.12   Chronic oophoritis ♀

     N70.13   Chronic salpingitis and oophoritis ♀

● **N70.9   Salpingitis and oophoritis, unspecified**

     N70.91   Salpingitis, unspecified ♀

     N70.92   Oophoritis, unspecified ♀

     N70.93   Salpingitis and oophoritis, unspecified ♀

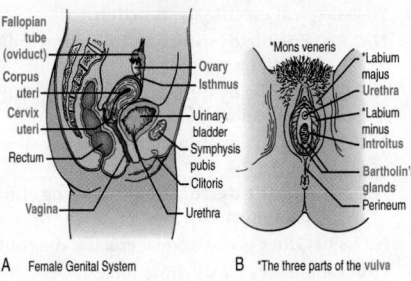

Figure 14-9   A. Female genital system. **B.** External female genital system. (From Buck CJ: Step-by-Step Medical Coding, ed 2011, Philadelphia, WB Saunders, 2011)

Item 14–10 Salpingitis is an infection of one or both fallopian tubes. **Oophoritis** is an infection of one or both ovaries.

● **N71   Inflammatory disease of uterus, except cervix**

     Includes   endo (myo) metritis

             metritis

             myometritis

             pyometra

             uterine abscess

     Use additional code (B95-B97), to identify infectious agent

     Excludes1   hyperplastic endometritis (N85.0-)

                 infection of uterus following delivery (O85, O86.-) ◄

     N71.0   Acute inflammatory disease of uterus ♀ 🔩

         Ex: A17.9, A18.10, A18.16-A18.18, A18.82, A18.84, A18.89, A54.03, A54.24, A54.82, A54.84, A54.89-A54.9, A59.00, A59.8-A59.9, B37.41-B37.49, N70.01-N71.9, N72, N73.0-N74, N75.9, N76.5, N76.81-N76.89, N85.8-N85.9, N90.810-N90.818, N94.818-N94.9, N96, Q55.0-Q55.4, Q55.7-Q55.9

     N71.1   Chronic inflammatory disease of uterus ♀

     N71.9   Inflammatory disease of uterus, unspecified ♀

     N72   Inflammatory disease of cervix uteri ♀

     Includes   cervicitis (with or without erosion or ectropion)

             endocervicitis (with or without erosion or ectropion)

             exocervicitis (with or without erosion or ectropion)

     Use additional code (B95-B97), to identify infectious agent

     Excludes1   erosion and ectropion of cervix without cervicitis (N86)

● **N73   Other female pelvic inflammatory diseases**

     Use additional code (B95-B97), to identify infectious agent

     N73.0   Acute parametritis and pelvic cellulitis ♀ 🔩

         Abscess of broad ligament

         Abscess of parametrium

         Pelvic cellulitis, female

         Ex: See N70.0

     N73.1   Chronic parametritis and pelvic cellulitis ♀

         Any condition in N73.0 specified as chronic

         Excludes1   tuberculous parametritis and pelvic cellultis (A18.17)

     N73.2   Unspecified parametritis and pelvic cellulitis ♀

         Any condition in N73.0 unspecified whether acute or chronic

     N73.3   Female acute pelvic peritonitis ♀ 🔩

         Ex: See N70.0

     N73.4   Female chronic pelvic peritonitis ♀ 🔩

         Excludes1   tuberculous pelvic (female) peritonitis (A18.17)

         Ex: See N70.0

     N73.5   Female pelvic peritonitis, unspecified ♀

     N73.6   Female pelvic peritoneal adhesions (postinfective) ♀

         Excludes2   postprocedural pelvic peritoneal adhesions (N99.4)

     N73.8   Other specified female pelvic inflammatory diseases ♀

     N73.9   Female pelvic inflammatory disease, unspecified ♀

         Female pelvic infection or inflammation NOS

◄ New   ◄ Revised   ~~deleted~~ Deleted   Excludes 1   Excludes 2   Includes   Use additional   Code first   Code also   Unspecified

OGCR Official Guidelines   ● Unacceptable Principal Diagnosis   X Assign placeholder X   ● Use Additional Character(s)   ▌ Manifestation Code   **Coding Clinic**

▌N74 *Female pelvic inflammatory disorders in diseases classified elsewhere* ♀

    Code first underlying disease

    Excludes1 ~~cervicitis:~~
        chlamydial cervicitis (A56.02) ◀▥
        ~~gonococcal (A54.03)~~
        ~~herpesviral [herpes simplex] (A60.03)~~
        ~~syphilitic (A52.76)~~
        ~~trichomonal (A59.09)~~
        ~~tuberculous (A18.16)~~
        ~~pelvic inflammatory disease:~~
        chlamydial pelvic inflammatory disease
          (A56.11) ◀▥
        gonococcal cervicitis (A54.03) ◀▥
        ~~herpesviral [herpes simplex] (A60.09)~~
        ~~syphilitic (A52.76)~~
        ~~tuberculous (A18.17)~~
        gonococcal pelvic inflammatory disease
          (A54.24) ◀
        herpesviral [herpes simplex] cervicitis (A60.03) ◀
        herpesviral [herpes simplex] pelvic inflammatory
          disease (A60.09) ◀
        syphilitic cervicitis (A52.76) ◀
        syphilitic pelvic inflammatory disease (A52.76) ◀
        trichomonal cervicitis (A59.09) ◀
        tuberculous cervicitis (A18.16) ◀
        tuberculous pelvic inflammatory disease
          (A18.17) ◀

●N75 **Diseases of Bartholin's gland**

  N75.0 Cyst of Bartholin's gland ♀
    Cysts filled with liquid or semisolid material.

  N75.1 Abscess of Bartholin's gland ♀ 🅒
    Localized collection of pus
    Ⓔⓧ A17.9, A18.10, A18.16-A18.18, A18.82, A18.84, A18.89, A59.00-A59.01,
    A59.8-A59.9, B37.3-B37.49, N75.0-N77.1, N84.3, N90.3, N90.6-N90.9,
    N94.810-N94.9, N96, Q55.0-Q55.4, Q55.7-Q55.9

  N75.8 Other diseases of Bartholin's gland ♀
    Bartholinitis

  N75.9 Disease of Bartholin's gland, unspecified ♀

●N76 **Other inflammation of vagina and vulva**
    Use additional code (B95-B97), to identify infectious agent
    Excludes2 senile (atrophic) vaginitis (N95.2)
              vulvar vestibulitis (N94.810)

  N76.0 Acute vaginitis ♀
    Acute vulvovaginitis
    Vaginitis NOS
    Vulvovaginitis NOS

  N76.1 Subacute and chronic vaginitis ♀
    Chronic vulvovaginitis
    Subacute vulvovaginitis

  N76.2 Acute vulvitis ♀
    Vulvitis NOS

  N76.3 Subacute and chronic vulvitis ♀

  N76.4 Abscess of vulva ♀ 🅒
    Furuncle of vulva
    Ⓔⓧ See N75.1

  N76.5 Ulceration of vagina ♀

  N76.6 Ulceration of vulva ♀

●**N76.8 Other specified inflammation of vagina and vulva**

    N76.81 Mucositis (ulcerative) of vagina and vulva ♀ 🅒
        Code also type of associated therapy, such as:
          antineoplastic and immunosuppressive
            drugs (T45.1X-) ◀▥
          radiological procedure and radiotherapy
            (Y84.2)
        Excludes2 gastrointestinal mucositis
              (ulcerative) (K92.81)
             nasal mucositis (ulcerative)
              (J34.81)
             oral mucositis (ulcerative) (K12.3-)
        Ⓔⓧ N72, N75.9, N76.5, N76.81-N76.89

    **N76.89 Other specified inflammation of vagina and
        vulva** ♀

●N77 **Vulvovaginal ulceration and inflammation in diseases classified elsewhere**

  ▌**N77.0 *Ulceration of vulva in diseases classified elsewhere*** ♀
    Code first underlying disease, such as:
    Behçet's disease (M35.2)
    Excludes1 ulceration of vulva in gonococcal
             infection (A54.02)
          ulceration of vulva in herpesviral [herpes
            simplex] infection (A60.04)
          ulceration of vulva in syphilis (A51.0)
          ulceration of vulva in tuberculosis (A18.18)

  ▌**N77.1 *Vaginitis, vulvitis and vulvovaginitis in diseases
    classified elsewhere*** ♀
    Code first underlying disease, such as:
    pinworm (B80)
    Excludes1 ~~vaginitis, vulvitis and vulvovaginitis (in):~~
          candidial vulvovaginitis (B37.3) ◀▥
          chlamydial vulvovaginitis (A56.02) ◀▥
          gonococcal vulvovaginitis (A54.02) ◀▥
          herpesviral [herpes simplex]
            vulvovaginitis (A60.04) ◀▥
          ~~syphilitic, early (A51.0)~~
          ~~syphilitic, late (A52.76)~~
          trichomonal vulvovaginitis (A59.01) ◀▥
          tuberculous vulvovaginitis (A18.18) ◀▥
          vulvovaginitis in early syphilis (A51.0) ◀
          vulvovaginitis in late syphilis (A52.76) ◀

NONINFLAMMATORY DISORDERS OF FEMALE GENITAL TRACT (N80-N98)

●N80 **Endometriosis**

  N80.0 Endometriosis of uterus ♀
    Adenomyosis
    Excludes1 stromal endometriosis (D39.0)

  N80.1 Endometriosis of ovary ♀

  N80.2 Endometriosis of fallopian tube ♀

  N80.3 Endometriosis of pelvic peritoneum ♀

  N80.4 Endometriosis of rectovaginal septum and vagina ♀

  N80.5 Endometriosis of intestine ♀

  N80.6 Endometriosis in cutaneous scar ♀

  N80.8 Other endometriosis ♀

  N80.9 Endometriosis, unspecified ♀

Item 14–11 Endometriosis is a condition for which no clear cause has been identified. Endometrial tissue is expelled from the uterus into the abdominal cavity and can implant onto a variety of organs. Classification is based on the site of implant of the endometrial tissue.

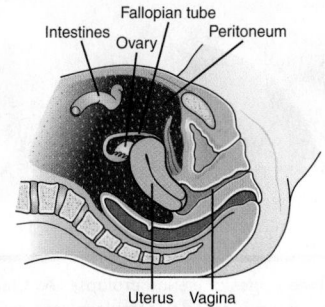

Figure 14-10 Sites of potential endometrial implants.

N Newborn Age: 0   **P** Pediatric Age: 0–17   **M** Maternity DX: 12–55   **A** Adult Age: 15–124   ♀ Females Only   ♂ Males Only

🅒 Complication\Comorbidity   🅜 Major C\C   Ⓔⓧ CC/MCC Exclusions   ▥ Present on Admission Requirement   🅗 Hospital-Acquired Condition

1187

CHAPTER 14 (N00-N99)

● **N81   Female genital prolapse**

    Excludes 1   genital prolapse complicating pregnancy, labor or delivery (O34.5-)

                  prolapse and hernia of ovary and fallopian tube (N83.4)

                  prolapse of vaginal vault after hysterectomy (N99.3)

  N81.0   Urethrocele ♀

      Excludes 1 urethrocele with cystocele (N81.1-)

               urethrocele with prolapse of uterus (N81.2-N81.4)

  ● **N81.1   Cystocele**

      Cystocele with urethrocele

      Cystourethrocele

      Excludes 1 cystocele with prolapse of uterus (N81.2-N81.4)

    N81.10   Cystocele, unspecified ♀

         Prolapse of (anterior) vaginal wall NOS

    N81.11   Cystocele, midline ♀

    N81.12   Cystocele, lateral ♀

         Paravaginal cystocele

  N81.2   Incomplete uterovaginal prolapse ♀

      First degree uterine prolapse

      Prolapse of cervix NOS

      Second degree uterine prolapse

      Excludes 1 cervical stump prolapse (N81.85)

  N81.3   Complete uterovaginal prolapse ♀

      Procidentia (uteri) NOS

      Third degree uterine prolapse

  N81.4   Uterovaginal prolapse, unspecified ♀

      Prolapse of uterus NOS

  N81.5   Vaginal enterocele ♀

      Excludes 1 enterocele with prolapse of uterus (N81.2-N81.4)

  N81.6   Rectocele ♀

      Prolapse of posterior vaginal wall

      Use additional code for any associated fecal incontinence, if applicable (R15.-) ◀▥

      Excludes 2 perineocele (N81.81) ◀▥

               rectal prolapse (K62.3)

               rectocele with prolapse of uterus (N81.2-N81.4)

  ● **N81.8   Other female genital prolapse**

    N81.81   Perineocele ♀

    N81.82   Incompetence or weakening of pubocervical tissue ♀

    N81.83   Incompetence or weakening of rectovaginal tissue ♀

    N81.84   Pelvic muscle wasting ♀

         Disuse atrophy of pelvic muscles and anal sphincter

    N81.85   Cervical stump prolapse ♀

    N81.89   Other female genital prolapse ♀

         Deficient perineum

         Old laceration of muscles of pelvic floor

  N81.9   Female genital prolapse, unspecified ♀

Figure 14-11   Three stages of uterine prolapse. **A.** Uterus is prolapsed. **B.** Vagina and uterus are prolapsed (incomplete uterovaginal prolapse). **C.** Vagina and uterus are completely prolapsed and are exposed through the external genitalia (complete uterovaginal prolapse).

● **N82   Fistulae involving female genital tract**

    Excludes 1 vesicointestinal fistulae (N32.1)

    (Ex) **For category N82 CC codes: N82.0-N82.9**

  N82.0   Vesicovaginal fistula ♀ ⊚

  N82.1   Other female urinary-genital tract fistulae ♀ ⊚

      Cervicovesical fistula

      Ureterovaginal fistula

      Urethrovaginal fistula

      Uteroureteric fistula

      Uterovesical fistula

  N82.2   Fistula of vagina to small intestine ♀ ⊚

  N82.3   Fistula of vagina to large intestine ♀ ⊚

      Rectovaginal fistula

  N82.4   Other female intestinal-genital tract fistulae ♀ ⊚

      Intestinouterine fistula

  N82.5   Female genital tract-skin fistulae ♀ ⊚

      Uterus to abdominal wall fistula

      Vaginoperineal fistula

  N82.8   Other female genital tract fistulae ♀ ⊚

  N82.9   Female genital tract fistula, unspecified ♀ ⊚

● **N83   Noninflammatory disorders of ovary, fallopian tube and broad ligament**

    Excludes 2 hydrosalpinx (N70.1-)

  N83.0   Follicular cyst of ovary ♀

      Cyst of graafian follicle

      Hemorrhagic follicular cyst (of ovary)

  N83.1   Corpus luteum cyst ♀

      Hemorrhagic corpus luteum cyst

  ● **N83.2   Other and unspecified ovarian cysts**

      Excludes 1 developmental ovarian cyst (Q50.1)

               neoplastic ovarian cyst (D27.-)

               polycystic ovarian syndrome (E28.2)

               Stein-Leventhal syndrome (E28.2)

    N83.20   Unspecified ovarian cysts ♀

    N83.29   Other ovarian cysts ♀

         Retention cyst of ovary

         Simple cyst of ovary

  ● **N83.3   Acquired atrophy of ovary and fallopian tube**

    N83.31   Acquired atrophy of ovary ♀

    N83.32   Acquired atrophy of fallopian tube ♀

    N83.33   Acquired atrophy of ovary and fallopian tube ♀

  N83.4   Prolapse and hernia of ovary and fallopian tube ♀

  ● **N83.5   Torsion of ovary, ovarian pedicle and fallopian tube**

      Torsion of accessory tube

      (Ex) **For category N83.5 CC codes: N83.0-N83.9, N99.83**

    N83.51   Torsion of ovary and ovarian pedicle ♀ ⊚

    N83.52   Torsion of fallopian tube ♀ ⊚

         Torsion of hydatid of Morgagni

    N83.53   Torsion of ovary, ovarian pedicle and fallopian tube ♀ ⊚

  N83.6   Hematosalpinx ♀

      Excludes 1 hematosalpinx (with) (in):

               hematocolpos (N89.7)

               hematometra (N85.7)

               tubal pregnancy (O00.1)

  N83.7   Hematoma of broad ligament ♀

  N83.8   Other noninflammatory disorders of ovary, fallopian tube and broad ligament ♀

      Broad ligament laceration syndrome [Allen-Masters]

  N83.9   Noninflammatory disorder of ovary, fallopian tube and broad ligament, unspecified ♀

◀ New   ◀▥ Revised   ~~deleted~~ Deleted   Excludes 1   Excludes 2   Includes   Use additional   Code first   Code also   Unspecified

OGCR Official Guidelines   ● Unacceptable Principal Diagnosis   X Assign placeholder X   ● Use Additional Character(s)   ▌ Manifestation Code   **Coding Clinic**

● **N84**   **Polyp of female genital tract**
    Excludes1   adenomatous polyp (D28.-)
                placental polyp (O90.89)

   N84.0   **Polyp of corpus uteri** ♀
       Polyp of endometrium
       Polyp of uterus NOS
       Excludes1   polypoid endometrial hyperplasia
                  (N85.0-)

   N84.1   **Polyp of cervix uteri** ♀
       Mucous polyp of cervix

   N84.2   **Polyp of vagina** ♀

   N84.3   **Polyp of vulva** ♀
       Polyp of labia

   N84.8   **Polyp of other parts of female genital tract** ♀

   N84.9   **Polyp of female genital tract, unspecified** ♀

● **N85**   **Other noninflammatory disorders of uterus, except cervix**
    Excludes1   endometriosis (N80.-)
                inflammatory diseases of uterus (N71.-)
                noninflammatory disorders of cervix, except
                  malposition (N86-N88)
                polyp of corpus uteri (N84.0)
                uterine prolapse (N81.-)

 ● **N85.0**   **Endometrial hyperplasia**
    N85.00   **Endometrial hyperplasia, unspecified** ♀
        Hyperplasia (adenomatous) (cystic)
          (glandular) of endometrium
        Hyperplastic endometritis

    N85.01   **Benign endometrial hyperplasia** ♀
        Endometrial hyperplasia (complex) (simple)
          without atypia

    N85.02   **Endometrial intraepithelial neoplasia [EIN]** ♀
        Endometrial hyperplasia with atypia
        Excludes1   malignant neoplasm of
                   endometrium (with
                   endometrial intraepithelial
                   neoplasia [EIN]) (C54.1)

   N85.2   **Hypertrophy of uterus** ♀
       Bulky or enlarged uterus
       Excludes1   puerperal hypertrophy of uterus (O90.89)

   N85.3   **Subinvolution of uterus** ♀
       Excludes1   puerperal subinvolution of uterus
                  (O90.89)

   N85.4   **Malposition of uterus** ♀
       Anteversion of uterus
       Retroflexion of uterus
       Retroversion of uterus
       Excludes1   malposition of uterus complicating
                  pregnancy, labor or delivery (O34.5-,
                  O65.5)

   N85.5   **Inversion of uterus** ♀
       Excludes1   current obstetric trauma (O71.2)
                postpartum inversion of uterus (O71.2)

   N85.6   **Intrauterine synechiae** ♀

   N85.7   **Hematometra** ♀
       Hematosalpinx with hematometra
       Excludes1   hematometra with hematocolpos (N89.7)

   N85.8   **Other specified noninflammatory disorders of uterus** ♀
       Atrophy of uterus, acquired
       Fibrosis of uterus NOS

   N85.9   **Noninflammatory disorder of uterus, unspecified** ♀
       Disorder of uterus NOS

● **N86**   **Erosion and ectropion of cervix uteri** ♀
       Decubitus (trophic) ulcer of cervix
       Eversion of cervix
    Excludes1   erosion and ectropion of cervix with cervicitis
                (N72)

● **N87**   **Dysplasia of cervix uteri**
    Excludes1   abnormal results from cervical cytologic
                examination without histologic confirmation
                (R87.61-)
                carcinoma in situ of cervix uteri (D06.-)
                cervical intraepithelial neoplasia III [CIN III]
                (D06.-)
                HGSIL of cervix (R87.613)
                severe dysplasia of cervix uteri (D06.-)

   N87.0   **Mild cervical dysplasia** ♀
       Cervical intraepithelial neoplasia I [CIN I]

   N87.1   **Moderate cervical dysplasia** ♀
       Cervical intraepithelial neoplasia II [CIN II]

   N87.9   **Dysplasia of cervix uteri, unspecified** ♀
       Anaplasia of cervix
       Cervical atypism
       Cervical dysplasia NOS

● **N88**   **Other noninflammatory disorders of cervix uteri**
    Excludes2   inflammatory disease of cervix (N72)
                polyp of cervix (N84.1)

   N88.0   **Leukoplakia of cervix uteri** ♀

   N88.1   **Old laceration of cervix uteri** ♀
       Adhesions of cervix
       Excludes1   current obstetric trauma (O71.3)

   N88.2   **Stricture and stenosis of cervix uteri** ♀
       Excludes1   stricture and stenosis of cervix uteri
                complicating labor (O65.5)

   N88.3   **Incompetence of cervix uteri** ♀
       Investigation and management of (suspected) cervical
         incompetence in a nonpregnant woman
       Excludes1   cervical incompetence complicating
                pregnancy (O34.3-)

   N88.4   **Hypertrophic elongation of cervix uteri** ♀

   N88.8   **Other specified noninflammatory disorders of cervix uteri** ♀
       Excludes1   current obstetric trauma (O71.3)

   N88.9   **Noninflammatory disorder of cervix uteri, unspecified** ♀

● **N89**   **Other noninflammatory disorders of vagina**
    Excludes1   abnormal results from vaginal cytologic
                examination without histologic confirmation
                (R87.62-)
                carcinoma in situ of vagina (D07.2)
                HGSIL of vagina (R87.623)
                inflammation of vagina (N76.-)
                senile (atrophic) vaginitis (N95.2)
                severe dysplasia of vagina (D07.2)
                trichomonal leukorrhea (A59.00)
                vaginal intraepithelial neoplasia [VAIN], grade
                III (D07.2)

   N89.0   **Mild vaginal dysplasia** ♀
       Vaginal intraepithelial neoplasia [VAIN], grade I

   N89.1   **Moderate vaginal dysplasia** ♀
       Vaginal intraepithelial neoplasia [VAIN], grade II

   N89.3   **Dysplasia of vagina, unspecified** ♀

   N89.4   **Leukoplakia of vagina** ♀

   N89.5   **Stricture and atresia of vagina** ♀
       Vaginal adhesions   Vaginal stenosis
       Excludes1   congenital atresia or stricture (Q52.4)
                postprocedural adhesions of vagina
                (N99.2)

   N89.6   **Tight hymenal ring** ♀
       Rigid hymen   Tight introitus
       Excludes1   imperforate hymen (Q52.3)

   N89.7   **Hematocolpos** ♀
       Hematocolpos with hematometra or hematosalpinx

N   Newborn Age: 0   **P**   Pediatric Age: 0–17   **M**   Maternity DX: 12–55   **A**   Adult Age: 15–124   ♀   Females Only   ♂   Males Only

  Complication\Comorbidity   Major C\C   (Ex)   CC/MCC Exclusions   Present on Admission Requirement   Hospital-Acquired Condition   **1189**

N89.8   Other specified noninflammatory disorders of vagina ♀
Leukorrhea NOS
Old vaginal laceration
Pessary ulcer of vagina

    Excludes1   current obstetric trauma (O70.-, O71.4,
O71.7-O71.8)
old laceration involving muscles of pelvic
floor (N81.8)

N89.9   Noninflammatory disorder of vagina, unspecified ♀

● **N90**   Other noninflammatory disorders of vulva and perineum
    Excludes1   anogenital (venereal) warts (A63.0)
carcinoma in situ of vulva (D07.1)
condyloma acuminatum (A63.0)
current obstetric trauma (O70.-, O71.7-O71.8)
inflammation of vulva (N76.-)
severe dysplasia of vulva (D07.1)
vulvar intraepithelial neoplasm III [VIN III]
(D07.1)

N90.0   Mild vulvar dysplasia ♀
Vulvar intraepithelial neoplasia [VIN], grade I

N90.1   Moderate vulvar dysplasia ♀
Vulvar intraepithelial neoplasia [VIN], grade II

N90.3   Dysplasia of vulva, unspecified ♀

N90.4   Leukoplakia of vulva ♀
Dystrophy of vulva
Kraurosis of vulva
Lichen sclerosus of external female genital organs

N90.5   Atrophy of vulva ♀
Stenosis of vulva

N90.6   Hypertrophy of vulva ♀
Hypertrophy of labia

N90.7   Vulvar cyst ♀

● **N90.8**   Other specified noninflammatory disorders of vulva and
perineum

   ● **N90.81**   Female genital mutilation status
Female genital cutting status

     N90.810   Female genital mutilation status,
unspecified ♀
Female genital cutting status,
unspecified
Female genital mutilation status
NOS

     N90.811   Female genital mutilation Type I
status ♀
Clitorectomy status
Female genital cutting Type I status

     N90.812   Female genital mutilation Type II
status ♀
Clitorectomy with excision of labia
minora status
Female genital cutting Type II status

     N90.813   Female genital mutilation Type III
status ♀
Female genital cutting Type III status
Infibulation status

     N90.818   Other female genital mutilation
status ♀
Female genital cutting Type IV
status
Female genital mutilation Type IV
status
Other female genital cutting status

   N90.89   Other specified noninflammatory disorders of
vulva and perineum ♀
Adhesions of vulva
Hypertrophy of clitoris

N90.9   Noninflammatory disorder of vulva and perineum,
unspecified ♀

● **N91**   Absent, scanty and rare menstruation
    Excludes1   ovarian dysfunction (E28.-)

N91.0   Primary amenorrhea ♀

N91.1   Secondary amenorrhea ♀

N91.2   Amenorrhea, unspecified ♀

N91.3   Primary oligomenorrhea ♀

N91.4   Secondary oligomenorrhea ♀

N91.5   Oligomenorrhea, unspecified ♀
Hypomenorrhea NOS

● **N92**   Excessive, frequent and irregular menstruation
    Excludes1   postmenopausal bleeding (N95.0)
precocious puberty (menstruation) (E30.1)

N92.0   Excessive and frequent menstruation with regular cycle ♀
Heavy periods NOS   Polymenorrhea
Menorrhagia NOS

N92.1   Excessive and frequent menstruation with irregular
cycle ♀
Irregular intermenstrual bleeding
Irregular, shortened intervals between menstrual
bleeding
Menometrorrhagia
Metrorrhagia

N92.2   Excessive menstruation at puberty ♀   P
Excessive bleeding associated with onset of menstrual
periods
Pubertal menorrhagia
Puberty bleeding

N92.3   Ovulation bleeding ♀
Regular intermenstrual bleeding

N92.4   Excessive bleeding in the premenopausal period ♀
Climacteric menorrhagia or metrorrhagia
Menopausal menorrhagia or metrorrhagia
Preclimacteric menorrhagia or metrorrhagia
Premenopausal menorrhagia or metrorrhagia

N92.5   Other specified irregular menstruation ♀

N92.6   Irregular menstruation, unspecified ♀
Irregular bleeding NOS
Irregular periods NOS

    Excludes1   irregular menstruation with:
lengthened intervals or scanty bleeding
(N91.3-N91.5)
shortened intervals or excessive
bleeding (N92.1)

● **N93**   Other abnormal uterine and vaginal bleeding
    Excludes1   neonatal vaginal hemorrhage (P54.6)
precocious puberty (menstruation) (E30.1)
pseudomenses (P54.6)

N93.0   Postcoital and contact bleeding ♀

N93.8   Other specified abnormal uterine and vaginal bleeding ♀
Dysfunctional or functional uterine or vaginal bleeding
NOS

N93.9   Abnormal uterine and vaginal bleeding, unspecified ♀

● **N94**   Pain and other conditions associated with female genital organs
and menstrual cycle

N94.0   Mittelschmerz ♀
Ovulation pain

N94.1   Dyspareunia ♀
Painful intercourse/coitus

    Excludes1   psychogenic dyspareunia (F52.6)

N94.2   Vaginismus ♀
Vagina tightness

    Excludes1   psychogenic vaginismus (F52.5)

N94.3   Premenstrual tension syndrome ♀
AKA: PMS
Premenstrual dysphoric disorder

    Code also associated menstrual migraine (G43.82-,
G43.83-)

N94.4　**Primary dysmenorrhea** ♀
Lifelong painful menstruation

N94.5　**Secondary dysmenorrhea** ♀
Later onset of painful menstruation

N94.6　**Dysmenorrhea, unspecified** ♀
　　　　Excludes1　psychogenic dysmenorrhea (F45.8)

● N94.8　**Other specified conditions associated with female genital organs and menstrual cycle**

　● N94.81　**Vulvodynia**
　　　　N94.810　**Vulvar vestibulitis** ♀
　　　　N94.818　**Other vulvodynia** ♀
　　　　N94.819　**Vulvodynia, unspecified** ♀
　　　　　　　　Vulvodynia NOS

　　　N94.89　**Other specified conditions associated with female genital organs and menstrual cycle** ♀

N94.9　**Unspecified condition associated with female genital organs and menstrual cycle** ♀

● N95　**Menopausal and other perimenopausal disorders**
　　　Menopausal and other perimenopausal disorders due to naturally occurring (age-related) menopause and perimenopause
　　　Excludes1　excessive bleeding in the premenopausal period (N92.4)
　　　　　　　　menopausal and perimenopausal disorders due to artificial or premature menopause (E89.4-, E28.31-)
　　　　　　　　premature menopause (E28.31-)
　　　Excludes2　postmenopausal osteoporosis (M81.0-)
　　　　　　　　postmenopausal osteoporosis with current pathological fracture (M80.0-)
　　　　　　　　postmenopausal urethritis (N34.2)

N95.0　**Postmenopausal bleeding** ♀

N95.1　**Menopausal and female climacteric states** ♀
　　　Symptoms such as flushing, sleeplessness, headache, lack of concentration, associated with natural (age-related) menopause
　　　Use additional code for associated symptoms
　　　Excludes1　asymptomatic menopausal state (Z78.0)
　　　　　　　　symptoms associated with artificial menopause (E89.41)
　　　　　　　　symptoms associated with premature menopause (E28.310)

N95.2　**Postmenopausal atrophic vaginitis** ♀
　　　Senile (atrophic) vaginitis

N95.8　**Other specified menopausal and perimenopausal disorders** ♀

N95.9　**Unspecified menopausal and perimenopausal disorder** ♀

N96　**Recurrent pregnancy loss** ♀
　　　Investigation or care in a nonpregnant woman with history of recurrent pregnancy loss
　　　Excludes1　recurrent pregnancy loss with current pregnancy (O26.2-)

● N97　**Female infertility**
　　　Includes　inability to achieve a pregnancy sterility, female NOS
　　　Excludes1　female infertility associated with:
　　　　　　　　hypopituitarism (E23.0)
　　　　　　　　Stein-Leventhal syndrome (E28.2)
　　　Excludes2　incompetence of cervix uteri (N88.3)

N97.0　**Female infertility associated with anovulation** ♀

N97.1　**Female infertility of tubal origin** ♀
　　　Female infertility associated with congenital anomaly of tube
　　　Female infertility due to tubal block
　　　Female infertility due to tubal occlusion
　　　Female infertility due to tubal stenosis

N97.2　**Female infertility of uterine origin** ♀
　　　Female infertility associated with congenital anomaly of uterus
　　　Female infertility due to nonimplantation of ovum

N97.8　**Female infertility of other origin** ♀

N97.9　**Female infertility, unspecified** ♀

● N98　**Complications associated with artificial fertilization**
　　　(Ex) **For category N98 CC codes unless otherwise indicated:** D78.81-D78.89, E36.8, E89.810-E89.89, H59.011-H59.019, H59.031-H59.099, H59.811-H59.89, H95.811-H95.89, I97.3, L76.81-L76.82, M96.89, N98.1-N98.9, T81.82X[A], T81.89X-T81.9XX[A]

N98.0　**Infection associated with artificial insemination** ♀ 🐾
　　　(Ex) N98.0, T80.211-T80.29X[A], T82.7XX[A], T88.0XX[A]

N98.1　**Hyperstimulation of ovaries** ♀ 🐾
　　　Hyperstimulation of ovaries NOS
　　　Hyperstimulation of ovaries associated with induced ovulation

N98.2　**Complications of attempted introduction of fertilized ovum following in vitro fertilization** ♀ 🐾

N98.3　**Complications of attempted introduction of embryo in embryo transfer** ♀ 🐾

N98.8　**Other complications associated with artificial fertilization** ♀ 🐾

N98.9　**Complication associated with artificial fertilization, unspecified** ♀ 🐾

INTRAOPERATIVE AND POSTPROCEDURAL COMPLICATIONS AND DISORDERS OF GENITOURINARY SYSTEM, NOT ELSEWHERE CLASSIFIED (N99)

● N99　**Intraoperative and postprocedural complications and disorders of genitourinary system, not elsewhere classified**
　　　Excludes2　irradiation cystitis (N30.4-)
　　　　　　　　postoophorectomy osteoporosis with current pathological fracture (M80.8-)
　　　　　　　　postoophorectomy osteoporosis without current pathological fracture (M81.8) ◀▥

N99.0　**Postprocedural (acute) (chronic) kidney failure**
　　　Use additional code to type of kidney disease

● N99.1　**Postprocedural urethral stricture**
　　　Postcatheterization urethral stricture

　● N99.11　**Postprocedural urethral stricture, male**
　　　　N99.110　**Postprocedural urethral stricture, male, meatal** ♂
　　　　N99.111　**Postprocedural bulbous urethral stricture**
　　　　N99.112　**Postprocedural membranous urethral stricture**
　　　　N99.113　**Postprocedural anterior urethral stricture**
　　　　N99.114　**Postprocedural urethral stricture, male, unspecified** ♂

　　　N99.12　**Postprocedural urethral stricture, female** ♀

N99.2　**Postprocedural adhesions of vagina** ♀

N99.3　**Prolapse of vaginal vault after hysterectomy** ♀

N99.4　**Postprocedural pelvic peritoneal adhesions**
　　　Excludes2　pelvic peritoneal adhesions NOS (N73.6)
　　　　　　　　postinfective pelvic peritoneal adhesions (N73.6)

N Newborn Age: 0　　**P** Pediatric Age: 0–17　　**M** Maternity DX: 12–55　　**A** Adult Age: 15–124　　♀ Females Only　　♂ Males Only

🐾 Complication\Comorbidity　　🐾 Major C\C　　(Ex) CC/MCC Exclusions　　🐾 Present on Admission Requirement　　🐾 Hospital-Acquired Condition

1191

● **N99.5   Complications of stoma of urinary tract**
      Excludes2 mechanical complication of urinary
               (indwelling) catheter (T83.0-)

● **N99.51   Complication of cystostomy**
    N99.510   Cystostomy hemorrhage 🔗
         (Ex:) D78.81-D78.89, E36.8, E89.810-E89.89,
             H59.011-H59.019, H59.031-H59.099,
             H59.811-H59.89, H95.811-H95.89, I97.3,
             L76.81-L76.82, M96.89, N32.89, N33,
             N98.1-N98.9, N99.510-N99.518, T81.82X[A],
             T81.89X-T81.9XX[A], T83.010[A], T83.020[A],
             T83.030[A], T83.090[A], T83.110-T83.29X[A],
             T83.410-T83.6XX[A], T83.718[A],
             T83.728-T83.9XX[A], T85.310-T85.311[A],
             T85.320-T85.321[A], T85.390-T85.391[A],
             T85.510-T85.9XX[A], T86.820-T86.829,
             T86.842-T86.849

    N99.511   Cystostomy infection 🔗
         (Ex:) D78.81-D78.89, E36.8, E89.810-E89.89,
              H59.011-H59.019, H59.031-H59.099,
              H59.811-H59.89, H95.811-H95.89, I97.3,
             L76.81-L76.82, M96.89, N32.89, N33, N39.0,
             N98.1-N98.9, N99.510-N99.518, T81.82X[A],
             T81.89X-T81.9XX[A], T83.010[A], T83.020[A],
             T83.030[A], T83.090[A], T83.110-T83.29X[A],
             T83.410-T83.6XX[A], T83.718[A],
             T83.728-T83.9XX[A], T85.310-T85.311[A],
             T85.320-T85.321[A], T85.390-T85.391[A],
             T85.510-T85.9XX[A], T86.842-T86.849

    N99.512   Cystostomy malfunction 🔗
         (Ex:) D78.81-D78.89, E36.8, E89.810-E89.89,
              H59.011-H59.019, H59.031-H59.099,
              H59.811-H59.89, H95.811-H95.89, I97.3,
             L76.81-L76.82, M96.89, N32.89, N33,
             N98.1-N98.9, N99.510-N99.518, T81.82XA,
             T81.89XA-T81.9XXA, T83.010[A], T83.020[A],
             T83.030[A], T83.090[A], T83.110-T83.29X[A],
             T83.410-T83.6XX[A], T83.718[A],
             T83.728-T83.9XX[A]

    N99.518   Other cystostomy complication 🔗
         (Ex:) See N99.510

● **N99.52   Complication of other external stoma of urinary tract**
    N99.520   Hemorrhage of other external stoma of urinary tract
    N99.521   Infection of other external stoma of urinary tract
    N99.522   Malfunction of other external stoma of urinary tract
    N99.528   Other complication of other external stoma of urinary tract

● **N99.53   Complication of other stoma of urinary tract**
    N99.530   Hemorrhage of other stoma of urinary tract
    N99.531   Infection of other stoma of urinary tract
    N99.532   Malfunction of other stoma of urinary tract
    N99.538   Other complication of other stoma of urinary tract

● **N99.6   Intraoperative hemorrhage and hematoma of a genitourinary system organ or structure complicating a procedure**
      Excludes1 intraoperative hemorrhage and
               hematoma of a genitourinary system
               organ or structure due to accidental
               puncture or laceration during a
               procedure (N99.7-)
      (Ex:) **For category N99.6 CC codes:** H95.811-H95.89, I85.01, I85.11, I97.3,
        K21.9, K22.8, K23-K25.0, K25.2, K25.4, K25.6, K26.0, K26.2, K26.4, K26.6,
        K27.0, K27.2, K27.4, K27.6, K28.0, K28.2, K28.4, K28.6, K29.01, K29.21,
        K29.31, K29.41, K29.51, K29.61, K29.71, K29.81, K29.91, K31.811,
        K55.21, K57.01, K57.11, K57.13, K57.21, K57.31, K57.33, K57.41, K57.51,
        K57.53, K57.81, K57.91, K57.93, K62.5, K92.0-K92.2, M96.89,
        N98.1-N98.9, N99.61-N99.62, N99.820-N99.821, P54.1-P54.3,
        T81.10X-T81.19X[A], T81.82X[A], T81.89X-T81.9XX[A]

    N99.61   Intraoperative hemorrhage and hematoma of a genitourinary system organ or structure complicating a genitourinary system procedure 🔗
    N99.62   Intraoperative hemorrhage and hematoma of a genitourinary system organ or structure complicating other procedure 🔗

● **N99.7   Accidental puncture and laceration of a genitourinary system organ or structure during a procedure**
    (Ex:) **For category N99.7 CC codes:** D78.11-D78.12, D78.81-D78.89,
      E36.11-E36.8, E89.810-E89.89, G96.11, G97.41-G97.49, H59.011-H59.019,
      H59.031-H59.099, H59.211-H59.229, H59.811-H59.89, H95.31-H95.32,
      H95.811-H95.89, I97.3, I97.51-I97.52, J95.71-J95.72, K91.71-K91.72,
      L76.11-L76.12, L76.81-L76.82, M96.820-M96.821, M96.89, N98.1-N98.9,
      N99.71-N99.72, T81.82X[A], T81.89X-T81.9XX[A]

    N99.71   Accidental puncture and laceration of a genitourinary system organ or structure during a genitourinary system procedure 🔗
    N99.72   Accidental puncture and laceration of a genitourinary system organ or structure during other procedure 🔗

● **N99.8   Other intraoperative and postprocedural complications and disorders of genitourinary system**
    N99.81   Other intraoperative complications of genitourinary system
  ● **N99.82   Postprocedural hemorrhage and hematoma of a genitourinary system organ or structure following a procedure**
      (Ex:) **For category N99.82 CC codes:** See N99.6
    N99.820   Postprocedural hemorrhage and hematoma of a genitourinary system organ or structure following a genitourinary system procedure 🔗
    N99.821   Postprocedural hemorrhage and hematoma of a genitourinary system organ or structure following other procedure 🔗

    N99.83   Residual ovary syndrome ♀
    N99.89   Other postprocedural complications and disorders of genitourinary system

◀ New   ◀▥ Revised   ~~deleted~~ Deleted   Excludes 1   Excludes 2   Includes   Use additional   Code first   Code also   Unspecified
OGCR Official Guidelines   ● Unacceptable Principal Diagnosis   X Assign placeholder X   ● Use Additional Character(s)   ▶ Manifestation Code   **Coding Clinic**

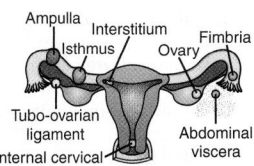

Figure 15-1 Implantation sites of ectopic pregnancy.

Item 15–1 Ectopic pregnancy most often occurs in the fallopian tube. Pregnancy outside the uterus may end in a lifethreatening rupture.

OGCR See Section I.C.15.

Chapter 15 Pregnancy, Childbirth, and the Puerperium

(See Plate 375 on page 52.)

CHAPTER 15

PREGNANCY, CHILDBIRTH AND THE PUERPERIUM (O00-O9A)

Note: CODES FROM THIS CHAPTER ARE FOR USE ONLY ON MATERNAL RECORDS, NEVER ON NEWBORN RECORDS

Codes from this chapter are for use for conditions related to or aggravated by the pregnancy, childbirth, or by the puerperium (maternal causes or obstetric causes)

Trimesters are counted from the first day of the last menstrual period. They are defined as follows:

1st trimester - less than 14 weeks 0 days

2nd trimester - 14 weeks 0 days to less than 28 weeks 0 days

3rd trimester - 28 weeks 0 days until delivery

Use additional code from category Z3A, Weeks of gestation, to identify the specific week of the pregnancy

Excludes1 supervision of normal pregnancy (Z34.-)

Excludes2 mental and behavioral disorders associated with the puerperium (F53)
obstetrical tetanus (A34)
postpartum necrosis of pituitary gland (E23.0)
puerperal osteomalacia (M83.0)

This chapter contains the following blocks:

O00-O08	Pregnancy with abortive outcome
O09	Supervision of high risk pregnancy
O10-O16	Edema, proteinuria and hypertensive disorders in pregnancy, childbirth and the puerperium
O20-O29	Other maternal disorders predominantly related to pregnancy
O30-O48	Maternal care related to the fetus and amniotic cavity and possible delivery problems
O60-O77	Complications of labor and delivery
O80, O82	Encounter for delivery
O85-O92	Complications predominantly related to the puerperium
O94-O9A	Other obstetric conditions, not elsewhere classified

PREGNANCY WITH ABORTIVE OUTCOME (O00-O08)

Excludes1 continuing pregnancy in multiple gestation after abortion of one fetus or more (O31.1-, O31.3-)

● **O00** **Ectopic pregnancy**

     Includes ruptured ectopic pregnancy

Use additional code from category O08 to identify any associated complication

Ⓔⓧ **For category O00 CC codes:** O00.0-O00.9

     O00.0 **Abdominal pregnancy** ♀ 🦠   M

         Excludes1 maternal care for viable fetus in abdominal pregnancy (O36.7-)

Item 15–2 A **hydatidiform** mole is a benign tumor of the placenta. The tumor secretes a hormone, chorionic gonadotropic hormone (CGH), that indicates a positive pregnancy test.

     O00.1 **Tubal pregnancy** ♀ 🦠   M
         Fallopian pregnancy
         Rupture of (fallopian) tube due to pregnancy
         Tubal abortion

     O00.2 **Ovarian pregnancy** ♀ 🦠   M

     O00.8 **Other ectopic pregnancy** ♀ 🦠   M
         Cervical pregnancy
         Cornual pregnancy
         Intraligamentous pregnancy
         Mural pregnancy

     O00.9 **Ectopic pregnancy, unspecified** ♀ 🦠   M

● **O01** **Hydatidiform mole**

     Use additional code from category O08 to identify any associated complication

         Excludes1 chorioadenoma (destruens) (D39.2)
                 malignant hydatidiform mole (D39.2)

     O01.0 **Classical hydatidiform mole** ♀   M
         Complete hydatidiform mole

     O01.1 **Incomplete and partial hydatidiform mole** ♀   M

     O01.9 **Hydatidiform mole, unspecified** ♀   M
         Trophoblastic disease NOS
         Vesicular mole NOS

● **O02** **Other abnormal products of conception**

     Use additional code from category O08 to identify any associated complication

         Excludes1 papyraceous fetus (O31.0-)

     O02.0 **Blighted ovum and nonhydatidiform mole** ♀   M
         Carneous mole   Molar pregnancy NEC
         Fleshy mole   Pathological ovum
         Intrauterine mole NOS

     O02.1 **Missed abortion** ♀   M
         Early fetal death, before completion of 20 weeks of gestation, with retention of dead fetus

         Excludes1 failed induced abortion (O07.-)
                 fetal death (intrauterine) (late) (O36.4)
                 missed abortion with blighted ovum (O02.0)
                 missed abortion with hydatidiform mole (O01.-)
                 missed abortion with nonhydatidiform (O02.0)
                 missed abortion with other abnormal products of conception (O02.8-)
                 missed delivery (O36.4)
                 stillbirth (P95)

● **O02.8** **Other specified abnormal products of conception**

         Excludes1 abnormal products of conception with blighted ovum (O02.0)
                 abnormal products of conception with hydatidiform mole (O01.-)
                 abnormal products of conception with nonhydatidiform mole (O02.0)

     O02.81 **Inappropriate change in quantitative human chorionic gonadotropin (hCG) in early pregnancy** ♀   M
         Biochemical pregnancy
         Chemical pregnancy
         Inappropriate level of quantitative human chorionic gonadotropin (hCG) for gestational age in early pregnancy

     O02.89 **Other abnormal products of conception** ♀   M

     O02.9 **Abnormal product of conception, unspecified** ♀   M

N Newborn Age: 0   **P** Pediatric Age: 0–17   **M** Maternity DX: 12–55   **A** Adult Age: 15–124   ♀ Females Only   ♂ Males Only

🦠 Complication\Comorbidity   🦠 Major C\C   Ⓔⓧ CC/MCC Exclusions   🦠 Present on Admission Requirement   🦠 Hospital-Acquired Condition

1193

● O03   **Spontaneous abortion**

Note: Incomplete abortion includes retained products of conception following spontaneous abortion.

Includes   miscarriage

O03.0   **Genital tract and pelvic infection following incomplete spontaneous abortion** ♀ 🦠   M

Endometritis following incomplete spontaneous abortion
Oophoritis following incomplete spontaneous abortion
Parametritis following incomplete spontaneous abortion
Pelvic peritonitis following incomplete spontaneous abortion
Salpingitis following incomplete spontaneous abortion
Salpingo-oophoritis following incomplete spontaneous abortion

Excludes1   sepsis following incomplete spontaneous abortion (O03.37)
urinary tract infection following incomplete spontaneous abortion (O03.38)

O03.1   **Delayed or excessive hemorrhage following incomplete spontaneous abortion** ♀   M

Afibrinogenemia following incomplete spontaneous abortion
Defibrination syndrome following incomplete spontaneous abortion
Hemolysis following incomplete spontaneous abortion
Intravascular coagulation following incomplete spontaneous abortion

O03.2   **Embolism following incomplete spontaneous abortion** ♀ 🦠   M

Air embolism following incomplete spontaneous abortion
Amniotic fluid embolism following incomplete spontaneous abortion
Blood-clot embolism following incomplete spontaneous abortion
Embolism NOS following incomplete spontaneous abortion
Fat embolism following incomplete spontaneous abortion
Pulmonary embolism following incomplete spontaneous abortion
Pyemic embolism following incomplete spontaneous abortion
Septic or septicopyemic embolism following incomplete spontaneous abortion
Soap embolism following incomplete spontaneous abortion

● O03.3   **Other and unspecified complications following incomplete spontaneous abortion**
(Ex) G70.1-G72.3, G72.81-G73.7

O03.30   **Unspecified** complication following incomplete spontaneous abortion ♀ 🦠   M

O03.31   **Shock following incomplete spontaneous abortion** ♀ 🦠   M

Circulatory collapse following incomplete spontaneous abortion
Shock (postprocedural) following incomplete spontaneous abortion

Excludes1   shock due to infection following incomplete spontaneous abortion (O03.37)

O03.32   **Renal failure following incomplete spontaneous abortion** ♀ 🦠   M

Kidney failure (acute) following incomplete spontaneous abortion
Oliguria following incomplete spontaneous abortion
Renal shutdown following incomplete spontaneous abortion
Renal tubular necrosis following incomplete spontaneous abortion
Uremia following incomplete spontaneous abortion

O03.33   **Metabolic disorder following incomplete spontaneous abortion** ♀ 🦠   M

O03.34   **Damage to pelvic organs following incomplete spontaneous abortion** ♀ 🦠   M

Laceration, perforation, tear or chemical damage of bladder following incomplete spontaneous abortion
Laceration, perforation, tear or chemical damage of bowel following incomplete spontaneous abortion
Laceration, perforation, tear or chemical damage of broad ligament following incomplete spontaneous abortion
Laceration, perforation, tear or chemical damage of cervix following incomplete spontaneous abortion
Laceration, perforation, tear or chemical damage of periurethral tissue following incomplete spontaneous abortion
Laceration, perforation, tear or chemical damage of uterus following incomplete spontaneous abortion
Laceration, perforation, tear or chemical damage of vagina following incomplete spontaneous abortion

O03.35   **Other venous complications following incomplete spontaneous abortion** ♀ 🦠   M

O03.36   **Cardiac arrest following incomplete spontaneous abortion** ♀ 🦠   M

O03.37   **Sepsis following incomplete spontaneous abortion** ♀ 🦠   M

Use additional code to identify infectious agent (B95-B97)

Use additional code to identify severe sepsis, if applicable (R65.2-)

Excludes1   septic or septicopyemic embolism following incomplete spontaneous abortion (O03.2)

O03.38   **Urinary tract infection following incomplete spontaneous abortion** ♀ 🦠   M

Cystitis following incomplete spontaneous abortion

O03.39   **Incomplete spontaneous abortion with other complications** ♀ 🦠   M

O03.4   **Incomplete spontaneous abortion without complication** ♀   M

O03.5 Genital tract and pelvic infection following complete or unspecified spontaneous abortion ♀ 🦠   **M**

Endometritis following complete or unspecified spontaneous abortion

Oophoritis following complete or unspecified spontaneous abortion

Parametritis following complete or unspecified spontaneous abortion

Pelvic peritonitis following complete or unspecified spontaneous abortion

Salpingitis following complete or unspecified spontaneous abortion

Salpingo-oophoritis following complete or unspecified spontaneous abortion

Excludes1   sepsis following complete or unspecified spontaneous abortion (O03.87)
urinary tract infection following complete or unspecified spontaneous abortion (O03.88)

O03.6 Delayed or excessive hemorrhage following complete or unspecified spontaneous abortion ♀   **M**

Afibrinogenemia following complete or unspecified spontaneous abortion

Defibrination syndrome following complete or unspecified spontaneous abortion

Hemolysis following complete or unspecified spontaneous abortion

Intravascular coagulation following complete or unspecified spontaneous abortion

O03.7 Embolism following complete or unspecified spontaneous abortion ♀ 🦠   **M**

Air embolism following complete or unspecified spontaneous abortion

Amniotic fluid embolism following complete or unspecified spontaneous abortion

Blood-clot embolism following complete or unspecified spontaneous abortion

Embolism NOS following complete or unspecified spontaneous abortion

Fat embolism following complete or unspecified spontaneous abortion

Pulmonary embolism following complete or unspecified spontaneous abortion

Pyemic embolism following complete or unspecified spontaneous abortion

Septic or septicopyemic embolism following complete or unspecified spontaneous abortion

Soap embolism following complete or unspecified spontaneous abortion

●**O03.8 Other and unspecified complications following complete or unspecified spontaneous abortion**

O03.80 Unspecified complication following complete or unspecified spontaneous abortion ♀ 🦠   **M**

O03.81 Shock following complete or unspecified spontaneous abortion ♀ 🦠   **M**

Circulatory collapse following complete or unspecified spontaneous abortion

Shock (postprocedural) following complete or unspecified spontaneous abortion

Excludes1   shock due to infection following complete or unspecified spontaneous abortion (O03.87)

O03.82 Renal failure following complete or unspecified spontaneous abortion ♀ 🦠   **M**

Kidney failure (acute) following complete or unspecified spontaneous abortion

Oliguria following complete or unspecified spontaneous abortion

Renal shutdown following complete or unspecified spontaneous abortion

Renal tubular necrosis following complete or unspecified spontaneous abortion

Uremia following complete or unspecified spontaneous abortion

O03.83 Metabolic disorder following complete or unspecified spontaneous abortion ♀ 🦠   **M**

O03.84 Damage to pelvic organs following complete or unspecified spontaneous abortion ♀ 🦠   **M**

Laceration, perforation, tear or chemical damage of bladder following complete or unspecified spontaneous abortion

Laceration, perforation, tear or chemical damage of bowel following complete or unspecified spontaneous abortion

Laceration, perforation, tear or chemical damage of broad ligament following complete or unspecified spontaneous abortion

Laceration, perforation, tear or chemical damage of cervix following complete or unspecified spontaneous abortion

Laceration, perforation, tear or chemical damage of periurethral tissue following complete or unspecified spontaneous abortion

Laceration, perforation, tear or chemical damage of uterus following complete or unspecified spontaneous abortion

Laceration, perforation, tear or chemical damage of vagina following complete or unspecified spontaneous abortion

O03.85 Other venous complications following complete or unspecified spontaneous abortion ♀ 🦠   **M**

O03.86 Cardiac arrest following complete or unspecified spontaneous abortion ♀ 🦠   **M**

O03.87 Sepsis following complete or unspecified spontaneous abortion ♀ 🦠   **M**

Use additional code to identify infectious agent (B95-B97)

Use additional code to identify severe sepsis, if applicable (R65.2-)

Excludes1   septic or septicopyemic embolism following complete or unspecified spontaneous abortion (O03.7)

O03.88 Urinary tract infection following complete or unspecified spontaneous abortion ♀ 🦠   **M**

Cystitis following complete or unspecified spontaneous abortion

O03.89 Complete or unspecified spontaneous abortion with other complications ♀ 🦠   **M**

O03.9 Complete or unspecified spontaneous abortion without complication ♀   **M**

Miscarriage NOS

Spontaneous abortion NOS

N Newborn Age: 0   **P** Pediatric Age: 0–17   **M** Maternity DX: 12–55   **A** Adult Age: 15–124   ♀ Females Only   ♂ Males Only
🦠 Complication\Comorbidity   Major C\C   (Exc) CC/MCC Exclusions   Present on Admission Requirement   Hospital-Acquired Condition

1195

CHAPTER 15 (O00-O9A)

CHAPTER 15 (O00-O9A)

● **O04   Complications following (induced) termination of pregnancy**

Includes   complications following (induced) termination of pregnancy

Excludes1   encounter for elective termination of pregnancy, uncomplicated (Z33.2)

failed attempted termination of pregnancy (O07.-)

(Ex) For category O04 CC codes unless otherwise indicated: See O03.3

O04.5   Genital tract and pelvic infection following (induced) termination of pregnancy ♀ 🐾   M

Endometritis following (induced) termination of pregnancy

Oophoritis following (induced) termination of pregnancy

Parametritis following (induced) termination of pregnancy

Pelvic peritonitis following (induced) termination of pregnancy

Salpingitis following (induced) termination of pregnancy

Salpingo-oophoritis following (induced) termination of pregnancy

Excludes1   sepsis following (induced) termination of pregnancy (O04.87)

urinary tract infection following (induced) termination of pregnancy (O04.88)

O04.6   Delayed or excessive hemorrhage following (induced) termination of pregnancy ♀   M

Afibrinogenemia following (induced) termination of pregnancy

Defibrination syndrome following (induced) termination of pregnancy

Hemolysis following (induced) termination of pregnancy

Intravascular coagulation following (induced) termination of pregnancy

O04.7   Embolism following (induced) termination of pregnancy ♀ 🐾   M

Air embolism following (induced) termination of pregnancy

Amniotic fluid embolism following (induced) termination of pregnancy

Blood-clot embolism following (induced) termination of pregnancy

Embolism NOS following (induced) termination of pregnancy

Fat embolism following (induced) termination of pregnancy

Pulmonary embolism following (induced) termination of pregnancy

Pyemic embolism following (induced) termination of pregnancy

Septic or septicopyemic embolism following (induced) termination of pregnancy

Soap embolism following (induced) termination of pregnancy

● **O04.8   (Induced) termination of pregnancy with other and unspecified complications**

O04.80   (Induced) termination of pregnancy with unspecified complications ♀ 🐾   M

O04.81   Shock following (induced) termination of pregnancy ♀ 🐾   M

Circulatory collapse following (induced) termination of pregnancy

Shock (postprocedural) following (induced) termination of pregnancy

Excludes1   shock due to infection following (induced) termination of pregnancy (O04.87)

O04.82   Renal failure following (induced) termination of pregnancy ♀ 🐾   M

Kidney failure (acute) following (induced) termination of pregnancy

Oliguria following (induced) termination of pregnancy

Renal shutdown following (induced) termination of pregnancy

Renal tubular necrosis following (induced) termination of pregnancy

Uremia following (induced) termination of pregnancy

O04.83   Metabolic disorder following (induced) termination of pregnancy ♀ 🐾   M

O04.84   Damage to pelvic organs following (induced) termination of pregnancy ♀ 🐾   M

Laceration, perforation, tear or chemical damage of bladder following (induced) termination of pregnancy

Laceration, perforation, tear or chemical damage of bowel following (induced) termination of pregnancy

Laceration, perforation, tear or chemical damage of broad ligament following (induced) termination of pregnancy

Laceration, perforation, tear or chemical damage of cervix following (induced) termination of pregnancy

Laceration, perforation, tear or chemical damage of periurethral tissue following (induced) termination of pregnancy

Laceration, perforation, tear or chemical damage of uterus following (induced) termination of pregnancy

Laceration, perforation, tear or chemical damage of vagina following (induced) termination of pregnancy

O04.85   Other venous complications following (induced) termination of pregnancy ♀ 🐾   M

O04.86   Cardiac arrest following (induced) termination of pregnancy ♀ 🐾   M

O04.87   Sepsis following (induced) termination of pregnancy ♀ 🐾   M

Use additional code to identify infectious agent (B95-B97)

Use additional code to identify severe sepsis, if applicable (R65.2-)

Excludes1   septic or septicopyemic embolism following (induced) termination of pregnancy (O04.7)

(Ex) O03.0-O07.4, O20.0-O20.9, O25.10-O25.53, O26.10-O26.13, O26.30-O26.43, O26.63-O26.819, O26.841-O26.86, O26.891-O26.93, O29.011-O29.93, O35.7XX0-O35.7XX9, O44.00-O44.13, O45.8X1-O45.93, O75.4, O75.81, O75.89-O75.9, O80, O90.89, O99.111-O99.285, O99.330-O99.335, O99.350-O99.355, O99.511-O99.73, O99.820-O99.825, O99.840-O9A.53, Z33.2

O04.88   Urinary tract infection following (induced) termination of pregnancy ♀ 🐾   M

Cystitis following (induced) termination of pregnancy

O04.89   (Induced) termination of pregnancy with other complications ♀ 🐾   M

◀ New   ◀▥ Revised   ~~deleted~~ Deleted   Excludes 1   Excludes 2   Includes   Use additional   Code first   Code also   Unspecified

OGCR Official Guidelines   ● Unacceptable Principal Diagnosis   X Assign placeholder X   ● Use Additional Character(s)   ▶ Manifestation Code   **Coding Clinic**

● **O07 Failed attempted termination of pregnancy**

     | Includes | failure of attempted induction of termination of pregnancy
                             incomplete elective abortion

     | Excludes1 | incomplete spontaneous abortion (O03.0-)

O07.0 Genital tract and pelvic infection following failed attempted termination of pregnancy ♀ 🦠   M

     Endometritis following failed attempted termination of pregnancy

     Oophoritis following failed attempted termination of pregnancy

     Parametritis following failed attempted termination of pregnancy

     Pelvic peritonitis following failed attempted termination of pregnancy

     Salpingitis following failed attempted termination of pregnancy

     Salpingo-oophoritis following failed attempted termination of pregnancy

     | Excludes1 | sepsis following failed attempted termination of pregnancy (O07.37)
                     urinary tract infection following failed attempted termination of pregnancy (O07.38)

     (Ex) 003.0-007.4, 020.0-020.9, 025.10-025.3, 026.10-026.13, 026.30-026.43, 026.63-026.819, 026.841-026.86, 026.891-026.93, 029.011-029.93, 035.7XX0-035.7XX9, 044.00-044.13, 045.8X1-045.93, 075.4, 075.81, 075.89-075.9, 080, 090.89, 099.111-099.285, 099.330-099.335, 099.350-099.355, 099.511-099.73, 099.820-099.825, 099.840-09A.53, Z33.2

O07.1 Delayed or excessive hemorrhage following failed attempted termination of pregnancy ♀ 🦠   M

     Afibrinogenemia following failed attempted termination of pregnancy

     Defibrination syndrome following failed attempted termination of pregnancy

     Hemolysis following failed attempted termination of pregnancy

     Intravascular coagulation following failed attempted termination of pregnancy

     (Ex) 003.0-007.4, 020.0-020.9, 025.10-025.3, 026.10-026.13, 026.30-026.43, 026.63-026.819, 026.841-026.86, 026.891-026.93, 029.011-029.93, 035.7XX0-035.7XX9, 044.00-044.13, 045.8X1-045.93, 075.4, 075.81, 075.89-075.9, 080, 090.89, 099.111-099.285, 099.330-099.335, 099.350-099.355, 099.511-099.73, 099.820-099.825, 099.840-09A.53, Z33.2

O07.2 Embolism following failed attempted termination of pregnancy ♀ 🦠   M

     Air embolism following failed attempted termination of pregnancy

     Amniotic fluid embolism following failed attempted termination of pregnancy

     Blood-clot embolism following failed attempted termination of pregnancy

     Embolism NOS following failed attempted termination of pregnancy

     Fat embolism following failed attempted termination of pregnancy

     Pulmonary embolism following failed attempted termination of pregnancy

     Pyemic embolism following failed attempted termination of pregnancy

     Septic or septicopyemic embolism following failed attempted termination of pregnancy

     Soap embolism following failed attempted termination of pregnancy

     (Ex) 003.0-007.4, 020.0-020.9, 025.10-025.3, 026.10-026.13, 026.30-026.43, 026.63-026.819, 026.841-026.86, 026.891-026.93, 029.011-029.93, 035.7XX0-035.7XX9, 044.00-044.13, 045.8X1-045.93, 075.4, 075.81, 075.89-075.9, 080, 090.89, 099.111-099.285, 099.330-099.335, 099.350-099.355, 099.511-099.73, 099.820-099.825, 099.840-09A.53, Z33.2

● **O07.3 Failed attempted termination of pregnancy with other and unspecified complications**

O07.30 Failed attempted termination of pregnancy with unspecified complications ♀ 🦠   M

     (Ex) See 000

O07.31 Shock following failed attempted termination of pregnancy ♀ 🦠   M

     Circulatory collapse following failed attempted termination of pregnancy

     Shock (postprocedural) following failed attempted termination of pregnancy

     | Excludes1 | shock due to infection following failed attempted termination of pregnancy (O07.37)

     (Ex) 003.0-007.4, 020.0-020.9, 025.10-025.3, 026.10-026.13, 026.30-026.43, 026.63-026.819, 026.841-026.86, 026.891-026.93, 029.011-029.93, 035.7XX0-035.7XX9, 044.00-044.13, 045.8X1-045.93, 075.4, 075.81, 075.89-075.9, 080, 090.89, 099.111-099.285, 099.330-099.335, 099.350-099.355, 099.511-099.73, 099.820-099.825, 099.840-09A.53, Z33.2

O07.32 Renal failure following failed attempted termination of pregnancy ♀ 🦠   M

     Kidney failure (acute) following failed attempted termination of pregnancy

     Oliguria following failed attempted termination of pregnancy

     Renal shutdown following failed attempted termination of pregnancy

     Renal tubular necrosis following failed attempted termination of pregnancy

     Uremia following failed attempted termination of pregnancy

     (Ex) 003.0-007.4, 020.0-020.9, 025.10-025.3, 026.10-026.13, 026.30-026.43, 026.63-026.819, 026.841-026.86, 026.891-026.93, 029.011-029.93, 035.7XX0-035.7XX9, 044.00-044.13, 045.8X1-045.93, 075.4, 075.81, 075.89-075.9, 080, 090.89, 099.111-099.285, 099.330-099.335, 099.350-099.355, 099.511-099.73, 099.820-099.825, 099.840-09A.53, Z33.2

O07.33 Metabolic disorder following failed attempted termination of pregnancy ♀ 🦠   M

     (Ex) See 003.3

O07.34 Damage to pelvic organs following failed attempted termination of pregnancy ♀ 🦠   M

     Laceration, perforation, tear or chemical damage of bladder following failed attempted termination of pregnancy

     Laceration, perforation, tear or chemical damage of bowel following failed attempted termination of pregnancy

     Laceration, perforation, tear or chemical damage of broad ligament following failed attempted termination of pregnancy

     Laceration, perforation, tear or chemical damage of cervix following failed attempted termination of pregnancy

     Laceration, perforation, tear or chemical damage of periurethral tissue following failed attempted termination of pregnancy

     Laceration, perforation, tear or chemical damage of uterus following failed attempted termination of pregnancy

     Laceration, perforation, tear or chemical damage of vagina following failed attempted termination of pregnancy

     (Ex) 003.0-007.4, 020.0-020.9, 025.10-025.3, 026.10-026.13, 026.30-026.43, 026.63-026.819, 026.841-026.86, 026.891-026.93, 029.011-029.93, 035.7XX0-035.7XX9, 044.00-044.13, 045.8X1-045.93, 075.4, 075.81, 075.89-075.9, 080, 090.89, 099.111-099.285, 099.330-099.335, 099.350-099.355, 099.511-099.73, 099.820-099.825, 099.840-09A.53, Z33.2

CHAPTER 15 (O00-O9A)

N Newborn Age: 0   **P** Pediatric Age: 0–17   **M** Maternity DX: 12–55   **A** Adult Age: 15–124   ♀ Females Only   ♂ Males Only

🦠 Complication\Comorbidity   🦠 Major C\C   (Ex) CC/MCC Exclusions   🦠 Present on Admission Requirement   🦠 Hospital-Acquired Condition

1197

CHAPTER 15 (O00-O9A)

O07.35 Other venous complications following failed attempted termination of pregnancy ♀ 🐾 **M**
(Ex:) See O03.3

O07.36 Cardiac arrest following failed attempted termination of pregnancy ♀ 🐾 **M**
(Ex:) See O03.3

O07.37 Sepsis following failed attempted termination of pregnancy ♀ 🐾 **M**
Use additional code (B95-B97), to identify infectious agent
Use additional code (R65.2-) to identify severe sepsis, if applicable
Excludes1 septic or septicopyemic embolism following failed attempted termination of pregnancy (O07.2)
(Ex:) See O07.0

O07.38 Urinary tract infection following failed attempted termination of pregnancy ♀ 🐾 **M**
Cystitis following failed attempted termination of pregnancy
(Ex:) See O03.3

O07.39 Failed attempted termination of pregnancy with other complications ♀ 🐾 **M**
(Ex:) See O03.3

O07.4 Failed attempted termination of pregnancy without complication ♀ **M**

● **O08 Complications following ectopic and molar pregnancy**
This category is for use with categories O00-O02 to identify any associated complications.
(Ex:) For category O08 CC codes unless otherwise indicated: 008.2-008.81, 008.83-008.9, 020.0-020.9, 025.10-025.3, 026.10-026.13, 026.30-026.43, 026.63-026.819, 026.841-026.86, 026.891-026.93, 029.011-029.93, 035.7XX0-035.7XX9, 044.00-044.13, 045.8X1-045.93, 075.4, 075.81, 075.89-075.9, 080, 090.89, 099.111-099.285, 099.330-099.335, 099.350-099.355, 099.511-099.73, 099.820-099.825, 099.840-09A.53

O08.0 Genital tract and pelvic infection following ectopic and molar pregnancy ♀ 🐾 **M**
Endometritis following ectopic and molar pregnancy
Oophoritis following ectopic and molar pregnancy
Parametritis following ectopic and molar pregnancy
Pelvic peritonitis following ectopic and molar pregnancy
Salpingitis following ectopic and molar pregnancy
Salpingo-oophoritis following ectopic and molar pregnancy
Excludes1 sepsis following ectopic and molar pregnancy (O08.82)
urinary tract infection (O08.83)
(Ex:) A34, 008.0, 008.2-008.9, 020.0-020.9, 025.10-025.3, 026.10-026.13, 026.30-026.43, 026.63-026.819, 026.841-026.86, 026.891-026.93, 029.011-029.93, 035.7XX0-035.7XX9, 044.00-044.13, 045.8X1-045.93, 075.4, 075.81, 075.89-075.9, 080, 090.89, 099.111-099.285, 099.330-099.335, 099.350-099.355, 099.511-099.73, 099.820-099.825, 099.840-09A.53

O08.1 Delayed or excessive hemorrhage following ectopic and molar pregnancy ♀ 🐾 **M**
Afibrinogenemia following ectopic and molar pregnancy
Defibrination syndrome following ectopic and molar pregnancy
Hemolysis following ectopic and molar pregnancy
Intravascular coagulation following ectopic and molar pregnancy
Excludes1 delayed or excessive hemorrhage due to incomplete abortion (O03.1)
(Ex:) 008.1-008.81, 008.83-008.9, 020.0-020.9, 025.10-025.3, 026.10-026.13, 026.30-026.43, 026.63-026.819, 026.841-026.86, 026.891-026.93, 029.011-029.93, 035.7XX0-035.7XX9, 044.00-044.13, 045.8X1-045.93, 075.4, 075.81, 075.89-075.9, 080, 090.89, 099.111-099.285, 099.330-099.335, 099.350-099.355, 099.511-099.73, 099.820-099.825, 099.840-09A.53

O08.2 Embolism following ectopic and molar pregnancy ♀ 🐾 M
Air embolism following ectopic and molar pregnancy
Amniotic fluid embolism following ectopic and molar pregnancy
Blood-clot embolism following ectopic and molar pregnancy
Embolism NOS following ectopic and molar pregnancy
Fat embolism following ectopic and molar pregnancy
Pulmonary embolism following ectopic and molar pregnancy
Pyemic embolism following ectopic and molar pregnancy
Septic or septicopyemic embolism following ectopic and molar pregnancy
Soap embolism following ectopic and molar pregnancy

O08.3 Shock following ectopic and molar pregnancy ♀ 🐾 **M**
Circulatory collapse following ectopic and molar pregnancy
Shock (postprocedural) following ectopic and molar pregnancy
Excludes1 shock due to infection following ectopic and molar pregnancy (O08.82)

O08.4 Renal failure following ectopic and molar pregnancy ♀ 🐾 **M**
Kidney failure (acute) following ectopic and molar pregnancy
Oliguria following ectopic and molar pregnancy
Renal shutdown following ectopic and molar pregnancy
Renal tubular necrosis following ectopic and molar pregnancy
Uremia following ectopic and molar pregnancy

O08.5 Metabolic disorders following an ectopic and molar pregnancy ♀ 🐾 **M**

O08.6 Damage to pelvic organs and tissues following an ectopic and molar pregnancy ♀ 🐾 **M**
Laceration, perforation, tear or chemical damage of bladder following an ectopic and molar pregnancy
Laceration, perforation, tear or chemical damage of bowel following an ectopic and molar pregnancy
Laceration, perforation, tear or chemical damage of broad ligament following an ectopic and molar pregnancy
Laceration, perforation, tear or chemical damage of cervix following an ectopic and molar pregnancy
Laceration, perforation, tear or chemical damage of periurethral tissue following an ectopic and molar pregnancy
Laceration, perforation, tear or chemical damage of uterus following an ectopic and molar pregnancy
Laceration, perforation, tear or chemical damage of vagina following an ectopic and molar pregnancy

O08.7 Other venous complications following an ectopic and molar pregnancy 🐾 **M**

● **O08.8 Other complications following an ectopic and molar pregnancy**
O08.81 Cardiac arrest following an ectopic and molar pregnancy ♀ 🐾 **M**
O08.82 Sepsis following ectopic and molar pregnancy ♀ 🐾 **M**
Use additional code (B95-B97), to identify infectious agent
Use additional code (R65.2-) to identify severe sepsis, if applicable
Excludes1 septic or septicopyemic embolism following ectopic and molar pregnancy (O08.2)
(Ex:) See O08.0

O08.83 Urinary tract infection following an ectopic and molar pregnancy ♀ 🐾 **M**
Cystitis following an ectopic and molar pregnancy

O08.89 Other complications following an ectopic and molar pregnancy ♀ 🐾 **M**

O08.9 Unspecified complication following an ectopic and molar pregnancy ♀ 🐾 **M**

SUPERVISION OF HIGH RISK PREGNANCY (O09)

● O09   Supervision of high risk pregnancy

   ● O09.0   Supervision of pregnancy with history of infertility

     ● O09.00   Supervision of pregnancy with history of infertility, unspecified trimester ♀   M

     ● O09.01   Supervision of pregnancy with history of infertility, first trimester ♀   M

     ● O09.02   Supervision of pregnancy with history of infertility, second trimester ♀   M

     ● O09.03   Supervision of pregnancy with history of infertility, third trimester ♀   M

   ● O09.1   Supervision of pregnancy with history of ectopic or molar pregnancy

     ● O09.10   Supervision of pregnancy with history of ectopic or molar pregnancy, unspecified trimester ♀   M

     ● O09.11   Supervision of pregnancy with history of ectopic or molar pregnancy, first trimester ♀   M

     ● O09.12   Supervision of pregnancy with history of ectopic or molar pregnancy, second trimester ♀   M

     ● O09.13   Supervision of pregnancy with history of ectopic or molar pregnancy, third trimester ♀   M

   ● O09.2   Supervision of pregnancy with other poor reproductive or obstetric history

     Excludes2   pregnancy care for patient with history of recurrent pregnancy loss (O26.2-)

     ● O09.21   Supervision of pregnancy with history of pre-term labor

       ● O09.211   Supervision of pregnancy with history of pre-term labor, first trimester ♀   M

       ● O09.212   Supervision of pregnancy with history of pre-term labor, second trimester ♀   M

       ● O09.213   Supervision of pregnancy with history of pre-term labor, third trimester ♀   M

       ● O09.219   Supervision of pregnancy with history of pre-term labor, unspecified trimester ♀   M

     ● O09.29   Supervision of pregnancy with other poor reproductive or obstetric history

         Supervision of pregnancy with history of neonatal death

         Supervision of pregnancy with history of stillbirth

       ● O09.291   Supervision of pregnancy with other poor reproductive or obstetric history, first trimester ♀   M

       ● O09.292   Supervision of pregnancy with other poor reproductive or obstetric history, second trimester ♀   M

       ● O09.293   Supervision of pregnancy with other poor reproductive or obstetric history, third trimester ♀   M

       ● O09.299   Supervision of pregnancy with other poor reproductive or obstetric history, unspecified trimester ♀   M

   ● O09.3   Supervision of pregnancy with insufficient antenatal care

         Supervision of concealed pregnancy

         Supervision of hidden pregnancy

     ● O09.30   Supervision of pregnancy with insufficient antenatal care, unspecified trimester ♀   M

     ● O09.31   Supervision of pregnancy with insufficient antenatal care, first trimester ♀   M

     ● O09.32   Supervision of pregnancy with insufficient antenatal care, second trimester ♀   M

     ● O09.33   Supervision of pregnancy with insufficient antenatal care, third trimester ♀   M

   ● O09.4   Supervision of pregnancy with grand multiparity

     ● O09.40   Supervision of pregnancy with grand multiparity, unspecified trimester ♀   M

     ● O09.41   Supervision of pregnancy with grand multiparity, first trimester ♀   M

     ● O09.42   Supervision of pregnancy with grand multiparity, second trimester ♀   M

     ● O09.43   Supervision of pregnancy with grand multiparity, third trimester ♀   M

   ● O09.5   Supervision of elderly primigravida and multigravida

     Pregnancy for a female 35 years and older at expected date of delivery

     ● O09.51   Supervision of elderly primigravida

       ● O09.511   Supervision of elderly primigravida, first trimester ♀   M

       ● O09.512   Supervision of elderly primigravida, second trimester ♀   M

       ● O09.513   Supervision of elderly primigravida, third trimester ♀   M

       ● O09.519   Supervision of elderly primigravida, unspecified trimester ♀   M

     ● O09.52   Supervision of elderly multigravida

       ● O09.521   Supervision of elderly multigravida, first trimester ♀   M

       ● O09.522   Supervision of elderly multigravida, second trimester ♀   M

       ● O09.523   Supervision of elderly multigravida, third trimester ♀   M

       ● O09.529   Supervision of elderly multigravida, unspecified trimester ♀   M

   ● O09.6   Supervision of young primigravida and multigravida

     Supervision of pregnancy for a female less than 16 years old at expected date of delivery

     ● O09.61   Supervision of young primigravida

       ● O09.611   Supervision of young primigravida, first trimester ♀   M

       ● O09.612   Supervision of young primigravida, second trimester ♀   M

       ● O09.613   Supervision of young primigravida, third trimester ♀   M

       ● O09.619   Supervision of young primigravida, unspecified trimester ♀   M

     ● O09.62   Supervision of young multigravida

       ● O09.621   Supervision of young multigravida, first trimester ♀   M

       ● O09.622   Supervision of young multigravida, second trimester ♀   M

       ● O09.623   Supervision of young multigravida, third trimester ♀   M

       ● O09.629   Supervision of young multigravida, unspecified trimester ♀   M

   ● O09.7   Supervision of high risk pregnancy due to social problems

     ● O09.70   Supervision of high risk pregnancy due to social problems, unspecified trimester ♀   M

     ● O09.71   Supervision of high risk pregnancy due to social problems, first trimester ♀   M

     ● O09.72   Supervision of high risk pregnancy due to social problems, second trimester ♀   M

     ● O09.73   Supervision of high risk pregnancy due to social problems, third trimester ♀   M

CHAPTER 15 (O00-O9A)

● O09.8   Supervision of other high risk pregnancies
  ● O09.81   Supervision of pregnancy resulting from assisted reproductive technology
            Supervision of pregnancy resulting from in-vitro fertilization
    ● O09.811   Supervision of pregnancy resulting from assisted reproductive technology, first trimester ♀ 🐾   M
    ● O09.812   Supervision of pregnancy resulting from assisted reproductive technology, second trimester ♀ 🐾   M
    ● O09.813   Supervision of pregnancy resulting from assisted reproductive technology, third trimester ♀ 🐾   M
    ● O09.819   Supervision of pregnancy resulting from assisted reproductive technology, unspecified trimester ♀   M
  ● O09.82   Supervision of pregnancy with history of in utero procedure during previous pregnancy
    ● O09.821   Supervision of pregnancy with history of in utero procedure during previous pregnancy, first trimester ♀ 🐾   M
    ● O09.822   Supervision of pregnancy with history of in utero procedure during previous pregnancy, second trimester ♀ 🐾   M
    ● O09.823   Supervision of pregnancy with history of in utero procedure during previous pregnancy, third trimester ♀ 🐾   M
    ● O09.829   Supervision of pregnancy with history of in utero procedure during previous pregnancy, unspecified trimester ♀ 🐾   M
              Excludes1   supervision of pregnancy affected by in utero procedure during current pregnancy (O35.7)
  ● O09.89   Supervision of other high risk pregnancies
    ● O09.891   Supervision of other high risk pregnancies, first trimester ♀ 🐾   M
    ● O09.892   Supervision of other high risk pregnancies, second trimester ♀ 🐾   M
    ● O09.893   Supervision of other high risk pregnancies, third trimester ♀ 🐾   M
    ● O09.899   Supervision of other high risk pregnancies, unspecified trimester ♀ 🐾   M
● O09.9   Supervision of high risk pregnancy, unspecified
  ● O09.90   Supervision of high risk pregnancy, unspecified, unspecified trimester ♀ 🐾   M
  ● O09.91   Supervision of high risk pregnancy, unspecified, first trimester ♀ 🐾   M
  ● O09.92   Supervision of high risk pregnancy, unspecified, second trimester ♀ 🐾   M
  ● O09.93   Supervision of high risk pregnancy, unspecified, third trimester ♀ 🐾   M

EDEMA, PROTEINURIA AND HYPERTENSIVE DISORDERS IN PREGNANCY, CHILDBIRTH AND THE PUERPERIUM (O10-O16)

● O10   Pre-existing hypertension complicating pregnancy, childbirth and the puerperium
    Includes   pre-existing hypertension with pre-existing proteinuria complicating pregnancy, childbirth and the puerperium
    Excludes2   pre-existing hypertension with superimposed pre-eclampsia complicating pregnancy, childbirth and the puerperium (O11.-)
    (Ex:) **For category O10 CC codes:** O10.011-O12.03, O12.20-O16.9, O25.10-O26.13, O26.30-O26.43, O26.63-O26.819, O26.841-O26.86, O26.891-O26.93, O29.011-O29.93, O35.7XX0-O35.7XX9, O75.4, O75.81, O75.89-O75.9, O80, O90.89, O99.111-O99.285, O99.330-O99.335, O99.350-O99.355, O99.511-O99.73, O99.820-O99.825, O99.840-O9A.53
  ● O10.0   Pre-existing essential hypertension complicating pregnancy, childbirth and the puerperium
            Any condition in I10 specified as a reason for obstetric care during pregnancy, childbirth or the puerperium
    ● O10.01   Pre-existing essential hypertension complicating pregnancy
        O10.011   Pre-existing essential hypertension complicating pregnancy, first trimester ♀ 🐾   M
        O10.012   Pre-existing essential hypertension complicating pregnancy, second trimester ♀ 🐾   M
        O10.013   Pre-existing essential hypertension complicating pregnancy, third trimester ♀ 🐾   M
        O10.019   Pre-existing essential hypertension complicating pregnancy, unspecified trimester ♀   M
      O10.02   Pre-existing essential hypertension complicating childbirth ♀ 🐾   M
      O10.03   Pre-existing essential hypertension complicating the puerperium ♀   M
  ● O10.1   Pre-existing hypertensive heart disease complicating pregnancy, childbirth and the puerperium
            Any condition in I11 specified as a reason for obstetric care during pregnancy, childbirth or the puerperium
            Use additional code from I11 to identify the type of hypertensive heart disease
    ● O10.11   Pre-existing hypertensive heart disease complicating pregnancy
        O10.111   Pre-existing hypertensive heart disease complicating pregnancy, first trimester ♀   M
        O10.112   Pre-existing hypertensive heart disease complicating pregnancy, second trimester ♀   M
        O10.113   Pre-existing hypertensive heart disease complicating pregnancy, third trimester ♀   M
        O10.119   Pre-existing hypertensive heart disease complicating pregnancy, unspecified trimester ♀   M
      O10.12   Pre-existing hypertensive heart disease complicating childbirth ♀   M
      O10.13   Pre-existing hypertensive heart disease complicating the puerperium ♀   M

● **O10.2**   **Pre-existing hypertensive chronic kidney disease complicating pregnancy, childbirth and the puerperium**
     Any condition in I12 specified as a reason for obstetric care during pregnancy, childbirth or the puerperium
     Use additional code from I12 to identify the type of hypertensive chronic kidney disease

   ● **O10.21**   **Pre-existing hypertensive chronic kidney disease complicating pregnancy**

     O10.211   Pre-existing hypertensive chronic kidney disease complicating pregnancy, first trimester ♀   M

     O10.212   Pre-existing hypertensive chronic kidney disease complicating pregnancy, second trimester ♀   M

     O10.213   Pre-existing hypertensive chronic kidney disease complicating pregnancy, third trimester ♀   M

     O10.219   Pre-existing hypertensive chronic kidney disease complicating pregnancy, unspecified trimester ♀   M

   O10.22   Pre-existing hypertensive chronic kidney disease complicating childbirth ♀   M

   O10.23   Pre-existing hypertensive chronic kidney disease complicating the puerperium ♀   M

● **O10.3**   **Pre-existing hypertensive heart and chronic kidney disease complicating pregnancy, childbirth and the puerperium**
     Any condition in I13 specified as a reason for obstetric care during pregnancy, childbirth or the puerperium
     Use additional code from I13 to identify the type of hypertensive heart and chronic kidney disease

   ● **O10.31**   **Pre-existing hypertensive heart and chronic kidney disease complicating pregnancy**

     O10.311   Pre-existing hypertensive heart and chronic kidney disease complicating pregnancy, first trimester ♀   M

     O10.312   Pre-existing hypertensive heart and chronic kidney disease complicating pregnancy, second trimester ♀   M

     O10.313   Pre-existing hypertensive heart and chronic kidney disease complicating pregnancy, third trimester ♀   M

     O10.319   Pre-existing hypertensive heart and chronic kidney disease complicating pregnancy, unspecified trimester ♀   M

   O10.32   Pre-existing hypertensive heart and chronic kidney disease complicating childbirth ♀   M

   O10.33   Pre-existing hypertensive heart and chronic kidney disease complicating the puerperium ♀   M

● **O10.4**   **Pre-existing secondary hypertension complicating pregnancy, childbirth and the puerperium**
     Any condition in I15 specified as a reason for obstetric care during pregnancy, childbirth or the puerperium
     Use additional code from I15 to identify the type of secondary hypertension

   ● **O10.41**   **Pre-existing secondary hypertension complicating pregnancy**

     O10.411   Pre-existing secondary hypertension complicating pregnancy, first trimester ♀ 🌕   M

     O10.412   Pre-existing secondary hypertension complicating pregnancy, second trimester ♀ 🌕   M

     O10.413   Pre-existing secondary hypertension complicating pregnancy, third trimester ♀ 🌕   M

     O10.419   Pre-existing secondary hypertension complicating pregnancy, unspecified trimester ♀   M

   O10.42   Pre-existing secondary hypertension complicating childbirth ♀ 🌕   M

   O10.43   Pre-existing secondary hypertension complicating the puerperium ♀ 🌕   M

● **O10.9**   **Unspecified pre-existing hypertension complicating pregnancy, childbirth and the puerperium**

   ● **O10.91**   **Unspecified pre-existing hypertension complicating pregnancy**

     O10.911   Unspecified pre-existing hypertension complicating pregnancy, first trimester ♀ 🌕   M

     O10.912   Unspecified pre-existing hypertension complicating pregnancy, second trimester ♀ 🌕   M

     O10.913   Unspecified pre-existing hypertension complicating pregnancy, third trimester ♀ 🌕   M

     O10.919   Unspecified pre-existing hypertension complicating pregnancy, unspecified trimester ♀   M

   O10.92   Unspecified pre-existing hypertension complicating childbirth ♀ 🌕   M

   O10.93   Unspecified pre-existing hypertension complicating the puerperium ♀   M

● **O11**   **Pre-existing hypertension with pre-eclampsia**
     Includes   conditions in O10 complicated by pre-eclampsia
        pre-eclampsia superimposed pre-existing hypertension
     Use additional code from O10 to identify the type of hypertension
     (Ex) For category O11 CC codes: See O10

   O11.1   Pre-existing hypertension with pre-eclampsia, first trimester ♀ 🌕   M

   O11.2   Pre-existing hypertension with pre-eclampsia, second trimester ♀ 🌕   M

   O11.3   Pre-existing hypertension with pre-eclampsia, third trimester ♀ 🌕   M

   O11.9   Pre-existing hypertension with pre-eclampsia, unspecified trimester ♀   M

● **O12**   **Gestational [pregnancy-induced] edema and proteinuria without hypertension**
     (Ex) For category O12 CC codes: O12.11-O12.13, O12.21-O12.23, O26.831-O26.833, O90.89

   ● **O12.0**   **Gestational edema**

     O12.00   Gestational edema, unspecified trimester ♀   M

     O12.01   Gestational edema, first trimester ♀   M

     O12.02   Gestational edema, second trimester ♀   M

     O12.03   Gestational edema, third trimester ♀   M

   ● **O12.1**   **Gestational proteinuria**

     O12.10   Gestational proteinuria, unspecified trimester ♀   M

     O12.11   Gestational proteinuria, first trimester ♀ 🌕   M

     O12.12   Gestational proteinuria, second trimester ♀ 🌕   M

     O12.13   Gestational proteinuria, third trimester ♀ 🌕   M

   ● **O12.2**   **Gestational edema with proteinuria**

     O12.20   Gestational edema with proteinuria, unspecified trimester ♀   M

     O12.21   Gestational edema with proteinuria, first trimester ♀ 🌕   M
        CC when PDx is its own CC

     O12.22   Gestational edema with proteinuria, second trimester ♀ 🌕   M
        CC when PDx is its own CC

     O12.23   Gestational edema with proteinuria, third trimester ♀ 🌕   M
        CC when PDx is its own CC

N   Newborn Age: 0   P   Pediatric Age: 0–17   M   Maternity DX: 12–55   A   Adult Age: 15–124   ♀   Females Only   ♂   Males Only

🌕   Complication\Comorbidity   🌕   Major C\C   (Ex)   CC/MCC Exclusions   🌕   Present on Admission Requirement   🌕   Hospital-Acquired Condition

1201

● O13   Gestational [pregnancy-induced] hypertension without significant proteinuria
>   **Includes**   gestational hypertension NOS

O13.1   Gestational [pregnancy-induced] hypertension without significant proteinuria, first trimester ♀   M

O13.2   Gestational [pregnancy-induced] hypertension without significant proteinuria, second trimester ♀   M

O13.3   Gestational [pregnancy-induced] hypertension without significant proteinuria, third trimester ♀   M

O13.9   Gestational [pregnancy-induced] hypertension without significant proteinuria, unspecified trimester ♀   M

● O14   Pre-eclampsia
>   **Excludes1**   pre-existing hypertension with pre-eclampsia (O11)
>   (Ex) For category O14 CC codes: See O10

● O14.0   Mild to moderate pre-eclampsia
O14.00   Mild to moderate pre-eclampsia, unspecified trimester ♀   M
O14.02   Mild to moderate pre-eclampsia, second trimester ♀ 🩺   M
O14.03   Mild to moderate pre-eclampsia, third trimester ♀ 🩺   M

● O14.1   Severe pre-eclampsia
>   **Excludes1**   HELLP syndrome (O14.2-)
>   *H=hemolysis, EL=elevated liver enzymes, LP=low platelet count*
O14.10   Severe pre-eclampsia, unspecified trimester ♀   M
O14.12   Severe pre-eclampsia, second trimester ♀ 🩺   M
O14.13   Severe pre-eclampsia, third trimester ♀🩺   M

● O14.2   HELLP syndrome
>   Severe pre-eclampsia with hemolysis, elevated liver enzymes and low platelet count (HELLP)
O14.20   HELLP syndrome (HELLP), unspecified trimester ♀   M
O14.22   HELLP syndrome (HELLP), second trimester ♀ 🩺   M
O14.23   HELLP syndrome (HELLP), third trimester ♀ 🩺   M

● O14.9   Unspecified pre-eclampsia
O14.90   Unspecified pre-eclampsia, unspecified trimester ♀   M
O14.92   Unspecified pre-eclampsia, second trimester ♀ 🩺   M
O14.93   Unspecified pre-eclampsia, third trimester ♀ 🩺   M

● O15   Eclampsia
>   **Includes**   convulsions following conditions in O10-O14 and O16
>   (Ex) For category O15 CC codes: See O10

● O15.0   Eclampsia in pregnancy
O15.00   Eclampsia in pregnancy, unspecified trimester ♀   M
O15.02   Eclampsia in pregnancy, second trimester ♀ 🩺M
O15.03   Eclampsia in pregnancy, third trimester ♀ 🩺   M
O15.1   Eclampsia in labor ♀ 🩺   M
O15.2   Eclampsia in the puerperium ♀ 🩺   M
O15.9   Eclampsia, unspecified as to time period ♀   M
>   Eclampsia NOS

● O16   Unspecified maternal hypertension
>   (Ex) For category O16 CC codes: See O10
O16.1   Unspecified maternal hypertension, first trimester ♀ 🩺 M
O16.2   Unspecified maternal hypertension, second trimester ♀ 🩺   M
O16.3   Unspecified maternal hypertension, third trimester ♀ 🩺   M
O16.9   Unspecified maternal hypertension, unspecified trimester ♀   M

OTHER MATERNAL DISORDERS PREDOMINANTLY RELATED TO PREGNANCY (O20-O29)

>   **Excludes2**   maternal care related to the fetus and amniotic cavity and possible delivery problems (O30-O48)
>   maternal diseases classifiable elsewhere but complicating pregnancy, labor and delivery, and the puerperium (O98-O99)

● O20   Hemorrhage in early pregnancy
>   **Includes**   hemorrhage before completion of 20 weeks gestation
>   **Excludes1**   pregnancy with abortive outcome (O00-O08)
>   (Ex) For category O20 CC codes: O20.0-O20.9, O25.10-O25.3, O26.10-O26.13, O26.30-O26.43, O26.63-O26.819, O26.841-O26.86, O26.891-O26.93, O29.011-O29.93, O35.7XX0-O35.7XX9, O44.00-O44.13, O75.4, O75.81, O75.89-O75.9, O80, O90.89, O99.111-O99.119, O99.12-O99.285, O99.330-O99.335, O99.350-O99.355, O99.511-O99.73, O99.820-O99.825, O99.840-O9A.53

O20.0   Threatened abortion ♀ 🩺   M
>   Hemorrhage specified as due to threatened abortion
O20.8   Other hemorrhage in early pregnancy ♀   M
O20.9   Hemorrhage in early pregnancy, unspecified ♀ 🩺   M

● O21   Excessive vomiting in pregnancy
O21.0   Mild hyperemesis gravidarum ♀   M
>   Hyperemesis gravidarum, mild or unspecified, starting before the end of the 20th week of gestation
O21.1   Hyperemesis gravidarum with metabolic disturbance ♀   M
>   Hyperemesis gravidarum, starting before the end of the 20th week of gestation, with metabolic disturbance such as carbohydrate depletion
>   Hyperemesis gravidarum, starting before the end of the 20th week of gestation, with metabolic disturbance such as dehydration
>   Hyperemesis gravidarum, starting before the end of the 20th week of gestation, with metabolic disturbance such as electrolyte imbalance
O21.2   Late vomiting of pregnancy ♀   M
>   Excessive vomiting starting after 20 completed weeks of gestation
O21.8   Other vomiting complicating pregnancy ♀   M
>   Vomiting due to diseases classified elsewhere, complicating pregnancy
>   Use additional code, to identify cause
O21.9   Vomiting of pregnancy, unspecified ♀   M

● O22   Venous complications and hemorrhoids in pregnancy
>   **Excludes1**   venous complications of:
>   abortion NOS (O03.9)
>   ectopic or molar pregnancy (O08.7)
>   failed attempted abortion (O07.35)
>   induced abortion (O04.85)
>   spontaneous abortion (O03.89)
>   **Excludes2**   obstetric pulmonary embolism (O88.-)
>   venous complications and hemorrhoids of childbirth and the puerperium (O87.-)
>   (Ex) For category O22 CC codes: O22.20-O22.93, O25.10-O25.3, O26.10-O26.13, O26.30-O26.43, O26.63-O26.819, O26.841-O26.86, O26.891-O26.93, O29.011-O29.93, O35.7XX0-O35.7XX9, O75.4, O75.81, O75.89-O75.9, O80, O87.0-O87.9, O90.89, O99.111-O99.119, O99.12-O99.285, O99.330-O99.335, O99.350-O99.355, O99.511-O99.73, O99.820-O99.825, O99.840-O9A.53

● O22.0   Varicose veins of lower extremity in pregnancy
>   Varicose veins NOS in pregnancy
O22.00   Varicose veins of lower extremity in pregnancy, unspecified trimester ♀   M
O22.01   Varicose veins of lower extremity in pregnancy, first trimester ♀   M
O22.02   Varicose veins of lower extremity in pregnancy, second trimester ♀   M
O22.03   Varicose veins of lower extremity in pregnancy, third trimester ♀   M

◀ New   ◀▬ Revised   ~~deleted~~ Deleted   Excludes 1   Excludes 2   Includes   Use additional   Code first   Code also   Unspecified
OGCR Official Guidelines   ● Unacceptable Principal Diagnosis   X Assign placeholder X   🩺 Use Additional Character(s)   ▶ Manifestation Code   **Coding Clinic**

● **O22.1**   **Genital varices in pregnancy**
Perineal varices in pregnancy
Vaginal varices in pregnancy
Vulval varices in pregnancy

    O22.10   Genital varices in pregnancy, unspecified
          trimester ♀   M

    O22.11   Genital varices in pregnancy, first trimester ♀ M

    O22.12   Genital varices in pregnancy, second
          trimester ♀   M

    O22.13   Genital varices in pregnancy, third trimester ♀ M

● **O22.2**   **Superficial thrombophlebitis in pregnancy**
Phlebitis in pregnancy NOS
Thrombophlebitis of legs in pregnancy
Thrombosis in pregnancy NOS
   Use additional code to identify the superficial
      thrombophlebitis (I80.0-)

    O22.20   Superficial thrombophlebitis in pregnancy,
          unspecified trimester ♀ 🖐   M

    O22.21   Superficial thrombophlebitis in pregnancy, first
          trimester ♀ 🖐   M

    O22.22   Superficial thrombophlebitis in pregnancy,
          second trimester ♀ 🖐   M

    O22.23   Superficial thrombophlebitis in pregnancy,
          third trimester ♀ 🖐   M

● **O22.3**   **Deep phlebothrombosis in pregnancy**
Deep vein thrombosis, antepartum
   Use additional code to identify the deep vein
      thrombosis (I82.4-, I82.5-, I82.62-. I82.72-)
   Use additional code, if applicable, for associated
      long-term (current) use of anticoagulants (Z79.01)

    O22.30   Deep phlebothrombosis in pregnancy,
          unspecified trimester ♀ 🖐   M

    O22.31   Deep phlebothrombosis in pregnancy,
          first trimester ♀ 🖐   M

    O22.32   Deep phlebothrombosis in pregnancy, second
          trimester ♀ 🖐   M

    O22.33   Deep phlebothrombosis in pregnancy, third
          trimester ♀ 🖐   M

● **O22.4**   **Hemorrhoids in pregnancy**

    O22.40   Hemorrhoids in pregnancy, unspecified
          trimester ♀ 🖐   M

    O22.41   Hemorrhoids in pregnancy, first trimester ♀ 🖐M

    O22.42   Hemorrhoids in pregnancy, second
          trimester ♀ 🖐   M

    O22.43   Hemorrhoids in pregnancy, third
          trimester ♀ 🖐   M

● **O22.5**   **Cerebral venous thrombosis in pregnancy**
Cerebrovenous sinus thrombosis in pregnancy

    O22.50   Cerebral venous thrombosis in pregnancy,
          unspecified trimester ♀ 🖐   M

    O22.51   Cerebral venous thrombosis in pregnancy, first
          trimester ♀ 🖐   M

    O22.52   Cerebral venous thrombosis in pregnancy,
          second trimester ♀ 🖐   M

    O22.53   Cerebral venous thrombosis in pregnancy, third
          trimester ♀ 🖐   M

● **O22.8**   **Other venous complications in pregnancy**

   ● **O22.8X**   **Other venous complications in pregnancy**

      O22.8X1   Other venous complications in
            pregnancy, first trimester ♀ 🖐   M

      O22.8X2   Other venous complications in
            pregnancy, second trimester ♀ 🖐   M

      O22.8X3   Other venous complications in
            pregnancy, third trimester ♀ 🖐   M

      O22.8X9   Other venous complications in
            pregnancy, unspecified
            trimester ♀ 🖐   M

● **O22.9**   **Venous complication in pregnancy, unspecified**
Gestational phlebitis NOS
Gestational phlebopathy NOS
Gestational thrombosis NOS

    O22.90   Venous complication in pregnancy, unspecified,
          unspecified trimester ♀ 🖐   M

    O22.91   Venous complication in pregnancy, unspecified,
          first trimester ♀   M

    O22.92   Venous complication in pregnancy, unspecified,
          second trimester ♀   M

    O22.93   Venous complication in pregnancy, unspecified,
          third trimester ♀   M

● **O23**   **Infections of genitourinary tract in pregnancy**
   Use additional code to identify organism (B95.-, B96.-)
   Excludes2   gonococcal infections complicating pregnancy,
           childbirth and the puerperium (O98.2)
          infections with a predominantly sexual mode of
           transmission NOS complicating pregnancy,
           childbirth and the puerperium (O98.3)
          syphilis complicating pregnancy, childbirth and
           the puerperium (O98.1)
          tuberculosis of genitourinary system
           complicating pregnancy, childbirth and the
           puerperium (O98.0)
          venereal disease NOS complicating pregnancy,
           childbirth and the puerperium (O98.3)

   ⓔ **For category O23 CC codes:** O23.00-O23.93, O25.10-O25.3, O26.10-O26.13,
      O26.30-O26.43, O26.63-O26.819, O26.841-O26.86, O26.891-O26.93, O29.011-O29.93,
      O35.7XX0-O35.7XX9, O75.4, O75.81, O75.89-O75.9, O80, O86.11, O86.13-O86.29,
      O90.89, O99.111-O99.285, O99.330-O99.335, O99.350-O99.355, O99.511-O99.73,
      O99.820-O99.825, O99.840-O9A.53

● **O23.0**   **Infections of kidney in pregnancy**
Pyelonephritis in pregnancy

    O23.00   Infections of kidney in pregnancy, unspecified
          trimester ♀   M

    O23.01   Infections of kidney in pregnancy, first
          trimester ♀ 🖐   M

    O23.02   Infections of kidney in pregnancy, second
          trimester ♀ 🖐   M

    O23.03   Infections of kidney in pregnancy, third
          trimester ♀ 🖐   M

● **O23.1**   **Infections of bladder in pregnancy**

    O23.10   Infections of bladder in pregnancy, unspecified
          trimester ♀   M

    O23.11   Infections of bladder in pregnancy, first
          trimester ♀ 🖐   M

    O23.12   Infections of bladder in pregnancy, second
          trimester ♀ 🖐   M

    O23.13   Infections of bladder in pregnancy, third
          trimester ♀ 🖐   M

● **O23.2**   **Infections of urethra in pregnancy**

    O23.20   Infections of urethra in pregnancy, unspecified
          trimester ♀   M

    O23.21   Infections of urethra in pregnancy, first
          trimester ♀ 🖐   M

    O23.22   Infections of urethra in pregnancy, second
          trimester ♀ 🖐   M

    O23.23   Infections of urethra in pregnancy, third
          trimester ♀ 🖐   M

● **O23.3**   **Infections of other parts of urinary tract in pregnancy**

    O23.30   Infections of other parts of urinary tract in
          pregnancy, unspecified trimester ♀   M

    O23.31   Infections of other parts of urinary tract in
          pregnancy, first trimester ♀ 🖐   M

    O23.32   Infections of other parts of urinary tract in
          pregnancy, second trimester ♀ 🖐   M

    O23.33   Infections of other parts of urinary tract in
          pregnancy, third trimester ♀ 🖐   M

N   Newborn Age: 0   P   Pediatric Age: 0–17   M   Maternity DX: 12–55   A   Adult Age: 15–124   ♀   Females Only   ♂   Males Only

🖐   Complication\Comorbidity   🖐   Major C\C   ⓔ   CC/MCC Exclusions   🖐   Present on Admission Requirement   🖐   Hospital-Acquired Condition

1203

● **O23.4**   **Unspecified infection of urinary tract in pregnancy**

    O23.40   Unspecified infection of urinary tract in pregnancy, unspecified trimester ♀   M

    O23.41   Unspecified infection of urinary tract in pregnancy, first trimester ♀ 🐾   M

    O23.42   Unspecified infection of urinary tract in pregnancy, second trimester ♀ 🐾   M

    O23.43   Unspecified infection of urinary tract in pregnancy, third trimester ♀ 🐾   M

● **O23.5**   **Infections of the genital tract in pregnancy**

   ● **O23.51**   **Infection of cervix in pregnancy**

     O23.511   Infections of cervix in pregnancy, first trimester ♀ 🐾   M

     O23.512   Infections of cervix in pregnancy, second trimester ♀ 🐾   M

     O23.513   Infections of cervix in pregnancy, third trimester ♀ 🐾   M

     O23.519   Infections of cervix in pregnancy, unspecified trimester ♀   M

   ● **O23.52**   **Salpingo-oophoritis in pregnancy**
     Oophoritis = inflammation of ovary
     Salpingitis = inflammation of fallopian tube
     Oophoritis in pregnancy
     Salpingitis in pregnancy

     O23.521   Salpingo-oophoritis in pregnancy, first trimester ♀ 🐾   M

     O23.522   Salpingo-oophoritis in pregnancy, second trimester ♀ 🐾   M

     O23.523   Salpingo-oophoritis in pregnancy, third trimester ♀ 🐾   M

     O23.529   Salpingo-oophoritis in pregnancy, unspecified trimester ♀   M

   ● **O23.59**   **Infection of other part of genital tract in pregnancy**

     O23.591   Infection of other part of genital tract in pregnancy, first trimester ♀ 🐾 M

     O23.592   Infection of other part of genital tract in pregnancy, second trimester ♀ 🐾 M

     O23.593   Infection of other part of genital tract in pregnancy, third trimester ♀ 🐾 M

     O23.599   Infection of other part of genital tract in pregnancy, unspecified trimester ♀   M

● **O23.9**   **Unspecified genitourinary tract infection in pregnancy**
    Genitourinary tract infection in pregnancy NOS

    O23.90   Unspecified genitourinary tract infection in pregnancy, unspecified trimester ♀   M

    O23.91   Unspecified genitourinary tract infection in pregnancy, first trimester ♀ 🐾   M

    O23.92   Unspecified genitourinary tract infection in pregnancy, second trimester ♀ 🐾   M

    O23.93   Unspecified genitourinary tract infection in pregnancy, third trimester ♀ 🐾   M

OGCR Section I.C.15.g.

g. Diabetes mellitus in pregnancy
Diabetes mellitus is a significant complicating factor in pregnancy. Pregnant women who are diabetic should be assigned a code from category O24, Diabetes mellitus in pregnancy, childbirth, and the puerperium, first, followed by the appropriate diabetes code(s) (E08-E13) from Chapter 4.

OGCR Section I.C.15.i.

i. Gestational (pregnancy induced) diabetes
Gestational (pregnancy induced) diabetes can occur during the second and third trimester of pregnancy in women who were not diabetic prior to pregnancy. Gestational diabetes can cause complications in the pregnancy similar to those of pre-existing diabetes mellitus. It also puts the woman at greater risk of developing diabetes after the pregnancy. Codes for gestational diabetes are in subcategory O24.4, Gestational diabetes mellitus. No other code from category O24, Diabetes mellitus in pregnancy, childbirth, and the puerperium, should be used with a code from O24.4

The codes under subcategory O24.4 include diet controlled and insulin controlled. If a patient with gestational diabetes is treated with both diet and insulin, only the code for insulin-controlled is required. Code Z79.4, Long-term (current) use of insulin, should not be assigned with codes from subcategory O24.4.

An abnormal glucose tolerance in pregnancy is assigned a code from subcategory O99.81, Abnormal glucose complicating pregnancy, childbirth, and the puerperium.

● **O24**   **Diabetes mellitus in pregnancy, childbirth, and the puerperium**
   (Ex:) **For category O24 CC codes:** 024.011-024.33, 024.811-025.3, 026.10-026.13, 026.30-026.43, 026.63-026.819, 026.841-026.86, 026.891-026.93, 029.011-029.93, 035.7XX0-035.7XX9, 075.4, 075.81, 075.89-075.9, 080, 090.89, 099.111-099.285, 099.330-099.335, 099.350-099.355, 099.511-099.73, 099.820-099.825, 099.840-09A.53

   ● **O24.0**   **Pre-existing diabetes mellitus, type 1, in pregnancy, childbirth and the puerperium**
     Juvenile onset diabetes mellitus, in pregnancy, childbirth and the puerperium
     Ketosis-prone diabetes mellitus in pregnancy, childbirth and the puerperium
     Use additional code from category E10 to further identify any manifestations

    ● **O24.01**   **Pre-existing diabetes mellitus, type 1, in pregnancy**

     O24.011   Pre-existing diabetes mellitus, type 1, in pregnancy, first trimester ♀ 🐾   M

     O24.012   Pre-existing diabetes mellitus, type 1, in pregnancy, second trimester ♀ 🐾 M

     O24.013   Pre-existing diabetes mellitus, type 1, in pregnancy, third trimester ♀ 🐾   M

     O24.019   Pre-existing diabetes mellitus, type 1, in pregnancy, unspecified trimester ♀   M

     O24.02   Pre-existing diabetes mellitus, type 1, in childbirth ♀ 🐾   M

     O24.03   Pre-existing diabetes mellitus, type 1, in the puerperium ♀ 🐾   M

   ● **O24.1**   **Pre-existing diabetes mellitus, type 2, in pregnancy, childbirth and the puerperium**
     Insulin-resistant diabetes mellitus in pregnancy, childbirth and the puerperium
     Use additional code (for):
       from category E11 to further identify any manifestations
       long-term (current) use of insulin (Z79.4)

    ● **O24.11**   **Pre-existing diabetes mellitus, type 2, in pregnancy**

     O24.111   Pre-existing diabetes mellitus, type 2, in pregnancy, first trimester ♀ 🐾   M

     O24.112   Pre-existing diabetes mellitus, type 2, in pregnancy, second trimester ♀ 🐾 M

     O24.113   Pre-existing diabetes mellitus, type 2, in pregnancy, third trimester ♀ 🐾   M

     O24.119   Pre-existing diabetes mellitus, type 2, in pregnancy, unspecified trimester ♀   M

     O24.12   Pre-existing diabetes mellitus, type 2, in childbirth ♀ 🐾   M

     O24.13   Pre-existing diabetes mellitus, type 2, in the puerperium ♀ 🐾   M

◀ New   ◀▥ Revised   ~~deleted~~ Deleted   Excludes 1   Excludes 2   Includes   Use additional   Code first   Code also   Unspecified

OGCR Official Guidelines   ● Unacceptable Principal Diagnosis   X Assign placeholder X   ● Use Additional Character(s)   ▶ Manifestation Code   **Coding Clinic**

● **O24.3 Unspecified pre-existing diabetes mellitus in pregnancy, childbirth and the puerperium**
  Use additional code (for):
      from category E11 to further identify any manifestation
      long-term (current) use of insulin (Z79.4)
  ● **O24.31 Unspecified pre-existing diabetes mellitus in pregnancy**
      O24.311 Unspecified pre-existing diabetes mellitus in pregnancy, first trimester ♀ 🐾   M
      O24.312 Unspecified pre-existing diabetes mellitus in pregnancy, second trimester ♀ 🐾   M
      O24.313 Unspecified pre-existing diabetes mellitus in pregnancy, third trimester ♀ 🐾   M
      O24.319 Unspecified pre-existing diabetes mellitus in pregnancy, unspecified trimester ♀ 🐾   M
  ● **O24.32 Unspecified pre-existing diabetes mellitus in childbirth ♀ 🐾**   M
  ● **O24.33 Unspecified pre-existing diabetes mellitus in the puerperium ♀ 🐾**   M

● **O24.4 Gestational diabetes mellitus**
      Diabetes mellitus arising in pregnancy
      Gestational diabetes mellitus NOS
  ● **O24.41 Gestational diabetes mellitus in pregnancy**
      O24.410 Gestational diabetes mellitus in pregnancy, diet controlled ♀   M
      O24.414 Gestational diabetes mellitus in pregnancy, insulin controlled ♀   M
      O24.419 Gestational diabetes mellitus in pregnancy, unspecified control ♀   M
  ● **O24.42 Gestational diabetes mellitus in childbirth**
      O24.420 Gestational diabetes mellitus in childbirth, diet controlled ♀   M
      O24.424 Gestational diabetes mellitus in childbirth, insulin controlled ♀   M
      O24.429 Gestational diabetes mellitus in childbirth, unspecified control ♀   M
  ● **O24.43 Gestational diabetes mellitus in the puerperium**
      O24.430 Gestational diabetes mellitus in the puerperium, diet controlled ♀   M
      O24.434 Gestational diabetes mellitus in the puerperium, insulin controlled ♀   M
      O24.439 Gestational diabetes mellitus in the puerperium, unspecified control ♀   M

● **O24.8 Other pre-existing diabetes mellitus in pregnancy, childbirth, and the puerperium**
      Use additional code (for):
          from categories E08, E09 and E13 to further identify any manifestation
          long-term (current) use of insulin (Z79.4)
  ● **O24.81 Other pre-existing diabetes mellitus in pregnancy**
      O24.811 Other pre-existing diabetes mellitus in pregnancy, first trimester ♀ 🐾   M
      O24.812 Other pre-existing diabetes mellitus in pregnancy, second trimester ♀ 🐾   M
      O24.813 Other pre-existing diabetes mellitus in pregnancy, third trimester ♀ 🐾   M
      O24.819 Other pre-existing diabetes mellitus in pregnancy, unspecified trimester ♀ 🐾   M
  ● **O24.82 Other pre-existing diabetes mellitus in childbirth ♀ 🐾**   M
  ● **O24.83 Other pre-existing diabetes mellitus in the puerperium ♀ 🐾**   M

● **O24.9 Unspecified diabetes mellitus in pregnancy, childbirth and the puerperium**
      Use additional code for long-term (current) use of insulin (Z79.4)
  ● **O24.91 Unspecified diabetes mellitus in pregnancy**
      O24.911 Unspecified diabetes mellitus in pregnancy, first trimester ♀ 🐾   M
      O24.912 Unspecified diabetes mellitus in pregnancy, second trimester ♀ 🐾   M
      O24.913 Unspecified diabetes mellitus in pregnancy, third trimester ♀ 🐾   M
      O24.919 Unspecified diabetes mellitus in pregnancy, unspecified trimester ♀ 🐾   M
  ● **O24.92 Unspecified diabetes mellitus in childbirth ♀** M
  ● **O24.93 Unspecified diabetes mellitus in the puerperium ♀ 🐾**   M

● **O25 Malnutrition in pregnancy, childbirth and the puerperium**
  ● **O25.1 Malnutrition in pregnancy**
      O25.10 Malnutrition in pregnancy, unspecified trimester ♀   M
      O25.11 Malnutrition in pregnancy, first trimester ♀   M
      O25.12 Malnutrition in pregnancy, second trimester ♀   M
      O25.13 Malnutrition in pregnancy, third trimester ♀   M
  O25.2 Malnutrition in childbirth ♀   M
  O25.3 Malnutrition in the puerperium ♀   M

● **O26 Maternal care for other conditions predominantly related to pregnancy**
  ● **O26.0 Excessive weight gain in pregnancy**
      Excludes2 gestational edema (O12.0, O12.2)
      O26.00 Excessive weight gain in pregnancy, unspecified trimester ♀   M
      O26.01 Excessive weight gain in pregnancy, first trimester ♀   M
      O26.02 Excessive weight gain in pregnancy, second trimester ♀   M
      O26.03 Excessive weight gain in pregnancy, third trimester ♀   M
  ● **O26.1 Low weight gain in pregnancy**
      O26.10 Low weight gain in pregnancy, unspecified trimester ♀   M
      O26.11 Low weight gain in pregnancy, first trimester ♀   M
      O26.12 Low weight gain in pregnancy, second trimester ♀   M
      O26.13 Low weight gain in pregnancy, third trimester ♀   M
  ● **O26.2 Pregnancy care for patient with recurrent pregnancy loss**
      O26.20 Pregnancy care for patient with recurrent pregnancy loss, unspecified trimester ♀   M
      O26.21 Pregnancy care for patient with recurrent pregnancy loss, first trimester ♀   M
      O26.22 Pregnancy care for patient with recurrent pregnancy loss, second trimester ♀   M
      O26.23 Pregnancy care for patient with recurrent pregnancy loss, third trimester ♀   M
  ● **O26.3 Retained intrauterine contraceptive device in pregnancy**
      O26.30 Retained intrauterine contraceptive device in pregnancy, unspecified trimester ♀   M
      O26.31 Retained intrauterine contraceptive device in pregnancy, first trimester ♀   M
      O26.32 Retained intrauterine contraceptive device in pregnancy, second trimester ♀   M
      O26.33 Retained intrauterine contraceptive device in pregnancy, third trimester ♀   M

CHAPTER 15 (O00-O9A)

N Newborn Age: 0   P Pediatric Age: 0–17   M Maternity DX: 12–55   A Adult Age: 15–124   ♀ Females Only   ♂ Males Only

🐾 Complication\Comorbidity   🐾 Major C\C   (Ex) CC/MCC Exclusions   🐾 Present on Admission Requirement   🐾 Hospital-Acquired Condition

1205

● **O26.4** **Herpes gestationis**
　　O26.40 Herpes gestationis, unspecified trimester ♀ M
　　O26.41 Herpes gestationis, first trimester ♀ M
　　O26.42 Herpes gestationis, second trimester ♀ M
　　O26.43 Herpes gestationis, third trimester ♀ M

● **O26.5** **Maternal hypotension syndrome**
　　Supine hypotensive syndrome
　　O26.50 Maternal hypotension syndrome, unspecified trimester ♀ M
　　O26.51 Maternal hypotension syndrome, first trimester ♀ M
　　O26.52 Maternal hypotension syndrome, second trimester ♀ M
　　O26.53 Maternal hypotension syndrome, third trimester ♀ M

● **O26.6** **Liver and biliary tract disorders in pregnancy, childbirth and the puerperium**
　　Use additional code to identify the specific disorder
　　Excludes2 hepatorenal syndrome following labor and delivery (O90.4)

　● **O26.61** **Liver and biliary tract disorders in pregnancy**
　　　(Ex:) For category O26.61 CC codes: 025.10-025.3, 026.10-026.13, 026.30-026.43, 026.611-026.819, 026.841-026.86, 026.891-026.93, 029.011-029.93, 035.7XX0-035.7XX9, 075.4, 075.81, 075.89-075.9, 080, 090.89, 099.111-099.285, 099.330-099.335, 099.350-099.355, 099.511-099.73, 099.820-099.825, 099.840-09A.53
　　　O26.611 Liver and biliary tract disorders in pregnancy, first trimester ♀ ◔ M
　　　O26.612 Liver and biliary tract disorders in pregnancy, second trimester ♀ ◔ M
　　　O26.613 Liver and biliary tract disorders in pregnancy, third trimester ♀ ◔ M
　　　O26.619 Liver and biliary tract disorders in pregnancy, unspecified trimester ♀ M
　　O26.62 Liver and biliary tract disorders in childbirth ♀ ◔ M
　　O26.63 Liver and biliary tract disorders in the puerperium ♀ M

● **O26.7** **Subluxation of symphysis (pubis) in pregnancy, childbirth and the puerperium**
　　Excludes1 traumatic separation of symphysis (pubis) during childbirth (O71.6)

　● **O26.71** **Subluxation of symphysis (pubis) in pregnancy**
　　　O26.711 Subluxation of symphysis (pubis) in pregnancy, first trimester ♀ M
　　　O26.712 Subluxation of symphysis (pubis) in pregnancy, second trimester ♀ M
　　　O26.713 Subluxation of symphysis (pubis) in pregnancy, third trimester ♀ M
　　　O26.719 Subluxation of symphysis (pubis) in pregnancy, unspecified trimester ♀ M
　　O26.72 Subluxation of symphysis (pubis) in childbirth ♀ M
　　O26.73 Subluxation of symphysis (pubis) in the puerperium ♀ M

● **O26.8** **Other specified pregnancy related conditions**
　● **O26.81** **Pregnancy related exhaustion and fatigue**
　　　O26.811 Pregnancy related exhaustion and fatigue, first trimester ♀ M
　　　O26.812 Pregnancy related exhaustion and fatigue, second trimester ♀ M
　　　O26.813 Pregnancy related exhaustion and fatigue, third trimester ♀ M
　　　O26.819 Pregnancy related exhaustion and fatigue, unspecified trimester ♀ M

● **O26.82** **Pregnancy related peripheral neuritis**
　　O26.821 Pregnancy related peripheral neuritis, first trimester ♀ M
　　O26.822 Pregnancy related peripheral neuritis, second trimester ♀ M
　　O26.823 Pregnancy related peripheral neuritis, third trimester ♀ M
　　O26.829 Pregnancy related peripheral neuritis, unspecified trimester ♀ M

● **O26.83** **Pregnancy related renal disease**
　　Use additional code to identify the specific disorder
　　(Ex:) For category O26.83 CC codes: 012.11-012.13, 012.21-012.23, 026.831-026.833, 090.89
　　O26.831 Pregnancy related renal disease, first trimester ♀ ◔ M
　　O26.832 Pregnancy related renal disease, second trimester ♀ ◔ M
　　O26.833 Pregnancy related renal disease, third trimester ♀ ◔ M
　　O26.839 Pregnancy related renal disease, unspecified trimester ♀ M

● **O26.84** **Uterine size-date discrepancy complicating pregnancy**
　　Excludes1 encounter for suspected problem with fetal growth ruled out (Z03.74)
　　O26.841 Uterine size-date discrepancy, first trimester ♀ M
　　O26.842 Uterine size-date discrepancy, second trimester ♀ M
　　O26.843 Uterine size-date discrepancy, third trimester ♀ M
　　O26.849 Uterine size-date discrepancy, unspecified trimester ♀ M

● **O26.85** **Spotting complicating pregnancy**
　　O26.851 Spotting complicating pregnancy, first trimester ♀ M
　　O26.852 Spotting complicating pregnancy, second trimester ♀ M
　　O26.853 Spotting complicating pregnancy, third trimester ♀ M
　　O26.859 Spotting complicating pregnancy, unspecified trimester ♀ M

　O26.86 **Pruritic urticarial papules and plaques of pregnancy (PUPPP)** ♀ M
　　Polymorphic eruption of pregnancy

● **O26.87** **Cervical shortening**
　　Excludes1 encounter for suspected cervical shortening ruled out (Z03.75)
　　(Ex:) For category O26.87 CC codes: 026.872-026.879, 034.31-034.33
　　O26.872 Cervical shortening, second trimester ♀ ◔ M
　　O26.873 Cervical shortening, third trimester ♀ ◔ M
　　O26.879 Cervical shortening, unspecified trimester ♀ ◔ M

● **O26.89** **Other specified pregnancy related conditions**
　　O26.891 Other specified pregnancy related conditions, first trimester ♀ M
　　O26.892 Other specified pregnancy related conditions, second trimester ♀ M
　　O26.893 Other specified pregnancy related conditions, third trimester ♀ M
　　O26.899 Other specified pregnancy related conditions, unspecified trimester ♀ M

● **O26.9 Pregnancy related conditions, unspecified**
     O26.90   Pregnancy related conditions, unspecified, unspecified trimester ♀   M
     O26.91   Pregnancy related conditions, unspecified, first trimester ♀   M
     O26.92   Pregnancy related conditions, unspecified, second trimester ♀   M
     O26.93   Pregnancy related conditions, unspecified, third trimester ♀   M

● **O28 Abnormal findings on antenatal screening of mother**
     Excludes1   diagnostic findings classified elsewhere - see Alphabetical Index
   O28.0   Abnormal hematological finding on antenatal screening of mother ♀   M
   O28.1   Abnormal biochemical finding on antenatal screening of mother ♀   M
   O28.2   Abnormal cytological finding on antenatal screening of mother ♀   M
   O28.3   Abnormal ultrasonic finding on antenatal screening of mother ♀   M
   O28.4   Abnormal radiological finding on antenatal screening of mother ♀   M
   O28.5   Abnormal chromosomal and genetic finding on antenatal screening of mother ♀   M
   O28.8   Other abnormal findings on antenatal screening of mother ♀   M
   O28.9   Unspecified abnormal findings on antenatal screening of mother ♀   M

● **O29 Complications of anesthesia during pregnancy**
     Includes   maternal complications arising from the administration of a general, regional or local anesthetic, analgesic or other sedation during pregnancy
     Use additional code, if necessary, to identify the complication
     Excludes2   complications of anesthesia during labor and delivery (O74.-)
         complications of anesthesia during the puerperium (O89.-)

   ● **O29.0 Pulmonary complications of anesthesia during pregnancy**
     ● **O29.01 Aspiration pneumonitis due to anesthesia during pregnancy**
         Inhalation of stomach contents or secretions NOS due to anesthesia during pregnancy
         Mendelson's syndrome due to anesthesia during pregnancy
         O29.011   Aspiration pneumonitis due to anesthesia during pregnancy, first trimester ♀   M
         O29.012   Aspiration pneumonitis due to anesthesia during pregnancy, second trimester ♀   M
         O29.013   Aspiration pneumonitis due to anesthesia during pregnancy, third trimester ♀   M
         O29.019   Aspiration pneumonitis due to anesthesia during pregnancy, unspecified trimester ♀   M
     ● **O29.02 Pressure collapse of lung due to anesthesia during pregnancy**
         O29.021   Pressure collapse of lung due to anesthesia during pregnancy, first trimester ♀   M
         O29.022   Pressure collapse of lung due to anesthesia during pregnancy, second trimester ♀   M

         O29.023   Pressure collapse of lung due to anesthesia during pregnancy, third trimester ♀   M
         O29.029   Pressure collapse of lung due to anesthesia during pregnancy, unspecified trimester ♀   M
     ● **O29.09 Other pulmonary complications of anesthesia during pregnancy**
         O29.091   Other pulmonary complications of anesthesia during pregnancy, first trimester ♀   M
         O29.092   Other pulmonary complications of anesthesia during pregnancy, second trimester ♀   M
         O29.093   Other pulmonary complications of anesthesia during pregnancy, third trimester ♀   M
         O29.099   Other pulmonary complications of anesthesia during pregnancy, unspecified trimester ♀   M

   ● **O29.1 Cardiac complications of anesthesia during pregnancy**
     ● **O29.11 Cardiac arrest due to anesthesia during pregnancy**
         O29.111   Cardiac arrest due to anesthesia during pregnancy, first trimester ♀   M
         O29.112   Cardiac arrest due to anesthesia during pregnancy, second trimester ♀   M
         O29.113   Cardiac arrest due to anesthesia during pregnancy, third trimester ♀   M
         O29.119   Cardiac arrest due to anesthesia during pregnancy, unspecified trimester ♀   M
     ● **O29.12 Cardiac failure due to anesthesia during pregnancy**
         O29.121   Cardiac failure due to anesthesia during pregnancy, first trimester ♀   M
         O29.122   Cardiac failure due to anesthesia during pregnancy, second trimester ♀   M
         O29.123   Cardiac failure due to anesthesia during pregnancy, third trimester ♀   M
         O29.129   Cardiac failure due to anesthesia during pregnancy, unspecified trimester ♀   M
     ● **O29.19 Other cardiac complications of anesthesia during pregnancy**
         O29.191   Other cardiac complications of anesthesia during pregnancy, first trimester ♀   M
         O29.192   Other cardiac complications of anesthesia during pregnancy, second trimester ♀   M
         O29.193   Other cardiac complications of anesthesia during pregnancy, third trimester ♀   M
         O29.199   Other cardiac complications of anesthesia during pregnancy, unspecified trimester ♀   M

   ● **O29.2 Central nervous system complications of anesthesia during pregnancy**
     ● **O29.21 Cerebral anoxia due to anesthesia during pregnancy**
         O29.211   Cerebral anoxia due to anesthesia during pregnancy, first trimester ♀   M
         O29.212   Cerebral anoxia due to anesthesia during pregnancy, second trimester ♀   M

N Newborn Age: 0   **P** Pediatric Age: 0–17   **M** Maternity DX: 12–55   **A** Adult Age: 15–124   ♀ Females Only   ♂ Males Only

Complication\Comorbidity   Major C\C   (Ex) CC/MCC Exclusions   Present on Admission Requirement   Hospital-Acquired Condition

1207

CHAPTER 15 (O00-O9A)

O29.213   Cerebral anoxia due to anesthesia during pregnancy, third trimester ♀ M

O29.219   Cerebral anoxia due to anesthesia during pregnancy, unspecified trimester ♀ M

● O29.29   Other central nervous system complications of anesthesia during pregnancy

O29.291   Other central nervous system complications of anesthesia during pregnancy, first trimester ♀ M

O29.292   Other central nervous system complications of anesthesia during pregnancy, second trimester ♀ M

O29.293   Other central nervous system complications of anesthesia during pregnancy, third trimester ♀ M

O29.299   Other central nervous system complications of anesthesia during pregnancy, unspecified trimester ♀ M

● O29.3   Toxic reaction to local anesthesia during pregnancy

● O29.3X   Toxic reaction to local anesthesia during pregnancy

O29.3X1   Toxic reaction to local anesthesia during pregnancy, first trimester ♀ M

O29.3X2   Toxic reaction to local anesthesia during pregnancy, second trimester ♀ M

O29.3X3   Toxic reaction to local anesthesia during pregnancy, third trimester ♀ M

O29.3X9   Toxic reaction to local anesthesia during pregnancy, unspecified trimester ♀ M

● O29.4   Spinal and epidural anesthesia induced headache during pregnancy

O29.40   Spinal and epidural anesthesia induced headache during pregnancy, unspecified trimester ♀ M

O29.41   Spinal and epidural anesthesia induced headache during pregnancy, first trimester ♀ M

O29.42   Spinal and epidural anesthesia induced headache during pregnancy, second trimester ♀ M

O29.43   Spinal and epidural anesthesia induced headache during pregnancy, third trimester ♀ M

● O29.5   Other complications of spinal and epidural anesthesia during pregnancy

● O29.5X   Other complications of spinal and epidural anesthesia during pregnancy

O29.5X1   Other complications of spinal and epidural anesthesia during pregnancy, first trimester ♀ M

O29.5X2   Other complications of spinal and epidural anesthesia during pregnancy, second trimester ♀ M

O29.5X3   Other complications of spinal and epidural anesthesia during pregnancy, third trimester ♀ M

O29.5X9   Other complications of spinal and epidural anesthesia during pregnancy, unspecified trimester ♀ M

● O29.6   Failed or difficult intubation for anesthesia during pregnancy

O29.60   Failed or difficult intubation for anesthesia during pregnancy, unspecified trimester ♀ M

O29.61   Failed or difficult intubation for anesthesia during pregnancy, first trimester ♀ M

O29.62   Failed or difficult intubation for anesthesia during pregnancy, second trimester ♀ M

O29.63   Failed or difficult intubation for anesthesia during pregnancy, third trimester ♀ M

● O29.8   Other complications of anesthesia during pregnancy

● O29.8X   Other complications of anesthesia during pregnancy

O29.8X1   Other complications of anesthesia during pregnancy, first trimester ♀ M

O29.8X2   Other complications of anesthesia during pregnancy, second trimester ♀ M

O29.8X3   Other complications of anesthesia during pregnancy, third trimester ♀ M

O29.8X9   Other complications of anesthesia during pregnancy, unspecified trimester ♀ M

● O29.9   Unspecified complication of anesthesia during pregnancy

O29.90   Unspecified complication of anesthesia during pregnancy, unspecified trimester ♀ M

O29.91   Unspecified complication of anesthesia during pregnancy, first trimester ♀ M

O29.92   Unspecified complication of anesthesia during pregnancy, second trimester ♀ M

O29.93   Unspecified complication of anesthesia during pregnancy, third trimester ♀ M

MATERNAL CARE RELATED TO THE FETUS AND AMNIOTIC CAVITY AND POSSIBLE DELIVERY PROBLEMS (O30-O48)

● O30   Multiple gestation

Code also any complications specific to multiple gestation

● O30.0   Twin pregnancy

● O30.00   Twin pregnancy, unspecified number of placenta and unspecified number of amniotic sacs

● O30.001   Twin pregnancy, unspecified number of placenta and unspecified number of amniotic sacs, first trimester ♀ M

● O30.002   Twin pregnancy, unspecified number of placenta and unspecified number of amniotic sacs, second trimester ♀ M

● O30.003   Twin pregnancy, unspecified number of placenta and unspecified number of amniotic sacs, third trimester ♀ M

● O30.009   Twin pregnancy, unspecified number of placenta and unspecified number of amniotic sacs, unspecified trimester ♀ M

● O30.01   Twin pregnancy, monochorionic/monoamniotic

Twin pregnancy, one placenta, one amniotic sac

Excludes1   conjoined twins (O30.02-)

● O30.011   Twin pregnancy, monochorionic/monoamniotic, first trimester ♀ M

● O30.012   Twin pregnancy, monochorionic/monoamniotic, second trimester ♀ M

● O30.013   Twin pregnancy, monochorionic/monoamniotic, third trimester ♀ M

● O30.019   Twin pregnancy, monochorionic/monoamniotic, unspecified trimester ♀ M

◀ New   ◀▥ Revised   ~~deleted~~ Deleted   Excludes 1   Excludes 2   Includes   Use additional   Code first   Code also   Unspecified

OGCR Official Guidelines   ● Unacceptable Principal Diagnosis   X Assign placeholder X   ● Use Additional Character(s)   ▶ Manifestation Code   **Coding Clinic**

● **O30.02**   Conjoined twin pregnancy

    O30.021   Conjoined twin pregnancy, first trimester ♀   **M**

    O30.022   Conjoined twin pregnancy, second trimester ♀   **M**

    O30.023   Conjoined twin pregnancy, third trimester ♀   **M**

    O30.029   Conjoined twin pregnancy, unspecified trimester ♀   **M**

● **O30.03**   Twin pregnancy, monochorionic/diamniotic
     Twin pregnancy, one placenta, two amniotic sacs

    ● O30.031   Twin pregnancy, monochorionic/diamniotic, first trimester ♀   **M**

    ● O30.032   Twin pregnancy, monochorionic/diamniotic, second trimester ♀   **M**

    ● O30.033   Twin pregnancy, monochorionic/diamniotic, third trimester ♀   **M**

    ● O30.039   Twin pregnancy, monochorionic/diamniotic, unspecified trimester ♀   **M**

● **O30.04**   Twin pregnancy, dichorionic/diamniotic
     Twin pregnancy, two placentae, two amniotic sacs

    ● O30.041   Twin pregnancy, dichorionic/diamniotic, first trimester ♀   **M**

    ● O30.042   Twin pregnancy, dichorionic/diamniotic, second trimester ♀   **M**

    ● O30.043   Twin pregnancy, dichorionic/diamniotic, third trimester ♀   **M**

    ● O30.049   Twin pregnancy, dichorionic/diamniotic, unspecified trimester ♀   **M**

● **O30.09**   Twin pregnancy, unable to determine number of placenta and number of amniotic sacs

    ● O30.091   Twin pregnancy, unable to determine number of placenta and number of amniotic sacs, first trimester ♀   **M**

    ● O30.092   Twin pregnancy, unable to determine number of placenta and number of amniotic sacs, second trimester ♀   **M**

    ● O30.093   Twin pregnancy, unable to determine number of placenta and number of amniotic sacs, third trimester ♀   **M**

    ● O30.099   Twin pregnancy, unable to determine number of placenta and number of amniotic sacs, unspecified trimester ♀   **M**

● **O30.1**   Triplet pregnancy
    (Ex) **For category O30.1 CC codes:** O30.001-O30.019, O30.031-O31.23X9, O31.31X0-O32.9XX9, O80

● **O30.10**   Triplet pregnancy, unspecified number of placenta and unspecified number of amniotic sacs

    ● O30.101   Triplet pregnancy, unspecified number of placenta and unspecified number of amniotic sacs, first trimester ♀ 🦠   **M**

    ● O30.102   Triplet pregnancy, unspecified number of placenta and unspecified number of amniotic sacs, second trimester ♀ 🦠   **M**

    ● O30.103   Triplet pregnancy, unspecified number of placenta and unspecified number of amniotic sacs, third trimester ♀ 🦠   **M**

    ● O30.109   Triplet pregnancy, unspecified number of placenta and unspecified number of amniotic sacs, unspecified trimester ♀   **M**

● **O30.11**   Triplet pregnancy with two or more monochorionic fetuses

    ● O30.111   Triplet pregnancy with two or more monochorionic fetuses, first trimester ♀ 🦠   **M**

    ● O30.112   Triplet pregnancy with two or more monochorionic fetuses, second trimester ♀ 🦠   **M**

    ● O30.113   Triplet pregnancy with two or more monochorionic fetuses, third trimester ♀ 🦠   **M**

    ● O30.119   Triplet pregnancy with two or more monochorionic fetuses, unspecified trimester ♀   **M**

● **O30.12**   Triplet pregnancy with two or more monoamniotic fetuses

    ● O30.121   Triplet pregnancy with two or more monoamniotic fetuses, first trimester ♀ 🦠   **M**

    ● O30.122   Triplet pregnancy with two or more monoamniotic fetuses, second trimester ♀ 🦠   **M**

    ● O30.123   Triplet pregnancy with two or more monoamniotic fetuses, third trimester ♀ 🦠   **M**

    ● O30.129   Triplet pregnancy with two or more monoamniotic fetuses, unspecified trimester ♀   **M**

● **O30.19**   Triplet pregnancy, unable to determine number of placenta and number of amniotic sacs

    ● O30.191   Triplet pregnancy, unable to determine number of placenta and number of amniotic sacs, first trimester ♀ 🦠   **M**

    ● O30.192   Triplet pregnancy, unable to determine number of placenta and number of amniotic sacs, second trimester ♀ 🦠   **M**

    ● O30.193   Triplet pregnancy, unable to determine number of placenta and number of amniotic sacs, third trimester ♀ 🦠   **M**

    ● O30.199   Triplet pregnancy, unable to determine number of placenta and number of amniotic sacs, unspecified trimester ♀   **M**

● **O30.2**   Quadruplet pregnancy
    (Ex) **For category O30.2 CC codes:** See O30.1

● **O30.20**   Quadruplet pregnancy, unspecified number of placenta and unspecified number of amniotic sacs

    ● O30.201   Quadruplet pregnancy, unspecified number of placenta and unspecified number of amniotic sacs, first trimester ♀ 🦠   **M**

    ● O30.202   Quadruplet pregnancy, unspecified number of placenta and unspecified number of amniotic sacs, second trimester ♀ 🦠   **M**

    ● O30.203   Quadruplet pregnancy, unspecified number of placenta and unspecified number of amniotic sacs, third trimester ♀ 🦠   **M**

    ● O30.209   Quadruplet pregnancy, unspecified number of placenta and unspecified number of amniotic sacs, unspecified trimester ♀   **M**

N   Newborn Age: 0   **P**   Pediatric Age: 0–17   **M**   Maternity DX: 12–55   **A**   Adult Age: 15–124   ♀   Females Only   ♂   Males Only

🦠   Complication\Comorbidity   🦠   Major C\C   (Ex)   CC/MCC Exclusions   🦠   Present on Admission Requirement   🦠   Hospital-Acquired Condition

1209

CHAPTER 15 (O00-O9A)

- O30.21   Quadruplet pregnancy with two or more monochorionic fetuses
  - O30.211   Quadruplet pregnancy with two or more monochorionic fetuses, first trimester ♀ 🐾   M
  - O30.212   Quadruplet pregnancy with two or more monochorionic fetuses, second trimester ♀ 🐾   M
  - O30.213   Quadruplet pregnancy with two or more monochorionic fetuses, third trimester ♀ 🐾   M
  - O30.219   Quadruplet pregnancy with two or more monochorionic fetuses, unspecified trimester ♀   M
- O30.22   Quadruplet pregnancy with two or more monoamniotic fetuses
  - O30.221   Quadruplet pregnancy with two or more monoamniotic fetuses, first trimester ♀ 🐾   M
  - O30.222   Quadruplet pregnancy with two or more monoamniotic fetuses, second trimester ♀ 🐾   M
  - O30.223   Quadruplet pregnancy with two or more monoamniotic fetuses, third trimester ♀ 🐾   M
  - O30.229   Quadruplet pregnancy with two or more monoamniotic fetuses, unspecified trimester ♀   M
- O30.29   Quadruplet pregnancy, unable to determine number of placenta and number of amniotic sacs
  - O30.291   Quadruplet pregnancy, unable to determine number of placenta and number of amniotic sacs, first trimester ♀ 🐾   M
  - O30.292   Quadruplet pregnancy, unable to determine number of placenta and number of amniotic sacs, second trimester ♀ 🐾   M
  - O30.293   Quadruplet pregnancy, unable to determine number of placenta and number of amniotic sacs, third trimester ♀ 🐾   M
  - O30.299   Quadruplet pregnancy, unable to determine number of placenta and number of amniotic sacs, unspecified trimester ♀   M
- O30.8   Other specified multiple gestation

  Multiple gestation pregnancy greater then quadruplets

  (Ex) For category O30.8 CC codes: See O30.1
  - O30.80   Other specified multiple gestation, unspecified number of placenta and unspecified number of amniotic sacs
    - O30.801   Other specified multiple gestation, unspecified number of placenta and unspecified number of amniotic sacs, first trimester ♀ 🐾   M
    - O30.802   Other specified multiple gestation, unspecified number of placenta and unspecified number of amniotic sacs, second trimester ♀ 🐾   M
    - O30.803   Other specified multiple gestation, unspecified number of placenta and unspecified number of amniotic sacs, third trimester ♀ 🐾   M
    - O30.809   Other specified multiple gestation, unspecified number of placenta and unspecified number of amniotic sacs, unspecified trimester ♀   M

- O30.81   Other specified multiple gestation with two or more monochorionic fetuses
  - O30.811   Other specified multiple gestation with two or more monochorionic fetuses, first trimester ♀ 🐾   M
  - O30.812   Other specified multiple gestation with two or more monochorionic fetuses, second trimester ♀ 🐾   M
  - O30.813   Other specified multiple gestation with two or more monochorionic fetuses, third trimester ♀ 🐾   M
  - O30.819   Other specified multiple gestation with two or more monochorionic fetuses, unspecified trimester ♀   M
- O30.82   Other specified multiple gestation with two or more monoamniotic fetuses
  - O30.821   Other specified multiple gestation with two or more monoamniotic fetuses, first trimester ♀ 🐾   M
  - O30.822   Other specified multiple gestation with two or more monoamniotic fetuses, second trimester ♀ 🐾   M
  - O30.823   Other specified multiple gestation with two or more monoamniotic fetuses, third trimester ♀ 🐾   M
  - O30.829   Other specified multiple gestation with two or more monoamniotic fetuses, unspecified trimester ♀   M
- O30.89   Other specified multiple gestation, unable to determine number of placenta and number of amniotic sacs
  - O30.891   Other specified multiple gestation, unable to determine number of placenta and number of amniotic sacs, first trimester ♀ 🐾   M
  - O30.892   Other specified multiple gestation, unable to determine number of placenta and number of amniotic sacs, second trimester ♀ 🐾   M
  - O30.893   Other specified multiple gestation, unable to determine number of placenta and number of amniotic sacs, third trimester ♀ 🐾   M
  - O30.899   Other specified multiple gestation, unable to determine number of placenta and number of amniotic sacs, unspecified trimester ♀   M
- O30.9   Multiple gestation, unspecified

  Multiple pregnancy NOS
  - O30.90   Multiple gestation, unspecified, unspecified trimester ♀   M
  - O30.91   Multiple gestation, unspecified, first trimester ♀   M
  - O30.92   Multiple gestation, unspecified, second trimester ♀   M
  - O30.93   Multiple gestation, unspecified, third trimester ♀   M

◀ New   ◀▥ Revised   ~~deleted~~ Deleted   Excludes 1   Excludes 2   Includes   Use additional   Code first   Code also   Unspecified

OGCR Official Guidelines   ● Unacceptable Principal Diagnosis   X Assign placeholder X   ● Use Additional Character(s)   ▶ Manifestation Code   Coding Clinic

● **O31　Complications specific to multiple gestation**

　　Excludes2　delayed delivery of second twin, triplet, etc. (O63.2)
　　　　　　　　malpresentation of one fetus or more (O32.9) ◀▥
　　　　　　　　placental transfusion syndromes (O43.0-)

　　Coding Clinic: 2012, Q4, P107

　　One of the following 7th characters is to be assigned to each code under category O31. 7th character 0 is for single gestations and multiple gestations where the fetus is unspecified. 7th characters 1 through 9 are for cases of multiple gestations to identify the fetus for which the code applies. The appropriate code from category O30, Multiple gestation, must also be assigned when assigning a code from category O31 that has a 7th character of 1 through 9.

0	not applicable or unspecified
1	fetus 1
2	fetus 2
3	fetus 3
4	fetus 4
5	fetus 5
9	other fetus

● **O31.0　Papyraceous fetus**
　　　　Fetus compressus
　X● O31.00　Papyraceous fetus, unspecified trimester ♀　M
　X● O31.01　Papyraceous fetus, first trimester ♀　M
　X● O31.02　Papyraceous fetus, second trimester ♀　M
　X● O31.03　Papyraceous fetus, third trimester ♀　M

● **O31.1　Continuing pregnancy after spontaneous abortion of one fetus or more**
　X● O31.10　Continuing pregnancy after spontaneous abortion of one fetus or more, unspecified trimester ♀　M
　X● O31.11　Continuing pregnancy after spontaneous abortion of one fetus or more, first trimester ♀　M
　X● O31.12　Continuing pregnancy after spontaneous abortion of one fetus or more, second trimester ♀　M
　X● O31.13　Continuing pregnancy after spontaneous abortion of one fetus or more, third trimester ♀　M

● **O31.2　Continuing pregnancy after intrauterine death of one fetus or more**
　X● O31.20　Continuing pregnancy after intrauterine death of one fetus or more, unspecified trimester ♀　M
　X● O31.21　Continuing pregnancy after intrauterine death of one fetus or more, first trimester ♀　M
　X● O31.22　Continuing pregnancy after intrauterine death of one fetus or more, second trimester ♀　M
　X● O31.23　Continuing pregnancy after intrauterine death of one fetus or more, third trimester ♀　M

● **O31.3　Continuing pregnancy after elective fetal reduction of one fetus or more**
　　　　Continuing pregnancy after selective termination of one fetus or more
　X● O31.30　Continuing pregnancy after elective fetal reduction of one fetus or more, unspecified trimester ♀　M
　X● O31.31　Continuing pregnancy after elective fetal reduction of one fetus or more, first trimester ♀　M
　X● O31.32　Continuing pregnancy after elective fetal reduction of one fetus or more, second trimester ♀　M
　X● O31.33　Continuing pregnancy after elective fetal reduction of one fetus or more, third trimester ♀　M

● **O31.8　Other complications specific to multiple gestation**
　　(Ex) For category O31.8 CC codes: See O30.1
　● **O31.8X　Other complications specific to multiple gestation**
　　● O31.8X1　Other complications specific to multiple gestation, first trimester ♀ 🆎　M
　　● O31.8X2　Other complications specific to multiple gestation, second trimester ♀ 🆎　M
　　● O31.8X3　Other complications specific to multiple gestation, third trimester ♀ 🆎　M
　　● O31.8X9　Other complications specific to multiple gestation, unspecified trimester ♀　M

● **O32　Maternal care for malpresentation of fetus**

　　Includes　the listed conditions as a reason for observation, hospitalization or other obstetric care of the mother, or for cesarean delivery before onset of labor

　　Excludes1　malpresentation of fetus with obstructed labor (O64.-)

　　Coding Clinic: 2012, Q4, P107

　　One of the following 7th characters is to be assigned to each code under category O32. 7th character 0 is for single gestations and multiple gestations where the fetus is unspecified. 7th characters 1 through 9 are for cases of multiple gestations to identify the fetus for which the code applies. The appropriate code from category O30, Multiple gestation, must also be assigned when assigning a code from category O32 that has a 7th character of 1 through 9.

0	not applicable or unspecified
1	fetus 1
2	fetus 2
3	fetus 3
4	fetus 4
5	fetus 5
9	other fetus

　X● O32.0　Maternal care for unstable lie ♀　M
　X● O32.1　Maternal care for breech presentation ♀　M
　　　　Maternal care for buttocks presentation
　　　　Maternal care for complete breech
　　　　Maternal care for frank breech
　　　Excludes1　footling presentation (O32.8)
　　　　　　　　incomplete breech (O32.8)
　X● O32.2　Maternal care for transverse and oblique lie ♀　M
　　　　Maternal care for oblique presentation
　　　　Maternal care for transverse presentation
　X● O32.3　Maternal care for face, brow and chin presentation ♀　M
　X● O32.4　Maternal care for high head at term ♀　M
　　　　Maternal care for failure of head to enter pelvic brim
　X● O32.6　Maternal care for compound presentation ♀　M
　X● O32.8　Maternal care for other malpresentation of fetus ♀　M
　　　　Maternal care for footling presentation
　　　　Maternal care for incomplete breech
　X● O32.9　Maternal care for malpresentation of fetus, unspecified ♀　M

N　Newborn Age: 0　　P　Pediatric Age: 0–17　　M　Maternity DX: 12–55　　A　Adult Age: 15–124　　♀　Females Only　　♂　Males Only
🆎 Complication\Comorbidity　　🆎 Major C\C　　(Ex) CC/MCC Exclusions　　🆎 Present on Admission Requirement　　🆎 Hospital-Acquired Condition

1211

● **O33 Maternal care for disproportion**

> **Includes** the listed conditions as a reason for observation, hospitalization or other obstetric care of the mother, or for cesarean delivery before onset of labor
>
> **Excludes1** disproportion with obstructed labor (O65-O66) ◄▥

O33.0 Maternal care for disproportion due to deformity of maternal pelvic bones ♀ ⓖ　　　　　　M
> Maternal care for disproportion due to pelvic deformity causing disproportion NOS
> ⒺⓍ O33.0

O33.1 Maternal care for disproportion due to generally contracted pelvis ♀　　　　　　　M
> Maternal care for disproportion due to contracted pelvis NOS causing disproportion

O33.2 Maternal care for disproportion due to inlet contraction of pelvis ♀　　　　　　　M
> Maternal care for disproportion due to inlet contraction (pelvis) causing disproportion

X ● **O33.3 Maternal care for disproportion due to outlet contraction of pelvis** ♀　　　　　　M
> Maternal care for disproportion due to mid-cavity contraction (pelvis)
> Maternal care for disproportion due to outlet contraction (pelvis)
>
> One of the following 7th characters is to be assigned to code O33.3. 7th character 0 is for single gestations and multiple gestations where the fetus is unspecified. 7th characters 1 through 9 are for cases of multiple gestations to identify the fetus for which the code applies. The appropriate code from category O30, Multiple gestation, must also be assigned when assigning code O33.3 with a 7th character of 1 through 9.

0	not applicable or unspecified
1	fetus 1
2	fetus 2
3	fetus 3
4	fetus 4
5	fetus 5
9	other fetus

X ● **O33.4 Maternal care for disproportion of mixed maternal and fetal origin** ♀　　　　　M
> One of the following 7th characters is to be assigned to code O33.4. 7th character 0 is for single gestations and multiple gestations where the fetus is unspecified. 7th characters 1 through 9 are for cases of multiple gestations to identify the fetus for which the code applies. The appropriate code from category O30, Multiple gestation, must also be assigned when assigning code O33.4 with a 7th character of 1 through 9.

0	not applicable or unspecified
1	fetus 1
2	fetus 2
3	fetus 3
4	fetus 4
5	fetus 5
9	other fetus

X ● **O33.5 Maternal care for disproportion due to unusually large fetus** ♀　　　　　　　M
> Maternal care for disproportion due to disproportion of fetal origin with normally formed fetus
> Maternal care for disproportion due to fetal disproportion NOS
>
> One of the following 7th characters is to be assigned to code O33.5. 7th character 0 is for single gestations and multiple gestations where the fetus is unspecified. 7th characters 1 through 9 are for cases of multiple gestations to identify the fetus for which the code applies. The appropriate code from category O30, Multiple gestation, must also be assigned when assigning code O33.5 with a 7th character of 1 through 9.

0	not applicable or unspecified
1	fetus 1
2	fetus 2
3	fetus 3
4	fetus 4
5	fetus 5
9	other fetus

X ● **O33.6 Maternal care for disproportion due to hydrocephalic fetus** ♀　　　　　　　　M
> One of the following 7th characters is to be assigned to code O33.6. 7th character 0 is for single gestations and multiple gestations where the fetus is unspecified. 7th characters 1 through 9 are for cases of multiple gestations to identify the fetus for which the code applies. The appropriate code from category O30, Multiple gestation, must also be assigned when assigning code O33.6 with a 7th character of 1 through 9.

0	not applicable or unspecified
1	fetus 1
2	fetus 2
3	fetus 3
4	fetus 4
5	fetus 5
9	other fetus

O33.7 Maternal care for disproportion due to other fetal deformities ♀　　　　　　　M
> Maternal care for disproportion due to fetal ascites
> Maternal care for disproportion due to fetal hydrops
> Maternal care for disproportion due to fetal meningomyelocele
> Maternal care for disproportion due to fetal sacral teratoma
> Maternal care for disproportion due to fetal tumor
>
> **Excludes1** obstructed labor due to other fetal deformities (O66.3)

O33.8 Maternal care for disproportion of other origin ♀　　　　　　　　M

O33.9 Maternal care for disproportion, unspecified ♀　　　　　　　M
> Maternal care for disproportion due to cephalopelvic disproportion NOS
> Maternal care for disproportion due to fetopelvic disproportion NOS

◄ New　◄▥ Revised　d̶e̶l̶e̶t̶e̶d̶ Deleted　Excludes 1　Excludes 2　Includes　Use additional　Code first　Code also　Unspecified
OGCR Official Guidelines　● Unacceptable Principal Diagnosis　X Assign placeholder X　● Use Additional Character(s)　▌ Manifestation Code　Coding Clinic

● **O34**   **Maternal care for abnormality of pelvic organs**

     Includes   the listed conditions as a reason for hospitalization or other obstetric care of the mother, or for cesarean delivery before onset of labor

     Code first any associated obstructed labor (O65.5)

     Use additional code for specific condition

● **O34.0**   Maternal care for congenital malformation of uterus

     O34.00   Maternal care for unspecified congenital malformation of uterus, unspecified trimester ♀   M

     O34.01   Maternal care for unspecified congenital malformation of uterus, first trimester ♀   M

     O34.02   Maternal care for unspecified congenital malformation of uterus, second trimester ♀   M

     O34.03   Maternal care for unspecified congenital malformation of uterus, third trimester ♀   M

● **O34.1**   Maternal care for benign tumor of corpus uteri

     Excludes2   maternal care for benign tumor of cervix (O34.4-)

               maternal care for malignant neoplasm of uterus (O9A.1-)

     O34.10   Maternal care for benign tumor of corpus uteri, unspecified trimester ♀   M

     O34.11   Maternal care for benign tumor of corpus uteri, first trimester ♀   M

     O34.12   Maternal care for benign tumor of corpus uteri, second trimester ♀   M

     O34.13   Maternal care for benign tumor of corpus uteri, third trimester ♀   M

● **O34.2**   Maternal care due to uterine scar from previous surgery

     O34.21   Maternal care for scar from previous cesarean delivery ♀   M

     O34.29   Maternal care due to uterine scar from other previous surgery ♀   M

● **O34.3**   Maternal care for cervical incompetence

     Maternal care for cerclage with or without cervical incompetence

     Maternal care for Shirodkar suture with or without cervical incompetence

     Ⓔⓧ For category **O34.3** **CC** codes: 026.872-026.879, 034.31-034.33

     O34.30   Maternal care for cervical incompetence, unspecified trimester ♀   M

     O34.31   Maternal care for cervical incompetence, first trimester ♀ 🏥   M

     O34.32   Maternal care for cervical incompetence, second trimester ♀ 🏥   M

     O34.33   Maternal care for cervical incompetence, third trimester ♀ 🏥   M

● **O34.4**   Maternal care for other abnormalities of cervix

     O34.40   Maternal care for other abnormalities of cervix, unspecified trimester ♀   M

     O34.41   Maternal care for other abnormalities of cervix, first trimester ♀   M

     O34.42   Maternal care for other abnormalities of cervix, second trimester ♀   M

     O34.43   Maternal care for other abnormalities of cervix, third trimester ♀   M

● **O34.5**   Maternal care for other abnormalities of gravid uterus

     ● **O34.51**   Maternal care for incarceration of gravid uterus

         O34.511   Maternal care for incarceration of gravid uterus, first trimester ♀   M

         O34.512   Maternal care for incarceration of gravid uterus, second trimester ♀   M

         O34.513   Maternal care for incarceration of gravid uterus, third trimester ♀   M

         O34.519   Maternal care for incarceration of gravid uterus, unspecified trimester ♀   M

● **O34.52**   Maternal care for prolapse of gravid uterus

     O34.521   Maternal care for prolapse of gravid uterus, first trimester ♀   M

     O34.522   Maternal care for prolapse of gravid uterus, second trimester ♀   M

     O34.523   Maternal care for prolapse of gravid uterus, third trimester ♀   M

     O34.529   Maternal care for prolapse of gravid uterus, unspecified trimester ♀   M

● **O34.53**   Maternal care for retroversion of gravid uterus

     O34.531   Maternal care for retroversion of gravid uterus, first trimester ♀   M

     O34.532   Maternal care for retroversion of gravid uterus, second trimester ♀   M

     O34.533   Maternal care for retroversion of gravid uterus, third trimester ♀   M

     O34.539   Maternal care for retroversion of gravid uterus, unspecified trimester ♀   M

● **O34.59**   Maternal care for other abnormalities of gravid uterus

     O34.591   Maternal care for other abnormalities of gravid uterus, first trimester ♀   M

     O34.592   Maternal care for other abnormalities of gravid uterus, second trimester ♀   M

     O34.593   Maternal care for other abnormalities of gravid uterus, third trimester ♀   M

     O34.599   Maternal care for other abnormalities of gravid uterus, unspecified trimester ♀   M

● **O34.6**   Maternal care for abnormality of vagina

     Excludes2   maternal care for vaginal varices in pregnancy (O22.1-)

     O34.60   Maternal care for abnormality of vagina, unspecified trimester ♀   M

     O34.61   Maternal care for abnormality of vagina, first trimester ♀   M

     O34.62   Maternal care for abnormality of vagina, second trimester ♀   M

     O34.63   Maternal care for abnormality of vagina, third trimester ♀   M

● **O34.7**   Maternal care for abnormality of vulva and perineum

     Excludes2   maternal care for perineal and vulval varices in pregnancy (O22.1-)

     O34.70   Maternal care for abnormality of vulva and perineum, unspecified trimester ♀   M

     O34.71   Maternal care for abnormality of vulva and perineum, first trimester ♀   M

     O34.72   Maternal care for abnormality of vulva and perineum, second trimester ♀   M

     O34.73   Maternal care for abnormality of vulva and perineum, third trimester ♀   M

● **O34.8**   Maternal care for other abnormalities of pelvic organs

     O34.80   Maternal care for other abnormalities of pelvic organs, unspecified trimester ♀   M

     O34.81   Maternal care for other abnormalities of pelvic organs, first trimester ♀   M

     O34.82   Maternal care for other abnormalities of pelvic organs, second trimester ♀   M

     O34.83   Maternal care for other abnormalities of pelvic organs, third trimester ♀   M

● **O34.9**   Maternal care for abnormality of pelvic organ, unspecified

     O34.90   Maternal care for abnormality of pelvic organ, unspecified, unspecified trimester ♀   M

     O34.91   Maternal care for abnormality of pelvic organ, unspecified, first trimester ♀   M

     O34.92   Maternal care for abnormality of pelvic organ, unspecified, second trimester ♀   M

     O34.93   Maternal care for abnormality of pelvic organ, unspecified, third trimester ♀   M

N Newborn Age: 0   **P** Pediatric Age: 0–17   **M** Maternity DX: 12–55   **A** Adult Age: 15–124   ♀ Females Only   ♂ Males Only

🔴 Complication\Comorbidity   🏥 Major C\C   Ⓔⓧ CC/MCC Exclusions   🅟 Present on Admission Requirement   🅗 Hospital-Acquired Condition

OGCR Section I.C.15.e.1.

Fetal Conditions Affecting the Management of the Mother

1) Code from categories O35 and O36

Codes from categories O35, Maternal care for known or suspected fetal abnormality and damage, and O36, Maternal care for other fetal problems, are assigned only when the fetal condition is actually responsible for modifying the management of the mother, i.e., by requiring diagnostic studies, additional observation, special care, or termination of pregnancy. The fact that the fetal condition exists does not justify assigning a code from this series to the mother's record.

2) In utero surgery

In cases when surgery is performed on the fetus, a diagnosis code from category O35, Maternal care for known or suspected fetal abnormality and damage, should be assigned identifying the fetal condition. Assign the appropriate procedure code for the procedure performed.

No code from Chapter 16, the perinatal codes, should be used on the mother's record to identify fetal conditions. Surgery performed in utero on a fetus is still to be coded as an obstetric encounter.

● **O35**   **Maternal care for known or suspected fetal abnormality and damage**

     Includes   the listed conditions in the fetus as a reason for hospitalization or other obstetric care to the mother, or for termination of pregnancy

     Code also any associated maternal condition

     Excludes1   encounter for suspected maternal and fetal conditions ruled out (Z03.7-)

     One of the following 7th characters is to be assigned to each code under category O35. 7th character 0 is for single gestations and multiple gestations where the fetus is unspecified. 7th characters 1 through 9 are for cases of multiple gestations to identify the fetus for which the code applies. The appropriate code from category O30, Multiple gestation, must also be assigned when assigning a code from category O35 that has a 7th character of 1 through 9.

0	not applicable or unspecified
1	fetus 1
2	fetus 2
3	fetus 3
4	fetus 4
5	fetus 5
9	other fetus

X● **O35.0**   **Maternal care for (suspected) central nervous system malformation in fetus** ♀   M

     Maternal care for fetal anencephaly
     Maternal care for fetal hydrocephalus
     Maternal care for fetal spina bifida

       Excludes2   chromosomal abnormality in fetus (O35.1)

X● **O35.1**   **Maternal care for (suspected) chromosomal abnormality in fetus** ♀   M

X● **O35.2**   **Maternal care for (suspected) hereditary disease in fetus** ♀   M

       Excludes2   chromosomal abnormality in fetus (O35.1)

X● **O35.3**   **Maternal care for (suspected) damage to fetus from viral disease in mother** ♀   M

     Maternal care for damage to fetus from maternal cytomegalovirus infection
     Maternal care for damage to fetus from maternal rubella

X● **O35.4**   **Maternal care for (suspected) damage to fetus from alcohol** ♀   M

X● **O35.5**   **Maternal care for (suspected) damage to fetus by drugs** ♀   M

     Maternal care for damage to fetus from drug addiction

X● **O35.6**   **Maternal care for (suspected) damage to fetus by radiation** ♀   M

X● **O35.7**   **Maternal care for (suspected) damage to fetus by other medical procedures** ♀   M

     Maternal care for damage to fetus by amniocentesis
     Maternal care for damage to fetus by biopsy procedures
     Maternal care for damage to fetus by hematological investigation
     Maternal care for damage to fetus by intrauterine contraceptive device
     Maternal care for damage to fetus by intrauterine surgery

X● **O35.8**   **Maternal care for other (suspected) fetal abnormality and damage** ♀   M

     Maternal care for damage to fetus from maternal listeriosis
     Maternal care for damage to fetus from maternal toxoplasmosis

X● **O35.9**   **Maternal care for (suspected) fetal abnormality and damage, unspecified** ♀   M

● **O36**   **Maternal care for other fetal problems**

     Includes   the listed conditions in the fetus as a reason for hospitalization or other obstetric care of the mother, or for termination of pregnancy

     Excludes1   encounter for suspected maternal and fetal conditions ruled out (Z03.7-)
       placental transfusion syndromes (O43.0-)

     Excludes2   labor and delivery complicated by fetal stress (O77.-)

     One of the following 7th characters is to be assigned to each code under category O36. 7th character 0 is for single gestations and multiple gestations where the fetus is unspecified. 7th characters 1 through 9 are for cases of multiple gestations to identify the fetus for which the code applies. The appropriate code from category O30, Multiple gestation, must also be assigned when assigning a code from category O36 that has a 7th character of 1 through 9.

0	not applicable or unspecified
1	fetus 1
2	fetus 2
3	fetus 3
4	fetus 4
5	fetus 5
9	other fetus

● **O36.0**   **Maternal care for rhesus isoimmunization**

     Maternal care for Rh incompatibility (with hydrops fetalis)

     Ⓔⓧ For category O36.0 CC codes: O36.0110-O36.0139, O36.0910-O36.0939

   ● **O36.01**   **Maternal care for anti-D [Rh] antibodies**

     ● **O36.011**   **Maternal care for anti-D [Rh] antibodies, first trimester** ♀ 🔖   M

     ● **O36.012**   **Maternal care for anti-D [Rh] antibodies, second trimester** ♀ 🔖   M

     ● **O36.013**   **Maternal care for anti-D [Rh] antibodies, third trimester** ♀ 🔖   M

     ● **O36.019**   **Maternal care for anti-D [Rh] antibodies, unspecified trimester** ♀   M

   ● **O36.09**   **Maternal care for other rhesus isoimmunization**

     ● **O36.091**   **Maternal care for other rhesus isoimmunization, first trimester** ♀ 🔖   M

     ● **O36.092**   **Maternal care for other rhesus isoimmunization, second trimester** ♀ 🔖   M

     ● **O36.093**   **Maternal care for other rhesus isoimmunization, third trimester** ♀ 🔖   M

     ● **O36.099**   **Maternal care for other rhesus isoimmunization, unspecified trimester** ♀   M

◄ New   ◄▥ Revised   ~~deleted~~ Deleted   Excludes 1   Excludes 2   Includes   Use additional   Code first   Code also   Unspecified

OGCR Official Guidelines   ● Unacceptable Principal Diagnosis   X Assign placeholder X   ● Use Additional Character(s)   ▶ Manifestation Code   **Coding Clinic**

● **O36.1**   **Maternal care for other isoimmunization**
Maternal care for ABO isoimmunization

   ● **O36.11**   **Maternal care for Anti-A sensitization**
Maternal care for isoimmunization NOS (with hydrops fetalis)

     ● **O36.111**   **Maternal care for Anti-A sensitization, first trimester** ♀   M

     ● **O36.112**   **Maternal care for Anti-A sensitization, second trimester** ♀   M

     ● **O36.113**   **Maternal care for Anti-A sensitization, third trimester** ♀   M

     ● **O36.119**   **Maternal care for Anti-A sensitization, unspecified trimester** ♀   M

   ● **O36.19**   **Maternal care for other isoimmunization**
Maternal care for Anti-B sensitization

     ● **O36.191**   **Maternal care for other isoimmunization, first trimester** ♀   M

     ● **O36.192**   **Maternal care for other isoimmunization, second trimester** ♀   M

     ● **O36.193**   **Maternal care for other isoimmunization, third trimester** ♀   M

     ● **O36.199**   **Maternal care for other isoimmunization, unspecified trimester** ♀   M

● **O36.2**   **Maternal care for hydrops fetalis**
Maternal care for hydrops fetalis NOS
Maternal care for hydrops fetalis not associated with isoimmunization

   Excludes1   hydrops fetalis associated with ABO isoimmunization (O36.1-)
hydrops fetalis associated with rhesus isoimmunization (O36.0-)

   ● **O36.20**   **Maternal care for hydrops fetalis, unspecified trimester** ♀   M

   ● **O36.21**   **Maternal care for hydrops fetalis, first trimester** ♀   M

   ● **O36.22**   **Maternal care for hydrops fetalis, second trimester** ♀   M

   ● **O36.23**   **Maternal care for hydrops fetalis, third trimester** ♀   M

● **O36.4**   **Maternal care for intrauterine death** ♀ 🦠   M
Maternal care for intrauterine fetal death NOS
Maternal care for intrauterine fetal death after completion of 20 weeks of gestation
Maternal care for late fetal death
Maternal care for missed delivery

   Excludes1   missed abortion (O02.1)
stillbirth (P95)

   (Ex) O36.4XX0-O36.4XX9

● **O36.5**   **Maternal care for known or suspected poor fetal growth**

   ● **O36.51**   **Maternal care for known or suspected placental insufficiency**

     ● **O36.511**   **Maternal care for known or suspected placental insufficiency, first trimester** ♀   M

     ● **O36.512**   **Maternal care for known or suspected placental insufficiency, second trimester** ♀   M

     ● **O36.513**   **Maternal care for known or suspected placental insufficiency, third trimester** ♀   M

     ● **O36.519**   **Maternal care for known or suspected placental insufficiency, unspecified trimester** ♀   M

● **O36.59**   **Maternal care for other known or suspected poor fetal growth**
Maternal care for known or suspected light-for-dates NOS
Maternal care for known or suspected small-for-dates NOS

   ● **O36.591**   **Maternal care for other known or suspected poor fetal growth, first trimester** ♀   M

   ● **O36.592**   **Maternal care for other known or suspected poor fetal growth, second trimester** ♀   M

   ● **O36.593**   **Maternal care for other known or suspected poor fetal growth, third trimester** ♀   M

   ● **O36.599**   **Maternal care for other known or suspected poor fetal growth, unspecified trimester** ♀   M

● **O36.6**   **Maternal care for excessive fetal growth**
Maternal care for known or suspected large-for-dates

   X ● **O36.60**   **Maternal care for excessive fetal growth, unspecified trimester** ♀   M

   X ● **O36.61**   **Maternal care for excessive fetal growth, first trimester** ♀   M

   X ● **O36.62**   **Maternal care for excessive fetal growth, second trimester** ♀   M

   X ● **O36.63**   **Maternal care for excessive fetal growth, third trimester** ♀   M

● **O36.7**   **Maternal care for viable fetus in abdominal pregnancy**

   X ● **O36.70**   **Maternal care for viable fetus in abdominal pregnancy, unspecified trimester** ♀   M

   X ● **O36.71**   **Maternal care for viable fetus in abdominal pregnancy, first trimester** ♀   M

   X ● **O36.72**   **Maternal care for viable fetus in abdominal pregnancy, second trimester** ♀   M

   X ● **O36.73**   **Maternal care for viable fetus in abdominal pregnancy, third trimester** ♀   M

● **O36.8**   **Maternal care for other specified fetal problems**

   ● X ● **O36.80**   **Pregnancy with inconclusive fetal viability** ♀ M
Encounter to determine fetal viability of pregnancy

   ● **O36.81**   **Decreased fetal movements**

     ● **O36.812**   **Decreased fetal movements, second trimester** ♀   M

     ● **O36.813**   **Decreased fetal movements, third trimester** ♀   M

     ● **O36.819**   **Decreased fetal movements, unspecified trimester** ♀   M

   ● **O36.82**   **Fetal anemia and thrombocytopenia**

     ● **O36.821**   **Fetal anemia and thrombocytopenia, first trimester** ♀   M

     ● **O36.822**   **Fetal anemia and thrombocytopenia, second trimester** ♀   M

     ● **O36.823**   **Fetal anemia and thrombocytopenia, third trimester** ♀   M

     ● **O36.829**   **Fetal anemia and thrombocytopenia, unspecified trimester** ♀   M

   ● **O36.89**   **Maternal care for other specified fetal problems**

     ● **O36.891**   **Maternal care for other specified fetal problems, first trimester** ♀   M

     ● **O36.892**   **Maternal care for other specified fetal problems, second trimester** ♀   M

     ● **O36.893**   **Maternal care for other specified fetal problems, third trimester** ♀   M

     ● **O36.899**   **Maternal care for other specified fetal problems, unspecified trimester** ♀   M

N Newborn Age: 0   **P** Pediatric Age: 0–17   **M** Maternity DX: 12–55   **A** Adult Age: 15–124   ♀ Females Only   ♂ Males Only

🦠 Complication\Comorbidity   🦠 Major C\C   (Ex) CC/MCC Exclusions   🦠 Present on Admission Requirement   🦠 Hospital-Acquired Condition

1215

CHAPTER 15 (O00-O9A)

CHAPTER 15 (O00-O9A)

● **O36.9**   Maternal care for fetal problem, unspecified

   X ● **O36.90**   Maternal care for fetal problem, unspecified, unspecified trimester ♀   M

   X ● **O36.91**   Maternal care for fetal problem, unspecified, first trimester ♀   M

   X ● **O36.92**   Maternal care for fetal problem, unspecified, second trimester ♀   M

   X ● **O36.93**   Maternal care for fetal problem, unspecified, third trimester ♀   M

● **O40**   **Polyhydramnios**

Overabundance of amniotic fluid

| **Includes** | hydramnios |
| **Excludes1** | encounter for suspected maternal and fetal conditions ruled out (Z03.7-) |

One of the following 7th characters is to be assigned to each code under category O40. 7th character 0 is for single gestations and multiple gestations where the fetus is unspecified. 7th characters 1 through 9 are for cases of multiple gestations to identify the fetus for which the code applies. The appropriate code from category O30, Multiple gestation, must also be assigned when assigning a code from category O40 that has a 7th character of 1 through 9.

0	not applicable or unspecified
1	fetus 1
2	fetus 2
3	fetus 3
4	fetus 4
5	fetus 5
9	other fetus

   X ● **O40.1**   Polyhydramnios, first trimester ♀   M

   X ● **O40.2**   Polyhydramnios, second trimester ♀   M

   X ● **O40.3**   Polyhydramnios, third trimester ♀   M

   X ● **O40.9**   Polyhydramnios, unspecified trimester ♀   M

● **O41**   **Other disorders of amniotic fluid and membranes**

| **Excludes1** | encounter for suspected maternal and fetal conditions ruled out (Z03.7-) |

One of the following 7th characters is to be assigned to each code under category O41. 7th character 0 is for single gestations and multiple gestations where the fetus is unspecified. 7th characters 1 through 9 are for cases of multiple gestations to identify the fetus for which the code applies. The appropriate code from category O30, Multiple gestation, must also be assigned when assigning a code from category O41 that has a 7th character of 1 through 9.

0	not applicable or unspecified
1	fetus 1
2	fetus 2
3	fetus 3
4	fetus 4
5	fetus 5
9	other fetus

● **O41.0**   **Oligohydramnios**

Scant volume of amniotic fluid

Oligohydramnios without rupture of membranes

(Ex) For category O41.0 CC codes: O41.01X0-O41.03X9

   X ● **O41.00**   Oligohydramnios, unspecified trimester ♀   M

   X ● **O41.01**   Oligohydramnios, first trimester ♀ 🔾   M

   X ● **O41.02**   Oligohydramnios, second trimester ♀ 🔾   M

   X ● **O41.03**   Oligohydramnios, third trimester ♀ 🔾   M

● **O41.1**   Infection of amniotic sac and membranes

(Ex) For category O41.1 CC codes: O41.1010-O41.1039, O41.1210-O41.1239, O41.1410-O41.1439

   ● **O41.10**   Infection of amniotic sac and membranes, unspecified

     ● **O41.101**   Infection of amniotic sac and membranes, unspecified, first trimester ♀ 🔾   M

     ● **O41.102**   Infection of amniotic sac and membranes, unspecified, second trimester ♀ 🔾   M

     ● **O41.103**   Infection of amniotic sac and membranes, unspecified, third trimester ♀ 🔾   M

     ● **O41.109**   Infection of amniotic sac and membranes, unspecified, unspecified trimester ♀   M

   ● **O41.12**   Chorioamnionitis

     ● **O41.121**   Chorioamnionitis, first trimester ♀ 🔾   M

     ● **O41.122**   Chorioamnionitis, second trimester ♀ 🔾   M

     ● **O41.123**   Chorioamnionitis, third trimester ♀ 🔾   M

     ● **O41.129**   Chorioamnionitis, unspecified trimester ♀   M

   ● **O41.14**   Placentitis

     ● **O41.141**   Placentitis, first trimester ♀ 🔾   M

     ● **O41.142**   Placentitis, second trimester ♀ 🔾   M

     ● **O41.143**   Placentitis, third trimester ♀ 🔾   M

     ● **O41.149**   Placentitis, unspecified trimester ♀   M

● **O41.8**   Other specified disorders of amniotic fluid and membranes

   ● **O41.8X**   Other specified disorders of amniotic fluid and membranes

     ● **O41.8X1**   Other specified disorders of amniotic fluid and membranes, first trimester ♀

     ● **O41.8X2**   Other specified disorders of amniotic fluid and membranes, second trimester ♀   M

     ● **O41.8X3**   Other specified disorders of amniotic fluid and membranes, third trimester ♀   M

     ● **O41.8X9**   Other specified disorders of amniotic fluid and membranes, unspecified trimester ♀

● **O41.9**   Disorder of amniotic fluid and membranes, unspecified

   X ● **O41.90**   Disorder of amniotic fluid and membranes, unspecified, unspecified trimester ♀   M

   X ● **O41.91**   Disorder of amniotic fluid and membranes, unspecified, first trimester ♀   M

   X ● **O41.92**   Disorder of amniotic fluid and membranes, unspecified, second trimester ♀   M

   X ● **O41.93**   Disorder of amniotic fluid and membranes, unspecified, third trimester ♀   M

1216

◀ New   ◀ Revised   ~~deleted~~ Deleted   Excludes 1   Excludes 2   Includes   Use additional   Code first   Code also   Unspecified

OGCR Official Guidelines   ● Unacceptable Principal Diagnosis   X Assign placeholder X   ● Use Additional Character(s)   ▶ Manifestation Code   **Coding Clinic**

● **O42**   **Premature rupture of membranes**
  ● **O42.0**   Premature rupture of membranes, onset of labor within 24 hours of rupture
     O42.00   Premature rupture of membranes, onset of labor within 24 hours of rupture, unspecified weeks of gestation ♀   M
    ● **O42.01**   Preterm premature rupture of membranes, onset of labor within 24 hours of rupture
         Premature rupture of membranes before 37 completed weeks of gestation
       O42.011   Preterm premature rupture of membranes, onset of labor within 24 hours of rupture, first trimester ♀   M
       O42.012   Preterm premature rupture of membranes, onset of labor within 24 hours of rupture, second trimester ♀ M
       O42.013   Preterm premature rupture of membranes, onset of labor within 24 hours of rupture, third trimester ♀   M
       O42.019   Preterm premature rupture of membranes, onset of labor within 24 hours of rupture, unspecified trimester ♀   M
     O42.02   Full-term premature rupture of membranes, onset of labor within 24 hours of rupture ♀   M
         Premature rupture of membranes after 37 completed weeks of gestation
  ● **O42.1**   Premature rupture of membranes, onset of labor more than 24 hours following rupture
     O42.10   Premature rupture of membranes, onset of labor more than 24 hours following rupture, unspecified weeks of gestation ♀   M
    ● **O42.11**   Preterm premature rupture of membranes, onset of labor more than 24 hours following rupture
         Premature rupture of membranes before 37 completed weeks of gestation
       O42.111   Preterm premature rupture of membranes, onset of labor more than 24 hours following rupture, first trimester ♀   M
       O42.112   Preterm premature rupture of membranes, onset of labor more than 24 hours following rupture, second trimester ♀   M
       O42.113   Preterm premature rupture of membranes, onset of labor more than 24 hours following rupture, third trimester ♀   M
       O42.119   Preterm premature rupture of membranes, onset of labor more than 24 hours following rupture, unspecified trimester ♀   M
     O42.12   Full-term premature rupture of membranes, onset of labor more than 24 hours following rupture ♀   M
         Premature rupture of membranes after 37 completed weeks of gestation

  ● **O42.9**   Premature rupture of membranes, unspecified as to length of time between rupture and onset of labor
     O42.90   Premature rupture of membranes, unspecified as to length of time between rupture and onset of labor, unspecified weeks of gestation ♀   M
    ● **O42.91**   Preterm premature rupture of membranes, unspecified as to length of time between rupture and onset of labor
         Premature rupture of membranes before 37 completed weeks of gestation
       O42.911   Preterm premature rupture of membranes, unspecified as to length of time between rupture and onset of labor, first trimester ♀   M
       O42.912   Preterm premature rupture of membranes, unspecified as to length of time between rupture and onset of labor, second trimester ♀   M
       O42.913   Preterm premature rupture of membranes, unspecified as to length of time between rupture and onset of labor, third trimester ♀   M
       O42.919   Preterm premature rupture of membranes, unspecified as to length of time between rupture and onset of labor, unspecified trimester ♀   M
     O42.92   Full-term premature rupture of membranes, unspecified as to length of time between rupture and onset of labor ♀   M
         Premature rupture of membranes after 37 completed weeks of gestation

● **O43**   **Placental disorders**
   Excludes2   maternal care for poor fetal growth due to placental insufficiency (O36.5-)
           placenta previa (O44.-)
           placental polyp (O90.89)
           placentitis (O41.14-)
           premature separation of placenta [abruptio placentae] (O45.-)
  ● **O43.0**   Placental transfusion syndromes
    ● **O43.01**   Fetomaternal placental transfusion syndrome
         Maternofetal placental transfusion syndrome
       O43.011   Fetomaternal placental transfusion syndrome, first trimester ♀   M
       O43.012   Fetomaternal placental transfusion syndrome, second trimester ♀   M
       O43.013   Fetomaternal placental transfusion syndrome, third trimester ♀   M
       O43.019   Fetomaternal placental transfusion syndrome, unspecified trimester ♀   M
    ● **O43.02**   Fetus-to-fetus placental transfusion syndrome
       O43.021   Fetus-to-fetus placental transfusion syndrome, first trimester ♀   M
       O43.022   Fetus-to-fetus placental transfusion syndrome, second trimester ♀   M
       O43.023   Fetus-to-fetus placental transfusion syndrome, third trimester ♀   M
       O43.029   Fetus-to-fetus placental transfusion syndrome, unspecified trimester ♀   M

CHAPTER 15 (O00-O9A)

CHAPTER 15 (O00-O9A)

● **O43.1 Malformation of placenta**
 ● **O43.10 Malformation of placenta, unspecified**
  Abnormal placenta NOS
  O43.101 Malformation of placenta, unspecified, first trimester ♀   M
  O43.102 Malformation of placenta, unspecified, second trimester ♀   M
  O43.103 Malformation of placenta, unspecified, third trimester ♀   M
  O43.109 Malformation of placenta, unspecified, unspecified trimester ♀   M
 ● **O43.11 Circumvallate placenta**
  O43.111 Circumvallate placenta, first trimester ♀   M
  O43.112 Circumvallate placenta, second trimester ♀   M
  O43.113 Circumvallate placenta, third trimester ♀   M
  O43.119 Circumvallate placenta, unspecified trimester ♀   M
 ● **O43.12 Velamentous insertion of umbilical cord**
  O43.121 Velamentous insertion of umbilical cord, first trimester ♀   M
  O43.122 Velamentous insertion of umbilical cord, second trimester ♀   M
  O43.123 Velamentous insertion of umbilical cord, third trimester ♀   M
  O43.129 Velamentous insertion of umbilical cord, unspecified trimester ♀   M
 ● **O43.19 Other malformation of placenta**
  O43.191 Other malformation of placenta, first trimester ♀   M
  O43.192 Other malformation of placenta, second trimester ♀   M
  O43.193 Other malformation of placenta, third trimester ♀   M
  O43.199 Other malformation of placenta, unspecified trimester ♀   M
● **O43.2 Morbidly adherent placenta**
 Code also associated third stage postpartum hemorrhage, if applicable (O72.0)
 Excludes1 retained placenta (O73.-)
 ● **O43.21 Placenta accreta**
  O43.211 Placenta accreta, first trimester ♀   M
  O43.212 Placenta accreta, second trimester ♀   M
  O43.213 Placenta accreta, third trimester ♀   M
  O43.219 Placenta accreta, unspecified trimester ♀   M
 ● **O43.22 Placenta increta**
  O43.221 Placenta increta, first trimester ♀   M
  O43.222 Placenta increta, second trimester ♀   M
  O43.223 Placenta increta, third trimester ♀   M
  O43.229 Placenta increta, unspecified trimester ♀   M
 ● **O43.23 Placenta percreta**
  O43.231 Placenta percreta, first trimester ♀   M
  O43.232 Placenta percreta, second trimester ♀ M
  O43.233 Placenta percreta, third trimester ♀   M
  O43.239 Placenta percreta, unspecified trimester ♀   M

● **O43.8 Other placental disorders**
 ● **O43.81 Placental infarction**
  O43.811 Placental infarction, first trimester ♀ M
  O43.812 Placental infarction, second trimester ♀   M
  O43.813 Placental infarction, third trimester ♀   M
  O43.819 Placental infarction, unspecified trimester ♀   M
 ● **O43.89 Other placental disorders**
  Placental dysfunction
  O43.891 Other placental disorders, first trimester ♀   M
  O43.892 Other placental disorders, second trimester ♀   M
  O43.893 Other placental disorders, third trimester ♀   M
  O43.899 Other placental disorders, unspecified trimester ♀   M
● **O43.9 Unspecified placental disorder**
 O43.90 Unspecified placental disorder, unspecified trimester ♀   M
 O43.91 Unspecified placental disorder, first trimester ♀   M
 O43.92 Unspecified placental disorder, second trimester ♀   M
 O43.93 Unspecified placental disorder, third trimester ♀   M

● **O44 Placenta previa**
 (Ex) **For category O44 CC codes:** O20.0-O20.9, O25.10-O25.3, O26.10-O26.13, O26.30-O26.43, O26.63-O26.819, O26.841-O26.86, O26.891-O26.93, O29.011-O29.93, O35.7XX0-O35.7XX9, O44.00-O44.13, O75.4, O75.81, O75.89-O75.9, O80, O90.89, O99.111-O99.119, O99.12-O99.285, O99.330-O99.335, O99.350-O99.355, O99.511-O99.73, O99.820-O99.825, O99.840-O9A.53

 ● **O44.0 Placenta previa specified as without hemorrhage**
  Low implantation of placenta specified as without hemorrhage
  O44.00 Placenta previa specified as without hemorrhage, unspecified trimester ♀   M
  O44.01 Placenta previa specified as without hemorrhage, first trimester ♀ 🔵   M
  O44.02 Placenta previa specified as without hemorrhage, second trimester ♀ 🔵   M
  O44.03 Placenta previa specified as without hemorrhage, third trimester ♀ 🔵   M

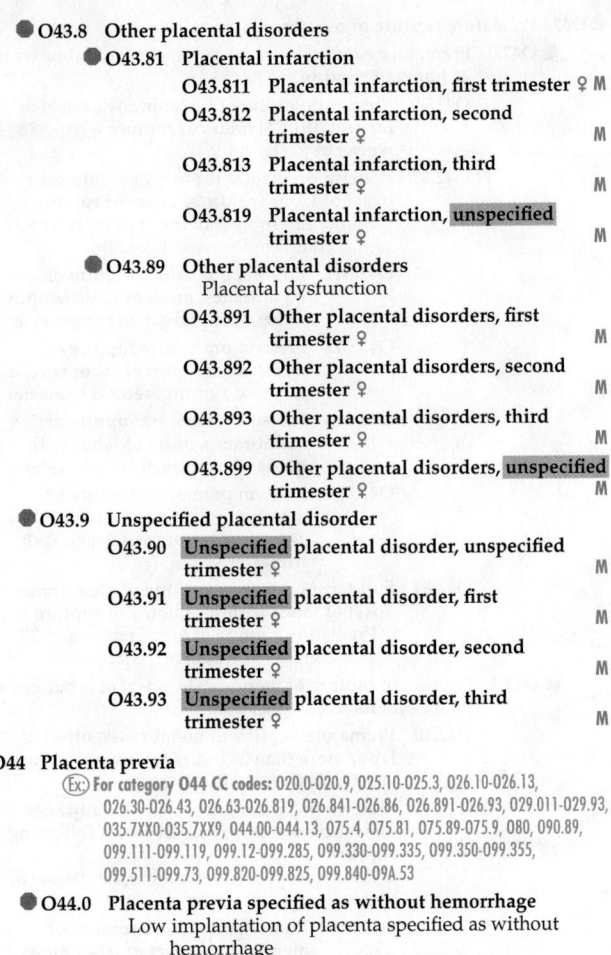

Figure 15-2 A. Marginal placento previa. **B.** Partial placenta previa. **C.** Total placento previa.

Item 15-3 Placenta previa is a condition in which the opening of the cervix is obstructed by the displaced placenta. The three types, marginal, partial, and total, are varying degrees of placenta displacement. Placenta abruption is the premature breaking away of the placenta from the site of the uterine implant before the delivery of the fetus.

◄ New   ◄▥ Revised   ~~deleted~~ Deleted   Excludes 1   Excludes 2   Includes   Use additional   Code first   Code also   Unspecified
OGCR Official Guidelines   ● Unacceptable Principal Diagnosis   X Assign placeholder X   ● Use Additional Character(s)   ▶ Manifestation Code   **Coding Clinic**

● O44.1   **Placenta previa with hemorrhage**
　　　　Low implantation of placenta, NOS or with hemorrhage
　　　　Marginal placenta previa, NOS or with hemorrhage
　　　　Partial placenta previa, NOS or with hemorrhage
　　　　Total placenta previa, NOS or with hemorrhage

　　　　Excludes1　labor and delivery complicated by
　　　　　　　hemorrhage from vasa previa
　　　　　　　(O69.4)

　　　O44.10　Placenta previa with hemorrhage, **unspecified**
　　　　　　trimester ♀　　　　　　　　　　M

　　　O44.11　Placenta previa with hemorrhage, first
　　　　　　trimester ♀ 🐾　　　　　　　　M

　　　O44.12　Placenta previa with hemorrhage, second
　　　　　　trimester ♀ 🐾　　　　　　　　M

　　　O44.13　Placenta previa with hemorrhage, third
　　　　　　trimester ♀ 🐾　　　　　　　　M

● O45   **Premature separation of placenta [abruptio placentae]**

　● O45.0　**Premature separation of placenta with coagulation
　　　　defect**
　　　　(Ex) For category O45.0 CC codes: 025.10-025.3, 026.10-026.13,
　　　　026.30-026.43, 026.63-026.819, 026.841-026.86, 026.891-026.93,
　　　　029.011-029.93, 035.7XX0-035.7XX9, 045.001-045.099, 046.001-046.93,
　　　　067.0-067.9, 075.4, 075.81, 075.89-075.9, 080, 090.89,
　　　　099.111-099.285, 099.330-099.335, 099.350-099.355, 099.511-099.73,
　　　　099.820-099.825, 099.840-09A.53

　　　● O45.00　**Premature separation of placenta with
　　　　　coagulation defect, unspecified**

　　　　　O45.001　Premature separation of placenta with
　　　　　　　coagulation defect, **unspecified**, first
　　　　　　　trimester ♀ 🐾　　　　　　　M

　　　　　O45.002　Premature separation of placenta with
　　　　　　　coagulation defect, **unspecified**,
　　　　　　　second trimester ♀ 🐾　　　　M

　　　　　O45.003　Premature separation of placenta with
　　　　　　　coagulation defect, **unspecified**, third
　　　　　　　trimester ♀ 🐾　　　　　　　M

　　　　　O45.009　Premature separation of placenta
　　　　　　　with coagulation defect, **unspecified**,
　　　　　　　unspecified trimester ♀　　　　M

　　　● O45.01　**Premature separation of placenta with
　　　　　afibrinogenemia**
　　　　　　Premature separation of placenta with
　　　　　　　hypofibrinogenemia

　　　　　O45.011　Premature separation of placenta with
　　　　　　　afibrinogenemia, first trimester ♀ 🐾 M

　　　　　O45.012　Premature separation of placenta with
　　　　　　　afibrinogenemia, second
　　　　　　　trimester ♀ 🐾　　　　　　　M

　　　　　O45.013　Premature separation of placenta with
　　　　　　　afibrinogenemia, third
　　　　　　　trimester ♀ 🐾　　　　　　　M

　　　　　O45.019　Premature separation of placenta
　　　　　　　with afibrinogenemia, **unspecified**
　　　　　　　trimester ♀　　　　　　　　M

Figure 15-3 Abruptio placentae is classified according to the grade
of separation of the placenta from the uterine wall. **A.** Mild separation
in which hemorrhage is internal. **B.** Moderate separation in which there
is external hemorrhage. **C.** Severe separation in which there is external
hemorrhage and extreme separation.

● O45.02　**Premature separation of placenta with
　　　　disseminated intravascular coagulation**

　　　O45.021　Premature separation of placenta with
　　　　　disseminated intravascular
　　　　　coagulation, first trimester ♀ 🐾　M

　　　O45.022　Premature separation of placenta with
　　　　　disseminated intravascular
　　　　　coagulation, second trimester ♀ 🐾　M

　　　O45.023　Premature separation of placenta with
　　　　　disseminated intravascular
　　　　　coagulation, third trimester ♀ 🐾　M

　　　O45.029　Premature separation of placenta
　　　　　with disseminated intravascular
　　　　　coagulation, **unspecified** trimester ♀ M

● O45.09　**Premature separation of placenta with other
　　　　coagulation defect**

　　　O45.091　Premature separation of placenta with
　　　　　other coagulation defect, first
　　　　　trimester ♀ 🐾　　　　　　　　M

　　　O45.092　Premature separation of placenta with
　　　　　other coagulation defect, second
　　　　　trimester ♀ 🐾　　　　　　　　M

　　　O45.093　Premature separation of placenta with
　　　　　other coagulation defect, third
　　　　　trimester ♀ 🐾　　　　　　　　M

　　　O45.099　Premature separation of placenta with
　　　　　other coagulation defect, **unspecified**
　　　　　trimester ♀　　　　　　　　　M

● O45.8　**Other premature separation of placenta**
　　　　(Ex) For category O45.8 CC codes: 020.0-020.9, 025.10-025.3,
　　　　026.10-026.13, 026.30-026.43, 026.63-026.819, 026.841-026.86,
　　　　026.891-026.93, 029.011-029.93, 035.7XX0-035.7XX9, 044.00-044.13,
　　　　045.8X1-045.8X3, 045.91-045.93, 075.4, 075.81, 075.89-075.9, 080,
　　　　090.89, 099.111-099.285, 099.330-099.335, 099.350-099.355,
　　　　099.511-099.73, 099.820-099.825, 099.840-09A.53

　　　● O45.8X　**Other premature separation of placenta**

　　　　　O45.8X1　Other premature separation of
　　　　　　　placenta, first trimester ♀ 🐾　M

　　　　　O45.8X2　Other premature separation of
　　　　　　　placenta, second trimester ♀ 🐾　M

　　　　　O45.8X3　Other premature separation of
　　　　　　　placenta, third trimester ♀ 🐾　M

　　　　　O45.8X9　Other premature separation of
　　　　　　　placenta, **unspecified** trimester ♀　M

● O45.9　**Premature separation of placenta, unspecified**
　　　　Abruptio placentae NOS
　　　　(Ex) For category O45.9 CC codes: See 045.8

　　　O45.90　Premature separation of placenta, **unspecified**,
　　　　　unspecified trimester ♀　　　　　M

　　　O45.91　Premature separation of placenta, **unspecified**,
　　　　　first trimester ♀ 🐾　　　　　　M

　　　O45.92　Premature separation of placenta, **unspecified**,
　　　　　second trimester ♀ 🐾　　　　　M

　　　O45.93　Premature separation of placenta, **unspecified**,
　　　　　third trimester ♀ 🐾　　　　　　M

● O46　**Antepartum hemorrhage, not elsewhere classified**

　　　Excludes1　hemorrhage in early pregnancy (O20.-)
　　　　　　intrapartum hemorrhage NEC (O67.-)
　　　　　　placenta previa (O44.-)
　　　　　　premature separation of placenta [abruptio
　　　　　　　placentae] (O45.-)

　● O46.0　**Antepartum hemorrhage with coagulation defect**
　　　　(Ex) For category O46.0 CC codes: See 045.0

　　　● O46.00　**Antepartum hemorrhage with coagulation
　　　　　defect, unspecified**

　　　　　O46.001　Antepartum hemorrhage with
　　　　　　　coagulation defect, **unspecified**, first
　　　　　　　trimester ♀ 🐾　　　　　　　M

　　　　　O46.002　Antepartum hemorrhage with
　　　　　　　coagulation defect, **unspecified**,
　　　　　　　second trimester ♀ 🐾　　　　M

N Newborn Age: 0　　P Pediatric Age: 0–17　　M Maternity DX: 12–55　　A Adult Age: 15–124　　♀ Females Only　　♂ Males Only
🐾 Complication\Comorbidity　　🐾 Major C\C　　(Ex) CC/MCC Exclusions　　🐾 Present on Admission Requirement　　🐾 Hospital-Acquired Condition

CHAPTER 15 (O00-O9A)

1219

CHAPTER 15 (O00–O9A)

O46.003   **Antepartum hemorrhage with coagulation defect, unspecified, third trimester** ♀ 🧬   M

O46.009   **Antepartum hemorrhage with coagulation defect, unspecified, unspecified trimester** ♀   M

● **O46.01 Antepartum hemorrhage with afibrinogenemia**
Antepartum hemorrhage with hypofibrinogenemia

O46.011   **Antepartum hemorrhage with afibrinogenemia, first trimester** ♀ 🧬 M

O46.012   **Antepartum hemorrhage with afibrinogenemia, second trimester** ♀ 🧬   M

O46.013   **Antepartum hemorrhage with afibrinogenemia, third trimester** ♀ 🧬   M

O46.019   **Antepartum hemorrhage with afibrinogenemia, unspecified trimester** ♀   M

● **O46.02 Antepartum hemorrhage with disseminated intravascular coagulation**

O46.021   **Antepartum hemorrhage with disseminated intravascular coagulation, first trimester** ♀ 🧬   M

O46.022   **Antepartum hemorrhage with disseminated intravascular coagulation, second trimester** ♀ 🧬   M

O46.023   **Antepartum hemorrhage with disseminated intravascular coagulation, third trimester** ♀ 🧬   M

O46.029   **Antepartum hemorrhage with disseminated intravascular coagulation, unspecified trimester** ♀ M

● **O46.09 Antepartum hemorrhage with other coagulation defect**

O46.091   **Antepartum hemorrhage with other coagulation defect, first trimester** ♀ 🧬   M

O46.092   **Antepartum hemorrhage with other coagulation defect, second trimester** ♀ 🧬   M

O46.093   **Antepartum hemorrhage with other coagulation defect, third trimester** ♀ 🧬   M

O46.099   **Antepartum hemorrhage with other coagulation defect, unspecified trimester** ♀   M

● **O46.8 Other antepartum hemorrhage**

  ● **O46.8x Other antepartum hemorrhage**

O46.8x1   **Other antepartum hemorrhage, first trimester** ♀   M

O46.8x2   **Other antepartum hemorrhage, second trimester** ♀   M

O46.8x3   **Other antepartum hemorrhage, third trimester** ♀   M

O46.8x9   **Other antepartum hemorrhage, unspecified trimester** ♀   M

● **O46.9 Antepartum hemorrhage, unspecified**

O46.90   **Antepartum hemorrhage, unspecified, unspecified trimester** ♀   M

O46.91   **Antepartum hemorrhage, unspecified, first trimester** ♀   M

O46.92   **Antepartum hemorrhage, unspecified, second trimester** ♀   M

O46.93   **Antepartum hemorrhage, unspecified, third trimester** ♀   M

● **O47 False labor**

  Includes   Braxton Hicks contractions
threatened labor

  Excludes1   preterm labor (O60.-)

ⒺⓍ **For category O47 CC codes:** O25.10-O25.3, O26.10-O26.13, O26.30-O26.43, O26.63-O26.819, O26.841-O26.86, O26.891-O26.93, O29.011-O29.93, O35.7XX0-O35.7XX9, O47.00-O47.9, O60.00-O60.23X9, O75.4, O75.81, O75.89-O75.9, O80, O90.89, O99.111-O99.285, O99.330-O99.335, O99.350-O99.355, O99.511-O99.73, O99.820-O99.825, O99.840-O9A.53

● **O47.0 False labor before 37 completed weeks of gestation**

O47.00   **False labor before 37 completed weeks of gestation, unspecified trimester** ♀   M

O47.02   **False labor before 37 completed weeks of gestation, second trimester** ♀ 🧬   M

O47.03   **False labor before 37 completed weeks of gestation, third trimester** ♀ 🧬   M

O47.1   **False labor at or after 37 completed weeks of gestation** ♀ 🧬   M

O47.9   **False labor, unspecified** ♀   M

● **O48 Late pregnancy**

O48.0   **Post-term pregnancy** ♀   M
Pregnancy over 40 completed weeks to 42 completed weeks gestation

O48.1   **Prolonged pregnancy** ♀   M
Pregnancy which has advanced beyond 42 completed weeks gestation

---

COMPLICATIONS OF LABOR AND DELIVERY (O60-O77)

● **O60 Preterm labor**

  Includes   onset (spontaneous) of labor before 37 completed weeks of gestation

  Excludes1   false labor (O47.0-)
threatened labor NOS (O47.0-)

ⒺⓍ **For category O60 CC codes:** O25.10-O25.3, O26.10-O26.13, O26.30-O26.43, O26.63-O26.819, O26.841-O26.86, O26.891-O26.93, O29.011-O29.93, O35.7XX0-O35.7XX9, O47.00-O47.9, O60.00-O60.23X9, O75.4, O75.81, O75.89-O75.9, O80, O90.89, O99.111-O99.285, O99.330-O99.335, O99.350-O99.355, O99.511-O99.73, O99.820-O99.825, O99.840-O9A.53

● **O60.0 Preterm labor without delivery**

O60.00   **Preterm labor without delivery, unspecified trimester** ♀   M

O60.02   **Preterm labor without delivery, second trimester** ♀ 🧬   M

O60.03   **Preterm labor without delivery, third trimester** ♀ 🧬   M

● **O60.1 Preterm labor with preterm delivery**

One of the following 7th characters is to be assigned to each code under subcategory O60.1. 7th character 0 is for single gestations and multiple gestations where the fetus is unspecified. 7th characters 1 through 9 are for cases of multiple gestations to identify the fetus for which the code applies. The appropriate code from category O30, Multiple gestation, must also be assigned when assigning a code from subcategory O60.1 that has a 7th character of 1 through 9.

0	not applicable or unspecified
1	fetus 1
2	fetus 2
3	fetus 3
4	fetus 4
5	fetus 5
9	other fetus

X ● O60.10   **Preterm labor with preterm delivery, unspecified trimester** ♀ 🧬   M
Preterm labor with delivery NOS

X ● O60.12   **Preterm labor second trimester with preterm delivery second trimester** ♀ 🧬   M

X ● O60.13   **Preterm labor second trimester with preterm delivery third trimester** ♀ 🧬   M

◀ New   ◀||| Revised   ~~deleted~~ Deleted   Excludes 1   Excludes 2   Includes   Use additional   Code first   Code also   Unspecified

OGCR Official Guidelines   ● Unacceptable Principal Diagnosis   X Assign placeholder X   ● Use Additional Character(s)   ⍒ Manifestation Code   **Coding Clinic**

X ● **O60.14**   **Preterm labor third trimester with preterm delivery third trimester** ♀ 🅶   M

● **O60.2**   **Term delivery with preterm labor**

One of the following 7th characters is to be assigned to each code under subcategory O60.2. 7th character 0 is for single gestations and multiple gestations where the fetus is unspecified. 7th characters 1 through 9 are for cases of multiple gestations to identify the fetus for which the code applies. The appropriate code from category O30, Multiple gestation, must also be assigned when assigning a code from subcategory O60.2 that has a 7th character of 1 through 9.

0	not applicable or unspecified
1	fetus 1
2	fetus 2
3	fetus 3
4	fetus 4
5	fetus 5
9	other fetus

X ● **O60.20**   **Term delivery with preterm labor, unspecified trimester** ♀ 🅶   M

X ● **O60.22**   **Term delivery with preterm labor, second trimester** ♀ 🅶   M

X ● **O60.23**   **Term delivery with preterm labor, third trimester** ♀ 🅶   M

● **O61**   **Failed induction of labor**

O61.0   **Failed medical induction of labor** ♀   M
Failed induction (of labor) by oxytocin
Failed induction (of labor) by prostaglandins

O61.1   **Failed instrumental induction of labor** ♀   M
Failed mechanical induction (of labor)
Failed surgical induction (of labor)

O61.8   **Other failed induction of labor** ♀   M

O61.9   **Failed induction of labor, unspecified** ♀   M

● **O62**   **Abnormalities of forces of labor**

O62.0   **Primary inadequate contractions** ♀   M
Failure of cervical dilatation
Primary hypotonic uterine dysfunction
Uterine inertia during latent phase of labor

O62.1   **Secondary uterine inertia** ♀   M
Arrested active phase of labor
Secondary hypotonic uterine dysfunction

O62.2   **Other uterine inertia** ♀   M
Atony of uterus without hemorrhage
Atony of uterus NOS
Desultory labor
Hypotonic uterine dysfunction NOS
Irregular labor
Poor contractions
Slow slope active phase of labor
Uterine inertia NOS

> **Excludes 1**   atony of uterus with hemorrhage (postpartum) (O72.1)
> postpartum atony of uterus without hemorrhage (O75.89)

O62.3   **Precipitate labor** ♀   M

O62.4   **Hypertonic, incoordinate, and prolonged uterine contractions** ♀   M
Cervical spasm
Contraction ring dystocia
Dyscoordinate labor
Hour-glass contraction of uterus
Hypertonic uterine dysfunction
Incoordinate uterine action
Tetanic contractions
Uterine dystocia NOS
Uterine spasm

> **Excludes 1**   dystocia (fetal) (maternal) NOS (O66.9)

O62.8   **Other abnormalities of forces of labor** ♀   M

O62.9   **Abnormality of forces of labor, unspecified** ♀   M

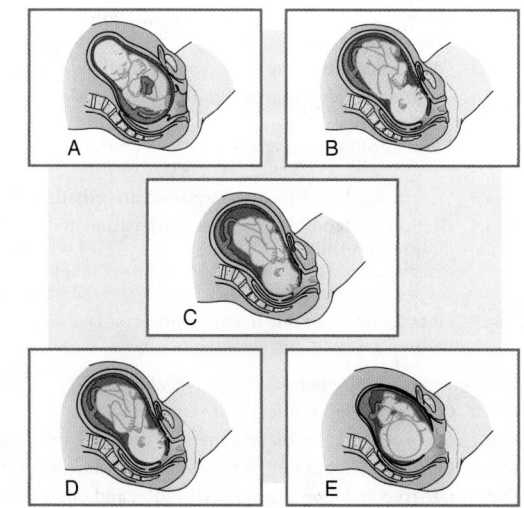

Figure 15-4   Five types of malposition and malpresentation of the fetus: **A.** Breech. **B.** Vertex. **C.** Face. **D.** Brow. **E.** Shoulder.

● **O63**   **Long labor**

O63.0   **Prolonged first stage (of labor)** ♀   M

O63.1   **Prolonged second stage (of labor)** ♀   M

O63.2   **Delayed delivery of second twin, triplet, etc.** ♀   M

O63.9   **Long labor, unspecified** ♀ 🅶   M
Prolonged labor NOS

> Ⓔⓧ O25.10-O25.3, O26.10-O26.13, O26.30-O26.43, O26.63-O26.819, O26.841-O26.86, O26.891-O26.93, O29.011-O29.93, O35.7XX0-O35.7XX9, O36.8120-O36.8199, O63.9, O71.00-O71.1, O71.5, O71.81, O71.89-O71.9, O75.4, O75.81, O75.89-O75.9, O80, O90.89, O99.111-O99.285, O99.330-O99.335, O99.350-O99.355, O99.511-O99.73, O99.820-O99.825, O99.840-O9A.53

● **O64**   **Obstructed labor due to malposition and malpresentation of fetus**

One of the following 7th characters is to be assigned to each code under category O64. 7th character 0 is for single gestations and multiple gestations where the fetus is unspecified. 7th characters 1 through 9 are for cases of multiple gestations to identify the fetus for which the code applies. The appropriate code from category O30, Multiple gestation, must also be assigned when assigning a code from category O64 that has a 7th character of 1 through 9.

0	not applicable or unspecified
1	fetus 1
2	fetus 2
3	fetus 3
4	fetus 4
5	fetus 5
9	other fetus

X ● **O64.0**   **Obstructed labor due to incomplete rotation of fetal head** ♀   M
Deep transverse arrest
Obstructed labor due to persistent occipitoiliac (position)
Obstructed labor due to persistent occipitoposterior (position)
Obstructed labor due to persistent occipitosacral (position)
Obstructed labor due to persistent occipitotransverse (position)

X ● **O64.1**   **Obstructed labor due to breech presentation** ♀   M
Obstructed labor due to buttocks presentation
Obstructed labor due to complete breech presentation
Obstructed labor due to frank breech presentation

N   Newborn Age: 0   P   Pediatric Age: 0–17   M   Maternity DX: 12–55   A   Adult Age: 15–124   ♀   Females Only   ♂   Males Only

🅲   Complication\Comorbidity   🅼   Major C\C   Ⓔⓧ   CC/MCC Exclusions   🅿   Present on Admission Requirement   🅷   Hospital-Acquired Condition

1221

CHAPTER 15 (O00-O9A)

X ● **O64.2** **Obstructed labor due to face presentation** ♀   M
Obstructed labor due to chin presentation

X ● **O64.3** **Obstructed labor due to brow presentation** ♀   M

X ● **O64.4** **Obstructed labor due to shoulder presentation** ♀   M
Prolapsed arm
Excludes1 impacted shoulders (O66.0)
shoulder dystocia (O66.0)

X ● **O64.5** **Obstructed labor due to compound presentation** ♀   M

X ● **O64.8** **Obstructed labor due to other malposition and
malpresentation** ♀   M
Obstructed labor due to footling presentation
Obstructed labor due to incomplete breech presentation

X ● **O64.9** **Obstructed labor due to malposition and
malpresentation, unspecified** ♀   M

● **O65** **Obstructed labor due to maternal pelvic abnormality**

O65.0 **Obstructed labor due to deformed pelvis** ♀   M

O65.1 **Obstructed labor due to generally contracted pelvis** ♀   M

O65.2 **Obstructed labor due to pelvic inlet contraction** ♀   M

O65.3 **Obstructed labor due to pelvic outlet and mid-cavity
contraction** ♀   M

O65.4 **Obstructed labor due to fetopelvic disproportion,
unspecified** ♀   M
Excludes1 dystocia due to abnormality of fetus
(O66.2-O66.3)

O65.5 **Obstructed labor due to abnormality of maternal pelvic
organs** ♀   M
Obstructed labor due to conditions listed in O34.-
Use additional code to identify abnormality of pelvic
organs O34.-

O65.8 **Obstructed labor due to other maternal pelvic
abnormalities** ♀   M

O65.9 **Obstructed labor due to maternal pelvic abnormality,
unspecified** ♀   M

● **O66** **Other obstructed labor**

O66.0 **Obstructed labor due to shoulder dystocia** ♀   M
Impacted shoulders

O66.1 **Obstructed labor due to locked twins** ♀   M

O66.2 **Obstructed labor due to unusually large fetus** ♀   M

O66.3 **Obstructed labor due to other abnormalities of fetus** ♀ M
Dystocia due to fetal ascites
Dystocia due to fetal hydrops
Dystocia due to fetal meningomyelocele
Dystocia due to fetal sacral teratoma
Dystocia due to fetal tumor
Dystocia due to hydrocephalic fetus
Use additional code to identify cause of obstruction

● **O66.4** **Failed trial of labor**

O66.40 **Failed trial of labor, unspecified** ♀   M

O66.41 **Failed attempted vaginal birth after previous
cesarean delivery** ♀   M
*Code first rupture of uterus, if applicable
(O71.0-, O71.1)*

O66.5 **Attempted application of vacuum extractor and
forceps** ♀ 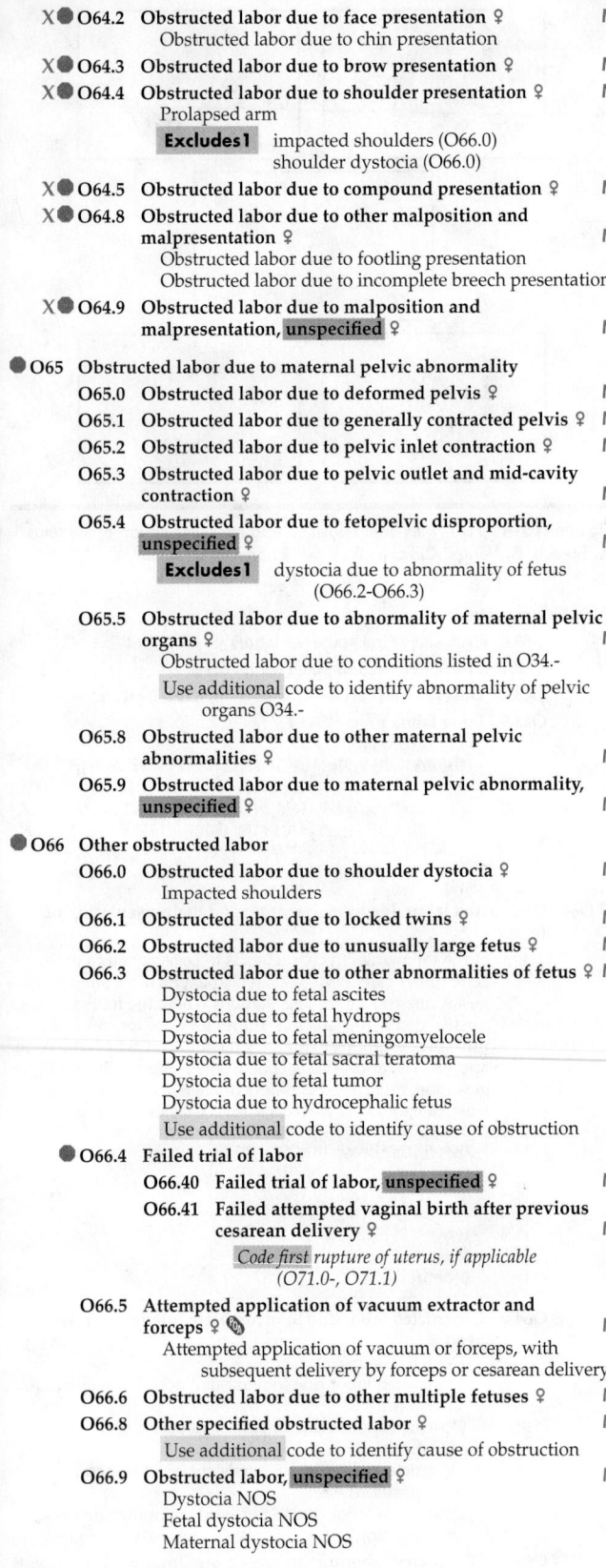   M
Attempted application of vacuum or forceps, with
subsequent delivery by forceps or cesarean delivery

O66.6 **Obstructed labor due to other multiple fetuses** ♀   M

O66.8 **Other specified obstructed labor** ♀   M
Use additional code to identify cause of obstruction

O66.9 **Obstructed labor, unspecified** ♀   M
Dystocia NOS
Fetal dystocia NOS
Maternal dystocia NOS

Figure 15-5 Hydrocephalic fetus causing
disproportion.

● **O67** **Labor and delivery complicated by intrapartum hemorrhage,
not elsewhere classified**
Excludes1 antepartum hemorrhage NEC (O46.-)
placenta previa (O44.-)
premature separation of placenta [abruptio
placentae] (O45.-)
Excludes2 postpartum hemorrhage (O72.-)

O67.0 **Intrapartum hemorrhage with coagulation defect** ♀ 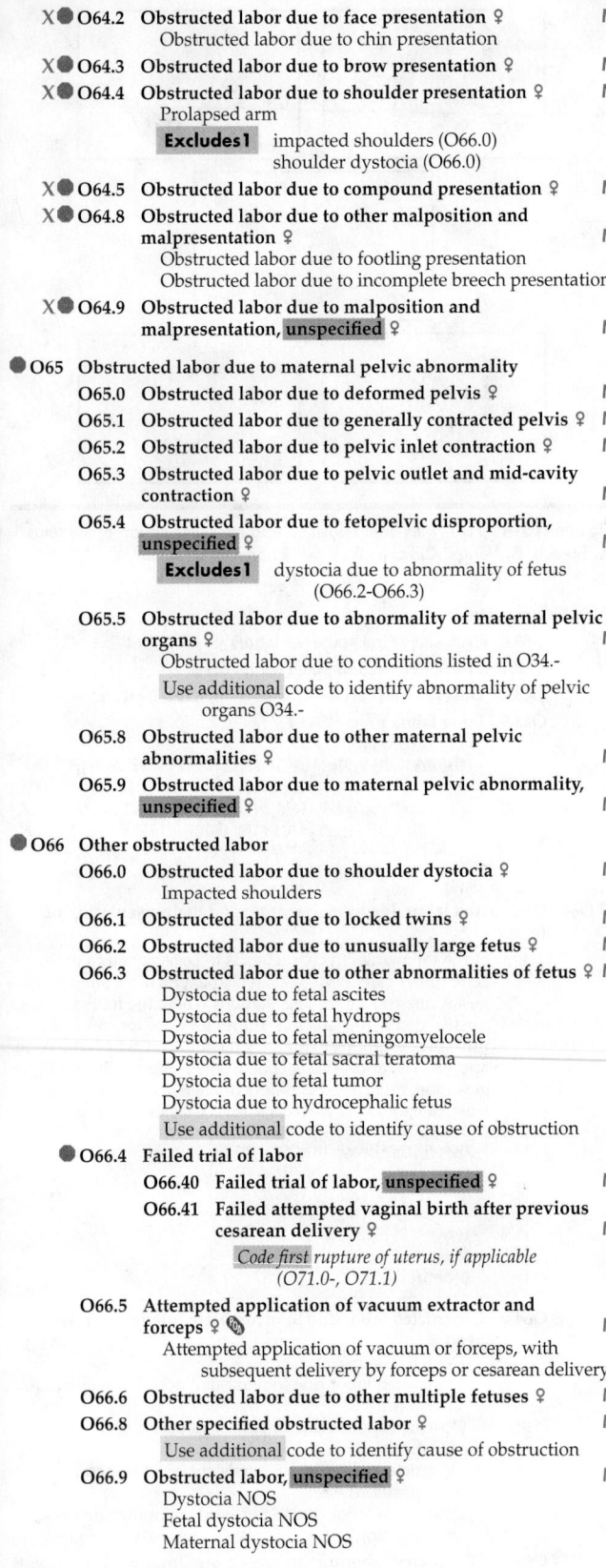 M
Intrapartum hemorrhage (excessive) associated with
afibrinogenemia
Intrapartum hemorrhage (excessive) associated with
disseminated intravascular coagulation
Intrapartum hemorrhage (excessive) associated with
hyperfibrinolysis
Intrapartum hemorrhage (excessive) associated with
hypofibrinogenemia
(Ex:) See 060

O67.8 **Other intrapartum hemorrhage** ♀   M
Excessive intrapartum hemorrhage

O67.9 **Intrapartum hemorrhage, unspecified** ♀   M

● **O68** **Labor and delivery complicated by abnormality of fetal
acid-base balance** ♀ 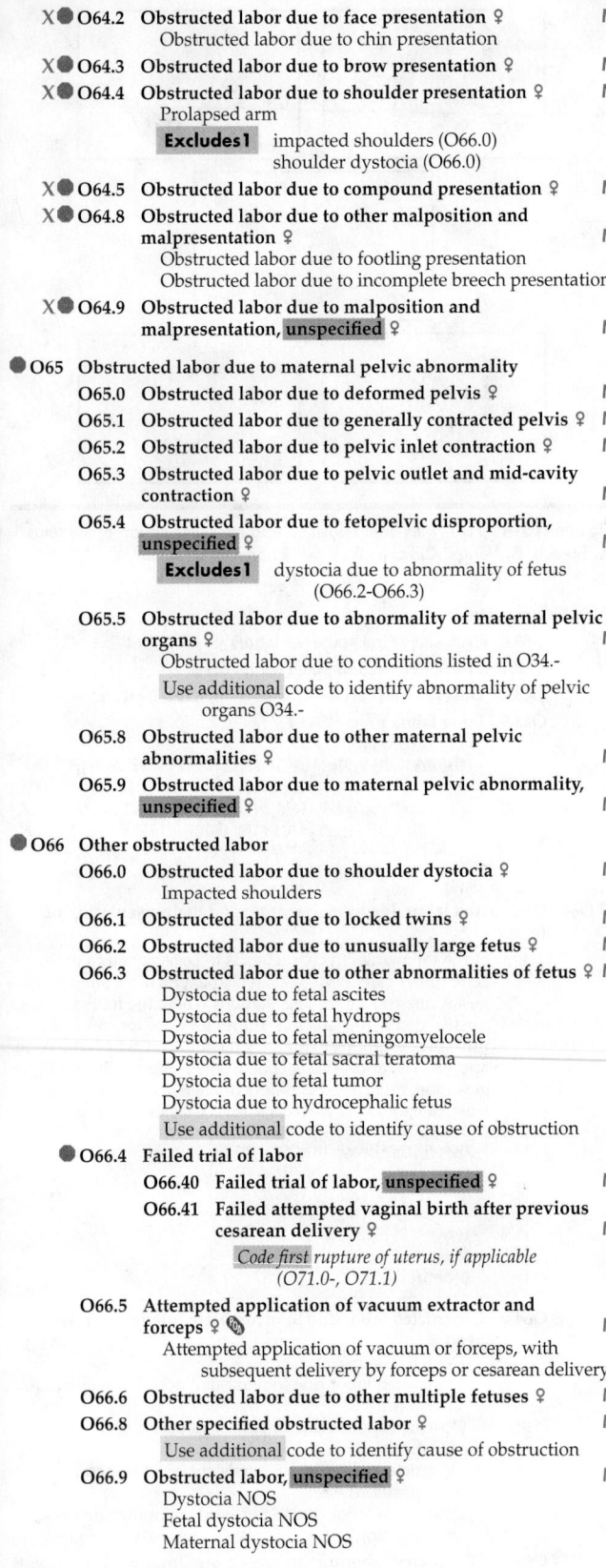   M
Fetal acidemia complicating labor and delivery
Fetal acidosis complicating labor and delivery
Fetal alkalosis complicating labor and delivery
Fetal metabolic acidemia complicating labor and delivery
Excludes1 fetal stress NOS (O77.9)
labor and delivery complicated by
electrocardiographic evidence of fetal
stress (O77.8)
labor and delivery complicated by ultrasonic
evidence of fetal stress (O77.8)
Excludes2 abnormality in fetal heart rate or rhythm (O76)
labor and delivery complicated by meconium in
amniotic fluid (O77.0)
(Ex:) 068, 076, P03.811

● **O69** **Labor and delivery complicated by umbilical cord
complications**
One of the following 7th characters is to be assigned to each
code under category O69. 7th character 0 is for single
gestations and multiple gestations where the fetus is
unspecified. 7th characters 1 through 9 are for cases of
multiple gestations to identify the fetus for which the code
applies. The appropriate code from category O30, Multiple
gestation, must also be assigned when assigning a code
from category O69 that has a 7th character of 1 through 9.

0	not applicable or unspecified
1	fetus 1
2	fetus 2
3	fetus 3
4	fetus 4
5	fetus 5
9	other fetus

X ● **O69.0** **Labor and delivery complicated by prolapse of cord** ♀ M

X ● **O69.1** **Labor and delivery complicated by cord around neck,
with compression** ♀   M
Excludes1 labor and delivery complicated by cord
around neck, without compression
(O69.81)

X ● **O69.2** **Labor and delivery complicated by other cord
entanglement, with compression** ♀   M
Labor and delivery complicated by compression of cord
NOS
Labor and delivery complicated by entanglement of
cords of twins in monoamniotic sac
Labor and delivery complicated by knot in cord
Excludes1 labor and delivery complicated by
other cord entanglement, without
compression (O69.82)

X ● **O69.3** **Labor and delivery complicated by short cord** ♀   M

◀ New ◀▬ Revised ~~deleted~~ Deleted Excludes 1 Excludes 2 Includes Use additional Code first Code also Unspecified
OGCR Official Guidelines ● Unacceptable Principal Diagnosis X Assign placeholder X ● Use Additional Character(s) ▌ Manifestation Code Coding Clinic

X ● **O69.4 Labor and delivery complicated by vasa previa** ♀   M
Labor and delivery complicated by hemorrhage from vasa previa

X ● **O69.5 Labor and delivery complicated by vascular lesion of cord** ♀   M
Labor and delivery complicated by cord bruising
Labor and delivery complicated by cord hematoma
Labor and delivery complicated by thrombosis of umbilical vessels

● **O69.8 Labor and delivery complicated by other cord complications**

X ● **O69.81 Labor and delivery complicated by cord around neck, without compression** ♀   M

X ● **O69.82 Labor and delivery complicated by other cord entanglement, without compression** ♀   M

X ● **O69.89 Labor and delivery complicated by other cord complications** ♀   M

X ● **O69.9 Labor and delivery complicated by cord complication, unspecified** ♀   M

● **O70 Perineal laceration during delivery**
    Includes   episiotomy extended by laceration
    Excludes1   obstetric high vaginal laceration alone (O71.4)

O70.0 First degree perineal laceration during delivery ♀   M
Perineal laceration, rupture or tear involving fourchette during delivery
Perineal laceration, rupture or tear involving labia during delivery
Perineal laceration, rupture or tear involving skin during delivery
Perineal laceration, rupture or tear involving vagina during delivery
Perineal laceration, rupture or tear involving vulva during delivery
Slight perineal laceration, rupture or tear during delivery

O70.1 Second degree perineal laceration during delivery ♀   M
Perineal laceration, rupture or tear during delivery as in O70.0, also involving pelvic floor
Perineal laceration, rupture or tear during delivery as in O70.0, also involving perineal muscles
Perineal laceration, rupture or tear during delivery as in O70.0, also involving vaginal muscles
    Excludes1   perineal laceration involving anal sphincter (O70.2)

O70.2 Third degree perineal laceration during delivery ♀ 🔵 M
Perineal laceration, rupture or tear during delivery as in O70.1, also involving anal sphincter
Perineal laceration, rupture or tear during delivery as in O70.1, also involving rectovaginal septum
Perineal laceration, rupture or tear during delivery as in O70.1, also involving sphincter NOS
    Excludes1   anal sphincter tear during delivery without third degree perineal laceration (O70.4)
             perineal laceration involving anal or rectal mucosa (O70.3)
   Ⓔ 025.10-025.3, 026.10-026.13, 026.30-026.43, 026.63-026.819, 026.841-026.86, 026.891-026.93, 029.011-029.93, 035.7XX0-035.7XX9, 036.8120-036.8199, 070.2, 070.4, 071.00-071.1, 071.5, 071.81, 071.89-071.9, 075.4, 075.81, 075.89-075.9, 080, 090.89, 099.111-099.285, 099.330-099.335, 099.350-099.355, 099.511-099.73, 099.820-099.825, 099.840-09A.53

O70.3 Fourth degree perineal laceration during delivery ♀ 🔵 M
Perineal laceration, rupture or tear during delivery as in O70.2, also involving anal mucosa
Perineal laceration, rupture or tear during delivery as in O70.2, also involving rectal mucosa
   Ⓔ 025.10-025.3, 026.10-026.13, 026.30-026.43, 026.63-026.819, 026.841-026.86, 026.891-026.93, 029.011-029.93, 035.7XX0-035.7XX9, 036.8120-036.8199, 070.3, 071.00-071.1, 071.5, 071.81, 071.89-071.9, 075.4, 075.81, 075.89-075.9, 080, 090.89, 099.111-099.285, 099.330-099.335, 099.350-099.355, 099.511-099.73, 099.820-099.825, 099.840-09A.53

Figure 15-6   Perineal lacerations: **A.** First-degree is laceration of superficial tissues. **B.** Second-degree is limited to the pelvic floor and may involve the perineal or vaginal muscles. **C.** Third-degree involves the anal sphincter. **D.** Fourth-degree involves anal or rectal mucosa.

O70.4 Anal sphincter tear complicating delivery, not associated with third degree laceration ♀ 🔵 M
    Excludes1   anal sphincter tear with third degree perineal laceration (O70.2)
   Ⓔ 025.10-025.3, 026.10-026.13, 026.30-026.43, 026.63-026.819, 026.841-026.86, 026.891-026.93, 029.011-029.93, 035.7XX0-035.7XX9, 036.8120-036.8199, 070.2, 070.4, 071.00-071.1, 071.5, 071.81, 071.89-071.9, 075.4, 075.81, 075.89-075.9, 080, 090.89, 099.111-099.285, 099.330-099.335, 099.350-099.355, 099.511-099.73, 099.820-099.825, 099.840-09A.53

O70.9 Perineal laceration during delivery, unspecified ♀   M

● **O71 Other obstetric trauma**
    Includes   obstetric damage from instruments

● **O71.0 Rupture of uterus (spontaneous) before onset of labor**
    Excludes1   disruption of (current) cesarean delivery wound (O90.0)
             laceration of uterus, NEC (O71.81)
   Ⓔ **For category O71.0 CC codes:** 025.10-025.3, 026.10-026.13, 026.30-026.43, 026.63-026.819, 026.841-026.86, 026.891-026.93, 029.011-029.93, 035.7XX0-035.7XX9, 036.8120-036.8199, 071.00-071.1, 071.5, 071.81, 071.89-071.9, 075.4, 075.81, 075.89-075.9, 080, 090.89, 099.111-099.285, 099.330-099.335, 099.350-099.355, 099.511-099.73, 099.820-099.825, 099.840-09A.53

O71.00 Rupture of uterus before onset of labor, unspecified trimester ♀   M

O71.02 Rupture of uterus before onset of labor, second trimester ♀ 🔵 M

O71.03 Rupture of uterus before onset of labor, third trimester ♀ 🔵 M

O71.1 Rupture of uterus during labor ♀ 🔵 M
Rupture of uterus not stated as occurring before onset of labor
    Excludes1   disruption of cesarean delivery wound (O90.0)
             laceration of uterus, NEC (O71.81)
   Ⓔ See 071.0

O71.2 Postpartum inversion of uterus ♀ 🔵 M
   Ⓔ 025.10-025.3, 026.10-026.13, 026.30-026.43, 026.63-026.819, 026.841-026.86, 026.891-026.93, 029.011-029.93, 035.7XX0-035.7XX9, 036.8120-036.8199, 071.00-071.2, 071.5, 071.81, 071.89-071.9, 075.4, 075.81, 075.89-075.9, 080, 090.89, 099.111-099.285, 099.330-099.335, 099.350-099.355, 099.511-099.73, 099.820-099.825, 099.840-09A.53

O71.3 Obstetric laceration of cervix ♀ 🔵 M
Annular detachment of cervix
   Ⓔ 025.10-025.3, 026.10-026.13, 026.30-026.43, 026.63-026.819, 026.841-026.86, 026.891-026.93, 029.011-029.93, 035.7XX0-035.7XX9, 036.8120-036.8199, 071.00-071.1, 071.3, 071.5, 071.81, 071.89-071.9, 075.4, 075.81, 075.89-075.9, 080, 090.89, 099.111-099.285, 099.330-099.335, 099.350-099.355, 099.511-099.73, 099.820-099.825, 099.840-09A.53

N   Newborn Age: 0   **P**   Pediatric Age: 0–17   **M**   Maternity DX: 12–55   **A**   Adult Age: 15–124   ♀   Females Only   ♂   Males Only

🔵   Complication\Comorbidity   🔵   Major C\C   Ⓔ   CC/MCC Exclusions   🔵   Present on Admission Requirement   🔵   Hospital-Acquired Condition

1223

CHAPTER 15 (O00-O9A)

O71.4   **Obstetric high vaginal laceration alone** ♀ 🐾   M
Laceration of vaginal wall without perineal laceration
> **Excludes1**   obstetric high vaginal laceration with perineal laceration (O70.-)
> (Ex:) O25.10-O25.3, O26.10-O26.13, O26.30-O26.43, O26.63-O26.819, O26.841-O26.86, O26.891-O26.93, O29.011-O29.93, O35.7XX0-O35.7XX9, O36.8120-O36.8199, O71.00-O71.1, O71.4, O71.5, O71.81, O71.89-O71.9, O75.4, O75.81, O75.89-O75.9, O80, O90.89, O99.111-O99.285, O99.330-O99.335, O99.350-O99.355, O99.511-O99.73, O99.820-O99.825, O99.840-O9A.53

O71.5   **Other obstetric injury to pelvic organs** ♀ 🐾   M
Obstetric injury to bladder
Obstetric injury to urethra
> **Excludes2**   obstetric periurethral trauma (O71.82)
> (Ex:) See O71.0

O71.6   **Obstetric damage to pelvic joints and ligaments** ♀ 🐾   M
Obstetric avulsion of inner symphyseal cartilage
Obstetric damage to coccyx
Obstetric traumatic separation of symphysis (pubis)
> (Ex:) O25.10-O25.3, O26.10-O26.13, O26.30-O26.43, O26.63-O26.819, O26.841-O26.86, O26.891-O26.93, O29.011-O29.93, O35.7XX0-O35.7XX9, O36.8120-O36.8199, O71.00-O71.1, O71.5-O71.6, O71.81, O71.89-O71.9, O75.4, O75.81, O75.89-O75.9, O80, O90.89, O99.111-O99.285, O99.330-O99.335, O99.350-O99.355, O99.511-O99.73, O99.820-O99.825, O99.840-O9A.53

O71.7   **Obstetric hematoma of pelvis** ♀ 🐾   M
Obstetric hematoma of perineum
Obstetric hematoma of vagina
Obstetric hematoma of vulva
> (Ex:) O25.10-O25.3, O26.10-O26.13, O26.30-O26.43, O26.63-O26.819, O26.841-O26.86, O26.891-O26.93, O29.011-O29.93, O35.7XX0-O35.7XX9, O36.8120-O36.8199, O71.00-O71.1, O71.5, O71.7, O71.81, O71.89-O71.9, O75.4, O75.81, O75.89-O75.9, O80, O90.89, O99.111-O99.285, O99.330-O99.335, O99.350-O99.355, O99.511-O99.73, O99.820-O99.825, O99.840-O9A.53

⬤ **O71.8**   **Other specified obstetric trauma**

    O71.81   **Laceration of uterus, not elsewhere classified** ♀   M

    O71.82   **Other specified trauma to perineum and vulva** ♀   M
       Obstetric periurethral trauma

    O71.89   **Other specified obstetric trauma** ♀   M

O71.9   **Obstetric trauma, unspecified** ♀   M

⬤ **O72**   **Postpartum hemorrhage**
> **Includes**   hemorrhage after delivery of fetus or infant

O72.0   **Third-stage hemorrhage** ♀ 🐾   M
Hemorrhage associated with retained, trapped or adherent placenta
Retained placenta NOS
> **Code also** type of adherent placenta (O43.2-)
> (Ex:) O25.10-O25.3, O26.10-O26.13, O26.30-O26.43, O26.63-O26.819, O26.841-O26.86, O26.891-O26.93, O29.011-O29.93, O35.7XX0-O35.7XX9, O36.8120-O36.8199, O71.00-O71.1, O71.5, O71.81, O71.89-O71.9, O72.0, O75.4, O75.81, O75.89-O75.9, O80, O90.89, O99.111-O99.285, O99.330-O99.335, O99.350-O99.355, O99.511-O99.73, O99.820-O99.825, O99.840-O9A.53

O72.1   **Other immediate postpartum hemorrhage** ♀ 🐾   M
Hemorrhage following delivery of placenta
Postpartum hemorrhage (atonic) NOS
Uterine atony with hemorrhage
> **Excludes1**   uterine atony NOS (O62.2)
>   uterine atony without hemorrhage (O62.2)
>   postpartum atony of uterus without hemorrhage (O75.89)
> (Ex:) O25.10-O25.3, O26.10-O26.13, O26.30-O26.43, O26.63-O26.819, O26.841-O26.86, O26.891-O26.93, O29.011-O29.93, O35.7XX0-O35.7XX9, O36.8120-O36.8199, O71.00-O71.1, O71.5, O71.81, O71.89-O71.9, O72.1, O75.4, O75.81, O75.89-O75.9, O80, O90.89, O99.111-O99.285, O99.330-O99.335, O99.350-O99.355, O99.511-O99.73, O99.820-O99.825, O99.840-O9A.53

O72.2   **Delayed and secondary postpartum hemorrhage** ♀ 🐾   M
Hemorrhage associated with retained portions of placenta or membranes after the first 24 hours following delivery of placenta
Retained products of conception NOS, following delivery
> (Ex:) O25.10-O25.3, O26.10-O26.13, O26.30-O26.43, O26.63-O26.819, O26.841-O26.86, O26.891-O26.93, O29.011-O29.93, O35.7XX0-O35.7XX9, O36.8120-O36.8199, O71.00-O71.1, O71.5, O71.81, O71.89-O71.9, O72.2, O75.4, O75.81, O75.89-O75.9, O80, O90.89, O99.111-O99.285, O99.330-O99.335, O99.350-O99.355, O99.511-O99.73, O99.820-O99.825, O99.840-O9A.53

O72.3   **Postpartum coagulation defects** ♀   M
Postpartum afibrinogenemia
Postpartum fibrinolysis

⬤ **O73**   **Retained placenta and membranes, without hemorrhage**
> **Excludes1**   placenta accreta (O43.21-)
>   placenta increta (O43.22-)
>   placenta percreta (O43.23-)

O73.0   **Retained placenta without hemorrhage** ♀   M
Adherent placenta, without hemorrhage
Trapped placenta without hemorrhage

O73.1   **Retained portions of placenta and membranes, without hemorrhage** ♀   M
Retained products of conception following delivery, without hemorrhage

⬤ **O74**   **Complications of anesthesia during labor and delivery**
> **Includes**   maternal complications arising from the administration of a general, regional or local anesthetic, analgesic or other sedation during labor and delivery
> **Use additional** code, if applicable, to identify specific complication

O74.0   **Aspiration pneumonitis due to anesthesia during labor and delivery** ♀   M
Inhalation of stomach contents or secretions NOS due to anesthesia during labor and delivery
Mendelson's syndrome due to anesthesia during labor and delivery

O74.1   **Other pulmonary complications of anesthesia during labor and delivery** ♀   M

O74.2   **Cardiac complications of anesthesia during labor and delivery** ♀   M

O74.3   **Central nervous system complications of anesthesia during labor and delivery** ♀   M

O74.4   **Toxic reaction to local anesthesia during labor and delivery** ♀   M

O74.5   **Spinal and epidural anesthesia-induced headache during labor and delivery** ♀   M

O74.6   **Other complications of spinal and epidural anesthesia during labor and delivery** ♀   M

O74.7   **Failed or difficult intubation for anesthesia during labor and delivery** ♀   M

O74.8   **Other complications of anesthesia during labor and delivery** ♀   M

O74.9   **Complication of anesthesia during labor and delivery, unspecified** ♀   M

⬤ **O75**   **Other complications of labor and delivery, not elsewhere classified**
> **Excludes2**   puerperal (postpartum) infection (O86.-)
>   puerperal (postpartum) sepsis (O85)

O75.0   **Maternal distress during labor and delivery** ♀   M

O75.1   **Shock during or following labor and delivery** ♀ 🐾   M
Obstetric shock following labor and delivery
> (Ex:) O25.10-O25.3, O26.10-O26.13, O26.30-O26.43, O26.63-O26.819, O26.841-O26.86, O26.891-O26.93, O29.011-O29.93, O35.7XX0-O35.7XX9, O75.1, O75.4, O75.81, O75.89-O75.9, O80, O90.89, O99.111-O99.285, O99.330-O99.335, O99.350-O99.355, O99.511-O99.73, O99.820-O99.825, O99.840-O9A.53

◀ New   ⬅ Revised   ~~deleted~~ Deleted   Excludes 1   Excludes 2   Includes   Use additional   Code first   Code also   Unspecified

OGCR Official Guidelines   ⬤ Unacceptable Principal Diagnosis   X Assign placeholder X   ⬤ Use Additional Character(s)   ▌ Manifestation Code   Coding Clinic

O75.2   **Pyrexia during labor, not elsewhere classified** ♀ 🔖   **M**
     (Ex) 075.2

O75.3   **Other infection during labor** ♀ 🔖   **M**
     Sepsis during labor
     Use additional code (B95-B97), to identify infectious
         agent
     (Ex) 025.10-025.3, 026.10-026.13, 026.30-026.43, 026.63-026.819,
          026.841-026.86, 026.891-026.93, 029.011-029.93, 035.7XX0-035.7XX9,
          075.3-075.4, 075.81, 075.89-075.9, 080, 090.89, 099.111-099.285,
          099.330-099.335, 099.350-099.355, 099.511-099.73, 099.820-099.825,
          099.840-09A.53

O75.4   **Other complications of obstetric surgery and** **procedures** ♀   **M**
     Cardiac arrest following obstetric surgery or procedures
     Cardiac failure following obstetric surgery or
         procedures
     Cerebral anoxia following obstetric surgery or procedures
     Pulmonary edema following obstetric surgery or
         procedures
     Use additional code to identify specific complication
     Excludes2   complications of anesthesia during labor
                and delivery (O74.-)
                disruption of obstetrical (surgical) wound
                    (O90.0-O90.1)
                hematoma of obstetrical (surgical) wound
                    (O90.2)
                infection of obstetrical (surgical) wound
                    (O86.0)

O75.5   **Delayed delivery after artificial rupture of** **membranes** ♀   **M**

● O75.8   **Other specified complications of labor and delivery**
     O75.81   **Maternal exhaustion complicating labor and** **delivery** ♀   **M**
     O75.82   **Onset (spontaneous) of labor after 37 completed** **weeks of gestation but before 39 completed** **weeks gestation, with delivery by (planned)** **cesarean section** ♀   **M**
                Delivery by (planned) cesarean section occurring
                    after 37 completed weeks of gestation but
                    before 39 completed weeks gestation due to
                    (spontaneous) onset of labor
                ~~Use additional code to specify reason for~~
                   ~~planned cesarean section such as:~~
                   ~~cephalopelvic disproportion (normally~~
                      ~~formed fetus) (O33.9)~~
                   ~~previous cesarean delivery (O34.21)~~
                Code first to specify reason for planned cesarean
                   section such as: ◄
                   cephalopelvic disproportion (normally
                      formed fetus) (O33.9) ◄
                   previous cesarean delivery (O34.21) ◄
     O75.89   **Other specified complications of labor and** **delivery** ♀   **M**

O75.9   **Complication of labor and delivery, unspecified** ♀   **M**

O76   **Abnormality in fetal heart rate and rhythm complicating labor** **and delivery** ♀   **M**
     Depressed fetal heart rate tones complicating labor and
         delivery
     Fetal bradycardia complicating labor and delivery
     Fetal heart rate decelerations complicating labor and delivery
     Fetal heart rate irregularity complicating labor and delivery
     Fetal heart rate abnormal variability complicating labor and
         delivery
     Fetal tachycardia complicating labor and delivery
     Non-reassuring fetal heart rate or rhythm complicating labor
         and delivery
     Excludes1   fetal stress NOS (O77.9)
                labor and delivery complicated by
                    electrocardiographic evidence of fetal stress
                    (O77.8)
                labor and delivery complicated by ultrasonic
                    evidence of fetal stress (O77.8)
     Excludes2   fetal metabolic acidemia (O68)
                other fetal stress (O77.0-O77.1)

● O77   **Other fetal stress complicating labor and delivery**
     O77.0   **Labor and delivery complicated by meconium in** **amniotic fluid** ♀   **M**
     O77.1   **Fetal stress in labor or delivery due to drug** **administration** ♀   **M**
     O77.8   **Labor and delivery complicated by other evidence of** **fetal stress** ♀   **M**
                Labor and delivery complicated by electrocardiographic
                    evidence of fetal stress
                Labor and delivery complicated by ultrasonic evidence
                    of fetal stress
              Excludes1   abnormality of fetal acid-base balance
                      (O68)
                    abnormality in fetal heart rate or rhythm
                      (O76)
                    fetal metabolic acidemia (O68)

     O77.9   **Labor and delivery complicated by fetal stress,** **unspecified** ♀   **M**
              Excludes1   abnormality of fetal acid-base balance
                      (O68)
                    abnormality in fetal heart rate or rhythm
                      (O76)
                    fetal metabolic acidemia (O68)

OGCR Section I.C., Chapter 15.m.

   Normal Delivery, Code O80

   1) Encounter for full term uncomplicated delivery

   Code O80 should be assigned when a woman is admitted for a full-term normal delivery and delivers a single, healthy infant without any complications antepartum, during the delivery, or postpartum during the delivery episode. Code O80 is always a principal diagnosis. It is not to be used if any other code from chapter 15 is needed to describe a current complication of the antenatal, delivery, or perinatal period. Additional codes from other chapters may be used with code O80 if they are not related to or are in any way complicating the pregnancy.

   2) Uncomplicated delivery with resolved antepartum complication

   Code O80 may be used if the patient had a complication at some point during the pregnancy, but the complication is not present at the time of the admission for delivery.

   3) Outcome of delivery for O80

   Z37.0, Single live brith, is the only outcome of delivery code appropriate for use with O80.

Figure 15-7   The four stages of normal delivery: **I.** Lightening, which occurs 2 to 4 weeks before birth, at which time the fetus turns with head toward the vagina. **II.** Regular contractions begin, the amniotic sac ruptures, and dilation is complete. **III.** Delivery of the head and rotation. **IV.** Expulsion of placenta.

N   Newborn Age: 0   **P**   Pediatric Age: 0–17   **M**   Maternity DX: 12–55   **A**   Adult Age: 15–124   ♀   Females Only   ♂   Males Only

🔖 Complication\Comorbidity   🔖 Major C\C   (Ex) CC/MCC Exclusions   🔖 Present on Admission Requirement   🔖 Hospital-Acquired Condition

1225

ENCOUNTER FOR DELIVERY (O80-O82)

O80   **Encounter for full-term uncomplicated delivery** ♀ 🦠   M

Delivery requiring minimal or no assistance, with or without episiotomy, without fetal manipulation [e.g., rotation version] or instrumentation [forceps] of a spontaneous, cephalic, vaginal, full-term, single, live-born infant. This code is for use as a single diagnosis code and is not to be used with any other code from chapter 15. ~~This code must be accompanied by a delivery code from the appropriate procedure classification.~~

Use additional code to indicate outcome of delivery (Z37.0)

O82   **Encounter for cesarean delivery without indication** ♀   M

~~This code must be accompanied by a delivery code from the appropriate procedure classification.~~

Use additional code to indicate outcome of delivery (Z37.0)

COMPLICATIONS PREDOMINANTLY RELATED TO THE PUERPERIUM (O85-O92)

> **Excludes2**   mental and behavioral disorders associated with the puerperium (F53)
> obstetrical tetanus (A34)
> puerperal osteomalacia (M83.0)

O85   **Puerperal sepsis** ♀ 🦠   M

Postpartum sepsis
Puerperal peritonitis
Puerperal pyemia

Use additional code (B95-B97), to identify infectious agent

Use additional code (R65.2-) to identify severe sepsis, if applicable

> **Excludes1**   fever of unknown origin following delivery (O86.4)
> genital tract infection following delivery (O86.1-)
> obstetric pyemic and septic embolism (O88.3-)
> puerperal septic thrombophlebitis (O86.81)
> urinary tract infection following delivery (O86.2-)

> **Excludes2**   sepsis during labor (O75.3)

Ⓔⓧ 025.10-025.3, 026.10-026.13, 026.30-026.43, 026.63-026.819, 026.841-026.86, 026.891-026.93, 026.899-026.93, 029.011-029.93, 035.7XX0-035.7XX9, 075.4, 075.81, 075.89, 075.9, 080, 085, 086.12, 086.81-086.89, 090.89, 099.111-099.285, 099.330-099.335, 099.350-099.355, 099.511-099.73, 099.820-099.825, 099.840-09A.53

● **O86**   **Other puerperal infections**

Use additional code (B95-B97), to identify infectious agent

> **Excludes2**   infection during labor (O75.3)
> obstetrical tetanus (A34)

Ⓔⓧ **For category O86 CC codes unless otherwise indicated:** 023.00-023.93, 025.10-025.3, 026.10-026.13, 026.30-026.43, 026.63-026.819, 026.841-026.86, 026.891-026.93, 029.011-029.93, 035.7XX0-035.7XX9, 075.4, 075.81, 075.89-075.9, 080, 086.11, 086.13-086.29, 090.89, 099.111-099.285, 099.330-099.335, 099.350-099.355, 099.511-099.73, 099.820-099.825, 099.840-09A.53

    O86.0   **Infection of obstetric surgical wound** ♀   M

Infected cesarean delivery wound following delivery
Infected perineal repair following delivery

●   **O86.1**   **Other infection of genital tract following delivery**

      O86.11   **Cervicitis following delivery** ♀ 🦠   M

      O86.12   **Endometritis following delivery** ♀ 🦠   M
         Ⓔⓧ See O85

      O86.13   **Vaginitis following delivery** ♀ 🦠   M

      O86.19   **Other infection of genital tract following delivery** ♀ 🦠   M

●   **O86.2**   **Urinary tract infection following delivery**

      O86.20   **Urinary tract infection following delivery, unspecified** ♀ 🦠   M
         Puerperal urinary tract infection NOS

      O86.21   **Infection of kidney following delivery** ♀ 🦠   M

      O86.22   **Infection of bladder following delivery** ♀ 🦠   M
         Infection of urethra following delivery

      O86.29   **Other urinary tract infection following delivery** ♀ 🦠   M

    O86.4   **Pyrexia of unknown origin following delivery** ♀ 🦠   M

Puerperal infection NOS following delivery
Puerperal pyrexia NOS following delivery

> **Excludes2**   pyrexia during labor (O75.2)

Ⓔⓧ 022.20-022.93, 025.10-025.3, 026.10-026.13, 026.30-026.43, 026.63-026.819, 026.841-026.86, 026.891-026.93, 029.011-029.93, 035.7XX0-035.7XX9, 075.4, 075.81, 075.89-075.9, 080, 086.4-087.9, 090.89, 099.111-099.285, 099.330-099.335, 099.350-099.355, 099.511-099.73, 099.820-099.825, 099.840-09A.53

●   **O86.8**   **Other specified puerperal infections**
      Ⓔⓧ **For category O86.8 CC codes:** See O85

      O86.81   **Puerperal septic thrombophlebitis** ♀ 🦠   M

      O86.89   **Other specified puerperal infections** ♀ 🦠   M

● **O87**   **Venous complications and hemorrhoids in the puerperium**

> **Includes**   venous complications in labor, delivery and the puerperium

> **Excludes2**   obstetric embolism (O88.-)
> puerperal septic thrombophlebitis (O86.81)
> venous complications in pregnancy (O22.-)

Ⓔⓧ **For category O87 CC codes:** 022.20-022.93, 025.10-025.3, 026.10-026.13, 026.30-026.43, 026.63-026.819, 026.841-026.86, 026.891-026.93, 029.011-029.93, 035.7XX0-035.7XX9, 075.4, 075.81, 075.89-075.9, 080, 087.0-087.9, 090.89, 099.111-099.119, 099.12-099.285, 099.330-099.335, 099.350-099.355, 099.511-099.73, 099.820-099.825, 099.840-09A.53

    O87.0   **Superficial thrombophlebitis in the puerperium** ♀ 🦠   M
Puerperal phlebitis NOS
Puerperal thrombosis NOS

    O87.1   **Deep phlebothrombosis in the puerperium** ♀ 🦠   M
Deep vein thrombosis, postpartum
Pelvic thrombophlebitis, postpartum

> Use additional code to identify the deep vein thrombosis (I82.4-, I82.5-, I82.62-. I82.72-)

> Use additional code, if applicable, for associated long-term (current) use of anticoagulants (Z79.01)

    O87.2   **Hemorrhoids in the puerperium** ♀ 🦠   M

    O87.3   **Cerebral venous thrombosis in the puerperium** ♀ 🦠   M
Cerebrovenous sinus thrombosis in the puerperium

    O87.4   **Varicose veins of lower extremity in the puerperium** ♀   M

    O87.8   **Other venous complications in the puerperium** ♀ 🦠   M
Genital varices in the puerperium

    O87.9   **Venous complication in the puerperium, unspecified** ♀   M
Puerperal phlebopathy NOS

O88   **Obstetric embolism**

> **Excludes1**   embolism complicating abortion NOS (O03.2)
> embolism complicating ectopic or molar pregnancy (O08.2)
> embolism complicating failed attempted abortion (O07.2) ◀
> embolism complicating induced abortion (O04.7)
> embolism complicating spontaneous abortion (O03.2, O03.7)

●   **O88.0**   **Obstetric air embolism**

●   **O88.01**   **Obstetric air embolism in pregnancy**

       O88.011   **Air embolism in pregnancy, first trimester** ♀ 🦠   M

       O88.012   **Air embolism in pregnancy, second trimester** ♀ 🦠   M

       O88.013   **Air embolism in pregnancy, third trimester** ♀ 🦠   M

       O88.019   **Air embolism in pregnancy, unspecified trimester** ♀   M

      O88.02   **Air embolism in childbirth** ♀ 🦠   M

      O88.03   **Air embolism in the puerperium** ♀ 🦠   M

● **O88.1 Amniotic fluid embolism**
  Anaphylactoid syndrome in pregnancy
  ● **O88.11 Amniotic fluid embolism in pregnancy**
    O88.111 Amniotic fluid embolism in
      pregnancy, first trimester ♀ 🐾 M
    O88.112 Amniotic fluid embolism in
      pregnancy, second trimester ♀ 🐾 M
    O88.113 Amniotic fluid embolism in
      pregnancy, third trimester ♀ 🐾 M
    O88.119 Amniotic fluid embolism in
      pregnancy, unspecified trimester ♀ M
  O88.12 Amniotic fluid embolism in childbirth ♀ 🐾 M
  O88.13 Amniotic fluid embolism in the
    puerperium ♀ 🐾 M
● **O88.2 Obstetric thromboembolism**
  ● **O88.21 Thromboembolism in pregnancy**
    Obstetric (pulmonary) embolism NOS
    O88.211 Thromboembolism in pregnancy, first
      trimester ♀ 🐾 M
    O88.212 Thromboembolism in pregnancy,
      second trimester ♀ 🐾 M
    O88.213 Thromboembolism in pregnancy,
      third trimester ♀ 🐾 M
    O88.219 Thromboembolism in pregnancy,
      unspecified trimester ♀ M
  O88.22 Thromboembolism in childbirth ♀ 🐾 M
  O88.23 Thromboembolism in the puerperium ♀ 🐾 M
    Puerperal (pulmonary) embolism NOS
● **O88.3 Obstetric pyemic and septic embolism**
  ● **O88.31 Pyemic and septic embolism in pregnancy**
    O88.311 Pyemic and septic embolism in
      pregnancy, first trimester ♀ 🐾 M
    O88.312 Pyemic and septic embolism in
      pregnancy, second trimester ♀ 🐾 M
    O88.313 Pyemic and septic embolism in
      pregnancy, third trimester ♀ 🐾 M
    O88.319 Pyemic and septic embolism in
      pregnancy, unspecified
      trimester ♀ 🐾 M
  O88.32 Pyemic and septic embolism in
    childbirth ♀ 🐾 M
  O88.33 Pyemic and septic embolism in the
    puerperium ♀ 🐾 M
● **O88.8 Other obstetric embolism**
  Obstetric fat embolism
  ● **O88.81 Other embolism in pregnancy**
    O88.811 Other embolism in pregnancy, first
      trimester ♀ 🐾 M
    O88.812 Other embolism in pregnancy, second
      trimester ♀ 🐾 M
    O88.813 Other embolism in pregnancy, third
      trimester ♀ 🐾 M
    O88.819 Other embolism in pregnancy,
      unspecified trimester ♀ M
  O88.82 Other embolism in childbirth ♀ 🐾 M
  O88.83 Other embolism in the puerperium ♀ 🐾 M

● **O89 Complications of anesthesia during the puerperium**
  Includes maternal complications arising from the
    administration of a general, regional or
    local anesthetic, analgesic or other sedation
    during the puerperium
  Use additional code, if applicable, to identify specific
  complication
  ● **O89.0 Pulmonary complications of anesthesia during the**
    puerperium
    O89.01 Aspiration pneumonitis due to anesthesia
      during the puerperium ♀ M
      Inhalation of stomach contents or secretions
        NOS due to anesthesia during the
        puerperium
      Mendelson's syndrome due to anesthesia
        during the puerperium
    O89.09 Other pulmonary complications of anesthesia
      during the puerperium ♀ M
  O89.1 Cardiac complications of anesthesia during the
    puerperium ♀ M
  O89.2 Central nervous system complications of anesthesia
    during the puerperium ♀ M
  O89.3 Toxic reaction to local anesthesia during the
    puerperium ♀ M
  O89.4 Spinal and epidural anesthesia-induced headache
    during the puerperium ♀ M
  O89.5 Other complications of spinal and epidural anesthesia
    during the puerperium ♀ M
  O89.6 Failed or difficult intubation for anesthesia during the
    puerperium ♀ M
  O89.8 Other complications of anesthesia during the
    puerperium ♀ M
  O89.9 Complication of anesthesia during the puerperium,
    unspecified ♀ M

● **O90 Complications of the puerperium, not elsewhere classified**
  O90.0 Disruption of cesarean delivery wound ♀ M
    Dehiscence of cesarean delivery wound
    Excludes1 rupture of uterus (spontaneous) before
      onset of labor (O71.0-)
      rupture of uterus during labor (O71.1)
  O90.1 Disruption of perineal obstetric wound ♀ M
    Disruption of wound of episiotomy
    Disruption of wound of perineal laceration
    Secondary perineal tear
  O90.2 Hematoma of obstetric wound ♀ M
  O90.3 Peripartum cardiomyopathy ♀ 🐾 M
    Conditions in I42.- arising during pregnancy and the
    puerperium
    Excludes1 pre-existing heart disease complicating
      pregnancy and the puerperium
      (O99.4-)
    (Ex) O25.10-O25.3, O26.10-O26.13, O26.30-O26.43, O26.63-O26.819,
    O26.841-O26.86, O26.891-O26.93, O29.011-O29.93, O35.7XX0-O35.7XX9,
    O75.4, O75.81, O75.89-O75.9, O80, O90.3, O90.89, O99.111-O99.285,
    O99.330-O99.335, O99.350-O99.73, O99.820-O99.825, O99.840-O9A.53
  O90.4 Postpartum acute kidney failure ♀ 🐾 M
    Hepatorenal syndrome following labor and delivery
    (Ex) O25.10-O25.3, O26.10-O26.13, O26.30-O26.43, O26.63-O26.819,
    O26.841-O26.86, O26.891-O26.93, O29.011-O29.93, O35.7XX0-O35.7XX9,
    O75.4, O75.81, O75.89-O75.9, O80, O90.4, O90.89, O99.111-O99.285,
    O99.330-O99.335, O99.350-O99.355, O99.511-O99.73, O99.820-O99.825,
    O99.840-O9A.53
  O90.5 Postpartum thyroiditis ♀ M
  O90.6 Postpartum mood disturbance ♀ M
    Postpartum blues   Postpartum sadness
    Postpartum dysphoria
    Excludes1 postpartum depression (F53)
      puerperal psychosis (F53)

CHAPTER 15 (O00-O9A)

● **O90.8**   **Other complications of the puerperium, not elsewhere classified**

    O90.81   **Anemia of the puerperium** ♀   M
        Postpartum anemia NOS

        Excludes1   pre-existing anemia complicating the puerperium (O99.03)

    O90.89   **Other complications of the puerperium, not elsewhere classified** ♀   M
        Placental polyp

   O90.9   **Complication of the puerperium, unspecified** ♀   M

● **O91**   **Infections of breast associated with pregnancy, the puerperium and lactation**

    Use additional code to identify infection

● **O91.0**   **Infection of nipple associated with pregnancy, the puerperium and lactation**

   ● **O91.01**   **Infection of nipple associated with pregnancy**
        Gestational abscess of nipple

      O91.011   **Infection of nipple associated with pregnancy, first trimester** ♀   M

      O91.012   **Infection of nipple associated with pregnancy, second trimester** ♀   M

      O91.013   **Infection of nipple associated with pregnancy, third trimester** ♀   M

      O91.019   **Infection of nipple associated with pregnancy, unspecified trimester** ♀   M

    O91.02   **Infection of nipple associated with the puerperium** ♀   M
        Puerperal abscess of nipple

    O91.03   **Infection of nipple associated with lactation** ♀ M
        Abscess of nipple associated with lactation

● **O91.1**   **Abscess of breast associated with pregnancy, the puerperium and lactation**

   ● **O91.11**   **Abscess of breast associated with pregnancy**
        Gestational mammary abscess
        Gestational purulent mastitis
        Gestational subareolar abscess

      O91.111   **Abscess of breast associated with pregnancy, first trimester** ♀   M

      O91.112   **Abscess of breast associated with pregnancy, second trimester** ♀   M

      O91.113   **Abscess of breast associated with pregnancy, third trimester** ♀   M

      O91.119   **Abscess of breast associated with pregnancy, unspecified trimester** ♀   M

    O91.12   **Abscess of breast associated with the puerperium** ♀   M
        Puerperal mammary abscess
        Puerperal purulent mastitis
        Puerperal subareolar abscess

    O91.13   **Abscess of breast associated with lactation** ♀   M
        Mammary abscess associated with lactation
        Purulent mastitis associated with lactation
        Subareolar abscess associated with lactation

● **O91.2**   **Nonpurulent mastitis associated with pregnancy, the puerperium and lactation**

   ● **O91.21**   **Nonpurulent mastitis associated with pregnancy**
        Gestational interstitial mastitis
        Gestational lymphangitis of breast
        Gestational mastitis NOS
        Gestational parenchymatous mastitis

      O91.211   **Nonpurulent mastitis associated with pregnancy, first trimester** ♀   M

      O91.212   **Nonpurulent mastitis associated with pregnancy, second trimester** ♀   M

      O91.213   **Nonpurulent mastitis associated with pregnancy, third trimester** ♀   M

      O91.219   **Nonpurulent mastitis associated with pregnancy, unspecified trimester** ♀   M

    O91.22   **Nonpurulent mastitis associated with the puerperium** ♀   M
        Puerperal interstitial mastitis
        Puerperal lymphangitis of breast
        Puerperal mastitis NOS
        Puerperal parenchymatous mastitis

    O91.23   **Nonpurulent mastitis associated with lactation** ♀   M
        Interstitial mastitis associated with lactation
        Lymphangitis of breast associated with lactation
        Mastitis NOS associated with lactation
        Parenchymatous mastitis associated with lactation

● **O92**   **Other disorders of breast and disorders of lactation associated with pregnancy and the puerperium**

● **O92.0**   **Retracted nipple associated with pregnancy, the puerperium, and lactation**

   ● **O92.01**   **Retracted nipple associated with pregnancy**

      O92.011   **Retracted nipple associated with pregnancy, first trimester** ♀   M

      O92.012   **Retracted nipple associated with pregnancy, second trimester** ♀   M

      O92.013   **Retracted nipple associated with pregnancy, third trimester** ♀   M

      O92.019   **Retracted nipple associated with pregnancy, unspecified trimester** ♀   M

    O92.02   **Retracted nipple associated with the puerperium** ♀   M

    O92.03   **Retracted nipple associated with lactation** ♀   M

● **O92.1**   **Cracked nipple associated with pregnancy, the puerperium, and lactation**
    Fissure of nipple, gestational or puerperal

   ● **O92.11**   **Cracked nipple associated with pregnancy**

      O92.111   **Cracked nipple associated with pregnancy, first trimester** ♀   M

      O92.112   **Cracked nipple associated with pregnancy, second trimester** ♀   M

      O92.113   **Cracked nipple associated with pregnancy, third trimester** ♀   M

      O92.119   **Cracked nipple associated with pregnancy, unspecified trimester** ♀   M

    O92.12   **Cracked nipple associated with the puerperium** ♀   M

    O92.13   **Cracked nipple associated with lactation** ♀   M

● **O92.2**   **Other and unspecified disorders of breast associated with pregnancy and the puerperium**

    O92.20   **Unspecified disorder of breast associated with pregnancy and the puerperium** ♀   M

    O92.29   **Other disorders of breast associated with pregnancy and the puerperium** ♀   M

   O92.3   **Agalactia** ♀   M
        Primary agalactia

        Excludes1   elective agalactia (O92.5)
                  secondary agalactia (O92.5)
                  therapeutic agalactia (O92.5)

   O92.4   **Hypogalactia** ♀   M

   O92.5   **Suppressed lactation** ♀   M
        Elective agalactia   Therapeutic agalactia
        Secondary agalactia

        Excludes1   primary agalactia (O92.3)

◄ New   ◄ Revised   ~~deleted~~ Deleted   Excludes 1   Excludes 2   Includes   Use additional   Code first   Code also   Unspecified

OGCR Official Guidelines   ● Unacceptable Principal Diagnosis   X Assign placeholder X   ▶ Use Additional Character(s)   ▶ Manifestation Code   **Coding Clinic**

O92.6   Galactorrhea ♀   M
● O92.7   Other and unspecified disorders of lactation
    O92.70   Unspecified disorders of lactation ♀   M
    O92.79   Other disorders of lactation ♀   M
            Puerperal galactocele

OGCR Section I.C.2.l.3.

Malignant neoplasm in a pregnant patient

When a pregnant woman has a malignant neoplasm, a code from subcategory O9A.1-, Malignant neoplasm complicating pregnancy, childbirth, and the puerperium, should be sequenced first, followed by the appropriate code from Chapter 2 to indicate the type of neoplasm.

OTHER OBSTETRIC CONDITIONS, NOT ELSEWHERE CLASSIFIED (O94-O9A)

O94   Sequelae of complication of pregnancy, childbirth, and the puerperium ♀ 🔖   M

Note: This category is to be used to indicate conditions in O00-O77.-, O85-O94 and O98-O9A.- as the cause of late effects. The 'sequelae' include conditions specified as such, or as late effects, which may occur at any time after the puerperium.

Code first condition resulting from (sequela) of complication of pregnancy, childbirth, and the puerperium

O98   Maternal infectious and parasitic diseases classifiable elsewhere but complicating pregnancy, childbirth and the puerperium
    Includes   the listed conditions when complicating the pregnant state, when aggravated by the pregnancy, or as a reason for obstetric care

    Use additional code (Chapter 1), to identify specific infectious or parasitic disease
    Excludes2   herpes gestationis (O26.4-)
            infectious carrier state (O99.82-, O99.83-)
            obstetrical tetanus (A34)
            puerperal infection (O86.-)
            puerperal sepsis (O85)
            when the reason for maternal care is that the disease is known or suspected to have affected the fetus (O35-O36)

● O98.0   Tuberculosis complicating pregnancy, childbirth and the puerperium
        Conditions in A15-A19
        (Ex) **For category O98.0 CC codes:** 025.10-025.3, 026.10-026.13, 026.30-026.43, 026.63-026.819, 026.841-026.86, 026.891-026.93, 029.011-029.93, 035.7XX0-035.7XX9, 075.4, 075.81, 075.89-075.9, 080, 090.89, 098.011-098.03, 099.111-099.285, 099.330-099.335, 099.350-099.355, 099.511-099.73, 099.820-099.825, 099.840-09A.53
    ● O98.01   Tuberculosis complicating pregnancy
        O98.011   Tuberculosis complicating pregnancy, first trimester ♀ 🔖   M
        O98.012   Tuberculosis complicating pregnancy, second trimester ♀ 🔖   M
        O98.013   Tuberculosis complicating pregnancy, third trimester ♀ 🔖   M
        O98.019   Tuberculosis complicating pregnancy, unspecified trimester ♀   M
    O98.02   Tuberculosis complicating childbirth ♀ 🔖   M
    O98.03   Tuberculosis complicating the puerperium ♀ 🔖   M

● O98.1   Syphilis complicating pregnancy, childbirth and the puerperium
        Conditions in A50-A53
        (Ex) **For category O98.1 CC codes:** 026.11-026.13, 026.31-026.33, 026.41-026.43, 026.63-026.713, 026.72-026.813, 026.86, 026.891-026.893, 026.90-026.93, 029.011-029.013, 029.021-029.023, 029.091-029.093, 029.111-029.113, 029.121-029.123, 029.191-029.193, 029.211-029.213, 029.291-029.293, 029.3X1-029.3X3, 029.41-029.5X3, 029.61-029.8X3, 029.91-029.93, 035.7XX0-035.7XX9, 098.111-098.33, 099.351-099.353, 099.355, 099.89
    ● O98.11   Syphilis complicating pregnancy
        O98.111   Syphilis complicating pregnancy, first trimester ♀ 🔖   M
        O98.112   Syphilis complicating pregnancy, second trimester ♀ 🔖   M
        O98.113   Syphilis complicating pregnancy, third trimester ♀ 🔖   M
        O98.119   Syphilis complicating pregnancy, unspecified trimester ♀   M
    O98.12   Syphilis complicating childbirth ♀ 🔖   M
    O98.13   Syphilis complicating the puerperium ♀ 🔖   M
● O98.2   Gonorrhea complicating pregnancy, childbirth and the puerperium
        Conditions in A54.-
        (Ex) **For category O98.2 CC codes:** See 098.1
    ● O98.21   Gonorrhea complicating pregnancy
        O98.211   Gonorrhea complicating pregnancy, first trimester ♀ 🔖   M
        O98.212   Gonorrhea complicating pregnancy, second trimester ♀ 🔖   M
        O98.213   Gonorrhea complicating pregnancy, third trimester ♀ 🔖   M
        O98.219   Gonorrhea complicating pregnancy, unspecified trimester ♀   M
    O98.22   Gonorrhea complicating childbirth ♀ 🔖   M
    O98.23   Gonorrhea complicating the puerperium ♀ 🔖   M
● O98.3   Other infections with a predominantly sexual mode of transmission complicating pregnancy, childbirth and the puerperium
        Conditions in A55-A64
        (Ex) **For category O98.3 CC codes:** See 098.1
    ● O98.31   Other infections with a predominantly sexual mode of transmission complicating pregnancy
        O98.311   Other infections with a predominantly sexual mode of transmission complicating pregnancy, first trimester ♀ 🔖   M
        O98.312   Other infections with a predominantly sexual mode of transmission complicating pregnancy, second trimester ♀ 🔖   M
        O98.313   Other infections with a predominantly sexual mode of transmission complicating pregnancy, third trimester ♀ 🔖   M
        O98.319   Other infections with a predominantly sexual mode of transmission complicating pregnancy, unspecified trimester ♀   M
    O98.32   Other infections with a predominantly sexual mode of transmission complicating childbirth ♀ 🔖   M
    O98.33   Other infections with a predominantly sexual mode of transmission complicating the puerperium ♀ 🔖   M

CHAPTER 15 (O00-O9A)

CHAPTER 15 (O00-O9A)

● **O98.4**   **Viral hepatitis complicating pregnancy, childbirth and the puerperium**
Conditions in B15-B19
Ⓔⓧ **For category O98.4 CC codes:** 098.411-098.613, 098.711-098.93, 099.830-099.835

● **O98.41**   **Viral hepatitis complicating pregnancy**

O98.411   Viral hepatitis complicating pregnancy, first trimester ♀ 🐾   M

O98.412   Viral hepatitis complicating pregnancy, second trimester ♀ 🐾   M

O98.413   Viral hepatitis complicating pregnancy, third trimester ♀ 🐾   M

O98.419   Viral hepatitis complicating pregnancy, unspecified trimester ♀   M

O98.42   Viral hepatitis complicating childbirth ♀ 🐾   M

O98.43   Viral hepatitis complicating the puerperium ♀ 🐾   M

● **O98.5**   **Other viral diseases complicating pregnancy, childbirth and the puerperium**
Conditions in A80-B09, B25-B34, R87.81-, R87.82-

Excludes:1   human immunodeficiency virus [HIV] disease complicating pregnancy, childbirth and the puerperium (O98.7-)

Ⓔⓧ **For category O98.5 CC codes:** See 098.4

● **O98.51**   **Other viral diseases complicating pregnancy**

O98.511   Other viral diseases complicating pregnancy, first trimester ♀ 🐾   M

O98.512   Other viral diseases complicating pregnancy, second trimester ♀ 🐾   M

O98.513   Other viral diseases complicating pregnancy, third trimester ♀ 🐾   M

O98.519   Other viral diseases complicating pregnancy, unspecified trimester ♀   M

O98.52   Other viral diseases complicating childbirth ♀ 🐾   M

O98.53   Other viral diseases complicating the puerperium ♀ 🐾   M

● **O98.6**   **Protozoal diseases complicating pregnancy, childbirth and the puerperium**
Conditions in B50-B64

● **O98.61**   **Protozoal diseases complicating pregnancy**
Ⓔⓧ **For category O98.61 CC codes:** 025.10-025.3, 026.10-026.13, 026.30-026.43, 026.63-026.819, 026.841-026.86, 026.891-026.93, 029.011-029.93, 035.7XX0-035.7XX9, 075.4, 075.81, 075.89-075.9, 080, 090.89, 098.411-098.93, 099.111-099.285, 099.330-099.335, 099.350-099.355, 099.511-099.73, 099.820-09A.53

O98.611   Protozoal diseases complicating pregnancy, first trimester ♀ 🐾   M

O98.612   Protozoal diseases complicating pregnancy, second trimester ♀ 🐾   M

O98.613   Protozoal diseases complicating pregnancy, third trimester ♀ 🐾   M

O98.619   Protozoal diseases complicating pregnancy, unspecified trimester ♀   M

O98.62   Protozoal diseases complicating childbirth ♀ 🐾   M
Ⓔⓧ 025.10-025.3, 026.10-026.13, 026.30-026.43, 026.63-026.819, 026.841-026.86, 026.891-026.93, 029.011-029.93, 035.7XX0-035.7XX9, 075.4, 075.81, 075.89-075.9, 080, 090.89, 098.611-098.63, 099.111-099.285, 099.330-099.335, 099.350-099.355, 099.511-099.73, 099.820-09A.53

O98.63   Protozoal diseases complicating the puerperium ♀ 🐾   M
Ⓔⓧ See 098.62

● **O98.7**   **Human immunodeficiency virus [HIV] disease complicating pregnancy, childbirth and the puerperium**
Use additional code to identify the type of HIV disease:
Acquired immune deficiency syndrome (AIDS) (B20)
Asymptomatic HIV status (Z21)
HIV positive NOS (Z21)
Symptomatic HIV disease (B20)

OGCR Section I.C.15.f.

HIV Infection in Pregnancy, Childbirth and the Puerperium
During pregnancy, childbirth or the puerperium, a patient admitted because of an HIV-related illness should receive a principal diagnosis from subcategory O98.7-. Human immunodeficiency [HIV] disease complicating pregnancy, childbirth and the puerperium, followed by the code(s) for the HIV-related illness(es).
Patients with asymptomatic HIV infection status admitted during pregnancy, childbirth, or the puerperium should receive codes of O98.7- and Z21, Asymptomatic human immunodeficiency virus [HIV] infection status.

Ⓔⓧ **For category O98.7 CC codes:** See 098.4

● **O98.71**   **Human immunodeficiency virus [HIV] disease complicating pregnancy**

O98.711   Human immunodeficiency virus [HIV] disease complicating pregnancy, first trimester ♀ 🐾   M

O98.712   Human immunodeficiency virus [HIV] disease complicating pregnancy, second trimester ♀ 🐾   M

O98.713   Human immunodeficiency virus [HIV] disease complicating pregnancy, third trimester ♀ 🐾   M

O98.719   Human immunodeficiency virus [HIV] disease complicating pregnancy, unspecified trimester ♀   M

O98.72   Human immunodeficiency virus [HIV] disease complicating childbirth ♀ 🐾   M

O98.73   Human immunodeficiency virus [HIV] disease complicating the puerperium ♀ 🐾   M

● **O98.8**   **Other maternal infectious and parasitic diseases complicating pregnancy, childbirth and the puerperium**
Ⓔⓧ **For category O98.8 CC codes:** See 098.4

● **O98.81**   **Other maternal infectious and parasitic diseases complicating pregnancy**

O98.811   Other maternal infectious and parasitic diseases complicating pregnancy, first trimester ♀ 🐾   M

O98.812   Other maternal infectious and parasitic diseases complicating pregnancy, second trimester ♀ 🐾   M

O98.813   Other maternal infectious and parasitic diseases complicating pregnancy, third trimester ♀ 🐾   M

O98.819   Other maternal infectious and parasitic diseases complicating pregnancy, unspecified trimester ♀   M

O98.82   Other maternal infectious and parasitic diseases complicating childbirth ♀ 🐾   M

O98.83   Other maternal infectious and parasitic diseases complicating the puerperium ♀ 🐾   M

◄ New   ◄ⅲ Revised   ~~deleted~~ Deleted   Excludes 1   Excludes 2   Includes   Use additional   Code first   Code also   Unspecified
OGCR Official Guidelines   ● Unacceptable Principal Diagnosis   X Assign placeholder X   ● Use Additional Character(s)   ▌ Manifestation Code   **Coding Clinic**

● **O98.9**   **Unspecified maternal infectious and parasitic disease complicating pregnancy, childbirth and the puerperium**
Ⓔ **For category O98.9 CC codes:** See O98.4

  ● **O98.91**   **Unspecified maternal infectious and parasitic disease complicating pregnancy**

     O98.911   Unspecified maternal infectious and parasitic disease complicating pregnancy, first trimester ♀ 🇦   M

     O98.912   Unspecified maternal infectious and parasitic disease complicating pregnancy, second trimester ♀ 🇦   M

     O98.913   Unspecified maternal infectious and parasitic disease complicating pregnancy, third trimester ♀ 🇦   M

     O98.919   Unspecified maternal infectious and parasitic disease complicating pregnancy, unspecified trimester ♀   M

   O98.92   Unspecified maternal infectious and parasitic disease complicating childbirth ♀ 🇦   M

   O98.93   Unspecified maternal infectious and parasitic disease complicating the puerperium ♀ 🇦   M

● **O99**   **Other maternal diseases classifiable elsewhere but complicating pregnancy, childbirth and the puerperium**

   Includes: conditions which complicate the pregnant state, are aggravated by the pregnancy or are a main reason for obstetric care

   Use additional code to identify specific condition

   Excludes2   when the reason for maternal care is that the condition is known or suspected to have affected the fetus (O35-O36)

  ● **O99.0**   **Anemia complicating pregnancy, childbirth and the puerperium**
     Conditions in D50-D64

     Excludes1   anemia arising in the puerperium (O90.81)
           postpartum anemia NOS (O90.81)

   ● **O99.01**   **Anemia complicating pregnancy**

     O99.011   Anemia complicating pregnancy, first trimester ♀   M

     O99.012   Anemia complicating pregnancy, second trimester ♀   M

     O99.013   Anemia complicating pregnancy, third trimester ♀   M

     O99.019   Anemia complicating pregnancy, unspecified trimester ♀   M

   O99.02   Anemia complicating childbirth ♀   M

   O99.03   Anemia complicating the puerperium ♀   M

     Excludes1   postpartum anemia not pre-existing prior to delivery (O90.81) ◀

  ● **O99.1**   **Other diseases of the blood and blood-forming organs and certain disorders involving the immune mechanism complicating pregnancy, childbirth and the puerperium**
     Conditions in D65-D89

     Excludes2   hemorrhage with coagulation defects (O45.-, O46.0-, O67.0, O72.3)

     Ⓔ **For category O99.1 CC codes unless otherwise indicated:** O25.11-O25.3, O99.281-O99.285, O99.511-O99.513, O99.52-O99.613, O99.62-O99.713, O99.72-O99.73, O99.820-O99.825, O9A.111-O9A.113, O9A.12-O9A.213, O9A.22-O9A.313, O9A.32-O9A.413, O9A.42-O9A.513, O9A.52-O9A.53

   ● **O99.11**   **Other diseases of the blood and blood-forming organs and certain disorders involving the immune mechanism complicating pregnancy**

     O99.111   Other diseases of the blood and blood-forming organs and certain disorders involving the immune mechanism complicating pregnancy, first trimester ♀ 🇦   M

     O99.112   Other diseases of the blood and blood-forming organs and certain disorders involving the immune mechanism complicating pregnancy, second trimester ♀ 🇦   M

     O99.113   Other diseases of the blood and blood-forming organs and certain disorders involving the immune mechanism complicating pregnancy, third trimester ♀   M

     O99.119   Other diseases of the blood and blood-forming organs and certain disorders involving the immune mechanism complicating pregnancy, unspecified trimester ♀ 🇦   M

       Ⓔ O25.10, O99.280, O99.519, O99.619, O99.719, O9A.119, O9A.219, O9A.319, O9A.419, O9A.519

   O99.12   Other diseases of the blood and blood-forming organs and certain disorders involving the immune mechanism complicating childbirth ♀ 🇦   M

   O99.13   Other diseases of the blood and blood-forming organs and certain disorders involving the immune mechanism complicating the puerperium ♀ 🇦   M

  ● **O99.2**   **Endocrine, nutritional and metabolic diseases complicating pregnancy, childbirth and the puerperium**
     Conditions in E00-E88

     Excludes2   diabetes mellitus (O24.-)
           malnutrition (O25.-)
           postpartum thyroiditis (O90.5)

   ● **O99.21**   **Obesity complicating pregnancy, childbirth, and the puerperium**

     Use additional code to identify the type of obesity (E66.-)

     O99.210   Obesity complicating pregnancy, unspecified trimester ♀   M

     O99.211   Obesity complicating pregnancy, first trimester ♀   M

     O99.212   Obesity complicating pregnancy, second trimester ♀   M

     O99.213   Obesity complicating pregnancy, third trimester ♀   M

     O99.214   Obesity complicating childbirth ♀   M

     O99.215   Obesity complicating the puerperium ♀   M

   ● **O99.28**   **Other endocrine, nutritional and metabolic diseases complicating pregnancy, childbirth and the puerperium**

     O99.280   Endocrine, nutritional and metabolic diseases complicating pregnancy, unspecified trimester ♀   M

     O99.281   Endocrine, nutritional and metabolic diseases complicating pregnancy, first trimester ♀   M

     O99.282   Endocrine, nutritional and metabolic diseases complicating pregnancy, second trimester ♀   M

     O99.283   Endocrine, nutritional and metabolic diseases complicating pregnancy, third trimester ♀   M

     O99.284   Endocrine, nutritional and metabolic diseases complicating childbirth ♀   M

     O99.285   Endocrine, nutritional and metabolic diseases complicating the puerperium ♀   M

  ● **O99.3**   **Mental disorders and diseases of the nervous system complicating pregnancy, childbirth and the puerperium**

   ● **O99.31**   **Alcohol use complicating pregnancy, childbirth, and the puerperium**

     Use additional code(s) from F10 to identify manifestations of the alcohol use

     O99.310   Alcohol use complicating pregnancy, unspecified trimester ♀   M

     O99.311   Alcohol use complicating pregnancy, first trimester ♀   M

N   Newborn Age: 0   **P**   Pediatric Age: 0–17   **M**   Maternity DX: 12–55   **A**   Adult Age: 15–124   ♀   Females Only   ♂   Males Only

🇦   Complication\Comorbidity   🇦   Major C\C   Ⓔ   CC/MCC Exclusions   🇦   Present on Admission Requirement   🇦   Hospital-Acquired Condition

1231

O99.312　Alcohol use complicating pregnancy, second trimester ♀　　M

O99.313　Alcohol use complicating pregnancy, third trimester ♀　　M

O99.314　Alcohol use complicating childbirth ♀　　M

O99.315　Alcohol use complicating the puerperium ♀　　M

● O99.32　Drug use complicating pregnancy, childbirth, and the puerperium

Use additional code(s) from F11-F16 and F18-F19 to identify manifestations of the drug use

(Ex) For category O99.32 CC codes: O25.10-O25.3, O26.10-O26.13, O26.30-O26.43, O26.63-O26.819, O26.841-O26.86, O26.891-O26.93, O29.011-O29.93, O35.7XX0-O35.7XX9, O75.4, O75.81, O75.89-O75.9, O80, O90.89, O99.111-O99.285, O99.320-O99.335, O99.350-O99.355, O99.511-O99.73, O99.820-O99.825, O99.840-O9A.53

O99.320　Drug use complicating pregnancy, unspecified trimester ♀　　M

O99.321　Drug use complicating pregnancy, first trimester ♀ 🔗　　M

O99.322　Drug use complicating pregnancy, second trimester ♀ 🔗　　M

O99.323　Drug use complicating pregnancy, third trimester ♀ 🔗　　M

O99.324　Drug use complicating childbirth ♀ 🔗　　M

O99.325　Drug use complicating the puerperium ♀ 🔗　　M

● O99.33　Smoking (tobacco) complicating pregnancy, childbirth, and the puerperium

Use additional code from F17 to identify type of tobacco

O99.330　Smoking (tobacco) complicating pregnancy, unspecified trimester ♀　　M

O99.331　Smoking (tobacco) complicating pregnancy, first trimester ♀　　M

O99.332　Smoking (tobacco) complicating pregnancy, second trimester ♀　　M

O99.333　Smoking (tobacco) complicating pregnancy, third trimester ♀　　M

O99.334　Smoking (tobacco) complicating childbirth ♀　　M

O99.335　Smoking (tobacco) complicating the puerperium ♀　　M

● O99.34　Other mental disorders complicating pregnancy, childbirth, and the puerperium
Conditions in F01-F09 and F20-F99

Excludes2　postpartum mood disturbance (O90.6)
postnatal psychosis (F53)
puerperal psychosis (F53)

O99.340　Other mental disorders complicating pregnancy, unspecified trimester ♀　M

O99.341　Other mental disorders complicating pregnancy, first trimester ♀　　M

O99.342　Other mental disorders complicating pregnancy, second trimester ♀　　M

O99.343　Other mental disorders complicating pregnancy, third trimester ♀　　M

O99.344　Other mental disorders complicating childbirth ♀　　M

O99.345　Other mental disorders complicating the puerperium ♀　　M

● O99.35　Diseases of the nervous system complicating pregnancy, childbirth, and the puerperium
Conditions in G00-G99

Excludes2　pregnancy related peripheral neuritis (O26.8-)

O99.350　Diseases of the nervous system complicating pregnancy, unspecified trimester ♀　　M

O99.351　Diseases of the nervous system complicating pregnancy, first trimester ♀　　M

O99.352　Diseases of the nervous system complicating pregnancy, second trimester ♀　　M

O99.353　Diseases of the nervous system complicating pregnancy, third trimester ♀　　M

O99.354　Diseases of the nervous system complicating childbirth ♀ 🔗　　M
(Ex) See O99.1

O99.355　Diseases of the nervous system complicating the puerperium ♀ 🔗　　M
(Ex) See O99.1

● O99.4　Diseases of the circulatory system complicating pregnancy, childbirth and the puerperium
Conditions in I00-I99

Excludes1　peripartum cardiomyopathy (O90.3)
Excludes2　hypertensive disorders (O10-O16)
obstetric embolism (O88.-)
venous complications and cerebrovenous sinus thrombosis in labor, childbirth and the puerperium (O87.-)
venous complications and cerebrovenous sinus thrombosis in pregnancy (O22.-)

(Ex) For category O99.4 CC codes unless otherwise indicated:
O25.10-O25.3, O26.10-O26.13, O26.30-O26.43, O26.63-O26.819, O26.841-O26.86, O26.891-O26.93, O29.011-O29.93, O35.7XX0-O35.7XX9, O75.4, O75.81, O75.89-O75.9, O80, O90.3, O90.89, O99.111-O99.285, O99.330-O99.335, O99.350-O99.73, O99.820-O99.825, O99.840-O9A.53

● O99.41　Diseases of the circulatory system complicating pregnancy

O99.411　Diseases of the circulatory system complicating pregnancy, first trimester ♀ 🔗　　M

O99.412　Diseases of the circulatory system complicating pregnancy, second trimester ♀ 🔗　　M

O99.413　Diseases of the circulatory system complicating pregnancy, third trimester ♀ 🔗　　M

O99.419　Diseases of the circulatory system complicating pregnancy, unspecified trimester ♀　　M

O99.42　Diseases of the circulatory system complicating childbirth ♀ 🔗　　M
(Ex) O25.10-O25.3, O26.10-O26.13, O26.30-O26.43, O26.63-O26.819, O26.841-O26.86, O26.891-O26.93, O29.011-O29.93, O35.7XX0-O35.7XX9, O75.4, O75.81, O75.89-O75.9, O80, O90.3, O90.89, O99.111-O99.285, O99.330-O99.335, O99.350-O99.73, O99.820-O99.825, O99.840-O9A.53

O99.43　Diseases of the circulatory system complicating the puerperium ♀ 🔗　　M

◀ New　◀▥ Revised　~~deleted~~ Deleted　Excludes 1　Excludes 2　Includes　Use additional　Code first　Code also　Unspecified

OGCR Official Guidelines　● Unacceptable Principal Diagnosis　X Assign placeholder X　● Use Additional Character(s)　▸ Manifestation Code　**Coding Clinic**

● **O99.5**   **Diseases of the respiratory system complicating pregnancy, childbirth and the puerperium**
Conditions in J00-J99

  ● **O99.51**   **Diseases of the respiratory system complicating pregnancy**

    O99.511   Diseases of the respiratory system complicating pregnancy, first trimester ♀   M

    O99.512   Diseases of the respiratory system complicating pregnancy, second trimester ♀   M

    O99.513   Diseases of the respiratory system complicating pregnancy, third trimester ♀   M

    O99.519   Diseases of the respiratory system complicating pregnancy, unspecified trimester ♀   M

  O99.52   Diseases of the respiratory system complicating childbirth ♀   M

  O99.53   Diseases of the respiratory system complicating the puerperium ♀   M

● **O99.6**   **Diseases of the digestive system complicating pregnancy, childbirth and the puerperium**
Conditions in K00-K93

    Excludes2   liver and biliary tract disorders in pregnancy, childbirth and the puerperium (O26.6-)

  ● **O99.61**   **Diseases of the digestive system complicating pregnancy**

    O99.611   Diseases of the digestive system complicating pregnancy, first trimester ♀   M

    O99.612   Diseases of the digestive system complicating pregnancy, second trimester ♀   M

    O99.613   Diseases of the digestive system complicating pregnancy, third trimester ♀   M

    O99.619   Diseases of the digestive system complicating pregnancy, unspecified trimester ♀   M

  O99.62   Diseases of the digestive system complicating childbirth ♀   M

  O99.63   Diseases of the digestive system complicating the puerperium ♀   M

● **O99.7**   **Diseases of the skin and subcutaneous tissue complicating pregnancy, childbirth and the puerperium**
Conditions in L00-L99

    Excludes2   herpes gestationis (O26.4)
pruritic urticarial papules and plaques of pregnancy (PUPPP) (O26.86)

  ● **O99.71**   **Diseases of the skin and subcutaneous tissue complicating pregnancy**

    O99.711   Diseases of the skin and subcutaneous tissue complicating pregnancy, first trimester ♀   M

    O99.712   Diseases of the skin and subcutaneous tissue complicating pregnancy, second trimester ♀   M

    O99.713   Diseases of the skin and subcutaneous tissue complicating pregnancy, third trimester ♀   M

    O99.719   Diseases of the skin and subcutaneous tissue complicating pregnancy, unspecified trimester ♀   M

  O99.72   Diseases of the skin and subcutaneous tissue complicating childbirth ♀   M

  O99.73   Diseases of the skin and subcutaneous tissue complicating the puerperium ♀   M

● **O99.8**   **Other specified diseases and conditions complicating pregnancy, childbirth and the puerperium**
Conditions in D00-D48, H00-H95, M00-N99, and Q00-Q99

  Use additional code to identify condition

    Excludes2   genitourinary infections in pregnancy (O23.-)
infection of genitourinary tract following delivery (O86.1-O86.3)
malignant neoplasm complicating pregnancy, childbirth and the puerperium (O9A.1-)
maternal care for known or suspected abnormality of maternal pelvic organs (O34.-)
postpartum acute kidney failure (O90.4)
traumatic injuries in pregnancy (O9A.2-)

  ● **O99.81**   **Abnormal glucose complicating pregnancy, childbirth and the puerperium**

    Excludes1   gestational diabetes (O24.4-)

    O99.810   Abnormal glucose complicating pregnancy ♀   M

    O99.814   Abnormal glucose complicating childbirth ♀   M

    O99.815   Abnormal glucose complicating the puerperium ♀   M

  ● **O99.82**   **Streptococcus B carrier state complicating pregnancy, childbirth and the puerperium**

    ● **O99.820**   Streptococcus B carrier state complicating pregnancy ♀   M

    O99.824   Streptococcus B carrier state complicating childbirth ♀   M

    ● **O99.825**   Streptococcus B carrier state complicating the puerperium ♀   M

  ● **O99.83**   **Other infection carrier state complicating pregnancy, childbirth and the puerperium**

  Use additional code to identify the carrier state (Z22.-)

    (Ex) For category O99.83 CC codes: O98.411-O98.613, O98.711-O98.93, O99.830-O99.835

    O99.830   Other infection carrier state complicating pregnancy ♀ 🖂   M

    O99.834   Other infection carrier state complicating childbirth ♀ 🖂   M

    O99.835   Other infection carrier state complicating the puerperium ♀ 🖂   M

  ● **O99.84**   **Bariatric surgery status complicating pregnancy, childbirth and the puerperium**
Gastric banding status complicating pregnancy, childbirth and the puerperium
Gastric bypass status for obesity complicating pregnancy, childbirth and the puerperium
Obesity surgery status complicating pregnancy, childbirth and the puerperium

    O99.840   Bariatric surgery status complicating pregnancy, unspecified trimester ♀ M

    O99.841   Bariatric surgery status complicating pregnancy, first trimester ♀   M

    O99.842   Bariatric surgery status complicating pregnancy, second trimester ♀   M

    O99.843   Bariatric surgery status complicating pregnancy, third trimester ♀   M

    O99.844   Bariatric surgery status complicating childbirth ♀   M

    O99.845   Bariatric surgery status complicating the puerperium ♀   M

  O99.89   Other specified diseases and conditions complicating pregnancy, childbirth and the puerperium ♀   M

N Newborn Age: 0   **P** Pediatric Age: 0–17   **M** Maternity DX: 12–55   **A** Adult Age: 15–124   ♀ Females Only   ♂ Males Only

🖂 Complication\Comorbidity   🖂 Major C\C   (Ex) CC/MCC Exclusions   🖂 Present on Admission Requirement   🖂 Hospital-Acquired Condition   **1233**

● **O9A**   **Maternal malignant neoplasms, traumatic injuries and abuse classifiable elsewhere but complicating pregnancy, childbirth and the puerperium**

  ● **O9A.1**   **Malignant neoplasm complicating pregnancy, childbirth and the puerperium**

     Conditions in C00-C96

     Use additional code to identify neoplasm

     Excludes2   maternal care for benign tumor of corpus uteri (O34.1-)

          maternal care for benign tumor of cervix (O34.4-)

    ● **O9A.11**   Malignant neoplasm complicating pregnancy

       O9A.111   Malignant neoplasm complicating pregnancy, first trimester ♀   M

       O9A.112   Malignant neoplasm complicating pregnancy, second trimester ♀   M

       O9A.113   Malignant neoplasm complicating pregnancy, third trimester ♀   M

       O9A.119   Malignant neoplasm complicating pregnancy, unspecified trimester ♀   M

     O9A.12   Malignant neoplasm complicating childbirth ♀   M

     O9A.13   Malignant neoplasm complicating the puerperium ♀   M

  ● **O9A.2**   **Injury, poisoning and certain other consequences of external causes complicating pregnancy, childbirth and the puerperium**

     Conditions in S00-T88, except T74 and T76

     Use additional code(s) to identify the injury or poisoning

     Excludes2   physical, sexual and psychological abuse complicating pregnancy, childbirth and the puerperium (O9A.3-, O9A.4-, O9A.5-)

    ● **O9A.21**   Injury, poisoning and certain other consequences of external causes complicating pregnancy

       O9A.211   Injury, poisoning and certain other consequences of external causes complicating pregnancy, first trimester ♀   M

       O9A.212   Injury, poisoning and certain other consequences of external causes complicating pregnancy, second trimester ♀   M

       O9A.213   Injury, poisoning and certain other consequences of external causes complicating pregnancy, third trimester ♀   M

       O9A.219   Injury, poisoning and certain other consequences of external causes complicating pregnancy, unspecified trimester ♀   M

     O9A.22   Injury, poisoning and certain other consequences of external causes complicating childbirth ♀   M

     O9A.23   Injury, poisoning and certain other consequences of external causes complicating the puerperium ♀   M

  ● **O9A.3**   **Physical abuse complicating pregnancy, childbirth and the puerperium**

     Conditions in T74.11 or T76.11

     Use additional code (if applicable):

     to identify any associated current injury due to physical abuse

     to identify the perpetrator of abuse (Y07.-)

     Excludes2   sexual abuse complicating pregnancy, childbirth and the puerperium (O9A.4)

    ● **O9A.31**   Physical abuse complicating pregnancy

       O9A.311   Physical abuse complicating pregnancy, first trimester ♀   M

       O9A.312   Physical abuse complicating pregnancy, second trimester ♀   M

       O9A.313   Physical abuse complicating pregnancy, third trimester ♀   M

       O9A.319   Physical abuse complicating pregnancy, unspecified trimester ♀   M

     O9A.32   Physical abuse complicating childbirth ♀   M

     O9A.33   Physical abuse complicating the puerperium ♀   M

  ● **O9A.4**   **Sexual abuse complicating pregnancy, childbirth and the puerperium**

     Conditions in T74.21 or T76.21

     Use additional code (if applicable):

     to identify any associated current injury due to sexual abuse

     to identify the perpetrator of abuse (Y07.-)

    ● **O9A.41**   Sexual abuse complicating pregnancy

       O9A.411   Sexual abuse complicating pregnancy, first trimester ♀   M

       O9A.412   Sexual abuse complicating pregnancy, second trimester ♀   M

       O9A.413   Sexual abuse complicating pregnancy, third trimester ♀   M

       O9A.419   Sexual abuse complicating pregnancy, unspecified trimester ♀   M

     O9A.42   Sexual abuse complicating childbirth ♀   M

     O9A.43   Sexual abuse complicating the puerperium ♀   M

  ● **O9A.5**   **Psychological abuse complicating pregnancy, childbirth and the puerperium**

     Conditions in T74.31 or T76.31

     Use additional code to identify the perpetrator of abuse (Y07.-)

    ● **O9A.51**   Psychological abuse complicating pregnancy

       O9A.511   Psychological abuse complicating pregnancy, first trimester ♀   M

       O9A.512   Psychological abuse complicating pregnancy, second trimester ♀   M

       O9A.513   Psychological abuse complicating pregnancy, third trimester ♀   M

       O9A.519   Psychological abuse complicating pregnancy, unspecified trimester ♀   M

     O9A.52   Psychological abuse complicating childbirth ♀ M

     O9A.53   Psychological abuse complicating the puerperium ♀   M

◀ New   ◀▥ Revised   ~~deleted~~ Deleted   Excludes 1   Excludes 2   Includes   Use additional   Code first   Code also   Unspecified

OGCR Official Guidelines   ● Unacceptable Principal Diagnosis   X Assign placeholder X   ● Use Additional Character(s)   ▌ Manifestation Code   **Coding Clinic**

OGCR See Section I.C., Chapter 16
Newborn (Perinatal) Guidelines

CHAPTER 16

CERTAIN CONDITIONS ORIGINATING IN THE PERINATAL PERIOD (P00-P96)

Note: Codes from this chapter are for use on newborn records only, never on maternal records.

Includes   conditions that have their origin in the fetal or perinatal period (before birth through the first 28 days after birth) even if morbidity occurs later

Excludes2   congenital malformations, deformations and chromosomal abnormalities (Q00-Q99)
endocrine, nutritional and metabolic diseases (E00-E88)
injury, poisoning and certain other consequences of external causes (S00-T88)
neoplasms (C00-D49)
tetanus neonatorum (A33)

This chapter contains the following blocks:

P00-P04	Newborn affected by maternal factors and by complications of pregnancy, labor, and delivery
P05-P08	Disorders of newborns related to length of gestation and fetal growth
P09	Abnormal findings on neonatal screening
P10-P15	Birth trauma
P19-P29	Respiratory and cardiovascular disorders specific to the perinatal period
P35-P39	Infections specific to the perinatal period
P50-P61	Hemorrhagic and hematological disorders of newborn
P70-P74	Transitory endocrine and metabolic disorders specific to newborn
P76-P78	Digestive system disorders of newborn
P80-P83	Conditions involving the integument and temperature regulation of newborn
P84	Other problems with newborn
P90-P96	Other disorders originating in the perinatal period

NEWBORN AFFECTED BY MATERNAL FACTORS AND BY COMPLICATIONS OF PREGNANCY, LABOR, AND DELIVERY (P00–P04)

Note: These codes are for use when the listed maternal conditions are specified as the cause of confirmed morbidity or potential morbidity which have their origin in the perinatal period (before birth through the first 28 days after birth). Codes from these categories are also for use for newborns who are suspected of having an abnormal condition resulting from exposure from the mother or the birth process, but without signs or symptoms, and, which after examination and observation, is found not to exist. These codes may be used even if treatment is begun for a suspected condition that is ruled out.

● **P00 Newborn (suspected to be) affected by maternal conditions that may be unrelated to present pregnancy**

Code first any current condition in newborn

Excludes2   newborn (suspected to be) affected by maternal complications of pregnancy (P01.-)
newborn affected by maternal endocrine and metabolic disorders (P70–P74)
newborn affected by noxious substances transmitted via placenta or breast milk (P04.-)

P00.0 Newborn (suspected to be) affected by maternal hypertensive disorders 🔍   N
Newborn (suspected to be) affected by maternal conditions classifiable to O10-O11, O13-O16

P00.1 Newborn (suspected to be) affected by maternal renal and urinary tract diseases 🔍   N
Newborn (suspected to be) affected by maternal conditions classifiable to N00-N39

P00.2 Newborn (suspected to be) affected by maternal infectious and parasitic diseases 🔍   N
Newborn (suspected to be) affected by maternal infectious disease classifiable to A00-B99, J09 and J10

Excludes1   infections specific to the perinatal period (P35-P39)
maternal genital tract or other localized infections (P00.8)

P00.3 Newborn (suspected to be) affected by other maternal circulatory and respiratory diseases 🔍   N
Newborn (suspected to be) affected by maternal conditions classifiable to I00-I99, J00-J99, Q20-Q34 and not included in P00.0, P00.2

P00.4 Newborn (suspected to be) affected by maternal nutritional disorders 🔍   N
Newborn (suspected to be) affected by maternal disorders classifiable to E40-E64
Maternal malnutrition NOS

P00.5 Newborn (suspected to be) affected by maternal injury 🔍   N
Newborn (suspected to be) affected by maternal conditions classifiable to O9A.2-

P00.6 Newborn (suspected to be) affected by surgical procedure on mother 🔍   N
Newborn (suspected to be) affected by amniocentesis

Excludes1   Cesarean delivery for present delivery (P03.4)
damage to placenta from amniocentesis, cesarean delivery or surgical induction (P02.1)
previous surgery to uterus or pelvic organs (P03.89)

Excludes2   newborn affected by complication of (fetal) intrauterine procedure (P96.5)

P00.7 Newborn (suspected to be) affected by other medical procedures on mother, not elsewhere classified 🔍   N
Newborn (suspected to be) affected by radiation to mother

Excludes1   damage to placenta from amniocentesis, cesarean delivery or surgical induction (P02.1)
newborn affected by other complications of labor and delivery (P03.-)

● **P00.8 Newborn (suspected to be) affected by other maternal conditions**

P00.81 Newborn (suspected to be) affected by periodontal disease in mother 🔍   N

P00.89 Newborn (suspected to be) affected by other maternal conditions 🔍   N
Newborn (suspected to be) affected by conditions classifiable to T80-T88
Newborn (suspected to be) affected by maternal genital tract or other localized infections
Newborn (suspected to be) affected by maternal systemic lupus erythematosus

P00.9 Newborn (suspected to be) affected by unspecified maternal condition 🔍   N

● **P01 Newborn (suspected to be) affected by maternal complications of pregnancy**

Code first any current condition in newborn

P01.0 Newborn (suspected to be) affected by incompetent cervix   N

P01.1 Newborn (suspected to be) affected by premature rupture of membranes   N

P01.2 Newborn (suspected to be) affected by oligohydramnios   N

Excludes1   oligohydramnios due to premature rupture of membranes (P01.1)

P01.3 Newborn (suspected to be) affected by polyhydramnios   N
Excess of amniotic fluid, usually > 2000 mL
Newborn (suspected to be) affected by hydramnios

N Newborn Age: 0   P Pediatric Age: 0–17   M Maternity DX: 12–55   A Adult Age: 15–124   ♀ Females Only   ♂ Males Only
🔍 Complication\Comorbidity   🔍 Major C\C   Ⓔ CC/MCC Exclusions   🔍 Present on Admission Requirement   🔍 Hospital-Acquired Condition

1235

CHAPTER 16 (P00-P96)

CHAPTER 16 (P00-P96)

P01.4   **Newborn (suspected to be) affected by ectopic pregnancy**   N
> Newborn (suspected to be) affected by abdominal pregnancy

P01.5   **Newborn (suspected to be) affected by multiple pregnancy**   N
> Newborn (suspected to be) affected by triplet (pregnancy)
> Newborn (suspected to be) affected by twin (pregnancy)

P01.6   **Newborn (suspected to be) affected by maternal death**   N

P01.7   **Newborn (suspected to be) affected by malpresentation before labor**   N
> Newborn (suspected to be) affected by breech presentation before labor
> Newborn (suspected to be) affected by external version before labor
> Newborn (suspected to be) affected by face presentation before labor
> Newborn (suspected to be) affected by transverse lie before labor
> Newborn (suspected to be) affected by unstable lie before labor

P01.8   **Newborn (suspected to be) affected by other maternal complications of pregnancy**   N

P01.9   **Newborn (suspected to be) affected by maternal complication of pregnancy, unspecified**   N

● **P02**   **Newborn (suspected to be) affected by complications of placenta, cord and membranes**
> *Code first* any current condition in newborn

P02.0   **Newborn (suspected to be) affected by placenta previa**   N

P02.1   **Newborn (suspected to be) affected by other forms of placental separation and hemorrhage**   N
> Newborn (suspected to be) affected by abruptio placenta
> Newborn (suspected to be) affected by accidental hemorrhage
> Newborn (suspected to be) affected by antepartum hemorrhage
> Newborn (suspected to be) affected by damage to placenta from amniocentesis, cesarean delivery or surgical induction
> Newborn (suspected to be) affected by maternal blood loss
> Newborn (suspected to be) affected by premature separation of placenta

● **P02.2**   **Newborn (suspected to be) affected by other and unspecified morphological and functional abnormalities of placenta**

P02.20   **Newborn (suspected to be) affected by unspecified morphological and functional abnormalities of placenta**   N

P02.29   **Newborn (suspected to be) affected by other morphological and functional abnormalities of placenta**   N
> Newborn (suspected to be) affected by placental dysfunction
> Newborn (suspected to be) affected by placental infarction
> Newborn (suspected to be) affected by placental insufficiency

P02.3   **Newborn (suspected to be) affected by placental transfusion syndromes**   N
> Newborn (suspected to be) affected by placental and cord abnormalities resulting in twin-to-twin or other transplacental transfusion

P02.4   **Newborn (suspected to be) affected by prolapsed cord**   N

P02.5   **Newborn (suspected to be) affected by other compression of umbilical cord**   N
> Newborn (suspected to be) affected by umbilical cord (tightly) around neck
> Newborn (suspected to be) affected by entanglement of umbilical cord
> Newborn (suspected to be) affected by knot in umbilical cord

● **P02.6**   **Newborn (suspected to be) affected by other and unspecified conditions of umbilical cord**

P02.60   **Newborn (suspected to be) affected by unspecified conditions of umbilical cord**   N

P02.69   **Newborn (suspected to be) affected by other conditions of umbilical cord**   N
> Newborn (suspected to be) affected by short umbilical cord
> Newborn (suspected to be) affected by vasa previa

> **Excludes1**   newborn affected by single umbilical artery (Q27.0)

P02.7   **Newborn (suspected to be) affected by chorioamnionitis**   N
> *Inflammation of chorion and amnion*
> Newborn (suspected to be) affected by amnionitis
> Newborn (suspected to be) affected by membranitis
> Newborn (suspected to be) affected by placentitis

P02.8   **Newborn (suspected to be) affected by other abnormalities of membranes**   N

P02.9   **Newborn (suspected to be) affected by abnormality of membranes, unspecified**   N

● **P03**   **Newborn (suspected to be) affected by other complications of labor and delivery**
> *Code first* any current condition in newborn

P03.0   **Newborn (suspected to be) affected by breech delivery and extraction**   N

P03.1   **Newborn (suspected to be) affected by other malpresentation, malposition and disproportion during labor and delivery**   N
> Newborn (suspected to be) affected by contracted pelvis
> Newborn (suspected to be) affected by conditions classifiable to O64-O66
> Newborn (suspected to be) affected by persistent occipitoposterior
> Newborn (suspected to be) affected by transverse lie

P03.2   **Newborn (suspected to be) affected by forceps delivery**   N

P03.3   **Newborn (suspected to be) affected by delivery by vacuum extractor [ventouse]**   N

P03.4   **Newborn (suspected to be) affected by Cesarean delivery**   N

P03.5   **Newborn (suspected to be) affected by precipitate delivery**   N
> Newborn (suspected to be) affected by rapid second stage

P03.6   **Newborn (suspected to be) affected by abnormal uterine contractions**   N
> Newborn (suspected to be) affected by conditions classifiable to O62.-, except O62.3
> Newborn (suspected to be) affected by hypertonic labor
> Newborn (suspected to be) affected by uterine inertia

● **P03.8**   **Newborn (suspected to be) affected by other specified complications of labor and delivery**

● **P03.81**   **Newborn (suspected to be) affected by abnormality in fetal (intrauterine) heart rate or rhythm**

> **Excludes1**   neonatal cardiac dysrhythmia (P29.1-)

P03.810   **Newborn (suspected to be) affected by abnormality in fetal (intrauterine) heart rate or rhythm before the onset of labor**   N

P03.811   **Newborn (suspected to be) affected by abnormality in fetal (intrauterine) heart rate or rhythm during labor**   N

P03.819   **Newborn (suspected to be) affected by abnormality in fetal (intrauterine) heart rate or rhythm, unspecified as to time of onset**   N

P03.82   **Meconium passage during delivery**   N

> **Excludes1**   meconium aspiration (P24.00, P24.01)
>   meconium staining (P96.83)

◄ New   ◄ Revised   ~~deleted~~ Deleted   Excludes 1   Excludes 2   Includes   Use additional   Code first   Code also   Unspecified

OGCR Official Guidelines   ● Unacceptable Principal Diagnosis   X Assign placeholder X   ● Use Additional Character(s)   ▌ Manifestation Code   Coding Clinic

P03.89 **Newborn (suspected to be) affected by other specified complications of labor and delivery** N
    Newborn (suspected to be) affected by abnormality of maternal soft tissues
    Newborn (suspected to be) affected by conditions classifiable to O60-O75 and by procedures used in labor and delivery not included in P02.- and P03.0-P03.6
    Newborn (suspected to be) affected by induction of labor

P03.9 **Newborn (suspected to be) affected by complication of labor and delivery, unspecified** N

● P04 **Newborn (suspected to be) affected by noxious substances transmitted via placenta or breast milk**
    Includes nonteratogenic effects of substances transmitted via placenta
    Excludes2 congenital malformations (Q00-Q99)
        neonatal jaundice from excessive hemolysis due to drugs or toxins transmitted from mother (P58.4)
        newborn in contact with and (suspected) exposures hazardous to health not transmitted via placenta or breast milk (Z77.-)

● P04.0 **Newborn (suspected to be) affected by maternal anesthesia and analgesia in pregnancy, labor and delivery** N
        Newborn (suspected to be) affected by reactions and intoxications from maternal opiates and tranquilizers administered during labor and delivery

P04.1 **Newborn (suspected to be) affected by other maternal medication** N
        Newborn (suspected to be) affected by cancer chemotherapy
        Newborn (suspected to be) affected by cytotoxic drugs
        Excludes1 dysmorphism due to warfarin (Q86.2)
            fetal hydantoin syndrome (Q86.1)
            maternal use of drugs of addiction (P04.4-)

P04.2 **Newborn (suspected to be) affected by maternal use of tobacco** N
        Newborn (suspected to be) affected by exposure in utero to tobacco smoke
        Excludes2 newborn exposure to environmental tobacco smoke (P96.81)

P04.3 **Newborn (suspected to be) affected by maternal use of alcohol** N
        Excludes1 fetal alcohol syndrome (Q86.0)

● P04.4 **Newborn (suspected to be) affected by maternal use of drugs of addiction**
    P04.41 **Newborn (suspected to be) affected by maternal use of cocaine** N
        'Crack baby'
    P04.49 **Newborn (suspected to be) affected by maternal use of other drugs of addiction** N
        Excludes2 newborn (suspected to be) affected by maternal anesthesia and analgesia (P04.0)
            withdrawal symptoms from maternal use of drugs of addiction (P96.1)

P04.5 **Newborn (suspected to be) affected by maternal use of nutritional chemical substances** N

P04.6 **Newborn (suspected to be) affected by maternal exposure to environmental chemical substances** N

P04.8 **Newborn (suspected to be) affected by other maternal noxious substances** N

P04.9 **Newborn (suspected to be) affected by maternal noxious substance, unspecified** N

OGCR Section I.C.16.d.

Prematurity and Fetal Growth Retardation
Providers utilize different criteria in determining prematurity. A code for prematurity should not be assigned unless it is documented. Assignment of codes in categories P05, Disorders of newborn related to slow fetal growth and fetal malnutrition, and P07, Disorders of newborn related to short gestation and low birth weight, not elsewhere classified, should be based on the recorded birth weight and estimated gestational age. Codes from category P05 should not be assigned with codes from category P07.

When both birth weight and gestational age are available, two codes from category P07 should be assigned, with the code for birth weight sequenced before the code for gestational age.

A code from P05 and codes from P07.2 and P07.3 may be used to specify weeks of gestation as documented by the provider in the record.

DISORDERS OF NEWBORN RELATED TO LENGTH OF GESTATION AND FETAL GROWTH (P05-P08)

● P05 **Disorders of newborn related to slow fetal growth and fetal malnutrition**

● P05.0 **Newborn light for gestational age**
        Newborn light-for-dates

    P05.00 **Newborn light for gestational age, unspecified weight** N

    P05.01 **Newborn light for gestational age, less than 500 grams** N

    P05.02 **Newborn light for gestational age, 500-749 grams** N

    P05.03 **Newborn light for gestational age, 750-999 grams** N

    P05.04 **Newborn light for gestational age, 1000-1249 grams** N

    P05.05 **Newborn light for gestational age, 1250-1499 grams** N

    P05.06 **Newborn light for gestational age, 1500-1749 grams** N

    P05.07 **Newborn light for gestational age, 1750-1999 grams** N

    P05.08 **Newborn light for gestational age, 2000-2499 grams** N

● P05.1 **Newborn small for gestational age**
        Newborn small-and-light-for-dates
        Newborn small-for-dates

    P05.10 **Newborn small for gestational age, unspecified weight** N

    P05.11 **Newborn small for gestational age, less than 500 grams** N

    P05.12 **Newborn small for gestational age, 500-749 grams** N

    P05.13 **Newborn small for gestational age, 750-999 grams** N

    P05.14 **Newborn small for gestational age, 1000-1249 grams** N

    P05.15 **Newborn small for gestational age, 1250-1499 grams** N

    P05.16 **Newborn small for gestational age, 1500-1749 grams** N

    P05.17 **Newborn small for gestational age, 1750-1999 grams** N

    P05.18 **Newborn small for gestational age, 2000-2499 grams** N

CHAPTER 16 (P00-P96)

N Newborn Age: 0   P Pediatric Age: 0–17   M Maternity DX: 12–55   A Adult Age: 15–124   ♀ Females Only   ♂ Males Only
⊗ Complication\Comorbidity   ⊗ Major C\C   (Ex) CC/MCC Exclusions   ⊗ Present on Admission Requirement   ⊗ Hospital-Acquired Condition

P05.2   **Newborn affected by fetal (intrauterine) malnutrition not light or small for gestational age**   N
> Infant, not light or small for gestational age, showing signs of fetal malnutrition, such as dry, peeling skin and loss of subcutaneous tissue
>> **Excludes1**   newborn affected by fetal malnutrition with light for gestational age (P05.0-)
>>> newborn affected by fetal malnutrition with small for gestational age (P05.1-)

P05.9   **Newborn affected by slow intrauterine growth, unspecified**   N
> Newborn affected by fetal growth retardation NOS

● **P07**   **Disorders of newborn related to short gestation and low birth weight, not elsewhere classified**
> **Note:** When both birth weight and gestational age of the newborn are available, both should be coded with birth weight sequenced before gestational age.
>> **Includes**   the listed conditions, without further specification, as the cause of morbidity or additional care, in newborn
>> **Excludes1**   low birth weight due to slow fetal growth and fetal malnutrition (P05.-)

● **P07.0**   **Extremely low birth weight newborn**
> Newborn birth weight 999 g. or less

P07.00   **Extremely low birth weight newborn, unspecified weight**   N

P07.01   **Extremely low birth weight newborn, less than 500 grams**   N

P07.02   **Extremely low birth weight newborn, 500-749 grams**   N

P07.03   **Extremely low birth weight newborn, 750-999 grams**   N

● **P07.1**   **Other low birth weight newborn**
> Newborn birth weight 1000-2499 g.

P07.10   **Other low birth weight newborn, unspecified weight**   N

P07.14   **Other low birth weight newborn, 1000-1249 grams**   N

P07.15   **Other low birth weight newborn, 1250-1499 grams**   N

P07.16   **Other low birth weight newborn, 1500-1749 grams**   N

P07.17   **Other low birth weight newborn, 1750-1999 grams**   N

P07.18   **Other low birth weight newborn, 2000-2499 grams**   N

● **P07.2**   **Extreme immaturity of newborn**
> Less than 28 completed weeks (less than 196 completed days) of gestation

P07.20   **Extreme immaturity of newborn, unspecified weeks of gestation**   N
> Gestational age less than 28 completed weeks NOS

P07.21   **Extreme immaturity of newborn, gestational age less than 23 completed weeks**   N
> Extreme immaturity of newborn, gestational age less than 23 weeks, 0 days

P07.22   **Extreme immaturity of newborn, gestational age 23 completed weeks**   N
> Extreme immaturity of newborn, gestational age 23 weeks, 0 days through 23 weeks, 6 days

P07.23   **Extreme immaturity of newborn, gestational age 24 completed weeks**   N
> Extreme immaturity of newborn, gestational age 24 weeks, 0 days through 24 weeks, 6 days

P07.24   **Extreme immaturity of newborn, gestational age 25 completed weeks**   N
> Extreme immaturity of newborn, gestational age 25 weeks, 0 days through 25 weeks, 6 days

P07.25   **Extreme immaturity of newborn, gestational age 26 completed weeks**   N
> Extreme immaturity of newborn, gestational age 26 weeks, 0 days through 26 weeks, 6 days

P07.26   **Extreme immaturity of newborn, gestational age 27 completed weeks**   N
> Extreme immaturity of newborn, gestational age 27 weeks, 0 days through 27 weeks, 6 days

● **P07.3**   **Preterm [premature] newborn [other]**
> 28 completed weeks or more but less than 37 completed weeks (196 completed days but less than 259 completed days) of gestation
> Prematurity NOS

P07.30   **Preterm newborn, unspecified weeks of gestation**   N

P07.31   **Preterm newborn, gestational age 28 completed weeks**   N
> Preterm newborn, gestational age 28 weeks, 0 days through 28 weeks, 6 days

P07.32   **Preterm newborn, gestational age 29 completed weeks**   N
> Preterm newborn, gestational age 29 weeks, 0 days through 29 weeks, 6 days

P07.33   **Preterm newborn, gestational age 30 completed weeks**   N
> Preterm newborn, gestational age 30 weeks, 0 days through 30 weeks, 6 days

P07.34   **Preterm newborn, gestational age 31 completed weeks**   N
> Preterm newborn, gestational age 31 weeks, 0 days through 31 weeks, 6 days

P07.35   **Preterm newborn, gestational age 32 completed weeks**   N
> Preterm newborn, gestational age 32 weeks, 0 days through 32 weeks, 6 days

P07.36   **Preterm newborn, gestational age 33 completed weeks**   N
> Preterm newborn, gestational age 33 weeks, 0 days through 33 weeks, 6 days

P07.37   **Preterm newborn, gestational age 34 completed weeks**   N
> Preterm newborn, gestational age 34 weeks, 0 days through 34 weeks, 6 days

P07.38   **Preterm newborn, gestational age 35 completed weeks**   N
> Preterm newborn, gestational age 35 weeks, 0 days through 35 weeks, 6 days

P07.39   **Preterm newborn, gestational age 36 completed weeks**   N
> Preterm newborn, gestational age 36 weeks, 0 days through 36 weeks, 6 days

◀ New   ◀▦ Revised   ~~deleted~~ Deleted   Excludes 1   Excludes 2   Includes   Use additional   Code first   Code also   Unspecified

OGCR Official Guidelines   ● Unacceptable Principal Diagnosis   X Assign placeholder X   ● Use Additional Character(s)   ▶ Manifestation Code   Coding Clinic

● **P08** **Disorders of newborn related to long gestation and high birth weight**

　　Note: When both birth weight and gestational age of the newborn are available, priority of assignment should be given to birth weight.

　　Includes　the listed conditions, without further specification, as causes of morbidity or additional care, in newborn

P08.0 **Exceptionally large newborn baby**　　　　　　N
　　Usually implies a birth weight of 4500 g. or more
　　Excludes1　syndrome of infant of diabetic mother (P70.1)
　　　　　　syndrome of infant of mother with gestational diabetes (P70.0)

P08.1 **Other heavy for gestational age newborn**　　　N
　　Other newborn heavy- or large-for-dates regardless of period of gestation
　　Usually implies a birth weight of 4000 g. to 4499 g.
　　Excludes1　newborn with a birth weight of 4500 or more (P08.0)
　　　　　　syndrome of infant of diabetic mother (P70.1)
　　　　　　syndrome of infant of mother with gestational diabetes (P70.0)

● **P08.2** **Late newborn, not heavy for gestational age**

　　P08.21　**Post-term newborn**　　　　　　　　　N
　　　　Newborn with gestation period over 40 completed weeks to 42 completed weeks

　　P08.22　**Prolonged gestation of newborn**　　　　N
　　　　Newborn with gestation period over 42 completed weeks (294 days or more), not heavy- or large-for-dates
　　　　Postmaturity NOS

ABNORMAL FINDINGS ON NEONATAL SCREENING (P09)

P09 **Abnormal findings on neonatal screening**　　　N
　　Use additional code to identify signs, symptoms and conditions associated with the screening
　　Excludes2　nonspecific serologic evidence of human immunodeficiency virus [HIV] (R75)

BIRTH TRAUMA (P10-P15)

● **P10** **Intracranial laceration and hemorrhage due to birth injury**
　　Excludes1　intracranial hemorrhage of newborn NOS (P52.9)
　　　　　　intracranial hemorrhage of newborn due to anoxia or hypoxia (P52.-)
　　　　　　nontraumatic intracranial hemorrhage of newborn (P52.-)
　　(Ex) **For category P10 CC codes unless otherwise indicated:** P10.0-P10.1, P10.4-P11.2, P11.9, P15.0-P15.9, P29.0-P29.2, P29.4, P29.89-P29.9, P52.4, P52.6-P52.9, P94.1-P94.9, P96.0, P96.3-P96.5, P96.82-P96.89

P10.0 **Subdural hemorrhage due to birth injury** 🐾　　N
　　Subdural hematoma (localized) due to birth injury
　　Excludes1　subdural hemorrhage accompanying tentorial tear (P10.4)

P10.1 **Cerebral hemorrhage due to birth injury** 🐾　　N

P10.2 **Intraventricular hemorrhage due to birth injury** 🐾　N
　　(Ex) P10.2-P10.3, P29.0-P29.2, P29.4, P29.89-P29.9, P50.0-P50.9, P52.0-P52.3, P52.5, P53-P54.0, P54.6-P54.9, P60-P61.9, P94.1-P94.9, P96.0, P96.3-P96.5, P96.82-P96.89

P10.3 **Subarachnoid hemorrhage due to birth injury** 🐾　N
　　(Ex) P10.2-P10.3, P29.0-P29.2, P29.4, P29.89-P29.9, P50.0-P50.9, P52.0-P52.3, P52.5, P53-P54.0, P54.6-P54.9, P60-P61.9, P91.2, P94.1-P94.9, P96.0, P96.3-P96.5, P96.82-P96.89

P10.4 **Tentorial tear due to birth injury** 🐾　　　　N
　　Pertaining to tentorium of cerebellum (extension of dura mater that separates cerebellum from inferior portion of occipital lobes)

P10.8 **Other intracranial lacerations and hemorrhages due to birth injury** 🐾　　　　　　　　　N

P10.9 **Unspecified intracranial laceration and hemorrhage due to birth injury** 🐾　　　　　　N

Item 16–1　The **peripheral nervous system** consists of 31 pairs of spinal nerves, 12 pairs of cranial nerves, and the autonomic nerves, which are divided into the parasympathetic and sympathetic nerves. The cranial nerves are: olfactory (I), optic (II), oculomotor (III), trochlear (IV), trigeminal (V), abducens (VI), facial (VII), vestibulocochlear (VIII), glossopharyngeal (IX), vagus (X), accessory (XI), and hypoglossal (XII).

Figure 16-1　A. Parasympathetic nervous system. **B.** Sympathetic nervous system. (From Buck CJ: Step-by-Step Medical Coding, Philadelphia, WB Saunders, 1998)

CHAPTER 16 (P00-P96)

N Newborn Age: 0　　**P** Pediatric Age: 0–17　　**M** Maternity DX: 12–55　　**A** Adult Age: 15–124　　♀ Females Only　　♂ Males Only

🐾 Complication\Comorbidity　　🐾 Major C\C　　(Ex) CC/MCC Exclusions　　🐾 Present on Admission Requirement　　🐾 Hospital-Acquired Condition

CHAPTER 16 (P00-P96)

● **P11**   **Other birth injuries to central nervous system**

    P11.0   Cerebral edema due to birth injury 🅦   N
       Ⓔ See P10

    P11.1   Other specified brain damage due to birth injury   N

    P11.2   Unspecified brain damage due to birth injury 🅦   N
       Ⓔ See P10

    P11.3   Birth injury to facial nerve   N
       Facial palsy due to birth injury

    P11.4   Birth injury to other cranial nerves   N

    P11.5   Birth injury to spine and spinal cord   N
       Fracture of spine due to birth injury

    P11.9   Birth injury to central nervous system, unspecified 🅦   N
       Ⓔ See P10

● **P12**   **Birth injury to scalp**

    P12.0   Cephalhematoma due to birth injury   N

    P12.1   Chignon (from vacuum extraction) due to birth injury   N

    P12.2   Epicranial subaponeurotic hemorrhage due to birth injury 🅦   N
       Subgaleal hemorrhage
       Ⓔ P10.0-P10.1, P10.4-P11.2, P11.9-P12.2, P15.0-P15.9, P29.0-P29.2, P29.4,
           P29.89-P29.9, P52.4, P52.6-P52.9, P94.1-P94.9, P96.0, P96.3-P96.5,
           P96.82-P96.89

    P12.3   Bruising of scalp due to birth injury   N

    P12.4   Injury of scalp of newborn due to monitoring equipment   N
       Sampling incision of scalp of newborn
       Scalp clip (electrode) injury of newborn

   ● **P12.8**   Other birth injuries to scalp

       P12.81   Caput succedaneum   N

       P12.89   Other birth injuries to scalp   N

    P12.9   Birth injury to scalp, unspecified   N

● **P13**   **Birth injury to skeleton**

    Excludes2   birth injury to spine (P11.5)

    P13.0   Fracture of skull due to birth injury   N

    P13.1   Other birth injuries to skull   N
       Excludes1   cephalhematoma (P12.0)

    P13.2   Birth injury to femur   N

    P13.3   Birth injury to other long bones   N

    P13.4   Fracture of clavicle due to birth injury   N

    P13.8   Birth injuries to other parts of skeleton   N

    P13.9   Birth injury to skeleton, unspecified   N

● **P14**   **Birth injury to peripheral nervous system**

    P14.0   Erb's paralysis due to birth injury   N

    P14.1   Klumpke's paralysis due to birth injury   N

    P14.2   Phrenic nerve paralysis due to birth injury   N

    P14.3   Other brachial plexus birth injuries   N

    P14.8   Birth injuries to other parts of peripheral nervous system   N

    P14.9   Birth injury to peripheral nervous system, unspecified   N

● **P15**   **Other birth injuries**

    P15.0   Birth injury to liver   N
       Rupture of liver due to birth injury

    P15.1   Birth injury to spleen   N
       Rupture of spleen due to birth injury

    P15.2   Sternomastoid injury due to birth injury   N

    P15.3   Birth injury to eye   N
       Subconjunctival hemorrhage due to birth injury
       Traumatic glaucoma due to birth injury

    P15.4   Birth injury to face   N
       Facial congestion due to birth injury

    P15.5   Birth injury to external genitalia   N

    P15.6   Subcutaneous fat necrosis due to birth injury   N

    P15.8   Other specified birth injuries   N

    P15.9   Birth injury, unspecified   N

RESPIRATORY AND CARDIOVASCULAR DISORDERS SPECIFIC TO THE PERINATAL PERIOD (P19-P29)

● **P19**   **Metabolic acidemia in newborn**

    Includes   metabolic acidemia in newborn

    P19.0   Metabolic acidemia in newborn first noted before onset of labor   N

    P19.1   Metabolic acidemia in newborn first noted during labor   N

    P19.2   Metabolic acidemia noted at birth   N

    P19.9   Metabolic acidemia, unspecified   N

● **P22**   **Respiratory distress of newborn**

    Excludes1   respiratory arrest of newborn (P28.81)
                 respiratory failure of newborn NOS (P28.5)

    P22.0   Respiratory distress syndrome of newborn   N
       Cardiorespiratory distress syndrome of newborn
       Hyaline membrane disease
       Idiopathic respiratory distress syndrome [IRDS or RDS] of newborn
       Pulmonary hypoperfusion syndrome
       Respiratory distress syndrome, type I
       Ⓔ J84.83-J84.848, P22.0-P28.5, P28.89-P29.2, P29.4, P29.89-P29.9, P84,
           P94.1-P96.0, P96.3-P96.5, P96.82-P96.89

    P22.1   Transient tachypnea of newborn   N
       Idiopathic tachypnea of newborn
       Respiratory distress syndrome, type II
       Wet lung syndrome

    P22.8   Other respiratory distress of newborn   N

    P22.9   Respiratory distress of newborn, unspecified   N

● **P23**   **Congenital pneumonia**

    Includes   infective pneumonia acquired in utero or during birth

    Excludes1   neonatal pneumonia resulting from aspiration (P24.-)

    Ⓔ For category P23 CC codes: See P22.0

    P23.0   Congenital pneumonia due to viral agent 🅦   N
       Use additional code (B97) to identify organism
       Excludes1   congenital rubella pneumonitis (P35.0)

    P23.1   Congenital pneumonia due to Chlamydia 🅦   N

    P23.2   Congenital pneumonia due to staphylococcus 🅦   N

    P23.3   Congenital pneumonia due to streptococcus, group B 🅦   N

    P23.4   Congenital pneumonia due to Escherichia coli 🅦   N

    P23.5   Congenital pneumonia due to Pseudomonas 🅦   N

    P23.6   Congenital pneumonia due to other bacterial agents 🅦   N
       Congenital pneumonia due to Hemophilus influenzae
       Congenital pneumonia due to Klebsiella pneumoniae
       Congenital pneumonia due to Mycoplasma
       Congenital pneumonia due to Streptococcus, except group B
       Use additional code (B95-B96) to identify organism

    P23.8   Congenital pneumonia due to other organisms 🅦   N

    P23.9   Congenital pneumonia, unspecified 🅦   N

● **P24**   **Neonatal aspiration**

    Includes   aspiration in utero and during delivery

   ● **P24.0**   Meconium aspiration

       Excludes1   meconium passage (without aspiration) during delivery (P03.82)
                 meconium staining (P96.83)

       P24.00   Meconium aspiration without respiratory symptoms   N
          Meconium aspiration NOS

       P24.01   Meconium aspiration with respiratory symptoms 🅦   N
          Meconium aspiration pneumonia
          Meconium aspiration pneumonitis
          Meconium aspiration syndrome NOS

          Use additional code to identify any secondary pulmonary hypertension, if applicable (I27.2)
          Ⓔ See P22.0

◀ New   ◀▦ Revised   ~~deleted~~ Deleted   Excludes 1   Excludes 2   Includes   Use additional   Code first   Code also   Unspecified

OGCR Official Guidelines   ● Unacceptable Principal Diagnosis   X Assign placeholder X   ● Use Additional Character(s)   ▌ Manifestation Code   **Coding Clinic**

● **P24.1**   **Neonatal aspiration of (clear) amniotic fluid and mucus**
Neonatal aspiration of liquor (amnii)

     P24.10   **Neonatal aspiration of (clear) amniotic fluid and mucus without respiratory symptoms**   N
Neonatal aspiration of amniotic fluid and mucus NOS

     P24.11   **Neonatal aspiration of (clear) amniotic fluid and mucus with respiratory symptoms** 🏥   N
Neonatal aspiration of amniotic fluid and mucus with pneumonia
Neonatal aspiration of amniotic fluid and mucus with pneumonitis
Use additional code to identify any secondary pulmonary hypertension, if applicable (I27.2)
Ⓔ See P22.0

● **P24.2**   **Neonatal aspiration of blood**

     P24.20   **Neonatal aspiration of blood without respiratory symptoms**   N
Neonatal aspiration of blood NOS

     P24.21   **Neonatal aspiration of blood with respiratory symptoms** 🏥   N
Neonatal aspiration of blood with pneumonia
Neonatal aspiration of blood with pneumonitis
Use additional code to identify any secondary pulmonary hypertension, if applicable (I27.2)
Ⓔ See P22.0

● **P24.3**   **Neonatal aspiration of milk and regurgitated food**
Neonatal aspiration of stomach contents

     P24.30   **Neonatal aspiration of milk and regurgitated food without respiratory symptoms**   N
Neonatal aspiration of milk and regurgitated food NOS

     P24.31   **Neonatal aspiration of milk and regurgitated food with respiratory symptoms** 🏥   N
Neonatal aspiration of milk and regurgitated food with pneumonia
Neonatal aspiration of milk and regurgitated food with pneumonitis
Use additional code to identify any secondary pulmonary hypertension, if applicable (I27.2)
Ⓔ See P22.0

● **P24.8**   **Other neonatal aspiration**

     P24.80   **Other neonatal aspiration without respiratory symptoms**   N
Neonatal aspiration NEC

     P24.81   **Other neonatal aspiration with respiratory symptoms** 🏥   N
Neonatal aspiration pneumonia NEC
Neonatal aspiration with pneumonitis NEC
Neonatal aspiration with pneumonia NOS
Neonatal aspiration with pneumonitis NOS
Use additional code to identify any secondary pulmonary hypertension, if applicable (I27.2)
Ⓔ See P22.0

     P24.9   **Neonatal aspiration, unspecified**   N

● **P25**   **Interstitial emphysema and related conditions originating in the perinatal period**
Ⓔ For category P25 CC codes: See P22.0

     P25.0   **Interstitial emphysema originating in the perinatal period** 🏥   N

     P25.1   **Pneumothorax originating in the perinatal period** 🏥   N

     P25.2   **Pneumomediastinum originating in the perinatal period** 🏥   N

     P25.3   **Pneumopericardium originating in the perinatal period** 🏥   N

     P25.8   **Other conditions related to interstitial emphysema originating in the perinatal period** 🏥   N

● **P26**   **Pulmonary hemorrhage originating in the perinatal period**
Excludes1   acute idiopathic hemorrhage in infants over 28 days old (R04.81)
Ⓔ For category P26 CC codes: See P22.0

     P26.0   **Tracheobronchial hemorrhage originating in the perinatal period** 🏥   N

     P26.1   **Massive pulmonary hemorrhage originating in the perinatal period** 🏥   N

     P26.8   **Other pulmonary hemorrhages originating in the perinatal period** 🏥   N

     P26.9   **Unspecified pulmonary hemorrhage originating in the perinatal period** 🏥   N

● **P27**   **Chronic respiratory disease originating in the perinatal period**
Excludes1   respiratory distress of newborn (P22.0-P22.9)
Ⓔ For category P27 CC codes: See P22.0

     P27.0   **Wilson-Mikity syndrome** 🏥
Pulmonary dysmaturity

     P27.1   **Bronchopulmonary dysplasia originating in the perinatal period** 🏥

     P27.8   **Other chronic respiratory diseases originating in the perinatal period** 🏥
Congenital pulmonary fibrosis
Ventilator lung in newborn

     P27.9   **Unspecified chronic respiratory disease originating in the perinatal period** 🏥

● **P28**   **Other respiratory conditions originating in the perinatal period**
Excludes1   congenital malformations of the respiratory system (Q30-Q34)

     P28.0   **Primary atelectasis of newborn** 🏥   N
Failure of lungs to expand properly at birth
Primary failure to expand terminal respiratory units
Pulmonary hypoplasia associated with short gestation
Pulmonary immaturity NOS
Ⓔ See P22.0

● **P28.1**   **Other and unspecified atelectasis of newborn**
Ⓔ For category P28.1 CC codes: See P22.0

     P28.10   **Unspecified atelectasis of newborn** 🏥   N
Atelectasis of newborn NOS

     P28.11   **Resorption atelectasis without respiratory distress syndrome** 🏥   N
Excludes1   resorption atelectasis with respiratory distress syndrome (P22.0)

     P28.19   **Other atelectasis of newborn** 🏥   N
Partial atelectasis of newborn
Secondary atelectasis of newborn

     P28.2   **Cyanotic attacks of newborn** 🏥   N
Excludes1   apnea of newborn (P28.3-P28.4)
Ⓔ P22.8-P22.9, P28.2-P28.4, P28.81-P28.9, R06.81, R23.0

     P28.3   **Primary sleep apnea of newborn** 🏥   N
Central sleep apnea of newborn
Obstructive sleep apnea of newborn
Sleep apnea of newborn NOS
Ⓔ P22.8-P22.9, P28.2, P28.4, P28.81-P28.9, R06.81

     P28.4   **Other apnea of newborn** 🏥   N
Apnea of prematurity
Obstructive apnea of newborn
Excludes1   obstructive sleep apnea of newborn (P28.3)
Ⓔ P22.8-P22.9, P28.2-P28.4, P28.81-P28.9, R06.81

     P28.5   **Respiratory failure of newborn** 🏥   N
Excludes1   respiratory arrest of newborn (P28.81)
respiratory distress of newborn (P22.0-)
Ⓔ See P22.0

N Newborn Age: 0   **P** Pediatric Age: 0–17   **M** Maternity DX: 12–55   **A** Adult Age: 15–124   ♀ Females Only   ♂ Males Only
🏥 Complication\Comorbidity   🏥 Major C\C   Ⓔ CC/MCC Exclusions   Present on Admission Requirement   🏥 Hospital-Acquired Condition

1241

● **P28.8**   **Other specified respiratory conditions of newborn**

     P28.81   **Respiratory arrest of newborn**   N
         (Ex) P22.1-P22.9, P24.00, P24.10, P24.20, P24.30, P24.80,
         P28.2-P28.5, P28.89-P28.9, P29.81, R06.81, R09.2

     P28.89   **Other specified respiratory conditions of newborn**   N
         Congenital laryngeal stridor
         Sniffles in newborn
         Snuffles in newborn
         Excludes1   early congenital syphilitic rhinitis (A50.05) ◀

P28.9   **Respiratory condition of newborn, unspecified**   N
     Respiratory depression in newborn

● **P29**   **Cardiovascular disorders originating in the perinatal period**
     Excludes1   congenital malformations of the circulatory system (Q20-Q28)

P29.0   **Neonatal cardiac failure**   N

● **P29.1**   **Neonatal cardiac dysrhythmia**

     P29.11   **Neonatal tachycardia**   N

     P29.12   **Neonatal bradycardia**   N

P29.2   **Neonatal hypertension**   N

P29.3   **Persistent fetal circulation**   N
     Delayed closure of ductus arteriosus
     (Persistent) pulmonary hypertension of newborn
     (Ex) I27.0, I27.2-I27.81, I27.89-I27.9

P29.4   **Transient myocardial ischemia in newborn**   N

● **P29.8**   **Other cardiovascular disorders originating in the perinatal period**

     P29.81   **Cardiac arrest of newborn**   N
         (Ex) P29.81

     P29.89   **Other cardiovascular disorders originating in the perinatal period**   N

P29.9   **Cardiovascular disorder originating in the perinatal period, unspecified**   N

INFECTIONS SPECIFIC TO THE PERINATAL PERIOD (P35-P39)

Infections acquired in utero, during birth via the umbilicus, or during the first 28 days after birth

Excludes2   asymptomatic human immunodeficiency virus [HIV] infection status (Z21)
     congenital gonococcal infection (A54.-)
     congenital pneumonia (P23.-)
     congenital syphilis (A50.-)
     human immunodeficiency virus [HIV] disease (B20)
     infant botulism (A48.51)
     infectious diseases not specific to the perinatal period (A00-B99, J09, J10.-)
     intestinal infectious disease (A00-A09)
     laboratory evidence of human immunodeficiency virus [HIV] (R75)
     tetanus neonatorum (A33)

● **P35**   **Congenital viral diseases**
     Includes   infections acquired in utero or during birth
     (Ex) A17.82, A28.1, A50.42, A52.14, A75.9, A79.9, A81.1, A81.82-A81.89, A83.0-A85.8,
     A87.2, A88.0, A88.8, A92.1-A92.8, A93.0, B00.4, B00.82, B01.11-B01.12, B04, B06.01,
     B08.09, B08.20-B08.22, B08.60-B08.79, B09, B10.01-B10.09, B26.2, B27.00-B27.99,
     B33.1, B45.0, B45.2-B45.9, B54, B58.2, B75, B97.10, B97.21, G04.00-G04.01, G04.31,
     G04.81-G05.4, G37.0, G37.4-G37.5, H66.40-H66.43, J09.X3-J09.X9, J10.2-J10.89,
     J11.2-J11.89, L44.4, M1A.10X0-M1A.19X1, M32.0-M32.9, P35.2-P35.9, P37.0-P37.9,
     T56.0X1-T56.0X4[A]

P35.0   **Congenital rubella syndrome**   N
     Congenital rubella pneumonitis
     (Ex) P29.0-P29.2, P29.4, P29.89-P35.9, P37.0-P37.4, P37.8-P37.9, P94.1-P94.9,
     P96.0, P96.3-P96.5, P96.82-P96.89

P35.1   **Congenital cytomegalovirus infection**   N
     Viruses transmitted by multiple routes that cause mild/ subclinical infection
     (Ex) See P35.0

P35.2   **Congenital herpesviral [herpes simplex] infection**   N

P35.3   **Congenital viral hepatitis**   N

P35.8   **Other congenital viral diseases**   N
     Congenital varicella [chickenpox]

P35.9   **Congenital viral disease, unspecified**   N

● **P36**   **Bacterial sepsis of newborn**
     Includes   congenital sepsis
     Use additional code(s), if applicable, to identify severe sepsis (R65.2-) and associated acute organ dysfunction(s)
     (Ex) For category P36 CC codes: P29.0-P29.2, P29.4, P29.89-P29.9, P36.0-P36.9, P37.5,
     P38.1-P39.9, P53, P60-P61.9, P94.1-P94.9, P96.0, P96.3-P96.5, P96.82-P96.89

P36.0   **Sepsis of newborn due to streptococcus, group B**   N

● **P36.1**   **Sepsis of newborn due to other and unspecified streptococci**

     P36.10   **Sepsis of newborn due to unspecified streptococci**   N

     P36.19   **Sepsis of newborn due to other streptococci**   N

P36.2   **Sepsis of newborn due to Staphylococcus aureus**   N

● **P36.3**   **Sepsis of newborn due to other and unspecified staphylococci**

     P36.30   **Sepsis of newborn due to unspecified staphylococci**   N

     P36.39   **Sepsis of newborn due to other staphylococci**   N

P36.4   **Sepsis of newborn due to Escherichia coli**   N

P36.5   **Sepsis of newborn due to anaerobes**   N

P36.8   **Other bacterial sepsis of newborn**   N
     Use additional code from category B96 to identify organism

P36.9   **Bacterial sepsis of newborn, unspecified**   N

● **P37**   **Other congenital infectious and parasitic diseases**
     Excludes2   congenital syphilis (A50.-)
     infectious neonatal diarrhea (A00-A09)
     necrotizing enterocolitis in newborn (P77.-)
     noninfectious neonatal diarrhea (P78.3)
     ophthalmia neonatorum due to gonococcus (A54.31)
     tetanus neonatorum (A33)
     (Ex) For category P37 CC codes: See P35

P37.0   **Congenital tuberculosis**   N

P37.1   **Congenital toxoplasmosis**   N
     Parasitic infection, often causing mild flu-like illness
     Hydrocephalus due to congenital toxoplasmosis

P37.2   **Neonatal (disseminated) listeriosis**   N
     Acquired transplacentally or during/after parturition in which symptoms are those of sepsis

P37.3   **Congenital falciparum malaria**   N

P37.4   **Other congenital malaria**   N

P37.5   **Neonatal candidiasis**   N

P37.8   **Other specified congenital infectious and parasitic diseases**   N

P37.9   **Congenital infectious or parasitic disease, unspecified**   N

● **P38**   **Omphalitis of newborn**
     Inflammation of umbilicus
     Excludes1   omphalitis not of newborn (L08.82)
     tetanus omphalitis (A33)
     umbilical hemorrhage of newborn (P51.-)
     (Ex) For category P38 CC codes: P39.2, P39.4-P39.9

P38.1   **Omphalitis with mild hemorrhage**   N

P38.9   **Omphalitis without hemorrhage**   N
     Omphalitis of newborn NOS

◀ New   ◀ Revised   ~~deleted~~ Deleted   Excludes 1   Excludes 2   Includes   Use additional   Code first   Code also   Unspecified

OGCR Official Guidelines   ● Unacceptable Principal Diagnosis   X Assign placeholder X   ● Use Additional Character(s)   ▸ Manifestation Code   **Coding Clinic**

● P39   Other infections specific to the perinatal period
        Use additional code to identify organism or specific infection
        (Ex:) **For category P39 CC codes unless otherwise indicated:** A02.1, A20.7, A22.7,
            A39.2-A39.4, A40.9-A41.59, A41.81-A41.9, A42.7, A48.2, A48.4, A48.8-A49.9, B00.7,
            B92, B94.2-B96.89, P39.2-P39.9, P95, P96.9, R78.81

    P39.0   Neonatal infective mastitis 🔾   N
            Excludes1   breast engorgement of newborn (P83.4)
                           noninfective mastitis of newborn (P83.4)
            (Ex:) See P38

    P39.1   Neonatal conjunctivitis and dacryocystitis   N
            Neonatal chlamydial conjunctivitis
            Ophthalmia neonatorum NOS
                Neonate = newborn
            Excludes1   gonococcal conjunctivitis (A54.31)

    P39.2   Intra-amniotic infection affecting newborn, not
            elsewhere classified 🔾   N

    P39.3   Neonatal urinary tract infection 🔾   N
            (Ex:) A49.9, N10-N11.0, N11.8-N12, N13.6, N15.1, N28.82, N28.84-N30.31,
                N30.80-N30.91, N36.9-N39.0, N39.9, N99.511, P39.2, P39.4-P39.9, R30.0,
                R30.9, T83.51X[A]

    P39.4   Neonatal skin infection 🔾   N
            Neonatal pyoderma
            Excludes1   pemphigus neonatorum (L00)
                           staphylococcal scalded skin syndrome
                               (L00)

    P39.8   Other specified infections specific to the perinatal
            period 🔾   N

    P39.9   Infection specific to the perinatal period, unspecified 🔾 N

HEMORRHAGIC AND HEMATOLOGICAL DISORDERS OF NEWBORN (P50-P61)

        Excludes1   congenital stenosis and stricture of bile ducts
                           (Q44.3)
                       Crigler-Najjar syndrome (E80.5)
                       Dubin-Johnson syndrome (E80.6)
                       Gilbert syndrome (E80.4)
                       hereditary hemolytic anemias (D55-D58)

● P50   Newborn affected by intrauterine (fetal) blood loss
        Excludes1   congenital anemia from intrauterine (fetal) blood
                           loss (P61.3)

    P50.0   Newborn affected by intrauterine (fetal) blood loss from
            vasa previa   N

    P50.1   Newborn affected by intrauterine (fetal) blood loss from
            ruptured cord   N

    P50.2   Newborn affected by intrauterine (fetal) blood loss from
            placenta   N

    P50.3   Newborn affected by hemorrhage into co-twin   N

    P50.4   Newborn affected by hemorrhage into maternal
            circulation   N

    P50.5   Newborn affected by intrauterine (fetal) blood loss from
            cut end of co-twin's cord   N

    P50.8   Newborn affected by other intrauterine (fetal) blood
            loss   N

    P50.9   Newborn affected by intrauterine (fetal) blood loss,
            unspecified   N
            Newborn affected by fetal hemorrhage NOS

● P51   Umbilical hemorrhage of newborn
        Excludes1   omphalitis with mild hemorrhage (P38.1)
                       umbilical hemorrhage from cut end of co-twins
                           cord (P50.5)

    P51.0   Massive umbilical hemorrhage of newborn   N

    P51.8   Other umbilical hemorrhages of newborn   N
            Slipped umbilical ligature NOS

    P51.9   Umbilical hemorrhage of newborn, unspecified   N

● P52   **Intracranial nontraumatic hemorrhage of newborn**
        Includes   intracranial hemorrhage due to anoxia or hypoxia
        Excludes1   intracranial hemorrhage due to birth injury
                           (P10.-)
                       intracranial hemorrhage due to other injury
                           (S06.-)

    P52.0   Intraventricular (nontraumatic) hemorrhage, grade 1,
            of newborn 🔾   N
            Subependymal hemorrhage (without intraventricular
                extension)
            Bleeding into germinal matrix
            (Ex:) P10.2-P10.3, P29.0-P29.2, P29.4, P29.89-P29.9, P50.0-P50.9, P52.0-P52.3,
                P52.5, P53-P54.0, P54.6-P54.9, P60-P61.9, P94.1-P94.9, P96.0,
                P96.3-P96.5, P96.82-P96.89

    P52.1   Intraventricular (nontraumatic) hemorrhage, grade 2,
            of newborn 🔾   N
            Subependymal hemorrhage with intraventricular
                extension
            Bleeding into ventricle
            (Ex:) See P52.0

● P52.2 Intraventricular (nontraumatic) hemorrhage, grade 3
        and grade 4, of newborn

    P52.21 Intraventricular (nontraumatic) hemorrhage,
            grade 3, of newborn 🔾   N
            Subependymal hemorrhage with
                intraventricular extension with
                enlargement of ventricle
            (Ex:) See P52.0

    P52.22 Intraventricular (nontraumatic) hemorrhage,
            grade 4, of newborn 🔾   N
            Bleeding into cerebral cortex
            Subependymal hemorrhage with intracerebral
                extension
            (Ex:) See P52.0

    P52.3   Unspecified intraventricular (nontraumatic) hemorrhage
            of newborn 🔾   N
            (Ex:) See P52.0

    P52.4   Intracerebral (nontraumatic) hemorrhage of
            newborn 🔾   N
            (Ex:) P10.0-P10.1, P10.4-P11.2, P11.9, P15.0-P15.9, P29.0-P29.2, P29.4,
                P29.89-P29.9, P52.4, P52.6-P52.9, P94.1-P94.9, P96.0, P96.3-P96.5,
                P96.82-P96.89

    P52.5   Subarachnoid (nontraumatic) hemorrhage of
            newborn 🔾   N
            (Ex:) P10.2-P10.3, P29.0-P29.2, P29.4, P29.89-P29.9, P50.0-P50.9, P52.0-P52.3,
                P52.5, P53-P54.0, P54.6-P54.9, P60-P61.9, P91.2, P94.1-P94.9, P96.0,
                P96.3-P96.5, P96.82-P96.89

    P52.6   Cerebellar (nontraumatic) and posterior fossa
            hemorrhage of newborn 🔾   N
            (Ex:) See P52.4

    P52.8   Other intracranial (nontraumatic) hemorrhages
            of newborn 🔾   N
            (Ex:) See P52.4

    P52.9   Intracranial (nontraumatic) hemorrhage of newborn,
            unspecified 🔾   N
            (Ex:) See P52.4

● P53   Hemorrhagic disease of newborn 🔾   N
        Vitamin K deficiency of newborn
        (Ex:) P29.0-P29.2, P29.4, P29.89-P29.9, P53, P60-P61.9, P94.1-P96.0, P96.3-P96.5,
            P96.82-P96.89

N Newborn Age: 0   **P** Pediatric Age: 0–17   **M** Maternity DX: 12–55   **A** Adult Age: 15–124   ♀ Females Only   ♂ Males Only

🔾 Complication\Comorbidity   🔾 Major C\C   (Ex:) CC/MCC Exclusions   🔾 Present on Admission Requirement   🔾 Hospital-Acquired Condition

1243

CHAPTER 16 (P00-P96)

● **P54** **Other neonatal hemorrhages**

> **Excludes1** newborn affected by (intrauterine) blood loss
> (P50.-)
> pulmonary hemorrhage originating in the
> perinatal period (P26.-)

　P54.0 **Neonatal hematemesis** N
　　　Vomiting of blood
> **Excludes1** neonatal hematemesis due to swallowed
> maternal blood (P78.2)

　P54.1 **Neonatal melena** 🔖 N
　　　Dark-colored feces stained with blood pigments
> **Excludes1** neonatal melena due to swallowed
> maternal blood (P78.2)
> Ⓔ P29.0-P29.2, P29.4, P29.89-P29.9, P50.0-P50.9, P53-P54.9, P60-P61.9,
> P94.1-P96.0, P96.3-P96.5, P96.82-P96.89

　P54.2 **Neonatal rectal hemorrhage** 🔖 N
　　　Ⓔ See P54.1

　P54.3 **Other neonatal gastrointestinal hemorrhage** 🔖 N
　　　Ⓔ See P54.1

　P54.4 **Neonatal adrenal hemorrhage** 🔖 N
　　　Ⓔ See P54.1

　P54.5 **Neonatal cutaneous hemorrhage** N
　　　Neonatal bruising
　　　Neonatal ecchymoses
　　　Neonatal petechiae
　　　Neonatal superficial hematomata
> **Excludes2** bruising of scalp due to birth injury
> (P12.3)
> cephalhematoma due to birth injury
> (P12.0)

　P54.6 **Neonatal vaginal hemorrhage** ♀ N
　　　Neonatal pseudomenses

　P54.8 **Other specified neonatal hemorrhages** N

　P54.9 **Neonatal hemorrhage, unspecified** N

● **P55** **Hemolytic disease of newborn**
　　AKA erythroblastosis fetalis and is due to Rh isoimmunization,
　　result of Rh blood factor incompatibilities between mother (Rh
　　negative) and fetus (Rh positive)

　P55.0 **Rh isoimmunization of newborn** N

　P55.1 **ABO isoimmunization of newborn** N

　P55.8 **Other hemolytic diseases of newborn** N

　P55.9 **Hemolytic disease of newborn, unspecified** N

● **P56** **Hydrops fetalis due to hemolytic disease**
　　Caused by maternal sensitization to fetal blood group antigen
> **Excludes1** hydrops fetalis NOS (P83.2)
> Ⓔ For category P56 CC codes: P29.0-P29.2, P29.4, P29.89-P29.9, P55.0-P57.0,
> P94.1-P96.0, P96.3-P96.5, P96.82-P96.89

　P56.0 **Hydrops fetalis due to isoimmunization** 🔖 N

● P56.9 **Hydrops fetalis due to other and unspecified hemolytic**
　　　disease
　　　P56.90 **Hydrops fetalis due to unspecified hemolytic**
　　　　　　disease 🔖 N
　　　P56.99 **Hydrops fetalis due to other hemolytic**
　　　　　　disease 🔖 N

● **P57** **Kernicterus**
　　High levels of bilirubin in blood, with severe neural symptoms
　　Ⓔ For category P57 CC codes unless otherwise indicated: P29.0-P29.2, P29.4,
　　P29.89-P29.9, P57.8-P59.9, P94.1-P96.0, P96.3-P96.5, P96.82-P96.89

　P57.0 **Kernicterus due to isoimmunization** 🔖 N
　　　Ⓔ See P56

　P57.8 **Other specified kernicterus** 🔖 N
> **Excludes1** Crigler-Najjar syndrome (E80.5)

　P57.9 **Kernicterus, unspecified** 🔖 N

● **P58** **Neonatal jaundice due to other excessive hemolysis**
> **Excludes1** jaundice due to isoimmunization (P55-P57)

　P58.0 **Neonatal jaundice due to bruising** N

　P58.1 **Neonatal jaundice due to bleeding** N

　P58.2 **Neonatal jaundice due to infection** N

　P58.3 **Neonatal jaundice due to polycythemia** N

● P58.4 **Neonatal jaundice due to drugs or toxins transmitted**
　　　from mother or given to newborn
　　　Code first poisoning due to drug or toxin, if applicable
　　　(T36-T65 with fifth or sixth character 1-4 or 6)
　　　Use additional code for adverse effect, if applicable,
　　　to identify drug (T36-T50 with fifth or sixth
　　　character 5)
　　　● P58.41 **Neonatal jaundice due to drugs or toxins**
　　　　　　transmitted from mother N
　　　● P58.42 **Neonatal jaundice due to drugs or toxins given**
　　　　　　to newborn N

　P58.5 **Neonatal jaundice due to swallowed maternal blood** N

　P58.8 **Neonatal jaundice due to other specified excessive**
　　　hemolysis N

　P58.9 **Neonatal jaundice due to excessive hemolysis,**
　　　unspecified N

● **P59** **Neonatal jaundice from other and unspecified causes**
> **Excludes1** jaundice due to inborn errors of metabolism
> (E70-E88)
> kernicterus (P57.-)

　P59.0 **Neonatal jaundice associated with preterm delivery** N
　　　Hyperbilirubinemia of prematurity
　　　Jaundice due to delayed conjugation associated with
　　　preterm delivery

　P59.1 **Inspissated bile syndrome** 🔖 N
　　　Ⓔ See P57

● P59.2 **Neonatal jaundice from other and unspecified**
　　　hepatocellular damage
> **Excludes1** congenital viral hepatitis (P35.3)
> Ⓔ For category P59.2 CC codes unless otherwise indicated: See P57
　　　P59.20 **Neonatal jaundice from unspecified**
　　　　　　hepatocellular damage 🔖 N
　　　P59.29 **Neonatal jaundice from other hepatocellular**
　　　　　　damage 🔖 N
　　　　　　Neonatal giant cell hepatitis
　　　　　　Neonatal (idiopathic) hepatitis

　P59.3 **Neonatal jaundice from breast milk inhibitor** N

　P59.8 **Neonatal jaundice from other specified causes** N

　P59.9 **Neonatal jaundice, unspecified** N
　　　Neonatal physiological jaundice (intense)(prolonged)
　　　NOS

　P60 **Disseminated intravascular coagulation of newborn** 🔖 N
　　　Defibrination syndrome of newborn
　　　Ⓔ See P53

● **P61** **Other perinatal hematological disorders**
> **Excludes1** transient hypogammaglobulinemia of infancy
> (D80.7)

　P61.0 **Transient neonatal thrombocytopenia** 🔖 N
　　　Lack of sufficient numbers of circulating thrombocytes
　　　(platelets)
　　　Neonatal thrombocytopenia due to exchange
　　　transfusion
　　　Neonatal thrombocytopenia due to idiopathic maternal
　　　thrombocytopenia
　　　Neonatal thrombocytopenia due to isoimmunization
　　　Ⓔ See P53

　P61.1 **Polycythemia neonatorum** N
　　　Neonate = newborn

◀ New　◀ⁱⁱⁱ Revised　deleted Deleted　Excludes 1　Excludes 2　Includes　Use additional　Code first　Code also　Unspecified
OGCR Official Guidelines　● Unacceptable Principal Diagnosis　X Assign placeholder X　● Use Additional Character(s)　▶ Manifestation Code　**Coding Clinic**

P61.2   **Anemia of prematurity** 🔹   N
    (Ex:) D50.0-D55.9, D56.4, D57.00-D57.3, D57.80-D64.9, D75.9, P61.2-P61.4

P61.3   **Congenital anemia from fetal blood loss** 🔹   N
    (Ex:) See P61.2

P61.4   **Other congenital anemias, not elsewhere classified** 🔹   N
    Congenital anemia NOS
    (Ex:) See P61.2

P61.5   **Transient neonatal neutropenia** 🔹   N
    Low levels of granulocytic neutrophilic white blood cells
    Excludes1   congenital neutropenia (nontransient)
            (D70.0)
    (Ex:) D50.1-D53.9, D56.4, D57.00-D57.20, D57.3, D57.811-D57.819, D58.2,
    D59.0-D59.1, D59.3, D60.0-D61.9, D63.0-D64.9, D75.9, P61.5, P61.8-P61.9

P61.6   **Other transient neonatal disorders of coagulation** 🔹   N
    (Ex:) See P53

P61.8   **Other specified perinatal hematological disorders**   N

P61.9   **Perinatal hematological disorder, unspecified**   N

TRANSITORY ENDOCRINE AND METABOLIC DISORDERS SPECIFIC TO NEWBORN (P70-P74)

Includes   transitory endocrine and metabolic disturbances caused by the infant's response to maternal endocrine and metabolic factors, or its adjustment to extrauterine environment

● **P70**   **Transitory disorders of carbohydrate metabolism specific to newborn**

P70.0   **Syndrome of infant of mother with gestational diabetes**   N
    Newborn (with hypoglycemia) affected by maternal gestational diabetes
    Excludes1   newborn (with hypoglycemia) affected by maternal (pre-existing) diabetes mellitus (P70.1)
            syndrome of infant of a diabetic mother (P70.1)

P70.1   **Syndrome of infant of a diabetic mother**   N
    Newborn (with hypoglycemia) affected by maternal (pre-existing) diabetes mellitus
    Excludes1   newborn (with hypoglycemia) affected by maternal gestational diabetes (P70.0)
            syndrome of infant of mother with gestational diabetes (P70.0)

P70.2   **Neonatal diabetes mellitus** 🔹   N
    (Ex:) P29.0-P29.2, P29.4, P29.89-P29.9, P70.0-P71.9, P72.1, P72.9-P74.4, P74.9,
    P94.0-P94.9, P96.0, P96.3-P96.5, P96.82-P96.89

P70.3   **Iatrogenic neonatal hypoglycemia**   N

P70.4   **Other neonatal hypoglycemia**   N
    Transitory neonatal hypoglycemia

P70.8   **Other transitory disorders of carbohydrate metabolism of newborn** 🔹   N
    (Ex:) P70.0-P70.4, P70.9-P71.9, P72.1, P72.9-P74.4, P74.9, P94.0

P70.9   **Transitory disorder of carbohydrate metabolism of newborn, unspecified**   N

● **P71**   **Transitory neonatal disorders of calcium and magnesium metabolism**
    (Ex:) For category P71 CC codes: See 70.2

P71.0   **Cow's milk hypocalcemia in newborn** 🔹   N

P71.1   **Other neonatal hypocalcemia** 🔹   N
    Excludes1   neonatal hypoparathyroidism (P71.4)

P71.2   **Neonatal hypomagnesemia** 🔹   N

P71.3   **Neonatal tetany without calcium or magnesium deficiency** 🔹   N
    Neonatal tetany NOS

P71.4   **Transitory neonatal hypoparathyroidism** 🔹   N

P71.8   **Other transitory neonatal disorders of calcium and magnesium metabolism** 🔹   N

P71.9   **Transitory neonatal disorder of calcium and magnesium metabolism, unspecified** 🔹   N

● **P72**   **Other transitory neonatal endocrine disorders**
    Excludes1   congenital hypothyroidism with or without goiter (E03.0-E03.1)
            dyshormogenetic goiter (E07.1)
            Pendred's syndrome (E07.1)
    (Ex:) For category P72 CC codes unless otherwise noted: See P70.8

P72.0   **Neonatal goiter, not elsewhere classified** 🔹   N
    Transitory congenital goiter with normal functioning

P72.1   **Transitory neonatal hyperthyroidism** 🔹   N
    Neonatal thyrotoxicosis
    (Ex:) See 70.2

P72.2   **Other transitory neonatal disorders of thyroid function, not elsewhere classified** 🔹   N
    Transitory neonatal hypothyroidism

P72.8   **Other specified transitory neonatal endocrine disorders** 🔹   N

P72.9   **Transitory neonatal endocrine disorder, unspecified**   N

● **P74**   **Other transitory neonatal electrolyte and metabolic disturbances**

P74.0   **Late metabolic acidosis of newborn** 🔹   N
    Excludes1   (fetal) metabolic acidosis of newborn (P19)
    (Ex:) See 70.2

P74.1   **Dehydration of newborn**   N

P74.2   **Disturbances of sodium balance of newborn**   N

P74.3   **Disturbances of potassium balance of newborn**   N

P74.4   **Other transitory electrolyte disturbances of newborn**   N

P74.5   **Transitory tyrosinemia of newborn** 🔹   N
    (Ex:) See 70.8

P74.6   **Transitory hyperammonemia of newborn** 🔹   N
    (Ex:) See 70.8

P74.8   **Other transitory metabolic disturbances of newborn** 🔹   N
    Amino-acid metabolic disorders described as transitory
    (Ex:) See 70.8

P74.9   **Transitory metabolic disturbance of newborn, unspecified**   N

DIGESTIVE SYSTEM DISORDERS OF NEWBORN (P76-P78)

● **P76**   **Other intestinal obstruction of newborn**

P76.0   **Meconium plug syndrome**   N
    Intestinal obstruction; most often seen in premature infants
    Meconium ileus NOS
    Excludes1   meconium ileus in cystic fibrosis (E84.11)

P76.1   **Transitory ileus of newborn** 🔹   N
    Temporary obstruction of ileus (small intestine)
    Excludes1   Hirschsprung's disease (Q43.1)
    (Ex:) P76.0-P78.9

P76.2   **Intestinal obstruction due to inspissated milk**   N
    Being thickened, dried, or made less fluid

P76.8   **Other specified intestinal obstruction of newborn**   N
    Excludes1   intestinal obstruction classifiable to K56.-

P76.9   **Intestinal obstruction of newborn, unspecified**   N

● **P77**   **Necrotizing enterocolitis of newborn**
    (Ex:) For category P77 CC codes: P29.0-P29.2, P29.4-P29.9, P76.0-P78.9, P94.1-P96.0,
    P96.3-P96.5, P96.82-P96.89

P77.1   **Stage 1 necrotizing enterocolitis in newborn** 🔹   N
    Necrotizing enterocolitis without pneumatosis, without perforation

P77.2   **Stage 2 necrotizing enterocolitis in newborn** 🔹   N
    Necrotizing enterocolitis with pneumatosis, without perforation

P77.3   **Stage 3 necrotizing enterocolitis in newborn** 🔹   N
    Necrotizing enterocolitis with perforation
    Necrotizing enterocolitis with pneumatosis and perforation

P77.9   **Necrotizing enterocolitis in newborn, unspecified** 🔹   N
    Necrotizing enterocolitis in newborn, NOS

CHAPTER 16 (P00-P96)

N Newborn Age: 0   P Pediatric Age: 0–17   M Maternity DX: 12–55   A Adult Age: 15–124   ♀ Females Only   ♂ Males Only

🔹 Complication\Comorbidity   🔹 Major C\C   (Ex:) CC/MCC Exclusions   🔹 Present on Admission Requirement   🔹 Hospital-Acquired Condition

1245

● **P78   Other perinatal digestive system disorders**
　　Excludes1　cystic fibrosis (E84.0-E84.9)
　　　　　　　　neonatal gastrointestinal hemorrhages
　　　　　　　　(P54.0-P54.3)

　　P78.0   Perinatal intestinal perforation 🐾   N
　　　　Meconium peritonitis
　　　　(Ex) See P77

　　P78.1   Other neonatal peritonitis
　　　　Neonatal peritonitis NOS

　　**P78.2   Neonatal hematemesis and melena due to swallowed
　　　　maternal blood**   N

　　P78.3   Noninfective neonatal diarrhea   N
　　　　Neonatal diarrhea NOS

● 　**P78.8   Other specified perinatal digestive system disorders**

　　　　P78.81   Congenital cirrhosis (of liver)   N

　　　　P78.82   Peptic ulcer of newborn   N

　　　　P78.83   Newborn esophageal reflux   N
　　　　　　Neonatal esophageal reflux

　　　　**P78.89   Other specified perinatal digestive system
　　　　　　disorders**   N

　　P78.9   Perinatal digestive system disorder, unspecified   N

CONDITIONS INVOLVING THE INTEGUMENT AND TEMPERATURE
REGULATION OF NEWBORN (P80-P83)

● **P80   Hypothermia of newborn**
　　P80.0   Cold injury syndrome   N
　　　　Severe and usually chronic hypothermia associated
　　　　　　with a pink flushed appearance, edema and
　　　　　　neurological and biochemical abnormalities.
　　　　Excludes1   mild hypothermia of newborn (P80.8)

　　P80.8   Other hypothermia of newborn   N
　　　　Mild hypothermia of newborn

　　P80.9   Hypothermia of newborn, unspecified   N

● **P81   Other disturbances of temperature regulation of newborn**
　　P81.0   Environmental hyperthermia of newborn   N

　　**P81.8   Other specified disturbances of temperature regulation
　　　　of newborn**   N

　　**P81.9   Disturbance of temperature regulation of newborn,
　　　　unspecified**   N
　　　　Fever of newborn NOS

● **P83   Other conditions of integument specific to newborn**
　　Excludes1   congenital malformations of skin and integument
　　　　　　　　(Q80-Q84)
　　　　　　　　hydrops fetalis due to hemolytic disease (P56.-)
　　　　　　　　neonatal skin infection (P39.4)
　　　　　　　　staphylococcal scalded skin syndrome (L00)
　　Excludes2   cradle cap (L21.0)
　　　　　　　　diaper [napkin] dermatitis (L22)

　　P83.0   Sclerema neonatorum 🐾   N
　　　　Neonate = newborn
　　　　(Ex) P83.0, P83.30-P83.39

　　P83.1   Neonatal erythema toxicum   N
　　　　*Benign, generalized, transient pustules that become firm
　　　　　vesicles*

　　P83.2   Hydrops fetalis not due to hemolytic disease 🐾   N
　　　　*Severe, life-threatening problem of severe edema (swelling)
　　　　　as result of too much fluid leaving blood and entering
　　　　　tissue*
　　　　Hydrops fetalis NOS
　　　　(Ex) P29.0-P29.2, P29.4, P29.89-P29.9, P83.2, P94.1-P96.0, P96.3-P96.5,
　　　　　P96.82-P96.89

● 　**P83.3   Other and unspecified edema specific to newborn**
　　　　(Ex) For category P83.3 CC codes: P80.0-P83.0, P83.30-P83.39

　　　　P83.30   Unspecified edema specific to newborn 🐾   N

　　　　P83.39   Other edema specific to newborn 🐾   N

　　P83.4   Breast engorgement of newborn   N
　　　　Noninfective mastitis of newborn

　　P83.5   Congenital hydrocele ♂

　　P83.6   Umbilical polyp of newborn   N

　　**P83.8   Other specified conditions of integument specific to
　　　　newborn**   N
　　　　Bronze baby syndrome
　　　　Neonatal scleroderma
　　　　Urticaria neonatorum

　　**P83.9   Condition of the integument specific to newborn,
　　　　unspecified**   N

OTHER PROBLEMS WITH NEWBORN (P84)

P84   Other problems with newborn 🐾   N
　　Acidemia of newborn
　　Acidosis of newborn
　　Anoxia of newborn NOS
　　Asphyxia of newborn NOS
　　Hypercapnia of newborn
　　Hypoxemia of newborn
　　Hypoxia of newborn NOS
　　Mixed metabolic and respiratory acidosis of newborn
　　Excludes1   intracranial hemorrhage due to anoxia or hypoxia
　　　　　　　　(P52.-)
　　　　　　　　hypoxic ischemic encephalopathy [HIE] (P91.6-)
　　　　　　　　late metabolic acidosis of newborn (P74.0)

OTHER DISORDERS ORIGINATING IN THE PERINATAL PERIOD (P90-P96)

P90   Convulsions of newborn 🐾   N
　　Excludes1   benign myoclonic epilepsy in infancy (G40.3-)
　　　　　　　　benign neonatal convulsions (familial) (G40.3-)
　　(Ex) P29.0-P29.2, P29.4, P29.89-P29.9, P90, P91.8-P91.9, P94.1-P96.0, P96.3-P96.5,
　　　　P96.82-P96.89

● **P91   Other disturbances of cerebral status of newborn**
　　P91.0   Neonatal cerebral ischemia 🐾   N
　　　　(Ex) P90-P91.1, P91.3-P91.5, P91.8-P91.9

　　P91.1   Acquired periventricular cysts of newborn 🐾   N
　　　　(Ex) See P91.0

　　P91.2   Neonatal cerebral leukomalacia 🐾   N
　　　　*Degeneration of white matter adjacent to cerebral ventricles
　　　　　following cerebral hypoxia or brain ischemia in neonates*
　　　　Periventricular leukomalacia
　　　　(Ex) P10.2-P10.3, P29.0-P29.2, P29.4, P29.89-P29.9, P50.0-P50.9, P52.0-P52.3,
　　　　　P52.5, P53-P54.0, P54.6-P54.9, P60-P61.9, P91.2, P94.1-P94.9, P96.0,
　　　　　P96.3-P96.5, P96.82-P96.89

　　P91.3   Neonatal cerebral irritability 🐾   N
　　　　(Ex) See P91.0

　　P91.4   Neonatal cerebral depression 🐾   N
　　　　(Ex) See P91.0

　　P91.5   Neonatal coma 🐾   N
　　　　(Ex) See P91.0

● 　**P91.6   Hypoxic ischemic encephalopathy [HIE]**
　　　　(Ex) For category P91.6 CC codes: P84, P91.60-P91.63

　　　　**P91.60   Hypoxic ischemic encephalopathy [HIE],
　　　　　　unspecified** 🐾   N

　　　　**P91.61   Mild hypoxic ischemic encephalopathy
　　　　　　[HIE]** 🐾   N

　　　　**P91.62   Moderate hypoxic ischemic encephalopathy
　　　　　　[HIE]** 🐾   N

　　　　**P91.63   Severe hypoxic ischemic encephalopathy
　　　　　　[HIE]** 🐾   N

　　**P91.8   Other specified disturbances of cerebral status of
　　　　newborn**   N

　　P91.9   Disturbance of cerebral status of newborn, unspecified N

◀ New　◀┅ Revised　~~deleted~~ Deleted　Excludes 1　Excludes 2　Includes　Use additional　Code first　Code also　Unspecified
OGCR Official Guidelines　● Unacceptable Principal Diagnosis　X Assign placeholder X　● Use Additional Character(s)　▶ Manifestation Code　Coding Clinic

● **P92   Feeding problems of newborn**

> **Excludes1**   feeding problems in child over 28 days old (R63.3)

● **P92.0   Vomiting of newborn**

> **Excludes1**   vomiting of child over 28 days old (R11.-)

P92.01   Bilious vomiting of newborn 🔷   N

> **Excludes1**   bilious vomiting in child over 28 days old (R11.14) ◀▦
>
> (Ex) P92.01-P92.09

P92.09   Other vomiting of newborn   N

> **Excludes1**   regurgitation of food in newborn (P92.1)

P92.1   Regurgitation and rumination of newborn   N

P92.2   Slow feeding of newborn   N

P92.3   Underfeeding of newborn   N

P92.4   Overfeeding of newborn   N

P92.5   Neonatal difficulty in feeding at breast   N

P92.6   Failure to thrive in newborn   N

> **Excludes1**   failure to thrive in child over 28 days old (R62.51)

P92.8   Other feeding problems of newborn   N

P92.9   Feeding problem of newborn, unspecified   N

● **P93   Reactions and intoxications due to drugs administered to newborn**

> **Includes**   reactions and intoxications due to drugs administered to fetus affecting newborn
>
> **Excludes1**   jaundice due to drugs or toxins transmitted from mother or given to newborn (P58.4-)
> reactions and intoxications from maternal opiates, tranquilizers and other medication (P04.0-P04.1, P04.4)
> withdrawal symptoms from maternal use of drugs of addiction (P96.1)
> withdrawal symptoms from therapeutic use of drugs in newborn (P96.2)
>
> (Ex) For category P93 CC codes: P93.0-P93.8, P96.1-P96.2

P93.0   Grey baby syndrome 🔷   N

> Grey syndrome from chloramphenicol administration in newborn

P93.8   Other reactions and intoxications due to drugs administered to newborn 🔷   N

> Use additional code for adverse effect, if applicable, to identify drug (T36-T50 with fifth or sixth character 5)

● **P94   Disorders of muscle tone of newborn**

P94.0   Transient neonatal myasthenia gravis 🔷   N

> **Excludes1**   myasthenia gravis (G70.0)
>
> (Ex) P29.0-P29.2, P29.4, P29.89-P29.9, P70.0-P71.9, P72.1, P72.9-P74.4, P74.9, P94.0-P94.9, P96.0, P96.3-P96.5, P96.82-P96.89

P94.1   Congenital hypertonia   N

P94.2   Congenital hypotonia   N

> Floppy baby syndrome, unspecified

P94.8   Other disorders of muscle tone of newborn   N

P94.9   Disorder of muscle tone of newborn, unspecified   N

P95   Stillbirth   N

> Deadborn fetus NOS
> Fetal death of unspecified cause
> Stillbirth NOS
>
> **Excludes1**   maternal care for intrauterine death (O36.4)
> missed abortion (O02.1)
> outcome of delivery, stillbirth (Z37.1, Z37.3, Z37.4, Z37.7)

OGCR   Section I.C.16.g.

> Stillbirth
> Code P95, Stillbirth, is only for use for institutions that maintain separate records for stillbirths. No other code should be used with P95. Code P95 should not be used on the mother's record.

● **P96   Other conditions originating in the perinatal period**

P96.0   Congenital renal failure   N

> Uremia of newborn

P96.1   Neonatal withdrawal symptoms from maternal use of drugs of addiction 🔷   N

> Drug withdrawal syndrome in infant of dependent mother
> Neonatal abstinence syndrome
>
> **Excludes1**   reactions and intoxications from maternal opiates and tranquilizers administered during labor and delivery (P04.0)
>
> (Ex) See P93

P96.2   Withdrawal symptoms from therapeutic use of drugs in newborn 🔷   N

> (Ex) See P93

P96.3   Wide cranial sutures of newborn   N

> Neonatal craniotabes

P96.5   Complication to newborn due to (fetal) intrauterine procedure   N

> **Excludes2**   newborn (suspected to be) affected by amniocentesis (P00.6)

● **P96.8   Other specified conditions originating in the perinatal period**

P96.81   Exposure to (parental) (environmental) tobacco smoke in the perinatal period

> **Excludes2**   newborn affected by in utero exposure to tobacco (P04.2)
> exposure to environmental tobacco smoke after the perinatal period (Z77.22)

P96.82   Delayed separation of umbilical cord   N

P96.83   Meconium staining   N

> **Excludes1**   meconium aspiration (P24.00, P24.01)
> meconium passage during delivery (P03.82)

P96.89   Other specified conditions originating in the perinatal period   N

> Use additional code to specify condition

P96.9   Condition originating in the perinatal period, unspecified   N

> Congenital debility NOS

CHAPTER 17

CONGENITAL MALFORMATIONS, DEFORMATIONS AND CHROMOSOMAL ABNORMALITIES (Q00-Q99)

Note: Codes from this chapter are not for use on maternal or fetal records

Excludes2 inborn errors of metabolism (E70-E88)

This chapter contains the following blocks:

Q00-Q07	Congenital malformations of the nervous system
Q10-Q18	Congenital malformations of eye, ear, face and neck
Q20-Q28	Congenital malformations of the circulatory system
Q30-Q34	Congenital malformations of the respiratory system
Q35-Q37	Cleft lip and cleft palate
Q38-Q45	Other congenital malformations of the digestive system
Q50-Q56	Congenital malformations of genital organs
Q60-Q64	Congenital malformations of the urinary system
Q65-Q79	Congenital malformations and deformations of the musculoskeletal system
Q80-Q89	Other congenital malformations
Q90-Q99	Chromosomal abnormalities, not elsewhere classified

Figure 17-1 An infant with a large occipital encephalocele. The large skin-covered encephalocele is visible. (From Townsend: Sabiston Textbook of Surgery, ed 19, Saunders, An Imprint of Elsevier, 2012)

CONGENITAL MALFORMATIONS OF THE NERVOUS SYSTEM (Q00–Q07)

● **Q00 Anencephaly and similar malformations**
Ⓔ For category Q00 CC codes: Q00.0-Q00.2

Q00.0 Anencephaly 🔲🔲
Absence of skull with cerebral hemispheres missing or reduced to small masses attached to base of cranium
Acephaly
Acrania
Amyelencephaly
Hemianencephaly
Hemicephaly

Q00.1 Craniorachischisis 🔲🔲
Developmental anomaly consisting of fissure of cranium and vertebral column

Q00.2 Iniencephaly 🔲🔲
Developmental anomaly characterized by enlargement of foramen magnum and absence of laminae and spinous processes of cervical, dorsal

● **Q01 Encephalocele**
Sac-like protrusions of brain and membranes visible through an opening in skull

Includes Arnold-Chiari syndrome, type III
encephalocystocele
encephalomyelocele
hydroencephalocele
hydromeningocele, cranial
meningocele, cerebral
meningoencephalocele

Excludes1 Meckel-Gruber syndrome (Q61.9)
Ⓔ For category Q01 CC codes: Q01.0-Q02, Q04.0-Q04.8

Q01.0 Frontal encephalocele 🔲🔲
Q01.1 Nasofrontal encephalocele 🔲🔲
Q01.2 Occipital encephalocele 🔲🔲
Q01.8 Encephalocele of other sites 🔲🔲
Q01.9 Encephalocele, unspecified 🔲🔲

● **Q02 Microcephaly** 🔲
Head size measures significantly below normal based on standardized charts

Includes hydromicrocephaly
micrencephalon

Excludes1 Meckel-Gruber syndrome (Q61.9)

● **Q03 Congenital hydrocephalus**
Accumulation of cerebrospinal fluid in ventricles resulting in swelling and enlargement

Includes hydrocephalus in newborn

Excludes1 Arnold-Chiari syndrome, type II (Q07.0-)
acquired hydrocephalus (G91.-)
hydrocephalus due to congenital toxoplasmosis (P37.1)
hydrocephalus with spina bifida (Q05.0-Q05.4)

Q03.0 Malformations of aqueduct of Sylvius 🔲
Anomaly of aqueduct of Sylvius
Obstruction of aqueduct of Sylvius, congenital
Stenosis of aqueduct of Sylvius

Q03.1 Atresia of foramina of Magendie and Luschka 🔲
Dandy-Walker syndrome

Q03.8 Other congenital hydrocephalus 🔲

Q03.9 Congenital hydrocephalus, unspecified 🔲

● **Q04 Other congenital malformations of brain**
Excludes1 cyclopia (Q87.0)
macrocephaly (Q75.3)
Ⓔ For category Q04 CC codes Q04.0-Q04.3: Q01.0-Q02, Q04.0-Q04.8
For category Q04 CC codes Q04.4-Q04.8: Q04.4-Q04.8

Q04.0 Congenital malformations of corpus callosum 🔲🔲
Agenesis of corpus callosum

Q04.1 Arhinencephaly 🔲🔲
Congenital absence of olfactory bulbs, tract, or nerves

Q04.2 Holoprosencephaly 🔲🔲
Failure of cleavage of forebrain (prosencephalon) resulting in incomplete or absent cortical separation and deficits in midline facial development

Q04.3 Other reduction deformities of brain 🔲🔲
Absence of part of brain   Agyria
Agenesis of part of brain
Cerebral cortex are not fully formed, brain surface is smooth
Aplasia of part of brain
Hydranencephaly
Hypoplasia of part of brain
Lissencephaly
Congenital malformation or absence of convolutions of cerebral cortex
Microgyria
Malformation of brain characterized by excessive number of small convolutions (gyri) on surface
Pachygyria
Reduction in number of sulci of cerebrum
Excludes1 congenital malformations of corpus callosum (Q04.0)

Q04.4 Septo-optic dysplasia of brain 🔲🔲

Q04.5 Megalencephaly 🔲🔲
Abnormally large brain

◀ New   ◀▥ Revised   ~~deleted~~ Deleted   Excludes 1   Excludes 2   Includes   Use additional   Code first   Code also   Unspecified
OGCR Official Guidelines   ● Unacceptable Principal Diagnosis   X Assign placeholder X   ◑ Use Additional Character(s)   ▶ Manifestation Code   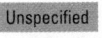 Coding Clinic

Q04.6 Congenital cerebral cysts 🔖🔖
    Porencephaly   Schizencephaly
     Excludes1   acquired porencephalic cyst (G93.0)

Q04.8 Other specified congenital malformations of brain 🔖🔖
    Arnold-Chiari syndrome, type IV
    Macrogyria

Q04.9 Congenital malformation of brain, unspecified 🔖
    Congenital anomaly NOS of brain
    Congenital deformity NOS of brain
    Congenital disease or lesion NOS of brain
    Multiple anomalies NOS of brain, congenital

● **Q05 Spina bifida**
    Developmental anomaly characterized by defective closure of vertebral arch, through which spinal cord and meninges may protrude
     Includes   hydromeningocele (spinal)
               meningocele (spinal)
               meningomyelocele
               myelocele
               myelomeningocele
               rachischisis
               spina bifida (aperta)(cystica)
               syringomyelocele

    Use additional code for any associated paraplegia (paraparesis) (G82.2-)
     Excludes1   Arnold-Chiari syndrome, type II (Q07.0-)
                 spina bifida occulta (Q76.0)
    (Ex) **For category Q05 CC codes:** E78.71-E78.72, G90.1, Q05.0-Q06.1, Q06.3, Q06.8-Q07.9, Q87.1-Q87.89, Q89.7-Q89.8, Q99.2

Q05.0 Cervical spina bifida with hydrocephalus 🔖🔖

Q05.1 Thoracic spina bifida with hydrocephalus 🔖🔖
    Dorsal spina bifida with hydrocephalus
    Thoracolumbar spina bifida with hydrocephalus

Q05.2 Lumbar spina bifida with hydrocephalus 🔖🔖
    Lumbosacral spina bifida with hydrocephalus

Q05.3 Sacral spina bifida with hydrocephalus 🔖🔖

Q05.4 Unspecified spina bifida with hydrocephalus 🔖🔖

Q05.5 Cervical spina bifida without hydrocephalus 🔖

Q05.6 Thoracic spina bifida without hydrocephalus 🔖
    Dorsal spina bifida NOS
    Thoracolumbar spina bifida NOS

Q05.7 Lumbar spina bifida without hydrocephalus 🔖
    Lumbosacral spina bifida NOS

Q05.8 Sacral spina bifida without hydrocephalus 🔖

Q05.9 Spina bifida, unspecified 🔖

● **Q06 Other congenital malformations of spinal cord**

Q06.0 Amyelia 🔖
    Congenital absence of spinal cord

Q06.1 Hypoplasia and dysplasia of spinal cord 🔖
    Underdevelopment of spinal cord
    Atelomyelia
       Congenitally incomplete development of spinal cord
    Myelatelia
    Myelodysplasia of spinal cord
       Defective development of spinal cord, especially lower segments

Q06.2 Diastematomyelia 🔖
    Congenital anomaly, associated with spina bifida, in which spinal cord is split into halves and surrounded by dural sac

Q06.3 Other congenital cauda equina malformations 🔖

Q06.4 Hydromyelia 🔖
    Dilation of central canal of spinal cord with increased fluid accumulation
    Hydrorachis

Q06.8 Other specified congenital malformations of spinal cord 🔖

Q06.9 Congenital malformation of spinal cord, unspecified 🔖
    Congenital anomaly NOS of spinal cord
    Congenital deformity NOS of spinal cord
    Congenital disease or lesion NOS of spinal cord

● **Q07 Other congenital malformations of nervous system**
     Excludes2   congenital central alveolar hypoventilation syndrome (G47.35)
                 familial dysautonomia [Riley-Day] (G90.1)
                 neurofibromatosis (nonmalignant) (Q85.0-)

● **Q07.0 Arnold-Chiari syndrome**
    Herniation of cerebellar tonsils and vermis through foramen magnum into spinal canal
    Arnold-Chiari syndrome, type II
     Excludes1   Arnold-Chiari syndrome, type III (Q01.-)
                 Arnold-Chiari syndrome, type IV (Q04.8)

Q07.00 Arnold-Chiari syndrome without spina bifida or hydrocephalus 🔖

Q07.01 Arnold-Chiari syndrome with spina bifida 🔖🔖
    (Ex) See Q05

Q07.02 Arnold-Chiari syndrome with hydrocephalus 🔖🔖
    (Ex) See Q05

Q07.03 Arnold-Chiari syndrome with spina bifida and hydrocephalus 🔖🔖
    (Ex) See Q05

Q07.8 Other specified congenital malformations of nervous system 🔖
    Agenesis of nerve
    Displacement of brachial plexus
    Jaw-winking syndrome
    Marcus Gunn's syndrome

Q07.9 Congenital malformation of nervous system, unspecified 🔖
    Congenital anomaly NOS of nervous system
    Congenital deformity NOS of nervous system
    Congenital disease or lesion NOS of nervous system

CONGENITAL MALFORMATIONS OF EYE, EAR, FACE AND NECK (Q10-Q18)

     Excludes2   cleft lip and cleft palate (Q35-Q37)
                 congenital malformation of cervical spine (Q05.0, Q05.5, Q67.5, Q76.0-Q76.4) ◄⫿⫿
                 ~~cervical spine (Q05.0, Q05.5, Q67.5, Q76.0-Q76.4)~~
                 congenital malformation of larynx (Q31.-) ◄⫿⫿
                 congenital malformation of lip NEC (Q38.0) ◄⫿⫿
                 congenital malformation of nose (Q30.-) ◄⫿⫿
                 congenital malformation of parathyroid gland (Q89.2) ◄⫿⫿
                 congenital malformation of thyroid gland (Q89.2) ◄⫿⫿

● **Q10 Congenital malformations of eyelid, lacrimal apparatus and orbit**
     Excludes1   cryptophthalmos NOS (Q11.2)
                 cryptophthalmos syndrome (Q87.0)

Q10.0 Congenital ptosis
    Prolapse or drooping of upper eyelid from paralysis of third nerve or from sympathetic innervations

Q10.1 Congenital ectropion 🔖
    Outward turning of eyelid

Q10.2 Congenital entropion 🔖
    Inward turning of eyelid

Q10.3 Other congenital malformations of eyelid 🔖
    Ablepharon
    Blepharophimosis, congenital
    Coloboma of eyelid
    Congenital absence or agenesis of cilia
    Congenital absence or agenesis of eyelid
    Congenital accessory eyelid
    Congenital accessory eye muscle
    Congenital malformation of eyelid NOS

Q10.4 Absence and agenesis of lacrimal apparatus 🔖
    Congenital absence of punctum lacrimale

Q10.5 Congenital stenosis and stricture of lacrimal duct 🔖

Q10.6 Other congenital malformations of lacrimal apparatus 🔖
    Congenital malformation of lacrimal apparatus NOS

Q10.7 Congenital malformation of orbit 🔖

N Newborn Age: 0   **P** Pediatric Age: 0–17   **M** Maternity DX: 12–55   **A** Adult Age: 15–124   ♀ Females Only   ♂ Males Only

 Complication\Comorbidity   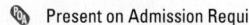 Major C\C   (Ex) CC/MCC Exclusions   Present on Admission Requirement   🔖 Hospital-Acquired Condition

1249

CHAPTER 17 (Q00-Q99)

Figure 17-2 Bilateral congenital **hydrophthalmia,** in which the eyes are very large in comparison to the other facial features due to glaucoma.

● **Q11 Anophthalmos, microphthalmos and macrophthalmos**
Absence of eye and optic pit

Q11.0 **Cystic eyeball** 🔍

Q11.1 **Other anophthalmos** 🔍
Anophthalmos NOS
Agenesis of eye
Absence of eye
Aplasia of eye

Q11.2 **Microphthalmos** 🔍
Partial absence of eye and optic pit
Cryptophthalmos NOS
Dysplasia of eye
Hypoplasia of eye
Rudimentary eye
Excludes1   cryptophthalmos syndrome (Q87.0)

Q11.3 **Macrophthalmos** 🔍
Congenital enlargement of eyes
Excludes1   macrophthalmos in congenital glaucoma (Q15.0)

● **Q12 Congenital lens malformations**

Q12.0 **Congenital cataract** 🔍

Q12.1 **Congenital displaced lens** 🔍

Q12.2 **Coloboma of lens** 🔍

Q12.3 **Congenital aphakia** 🔍

Q12.4 **Spherophakia** 🔍
Smaller, more spherical optic lens than normal

Q12.8 **Other congenital lens malformations** 🔍
Microphakia

Q12.9 **Congenital lens malformation, unspecified** 🔍

● **Q13 Congenital malformations of anterior segment of eye**

Q13.0 **Coloboma of iris** 🔍
Coloboma NOS

Q13.1 **Absence of iris** 🔍
Aniridia
Use additional code for associated glaucoma (H42)

Q13.2 **Other congenital malformations of iris** 🔍
Anisocoria, congenital
Atresia of pupil
Congenital malformation of iris NOS
Corectopia

Q13.3 **Congenital corneal opacity** 🔍

Q13.4 **Other congenital corneal malformations** 🔍
Congenital malformation of cornea NOS
Microcornea
Peter's anomaly

Q13.5 **Blue sclera** 🔍
Condition of unusual blueness of sclera; not harmful

● Q13.8 **Other congenital malformations of anterior segment of eye**

Q13.81 **Rieger's anomaly** 🔍
Use additional code for associated glaucoma (H42)

Q13.89 **Other congenital malformations of anterior segment of eye** 🔍

Q13.9 **Congenital malformation of anterior segment of eye, unspecified** 🔍

● **Q14 Congenital malformations of posterior segment of eye**
Excludes2   optic nerve hypoplasia (H47.03-)

Q14.0 **Congenital malformation of vitreous humor** 🔍
Congenital vitreous opacity

Q14.1 **Congenital malformation of retina** 🔍
Congenital retinal aneurysm

Q14.2 **Congenital malformation of optic disc** 🔍
Coloboma of optic disc

Q14.3 **Congenital malformation of choroid** 🔍

Q14.8 **Other congenital malformations of posterior segment of eye** 🔍
Coloboma of the fundus

Q14.9 **Congenital malformation of posterior segment of eye, unspecified** 🔍

● **Q15 Other congenital malformations of eye**
Excludes1   congenital nystagmus (H55.01)
ocular albinism (E70.31-)
optic nerve hypoplasia (H47.03-)
retinitis pigmentosa (H35.52)

Q15.0 **Congenital glaucoma** 🔍
Axenfeld's anomaly
Buphthalmos
Congenital syndrome characterized by port-wine nevus covering portions of face and cranium
Glaucoma of childhood
Glaucoma of newborn
Hydrophthalmos
Keratoglobus, congenital, with glaucoma
Macrocornea with glaucoma
Macrophthalmos in congenital glaucoma
Megalocornea with glaucoma

Q15.8 **Other specified congenital malformations of eye** 🔍

Q15.9 **Congenital malformation of eye, unspecified** 🔍
Congenital anomaly of eye
Congenital deformity of eye

● **Q16 Congenital malformations of ear causing impairment of hearing**
Excludes1   congenital deafness (H90.-)

Q16.0 **Congenital absence of (ear) auricle** 🔍

Q16.1 **Congenital absence, atresia and stricture of auditory canal (external)** 🔍
Congenital atresia or stricture of osseous meatus

Q16.2 **Absence of eustachian tube** 🔍

Q16.3 **Congenital malformation of ear ossicles** 🔍
Congenital fusion of ear ossicles

Q16.4 **Other congenital malformations of middle ear** 🔍
Congenital malformation of middle ear NOS

Q16.5 **Congenital malformation of inner ear** 🔍
Congenital anomaly of membranous labyrinth
Congenital anomaly of organ of Corti

Q16.9 **Congenital malformation of ear causing impairment of hearing, unspecified** 🔍
Congenital absence of ear NOS

● **Q17 Other congenital malformations of ear**
Excludes1   congenital malformations of ear with impairment of hearing (Q16.0-Q16.9)
preauricular sinus (Q18.1)

Q17.0 **Accessory auricle** 🔍
Accessory tragus
Polyotia
Preauricular appendage or tag
Supernumerary ear
Supernumerary lobule

Q17.1 **Macrotia** 🔍
Enlarged ears

Q17.2 **Microtia** 🔍
An abnormally small or underdeveloped external ear

Q17.3 **Other misshapen ear** 🔍
Pointed ear

◀ New   ◀░ Revised   ~~deleted~~ Deleted   Excludes 1   Excludes 2   Includes   Use additional   Code first   Code also   Unspecified
OGCR Official Guidelines   ● Unacceptable Principal Diagnosis   X Assign placeholder X   ▶ Use Additional Character(s)   ▶ Manifestation Code   **Coding Clinic**

Q17.4   **Misplaced ear** 🔖
Low-set ears
Excludes1   cervical auricle (Q18.2)

Q17.5   **Prominent ear** 🔖
Bat ear

Q17.8   **Other specified congenital malformations of ear** 🔖
Congenital absence of lobe of ear

Q17.9   **Congenital malformation of ear, unspecified** 🔖
Congenital anomaly of ear NOS

● Q18   **Other congenital malformations of face and neck**
Excludes1   cleft lip and cleft palate (Q35-Q37)
conditions classified to Q67.0-Q67.4
congenital malformations of skull and face bones
(Q75.-)
cyclopia (Q87.0)
dentofacial anomalies [including malocclusion]
(M26.-)
malformation syndromes affecting facial
appearance (Q87.0)
persistent thyroglossal duct (Q89.2)

Q18.0   **Sinus, fistula and cyst of branchial cleft** 🔖
Branchial vestige
Branchial remnants (cysts, fistula, skin tags) that are
developmental anomalies

Q18.1   **Preauricular sinus and cyst** 🔖
Fistula of auricle, congenital
Cervicoaural fistula
Abnormal passage in neck originating from first branchial
cleft

Q18.2   **Other branchial cleft malformations** 🔖
Branchial cleft malformation NOS
Cervical auricle
Otocephaly

Q18.3   **Webbing of neck** 🔖
Pterygium colli
Thick fold of skin on side of neck

Q18.4   **Macrostomia** 🔖
Results from failure of union of maxillary and mandibular
processes, results in abnormally large mouth

Q18.5   **Microstomia** 🔖

Q18.6   **Macrocheilia** 🔖
Excessive size of lips
Hypertrophy of lip, congenital

Q18.7   **Microcheilia** 🔖
Abnormal smallness of lips

Q18.8   **Other specified congenital malformations of face and
neck** 🔖
Medial cyst of face and neck
Medial fistula of face and neck
Medial sinus of face and neck

Q18.9   **Congenital malformation of face and neck,
unspecified** 🔖
Congenital anomaly NOS of face and neck

CONGENITAL MALFORMATIONS OF THE CIRCULATORY SYSTEM (Q20-Q28)

● Q20   **Congenital malformations of cardiac chambers and connections**
Excludes1   dextrocardia with situs inversus (Q89.3)
mirror-image atrial arrangement with situs
inversus (Q89.3)
(Ex) **For category Q20 CC codes:** E78.71-E78.72, I23.0-I23.3, I23.6-I23.8, I51.0, I51.3,
P29.3, Q20.0-Q21.9, Q23.8-Q23.9, Q24.8-Q24.9, Q27.30, Q27.4, Q28.0-Q28.1,
Q28.8-Q28.9, Q87.1-Q87.89, Q89.7-Q89.8, Q99.2

Q20.0   **Common arterial trunk** 🔖 🔖
Persistent truncus arteriosus
Excludes1   aortic septal defect (Q21.4)

Q20.1   **Double outlet right ventricle** 🔖 🔖
Taussig-Bing syndrome

Q20.2   **Double outlet left ventricle** 🔖 🔖

Q20.3   **Discordant ventriculoarterial connection** 🔖 🔖
Dextrotransposition of aorta
Transposition of great vessels (complete)

Q20.4   **Double inlet ventricle** 🔖 🔖
Common ventricle
Cor triloculare biatriatum
Single ventricle

Q20.5   **Discordant atrioventricular connection** 🔖 🔖
Corrected transposition
Levotransposition
Ventricular inversion

Q20.6   **Isomerism of atrial appendages** 🔖
Isomerism of atrial appendages with asplenia or
polysplenia

Q20.8   **Other congenital malformations of cardiac chambers
and connections** 🔖
Cor binoculare

Q20.9   **Congenital malformation of cardiac chambers and
connections, unspecified** 🔖

● Q21   **Congenital malformations of cardiac septa**
Excludes1   acquired cardiac septal defect (I51.0)

Q21.0   **Ventricular septal defect** 🔖 🔖
Roger's disease
(Ex) See Q20

Q21.1   **Atrial septal defect** 🔖 🔖
Coronary sinus defect
Patent or persistent foramen ovale
Patent or persistent ostium secundum defect (type II)
Patent or persistent sinus venosus defect
(Ex) E78.71-E78.72, I23.0-I23.3, I23.6-I23.8, I51.0, I51.3, Q20.0-Q20.9,
Q21.1-Q21.9, Q23.8-Q23.9, Q24.8-Q24.9, Q27.30, Q27.4, Q28.0-Q28.1,
Q28.8-Q28.9, Q87.2-Q87.3, Q87.5-Q87.89, Q89.7-Q89.8

Q21.2   **Atrioventricular septal defect** 🔖 🔖
Common atrioventricular canal
Endocardial cushion defect
Ostium primum atrial septal defect (type I)
(Ex) See Q20

Q21.3   **Tetralogy of Fallot** 🔖 🔖
Ventricular septal defect with pulmonary stenosis or
atresia, dextroposition of aorta and hypertrophy of
right ventricle.
(Ex) See Q20

Q21.4   **Aortopulmonary septal defect** 🔖
Aortic septal defect
Aortopulmonary window

Q21.8   **Other congenital malformations of cardiac septa** 🔖
Eisenmenger's defect
Pentalogy of Fallot
Excludes1   Eisenmenger's complex (I27.8)
Eisenmenger's syndrome (I27.8)

Q21.9   **Congenital malformation of cardiac septum,
unspecified** 🔖
Septal (heart) defect NOS

● Q22   **Congenital malformations of pulmonary and tricuspid valves**
(Ex) **For category Q22 CC codes unless otherwise indicated:** E78.71-E78.72, P29.3,
Q20.9, Q22.4-Q23.9, Q24.8-Q24.9, Q27.30, Q27.4, Q28.0-Q28.1, Q28.8-Q28.9,
Q87.1-Q87.89, Q89.7-Q89.8, Q99.2

Q22.0   **Pulmonary valve atresia** 🔖 🔖
(Ex) E78.71-E78.72, P29.3, Q20.9, Q22.0-Q22.3, Q23.8-Q23.9, Q24.8-Q24.9,
Q27.30, Q27.4, Q28.0-Q28.1, Q28.8-Q28.9, Q87.1-Q87.89, Q89.7-Q89.8,
Q99.2

Q22.1   **Congenital pulmonary valve stenosis** 🔖 🔖
(Ex) See Q22.0

Q22.2   **Congenital pulmonary valve insufficiency** 🔖 🔖
Congenital pulmonary valve regurgitation
(Ex) E78.71-E78.72, Q20.9, Q22.0-Q22.3, Q23.8-Q23.9, Q24.8-Q24.9, Q27.30,
Q27.4, Q28.0-Q28.1, Q28.8-Q28.9, Q87.2-Q87.3, Q87.5-Q87.89,
Q89.7-Q89.8

Q22.3   **Other congenital malformations of pulmonary
valve** 🔖 🔖
Congenital malformation of pulmonary valve NOS
Supernumerary cusps of pulmonary valve
(Ex) See Q22.2

N Newborn Age: 0   P Pediatric Age: 0-17   M Maternity DX: 12-55   A Adult Age: 15-124   ♀ Females Only   ♂ Males Only

🔖 Complication\Comorbidity   🔖 Major C\C   (Ex) CC/MCC Exclusions   🔖 Present on Admission Requirement   🔖 Hospital-Acquired Condition

1251

CHAPTER 17 (Q00-Q99)

Q22.4 Congenital tricuspid stenosis
Congenital tricuspid atresia

Q22.5 Ebstein's anomaly
Malformation of tricuspid valve

Q22.6 Hypoplastic right heart syndrome

Q22.8 Other congenital malformations of tricuspid valve

Q22.9 Congenital malformation of tricuspid valve, unspecified

● **Q23 Congenital malformations of aortic and mitral valves**
Ⓔ For category Q23 CC codes unless otherwise indicated: See Q22

Q23.0 Congenital stenosis of aortic valve
Congenital aortic atresia
Congenital aortic stenosis NOS

    Excludes1 congenital stenosis of aortic valve in hypoplastic left heart syndrome (Q23.4)
    congenital subaortic stenosis (Q24.4)
    supravalvular aortic stenosis (congenital) (Q25.3)

Q23.1 Congenital insufficiency of aortic valve
Bicuspid aortic valve
Congenital aortic insufficiency

Q23.2 Congenital mitral stenosis
Congenital mitral atresia

Q23.3 Congenital mitral insufficiency

Q23.4 Hypoplastic left heart syndrome

Q23.8 Other congenital malformations of aortic and mitral valves

Q23.9 Congenital malformation of aortic and mitral valves, unspecified

● **Q24 Other congenital malformations of heart**
    Excludes1 endocardial fibroelastosis (I42.4)

Q24.0 Dextrocardia
Heart is located in right hemithorax

    Excludes1 dextrocardia with situs inversus (Q89.3)
    isomerism of atrial appendages (with asplenia or polysplenia) (Q20.6)
    mirror-image atrial arrangement with situs inversus (Q89.3)
Ⓔ E78.71-E78.72, Q20.9, Q23.8-Q24.4, Q24.8-Q24.9, Q27.30, Q27.4, Q28.0-Q28.1, Q28.8-Q28.9, Q87.2-Q87.3, Q87.5-Q87.89, Q89.7-Q89.8

Q24.1 Levocardia
Normal position of heart but related structures on wrong side
Ⓔ See Q24.0

Q24.2 Cor triatriatum
Congenital heart defect; left atrium is subdivided
Ⓔ E78.71-E78.72, P29.3, Q20.9, Q23.8-Q23.9, Q24.2-Q24.4, Q24.8-Q24.9, Q27.30, Q27.4, Q28.0-Q28.1, Q28.8-Q28.9, Q87.1-Q87.89, Q89.7-Q89.8, Q99.2

Q24.3 Pulmonary infundibular stenosis
Subvalvular pulmonic stenosis
Ⓔ See Q24.3

Q24.4 Congenital subaortic stenosis
Ⓔ See Q24.3

Q24.5 Malformation of coronary vessels
Congenital coronary (artery) aneurysm
Ⓔ Q20.9, Q23.8-Q23.9, Q24.5, Q24.8-Q24.9

Q24.6 Congenital heart block
Ⓔ E78.71-E78.72, P29.3, Q20.9, Q23.8-Q23.9, Q24.6-Q24.9, Q27.30, Q27.4, Q28.0-Q28.1, Q28.8-Q28.9, Q87.1-Q87.89, Q89.7-Q89.8, Q99.2

Q24.8 Other specified congenital malformations of heart
Congenital diverticulum of left ventricle
Congenital malformation of myocardium
Congenital malformation of pericardium
Malposition of heart
Uhl's disease

Q24.9 Congenital malformation of heart, unspecified
Congenital anomaly of heart
Congenital disease of heart

● **Q25 Congenital malformations of great arteries**

Q25.0 Patent ductus arteriosus
Fetal blood vessel connecting left pulmonary artery directly to descending aorta
Patent ductus Botallo
Persistent ductus arteriosus
Ⓔ Q25.0, Q27.30, Q27.4, Q28.0-Q28.1, Q28.8

Q25.1 Coarctation of aorta
Coarctation of aorta (preductal) (postductal)
Ⓔ E78.71-E78.72, Q25.1-Q25.3, Q27.30, Q27.4, Q28.0-Q28.1, Q28.8-Q28.9, Q87.2-Q87.3, Q87.5-Q87.89, Q89.7-Q89.8

Q25.2 Atresia of aorta
Ⓔ E78.71-E78.72, P29.3, Q25.1-Q25.3, Q27.30, Q27.4, Q28.0-Q28.1, Q28.8-Q28.9, Q87.1-Q87.89, Q89.7-Q89.8, Q99.2

Q25.3 Supravalvular aortic stenosis
    Excludes1 congenital aortic stenosis NOS (Q23.0)
    congenital stenosis of aortic valve (Q23.0)
Ⓔ See Q25.2

Q25.4 Other congenital malformations of aorta
Absence of aorta
Aneurysm of sinus of Valsalva (ruptured)
Aplasia of aorta
Congenital aneurysm of aorta
Congenital malformations of aorta
Congenital dilatation of aorta
Double aortic arch [vascular ring of aorta]
Hypoplasia of aorta
Persistent convolutions of aortic arch
Persistent right aortic arch

    Excludes1 hypoplasia of aorta in hypoplastic left heart syndrome (Q23.4)
Ⓔ E78.71-E78.72, Q25.1-Q25.4, Q25.8-Q25.9, Q27.30, Q27.4, Q28.0-Q28.1, Q28.8-Q28.9, Q87.2-Q87.3, Q87.5-Q87.89, Q89.7-Q89.8

Q25.5 Atresia of pulmonary artery
Ⓔ Q25.5-Q25.79, Q27.30, Q27.4, Q28.0-Q28.1, Q28.8-Q28.9

Q25.6 Stenosis of pulmonary artery
Supravalvular pulmonary stenosis
Ⓔ See Q25.5

● **Q25.7 Other congenital malformations of pulmonary artery**
Ⓔ For category Q25.7 CC codes: See Q25.5

Q25.71 Coarctation of pulmonary artery

Q25.72 Congenital pulmonary arteriovenous malformation
Congenital pulmonary arteriovenous aneurysm

Q25.79 Other congenital malformations of pulmonary artery
Aberrant pulmonary artery
Agenesis of pulmonary artery
Congenital aneurysm of pulmonary artery
Congenital anomaly of pulmonary artery
Hypoplasia of pulmonary artery

Q25.8 Other congenital malformations of other great arteries
Ⓔ See Q25.4

Q25.9 Congenital malformation of great arteries, unspecified
Ⓔ See Q25.4

● **Q26 Congenital malformations of great veins**

Q26.0 Congenital stenosis of vena cava
Congenital stenosis of vena cava (inferior)(superior)
Ⓔ Q26.0-Q26.1, Q26.8, Q27.30, Q27.4, Q28.0-Q28.1, Q28.8-Q28.9

Q26.1 Persistent left superior vena cava
Ⓔ See Q26.0

Q26.2 Total anomalous pulmonary venous connection
Total anomalous pulmonary venous return [TAPVR], subdiaphragmatic
Total anomalous pulmonary venous return [TAPVR], supradiaphragmatic
Ⓔ Q26.2, Q27.30, Q27.4, Q28.0-Q28.1, Q28.8-Q28.9

◄ New   ◄ Revised   ~~deleted~~ Deleted   Excludes 1   Excludes 2   Includes   Use additional   Code first   Code also   Unspecified
 OGCR Official Guidelines   ● Unacceptable Principal Diagnosis   X Assign placeholder X   ● Use Additional Character(s)   ▶ Manifestation Code   **Coding Clinic**

Q26.3   **Partial anomalous pulmonary venous connection**
Partial anomalous pulmonary venous return
(Ex:) Q26.3-Q26.4, Q27.30, Q27.4, Q28.0-Q28.1, Q28.8-Q28.9

Q26.4   **Anomalous pulmonary venous connection, unspecified**
(Ex:) See Q26.3

Q26.5   **Anomalous portal venous connection**

Q26.6   **Portal vein-hepatic artery fistula**

Q26.8   **Other congenital malformations of great veins**
Absence of vena cava (inferior) (superior)
Azygos continuation of inferior vena cava
Persistent left posterior cardinal vein
Scimitar syndrome
(Ex:) See Q26.0

Q26.9   **Congenital malformation of great vein, unspecified**
Congenital anomaly of vena cava (inferior) (superior) NOS
(Ex:) Q26.9, Q27.30, Q27.4, Q28.0-Q28.1, Q28.8-Q28.9

● **Q27**   **Other congenital malformations of peripheral vascular system**
    Excludes2   anomalies of cerebral and precerebral vessels (Q28.0-Q28.3)
anomalies of coronary vessels (Q24.5)
anomalies of pulmonary artery (Q25.5-Q25.7)
congenital retinal aneurysm (Q14.1)
hemangioma and lymphangioma (D18.-)

Q27.0   **Congenital absence and hypoplasia of umbilical artery**
Single umbilical artery

Q27.1   **Congenital renal artery stenosis**

Q27.2   **Other congenital malformations of renal artery**
Congenital malformation of renal artery NOS
Multiple renal arteries

● **Q27.3**   **Arteriovenous malformation (peripheral)**
Arteriovenous aneurysm
    Excludes1   acquired arteriovenous aneurysm (I77.0)
    Excludes2   arteriovenous malformation of cerebral vessels (Q28.2)
arteriovenous malformation of precerebral vessels (Q28.0)

Q27.30   **Arteriovenous malformation, site unspecified**
(Ex:) Q20.0-Q20.8, Q21.0-Q21.9, Q27.30, Q27.4, Q28.0-Q28.1, Q28.8

Q27.31   **Arteriovenous malformation of vessel of upper limb**

Q27.32   **Arteriovenous malformation of vessel of lower limb**

Q27.33   **Arteriovenous malformation of digestive system vessel**

Q27.34   **Arteriovenous malformation of renal vessel**

Q27.39   **Arteriovenous malformation, other site**

Q27.4   **Congenital phlebectasia**
(Ex:) See Q27.30

Q27.8   **Other specified congenital malformations of peripheral vascular system**
Absence of peripheral vascular system
Atresia of peripheral vascular system
Congenital aneurysm (peripheral)
Congenital stricture, artery
Congenital varix
    Excludes1   arteriovenous malformation (Q27.3-)

Q27.9   **Congenital malformation of peripheral vascular system, unspecified**
Anomaly of artery or vein NOS

● **Q28**   **Other congenital malformations of circulatory system**
    Excludes1   congenital aneurysm NOS (Q27.8)
congenital coronary aneurysm (Q24.5)
ruptured cerebral arteriovenous malformation (I60.8)
ruptured malformation of precerebral vessels (I72.0)
    Excludes2   congenital peripheral aneurysm (Q27.8)
congenital pulmonary aneurysm (Q25.79)
congenital retinal aneurysm (Q14.1)

Q28.0   **Arteriovenous malformation of precerebral vessels**
Congenital arteriovenous precerebral aneurysm (nonruptured)
(Ex:) See Q27.30

Q28.1   **Other malformations of precerebral vessels**
Congenital malformation of precerebral vessels NOS
Congenital precerebral aneurysm (nonruptured)
(Ex:) See Q27.30

Q28.2   **Arteriovenous malformation of cerebral vessels**
Arteriovenous malformation of brain NOS
Congenital arteriovenous cerebral aneurysm (nonruptured)
(Ex:) Q27.30, Q27.4, Q28.0-Q28.9

Q28.3   **Other malformations of cerebral vessels**
Congenital cerebral aneurysm (nonruptured)
Congenital malformation of cerebral vessels NOS
Developmental venous anomaly
(Ex:) See Q28.2

Q28.8   **Other specified congenital malformations of circulatory system**
Congenital aneurysm, specified site NEC
Spinal vessel anomaly
(Ex:) See Q27.30

Q28.9   **Congenital malformation of circulatory system, unspecified**
(Ex:) Q20.0-Q28.9

CONGENITAL MALFORMATIONS OF THE RESPIRATORY SYSTEM (Q30-Q34)

● **Q30**   **Congenital malformations of nose**
    Excludes1   congenital deviation of nasal septum (Q67.4)

Q30.0   **Choanal atresia**
Atresia of nares (anterior) (posterior)
Congenital stenosis of nares (anterior) (posterior)

Q30.1   **Agenesis and underdevelopment of nose**
Congenital absent of nose

Q30.2   **Fissured, notched and cleft nose**

Q30.3   **Congenital perforated nasal septum**

Q30.8   **Other congenital malformations of nose**
Accessory nose
Congenital anomaly of nasal sinus wall

Q30.9   **Congenital malformation of nose, unspecified**

● **Q31**   **Congenital malformations of larynx**
    Excludes1   congenital laryngeal stridor NOS (P28.89)
(Ex:) **For category Q31 CC codes:** J39.8, J45.990, J98.09, Q31.1-Q32.4, Q34.0-Q34.9

Q31.0   **Web of larynx**
Glottic web of larynx
Subglottic web of larynx
Web of larynx NOS

Q31.1   **Congenital subglottic stenosis**

Q31.2   **Laryngeal hypoplasia**

Q31.3   **Laryngocele**

Q31.5   **Congenital laryngomalacia**

Q31.8   **Other congenital malformations of larynx**
Absence of larynx
Agenesis of larynx
Atresia of larynx
Congenital cleft thyroid cartilage
Congenital fissure of epiglottis
Congenital stenosis of larynx NEC
Posterior cleft of cricoid cartilage

Q31.9   **Congenital malformation of larynx, unspecified**

N Newborn Age: 0   **P** Pediatric Age: 0–17   **M** Maternity DX: 12–55   **A** Adult Age: 15–124   ♀ Females Only   ♂ Males Only

 Complication\Comorbidity   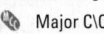 Major C\C   (Ex:) CC/MCC Exclusions   Present on Admission Requirement   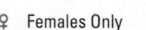 Hospital-Acquired Condition

1253

CHAPTER 17 (Q00-Q99)

● **Q32   Congenital malformations of trachea and bronchus**

> **Excludes1**   congenital bronchiectasis (Q33.4)

Ⓔ For category Q32 CC codes: See Q31

Q32.0   Congenital tracheomalacia 🔹🔹

Q32.1   Other congenital malformations of trachea 🔹🔹
Atresia of trachea
Congenital anomaly of tracheal cartilage
Congenital dilatation of trachea
Congenital malformation of trachea
Congenital stenosis of trachea
Congenital tracheocele

Q32.2   Congenital bronchomalacia 🔹🔹

Q32.3   Congenital stenosis of bronchus 🔹🔹

Q32.4   Other congenital malformations of bronchus 🔹🔹
Absence of bronchus
Agenesis of bronchus
Atresia of bronchus
Congenital diverticulum of bronchus
Congenital malformation of bronchus NOS

● **Q33   Congenital malformations of lung**

Q33.0   Congenital cystic lung 🔹🔹
Congenital cystic lung disease
Congenital honeycomb lung
Congenital polycystic lung disease

> **Excludes1**   cystic fibrosis (E84.0)
> cystic lung disease, acquired or
> unspecified (J98.4)

Ⓔ Q33.0-Q34.9

Q33.1   Accessory lobe of lung 🔹
Azygos lobe (fissured), lung

Q33.2   Sequestration of lung 🔹🔹
Ⓔ Q33.0-Q34.9

Q33.3   Agenesis of lung 🔹🔹
Congenital absence of lung (lobe)
Ⓔ Q33.0-Q34.9

Q33.4   Congenital bronchiectasis 🔹🔹
Ⓔ J44.9, J47.0-J47.9, J68.1, J68.4-J68.9, Q33.4

Q33.5   Ectopic tissue in lung 🔹

Q33.6   Congenital hypoplasia and dysplasia of lung 🔹🔹

> **Excludes1**   pulmonary hypoplasia associated with
> short gestation (P28.0)

Ⓔ Q33.0-Q34.9

Q33.8   Other congenital malformations of lung 🔹

Q33.9   Congenital malformation of lung, unspecified 🔹

● **Q34   Other congenital malformations of respiratory system**

> **Excludes2**   congenital central alveolar hypoventilation
> syndrome (G47.35)

Q34.0   Anomaly of pleura 🔹

Q34.1   Congenital cyst of mediastinum 🔹

Q34.8   Other specified congenital malformations of respiratory system 🔹
Atresia of nasopharynx

Q34.9   Congenital malformation of respiratory system, unspecified 🔹
Congenital absence of respiratory system
Congenital anomaly of respiratory system NOS

CLEFT LIP AND CLEFT PALATE (Q35-Q37)

Use additional code to identify associated malformation of the
nose (Q30.2)

> **Excludes1**   Robin's syndrome (Q87.0)

● **Q35   Cleft palate**

> **Includes**   fissure of palate
> palatoschisis

> **Excludes1**   cleft palate with cleft lip (Q37.-)

Q35.1   Cleft hard palate 🔹

Q35.3   Cleft soft palate 🔹

Figure 17-3   Cleft palate.

Q35.5   Cleft hard palate with cleft soft palate 🔹

Q35.7   Cleft uvula 🔹

Q35.9   Cleft palate, unspecified 🔹
Cleft palate NOS

● **Q36   Cleft lip**

> **Includes**   cheiloschisis
> congenital fissure of lip
> harelip
> labium leporinum

> **Excludes1**   cleft lip with cleft palate (Q37.-)

Q36.0   Cleft lip, bilateral 🔹

Q36.1   Cleft lip, median 🔹

Q36.9   Cleft lip, unilateral 🔹
Cleft lip NOS

● **Q37   Cleft palate with cleft lip**

> **Includes**   cheilopalatoschisis

Q37.0   Cleft hard palate with bilateral cleft lip 🔹

Q37.1   Cleft hard palate with unilateral cleft lip 🔹
Cleft hard palate with cleft lip NOS

Q37.2   Cleft soft palate with bilateral cleft lip 🔹

Q37.3   Cleft soft palate with unilateral cleft lip 🔹
Cleft soft palate with cleft lip NOS

Q37.4   Cleft hard and soft palate with bilateral cleft lip 🔹

Q37.5   Cleft hard and soft palate with unilateral cleft lip 🔹
Cleft hard and soft palate with cleft lip NOS

Q37.8   Unspecified cleft palate with bilateral cleft lip 🔹

Q37.9   Unspecified cleft palate with unilateral cleft lip 🔹
Cleft palate with cleft lip NOS

OTHER CONGENITAL MALFORMATIONS OF THE DIGESTIVE SYSTEM (Q38-Q45)

● **Q38   Other congenital malformations of tongue, mouth and pharynx**

> **Excludes1**   dentofacial anomalies (M26.-)
> macrostomia (Q18.4)
> microstomia (Q18.5)

Q38.0   Congenital malformations of lips, not elsewhere classified 🔹
Congenital fistula of lip
Congenital malformation of lip NOS
Van der Woude's syndrome

> **Excludes1**   cleft lip (Q36.-)
> cleft lip with cleft palate (Q37.-)
> macrocheilia (Q18.6)
> microcheilia (Q18.7)

Q38.1   Ankyloglossia 🔹
Restricted movement of tongue resulting in speech difficulty
Tongue tie

Q38.2   Macroglossia 🔹
Excessive size of tongue
Congenital hypertrophy of tongue

Q38.3 Other congenital malformations of tongue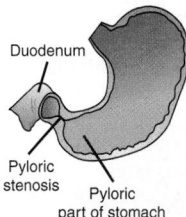
     Aglossia
     Bifid tongue
     Congenital adhesion of tongue
     Congenital fissure of tongue
     Congenital malformation of tongue NOS
     Double tongue
     Hypoglossia
     Hypoplasia of tongue
     Microglossia

Q38.4 Congenital malformations of salivary glands and ducts
     Atresia of salivary glands and ducts
     Congenital absence of salivary glands and ducts
     Congenital accessory salivary glands and ducts
     Congenital fistula of salivary gland

Q38.5 Congenital malformations of palate, not elsewhere classified
     Congenital absence of uvula
     Congenital malformation of palate NOS
     Congenital high arched palate
     Excludes1   cleft palate (Q35.-)
                 cleft palate with cleft lip (Q37.-)

Q38.6 Other congenital malformations of mouth
     Congenital malformation of mouth NOS

Q38.7 Congenital pharyngeal pouch
     Congenital diverticulum of pharynx
     Excludes1   pharyngeal pouch syndrome (D82.1)

Q38.8 Other congenital malformations of pharynx
     Congenital malformation of pharynx NOS
     Imperforate pharynx

● **Q39 Congenital malformations of esophagus**
     (Ex) **For category Q39 CC codes Q39.0-Q39.4:** Q39.0-Q39.9, Q45.8-Q45.9
          For category Q39 CC codes Q39.5-Q39.9: Q39.5-Q39.9, Q45.8-Q45.9

Q39.0 Atresia of esophagus without fistula
     Atresia of esophagus NOS

Q39.1 Atresia of esophagus with tracheo-esophageal fistula
     Atresia of esophagus with broncho-esophageal fistula

Q39.2 Congenital tracheo-esophageal fistula without atresia
     Congenital tracheo-esophageal fistula NOS

Q39.3 Congenital stenosis and stricture of esophagus

Q39.4 Esophageal web

Q39.5 Congenital dilatation of esophagus
     Congenital cardiospasm

Q39.6 Congenital diverticulum of esophagus
     Congenital esophageal pouch

Q39.8 Other congenital malformations of esophagus
     Congenital absence of esophagus
     Congenital displacement of esophagus
     Congenital duplication of esophagus

Q39.9 Congenital malformation of esophagus, unspecified

● **Q40 Other congenital malformations of upper alimentary tract**

Q40.0 Congenital hypertrophic pyloric stenosis
     Congenital or infantile constriction
     Congenital or infantile hypertrophy
     Congenital or infantile spasm
     Congenital or infantile stenosis
     Congenital or infantile stricture

Q40.1 Congenital hiatus hernia
     Congenital displacement of cardia through esophageal hiatus
     Excludes1   congenital diaphragmatic hernia (Q79.0)

Figure 17-4   Pyloric stenosis.

Q40.2 Other specified congenital malformations of stomach
     Congenital displacement of stomach
     Congenital diverticulum of stomach
     Congenital hourglass stomach
     Congenital duplication of stomach
     Megalogastria
     Microgastria

Q40.3 Congenital malformation of stomach, unspecified

Q40.8 Other specified congenital malformations of upper alimentary tract

Q40.9 Congenital malformation of upper alimentary tract, unspecified
     Congenital anomaly of upper alimentary tract
     Congenital deformity of upper alimentary tract

● **Q41 Congenital absence, atresia and stenosis of small intestine**
     Includes   congenital obstruction, occlusion or stricture of small intestine or intestine NOS
     Excludes1   cystic fibrosis with intestinal manifestation (E84.11)
                 meconium ileus NOS (without cystic fibrosis) (P76.0)
     (Ex) **For category Q41 CC codes:** Q41.0-Q41.9, Q45.8-Q45.9

Q41.0 Congenital absence, atresia and stenosis of duodenum

Q41.1 Congenital absence, atresia and stenosis of jejunum
     Apple peel syndrome
     Imperforate jejunum

Q41.2 Congenital absence, atresia and stenosis of ileum

Q41.8 Congenital absence, atresia and stenosis of other specified parts of small intestine

Q41.9 Congenital absence, atresia and stenosis of small intestine, part unspecified
     Congenital absence, atresia and stenosis of intestine NOS

● **Q42 Congenital absence, atresia and stenosis of large intestine**
     Includes   congenital obstruction, occlusion and stricture of large intestine
     (Ex) **For category Q42 CC codes:** Q42.0-Q42.9, Q45.8-Q45.9

Q42.0 Congenital absence, atresia and stenosis of rectum with fistula

Q42.1 Congenital absence, atresia and stenosis of rectum without fistula
     Imperforate rectum

Q42.2 Congenital absence, atresia and stenosis of anus with fistula

Q42.3 Congenital absence, atresia and stenosis of anus without fistula
     Imperforate anus

Q42.8 Congenital absence, atresia and stenosis of other parts of large intestine

Q42.9 Congenital absence, atresia and stenosis of large intestine, part unspecified

● **Q43   Other congenital malformations of intestine**
(Ex) For category Q43 CC codes unless otherwise indicated: Q41.0-Q43.9

Q43.0   Meckel's diverticulum (displaced) (hypertrophic) 🔖
Congenital abnormality in which a pouch remains on the lower end of the small intestine
Persistent omphalomesenteric duct
Persistent vitelline duct

Q43.1   Hirschsprung's disease 🔖🔖
Developmental disorder of enteric nervous system characterized by absence of ganglion cells in distal colon resulting in functional obstruction.
Aganglionosis
Congenital (aganglionic) megacolon
(Ex) Q43.1-Q43.2, Q45.8-Q45.9

Q43.2   Other congenital functional disorders of colon 🔖🔖
Congenital dilatation of colon
(Ex) Q43.1-Q43.2, Q45.8-Q45.9

Q43.3   Congenital malformations of intestinal fixation 🔖🔖
Congenital omental, anomalous adhesions [bands]
Congenital peritoneal adhesions [bands]
Incomplete rotation of cecum and colon
Insufficient rotation of cecum and colon
Jackson's membrane
Malrotation of colon
Rotation failure of cecum and colon
Universal mesentery
(Ex) Q43.3-Q43.9

Q43.4   Duplication of intestine 🔖🔖

Q43.5   Ectopic anus 🔖🔖
Anal opening in abnormal location

Q43.6   Congenital fistula of rectum and anus 🔖🔖
Excludes1   congenital fistula of anus with absence, atresia and stenosis (Q42.2)
congenital fistula of rectum with absence, atresia and stenosis (Q42.0)
congenital rectovaginal fistula (Q52.2)
congenital urethrorectal fistula (Q64.73) ◀⏸
pilonidal fistula or sinus (L05.-)

Q43.7   Persistent cloaca 🔖🔖
Malformation in which rectum, vagina, and urinary tract form one channel AKA congenital cloaca
Cloaca NOS

Q43.8   Other specified congenital malformations of intestine 🔖🔖
Congenital blind loop syndrome
Congenital diverticulitis, colon
Congenital diverticulum, intestine
Dolichocolon
Megaloappendix
Megaloduodenum
Microcolon
Transposition of appendix
Transposition of colon
Transposition of intestine

Q43.9   Congenital malformation of intestine, unspecified 🔖🔖

● **Q44   Congenital malformations of gallbladder, bile ducts and liver**
(Ex) For category Q44 CC codes unless otherwise indicated: Q44.0-Q44.7

Q44.0   Agenesis, aplasia and hypoplasia of gallbladder 🔖🔖
Congenital absence of gallbladder

Q44.1   Other congenital malformations of gallbladder 🔖🔖
Congenital malformation of gallbladder NOS
Intrahepatic gallbladder

Q44.2   Atresia of bile ducts 🔖🔖
(Ex) Q44.2-Q44.3, Q45.8-Q45.9

Q44.3   Congenital stenosis and stricture of bile ducts 🔖🔖
(Ex) Q44.2-Q44.3, Q45.8-Q45.9

Q44.4   Choledochal cyst 🔖🔖

Q44.5   Other congenital malformations of bile ducts 🔖🔖
Accessory hepatic duct
Biliary duct duplication
Congenital malformation of bile duct NOS
Cystic duct duplication

Q44.6   Cystic disease of liver 🔖🔖
Fibrocystic disease of liver
(Ex) Q44.0-Q44.1, Q44.4-Q44.7

Q44.7   Other congenital malformations of liver 🔖🔖
Accessory liver
Alagille's syndrome
Congenital absence of liver
Congenital hepatomegaly
Congenital malformation of liver NOS

● **Q45   Other congenital malformations of digestive system**
Excludes2   congenital diaphragmatic hernia (Q79.0)
congenital hiatus hernia (Q40.1)
(Ex) For category Q45 CC codes: Q45.0-Q45.9

Q45.0   Agenesis, aplasia and hypoplasia of pancreas 🔖🔖
Congenital absence of pancreas

Q45.1   Annular pancreas 🔖🔖

Q45.2   Congenital pancreatic cyst 🔖🔖

Q45.3   Other congenital malformations of pancreas and pancreatic duct 🔖🔖
Accessory pancreas
Congenital malformation of pancreas or pancreatic duct NOS
Excludes1   congenital diabetes mellitus (E10.-)
cystic fibrosis (E84.0-E84.9)
fibrocystic disease of pancreas (E84.-)
neonatal diabetes mellitus (P70.2)

Q45.8   Other specified congenital malformations of digestive system 🔖
Absence (complete) (partial) of alimentary tract NOS
Duplication of digestive system
Malposition, congenital of digestive system

Q45.9   Congenital malformation of digestive system, unspecified 🔖
Congenital anomaly of digestive system
Congenital deformity of digestive system

CONGENITAL MALFORMATIONS OF GENITAL ORGANS (Q50-Q56)

Excludes1   androgen insensitivity syndrome (E34.5-)
syndromes associated with anomalies in the number and form of chromosomes (Q90-Q99)

● **Q50   Congenital malformations of ovaries, fallopian tubes and broad ligaments**

● **Q50.0   Congenital absence of ovary**
Excludes1   Turner's syndrome (Q96.-)

Q50.01   Congenital absence of ovary, unilateral ♀ 🔖

Q50.02   Congenital absence of ovary, bilateral ♀ 🔖

Q50.1   Developmental ovarian cyst ♀ 🔖

Q50.2   Congenital torsion of ovary ♀ 🔖

● **Q50.3   Other congenital malformations of ovary**

Q50.31   Accessory ovary ♀ 🔖

Q50.32   Ovarian streak ♀ 🔖
Inadequate ovaries with absent follicular and hormonal function
46, XX with streak gonads

Q50.39   Other congenital malformation of ovary ♀ 🔖
Congenital malformation of ovary NOS

Q50.4   Embryonic cyst of fallopian tube ♀ 🔖
Fimbrial cyst

Q50.5   Embryonic cyst of broad ligament ♀ 🔖
Epoophoron cyst
Parovarian cyst

Q50.6   Other congenital malformations of fallopian tube and broad ligament ♀ 🔖
Absence of fallopian tube and broad ligament
Accessory fallopian tube and broad ligament
Atresia of fallopian tube and broad ligament
Congenital malformation of fallopian tube or broad ligament NOS

◀ New   ◀⏸ Revised   ~~deleted~~ Deleted   Excludes 1   Excludes 2   Includes   Use additional   Code first   Code also   Unspecified
OGCR Official Guidelines   ● Unacceptable Principal Diagnosis   X Assign placeholder X   ● Use Additional Character(s)   ▌ Manifestation Code   **Coding Clinic**

- **Q51   Congenital malformations of uterus and cervix**
  - **Q51.0   Agenesis and aplasia of uterus** ♀ 🐾
    - Congenital absence of uterus
  - **Q51.1   Doubling of uterus with doubling of cervix and vagina**
    - **Q51.10   Doubling of uterus with doubling of cervix and vagina without obstruction** ♀ 🐾
      - Doubling of uterus with doubling of cervix and vagina NOS
    - **Q51.11   Doubling of uterus with doubling of cervix and vagina with obstruction** ♀ 🐾
  - **Q51.2   Other doubling of uterus** ♀ 🐾
    - Doubling of uterus NOS
    - Septate uterus, complete or partial
  - **Q51.3   Bicornate uterus** ♀ 🐾
    - Bicornate uterus, complete or partial
    - *Birth defect in which uterus has two separate 'horns' that form top of uterus*
  - **Q51.4   Unicornate uterus** ♀ 🐾
    - Unicornate uterus with or without a separate uterine horn
    - Uterus with only one functioning horn
    - *Uterus with half being undeveloped*
  - **Q51.5   Agenesis and aplasia of cervix** ♀ 🐾
    - Congenital absence of cervix
  - **Q51.6   Embryonic cyst of cervix** ♀ 🐾
  - **Q51.7   Congenital fistulae between uterus and digestive and urinary tracts** ♀ 🐾
  - **Q51.8   Other congenital malformations of uterus and cervix**
    - **Q51.81   Other congenital malformations of uterus**
      - **Q51.810   Arcuate uterus** ♀ 🐾
        - Arcuatus uterus
      - **Q51.811   Hypoplasia of uterus** ♀ 🐾
      - **Q51.818   Other congenital malformations of uterus** ♀ 🐾
        - Müllerian anomaly of uterus NEC
    - **Q51.82   Other congenital malformations of cervix**
      - **Q51.820   Cervical duplication** ♀ 🐾
      - **Q51.821   Hypoplasia of cervix** ♀ 🐾
      - **Q51.828   Other congenital malformations of cervix** ♀ 🐾
  - **Q51.9   Congenital malformation of uterus and cervix, unspecified** ♀ 🐾

- **Q52   Other congenital malformations of female genitalia**
  - **Q52.0   Congenital absence of vagina** ♀ 🐾
    - Vaginal agenesis, total or partial
  - **Q52.1   Doubling of vagina**
    - **Excludes1**   doubling of vagina with doubling of uterus and cervix (Q51.1-)
    - **Q52.10   Doubling of vagina, unspecified** ♀ 🐾
      - Septate vagina NOS
    - **Q52.11   Transverse vaginal septum** ♀ 🐾
    - **Q52.12   Longitudinal vaginal septum** ♀ 🐾
      - Longitudinal vaginal septum with or without obstruction
  - **Q52.2   Congenital rectovaginal fistula** ♀ 🐾
    - **Excludes1**   cloaca (Q43.7)
  - **Q52.3   Imperforate hymen** ♀ 🐾
    - *Membrane (hymen) completely closes vaginal orifice*
  - **Q52.4   Other congenital malformations of vagina** ♀ 🐾
    - Canal of Nuck cyst, congenital
    - Congenital malformation of vagina NOS
    - Embryonic vaginal cyst
    - Gartner's duct cyst
  - **Q52.5   Fusion of labia** ♀ 🐾
  - **Q52.6   Congenital malformation of clitoris** ♀ 🐾

Item 17–1   Testes form in the abdomen of the male and only descend into the scrotum during normal embryonic development. "Ectopic" testes are out of their normal place or "retained" (left behind) in the abdomen. Crypto (hidden) orchism (testicle) is a major risk factor for testicular cancer.

ECTOPIC TESTES	CRYPTORCHID TESTES
Penile	Abdominal
Superficial inguinal	Inguinal
(most common)	Prepubic
Femoral	(most common)

Figure 17-5   Undescended testes and the positions of the testes in various types of cryptorchidism or abnormal paths of descent.

- **Q52.7   Other and unspecified congenital malformations of vulva**
  - **Q52.70   Unspecified congenital malformations of vulva** ♀ 🐾
    - Congenital malformation of vulva NOS
  - **Q52.71   Congenital absence of vulva** ♀ 🐾
  - **Q52.79   Other congenital malformations of vulva** ♀ 🐾
    - Congenital cyst of vulva
- **Q52.8   Other specified congenital malformations of female genitalia** ♀ 🐾
- **Q52.9   Congenital malformation of female genitalia, unspecified** ♀ 🐾

- **Q53   Undescended and ectopic testicle**
  - **Q53.0   Ectopic testis**
    - **Q53.00   Ectopic testis, unspecified** ♂ 🐾
    - **Q53.01   Ectopic testis, unilateral** ♂ 🐾
    - **Q53.02   Ectopic testes, bilateral** ♂ 🐾
  - **Q53.1   Undescended testicle, unilateral**
    - **Q53.10   Unspecified undescended testicle, unilateral** ♂ 🐾
    - **Q53.11   Abdominal testis, unilateral** ♂ 🐾
    - **Q53.12   Ectopic perineal testis, unilateral** ♂ 🐾
  - **Q53.2   Undescended testicle, bilateral**
    - **Q53.20   Undescended testicle, unspecified, bilateral** ♂ 🐾
    - **Q53.21   Abdominal testis, bilateral** ♂ 🐾
    - **Q53.22   Ectopic perineal testis, bilateral** ♂ 🐾
  - **Q53.9   Undescended testicle, unspecified** ♂ 🐾
    - Cryptorchism NOS

- **Q54   Hypospadias**
  - *Birth defect of male; urethra opens in abnormal location on shaft*
  - **Excludes1**   epispadias (Q64.0)
  - **Q54.0   Hypospadias, balanic** ♂ 🐾
    - Hypospadias, coronal
    - Hypospadias, glandular
  - **Q54.1   Hypospadias, penile** ♂ 🐾
  - **Q54.2   Hypospadias, penoscrotal** ♂ 🐾
  - **Q54.3   Hypospadias, perineal** ♂ 🐾
  - **Q54.4   Congenital chordee** ♂ 🐾
    - Chordee without hypospadias
  - **Q54.8   Other hypospadias** ♂ 🐾
    - Hypospadias with intersex state
  - **Q54.9   Hypospadias, unspecified** ♂ 🐾

CHAPTER 17 (Q00-Q99)

N Newborn Age: 0	P Pediatric Age: 0–17	M Maternity DX: 12–55	A Adult Age: 15–124	♀ Females Only	♂ Males Only
🐾 Complication\Comorbidity	🐾 Major C\C	(Ex) CC/MCC Exclusions	🐾 Present on Admission Requirement	🐾 Hospital-Acquired Condition	

CHAPTER 17 (Q00-Q99)

● **Q55   Other congenital malformations of male genital organs**

     Excludes1   congenital hydrocele (P83.5)
                      hypospadias (Q54.-)

   Q55.0   Absence and aplasia of testis ♂ 🐾
          Monorchism

   Q55.1   Hypoplasia of testis and scrotum ♂ 🐾
          Fusion of testes

●   **Q55.2   Other and unspecified congenital malformations of testis and scrotum**

     Q55.20   Unspecified congenital malformations of testis and scrotum ♂ 🐾
            Congenital malformation of testis or scrotum NOS

     Q55.21   Polyorchism ♂ 🐾
            Developmental anomaly characterized by presence of more than two testes

     Q55.22   Retractile testis ♂ 🐾

     Q55.23   Scrotal transposition ♂ 🐾

     Q55.29   Other congenital malformations of testis and scrotum ♂ 🐾

   Q55.3   Atresia of vas deferens ♂ 🐾
         Code first any associated cystic fibrosis (E84.-)

   Q55.4   Other congenital malformations of vas deferens, epididymis, seminal vesicles and prostate ♂
         Absence or aplasia of prostate
         Absence or aplasia of spermatic cord
         Congenital malformation of vas deferens, epididymis, seminal vesicles or prostate NOS

   Q55.5   Congenital absence and aplasia of penis ♂ 🐾

●   **Q55.6   Other congenital malformations of penis**

     Q55.61   Curvature of penis (lateral) ♂ 🐾

     Q55.62   Hypoplasia of penis ♂ 🐾
            Underdevelopment penis
            Micropenis

     Q55.63   Congenital torsion of penis ♂ 🐾
            Excludes1   acquired torsion of penis (N48.82)

     Q55.64   Hidden penis ♂ 🐾
            Buried penis
            Concealed penis
            Excludes1   acquired buried penis (N48.83)

     Q55.69   Other congenital malformation of penis ♂ 🐾
            Congenital malformation of penis NOS

   Q55.7   Congenital vasocutaneous fistula ♂ 🐾
         Abnormal opening between vas deferens and skin

   Q55.8   Other specified congenital malformations of male genital organs ♂ 🐾

   Q55.9   Congenital malformation of male genital organ, unspecified ♂ 🐾
         Congenital anomaly of male genital organ
         Congenital deformity of male genital organ

● **Q56   Indeterminate sex and pseudohermaphroditism**
     Internal reproductive organs are opposite external physical characteristics.

     Excludes1   46,XX true hermaphrodite (Q99.1)
                   androgen insensitivity syndrome (E34.5-)
                   chimera 46,XX/46,XY true hermaphrodite (Q99.0)
                   female pseudohermaphroditism with adrenocortical disorder (E25.-)
                   pseudohermaphroditism with specified chromosomal anomaly (Q96-Q99)
                   pure gonadal dysgenesis (Q99.1)

   Q56.0   Hermaphroditism, not elsewhere classified 🐾
         Ovotestis

   Q56.1   Male pseudohermaphroditism, not elsewhere classified ♂ 🐾
         46, XY with streak gonads
         Male pseudohermaphroditism NOS

   Q56.2   Female pseudohermaphroditism, not elsewhere classified ♀ 🐾
         Female pseudohermaphroditism NOS

   Q56.3   Pseudohermaphroditism, unspecified 🐾

   Q56.4   Indeterminate sex, unspecified 🐾
         Ambiguous genitalia

CONGENITAL MALFORMATIONS OF THE URINARY SYSTEM (Q60-Q64)

● **Q60   Renal agenesis and other reduction defects of kidney**

     Includes   congenital absence of kidney
                 congenital atrophy of kidney
                 infantile atrophy of kidney
     (Ex) For category Q60 CC codes: N13.9, Q60.0-Q60.6

   Q60.0   Renal agenesis, unilateral 🐾 🐾

   Q60.1   Renal agenesis, bilateral 🐾 🐾

   Q60.2   Renal agenesis, unspecified 🐾 🐾

   Q60.3   Renal hypoplasia, unilateral 🐾 🐾

   Q60.4   Renal hypoplasia, bilateral 🐾 🐾

   Q60.5   Renal hypoplasia, unspecified 🐾 🐾

   Q60.6   Potter's syndrome 🐾 🐾

● **Q61   Cystic kidney disease**
     Cysts that develop in failing kidney due to end-stage renal disease

     Excludes1   acquired cyst of kidney (N28.1)
                   Potter's syndrome (Q60.6)

●   **Q61.0   Congenital renal cyst**

     Q61.00   Congenital renal cyst, unspecified 🐾 🐾
            Cyst of kidney NOS (congenital)
            (Ex) N13.9, Q61.00, Q61.9

     Q61.01   Congenital single renal cyst 🐾 🐾
            (Ex) N13.9, Q61.01

     Q61.02   Congenital multiple renal cysts 🐾 🐾
            (Ex) N13.9, Q61.02, Q61.5-Q61.8

●   **Q61.1   Polycystic kidney, infantile type**
         Polycystic kidney, autosomal recessive
     (Ex) For category Q61.1 CC codes: N13.9, Q61.11-Q61.3

     Q61.11   Cystic dilatation of collecting ducts 🐾 🐾

     Q61.19   Other polycystic kidney, infantile type 🐾 🐾

   Q61.2   Polycystic kidney, adult type 🐾 🐾
         Polycystic kidney, autosomal dominant
         (Ex) N13.9, Q61.11-Q61.3

   Q61.3   Polycystic kidney, unspecified 🐾 🐾
         (Ex) N13.9, Q61.11-Q61.3

   Q61.4   Renal dysplasia 🐾 🐾
         Multicystic dysplastic kidney
         Multicystic kidney (development)
         Multicystic kidney disease
         Multicystic renal dysplasia
         Excludes1   polycystic kidney disease (Q61.11-Q61.3)
         (Ex) N13.9, Q61.4

   Q61.5   Medullary cystic kidney 🐾 🐾
         Nephronopthisis
         Sponge kidney NOS
         (Ex) N13.9, Q61.02, Q61.5-Q61.8

   Q61.8   Other cystic kidney diseases 🐾 🐾
         Fibrocystic kidney
         Fibrocystic renal degeneration or disease
         (Ex) N13.9, Q61.02, Q61.5-Q61.8

   Q61.9   Cystic kidney disease, unspecified 🐾 🐾
         Meckel-Gruber syndrome
         (Ex) N13.9, Q61.00, Q61.9

◄ New   ◄▥ Revised   ~~deleted~~ Deleted   Excludes 1   Excludes 2   Includes   Use additional   Code first   Code also   Unspecified

OGCR Official Guidelines   ● Unacceptable Principal Diagnosis   X Assign placeholder X   ● Use Additional Character(s)   ▶ Manifestation Code   **Coding Clinic**

● **Q62   Congenital obstructive defects of renal pelvis and congenital malformations of ureter**

Q62.0   **Congenital hydronephrosis** 🔹🔹
     (Ex) N13.9, Q62.0-Q62.2, Q62.39

● Q62.1   **Congenital occlusion of ureter**
     Atresia and stenosis of ureter
     (Ex) **For category Q62.1 CC codes:** See Q62.0

     Q62.10   **Congenital occlusion of ureter,** unspecified 🔹🔹

     Q62.11   **Congenital occlusion of ureteropelvic junction** 🔹🔹

     Q62.12   **Congenital occlusion of ureterovesical orifice** 🔹🔹

Q62.2   **Congenital megaureter** 🔹🔹
     Congenital dilatation of ureter
     (Ex) See Q62.0

● Q62.3   **Other obstructive defects of renal pelvis and ureter**
     (Ex) **For category Q62.3 CC codes:** See Q62.0

     Q62.31   **Congenital ureterocele, orthotopic** 🔹🔹

     Q62.32   **Cecoureterocele** 🔹🔹
        Ectopic ureterocele

     Q62.39   **Other obstructive defects of renal pelvis and ureter** 🔹🔹
        Ureteropelvic junction obstruction NOS

Q62.4   **Agenesis of ureter** 🔹
     Congenital absence ureter

Q62.5   **Duplication of ureter** 🔹
     Accessory ureter
     Double ureter

● Q62.6   **Malposition of ureter**

     Q62.60   **Malposition of ureter,** unspecified 🔹

     Q62.61   **Deviation of ureter** 🔹

     Q62.62   **Displacement of ureter** 🔹

     Q62.63   **Anomalous implantation of ureter** 🔹
        Ectopia of ureter
        Ectopic ureter

     Q62.69   **Other malposition of ureter** 🔹

Q62.7   **Congenital vesico-uretero-renal reflux** 🔹

Q62.8   **Other congenital malformations of ureter** 🔹
     Anomaly of ureter NOS

● **Q63   Other congenital malformations of kidney**

     Excludes1   congenital nephrotic syndrome (N04.-)

Q63.0   **Accessory kidney** 🔹

Q63.1   **Lobulated, fused and horseshoe kidney** 🔹

Q63.2   **Ectopic kidney** 🔹
     Congenital displaced kidney
     Malrotation of kidney

Q63.3   **Hyperplastic and giant kidney** 🔹
     Compensatory hypertrophy of kidney

Q63.8   **Other specified congenital malformations of kidney** 🔹
     Congenital renal calculi

Q63.9   **Congenital malformation of kidney,** unspecified 🔹

● **Q64   Other congenital malformations of urinary system**

Q64.0   **Epispadias** ♂ 🔹
     Urethral opening somewhere on dorsum of penis

     Excludes1   hypospadias (Q54.-)

● Q64.1   **Exstrophy of urinary bladder**
     Bladder is exposed, inside out, and protrudes through abdominal wall
     (Ex) **For category Q64.1 CC codes:** N13.9, Q64.10-Q64.19, Q64.8-Q64.9

     Q64.10   **Exstrophy of urinary bladder,** unspecified 🔹🔹
        Ectopia vesicae

     Q64.11   **Supravesical fissure of urinary bladder** 🔹🔹

     Q64.12   **Cloacal extrophy of urinary bladder** 🔹🔹

     Q64.19   **Other exstrophy of urinary bladder** 🔹🔹
        Extroversion of bladder

Q64.2   **Congenital posterior urethral valves** 🔹🔹
     (Ex) N13.9, Q64.2-Q64.39, Q64.8-Q64.9

● Q64.3   **Other atresia and stenosis of urethra and bladder neck**
     (Ex) **For category Q64.3 CC codes:** See Q64.2

     Q64.31   **Congenital bladder neck obstruction** 🔹🔹
        Congenital obstruction of vesicourethral orifice

     Q64.32   **Congenital stricture of urethra** 🔹🔹

     Q64.33   **Congenital stricture of urinary meatus** 🔹🔹

     Q64.39   **Other atresia and stenosis of urethra and bladder neck** 🔹🔹
        Atresia and stenosis of urethra and bladder neck NOS

Q64.4   **Malformation of urachus** 🔹
     Cyst of urachus
     Patent urachus
     Prolapse of urachus

Q64.5   **Congenital absence of bladder and urethra** 🔹

Q64.6   **Congenital diverticulum of bladder** 🔹

● Q64.7   **Other and unspecified congenital malformations of bladder and urethra**

     Excludes1   congenital prolapse of bladder (mucosa) (Q79.4)

     Q64.70   unspecified **congenital malformation of bladder and urethra** 🔹
        Malformation of bladder or urethra NOS

     Q64.71   **Congenital prolapse of urethra** 🔹

     Q64.72   **Congenital prolapse of urinary meatus** 🔹

     Q64.73   **Congenital urethrorectal fistula** 🔹

     Q64.74   **Double urethra** 🔹

     Q64.75   **Double urinary meatus** 🔹

     Q64.79   **Other congenital malformations of bladder and urethra** 🔹

Q64.8   **Other specified congenital malformations of urinary system** 🔹

Q64.9   **Congenital malformation of urinary system,** unspecified 🔹
     Congenital anomaly NOS of urinary system
     Congenital deformity NOS of urinary system

CONGENITAL MALFORMATIONS AND DEFORMATIONS OF THE MUSCULOSKELETAL SYSTEM (Q65-Q79)

● **Q65   Congenital deformities of hip**

     Excludes1   clicking hip (R29.4)

● Q65.0   **Congenital dislocation of hip, unilateral**

     Q65.00   **Congenital dislocation of** unspecified **hip, unilateral** 🔹

     Q65.01   **Congenital dislocation of right hip, unilateral** 🔹

     Q65.02   **Congenital dislocation of left hip, unilateral** 🔹

Q65.1   **Congenital dislocation of hip, bilateral** 🔹

Q65.2   **Congenital dislocation of hip,** unspecified 🔹

● Q65.3   **Congenital partial dislocation of hip, unilateral**

     Q65.30   **Congenital partial dislocation of** unspecified **hip, unilateral** 🔹

     Q65.31   **Congenital partial dislocation of right hip, unilateral** 🔹

     Q65.32   **Congenital partial dislocation of left hip, unilateral** 🔹

Q65.4   **Congenital partial dislocation of hip, bilateral** 🔹

Q65.5   **Congenital partial dislocation of hip,** unspecified 🔹

Q65.6   **Congenital unstable hip** 🔹
     Congenital dislocatable hip

● Q65.8   **Other congenital deformities of hip**

     Q65.81   **Congenital coxa valga** 🔹

     Q65.82   **Congenital coxa vara** 🔹

     Q65.89   **Other specified congenital deformities of hip** 🔹
        Anteversion of femoral neck
        Congenital acetabular dysplasia

Q65.9   **Congenital deformity of hip,** unspecified 🔹

CHAPTER 17 (Q00-Q99)

N   Newborn Age: 0   P   Pediatric Age: 0–17   M   Maternity DX: 12–55   A   Adult Age: 15–124   ♀   Females Only   ♂   Males Only

🔹 Complication\Comorbidity   🔹 Major C\C   (Ex) CC/MCC Exclusions   🔹 Present on Admission Requirement   🔹 Hospital-Acquired Condition

1259

CHAPTER 17 (Q00-Q99)

Item 17-2 Equinus foot is a term referring to the hoof of a horse. The deformity is usually congenital or spastic. Talipes equinovarus is referred to as clubfoot. The foot tends to be smaller than normal, with the heel pointing downward and the forefoot turning inward. The heel cord (Achilles tendon) is tight, causing the heel to be drawn up toward the leg.

Figure 17-6 Supination and cavus deformity of forefoot. *(Courtesy Jay Cummings, MD.)* (From Canale: Campbell's Operative Orthopaedics, ed 11, Mosby, Inc., 2007)

Q66   Congenital deformities of feet
Excludes1   reduction defects of feet (Q72.-)
               valgus deformities (acquired) (M21.0-)
               varus deformities (acquired) (M21.1-)

Q66.0   Congenital talipes equinovarus
Heel is turned inward from midline and foot is plantar flexed; AKA clubfoot

Q66.1   Congenital talipes calcaneovarus
Deformity of foot in which heel is turned toward midline of body and anterior of foot is elevated

Q66.2   Congenital metatarsus (primus) varus
Angulation of first metatarsal bone toward midline of body

Q66.3   Other congenital varus deformities of feet
Hallux varus, congenital

Q66.4   Congenital talipes calcaneovalgus

Q66.5   Congenital pes planus
Congenital flat foot
Congenital rigid flat foot
Congenital spastic (everted) flat foot
Excludes1   pes planus, acquired (M21.4)

Q66.50   Congenital pes planus, unspecified foot

Q66.51   Congenital pes planus, right foot

Q66.52   Congenital pes planus, left foot

Q66.6   Other congenital valgus deformities of feet
Inward angulation
Congenital metatarsus valgus

Q66.7   Congenital pes cavus

Q66.8   Other congenital deformities of feet

Q66.80   Congenital vertical talus deformity, unspecified foot

Q66.81   Congenital vertical talus deformity, right foot

Q66.82   Congenital vertical talus deformity, left foot

Q66.89   Other specified congenital deformities of feet
Congenital asymmetric talipes
Congenital clubfoot NOS
Congenital talipes NOS
Congenital tarsal coalition
Hammer toe, congenital

Q66.9   Congenital deformity of feet, unspecified

Q67   Congenital musculoskeletal deformities of head, face, spine and chest
Excludes1   congenital malformation syndromes classified to Q87.-
               Potter's syndrome (Q60.6)

Q67.0   Congenital facial asymmetry

Q67.1   Congenital compression facies

Q67.2   Dolichocephaly
Long head dimension

Q67.3   Plagiocephaly
Asymmetric shape of head resulting from irregular closure of cranial sutures

Q67.4   Other congenital deformities of skull, face and jaw
Congenital depressions in skull
Congenital hemifacial atrophy or hypertrophy
Deviation of nasal septum, congenital
Squashed or bent nose, congenital
Excludes1   dentofacial anomalies [including malocclusion] (M26.-)
               syphilitic saddle nose (A50.5)

Q67.5   Congenital deformity of spine
Congenital postural scoliosis
Congenital scoliosis NOS
Excludes1   infantile idiopathic scoliosis (M41.0)
               scoliosis due to congenital bony malformation (Q76.3)
(Ex) Q67.5, Q76.3, Q76.425-Q76.429

Q67.6   Pectus excavatum
Congenital funnel chest
Funnel-shaped chest depression

Q67.7   Pectus carinatum
Congenital pigeon chest

Q67.8   Other congenital deformities of chest
Congenital deformity of chest wall NOS
(Ex) Q67.6-Q67.8, Q68.1, Q74.3

Q68   Other congenital musculoskeletal deformities
Excludes1   reduction defects of limb(s) (Q71-Q73)
Excludes2   congenital myotonic chondrodystrophy (G71.13)

Q68.0   Congenital deformity of sternocleidomastoid muscle
Congenital contracture of sternocleidomastoid (muscle)
Congenital (sternomastoid) torticollis
Sternomastoid tumor (congenital)

Q68.1   Congenital deformity of finger(s) and hand
Congenital clubfinger
Spade-like hand (congenital)
(Ex) Q67.6-Q67.8, Q68.1, Q74.3

Q68.2   Congenital deformity of knee
Congenital dislocation of knee
Congenital genu recurvatum
Hyperextension of knee resulting from hypermobility

Talipes cavus
Talipes equinus
Talipes calcaneus
Talipes valgus
Talipes equinovalgus
Talipes calcaneovalgus
Talipes varus
Talipes cavovarus
Talipes equinovarus
Talipes calcaneocavus

Figure 17-7 Talipes. (From Dorland: Dorland's Illustrated Medical Dictionary, ed 31, Saunders, 2007, p 1893)

◄ New   ◄ Revised   ~~deleted~~ Deleted   Excludes 1   Excludes 2   Includes   Use additional   Code first   Code also   Unspecified
OGCR Official Guidelines   ● Unacceptable Principal Diagnosis   X Assign placeholder X   ● Use Additional Character(s)   ▌ Manifestation Code   **Coding Clinic**

Figure 17-8 Mild to moderate inbowing of the lower leg. (From Jones KL: Smith's Recognizable Patterns of Human Malformation, ed 6, Philadelphia, Saunders, 2005)

Q68.3   Congenital bowing of femur
   Excludes1   anteversion of femur (neck) (Q65.89)
Q68.4   Congenital bowing of tibia and fibula
Q68.5   Congenital bowing of long bones of leg, unspecified
Q68.6   Discoid meniscus
Q68.8   Other specified congenital musculoskeletal deformities
    Congenital deformity of clavicle
    Congenital deformity of elbow
    Congenital deformity of forearm
    Congenital deformity of scapula
    Congenital deformity of wrist
    Congenital dislocation of elbow
    Congenital dislocation of shoulder
    Congenital dislocation of wrist

Q69   Polydactyly
AKA hyperdactyly, consists of supernumerary fingers or toes
Q69.0   Accessory finger(s)
Q69.1   Accessory thumb(s)
Q69.2   Accessory toe(s)
    Accessory hallux
Q69.9   Polydactyly, unspecified
    Supernumerary digit(s) NOS

Q70   Syndactyly
Webbing between distal phalanges of adjacent digits
Q70.0   Fused fingers
    Complex syndactyly of fingers with synostosis
Q70.00   Fused fingers, unspecified hand
Q70.01   Fused fingers, right hand
Q70.02   Fused fingers, left hand
Q70.03   Fused fingers, bilateral
Q70.1   Webbed fingers
    Simple syndactyly of fingers without synostosis
Q70.10   Webbed fingers, unspecified hand
Q70.11   Webbed fingers, right hand
Q70.12   Webbed fingers, left hand
Q70.13   Webbed fingers, bilateral
Q70.2   Fused toes
    Complex syndactyly of toes with synostosis
Q70.20   Fused toes, unspecified foot
Q70.21   Fused toes, right foot
Q70.22   Fused toes, left foot
Q70.23   Fused toes, bilateral
Q70.3   Webbed toes
    Simple syndactyly of toes without synostosis
Q70.30   Webbed toes, unspecified foot
Q70.31   Webbed toes, right foot
Q70.32   Webbed toes, left foot
Q70.33   Webbed toes, bilateral

Figure 17-9 Polydactyly, congenital duplicated thumb. (From DeLee: DeLee and Drez's Orthopaedic Sports Medicine, ed 3, Saunders, An Imprint of Elsevier, 2009)

Q70.4   Polysyndactyly, unspecified
   Excludes1   specified syndactyly of hand and feet - code to specified conditions (Q70.0- -Q70.3-)
Extra and webbed digits
Q70.9   Syndactyly, unspecified
    Symphalangy NOS

Q71   Reduction defects of upper limb
Q71.0   Congenital complete absence of upper limb
Q71.00   Congenital complete absence of unspecified upper limb
Q71.01   Congenital complete absence of right upper limb
Q71.02   Congenital complete absence of left upper limb
Q71.03   Congenital complete absence of upper limb, bilateral
Q71.1   Congenital absence of upper arm and forearm with hand present
Q71.10   Congenital absence of unspecified upper arm and forearm with hand present
Q71.11   Congenital absence of right upper arm and forearm with hand present
Q71.12   Congenital absence of left upper arm and forearm with hand present
Q71.13   Congenital absence of upper arm and forearm with hand present, bilateral
Q71.2   Congenital absence of both forearm and hand
Q71.20   Congenital absence of both forearm and hand, unspecified upper limb
Q71.21   Congenital absence of both forearm and hand, right upper limb
Q71.22   Congenital absence of both forearm and hand, left upper limb
Q71.23   Congenital absence of both forearm and hand, bilateral
Q71.3   Congenital absence of hand and finger
Q71.30   Congenital absence of unspecified hand and finger
Q71.31   Congenital absence of right hand and finger
Q71.32   Congenital absence of left hand and finger
Q71.33   Congenital absence of hand and finger, bilateral
Q71.4   Longitudinal reduction defect of radius
    Clubhand (congenital)
    Radial clubhand
Q71.40   Longitudinal reduction defect of unspecified radius
Q71.41   Longitudinal reduction defect of right radius
Q71.42   Longitudinal reduction defect of left radius
Q71.43   Longitudinal reduction defect of radius, bilateral
Q71.5   Longitudinal reduction defect of ulna
Q71.50   Longitudinal reduction defect of unspecified ulna
Q71.51   Longitudinal reduction defect of right ulna
Q71.52   Longitudinal reduction defect of left ulna
Q71.53   Longitudinal reduction defect of ulna, bilateral
Q71.6   Lobster-claw hand
Q71.60   Lobster-claw hand, unspecified hand
Q71.61   Lobster-claw right hand
Q71.62   Lobster-claw left hand
Q71.63   Lobster-claw hand, bilateral

CHAPTER 17 (Q00-Q99)

N Newborn Age: 0   P Pediatric Age: 0–17   M Maternity DX: 12–55   A Adult Age: 15–124   ♀ Females Only   ♂ Males Only
Complication\Comorbidity   Major C\C   (Ex) CC/MCC Exclusions   Present on Admission Requirement   Hospital-Acquired Condition
1261

- Q71.8   Other reduction defects of upper limb
  - Q71.81   Congenital shortening of upper limb
    - Q71.811   Congenital shortening of right upper limb
    - Q71.812   Congenital shortening of left upper limb
    - Q71.813   Congenital shortening of upper limb, bilateral
    - Q71.819   Congenital shortening of unspecified upper limb
  - Q71.89   Other reduction defects of upper limb
    - Q71.891   Other reduction defects of right upper limb
    - Q71.892   Other reduction defects of left upper limb
    - Q71.893   Other reduction defects of upper limb, bilateral
    - Q71.899   Other reduction defects of unspecified upper limb
  - Q71.9   Unspecified reduction defect of upper limb
    - Q71.90   Unspecified reduction defect of unspecified upper limb
    - Q71.91   Unspecified reduction defect of right upper limb
    - Q71.92   Unspecified reduction defect of left upper limb
    - Q71.93   Unspecified reduction defect of upper limb, bilateral

- Q72   Reduction defects of lower limb
  - Q72.0   Congenital complete absence of lower limb
    - Q72.00   Congenital complete absence of unspecified lower limb
    - Q72.01   Congenital complete absence of right lower limb
    - Q72.02   Congenital complete absence of left lower limb
    - Q72.03   Congenital complete absence of lower limb, bilateral
  - Q72.1   Congenital absence of thigh and lower leg with foot present
    - Q72.10   Congenital absence of unspecified thigh and lower leg with foot present
    - Q72.11   Congenital absence of right thigh and lower leg with foot present
    - Q72.12   Congenital absence of left thigh and lower leg with foot present
    - Q72.13   Congenital absence of thigh and lower leg with foot present, bilateral
  - Q72.2   Congenital absence of both lower leg and foot
    - Q72.20   Congenital absence of both lower leg and foot, unspecified lower limb
    - Q72.21   Congenital absence of both lower leg and foot, right lower limb
    - Q72.22   Congenital absence of both left lower leg and foot, left lower limb
    - Q72.23   Congenital absence of both lower leg and foot, bilateral
  - Q72.3   Congenital absence of foot and toe(s)
    - Q72.30   Congenital absence of unspecified foot and toe(s)
    - Q72.31   Congenital absence of right foot and toe(s)
    - Q72.32   Congenital absence of left foot and toe(s)
    - Q72.33   Congenital absence of foot and toe(s), bilateral

- Q72.4   Longitudinal reduction defect of femur
  Proximal femoral focal deficiency
    - Q72.40   Longitudinal reduction defect of unspecified femur
    - Q72.41   Longitudinal reduction defect of right femur
    - Q72.42   Longitudinal reduction defect of left femur
    - Q72.43   Longitudinal reduction defect of femur, bilateral
  - Q72.5   Longitudinal reduction defect of tibia
    - Q72.50   Longitudinal reduction defect of unspecified tibia
    - Q72.51   Longitudinal reduction defect of right tibia
    - Q72.52   Longitudinal reduction defect of left tibia
    - Q72.53   Longitudinal reduction defect of tibia, bilateral
  - Q72.6   Longitudinal reduction defect of fibula
    - Q72.60   Longitudinal reduction defect of unspecified fibula
    - Q72.61   Longitudinal reduction defect of right fibula
    - Q72.62   Longitudinal reduction defect of left fibula
    - Q72.63   Longitudinal reduction defect of fibula, bilateral
  - Q72.7   Split foot
    - Q72.70   Split foot, unspecified lower limb
    - Q72.71   Split foot, right lower limb
    - Q72.72   Split foot, left lower limb
    - Q72.73   Split foot, bilateral
  - Q72.8   Other reduction defects of lower limb
    - Q72.81   Congenital shortening of lower limb
      - Q72.811   Congenital shortening of right lower limb
      - Q72.812   Congenital shortening of left lower limb
      - Q72.813   Congenital shortening of lower limb, bilateral
      - Q72.819   Congenital shortening of unspecified lower limb
    - Q72.89   Other reduction defects of lower limb
      - Q72.891   Other reduction defects of right lower limb
      - Q72.892   Other reduction defects of left lower limb
      - Q72.893   Other reduction defects of lower limb, bilateral
      - Q72.899   Other reduction defects of unspecified lower limb
  - Q72.9   Unspecified reduction defect of lower limb
    - Q72.90   Unspecified reduction defect of unspecified lower limb
    - Q72.91   Unspecified reduction defect of right lower limb
    - Q72.92   Unspecified reduction defect of left lower limb
    - Q72.93   Unspecified reduction defect of lower limb, bilateral

◀ New   ◀⫶ Revised   ~~deleted~~ Deleted   Excludes 1   Excludes 2   Includes   Use additional   Code first   Code also   Unspecified

OGCR Official Guidelines   ● Unacceptable Principal Diagnosis   X Assign placeholder X   ● Use Additional Character(s)   ▌Manifestation Code   **Coding Clinic**

● **Q73** **Reduction defects of unspecified limb**

Q73.0 **Congenital absence of unspecified limb(s)** 🔷
   Amelia NOS

Q73.1 **Phocomelia, unspecified limb(s)** 🔷
   Phocomelia NOS
   Absence/shortening of long bones primarily as a result of thalidomide

Q73.8 **Other reduction defects of unspecified limb(s)** 🔷
   Longitudinal reduction deformity of unspecified limb(s)
   Ectromelia of limb NOS
   Gross hypoplasia or aplasia of one or more long bones of limb(s)
   Hemimelia of limb NOS
   Absence of one-half of long bone
   Reduction defect of limb NOS

● **Q74** **Other congenital malformations of limb(s)**

Excludes1 polydactyly (Q69.-)
   reduction defect of limb (Q71-Q73)
   syndactyly (Q70.-)

Q74.0 **Other congenital malformations of upper limb(s), including shoulder girdle** 🔷
   Accessory carpal bones
   Cleidocranial dysostosis
   Congenital pseudarthrosis of clavicle
   Macrodactylia (fingers)
   Madelung's deformity
   Radioulnar synostosis
   Sprengel's deformity
   Triphalangeal thumb

Q74.1 **Congenital malformation of knee** 🔷
   Congenital absence of patella
   Congenital dislocation of patella
   Congenital genu valgum
   Congenital genu varum
   Rudimentary patella

   Excludes1 congenital dislocation of knee (Q68.2)
      congenital genu recurvatum (Q68.2)
      nail patella syndrome (Q87.2)

Q74.2 **Other congenital malformations of lower limb(s), including pelvic girdle** 🔷
   Congenital fusion of sacroiliac joint
   Congenital malformation of ankle joint
   Congenital malformation of sacroiliac joint

   Excludes1 anteversion of femur (neck) (Q65.89)

Q74.3 **Arthrogryposis multiplex congenita** 🔷 🔷
   (Ex) Q67.6-Q67.8, Q68.1, Q74.3

Q74.8 **Other specified congenital malformations of limb(s)** 🔷

Q74.9 **Unspecified congenital malformation of limb(s)** 🔷
   Congenital anomaly of limb(s) NOS

● **Q75** **Other congenital malformations of skull and face bones**

Excludes1 congenital malformation of face NOS (Q18.-)
   congenital malformation syndromes classified to Q87.-
   dentofacial anomalies [including malocclusion] (M26.-)
   musculoskeletal deformities of head and face (Q67.0-Q67.4)
   skull defects associated with congenital anomalies of brain such as:
      anencephaly (Q00.0)
      encephalocele (Q01.-)
      hydrocephalus (Q03.-)
      microcephaly (Q02)

Q75.0 **Craniosynostosis** 🔷
   Premature closure of sutures of skull
   Acrocephaly
   Imperfect fusion of skull
   Oxycephaly
   Trigonocephaly

Q75.1 **Craniofacial dysostosis** 🔷
   Congenital deformity of head
   Crouzon's disease

Item 17-3 **Anencephalus** is a congenital deformity of the cranial vault. **Craniosynostosis,** also known as craniostenosis and stenocephaly, signifies any form of congenital deformity of the skull that results from the premature closing of the sutures of the skull. **Iniencephaly** is a deformity in which the head and neck are flexed backward to a great extent and the head is very large in comparison to the shortened body.

Figure 17-10 Generalized craniosynostosis in a 4-year-old girl without symptoms or signs of increased intracranial pressure. (From Bell WE, McCormick WF: Increased Intracranial Pressure in Children, ed 2, Philadelphia, WB Saunders, 1978, p 116)

Q75.2 **Hypertelorism** 🔷

Q75.3 **Macrocephaly** 🔷
   Unusually large size of head; AKA megalocephaly

Q75.4 **Mandibulofacial dysostosis** 🔷
   Franceschetti syndrome
   Treacher Collins syndrome

Q75.5 **Oculomandibular dysostosis** 🔷
   Ossification of occular and mandibular bones

Q75.8 **Other specified congenital malformations of skull and face bones** 🔷
   Absence of skull bone, congenital
   Congenital deformity of forehead
   Platybasia

Q75.9 **Congenital malformation of skull and face bones, unspecified** 🔷
   Congenital anomaly of face bones NOS
   Congenital anomaly of skull NOS

● **Q76** **Congenital malformations of spine and bony thorax**

Excludes1 congenital musculoskeletal deformities of spine and chest (Q67.5-Q67.8)

Q76.0 **Spina bifida occulta** 🔷

   Excludes1 meningocele (spinal) (Q05.-)
      spina bifida (aperta) (cystica) (Q05.-)

Q76.1 **Klippel-Feil syndrome** 🔷
   Cervical fusion syndrome

Q76.2 **Congenital spondylolisthesis** 🔷
   Congenital spondylolysis

   Excludes1 spondylolisthesis (acquired) (M43.1-)
      spondylolysis (acquired) (M43.0-)

Q76.3 **Congenital scoliosis due to congenital bony malformation** 🔷 🔷
   Hemivertebra fusion or failure of segmentation with scoliosis
   (Ex) Q67.5, Q76.3, Q76.425-Q76.429

● **Q76.4** **Other congenital malformations of spine, not associated with scoliosis**

● **Q76.41** **Congenital kyphosis**
   Abnormal increase in convexity curvature of thoracic spinal column; AKA humpback

   Q76.411 **Congenital kyphosis, occipito-atlanto-axial region** 🔷

   Q76.412 **Congenital kyphosis, cervical region** 🔷

   Q76.413 **Congenital kyphosis, cervicothoracic region** 🔷

   Q76.414 **Congenital kyphosis, thoracic region** 🔷

   Q76.415 **Congenital kyphosis, thoracolumbar region** 🔷

   Q76.419 **Congenital kyphosis, unspecified region** 🔷

N Newborn Age: 0   **P** Pediatric Age: 0–17   **M** Maternity DX: 12–55   **A** Adult Age: 15–124   ♀ Females Only   ♂ Males Only

🔷 Complication\Comorbidity   🔷 Major C\C   (Ex) CC/MCC Exclusions   🔷 Present on Admission Requirement   🔷 Hospital-Acquired Condition

Figure 17-11 **A.** Spina bifida occulta. **B.** Meningocele.
C. Myelomeningocele. **D.** Myelocystocele (syringomyelocele)
or hydromyelia.

Item 17–4 Spina bifida is a midline spinal defect in which one or more vertebrae fail to fuse, leaving an opening in the vertebral canal. When the defect is not visible, it is called spina bifida occulta, and when it is visible, it is called spina bifida cystica.

● **Q76.42 Congenital lordosis**
An abnormal increase in curvature of lumbar spine (sway back)
Ⓔ **For category Q76.42 CC codes:** Q67.5, Q76.3, Q76.425-Q76.429

    Q76.425 Congenital lordosis, thoracolumbar region 🔹🔹

    Q76.426 Congenital lordosis, lumbar region 🔹🔹

    Q76.427 Congenital lordosis, lumbosacral region 🔹🔹

    Q76.428 Congenital lordosis, sacral and sacrococcygeal region 🔹🔹

    Q76.429 Congenital lordosis, unspecified region 🔹🔹

    Q76.49 Other congenital malformations of spine, not associated with scoliosis 🔹
Congenital absence of vertebra NOS
Congenital fusion of spine NOS
Congenital malformation of lumbosacral (joint) (region) NOS
Congenital malformation of spine NOS
Hemivertebra NOS
Malformation of spine NOS
Platyspondylisis NOS
Supernumerary vertebra NOS

Q76.5 Cervical rib 🔹
Supernumerary rib in cervical region

Q76.6 Other congenital malformations of ribs 🔹🔹
Accessory rib
Congenital absence of rib
Congenital fusion of ribs
Congenital malformation of ribs NOS
    Excludes1 short rib syndrome (Q77.2)
Ⓔ Q76.5-Q76.9, Q77.2

Q76.7 Congenital malformation of sternum 🔹🔹
Congenital absence of sternum
Sternum bifidum
Ⓔ Q76.5-Q76.9, Q77.2

Q76.8 Other congenital malformations of bony thorax 🔹🔹
Ⓔ Q76.5-Q76.9, Q77.2

Q76.9 Congenital malformation of bony thorax, unspecified 🔹🔹
Ⓔ Q76.5-Q76.9, Q77.2

● **Q77 Osteochondrodysplasia with defects of growth of tubular bones and spine**
    Excludes1 mucopolysaccharidosis (E76.0-E76.3)
    Excludes2 congenital myotonic chondrodystrophy (G71.13)

Q77.0 Achondrogenesis 🔹
Hypochondrogenesis

Q77.1 Thanatophoric short stature 🔹

Q77.2 Short rib syndrome 🔹🔹
Asphyxiating thoracic dysplasia [Jeune]
Ⓔ Q76.5-Q76.9, Q77.2

Q77.3 Chondrodysplasia punctata 🔹
Benign cartilaginous neoplasms
    Excludes1 rhizomelic chondrodysplasia punctata (E71.43)

Q77.4 Achondroplasia 🔹
Disturbance of epiphyseal chondroblastic growth and maturation, results in dwarfism
Hypochondroplasia
Osteosclerosis congenita

Q77.5 Diastrophic dysplasia 🔹

Q77.6 Chondroectodermal dysplasia 🔹
Defective development of skin, hair, teeth, with polydactyly and defect of cardiac septum
Ellis-van Creveld syndrome

Q77.7 Spondyloepiphyseal dysplasia 🔹

Q77.8 Other osteochondrodysplasia with defects of growth of tubular bones and spine 🔹

Q77.9 Osteochondrodysplasia with defects of growth of tubular bones and spine, unspecified 🔹

● **Q78 Other osteochondrodysplasias**
Disorder of development of bone and cartilage; common cause of dwarfism
    Excludes2 congenital myotonic chondrodystrophy (G71.13)

Q78.0 Osteogenesis imperfecta 🔹🔹
Fragilitas ossium
Osteopsathyrosis
Ⓔ Q77.3, Q77.6, Q78.0-Q78.3, Q78.5-Q78.9

Q78.1 Polyostotic fibrous dysplasia 🔹
Albright(-McCune)(-Sternberg) syndrome
Ⓔ See Q78.0

Q78.2 Osteopetrosis 🔹🔹
Abnormally dense bone; AKA marble bones disease, ivory bones
Albers-Schönberg syndrome
Osteosclerosis NOS

Q78.3 Progressive diaphyseal dysplasia 🔹
Camurati-Engelmann syndrome

Q78.4 Enchondromatosis 🔹
Thinning of overlying cortex of bone and distorted length
Maffucci's syndrome
Ollier's disease

Q78.5 Metaphyseal dysplasia 🔹
Disturbance in enchondral bone growth, causing ends of shafts to remain larger than normal in circumference
Pyle's syndrome

Q78.6 Multiple congenital exostoses 🔹
Diaphyseal aclasis

Q78.8 Other specified osteochondrodysplasias 🔹
Osteopoikilosis

Q78.9 Osteochondrodysplasia, unspecified 🔹
Chondrodystrophy NOS
AKA skeletal dysplasia (dwarfism) caused by genetic mutations affecting hyaline cartilage capping long bones and vertebrae
Osteodystrophy NOS

◀ New   ◀ Revised   ~~deleted~~ Deleted   Excludes 1   Excludes 2   Includes   Use additional   Code first   Code also   Unspecified

OGCR Official Guidelines   ● Unacceptable Principal Diagnosis   **X** Assign placeholder X   ◗ Use Additional Character(s)   ▌ Manifestation Code   **Coding Clinic**

● **Q79** **Congenital malformations of musculoskeletal system, not elsewhere classified**

　　Excludes2　congenital (sternomastoid) torticollis (Q68.0)

Q79.0 **Congenital diaphragmatic hernia** 🕮🕮🕮

　　Excludes1　congenital hiatus hernia (Q40.1)

　　Ⓔⓧ Q40.1, Q79.0-Q79.1

Q79.1 **Other congenital malformations of diaphragm** 🕮🕮

　　Absence of diaphragm
　　Congenital malformation of diaphragm NOS
　　Eventration of diaphragm

　　Ⓔⓧ Q40.1, Q79.0-Q79.1

Q79.2 **Exomphalos** 🕮🕮

　　Abdominal hernia in which part of intestine protrudes at umbilicus; AKA exomphalos and exumbilication
　　Omphalocele

　　Excludes1　umbilical hernia (K42.-)

　　Ⓔⓧ Q79.2-Q79.59

Q79.3 **Gastroschisis** 🕮🕮

　　Congenital fissure of anterior abdominal wall often with protrusion of small/large intestine

　　Ⓔⓧ Q79.2-Q79.59

Q79.4 **Prune belly syndrome** 🕮🕮

　　Congenital prolapse of bladder mucosa
　　Eagle-Barrett syndrome

　　Ⓔⓧ Q79.2-Q79.59

● **Q79.5** **Other congenital malformations of abdominal wall**

　　Excludes1　umbilical hernia (K42.-)

　　Ⓔⓧ For category Q79.5 CC codes: Q79.2-Q79.59

　　Q79.51 **Congenital hernia of bladder** 🕮🕮

　　Q79.59 **Other congenital malformations of abdominal wall** 🕮🕮

Q79.6 **Ehlers-Danlos syndrome** 🕮🕮

　　Ⓔⓧ Q79.6

　　Group of inherited disorders of connective tissue; AKA cutis hyperelastica

Q79.8 **Other congenital malformations of musculoskeletal system** 🕮

　　Absence of muscle
　　Absence of tendon
　　Accessory muscle
　　Amyotrophia congenita
　　Congenital constricting bands
　　Congenital shortening of tendon
　　Poland syndrome

Q79.9 **Congenital malformation of musculoskeletal system, unspecified** 🕮

　　Congenital anomaly of musculoskeletal system NOS
　　Congenital deformity of musculoskeletal system NOS

OTHER CONGENITAL MALFORMATIONS (Q80-Q89)

● **Q80** **Congenital ichthyosis**

　　Characterized by increased keratinization, resulting in noninflammatory scaling of skin

　　Excludes1　Refsum's disease (G60.1)

Q80.0 **Ichthyosis vulgaris** 🕮

Q80.1 **X-linked ichthyosis** 🕮

Q80.2 **Lamellar ichthyosis** 🕮

　　Collodion baby

Q80.3 **Congenital bullous ichthyosiform erythroderma** 🕮

Q80.4 **Harlequin fetus** 🕮

Q80.8 **Other congenital ichthyosis** 🕮

Q80.9 **Congenital ichthyosis, unspecified** 🕮

● **Q81** **Epidermolysis bullosa**

　　Loosening of epidermis

Q81.0 **Epidermolysis bullosa simplex** 🕮

　　Excludes1　Cockayne's syndrome (Q87.1)

Q81.1 **Epidermolysis bullosa letalis** 🕮

　　Herlitz' syndrome

Q81.2 **Epidermolysis bullosa dystrophica** 🕮

Q81.8 **Other epidermolysis bullosa** 🕮

Q81.9 **Epidermolysis bullosa, unspecified** 🕮

● **Q82** **Other congenital malformations of skin**

　　Excludes1　acrodermatitis enteropathica (E83.2)
　　　　　　　congenital erythropoietic porphyria (E80.0)
　　　　　　　pilonidal cyst or sinus (L05.-)
　　　　　　　Sturge-Weber (-Dimitri) syndrome (Q85.8)

Q82.0 **Hereditary lymphedema** 🕮

　　Characterized by swelling of subcutaneous tissue caused by obstruction of lymphatic vessels and resulting edema of lymph fluid

Q82.1 **Xeroderma pigmentosum** 🕮

　　Dry, rough, discolored state of skin, and formation of scaly desquamation

Q82.2 **Mastocytosis** 🕮

　　Characterized by infiltrates of mast cells in tissues/organs
　　Urticaria pigmentosa

　　Excludes1　malignant mastocytosis (C96.2)

Q82.3 **Incontinentia pigmenti** 🕮

　　Characterized by hyperpigmented cutaneous

Q82.4 **Ectodermal dysplasia (anhidrotic)** 🕮

　　Absence/deficiency of tissues/structures, including teeth, hair, nails, and certain glands

　　Excludes1　Ellis-van Creveld syndrome (Q77.6)

Q82.5 **Congenital non-neoplastic nevus** 🕮

　　Birthmark NOS
　　Flammeus Nevus
　　Portwine Nevus
　　Sanguineous Nevus
　　Strawberry Nevus
　　Vascular Nevus NOS
　　Verrucous Nevus

　　Excludes2　Café au lait spots (L81.3)
　　　　　　　lentigo (L81.4)
　　　　　　　nevus NOS (D22.-)
　　　　　　　araneus nevus (I78.1)
　　　　　　　melanocytic nevus (D22.-)
　　　　　　　pigmented nevus (D22.-)
　　　　　　　spider nevus (I78.1)
　　　　　　　stellar nevus (I78.1)

Q82.8 **Other specified congenital malformations of skin** 🕮

　　Abnormal palmar creases
　　Accessory skin tags
　　Benign familial pemphigus [Hailey-Hailey]
　　Congenital poikiloderma
　　Cutis laxa (hyperelastica)
　　Dermatoglyphic anomalies
　　Inherited keratosis palmaris et plantaris
　　Keratosis follicularis [Darier-White]

　　Excludes1　Ehlers-Danlos syndrome (Q79.6)

Q82.9 **Congenital malformation of skin, unspecified** 🕮

● **Q83** **Congenital malformations of breast**

　　Excludes2　absence of pectoral muscle (Q79.8)
　　　　　　　hypoplasia of breast (N64.82)
　　　　　　　micromastia (N64.82)

Q83.0 **Congenital absence of breast with absent nipple** 🕮

Q83.1 **Accessory breast** 🕮

　　Supernumerary breast

Q83.2 **Absent nipple** 🕮

Q83.3 **Accessory nipple** 🕮

　　Supernumerary nipple

Q83.8 **Other congenital malformations of breast** 🕮

Q83.9 **Congenital malformation of breast, unspecified** 🕮

CHAPTER 17 (Q00-Q99)

N Newborn Age: 0　　　**P** Pediatric Age: 0–17　　　**M** Maternity DX: 12–55　　　**A** Adult Age: 15–124　　　♀ Females Only　　　♂ Males Only

🕮 Complication\Comorbidity　　　🕮 Major C\C　　　Ⓔⓧ CC/MCC Exclusions　　　🕮 Present on Admission Requirement　　　🕮 Hospital-Acquired Condition

1265

● **Q84   Other congenital malformations of integument**

Q84.0   **Congenital alopecia** 🔗
Congenital atrichosis

Q84.1   **Congenital morphological disturbances of hair, not elsewhere classified** 🔗
Beaded hair
Monilethrix
Pili annulati
Excludes1   Menkes' kinky hair syndrome (E83.0)

Q84.2   **Other congenital malformations of hair** 🔗
Congenital hypertrichosis
Congenital malformation of hair NOS
Persistent lanugo

Q84.3   **Anonychia** 🔗
Absence of nail
Excludes1   nail patella syndrome (Q87.2)

Q84.4   **Congenital leukonychia** 🔗
Opaque, whitish discoloration of nails; AKA leukopathia unguium

Q84.5   **Enlarged and hypertrophic nails** 🔗
Congenital onychauxis
Pachyonychia

Q84.6   **Other congenital malformations of nails** 🔗
Congenital clubnail
Congenital koilonychia
Congenital malformation of nail NOS

Q84.8   **Other specified congenital malformations of integument** 🔗
Aplasia cutis congenita

Q84.9   **Congenital malformation of integument, unspecified** 🔗
Congenital anomaly of integument NOS
Congenital deformity of integument NOS

● **Q85   Phakomatoses, not elsewhere classified**
Excludes1   ataxia telangiectasia [Louis-Bar] (G11.3)
familial dysautonomia [Riley-Day] (G90.1)

● Q85.0   **Neurofibromatosis (nonmalignant)**
Developmental changes in nervous system and other structures, with formation of neurofibromas

Q85.00   **Neurofibromatosis, unspecified** 🔗

Q85.01   **Neurofibromatosis, type 1** 🔗
Von Recklinghausen disease

Q85.02   **Neurofibromatosis, type 2** 🔗
Acoustic neurofibromatosis

Q85.03   **Schwannomatosis** 🔗

Q85.09   **Other neurofibromatosis** 🔗

Q85.1   **Tuberous sclerosis** 🔗🔗
Bourneville's disease
Epiloia
Ⓔ Q85.1-Q85.9, Q89.7, Q89.9

Q85.8   **Other phakomatoses, not elsewhere classified** 🔗🔗
Peutz-Jeghers Syndrome
Sturge-Weber(-Dimitri) syndrome
von Hippel-Lindau syndrome
Excludes1   Meckel-Gruber syndrome (Q61.9)
Ⓔ Q85.8-Q85.9, Q89.9

Q85.9   **Phakomatosis, unspecified** 🔗🔗
Hamartosis NOS
Ⓔ Q85.8-Q85.9, Q89.9

● **Q86   Congenital malformation syndromes due to known exogenous causes, not elsewhere classified**
Excludes2   iodine-deficiency-related hypothyroidism (E00-E02)
nonteratogenic effects of substances transmitted via placenta or breast milk (P04.-)

Q86.0   **Fetal alcohol syndrome (dysmorphic)** 🔗

Q86.1   **Fetal hydantoin syndrome** 🔗   N
Meadow's syndrome

Q86.2   **Dysmorphism due to warfarin** 🔗

Q86.8   **Other congenital malformation syndromes due to known exogenous causes** 🔗

● **Q87   Other specified congenital malformation syndromes affecting multiple systems**
Use additional code(s) to identify all associated manifestations

Q87.0   **Congenital malformation syndromes predominantly affecting facial appearance** 🔗
Acrocephalopolysyndactyly
Acrocephalosyndactyly [Apert]
Cryptophthalmos syndrome
Cyclopia
Goldenhar syndrome
Moebius syndrome
Oro-facial-digital syndrome
Robin syndrome
Whistling face

Q87.1   **Congenital malformation syndromes predominantly associated with short stature** 🔗🔗
Aarskog syndrome
Cockayne syndrome
De Lange syndrome
Dubowitz syndrome
Noonan syndrome
Prader-Willi syndrome
Robinow-Silverman-Smith syndrome
Russell-Silver syndrome
Seckel syndrome
Excludes1   Ellis-van Creveld syndrome (Q77.6)
Smith-Lemli-Opitz syndrome (E78.72)
Ⓔ E78.71-E78.72, Q85.8-Q85.9, Q87.1-Q87.89, Q89.7-Q89.9, Q99.2

Q87.2   **Congenital malformation syndromes predominantly involving limbs** 🔗🔗
Holt-Oram syndrome
Klippel-Trenaunay-Weber syndrome
Nail patella syndrome
Rubinstein-Taybi syndrome
Sirenomelia syndrome
Thrombocytopenia with absent radius [TAR] syndrome
VATER syndrome
Ⓔ E78.71-E78.72, Q87.1-Q87.89, Q89.8, Q99.2

Q87.3   **Congenital malformation syndromes involving early overgrowth**
Beckwith-Wiedemann syndrome
Sotos' syndrome
Weaver syndrome
Ⓔ See Q87.2

● Q87.4   **Marfan's syndrome**
Ⓔ For category Q87.4 CC codes: See Q87.1

Q87.40   **Marfan's syndrome, unspecified** 🔗🔗

● Q87.41   **Marfan's syndrome with cardiovascular manifestations**

Q87.410   **Marfan's syndrome with aortic dilation** 🔗🔗

Q87.418   **Marfan's syndrome with other cardiovascular manifestations** 🔗🔗

Q87.42   **Marfan's syndrome with ocular manifestations** 🔗🔗

Q87.43   **Marfan's syndrome with skeletal manifestation** 🔗🔗

Q87.5   **Other congenital malformation syndromes with other skeletal changes** 🔗🔗
Ⓔ See Q87.2

● Q87.8   **Other specified congenital malformation syndromes, not elsewhere classified**
Excludes1   Zellweger syndrome (E71.510)
Ⓔ For category Q87.8 CC codes: See Q87.2

Q87.81   **Alport syndrome** 🔗🔗
Progressive sensorineural hearing loss, progressive pyelonephritis or glomerulonephritis, and ocular defects
Use additional code to identify stage of chronic kidney disease (N18.1-N18.6)

Q87.89   **Other specified congenital malformation syndromes, not elsewhere classified** 🔗🔗
Laurence-Moon (-Bardet)-Biedl syndrome

◄ New   ⬕ Revised   ~~deleted~~ Deleted   Excludes 1   Excludes 2   Includes   Use additional   Code first   Code also   Unspecified
OGCR Official Guidelines   ● Unacceptable Principal Diagnosis   X Assign placeholder X   ● Use Additional Character(s)   ▶ Manifestation Code   **Coding Clinic**

● **Q89 Other congenital malformations, not elsewhere classified**
  ● **Q89.0 Congenital absence and malformations of spleen**
      Excludes1   isomerism of atrial appendages (with asplenia or polysplenia) (Q20.6)
      (Ex) **For category Q87.8 CC codes:** Q89.01-Q89.09, Q89.9

      Q89.01   Asplenia (congenital) 🖐🖐
      Q89.09   Congenital malformations of spleen 🖐🖐
              Congenital splenomegaly
  Q89.1 Congenital malformations of adrenal gland 🖐
      Excludes1   adrenogenital disorders (E25.-)
              congenital adrenal hyperplasia (E25.0)
  Q89.2 Congenital malformations of other endocrine glands 🖐
          Congenital malformation of parathyroid or thyroid
              gland
          Persistent thyroglossal duct
          Thyroglossal cyst
      Excludes1   congenital goiter (E03.0)
              congenital hypothyroidism (E03.1)
  Q89.3 Situs inversus 🖐🖐
          Lateral transposition of viscera of thorax and abdomen
          Dextrocardia with situs inversus
          Mirror-image atrial arrangement with situs inversus
          Situs inversus or transversus abdominalis
          Situs inversus or transversus thoracis
          Transposition of abdominal viscera
          Transposition of thoracic viscera
      Excludes1   dextrocardia NOS (Q24.0)
          (Ex) Q89.3, Q89.7, Q89.9
  Q89.4 Conjoined twins 🖐🖐
          Craniopagus
          Dicephaly
          Pygopagus
          Thoracopagus
          (Ex) Q89.4-Q89.7, Q89.9
  Q89.7 Multiple congenital malformations, not elsewhere classified 🖐🖐
          Multiple congenital anomalies NOS
          Multiple congenital deformities NOS
      Excludes1   congenital malformation syndromes affecting multiple systems (Q87.-)
          (Ex) Q89.3, Q89.7, Q89.9
  Q89.8 Other specified congenital malformations 🖐🖐
          Use additional code(s) to identify all associated manifestations
          (Ex) See Q87.2
  Q89.9 Congenital malformation, unspecified 🖐
          Congenital anomaly NOS
          Congenital deformity NOS

CHROMOSOMAL ABNORMALITIES, NOT ELSEWHERE CLASSIFIED (Q90-Q99)

      Excludes2   mitochondrial metabolic disorders (E88.4-)

● **Q90 Down syndrome**
          Use additional code(s) to identify any associated physical conditions and degree of intellectual disabilities (F70-F79)
  Q90.0 Trisomy 21, nonmosaicism (meiotic nondisjunction) 🖐
  Q90.1 Trisomy 21, mosaicism (mitotic nondisjunction) 🖐
  Q90.2 Trisomy 21, translocation 🖐
  Q90.9 Down syndrome, unspecified 🖐
          Trisomy 21 NOS

● **Q91 Trisomy 18 and Trisomy 13**
      (Ex) **For category Q91 CC codes:** Q90.0-Q99.1, Q99.8-Q99.9
  Q91.0 Trisomy 18, nonmosaicism (meiotic nondisjunction) 🖐🖐
  Q91.1 Trisomy 18, mosaicism (mitotic nondisjunction) 🖐🖐
  Q91.2 Trisomy 18, translocation 🖐🖐
  Q91.3 Trisomy 18, unspecified 🖐🖐
  Q91.4 Trisomy 13, nonmosaicism (meiotic nondisjunction) 🖐🖐
  Q91.5 Trisomy 13, mosaicism (mitotic nondisjunction) 🖐🖐
  Q91.6 Trisomy 13, translocation 🖐🖐
  Q91.7 Trisomy 13, unspecified 🖐🖐

● **Q92 Other trisomies and partial trisomies of the autosomes, not elsewhere classified**
      Includes   unbalanced translocations and insertions
      Excludes1   trisomies of chromosomes 13, 18, 21 (Q90-Q91)
  Q92.0 Whole chromosome trisomy, nonmosaicism (meiotic nondisjunction) 🖐
  Q92.1 Whole chromosome trisomy, mosaicism (mitotic nondisjunction) 🖐
  Q92.2 Partial trisomy 🖐
          Less than whole arm duplicated
          Whole arm or more duplicated
      Excludes1   partial trisomy due to unbalanced translocation (Q92.5)
  Q92.5 Duplications with other complex rearrangements 🖐
          Partial trisomy due to unbalanced translocations
          Code also any associated deletions due to unbalanced translocations, inversions and insertions (Q93.7)
  ● **Q92.6 Marker chromosomes**
          Trisomies due to dicentrics
          Trisomies due to extra rings
          Trisomies due to isochromosomes
          Individual with marker heterochromatin
      Q92.61   Marker chromosomes in normal individual 🖐
      Q92.62   Marker chromosomes in abnormal individual 🖐
  Q92.7 Triploidy and polyploidy 🖐
  Q92.8 Other specified trisomies and partial trisomies of autosomes 🖐
          Duplications identified by fluorescence in situ hybridization (FISH)
          Duplications identified by in situ hybridization (ISH)
          Duplications seen only at prometaphase
  Q92.9 Trisomy and partial trisomy of autosomes, unspecified 🖐

● **Q93 Monosomies and deletions from the autosomes, not elsewhere classified**
      (Ex) **For category Q93 CC codes unless otherwise indicated:** Q90.0-Q99.1, Q99.8-Q99.9
  Q93.0 Whole chromosome monosomy, nonmosaicism (meiotic nondisjunction) 🖐
  Q93.1 Whole chromosome monosomy, mosaicism (mitotic nondisjunction) 🖐
  Q93.2 Chromosome replaced with ring, dicentric or isochromosome 🖐
  Q93.3 Deletion of short arm of chromosome 4 🖐🖐
          Wolff-Hirschorn syndrome
  Q93.4 Deletion of short arm of chromosome 5 🖐🖐
          Cri-du-chat syndrome
          (Ex) Q90.0-Q99.1, Q99.8-Q99.9
  Q93.5 Other deletions of part of a chromosome 🖐🖐
          Angelman syndrome
  Q93.7 Deletions with other complex rearrangements 🖐🖐
          Deletions due to unbalanced translocations, inversions and insertions
          Code also any associated duplications due to unbalanced translocations, inversions and insertions (Q92.5)

CHAPTER 17 (Q00-Q99)

N	Newborn Age: 0	P	Pediatric Age: 0–17	M	Maternity DX: 12–55	A	Adult Age: 15–124	♀	Females Only	♂	Males Only
🖐 Complication\Comorbidity		🖐 Major C\C		(Ex) CC/MCC Exclusions		Present on Admission Requirement		🖐 Hospital-Acquired Condition			

● **Q93.8   Other deletions from the autosomes**

     Q93.81   Velo-cardio-facial syndrome 🐾 🐾

           Deletion 22q11.2

           (Ex:) Q90.0-Q99.1, Q99.8-Q99.9

     Q93.88   Other microdeletions Miller-Dieker syndrome 🐾 🐾

           Smith-Magenis syndrome

           (Ex:) Q90.0-Q99.1, Q99.8-Q99.9

     Q93.89   Other deletions from the autosomes 🐾 🐾

           Deletions identified by fluorescence in situ hybridization (FISH)

           Deletions identified by in situ hybridization (ISH)

           Deletions seen only at prometaphase

    Q93.9   Deletion from autosomes, unspecified 🐾 🐾

● **Q95   Balanced rearrangements and structural markers, not elsewhere classified**

     Includes   Robertsonian and balanced reciprocal translocations and insertions

    Q95.0   Balanced translocation and insertion in normal individual 🐾

    Q95.1   Chromosome inversion in normal individual 🐾

    Q95.2   Balanced autosomal rearrangement in abnormal individual 🐾

    Q95.3   Balanced sex/autosomal rearrangement in abnormal individual 🐾

    Q95.5   Individual with autosomal fragile site 🐾

    Q95.8   Other balanced rearrangements and structural markers 🐾

    Q95.9   Balanced rearrangement and structural marker, unspecified 🐾

● **Q96   Turner's syndrome**

     Caused by missing or incomplete X chromosome affecting growth and sexual development

     Excludes1   Noonan syndrome (Q87.1)

    Q96.0   Karyotype 45, X ♀ 🐾

    Q96.1   Karyotype 46, X iso (Xq) ♀ 🐾

           Karyotype 46, isochromosome Xq

    Q96.2   Karyotype 46, X with abnormal sex chromosome, except iso (Xq) ♀ 🐾

           Karyotype 46, X with abnormal sex chromosome, except isochromosome Xq

    Q96.3   Mosaicism, 45, X/46, XX or XY ♀ 🐾

    Q96.4   Mosaicism, 45, X/other cell line(s) with abnormal sex chromosome ♀ 🐾

    Q96.8   Other variants of Turner's syndrome ♀ 🐾

    Q96.9   Turner's syndrome, unspecified ♀ 🐾

● **Q97   Other sex chromosome abnormalities, female phenotype, not elsewhere classified**

     Excludes1   Turner's syndrome (Q96.-)

    Q97.0   Karyotype 47, XXX ♀ 🐾

    Q97.1   Female with more than three X chromosomes ♀ 🐾

    Q97.2   Mosaicism, lines with various numbers of X chromosomes ♀ 🐾

    Q97.3   Female with 46, XY karyotype ♀ 🐾

    Q97.8   Other specified sex chromosome abnormalities, female phenotype ♀ 🐾

    Q97.9   Sex chromosome abnormality, female phenotype, unspecified ♀ 🐾

● **Q98   Other sex chromosome abnormalities, male phenotype, not elsewhere classified**

    Q98.0   Klinefelter syndrome karyotype 47, XXY ♂ 🐾

    Q98.1   Klinefelter syndrome, male with more than two X chromosomes ♂ 🐾

    Q98.3   Other male with 46, XX karyotype ♂ 🐾

    Q98.4   Klinefelter syndrome, unspecified ♂ 🐾

    Q98.5   Karyotype 47, XYY 🐾

    Q98.6   Male with structurally abnormal sex chromosome ♂ 🐾

    Q98.7   Male with sex chromosome mosaicism ♂ 🐾

    Q98.8   Other specified sex chromosome abnormalities, male phenotype ♂ 🐾

    Q98.9   Sex chromosome abnormality, male phenotype, unspecified ♂ 🐾

● **Q99   Other chromosome abnormalities, not elsewhere classified**

    Q99.0   Chimera 46, XX/46, XY 🐾

           Chimera 46, XX/46, XY true hermaphrodite

    Q99.1   46, XX true hermaphrodite 🐾

           46, XX with streak gonads

           46, XY with streak gonads

           Pure gonadal dysgenesis

    Q99.2   Fragile X chromosome 🐾

           Fragile X syndrome

    Q99.8   Other specified chromosome abnormalities 🐾

    Q99.9   Chromosomal abnormality, unspecified 🐾

CHAPTER 17 (Q00-Q99)

◀ New   ◀━ Revised   ~~deleted~~ Deleted   Excludes 1   Excludes 2   Includes   Use additional   Code first   Code also   Unspecified

OGCR Official Guidelines   ● Unacceptable Principal Diagnosis   X Assign placeholder X   ● Use Additional Character(s)   ▌ Manifestation Code   **Coding Clinic**

OGCR Section I.B.4.

Signs and symptoms

Codes that describe symptoms and signs, as opposed to diagnoses, are acceptable for reporting purposes when a related definitive diagnosis has not been established (confirmed) by the provider. Chapter 18 of ICD-10-CM, Symptoms, Signs, and Abnormal Clinical and Laboratory Findings, Not Elsewhere Classified (codes R00.0-R99) contains many, but not all codes for symptoms.

Section I.C.18.a. to c.

Symptoms, signs, and abnormal clinical and laboratory findings, not elsewhere classified.

Chapter 18 includes symptoms, signs, abnormal results of clinical or other investigative procedures, and ill-defined conditions regarding which no diagnosis classifiable elsewhere is recorded. Signs and symptoms that point to a specific diagnosis have been assigned to a category in other chapters of the classification.

a. Use of symptom codes

Codes that describe symptoms and signs are acceptable for reporting purposes when a related definitive diagnosis has not been established (confirmed) by the provider.

b. Use of a symptom code with a definitive diagnosis code

Codes for signs and symptoms may be reported in addition to a related definitive diagnosis when the sign or symptom is not routinely associated with that diagnosis, such as the various signs and symptoms associated with complex syndromes. The definitive diagnosis code should be sequenced before the symptom code.

Signs or symptoms that are associated routinely with a disease process should not be assigned as additional codes, unless otherwise instructed by the classification.

c. Combination codes that include symptoms

ICD-10-CM contains a number of combination codes that identify both the definitive diagnosis and common symptoms of that diagnosis. When using one of these combination codes, an additional code should not be assigned for the symptom.

CHAPTER 18

SYMPTOMS, SIGNS AND ABNORMAL CLINICAL AND LABORATORY FINDINGS, NOT ELSEWHERE CLASSIFIED (R00-R99)

Note: This chapter includes symptoms, signs, abnormal results of clinical or other investigative procedures, and ill-defined conditions regarding which no diagnosis classifiable elsewhere is recorded.

Signs and symptoms that point rather definitely to a given diagnosis have been assigned to a category in other chapters of the classification. In general, categories in this chapter include the less well-defined conditions and symptoms that, without the necessary study of the case to establish a final diagnosis, point perhaps equally to two or more diseases or to two or more systems of the body. Practically all categories in the chapter could be designated 'not otherwise specified', 'unknown etiology' or 'transient'. The Alphabetical Index should be consulted to determine which symptoms and signs are to be allocated here and which to other chapters. The residual subcategories, numbered .8, are generally provided for other relevant symptoms that cannot be allocated elsewhere in the classification.

The conditions and signs or symptoms included in categories R00-R94 consist of:
(a) cases for which no more specific diagnosis can be made even after all the facts bearing on the case have been investigated; ◀━━
(b) signs or symptoms existing at the time of initial encounter that proved to be transient and whose causes could not be determined;
(c) provisional diagnosis in a patient who failed to return for further investigation or care;

(d) cases referred elsewhere for investigation or treatment before the diagnosis was made;
(e) cases in which a more precise diagnosis was not available for any other reason;
(f) certain symptoms, for which supplementary information is provided, that represent important problems in medical care in their own right.

  Excludes2   abnormal findings on antenatal screening of mother (O28.-)
                  certain conditions originating in the perinatal period (P04-P96)
                  signs and symptoms classified in the body system chapters
                  signs and symptoms of breast (N63, N64.5)

This chapter contains the following blocks:

R00-R09	Symptoms and signs involving the circulatory and respiratory systems
R10-R19	Symptoms and signs involving the digestive system and abdomen
R20-R23	Symptoms and signs involving the skin and subcutaneous tissue
R25-R29	Symptoms and signs involving the nervous and musculoskeletal systems
R30-R39	Symptoms and signs involving the genitourinary system
R40-R46	Symptoms and signs involving cognition, perception, emotional state and behavior
R47-R49	Symptoms and signs involving speech and voice
R50-R69	General symptoms and signs
R70-R79	Abnormal findings on examination of blood, without diagnosis
R80-R82	Abnormal findings on examination of urine, without diagnosis
R83-R89	Abnormal findings on examination of other body fluids, substances and tissues, without diagnosis
R90-R94	Abnormal findings on diagnostic imaging and in function studies, without diagnosis
R97	Abnormal tumor markers
R99	Ill-defined and unknown cause of mortality

SYMPTOMS AND SIGNS INVOLVING THE CIRCULATORY AND RESPIRATORY SYSTEMS (R00-R09)

● **R00**   **Abnormalities of heart beat**
  Excludes1   abnormalities originating in the perinatal period (P29.1-)
                  specified arrhythmias (I47-I49)

R00.0   **Tachycardia, unspecified**
            Rapid heart rate >100 beats
            Rapid heart beat
            Sinoauricular tachycardia NOS
            Sinus [sinusal] tachycardia NOS
  Excludes1   neonatal tachycardia (P29.11)
                  paroxysmal tachycardia (I47.-)

R00.1   **Bradycardia, unspecified**
            Slow heart rate, <60
            Sinoatrial bradycardia
            Sinus bradycardia
            Slow heart beat
            Vagal bradycardia
            Use additional code for adverse effect, if applicable, to identify drug (T36-T50 with fifth or sixth character 5)
  Excludes1   neonatal bradycardia (P29.12)

R00.2   **Palpitations**
            Awareness of heart beat

R00.8   **Other abnormalities of heart beat**

R00.9   **Unspecified abnormalities of heart beat**

CHAPTER 18 (R00-R99)

R01 Cardiac murmurs and other cardiac sounds

Excludes1 cardiac murmurs and sounds originating in the perinatal period (P29.8)

R01.0 Benign and innocent cardiac murmurs
Functional cardiac murmur

R01.1 Cardiac murmur, unspecified
Cardiac bruit NOS
Heart murmur NOS

R01.2 Other cardiac sounds
Cardiac dullness, increased or decreased
Precordial friction

OGCR Section I.C.9.a.7.

Hypertension, Transient
Assign code R03.0, Elevated blood pressure reading without diagnosis of hypertension, unless patient has an established diagnosis of hypertension. Assign code O13.-, Gestational [pregnancy-induced] hypertension with significant proteinuria, or O14.-, Pre-eclampsia, for transient hypertension of pregnancy.

R03 Abnormal blood-pressure reading, without diagnosis

R03.0 Elevated blood-pressure reading, without diagnosis of hypertension
Note: This category is to be used to record an episode of elevated blood pressure in a patient in whom no formal diagnosis of hypertension has been made, or as an isolated incidental finding.
MCE: Questionable admission when principal dx

R03.1 Nonspecific low blood-pressure reading
Excludes1 hypotension (I95.-)
maternal hypotension syndrome (O26.5-)
neurogenic orthostatic hypotension (G90.3)

R04 Hemorrhage from respiratory passages

(Ex) For category R04 CC codes: R04.2-R04.9, R09.3, R68.13

R04.0 Epistaxis
Hemorrhage from nose
Nosebleed

R04.1 Hemorrhage from throat
Excludes2 hemoptysis (R04.2)

R04.2 Hemoptysis
Blood-stained sputum
Cough with hemorrhage

R04.8 Hemorrhage from other sites in respiratory passages

R04.81 Acute idiopathic pulmonary hemorrhage in infants P
AIPHI
Acute idiopathic hemorrhage in infants over 28 days old
Excludes1 perinatal pulmonary hemorrhage (P26.-)
von Willebrand's disease (D68.0)

R04.89 Hemorrhage from other sites in respiratory passages
Pulmonary hemorrhage NOS

R04.9 Hemorrhage from respiratory passages, unspecified

R05 Cough

Excludes1 cough with hemorrhage (R04.2)
smoker's cough (J41.0)

R06 Abnormalities of breathing

Excludes1 acute respiratory distress syndrome (J80)
respiratory arrest (R09.2)
respiratory arrest of newborn (P28.81)
respiratory distress syndrome of newborn (P22.-)
respiratory failure (J96.-)
respiratory failure of newborn (P28.5)

R06.0 Dyspnea

Excludes1 tachypnea NOS (R06.82)
transient tachypnea of newborn (P22.1)

R06.00 Dyspnea, unspecified
R06.01 Orthopnea
R06.02 Shortness of breath
R06.09 Other forms of dyspnea

R06.1 Stridor
Harsh, high-pitched breath sound
Excludes1 congenital laryngeal stridor (P28.89)
laryngismus (stridulus) (J38.5)

R06.2 Wheezing
Excludes1 Asthma (J45.-)

R06.3 Periodic breathing
Cheyne-Stokes breathing
An abnormal pattern of breathing with gradually increasing and decreasing tidal volume with some periods of apnea
(Ex) J22, J80, J96.00-J96.92, J98.8-J98.9, R06.3, R06.81, R09.2

R06.4 Hyperventilation
Excludes1 psychogenic hyperventilation (F45.8)

R06.5 Mouth breathing
Excludes2 dry mouth NOS (R68.2)

R06.6 Hiccough
Excludes1 psychogenic hiccough (F45.8)

R06.7 Sneezing

R06.8 Other abnormalities of breathing

R06.81 Apnea, not elsewhere classified
Apnea NOS
Excludes1 apnea (of) newborn (P28.4)
sleep apnea (G47.3-)
sleep apnea of newborn (primary) (P28.3)

R06.82 Tachypnea, not elsewhere classified
Tachypnea NOS
Excludes1 transitory tachypnea of newborn (P22.1)

R06.83 Snoring
R06.89 Other abnormalities of breathing
Breath-holding (spells)
Sighing

R06.9 Unspecified abnormalities of breathing

R07 Pain in throat and chest

Excludes1 epidemic myalgia (B33.0)
Excludes2 jaw pain R68.84
pain in breast (N64.4)

R07.0 Pain in throat
Excludes1 chronic sore throat (J31.2)
sore throat (acute) NOS (J02.9)
Excludes2 dysphagia (R13.1-)
pain in neck (M54.2)

R07.1 Chest pain on breathing
Painful respiration

R07.2 Precordial pain

R07.8 Other chest pain

R07.81 Pleurodynia
Pleurodynia NOS
Excludes1 epidemic pleurodynia (B33.0)

R07.82 Intercostal pain
R07.89 Other chest pain
Anterior chest-wall pain NOS

R07.9 Chest pain, unspecified

Legend: New | Revised | deleted Deleted | Excludes 1 | Excludes 2 | Includes | Use additional | Code first | Code also | Unspecified | OGCR Official Guidelines | Unacceptable Principal Diagnosis | X Assign placeholder X | Use Additional Character(s) | Manifestation Code | Coding Clinic

● **R09**   **Other symptoms and signs involving the circulatory and respiratory system**

> **Excludes1**   acute respiratory distress syndrome (J80)
> respiratory arrest of newborn (P28.81)
> respiratory distress syndrome of newborn (P22.0)
> respiratory failure (J96.-)
> respiratory failure of newborn (P28.5)

● **R09.0**   **Asphyxia and hypoxemia**

> **Excludes1**   asphyxia due to carbon monoxide (T58.-)
> asphyxia due to foreign body in respiratory tract (T17.-)
> birth (intrauterine) asphyxia (P84)
> hypercapnia (R06.4)
> hyperventilation (R06.4)
> traumatic asphyxia (T71.-) ◀▥▥

     R09.01   **Asphyxia** 🅟

> (Ex:) G89.0-G89.4, J80, J96.00-J96.92, R09.01-R09.02, R09.2,
> R41.0-R41.3, R41.82, R41.9, R44.8-R44.9, R45.83-R45.84,
> R46.0-R46.89, R52, R68.0-R68.19, R68.81-R68.83, R68.89-R69

     R09.02   **Hypoxemia**

R09.1   **Pleurisy**

> *Occurs when double membrane (pleura) lining chest cavity
> and lung surface becomes inflamed causing sharp pain
> on inspiration/expiration.*

> **Excludes1**   pleurisy with effusion (J90)

R09.2   **Respiratory arrest** 🅟
Cardiorespiratory failure

> **Excludes1**   cardiac arrest (I46.-)
> respiratory arrest of newborn (P28.81)
> respiratory distress of newborn (P22.0)
> respiratory failure (J96.-)
> respiratory failure of newborn (P28.5)
> respiratory insufficiency (R06.89)
> respiratory insufficiency of newborn (P28.5)

> MCC: *Only if patient discharged alive*
> (Ex:) *See R09.01*

R09.3   **Abnormal sputum**
Abnormal amount of sputum
Abnormal color of sputum
Abnormal odor of sputum
Excessive sputum

> **Excludes1**   blood-stained sputum (R04.2)

● **R09.8**   **Other specified symptoms and signs involving the circulatory and respiratory systems**

     R09.81   **Nasal congestion**

     R09.82   **Postnasal drip**

     R09.89   **Other specified symptoms and signs involving the circulatory and respiratory systems**
Bruit (arterial)
Abnormal chest percussion
Feeling of foreign body in throat
Friction sounds in chest
Chest tympany
Choking sensation
Rales
> *Wet rattling, clicking, crackling sounds on auscultation*
Weak pulse

> **Excludes2**   foreign body in throat (T17.2-)
> wheezing (R06.2)

**SYMPTOMS AND SIGNS INVOLVING THE DIGESTIVE
SYSTEM AND ABDOMEN (R10-R19)**

> **Excludes1**   congenital or infantile pylorospasm (Q40.0)
> gastrointestinal hemorrhage (K92.0-K92.2)
> intestinal obstruction (K56.-)
> newborn gastrointestinal hemorrhage (P54.0-P54.3)
> newborn intestinal obstruction (P76.-)
> pylorospasm (K31.3)
> signs and symptoms involving the urinary system (R30-R39)
> symptoms referable to female genital organs (N94.-)
> symptoms referable to male genital organs male (N48-N50)

● **R10**   **Abdominal and pelvic pain**

> **Excludes1**   renal colic (N23)
> **Excludes2**   dorsalgia (M54.-)
> flatulence and related conditions (R14.-)

R10.0   **Acute abdomen**
Severe abdominal pain (generalized) (with abdominal rigidity)

> **Excludes1**   abdominal rigidity NOS (R19.3)
> generalized abdominal pain NOS (R10.84)
> localized abdominal pain (R10.1-R10.3-)

● **R10.1**   **Pain localized to upper abdomen**

     R10.10   Upper abdominal pain, unspecified

     R10.11   Right upper quadrant pain

     R10.12   Left upper quadrant pain

     R10.13   Epigastric pain
Dyspepsia
> **Excludes1**   functional dyspepsia (K30)

● **R10.2**   **Pelvic and perineal pain**

> **Excludes1**   vulvodynia (N94.81)

● **R10.3**   **Pain localized to other parts of lower abdomen**

     R10.30   Lower abdominal pain, unspecified

     R10.31   Right lower quadrant pain

     R10.32   Left lower quadrant pain

     R10.33   Periumbilical pain

● **R10.8**   **Other abdominal pain**

     ● **R10.81**   **Abdominal tenderness**
Abdominal tenderness NOS

         R10.811   **Right upper quadrant abdominal tenderness**

         R10.812   **Left upper quadrant abdominal tenderness**

         R10.813   **Right lower quadrant abdominal tenderness**

         R10.814   **Left lower quadrant abdominal tenderness**

         R10.815   **Periumbilic abdominal tenderness**

         R10.816   **Epigastric abdominal tenderness**

         R10.817   **Generalized abdominal tenderness**

         R10.819   **Abdominal tenderness, unspecified site**

     ● **R10.82**   **Rebound abdominal tenderness**

         R10.821   **Right upper quadrant rebound abdominal tenderness**

         R10.822   **Left upper quadrant rebound abdominal tenderness**

         R10.823   **Right lower quadrant rebound abdominal tenderness**

CHAPTER 18 (R00-R99)

N Newborn Age: 0   **P** Pediatric Age: 0–17   **M** Maternity DX: 12–55   **A** Adult Age: 15–124   ♀ Females Only   ♂ Males Only

🅒 Complication\Comorbidity   🅒 Major C\C   (Ex:) CC/MCC Exclusions   🅟 Present on Admission Requirement   🅗 Hospital-Acquired Condition

1271

    R10.824   Left lower quadrant rebound abdominal tenderness

    R10.825   Periumbilic rebound abdominal tenderness

    R10.826   Epigastric rebound abdominal tenderness

    R10.827   Generalized rebound abdominal tenderness

    R10.829   Rebound abdominal tenderness, unspecified site

R10.83   Colic   P
    Colic NOS
    Infantile colic
    Excludes1   colic in adult and child over 12 months old (R10.84)

R10.84   Generalized abdominal pain
    Excludes1   generalized abdominal pain associated with acute abdomen (R10.0)

R10.9   Unspecified abdominal pain

● **R11**   **Nausea and vomiting**
    Excludes1   cyclical vomiting associated with migraine (G43.A-)
             excessive vomiting in pregnancy (O21.-)
             hematemesis (K92.0)
             neonatal hematemesis (P54.0)
             newborn vomiting (P92.0-)
             psychogenic vomiting (F50.8)
             vomiting associated with bulimia nervosa (F50.2)
             vomiting following gastrointestinal surgery (K91.0)

● **R11.0**   Nausea
    Nausea NOS
    Nausea without vomiting

● **R11.1**   Vomiting
    R11.10   Vomiting, unspecified
        Vomiting NOS
    R11.11   Vomiting without nausea
    R11.12   Projectile vomiting
    R11.13   Vomiting of fecal matter
    R11.14   Bilious vomiting
        Bilious emesis

R11.2   Nausea with vomiting, unspecified
    Persistent nausea with vomiting NOS

R12   **Heartburn**
    Excludes1   dyspepsia NOS (R10.13)
             functional dyspepsia (K30)

● **R13**   **Aphagia and dysphagia**
    R13.0   Aphagia
        Inability to swallow
        Excludes1   psychogenic aphagia (F50.9)

● **R13.1**   Dysphagia
    Difficulty swallowing
    Code first, if applicable, dysphagia following cerebrovascular disease (I69. with final characters -91)
    Excludes1   psychogenic dysphagia (F45.8)
    R13.10   Dysphagia, unspecified
        Difficulty in swallowing NOS
    R13.11   Dysphagia, oral phase
    R13.12   Dysphagia, oropharyngeal phase
    R13.13   Dysphagia, pharyngeal phase
    R13.14   Dysphagia, pharyngoesophageal phase
    R13.19   Other dysphagia
        Cervical dysphagia
        Neurogenic dysphagia

● **R14**   **Flatulence and related conditions**
    Excludes1   psychogenic aerophagy (F45.8)
    R14.0   Abdominal distension (gaseous)
        Bloating
        Tympanites (abdominal) (intestinal)
    R14.1   Gas pain
    R14.2   Eructation
        Belching air from stomach through mouth
    R14.3   Flatulence

● **R15**   **Fecal incontinence**
    Includes   encopresis NOS
    Excludes1   fecal incontinence of nonorganic origin (F98.1)
    R15.0   Incomplete defecation
        Excludes1   constipation (K59.0-)
               fecal impaction (K56.41)
    R15.1   Fecal smearing
        Fecal soiling
    R15.2   Fecal urgency
    R15.9   Full incontinence of feces
        Fecal incontinence NOS

● **R16**   **Hepatomegaly and splenomegaly, not elsewhere classified**
    Enlargement of liver or spleen
    R16.0   Hepatomegaly, not elsewhere classified
        Hepatomegaly NOS
    R16.1   Splenomegaly, not elsewhere classified
        Splenomegaly NOS
    R16.2   Hepatomegaly with splenomegaly, not elsewhere classified
        Hepatosplenomegaly NOS

R17   Unspecified jaundice
    Excludes1   neonatal jaundice (P55, P57-P59)
    (Ex:) P57.8-P59.9, R17, R23.8-R23.9

● **R18**   **Ascites**
    Includes   fluid in peritoneal cavity
    Excludes1   ascites in alcoholic cirrhosis (K70.31)
             ascites in alcoholic hepatitis (K70.11)
             ascites in toxic liver disease with chronic active hepatitis (K71.51)
    (Ex:) For category R18 CC codes: G89.0-G89.4, R18.0-R19.09, R19.30-R19.37, R41.0-R41.3, R41.82, R41.9, R44.8-R44.9, R45.83-R45.84, R46.0-R46.89, R52, R68.0-R68.19, R68.81-R68.83, R68.89-R69

● **R18.0**   Malignant ascites
    Code first malignancy, such as:
        malignant neoplasm of ovary (C56.-)
        secondary malignant neoplasm of retroperitoneum and peritoneum (C78.6)

    R18.8   Other ascites
        Ascites NOS
        Peritoneal effusion (chronic)

● **R19**   **Other symptoms and signs involving the digestive system and abdomen**
    Excludes1   acute abdomen (R10.0)
● **R19.0**   Intra-abdominal and pelvic swelling, mass and lump
    Excludes1   abdominal distension (gaseous) (R14.-)
             ascites (R18.-)
    R19.00   Intra-abdominal and pelvic swelling, mass and lump, unspecified site
    R19.01   Right upper quadrant abdominal swelling, mass and lump
    R19.02   Left upper quadrant abdominal swelling, mass and lump
    R19.03   Right lower quadrant abdominal swelling, mass and lump
    R19.04   Left lower quadrant abdominal swelling, mass and lump

◀ New   ◀ Revised   ~~deleted~~ Deleted   Excludes 1   Excludes 2   Includes   Use additional   Code first   Code also   Unspecified

OGCR Official Guidelines   ● Unacceptable Principal Diagnosis   X Assign placeholder X   ● Use Additional Character(s)   ▌ Manifestation Code   **Coding Clinic**

R19.05 **Periumbilic swelling, mass or lump**
     Diffuse or generalized umbilical swelling or mass

R19.06 **Epigastric swelling, mass or lump**

R19.07 **Generalized intra-abdominal and pelvic swelling, mass and lump**
     Diffuse or generalized intra-abdominal swelling or mass NOS
     Diffuse or generalized pelvic swelling or mass NOS

R19.09 **Other intra-abdominal and pelvic swelling, mass and lump**

● R19.1 **Abnormal bowel sounds**

R19.11 **Absent bowel sounds**

R19.12 **Hyperactive bowel sounds**

R19.15 **Other abnormal bowel sounds**
     Abnormal bowel sounds NOS

R19.2 **Visible peristalsis**
     Hyperperistalsis

● R19.3 **Abdominal rigidity**
     Excludes1   abdominal rigidity with severe abdominal pain (R10.0)

R19.30 **Abdominal rigidity, unspecified site**

R19.31 **Right upper quadrant abdominal rigidity**

R19.32 **Left upper quadrant abdominal rigidity**

R19.33 **Right lower quadrant abdominal rigidity**

R19.34 **Left lower quadrant abdominal rigidity**

R19.35 **Periumbilic abdominal rigidity**

R19.36 **Epigastric abdominal rigidity**

R19.37 **Generalized abdominal rigidity**

R19.4 **Change in bowel habit**
     Excludes1   constipation (K59.0-)
                   functional diarrhea (K59.1)

R19.5 **Other fecal abnormalities**
     Abnormal stool color
     Bulky stools
     Mucus in stools
     Occult blood in feces
     Occult blood in stools
     Excludes1   melena (K92.1)
                   neonatal melena (P54.1)

R19.6 **Halitosis**

R19.7 **Diarrhea, unspecified**
     Diarrhea NOS
     Excludes1   functional diarrhea (K59.1)
                   neonatal diarrhea (P78.3)
                   psychogenic diarrhea (F45.8)

R19.8 **Other specified symptoms and signs involving the digestive system and abdomen**

SYMPTOMS AND SIGNS INVOLVING THE SKIN AND SUBCUTANEOUS TISSUE (R20-R23)

     Excludes2   symptoms relating to breast (N64.4-N64.5)

● R20 **Disturbances of skin sensation**
     Excludes1   dissociative anesthesia and sensory loss (F44.6)
                   psychogenic disturbances (F45.8)

R20.0 **Anesthesia of skin**
     Loss of sensation

R20.1 **Hypoesthesia of skin**
     Unpleasant abnormal sensation

R20.2 **Paresthesia of skin**
     Abnormal touch sensation, including burning, prickling, often in absence of external stimulus
     Formication   Tingling skin
     Pins and needles
     Excludes1   acroparesthesia (I73.8)

R20.3 **Hyperesthesia**

R20.8 **Other disturbances of skin sensation**

R20.9 **Unspecified disturbances of skin sensation**

R21 **Rash and other nonspecific skin eruption**
     Includes   rash NOS
     Excludes1   specified type of rash- code to condition
                   vesicular eruption (R23.8)

● R22 **Localized swelling, mass and lump of skin and subcutaneous tissue**
     Includes   subcutaneous nodules (localized) (superficial)
     Excludes1   abnormal findings on diagnostic imaging (R90-R93)
                   edema (R60.-)
                   enlarged lymph nodes (R59.-)
                   localized adiposity (E65)
                   swelling of joint (M25.4-)

R22.0 **Localized swelling, mass and lump, head**

R22.1 **Localized swelling, mass and lump, neck**

R22.2 **Localized swelling, mass and lump, trunk**
     Excludes1   intra-abdominal or pelvic mass and lump (R19.0-)
                   intra-abdominal or pelvic swelling (R19.0-)
     Excludes2   breast mass and lump (N63)

● R22.3 **Localized swelling, mass and lump, upper limb**

R22.30 **Localized swelling, mass and lump, unspecified upper limb**

R22.31 **Localized swelling, mass and lump, right upper limb**

R22.32 **Localized swelling, mass and lump, left upper limb**

R22.33 **Localized swelling, mass and lump, upper limb, bilateral**

● R22.4 **Localized swelling, mass and lump, lower limb**

R22.40 **Localized swelling, mass and lump, unspecified lower limb**

R22.41 **Localized swelling, mass and lump, right lower limb**

R22.42 **Localized swelling, mass and lump, left lower limb**

R22.43 **Localized swelling, mass and lump, lower limb, bilateral**

R22.9 **Localized swelling, mass and lump, unspecified**

● R23 **Other skin changes**

R23.0 **Cyanosis**
     Excludes1   acrocyanosis (I73.8)
                   cyanotic attacks of newborn (P28.2)

R23.1 **Pallor**
     Clammy skin

R23.2 **Flushing**
     Excessive blushing
     Code first, if applicable, menopausal and female climacteric states (N95.1)

R23.3 **Spontaneous ecchymoses**
     Small hemorrhagic spot of skin; AKA black and blue spot
     Petechiae
     Excludes1   ecchymoses of newborn (P54.5)
                   purpura (D69.-)

R23.4 **Changes in skin texture**
     Desquamation of skin   Scaling of skin
     Induration of skin
     Excludes1   epidermal thickening NOS (L85.9)

R23.8 **Other skin changes**

R23.9 **Unspecified skin changes**

CHAPTER 18 (R00-R99)

N Newborn Age: 0   **P** Pediatric Age: 0–17   **M** Maternity DX: 12–55   **A** Adult Age: 15–124   ♀ Females Only   ♂ Males Only

Complication\Comorbidity   Major C\C   (Ex) CC/MCC Exclusions   Present on Admission Requirement   Hospital-Acquired Condition   **1273**

CHAPTER 18 (R00-R99)

SYMPTOMS AND SIGNS INVOLVING THE NERVOUS AND MUSCULOSKELETAL SYSTEMS (R25-R29)

● **R25   Abnormal involuntary movements**
> **Excludes1**   specific movement disorders (G20-G26)
> stereotyped movement disorders (F98.4)
> tic disorders (F95.-)

R25.0   Abnormal head movements

R25.1   Tremor, unspecified
> **Excludes1**   chorea NOS (G25.5)
> essential tremor (G25.0)
> hysterical tremor (F44.4)
> intention tremor (G25.2)

R25.2   Cramp and spasm
> **Excludes2**   carpopedal spasm (R29.0)
> charley-horse (M62.831)
> infantile spasms (G40.4-)
> muscle spasm of back (M62.830)
> muscle spasm of calf (M62.831)

R25.3   Fasciculation
> Twitching NOS

R25.8   Other abnormal involuntary movements

R25.9   Unspecified abnormal involuntary movements

● **R26   Abnormalities of gait and mobility**
> **Excludes1**   ataxia NOS (R27.0)
> hereditary ataxia (G11.-)
> locomotor (syphilitic) ataxia (A52.11)
> immobility syndrome (paraplegic) (M62.3)

R26.0   Ataxic gait
> Staggering gait

R26.1   Paralytic gait
> Spastic gait

R26.2   Difficulty in walking, not elsewhere classified
> **Excludes1**   falling (R29.6)
> unsteadiness on feet (R26.81)

● **R26.8   Other abnormalities of gait and mobility**

R26.81   Unsteadiness on feet

R26.89   Other abnormalities of gait and mobility

R26.9   Unspecified abnormalities of gait and mobility

● **R27   Other lack of coordination**
> **Excludes1**   ataxic gait (R26.0)
> hereditary ataxia (G11.-)
> vertigo NOS (R42)

R27.0   Ataxia, unspecified
> **Excludes1**   ataxia following cerebrovascular disease (I69. with final characters -93)

R27.8   Other lack of coordination

R27.9   Unspecified lack of coordination

● **R29   Other symptoms and signs involving the nervous and musculoskeletal systems**

R29.0   Tetany
> *Hyperexcitability of nerves and muscles characterized by spasm, twitching, and cramps*
> Carpopedal spasm
> **Excludes1**   hysterical tetany (F44.5)
> neonatal tetany (P71.3)
> parathyroid tetany (E20.9)
> post-thyroidectomy tetany (E89.2)
> (Ex:) A33, A35, G10-G11.2, G11.4, G20-G25.79, G25.82-G26, G32.81, G80.3, G81.10-G81.14, G89.0-G89.4, G90.3, R29.0, R41.0-R41.3, R41.82, R41.9, R44.8-R44.9, R45.83-R45.84, R46.0-R46.89, R52, R68.0-R68.19, R68.81-R68.83, R68.89-R69

R29.1   Meningismus
> (Ex:) R29.1, R29.810

R29.2   Abnormal reflex
> **Excludes2**   abnormal pupillary reflex (H57.0)
> hyperactive gag reflex (J39.2)
> vasovagal reaction or syncope (R55)

R29.3   Abnormal posture

R29.4   Clicking hip
> **Excludes1**   congenital deformities of hip (Q65.-)

R29.5   Transient paralysis
> *Code first any associated spinal cord injury (S14.0, S14.1-, S24.0, S24.1-, S34.0-, S34.1-)*
> **Excludes1**   transient ischemic attack (G45.9)
> (Ex:) R29.5, R29.810

R29.6   Repeated falls
> Falling
> Tendency to fall
> **Excludes2**   at risk for falling (Z91.81)
> history of falling (Z91.81)

OGCR Section I.C.18.d.

Repeated falls

Code R29.6, Repeated falls, is for use for encounters when a patient has recently fallen and the reason for the fall is being investigated.

Code Z91.81, History of falling, is for use when a patient has fallen in the past and is at risk for future falls. When appropriate, both codes R29.6 and Z91.81 may be assigned together.

● **R29.8   Other symptoms and signs involving the nervous and musculoskeletal systems**

● **R29.81   Other symptoms and signs involving the nervous system**

R29.810   Facial weakness
> Facial droop
> **Excludes1**   Bell's palsy (G51.0)
> facial weakness following cerebrovascular disease (I69. with final characters -92)

R29.818   Other symptoms and signs involving the nervous system

● **R29.89   Other symptoms and signs involving the musculoskeletal system**
> **Excludes2**   pain in limb (M79.6-)

R29.890   Loss of height
> **Excludes1**   osteoporosis (M80-M81)

R29.891   Ocular torticollis
> **Excludes1**   congenital (sterno-mastoid) torticollis Q68.0
> psychogenic torticollis (F45.8)
> spasmodic torticollis (G24.3)
> torticollis due to birth injury (P15.8)
> torticollis NOS M43.6

R29.898   Other symptoms and signs involving the musculoskeletal system

● **R29.9   Unspecified symptoms and signs involving the nervous and musculoskeletal systems**

R29.90   Unspecified symptoms and signs involving the nervous system

R29.91   Unspecified symptoms and signs involving the musculoskeletal system

◄ New   ◄ Revised   ~~deleted~~ Deleted   Excludes 1   Excludes 2   Includes   Use additional   Code first   Code also   Unspecified

OGCR Official Guidelines   ● Unacceptable Principal Diagnosis   X Assign placeholder X   Use Additional Character(s)   ▶ Manifestation Code   **Coding Clinic**

SYMPTOMS AND SIGNS INVOLVING THE GENITOURINARY SYSTEM (R30-R39)

● **R30**   **Pain associated with micturition**
> **Excludes1**   psychogenic pain associated with micturition (F45.8)

    R30.0   **Dysuria**
> *Painful urination*
> Strangury

    R30.1   **Vesical tenesmus**
> *Straining to urinate*

    R30.9   **Painful micturition, unspecified**
> Painful urination NOS

● **R31**   **Hematuria**
> **Excludes1**   hematuria included with underlying conditions, such as:
>   acute cystitis with hematuria (N30.01)
>   ~~acute prostatitis with hematuria (N41.01)~~
>   recurrent and persistent hematuria in glomerular diseases (N02.-)

    R31.0   **Gross hematuria**

    R31.1   **Benign essential microscopic hematuria**

    R31.2   **Other microscopic hematuria**

    R31.9   **Hematuria, unspecified**

  R32   **Unspecified urinary incontinence**
> Enuresis NOS
> **Excludes1**   functional urinary incontinence (R39.81)
>   nonorganic enuresis (F98.0)
>   stress incontinence and other specified urinary incontinence (N39.3-N39.4-)
>   urinary incontinence associated with cognitive impairment (R39.81)

● **R33**   **Retention of urine**
> **Excludes1**   psychogenic retention of urine (F45.8)

    R33.0   **Drug induced retention of urine**
> Use additional code for adverse effect, if applicable, to identify drug (T36-T50 with fifth or sixth character 5)

    R33.8   **Other retention of urine**
> *Code first, if applicable, any causal condition, such as:*
>   enlarged prostate (N40.1)

    R33.9   **Retention of urine, unspecified**

  R34   **Anuria and oliguria**
> **Excludes1**   anuria and oliguria complicating abortion or ectopic or molar pregnancy (O00-O07, O08.4)
>   anuria and oliguria complicating pregnancy (O26.83-)
>   anuria and oliguria complicating the puerperium (O90.4)

● **R35**   **Polyuria**
> *Passage of excessive volume of urine*
> *Code first, if applicable, any causal condition, such as:*
>   enlarged prostate (N40.1)
> **Excludes1**   psychogenic polyuria (F45.8)

    R35.0   **Frequency of micturition**
> *Discharge or passage of urine; AKA uresis*

    R35.1   **Nocturia**
> *Urinary frequency at night*

    R35.8   **Other polyuria**
> Polyuria NOS

● **R36**   **Urethral discharge**

    R36.0   **Urethral discharge without blood**

    R36.1   **Hematospermia** ♂
> *Presence of blood in semen*

    R36.9   **Urethral discharge, unspecified**
> Penile discharge NOS
> Urethrorrhea

  R37   **Sexual dysfunction, unspecified**

● **R39**   **Other and unspecified symptoms and signs involving the genitourinary system**

    R39.0   **Extravasation of urine** 🔵
> *Leakage, discharge*
> (Ex) R30.1, R39.0, R39.2-R39.9

●   **R39.1**   **Other difficulties with micturition**
> *Code first, if applicable, any causal condition, such as:*
>   enlarged prostate (N40.1)

      R39.11   **Hesitancy of micturition**

      R39.12   **Poor urinary stream**
> Weak urinary steam

      R39.13   **Splitting of urinary stream**

      R39.14   **Feeling of incomplete bladder emptying**

      R39.15   **Urgency of urination**
> **Excludes1**   urge incontinence (N39.41, N39.46)

      R39.16   **Straining to void**

      R39.19   **Other difficulties with micturition**

    R39.2   **Extrarenal uremia**
> Prerenal uremia
> **Excludes1**   uremia NOS (N19)

●   **R39.8**   **Other symptoms and signs involving the genitourinary system**

      R39.81   **Functional urinary incontinence**
> Urinary incontinence due to cognitive impairment, or severe physical disability or immobility
> **Excludes1**   stress incontinence and other specified urinary incontinence (N39.3-N39.4-)
>   urinary incontinence NOS (R32)

      R39.89   **Other symptoms and signs involving the genitourinary system**

    R39.9   **Unspecified symptoms and signs involving the genitourinary system**

SYMPTOMS AND SIGNS INVOLVING COGNITION, PERCEPTION, EMOTIONAL STATE AND BEHAVIOR (R40-R46)

> **Excludes1**   symptoms and signs constituting part of a pattern of mental disorder (F01-F99)

● **R40**   **Somnolence, stupor and coma**
> **Excludes1**   neonatal coma (P91.5)
>   somnolence, stupor and coma in diabetes (E08-E13)
>   somnolence, stupor and coma in hepatic failure (K72.-)
>   somnolence, stupor and coma in hypoglycemia (nondiabetic) (E15)

    R40.0   **Somnolence**
> Drowsiness
> **Excludes1**   coma (R40.2-)

    R40.1   **Stupor**
> *Lowered level of consciousness*
> Catatonic stupor
> Semicoma
> **Excludes1**   catatonic schizophrenia (F20.2)
>   coma (R40.2-)
>   depressive stupor (F31-F33)
>   dissociative stupor (F44.2)
>   manic stupor (F30.2)

N   Newborn Age: 0   P   Pediatric Age: 0–17   M   Maternity DX: 12–55   A   Adult Age: 15–124   ♀   Females Only   ♂   Males Only

🔵 Complication\Comorbidity   🔵 Major C\C   (Ex) CC/MCC Exclusions   🔵 Present on Admission Requirement   🔵 Hospital-Acquired Condition

1275

OGCR Section I.C.18.e.

Coma scale

The coma scale codes (R40.2-) can be used in conjunction with traumatic brain injury codes, acute cerebrovascular disease or sequelae of cerebrovascular disease codes. These codes are primarily for use by trauma registries, but they may be used in any setting where this information is collected. The coma scale codes should be sequenced after the diagnosis code(s).

These codes, one from each subcategory, are needed to complete the scale. The 7th character indicates when the scale was recorded. The 7th character should match for all three codes.

At a minimum, report the initial score documented on presentation at your facility. This may be a score from the emergency medicine technician (EMT) or in the emergency department. If desired, a facility may choose to capture multiple coma scale scores.

Assign code R40.24, Glasgow coma scale, total score, when only the total score is documented in the medical record and not the individual score(s).

● **R40.2   Coma**

Code first any associated:
    fracture of skull (S02.-) ◀▦
    intracranial injury (S06.-) ◀▦

~~The appropriate 7th character is to be added to each code from subcategory R40.21-, R40.22-, R40.23-:~~

0	unspecified time
1	in the field [EMT or ambulance]
2	at arrival to emergency department
3	at hospital admission
4	24 hours or more after hospital admission

Note: One code from subcategories R40.21-R40.23 is required to complete the coma scale ◀▦

(Ex) **For category R40.2 CC codes:** B15.0-B19.9, E03.5, E08.00-E08.59, E08.618-E09.59, E09.618-E10.59, E10.618-E10.649, E10.69-E11.59, E11.618-E11.649, E11.69-E13.59, E13.618-E16.2, E89.1, G32.89, G89.0-G89.4, G93.81-G93.9, G96.8-G96.9, G98.0-G98.8, G99.8, I60.00-I62.9, K72.91, R40.0-R40.2124, R40.2210-R40.2224, R40.2310-R40.2324, R40.2340-R40.2344, R40.3-R41.3, R41.82, R41.9-R42, R44.8-R44.9, R45.83-R45.84, R46.0-R46.89, R52, R55, R68.0-R68.83, R68.89-R69, S02.0XX-S02.19X[A,B], S02.91X[A,B], S06.0X0-S06.9X9[A]

R40.20   Unspecified coma 🦠
    Coma NOS
    Unconsciousness NOS

● **R40.21   Coma scale, eyes open**

The following appropriate 7th character is to be added to subcategory R40.21-: ◀

0	unspecified time ◀
1	in the field [EMT or ambulance] ◀
2	at arrival to emergency department ◀
3	at hospital admission ◀
4	24 hours or more after hospital admission ◀

  ● **R40.211   Coma scale, eyes open, never** 🦠
  ● **R40.212   Coma scale, eyes open, to pain** 🦠
  ● **R40.213   Coma scale, eyes open, to sound** 🦠
  ● **R40.214   Coma scale, eyes open, spontaneous** 🦠

● **R40.22   Coma scale, best verbal response**

The following appropriate 7th character is to be added to subcategory R40.22-: ◀

0	unspecified time ◀
1	in the field [EMT or ambulance] ◀
2	at arrival to emergency department ◀
3	at hospital admission ◀
4	24 hours or more after hospital admission ◀

  ● **R40.221   Coma scale, best verbal response, none** 🦠
  ● **R40.222   Coma scale, best verbal response, incomprehensible words** 🦠

Glasgow Coma Scale

Eye Opening Response	
• Spontaneous--open with blinking at baseline	4 points
• To verbal stimuli, command, speech	3 points
• To pain only (not applied to face)	2 points
• No response	1 point
Verbal Response	
• Oriented	5 points
• Confused conversation, but able to answer questions	4 points
• Inappropriate words	3 points
• Incomprehensible speech	2 points
• No response	1 point
Motor Response	
• Obeys commands for movement	6 points
• Purposeful movement to painful stimulus	5 points
• Withdraws in response to pain	4 points
• Flexion in response to pain (decorticate posturing)	3 points
• Extension response in response to pain (decerebrate posturing)	2 points
• No response	1 point

Categorization:
Coma: No eye opening, no ability to follow commands, no word verbalizations (3-8)

Head Injury Classification:
Severe Head Injury--GCS score of 8 or less
Moderate Head Injury--GCS score of 9 to 12
Mild head injury--GCS score of 13 to 15

(Adapted from: Advanced Trauma Life Support: Course for Physicians, American College of Surgeons, 1993).
http://www.bt.cdc.gov/masscasulatires/gscale.asp

Figure 18-1

  ● **R40.223   Coma scale, best verbal response, inappropriate words** 🦠
  ● **R40.224   Coma scale, best verbal response, confused conversation** 🦠
  ● **R40.225   Coma scale, best verbal response, oriented** 🦠

● **R40.23   Coma scale, best motor response**

The following appropriate 7th character is to be added to subcategory R40.23-: ◀

0	unspecified time ◀
1	in the field [EMT or ambulance] ◀
2	at arrival to emergency department ◀
3	at hospital admission ◀
4	24 hours or more after hospital admission ◀

  ● **R40.231   Coma scale, best motor response, none** 🦠
  ● **R40.232   Coma scale, best motor response, extension** 🦠
  ● **R40.233   Coma scale, best motor response, abnormal** 🦠
  ● **R40.234   Coma scale, best motor response, flexion withdrawal** 🦠
  ● **R40.235   Coma scale, best motor response, localizes pain** 🦠
  ● **R40.236   Coma scale, best motor response, obeys commands** 🦠

◀ New   ◀▦ Revised   ~~deleted~~ Deleted   Excludes 1   Excludes 2   Includes   Use additional   Code first   Code also   Unspecified
OGCR Official Guidelines   ● Unacceptable Principal Diagnosis   X Assign placeholder X   🦠 Use Additional Character(s)   ▶ Manifestation Code   **Coding Clinic**

● **R40.24**   **Glasgow coma scale, total score**
Use codes R40.21- through R40.23- only when the individual score(s) are documented

     R40.241   **Glasgow coma scale score 13-15** 🔖

     R40.242   **Glasgow coma scale score 9-12** 🔖

     R40.243   **Glasgow coma scale score 3-8** 🔖

     R40.244   **Other coma, without documented Glasgow coma scale score, or with partial score reported** 🔖

R40.3   **Persistent vegetative state** 🔖
    (Ex) See R40.2

R40.4   **Transient alteration of awareness**

● **R41**   **Other symptoms and signs involving cognitive functions and awareness**

     Excludes1   dissociative [conversion] disorders (F44.-)
mild cognitive impairment, so stated (G31.84)

R41.0   **Disorientation, unspecified**
Confusion NOS   Delirium NOS

R41.1   **Anterograde amnesia**

R41.2   **Retrograde amnesia**

R41.3   **Other amnesia**
Amnesia NOS
Memory loss NOS

     Excludes1   amnestic disorder due to known physiologic condition (F04)
amnestic syndrome due to psychoactive substance use (F10-F19 with 5th character .6)
mild memory disturbance due to known physiological condition (F06.8)
transient global amnesia (G45.4)

R41.4   **Neurologic neglect syndrome** 🔖
Asomatognosia   Left-sided neglect
Hemi-akinesia   Sensory neglect
Hemi-inattention   Visuospatial neglect
Hemispatial neglect

     Excludes1   visuospatial deficit (R41.842)
    (Ex) R29.3, R29.6-R29.890, R29.90-R29.91, R41.4

● **R41.8**   **Other symptoms and signs involving cognitive functions and awareness**

     R41.81   **Age-related cognitive decline**   A
Senility NOS

     R41.82   **Altered mental status, unspecified**
Change in mental status NOS

        Excludes1   altered level of consciousness (R40.-)
altered mental status due to known condition - code to condition
delirium NOS (R41.0)

        Coding Clinic: 2012, Q4, P98

●   **R41.83**   **Borderline intellectual functioning**
IQ level 71 to 84

        Excludes1   intellectual disabilities (F70-F79)

●   **R41.84**   **Other specified cognitive deficit**

     R41.840   **Attention and concentration deficit**

        Excludes1   attention-deficit hyperactivity disorders (F90.-)

     R41.841   **Cognitive communication deficit**

     R41.842   **Visuospatial deficit**

     R41.843   **Psychomotor deficit**

     R41.844   **Frontal lobe and executive function deficit**

     R41.89   **Other symptoms and signs involving cognitive functions and awareness**
Anosognosia

R41.9   **Unspecified symptoms and signs involving cognitive functions and awareness**

R42   **Dizziness and giddiness**
Light-headedness
Vertigo NOS

     Excludes1   vertiginous syndromes (H81.-)
vertigo from infrasound (T75.23)

● **R43**   **Disturbances of smell and taste**

R43.0   **Anosmia**
Absence of sense of smell; AKA anosphresia and olfactory anesthesia

R43.1   **Parosmia**

R43.2   **Parageusia**
Perversion of sense of taste or bad taste in mouth; AKA dysgeusia

R43.8   **Other disturbances of smell and taste**
Mixed disturbance of smell and taste

R43.9   **Unspecified disturbances of smell and taste**

● **R44**   **Other symptoms and signs involving general sensations and perceptions**

     Excludes1   alcoholic hallucinations (F1.5)
hallucinations in drug psychosis (F11-F19 with .5)
hallucinations in mood disorders with psychotic symptoms (F30.2, F31.5, F32.3, F33.3)
hallucinations in schizophrenia, schizotypal and delusional disorders (F20-F29)

     Excludes2   disturbances of skin sensation (R20.-)

R44.0   **Auditory hallucinations** 🔖
    (Ex) G89.0-G89.4, R41.0-R41.3, R41.82, R41.9-R42, R44.0, R44.2-R44.9, R45.83-R45.84, R46.0-R46.89, R52, R68.0-R68.19, R68.81-R68.83, R68.89-R69

R44.1   **Visual hallucinations**

R44.2   **Other hallucinations** 🔖
    (Ex) See R44.0

R44.3   **Hallucinations, unspecified** 🔖
    (Ex) See R44.0

R44.8   **Other symptoms and signs involving general sensations and perceptions**

R44.9   **Unspecified symptoms and signs involving general sensations and perceptions**

● **R45**   **Symptoms and signs involving emotional state**

R45.0   **Nervousness**
Nervous tension

R45.1   **Restlessness and agitation**

R45.2   **Unhappiness**

R45.3   **Demoralization and apathy**
     Excludes1   anhedonia (R45.84)

R45.4   **Irritability and anger**

R45.5   **Hostility**

R45.6   **Violent behavior**

R45.7   **State of emotional shock and stress, unspecified**

● **R45.8**   **Other symptoms and signs involving emotional state**

     R45.81   **Low self-esteem**

     R45.82   **Worries**

     R45.83   **Excessive crying of child, adolescent or adult**

        Excludes1   excessive crying of infant (baby) R68.11

     R45.84   **Anhedonia**
Total loss of feeling of pleasure in pleasurable acts

●   **R45.85**   **Homicidal and suicidal ideations**

        Excludes1   suicide attempt (T14.91)

      ● **R45.850**   **Homicidal ideations**

       R45.851   **Suicidal ideations** 🔖
        (Ex) F05

     R45.86   **Emotional lability**

     R45.87   **Impulsiveness**

     R45.89   **Other symptoms and signs involving emotional state**

CHAPTER 18 (R00-R99)

N Newborn Age: 0   **P** Pediatric Age: 0–17   **M** Maternity DX: 12–55   **A** Adult Age: 15–124   ♀ Females Only   ♂ Males Only

🔖 Complication\Comorbidity   🔖 Major C\C   (Ex) CC/MCC Exclusions   🔖 Present on Admission Requirement   🔖 Hospital-Acquired Condition   **1277**

● **R46**   **Symptoms and signs involving appearance and behavior**
> **Excludes1**   appearance and behavior in schizophrenia, schizotypal and delusional disorders (F20-F29)
> mental and behavioral disorders (F01-F99)

   R46.0   **Very low level of personal hygiene**

   R46.1   **Bizarre personal appearance**

   R46.2   **Strange and inexplicable behavior**

   R46.3   **Overactivity**

   R46.4   **Slowness and poor responsiveness**
> **Excludes1**   stupor (R40.1)

   R46.5   **Suspiciousness and marked evasiveness**

   R46.6   **Undue concern and preoccupation with stressful events**

   R46.7   **Verbosity and circumstantial detail obscuring reason for contact**

●   **R46.8**   **Other symptoms and signs involving appearance and behavior**

     ● **R46.81**   **Obsessive-compulsive behavior**
> **Excludes1**   obsessive-compulsive disorder (F42)

     ● **R46.89**   **Other symptoms and signs involving appearance and behavior**

SYMPTOMS AND SIGNS INVOLVING SPEECH AND VOICE (R47-R49)

● **R47**   **Speech disturbances, not elsewhere classified**
> **Excludes1**   autism (F84.0)
> cluttering (F80.81)
> specific developmental disorders of speech and language (F80.-)
> stuttering (F80.81)

●   **R47.0**   **Dysphasia and aphasia**

     R47.01   **Aphasia** 🚫
> **Excludes1**   aphasia following cerebrovascular disease (I69. with final characters -20)
> progressive isolated aphasia (G31.01)
> (Ex) F80.1, F80.81, I62.00-I66.9, R47.01-R47.9, R49.0-R49.9

     R47.02   **Dysphasia**
> *Impairment in comprehension of speech, caused by left-sided brain damage*
> **Excludes1**   dysphasia following cerebrovascular disease (I69. with final characters -21)

   R47.1   **Dysarthria and anarthria**
> *Motor speech disorder*
> **Excludes1**   dysarthria following cerebrovascular disease (I69. with final characters -22)

●   **R47.8**   **Other speech disturbances**
> **Excludes1**   dysarthria following cerebrovascular disease (I69. with final characters -28)

     R47.81   **Slurred speech**

     ▷ **R47.82**   *Fluency disorder in conditions classified elsewhere*
> Stuttering in conditions classified elsewhere
> *Code first underlying disease or condition, such as:*
> Parkinson's disease (G20)
> **Excludes1**   adult onset fluency disorder (F98.5)
> childhood onset fluency disorder (F80.81)
> fluency disorder (stuttering) following cerebrovascular disease (I69. with final characters -23)

     R47.89   **Other speech disturbances**

   R47.9   **Unspecified speech disturbances**

● **R48**   **Dyslexia and other symbolic dysfunctions, not elsewhere classified**
> **Excludes1**   specific developmental disorders of scholastic skills (F81.-)

   R48.0   **Dyslexia and alexia**

   R48.1   **Agnosia**
> *Loss of ability to recognize objects, persons, sounds, shapes, or smells*
> Astereognosia (astereognosis)
> Autotopagnosia
> **Excludes1**   visual object agnosia (R48.3)

   R48.2   **Apraxia**
> *Loss of ability to execute or carry out learned purposeful movements*
> **Excludes1**   apraxia following cerebrovascular disease (I69. with final characters -90)

   R48.3   **Visual agnosia**
> Prosopagnosia
> Simultanagnosia (asimultagnosia)

   R48.8   **Other symbolic dysfunctions**
> Acalculia
> *Difficulty performing simple mathematical tasks resulting from neurological injury*
> Agraphia

   R48.9   **Unspecified symbolic dysfunctions**

● **R49**   **Voice and resonance disorders**
> **Excludes1**   psychogenic voice and resonance disorders (F44.4)

   R49.0   **Dysphonia**
> Hoarseness

   R49.1   **Aphonia**
> Loss of voice

●   **R49.2**   **Hypernasality and hyponasality**

     R49.21   **Hypernasality**

     R49.22   **Hyponasality**

   R49.8   **Other voice and resonance disorders**

   R49.9   **Unspecified voice and resonance disorder**
> Change in voice NOS
> Resonance disorder NOS

GENERAL SYMPTOMS AND SIGNS (R50-R69)

● **R50**   **Fever of other and unknown origin**
> **Excludes1**   chills without fever (R68.83)
> febrile convulsions (R56.0-)
> fever of unknown origin during labor (O75.2)
> fever of unknown origin in newborn (P81.9)
> hypothermia due to illness (R68.0)
> malignant hyperthermia due to anesthesia (T88.3)
> puerperal pyrexia NOS (O86.4)

   R50.2   **Drug induced fever**
> Use additional code for adverse effect, if applicable, to identify drug (T36-T50 with fifth or sixth character 5)
> **Excludes1**   postvaccination (postimmunization) fever (R50.83)

●   **R50.8**   **Other specified fever**

     ▷ **R50.81**   *Fever presenting with conditions classified elsewhere*
> *Code first underlying condition when associated fever is present, such as with:*
> leukemia (C91-C95)
> neutropenia (D70.-)
> sickle-cell disease (D57.-)

     R50.82   **Postprocedural fever**
> **Excludes1**   postprocedural infection (T81.4)
> posttransfusion fever (R50.84)
> postvaccination (postimmunization) fever (R50.83)

◀ New   ◀▥ Revised   ~~deleted~~ Deleted   Excludes 1   Excludes 2   Includes   Use additional   Code first   Code also   Unspecified

OGCR Official Guidelines   ● Unacceptable Principal Diagnosis   X Assign placeholder X   ● Use Additional Character(s)   ▷ Manifestation Code   **Coding Clinic**

R50.83   **Postvaccination fever**
    Postimmunization fever

R50.84   **Febrile nonhemolytic transfusion reaction**
    FNHTR
    Posttransfusion fever

R50.9   **Fever, `unspecified`**
    Fever NOS
    Fever of unknown origin [FUO]
    Fever with chills
    Fever with rigors
    Hyperpyrexia NOS
    Persistent fever
    Pyrexia NOS

R51   Headache
    Facial pain NOS

    Excludes1   atypical face pain (G50.1)
        migraine and other headache syndromes
          (G43-G44)
        trigeminal neuralgia (G50.0)

R52   Pain, `unspecified`
    Acute pain NOS   Pain NOS
    Generalized pain NOS

    Excludes1   acute and chronic pain, not elsewhere classified
          (G89.-)
        localized pain, unspecified type - code to pain by
          site, such as:
          abdomen pain (R10.-)
          back pain (M54.9)
          breast pain (N64.4)
          chest pain (R07.1-R07.9)
          ear pain (H92.0-)
          eye pain (H57.1)
          headache (R51)
          joint pain (M25.5-)
          limb pain (M79.6-)
          lumbar region pain (M54.5)
          pelvic and perineal pain (R10.2)
          shoulder pain (M25.51-)
          spine pain (M54.-)
          throat pain (R07.0)
          tongue pain (K14.6)
          tooth pain (K08.8)
          renal colic (N23)
        pain disorders exclusively related to
          psychological factors (F45.41)

⬤ **R53   Malaise and fatigue**

R53.0   **Neoplastic (malignant) related fatigue**
    Code first associated neoplasm

R53.1   **Weakness**
    Asthenia NOS

    Excludes1   age-related weakness (R54)
        muscle weakness (M62.8-)
        senile asthenia (R54)

R53.2   **Functional quadriplegia** 🔖
    Complete immobility due to severe physical disability
      or frailty

    Excludes1   frailty NOS (R54)
        hysterical paralysis (F44.4)
        immobility syndrome (M62.3)
        neurologic quadriplegia (G82.5-)
        quadriplegia (G82.50)

Ⓔ⨯ E08.40-E08.49, E08.618-E08.638, E08.649-E08.8, E09.40-E09.49,
    E09.618-E09.638, E09.649-E09.8, E10.40-E10.49, E10.618-E10.638,
    E10.649, E10.69-E10.8, E11.40-E11.49, E11.618-E11.638, E11.649,
    E11.69-E11.8, E13.40-E13.49, E13.618-E13.638, E13.649-E13.8, G04.1,
    G32.89, G80.0-G80.2, G80.4-G83.9, G90.1, G93.81, G93.89-G93.9,
    G96.8-G96.9, G98.0-G98.8, G99.8, Q06.0-Q06.1, Q06.3, Q06.8-Q06.9,
    Q07.8-Q07.9, R53.2

⬤ R53.8   **Other malaise and fatigue**

    Excludes1   combat exhaustion and fatigue (F43.0)
        congenital debility (P96.9)
        exhaustion and fatigue due to depressive
          episode (F32.-) ◀▥
        ~~depressive episode (F32.-)~~
        exhaustion and fatigue due to excessive
          exertion (T73.3) ◀▥
        exhaustion and fatigue due to exposure
          (T73.2) ◀▥
        exhaustion and fatigue due to heat
          (T67.-) ◀▥
        exhaustion and fatigue due to pregnancy
          (O26.8-) ◀▥
        exhaustion and fatigue due to recurrent
          depressive episode (F33) ◀▥
        exhaustion and fatigue due to senile
          debility (R54) ◀▥

R53.81   **Other malaise**
    Chronic debility
    Debility NOS
    General physical deterioration
    Malaise NOS
    Nervous debility

    Excludes1   age-related physical debility
        (R54)

R53.82   **Chronic fatigue, `unspecified`**
    Chronic fatigue syndrome NOS

    Excludes1   postviral fatigue syndrome
        (G93.3)

R53.83   **Other fatigue**
    Fatigue NOS   Lethargy
    Lack of energy   Tiredness

R54   Age-related physical debility   A
    Frailty   Senile asthenia
    Old age   Senile debility
    Senescence

    Excludes1   age-related cognitive decline (R41.81)
        senile psychosis (F03)
        senility NOS (R41.81)

R55   Syncope and collapse
    Blackout
    Fainting
    Vasovagal attack

    Excludes1   cardiogenic shock (R57.0)
        carotid sinus syncope (G90.01)
        heat syncope (T67.1)
        neurocirculatory asthenia (F45.8)
        neurogenic orthostatic hypotension (G90.3)
        orthostatic hypotension (I95.1)
        postprocedural shock (T81.1-)
        psychogenic syncope (F48.8)
        shock NOS (R57.9)
        shock complicating or following abortion or
          ectopic or molar pregnancy (O00-O07, O08.3)
        shock complicating or following labor and
          delivery (O75.1)
        Stokes-Adams attack (I45.9)
        unconsciousness NOS (R40.2-)

CHAPTER 18 (R00-R99)

N Newborn Age: 0   **P** Pediatric Age: 0–17   **M** Maternity DX: 12–55   **A** Adult Age: 15–124   ♀ Females Only   ♂ Males Only

🔖 Complication\Comorbidity   🔖 Major C\C   Ⓔ⨯ CC/MCC Exclusions   🔖 Present on Admission Requirement   🔖 Hospital-Acquired Condition

1279

CHAPTER 18 (R00-R99)

● **R56   Convulsions, not elsewhere classified**

> **Excludes1**   dissociative convulsions and seizures (F44.5)
> epileptic convulsions and seizures (G40.-)
> newborn convulsions and seizures (P90)

  ● **R56.0   Febrile convulsions**

> (Ex) **For category R56.0 CC codes:** G32.89, G40.001-G40.319,
> G40.401-G40.919, G40.A01-G40.B19, G89.0-G89.4, G93.81, G93.89-G93.9,
> G96.8-G96.9, G98.0-G98.8, P90, P91.8-P91.9, R41.0-R41.3, R41.82, R41.9,
> R44.8-R44.9, R45.83-R45.84, R46.0-R46.89, R52, R56.00-R56.9,
> R68.0-R68.19, R68.81-R68.83, R68.89-R69

     R56.00   Simple febrile convulsions 🔗
> Febrile convulsion NOS
> Febrile seizure NOS

     R56.01   Complex febrile convulsions 🔗
> Atypical febrile seizure
> Complex febrile seizure
> Complicated febrile seizure

> > **Excludes1**   status epilepticus (G40.901)

  ● **R56.1   Post traumatic seizures** 🔗

> **Excludes1**   post traumatic epilepsy (G40.-)

> (Ex) E08.40-E08.49, E09.40-E09.49, E10.40-E10.49, E11.40-E11.49,
> E13.40-E13.49, G32.89, G40.001-G40.319, G40.401-G40.919, G40.
> A01-G40.A19, G40.B01-G40.B19, G93.81, G93.89-G93.9, G96.8-G96.9,
> G98.0-G98.8, G99.8, R56.1

  ● **R56.9   Unspecified convulsions**

> Convulsion disorder   Recurrent convulsions
> Fit NOS   Seizure(s) (convulsive) NOS

● **R57   Shock, not elsewhere classified**

> **Excludes1**   anaphylactic shock NOS (T78.2)
> anaphylactic reaction or shock due to adverse
>   food reaction (T78.0-)
> anaphylactic shock due to adverse effect of
>   correct drug or medicament properly
>   administered (T88.6)
> anaphylactic shock due to serum (T80.5-)
> anesthetic shock (T88.3)
> electric shock (T75.4)
> obstetric shock (O75.1)
> postprocedural shock (T81.1-)
> psychic shock (F43.0)
> septic shock (R65.21)
> shock complicating or following ectopic or molar
>   pregnancy (O00-O07, O08.3)
> shock due to lightning (T75.01)
> traumatic shock (T79.4)
> toxic shock syndrome (A48.3)

> (Ex) **For category R57 CC codes:** G89.0-G89.4, R09.89, R41.0-R41.3, R41.82, R41.9,
> R44.8-R44.9, R45.83-R45.84, R46.0-R46.89, R52, R57.0-R57.9, R65.21, R68.0-R68.19,
> R68.81-R68.83, R68.89-R69

   R57.0   Cardiogenic shock 🔗
> MCC: Only if patient discharged alive

   R57.1   Hypovolemic shock 🔗
> *Decreased blood volume (loss)*
> MCC: Only if patient discharged alive

   R57.8   Other shock 🔗
> MCC: Only if patient discharged alive

   R57.9   Shock, unspecified 🔗
> Failure of peripheral circulation NOS
> *Resulting in significant blood pressure drop*

R58   Hemorrhage, not elsewhere classified
> Hemorrhage NOS

> **Excludes1**   hemorrhage included with underlying
>   conditions, such as:
>   acute duodenal ulcer with hemorrhage (K26.0)
>   acute gastritis with bleeding (K29.01)
>   ulcerative enterocolitis with rectal bleeding
>   (K51.01)

● **R59   Enlarged lymph nodes**

> **Includes**   swollen glands

> **Excludes1**   lymphadenitis NOS (I88.9)
> acute lymphadenitis (L04.-)
> chronic lymphadenitis (I88.1)
> mesenteric (acute) (chronic) lymphadenitis (I88.0)

   R59.0   Localized enlarged lymph nodes

   R59.1   Generalized enlarged lymph nodes
> Lymphadenopathy NOS

   R59.9   Enlarged lymph nodes, unspecified

● **R60   Edema, not elsewhere classified**

> **Excludes1**   angioneurotic edema (T78.3)
> ascites (R18.-)
> cerebral edema (G93.6)
> cerebral edema due to birth injury (P11.0)
> edema of larynx (J38.4)
> edema of nasopharynx (J39.2)
> edema of pharynx (J39.2)
> gestational edema (O12.0-)
> hereditary edema (Q82.0)
> hydrops fetalis NOS (P83.2)
> hydrothorax (J94.8)
> nutritional edema (E40-E46)
> hydrops fetalis NOS (P83.2)
> newborn edema (P83.3)
> pulmonary edema (J81.-)

   R60.0   Localized edema

   R60.1   Generalized edema

   R60.9   Edema, unspecified
> Fluid retention NOS

   R61   Generalized hyperhidrosis
> Excessive sweating
> Night sweats
> Secondary hyperhidrosis

> *Code first, if applicable, menopausal and female climacteric states*
> *(N95.1)*

> **Excludes1**   focal (primary) (secondary) hyperhidrosis (L74.5-)
> Frey's syndrome (L74.52)
> localized (primary) (secondary) hyperhidrosis
>   (L74.5-)

● **R62   Lack of expected normal physiological development in childhood and adults**

> **Excludes1**   delayed puberty (E30.0)
> gonadal dysgenesis (Q99.1)
> hypopituitarism (E23.0)

   R62.0   Delayed milestone in childhood   P
> Delayed attainment of expected physiological
>   developmental stage
> Late talker
> Late walker

  ● **R62.5   Other and unspecified lack of expected normal physiological development in childhood**

> **Excludes1**   HIV disease resulting in failure to thrive
>   (B20)
>   physical retardation due to malnutrition
>   (E45)

     R62.50   Unspecified lack of expected normal physiological development in childhood   P
> Infantilism NOS

     R62.51   Failure to thrive (child)   P
> Failure to gain weight

> > **Excludes1**   failure to thrive in child under 28
> > days old (P92.6)

     R62.52   Short stature (child)   P
> Lack of growth   Short stature NOS
> Physical retardation

> > **Excludes1**   short stature due to endocrine
> > disorder (E34.3)

     R62.59   Other lack of expected normal physiological development in childhood   P

   R62.7   Adult failure to thrive   A

◀ New   ◀ Revised   ~~deleted~~ Deleted   Excludes 1   Excludes 2   Includes   Use additional   Code first   Code also   Unspecified

OGCR Official Guidelines   ● Unacceptable Principal Diagnosis   X Assign placeholder X   ● Use Additional Character(s)   ▶ Manifestation Code   **Coding Clinic**

● **R63 Symptoms and signs concerning food and fluid intake**

> **Excludes1**   bulimia NOS (F50.2)
> eating disorders of nonorganic origin (F50.-)
> malnutrition (E40-E46)

R63.0 Anorexia
> Loss of appetite
> **Excludes1**   anorexia nervosa (F50.0-)
> loss of appetite of nonorganic origin (F50.8)

R63.1 Polydipsia
> Excessive thirst

R63.2 Polyphagia
> Excessive eating   Hyperalimentation NOS

R63.3 Feeding difficulties
> Feeding problem (elderly) (infant) NOS
> **Excludes1**   feeding problems of newborn (P92.-)
> infant feeding disorder of nonorganic origin (F98.2-)

R63.4 Abnormal weight loss

R63.5 Abnormal weight gain
> **Excludes1**   excessive weight gain in pregnancy (O26.0-)
> obesity (E66.-)

R63.6 Underweight
> Use additional code to identify body mass index (BMI), if known (Z68.-)
> **Excludes1**   abnormal weight loss (R63.4)
> anorexia nervosa (F50.0-)
> malnutrition (E40-E46)

R63.8 Other symptoms and signs concerning food and fluid intake

● **R64 Cachexia** 🖫
> Wasting syndrome
> *Code first* underlying condition, if known
> **Excludes1**   abnormal weight loss (R63.4)
> nutritional marasmus (E41)
> Ⓔ G89.0-G89.4, R41.0-R41.3, R41.82, R41.9, R44.8-R44.9, R45.83-R45.84, R46.0-R46.89, R52, R64, R68.0-R68.19, R68.81-R68.83, R68.89-R69

OGCR Section I.C.18.g.

> SIRS due to Non-Infectious Process
>
> The systemic inflammatory response syndrome (SIRS) can develop as a result of certain non-infectious disease processes, such as trauma, malignant neoplasm, or pancreatitis. When SIRS is documented with a noninfectious condition, and no subsequent infection is documented, the code for the underlying condition, such as an injury, should be assigned, followed by code R65.10, Systemic inflammatory response syndrome (SIRS) of non-infectious origin without acute organ dysfunction, or code R65.11, Systemic inflammatory response syndrome (SIRS) of non-infectious origin with acute organ dysfunction. If an associated acute organ dysfunction is documented, the appropriate code(s) for the specific type of organ dysfunction(s) should be assigned in addition to code R65.11. If acute organ dysfunction is documented, but it cannot be determined if the acute organ dysfunction is associated with SIRS or due to another condition (e.g., directly due to the trauma), the provider should be queried.

● **R65 Symptoms and signs specifically associated with systemic inflammation and infection**
> Ⓔ **For category R65 CC codes unless otherwise indicated:** A02.1, A20.7, A22.7, A26.7, A32.7, A39.2-A39.4, A40.0-A40.1, A40.8-A41.9, A42.7, A48.2-A48.4, A48.8-A49.9, A54.86, B00.7, B3.77, B92, B94.2-B96.89, R65.10-R65.20, Z16.10-Z16.39

● **R65.1 Systemic inflammatory response syndrome (SIRS) of non-infectious origin**
> *Code first* underlying condition, such as:
> heatstroke (T67.0)
> injury and trauma (S00-T88)
> **Excludes1**   sepsis - code to infection
> severe sepsis (R65.2)

R65.10 Systemic inflammatory response syndrome (SIRS) of non-infectious origin without acute organ dysfunction 🖫
> Systemic inflammatory response syndrome (SIRS) NOS

R65.11 Systemic inflammatory response syndrome (SIRS) of non-infectious origin with acute organ dysfunction 🖫
> Use additional code to identify specific acute organ dysfunction, such as:
> acute kidney failure (N17.-)
> acute respiratory failure (J96.0-)
> critical illness myopathy (G72.81)
> critical illness polyneuropathy (G62.81)
> disseminated intravascular coagulopathy [DIC] (D65)
> encephalopathy (metabolic) (septic) (G93.41)
> hepatic failure (K72.0-)

● **R65.2 Severe sepsis**
> Infection with associated acute organ dysfunction
> Sepsis with acute organ dysfunction
> Sepsis with multiple organ dysfunction
> Systemic inflammatory response syndrome due to infectious process with acute organ dysfunction
> *Code first* underlying infection, such as:
> infection following a procedure (T81.4)
> infections following infusion, transfusion and therapeutic injection (T80.2-)
> puerperal sepsis (O85)
> sepsis following complete or unspecified spontaneous abortion (O03.87)
> sepsis following ectopic and molar pregnancy (O08.82)
> sepsis following incomplete spontaneous abortion (O03.37)
> sepsis following (induced) termination of pregnancy (O04.87)
> sepsis NOS (A41.9) ◄▥
> Use additional code to identify specific acute organ dysfunction, such as:
> acute kidney failure (N17.-)
> acute respiratory failure (J96.0-)
> critical illness myopathy (G72.81)
> critical illness polyneuropathy (G62.81)
> disseminated intravascular coagulopathy [DIC] (D65)
> encephalopathy (metabolic) (septic) (G93.41)
> hepatic failure (K72.0-)

R65.20 Severe sepsis without septic shock 🖫
> Severe sepsis NOS

R65.21 Severe sepsis with septic shock 🖫
> MCC when PDx is its own MCC
> Ⓔ See R57

N   Newborn Age: 0   P   Pediatric Age: 0–17   M   Maternity DX: 12–55   A   Adult Age: 15–124   ♀   Females Only   ♂   Males Only

🖫 Complication\Comorbidity   🖫 Major C\C   Ⓔ CC/MCC Exclusions   🖫 Present on Admission Requirement   🖫 Hospital-Acquired Condition   **1281**

CHAPTER 18 (R00-R99)

CHAPTER 18 (R00-R99)

● **R68 Other general symptoms and signs**

R68.0 Hypothermia, not associated with low environmental temperature

Excludes1 hypothermia NOS (accidental) (T68)
hypothermia due to anesthesia (T88.51)
hypothermia due to low environmental temperature (T68)
newborn hypothermia (P80.-)

● **R68.1 Nonspecific symptoms peculiar to infancy**

Excludes1 colic, infantile (R10.83)
neonatal cerebral irritability (P91.3)
teething syndrome (K00.7)

R68.11 Excessive crying of infant (baby) P

Excludes1 excessive crying of child, adolescent, or adult (R45.83)

R68.12 Fussy infant (baby) P
Irritable infant

R68.13 Apparent life threatening event in infant (ALTE) P
Apparent life threatening event in newborn
Code first confirmed diagnosis, if known
Use additional code(s) for associated signs and symptoms if no confirmed diagnosis established, or if signs and symptoms are not associated routinely with confirmed diagnosis, or provide additional information for cause of ALTE

R68.19 Other nonspecific symptoms peculiar to infancy P

R68.2 Dry mouth, unspecified

Excludes1 dry mouth due to dehydration (E86.0)
dry mouth due to sicca syndrome [Sjögren] (M35.0-)
salivary gland hyposecretion (K11.7)

R68.3 Clubbing of fingers
Clubbing of nails

Excludes1 congenital clubfinger (Q68.1)

● **R68.8 Other general symptoms and signs**

R68.81 Early satiety

R68.82 Decreased libido A
Decreased sexual desire

R68.83 Chills (without fever)
Chills NOS

Excludes1 chills with fever (R50.9)

R68.84 Jaw pain
Mandibular pain
Maxilla pain

Excludes1 temporomandibular joint arthralgia (M26.62)

R68.89 Other general symptoms and signs

R69 Illness, unspecified
Unknown and unspecified cases of morbidity

ABNORMAL FINDINGS ON EXAMINATION OF BLOOD, WITHOUT DIAGNOSIS (R70-R79)

Excludes1 abnormalities (of)(on):
abnormal findings on antenatal screening of mother (O28.-)
coagulation hemorrhagic disorders (D65-D68)
lipids (E78.-)
platelets and thrombocytes (D69.-)
white blood cells classified elsewhere (D70-D72)
diagnostic abnormal findings classified elsewhere - see Alphabetical Index
hemorrhagic and hematological disorders of newborn (P50-P61)

● **R70 Elevated erythrocyte sedimentation rate and abnormality of plasma viscosity**

R70.0 Elevated erythrocyte sedimentation rate

R70.1 Abnormal plasma viscosity

● **R71 Abnormality of red blood cells**

Excludes1 anemias (D50-D64)
anemia of premature infant (P61.2)
benign (familial) polycythemia (D75.0)
congenital anemias (P61.2-P61.4)
newborn anemia due to isoimmunization (P55.-)
polycythemia neonatorum (P61.1)
polycythemia NOS (D75.1)
polycythemia vera (D45)
secondary polycythemia (D75.1)

R71.0 Precipitous drop in hematocrit 🔾
Drop (precipitous) in hemoglobin
Drop in hematocrit
Blood volume that is red blood cells
(Ex) D62, D64.4-D64.9

R71.8 Other abnormality of red blood cells
Abnormal red-cell morphology NOS
Abnormal red-cell volume NOS
Anisocytosis
Red blood cells of unequal size
Poikilocytosis
Red blood cells of abnormal shape

● **R73 Elevated blood glucose level**

Excludes1 diabetes mellitus (E08-E13)
diabetes mellitus in pregnancy, childbirth and the puerperium (O24.-)
neonatal disorders (P70.0-P70.2)
postsurgical hypoinsulinemia (E89.1)

● **R73.0 Abnormal glucose**

Excludes1 abnormal glucose in pregnancy (O99.81-)
diabetes mellitus (E08-E13)
dysmetabolic syndrome X (E88.81)
gestational diabetes (O24.4-)
glycosuria (R81)
hypoglycemia (E16.2)

R73.01 Impaired fasting glucose
Elevated fasting glucose

R73.02 Impaired glucose tolerance (oral)
Elevated glucose tolerance

R73.09 Other abnormal glucose
Abnormal glucose NOS
Abnormal non-fasting glucose tolerance
Latent diabetes
Prediabetes

R73.9 Hyperglycemia, unspecified

● **R74 Abnormal serum enzyme levels**

R74.0 Nonspecific elevation of levels of transaminase and lactic acid dehydrogenase [LDH]

R74.8 Abnormal levels of other serum enzymes
Abnormal level of acid phosphatase
Abnormal level of alkaline phosphatase
Abnormal level of amylase
Abnormal level of lipase [triacylglycerol lipase]

R74.9 Abnormal serum enzyme level, unspecified

OGCR Section I.C.1.2.e and f.

Patients with inconclusive HIV serology

e. Patients with inconclusive HIV serology, but no definitive diagnosis or manifestations of the illness, may be assigned code R75, Inconclusive laboratory evidence of human immunodeficiency virus [HIV].

f. Previously diagnosed HIV-related illness

Patients with any known prior diagnosis of an HIV-related illness should be coded to B20. Once a patient has developed an HIV-related illness, the patient should always be assigned code B20 on every subsequent admission/encounter. Patients previously diagnosed with any HIV illness (B20) should never be assigned to R75 or Z21, Asymptomatic human immunodeficiency virus [HIV] infection status.

◄ New ◄ Revised ~~deleted~~ Deleted Excludes 1 Excludes 2 Includes Use additional Code first Code also Unspecified

1282 OGCR Official Guidelines ● Unacceptable Principal Diagnosis X Assign placeholder X ● Use Additional Character(s) ▶ Manifestation Code **Coding Clinic**

R75 Inconclusive laboratory evidence of human immunodeficiency virus [HIV]
    Nonconclusive HIV-test finding in infants
    Excludes1 asymptomatic human immunodeficiency virus [HIV] infection status (Z21)
                 human immunodeficiency virus [HIV] disease (B20)

● R76 Other abnormal immunological findings in serum
  R76.0 Raised antibody titer
    Excludes1 isoimmunization in pregnancy (O36.0-O36.1)
                 isoimmunization affecting newborn (P55.-)

  ● R76.1 Nonspecific reaction to test for tuberculosis
    R76.11 Nonspecific reaction to tuberculin skin test without active tuberculosis
      Abnormal result of Mantoux test
      PPD positive
      Tuberculin (skin test) positive
      Tuberculin (skin test) reactor
      Excludes1 nonspecific reaction to cell mediated immunity measurement of gamma interferon antigen response without active tuberculosis (R76.12)
    R76.12 Nonspecific reaction to cell mediated immunity measurement of gamma interferon antigen response without active tuberculosis
      Nonspecific reaction to QuantiFERON-TB test (QFT) without active tuberculosis
      Excludes1 nonspecific reaction to tuberculin skin test without active tuberculosis (R76.11)
                 positive tuberculin skin test (R76.11)

  R76.8 Other specified abnormal immunological findings in serum
    Raised level of immunoglobulins NOS
  R76.9 Abnormal immunological finding in serum, unspecified

● R77 Other abnormalities of plasma proteins
    Excludes1 disorders of plasma-protein metabolism (E88.0)
  R77.0 Abnormality of albumin
  R77.1 Abnormality of globulin
    Hyperglobulinemia NOS
  R77.2 Abnormality of alphafetoprotein
  R77.8 Other specified abnormalities of plasma proteins
  R77.9 Abnormality of plasma protein, unspecified

● R78 Findings of drugs and other substances, not normally found in blood
    Use additional code to identify any retained foreign body, if applicable (Z18.-)
    Excludes1 mental or behavioral disorders due to psychoactive substance use (F10-F19)
  R78.0 Finding of alcohol in blood
    Use additional external cause code (Y90.-), for detail regarding alcohol level.
  R78.1 Finding of opiate drug in blood
  R78.2 Finding of cocaine in blood
  R78.3 Finding of hallucinogen in blood
  R78.4 Finding of other drugs of addictive potential in blood
  R78.5 Finding of other psychotropic drug in blood
  R78.6 Finding of steroid agent in blood

● R78.7 Finding of abnormal level of heavy metals in blood
  R78.71 Abnormal lead level in blood
    Excludes1 lead poisoning (T56.0-)
  R78.79 Finding of abnormal level of heavy metals in blood

● R78.8 Finding of other specified substances, not normally found in blood
  R78.81 Bacteremia 🔧
    Blood poisoning/bacteremia
    Excludes1 sepsis-code to specified infection (A00-B99)
    (Ex) B34.9, E07.81, G89.0-G89.4, R41.0-R41.3, R41.82, R41.9, R44.8-R44.9, R45.83-R45.84, R46.0-R46.89, R52, R68.0-R68.19, R68.81-R68.83, R68.89-R69, R70.1, R77.0-R77.9, R78.1-R78.6, R78.81, R78.9, R79.1-R79.89, R97.2
  R78.89 Finding of other specified substances, not normally found in blood
    Finding of abnormal level of lithium in blood
  R78.9 Finding of unspecified substance, not normally found in blood

● R79 Other abnormal findings of blood chemistry
    Use additional code to identify any retained foreign body, if applicable (Z18.-)
    Excludes1 abnormality of fluid, electrolyte or acid-base balance (E86-E87)
                 asymptomatic hyperuricemia (E79.0)
                 hyperglycemia NOS (R73.9)
                 hypoglycemia NOS (E16.2)
                 neonatal hypoglycemia (P70.3-P70.4)
                 specific findings indicating disorder of amino-acid metabolism (E70-E72) ◀▦
                 ~~amino-acid metabolism (E70-E72)~~
                 specific findings indicating disorder of carbohydrate metabolism (E73-E74) ◀▦
                 specific findings indicating disorder of lipid metabolism (E75.-) ◀▦

  R79.0 Abnormal level of blood mineral
    Abnormal blood level of cobalt
    Abnormal blood level of copper
    Abnormal blood level of iron
    Abnormal blood level of magnesium
    Abnormal blood level of mineral NEC
    Abnormal blood level of zinc
    Excludes1 abnormal level of lithium (R78.89)
                 disorders of mineral metabolism (E83.-)
                 neonatal hypomagnesemia (P71.2)
                 nutritional mineral deficiency (E58-E61)

  R79.1 Abnormal coagulation profile
    Abnormal or prolonged bleeding time
    Abnormal or prolonged coagulation time
    Abnormal or prolonged partial thromboplastin time [PTT]
    Abnormal or prolonged prothrombin time [PT]
    Excludes1 coagulation defects (D68.-)

● R79.8 Other specified abnormal findings of blood chemistry
  R79.81 Abnormal blood-gas level
  R79.82 Elevated C-reactive protein (CRP)
  R79.89 Other specified abnormal findings of blood chemistry

  R79.9 Abnormal finding of blood chemistry, unspecified

N Newborn Age: 0   **P** Pediatric Age: 0–17   **M** Maternity DX: 12–55   **A** Adult Age: 15–124   ♀ Females Only   ♂ Males Only

🔧 Complication\Comorbidity   🔧 Major C\C   (Ex) CC/MCC Exclusions   🔧 Present on Admission Requirement   🔧 Hospital-Acquired Condition   **1283**

ABNORMAL FINDINGS ON EXAMINATION OF URINE, WITHOUT DIAGNOSIS (R80-R82)

Excludes1   abnormal findings on antenatal screening of mother (O28.-)
diagnostic abnormal findings classified elsewhere - see Alphabetical Index
specific findings indicating disorder of amino-acid metabolism (E70-E72) ◄▦
~~amino-acid metabolism (E70-E72)~~
specific findings indicating disorder of carbohydrate metabolism (E73-E74) ◄▦

● **R80   Proteinuria**

Excludes1   gestational proteinuria (O12.1-)

R80.0   Isolated proteinuria
Idiopathic proteinuria

Excludes1   isolated proteinuria with specific morphological lesion (N06.-)

R80.1   Persistent proteinuria, unspecified

R80.2   Orthostatic proteinuria, unspecified
Postural proteinuria

R80.3   Bence Jones proteinuria

R80.8   Other proteinuria

R80.9   Proteinuria, unspecified
Albuminuria NOS

R81   Glycosuria

Excludes1   renal glycosuria (E74.8)

● **R82   Other and unspecified abnormal findings in urine**

Includes   chromoabnormalities in urine

Use additional code to identify any retained foreign body, if applicable (Z18.-)

Excludes2   hematuria (R31.-)

R82.0   Chyluria 🔊
White milky urine

Excludes1   filarial chyluria (B74.-)

(Ex:) G89.0-G89.4, R41.0-R41.3, R41.82, R41.9, R44.8-R44.9, R45.83-R45.84, R46.0-R46.89, R52, R68.0-R68.19, R68.81-R68.83, R68.89-R69, R82.0, R82.5-R82.99

R82.1   Myoglobinuria 🔊
Presence of myoglobin (iron containing protein) in urine
(Ex:) G89.0-G89.4, R41.0-R41.3, R41.82, R41.9, R44.8-R44.9, R45.83-R45.84, R46.0-R46.89, R52, R68.0-R68.19, R68.81-R68.83, R68.89-R69, R82.1, R82.3, R82.5-R82.99

R82.2   Biliuria
Presence of bile pigments/salts in urine

R82.3   Hemoglobinuria
Presence of hemoglobin in urine

Excludes1   hemoglobinuria due to hemolysis from external causes NEC (D59.6)
hemoglobinuria due to paroxysmal nocturnal [Marchiafava-Micheli] (D59.5)

R82.4   Acetonuria
Ketonuria

R82.5   Elevated urine levels of drugs, medicaments and biological substances
Elevated urine levels of catecholamines
Elevated urine levels of indoleacetic acid
Elevated urine levels of 17-ketosteroids
Elevated urine levels of steroids

R82.6   Abnormal urine levels of substances chiefly nonmedicinal as to source
Abnormal urine level of heavy metals

R82.7   Abnormal findings on microbiological examination of urine
Positive culture findings of urine

Excludes1   colonization status (Z22.-)

R82.8   Abnormal findings on cytological and histological examination of urine

R82.9   Other and unspecified abnormal findings in urine

R82.90   Unspecified abnormal findings in urine

R82.91   Other chromoabnormalities of urine
Chromoconversion (dipstick)
Idiopathic dipstick converts positive for blood with no cellular forms in sediment

Excludes1   hemoglobinuria (R82.3)
myoglobinuria (R82.1)

R82.99   Other abnormal findings in urine
Cells and casts in urine
Crystalluria
Melanuria

ABNORMAL FINDINGS ON EXAMINATION OF OTHER BODY FLUIDS, SUBSTANCES AND TISSUES, WITHOUT DIAGNOSIS (R83-R89)

Excludes1   abnormal findings on antenatal screening of mother (O28.-)
diagnostic abnormal findings classified elsewhere - see Alphabetical Index

Excludes2   abnormal findings on examination of blood, without diagnosis (R70-R79)
abnormal findings on examination of urine, without diagnosis (R80-R82)
abnormal tumor markers (R97.-)

● **R83   Abnormal findings in cerebrospinal fluid**

R83.0   Abnormal level of enzymes in cerebrospinal fluid

R83.1   Abnormal level of hormones in cerebrospinal fluid

R83.2   Abnormal level of other drugs, medicaments and biological substances in cerebrospinal fluid

R83.3   Abnormal level of substances chiefly nonmedicinal as to source in cerebrospinal fluid

R83.4   Abnormal immunological findings in cerebrospinal fluid

R83.5   Abnormal microbiological findings in cerebrospinal fluid
Positive culture findings in cerebrospinal fluid

Excludes1   colonization status (Z22.-)

R83.6   Abnormal cytological findings in cerebrospinal fluid

R83.8   Other abnormal findings in cerebrospinal fluid
Abnormal chromosomal findings in cerebrospinal fluid

R83.9   Unspecified abnormal finding in cerebrospinal fluid

● **R84   Abnormal findings in specimens from respiratory organs and thorax**

Includes   abnormal findings in bronchial washings
abnormal findings in nasal secretions
abnormal findings in pleural fluid
abnormal findings in sputum
abnormal findings in throat scrapings

Excludes1   blood-stained sputum (R04.2)

R84.0   Abnormal level of enzymes in specimens from respiratory organs and thorax

R84.1   Abnormal level of hormones in specimens from respiratory organs and thorax

R84.2   Abnormal level of other drugs, medicaments and biological substances in specimens from respiratory organs and thorax

R84.3   Abnormal level of substances chiefly nonmedicinal as to source in specimens from respiratory organs and thorax

R84.4   Abnormal immunological findings in specimens from respiratory organs and thorax

R84.5   Abnormal microbiological findings in specimens from respiratory organs and thorax
Positive culture findings in specimens from respiratory organs and thorax

Excludes1   colonization status (Z22.-)

R84.6   Abnormal cytological findings in specimens from respiratory organs and thorax

R84.7   Abnormal histological findings in specimens from respiratory organs and thorax

R84.8   **Other abnormal findings in specimens from respiratory organs and thorax**
    Abnormal chromosomal findings in specimens from respiratory organs and thorax

R84.9   Unspecified **abnormal finding in specimens from respiratory organs and thorax**

● **R85   Abnormal findings in specimens from digestive organs and abdominal cavity**

    Includes   abnormal findings in peritoneal fluid
                abnormal findings in saliva

    Excludes1   cloudy peritoneal dialysis effluent (R88.0)
                  fecal abnormalities (R19.5)

R85.0   **Abnormal level of enzymes in specimens from digestive organs and abdominal cavity**

R85.1   **Abnormal level of hormones in specimens from digestive organs and abdominal cavity**

R85.2   **Abnormal level of other drugs, medicaments and biological substances in specimens from digestive organs and abdominal cavity**

R85.3   **Abnormal level of substances chiefly nonmedicinal as to source in specimens from digestive organs and abdominal cavity**

R85.4   **Abnormal immunological findings in specimens from digestive organs and abdominal cavity**

R85.5   **Abnormal microbiological findings in specimens from digestive organs and abdominal cavity**
    Positive culture findings in specimens from digestive organs and abdominal cavity

    Excludes1   colonization status (Z22.-)

● R85.6   **Abnormal cytological findings in specimens from digestive organs and abdominal cavity**

  ● R85.61   **Abnormal cytologic smear of anus**

        Excludes1   abnormal cytological findings in specimens from other digestive organs and abdominal cavity (R85.69)
                carcinoma in situ of anus (histologically confirmed) (D01.3)
                anal intraepithelial neoplasia I [AIN I] (K62.82)
                anal intraepithelial neoplasia II [AIN II] (K62.82)
                anal intraepithelial neoplasia III [AIN III] (D01.3)
                dysplasia (mild) (moderate) of anus (histologically confirmed) (K62.82)
                severe dysplasia of anus (histologically confirmed) (D01.3)

        Excludes2   anal high risk human papillomavirus (HPV) DNA test positive (R85.81)
                anal low risk human papillomavirus (HPV) DNA test positive (R85.82)

    R85.610   **Atypical squamous cells of undetermined significance on cytologic smear of anus (ASC-US)**

    R85.611   **Atypical squamous cells cannot exclude high grade squamous intraepithelial lesion on cytologic smear of anus (ASC-H)**

    R85.612   **Low grade squamous intraepithelial lesion on cytologic smear of anus (LGSIL)**

    R85.613   **High grade squamous intraepithelial lesion on cytologic smear of anus (HGSIL)**

    R85.614   **Cytologic evidence of malignancy on smear of anus**

    R85.615   **Unsatisfactory cytologic smear of anus**
        Inadequate sample of cytologic smear of anus

    R85.616   **Satisfactory anal smear but lacking transformation zone**

    R85.618   **Other abnormal cytological findings on specimens from anus**

    R85.619   Unspecified **abnormal cytological findings in specimens from anus**
        Abnormal anal cytology NOS
        Atypical glandular cells of anus NOS

  R85.69   **Abnormal cytological findings in specimens from other digestive organs and abdominal cavity**

R85.7   **Abnormal histological findings in specimens from digestive organs and abdominal cavity**

● R85.8   **Other abnormal findings in specimens from digestive organs and abdominal cavity**

  R85.81   **Anal high risk human papillomavirus (HPV) DNA test positive**

        Excludes1   anogenital warts due to human papillomavirus (HPV) (A63.0)
                condyloma acuminatum (A63.0)

  R85.82   **Anal low risk human papillomavirus (HPV) DNA test positive**
    Use additional code for associated human papillomavirus (B97.7)

  R85.89   **Other abnormal findings in specimens from digestive organs and abdominal cavity**
    Abnormal chromosomal findings in specimens from digestive organs and abdominal cavity

R85.9   Unspecified **abnormal finding in specimens from digestive organs and abdominal cavity**

● **R86   Abnormal findings in specimens from male genital organs**

    Includes   abnormal findings in prostatic secretions
                abnormal findings in semen, seminal fluid
                abnormal spermatozoa

    Excludes1   azoospermia (N46.0-)
                  oligospermia (N46.1-)

R86.0   **Abnormal level of enzymes in specimens from male genital organs** ♂

R86.1   **Abnormal level of hormones in specimens from male genital organs** ♂

R86.2   **Abnormal level of other drugs, medicaments and biological substances in specimens from male genital organs** ♂

R86.3   **Abnormal level of substances chiefly nonmedicinal as to source in specimens from male genital organs** ♂

R86.4   **Abnormal immunological findings in specimens from male genital organs** ♂

R86.5   **Abnormal microbiological findings in specimens from male genital organs** ♂
    Positive culture findings in specimens from male genital organs

    Excludes1   colonization status (Z22.-)

R86.6   **Abnormal cytological findings in specimens from male genital organs** ♂

R86.7   **Abnormal histological findings in specimens from male genital organs** ♂

R86.8   **Other abnormal findings in specimens from male genital organs** ♂
    Abnormal chromosomal findings in specimens from male genital organs

R86.9   Unspecified **abnormal finding in specimens from male genital organs** ♂

N   Newborn Age: 0   P   Pediatric Age: 0–17   M   Maternity DX: 12–55   A   Adult Age: 15–124   ♀   Females Only   ♂   Males Only

🔴 Complication\Comorbidity   🔴 Major C\C   (Ex) CC/MCC Exclusions   🔴 Present on Admission Requirement   🔴 Hospital-Acquired Condition   **1285**

CHAPTER 18 (R00-R99)

● **R87**   **Abnormal findings in specimens from female genital organs**

      Includes   abnormal findings in secretion and smears from cervix uteri

                      abnormal findings in secretion and smears from vagina

                      abnormal findings in secretion and smears from vulva

  R87.0   **Abnormal level of enzymes in specimens from female genital organs** ♀

  R87.1   **Abnormal level of hormones in specimens from female genital organs** ♀

  R87.2   **Abnormal level of other drugs, medicaments and biological substances in specimens from female genital organs** ♀

  R87.3   **Abnormal level of substances chiefly nonmedicinal as to source in specimens from female genital organs** ♀

  R87.4   **Abnormal immunological findings in specimens from female genital organs** ♀

  R87.5   **Abnormal microbiological findings in specimens from female genital organs** ♀

      Positive culture findings in specimens from female genital organs

      Excludes1   colonization status (Z22.-)

● **R87.6**   **Abnormal cytological findings in specimens from female genital organs**

  ● **R87.61**   **Abnormal cytological findings in specimens from cervix uteri**

      Excludes1   abnormal cytological findings in specimens from other female genital organs (R87.69)

                  abnormal cytological findings in specimens from vagina (R87.62-)

                  carcinoma in situ of cervix uteri (histologically confirmed) (D06.-)

                  cervical intraepithelial neoplasia I [CIN I] (N87.0)

                  cervical intraepithelial neoplasia II [CIN II] (N87.1)

                  cervical intraepithelial neoplasia III [CIN III] (D06.-)

                  dysplasia (mild) (moderate) of cervix uteri (histologically confirmed) (N87.-)

                  severe dysplasia of cervix uteri (histologically confirmed) (D06.-)

      Excludes2   cervical high risk human papillomavirus (HPV) DNA test positive (R87.810)

                  cervical low risk human papillomavirus (HPV) DNA test positive (R87.820)

    R87.610   **Atypical squamous cells of undetermined significance on cytologic smear of cervix (ASC-US)** ♀

    R87.611   **Atypical squamous cells cannot exclude high grade squamous intraepithelial lesion on cytologic smear of cervix (ASC-H)** ♀

    R87.612   **Low grade squamous intraepithelial lesion on cytologic smear of cervix (LGSIL)** ♀

    R87.613   **High grade squamous intraepithelial lesion on cytologic smear of cervix (HGSIL)** ♀

    R87.614   **Cytologic evidence of malignancy on smear of cervix** ♀

    R87.615   **Unsatisfactory cytologic smear of cervix** ♀

      Inadequate sample of cytologic smear of cervix

    R87.616   **Satisfactory cervical smear but lacking transformation zone** ♀

    R87.618   **Other abnormal cytological findings on specimens from cervix uteri** ♀

    R87.619   **Unspecified abnormal cytological findings in specimens from cervix uteri** ♀

      Abnormal cervical cytology NOS

      Abnormal Papanicolaou smear of cervix NOS

      Abnormal thin preparation smear of cervix NOS

      Atypical endocervical cells of cervix NOS

      Atypical endometrial cells of cervix NOS

      Atypical glandular cells of cervix NOS

  ● **R87.62**   **Abnormal cytological findings in specimens from vagina**

      Use additional code to identify acquired absence of uterus and cervix, if applicable (Z90.71-)

      Excludes1   abnormal cytological findings in specimens from cervix uteri (R87.61-)

                  abnormal cytological findings in specimens from other female genital organs (R87.69)

                  carcinoma in situ of vagina (histologically confirmed) (D07.2)

                  vaginal intraepithelial neoplasia I [VAIN I] (N89.0)

                  vaginal intraepithelial neoplasia II [VAIN II] (N89.1)

                  vaginal intraepithelial neoplasia III [VAIN III] (D07.2)

                  dysplasia (mild) (moderate) of vagina (histologically confirmed) (N89.-)

                  severe dysplasia of vagina (histologically confirmed) (D07.2)

      Excludes2   vaginal high risk human papillomavirus (HPV) DNA test positive (R87.811)

                  vaginal low risk human papillomavirus (HPV) DNA test positive (R87.821)

    R87.620   **Atypical squamous cells of undetermined significance on cytologic smear of vagina (ASC-US)** ♀

    R87.621   **Atypical squamous cells cannot exclude high grade squamous intraepithelial lesion on cytologic smear of vagina (ASC-H)** ♀

    R87.622   **Low grade squamous intraepithelial lesion on cytologic smear of vagina (LGSIL)** ♀

    R87.623   **High grade squamous intraepithelial lesion on cytologic smear of vagina (HGSIL)** ♀

    R87.624   **Cytologic evidence of malignancy on smear of vagina** ♀

    R87.625   **Unsatisfactory cytologic smear of vagina** ♀

      Inadequate sample of cytologic smear of vagina

    R87.628   **Other abnormal cytological findings on specimens from vagina** ♀

R87.629   Unspecified abnormal cytological findings in specimens from vagina ♀
     Abnormal Papanicolaou smear of vagina NOS
     Abnormal thin preparation smear of vagina NOS
     Abnormal vaginal cytology NOS
     Atypical endocervical cells of vagina NOS
     Atypical endometrial cells of vagina NOS
     Atypical glandular cells of vagina NOS

R87.69   Abnormal cytological findings in specimens from other female genital organs ♀
     Abnormal cytological findings in specimens from female genital organs NOS

     Excludes1   dysplasia of vulva (histologically confirmed) (N90.0-N90.3)

R87.7   Abnormal histological findings in specimens from female genital organs ♀

     Excludes1   carcinoma in situ (histologically confirmed) of female genital organs (D06-D07.3)
       cervical intraepithelial neoplasia I [CIN I] (N87.0)
       cervical intraepithelial neoplasia II [CIN II] (N87.1)
       cervical intraepithelial neoplasia III [CIN III] (D06.-)
       dysplasia (mild) (moderate) of cervix uteri (histologically confirmed) (N87.-)
       dysplasia (mild) (moderate) of vagina (histologically confirmed) (N89.-)
       vaginal intraepithelial neoplasia I [VAIN I] (N89.0)
       vaginal intraepithelial neoplasia II [VAIN II] (N89.1)
       vaginal intraepithelial neoplasia III [VAIN III] (D07.2)
       severe dysplasia of cervix uteri (histologically confirmed) (D06.-)
       severe dysplasia of vagina (histologically confirmed) (D07.2)

● R87.8   Other abnormal findings in specimens from female genital organs

   ● R87.81   High risk human papillomavirus (HPV) DNA test positive from female genital organs

       Excludes1   anogenital warts due to human papillomavirus (HPV) (A63.0)
         condyloma acuminatum (A63.0)

     R87.810   Cervical high risk human papillomavirus (HPV) DNA test positive ♀

     R87.811   Vaginal high risk human papillomavirus (HPV) DNA test positive ♀

   ● R87.82   Low risk human papillomavirus (HPV) DNA test positive from female genital organs

       Use additional code for associated human papillomavirus (B97.7)

     R87.820   Cervical low risk human papillomavirus (HPV) DNA test positive ♀

     R87.821   Vaginal low risk human papillomavirus (HPV) DNA test positive ♀

   R87.89   Other abnormal findings in specimens from female genital organs ♀
     Abnormal chromosomal findings in specimens from female genital organs

R87.9   Unspecified abnormal finding in specimens from female genital organs ♀

● R88   Abnormal findings in other body fluids and substances
   R88.0   Cloudy (hemodialysis) (peritoneal) dialysis effluent
   R88.8   Abnormal findings in other body fluids and substances

● R89   Abnormal findings in specimens from other organs, systems and tissues

   Includes   abnormal findings in nipple discharge
     abnormal findings in synovial fluid
     abnormal findings in wound secretions

   R89.0   Abnormal level of enzymes in specimens from other organs, systems and tissues
   R89.1   Abnormal level of hormones in specimens from other organs, systems and tissues
   R89.2   Abnormal level of other drugs, medicaments and biological substances in specimens from other organs, systems and tissues
   R89.3   Abnormal level of substances chiefly nonmedicinal as to source in specimens from other organs, systems and tissues
   R89.4   Abnormal immunological findings in specimens from other organs, systems and tissues
   R89.5   Abnormal microbiological findings in specimens from other organs, systems and tissues
     Positive culture findings in specimens from other organs, systems and tissues

     Excludes1   colonization status (Z22.-)

   R89.6   Abnormal cytological findings in specimens from other organs, systems and tissues
   R89.7   Abnormal histological findings in specimens from other organs, systems and tissues
   R89.8   Other abnormal findings in specimens from other organs, systems and tissues
     Abnormal chromosomal findings in specimens from other organs, systems and tissues
   R89.9   Unspecified abnormal finding in specimens from other organs, systems and tissues

---

ABNORMAL FINDINGS ON DIAGNOSTIC IMAGING AND IN FUNCTION STUDIES, WITHOUT DIAGNOSIS (R90-R94)

   Includes   nonspecific abnormal findings on diagnostic imaging by computerized axial tomography [CAT scan]
     nonspecific abnormal findings on diagnostic imaging by magnetic resonance imaging [MRI][NMR]
     nonspecific abnormal findings on diagnostic imaging by positron emission tomography [PET scan]
     nonspecific abnormal findings on diagnostic imaging by thermography
     nonspecific abnormal findings on diagnostic imaging by ultrasound [echogram]
     nonspecific abnormal findings on diagnostic imaging by X-ray examination

   Excludes1   abnormal findings on antenatal screening of mother (O28.-)
     diagnostic abnormal findings classified elsewhere - see Alphabetical Index

● R90   Abnormal findings on diagnostic imaging of central nervous system
   R90.0   Intracranial space-occupying lesion found on diagnostic imaging of central nervous system
   ● R90.8   Other abnormal findings on diagnostic imaging of central nervous system
     R90.81   Abnormal echoencephalogram
     R90.82   White matter disease, unspecified
     R90.89   Other abnormal findings on diagnostic imaging of central nervous system
       Other cerebrovascular abnormality found on diagnostic imaging of central nervous system

● **R91**   **Abnormal findings on diagnostic imaging of lung**

    R91.1   **Solitary pulmonary nodule**
         Coin lesion lung
         Solitary pulmonary nodule, subsegmental branch of the bronchial tree

    R91.8   **Other nonspecific abnormal finding of lung field**
         Lung mass NOS found on diagnostic imaging of lung
         Pulmonary infiltrate NOS
         Shadow, lung

● **R92**   **Abnormal and inconclusive findings on diagnostic imaging of breast**

    R92.0   **Mammographic microcalcification found on diagnostic imaging of breast**
         Excludes2   mammographic calcification (calculus) found on diagnostic imaging of breast (R92.1)

    R92.1   **Mammographic calcification found on diagnostic imaging of breast**
         Mammographic calculus found on diagnostic imaging of breast

    R92.2   **Inconclusive mammogram**
         Dense breasts NOS
         Inconclusive mammogram NEC
         Inconclusive mammography due to dense breasts
         Inconclusive mammography NEC

    R92.8   **Other abnormal and inconclusive findings on diagnostic imaging of breast**

● **R93**   **Abnormal findings on diagnostic imaging of other body structures**

    R93.0   **Abnormal findings on diagnostic imaging of skull and head, not elsewhere classified**
         Excludes1   intracranial space-occupying lesion found on diagnostic imaging (R90.0)

    R93.1   **Abnormal findings on diagnostic imaging of heart and coronary circulation**
         Abnormal echocardiogram NOS
         Abnormal heart shadow

    R93.2   **Abnormal findings on diagnostic imaging of liver and biliary tract**
         Nonvisualization of gallbladder

    R93.3   **Abnormal findings on diagnostic imaging of other parts of digestive tract**

    R93.4   **Abnormal findings on diagnostic imaging of urinary organs**
         Filling defect of bladder found on diagnostic imaging
         Filling defect of kidney found on diagnostic imaging
         Filling defect of ureter found on diagnostic imaging
         Excludes1   hypertrophy of kidney (N28.81)

    R93.5   **Abnormal findings on diagnostic imaging of other abdominal regions, including retroperitoneum**

    R93.6   **Abnormal findings on diagnostic imaging of limbs**
         Excludes2   abnormal finding in skin and subcutaneous tissue (R93.8)

    R93.7   **Abnormal findings on diagnostic imaging of other parts of musculoskeletal system**
         Excludes2   abnormal findings on diagnostic imaging of skull (R93.0)

    R93.8   **Abnormal findings on diagnostic imaging of other specified body structures**
         Abnormal finding by radioisotope localization of placenta
         Abnormal radiological finding in skin and subcutaneous tissue
         Mediastinal shift

    R93.9   **Diagnostic imaging inconclusive due to excess body fat of patient**

● **R94**   **Abnormal results of function studies**
      Includes   abnormal results of radionuclide [radioisotope] uptake studies
                 abnormal results of scintigraphy

    ● **R94.0**   **Abnormal results of function studies of central nervous system**

       R94.01   **Abnormal electroencephalogram [EEG]**

       R94.02   **Abnormal brain scan**

       R94.09   **Abnormal results of other function studies of central nervous system**

    ● **R94.1**   **Abnormal results of function studies of peripheral nervous system and special senses**

       ● **R94.11**   **Abnormal results of function studies of eye**

          R94.110   **Abnormal electro-oculogram [EOG]**

          R94.111   **Abnormal electroretinogram [ERG]**
                Abnormal retinal function study

          R94.112   **Abnormal visually evoked potential [VEP]**

CHAPTER 18 (R00-R99)

Figure 18-2   A. Parasympathetic nervous system. **B.** Sympathetic nervous system. (From Buck CJ: Step-by-Step Medical Coding, Philadelphia, WB Saunders, 1998)

◀ New   ⬅ Revised   ~~deleted~~ Deleted   Excludes 1   Excludes 2   Includes   Use additional   Code first   Code also   Unspecified

OGCR Official Guidelines   ● Unacceptable Principal Diagnosis   X Assign placeholder X   ▶ Use Additional Character(s)   ▶ Manifestation Code   **Coding Clinic**

Item 18-1 The **peripheral nervous system** consists of 31 pairs of spinal nerves, 12 pairs of cranial nerves, and the autonomic nerves, which are divided into the parasympathetic and sympathetic nerves. The cranial nerves are: olfactory (I), optic (II), oculomotor (III), trochlear (IV), trigeminal (V), abducens (VI), facial (VII), vestibulocochlear (VIII), glossopharyngeal (IX), vagus (X), accessory (XI), and hypoglossal (XII).

     R94.113   Abnormal oculomotor study

     R94.118   Abnormal results of other function studies of eye

● R94.12   Abnormal results of function studies of ear and other special senses

     R94.120   Abnormal auditory function study

     R94.121   Abnormal vestibular function study

     R94.128   Abnormal results of other function studies of ear and other special senses

● R94.13   Abnormal results of function studies of peripheral nervous system

     R94.130   Abnormal response to nerve stimulation, unspecified

     R94.131   Abnormal electromyogram [EMG]
             Excludes1   electromyogram of eye (R94.113)

     R94.138   Abnormal results of other function studies of peripheral nervous system

R94.2   Abnormal results of pulmonary function studies
     Reduced ventilatory capacity
     Reduced vital capacity

● R94.3   Abnormal results of cardiovascular function studies

     R94.30   Abnormal result of cardiovascular function study, unspecified

     R94.31   Abnormal electrocardiogram [ECG] [EKG]
             Excludes1   long QT syndrome (I45.81)

     R94.39   Abnormal result of other cardiovascular function study
     Abnormal electrophysiological intracardiac studies
     Abnormal phonocardiogram
     Abnormal vectorcardiogram

R94.4   Abnormal results of kidney function studies
     Abnormal renal function test

R94.5   Abnormal results of liver function studies

R94.6   Abnormal results of thyroid function studies

R94.7   Abnormal results of other endocrine function studies
     Excludes2   abnormal glucose (R73.0-)

R94.8   Abnormal results of function studies of other organs and systems
     Abnormal basal metabolic rate [BMR]
     Abnormal bladder function test
     Abnormal splenic function test

ABNORMAL TUMOR MARKERS (R97)

● R97   Abnormal tumor markers
     Elevated tumor associated antigens [TAA]
     Elevated tumor specific antigens [TSA]

R97.0   Elevated carcinoembryonic antigen [CEA]

R97.1   Elevated cancer antigen 125 [CA 125] ♀

R97.2   Elevated prostate specific antigen [PSA] ♂   A
     MCE: Questionable admission when principal dx

R97.8   Other abnormal tumor markers

ILL-DEFINED AND UNKNOWN CAUSE OF MORTALITY (R99)

R99   Ill-defined and unknown cause of mortality
     Death (unexplained) NOS
     Unspecified cause of mortality

OGCR   Section I.C.18.h.

18.6 Death NOS

Code R99, Ill-defined and unknown cause of mortality, is only for use in the very limited circumstance when a patient who has already died is brought into the emergency department or other healthcare facility and is pronounced dead upon arrival. It does not represent the discharge disposition of death.

CHAPTER 18 (R00-R99)

| N Newborn Age: 0 | P Pediatric Age: 0–17 | M Maternity DX: 12–55 | A Adult Age: 15–124 | ♀ Females Only | ♂ Males Only |

Complication\Comorbidity   Major C\C   (Ex.) CC/MCC Exclusions   Present on Admission Requirement   Hospital-Acquired Condition

1289

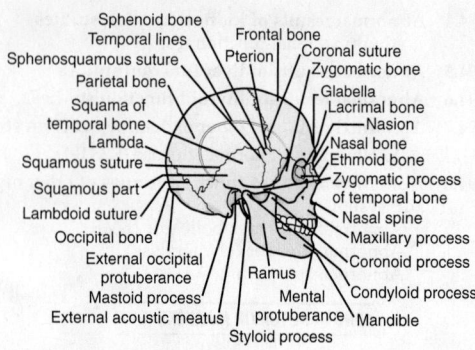

Figure 19-1 Lateral view of skull.

Figure 19-2 Frontal view of skull.

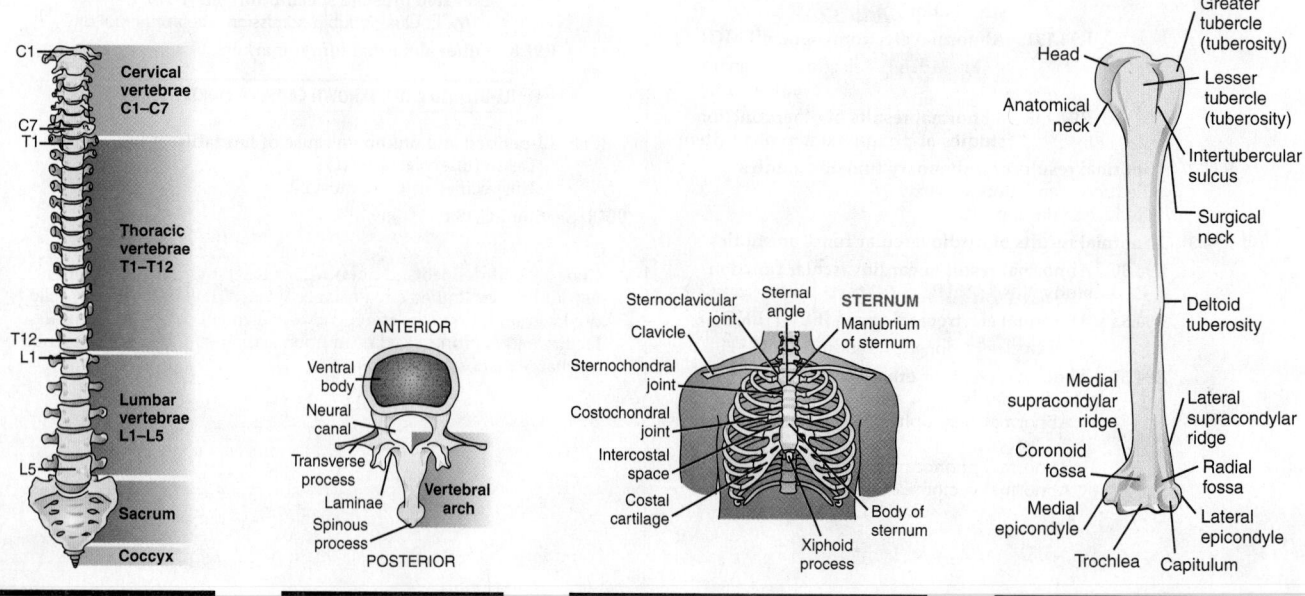

CHAPTER 19 (S00-T88)

Figure 19-3 Anterior view of vertebral column.

Figure 19-4 Vertebra viewed from above.

Figure 19-5 Anterior view of rib cage.

Figure 19-6 Anterior aspect of left humerus.

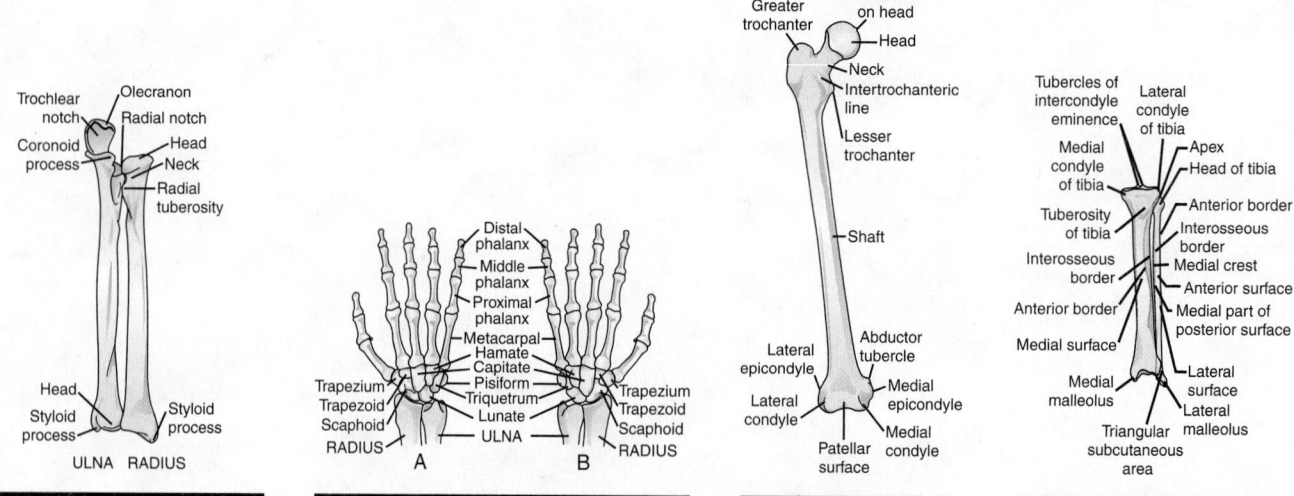

Figure 19-7 Anterior aspect of left radius and ulna.

Figure 19-8 Right hand and wrist: **A.** Dorsal surface. **B.** Palmar surface.

Figure 19-9 Anterior aspect of right femur.

Figure 19-10 Anterior aspect of left tibia and fibula.

◀ New　◀▥ Revised　d̶e̶l̶e̶t̶e̶d̶ Deleted　Excludes 1　Excludes 2　Includes　Use additional　Code first　Code also　Unspecified

OGCR Official Guidelines　● Unacceptable Principal Diagnosis　X Assign placeholder X　● Use Additional Character(s)　▸ Manifestation Code　**Coding Clinic**

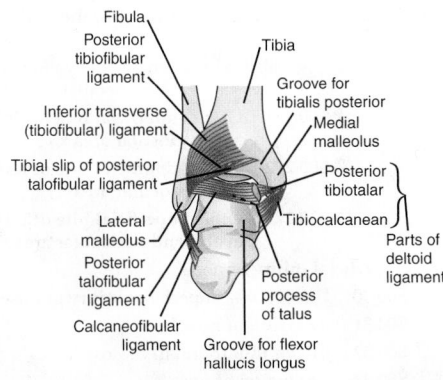

Figure 19-11 Posterior aspect of the left ankle joint.

Figure 19-12 Right foot viewed from above.

OGCR Chapter Guidelines are located in **Section I.9.**

CHAPTER 19

INJURY, POISONING AND CERTAIN OTHER CONSEQUENCES OF EXTERNAL CAUSES (S00-T88)

Note: Use secondary code(s) from Chapter 20, External causes of morbidity, to indicate cause of injury. Codes within the T section that include the external cause do not require an additional external cause code.

Use additional code to identify any retained foreign body, if applicable (Z18.-)

Excludes1 birth trauma (P10-P15)
obstetric trauma (O70-O71)

Note: The chapter uses the S-section for coding different types of injuries related to single body regions and the T-section to cover injuries to unspecified body regions as well as poisoning and certain other consequences of external causes.

This chapter contains the following blocks:

S00-S09	Injuries to the head
S10-S19	Injuries to the neck
S20-S29	Injuries to the thorax
S30-S39	Injuries to the abdomen, lower back, lumbar spine, pelvis and external genitals
S40-S49	Injuries to the shoulder and upper arm
S50-S59	Injuries to the elbow and forearm
S60-S69	Injuries to the wrist, hand, and fingers
S70-S79	Injuries to the hip and thigh
S80-S89	Injuries to the knee and lower leg
S90-S99	Injuries to the ankle and foot

T07	Injuries involving multiple body regions
T14	Injury of unspecified body region
T15-T19	Effects of foreign body entering through natural orifice
T20-T32	Burns and corrosions
T20-T25	Burns and corrosions of external body surface, specified by site
T26-T28	Burns and corrosions confined to eye and internal organs
T30-T32	Burns and corrosions of multiple and unspecified body regions
T33-T34	Frostbite
T36-T50	Poisoning by, adverse effect of and underdosing of drugs, medicaments and biological substances
T51-T65	Toxic effects of substances chiefly nonmedicinal as to source
T66-T78	Other and unspecified effects of external causes
T79	Certain early complications of trauma
T80-T88	Complications of surgical and medical care, not elsewhere classified

INJURIES TO THE HEAD (S00-S09)

Includes injuries of ear
injuries of eye
injuries of face [any part]
injuries of gum
injuries of jaw
injuries of oral cavity
injuries of palate
injuries of periocular area
injuries of scalp
injuries of temporomandibular joint area
injuries of tongue
injuries of tooth

Code also for any associated infection

Excludes2 burns and corrosions (T20-T32)
effects of foreign body in ear (T16)
effects of foreign body in larynx (T17.3)
effects of foreign body in mouth NOS (T18.0)
effects of foreign body in nose (T17.0-T17.1)
effects of foreign body in pharynx (T17.2)
effects of foreign body on external eye (T15.-)
frostbite (T33-T34)
insect bite or sting, venomous (T63.4)

● **S00 Superficial injury of head**
   Excludes1 diffuse cerebral contusion (S06.2-)
   focal cerebral contusion (S06.3-)
   injury of eye and orbit (S05.-)
   open wound of head (S01.-)

The appropriate 7th character is to be added to each code from category S00

A	initial encounter
D	subsequent encounter
S	sequela

● **S00.0 Superficial injury of scalp**
   X ● **S00.00 Unspecified superficial injury of scalp** 🔎
   X ● **S00.01 Abrasion of scalp** 🔎
   X ● **S00.02 Blister (nonthermal) of scalp** 🔎
   X ● **S00.03 Contusion of scalp** 🔎
      Bruise of scalp
      Hematoma of scalp
   X ● **S00.04 External constriction of part of scalp** 🔎
   X ● **S00.05 Superficial foreign body of scalp** 🔎
      Splinter in the scalp
   X ● **S00.06 Insect bite (nonvenomous) of scalp** 🔎
   X ● **S00.07 Other superficial bite of scalp** 🔎
      Excludes1 open bite of scalp (S01.05)

N Newborn Age: 0   P Pediatric Age: 0–17   M Maternity DX: 12–55   A Adult Age: 15–124   ♀ Females Only   ♂ Males Only

🔎 Complication\Comorbidity   🔎 Major C\C   (Ex) CC/MCC Exclusions   🔎 Present on Admission Requirement   🔎 Hospital-Acquired Condition   1291

● S00.1   Contusion of eyelid and periocular area
    Black eye
    Excludes2   contusion of eyeball and orbital tissues (S05.1)
X ● S00.10   Contusion of unspecified eyelid and periocular area 🔍
X ● S00.11   Contusion of right eyelid and periocular area 🔍
X ● S00.12   Contusion of left eyelid and periocular area 🔍

● S00.2   Other and unspecified superficial injuries of eyelid and periocular area
    Excludes2   superficial injury of conjunctiva and cornea (S05.0-)
   ● S00.20   Unspecified superficial injury of eyelid and periocular area
     ● S00.201   Unspecified superficial injury of right eyelid and periocular area 🔍
     ● S00.202   Unspecified superficial injury of left eyelid and periocular area 🔍
     ● S00.209   Unspecified superficial injury of unspecified eyelid and periocular area 🔍
   ● S00.21   Abrasion of eyelid and periocular area
     ● S00.211   Abrasion of right eyelid and periocular area 🔍
     ● S00.212   Abrasion of left eyelid and periocular area 🔍
     ● S00.219   Abrasion of unspecified eyelid and periocular area 🔍
   ● S00.22   Blister (nonthermal) of eyelid and periocular area
     ● S00.221   Blister (nonthermal) of right eyelid and periocular area 🔍
     ● S00.222   Blister (nonthermal) of left eyelid and periocular area 🔍
     ● S00.229   Blister (nonthermal) of unspecified eyelid and periocular area 🔍
   ● S00.24   External constriction of eyelid and periocular area
     ● S00.241   External constriction of right eyelid and periocular area 🔍
     ● S00.242   External constriction of left eyelid and periocular area 🔍
     ● S00.249   External constriction of unspecified eyelid and periocular area 🔍
   ● S00.25   Superficial foreign body of eyelid and periocular area
     Splinter of eyelid and periocular area
     Excludes2   retained foreign body in eyelid (H02.81-)
     ● S00.251   Superficial foreign body of right eyelid and periocular area 🔍
     ● S00.252   Superficial foreign body of left eyelid and periocular area 🔍
     ● S00.259   Superficial foreign body of unspecified eyelid and periocular area 🔍
   ● S00.26   Insect bite (nonvenomous) of eyelid and periocular area
     ● S00.261   Insect bite (nonvenomous) of right eyelid and periocular area 🔍
     ● S00.262   Insect bite (nonvenomous) of left eyelid and periocular area 🔍
     ● S00.269   Insect bite (nonvenomous) of unspecified eyelid and periocular area 🔍

● S00.27   Other superficial bite of eyelid and periocular area
    Excludes1   open bite of eyelid and periocular area (S01.15)
     ● S00.271   Other superficial bite of right eyelid and periocular area 🔍
     ● S00.272   Other superficial bite of left eyelid and periocular area 🔍
     ● S00.279   Other superficial bite of unspecified eyelid and periocular area 🔍

● S00.3   Superficial injury of nose
X ● S00.30   Unspecified superficial injury of nose 🔍
X ● S00.31   Abrasion of nose 🔍
X ● S00.32   Blister (nonthermal) of nose 🔍
X ● S00.33   Contusion of nose 🔍
    Bruise of nose
    Hematoma of nose
X ● S00.34   External constriction of nose 🔍
X ● S00.35   Superficial foreign body of nose 🔍
    Splinter in the nose
X ● S00.36   Insect bite (nonvenomous) of nose 🔍
X ● S00.37   Other superficial bite of nose 🔍
    Excludes1   open bite of nose (S01.25)

● S00.4   Superficial injury of ear
   ● S00.40   Unspecified superficial injury of ear
     ● S00.401   Unspecified superficial injury of right ear 🔍
     ● S00.402   Unspecified superficial injury of left ear 🔍
     ● S00.409   Unspecified superficial injury of unspecified ear 🔍
   ● S00.41   Abrasion of ear
     ● S00.411   Abrasion of right ear 🔍
     ● S00.412   Abrasion of left ear 🔍
     ● S00.419   Abrasion of unspecified ear 🔍
   ● S00.42   Blister (nonthermal) of ear
     ● S00.421   Blister (nonthermal) of right ear 🔍
     ● S00.422   Blister (nonthermal) of left ear 🔍
     ● S00.429   Blister (nonthermal) of unspecified ear 🔍
   ● S00.43   Contusion of ear
     Bruise of ear
     Hematoma of ear
     ● S00.431   Contusion of right ear 🔍
     ● S00.432   Contusion of left ear 🔍
     ● S00.439   Contusion of unspecified ear 🔍
   ● S00.44   External constriction of ear
     ● S00.441   External constriction of right ear 🔍
     ● S00.442   External constriction of left ear 🔍
     ● S00.449   External constriction of unspecified ear 🔍
   ● S00.45   Superficial foreign body of ear
     Splinter in the ear
     ● S00.451   Superficial foreign body of right ear 🔍
     ● S00.452   Superficial foreign body of left ear 🔍
     ● S00.459   Superficial foreign body of unspecified ear 🔍
   ● S00.46   Insect bite (nonvenomous) of ear
     ● S00.461   Insect bite (nonvenomous) of right ear 🔍
     ● S00.462   Insect bite (nonvenomous) of left ear 🔍
     ● S00.469   Insect bite (nonvenomous) of unspecified ear 🔍

● S00.47   Other superficial bite of ear
    Excludes1   open bite of ear (S01.35)
   ● S00.471   Other superficial bite of right ear 🔖
   ● S00.472   Other superficial bite of left ear 🔖
   ● S00.479   Other superficial bite of unspecified ear 🔖

● S00.5   Superficial injury of lip and oral cavity
  ● S00.50   Unspecified superficial injury of lip and oral cavity
   ● S00.501   Unspecified superficial injury of lip 🔖
   ● S00.502   Unspecified superficial injury of oral cavity 🔖
  ● S00.51   Abrasion of lip and oral cavity
   ● S00.511   Abrasion of lip 🔖
   ● S00.512   Abrasion of oral cavity 🔖
  ● S00.52   Blister (nonthermal) of lip and oral cavity
   ● S00.521   Blister (nonthermal) of lip 🔖
   ● S00.522   Blister (nonthermal) of oral cavity 🔖
  ● S00.53   Contusion of lip and oral cavity
   ● S00.531   Contusion of lip 🔖
     Bruise of lip
     Hematoma of oral cavity
   ● S00.532   Contusion of oral cavity 🔖
     Bruise of lip
     Hematoma of oral cavity
  ● S00.54   External constriction of lip and oral cavity
   ● S00.541   External constriction of lip 🔖
   ● S00.542   External constriction of oral cavity 🔖
  ● S00.55   Superficial foreign body of lip and oral cavity
   ● S00.551   Superficial foreign body of lip 🔖
     Splinter of lip and oral cavity
   ● S00.552   Superficial foreign body of oral cavity 🔖
     Splinter of lip and oral cavity
  ● S00.56   Insect bite (nonvenomous) of lip and oral cavity
   ● S00.561   Insect bite (nonvenomous) of lip 🔖
   ● S00.562   Insect bite (nonvenomous) of oral cavity 🔖
  ● S00.57   Other superficial bite of lip and oral cavity
   ● S00.571   Other superficial bite of lip 🔖
     Excludes1   open bite of lip (S01.551)
   ● S00.572   Other superficial bite of oral cavity 🔖
     Excludes1   open bite of oral cavity (S01.552)

● S00.8   Superficial injury of other parts of head
  X ● S00.80   Unspecified superficial injury of other part of head 🔖
  X ● S00.81   Abrasion of other part of head 🔖
  X ● S00.82   Blister (nonthermal) of other part of head 🔖
  X ● S00.83   Contusion of other part of head 🔖
     Bruise of other part of head
     Hematoma of other part of head
  X ● S00.84   External constriction of other part of head 🔖
  X ● S00.85   Superficial foreign body of other part of head 🔖
     Splinter in other part of head
  X ● S00.86   Insect bite (nonvenomous) of other part of head 🔖
  X ● S00.87   Other superficial bite of other part of head 🔖
     Excludes1   open bite of other part of head (S01.85)

● S00.9   Superficial injury of unspecified part of head
  X ● S00.90   Unspecified superficial injury of unspecified part of head 🔖
  X ● S00.91   Abrasion of unspecified part of head 🔖
  X ● S00.92   Blister (nonthermal) of unspecified part of head 🔖
  X ● S00.93   Contusion of unspecified part of head 🔖
     Bruise of head
     Hematoma of head
  X ● S00.94   External constriction of unspecified part of head 🔖
  X ● S00.95   Superficial foreign body of unspecified part of head 🔖
     Splinter of head
  X ● S00.96   Insect bite (nonvenomous) of unspecified part of head 🔖
  X ● S00.97   Other superficial bite of unspecified part of head 🔖
     Excludes1   open bite of head (S01.95)

● S01   **Open wound of head**
   Code also any associated:
     injury of cranial nerve (S04.-)
     injury of muscle and tendon of head (S09.1-)
     intracranial injury (S06.-)
     wound infection
   Excludes1   open skull fracture (S02.- with 7th character B)
   Excludes2   injury of eye and orbit (S05.-)
     traumatic amputation of part of head (S08.-)
   The appropriate 7th character is to be added to each code from category S01

    | | |
    A   initial encounter
    D   subsequent encounter
    S   sequela

  ● S01.0   Open wound of scalp
     Excludes1   avulsion of scalp (S08.0)
  X ● S01.00   Unspecified open wound of scalp 🔖
  X ● S01.01   Laceration without foreign body of scalp 🔖
  X ● S01.02   Laceration with foreign body of scalp 🔖
  X ● S01.03   Puncture wound without foreign body of scalp 🔖
  X ● S01.04   Puncture wound with foreign body of scalp 🔖
  X ● S01.05   Open bite of scalp 🔖
     Bite of scalp NOS
     Excludes1   superficial bite of scalp (S00.06, S00.07-)

  ● S01.1   Open wound of eyelid and periocular area
     Open wound of eyelid and periocular area with or without involvement of lacrimal passages
   ● S01.10   Unspecified open wound of eyelid and periocular area
     (Ex) **For category S01.10 CC codes:** S01.101-S01.159[A], S05.20X-S05.8X9[A], S05.91X-S05.92X[A], S38.3XX[A], T14.8-T14.91, T79.A0X-T79.9XX[A]
    ● S01.101   Unspecified open wound of right eyelid and periocular area A 🔖, 🔖
    ● S01.102   Unspecified open wound of left eyelid and periocular area A 🔖, 🔖
    ● S01.109   Unspecified open wound of unspecified eyelid and periocular area A 🔖, 🔖
   ● S01.11   Laceration without foreign body of eyelid and periocular area
    ● S01.111   Laceration without foreign body of right eyelid and periocular area 🔖
    ● S01.112   Laceration without foreign body of left eyelid and periocular area 🔖
    ● S01.119   Laceration without foreign body of unspecified eyelid and periocular area 🔖

N   Newborn Age: 0   P   Pediatric Age: 0–17   M   Maternity DX: 12–55   A   Adult Age: 15–124   ♀   Females Only   ♂   Males Only

🔖 Complication\Comorbidity   🔖 Major C\C   (Ex) CC/MCC Exclusions   🔖 Present on Admission Requirement   🔖 Hospital-Acquired Condition

1293

CHAPTER 19 (S00–T88)

- S01.12 Laceration with foreign body of eyelid and periocular area
  - S01.121 Laceration with foreign body of right eyelid and periocular area 🖉
  - S01.122 Laceration with foreign body of left eyelid and periocular area 🖉
  - S01.129 Laceration with foreign body of unspecified eyelid and periocular area 🖉
- S01.13 Puncture wound without foreign body of eyelid and periocular area
  - S01.131 Puncture wound without foreign body of right eyelid and periocular area 🖉
  - S01.132 Puncture wound without foreign body of left eyelid and periocular area 🖉
  - S01.139 Puncture wound without foreign body of unspecified eyelid and periocular area 🖉
- S01.14 Puncture wound with foreign body of eyelid and periocular area
  - S01.141 Puncture wound with foreign body of right eyelid and periocular area 🖉
  - S01.142 Puncture wound with foreign body of left eyelid and periocular area 🖉
  - S01.149 Puncture wound with foreign body of unspecified eyelid and periocular area 🖉
- S01.15 Open bite of eyelid and periocular area
  Bite of eyelid and periocular area NOS
  Excludes1 superficial bite of eyelid and periocular area (S00.26, S00.27)
  - S01.151 Open bite of right eyelid and periocular area 🖉
  - S01.152 Open bite of left eyelid and periocular area 🖉
  - S01.159 Open bite of unspecified eyelid and periocular area 🖉
- S01.2 Open wound of nose
  - X S01.20 Unspecified open wound of nose 🖉
  - X S01.21 Laceration without foreign body of nose 🖉
  - X S01.22 Laceration with foreign body of nose 🖉
  - X S01.23 Puncture wound without foreign body of nose 🖉
  - X S01.24 Puncture wound with foreign body of nose 🖉
  - X S01.25 Open bite of nose 🖉
    Bite of nose NOS
    Excludes1 superficial bite of nose (S00.36, S00.37)
- S01.3 Open wound of ear
  - S01.30 Unspecified open wound of ear
    - S01.301 Unspecified open wound of right ear 🖉
    - S01.302 Unspecified open wound of left ear 🖉
    - S01.309 Unspecified open wound of unspecified ear 🖉
  - S01.31 Laceration without foreign body of ear
    - S01.311 Laceration without foreign body of right ear 🖉
    - S01.312 Laceration without foreign body of left ear 🖉
    - S01.319 Laceration without foreign body of unspecified ear 🖉

- S01.32 Laceration with foreign body of ear
  - S01.321 Laceration with foreign body of right ear 🖉
  - S01.322 Laceration with foreign body of left ear 🖉
  - S01.329 Laceration with foreign body of unspecified ear 🖉
- S01.33 Puncture wound without foreign body of ear
  - S01.331 Puncture wound without foreign body of right ear 🖉
  - S01.332 Puncture wound without foreign body of left ear 🖉
  - S01.339 Puncture wound without foreign body of unspecified ear 🖉
- S01.34 Puncture wound with foreign body of ear
  - S01.341 Puncture wound with foreign body of right ear 🖉
  - S01.342 Puncture wound with foreign body of left ear 🖉
  - S01.349 Puncture wound with foreign body of unspecified ear 🖉
- S01.35 Open bite of ear
  Bite of ear NOS
  Excludes1 superficial bite of ear (S00.46, S00.47)
  - S01.351 Open bite of right ear 🖉
  - S01.352 Open bite of left ear 🖉
  - S01.359 Open bite of unspecified ear 🖉
- S01.4 Open wound of cheek and temporomandibular area
  - S01.40 Unspecified open wound of cheek and temporomandibular area
    - S01.401 Unspecified open wound of right cheek and temporomandibular area 🖉
    - S01.402 Unspecified open wound of left cheek and temporomandibular area 🖉
    - S01.409 Unspecified open wound of unspecified cheek and temporomandibular area 🖉
  - S01.41 Laceration without foreign body of cheek and temporomandibular area
    - S01.411 Laceration without foreign body of right cheek and temporomandibular area 🖉
    - S01.412 Laceration without foreign body of left cheek and temporomandibular area 🖉
    - S01.419 Laceration without foreign body of unspecified cheek and temporomandibular area 🖉
  - S01.42 Laceration with foreign body of cheek and temporomandibular area
    - S01.421 Laceration with foreign body of right cheek and temporomandibular area 🖉
    - S01.422 Laceration with foreign body of left cheek and temporomandibular area 🖉
    - S01.429 Laceration with foreign body of unspecified cheek and temporomandibular area 🖉

◀ New ◀⁞⁞ Revised ~~deleted~~ Deleted | Excludes 1 | Excludes 2 | Includes | Use additional | Code first | Code also | Unspecified |

OGCR Official Guidelines ● Unacceptable Principal Diagnosis X Assign placeholder X ● Use Additional Character(s) ▶ Manifestation Code **Coding Clinic**

● **S01.43**   Puncture wound without foreign body of cheek and temporomandibular area
  ● **S01.431**   Puncture wound without foreign body of right cheek and temporomandibular area 🐾
  ● **S01.432**   Puncture wound without foreign body of left cheek and temporomandibular area 🐾
  ● **S01.439**   Puncture wound without foreign body of unspecified cheek and temporomandibular area 🐾

● **S01.44**   Puncture wound with foreign body of cheek and temporomandibular area
  ● **S01.441**   Puncture wound with foreign body of right cheek and temporomandibular area 🐾
  ● **S01.442**   Puncture wound with foreign body of left cheek and temporomandibular area 🐾
  ● **S01.449**   Puncture wound with foreign body of unspecified cheek and temporomandibular area 🐾

● **S01.45**   Open bite of cheek and temporomandibular area
   Bite of cheek and temporomandibular area NOS
   Excludes2   superficial bite of cheek and temporomandibular area (S00.86, S00.87)
  ● **S01.451**   Open bite of right cheek and temporomandibular area 🐾
  ● **S01.452**   Open bite of left cheek and temporomandibular area 🐾
  ● **S01.459**   Open bite of unspecified cheek and temporomandibular area 🐾

● **S01.5**   Open wound of lip and oral cavity
   Excludes2   tooth dislocation (S03.2)
               tooth fracture (S02.5)
  ● **S01.50**   Unspecified open wound of lip and oral cavity
    ● **S01.501**   Unspecified open wound of lip 🐾
    ● **S01.502**   Unspecified open wound of oral cavity 🐾
  ● **S01.51**   Laceration of lip and oral cavity without foreign body
    ● **S01.511**   Laceration without foreign body of lip 🐾
    ● **S01.512**   Laceration without foreign body of oral cavity 🐾
  ● **S01.52**   Laceration of lip and oral cavity with foreign body
    ● **S01.521**   Laceration with foreign body of lip 🐾
    ● **S01.522**   Laceration with foreign body of oral cavity 🐾
  ● **S01.53**   Puncture wound of lip and oral cavity without foreign body
    ● **S01.531**   Puncture wound without foreign body of lip 🐾
    ● **S01.532**   Puncture wound without foreign body of oral cavity 🐾
  ● **S01.54**   Puncture wound of lip and oral cavity with foreign body
    ● **S01.541**   Puncture wound with foreign body of lip 🐾
    ● **S01.542**   Puncture wound with foreign body of oral cavity 🐾

● **S01.55**   Open bite of lip and oral cavity
  ● **S01.551**   Open bite of lip 🐾
     Bite of lip NOS
     Excludes1   superficial bite of lip (S00.571)
  ● **S01.552**   Open bite of oral cavity 🐾
     Bite of oral cavity NOS
     Excludes1   superficial bite of oral cavity (S00.572)

● **S01.8**   Open wound of other parts of head
  X ● **S01.80**   Unspecified open wound of other part of head 🐾
  X ● **S01.81**   Laceration without foreign body of other part of head 🐾
  X ● **S01.82**   Laceration with foreign body of other part of head 🐾
  X ● **S01.83**   Puncture wound without foreign body of other part of head 🐾
  X ● **S01.84**   Puncture wound with foreign body of other part of head 🐾
  X ● **S01.85**   Open bite of other part of head 🐾
     Bite of other part of head NOS
     Excludes1   superficial bite of other part of head (S00.85)

● **S01.9**   Open wound of unspecified part of head
  X ● **S01.90**   Unspecified open wound of unspecified part of head 🐾
  X ● **S01.91**   Laceration without foreign body of unspecified part of head 🐾
  X ● **S01.92**   Laceration with foreign body of unspecified part of head 🐾
  X ● **S01.93**   Puncture wound without foreign body of unspecified part of head 🐾
  X ● **S01.94**   Puncture wound with foreign body of unspecified part of head 🐾
  X ● **S01.95**   Open bite of unspecified part of head 🐾
     Bite of head NOS
     Excludes1   superficial bite of head NOS (S00.97)

● **S02**   Fracture of skull and facial bones
   Note: A fracture not indicated as open or closed should be coded to closed
        The appropriate 7th character is to be added to each code from category S02

A	initial encounter for closed fracture
B	initial encounter for open fracture
D	subsequent encounter for fracture with routine healing
G	subsequent encounter for fracture with delayed healing
K	subsequent encounter for fracture with nonunion
S	sequela

   Code also any associated intracranial injury (S06.-)
  X ● **S02.0**   Fracture of vault of skull A, K 🐾, B 🐾, 🐾, A, B 🐾
     Fracture of frontal bone
     Fracture of parietal bone
     (Ex) **For category S02.0 CC codes S02.0[A,B]:** S01.90X-S01.95X[A], S02.0XX-S02.19X[A,B,S], S02.2XX-S02.8XX[S], S02.91X[A,B,S], S02.92X[S], S06.0X0-S07.9XX[A], S08.89X[A], S09.10X-S09.19X[A], S09.8XX-S09.90X[A], S09.92X-S09.93X[A], S16.8XX-S19.9XX[A], S38.3XX[A], T14.8-T14.91, T79.A0XA-T79.9XX[A] **For S02.0[K]:** M80.00X-M80.88X[K,P], M84.30X-M84.68X[K,P], S02.0XX-S02.92X[K], S12.000-S12.691[K], S22.000-S22.9XX[K], S32.000-S32.9XX[K], S42.001-S42.92X[K,P], S49.001-S49.199[K,P], S52.001-S52.92X[K,M,N,P,Q,R], S59.001-S59.299[K,P], S62.001-S62.92X[K,P], S72.001-S72.92X[K,M,N,P,Q,R], S79.001-S79.199[K,P], S82.001-S82.92X[K,M,N,P,Q,R], S89.001-S89.399[K,P], S92.001-S92.919[K,P]

N Newborn Age: 0   **P** Pediatric Age: 0–17   **M** Maternity DX: 12–55   **A** Adult Age: 15–124   ♀ Females Only   ♂ Males Only

🐾 Complication\Comorbidity   🐾 Major C\C   (Ex) CC/MCC Exclusions   🐾 Present on Admission Requirement   🐾 Hospital-Acquired Condition

1295

● S02.1   Fracture of base of skull
     Excludes1   orbit NOS (S02.8)
     Excludes2   orbital floor (S02.3-)
     (Ex:) For category S02.1 CC codes S02.1[A,B]: See S02.0[A,B] For S02.1[K]: See S02.0[K]

X ● S02.10   Unspecified fracture of base of skull A, K , B , , A, B

   ● S02.11   Fracture of occiput

     ● S02.110   Type I occipital condyle fracture A, K , B , , A, B

     ● S02.111   Type II occipital condyle fracture A, K , B , , A, B

     ● S02.112   Type III occipital condyle fracture A, K , B , , A, B

     ● S02.113   Unspecified occipital condyle fracture A, K , B , , A, B

     ● S02.118   Other fracture of occiput A, K , B , , A, B

     ● S02.119   Unspecified fracture of occiput A, K , B , , A, B

X ● S02.19   Other fracture of base of skull A, K , B , , A, B
     Fracture of anterior fossa of base of skull
     Fracture of ethmoid sinus
     Fracture of frontal sinus
     Fracture of middle fossa of base of skull
     Fracture of orbital roof
     Fracture of posterior fossa of base of skull
     Fracture of sphenoid
     Fracture of temporal bone

X ● S02.2   Fracture of nasal bones B, K , , B
     (Ex:) For category S02.2 CC codes S02.2[B]: S01.90X-S01.95X[A], S02.0XX-S02.2XX[A,B,S], S02.3XX-S02.413[S], S02.42XS-S02.8XX[S], S02.91X[A,B,S], S02.92X[S], S06.0X0-S07.9XX[A], S08.89X[A], S09.10X-S09.19X[A], S09.8XX-S09.90X[A], S09.92XA-S09.93X[A], S16.8XX-S19.9XX[A], S38.3XX[A], T14.8-T14.91, T79.A0X-T79.8XX[A] For S02.2[K]: See S02.0[K]

X ● S02.3   Fracture of orbital floor A, B, K , , A, B
     Excludes1   orbit NOS (S02.8)
     Excludes2   orbital roof (S02.1-)
     (Ex:) For category S02.3 CC codes S02.3[A,B]: S01.90X-S01.95X[A], S02.0XX-S02.2XX[A,B,S], S02.3XX-S02.413[S], S02.42XS-S02.8XX[S], S02.91X[A,B,S], S06.0X0-S07.9XX[A], S08.89X[A], S09.10X-S09.19X[A], S09.8XX-S09.90X[A], S09.92X-S09.93X[A], S16.8XX-S19.9XX[A], S38.3XX[A], T14.8-T14.91, T79.8XX-T79.9XX[A], T79.A0X-T79.A9X[A] For S02.3[K]: See S02.0[K]

● S02.4   Fracture of malar, maxillary and zygoma bones
     Fracture of superior maxilla
     Fracture of upper jaw (bone)
     Fracture of zygomatic process of temporal bone
     (Ex:) For category S02.4 CC codes S02.43[A,B]: S01.90X- S01.95X[A], S02.0XX-S02.2XX[A,B,S], S02.3XX-S02.413[S], S02.42XS-S02.8XX[S], S02.91X[A,B,S], S02.92X[S], S03.0XX[A], S06.0X0-S07.9XX[A], S08.89X[A], S09.10X-S09.19X[A], S09.8XX-S09.90X[A], S09.92X-S09.93X[A], S16.8XX-S19.9XX[A], S38.3XX[A], T14.8-T14.91, T79.8XX-T79.9XX[A], T79.A0X-T79.A9X[A] For S02.4[K]: See S02.0[K] unless otherwise indicated

   ● S02.40   Fracture of malar, maxillary and zygoma bones, unspecified

     ● S02.400   Malar fracture unspecified A, B, K , , A, B

     ● S02.401   Maxillary fracture, unspecified A, B, K , , A, B

     ● S02.402   Zygomatic fracture, unspecified A, B, K , , A, B

   ● S02.41   LeFort fracture

     ● S02.411   LeFort I fracture A, B, K , , A, B

     ● S02.412   LeFort II fracture A, B, K , , A, B

     ● S02.413   LeFort III fracture A, B, K , , A, B

X ● S02.42   Fracture of alveolus of maxilla A, B, K , , A, B
     (Ex:) For S02.42[A,B]: See S02.3[A,B] For S02.42[K]: See S02.0[K]

X ● S02.5   Fracture of tooth (traumatic) Broken tooth K ,
     Excludes1   cracked tooth (nontraumatic) (K03.81)
     (Ex:) See S02.0[K]

● S02.6   Fracture of mandible
     Fracture of lower jaw (bone)
     (Ex:) For category S02.6 CC codes S02.6[A,B]: See S02.4[A,B] For S02.6[K]: See S02.0[K]

   ● S02.60   Fracture of mandible of unspecified site

     ● S02.600   Fracture of unspecified part of body of mandible A, B, K , , A, B

     ● S02.609   Fracture of mandible, unspecified A, B, K , , A, B

X ● S02.61   Fracture of condylar process of mandible A, B, K , , A, B

X ● S02.62   Fracture of subcondylar process of mandible A, B, K , , A, B

X ● S02.63   Fracture of coronoid process of mandible A, B, K , , A, B

X ● S02.64   Fracture of ramus of mandible A, B, K , , A, B

X ● S02.65   Fracture of angle of mandible A, B, K , , A, B

X ● S02.66   Fracture of symphysis of mandible A, B, K , , A, B

X ● S02.67   Fracture of alveolus of mandible A, B, K , , A, B

X ● S02.69   Fracture of mandible of other specified site A, B, K , , A, B

X ● S02.8   Fractures of other specified skull and facial bones A, B, K , , A, B
     Fracture of orbit NOS
     Fracture of palate
     Excludes1   fracture of orbital floor (S02.3-)
                   fracture of orbital roof (S02.1-)
     (Ex:) For category S02.8 CC codes S02.8[A,B]: See S02.3[A,B] For S02.8[K]: See S02.0[K]

● S02.9   Fracture of unspecified skull and facial bones

X ● S02.91   Unspecified fracture of skull A, K , B , , A, B
     (Ex:) For category S02.91 CC codes S02.91[A,B]: See S02.0[A,B] For S02.91[K]: See S02.0[K]

X ● S02.92   Unspecified fracture of facial bones A, B, K , , A, B
     (Ex:) For category S02.92 CC codes S02.92[A,B]: See S02.3[A,B] For S02.92[K]: See S02.0[K]

◀ New   ◀▥ Revised   ~~deleted~~ Deleted   Excludes 1   Excludes 2   Includes   Use additional   Code first   Code also   Unspecified
OGCR Official Guidelines   ● Unacceptable Principal Diagnosis   X Assign placeholder X   ● Use Additional Character(s)   ▶ Manifestation Code   **Coding Clinic**

● **S03** **Dislocation and sprain of joints and ligaments of head**

    Includes avulsion of joint (capsule) or ligament of head
        laceration of cartilage, joint (capsule) or ligament of head
        sprain of cartilage, joint (capsule) or ligament of head
        traumatic hemarthrosis of joint or ligament of head
        traumatic rupture of joint or ligament of head
        traumatic subluxation of joint or ligament of head
        traumatic tear of joint or ligament of head

    Code also any associated open wound

    Excludes2 Strain of muscle or tendon of head (S09.1)

    The appropriate 7th character is to be added to each code from category S03

> A   initial encounter
> D   subsequent encounter
> S   sequela

X ● **S03.0** **Dislocation of jaw**
    Dislocation of jaw (cartilage) (meniscus)
    Dislocation of mandible
    Dislocation of temporomandibular (joint)

X ● **S03.1** **Dislocation of septal cartilage of nose**

X ● **S03.2** **Dislocation of tooth**

X ● **S03.4** **Sprain of jaw**
    Sprain of temporomandibular (joint) (ligament)

X ● **S03.8** **Sprain of joints and ligaments of other parts of head**

X ● **S03.9** **Sprain of joints and ligaments of unspecified parts of head**

● **S04** **Injury of cranial nerve**

    The selection of side should be based on the side of the body being affected

    Code first any associated intracranial injury (S06.-)

    Code also any associated:
    open wound of head (S01.-)
    skull fracture (S02.-)

    The appropriate 7th character is to be added to each code from category S04

> A   initial encounter
> D   subsequent encounter
> S   sequela

● **S04.0** **Injury of optic nerve and pathways**

    Use additional code to identify any visual field defect or blindness (H53.4-, H54)
    (Ex) For category **S04.0** CC codes: S04.011-S04.049[A], S04.811A-S04.9XX[A]

  ● **S04.01** **Injury of optic nerve**
    Injury of 2nd cranial nerve

    ● **S04.011** **Injury of optic nerve, right eye** A

    ● **S04.012** **Injury of optic nerve, left eye** A

    ● **S04.019** **Injury of optic nerve, unspecified eye** A
        Injury of optic nerve NOS

  X ● **S04.02** **Injury of optic chiasm** A

  ● **S04.03** **Injury of optic tract and pathways**
    Injury of optic radiation

    ● **S04.031** **Injury of optic tract and pathways, right eye** A

    ● **S04.032** **Injury of optic tract and pathways, left eye** A

    ● **S04.039** **Injury of optic tract and pathways, unspecified eye** A
        Injury of optic tract and pathways NOS

● **S04.04** **Injury of visual cortex**

  ● **S04.041** **Injury of visual cortex, right eye** A

  ● **S04.042** **Injury of visual cortex, left eye** A

  ● **S04.049** **Injury of visual cortex, unspecified eye** A
    Injury of visual cortex NOS

● **S04.1** **Injury of oculomotor nerve**
    Injury of 3rd cranial nerve
    (Ex) For category **S04.1** CC codes: S04.10X-S04.12X[A], S04.811-S04.9XX[A]

X ● **S04.10** **Injury of oculomotor nerve, unspecified side** A

X ● **S04.11** **Injury of oculomotor nerve, right side** A

X ● **S04.12** **Injury of oculomotor nerve, left side** A

● **S04.2** **Injury of trochlear nerve**
    Injury of 4th cranial nerve
    (Ex) For category **S04.2** CC codes: S04.20X-S04.22X[A], S04.811-S04.9XX[A]

X ● **S04.20** **Injury of trochlear nerve, unspecified side** A

X ● **S04.21** **Injury of trochlear nerve, right side** A

X ● **S04.22** **Injury of trochlear nerve, left side** A

● **S04.3** **Injury of trigeminal nerve**
    Injury of 5th cranial nerve
    (Ex) For category **S04.3** CC codes: S04.30XA-S04.32X[A], S04.811-S04.9XX[A]

X ● **S04.30** **Injury of trigeminal nerve, unspecified side** A

X ● **S04.31** **Injury of trigeminal nerve, right side** A

X ● **S04.32** **Injury of trigeminal nerve, left side** A

● **S04.4** **Injury of abducent nerve**
    Injury of 6th cranial nerve
    (Ex) For category **S04.4** CC codes: S04.40X-S04.42X[A], S04.811-S04.9XX[A]

X ● **S04.40** **Injury of abducent nerve, unspecified side** A

X ● **S04.41** **Injury of abducent nerve, right side** A

X ● **S04.42** **Injury of abducent nerve, left side** A

● **S04.5** **Injury of facial nerve**
    Injury of 7th cranial nerve
    (Ex) For category **S04.5** CC codes: S04.50X-S04.52X[A], S04.811-S04.9XX[A]

X ● **S04.50** **Injury of facial nerve, unspecified side** A

X ● **S04.51** **Injury of facial nerve, right side** A

X ● **S04.52** **Injury of facial nerve, left side** A

● **S04.6** **Injury of acoustic nerve**
    Injury of auditory nerve
    Injury of 8th cranial nerve
    (Ex) For category **S04.6** CC codes: S04.60X-S04.62X[A], S04.811-S04.9XX[A]

X ● **S04.60** **Injury of acoustic nerve, unspecified side** A

X ● **S04.61** **Injury of acoustic nerve, right side** A

X ● **S04.62** **Injury of acoustic nerve, left side** A

● **S04.7** **Injury of accessory nerve**
    Injury of 11th cranial nerve
    (Ex) For category **S04.7** CC codes: S04.70X-S04.9XX[A]

X ● **S04.70** **Injury of accessory nerve, unspecified side** A

X ● **S04.71** **Injury of accessory nerve, right side** A

X ● **S04.72** **Injury of accessory nerve, left side** A

● **S04.8** **Injury of other cranial nerves**
    (Ex) For category **S04.8** CC codes: S04.811-S04.9XX[A]

  ● **S04.81** **Injury of olfactory [1st] nerve**

    ● **S04.811** **Injury of olfactory [1st] nerve, right side** A

    ● **S04.812** **Injury of olfactory [1st] nerve, left side** A

    ● **S04.819** **Injury of olfactory [1st] nerve, unspecified side** A

CHAPTER 19 (S00-T88)

N Newborn Age: 0   **P** Pediatric Age: 0–17   **M** Maternity DX: 12–55   **A** Adult Age: 15–124   ♀ Females Only   ♂ Males Only

 Complication\Comorbidity   Major C\C   (Ex) CC/MCC Exclusions   Present on Admission Requirement   Hospital-Acquired Condition

1297

● S04.89   **Injury of other cranial nerves**
Injury of vagus [10th] nerve

   ● S04.891   **Injury of other cranial nerves, right side** A 🔖, 🔖

   ● S04.892   **Injury of other cranial nerves, left side** A 🔖, 🔖

   ● S04.899   **Injury of other cranial nerves, unspecified side** A 🔖, 🔖

X ● S04.9   **Injury of unspecified cranial nerve** A 🔖, 🔖
   (Ex:) S04.811-S04.9XX[A]

● **S05**   **Injury of eye and orbit**

  Includes   open wound of eye and orbit

  Excludes2   2nd cranial [optic] nerve injury (S04.0-)
       3rd cranial [oculomotor] nerve injury (S04.1-)
       open wound of eyelid and periocular area (S01.1-)
       orbital bone fracture (S02.1-, S02.3-, S02.8-)
       superficial injury of eyelid (S00.1-S00.2)

The appropriate 7th character is to be added to each code from category S05

> A   initial encounter
> D   subsequent encounter
> S   sequela

● S05.0   **Injury of conjunctiva and corneal abrasion without foreign body**

  Excludes1   foreign body in conjunctival sac (T15.1)
       foreign body in cornea (T15.0)

  (Ex:) **For category S05 CC codes unless otherwise indicated:** S01.101-S01.159[A], S05.20X-S05.8X9[A], S05.91X-S05.92X[A], S38.3XX[A], T14.8-T14.91, T79.A0X-T79.9XX[A]

X ● S05.00   **Injury of conjunctiva and corneal abrasion without foreign body, unspecified eye** 🔖

X ● S05.01   **Injury of conjunctiva and corneal abrasion without foreign body, right eye** 🔖

X ● S05.02   **Injury of conjunctiva and corneal abrasion without foreign body, left eye** 🔖

● S05.1   **Contusion of eyeball and orbital tissues**
Traumatic hyphema

  Excludes2   black eye NOS (S00.1)
       contusion of eyelid and periocular area (S00.1)

X ● S05.10   **Contusion of eyeball and orbital tissues, unspecified eye** 🔖

X ● S05.11   **Contusion of eyeball and orbital tissues, right eye** 🔖

X ● S05.12   **Contusion of eyeball and orbital tissues, left eye** 🔖

● S05.2   **Ocular laceration and rupture with prolapse or loss of intraocular tissue**

X ● S05.20   **Ocular laceration and rupture with prolapse or loss of intraocular tissue, unspecified eye** A 🔖, 🔖

X ● S05.21   **Ocular laceration and rupture with prolapse or loss of intraocular tissue, right eye** A 🔖, 🔖

X ● S05.22   **Ocular laceration and rupture with prolapse or loss of intraocular tissue, left eye** A 🔖, 🔖

● S05.3   **Ocular laceration without prolapse or loss of intraocular tissue**
Laceration of eye NOS

X ● S05.30   **Ocular laceration without prolapse or loss of intraocular tissue, unspecified eye** A 🔖, 🔖

X ● S05.31   **Ocular laceration without prolapse or loss of intraocular tissue, right eye** A 🔖, 🔖

X ● S05.32   **Ocular laceration without prolapse or loss of intraocular tissue, left eye** A 🔖, 🔖

● S05.4   **Penetrating wound of orbit with or without foreign body**

  Excludes2   retained (old) foreign body following penetrating wound in orbit (H05.5-)

X ● S05.40   **Penetrating wound of orbit with or without foreign body, unspecified eye** A 🔖, 🔖

X ● S05.41   **Penetrating wound of orbit with or without foreign body, right eye** A 🔖, 🔖

X ● S05.42   **Penetrating wound of orbit with or without foreign body, left eye** A 🔖, 🔖

● S05.5   **Penetrating wound with foreign body of eyeball**

  Excludes2   retained (old) intraocular foreign body (H44.6-, H44.7)

  (Ex:) **For category S05.5 CC codes:** S01.101-S01.159[A], S05.20X-S05.8X9[A], S05.91X-S05.92X[A], S38.3XX[A], T14.8-T14.91, T79.8XX-T79.9XX[A]

X ● S05.50   **Penetrating wound with foreign body of unspecified eyeball** A 🔖, 🔖

X ● S05.51   **Penetrating wound with foreign body of right eyeball** A 🔖, 🔖

X ● S05.52   **Penetrating wound with foreign body of left eyeball** A 🔖, 🔖

● S05.6   **Penetrating wound without foreign body of eyeball**
Ocular penetration NOS

X ● S05.60   **Penetrating wound without foreign body of unspecified eyeball** 🔖

X ● S05.61   **Penetrating wound without foreign body of right eyeball** 🔖

X ● S05.62   **Penetrating wound without foreign body of left eyeball** 🔖

● S05.7   **Avulsion of eye**
Traumatic enucleation

X ● S05.70   **Avulsion of unspecified eye** A 🔖, 🔖

X ● S05.71   **Avulsion of right eye** A 🔖, 🔖

X ● S05.72   **Avulsion of left eye** A 🔖, 🔖

● S05.8   **Other injuries of eye and orbit**
Lacrimal duct injury

  ● S05.8X   **Other injuries of eye and orbit**

     ● S05.8X1   **Other injuries of right eye and orbit** A 🔖, 🔖

     ● S05.8X2   **Other injuries of left eye and orbit** A 🔖, 🔖

     ● S05.8X9   **Other injuries of unspecified eye and orbit** A 🔖, 🔖

● S05.9   **Unspecified injury of eye and orbit**
Injury of eye NOS

X ● S05.90   **Unspecified injury of unspecified eye and orbit** 🔖

X ● S05.91   **Unspecified injury of right eye and orbit** A 🔖, 🔖

X ● S05.92   **Unspecified injury of left eye and orbit** A 🔖, 🔖

● **S06**   **Intracranial injury**

    Includes   traumatic brain injury

    Code also any associated:
      open wound of head (S01.-)
      skull fracture (S02.-)

    Excludes1   head injury NOS (S09.90)

    The appropriate 7th character is to be added to each code from
      category S06

> A   initial encounter
> D   subsequent encounter
> S   sequela

    (Ex) **For category S06 CC codes unless otherwise indicated:** S01.90X-S01.95X[A],
     S02.0XX-S02.19X[A,B,S], S02.2XX-S02.8XX[S], S02.91X[A,B,S], S02.92X[S], S06.0X0-
     S07.9XX[A], S08.89X-S09.19X[A], S09.8XX-S09.90X[A], S09.92X-S09.93X[A], S16.8XX-
     S19.9XX[A], S38.3XX[A], T14.8-T14.91, T79.8XX-T79.9XX[A], T79.A0X-T79.A9X[A]

● **S06.0**   **Concussion**
    Commotio cerebri

    Excludes1   concussion with other intracranial
                injuries classified in category S06-
                code to specified intracranial injury

   ● **S06.0X**   **Concussion**

     ● **S06.0X0**   Concussion without loss of
                 consciousness

     ● **S06.0X1**   Concussion with loss of
                 consciousness of 30 minutes or less
                 A, A

     ● **S06.0X2**   Concussion with loss of
                 consciousness of 31 minutes to
                 59 minutes A, A

     ● **S06.0X3**   Concussion with loss of
                 consciousness of 1 hour to 5 hours
                 59 minutes A, A

     ● **S06.0X4**   Concussion with loss of
                 consciousness of 6 hours to 24 hours
                 A, A

     ● **S06.0X5**   Concussion with loss of
                 consciousness greater than 24 hours
                 with return to pre-existing conscious
                 level A, A

     ● **S06.0X6**   Concussion with loss of
                 consciousness greater than 24 hours
                 without return to pre-existing
                 conscious level with patient surviving
                 A, A

     ● **S06.0X7**   Concussion with loss of
                 consciousness of any duration with
                 death due to brain injury prior to
                 regaining consciousness A,
                 A

     ● **S06.0X8**   Concussion with loss of
                 consciousness of any duration with
                 death due to other cause prior to
                 regaining consciousness A,
                 A

     ● **S06.0X9**   Concussion with loss of
                 consciousness of unspecified duration
                 A, A
                 Concussion NOS

● **S06.1**   **Traumatic cerebral edema**
    Diffuse traumatic cerebral edema
    Focal traumatic cerebral edema

   ● **S06.1X**   **Traumatic cerebral edema**

     ● **S06.1X0**   Traumatic cerebral edema without
                 loss of consciousness A,
                 MCC when PDx is its own MCC
                 (Ex) G93.6, G93.82

     ● **S06.1X1**   Traumatic cerebral edema with loss of
                 consciousness of 30 minutes or less
                 A, A
                 MCC when PDx is its own MCC
                 (Ex) G93.6, G93.82, S01.90X-S01.95X[A], S02.0XX-
                      S02.19X[A,B,S], S02.2XXS-S02.8XX[S],
                      S02.91X[A,B,S], S02.92X[S], S06.0X0-
                      S07.9XX[A], S08.89X-S09.19X[A], S09.8XX-
                      S09.90X[A], S09.92X-S09.93X[A], S16.8XX-
                      S19.9XX[A], S38.3XX[A], T14.8-T14.91,
                      T79.8XX-T79.9XX[A], T79.A0X-T79.A9X[A]

     ● **S06.1X2**   Traumatic cerebral edema with loss of
                 consciousness of 31 minutes to
                 59 minutes A, A
                 MCC when PDx is its own MCC
                 (Ex) See S06.1X1

     ● **S06.1X3**   Traumatic cerebral edema with loss of
                 consciousness of 1 hour to 5 hours
                 59 minutes A, A
                 MCC when PDx is its own MCC
                 (Ex) See S06.1X1

     ● **S06.1X4**   Traumatic cerebral edema with loss of
                 consciousness of 6 hours to 24 hours
                 A, A
                 MCC when PDx is its own MCC
                 (Ex) See S06.1X1

     ● **S06.1X5**   Traumatic cerebral edema with loss of
                 consciousness greater than 24 hours
                 with return to pre-existing conscious
                 level A, A
                 MCC when PDx is its own MCC
                 (Ex) See S06.1X1

     ● **S06.1X6**   Traumatic cerebral edema with loss of
                 consciousness greater than 24 hours
                 without return to pre-existing
                 conscious level with patient surviving
                 A, A
                 MCC when PDx is its own MCC

     ● **S06.1X7**   Traumatic cerebral edema with loss of
                 consciousness of any duration with
                 death due to brain injury prior to
                 regaining consciousness A,
                 A
                 MCC when PDx is its own MCC

     ● **S06.1X8**   Traumatic cerebral edema with loss of
                 consciousness of any duration with
                 death due to other cause prior to
                 regaining consciousness A,
                 A
                 MCC when PDx is its own MCC

     ● **S06.1X9**   Traumatic cerebral edema with loss of
                 consciousness of unspecified duration
                 A, A
                 Traumatic cerebral edema NOS
                 MCC when PDx is its own MCC
                 (Ex) See S06.1X1

N Newborn Age: 0   **P** Pediatric Age: 0–17   **M** Maternity DX: 12–55   **A** Adult Age: 15–124   ♀ Females Only   ♂ Males Only

Complication\Comorbidity   Major C\C   (Ex) CC/MCC Exclusions   Present on Admission Requirement   Hospital-Acquired Condition

1299

CHAPTER 19 (S00-T88)

● **S06.2**   **Diffuse traumatic brain injury**
Diffuse axonal brain injury
Excludes1   traumatic diffuse cerebral edema (S06.1X-) ◀▥

  ● **S06.2X**   **Diffuse traumatic brain injury**

    ● **S06.2X0**   Diffuse traumatic brain injury without loss of consciousness ▥

    ● **S06.2X1**   Diffuse traumatic brain injury with loss of consciousness of 30 minutes or less A ▥, ▥, A ▥

    ● **S06.2X2**   Diffuse traumatic brain injury with loss of consciousness of 31 minutes to 59 minutes A ▥, ▥, A ▥

    ● **S06.2X3**   Diffuse traumatic brain injury with loss of consciousness of 1 hour to 5 hours 59 minutes A ▥, ▥, A ▥

    ● **S06.2X4**   Diffuse traumatic brain injury with loss of consciousness of 6 hours to 24 hours A ▥, ▥, A ▥

    ● **S06.2X5**   Diffuse traumatic brain injury with loss of consciousness greater than 24 hours with return to pre-existing conscious levels A ▥, ▥, A ▥

    ● **S06.2X6**   Diffuse traumatic brain injury with loss of consciousness greater than 24 hours without return to pre-existing conscious level with patient surviving A ▥, ▥, A ▥

    ● **S06.2X7**   Diffuse traumatic brain injury with loss of consciousness of any duration with death due to brain injury prior to regaining consciousness A ▥, ▥, A ▥

    ● **S06.2X8**   Diffuse traumatic brain injury with loss of consciousness of any duration with death due to other cause prior to regaining consciousness A ▥, ▥, A ▥

    ● **S06.2X9**   Diffuse traumatic brain injury with loss of consciousness of unspecified duration A ▥, ▥, A ▥
Diffuse traumatic brain injury NOS

● **S06.3**   **Focal traumatic brain injury**
Excludes1   any condition classifiable to S06.4-S06.6 focal cerebral edema (S06.1)

  ● **S06.30**   **Unspecified focal traumatic brain injury**

    ● **S06.300**   Unspecified focal traumatic brain injury without loss of consciousness ▥

    ● **S06.301**   Unspecified focal traumatic brain injury with loss of consciousness of 30 minutes or less A ▥, ▥, A ▥

    ● **S06.302**   Unspecified focal traumatic brain injury with loss of consciousness of 31 minutes to 59 minutes A ▥, ▥, A ▥

    ● **S06.303**   Unspecified focal traumatic brain injury with loss of consciousness of 1 hour to 5 hours 59 minutes A ▥, ▥, A ▥

    ● **S06.304**   Unspecified focal traumatic brain injury with loss of consciousness of 6 hours to 24 hours A ▥, ▥, A ▥

    ● **S06.305**   Unspecified focal traumatic brain injury with loss of consciousness greater than 24 hours with return to pre-existing conscious level A ▥, ▥, A ▥

    ● **S06.306**   Unspecified focal traumatic brain injury with loss of consciousness greater than 24 hours without return to pre-existing conscious level with patient surviving A ▥, ▥, A ▥

    ● **S06.307**   Unspecified focal traumatic brain injury with loss of consciousness of any duration with death due to brain injury prior to regaining consciousness A ▥, ▥, A ▥

    ● **S06.308**   Unspecified focal traumatic brain injury with loss of consciousness of any duration with death due to other cause prior to regaining consciousness A ▥, ▥, A ▥

    ● **S06.309**   Unspecified focal traumatic brain injury with loss of consciousness of unspecified duration A ▥, ▥, A ▥
Unspecified focal traumatic brain injury NOS

  ● **S06.31**   **Contusion and laceration of right cerebrum**

    ● **S06.310**   Contusion and laceration of right cerebrum without loss of consciousness A ▥, ▥, A ▥

    ● **S06.311**   Contusion and laceration of right cerebrum with loss of consciousness of 30 minutes or less A ▥, ▥, A ▥

    ● **S06.312**   Contusion and laceration of right cerebrum with loss of consciousness of 31 minutes to 59 minutes A ▥, ▥, A ▥

    ● **S06.313**   Contusion and laceration of right cerebrum with loss of consciousness of 1 hour to 5 hours 59 minutes A ▥, ▥, A ▥

    ● **S06.314**   Contusion and laceration of right cerebrum with loss of consciousness of 6 hours to 24 hours A ▥, ▥, A ▥

    ● **S06.315**   Contusion and laceration of right cerebrum with loss of consciousness greater than 24 hours with return to pre-existing conscious level A ▥, ▥, A ▥

    ● **S06.316**   Contusion and laceration of right cerebrum with loss of consciousness greater than 24 hours without return to pre-existing conscious level with patient surviving A ▥, ▥, A ▥

    ● **S06.317**   Contusion and laceration of right cerebrum with loss of consciousness of any duration with death due to brain injury prior to regaining consciousness A ▥, ▥, A ▥

    ● **S06.318**   Contusion and laceration of right cerebrum with loss of consciousness of any duration with death due to other cause prior to regaining consciousness A ▥, ▥, A ▥

    ● **S06.319**   Contusion and laceration of right cerebrum with loss of consciousness of unspecified duration A ▥, ▥, A ▥
Contusion and laceration of right cerebrum NOS

◀ New   ◀▥ Revised   ~~deleted~~ Deleted   Excludes 1   Excludes 2   Includes   Use additional   Code first   Code also   Unspecified
OGCR Official Guidelines   ● Unacceptable Principal Diagnosis   X Assign placeholder X   ● Use Additional Character(s)   ▌Manifestation Code   **Coding Clinic**

● S06.32   Contusion and laceration of left cerebrum
   ● S06.320   Contusion and laceration of left cerebrum without loss of consciousness A 🐾, 🐾, A 🐾
   ● S06.321   Contusion and laceration of left cerebrum with loss of consciousness of 30 minutes or less A 🐾, 🐾, A 🐾
   ● S06.322   Contusion and laceration of left cerebrum with loss of consciousness of 31 minutes to 59 minutes A 🐾, 🐾, A 🐾
   ● S06.323   Contusion and laceration of left cerebrum with loss of consciousness of 1 hour to 5 hours 59 minutes A 🐾, 🐾, A 🐾
   ● S06.324   Contusion and laceration of left cerebrum with loss of consciousness of 6 hours to 24 hours A 🐾, 🐾, A 🐾
   ● S06.325   Contusion and laceration of left cerebrum with loss of consciousness greater than 24 hours with return to pre-existing conscious level A 🐾, 🐾, A 🐾
   ● S06.326   Contusion and laceration of left cerebrum with loss of consciousness greater than 24 hours without return to pre-existing conscious level with patient surviving A 🐾, 🐾, A 🐾
   ● S06.327   Contusion and laceration of left cerebrum with loss of consciousness of any duration with death due to brain injury prior to regaining consciousness A 🐾, 🐾, A 🐾
   ● S06.328   Contusion and laceration of left cerebrum with loss of consciousness of any duration with death due to other cause prior to regaining consciousness A 🐾, 🐾, A 🐾
   ● S06.329   Contusion and laceration of left cerebrum with loss of consciousness of unspecified duration A 🐾, 🐾, A 🐾
      Contusion and laceration of left cerebrum NOS

● S06.33   Contusion and laceration of cerebrum, unspecified
   ● S06.330   Contusion and laceration of cerebrum, unspecified, without loss of consciousness A 🐾, 🐾, A 🐾
   ● S06.331   Contusion and laceration of cerebrum, unspecified, with loss of consciousness of 30 minutes or less A 🐾, 🐾, A 🐾
   ● S06.332   Contusion and laceration of cerebrum, unspecified, with loss of consciousness of 31 minutes to 59 minutes A 🐾, 🐾, A 🐾
   ● S06.333   Contusion and laceration of cerebrum, unspecified, with loss of consciousness of 1 hour to 5 hours 59 minutes A 🐾, 🐾, A 🐾
   ● S06.334   Contusion and laceration of cerebrum, unspecified, with loss of consciousness of 6 hours to 24 hours A 🐾, 🐾, A 🐾
   ● S06.335   Contusion and laceration of cerebrum, unspecified, with loss of consciousness greater than 24 hours with return to pre-existing conscious level A 🐾, 🐾, A 🐾

● S06.336   Contusion and laceration of cerebrum, unspecified, with loss of consciousness greater than 24 hours without return to pre-existing conscious level with patient surviving A 🐾, 🐾, A 🐾
● S06.337   Contusion and laceration of cerebrum, unspecified, with loss of consciousness of any duration with death due to brain injury prior to regaining consciousness A 🐾, 🐾, A 🐾
● S06.338   Contusion and laceration of cerebrum, unspecified, with loss of consciousness of any duration with death due to other cause prior to regaining consciousness A 🐾, 🐾, A 🐾
● S06.339   Contusion and laceration of cerebrum, unspecified, with loss of consciousness of unspecified duration A 🐾, 🐾, A 🐾
      Contusion and laceration of cerebrum NOS

● S06.34   Traumatic hemorrhage of right cerebrum
   Traumatic intracerebral hemorrhage and hematoma of right cerebrum
   ● S06.340   Traumatic hemorrhage of right cerebrum without loss of consciousness A 🐾, 🐾, A 🐾
   ● S06.341   Traumatic hemorrhage of right cerebrum with loss of consciousness of 30 minutes or less A 🐾, 🐾, A 🐾
   ● S06.342   Traumatic hemorrhage of right cerebrum with loss of consciousness of 31 minutes to 59 minutes A 🐾, 🐾, A 🐾
   ● S06.343   Traumatic hemorrhage of right cerebrum with loss of consciousness of 1 hours to 5 hours 59 minutes A 🐾, 🐾, A 🐾
   ● S06.344   Traumatic hemorrhage of right cerebrum with loss of consciousness of 6 hours to 24 hours A 🐾, 🐾, A 🐾
   ● S06.345   Traumatic hemorrhage of right cerebrum with loss of consciousness greater than 24 hours with return to pre-existing conscious level A 🐾, 🐾, A 🐾
   ● S06.346   Traumatic hemorrhage of right cerebrum with loss of consciousness greater than 24 hours without return to pre-existing conscious level with patient surviving A 🐾, 🐾, A 🐾
   ● S06.347   Traumatic hemorrhage of right cerebrum with loss of consciousness of any duration with death due to brain injury prior to regaining consciousness A 🐾, 🐾, A 🐾
   ● S06.348   Traumatic hemorrhage of right cerebrum with loss of consciousness of any duration with death due to other cause prior to regaining consciousness A 🐾, 🐾, A 🐾
   ● S06.349   Traumatic hemorrhage of right cerebrum with loss of consciousness of unspecified duration A 🐾, 🐾, A 🐾
      Traumatic hemorrhage of right cerebrum NOS

CHAPTER 19 (S00–T88)

N Newborn Age: 0   P Pediatric Age: 0–17   M Maternity DX: 12–55   A Adult Age: 15–124   ♀ Females Only   ♂ Males Only

🐾 Complication\Comorbidity   🐾 Major C\C   Ⓔ CC/MCC Exclusions   🐾 Present on Admission Requirement   🐾 Hospital-Acquired Condition

1301

● **S06.35**   **Traumatic hemorrhage of left cerebrum**
Traumatic intracerebral hemorrhage and hematoma of left cerebrum

  ● **S06.350**   Traumatic hemorrhage of left cerebrum without loss of consciousness A 🖉, 🖉, A 🖉

  ● **S06.351**   Traumatic hemorrhage of left cerebrum with loss of consciousness of 30 minutes or less A 🖉, 🖉, A 🖉

  ● **S06.352**   Traumatic hemorrhage of left cerebrum with loss of consciousness of 31 minutes to 59 minutes A 🖉, 🖉, A 🖉

  ● **S06.353**   Traumatic hemorrhage of left cerebrum with loss of consciousness of 1 hours to 5 hours 59 minutes A 🖉, 🖉, A 🖉

  ● **S06.354**   Traumatic hemorrhage of left cerebrum with loss of consciousness of 6 hours to 24 hours A 🖉, 🖉, A 🖉

  ● **S06.355**   Traumatic hemorrhage of left cerebrum with loss of consciousness greater than 24 hours with return to pre-existing conscious level A 🖉, 🖉, A 🖉

  ● **S06.356**   Traumatic hemorrhage of left cerebrum with loss of consciousness greater than 24 hours without return to pre-existing conscious level with patient surviving A 🖉, 🖉, A 🖉

  ● **S06.357**   Traumatic hemorrhage of left cerebrum with loss of consciousness of any duration with death due to brain injury prior to regaining consciousness A 🖉, 🖉, A 🖉

  ● **S06.358**   Traumatic hemorrhage of left cerebrum with loss of consciousness of any duration with death due to other cause prior to regaining consciousness A 🖉, 🖉, A 🖉

  ● **S06.359**   Traumatic hemorrhage of left cerebrum with loss of consciousness of unspecified duration A 🖉, 🖉, A 🖉
       Traumatic hemorrhage of left cerebrum NOS

● **S06.36**   **Traumatic hemorrhage of cerebrum, unspecified**
Traumatic intracerebral hemorrhage and hematoma, unspecified

  ● **S06.360**   Traumatic hemorrhage of cerebrum, unspecified, without loss of consciousness A 🖉, 🖉, A 🖉

  ● **S06.361**   Traumatic hemorrhage of cerebrum, unspecified, with loss of consciousness of 30 minutes or less A 🖉, 🖉, A 🖉

  ● **S06.362**   Traumatic hemorrhage of cerebrum, unspecified, with loss of consciousness of 31 minutes to 59 minutes A 🖉, 🖉, A 🖉

  ● **S06.363**   Traumatic hemorrhage of cerebrum, unspecified, with loss of consciousness of 1 hours to 5 hours 59 minutes A 🖉, 🖉, A 🖉

  ● **S06.364**   Traumatic hemorrhage of cerebrum, unspecified, with loss of consciousness of 6 hours to 24 hours A 🖉, 🖉, A 🖉

  ● **S06.365**   Traumatic hemorrhage of cerebrum, unspecified, with loss of consciousness greater than 24 hours with return to pre-existing conscious level A 🖉, 🖉, A 🖉

  ● **S06.366**   Traumatic hemorrhage of cerebrum, unspecified, with loss of consciousness greater than 24 hours without return to pre-existing conscious level with patient surviving A 🖉, 🖉, A 🖉

  ● **S06.367**   Traumatic hemorrhage of cerebrum, unspecified, with loss of consciousness of any duration with death due to brain injury prior to regaining consciousness A 🖉, 🖉, A 🖉

  ● **S06.368**   Traumatic hemorrhage of cerebrum, unspecified, with loss of consciousness of any duration with death due to other cause prior to regaining consciousness A 🖉, 🖉, A 🖉

  ● **S06.369**   Traumatic hemorrhage of cerebrum, unspecified, with loss of consciousness of unspecified duration A 🖉, 🖉, A 🖉
       Traumatic hemorrhage of cerebrum NOS

● **S06.37**   **Contusion, laceration, and hemorrhage of cerebellum**

  ● **S06.370**   Contusion, laceration, and hemorrhage of cerebellum without loss of consciousness A 🖉, 🖉, A 🖉
       Ⓔⓧ No exclusions

  ● **S06.371**   Contusion, laceration, and hemorrhage of cerebellum with loss of consciousness of 30 minutes or less A 🖉, 🖉, A 🖉

  ● **S06.372**   Contusion, laceration, and hemorrhage of cerebellum with loss of consciousness of 31 minutes to 59 minutes A 🖉, 🖉, A 🖉

  ● **S06.373**   Contusion, laceration, and hemorrhage of cerebellum with loss of consciousness of 1 hour to 5 hours 59 minutes A 🖉, 🖉, A 🖉

  ● **S06.374**   Contusion, laceration, and hemorrhage of cerebellum with loss of consciousness of 6 hours to 24 hours A 🖉, 🖉, A 🖉

  ● **S06.375**   Contusion, laceration, and hemorrhage of cerebellum with loss of consciousness greater than 24 hours with return to pre-existing conscious level A 🖉, 🖉, A 🖉

  ● **S06.376**   Contusion, laceration, and hemorrhage of cerebellum with loss of consciousness greater than 24 hours without return to pre-existing conscious level with patient surviving A 🖉, 🖉, A 🖉

  ● **S06.377**   Contusion, laceration, and hemorrhage of cerebellum with loss of consciousness of any duration with death due to brain injury prior to regaining consciousness A 🖉, 🖉, A 🖉

  ● **S06.378**   Contusion, laceration, and hemorrhage of cerebellum with loss of consciousness of any duration with death due to other cause prior to regaining consciousness A 🖉, 🖉, A 🖉

  ● **S06.379**   Contusion, laceration, and hemorrhage of cerebellum with loss of consciousness of unspecified duration A 🖉, 🖉, A 🖉
       Contusion, laceration, and hemorrhage of cerebellum NOS

◀ New   ◀▥ Revised   ~~deleted~~ Deleted   Excludes 1   Excludes 2   Includes   Use additional   Code first   Code also   Unspecified
OGCR Official Guidelines   ● Unacceptable Principal Diagnosis   X Assign placeholder X   ● Use Additional Character(s)   ▶ Manifestation Code   **Coding Clinic**

- ● S06.38   Contusion, laceration, and hemorrhage of brainstem
  - ● S06.380   Contusion, laceration, and hemorrhage of brainstem without loss of consciousness A 🔹, 🔹, A 🔹
    - (Ex:) No exclusions
  - ● S06.381   Contusion, laceration, and hemorrhage of brainstem with loss of consciousness of 30 minutes or less A 🔹, 🔹, A 🔹
  - ● S06.382   Contusion, laceration, and hemorrhage of brainstem with loss of consciousness of 31 minutes to 59 minutes A 🔹, 🔹, A 🔹
  - ● S06.383   Contusion, laceration, and hemorrhage of brainstem with loss of consciousness of 1 hour to 5 hours 59 minutes A 🔹, 🔹, A 🔹
  - ● S06.384   Contusion, laceration, and hemorrhage of brainstem with loss of consciousness of 6 hours to 24 hours A 🔹, 🔹, A 🔹
  - ● S06.385   Contusion, laceration, and hemorrhage of brainstem with loss of consciousness greater than 24 hours with return to pre-existing conscious level A 🔹, 🔹, A 🔹
  - ● S06.386   Contusion, laceration, and hemorrhage of brainstem with loss of consciousness greater than 24 hours without return to pre-existing conscious level with patient surviving A 🔹, 🔹, A 🔹
  - ● S06.387   Contusion, laceration, and hemorrhage of brainstem with loss of consciousness of any duration with death due to brain injury prior to regaining consciousness A 🔹, 🔹, A 🔹
  - ● S06.388   Contusion, laceration, and hemorrhage of brainstem with loss of consciousness of any duration with death due to other cause prior to regaining consciousness A 🔹, 🔹, A 🔹
  - ● S06.389   Contusion, laceration, and hemorrhage of brainstem with loss of consciousness of unspecified duration A 🔹, 🔹, A 🔹
    - Contusion, laceration, and hemorrhage of brainstem NOS
- ● S06.4   **Epidural hemorrhage**
  - *Situated outside dura mater*
  - Extradural hemorrhage NOS
  - *Intracranial hemorrhage due to trauma*
  - Extradural hemorrhage (traumatic)
  - ● S06.4X   **Epidural hemorrhage**
    - ● S06.4X0   Epidural hemorrhage without loss of consciousness A 🔹, 🔹, A 🔹
    - ● S06.4X1   Epidural hemorrhage with loss of consciousness of 30 minutes or less A 🔹, 🔹, A 🔹
    - ● S06.4X2   Epidural hemorrhage with loss of consciousness of 31 minutes to 59 minutes A 🔹, 🔹, A 🔹
    - ● S06.4X3   Epidural hemorrhage with loss of consciousness of 1 hour to 5 hours 59 minutes A 🔹, 🔹, A 🔹
    - ● S06.4X4   Epidural hemorrhage with loss of consciousness of 6 hours to 24 hours A 🔹, 🔹, A 🔹
    - ● S06.4X5   Epidural hemorrhage with loss of consciousness greater than 24 hours with return to pre-existing conscious level A 🔹, 🔹, A 🔹

- ● S06.4X6   Epidural hemorrhage with loss of consciousness greater than 24 hours without return to pre-existing conscious level with patient surviving A 🔹, 🔹, A 🔹
- ● S06.4X7   Epidural hemorrhage with loss of consciousness of any duration with death due to brain injury prior to regaining consciousness A 🔹, 🔹, A 🔹
- ● S06.4X8   Epidural hemorrhage with loss of consciousness of any duration with death due to other causes prior to regaining consciousness A 🔹, 🔹, A 🔹
- ● S06.4X9   Epidural hemorrhage with loss of consciousness of unspecified duration A 🔹, 🔹, A 🔹
  - Epidural hemorrhage NOS
- ● S06.5   **Traumatic subdural hemorrhage**
  - ● S06.5X   **Traumatic subdural hemorrhage**
    - ● S06.5X0   Traumatic subdural hemorrhage without loss of consciousness A 🔹, 🔹, A 🔹
    - ● S06.5X1   Traumatic subdural hemorrhage with loss of consciousness of 30 minutes or less A 🔹, 🔹, A 🔹
    - ● S06.5X2   Traumatic subdural hemorrhage with loss of consciousness of 31 minutes to 59 minutes A 🔹, 🔹, A 🔹
    - ● S06.5X3   Traumatic subdural hemorrhage with loss of consciousness of 1 hour to 5 hours 59 minutes A 🔹, 🔹, A 🔹
    - ● S06.5X4   Traumatic subdural hemorrhage with loss of consciousness of 6 hours to 24 hours A 🔹, 🔹, A 🔹
    - ● S06.5X5   Traumatic subdural hemorrhage with loss of consciousness greater than 24 hours with return to pre-existing conscious level A 🔹, 🔹, A 🔹
    - ● S06.5X6   Traumatic subdural hemorrhage with loss of consciousness greater than 24 hours without return to pre-existing conscious level with patient surviving A 🔹, 🔹, A 🔹
    - ● S06.5X7   Traumatic subdural hemorrhage with loss of consciousness of any duration with death due to brain injury before regaining consciousness A 🔹, 🔹, A 🔹
    - ● S06.5X8   Traumatic subdural hemorrhage with loss of consciousness of any duration with death due to other cause before regaining consciousness A 🔹, 🔹, A 🔹
    - ● S06.5X9   Traumatic subdural hemorrhage with loss of consciousness of unspecified duration A 🔹, 🔹, A 🔹
      - Traumatic subdural hemorrhage NOS
- ● S06.6   **Traumatic subarachnoid hemorrhage**
  - *Between arachnoid and pia mater*
  - ● S06.6X   **Traumatic subarachnoid hemorrhage**
    - ● S06.6X0   Traumatic subarachnoid hemorrhage without loss of consciousness A 🔹, 🔹, A 🔹
    - ● S06.6X1   Traumatic subarachnoid hemorrhage with loss of consciousness of 30 minutes or less A 🔹, 🔹, A 🔹
    - ● S06.6X2   Traumatic subarachnoid hemorrhage with loss of consciousness of 31 minutes to 59 minutes A 🔹, 🔹, A 🔹

CHAPTER 19 (S00-T88)

N Newborn Age: 0	P Pediatric Age: 0–17	M Maternity DX: 12–55	A Adult Age: 15–124	♀ Females Only	♂ Males Only
🔹 Complication\Comorbidity	🔹 Major C\C	(Ex) CC/MCC Exclusions	🔹 Present on Admission Requirement	🔹 Hospital-Acquired Condition	

1303

● S06.6X3   Traumatic subarachnoid hemorrhage with loss of consciousness of 1 hour to 5 hours 59 minutes A 🔖, 🔖, A 🔖

● S06.6X4   Traumatic subarachnoid hemorrhage with loss of consciousness of 6 hours to 24 hours A 🔖, 🔖, A 🔖

● S06.6X5   Traumatic subarachnoid hemorrhage with loss of consciousness greater than 24 hours with return to pre-existing conscious level A 🔖, 🔖, A 🔖

● S06.6X6   Traumatic subarachnoid hemorrhage with loss of consciousness greater than 24 hours without return to pre-existing conscious level with patient surviving A 🔖, 🔖, A 🔖

● S06.6X7   Traumatic subarachnoid hemorrhage with loss of consciousness of any duration with death due to brain injury prior to regaining consciousness A 🔖, 🔖, A 🔖

● S06.6X8   Traumatic subarachnoid hemorrhage with loss of consciousness of any duration with death due to other cause prior to regaining consciousness A 🔖, 🔖, A 🔖

● S06.6X9   Traumatic subarachnoid hemorrhage with loss of consciousness of unspecified duration A 🔖, 🔖, A 🔖
     Traumatic subarachnoid hemorrhage NOS

● S06.8   **Other specified intracranial injuries**

● S06.81   Injury of right internal carotid artery, intracranial portion, not elsewhere classified

● S06.810   Injury of right internal carotid artery, intracranial portion, not elsewhere classified without loss of consciousness 🔖

● S06.811   Injury of right internal carotid artery, intracranial portion, not elsewhere classified with loss of consciousness of 30 minutes or less A 🔖, 🔖, A 🔖

● S06.812   Injury of right internal carotid artery, intracranial portion, not elsewhere classified with loss of consciousness of 31 minutes to 59 minutes A 🔖, 🔖, A 🔖

● S06.813   Injury of right internal carotid artery, intracranial portion, not elsewhere classified with loss of consciousness of 1 hour to 5 hours 59 minutes A 🔖, 🔖, A 🔖

● S06.814   Injury of right internal carotid artery, intracranial portion, not elsewhere classified with loss of consciousness of 6 hours to 24 hours A 🔖, 🔖, A 🔖

● S06.815   Injury of right internal carotid artery, intracranial portion, not elsewhere classified with loss of consciousness greater than 24 hours with return to pre-existing conscious level A 🔖, 🔖, A 🔖

● S06.816   Injury of right internal carotid artery, intracranial portion, not elsewhere classified with loss of consciousness greater than 24 hours without return to pre-existing conscious level with patient surviving A 🔖, 🔖, A 🔖

● S06.817   Injury of right internal carotid artery, intracranial portion, not elsewhere classified with loss of consciousness of any duration with death due to brain injury prior to regaining consciousness A 🔖, 🔖, A 🔖

● S06.818   Injury of right internal carotid artery, intracranial portion, not elsewhere classified with loss of consciousness of any duration with death due to other cause prior to regaining consciousness A 🔖, 🔖, A 🔖

● S06.819   Injury of right internal carotid artery, intracranial portion, not elsewhere classified with loss of consciousness of unspecified duration A 🔖, 🔖, A 🔖
     Injury of right internal carotid artery, intracranial portion, not elsewhere classified NOS

● S06.82   Injury of left internal carotid artery, intracranial portion, not elsewhere classified

● S06.820   Injury of left internal carotid artery, intracranial portion, not elsewhere classified without loss of consciousness 🔖

● S06.821   Injury of left internal carotid artery, intracranial portion, not elsewhere classified with loss of consciousness of 30 minutes or less A 🔖, 🔖, A 🔖

● S06.822   Injury of left internal carotid artery, intracranial portion, not elsewhere classified with loss of consciousness of 31 minutes to 59 minutes A 🔖, 🔖, A 🔖

● S06.823   Injury of left internal carotid artery, intracranial portion, not elsewhere classified with loss of consciousness of 1 hour to 5 hours 59 minutes A 🔖, 🔖, A 🔖

● S06.824   Injury of left internal carotid artery, intracranial portion, not elsewhere classified with loss of consciousness of 6 hours to 24 hours A 🔖, 🔖, A 🔖

● S06.825   Injury of left internal carotid artery, intracranial portion, not elsewhere classified with loss of consciousness greater than 24 hours with return to pre-existing conscious level A 🔖, 🔖, A 🔖

● S06.826   Injury of left internal carotid artery, intracranial portion, not elsewhere classified with loss of consciousness greater than 24 hours without return to pre-existing conscious level with patient surviving A 🔖, 🔖, A 🔖

● S06.827   Injury of left internal carotid artery, intracranial portion, not elsewhere classified with loss of consciousness of any duration with death due to brain injury prior to regaining consciousness A 🔖, 🔖, A 🔖

● S06.828   Injury of left internal carotid artery, intracranial portion, not elsewhere classified with loss of consciousness of any duration with death due to other cause prior to regaining consciousness A 🔖, 🔖, A 🔖

● S06.829   Injury of left internal carotid artery, intracranial portion, not elsewhere classified with loss of consciousness of unspecified duration A 🔖, 🔖, A 🔖
     Injury of left internal carotid artery, intracranial portion, not elsewhere classified NOS

● S06.89   Other specified intracranial injury

  ● S06.890   Other specified intracranial injury without loss of consciousness 🦠

  ● S06.891   Other specified intracranial injury with loss of consciousness of 30 minutes or less A 🦠, 🦠, A 🦠

  ● S06.892   Other specified intracranial injury with loss of consciousness of 31 minutes to 59 minutes A 🦠, 🦠, A 🦠

  ● S06.893   Other specified intracranial injury with loss of consciousness of 1 hour to 5 hours 59 minutes A 🦠, 🦠, A 🦠

  ● S06.894   Other specified intracranial injury with loss of consciousness of 6 hours to 24 hours A 🦠, 🦠, A 🦠

  ● S06.895   Other specified intracranial injury with loss of consciousness greater than 24 hours with return to pre-existing conscious level A 🦠, 🦠, A 🦠

  ● S06.896   Other specified intracranial injury with loss of consciousness greater than 24 hours without return to pre-existing conscious level with patient surviving A 🦠, 🦠, A 🦠

  ● S06.897   Other specified intracranial injury with loss of consciousness of any duration with death due to brain injury prior to regaining consciousness A 🦠, 🦠, A 🦠

  ● S06.898   Other specified intracranial injury with loss of consciousness of any duration with death due to other cause prior to regaining consciousness A 🦠, 🦠, A 🦠

  ● S06.899   Other specified intracranial injury with loss of consciousness of unspecified duration A 🦠, 🦠, A 🦠

● S06.9   Unspecified intracranial injury

   Brain injury NOS

   Head injury NOS with loss of consciousness

   Excludes1   head injury NOS (S09.90)

  ● S06.9X   Unspecified intracranial injury

    ● S06.9X0   Unspecified intracranial injury without loss of consciousness 🦠

    ● S06.9X1   Unspecified intracranial injury with loss of consciousness of 30 minutes or less A 🦠, 🦠, A 🦠

    ● S06.9X2   Unspecified intracranial injury with loss of consciousness of 31 minutes to 59 minutes A 🦠, 🦠, A 🦠

    ● S06.9X3   Unspecified intracranial injury with loss of consciousness of 1 hour to 5 hours 59 minutes A 🦠, 🦠, A 🦠

    ● S06.9X4   Unspecified intracranial injury with loss of consciousness of 6 hours to 24 hours A 🦠, 🦠, A 🦠

    ● S06.9X5   Unspecified intracranial injury with loss of consciousness greater than 24 hours with return to pre-existing conscious level A 🦠, 🦠, A 🦠

    ● S06.9X6   Unspecified intracranial injury with loss of consciousness greater than 24 hours without return to pre-existing conscious level with patient surviving A 🦠, 🦠, A 🦠

    ● S06.9X7   Unspecified intracranial injury with loss of consciousness of any duration with death due to brain injury prior to regaining consciousness A 🦠, 🦠, A 🦠

    ● S06.9X8   Unspecified intracranial injury with loss of consciousness of any duration with death due to other cause prior to regaining consciousness A 🦠, 🦠, A 🦠

    ● S06.9X9   Unspecified intracranial injury with loss of consciousness of unspecified duration A 🦠, 🦠, A 🦠

● S07   Crushing injury of head

   Use additional code for all associated injuries, such as:

     intracranial injuries (S06.-) ◀▥

     skull fractures (S02.-)

   The appropriate 7th character is to be added to each code from category S07

   A   initial encounter
   D   subsequent encounter
   S   sequela

   (Ex:) **For category S07 CC codes:** S01.90X-S01.95X[A], S02.0XX-S02.92X[S], S07.0XX-S07.9XX[A], S08.89X-S09.19X[A], S09.8XXA-S09.90X[A], S09.92XA-S09.93X[A], S16.8XX-S19.9XX[A], T14.8-T14.91, T79.8XX-T79.9XX[A], T79.A0X-T79.A9X[A]

  X ● S07.0   Crushing injury of face A 🦠, 🦠, A 🦠

  X ● S07.1   Crushing injury of skull A 🦠, 🦠, A 🦠

  X ● S07.8   Crushing injury of other parts of head A 🦠, 🦠, A 🦠

  X ● S07.9   Crushing injury of head, part unspecified A 🦠, 🦠, A 🦠

● S08   Avulsion and traumatic amputation of part of head

   An amputation not identified as partial or complete should be coded to complete

   The appropriate 7th character is to be added to each code from category S08

   A   initial encounter
   D   subsequent encounter
   S   sequela

  X ● S08.0   Avulsion of scalp 🦠

  ● S08.1   Traumatic amputation of ear

    ● S08.11   Complete traumatic amputation of ear

      ● S08.111   Complete traumatic amputation of right ear 🦠

      ● S08.112   Complete traumatic amputation of left ear 🦠

      ● S08.119   Complete traumatic amputation of unspecified ear 🦠

    ● S08.12   Partial traumatic amputation of ear

      ● S08.121   Partial traumatic amputation of right ear 🦠

      ● S08.122   Partial traumatic amputation of left ear 🦠

      ● S08.129   Partial traumatic amputation of unspecified ear 🦠

  ● S08.8   Traumatic amputation of other parts of head

    ● S08.81   Traumatic amputation of nose

      ● S08.811   Complete traumatic amputation of nose 🦠

      ● S08.812   Partial traumatic amputation of nose 🦠

  X ● S08.89   Traumatic amputation of other parts of head 🦠

CHAPTER 19 (S00–T88)

N Newborn Age: 0   **P** Pediatric Age: 0–17   **M** Maternity DX: 12–55   **A** Adult Age: 15–124   ♀ Females Only   ♂ Males Only

🦠 Complication\Comorbidity   🦠 Major C\C   (Ex:) CC/MCC Exclusions   🦠 Present on Admission Requirement   🦠 Hospital-Acquired Condition

1305

● **S09　Other and unspecified injuries of head**

The appropriate 7th character is to be added to each code from category S09

A	initial encounter
D	subsequent encounter
S	sequela

X● **S09.0　Injury of blood vessels of head, not elsewhere classified**
A

    Excludes1　injury of cerebral blood vessels (S06.-)
                injury of precerebral blood vessels (S15.-)
    (Ex:) S09.0XX[A], S15.101-S15.199[A], S15.8XX-S15.9XX[A], T14.8-T14.91,
      T79.8XX-T79.9XX[A], T79.A0X-T79.A9X[A]

● **S09.1　Injury of muscle and tendon of head**
Code also any associated open wound (S01.-)
    Excludes2　sprain to joints and ligament of head (S03.9)

X● **S09.10　Unspecified injury of muscle and tendon of head**
Injury of muscle and tendon of head NOS

X● **S09.11　Strain of muscle and tendon of head**

X● **S09.12　Laceration of muscle and tendon of head**

X● **S09.19　Other specified injury of muscle and tendon of head**

● **S09.2　Traumatic rupture of ear drum**
    Excludes1　traumatic rupture of ear drum due to blast injury (S09.31-)
    (Ex:) **For category S09.2 CC codes:** S01.301-S01.359[A], S08.111-S08.129[A],
      S09.20X-S09.399[A], S09.91X[A], S38.3XX[A], T14.8-T14.91, T79.8XX-
      T79.9XX[A]

X● **S09.20　Traumatic rupture of unspecified ear drum**
A

X● **S09.21　Traumatic rupture of right ear drum** A

X● **S09.22　Traumatic rupture of left ear drum** A

● **S09.3　Other specified and unspecified injury of middle and inner ear**
    Excludes1　injury to ear NOS (S09.91-)
    Excludes2　injury to external ear (S00.4-, S01.3-, S08.1-)
    (Ex:) **For category S09.3 CC codes: See S09.2**

● **S09.30　Unspecified injury of middle and inner ear**

  ● **S09.301　Unspecified injury of right middle and inner ear** A

  ● **S09.302　Unspecified injury of left middle and inner ear** A

  ● **S09.309　Unspecified injury of unspecified middle and inner ear** A

● **S09.31　Primary blast injury of ear**
Blast injury of ear NOS

  ● **S09.311　Primary blast injury of right ear** A

  ● **S09.312　Primary blast injury of left ear** A

  ● **S09.313　Primary blast injury of ear, bilateral** A

  ● **S09.319　Primary blast injury of unspecified ear** A

● **S09.39　Other specified injury of middle and inner ear**
Secondary blast injury to ear

  ● **S09.391　Other specified injury of right middle and inner ear** A

  ● **S09.392　Other specified injury of left middle and inner ear** A

  ● **S09.399　Other specified injury of unspecified middle and inner ear** A

X● **S09.8　Other specified injuries of head**

● **S09.9　Unspecified injury of face and head**

X● **S09.90　Unspecified injury of head**
Head injury NOS
    Excludes1　brain injury NOS (S06.9-)
                head injury NOS with loss of consciousness (S06.9-)
                intracranial injury NOS (S06.9-)

X● **S09.91　Unspecified injury of ear**
Injury of ear NOS

X● **S09.92　Unspecified injury of nose**
Injury of nose NOS

X● **S09.93　Unspecified injury of face**
Injury of face NOS

INJURIES TO THE NECK (S10-S19)

Includes　injuries of nape
          injuries of supraclavicular region
          injuries of throat

Excludes2　burns and corrosions (T20-T32)
          effects of foreign body in esophagus (T18.1)
          effects of foreign body in larynx (T17.3)
          effects of foreign body in pharynx (T17.2)
          effects of foreign body in trachea (T17.4)
          frostbite (T33-T34)
          insect bite or sting, venomous (T63.4)

● **S10　Superficial injury of neck**

The appropriate 7th character is to be added to each code from category S10

A	initial encounter
D	subsequent encounter
S	sequela

X● **S10.0　Contusion of throat**
Contusion of cervical esophagus
Contusion of larynx
Contusion of pharynx
Contusion of trachea

● **S10.1　Other and unspecified superficial injuries of throat**

X● **S10.10　Unspecified superficial injuries of throat**

X● **S10.11　Abrasion of throat**

X● **S10.12　Blister (nonthermal) of throat**

X● **S10.14　External constriction of part of throat**

X● **S10.15　Superficial foreign body of throat**
Splinter in the throat

X● **S10.16　Insect bite (nonvenomous) of throat**

X● **S10.17　Other superficial bite of throat**
    Excludes1　open bite of throat (S11.85)

● **S10.8　Superficial injury of other specified parts of neck**

X● **S10.80　Unspecified superficial injury of other specified part of neck**

X● **S10.81　Abrasion of other specified part of neck**

X● **S10.82　Blister (nonthermal) of other specified part of neck**

X● **S10.83　Contusion of other specified part of neck**

X● **S10.84　External constriction of other specified part of neck**

X● **S10.85　Superficial foreign body of other specified part of neck**
Splinter in other part of neck

X● **S10.86　Insect bite of other specified part of neck**

X● **S10.87　Other superficial bite of other specified part of neck**
    Excludes1　open bite of other specified parts of neck (S11.85)

● S10.9　Superficial injury of unspecified part of neck
　X ● S10.90　Unspecified superficial injury of unspecified part of neck 🔖
　X ● S10.91　Abrasion of unspecified part of neck 🔖
　X ● S10.92　Blister (nonthermal) of unspecified part of neck 🔖
　X ● S10.93　Contusion of unspecified part of neck 🔖
　X ● S10.94　External constriction of unspecified part of neck 🔖
　X ● S10.95　Superficial foreign body of unspecified part of neck 🔖
　X ● S10.96　Insect bite of unspecified part of neck 🔖
　X ● S10.97　Other superficial bite of unspecified part of neck 🔖

● S11　Open wound of neck
　Code also any associated:
　　spinal cord injury (S14.0, S14.1-)
　　wound infection
　　Excludes2　open fracture of vertebra (S12.- with 7th character B)

　The appropriate 7th character is to be added to each code from category S11

　┌─────────────────────────────────┐
　│ A　initial encounter   │
　│ D　subsequent encounter   │
　│ S　sequela   │
　└─────────────────────────────────┘

　● S11.0　Open wound of larynx and trachea
　　　(Ex) **For category S11.0 CC codes:** S11.011-S11.039[A], S11.80X-S11.95X[A], S13.4XX[A], S13.8XX[A], S16.1XX-S16.2XX[A], S38.3XX[A], T14.8-T14.91, T79.8XX-T79.9XX[A], T79.A0X-T79.A9X[A]

　　● S11.01　Open wound of larynx
　　　　Excludes2　open wound of vocal cord (S11.03)
　　　● S11.011　Laceration without foreign body of larynx A 🔖, 🔖
　　　● S11.012　Laceration with foreign body of larynx A 🔖, 🔖
　　　● S11.013　Puncture wound without foreign body of larynx A 🔖, 🔖
　　　● S11.014　Puncture wound with foreign body of larynx A 🔖, 🔖
　　　● S11.015　Open bite of larynx A 🔖, 🔖
　　　　　　Bite of larynx NOS
　　　● S11.019　Unspecified open wound of larynx A 🔖, 🔖

　　● S11.02　Open wound of trachea
　　　　Open wound of cervical trachea
　　　　Open wound of trachea NOS
　　　　Excludes2　open wound of thoracic trachea (S27.5-)
　　　● S11.021　Laceration without foreign body of trachea A 🔖, 🔖
　　　● S11.022　Laceration with foreign body of trachea A 🔖, 🔖
　　　● S11.023　Puncture wound without foreign body of trachea A 🔖, 🔖
　　　● S11.024　Puncture wound with foreign body of trachea A 🔖, 🔖
　　　● S11.025　Open bite of trachea A 🔖, 🔖
　　　　　　Bite of trachea NOS
　　　● S11.029　Unspecified open wound of trachea A 🔖, 🔖

　　● S11.03　Open wound of vocal cord
　　　● S11.031　Laceration without foreign body of vocal cord A 🔖, 🔖
　　　● S11.032　Laceration with foreign body of vocal cord A 🔖, 🔖

　　　● S11.033　Puncture wound without foreign body of vocal cord A 🔖, 🔖
　　　● S11.034　Puncture wound with foreign body of vocal cord A 🔖, 🔖
　　　● S11.035　Open bite of vocal cord A 🔖, 🔖
　　　　　　Bite of vocal cord NOS
　　　● S11.039　Unspecified open wound of vocal cord A 🔖, 🔖

　● S11.1　Open wound of thyroid gland
　　　(Ex) **For category S11.1 CC codes unless otherwise indicated:** S11.10X-S11.15X[A], S11.80X-S11.95X[A], S13.4XX[A], S13.8XX[A], S16.1XX-S16.2XX[A], S38.3XX[A], T14.8-T14.91, T79.8XX-T79.9XX[A]

　　X ● S11.10　Unspecified open wound of thyroid gland A 🔖, 🔖
　　X ● S11.11　Laceration without foreign body of thyroid gland A 🔖, 🔖
　　X ● S11.12　Laceration with foreign body of thyroid gland A 🔖, 🔖
　　　　(Ex) S11.10X-S11.15X[A], S11.80X-S11.95X[A], S13.4XX[A], S13.8XX[A], S16.1XX-S16.2XX[A], S38.3XX[A], T14.8-T14.91, T79.8XX-T79.9XX[A], T79.A0XA-T79.A9X[A]
　　X ● S11.13　Puncture wound without foreign body of thyroid gland A 🔖, 🔖
　　X ● S11.14　Puncture wound with foreign body of thyroid gland A 🔖, 🔖
　　　　(Ex) See S11.12
　　X ● S11.15　Open bite of thyroid gland A 🔖, 🔖
　　　　　　Bite of thyroid gland NOS

　● S11.2　Open wound of pharynx and cervical esophagus
　　　Excludes1　open wound of esophagus NOS (S27.8-)
　　　(Ex) **For category S11.2 CC codes unless otherwise indicated:** S11.20X-S11.95X[A], S13.4XX[A], S13.8XX[A], S16.1XX-S16.2XX[A], S38.3XX[A], T14.8-T14.91, T79.8XX-T79.9XX[A]

　　X ● S11.20　Unspecified open wound of pharynx and cervical esophagus A 🔖, 🔖
　　X ● S11.21　Laceration without foreign body of pharynx and cervical esophagus A 🔖, 🔖
　　X ● S11.22　Laceration with foreign body of pharynx and cervical esophagus A 🔖, 🔖
　　　　(Ex) S11.20X-S11.95X[A], S13.4XX[A], S13.8XX[A], S16.1XX-S16.2XX[A], S38.3XX[A], T14.8-T14.91, T79.8XX-T79.9XX[A], T79.A0X-T79.A9X[A]
　　X ● S11.23　Puncture wound without foreign body of pharynx and cervical esophagus A 🔖, 🔖
　　X ● S11.24　Puncture wound with foreign body of pharynx and cervical esophagus A 🔖, 🔖
　　　　(Ex) See S11.22
　　X ● S11.25　Open bite of pharynx and cervical esophagus A 🔖, 🔖
　　　　　　Bite of pharynx and cervical esophagus NOS

　● S11.8　Open wound of other specified parts of neck
　　X ● S11.80　Unspecified open specified wound of other part of neck 🔖
　　X ● S11.81　Laceration without foreign body of other specified part of neck 🔖
　　X ● S11.82　Laceration with foreign body of other specified part of neck 🔖
　　X ● S11.83　Puncture wound without foreign body of other specified part of neck 🔖
　　X ● S11.84　Puncture wound with foreign body of other specified part of neck 🔖
　　X ● S11.85　Open bite of other specified part of neck 🔖
　　　　　　Bite of other part of neck NOS
　　　　　Excludes1　superficial bite of other specified part of neck (S10.87)
　　X ● S11.89　Other open wound of other part of neck 🔖

N　Newborn Age: 0　　P　Pediatric Age: 0–17　　M　Maternity DX: 12–55　　A　Adult Age: 15–124　　♀　Females Only　　♂　Males Only

🔖　Complication\Comorbidity　　🔖　Major C\C　　(Ex) CC/MCC Exclusions　　🔖　Present on Admission Requirement　　🔖　Hospital-Acquired Condition

1307

● **S11.9**   **Open wound of unspecified part of neck**

X ● **S11.90**   Unspecified open wound of unspecified part of neck 🖻

X ● **S11.91**   Laceration without foreign body of unspecified part of neck 🖻

X ● **S11.92**   Laceration with foreign body of unspecified part of neck 🖻

X ● **S11.93**   Puncture wound without foreign body of unspecified part of neck 🖻

X ● **S11.94**   Puncture wound with foreign body of unspecified part of neck 🖻

X ● **S11.95**   Open bite of unspecified part of neck 🖻
     Bite of neck NOS

> **Excludes1**   superficial bite of neck (S10.97)

● **S12**   **Fracture of cervical vertebra and other parts of neck**

> **Note:** A fracture not indicated as displaced or nondisplaced should be coded to displaced
>
> A fracture not indicated as open or closed should be coded to closed

> **Includes**   fracture of cervical neural arch
> fracture of cervical spine
> fracture of cervical spinous process
> fracture of cervical transverse process
> fracture of cervical vertebral arch
> fracture of neck

Code first any associated cervical spinal cord injury
     (S14.0, S14.1-) ◀

The appropriate 7th character is to be added to all codes from subcategories S12.0-S12.6

> A   initial encounter for closed fracture
> B   initial encounter for open fracture
> D   subsequent encounter for fracture with routine healing
> G   subsequent encounter for fracture with delayed healing
> K   subsequent encounter for fracture with nonunion
> S   sequela

~~Code also any associated cervical spinal cord injury (S14.0, S14.1-)~~

(Ex:) **For category S12 CC codes S12[A,B]:** M48.40X-M48.58X[S], M80.08X[S], M80.88X[S], M84.350[S], M84.454[S], M84.550[S], M84.58X[S], M84.650[S], M99.10-M99.11, M99.15-M99.17, M99.19, S03.8XX-S03.9XX[A], S12.000-S12.691{A,B,S], S12.8XX[S], S12.9XX[A,S], S13.0XX-S13.4XX[A], S13.8XXA-S14.159[A], S16.1XX[A], S22.000-S22.9XX[S], S23.20X-S23.29X[A], S23.9XX[A], S24.109[A], S24.119[A], S24.139[A], S24.149[A], S24.159[A], S29.001-S29.019[A], S29.091-S29.9XX[A], S32.000-S32.9XX[S], S33.30X-S33.39X[A], S33.9XX[A], S38.1XX[A], S38.3XX-S39.013[A], S39.091-S39.94X[A], T14.8-T14.91, T79.8XX-T79.9XX[A], T79.A0X-T79.A9X[A] **For S12[K]:** M80.00X-M80.88X[K,P], M84.30X-M84.68X[K,P], S02.0XX-S02.92X[K], S12.000-S12.691[K], S22.000-S22.9XX[K], S32.000-S32.9XX[K], S42.001-S42.92X[K,P], S49.001-S49.199[K,P], S52.001-S52.92X[K,M,N,P,Q,R], S59.001-S59.299[K,P], S62.001-S62.92X[K,P], S72.001-S72.92X[K,M,N,P,Q,R], S79.001-S79.199[K,P], S82.001-S82.92X[K,M,N,P,Q,R], S89.001-S89.399[K,P], S92.001-S92.919[K,P] **unless otherwise indicated**

● **S12.0**   **Fracture of first cervical vertebra**
     Atlas

● **S12.00**   Unspecified fracture of first cervical vertebra

● **S12.000**   Unspecified displaced fracture of first cervical vertebra A, K 🖻, B 🖻, 🖻, A, B 🖻

● **S12.001**   Unspecified nondisplaced fracture of first cervical vertebra A, K 🖻, B 🖻, 🖻, A, B 🖻

X ● **S12.01**   Stable burst fracture of first cervical vertebra A, K 🖻, B 🖻, 🖻, A, B 🖻

X ● **S12.02**   Unstable burst fracture of first cervical vertebra A, K 🖻, B 🖻, 🖻, A, B

● **S12.03**   Posterior arch fracture of first cervical vertebra

● **S12.030**   Displaced posterior arch fracture of first cervical vertebra A, K 🖻, B 🖻, 🖻, A, B 🖻

● **S12.031**   Nondisplaced posterior arch fracture of first cervical vertebra A, K 🖻, B 🖻, 🖻, A, B 🖻

● **S12.04**   Lateral mass fracture of first cervical vertebra

● **S12.040**   Displaced lateral mass fracture of first cervical vertebra A, K 🖻, B 🖻, 🖻, A, B 🖻

● **S12.041**   Nondisplaced lateral mass fracture of first cervical vertebra A, K 🖻, B 🖻, 🖻, A, B 🖻

● **S12.09**   Other fracture of first cervical vertebra

● **S12.090**   Other displaced fracture of first cervical vertebra A, K 🖻, B 🖻, 🖻, A, B 🖻

● **S12.091**   Other nondisplaced fracture of first cervical vertebra A, K 🖻, B 🖻, 🖻, A, B 🖻

● **S12.1**   **Fracture of second cervical vertebra**
     Axis

● **S12.10**   Unspecified fracture of second cervical vertebra

● **S12.100**   Unspecified displaced fracture of second cervical vertebra A, K 🖻, B 🖻, 🖻, A, B 🖻

● **S12.101**   Unspecified nondisplaced fracture of second cervical vertebra A, K 🖻, B 🖻, 🖻, A, B 🖻

● **S12.11**   Type II dens fracture

● **S12.110**   Anterior displaced Type II dens fracture A, K 🖻, B 🖻, 🖻, A, B 🖻

● **S12.111**   Posterior displaced Type II dens fracture A, K 🖻, B 🖻, 🖻, A, B 🖻

● **S12.112**   Nondisplaced Type II dens fracture A, K 🖻, B 🖻, 🖻, A, B 🖻

● **S12.12**   Other dens fracture

● **S12.120**   Other displaced dens fracture A, K 🖻, B 🖻, 🖻, A, B 🖻

● **S12.121**   Other nondisplaced dens fracture A, K 🖻, B 🖻, 🖻, A, B 🖻

● **S12.13**   Unspecified traumatic spondylolisthesis of second cervical vertebra

● **S12.130**   Unspecified traumatic displaced spondylolisthesis of second cervical vertebra A, K 🖻, B 🖻, 🖻, A, B 🖻

● **S12.131**   Unspecified traumatic nondisplaced spondylolisthesis of second cervical vertebra A, K 🖻, B 🖻, 🖻, A, B 🖻

X ● **S12.14**   Type III traumatic spondylolisthesis of second cervical vertebra A, K 🖻, B 🖻, 🖻, A, B 🖻

● **S12.15**   Other traumatic spondylolisthesis of second cervical vertebra

● **S12.150**   Other traumatic displaced spondylolisthesis of second cervical vertebra A, K 🖻, B 🖻, 🖻, A, B 🖻

● **S12.151**   Other traumatic nondisplaced spondylolisthesis of second cervical vertebra A, K 🖻, B 🖻, 🖻, A, B 🖻

● **S12.19**   Other fracture of second cervical vertebra

● **S12.190**   Other displaced fracture of second cervical vertebra A, K 🖻, B 🖻, 🖻, A, B 🖻

● **S12.191**   Other nondisplaced fracture of second cervical vertebra A, K 🖻, B 🖻, 🖻, A, B 🖻

◀ New   ◀⁞⁞⁞ Revised   ~~deleted~~ Deleted   Excludes 1   Excludes 2   Includes   Use additional   Code first   Code also   Unspecified

OGCR Official Guidelines   ● Unacceptable Principal Diagnosis   X Assign placeholder X   ● Use Additional Character(s)   ▌ Manifestation Code   **Coding Clinic**

● **S12.2**   Fracture of third cervical vertebra
   ● **S12.20**   Unspecified fracture of third cervical vertebra
     ● **S12.200**   Unspecified displaced fracture of third cervical vertebra A, K 🖉, B 🖉, 🖉, A, B 🖉
     ● **S12.201**   Unspecified nondisplaced fracture of third cervical vertebra A, K 🖉, B 🖉, 🖉, A, B 🖉
   ● **S12.23**   Unspecified traumatic spondylolisthesis of third cervical vertebra
     ● **S12.230**   Unspecified traumatic displaced spondylolisthesis of third cervical vertebra A, K 🖉, B 🖉, 🖉, A, B 🖉
     ● **S12.231**   Unspecified traumatic nondisplaced spondylolisthesis of third cervical vertebra A, K 🖉, B 🖉, 🖉, A, B 🖉
   X ● **S12.24**   Type III traumatic spondylolisthesis of third cervical vertebra A, K 🖉, B 🖉, 🖉, A, B 🖉
   ● **S12.25**   Other traumatic spondylolisthesis of third cervical vertebra
     ● **S12.250**   Other traumatic displaced spondylolisthesis of third cervical vertebra A, K 🖉, B 🖉, 🖉, A, B 🖉
     ● **S12.251**   Other traumatic nondisplaced spondylolisthesis of third cervical vertebra A, K 🖉, B 🖉, 🖉, A, B 🖉
   ● **S12.29**   Other fracture of third cervical vertebra
     ● **S12.290**   Other displaced fracture of third cervical vertebra A, K 🖉, B 🖉, 🖉, A, B 🖉
     ● **S12.291**   Other nondisplaced fracture of third cervical vertebra A, K 🖉, B 🖉, 🖉, A, B 🖉

● **S12.3**   Fracture of fourth cervical vertebra
   ● **S12.30**   Unspecified fracture of fourth cervical vertebra
     ● **S12.300**   Unspecified displaced fracture of fourth cervical vertebra A, K 🖉, B 🖉, 🖉, A, B 🖉
     ● **S12.301**   Unspecified nondisplaced fracture of fourth cervical vertebra A, K 🖉, B 🖉, 🖉, A, B 🖉
   ● **S12.33**   Unspecified traumatic spondylolisthesis of fourth cervical vertebra
     ● **S12.330**   Unspecified traumatic displaced spondylolisthesis of fourth cervical vertebra A, K 🖉, B 🖉, 🖉, A, B 🖉
     ● **S12.331**   Unspecified traumatic nondisplaced spondylolisthesis of fourth cervical vertebra A, K 🖉, B 🖉, 🖉, A, B 🖉
   X ● **S12.34**   Type III traumatic spondylolisthesis of fourth cervical vertebra A, K 🖉, B 🖉, 🖉, A, B 🖉
   ● **S12.35**   Other traumatic spondylolisthesis of fourth cervical vertebra
     ● **S12.350**   Other traumatic displaced spondylolisthesis of fourth cervical vertebra A, K 🖉, B 🖉, 🖉, A, B 🖉
     ● **S12.351**   Other traumatic nondisplaced spondylolisthesis of fourth cervical vertebra A, K 🖉, B 🖉, 🖉, A, B 🖉
   ● **S12.39**   Other fracture of fourth cervical vertebra
     ● **S12.390**   Other displaced fracture of fourth cervical vertebra A, K 🖉, B 🖉, 🖉, A, B 🖉
     ● **S12.391**   Other nondisplaced fracture of fourth cervical vertebra A, K 🖉, B 🖉, 🖉, A, B 🖉

● **S12.4**   Fracture of fifth cervical vertebra
   ● **S12.40**   Unspecified fracture of fifth cervical vertebra
     ● **S12.400**   Unspecified displaced fracture of fifth cervical vertebra A, K 🖉, B 🖉, 🖉, A, B 🖉
     ● **S12.401**   Unspecified nondisplaced fracture of fifth cervical vertebra A, K 🖉, B 🖉, 🖉, A, B 🖉
   ● **S12.43**   Unspecified traumatic spondylolisthesis of fifth cervical vertebra
     ● **S12.430**   Unspecified traumatic displaced spondylolisthesis of fifth cervical vertebra A, K 🖉, B 🖉, 🖉, A, B 🖉
     ● **S12.431**   Unspecified traumatic nondisplaced spondylolisthesis of fifth cervical vertebra A, K 🖉, B 🖉, 🖉, A, B 🖉
   X ● **S12.44**   Type III traumatic spondylolisthesis of fifth cervical vertebra A, K 🖉, B 🖉, 🖉, A, B 🖉
   ● **S12.45**   Other traumatic spondylolisthesis of fifth cervical vertebra
     ● **S12.450**   Other traumatic displaced spondylolisthesis of fifth cervical vertebra A, K 🖉, B 🖉, 🖉, A, B 🖉
     ● **S12.451**   Other traumatic nondisplaced spondylolisthesis of fifth cervical vertebra A, K 🖉, B 🖉, 🖉, A, B 🖉
   ● **S12.49**   Other fracture of fifth cervical vertebra
     ● **S12.490**   Other displaced fracture of fifth cervical vertebra A, K 🖉, B 🖉, 🖉, A, B 🖉
     ● **S12.491**   Other nondisplaced fracture of fifth cervical vertebra A, K 🖉, B 🖉, 🖉, A, B 🖉

● **S12.5**   Fracture of sixth cervical vertebra
   ● **S12.50**   Unspecified fracture of sixth cervical vertebra
     ● **S12.500**   Unspecified displaced fracture of sixth cervical vertebra A, K 🖉, B 🖉, 🖉, A, B 🖉
     ● **S12.501**   Unspecified nondisplaced fracture of sixth cervical vertebra A, K 🖉, B 🖉, 🖉, A, B 🖉
   ● **S12.53**   Unspecified traumatic spondylolisthesis of sixth cervical vertebra
     ● **S12.530**   Unspecified traumatic displaced spondylolisthesis of sixth cervical vertebra A, K 🖉, B 🖉, 🖉, A, B 🖉
     ● **S12.531**   Unspecified traumatic nondisplaced spondylolisthesis of sixth cervical vertebra A, K 🖉, B 🖉, 🖉, A, B 🖉
   X ● **S12.54**   Type III traumatic spondylolisthesis of sixth cervical vertebra A, K 🖉, B 🖉, 🖉, A, B 🖉
   ● **S12.55**   Other traumatic spondylolisthesis of sixth cervical vertebra
     ● **S12.550**   Other traumatic displaced spondylolisthesis of sixth cervical vertebra A, K 🖉, B 🖉, 🖉, A, B 🖉
     ● **S12.551**   Other traumatic nondisplaced spondylolisthesis of sixth cervical vertebra A, K 🖉, B 🖉, 🖉, A, B 🖉
   ● **S12.59**   Other fracture of sixth cervical vertebra
     ● **S12.590**   Other displaced fracture of sixth cervical vertebra A, K 🖉, B 🖉, 🖉, A, B 🖉
     ● **S12.591**   Other nondisplaced fracture of sixth cervical vertebra A, K 🖉, B 🖉, 🖉, A, B 🖉

CHAPTER 19 (S00-T88)

N   Newborn Age: 0   **P**   Pediatric Age: 0–17   **M**   Maternity DX: 12–55   **A**   Adult Age: 15–124   ♀   Females Only   ♂   Males Only

🖉   Complication\Comorbidity   🖉   Major C\C   (Ex)   CC/MCC Exclusions   🖉   Present on Admission Requirement   🖉   Hospital-Acquired Condition

1309

● **S12.6**   **Fracture of seventh cervical vertebra**

    S12.60   **Unspecified fracture of seventh cervical vertebra**

      ● **S12.600**   Unspecified displaced fracture of seventh cervical vertebra A, K ▥, B ▥, ▥, A, B ▥

      ● **S12.601**   Unspecified nondisplaced fracture of seventh cervical vertebra A, K ▥, B ▥, ▥, A, B ▥

    ● **S12.63**   Unspecified traumatic spondylolisthesis of seventh cervical vertebra

      ● **S12.630**   Unspecified traumatic displaced spondylolisthesis of seventh cervical vertebra A, K ▥, B ▥, ▥, A, B ▥

      ● **S12.631**   Unspecified traumatic nondisplaced spondylolisthesis of seventh cervical vertebra A, K ▥, B ▥, ▥, A, B ▥

  X **S12.64**   Type III traumatic spondylolisthesis of seventh cervical vertebra A, K ▥, B ▥, ▥, A, B ▥

    ● **S12.65**   Other traumatic spondylolisthesis of seventh cervical vertebra

      ● **S12.650**   Other traumatic displaced spondylolisthesis of seventh cervical vertebra A, K ▥, B ▥, ▥, A, B ▥

      ● **S12.651**   Other traumatic nondisplaced spondylolisthesis of seventh cervical vertebra A, K ▥, B ▥, ▥, A, B ▥

    ● **S12.69**   Other fracture of seventh cervical vertebra

      ● **S12.690**   Other displaced fracture of seventh cervical vertebra A, K ▥, B ▥, ▥, A, B ▥

      ● **S12.691**   Other nondisplaced fracture of seventh cervical vertebra A, K ▥, B ▥, ▥, A, B ▥

  X● **S12.8**   **Fracture of other parts of neck** A ▥, ▥, A ▥

    Hyoid bone ◀   Thyroid cartilage ◀

    Larynx ◀   Trachea ◀

    The appropriate 7th character is to be added to code S12.8

> A   initial encounter
> D   subsequent encounter
> S   sequela

    ~~Hyoid bone~~   ~~Thyroid cartilage~~

    ~~Larynx~~   ~~Trachea~~

    (Ex) S03.8XX-S03.9XX[A], S12.8XX[A], S29.011-S29.019[A], S38.3XX[A], S39.011-S39.013[A], T14.8-T14.91, T79.8XX-T79.9XX[A], T79.A0XA-T79.A9X[A]

  X● **S12.9**   **Fracture of neck, unspecified** A ▥, ▥, A ▥

    Fracture of neck NOS ◀

    Fracture of cervical spine NOS ◀

    Fracture of cervical vertebra NOS ◀

    The appropriate 7th character is to be added to code S12.9

> A   initial encounter
> D   subsequent encounter
> S   sequela

    ~~Fracture of neck NOS~~

    ~~Fracture of cervical spine NOS~~

    ~~Fracture of cervical vertebra NOS~~

● **S13**   **Dislocation and sprain of joints and ligaments at neck level**

    Includes   avulsion of joint or ligament at neck level

         laceration of cartilage, joint or ligament at neck level

         sprain of cartilage, joint or ligament at neck level

         traumatic hemarthrosis of joint or ligament at neck level

         traumatic rupture of joint or ligament at neck level

         traumatic subluxation of joint or ligament at neck level

         traumatic tear of joint or ligament at neck level

    Code also any associated open wound

    Excludes2   strain of muscle or tendon at neck level (S16.1)

    The appropriate 7th character is to be added to each code from category S13

> A   initial encounter
> D   subsequent encounter
> S   sequela

    (Ex) M99.10-M99.11, S03.8XX-S03.9XX[A], S12.000-S12.691[A,B], S12.9XX-S13.4XX[A], S13.8XX[A], S14.0XX-S14.108[A], S14.111-S14.118[A], S14.121-S14.128[A], S14.131-S14.138[A], S14.141-S14.148[A], S14.151-S14.158[A], S16.1XX[A], S29.011-S29.019[A], S38.3XX[A], S39.011-S39.013[A], T14.8-T14.91, T79.A0X-T79.9XX[A]

  X● **S13.0**   **Traumatic rupture of cervical intervertebral disc** A ▥, ▥, A ▥

      Excludes1   rupture or displacement (nontraumatic) of cervical intervertebral disc NOS (M50.-)

  ● **S13.1**   **Subluxation and dislocation of cervical vertebrae**

    Code also any associated:

      open wound of neck (S11.-)

      spinal cord injury (S14.1-)

    Excludes2   fracture of cervical vertebrae (S12.0-S12.3-)

    ● **S13.10**   **Subluxation and dislocation of unspecified cervical vertebrae**

      ● **S13.100**   Subluxation of unspecified cervical vertebrae A ▥, ▥, A ▥

      ● **S13.101**   Dislocation of unspecified cervical vertebrae A ▥, ▥, A ▥

    ● **S13.11**   **Subluxation and dislocation of C_0/C_1 cervical vertebrae**

      Subluxation and dislocation of atlantooccipital joint

      Subluxation and dislocation of atloidooccipital joint

      Subluxation and dislocation of occipitoatloid joint

      ● **S13.110**   Subluxation of C_0/C_1 cervical vertebrae A ▥, ▥, A ▥

      ● **S13.111**   Dislocation of C_0/C_1 cervical vertebrae A ▥, ▥, A ▥

    ● **S13.12**   **Subluxation and dislocation of C_1/C_2 cervical vertebrae**

      Subluxation and dislocation of atlantoaxial joint

      ● **S13.120**   Subluxation of C_1/C_2 cervical vertebrae A ▥, ▥, A ▥

      ● **S13.121**   Dislocation of C_1/C_2 cervical vertebrae A ▥, ▥, A ▥

◀ New   ◀▥ Revised   ~~deleted~~ Deleted   Excludes 1   Excludes 2   Includes   Use additional   Code first   Code also   Unspecified

OGCR Official Guidelines   ● Unacceptable Principal Diagnosis   X Assign placeholder X   ● Use Additional Character(s)   ▶ Manifestation Code   **Coding Clinic**

- **S13.13** Subluxation and dislocation of C_2/C_3 cervical vertebrae
    - **S13.130** Subluxation of C_2/C_3 cervical vertebrae A 🐾, 🐾, A 🐾
    - **S13.131** Dislocation of C_2/C_3 cervical vertebrae A 🐾, 🐾, A 🐾
- **S13.14** Subluxation and dislocation of C_3/C_4 cervical vertebrae
    - **S13.140** Subluxation of C_3/C_4 cervical vertebrae A 🐾, 🐾, A 🐾
    - **S13.141** Dislocation of C_3/C_4 cervical vertebrae A 🐾, 🐾, A 🐾
- **S13.15** Subluxation and dislocation of C_4/C_5 cervical vertebrae
    - **S13.150** Subluxation of C_4/C_5 cervical vertebrae A 🐾, 🐾, A 🐾
    - **S13.151** Dislocation of C_4/C_5 cervical vertebrae A 🐾, 🐾, A 🐾
- **S13.16** Subluxation and dislocation of C_5/C_6 cervical vertebrae
    - **S13.160** Subluxation of C_5/C_6 cervical vertebrae A 🐾, 🐾, A 🐾
    - **S13.161** Dislocation of C_5/C_6 cervical vertebrae A 🐾, 🐾, A 🐾
- **S13.17** Subluxation and dislocation of C_6/C_7 cervical vertebrae
    - **S13.170** Subluxation of C_6/C_7 cervical vertebrae A 🐾, 🐾, A 🐾
    - **S13.171** Dislocation of C_6/C_7 cervical vertebrae A 🐾, 🐾, A 🐾
- **S13.18** Subluxation and dislocation of C_7/T_1 cervical vertebrae
    - **S13.180** Subluxation of C_7/T_1 cervical vertebrae A 🐾, 🐾, A 🐾
    - **S13.181** Dislocation of C_7/T_1 cervical vertebrae A 🐾, 🐾, A 🐾
- **S13.2** Dislocation of other and unspecified parts of neck
    - X **S13.20** Dislocation of unspecified parts of neck A 🐾, 🐾, A 🐾
    - X **S13.29** Dislocation of other parts of neck A 🐾, 🐾, A 🐾
- X **S13.4** Sprain of ligaments of cervical spine 🐾
    Sprain of anterior longitudinal (ligament), cervical
    Sprain of atlanto-axial (joints)
    Sprain of atlanto-occipital (joints)
    Whiplash injury of cervical spine
- X **S13.5** Sprain of thyroid region 🐾
    Sprain of cricoarytenoid (joint) (ligament)
    Sprain of cricothyroid (joint) (ligament)
    Sprain of thyroid cartilage
- X **S13.8** Sprain of joints and ligaments of other parts of neck 🐾
- X **S13.9** Sprain of joints and ligaments of unspecified parts of neck 🐾

- **S14** Injury of nerves and spinal cord at neck level
    Note: Code to highest level of cervical cord injury
    Code also any associated:
    fracture of cervical vertebra (S12.0--S12.6.-)
    open wound of neck (S11.-) ◄▥
    transient paralysis (R29.5)

    The appropriate 7th character is to be added to each code from category S14

A	initial encounter
D	subsequent encounter
S	sequela

    (Ex) **For category S14 CC codes:** M48.40X-M48.58X[S], M80.08X[S], M80.88X[S], M84.350[S], M84.454[S], M84.550[S], M84.58X[S], M84.650[S], M99.10-M99.11, M99.15-M99.17, M99.19, S12.000-S12.691[A,B,S], S12.8XX[S], S12.9XX[A, S], S13.0XX-S13.29X[A], S13.9XX-S14.159[A], S22.000-S22.9XX[S], S23.20X-S23.29X[A], S23.9XX[A], S24.109[A], S24.119[A], S24.139[A], S24.149[A], S24.159[A], S29.001-S29.009[A], S29.091-S29.9XX[A], S32.000-S32.9XX[S], S33.30X-S33.39X[A], S33.9XX[A], S38.1XX[A], S39.001-S39.003[A], S39.091-S39.94X[A], T14.8-T14.91, T79.8XX-T79.9XX[A], T79.A0X-T79.A9X[A]

- X **S14.0** Concussion and edema of cervical spinal cord A 🐾, 🐾
- **S14.1** Other and unspecified injuries of cervical spinal cord
    - **S14.10** Unspecified injury of cervical spinal cord
        - **S14.101** Unspecified injury at C_1 level of cervical spinal cord A 🐾, 🐾, A 🐾
        - **S14.102** Unspecified injury at C_2 level of cervical spinal cord A 🐾, 🐾, A 🐾
        - **S14.103** Unspecified injury at C_3 level of cervical spinal cord A 🐾, 🐾, A 🐾
        - **S14.104** Unspecified injury at C_4 level of cervical spinal cord A 🐾, 🐾, A 🐾
        - **S14.105** Unspecified injury at C_5 level of cervical spinal cord A 🐾, 🐾, A 🐾
        - **S14.106** Unspecified injury at C_6 level of cervical spinal cord A 🐾, 🐾, A 🐾
        - **S14.107** Unspecified injury at C_7 level of cervical spinal cord A 🐾, 🐾, A 🐾
        - **S14.108** Unspecified injury at C_8 level of cervical spinal cord A 🐾, 🐾
        - **S14.109** Unspecified injury at unspecified level of cervical spinal cord 🐾, A 🐾
            Injury of cervical spinal cord NOS
    - **S14.11** Complete lesion of cervical spinal cord
        - **S14.111** Complete lesion at C_1 level of cervical spinal cord A 🐾, 🐾, A 🐾
        - **S14.112** Complete lesion at C_2 level of cervical spinal cord A 🐾, 🐾, A 🐾
        - **S14.113** Complete lesion at C_3 level of cervical spinal cord A 🐾, 🐾, A 🐾
        - **S14.114** Complete lesion at C_4 level of cervical spinal cord A 🐾, 🐾, A 🐾
        - **S14.115** Complete lesion at C_5 level of cervical spinal cord A 🐾, 🐾, A 🐾
        - **S14.116** Complete lesion at C_6 level of cervical spinal cord A 🐾, 🐾, A 🐾
        - **S14.117** Complete lesion at C_7 level of cervical spinal cord A 🐾, 🐾, A 🐾
        - **S14.118** Complete lesion at C_8 level of cervical spinal cord A 🐾, 🐾
        - **S14.119** Complete lesion at unspecified level of cervical spinal cord 🐾

| N | Newborn Age: 0 | P | Pediatric Age: 0–17 | M | Maternity DX: 12–55 | A | Adult Age: 15–124 | ♀ | Females Only | ♂ | Males Only |

🐾 Complication\Comorbidity 🐾 Major C\C (Ex) CC/MCC Exclusions 🐾 Present on Admission Requirement 🐾 Hospital-Acquired Condition

1311

● S14.12　Central cord syndrome of cervical spinal cord

● S14.121　Central cord syndrome at C_1 level of cervical spinal cord A 🦠, 🦠, A 🦠

● S14.122　Central cord syndrome at C_2 level of cervical spinal cord A 🦠, 🦠, A 🦠

● S14.123　Central cord syndrome at C_3 level of cervical spinal cord A 🦠, 🦠, A 🦠

● S14.124　Central cord syndrome at C_4 level of cervical spinal cord A 🦠, 🦠, A 🦠

● S14.125　Central cord syndrome at C_5 level of cervical spinal cord A 🦠, 🦠, A 🦠

● S14.126　Central cord syndrome at C_6 level of cervical spinal cord A 🦠, 🦠, A 🦠

● S14.127　Central cord syndrome at C_7 level of cervical spinal cord A 🦠, 🦠, A 🦠

● S14.128　Central cord syndrome at C_8 level of cervical spinal cord A 🦠, 🦠

● S14.129　Central cord syndrome at unspecified level of cervical spinal cord 🦠

● S14.13　Anterior cord syndrome of cervical spinal cord

● S14.131　Anterior cord syndrome at C_1 level of cervical spinal cord A 🦠, 🦠, A 🦠

● S14.132　Anterior cord syndrome at C_2 level of cervical spinal cord A 🦠, 🦠, A 🦠

● S14.133　Anterior cord syndrome at C_3 level of cervical spinal cord A 🦠, 🦠, A 🦠

● S14.134　Anterior cord syndrome at C_4 level of cervical spinal cord A 🦠, 🦠, A 🦠

● S14.135　Anterior cord syndrome at C_5 level of cervical spinal cord A 🦠, 🦠, A 🦠

● S14.136　Anterior cord syndrome at C_6 level of cervical spinal cord A 🦠, 🦠, A 🦠

● S14.137　Anterior cord syndrome at C_7 level of cervical spinal cord A 🦠, 🦠, A 🦠

● S14.138　Anterior cord syndrome at C_8 level of cervical spinal cord A 🦠, 🦠

● S14.139　Anterior cord syndrome at unspecified level of cervical spinal cord 🦠

● S14.14　Brown-Séquard syndrome of cervical spinal cord

● S14.141　Brown-Séquard syndrome at C_1 level of cervical spinal cord A 🦠, 🦠

● S14.142　Brown-Séquard syndrome at C_2 level of cervical spinal cord A 🦠, 🦠

● S14.143　Brown-Séquard syndrome at C_3 level of cervical spinal cord A 🦠, 🦠

● S14.144　Brown-Séquard syndrome at C_4 level of cervical spinal cord A 🦠, 🦠

● S14.145　Brown-Séquard syndrome at C_5 level of cervical spinal cord A 🦠, 🦠

● S14.146　Brown-Séquard syndrome at C_6 level of cervical spinal cord A 🦠, 🦠

● S14.147　Brown-Séquard syndrome at C_7 level of cervical spinal cord A 🦠, 🦠

● S14.148　Brown-Séquard syndrome at C_8 level of cervical spinal cord A 🦠, 🦠

● S14.149　Brown-Séquard syndrome at unspecified level of cervical spinal cord 🦠

● S14.15　Other incomplete lesions of cervical spinal cord
Incomplete lesion of cervical spinal cord NOS
Posterior cord syndrome of cervical spinal cord

● S14.151　Other incomplete lesion at C_1 level of cervical spinal cord A 🦠, 🦠, A 🦠

● S14.152　Other incomplete lesion at C_2 level of cervical spinal cord A 🦠, 🦠, A 🦠

● S14.153　Other incomplete lesion at C_3 level of cervical spinal cord A 🦠, 🦠, A 🦠

● S14.154　Other incomplete lesion at C_4 level of cervical spinal cord A 🦠, 🦠, A 🦠

● S14.155　Other incomplete lesion at C_5 level of cervical spinal cord A 🦠, 🦠, A 🦠

● S14.156　Other incomplete lesion at C_6 level of cervical spinal cord A 🦠, 🦠, A 🦠

● S14.157　Other incomplete lesion at C_7 level of cervical spinal cord A 🦠, 🦠, A 🦠

● S14.158　Other incomplete lesion at C_8 level of cervical spinal cord A 🦠, 🦠

● S14.159　Other incomplete lesion at unspecified level of cervical spinal cord 🦠

X ● S14.2　Injury of nerve root of cervical spine 🦠

X ● S14.3　Injury of brachial plexus 🦠

X ● S14.4　Injury of peripheral nerves of neck 🦠

X ● S14.5　Injury of cervical sympathetic nerves 🦠

X ● S14.8　Injury of other specified nerves of neck 🦠

X ● S14.9　Injury of unspecified nerves of neck 🦠

● S15　Injury of blood vessels at neck level
Code also any associated open wound (S11.-)

The appropriate 7th character is to be added to each code from category S15

A	initial encounter
D	subsequent encounter
S	sequela

● S15.0　Injury of carotid artery of neck
Injury of carotid artery (common) (external) (internal, extracranial portion)
Injury of carotid artery NOS

Excludes1　injury of internal carotid artery, intracranial portion (S06.8)

Ex: For category S15.0 CC codes: S09.0XX[A], S15.009[A], S15.029[A], S15.099-S15.199[A], S15.8XX-S15.9XX[A], T14.8-T14.91, T79.8XX-T79.9XX[A], T79.A0X-T79.A9X[A]

● S15.00　Unspecified injury of carotid artery

● S15.001　Unspecified injury of right carotid artery A 🦠, 🦠

● S15.002　Unspecified injury of left carotid artery A 🦠, 🦠

● S15.009　Unspecified injury of unspecified carotid artery A 🦠, 🦠

● S15.01　Minor laceration of carotid artery
Incomplete transection of carotid artery
Laceration of carotid artery NOS
Superficial laceration of carotid artery

● S15.011　Minor laceration of right carotid artery A 🦠, 🦠

● S15.012　Minor laceration of left carotid artery A 🦠, 🦠

● S15.019　Minor laceration of unspecified carotid artery A 🦠, 🦠

● S15.02　Major laceration of carotid artery
Complete transection of carotid artery
Traumatic rupture of carotid artery

● S15.021　Major laceration of right carotid artery A 🦠, 🦠

● S15.022　Major laceration of left carotid artery A 🦠, 🦠

● S15.029　Major laceration of unspecified carotid artery A 🦠, 🦠

● S15.09　Other specified injury of carotid artery

● S15.091　Other specified injury of right carotid artery A 🦠, 🦠

● S15.092　Other specified injury of left carotid artery A 🦠, 🦠

● S15.099　Other specified injury of unspecified carotid artery A 🦠, 🦠

◀ New　◀ⅲ Revised　d̶e̶l̶e̶t̶e̶d̶ Deleted　Excludes 1　Excludes 2　Includes　Use additional　Code first　Code also　Unspecified
OGCR Official Guidelines　● Unacceptable Principal Diagnosis　X Assign placeholder X　● Use Additional Character(s)　▌ Manifestation Code　Coding Clinic

- **S15.1**   **Injury of vertebral artery**
  - (Ex:) **For category S15.1 CC codes:** S09.0XX[A], S15.101-S15.199[A], S15.8XX-S15.9XX[A], T14.8-T14.91, T79.8XX-T79.9XX[A], T79.A0X-T79.A9X[A]
  - **S15.10**   **Unspecified injury of vertebral artery**
    - **S15.101**   Unspecified injury of right vertebral artery A 🔵, 🔵
    - **S15.102**   Unspecified injury of left vertebral artery A 🔵, 🔵
    - **S15.109**   Unspecified injury of unspecified vertebral artery A 🔵, 🔵
  - **S15.11**   **Minor laceration of vertebral artery**
    Incomplete transection of vertebral artery
    Laceration of vertebral artery NOS
    Superficial laceration of vertebral artery
    - **S15.111**   Minor laceration of right vertebral artery A 🔵, 🔵
    - **S15.112**   Minor laceration of left vertebral artery A 🔵, 🔵
    - **S15.119**   Minor laceration of unspecified vertebral artery A 🔵, 🔵
  - **S15.12**   **Major laceration of vertebral artery**
    Complete transection of vertebral artery
    Traumatic rupture of vertebral artery
    - **S15.121**   Major laceration of right vertebral artery A 🔵, 🔵
    - **S15.122**   Major laceration of left vertebral artery A 🔵, 🔵
    - **S15.129**   Major laceration of unspecified vertebral artery A 🔵, 🔵
  - **S15.19**   **Other specified injury of vertebral artery**
    - **S15.191**   Other specified injury of right vertebral artery A 🔵, 🔵
    - **S15.192**   Other specified injury of left vertebral artery A 🔵, 🔵
    - **S15.199**   Other specified injury of unspecified vertebral artery A 🔵, 🔵
- **S15.2**   **Injury of external jugular vein**
  - (Ex:) **For category S15.2 CC codes:** See S15.1
  - **S15.20**   **Unspecified injury of external jugular vein**
    - **S15.201**   Unspecified injury of right external jugular vein A 🔵, 🔵
    - **S15.202**   Unspecified injury of left external jugular vein A 🔵, 🔵
    - **S15.209**   Unspecified injury of unspecified external jugular vein A 🔵, 🔵
  - **S15.21**   **Minor laceration of external jugular vein**
    Incomplete transection of external jugular vein
    Laceration of external jugular vein NOS
    Superficial laceration of external jugular vein
    - **S15.211**   Minor laceration of right external jugular vein A 🔵, 🔵
    - **S15.212**   Minor laceration of left external jugular vein A 🔵, 🔵
    - **S15.219**   Minor laceration of unspecified external jugular vein A 🔵, 🔵
  - **S15.22**   **Major laceration of external jugular vein**
    Complete transection of external jugular vein
    Traumatic rupture of external jugular vein
    - **S15.221**   Major laceration of right external jugular vein A 🔵, 🔵
    - **S15.222**   Major laceration of left external jugular vein A 🔵, 🔵
    - **S15.229**   Major laceration of unspecified external jugular vein A 🔵, 🔵

- **S15.29**   **Other specified injury of external jugular vein**
  - **S15.291**   Other specified injury of right external jugular vein A 🔵, 🔵
  - **S15.292**   Other specified injury of left external jugular vein A 🔵, 🔵
  - **S15.299**   Other specified injury of unspecified external jugular vein A 🔵, 🔵
- **S15.3**   **Injury of internal jugular vein**
  - (Ex:) **For category S15.3 CC codes:** See S15.1
  - **S15.30**   **Unspecified injury of internal jugular vein**
    - **S15.301**   Unspecified injury of right internal jugular vein A 🔵, 🔵
    - **S15.302**   Unspecified injury of left internal jugular vein A 🔵, 🔵
    - **S15.309**   Unspecified injury of unspecified internal jugular vein A 🔵, 🔵
  - **S15.31**   **Minor laceration of internal jugular vein**
    Incomplete transection of internal jugular vein
    Laceration of internal jugular vein NOS
    Superficial laceration of internal jugular vein
    - **S15.311**   Minor laceration of right internal jugular vein A 🔵, 🔵
    - **S15.312**   Minor laceration of left internal jugular vein A 🔵, 🔵
    - **S15.319**   Minor laceration of unspecified internal jugular vein A 🔵, 🔵
  - **S15.32**   **Major laceration of internal jugular vein**
    Complete transection of internal jugular vein
    Traumatic rupture of internal jugular vein
    - **S15.321**   Major laceration of right internal jugular vein A 🔵, 🔵
    - **S15.322**   Major laceration of left internal jugular vein A 🔵, 🔵
    - **S15.329**   Major laceration of unspecified internal jugular vein A 🔵, 🔵
  - **S15.39**   **Other specified injury of internal jugular vein**
    - **S15.391**   Other specified injury of right internal jugular vein A 🔵, 🔵
    - **S15.392**   Other specified injury of left internal jugular vein A 🔵, 🔵
    - **S15.399**   Other specified injury of unspecified internal jugular vein A 🔵, 🔵
- X **S15.8**   **Injury of other specified blood vessels at neck level** A 🔵, 🔵
  - (Ex:) See S15.1
- X **S15.9**   **Injury of unspecified blood vessel at neck level** A 🔵, 🔵
  - (Ex:) See S15.1

- **S16**   **Injury of muscle, fascia and tendon at neck level**
  Code also any associated open wound (S11.-)
  Excludes2   sprain of joint or ligament at neck level (S13.9)
  The appropriate 7th character is to be added to each code from category S16

A	initial encounter
D	subsequent encounter
S	sequela

- X **S16.1**   Strain of muscle, fascia and tendon at neck level 🔵
- X **S16.2**   Laceration of muscle, fascia and tendon at neck level 🔵
- X **S16.8**   Other specified injury of muscle, fascia and tendon at neck level 🔵
- X **S16.9**   Unspecified injury of muscle, fascia and tendon at neck level 🔵

CHAPTER 19 (S00-T88)

| N | Newborn Age: 0 | P | Pediatric Age: 0–17 | M | Maternity DX: 12–55 | A | Adult Age: 15–124 | ♀ Females Only | ♂ Males Only |

🔵 Complication\Comorbidity   🔵 Major C\C   (Ex:) CC/MCC Exclusions   🔵 Present on Admission Requirement   🔵 Hospital-Acquired Condition

1313

● **S17   Crushing injury of neck**

Use additional code for all associated injuries, such as:
injury of blood vessels (S15.-)
open wound of neck (S11.-)
spinal cord injury (S14.0, S14.1-)
vertebral fracture (S12.0--S12.3-)

The appropriate 7th character is to be added to each code from category S17

A	initial encounter
D	subsequent encounter
S	sequela

(Ex) **For category S17 CC codes:** S01.90X-S01.95X[A], S02.0XX-S02.92X[S], S07.0XX-S07.9XX[A], S08.89X-S09.19X[A], S09.8XXA-S09.90X[A], S09.92XA-S09.93X[A], S16.8XX-S19.9XX[A], T14.8-T14.91, T79.8XX-T79.9XX[A], T79.A0X-T79.A9X[A]

X ● **S17.0   Crushing injury of larynx and trachea** A 🖉, 🖉, A 🖉

X ● **S17.8   Crushing injury of other specified parts of neck** A 🖉, 🖉, A 🖉

X ● **S17.9   Crushing injury of neck, part** unspecified A 🖉, 🖉, A 🖉

● **S19   Other and unspecified injuries of neck**

The appropriate 7th character is to be added to each code from category S19

A	initial encounter
D	subsequent encounter
S	sequela

● **S19.8   Other specified injuries of neck**

X ● **S19.80   Other specified injuries of** unspecified **part of neck** 🖉

X ● **S19.81   Other specified injuries of larynx** 🖉

X ● **S19.82   Other specified injuries of cervical trachea** 🖉

     Excludes2   other specified injury of thoracic trachea (S27.5-)

X ● **S19.83   Other specified injuries of vocal cord** 🖉

X ● **S19.84   Other specified injuries of thyroid gland** 🖉

X ● **S19.85   Other specified injuries of pharynx and cervical esophagus** 🖉

X ● **S19.89   Other specified injuries of other specified part of neck** 🖉

X ● **S19.9   Unspecified injury of neck** 🖉

INJURIES TO THE THORAX (S20-S29)

Includes	injuries of breast
	injuries of chest (wall)
	injuries of interscapular area
Excludes2	burns and corrosions (T20-T32)
	effects of foreign body in bronchus (T17.5)
	effects of foreign body in esophagus (T18.1)
	effects of foreign body in lung (T17.8)
	effects of foreign body in trachea (T17.4)
	frostbite (T33-T34)
	injuries of axilla
	injuries of clavicle
	injuries of scapular region
	injuries of shoulder
	insect bite or sting, venomous (T63.4)

● **S20   Superficial injury of thorax**

The appropriate 7th character is to be added to each code from category S20

A	initial encounter
D	subsequent encounter
S	sequela

● **S20.0   Contusion of breast**

X ● **S20.00   Contusion of breast,** unspecified **breast** 🖉

X ● **S20.01   Contusion of right breast** 🖉

X ● **S20.02   Contusion of left breast** 🖉

● **S20.1   Other and unspecified superficial injuries of breast**

● **S20.10   Unspecified superficial injuries of breast**

● **S20.101 ** Unspecified **superficial injuries of breast, right breast** 🖉

● **S20.102 ** Unspecified **superficial injuries of breast, left breast** 🖉

● **S20.109 ** Unspecified **superficial injuries of breast, unspecified breast** 🖉

● **S20.11   Abrasion of breast**

● **S20.111   Abrasion of breast, right breast** 🖉

● **S20.112   Abrasion of breast, left breast** 🖉

● **S20.119   Abrasion of breast,** unspecified **breast** 🖉

● **S20.12   Blister (nonthermal) of breast**

● **S20.121   Blister (nonthermal) of breast, right breast** 🖉

● **S20.122   Blister (nonthermal) of breast, left breast** 🖉

● **S20.129   Blister (nonthermal) of breast,** unspecified **breast** 🖉

● **S20.14   External constriction of part of breast**

● **S20.141   External constriction of part of breast, right breast** 🖉

● **S20.142   External constriction of part of breast, left breast** 🖉

● **S20.149   External constriction of part of breast,** unspecified **breast** 🖉

● **S20.15   Superficial foreign body of breast**
     Splinter in the breast

● **S20.151   Superficial foreign body of breast, right breast** 🖉

● **S20.152   Superficial foreign body of breast, left breast** 🖉

● **S20.159   Superficial foreign body of breast,** unspecified **breast** 🖉

● **S20.16   Insect bite (nonvenomous) of breast**

● **S20.161   Insect bite (nonvenomous) of breast, right breast** 🖉

● **S20.162   Insect bite (nonvenomous) of breast, left breast** 🖉

● **S20.169   Insect bite (nonvenomous) of breast,** unspecified **breast** 🖉

● **S20.17   Other superficial bite of breast**

     Excludes1   open bite of breast (S21.05-)

● **S20.171   Other superficial bite of breast, right breast** 🖉

● **S20.172   Other superficial bite of breast, left breast** 🖉

● **S20.179   Other superficial bite of breast,** unspecified **breast** 🖉

● **S20.2   Contusion of thorax**

X ● **S20.20   Contusion of thorax,** unspecified 🖉

● **S20.21   Contusion of front wall of thorax**

● **S20.211   Contusion of right front wall of thorax** 🖉

● **S20.212   Contusion of left front wall of thorax** 🖉

● **S20.219   Contusion of** unspecified **front wall of thorax** 🖉

● **S20.22   Contusion of back wall of thorax**

● **S20.221   Contusion of right back wall of thorax** 🖉

● **S20.222   Contusion of left back wall of thorax** 🖉

● **S20.229   Contusion of** unspecified **back wall of thorax** 🖉

◀ New   ◀▥ Revised   ~~deleted~~ Deleted   Excludes 1   Excludes 2   Includes   Use additional   Code first   Code also   Unspecified

OGCR Official Guidelines   ● Unacceptable Principal Diagnosis   X Assign placeholder X   ● Use Additional Character(s)   ▶ Manifestation Code   **Coding Clinic**

● **S20.3**   **Other and unspecified superficial injuries of front wall of thorax**
  ● **S20.30**   **Unspecified superficial injuries of front wall of thorax**
    ● **S20.301**   Unspecified superficial injuries of right front wall of thorax 🔲
    ● **S20.302**   Unspecified superficial injuries of left front wall of thorax 🔲
    ● **S20.309**   Unspecified superficial injuries of unspecified front wall of thorax 🔲
  ● **S20.31**   **Abrasion of front wall of thorax**
    ● **S20.311**   Abrasion of right front wall of thorax 🔲
    ● **S20.312**   Abrasion of left front wall of thorax 🔲
    ● **S20.319**   Abrasion of unspecified front wall of thorax 🔲
  ● **S20.32**   **Blister (nonthermal) of front wall of thorax**
    ● **S20.321**   Blister (nonthermal) of right front wall of thorax 🔲
    ● **S20.322**   Blister (nonthermal) of left front wall of thorax 🔲
    ● **S20.329**   Blister (nonthermal) of unspecified front wall of thorax 🔲
  ● **S20.34**   **External constriction of front wall of thorax**
    ● **S20.341**   External constriction of right front wall of thorax 🔲
    ● **S20.342**   External constriction of left front wall of thorax 🔲
    ● **S20.349**   External constriction of unspecified front wall of thorax 🔲
  ● **S20.35**   **Superficial foreign body of front wall of thorax**
       Splinter in front wall of thorax
    ● **S20.351**   Superficial foreign body of right front wall of thorax 🔲
    ● **S20.352**   Superficial foreign body of left front wall of thorax 🔲
    ● **S20.359**   Superficial foreign body of unspecified front wall of thorax 🔲
  ● **S20.36**   **Insect bite (nonvenomous) of front wall of thorax**
    ● **S20.361**   Insect bite (nonvenomous) of right front wall of thorax 🔲
    ● **S20.362**   Insect bite (nonvenomous) of left front wall of thorax 🔲
    ● **S20.369**   Insect bite (nonvenomous) of unspecified front wall of thorax 🔲
  ● **S20.37**   **Other superficial bite of front wall of thorax**
       Excludes1   open bite of front wall of thorax (S21.14)
    ● **S20.371**   Other superficial bite of right front wall of thorax 🔲
    ● **S20.372**   Other superficial bite of left front wall of thorax 🔲
    ● **S20.379**   Other superficial bite of unspecified front wall of thorax 🔲
● **S20.4**   **Other and unspecified superficial injuries of back wall of thorax**
  ● **S20.40**   **Unspecified superficial injuries of back wall of thorax**
    ● **S20.401**   Unspecified superficial injuries of right back wall of thorax 🔲
    ● **S20.402**   Unspecified superficial injuries of left back wall of thorax 🔲
    ● **S20.409**   Unspecified superficial injuries of unspecified back wall of thorax 🔲

● **S20.41**   **Abrasion of back wall of thorax**
  ● **S20.411**   Abrasion of right back wall of thorax 🔲
  ● **S20.412**   Abrasion of left back wall of thorax 🔲
  ● **S20.419**   Abrasion of unspecified back wall of thorax 🔲
● **S20.42**   **Blister (nonthermal) of back wall of thorax**
  ● **S20.421**   Blister (nonthermal) of right back wall of thorax 🔲
  ● **S20.422**   Blister (nonthermal) of left back wall of thorax 🔲
  ● **S20.429**   Blister (nonthermal) of unspecified back wall of thorax 🔲
● **S20.44**   **External constriction of back wall of thorax**
  ● **S20.441**   External constriction of right back wall of thorax 🔲
  ● **S20.442**   External constriction of left back wall of thorax 🔲
  ● **S20.449**   External constriction of unspecified back wall of thorax 🔲
● **S20.45**   **Superficial foreign body of back wall of thorax**
     Splinter of back wall of thorax
  ● **S20.451**   Superficial foreign body of right back wall of thorax 🔲
  ● **S20.452**   Superficial foreign body of left back wall of thorax 🔲
  ● **S20.459**   Superficial foreign body of unspecified back wall of thorax 🔲
● **S20.46**   **Insect bite (nonvenomous) of back wall of thorax**
  ● **S20.461**   Insect bite (nonvenomous) of right back wall of thorax 🔲
  ● **S20.462**   Insect bite (nonvenomous) of left back wall of thorax 🔲
  ● **S20.469**   Insect bite (nonvenomous) of unspecified back wall of thorax 🔲
● **S20.47**   **Other superficial bite of back wall of thorax**
     Excludes1   open bite of back wall of thorax (S21.24)
  ● **S20.471**   Other superficial bite of right back wall of thorax 🔲
  ● **S20.472**   Other superficial bite of left back wall of thorax 🔲
  ● **S20.479**   Other superficial bite of unspecified back wall of thorax 🔲
● **S20.9**   **Superficial injury of unspecified parts of thorax**
     Excludes1   contusion of thorax NOS (S20.20)
  X ● **S20.90**   Unspecified superficial injury of unspecified parts of thorax 🔲
       Superficial injury of thoracic wall NOS
  X ● **S20.91**   Abrasion of unspecified parts of thorax 🔲
  X ● **S20.92**   Blister (nonthermal) of unspecified parts of thorax 🔲
  X ● **S20.94**   External constriction of unspecified parts of thorax 🔲
  X ● **S20.95**   Superficial foreign body of unspecified parts of thorax 🔲
       Splinter in thorax NOS
  X ● **S20.96**   Insect bite (nonvenomous) of unspecified parts of thorax 🔲
  X ● **S20.97**   Other superficial bite of unspecified parts of thorax 🔲
       Excludes1   open bite of thorax NOS (S21.95)

N Newborn Age: 0   P Pediatric Age: 0–17   M Maternity DX: 12–55   A Adult Age: 15–124   ♀ Females Only   ♂ Males Only

🔲 Complication\Comorbidity   🔲 Major C\C   (Ex) CC/MCC Exclusions   🔲 Present on Admission Requirement   🔲 Hospital-Acquired Condition

CHAPTER 19 (S00-T88)

1315

Item 19–1   Pneumothorax is a collection of gas (positive air pressure) in the pleural space resulting in the lung collapsing. A tension pneumothorax is life-threatening and is a result of air in the pleural space causing a displacement in the mediastinal structures and cardiopulmonary function compromise. A traumatic pneumothorax results from blunt or penetrating injury that disrupts the parietal/visceral pleura. **Hemothorax** is blood or bloody fluid in the pleural cavity as a result of traumatic blood vessel rupture or inflammation of the lungs from pneumonia.

● **S21   Open wound of thorax**

　　Code also any associated injury such as: ◀▥
　　　　injury of heart (S26.-) ◀▥
　　　　injury of intrathoracic organs (S27.-) ◀▥
　　　　rib fracture (S22.3-, S22.4-)
　　　　spinal cord injury (S24.0-, S24.1-)
　　　　traumatic hemothorax (S27.1)
　　　　traumatic hemopneumothorax (S27.3)
　　　　traumatic pneumothorax (S27.0)
　　　　wound infection

　　Excludes1   traumatic amputation (partial) of thorax (S28.1)

　　The appropriate 7th character is to be added to each code from category S21

A	initial encounter
D	subsequent encounter
S	sequela

● **S21.0   Open wound of breast**

　● **S21.00   Unspecified open wound of breast**

　　● **S21.001   Unspecified** open wound of right breast ▨

　　● **S21.002   Unspecified** open wound of left breast ▨

　　● **S21.009   Unspecified** open wound of unspecified breast ▨

　● **S21.01   Laceration without foreign body of breast**

　　● **S21.011   Laceration without foreign body of right breast ▨**

　　● **S21.012   Laceration without foreign body of left breast ▨**

　　● **S21.019   Laceration without foreign body of unspecified breast ▨**

　● **S21.02   Laceration with foreign body of breast**

　　● **S21.021   Laceration with foreign body of right breast ▨**

　　● **S21.022   Laceration with foreign body of left breast ▨**

　　● **S21.029   Laceration with foreign body of unspecified breast ▨**

　● **S21.03   Puncture wound without foreign body of breast**

　　● **S21.031   Puncture wound without foreign body of right breast ▨**

　　● **S21.032   Puncture wound without foreign body of left breast ▨**

　　● **S21.039   Puncture wound without foreign body of unspecified breast ▨**

　● **S21.04   Puncture wound with foreign body of breast**

　　● **S21.041   Puncture wound with foreign body of right breast ▨**

　　● **S21.042   Puncture wound with foreign body of left breast ▨**

　　● **S21.049   Puncture wound with foreign body of unspecified breast ▨**

　● **S21.05   Open bite of breast**
　　　Bite of breast NOS

　　Excludes1   superficial bite of breast (S20.17)

　　● **S21.051   Open bite of right breast ▨**

　　● **S21.052   Open bite of left breast ▨**

　　● **S21.059   Open bite of unspecified breast ▨**

● **S21.1   Open wound of front wall of thorax without penetration into thoracic cavity**

　　Open wound of chest without penetration into thoracic cavity

　　Ⓔⓧ **For category S21.1 CC codes:** S21.101-S21.159[A], S21.301-S21.95X[A], S23.3XX[A], S23.8XX[A], S27.50X-S27.69X[A], S27.892A-S28.1XX[A], S29.021[A], S29.029[A], S38.3XX[A], T14.8-T14.91, T79.7XX[A], T79.8XX-T79.9XX[A], T79.A0X-T79.A9X[A]

　● **S21.10   Unspecified open wound of front wall of thorax without penetration into thoracic cavity**

　　● **S21.101   Unspecified** open wound of right front wall of thorax without penetration into thoracic cavity A ▨, ▨

　　● **S21.102   Unspecified** open wound of left front wall of thorax without penetration into thoracic cavity A ▨, ▨

　　● **S21.109   Unspecified** open wound of unspecified front wall of thorax without penetration into thoracic cavity A ▨, ▨

　● **S21.11   Laceration without foreign body of front wall of thorax without penetration into thoracic cavity**

　　● **S21.111   Laceration without foreign body of right front wall of thorax without penetration into thoracic cavity A ▨, ▨**

　　● **S21.112   Laceration without foreign body of left front wall of thorax without penetration into thoracic cavity A ▨, ▨**

　　● **S21.119   Laceration without foreign body of unspecified front wall of thorax without penetration into thoracic cavity A ▨, ▨**

　● **S21.12   Laceration with foreign body of front wall of thorax without penetration into thoracic cavity**

　　● **S21.121   Laceration with foreign body of right front wall of thorax without penetration into thoracic cavity A ▨, ▨**

　　● **S21.122   Laceration with foreign body of left front wall of thorax without penetration into thoracic cavity A ▨, ▨**

　　● **S21.129   Laceration with foreign body of unspecified front wall of thorax without penetration into thoracic cavity A ▨, ▨**

　● **S21.13   Puncture wound without foreign body of front wall of thorax without penetration into thoracic cavity**

　　● **S21.131   Puncture wound without foreign body of right front wall of thorax without penetration into thoracic cavity A ▨, ▨**

　　● **S21.132   Puncture wound without foreign body of left front wall of thorax without penetration into thoracic cavity A ▨, ▨**

　　● **S21.139   Puncture wound without foreign body of unspecified front wall of thorax without penetration into thoracic cavity A ▨, ▨**

◀ New   ◀▥ Revised   ~~deleted~~ Deleted   │Excludes 1│   │Excludes 2│   │Includes│   │Use additional│   │Code first│   │Code also│   │Unspecified│

OGCR Official Guidelines   ● Unacceptable Principal Diagnosis   X Assign placeholder X   ● Use Additional Character(s)   ▶ Manifestation Code   **Coding Clinic**

S21.14   Puncture wound with foreign body of front wall of thorax without penetration into thoracic cavity

- S21.141   Puncture wound with foreign body of right front wall of thorax without penetration into thoracic cavity A 🔾, 🔾
- S21.142   Puncture wound with foreign body of left front wall of thorax without penetration into thoracic cavity A 🔾, 🔾
- S21.149   Puncture wound with foreign body of unspecified front wall of thorax without penetration into thoracic cavity A 🔾, 🔾

S21.15   Open bite of front wall of thorax without penetration into thoracic cavity
   Bite of front wall of thorax NOS

   Excludes1   superficial bite of front wall of thorax (S20.37)

- S21.151   Open bite of right front wall of thorax without penetration into thoracic cavity A 🔾, 🔾
- S21.152   Open bite of left front wall of thorax without penetration into thoracic cavity A 🔾, 🔾
- S21.159   Open bite of unspecified front wall of thorax without penetration into thoracic cavity A 🔾, 🔾

S21.2   Open wound of back wall of thorax without penetration into thoracic cavity

- S21.20   Unspecified open wound of back wall of thorax without penetration into thoracic cavity
  - S21.201   Unspecified open wound of right back wall of thorax without penetration into thoracic cavity 🔾
  - S21.202   Unspecified open wound of left back wall of thorax without penetration into thoracic cavity 🔾
  - S21.209   Unspecified open wound of unspecified back wall of thorax without penetration into thoracic cavity 🔾

- S21.21   Laceration without foreign body of back wall of thorax without penetration into thoracic cavity
  - S21.211   Laceration without foreign body of right back wall of thorax without penetration into thoracic cavity 🔾
  - S21.212   Laceration without foreign body of left back wall of thorax without penetration into thoracic cavity 🔾
  - S21.219   Laceration without foreign body of unspecified back wall of thorax without penetration into thoracic cavity 🔾

- S21.22   Laceration with foreign body of back wall of thorax without penetration into thoracic cavity
  - S21.221   Laceration with foreign body of right back wall of thorax without penetration into thoracic cavity 🔾
  - S21.222   Laceration with foreign body of left back wall of thorax without penetration into thoracic cavity 🔾
  - S21.229   Laceration with foreign body of unspecified back wall of thorax without penetration into thoracic cavity 🔾

S21.23   Puncture wound without foreign body of back wall of thorax without penetration into thoracic cavity

- S21.231   Puncture wound without foreign body of right back wall of thorax without penetration into thoracic cavity 🔾
- S21.232   Puncture wound without foreign body of left back wall of thorax without penetration into thoracic cavity 🔾
- S21.239   Puncture wound without foreign body of unspecified back wall of thorax without penetration into thoracic cavity 🔾

S21.24   Puncture wound with foreign body of back wall of thorax without penetration into thoracic cavity

- S21.241   Puncture wound with foreign body of right back wall of thorax without penetration into thoracic cavity 🔾
- S21.242   Puncture wound with foreign body of left back wall of thorax without penetration into thoracic cavity 🔾
- S21.249   Puncture wound with foreign body of unspecified back wall of thorax without penetration into thoracic cavity 🔾

S21.25   Open bite of back wall of thorax without penetration into thoracic cavity
   Bite of back wall of thorax NOS

   Excludes1   superficial bite of back wall of thorax (S20.47)

- S21.251   Open bite of right back wall of thorax without penetration into thoracic cavity 🔾
- S21.252   Open bite of left back wall of thorax without penetration into thoracic cavity 🔾
- S21.259   Open bite of unspecified back wall of thorax without penetration into thoracic cavity 🔾

S21.3   Open wound of front wall of thorax with penetration into thoracic cavity
   Open wound of chest with penetration into thoracic cavity

   (Ex) For category S21.3 CC codes unless otherwise indicated: S21.101-S21.159[A], S21.301A-S21.95X[A], S27.50X-S27.69X[A], S27.892-S27.9XX[A], S28.1XX[A], S29.021[A], S29.029[A], S38.3XX[A], T14.8-T14.91, T79.7XX[A], T79.8XX-T79.9XX[A], T79.A0X-T79.A9X[A]

- S21.30   Unspecified open wound of front wall of thorax with penetration into thoracic cavity
  - S21.301   Unspecified open wound of right front wall of thorax with penetration into thoracic cavity A 🔾, 🔾
  - S21.302   Unspecified open wound of left front wall of thorax with penetration into thoracic cavity A 🔾, 🔾
  - S21.309   Unspecified open wound of unspecified front wall of thorax with penetration into thoracic cavity A 🔾, 🔾
      (Ex) S21.101A-S21.159[A], S21.301-S21.95X[A], S27.0XX-S27.2XX[A], S27.309[A], S27.329[A], S27.339[A], S27.409[A], S27.50X-S27.69X[A], S27.803[A], S27.892-S28.1XX[A], S29.021[A], S29.029[A], S38.3XX[A], T14.8-T14.91, T79.7XX[A], T79.8XX-T79.9XX[A], T79.A0X-T79.A9X[A]

N Newborn Age: 0   P Pediatric Age: 0–17   M Maternity DX: 12–55   A Adult Age: 15–124   ♀ Females Only   ♂ Males Only

🔾 Complication\Comorbidity   🔾 Major C\C   (Ex) CC/MCC Exclusions   🔾 Present on Admission Requirement   🔾 Hospital-Acquired Condition

1317

● **S21.31** Laceration without foreign body of front wall of thorax with penetration into thoracic cavity

  ● **S21.311** Laceration without foreign body of right front wall of thorax with penetration into thoracic cavity A

  ● **S21.312** Laceration without foreign body of left front wall of thorax with penetration into thoracic cavity A

  ● **S21.319** Laceration without foreign body of unspecified front wall of thorax with penetration into thoracic cavity A

● **S21.32** Laceration with foreign body of front wall of thorax with penetration into thoracic cavity

  ● **S21.321** Laceration with foreign body of right front wall of thorax with penetration into thoracic cavity A

  ● **S21.322** Laceration with foreign body of left front wall of thorax with penetration into thoracic cavity A

  ● **S21.329** Laceration with foreign body of unspecified front wall of thorax with penetration into thoracic cavity A

● **S21.33** Puncture wound without foreign body of front wall of thorax with penetration into thoracic cavity

  ● **S21.331** Puncture wound without foreign body of right front wall of thorax with penetration into thoracic cavity A

  ● **S21.332** Puncture wound without foreign body of left front wall of thorax with penetration into thoracic cavity A

  ● **S21.339** Puncture wound without foreign body of unspecified front wall of thorax with penetration into thoracic cavity A

● **S21.34** Puncture wound with foreign body of front wall of thorax with penetration into thoracic cavity

  ● **S21.341** Puncture wound with foreign body of right front wall of thorax with penetration into thoracic cavity A

  ● **S21.342** Puncture wound with foreign body of left front wall of thorax with penetration into thoracic cavity A

  ● **S21.349** Puncture wound with foreign body of unspecified front wall of thorax with penetration into thoracic cavity A

● **S21.35** Open bite of front wall of thorax with penetration into thoracic cavity

  Excludes1 superficial bite of front wall of thorax (S20.37)

  ● **S21.351** Open bite of right front wall of thorax with penetration into thoracic cavity A

  ● **S21.352** Open bite of left front wall of thorax with penetration into thoracic cavity A

  ● **S21.359** Open bite of unspecified front wall of thorax with penetration into thoracic cavity A

● **S21.4** Open wound of back wall of thorax with penetration into thoracic cavity

  Ex For category S21.4 CC codes: See S21.3

  ● **S21.40** Unspecified open wound of back wall of thorax with penetration into thoracic cavity

    ● **S21.401** Unspecified open wound of right back wall of thorax with penetration into thoracic cavity A

    ● **S21.402** Unspecified open wound of left back wall of thorax with penetration into thoracic cavity A

    ● **S21.409** Unspecified open wound of unspecified back wall of thorax with penetration into thoracic cavity A

  ● **S21.41** Laceration without foreign body of back wall of thorax with penetration into thoracic cavity

    ● **S21.411** Laceration without foreign body of right back wall of thorax with penetration into thoracic cavity A

    ● **S21.412** Laceration without foreign body of left back wall of thorax with penetration into thoracic cavity A

    ● **S21.419** Laceration without foreign body of unspecified back wall of thorax with penetration into thoracic cavity A

  ● **S21.42** Laceration with foreign body of back wall of thorax with penetration into thoracic cavity

    ● **S21.421** Laceration with foreign body of right back wall of thorax with penetration into thoracic cavity A

    ● **S21.422** Laceration with foreign body of left back wall of thorax with penetration into thoracic cavity A

    ● **S21.429** Laceration with foreign body of unspecified back wall of thorax with penetration into thoracic cavity A

● **S21.43** **Puncture wound without foreign body of back wall of thorax with penetration into thoracic cavity**

  ● **S21.431** Puncture wound without foreign body of right back wall of thorax with penetration into thoracic cavity A 🐾, 🐾

  ● **S21.432** Puncture wound without foreign body of left back wall of thorax with penetration into thoracic cavity A 🐾, 🐾

  ● **S21.439** Puncture wound without foreign body of unspecified back wall of thorax with penetration into thoracic cavity A 🐾, 🐾

● **S21.44** **Puncture wound with foreign body of back wall of thorax with penetration into thoracic cavity**

  ● **S21.441** Puncture wound with foreign body of right back wall of thorax with penetration into thoracic cavity A 🐾, 🐾

  ● **S21.442** Puncture wound with foreign body of left back wall of thorax with penetration into thoracic cavity A 🐾, 🐾

  ● **S21.449** Puncture wound with foreign body of unspecified back wall of thorax with penetration into thoracic cavity A 🐾, 🐾

● **S21.45** **Open bite of back wall of thorax with penetration into thoracic cavity**
    Bite of back wall of thorax NOS

    Excludes1 superficial bite of back wall of thorax (S20.47)

  ● **S21.451** Open bite of right back wall of thorax with penetration into thoracic cavity A 🐾, 🐾

  ● **S21.452** Open bite of left back wall of thorax with penetration into thoracic cavity A 🐾, 🐾

  ● **S21.459** Open bite of unspecified back wall of thorax with penetration into thoracic cavity A 🐾, 🐾

● **S21.9** **Open wound of unspecified part of thorax**
    Open wound of thoracic wall NOS
    (Ex) For category S21.9 CC codes: See S21.1

X ● **S21.90** Unspecified open wound of unspecified part of thorax A 🐾, 🐾

X ● **S21.91** Laceration without foreign body of unspecified part of thorax A 🐾, 🐾

X ● **S21.92** Laceration with foreign body of unspecified part of thorax A 🐾, 🐾

X ● **S21.93** Puncture wound without foreign body of unspecified part of thorax A 🐾, 🐾

X ● **S21.94** Puncture wound with foreign body of unspecified part of thorax A 🐾, 🐾

X ● **S21.95** Open bite of unspecified part of thorax A 🐾, 🐾
    Excludes1 superficial bite of thorax (S20.97)

● **S22** **Fracture of rib(s), sternum and thoracic spine**

  Note: A fracture not indicated as displaced or nondisplaced should be coded to displaced

    A fracture not indicated as open or closed should be coded to closed

  Includes fracture of thoracic neural arch
       fracture of thoracic spinous process
       fracture of thoracic transverse process
       fracture of thoracic vertebra
       fracture of thoracic vertebral arch

  Code first any associated:
    injury of intrathoracic organ (S27.-)
    spinal cord injury (S24.0-, S24.1-)

  Excludes1 transection of thorax (S28.1)
  Excludes2 fracture of clavicle (S42.0-)
        fracture of scapula (S42.1-)

The appropriate 7th character is to be added to each code from category S22

A	initial encounter for closed fracture
B	initial encounter for open fracture
D	subsequent encounter for fracture with routine healing
G	subsequent encounter for fracture with delayed healing
K	subsequent encounter for fracture with nonunion
S	sequela

● **S22.0** **Fracture of thoracic vertebra**
  (Ex) For category **S22.0 CC codes S22.0[A,B]:** M48.40X-M48.58X[S], M80.08X[S], M80.88X[S], M83.50[S], M84.454[S], M84.550[S], M84.58X[S], M84.650[S], M99.12, M99.15-M99.17, M99.19, S03.8XX-S03.9XX[A], S12.000-S12.9XX[S], S13.9XX[A], S14.109[A], S14.119[A], S14.129[A], S14.139[A], S14.149[A], S14.159[A], S22.000-S22.089[A,B,S], S22.20XS-S23.3XX[A], S23.8XX-S24.159[A], S29.001-S29.019[A], S29.091-S29.9XX[A], S32.000-S32.9XX[S], S32.9XX[S], S33.30X-S33.39X[A], S33.9XX[A], S38.1XX[A], S38.3XX[A], S39.001-S39.013[A], S39.091A-S39.94X[A], T14.8-T14.91, T79.8XX-T79.9XX[A], T79.A0X-T79.A9X[A] For **S22.0[K]:** M80.00X-M80.88X[K,P], M84.30X-M84.68X[K,P], S02.0XX-S02.92X[K], S12.000-S12.691[K], S22.000-S22.9XX[K], S32.000-S32.9XX[K], S42.001-S42.92X[K,P], S49.001-S49.199[K,P], S52.001-S52.92X[K,M,N,P,Q,R], S59.001-S59.299[K,P], S62.001-S62.92X[K,P], S72.001-S72.92X[K,M,N,P,Q,R]; S79.001-S79.199[K,P], S82.001-S82.92X[K,M,N,P,Q,R], S89.001-S89.399[K,P], S92.001-S92.919[K,P]

  ● **S22.00** **Fracture of unspecified thoracic vertebra**

    ● **S22.000** Wedge compression fracture of unspecified thoracic vertebra A, K 🐾, B 🐾, 🐾, A, B 🐾

    ● **S22.001** Stable burst fracture of unspecified thoracic vertebra A, K 🐾, B 🐾, 🐾, A, B 🐾

    ● **S22.002** Unstable burst fracture of unspecified thoracic vertebra A, K 🐾, B 🐾, 🐾, A, B 🐾

    ● **S22.008** Other fracture of unspecified thoracic vertebra A, K 🐾, B 🐾, 🐾, A, B 🐾

    ● **S22.009** Unspecified fracture of unspecified thoracic vertebra A, K 🐾, B 🐾, 🐾, A, B 🐾

  ● **S22.01** **Fracture of first thoracic vertebra**

    ● **S22.010** Wedge compression fracture of first thoracic vertebra A, K 🐾, B 🐾, 🐾, A, B 🐾

    ● **S22.011** Stable burst fracture of first thoracic vertebra A, K 🐾, B 🐾, 🐾, A, B 🐾

    ● **S22.012** Unstable burst fracture of first thoracic vertebra A, K 🐾, B 🐾, 🐾, A, B 🐾

    ● **S22.018** Other fracture of first thoracic vertebra A, K 🐾, B 🐾, 🐾, A, B 🐾

    ● **S22.019** Unspecified fracture of first thoracic vertebra A, K 🐾, B 🐾, 🐾, A, B 🐾

N Newborn Age: 0   **P** Pediatric Age: 0–17   **M** Maternity DX: 12–55   **A** Adult Age: 15–124   ♀ Females Only   ♂ Males Only

🐾 Complication\Comorbidity   🐾 Major C\C   (Ex) CC/MCC Exclusions   🐾 Present on Admission Requirement   🐾 Hospital-Acquired Condition

1319

● S22.02   Fracture of second thoracic vertebra
  ● S22.020   Wedge compression fracture of second thoracic vertebra A, K ▸, B ▸, ▸, A, B ▸
  ● S22.021   Stable burst fracture of second thoracic vertebra A, K ▸, B ▸, ▸, A, B ▸
  ● S22.022   Unstable burst fracture of second thoracic vertebra A, K ▸, B ▸, ▸, A, B ▸
  ● S22.028   Other fracture of second thoracic vertebra A, K ▸, B ▸, ▸, A, B ▸
  ● S22.029   Unspecified fracture of second thoracic vertebra A, K ▸, B ▸, ▸, A, B ▸

● S22.03   Fracture of third thoracic vertebra
  ● S22.030   Wedge compression fracture of third thoracic vertebra A, K ▸, B ▸, ▸, A, B ▸
  ● S22.031   Stable burst fracture of third thoracic vertebra A, K ▸, B ▸, ▸, A, B ▸
  ● S22.032   Unstable burst fracture of third thoracic vertebra A, K ▸, B ▸, ▸, A, B ▸
  ● S22.038   Other fracture of third thoracic vertebra A, K ▸, B ▸, ▸, A, B ▸
  ● S22.039   Unspecified fracture of third thoracic vertebra A, K ▸, B ▸, ▸, A, B ▸

● S22.04   Fracture of fourth thoracic vertebra
  ● S22.040   Wedge compression fracture of fourth thoracic vertebra A, K ▸, B ▸, ▸, A, B ▸
  ● S22.041   Stable burst fracture of fourth thoracic vertebra A, K ▸, B ▸, ▸, A, B ▸
  ● S22.042   Unstable burst fracture of fourth thoracic vertebra A, K ▸, B ▸, ▸, A, B ▸
  ● S22.048   Other fracture of fourth thoracic vertebra A, K ▸, B ▸, ▸, A, B ▸
  ● S22.049   Unspecified fracture of fourth thoracic vertebra A, K ▸, B ▸, ▸, A, B ▸

● S22.05   Fracture of T_5-T_6 vertebra
  ● S22.050   Wedge compression fracture of T_5-T_6 vertebra A, K ▸, B ▸, ▸, A, B ▸
  ● S22.051   Stable burst fracture of T_5-T_6 vertebra A, K ▸, B ▸, ▸, A, B ▸
  ● S22.052   Unstable burst fracture of T_5-T_6 vertebra A, K ▸, B ▸, ▸, A, B ▸
  ● S22.058   Other fracture of T_5-T_6 vertebra A, K ▸, B ▸, ▸, A, B ▸
  ● S22.059   Unspecified fracture of T_5-T_6 vertebra A, K ▸, B ▸, ▸, A, B ▸

● S22.06   Fracture of T_7-T_8 vertebra
  ● S22.060   Wedge compression fracture of T_7-T_8 vertebra A, K ▸, B ▸, ▸, A, B ▸
  ● S22.061   Stable burst fracture of T_7-T_8 vertebra A, K ▸, B ▸, ▸, A, B ▸
  ● S22.062   Unstable burst fracture of T_7-T_8 vertebra A, K ▸, B ▸, ▸, A, B ▸
  ● S22.068   Other fracture of T_7-T_8 thoracic vertebra A, K ▸, B ▸, ▸, A, B ▸
  ● S22.069   Unspecified fracture of T_7-T_8 vertebra A, K ▸, B ▸, ▸, A, B ▸

● S22.07   Fracture of T_9-T_{10} vertebra
  ● S22.070   Wedge compression fracture of T_9-T_{10} vertebra A, K ▸, B ▸, ▸, A, B ▸
  ● S22.071   Stable burst fracture of T_9-T_{10} vertebra A, K ▸, B ▸, ▸, A, B ▸
  ● S22.072   Unstable burst fracture of T_9-T_{10} vertebra A, K ▸, B ▸, ▸, A, B ▸
  ● S22.078   Other fracture of T_9-T_{10} vertebra A, K ▸, B ▸, ▸, A, B ▸
  ● S22.079   Unspecified fracture of T_9-T_{10} vertebra A, K ▸, B ▸, ▸, A, B ▸

● S22.08   Fracture of T_{11}-T_{12} vertebra
  ● S22.080   Wedge compression fracture of T_{11}-T_{12} vertebra A, K ▸, B ▸, ▸, A, B ▸
  ● S22.081   Stable burst fracture of T_{11}-T_{12} vertebra A, K ▸, B ▸, ▸, A, B ▸
  ● S22.082   Unstable burst fracture of T_{11}-T_{12} vertebra A, K ▸, B ▸, ▸, A, B ▸
  ● S22.088   Other fracture of T_{11}-T_{12} vertebra A, K ▸, B ▸, ▸, A, B ▸
  ● S22.089   Unspecified fracture of T_{11}-T_{12} vertebra A, K ▸, B ▸, ▸, A, B ▸

● S22.2   Fracture of sternum
  Ⓔ For category S22.2 CC codes S22.2[A,B]: S03.8XX-S03.9XX[A], S22.20X-
  S22.24X[A,B], S22.5XX[A,B], S29.011-S29.019[A], S38.3XX[A], S39.011-
  S39.013[A], T14.8-T14.91, T79.8XX-T79.9XX[A], T79.A0X-T79.A9X[A] For
  S22.2[K]: See S22.0[K]
  X ● S22.20   Unspecified fracture of sternum A, K ▸, B ▸, ▸, A, B ▸
  X ● S22.21   Fracture of manubrium A, K ▸, B ▸, ▸, A, B ▸
  X ● S22.22   Fracture of body of sternum A, K ▸, B ▸, ▸, A, B ▸
  X ● S22.23   Sternal manubrial dissociation A, K ▸, B ▸, ▸, A, B ▸
  X ● S22.24   Fracture of xiphoid process A, K ▸, B ▸, ▸, A, B ▸

● S22.3   Fracture of one rib
  Ⓔ For category S22.3 CC codes S22.3[A]: S03.8XX-S03.9XX[A], S22.20X-
  S22.5XX[A,B], S29.011-S29.019[A], S38.3XX[A], S39.011-S39.013[A],
  T14.8-T14.91, T79.8XX-T79.9XX[A], T79.A0X-T79.A9X[A] For S22.3[B]:
  S03.8XX-S03.9XX[A], S22.31X-S22.5XX[A,B], S29.011-S29.019[A],
  S38.3XX[A], S39.011-S39.013[A], T14.8-T14.91, T79.8XX-T79.9XX[A], T79.
  A0X-T79.A9X[A] For S22.3[K]: See S22.0[K]
  X ● S22.31   Fracture of one rib, right side A, K ▸, B ▸, ▸, A, B ▸
  X ● S22.32   Fracture of one rib, left side A, K ▸, B ▸, ▸, A, B ▸
  X ● S22.39   Fracture of one rib, unspecified side A, K ▸, B ▸, ▸, A, B ▸

● S22.4   Multiple fractures of ribs
  Fractures of two or more ribs
  Excludes1   flail chest (S22.5-)
  Ⓔ For category S22.4 CC codes S22.4[A,B]: See S22.3[B] For S22.49[B]:
  No exclusions For S22.4[K]: See S22.0[K]
  X ● S22.41   Multiple fractures of ribs, right side A, K ▸, B ▸, ▸, A, B ▸
  X ● S22.42   Multiple fractures of ribs, left side A, K ▸, B ▸, ▸, A, B ▸
  X ● S22.43   Multiple fractures of ribs, bilateral A, K ▸, B ▸, ▸, A, B ▸
  X ● S22.49   Multiple fractures of ribs, unspecified side A, K ▸, B ▸, ▸, A, B ▸

◀ New   ◀ Revised   deleted Deleted   Excludes 1   Excludes 2   Includes   Use additional   Code first   Code also   Unspecified
OGCR Official Guidelines   ● Unacceptable Principal Diagnosis   X Assign placeholder X   ● Use Additional Character(s)   ▸ Manifestation Code   Coding Clinic

X ● **S22.5**   **Flail chest** K 🖐, A, B 🖐, 🖐, A, B 🖐
Unstable chest due to sternum and/or rib fracture
Ⓔ For category S22.5 CC codes S22.5[A,B]: S03.8XX-S03.9XX[A], S22.20X-
S22.5XX[A,B], S29.011-S29.019[A], S38.3XX[A], S39.011-S39.013[A],
T14.8-T14.91, T79.8XX-T79.9XX[A], T79.A0X-T79.A9X[A] For S22.5[K]:
See S22.0[K]

X ● **S22.9**   **Fracture of bony thorax, part** unspecified **A, K** 🖐, **B** 🖐,
🖐, **A, B** 🖐
Ⓔ For category S22.9 CC codes S22.9[A,B]: M80.00X-M80.019[A],
M80.041A-M80.049[A], M80.80X-M80.819[A], M80.841-M80.849[A],
M84.40X-M84.419[A], M84.441-M84.446[A], M84.454[A], M84.474-
M84.519[A], M84.541-M84.550[A], M84.574-M84.576[A], M84.60X-
M84.619[A], M84.641-M84.650[A], M84.674-M84.68X[A], S03.8XX-
S03.9XX[A], S22.9XX-S22.9XX[A,B], S29.011A-S29.019[A], S32.301-
S32.9XX[A,B], S33.4XX[A], S33.6XX-S33.8XX[A], S38.3XX[A], S39.011-
S39.013[A], S73.001-S73.199[A], S76.001-S76.019[A], S76.091-
S76.119[A], S76.191-S76.219[A], S76.291-S76.319[A], S76.391-
S76.819[A], S76.891-S76.919[A], S76.991-S76.999[A], S79.811-
S79.929[A], T14.8-T14.91, T79.8XX-T79.9XX[A], T79.A9X[A] For S22.9[K]:
See S22.0[K]

● **S23**   **Dislocation and sprain of joints and ligaments of thorax**

> **Includes**   avulsion of joint or ligament of thorax
> laceration of cartilage, joint or ligament of thorax
> sprain of cartilage, joint or ligament of thorax
> traumatic hemarthrosis of joint or ligament of
> thorax
> traumatic rupture of joint or ligament of thorax
> traumatic subluxation of joint or ligament of
> thorax
> traumatic tear of joint or ligament of thorax

Code also any associated open wound

> **Excludes2**   dislocation, sprain of sternoclavicular joint (S43.2,
> S43.6)
> strain of muscle or tendon of thorax (S29.01-)

The appropriate 7th character is to be added to each code from
category S23

> A   initial encounter
> D   subsequent encounter
> S   sequela

X ● **S23.0**   **Traumatic rupture of thoracic intervertebral disc** 🖐

> **Excludes1**   rupture or displacement (nontraumatic)
> of thoracic intervertebral disc NOS
> (M51.- with fifth character 4)

● **S23.1**   **Subluxation and dislocation of thoracic vertebra**

> Code also any associated
> open wound of thorax (S21.-)
> spinal cord injury (S24.0-, S24.1-)

> **Excludes2**   fracture of thoracic vertebrae (S22.0-)

● **S23.10**   **Subluxation and dislocation of unspecified**
thoracic vertebra

     ● **S23.100**   Subluxation of unspecified thoracic
vertebra 🖐

     ● **S23.101**   Dislocation of unspecified thoracic
vertebra 🖐

● **S23.11**   **Subluxation and dislocation of T$_1$/T$_2$ thoracic**
vertebra

     ● **S23.110**   Subluxation of T$_1$/T$_2$ thoracic
vertebra 🖐

     ● **S23.111**   Dislocation of T$_1$/T$_2$ thoracic
vertebra 🖐

● **S23.12**   **Subluxation and dislocation of T$_2$/T$_3$-T$_3$/T$_4$**
thoracic vertebra

     ● **S23.120**   Subluxation of T$_2$/T$_3$ thoracic
vertebra 🖐

     ● **S23.121**   Dislocation of T$_2$/T$_3$ thoracic
vertebra 🖐

     ● **S23.122**   Subluxation of T$_3$/T$_4$ thoracic
vertebra 🖐

     ● **S23.123**   Dislocation of T$_3$/T$_4$ thoracic
vertebra 🖐

● **S23.13**   **Subluxation and dislocation of T$_4$/T$_5$-T$_5$/T$_6$**
thoracic vertebra

     ● **S23.130**   Subluxation of T$_4$/T$_5$ thoracic
vertebra 🖐

     ● **S23.131**   Dislocation of T$_4$/T$_5$ thoracic
vertebra 🖐

     ● **S23.132**   Subluxation of T$_5$/T$_6$ thoracic
vertebra 🖐

     ● **S23.133**   Dislocation of T$_5$/T$_6$ thoracic
vertebra 🖐

● **S23.14**   **Subluxation and dislocation of T$_6$/T$_7$-T$_7$/T$_8$**
thoracic vertebra

     ● **S23.140**   Subluxation of T$_6$/T$_7$ thoracic
vertebra 🖐

     ● **S23.141**   Dislocation of T$_6$/T$_7$ thoracic
vertebra 🖐

     ● **S23.142**   Subluxation of T$_7$/T$_8$ thoracic
vertebra 🖐

     ● **S23.143**   Dislocation of T$_7$/T$_8$ thoracic
vertebra 🖐

● **S23.15**   **Subluxation and dislocation of T$_8$/T$_9$-T$_9$/T$_{10}$**
thoracic vertebra

     ● **S23.150**   Subluxation of T$_8$/T$_9$ thoracic
vertebra 🖐

     ● **S23.151**   Dislocation of T$_8$/T$_9$ thoracic
vertebra 🖐

     ● **S23.152**   Subluxation of T$_9$/T$_{10}$ thoracic
vertebra 🖐

     ● **S23.153**   Dislocation of T$_9$/T$_{10}$ thoracic
vertebra 🖐

● **S23.16**   **Subluxation and dislocation of T$_{10}$/T$_{11}$-T$_{11}$/T$_{12}$**
thoracic vertebra

     ● **S23.160**   Subluxation of T$_{10}$/T$_{11}$ thoracic
vertebra 🖐

     ● **S23.161**   Dislocation of T$_{10}$/T$_{11}$ thoracic
vertebra 🖐

     ● **S23.162**   Subluxation of T$_{11}$/T$_{12}$ thoracic
vertebra 🖐

     ● **S23.163**   Dislocation of T$_{11}$/T$_{12}$ thoracic
vertebra 🖐

● **S23.17**   **Subluxation and dislocation of T$_{12}$/L$_1$ thoracic**
vertebra

     ● **S23.170**   Subluxation of T$_{12}$/L$_1$ thoracic
vertebra 🖐

     ● **S23.171**   Dislocation of T$_{12}$/L$_1$ thoracic
vertebra 🖐

● **S23.2**   **Dislocation of other and unspecified parts of thorax**

X ● **S23.20**   Dislocation of unspecified part of thorax 🖐

X ● **S23.29**   Dislocation of other parts of thorax 🖐

X ● **S23.3**   **Sprain of ligaments of thoracic spine** 🖐

● **S23.4**   **Sprain of ribs and sternum**

X ● **S23.41**   Sprain of ribs 🖐

● **S23.42**   Sprain of sternum

     ● **S23.420**   Sprain of sternoclavicular (joint)
(ligament) 🖐

     ● **S23.421**   Sprain of chondrosternal joint 🖐

     ● **S23.428**   Other sprain of sternum 🖐

     ● **S23.429**   Unspecified sprain of sternum 🖐

X ● **S23.8**   **Sprain of other specified parts of thorax** 🖐

X ● **S23.9**   **Sprain of** unspecified **parts of thorax** 🖐

N Newborn Age: 0   **P** Pediatric Age: 0–17   **M** Maternity DX: 12–55   **A** Adult Age: 15–124   ♀ Females Only   ♂ Males Only

🖐 Complication\Comorbidity   🖐 Major C\C   Ⓔ CC/MCC Exclusions   🖐 Present on Admission Requirement   🖐 Hospital-Acquired Condition

1321

CHAPTER 19 (S00-T88)

● **S24**   **Injury of nerves and spinal cord at thorax level**

Note: Code to highest level of thoracic spinal cord injury.

Injuries to the spinal cord (S24.0 and S24.1) refer to the cord level and not bone level injury, and can affect nerve roots at and below the level given. ◀

Code also any associated:
fracture of thoracic vertebra (S22.0-)
open wound of thorax (S21.-)
transient paralysis (R29.5)

Excludes2   injury of brachial plexus (S14.3)

The appropriate 7th character is to be added to each code from category S24

A	initial encounter
D	subsequent encounter
S	sequela

(Ex:) **For category S24 CC codes:** M48.40X-M48.58X[S], M80.08X[S], M80.88X[S], M84.350[S], M84.454[S], M84.550[S], M84.58[S], M84.650[S], M99.15-M99.17, M99.19, S12.000-S12.9XX[S], S13.9XX[A], S14.109[A], S14.119[A], S14.129[A], S14.139[A], S14.149[A], S14.159[A], S22.000-S22.9XX[S], S23.20X-S23.29X[A], S23.9XX-S24.159[A], S29.001-S29.009[A], S29.091-S29.9XX[A], S32.000-S32.9XX[S], S33.30X-S33.39X[A], S33.9XX[A], S38.1XX[A], S39.001-S39.003[A], S39.091-S39.94X[A], T14.8-T14.91, T79.8XX-T79.9XX[A], T79.A0X-T79.A9X[A]

X ● **S24.0**   **Concussion and edema of thoracic spinal cord** A 🔏, 🔏

● **S24.1**   **Other and unspecified injuries of thoracic spinal cord**

   ● **S24.10**   Unspecified injury of thoracic spinal cord

     ● **S24.101**   Unspecified injury at T_1 level of thoracic spinal cord A 🔏, 🔏, A 🔏

     ● **S24.102**   Unspecified injury at T_2-T_6 level of thoracic spinal cord A 🔏, 🔏, A 🔏

     ● **S24.103**   Unspecified injury at T_7-T_{10} level of thoracic spinal cord A 🔏, 🔏, A 🔏

     ● **S24.104**   Unspecified injury at T_{11}-T_{12} level of thoracic spinal cord A 🔏, 🔏, A 🔏

     ● **S24.109**   Unspecified injury at unspecified level of thoracic spinal cord 🔏, A 🔏
       Injury of thoracic spinal cord NOS

   ● **S24.11**   Complete lesion of thoracic spinal cord

     ● **S24.111**   Complete lesion at T_1 level of thoracic spinal cord A 🔏, 🔏, A 🔏

     ● **S24.112**   Complete lesion at T_2-T_6 level of thoracic spinal cord A 🔏, 🔏, A 🔏

     ● **S24.113**   Complete lesion at T_7-T_{10} level of thoracic spinal cord A 🔏, 🔏, A 🔏

     ● **S24.114**   Complete lesion at T_{11}-T_{12} level of thoracic spinal cord A 🔏, 🔏, A 🔏

     ● **S24.119**   Complete lesion at unspecified level of thoracic spinal cord 🔏

   ● **S24.13**   Anterior cord syndrome of thoracic spinal cord

     ● **S24.131**   Anterior cord syndrome at T_1 level of thoracic spinal cord A 🔏, 🔏, A 🔏

     ● **S24.132**   Anterior cord syndrome at T_2-T_6 level of thoracic spinal cord A 🔏, 🔏, A 🔏

     ● **S24.133**   Anterior cord syndrome at T_7-T_{10} level of thoracic spinal cord A 🔏, 🔏, A 🔏

     ● **S24.134**   Anterior cord syndrome at T_{11}-T_{12} level of thoracic spinal cord A 🔏, 🔏, A 🔏

     ● **S24.139**   Anterior cord syndrome at unspecified level of thoracic spinal cord 🔏

   ● **S24.14**   Brown-Séquard syndrome of thoracic spinal cord

     ● **S24.141**   Brown-Séquard syndrome at T_1 level of thoracic spinal cord A 🔏, 🔏

     ● **S24.142**   Brown-Séquard syndrome at T_2-T_6 level of thoracic spinal cord A 🔏

     ● **S24.143**   Brown-Séquard syndrome at T_7-T_{10} level of thoracic spinal cord A 🔏, 🔏

     ● **S24.144**   Brown-Séquard syndrome at T_{11}-T_{12} level of thoracic spinal cord A 🔏, 🔏

     ● **S24.149**   Brown-Séquard syndrome at unspecified level of thoracic spinal cord 🔏

   ● **S24.15**   Other incomplete lesions of thoracic spinal cord
     Incomplete lesion of thoracic spinal cord NOS
     Posterior cord syndrome of thoracic spinal cord

     ● **S24.151**   Other incomplete lesion at T_1 level of thoracic spinal cord A 🔏, 🔏, A 🔏

     ● **S24.152**   Other incomplete lesion at T_2-T_6 level of thoracic spinal cord A 🔏, 🔏, A 🔏

     ● **S24.153**   Other incomplete lesion at T_7-T_{10} level of thoracic spinal cord A 🔏, 🔏, A 🔏

     ● **S24.154**   Other incomplete lesion at T_{11}-T_{12} level of thoracic spinal cord A 🔏, 🔏, A 🔏

     ● **S24.159**   Other incomplete lesion at unspecified level of thoracic spinal cord 🔏

X ● **S24.2**   **Injury of nerve root of thoracic spine** 🔏

X ● **S24.3**   **Injury of peripheral nerves of thorax** 🔏

X ● **S24.4**   **Injury of thoracic sympathetic nervous system** 🔏
   Injury of cardiac plexus
   Injury of esophageal plexus
   Injury of pulmonary plexus
   Injury of stellate ganglion
   Injury of thoracic sympathetic ganglion

X ● **S24.8**   **Injury of other specified nerves of thorax** 🔏

X ● **S24.9**   **Injury of unspecified nerve of thorax** 🔏

● **S25**   **Injury of blood vessels of thorax**

The appropriate 7th character is to be added to each code from category S25

A	initial encounter
D	subsequent encounter
S	sequela

Code also any associated open wound (S21.-)

● **S25.0**   **Injury of thoracic aorta**
   Injury of aorta NOS

   (Ex:) **For category S25.0 CC codes:** S25.00XA-S25.09X[A], T14.8-T14.91, T79.8XX-T79.9XX[A], T79.A0X-T79.A9X[A]

X ● **S25.00**   Unspecified injury of thoracic aorta A 🔏, 🔏

X ● **S25.01**   Minor laceration of thoracic aorta A 🔏, 🔏
     Incomplete transection of thoracic aorta
     Laceration of thoracic aorta NOS
     Superficial laceration of thoracic aorta

X ● **S25.02**   Major laceration of thoracic aorta A 🔏, 🔏
     Complete transection of thoracic aorta
     Traumatic rupture of thoracic aorta

X ● **S25.09**   Other specified injury of thoracic aorta A 🔏, 🔏

● **S25.1**   **Injury of innominate or subclavian artery**

   (Ex:) **For category S25.1 CC codes:** S25.101-S25.199[A], T14.8-T14.91, T79.8XX-T79.9XX[A], T79.A0X-T79.A9X[A]

   ● **S25.10**   Unspecified injury of innominate or subclavian artery

     ● **S25.101**   Unspecified injury of right innominate or subclavian artery A 🔏, 🔏

     ● **S25.102**   Unspecified injury of left innominate or subclavian artery A 🔏, 🔏

     ● **S25.109**   Unspecified injury of unspecified innominate or subclavian artery A 🔏, 🔏

◀ New   ◀▒▒ Revised   ~~deleted~~ Deleted   Excludes 1   Excludes 2   Includes   Use additional   Code first   Code also   Unspecified

OGCR Official Guidelines   ● Unacceptable Principal Diagnosis   X Assign placeholder X   ● Use Additional Character(s)   ▌ Manifestation Code   **Coding Clinic**

● **S25.11**   **Minor laceration of innominate or subclavian artery**
　　Incomplete transection of innominate or subclavian artery
　　Laceration of innominate or subclavian artery NOS
　　Superficial laceration of innominate or subclavian artery

　　● **S25.111**   **Minor laceration of right innominate or subclavian artery** A 🐾, 🐾

　　● **S25.112**   **Minor laceration of left innominate or subclavian artery** A 🐾, 🐾

　　● **S25.119**   **Minor laceration of** unspecified **innominate or subclavian artery** A 🐾, 🐾

● **S25.12**   **Major laceration of innominate or subclavian artery**
　　Complete transection of innominate or subclavian artery
　　Traumatic rupture of innominate or subclavian artery

　　● **S25.121**   **Major laceration of right innominate or subclavian artery** A 🐾, 🐾

　　● **S25.122**   **Major laceration of left innominate or subclavian artery** A 🐾, 🐾

　　● **S25.129**   **Major laceration of** unspecified **innominate or subclavian artery** A 🐾, 🐾

● **S25.19**   **Other specified injury of innominate or subclavian artery**

　　● **S25.191**   **Other specified injury of right innominate or subclavian artery** A 🐾, 🐾

　　● **S25.192**   **Other specified injury of left innominate or subclavian artery** A 🐾, 🐾

　　● **S25.199**   **Other specified injury of** unspecified **innominate or subclavian artery** A 🐾, 🐾

● **S25.2**   **Injury of superior vena cava**
　　Injury of vena cava NOS
　　(Ex) **For category S25.2 CC codes:** S25.20X-S25.29X[A], T14.8-T14.91, T79.8XX-T79.9XX[A], T79.A0XA-T79.A9X[A]

X ● **S25.20**   Unspecified **injury of superior vena cava** A 🐾, 🐾

X ● **S25.21**   **Minor laceration of superior vena cava** A 🐾, 🐾
　　Incomplete transection of superior vena cava
　　Laceration of superior vena cava NOS
　　Superficial laceration of superior vena cava

X ● **S25.22**   **Major laceration of superior vena cava** A 🐾, 🐾
　　Complete transection of superior vena cava
　　Traumatic rupture of superior vena cava

X ● **S25.29**   **Other specified injury of superior vena cava** A 🐾, 🐾

● **S25.3**   **Injury of innominate or subclavian vein**
　　(Ex) **For category S25.3 CC codes:** S25.301-S25.399[A], T14.8-T14.91, T79.8XX-T79.9XX[A], T79.A0X-T79.A9X[A]

● **S25.30**   **Unspecified injury of innominate or subclavian vein**

　　● **S25.301**   Unspecified **injury of right innominate or subclavian vein** A 🐾, 🐾

　　● **S25.302**   Unspecified **injury of left innominate or subclavian vein** A 🐾, 🐾

　　● **S25.309**   Unspecified **injury of unspecified innominate or subclavian vein** A 🐾, 🐾

● **S25.31**   **Minor laceration of innominate or subclavian vein**
　　Incomplete transection of innominate or subclavian vein
　　Laceration of innominate or subclavian vein NOS
　　Superficial laceration of innominate or subclavian vein

　　● **S25.311**   **Minor laceration of right innominate or subclavian vein** A 🐾, 🐾

　　● **S25.312**   **Minor laceration of left innominate or subclavian vein** A 🐾, 🐾

　　● **S25.319**   **Minor laceration of** unspecified **innominate or subclavian vein** A 🐾, 🐾

● **S25.32**   **Major laceration of innominate or subclavian vein**
　　Complete transection of innominate or subclavian vein
　　Traumatic rupture of innominate or subclavian vein

　　● **S25.321**   **Major laceration of right innominate or subclavian vein** A 🐾, 🐾

　　● **S25.322**   **Major laceration of left innominate or subclavian vein** A 🐾, 🐾

　　● **S25.329**   **Major laceration of** unspecified **innominate or subclavian vein** A 🐾, 🐾

● **S25.39**   **Other specified injury of innominate or subclavian vein**

　　● **S25.391**   **Other specified injury of right innominate or subclavian vein** A 🐾, 🐾

　　● **S25.392**   **Other specified injury of left innominate or subclavian vein** A 🐾, 🐾

　　● **S25.399**   **Other specified injury of** unspecified **innominate or subclavian vein** A 🐾, 🐾

● **S25.4**   **Injury of pulmonary blood vessels**
　　(Ex) **For category S25.4 CC codes:** S25.401-S25.499[A], T14.8-T14.91, T79.8XX-T79.9XX[A], T79.A0X-T79.A9X[A]

● **S25.40**   **Unspecified injury of pulmonary blood vessels**

　　● **S25.401**   Unspecified **injury of right pulmonary blood vessels** A 🐾, 🐾

　　● **S25.402**   Unspecified **injury of left pulmonary blood vessels** A 🐾, 🐾

　　● **S25.409**   Unspecified **injury of unspecified pulmonary blood vessels** A 🐾, 🐾

● **S25.41**   **Minor laceration of pulmonary blood vessels**
　　Incomplete transection of pulmonary blood vessels
　　Laceration of pulmonary blood vessels NOS
　　Superficial laceration of pulmonary blood vessels

　　● **S25.411**   **Minor laceration of right pulmonary blood vessels** A 🐾, 🐾

　　● **S25.412**   **Minor laceration of left pulmonary blood vessels** A 🐾, 🐾

　　● **S25.419**   **Minor laceration of** unspecified **pulmonary blood vessels** A 🐾, 🐾

CHAPTER 19 (S00-T88)

N Newborn Age: 0   P Pediatric Age: 0–17   M Maternity DX: 12–55   A Adult Age: 15–124   ♀ Females Only   ♂ Males Only

🐾 Complication\Comorbidity   🐾 Major C\C   (Ex) CC/MCC Exclusions   🐾 Present on Admission Requirement   🐾 Hospital-Acquired Condition   **1323**

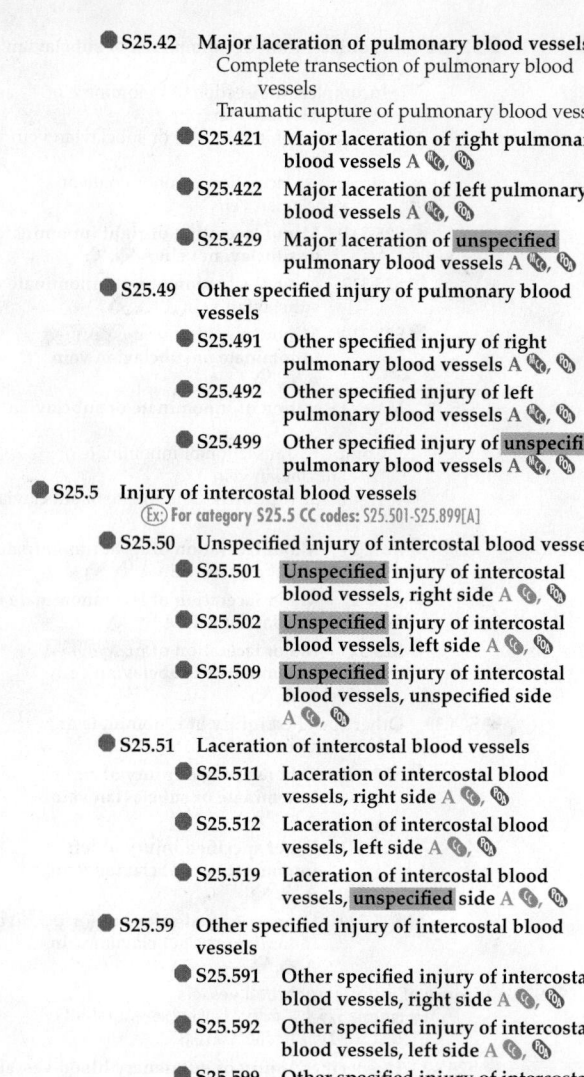

● **S25.42   Major laceration of pulmonary blood vessels**
Complete transection of pulmonary blood vessels
Traumatic rupture of pulmonary blood vessels

  ● S25.421   Major laceration of right pulmonary blood vessels A 🔖, 🔖
  ● S25.422   Major laceration of left pulmonary blood vessels A 🔖, 🔖
  ● S25.429   Major laceration of unspecified pulmonary blood vessels A 🔖, 🔖

● **S25.49   Other specified injury of pulmonary blood vessels**

  ● S25.491   Other specified injury of right pulmonary blood vessels A 🔖, 🔖
  ● S25.492   Other specified injury of left pulmonary blood vessels A 🔖, 🔖
  ● S25.499   Other specified injury of unspecified pulmonary blood vessels A 🔖, 🔖

● **S25.5   Injury of intercostal blood vessels**
Ⓔ𝕩 For category S25.5 CC codes: S25.501-S25.899[A]

  ● **S25.50   Unspecified injury of intercostal blood vessels**
    ● S25.501   Unspecified injury of intercostal blood vessels, right side A 🔖, 🔖
    ● S25.502   Unspecified injury of intercostal blood vessels, left side A 🔖, 🔖
    ● S25.509   Unspecified injury of intercostal blood vessels, unspecified side A 🔖, 🔖

  ● **S25.51   Laceration of intercostal blood vessels**
    ● S25.511   Laceration of intercostal blood vessels, right side A 🔖, 🔖
    ● S25.512   Laceration of intercostal blood vessels, left side A 🔖, 🔖
    ● S25.519   Laceration of intercostal blood vessels, unspecified side A 🔖, 🔖

  ● **S25.59   Other specified injury of intercostal blood vessels**
    ● S25.591   Other specified injury of intercostal blood vessels, right side A 🔖, 🔖
    ● S25.592   Other specified injury of intercostal blood vessels, left side A 🔖, 🔖
    ● S25.599   Other specified injury of intercostal blood vessels, unspecified side A 🔖, 🔖

● **S25.8   Injury of other blood vessels of thorax**
Injury of azygos vein
Injury of mammary artery or vein
Ⓔ𝕩 For category S25.8 CC codes: S25.00X-S25.99X[A]

  ● **S25.80   Unspecified injury of other blood vessels of thorax**
    ● S25.801   Unspecified injury of other blood vessels of thorax, right side A 🔖, 🔖
    ● S25.802   Unspecified injury of other blood vessels of thorax, left side A 🔖, 🔖
    ● S25.809   Unspecified injury of other blood vessels of thorax, unspecified side A 🔖, 🔖

  ● **S25.81   Laceration of other blood vessels of thorax**
    ● S25.811   Laceration of other blood vessels of thorax, right side A 🔖, 🔖
    ● S25.812   Laceration of other blood vessels of thorax, left side A 🔖, 🔖
    ● S25.819   Laceration of other blood vessels of thorax, unspecified side A 🔖, 🔖

● **S25.89   Other specified injury of other blood vessels of thorax**
  ● S25.891   Other specified injury of other blood vessels of thorax, right side A 🔖, 🔖
  ● S25.892   Other specified injury of other blood vessels of thorax, left side A 🔖, 🔖
  ● S25.899   Other specified injury of other blood vessels of thorax, unspecified side A 🔖, 🔖

● **S25.9   Injury of unspecified blood vessel of thorax**
Ⓔ𝕩 For category S25.9 CC codes: S25.00X-S25.99X[A]

  X ● S25.90   Unspecified injury of unspecified blood vessel of thorax A 🔖, 🔖
  X ● S25.91   Laceration of unspecified blood vessel of thorax A 🔖, 🔖
  X ● S25.99   Other specified injury of unspecified blood vessel of thorax A 🔖, 🔖

● **S26   Injury of heart**
The appropriate 7th character is to be added to each code from category S26

A	initial encounter
D	subsequent encounter
S	sequela

Code also any associated:
    open wound of thorax (S21.-)
    traumatic hemopneumothorax (S27.2)
    traumatic hemothorax (S27.1)
    traumatic pneumothorax (S27.0)

● **S26.0   Injury of heart with hemopericardium**
Hemopericardium: effusion of blood within pericardium
Ⓔ𝕩 For category S26.0 CC codes unless otherwise indicated: S21.101-S21.159[A], S21.301-S21.95X[A], S26.00X-S26.99X[A], S27.50X-S27.69X[A], S27.892-S27.9XX[A], S28.1XX[A], S29.021[A], S29.029[A], S38.3XX[A], T14.8-T14.91, T79.7XX-T79.9XX[A], T79.A0X-T79.A9X[A]

  X ● S26.00   Unspecified injury of heart with hemopericardium A 🔖, 🔖
    Ⓔ𝕩 S21.301-S21.459[A], S26.00X-S26.99X[A], S27.50X-S27.69X[A], S27.892-S27.9XX[A], T14.8-T14.91

  X ● S26.01   Contusion of heart with hemopericardium A 🔖, 🔖

  ● **S26.02   Laceration of heart with hemopericardium**
    ● S26.020   Mild laceration of heart with hemopericardium A 🔖, 🔖
        Laceration of heart without penetration of heart chamber
    ● S26.021   Moderate laceration of heart with hemopericardium A 🔖, 🔖
        Laceration of heart with penetration of heart chamber
    ● S26.022   Major laceration of heart with hemopericardium A 🔖, 🔖
        Laceration of heart with penetration of multiple heart chambers

  X ● S26.09   Other injury of heart with hemopericardium A 🔖, 🔖
        Ⓔ𝕩 See 26.00

Item 19–2 Pneumothorax is a collection of gas (positive air pressure) in the pleural space resulting in the lung collapsing. A tension pneumothorax is life-threatening and is a result of air in the pleural space causing a displacement in the mediastinal structures and cardiopulmonary function compromise. A traumatic pneumothorax results from blunt or penetrating injury that disrupts the parietal/visceral pleura. **Hemothorax** is blood or bloody fluid in the pleural cavity as a result of traumatic blood vessel rupture or inflammation of the lungs from pneumonia.

◄ New   ◄ Revised   ~~deleted~~ Deleted   Excludes 1   Excludes 2   Includes   Use additional   Code first   Code also   Unspecified
OGCR Official Guidelines   ● Unacceptable Principal Diagnosis   X Assign placeholder X   ● Use Additional Character(s)   ▌ Manifestation Code   **Coding Clinic**

● **S26.1**   **Injury of heart without hemopericardium**
Hemopericardium: effusion of blood within pericardium

X ● **S26.10**   Unspecified injury of heart without hemopericardium A 🔵, 🔵
(Ex) See S26.00

X ● **S26.11**   Contusion of heart without hemopericardium A 🔵, 🔵
(Ex) See S26.0

X ● **S26.12**   Laceration of heart without hemopericardium A 🔵, 🔵
(Ex) See S26.0

X ● **S26.19**   Other injury of heart without hemopericardium A 🔵, 🔵
(Ex) See S26.00

● **S26.9**   **Injury of heart, unspecified with or without hemopericardium**
Hemopericardium: effusion of blood within pericardium

X ● **S26.90**   Unspecified injury of heart, unspecified with or without hemopericardium A 🔵, 🔵
(Ex) See S26.00

X ● **S26.91**   Contusion of heart, unspecified with or without hemopericardium A 🔵, 🔵
(Ex) See S26.0

X ● **S26.92**   Laceration of heart, unspecified with or without hemopericardium A 🔵, 🔵
Laceration of heart NOS
(Ex) See S26.0

X ● **S26.99**   Other injury of heart, unspecified with or without hemopericardium A 🔵, 🔵
(Ex) See S26.00

● **S27**   **Injury of other and unspecified intrathoracic organs**
Code also any associated open wound of thorax (S21.-)
   Excludes2   injury of cervical esophagus (S10-S19)
                injury of trachea (cervical) (S10-S19)

The appropriate 7th character is to be added to each code from category S27

A	initial encounter
D	subsequent encounter
S	sequela

X ● **S27.0**   Traumatic pneumothorax A 🔵, 🔵
   Excludes1   spontaneous pneumothorax (J93.-)
(Ex) S21.101-S21.159[A], S21.301-S21.95X[A], S27.0XX-S27.399[A], S27.50X-S27.69X[A], S27.892-S27.9XX[A], S28.1XX[A], S29.021[A], S29.029[A], S38.3XX[A], T14.8-T14.91, T79.7XX-T79.9XX[A], T79.A0X-T79.A9X[A]

X ● **S27.1**   Traumatic hemothorax A 🔵, 🔵
(Ex) See S27.0

X ● **S27.2**   Traumatic hemopneumothorax A 🔵, 🔵
(Ex) See S27.0

X ● **S27.3**   Other and unspecified injuries of lung
(Ex) For category S27.3 CC codes unless otherwise indicated: S21.101-S21.159[A], S21.301-S21.95X[A], S27.301-S27.399[A], S27.50X-S27.69X[A], S27.892-S27.9XX[A], S28.1XX[A], S29.021[A], S29.029[A], S38.3XX[A], T14.8-T14.91, T79.7XX-T79.9XX[A], T79.A9X[A]

● **S27.30**   Unspecified injury of lung

● **S27.301**   Unspecified injury of lung, unilateral A 🔵, 🔵

● **S27.302**   Unspecified injury of lung, bilateral A 🔵, 🔵

● **S27.309**   Unspecified injury of lung, unspecified A 🔵, 🔵

● **S27.31**   Primary blast injury of lung
Blast injury of lung NOS

● **S27.311**   Primary blast injury of lung, unilateral A 🔵, 🔵

● **S27.312**   Primary blast injury of lung, bilateral A 🔵, 🔵

● **S27.319**   Primary blast injury of lung, unspecified A 🔵, 🔵

● **S27.32**   Contusion of lung

● **S27.321**   Contusion of lung, unilateral A 🔵, 🔵

● **S27.322**   Contusion of lung, bilateral A 🔵, 🔵

● **S27.329**   Contusion of lung, unspecified A 🔵, 🔵

● **S27.33**   Laceration of lung
(Ex) For category S27.33 CC codes: S21.101-S21.159[A], S21.301-S21.95X[A], S21.301-S27.399[A], S27.50X-S27.69X[A], S27.892-S27.9XX[A], S28.1XX[A], S29.021[A], S29.029[A], S38.3XX[A], T14.8-T14.91, T79.7XX-T79.9XX[A], T79.A0X-T79.A9X[A]

● **S27.331**   Laceration of lung, unilateral A 🔵, 🔵

● **S27.332**   Laceration of lung, bilateral A 🔵, 🔵

● **S27.339**   Laceration of lung, unspecified A 🔵, 🔵

● **S27.39**   Other injuries of lung
Secondary blast injury of lung

● **S27.391**   Other injuries of lung, unilateral A 🔵, 🔵

● **S27.392**   Other injuries of lung, bilateral A 🔵, 🔵

● **S27.399**   Other injuries of lung, unspecified A 🔵, 🔵

● **S27.4**   **Injury of bronchus**
(Ex) For category S27.4 CC codes: S21.101-S21.159[A], S21.301-S21.95X[A], S27.401-S27.69X[A], S27.892-S27.9XX[A], S28.1XX[A], S29.021[A], S29.029[A], S38.3XX[A], T14.8-T14.91, T79.7XX-T79.9XX[A], T79.A0X-T79.A9X[A]

● **S27.40**   Unspecified injury of bronchus

● **S27.401**   Unspecified injury of bronchus, unilateral A 🔵, 🔵

● **S27.402**   Unspecified injury of bronchus, bilateral A 🔵, 🔵

● **S27.409**   Unspecified injury of bronchus, unspecified A 🔵, 🔵

● **S27.41**   Primary blast injury of bronchus
Blast injury of bronchus NOS

● **S27.411**   Primary blast injury of bronchus, unilateral A 🔵, 🔵

● **S27.412**   Primary blast injury of bronchus, bilateral A 🔵, 🔵

● **S27.419**   Primary blast injury of bronchus, unspecified A 🔵, 🔵

● **S27.42**   Contusion of bronchus

● **S27.421**   Contusion of bronchus, unilateral A 🔵, 🔵

● **S27.422**   Contusion of bronchus, bilateral A 🔵, 🔵

● **S27.429**   Contusion of bronchus, unspecified A 🔵, 🔵

● **S27.43**   Laceration of bronchus

● **S27.431**   Laceration of bronchus, unilateral A 🔵, 🔵

● **S27.432**   Laceration of bronchus, bilateral A 🔵, 🔵

● **S27.439**   Laceration of bronchus, unspecified A 🔵, 🔵

● **S27.49**   Other injury of bronchus
Secondary blast injury of bronchus

● **S27.491**   Other injury of bronchus, unilateral A 🔵, 🔵

● **S27.492**   Other injury of bronchus, bilateral A 🔵, 🔵

● **S27.499**   Other injury of bronchus, unspecified A 🔵, 🔵

CHAPTER 19 (S00-T88)

N   Newborn Age: 0   P   Pediatric Age: 0–17   M   Maternity DX: 12–55   A   Adult Age: 15–124   ♀   Females Only   ♂   Males Only

🔵   Complication\Comorbidity   🔵   Major C\C   (Ex)   CC/MCC Exclusions   🔵   Present on Admission Requirement   🔵   Hospital-Acquired Condition

1325

● **S27.5   Injury of thoracic trachea**
    (Ex) **For category S27.5 CC codes:** S21.101-S21.159[A], S21.301A-S21.95X[A], S27.50X-S27.69X[A], S27.892-S27.9XX[A], S28.1XX[A], S29.021[A], S29.029[A], S38.3XX[A], T14.8-T14.91, T79.7XX[A], T79.8XX-T79.9XX[A], T79.A0X-T79.A9X[A]

X● **S27.50   Unspecified** injury of thoracic trachea A 🔖, 🔖

X● **S27.51   Primary blast injury of thoracic trachea** A 🔖, 🔖
      Blast injury of thoracic trachea NOS

X● **S27.52   Contusion of thoracic trachea** A 🔖, 🔖

X● **S27.53   Laceration of thoracic trachea** A 🔖, 🔖

X● **S27.59   Other injury of thoracic trachea** A 🔖, 🔖
      Secondary blast injury of thoracic trachea

● **S27.6   Injury of pleura**
    (Ex) **For category S27.6 CC codes:** See S27.5

X● **S27.60   Unspecified** injury of pleura A 🔖, 🔖

X● **S27.63   Laceration of pleura** A 🔖, 🔖

X● **S27.69   Other injury of pleura** A 🔖, 🔖

● **S27.8   Injury of other specified intrathoracic organs**

● **S27.80   Injury of diaphragm**
    (Ex) **For category S27.80 CC codes:** S21.101-S21.159[A], S21.301-S21.95X[A], S27.50X-S27.809[A], S27.892-S27.9XX[A], S28.1XX[A], S29.021[A], S29.029[A], S38.3XX[A], T14.8-T14.91, T79.7XX-T79.9XX[A], T79.A9X[A]

    ● **S27.802   Contusion of diaphragm** A 🔖, 🔖
    ● **S27.803   Laceration of diaphragm** A 🔖, 🔖
    ● **S27.808   Other injury of diaphragm** A 🔖, 🔖
    ● **S27.809   Unspecified** injury of diaphragm A 🔖, 🔖

● **S27.81   Injury of esophagus (thoracic part)**
    (Ex) **For category S27.81 CC codes:** S21.101-S21.159[A], S21.301-S21.95X[A], S27.50X-S27.69X[A], S27.812-S27.9XX[A], S28.1XX[A], S29.021[A], S29.029[A], S38.3XX[A], T14.8-T14.91, T79.7XX-T79.9XX[A], T79.A0X-T79.A9X[A]

    ● **S27.812   Contusion of esophagus (thoracic part)** A 🔖, 🔖
    ● **S27.813   Laceration of esophagus (thoracic part)** A 🔖, 🔖
    ● **S27.818   Other injury of esophagus (thoracic part)** A 🔖, 🔖
    ● **S27.819   Unspecified** injury of esophagus (thoracic part) A 🔖, 🔖

● **S27.89   Injury of other specified intrathoracic organs**
    Injury of lymphatic thoracic duct
    Injury of thymus gland
    (Ex) **For category S27.89 CC codes:** See S27.5

    ● **S27.892   Contusion of other specified intrathoracic organs** A 🔖, 🔖
    ● **S27.893   Laceration of other specified intrathoracic organs** A 🔖, 🔖
    ● **S27.898   Other injury of other specified intrathoracic organs** A 🔖, 🔖
    ● **S27.899   Unspecified** injury of other specified intrathoracic organs A 🔖, 🔖

X● **S27.9   Injury of unspecified intrathoracic organ** A 🔖, 🔖
    (Ex) S21.101-S21.159[A], S21.301-S21.95X[A], S27.50X-S27.69X[A], S27.892-S27.9XX[A], S28.1XX[A], S29.021[A], S29.029[A], S38.3XX[A], T14.8-T14.91, T79.7XX-T79.9XX[A], T79.A3X-T79.A9X[A]

● **S28   Crushing injury of thorax, and traumatic amputation of part of thorax**
    The appropriate 7th character is to be added to each code from category S28

A	initial encounter
D	subsequent encounter
S	sequela

X● **S28.0   Crushed chest** 🔖
    Use additional code for all associated injuries
    Excludes 1   flail chest (S22.5)

X● **S28.1   Traumatic amputation (partial) of part of thorax, except breast** A 🔖, 🔖
    (Ex) **For category S28.1 CC codes:** S21.101-S21.159[A], S21.301-S21.95X[A], S23.3XX[A], S23.8XX[A], S27.50X-S27.69X[A], S27.892a-S28.1XX[A], S29.021[A], S29.029[A], S38.3XX[A], T14.8-T14.91, T79.7XX[A], T79.8XX-T79.9XX[A], T79.A0X-T79.A9X[A]

● **S28.2   Traumatic amputation of breast**

    ● **S28.21   Complete traumatic amputation of breast**
      Traumatic amputation of breast NOS

      ● **S28.211   Complete traumatic amputation of right breast** 🔖
      ● **S28.212   Complete traumatic amputation of left breast** 🔖
      ● **S28.219   Complete traumatic amputation of unspecified breast** 🔖

    ● **S28.22   Partial traumatic amputation of breast**

      ● **S28.221   Partial traumatic amputation of right breast** 🔖
      ● **S28.222   Partial traumatic amputation of left breast** 🔖
      ● **S28.229   Partial traumatic amputation of unspecified breast** 🔖

● **S29   Other and unspecified injuries of thorax**
    Code also any associated open wound (S21.-)
    The appropriate 7th character is to be added to each code from category S29

A	initial encounter
D	subsequent encounter
S	sequela

● **S29.0   Injury of muscle and tendon at thorax level**

    ● **S29.00   Unspecified injury of muscle and tendon of thorax**

      ● **S29.001   Unspecified** injury of muscle and tendon of front wall of thorax 🔖
      ● **S29.002   Unspecified** injury of muscle and tendon of back wall of thorax 🔖
      ● **S29.009   Unspecified** injury of muscle and tendon of unspecified wall of thorax 🔖

    ● **S29.01   Strain of muscle and tendon of thorax**

      ● **S29.011   Strain of muscle and tendon of front wall of thorax** 🔖
      ● **S29.012   Strain of muscle and tendon of back wall of thorax** 🔖
      ● **S29.019   Strain of muscle and tendon of unspecified wall of thorax** 🔖

    ● **S29.02   Laceration of muscle and tendon of thorax**
      (Ex) **For category S29.02 CC codes:** See S28.1

      ● **S29.021   Laceration of muscle and tendon of front wall of thorax** A 🔖, 🔖
      ● **S29.022   Laceration of muscle and tendon of back wall of thorax** 🔖
      ● **S29.029   Laceration of muscle and tendon of unspecified wall of thorax** A 🔖, 🔖

◀ New   ◀═ Revised   ~~deleted~~ Deleted   Excludes 1   Excludes 2   Includes   Use additional   Code first   Code also   Unspecified

OGCR Official Guidelines   ● Unacceptable Principal Diagnosis   X Assign placeholder X   🔖 Use Additional Character(s)   ▌ Manifestation Code   **Coding Clinic**

● S29.09   Other injury of muscle and tendon of thorax
     ● S29.091   Other injury of muscle and tendon of front wall of thorax 🔟
     ● S29.092   Other injury of muscle and tendon of back wall of thorax 🔟
     ● S29.099   Other injury of muscle and tendon of unspecified wall of thorax 🔟
X ● S29.8   Other specified injuries of thorax 🔟
X ● S29.9   Unspecified injury of thorax 🔟

INJURIES TO THE ABDOMEN, LOWER BACK, LUMBAR SPINE, PELVIS AND EXTERNAL GENITALS (S30-S39)

Includes	injuries to the abdominal wall
	injuries to the anus
	injuries to the buttock
	injuries to the external genitalia
	injuries to the flank
	injuries to the groin
Excludes2	burns and corrosions (T20-T32)
	effects of foreign body in anus and rectum (T18.5)
	effects of foreign body in genitourinary tract (T19.-)
	effects of foreign body in stomach, small intestine and colon (T18.2-T18.4)
	frostbite (T33-T34)
	insect bite or sting, venomous (T63.4)

● S30   Superficial injury of abdomen, lower back, pelvis and external genitals

    Excludes2   superficial injury of hip (S70.-)

    The appropriate 7th character is to be added to each code from category S30

A	initial encounter
D	subsequent encounter
S	sequela

X ● S30.0   Contusion of lower back and pelvis 🔟
     Contusion of buttock
X ● S30.1   Contusion of abdominal wall 🔟
     Contusion of flank
     Contusion of groin
● S30.2   Contusion of external genital organs
     ● S30.20   Contusion of unspecified external genital organ
         ● S30.201   Contusion of unspecified external genital organ, male ♂ 🔟
         ● S30.202   Contusion of unspecified external genital organ, female ♀ 🔟
     X ● S30.21   Contusion of penis ♂ 🔟
     X ● S30.22   Contusion of scrotum and testes ♂ 🔟
     X ● S30.23   Contusion of vagina and vulva ♀ 🔟
X ● S30.3   Contusion of anus 🔟
● S30.8   Other superficial injuries of abdomen, lower back, pelvis and external genitals
     ● S30.81   Abrasion of abdomen, lower back, pelvis and external genitals
         ● S30.810   Abrasion of lower back and pelvis 🔟
         ● S30.811   Abrasion of abdominal wall 🔟
         ● S30.812   Abrasion of penis ♂ 🔟
         ● S30.813   Abrasion of scrotum and testes ♂ 🔟
         ● S30.814   Abrasion of vagina and vulva ♀ 🔟
         ● S30.815   Abrasion of unspecified external genital organs, male ♂ 🔟
         ● S30.816   Abrasion of unspecified external genital organs, female ♀ 🔟
         ● S30.817   Abrasion of anus 🔟
     ● S30.82   Blister (nonthermal) of abdomen, lower back, pelvis and external genitals
         ● S30.820   Blister (nonthermal) of lower back and pelvis 🔟
         ● S30.821   Blister (nonthermal) of abdominal wall 🔟

● S30.822   Blister (nonthermal) of penis ♂ 🔟
● S30.823   Blister (nonthermal) of scrotum and testes ♂ 🔟
● S30.824   Blister (nonthermal) of vagina and vulva ♀ 🔟
● S30.825   Blister (nonthermal) of unspecified external genital organs, male ♂ 🔟
● S30.826   Blister (nonthermal) of unspecified external genital organs, female ♀ 🔟
● S30.827   Blister (nonthermal) of anus 🔟
● S30.84   External constriction of abdomen, lower back, pelvis and external genitals
     ● S30.840   External constriction of lower back and pelvis 🔟
     ● S30.841   External constriction of abdominal wall 🔟
     ● S30.842   External constriction of penis ♂ 🔟
         Hair tourniquet syndrome of penis
         Use additional cause code to identify the constricting item (W49.0-)
     ● S30.843   External constriction of scrotum and testes ♂ 🔟
     ● S30.844   External constriction of vagina and vulva ♀ 🔟
     ● S30.845   External constriction of unspecified external genital organs, male ♂ 🔟
     ● S30.846   External constriction of unspecified external genital organs, female ♀ 🔟
● S30.85   Superficial foreign body of abdomen, lower back, pelvis and external genitals
     Splinter in the abdomen, lower back, pelvis and external genitals
     ● S30.850   Superficial foreign body of lower back and pelvis 🔟
     ● S30.851   Superficial foreign body of abdominal wall 🔟
     ● S30.852   Superficial foreign body of penis ♂ 🔟
     ● S30.853   Superficial foreign body of scrotum and testes ♂ 🔟
     ● S30.854   Superficial foreign body of vagina and vulva ♀ 🔟
     ● S30.855   Superficial foreign body of unspecified external genital organs, male ♂ 🔟
     ● S30.856   Superficial foreign body of unspecified external genital organs, female ♀ 🔟
     ● S30.857   Superficial foreign body of anus 🔟
● S30.86   Insect bite (nonvenomous) of abdomen, lower back, pelvis and external genitals
     ● S30.860   Insect bite (nonvenomous) of lower back and pelvis 🔟
     ● S30.861   Insect bite (nonvenomous) of abdominal wall 🔟
     ● S30.862   Insect bite (nonvenomous) of penis ♂ 🔟
     ● S30.863   Insect bite (nonvenomous) of scrotum and testes ♂ 🔟
     ● S30.864   Insect bite (nonvenomous) of vagina and vulva ♀ 🔟
     ● S30.865   Insect bite (nonvenomous) of unspecified external genital organs, male ♂ 🔟
     ● S30.866   Insect bite (nonvenomous) of unspecified external genital organs, female ♀ 🔟
     ● S30.867   Insect bite (nonvenomous) of anus 🔟

CHAPTER 19 (S00-T88)

N Newborn Age: 0   **P** Pediatric Age: 0–17   **M** Maternity DX: 12–55   **A** Adult Age: 15–124   ♀ Females Only   ♂ Males Only

🔟 Complication\Comorbidity   🔟 Major C\C   (Ex) CC/MCC Exclusions   🔟 Present on Admission Requirement   🔟 Hospital-Acquired Condition

1327

● S30.87   Other superficial bite of abdomen, lower back, pelvis and external genitals

> **Excludes1**   open bite of abdomen, lower back, pelvis and external genitals (S31.05, S31.15, S31.25, S31.35, S31.45, S31.55)

● S30.870   Other superficial bite of lower back and pelvis 🐾

● S30.871   Other superficial bite of abdominal wall 🐾

● S30.872   Other superficial bite of penis ♂ 🐾

● S30.873   Other superficial bite of scrotum and testes ♂ 🐾

● S30.874   Other superficial bite of vagina and vulva ♀ 🐾

● S30.875   Other superficial bite of unspecified external genital organs, male ♂ 🐾

● S30.876   Other superficial bite of unspecified external genital organs, female ♀ 🐾

● S30.877   Other superficial bite of anus 🐾

● S30.9   Unspecified superficial injury of abdomen, lower back, pelvis and external genitals

X ● S30.91   Unspecified superficial injury of lower back and pelvis 🐾

X ● S30.92   Unspecified superficial injury of abdominal wall 🐾

X ● S30.93   Unspecified superficial injury of penis ♂ 🐾

X ● S30.94   Unspecified superficial injury of scrotum and testes ♂ 🐾

X ● S30.95   Unspecified superficial injury of vagina and vulva ♀ 🐾

X ● S30.96   Unspecified superficial injury of unspecified external genital organs, male ♂ 🐾

X ● S30.97   Unspecified superficial injury of unspecified external genital organs, female ♀ 🐾

X ● S30.98   Unspecified superficial injury of anus 🐾

● S31   Open wound of abdomen, lower back, pelvis and external genitals

Code also any associated:
spinal cord injury (S24.0, S24.1-, S34.0-, S34.1-)
wound infection

> **Excludes1**   traumatic amputation of part of abdomen, lower back and pelvis (S38.2-, S38.3)

> **Excludes2**   open wound of hip (S71.00-S71.02)
> open fracture of pelvis (S32.1--S32.9 with 7th character B)

The appropriate 7th character is to be added to each code from category S31

A	initial encounter
D	subsequent encounter
S	sequela

● S31.0   Open wound of lower back and pelvis

(Ex:) For category S31.0 CC codes: S31.001[A], S31.011[A], S31.021[A], S31.031[A], S31.041[A], S31.051[A], S31.100-S31.159[A], S31.600-S31.659[A], S31.831-S31.839[A], S36.81X-S36.99X[A], S38.3XX[A], S39.021-S39.023[A], T14.8-T14.91, T79.8XX-T79.9XX[A], T79.A0X-T79.A9X[A]

● S31.00   Unspecified open wound of lower back and pelvis

● S31.000   Unspecified open wound of lower back and pelvis without penetration into retroperitoneum 🐾
Unspecified open wound of lower back and pelvis NOS

● S31.001   Unspecified open wound of lower back and pelvis with penetration into retroperitoneum A 🐾, 🐾

● S31.01   Laceration without foreign body of lower back and pelvis

● S31.010   Laceration without foreign body of lower back and pelvis without penetration into retroperitoneum 🐾
Laceration without foreign body of lower back and pelvis NOS

● S31.011   Laceration without foreign body of lower back and pelvis with penetration into retroperitoneum A 🐾, 🐾

● S31.02   Laceration with foreign body of lower back and pelvis

● S31.020   Laceration with foreign body of lower back and pelvis without penetration into retroperitoneum 🐾
Laceration with foreign body of lower back and pelvis NOS

● S31.021   Laceration with foreign body of lower back and pelvis with penetration into retroperitoneum A 🐾, 🐾

● S31.03   Puncture wound without foreign body of lower back and pelvis

● S31.030   Puncture wound without foreign body of lower back and pelvis without penetration into retroperitoneum 🐾
Puncture wound without foreign body of lower back and pelvis NOS

● S31.031   Puncture wound without foreign body of lower back and pelvis with penetration into retroperitoneum A 🐾, 🐾

● S31.04   Puncture wound with foreign body of lower back and pelvis

● S31.040   Puncture wound with foreign body of lower back and pelvis without penetration into retroperitoneum 🐾
Puncture wound with foreign body of lower back and pelvis NOS

● S31.041   Puncture wound with foreign body of lower back and pelvis with penetration into retroperitoneum A 🐾, 🐾

● S31.05   Open bite of lower back and pelvis
Bite of lower back and pelvis NOS

> **Excludes1**   superficial bite of lower back and pelvis (S30.860, S30.870)

● S31.050   Open bite of lower back and pelvis without penetration into retroperitoneum 🐾
Open bite of lower back and pelvis NOS

● S31.051   Open bite of lower back and pelvis with penetration into retroperitoneum A 🐾, 🐾

● S31.1   Open wound of abdominal wall without penetration into peritoneal cavity
Open wound of abdominal wall NOS

> **Excludes2**   open wound of abdominal wall with penetration into peritoneal cavity (S31.6-)

● S31.10   Unspecified open wound of abdominal wall without penetration into peritoneal cavity

● S31.100   Unspecified open wound of abdominal wall, right upper quadrant without penetration into peritoneal cavity 🐾

● S31.101   Unspecified open wound of abdominal wall, left upper quadrant without penetration into peritoneal cavity 🐾

◀ New   ◀⋯ Revised   deleted Deleted   Excludes 1   Excludes 2   Includes   Use additional   Code first   Code also   Unspecified

OGCR Official Guidelines   ● Unacceptable Principal Diagnosis   X Assign placeholder X   ● Use Additional Character(s)   ▶ Manifestation Code   Coding Clinic

● S31.102   Unspecified open wound of
             abdominal wall, epigastric region
             without penetration into peritoneal
             cavity 🔖

● S31.103   Unspecified open wound of
             abdominal wall, right lower quadrant
             without penetration into peritoneal
             cavity 🔖

● S31.104   Unspecified open wound of
             abdominal wall, left lower quadrant
             without penetration into peritoneal
             cavity 🔖

● S31.105   Unspecified open wound of
             abdominal wall, periumbilic region
             without penetration into peritoneal
             cavity 🔖

● S31.109   Unspecified open wound of
             abdominal wall, unspecified quadrant
             without penetration into peritoneal
             cavity 🔖
                 Unspecified open wound of
                 abdominal wall NOS

● S31.11 Laceration without foreign body of abdominal
          wall without penetration into peritoneal cavity

● S31.110   Laceration without foreign body of
             abdominal wall, right upper quadrant
             without penetration into peritoneal
             cavity 🔖

● S31.111   Laceration without foreign body of
             abdominal wall, left upper quadrant
             without penetration into peritoneal
             cavity 🔖

● S31.112   Laceration without foreign body of
             abdominal wall, epigastric region
             without penetration into peritoneal
             cavity 🔖

● S31.113   Laceration without foreign body of
             abdominal wall, right lower quadrant
             without penetration into peritoneal
             cavity 🔖

● S31.114   Laceration without foreign body of
             abdominal wall, left lower quadrant
             without penetration into peritoneal
             cavity 🔖

● S31.115   Laceration without foreign body of
             abdominal wall, periumbilic region
             without penetration into peritoneal
             cavity 🔖

● S31.119   Laceration without foreign body of
             abdominal wall, unspecified quadrant
             without penetration into peritoneal
             cavity 🔖

● S31.12 Laceration with foreign body of abdominal
          wall without penetration into peritoneal cavity

● S31.120   Laceration of abdominal wall with
             foreign body, right upper quadrant
             without penetration into peritoneal
             cavity 🔖

● S31.121   Laceration of abdominal wall with
             foreign body, left upper quadrant
             without penetration into peritoneal
             cavity 🔖

● S31.122   Laceration of abdominal wall with
             foreign body, epigastric region
             without penetration into peritoneal
             cavity 🔖

● S31.123   Laceration of abdominal wall with
             foreign body, right lower quadrant
             without penetration into peritoneal
             cavity 🔖

● S31.124   Laceration of abdominal wall with
             foreign body, left lower quadrant
             without penetration into peritoneal
             cavity 🔖

● S31.125   Laceration of abdominal wall with
             foreign body, periumbilic region
             without penetration into peritoneal
             cavity 🔖

● S31.129   Laceration of abdominal wall with
             foreign body, unspecified quadrant
             without penetration into peritoneal
             cavity 🔖

● S31.13 Puncture wound of abdominal wall without
          foreign body without penetration into
          peritoneal cavity

● S31.130   Puncture wound of abdominal wall
             without foreign body, right upper
             quadrant without penetration into
             peritoneal cavity 🔖

● S31.131   Puncture wound of abdominal wall
             without foreign body, left upper
             quadrant without penetration into
             peritoneal cavity 🔖

● S31.132   Puncture wound of abdominal wall
             without foreign body, epigastric
             region without penetration into
             peritoneal cavity 🔖

● S31.133   Puncture wound of abdominal wall
             without foreign body, right lower
             quadrant without penetration into
             peritoneal cavity 🔖

● S31.134   Puncture wound of abdominal wall
             without foreign body, left lower
             quadrant without penetration into
             peritoneal cavity 🔖

● S31.135   Puncture wound of abdominal wall
             without foreign body, periumbilic
             region without penetration into
             peritoneal cavity 🔖

● S31.139   Puncture wound of abdominal wall
             without foreign body, unspecified
             quadrant without penetration into
             peritoneal cavity 🔖

● S31.14 Puncture wound of abdominal wall with
          foreign body without penetration into
          peritoneal cavity

● S31.140   Puncture wound of abdominal wall
             with foreign body, right upper
             quadrant without penetration into
             peritoneal cavity 🔖

● S31.141   Puncture wound of abdominal wall
             with foreign body, left upper
             quadrant without penetration into
             peritoneal cavity 🔖

● S31.142   Puncture wound of abdominal wall
             with foreign body, epigastric region
             without penetration into peritoneal
             cavity 🔖

● S31.143   Puncture wound of abdominal wall
             with foreign body, right lower
             quadrant without penetration into
             peritoneal cavity 🔖

● S31.144   Puncture wound of abdominal wall
             with foreign body, left lower
             quadrant without penetration into
             peritoneal cavity 🔖

● S31.145   Puncture wound of abdominal wall
             with foreign body, periumbilic region
             without penetration into peritoneal
             cavity 🔖

● S31.149   Puncture wound of abdominal wall
             with foreign body, unspecified
             quadrant without penetration into
             peritoneal cavity 🔖

N Newborn Age: 0   P Pediatric Age: 0–17   M Maternity DX: 12–55   A Adult Age: 15–124   ♀ Females Only   ♂ Males Only

🔖 Complication\Comorbidity   🔖 Major C\C   (Ex) CC/MCC Exclusions   🔖 Present on Admission Requirement   🔖 Hospital-Acquired Condition

1329

● S31.15 **Open bite of abdominal wall without penetration into peritoneal cavity**
Bite of abdominal wall NOS

> **Excludes1** superficial bite of abdominal wall (S30.871)

● S31.150 **Open bite of abdominal wall, right upper quadrant without penetration into peritoneal cavity** 🖐

● S31.151 **Open bite of abdominal wall, left upper quadrant without penetration into peritoneal cavity** 🖐

● S31.152 **Open bite of abdominal wall, epigastric region without penetration into peritoneal cavity** 🖐

● S31.153 **Open bite of abdominal wall, right lower quadrant without penetration into peritoneal cavity** 🖐

● S31.154 **Open bite of abdominal wall, left lower quadrant without penetration into peritoneal cavity** 🖐

● S31.155 **Open bite of abdominal wall, periumbilic region without penetration into peritoneal cavity** 🖐

● S31.159 **Open bite of abdominal wall, unspecified quadrant without penetration into peritoneal cavity** 🖐

● S31.2 **Open wound of penis**

X● S31.20 Unspecified **open wound of penis** ♂ 🖐

X● S31.21 **Laceration without foreign body of penis** ♂ 🖐

X● S31.22 **Laceration with foreign body of penis** ♂ 🖐

X● S31.23 **Puncture wound without foreign body of penis** ♂ 🖐

X● S31.24 **Puncture wound with foreign body of penis** ♂ 🖐

X● S31.25 **Open bite of penis** ♂ 🖐
Bite of penis NOS

> **Excludes1** superficial bite of penis (S30.862, S30.872)

● S31.3 **Open wound of scrotum and testes**

X● S31.30 Unspecified **open wound of scrotum and testes** ♂ 🖐

X● S31.31 **Laceration without foreign body of scrotum and testes** ♂ 🖐

X● S31.32 **Laceration with foreign body of scrotum and testes** ♂ 🖐

X● S31.33 **Puncture wound without foreign body of scrotum and testes** ♂ 🖐

X● S31.34 **Puncture wound with foreign body of scrotum and testes** ♂ 🖐

X● S31.35 **Open bite of scrotum and testes** ♂ 🖐
Bite of scrotum and testes NOS

> **Excludes1** superficial bite of scrotum and testes (S30.863, S30.873)

● S31.4 **Open wound of vagina and vulva**

> **Excludes1** injury to vagina and vulva during delivery (O70.-, O71.4)

X● S31.40 Unspecified **open wound of vagina and vulva** ♀ 🖐

X● S31.41 **Laceration without foreign body of vagina and vulva** ♀ 🖐

X● S31.42 **Laceration with foreign body of vagina and vulva** ♀ 🖐

X● S31.43 **Puncture wound without foreign body of vagina and vulva** ♀ 🖐

X● S31.44 **Puncture wound with foreign body of vagina and vulva** ♀ 🖐

X● S31.45 **Open bite of vagina and vulva** ♀ 🖐
Bite of vagina and vulva NOS

> **Excludes1** superficial bite of vagina and vulva (S30.864, S30.874)

● S31.5 **Open wound of unspecified external genital organs**

> **Excludes1** traumatic amputation of external genital organs (S38.21, S38.22)

● S31.50 **Unspecified open wound of unspecified external genital organs**

● S31.501 Unspecified **open wound of unspecified external genital organs, male** ♂ 🖐

● S31.502 Unspecified **open wound of unspecified external genital organs, female** ♀ 🖐

● S31.51 **Laceration without foreign body of unspecified external genital organs**

● S31.511 **Laceration without foreign body of** unspecified **external genital organs, male** ♂ 🖐

● S31.512 **Laceration without foreign body of** unspecified **external genital organs, female** ♀ 🖐

● S31.52 **Laceration with foreign body of unspecified external genital organs**

● S31.521 **Laceration with foreign body of** unspecified **external genital organs, male** ♂ 🖐

● S31.522 **Laceration with foreign body of** unspecified **external genital organs, female** ♀ 🖐

● S31.53 **Puncture wound without foreign body of unspecified external genital organs**

● S31.531 **Puncture wound without foreign body of** unspecified **external genital organs, male** ♂ 🖐

● S31.532 **Puncture wound without foreign body of** unspecified **external genital organs, female** ♀ 🖐

● S31.54 **Puncture wound with foreign body of unspecified external genital organs**

● S31.541 **Puncture wound with foreign body of** unspecified **external genital organs, male** ♂ 🖐

● S31.542 **Puncture wound with foreign body of** unspecified **external genital organs, female** ♀ 🖐

● S31.55 **Open bite of unspecified external genital organs**
Bite of unspecified external genital organs NOS

> **Excludes1** superficial bite of unspecified external genital organs (S30.865, S30.866, S30.875, S30.876)

● S31.551 **Open bite of** unspecified **external genital organs, male** ♂ 🖐

● S31.552 **Open bite of** unspecified **external genital organs, female** ♀ 🖐

● S31.6 **Open wound of abdominal wall with penetration into peritoneal cavity**
(Ex) For category **S31.6 CC codes:** S31.001[A], S31.011[A], S31.021[A], S31.031[A], S31.041[A], S31.051[A], S31.100-S31.159[A], S31.600-S31.659[A], S31.831-S31.839[A], S36.81X-S36.99X[A], S38.3XX[A], S39.021-S39.023[A], T14.8-T14.91, T79.8XX-T79.9XX[A], T79.A0X-T79.A9X[A]

● S31.60 **Unspecified open wound of abdominal wall with penetration into peritoneal cavity**

● S31.600 Unspecified **open wound of abdominal wall, right upper quadrant with penetration into peritoneal cavity** A 🖐, 🖐

● S31.601 Unspecified **open wound of abdominal wall, left upper quadrant with penetration into peritoneal cavity** A 🖐, 🖐

● S31.602   Unspecified open wound of abdominal wall, epigastric region with penetration into peritoneal cavity A 🦠, 🦠

● S31.603   Unspecified open wound of abdominal wall, right lower quadrant with penetration into peritoneal cavity A 🦠, 🦠

● S31.604   Unspecified open wound of abdominal wall, left lower quadrant with penetration into peritoneal cavity A 🦠, 🦠

● S31.605   Unspecified open wound of abdominal wall, periumbilic region with penetration into peritoneal cavity A 🦠, 🦠

● S31.609   Unspecified open wound of abdominal wall, unspecified quadrant with penetration into peritoneal cavity A 🦠, 🦠

● S31.61   Laceration without foreign body of abdominal wall with penetration into peritoneal cavity

● S31.610   Laceration without foreign body of abdominal wall, right upper quadrant with penetration into peritoneal cavity A 🦠, 🦠

● S31.611   Laceration without foreign body of abdominal wall, left upper quadrant with penetration into peritoneal cavity A 🦠, 🦠

● S31.612   Laceration without foreign body of abdominal wall, epigastric region with penetration into peritoneal cavity A 🦠, 🦠

● S31.613   Laceration without foreign body of abdominal wall, right lower quadrant with penetration into peritoneal cavity A 🦠, 🦠

● S31.614   Laceration without foreign body of abdominal wall, left lower quadrant with penetration into peritoneal cavity A 🦠, 🦠

● S31.615   Laceration without foreign body of abdominal wall, periumbilic region with penetration into peritoneal cavity A 🦠, 🦠

● S31.619   Laceration without foreign body of abdominal wall, unspecified quadrant with penetration into peritoneal cavity A 🦠, 🦠

● S31.62   Laceration with foreign body of abdominal wall with penetration into peritoneal cavity

● S31.620   Laceration with foreign body of abdominal wall, right upper quadrant with penetration into peritoneal cavity A 🦠, 🦠

● S31.621   Laceration with foreign body of abdominal wall, left upper quadrant with penetration into peritoneal cavity A 🦠, 🦠

● S31.622   Laceration with foreign body of abdominal wall, epigastric region with penetration into peritoneal cavity A 🦠, 🦠

● S31.623   Laceration with foreign body of abdominal wall, right lower quadrant with penetration into peritoneal cavity A 🦠, 🦠

● S31.624   Laceration with foreign body of abdominal wall, left lower quadrant with penetration into peritoneal cavity A 🦠, 🦠

● S31.625   Laceration with foreign body of abdominal wall, periumbilic region with penetration into peritoneal cavity A 🦠, 🦠

● S31.629   Laceration with foreign body of abdominal wall, unspecified quadrant with penetration into peritoneal cavity A 🦠, 🦠

● S31.63   Puncture wound without foreign body of abdominal wall with penetration into peritoneal cavity

● S31.630   Puncture wound without foreign body of abdominal wall, right upper quadrant with penetration into peritoneal cavity A 🦠, 🦠

● S31.631   Puncture wound without foreign body of abdominal wall, left upper quadrant with penetration into peritoneal cavity A 🦠, 🦠

● S31.632   Puncture wound without foreign body of abdominal wall, epigastric region with penetration into peritoneal cavity A 🦠, 🦠

● S31.633   Puncture wound without foreign body of abdominal wall, right lower quadrant with penetration into peritoneal cavity A 🦠, 🦠

● S31.634   Puncture wound without foreign body of abdominal wall, left lower quadrant with penetration into peritoneal cavity A 🦠, 🦠

● S31.635   Puncture wound without foreign body of abdominal wall, periumbilic region with penetration into peritoneal cavity A 🦠, 🦠

● S31.639   Puncture wound without foreign body of abdominal wall, unspecified quadrant with penetration into peritoneal cavity A 🦠, 🦠

● S31.64   Puncture wound with foreign body of abdominal wall with penetration into peritoneal cavity

● S31.640   Puncture wound with foreign body of abdominal wall, right upper quadrant with penetration into peritoneal cavity A 🦠, 🦠

● S31.641   Puncture wound with foreign body of abdominal wall, left upper quadrant with penetration into peritoneal cavity A 🦠, 🦠

● S31.642   Puncture wound with foreign body of abdominal wall, epigastric region with penetration into peritoneal cavity A 🦠, 🦠

● S31.643   Puncture wound with foreign body of abdominal wall, right lower quadrant with penetration into peritoneal cavity A 🦠, 🦠

● S31.644   Puncture wound with foreign body of abdominal wall, left lower quadrant with penetration into peritoneal cavity A 🦠, 🦠

● S31.645   Puncture wound with foreign body of abdominal wall, periumbilic region with penetration into peritoneal cavity A 🦠, 🦠

● S31.649   Puncture wound with foreign body of abdominal wall, unspecified quadrant with penetration into peritoneal cavity A 🦠, 🦠

N   Newborn Age: 0   P   Pediatric Age: 0–17   M   Maternity DX: 12–55   A   Adult Age: 15–124   ♀   Females Only   ♂   Males Only

🦠   Complication\Comorbidity   🦠   Major C\C   (Ex)   CC/MCC Exclusions   🦠   Present on Admission Requirement   🦠   Hospital-Acquired Condition

1331

● S31.65   **Open bite of abdominal wall with penetration into peritoneal cavity**

> **Excludes1**   superficial bite of abdominal wall (S30.861, S30.871)

  ● S31.650   **Open bite of abdominal wall, right upper quadrant with penetration into peritoneal cavity** A 🖐, 🖐

  ● S31.651   **Open bite of abdominal wall, left upper quadrant with penetration into peritoneal cavity** A 🖐, 🖐

  ● S31.652   **Open bite of abdominal wall, epigastric region with penetration into peritoneal cavity** A 🖐, 🖐

  ● S31.653   **Open bite of abdominal wall, right lower quadrant with penetration into peritoneal cavity** A 🖐, 🖐

  ● S31.654   **Open bite of abdominal wall, left lower quadrant with penetration into peritoneal cavity** A 🖐, 🖐

  ● S31.655   **Open bite of abdominal wall, periumbilic region with penetration into peritoneal cavity** A 🖐, 🖐

  ● S31.659   **Open bite of abdominal wall, unspecified quadrant with penetration into peritoneal cavity** A 🖐, 🖐

● S31.8   **Open wound of other parts of abdomen, lower back and pelvis**

 ● S31.80   **Open wound of unspecified buttock**

  ● S31.801   **Laceration without foreign body of unspecified buttock** 🖐

  ● S31.802   **Laceration with foreign body of unspecified buttock** 🖐

  ● S31.803   **Puncture wound without foreign body of unspecified buttock** 🖐

  ● S31.804   **Puncture wound with foreign body of unspecified buttock** 🖐

  ● S31.805   **Open bite of unspecified buttock** 🖐
Bite of buttock NOS

> **Excludes1**   superficial bite of buttock (S30.870)

  ● S31.809   **Unspecified open wound of unspecified buttock** 🖐

 ● S31.81   **Open wound of right buttock**

  ● S31.811   **Laceration without foreign body of right buttock** 🖐

  ● S31.812   **Laceration with foreign body of right buttock** 🖐

  ● S31.813   **Puncture wound without foreign body of right buttock** 🖐

  ● S31.814   **Puncture wound with foreign body of right buttock** 🖐

  ● S31.815   **Open bite of right buttock** 🖐
Bite of right buttock NOS

> **Excludes1**   superficial bite of buttock (S30.870)

  ● S31.819   **Unspecified open wound of right buttock** 🖐

 ● S31.82   **Open wound of left buttock**

  ● S31.821   **Laceration without foreign body of left buttock** 🖐

  ● S31.822   **Laceration with foreign body of left buttock** 🖐

  ● S31.823   **Puncture wound without foreign body of left buttock** 🖐

  ● S31.824   **Puncture wound with foreign body of left buttock** 🖐

  ● S31.825   **Open bite of left buttock** 🖐
Bite of left buttock NOS

> **Excludes1**   superficial bite of buttock (S30.870)

  ● S31.829   **Unspecified open wound of left buttock** 🖐

 ● S31.83   **Open wound of anus**

  ● S31.831   **Laceration without foreign body of anus** 🖐

  ● S31.832   **Laceration with foreign body of anus** 🖐

  ● S31.833   **Puncture wound without foreign body of anus** 🖐

  ● S31.834   **Puncture wound with foreign body of anus** 🖐

  ● S31.835   **Open bite of anus** 🖐
Bite of anus NOS

> **Excludes1**   superficial bite of anus (S30.877)

  ● S31.839   **Unspecified open wound of anus** 🖐

● S32   **Fracture of lumbar spine and pelvis**

Note: A fracture not indicated as displaced or nondisplaced should be coded to displaced

A fracture not indicated as opened or closed should be coded to closed

> **Includes**   fracture of lumbosacral neural arch
> fracture of lumbosacral spinous process
> fracture of lumbosacral transverse process
> fracture of lumbosacral vertebra
> fracture of lumbosacral vertebral arch

Code first any associated spinal cord and spinal nerve injury (S34.-) ◄▦

> **Excludes1**   transection of abdomen (S38.3)
> **Excludes2**   fracture of hip NOS (S72.0-)

The appropriate 7th character is to be added to each code from category S32

A	initial encounter for closed fracture
B	initial encounter for open fracture
D	subsequent encounter for fracture with routine healing
G	subsequent encounter for fracture with delayed healing
K	subsequent encounter for fracture with nonunion
S	sequela

● S32.0   **Fracture of lumbar vertebra**
Fracture of lumbar spine NOS

(Ex) **For category S32.0 CC codes S32.0[A,B]:** M48.40X-M48.58X[S], M80.08X[S], M80.88X[S], M84.350[S], M84.454[S], M84.550[S], M84.58X[S], M84.650[S], M99.13, M99.15-M99.17, M99.19, S03.8XX-S03.9XX[A], S12.000-S12.9XX[S], S13.9XX[A], S14.109[A], S14.119[A], S14.129[A], S14.139[A], S14.149[A], S14.159[A], S22.000-S22.9XX[S], S23.20X-S23.29X[A], S23.9XX[A], S24.109[A], S24.119[A], S24.139[A], S24.149[A], S24.159[A], S29.001-S29.019[A], S29.091-S29.9XX[A], S32.000-S32.059[A,B,S], S32.10X-S32.9XX[S], S33.0XX-S33.141[A], S33.30X-S33.39X[A], S33.5XX[A], S33.9XX[A], S34.01X[A], S34.101-S34.129[A], S38.1XX[A], S38.3XX-S39.013[A], S39.091-S39.94X[A], T14.8-T14.91, T79.8XX-T79.9XX[A], T79.A0X-T79.A9X[A] **For S32.0[K]:** M80.00X-M80.88X[K,P], M84.30X-M84.68X[K,P], S02.0XX-S02.92X[K], S12.000-S12.691[K], S22.000-S22.9XX[K], S32.000-S32.9XX[K], S42.001-S42.92X[K,P], S49.001-S49.199[K,P], S52.001-S52.92X[K,M,N,P,Q,R], S59.001-S59.299[K,P], S62.001-S62.92X[K,P], S72.001-S72.92X[K,M,N,P,Q,R], S79.001-S79.199[K,P], S82.001-S82.92X[K,M,N,P,Q,R], S89.001-S89.399[K,P], S92.001-S92.919[K,P]

 ● S32.00   **Fracture of unspecified lumbar vertebra**

  ● S32.000   **Wedge compression fracture of unspecified lumbar vertebra** A, K 🖐, B 🖐, 🖐, A, B 🖐

  ● S32.001   **Stable burst fracture of unspecified lumbar vertebra** A, K 🖐, B 🖐, 🖐, A, B 🖐

◄ New   ◄▦ Revised   ~~deleted~~ Deleted   Excludes 1   Excludes 2   Includes   Use additional   Code first   Code also   Unspecified

OGCR Official Guidelines   ● Unacceptable Principal Diagnosis   X Assign placeholder X   ● Use Additional Character(s)   ▶ Manifestation Code   **Coding Clinic**

● S32.002   Unstable burst fracture of unspecified lumbar vertebra A, K 🦠, B 🦠, 🦠, A, B 🦠

● S32.008   Other fracture of unspecified lumbar vertebra A, K 🦠, B 🦠, 🦠, A, B 🦠

● S32.009   Unspecified fracture of unspecified lumbar vertebra A, K 🦠, B 🦠, 🦠, A, B 🦠

● S32.01   **Fracture of first lumbar vertebra**

  ● S32.010   Wedge compression fracture of first lumbar vertebra A, K 🦠, B 🦠, 🦠, A, B 🦠

  ● S32.011   Stable burst fracture of first lumbar vertebra A, K 🦠, B 🦠, 🦠, A, B 🦠

  ● S32.012   Unstable burst fracture of first lumbar vertebra A, K 🦠, B 🦠, 🦠, A, B 🦠

  ● S32.018   Other fracture of first lumbar vertebra A, K 🦠, B 🦠, 🦠, A, B 🦠

  ● S32.019   Unspecified fracture of first lumbar vertebra A, K 🦠, B 🦠, 🦠, A, B 🦠

● S32.02   **Fracture of second lumbar vertebra**

  ● S32.020   Wedge compression fracture of second lumbar vertebra A, K 🦠, B 🦠, 🦠, A, B 🦠

  ● S32.021   Stable burst fracture of second lumbar vertebra A, K 🦠, B 🦠, 🦠, A, B 🦠

  ● S32.022   Unstable burst fracture of second lumbar vertebra A, K 🦠, B 🦠, 🦠, A, B 🦠

  ● S32.028   Other fracture of second lumbar vertebra A, K 🦠, B 🦠, 🦠, A, B 🦠

  ● S32.029   Unspecified fracture of second lumbar vertebra A, K 🦠, B 🦠, 🦠, A, B 🦠

● S32.03   **Fracture of third lumbar vertebra**

  ● S32.030   Wedge compression fracture of third lumbar vertebra A, K 🦠, B 🦠, 🦠, A, B 🦠

  ● S32.031   Stable burst fracture of third lumbar vertebra A, K 🦠, B 🦠, 🦠, A, B 🦠

  ● S32.032   Unstable burst fracture of third lumbar vertebra A, K 🦠, B 🦠, 🦠, A, B 🦠

  ● S32.038   Other fracture of third lumbar vertebra A, K 🦠, B 🦠, 🦠, A, B 🦠

  ● S32.039   Unspecified fracture of third lumbar vertebra A, K 🦠, B 🦠, 🦠, A, B 🦠

● S32.04   **Fracture of fourth lumbar vertebra**

  ● S32.040   Wedge compression fracture of fourth lumbar vertebra A, K 🦠, B 🦠, 🦠, A, B 🦠

  ● S32.041   Stable burst fracture of fourth lumbar vertebra A, K 🦠, B 🦠, 🦠, A, B 🦠

  ● S32.042   Unstable burst fracture of fourth lumbar vertebra A, K 🦠, B 🦠, 🦠, A, B 🦠

  ● S32.048   Other fracture of fourth lumbar vertebra A, K 🦠, B 🦠, 🦠, A, B 🦠

  ● S32.049   Unspecified fracture of fourth lumbar vertebra A, K 🦠, B 🦠, 🦠, A, B 🦠

● S32.05   **Fracture of fifth lumbar vertebra**

  ● S32.050   Wedge compression fracture of fifth lumbar vertebra A, K 🦠, B 🦠, 🦠, A, B 🦠

  ● S32.051   Stable burst fracture of fifth lumbar vertebra A, K 🦠, B 🦠, 🦠, A, B 🦠

  ● S32.052   Unstable burst fracture of fifth lumbar vertebra A, K 🦠, B 🦠, 🦠, A, B 🦠

  ● S32.058   Other fracture of fifth lumbar vertebra A, K 🦠, B 🦠, 🦠, A, B 🦠

  ● S32.059   Unspecified fracture of fifth lumbar vertebra A, K 🦠, B 🦠, 🦠, A, B 🦠

● S32.1   **Fracture of sacrum**

For vertical fractures, code to most medial fracture extension

Use two codes if both a vertical and transverse fracture are present

Code also any associated fracture of pelvic ring (S32.8-)

(Ex) **For category S32.1 CC codes S32.1[A,B]:** M48.40X-M48.58X[S], M80.08X[S], M80.88X[S], M84.350[S], M84.454[S], M84.550[S], M84.58X[S], M84.650[S], M99.14-M99.17, M99.19, S03.8XX-S03.9XX[A], S12.000-S12.9XX[S], S13.9XX[A], S14.109[A], S14.119[A], S14.129[A], S14.139[A], S14.149[A], S14.159[A], S22.000-S22.9XX[S], S23.20X[A], S23.29X[A], S23.9XX[A], S24.109[A], S24.119[A], S24.139[A], S24.149[A], S24.159[A], S29.001-S29.019[A], S29.091-S29.9XX[A], S32.000-S32.059[S], S32.10X-S32.2XX[A,B,S], S32.301-S32.9XX[S], S33.2XX-S33.4XX[A], S33.6XX-S33.9XX[A], S34.02X[A], S34.131-S34.3XX[A], S38.1XX[A], S38.3XX[A], S39.001-S39.013[A], S39.091-39.94X[A], T14.8-T14.91, T79.8XX-T79.9XX[A], T79.A0X-T79.A9X[A] **For S32.1[K]:** See S32.0[K]

X ● S32.10   Unspecified fracture of sacrum A, K 🦠, B 🦠, 🦠, A, B 🦠

● S32.11   **Zone I fracture of sacrum**

Vertical sacral ala fracture of sacrum

  ● S32.110   Nondisplaced Zone I fracture of sacrum A, K 🦠, B 🦠, 🦠, A, B 🦠

  ● S32.111   Minimally displaced Zone I fracture of sacrum A, K 🦠, B 🦠, 🦠, A, B 🦠

  ● S32.112   Severely displaced Zone I fracture of sacrum A, K 🦠, B 🦠, 🦠, A, B 🦠

  ● S32.119   Unspecified Zone I fracture of sacrum A, K 🦠, B 🦠, 🦠, A, B 🦠

● S32.12   **Zone II fracture of sacrum**

Vertical foraminal region fracture of sacrum

  ● S32.120   Nondisplaced Zone II fracture of sacrum A, K 🦠, B 🦠, 🦠, A, B 🦠

  ● S32.121   Minimally displaced Zone II fracture of sacrum A, K 🦠, B 🦠, 🦠, A, B 🦠

  ● S32.122   Severely displaced Zone II fracture of sacrum A, K 🦠, B 🦠, 🦠, A, B 🦠

  ● S32.129   Unspecified Zone II fracture of sacrum A, K 🦠, B 🦠, 🦠, A, B 🦠

● S32.13   **Zone III fracture of sacrum**

Vertical fracture into spinal canal region of sacrum

  ● S32.130   Nondisplaced Zone III fracture of sacrum A, K 🦠, B 🦠, 🦠, A, B 🦠

  ● S32.131   Minimally displaced Zone III fracture of sacrum A, K 🦠, B 🦠, 🦠, A, B 🦠

  ● S32.132   Severely displaced Zone III fracture of sacrum A, K 🦠, B 🦠, 🦠, A, B 🦠

  ● S32.139   Unspecified Zone III fracture of sacrum A, K 🦠, B 🦠, 🦠, A, B 🦠

X ● S32.14   Type 1 fracture of sacrum A, K 🦠, B 🦠, 🦠, A, B 🦠

Transverse flexion fracture of sacrum without displacement

X ● S32.15   Type 2 fracture of sacrum A, K 🦠, B 🦠, 🦠, A, B 🦠

Transverse flexion fracture of sacrum with posterior displacement

X ● S32.16   Type 3 fracture of sacrum A, K 🦠, B 🦠, 🦠, A, B 🦠

Transverse extension fracture of sacrum with anterior displacement

X ● S32.17   Type 4 fracture of sacrum A, K 🦠, B 🦠, 🦠, A, B 🦠

Transverse segmental comminution of upper sacrum

X ● S32.19   Other fracture of sacrum A, K 🦠, B 🦠, 🦠, A, B 🦠

N Newborn Age: 0   **P** Pediatric Age: 0–17   **M** Maternity DX: 12–55   **A** Adult Age: 15–124   ♀ Females Only   ♂ Males Only

🦠 Complication\Comorbidity   🦠 Major C\C   (Ex) CC/MCC Exclusions   🦠 Present on Admission Requirement   🦠 Hospital-Acquired Condition

1333

X ● **S32.2**   Fracture of coccyx A, K 🔖, B 🔖, 🔖, A, B 🔖
   🄴x For category S32.2 CC codes **S32.2[A,B]:** See S32.1 [A,B]
   For **S32.2[K]:** See S32.0[K]

● **S32.3**   Fracture of ilium

   Excludes1   fracture of ilium with associated disruption of pelvic ring (S32.8-)
   🄴x For category S32.3 CC codes **S32.3[A]:** M80.00X-M80.019[A], M80.041A-M80.049[A], M80.80X-M80.819[A], M80.841-M80.849[A], M84.40X-M84.419[A], M84.441-M84.446[A], M84.454[A], M84.474-M84.519[A], M84.541-M84.550[A], M84.574-M84.576[A], M84.60X-M84.619[A], M84.641-M84.650[A], M84.674-M84.68X[A], S03.8XX-S03.9XX[A], S22.9XX-S22.9XX[A,B], S29.011A-S29.019[A], S32.301-S32.9XX[A,B], S33.4XX[A], S33.6XX-S33.8XX[A], S38.3XX[A], S39.011-S39.013[A], S73.001-S73.199[A], S76.001-S76.019[A], S76.091-S76.119[A], S76.191-S76.219[A], S76.291-S76.319[A], S76.391-S76.819[A], S76.891-S76.919[A], S76.991-S76.999[A], S79.811-S79.929[A], T14.8-T14.91, T79.8XX-T79.9XX[A], T79.A9X[A] **For S32.3[B]:** M48.40X-M48.58X[A], M80.00X-M80.88X[A], M84.30X-M84.68X[A], S03.8XX-S03.9XX[A], S22.9XX[A,B], S29.011-S29.019[A], S32.301-S32.399[A,B], S32.810-S32.9XX[A,B], S33.4XX[A], S33.6XX-S33.8XX[A], S38.3XX[A], S39.011-S39.013[A], S73.001-S73.199[A], S76.001-S76.019[A], S76.091-S76.119[A], S76.191-S76.219[A], S76.291-S76.319[A], S76.391-S76.819[A], S76.891-S76.919[A], S76.991-S76.999[A], S79.811-S79.929[A], T14.8-T14.91, T79.8XX-T79.9XX[A], T79.A0X-T79.A9X[A] **For S32.3[K]:** See S32.0[K]

   ● **S32.30**   Unspecified fracture of ilium
      ● **S32.301**   Unspecified fracture of right ilium A, K 🔖, B 🔖, 🔖, A, B 🔖
      ● **S32.302**   Unspecified fracture of left ilium A, K 🔖, B 🔖, 🔖, A, B 🔖
      ● **S32.309**   Unspecified fracture of unspecified ilium A, K 🔖, B 🔖, 🔖, A, B 🔖

   ● **S32.31**   Avulsion fracture of ilium
      ● **S32.311**   Displaced avulsion fracture of right ilium A, K 🔖, B 🔖, 🔖, A, B 🔖
      ● **S32.312**   Displaced avulsion fracture of left ilium A, K 🔖, B 🔖, 🔖, A, B 🔖
      ● **S32.313**   Displaced avulsion fracture of unspecified ilium A, K 🔖, B 🔖, 🔖, A, B 🔖
      ● **S32.314**   Nondisplaced avulsion fracture of right ilium A, K 🔖, B 🔖, 🔖, A, B 🔖
      ● **S32.315**   Nondisplaced avulsion fracture of left ilium A, K 🔖, B 🔖, 🔖, A, B 🔖
      ● **S32.316**   Nondisplaced avulsion fracture of unspecified ilium A, K 🔖, B 🔖, 🔖, A, B 🔖

   ● **S32.39**   Other fracture of ilium
      ● **S32.391**   Other fracture of right ilium A, K 🔖, B 🔖, 🔖, A, B 🔖
      ● **S32.392**   Other fracture of left ilium A, K 🔖, B 🔖, 🔖, A, B 🔖
      ● **S32.399**   Other fracture of unspecified ilium A, K 🔖, B 🔖, 🔖, A, B 🔖

● **S32.4**   Fracture of acetabulum
   Code also any associated fracture of pelvic ring (S32.8-)
   🄴x For category S32.4 CC codes **S32.4[A]:** M48.40X-M48.58X[A], M80.00X-M80.88X[A], M84.30X-M84.68X[A], S03.8XX-S03.9XX[A], S22.9XX [A,B], S29.011-S29.019[A], S32.401-S32.499[A,B], S32.810-S32.811[A,B], S32.89X-S32.9XX[A,B], S33.4XX[A], S33.6XX-S33.8XX[A], S38.3XX[A], S39.011-S39.013[A], S73.001-S73.199[A], S76.001-S76.019[A], S76.091-S76.119[A], S76.191-S76.219[A], S76.291-S76.319[A], S76.391-S76.819[A], S76.891-S76.919[A], S76.991-S76.999[A], S79.811-S79.829[A], S79.911-S79.929[A], T14.8-T14.91, T79.8XX-T79.9XX[A], T79.A0X-T79.A9X[A] **For S32.4[B]:** S03.8XX-S03.9XX[A], S22.9XX [A,B], S29.011-S29.019[A], S32.401-S32.499[A,B], S32.810-S32.811 [A,B], S32.89X-S32.9XX[A,B], S33.4XX[A], S33.6XX-S33.8XX[A], S38.3XX[A], S39.011-S39.013[A], S73.001-S73.199[A], S76.001-S76.019[A], S76.091-S76.119[A], S76.191-S76.219[A], S76.291-S76.319[A], S76.391-S76.819[A], S76.891-S76.919[A], S76.991-S76.999[A], S79.811-S79.929[A], T14.8-T14.91, T79.A0X-T79.A9X[A], T79.8XX-T79.9XX[A] **For S32.4[K]:** See S32.0[K]

● **S32.40**   Unspecified fracture of acetabulum
   ● **S32.401**   Unspecified fracture of right acetabulum K 🔖, A, B 🔖, 🔖, A, B 🔖
   ● **S32.402**   Unspecified fracture of left acetabulum K 🔖, A, B 🔖, 🔖, A, B 🔖
   ● **S32.409**   Unspecified fracture of unspecified acetabulum K 🔖, A, B 🔖, 🔖, A, B 🔖

● **S32.41**   Fracture of anterior wall of acetabulum
   ● **S32.411**   Displaced fracture of anterior wall of right acetabulum K 🔖, A, B 🔖, 🔖, A, B 🔖
   ● **S32.412**   Displaced fracture of anterior wall of left acetabulum K 🔖, A, B 🔖, 🔖, A, B 🔖
   ● **S32.413**   Displaced fracture of anterior wall of unspecified acetabulum K 🔖, A, B 🔖, 🔖, A, B 🔖
   ● **S32.414**   Nondisplaced fracture of anterior wall of right acetabulum K 🔖, A, B 🔖, 🔖, A, B 🔖
   ● **S32.415**   Nondisplaced fracture of anterior wall of left acetabulum K 🔖, A, B 🔖, 🔖, A, B 🔖
   ● **S32.416**   Nondisplaced fracture of anterior wall of unspecified acetabulum K 🔖, A, B 🔖, 🔖, A, B 🔖

● **S32.42**   Fracture of posterior wall of acetabulum
   ● **S32.421**   Displaced fracture of posterior wall of right acetabulum K 🔖, A, B 🔖, 🔖, A, B 🔖
   ● **S32.422**   Displaced fracture of posterior wall of left acetabulum K 🔖, A, B 🔖, 🔖, A, B 🔖
   ● **S32.423**   Displaced fracture of posterior wall of unspecified acetabulum K 🔖, A, B 🔖, 🔖, A, B 🔖
   ● **S32.424**   Nondisplaced fracture of posterior wall of right acetabulum K 🔖, A, B 🔖, 🔖, A, B 🔖
   ● **S32.425**   Nondisplaced fracture of posterior wall of left acetabulum K 🔖, A, B 🔖, 🔖, A, B 🔖
   ● **S32.426**   Nondisplaced fracture of posterior wall of unspecified acetabulum K 🔖, A, B 🔖, 🔖, A, B 🔖

● **S32.43**   Fracture of anterior column [iliopubic] of acetabulum
   ● **S32.431**   Displaced fracture of anterior column [iliopubic] of right acetabulum K 🔖, A, B 🔖, 🔖, A, B 🔖
   ● **S32.432**   Displaced fracture of anterior column [iliopubic] of left acetabulum K 🔖, A, B 🔖, 🔖, A, B 🔖
   ● **S32.433**   Displaced fracture of anterior column [iliopubic] of unspecified acetabulum K 🔖, A, B 🔖, 🔖, A, B 🔖
   ● **S32.434**   Nondisplaced fracture of anterior column [iliopubic] of right acetabulum K 🔖, A, B 🔖, 🔖, A, B 🔖
   ● **S32.435**   Nondisplaced fracture of anterior column [iliopubic] of left acetabulum K 🔖, A, B 🔖, 🔖, A, B 🔖
   ● **S32.436**   Nondisplaced fracture of anterior column [iliopubic] of unspecified acetabulum K 🔖, A, B 🔖, 🔖, A, B 🔖

◀ New   ◀⃥ Revised   ~~deleted~~ Deleted   Excludes 1   Excludes 2   Includes   Use additional   Code first   Code also   Unspecified
OGCR Official Guidelines   ● Unacceptable Principal Diagnosis   X Assign placeholder X   ● Use Additional Character(s)   ▶ Manifestation Code   **Coding Clinic**

● S32.44   Fracture of posterior column [ilioischial] of
         acetabulum
   ● S32.441   Displaced fracture of posterior
          column [ilioischial] of right
          acetabulum K ⊛, A, B ⊛, ⊛, A, B ⊛
   ● S32.442   Displaced fracture of posterior
          column [ilioischial] of left
          acetabulum K ⊛, A, B ⊛, ⊛, A, B ⊛
   ● S32.443   Displaced fracture of posterior
          column [ilioischial] of unspecified
          acetabulum K ⊛, A, B ⊛, ⊛, A, B ⊛
   ● S32.444   Nondisplaced fracture of posterior
          column [ilioischial] of right
          acetabulum K ⊛, A, B ⊛, ⊛, A, B ⊛
   ● S32.445   Nondisplaced fracture of posterior
          column [ilioischial] of left
          acetabulum K ⊛, A, B ⊛, ⊛, A, B ⊛
   ● S32.446   Nondisplaced fracture of posterior
          column [ilioischial] of unspecified
          acetabulum K ⊛, A, B ⊛, ⊛, A, B ⊛

● S32.45   Transverse fracture of acetabulum
   ● S32.451   Displaced transverse fracture of right
          acetabulum K ⊛, A, B ⊛, ⊛, A, B ⊛
   ● S32.452   Displaced transverse fracture of left
          acetabulum K ⊛, A, B ⊛, ⊛, A, B ⊛
   ● S32.453   Displaced transverse fracture of
          unspecified acetabulum K ⊛, A, B ⊛,
          ⊛, A, B ⊛
   ● S32.454   Nondisplaced transverse fracture of
          right acetabulum K ⊛, A, B ⊛, ⊛, A,
          B ⊛
   ● S32.455   Nondisplaced transverse fracture of
          left acetabulum K ⊛, A, B ⊛, ⊛, A,
          B ⊛
   ● S32.456   Nondisplaced transverse fracture of
          unspecified acetabulum K ⊛, A, B ⊛,
          ⊛, A, B ⊛

● S32.46   Associated transverse-posterior fracture of
         acetabulum
   ● S32.461   Displaced associated
          transverse-posterior fracture of right
          acetabulum K ⊛, A, B ⊛, ⊛, A, B ⊛
   ● S32.462   Displaced associated
          transverse-posterior fracture of left
          acetabulum K ⊛, A, B ⊛, ⊛, A, B ⊛
   ● S32.463   Displaced associated
          transverse-posterior fracture of
          unspecified acetabulum K ⊛, A, B ⊛,
          ⊛, A, B ⊛
   ● S32.464   Nondisplaced associated
          transverse-posterior fracture of right
          acetabulum K ⊛, A, B ⊛, ⊛, A, B ⊛
   ● S32.465   Nondisplaced associated
          transverse-posterior fracture of left
          acetabulum K ⊛, A, B ⊛, ⊛, A, B ⊛
   ● S32.466   Nondisplaced associated
          transverse-posterior fracture of
          unspecified acetabulum K ⊛, A, B ⊛,
          ⊛, A, B ⊛

● S32.47   Fracture of medial wall of acetabulum
   ● S32.471   Displaced fracture of medial wall of
          right acetabulum K ⊛, A, B ⊛, ⊛, A,
          B ⊛
   ● S32.472   Displaced fracture of medial wall of
          left acetabulum K ⊛, A, B ⊛, ⊛, A,
          B ⊛
   ● S32.473   Displaced fracture of medial wall of
          unspecified acetabulum K ⊛, A, B ⊛,
          ⊛, A, B ⊛

   ● S32.474   Nondisplaced fracture of medial wall
          of right acetabulum K ⊛, A, B ⊛, ⊛,
          A, B ⊛
   ● S32.475   Nondisplaced fracture of medial wall
          of left acetabulum K ⊛, A, B ⊛, ⊛, A,
          B ⊛
   ● S32.476   Nondisplaced fracture of medial wall
          of unspecified acetabulum K ⊛,
          A, B ⊛, ⊛, A, B ⊛

● S32.48   Dome fracture of acetabulum
   ● S32.481   Displaced dome fracture of right
          acetabulum K ⊛, A, B ⊛, ⊛, A, B ⊛
   ● S32.482   Displaced dome fracture of left
          acetabulum K ⊛, A, B ⊛, ⊛, A, B ⊛
   ● S32.483   Displaced dome fracture of
          unspecified acetabulum K ⊛, A, B ⊛,
          ⊛, A, B ⊛
   ● S32.484   Nondisplaced dome fracture of right
          acetabulum K ⊛, A, B ⊛, ⊛, A, B ⊛
   ● S32.485   Nondisplaced dome fracture of left
          acetabulum K ⊛, A, B ⊛, ⊛, A, B ⊛
   ● S32.486   Nondisplaced dome fracture of
          unspecified acetabulum K ⊛, A, B ⊛,
          ⊛, A, B ⊛

● S32.49   Other fracture of acetabulum
   ● S32.491   Other fracture of right acetabulum
          K ⊛, A, B ⊛, ⊛, A, B ⊛
   ● S32.492   Other fracture of left acetabulum
          K ⊛, A, B ⊛, ⊛, A, B ⊛
   ● S32.499   Other fracture of unspecified
          acetabulum K ⊛, A, B ⊛, ⊛, A, B ⊛

● S32.5   Fracture of pubis
    Excludes1   fracture of pubis with associated
         disruption of pelvic ring (S32.8-)
    (Ex): **For category S32.5 CC codes S32.5[A,B]:** M48.40X-M48.58X[A],
    M80.00X-M80.88X[A], M84.30X-M84.68X[A], S03.8XX-S03.9XX[A], S22.9XX
    [A,B], S29.011-S29.019[A], S32.501A-S32.599[A,B], S32.810-S32.811[A,B],
    S32.89X-S32.9XX[A,B], S33.4XX[A], S33.6XX-S33.8XX[A],
    S38.3XX-S39.013[A], S73.001-S73.199[A], S76.001-S76.019[A],
    S76.091-S76.119[A], S76.191-S76.219[A], S76.291-S76.319[A],
    S76.391-S76.819[A], S76.891-S76.919[A], S76.991-S76.999[A],
    S79.811-S79.929[A], T14.8-T14.91,T79.A0X-T79.A9X[A],
    T79.8XX-T79.9XX[A] **For S32.5[K]:** See S32.0[K]

  ● S32.50   Unspecified fracture of pubis
   ● S32.501   Unspecified fracture of right pubis
          A, K ⊛, B ⊛, ⊛, A, B ⊛
   ● S32.502   Unspecified fracture of left pubis
          A, K ⊛, B ⊛, ⊛, A, B ⊛
   ● S32.509   Unspecified fracture of unspecified
          pubis A, K ⊛, B ⊛, ⊛, A, B ⊛

  ● S32.51   Fracture of superior rim of pubis
   ● S32.511   Fracture of superior rim of right pubis
          A, K ⊛, B ⊛, ⊛, A, B ⊛
   ● S32.512   Fracture of superior rim of left pubis
          A, K ⊛, B ⊛, ⊛, A, B ⊛
   ● S32.519   Fracture of superior rim of
          unspecified pubis A, K ⊛, B ⊛, ⊛,
          A, B ⊛

  ● S32.59   Other specified fracture of pubis
   ● S32.591   Other specified fracture of right pubis
          A, K ⊛, B ⊛, ⊛, A, B ⊛
   ● S32.592   Other specified fracture of left pubis
          A, K ⊛, B ⊛, ⊛, A, B ⊛
   ● S32.599   Other specified fracture of
          unspecified pubis A, K ⊛, B ⊛, ⊛,
          A, B ⊛

CHAPTER 19 (S00-T88)

N   Newborn Age: 0   P   Pediatric Age: 0–17   M   Maternity DX: 12–55   A   Adult Age: 15–124   ♀ Females Only   ♂ Males Only

⊛ Complication\Comorbidity   ⊛ Major C\C   (Ex) CC/MCC Exclusions   ⊛ Present on Admission Requirement   ⊛ Hospital-Acquired Condition

1335

● S32.6   Fracture of ischium
         Excludes1   fracture of ischium with associated
                         disruption of pelvic ring (S32.8-)
         (Ex:) For category S32.6 CC codes S32.6[A]: S32.601-S32.699[A]
              For S32.6[B]: M48.40X-M48.58X[A], M80.00X-M80.88X[A],
              M84.30X-M84.68X[A], S03.8XX-S03.9XX[A], S22.9XX[A,B],
              S29.011-S29.019[A], S32.601-S32.811[A,B], S32.89X-S32.9XX[A,B],
              S33.4XX[A], S33.6XX-S33.8XX[A], S38.3XX[A], S39.011-S39.013[A],
              S73.001-S73.199[A], S76.001-S76.019[A], S76.091-S76.119[A],
              S76.191-S76.219[A], S76.291-S76.319[A], S76.391-S76.819[A],
              S76.891-S76.919[A], S76.991-S76.999[A], S79.811-S79.929[A],
              T14.8-T14.91, T79.A0X-T79.A9X[A], T79.8XX-T79.9XX[A] For S32.5[K]: See
              S32.0[K]

   ● S32.60   Unspecified fracture of ischium
      ● S32.601   **Unspecified** fracture of right ischium
                  A, K 🔲, B 🔲, 🔲, A, B 🔲
      ● S32.602   **Unspecified** fracture of left ischium
                  A, K 🔲, B 🔲, 🔲, A, B 🔲
      ● S32.609   **Unspecified** fracture of unspecified
                  ischium A, K 🔲, B 🔲, 🔲, A, B 🔲

   ● S32.61   Avulsion fracture of ischium
      ● S32.611   Displaced avulsion fracture of right
                  ischium A, K 🔲, B 🔲, 🔲, A, B 🔲
      ● S32.612   Displaced avulsion fracture of left
                  ischium A, K 🔲, B 🔲, 🔲, A, B 🔲
      ● S32.613   Displaced avulsion fracture of
                  unspecified ischium A, K 🔲, B 🔲, 🔲,
                  A, B 🔲
      ● S32.614   Nondisplaced avulsion fracture of
                  right ischium A, K 🔲, B 🔲, 🔲, A, B 🔲
      ● S32.615   Nondisplaced avulsion fracture of left
                  ischium A, K 🔲, B 🔲, 🔲, A, B 🔲
      ● S32.616   Nondisplaced avulsion fracture of
                  unspecified ischium A, K 🔲, B 🔲, 🔲,
                  A, B 🔲

   ● S32.69   Other specified fracture of ischium
      ● S32.691   Other specified fracture of right
                  ischium A, K 🔲, B 🔲, 🔲, A, B 🔲
      ● S32.692   Other specified fracture of left
                  ischium A, K 🔲, B 🔲, 🔲, A, B 🔲
      ● S32.699   Other specified fracture of
                  unspecified ischium A, K 🔲, B 🔲, 🔲,
                  A, B 🔲

● S32.8   Fracture of other parts of pelvis
         Code also any associated:
            fracture of acetabulum (S32.4-)
            sacral fracture (S32.1-)

   ● S32.81   Multiple fractures of pelvis with disruption of
              pelvic ring
              Multiple pelvic fractures with disruption of
              pelvic circle
              (Ex:) For category S32.81 CC codes S32.81[A,B]:
                   M48.40X-M48.58X[A], M80.00X-M80.88X[A],
                   M84.30X-M84.68X[A], S03.8XX-S03.9XX[A], S22.9XX[A,B],
                   S29.011-S29.019[A], S32.301-S32.811[A,B],
                   S32.89X-S32.9XX[A,B], S33.4XX[A], S33.6XX-S33.8XX[A],
                   S38.3XX[A], S39.011-S39.013[A], S73.001-S73.199[A],
                   S76.001-S76.019[A], S76.091-S76.119[A],
                   S76.191-S76.219[A], S76.291-S76.319[A],
                   S76.391-S76.819[A], S76.891-S76.919[A],
                   S76.991-S76.999[A], S79.811-S79.929[A], T14.8-T14.91, T79.
                   A0X-T79.A9X[A], T79.8XX-T79.9XX[A] For S32.81[K]: See
                   S32.0[K]

      ● S32.810   Multiple fractures of pelvis with
                  stable disruption of pelvic ring
                  A, K 🔲, B 🔲, 🔲, A, B 🔲
      ● S32.811   Multiple fractures of pelvis with
                  unstable disruption of pelvic ring
                  A, K 🔲, B 🔲, 🔲, A, B 🔲

X ● S32.82   Multiple fractures of pelvis without disruption
             of pelvic ring A, K 🔲, B 🔲, 🔲, A, B 🔲
             Multiple pelvic fractures without disruption of
             pelvic circle
             (Ex:) For category S32.82 CC codes S32.82[A,B]: S32.89X[A]
                  For S32.81[K]: See S32.0[K]

X ● S32.89   Fracture of other parts of pelvis A, K 🔲, B 🔲,
             🔲, A, B 🔲
             (Ex:) For category S32.89 CC codes S32.89[A,B]:
                  M48.40X-M48.58X[A], M80.00X-M80.88X[A],
                  M84.30X-M84.68X[A], S03.8XX-S03.9XX[A], S22.9XX[A,B],
                  S29.011-S29.019[A], S32.301-S32.9XX[A,B], S33.4XX[A],
                  S33.6XX-S33.8XX[A], S38.3XX[A], S39.011-S39.013[A],
                  S73.001-S73.199[A], S76.001-S76.019[A],
                  S76.091-S76.119[A], S76.191-S76.219[A], 76.291-S76.319[A],
                  S76.391-S76.819[A], S76.891-S76.919[A],
                  S76.991-S76.999[A], S79.811-S79.929[A], T14.8-T14.91, T79.
                  A0X-T79.A9X[A], T79.8XX-T79.9XX[A] For S32.89[K]: See
                  S32.0[K]

X ● S32.9   Fracture of **unspecified** parts of lumbosacral spine and
            pelvis A, K 🔲, B 🔲, 🔲, A, B 🔲
            Fracture of lumbosacral spine NOS
            Fracture of pelvis NOS
            (Ex:) For category S32.9 CC codes S32.9[A,B]: See S32.81 For S32.9[K]:
                 See S32.0[K]
            Coding Clinic: 2012, Q4, P93

● S33   Dislocation and sprain of joints and ligaments of lumbar spine
        and pelvis
        Includes   avulsion of joint or ligament of lumbar spine and
                       pelvis
                       laceration of cartilage, joint or ligament of lumbar
                          spine and pelvis
                       sprain of cartilage, joint or ligament of lumbar
                          spine and pelvis
                       traumatic hemarthrosis of joint or ligament of
                          lumbar spine and pelvis
                       traumatic rupture of joint or ligament of lumbar
                          spine and pelvis
                       traumatic subluxation of joint or ligament of
                          lumbar spine and pelvis
                       traumatic tear of joint or ligament of lumbar
                          spine and pelvis
        Code also any associated open wound
        Excludes1   nontraumatic rupture or displacement of lumbar
                        intervertebral disc NOS (M51.-)
                        obstetric damage to pelvic joints and ligaments
                        (O71.6)

        Excludes2   dislocation and sprain of joints and ligaments of
                        hip (S73.-)
                        strain of muscle of lower back and pelvis
                        (S39.01-)
        The appropriate 7th character is to be added to each code from
        category S33

A	initial encounter
D	subsequent encounter
S	sequela

X ● S33.0   Traumatic rupture of lumbar intervertebral disc 🔲
            Excludes1   rupture or displacement (nontraumatic)
                            of lumbar intervertebral disc NOS
                            (M51.- with fifth character 6)

◄ New   ◄ Revised   ̶d̶e̶l̶e̶t̶e̶d̶ Deleted   Excludes 1   Excludes 2   Includes   Use additional   Code first   Code also   Unspecified
OGCR Official Guidelines   ● Unacceptable Principal Diagnosis   X Assign placeholder X   ● Use Additional Character(s)   ▶ Manifestation Code   Coding Clinic

● **S33.1**   **Subluxation and dislocation of lumbar vertebra**
    Code also any associated:
       open wound of abdomen, lower back and pelvis (S31)
       spinal cord injury (S24.0, S24.1-, S34.0-, S34.1-)
    Excludes2   fracture of lumbar vertebrae (S32.0-)

   ● **S33.10**   Subluxation and dislocation of unspecified lumbar vertebra
     ● **S33.100**   Subluxation of unspecified lumbar vertebra 🖐
     ● **S33.101**   Dislocation of unspecified lumbar vertebra 🖐

   ● **S33.11**   Subluxation and dislocation of L$_1$/L$_2$ lumbar vertebra
     ● **S33.110**   Subluxation of L$_1$/L$_2$ lumbar vertebra 🖐
     ● **S33.111**   Dislocation of L$_1$/L$_2$ lumbar vertebra 🖐

   ● **S33.12**   Subluxation and dislocation of L$_2$/L$_3$ lumbar vertebra
     ● **S33.120**   Subluxation of L$_2$/L$_3$ lumbar vertebra 🖐
     ● **S33.121**   Dislocation of L$_2$/L$_3$ lumbar vertebra 🖐

   ● **S33.13**   Subluxation and dislocation of L$_3$/L$_4$ lumbar vertebra
     ● **S33.130**   Subluxation of L$_3$/L$_4$ lumbar vertebra 🖐
     ● **S33.131**   Dislocation of L$_3$/L$_4$ lumbar vertebra 🖐

   ● **S33.14**   Subluxation and dislocation of L$_4$/L$_5$ lumbar vertebra
     ● **S33.140**   Subluxation of L$_4$/L$_5$ lumbar vertebra 🖐
     ● **S33.141**   Dislocation of L$_4$/L$_5$ lumbar vertebra 🖐

X ● **S33.2**   Dislocation of sacroiliac and sacrococcygeal joint 🖐
● **S33.3**   Dislocation of other and unspecified parts of lumbar spine and pelvis
   X ● **S33.30**   Dislocation of unspecified parts of lumbar spine and pelvis 🖐
   X ● **S33.39**   Dislocation of other parts of lumbar spine and pelvis 🖐
X ● **S33.4**   Traumatic rupture of symphysis pubis 🖐
X ● **S33.5**   Sprain of ligaments of lumbar spine 🖐
X ● **S33.6**   Sprain of sacroiliac joint 🖐
X ● **S33.8**   Sprain of other parts of lumbar spine and pelvis 🖐
X ● **S33.9**   Sprain of unspecified parts of lumbar spine and pelvis 🖐

● **S34**   **Injury of lumbar and sacral spinal cord and nerves at abdomen, lower back and pelvis level**
   Note: Code to highest level of lumbar cord injury
     Injuries to the spinal cord (S34.0 and S34.1) refer to the cord level and not bone level injury, and can affect nerve roots at and below the level given. ◄
   The appropriate 7th character is to be added to each code from category S34

A	initial encounter
D	subsequent encounter
S	sequela

   Code also any associated:
     fracture of vertebra (S22.0-, S32.0-)
     open wound of abdomen, lower back and pelvis (S31.-)
     transient paralysis (R29.5)
   (Ex) For category S34 CC codes unless otherwise indicated: M48.40X-M48.58X[S], M80.08X[S], M80.88X[S], M84.350[S], M84.454[S], M84.550[S], M84.58X[S], M84.650[S], M99.15-M99.17, M99.19, S12.000-S12.9XX[S], S13.9XX[A], S14.109[A], S14.119[A], S14.129[A], S14.139[A], S14.149[A], S14.159[A], S22.000-S22.9XX[S], S23.20X[A], S23.29X[A], S23.9XX[A], S24.109[A], S24.119[A], S24.139[A], S24.149[A], S24.159[A], S29.001-S29.009[A], S29.091-S29.9XX[A], S32.000-S32.9XX[S], S33.30X-S33.39X[A], S33.9XX-S34.01X[A], S34.101-S34.129[A], S38.1XX[A], S39.001-S39.003[A], S39.091-S39.94X[A], T14.8-T14.91, T79.A0X-T79.A9X[A], T79.8XX-T79.9XX[A]

● **S34.0**   **Concussion and edema of lumbar and sacral spinal cord**
   X ● **S34.01**   Concussion and edema of lumbar spinal cord A 🖐, 🖐
   X ● **S34.02**   Concussion and edema of sacral spinal cord A 🖐, 🖐
     Concussion and edema of conus medullaris
     (Ex) M48.40X-M48.58X[S], M80.08X[S], M80.88X[S], M84.350[S], M84.454[S], M84.550[S], M84.58X[S], M84.650[S], M99.15-M99.17, M99.19, S12.000-S12.9XX[S], S13.9XX[A], S14.109[A], S14.119[A], S14.129[A], S14.139[A], S14.149[A], S14.159[A], S22.000-S22.9XX[S], S23.20X-S23.29X[A], S23.9XX[A], S24.109[A], S24.119[A], S24.139[A], S24.149[A], S24.159[A], S29.001-S29.009[A], S29.091-S29.9XX[A], S32.000-S32.9XX[S], S33.30X-S33.39X[A], S33.9XX[A], S34.02X[A], S34.131-S34.139[A], S34.3XX[A], S38.1XX[A], S39.001-S39.003[A], S39.091-S39.94X[A], T14.8-T14.91, T79.A0X-T79.A9X[A], T79.8XX-T79.9XX[A]

● **S34.1**   **Other and unspecified injury of lumbar and sacral spinal cord**
   ● **S34.10**   Unspecified injury to lumbar spinal cord
     ● **S34.101**   Unspecified injury to L$_1$ level of lumbar spinal cord A 🖐, 🖐, A 🖐
     ● **S34.102**   Unspecified injury to L$_2$ level of lumbar spinal cord A 🖐, 🖐, A 🖐
     ● **S34.103**   Unspecified injury to L$_3$ level of lumbar spinal cord A 🖐, 🖐, A 🖐
     ● **S34.104**   Unspecified injury to L$_4$ level of lumbar spinal cord A 🖐, 🖐, A 🖐
     ● **S34.105**   Unspecified injury to L$_5$ level of lumbar spinal cord A 🖐, 🖐, A 🖐
     ● **S34.109**   Unspecified injury to unspecified level of lumbar spinal cord A 🖐, 🖐, A 🖐

   ● **S34.11**   Complete lesion of lumbar spinal cord
     ● **S34.111**   Complete lesion of L$_1$ level of lumbar spinal cord A 🖐, 🖐, A 🖐
     ● **S34.112**   Complete lesion of L$_2$ level of lumbar spinal cord A 🖐, 🖐, A 🖐
     ● **S34.113**   Complete lesion of L$_3$ level of lumbar spinal cord A 🖐, 🖐, A 🖐
     ● **S34.114**   Complete lesion of L$_4$ level of lumbar spinal cord A 🖐, 🖐, A 🖐
     ● **S34.115**   Complete lesion of L$_5$ level of lumbar spinal cord A 🖐, 🖐, A 🖐
     ● **S34.119**   Complete lesion of unspecified level of lumbar spinal cord A 🖐, 🖐, A 🖐

N Newborn Age: 0   **P** Pediatric Age: 0–17   **M** Maternity DX: 12–55   **A** Adult Age: 15–124   ♀ Females Only   ♂ Males Only

🖐 Complication\Comorbidity   🖐 Major C\C   (Ex) CC/MCC Exclusions   🖐 Present on Admission Requirement   🖐 Hospital-Acquired Condition

1337

CHAPTER 19 (S00–T88)

CHAPTER 19 (S00–T88)

● S34.12   Incomplete lesion of lumbar spinal cord
     ● S34.121   Incomplete lesion of L$_1$ level of lumbar spinal cord A 🔊, 🔊, A 🔊
     ● S34.122   Incomplete lesion of L$_2$ level of lumbar spinal cord A 🔊, 🔊, A 🔊
     ● S34.123   Incomplete lesion of L$_3$ level of lumbar spinal cord A 🔊, 🔊, A 🔊
     ● S34.124   Incomplete lesion of L$_4$ level of lumbar spinal cord A 🔊, 🔊, A 🔊
     ● S34.125   Incomplete lesion of L$_5$ level of lumbar spinal cord A 🔊, 🔊, A 🔊
     ● S34.129   Incomplete lesion of unspecified level of lumbar spinal cord A 🔊, 🔊, A 🔊

● S34.13   Other and unspecified injury to sacral spinal cord
     Other injury to conus medullaris
     (Ex) For category S34.13 CC codes: See S32.04
     ● S34.131   Complete lesion of sacral spinal cord A 🔊, 🔊, A 🔊
         Complete lesion of conus medullaris
     ● S34.132   Incomplete lesion of sacral spinal cord A 🔊, 🔊, A 🔊
         Incomplete lesion of conus medullaris
     ● S34.139   Unspecified injury to sacral spinal cord A 🔊, 🔊, A 🔊
         Unspecified injury of conus medullaris

● S34.2   Injury of nerve root of lumbar and sacral spine
   X ● S34.21   Injury of nerve root of lumbar spine 🔊
   X ● S34.22   Injury of nerve root of sacral spine 🔊
X ● S34.3   Injury of cauda equina A 🔊, 🔊, A 🔊
     (Ex) See S32.04
X ● S34.4   Injury of lumbosacral plexus 🔊
X ● S34.5   Injury of lumbar, sacral and pelvic sympathetic nerves 🔊
     Injury of celiac ganglion or plexus
     Injury of hypogastric plexus
     Injury of mesenteric plexus (inferior) (superior)
     Injury of splanchnic nerve
X ● S34.6   Injury of peripheral nerve(s) at abdomen, lower back and pelvis level 🔊
X ● S34.8   Injury of other nerves at abdomen, lower back and pelvis level 🔊
X ● S34.9   Injury of unspecified nerves at abdomen, lower back and pelvis level 🔊

● S35   Injury of blood vessels at abdomen, lower back and pelvis level
     The appropriate 7th character is to be added to each code from category S35

> A   initial encounter
> D   subsequent encounter
> S   sequela

     Code also any associated open wound (S31.-)

● S35.0   Injury of abdominal aorta
     Excludes1   injury of aorta NOS (S25.0)
     (Ex) For category S35.0 CC codes: S35.00X–S35.09X[A], S35.8X1–S35.99X[A], T14.8–T14.91, T79.A0X–T79.A9X[A], T79.8XX–T79.9XX[A]
   X ● S35.00   Unspecified injury of abdominal aorta A 🔊, 🔊
   X ● S35.01   Minor laceration of abdominal aorta A 🔊, 🔊
         Incomplete transection of abdominal aorta
         Laceration of abdominal aorta NOS
         Superficial laceration of abdominal aorta
   X ● S35.02   Major laceration of abdominal aorta A 🔊, 🔊
         Complete transection of abdominal aorta
         Traumatic rupture of abdominal aorta
   X ● S35.09   Other injury of abdominal aorta A 🔊, 🔊

● S35.1   Injury of inferior vena cava
     Injury of hepatic vein
     Excludes1   injury of vena cava NOS (S25.2)
     (Ex) For category S35.1 CC codes: S35.10X–S35.19X[A], S35.8X1–S35.99X[A], T14.8–T14.91, T79.A0X–T79.A9X[A], T79.8XX–T79.9XX[A]
   X ● S35.10   Unspecified injury of inferior vena cava A 🔊, 🔊
   X ● S35.11   Minor laceration of inferior vena cava A 🔊, 🔊
         Incomplete transection of inferior vena cava
         Laceration of inferior vena cava NOS
         Superficial laceration of inferior vena cava
   X ● S35.12   Major laceration of inferior vena cava A 🔊, 🔊
         Complete transection of inferior vena cava
         Traumatic rupture of inferior vena cava
   X ● S35.19   Other injury of inferior vena cava A 🔊, 🔊

● S35.2   Injury of celiac or mesenteric artery and branches
   ● S35.21   Injury of celiac artery
     (Ex) For category S35.21 CC codes: S35.211–S35.219[A], S35.8X1–S35.99X[A], T14.8–T14.91, T79.A0X–T79.A9X[A], T79.8XX–T79.9XX[A]
     ● S35.211   Minor laceration of celiac artery A 🔊, 🔊
         Incomplete transection of celiac artery
         Laceration of celiac artery NOS
         Superficial laceration of celiac artery
     ● S35.212   Major laceration of celiac artery A 🔊, 🔊
         Complete transection of celiac artery
         Traumatic rupture of celiac artery
     ● S35.218   Other injury of celiac artery A 🔊, 🔊
     ● S35.219   Unspecified injury of celiac artery A 🔊, 🔊
   ● S35.22   Injury of superior mesenteric artery
     (Ex) For category S35.22 CC codes: S35.221–S35.229[A], S35.8X1–S35.99X[A], T14.8–T14.91, T79.A0X–T79.A9X[A], T79.8XX–T79.9XX[A]
     ● S35.221   Minor laceration of superior mesenteric artery A 🔊, 🔊
         Incomplete transection of superior mesenteric artery
         Laceration of superior mesenteric artery NOS
         Superficial laceration of superior mesenteric artery
     ● S35.222   Major laceration of superior mesenteric artery A 🔊, 🔊
         Complete transection of superior mesenteric artery
         Traumatic rupture of superior mesenteric artery
     ● S35.228   Other injury of superior mesenteric artery A 🔊, 🔊
     ● S35.229   Unspecified injury of superior mesenteric artery A 🔊, 🔊
   ● S35.23   Injury of inferior mesenteric artery
     (Ex) For category S35.23 CC codes: S35.231–S35.239[A], S35.8X1–S35.99X[A], T14.8–T14.91, T79.A0X–T79.A9X[A], T79.8XX–T79.9XX[A]
     ● S35.231   Minor laceration of inferior mesenteric artery A 🔊, 🔊
         Incomplete transection of inferior mesenteric artery
         Laceration of inferior mesenteric artery NOS
         Superficial laceration of inferior mesenteric artery
     ● S35.232   Major laceration of inferior mesenteric artery A 🔊, 🔊
         Complete transection of inferior mesenteric artery
         Traumatic rupture of inferior mesenteric artery

◀ New   ◀━ Revised   ~~deleted~~ Deleted   Excludes 1   Excludes 2   Includes   Use additional   Code first   Code also   Unspecified
OGCR Official Guidelines   ● Unacceptable Principal Diagnosis   X Assign placeholder X   ● Use Additional Character(s)   ▶ Manifestation Code   **Coding Clinic**

● S35.238   Other injury of inferior mesenteric artery A 🐾, 🐾

● S35.239   Unspecified injury of inferior mesenteric artery A 🐾, 🐾

● S35.29   Injury of branches of celiac and mesenteric artery
    Injury of gastric artery
    Injury of gastroduodenal artery
    Injury of hepatic artery
    Injury of splenic artery
    (Ex:) For category **S35.29 CC** codes unless otherwise indicated: S35.292-S35.298[A], S35.8X1-S35.99X[A], T14.8-T14.91, T79.A0X-T79.A9X[A], T79.8XX-T79.9XX[A]

● S35.291   Minor laceration of branches of celiac and mesenteric artery A 🐾, 🐾
    Incomplete transection of branches of celiac and mesenteric artery
    Laceration of branches of celiac and mesenteric artery NOS
    Superficial laceration of branches of celiac and mesenteric artery
    (Ex:) S35.291[A], S35.8X1-S35.99X[A], T14.8-T14.91, T79.8XX-T79.9XX[A], T79.A0X[A], T79.A3X-T79.A9X[A]

● S35.292   Major laceration of branches of celiac and mesenteric artery A 🐾, 🐾
    Complete transection of branches of celiac and mesenteric artery
    Traumatic rupture of branches of celiac and mesenteric artery

● S35.298   Other injury of branches of celiac and mesenteric artery A 🐾, 🐾

● S35.299   Unspecified injury of branches of celiac and mesenteric artery A 🐾, 🐾
    (Ex:) S35.299[A], S35.8X1-S35.99X[A], T14.8-T14.91, T79.A0X-T79.A9X[A], T79.8XX-T79.9XX[A]

● S35.3   Injury of portal or splenic vein and branches

● S35.31   Injury of portal vein
    (Ex:) For category **S35.31 CC** codes: S35.311-S35.319[A], S35.8X1-S35.99X[A], T14.8-T14.91, T79.A0X-T79.A9X[A], T79.8XX-T79.9XX[A]

   ● S35.311   Laceration of portal vein A 🐾, 🐾

   ● S35.318   Other specified injury of portal vein A 🐾, 🐾

   ● S35.319   Unspecified injury of portal vein A 🐾, 🐾

● S35.32   Injury of splenic vein
    (Ex:) For category **S35.32 CC** codes: S35.321-S35.329[A], S35.8X1-S35.99X[A], T14.8-T14.91, T79.A0X-T79.A9X[A], T79.8XX-T79.9XX[A]

   ● S35.321   Laceration of splenic vein A 🐾, 🐾

   ● S35.328   Other specified injury of splenic vein A 🐾, 🐾

   ● S35.329   Unspecified injury of splenic vein A 🐾, 🐾

● S35.33   Injury of superior mesenteric vein
    (Ex:) For category **S35.33 CC** codes: S35.331-S35.339[A], S35.8X1-S35.99X[A], T14.8-T14.91, T79.A0X-T79.A9X[A], T79.8XX-T79.9XX[A]

   ● S35.331   Laceration of superior mesenteric vein A 🐾, 🐾

   ● S35.338   Other specified injury of superior mesenteric vein A 🐾, 🐾

   ● S35.339   Unspecified injury of superior mesenteric vein A 🐾, 🐾

● S35.34   Injury of inferior mesenteric vein
    (Ex:) For category **S35.34 CC** codes: S35.341-S35.349[A], S35.8X1-S35.99X[A], T14.8-T14.91, T79.A0X-T79.A9X[A], T79.8XX-T79.9XX[A]

   ● S35.341   Laceration of inferior mesenteric vein A 🐾, 🐾

   ● S35.348   Other specified injury of inferior mesenteric vein A 🐾, 🐾

   ● S35.349   Unspecified injury of inferior mesenteric vein A 🐾, 🐾

● S35.4   Injury of renal blood vessels

● S35.40   Unspecified injury of renal blood vessel
    (Ex:) For category **S35.40 CC** codes S35.401-S35.403: S35.401-S35.403[A], S35.411-S35.413[A], S35.491-S35.493[A], S35.8X1-S35.99X[A], T14.8-T14.91, T79.A0X-T79.A9X[A], T79.8XX-T79.9XX[A] For category **S35.40 CC** codes S35.404-S35.406: S35.404-S35.406[A], S35.414-S35.416[A], S35.494-S35.496[A], S35.8X1-S35.99X[A], T14.8-T14.91, T79.A0X-T79.A9X[A], T79.8XX-T79.9XX[A]

   ● S35.401   Unspecified injury of right renal artery A 🐾, 🐾

   ● S35.402   Unspecified injury of left renal artery A 🐾, 🐾

   ● S35.403   Unspecified injury of unspecified renal artery A 🐾, 🐾

   ● S35.404   Unspecified injury of right renal vein A 🐾, 🐾

   ● S35.405   Unspecified injury of left renal vein A 🐾, 🐾

   ● S35.406   Unspecified injury of unspecified renal vein A 🐾, 🐾

● S35.41   Laceration of renal blood vessel
    (Ex:) For category **S35.41 CC** codes S35.411-S35.413: See S35.401-S35.403 For category **S35.41 CC** codes S35.414-S35.416: See 35.404-S35.406

   ● S35.411   Laceration of right renal artery A 🐾, 🐾

   ● S35.412   Laceration of left renal artery A 🐾, 🐾

   ● S35.413   Laceration of unspecified renal artery A 🐾, 🐾

   ● S35.414   Laceration of right renal vein A 🐾, 🐾

   ● S35.415   Laceration of left renal vein A 🐾, 🐾

   ● S35.416   Laceration of unspecified renal vein A 🐾, 🐾

● S35.49   Other specified injury of renal blood vessel
    (Ex:) For category **S35.49 CC** codes S35.491-S35.493: See S35.401-S35.403 For category **S35.49 CC** codes S35.494-S35.496: See 35.404-S35.406

   ● S35.491   Other specified injury of right renal artery A 🐾, 🐾

   ● S35.492   Other specified injury of left renal artery A 🐾, 🐾

   ● S35.493   Other specified injury of unspecified renal artery A 🐾, 🐾

   ● S35.494   Other specified injury of right renal vein A 🐾, 🐾

   ● S35.495   Other specified injury of left renal vein A 🐾, 🐾

   ● S35.496   Other specified injury of unspecified renal vein A 🐾, 🐾

N Newborn Age: 0   **P** Pediatric Age: 0–17   **M** Maternity DX: 12–55   **A** Adult Age: 15–124   ♀ Females Only   ♂ Males Only

🐾 Complication\Comorbidity   🐾 Major C\C   (Ex:) CC/MCC Exclusions   🐾 Present on Admission Requirement   🐾 Hospital-Acquired Condition

● **S35.5**   **Injury of iliac blood vessels**

X ● **S35.50**   Injury of unspecified iliac blood vessel(s) A 🔍, 🔍
> (Ex:) S35.50X-S35.516[A], S35.59X-S35.99X[A], T14.8-T14.91, T79.A0X-T79.A9X[A], T79.8XX-T79.9XX[A]

● **S35.51**   Injury of iliac artery or vein
> Injury of hypogastric artery or vein
> (Ex:) For category S35.51 CC codes S35.511-S35.513: S35.50X-S35.513[A], S35.59X-S35.99X[A], T14.8-T14.91, T79.A0X-T79.A9X[A], T79.8XX-T79.9XX[A] For category S35.51 CC codes S35.514-S35.516: S35.50X[A], S35.514-S35.516[A], S35.59X-S35.99X[A], T14.8-T14.91, T79.A0X-T79.A9X[A], T79.8XX-T79.9XX[A]

   ● **S35.511**   Injury of right iliac artery A 🔍, 🔍
   ● **S35.512**   Injury of left iliac artery A 🔍, 🔍
   ● **S35.513**   Injury of unspecified iliac artery A 🔍, 🔍
   ● **S35.514**   Injury of right iliac vein A 🔍, 🔍
   ● **S35.515**   Injury of left iliac vein A 🔍, 🔍
   ● **S35.516**   Injury of unspecified iliac vein A 🔍, 🔍

● **S35.53**   Injury of uterine artery or vein
> (Ex:) For category S35.53 CC codes S35.531-S35.533: S35.50X[A], S35.531-S35.533[A], S35.59X-S35.99X[A], T14.8-T14.91, T79.8XX-T79.9XX[A], T79.A0X-T79.A9X[A] For category S35.53 CC codes S35.534-S35.536: S35.50X[A], S35.534-S35.536[A], S35.59X-S35.99X[A], T79.8XX-T79.9XX[A], T79.A0X-T79.A3X-T79.A9X[A]

   ● **S35.531**   Injury of right uterine artery ♀ A 🔍, 🔍
   ● **S35.532**   Injury of left uterine artery ♀ A 🔍, 🔍
   ● **S35.533**   Injury of unspecified uterine artery ♀ A 🔍, 🔍
   ● **S35.534**   Injury of right uterine vein ♀ A 🔍, 🔍
   ● **S35.535**   Injury of left uterine vein ♀ A 🔍, 🔍
   ● **S35.536**   Injury of unspecified uterine vein ♀ A 🔍, 🔍

X ● **S35.59**   Injury of other iliac blood vessels A 🔍, 🔍
> (Ex:) See S35.50

● **S35.8**   **Injury of other blood vessels at abdomen, lower back and pelvis level**
> Injury of ovarian artery or vein
> (Ex:) For category S35.8 CC codes: S35.8X1-S35.99X[A], T14.8-T14.91, T79.8XX-T79.9XX[A], T79.A0X[A], T79.A3X-T79.A9X[A]

● **S35.8X**   Injury of other blood vessels at abdomen, lower back and pelvis level

   ● **S35.8X1**   Laceration of other blood vessels at abdomen, lower back and pelvis level A 🔍, 🔍
   ● **S35.8X8**   Other specified injury of other blood vessels at abdomen, lower back and pelvis level A 🔍, 🔍
   ● **S35.8X9**   Unspecified injury of other blood vessels at abdomen, lower back and pelvis level A 🔍, 🔍

● **S35.9**   **Injury of unspecified blood vessel at abdomen, lower back and pelvis level**
> (Ex:) For category S35.9 CC codes: S35.00X-S35.99X[A], T14.8-T14.91, T79.8XX-T79.9XX[A], T79.A0X[A], T79.A3X-T79.A9X[A]

X ● **S35.90**   Unspecified injury of unspecified blood vessel at abdomen, lower back and pelvis level A 🔍, 🔍
X ● **S35.91**   Laceration of unspecified blood vessel at abdomen, lower back and pelvis level A 🔍, 🔍
X ● **S35.99**   Other specified injury of unspecified blood vessel at abdomen, lower back and pelvis level A 🔍, 🔍

● **S36**   **Injury of intra-abdominal organs**
> The appropriate 7th character is to be added to each code from category S36

A	initial encounter
D	subsequent encounter
S	sequela

> Code also any associated open wound (S31.-)

● **S36.0**   **Injury of spleen**
> (Ex:) For category S36.0 CC codes: S31.001[A], S31.011[A], S31.021[A], S31.031[A], S31.041[A], S31.051[A], S31.100-S31.159[A], S31.600-S31.659[A], S31.831-S31.839[A], S36.00X-S36.09X[A], S36.81X-S36.99X[A], S38.3XX[A], S39.021-S39.023[A], T14.8-T14.91, T79.8XX-T79.9XX[A], T79.A0X-T79.A9X[A]

X ● **S36.00**   Unspecified injury of spleen A 🔍, 🔍
● **S36.02**   Contusion of spleen

   ● **S36.020**   Minor contusion of spleen A 🔍, 🔍
     Contusion of spleen less than 2 cm
   ● **S36.021**   Major contusion of spleen A 🔍, 🔍
     Contusion of spleen greater than 2 cm
   ● **S36.029**   Unspecified contusion of spleen A 🔍, 🔍

● **S36.03**   Laceration of spleen

   ● **S36.030**   Superficial (capsular) laceration of spleen A 🔍, 🔍
     Laceration of spleen less than 1 cm
     Minor laceration of spleen
   ● **S36.031**   Moderate laceration of spleen A 🔍, 🔍
     Laceration of spleen 1 to 3 cm
   ● **S36.032**   Major laceration of spleen A 🔍, 🔍
     Avulsion of spleen
     Laceration of spleen greater than 3 cm
     Massive laceration of spleen
     Multiple moderate lacerations of spleen
     Stellate laceration of spleen
   ● **S36.039**   Unspecified laceration of spleen A 🔍, 🔍

X ● **S36.09**   Other injury of spleen A 🔍, 🔍

● **S36.1**   **Injury of liver and gallbladder and bile duct**

● **S36.11**   Injury of liver
> (Ex:) For category S36.11 CC codes: S31.001[A], S31.011[A], S31.021[A], S31.031[A], S31.041[A], S31.051[A], S31.100-S31.159[A], S31.600-S31.659[A], S31.831-S31.839[A], S36.112-S36.119[A], S36.81X-S36.99X[A], S38.3XX[A], S39.021-S39.023[A], T14.8-T14.91, T79.8XX-T79.9XX[A], T79.A0XA-T79.A9X[A]

   ● **S36.112**   Contusion of liver A 🔍, 🔍
   ● **S36.113**   Laceration of liver, unspecified degree A 🔍, 🔍
   ● **S36.114**   Minor laceration of liver A 🔍, 🔍
     Laceration involving capsule only, or, without significant involvement of hepatic parenchyma [i.e., less than 1 cm deep]
   ● **S36.115**   Moderate laceration of liver A 🔍, 🔍
     Laceration involving parenchyma but without major disruption of parenchyma [i.e., less than 10 cm long and less than 3 cm deep]

◀ New   ◀▥ Revised   ~~deleted~~ Deleted   Excludes 1   Excludes 2   Includes   Use additional   Code first   Code also   Unspecified

OGCR Official Guidelines   ● Unacceptable Principal Diagnosis   X Assign placeholder X   ● Use Additional Character(s)   ▷ Manifestation Code   **Coding Clinic**

- ● S36.116   Major laceration of liver A 🔹, 🔹
  Laceration with significant disruption of hepatic parenchyma [i.e., greater than 10 cm long and 3 cm deep]
  Multiple moderate lacerations, with or without hematoma
  Stellate laceration of liver
- ● S36.118   Other injury of liver A 🔹, 🔹
- ● S36.119   Unspecified injury of liver A 🔹, 🔹
- ● S36.12   Injury of gallbladder
  - (Ex:) For category S36.12 CC codes: S31.001[A], S31.011[A], S31.021[A], S31.031[A], S31.041[A], S31.051[A], S31.100-S31.159[A], S31.600-S31.659[A], S31.831-S31.839[A], S36.122-S36.13X[A], S36.81X-S36.99X[A], S38.3XX[A], S39.021-S39.023[A], T14.8-T14.91, T79.8XX-T79.9XX[A], T79.A0X-T79.A9X[A]
  - ● S36.122   Contusion of gallbladder A 🔹, 🔹
  - ● S36.123   Laceration of gallbladder A 🔹, 🔹
  - ● S36.128   Other injury of gallbladder A 🔹, 🔹
  - ● S36.129   Unspecified injury of gallbladder A 🔹, 🔹
- X ● S36.13   Injury of bile duct A 🔹, 🔹
  - (Ex:) See S36.12
- ● S36.2   Injury of pancreas
  - (Ex:) For category S36.2 CC codes: M79.A3, S31.001[A], S31.011[A], S31.021[A], S31.031[A], S31.041[A], S31.051[A], S31.100-S31.159[A], S31.600-S31.659[A], S31.831-S31.839[A], S36.200-S36.299[A], S36.81X-S36.99X[A], S38.3XX[A], S39.021-S39.023[A], T14.8-T14.91, T79.8XX-T79.9XX[A], T79.A3X-T79.A9X[A]
  - S36.20   Unspecified injury of pancreas
    - ● S36.200   Unspecified injury of head of pancreas A 🔹, 🔹
    - ● S36.201   Unspecified injury of body of pancreas A 🔹, 🔹
    - ● S36.202   Unspecified injury of tail of pancreas A 🔹, 🔹
    - ● S36.209   Unspecified injury of unspecified part of pancreas A 🔹, 🔹
  - ● S36.22   Contusion of pancreas
    - ● S36.220   Contusion of head of pancreas A 🔹, 🔹
    - ● S36.221   Contusion of body of pancreas A 🔹, 🔹
    - ● S36.222   Contusion of tail of pancreas A 🔹, 🔹
    - ● S36.229   Contusion of unspecified part of pancreas A 🔹, 🔹
  - ● S36.23   Laceration of pancreas, unspecified degree
    - ● S36.230   Laceration of head of pancreas, unspecified degree A 🔹, 🔹
    - ● S36.231   Laceration of body of pancreas, unspecified degree A 🔹, 🔹
    - ● S36.232   Laceration of tail of pancreas, unspecified degree A 🔹, 🔹
    - ● S36.239   Laceration of unspecified part of pancreas, unspecified degree A 🔹, 🔹
  - ● S36.24   Minor laceration of pancreas
    - ● S36.240   Minor laceration of head of pancreas A 🔹, 🔹
    - ● S36.241   Minor laceration of body of pancreas A 🔹, 🔹
    - ● S36.242   Minor laceration of tail of pancreas A 🔹, 🔹
    - ● S36.249   Minor laceration of unspecified part of pancreas A 🔹, 🔹

- ● S36.25   Moderate laceration of pancreas
  - ● S36.250   Moderate laceration of head of pancreas A 🔹, 🔹
  - ● S36.251   Moderate laceration of body of pancreas A 🔹, 🔹
  - ● S36.252   Moderate laceration of tail of pancreas A 🔹, 🔹
  - ● S36.259   Moderate laceration of unspecified part of pancreas A 🔹, 🔹
- ● S36.26   Major laceration of pancreas
  - ● S36.260   Major laceration of head of pancreas A 🔹, 🔹
  - ● S36.261   Major laceration of body of pancreas A 🔹, 🔹
  - ● S36.262   Major laceration of tail of pancreas A 🔹, 🔹
  - ● S36.269   Major laceration of unspecified part of pancreas A 🔹, 🔹
- ● S36.29   Other injury of pancreas
  - ● S36.290   Other injury of head of pancreas A 🔹, 🔹
  - ● S36.291   Other injury of body of pancreas A 🔹, 🔹
  - ● S36.292   Other injury of tail of pancreas A 🔹, 🔹
  - ● S36.299   Other injury of unspecified part of pancreas A 🔹, 🔹
- ● S36.3   Injury of stomach
  - (Ex:) For category S36.3 CC codes: M79.A3, S31.001[A], S31.011[A], S31.021[A], S31.031[A], S31.041[A], S31.051[A], S31.100-S31.159[A], S31.600-S31.659[A], S31.831-S31.839[A], S36.30X-S36.39X[A], S36.81X-S36.99X[A], S38.3XX[A], S39.021-S39.023[A], T14.8-T14.91, T79.8XX-T799.XX[A], T79.A3X-T79.A9X[A]
  - X ● S36.30   Unspecified injury of stomach A 🔹, 🔹
  - X ● S36.32   Contusion of stomach A 🔹, 🔹
  - X ● S36.33   Laceration of stomach A 🔹, 🔹
  - X ● S36.39   Other injury of stomach A 🔹, 🔹
- ● S36.4   Injury of small intestine
  - (Ex:) For category S36.4 CC codes: M79.A3, S31.001[A], S31.011[A], S31.021[A], S31.031[A], S31.041[A], S31.051[A], S31.100-S31.159[A], S31.600-S31.659[A], S31.831-S31.839[A], S36.400-S36.499[A], S36.81X-S36.99X[A], S38.3XX[A], S39.021-S39.023[A], T14.8-T14.91, T79.8XX-T79.9XX[A], T79.A3X-T79.A9X[A]
  - ● S36.40   Unspecified injury of small intestine
    - ● S36.400   Unspecified injury of duodenum A 🔹, 🔹
    - ● S36.408   Unspecified injury of other part of small intestine A 🔹, 🔹
    - ● S36.409   Unspecified injury of unspecified part of small intestine A 🔹, 🔹
  - ● S36.41   Primary blast injury of small intestine
    Blast injury of small intestine NOS
    - ● S36.410   Primary blast injury of duodenum A 🔹, 🔹
    - ● S36.418   Primary blast injury of other part of small intestine A 🔹, 🔹
    - ● S36.419   Primary blast injury of unspecified part of small intestine A 🔹, 🔹
  - ● S36.42   Contusion of small intestine
    - ● S36.420   Contusion of duodenum A 🔹, 🔹
    - ● S36.428   Contusion of other part of small intestine A 🔹, 🔹
    - ● S36.429   Contusion of unspecified part of small intestine A 🔹, 🔹

N Newborn Age: 0   **P** Pediatric Age: 0–17   **M** Maternity DX: 12–55   **A** Adult Age: 15–124   ♀ Females Only   ♂ Males Only

🔹 Complication\Comorbidity   🔹 Major C\C   (Ex:) CC/MCC Exclusions   Present on Admission Requirement   🔹 Hospital-Acquired Condition

1341

CHAPTER 19 (S00-T88)

● **S36.43** Laceration of small intestine
  ● **S36.430** Laceration of duodenum A 🦠, 🦠
  ● **S36.438** Laceration of other part of small intestine A 🦠, 🦠
  ● **S36.439** Laceration of unspecified part of small intestine A 🦠, 🦠
● **S36.49** Other injury of small intestine
  ● **S36.490** Other injury of duodenum A 🦠, 🦠
  ● **S36.498** Other injury of other part of small intestine A 🦠, 🦠
  ● **S36.499** Other injury of unspecified part of small intestine A 🦠, 🦠
● **S36.5** Injury of colon
  Excludes2 injury of rectum (S36.6-)
  Ⓔⓧ **For category S36.5 CC codes:** M79.A3, S31.001[A], S31.011[A], S31.021[A], S31.031[A], S31.041[A], S31.051[A], S31.100-S31.159[A], S31.600-S31.659[A], S31.831-S31.839[A], S36.500-S36.99X[A], S38.3XX[A], S39.021-S39.023[A], T14.8-T14.91, T79.8XX-T79.9XX[A], T79.A3X-T79.A9X[A]
● **S36.50** Unspecified injury of colon
  ● **S36.500** Unspecified injury of ascending [right] colon A 🦠, 🦠
  ● **S36.501** Unspecified injury of transverse colon A 🦠, 🦠
  ● **S36.502** Unspecified injury of descending [left] colon A 🦠, 🦠
  ● **S36.503** Unspecified injury of sigmoid colon A 🦠, 🦠
  ● **S36.508** Unspecified injury of other part of colon A 🦠, 🦠
  ● **S36.509** Unspecified injury of unspecified part of colon A 🦠, 🦠
● **S36.51** Primary blast injury of colon
  Blast injury of colon NOS
  ● **S36.510** Primary blast injury of ascending [right] colon A 🦠, 🦠
  ● **S36.511** Primary blast injury of transverse colon A 🦠, 🦠
  ● **S36.512** Primary blast injury of descending [left] colon A 🦠, 🦠
  ● **S36.513** Primary blast injury of sigmoid colon A 🦠, 🦠
  ● **S36.518** Primary blast injury of other part of colon A 🦠, 🦠
  ● **S36.519** Primary blast injury of unspecified part of colon A 🦠, 🦠
● **S36.52** Contusion of colon
  ● **S36.520** Contusion of ascending [right] colon A 🦠, 🦠
  ● **S36.521** Contusion of transverse colon A 🦠, 🦠
  ● **S36.522** Contusion of descending [left] colon A 🦠, 🦠
  ● **S36.523** Contusion of sigmoid colon A 🦠, 🦠
  ● **S36.528** Contusion of other part of colon A 🦠, 🦠
  ● **S36.529** Contusion of unspecified part of colon A 🦠, 🦠

● **S36.53** Laceration of colon
  ● **S36.530** Laceration of ascending [right] colon A 🦠, 🦠
  ● **S36.531** Laceration of transverse colon A 🦠, 🦠
  ● **S36.532** Laceration of descending [left] colon A 🦠, 🦠
  ● **S36.533** Laceration of sigmoid colon A 🦠, 🦠
  ● **S36.538** Laceration of other part of colon A 🦠, 🦠
  S36.539 Laceration of unspecified part of colon A 🦠, 🦠
● **S36.59** Other injury of colon
  Secondary blast injury of colon
  ● **S36.590** Other injury of ascending [right] colon A 🦠, 🦠
  ● **S36.591** Other injury of transverse colon A 🦠, 🦠
  ● **S36.592** Other injury of descending [left] colon A 🦠, 🦠
  ● **S36.593** Other injury of sigmoid colon A 🦠, 🦠
  ● **S36.598** Other injury of other part of colon A 🦠, 🦠
  ● **S36.599** Other injury of unspecified part of colon A 🦠, 🦠
● **S36.6** Injury of rectum
  Ⓔⓧ **For category S36.6 CC codes:** See S36.5
  X ● **S36.60** Unspecified injury of rectum A 🦠, 🦠
  X ● **S36.61** Primary blast injury of rectum A 🦠, 🦠
        Blast injury of rectum NOS
  X ● **S36.62** Contusion of rectum A 🦠, 🦠
  X ● **S36.63** Laceration of rectum A 🦠, 🦠
  X ● **S36.69** Other injury of rectum A 🦠, 🦠
        Secondary blast injury of rectum
● **S36.8** Injury of other intra-abdominal organs
  Ⓔⓧ **For category S36.8 CC codes:** S31.001[A], S31.011[A], S31.021[A], S31.031[A], S31.041[A], S31.051[A], S31.100-S31.159[A], S31.600-S31.659[A], S31.831-S31.839[A], S36.81X-S36.99X[A], S38.3XX[A], S39.021-S39.023[A], T14.8-T14.91, T79.8XX-T79.9XX[A], T79.A0X-T79.A9X[A]
  ● **S36.81** Injury of peritoneum A 🦠, 🦠
  ● **S36.89** Injury of other intra-abdominal organs
        Injury of retroperitoneum
    ● **S36.892** Contusion of other intra-abdominal organs A 🦠, 🦠
    ● **S36.893** Laceration of other intra-abdominal organs A 🦠, 🦠
    ● **S36.898** Other injury of other intra-abdominal organs A 🦠, 🦠
    S36.899 Unspecified injury of other intra-abdominal organs A 🦠, 🦠
● **S36.9** Injury of unspecified intra-abdominal organ
  Ⓔⓧ **For category S36.9 CC codes:** See S36.8
  X ● **S36.90** Unspecified injury of unspecified intra-abdominal organ A 🦠, 🦠
  X ● **S36.92** Contusion of unspecified intra-abdominal organ A 🦠, 🦠
  X ● **S36.93** Laceration of unspecified intra-abdominal organ A 🦠, 🦠
  X ● **S36.99** Other injury of unspecified intra-abdominal organ A 🦠, 🦠

CHAPTER 19 (S00-T88)

◀ New   ◀ⁿ Revised   ~~deleted~~ Deleted | Excludes 1 | | Excludes 2 | | Includes | | Use additional | | Code first | | Code also | | Unspecified |
OGCR Official Guidelines   ● Unacceptable Principal Diagnosis   X Assign placeholder X   ● Use Additional Character(s)   ▶ Manifestation Code   **Coding Clinic**

● S37   **Injury of urinary and pelvic organs**
    Code also any associated open wound (S31.-)
    Excludes1   obstetric trauma to pelvic organs (O71.-) ◄▦
    Excludes2   injury of peritoneum (S36.81)
                injury of retroperitoneum (S36.89-)

    The appropriate 7th character is to be added to each code from
      category S37

> A   initial encounter
> D   subsequent encounter
> S   sequela

● S37.0   **Injury of kidney**
    Excludes2   acute kidney injury (nontraumatic)
                (N17.9)
    Ⓔⓧ For category S37.0 CC codes: S31.001[A], S31.011[A], S31.021[A],
        S31.031[A], S31.041[A], S31.051[A], S31.100-S31.159[A],
        S31.600-S31.659[A], S31.831-S31.839[A], S36.81X-S37.099[A],
        S38.3XX[A], S39.021-S39.023[A], T14.8-T14.91, T79.8XX-T79.9XX[A], T79.
        A0X-T79.A9X[A]

    ● S37.00   **Unspecified injury of kidney**
       ● S37.001   Unspecified injury of right kidney
                A 🝕, 🝕
       ● S37.002   Unspecified injury of left kidney
                A 🝕, 🝕
       ● S37.009   Unspecified injury of unspecified
                kidney A 🝕, 🝕

    ● S37.01   **Minor contusion of kidney**
       Contusion of kidney less than 2 cm
       Contusion of kidney NOS
       ● S37.011   Minor contusion of right kidney
                A 🝕, 🝕
       ● S37.012   Minor contusion of left kidney
                A 🝕, 🝕
       ● S37.019   Minor contusion of unspecified
                kidney A 🝕, 🝕

    ● S37.02   **Major contusion of kidney**
       Contusion of kidney greater than 2 cm
       ● S37.021   Major contusion of right kidney
                A 🝕, 🝕
       ● S37.022   Major contusion of left kidney
                A 🝕, 🝕
       ● S37.029   Major contusion of unspecified
                kidney A 🝕, 🝕

    ● S37.03   **Laceration of kidney, unspecified degree**
       ● S37.031   Laceration of right kidney,
                unspecified degree A 🝕, 🝕
       ● S37.032   Laceration of left kidney, unspecified
                degree A 🝕, 🝕
       ● S37.039   Laceration of unspecified kidney,
                unspecified degree A 🝕, 🝕

    ● S37.04   **Minor laceration of kidney**
       Laceration of kidney less than 1 cm
       ● S37.041   Minor laceration of right kidney
                A 🝕, 🝕
       ● S37.042   Minor laceration of left kidney
                A 🝕, 🝕
       ● S37.049   Minor laceration of unspecified
                kidney A 🝕, 🝕

    ● S37.05   **Moderate laceration of kidney**
       Laceration of kidney 1 to 3 cm
       ● S37.051   Moderate laceration of right kidney
                A 🝕, 🝕
       ● S37.052   Moderate laceration of left kidney
                A 🝕, 🝕
       ● S37.059   Moderate laceration of unspecified
                kidney A 🝕, 🝕

    ● S37.06   **Major laceration of kidney**
       Avulsion of kidney
       Laceration of kidney greater than 3 cm
       Massive laceration of kidney
       Multiple moderate lacerations of kidney
       Stellate laceration of kidney
       ● S37.061   Major laceration of right kidney
                A 🝕, 🝕
       ● S37.062   Major laceration of left kidney
                A 🝕, 🝕
       ● S37.069   Major laceration of unspecified
                kidney A 🝕, 🝕

    ● S37.09   **Other injury of kidney**
       ● S37.091   Other injury of right kidney A 🝕, 🝕
       ● S37.092   Other injury of left kidney A 🝕, 🝕
       ● S37.099   Other injury of unspecified kidney
                A 🝕, 🝕

● S37.1   **Injury of ureter**
    Ⓔⓧ For category S37.1 CC codes: S31.001[A], S31.011[A], S31.021[A],
        S31.031[A], S31.041[A], S31.051[A], S31.100-S31.159[A],
        S31.600-S31.659[A], S31.831-S31.839[A], S36.81X-S36.99X[A],
        S37.10X-S37.19X[A], S37.401-S37.599[A], S37.822-S37.99X[A],
        S38.3XX[A], S39.021-S39.023[A], T14.8-T14.91, T79.8XX-T79.9XX[A], T79.
        A0X-T79.A9X[A]

    X ● S37.10   Unspecified injury of ureter A 🝕, 🝕
    X ● S37.12   Contusion of ureter A 🝕, 🝕
    X ● S37.13   Laceration of ureter A 🝕, 🝕
    X ● S37.19   Other injury of ureter A 🝕, 🝕

● S37.2   **Injury of bladder**
    Ⓔⓧ For category S37.2 CC codes: S31.001[A], S31.011[A], S31.021[A],
        S31.031[A], S31.041[A], S31.051[A], S31.100-S31.159[A],
        S31.600-S31.659[A], S31.831-S31.839[A], S36.81X-S36.99X[A],
        S37.20X-S37.599[A], S37.822-S37.99X[A], S38.3XX[A],
        S39.021-S39.023[A], T14.8-T14.91, T79.8XX-T79.9XX[A], T79.A0X-T79.
        A9X[A]

    X ● S37.20   Unspecified injury of bladder A 🝕, 🝕
    X ● S37.22   Contusion of bladder A 🝕, 🝕
    X ● S37.23   Laceration of bladder A 🝕, 🝕
    X ● S37.29   Other injury of bladder A 🝕, 🝕

● S37.3   **Injury of urethra**
    Ⓔⓧ For category S37.3 CC codes: See S37.2
    X ● S37.30   Unspecified injury of urethra A 🝕, 🝕
    X ● S37.32   Contusion of urethra A 🝕, 🝕
    X ● S37.33   Laceration of urethra A 🝕, 🝕
    X ● S37.39   Other injury of urethra A 🝕, 🝕

● S37.4   **Injury of ovary**
    ● S37.40   **Unspecified injury of ovary**
       ● S37.401   Unspecified injury of ovary,
                unilateral ♀🝕
       ● S37.402   Unspecified injury of ovary,
                bilateral ♀🝕
       ● S37.409   Unspecified injury of ovary,
                unspecified ♀🝕

    ● S37.42   **Contusion of ovary**
       ● S37.421   Contusion of ovary, unilateral ♀🝕
       ● S37.422   Contusion of ovary, bilateral ♀🝕
       ● S37.429   Contusion of ovary, unspecified ♀🝕

    ● S37.43   **Laceration of ovary**
       ● S37.431   Laceration of ovary, unilateral ♀🝕
       ● S37.432   Laceration of ovary, bilateral ♀🝕
       ● S37.439   Laceration of ovary, unspecified ♀🝕

    ● S37.49   **Other injury of ovary**
       ● S37.491   Other injury of ovary, unilateral ♀🝕
       ● S37.492   Other injury of ovary, bilateral ♀🝕
       ● S37.499   Other injury of ovary, unspecified ♀🝕

N   Newborn Age: 0   **P**   Pediatric Age: 0–17   **M**   Maternity DX: 12–55   **A**   Adult Age: 15–124   ♀   Females Only   ♂   Males Only

🝕 Complication\Comorbidity   🝕 Major C\C   Ⓔⓧ CC/MCC Exclusions   🝕 Present on Admission Requirement   🝕 Hospital-Acquired Condition   **1343**

● **S37.5**   **Injury of fallopian tube**

  ● **S37.50**   Unspecified injury of fallopian tube

    ● **S37.501**   Unspecified injury of fallopian tube, unilateral ♀ 🅒

    ● **S37.502**   Unspecified injury of fallopian tube, bilateral ♀ 🅒

    ● **S37.509**   Unspecified injury of fallopian tube, unspecified ♀ 🅒

  ● **S37.51**   Primary blast injury of fallopian tube

    Blast injury of fallopian tube NOS

    ● **S37.511**   Primary blast injury of fallopian tube, unilateral ♀ 🅒

    ● **S37.512**   Primary blast injury of fallopian tube, bilateral ♀ 🅒

    ● **S37.519**   Primary blast injury of fallopian tube, unspecified ♀ 🅒

  ● **S37.52**   Contusion of fallopian tube

    ● **S37.521**   Contusion of fallopian tube, unilateral ♀ 🅒

    ● **S37.522**   Contusion of fallopian tube, bilateral ♀ 🅒

    ● **S37.529**   Contusion of fallopian tube, unspecified ♀ 🅒

  ● **S37.53**   Laceration of fallopian tube

    ● **S37.531**   Laceration of fallopian tube, unilateral ♀ 🅒

    ● **S37.532**   Laceration of fallopian tube, bilateral ♀ 🅒

    ● **S37.539**   Laceration of fallopian tube, unspecified ♀ 🅒

  ● **S37.59**   Other injury of fallopian tube

    Secondary blast injury of fallopian tube

    ● **S37.591**   Other injury of fallopian tube, unilateral ♀ 🅒

    ● **S37.592**   Other injury of fallopian tube, bilateral ♀ 🅒

    ● **S37.599**   Other injury of fallopian tube, unspecified ♀ 🅒

● **S37.6**   **Injury of uterus**

  Excludes1   injury to gravid uterus (O9A.2-)

    injury to uterus during delivery (O71.-)

  Ⓔ **For category S37.6 CC codes:** S31.001[A], S31.011[A], S31.021[A], S31.031[A], S31.041[A], S31.051[A], S31.100-S31.159[A], S31.600-S31.659[A], S31.831-S31.839[A], S36.81X-S36.99X[A], S37.401-S37.69X[A], S37.822-S37.99X[A], S38.3XX[A], S39.021-S39.023[A], T14.8-T14.91, T79.8XX-T79.9XX[A], T79.A0X-T79.A9X[A]

  X ● **S37.60**   Unspecified injury of uterus ♀ A 🅒, 🅒

  X ● **S37.62**   Contusion of uterus ♀ A 🅒, 🅒

  X ● **S37.63**   Laceration of uterus ♀ A 🅒, 🅒

  X ● **S37.69**   Other injury of uterus ♀ A 🅒, 🅒

● **S37.8**   **Injury of other urinary and pelvic organs**

  ● **S37.81**   Injury of adrenal gland

    Ⓔ **For category S37.81 CC codes:** S31.001[A], S31.011[A], S31.021[A], S31.031[A], S31.041[A], S31.051[A], S31.100-S31.159[A], S31.600-S31.659[A], S31.831-S31.839[A], S36.81X-S36.99X[A], S37.812-S37.819[A], S38.3XX[A], S39.021-S39.023[A], T14.8-T14.91, T79.8XX-T79.9XX[A], T79.A0X-T79.A9X[A]

    ● **S37.812**   Contusion of adrenal gland A 🅒, 🅒

    ● **S37.813**   Laceration of adrenal gland A 🅒, 🅒

    ● **S37.818**   Other injury of adrenal gland A 🅒, 🅒

    ● **S37.819**   Unspecified injury of adrenal gland A 🅒, 🅒

  ● **S37.82**   Injury of prostate

    ● **S37.822**   Contusion of prostate ♂ 🅒

    ● **S37.823**   Laceration of prostate ♂ 🅒

    ● **S37.828**   Other injury of prostate ♂ 🅒

    ● **S37.829**   Unspecified injury of prostate ♂ 🅒

● **S37.89**   **Injury of other urinary and pelvic organ**

  Ⓔ **For category S37.89 CC codes:** S31.001[A], S31.011[A], S31.021[A], S31.031[A], S31.041[A], S31.051[A], S31.100-S31.159[A], S31.600-S31.659[A], S31.831-S31.839[A], S36.81X-S36.99X[A], S37.401-S37.599[A], S37.822-S37.99[A], S38.3XX[A], S39.021-S39.023[A], T14.8-T14.91, T79.8XX-T79.9XX[A], T79.A0X-T79.A9X[A]

  ● **S37.892**   Contusion of other urinary and pelvic organ A 🅒, 🅒

  ● **S37.893**   Laceration of other urinary and pelvic organ A 🅒, 🅒

  ● **S37.898**   Other injury of other urinary and pelvic organ A 🅒, 🅒

  ● **S37.899**   Unspecified injury of other urinary and pelvic organ A 🅒, 🅒

● **S37.9**   **Injury of unspecified urinary and pelvic organ**

  Ⓔ **For category S37.9 CC codes:** See S37.89

  X ● **S37.90**   Unspecified injury of unspecified urinary and pelvic organ A 🅒, 🅒

  X ● **S37.92**   Contusion of unspecified urinary and pelvic organ A 🅒, 🅒

  X ● **S37.93**   Laceration of unspecified urinary and pelvic organ A 🅒, 🅒

  X ● **S37.99**   Other injury of unspecified urinary and pelvic organ A 🅒, 🅒

● **S38**   **Crushing injury and traumatic amputation of abdomen, lower back, pelvis and external genitals**

  An amputation not identified as partial or complete should be coded to complete

  The appropriate 7th character is to be added to each code from category S38

A	initial encounter
D	subsequent encounter
S	sequela

● **S38.0**   **Crushing injury of external genital organs**

  Use additional code for any associated injuries

  ● **S38.00**   Crushing injury of unspecified external genital organs

    ● **S38.001**   Crushing injury of unspecified external genital organs, male ♂ 🅒

    ● **S38.002**   Crushing injury of unspecified external genital organs, female ♀ 🅒

  X ● **S38.01**   Crushing injury of penis ♂ 🅒

  X ● **S38.02**   Crushing injury of scrotum and testis ♂ 🅒

  X ● **S38.03**   Crushing injury of vulva ♀ 🅒

X ● **S38.1**   **Crushing injury of abdomen, lower back, and pelvis** 🅒

  Use additional code for all associated injuries, such as:

    fracture of thoracic or lumbar spine and pelvis (S22.0-, S32.-)

    injury to intra-abdominal organs (S36.-)

    injury to urinary and pelvic organs (S37.-)

    open wound of abdominal wall (S31.-) ◀▥

    spinal cord injury (S34.0, S34.1-)

  Excludes2   crushing injury of external genital organs (S38.0-) ◀▥

● **S38.2**   **Traumatic amputation of external genital organs**

  ● **S38.21**   Traumatic amputation of female external genital organs

    Traumatic amputation of clitoris

    Traumatic amputation of labium (majus) (minus)

    Traumatic amputation of vulva

    ● **S38.211**   Complete traumatic amputation of female external genital organs ♀ 🅒

    ● **S38.212**   Partial traumatic amputation of female external genital organs ♀ 🅒

◀ New   ◀▥ Revised   ~~deleted~~ Deleted   Excludes 1   Excludes 2   Includes   Use additional   Code first   Code also   Unspecified

OGCR Official Guidelines   ● Unacceptable Principal Diagnosis   X Assign placeholder X   ● Use Additional Character(s)   ▸ Manifestation Code   **Coding Clinic**

- S38.22   Traumatic amputation of penis
  - S38.221   Complete traumatic amputation of penis ♂
  - S38.222   Partial traumatic amputation of penis ♂
- S38.23   Traumatic amputation of scrotum and testis
  - S38.231   Complete traumatic amputation of scrotum and testis ♂
  - S38.232   Partial traumatic amputation of scrotum and testis ♂
- X ● S38.3   Transection (partial) of abdomen

- ● S39   **Other and unspecified injuries of abdomen, lower back, pelvis and external genitals**

  Code also any associated open wound (S31.-)

  Excludes2   sprain of joints and ligaments of lumbar spine and pelvis (S33.-)

  The appropriate 7th character is to be added to each code from category S39

A	initial encounter
D	subsequent encounter
S	sequela

  - S39.0   Injury of muscle, fascia and tendon of abdomen, lower back and pelvis
    - S39.00   Unspecified injury of muscle, fascia and tendon of abdomen, lower back and pelvis
      - S39.001   Unspecified injury of muscle, fascia and tendon of abdomen
      - S39.002   Unspecified injury of muscle, fascia and tendon of lower back
      - S39.003   Unspecified injury of muscle, fascia and tendon of pelvis
    - S39.01   Strain of muscle, fascia and tendon of abdomen, lower back and pelvis
      - S39.011   Strain of muscle, fascia and tendon of abdomen
      - S39.012   Strain of muscle, fascia and tendon of lower back
      - S39.013   Strain of muscle, fascia and tendon of pelvis
    - S39.02   Laceration of muscle, fascia and tendon of abdomen, lower back and pelvis
      - S39.021   Laceration of muscle, fascia and tendon of abdomen
      - S39.022   Laceration of muscle, fascia and tendon of lower back
      - S39.023   Laceration of muscle, fascia and tendon of pelvis
    - S39.09   Other injury of muscle, fascia and tendon of abdomen, lower back and pelvis
      - S39.091   Other injury of muscle, fascia and tendon of abdomen
      - S39.092   Other injury of muscle, fascia and tendon of lower back
      - S39.093   Other injury of muscle, fascia and tendon of pelvis
  - S39.8   Other specified injuries of abdomen, lower back, pelvis and external genitals
    - X ● S39.81   Other specified injuries of abdomen
    - X ● S39.82   Other specified injuries of lower back
    - X ● S39.83   Other specified injuries of pelvis
    - S39.84   Other specified injuries of external genitals
      - S39.840   Fracture of corpus cavernosum penis ♂
      - S39.848   Other specified injuries of external genitals

- ● S39.9   Unspecified injury of abdomen, lower back, pelvis and external genitals
  - X ● S39.91   Unspecified injury of abdomen
  - X ● S39.92   Unspecified injury of lower back
  - X ● S39.93   Unspecified injury of pelvis
  - X ● S39.94   Unspecified injury of external genitals

INJURIES TO THE SHOULDER AND UPPER ARM (S40-S49)

Includes	injuries of axilla injuries of scapular region
Excludes2	burns and corrosions (T20-T32)
	frostbite (T33-T34)
	injuries of elbow (S50-S59)
	insect bite or sting, venomous (T63.4)

- ● S40   **Superficial injury of shoulder and upper arm**

  The appropriate 7th character is to be added to each code from category S40

A	initial encounter
D	subsequent encounter
S	sequela

  - S40.0   Contusion of shoulder and upper arm
    - S40.01   Contusion of shoulder
      - S40.011   Contusion of right shoulder
      - S40.012   Contusion of left shoulder
      - S40.019   Contusion of unspecified shoulder
    - S40.02   Contusion of upper arm
      - S40.021   Contusion of right upper arm
      - S40.022   Contusion of left upper arm
      - S40.029   Contusion of unspecified upper arm
  - S40.2   Other superficial injuries of shoulder
    - S40.21   Abrasion of shoulder
      - S40.211   Abrasion of right shoulder
      - S40.212   Abrasion of left shoulder
      - S40.219   Abrasion of unspecified shoulder
    - S40.22   Blister (nonthermal) of shoulder
      - S40.221   Blister (nonthermal) of right shoulder
      - S40.222   Blister (nonthermal) of left shoulder
      - S40.229   Blister (nonthermal) of unspecified shoulder
    - S40.24   External constriction of shoulder
      - S40.241   External constriction of right shoulder
      - S40.242   External constriction of left shoulder
      - S40.249   External constriction of unspecified shoulder
    - S40.25   Superficial foreign body of shoulder
      Splinter in the shoulder
      - S40.251   Superficial foreign body of right shoulder
      - S40.252   Superficial foreign body of left shoulder
      - S40.259   Superficial foreign body of unspecified shoulder
    - S40.26   Insect bite (nonvenomous) of shoulder
      - S40.261   Insect bite (nonvenomous) of right shoulder
      - S40.262   Insect bite (nonvenomous) of left shoulder
      - S40.269   Insect bite (nonvenomous) of unspecified shoulder

CHAPTER 19 (S00-T88)

● S40.27   Other superficial bite of shoulder
> **Excludes1**   open bite of shoulder (S41.05)

     ● S40.271   Other superficial bite of right shoulder

     ● S40.272   Other superficial bite of left shoulder

     ● S40.279   Other superficial bite of unspecified shoulder

● S40.8   Other superficial injuries of upper arm

   ● S40.81   Abrasion of upper arm

     ● S40.811   Abrasion of right upper arm

     ● S40.812   Abrasion of left upper arm

     ● S40.819   Abrasion of unspecified upper arm

   ● S40.82   Blister (nonthermal) of upper arm

     ● S40.821   Blister (nonthermal) of right upper arm

     ● S40.822   Blister (nonthermal) of left upper arm

     ● S40.829   Blister (nonthermal) of unspecified upper arm

   ● S40.84   External constriction of upper arm

     ● S40.841   External constriction of right upper arm

     ● S40.842   External constriction of left upper arm

     ● S40.849   External constriction of unspecified upper arm

   ● S40.85   Superficial foreign body of upper arm
> Splinter in the upper arm

     ● S40.851   Superficial foreign body of right upper arm

     ● S40.852   Superficial foreign body of left upper arm

     ● S40.859   Superficial foreign body of unspecified upper arm

   ● S40.86   Insect bite (nonvenomous) of upper arm

     ● S40.861   Insect bite (nonvenomous) of right upper arm

     ● S40.862   Insect bite (nonvenomous) of left upper arm

     ● S40.869   Insect bite (nonvenomous) of unspecified upper arm

   ● S40.87   Other superficial bite of upper arm
> **Excludes1**   open bite of upper arm (S41.14)
> **Excludes2**   other superficial bite of shoulder (S40.27-)

     ● S40.871   Other superficial bite of right upper arm

     ● S40.872   Other superficial bite of left upper arm

     ● S40.879   Other superficial bite of unspecified upper arm

● S40.9   Unspecified superficial injury of shoulder and upper arm

   ● S40.91   Unspecified superficial injury of shoulder

     ● S40.911   Unspecified superficial injury of right shoulder

     ● S40.912   Unspecified superficial injury of left shoulder

     ● S40.919   Unspecified superficial injury of unspecified shoulder

   ● S40.92   Unspecified superficial injury of upper arm

     ● S40.921   Unspecified superficial injury of right upper arm

     ● S40.922   Unspecified superficial injury of left upper arm

     ● S40.929   Unspecified superficial injury of unspecified upper arm

● S41   Open wound of shoulder and upper arm
> Code also any associated wound infection
> **Excludes1**   traumatic amputation of shoulder and upper arm (S48.-)
> **Excludes2**   open fracture of shoulder and upper arm (S42.- with 7th character B or C)

The appropriate 7th character is to be added to each code from category S41

> A   initial encounter
> D   subsequent encounter
> S   sequela

   ● S41.0   Open wound of shoulder

     ● S41.00   Unspecified open wound of shoulder

       ● S41.001   Unspecified open wound of right shoulder

       ● S41.002   Unspecified open wound of left shoulder

       ● S41.009   Unspecified open wound of unspecified shoulder

     ● S41.01   Laceration without foreign body of shoulder

       ● S41.011   Laceration without foreign body of right shoulder

       ● S41.012   Laceration without foreign body of left shoulder

       ● S41.019   Laceration without foreign body of unspecified shoulder

     ● S41.02   Laceration with foreign body of shoulder

       ● S41.021   Laceration with foreign body of right shoulder

       ● S41.022   Laceration with foreign body of left shoulder

       ● S41.029   Laceration with foreign body of unspecified shoulder

     ● S41.03   Puncture wound without foreign body of shoulder

       ● S41.031   Puncture wound without foreign body of right shoulder

       ● S41.032   Puncture wound without foreign body of left shoulder

       ● S41.039   Puncture wound without foreign body of unspecified shoulder

● S41.04   Puncture wound with foreign body of shoulder
   ● S41.041   Puncture wound with foreign body of right shoulder🖐
   ● S41.042   Puncture wound with foreign body of left shoulder🖐
   ● S41.049   Puncture wound with foreign body of unspecified shoulder🖐
● S41.05   Open bite of shoulder
     Bite of shoulder NOS
     Excludes1   superficial bite of shoulder (S40.27)
   ● S41.051   Open bite of right shoulder🖐
   ● S41.052   Open bite of left shoulder🖐
   ● S41.059   Open bite of unspecified shoulder🖐

● S41.1   Open wound of upper arm
  ● S41.10   Unspecified open wound of upper arm
   ● S41.101   Unspecified open wound of right upper arm🖐
   ● S41.102   Unspecified open wound of left upper arm🖐
   ● S41.109   Unspecified open wound of unspecified upper arm🖐
  ● S41.11   Laceration without foreign body of upper arm
   ● S41.111   Laceration without foreign body of right upper arm🖐
   ● S41.112   Laceration without foreign body of left upper arm🖐
   ● S41.119   Laceration without foreign body of unspecified upper arm🖐
  ● S41.12   Laceration with foreign body of upper arm
   ● S41.121   Laceration with foreign body of right upper arm🖐
   ● S41.122   Laceration with foreign body of left upper arm🖐
   ● S41.129   Laceration with foreign body of unspecified upper arm🖐
  ● S41.13   Puncture wound without foreign body of upper arm
   ● S41.131   Puncture wound without foreign body of right upper arm🖐
   ● S41.132   Puncture wound without foreign body of left upper arm🖐
   ● S41.139   Puncture wound without foreign body of unspecified upper arm🖐
  ● S41.14   Puncture wound with foreign body of upper arm
   ● S41.141   Puncture wound with foreign body of right upper arm🖐
   ● S41.142   Puncture wound with foreign body of left upper arm🖐
   ● S41.149   Puncture wound with foreign body of unspecified upper arm🖐
  ● S41.15   Open bite of upper arm
     Bite of upper arm NOS
     Excludes1   superficial bite of upper arm (S40.87)
   ● S41.151   Open bite of right upper arm🖐
   ● S41.152   Open bite of left upper arm🖐
   ● S41.159   Open bite of unspecified upper arm🖐

● S42   Fracture of shoulder and upper arm
   Note: A fracture not indicated as displaced or nondisplaced should be coded to displaced
     A fracture not indicated as open or closed should be coded to closed
   Excludes1   traumatic amputation of shoulder and upper arm (S48.-)
   The appropriate 7th character is to be added to all codes from category S42

A	initial encounter for closed fracture
B	initial encounter for open fracture
D	subsequent encounter for fracture with routine healing
G	subsequent encounter for fracture with delayed healing
K	subsequent encounter for fracture with nonunion
P	subsequent encounter for fracture with malunion
S	sequela

● S42.0   Fracture of clavicle
   (Ex) For S42.0[B]: S42.001-S42.036[A,B], S62.90X[B] For S42.0[K,P]: M80.00X-M80.88X[K,P], M84.30X-M84.68X[K,P], S02.0XX-S02.92X[K], S12.000-S12.691[K], S22.000-S22.9XX[K], S32.000-S32.9XX[K], S42.001-S42.92X[K,P], S49.001-S49.199[K,P], S52.001-S52.92X[K,M,N,P,Q,R], S59.001-S59.299[K,P], S62.001-S62.92X[K,P], S72.001-S72.92X[K,M,N,P,Q,R], S79.001-S79.199[K,P], S82.001-S82.92X[K,M,N,P,Q,R], S89.001-S89.399[K,P], S92.001-S92.919[K,P]

  ● S42.00   Fracture of unspecified part of clavicle
   ● S42.001   Fracture of unspecified part of right clavicle B, K, P 🖐, 🖐, B 🖐
   ● S42.002   Fracture of unspecified part of left clavicle B, K, P 🖐, 🖐, B 🖐
   ● S42.009   Fracture of unspecified part of unspecified clavicle B, K, P 🖐, 🖐, B 🖐
     Coding Clinic: 2012, Q4, P3
  ● S42.01   Fracture of sternal end of clavicle
   ● S42.011   Anterior displaced fracture of sternal end of right clavicle B, K, P 🖐, 🖐, B 🖐
   ● S42.012   Anterior displaced fracture of sternal end of left clavicle B, K, P 🖐, 🖐, B 🖐
   ● S42.013   Anterior displaced fracture of sternal end of unspecified clavicle B, K, P 🖐, 🖐, B 🖐
     Displaced fracture of sternal end of clavicle NOS
   ● S42.014   Posterior displaced fracture of sternal end of right clavicle B, K, P 🖐, 🖐, B 🖐
   ● S42.015   Posterior displaced fracture of sternal end of left clavicle B, K, P 🖐, 🖐, B 🖐
   ● S42.016   Posterior displaced fracture of sternal end of unspecified clavicle B, K, P 🖐, 🖐, B 🖐
   ● S42.017   Nondisplaced fracture of sternal end of right clavicle B, K, P 🖐, 🖐, B 🖐
   ● S42.018   Nondisplaced fracture of sternal end of left clavicle B, K, P 🖐, 🖐, B 🖐
   ● S42.019   Nondisplaced fracture of sternal end of unspecified clavicle B, K, P 🖐, 🖐, B 🖐
  ● S42.02   Fracture of shaft of clavicle
   ● S42.021   Displaced fracture of shaft of right clavicle B, K, P 🖐, 🖐, B 🖐
   ● S42.022   Displaced fracture of shaft of left clavicle B, K, P 🖐, 🖐, B 🖐
   ● S42.023   Displaced fracture of shaft of unspecified clavicle B, K, P 🖐, 🖐, B 🖐

N   Newborn Age: 0   P   Pediatric Age: 0–17   M   Maternity DX: 12–55   A   Adult Age: 15–124   ♀   Females Only   ♂   Males Only

🖐 Complication\Comorbidity   🖐 Major C\C   (Ex) CC/MCC Exclusions   🖐 Present on Admission Requirement   🖐 Hospital-Acquired Condition

1347

CHAPTER 19 (S00-T88)

● S42.024   Nondisplaced fracture of shaft of right clavicle B, K, P 🔘, 🔘, B 🔘

● S42.025   Nondisplaced fracture of shaft of left clavicle B, K, P 🔘, 🔘, B 🔘

● S42.026   Nondisplaced fracture of shaft of unspecified clavicle B, K, P 🔘, 🔘, B 🔘

● S42.03   Fracture of lateral end of clavicle
Fracture of acromial end of clavicle

● S42.031   Displaced fracture of lateral end of right clavicle B, K, P 🔘, 🔘, B 🔘

● S42.032   Displaced fracture of lateral end of left clavicle B, K, P 🔘, 🔘, B 🔘

● S42.033   Displaced fracture of lateral end of unspecified clavicle B, K, P 🔘, 🔘, B 🔘

● S42.034   Nondisplaced fracture of lateral end of right clavicle B, K, P 🔘, 🔘, B 🔘

● S42.035   Nondisplaced fracture of lateral end of left clavicle B, K, P 🔘, 🔘, B 🔘

● S42.036   Nondisplaced fracture of lateral end of unspecified clavicle B, K, P 🔘, 🔘, B 🔘

● S42.1   Fracture of scapula
Ⓔⓧ **For S42.1[B]:** S42.101-S42.199[A,B], S62.90X[B] **For S42.1[K,P]:** See S42.0[K,P]

● S42.10   Fracture of unspecified part of scapula

● S42.101   Fracture of unspecified part of scapula, right shoulder B, K, P 🔘, 🔘, B 🔘

● S42.102   Fracture of unspecified part of scapula, left shoulder B, K, P 🔘, 🔘, B 🔘

● S42.109   Fracture of unspecified part of scapula, unspecified shoulder B, K, P 🔘, 🔘, B 🔘

● S42.11   Fracture of body of scapula

● S42.111   Displaced fracture of body of scapula, right shoulder B, K, P 🔘, 🔘, B 🔘

● S42.112   Displaced fracture of body of scapula, left shoulder B, K, P 🔘, 🔘, B 🔘

● S42.113   Displaced fracture of body of scapula, unspecified shoulder B, K, P 🔘, 🔘, B 🔘

● S42.114   Nondisplaced fracture of body of scapula, right shoulder B, K, P 🔘, 🔘, B 🔘

● S42.115   Nondisplaced fracture of body of scapula, left shoulder B, K, P 🔘, 🔘, B 🔘

● S42.116   Nondisplaced fracture of body of scapula, unspecified shoulder B, K, P 🔘, 🔘, B 🔘

● S42.12   Fracture of acromial process

● S42.121   Displaced fracture of acromial process, right shoulder B, K, P 🔘, 🔘, B 🔘

● S42.122   Displaced fracture of acromial process, left shoulder B, K, P 🔘, 🔘, B 🔘

● S42.123   Displaced fracture of acromial process, unspecified shoulder B, K, P 🔘, 🔘, B 🔘

● S42.124   Nondisplaced fracture of acromial process, right shoulder B, K, P 🔘, 🔘, B 🔘

● S42.125   Nondisplaced fracture of acromial process, left shoulder B, K, P 🔘, 🔘, B 🔘

● S42.126   Nondisplaced fracture, of acromial process, unspecified shoulder B, K, P 🔘, 🔘, B 🔘

● S42.13   Fracture of coracoid process

● S42.131   Displaced fracture of coracoid process, right shoulder B, K, P 🔘, 🔘, B 🔘

● S42.132   Displaced fracture of coracoid process, left shoulder B, K, P 🔘, 🔘, B 🔘

● S42.133   Displaced fracture of coracoid process, unspecified shoulder B, K, P 🔘, 🔘, B 🔘

● S42.134   Nondisplaced fracture of coracoid process, right shoulder B, K, P 🔘, 🔘, B 🔘

● S42.135   Nondisplaced fracture of coracoid process, left shoulder B, K, P 🔘, 🔘, B 🔘

● S42.136   Nondisplaced fracture of coracoid process, unspecified shoulder B, K, P 🔘, 🔘, B 🔘

● S42.14   Fracture of glenoid cavity of scapula

● S42.141   Displaced fracture of glenoid cavity of scapula, right shoulder B, K, P 🔘, 🔘, B 🔘

● S42.142   Displaced fracture of glenoid cavity of scapula, left shoulder B, K, P 🔘, 🔘, B 🔘

● S42.143   Displaced fracture of glenoid cavity of scapula, unspecified shoulder B, K, P 🔘, 🔘, B 🔘

● S42.144   Nondisplaced fracture of glenoid cavity of scapula, right shoulder B, K, P 🔘, 🔘, B 🔘

● S42.145   Nondisplaced fracture of glenoid cavity of scapula, left shoulder B, K, P 🔘, 🔘, B 🔘

● S42.146   Nondisplaced fracture of glenoid cavity of scapula, unspecified shoulder B, K, P 🔘, 🔘, B 🔘

● S42.15   Fracture of neck of scapula

● S42.151   Displaced fracture of neck of scapula, right shoulder B, K, P 🔘, 🔘, B 🔘

● S42.152   Displaced fracture of neck of scapula, left shoulder B, K, P 🔘, 🔘, B 🔘

● S42.153   Displaced fracture of neck of scapula, unspecified shoulder B, K, P 🔘, 🔘, B 🔘

● S42.154   Nondisplaced fracture of neck of scapula, right shoulder B, K, P 🔘, 🔘, B 🔘

● S42.155   Nondisplaced fracture of neck of scapula, left shoulder B, K, P 🔘, 🔘, B 🔘

● S42.156   Nondisplaced fracture of neck of scapula, unspecified shoulder B, K, P 🔘, 🔘, B 🔘

● S42.19   Fracture of other part of scapula

● S42.191   Fracture of other part of scapula, right shoulder B, K, P 🔘, 🔘, B 🔘

● S42.192   Fracture of other part of scapula, left shoulder B, K, P 🔘, 🔘, B 🔘

● S42.199   Fracture of other part of scapula, unspecified shoulder B, K, P 🔘, 🔘, B 🔘

● **S42.2** **Fracture of upper end of humerus**
  Fracture of proximal end of humerus
  Excludes2   fracture of shaft of humerus (S42.3-)
            physeal fracture of upper end of humerus
              (S49.0-)

● **S42.20** **Unspecified fracture of upper end of humerus**

  ● **S42.201** Unspecified fracture of upper end of
          right humerus A, K, P 🔹, B 🔹, 🔹,
          A, B 🔹
      (Ex) **For S42.201[A]:** S42.201[A,B], S42.202[B],
          S42.209-S42.211[A,B], S42.212[B],
          S42.213-S42.214[A,B], S42.215[B],
          S42.216-S42.221[A,B], S42.222[B],
          S42.223-S42.224[A,B], S42.225[B],
          S42.226-S42.231[A,B], S42.232[B],
          S42.239-S42.241[A,B], S42.242[B],
          S42.249-S42.251[A,B], S42.252[B],
          S42.253-S42.254[A,B], S42.255[B],
          S42.256-S42.261[A,B], S42.262[B],
          S42.263-S42.264[A,B], S42.265[B],
          S42.266[A,B], S42.271[A], S42.279[A],
          S42.291[A,B], S42.292[B],
          S42.293-S42.294[A,B], S42.295[B],
          S42.296-S42.301[A,B], S42.302[B],
          S42.309[A,B], S42.311[A], S42.319[A],
          S42.321[A,B], S42.322[B],
          S42.323-S42.324[A,B], S42.325[B],
          S42.326-S42.331[A,B], S42.332[B],
          S42.333-S42.334[A,B], S42.335[B],
          S42.336-S42.341[A,B], S42.342[B],
          S42.343-S42.344[A,B], S42.345[B],
          S42.346-S42.351[A,B], S42.352[B],
          S42.353-S42.354[A,B], S42.355[B],
          S42.356-S42.361[A,B], S42.362[B],
          S42.363-S42.364[A,B], S42.365[B],
          S42.366-S42.391[A,B], S42.392[B],
          S42.399-S42.401[A,B], S42.402[B],
          S42.409-S42.411[A,B], S42.412[B],
          S42.413-S42.414[A,B], S42.415[B],
          S42.416-S42.421[A,B], S42.422[B],
          S42.423-S42.424[A,B], S42.425[B],
          S42.426-S42.431[A,B], S42.432[B],
          S42.433-S42.434[A,B], S42.435[B],
          S42.436-S42.441[A,B], S42.442[B],
          S42.443-S42.444[A,B], S42.445[B],
          S42.446-S42.447[A,B], S42.448[B],
          S42.449-S42.451[A,B], S42.452[B],
          S42.453-S42.454[A,B], S42.455[B],
          S42.456-S42.461[A,B], S42.462[B],
          S42.463-S42.464[A,B], S42.465[B],
          S42.466-S42.471[A,B], S42.472[B],
          S42.473-S42.474[A,B], S42.475[B], S42.476
          [A,B], S42.481[A], S42.489[A], S42.491[A,B],
          S42.492[B], S42.493-S42.494[A,B],
          S42.495[B], S42.496-S42.92X[A,B],
          S49.001[A], S49.009-S49.011[A],
          S49.019-S49.021[A], S49.029-S49.031[A],
          S49.039-S49.041[A], S49.049-S49.091[A],
          S49.099-S49.101[A], S49.109-S49.111[A],
          S49.119-S49.121[A], S49.129-S49.131[A],
          S49.139-S49.141[A], S49.149-S49.191[A],
          S49.199[A] **For S42.201[B]:**
          S42.201-S42.266[B], S42.291-S42.296[B],
          S42.301-S42.309[A,B], S42.311-S42.319[A],
          S42.321-S42.476[A,B], S42.481-S42.489[A],
          S42.491-S42.92X[A,B], S49.101-S49.199[A],
          S62.90X[B] **For S42.201[K,P]:** See
          S42.0[K,P]

● **S42.202** Unspecified fracture of upper end of
          left humerus A, K, P 🔹, B 🔹, 🔹,
          A, B 🔹
      (Ex) **For category S42.202 CC codes**
          S42.202[A]: S42.201[B],
          S42.202-S42.209[A,B], S42.211[B],
          S42.212-S42.213[A,B], S42.214[B],
          S42.215-S42.216[A,B], S42.221[B],
          S42.222-S42.223[A,B], S42.224[B],
          S42.225-S42.226[A,B], S42.231[B],
          S42.232-S42.239[A,B], S42.241[B],
          S42.242-S42.249[A,B], S42.251[B],
          S42.252-S42.253[A,B], S42.254[B],
          S42.255-S42.256[A,B], S42.261[B],
          S42.262-S42.263[A,B], S42.264[B],
          S42.265-S42.266[A,B], S42.272-S42.279[A],
          S42.291[B], S42.292-S42.293[A,B],
          S42.294[B], S42.295-S42.296[A,B],
          S42.301[B], S42.302-S42.309[A,B],
          S42.312-S42.319[A], S42.321[B],
          S42.322-S42.323[A,B], S42.324[B],
          S42.325-S42.326[A,B], S42.331[B],
          S42.332-S42.333[A,B], S42.334[B],
          S42.335-S42.336[A,B], S42.341[B],
          S42.342-S42.343[A,B], S42.344[B],
          S42.345-S42.346[A,B], S42.351[B],
          S42.352-S42.353[A,B], S42.354[B],
          S42.355-S42.356[A,B], S42.361[B],
          S42.362-S42.363[A,B], S42.364[B],
          S42.365-S42.366[A,B], S42.391[B],
          S42.392-S42.399[A,B], S42.401[B],
          S42.402-S42.409[A,B], S42.411[B],
          S42.412-S42.413[A,B], S42.414[B],
          S42.415-S42.416[A,B], S42.421[B],
          S42.422-S42.423[A,B], S42.424[B],
          S42.425-S42.426[A,B], S42.431[B],
          S42.432-S42.433[A,B], S42.434[B],
          S42.435-S42.436[A,B], S42.441[B],
          S42.442-S42.443[A,B], S42.444[B],
          S42.445-S42.446[A,B], S42.447[B],
          S42.448-S42.449[A,B], S42.451[B],
          S42.452-S42.453[A,B], S42.454[B],
          S42.455-S42.456[A,B], S42.461[B],
          S42.462-S42.463[A,B], S42.464[B],
          S42.465-S42.466[A,B], S42.471[B],
          S42.472-S42.473[A,B], S42.474[B],
          S42.475-S42.476[A,B], S42.482-S42.489[A],
          S42.491[B], S42.492-S42.493[A,B],
          S42.494[B], S42.495-S42.92X[A,B],
          S49.002-S49.009[A], S49.012-S49.019[A],
          S49.022-S49.029[A], S49.032-S49.039[A],
          S49.042-S49.049[A], S49.092-S49.099[A],
          S49.102-S49.109[A], S49.112-S49.119[A],
          S49.122-S49.129[A], S49.132-S49.139[A],
          S49.142-S49.149[A], S49.192-S49.199[A]
          For S42.202[B]: See S42.201[B]
          For S42.202[K,P]: See S42.0[K,P]

● **S42.209** Unspecified fracture of upper end of
          unspecified humerus A, K, P 🔹, B 🔹,
          🔹, A, B 🔹
      (Ex) **For S42.209[A]:** S42.201-S42.266[A,B],
          S42.271-S42.279[A], S42.291-S42.309[A,B],
          S42.311-S42.319[A], S42.321-S42.476[A,B],
          S42.481-S42.489[A], S42.491-S42.92X[A,B],
          S49.001-S49.199[A] **For S42.202[B]:** See
          S42.201[B] **For S42.202[K,P]:** See
          S42.0[K,P]

N Newborn Age: 0   **P** Pediatric Age: 0–17   **M** Maternity DX: 12–55   **A** Adult Age: 15–124   ♀ Females Only   ♂ Males Only

🔹 Complication\Comorbidity   🔹 Major C\C   (Ex) CC/MCC Exclusions   🔹 Present on Admission Requirement   🔹 Hospital-Acquired Condition

● **S42.21** Unspecified fracture of surgical neck of humerus
    Fracture of neck of humerus NOS

● **S42.211** Unspecified displaced fracture of surgical neck of right humerus
    A, K, P 🔒, B 🔒, 🔒, A, B 🔒
    Ex: For S42.211[A]: See S42.201[A]
      For S42.211[B]: See S42.201[B]
      For S42.211[K,P]: See S42.0[K,P]

● **S42.212** Unspecified displaced fracture of surgical neck of left humerus
    A, K, P 🔒, B 🔒, 🔒, A, B 🔒
    Ex: For S42.212[A]: See S42.202[A]
      For S42.212[B]: See S42.201[B]
      For S42.212[K,P]: See S42.0[K,P]

● **S42.213** Unspecified displaced fracture of surgical neck of unspecified humerus
    A, K, P 🔒, B 🔒, 🔒, A, B 🔒
    Ex: For S42.213[A]: See S42.209
      For S42.213[B]: See S42.201[B]
      For S42.213[K,P]: See S42.0[K,P]

● **S42.214** Unspecified nondisplaced fracture of surgical neck of right humerus
    A, K, P 🔒, B 🔒, 🔒, A, B 🔒
    Ex: For S42.214[A]: See S42.201[A]
      For S42.214[B]: See S42.201[B]
      For S42.214[K,P]: See S42.0[K,P]

● **S42.215** Unspecified nondisplaced fracture of surgical neck of left humerus
    A, K, P 🔒, B 🔒, 🔒, A, B 🔒
    Ex: For S42.215[A]: See S42.202[A]
      For S42.215[B]: See S42.201[B]
      For S42.215[K,P]: See S42.0[K,P]

● **S42.216** Unspecified nondisplaced fracture of surgical neck of unspecified humerus
    A, K, P 🔒, B 🔒, 🔒, A, B 🔒
    Ex: For S42.216[A]: See S42.209
      For S42.216[B]: See S42.201[B]
      For S42.216[K,P]: See S42.0[K,P]

● **S42.22** 2-part fracture of surgical neck of humerus

● **S42.221** 2-part displaced fracture of surgical neck of right humerus A, K, P 🔒, B 🔒, 🔒, A, B 🔒
    Ex: For S42.221[A]: See S42.201[A]
      For S42.221[B]: See S42.201[B]
      For S42.221[K,P]: See S42.0[K,P]

● **S42.222** 2-part displaced fracture of surgical neck of left humerus A, K, P 🔒, B 🔒, 🔒, A, B 🔒
    Ex: For S42.222[A]: See S42.202[A]
      For S42.222[B]: See S42.201[B]
      For S42.222[K,P]: See S42.0[K,P]

● **S42.223** 2-part displaced fracture of surgical neck of unspecified humerus
    A, K, P 🔒, B 🔒, 🔒, A, B 🔒
    Ex: For S42.223[A]: See S42.209
      For S42.223[B]: See S42.201[B]
      For S42.223[K,P]: See S42.0[K,P]

● **S42.224** 2-part nondisplaced fracture of surgical neck of right humerus
    A, K, P 🔒, B 🔒, 🔒, A, B 🔒
    Ex: For S42.224[A]: See S42.201[A]
      For S42.224[B]: See S42.201[B]
      For S42.224[K,P]: See S42.0[K,P]

● **S42.225** 2-part nondisplaced fracture of surgical neck of left humerus
    A, K, P 🔒, B 🔒, 🔒, A, B 🔒
    Ex: For S42.225[A]: See S42.202[A]
      For S42.225[B]: See S42.201[B]
      For S42.225[K,P]: See S42.0[K,P]

● **S42.226** 2-part nondisplaced fracture of surgical neck of unspecified humerus
    A, K, P 🔒, B 🔒, 🔒, A, B 🔒
    Ex: For S42.226[A]: See S42.209
      For S42.226[B]: See S42.201[B]
      For S42.226[K,P]: See S42.0[K,P]

● **S42.23** 3-part fracture of surgical neck of humerus

● **S42.231** 3-part fracture of surgical neck of right humerus A, K, P 🔒, B 🔒, 🔒, A, B 🔒
    Ex: For S42.231[A]: See S42.201[A]
      For S42.231[B]: See S42.201[B]
      For S42.231[K,P]: See S42.0[K,P]

● **S42.232** 3-part fracture of surgical neck of left humerus A, K, P 🔒, B 🔒, 🔒, A, B 🔒
    Ex: For S42.232[A]: See S42.202[A]
      For S42.232[B]: See S42.201[B]
      For S42.232[K,P]: See S42.0[K,P]

● **S42.239** 3-part fracture of surgical neck of unspecified humerus A, K, P 🔒, B 🔒, 🔒, A, B 🔒
    Ex: For S42.239[A]: See S42.209
      For S42.239[B]: See S42.201[B]
      For S42.239[K,P]: See S42.0[K,P]

● **S42.24** 4-part fracture of surgical neck of humerus

● **S42.241** 4-part fracture of surgical neck of right humerus A, K, P 🔒, B 🔒, 🔒, A, B 🔒
    Ex: For S42.241[A]: See S42.201[A]
      For S42.241[B]: See S42.201[B]
      For S42.241[K,P]: See S42.0[K,P]

● **S42.242** 4-part fracture of surgical neck of left humerus A, K, P 🔒, B 🔒, 🔒, A, B 🔒
    Ex: For S42.242[A]: See S42.202[A]
      For S42.242[B]: See S42.201[B]
      For S42.242[K,P]: See S42.0[K,P]

● **S42.249** 4-part fracture of surgical neck of unspecified humerus A, K, P 🔒, B 🔒, 🔒, A, B 🔒
    Ex: For S42.249[A]: See S42.209
      For S42.249[B]: See S42.201[B]
      For S42.249[K,P]: See S42.0[K,P]

● **S42.25** Fracture of greater tuberosity of humerus

● **S42.251** Displaced fracture of greater tuberosity of right humerus
    A, K, P 🔒, B 🔒, 🔒, A, B 🔒
    Ex: For S42.251[A]: See S42.201[A]
      For S42.251[B]: See S42.201[B]
      For S42.251[K,P]: See S42.0[K,P]

● **S42.252** Displaced fracture of greater tuberosity of left humerus A, K, P 🔒, B 🔒, 🔒, A, B 🔒
    Ex: For S42.252[A]: See S42.202[A]
      For S42.252[B]: See S42.201[B]
      For S42.252[K,P]: See S42.0[K,P]

● **S42.253** Displaced fracture of greater tuberosity of unspecified humerus
    A, K, P 🔒, B 🔒, 🔒, A, B 🔒
    Ex: For category S42.253 CC codes
    S42.253[A]: See S42.209 For S42.253[B]:
    See S42.201[B] For S42.253[K,P]: See
    S42.0[K,P]

● **S42.254** Nondisplaced fracture of greater tuberosity of right humerus
    A, K, P 🔒, B 🔒, 🔒, A, B 🔒
    Ex: For S42.254[A]: See S42.201[A]
      For S42.254[B]: See S42.201[B]
      For S42.254[K,P]: See S42.0[K,P]

● **S42.255** Nondisplaced fracture of greater tuberosity of left humerus A, K, P 🔒, B 🔒, 🔒, A, B 🔒
    Ex: For S42.255[A]: See S42.202[A]
      For S42.255[B]: See S42.201[B]
      For S42.255[K,P]: See S42.0[K,P]

● **S42.256** Nondisplaced fracture of greater tuberosity of unspecified humerus
    A, K, P 🔒, B 🔒, 🔒, A, B 🔒
    Ex: For S42.256[A]: See S42.209
      For S42.256[B]: See S42.201[B]
      For S42.256[K,P]: See S42.0[K,P]

◄ New ◄▦ Revised ~~deleted~~ Deleted | Excludes 1 | Excludes 2 | Includes | Use additional | Code first | Code also | Unspecified
OGCR Official Guidelines ● Unacceptable Principal Diagnosis X Assign placeholder X ● Use Additional Character(s) ▶ Manifestation Code **Coding Clinic**

● **S42.26**   Fracture of lesser tuberosity of humerus

  ● **S42.261**   Displaced fracture of lesser tuberosity of right humerus A, K, P 🪙, B 🪙, 🪙, A, B 🪙

     Ⓔˣ For S42.261[A]: See S42.201[A]
        For S42.261[B]: See S42.201[B]
        For S42.261[K,P]: See S42.0[K,P]

  ● **S42.262**   Displaced fracture of lesser tuberosity of left humerus A, K, P 🪙, B 🪙, 🪙, A, B 🪙

     Ⓔˣ For S42.262[A]: See S42.202[A]
        For S42.262[B]: See S42.201[B]
        For S42.262[K,P]: See S42.0[K,P]

  ● **S42.263**   Displaced fracture of lesser tuberosity of unspecified humerus A, K, P 🪙, B 🪙, 🪙, A, B 🪙

     Ⓔˣ For S42.263[A]: See S42.209
        For S42.263[B]: See S42.201[B]
        For S42.263[K,P]: See S42.0[K,P]

  ● **S42.264**   Nondisplaced fracture of lesser tuberosity of right humerus A, K, P 🪙, B 🪙, 🪙, A, B 🪙

     Ⓔˣ For S42.264[A]: See S42.201[A]
        For S42.264[B]: See S42.201[B]
        For S42.264[K,P]: See S42.0[K,P]

  ● **S42.265**   Nondisplaced fracture of lesser tuberosity of left humerus A, K, P 🪙, B 🪙, 🪙, A, B 🪙

     Ⓔˣ For S42.265[A]: See S42.202[A]
        For S42.265[B]: See S42.201[B]
        For S42.265[K,P]: See S42.0[K,P]

  ● **S42.266**   Nondisplaced fracture of lesser tuberosity of unspecified humerus A, K, P 🪙, B 🪙, 🪙, A, B 🪙

     Ⓔˣ For S42.266[A]: See S42.209
        For S42.266[B]: See S42.201[B]
        For S42.266[K,P]: See S42.0[K,P]

● **S42.27**   Torus fracture of upper end of humerus

   The appropriate 7th character is to be added to all codes in subcategory S42.27

A	initial encounter for closed fracture
D	subsequent encounter for fracture with routine healing
G	subsequent encounter for fracture with delayed healing
K	subsequent encounter for fracture with nonunion
P	subsequent encounter for fracture with malunion
S	sequela

  ● **S42.271**   Torus fracture of upper end of right humerus A, K, P 🪙, 🪙, A 🪙

     Ⓔˣ For S42.271[A]: See S42.201[A]
        For S42.271[K,P]: See S42.0[K,P]

  ● **S42.272**   Torus fracture of upper end of left humerus A, K, P 🪙, 🪙, A 🪙

     Ⓔˣ For S42.272[A]: See S42.202[A]
        For S42.272[K,P]: See S42.0[K,P]

  ● **S42.279**   Torus fracture of upper end of unspecified humerus A, K, P 🪙, 🪙, A 🪙

     Ⓔˣ For S42.279[A]: See S42.209
        For S42.279[K,P]: See S42.0[K,P]

● **S42.29**   Other fracture of upper end of humerus
     Fracture of anatomical neck of humerus
     Fracture of articular head of humerus

  ● **S42.291**   Other displaced fracture of upper end of right humerus A, K, P 🪙, B 🪙, 🪙, A, B 🪙

     Ⓔˣ For S42.291[A]: See S42.201[A]
        For S42.291[B]: See S42.201[B]
        For S42.291[K,P]: See S42.0[K,P]

  ● **S42.292**   Other displaced fracture of upper end of left humerus A, K, P 🪙, B 🪙, 🪙, A, B 🪙

     Ⓔˣ For S42.292[A]: See S42.202[A]
        For S42.292[B]: See S42.201[B]
        For S42.292[K,P]: See S42.0[K,P]

  ● **S42.293**   Other displaced fracture of upper end of unspecified humerus A, K, P 🪙, B 🪙, 🪙, A, B 🪙

     Ⓔˣ For S42.293[A]: See S42.209
        For S42.293[B]: See S42.201[B]
        For S42.293[K,P]: See S42.0[K,P]

  ● **S42.294**   Other nondisplaced fracture of upper end of right humerus A, K, P 🪙, B 🪙, 🪙, A, B 🪙

     Ⓔˣ For S42.294[A]: See S42.201[A]
        For S42.294[B]: See S42.201[B]
        For S42.294[K,P]: See S42.0[K,P]

  ● **S42.295**   Other nondisplaced fracture of upper end of left humerus A, K, P 🪙, B 🪙, 🪙, A, B 🪙

     Ⓔˣ For S42.295[A]: See S42.202[A]
        For S42.295[B]: See S42.201[B]
        For S42.295[K,P]: See S42.0[K,P]

  ● **S42.296**   Other nondisplaced fracture of upper end of unspecified humerus A, K, P 🪙, B 🪙, 🪙, A, B 🪙

     Ⓔˣ For S42.296[A]: See S42.209
        For S42.296[B]: See S42.201[B]
        For S42.296[K,P]: See S42.0[K,P]

● **S42.3**   Fracture of shaft of humerus
     Fracture of humerus NOS
     Fracture of upper arm NOS

   Excludes2   physeal fractures of upper end of humerus (S49.0-)
         physeal fractures of lower end of humerus (S49.1-)

● **S42.30**   Unspecified fracture of shaft of humerus

  ● **S42.301**   Unspecified fracture of shaft of humerus, right arm A, K, P 🪙, B 🪙, 🪙, A, B 🪙

     Ⓔˣ For S42.301[A]: See S42.201[A]
        For S42.301[B]: See S42.201[B]
        For S42.301[K,P]: See S42.0[K,P]

  ● **S42.302**   Unspecified fracture of shaft of humerus, left arm A, K, P 🪙, B 🪙, 🪙, A, B 🪙

     Ⓔˣ For S42.302[A]: See S42.202[A]
        For S42.302[B]: See S42.201[B]
        For S42.302[K,P]: See S42.0[K,P]

  ● **S42.309**   Unspecified fracture of shaft of humerus, unspecified arm A, K, P 🪙, B 🪙, 🪙, A, B 🪙

     Ⓔˣ For S42.309[A]: See S42.209
        For S42.309[B]: See S42.201[B]
        For S42.309[K,P]: See S42.0[K,P]

CHAPTER 19 (S00-T88)

N   Newborn Age: 0   P   Pediatric Age: 0–17   M   Maternity DX: 12–55   A   Adult Age: 15–124   ♀   Females Only   ♂   Males Only
🪙   Complication\Comorbidity   🪙   Major C\C   Ⓔˣ   CC/MCC Exclusions   🪙   Present on Admission Requirement   🪙   Hospital-Acquired Condition

1351

CHAPTER 19 (S00-T88)

- ● **S42.31**   **Greenstick fracture of shaft of humerus**

  The appropriate 7th character is to be added to all codes in subcategory S42.31

A	initial encounter for closed fracture
D	subsequent encounter for fracture with routine healing
G	subsequent encounter for fracture with delayed healing
K	subsequent encounter for fracture with nonunion
P	subsequent encounter for fracture with malunion
S	sequela

  - ● **S42.311**   **Greenstick fracture of shaft of humerus, right arm** A, K, P 🔵, 🔵, A 🔵

    Ⓔⓧ For category S42.311 CC codes
    S42.311[A]: S42.311[A],
    S42.319-S42.321[A], S42.323-S42.324[A],
    S42.326-S42.331[A], S42.333-S42.334[A],
    S42.336-S42.341[A], S42.343-S42.344[A],
    S42.346-S42.351[A], S42.353-S42.354[A],
    S42.356-S42.361[A], S42.363-S42.364[A],
    S42.366-S42.391[A], S42.399[A]
    For S42.311[K,P]: See S42.0[K,P]

  - ● **S42.312**   **Greenstick fracture of shaft of humerus, left arm** A, K, P 🔵, 🔵, A 🔵

    Ⓔⓧ For category S42.312 CC codes
    S42.312[A]: S42.312-S42.319[A],
    S42.322-S42.323[A], S42.325-S42.326[A],
    S42.332-S42.333[A], S42.335-S42.336[A],
    S42.342-S42.343[A], S42.345-S42.346[A],
    S42.352-S42.353[A], S42.355-S42.356[A],
    S42.362-S42.363[A], S42.365-S42.366[A],
    S42.392-S42.399[A] For S42.312[K,P]: See
    S42.0[K,P]

  - ● **S42.319**   **Greenstick fracture of shaft of humerus, unspecified arm** A, K, P 🔵, 🔵, A 🔵

    Ⓔⓧ For category S42.319 CC codes
    S42.319[A]: S42.311-S42.399[A]
    For S42.319[K,P]: See S42.0[K,P]

- ● **S42.32**   **Transverse fracture of shaft of humerus**

  - ● **S42.321**   **Displaced transverse fracture of shaft of humerus, right arm** A, K, P 🔵, B 🔵, 🔵, A, B 🔵

    Ⓔⓧ For category S42.321 CC codes
    S42.321[A]: See S42.311[A]
    For S42.321[B]: See S42.201[B]
    For S42.321[K,P]: See S42.0[K,P]

  - ● **S42.322**   **Displaced transverse fracture of shaft of humerus, left arm** A, K, P 🔵, B 🔵, 🔵, A, B 🔵

    Ⓔⓧ For category S42.322 CC codes
    S42.322[A]: See S42.312[A]
    For S42.322[B]: See S42.201[B]
    For S42.322[K,P]: See S42.0[K,P]

  - ● **S42.323**   **Displaced transverse fracture of shaft of humerus, unspecified arm** A, K, P 🔵, B 🔵, 🔵, A, B 🔵

    Ⓔⓧ For category S42.323 CC codes
    S42.323[A]: S42.311-S42.399[A]
    For S42.323[B]: See S42.201[B]
    For S42.313[K,P]: See S42.0[K,P]

  - ● **S42.324**   **Nondisplaced transverse fracture of shaft of humerus, right arm** A, K, P 🔵, B 🔵, 🔵, A, B 🔵

    Ⓔⓧ For category S42.324 CC codes
    S42.324[A]: See S42.311[A]
    For S42.324[B]: See S42.201[B]
    For S42.324[K,P]: See S42.0[K,P]

- ● **S42.325**   **Nondisplaced transverse fracture of shaft of humerus, left arm** A, K, P 🔵, B 🔵, 🔵, A, B 🔵

  Ⓔⓧ For category S42.325 CC codes
  S42.325[A]: See S42.312[A]
  For S42.325[B]: See S42.201[B]
  For S42.325[K,P]: See S42.0[K,P]

- ● **S42.326**   **Nondisplaced transverse fracture of shaft of humerus, unspecified arm** A, K, P 🔵, B 🔵, 🔵, A, B 🔵

  Ⓔⓧ For category S42.326 CC codes
  S42.326[A]: S42.311-S42.399[A]
  For S42.326[B]: See S42.201[B]
  For S42.316[K,P]: See S42.0[K,P]

- ● **S42.33**   **Oblique fracture of shaft of humerus**

  - ● **S42.331**   **Displaced oblique fracture of shaft of humerus, right arm** A, K, P 🔵, B 🔵, 🔵, A, B 🔵

    Ⓔⓧ For category S42.331 CC codes
    S42.331[A]: See S42.311[A]
    For S42.331[B]: See S42.201[B]
    For S42.331[K,P]: See S42.0[K,P]

  - ● **S42.332**   **Displaced oblique fracture of shaft of humerus, left arm** A, K, P 🔵, B 🔵, 🔵, A, B 🔵

    Ⓔⓧ For category S42.332 CC codes
    S42.332[A]: See S42.312[A]
    For S42.332[B]: See S42.201[B]
    For S42.332[K,P]: See S42.0[K,P]

  - ● **S42.333**   **Displaced oblique fracture of shaft of humerus, unspecified arm** A, K, P 🔵, B 🔵, A, B 🔵

    Ⓔⓧ For category S42.333 CC codes
    S42.333[A]: S42.311-S42.399[A]
    For S42.333[B]: See S42.201[B]
    For S42.333[K,P]: See S42.0[K,P]

  - ● **S42.334**   **Nondisplaced oblique fracture of shaft of humerus, right arm** A, K, P 🔵, B 🔵, 🔵, A, B 🔵

    Ⓔⓧ For category S42.334 CC codes
    S42.334[A]: See S42.311[A]
    For S42.334[B]: See S42.201[B]
    For S42.334[K,P]: See S42.0[K,P]

  - ● **S42.335**   **Nondisplaced oblique fracture of shaft of humerus, left arm** A, K, P 🔵, B 🔵, 🔵, A, B 🔵

    Ⓔⓧ For category S42.335 CC codes
    S42.335[A]: See S42.312[A]
    For S42.335[B]: See S42.201[B]
    For S42.335[K,P]: See S42.0[K,P]

  - ● **S42.336**   **Nondisplaced oblique fracture of shaft of humerus, unspecified arm** A, K, P 🔵, B 🔵, 🔵, A, B 🔵

    Ⓔⓧ For category S42.336 CC codes
    S42.336[A]: S42.311-S42.399[A]
    For S42.336[B]: See S42.201[B]
    For S42.336[K,P]: See S42.0[K,P]

- ● **S42.34**   **Spiral fracture of shaft of humerus**

  - ● **S42.341**   **Displaced spiral fracture of shaft of humerus, right arm** A, K, P 🔵, B 🔵, 🔵, A, B 🔵

    Ⓔⓧ For category S42.341 CC codes
    S42.341[A]: See S42.311[A]
    For S42.341[B]: See S42.201[B]
    For S42.341[K,P]: See S42.0[K,P]

  - ● **S42.342**   **Displaced spiral fracture of shaft of humerus, left arm** A, K, P 🔵, B 🔵, 🔵, A, B 🔵

    Ⓔⓧ For category S42.342 CC codes
    S42.342[A]: See S42.312[A]
    For S42.342[B]: See S42.201[B]
    For S42.342[K,P]: See S42.0[K,P]

◀ New   ◀▥ Revised   ~~deleted~~ Deleted   Excludes 1   Excludes 2   Includes   Use additional   Code first   Code also   Unspecified

OGCR Official Guidelines   ● Unacceptable Principal Diagnosis   X Assign placeholder X   ▶ Use Additional Character(s)   ▌ Manifestation Code   **Coding Clinic**

● **S42.343** Displaced spiral fracture of shaft of
humerus, unspecified arm A, K, P 🪙,
B 🪙, 🪙, A, B 🪙
(Ex:) For category S42.343 CC codes
S42.343[A]: S42.311-S42.399[A]
For S42.343[B]: See S42.201[B]
For S42.343[K,P]: See S42.0[K,P]

● **S42.344** Nondisplaced spiral fracture of shaft
of humerus, right arm A, K, P 🪙, B 🪙,
🪙, A, B 🪙
(Ex:) For category S42.344 CC codes
S42.344[A]: See S42.311[A]
For S42.344[B]: See S42.201[B]
For S42.344[K,P]: See S42.0[K,P]

● **S42.345** Nondisplaced spiral fracture of shaft
of humerus, left arm A, K, P 🪙, B 🪙,
🪙, A, B 🪙
(Ex:) For category S42.345 CC codes
S42.345[A]: See S42.312[A]
For S42.345[B]: See S42.201[B]
For S42.345[K,P]: See S42.0[K,P]

● **S42.346** Nondisplaced spiral fracture of shaft
of humerus, unspecified arm
A, K, P 🪙, B 🪙, 🪙, A, B 🪙
(Ex:) For category S42.346 CC codes
S42.346[A]: S42.311-S42.399[A]
For S42.346[B]: See S42.201[B]
For S42.346[K,P]: See S42.0[K,P]

● **S42.35** Comminuted fracture of shaft of humerus
● **S42.351** Displaced comminuted fracture of
shaft of humerus, right arm A, K, P 🪙,
B 🪙, 🪙, A, B 🪙
(Ex:) For category S42.351 CC codes
S42.351[A]: See S42.311[A]
For S42.351[B]: See S42.201[B]
For S42.351[K,P]: See S42.0[K,P]

● **S42.352** Displaced comminuted fracture of
shaft of humerus, left arm A, K, P 🪙,
B 🪙, 🪙, A, B 🪙
(Ex:) For category S42.352 CC codes
S42.352[A]: See S42.312[A]
For S42.352[B]: See S42.201[B]
For S42.352[K,P]: See S42.0[K,P]

● **S42.353** Displaced comminuted fracture of
shaft of humerus, unspecified arm
A, K, P 🪙, B 🪙, 🪙, A, B 🪙
(Ex:) For category S42.353 CC codes
S42.353[A]: S42.311-S42.399[A]
For S42.353[B]: See S42.201[B]
For S42.353[K,P]: See S42.0[K,P]

● **S42.354** Nondisplaced comminuted fracture of
shaft of humerus, right arm A, K, P 🪙,
B 🪙, 🪙, A, B 🪙
(Ex:) For category S42.354 CC codes
S42.354[A]: See S42.311[A]
For S42.354[B]: See S42.201[B]
For S42.354[K,P]: See S42.0[K,P]

● **S42.355** Nondisplaced comminuted fracture of
shaft of humerus, left arm A, K, P 🪙,
B 🪙, 🪙, A, B 🪙
(Ex:) For category S42.355 CC codes
S42.355[A]: See S42.312[A]
For S42.355[B]: See S42.201[B]
For S42.355[K,P]: See S42.0[K,P]

● **S42.356** Nondisplaced comminuted fracture of
shaft of humerus, unspecified arm
A, K, P 🪙, B 🪙, 🪙, A, B 🪙
(Ex:) For category S42.356 CC codes
S42.356[A]: S42.311-S42.399[A]
For S42.356[B]: See S42.201[B]
For S42.356[K,P]: See S42.0[K,P]

● **S42.36** Segmental fracture of shaft of humerus
● **S42.361** Displaced segmental fracture of shaft
of humerus, right arm A, K, P 🪙, B 🪙,
🪙, A, B 🪙
(Ex:) For category S42.361 CC codes
S42.361[A]: See S42.311[A]
For S42.361[B]: See S42.201[B]
For S42.361[K,P]: See S42.0[K,P]

● **S42.362** Displaced segmental fracture of shaft
of humerus, left arm A, K, P 🪙, B 🪙,
🪙, A, B 🪙
(Ex:) For category S42.362 CC codes
S42.362[A]: See S42.312[A]
For S42.362[B]: See S42.201[B]
For S42.362[K,P]: See S42.0[K,P]

● **S42.363** Displaced segmental fracture of shaft
of humerus, unspecified arm
A, K, P 🪙, B 🪙, 🪙, A, B 🪙
(Ex:) For category S42.363 CC codes
S42.363[A]: S42.311-S42.399[A]
For S42.363[B]: See S42.201[B]
For S42.363[K,P]: See S42.0[K,P]

● **S42.364** Nondisplaced segmental fracture of
shaft of humerus, right arm A, K, P 🪙,
B 🪙, 🪙, A, B 🪙
(Ex:) For category S42.364 CC codes
S42.364[A]: See S42.311[A]
For S42.364[B]: See S42.201[B]
For S42.364[K,P]: See S42.0[K,P]

● **S42.365** Nondisplaced segmental fracture of
shaft of humerus, left arm A, K, P 🪙,
B 🪙, 🪙, A, B 🪙
(Ex:) For category S42.365 CC codes
S42.365[A]: See S42.312[A]
For S42.365[B]: See S42.201[B]
For S42.365[K,P]: See S42.0[K,P]

● **S42.366** Nondisplaced segmental fracture of
shaft of humerus, unspecified arm
A, K, P 🪙, B 🪙, 🪙, A, B 🪙
(Ex:) For category S42.366 CC codes
S42.366[A]: S42.311-S42.399[A]
For S42.366[B]: See S42.201[B]
For S42.366[K,P]: See S42.0[K,P]

● **S42.39** Other fracture of shaft of humerus
● **S42.391** Other fracture of shaft of right
humerus A, K, P 🪙, B 🪙, 🪙, A, B 🪙
(Ex:) For category S42.391 CC codes
S42.391[A]: See S42.311[A]
For S42.391[B]: See S42.201[B]
For S42.391[K,P]: See S42.0[K,P]

● **S42.392** Other fracture of shaft of left
humerus A, K, P 🪙, B 🪙, 🪙, A, B 🪙
(Ex:) For category S42.392 CC codes
S42.392[A]: See S42.312[A]
For S42.392[B]: See S42.201[B]
For S42.392[K,P]: See S42.0[K,P]

● **S42.399** Other fracture of shaft of unspecified
humerus A, K, P 🪙, B 🪙, 🪙, A, B 🪙
(Ex:) For category S42.399 CC codes
S42.399[A]: S42.311-S42.399[A]
For S42.399[B]: See S42.201[B]
For S42.399[K,P]: See S42.0[K,P]

CHAPTER 19 (S00-T88)

N Newborn Age: 0   P Pediatric Age: 0–17   M Maternity DX: 12–55   A Adult Age: 15–124   ♀ Females Only   ♂ Males Only

🪙 Complication\Comorbidity   🪙 Major C\C   (Ex:) CC/MCC Exclusions   🪙 Present on Admission Requirement   🪙 Hospital-Acquired Condition

1353

S42.4   Fracture of lower end of humerus
Fracture of distal end of humerus

> **Excludes2**   fracture of shaft of humerus (S42.3-)
> physeal fracture of lower end of humerus (S49.1-)

S42.40   Unspecified fracture of lower end of humerus
Fracture of elbow NOS

S42.401   Unspecified fracture of lower end of right humerus A, K, P 🔖, B 🔖, 🔖, A, B 🔖
> Ex: For S42.401[A]: See S42.201[A]
> For S42.401[B]: See S42.201[B]
> For S42.401[K,P]: See S42.0[K,P]

S42.402   Unspecified fracture of lower end of left humerus A, K, P 🔖, B 🔖, 🔖, A, B 🔖
> Ex: For S42.402[A]: See S42.202[A]
> For S42.402[B]: See S42.201[B]
> For S42.402[K,P]: See S42.0[K,P]

S42.409   Unspecified fracture of lower end of unspecified humerus A, K, P 🔖, B 🔖, 🔖, A, B 🔖
> Ex: For S42.409[A]: See S42.209
> For S42.409[B]: See S42.201[B]
> For S42.409[K,P]: See S42.0[K,P]

S42.41   Simple supracondylar fracture without intercondylar fracture of humerus

S42.411   Displaced simple supracondylar fracture without intercondylar fracture of right humerus A, K, P 🔖, B 🔖, 🔖, A, B 🔖
> Ex: For S42.411[A]: See S42.201[A]
> For S42.411[B]: See S42.201[B]
> For S42.411[K,P]: See S42.0[K,P]

S42.412   Displaced simple supracondylar fracture without intercondylar fracture of left humerus A, K, P 🔖, B 🔖, 🔖, A, B 🔖
> Ex: For S42.412[A]: See S42.202[A]
> For S42.412[B]: See S42.201[B]
> For S42.412[K,P]: See S42.0[K,P]

S42.413   Displaced simple supracondylar fracture without intercondylar fracture of unspecified humerus A, K, P 🔖, B 🔖, 🔖, A, B 🔖
> Ex: For S42.413[A]: See S42.209
> For S42.413[B]: See S42.201[B]
> For S42.413[K,P]: See S42.0[K,P]

S42.414   Nondisplaced simple supracondylar fracture without intercondylar fracture of right humerus A, K, P 🔖, B 🔖, 🔖, A, B 🔖
> Ex: For S42.414[A]: See S42.201[A]
> For S42.414[B]: See S42.201[B]
> For S42.414[K,P]: See S42.0[K,P]

S42.415   Nondisplaced simple supracondylar fracture without intercondylar fracture of left humerus A, K, P 🔖, B 🔖, 🔖, A, B 🔖
> Ex: For S42.415[A]: See S42.202[A]
> For S42.415[B]: See S42.201[B]
> For S42.415[K,P]: See S42.0[K,P]

S42.416   Nondisplaced simple supracondylar fracture without intercondylar fracture of unspecified humerus A, K, P 🔖, B 🔖, 🔖, A, B 🔖
> Ex: For S42.416[A]: See S42.209
> For S42.416[B]: See S42.201[B]
> For S42.416[K,P]: See S42.0[K,P]

S42.42   Comminuted supracondylar fracture without intercondylar fracture of humerus

S42.421   Displaced comminuted supracondylar fracture without intercondylar fracture of right humerus A, K, P 🔖, B 🔖, 🔖, A, B 🔖
> Ex: For S42.421[A]: See S42.201[A]
> For S42.421[B]: See S42.201[B]
> For S42.421[K,P]: See S42.0[K,P]

S42.422   Displaced comminuted supracondylar fracture without intercondylar fracture of left humerus A, K, P 🔖, B 🔖, 🔖, A, B 🔖
> Ex: For S42.422[A]: See S42.202[A]
> For S42.422[B]: See S42.201[B]
> For S42.422[K,P]: See S42.0[K,P]

S42.423   Displaced comminuted supracondylar fracture without intercondylar fracture of unspecified humerus A, K, P 🔖, B 🔖, 🔖, A, B 🔖
> Ex: For S42.423[A]: See S42.209
> For S42.423[B]: See S42.201[B]
> For S42.423[K,P]: See S42.0[K,P]

S42.424   Nondisplaced comminuted supracondylar fracture without intercondylar fracture of right humerus A, K, P 🔖, B 🔖, 🔖, A, B 🔖
> Ex: For S42.424[A]: See S42.201[A]
> For S42.424[B]: See S42.201[B]
> For S42.424[K,P]: See S42.0[K,P]

S42.425   Nondisplaced comminuted supracondylar fracture without intercondylar fracture of left humerus A, K, P 🔖, B 🔖, 🔖, A, B 🔖
> Ex: For S42.425[A]: See S42.202[A]
> For S42.425[B]: See S42.201[B]
> For S42.425[K,P]: See S42.0[K,P]

S42.426   Nondisplaced comminuted supracondylar fracture without intercondylar fracture of unspecified humerus A, K, P 🔖, B 🔖, 🔖, A, B 🔖
> Ex: For S42.426[A]: See S42.209
> For S42.426[B]: See S42.201[B]
> For S42.426[K,P]: See S42.0[K,P]

S42.43   Fracture (avulsion) of lateral epicondyle of humerus

S42.431   Displaced fracture (avulsion) of lateral epicondyle of right humerus A, K, P 🔖, B 🔖, 🔖, A, B 🔖
> Ex: For S42.431[A]: See S42.201[A]
> For S42.431[B]: See S42.201[B]
> For S42.431[K,P]: See S42.0[K,P]

S42.432   Displaced fracture (avulsion) of lateral epicondyle of left humerus A, K, P 🔖, B 🔖, 🔖, A, B 🔖
> Ex: For S42.432[A]: See S42.202[A]
> For S42.432[B]: See S42.201[B]
> For S42.432[K,P]: See S42.0[K,P]

S42.433   Displaced fracture (avulsion) of lateral epicondyle of unspecified humerus A, K, P 🔖, B 🔖, 🔖, A, B 🔖
> Ex: For S42.433[A]: See S42.209
> For S42.433[B]: See S42.201[B]
> For S42.433[K,P]: See S42.0[K,P]

S42.434   Nondisplaced fracture (avulsion) of lateral epicondyle of right humerus A, K, P 🔖, B 🔖, 🔖, A, B 🔖
> Ex: For S42.434[A]: See S42.201[A]
> For S42.434[B]: See S42.201[B]
> For S42.434[K,P]: See S42.0[K,P]

● S42.435　Nondisplaced fracture (avulsion) of
　　　　　　lateral epicondyle of left humerus
　　　　　　A, K, P 🔵, B 🔵🔵, 🔵, A, B 🔵🔵
　　　　　　(Ex:) For S42.435[A]: See S42.202[A]
　　　　　　　　　For S42.435[B]: See S42.201[B]
　　　　　　　　　For S42.435[K,P]: See S42.0[K,P]

● S42.436　Nondisplaced fracture (avulsion) of
　　　　　　lateral epicondyle of unspecified
　　　　　　humerus A, K, P 🔵, B 🔵🔵, 🔵, A, B 🔵🔵
　　　　　　(Ex:) For S42.436[A]: See S42.209
　　　　　　　　　For S42.436[B]: See S42.201[B]
　　　　　　　　　For S42.436[K,P]: See S42.0[K,P]

● S42.44　Fracture (avulsion) of medial epicondyle of
　　　　　　humerus

● S42.441　Displaced fracture (avulsion) of
　　　　　　medial epicondyle of right humerus
　　　　　　A, K, P 🔵, B 🔵🔵, 🔵, A, B 🔵🔵
　　　　　　(Ex:) For S42.441[A]: See S42.201[A]
　　　　　　　　　For S42.441[B]: See S42.201[B]
　　　　　　　　　For S42.441[K,P]: See S42.0[K,P]

● S42.442　Displaced fracture (avulsion) of
　　　　　　medial epicondyle of left humerus
　　　　　　A, K, P 🔵, B 🔵🔵, 🔵, A, B 🔵🔵
　　　　　　(Ex:) For S42.442[A]: See S42.202[A]
　　　　　　　　　For S42.442[B]: See S42.201[B]
　　　　　　　　　For S42.442[K,P]: See S42.0[K,P]

● S42.443　Displaced fracture (avulsion) of
　　　　　　medial epicondyle of unspecified
　　　　　　humerus A, K, P 🔵, B 🔵🔵, 🔵, A, B 🔵🔵
　　　　　　(Ex:) For S42.443[A]: See S42.209
　　　　　　　　　For S42.443[B]: See S42.201[B]
　　　　　　　　　For S42.443[K,P]: See S42.0[K,P]

● S42.444　Nondisplaced fracture (avulsion) of
　　　　　　medial epicondyle of right humerus
　　　　　　A, K, P 🔵, B 🔵🔵, 🔵, A, B 🔵🔵
　　　　　　(Ex:) For S42.444[A]: See S42.201[A]
　　　　　　　　　For S42.444[B]: See S42.201[B]
　　　　　　　　　For S42.444[K,P]: See S42.0[K,P]

● S42.445　Nondisplaced fracture (avulsion) of
　　　　　　medial epicondyle of left humerus
　　　　　　A, K, P 🔵, B 🔵🔵, 🔵, A, B 🔵🔵
　　　　　　(Ex:) For S42.445[A]: See S42.202[A]
　　　　　　　　　For S42.445[B]: See S42.201[B]
　　　　　　　　　For S42.445[K,P]: See S42.0[K,P]

● S42.446　Nondisplaced fracture (avulsion) of
　　　　　　medial epicondyle of unspecified
　　　　　　humerus A, K, P 🔵, B 🔵🔵, 🔵, A, B 🔵🔵
　　　　　　(Ex:) For S42.446[A]: See S42.209
　　　　　　　　　For S42.446[B]: See S42.201[B]
　　　　　　　　　For S42.446[K,P]: See S42.0[K,P]

● S42.447　Incarcerated fracture (avulsion) of
　　　　　　medial epicondyle of right humerus
　　　　　　A, K, P 🔵, B 🔵🔵, 🔵, A, B 🔵🔵
　　　　　　(Ex:) For S42.447[A]: See S42.201[A]
　　　　　　　　　For S42.447[B]: See S42.201[B]
　　　　　　　　　For S42.447[K,P]: See S42.0[K,P]

● S42.448　Incarcerated fracture (avulsion) of
　　　　　　medial epicondyle of left humerus
　　　　　　A, K, P 🔵, B 🔵🔵, 🔵, A, B 🔵🔵
　　　　　　(Ex:) For S42.448[A]: See S42.202[A]
　　　　　　　　　For S42.448[B]: See S42.201[B]
　　　　　　　　　For S42.448[K,P]: See S42.0[K,P]

● S42.449　Incarcerated fracture (avulsion) of
　　　　　　medial epicondyle of unspecified
　　　　　　humerus A, K, P 🔵, B 🔵🔵, 🔵, A, B 🔵🔵
　　　　　　(Ex:) For S42.449[A]: See S42.209
　　　　　　　　　For S42.449[B]: See S42.201[B]
　　　　　　　　　For S42.449[K,P]: See S42.0[K,P]

● S42.45　Fracture of lateral condyle of humerus
　　　　　　Fracture of capitellum of humerus

● S42.451　Displaced fracture of lateral condyle
　　　　　　of right humerus A, K, P 🔵, B 🔵🔵, 🔵,
　　　　　　A, B 🔵🔵
　　　　　　(Ex:) For S42.451[A]: See S42.201[A]
　　　　　　　　　For S42.451[B]: See S42.201[B]
　　　　　　　　　For S42.451[K,P]: See S42.0[K,P]

● S42.452　Displaced fracture of lateral condyle
　　　　　　of left humerus A, K, P 🔵, B 🔵🔵, 🔵,
　　　　　　A, B 🔵🔵
　　　　　　(Ex:) For S42.452[A]: See S42.202[A]
　　　　　　　　　For S42.452[B]: See S42.201[B]
　　　　　　　　　For S42.452[K,P]: See S42.0[K,P]

● S42.453　Displaced fracture of lateral condyle
　　　　　　of unspecified humerus A, K, P 🔵,
　　　　　　B 🔵🔵, 🔵, A, B 🔵🔵
　　　　　　(Ex:) For S42.453[A]: See S42.209
　　　　　　　　　For S42.453[B]: See S42.201[B]
　　　　　　　　　For S42.453[K,P]: See S42.0[K,P]

● S42.454　Nondisplaced fracture of lateral
　　　　　　condyle of right humerus A, K, P 🔵,
　　　　　　B 🔵🔵, 🔵, A, B 🔵🔵
　　　　　　(Ex:) For S42.454[A]: See S42.201[A]
　　　　　　　　　For S42.454[B]: See S42.201[B]
　　　　　　　　　For S42.454[K,P]: See S42.0[K,P]

● S42.455　Nondisplaced fracture of lateral
　　　　　　condyle of left humerus A, K, P 🔵,
　　　　　　B 🔵🔵, 🔵, A, B 🔵🔵
　　　　　　(Ex:) For S42.455[A]: See S42.202[A]
　　　　　　　　　For S42.455[B]: See S42.201[B]
　　　　　　　　　For S42.455[K,P]: See S42.0[K,P]

● S42.456　Nondisplaced fracture of lateral
　　　　　　condyle of unspecified humerus
　　　　　　A, K, P 🔵, B 🔵🔵, 🔵, A, B 🔵🔵
　　　　　　(Ex:) For S42.456[A]: See S42.209
　　　　　　　　　For S42.456[B]: See S42.201[B]
　　　　　　　　　For S42.456[K,P]: See S42.0[K,P]

● S42.46　Fracture of medial condyle of humerus
　　　　　　Trochlea fracture of humerus

● S42.461　Displaced fracture of medial condyle
　　　　　　of right humerus A, K, P 🔵, B 🔵🔵, 🔵,
　　　　　　A, B 🔵🔵
　　　　　　(Ex:) For S42.461[A]: See S42.201[A]
　　　　　　　　　For S42.461[B]: See S42.201[B]
　　　　　　　　　For S42.461[K,P]: See S42.0[K,P]

● S42.462　Displaced fracture of medial condyle
　　　　　　of left humerus A, K, P 🔵, B 🔵🔵, 🔵,
　　　　　　A, B 🔵🔵
　　　　　　(Ex:) For S42.462[A]: See S42.202[A]
　　　　　　　　　For S42.462[B]: See S42.201[B]
　　　　　　　　　For S42.462[K,P]: See S42.0[K,P]

● S42.463　Displaced fracture of medial condyle
　　　　　　of unspecified humerus A, K, P 🔵,
　　　　　　B 🔵🔵, 🔵, A, B 🔵🔵
　　　　　　(Ex:) For S42.463[A]: See S42.209
　　　　　　　　　For S42.463[B]: See S42.201[B]
　　　　　　　　　For S42.463[K,P]: See S42.0[K,P]

● S42.464　Nondisplaced fracture of medial
　　　　　　condyle of right humerus A, K, P 🔵,
　　　　　　B 🔵🔵, 🔵, A, B 🔵🔵
　　　　　　(Ex:) For S42.464[A]: See S42.201[A]
　　　　　　　　　For S42.464[B]: See S42.201[B]
　　　　　　　　　For S42.464[K,P]: See S42.0[K,P]

● S42.465　Nondisplaced fracture of medial
　　　　　　condyle of left humerus A, K, P 🔵,
　　　　　　B 🔵🔵, 🔵, A, B 🔵🔵
　　　　　　(Ex:) For S42.465[A]: See S42.202[A]
　　　　　　　　　For S42.465[B]: See S42.201[B]
　　　　　　　　　For S42.465[K,P]: See S42.0[K,P]

● S42.466　Nondisplaced fracture of medial
　　　　　　condyle of unspecified humerus
　　　　　　A, K, P 🔵, B 🔵🔵, 🔵, A, B 🔵🔵
　　　　　　(Ex:) For S42.466[A]: See S42.209
　　　　　　　　　For S42.466[B]: See S42.201[B]
　　　　　　　　　For S42.466[K,P]: See S42.0[K,P]

CHAPTER 19 (S00-T88)

N　Newborn Age: 0　　P　Pediatric Age: 0–17　　M　Maternity DX: 12–55　　A　Adult Age: 15–124　　♀　Females Only　　♂　Males Only

🔵　Complication\Comorbidity　　🔵　Major C\C　　(Ex:)　CC/MCC Exclusions　　🔵　Present on Admission Requirement　　🔵🔵　Hospital-Acquired Condition

● **S42.47　Transcondylar fracture of humerus**

● S42.471　Displaced transcondylar fracture of right humerus A, K, P 🖉, B 🖉, 🖉, A, B 🖉

> Ⓔⓧ For S42.471[A]: See S42.201[A]
> For S42.471[B]: See S42.201[B]
> For S42.471[K,P]: See S42.0[K,P]

● S42.472　Displaced transcondylar fracture of left humerus A, K, P 🖉, B 🖉, 🖉, A, B 🖉

> Ⓔⓧ For S42.472[A]: See S42.202[A]
> For S42.472[B]: See S42.201[B]
> For S42.472[K,P]: See S42.0[K,P]

● S42.473　Displaced transcondylar fracture of unspecified humerus A, K, P 🖉, B 🖉, A, B 🖉

> Ⓔⓧ For S42.473[A]: See S42.209
> For S42.473[B]: See S42.201[B]
> For S42.473[K,P]: See S42.0[K,P]

● S42.474　Nondisplaced transcondylar fracture of right humerus A, K, P 🖉, B 🖉, 🖉, A, B 🖉

> Ⓔⓧ For S42.474[A]: See S42.201[A]
> For S42.474[B]: See S42.201[B]
> For S42.474[K,P]: See S42.0[K,P]

● S42.475　Nondisplaced transcondylar fracture of left humerus A, K, P 🖉, B 🖉, 🖉, A, B 🖉

> Ⓔⓧ For S42.475[A]: See S42.202[A]
> For S42.475[B]: See S42.201[B]
> For S42.475[K,P]: See S42.0[K,P]

● S42.476　Nondisplaced transcondylar fracture of unspecified humerus A, K, P 🖉, B 🖉, A, B 🖉

> Ⓔⓧ For S42.476[A]: See S42.209
> For S42.476[B]: See S42.201[B]
> For S42.476[K,P]: See S42.0[K,P]

● **S42.48　Torus fracture of lower end of humerus**

The appropriate 7th character is to be added to all codes in subcategory S42.48

A	initial encounter for closed fracture
D	subsequent encounter for fracture with routine healing
G	subsequent encounter for fracture with delayed healing
K	subsequent encounter for fracture with nonunion
P	subsequent encounter for fracture with malunion
S	sequela

● S42.481　Torus fracture of lower end of right humerus A, K, P 🖉, 🖉, A 🖉

> Ⓔⓧ For S42.481[A]: See S42.201[A]
> For S42.481[K,P]: See S42.0[K,P]

● S42.482　Torus fracture of lower end of left humerus A, K, P 🖉, 🖉, A 🖉

> Ⓔⓧ For S42.482[A]: See S42.202[A]
> For S42.482[K,P]: See S42.0[K,P]

● S42.489　Torus fracture of lower end of unspecified humerus A, K, P 🖉, 🖉, A 🖉

> Ⓔⓧ For S42.489[A]: See S42.209
> For S42.489[K,P]: See S42.0[K,P]

● **S42.49　Other fracture of lower end of humerus**

● S42.491　Other displaced fracture of lower end of right humerus A, K, P 🖉, B 🖉, 🖉, A, B 🖉

> Ⓔⓧ For S42.491[A]: See S42.201[A]
> For S42.491[B]: See S42.201[B]
> For S42.491[K,P]: See S42.0[K,P]

● S42.492　Other displaced fracture of lower end of left humerus A, K, P 🖉, B 🖉, 🖉, A, B 🖉

> Ⓔⓧ For S42.492[A]: See S42.202[A]
> For S42.492[B]: See S42.201[B]
> For S42.492[K,P]: See S42.0[K,P]

● S42.493　Other displaced fracture of lower end of unspecified humerus A, K, P 🖉, B 🖉, 🖉, A, B 🖉

> Ⓔⓧ For S42.493[A]: See S42.209
> For S42.493[B]: See S42.201[B]
> For S42.493[K,P]: See S42.0[K,P]

● S42.494　Other nondisplaced fracture of lower end of right humerus A, K, P 🖉, B 🖉, 🖉, A, B 🖉

> Ⓔⓧ For S42.494[A]: See S42.201[A]
> For S42.494[B]: See S42.201[B]
> For S42.494[K,P]: See S42.0[K,P]

● S42.495　Other nondisplaced fracture of lower end of left humerus A, K, P 🖉, B 🖉, 🖉, A, B 🖉

> Ⓔⓧ For S42.495[A]: See S42.202[A]
> For S42.495[B]: See S42.201[B]
> For S42.495[K,P]: See S42.0[K,P]

● S42.496　Other nondisplaced fracture of lower end of unspecified humerus A, K, P 🖉, B 🖉, A, B 🖉

> Ⓔⓧ For S42.496[A]: See S42.209
> For S42.496[B]: See S42.201[B]
> For S42.496[K,P]: See S42.0[K,P]

● **S42.9　Fracture of shoulder girdle, part unspecified**
　　Fracture of shoulder NOS

> Ⓔⓧ For category S42.9 CC codes S42.9[A]: See S42.209 For S42.9[B]: See S42.201[B] For S42.9[K,P]: See S42.0[K,P]

● S42.90　Fracture of unspecified shoulder girdle, part unspecified A, K, P 🖉, B 🖉, 🖉, A, B 🖉

● S42.91　Fracture of right shoulder girdle, part unspecified A, K, P 🖉, B 🖉, 🖉, A, B 🖉

● S42.92　Fracture of left shoulder girdle, part unspecified A, K, P 🖉, B 🖉, 🖉, A, B 🖉

◀ New　　◀▥ Revised　　deleted Deleted　　Excludes 1　　Excludes 2　　Includes　　Use additional　　Code first　　Code also　　Unspecified

OGCR Official Guidelines　　● Unacceptable Principal Diagnosis　　X Assign placeholder X　　● Use Additional Character(s)　　▸ Manifestation Code　　Coding Clinic

● **S43**   **Dislocation and sprain of joints and ligaments of shoulder girdle**

> **Includes**   avulsion of joint or ligament of shoulder girdle
>
> laceration of cartilage, joint or ligament of shoulder girdle
>
> sprain of cartilage, joint or ligament of shoulder girdle
>
> traumatic hemarthrosis of joint or ligament of shoulder girdle
>
> traumatic rupture of joint or ligament of shoulder girdle
>
> traumatic subluxation of joint or ligament of shoulder girdle
>
> traumatic tear of joint or ligament of shoulder girdle

Code also any associated open wound

> **Excludes2**   strain of muscle, fascia and tendon of shoulder and upper arm (S46.-)

The appropriate 7th character is to be added to each code from category S43

> A   initial encounter
> D   subsequent encounter
> S   sequela

● **S43.0**   **Subluxation and dislocation of shoulder joint**
> Dislocation of glenohumeral joint
> Subluxation of glenohumeral joint

   ● **S43.00**   **Unspecified subluxation and dislocation of shoulder joint**
> Dislocation of humerus NOS
> Subluxation of humerus NOS

     ● S43.001   Unspecified subluxation of right shoulder joint 🔍

     ● S43.002   Unspecified subluxation of left shoulder joint 🔍

     ● S43.003   Unspecified subluxation of unspecified shoulder joint 🔍

     ● S43.004   Unspecified dislocation of right shoulder joint 🔍

     ● S43.005   Unspecified dislocation of left shoulder joint 🔍

     ● S43.006   Unspecified dislocation of unspecified shoulder joint 🔍

   ● **S43.01**   **Anterior subluxation and dislocation of humerus**

     ● S43.011   Anterior subluxation of right humerus 🔍

     ● S43.012   Anterior subluxation of left humerus 🔍

     ● S43.013   Anterior subluxation of unspecified humerus 🔍

     ● S43.014   Anterior dislocation of right humerus 🔍

     ● S43.015   Anterior dislocation of left humerus 🔍

     ● S43.016   Anterior dislocation of unspecified humerus 🔍

● **S43.02**   **Posterior subluxation and dislocation of humerus**

   ● S43.021   Posterior subluxation of right humerus 🔍

   ● S43.022   Posterior subluxation of left humerus 🔍

   ● S43.023   Posterior subluxation of unspecified humerus 🔍

   ● S43.024   Posterior dislocation of right humerus 🔍

   ● S43.025   Posterior dislocation of left humerus 🔍

   ● S43.026   Posterior dislocation of unspecified humerus 🔍

● **S43.03**   **Inferior subluxation and dislocation of humerus**

   ● S43.031   Inferior subluxation of right humerus 🔍

   ● S43.032   Inferior subluxation of left humerus 🔍

   ● S43.033   Inferior subluxation of unspecified humerus 🔍

   ● S43.034   Inferior dislocation of right humerus 🔍

   ● S43.035   Inferior dislocation of left humerus 🔍

   ● S43.036   Inferior dislocation of unspecified humerus 🔍

● **S43.08**   **Other subluxation and dislocation of shoulder joint**

   ● S43.081   Other subluxation of right shoulder joint 🔍

   ● S43.082   Other subluxation of left shoulder joint 🔍

   ● S43.083   Other subluxation of unspecified shoulder joint 🔍

   ● S43.084   Other dislocation of right shoulder joint 🔍

   ● S43.085   Other dislocation of left shoulder joint 🔍

   ● S43.086   Other dislocation of unspecified shoulder joint 🔍

● **S43.1**   **Subluxation and dislocation of acromioclavicular joint**

   ● **S43.10**   **Unspecified dislocation of acromioclavicular joint**

     ● S43.101   Unspecified dislocation of right acromioclavicular joint 🔍

     ● S43.102   Unspecified dislocation of left acromioclavicular joint 🔍

     ● S43.109   Unspecified dislocation of unspecified acromioclavicular joint 🔍

   ● **S43.11**   **Subluxation of acromioclavicular joint**

     ● S43.111   Subluxation of right acromioclavicular joint 🔍

     ● S43.112   Subluxation of left acromioclavicular joint 🔍

     ● S43.119   Subluxation of unspecified acromioclavicular joint 🔍

N   Newborn Age: 0   P   Pediatric Age: 0–17   M   Maternity DX: 12–55   A   Adult Age: 15–124   ♀   Females Only   ♂   Males Only

🔍 Complication\Comorbidity   🔍 Major C\C   (Ex)   CC/MCC Exclusions   🔍 Present on Admission Requirement   🔍 Hospital-Acquired Condition

1357

● S43.12   Dislocation of acromioclavicular joint, 100%-200% displacement
     ● S43.121   Dislocation of right acromioclavicular joint, 100%-200% displacement
     ● S43.122   Dislocation of left acromioclavicular joint, 100%-200% displacement 🔊
     ● S43.129   Dislocation of unspecified acromioclavicular joint, 100%-200% displacement 🔊

● S43.13   Dislocation of acromioclavicular joint, greater than 200% displacement
     ● S43.131   Dislocation of right acromioclavicular joint, greater than 200% displacement
     ● S43.132   Dislocation of left acromioclavicular joint, greater than 200% displacement 🔊
     ● S43.139   Dislocation of unspecified acromioclavicular joint, greater than 200% displacement 🔊

● S43.14   Inferior dislocation of acromioclavicular joint
     ● S43.141   Inferior dislocation of right acromioclavicular joint 🔊
     ● S43.142   Inferior dislocation of left acromioclavicular joint 🔊
     ● S43.149   Inferior dislocation of unspecified acromioclavicular joint 🔊

● S43.15   Posterior dislocation of acromioclavicular joint
     ● S43.151   Posterior dislocation of right acromioclavicular joint 🔊
     ● S43.152   Posterior dislocation of left acromioclavicular joint 🔊
     ● S43.159   Posterior dislocation of unspecified acromioclavicular joint 🔊

● S43.2   Subluxation and dislocation of sternoclavicular joint
   ● S43.20   Unspecified subluxation and dislocation of sternoclavicular joint
     ● S43.201   Unspecified subluxation of right sternoclavicular joint A 🔊, 🔊, A 🔊
       (Ex:) M99.18, S43.201[A], S43.203-S43.204[A], S43.206[A], S43.211[A], S43.213-S43.214[A], S43.216[A], S43.221[A], S43.223-S43.224[A], S43.226[A]
     ● S43.202   Unspecified subluxation of left sternoclavicular joint A 🔊, 🔊, A 🔊
       (Ex:) M99.18, S43.202-S43.203[A], S43.205-S43.206[A], S43.212-S43.213[A], S43.215-S43.216[A], S43.222-S43.223[A], S43.225-S43.226[A]
     ● S43.203   Unspecified subluxation of unspecified sternoclavicular joint A 🔊, 🔊, A 🔊
       (Ex:) M99.18, S43.201-S43.226[A]
     ● S43.204   Unspecified dislocation of right sternoclavicular joint A 🔊, 🔊, A 🔊
       (Ex:) See S43.201
     ● S43.205   Unspecified dislocation of left sternoclavicular joint A 🔊, 🔊, A 🔊
       (Ex:) See S43.202
     ● S43.206   Unspecified dislocation of unspecified sternoclavicular joint A 🔊, 🔊, A 🔊
       (Ex:) See S43.203

   ● S43.21   Anterior subluxation and dislocation of sternoclavicular joint
     ● S43.211   Anterior subluxation of right sternoclavicular joint A 🔊, 🔊, A 🔊
       (Ex:) See S43.201
     ● S43.212   Anterior subluxation of left sternoclavicular joint A 🔊, 🔊, A 🔊
       (Ex:) See S43.202
     ● S43.213   Anterior subluxation of unspecified sternoclavicular joint A 🔊, 🔊, A 🔊
       (Ex:) See S43.203
     ● S43.214   Anterior dislocation of right sternoclavicular joint A 🔊, 🔊, A 🔊
       (Ex:) See S43.201
     ● S43.215   Anterior dislocation of left sternoclavicular joint A 🔊, 🔊, A 🔊
       (Ex:) See S43.202
     ● S43.216   Anterior dislocation of unspecified sternoclavicular joint A 🔊, 🔊, A 🔊
       (Ex:) See S43.203

   ● S43.22   Posterior subluxation and dislocation of sternoclavicular joint
     ● S43.221   Posterior subluxation of right sternoclavicular joint A 🔊, 🔊, A 🔊
       (Ex:) See S43.201
     ● S43.222   Posterior subluxation of left sternoclavicular joint A 🔊, 🔊, A 🔊
       (Ex:) See S43.202
     ● S43.223   Posterior subluxation of unspecified sternoclavicular joint A 🔊, 🔊, A 🔊
       (Ex:) See S43.203
     ● S43.224   Posterior dislocation of right sternoclavicular joint A 🔊, 🔊, A 🔊
       (Ex:) See S43.201
     ● S43.225   Posterior dislocation of left sternoclavicular joint A 🔊, 🔊, A 🔊
       (Ex:) See S43.202
     ● S43.226   Posterior dislocation of unspecified sternoclavicular joint A 🔊, 🔊, A 🔊
       (Ex:) See S43.203

● S43.3   Subluxation and dislocation of other and unspecified parts of shoulder girdle
   ● S43.30   Subluxation and dislocation of unspecified parts of shoulder girdle
     Dislocation of shoulder girdle NOS
     Subluxation of shoulder girdle NOS
     ● S43.301   Subluxation of unspecified parts of right shoulder girdle 🔊
     ● S43.302   Subluxation of unspecified parts of left shoulder girdle 🔊
     ● S43.303   Subluxation of unspecified parts of unspecified shoulder girdle 🔊
     ● S43.304   Dislocation of unspecified parts of right shoulder girdle 🔊
     ● S43.305   Dislocation of unspecified parts of left shoulder girdle 🔊
     ● S43.306   Dislocation of unspecified parts of unspecified shoulder girdle 🔊

   ● S43.31   Subluxation and dislocation of scapula
     ● S43.311   Subluxation of right scapula 🔊
     ● S43.312   Subluxation of left scapula 🔊
     ● S43.313   Subluxation of unspecified scapula 🔊
     ● S43.314   Dislocation of right scapula 🔊
     ● S43.315   Dislocation of left scapula 🔊
     ● S43.316   Dislocation of unspecified scapula 🔊

◀ New   ◀ Revised   ~~deleted~~ Deleted   Excludes 1   Excludes 2   Includes   Use additional   Code first   Code also   Unspecified
OGCR Official Guidelines   ● Unacceptable Principal Diagnosis   X Assign placeholder X   ● Use Additional Character(s)   ▶ Manifestation Code   **Coding Clinic**

● S43.39   Subluxation and dislocation of other parts of shoulder girdle
    ● S43.391   Subluxation of other parts of right shoulder girdle 🖐
    ● S43.392   Subluxation of other parts of left shoulder girdle 🖐
    ● S43.393   Subluxation of other parts of unspecified shoulder girdle 🖐
    ● S43.394   Dislocation of other parts of right shoulder girdle 🖐
    ● S43.395   Dislocation of other parts of left shoulder girdle 🖐
    ● S43.396   Dislocation of other parts of unspecified shoulder girdle 🖐

● S43.4   Sprain of shoulder joint
   ● S43.40   Unspecified sprain of shoulder joint
    ● S43.401   Unspecified sprain of right shoulder joint 🖐
    ● S43.402   Unspecified sprain of left shoulder joint 🖐
    ● S43.409   Unspecified sprain of unspecified shoulder joint 🖐
   ● S43.41   Sprain of coracohumeral (ligament)
    ● S43.411   Sprain of right coracohumeral (ligament) 🖐
    ● S43.412   Sprain of left coracohumeral (ligament) 🖐
    ● S43.419   Sprain of unspecified coracohumeral (ligament) 🖐
   ● S43.42   Sprain of rotator cuff capsule
     Excludes1   rotator cuff syndrome (complete) (incomplete), not specified as traumatic (M75.1-)
     Excludes2   injury of tendon of rotator cuff (S46.0-)
    ● S43.421   Sprain of right rotator cuff capsule 🖐
    ● S43.422   Sprain of left rotator cuff capsule 🖐
    ● S43.429   Sprain of unspecified rotator cuff capsule 🖐
   ● S43.43   Superior glenoid labrum lesion
     SLAP lesion
    ● S43.431   Superior glenoid labrum lesion of right shoulder 🖐
    ● S43.432   Superior glenoid labrum lesion of left shoulder 🖐
    ● S43.439   Superior glenoid labrum lesion of unspecified shoulder 🖐
   ● S43.49   Other sprain of shoulder joint
    ● S43.491   Other sprain of right shoulder joint 🖐
    ● S43.492   Other sprain of left shoulder joint 🖐
    ● S43.499   Other sprain of unspecified shoulder joint 🖐

● S43.5   Sprain of acromioclavicular joint
    Sprain of acromioclavicular ligament
   X ● S43.50   Sprain of unspecified acromioclavicular joint 🖐
   X ● S43.51   Sprain of right acromioclavicular joint 🖐
   X ● S43.52   Sprain of left acromioclavicular joint 🖐

● S43.6   Sprain of sternoclavicular joint
   X ● S43.60   Sprain of unspecified sternoclavicular joint 🖐
   X ● S43.61   Sprain of right sternoclavicular joint 🖐
   X ● S43.62   Sprain of left sternoclavicular joint 🖐

● S43.8   Sprain of other specified parts of shoulder girdle
   X ● S43.80   Sprain of other specified parts of unspecified shoulder girdle 🖐
   X ● S43.81   Sprain of other specified parts of right shoulder girdle 🖐
   X ● S43.82   Sprain of other specified parts of left shoulder girdle 🖐

● S43.9   Sprain of unspecified parts of shoulder girdle
   X ● S43.90   Sprain of unspecified parts of unspecified shoulder girdle 🖐
     Sprain of shoulder girdle NOS
   X ● S43.91   Sprain of unspecified parts of right shoulder girdle 🖐
   X ● S43.92   Sprain of unspecified parts of left shoulder girdle 🖐

● S44   **Injury of nerves at shoulder and upper arm level**
    Code also any associated open wound (S41.-)
    Excludes2   injury of brachial plexus (S14.3-)
    The appropriate 7th character is to be added to each code from category S44

> A   initial encounter
> D   subsequent encounter
> S   sequela

● S44.0   Injury of ulnar nerve at upper arm level
     Excludes1   ulnar nerve NOS (S54.0)
   X ● S44.00   Injury of ulnar nerve at upper arm level, unspecified arm 🖐
   X ● S44.01   Injury of ulnar nerve at upper arm level, right arm 🖐
   X ● S44.02   Injury of ulnar nerve at upper arm level, left arm 🖐

● S44.1   Injury of median nerve at upper arm level
     Excludes1   median nerve NOS (S54.1)
   X ● S44.10   Injury of median nerve at upper arm level, unspecified arm 🖐
   X ● S44.11   Injury of median nerve at upper arm level, right arm 🖐
   X ● S44.12   Injury of median nerve at upper arm level, left arm 🖐

● S44.2   Injury of radial nerve at upper arm level
     Excludes1   radial nerve NOS (S54.2)
   X ● S44.20   Injury of radial nerve at upper arm level, unspecified arm 🖐
   X ● S44.21   Injury of radial nerve at upper arm level, right arm 🖐
   X ● S44.22   Injury of radial nerve at upper arm level, left arm 🖐

● S44.3   Injury of axillary nerve
   X ● S44.30   Injury of axillary nerve, unspecified arm 🖐
   X ● S44.31   Injury of axillary nerve, right arm 🖐
   X ● S44.32   Injury of axillary nerve, left arm 🖐

● S44.4   Injury of musculocutaneous nerve
   X ● S44.40   Injury of musculocutaneous nerve, unspecified arm 🖐
   X ● S44.41   Injury of musculocutaneous nerve, right arm 🖐
   X ● S44.42   Injury of musculocutaneous nerve, left arm 🖐

● S44.5   Injury of cutaneous sensory nerve at shoulder and upper arm level
   X ● S44.50   Injury of cutaneous sensory nerve at shoulder and upper arm level, unspecified arm 🖐
   X ● S44.51   Injury of cutaneous sensory nerve at shoulder and upper arm level, right arm 🖐
   X ● S44.52   Injury of cutaneous sensory nerve at shoulder and upper arm level, left arm 🖐

CHAPTER 19 (S00-T88)

N   Newborn Age: 0   P   Pediatric Age: 0–17   M   Maternity DX: 12–55   A   Adult Age: 15–124   ♀   Females Only   ♂   Males Only

🖐   Complication\Comorbidity   🖐   Major C\C   (Ex)   CC/MCC Exclusions   🖐   Present on Admission Requirement   🖐   Hospital-Acquired Condition

1359

● **S44.8**   Injury of other nerves at shoulder and upper arm level
  ● **S44.8X**   Injury of other nerves at shoulder and upper arm level
    ● **S44.8X1**   Injury of other nerves at shoulder and upper arm level, right arm
    ● **S44.8X2**   Injury of other nerves at shoulder and upper arm level, left arm
    ● **S44.8X9**   Injury of other nerves at shoulder and upper arm level, unspecified arm

● **S44.9**   Injury of unspecified nerve at shoulder and upper arm level
  X ● **S44.90**   Injury of unspecified nerve at shoulder and upper arm level, unspecified arm
  X ● **S44.91**   Injury of unspecified nerve at shoulder and upper arm level, right arm
  X ● **S44.92**   Injury of unspecified nerve at shoulder and upper arm level, left arm

● **S45**   Injury of blood vessels at shoulder and upper arm level
    Code also any associated open wound (S41.-)
    Excludes2   injury of subclavian artery (S25.1)
                 injury of subclavian vein (S25.3)

    The appropriate 7th character is to be added to each code from category S45

    A   initial encounter
    D   subsequent encounter
    S   sequela

● **S45.0**   Injury of axillary artery
  ● **S45.00**   Unspecified injury of axillary artery
    ● **S45.001**   Unspecified injury of axillary artery, right side A
      (Ex:) S45.001[A], S45.009-S45.011[A], S45.019-S45.091[A], S45.099[A], S45.301[A], S45.309-S45.311[A], S45.319-S45.391[A], S45.399-S45.801[A], S45.809-S45.811[A], S45.819-S45.891[A], S45.899-S45.901[A], S45.909-S45.911[A], S45.919-S45.991[A], S45.999[A], S55.201[A], S55.209-S55.211[A], S55.219-S55.291[A], S55.299-S55.801[A], S55.809-S55.811[A], S55.819-S55.891[A], S55.899-S55.901[A], S55.909-S55.911[A], S55.919-S55.991[A], S55.999[A], S65.801[A], S65.809-S65.811[A], S65.819-S65.891[A], S65.899-S65.901[A], S65.909-S65.911[A], S65.919-S65.991[A], S65.999[A]

    ● **S45.002**   Unspecified injury of axillary artery, left side A
      (Ex:) S45.002-S45.009[A], S45.012-S45.019[A], S45.092-S45.099[A], S45.302-S45.309[A], S45.312-S45.319[A], S45.392-S45.399[A], S45.802-S45.809[A], S45.812-S45.819[A], S45.892-S45.899[A], S45.902-S45.909[A], S45.912-S45.919[A], S45.992-S45.999[A], S55.202-S55.209[A], S55.212-S55.219[A], S55.292-S55.299[A], S55.802-S55.809[A], S55.812-S55.819[A], S55.892-S55.899[A], S55.902-S55.909[A], S55.912-S55.919[A], S55.992-S55.999[A], S65.802-S65.809[A], S65.812-S65.819[A], S65.892-S65.899[A], S65.902-S65.909[A], S65.912-S65.919[A], S65.992-S65.999[A]

    ● **S45.009**   Unspecified injury of axillary artery, unspecified side A
      (Ex:) S45.001-S45.099[A], S45.301-S45.399[A], S45.801-S45.999[A], S55.201-S55.999[A], S65.801-S65.999[A]

● **S45.01**   Laceration of axillary artery
  ● **S45.011**   Laceration of axillary artery, right side A
    (Ex:) See S45.001
  ● **S45.012**   Laceration of axillary artery, left side A
    (Ex:) See S45.002
  ● **S45.019**   Laceration of axillary artery, unspecified side A
    (Ex:) See S45.009

● **S45.09**   Other specified injury of axillary artery
  ● **S45.091**   Other specified injury of axillary artery, right side A
    (Ex:) See S45.001
  ● **S45.092**   Other specified injury of axillary artery, left side A
    (Ex:) See S45.002
  ● **S45.099**   Other specified injury of axillary artery, unspecified side A
    (Ex:) See S45.009

● **S45.1**   Injury of brachial artery
  ● **S45.10**   Unspecified injury of brachial artery
    ● **S45.101**   Unspecified injury of brachial artery, right side A
      (Ex:) S45.101[A], S45.109-S45.111[A], S45.119-S45.191[A], S45.199-S45.201[A], S45.209A-S45.211[A], S45.219-S45.291[A], S45.299-S45.301[A], S45.309-S45.311[A], S45.319-S45.391[A], S45.399-S45.801[A], S45.809-S45.811[A], S45.819-S45.891[A], S45.899-S45.901[A], S45.909-S45.911[A], S45.919-S45.991[A], S45.999[A], S55.201[A], S55.209-S55.211[A], S55.219-S55.291[A], S55.299-S55.801[A], S55.809-S55.811[A], S55.819-S55.891[A], S55.899-S55.901[A], S55.909-S55.911[A], S55.919-S55.991[A], S55.999[A], S65.801[A], S65.809-S65.811[A], S65.819-S65.891[A], S65.899-S65.901[A], S65.909-S65.911[A], S65.919-S65.991[A], S65.999[A]

    ● **S45.102**   Unspecified injury of brachial artery, left side A
      (Ex:) S45.102-S45.109[A], S45.112-S45.119[A], S45.192-S45.199[A], S45.202-S45.209[A], S45.212-S45.219[A], S45.292-S45.299[A], S45.302-S45.309[A], S45.312-S45.319[A], S45.392-S45.399[A], S45.802-S45.809[A], S45.812-S45.819[A], S45.892-S45.899[A], S45.902-S45.909[A], S45.912-S45.919[A], S45.992-S45.999[A], S55.202-S55.209[A], S55.212-S55.219[A], S55.292-S55.299[A], S55.802-S55.809[A], S55.812-S55.819[A], S55.892-S55.899[A], S55.902-S55.909[A], S55.912-S55.919[A], S55.992-S55.999[A], S65.802-S65.809[A], S65.812-S65.819[A], S65.892-S65.899[A], S65.902-S65.909[A], S65.912-S65.919[A], S65.992-S65.999[A]

    ● **S45.109**   Unspecified injury of brachial artery, unspecified side A
      (Ex:) S45.101-S45.999[A], S55.201-S55.999[A], S65.801-S65.999[A]

◀ New   ◀ Revised   ~~deleted~~ Deleted   Excludes 1   Excludes 2   Includes   Use additional   Code first   Code also   Unspecified
OGCR Official Guidelines   ● Unacceptable Principal Diagnosis   X Assign placeholder X   ● Use Additional Character(s)   ▶ Manifestation Code   Coding Clinic

● S45.11   Laceration of brachial artery

    ● S45.111   Laceration of brachial artery, right side A 🩸, 🩸
           (Ex) See S45.101

    ● S45.112   Laceration of brachial artery, left side A 🩸, 🩸
           (Ex) See S45.102

    ● S45.119   Laceration of brachial artery, unspecified side A 🩸, 🩸
           (Ex) See S45.109

● S45.19   Other specified injury of brachial artery

    ● S45.191   Other specified injury of brachial artery, right side A 🩸, 🩸
           (Ex) See S45.101

    ● S45.192   Other specified injury of brachial artery, left side A 🩸, 🩸
           (Ex) See S45.102

    ● S45.199   Other specified injury of brachial artery, unspecified side A 🩸, 🩸
           (Ex) See S45.109

● S45.2   Injury of axillary or brachial vein

    ● S45.20   Unspecified injury of axillary or brachial vein

       ● S45.201   Unspecified injury of axillary or brachial vein, right side A 🩸, 🩸
              (Ex) See S45.101

       ● S45.202   Unspecified injury of axillary or brachial vein, left side A 🩸, 🩸
              (Ex) See S45.102

       ● S45.209   Unspecified injury of axillary or brachial vein, unspecified side A 🩸, 🩸
              (Ex) See S45.109

    ● S45.21   Laceration of axillary or brachial vein

       ● S45.211   Laceration of axillary or brachial vein, right side A 🩸, 🩸
              (Ex) See S45.101

       ● S45.212   Laceration of axillary or brachial vein, left side A 🩸, 🩸
              (Ex) See S45.102

       ● S45.219   Laceration of axillary or brachial vein, unspecified side A 🩸, 🩸
              (Ex) See S45.109

    ● S45.29   Other specified injury of axillary or brachial vein

       ● S45.291   Other specified injury of axillary or brachial vein, right side A 🩸, 🩸
              (Ex) See S45.101

       ● S45.292   Other specified injury of axillary or brachial vein, left side A 🩸, 🩸
              (Ex) See S45.102

       ● S45.299   Other specified injury of axillary or brachial vein, unspecified side A 🩸, 🩸
              (Ex) See S45.109

● S45.3   Injury of superficial vein at shoulder and upper arm level

    ● S45.30   Unspecified injury of superficial vein at shoulder and upper arm level

       ● S45.301   Unspecified injury of superficial vein at shoulder and upper arm level, right arm A 🩸, 🩸
              (Ex) S45.301[A], S45.309-S45.311[A], S45.319-S45.391[A], S45.399-S45.801[A], S45.809-S45.811[A], S45.819-S45.891[A], S45.899-S45.901[A], S45.909-S45.911[A], S45.919-S45.991[A], S45.999[A], S55.001[A], S55.009-S55.011[A], S55.019-S55.091[A], S55.099[A], S55.201[A], S55.209-S55.211[A], S55.219-S55.291[A], S55.299-S55.801[A], S55.809-S55.811[A], S55.819-S55.891[A], S55.899-S55.901[A], S55.909-S55.911[A], S55.919-S55.991[A], S55.999[A], S65.001[A], S65.009-S65.011[A], S65.019-S65.091[A], S65.099[A], S65.201[A], S65.209-S65.211[A], S65.219-S65.291[A], S65.299-S65.301[A], S65.309-S65.311[A], S65.319-S65.391[A], S65.399-S65.401[A], S65.409-S65.411[A], S65.419-S65.491[A], S65.499-S65.500[A], S65.502[A], S65.504[A], S65.506[A], S65.508-S65.510[A], S65.512[A], S65.514[A], S65.516[A], S65.518-S65.590[A], S65.592[A], S65.594[A], S65.596[A], S65.598-S65.801[A], S65.809-S65.811[A], S65.819-S65.891[A], S65.899-S65.901[A], S65.909-S65.911[A], S65.919-S65.991[A], S65.999[A]

       ● S45.302   Unspecified injury of superficial vein at shoulder and upper arm level, left arm A 🩸, 🩸
              (Ex) S45.302-S45.309[A], S45.312-S45.319[A], S45.392-S45.399[A], S45.802-S45.809[A], S45.812-S45.819[A], S45.892-S45.899[A], S45.902-S45.909[A], S45.912-S45.919[A], S45.992-S45.999[A], S55.002-S55.009[A], S55.012-S55.019[A], S55.092-S55.099[A], S55.202-S55.209[A], S55.212-S55.219[A], S55.292-S55.299[A], S55.802-S55.809[A], S55.812-S55.819[A], S55.892-S55.899[A], S55.902-S55.909[A], S55.912-S55.919[A], S55.992-S55.999[A], S65.002-S65.009[A], S65.012-S65.019[A], S65.092-S65.099[A], S65.202-S65.209[A], S65.212-S65.219[A], S65.292-S65.299[A], S65.302-S65.309[A], S65.312-S65.319[A]. S65.392-S65.399[A], S65.402-S65.409[A], S65.412-S65.419[A], S65.492-S65.499[A], S65.501[A], S65.503[A], S65.505[A], S65.507-S65.509[A], S65.511[A], S65.513[A], S65.515[A], S65.517-S65.519[A], S65.591[A], S65.593[A], S65.595[A], S65.597-S65.599[A], S65.802-S65.809[A], S65.812-S65.819[A], S65.892-S65.899[A], S65.902-S65.909[A], S65.912-S65.919[A], S65.992-S65.999[A]

       ● S45.309   Unspecified injury of superficial vein at shoulder and upper arm level, unspecified arm A 🩸, 🩸
              (Ex) S45.301-S45.999[A], S55.001-S55.099[A], S55.201-S55.999[A], S65.001-S65.099[A], S65.201-S65.999[A]

N Newborn Age: 0   **P** Pediatric Age: 0–17   **M** Maternity DX: 12–55   **A** Adult Age: 15–124   ♀ Females Only   ♂ Males Only

🩸 Complication\Comorbidity   🩸 Major C\C   (Ex) CC/MCC Exclusions   🩸 Present on Admission Requirement   🩸 Hospital-Acquired Condition

1361

● **S45.31**   Laceration of superficial vein at shoulder and upper arm level

  ● **S45.311**   Laceration of superficial vein at shoulder and upper arm level, right arm A 🔖, 🔖
     (Ex:) See S45.301

  ● **S45.312**   Laceration of superficial vein at shoulder and upper arm level, left arm A 🔖, 🔖
     (Ex:) See S45.302

  ● **S45.319**   Laceration of superficial vein at shoulder and upper arm level, unspecified arm A 🔖, 🔖
     (Ex:) See S45.309

● **S45.39**   Other specified injury of superficial vein at shoulder and upper arm level

  ● **S45.391**   Other specified injury of superficial vein at shoulder and upper arm level, right arm A 🔖, 🔖
     (Ex:) See S45.301

  ● **S45.392**   Other specified injury of superficial vein at shoulder and upper arm level, left arm A 🔖, 🔖
     (Ex:) See S45.302

  ● **S45.399**   Other specified injury of superficial vein at shoulder and upper arm level, unspecified arm A 🔖, 🔖
     (Ex:) See S45.309

● **S45.8**   Injury of other specified blood vessels at shoulder and upper arm level

  ● **S45.80**   Unspecified injury of other specified blood vessels at shoulder and upper arm level

    ● **S45.801**   Unspecified injury of other specified blood vessels at shoulder and upper arm level, right arm A 🔖, 🔖
       (Ex:) See S45.301

    ● **S45.802**   Unspecified injury of other specified blood vessels at shoulder and upper arm level, left arm A 🔖, 🔖
       (Ex:) See S45.302

    ● **S45.809**   Unspecified injury of other specified blood vessels at shoulder and upper arm level, unspecified arm A 🔖, 🔖
       (Ex:) See S45.309

  ● **S45.81**   Laceration of other specified blood vessels at shoulder and upper arm level

    ● **S45.811**   Laceration of other specified blood vessels at shoulder and upper arm level, right arm A 🔖, 🔖
       (Ex:) See S45.301

    ● **S45.812**   Laceration of other specified blood vessels at shoulder and upper arm level, left arm A 🔖, 🔖
       (Ex:) See S45.302

    ● **S45.819**   Laceration of other specified blood vessels at shoulder and upper arm level, unspecified arm A 🔖, 🔖
       (Ex:) See S45.309

● **S45.89**   Other specified injury of other specified blood vessels at shoulder and upper arm level

  ● **S45.891**   Other specified injury of other specified blood vessels at shoulder and upper arm level, right arm A 🔖, 🔖
     (Ex:) See S45.301

  ● **S45.892**   Other specified injury of other specified blood vessels at shoulder and upper arm level, left arm A 🔖, 🔖
     (Ex:) See S45.302

  ● **S45.899**   Other specified injury of other specified blood vessels at shoulder and upper arm level, unspecified arm A 🔖, 🔖
     (Ex:) See S45.309

● **S45.9**   Injury of unspecified blood vessel at shoulder and upper arm level

  ● **S45.90**   Unspecified injury of unspecified blood vessel at shoulder and upper arm level

    ● **S45.901**   Unspecified injury of unspecified blood vessel at shoulder and upper arm level, right arm A 🔖, 🔖
       (Ex:) See S45.301

    ● **S45.902**   Unspecified injury of unspecified blood vessel at shoulder and upper arm level, left arm A 🔖, 🔖
       (Ex:) See S45.302

    ● **S45.909**   Unspecified injury of unspecified blood vessel at shoulder and upper arm level, unspecified arm A 🔖, 🔖
       (Ex:) See S45.309

  ● **S45.91**   Laceration of unspecified blood vessel at shoulder and upper arm level

    ● **S45.911**   Laceration of unspecified blood vessel at shoulder and upper arm level, right arm A 🔖, 🔖
       (Ex:) See S45.301

    ● **S45.912**   Laceration of unspecified blood vessel at shoulder and upper arm level, left arm A 🔖, 🔖
       (Ex:) See S45.302

    ● **S45.919**   Laceration of unspecified blood vessel at shoulder and upper arm level, unspecified arm A 🔖, 🔖
       (Ex:) See S45.309

  ● **S45.99**   Other specified injury of unspecified blood vessel at shoulder and upper arm level

    ● **S45.991**   Other specified injury of unspecified blood vessel at shoulder and upper arm level, right arm A 🔖, 🔖
       (Ex:) See S45.301

    ● **S45.992**   Other specified injury of unspecified blood vessel at shoulder and upper arm level, left arm A 🔖, 🔖
       (Ex:) See S45.302

    ● **S45.999**   Other specified injury of unspecified blood vessel at shoulder and upper arm level, unspecified arm A 🔖, 🔖
       (Ex:) See S45.309

◀ New   ◀▦ Revised   ~~deleted~~ Deleted   Excludes 1   Excludes 2   Includes   Use additional   Code first   Code also   Unspecified

OGCR Official Guidelines   ● Unacceptable Principal Diagnosis   X Assign placeholder X   ● Use Additional Character(s)   ▌ Manifestation Code   **Coding Clinic**

● **S46** Injury of muscle, fascia and tendon at shoulder and upper arm level

Code also any associated open wound (S41.-)

Excludes2 injury of muscle, fascia and tendon at elbow (S56.-)

sprain of joints and ligaments of shoulder girdle (S43.9)

The appropriate 7th character is to be added to each code from category S46

A	initial encounter
D	subsequent encounter
S	sequela

● **S46.0** Injury of muscle(s) and tendon(s) of the rotator cuff of shoulder

● **S46.00** Unspecified injury of muscle(s) and tendon(s) of the rotator cuff of shoulder

● **S46.001** Unspecified injury of muscle(s) and tendon(s) of the rotator cuff of right shoulder 🏵

● **S46.002** Unspecified injury of muscle(s) and tendon(s) of the rotator cuff of left shoulder 🏵

● **S46.009** Unspecified injury of muscle(s) and tendon(s) of the rotator cuff of unspecified shoulder 🏵

● **S46.01** Strain of muscle(s) and tendon(s) of the rotator cuff of shoulder

● **S46.011** Strain of muscle(s) and tendon(s) of the rotator cuff of right shoulder 🏵

● **S46.012** Strain of muscle(s) and tendon(s) of the rotator cuff of left shoulder 🏵

● **S46.019** Strain of muscle(s) and tendon(s) of the rotator cuff of unspecified shoulder 🏵

● **S46.02** Laceration of muscle(s) and tendon(s) of the rotator cuff of shoulder

● **S46.021** Laceration of muscle(s) and tendon(s) of the rotator cuff of right shoulder A 🏵, 🏵

Ex: S41.001[A], S41.009-S41.011[A], S41.019-S41.021[A], S41.029-S41.031[A], S41.039-S41.041[A], S41.049-S41.051[A], S41.059-S41.101[A], S41.109-S41.111[A], S41.119-S41.121[A], S41.129-S41.131[A], S41.139-S41.141[A], S41.149-S41.151[A], S41.159[A], S46.021[A], S46.029[A], S46.121[A], S46.129[A], S46.221[A], S46.229[A], S46.321[A], S46.329[A], S46.821[A], S46.829[A], S46.921[A], S46.929[A]

● **S46.022** Laceration of muscle(s) and tendon(s) of the rotator cuff of left shoulder A 🏵, 🏵

Ex: S41.002-S41.009[A], S41.012-S41.019[A], S41.022-S41.029[A], S41.032-S41.039[A], S41.042-S41.049[A], S41.052-S41.059[A], S41.102-S41.109[A], S41.112-S41.119[A], S41.122-S41.129[A], S41.132-S41.139[A], S41.142-S41.149[A], S41.152-S41.159[A], S46.022-S46.029[A], S46.122-S46.129[A], S46.222-S46.229[A], S46.322-S46.329[A], S46.822-S46.829[A], S46.922-S46.929[A]

● **S46.029** Laceration of muscle(s) and tendon(s) of the rotator cuff of unspecified shoulder A 🏵, 🏵

Ex: S41.001-S41.159[A], S46.021-S46.029[A], S46.121-S46.129[A], S46.221-S46.229[A], S46.321-S46.329[A], S46.821-S46.829[A], S46.921-S46.929[A]

● **S46.09** Other injury of muscle(s) and tendon(s) of the rotator cuff of shoulder

● **S46.091** Other injury of muscle(s) and tendon(s) of the rotator cuff of right shoulder 🏵

● **S46.092** Other injury of muscle(s) and tendon(s) of the rotator cuff of left shoulder 🏵

● **S46.099** Other injury of muscle(s) and tendon(s) of the rotator cuff of unspecified shoulder 🏵

● **S46.1** Injury of muscle, fascia and tendon of long head of biceps

● **S46.10** Unspecified injury of muscle, fascia and tendon of long head of biceps

● **S46.101** Unspecified injury of muscle, fascia and tendon of long head of biceps, right arm 🏵

● **S46.102** Unspecified injury of muscle, fascia and tendon of long head of biceps, left arm 🏵

● **S46.109** Unspecified injury of muscle, fascia and tendon of long head of biceps, unspecified arm 🏵

● **S46.11** Strain of muscle, fascia and tendon of long head of biceps

● **S46.111** Strain of muscle, fascia and tendon of long head of biceps, right arm 🏵

● **S46.112** Strain of muscle, fascia and tendon of long head of biceps, left arm 🏵

● **S46.119** Strain of muscle, fascia and tendon of long head of biceps, unspecified arm 🏵

● **S46.12** Laceration of muscle, fascia and tendon of long head of biceps

● **S46.121** Laceration of muscle, fascia and tendon of long head of biceps, right arm A 🏵, 🏵

Ex: See S46.021

● **S46.122** Laceration of muscle, fascia and tendon of long head of biceps, left arm A 🏵, 🏵

Ex: See S46.022

● **S46.129** Laceration of muscle, fascia and tendon of long head of biceps, unspecified arm A 🏵, 🏵

Ex: See S46.029

● **S46.19** Other injury of muscle, fascia and tendon of long head of biceps

● **S46.191** Other injury of muscle, fascia and tendon of long head of biceps, right arm 🏵

● **S46.192** Other injury of muscle, fascia and tendon of long head of biceps, left arm 🏵

● **S46.199** Other injury of muscle, fascia and tendon of long head of biceps, unspecified arm 🏵

● **S46.2** Injury of muscle, fascia and tendon of other parts of biceps

● **S46.20** Unspecified injury of muscle, fascia and tendon of other parts of biceps

● **S46.201** Unspecified injury of muscle, fascia and tendon of other parts of biceps, right arm 🏵

● **S46.202** Unspecified injury of muscle, fascia and tendon of other parts of biceps, left arm 🏵

● **S46.209** Unspecified injury of muscle, fascia and tendon of other parts of biceps, unspecified arm 🏵

N Newborn Age: 0   P Pediatric Age: 0–17   M Maternity DX: 12–55   A Adult Age: 15–124   ♀ Females Only   ♂ Males Only

🏵 Complication\Comorbidity   🏵 Major C\C   Ex CC/MCC Exclusions   🏵 Present on Admission Requirement   🏵 Hospital-Acquired Condition

1363

CHAPTER 19 (S00-T88)

● S46.21   Strain of muscle, fascia and tendon of other parts of biceps
- ● S46.211   Strain of muscle, fascia and tendon of other parts of biceps, right arm 🔲
- ● S46.212   Strain of muscle, fascia and tendon of other parts of biceps, left arm 🔲
- ● S46.219   Strain of muscle, fascia and tendon of other parts of biceps, unspecified arm 🔲

● S46.22   Laceration of muscle, fascia and tendon of other parts of biceps
- ● S46.221   Laceration of muscle, fascia and tendon of other parts of biceps, right arm A 🔲, 🔲
  (Ex) See S46.021
- ● S46.222   Laceration of muscle, fascia and tendon of other parts of biceps, left arm A 🔲, 🔲
  (Ex) See S46.022
- ● S46.229   Laceration of muscle, fascia and tendon of other parts of biceps, unspecified arm A 🔲, 🔲
  (Ex) See S46.029

● S46.29   Other injury of muscle, fascia and tendon of other parts of biceps
- ● S46.291   Other injury of muscle, fascia and tendon of other parts of biceps, right arm 🔲
- ● S46.292   Other injury of muscle, fascia and tendon of other parts of biceps, left arm 🔲
- ● S46.299   Other injury of muscle, fascia and tendon of other parts of biceps, unspecified arm 🔲

● S46.3   Injury of muscle, fascia and tendon of triceps
● S46.30   Unspecified injury of muscle, fascia and tendon of triceps
- ● S46.301   Unspecified injury of muscle, fascia and tendon of triceps, right arm 🔲
- ● S46.302   Unspecified injury of muscle, fascia and tendon of triceps, left arm 🔲
- ● S46.309   Unspecified injury of muscle, fascia and tendon of triceps, unspecified arm 🔲

● S46.31   Strain of muscle, fascia and tendon of triceps
- ● S46.311   Strain of muscle, fascia and tendon of triceps, right arm 🔲
- ● S46.312   Strain of muscle, fascia and tendon of triceps, left arm 🔲
- ● S46.319   Strain of muscle, fascia and tendon of triceps, unspecified arm 🔲

● S46.32   Laceration of muscle, fascia and tendon of triceps
- ● S46.321   Laceration of muscle, fascia and tendon of triceps, right arm A 🔲, 🔲
  (Ex) See S46.021
- ● S46.322   Laceration of muscle, fascia and tendon of triceps, left arm A 🔲, 🔲
  (Ex) See S46.022
- ● S46.329   Laceration of muscle, fascia and tendon of triceps, unspecified arm A 🔲, 🔲
  (Ex) See S46.029

● S46.39   Other injury of muscle, fascia and tendon of triceps
- ● S46.391   Other injury of muscle, fascia and tendon of triceps, right arm 🔲
- ● S46.392   Other injury of muscle, fascia and tendon of triceps, left arm 🔲
- ● S46.399   Other injury of muscle, fascia and tendon of triceps, unspecified arm 🔲

● S46.8   Injury of other muscles, fascia and tendons at shoulder and upper arm level
● S46.80   Unspecified injury of other muscles, fascia and tendons at shoulder and upper arm level
- ● S46.801   Unspecified injury of other muscles, fascia and tendons at shoulder and upper arm level, right arm 🔲
- ● S46.802   Unspecified injury of other muscles, fascia and tendons at shoulder and upper arm level, left arm 🔲
- ● S46.809   Unspecified injury of other muscles, fascia and tendons at shoulder and upper arm level, unspecified arm 🔲

● S46.81   Strain of other muscles, fascia and tendons at shoulder and upper arm level
- ● S46.811   Strain of other muscles, fascia and tendons at shoulder and upper arm level, right arm 🔲
- ● S46.812   Strain of other muscles, fascia and tendons at shoulder and upper arm level, left arm 🔲
- ● S46.819   Strain of other muscles, fascia and tendons at shoulder and upper arm level, unspecified arm 🔲

● S46.82   Laceration of other muscles, fascia and tendons at shoulder and upper arm level
- ● S46.821   Laceration of other muscles, fascia and tendons at shoulder and upper arm level, right arm A 🔲, 🔲
  (Ex) See S46.021
- ● S46.822   Laceration of other muscles, fascia and tendons at shoulder and upper arm level, left arm A 🔲, 🔲
  (Ex) See S46.022
- ● S46.829   Laceration of other muscles, fascia and tendons at shoulder and upper arm level, unspecified arm A 🔲, 🔲
  (Ex) See S46.029

● S46.89   Other injury of other muscles, fascia and tendons at shoulder and upper arm level
- ● S46.891   Other injury of other muscles, fascia and tendons at shoulder and upper arm level, right arm 🔲
- ● S46.892   Other injury of other muscles, fascia and tendons at shoulder and upper arm level, left arm 🔲
- ● S46.899   Other injury of other muscles, fascia and tendons at shoulder and upper arm level, unspecified arm 🔲

● S46.9   Injury of unspecified muscle, fascia and tendon at shoulder and upper arm level
● S46.90   Unspecified injury of unspecified muscle, fascia and tendon at shoulder and upper arm level
- ● S46.901   Unspecified injury of unspecified muscle, fascia and tendon at shoulder and upper arm level, right arm 🔲
- ● S46.902   Unspecified injury of unspecified muscle, fascia and tendon at shoulder and upper arm level, left arm 🔲
- ● S46.909   Unspecified injury of unspecified muscle, fascia and tendon at shoulder and upper arm level, unspecified arm 🔲

◀ New   ◀▥ Revised   ~~deleted~~ Deleted   Excludes 1   Excludes 2   Includes   Use additional   Code first   Code also   Unspecified
OGCR Official Guidelines   ● Unacceptable Principal Diagnosis   X Assign placeholder X   ● Use Additional Character(s)   ▌ Manifestation Code   **Coding Clinic**

● **S46.91 Strain of unspecified muscle, fascia and tendon at shoulder and upper arm level**

  ● **S46.911 Strain of unspecified muscle, fascia and tendon at shoulder and upper arm level, right arm** 🔾

  ● **S46.912 Strain of unspecified muscle, fascia and tendon at shoulder and upper arm level, left arm** 🔾

  ● **S46.919 Strain of unspecified muscle, fascia and tendon at shoulder and upper arm level, unspecified arm** 🔾

 ● **S46.92 Laceration of unspecified muscle, fascia and tendon at shoulder and upper arm level**

  ● **S46.921 Laceration of unspecified muscle, fascia and tendon at shoulder and upper arm level, right arm** A 🔾, 🔾
    (Ex) See S46.021

  ● **S46.922 Laceration of unspecified muscle, fascia and tendon at shoulder and upper arm level, left arm** A 🔾, 🔾
    (Ex) See S46.022

  ● **S46.929 Laceration of unspecified muscle, fascia and tendon at shoulder and upper arm level, unspecified arm** A 🔾, 🔾
    (Ex) See S46.029

 ● **S46.99 Other injury of unspecified muscle, fascia and tendon at shoulder and upper arm level**

  ● **S46.991 Other injury of unspecified muscle, fascia and tendon at shoulder and upper arm level, right arm** 🔾

  ● **S46.992 Other injury of unspecified muscle, fascia and tendon at shoulder and upper arm level, left arm** 🔾

  ● **S46.999 Other injury of unspecified muscle, fascia and tendon at shoulder and upper arm level, unspecified arm** 🔾

● **S47 Crushing injury of shoulder and upper arm**

Use additional code for all associated injuries

Excludes2   crushing injury of elbow (S57.0-)

The appropriate 7th character is to be added to each code from category S47

A	initial encounter
D	subsequent encounter
S	sequela

X ● **S47.1 Crushing injury of right shoulder and upper arm** 🔾

X ● **S47.2 Crushing injury of left shoulder and upper arm** 🔾

X ● **S47.9 Crushing injury of shoulder and upper arm, unspecified arm** 🔾

● **S48 Traumatic amputation of shoulder and upper arm**

An amputation not identified as partial or complete should be coded to complete

Excludes1   traumatic amputation at elbow level (S58.0)

The appropriate 7th character is to be added to each code from category S48

A	initial encounter
D	subsequent encounter
S	sequela

 ● **S48.0 Traumatic amputation at shoulder joint**

  ● **S48.01 Complete traumatic amputation at shoulder joint**

● **S48.011 Complete traumatic amputation at right shoulder joint** A 🔾, 🔾
(Ex) S41.001[A], S41.009-S41.011[A], S41.019-S41.021[A], S41.029-S41.031[A], S41.039-S41.041[A], S41.049-S41.051[A], S41.059-S41.101[A], S41.109-S41.111[A], S41.119-S41.121[A], S41.129-S41.131[A], S41.139-S41.141[A], S41.149-S41.151[A], S41.159[A], S46.021[A], S46.029[A], S46.121[A], S46.129[A], S46.221[A], S46.229[A], S46.321[A], S46.329[A], S46.821[A], S46.829[A], S46.921[A], S46.929[A], S48.011[A], S48.019-S48.021[A], S48.029-S48.111[A], S48.119-S48.121[A], S48.129-S48.911[A], S48.919-S48.921[A], S48.929[A], S51.001[A], S51.009-S51.011[A], S51.019-S51.021[A], S51.029-S51.031[A], S51.039-S51.041[A], S51.049-S51.051[A], S51.059-S51.801[A], S51.809-S51.811[A], S51.819-S51.821[A], S51.829-S51.831[A], S51.839-S51.841[A], S51.849-S51.851[A], S51.859[A], S56.021[A], S56.029[A], S56.121[A], S56.123[A], S56.125[A], S56.127[A], S56.129[A], S56.221[A], S56.229[A], S56.321[A], S56.329[A], S56.421[A], S56.423[A], S56.425[A], S56.427[A], S56.429[A], S56.521[A], S56.529[A], S56.821[A], S56.829[A], S56.921[A], S56.929[A], S58.011[A], S58.019-S58.021[A], S58.029-S58.111[A], S58.119-S58.121[A], S58.129-S58.911[A], S58.919-S58.921[A], S58.929[A], S61.001[A], S61.009-S61.011[A], S61.019-S61.021[A], S61.029-S61.031[A], S61.039-S61.041[A], S61.049-S61.051[A], S61.059-S61.101[A], S61.109-S61.111[A], S61.119-S61.121[A], S61.129-S61.131[A], S61.139-S61.141[A], S61.149-S61.151[A], S61.159-S61.200[A], S61.202[A], S61.204[A], S61.206[A], S61.208-S61.210[A], S61.212[A], S61.214[A], S61.216[A], S61.218-S61.220[A], S61.222[A], S61.224[A], S61.226[A], S61.228-S61.230[A], S61.232[A], S61.234[A], S61.236[A], S61.238-S61.240[A], S61.242[A], S61.244[A], S61.246[A], S61.248-S61.250[A], S61.252[A], S61.254[A], S61.256[A], S61.258-S61.300[A], S61.302[A], S61.304[A], S61.306[A], S61.308-S61.310[A], S61.312[A], S61.314[A], S61.316[A], S61.318-S61.320[A], S61.322[A], S61.324[A], S61.326[A], S61.328-S61.330[A], S61.332[A], S61.334[A], S61.336[A], S61.338-S61.340[A], S61.342[A], S61.344[A], S61.346[A], S61.348-S61.350[A], S61.352[A], S61.354[A], S61.356[A], S61.358-S61.401[A], S61.409-S61.411[A], S61.419-S61.421[A], S61.429-S61.431[A], S61.439-S61.441[A], S61.449-S61.451[A], S61.459-S61.501[A], S61.509-S61.511[A], S61.519-S61.521[A], S61.529-S61.531[A], S61.539-S61.541[A], S61.549-S61.551[A], S61.559[A], S66.021[A], S66.029[A], S66.120[A], S66.122[A], S66.124[A], S66.126[A], S66.128-S66.129[A], S66.221[A], S66.229[A], S66.320[A], S66.322[A], S66.324[A], S66.326[A], S66.328-S66.329[A], S66.421[A], S66.429[A], S66.520[A], S66.522[A], S66.524[A], S66.526[A], S66.528-S66.529[A], S66.821[A], S66.829[A], S66.921[A], S66.929[A], S68.011[A], S68.019-S68.021[A], S68.029-S68.110[A], S68.112[A], S68.114[A], S68.116[A], S68.118-S68.120[A], S68.122[A], S68.124[A], S68.126[A], S68.128-S68.411[A], S68.419-S68.421[A], S68.429-S68.511[A], S68.519-S68.521[A], S68.529-S68.610[A], S68.612[A], S68.614[A], S68.616[A], S68.618-S68.620[A], S68.622[A], S68.624[A], S68.626[A], S68.628-S68.711[A], S68.719-S68.721[A], S68.729[A], T14.8-T14.91, T79.A0X-T79.9XX[A]

N   Newborn Age: 0   P   Pediatric Age: 0–17   M   Maternity DX: 12–55   A   Adult Age: 15–124   ♀   Females Only   ♂   Males Only

🔾 Complication\Comorbidity   🔾 Major C\C   (Ex) CC/MCC Exclusions   🔾 Present on Admission Requirement   🔾 Hospital-Acquired Condition

1365

CHAPTER 19 (S00-T88)

CHAPTER 19 (S00-T88)

● **S48.012**   **Complete traumatic amputation at left shoulder joint** A
    Ex: S41.002-S41.009[A], S41.012-S41.019[A],
    S41.022-S41.029[A], S41.032-S41.039[A],
    S41.042-S41.049[A], S41.052-S41.059[A],
    S41.102-S41.109[A], S41.112-S41.119[A],
    S41.122-S41.129[A], S41.132-S41.139[A],
    S41.142-S41.149[A], S41.152-S41.159[A],
    S46.022-S46.029[A], S46.122-S46.129[A],
    S46.222-S46.229[A], S46.322-S46.329[A],
    S46.822-S46.829[A], S46.922-S46.929[A],
    S48.012-S48.019[A], S48.022-S48.029[A],
    S48.112-S48.119[A], S48.122-S48.129[A],
    S48.912-S48.919[A], S48.922-S48.929[A],
    S51.002-S51.009[A], S51.012-S51.019[A],
    S51.022-S51.029[A], S51.032-S51.039[A],
    S51.042-S51.049[A], S51.052-S51.059[A],
    S51.802-S51.809[A], S51.812-S51.819[A],
    S51.822-S51.829[A], S51.832-S51.839[A],
    S51.842-S51.849[A], S51.852-S51.859[A],
    S56.022-S56.029[A], S56.122[A], S56.124[A],
    S56.126[A], S56.128-S56.129[A],
    S56.222-S56.229[A], S56.322-S56.329[A],
    S56.422[A], S56.424[A], S56.426[A],
    S56.428-S56.429[A], S56.522-S56.529[A],
    S56.822-S56.829[A], S56.922-S56.929[A],
    S58.012-S58.019[A], S58.022-S58.029[A],
    S58.112-S58.119[A], S58.122-S58.129[A],
    S58.912-S58.919[A], S58.922-S58.929[A],
    S61.002-S61.009[A], S61.012-S61.019[A],
    S61.022-S61.029[A], S61.032-S61.039[A],
    S61.042-S61.049[A], S61.052-S61.059[A],
    S61.102-S61.109[A], S61.112-S61.119[A],
    S61.122-S61.129[A], S61.132-S61.139[A],
    S61.142-S61.149[A], S61.152-S61.159[A],
    S61.201[A], S61.203[A], S61.205[A],
    S61.207-S61.209[A], S61.211[A], S61.213[A],
    S61.215[A], S61.217-S61.219[A], S61.221[A],
    S61.223[A], S61.225[A], S61.227-S61.229[A],
    S61.231[A], S61.233[A], S61.235[A],
    S61.237-S61.239[A], S61.241[A], S61.243[A],
    S61.245[A], S61.247-S61.249[A], S61.251[A],
    S61.253[A], S61.255[A], S61.257-S61.259[A],
    S61.301[A], S61.303[A], S61.305[A],
    S61.307-S61.309[A], S61.311[A], S61.313[A],
    S61.315[A], S61.317-S61.319[A], S61.321[A],
    S61.323[A], S61.325[A], S61.327-S61.329[A],
    S61.331[A], S61.333[A], S61.335[A],
    S61.337-S61.339[A], S61.341[A], S61.343[A],
    S61.345[A], S61.347-S61.349[A], S61.351[A],
    S61.353[A], S61.355[A], S61.357-S61.359[A],
    S61.402-S61.409[A], S61.412-S61.419[A],
    S61.422-S61.429[A], S61.432-S61.439[A],
    S61.442-S61.449[A], S61.452-S61.459[A],
    S61.502-S61.509[A], S61.512-S61.519[A],
    S61.522-S61.529[A], S61.532-S61.539[A],
    S61.542-S61.549[A], S61.552-S61.559[A],
    S66.022-S66.029[A], S66.121[A], S66.123[A],
    S66.125[A], S66.127-S66.129[A],
    S66.222-S66.229[A], S66.321[A], S66.323[A],
    S66.325[A], S66.327-S66.329[A],
    S66.422-S66.429[A], S66.521[A], S66.523[A],
    S66.525[A], S66.527-S66.529[A],
    S66.822-S66.829[A], S66.922-S66.929[A],
    S68.012-S68.019[A], S68.022-S68.029[A],
    S68.111[A], S68.113[A], S68.115[A],
    S68.117-S68.119[A], S68.121[A], S68.123[A],
    S68.125[A], S68.127-S68.129[A],
    S68.412-S68.419[A], S68.422-S68.429[A],
    S68.512-S68.519[A], S68.522-S68.529[A],
    S68.611[A], S68.613[A], S68.615[A],
    S68.617-S68.619[A], S68.621[A], S68.623[A],
    S68.625[A], S68.627-S68.629[A],
    S68.712-S68.719[A], S68.722-S68.729[A],
    T14.8-T14.91, T79.A0X-T79.9XX[A]

● **S48.019**   **Complete traumatic amputation at unspecified shoulder joint** A
    Ex: S41.001-S41.159[A], S46.021-S46.029[A],
    S46.121-S46.129[A], S46.221-S46.229[A],
    S46.321-S46.329[A], S46.821-S46.829[A],
    S46.921-S46.929[A], S48.011-S48.929[A],
    S51.001-S51.859[A], S56.021-S56.029[A],
    S56.121-S56.129[A], S56.221-S56.229[A],
    S56.321-S56.329[A], S56.421-S56.429[A],
    S56.521-S56.529[A], S56.821-S56.829[A],
    S56.921-S56.929[A], S58.011-S58.929[A],
    S61.001-S61.559[A], S66.021-S66.029[A],
    S66.120-S66.129[A], S66.221-S66.229[A],
    S66.320-S66.329[A], S66.421-S66.429[A],
    S66.520-S66.529[A], S66.821-S66.829[A],
    S66.921-S66.929[A], S68.011-S68.729[A],
    T14.8-T14.91, T79.A0X-T79.9XX[A]

● **S48.02**   **Partial traumatic amputation at shoulder joint**

● **S48.021**   **Partial traumatic amputation at right shoulder joint** A
    Ex: See S48.011

● **S48.022**   **Partial traumatic amputation at left shoulder joint** A
    Ex: See S48.012

● **S48.029**   **Partial traumatic amputation at unspecified shoulder joint** A
    Ex: See S48.019

● **S48.1**   **Traumatic amputation at level between shoulder and elbow**

● **S48.11**   **Complete traumatic amputation at level between shoulder and elbow**

● **S48.111**   **Complete traumatic amputation at level between right shoulder and elbow** A
    Ex: See S48.011

● **S48.112**   **Complete traumatic amputation at level between left shoulder and elbow** A
    Ex: See S48.012

● **S48.119**   **Complete traumatic amputation at level between unspecified shoulder and elbow** A
    Ex: See S48.019

● **S48.12**   **Partial traumatic amputation at level between shoulder and elbow**

● **S48.121**   **Partial traumatic amputation at level between right shoulder and elbow** A
    Ex: See S48.011

● **S48.122**   **Partial traumatic amputation at level between left shoulder and elbow** A
    Ex: See S48.012

● **S48.129**   **Partial traumatic amputation at level between unspecified shoulder and elbow** A
    Ex: See S48.019

● **S48.9**   **Traumatic amputation of shoulder and upper arm, level unspecified**

● **S48.91**   **Complete traumatic amputation of shoulder and upper arm, level unspecified**

● **S48.911**   **Complete traumatic amputation of right shoulder and upper arm, level unspecified** A
    Ex: See S48.011

● **S48.912**   **Complete traumatic amputation of left shoulder and upper arm, level unspecified** A
    Ex: See S48.012

● **S48.919**   **Complete traumatic amputation of unspecified shoulder and upper arm, level unspecified** A
    Ex: See S48.019

● **S48.92**   **Partial traumatic amputation of shoulder and upper arm, level unspecified**

    ● **S48.921**   **Partial traumatic amputation of right shoulder and upper arm, level unspecified** A 🔾, 🔾
         (Ex) See S48.011

    ● **S48.922**   **Partial traumatic amputation of left shoulder and upper arm, level unspecified** A 🔾, 🔾
         (Ex) See S48.012

    ● **S48.929**   **Partial traumatic amputation of unspecified shoulder and upper arm, level unspecified** A 🔾, 🔾
         (Ex) See S48.019

● **S49**   **Other and unspecified injuries of shoulder and upper arm**

    The appropriate 7th character is to be added to each code from subcategories S49.0 and S49.1

A	initial encounter for closed fracture
D	subsequent encounter for fracture with routine healing
G	subsequent encounter for fracture with delayed healing
K	subsequent encounter for fracture with nonunion
P	subsequent encounter for fracture with malunion
S	sequela

● **S49.0**   **Physeal fracture of upper end of humerus**

    ● **S49.00**   **Unspecified physeal fracture of upper end of humerus**

       ● **S49.001**   **Unspecified physeal fracture of upper end of humerus, right arm** A, K, P 🔾, 🔾, A 🔾
           (Ex) For S49.001[A]: S42.201[A,B], S42.202[B], S42.209-S42.211[A,B], S42.212[B], S42.213-S42.214[A,B], S42.215[B], S42.216-S42.221[A,B], S42.222[B], S42.223-S42.224[A,B], S42.225[B], S42.226-S42.231[A,B], S42.232[B], S42.239-S42.241[A,B], S42.242[B], S42.249-S42.251[A,B], S42.252[B], S42.253-S42.254[A,B], S42.255[B], S42.256-S42.261[A,B], S42.262[B], S42.263-S42.264[A,B], S42.265[B], S42.266[A,B], S42.271[A], S42.279[A], S42.291[A,B], S42.292[B], S42.293-S42.294[A,B], S42.295[B], S42.296-S42.301[A,B], S42.302[B], S42.309[A,B], S42.311[A], S42.319[A], S42.321[A,B], S42.322[B], S42.323-S42.324[A,B], S42.325[B], S42.326-S42.331[A,B], S42.332[B], S42.333-S42.334[A,B], S42.335[B], S42.336-S42.341[A,B], S42.342[B], S42.343-S42.344[A,B], S42.345[B], S42.346-S42.351[A,B], S42.352[B], S42.353-S42.354[A,B], S42.355[B], S42.356-S42.361[A,B], S42.362[B], S42.363-S42.364[A,B], S42.365[B], S42.366-S42.391[A,B], S42.392[B], S42.399-S42.401[A,B], S42.402[B], S42.409-S42.411[A,B], S42.412[B], S42.413-S42.414[A,B], S42.415[B], S42.416-S42.421[A,B], S42.422[B], S42.423-S42.424[A,B], S42.425[B], S42.426-S42.431[A,B], S42.432[B], S42.433-S42.434[A,B], S42.435[B], S42.436-S42.441[A,B], S42.442[B], S42.443-S42.444[A,B], S42.445[B], S42.446-S42.447[A,B], S42.448[B], S42.449-S42.451[A,B], S42.452[B], S42.453-S42.454[A,B], S42.455[B], S42.456-S42.461[A,B], S42.462[B], S42.463-S42.464[A,B], S42.465[B], S42.466-S42.471[A,B], S42.472[B],

S42.473-S42.474[A,B], S42.475[B], S42.476[A,B], S42.481[A], S42.489[A], S42.491[A,B], S42.492[B], S42.493-S42.494[A,B], S42.495[B], S42.496-S42.92X[A,B], S49.001[A], S49.009-S49.011[A], S49.019-S49.021[A], S49.029-S49.031[A], S49.039-S49.041[A], S49.049-S49.091[A], S49.099-S49.101[A], S49.109-S49.111[A], S49.119-S49.121[A], S49.129-S49.131[A], S49.139-S49.141[A], S49.149-S49.191[A], S49.199[A]
For S49.001[K,P]: M80.00X-M80.88X[K,P], M84.30X-M84.68X[K,P], S02.0XX-S02.92X[K], S12.000-S12.691[K], S22.000-S22.9XX[K], S32.000-S32.9XX[K], S42.001-S42.92X[K,P], S49.001-S49.199[K,P], S52.001-S52.92X[K,M,N,P,Q,R], S59.001-S59.299[K,P], S62.001-S62.92X[K,P], S72.001-S72.92X[K,M,N,P,Q,R], S79.001-S79.199[K,P], S82.001-S82.92X[K,M,N,P,Q,R], S89.001-S89.399[K,P], S92.001-S92.919[K,P]

       ● **S49.002**   **Unspecified physeal fracture of upper end of humerus, left arm** A, K, P 🔾, 🔾, A 🔾
           (Ex) For S49.002[A]: S42.201[B], S42.202-S42.209[A,B], S42.211[B], S42.212-S42.213[A,B], S42.214[B], S42.215-S42.216[A,B], S42.221[B], S42.222-S42.223[A,B], S42.224[B], S42.225-S42.226[A,B], S42.231[B], S42.232-S42.239[A,B], S42.241[B], S42.242-S42.249[A,B], S42.251[B], S42.252-S42.253[A,B], S42.254[B], S42.255-S42.256[A,B], S42.261[B], S42.262-S42.263[A,B], S42.264[B], S42.265-S42.266[A,B], S42.272-S42.279[A], S42.291[B], S42.292-S42.293[A,B], S42.294[B], S42.295-S42.296[A,B], S42.301[B], S42.302-S42.309[A,B], S42.312-S42.319[A], S42.321[B], S42.322-S42.323[A,B], S42.324[B], S42.325-S42.326[A,B], S42.331[B], S42.332-S42.333[A,B], S42.334[B], S42.335-S42.336[A,B], S42.341[B], S42.342-S42.343[A,B], S42.344[B], S42.345-S42.346[A,B], S42.351[B], S42.352-S42.353[A,B], S42.354[B], S42.355-S42.356[A,B], S42.361[B], S42.362-S42.363[A,B], S42.364[B], S42.365-S42.366[A,B], S42.391[B], S42.392-S42.399[A,B], S42.401[B], S42.402-S42.409[A,B], S42.411[B], S42.412-S42.413[A,B], S42.414[B], S42.415-S42.416[A,B], S42.421[B], S42.422-S42.423[A,B], S42.424[B], S42.425-S42.426[A,B], S42.431[B], S42.432-S42.433[A,B], S42.434[B], S42.435-S42.436[A,B], S42.441[B], S42.442-S42.443[A,B], S42.444[B], S42.445-S42.446[A,B], S42.447[B], S42.448-S42.449[A,B], S42.451[B], S42.452-S42.453[A,B], S42.454[B], S42.455-S42.456[A,B], S42.461[B], S42.462-S42.463[A,B], S42.464[B], S42.465-S42.466[A,B], S42.471[B], S42.472-S42.473[A,B], S42.474[B], S42.475-S42.476[A,B], S42.482-S42.489[A], S42.491[B], S42.492-S42.493[A,B], S42.494[B], S42.495-S42.92X[A,B], S49.002-S49.009[A], S49.012-S49.019[A], S49.022-S49.029[A], S49.032-S49.039[A], S49.042-S49.049[A], S49.092-S49.099[A], S49.102-S49.109[A], S49.112-S49.119[A], S49.122-S49.129[A], S49.132-S49.139[A], S49.142-S49.149[A], S49.192-S49.199[A]
For S49.002[K,P]: See S49.001

N   Newborn Age: 0   P   Pediatric Age: 0–17   M   Maternity DX: 12–55   A   Adult Age: 15–124   ♀   Females Only   ♂   Males Only

🔾   Complication\Comorbidity   🔾   Major C\C   (Ex)   CC/MCC Exclusions   🔾   Present on Admission Requirement   🔾   Hospital-Acquired Condition

1367

Item 19-3 SALTER-HARRIS TYPE 1: epiphysis is completely separated from end of bone, or metaphysic growth plate remains attached to epiphysis

    SALTER-HARRIS TYPE 2: epiphysis and growth plate are partially separated from metaphysis, which is cracked—most common type

    SALTER-HARRIS TYPE 3: fracture occurring through epiphysis and separates part of epiphysis and growth plate from metaphysis fracture, usually at distal end of tibia

    SALTER-HARRIS TYPE 4: fracture runs through epiphysis, across growth plate, into metaphysic, surgery is required to restore joint surface to normal and align growth plate

● S49.009   Unspecified physeal fracture of upper end of humerus, unspecified arm A, K, P, A
    (Ex:) For S49.009[A]: S42.201-S42.266[A,B], S42.271-S42.279[A], S42.291-S42.309[A,B], S42.311-S42.319[A], S42.321-S42.476[A,B], S42.481-S42.489[A], S42.491-S42.92X[A,B], S49.001-S49.199[A] For S49.009[K,P]: See S49.001

● S49.01   Salter-Harris Type I physeal fracture of upper end of humerus

  ● S49.011   Salter-Harris Type I physeal fracture of upper end of humerus, right arm A, K, P, A
      (Ex:) For S49.011[A]: See S49.001[A]
      For S49.011[K,P]: See S49.001[K,P]

  ● S49.012   Salter-Harris Type I physeal fracture of upper end of humerus, left arm A, K, P, A
      (Ex:) For S49.012[A]: See S49.002[A]
      For S49.012[K,P]: See S49.001[K,P]

  ● S49.019   Salter-Harris Type I physeal fracture of upper end of humerus, unspecified arm A, K, P, A
      (Ex:) For S49.019[A]: See S49.009
      For S49.019[K,P]: See S49.001

● S49.02   Salter-Harris Type II physeal fracture of upper end of humerus

  ● S49.021   Salter-Harris Type II physeal fracture of upper end of humerus, right arm A, K, P, A
      (Ex:) For S49.021[A]: See S49.001[A]
      For S49.021[K,P]: See S49.001[K,P]

  ● S49.022   Salter-Harris Type II physeal fracture of upper end of humerus, left arm A, K, P, A
      (Ex:) For S49.022[A]: See S49.002[A]
      For S49.022[K,P]: See S49.001[K,P]

  ● S49.029   Salter-Harris Type II physeal fracture of upper end of humerus, unspecified arm A, K, P, A
      (Ex:) For S49.029[A]: See S49.009
      For S49.029[K,P]: See S49.001

● S49.03   Salter-Harris Type III physeal fracture of upper end of humerus

  ● S49.031   Salter Harris Type III physeal fracture of upper end of humerus, right arm A, K, P, A
      (Ex:) For S49.031[A]: See S49.001[A]
      For S49.031[K,P]: See S49.001[K,P]

  ● S49.032   Salter Harris Type III physeal fracture of upper end of humerus, left arm A, K, P, A
      (Ex:) For S49.032[A]: See S49.002[A]
      For S49.032[K,P]: See S49.001[K,P]

  ● S49.039   Salter Harris Type III physeal fracture of upper end of humerus, unspecified arm A, K, P, A
      (Ex:) For S49.039[A]: See S49.009
      For S49.039[K,P]: See S49.001

● S49.04   Salter-Harris Type IV physeal fracture of upper end of humerus

  ● S49.041   Salter-Harris Type IV physeal fracture of upper end of humerus, right arm A, K, P, A
      (Ex:) For S49.041[A]: See S49.001[A]
      For S49.041[K,P]: See S49.001[K,P]

  ● S49.042   Salter-Harris Type IV physeal fracture of upper end of humerus, left arm A, K, P, A
      (Ex:) For S49.042[A]: See S49.002[A]
      For S49.042[K,P]: See S49.001[K,P]

  ● S49.049   Salter-Harris Type IV physeal fracture of upper end of humerus, unspecified arm A, K, P, A
      (Ex:) For S49.049[A]: See S49.009
      For S49.049[K,P]: See S49.001

● S49.09   Other physeal fracture of upper end of humerus

  ● S49.091   Other physeal fracture of upper end of humerus, right arm A, K, P, A
      (Ex:) For S49.091[A]: See S49.001[A]
      For S49.091[K,P]: See S49.001[K,P]

  ● S49.092   Other physeal fracture of upper end of humerus, left arm A, K, P, A
      (Ex:) For S49.092[A]: See S49.002[A]
      For S49.092[K,P]: See S49.001[K,P]

  ● S49.099   Other physeal fracture of upper end of humerus, unspecified arm A, K, P, A
      (Ex:) For S49.099[A]: See S49.009
      For S49.099[K,P]: See S49.001

● S49.1   Physeal fracture of lower end of humerus

  ● S49.10   Unspecified physeal fracture of lower end of humerus

    ● S49.101   Unspecified physeal fracture of lower end of humerus, right arm A, K, P, A
      (Ex:) For S49.101[A]: See S49.001[A]
      For S49.101[K,P]: See S49.001[K,P]

    ● S49.102   Unspecified physeal fracture of lower end of humerus, left arm A, K, P, A
      (Ex:) For S49.102[A]: See S49.002[A]
      For S49.102[K,P]: See S49.001[K,P]

    ● S49.109   Unspecified physeal fracture of lower end of humerus, unspecified arm A, K, P, A
      (Ex:) For S49.109[A]: See S49.009
      For S49.109[K,P]: See S49.001

  ● S49.11   Salter-Harris Type I physeal fracture of lower end of humerus

    ● S49.111   Salter-Harris Type I physeal fracture of lower end of humerus, right arm A, K, P, A
      (Ex:) For S49.111[A]: See S49.001[A]
      For S49.111[K,P]: See S49.001[K,P]

    ● S49.112   Salter-Harris Type I physeal fracture of lower end of humerus, left arm A, K, P, A
      (Ex:) For S49.112[A]: See S49.002[A]
      For S49.112[K,P]: See S49.001[K,P]

    ● S49.119   Salter-Harris Type I physeal fracture of lower end of humerus, unspecified arm A, K, P, A
      (Ex:) For S49.119[A]: See S49.009
      For S49.119[K,P]: See S49.001

◀ New   ◀ Revised   ~~deleted~~ Deleted   Excludes 1   Excludes 2   Includes   Use additional   Code first   Code also   Unspecified

OGCR Official Guidelines   ● Unacceptable Principal Diagnosis   X Assign placeholder X   ● Use Additional Character(s)   ▶ Manifestation Code   **Coding Clinic**

● **S49.12**   Salter-Harris Type II physeal fracture of lower end of humerus

  ● **S49.121**   Salter-Harris Type II physeal fracture of lower end of humerus, right arm
A, K, P 🐾, 🐾, A 🐾
    (Ex) For S49.121[A]: See S49.001[A]
    For S49.121[K,P]: See S49.001[K,P]

  ● **S49.122**   Salter-Harris Type II physeal fracture of lower end of humerus, left arm
A, K, P 🐾, 🐾, A 🐾
    (Ex) For S49.122[A]: See S49.002[A]
    For S49.122[K,P]: See S49.001[K,P]

  ● **S49.129**   Salter-Harris Type II physeal fracture of lower end of humerus, unspecified arm A, K, P 🐾, 🐾, A 🐾
    (Ex) For S49.129[A]: See S49.009
    For S49.129[K,P]: See S49.001

● **S49.13**   Salter Harris Type III physeal fracture of lower end of humerus

  ● **S49.131**   Salter-Harris Type III physeal fracture of lower end of humerus, right arm
A, K, P 🐾, 🐾, A 🐾
    (Ex) For S49.131[A]: See S49.001[A]
    For S49.131[K,P]: See S49.001[K,P]

  ● **S49.132**   Salter Harris Type III physeal fracture of lower end of humerus, left arm
A, K, P 🐾, 🐾, A 🐾
    (Ex) For S49.132[A]: See S49.002[A]
    For S49.132[K,P]: See S49.001[K,P]

  ● **S49.139**   Salter-Harris Type III physeal fracture of lower end of humerus, unspecified arm A, K, P 🐾, 🐾, A 🐾
    (Ex) For S49.139[A]: See S49.009
    For S49.139[K,P]: See S49.001

● **S49.14**   Salter-Harris Type IV physeal fracture of lower end of humerus

  ● **S49.141**   Salter-Harris Type IV physeal fracture of lower end of humerus, right arm
A, K, P 🐾, 🐾, A 🐾
    (Ex) For S49.141[A]: See S49.001[A]
    For S49.141[K,P]: See S49.001[K,P]

  ● **S49.142**   Salter-Harris Type IV physeal fracture of lower end of humerus, left arm
A, K, P 🐾, 🐾, A 🐾
    (Ex) For S49.142[A]: See S49.002[A]
    For S49.142[K,P]: See S49.001[K,P]

  ● **S49.149**   Salter-Harris Type IV physeal fracture of lower end of humerus, unspecified arm A, K, P 🐾, 🐾, A 🐾
    (Ex) For S49.149[A]: See S49.009
    For S49.149[K,P]: See S49.001

● **S49.19**   Other physeal fracture of lower end of humerus

  ● **S49.191**   Other physeal fracture of lower end of humerus, right arm A, K, P 🐾, 🐾, A 🐾
    (Ex) For S49.191[A]: See S49.001[A]
    For S49.191[K,P]: See S49.001[K,P]

  ● **S49.192**   Other physeal fracture of lower end of humerus, left arm A, K, P 🐾, 🐾, A 🐾
    (Ex) For S49.192[A]: See S49.002[A]
    For S49.192[K,P]: See S49.001[K,P]

  ● **S49.199**   Other physeal fracture of lower end of humerus, unspecified arm A, K, P 🐾, 🐾, A 🐾
    (Ex) For S49.199[A]: See S49.009
    For S49.199[K,P]: See S49.001

● **S49.8**   Other specified injuries of shoulder and upper arm
The appropriate 7th character is to be added to each code in subcategory S49.8

A	initial encounter
D	subsequent encounter
S	sequela

  X ● **S49.80**   Other specified injuries of shoulder and upper arm, unspecified arm 🐾

  X ● **S49.81**   Other specified injuries of right shoulder and upper arm 🐾

  X ● **S49.82**   Other specified injuries of left shoulder and upper arm 🐾

● **S49.9**   Unspecified injury of shoulder and upper arm
The appropriate 7th character is to be added to each code in subcategory S49.9

A	initial encounter
D	subsequent encounter
S	sequela

  X ● **S49.90**   Unspecified injury of shoulder and upper arm, unspecified arm 🐾

  X ● **S49.91**   Unspecified injury of right shoulder and upper arm 🐾

  X ● **S49.92**   Unspecified injury of left shoulder and upper arm 🐾

INJURIES TO THE ELBOW AND FOREARM (S50-S59)

Excludes2   burns and corrosions (T20-T32)
frostbite (T33-T34)
injuries of wrist and hand (S60-S69)
insect bite or sting, venomous (T63.4)

● **S50**   Superficial injury of elbow and forearm
Excludes2   superficial injury of wrist and hand (S60.-)
The appropriate 7th character is to be added to each code from category S50

A	initial encounter
D	subsequent encounter
S	sequela

● **S50.0**   Contusion of elbow
  X ● **S50.00**   Contusion of unspecified elbow 🐾
  X ● **S50.01**   Contusion of right elbow 🐾
  X ● **S50.02**   Contusion of left elbow 🐾

● **S50.1**   Contusion of forearm
  X ● **S50.10**   Contusion of unspecified forearm 🐾
  X ● **S50.11**   Contusion of right forearm 🐾
  X ● **S50.12**   Contusion of left forearm 🐾

● **S50.3**   Other superficial injuries of elbow
  ● **S50.31**   Abrasion of elbow
    ● **S50.311**   Abrasion of right elbow 🐾
    ● **S50.312**   Abrasion of left elbow 🐾
    ● **S50.319**   Abrasion of unspecified elbow 🐾

  ● **S50.32**   Blister (nonthermal) of elbow
    ● **S50.321**   Blister (nonthermal) of right elbow 🐾
    ● **S50.322**   Blister (nonthermal) of left elbow 🐾
    ● **S50.329**   Blister (nonthermal) of unspecified elbow 🐾

  ● **S50.34**   External constriction of elbow
    ● **S50.341**   External constriction of right elbow 🐾
    ● **S50.342**   External constriction of left elbow 🐾
    ● **S50.349**   External constriction of unspecified elbow 🐾

N Newborn Age: 0   **P** Pediatric Age: 0–17   **M** Maternity DX: 12–55   **A** Adult Age: 15–124   ♀ Females Only   ♂ Males Only

🐾 Complication\Comorbidity   🐾 Major C\C   (Ex) CC/MCC Exclusions   🐾 Present on Admission Requirement   🐾 Hospital-Acquired Condition

● S50.35   Superficial foreign body of elbow
     Splinter in the elbow
   ● S50.351   Superficial foreign body of right elbow 🔍
   ● S50.352   Superficial foreign body of left elbow 🔍
   ● S50.359   Superficial foreign body of unspecified elbow 🔍

● S50.36   Insect bite (nonvenomous) of elbow
   ● S50.361   Insect bite (nonvenomous) of right elbow 🔍
   ● S50.362   Insect bite (nonvenomous) of left elbow 🔍
   ● S50.369   Insect bite (nonvenomous) of unspecified elbow 🔍

● S50.37   Other superficial bite of elbow
    Excludes1   open bite of elbow (S51.04)
   ● S50.371   Other superficial bite of right elbow 🔍
   ● S50.372   Other superficial bite of left elbow 🔍
   ● S50.379   Other superficial bite of unspecified elbow 🔍

● S50.8   Other superficial injuries of forearm
   ● S50.81   Abrasion of forearm
     ● S50.811   Abrasion of right forearm 🔍
     ● S50.812   Abrasion of left forearm 🔍
     ● S50.819   Abrasion of unspecified forearm 🔍

   ● S50.82   Blister (nonthermal) of forearm
     ● S50.821   Blister (nonthermal) of right forearm 🔍
     ● S50.822   Blister (nonthermal) of left forearm 🔍
     ● S50.829   Blister (nonthermal) of unspecified forearm 🔍

   ● S50.84   External constriction of forearm
     ● S50.841   External constriction of right forearm 🔍
     ● S50.842   External constriction of left forearm 🔍
     ● S50.849   External constriction of unspecified forearm 🔍

   ● S50.85   Superficial foreign body of forearm
     Splinter in the forearm
     ● S50.851   Superficial foreign body of right forearm 🔍
     ● S50.852   Superficial foreign body of left forearm 🔍
     ● S50.859   Superficial foreign body of unspecified forearm 🔍

   ● S50.86   Insect bite (nonvenomous) of forearm
     ● S50.861   Insect bite (nonvenomous) of right forearm 🔍
     ● S50.862   Insect bite (nonvenomous) of left forearm 🔍
     ● S50.869   Insect bite (nonvenomous) of unspecified forearm 🔍

   ● S50.87   Other superficial bite of forearm
     Excludes1   open bite of forearm (S51.84)
     ● S50.871   Other superficial bite of right forearm 🔍
     ● S50.872   Other superficial bite of left forearm 🔍
     ● S50.879   Other superficial bite of unspecified forearm 🔍

● S50.9   Unspecified superficial injury of elbow and forearm
   ● S50.90   Unspecified superficial injury of elbow
     ● S50.901   Unspecified superficial injury of right elbow 🔍
     ● S50.902   Unspecified superficial injury of left elbow 🔍
     ● S50.909   Unspecified superficial injury of unspecified elbow 🔍

   ● S50.91   Unspecified superficial injury of forearm
     ● S50.911   Unspecified superficial injury of right forearm 🔍
     ● S50.912   Unspecified superficial injury of left forearm 🔍
     ● S50.919   Unspecified superficial injury of unspecified forearm 🔍

● S51   Open wound of elbow and forearm
   Code also any associated wound infection
   Excludes1   open fracture of elbow and forearm (S52.- with open fracture 7th character)
         traumatic amputation of elbow and forearm (S58.-)
   Excludes2   open wound of wrist and hand (S61.-)
   The appropriate 7th character is to be added to each code from category S51

    | | |
    A   initial encounter
    D   subsequent encounter
    S   sequela

● S51.0   Open wound of elbow
   ● S51.00   Unspecified open wound of elbow
     ● S51.001   Unspecified open wound of right elbow 🔍
        Coding Clinic: 2012, Q4, P108
     ● S51.002   Unspecified open wound of left elbow 🔍
     ● S51.009   Unspecified open wound of unspecified elbow 🔍
        Open wound of elbow NOS

   ● S51.01   Laceration without foreign body of elbow
     ● S51.011   Laceration without foreign body of right elbow 🔍
     ● S51.012   Laceration without foreign body of left elbow 🔍
     ● S51.019   Laceration without foreign body of unspecified elbow 🔍

   ● S51.02   Laceration with foreign body of elbow
     ● S51.021   Laceration with foreign body of right elbow 🔍
     ● S51.022   Laceration with foreign body of left elbow 🔍
     ● S51.029   Laceration with foreign body of unspecified elbow 🔍

   ● S51.03   Puncture wound without foreign body of elbow
     ● S51.031   Puncture wound without foreign body of right elbow 🔍
     ● S51.032   Puncture wound without foreign body of left elbow 🔍
     ● S51.039   Puncture wound without foreign body of unspecified elbow 🔍

- S51.04   Puncture wound with foreign body of elbow
    - S51.041   Puncture wound with foreign body of right elbow 🖐
    - S51.042   Puncture wound with foreign body of left elbow 🖐
    - S51.049   Puncture wound with foreign body of unspecified elbow 🖐
- S51.05   Open bite of elbow
        Bite of elbow NOS
        Excludes1   superficial bite of elbow (S50.36, S50.37)
    - S51.051   Open bite, right elbow 🖐
    - S51.052   Open bite, left elbow 🖐
    - S51.059   Open bite, unspecified elbow 🖐
- S51.8   Open wound of forearm
    Excludes2   open wound of elbow (S51.0-)
    - S51.80   Unspecified open wound of forearm
        - S51.801   Unspecified open wound of right forearm 🖐
        - S51.802   Unspecified open wound of left forearm 🖐
        - S51.809   Unspecified open wound of unspecified forearm 🖐
                Open wound of forearm NOS
    - S51.81   Laceration without foreign body of forearm
        - S51.811   Laceration without foreign body of right forearm 🖐
        - S51.812   Laceration without foreign body of left forearm 🖐
        - S51.819   Laceration without foreign body of unspecified forearm 🖐
    - S51.82   Laceration with foreign body of forearm
        - S51.821   Laceration with foreign body of right forearm 🖐
        - S51.822   Laceration with foreign body of left forearm 🖐
        - S51.829   Laceration with foreign body of unspecified forearm 🖐
    - S51.83   Puncture wound without foreign body of forearm
        - S51.831   Puncture wound without foreign body of right forearm 🖐
        - S51.832   Puncture wound without foreign body of left forearm 🖐
        - S51.839   Puncture wound without foreign body of unspecified forearm 🖐
    - S51.84   Puncture wound with foreign body of forearm
        - S51.841   Puncture wound with foreign body of right forearm 🖐
        - S51.842   Puncture wound with foreign body of left forearm 🖐
        - S51.849   Puncture wound with foreign body of unspecified forearm 🖐
    - S51.85   Open bite of forearm
            Bite of forearm NOS
            Excludes1   superficial bite of forearm (S50.86, S50.87)
        - S51.851   Open bite of right forearm 🖐
        - S51.852   Open bite of left forearm 🖐
        - S51.859   Open bite of unspecified forearm 🖐

- S52   Fracture of forearm
    Note: A fracture not identified as displaced or nondisplaced should be coded to displaced

    A fracture not designated as open or closed should be coded to closed

    The open fracture designations are based on the Gustilo open fracture classification

    Excludes1   traumatic amputation of forearm (S58.-)
    Excludes2   fracture at wrist and hand level (S62.-)

    The appropriate 7th character is to be added to all codes from category S52

A	initial encounter for closed fracture
B	initial encounter for open fracture type I or II
	initial encounter for open fracture NOS
C	initial encounter for open fracture type IIIA, IIIB, or IIIC
D	subsequent encounter for closed fracture with routine healing
E	subsequent encounter for open fracture type I or II with routine healing
F	subsequent encounter for open fracture type IIIA, IIIB, or IIIC with routine healing
G	subsequent encounter for closed fracture with delayed healing
H	subsequent encounter for open fracture type I or II with delayed healing
J	subsequent encounter for open fracture type IIIA, IIIB, or IIIC with delayed healing
K	subsequent encounter for closed fracture with nonunion
M	subsequent encounter for open fracture type I or II with nonunion
N	subsequent encounter for open fracture type IIIA, IIIB, or IIIC with nonunion
P	subsequent encounter for closed fracture with malunion
Q	subsequent encounter for open fracture type I or II with malunion
R	subsequent encounter for open fracture type IIIA, IIIB, or IIIC with malunion
S	sequela

    - S52.0   Fracture of upper end of ulna
            Fracture of proximal end of ulna
            Excludes2   fracture of elbow NOS (S42.40-)
                    fractures of shaft of ulna (S52.2-)
        - S52.00   Unspecified fracture of upper end of ulna
            (Ex) For category S52.00 CC codes S52.00[B,C]:
            S52.001-S52.009[B,C], S52.021-S52.109[B,C],
            S52.121-S52.189[B,C], S52.201-S52.209[A,B,C],
            S52.211-S52.219[A], S52.221-S52.266[A,B,C],
            S52.271-S52.279[B,C], S52.281-S52.309[A,B,C],
            S52.311-S52.319[A], S52.321-S52.516[A,B,C],
            S52.531-S52.616[A,B,C], S52.691-S52.92X[A,B,C],
            S59.001-S59.099[A], S59.201-S59.299[A], S62.90X[B]
            For S52.00[K,M,N,P,Q,R]: M80.00X-M80.88X[K,P],
            M84.30X-M84.68X[K,P], S02.0XX-S02.92X[K],
            S12.000-S12.691[K], S22.000-S22.9XX[K],
            S32.000-S32.9XX[K], S42.001-S42.92X[K,P],
            S49.001-S49.199[K,P], S52.001-S52.92X[K,M,N,P,Q,R],
            S59.001-S59.299[K,P], S62.001-S62.92X[K,P],
            S72.001-S72.92X[K,M,N,P,Q,R], S79.001-S79.199[K,P],
            S82.001-S82.92X[K,M,N,P,Q,R], S89.001-S89.399[K,P],
            S92.001-S92.919[K,P]

            - S52.001   Unspecified fracture of upper end of right ulna K, M, N, P, Q, R 🖐 **B, C** 🖐, 🖐, B, C 🖐
            - S52.002   Unspecified fracture of upper end of left ulna K, M, N, P, Q, R 🖐 **B, C** 🖐, 🖐, B, C 🖐
            - S52.009   Unspecified fracture of upper end of unspecified ulna K, M, N, P, Q, R 🖐 **B, C** 🖐, 🖐, B, C 🖐

N Newborn Age: 0   P Pediatric Age: 0–17   M Maternity DX: 12–55   A Adult Age: 15–124   ♀ Females Only   ♂ Males Only

🖐 Complication\Comorbidity   🖐 Major C\C   (Ex) CC/MCC Exclusions   🖐 Present on Admission Requirement   🖐 Hospital-Acquired Condition

1371

CHAPTER 19 (S00–T88)

● **S52.01**   Torus fracture of upper end of ulna

The appropriate 7th character is to be added to all codes in subcategory S52.01

A	initial encounter for closed fracture
D	subsequent encounter for fracture with routine healing
G	subsequent encounter for fracture with delayed healing
K	subsequent encounter for fracture with nonunion
P	subsequent encounter for fracture with malunion
S	sequela

● S52.011   Torus fracture of upper end of right
ulna A, K, P , , A
Ex For code S52.011[A]: S52.001 [A,B,C], S52.002
[B,C], S52.009 [A,B,C], S52.011[A], S52.019[A],
S52.021[A,B,C], S52.022[B,C],
S52.023-S52.024[A,B,C], S52.025[B,C],
S52.026-S52.031[A,B,C], S52.032[B,C],
S52.033-S52.034[A,B,C], S52.035[B,C],
S52.036-S52.041[A,B,C], S52.042[B,C],
S52.043-S52.044[A,B,C], S52.045[B,C],
S52.046-S52.091[A,B,C], S52.092[B,C],
S52.099-S52.101[A,B,C], S52.102[B,C],
S52.109[A,B,C], S52.111[A], S52.119[A],
S52.121[A,B,C], S52.122[B,C],
S52.123-S52.124[A,B,C], S52.125[B,C],
S52.126-S52.131[A,B,C], S52.132[B,C],
S52.133-S52.134[A,B,C], S52.135[B, C],
S52.136-S52.181[A,B,C], S52.182[B,C],
S52.189-S52.201[A,B,C], S52.202[B,C],
S52.209[A,B,C], S52.211[A], S52.219[A],
S52.221[A,B,C], S52.222[B,C],
S52.223-S52.224[A,B,C], S52.225[B,C],
S52.226-S52.231[C], S52.232[B,C],
S52.233-S52.234[A,B,C], S52.235[B,C],
S52.236-S52.241[C], S52.242[B,C],
S52.243-S52.244[A,B,C], S52.245[B,C],
S52.246-S52.251[A,B,C], S52.252[B,C],
S52.253-S52.254[A,B,C], S52.255[B,C],
S52.256-S52.261[A,B,C], S52.262[BC],
S52.263-S52.264[A,B,C], S52.265[B,C],
S52.266-S52.271[A,B,C], S52.272[B,C],
S52.279-S52.281[A,B,C], S52.282[B,C],
S52.283-S52.291[A,B,C], S52.292[B,C],
S52.299-S52.301[A,B,C], S52.302[B,C],
S52.309[A,B,C], S52.311[A], S52.319[A],
S52.321[A,B,C], S52.322[B,C],
S52.323-S52.324[A,B,C], S52.325[B,C],
S52.326-S52.331[A,B,C], S52.332[B,C],
S52.333-S52.334[A,B,C], S52.335[B,C],
S52.336-S52.341[A,B,C], S52.342[B,C],
S52.343-S52.344[A,B,C], S52.345[B,C],
S52.346-S52.351[A,B,C], S52.352[B,C],
S52.353-S52.354[A,B,C], S52.355[B,C],
S52.356-S52.361[A,B,C], S52.362[B,C],
S52.363-S52.364[A,B,C], S52.365[B,C],
S52.366-S52.371[A,B,C], S52.372[B,C],
S52.379-S52.381[A,B,C], S52.382[B,C],
S52.389-S52.391[A,B,C], S52.392[B,C],
S52.399-S52.501[A,B,C], S52.502[B,C],
S52.509-S52.511[A,B,C], S52.512[B,C],
S52.513-S52.514[A,B,C], S52.515[B,C],
S52.16[A,B,C], S52.521[A], S52.529[A],
S52.531[A,B,C], S52.532[B,C],
S52.539-S52.541[A,B,C], S52.542[B,C],
S52.549-S52.551[A,B,C], S52.552[B,C],
S52.559-S52.561[A,B,C], S52.562[B,C],
S52.569-S52.571[A,B,C], S52.572[B,C],
S52.579-S52.591[A,B,C], S52.592[B,C],
S52.599-S52.601[A,B,C], S52.602[B,C],
S52.609-S52.611[A,B,C], S52.612[B,C],
S52.613-S52.614[A,B,C], S52.615[B,C],
S52.616[A,B,C], S52.621[A], S52.629[A],
S52.691[A,B,C], S52.692[B,C],
S52.699-S52.92X[A,B,C], S59.001[A],
S59.009-S59.011[A], S59.019-S59.021[A],

S59.029-S59.031[A], S59.039-S59.041[A],
S59.049-S59.091[A], S59.099-S59.101[A],
S59.109-S59.111[A], S59.119-S59.121[A],
S59.129-S59.131[A], S59.139-S59.141[A],
S59.149-S59.191[A], S59.199-S59.201[A],
S59.209-S59.211[A], S59.219-S59.221[A],
S59.229-S59.231[A], S59.239-S59.241[A],
S59.249-S59.291[A], S59.299[A]
For S52.011[K,P]: See S52.00[L,M,N,P,Q,R]

● S52.012   Torus fracture of upper end of left
ulna A, K, P , , A
Ex For code S52.012[A]: S52.001[B,C],
S52.002-S52.009[A,B,C], S52.012-S52.019[A],
S52.021[B,C], S52.022-S52.023[A,B,C],
S52.024[B,C], S52.025-S52.026[A,B,C],
S52.031[B,C], S52.032-S52.033[A,B,C],
S52.034[B,C], S52.035-S52.036[A,B,C],
S52.041[B,C], S52.042-S52.043[A,B,C],
S52.044[B,C], S52.045-S52.046[A,B,C],
S52.091[B,C], S52.092-S52.099[A,B,C],
S52.101[B,C], S52.102-S52.109[A,B,C],
S52.112-S52.119[A], S52.121[B,C],
S52.122-S52.123[A,B,C], S52.124[B,C],
S52.125-S52.126[A,B,C], S52.131[B,C],
S52.132-S52.133[A,B,C], S52.134[B,C],
S52.135-S52.136[A,B,C], S52.181[B,C],
S52.182-S52.189[A,B,C], S52.201[B,C],
S52.202-S52.209[A,B,C], S52.212-S52.219[A],
S52.221[B,C], S52.222-S52.223[A,B,C],
S52.224[B,C], S52.225-S52.226[A,B,C],
S52.231[B,C], S52.232-S52.233[A,B,C],
S52.234[B,C], S52.235-S52.236[A,B,C],
S52.241[B,C], S52.242-S52.243[A,B,C],
S52.244[B,C], S52.245-S52.246[A,B,C],
S52.251[B,C], S52.252-S52.253[A,B,C],
S52.254[B,C], S52.255-S52.256[A,B,C],
S52.261[B,C], S52.262-S52.263[A,B,C],
S52.264[B,C], S52.265-S52.266[A,B,C],
S52.271[B,C], S52.272-S52.279[A,B,C],
S52.281[B,C], S52.282-S52.283[A,B,C],
S52.291[B,C], S52.292-S52.299[A,B,C],
S52.301[B,C], S52.302-S52.309[A,B,C],
S52.312-S52.319[A], S52.321[B,C],
S52.322-S52.323[A,B,C], S52.324[B,C],
S52.325-S52.326[A,B,C], S52.331[B,C],
S52.332-S52.333[A,B,C], S52.334[B,C],
S52.335-S52.336[A,B,C], S52.341[B,C],
S52.342-S52.343[A,B,C], S52.344[B,C],
S52.345-S52.346[A,B,C], S52.351[B,C],
S52.352-S52.353[A,B,C], S52.354[B,C],
S52.355-S52.356[A,B,C], S52.361[B,C],
S52.362-S52.363[A,B,C], S52.364[B,C],
S52.365-S52.366[A,B,C], S52.371[B,C],
S52.372-S52.379[A,B,C], S52.381[B,C],
S52.382-S52.389[A,B,C], S52.391[B,C],
S52.392-S52.399[A,B,C], S52.501[B,C],
S52.502-S52.509[A,B,C], S52.511[B,C],
S52.512-S52.513[A,B,C], S52.514[B,C],
S52.515-S52.516[A,B,C], S52.522-S52.529[A],
S52.531[B,C], S52.532-S52.539[A,B,C],
S52.541[B,C], S52.542-S52.549[A,B,C],
S52.551[B,C], S52.552-S52.559[A,B,C],
S52.561[B,C], S52.562-S52.569[A,B,C],
S52.571[B,C], S52.572-S52.579[A,B,C],
S52.591[B,C], S52.592-S52.599[A,B,C],
S52.601[B,C], S52.602-S52.609[A,B,C],
S52.611[B,C], S52.612-S52.613[A,B,C],
S52.614[B,C], S52.615-S52.616[A,B,C],
S52.622-S52.629[A], S52.691[B,C],
S52.692-S52.92X[A,B,C], S59.002-S59.009[A],
S59.012-S59.019[A], S59.022-S59.029[A],
S59.032-S59.039[A], S59.042-S59.049[A],
S59.092-S59.099[A], S59.102-S59.109[A],
S59.112-S59.119[A], S59.122-S59.129[A],
S59.132-S59.139[A], S59.142-S59.149[A],
S59.192-S59.199[A], S59.202-S59.209[A],
S59.212-S59.219[A], S59.222-S59.229[A],
S59.232-S59.239[A], S59.242-S59.249[A],
S59.292-S59.299[A] For S52.012[K,P]: See
S52.00[L,M,N,P,Q,R]

◀ New   ◀▥ Revised   ~~deleted~~ Deleted   Excludes 1   Excludes 2   Includes   Use additional   Code first   Code also   Unspecified
OGCR Official Guidelines   ● Unacceptable Principal Diagnosis   X Assign placeholder X   ● Use Additional Character(s)   ▷ Manifestation Code   Coding Clinic

● **S52.019**   Torus fracture of upper end of
  unspecified ulna A, K, P 🔖, 🔖, A 🔖
  (Ex) **For code S52.019[A]:** S52.001-S52.009[A,B,C],
  S52.011-S52.019[A], S52.021-S52.109[A,B,C],
  S52.111-S52.119[A], S52.121-S52.209[A,B,C],
  S52.211-S52.219[A], S52.221-S52.309[A,B,C],
  S52.311-S52.319[A], S52.321-S52.516[A,B,C],
  S52.521-S52.529[A], S52.531-S52.616[A,B,C],
  S52.621-S52.629[A], S52.691-S52.92X[A,B,C],
  S59.001-S59.299[A] **For S52.019[K,P]:** See
  S52.00[L,M,N,P,Q,R]

● **S52.02**   Fracture of olecranon process without
  intraarticular extension of ulna
  (Ex) **For category S52.02 CC codes S52.02[B,C]:**
  S52.001-S52.009[B,C], S52.021-S52.109[B,C],
  S52.121-S52.189[B,C], S52.201-S52.209[A,B,C],
  S52.211-S52.219[A], S52.221-S52.266[A,B,C],
  S52.271-S52.279[B,C], S52.281-S52.309[A,B,C],
  S52.311-S52.319[A], S52.321-S52.516[A,B,C],
  S52.531-S52.539[B,C], S52.541-S52.616[A,B,C],
  S52.691-S52.92X[A,B,C], S59.001-S59.099[A],
  S59.201-S59.299[A], S62.90X[B] **For S52.02[K,M,N,P,Q,R]:**
  See S52.00[L,M,N,P,Q,R]

● **S52.021**   Displaced fracture of olecranon
  process without intraarticular
  extension of right ulna
  K, M, N, P, Q, R 🔖, B, C 🔖, 🔖, B, C 🔖

● **S52.022**   Displaced fracture of olecranon
  process without intraarticular
  extension of left ulna
  K, M, N, P, Q, R 🔖, B, C 🔖, 🔖, B, C 🔖

● **S52.023**   Displaced fracture of olecranon
  process without intraarticular
  extension of unspecified ulna
  K, M, N, P, Q, R 🔖, B, C 🔖, 🔖, B, C 🔖

● **S52.024**   Nondisplaced fracture of olecranon
  process without intraarticular
  extension of right ulna
  K, M, N, P, Q, R 🔖, B, C 🔖, 🔖, B, C 🔖

● **S52.025**   Nondisplaced fracture of olecranon
  process without intraarticular
  extension of left ulna
  K, M, N, P, Q, R 🔖, B, C 🔖, 🔖, B, C 🔖

● **S52.026**   Nondisplaced fracture of olecranon
  process without intraarticular
  extension of unspecified ulna
  K, M, N, P, Q, R 🔖, B, C 🔖, 🔖, B, C 🔖

● **S52.03**   Fracture of olecranon process with intraarticular
  extension of ulna
  (Ex) **For category S52.03 CC codes S52.03[B,C]:** See
  S52.02[B,C] **For S52.03[K,M,N,P,Q,R]:** See
  S52.00[L,M,N,P,Q,R]

● **S52.031**   Displaced fracture of olecranon
  process with intraarticular extension
  of right ulna K, M, N, P, Q, R 🔖,
  B, C 🔖, 🔖, B, C 🔖

● **S52.032**   Displaced fracture of olecranon
  process with intraarticular extension
  of left ulna K, M, N, P, Q, R 🔖,
  B, C 🔖, 🔖, B, C 🔖

● **S52.033**   Displaced fracture of olecranon
  process with intraarticular extension
  of unspecified ulna
  K, M, N, P, Q, R 🔖, B, C 🔖, 🔖, B, C 🔖

● **S52.034**   Nondisplaced fracture of olecranon
  process with intraarticular extension
  of right ulna K, M, N, P, Q, R 🔖,
  B, C 🔖, 🔖, B, C 🔖

● **S52.035**   Nondisplaced fracture of olecranon
  process with intraarticular extension
  of left ulna K, M, N, P, Q, R 🔖,
  B, C 🔖, 🔖, B, C 🔖

● **S52.036**   Nondisplaced fracture of olecranon
  process with intraarticular extension of
  unspecified ulna K, M, N, P, Q, R 🔖,
  B, C 🔖, 🔖, B, C 🔖

● **S52.04**   Fracture of coronoid process of ulna
  (Ex) **For category S52.04 CC codes S52.04[B,C]:** See
  S52.00[B,C] **For S52.04[K,M,N,P,Q,R]:** See
  S52.00[K,M,N,P,Q,R]

● **S52.041**   Displaced fracture of coronoid
  process of right ulna
  K, M, N, P, Q, R 🔖, B, C 🔖, 🔖, B, C 🔖

● **S52.042**   Displaced fracture of coronoid
  process of left ulna
  K, M, N, P, Q, R 🔖, B, C 🔖, 🔖, B, C 🔖

● **S52.043**   Displaced fracture of coronoid
  process of unspecified ulna
  K, M, N, P, Q, R 🔖, B, C 🔖, 🔖, B, C 🔖

● **S52.044**   Nondisplaced fracture of coronoid
  process of right ulna
  K, M, N, P, Q, R 🔖, B, C 🔖, 🔖, B, C 🔖

● **S52.045**   Nondisplaced fracture of coronoid
  process of left ulna
  K, M, N, P, Q, R 🔖, B, C 🔖, 🔖, B, C 🔖

● **S52.046**   Nondisplaced fracture of coronoid
  process of unspecified ulna
  K, M, N, P, Q, R 🔖, B, C 🔖, 🔖, B, C 🔖

● **S52.09**   Other fracture of upper end of ulna
  (Ex) **For category S52.09 CC codes S52.09[B,C]:** See
  S52.00[B,C] **For S52.09[K,M,N,P,Q,R]:** See
  S52.00[K,M,N,P,Q,R]

● **S52.091**   Other fracture of upper end of right
  ulna K, M, N, P, Q, R 🔖, B, C 🔖, 🔖,
  B, C 🔖

● **S52.092**   Other fracture of upper end of left
  ulna K, M, N, P, Q, R 🔖, B, C 🔖, 🔖,
  B, C 🔖

● **S52.099**   Other fracture of upper end of
  unspecified ulna K, M, N, P, Q, R 🔖,
  B, C 🔖, 🔖, B, C 🔖

● **S52.1**   Fracture of upper end of radius
  Fracture of proximal end of radius
  Excludes2   physeal fractures of upper end of radius
  (S59.2-)
  fracture of shaft of radius (S52.3-)

● **S52.10**   Unspecified fracture of upper end of radius
  (Ex) **For category S52.10 CC codes S52.10[B,C]:** See
  S52.00[B,C] **For S52.10[K,M,N,P,Q,R]:** See
  S52.00[K,M,N,P,Q,R]

● **S52.101**   Unspecified fracture of upper end of
  right radius K, M, N, P, Q, R 🔖,
  B, C 🔖, 🔖, B, C 🔖

● **S52.102**   Unspecified fracture of upper end of
  left radius K, M, N, P, Q, R 🔖, B, C 🔖,
  🔖, B, C 🔖

● **S52.109**   Unspecified fracture of upper end of
  unspecified radius K, M, N, P, Q, R 🔖,
  B, C 🔖, 🔖, B, C 🔖

N Newborn Age: 0   **P** Pediatric Age: 0–17   **M** Maternity DX: 12–55   **A** Adult Age: 15–124   ♀ Females Only   ♂ Males Only
🔖 Complication\Comorbidity   🔖 Major C\C   (Ex) CC/MCC Exclusions   🔖 Present on Admission Requirement   🔖 Hospital-Acquired Condition

CHAPTER 19 (S00-T88)

1373

● **S52.11　Torus fracture of upper end of radius**

The appropriate 7th character is to be added to all codes in subcategory S52.11

A	initial encounter for closed fracture
D	subsequent encounter for fracture with routine healing
G	subsequent encounter for fracture with delayed healing
K	subsequent encounter for fracture with nonunion
P	subsequent encounter for fracture with malunion
S	sequela

● **S52.111　Torus fracture of upper end of right radius** A, K, P 🦠, 🦠, A 🦠
　(Ex:) For code S52.111[A]: See S52.011[A]
　　For S52.111[K,P]: See S52.00[L,M,N,P,Q,R]

● **S52.112　Torus fracture of upper end of left radius** A, K, P 🦠, 🦠, A 🦠
　(Ex:) For code S52.112[A]: See S52.012[A]
　　For S52.112[K,P]: See S52.00[L,M,N,P,Q,R]

● **S52.119　Torus fracture of upper end of unspecified radius** A, K, P 🦠, 🦠, A 🦠
　(Ex:) For code S52.119[A]: See S52.019[A]
　　For S52.119[K,P]: See S52.00[L,M,N,P,Q,R]

● **S52.12　Fracture of head of radius**
　(Ex:) For category S52.12 CC codes S52.12[B,C]: See S52.00[B,C] For S52.12[K,M,N,P,Q,R]: See S52.00[K,M,N,P,Q,R]

● **S52.121　Displaced fracture of head of right radius** K, M, N, P, Q, R 🦠, B, C 🦠, 🦠, B, C 🦠

● **S52.122　Displaced fracture of head of left radius** K, M, N, P, Q, R 🦠, B, C 🦠, 🦠, B, C 🦠

● **S52.123　Displaced fracture of head of unspecified radius** K, M, N, P, Q, R 🦠, B, C 🦠, 🦠, B, C 🦠

● **S52.124　Nondisplaced fracture of head of right radius** K, M, N, P, Q, R 🦠, B, C 🦠, 🦠, B, C 🦠

● **S52.125　Nondisplaced fracture of head of left radius** K, M, N, P, Q, R 🦠, B, C 🦠, 🦠, B, C 🦠

● **S52.126　Nondisplaced fracture of head of unspecified radius** K, M, N, P, Q, R 🦠, B, C 🦠, 🦠, B, C 🦠

● **S52.13　Fracture of neck of radius**
　(Ex:) For category S52.13 CC codes S52.13[B,C]: See S52.00[B,C] For S52.13[K,M,N,P,Q,R]: See S52.00[K,M,N,P,Q,R]

● **S52.131　Displaced fracture of neck of right radius** K, M, N, P, Q, R 🦠, B, C 🦠, 🦠, B, C 🦠

● **S52.132　Displaced fracture of neck of left radius** K, M, N, P, Q, R 🦠, B, C 🦠, 🦠, B, C 🦠

● **S52.133　Displaced fracture of neck of unspecified radius** K, M, N, P, Q, R 🦠, B, C 🦠, 🦠, B, C 🦠

● **S52.134　Nondisplaced fracture of neck of right radius** K, M, N, P, Q, R 🦠, B, C 🦠, 🦠, B, C 🦠

● **S52.135　Nondisplaced fracture of neck of left radius** K, M, N, P, Q, R 🦠, B, C 🦠, 🦠, B, C 🦠

● **S52.136　Nondisplaced fracture of neck of unspecified radius** K, M, N, P, Q, R 🦠, B, C 🦠, 🦠, B, C 🦠

● **S52.18　Other fracture of upper end of radius**
　(Ex:) For category S52.18 CC codes S52.18[B,C]: See S52.00[B,C] For S52.18[K,M,N,P,Q,R]: See S52.00[K,M,N,P,Q,R]

● **S52.181　Other fracture of upper end of right radius** K, M, N, P, Q, R 🦠, B, C 🦠, 🦠, B, C 🦠

● **S52.182　Other fracture of upper end of left radius** K, M, N, P, Q, R 🦠, B, C 🦠, 🦠, B, C 🦠

● **S52.189　Other fracture of upper end of unspecified radius** K, M, N, P, Q, R 🦠, B, C 🦠, 🦠, B, C 🦠

● **S52.2　Fracture of shaft of ulna**

● **S52.20　Unspecified fracture of shaft of ulna**
　Fracture of ulna NOS

● **S52.201　Unspecified fracture of shaft of right ulna** A, K, M, N, P, Q, R 🦠, B, C 🦠, 🦠, A, B, C 🦠
　(Ex:) For code S52.201[A]: See S52.011[A]
　　For S52.201[B,C]: See S52.00[B,C]
　　For S52.201[K,M,N,P,Q,R]: See S52.00[L,M,N,P,Q,R]

● **S52.202　Unspecified fracture of shaft of left ulna** A, K, M, N, P, Q, R 🦠, B, C 🦠, 🦠, A, B, C 🦠
　(Ex:) For code S52.202[A]: See S52.012[A] For code S52.202[B,C]: See S52.00[B,C]
　　For S52.202[K,M,N,P,Q,R]: See S52.00[L,M,N,P,Q,R]

● **S52.209　Unspecified fracture of shaft of unspecified ulna** A, K, M, N, P, Q, R 🦠, B, C 🦠, 🦠, A, B, C 🦠
　(Ex:) For code S52.209[A]: See S52.019[A] For code S52.209[B,C]: See S52.00[B,C]
　　For S52.209[K,M,N,P,Q,R]: See S52.00[L,M,N,P,Q,R]

● **S52.21　Greenstick fracture of shaft of ulna**

The appropriate 7th character is to be added to all codes in subcategory S52.21

A	initial encounter for closed fracture
D	subsequent encounter for fracture with routine healing
G	subsequent encounter for fracture with delayed healing
K	subsequent encounter for fracture with nonunion
P	subsequent encounter for fracture with malunion
S	sequela

● **S52.211　Greenstick fracture of shaft of right ulna** A, K, P 🦠, 🦠, A 🦠
　(Ex:) For code S52.211[A]: See S52.011[A]
　　For S52.211[K,P]: See S52.00[L,M,N,P,Q,R]

● **S52.212　Greenstick fracture of shaft of left ulna** A, K, P 🦠, 🦠, A 🦠
　(Ex:) For code S52.212[A]: See S52.012[A]
　　For S52.202[K,P]: See S52.00[L,M,N,P,Q,R]

● **S52.219　Greenstick fracture of shaft of unspecified ulna** A, K, P 🦠, 🦠, A 🦠
　(Ex:) For code S52.219[A]: See S52.019[A]
　　For S52.219[K,P]: See S52.00[L,M,N,P,Q,R]

CHAPTER 19 (S00-T88)

◀ New　◀|||| Revised　~~deleted~~ Deleted　Excludes 1　Excludes 2　Includes　Use additional　Code first　Code also　Unspecified

OGCR Official Guidelines　● Unacceptable Principal Diagnosis　X Assign placeholder X　● Use Additional Character(s)　▶ Manifestation Code　**Coding Clinic**

● **S52.22**   Transverse fracture of shaft of ulna

  ● **S52.221**   Displaced transverse fracture of shaft of right ulna A, K, M, N, P, Q, R 🪙, B, C 🪙, 🪙, A, B, C 🪙
     (Ex) For code S52.221[A]: See S52.011[A]
     For S52.221[B,C]: See S52.00[B,C]
     For S52.221[K,M,N,P,Q,R]: See S52.00[L,M,N,P,Q,R]

  ● **S52.222**   Displaced transverse fracture of shaft of left ulna A, K, M, N, P, Q, R 🪙, B, C 🪙, 🪙, A, B, C 🪙
     (Ex) For code S52.222[A]: See S52.012[A] For code S52.222[B,C]: See S52.00[B,C]
     For S52.222[K,M,N,P,Q,R]: See S52.00[L,M,N,P,Q,R]

  ● **S52.223**   Displaced transverse fracture of shaft of unspecified ulna A, K, M, N, P, Q, R 🪙, B, C 🪙, 🪙, A, B, C 🪙
     (Ex) For code S52.223[A]: See S52.019[A] For code S52.223[B,C]: See S52.00[B,C]
     For S52.223[K,M,N,P,Q,R]: See S52.00[L,M,N,P,Q,R]

  ● **S52.224**   Nondisplaced transverse fracture of shaft of right ulna A, K, M, N, P, Q, R 🪙, B, C 🪙, 🪙, A, B, C 🪙
     (Ex) For code S52.224[A]: See S52.011[A]
     For S52.224[B,C]: See S52.00[B,C]
     For S52.224[K,M,N,P,Q,R]: See S52.00[L,M,N,P,Q,R]

  ● **S52.225**   Nondisplaced transverse fracture of shaft of left ulna A, K, M, N, P, Q, R 🪙, B, C 🪙, 🪙, A, B, C 🪙
     (Ex) For code S52.225[A]: See S52.012[A] For code S52.225[B,C]: See S52.00[B,C]
     For S52.225[K,M,N,P,Q,R]: See S52.00[L,M,N,P,Q,R]

  ● **S52.226**   Nondisplaced transverse fracture of shaft of unspecified ulna A, K, M, N, P, Q, R 🪙, B, C 🪙, 🪙, A, B, C 🪙
     (Ex) For code S52.226[A]: See S52.019[A] For code S52.226[B,C]: See S52.00[B,C]
     For S52.226[K,M,N,P,Q,R]: See S52.00[L,M,N,P,Q,R]

● **S52.23**   Oblique fracture of shaft of ulna

  ● **S52.231**   Displaced oblique fracture of shaft of right ulna A, K, M, N, P, Q, R 🪙, B, C 🪙, 🪙, A, B, C 🪙
     (Ex) For code S52.231[A]: See S52.011[A]
     For S52.231[B,C]: See S52.00[B,C]
     For S52.231[K,M,N,P,Q,R]: See S52.00[L,M,N,P,Q,R]

  ● **S52.232**   Displaced oblique fracture of shaft of left ulna A, K, M, N, P, Q, R 🪙, B, C 🪙, 🪙, A, B, C 🪙
     (Ex) For code S52.232[A]: See S52.012[A] For code S52.232[B,C]: See S52.00[B,C]
     For S52.232[K,M,N,P,Q,R]: See S52.00[L,M,N,P,Q,R]

  ● **S52.233**   Displaced oblique fracture of shaft of unspecified ulna A, K, M, N, P, Q, R 🪙, B, C 🪙, 🪙, A, B, C 🪙
     (Ex) For code S52.233[A]: See S52.019[A] For code S52.233[B,C]: See S52.00[B,C]
     For S52.233[K,M,N,P,Q,R]: See S52.00[L,M,N,P,Q,R]

  ● **S52.234**   Nondisplaced oblique fracture of shaft of right ulna A, K, M, N, P, Q, R 🪙, B, C 🪙, 🪙, A, B, C 🪙
     (Ex) For code S52.234[A]: See S52.011[A]
     For S52.234[B,C]: See S52.00[B,C]
     For S52.234[K,M,N,P,Q,R]: See S52.00[L,M,N,P,Q,R]

  ● **S52.235**   Nondisplaced oblique fracture of shaft of left ulna A, K, M, N, P, Q, R 🪙, B, C 🪙, 🪙, A, B, C 🪙
     (Ex) For code S52.235[A]: See S52.012[A] For code S52.235[B,C]: See S52.00[B,C]
     For S52.235[K,M,N,P,Q,R]: See S52.00[L,M,N,P,Q,R]

  ● **S52.236**   Nondisplaced oblique fracture of shaft of unspecified ulna A, K, M, N, P, Q, R 🪙, B, C 🪙, 🪙, A, B, C 🪙
     (Ex) For code S52.236[A]: See S52.019[A] For code S52.236[B,C]: See S52.00[B,C]
     For S52.236[K,M,N,P,Q,R]: See S52.00[L,M,N,P,Q,R]

● **S52.24**   Spiral fracture of shaft of ulna

  ● **S52.241**   Displaced spiral fracture of shaft of ulna, right arm A, K, M, N, P, Q, R 🪙, B, C 🪙, 🪙, A, B, C 🪙
     (Ex) For code S52.241[A]: See S52.011[A]
     For S52.241[B,C]: See S52.00[B,C]
     For S52.241[K,M,N,P,Q,R]: See S52.00[L,M,N,P,Q,R]

  ● **S52.242**   Displaced spiral fracture of shaft of ulna, left arm A, K, M, N, P, Q, R 🪙, B, C 🪙, 🪙, A, B, C 🪙
     (Ex) For code S52.242[A]: See S52.012[A] For code S52.242[B,C]: See S52.00[B,C]
     For S52.242[K,M,N,P,Q,R]: See S52.00[L,M,N,P,Q,R]

  ● **S52.243**   Displaced spiral fracture of shaft of ulna, unspecified arm A, K, M, N, P, Q, R 🪙, B, C 🪙, 🪙, A, B, C 🪙
     (Ex) For code S52.243[A]: See S52.019[A] For code S52.243[B,C]: See S52.00[B,C]
     For S52.243[K,M,N,P,Q,R]: See S52.00[L,M,N,P,Q,R]

  ● **S52.244**   Nondisplaced spiral fracture of shaft of ulna, right arm A, K, M, N, P, Q, R 🪙, B, C 🪙, 🪙, A, B, C 🪙
     (Ex) For code S52.244[A]: See S52.011[A]
     For S52.244[B,C]: See S52.00[B,C]
     For S52.244[K,M,N,P,Q,R]: See S52.00[L,M,N,P,Q,R]

  ● **S52.245**   Nondisplaced spiral fracture of shaft of ulna, left arm A, K, M, N, P, Q, R 🪙, B, C 🪙, 🪙, A, B, C 🪙
     (Ex) For code S52.245[A]: See S52.012[A] For code S52.245[B,C]: See S52.00[B,C]
     For S52.245[K,M,N,P,Q,R]: See S52.00[L,M,N,P,Q,R]

  ● **S52.246**   Nondisplaced spiral fracture of shaft of ulna, unspecified arm A, K, M, N, P, Q, R 🪙, B, C 🪙, 🪙, A, B, C 🪙
     (Ex) For code S52.246[A]: See S52.019[A] For code S52.246[B,C]: See S52.00[B,C]
     For S52.246[K,M,N,P,Q,R]: See S52.00[L,M,N,P,Q,R]

CHAPTER 19 (S00-T88)

N Newborn Age: 0   **P** Pediatric Age: 0–17   **M** Maternity DX: 12–55   **A** Adult Age: 15–124   ♀ Females Only   ♂ Males Only

🪙 Complication\Comorbidity   🪙 Major C\C   (Ex) CC/MCC Exclusions   🪙 Present on Admission Requirement   🪙 Hospital-Acquired Condition

1375

● **S52.25** Comminuted fracture of shaft of ulna

● **S52.251** Displaced comminuted fracture of shaft of ulna, right arm
A, K, M, N, P, Q, R 🔧, B, C 🔧, 🔧, A, B, C 🔧
Ⓔⓧ For code S52.251[A]: See S52.011[A]
For S52.251[B,C]: See S52.00[B,C]
For S52.251[K,M,N,P,Q,R]: See S52.00[L,M,N,P,Q,R]

● **S52.252** Displaced comminuted fracture of shaft of ulna, left arm
A, K, M, N, P, Q, R 🔧, B, C 🔧, 🔧, A, B, C 🔧
Ⓔⓧ For code S52.252[A]: See S52.012[A] For code S52.252[B,C]: See S52.00[B,C]
For S52.252[K,M,N,P,Q,R]: See S52.00[L,M,N,P,Q,R]

● **S52.253** Displaced comminuted fracture of shaft of ulna, unspecified arm
A, K, M, N, P, Q, R 🔧, B, C 🔧, 🔧, A, B, C 🔧
Ⓔⓧ For code S52.253[A]: See S52.019[A] For code S52.253[B,C]: See S52.00[B,C]
For S52.253[K,M,N,P,Q,R]: See S52.00[L,M,N,P,Q,R]

● **S52.254** Nondisplaced comminuted fracture of shaft of ulna, right arm
A, K, M, N, P, Q, R 🔧, B, C 🔧, 🔧, A, B, C 🔧
Ⓔⓧ For code S52.254[A]: See S52.011[A]
For S52.254[B,C]: See S52.00[B,C]
For S52.254[K,M,N,P,Q,R]: See S52.00[L,M,N,P,Q,R]

● **S52.255** Nondisplaced comminuted fracture of shaft of ulna, left arm
A, K, M, N, P, Q, R 🔧, B, C 🔧, 🔧, A, B, C 🔧
Ⓔⓧ For code S52.255[A]: See S52.012[A] For code S52.255[B,C]: See S52.00[B,C]
For S52.255[K,M,N,P,Q,R]: See S52.00[L,M,N,P,Q,R]

● **S52.256** Nondisplaced comminuted fracture of shaft of ulna, unspecified arm
A, K, M, N, P, Q, R 🔧, B, C 🔧, 🔧, A, B, C 🔧
Ⓔⓧ For code S52.256[A]: See S52.019[A] For code S52.256[B,C]: See S52.00[B,C]
For S52.256[K,M,N,P,Q,R]: See S52.00[L,M,N,P,Q,R]

● **S52.26** Segmental fracture of shaft of ulna

● **S52.261** Displaced segmental fracture of shaft of ulna, right arm
A, K, M, N, P, Q, R 🔧, B, C 🔧, 🔧, A, B, C 🔧
Ⓔⓧ For code S52.261[A]: See S52.011[A]
For S52.261[B,C]: See S52.00[B,C]
For S52.261[K,M,N,P,Q,R]: See S52.00[L,M,N,P,Q,R]

● **S52.262** Displaced segmental fracture of shaft of ulna, left arm A, K, M, N, P, Q, R 🔧, B, C 🔧, 🔧, A, B, C 🔧
Ⓔⓧ For code S52.262[A]: See S52.012[A] For code S52.262[B,C]: See S52.00[B,C]
For S52.262[K,M,N,P,Q,R]: See S52.00[L,M,N,P,Q,R]

● **S52.263** Displaced segmental fracture of shaft of ulna, unspecified arm
A, K, M, N, P, Q, R 🔧, B, C 🔧, 🔧, A, B, C 🔧
Ⓔⓧ For code S52.263[A]: See S52.019[A] For code S52.263[B,C]: See S52.00[B,C]
For S52.263[K,M,N,P,Q,R]: See S52.00[L,M,N,P,Q,R]

● **S52.264** Nondisplaced segmental fracture of shaft of ulna, right arm
A, K, M, N, P, Q, R 🔧, B, C 🔧, 🔧, A, B, C 🔧
Ⓔⓧ For code S52.264[A]: See S52.011[A]
For S52.264[B,C]: See S52.00[B,C]
For S52.264[K,M,N,P,Q,R]: See S52.00[L,M,N,P,Q,R]

● **S52.265** Nondisplaced segmental fracture of shaft of ulna, left arm
A, K, M, N, P, Q, R 🔧, B, C 🔧, 🔧, A, B, C 🔧
Ⓔⓧ For code S52.265[A]: See S52.012[A] For code S52.265[B,C]: See S52.00[B,C]
For S52.265[K,M,N,P,Q,R]: See S52.00[L,M,N,P,Q,R]

● **S52.266** Nondisplaced segmental fracture of shaft of ulna, unspecified arm
A, K, M, N, P, Q, R 🔧, B, C 🔧, 🔧, A, B, C 🔧
Ⓔⓧ For code S52.266[A]: See S52.019[A] For code S52.266[B,C]: See S52.00[B,C]
For S52.266[K,M,N,P,Q,R]: See S52.00[L,M,N,P,Q,R]

● **S52.27** Monteggia's fracture of ulna
Fracture of upper shaft of ulna with dislocation of radial head
Ⓔⓧ For category S52.27 CC codes S52.27[B,C]: See S52.00[B,C] For S52.27[K,M,N,P,Q,R]: See S52.00[K,M,N,P,Q,R]

● **S52.271** Monteggia's fracture of right ulna
K, M, N, P, Q, R 🔧, B, C 🔧, 🔧, B, C 🔧

● **S52.272** Monteggia's fracture of left ulna
K, M, N, P, Q, R 🔧, B, C 🔧, 🔧, B, C 🔧

● **S52.279** Monteggia's fracture of unspecified ulna K, M, N, P, Q, R 🔧, B, C 🔧, 🔧, B, C 🔧

● **S52.28** Bent bone of ulna

● **S52.281** Bent bone of right ulna
A, K, M, N, P, Q, R 🔧, B, C 🔧, 🔧, A, B, C 🔧
Ⓔⓧ For code S52.281[A]: See S52.011[A]
For S52.281[B,C]: See S52.00[B,C]
For S52.281[K,M,N,P,Q,R]: See S52.00[L,M,N,P,Q,R]

● **S52.282** Bent bone of left ulna
A, K, M, N, P, Q, R 🔧, B, C 🔧, 🔧, A, B, C 🔧
Ⓔⓧ For code S52.282[A]: See S52.012[A] For code S52.282[B,C]: See S52.00[B,C]
For S52.282[K,M,N,P,Q,R]: See S52.00[L,M,N,P,Q,R]

● **S52.283** Bent bone of unspecified ulna
A, K, M, N, P, Q, R 🔧, B, C 🔧, 🔧, A, B, C 🔧
Ⓔⓧ For code S52.283[A]: See S52.019[A] For code S52.283[B,C]: See S52.00[B,C]
For S52.283[K,M,N,P,Q,R]: See S52.00[L,M,N,P,Q,R]

◀ New   ◀▥ Revised   ~~deleted~~ Deleted   Excludes 1   Excludes 2   Includes   Use additional   Code first   Code also   Unspecified
OGCR Official Guidelines   ● Unacceptable Principal Diagnosis   X Assign placeholder X   ● Use Additional Character(s)   ▶ Manifestation Code   **Coding Clinic**

● **S52.29**   Other fracture of shaft of ulna

  ● **S52.291**   Other fracture of shaft of right ulna
A, K, M, N, P, Q, R 🅒, B, C 🅜, 🅟,
A, B, C 🅗
     Ⓔ **For code S52.291[A]:** See S52.011[A]
       For S52.291[B,C]: See S52.00[B,C]
       For S52.291[K,M,N,P,Q,R]: See
       S52.00[L,M,N,P,Q,R]

  ● **S52.292**   Other fracture of shaft of left ulna
A, K, M, N, P, Q, R 🅒, B, C 🅜, 🅟,
A, B, C 🅗
     Ⓔ **For code S52.292[A]:** See S52.012[A] For
       code S52.292[B,C]: See S52.00[B,C]
       For S52.292[K,M,N,P,Q,R]: See
       S52.00[L,M,N,P,Q,R]

  ● **S52.299**   Other fracture of shaft of unspecified
ulna A, K, M, N, P, Q, R 🅒, B, C 🅜, 🅟,
A, B, C 🅗
     Ⓔ **For code S52.299[A]:** See S52.019[A] For
       code S52.299[B,C]: See S52.00[B,C]
       For S52.299[K,M,N,P,Q,R]: See
       S52.00[L,M,N,P,Q,R]

● **S52.3**   Fracture of shaft of radius

  ● **S52.30**   Unspecified fracture of shaft of radius

    ● **S52.301**   Unspecified fracture of shaft of right
radius A, K, M, N, P, Q, R 🅒, B, C 🅜,
🅟, A, B, C 🅗
     Ⓔ **For code S52.301[A]:** See S52.011[A]
       For S52.301[B,C]: See S52.00[B,C]
       For S52.301[K,M,N,P,Q,R]: See
       S52.00[L,M,N,P,Q,R]

    ● **S52.302**   Unspecified fracture of shaft of left
radius A, K, M, N, P, Q, R 🅒, B, C 🅜,
🅟, A, B, C 🅗
     Ⓔ **For code S52.302[A]:** See S52.012[A] For
       code S52.302[B,C]: See S52.00[B,C]
       For S52.302[K,M,N,P,Q,R]: See
       S52.00[L,M,N,P,Q,R]

    ● **S52.309**   Unspecified fracture of shaft of
unspecified radius
A, K, M, N, P, Q, R 🅒, B, C 🅜, 🅟,
A, B, C 🅗
     Ⓔ **For code S52.309[A]:** See S52.019[A] For
       code S52.309[B,C]: See S52.00[B,C]
       For S52.309[K,M,N,P,Q,R]: See
       S52.00[L,M,N,P,Q,R]

  ● **S52.31**   Greenstick fracture of shaft of radius

     The appropriate 7th character is to be added to
all codes in subcategory S52.31

A	initial encounter for closed fracture
D	subsequent encounter for fracture with routine healing
G	subsequent encounter for fracture with delayed healing
K	subsequent encounter for fracture with nonunion
P	subsequent encounter for fracture with malunion
S	sequela

    ● **S52.311**   Greenstick fracture of shaft of radius,
right arm A, K, P 🅒, 🅟, A 🅗
     Ⓔ **For code S52.311[A]:** See S52.011[A]
       For S52.311[K,P]: See S52.00[L,M,N,P,Q,R]

    ● **S52.312**   Greenstick fracture of shaft of radius,
left arm A, K, P 🅒, 🅟, A 🅗
     Ⓔ **For code S52.312[A]:** See S52.012[A]
       For S52.312[K,P]: See S52.00[L,M,N,P,Q,R]

    ● **S52.319**   Greenstick fracture of shaft of radius,
unspecified arm A, K, P 🅒, 🅟, A 🅗
     Ⓔ **For code S52.319[A]:** See S52.019[A]
       For S52.319[K,P]: See S52.00[L,M,N,P,Q,R]

● **S52.32**   Transverse fracture of shaft of radius

  ● **S52.321**   Displaced transverse fracture of shaft
of right radius A, K, M, N, P, Q, R 🅒,
B, C 🅜, 🅟, A, B, C 🅗
     Ⓔ **For code S52.321[A]:** See S52.011[A]
       For S52.321[B,C]: See S52.00[B,C]
       For S52.321[K,M,N,P,Q,R]: See
       S52.00[L,M,N,P,Q,R]

  ● **S52.322**   Displaced transverse fracture of shaft
of left radius A, K, M, N, P, Q, R 🅒,
B, C 🅜, 🅟, A, B, C 🅗
     Ⓔ **For code S52.322[A]:** See S52.012[A] For
       code S52.322[B,C]: See S52.00[B,C]
       For S52.322[K,M,N,P,Q,R]: See
       S52.00[L,M,N,P,Q,R]

  ● **S52.323**   Displaced transverse fracture of shaft
of unspecified radius
A, K, M, N, P, Q, R 🅒, B, C 🅜, 🅟,
A, B, C 🅗
     Ⓔ **For code S52.323[A]:** See S52.019[A] For
       code S52.323[B,C]: See S52.00[B,C]
       For S52.323[K,M,N,P,Q,R]: See
       S52.00[L,M,N,P,Q,R]

  ● **S52.324**   Nondisplaced transverse fracture of
shaft of right radius
A, K, M, N, P, Q, R 🅒, B, C 🅜, 🅟,
A, B, C 🅗
     Ⓔ **For code S52.324[A]:** See S52.011[A]
       For S52.324[B,C]: See S52.00[B,C]
       For S52.324[K,M,N,P,Q,R]: See
       S52.00[L,M,N,P,Q,R]

  ● **S52.325**   Nondisplaced transverse fracture of
shaft of left radius
A, K, M, N, P, Q, R 🅒, B, C 🅜, 🅟,
A, B, C 🅗
     Ⓔ **For code S52.325[A]:** See S52.012[A] For
       code S52.325[B,C]: See S52.00[B,C]
       For S52.325[K,M,N,P,Q,R]: See
       S52.00[L,M,N,P,Q,R]

  ● **S52.326**   Nondisplaced transverse fracture of
shaft of unspecified radius
A, K, M, N, P, Q, R 🅒, B, C 🅜, 🅟,
A, B, C 🅗
     Ⓔ **For code S52.326[A]:** See S52.019[A] For
       code S52.326[B,C]: See S52.00[B,C]
       For S52.326[K,M,N,P,Q,R]: See
       S52.00[L,M,N,P,Q,R]

● **S52.33**   Oblique fracture of shaft of radius

  ● **S52.331**   Displaced oblique fracture of shaft of
right radius A, K, M, N, P, Q, R 🅒,
B, C 🅜, 🅟, A, B, C 🅗
     Ⓔ **For code S52.331[A]:** See S52.011[A]
       For S52.331[B,C]: See S52.00[B,C]
       For S52.331[K,M,N,P,Q,R]: See
       S52.00[L,M,N,P,Q,R]

  ● **S52.332**   Displaced oblique fracture of shaft of
left radius A, K, M, N, P, Q, R 🅒,
B, C 🅜, 🅟, A, B, C 🅗
     Ⓔ **For code S52.332[A]:** See S52.012[A] For
       code S52.332[B,C]: See S52.00[B,C]
       For S52.332[K,M,N,P,Q,R]: See
       S52.00[L,M,N,P,Q,R]

  ● **S52.333**   Displaced oblique fracture of shaft of
unspecified radius
A, K, M, N, P, Q, R 🅒, B, C 🅜, 🅟,
A, B, C 🅗
     Ⓔ **For code S52.333[A]:** See S52.019[A] For
       code S52.333[B,C]: See S52.00[B,C]
       For S52.333[K,M,N,P,Q,R]: See
       S52.00[L,M,N,P,Q,R]

CHAPTER 19 (S00–T88)

N Newborn Age: 0   **P** Pediatric Age: 0–17   **M** Maternity DX: 12–55   **A** Adult Age: 15–124   ♀ Females Only   ♂ Males Only

🅒 Complication\Comorbidity   🅜 Major C\C   Ⓔ CC/MCC Exclusions   🅟 Present on Admission Requirement   🅗 Hospital-Acquired Condition

1377

● S52.334   Nondisplaced oblique fracture of shaft of right radius
A, K, M, N, P, Q, R 🪙, B, C 🪙, 🪙, A, B, C 🪙
(Ex:) For code S52.334[A]: See S52.011[A]
For S52.334[B,C]: See S52.00[B,C]
For S52.334[K,M,N,P,Q,R]: See S52.00[L,M,N,P,Q,R]

● S52.335   Nondisplaced oblique fracture of shaft of left radius
A, K, M, N, P, Q, R 🪙, B, C 🪙, 🪙, A, B, C 🪙
(Ex:) For code S52.335[A]: See S52.012[A] For code S52.335[B,C]: See S52.00[B,C]
For S52.335[K,M,N,P,Q,R]: See S52.00[L,M,N,P,Q,R]

● S52.336   Nondisplaced oblique fracture of shaft of unspecified radius
A, K, M, N, P, Q, R 🪙, B, C 🪙, 🪙, A, B, C 🪙
(Ex:) For code S52.336[A]: See S52.019[A] For code S52.336[B,C]: See S52.00[B,C]
For S52.336[K,M,N,P,Q,R]: See S52.00[L,M,N,P,Q,R]

● S52.34   Spiral fracture of shaft of radius

● S52.341   Displaced spiral fracture of shaft of radius, right arm
A, K, M, N, P, Q, R 🪙, B, C 🪙, 🪙, A, B, C 🪙
(Ex:) For code S52.341[A]: See S52.011[A]
For S52.341[B,C]: See S52.00[B,C]
For S52.341[K,M,N,P,Q,R]: See S52.00[L,M,N,P,Q,R]

● S52.342   Displaced spiral fracture of shaft of radius, left arm A, K, M, N, P, Q, R 🪙, B, C 🪙, 🪙, A, B, C 🪙
(Ex:) For code S52.342[A]: See S52.012[A] For code S52.342[B,C]: See S52.00[B,C]
For S52.342[K,M,N,P,Q,R]: See S52.00[L,M,N,P,Q,R]

● S52.343   Displaced spiral fracture of shaft of radius, unspecified arm
A, K, M, N, P, Q, R 🪙, B, C 🪙, 🪙, A, B, C 🪙
(Ex:) For code S52.343[A]: See S52.019[A] For code S52.343[B,C]: See S52.00[B,C]
For S52.343[K,M,N,P,Q,R]: See S52.00[L,M,N,P,Q,R]

● S52.344   Nondisplaced spiral fracture of shaft of radius, right arm
A, K, M, N, P, Q, R 🪙, B, C 🪙, 🪙, A, B, C 🪙
(Ex:) For code S52.344[A]: See S52.011[A]
For S52.344[B,C]: See S52.00[B,C]
For S52.344[K,M,N,P,Q,R]: See S52.00[L,M,N,P,Q,R]

● S52.345   Nondisplaced spiral fracture of shaft of radius, left arm
A, K, M, N, P, Q, R 🪙, B, C 🪙, 🪙, A, B, C 🪙
(Ex:) For code S52.345[A]: See S52.012[A] For code S52.345[B,C]: See S52.00[B,C]
For S52.345[K,M,N,P,Q,R]: See S52.00[L,M,N,P,Q,R]

● S52.346   Nondisplaced spiral fracture of shaft of radius, unspecified arm
A, K, M, N, P, Q, R 🪙, B, C 🪙, 🪙, A, B, C 🪙
(Ex:) For code S52.346[A]: See S52.019[A] For code S52.346[B,C]: See S52.00[B,C]
For S52.346[K,M,N,P,Q,R]: See S52.00[L,M,N,P,Q,R]

● S52.35   Comminuted fracture of shaft of radius

● S52.351   Displaced comminuted fracture of shaft of radius, right arm
A, K, M, N, P, Q, R 🪙, B, C 🪙, 🪙, A, B, C 🪙
(Ex:) For code S52.351[A]: See S52.011[A]
For S52.351[B,C]: See S52.00[B,C]
For S52.351[K,M,N,P,Q,R]: See S52.00[L,M,N,P,Q,R]

● S52.352   Displaced comminuted fracture of shaft of radius, left arm
A, K, M, N, P, Q, R 🪙, B, C 🪙, 🪙, A, B, C 🪙
(Ex:) For code S52.352[A]: See S52.012[A] For code S52.352[B,C]: See S52.00[B,C]
For S52.352[K,M,N,P,Q,R]: See S52.00[L,M,N,P,Q,R] ·

● S52.353   Displaced comminuted fracture of shaft of radius, unspecified arm
A, K, M, N, P, Q, R 🪙, B, C 🪙, 🪙, A, B, C 🪙
(Ex:) For code S52.353[A]: See S52.019[A] For code S52.353[B,C]: See S52.00[B,C]
For S52.353[K,M,N,P,Q,R]: See S52.00[L,M,N,P,Q,R]

● S52.354   Nondisplaced comminuted fracture of shaft of radius, right arm
A, K, M, N, P, Q, R 🪙, B, C 🪙, 🪙, A, B, C 🪙
(Ex:) For code S52.354[A]: See S52.011[A]
For S52.354[B,C]: See S52.00[B,C]
For S52.354[K,M,N,P,Q,R]: See S52.00[L,M,N,P,Q,R]

● S52.355   Nondisplaced comminuted fracture of shaft of radius, left arm
A, K, M, N, P, Q, R 🪙, B, C 🪙, 🪙, A, B, C 🪙
(Ex:) For code S52.355[A]: See S52.012[A] For code S52.355[B,C]: See S52.00[B,C]
For S52.355[K,M,N,P,Q,R]: See S52.00[L,M,N,P,Q,R]

● S52.356   Nondisplaced comminuted fracture of shaft of radius, unspecified arm
A, K, M, N, P, Q, R 🪙, B, C 🪙, 🪙, A, B, C 🪙
(Ex:) For code S52.356[A]: See S52.019[A] For code S52.356[B,C]: See S52.00[B,C]
For S52.356[K,M,N,P,Q,R]: See S52.00[L,M,N,P,Q,R]

● S52.36   Segmental fracture of shaft of radius

● S52.361   Displaced segmental fracture of shaft of radius, right arm
A, K, M, N, P, Q, R 🪙, B, C 🪙, 🪙, A, B, C 🪙
(Ex:) For code S52.361[A]: See S52.011[A]
For S52.361[B,C]: See S52.00[B,C]
For S52.361[K,M,N,P,Q,R]: See S52.00[L,M,N,P,Q,R]

● S52.362   Displaced segmental fracture of shaft of radius, left arm
A, K, M, N, P, Q, R 🪙, B, C 🪙, 🪙, A, B, C 🪙
(Ex:) For code S52.362[A]: See S52.012[A] For code S52.362[B,C]: See S52.00[B,C]
For S52.362[K,M,N,P,Q,R]: See S52.00[L,M,N,P,Q,R]

● S52.363   Displaced segmental fracture of shaft of radius, unspecified arm
A, K, M, N, P, Q, R 🪙, B, C 🪙, 🪙, A, B, C 🪙
(Ex:) For code S52.363[A]: See S52.019[A] For code S52.363[B,C]: See S52.00[B,C]
For S52.363[K,M,N,P,Q,R]: See S52.00[L,M,N,P,Q,R]

◀ New   ◀▥ Revised   ~~deleted~~ Deleted   Excludes 1   Excludes 2   Includes   Use additional   Code first   Code also   Unspecified
OGCR Official Guidelines   ● Unacceptable Principal Diagnosis   X Assign placeholder X   ▶ Use Additional Character(s)   ▶ Manifestation Code   **Coding Clinic**

● **S52.364**   Nondisplaced segmental fracture of shaft of radius, right arm
A, K, M, N, P, Q, R 🗫, B, C 🗫, 🗫, A, B, C 🗫

> (Ex:) For code S52.364[A]: See S52.011[A]
> For S52.364[B,C]: See S52.00[B,C]
> For S52.364[K,M,N,P,Q,R]: See S52.00[L,M,N,P,Q,R]

● **S52.365**   Nondisplaced segmental fracture of shaft of radius, left arm
A, K, M, N, P, Q, R 🗫, B, C 🗫, 🗫, A, B, C 🗫

> (Ex:) For code S52.365[A]: See S52.012[A] For code S52.365[B,C]: See S52.00[B,C]
> For S52.365[K,M,N,P,Q,R]: See S52.00[L,M,N,P,Q,R]

● **S52.366**   Nondisplaced segmental fracture of shaft of radius, unspecified arm
A, K, M, N, P, Q, R 🗫, B, C 🗫, 🗫, A, B, C 🗫

> (Ex:) For code S52.366[A]: See S52.019[A] For code S52.366[B,C]: See S52.00[B,C]
> For S52.366[K,M,N,P,Q,R]: See S52.00[L,M,N,P,Q,R]

● **S52.37**   Galeazzi's fracture
Fracture of lower shaft of radius with radioulnar joint dislocation

● **S52.371**   Galeazzi's fracture of right radius
A, K, M, N, P, Q, R 🗫, B, C 🗫, 🗫, A, B, C 🗫

> (Ex:) For code S52.371[A]: See S52.011[A]
> For S52.371[B,C]: See S52.00[B,C]
> For S52.371[K,M,N,P,Q,R]: See S52.00[L,M,N,P,Q,R]

● **S52.372**   Galeazzi's fracture of left radius
A, K, M, N, P, Q, R 🗫, B, C 🗫, 🗫, A, B, C 🗫

> (Ex:) For code S52.372[A]: See S52.012[A] For code S52.372[B,C]: See S52.00[B,C]
> For S52.372[K,M,N,P,Q,R]: See S52.00[L,M,N,P,Q,R]

● **S52.379**   Galeazzi's fracture of unspecified radius
A, K, M, N, P, Q, R 🗫, B, C 🗫, 🗫, A, B, C 🗫

> (Ex:) For code S52.379[A]: See S52.019[A] For code S52.379[B,C]: See S52.00[B,C]
> For S52.379[K,M,N,P,Q,R]: See S52.00[L,M,N,P,Q,R]

● **S52.38**   Bent bone of radius

● **S52.381**   Bent bone of right radius
A, K, M, N, P, Q, R 🗫, B, C 🗫, 🗫, A, B, C 🗫

> (Ex:) For code S52.381[A]: See S52.011[A]
> For S52.381[B,C]: See S52.00[B,C]
> For S52.381[K,M,N,P,Q,R]: See S52.00[L,M,N,P,Q,R]

● **S52.382**   Bent bone of left radius
A, K, M, N, P, Q, R 🗫, B, C 🗫, 🗫, A, B, C 🗫

> (Ex:) For code S52.382[A]: See S52.012[A] For code S52.382[B,C]: See S52.00[B,C]
> For S52.382[K,M,N,P,Q,R]: See S52.00[L,M,N,P,Q,R]

● **S52.389**   Bent bone of unspecified radius
A, K, M, N, P, Q, R 🗫, B, C 🗫, 🗫, A, B, C 🗫

> (Ex:) For code S52.389[A]: See S52.019[A] For code S52.389[B,C]: See S52.00[B,C]
> For S52.389[K,M,N,P,Q,R]: See S52.00[L,M,N,P,Q,R]

● **S52.39**   Other fracture of shaft of radius

● **S52.391**   Other fracture of shaft of radius, right arm
A, K, M, N, P, Q, R 🗫, B, C 🗫, 🗫, A, B, C 🗫

> (Ex:) For code S52.391[A]: See S52.011[A]
> For S52.391[B,C]: See S52.00[B,C]
> For S52.391[K,M,N,P,Q,R]: See S52.00[L,M,N,P,Q,R]

● **S52.392**   Other fracture of shaft of radius, left arm
A, K, M, N, P, Q, R 🗫, B, C 🗫, 🗫, A, B, C 🗫

> (Ex:) For code S52.392[A]: See S52.012[A] For code S52.392[B,C]: See S52.00[B,C]
> For S52.392[K,M,N,P,Q,R]: See S52.00[L,M,N,P,Q,R]

● **S52.399**   Other fracture of shaft of radius, unspecified arm A, K, M, N, P, Q, R 🗫, B, C 🗫, 🗫, A, B, C 🗫

> (Ex:) For code S52.399[A]: See S52.019[A] For code S52.399[B,C]: See S52.00[B,C]
> For S52.399[K,M,N,P,Q,R]: See S52.00[L,M,N,P,Q,R]

● **S52.5**   Fracture of lower end of radius
Fracture of distal end of radius

> **Excludes2**   physeal fractures of lower end of radius (S59.2-)

● **S52.50**   Unspecified fracture of the lower end of radius

● **S52.501**   Unspecified fracture of the lower end of right radius A, K, M, N, P, Q, R 🗫, B, C 🗫, 🗫, A, B, C 🗫

> (Ex:) For code S52.501[A]: See S52.011[A]
> For S52.501[B,C]: See S52.00[B,C]
> For S52.501[K,M,N,P,Q,R]: See S52.00[L,M,N,P,Q,R]

● **S52.502**   Unspecified fracture of the lower end of left radius A, K, M, N, P, Q, R 🗫, B, C 🗫, 🗫, A, B, C 🗫

> (Ex:) For code S52.502[A]: See S52.012[A] For code S52.502[B,C]: See S52.00[B,C]
> For S52.502[K,M,N,P,Q,R]: See S52.00[L,M,N,P,Q,R]

● **S52.509**   Unspecified fracture of the lower end of unspecified radius
A, K, M, N, P, Q, R 🗫, B, C 🗫, 🗫, A, B, C 🗫

> (Ex:) For code S52.509[A]: See S52.019[A] For code S52.509[B,C]: See S52.00[B,C]
> For S52.509[K,M,N,P,Q,R]: See S52.00[L,M,N,P,Q,R]

● **S52.51**   Fracture of radial styloid process

● **S52.511**   Displaced fracture of right radial styloid process A, K, M, N, P, Q, R 🗫, B, C 🗫, 🗫, A, B, C 🗫

> (Ex:) For code S52.511[A]: See S52.011[A]
> For S52.511[B,C]: See S52.00[B,C]
> For S52.511[K,M,N,P,Q,R]: See S52.00[L,M,N,P,Q,R]

● **S52.512**   Displaced fracture of left radial styloid process A, K, M, N, P, Q, R 🗫, B, C 🗫, 🗫, A, B, C 🗫

> (Ex:) For code S52.512[A]: See S52.012[A] For code S52.512[B,C]: See S52.00[B,C]
> For S52.512[K,M,N,P,Q,R]: See S52.00[L,M,N,P,Q,R]

● **S52.513**   Displaced fracture of unspecified radial styloid process
A, K, M, N, P, Q, R 🗫, B, C 🗫, 🗫, A, B, C 🗫

> (Ex:) For code S52.513[A]: See S52.019[A] For code S52.513[B,C]: See S52.00[B,C]
> For S52.513[K,M,N,P,Q,R]: See S52.00[L,M,N,P,Q,R]

N   Newborn Age: 0   P   Pediatric Age: 0–17   M   Maternity DX: 12–55   A   Adult Age: 15–124   ♀ Females Only   ♂ Males Only

🗫 Complication\Comorbidity   🗫 Major C\C   (Ex:) CC/MCC Exclusions   🗫 Present on Admission Requirement   🗫 Hospital-Acquired Condition

● **S52.514** **Nondisplaced fracture of right radial styloid process** A, K, M, N, P, Q, R 🔖, B, C 🔖, 🔖, A, B, C 🔖
　　Ⓔⓧ For code S52.514[A]: See S52.011[A]
　　　For S52.514[B,C]: See S52.00[B,C]
　　　For S52.514[K,M,N,P,Q,R]: See
　　　S52.00[L,M,N,P,Q,R]

● **S52.515** **Nondisplaced fracture of left radial styloid process** A, K, M, N, P, Q, R 🔖, B, C 🔖, 🔖, A, B, C 🔖
　　Ⓔⓧ For code S52.515[A]: See S52.012[A] For code S52.515[B,C]: See S52.00[B,C]
　　　For S52.515[K,M,N,P,Q,R]: See
　　　S52.00[L,M,N,P,Q,R]

● **S52.516** **Nondisplaced fracture of unspecified radial styloid process**
　　A, K, M, N, P, Q, R 🔖, B, C 🔖, 🔖, A, B, C 🔖
　　Ⓔⓧ For code S52.516[A]: See S52.019[A] For code S52.516[B,C]: See S52.00[B,C]
　　　For S52.516[K,M,N,P,Q,R]: See
　　　S52.00[L,M,N,P,Q,R]

● **S52.52** **Torus fracture of lower end of radius**
　The appropriate 7th character is to be added to all codes in subcategory S52.52

A	initial encounter for closed fracture
D	subsequent encounter for fracture with routine healing
G	subsequent encounter for fracture with delayed healing
K	subsequent encounter for fracture with nonunion
P	subsequent encounter for fracture with malunion
S	sequela

● **S52.521** **Torus fracture of lower end of right radius** A, K, P 🔖, 🔖, A 🔖
　　Ⓔⓧ For code S52.521[A]: See S52.011[A]
　　　For S52.521[K,P]: See S52.00[L,M,N,P,Q,R]

● **S52.522** **Torus fracture of lower end of left radius** A, K, P 🔖, 🔖, A 🔖
　　Ⓔⓧ For code S52.522[A]: See S52.012[A]
　　　For S52.522[K,P]: See S52.00[L,M,N,P,Q,R]

● **S52.529** **Torus fracture of lower end of unspecified radius** A, K, P 🔖, 🔖, A 🔖
　　Ⓔⓧ For code S52.529[A]: See S52.019[A]
　　　For S52.529[K,P]: See S52.00[L,M,N,P,Q,R]

● **S52.53** **Colles' fracture**

● **S52.531** **Colles' fracture of right radius**
　　A, K, M, N, P, Q, R 🔖, B, C 🔖, 🔖, A, B, C 🔖
　　Ⓔⓧ For code S52.531[A]: See S52.011[A]
　　　For S52.531[B,C]: See S52.00[B,C]
　　　For S52.531[K,M,N,P,Q,R]: See
　　　S52.00[L,M,N,P,Q,R]

● **S52.532** **Colles' fracture of left radius**
　　A, K, M, N, P, Q, R 🔖, B, C 🔖, 🔖, A, B, C 🔖
　　Ⓔⓧ For code S52.532[A]: See S52.012[A] For code S52.532[B,C]: See S52.00[B,C]
　　　For S52.532[K,M,N,P,Q,R]: See
　　　S52.00[L,M,N,P,Q,R]

● **S52.539** **Colles' fracture of unspecified radius**
　　A, K, M, N, P, Q, R 🔖, B, C 🔖, 🔖, A, B, C 🔖
　　Ⓔⓧ For code S52.539[A]: See S52.019[A] For code S52.539[B,C]: See S52.00[B,C]
　　　For S52.539[K,M,N,P,Q,R]: See
　　　S52.00[L,M,N,P,Q,R]

● **S52.54** **Smith's fracture**

● **S52.541** **Smith's fracture of right radius**
　　A, K, M, N, P, Q, R 🔖, B, C 🔖, 🔖, A, B, C 🔖
　　Ⓔⓧ For code S52.541[A]: See S52.011[A]
　　　For S52.541[B,C]: See S52.00[B,C]
　　　For S52.541[K,M,N,P,Q,R]: See
　　　S52.00[L,M,N,P,Q,R]

● **S52.542** **Smith's fracture of left radius**
　　A, K, M, N, P, Q, R 🔖, B, C 🔖, 🔖, A, B, C 🔖
　　Ⓔⓧ For code S52.542[A]: See S52.012[A] For code S52.542[B,C]: See S52.00[B,C]
　　　For S52.542[K,M,N,P,Q,R]: See
　　　S52.00[L,M,N,P,Q,R]

● **S52.549** **Smith's fracture of unspecified radius**
　　A, K, M, N, P, Q, R 🔖, B, C 🔖, 🔖, A, B, C 🔖
　　Ⓔⓧ For code S52.549[A]: See S52.019[A] For code S52.549[B,C]: See S52.00[B,C]
　　　For S52.549[K,M,N,P,Q,R]: See
　　　S52.00[L,M,N,P,Q,R]

● **S52.55** **Other extraarticular fracture of lower end of radius**

● **S52.551** **Other extraarticular fracture of lower end of right radius**
　　A, K, M, N, P, Q, R 🔖, B, C 🔖, 🔖, A, B, C 🔖
　　Ⓔⓧ For code S52.551[A]: See S52.011[A]
　　　For S52.551[B,C]: See S52.00[B,C]
　　　For S52.551[K,M,N,P,Q,R]: See
　　　S52.00[L,M,N,P,Q,R]

● **S52.552** **Other extraarticular fracture of lower end of left radius**
　　A, K, M, N, P, Q, R 🔖, B, C 🔖, 🔖, A, B, C 🔖
　　Ⓔⓧ For code S52.552[A]: See S52.012[A] For code S52.552[B,C]: See S52.00[B,C]
　　　For S52.552[K,M,N,P,Q,R]: See
　　　S52.00[L,M,N,P,Q,R]

● **S52.559** **Other extraarticular fracture of lower end of unspecified radius**
　　A, K, M, N, P, Q, R 🔖, B, C 🔖, 🔖, A, B, C 🔖
　　Ⓔⓧ For code S52.559[A]: See S52.019[A] For code S52.559[B,C]: See S52.00[B,C]
　　　For S52.559[K,M,N,P,Q,R]: See
　　　S52.00[L,M,N,P,Q,R]

● **S52.56** **Barton's fracture**

● **S52.561** **Barton's fracture of right radius**
　　A, K, M, N, P, Q, R 🔖, B, C 🔖, 🔖, A, B, C 🔖
　　Ⓔⓧ For code S52.561[A]: See S52.011[A]
　　　For S52.561[B,C]: See S52.00[B,C]
　　　For S52.561[K,M,N,P,Q,R]: See
　　　S52.00[L,M,N,P,Q,R]

● **S52.562** **Barton's fracture of left radius**
　　A, K, M, N, P, Q, R 🔖, B, C 🔖, 🔖, A, B, C 🔖
　　Ⓔⓧ For code S52.562[A]: See S52.012[A] For code S52.562[B,C]: See S52.00[B,C]
　　　For S52.562[K,M,N,P,Q,R]: See
　　　S52.00[L,M,N,P,Q,R]

● **S52.569** **Barton's fracture of unspecified radius**
　　A, K, M, N, P, Q, R 🔖, B, C 🔖, 🔖, A, B, C 🔖
　　Ⓔⓧ For code S52.569[A]: See S52.019[A] For code S52.569[B,C]: See S52.00[B,C]
　　　For S52.569[K,M,N,P,Q,R]: See
　　　S52.00[L,M,N,P,Q,R]

◀ New　◀ Revised　~~deleted~~ Deleted　Excludes 1　Excludes 2　Includes　Use additional　Code first　Code also　Unspecified
OGCR Official Guidelines　● Unacceptable Principal Diagnosis　X Assign placeholder X　● Use Additional Character(s)　▶ Manifestation Code　**Coding Clinic**

● **S52.57**   Other intraarticular fracture of lower end of radius

    ● **S52.571**   Other intraarticular fracture of lower end of right radius A, K, M, N, P, Q, R 🪙, B, C 🪙, 🪙, A, B, C 🪙
         (Ex) For code S52.571[A]: See S52.011[A] For S52.571[B,C]: See S52.00[B,C] For S52.571[K,M,N,P,Q,R]: See S52.00[L,M,N,P,Q,R]

    ● **S52.572**   Other intraarticular fracture of lower end of left radius A, K, M, N, P, Q, R 🪙, B, C 🪙, 🪙, A, B, C 🪙
         (Ex) For code S52.572[A]: See S52.012[A] For code S52.572[B,C]: See S52.00[B,C] For S52.572[K,M,N,P,Q,R]: See S52.00[L,M,N,P,Q,R]

    ● **S52.579**   Other intraarticular fracture of lower end of unspecified radius A, K, M, N, P, Q, R 🪙, B, C 🪙, 🪙, A, B, C 🪙
         (Ex) For code S52.579[A]: See S52.019[A] For code S52.579[B,C]: See S52.00[B,C] For S52.579[K,M,N,P,Q,R]: See S52.00[L,M,N,P,Q,R]

   ● **S52.59**   Other fractures of lower end of radius

    ● **S52.591**   Other fractures of lower end of right radius A, K, M, N, P, Q, R 🪙, B, C 🪙, 🪙, A, B, C 🪙
         (Ex) For code S52.591[A]: See S52.011[A] For S52.591[B,C]: See S52.00[B,C] For S52.591[K,M,N,P,Q,R]: See S52.00[L,M,N,P,Q,R]

    ● **S52.592**   Other fractures of lower end of left radius A, K, M, N, P, Q, R 🪙, B, C 🪙, 🪙, A, B, C 🪙
         (Ex) For code S52.592[A]: See S52.012[A] For code S52.592[B,C]: See S52.00[B,C] For S52.592[K,M,N,P,Q,R]: See S52.00[L,M,N,P,Q,R]

    ● **S52.599**   Other fractures of lower end of unspecified radius A, K, M, N, P, Q, R 🪙, B, C 🪙, 🪙, A, B, C 🪙
         (Ex) For code S52.599[A]: See S52.019[A] For code S52.599[B,C]: See S52.00[B,C] For S52.599[K,M,N,P,Q,R]: See S52.00[L,M,N,P,Q,R]

● **S52.6**   Fracture of lower end of ulna

   ● **S52.60**   Unspecified fracture of lower end of ulna

    ● **S52.601**   Unspecified fracture of lower end of right ulna A, K, M, N, P, Q, R 🪙, B, C 🪙, 🪙, A, B, C 🪙
         (Ex) For code S52.601[A]: See S52.011[A] For S52.601[B,C]: See S52.00[B,C] For S52.601[K,M,N,P,Q,R]: See S52.00[L,M,N,P,Q,R]

    ● **S52.602**   Unspecified fracture of lower end of left ulna A, K, M, N, P, Q, R 🪙, B, C 🪙, 🪙, A, B, C 🪙
         (Ex) For code S52.602[A]: See S52.012[A] For code S52.602[B,C]: See S52.00[B,C] For S52.602[K,M,N,P,Q,R]: See S52.00[L,M,N,P,Q,R]

    ● **S52.609**   Unspecified fracture of lower end of unspecified ulna A, K, M, N, P, Q, R 🪙, B, C 🪙, 🪙, A, B, C 🪙
         (Ex) For code S52.609[A]: See S52.019[A] For code S52.609[B,C]: See S52.00[B,C] For S52.609[K,M,N,P,Q,R]: See S52.00[L,M,N,P,Q,R]

● **S52.61**   Fracture of ulna styloid process

   ● **S52.611**   Displaced fracture of right ulna styloid process A, K, M, N, P, Q, R 🪙, B, C 🪙, 🪙, A, B, C 🪙
         (Ex) For code S52.611[A]: See S52.011[A] For S52.611[B,C]: See S52.00[B,C] For S52.611[K,M,N,P,Q,R]: See S52.00[L,M,N,P,Q,R]

   ● **S52.612**   Displaced fracture of left ulna styloid process A, K, M, N, P, Q, R 🪙, B, C 🪙, 🪙, A, B, C 🪙
         (Ex) For code S52.612[A]: See S52.012[A] For code S52.612[B,C]: See S52.00[B,C] For S52.612[K,M,N,P,Q,R]: See S52.00[L,M,N,P,Q,R]

   ● **S52.613**   Displaced fracture of unspecified ulna styloid process A, K, M, N, P, Q, R 🪙, B, C 🪙, 🪙, A, B, C 🪙
         (Ex) For code S52.613[A]: See S52.019[A] For code S52.613[B,C]: See S52.00[B,C] For S52.613[K,M,N,P,Q,R]: See S52.00[L,M,N,P,Q,R]

   ● **S52.614**   Nondisplaced fracture of right ulna styloid process A, K, M, N, P, Q, R 🪙, B, C 🪙, 🪙, A, B, C 🪙
         (Ex) For code S52.614[A]: See S52.011[A] For S52.614[B,C]: See S52.00[B,C] For S52.614[K,M,N,P,Q,R]: See S52.00[L,M,N,P,Q,R]

   ● **S52.615**   Nondisplaced fracture of left ulna styloid process A, K, M, N, P, Q, R 🪙, B, C 🪙, 🪙, A, B, C 🪙
         (Ex) For code S52.615[A]: See S52.012[A] For code S52.615[B,C]: See S52.00[B,C] For S52.615[K,M,N,P,Q,R]: See S52.00[L,M,N,P,Q,R]

   ● **S52.616**   Nondisplaced fracture of unspecified ulna styloid process A, K, M, N, P, Q, R 🪙, B, C 🪙, 🪙, A, B, C 🪙
         (Ex) For code S52.616[A]: See S52.019[A] For code S52.616[B,C]: See S52.00[B,C] For S52.616[K,M,N,P,Q,R]: See S52.00[L,M,N,P,Q,R]

● **S52.62**   Torus fracture of lower end of ulna

     The appropriate 7th character is to be added to all codes in subcategory S52.62

A	initial encounter for closed fracture
D	subsequent encounter for fracture with routine healing
G	subsequent encounter for fracture with delayed healing
K	subsequent encounter for fracture with nonunion
P	subsequent encounter for fracture with malunion
S	sequela

   ● **S52.621**   Torus fracture of lower end of right ulna A, K, P 🪙, 🪙, A 🪙
         (Ex) For code S52.621[A]: See S52.011[A] For S52.621[K,P]: See S52.00[L,M,N,P,Q,R]

   ● **S52.622**   Torus fracture of lower end of left ulna A, K, P 🪙, 🪙, A 🪙
         (Ex) For code S52.622[A]: See S52.012[A] For S52.622[K,P]: See S52.00[L,M,N,P,Q,R]

   ● **S52.629**   Torus fracture of lower end of unspecified ulna A, K, P 🪙, 🪙, A 🪙
         (Ex) For code S52.629[A]: See S52.019[A] For S52.629[K,P]: See S52.00[L,M,N,P,Q,R]

N   Newborn Age: 0   P   Pediatric Age: 0–17   M   Maternity DX: 12–55   A   Adult Age: 15–124   ♀   Females Only   ♂   Males Only

🪙 Complication\Comorbidity   🪙 Major C\C   (Ex) CC/MCC Exclusions   🪙 Present on Admission Requirement   🪙 Hospital-Acquired Condition

1381

S52.69 Other fracture of lower end of ulna

● S52.691 Other fracture of lower end of right ulna A, K, M, N, P, Q, R , B, C , , A, B, C

(Ex) For code S52.691[A]: See S52.011[A]
For S52.691[B,C]: See S52.00[B,C]
For S52.691[K,M,N,P,Q,R]: See S52.00[L,M,N,P,Q,R]

● S52.692 Other fracture of lower end of left ulna A, K, M, N, P, Q, R , B, C , , A, B, C

(Ex) For code S52.692[A]: See S52.012[A] For code S52.692[B,C]: See S52.00[B,C]
For S52.692[K,M,N,P,Q,R]: See S52.00[L,M,N,P,Q,R]

● S52.699 Other fracture of lower end of unspecified ulna
A, K, M, N, P, Q, R , B, C , , A, B, C

(Ex) For code S52.699[A]: See S52.019[A] For code S52.699[B,C]: See S52.00[B,C]
For S52.699[K,M,N,P,Q,R]: See S52.00[L,M,N,P,Q,R]

● S52.9 Unspecified fracture of forearm

(Ex) For category S52.9 CC codes S52.9[A]: See S52.019[A] For code S52.9[B,C]: See S52.00[B,C] For S52.9[K,M,N,P,Q,R]: See S52.00[L,M,N,P,Q,R]

X ● S52.90 Unspecified fracture of unspecified forearm
A, K, M, N, P, Q, R , B, C , , A, B, C

X ● S52.91 Unspecified fracture of right forearm
A, K, M, N, P, Q, R , B, C , , A, B, C

X ● S52.92 Unspecified fracture of left forearm
A, K, M, N, P, Q, R , B, C , , A, B, C

● S53 Dislocation and sprain of joints and ligaments of elbow

Includes avulsion of joint or ligament of elbow
laceration of cartilage, joint or ligament of elbow
sprain of cartilage, joint or ligament of elbow
traumatic hemarthrosis of joint or ligament of elbow
traumatic rupture of joint or ligament of elbow
traumatic subluxation of joint or ligament of elbow
traumatic tear of joint or ligament of elbow

Code also any associated open wound

Excludes2 strain of muscle, fascia and tendon at forearm level (S56.-)

The appropriate 7th character is to be added to each code from category S53

A	initial encounter
D	subsequent encounter
S	sequela

● S53.0 Subluxation and dislocation of radial head
Dislocation of radiohumeral joint
Subluxation of radiohumeral joint

Excludes1 Monteggia's fracture-dislocation (S52.27-)

● S53.00 Unspecified subluxation and dislocation of radial head

● S53.001 Unspecified subluxation of right radial head

● S53.002 Unspecified subluxation of left radial head

● S53.003 Unspecified subluxation of unspecified radial head

● S53.004 Unspecified dislocation of right radial head

● S53.005 Unspecified dislocation of left radial head

● S53.006 Unspecified dislocation of unspecified radial head

● S53.01 Anterior subluxation and dislocation of radial head
Anteriomedial subluxation and dislocation of radial head

● S53.011 Anterior subluxation of right radial head

● S53.012 Anterior subluxation of left radial head

● S53.013 Anterior subluxation of unspecified radial head

● S53.014 Anterior dislocation of right radial head

● S53.015 Anterior dislocation of left radial head

● S53.016 Anterior dislocation of unspecified radial head

● S53.02 Posterior subluxation and dislocation of radial head
Posteriolateral subluxation and dislocation of radial head

● S53.021 Posterior subluxation of right radial head

● S53.022 Posterior subluxation of left radial head

● S53.023 Posterior subluxation of unspecified radial head

● S53.024 Posterior dislocation of right radial head

● S53.025 Posterior dislocation of left radial head

● S53.026 Posterior dislocation of unspecified radial head

● S53.03 Nursemaid's elbow

● S53.031 Nursemaid's elbow, right elbow

● S53.032 Nursemaid's elbow, left elbow

● S53.033 Nursemaid's elbow, unspecified elbow

● S53.09 Other subluxation and dislocation of radial head

● S53.091 Other subluxation of right radial head

● S53.092 Other subluxation of left radial head

● S53.093 Other subluxation of unspecified radial head

● S53.094 Other dislocation of right radial head

● S53.095 Other dislocation of left radial head

● S53.096 Other dislocation of unspecified radial head

● S53.1 Subluxation and dislocation of ulnohumeral joint
Subluxation and dislocation of elbow NOS

Excludes1 dislocation of radial head alone (S53.0-)

● S53.10 Unspecified subluxation and dislocation of ulnohumeral joint

● S53.101 Unspecified subluxation of right ulnohumeral joint

● S53.102 Unspecified subluxation of left ulnohumeral joint

● S53.103 Unspecified subluxation of unspecified ulnohumeral joint

● S53.104 Unspecified dislocation of right ulnohumeral joint

● S53.105 Unspecified dislocation of left ulnohumeral joint

● S53.106 Unspecified dislocation of unspecified ulnohumeral joint

◀ New   ◀ᴵᴵᴵ Revised   ~~deleted~~ Deleted   Excludes 1   Excludes 2   Includes   Use additional   Code first   Code also   Unspecified

OGCR Official Guidelines   ● Unacceptable Principal Diagnosis   X Assign placeholder X   ● Use Additional Character(s)   ▶ Manifestation Code   **Coding Clinic**

CHAPTER 19 (S00-T88)

● **S53.11**   Anterior subluxation and dislocation of ulnohumeral joint
   ● **S53.111**   Anterior subluxation of right ulnohumeral joint ✍
   ● **S53.112**   Anterior subluxation of left ulnohumeral joint ✍
   ● **S53.113**   Anterior subluxation of unspecified ulnohumeral joint ✍
   ● **S53.114**   Anterior dislocation of right ulnohumeral joint ✍
       Coding Clinic: 2012, Q4, P108
   ● **S53.115**   Anterior dislocation of left ulnohumeral joint ✍
   ● **S53.116**   Anterior dislocation of unspecified ulnohumeral joint ✍
● **S53.12**   Posterior subluxation and dislocation of ulnohumeral joint
   ● **S53.121**   Posterior subluxation of right ulnohumeral joint ✍
   ● **S53.122**   Posterior subluxation of left ulnohumeral joint ✍
   ● **S53.123**   Posterior subluxation of unspecified ulnohumeral joint ✍
   ● **S53.124**   Posterior dislocation of right ulnohumeral joint ✍
   ● **S53.125**   Posterior dislocation of left ulnohumeral joint ✍
   ● **S53.126**   Posterior dislocation of unspecified ulnohumeral joint ✍
● **S53.13**   Medial subluxation and dislocation of ulnohumeral joint
   ● **S53.131**   Medial subluxation of right ulnohumeral joint ✍
   ● **S53.132**   Medial subluxation of left ulnohumeral joint ✍
   ● **S53.133**   Medial subluxation of unspecified ulnohumeral joint ✍
   ● **S53.134**   Medial dislocation of right ulnohumeral joint ✍
   ● **S53.135**   Medial dislocation of left ulnohumeral joint ✍
   ● **S53.136**   Medial dislocation of unspecified ulnohumeral joint ✍
● **S53.14**   Lateral subluxation and dislocation of ulnohumeral joint
   ● **S53.141**   Lateral subluxation of right ulnohumeral joint ✍
   ● **S53.142**   Lateral subluxation of left ulnohumeral joint ✍
   ● **S53.143**   Lateral subluxation of unspecified ulnohumeral joint ✍
   ● **S53.144**   Lateral dislocation of right ulnohumeral joint ✍
   ● **S53.145**   Lateral dislocation of left ulnohumeral joint ✍
   ● **S53.146**   Lateral dislocation of unspecified ulnohumeral joint ✍
● **S53.19**   Other subluxation and dislocation of ulnohumeral joint
   ● **S53.191**   Other subluxation of right ulnohumeral joint ✍
   ● **S53.192**   Other subluxation of left ulnohumeral joint ✍
   ● **S53.193**   Other subluxation of unspecified ulnohumeral joint ✍
   ● **S53.194**   Other dislocation of right ulnohumeral joint ✍
   ● **S53.195**   Other dislocation of left ulnohumeral joint ✍
   ● **S53.196**   Other dislocation of unspecified ulnohumeral joint ✍

● **S53.2**   Traumatic rupture of radial collateral ligament
   Excludes1   sprain of radial collateral ligament NOS (S53.43-)
   X ● **S53.20**   Traumatic rupture of unspecified radial collateral ligament ✍
   X ● **S53.21**   Traumatic rupture of right radial collateral ligament ✍
   X ● **S53.22**   Traumatic rupture of left radial collateral ligament ✍
● **S53.3**   Traumatic rupture of ulnar collateral ligament
   Excludes1   sprain of ulnar collateral ligament (S53.44-)
   X ● **S53.30**   Traumatic rupture of unspecified ulnar collateral ligament ✍
   X ● **S53.31**   Traumatic rupture of right ulnar collateral ligament ✍
   X ● **S53.32**   Traumatic rupture of left ulnar collateral ligament ✍
● **S53.4**   Sprain of elbow
   Excludes2   traumatic rupture of radial collateral ligament (S53.2-)
             traumatic rupture of ulnar collateral ligament (S53.3-)
   ● **S53.40**   Unspecified sprain of elbow
     ● **S53.401**   Unspecified sprain of right elbow ✍
     ● **S53.402**   Unspecified sprain of left elbow ✍
     ● **S53.409**   Unspecified sprain of unspecified elbow ✍
         Sprain of elbow NOS
   ● **S53.41**   Radiohumeral (joint) sprain
     ● **S53.411**   Radiohumeral (joint) sprain of right elbow ✍
     ● **S53.412**   Radiohumeral (joint) sprain of left elbow ✍
     ● **S53.419**   Radiohumeral (joint) sprain of unspecified elbow ✍
   ● **S53.42**   Ulnohumeral (joint) sprain
     ● **S53.421**   Ulnohumeral (joint) sprain of right elbow ✍
     ● **S53.422**   Ulnohumeral (joint) sprain of left elbow ✍
     ● **S53.429**   Ulnohumeral (joint) sprain of unspecified elbow ✍
   ● **S53.43**   Radial collateral ligament sprain
     ● **S53.431**   Radial collateral ligament sprain of right elbow ✍
     ● **S53.432**   Radial collateral ligament sprain of left elbow ✍
     ● **S53.439**   Radial collateral ligament sprain of unspecified elbow ✍
   ● **S53.44**   Ulnar collateral ligament sprain
     ● **S53.441**   Ulnar collateral ligament sprain of right elbow ✍
     ● **S53.442**   Ulnar collateral ligament sprain of left elbow ✍
     ● **S53.449**   Ulnar collateral ligament sprain of unspecified elbow ✍
   ● **S53.49**   Other sprain of elbow
     ● **S53.491**   Other sprain of right elbow ✍
     ● **S53.492**   Other sprain of left elbow ✍
     ● **S53.499**   Other sprain of unspecified elbow ✍

CHAPTER 19 (S00-T88)

N   Newborn Age: 0   P   Pediatric Age: 0–17   M   Maternity DX: 12–55   A   Adult Age: 15–124   ♀   Females Only   ♂   Males Only

✍   Complication\Comorbidity   ✍   Major C\C   (Ex)   CC/MCC Exclusions   ✍   Present on Admission Requirement   ✍   Hospital-Acquired Condition   **1383**

CHAPTER 19 (S00-T88)

● **S54 Injury of nerves at forearm level**

Code also any associated open wound (S51.-)

Excludes2 injury of nerves at wrist and hand level (S64.-)

The appropriate 7th character is to be added to each code from category S54

A	initial encounter
D	subsequent encounter
S	sequela

● **S54.0 Injury of ulnar nerve at forearm level**
Injury of ulnar nerve NOS

X● **S54.00 Injury of ulnar nerve at forearm level, unspecified arm** 🖉

X● **S54.01 Injury of ulnar nerve at forearm level, right arm** 🖉

X● **S54.02 Injury of ulnar nerve at forearm level, left arm** 🖉

● **S54.1 Injury of median nerve at forearm level**
Injury of median nerve NOS

X● **S54.10 Injury of median nerve at forearm level, unspecified arm** 🖉

X● **S54.11 Injury of median nerve at forearm level, right arm** 🖉

X● **S54.12 Injury of median nerve at forearm level, left arm** 🖉

● **S54.2 Injury of radial nerve at forearm level**
Injury of radial nerve NOS

X● **S54.20 Injury of radial nerve at forearm level, unspecified arm** 🖉

X● **S54.21 Injury of radial nerve at forearm level, right arm** 🖉

X● **S54.22 Injury of radial nerve at forearm level, left arm** 🖉

● **S54.3 Injury of cutaneous sensory nerve at forearm level**

X● **S54.30 Injury of cutaneous sensory nerve at forearm level, unspecified arm** 🖉

X● **S54.31 Injury of cutaneous sensory nerve at forearm level, right arm** 🖉

X● **S54.32 Injury of cutaneous sensory nerve at forearm level, left arm** 🖉

● **S54.8 Injury of other nerves at forearm level**

● **S54.8X Unspecified injury of other nerves at forearm level** ◀◀

● **S54.8X1 Unspecified injury of other nerves at forearm level, right arm** 🖉

● **S54.8X2 Unspecified injury of other nerves at forearm level, left arm** 🖉

● **S54.8X9 Unspecified injury of other nerves at forearm level, unspecified arm** 🖉

● **S54.9 Injury of unspecified nerve at forearm level**

X● **S54.90 Injury of unspecified nerve at forearm level, unspecified arm** 🖉

X● **S54.91 Injury of unspecified nerve at forearm level, right arm** 🖉

X● **S54.92 Injury of unspecified nerve at forearm level, left arm** 🖉

● **S55 Injury of blood vessels at forearm level**

Code also any associated open wound (S51.-)

Excludes2 injury of blood vessels at wrist and hand level (S65.-)
injury of brachial vessels (S45.1-S45.2)

The appropriate 7th character is to be added to each code from category S55

A	initial encounter
D	subsequent encounter
S	sequela

● **S55.0 Injury of ulnar artery at forearm level**

● **S55.00 Unspecified injury of ulnar artery at forearm level**

● **S55.001 Unspecified injury of ulnar artery at forearm level, right arm** A 🖉, 🖉
(Ex:) S45.301[A], S45.309-S45.311[A], S45.319-S45.391[A], S45.399-S45.801[A], S45.809-S45.811[A], S45.819-S45.891[A], S45.899-S45.901[A], S45.909-S45.911[A], S45.919-S45.991[A], S45.999[A], S55.001[A], S55.009-S55.011[A], S55.019-S55.091[A], S55.099[A], S55.201[A], S55.209-S55.211[A], S55.219-S55.291[A], S55.299-S55.801[A], S55.809-S55.811[A], S55.819-S55.891[A], S55.899-S55.901[A], S55.909-S55.911[A], S55.919-S55.991[A], S55.999[A], S65.001[A], S65.009-S65.011[A], S65.019-S65.091[A], S65.099[A], S65.801[A], S65.809-S65.811[A], S65.819-S65.891[A], S65.899-S65.901[A], S65.909-S65.911[A], S65.919-S65.991[A], S65.999[A]

● **S55.002 Unspecified injury of ulnar artery at forearm level, left arm** A 🖉, 🖉
(Ex:) S45.302-S45.309[A], S45.312-S45.319[A], S45.392-S45.399[A], S45.802-S45.809[A], S45.812-S45.819[A], S45.892-S45.899[A], S45.902-S45.909[A], S45.912-S45.919[A], S45.992-S45.999[A], S55.002-S55.009[A], S55.012-S55.019[A], S55.092-S55.099[A], S55.202-S55.209[A], S55.212-S55.219[A], S55.292-S55.299[A], S55.802-S55.809[A], S55.812-S55.819[A], S55.892-S55.899[A], S55.902-S55.909[A], S55.912-S55.919[A], S55.992-S55.999[A], S65.002-S65.009[A], S65.012-S65.019[A], S65.092-S65.099[A], S65.802-S65.809[A] S65.812-S65.819[A], S65.892-S65.899[A], S65.902-S65.909[A], S65.912-S65.919[A], S65.992-S65.999[A]

● **S55.009 Unspecified injury of ulnar artery at forearm level, unspecified arm** A 🖉, 🖉
(Ex:) S45.301-S45.999[A], S55.001-S55.099[A], S55.201-S55.999[A], S65.001-S65.099[A], S65.801-S65.999[A]

● **S55.01 Laceration of ulnar artery at forearm level**

● **S55.011 Laceration of ulnar artery at forearm level, right arm** A 🖉, 🖉
(Ex:) See S55.001

● **S55.012 Laceration of ulnar artery at forearm level, left arm** A 🖉, 🖉
(Ex:) See S55.002

● **S55.019 Laceration of ulnar artery at forearm level, unspecified arm** A 🖉, 🖉
(Ex:) See S55.009

◀ New	◀◀ Revised	~~deleted~~ Deleted	Excludes 1	Excludes 2	Includes	Use additional	Code first	Code also	Unspecified

OGCR Official Guidelines   ● Unacceptable Principal Diagnosis   X Assign placeholder X   ● Use Additional Character(s)   ▌ Manifestation Code   **Coding Clinic**

● **S55.09**   **Other specified injury of ulnar artery at forearm level**

     ● **S55.091**   Other specified injury of ulnar artery at forearm level, right arm A 🖉, 🖉
           Ⓔⓧ See S55.001

     ● **S55.092**   Other specified injury of ulnar artery at forearm level, left arm A 🖉, 🖉
           Ⓔⓧ See S55.002

     ● **S55.099**   Other specified injury of ulnar artery at forearm level, unspecified arm A 🖉, 🖉
           Ⓔⓧ See S55.009

● **S55.1**   Injury of radial artery at forearm level

   ● **S55.10**   Unspecified injury of radial artery at forearm level

     ● **S55.101**   Unspecified injury of radial artery at forearm level, right arm A 🖉, 🖉
           Ⓔⓧ S45.301[A], S45.309-S45.311[A], S45.319-S45.391[A], S45.399-S45.801[A], S45.809-S45.811[A], S45.819-S45.891[A], S45.899-S45.901[A], S45.909-S45.911[A], S45.919-S45.991[A], S45.999[A], S55.101[A], S55.109-S55.111[A], S55.119-S55.191[A], S55.199-S55.201[A], S55.209-S55.211[A], S55.219-S55.291[A], S55.299-S55.801[A], S55.809-S55.811[A], S55.819-S55.891[A], S55.899-S55.901[A], S55.909-S55.911[A], S55.919-S55.991[A], S55.999[A], S65.101[A], S65.109-S65.111[A], S65.119-S65.191[A], S65.199[A], S65.801[A], S65.809-S65.811[A], S65.819-S65.891[A], S65.899-S65.901[A], S65.909-S65.911[A], S65.919-S65.991[A], S65.999[A]

     ● **S55.102**   Unspecified injury of radial artery at forearm level, left arm A 🖉, 🖉
           Ⓔⓧ S45.302-S45.309[A], S45.312-S45.319[A], S45.392-S45.399[A], S45.802-S45.809[A], S45.812-S45.819[A], S45.892-S45.899[A], S45.902-S45.909[A], S45.912-S45.919[A], S45.992-S45.999[A], S55.102-S55.109[A], S55.112-S55.119[A], S55.192-S55.199[A], S55.202-S55.209[A], S55.212-S55.219[A], S55.292-S55.299[A], S55.802A-S55.809[A], S55.812-S55.819[A], S55.892-S55.899[A], S55.902-S55.909[A], S55.912-S55.919[A], S55.992-S55.999[A], S65.102-S65.109[A], S65.112-S65.119[A], S65.192-S65.199[A], S65.802-S65.809[A], S65.812-S65.819[A], S65.892-S65.899[A], S65.902-S65.909[A], S65.912-S65.919[A], S65.992-S65.999[A]

     ● **S55.109**   Unspecified injury of radial artery at forearm level, unspecified arm A 🖉, 🖉
           Ⓔⓧ S45.301-S45.999[A], S55.101-S55.999[A], S65.101-S65.199[A], S65.801-S65.999[A]

   ● **S55.11**   Laceration of radial artery at forearm level

     ● **S55.111**   Laceration of radial artery at forearm level, right arm A 🖉, 🖉
           Ⓔⓧ See S55.101

     ● **S55.112**   Laceration of radial artery at forearm level, left arm A 🖉, 🖉
           Ⓔⓧ See S55.102

     ● **S55.119**   Laceration of radial artery at forearm level, unspecified arm A 🖉, 🖉
           Ⓔⓧ See S55.109

● **S55.19**   **Other specified injury of radial artery at forearm level**

     ● **S55.191**   Other specified injury of radial artery at forearm level, right arm A 🖉, 🖉
           Ⓔⓧ See S55.101

     ● **S55.192**   Other specified injury of radial artery at forearm level, left arm A 🖉, 🖉
           Ⓔⓧ See S55.102

     ● **S55.199**   Other specified injury of radial artery at forearm level, unspecified arm A 🖉, 🖉
           Ⓔⓧ See S55.109

● **S55.2**   Injury of vein at forearm level

   ● **S55.20**   Unspecified injury of vein at forearm level

     ● **S55.201**   Unspecified injury of vein at forearm level, right arm A 🖉, 🖉
           Ⓔⓧ S45.301[A], S45.309-S45.311[A], S45.319-S45.391[A], S45.399-S45.801[A], S45.809-S45.811[A], S45.819-S45.891[A], S45.899-S45.901[A], S45.909-S45.911[A], S45.919-S45.991[A], S45.999[A], S55.001[A], S55.009-S55.011[A], S55.019-S55.091[A], S55.099[A], S55.201[A], S55.209-S55.211[A], S55.219-S55.291[A], S55.299-S55.801[A], S55.809-S55.811[A], S55.819-S55.891[A], S55.899-S55.901[A], S55.909-S55.911[A], S55.919-S55.991[A], S55.999[A], S65.001[A], S65.009-S65.011[A], S65.019-S65.091[A], S65.099[A], S65.201[A], S65.209-S65.211[A], S65.219-S65.291[A], S65.299-S65.301[A], S65.309-S65.311[A], S65.319-S65.391[A], S65.399-S65.401[A], S65.409-S65.411[A], S65.419-S65.491[A], S65.499-S65.500[A], S65.502[A], S65.504[A], S65.506[A], S65.508-S65.510[A], S65.512[A], S65.514[A], S65.516[A], S65.518-S65.590[A], S65.592[A], S65.594[A], S65.596[A], S65.598-S65.801[A], S65.809-S65.811[A], S65.819-S65.891[A], S65.899-S65.901[A], S65.909-S65.911[A], S65.919-S65.991[A], S65.999[A]

     ● **S55.202**   Unspecified injury of vein at forearm level, left arm A 🖉, 🖉
           Ⓔⓧ S45.302-S45.309[A], S45.312-S45.319[A], S45.392-S45.399[A], S45.802-S45.809[A], S45.812-S45.819[A], S45.892-S45.899[A], S45.902-S45.909[A], S45.912-S45.919[A], S45.992-S45.999[A], S55.002-S55.009[A], S55.012-S55.019[A], S55.092-S55.099[A], S55.202-S55.209[A], S55.212-S55.219[A], S55.292-S55.299[A], S55.802-S55.809[A], S55.812-S55.819[A], S55.892-S55.899[A], S55.902-S55.909[A], S55.912-S55.919[A], S55.992-S55.999[A], S65.002-S65.009[A], S65.012-S65.019[A], S65.092-S65.099[A], S65.202-S65.209[A], S65.212-S65.219[A], S65.292-S65.299[A], S65.302-S65.309[A], S65.312-S65.319[A]. S65.392-S65.399[A], S65.402-S65.409[A], S65.412-S65.419[A], S65.492-S65.499[A], S65.501[A], S65.503[A], S65.505[A], S65.507-S65.509[A], S65.511[A], S65.513[A], S65.515[A], S65.517-S65.519[A], S65.591[A], S65.593[A], S65.595[A], S65.597-S65.599[A], S65.802-S65.809[A], S65.812-S65.819[A], S65.892-S65.899[A], S65.902-S65.909[A], S65.912-S65.919[A], S65.992-S65.999[A]

     ● **S55.209**   Unspecified injury of vein at forearm level, unspecified arm A 🖉, 🖉
           Ⓔⓧ S45.301-S45.999[A], S55.001-S55.099[A], S55.201-S55.999[A], S65.001-S65.099[A], S65.201-S65.999[A]

- S55.21 Laceration of vein at forearm level
  - S55.211 Laceration of vein at forearm level, right arm A 🔖, 🔖
    (Ex:) See S55.201
  - S55.212 Laceration of vein at forearm level, left arm A 🔖, 🔖
    (Ex:) See S55.202
  - S55.219 Laceration of vein at forearm level, unspecified arm A 🔖, 🔖
    (Ex:) See S55.209
- S55.29 Other specified injury of vein at forearm level
  - S55.291 Other specified injury of vein at forearm level, right arm A 🔖, 🔖
    (Ex:) See S55.201
  - S55.292 Other specified injury of vein at forearm level, left arm A 🔖, 🔖
    (Ex:) See S55.202
  - S55.299 Other specified injury of vein at forearm level, unspecified arm A 🔖, 🔖
    (Ex:) See S55.209
- S55.8 Injury of other blood vessels at forearm level
  - S55.80 Unspecified injury of other blood vessels at forearm level
    - S55.801 Unspecified injury of other blood vessels at forearm level, right arm A 🔖, 🔖
      (Ex:) See S55.201
    - S55.802 Unspecified injury of other blood vessels at forearm level, left arm A 🔖, 🔖
      (Ex:) See S55.202
    - S55.809 Unspecified injury of other blood vessels at forearm level, unspecified arm A 🔖, 🔖
      (Ex:) See S55.209
  - S55.81 Laceration of other blood vessels at forearm level
    - S55.811 Laceration of other blood vessels at forearm level, right arm A 🔖, 🔖
      (Ex:) See S55.201
    - S55.812 Laceration of other blood vessels at forearm level, left arm A 🔖, 🔖
      (Ex:) See S55.202
    - S55.819 Laceration of other blood vessels at forearm level, unspecified arm A 🔖, 🔖
      (Ex:) See S55.209
  - S55.89 Other specified injury of other blood vessels at forearm level
    - S55.891 Other specified injury of other blood vessels at forearm level, right arm A 🔖, 🔖
      (Ex:) See S55.201
    - S55.892 Other specified injury of other blood vessels at forearm level, left arm A 🔖, 🔖
      (Ex:) See S55.202
    - S55.899 Other specified injury of other blood vessels at forearm level, unspecified arm A 🔖, 🔖
      (Ex:) See S55.209

- S55.9 Injury of unspecified blood vessel at forearm level
  - S55.90 Unspecified injury of unspecified blood vessel at forearm level
    - S55.901 Unspecified injury of unspecified blood vessel at forearm level, right arm A 🔖, 🔖
      (Ex:) See S55.201
    - S55.902 Unspecified injury of unspecified blood vessel at forearm level, left arm A 🔖, 🔖
      (Ex:) See S55.202
    - S55.909 Unspecified injury of unspecified blood vessel at forearm level, unspecified arm A 🔖, 🔖
      (Ex:) See S55.209
  - S55.91 Laceration of unspecified blood vessel at forearm level
    - S55.911 Laceration of unspecified blood vessel at forearm level, right arm A 🔖, 🔖
      (Ex:) See S55.201
    - S55.912 Laceration of unspecified blood vessel at forearm level, left arm A 🔖, 🔖
      (Ex:) See S55.202
    - S55.919 Laceration of unspecified blood vessel at forearm level, unspecified arm A 🔖, 🔖
      (Ex:) See S55.209
  - S55.99 Other specified injury of unspecified blood vessel at forearm level
    - S55.991 Other specified injury of unspecified blood vessel at forearm level, right arm A 🔖, 🔖
      (Ex:) See S55.201
    - S55.992 Other specified injury of unspecified blood vessel at forearm level, left arm A 🔖, 🔖
      (Ex:) See S55.202
    - S55.999 Other specified injury of unspecified blood vessel at forearm level, unspecified arm A 🔖, 🔖
      (Ex:) See S55.209

- S56 Injury of muscle, fascia and tendon at forearm level

  Code also any associated open wound (S51.-)

  Excludes2 injury of muscle, fascia and tendon at or below wrist (S66.-)

  sprain of joints and ligaments of elbow (S53.4-)

  The appropriate 7th character is to be added to each code from category S56

A	initial encounter
D	subsequent encounter
S	sequela

  - S56.0 Injury of flexor muscle, fascia and tendon of thumb at forearm level
    - S56.00 Unspecified injury of flexor muscle, fascia and tendon of thumb at forearm level
      - S56.001 Unspecified injury of flexor muscle, fascia and tendon of right thumb at forearm level 🔖
      - S56.002 Unspecified injury of flexor muscle, fascia and tendon of left thumb at forearm level 🔖
      - S56.009 Unspecified injury of flexor muscle, fascia and tendon of unspecified thumb at forearm level 🔖

● **S56.01**   Strain of flexor muscle, fascia and tendon of thumb at forearm level
   ● **S56.011**   Strain of flexor muscle, fascia and tendon of right thumb at forearm level 🔖
   ● **S56.012**   Strain of flexor muscle, fascia and tendon of left thumb at forearm level 🔖
   ● **S56.019**   Strain of flexor muscle, fascia and tendon of unspecified thumb at forearm level 🔖
● **S56.02**   Laceration of flexor muscle, fascia and tendon of thumb at forearm level
   ● **S56.021**   Laceration of flexor muscle, fascia and tendon of right thumb at forearm level A 🔖, 🔖
     (Ex:) S51.001[A], S51.009-S51.011[A], S51.019-S51.021[A], S51.029-S51.031[A], S51.039-S51.041[A], S51.049-S51.051[A], S51.059-S51.801[A], S51.809-S51.811[A], S51.819-S51.821[A]. S51.829-S51.831[A], S51.839-S51.841[A], S51.849-S51.851[A], S51.859[A], S56.021[A], S56.029[A], S56.121[A], S56.123[A], S56.125[A], S56.127[A], S56.129[A], S56.221[A], S56.229[A], S56.321[A], S56.329[A], S56.421[A], S56.423[A], S56.425[A], S56.427[A], S56.429[A], S56.521[A], S56.529[A], S56.821[A], S56.829[A], S56.921[A], S56.929[A], S61.501[A], S61.509-S61.511[A], S61.519-S61.521[A], S61.529-S61.531[A], S61.539-S61.541[A], S61.549-S61.551[A], S61.559[A]
   ● **S56.022**   Laceration of flexor muscle, fascia and tendon of left thumb at forearm level A 🔖, 🔖
     (Ex:) S51.002-S51.009[A], S51.012-S51.019[A], S51.022-S51.029[A], S51.032-S51.039[A], S51.042-S51.049[A], S51.052-S51.059[A], S51.802-S51.809[A], S51.812-S51.819[A], S51.822-S51.829[A], S51.832-S51.839[A], S51.842-S51.849[A], S51.852-S51.859[A], S56.022-S56.029[A], S56.122[A], S56.124[A], S56.126[A], S56.128-S56.129[A], S56.222-S56.229[A], S56.322-S56.329[A], S56.422[A], S56.424[A], S56.426[A], S56.428-S56.429[A], S56.522-S56.529[A], S56.822-S56.829[A], S56.922-S56.929[A], S61.502-S61.509[A], S61.512-S61.519[A], S61.522-S61.529[A], S61.532-S61.539[A], S61.542-S61.549[A], S61.552-S61.559[A]
   ● **S56.029**   Laceration of flexor muscle, fascia and tendon of unspecified thumb at forearm level A 🔖, 🔖
     (Ex:) S51.001-S51.859[A], S56.021-S56.029[A], S56.121-S56.129[A], S56.221-S56.229[A], S56.321-S56.329[A], S56.421-S56.429[A], S56.521-S56.529[A], S56.821-S56.829[A], S56.921-S56.929[A], S61.501-S61.559[A]
● **S56.09**   Other injury of flexor muscle, fascia and tendon of thumb at forearm level
   ● **S56.091**   Other injury of flexor muscle, fascia and tendon of right thumb at forearm level 🔖
   ● **S56.092**   Other injury of flexor muscle, fascia and tendon of left thumb at forearm level 🔖
   ● **S56.099**   Other injury of flexor muscle, fascia and tendon of unspecified thumb at forearm level 🔖

● **S56.1**   Injury of flexor muscle, fascia and tendon of other and unspecified finger at forearm level
   ● **S56.10**   Unspecified injury of flexor muscle, fascia and tendon of other and unspecified finger at forearm level
     ● **S56.101**   Unspecified injury of flexor muscle, fascia and tendon of right index finger at forearm level 🔖
     ● **S56.102**   Unspecified injury of flexor muscle, fascia and tendon of left index finger at forearm level 🔖
     ● **S56.103**   Unspecified injury of flexor muscle, fascia and tendon of right middle finger at forearm level 🔖
     ● **S56.104**   Unspecified injury of flexor muscle, fascia and tendon of left middle finger at forearm level 🔖
     ● **S56.105**   Unspecified injury of flexor muscle, fascia and tendon of right ring finger at forearm level 🔖
     ● **S56.106**   Unspecified injury of flexor muscle, fascia and tendon of left ring finger at forearm level 🔖
     ● **S56.107**   Unspecified injury of flexor muscle, fascia and tendon of right little finger at forearm level 🔖
     ● **S56.108**   Unspecified injury of flexor muscle, fascia and tendon of left little finger at forearm level 🔖
     ● **S56.109**   Unspecified injury of flexor muscle, fascia and tendon of unspecified finger at forearm level 🔖
   ● **S56.11**   Strain of flexor muscle, fascia and tendon of other and unspecified finger at forearm level
     ● **S56.111**   Strain of flexor muscle, fascia and tendon of right index finger at forearm level 🔖
     ● **S56.112**   Strain of flexor muscle, fascia and tendon of left index finger at forearm level 🔖
     ● **S56.113**   Strain of flexor muscle, fascia and tendon of right middle finger at forearm level 🔖
     ● **S56.114**   Strain of flexor muscle, fascia and tendon of left middle finger at forearm level 🔖
     ● **S56.115**   Strain of flexor muscle, fascia and tendon of right ring finger at forearm level 🔖
     ● **S56.116**   Strain of flexor muscle, fascia and tendon of left ring finger at forearm level 🔖
     ● **S56.117**   Strain of flexor muscle, fascia and tendon of right little finger at forearm level 🔖
     ● **S56.118**   Strain of flexor muscle, fascia and tendon of left little finger at forearm level 🔖
     ● **S56.119**   Strain of flexor muscle, fascia and tendon of finger of unspecified finger at forearm level 🔖

N Newborn Age: 0   **P** Pediatric Age: 0–17   **M** Maternity DX: 12–55   **A** Adult Age: 15–124   ♀ Females Only   ♂ Males Only

🔖 Complication\Comorbidity   🔖 Major C\C   (Ex:) CC/MCC Exclusions   🔖 Present on Admission Requirement   🔖 Hospital-Acquired Condition

1387

CHAPTER 19 (S00-T88)

CHAPTER 19 (S00-T88)

● S56.12   Laceration of flexor muscle, fascia and tendon of other and unspecified finger at forearm level

   ● S56.121   Laceration of flexor muscle, fascia and tendon of right index finger at forearm level A 🕭, 🕭
      (Ex:) See S56.021

   ● S56.122   Laceration of flexor muscle, fascia and tendon of left index finger at forearm level A 🕭, 🕭
      (Ex:) See S56.022

   ● S56.123   Laceration of flexor muscle, fascia and tendon of right middle finger at forearm level A 🕭, 🕭
      (Ex:) See S56.021

   ● S56.124   Laceration of flexor muscle, fascia and tendon of left middle finger at forearm level A 🕭, 🕭
      (Ex:) See S56.022

   ● S56.125   Laceration of flexor muscle, fascia and tendon of right ring finger at forearm level A 🕭, 🕭
      (Ex:) See S56.021

   ● S56.126   Laceration of flexor muscle, fascia and tendon of left ring finger at forearm level A 🕭, 🕭
      (Ex:) See S56.022

   ● S56.127   Laceration of flexor muscle, fascia and tendon of right little finger at forearm level A 🕭, 🕭
      (Ex:) See S56.021

   ● S56.128   Laceration of flexor muscle, fascia and tendon of left little finger at forearm level A 🕭, 🕭
      (Ex:) See S56.022

   ● S56.129   Laceration of flexor muscle, fascia and tendon of unspecified finger at forearm level A 🕭, 🕭
      (Ex:) See S56.029

● S56.19   Other injury of flexor muscle, fascia and tendon of other and unspecified finger at forearm level

   ● S56.191   Other injury of flexor muscle, fascia and tendon of right index finger at forearm level 🕭

   ● S56.192   Other injury of flexor muscle, fascia and tendon of left index finger at forearm level 🕭

   ● S56.193   Other injury of flexor muscle, fascia and tendon of right middle finger at forearm level 🕭

   ● S56.194   Other injury of flexor muscle, fascia and tendon of left middle finger at forearm level 🕭

   ● S56.195   Other injury of flexor muscle, fascia and tendon of right ring finger at forearm level 🕭

   ● S56.196   Other injury of flexor muscle, fascia and tendon of left ring finger at forearm level 🕭

   ● S56.197   Other injury of flexor muscle, fascia and tendon of right little finger at forearm level 🕭

   ● S56.198   Other injury of flexor muscle, fascia and tendon of left little finger at forearm level 🕭

   ● S56.199   Other injury of flexor muscle, fascia and tendon of unspecified finger at forearm level 🕭

● S56.2   Injury of other flexor muscle, fascia and tendon at forearm level

  ● S56.20   Unspecified injury of other flexor muscle, fascia and tendon at forearm level

   ● S56.201   Unspecified injury of other flexor muscle, fascia and tendon at forearm level, right arm 🕭

   ● S56.202   Unspecified injury of other flexor muscle, fascia and tendon at forearm level, left arm 🕭

   ● S56.209   Unspecified injury of other flexor muscle, fascia and tendon at forearm level, unspecified arm 🕭

  ● S56.21   Strain of other flexor muscle, fascia and tendon at forearm level

   ● S56.211   Strain of other flexor muscle, fascia and tendon at forearm level, right arm 🕭

   ● S56.212   Strain of other flexor muscle, fascia and tendon at forearm level, left arm 🕭

   ● S56.219   Strain of other flexor muscle, fascia and tendon at forearm level, unspecified arm 🕭

  ● S56.22   Laceration of other flexor muscle, fascia and tendon at forearm level

   ● S56.221   Laceration of other flexor muscle, fascia and tendon at forearm level, right arm A 🕭, 🕭
      (Ex:) See S56.021

   ● S56.222   Laceration of other flexor muscle, fascia and tendon at forearm level, left arm A 🕭, 🕭
      (Ex:) See S56.022

   ● S56.229   Laceration of other flexor muscle, fascia and tendon at forearm level, unspecified arm A 🕭, 🕭
      (Ex:) See S56.029

  ● S56.29   Other injury of other flexor muscle, fascia and tendon at forearm level

   ● S56.291   Other injury of other flexor muscle, fascia and tendon at forearm level, right arm 🕭

   ● S56.292   Other injury of other flexor muscle, fascia and tendon at forearm level, left arm 🕭

   ● S56.299   Other injury of other flexor muscle, fascia and tendon at forearm level, unspecified arm 🕭

● S56.3   Injury of extensor or abductor muscles, fascia and tendons of thumb at forearm level

  ● S56.30   Unspecified injury of extensor or abductor muscles, fascia and tendons of thumb at forearm level

   ● S56.301   Unspecified injury of extensor or abductor muscles, fascia and tendons of right thumb at forearm level 🕭

   ● S56.302   Unspecified injury of extensor or abductor muscles, fascia and tendons of left thumb at forearm level 🕭

   ● S56.309   Unspecified injury of extensor or abductor muscles, fascia and tendons of unspecified thumb at forearm level 🕭

● S56.31   Strain of extensor or abductor muscles, fascia and tendons of thumb at forearm level
    ● S56.311   Strain of extensor or abductor muscles, fascia and tendons of right thumb at forearm level 🅖
    ● S56.312   Strain of extensor or abductor muscles, fascia and tendons of left thumb at forearm level 🅖
    ● S56.319   Strain of extensor or abductor muscles, fascia and tendons of unspecified thumb at forearm level 🅖

● S56.32   Laceration of extensor or abductor muscles, fascia and tendons of thumb at forearm level
    ● S56.321   Laceration of extensor or abductor muscles, fascia and tendons of right thumb at forearm level A 🅖, 🅖
         (Ex) See S56.021
    ● S56.322   Laceration of extensor or abductor muscles, fascia and tendons of left thumb at forearm level A 🅖, 🅖
         (Ex) See S56.022
    ● S56.329   Laceration of extensor or abductor muscles, fascia and tendons of unspecified thumb at forearm level A 🅖, 🅖
         (Ex) See S56.029

● S56.39   Other injury of extensor or abductor muscles, fascia and tendons of thumb at forearm level
    ● S56.391   Other injury of extensor or abductor muscles, fascia and tendons of right thumb at forearm level 🅖
    ● S56.392   Other injury of extensor or abductor muscles, fascia and tendons of left thumb at forearm level 🅖
    ● S56.399   Other injury of extensor or abductor muscles, fascia and tendons of unspecified thumb at forearm level 🅖

● S56.4   Injury of extensor muscle, fascia and tendon of other and unspecified finger at forearm level
   ● S56.40   Unspecified injury of extensor muscle, fascia and tendon of other and unspecified finger at forearm level
    ● S56.401   Unspecified injury of extensor muscle, fascia and tendon of right index finger at forearm level 🅖
    ● S56.402   Unspecified injury of extensor muscle, fascia and tendon of left index finger at forearm level 🅖
    ● S56.403   Unspecified injury of extensor muscle, fascia and tendon of right middle finger at forearm level 🅖
    ● S56.404   Unspecified injury of extensor muscle, fascia and tendon of left middle finger at forearm level 🅖
    ● S56.405   Unspecified injury of extensor muscle, fascia and tendon of right ring finger at forearm level 🅖
    ● S56.406   Unspecified injury of extensor muscle, fascia and tendon of left ring finger at forearm level 🅖
    ● S56.407   Unspecified injury of extensor muscle, fascia and tendon of right little finger at forearm level 🅖
    ● S56.408   Unspecified injury of extensor muscle, fascia and tendon of left little finger at forearm level 🅖
    ● S56.409   Unspecified injury of extensor muscle, fascia and tendon of unspecified finger at forearm level 🅖

● S56.41   Strain of extensor muscle, fascia and tendon of other and unspecified finger at forearm level
    ● S56.411   Strain of extensor muscle, fascia and tendon of right index finger at forearm level 🅖
    ● S56.412   Strain of extensor muscle, fascia and tendon of left index finger at forearm level 🅖
    ● S56.413   Strain of extensor muscle, fascia and tendon of right middle finger at forearm level 🅖
    ● S56.414   Strain of extensor muscle, fascia and tendon of left middle finger at forearm level 🅖
    ● S56.415   Strain of extensor muscle, fascia and tendon of right ring finger at forearm level 🅖
    ● S56.416   Strain of extensor muscle, fascia and tendon of left ring finger at forearm level 🅖
    ● S56.417   Strain of extensor muscle, fascia and tendon of right little finger at forearm level 🅖
    ● S56.418   Strain of extensor muscle, fascia and tendon of left little finger at forearm level 🅖
    ● S56.419   Strain of extensor muscle, fascia and tendon of finger, unspecified finger at forearm level 🅖

● S56.42   Laceration of extensor muscle, fascia and tendon of other and unspecified finger at forearm level
    ● S56.421   Laceration of extensor muscle, fascia and tendon of right index finger at forearm level A 🅖, 🅖
         (Ex) See S56.021
    ● S56.422   Laceration of extensor muscle, fascia and tendon of left index finger at forearm level A 🅖, 🅖
         (Ex) See S56.022
    ● S56.423   Laceration of extensor muscle, fascia and tendon of right middle finger at forearm level A 🅖, 🅖
         (Ex) See S56.021
    ● S56.424   Laceration of extensor muscle, fascia and tendon of left middle finger at forearm level A 🅖, 🅖
         (Ex) See S56.022
    ● S56.425   Laceration of extensor muscle, fascia and tendon of right ring finger at forearm level A 🅖, 🅖
         (Ex) See S56.021
    ● S56.426   Laceration of extensor muscle, fascia and tendon of left ring finger at forearm level A 🅖, 🅖
         (Ex) See S56.022
    ● S56.427   Laceration of extensor muscle, fascia and tendon of right little finger at forearm level A 🅖, 🅖
         (Ex) See S56.021
    ● S56.428   Laceration of extensor muscle, fascia and tendon of left little finger at forearm level A 🅖, 🅖
         (Ex) See S56.022
    ● S56.429   Laceration of extensor muscle, fascia and tendon of unspecified finger at forearm level A 🅖, 🅖
         (Ex) See S56.029

CHAPTER 19 (S00-T88)

N   Newborn Age: 0   P   Pediatric Age: 0–17   M   Maternity DX: 12–55   A   Adult Age: 15–124   ♀   Females Only   ♂   Males Only

🅖 Complication\Comorbidity   🅖 Major C\C   (Ex) CC/MCC Exclusions   🅖 Present on Admission Requirement   🅖 Hospital-Acquired Condition

1389

CHAPTER 19 (S00-T88)

● **S56.49**   Other injury of extensor muscle, fascia and tendon of other and unspecified finger at forearm level

● **S56.491**   Other injury of extensor muscle, fascia and tendon of right index finger at forearm level 🖎

● **S56.492**   Other injury of extensor muscle, fascia and tendon of left index finger at forearm level 🖎

● **S56.493**   Other injury of extensor muscle, fascia and tendon of right middle finger at forearm level 🖎

● **S56.494**   Other injury of extensor muscle, fascia and tendon of left middle finger at forearm level 🖎

● **S56.495**   Other injury of extensor muscle, fascia and tendon of right ring finger at forearm level 🖎

● **S56.496**   Other injury of extensor muscle, fascia and tendon of left ring finger at forearm level 🖎

● **S56.497**   Other injury of extensor muscle, fascia and tendon of right little finger at forearm level 🖎

● **S56.498**   Other injury of extensor muscle, fascia and tendon of left little finger at forearm level 🖎

● **S56.499**   Other injury of extensor muscle, fascia and tendon of unspecified finger at forearm level 🖎

● **S56.5**   Injury of other extensor muscle, fascia and tendon at forearm level

● **S56.50**   Unspecified injury of other extensor muscle, fascia and tendon at forearm level

● **S56.501**   Unspecified injury of other extensor muscle, fascia and tendon at forearm level, right arm 🖎

● **S56.502**   Unspecified injury of other extensor muscle, fascia and tendon at forearm level, left arm 🖎

● **S56.509**   Unspecified injury of other extensor muscle, fascia and tendon at forearm level, unspecified arm 🖎

● **S56.51**   Strain of other extensor muscle, fascia and tendon at forearm level

● **S56.511**   Strain of other extensor muscle, fascia and tendon at forearm level, right arm 🖎

● **S56.512**   Strain of other extensor muscle, fascia and tendon at forearm level, left arm 🖎

● **S56.519**   Strain of other extensor muscle, fascia and tendon at forearm level, unspecified arm 🖎

● **S56.52**   Laceration of other extensor muscle, fascia and tendon at forearm level

● **S56.521**   Laceration of other extensor muscle, fascia and tendon at forearm level, right arm A 🖎, 🖎
Ⓔⓧ See S56.021

● **S56.522**   Laceration of other extensor muscle, fascia and tendon at forearm level, left arm A 🖎, 🖎
Ⓔⓧ See S56.022

● **S56.529**   Laceration of other extensor muscle, fascia and tendon at forearm level, unspecified arm A 🖎, 🖎
Ⓔⓧ See S56.029

● **S56.59**   Other injury of other extensor muscle, fascia and tendon at forearm level

● **S56.591**   Other injury of other extensor muscle, fascia and tendon at forearm level, right arm 🖎

● **S56.592**   Other injury of other extensor muscle, fascia and tendon at forearm level, left arm 🖎

● **S56.599**   Other injury of other extensor muscle, fascia and tendon at forearm level, unspecified arm 🖎

● **S56.8**   Injury of other muscles, fascia and tendons at forearm level

● **S56.80**   Unspecified injury of other muscles, fascia and tendons at forearm level

● **S56.801**   Unspecified injury of other muscles, fascia and tendons at forearm level, right arm 🖎

● **S56.802**   Unspecified injury of other muscles, fascia and tendons at forearm level, left arm 🖎

● **S56.809**   Unspecified injury of other muscles, fascia and tendons at forearm level, unspecified arm 🖎

● **S56.81**   Strain of other muscles, fascia and tendons at forearm level

● **S56.811**   Strain of other muscles, fascia and tendons at forearm level, right arm 🖎

● **S56.812**   Strain of other muscles, fascia and tendons at forearm level, left arm 🖎

● **S56.819**   Strain of other muscles, fascia and tendons at forearm level, unspecified arm 🖎

● **S56.82**   Laceration of other muscles, fascia and tendons at forearm level

● **S56.821**   Laceration of other muscles, fascia and tendons at forearm level, right arm A 🖎, 🖎
Ⓔⓧ See S56.021

● **S56.822**   Laceration of other muscles, fascia and tendons at forearm level, left arm A 🖎, 🖎
Ⓔⓧ See S56.022

● **S56.829**   Laceration of other muscles, fascia and tendons at forearm level, unspecified arm A 🖎, 🖎
Ⓔⓧ See S56.029

● **S56.89**   Other injury of other muscles, fascia and tendons at forearm level

● **S56.891**   Other injury of other muscles, fascia and tendons at forearm level, right arm 🖎

● **S56.892**   Other injury of other muscles, fascia and tendons at forearm level, left arm 🖎

● **S56.899**   Other injury of other muscles, fascia and tendons at forearm level, unspecified arm 🖎

● **S56.9**   Injury of unspecified muscles, fascia and tendons at forearm level

● **S56.90**   Unspecified injury of unspecified muscles, fascia and tendons at forearm level

● **S56.901**   Unspecified injury of unspecified muscles, fascia and tendons at forearm level, right arm 🖎

● **S56.902**   Unspecified injury of unspecified muscles, fascia and tendons at forearm level, left arm 🖎

● **S56.909**   Unspecified injury of unspecified muscles, fascia and tendons at forearm level, unspecified arm 🖎

◀ New   ◀▥ Revised   d̶e̶l̶e̶t̶e̶d̶ Deleted   Excludes 1   Excludes 2   Includes   Use additional   Code first   Code also   Unspecified

OGCR Official Guidelines   ● Unacceptable Principal Diagnosis   X Assign placeholder X   ● Use Additional Character(s)   ▶ Manifestation Code   **Coding Clinic**

- **S56.91** Strain of unspecified muscles, fascia and tendons at forearm level
  - **S56.911** Strain of unspecified muscles, fascia and tendons at forearm level, right arm 🔖
  - **S56.912** Strain of unspecified muscles, fascia and tendons at forearm level, left arm 🔖
  - **S56.919** Strain of unspecified muscles, fascia and tendons at forearm level, unspecified arm 🔖
- **S56.92** Laceration of unspecified muscles, fascia and tendons at forearm level
  - **S56.921** Laceration of unspecified muscles, fascia and tendons at forearm level, right arm A 🔖, 🔖
    - (Ex:) See S56.021
  - **S56.922** Laceration of unspecified muscles, fascia and tendons at forearm level, left arm A 🔖, 🔖
    - (Ex:) See S56.022
  - **S56.929** Laceration of unspecified muscles, fascia and tendons at forearm level, unspecified arm A 🔖, 🔖
    - (Ex:) See S56.029
- **S56.99** Other injury of unspecified muscles, fascia and tendons at forearm level
  - **S56.991** Other injury of unspecified muscles, fascia and tendons at forearm level, right arm 🔖
  - **S56.992** Other injury of unspecified muscles, fascia and tendons at forearm level, left arm 🔖
  - **S56.999** Other injury of unspecified muscles, fascia and tendons at forearm level, unspecified arm 🔖

- **S57**   **Crushing injury of elbow and forearm**
  Use additional code(s) for all associated injuries
  Excludes2   crushing injury of wrist and hand (S67.-)
  The appropriate 7th character is to be added to each code from category S57

A	initial encounter
D	subsequent encounter
S	sequela

  - **S57.0**   Crushing injury of elbow
    - X **S57.00** Crushing injury of unspecified elbow 🔖
    - X **S57.01** Crushing injury of right elbow 🔖
    - X **S57.02** Crushing injury of left elbow 🔖
  - **S57.8**   Crushing injury of forearm
    - X **S57.80** Crushing injury of unspecified forearm 🔖
    - X **S57.81** Crushing injury of right forearm 🔖
    - X **S57.82** Crushing injury of left forearm 🔖

- **S58**   **Traumatic amputation of elbow and forearm**
  An amputation not identified as partial or complete should be coded to complete
  Excludes1   traumatic amputation of wrist and hand (S68.-)
  The appropriate 7th character is to be added to each code from category S58

A	initial encounter
D	subsequent encounter
S	sequela

  - **S58.0**   Traumatic amputation at elbow level
    - **S58.01** Complete traumatic amputation at elbow level

- **S58.011**   Complete traumatic amputation at elbow level, right arm A 🔖, 🔖
  (Ex:) S41.001[A], S41.009-S41.011[A], S41.019-S41.021[A], S41.029-S41.031[A], S41.039-S41.041[A], S41.049-S41.051[A], S41.059-S41.101[A], S41.109-S41.111[A], S41.119-S41.121[A], S41.129-S41.131[A], S41.139-S41.141[A], S41.149-S41.151[A], S41.159[A], S46.021[A], S46.029[A], S46.121[A], S46.129[A], S46.221[A], S46.229[A], S46.321[A], S46.329[A], S46.821[A], S46.829[A], S46.921[A], S46.929[A], S48.011[A], S48.019-S48.021[A], S48.029-S48.111[A], S48.119-S48.121[A], S48.129-S48.911[A], S48.919-S48.921[A], S48.929[A], S51.001[A], S51.009-S51.011[A], S51.019-S51.021[A], S51.029-S51.031[A], S51.039-S51.041[A], S51.049-S51.051[A], S51.059-S51.801[A], S51.809-S51.811[A], S51.819-S51.821[A], S51.829-S51.831[A], S51.839-S51.841[A], S51.849-S51.851[A], S51.859[A], S56.021[A], S56.029[A], S56.121[A], S56.123[A], S56.125[A], S56.127[A], S56.129[A], S56.221[A], S56.229[A], S56.321[A], S56.329[A], S56.421[A], S56.423[A], S56.425[A], S56.427[A], S56.429[A], S56.521[A], S56.529[A], S56.821[A], S56.829[A], S56.921[A], S56.929[A], S58.011[A], S58.019-S58.021[A], S58.029-S58.111[A], S58.119-S58.121[A], S58.129-S58.911[A], S58.919-S58.921[A], S58.929[A], S61.001[A], S61.009-S61.011[A], S61.019-S61.021[A], S61.029-S61.031[A], S61.039-S61.041[A], S61.049-S61.051[A], S61.059-S61.101[A], S61.109-S61.111[A], S61.119-S61.121[A], S61.129-S61.131[A], S61.139-S61.141[A], S61.149-S61.151[A], S61.159-S61.200[A], S61.202[A], S61.204[A], S61.206[A], S61.208-S61.210[A], S61.212[A], S61.214[A], S61.216[A], S61.218-S61.220[A], S61.222[A], S61.224[A], S61.226[A], S61.228-S61.230[A], S61.232[A], S61.234[A], S61.236[A], S61.238-S61.240[A], S61.242[A], S61.244[A], S61.246[A], S61.248-S61.250[A], S61.252[A], S61.254[A], S61.256[A], S61.258-S61.300[A], S61.302[A], S61.304[A], S61.306[A], S61.308-S61.310[A], S61.312[A], S61.314[A], S61.316[A], S61.318-S61.320[A], S61.322[A], S61.324[A], S61.326[A], S61.328-S61.330[A], S61.332[A], S61.334[A], S61.336[A], S61.338-S61.340[A], S61.342[A], S61.344[A], S61.346[A], S61.348-S61.350[A], S61.352[A], S61.354[A], S61.356[A], S61.358-S61.401[A], S61.409-S61.411[A], S61.419-S61.421[A], S61.429-S61.431[A], S61.439-S61.441[A], S61.449-S61.451[A], S61.459-S61.501[A], S61.509-S61.511[A], S61.519-S61.521[A], S61.529-S61.531[A], S61.539-S61.541[A], S61.549-S61.551[A], S61.559[A], S66.021[A], S66.029[A], S66.120[A], S66.122[A], S66.124[A], S66.126[A], S66.128-S66.129[A], S66.221[A], S66.229[A], S66.320[A], S66.322[A], S66.324[A], S66.326[A], S66.328-S66.329[A], S66.421[A], S66.429[A], S66.520[A], S66.522[A], S66.524[A], S66.526[A], S66.528-S66.529[A], S66.821[A], S66.829[A], S66.921[A], S66.929[A], S68.011[A], S68.019-S68.021[A], S68.029-S68.110[A], S68.112[A], S68.114[A], S68.116[A], S68.118-S68.120[A], S68.122[A], S68.124[A], S68.126[A], S68.128-S68.411[A], S68.419-S68.421[A], S68.429-S68.511[A], S68.519-S68.521[A], S68.529-S68.610[A], S68.612[A], S68.614[A], S68.616[A], S68.618-S68.620[A], S68.622[A], S68.624[A], S68.626[A], S68.628-S68.711[A], S68.719-S68.721[A], S68.729[A], T14.8-T14.91, T79.A0X-T79.9XX[A]

CHAPTER 19 (S00-T88)

N   Newborn Age: 0   P   Pediatric Age: 0–17   M   Maternity DX: 12–55   A   Adult Age: 15–124   ♀   Females Only   ♂   Males Only

🔖 Complication\Comorbidity   🔖 Major C\C   (Ex:) CC/MCC Exclusions   🔖 Present on Admission Requirement   🔖 Hospital-Acquired Condition

1391

● **S58.012**   Complete traumatic amputation at elbow level, left arm A 🔾, 🔾

   Ex: S41.002-S41.009[A], S41.012-S41.019[A],
     S41.022-S41.029[A], S41.032-S41.039[A],
     S41.042-S41.049[A], S41.052-S41.059[A],
     S41.102-S41.109[A], S41.112-S41.119[A],
     S41.122-S41.129[A], S41.132-S41.139[A],
     S41.142-S41.149[A], S41.152-S41.159[A],
     S46.022-S46.029[A], S46.122-S46.129[A],
     S46.222-S46.229[A], S46.322-S46.329[A],
     S46.822-S46.829[A], S46.922-S46.929[A],
     S48.012-S48.019[A], S48.022-S48.029[A],
     S48.112-S48.119[A], S48.122-S48.129[A],
     S48.912-S48.919[A], S48.922-S48.929[A],
     S51.002-S51.009[A], S51.012-S51.019[A],
     S51.022-S51.029[A], S51.032-S51.039[A],
     S51.042-S51.049[A], S51.052-S51.059[A],
     S51.802-S51.809[A], S51.812-S51.819[A],
     S51.822-S51.829[A], S51.832-S51.839[A],
     S51.842-S51.849[A], S51.852-S51.859[A],
     S56.022-S56.029[A], S56.122[A], S56.124[A],
     S56.126[A], S56.128-S56.129[A],
     S56.222-S56.229[A], S56.322-S56.329[A],
     S56.422[A], S56.424[A], S56.426[A],
     S56.428-S56.429[A], S56.522-S56.529[A],
     S56.822-S56.829[A], S56.922-S56.929[A],
     S58.012-S58.019[A], S58.022-S58.029[A],
     S58.112-S58.119[A], S58.122-S58.129[A],
     S58.912-S58.919[A], S58.922-S58.929[A],
     S61.002-S61.009[A], S61.012-S61.019[A],
     S61.022-S61.029[A], S61.032-S61.039[A],
     S61.042-S61.049[A], S61.052-S61.059[A],
     S61.102-S61.109[A], S61.112-S61.119[A],
     S61.122-S61.129[A], S61.132-S61.139[A],
     S61.142-S61.149[A], S61.152-S61.159[A],
     S61.201[A], S61.203[A], S61.205[A],
     S61.207-S61.209[A], S61.211[A], S61.213[A],
     S61.215[A], S61.217-S61.219[A], S61.221[A],
     S61.223[A], S61.225[A], S61.227-S61.229[A],
     S61.231[A], S61.233[A], S61.235[A],
     S61.237-S61.239[A], S61.241[A], S61.243[A],
     S61.245[A], S61.247-S61.249[A], S61.251[A],
     S61.253[A], S61.255[A], S61.257-S61.259[A],
     S61.301[A], S61.303[A], S61.305[A],
     S61.307-S61.309[A], S61.311[A], S61.313[A],
     S61.315[A], S61.317-S61.319[A], S61.321[A],
     S61.323[A], S61.325[A], S61.327-S61.329[A],
     S61.331[A], S61.333[A], S61.335[A],
     S61.337-S61.339[A], S61.341[A], S61.343[A],
     S61.345[A], S61.347-S61.349[A], S61.351[A],
     S61.353[A], S61.355[A], S61.357-S61.359[A],
     S61.402-S61.409[A], S61.412-S61.419[A],
     S61.422-S61.429[A], S61.432-S61.439[A],
     S61.442-S61.449[A], S61.452-S61.459[A],
     S61.502-S61.509[A], S61.512-S61.519[A],
     S61.522-S61.529[A], S61.532-S61.539[A],
     S61.542-S61.549[A], S61.552-S61.559[A],
     S66.022-S66.029[A], S66.121[A], S66.123[A],
     S66.125[A], S66.127-S66.129[A],
     S66.222-S66.229[A], S66.321[A], S66.323[A],
     S66.325[A], S66.327-S66.329[A],
     S66.422-S66.429[A], S66.521[A], S66.523[A],
     S66.525[A], S66.527-S66.529[A],
     S66.822-S66.829[A], S66.922-S66.929[A],
     S68.012-S68.019[A], S68.022-S68.029[A],
     S68.111[A], S68.113[A], S68.115[A],
     S68.117-S68.119[A], S68.121[A], S68.123[A],
     S68.125[A], S68.127-S68.129[A],
     S68.412-S68.419[A], S68.422-S68.429[A],
     S68.512-S68.519[A], S68.522-S68.529[A],
     S68.611[A], S68.613[A], S68.615[A],
     S68.617-S68.619[A], S68.621[A], S68.623[A],
     S68.625[A], S68.627-S68.629[A],
     S68.712-S68.719[A], S68.722-S68.729[A],
     T14.8-T14.91, T79.A0X-T79.9XX[A]

● **S58.019**   Complete traumatic amputation at elbow level, unspecified arm A 🔾, 🔾

   Ex: S41.001-S41.159[A], S46.021-S46.029[A],
     S46.121-S46.129[A], S46.221-S46.229[A],
     S46.321-S46.329[A], S46.821-S46.829[A],
     S46.921-S46.929[A], S48.011-S48.929[A],
     S51.001-S51.859[A], S56.021-S56.029[A],
     S56.121-S56.129[A], S56.221-S56.229[A],
     S56.321-S56.329[A], S56.421-S56.429[A],
     S56.521-S56.529[A], S56.821-S56.829[A],
     S56.921-S56.929[A], S58.011-S58.929[A],
     S61.001-S61.559[A], S66.021-S66.029[A],
     S66.120-S66.129[A], S66.221-S66.229[A],
     S66.320-S66.329[A], S66.421-S66.429[A],
     S66.520-S66.529[A], S66.821-S66.829[A],
     S66.921-S66.929[A], S68.011-S68.729[A],
     T14.8-T14.91, T79.A0X-T79.9XX[A]

● **S58.02**   Partial traumatic amputation at elbow level

    ● **S58.021**   Partial traumatic amputation at elbow level, right arm A 🔾, 🔾
       Ex: See S56.011

    ● **S58.022**   Partial traumatic amputation at elbow level, left arm A 🔾, 🔾
       Ex: See S56.012

    ● **S58.029**   Partial traumatic amputation at elbow level, unspecified arm A 🔾, 🔾
       Ex: See S56.019

● **S58.1**   Traumatic amputation at level between elbow and wrist

   ● **S58.11**   Complete traumatic amputation at level between elbow and wrist

    ● **S58.111**   Complete traumatic amputation at level between elbow and wrist, right arm A 🔾, 🔾
       Ex: See S56.011

    ● **S58.112**   Complete traumatic amputation at level between elbow and wrist, left arm A 🔾, 🔾
       Ex: See S56.012

    ● **S58.119**   Complete traumatic amputation at level between elbow and wrist, unspecified arm A 🔾, 🔾
       Ex: See S56.019

   ● **S58.12**   Partial traumatic amputation at level between elbow and wrist

    ● **S58.121**   Partial traumatic amputation at level between elbow and wrist, right arm A 🔾, 🔾
       Ex: See S56.011

    ● **S58.122**   Partial traumatic amputation at level between elbow and wrist, left arm A 🔾, 🔾
       Ex: See S56.012

    ● **S58.129**   Partial traumatic amputation at level between elbow and wrist, unspecified arm A 🔾, 🔾
       Ex: See S56.019

● **S58.9**   Traumatic amputation of forearm, level unspecified

    Excludes1   traumatic amputation of wrist (S68.-)

   ● **S58.91**   Complete traumatic amputation of forearm, level unspecified

    ● **S58.911**   Complete traumatic amputation of right forearm, level unspecified A 🔾, 🔾
       Ex: See S56.011

    ● **S58.912**   Complete traumatic amputation of left forearm, level unspecified A 🔾, 🔾
       Ex: See S56.012

    ● **S58.919**   Complete traumatic amputation of unspecified forearm, level unspecified A 🔾, 🔾
       Ex: See S56.019

◀ New   ◀═ Revised   ~~deleted~~ Deleted   Excludes 1   Excludes 2   Includes   Use additional   Code first   Code also   Unspecified

OGCR Official Guidelines   ● Unacceptable Principal Diagnosis   X Assign placeholder X   🔾 Use Additional Character(s)   🔾 Manifestation Code   Coding Clinic

● **S58.92**   Partial traumatic amputation of forearm, level unspecified

    ● **S58.921**   Partial traumatic amputation of right forearm, level unspecified A ⊚, ⊚
        Ⓔ See S56.011

    ● **S58.922**   Partial traumatic amputation of left forearm, level unspecified A ⊚, ⊚
        Ⓔ See S56.012

    ● **S58.929**   Partial traumatic amputation of unspecified forearm, level unspecified A ⊚, ⊚
        Ⓔ See S56.019

● **S59**   Other and unspecified injuries of elbow and forearm

    Excludes2   other and unspecified injuries of wrist and hand (S69.-)

    The appropriate 7th character is to be added to each code from subcategories S59.0, S59.1, and S59.2

A	initial encounter for closed fracture
D	subsequent encounter for fracture with routine healing
G	subsequent encounter for fracture with delayed healing
K	subsequent encounter for fracture with nonunion
P	subsequent encounter for fracture with malunion
S	sequela

● **S59.0**   Physeal fracture of lower end of ulna

    ● **S59.00**   Unspecified physeal fracture of lower end of ulna

       ● **S59.001**   Unspecified physeal fracture of lower end of ulna, right arm A, K, P ⊚, ⊚, A ⊚
          Ⓔ For code S59.001[A]: See S52.011[A]
            For S59.001[K,P]: See S52.00[L,M,N,P,Q,R]

       ● **S59.002**   Unspecified physeal fracture of lower end of ulna, left arm A, K, P ⊚, ⊚, A ⊚
          Ⓔ For code S59.002[A]: See S52.012[A]
            For S59.002[K,P]: See S52.00[L,M,N,P,Q,R]

       ● **S59.009**   Unspecified physeal fracture of lower end of ulna, unspecified arm A, K, P ⊚, ⊚, A ⊚
          Ⓔ For code S59.009[A]: See S52.019[A]
            For S59.009[K,P]: See S52.00[L,M,N,P,Q,R]

    ● **S59.01**   Salter-Harris Type I physeal fracture of lower end of ulna

       ● **S59.011**   Salter-Harris Type I physeal fracture of lower end of ulna, right arm A, K, P ⊚, ⊚, A ⊚
          Ⓔ For code S59.011[A]: See S52.011[A]
            For S59.011[K,P]: See S52.00[L,M,N,P,Q,R]

       ● **S59.012**   Salter-Harris Type I physeal fracture of lower end of ulna, left arm A, K, P ⊚, ⊚, A ⊚
          Ⓔ For code S59.012[A]: See S52.012[A]
            For S59.012[K,P]: See S52.00[L,M,N,P,Q,R]

       ● **S59.019**   Salter-Harris Type I physeal fracture of lower end of ulna, unspecified arm A, K, P ⊚, ⊚, A ⊚
          Ⓔ For code S59.019[A]: See S52.019[A]
            For S59.019[K,P]: See S52.00[L,M,N,P,Q,R]

Item 19-4   **SALTER-HARRIS TYPE 1:** epiphysis is completely separated from end of bone, or metaphysic growth plate remains attached to epiphysis
    SALTER-HARRIS TYPE 2: epiphysis and growth plate are partially separated from metaphysis, which is cracked—most common type
    SALTER-HARRIS TYPE 3: fracture occurring through epiphysis and separates part of epiphysis and growth plate from metaphysis fracture, usually at distal end of tibia
    SALTER-HARRIS TYPE 4: fracture runs through epiphysis, across growth plate, into metaphysic, surgery is required to restore joint surface to normal and align growth plate

● **S59.02**   Salter-Harris Type II physeal fracture of lower end of ulna

    ● **S59.021**   Salter-Harris Type II physeal fracture of lower end of ulna, right arm A, K, P ⊚, ⊚, A ⊚
        Ⓔ For code S59.021[A]: See S52.011[A]
          For S59.021[K,P]: See S52.0[L,M,N,P,Q,R]

    ● **S59.022**   Salter-Harris Type II physeal fracture of lower end of ulna, left arm A, K, P ⊚, ⊚, A ⊚
        Ⓔ For code S59.022[A]: See S52.012[A]
          For S59.022[K,P]: See S52.0[L,M,N,P,Q,R]

    ● **S59.029**   Salter-Harris Type II physeal fracture of lower end of ulna, unspecified arm A, K, P ⊚, ⊚, A ⊚
        Ⓔ For code S59.029[A]: See S52.019[A]
          For S59.029[K,P]: See S52.0[L,M,N,P,Q,R]

● **S59.03**   Salter-Harris Type III physeal fracture of lower end of ulna

    ● **S59.031**   Salter-Harris Type III physeal fracture of lower end of ulna, right arm A, K, P ⊚, ⊚, A ⊚
        Ⓔ For code S59.031[A]: See S52.011[A]
          For S59.031[K,P]: See S52.0[L,M,N,P,Q,R]

    ● **S59.032**   Salter-Harris Type III physeal fracture of lower end of ulna, left arm A, K, P ⊚, ⊚, A ⊚
        Ⓔ For code S59.032[A]: See S52.012[A]
          For S59.032[K,P]: See S52.0[L,M,N,P,Q,R]

    ● **S59.039**   Salter-Harris Type III physeal fracture of lower end of ulna, unspecified arm A, K, P ⊚, ⊚, A ⊚
        Ⓔ For code S59.039[A]: See S52.019[A]
          For S59.039[K,P]: See S52.0[L,M,N,P,Q,R]

● **S59.04**   Salter-Harris Type IV physeal fracture of lower end of ulna

    ● **S59.041**   Salter-Harris Type IV physeal fracture of lower end of ulna, right arm A, K, P ⊚, ⊚, A ⊚
        Ⓔ For code S59.041[A]: See S52.011[A]
          For S59.041[K,P]: See S52.0[L,M,N,P,Q,R]

    ● **S59.042**   Salter-Harris Type IV physeal fracture of lower end of ulna, left arm A, K, P ⊚, ⊚, A ⊚
        Ⓔ For code S59.042[A]: See S52.012[A]
          For S59.042[K,P]: See S52.0[L,M,N,P,Q,R]

    ● **S59.049**   Salter-Harris Type IV physeal fracture of lower end of ulna, unspecified arm A, K, P ⊚, ⊚, A ⊚
        Ⓔ For code S59.049[A]: See S52.019[A]
          For S59.049[K,P]: See S52.0[L,M,N,P,Q,R]

N Newborn Age: 0   **P** Pediatric Age: 0–17   **M** Maternity DX: 12–55   **A** Adult Age: 15–124   ♀ Females Only   ♂ Males Only

⊚ Complication\Comorbidity   ⊚ Major C\C   Ⓔ CC/MCC Exclusions   ⊚ Present on Admission Requirement   ⊚ Hospital-Acquired Condition

1393

CHAPTER 19 (S00-T88)

● S59.09   Other physeal fracture of lower end of ulna
   ● S59.091   Other physeal fracture of lower end of ulna, right arm A, K, P 🔵, 🔵, A 🔵
     Ⓔ For code S59.091[A]: See S52.011[A]
     For S59.091[K,P]: See S52.00[L,M,N,P,Q,R]
   ● S59.092   Other physeal fracture of lower end of ulna, left arm A, K, P 🔵, 🔵, A 🔵
     Ⓔ For code S59.092[A]: See S52.012[A]
     For S59.092[K,P]: See S52.00[L,M,N,P,Q,R]
   ● S59.099   Other physeal fracture of lower end of ulna, unspecified arm A, K, P 🔵, 🔵, A 🔵
     Ⓔ For code S59.099[A]: See S52.019[A]
     For S59.099[K,P]: See S52.00[L,M,N,P,Q,R]

● S59.1   Physeal fracture of upper end of radius
   Ⓔ For category S59.1 CC codes: See S52.00[L,M,N,P,Q,R]
   ● S59.10   Unspecified physeal fracture of upper end of radius
     ● S59.101   Unspecified physeal fracture of upper end of radius, right arm K, P 🔵, 🔵
     ● S59.102   Unspecified physeal fracture of upper end of radius, left arm K, P 🔵, 🔵
     ● S59.109   Unspecified physeal fracture of upper end of radius, unspecified arm K, P 🔵, 🔵
   ● S59.11   Salter-Harris Type I physeal fracture of upper end of radius
     ● S59.111   Salter-Harris Type I physeal fracture of upper end of radius, right arm K, P 🔵, 🔵
     ● S59.112   Salter-Harris Type I physeal fracture of upper end of radius, left arm K, P 🔵, 🔵
     ● S59.119   Salter-Harris Type I physeal fracture of upper end of radius, unspecified arm K, P 🔵, 🔵
   ● S59.12   Salter-Harris Type II physeal fracture of upper end of radius
     ● S59.121   Salter-Harris Type II physeal fracture of upper end of radius, right arm K, P 🔵, 🔵
     ● S59.122   Salter-Harris Type II physeal fracture of upper end of radius, left arm K, P 🔵, 🔵
     ● S59.129   Salter-Harris Type II physeal fracture of upper end of radius, unspecified arm K, P 🔵, 🔵
   ● S59.13   Salter-Harris Type III physeal fracture of upper end of radius
     ● S59.131   Salter-Harris Type III physeal fracture of upper end of radius, right arm K, P 🔵, 🔵
     ● S59.132   Salter-Harris Type III physeal fracture of upper end of radius, left arm K, P 🔵, 🔵
     ● S59.139   Salter-Harris Type III physeal fracture of upper end of radius, unspecified arm K, P 🔵, 🔵
   ● S59.14   Salter-Harris Type IV physeal fracture of upper end of radius
     ● S59.141   Salter-Harris Type IV physeal fracture of upper end of radius, right arm K, P 🔵, 🔵
     ● S59.142   Salter-Harris Type IV physeal fracture of upper end of radius, left arm K, P 🔵, 🔵
     ● S59.149   Salter-Harris Type IV physeal fracture of upper end of radius, unspecified arm K, P 🔵, 🔵

● S59.19   Other physeal fracture of upper end of radius
   ● S59.191   Other physeal fracture of upper end of radius, right arm K, P 🔵, 🔵
   ● S59.192   Other physeal fracture of upper end of radius, left arm K, P 🔵, 🔵
   ● S59.199   Other physeal fracture of upper end of radius, unspecified arm K, P 🔵, 🔵

● S59.2   Physeal fracture of lower end of radius
   ● S59.20   Unspecified physeal fracture of lower end of radius
     ● S59.201   Unspecified physeal fracture of lower end of radius, right arm A, K, P 🔵, 🔵, A 🔵
      Ⓔ For code S59.201[A]: See S52.011[A]
      For S59.201[K,P]: See S52.00[L,M,N,P,Q,R]
     ● S59.202   Unspecified physeal fracture of lower end of radius, left arm A, K, P 🔵, 🔵, A 🔵
      Ⓔ For code S59.202[A]: See S52.012[A]
      For S59.202[K,P]: See S52.00[L,M,N,P,Q,R]
     ● S59.209   Unspecified physeal fracture of lower end of radius, unspecified arm A, K, P 🔵, 🔵, A 🔵
      Ⓔ For code S59.209[A]: See S52.019[A]
      For S59.209[K,P]: See S52.00[L,M,N,P,Q,R]

   ● S59.21   Salter-Harris Type I physeal fracture of lower end of radius
     ● S59.211   Salter-Harris Type I physeal fracture of lower end of radius, right arm A, K, P 🔵, 🔵, A 🔵
      Ⓔ For code S59.211[A]: See S52.011[A]
      For S59.211[K,P]: See S52.00[L,M,N,P,Q,R]
     ● S59.212   Salter-Harris Type I physeal fracture of lower end of radius, left arm A, K, P 🔵, 🔵, A 🔵
      Ⓔ For code S59.212[A]: See S52.012[A]
      For S59.212[K,P]: See S52.00[L,M,N,P,Q,R]
     ● S59.219   Salter-Harris Type I physeal fracture of lower end of radius, unspecified arm A, K, P 🔵, 🔵, A 🔵
      Ⓔ For code S59.219[A]: See S52.019[A]
      For S59.219[K,P]: See S52.00[L,M,N,P,Q,R]

   ● S59.22   Salter-Harris Type II physeal fracture of lower end of radius
     ● S59.221   Salter-Harris Type II physeal fracture of lower end of radius, right arm A, K, P 🔵, 🔵, A 🔵
      Ⓔ For code S59.221[A]: See S52.011[A]
      For S59.221[K,P]: See S52.00[L,M,N,P,Q,R]
     ● S59.222   Salter-Harris Type II physeal fracture of lower end of radius, left arm A, K, P 🔵, 🔵, A 🔵
      Ⓔ For code S59.222[A]: See S52.012[A]
      For S59.222[K,P]: See S52.00[L,M,N,P,Q,R]
     ● S59.229   Salter-Harris Type II physeal fracture of lower end of radius, unspecified arm A, K, P 🔵, 🔵, A 🔵
      Ⓔ For code S59.229[A]: See S52.019[A]
      For S59.229[K,P]: See S52.00[L,M,N,P,Q,R]

◀ New   ◀⁞⁞ Revised   ~~deleted~~ Deleted   Excludes 1   Excludes 2   Includes   Use additional   Code first   Code also   Unspecified
OGCR Official Guidelines   ● Unacceptable Principal Diagnosis   X Assign placeholder X   ● Use Additional Character(s)   ▶ Manifestation Code   **Coding Clinic**

● S59.23 Salter-Harris Type III physeal fracture of lower end of radius
  ● S59.231 Salter-Harris Type III physeal fracture of lower end of radius, right arm A, K, P 🔹, 🔹, A 🔹
    (Ex) For code S59.231[A]: See S52.011[A]
    For S59.231[K,P]: See S52.00[L,M,N,P,Q,R]
  ● S59.232 Salter-Harris Type III physeal fracture of lower end of radius, left arm A, K, P 🔹, 🔹, A 🔹
    (Ex) For code S59.232[A]: See S52.012[A]
    For S59.232[K,P]: See S52.00[L,M,N,P,Q,R]
  ● S59.239 Salter-Harris Type III physeal fracture of lower end of radius, unspecified arm A, K, P 🔹, 🔹, A 🔹
    (Ex) For code S59.239[A]: See S52.019[A]
    For S59.239[K,P]: See S52.00[L,M,N,P,Q,R]

● S59.24 Salter-Harris Type IV physeal fracture of lower end of radius
  ● S59.241 Salter-Harris Type IV physeal fracture of lower end of radius, right arm A, K, P 🔹, 🔹, A 🔹
    (Ex) For code S59.241[A]: See S52.011[A]
    For S59.241[K,P]: See S52.00[L,M,N,P,Q,R]
  ● S59.242 Salter-Harris Type IV physeal fracture of lower end of radius, left arm A, K, P 🔹, 🔹, A 🔹
    (Ex) For code S59.242[A]: See S52.012[A]
    For S59.242[K,P]: See S52.00[L,M,N,P,Q,R]
  ● S59.249 Salter-Harris Type IV physeal fracture of lower end of radius, unspecified arm A, K, P 🔹, 🔹, A 🔹
    (Ex) For code S59.249[A]: See S52.019[A]
    For S59.249[K,P]: See S52.00[L,M,N,P,Q,R]

● S59.29 Other physeal fracture of lower end of radius
  ● S59.291 Other physeal fracture of lower end of radius, right arm A, K, P 🔹, 🔹, A 🔹
    (Ex) For code S59.291[A]: See S52.011[A]
    For S59.291[K,P]: See S52.00[L,M,N,P,Q,R]
  ● S59.292 Other physeal fracture of lower end of radius, left arm A, K, P 🔹, 🔹, A 🔹
    (Ex) For code S59.292[A]: See S52.012[A]
    For S59.292[K,P]: See S52.00[L,M,N,P,Q,R]
  ● S59.299 Other physeal fracture of lower end of radius, unspecified arm A, K, P 🔹, 🔹, A 🔹
    (Ex) For code S59.299[A]: See S52.019[A]
    For S59.299[K,P]: See S52.00[L,M,N,P,Q,R]

● S59.8 Other specified injuries of elbow and forearm
The appropriate 7th character is to be added to each code in subcategory S59.8
  A initial encounter
  D subsequent encounter
  S sequela

● S59.80 Other specified injuries of elbow
  ● S59.801 Other specified injuries of right elbow 🔹
  ● S59.802 Other specified injuries of left elbow 🔹
  ● S59.809 Other specified injuries of unspecified elbow 🔹
● S59.81 Other specified injuries of forearm
  ● S59.811 Other specified injuries right forearm 🔹
  ● S59.812 Other specified injuries left forearm 🔹
  ● S59.819 Other specified injuries unspecified forearm 🔹

● S59.9 Unspecified injury of elbow and forearm
The appropriate 7th character is to be added to each code in subcategory S59.9
  A initial encounter
  D subsequent encounter
  S sequela

● S59.90 Unspecified injury of elbow
  ● S59.901 Unspecified injury of right elbow 🔹
  ● S59.902 Unspecified injury of left elbow 🔹
  ● S59.909 Unspecified injury of unspecified elbow 🔹
● S59.91 Unspecified injury of forearm
  ● S59.911 Unspecified injury of right forearm 🔹
  ● S59.912 Unspecified injury of left forearm 🔹
  ● S59.919 Unspecified injury of unspecified forearm 🔹

INJURIES TO THE WRIST, HAND AND FINGERS (S60-S69)

Excludes2 burns and corrosions (T20-T32)
frostbite (T33-T34)
insect bite or sting, venomous (T63.4)

● S60 Superficial injury of wrist, hand and fingers
The appropriate 7th character is to be added to each code from category S60
  A initial encounter
  D subsequent encounter
  S sequela

● S60.0 Contusion of finger without damage to nail
  Excludes1 contusion involving nail (matrix) (S60.1)
X ● S60.00 Contusion of unspecified finger without damage to nail 🔹
  Contusion of finger(s) NOS
● S60.01 Contusion of thumb without damage to nail
  ● S60.011 Contusion of right thumb without damage to nail 🔹
  ● S60.012 Contusion of left thumb without damage to nail 🔹
  ● S60.019 Contusion of unspecified thumb without damage to nail 🔹
● S60.02 Contusion of index finger without damage to nail
  ● S60.021 Contusion of right index finger without damage to nail 🔹
  ● S60.022 Contusion of left index finger without damage to nail 🔹
  ● S60.029 Contusion of unspecified index finger without damage to nail 🔹
● S60.03 Contusion of middle finger without damage to nail
  ● S60.031 Contusion of right middle finger without damage to nail 🔹
  ● S60.032 Contusion of left middle finger without damage to nail 🔹
  ● S60.039 Contusion of unspecified middle finger without damage to nail 🔹
● S60.04 Contusion of ring finger without damage to nail
  ● S60.041 Contusion of right ring finger without damage to nail 🔹
  ● S60.042 Contusion of left ring finger without damage to nail 🔹
  ● S60.049 Contusion of unspecified ring finger without damage to nail 🔹

N Newborn Age: 0   P Pediatric Age: 0–17   M Maternity DX: 12–55   A Adult Age: 15–124   ♀ Females Only   ♂ Males Only
🔹 Complication\Comorbidity   🔹 Major C\C   (Ex) CC/MCC Exclusions   🔹 Present on Admission Requirement   🔹 Hospital-Acquired Condition

1395

CHAPTER 19 (S00-T88)

- ● S60.05   Contusion of little finger without damage to nail
  - ● S60.051   Contusion of right little finger without damage to nail 🖉
  - ● S60.052   Contusion of left little finger without damage to nail 🖉
  - ● S60.059   Contusion of unspecified little finger without damage to nail 🖉
- ● S60.1   Contusion of finger with damage to nail
  - X ● S60.10   Contusion of unspecified finger with damage to nail 🖉
  - ● S60.11   Contusion of thumb with damage to nail
    - ● S60.111   Contusion of right thumb with damage to nail 🖉
    - ● S60.112   Contusion of left thumb with damage to nail 🖉
    - ● S60.119   Contusion of unspecified thumb with damage to nail 🖉
  - ● S60.12   Contusion of index finger with damage to nail
    - ● S60.121   Contusion of right index finger with damage to nail 🖉
    - ● S60.122   Contusion of left index finger with damage to nail 🖉
    - ● S60.129   Contusion of unspecified index finger with damage to nail 🖉
  - ● S60.13   Contusion of middle finger with damage to nail
    - ● S60.131   Contusion of right middle finger with damage to nail 🖉
    - ● S60.132   Contusion of left middle finger with damage to nail 🖉
    - ● S60.139   Contusion of unspecified middle finger with damage to nail 🖉
  - ● S60.14   Contusion of ring finger with damage to nail
    - ● S60.141   Contusion of right ring finger with damage to nail 🖉
    - ● S60.142   Contusion of left ring finger with damage to nail 🖉
    - ● S60.149   Contusion of unspecified ring finger with damage to nail 🖉
  - ● S60.15   Contusion of little finger with damage to nail
    - ● S60.151   Contusion of right little finger with damage to nail 🖉
    - ● S60.152   Contusion of left little finger with damage to nail 🖉
    - ● S60.159   Contusion of unspecified little finger with damage to nail 🖉
- ● S60.2   Contusion of wrist and hand
  - Excludes2   contusion of fingers (S60.0-, S60.1-)
  - ● S60.21   Contusion of wrist
    - ● S60.211   Contusion of right wrist 🖉
    - ● S60.212   Contusion of left wrist 🖉
    - ● S60.219   Contusion of unspecified wrist 🖉
  - ● S60.22   Contusion of hand
    - ● S60.221   Contusion of right hand 🖉
    - ● S60.222   Contusion of left hand 🖉
    - ● S60.229   Contusion of unspecified hand 🖉
- ● S60.3   Other superficial injuries of thumb
  - ● S60.31   Abrasion of thumb
    - ● S60.311   Abrasion of right thumb 🖉
    - ● S60.312   Abrasion of left thumb 🖉
    - ● S60.319   Abrasion of unspecified thumb 🖉
  - ● S60.32   Blister (nonthermal) of thumb
    - ● S60.321   Blister (nonthermal) of right thumb 🖉
    - ● S60.322   Blister (nonthermal) of left thumb 🖉
    - ● S60.329   Blister (nonthermal) of unspecified thumb 🖉

- ● S60.34   External constriction of thumb
  - Hair tourniquet syndrome of thumb
  - Use additional cause code to identify the constricting item (W49.0-)
  - ● S60.341   External constriction of right thumb 🖉
  - ● S60.342   External constriction of left thumb 🖉
  - ● S60.349   External constriction of unspecified thumb 🖉
- ● S60.35   Superficial foreign body of thumb
  - Splinter in the thumb
  - ● S60.351   Superficial foreign body of right thumb 🖉
  - ● S60.352   Superficial foreign body of left thumb 🖉
  - ● S60.359   Superficial foreign body of unspecified thumb 🖉
- ● S60.36   Insect bite (nonvenomous) of thumb
  - ● S60.361   Insect bite (nonvenomous) of right thumb 🖉
  - ● S60.362   Insect bite (nonvenomous) of left thumb 🖉
  - ● S60.369   Insect bite (nonvenomous) of unspecified thumb 🖉
- ● S60.37   Other superficial bite of thumb
  - Excludes1   open bite of thumb (S61.05-, S61.15-)
  - ● S60.371   Other superficial bite of right thumb 🖉
  - ● S60.372   Other superficial bite of left thumb 🖉
  - ● S60.379   Other superficial bite of unspecified thumb 🖉
- ● S60.39   Other superficial injuries of thumb
  - ● S60.391   Other superficial injuries of right thumb 🖉
  - ● S60.392   Other superficial injuries of left thumb 🖉
  - ● S60.399   Other superficial injuries of unspecified thumb 🖉
- ● S60.4   Other superficial injuries of other fingers
  - ● S60.41   Abrasion of fingers
    - ● S60.410   Abrasion of right index finger 🖉
    - ● S60.411   Abrasion of left index finger 🖉
    - ● S60.412   Abrasion of right middle finger 🖉
    - ● S60.413   Abrasion of left middle finger 🖉
    - ● S60.414   Abrasion of right ring finger 🖉
    - ● S60.415   Abrasion of left ring finger 🖉
    - ● S60.416   Abrasion of right little finger 🖉
    - ● S60.417   Abrasion of left little finger 🖉
    - ● S60.418   Abrasion of other finger 🖉
      - Abrasion of specified finger with unspecified laterality
    - ● S60.419   Abrasion of unspecified finger 🖉
  - ● S60.42   Blister (nonthermal) of fingers
    - ● S60.420   Blister (nonthermal) of right index finger 🖉
    - ● S60.421   Blister (nonthermal) of left index finger 🖉
    - ● S60.422   Blister (nonthermal) of right middle finger 🖉
    - ● S60.423   Blister (nonthermal) of left middle finger 🖉
    - ● S60.424   Blister (nonthermal) of right ring finger 🖉
    - ● S60.425   Blister (nonthermal) of left ring finger 🖉

◀ New   ◀▥ Revised   ~~deleted~~ Deleted   Excludes 1   Excludes 2   Includes   Use additional   Code first   Code also   Unspecified

OGCR Official Guidelines   ● Unacceptable Principal Diagnosis   X Assign placeholder X   ● Use Additional Character(s)   ▶ Manifestation Code   Coding Clinic

● S60.426　Blister (nonthermal) of right little finger 🐾

● S60.427　Blister (nonthermal) of left little finger 🐾

● S60.428　Blister (nonthermal) of other finger 🐾
　　　　　　Blister (nonthermal) of specified finger with unspecified laterality

● S60.429　Blister (nonthermal) of unspecified finger 🐾

● S60.44　External constriction of fingers
　　　　　Hair tourniquet syndrome of finger
　　　　　Use additional cause code to identify the constricting item (W49.0-)

● S60.440　External constriction of right index finger 🐾

● S60.441　External constriction of left index finger 🐾

● S60.442　External constriction of right middle finger 🐾

● S60.443　External constriction of left middle finger 🐾

● S60.444　External constriction of right ring finger 🐾

● S60.445　External constriction of left ring finger 🐾

● S60.446　External constriction of right little finger 🐾

● S60.447　External constriction of left little finger 🐾

● S60.448　External constriction of other finger 🐾
　　　　　　External constriction of specified finger with unspecified laterality

● S60.449　External constriction of unspecified finger 🐾

● S60.45　Superficial foreign body of fingers
　　　　　Splinter in the finger(s)

● S60.450　Superficial foreign body of right index finger 🐾

● S60.451　Superficial foreign body of left index finger 🐾

● S60.452　Superficial foreign body of right middle finger 🐾

● S60.453　Superficial foreign body of left middle finger 🐾

● S60.454　Superficial foreign body of right ring finger 🐾

● S60.455　Superficial foreign body of left ring finger 🐾

● S60.456　Superficial foreign body of right little finger 🐾

● S60.457　Superficial foreign body of left little finger 🐾

● S60.458　Superficial foreign body of other finger 🐾
　　　　　　Superficial foreign body of specified finger with unspecified laterality

● S60.459　Superficial foreign body of unspecified finger 🐾

● S60.46　Insect bite (nonvenomous) of fingers

● S60.460　Insect bite (nonvenomous) of right index finger 🐾

● S60.461　Insect bite (nonvenomous) of left index finger 🐾

● S60.462　Insect bite (nonvenomous) of right middle finger 🐾

● S60.463　Insect bite (nonvenomous) of left middle finger 🐾

● S60.464　Insect bite (nonvenomous) of right ring finger 🐾

● S60.465　Insect bite (nonvenomous) of left ring finger 🐾

● S60.466　Insect bite (nonvenomous) of right little finger 🐾

● S60.467　Insect bite (nonvenomous) of left little finger 🐾

● S60.468　Insect bite (nonvenomous) of other finger 🐾
　　　　　　Insect bite (nonvenomous) of specified finger with unspecified laterality

● S60.469　Insect bite (nonvenomous) of unspecified finger 🐾

● S60.47　Other superficial bite of fingers
　　　　　Excludes1　open bite of fingers (S61.25-, S61.35-)

● S60.470　Other superficial bite of right index finger 🐾

● S60.471　Other superficial bite of left index finger 🐾

● S60.472　Other superficial bite of right middle finger 🐾

● S60.473　Other superficial bite of left middle finger 🐾

● S60.474　Other superficial bite of right ring finger 🐾

● S60.475　Other superficial bite of left ring finger 🐾

● S60.476　Other superficial bite of right little finger 🐾

● S60.477　Other superficial bite of left little finger 🐾

● S60.478　Other superficial bite of other finger 🐾
　　　　　　Other superficial bite of specified finger with unspecified laterality

● S60.479　Other superficial bite of unspecified finger 🐾

● S60.5　Other superficial injuries of hand
　　　　　Excludes2　superficial injuries of fingers (S60.3-, S60.4-)

● S60.51　Abrasion of hand

　　● S60.511　Abrasion of right hand 🐾

　　● S60.512　Abrasion of left hand 🐾

　　● S60.519　Abrasion of unspecified hand 🐾

● S60.52　Blister (nonthermal) of hand

　　● S60.521　Blister (nonthermal) of right hand 🐾

　　● S60.522　Blister (nonthermal) of left hand 🐾

　　● S60.529　Blister (nonthermal) of unspecified hand 🐾

● S60.54　External constriction of hand

　　● S60.541　External constriction of right hand 🐾

　　● S60.542　External constriction of left hand 🐾

　　● S60.549　External constriction of unspecified hand 🐾

● S60.55　Superficial foreign body of hand
　　　　　Splinter in the hand

　　● S60.551　Superficial foreign body of right hand 🐾

　　● S60.552　Superficial foreign body of left hand 🐾

　　● S60.559　Superficial foreign body of unspecified hand 🐾

N Newborn Age: 0　　**P** Pediatric Age: 0–17　　**M** Maternity DX: 12–55　　**A** Adult Age: 15–124　　♀ Females Only　　♂ Males Only

🐾 Complication\Comorbidity　　🐾 Major C\C　　(Ex) CC/MCC Exclusions　　🐾 Present on Admission Requirement　　🐾 Hospital-Acquired Condition

1397

● S60.56   Insect bite (nonvenomous) of hand
   ● S60.561   Insect bite (nonvenomous) of right hand
   ● S60.562   Insect bite (nonvenomous) of left hand
   ● S60.569   Insect bite (nonvenomous) of unspecified hand
● S60.57   Other superficial bite of hand
   Excludes1   open bite of hand (S61.45-)
   ● S60.571   Other superficial bite of hand of right hand
   ● S60.572   Other superficial bite of hand of left hand
   ● S60.579   Other superficial bite of hand of unspecified hand
● S60.8   Other superficial injuries of wrist
  ● S60.81   Abrasion of wrist
   ● S60.811   Abrasion of right wrist
   ● S60.812   Abrasion of left wrist
   ● S60.819   Abrasion of unspecified wrist
  ● S60.82   Blister (nonthermal) of wrist
   ● S60.821   Blister (nonthermal) of right wrist
   ● S60.822   Blister (nonthermal) of left wrist
   ● S60.829   Blister (nonthermal) of unspecified wrist
  ● S60.84   External constriction of wrist
   ● S60.841   External constriction of right wrist
   ● S60.842   External constriction of left wrist
   ● S60.849   External constriction of unspecified wrist
  ● S60.85   Superficial foreign body of wrist
   Splinter in the wrist
   ● S60.851   Superficial foreign body of right wrist
   ● S60.852   Superficial foreign body of left wrist
   ● S60.859   Superficial foreign body of unspecified wrist
  ● S60.86   Insect bite (nonvenomous) of wrist
   ● S60.861   Insect bite (nonvenomous) of right wrist
   ● S60.862   Insect bite (nonvenomous) of left wrist
   ● S60.869   Insect bite (nonvenomous) of unspecified wrist
  ● S60.87   Other superficial bite of wrist
   Excludes1   open bite of wrist (S61.55)
   ● S60.871   Other superficial bite of right wrist
   ● S60.872   Other superficial bite of left wrist
   ● S60.879   Other superficial bite of unspecified wrist
● S60.9   Unspecified superficial injury of wrist, hand and fingers
  ● S60.91   Unspecified superficial injury of wrist
   ● S60.911   Unspecified superficial injury of right wrist
   ● S60.912   Unspecified superficial injury of left wrist
   ● S60.919   Unspecified superficial injury of unspecified wrist
  ● S60.92   Unspecified superficial injury of hand
   ● S60.921   Unspecified superficial injury of right hand
   ● S60.922   Unspecified superficial injury of left hand
   ● S60.929   Unspecified superficial injury of unspecified hand

● S60.93   Unspecified superficial injury of thumb
   ● S60.931   Unspecified superficial injury of right thumb
   ● S60.932   Unspecified superficial injury of left thumb
   ● S60.939   Unspecified superficial injury of unspecified thumb
● S60.94   Unspecified superficial injury of other fingers
   ● S60.940   Unspecified superficial injury of right index finger
   ● S60.941   Unspecified superficial injury of left index finger
   ● S60.942   Unspecified superficial injury of right middle finger
   ● S60.943   Unspecified superficial injury of left middle finger
   ● S60.944   Unspecified superficial injury of right ring finger
   ● S60.945   Unspecified superficial injury of left ring finger
   ● S60.946   Unspecified superficial injury of right little finger
   ● S60.947   Unspecified superficial injury of left little finger
   ● S60.948   Unspecified superficial injury of other finger
     Unspecified superficial injury of specified finger with unspecified laterality
   ● S60.949   Unspecified superficial injury of unspecified finger
● S61   **Open wound of wrist, hand and fingers**
  Code also any associated wound infection
  Excludes1   open fracture of wrist, hand and finger (S62.- with 7th character B)
     traumatic amputation of wrist and hand (S68.-)
  The appropriate 7th character is to be added to each code from category S61

A	initial encounter
D	subsequent encounter
S	sequela

● S61.0   Open wound of thumb without damage to nail
  Excludes1   open wound of thumb with damage to nail (S61.1-)
  ● S61.00   Unspecified open wound of thumb without damage to nail
   ● S61.001   Unspecified open wound of right thumb without damage to nail
   ● S61.002   Unspecified open wound of left thumb without damage to nail
   ● S61.009   Unspecified open wound of unspecified thumb without damage to nail
  ● S61.01   Laceration without foreign body of thumb without damage to nail
   ● S61.011   Laceration without foreign body of right thumb without damage to nail
   ● S61.012   Laceration without foreign body of left thumb without damage to nail
   ● S61.019   Laceration without foreign body of unspecified thumb without damage to nail

● **S61.02** Laceration with foreign body of thumb without damage to nail
  ● **S61.021** Laceration with foreign body of right thumb without damage to nail ⚕
  ● **S61.022** Laceration with foreign body of left thumb without damage to nail ⚕
  ● **S61.029** Laceration with foreign body of unspecified thumb without damage to nail ⚕

● **S61.03** Puncture wound without foreign body of thumb without damage to nail
  ● **S61.031** Puncture wound without foreign body of right thumb without damage to nail ⚕
  ● **S61.032** Puncture wound without foreign body of left thumb without damage to nail ⚕
  ● **S61.039** Puncture wound without foreign body of unspecified thumb without damage to nail ⚕

● **S61.04** Puncture wound with foreign body of thumb without damage to nail
  ● **S61.041** Puncture wound with foreign body of right thumb without damage to nail ⚕
  ● **S61.042** Puncture wound with foreign body of left thumb without damage to nail ⚕
  ● **S61.049** Puncture wound with foreign body of unspecified thumb without damage to nail ⚕

● **S61.05** Open bite of thumb without damage to nail
       Bite of thumb NOS
       Excludes1 superficial bite of thumb (S60.36-, S60.37-)
  ● **S61.051** Open bite of right thumb without damage to nail ⚕
  ● **S61.052** Open bite of left thumb without damage to nail ⚕
  ● **S61.059** Open bite of unspecified thumb without damage to nail ⚕

● **S61.1** Open wound of thumb with damage to nail
  ● **S61.10** Unspecified open wound of thumb with damage to nail
    ● **S61.101** Unspecified open wound of right thumb with damage to nail ⚕
    ● **S61.102** Unspecified open wound of left thumb with damage to nail ⚕
    ● **S61.109** Unspecified open wound of unspecified thumb with damage to nail ⚕

  ● **S61.11** Laceration without foreign body of thumb with damage to nail
    ● **S61.111** Laceration without foreign body of right thumb with damage to nail ⚕
    ● **S61.112** Laceration without foreign body of left thumb with damage to nail ⚕
    ● **S61.119** Laceration without foreign body of unspecified thumb with damage to nail ⚕

  ● **S61.12** Laceration with foreign body of thumb with damage to nail
    ● **S61.121** Laceration with foreign body of right thumb with damage to nail ⚕
    ● **S61.122** Laceration with foreign body of left thumb with damage to nail ⚕
    ● **S61.129** Laceration with foreign body of unspecified thumb with damage to nail ⚕

● **S61.13** Puncture wound without foreign body of thumb with damage to nail
  ● **S61.131** Puncture wound without foreign body of right thumb with damage to nail ⚕
  ● **S61.132** Puncture wound without foreign body of left thumb with damage to nail ⚕
  ● **S61.139** Puncture wound without foreign body of unspecified thumb with damage to nail ⚕

● **S61.14** Puncture wound with foreign body of thumb with damage to nail
  ● **S61.141** Puncture wound with foreign body of right thumb with damage to nail ⚕
  ● **S61.142** Puncture wound with foreign body of left thumb with damage to nail ⚕
  ● **S61.149** Puncture wound with foreign body of unspecified thumb with damage to nail ⚕

● **S61.15** Open bite of thumb with damage to nail
       Bite of thumb with damage to nail NOS
       Excludes1 superficial bite of thumb (S60.36-, S60.37-)
  ● **S61.151** Open bite of right thumb with damage to nail ⚕
  ● **S61.152** Open bite of left thumb with damage to nail ⚕
  ● **S61.159** Open bite of unspecified thumb with damage to nail ⚕

● **S61.2** Open wound of other finger without damage to nail
       Excludes1 open wound of finger involving nail (matrix) (S61.3-)
       Excludes2 open wound of thumb without damage to nail (S61.0-)
  ● **S61.20** Unspecified open wound of other finger without damage to nail
    ● **S61.200** Unspecified open wound of right index finger without damage to nail ⚕
    ● **S61.201** Unspecified open wound of left index finger without damage to nail ⚕
    ● **S61.202** Unspecified open wound of right middle finger without damage to nail ⚕
    ● **S61.203** Unspecified open wound of left middle finger without damage to nail ⚕
    ● **S61.204** Unspecified open wound of right ring finger without damage to nail ⚕
    ● **S61.205** Unspecified open wound of left ring finger without damage to nail ⚕
    ● **S61.206** Unspecified open wound of right little finger without damage to nail ⚕
    ● **S61.207** Unspecified open wound of left little finger without damage to nail ⚕
    ● **S61.208** Unspecified open wound of other finger without damage to nail ⚕
         Unspecified open wound of specified finger with unspecified laterality without damage to nail
    ● **S61.209** Unspecified open wound of unspecified finger without damage to nail ⚕

N Newborn Age: 0   P Pediatric Age: 0–17   M Maternity DX: 12–55   A Adult Age: 15–124   ♀ Females Only   ♂ Males Only
⚕ Complication\Comorbidity   ⚕ Major C\C   (Ex) CC/MCC Exclusions   ⚕ Present on Admission Requirement   ⚕ Hospital-Acquired Condition

1399

● S61.21   Laceration without foreign body of finger without damage to nail

● S61.210   Laceration without foreign body of right index finger without damage to nail 🖐

● S61.211   Laceration without foreign body of left index finger without damage to nail 🖐

● S61.212   Laceration without foreign body of right middle finger without damage to nail 🖐

● S61.213   Laceration without foreign body of left middle finger without damage to nail 🖐

● S61.214   Laceration without foreign body of right ring finger without damage to nail 🖐

● S61.215   Laceration without foreign body of left ring finger without damage to nail 🖐

● S61.216   Laceration without foreign body of right little finger without damage to nail 🖐

● S61.217   Laceration without foreign body of left little finger without damage to nail 🖐

● S61.218   Laceration without foreign body of other finger without damage to nail 🖐
          Laceration without foreign body of specified finger with unspecified laterality without damage to nail

● S61.219   Laceration without foreign body of unspecified finger without damage to nail 🖐

● S61.22   Laceration with foreign body of finger without damage to nail

● S61.220   Laceration with foreign body of right index finger without damage to nail 🖐

● S61.221   Laceration with foreign body of left index finger without damage to nail 🖐

● S61.222   Laceration with foreign body of right middle finger without damage to nail 🖐

● S61.223   Laceration with foreign body of left middle finger without damage to nail 🖐

● S61.224   Laceration with foreign body of right ring finger without damage to nail 🖐

● S61.225   Laceration with foreign body of left ring finger without damage to nail 🖐

● S61.226   Laceration with foreign body of right little finger without damage to nail 🖐

● S61.227   Laceration with foreign body of left little finger without damage to nail 🖐

● S61.228   Laceration with foreign body of other finger without damage to nail 🖐
          Laceration with foreign body of specified finger with unspecified laterality without damage to nail

● S61.229   Laceration with foreign body of unspecified finger without damage to nail 🖐

● S61.23   Puncture wound without foreign body of finger without damage to nail

● S61.230   Puncture wound without foreign body of right index finger without damage to nail 🖐

● S61.231   Puncture wound without foreign body of left index finger without damage to nail 🖐

● S61.232   Puncture wound without foreign body of right middle finger without damage to nail 🖐

● S61.233   Puncture wound without foreign body of left middle finger without damage to nail 🖐

● S61.234   Puncture wound without foreign body of right ring finger without damage to nail 🖐

● S61.235   Puncture wound without foreign body of left ring finger without damage to nail 🖐

● S61.236   Puncture wound without foreign body of right little finger without damage to nail 🖐

● S61.237   Puncture wound without foreign body of left little finger without damage to nail 🖐

● S61.238   Puncture wound without foreign body of other finger without damage to nail 🖐
          Puncture wound without foreign body of specified finger with unspecified laterality without damage to nail

● S61.239   Puncture wound without foreign body of unspecified finger without damage to nail 🖐

● S61.24   Puncture wound with foreign body of finger without damage to nail

● S61.240   Puncture wound with foreign body of right index finger without damage to nail 🖐

● S61.241   Puncture wound with foreign body of left index finger without damage to nail 🖐

● S61.242   Puncture wound with foreign body of right middle finger without damage to nail 🖐

● S61.243   Puncture wound with foreign body of left middle finger without damage to nail 🖐

● S61.244   Puncture wound with foreign body of right ring finger without damage to nail 🖐

● S61.245   Puncture wound with foreign body of left ring finger without damage to nail 🖐

● S61.246   Puncture wound with foreign body of right little finger without damage to nail 🖐

● S61.247   Puncture wound with foreign body of left little finger without damage to nail 🖐

● S61.248   Puncture wound with foreign body of other finger without damage to nail 🖐
          Puncture wound with foreign body of specified finger with unspecified laterality without damage to nail

● S61.249   Puncture wound with foreign body of unspecified finger without damage to nail 🖐

◀ New   ◀▥ Revised   d̶e̶l̶e̶t̶e̶d̶ Deleted   Excludes 1   Excludes 2   Includes   Use additional   Code first   Code also   Unspecified

OGCR Official Guidelines   ● Unacceptable Principal Diagnosis   X Assign placeholder X   ● Use Additional Character(s)   ▶ Manifestation Code   Coding Clinic

● S61.25 **Open bite of finger without damage to nail**
Bite of finger without damage to nail NOS
Excludes1 superficial bite of finger (S60.46-, S60.47-)

● S61.250 **Open bite of right index finger without damage to nail** 🔗

● S61.251 **Open bite of left index finger without damage to nail** 🔗

● S61.252 **Open bite of right middle finger without damage to nail** 🔗

● S61.253 **Open bite of left middle finger without damage to nail** 🔗

● S61.254 **Open bite of right ring finger without damage to nail** 🔗

● S61.255 **Open bite of left ring finger without damage to nail** 🔗

● S61.256 **Open bite of right little finger without damage to nail** 🔗

● S61.257 **Open bite of left little finger without damage to nail** 🔗

● S61.258 **Open bite of other finger without damage to nail** 🔗
Open bite of specified finger with unspecified laterality without damage to nail

● S61.259 **Open bite of unspecified finger without damage to nail** 🔗

● S61.3 **Open wound of other finger with damage to nail**

● S61.30 **Unspecified open wound of finger with damage to nail**

● S61.300 **Unspecified open wound of right index finger with damage to nail** 🔗

● S61.301 **Unspecified open wound of left index finger with damage to nail** 🔗

● S61.302 **Unspecified open wound of right middle finger with damage to nail** 🔗

● S61.303 **Unspecified open wound of left middle finger with damage to nail** 🔗

● S61.304 **Unspecified open wound of right ring finger with damage to nail** 🔗

● S61.305 **Unspecified open wound of left ring finger with damage to nail** 🔗

● S61.306 **Unspecified open wound of right little finger with damage to nail** 🔗

● S61.307 **Unspecified open wound of left little finger with damage to nail** 🔗

● S61.308 **Unspecified open wound of other finger with damage to nail** 🔗
Unspecified open wound of specified finger with unspecified laterality with damage to nail

● S61.309 **Unspecified open wound of unspecified finger with damage to nail** 🔗

● S61.31 **Laceration without foreign body of finger with damage to nail**

● S61.310 **Laceration without foreign body of right index finger with damage to nail** 🔗

● S61.311 **Laceration without foreign body of left index finger with damage to nail** 🔗

● S61.312 **Laceration without foreign body of right middle finger with damage to nail** 🔗

● S61.313 **Laceration without foreign body of left middle finger with damage to nail** 🔗

● S61.314 **Laceration without foreign body of right ring finger with damage to nail** 🔗

● S61.315 **Laceration without foreign body of left ring finger with damage to nail** 🔗

● S61.316 **Laceration without foreign body of right little finger with damage to nail** 🔗

● S61.317 **Laceration without foreign body of left little finger with damage to nail** 🔗

● S61.318 **Laceration without foreign body of other finger with damage to nail** 🔗
Laceration without foreign body of specified finger with unspecified laterality with damage to nail

● S61.319 **Laceration without foreign body of unspecified finger with damage to nail** 🔗

● S61.32 **Laceration with foreign body of finger with damage to nail**

● S61.320 **Laceration with foreign body of right index finger with damage to nail** 🔗

● S61.321 **Laceration with foreign body of left index finger with damage to nail** 🔗

● S61.322 **Laceration with foreign body of right middle finger with damage to nail** 🔗

● S61.323 **Laceration with foreign body of left middle finger with damage to nail** 🔗

● S61.324 **Laceration with foreign body of right ring finger with damage to nail** 🔗

● S61.325 **Laceration with foreign body of left ring finger with damage to nail** 🔗

● S61.326 **Laceration with foreign body of right little finger with damage to nail** 🔗

● S61.327 **Laceration with foreign body of left little finger with damage to nail** 🔗

● S61.328 **Laceration with foreign body of other finger with damage to nail** 🔗
Laceration with foreign body of specified finger with unspecified laterality with damage to nail

● S61.329 **Laceration with foreign body of unspecified finger with damage to nail** 🔗

● S61.33 **Puncture wound without foreign body of finger with damage to nail**

● S61.330 **Puncture wound without foreign body of right index finger with damage to nail** 🔗

● S61.331 **Puncture wound without foreign body of left index finger with damage to nail** 🔗

● S61.332 **Puncture wound without foreign body of right middle finger with damage to nail** 🔗

● S61.333 **Puncture wound without foreign body of left middle finger with damage to nail** 🔗

● S61.334 **Puncture wound without foreign body of right ring finger with damage to nail** 🔗

● S61.335 **Puncture wound without foreign body of left ring finger with damage to nail** 🔗

● S61.336 **Puncture wound without foreign body of right little finger with damage to nail** 🔗

● S61.337 **Puncture wound without foreign body of left little finger with damage to nail** 🔗

N Newborn Age: 0   P Pediatric Age: 0–17   M Maternity DX: 12–55   A Adult Age: 15–124   ♀ Females Only   ♂ Males Only
🔗 Complication\Comorbidity   🔗 Major C\C   Ⓔⱼ CC/MCC Exclusions   🔗 Present on Admission Requirement   🔗 Hospital-Acquired Condition

1401

● S61.338　Puncture wound without foreign body of other finger with damage to nail 🖏
　　　　Puncture wound without foreign body of specified finger with unspecified laterality with damage to nail

● S61.339　Puncture wound without foreign body of unspecified finger with damage to nail 🖏

● S61.34　Puncture wound with foreign body of finger with damage to nail

● S61.340　Puncture wound with foreign body of right index finger with damage to nail 🖏

● S61.341　Puncture wound with foreign body of left index finger with damage to nail 🖏

● S61.342　Puncture wound with foreign body of right middle finger with damage to nail 🖏

● S61.343　Puncture wound with foreign body of left middle finger with damage to nail 🖏

● S61.344　Puncture wound with foreign body of right ring finger with damage to nail 🖏

● S61.345　Puncture wound with foreign body of left ring finger with damage to nail 🖏

● S61.346　Puncture wound with foreign body of right little finger with damage to nail 🖏

● S61.347　Puncture wound with foreign body of left little finger with damage to nail 🖏

● S61.348　Puncture wound with foreign body of other finger with damage to nail 🖏
　　　　Puncture wound with foreign body of specified finger with unspecified laterality with damage to nail

● S61.349　Puncture wound with foreign body of unspecified finger with damage to nail 🖏

● S61.35　Open bite of finger with damage to nail
　　　　Bite of finger with damage to nail NOS
　　　　Excludes1　superficial bite of finger (S60.46-, S60.47-)

● S61.350　Open bite of right index finger with damage to nail 🖏

● S61.351　Open bite of left index finger with damage to nail 🖏

● S61.352　Open bite of right middle finger with damage to nail 🖏

● S61.353　Open bite of left middle finger with damage to nail 🖏

● S61.354　Open bite of right ring finger with damage to nail 🖏

● S61.355　Open bite of left ring finger with damage to nail 🖏

● S61.356　Open bite of right little finger with damage to nail 🖏

● S61.357　Open bite of left little finger with damage to nail 🖏

● S61.358　Open bite of other finger with damage to nail 🖏
　　　　Open bite of specified finger with unspecified laterality with damage to nail

● S61.359　Open bite of unspecified finger with damage to nail 🖏

● S61.4　Open wound of hand

● S61.40　Unspecified open wound of hand

● S61.401　Unspecified open wound of right hand 🖏

● S61.402　Unspecified open wound of left hand 🖏

● S61.409　Unspecified open wound of unspecified hand 🖏

● S61.41　Laceration without foreign body of hand

● S61.411　Laceration without foreign body of right hand 🖏

● S61.412　Laceration without foreign body of left hand 🖏

● S61.419　Laceration without foreign body of unspecified hand 🖏

● S61.42　Laceration with foreign body of hand

● S61.421　Laceration with foreign body of right hand 🖏

● S61.422　Laceration with foreign body of left hand 🖏

● S61.429　Laceration with foreign body of unspecified hand 🖏

● S61.43　Puncture wound without foreign body of hand

● S61.431　Puncture wound without foreign body of right hand 🖏

● S61.432　Puncture wound without foreign body of left hand 🖏

● S61.439　Puncture wound without foreign body of unspecified hand 🖏

● S61.44　Puncture wound with foreign body of hand

● S61.441　Puncture wound with foreign body of right hand 🖏

● S61.442　Puncture wound with foreign body of left hand 🖏

● S61.449　Puncture wound with foreign body of unspecified hand 🖏

● S61.45　Open bite of hand
　　　　Bite of hand NOS
　　　　Excludes1　superficial bite of hand (S60.56-, S60.57-)

● S61.451　Open bite of right hand 🖏

● S61.452　Open bite of left hand 🖏

● S61.459　Open bite of unspecified hand 🖏

● S61.5　Open wound of wrist

● S61.50　Unspecified open wound of wrist

● S61.501　Unspecified open wound of right wrist 🖏

● S61.502　Unspecified open wound of left wrist 🖏

● S61.509　Unspecified open wound of unspecified wrist 🖏

● S61.51　Laceration without foreign body of wrist

● S61.511　Laceration without foreign body of right wrist 🖏

● S61.512　Laceration without foreign body of left wrist 🖏

● S61.519　Laceration without foreign body of unspecified wrist 🖏

● S61.52　Laceration with foreign body of wrist

● S61.521　Laceration with foreign body of right wrist 🖏

● S61.522　Laceration with foreign body of left wrist 🖏

● S61.529　Laceration with foreign body of unspecified wrist 🖏

◀ New　◀⊪ Revised　deleted Deleted　Excludes 1　Excludes 2　Includes　Use additional　Code first　Code also　Unspecified

1402　OGCR Official Guidelines　● Unacceptable Principal Diagnosis　X Assign placeholder X　● Use Additional Character(s)　▌ Manifestation Code　Coding Clinic

● **S61.53**   Puncture wound without foreign body of wrist
- ● **S61.531**   Puncture wound without foreign body of right wrist 🔊
- ● **S61.532**   Puncture wound without foreign body of left wrist 🔊
- ● **S61.539**   Puncture wound without foreign body of unspecified wrist 🔊

● **S61.54**   Puncture wound with foreign body of wrist
- ● **S61.541**   Puncture wound with foreign body of right wrist 🔊
- ● **S61.542**   Puncture wound with foreign body of left wrist 🔊
- ● **S61.549**   Puncture wound with foreign body of unspecified wrist 🔊

● **S61.55**   Open bite of wrist
> Bite of wrist NOS
>
> **Excludes1**   superficial bite of wrist (S60.86-, S60.87-)
- ● **S61.551**   Open bite of right wrist 🔊
- ● **S61.552**   Open bite of left wrist 🔊
- ● **S61.559**   Open bite of unspecified wrist 🔊

● **S62**   **Fracture at wrist and hand level**
> **Note:** A fracture not indicated as displaced or nondisplaced should be coded to displaced
>
> A fracture not indicated as open or closed should be coded to closed
>
> **Excludes1**   traumatic amputation of wrist and hand (S68.-)
>
> **Excludes2**   fracture of distal parts of ulna and radius (S52.-)
>
> The appropriate 7th character is to be added to each code from category S62

A	initial encounter for closed fracture
B	initial encounter for open fracture
D	subsequent encounter for fracture with routine healing
G	subsequent encounter for fracture with delayed healing
K	subsequent encounter for fracture with nonunion
P	subsequent encounter for fracture with malunion
S	sequela

● **S62.0**   **Fracture of navicular [scaphoid] bone of wrist**
> (Ex) For category S62.0 CC codes S62.0[B]: S62.001-S62.186[A,B]
> For S62.0[K,P]: M80.00X-M80.88X[K,P], M84.30X-M84.68X[K,P], S02.0XX-S02.92X[K], S12.000-S12.691[K], S22.000-S22.9XX[K], S32.000-S32.9XX[K], S42.001-S42.92X[K,P], S49.001-S49.199[K,P], S52.001-S52.92X[K,M,N,P,Q,R], S59.001-S59.299[K,P], S62.001-S62.92X[K,P], S72.001-S72.92X[K,M,N,P,Q,R], S79.001-S79.199[K,P], S82.001-S82.92X[K,M,N,P,Q,R], S89.001-S89.399[K,P], S92.001-S92.919[K,P]

- ● **S62.00**   Unspecified fracture of navicular [scaphoid] bone of wrist
  - ● **S62.001**   Unspecified fracture of navicular [scaphoid] bone of right wrist B, K, P 🔊, 🔊, B 🔊
  - ● **S62.002**   Unspecified fracture of navicular [scaphoid] bone of left wrist B, K, P 🔊, 🔊, B 🔊
    > **Coding Clinic: 2012, Q4, P106**
  - ● **S62.009**   Unspecified fracture of navicular [scaphoid] bone of unspecified wrist B, K, P 🔊, 🔊, B 🔊

- ● **S62.01**   Fracture of distal pole of navicular [scaphoid] bone of wrist
  > Fracture of volar tuberosity of navicular [scaphoid] bone of wrist
  - ● **S62.011**   Displaced fracture of distal pole of navicular [scaphoid] bone of right wrist B, K, P 🔊, 🔊, B 🔊
  - ● **S62.012**   Displaced fracture of distal pole of navicular [scaphoid] bone of left wrist B, K, P 🔊, 🔊, B 🔊

- ● **S62.013**   Displaced fracture of distal pole of navicular [scaphoid] bone of unspecified wrist B, K, P 🔊, 🔊, B 🔊
- ● **S62.014**   Nondisplaced fracture of distal pole of navicular [scaphoid] bone of right wrist B, K, P 🔊, 🔊, B 🔊
- ● **S62.015**   Nondisplaced fracture of distal pole of navicular [scaphoid] bone of left wrist B, K, P 🔊, 🔊, B 🔊
- ● **S62.016**   Nondisplaced fracture of distal pole of navicular [scaphoid] bone of unspecified wrist B, K, P 🔊, 🔊, B 🔊

● **S62.02**   Fracture of middle third of navicular [scaphoid] bone of wrist
- ● **S62.021**   Displaced fracture of middle third of navicular [scaphoid] bone of right wrist B, K, P 🔊, 🔊, B 🔊
- ● **S62.022**   Displaced fracture of middle third of navicular [scaphoid] bone of left wrist B, K, P 🔊, 🔊, B 🔊
- ● **S62.023**   Displaced fracture of middle third of navicular [scaphoid] bone of unspecified wrist B, K, P 🔊, 🔊, B 🔊
- ● **S62.024**   Nondisplaced fracture of middle third of navicular [scaphoid] bone of right wrist B, K, P 🔊, 🔊, B 🔊
- ● **S62.025**   Nondisplaced fracture of middle third of navicular [scaphoid] bone of left wrist B, K, P 🔊, 🔊, B 🔊
- ● **S62.026**   Nondisplaced fracture of middle third of navicular [scaphoid] bone of unspecified wrist B, K, P 🔊, 🔊, B 🔊

● **S62.03**   Fracture of proximal third of navicular [scaphoid] bone of wrist
- ● **S62.031**   Displaced fracture of proximal third of navicular [scaphoid] bone of right wrist B, K, P 🔊, 🔊, B 🔊
- ● **S62.032**   Displaced fracture of proximal third of navicular [scaphoid] bone of left wrist B, K, P 🔊, 🔊, B 🔊
- ● **S62.033**   Displaced fracture of proximal third of navicular [scaphoid] bone of unspecified wrist B, K, P 🔊, 🔊, B 🔊
- ● **S62.034**   Nondisplaced fracture of proximal third of navicular [scaphoid] bone of right wrist B, K, P 🔊, 🔊, B 🔊
- ● **S62.035**   Nondisplaced fracture of proximal third of navicular [scaphoid] bone of left wrist B, K, P 🔊, 🔊, B 🔊
- ● **S62.036**   Nondisplaced fracture of proximal third of navicular [scaphoid] bone of unspecified wrist B, K, P 🔊, 🔊, B 🔊

● **S62.1**   Fracture of other and unspecified carpal bone(s)
> **Excludes2**   fracture of scaphoid of wrist (S62.0-)
>
> (Ex) For category S62.1 CC codes S62.1[B]: S62.001-S62.186[A,B]
> For S62.0[K,P]: See S62.0[K,P]

- ● **S62.10**   Fracture of unspecified carpal bone
  > Fracture of wrist NOS
  - ● **S62.101**   Fracture of unspecified carpal bone, right wrist B, K, P 🔊, 🔊, B 🔊
  - ● **S62.102**   Fracture of unspecified carpal bone, left wrist B, K, P 🔊, 🔊, B 🔊
    > **Coding Clinic: 2012, Q4, P95**
  - ● **S62.109**   Fracture of unspecified carpal bone, unspecified wrist B, K, P 🔊, 🔊, B 🔊

N   Newborn Age: 0   P   Pediatric Age: 0–17   M   Maternity DX: 12–55   A   Adult Age: 15–124   ♀   Females Only   ♂   Males Only

🔊   Complication\Comorbidity   🔊   Major C\C   (Ex)   CC/MCC Exclusions   🔊   Present on Admission Requirement   🔊   Hospital-Acquired Condition

1403

CHAPTER 19 (S00-T88)

- ● S62.11 Fracture of triquetrum [cuneiform] bone of wrist
  - ● S62.111 Displaced fracture of triquetrum [cuneiform] bone, right wrist B, K, P 🐾, 🐾, B 🐾
  - ● S62.112 Displaced fracture of triquetrum [cuneiform] bone, left wrist B, K, P 🐾, 🐾, B 🐾
  - ● S62.113 Displaced fracture of triquetrum [cuneiform] bone, unspecified wrist B, K, P 🐾, 🐾, B 🐾
  - ● S62.114 Nondisplaced fracture of triquetrum [cuneiform] bone, right wrist B, K, P 🐾, 🐾, B 🐾
  - ● S62.115 Nondisplaced fracture of triquetrum [cuneiform] bone, left wrist B, K, P 🐾, 🐾, B 🐾
  - ● S62.116 Nondisplaced fracture of triquetrum [cuneiform] bone, unspecified wrist B, K, P 🐾, 🐾, B 🐾
- ● S62.12 Fracture of lunate [semilunar]
  - ● S62.121 Displaced fracture of lunate [semilunar], right wrist B, K, P 🐾, 🐾, B 🐾
  - ● S62.122 Displaced fracture of lunate [semilunar], left wrist B, K, P 🐾, 🐾, B 🐾
  - ● S62.123 Displaced fracture of lunate [semilunar], unspecified wrist B, K, P 🐾, 🐾, B 🐾
  - ● S62.124 Nondisplaced fracture of lunate [semilunar], right wrist B, K, P 🐾, 🐾, B 🐾
  - ● S62.125 Nondisplaced fracture of lunate [semilunar], left wrist B, K, P 🐾, 🐾, B 🐾
  - ● S62.126 Nondisplaced fracture of lunate [semilunar], unspecified wrist B, K, P 🐾, 🐾, B 🐾
- ● S62.13 Fracture of capitate [os magnum] bone
  - ● S62.131 Displaced fracture of capitate [os magnum] bone, right wrist B, K, P 🐾, 🐾, B 🐾
  - ● S62.132 Displaced fracture of capitate [os magnum] bone, left wrist B, K, P 🐾, 🐾, B 🐾
  - ● S62.133 Displaced fracture of capitate [os magnum] bone, unspecified wrist B, K, P 🐾, 🐾, B 🐾
  - ● S62.134 Nondisplaced fracture of capitate [os magnum] bone, right wrist B, K, P 🐾, 🐾, B 🐾
  - ● S62.135 Nondisplaced fracture of capitate [os magnum] bone, left wrist B, K, P 🐾, 🐾, B 🐾
  - ● S62.136 Nondisplaced fracture of capitate [os magnum] bone, unspecified wrist B, K, P 🐾, 🐾, B 🐾
- ● S62.14 Fracture of body of hamate [unciform] bone
  Fracture of hamate [unciform] bone NOS
  - ● S62.141 Displaced fracture of body of hamate [unciform] bone, right wrist B, K, P 🐾, 🐾, B 🐾
  - ● S62.142 Displaced fracture of body of hamate [unciform] bone, left wrist B, K, P 🐾, 🐾, B 🐾
  - ● S62.143 Displaced fracture of body of hamate [unciform] bone, unspecified wrist B, K, P 🐾, 🐾, B 🐾
  - ● S62.144 Nondisplaced fracture of body of hamate [unciform] bone, right wrist B, K, P 🐾, 🐾, B 🐾
  - ● S62.145 Nondisplaced fracture of body of hamate [unciform] bone, left wrist B, K, P 🐾, 🐾, B 🐾
  - ● S62.146 Nondisplaced fracture of body of hamate [unciform] bone, unspecified wrist B, K, P 🐾, 🐾, B 🐾
- ● S62.15 Fracture of hook process of hamate [unciform] bone
  Fracture of unciform process of hamate [unciform] bone
  - ● S62.151 Displaced fracture of hook process of hamate [unciform] bone, right wrist B, K, P 🐾, 🐾, B 🐾
  - ● S62.152 Displaced fracture of hook process of hamate [unciform] bone, left wrist B, K, P 🐾, 🐾, B 🐾
  - ● S62.153 Displaced fracture of hook process of hamate [unciform] bone, unspecified wrist B, K, P 🐾, 🐾, B 🐾
  - ● S62.154 Nondisplaced fracture of hook process of hamate [unciform] bone, right wrist B, K, P 🐾, 🐾, B 🐾
  - ● S62.155 Nondisplaced fracture of hook process of hamate [unciform] bone, left wrist B, K, P 🐾, 🐾, B 🐾
  - ● S62.156 Nondisplaced fracture of hook process of hamate [unciform] bone, unspecified wrist B, K, P 🐾, 🐾, B 🐾
- ● S62.16 Fracture of pisiform
  - ● S62.161 Displaced fracture of pisiform, right wrist B, K, P 🐾, 🐾, B 🐾
  - ● S62.162 Displaced fracture of pisiform, left wrist B, K, P 🐾, 🐾, B 🐾
  - ● S62.163 Displaced fracture of pisiform, unspecified wrist B, K, P 🐾, 🐾, B 🐾
  - ● S62.164 Nondisplaced fracture of pisiform, right wrist B, K, P 🐾, 🐾, B 🐾
  - ● S62.165 Nondisplaced fracture of pisiform, left wrist B, K, P 🐾, 🐾, B 🐾
  - ● S62.166 Nondisplaced fracture of pisiform, unspecified wrist B, K, P 🐾, 🐾, B 🐾
- ● S62.17 Fracture of trapezium [larger multangular]
  - ● S62.171 Displaced fracture of trapezium [larger multangular], right wrist B, K, P 🐾, 🐾, B 🐾
  - ● S62.172 Displaced fracture of trapezium [larger multangular], left wrist B, K, P 🐾, 🐾, B 🐾
  - ● S62.173 Displaced fracture of trapezium [larger multangular], unspecified wrist B, K, P 🐾, 🐾, B 🐾
  - ● S62.174 Nondisplaced fracture of trapezium [larger multangular], right wrist B, K, P 🐾, 🐾, B 🐾
  - ● S62.175 Nondisplaced fracture of trapezium [larger multangular], left wrist B, K, P 🐾, 🐾, B 🐾
  - ● S62.176 Nondisplaced fracture of trapezium [larger multangular], unspecified wrist B, K, P 🐾, 🐾, B 🐾

◀ New   ◀▥ Revised   ~~deleted~~ Deleted   Excludes 1   Excludes 2   Includes   Use additional   Code first   Code also   Unspecified

OGCR Official Guidelines   ● Unacceptable Principal Diagnosis   X Assign placeholder X   ▶ Use Additional Character(s)   ▶ Manifestation Code   **Coding Clinic**

● S62.18   Fracture of trapezoid [smaller multangular]

   ● S62.181   Displaced fracture of trapezoid [smaller multangular], right wrist B, K, P 🪙, 🪙, B 🪙

   ● S62.182   Displaced fracture of trapezoid [smaller multangular], left wrist B, K, P 🪙, 🪙, B 🪙

   ● S62.183   Displaced fracture of trapezoid [smaller multangular], unspecified wrist B, K, P 🪙, 🪙, B 🪙

   ● S62.184   Nondisplaced fracture of trapezoid [smaller multangular], right wrist B, K, P 🪙, 🪙, B 🪙

   ● S62.185   Nondisplaced fracture of trapezoid [smaller multangular], left wrist B, K, P 🪙, 🪙, B 🪙

   ● S62.186   Nondisplaced fracture of trapezoid [smaller multangular], unspecified wrist B, K, P 🪙, 🪙, B 🪙

● S62.2   Fracture of first metacarpal bone

   (Ex) For category S62.2 CC codes S62.2[B]: S62.201-S62.399[B], S62.90X[A]
   For S62.2[K,P]: See S62.0[K,P]

  ● S62.20   Unspecified fracture of first metacarpal bone

   ● S62.201   Unspecified fracture of first metacarpal bone, right hand B, K, P 🪙, 🪙, B 🪙

   ● S62.202   Unspecified fracture of first metacarpal bone, left hand B, K, P 🪙, 🪙, B 🪙

   ● S62.209   Unspecified fracture of first metacarpal bone, unspecified hand B, K, P 🪙, 🪙, B 🪙

  ● S62.21   Bennett's fracture

   ● S62.211   Bennett's fracture, right hand B, K, P 🪙, 🪙, B 🪙

   ● S62.212   Bennett's fracture, left hand B, K, P 🪙, 🪙, B 🪙

   ● S62.213   Bennett's fracture, unspecified hand B, K, P 🪙, 🪙, B 🪙

  ● S62.22   Rolando's fracture

   ● S62.221   Displaced Rolando's fracture, right hand B, K, P 🪙, 🪙, B 🪙

   ● S62.222   Displaced Rolando's fracture, left hand B, K, P 🪙, 🪙, B 🪙

   ● S62.223   Displaced Rolando's fracture, unspecified hand B, K, P 🪙, 🪙, B 🪙

   ● S62.224   Nondisplaced Rolando's fracture, right hand B, K, P 🪙, 🪙, B 🪙

   ● S62.225   Nondisplaced Rolando's fracture, left hand B, K, P 🪙, 🪙, B 🪙

   ● S62.226   Nondisplaced Rolando's fracture, unspecified hand B, K, P 🪙, 🪙, B 🪙

  ● S62.23   Other fracture of base of first metacarpal bone

   ● S62.231   Other displaced fracture of base of first metacarpal bone, right hand B, K, P 🪙, 🪙, B 🪙

   ● S62.232   Other displaced fracture of base of first metacarpal bone, left hand B, K, P 🪙, 🪙, B 🪙

   ● S62.233   Other displaced fracture of base of first metacarpal bone, unspecified hand B, K, P 🪙, 🪙, B 🪙

   ● S62.234   Other nondisplaced fracture of base of first metacarpal bone, right hand B, K, P 🪙, 🪙, B 🪙

   ● S62.235   Other nondisplaced fracture of base of first metacarpal bone, left hand B, K, P 🪙, 🪙, B 🪙

   ● S62.236   Other nondisplaced fracture of base of first metacarpal bone, unspecified hand B, K, P 🪙, 🪙, B 🪙

● S62.24   Fracture of shaft of first metacarpal bone

   ● S62.241   Displaced fracture of shaft of first metacarpal bone, right hand B, K, P 🪙, 🪙, B 🪙

   ● S62.242   Displaced fracture of shaft of first metacarpal bone, left hand B, K, P 🪙, 🪙, B 🪙

   ● S62.243   Displaced fracture of shaft of first metacarpal bone, unspecified hand B, K, P 🪙, 🪙, B 🪙

   ● S62.244   Nondisplaced fracture of shaft of first metacarpal bone, right hand B, K, P 🪙, 🪙, B 🪙

   ● S62.245   Nondisplaced fracture of shaft of first metacarpal bone, left hand B, K, P 🪙, 🪙, B 🪙

   ● S62.246   Nondisplaced fracture of shaft of first metacarpal bone, unspecified hand B, K, P 🪙, 🪙, B 🪙

● S62.25   Fracture of neck of first metacarpal bone

   ● S62.251   Displaced fracture of neck of first metacarpal bone, right hand B, K, P 🪙, 🪙, B 🪙

   ● S62.252   Displaced fracture of neck of first metacarpal bone, left hand B, K, P 🪙, 🪙, B 🪙

   ● S62.253   Displaced fracture of neck of first metacarpal bone, unspecified hand B, K, P 🪙, 🪙, B 🪙

   ● S62.254   Nondisplaced fracture of neck of first metacarpal bone, right hand B, K, P 🪙, 🪙, B 🪙

   ● S62.255   Nondisplaced fracture of neck of first metacarpal bone, left hand B, K, P 🪙, 🪙, B 🪙

   ● S62.256   Nondisplaced fracture of neck of first metacarpal bone, unspecified hand B, K, P 🪙, 🪙, B 🪙

  ● S62.29   Other fracture of first metacarpal bone

   ● S62.291   Other fracture of first metacarpal bone, right hand B, K, P 🪙, 🪙, B 🪙

   ● S62.292   Other fracture of first metacarpal bone, left hand B, K, P 🪙, 🪙, B 🪙

   ● S62.299   Other fracture of first metacarpal bone, unspecified hand B, K, P 🪙, 🪙, B 🪙

● S62.3   Fracture of other and unspecified metacarpal bone

   Excludes2   fracture of first metacarpal bone (S62.2-)

   (Ex) For category S62.3 CC codes S62.3[B]: See S62.2[B] For S62.3[K,P]: See S62.0[K,P]

  ● S62.30   Unspecified fracture of other metacarpal bone

   ● S62.300   Unspecified fracture of second metacarpal bone, right hand B, K, P 🪙, 🪙, B 🪙

   ● S62.301   Unspecified fracture of second metacarpal bone, left hand B, K, P 🪙, 🪙, B 🪙

   ● S62.302   Unspecified fracture of third metacarpal bone, right hand B, K, P 🪙, 🪙, B 🪙

   ● S62.303   Unspecified fracture of third metacarpal bone, left hand B, K, P 🪙, 🪙, B 🪙

   ● S62.304   Unspecified fracture of fourth metacarpal bone, right hand B, K, P 🪙, 🪙, B 🪙

   ● S62.305   Unspecified fracture of fourth metacarpal bone, left hand B, K, P 🪙, 🪙, B 🪙

N Newborn Age: 0   **P** Pediatric Age: 0–17   **M** Maternity DX: 12–55   **A** Adult Age: 15–124   ♀ Females Only   ♂ Males Only

🪙 Complication\Comorbidity   🪙 Major C\C   (Ex) CC/MCC Exclusions   🪙 Present on Admission Requirement   🪙 Hospital-Acquired Condition

1405

● S62.306   Unspecified fracture of fifth metacarpal bone, right hand B, K, P 🔹, 🔹, B 🔹

● S62.307   Unspecified fracture of fifth metacarpal bone, left hand B, K, P 🔹, 🔹, B 🔹

● S62.308   Unspecified fracture of other metacarpal bone B, K, P 🔹, 🔹, B 🔹
      Unspecified fracture of specified metacarpal bone with unspecified laterality

● S62.309   Unspecified fracture of unspecified metacarpal bone B, K, P 🔹, 🔹, B 🔹

● S62.31   Displaced fracture of base of other metacarpal bone

● S62.310   Displaced fracture of base of second metacarpal bone, right hand B, K, P 🔹, 🔹, B 🔹

● S62.311   Displaced fracture of base of second metacarpal bone, left hand B, K, P 🔹, 🔹, B 🔹

● S62.312   Displaced fracture of base of third metacarpal bone, right hand B, K, P 🔹, 🔹, B 🔹

● S62.313   Displaced fracture of base of third metacarpal bone, left hand B, K, P 🔹, 🔹, B 🔹

● S62.314   Displaced fracture of base of fourth metacarpal bone, right hand B, K, P 🔹, 🔹, B 🔹

● S62.315   Displaced fracture of base of fourth metacarpal bone, left hand B, K, P 🔹, 🔹, B 🔹

● S62.316   Displaced fracture of base of fifth metacarpal bone, right hand B, K, P 🔹, 🔹, B 🔹

● S62.317   Displaced fracture of base of fifth metacarpal bone, left hand B, K, P 🔹, 🔹, B 🔹

● S62.318   Displaced fracture of base of other metacarpal bone B, K, P 🔹, 🔹, B 🔹
      Displaced fracture of base of specified metacarpal bone with unspecified laterality

● S62.319   Displaced fracture of base of unspecified metacarpal bone B, K, P 🔹, 🔹, B 🔹

● S62.32   Displaced fracture of shaft of other metacarpal bone

● S62.320   Displaced fracture of shaft of second metacarpal bone, right hand B, K, P 🔹, 🔹, B 🔹

● S62.321   Displaced fracture of shaft of second metacarpal bone, left hand B, K, P 🔹, 🔹, B 🔹

● S62.322   Displaced fracture of shaft of third metacarpal bone, right hand B, K, P 🔹, 🔹, B 🔹

● S62.323   Displaced fracture of shaft of third metacarpal bone, left hand B, K, P 🔹, 🔹, B 🔹

● S62.324   Displaced fracture of shaft of fourth metacarpal bone, right hand B, K, P 🔹, 🔹, B 🔹

● S62.325   Displaced fracture of shaft of fourth metacarpal bone, left hand B, K, P 🔹, 🔹, B 🔹

● S62.326   Displaced fracture of shaft of fifth metacarpal bone, right hand B, K, P 🔹, 🔹, B 🔹

● S62.327   Displaced fracture of shaft of fifth metacarpal bone, left hand B, K, P 🔹, 🔹, B 🔹

● S62.328   Displaced fracture of shaft of other metacarpal bone B, K, P 🔹, 🔹, B 🔹
      Displaced fracture of shaft of specified metacarpal bone with unspecified laterality

● S62.329   Displaced fracture of shaft of unspecified metacarpal bone B, K, P 🔹, 🔹, B 🔹

● S62.33   Displaced fracture of neck of other metacarpal bone

● S62.330   Displaced fracture of neck of second metacarpal bone, right hand B, K, P 🔹, 🔹, B 🔹

● S62.331   Displaced fracture of neck of second metacarpal bone, left hand B, K, P 🔹, 🔹, B 🔹

● S62.332   Displaced fracture of neck of third metacarpal bone, right hand B, K, P 🔹, 🔹, B 🔹

● S62.333   Displaced fracture of neck of third metacarpal bone, left hand B, K, P 🔹, 🔹, B 🔹

● S62.334   Displaced fracture of neck of fourth metacarpal bone, right hand B, K, P 🔹, 🔹, B 🔹

● S62.335   Displaced fracture of neck of fourth metacarpal bone, left hand B, K, P 🔹, 🔹, B 🔹

● S62.336   Displaced fracture of neck of fifth metacarpal bone, right hand B, K, P 🔹, 🔹, B 🔹

● S62.337   Displaced fracture of neck of fifth metacarpal bone, left hand B, K, P 🔹, 🔹, B 🔹

● S62.338   Displaced fracture of neck of other metacarpal bone B, K, P 🔹, 🔹, B 🔹
      Displaced fracture of neck of specified metacarpal bone with unspecified laterality

● S62.339   Displaced fracture of neck of unspecified metacarpal bone B, K, P 🔹, 🔹, B 🔹

● S62.34   Nondisplaced fracture of base of other metacarpal bone

● S62.340   Nondisplaced fracture of base of second metacarpal bone, right hand B, K, P 🔹, 🔹, B 🔹

● S62.341   Nondisplaced fracture of base of second metacarpal bone, left hand B, K, P 🔹, 🔹, B 🔹

● S62.342   Nondisplaced fracture of base of third metacarpal bone, right hand B, K, P 🔹, 🔹, B 🔹

● S62.343   Nondisplaced fracture of base of third metacarpal bone, left hand B, K, P 🔹, 🔹, B 🔹

● S62.344   Nondisplaced fracture of base of fourth metacarpal bone, right hand B, K, P 🔹, 🔹, B 🔹

● S62.345   Nondisplaced fracture of base of fourth metacarpal bone, left hand B, K, P 🔹, 🔹, B 🔹

● S62.346   Nondisplaced fracture of base of fifth metacarpal bone, right hand B, K, P 🔹, 🔹, B 🔹

● S62.347   Nondisplaced fracture of base of fifth metacarpal bone, left hand B, K, P 🔹, 🔹, B 🔹

● S62.348 Nondisplaced fracture of base of other metacarpal bone B, K, P 🪙 🪙, B 🪙

    Nondisplaced fracture of base of specified metacarpal bone with unspecified laterality

● S62.349 Nondisplaced fracture of base of unspecified metacarpal bone B, K, P 🪙, 🪙, B 🪙

● S62.35 Nondisplaced fracture of shaft of other metacarpal bone

● S62.350 Nondisplaced fracture of shaft of second metacarpal bone, right hand B, K, P 🪙, 🪙, B 🪙

● S62.351 Nondisplaced fracture of shaft of second metacarpal bone, left hand B, K, P 🪙, 🪙, B 🪙

● S62.352 Nondisplaced fracture of shaft of third metacarpal bone, right hand B, K, P 🪙, 🪙, B 🪙

● S62.353 Nondisplaced fracture of shaft of third metacarpal bone, left hand B, K, P 🪙, 🪙, B 🪙

● S62.354 Nondisplaced fracture of shaft of fourth metacarpal bone, right hand B, K, P 🪙, 🪙, B 🪙

● S62.355 Nondisplaced fracture of shaft of fourth metacarpal bone, left hand B, K, P 🪙, 🪙, B 🪙

● S62.356 Nondisplaced fracture of shaft of fifth metacarpal bone, right hand B, K, P 🪙, 🪙, B 🪙

● S62.357 Nondisplaced fracture of shaft of fifth metacarpal bone, left hand B, K, P 🪙, 🪙, B 🪙

● S62.358 Nondisplaced fracture of shaft of other metacarpal bone B, K, P 🪙, 🪙, B 🪙

    Nondisplaced fracture of shaft of specified metacarpal bone with unspecified laterality

● S62.359 Nondisplaced fracture of shaft of unspecified metacarpal bone B, K, P 🪙, 🪙, B 🪙

● S62.36 Nondisplaced fracture of neck of other metacarpal bone

● S62.360 Nondisplaced fracture of neck of second metacarpal bone, right hand B, K, P 🪙, 🪙, B 🪙

● S62.361 Nondisplaced fracture of neck of second metacarpal bone, left hand B, K, P 🪙, 🪙, B 🪙

● S62.362 Nondisplaced fracture of neck of third metacarpal bone, right hand B, K, P 🪙, 🪙, B 🪙

● S62.363 Nondisplaced fracture of neck of third metacarpal bone, left hand B, K, P 🪙, 🪙, B 🪙

● S62.364 Nondisplaced fracture of neck of fourth metacarpal bone, right hand B, K, P 🪙, 🪙, B 🪙

● S62.365 Nondisplaced fracture of neck of fourth metacarpal bone, left hand B, K, P 🪙, 🪙, B 🪙

● S62.366 Nondisplaced fracture of neck of fifth metacarpal bone, right hand B, K, P 🪙, 🪙, B 🪙

● S62.367 Nondisplaced fracture of neck of fifth metacarpal bone, left hand B, K, P 🪙, 🪙, B 🪙

● S62.368 Nondisplaced fracture of neck of other metacarpal bone B, K, P 🪙 🪙, B 🪙

    Nondisplaced fracture of neck of specified metacarpal bone with unspecified laterality

● S62.369 Nondisplaced fracture of neck of unspecified metacarpal bone B, K, P 🪙, 🪙, B 🪙

● S62.39 Other fracture of other metacarpal bone

● S62.390 Other fracture of second metacarpal bone, right hand B, K, P 🪙, 🪙, B 🪙

● S62.391 Other fracture of second metacarpal bone, left hand B, K, P 🪙, 🪙, B 🪙

● S62.392 Other fracture of third metacarpal bone, right hand B, K, P 🪙, 🪙, B 🪙

● S62.393 Other fracture of third metacarpal bone, left hand B, K, P 🪙, 🪙, B 🪙

● S62.394 Other fracture of fourth metacarpal bone, right hand B, K, P 🪙, 🪙, B 🪙

● S62.395 Other fracture of fourth metacarpal bone, left hand B, K, P 🪙, 🪙, B 🪙

● S62.396 Other fracture of fifth metacarpal bone, right hand B, K, P 🪙, 🪙, B 🪙

● S62.397 Other fracture of fifth metacarpal bone, left hand B, K, P 🪙, 🪙, B 🪙

● S62.398 Other fracture of other metacarpal bone B, K, P 🪙, 🪙, B 🪙

    Other fracture of specified metacarpal bone with unspecified laterality

● S62.399 Other fracture of unspecified metacarpal bone B, K, P 🪙, 🪙, B 🪙

● S62.5 Fracture of thumb

    Ⓔˣ **For category S62.5 CC codes S62.5[B]:** S62.501-S62.669[A,B], S62.90X[A], S62.91X-S62.92X[A,B] **For S62.5[K,P]:** See S62.0[K,P]

● S62.50 Fracture of unspecified phalanx of thumb

● S62.501 Fracture of unspecified phalanx of right thumb B, K, P 🪙, 🪙, B 🪙

● S62.502 Fracture of unspecified phalanx of left thumb B, K, P 🪙, 🪙, B 🪙

● S62.509 Fracture of unspecified phalanx of unspecified thumb B, K, P 🪙, 🪙, B 🪙

● S62.51 Fracture of proximal phalanx of thumb

● S62.511 Displaced fracture of proximal phalanx of right thumb B, K, P 🪙, 🪙, B 🪙

● S62.512 Displaced fracture of proximal phalanx of left thumb B, K, P 🪙, 🪙, B 🪙

● S62.513 Displaced fracture of proximal phalanx of unspecified thumb B, K, P 🪙, 🪙, B 🪙

● S62.514 Nondisplaced fracture of proximal phalanx of right thumb B, K, P 🪙, 🪙, B 🪙

● S62.515 Nondisplaced fracture of proximal phalanx of left thumb B, K, P 🪙, 🪙, B 🪙

● S62.516 Nondisplaced fracture of proximal phalanx of unspecified thumb B, K, P 🪙, 🪙, B 🪙

● S62.52 Fracture of distal phalanx of thumb

● S62.521 Displaced fracture of distal phalanx of right thumb B, K, P 🪙, 🪙, B 🪙

● S62.522 Displaced fracture of distal phalanx of left thumb B, K, P 🪙, 🪙, B 🪙

N Newborn Age: 0   P Pediatric Age: 0–17   M Maternity DX: 12–55   A Adult Age: 15–124   ♀ Females Only   ♂ Males Only

🪙 Complication\Comorbidity   🪙 Major C\C   Ⓔˣ CC/MCC Exclusions   🪙 Present on Admission Requirement   🪙 Hospital-Acquired Condition

1407

CHAPTER 19 (S00-T88)

- S62.523   Displaced fracture of distal phalanx of unspecified thumb B, K, P 🔾, 🔾, B 🔾
- S62.524   Nondisplaced fracture of distal phalanx of right thumb B, K, P 🔾, 🔾, B 🔾
- S62.525   Nondisplaced fracture of distal phalanx of left thumb B, K, P 🔾, 🔾, B 🔾
- S62.526   Nondisplaced fracture of distal phalanx of unspecified thumb B, K, P 🔾, B 🔾

● S62.6   Fracture of other and unspecified finger(s)

     Excludes2   fracture of thumb (S62.5-)

     (Ex) **For category S62.6 CC codes S62.6[B]:** See S62.5[B] **For S62.5[K,P]:** See S62.0[K,P]

     ● S62.60   Fracture of unspecified phalanx of finger

- S62.600   Fracture of unspecified phalanx of right index finger B, K, P 🔾, 🔾, B 🔾
- S62.601   Fracture of unspecified phalanx of left index finger B, K, P 🔾, 🔾, B 🔾
- S62.602   Fracture of unspecified phalanx of right middle finger B, K, P 🔾, 🔾, B 🔾
- S62.603   Fracture of unspecified phalanx of left middle finger B, K, P 🔾, 🔾, B 🔾
- S62.604   Fracture of unspecified phalanx of right ring finger B, K, P 🔾, 🔾, B 🔾
- S62.605   Fracture of unspecified phalanx of left ring finger B, K, P 🔾, 🔾, B 🔾
- S62.606   Fracture of unspecified phalanx of right little finger B, K, P 🔾, 🔾, B 🔾
- S62.607   Fracture of unspecified phalanx of left little finger B, K, P 🔾, 🔾, B 🔾
- S62.608   Fracture of unspecified phalanx of other finger B, K, P 🔾, 🔾, B 🔾

     Fracture of unspecified phalanx of specified finger with unspecified laterality

- S62.609   Fracture of unspecified phalanx of unspecified finger B, K, P 🔾, 🔾, B 🔾

     ● S62.61   Displaced fracture of proximal phalanx of finger

- S62.610   Displaced fracture of proximal phalanx of right index finger B, K, P 🔾, 🔾, B 🔾
- S62.611   Displaced fracture of proximal phalanx of left index finger B, K, P 🔾, 🔾, B 🔾
- S62.612   Displaced fracture of proximal phalanx of right middle finger B, K, P 🔾, 🔾, B 🔾
- S62.613   Displaced fracture of proximal phalanx of left middle finger B, K, P 🔾, 🔾, B 🔾
- S62.614   Displaced fracture of proximal phalanx of right ring finger B, K, P 🔾, 🔾, B 🔾
- S62.615   Displaced fracture of proximal phalanx of left ring finger B, K, P 🔾, 🔾, B 🔾
- S62.616   Displaced fracture of proximal phalanx of right little finger B, K, P 🔾, 🔾, B 🔾
- S62.617   Displaced fracture of proximal phalanx of left little finger B, K, P 🔾, 🔾, B 🔾
- S62.618   Displaced fracture of proximal phalanx of other finger B, K, P 🔾, 🔾, B 🔾

     Displaced fracture of proximal phalanx of specified finger with unspecified laterality

- S62.619   Displaced fracture of proximal phalanx of unspecified finger B, K, P 🔾, 🔾, B 🔾

     ● S62.62   Displaced fracture of medial phalanx of finger

- S62.620   Displaced fracture of medial phalanx of right index finger B, K, P 🔾, 🔾, B 🔾
- S62.621   Displaced fracture of medial phalanx of left index finger B, K, P 🔾, 🔾, B 🔾
- S62.622   Displaced fracture of medial phalanx of right middle finger B, K, P 🔾, 🔾, B 🔾
- S62.623   Displaced fracture of medial phalanx of left middle finger B, K, P 🔾, 🔾, B 🔾
- S62.624   Displaced fracture of medial phalanx of right ring finger B, K, P 🔾, 🔾, B 🔾
- S62.625   Displaced fracture of medial phalanx of left ring finger B, K, P 🔾, 🔾, B 🔾
- S62.626   Displaced fracture of medial phalanx of right little finger B, K, P 🔾, 🔾, B 🔾
- S62.627   Displaced fracture of medial phalanx of left little finger B, K, P 🔾, 🔾, B 🔾
- S62.628   Displaced fracture of medial phalanx of other finger B, K, P 🔾, 🔾, B 🔾

     Displaced fracture of medial phalanx of specified finger with unspecified laterality

- S62.629   Displaced fracture of medial phalanx of unspecified finger B, K, P 🔾, 🔾, B 🔾

     ● S62.63   Displaced fracture of distal phalanx of finger

- S62.630   Displaced fracture of distal phalanx of right index finger B, K, P 🔾, 🔾, B 🔾
- S62.631   Displaced fracture of distal phalanx of left index finger B, K, P 🔾, 🔾, B 🔾
- S62.632   Displaced fracture of distal phalanx of right middle finger B, K, P 🔾, 🔾, B 🔾
- S62.633   Displaced fracture of distal phalanx of left middle finger B, K, P 🔾, 🔾, B 🔾
- S62.634   Displaced fracture of distal phalanx of right ring finger B, K, P 🔾, 🔾, B 🔾
- S62.635   Displaced fracture of distal phalanx of left ring finger B, K, P 🔾, 🔾, B 🔾
- S62.636   Displaced fracture of distal phalanx of right little finger B, K, P 🔾, 🔾, B 🔾
- S62.637   Displaced fracture of distal phalanx of left little finger B, K, P 🔾, 🔾, B 🔾
- S62.638   Displaced fracture of distal phalanx of other finger B, K, P 🔾, 🔾, B 🔾

     Displaced fracture of distal phalanx of specified finger with unspecified laterality

- S62.639   Displaced fracture of distal phalanx of unspecified finger B, K, P 🔾, B 🔾

● **S62.64   Nondisplaced fracture of proximal phalanx of finger**

　● **S62.640   Nondisplaced fracture of proximal phalanx of right index finger** B, K, P 🅲🅲, 🅼🅲, B 🅟

　● **S62.641   Nondisplaced fracture of proximal phalanx of left index finger** B, K, P 🅲🅲, 🅼🅲, B 🅟

　● **S62.642   Nondisplaced fracture of proximal phalanx of right middle finger** B, K, P 🅲🅲, 🅼🅲, B 🅟

　● **S62.643   Nondisplaced fracture of proximal phalanx of left middle finger** B, K, P 🅲🅲, 🅼🅲, B 🅟

　● **S62.644   Nondisplaced fracture of proximal phalanx of right ring finger** B, K, P 🅲🅲, 🅼🅲, B 🅟

　● **S62.645   Nondisplaced fracture of proximal phalanx of left ring finger** B, K, P 🅲🅲, 🅼🅲, B 🅟

　● **S62.646   Nondisplaced fracture of proximal phalanx of right little finger** B, K, P 🅲🅲, 🅼🅲, B 🅟

　● **S62.647   Nondisplaced fracture of proximal phalanx of left little finger** B, K, P 🅲🅲, 🅼🅲, B 🅟

　● **S62.648   Nondisplaced fracture of proximal phalanx of other finger** B, K, P 🅲🅲, 🅼🅲, B 🅟

　　　Nondisplaced fracture of proximal phalanx of specified finger with unspecified laterality

　● **S62.649   Nondisplaced fracture of proximal phalanx of unspecified finger** B, K, P 🅲🅲, 🅼🅲, B 🅟

● **S62.65   Nondisplaced fracture of medial phalanx of finger**

　● **S62.650   Nondisplaced fracture of medial phalanx of right index finger** B, K, P 🅲🅲, 🅼🅲, B 🅟

　● **S62.651   Nondisplaced fracture of medial phalanx of left index finger** B, K, P 🅲🅲, 🅼🅲, B 🅟

　● **S62.652   Nondisplaced fracture of medial phalanx of right middle finger** B, K, P 🅲🅲, 🅼🅲, B 🅟

　● **S62.653   Nondisplaced fracture of medial phalanx of left middle finger** B, K, P 🅲🅲, 🅼🅲, B 🅟

　● **S62.654   Nondisplaced fracture of medial phalanx of right ring finger** B, K, P 🅲🅲, 🅼🅲, B 🅟

　● **S62.655   Nondisplaced fracture of medial phalanx of left ring finger** B, K, P 🅲🅲, 🅼🅲, B 🅟

　● **S62.656   Nondisplaced fracture of medial phalanx of right little finger** B, K, P 🅲🅲, 🅼🅲, B 🅟

　● **S62.657   Nondisplaced fracture of medial phalanx of left little finger** B, K, P 🅲🅲, 🅼🅲, B 🅟

　● **S62.658   Nondisplaced fracture of medial phalanx of other finger** B, K, P 🅲🅲, 🅼🅲, B 🅟

　　　Nondisplaced fracture of medial phalanx of specified finger with unspecified laterality

　● **S62.659   Nondisplaced fracture of medial phalanx of unspecified finger** B, K, P 🅲🅲, 🅼🅲, B 🅟

● **S62.66   Nondisplaced fracture of distal phalanx of finger**

　● **S62.660   Nondisplaced fracture of distal phalanx of right index finger** B, K, P 🅲🅲, 🅼🅲, B 🅟

　● **S62.661   Nondisplaced fracture of distal phalanx of left index finger** B, K, P 🅲🅲, 🅼🅲, B 🅟

　● **S62.662   Nondisplaced fracture of distal phalanx of right middle finger** B, K, P 🅲🅲, 🅼🅲, B 🅟

　● **S62.663   Nondisplaced fracture of distal phalanx of left middle finger** B, K, P 🅲🅲, 🅼🅲, B 🅟

　● **S62.664   Nondisplaced fracture of distal phalanx of right ring finger** B, K, P 🅲🅲, 🅼🅲, B 🅟

　● **S62.665   Nondisplaced fracture of distal phalanx of left ring finger** B, K, P 🅲🅲, 🅼🅲, B 🅟

　● **S62.666   Nondisplaced fracture of distal phalanx of right little finger** B, K, P 🅲🅲, 🅼🅲, B 🅟

　● **S62.667   Nondisplaced fracture of distal phalanx of left little finger** B, K, P 🅲🅲, 🅼🅲, B 🅟

　● **S62.668   Nondisplaced fracture of distal phalanx of other finger** B, K, P 🅲🅲, 🅼🅲, B 🅟

　　　Nondisplaced fracture of distal phalanx of specified finger with unspecified laterality

　● **S62.669   Nondisplaced fracture of distal phalanx of unspecified finger** B, K, P 🅲🅲, 🅼🅲, B 🅟

● **S62.9   Unspecified fracture of wrist and hand**

　X● **S62.90   Unspecified fracture of unspecified wrist and hand** B, K, P 🅲🅲, 🅼🅲, B 🅟
　　　(Ex) **For S62.90[B]:** S42.201-S42.266[A,B], S42.271-S42.279[A], S42.291-S42.309[A,B], S42.311-S42.319[A], S42.321-S42.476[A,B], S42.481-S42.489[A], S42.491-S42.92X[A,B], S49.001-S49.199[A], S52.001-S52.009[A,B,C], S52.021-S52.109[A,B,C], S52.121-S52.209[A,B,C], S52.211-S52.219[A], S52.221-S52.309[A,B,C], S52.311-S52.319[A], S52.321-S52.616[A,B,C], S52.691-S52.92X[A,B,C], S59.001-S59.299[A], S62.001-S62.92X[A,B]
　　　For S62.90[K,P]: See S62.0[K,P]

　X● **S62.91   Unspecified fracture of right wrist and hand** B, K, P 🅲🅲, 🅼🅲, B 🅟
　　　(Ex) **For S62.91[B]:** S62.501-S62.669[A,B], S62.90X[B], S62.91X-S62.92X[A,B] **For S62.91[K,P]:** See S62.0[K,P]

　X● **S62.92   Unspecified fracture of left wrist and hand** B, K, P 🅲🅲, 🅼🅲, B 🅟
　　　(Ex) **For S62.92[B]:** S62.91[B] **For S62.92[K,P]:** See S62.0[K,P]

N Newborn Age: 0   **P** Pediatric Age: 0–17   **M** Maternity DX: 12–55   **A** Adult Age: 15–124   ♀ Females Only   ♂ Males Only

🅲🅲 Complication\Comorbidity   🅼🅲 Major C\C   (Ex) CC/MCC Exclusions   🅟 Present on Admission Requirement   🅗🅒 Hospital-Acquired Condition

1409

Figure 19-13   Dislocation including displacement and subluxation. (From Grainger & Allison's Diagnostic Radiology: A Textbook of Medical Imaging, ed 4, Churchill Livingstone, 2001)

● S63   **Dislocation and sprain of joints and ligaments at wrist and hand level**

     Includes   avulsion of joint or ligament at wrist and hand level

                 laceration of cartilage, joint or ligament at wrist and hand level

                 sprain of cartilage, joint or ligament at wrist and hand level

                 traumatic hemarthrosis of joint or ligament at wrist and hand level

                 traumatic rupture of joint or ligament at wrist and hand level

                 traumatic subluxation of joint or ligament at wrist and hand level

                 traumatic tear of joint or ligament at wrist and hand level

     Code also any associated open wound

     Excludes2   strain of muscle, fascia and tendon of wrist and hand (S66.-)

     The appropriate 7th character is to be added to each code from category S63

       A   initial encounter
       D   subsequent encounter
       S   sequela

   ● S63.0   **Subluxation and dislocation of wrist and hand joints**

     ● S63.00   **Unspecified subluxation and dislocation of wrist and hand**
           Dislocation of carpal bone NOS
           Dislocation of distal end of radius NOS
           Subluxation of carpal bone NOS
           Subluxation of distal end of radius NOS

       ● S63.001   **Unspecified** subluxation of right wrist and hand 🔍

       ● S63.002   **Unspecified** subluxation of left wrist and hand 🔍

       ● S63.003   **Unspecified** subluxation of unspecified wrist and hand 🔍

       ● S63.004   **Unspecified** dislocation of right wrist and hand 🔍

       ● S63.005   **Unspecified** dislocation of left wrist and hand 🔍

       ● S63.006   **Unspecified** dislocation of unspecified wrist and hand 🔍

     ● S63.01   **Subluxation and dislocation of distal radioulnar joint**

       ● S63.011   **Subluxation of distal radioulnar joint of right wrist** 🔍

       ● S63.012   **Subluxation of distal radioulnar joint of left wrist** 🔍

       ● S63.013   **Subluxation of distal radioulnar joint of unspecified wrist** 🔍

       ● S63.014   **Dislocation of distal radioulnar joint of right wrist** 🔍

       ● S63.015   **Dislocation of distal radioulnar joint of left wrist** 🔍

       ● S63.016   **Dislocation of distal radioulnar joint of unspecified wrist** 🔍

     ● S63.02   **Subluxation and dislocation of radiocarpal joint**

       ● S63.021   **Subluxation of radiocarpal joint of right wrist** 🔍

       ● S63.022   **Subluxation of radiocarpal joint of left wrist** 🔍

       ● S63.023   **Subluxation of radiocarpal joint of unspecified wrist** 🔍

       ● S63.024   **Dislocation of radiocarpal joint of right wrist** 🔍

       ● S63.025   **Dislocation of radiocarpal joint of left wrist** 🔍

       ● S63.026   **Dislocation of radiocarpal joint of unspecified wrist** 🔍

     ● S63.03   **Subluxation and dislocation of midcarpal joint**

       ● S63.031   **Subluxation of midcarpal joint of right wrist** 🔍

       ● S63.032   **Subluxation of midcarpal joint of left wrist** 🔍

       ● S63.033   **Subluxation of midcarpal joint of unspecified wrist** 🔍

       ● S63.034   **Dislocation of midcarpal joint of right wrist** 🔍

       ● S63.035   **Dislocation of midcarpal joint of left wrist** 🔍

       ● S63.036   **Dislocation of midcarpal joint of unspecified wrist** 🔍

     ● S63.04   **Subluxation and dislocation of carpometacarpal joint of thumb**

       Excludes2   interphalangeal subluxation and dislocation of thumb (S63.1-)

       ● S63.041   **Subluxation of carpometacarpal joint of right thumb** 🔍

       ● S63.042   **Subluxation of carpometacarpal joint of left thumb** 🔍

       ● S63.043   **Subluxation of carpometacarpal joint of unspecified thumb** 🔍

       ● S63.044   **Dislocation of carpometacarpal joint of right thumb** 🔍

       ● S63.045   **Dislocation of carpometacarpal joint of left thumb** 🔍

       ● S63.046   **Dislocation of carpometacarpal joint of unspecified thumb** 🔍

     ● S63.05   **Subluxation and dislocation of other carpometacarpal joint**

       Excludes2   subluxation and dislocation of carpometacarpal joint of thumb (S63.04-)

       ● S63.051   **Subluxation of other carpometacarpal joint of right hand** 🔍

       ● S63.052   **Subluxation of other carpometacarpal joint of left hand** 🔍

       ● S63.053   **Subluxation of other carpometacarpal joint of unspecified hand** 🔍

       ● S63.054   **Dislocation of other carpometacarpal joint of right hand** 🔍

       ● S63.055   **Dislocation of other carpometacarpal joint of left hand** 🔍

       ● S63.056   **Dislocation of other carpometacarpal joint of unspecified hand** 🔍

◀ New   ◀▥ Revised   ~~deleted~~ Deleted   Excludes 1   Excludes 2   Includes   Use additional   Code first   Code also   Unspecified

OGCR Official Guidelines   ● Unacceptable Principal Diagnosis   X Assign placeholder X   ▶ Use Additional Character(s)   ▌ Manifestation Code   **Coding Clinic**

1410

● S63.06   Subluxation and dislocation of metacarpal (bone), proximal end
   ● S63.061   Subluxation of metacarpal (bone), proximal end of right hand ✎
   ● S63.062   Subluxation of metacarpal (bone), proximal end of left hand ✎
   ● S63.063   Subluxation of metacarpal (bone), proximal end of unspecified hand ✎
   ● S63.064   Dislocation of metacarpal (bone), proximal end of right hand ✎
   ● S63.065   Dislocation of metacarpal (bone), proximal end of left hand ✎
   ● S63.066   Dislocation of metacarpal (bone), proximal end of unspecified hand ✎

● S63.07   Subluxation and dislocation of distal end of ulna
   ● S63.071   Subluxation of distal end of right ulna ✎
   ● S63.072   Subluxation of distal end of left ulna ✎
   ● S63.073   Subluxation of distal end of unspecified ulna ✎
   ● S63.074   Dislocation of distal end of right ulna ✎
   ● S63.075   Dislocation of distal end of left ulna ✎
   ● S63.076   Dislocation of distal end of unspecified ulna ✎

● S63.09   Other subluxation and dislocation of wrist and hand
   ● S63.091   Other subluxation of right wrist and hand ✎
   ● S63.092   Other subluxation of left wrist and hand ✎
   ● S63.093   Other subluxation of unspecified wrist and hand ✎
   ● S63.094   Other dislocation of right wrist and hand ✎
   ● S63.095   Other dislocation of left wrist and hand ✎
   ● S63.096   Other dislocation of unspecified wrist and hand ✎

● S63.1   Subluxation and dislocation of thumb
  ● S63.10   Unspecified subluxation and dislocation of thumb
   ● S63.101   Unspecified subluxation of right thumb ✎
   ● S63.102   Unspecified subluxation of left thumb ✎
   ● S63.103   Unspecified subluxation of unspecified thumb ✎
   ● S63.104   Unspecified dislocation of right thumb ✎
   ● S63.105   Unspecified dislocation of left thumb ✎
   ● S63.106   Unspecified dislocation of unspecified thumb ✎

  ● S63.11   Subluxation and dislocation of metacarpophalangeal joint of thumb
   ● S63.111   Subluxation of metacarpophalangeal joint of right thumb ✎
   ● S63.112   Subluxation of metacarpophalangeal joint of left thumb ✎
   ● S63.113   Subluxation of metacarpophalangeal joint of unspecified thumb ✎
   ● S63.114   Dislocation of metacarpophalangeal joint of right thumb ✎
   ● S63.115   Dislocation of metacarpophalangeal joint of left thumb ✎
   ● S63.116   Dislocation of metacarpophalangeal joint of unspecified thumb ✎

● S63.12   Subluxation and dislocation of unspecified interphalangeal joint of thumb
   ● S63.121   Subluxation of unspecified interphalangeal joint of right thumb ✎
   ● S63.122   Subluxation of unspecified interphalangeal joint of left thumb ✎
   ● S63.123   Subluxation of unspecified interphalangeal joint of unspecified thumb ✎
   ● S63.124   Dislocation of unspecified interphalangeal joint of right thumb ✎
   ● S63.125   Dislocation of unspecified interphalangeal joint of left thumb ✎
   ● S63.126   Dislocation of unspecified interphalangeal joint of unspecified thumb ✎

● S63.13   Subluxation and dislocation of proximal interphalangeal joint of thumb
   ● S63.131   Subluxation of proximal interphalangeal joint of right thumb ✎
   ● S63.132   Subluxation of proximal interphalangeal joint of left thumb ✎
   ● S63.133   Subluxation of proximal interphalangeal joint of unspecified thumb ✎
   ● S63.134   Dislocation of proximal interphalangeal joint of right thumb ✎
   ● S63.135   Dislocation of proximal interphalangeal joint of left thumb ✎
   ● S63.136   Dislocation of proximal interphalangeal joint of unspecified thumb ✎

● S63.14   Subluxation and dislocation of distal interphalangeal joint of thumb
   ● S63.141   Subluxation of distal interphalangeal joint of right thumb ✎
   ● S63.142   Subluxation of distal interphalangeal joint of left thumb ✎
   ● S63.143   Subluxation of distal interphalangeal joint of unspecified thumb ✎
   ● S63.144   Dislocation of distal interphalangeal joint of right thumb ✎
   ● S63.145   Dislocation of distal interphalangeal joint of left thumb ✎
   ● S63.146   Dislocation of distal interphalangeal joint of unspecified thumb ✎

● S63.2   Subluxation and dislocation of other finger(s)
  Excludes2   subluxation and dislocation of thumb (S63.1-)
  ● S63.20   Unspecified subluxation of other finger
   ● S63.200   Unspecified subluxation of right index finger ✎
   ● S63.201   Unspecified subluxation of left index finger ✎
   ● S63.202   Unspecified subluxation of right middle finger ✎
   ● S63.203   Unspecified subluxation of left middle finger ✎
   ● S63.204   Unspecified subluxation of right ring finger ✎
   ● S63.205   Unspecified subluxation of left ring finger ✎
   ● S63.206   Unspecified subluxation of right little finger ✎
   ● S63.207   Unspecified subluxation of left little finger ✎

CHAPTER 19 (S00–T88)

N   Newborn Age: 0   P   Pediatric Age: 0–17   M   Maternity DX: 12–55   A   Adult Age: 15–124   ♀   Females Only   ♂   Males Only

✎ Complication\Comorbidity   ✎ Major C\C   (Exc) CC/MCC Exclusions   ✎ Present on Admission Requirement   ✎ Hospital-Acquired Condition

1411

● S63.208 **Unspecified** subluxation of other
          finger 🖐
          Unspecified subluxation of specified
          finger with unspecified
          laterality
● S63.209 **Unspecified** subluxation of
          unspecified finger 🖐
● S63.21 Subluxation of metacarpophalangeal joint of
         finger
● S63.210 Subluxation of metacarpophalangeal
          joint of right index finger 🖐
● S63.211 Subluxation of metacarpophalangeal
          joint of left index finger 🖐
● S63.212 Subluxation of metacarpophalangeal
          joint of right middle finger 🖐
● S63.213 Subluxation of metacarpophalangeal
          joint of left middle finger 🖐
● S63.214 Subluxation of metacarpophalangeal
          joint of right ring finger 🖐
● S63.215 Subluxation of metacarpophalangeal
          joint of left ring finger 🖐
● S63.216 Subluxation of metacarpophalangeal
          joint of right little finger 🖐
● S63.217 Subluxation of metacarpophalangeal
          joint of left little finger 🖐
● S63.218 Subluxation of metacarpophalangeal
          joint of other finger 🖐
          Subluxation of metacarpophalangeal
          joint of specified finger with
          unspecified laterality
● S63.219 Subluxation of metacarpophalangeal
          joint of **unspecified** finger 🖐
● S63.22 Subluxation of unspecified interphalangeal
         joint of finger
● S63.220 Subluxation of **unspecified**
          interphalangeal joint of right index
          finger 🖐
● S63.221 Subluxation of **unspecified**
          interphalangeal joint of left index
          finger 🖐
● S63.222 Subluxation of **unspecified**
          interphalangeal joint of right middle
          finger 🖐
● S63.223 Subluxation of **unspecified**
          interphalangeal joint of left middle
          finger 🖐
● S63.224 Subluxation of **unspecified**
          interphalangeal joint of right ring
          finger 🖐
● S63.225 Subluxation of **unspecified**
          interphalangeal joint of left ring
          finger 🖐
● S63.226 Subluxation of **unspecified**
          interphalangeal joint of right little
          finger 🖐
● S63.227 Subluxation of **unspecified**
          interphalangeal joint of left little
          finger 🖐
● S63.228 Subluxation of **unspecified**
          interphalangeal joint of other
          finger 🖐
          Subluxation of unspecified
          interphalangeal joint
          of specified finger with
          unspecified laterality
● S63.229 Subluxation of **unspecified**
          interphalangeal joint of unspecified
          finger 🖐

● S63.23 Subluxation of proximal interphalangeal joint
         of finger
● S63.230 Subluxation of proximal
          interphalangeal joint of right index
          finger 🖐
● S63.231 Subluxation of proximal
          interphalangeal joint of left index
          finger 🖐
● S63.232 Subluxation of proximal
          interphalangeal joint of right middle
          finger 🖐
● S63.233 Subluxation of proximal
          interphalangeal joint of left middle
          finger 🖐
● S63.234 Subluxation of proximal
          interphalangeal joint of right ring
          finger 🖐
● S63.235 Subluxation of proximal
          interphalangeal joint of left ring
          finger 🖐
● S63.236 Subluxation of proximal
          interphalangeal joint of right little
          finger 🖐
● S63.237 Subluxation of proximal
          interphalangeal joint of left little
          finger 🖐
● S63.238 Subluxation of proximal
          interphalangeal joint of other
          finger 🖐
          Subluxation of proximal
          interphalangeal joint
          of specified finger with
          unspecified laterality
● S63.239 Subluxation of proximal
          interphalangeal joint of **unspecified**
          finger 🖐
● S63.24 Subluxation of distal interphalangeal joint of
         finger
● S63.240 Subluxation of distal interphalangeal
          joint of right index finger 🖐
● S63.241 Subluxation of distal interphalangeal
          joint of left index finger 🖐
● S63.242 Subluxation of distal interphalangeal
          joint of right middle finger 🖐
● S63.243 Subluxation of distal interphalangeal
          joint of left middle finger 🖐
● S63.244 Subluxation of distal interphalangeal
          joint of right ring finger 🖐
● S63.245 Subluxation of distal interphalangeal
          joint of left ring finger 🖐
● S63.246 Subluxation of distal interphalangeal
          joint of right little finger 🖐
● S63.247 Subluxation of distal interphalangeal
          joint of left little finger 🖐
● S63.248 Subluxation of distal interphalangeal
          joint of other finger 🖐
          Subluxation of distal interphalangeal
          joint of specified finger with
          unspecified laterality
● S63.249 Subluxation of distal interphalangeal
          joint of **unspecified** finger 🖐
● S63.25 Unspecified dislocation of other finger
● S63.250 **Unspecified** dislocation of right index
          finger 🖐
● S63.251 **Unspecified** dislocation of left index
          finger 🖐
● S63.252 **Unspecified** dislocation of right
          middle finger 🖐

◀ New   ◀▥ Revised   ~~deleted~~ Deleted   Excludes 1   Excludes 2   Includes   Use additional   Code first   Code also   Unspecified
OGCR Official Guidelines   ● Unacceptable Principal Diagnosis   X Assign placeholder X   ● Use Additional Character(s)   ▶ Manifestation Code   Coding Clinic

● S63.253   Unspecified dislocation of left middle finger 🔍

● S63.254   Unspecified dislocation of right ring finger 🔍

● S63.255   Unspecified dislocation of left ring finger 🔍

● S63.256   Unspecified dislocation of right little finger 🔍

● S63.257   Unspecified dislocation of left little finger 🔍

● S63.258   Unspecified dislocation of other finger 🔍
             Unspecified dislocation of specified finger with unspecified laterality

● S63.259   Unspecified dislocation of unspecified finger 🔍
             Unspecified dislocation of specified finger with unspecified laterality

● S63.26   Dislocation of metacarpophalangeal joint of finger

● S63.260   Dislocation of metacarpophalangeal joint of right index finger 🔍

● S63.261   Dislocation of metacarpophalangeal joint of left index finger 🔍

● S63.262   Dislocation of metacarpophalangeal joint of right middle finger 🔍

● S63.263   Dislocation of metacarpophalangeal joint of left middle finger 🔍

● S63.264   Dislocation of metacarpophalangeal joint of right ring finger 🔍

● S63.265   Dislocation of metacarpophalangeal joint of left ring finger 🔍

● S63.266   Dislocation of metacarpophalangeal joint of right little finger 🔍

● S63.267   Dislocation of metacarpophalangeal joint of left little finger 🔍

● S63.268   Dislocation of metacarpophalangeal joint of other finger 🔍
             Dislocation of metacarpophalangeal joint of specified finger with unspecified laterality

● S63.269   Dislocation of metacarpophalangeal joint of unspecified finger 🔍

● S63.27   Dislocation of unspecified interphalangeal joint of finger

● S63.270   Dislocation of unspecified interphalangeal joint of right index finger 🔍

● S63.271   Dislocation of unspecified interphalangeal joint of left index finger 🔍

● S63.272   Dislocation of unspecified interphalangeal joint of right middle finger 🔍

● S63.273   Dislocation of unspecified interphalangeal joint of left middle finger 🔍

● S63.274   Dislocation of unspecified interphalangeal joint of right ring finger 🔍

● S63.275   Dislocation of unspecified interphalangeal joint of left ring finger 🔍

● S63.276   Dislocation of unspecified interphalangeal joint of right little finger 🔍

● S63.277   Dislocation of unspecified interphalangeal joint of left little finger 🔍

● S63.278   Dislocation of unspecified interphalangeal joint of other finger 🔍
             Dislocation of unspecified interphalangeal joint of specified finger with unspecified laterality

● S63.279   Dislocation of unspecified interphalangeal joint of unspecified finger 🔍
             Dislocation of unspecified interphalangeal joint of specified finger without specified laterality

● S63.28   Dislocation of proximal interphalangeal joint of finger

● S63.280   Dislocation of proximal interphalangeal joint of right index finger 🔍

● S63.281   Dislocation of proximal interphalangeal joint of left index finger 🔍

● S63.282   Dislocation of proximal interphalangeal joint of right middle finger 🔍

● S63.283   Dislocation of proximal interphalangeal joint of left middle finger 🔍

● S63.284   Dislocation of proximal interphalangeal joint of right ring finger 🔍

● S63.285   Dislocation of proximal interphalangeal joint of left ring finger 🔍

● S63.286   Dislocation of proximal interphalangeal joint of right little finger 🔍

● S63.287   Dislocation of proximal interphalangeal joint of left little finger 🔍

● S63.288   Dislocation of proximal interphalangeal joint of other finger 🔍
             Dislocation of proximal interphalangeal joint of specified finger with unspecified laterality

● S63.289   Dislocation of proximal interphalangeal joint of unspecified finger 🔍

● S63.29   Dislocation of distal interphalangeal joint of finger

● S63.290   Dislocation of distal interphalangeal joint of right index finger 🔍

● S63.291   Dislocation of distal interphalangeal joint of left index finger 🔍

● S63.292   Dislocation of distal interphalangeal joint of right middle finger 🔍

● S63.293   Dislocation of distal interphalangeal joint of left middle finger 🔍

● S63.294   Dislocation of distal interphalangeal joint of right ring finger 🔍

● S63.295   Dislocation of distal interphalangeal joint of left ring finger 🔍

● S63.296   Dislocation of distal interphalangeal joint of right little finger 🔍

CHAPTER 19 (S00–T88)

N Newborn Age: 0   **P** Pediatric Age: 0–17   **M** Maternity DX: 12–55   **A** Adult Age: 15–124   ♀ Females Only   ♂ Males Only

🔍 Complication\Comorbidity   🔍 Major C\C   (Ex) CC/MCC Exclusions   🔍 Present on Admission Requirement   🔍 Hospital-Acquired Condition

1413

S63.297 Dislocation of distal interphalangeal joint of left little finger 🔍

S63.298 Dislocation of distal interphalangeal joint of other finger 🔍
> Dislocation of distal interphalangeal joint of specified finger with unspecified laterality

S63.299 Dislocation of distal interphalangeal joint of unspecified finger 🔍

● **S63.3** Traumatic rupture of ligament of wrist

● **S63.30** Traumatic rupture of unspecified ligament of wrist

S63.301 Traumatic rupture of unspecified ligament of right wrist 🔍

S63.302 Traumatic rupture of unspecified ligament of left wrist 🔍

S63.309 Traumatic rupture of unspecified ligament of unspecified wrist 🔍

● **S63.31** Traumatic rupture of collateral ligament of wrist

S63.311 Traumatic rupture of collateral ligament of right wrist 🔍

S63.312 Traumatic rupture of collateral ligament of left wrist 🔍

S63.319 Traumatic rupture of collateral ligament of unspecified wrist 🔍

● **S63.32** Traumatic rupture of radiocarpal ligament

S63.321 Traumatic rupture of right radiocarpal ligament 🔍

S63.322 Traumatic rupture of left radiocarpal ligament 🔍

S63.329 Traumatic rupture of unspecified radiocarpal ligament 🔍

● **S63.33** Traumatic rupture of ulnocarpal (palmar) ligament

S63.331 Traumatic rupture of right ulnocarpal (palmar) ligament 🔍

S63.332 Traumatic rupture of left ulnocarpal (palmar) ligament 🔍

S63.339 Traumatic rupture of unspecified ulnocarpal (palmar) ligament 🔍

● **S63.39** Traumatic rupture of other ligament of wrist

S63.391 Traumatic rupture of other ligament of right wrist 🔍

S63.392 Traumatic rupture of other ligament of left wrist 🔍

S63.399 Traumatic rupture of other ligament of unspecified wrist 🔍

● **S63.4** Traumatic rupture of ligament of finger at metacarpophalangeal and interphalangeal joint(s)

● **S63.40** Traumatic rupture of unspecified ligament of finger at metacarpophalangeal and interphalangeal joint

S63.400 Traumatic rupture of unspecified ligament of right index finger at metacarpophalangeal and interphalangeal joint 🔍

S63.401 Traumatic rupture of unspecified ligament of left index finger at metacarpophalangeal and interphalangeal joint 🔍

S63.402 Traumatic rupture of unspecified ligament of right middle finger at metacarpophalangeal and interphalangeal joint 🔍

S63.403 Traumatic rupture of unspecified ligament of left middle finger at metacarpophalangeal and interphalangeal joint 🔍

S63.404 Traumatic rupture of unspecified ligament of right ring finger at metacarpophalangeal and interphalangeal joint 🔍

S63.405 Traumatic rupture of unspecified ligament of left ring finger at metacarpophalangeal and interphalangeal joint 🔍

S63.406 Traumatic rupture of unspecified ligament of right little finger at metacarpophalangeal and interphalangeal joint 🔍

S63.407 Traumatic rupture of unspecified ligament of left little finger at metacarpophalangeal and interphalangeal joint 🔍

S63.408 Traumatic rupture of unspecified ligament of other finger at metacarpophalangeal and interphalangeal joint 🔍
> Traumatic rupture of unspecified ligament of specified finger with unspecified laterality at metacarpophalangeal and interphalangeal joint

S63.409 Traumatic rupture of unspecified ligament of unspecified finger at metacarpophalangeal and interphalangeal joint 🔍

● **S63.41** Traumatic rupture of collateral ligament of finger at metacarpophalangeal and interphalangeal joint

S63.410 Traumatic rupture of collateral ligament of right index finger at metacarpophalangeal and interphalangeal joint 🔍

S63.411 Traumatic rupture of collateral ligament of left index finger at metacarpophalangeal and interphalangeal joint 🔍

S63.412 Traumatic rupture of collateral ligament of right middle finger at metacarpophalangeal and interphalangeal joint 🔍

S63.413 Traumatic rupture of collateral ligament of left middle finger at metacarpophalangeal and interphalangeal joint 🔍

S63.414 Traumatic rupture of collateral ligament of right ring finger at metacarpophalangeal and interphalangeal joint 🔍

S63.415 Traumatic rupture of collateral ligament of left ring finger at metacarpophalangeal and interphalangeal joint 🔍

S63.416 Traumatic rupture of collateral ligament of right little finger at metacarpophalangeal and interphalangeal joint 🔍

S63.417 Traumatic rupture of collateral ligament of left little finger at metacarpophalangeal and interphalangeal joint 🔍

● S63.418   Traumatic rupture of collateral ligament of other finger at metacarpophalangeal and interphalangeal joint ✇
     Traumatic rupture of collateral ligament of specified finger with unspecified laterality at metacarpophalangeal and interphalangeal joint

● S63.419   Traumatic rupture of collateral ligament of unspecified finger at metacarpophalangeal and interphalangeal joint ✇

● S63.42   Traumatic rupture of palmar ligament of finger at metacarpophalangeal and interphalangeal joint

● S63.420   Traumatic rupture of palmar ligament of right index finger at metacarpophalangeal and interphalangeal joint ✇

● S63.421   Traumatic rupture of palmar ligament of left index finger at metacarpophalangeal and interphalangeal joint ✇

● S63.422   Traumatic rupture of palmar ligament of right middle finger at metacarpophalangeal and interphalangeal joint ✇

● S63.423   Traumatic rupture of palmar ligament of left middle finger at metacarpophalangeal and interphalangeal joint ✇

● S63.424   Traumatic rupture of palmar ligament of right ring finger at metacarpophalangeal and interphalangeal joint ✇

● S63.425   Traumatic rupture of palmar ligament of left ring finger at metacarpophalangeal and interphalangeal joint ✇

● S63.426   Traumatic rupture of palmar ligament of right little finger at metacarpophalangeal and interphalangeal joint ✇

● S63.427   Traumatic rupture of palmar ligament of left little finger at metacarpophalangeal and interphalangeal joint ✇

● S63.428   Traumatic rupture of palmar ligament of other finger at metacarpophalangeal and interphalangeal joint ✇
     Traumatic rupture of palmar ligament of specified finger with unspecified laterality at metacarpophalangeal and interphalangeal joint

● S63.429   Traumatic rupture of palmar ligament of unspecified finger at metacarpophalangeal and interphalangeal joint ✇

● S63.43   Traumatic rupture of volar plate of finger at metacarpophalangeal and interphalangeal joint

● S63.430   Traumatic rupture of volar plate of right index finger at metacarpophalangeal and interphalangeal joint ✇

● S63.431   Traumatic rupture of volar plate of left index finger at metacarpophalangeal and interphalangeal joint ✇

● S63.432   Traumatic rupture of volar plate of right middle finger at metacarpophalangeal and interphalangeal joint ✇

● S63.433   Traumatic rupture of volar plate of left middle finger at metacarpophalangeal and interphalangeal joint ✇

● S63.434   Traumatic rupture of volar plate of right ring finger at metacarpophalangeal and interphalangeal joint ✇

● S63.435   Traumatic rupture of volar plate of left ring finger at metacarpophalangeal and interphalangeal joint ✇

● S63.436   Traumatic rupture of volar plate of right little finger at metacarpophalangeal and interphalangeal joint ✇

● S63.437   Traumatic rupture of volar plate of left little finger at metacarpophalangeal and interphalangeal joint ✇

● S63.438   Traumatic rupture of volar plate of other finger at metacarpophalangeal and interphalangeal joint ✇
     Traumatic rupture of volar plate of specified finger with unspecified laterality at metacarpophalangeal and interphalangeal joint

● S63.439   Traumatic rupture of volar plate of unspecified finger at metacarpophalangeal and interphalangeal joint ✇

● S63.49   Traumatic rupture of other ligament of finger at metacarpophalangeal and interphalangeal joint

● S63.490   Traumatic rupture of other ligament of right index finger at metacarpophalangeal and interphalangeal joint ✇

● S63.491   Traumatic rupture of other ligament of left index finger at metacarpophalangeal and interphalangeal joint ✇

● S63.492   Traumatic rupture of other ligament of right middle finger at metacarpophalangeal and interphalangeal joint ✇

● S63.493   Traumatic rupture of other ligament of left middle finger at metacarpophalangeal and interphalangeal joint ✇

● S63.494   Traumatic rupture of other ligament of right ring finger at metacarpophalangeal and interphalangeal joint ✇

● S63.495   Traumatic rupture of other ligament of left ring finger at metacarpophalangeal and interphalangeal joint ✇

● S63.496   Traumatic rupture of other ligament of right little finger at metacarpophalangeal and interphalangeal joint ✇

● S63.497   Traumatic rupture of other ligament of left little finger at metacarpophalangeal and interphalangeal joint ✇

N   Newborn Age: 0   P   Pediatric Age: 0–17   M   Maternity DX: 12–55   A   Adult Age: 15–124   ♀   Females Only   ♂   Males Only

✇ Complication\Comorbidity   ✇ Major C\C   (Ex) CC/MCC Exclusions   ✇ Present on Admission Requirement   ✇ Hospital-Acquired Condition   **1415**

● S63.498   **Traumatic rupture of other ligament of other finger at metacarpophalangeal and interphalangeal joint** 🔍
    Traumatic rupture of ligament of specified finger with unspecified laterality at metacarpophalangeal and interphalangeal joint

● S63.499   **Traumatic rupture of other ligament of unspecified finger at metacarpophalangeal and interphalangeal joint** 🔍

● S63.5   Other and unspecified sprain of wrist

   ● S63.50   Unspecified sprain of wrist

     ● S63.501   Unspecified sprain of right wrist 🔍

     ● S63.502   Unspecified sprain of left wrist 🔍

     ● S63.509   Unspecified sprain of unspecified wrist 🔍

   ● S63.51   Sprain of carpal (joint)

     ● S63.511   Sprain of carpal joint of right wrist 🔍

     ● S63.512   Sprain of carpal joint of left wrist 🔍

     ● S63.519   Sprain of carpal joint of unspecified wrist 🔍

   ● S63.52   Sprain of radiocarpal joint

     Excludes1   traumatic rupture of radiocarpal ligament (S63.32-)

     ● S63.521   Sprain of radiocarpal joint of right wrist 🔍

     ● S63.522   Sprain of radiocarpal joint of left wrist 🔍

     ● S63.529   Sprain of radiocarpal joint of unspecified wrist 🔍

   ● S63.59   Other specified sprain of wrist

     ● S63.591   Other specified sprain of right wrist 🔍

     ● S63.592   Other specified sprain of left wrist 🔍

     ● S63.599   Other specified sprain of unspecified wrist 🔍

● S63.6   Other and unspecified sprain of finger(s)

    Excludes1   traumatic rupture of ligament of finger at metacarpophalangeal and interphalangeal joint(s) (S63.4-)

   ● S63.60   Unspecified sprain of thumb

     ● S63.601   Unspecified sprain of right thumb 🔍

     ● S63.602   Unspecified sprain of left thumb 🔍

     ● S63.609   Unspecified sprain of unspecified thumb 🔍

   ● S63.61   Unspecified sprain of other and unspecified finger(s)

     ● S63.610   Unspecified sprain of right index finger 🔍

     ● S63.611   Unspecified sprain of left index finger 🔍

     ● S63.612   Unspecified sprain of right middle finger 🔍

     ● S63.613   Unspecified sprain of left middle finger 🔍

     ● S63.614   Unspecified sprain of right ring finger 🔍

     ● S63.615   Unspecified sprain of left ring finger 🔍

     ● S63.616   Unspecified sprain of right little finger 🔍

     ● S63.617   Unspecified sprain of left little finger 🔍

● S63.618   Unspecified sprain of other finger 🔍
    Unspecified sprain of specified finger with unspecified laterality

● S63.619   Unspecified sprain of unspecified finger 🔍

● S63.62   Sprain of interphalangeal joint of thumb

     ● S63.621   Sprain of interphalangeal joint of right thumb 🔍

     ● S63.622   Sprain of interphalangeal joint of left thumb 🔍

     ● S63.629   Sprain of interphalangeal joint of unspecified thumb 🔍

● S63.63   Sprain of interphalangeal joint of other and unspecified finger(s)

     ● S63.630   Sprain of interphalangeal joint of right index finger 🔍

     ● S63.631   Sprain of interphalangeal joint of left index finger 🔍

     ● S63.632   Sprain of interphalangeal joint of right middle finger 🔍

     ● S63.633   Sprain of interphalangeal joint of left middle finger 🔍

     ● S63.634   Sprain of interphalangeal joint of right ring finger 🔍

     ● S63.635   Sprain of interphalangeal joint of left ring finger 🔍

     ● S63.636   Sprain of interphalangeal joint of right little finger 🔍

     ● S63.637   Sprain of interphalangeal joint of left little finger 🔍

     ● S63.638   Sprain of interphalangeal joint of other finger 🔍

     ● S63.639   Sprain of interphalangeal joint of unspecified finger 🔍

● S63.64   Sprain of metacarpophalangeal joint of thumb

     ● S63.641   Sprain of metacarpophalangeal joint of right thumb 🔍

     ● S63.642   Sprain of metacarpophalangeal joint of left thumb 🔍

     ● S63.649   Sprain of metacarpophalangeal joint of unspecified thumb 🔍

● S63.65   Sprain of metacarpophalangeal joint of other and unspecified finger(s)

     ● S63.650   Sprain of metacarpophalangeal joint of right index finger 🔍

     ● S63.651   Sprain of metacarpophalangeal joint of left index finger 🔍

     ● S63.652   Sprain of metacarpophalangeal joint of right middle finger 🔍

     ● S63.653   Sprain of metacarpophalangeal joint of left middle finger 🔍

     ● S63.654   Sprain of metacarpophalangeal joint of right ring finger 🔍

     ● S63.655   Sprain of metacarpophalangeal joint of left ring finger 🔍

     ● S63.656   Sprain of metacarpophalangeal joint of right little finger 🔍

     ● S63.657   Sprain of metacarpophalangeal joint of left little finger 🔍

     ● S63.658   Sprain of metacarpophalangeal joint of other finger 🔍
      Sprain of metacarpophalangeal joint of specified finger with unspecified laterality

     ● S63.659   Sprain of metacarpophalangeal joint of unspecified finger 🔍

◀ New   ◀▦ Revised   ~~deleted~~ Deleted   Excludes 1   Excludes 2   Includes   Use additional   Code first   Code also   Unspecified

OGCR Official Guidelines   ● Unacceptable Principal Diagnosis   X Assign placeholder X   ● Use Additional Character(s)   ▌ Manifestation Code   **Coding Clinic**

● S63.68   Other sprain of thumb
    ● S63.681   Other sprain of right thumb 🔖
    ● S63.682   Other sprain of left thumb 🔖
    ● S63.689   Other sprain of unspecified thumb 🔖
● S63.69   Other sprain of other and unspecified finger(s)
    ● S63.690   Other sprain of right index finger 🔖
    ● S63.691   Other sprain of left index finger 🔖
    ● S63.692   Other sprain of right middle finger 🔖
    ● S63.693   Other sprain of left middle finger 🔖
    ● S63.694   Other sprain of right ring finger 🔖
    ● S63.695   Other sprain of left ring finger 🔖
    ● S63.696   Other sprain of right little finger 🔖
    ● S63.697   Other sprain of left little finger 🔖
    ● S63.698   Other sprain of other finger 🔖
            Other sprain of specified finger with unspecified laterality
    ● S63.699   Other sprain of unspecified finger 🔖
● S63.8   Sprain of other part of wrist and hand
  ● S63.8X   Sprain of other part of wrist and hand
    ● S63.8X1   Sprain of other part of right wrist and hand 🔖
    ● S63.8X2   Sprain of other part of left wrist and hand 🔖
    ● S63.8X9   Sprain of other part of unspecified wrist and hand 🔖
● S63.9   Sprain of unspecified part of wrist and hand
  X ● S63.90   Sprain of unspecified part of unspecified wrist and hand 🔖
  X ● S63.91   Sprain of unspecified part of right wrist and hand 🔖
  X ● S63.92   Sprain of unspecified part of left wrist and hand 🔖

● S64   Injury of nerves at wrist and hand level
    The appropriate 7th character is to be added to each code from category S64

> | | |
> |---|---|
> | A | initial encounter |
> | D | subsequent encounter |
> | S | sequela |

    Code also any associated open wound (S61.-)
● S64.0   Injury of ulnar nerve at wrist and hand level
  X ● S64.00   Injury of ulnar nerve at wrist and hand level of unspecified arm 🔖
  X ● S64.01   Injury of ulnar nerve at wrist and hand level of right arm 🔖
  X ● S64.02   Injury of ulnar nerve at wrist and hand level of left arm 🔖
● S64.1   Injury of median nerve at wrist and hand level
  X ● S64.10   Injury of median nerve at wrist and hand level of unspecified arm 🔖
  X ● S64.11   Injury of median nerve at wrist and hand level of right arm 🔖
  X ● S64.12   Injury of median nerve at wrist and hand level of left arm 🔖
● S64.2   Injury of radial nerve at wrist and hand level
  X ● S64.20   Injury of radial nerve at wrist and hand level of unspecified arm 🔖
  X ● S64.21   Injury of radial nerve at wrist and hand level of right arm 🔖
  X ● S64.22   Injury of radial nerve at wrist and hand level of left arm 🔖
● S64.3   Injury of digital nerve of thumb
  X ● S64.30   Injury of digital nerve of unspecified thumb 🔖
  X ● S64.31   Injury of digital nerve of right thumb 🔖
  X ● S64.32   Injury of digital nerve of left thumb 🔖

● S64.4   Injury of digital nerve of other and unspecified finger
  X ● S64.40   Injury of digital nerve of unspecified finger 🔖
  ● S64.49   Injury of digital nerve of other finger
    ● S64.490   Injury of digital nerve of right index finger 🔖
    ● S64.491   Injury of digital nerve of left index finger 🔖
    ● S64.492   Injury of digital nerve of right middle finger 🔖
    ● S64.493   Injury of digital nerve of left middle finger 🔖
    ● S64.494   Injury of digital nerve of right ring finger 🔖
    ● S64.495   Injury of digital nerve of left ring finger 🔖
    ● S64.496   Injury of digital nerve of right little finger 🔖
    ● S64.497   Injury of digital nerve of left little finger 🔖
    ● S64.498   Injury of digital nerve of other finger 🔖
            Injury of digital nerve of specified finger with unspecified laterality
● S64.8   Injury of other nerves at wrist and hand level
  ● S64.8X   Injury of other nerves at wrist and hand level
    ● S64.8X1   Injury of other nerves at wrist and hand level of right arm 🔖
    ● S64.8X2   Injury of other nerves at wrist and hand level of left arm 🔖
    ● S64.8X9   Injury of other nerves at wrist and hand level of unspecified arm 🔖
● S64.9   Injury of unspecified nerve at wrist and hand level
  X ● S64.90   Injury of unspecified nerve at wrist and hand level of unspecified arm 🔖
  X ● S64.91   Injury of unspecified nerve at wrist and hand level of right arm 🔖
  X ● S64.92   Injury of unspecified nerve at wrist and hand level of left arm 🔖

● S65   Injury of blood vessels at wrist and hand level
    The appropriate 7th character is to be added to each code from category S65

> | | |
> |---|---|
> | A | initial encounter |
> | D | subsequent encounter |
> | S | sequela |

    Code also any associated open wound (S61.-)
● S65.0   Injury of ulnar artery at wrist and hand level
  ● S65.00   Unspecified injury of ulnar artery at wrist and hand level
    ● S65.001   Unspecified injury of ulnar artery at wrist and hand level of right arm
        A 🔖, 🔖
        (Ex) S45.301[A], S45.309-S45.311[A],
            S45.319-S45.391[A], S45.399-S45.801[A],
            S45.809-S45.811[A], S45.819-S45.891[A],
            S45.899-S45.901[A], S45.909-S45.911[A],
            S45.919-S45.991[A], S45.999[A], S55.001[A],
            S55.009-S55.011[A], S55.019-S55.091[A],
            S55.099[A], S55.201[A], S55.209-S55.211[A],
            S55.219-S55.291[A], S55.299-S55.801[A],
            S55.809-S55.811[A], S55.819-S55.891[A],
            S55.899-S55.901[A], S55.909-S55.911[A],
            S55.919-S55.991[A], S55.999[A], S65.001[A],
            S65.009-S65.011[A], S65.019-S65.091[A],
            S65.099[A], S65.801[A], S65.809-S65.811[A],
            S65.819-S65.891[A], S65.899-S65.901[A],
            S65.909-S65.911[A], S65.919-S65.991[A],
            S65.999[A]

CHAPTER 19 (S00-T88)

N Newborn Age: 0   P Pediatric Age: 0–17   M Maternity DX: 12–55   A Adult Age: 15–124   ♀ Females Only   ♂ Males Only

🔖 Complication\Comorbidity   🔖 Major C\C   (Ex) CC/MCC Exclusions   🔖 Present on Admission Requirement   🔖 Hospital-Acquired Condition   **1417**

● S65.002   Unspecified injury of ulnar artery at wrist and hand level of left arm A 🖋, 🖋
     (Ex:) S45.302-S45.309[A], S45.312-S45.319[A],
     S45.392-S45.399[A], S45.802-S45.809[A],
     S45.812-S45.819[A], S45.892-S45.899[A],
     S45.902-S45.909[A], S45.912-S45.919[A],
     S45.992-S45.999[A], S55.002-S55.009[A],
     S55.012-S55.019[A], S55.092-S55.099[A],
     S55.202-S55.209[A], S55.212-S55.219[A],
     S55.292-S55.299[A], S55.802-S55.809[A],
     S55.812-S55.819[A], S55.892-S55.899[A],
     S55.902-S55.909[A], S55.912-S55.919[A],
     S55.992-S55.999[A], S65.002-S65.009[A],
     S65.012-S65.019[A], S65.092-S65.099[A],
     S65.802-S65.809[A] S65.812-S65.819[A],
     S65.892-S65.899[A], S65.902-S65.909[A],
     S65.912-S65.919[A], S65.992-S65.999[A]

● S65.009   Unspecified injury of ulnar artery at wrist and hand level of unspecified arm A 🖋, 🖋
     (Ex:) S45.301-S45.999[A], S55.001-S55.099[A],
     S55.201-S55.999[A], S65.001-S65.099[A],
     S65.801-S65.999[A]

● S65.01   Laceration of ulnar artery at wrist and hand level

● S65.011   Laceration of ulnar artery at wrist and hand level of right arm A 🖋, 🖋
     (Ex:) See S65.001

● S65.012   Laceration of ulnar artery at wrist and hand level of left arm A 🖋, 🖋
     (Ex:) See S65.002

● S65.019   Laceration of ulnar artery at wrist and hand level of unspecified arm A 🖋, 🖋
     (Ex:) See S65.009

● S65.09   Other specified injury of ulnar artery at wrist and hand level

● S65.091   Other specified injury of ulnar artery at wrist and hand level of right arm A 🖋, 🖋
     (Ex:) See S65.001

● S65.092   Other specified injury of ulnar artery at wrist and hand level of left arm A 🖋, 🖋
     (Ex:) See S65.002

● S65.099   Other specified injury of ulnar artery at wrist and hand level of unspecified arm A 🖋, 🖋
     (Ex:) See S65.009

● S65.1   Injury of radial artery at wrist and hand level

● S65.10   Unspecified injury of radial artery at wrist and hand level

● S65.101   Unspecified injury of radial artery at wrist and hand level of right arm A 🖋, 🖋
     (Ex:) S45.301[A], S45.309-S45.311[A],
     S45.319-S45.391[A], S45.399-S45.801[A],
     S45.809-S45.811[A], S45.819-S45.891[A],
     S45.899-S45.901[A], S45.909-S45.911[A],
     S45.919-S45.991[A], S45.999[A], S55.101[A],
     S55.109-S55.111[A], S55.119-S55.191[A],
     S55.199-S55.201[A], S55.209-S55.211[A],
     S55.219-S55.291[A], S55.299-S55.801[A],
     S55.809-S55.811[A], S55.819-S55.891[A],
     S55.899-S55.901[A], S55.909-S55.911[A],
     S55.919-S55.991[A], S55.999[A], S65.101[A],
     S65.109-S65.111[A], S65.119-S65.191[A],
     S65.199[A], S65.801[A], S65.809-S65.811[A],
     S65.819-S65.891[A], S65.899-S65.901[A],
     S65.909-S65.911[A], S65.919-S65.991[A],
     S65.999[A]

● S65.102   Unspecified injury of radial artery at wrist and hand level of left arm A 🖋, 🖋
     (Ex:) S45.302-S45.309[A], S45.312-S45.319[A],
     S45.392-S45.399[A], S45.802-S45.809[A],
     S45.812-S45.819[A], S45.892-S45.899[A],
     S45.902-S45.909[A], S45.912-S45.919[A],
     S45.992-S45.999[A], S55.102-S55.109[A],
     S55.112-S55.119[A], S55.192-S55.199[A],
     S55.202-S55.209[A], S55.212-S55.219[A],
     S55.292-S55.299[A], S55.802A-S55.809[A],
     S55.812-S55.819[A], S55.892-S55.899[A],
     S55.902-S55.909[A], S55.912-S55.919[A],
     S55.992-S55.999[A], S65.102-S65.109[A],
     S65.112-S65.119[A], S65.192-S65.199[A],
     S65.802-S65.809[A], S65.812-S65.819[A],
     S65.892-S65.899[A], S65.902-S65.909[A],
     S65.912-S65.919[A], S65.992-S65.999[A]

● S65.109   Unspecified injury of radial artery at wrist and hand level of unspecified arm A 🖋, 🖋
     (Ex:) S45.301-S45.999[A], S55.101-S55.999[A],
     S65.101-S65.199[A], S65.801-S65.999[A]

● S65.11   Laceration of radial artery at wrist and hand level

● S65.111   Laceration of radial artery at wrist and hand level of right arm A 🖋, 🖋
     (Ex:) See S65.101

● S65.112   Laceration of radial artery at wrist and hand level of left arm A 🖋, 🖋
     (Ex:) See S65.102

● S65.119   Laceration of radial artery at wrist and hand level of unspecified arm A 🖋, 🖋
     (Ex:) See S65.109

● S65.19   Other specified injury of radial artery at wrist and hand level

● S65.191   Other specified injury of radial artery at wrist and hand level of right arm A 🖋, 🖋
     (Ex:) See S65.101

● S65.192   Other specified injury of radial artery at wrist and hand level of left arm A 🖋, 🖋
     (Ex:) See S65.102

● S65.199   Other specified injury of radial artery at wrist and hand level of unspecified arm A 🖋, 🖋
     (Ex:) See S65.109

● S65.2   Injury of superficial palmar arch

● S65.20   Unspecified injury of superficial palmar arch

● S65.201   Unspecified injury of superficial palmar arch of right hand A 🖋, 🖋
     (Ex:) S45.301[A], S45.309-S45.311[A],
     S45.319-S45.391[A], S45.399-S45.801[A],
     S45.809-S45.811[A], S45.819-S45.891[A],
     S45.899-S45.901[A], S45.909-S45.911[A],
     S45.919-S45.991[A], S45.999[A], S55.201[A],
     S55.209-S55.211[A], S55.219-S55.291[A],
     S55.299-S55.801[A], S55.809-S55.811[A],
     S55.819-S55.891[A], S55.899-S55.901[A],
     S55.909-S55.911[A], S55.919-S55.991[A],
     S55.999[A], S65.201[A], S65.209-S65.211[A],
     S65.219-S65.291[A], S65.299-S65.301[A],
     S65.309-S65.311[A], S65.319- S65.391[A],
     S65.399[A], S65.801[A], S65.809-S65.811[A],
     S65.819-S65.891[A], S65.899-S65.901[A],
     S65.909-S65.911[A], S65.919-S65.991[A],
     S65.999[A]

● S65.202   Unspecified injury of superficial
palmar arch of left hand A 🏥, 🏥
(Ex:) S45.302-S45.309[A], S45.312-S45.319[A],
S45.392-S45.399[A], S45.802-S45.809[A],
S45.812-S45.819[A], S45.892-S45.899[A],
S45.902-S45.909[A], S45.912-S45.919[A],
S45.992-S45.999[A], S55.202-S55.209[A],
S55.212-S55.219[A], S55.292-S55.299[A],
S55.802-S55.809[A], S55.812-S55.819[A],
S55.892-S55.899[A], S55.902-S55.909[A],
S55.912-S55.919[A], S55.992-S55.999[A],
S65.202-S65.209[A], S65.212-S65.219[A],
S65.292-S65.299[A], S65.302-S65.309[A],
S65.312-S65.319[A], S65.392-S65.399[A],
S65.802-S65.809[A], S65.812-S65.819[A],
S65.892-S65.899[A], S65.902-S65.909[A],
S65.912-S65.919[A], S65.992-S65.999[A]

● S65.209   Unspecified injury of superficial
palmar arch of unspecified hand
A 🏥, 🏥
(Ex:) S45.301-S45.999[A], S55.201-S55.999[A],
S65.201-S65.399[A], S65.801-S65.999[A]

● S65.21   Laceration of superficial palmar arch

● S65.211   Laceration of superficial palmar arch
of right hand A 🏥, 🏥
(Ex:) See S65.201

● S65.212   Laceration of superficial palmar arch
of left hand A 🏥, 🏥
(Ex:) See S65.202

● S65.219   Laceration of superficial palmar arch
of unspecified hand A 🏥, 🏥
(Ex:) See S65.209

● S65.29   Other specified injury of superficial palmar
arch

● S65.291   Other specified injury of superficial
palmar arch of right hand A 🏥, 🏥
(Ex:) See S65.201

● S65.292   Other specified injury of superficial
palmar arch of left hand A 🏥, 🏥
(Ex:) See S65.202

● S65.299   Other specified injury of superficial
palmar arch of unspecified hand
A 🏥, 🏥
(Ex:) See S65.209

● S65.3   Injury of deep palmar arch

● S65.30   Unspecified injury of deep palmar arch

● S65.301   Unspecified injury of deep palmar
arch of right hand A 🏥, 🏥
(Ex:) See S65.201

● S65.302   Unspecified injury of deep palmar
arch of left hand A 🏥, 🏥
(Ex:) See S65.202

● S65.309   Unspecified injury of deep palmar
arch of unspecified hand A 🏥, 🏥
(Ex:) See S65.209

● S65.31   Laceration of deep palmar arch

● S65.311   Laceration of deep palmar arch of
right hand A 🏥, 🏥
(Ex:) See S65.201

● S65.312   Laceration of deep palmar arch of left
hand A 🏥, 🏥
(Ex:) See S65.202

● S65.319   Laceration of deep palmar arch of
unspecified hand A 🏥, 🏥
(Ex:) See S65.209

● S65.39   Other specified injury of deep palmar arch

● S65.391   Other specified injury of deep palmar
arch of right hand A 🏥, 🏥
(Ex:) See S65.201

● S65.392   Other specified injury of deep palmar
arch of left hand A 🏥, 🏥
(Ex:) See S65.202

● S65.399   Other specified injury of deep palmar
arch of unspecified hand A 🏥, 🏥
(Ex:) See S65.209

● S65.4   Injury of blood vessel of thumb

● S65.40   Unspecified injury of blood vessel of thumb

● S65.401   Unspecified injury of blood vessel of
right thumb A 🏥, 🏥
(Ex:) S45.301[A], S45.309-S45.311[A],
S45.319-S45.391[A], S45.399-S45.801[A],
S45.809-S45.811[A], S45.819-S45.891[A],
S45.899-S45.901[A], S45.909-S45.911[A],
S45.919-S45.991[A], S45.999[A], S55.201[A],
S55.209-S55.211[A], S55.219-S55.291[A],
S55.299-S55.801[A], S55.809-S55.811[A],
S55.819-S55.891[A], S55.899-S55.901[A],
S55.909-S55.911[A], S55.919-S55.991[A],
S55.999[A], S65.401[A], S65.409-S65.411[A],
S65.419-S65.491[A], S65.499-S65.500[A],
S65.502[A], S65.504[A], S65.506[A],
S65.508-S65.510[A], S65.512[A], S65.514[A],
S65.516[A], S65.518-S65.590[A], S65.592[A],
S65.594[A], S65.596[A], S65.598-S65.801[A],
S65.809-S65.811[A], S65.819-S65.891[A],
S65.899-S65.901[A], S65.909-S65.911[A],
S65.919-S65.991[A], S65.999[A]

● S65.402   Unspecified injury of blood vessel of
left thumb A 🏥, 🏥
(Ex:) S45.302-S45.309[A], S45.312-S45.319[A],
S45.392-S45.399[A], S45.802-S45.809[A],
S45.812-S45.819[A], S45.892-S45.899[A],
S45.902-S45.909[A], S45.912-S45.919[A],
S45.992-S45.999[A], S55.202-S55.209[A],
S55.212-S55.219[A], S55.292-S55.299[A],
S55.802-S55.809[A], S55.812-S55.819[A],
S55.892-S55.899[A], S55.902-S55.909[A],
S55.912-S55.919[A], S55.992-S55.999[A],
S65.402-S65.409[A], S65.412-S65.419[A],
S65.492-S65.499[A], S65.501[A], S65.503[A],
S65.505[A], S65.507-S65.509[A], S65.511[A],
S65.513[A], S65.515[A], S65.517-S65.519[A],
S65.591[A], S65.593[A], S65.595[A],
S65.597-S65.599[A], S65.802-S65.809[A],
S65.812-S65.819[A], S65.892-S65.899[A],
S65.902-S65.909[A], S65.912-S65.919[A],
S65.992-S65.999[A]

● S65.409   Unspecified injury of blood vessel of
unspecified thumb A 🏥, 🏥
(Ex:) S45.301-S45.999[A], S55.201-S55.999[A],
S65.401-S65.999[A]

● S65.41   Laceration of blood vessel of thumb

● S65.411   Laceration of blood vessel of right
thumb A 🏥, 🏥
(Ex:) See S65.401

● S65.412   Laceration of blood vessel of left
thumb A 🏥, 🏥
(Ex:) See S65.402

● S65.419   Laceration of blood vessel of
unspecified thumb A 🏥, 🏥
(Ex:) See S65.409

● S65.49   Other specified injury of blood vessel of thumb

● S65.491   Other specified injury of blood vessel
of right thumb A 🏥, 🏥
(Ex:) See S65.401

● S65.492   Other specified injury of blood vessel
of left thumb A 🏥, 🏥
(Ex:) See S65.402

● S65.499   Other specified injury of blood vessel
of unspecified thumb A 🏥, 🏥
(Ex:) See S65.409

N   Newborn Age: 0   P   Pediatric Age: 0–17   M   Maternity DX: 12–55   A   Adult Age: 15–124   ♀   Females Only   ♂   Males Only

🏥   Complication\Comorbidity   🏥   Major C\C   (Ex:)   CC/MCC Exclusions   🏥   Present on Admission Requirement   🏥   Hospital-Acquired Condition

1419

● S65.5 Injury of blood vessel of other and unspecified finger
  ● S65.50 Unspecified injury of blood vessel of other and
    unspecified finger
    ● S65.500 Unspecified injury of blood vessel of
      right index finger A ◐, ◐
      Ex: See S65.401
    ● S65.501 Unspecified injury of blood vessel of
      left index finger A ◐, ◐
      Ex: See S65.402
    ● S65.502 Unspecified injury of blood vessel of
      right middle finger A ◐, ◐
      Ex: See S65.401
    ● S65.503 Unspecified injury of blood vessel of
      left middle finger A ◐, ◐
      Ex: See S65.402
    ● S65.504 Unspecified injury of blood vessel of
      right ring finger A ◐, ◐
      Ex: See S65.401
    ● S65.505 Unspecified injury of blood vessel of
      left ring finger A ◐, ◐
      Ex: See S65.409
    ● S65.506 Unspecified injury of blood vessel of
      right little finger A ◐, ◐
      Ex: See S65.401
    ● S65.507 Unspecified injury of blood vessel of
      left little finger A ◐, ◐
      Ex: See S65.402
    ● S65.508 Unspecified injury of blood vessel of
      other finger A ◐, ◐
        Unspecified injury of blood vessel
          of specified finger with
          unspecified laterality
      Ex: See S65.409
    ● S65.509 Unspecified injury of blood vessel of
      unspecified finger A ◐, ◐
      Ex: See S65.409
  ● S65.51 Laceration of blood vessel of other and
    unspecified finger
    ● S65.510 Laceration of blood vessel of right
      index finger A ◐, ◐
      Ex: See S65.401
    ● S65.511 Laceration of blood vessel of left
      index finger A ◐, ◐
      Ex: See S65.402
    ● S65.512 Laceration of blood vessel of right
      middle finger A ◐, ◐
      Ex: See S65.401
    ● S65.513 Laceration of blood vessel of left
      middle finger A ◐, ◐
      Ex: See S65.402
    ● S65.514 Laceration of blood vessel of right
      ring finger A ◐, ◐
      Ex: See S65.401
    ● S65.515 Laceration of blood vessel of left ring
      finger A ◐, ◐
      Ex: See S65.402
    ● S65.516 Laceration of blood vessel of right
      little finger A ◐, ◐
      Ex: See S65.401
    ● S65.517 Laceration of blood vessel of left little
      finger A ◐, ◐
      Ex: See S65.402
    ● S65.518 Laceration of blood vessel of other
      finger A ◐, ◐
        Laceration of blood vessel
          of specified finger with
          unspecified laterality
      Ex: See S65.409
    ● S65.519 Laceration of blood vessel of
      unspecified finger A ◐, ◐
      Ex: See S65.409

● S65.59 Other specified injury of blood vessel of other
  and unspecified finger
    ● S65.590 Other specified injury of blood vessel
      of right index finger A ◐, ◐
      Ex: See S65.401
    ● S65.591 Other specified injury of blood vessel
      of left index finger A ◐, ◐
      Ex: See S65.402
    ● S65.592 Other specified injury of blood vessel
      of right middle finger A ◐, ◐
      Ex: See S65.401
    ● S65.593 Other specified injury of blood vessel
      of left middle finger A ◐, ◐
      Ex: See S65.402
    ● S65.594 Other specified injury of blood vessel
      of right ring finger A ◐, ◐
      Ex: See S65.401
    ● S65.595 Other specified injury of blood vessel
      of left ring finger A ◐, ◐
      Ex: See S65.402
    ● S65.596 Other specified injury of blood vessel
      of right little finger A ◐, ◐
      Ex: See S65.401
    ● S65.597 Other specified injury of blood vessel
      of left little finger A ◐, ◐
      Ex: See S65.402
    ● S65.598 Other specified injury of blood vessel
      of other finger A ◐, ◐
        Other specified injury of blood
          vessel of specified finger with
          unspecified laterality
      Ex: See S65.409
    ● S65.599 Other specified injury of blood vessel
      of unspecified finger A ◐, ◐
      Ex: See S65.409

● S65.8 Injury of other blood vessels at wrist and hand level
  ● S65.80 Unspecified injury of other blood vessels at
    wrist and hand level
    ● S65.801 Unspecified injury of other blood
      vessels at wrist and hand level of
      right arm A ◐, ◐
      Ex: S45.301[A], S45.309-S45.311[A],
        S45.319-S45.391[A], S45.399-S45.801[A],
        S45.809-S45.811[A], S45.819-S45.891[A],
        S45.899-S45.901[A], S45.909-S45.911[A],
        S45.919-S45.991[A], S45.999[A], S55.001[A],
        S55.009-S55.011[A], S55.019-S55.091[A],
        S55.099[A], S55.201[A], S55.209-S55.211[A],
        S55.219-S55.291[A], S55.299-S55.801[A],
        S55.809-S55.811[A], S55.819-S55.891[A],
        S55.899-S55.901[A], S55.909-S55.911[A],
        S55.919-S55.991[A], S55.999[A], S65.001[A],
        S65.009-S65.011[A], S65.019-S65.091[A],
        S65.099[A], S65.201[A], S65.209-S65.211[A],
        S65.219-S65.291[A], S65.299-S65.301[A],
        S65.309-S65.311[A], S65.319-S65.391[A],
        S65.399-S65.401[A], S65.409-S65.411[A],
        S65.419-S65.491[A], S65.499-S65.500[A],
        S65.502[A], S65.504[A], S65.506[A],
        S65.508-S65.510[A], S65.512[A], S65.514[A],
        S65.516[A], S65.518-S65.590[A], S65.592[A],
        S65.594[A], S65.596[A], S65.598-S65.801[A],
        S65.809-S65.811[A], S65.819-S65.891[A],
        S65.899-S65.901[A], S65.909-S65.911[A],
        S65.919-S65.991[A], S65.999[A]

◀ New   ◀ Revised   deleted Deleted   Excludes 1   Excludes 2   Includes   Use additional   Code first   Code also   Unspecified
OGCR Official Guidelines   ● Unacceptable Principal Diagnosis   X Assign placeholder X   ● Use Additional Character(s)   ▶ Manifestation Code   Coding Clinic

● S65.802 Unspecified injury of other blood
vessels at wrist and hand level of left
arm A 🔵, 🔵
(Ex:) S45.302-S45.309[A], S45.312-S45.319[A],
S45.392-S45.399[A], S45.802-S45.809[A],
S45.812-S45.819[A], S45.892-S45.899[A],
S45.902-S45.909[A], S45.912-S45.919[A],
S45.992-S45.999[A], S55.002-S55.009[A],
S55.012-S55.019[A], S55.092-S55.099[A],
S55.202-S55.209[A], S55.212-S55.219[A],
S55.292-S55.299[A], S55.802-S55.809[A],
S55.812-S55.819[A], S55.892-S55.899[A],
S55.902-S55.909[A], S55.912-S55.919[A],
S55.992-S55.999[A], S65.002-S65.009[A],
S65.012-S65.019[A], S65.092-S65.099[A],
S65.202-S65.209[A], S65.212-S65.219[A],
S65.292-S65.299[A], S65.302-S65.309[A],
S65.312-S65.319[A], S65.392-S65.399[A],
S65.402-S65.409[A], S65.412-S65.419[A],
S65.492-S65.499[A], S65.501[A], S65.503[A],
S65.505[A], S65.507-S65.509[A], S65.511[A],
S65.513[A], S65.515[A], S65.517-S65.519[A],
S65.591[A], S65.593[A], S65.595[A],
S65.597-S65.599[A], S65.802-S65.809[A],
S65.812-S65.819[A], S65.892-S65.899[A],
S65.902-S65.909[A], S65.912-S65.919[A],
S65.992-S65.999[A]

● S65.809 Unspecified injury of other blood
vessels at wrist and hand level of
unspecified arm A 🔵, 🔵
(Ex:) S45.301-S45.999[A], S55.001-S55.099[A],
S55.201-S55.999[A], S65.001-S65.099[A],
S65.201-S65.999[A]

● S65.81 Laceration of other blood vessels at wrist and
hand level

● S65.811 Laceration of other blood vessels at
wrist and hand level of right arm
A 🔵, 🔵
(Ex:) See S65.801

● S65.812 Laceration of other blood vessels at
wrist and hand level of left arm
A 🔵, 🔵
(Ex:) See S65.802

● S65.819 Laceration of other blood vessels at
wrist and hand level of unspecified
arm A 🔵, 🔵
(Ex:) See S65.809

● S65.89 Other specified injury of other blood vessels at
wrist and hand level

● S65.891 Other specified injury of other blood
vessels at wrist and hand level of
right arm A 🔵, 🔵
(Ex:) See S65.801

● S65.892 Other specified injury of other blood
vessels at wrist and hand level of left
arm A 🔵, 🔵
(Ex:) See S65.802

● S65.899 Other specified injury of other blood
vessels at wrist and hand level of
unspecified arm A 🔵, 🔵
(Ex:) See S65.809

● S65.9 Injury of unspecified blood vessel at wrist and hand
level

● S65.90 Unspecified injury of unspecified blood vessel
at wrist and hand level

● S65.901 Unspecified injury of unspecified
blood vessel at wrist and hand level
of right arm A 🔵, 🔵
(Ex:) See S65.801

● S65.902 Unspecified injury of unspecified
blood vessel at wrist and hand level
of left arm A 🔵, 🔵
(Ex:) See S65.802

● S65.909 Unspecified injury of unspecified
blood vessel at wrist and hand level
of unspecified arm A 🔵, 🔵
(Ex:) See S65.809

● S65.91 Laceration of unspecified blood vessel at wrist
and hand level

● S65.911 Laceration of unspecified blood vessel
at wrist and hand level of right arm
A 🔵, 🔵
(Ex:) See S65.801

● S65.912 Laceration of unspecified blood vessel
at wrist and hand level of left arm
A 🔵, 🔵
(Ex:) See S65.802

● S65.919 Laceration of unspecified blood vessel
at wrist and hand level of unspecified
arm A 🔵, 🔵
(Ex:) See S65.809

● S65.99 Other specified injury of unspecified blood
vessel at wrist and hand level

● S65.991 Other specified injury of unspecified
blood vessel at wrist and hand of
right arm A 🔵, 🔵
(Ex:) See S65.801

● S65.992 Other specified injury of unspecified
blood vessel at wrist and hand of left
arm A 🔵, 🔵
(Ex:) See S65.802

● S65.999 Other specified injury of unspecified
blood vessel at wrist and hand of
unspecified arm A 🔵, 🔵
(Ex:) See S65.809

● S66 Injury of muscle, fascia and tendon at wrist and hand level
Code also any associated open wound (S61.-)
Excludes2 sprain of joints and ligaments of wrist and hand
(S63.-)
The appropriate 7th character is to be added to each code from
category S66

A	initial encounter
D	subsequent encounter
S	sequela

● S66.0 Injury of long flexor muscle, fascia and tendon of thumb
at wrist and hand level

● S66.00 Unspecified injury of long flexor muscle, fascia
and tendon of thumb at wrist and hand level

● S66.001 Unspecified injury of long flexor
muscle, fascia and tendon of right
thumb at wrist and hand level 🔵

● S66.002 Unspecified injury of long flexor
muscle, fascia and tendon of left
thumb at wrist and hand level 🔵

● S66.009 Unspecified injury of long flexor
muscle, fascia and tendon of
unspecified thumb at wrist and hand
level 🔵

N Newborn Age: 0   P Pediatric Age: 0–17   M Maternity DX: 12–55   A Adult Age: 15–124   ♀ Females Only   ♂ Males Only

🔵 Complication\Comorbidity   🔵 Major C\C   (Ex:) CC/MCC Exclusions   🔵 Present on Admission Requirement   🔵 Hospital-Acquired Condition

1421

CHAPTER 19 (S00-T88)

● **S66.01** Strain of long flexor muscle, fascia and tendon of thumb at wrist and hand level

● **S66.011** Strain of long flexor muscle, fascia and tendon of right thumb at wrist and hand level 🔍

● **S66.012** Strain of long flexor muscle, fascia and tendon of left thumb at wrist and hand level 🔍

● **S66.019** Strain of long flexor muscle, fascia and tendon of unspecified thumb at wrist and hand level 🔍

● **S66.02** Laceration of long flexor muscle, fascia and tendon of thumb at wrist and hand level

● **S66.021** Laceration of long flexor muscle, fascia and tendon of right thumb at wrist and hand level A 🔍 🔍

Ex: S61.401[A], S61.409-S61.411[A], S61.419-S61.421[A], S61.429-S61.431[A], S61.439-S61.441[A], S61.449-S61.451[A], S61.459[A], S66.021[A], S66.029[A], S66.120[A], S66.122[A], S66.124[A], S66.126[A], S66.128-S66.129[A], S66.221[A], S66.229[A], S66.320[A], S66.322[A], S66.324[A], S66.326[A], S66.328-S66.329[A], S66.421[A], S66.429[A], S66.520[A], S66.522[A], S66.524[A], S66.526[A], S66.528-S66.529[A], S66.821[A], S66.829[A], S66.921[A], S66.929[A]

● **S66.022** Laceration of long flexor muscle, fascia and tendon of left thumb at wrist and hand level A 🔍, 🔍

Ex: S61.402-S61.409[A], S61.412-S61.419[A], S61.422-S61.429[A], S61.432-S61.439[A], S61.442-S61.449[A], S61.452-S61.459[A], S66.022-S66.029[A], S66.121[A], S66.123[A], S66.125[A], S66.127-S66.129[A], S66.222-S66.229[A], S66.321[A], S66.323[A], S66.325[A], S66.327-S66.329[A], S66.422-S66.429[A], S66.521[A], S66.523[A], S66.525[A], S66.527-S66.529[A], S66.822-S66.829[A], S66.922-S66.929[A]

● **S66.029** Laceration of long flexor muscle, fascia and tendon of unspecified thumb at wrist and hand level A 🔍, 🔍

Ex: S61.401-S61.459[A], S66.021-S66.029[A], S66.120-S66.129[A], S66.221-S66.229[A], S66.320-S66.329[A], S66.421-S66.429[A], S66.520-S66.529[A], S66.821-S66.829[A], S66.921-S66.929[A]

● **S66.09** Other specified injury of long flexor muscle, fascia and tendon of thumb at wrist and hand level

● **S66.091** Other specified injury of long flexor muscle, fascia and tendon of right thumb at wrist and hand level 🔍

● **S66.092** Other specified injury of long flexor muscle, fascia and tendon of left thumb at wrist and hand level 🔍

● **S66.099** Other specified injury of long flexor muscle, fascia and tendon of unspecified thumb at wrist and hand level 🔍

● **S66.1** Injury of flexor muscle, fascia and tendon of other and unspecified finger at wrist and hand level

Excludes2 injury of long flexor muscle, fascia and tendon of thumb at wrist and hand level (S66.0-)

● **S66.10** Unspecified injury of flexor muscle, fascia and tendon of other and unspecified finger at wrist and hand level

● **S66.100** Unspecified injury of flexor muscle, fascia and tendon of right index finger at wrist and hand level 🔍

● **S66.101** Unspecified injury of flexor muscle, fascia and tendon of left index finger at wrist and hand level 🔍

● **S66.102** Unspecified injury of flexor muscle, fascia and tendon of right middle finger at wrist and hand level 🔍

● **S66.103** Unspecified injury of flexor muscle, fascia and tendon of left middle finger at wrist and hand level 🔍

● **S66.104** Unspecified injury of flexor muscle, fascia and tendon of right ring finger at wrist and hand level 🔍

● **S66.105** Unspecified injury of flexor muscle, fascia and tendon of left ring finger at wrist and hand level 🔍

● **S66.106** Unspecified injury of flexor muscle, fascia and tendon of right little finger at wrist and hand level 🔍

● **S66.107** Unspecified injury of flexor muscle, fascia and tendon of left little finger at wrist and hand level 🔍

● **S66.108** Unspecified injury of flexor muscle, fascia and tendon of other finger at wrist and hand level 🔍

Unspecified injury of flexor muscle, fascia and tendon of specified finger with unspecified laterality at wrist and hand level

● **S66.109** Unspecified injury of flexor muscle, fascia and tendon of unspecified finger at wrist and hand level 🔍

● **S66.11** Strain of flexor muscle, fascia and tendon of other and unspecified finger at wrist and hand level

● **S66.110** Strain of flexor muscle, fascia and tendon of right index finger at wrist and hand level 🔍

● **S66.111** Strain of flexor muscle, fascia and tendon of left index finger at wrist and hand level 🔍

● **S66.112** Strain of flexor muscle, fascia and tendon of right middle finger at wrist and hand level 🔍

● **S66.113** Strain of flexor muscle, fascia and tendon of left middle finger at wrist and hand level 🔍

● **S66.114** Strain of flexor muscle, fascia and tendon of right ring finger at wrist and hand level 🔍

● **S66.115** Strain of flexor muscle, fascia and tendon of left ring finger at wrist and hand level 🔍

● **S66.116** Strain of flexor muscle, fascia and tendon of right little finger at wrist and hand level 🔍

● **S66.117** Strain of flexor muscle, fascia and tendon of left little finger at wrist and hand level 🔍

◄ New ◄█ Revised ~~deleted~~ Deleted Excludes 1 Excludes 2 Includes Use additional Code first Code also Unspecified

OGCR Official Guidelines ● Unacceptable Principal Diagnosis X Assign placeholder X 🔍 Use Additional Character(s) ▶ Manifestation Code Coding Clinic

● S66.118   Strain of flexor muscle, fascia and tendon of other finger at wrist and hand level 🅿

    Strain of flexor muscle, fascia and tendon of specified finger with unspecified laterality at wrist and hand level

● S66.119   Strain of flexor muscle, fascia and tendon of unspecified finger at wrist and hand level 🅿

● S66.12   Laceration of flexor muscle, fascia and tendon of other and unspecified finger at wrist and hand level

● S66.120   Laceration of flexor muscle, fascia and tendon of right index finger at wrist and hand level A 🅒, 🅟
    (Ex) See S65.021

● S66.121   Laceration of flexor muscle, fascia and tendon of left index finger at wrist and hand level A 🅒, 🅟
    (Ex) See S65.022

● S66.122   Laceration of flexor muscle, fascia and tendon of right middle finger at wrist and hand level A 🅒, 🅟
    (Ex) See S65.021

● S66.123   Laceration of flexor muscle, fascia and tendon of left middle finger at wrist and hand level A 🅒, 🅟
    (Ex) See S65.022

● S66.124   Laceration of flexor muscle, fascia and tendon of right ring finger at wrist and hand level A 🅒, 🅟
    (Ex) See S65.021

● S66.125   Laceration of flexor muscle, fascia and tendon of left ring finger at wrist and hand level A 🅒, 🅟
    (Ex) See S65.022

● S66.126   Laceration of flexor muscle, fascia and tendon of right little finger at wrist and hand level A 🅒, 🅟
    (Ex) See S65.021

● S66.127   Laceration of flexor muscle, fascia and tendon of left little finger at wrist and hand level A 🅒, 🅟
    (Ex) See S65.022

● S66.128   Laceration of flexor muscle, fascia and tendon of other finger at wrist and hand level A 🅒, 🅟

    Laceration of flexor muscle, fascia and tendon of specified finger with unspecified laterality at wrist and hand level
    (Ex) See S65.029

● S66.129   Laceration of flexor muscle, fascia and tendon of unspecified finger at wrist and hand level A 🅒, 🅟
    (Ex) See S65.029

● S66.19   Other injury of flexor muscle, fascia and tendon of other and unspecified finger at wrist and hand level

● S66.190   Other injury of flexor muscle, fascia and tendon of right index finger at wrist and hand level 🅟

● S66.191   Other injury of flexor muscle, fascia and tendon of left index finger at wrist and hand level 🅟

● S66.192   Other injury of flexor muscle, fascia and tendon of right middle finger at wrist and hand level 🅟

● S66.193   Other injury of flexor muscle, fascia and tendon of left middle finger at wrist and hand level 🅟

● S66.194   Other injury of flexor muscle, fascia and tendon of right ring finger at wrist and hand level 🅟

● S66.195   Other injury of flexor muscle, fascia and tendon of left ring finger at wrist and hand level 🅟

● S66.196   Other injury of flexor muscle, fascia and tendon of right little finger at wrist and hand level 🅟

● S66.197   Other injury of flexor muscle, fascia and tendon of left little finger at wrist and hand level 🅟

● S66.198   Other injury of flexor muscle, fascia and tendon of other finger at wrist and hand level 🅟

    Other injury of flexor muscle, fascia and tendon of specified finger with unspecified laterality at wrist and hand level

● S66.199   Other injury of flexor muscle, fascia and tendon of unspecified finger at wrist and hand level 🅟

● **S66.2**   Injury of extensor muscle, fascia and tendon of thumb at wrist and hand level

● S66.20   Unspecified injury of extensor muscle, fascia and tendon of thumb at wrist and hand level

● S66.201   Unspecified injury of extensor muscle, fascia and tendon of right thumb at wrist and hand level 🅟

● S66.202   Unspecified injury of extensor muscle, fascia and tendon of left thumb at wrist and hand level 🅟

● S66.209   Unspecified injury of extensor muscle, fascia and tendon of unspecified thumb at wrist and hand level 🅟

● S66.21   Strain of extensor muscle, fascia and tendon of thumb at wrist and hand level

● S66.211   Strain of extensor muscle, fascia and tendon of right thumb at wrist and hand level 🅟

● S66.212   Strain of extensor muscle, fascia and tendon of left thumb at wrist and hand level 🅟

● S66.219   Strain of extensor muscle, fascia and tendon of unspecified thumb at wrist and hand level 🅟

● S66.22   Laceration of extensor muscle, fascia and tendon of thumb at wrist and hand level

● S66.221   Laceration of extensor muscle, fascia and tendon of right thumb at wrist and hand level A 🅒, 🅟
    (Ex) See S65.021

● S66.222   Laceration of extensor muscle, fascia and tendon of left thumb at wrist and hand level A 🅒, 🅟
    (Ex) See S65.022

● S66.229   Laceration of extensor muscle, fascia and tendon of unspecified thumb at wrist and hand level A 🅒, 🅟
    (Ex) See S65.029

● S66.29   Other specified injury of extensor muscle, fascia and tendon of thumb at wrist and hand level

● S66.291   Other specified injury of extensor muscle, fascia and tendon of right thumb at wrist and hand level 🅟

● S66.292   Other specified injury of extensor muscle, fascia and tendon of left thumb at wrist and hand level 🅟

● S66.299   Other specified injury of extensor muscle, fascia and tendon of unspecified thumb at wrist and hand level 🅟

N Newborn Age: 0   **P** Pediatric Age: 0–17   **M** Maternity DX: 12–55   **A** Adult Age: 15–124   ♀ Females Only   ♂ Males Only

🅒 Complication\Comorbidity   🅜 Major C\C   (Ex) CC/MCC Exclusions   🅟 Present on Admission Requirement   🅗 Hospital-Acquired Condition

1423

● **S66.3 Injury of extensor muscle, fascia and tendon of other and unspecified finger at wrist and hand level**

> **Excludes2**   injury of extensor muscle, fascia and tendon of thumb at wrist and hand level (S66.2-)

● **S66.30 Unspecified injury of extensor muscle, fascia and tendon of other and unspecified finger at wrist and hand level**

● **S66.300** Unspecified injury of extensor muscle, fascia and tendon of right index finger at wrist and hand level 🔍

● **S66.301** Unspecified injury of extensor muscle, fascia and tendon of left index finger at wrist and hand level 🔍

● **S66.302** Unspecified injury of extensor muscle, fascia and tendon of right middle finger at wrist and hand level 🔍

● **S66.303** Unspecified injury of extensor muscle, fascia and tendon of left middle finger at wrist and hand level 🔍

● **S66.304** Unspecified injury of extensor muscle, fascia and tendon of right ring finger at wrist and hand level 🔍

● **S66.305** Unspecified injury of extensor muscle, fascia and tendon of left ring finger at wrist and hand level 🔍

● **S66.306** Unspecified injury of extensor muscle, fascia and tendon of right little finger at wrist and hand level 🔍

● **S66.307** Unspecified injury of extensor muscle, fascia and tendon of left little finger at wrist and hand level 🔍

● **S66.308** Unspecified injury of extensor muscle, fascia and tendon of other finger at wrist and hand level 🔍

> Unspecified injury of extensor muscle, fascia and tendon of specified finger with unspecified laterality at wrist and hand level

● **S66.309** Unspecified injury of extensor muscle, fascia and tendon of unspecified finger at wrist and hand level 🔍

● **S66.31 Strain of extensor muscle, fascia and tendon of other and unspecified finger at wrist and hand level**

● **S66.310** Strain of extensor muscle, fascia and tendon of right index finger at wrist and hand level 🔍

● **S66.311** Strain of extensor muscle, fascia and tendon of left index finger at wrist and hand level 🔍

● **S66.312** Strain of extensor muscle, fascia and tendon of right middle finger at wrist and hand level 🔍

● **S66.313** Strain of extensor muscle, fascia and tendon of left middle finger at wrist and hand level 🔍

● **S66.314** Strain of extensor muscle, fascia and tendon of right ring finger at wrist and hand level 🔍

● **S66.315** Strain of extensor muscle, fascia and tendon of left ring finger at wrist and hand level 🔍

● **S66.316** Strain of extensor muscle, fascia and tendon of right little finger at wrist and hand level 🔍

● **S66.317** Strain of extensor muscle, fascia and tendon of left little finger at wrist and hand level 🔍

● **S66.318** Strain of extensor muscle, fascia and tendon of other finger at wrist and hand level 🔍

> Strain of extensor muscle, fascia and tendon of specified finger with unspecified laterality at wrist and hand level

● **S66.319** Strain of extensor muscle, fascia and tendon of unspecified finger at wrist and hand level 🔍

● **S66.32 Laceration of extensor muscle, fascia and tendon of other and unspecified finger at wrist and hand level**

● **S66.320** Laceration of extensor muscle, fascia and tendon of right index finger at wrist and hand level A 🔍, 🔍
> (Ex:) See S65.021

● **S66.321** Laceration of extensor muscle, fascia and tendon of left index finger at wrist and hand level A 🔍, 🔍
> (Ex:) See S65.022

● **S66.322** Laceration of extensor muscle, fascia and tendon of right middle finger at wrist and hand level A 🔍, 🔍
> (Ex:) See S65.021

● **S66.323** Laceration of extensor muscle, fascia and tendon of left middle finger at wrist and hand level A 🔍, 🔍
> (Ex:) See S65.022

● **S66.324** Laceration of extensor muscle, fascia and tendon of right ring finger at wrist and hand level A 🔍, 🔍
> (Ex:) See S65.021

● **S66.325** Laceration of extensor muscle, fascia and tendon of left ring finger at wrist and hand level A 🔍, 🔍
> (Ex:) See S65.022

● **S66.326** Laceration of extensor muscle, fascia and tendon of right little finger at wrist and hand level A 🔍, 🔍
> (Ex:) See S65.021

● **S66.327** Laceration of extensor muscle, fascia and tendon of left little finger at wrist and hand level A 🔍, 🔍
> (Ex:) See S65.022

● **S66.328** Laceration of extensor muscle, fascia and tendon of other finger at wrist and hand level A 🔍, 🔍

> Laceration of extensor muscle, fascia and tendon of specified finger with unspecified laterality at wrist and hand level
> (Ex:) See S65.029

● **S66.329** Laceration of extensor muscle, fascia and tendon of unspecified finger at wrist and hand level A 🔍, 🔍
> (Ex:) See S65.029

● **S66.39 Other injury of extensor muscle, fascia and tendon of other and unspecified finger at wrist and hand level**

● **S66.390** Other injury of extensor muscle, fascia and tendon of right index finger at wrist and hand level 🔍

● **S66.391** Other injury of extensor muscle, fascia and tendon of left index finger at wrist and hand level 🔍

● **S66.392** Other injury of extensor muscle, fascia and tendon of right middle finger at wrist and hand level 🔍

● **S66.393** Other injury of extensor muscle, fascia and tendon of left middle finger at wrist and hand level 🔍

● **S66.394** Other injury of extensor muscle, fascia and tendon of right ring finger at wrist and hand level 🔍

● S66.395　Other injury of extensor muscle, fascia and tendon of left ring finger at wrist and hand level 🖐

● S66.396　Other injury of extensor muscle, fascia and tendon of right little finger at wrist and hand level 🖐

● S66.397　Other injury of extensor muscle, fascia and tendon of left little finger at wrist and hand level 🖐

● S66.398　Other injury of extensor muscle, fascia and tendon of other finger at wrist and hand level 🖐

　　　　Other injury of extensor muscle, fascia and tendon of specified finger with unspecified laterality at wrist and hand level

● S66.399　Other injury of extensor muscle, fascia and tendon of unspecified finger at wrist and hand level 🖐

● S66.4　Injury of intrinsic muscle, fascia and tendon of thumb at wrist and hand level

● S66.40　Unspecified injury of intrinsic muscle, fascia and tendon of thumb at wrist and hand level

● S66.401　Unspecified injury of intrinsic muscle, fascia and tendon of right thumb at wrist and hand level 🖐

● S66.402　Unspecified injury of intrinsic muscle, fascia and tendon of left thumb at wrist and hand level 🖐

● S66.409　Unspecified injury of intrinsic muscle, fascia and tendon of unspecified thumb at wrist and hand level 🖐

● S66.41　Strain of intrinsic muscle, fascia and tendon of thumb at wrist and hand level

● S66.411　Strain of intrinsic muscle, fascia and tendon of right thumb at wrist and hand level 🖐

● S66.412　Strain of intrinsic muscle, fascia and tendon of left thumb at wrist and hand level 🖐

● S66.419　Strain of intrinsic muscle, fascia and tendon of unspecified thumb at wrist and hand level 🖐

● S66.42　Laceration of intrinsic muscle, fascia and tendon of thumb at wrist and hand level

● S66.421　Laceration of intrinsic muscle, fascia and tendon of right thumb at wrist and hand level A 🖐, 🖐
　　　　　Ex: See S65.021

● S66.422　Laceration of intrinsic muscle, fascia and tendon of left thumb at wrist and hand level A 🖐, 🖐
　　　　　Ex: See S65.022

● S66.429　Laceration of intrinsic muscle, fascia and tendon of unspecified thumb at wrist and hand level A 🖐, 🖐
　　　　　Ex: See S65.029

● S66.49　Other specified injury of intrinsic muscle, fascia and tendon of thumb at wrist and hand level

● S66.491　Other specified injury of intrinsic muscle, fascia and tendon of right thumb at wrist and hand level 🖐

● S66.492　Other specified injury of intrinsic muscle, fascia and tendon of left thumb at wrist and hand level 🖐

● S66.499　Other specified injury of intrinsic muscle, fascia and tendon of unspecified thumb at wrist and hand level 🖐

● S66.5　Injury of intrinsic muscle, fascia and tendon of other and unspecified finger at wrist and hand level

　　Excludes2　injury of intrinsic muscle, fascia and tendon of thumb at wrist and hand level (S66.4-)

● S66.50　Unspecified injury of intrinsic muscle, fascia and tendon of other and unspecified finger at wrist and hand level

● S66.500　Unspecified injury of intrinsic muscle, fascia and tendon of right index finger at wrist and hand level 🖐

● S66.501　Unspecified injury of intrinsic muscle, fascia and tendon of left index finger at wrist and hand level 🖐

● S66.502　Unspecified injury of intrinsic muscle, fascia and tendon of right middle finger at wrist and hand level 🖐

● S66.503　Unspecified injury of intrinsic muscle, fascia and tendon of left middle finger at wrist and hand level 🖐

● S66.504　Unspecified injury of intrinsic muscle, fascia and tendon of right ring finger at wrist and hand level 🖐

● S66.505　Unspecified injury of intrinsic muscle, fascia and tendon of left ring finger at wrist and hand level 🖐

● S66.506　Unspecified injury of intrinsic muscle, fascia and tendon of right little finger at wrist and hand level 🖐

● S66.507　Unspecified injury of intrinsic muscle, fascia and tendon of left little finger at wrist and hand level 🖐

● S66.508　Unspecified injury of intrinsic muscle, fascia and tendon of other finger at wrist and hand level 🖐

　　　　Unspecified injury of intrinsic muscle, fascia and tendon of specified finger with unspecified laterality at wrist and hand level

● S66.509　Unspecified injury of intrinsic muscle, fascia and tendon of unspecified finger at wrist and hand level 🖐

● S66.51　Strain of intrinsic muscle, fascia and tendon of other and unspecified finger at wrist and hand level

● S66.510　Strain of intrinsic muscle, fascia and tendon of right index finger at wrist and hand level 🖐

● S66.511　Strain of intrinsic muscle, fascia and tendon of left index finger at wrist and hand level 🖐

● S66.512　Strain of intrinsic muscle, fascia and tendon of right middle finger at wrist and hand level 🖐

● S66.513　Strain of intrinsic muscle, fascia and tendon of left middle finger at wrist and hand level 🖐

● S66.514　Strain of intrinsic muscle, fascia and tendon of right ring finger at wrist and hand level 🖐

● S66.515　Strain of intrinsic muscle, fascia and tendon of left ring finger at wrist and hand level 🖐

● S66.516　Strain of intrinsic muscle, fascia and tendon of right little finger at wrist and hand level 🖐

N　Newborn Age: 0　　P　Pediatric Age: 0–17　　M　Maternity DX: 12–55　　A　Adult Age: 15–124　　♀　Females Only　　♂　Males Only

🖐 Complication\Comorbidity　　🖐 Major C\C　　Ex: CC/MCC Exclusions　　🖐 Present on Admission Requirement　　🖐 Hospital-Acquired Condition

1425

● S66.517   Strain of intrinsic muscle, fascia and tendon of left little finger at wrist and hand level 🔖

● S66.518   Strain of intrinsic muscle, fascia and tendon of other finger at wrist and hand level 🔖

Strain of intrinsic muscle, fascia and tendon of specified finger with unspecified laterality at wrist and hand level

● S66.519   Strain of intrinsic muscle, fascia and tendon of unspecified finger at wrist and hand level 🔖

● S66.52   Laceration of intrinsic muscle, fascia and tendon of other and unspecified finger at wrist and hand level

● S66.520   Laceration of intrinsic muscle, fascia and tendon of right index finger at wrist and hand level A 🔖, 🔖
Ex: See S65.021

● S66.521   Laceration of intrinsic muscle, fascia and tendon of left index finger at wrist and hand level A 🔖, 🔖
Ex: See S65.022

● S66.522   Laceration of intrinsic muscle, fascia and tendon of right middle finger at wrist and hand level A 🔖, 🔖
Ex: See S65.021

● S66.523   Laceration of intrinsic muscle, fascia and tendon of left middle finger at wrist and hand level A 🔖, 🔖
Ex: See S65.022

● S66.524   Laceration of intrinsic muscle, fascia and tendon of right ring finger at wrist and hand level A 🔖, 🔖
Ex: See S65.021

● S66.525   Laceration of intrinsic muscle, fascia and tendon of left ring finger at wrist and hand level A 🔖, 🔖
Ex: See S65.022

● S66.526   Laceration of intrinsic muscle, fascia and tendon of right little finger at wrist and hand level A 🔖, 🔖
Ex: See S65.021

● S66.527   Laceration of intrinsic muscle, fascia and tendon of left little finger at wrist and hand level A 🔖, 🔖
Ex: See S65.022

● S66.528   Laceration of intrinsic muscle, fascia and tendon of other finger at wrist and hand level A 🔖, 🔖

Laceration of intrinsic muscle, fascia and tendon of specified finger with unspecified laterality at wrist and hand level
Ex: See S65.029

● S66.529   Laceration of intrinsic muscle, fascia and tendon of unspecified finger at wrist and hand level A 🔖, 🔖
Ex: See S65.029

● S66.59   Other injury of intrinsic muscle, fascia and tendon of other and unspecified finger at wrist and hand level

● S66.590   Other injury of intrinsic muscle, fascia and tendon of right index finger at wrist and hand level 🔖

● S66.591   Other injury of intrinsic muscle, fascia and tendon of left index finger at wrist and hand level 🔖

● S66.592   Other injury of intrinsic muscle, fascia and tendon of right middle finger at wrist and hand level 🔖

● S66.593   Other injury of intrinsic muscle, fascia and tendon of left middle finger at wrist and hand level 🔖

● S66.594   Other injury of intrinsic muscle, fascia and tendon of right ring finger at wrist and hand level 🔖

● S66.595   Other injury of intrinsic muscle, fascia and tendon of left ring finger at wrist and hand level 🔖

● S66.596   Other injury of intrinsic muscle, fascia and tendon of right little finger at wrist and hand level 🔖

● S66.597   Other injury of intrinsic muscle, fascia and tendon of left little finger at wrist and hand level 🔖

● S66.598   Other injury of intrinsic muscle, fascia and tendon of other finger at wrist and hand level 🔖

Other injury of intrinsic muscle, fascia and tendon of specified finger with unspecified laterality at wrist and hand level

● S66.599   Other injury of intrinsic muscle, fascia and tendon of unspecified finger at wrist and hand level 🔖

● S66.8   Injury of other specified muscles, fascia and tendons at wrist and hand level

● S66.80   Unspecified injury of other specified muscles, fascia and tendons at wrist and hand level

● S66.801   Unspecified injury of other specified muscles, fascia and tendons at wrist and hand level, right hand 🔖

● S66.802   Unspecified injury of other specified muscles, fascia and tendons at wrist and hand level, left hand 🔖

● S66.809   Unspecified injury of other specified muscles, fascia and tendons at wrist and hand level, unspecified hand 🔖

● S66.81   Strain of other specified muscles, fascia and tendons at wrist and hand level

● S66.811   Strain of other specified muscles, fascia and tendons at wrist and hand level, right hand 🔖

● S66.812   Strain of other specified muscles, fascia and tendons at wrist and hand level, left hand 🔖

● S66.819   Strain of other specified muscles, fascia and tendons at wrist and hand level, unspecified hand 🔖

● S66.82   Laceration of other specified muscles, fascia and tendons at wrist and hand level

● S66.821   Laceration of other specified muscles, fascia and tendons at wrist and hand level, right hand A 🔖, 🔖
Ex: See S65.021

● S66.822   Laceration of other specified muscles, fascia and tendons at wrist and hand level, left hand A 🔖, 🔖
Ex: See S65.022

● S66.829   Laceration of other specified muscles, fascia and tendons at wrist and hand level, unspecified hand A 🔖, 🔖
Ex: See S65.029

◀ New   ◀▦ Revised   ~~deleted~~ Deleted   Excludes 1   Excludes 2   Includes   Use additional   Code first   Code also   Unspecified

OGCR Official Guidelines   ● Unacceptable Principal Diagnosis   X Assign placeholder X   ● Use Additional Character(s)   ▶ Manifestation Code   **Coding Clinic**

● S66.89   Other injury of other specified muscles, fascia and tendons at wrist and hand level

     ● S66.891   Other injury of other specified muscles, fascia and tendons at wrist and hand level, right hand 🗞

     ● S66.892   Other injury of other specified muscles, fascia and tendons at wrist and hand level, left hand 🗞

     ● S66.899   Other injury of other specified muscles, fascia and tendons at wrist and hand level, ==unspecified== hand 🗞

● S66.9   Injury of unspecified muscle, fascia and tendon at wrist and hand level

   ● S66.90   Unspecified injury of unspecified muscle, fascia and tendon at wrist and hand level

     ● S66.901   ==Unspecified== injury of unspecified muscle, fascia and tendon at wrist and hand level, right hand 🗞

     ● S66.902   ==Unspecified== injury of unspecified muscle, fascia and tendon at wrist and hand level, left hand 🗞

     ● S66.909   ==Unspecified== injury of unspecified muscle, fascia and tendon at wrist and hand level, unspecified hand 🗞

   ● S66.91   Strain of unspecified muscle, fascia and tendon at wrist and hand level

     ● S66.911   Strain of ==unspecified== muscle, fascia and tendon at wrist and hand level, right hand 🗞

     ● S66.912   Strain of ==unspecified== muscle, fascia and tendon at wrist and hand level, left hand 🗞

     ● S66.919   Strain of ==unspecified== muscle, fascia and tendon at wrist and hand level, unspecified hand 🗞

   ● S66.92   Laceration of unspecified muscle, fascia and tendon at wrist and hand level

     ● S66.921   Laceration of ==unspecified== muscle, fascia and tendon at wrist and hand level, right hand A 🗞, 🗞
         (Ex) See S65.021

     ● S66.922   Laceration of ==unspecified== muscle, fascia and tendon at wrist and hand level, left hand A 🗞, 🗞
         (Ex) See S65.022

     ● S66.929   Laceration of ==unspecified== muscle, fascia and tendon at wrist and hand level, unspecified hand A 🗞, 🗞
         (Ex) See S65.029

   ● S66.99   Other injury of unspecified muscle, fascia and tendon at wrist and hand level

     ● S66.991   Other injury of ==unspecified== muscle, fascia and tendon at wrist and hand level, right hand 🗞

     ● S66.992   Other injury of ==unspecified== muscle, fascia and tendon at wrist and hand level, left hand 🗞

     ● S66.999   Other injury of ==unspecified== muscle, fascia and tendon at wrist and hand level, unspecified hand 🗞

● S67   Crushing injury of wrist, hand and fingers

     Use additional code for all associated injuries, such as:
       fracture of wrist and hand (S62.-)
       open wound of wrist and hand (S61.-)

     The appropriate 7th character is to be added to each code from category S67

A	initial encounter
D	subsequent encounter
S	sequela

● S67.0   Crushing injury of thumb

   X ● S67.00   Crushing injury of ==unspecified== thumb 🗞

   X ● S67.01   Crushing injury of right thumb 🗞

   X ● S67.02   Crushing injury of left thumb 🗞

● S67.1   Crushing injury of other and unspecified finger(s)

     Excludes2   crushing injury of thumb (S67.0-)

   ● S67.10   Crushing injury of ==unspecified== finger(s) 🗞

   ● S67.19   Crushing injury of other finger(s)

     ● S67.190   Crushing injury of right index finger 🗞

     ● S67.191   Crushing injury of left index finger 🗞

     ● S67.192   Crushing injury of right middle finger 🗞

     ● S67.193   Crushing injury of left middle finger 🗞

     ● S67.194   Crushing injury of right ring finger 🗞

     ● S67.195   Crushing injury of left ring finger 🗞

     ● S67.196   Crushing injury of right little finger 🗞

     ● S67.197   Crushing injury of left little finger 🗞

     ● S67.198   Crushing injury of other finger 🗞
         Crushing injury of specified finger with unspecified laterality

● S67.2   Crushing injury of hand

     Excludes2   crushing injury of fingers (S67.1-)
                 crushing injury of thumb (S67.0-)

   X ● S67.20   Crushing injury of ==unspecified== hand 🗞

   X ● S67.21   Crushing injury of right hand 🗞

   X ● S67.22   Crushing injury of left hand 🗞

● S67.3   Crushing injury of wrist

   X ● S67.30   Crushing injury of ==unspecified== wrist 🗞

   X ● S67.31   Crushing injury of right wrist 🗞

   X ● S67.32   Crushing injury of left wrist 🗞

● S67.4   Crushing injury of wrist and hand

     Excludes1   crushing injury of hand alone (S67.2-)
                 crushing injury of wrist alone (S67.3-)

     Excludes2   crushing injury of fingers (S67.1-)
                 crushing injury of thumb (S67.0-)

   X ● S67.40   Crushing injury of ==unspecified== wrist and hand 🗞

   X ● S67.41   Crushing injury of right wrist and hand 🗞

   X ● S67.42   Crushing injury of left wrist and hand 🗞

● S67.9   Crushing injury of unspecified part(s) of wrist, hand and fingers

   X ● S67.90   Crushing injury of ==unspecified== part(s) of unspecified wrist, hand and fingers 🗞

   X ● S67.91   Crushing injury of ==unspecified== part(s) of right wrist, hand and fingers 🗞

   X ● S67.92   Crushing injury of ==unspecified== part(s) of left wrist, hand and fingers 🗞

● **S68**   **Traumatic amputation of wrist, hand and fingers**

An amputation not identified as partial or complete should be coded to complete

The appropriate 7th character is to be added to each code from category S68

> A   initial encounter
> D   subsequent encounter
> S   sequela

● **S68.0**   **Traumatic metacarpophalangeal amputation of thumb**
Traumatic amputation of thumb NOS

   ● **S68.01**   **Complete traumatic metacarpophalangeal amputation of thumb**

     ● **S68.011**   Complete traumatic metacarpophalangeal amputation of right thumb 🖐

     ● **S68.012**   Complete traumatic metacarpophalangeal amputation of left thumb 🖐

     ● **S68.019**   Complete traumatic metacarpophalangeal amputation of <mark>unspecified</mark> thumb 🖐

   ● **S68.02**   **Partial traumatic metacarpophalangeal amputation of thumb**

     ● **S68.021**   Partial traumatic metacarpophalangeal amputation of right thumb 🖐

     ● **S68.022**   Partial traumatic metacarpophalangeal amputation of left thumb 🖐

     ● **S68.029**   Partial traumatic metacarpophalangeal amputation of <mark>unspecified</mark> thumb 🖐

● **S68.1**   **Traumatic metacarpophalangeal amputation of other and unspecified finger**
Traumatic amputation of finger NOS

> **Excludes2**   traumatic metacarpophalangeal amputation of thumb (S68.0-)

   ● **S68.11**   **Complete traumatic metacarpophalangeal amputation of other and unspecified finger**

     ● **S68.110**   Complete traumatic metacarpophalangeal amputation of right index finger 🖐

     ● **S68.111**   Complete traumatic metacarpophalangeal amputation of left index finger 🖐

     ● **S68.112**   Complete traumatic metacarpophalangeal amputation of right middle finger 🖐

     ● **S68.113**   Complete traumatic metacarpophalangeal amputation of left middle finger 🖐

     ● **S68.114**   Complete traumatic metacarpophalangeal amputation of right ring finger 🖐

     ● **S68.115**   Complete traumatic metacarpophalangeal amputation of left ring finger 🖐

     ● **S68.116**   Complete traumatic metacarpophalangeal amputation of right little finger 🖐

     ● **S68.117**   Complete traumatic metacarpophalangeal amputation of left little finger 🖐

     ● **S68.118**   Complete traumatic metacarpophalangeal amputation of other finger 🖐
Complete traumatic metacarpophalangeal amputation of specified finger with unspecified laterality

     ● **S68.119**   Complete traumatic metacarpophalangeal amputation of <mark>unspecified</mark> finger 🖐

   ● **S68.12**   **Partial traumatic metacarpophalangeal amputation of other and unspecified finger**

     ● **S68.120**   Partial traumatic metacarpophalangeal amputation of right index finger 🖐

     ● **S68.121**   Partial traumatic metacarpophalangeal amputation of left index finger 🖐

     ● **S68.122**   Partial traumatic metacarpophalangeal amputation of right middle finger 🖐

     ● **S68.123**   Partial traumatic metacarpophalangeal amputation of left middle finger 🖐

     ● **S68.124**   Partial traumatic metacarpophalangeal amputation of right ring finger 🖐

     ● **S68.125**   Partial traumatic metacarpophalangeal amputation of left ring finger 🖐

     ● **S68.126**   Partial traumatic metacarpophalangeal amputation of right little finger 🖐

     ● **S68.127**   Partial traumatic metacarpophalangeal amputation of left little finger 🖐

     ● **S68.128**   Partial traumatic metacarpophalangeal amputation of other finger 🖐
Partial traumatic metacarpophalangeal amputation of specified finger with unspecified laterality

     ● **S68.129**   Partial traumatic metacarpophalangeal amputation of <mark>unspecified</mark> finger 🖐

● **S68.4**   **Traumatic amputation of hand at wrist level**
Traumatic amputation of hand NOS
Traumatic amputation of wrist

   ● **S68.41**   **Complete traumatic amputation of hand at wrist level**

     ● **S68.411**   Complete traumatic amputation of right hand at wrist level A 🖐, 🖐
       (Ex:) See S48.011

     ● **S68.412**   Complete traumatic amputation of left hand at wrist level A 🖐, 🖐
       (Ex:) See S48.012

     ● **S68.419**   Complete traumatic amputation of <mark>unspecified</mark> hand at wrist level A 🖐, 🖐
       (Ex:) See S48.019

◀ New   ◀▥ Revised   ~~deleted~~ Deleted   Excludes 1   Excludes 2   Includes   Use additional   Code first   Code also   <mark>Unspecified</mark>

OGCR Official Guidelines   ● Unacceptable Principal Diagnosis   X Assign placeholder X   ● Use Additional Character(s)   ▶ Manifestation Code   **Coding Clinic**

● **S68.42**   **Partial traumatic amputation of hand at wrist level**
- ● **S68.421**   Partial traumatic amputation of right hand at wrist level A 🖐, 🖐
  - (Ex:) See S48.011
- ● **S68.422**   Partial traumatic amputation of left hand at wrist level A 🖐, 🖐
  - (Ex:) See S48.012
- ● **S68.429**   Partial traumatic amputation of unspecified hand at wrist level A 🖐, 🖐
  - (Ex:) See S48.019

● **S68.5**   **Traumatic transphalangeal amputation of thumb**
Traumatic interphalangeal joint amputation of thumb
- ● **S68.51**   Complete traumatic transphalangeal amputation of thumb
  - ● **S68.511**   Complete traumatic transphalangeal amputation of right thumb 🖐
  - ● **S68.512**   Complete traumatic transphalangeal amputation of left thumb 🖐
  - ● **S68.519**   Complete traumatic transphalangeal amputation of unspecified thumb 🖐
- ● **S68.52**   Partial traumatic transphalangeal amputation of thumb
  - ● **S68.521**   Partial traumatic transphalangeal amputation of right thumb 🖐
  - ● **S68.522**   Partial traumatic transphalangeal amputation of left thumb 🖐
  - ● **S68.529**   Partial traumatic transphalangeal amputation of unspecified thumb 🖐

● **S68.6**   **Traumatic transphalangeal amputation of other and unspecified finger**
- ● **S68.61**   Complete traumatic transphalangeal amputation of other and unspecified finger(s)
  - ● **S68.610**   Complete traumatic transphalangeal amputation of right index finger 🖐
  - ● **S68.611**   Complete traumatic transphalangeal amputation of left index finger 🖐
  - ● **S68.612**   Complete traumatic transphalangeal amputation of right middle finger 🖐
  - ● **S68.613**   Complete traumatic transphalangeal amputation of left middle finger 🖐
  - ● **S68.614**   Complete traumatic transphalangeal amputation of right ring finger 🖐
  - ● **S68.615**   Complete traumatic transphalangeal amputation of left ring finger 🖐
  - ● **S68.616**   Complete traumatic transphalangeal amputation of right little finger 🖐
  - ● **S68.617**   Complete traumatic transphalangeal amputation of left little finger 🖐
  - ● **S68.618**   Complete traumatic transphalangeal amputation of other finger 🖐
    Complete traumatic transphalangeal amputation of specified finger with unspecified laterality
  - ● **S68.619**   Complete traumatic transphalangeal amputation of unspecified finger 🖐
- ● **S68.62**   Partial traumatic transphalangeal amputation of other and unspecified finger
  - ● **S68.620**   Partial traumatic transphalangeal amputation of right index finger 🖐
  - ● **S68.621**   Partial traumatic transphalangeal amputation of left index finger 🖐
  - ● **S68.622**   Partial traumatic transphalangeal amputation of right middle finger 🖐

- ● **S68.623**   Partial traumatic transphalangeal amputation of left middle finger 🖐
- ● **S68.624**   Partial traumatic transphalangeal amputation of right ring finger 🖐
- ● **S68.625**   Partial traumatic transphalangeal amputation of left ring finger 🖐
- ● **S68.626**   Partial traumatic transphalangeal amputation of right little finger 🖐
- ● **S68.627**   Partial traumatic transphalangeal amputation of left little finger 🖐
- ● **S68.628**   Partial traumatic transphalangeal amputation of other finger 🖐
  Partial traumatic transphalangeal amputation of specified finger with unspecified laterality
- ● **S68.629**   Partial traumatic transphalangeal amputation of unspecified finger 🖐

● **S68.7**   **Traumatic transmetacarpal amputation of hand**
- ● **S68.71**   Complete traumatic transmetacarpal amputation of hand
  - ● **S68.711**   Complete traumatic transmetacarpal amputation of right hand A 🖐, 🖐
    - (Ex:) See S48.011
  - ● **S68.712**   Complete traumatic transmetacarpal amputation of left hand A 🖐, 🖐
    - (Ex:) See S48.012
  - ● **S68.719**   Complete traumatic transmetacarpal amputation of unspecified hand A 🖐, 🖐
    - (Ex:) See S48.019
- ● **S68.72**   Partial traumatic transmetacarpal amputation of hand
  - ● **S68.721**   Partial traumatic transmetacarpal amputation of right hand A 🖐, 🖐
    - (Ex:) See S48.011
  - ● **S68.722**   Partial traumatic transmetacarpal amputation of left hand A 🖐, 🖐
    - (Ex:) See S48.012
  - ● **S68.729**   Partial traumatic transmetacarpal amputation of unspecified hand A 🖐, 🖐
    - (Ex:) See S48.019

● **S69**   **Other and unspecified injuries of wrist, hand and finger(s)**
The appropriate 7th character is to be added to each code from category S69

A	initial encounter
D	subsequent encounter
S	sequela

● **S69.8**   **Other specified injuries of wrist, hand and finger(s)**
- X ● **S69.80**   Other specified injuries of unspecified wrist, hand and finger(s) 🖐
- X ● **S69.81**   Other specified injuries of right wrist, hand and finger(s) 🖐
- X ● **S69.82**   Other specified injuries of left wrist, hand and finger(s) 🖐

● **S69.9**   **Unspecified injury of wrist, hand and finger(s)**
- X ● **S69.90**   Unspecified injury of unspecified wrist, hand and finger(s) 🖐
- X ● **S69.91**   Unspecified injury of right wrist, hand and finger(s) 🖐
- X ● **S69.92**   Unspecified injury of left wrist, hand and finger(s) 🖐

CHAPTER 19 (S00-T88)

N   Newborn Age: 0   **P**   Pediatric Age: 0–17   **M**   Maternity DX: 12–55   **A**   Adult Age: 15–124   ♀ Females Only   ♂ Males Only

 Complication\Comorbidity   🖐 Major C\C   (Ex:) CC/MCC Exclusions   🖐 Present on Admission Requirement   🖐 Hospital-Acquired Condition

1429

INJURIES TO THE HIP AND THIGH (S70-S79)

Excludes2　burns and corrosions (T20-T32)
　　　　　　　frostbite (T33-T34)
　　　　　　　snake bite (T63.0-)
　　　　　　　venomous insect bite or sting (T63.4-)

● **S70**　**Superficial injury of hip and thigh**
　　　The appropriate 7th character is to be added to each code from category S70

A	initial encounter
D	subsequent encounter
S	sequela

● **S70.0**　**Contusion of hip**
　　X ● S70.00　Contusion of unspecified hip 🖉
　　X ● S70.01　Contusion of right hip 🖉
　　X ● S70.02　Contusion of left hip 🖉

● **S70.1**　**Contusion of thigh**
　　X ● S70.10　Contusion of unspecified thigh 🖉
　　X ● S70.11　Contusion of right thigh 🖉
　　X ● S70.12　Contusion of left thigh 🖉

● **S70.2**　**Other superficial injuries of hip**
　● **S70.21**　Abrasion of hip
　　● S70.211　Abrasion, right hip 🖉
　　● S70.212　Abrasion, left hip 🖉
　　● S70.219　Abrasion, unspecified hip 🖉
　● **S70.22**　Blister (nonthermal) of hip
　　● S70.221　Blister (nonthermal), right hip 🖉
　　● S70.222　Blister (nonthermal), left hip 🖉
　　● S70.229　Blister (nonthermal), unspecified hip 🖉
　● **S70.24**　External constriction of hip
　　● S70.241　External constriction, right hip 🖉
　　● S70.242　External constriction, left hip 🖉
　　● S70.249　External constriction, unspecified hip 🖉
　● **S70.25**　Superficial foreign body of hip
　　　Splinter in the hip
　　● S70.251　Superficial foreign body, right hip 🖉
　　● S70.252　Superficial foreign body, left hip 🖉
　　● S70.259　Superficial foreign body, unspecified hip 🖉
　● **S70.26**　Insect bite (nonvenomous) of hip
　　● S70.261　Insect bite (nonvenomous), right hip 🖉
　　● S70.262　Insect bite (nonvenomous), left hip 🖉
　　● S70.269　Insect bite (nonvenomous), unspecified hip 🖉
　● **S70.27**　Other superficial bite of hip
　　　Excludes1　open bite of hip (S71.05-)
　　● S70.271　Other superficial bite of hip, right hip 🖉
　　● S70.272　Other superficial bite of hip, left hip 🖉
　　● S70.279　Other superficial bite of hip, unspecified hip 🖉

● **S70.3**　**Other superficial injuries of thigh**
　● **S70.31**　Abrasion of thigh
　　● S70.311　Abrasion, right thigh 🖉
　　● S70.312　Abrasion, left thigh 🖉
　　● S70.319　Abrasion, unspecified thigh 🖉
　● **S70.32**　Blister (nonthermal) of thigh
　　● S70.321　Blister (nonthermal), right thigh 🖉
　　● S70.322　Blister (nonthermal), left thigh 🖉
　　● S70.329　Blister (nonthermal), unspecified thigh 🖉
　● **S70.34**　External constriction of thigh
　　● S70.341　External constriction, right thigh 🖉
　　● S70.342　External constriction, left thigh 🖉
　　● S70.349　External constriction, unspecified thigh 🖉
　● **S70.35**　Superficial foreign body of thigh
　　　Splinter in the thigh
　　● S70.351　Superficial foreign body, right thigh 🖉
　　● S70.352　Superficial foreign body, left thigh 🖉
　　● S70.359　Superficial foreign body, unspecified thigh 🖉
　● **S70.36**　Insect bite (nonvenomous) of thigh
　　● S70.361　Insect bite (nonvenomous), right thigh 🖉
　　● S70.362　Insect bite (nonvenomous), left thigh 🖉
　　● S70.369　Insect bite (nonvenomous), unspecified thigh 🖉
　● **S70.37**　Other superficial bite of thigh
　　　Excludes1　open bite of thigh (S71.15)
　　● S70.371　Other superficial bite of right thigh 🖉
　　● S70.372　Other superficial bite of left thigh 🖉
　　● S70.379　Other superficial bite of unspecified thigh 🖉

● **S70.9**　**Unspecified superficial injury of hip and thigh**
　● **S70.91**　Unspecified superficial injury of hip
　　● S70.911　Unspecified superficial injury of right hip 🖉
　　● S70.912　Unspecified superficial injury of left hip 🖉
　　● S70.919　Unspecified superficial injury of unspecified hip 🖉
　● **S70.92**　Unspecified superficial injury of thigh
　　● S70.921　Unspecified superficial injury of right thigh 🖉
　　● S70.922　Unspecified superficial injury of left thigh 🖉
　　● S70.929　Unspecified superficial injury of unspecified thigh 🖉

◀ New　　◀▥ Revised　　~~deleted~~ Deleted　　Excludes 1　　Excludes 2　　Includes　　Use additional　　Code first　　Code also　　Unspecified
OGCR Official Guidelines　● Unacceptable Principal Diagnosis　X Assign placeholder X　● Use Additional Character(s)　▸ Manifestation Code　**Coding Clinic**

CHAPTER 19 (S00-T88)

● **S71   Open wound of hip and thigh**

    Code also any associated wound infection

    Excludes1 open fracture of hip and thigh (S72.-)
                  traumatic amputation of hip and thigh (S78.-)

    Excludes2 bite of venomous animal (T63.-)
                  open wound of ankle, foot and toes (S91.-)
                  open wound of knee and lower leg (S81.-)

    The appropriate 7th character is to be added to each code from category S71

> A   initial encounter
> D   subsequent encounter
> S   sequela

● **S71.0   Open wound of hip**

  ● **S71.00   Unspecified open wound of hip**

    ● **S71.001**   Unspecified open wound, right hip 🐾

    ● **S71.002**   Unspecified open wound, left hip 🐾

    ● **S71.009**   Unspecified open wound, unspecified hip 🐾

  ● **S71.01   Laceration without foreign body of hip**

    ● **S71.011**   Laceration without foreign body, right hip 🐾

    ● **S71.012**   Laceration without foreign body, left hip 🐾

    ● **S71.019**   Laceration without foreign body, unspecified hip 🐾

  ● **S71.02   Laceration with foreign body of hip**

    ● **S71.021**   Laceration with foreign body, right hip 🐾

    ● **S71.022**   Laceration with foreign body, left hip 🐾

    ● **S71.029**   Laceration with foreign body, unspecified hip 🐾

  ● **S71.03   Puncture wound without foreign body of hip**

    ● **S71.031**   Puncture wound without foreign body, right hip 🐾

    ● **S71.032**   Puncture wound without foreign body, left hip 🐾

    ● **S71.039**   Puncture wound without foreign body, unspecified hip 🐾

  ● **S71.04   Puncture wound with foreign body of hip**

    ● **S71.041**   Puncture wound with foreign body, right hip 🐾

    ● **S71.042**   Puncture wound with foreign body, left hip 🐾

    ● **S71.049**   Puncture wound with foreign body, unspecified hip 🐾

  ● **S71.05   Open bite of hip**

    Bite of hip NOS

    Excludes1 superficial bite of hip (S70.26, S70.27)

    ● **S71.051**   Open bite, right hip 🐾

    ● **S71.052**   Open bite, left hip 🐾

    ● **S71.059**   Open bite, unspecified hip 🐾

● **S71.1   Open wound of thigh**

  ● **S71.10   Unspecified open wound of thigh**

    ● **S71.101**   Unspecified open wound, right thigh 🐾

    ● **S71.102**   Unspecified open wound, left thigh 🐾

    ● **S71.109**   Unspecified open wound, unspecified thigh 🐾

  ● **S71.11   Laceration without foreign body of thigh**

    ● **S71.111**   Laceration without foreign body, right thigh 🐾

    ● **S71.112**   Laceration without foreign body, left thigh 🐾

    ● **S71.119**   Laceration without foreign body, unspecified thigh 🐾

  ● **S71.12   Laceration with foreign body of thigh**

    ● **S71.121**   Laceration with foreign body, right thigh 🐾

    ● **S71.122**   Laceration with foreign body, left thigh 🐾

    ● **S71.129**   Laceration with foreign body, unspecified thigh 🐾

  ● **S71.13   Puncture wound without foreign body of thigh**

    ● **S71.131**   Puncture wound without foreign body, right thigh 🐾

    ● **S71.132**   Puncture wound without foreign body, left thigh 🐾

    ● **S71.139**   Puncture wound without foreign body, unspecified thigh 🐾

  ● **S71.14   Puncture wound with foreign body of thigh**

    ● **S71.141**   Puncture wound with foreign body, right thigh 🐾

    ● **S71.142**   Puncture wound with foreign body, left thigh 🐾

    ● **S71.149**   Puncture wound with foreign body, unspecified thigh 🐾

  ● **S71.15   Open bite of thigh**

    Bite of thigh NOS

    Excludes1 superficial bite of thigh (S70.37-)

    ● **S71.151**   Open bite, right thigh 🐾

    ● **S71.152**   Open bite, left thigh 🐾

    ● **S71.159**   Open bite, unspecified thigh 🐾

CHAPTER 19 (S00-T88)

N Newborn Age: 0   P Pediatric Age: 0–17   M Maternity DX: 12–55   A Adult Age: 15–124   ♀ Females Only   ♂ Males Only

🐾 Complication\Comorbidity   🐾 Major C\C   (Ex) CC/MCC Exclusions   🐾 Present on Admission Requirement   🐾 Hospital-Acquired Condition

1431

S72 Fracture of femur

Note: A fracture not indicated as displaced or nondisplaced should be coded to displaced

A fracture not indicated as open or closed should be coded to closed

The open fracture designations are based on the Gustilo open fracture classification

Excludes1	traumatic amputation of hip and thigh (S78.-)
Excludes2	fracture of lower leg and ankle (S82.-)
	fracture of foot (S92.-)
	periprosthetic fracture of prosthetic implant of hip (T84.040, T84.041)

The appropriate 7th character is to be added to all codes from category S72

A	initial encounter for closed fracture
B	initial encounter for open fracture type I or II
	initial encounter for open fracture NOS
C	initial encounter for open fracture type IIIA, IIIB, or IIIC
D	subsequent encounter for closed fracture with routine healing
E	subsequent encounter for open fracture type I or II with routine healing
F	subsequent encounter for open fracture type IIIA, IIIB, or IIIC with routine healing
G	subsequent encounter for closed fracture with delayed healing
H	subsequent encounter for open fracture type I or II with delayed healing
J	subsequent encounter for open fracture type IIIA, IIIB, or IIIC with delayed healing
K	subsequent encounter for closed fracture with nonunion
M	subsequent encounter for open fracture type I or II with nonunion
N	subsequent encounter for open fracture type IIIA, IIIB, or IIIC with nonunion
P	subsequent encounter for closed fracture with malunion
Q	subsequent encounter for open fracture type I or II with malunion
R	subsequent encounter for open fracture type IIIA, IIIB, or IIIC with malunion
S	sequela

● S72.0 Fracture of head and neck of femur

| Excludes2 | physeal fracture of upper end of femur (S79.0-) |

● S72.00 Fracture of unspecified part of neck of femur
Fracture of hip NOS
Fracture of neck of femur NOS

● S72.001 Fracture of unspecified part of neck of right femur K, M, N, P, Q, R 🗪, A, B, C 🗪, 🗪, A, B, C 🗪

Ⓔⓧ For S72.001[A]: M48.40X-M48.58X[A], M80.00X-M80.88X[A], M84.30X-M84.68X[A], S03.8XX-S03.9XX[A], S29.011-S29.019[A], S38.3XX[A], S39.011-S39.013[A], S72.001[A,B,C], S72.002[B,C], S72.009-S72.011[A,B,C], S72.012[B,C], S72.019-S72.021[A,B,C], S72.022[B,C], S72.023-S72.024[A,B,C], S72.025[B,C], S72.026-S72.031[A,B,C], S72.032[B,C], S72.033-S72.034[A,B,C], S72.035[B,C], S72.036-S72.041[A,B,C], S72.042[B,C], S72.043-S72.044[A,B,C], S72.045[B,C], S72.046-S72.051[A,B,C], S72.052[B,C], S72.059-S72.061[A,B,C], S72.062[B,C], S72.063-S72.064[A,B,C], S72.065[B,C], S72.066-S72.091[A,B,C], S72.092[B,C], S72.099-S72.101[A,B,C], S72.102[B,C], S72.109-S72.111[A,B,C], S72.112[B,C], S72.113-S72.114[A,B,C], S72.115[B,C], S72.116-S72.121[A,B,C], S72.122[B,C],

S72.123-S72.124[A,B,C], S72.125[B,C], S72.126-S72.131[A,B,C], S72.132[B,C], S72.133-S72.134[A,B,C], S72.135[B,C], S72.136-S72.141[A,B,C], S72.142[B,C], S72.143-S72.144[A,B,C], S72.145[B,C], S72.146-S72.301[A,B,C], S72.302[B,C], S72.309-S72.321[A,B,C], S72.322[B,C], S72.323-S72.324[A,B,C], S72.325[B,C], S72.326-S72.331[A,B,C], S72.332[B,C], S72.333-S72.334[A,B,C], S72.335[B,C], S72.336-S72.341[A,B,C], S72.342[B,C], S72.343-S72.344[A,B,C], S72.345[B,C], S72.346-S72.351[A,B,C], S72.352[B,C], S72.353-S72.354[A,B,C], S72.355[B,C], S72.356-S72.361[A,B,C], S72.362[B,C], S72.363-S72.364[A,B,C], S72.365[B,C], S72.366-S72.391[A,B,C], S72.392[B,C], S72.399-S72.401[A,B,C], S72.402[B,C], S72.409-S72.411[A,B,C], S72.412[B,C], S72.413-S72.414[A,B,C], S72.415[B,C], S72.416-S72.421[A,B,C], S72.422[B,C], S72.423-S72.424[A,B,C], S72.425[B,C], S72.426-S72.431[A,B,C], S72.432[B,C], S72.433-S72.434[A,B,C], S72.435[B,C], S72.436-S72.441[A,B,C], S72.442[B,C], S72.443-S72.444[A,B,C], S72.445[B,C], S72.446-S72.451[A,B,C], S72.452[B,C], S72.453-S72.454[A,B,C], S72.455[B,C], S72.456-S72.461[A,B,C], S72.462[B,C], S72.463-S72.464[A,B,C], S72.465[B,C], S72.466[A,B,C], S72.471[A], S72.479[A], S72.491[A,B,C], S72.492[B,C], S72.499-S72.92X[A,B,C], S73.101[A], S73.109-S73.111[A], S73.119-S73.121[A], S73.129-S73.191[A], S73.199[A], S76.001[A], S76.009-S76.011[A], S76.019[A], S76.091[A], S76.099-S76.101[A], S76.109-S76.111[A], S76.119[A], S76.191[A], S76.199-S76.201[A], S76.209-S76.211[A], S76.219[A], S76.291[A], S76.299-S76.301[A], S76.309-S76.311[A], S76.319[A], S76.391[A], S76.399-S76.801[A], S76.809-S76.811[A], S76.819[A], S76.891[A], S76.899-S76.901[A], S76.909-S76.911[A], S76.919[A], S76.991[A], S76.999[A], S79.001[A], S79.009-S79.011[A], S79.019-S79.091[A], S79.099-S79.101[A], S79.109-S79.111[A], S79.119-S79.121[A], S79.129-S79.131[A], S79.139-S79.141[A], S79.149-S79.191[A], S79.199-S79.811[A], S79.819-S79.821[A], S79.829-S79.911[A], S79.919-S79.921[A], S79.929[A], S82.90X-S82.92X[A,B,C], T14.8-T14.91, T79. A0X-T79.9XX[A] **For S72.001[B,C]:** M48.40X-M48.58X[A], M80.00X-M80.88X[A], M84.30X-M84.68X[A], S03.8XX-S03.9XX[A], S29.011-S29.019[A], S38.3XX[A], S39.011-S39.013[A], S72.001-S72.466[A,B,C], S72.471-S72.479[A], S72.491-S72.92X[A,B,C], S73.101-S73.199[A], S76.001-S76.019[A], S76.091-S76.119[A], S76.191-S76.219[A], S76.291-S76.319[A], S76.391-S76.819[A], S76.891-S76.919[A], S76.991-S76.999[A], S79.001-S79.929[A], S82.90X-S82.92X[A,B,C], T14.8-T14.91, T79.A0X-T79.9XX[A] **For S72.001[K,M,N,P,Q,R]:** M80.00X-M80.88X[K,P], M84.30X-M84.68X[K,P], S02.0XX-S02.92X[K], S12.000-S12.691[K], S22.000-S22.9XX[K], S32.000-S32.9XX[K], S42.001-S42.92X[K,P], S49.001-S49.199[K,P], S52.001-S52.92X[K,M,N,P,Q,R], S59.001-S59.299[K,P], S62.001-S62.92X[K,P], S72.001-S72.92X[K,M,N,P,Q,R], S79.001-S79.199[K,P], S82.001-S82.92X[K,M,N,P,Q,R], S89.001-S89.399[K,P], S92.001-S92.919[K,P]

◀ New   ◀═ Revised   d̶e̶l̶e̶t̶e̶d̶ Deleted   Excludes 1   Excludes 2   Includes   Use additional   Code first   Code also   Unspecified

OGCR Official Guidelines   ● Unacceptable Principal Diagnosis   X Assign placeholder X   ● Use Additional Character(s)   ▶ Manifestation Code   **Coding Clinic**

CHAPTER 19 (S00-T88)

● S72.002 Fracture of unspecified part of neck of
left femur K, M, N, P, Q, R 🔵,
A, B, C 🔵, 🔵, A, B, C 🔵
⊕ **For S72.002[A]:** M48.40X-M48.58X[A],
M80.00X-M80.88X[A], M84.30X-M84.68X[A],
S03.8XX-S03.9XX[A], S29.011-S29.019[A],
S38.3XX[A], S39.011-S39.013[A],
S72.001[B,C], S72.002-S72.009[A,B,C],
S72.011[B,C], S72.012-S72.019[A,B,C],
S72.021[B,C], S72.022-S72.023[A,B,C],
S72.024[B,C], S72.025-S72.026[A,B,C],
S72.031[B,C], S72.032-S72.033[A,B,C],
S72.034[B,C], S72.035-S72.036[A,B,C],
S72.041[B,C], S72.042-S72.043[A,B,C],
S72.044[B,C], S72.045-S72.046[A,B,C],
S72.051[B,C], S72.052-S72.059[A,B,C],
S72.061[B,C], S72.062-S72.063[A,B,C],
S72.064[B,C], S72.065-S72.066[A,B,C],
S72.091[B,C], S72.092-S72.099[A,B,C],
S72.101[B,C], S72.102-S72.109[A,B,C],
S72.111[B,C], S72.112-S72.113[A,B,C],
S72.114[B,C], S72.115-S72.116[A,B,C],
S72.121[B,C], S72.122-S72.123[A,B,C],
S72.124[B,C], S72.125-S72.126[A,B,C],
S72.131[B,C], S72.132-S72.133[A,B,C],
S72.134[B,C], S72.135-S72.136[A,B,C],
S72.141[B,C], S72.142-S72.143[C],
S72.144[B,C], S72.145-S72.146[A,B,C],
S72.21X-S72.26X[A,B,C], S72.301[B,C],
S72.302-S72.309[A,B,C], S72.311[B,C],
S72.322-S72.323[A,B,C], S72.324[B,C],
S72.325-S72.326[A,B,C], S72.331[B,C],
S72.332-S72.333[A,B,C], S72.334[B,C],
S72.335-S72.336[A,B,C], S72.341[B,C],
S72.342-S72.343[A,B,C], S72.344[B,C],
S72.345-S72.346[A,B,C], S72.351[B,C],
S72.352-S72.353[A,B,C], S72.354[B,C],
S72.355-S72.356[A,B,C], S72.361[B,C],
S72.362-S72.363[A,B,C], S72.364[B,C],
S72.365-S72.366[A,B,C], S72.391[B,C],
S72.392-S72.399[A,B,C], S72.401[B,C],
S72.402-S72.409[A,B,C], S72.411[B,C],
S72.412-S72.413[A,B,C], S72.414[B,C],
S72.415-S72.416[A,B,C], S72.421[B,C],
S72.422-S72.423[A,B,C], S72.424[B,C],
S72.425-S72.426[A,B,C], S72.431[B,C],
S72.432-S72.433[A,B,C], S72.434[B,C],
S72.435-S72.436[A,B,C], S72.441[B,C],
S72.442-S72.443[A,B,C], S72.444[B,C],
S72.445-S72.446[A,B,C], S72.451[B,C],
S72.452-S72.453[A,B,C], S72.454[B,C],
S72.455-S72.456[A,B,C], S72.461[B,C],
S72.462-S72.463[A,B,C], S72.464[B,C],
S72.465-S72.466[A,B,C], S72.472-S72.479[A],
S72.491[B,C], S72.492-S72.92X[A,B,C],
S73.102-S73.109[A], S73.112-S73.119[A],
S73.122-S73.129[A], S73.192-S73.199[A],
S76.002-S76.009[A], S76.012-S76.019[A],
S76.092-S76.099[A], S76.102-S76.109[A],
S76.112-S76.119[A], S76.192-S76.199[A],
S76.202-S76.209[A], S76.212-S76.219[A],
S76.292-S76.299[A], S76.302-S76.309[A],
S76.312-S76.319[A], S76.392-S76.399[A],
S76.802-S76.809[A], S76.812-S76.819[A],
S76.892-S76.899[A], S76.902-S76.909[A],
S76.912-S76.919[A], S76.992-S76.999[A],
S79.002-S79.009[A], S79.012-S79.019[A],
S79.092-S79.099[A], S79.102-S79.109[A],
S79.112-S79.119[A], S79.122-S79.129[A],
S79.132-S79.139[A], S79.142-S79.149[A],
S79.192-S79.199[A], S79.812-S79.819[A],
S79.822-S79.829[A], S79.912-S79.919[A],
S79.922-S79.929[A], S82.90X-S82.92X[A,B,C],
T14.8-T14.91, T79.8XXA T79.A0X-T79.9XX[A]
For S72.002[B,C]: See S72.001[B,C]
For S72.002[K,M,N,P,Q,R]: See
S72.001[K,M,N,P,Q,R]

● S72.009 Fracture of unspecified part of neck of
unspecified femur K, M, N, P, Q, R 🔵,
A, B, C 🔵, 🔵, A, B, C 🔵
⊕ **For S72.009[A,B,C]:** See S72.001[B,C]
For S72.009[K,M,N,P,Q,R]: See
S72.001[K,M,N,P,Q,R]

● S72.01 Unspecified intracapsular fracture of femur
Subcapital fracture of femur

● S72.011 Unspecified intracapsular fracture of
right femur K, M, N, P, Q, R 🔵,
A, B, C 🔵, 🔵, A, B, C 🔵
⊕ **For S72.011[A]:** See S72.001 [A]
For S72.011[B,C]: See S72.001[B,C]
For S72.011[K,M,N,P,Q,R]: See
S72.001K,M,N,P,Q,R]

● S72.012 Unspecified intracapsular fracture of
left femur K, M, N, P, Q, R 🔵,
A, B, C 🔵, 🔵, A, B, C 🔵
⊕ **For S72.012[A]:** See S72.002[A]
For S72.012[B,C]: See S72.001[B,C]
For S72.012[K,M,N,P,Q,R]: See
S72.001[K,M,N,P,Q,R]

● S72.019 Unspecified intracapsular fracture of
unspecified femur K, M, N, P, Q, R 🔵,
A, B, C 🔵, 🔵, A, B, C 🔵
⊕ **For S72.019[A,B,C]:** See S72.001[B,C]
For S72.019[K,M,N,P,Q,R]: See
S72.001[K,M,N,P,Q,R]

● S72.02 Fracture of epiphysis (separation) (upper) of
femur
Transepiphyseal fracture of femur
Fracture and separation across growth plate
Excludes1 capital femoral epiphyseal
fracture (pediatric) of femur
(S79.01-)
Salter-Harris Type I physeal
fracture of upper end of
femur (S79.01-)

● S72.021 Displaced fracture of epiphysis
(separation) (upper) of right femur
K, M, N, P, Q, R 🔵, A, B, C 🔵, 🔵,
A, B, C 🔵
⊕ **For S72.021[A]:** See S72.001[A]
For S72.021[B,C]: See S72.001[B,C]
For S72.021[K,M,N,P,Q,R]: See
S72.001[K,M,N,P,Q,R]

● S72.022 Displaced fracture of epiphysis
(separation) (upper) of left femur
K, M, N, P, Q, R 🔵, A, B, C 🔵, 🔵,
A, B, C 🔵
⊕ **For S72.022[A]:** See S72.002[A]
For S72.022[B,C]: See S72.001[B,C]
For S72.022[K,M,N,P,Q,R]: See
S72.001[K,M,N,P,Q,R]

● S72.023 Displaced fracture of epiphysis
(separation) (upper) of unspecified
femur K, M, N, P, Q, R 🔵, A, B, C 🔵,
🔵, A, B, C 🔵
⊕ **For S72.023[A,B,C]:** See S72.001[B,C]
For S72.023[K,M,N,P,Q,R]: See
S72.001[K,M,N,P,Q,R]

● S72.024 Nondisplaced fracture of epiphysis
(separation) (upper) of right femur
K, M, N, P, Q, R 🔵, A, B, C 🔵, 🔵,
A, B, C 🔵
⊕ **For S72.024[A]:** See S72.004[A]
For S72.024[B,C]: See S72.001[B,C]
For S72.024[K,M,N,P,Q,R]: See
S72.001[K,M,N,P,Q,R]

CHAPTER 19 (S00-T88)

N   Newborn Age: 0   P   Pediatric Age: 0–17   M   Maternity DX: 12–55   A   Adult Age: 15–124   ♀   Females Only   ♂   Males Only
🔵 Complication\Comorbidity   🔵   Major C\C   ⊕   CC/MCC Exclusions   🔵   Present on Admission Requirement   🔵   Hospital-Acquired Condition

1433

CHAPTER 19 (S00–T88)

● S72.025   Nondisplaced fracture of epiphysis (separation) (upper) of left femur K, M, N, P, Q, R ◉, A, B, C ◉, ◉, A, B, C ◉
    Ⓔⓧ For S72.025[A]: See S72.002[A]
       For S72.025[B,C]: See S72.001[B,C]
       For S72.025[K,M,N,P,Q,R]:
         See S72.001[K,M,N,P,Q,R]

● S72.026   Nondisplaced fracture of epiphysis (separation) (upper) of unspecified femur K, M, N, P, Q, R ◉, A, B, C ◉, ◉, A, B, C ◉
    Ⓔⓧ For S72.026[A,B,C]: See S72.001[B,C]
       For S72.026[K,M,N,P,Q,R]:
         See S72.001[K,M,N,P,Q,R]

● S72.03   Midcervical fracture of femur
    Transcervical fracture of femur NOS

● S72.031   Displaced midcervical fracture of right femur K, M, N, P, Q, R ◉, A, B, C ◉, ◉, A, B, C ◉
    Ⓔⓧ For S72.031[A]: See S72.004[A]
       For S72.031[B,C]: See S72.001[B,C]
       For S72.031[K,M,N,P,Q,R]:
         See S72.001[K,M,N,P,Q,R]

● S72.032   Displaced midcervical fracture of left femur K, M, N, P, Q, R ◉, A, B, C ◉, ◉, A, B, C ◉
    Ⓔⓧ For S72.032[A]: See S72.002[A]
       For S72.032[B,C]: See S72.001[B,C]
       For S72.032[K,M,N,P,Q,R]:
         See S72.001[K,M,N,P,Q,R]

● S72.033   Displaced midcervical fracture of unspecified femur K, M, N, P, Q, R ◉, A, B, C ◉, ◉, A, B, C ◉
    Ⓔⓧ For S72.033[A,B,C]: See S72.001[B,C]
       For S72.033[K,M,N,P,Q,R]:
         See S72.001[K,M,N,P,Q,R]

● S72.034   Nondisplaced midcervical fracture of right femur K, M, N, P, Q, R ◉, A, B, C ◉, ◉, A, B, C ◉
    Ⓔⓧ For S72.034[A]: See S72.004[A]
       For S72.034[B,C]: See S72.001[B,C]
       For S72.034[K,M,N,P,Q,R]:
         See S72.001[K,M,N,P,Q,R]

● S72.035   Nondisplaced midcervical fracture of left femur K, M, N, P, Q, R ◉, A, B, C ◉, ◉, A, B, C ◉
    Ⓔⓧ For S72.035[A]: See S72.002[A]
       For S72.035[B,C]: See S72.001[B,C]
       For S72.035[K,M,N,P,Q,R]:
         See S72.001[K,M,N,P,Q,R]

● S72.036   Nondisplaced midcervical fracture of unspecified femur K, M, N, P, Q, R ◉, A, B, C ◉, ◉, A, B, C ◉
    Ⓔⓧ For S72.036[A,B,C]: See S72.001[B,C]
       For S72.036[K,M,N,P,Q,R]:
         See S72.001[K,M,N,P,Q,R]

● S72.04   Fracture of base of neck of femur
    Cervicotrochanteric fracture of femur

● S72.041   Displaced fracture of base of neck of right femur K, M, N, P, Q, R ◉, A, B, C ◉, ◉, A, B, C ◉
    Ⓔⓧ For S72.041[A]: See S72.004[A]
       For S72.041[B,C]: See S72.001[B,C]
       For S72.041[K,M,N,P,Q,R]:
         See S72.001[K,M,N,P,Q,R]

● S72.042   Displaced fracture of base of neck of left femur K, M, N, P, Q, R ◉, A, B, C ◉, ◉, A, B, C ◉
    Ⓔⓧ For S72.042[A]: See S72.002[A]
       For S72.042[B,C]: See S72.001[B,C]
       For S72.042[K,M,N,P,Q,R]:
         See S72.001[K,M,N,P,Q,R]

● S72.043   Displaced fracture of base of neck of unspecified femur K, M, N, P, Q, R ◉, A, B, C ◉, ◉, A, B, C ◉
    Ⓔⓧ For S72.043[A,B,C]: See S72.001[B,C]
       For S72.043[K,M,N,P,Q,R]:
         See S72.001[K,M,N,P,Q,R]

● S72.044   Nondisplaced fracture of base of neck of right femur K, M, N, P, Q, R ◉, A, B, C ◉, ◉, A, B, C ◉
    Ⓔⓧ For S72.044[A]: See S72.004[A]
       For S72.044[B,C]: See S72.001[B,C]
       For S72.044[K,M,N,P,Q,R]:
         See S72.001[K,M,N,P,Q,R]

● S72.045   Nondisplaced fracture of base of neck of left femur K, M, N, P, Q, R ◉, A, B, C ◉, ◉, A, B, C ◉
    Ⓔⓧ For S72.045[A]: See S72.002[A]
       For S72.045[B,C]: See S72.001[B,C]
       For S72.045[K,M,N,P,Q,R]:
         See S72.001[K,M,N,P,Q,R]

● S72.046   Nondisplaced fracture of base of neck of unspecified femur K, M, N, P, Q, R ◉, A, B, C ◉, ◉, A, B, C ◉
    Ⓔⓧ For S72.046[A,B,C]: See S72.001[B,C]
       For S72.046[K,M,N,P,Q,R]:
         See S72.001[K,M,N,P,Q,R]

● S72.05   Unspecified fracture of head of femur
    Fracture of head of femur NOS

● S72.051   Unspecified fracture of head of right femur K, M, N, P, Q, R ◉, A, B, C ◉, ◉, A, B, C ◉
    Ⓔⓧ For S72.051[A]: See S72.004[A]
       For S72.051[B,C]: See S72.001[B,C]
       For S72.051[K,M,N,P,Q,R]:
         See S72.001[K,M,N,P,Q,R]

● S72.052   Unspecified fracture of head of left femur K, M, N, P, Q, R ◉, A, B, C ◉, ◉, A, B, C ◉
    Ⓔⓧ For S72.052[A]: See S72.002[A]
       For S72.052[B,C]: See S72.001[B,C]
       For S72.052[K,M,N,P,Q,R]:
         See S72.001[K,M,N,P,Q,R]

● S72.059   Unspecified fracture of head of unspecified femur K, M, N, P, Q, R ◉, A, B, C ◉, ◉, A, B, C ◉
    Ⓔⓧ For S72.059[A,B,C]: See S72.001[B,C]
       For S72.059[K,M,N,P,Q,R]:
         See S72.001[K,M,N,P,Q,R]

● S72.06   Articular fracture of head of femur

● S72.061   Displaced articular fracture of head of right femur K, M, N, P, Q, R ◉, A, B, C ◉, ◉, A, B, C ◉
    Ⓔⓧ For S72.061[A]: See S72.004[A]
       For S72.061[B,C]: See S72.001[B,C]
       For S72.061[K,M,N,P,Q,R]:
         See S72.001[K,M,N,P,Q,R]

● S72.062   Displaced articular fracture of head of left femur K, M, N, P, Q, R ◉, A, B, C ◉, ◉, A, B, C ◉
    Ⓔⓧ For S72.062[A]: See S72.002[A]
       For S72.062[B,C]: See S72.001[B,C]
       For S72.062[K,M,N,P,Q,R]:
         See S72.001[K,M,N,P,Q,R]

● S72.063   Displaced articular fracture of head of unspecified femur K, M, N, P, Q, R ◉, A, B, C ◉, ◉, A, B, C ◉
    Ⓔⓧ For S72.063[A,B,C]: See S72.001[B,C]
       For S72.063[K,M,N,P,Q,R]:
         See S72.001[K,M,N,P,Q,R]

● S72.064   Nondisplaced articular fracture of head of right femur K, M, N, P, Q, R ◉, A, B, C ◉, ◉, A, B, C ◉
    Ⓔⓧ For S72.064[A]: See S72.004[A]
       For S72.064[B,C]: See S72.001[B,C]
       For S72.064[K,M,N,P,Q,R]:
         See S72.001[K,M,N,P,Q,R]

◀ New   ◀▥ Revised   ~~deleted~~ Deleted   Excludes 1   Excludes 2   Includes   Use additional   Code first   Code also   Unspecified
OGCR Official Guidelines   ● Unacceptable Principal Diagnosis   X Assign placeholder X   ◉ Use Additional Character(s)   ▸ Manifestation Code   Coding Clinic

● S72.065   Nondisplaced articular fracture of head of left femur K, M, N, P, Q, R 🝝, A, B, C 🝝, 🝝, A, B, C 🝝
   Ⓔ For S72.065[A]: See S72.002[A]
     For S72.065[B,C]: See S72.001[B,C]
     For S72.065[K,M,N,P,Q,R]:
     See S72.001[K,M,N,P,Q,R]

● S72.066   Nondisplaced articular fracture of head of unspecified femur K, M, N, P, Q, R 🝝, A, B, C 🝝, 🝝, A, B, C 🝝
   Ⓔ For S72.066[A,B,C]: See S72.001[B,C]
     For S72.066[K,M,N,P,Q,R]:
     See S72.001[K,M,N,P,Q,R]

● S72.09   Other fracture of head and neck of femur

● S72.091   Other fracture of head and neck of right femur K, M, N, P, Q, R 🝝, A, B, C 🝝, 🝝, A, B, C 🝝
   Ⓔ For S72.091[A]: See S72.004[A]
     For S72.091[B,C]: See S72.001[B,C]
     For S72.091[K,M,N,P,Q,R]:
     See S72.001K,M,N,P,Q,R]

● S72.092   Other fracture of head and neck of left femur K, M, N, P, Q, R 🝝, A, B, C 🝝, 🝝, A, B, C 🝝
   Ⓔ For S72.092[A]: See S72.002[A]
     For S72.092[B,C]: See S72.001[B,C]
     For S72.092[K,M,N,P,Q,R]:
     See S72.001[K,M,N,P,Q,R]

● S72.099   Other fracture of head and neck of unspecified femur K, M, N, P, Q, R 🝝, A, B, C 🝝, 🝝, A, B, C 🝝
   Ⓔ For S72.099[A,B,C]: See S72.001[B,C]
     For S72.099[K,M,N,P,Q,R]:
     See S72.001[K,M,N,P,Q,R]

● S72.1   **Pertrochanteric fracture**
Fracture extending close to, but not into, joint

● S72.10   Unspecified trochanteric fracture of femur
Fracture of trochanter NOS

● S72.101   Unspecified trochanteric fracture of right femur K, M, N, P, Q, R 🝝, A, B, C 🝝, 🝝, A, B, C 🝝
   Ⓔ For S72.101[A]: See S72.004[A]
     For S72.101[B,C]: See S72.001[B,C]
     For S72.101[K,M,N,P,Q,R]:
     See S72.001[K,M,N,P,Q,R]

● S72.102   Unspecified trochanteric fracture of left femur K, M, N, P, Q, R 🝝, A, B, C 🝝, 🝝, A, B, C 🝝
   Ⓔ For S72.102[A]: See S72.002[A]
     For S72.102[B,C]: See S72.001[B,C]
     For S72.102[K,M,N,P,Q,R]:
     See S72.001[K,M,N,P,Q,R]

● S72.109   Unspecified trochanteric fracture of unspecified femur K, M, N, P, Q, R 🝝, A, B, C 🝝
   Ⓔ For S72.109[A,B,C]: See S72.001[B,C]
     For S72.109[K,M,N,P,Q,R]:
     See S72.001[K,M,N,P,Q,R]

● S72.11   Fracture of greater trochanter of femur

● S72.111   Displaced fracture of greater trochanter of right femur K, M, N, P, Q, R 🝝, A, B, C 🝝, 🝝, A, B, C 🝝
   Ⓔ For S72.111[A]: See S72.004[A]
     For S72.111[B,C]: See S72.001[B,C]
     For S72.111[K,M,N,P,Q,R]:
     See S72.001[K,M,N,P,Q,R]

● S72.112   Displaced fracture of greater trochanter of left femur K, M, N, P, Q, R 🝝, A, B, C 🝝, 🝝, A, B, C 🝝
   Ⓔ For S72.112[A]: See S72.002[A]
     For S72.112[B,C]: See S72.001[B,C]
     For S72.112[K,M,N,P,Q,R]:
     See S72.001[K,M,N,P,Q,R]

● S72.113   Displaced fracture of greater trochanter of unspecified femur K, M, N, P, Q, R 🝝, A, B, C 🝝, 🝝, A, B, C 🝝
   Ⓔ For S72.113[A,B,C]: See S72.001[B,C]
     For S72.113[K,M,N,P,Q,R]:
     See S72.001[K,M,N,P,Q,R]

● S72.114   Nondisplaced fracture of greater trochanter of right femur K, M, N, P, Q, R 🝝, A, B, C 🝝, 🝝, A, B, C 🝝
   Ⓔ For S72.114[A]: See S72.004[A]
     For S72.114[B,C]: See S72.001[B,C]
     For S72.114[K,M,N,P,Q,R]:
     See S72.001[K,M,N,P,Q,R]

● S72.115   Nondisplaced fracture of greater trochanter of left femur K, M, N, P, Q, R 🝝, A, B, C 🝝, 🝝, A, B, C 🝝
   Ⓔ For S72.115[A]: See S72.002[A]
     For S72.115[B,C]: See S72.001[B,C]
     For S72.115[K,M,N,P,Q,R]:
     See S72.001[K,M,N,P,Q,R]

● S72.116   Nondisplaced fracture of greater trochanter of unspecified femur K, M, N, P, Q, R 🝝, A, B, C 🝝
   Ⓔ For S72.116[A,B,C]: See S72.001[B,C]
     For S72.116[K,M,N,P,Q,R]:
     See S72.001[K,M,N,P,Q,R]

● S72.12   Fracture of lesser trochanter of femur

● S72.121   Displaced fracture of lesser trochanter of right femur K, M, N, P, Q, R 🝝, A, B, C 🝝, 🝝, A, B, C 🝝
   Ⓔ For S72.121[A]: See S72.004[A]
     For S72.121[B,C]: See S72.001[B,C]
     For S72.121[K,M,N,P,Q,R]:
     See S72.001[K,M,N,P,Q,R]

● S72.122   Displaced fracture of lesser trochanter of left femur K, M, N, P, Q, R 🝝, A, B, C 🝝, 🝝, A, B, C 🝝
   Ⓔ For S72.122[A]: See S72.002[A]
     For S72.122[B,C]: See S72.001[B,C]
     For S72.122[K,M,N,P,Q,R]:
     See S72.001[K,M,N,P,Q,R]

● S72.123   Displaced fracture of lesser trochanter of unspecified femur K, M, N, P, Q, R 🝝, A, B, C 🝝, 🝝, A, B, C 🝝
   Ⓔ For S72.123[A,B,C]: See S72.001[B,C]
     For S72.123[K,M,N,P,Q,R]:
     See S72.001[K,M,N,P,Q,R]

● S72.124   Nondisplaced fracture of lesser trochanter of right femur K, M, N, P, Q, R 🝝, A, B, C 🝝, 🝝, A, B, C 🝝
   Ⓔ For S72.124[A]: See S72.004[A]
     For S72.124[B,C]: See S72.001[B,C]
     For S72.124[K,M,N,P,Q,R]:
     See S72.001[K,M,N,P,Q,R]

● S72.125   Nondisplaced fracture of lesser trochanter of left femur K, M, N, P, Q, R 🝝, A, B, C 🝝, 🝝, A, B, C 🝝
   Ⓔ For S72.125[A]: See S72.002[A]
     For S72.125[B,C]: See S72.001[B,C]
     For S72.125[K,M,N,P,Q,R]:
     See S72.001[K,M,N,P,Q,R]

● S72.126   Nondisplaced fracture of lesser trochanter of unspecified femur K, M, N, P, Q, R 🝝, A, B, C 🝝, 🝝, A, B, C 🝝
   Ⓔ For S72.126[A,B,C]: See S72.001[B,C]
     For S72.126[K,M,N,P,Q,R]:
     See S72.001[K,M,N,P,Q,R]

CHAPTER 19 (S00–T88)

N Newborn Age: 0   P Pediatric Age: 0–17   M Maternity DX: 12–55   A Adult Age: 15–124   ♀ Females Only   ♂ Males Only
🝝 Complication\Comorbidity   🝝 Major C\C   Ⓔ CC/MCC Exclusions   🝝 Present on Admission Requirement   🝝 Hospital-Acquired Condition

1435

● S72.13 Apophyseal fracture of femur
Pertaining to articulations between articular facets of adjacent vertebrae

Excludes1 chronic (nontraumatic) slipped upper femoral epiphysis (M93.0-)

● S72.131 Displaced apophyseal fracture of right femur K, M, N, P, Q, R 🔖, A, B, C 🔖, 🔖, A, B, C 🔖
(Ex:) For S72.131[A]: See S72.004[A]
For S72.131[B,C]: See S72.001[B,C]
For S72.131[K,M,N,P,Q,R]: See S72.001[K,M,N,P,Q,R]

● S72.132 Displaced apophyseal fracture of left femur K, M, N, P, Q, R 🔖, A, B, C 🔖, 🔖, A, B, C 🔖
(Ex:) For S72.132[A]: See S72.002[A]
For S72.132[B,C]: See S72.001[B,C]
For S72.132[K,M,N,P,Q,R]: See S72.001[K,M,N,P,Q,R]

● S72.133 Displaced apophyseal fracture of unspecified femur K, M, N, P, Q, R 🔖, A, B, C 🔖, 🔖, A, B, C 🔖
(Ex:) For S72.133[A,B,C]: See S72.001[B,C]
For S72.133[K,M,N,P,Q,R]: See S72.001[K,M,N,P,Q,R]

● S72.134 Nondisplaced apophyseal fracture of right femur K, M, N, P, Q, R 🔖, A, B, C 🔖, 🔖, A, B, C 🔖
(Ex:) For S72.134[A]: See S72.004[A]
For S72.134[B,C]: See S72.001[B,C]
For S72.134[K,M,N,P,Q,R]: See S72.001[K,M,N,P,Q,R]

● S72.135 Nondisplaced apophyseal fracture of left femur K, M, N, P, Q, R 🔖, A, B, C 🔖, 🔖, A, B, C 🔖
(Ex:) For S72.135[A]: See S72.002[A]
For S72.135[B,C]: See S72.001[B,C]
For S72.135[K,M,N,P,Q,R]: See S72.001[K,M,N,P,Q,R]

● S72.136 Nondisplaced apophyseal fracture of unspecified femur K, M, N, P, Q, R 🔖, A, B, C 🔖, 🔖, A, B, C 🔖
(Ex:) For S72.136[A,B,C]: See S72.001[B,C]
For S72.136[K,M,N,P,Q,R]: See S72.001[K,M,N,P,Q,R]

● S72.14 Intertrochanteric fracture of femur

● S72.141 Displaced intertrochanteric fracture of right femur K, M, N, P, Q, R 🔖, A, B, C 🔖, 🔖, A, B, C 🔖
(Ex:) For S72.141[A]: See S72.004[A]
For S72.141[B,C]: See S72.001[B,C]
For S72.141[K,M,N,P,Q,R]: See S72.001[K,M,N,P,Q,R]

● S72.142 Displaced intertrochanteric fracture of left femur K, M, N, P, Q, R 🔖, A, B, C 🔖, 🔖, A, B, C 🔖
(Ex:) For S72.142[A]: See S72.002[A]
For S72.142[B,C]: See S72.001[B,C]
For S72.142[K,M,N,P,Q,R]: See S72.001[K,M,N,P,Q,R]

● S72.143 Displaced intertrochanteric fracture of unspecified femur K, M, N, P, Q, R 🔖, A, B, C 🔖, 🔖, A, B, C 🔖
(Ex:) For S72.143[A,B,C]: See S72.001[B,C]
For S72.143[K,M,N,P,Q,R]: See S72.001[K,M,N,P,Q,R]

● S72.144 Nondisplaced intertrochanteric fracture of right femur K, M, N, P, Q, R 🔖, A, B, C 🔖, 🔖, A, B, C 🔖
(Ex:) For S72.144[A]: See S72.004[A]
For S72.144[B,C]: See S72.001[B,C]
For S72.144[K,M,N,P,Q,R]: See S72.001[K,M,N,P,Q,R]

● S72.145 Nondisplaced intertrochanteric fracture of left femur K, M, N, P, Q, R 🔖, A, B, C 🔖, 🔖, A, B, C 🔖
(Ex:) For S72.145[A]: See S72.002[A]
For S72.145[B,C]: See S72.001[B,C]
For S72.145[K,M,N,P,Q,R]: See S72.001[K,M,N,P,Q,R]

● S72.146 Nondisplaced intertrochanteric fracture of unspecified femur K, M, N, P, Q, R 🔖, A, B, C 🔖, 🔖, A, B, C 🔖
(Ex:) For S72.146[A,B,C]: See S72.001[B,C]
For S72.146[K,M,N,P,Q,R]: See S72.001[K,M,N,P,Q,R]

● S72.2 Subtrochanteric fracture of femur
Subtrochanteric: inferior to trochanter
(Ex:) For category S72.2 CC codes S72.2[A,B,C]: See S72.001[B,C]
For S72.2[K,M,N,P,Q,R]: See S72.001[K,M,N,P,Q,R]

X ● S72.21 Displaced subtrochanteric fracture of right femur K, M, N, P, Q, R 🔖, A, B, C 🔖, A, B, C 🔖

X ● S72.22 Displaced subtrochanteric fracture of left femur K, M, N, P, Q, R 🔖, A, B, C 🔖, 🔖, A, B, C 🔖

X ● S72.23 Displaced subtrochanteric fracture of unspecified femur K, M, N, P, Q, R 🔖, A, B, C 🔖, 🔖, A, B, C 🔖

X ● S72.24 Nondisplaced subtrochanteric fracture of right femur K, M, N, P, Q, R 🔖, A, B, C 🔖, 🔖, A, B, C 🔖

X ● S72.25 Nondisplaced subtrochanteric fracture of left femur K, M, N, P, Q, R 🔖, A, B, C 🔖, 🔖, A, B, C 🔖

X ● S72.26 Nondisplaced subtrochanteric fracture of unspecified femur K, M, N, P, Q, R 🔖, A, B, C 🔖, A, B, C 🔖

● S72.3 Fracture of shaft of femur

● S72.30 Unspecified fracture of shaft of femur

● S72.301 Unspecified fracture of shaft of right femur K, M, N, P, Q, R 🔖, A, B, C 🔖, 🔖, A, B, C 🔖
(Ex:) For S72.301[A]: See S72.004[A]
For S72.301[B,C]: See S72.001[B,C]
For S72.301[K,M,N,P,Q,R]: See S72.001[K,M,N,P,Q,R]

● S72.302 Unspecified fracture of shaft of left femur K, M, N, P, Q, R 🔖, A, B, C 🔖, 🔖, A, B, C 🔖
(Ex:) For S72.302[A]: See S72.002[A]
For S72.302[B,C]: See S72.001[B,C]
For S72.302[K,M,N,P,Q,R]: See S72.001[K,M,N,P,Q,R]

● S72.309 Unspecified fracture of shaft of unspecified femur K, M, N, P, Q, R 🔖, A, B, C 🔖, 🔖, A, B, C 🔖
(Ex:) For S72.309[A,B,C]: See S72.001[B,C]
For S72.309[K,M,N,P,Q,R]: See S72.001[K,M,N,P,Q,R]

● S72.32 Transverse fracture of shaft of femur

● S72.321 Displaced transverse fracture of shaft of right femur K, M, N, P, Q, R 🔖, A, B, C 🔖, 🔖, A, B, C 🔖
(Ex:) For S72.321[A]: See S72.004[A]
For S72.321[B,C]: See S72.001[B,C]
For S72.321[K,M,N,P,Q,R]: See S72.001[K,M,N,P,Q,R]

● S72.322 Displaced transverse fracture of shaft of left femur K, M, N, P, Q, R 🔖, A, B, C 🔖, 🔖, A, B, C 🔖
(Ex:) For S72.322[A]: See S72.002[A]
For S72.322[B,C]: See S72.001[B,C]
For S72.322[K,M,N,P,Q,R]: See S72.001[K,M,N,P,Q,R]

◀ New ◀‖‖ Revised ~~deleted~~ Deleted | Excludes 1 | Excludes 2 | Includes | Use additional | Code first | Code also | Unspecified
OGCR Official Guidelines ● Unacceptable Principal Diagnosis X Assign placeholder X ● Use Additional Character(s) ▌ Manifestation Code **Coding Clinic**

CHAPTER 19 (S00-T88)

● S72.323   Displaced transverse fracture of shaft of unspecified femur K, M, N, P, Q, R 🝔, A, B, C 🝔, 🝔, A, B, C 🝔
    (Ex) For S72.323[A,B,C]: See S72.001[B,C]
      For S72.323[K,M,N,P,Q,R]:
      See S72.001[K,M,N,P,Q,R]

● S72.324   Nondisplaced transverse fracture of shaft of right femur K, M, N, P, Q, R 🝔, A, B, C 🝔, 🝔, A, B, C 🝔
    (Ex) For S72.324[A]: See S72.004[A]
      For S72.324[B,C]: See S72.001[B,C]
      For S72.324[K,M,N,P,Q,R]:
      See S72.001[K,M,N,P,Q,R]

● S72.325   Nondisplaced transverse fracture of shaft of left femur K, M, N, P, Q, R 🝔, A, B, C 🝔, 🝔, A, B, C 🝔
    (Ex) For S72.325[A]: See S72.002[A]
      For S72.325[B,C]: See S72.001[B,C]
      For S72.325[K,M,N,P,Q,R]:
      See S72.001[K,M,N,P,Q,R]

● S72.326   Nondisplaced transverse fracture of shaft of unspecified femur K, M, N, P, Q, R 🝔, A, B, C 🝔, 🝔, A, B, C 🝔
    (Ex) For S72.326[A,B,C]: See S72.001[B,C]
      For S72.326[K,M,N,P,Q,R]:
      See S72.001[K,M,N,P,Q,R]

● S72.33   Oblique fracture of shaft of femur

● S72.331   Displaced oblique fracture of shaft of right femur K, M, N, P, Q, R 🝔, A, B, C 🝔, 🝔, A, B, C 🝔
    (Ex) For S72.331[A]: See S72.004[A]
      For S72.331[B,C]: See S72.001[B,C]
      For S72.331[K,M,N,P,Q,R]:
      See S72.001[K,M,N,P,Q,R]

● S72.332   Displaced oblique fracture of shaft of left femur K, M, N, P, Q, R 🝔, A, B, C 🝔, 🝔, A, B, C 🝔
    (Ex) For S72.332[A]: See S72.002[A]
      For S72.332[B,C]: See S72.001[B,C]
      For S72.332[K,M,N,P,Q,R]:
      See S72.001[K,M,N,P,Q,R]

● S72.333   Displaced oblique fracture of shaft of unspecified femur K, M, N, P, Q, R 🝔, A, B, C 🝔, 🝔, A, B, C 🝔
    (Ex) For S72.333[A,B,C]: See S72.001[B,C]
      For S72.333[K,M,N,P,Q,R]:
      See S72.001[K,M,N,P,Q,R]

● S72.334   Nondisplaced oblique fracture of shaft of right femur K, M, N, P, Q, R 🝔, A, B, C 🝔, 🝔, A, B, C 🝔
    (Ex) For S72.334[A]: See S72.004[A]
      For S72.334[B,C]: See S72.001[B,C]
      For S72.334[K,M,N,P,Q,R]:
      See S72.001[K,M,N,P,Q,R]

● S72.335   Nondisplaced oblique fracture of shaft of left femur K, M, N, P, Q, R 🝔, A, B, C 🝔, 🝔, A, B, C 🝔
    (Ex) For S72.335[A]: See S72.002[A]
      For S72.335[B,C]: See S72.001[B,C]
      For S72.335[K,M,N,P,Q,R]:
      See S72.001[K,M,N,P,Q,R]

● S72.336   Nondisplaced oblique fracture of shaft of unspecified femur K, M, N, P, Q, R 🝔, A, B, C 🝔, 🝔, A, B, C 🝔
    (Ex) For S72.336[A,B,C]: See S72.001 [B,C]
      For S72.336[K,M,N,P,Q,R]:
      See S72.001[K,M,N,P,Q,R]

● S72.34   Spiral fracture of shaft of femur

● S72.341   Displaced spiral fracture of shaft of right femur K, M, N, P, Q, R 🝔, A, B, C 🝔, 🝔, A, B, C 🝔
    (Ex) For S72.341[A]: See S72.004[A]
      For S72.341[B,C]: See S72.001[B,C]
      For S72.341[K,M,N,P,Q,R]:
      See S72.001[K,M,N,P,Q,R]

● S72.342   Displaced spiral fracture of shaft of left femur K, M, N, P, Q, R 🝔, A, B, C 🝔, 🝔, A, B, C 🝔
    (Ex) For S72.342[A]: See S72.002[A]
      For S72.342[B,C]: See S72.001[B,C]
      For S72.342[K,M,N,P,Q,R]:
      See S72.001[K,M,N,P,Q,R]

● S72.343   Displaced spiral fracture of shaft of unspecified femur K, M, N, P, Q, R 🝔, A, B, C 🝔, 🝔, A, B, C 🝔
    (Ex) For S72.343[A,B,C]: See S72.001[B,C]
      For S72.343[K,M,N,P,Q,R]:
      See S72.001[K,M,N,P,Q,R]

● S72.344   Nondisplaced spiral fracture of shaft of right femur K, M, N, P, Q, R 🝔, A, B, C 🝔, 🝔, A, B, C 🝔
    (Ex) For S72.344[A]: See S72.004[A]
      For S72.344[B,C]: See S72.001[B,C]
      For S72.344[K,M,N,P,Q,R]:
      See S72.001[K,M,N,P,Q,R]

● S72.345   Nondisplaced spiral fracture of shaft of left femur K, M, N, P, Q, R 🝔, A, B, C 🝔, 🝔, A, B, C 🝔
    (Ex) For S72.345[A]: See S72.002[A]
      For S72.345[B,C]: See S72.001[B,C]
      For S72.345[K,M,N,P,Q,R]:
      See S72.001[K,M,N,P,Q,R]

● S72.346   Nondisplaced spiral fracture of shaft of unspecified femur K, M, N, P, Q, R 🝔, A, B, C 🝔, 🝔, A, B, C 🝔
    (Ex) For S72.346[A,B,C]: See S72.001[B,C]
      For S72.346[K,M,N,P,Q,R]:
      See S72.001[K,M,N,P,Q,R]

● S72.35   Comminuted fracture of shaft of femur

● S72.351   Displaced comminuted fracture of shaft of right femur K, M, N, P, Q, R 🝔, A, B, C 🝔, 🝔, A, B, C 🝔
    (Ex) For S72.351[A]: See S72.004[A]
      For S72.351[B,C]: See S72.001[B,C]
      For S72.351[K,M,N,P,Q,R]:
      See S72.001[K,M,N,P,Q,R]

● S72.352   Displaced comminuted fracture of shaft of left femur K, M, N, P, Q, R 🝔, A, B, C 🝔, 🝔, A, B, C 🝔
    (Ex) For S72.352[A]: See S72.002[A]
      For S72.352[B,C]: See S72.001[B,C]
      For S72.352[K,M,N,P,Q,R]:
      See S72.001[K,M,N,P,Q,R]

● S72.353   Displaced comminuted fracture of shaft of unspecified femur K, M, N, P, Q, R 🝔, A, B, C 🝔, 🝔, A, B, C 🝔
    (Ex) For S72.353[A,B,C]: See S72.001[B,C]
      For S72.353[K,M,N,P,Q,R]:
      See S72.001[K,M,N,P,Q,R]

● S72.354   Nondisplaced comminuted fracture of shaft of right femur K, M, N, P, Q, R 🝔, A, B, C 🝔, 🝔, A, B, C 🝔
    (Ex) For S72.354[A]: See S72.004[A]
      For S72.354[B,C]: See S72.001[B,C]
      For S72.354[K,M,N,P,Q,R]:
      See S72.001[K,M,N,P,Q,R]

CHAPTER 19 (S00-T88)

N   Newborn Age: 0   P   Pediatric Age: 0–17   M   Maternity DX: 12–55   A   Adult Age: 15–124   ♀   Females Only   ♂   Males Only
🝔 Complication\Comorbidity   🝔 Major C\C   (Ex) CC/MCC Exclusions   ● Present on Admission Requirement   🝔 Hospital-Acquired Condition

1437

CHAPTER 19 (S00–T88)

● S72.355   **Nondisplaced comminuted fracture of shaft of left femur** K, M, N, P, Q, R ⬡, A, B, C ⬡, ⬡, A, B, C ⬡
    (Ex) For S72.355[A]: See S72.002[A]
      For S72.355[B,C]: See S72.001[B,C]
      For S72.355[K,M,N,P,Q,R]:
      See S72.001[K,M,N,P,Q,R]

● S72.356   **Nondisplaced comminuted fracture of shaft of unspecified femur** K, M, N, P, Q, R ⬡, A, B, C ⬡, ⬡, A, B, C ⬡
    (Ex) For S72.356[A,B,C]: See S72.001[B,C]
      For S72.356[K,M,N,P,Q,R]:
      See S72.001[K,M,N,P,Q,R]

● S72.36   **Segmental fracture of shaft of femur**

● S72.361   **Displaced segmental fracture of shaft of right femur** K, M, N, P, Q, R ⬡, A, B, C ⬡, ⬡, A, B, C ⬡
    (Ex) For S72.361[A]: See S72.004[A]
      For S72.361[B,C]: See S72.001[B,C]
      For S72.361[K,M,N,P,Q,R]:
      See S72.001[K,M,N,P,Q,R]

● S72.362   **Displaced segmental fracture of shaft of left femur** K, M, N, P, Q, R ⬡, A, B, C ⬡, ⬡, A, B, C ⬡
    (Ex) For S72.362[A]: See S72.002[A]
      For S72.362[B,C]: See S72.001[B,C]
      For S72.362[K,M,N,P,Q,R]:
      See S72.001[K,M,N,P,Q,R]

● S72.363   **Displaced segmental fracture of shaft of unspecified femur** K, M, N, P, Q, R ⬡, A, B, C ⬡, ⬡, A, B, C ⬡
    (Ex) For S72.363[A,B,C]: See S72.001[B,C]
      For S72.363[K,M,N,P,Q,R]:
      See S72.001[K,M,N,P,Q,R]

● S72.364   **Nondisplaced segmental fracture of shaft of right femur** K, M, N, P, Q, R ⬡, A, B, C ⬡, ⬡, A, B, C ⬡
    (Ex) For S72.364[A]: See S72.004[A]
      For S72.364[B,C]: See S72.001[B,C]
      For S72.364[K,M,N,P,Q,R]:
      See S72.001[K,M,N,P,Q,R]

● S72.365   **Nondisplaced segmental fracture of shaft of left femur** K, M, N, P, Q, R ⬡, A, B, C ⬡, ⬡, A, B, C ⬡
    (Ex) For S72.365[A]: See S72.002[A]
      For S72.365[B,C]: See S72.001[B,C]
      For S72.365[K,M,N,P,Q,R]:
      See S72.001[K,M,N,P,Q,R]

● S72.366   **Nondisplaced segmental fracture of shaft of unspecified femur** K, M, N, P, Q, R ⬡, A, B, C ⬡, ⬡, A, B, C ⬡
    (Ex) For S72.366[A,B,C]: See S72.001[B,C]
      For S72.366[K,M,N,P,Q,R]:
      See S72.001[K,M,N,P,Q,R]

● S72.39   **Other fracture of shaft of femur**

● S72.391   **Other fracture of shaft of right femur** K, M, N, P, Q, R ⬡, A, B, C ⬡, ⬡, A, B, C ⬡
    (Ex) For S72.391[A]: See S72.004[A]
      For S72.391[B,C]: See S72.001[B,C]
      For S72.391[K,M,N,P,Q,R]:
      See S72.001[K,M,N,P,Q,R]

● S72.392   **Other fracture of shaft of left femur** K, M, N, P, Q, R ⬡, A, B, C ⬡, ⬡, A, B, C ⬡
    (Ex) For S72.392[A]: See S72.002[A]
      For S72.392[B,C]: See S72.001[B,C]
      For S72.392[K,M,N,P,Q,R]:
      See S72.001[K,M,N,P,Q,R]

● S72.399   **Other fracture of shaft of unspecified femur** K, M, N, P, Q, R ⬡, A, B, C ⬡, ⬡, A, B, C ⬡
    (Ex) For S72.399[A,B,C]: See S72.001[B,C]
      For S72.399[K,M,N,P,Q,R]:
      See S72.001[K,M,N,P,Q,R]

● S72.4   **Fracture of lower end of femur**
Fracture of distal end of femur
Excludes2   fracture of shaft of femur (S72.3-)
      physeal fracture of lower end of femur
      (S79.1-)

● S72.40   **Unspecified fracture of lower end of femur**

● S72.401   Unspecified **fracture of lower end of right femur** A, K, M, N, P, Q, R ⬡, B, C ⬡, ⬡, A, B, C ⬡
    (Ex) For S72.401[A]: M80.00X-M80.019[A],
      M80.041-M80.059[A], M80.80X-M80.819[A],
      M80.841-M80.859[A], M84.40X-M84.419[A],
      M84.441-M84.459[A], M84.474-M84.519[A],
      M84.541-M84.559[A], M84.574-M84.576[A],
      M84.60X-M84.619[A], M84.641-M84.659[A],
      M84.674-M84.68X[A], S03.8XX-S03.9XX[A],
      S29.011-S29.019[A], S38.3XX[A],
      S39.011-S39.013[A], S72.001[A,B,C],
      S72.002[B,C], S72.009-S72.011[A,B,C],
      S72.012[B,C], S72.019-S72.021[A,B,C],
      S72.022[B,C], S72.023-S72.024[A,B,C],
      S72.025[B,C], S72.026-S72.031[A,B,C],
      S72.032[B,C], S72.033-S72.034[A,B,C],
      S72.035[B,C], S72.036-S72.041[A,B,C],
      S72.042[B,C], S72.043-S72.044[A,B,C],
      S72.045[B,C], S72.046-S72.051[A,B,C],
      S72.052[B,C], S72.059-S72.061[A,B,C],
      S72.062[B,C], S72.063-S72.064[A,B,C],
      S72.065[B,C], S72.066-S72.091[A,B,C],
      S72.092[B,C], S72.099-S72.101[C],
      S72.102[B,C], S72.109-S72.111[A,B,C],
      S72.112[B,C], S72.113-S72.114[A,B,C],
      S72.115[B,C], S72.116-S72.121[A,B,C],
      S72.122[B,C], S72.123-S72.124[A,B,C],
      S72.125[B,C], S72.126-S72.131[A,B,C],
      S72.132[B,C], S72.133-S72.134[A,B,C],
      S72.135[B,C], S72.136-S72.141[A,B,C],
      S72.142[B,C], S72.143-S72.144[A,B,C],
      S72.145[B,C], S72.146-S72.301[A,B,C],
      S72.302[B,C], S72.309-S72.321[A,B,C],
      S72.322[B,C], S72.323-S72.324[A,B,C],
      S72.325[B,C], S72.326-S72.331[A,B,C],
      S72.332[B,C], S72.333-S72.334[A,B,C],
      S72.335[B,C], S72.336-S72.341[A,B,C],
      S72.342[B,C], S72.343-S72.344[A,B,C],
      S72.345[B,C], S72.346-S72.351[A,B,C],
      S72.352[B,C], S72.353-S72.354[A,B,C],
      S72.355[B,C], S72.356-S72.361[A,B,C],
      S72.362[B,C], S72.363-S72.364[A,B,C],
      S72.365[B,C], S72.366-S72.391[A,B,C],
      S72.392[B,C], S72.399-S72.401[A,B,C],
      S72.402[B,C], S72.409-S72.411[A,B,C],
      S72.412[B,C], S72.413-S72.414[A,B,C],
      S72.415[B,C], S72.416-S72.421[A,B,C],
      S72.422[B,C], S72.423-S72.424[A,B,C],
      S72.425[B,C], S72.426-S72.431[A,B,C],
      S72.432[B,C], S72.433-S72.434[A,B,C],
      S72.435[B,C], S72.436-S72.441[A,B,C],
      S72.442[B,C], S72.443-S72.444[A,B,C],
      S72.445[B,C], S72.446-S72.451[A,B,C],
      S72.452[B,C], S72.453-S72.454[A,B,C],
      S72.455[B,C], S72.456-S72.461[A,B,C],
      S72.462[B,C], S72.463-S72.464[A,B,C],
      S72.465[B,C], S72.466[A,B,C], S72.471[A],
      S72.479[A], S72.491[A,B,C], S72.492[B,C],
      S72.499-S72.92X[A,B,C], S73.101[A],
      S73.109-S73.111[A], S73.119-S73.121[A],
      S73.129-S73.191[A], S73.199[A], S76.001[A],
      S76.009-S76.011[A], S76.019[A], S76.091[A],
      S76.099-S76.101[A], S76.109-S76.111[A],
      S76.119[A], S76.191[A], S76.199-S76.201[A],
      S76.209-S76.211[A], S76.219[A], S76.291[A],
      S76.299-S76.301[A], S76.309-S76.311[A],

S76.319[A], S76.391[A], S76.399-S76.801[A],
S76.809-S76.811[A], S76.819[A], S76.891[A],
S76.899-S76.901[A], S76.909-S76.911[A],
S76.919[A], S76.991[A], S76.999[A],
S79.001[A], S79.009-S79.011[A],
S79.019-S79.091[A], S79.099-S79.101[A],
S79.109-S79.111[A], S79.119-S79.121[A],
S79.129-S79.131[A], S79.139-S79.141[A],
S79.149-S79.191[A], S79.199-S79.811[A],
S79.819-S79.821[A], S79.829-S79.911[A],
S79.919-S79.921[A], S79.929[A],
S82.90X-S82.92X[A,B,C], T14.8-T14.91, T79.
A9X-T79.9XX[A] **For S72.401[B,C]:**
M80.00X-M80.019[A], M80.041-M80.059[A],
M80.80X-M80.819[A], M80.841-M80.859[A],
M84.40X-M84.419[A], M84.441-M84.459[A],
M84.474-M84.519[A], M84.541-M84.559[A],
M84.574-M84.576[A], M84.60X-M84.619[A],
M84.641-M84.659[A], M84.674-M84.68X[A],
S03.8XX-S03.9XX[A], S29.011-S29.019[A],
S38.3XX[A], S39.011-S39.013[A],
S72.001-S72.466[A,B,C], S72.471-S72.479[A],
S72.491-S72.92X[A,B,C], S73.101-S73.199[A],
S76.001-S76.019[A], S76.091-S76.119[A],
S76.191-S76.219[A], S76.291-S76.319[A],
S76.391-S76.819[A], S76.891-S76.919[A],
S76.991-S76.999[A], S79.001-S79.929[A],
S82.90X-S82.92X[A,B,C], T14.8-T14.91, T79.
A9X-T79.9XX[A] **For S72.401[K,M,N,P,Q,R]:**
See S72.001[K,M,N,P,Q,R]

● **S72.402 Unspecified fracture of lower end of**
left femur A, K, M, N, P, Q, R 🅒,
B, C 🅜, **A, B, C** 🅟
(Ex) **For S72.402[A]:** M80.00X-M80.019[A],
M80.041-M80.059[A], M80.80X-M80.819[A],
M80.841-M80.859[A], M84.40X-M84.419[A],
M84.441-M84.459[A], M84.474-M84.519[A],
M84.541-M84.559[A], M84.574-M84.576[A],
M84.60X-M84.619[A], M84.641-M84.659[A],
M84.674-M84.68X[A], S03.8XX-S03.9XX[A],
S29.011-S29.019[A], S38.3XX[A],
S39.011-S39.013[A], S72.001[B,C],
S72.002-S72.009[A,B,C], S72.011[B,C],
S72.012-S72.019[A,B,C], S72.021[B,C],
S72.022-S72.023[A,B,C], S72.024[B,C],
S72.025-S72.026[A,B,C], S72.031[B,C],
S72.032-S72.033[A,B,C], S72.034[B,C],
S72.035-S72.036[A,B,C], S72.041[B,C],
S72.042-S72.043[A,B,C], S72.044[B,C],
S72.045-S72.046[A,B,C], S72.051[B,C],
S72.052-S72.059[A,B,C], S72.061[B,C],
S72.062-S72.063[A,B,C], S72.064[B,C],
S72.065-S72.066[A,B,C], S72.091[B,C],
S72.092-S72.099[A,B,C], S72.101[B,C],
S72.102-S72.109[A,B,C], S72.111[B,C],
S72.112-S72.113[A,B,C], S72.114[B,C],
S72.115-S72.116[A,B,C], S72.121[B,C],
S72.122-S72.123[A,B,C], S72.124[B,C],
S72.125-S72.126[A,B,C], S72.131[B,C],
S72.132-S72.133[A,B,C], S72.134[B,C],
S72.135-S72.136[A,B,C], S72.141[B,C],
S72.142-S72.143[A,B,C], S72.144[B,C],
S72.145-S72.146[A,B,C],
S72.21X-S72.26X[A,B,C], S72.301[B,C],
S72.302-S72.309[A,B,C], S72.321[B,C],
S72.322-S72.323[A,B,C], S72.324[B,C],
S72.325-S72.326[A,B,C], S72.331[B,C],
S72.332-S72.333[A,B,C], S72.334[B,C],
S72.335-S72.336[A,B,C], S72.341[B,C],
S72.342-S72.343[A,B,C], S72.344[B,C],
S72.345-S72.346[A,B,C], S72.351[B,C],
S72.352-S72.353[A,B,C], S72.354[B,C],
S72.355-S72.356[A,B,C], S72.361[B,C],
S72.362-S72.363[A,B,C], S72.364[B,C],

S72.365-S72.366[A,B,C], S72.391[B,C],
S72.392-S72.399[A,B,C], S72.401[B,C],
S72.402-S72.409[A,B,C], S72.411[B,C],
S72.412-S72.413[A,B,C], S72.414[B,C],
S72.415-S72.416[A,B,C], S72.421[B,C],
S72.422-S72.423[A,B,C], S72.424[B,C],
S72.425-S72.426[A,B,C], S72.431[B,C],
S72.432-S72.433[A,B,C], S72.434[B,C],
S72.435-S72.436[A,B,C], S72.441[B,C],
S72.442-S72.443[A,B,C], S72.444[B,C],
S72.445-S72.446[A,B,C], S72.451[B,C],
S72.452-S72.453[A,B,C], S72.454[B,C],
S72.455-S72.456[A,B,C], S72.461[B,C],
S72.462-S72.463[A,B,C], S72.464[B,C],
S72.465-S72.466[A,B,C], S72.472-S72.479[A],
S72.491[B,C], S72.492-S72.92X[A,B,C],
S73.102-S73.109[A], S73.112-S73.119[A],
S73.122-S73.129[A], S73.192-S73.199[A],
S76.002-S76.009[A], S76.012-S76.019[A],
S76.092-S76.099[A], S76.102-S76.109[A],
S76.112-S76.119[A], S76.192-S76.199[A],
S76.202-S76.209[A], S76.212-S76.219[A],
S76.292-S76.299[A], S76.302-S76.309[A],
S76.312-S76.319[A], S76.392-S76.399[A],
S76.802-S76.809[A], S76.812-S76.819[A],
S76.892-S76.899[A], S76.902-S76.909[A],
S76.912-S76.919[A], S76.992-S76.999[A],
S79.002-S79.009[A], S79.012-S79.019[A],
S79.092-S79.099[A], S79.102-S79.109[A],
S79.112-S79.119[A], S79.122-S79.129[A],
S79.132-S79.139[A], S79.142-S79.149[A],
S79.192-S79.199[A], S79.812-S79.819[A],
S79.822-S79.829[A], S79.912-S79.919[A],
S79.922-S79.929[A], S82.90X-S82.92X[A,B,C],
T14.8-T14.91, T79.A9X- T79.9XX[A]
For S72.402[B,C]: See S72.401[B,C]
For S72.401[K,M,N,P,Q,R]:
See S72.001[K,M,N,P,Q,R]

● **S72.409 Unspecified fracture of lower end of**
unspecified femur
A, K, M, N, P, Q, R 🅒, **B, C** 🅜, 🅒,
A, B, C 🅟
(Ex) **For S72.409[A,B,C]:** See S72.401[B,C]
For S72.401[K,M,N,P,Q,R]:
See S72.001[K,M,N,P,Q,R]

● **S72.41   Unspecified condyle fracture of lower end of**
femur
Condyle fracture of femur NOS

● **S72.411 Displaced unspecified condyle**
fracture of lower end of right femur
A, K, M, N, P, Q, R 🅒, **B, C** 🅜,
A, B, C 🅟
(Ex) **For S72.411[A]:** See S72.401[A]
For S72.411[B,C]: See S72.401[B,C]
For S72.411[K,M,N,P,Q,R]:
See S72.001[K,M,N,P,Q,R]

● **S72.412 Displaced unspecified condyle**
fracture of lower end of left femur
A, K, M, N, P, Q, R 🅒, **B, C** 🅜, 🅒,
A, B, C 🅟
(Ex) **For S72.412[A]:** See S72.402[A]
For S72.412[B,C]: See S72.401[B,C]
For S72.411[K,M,N,P,Q,R]:
See S72.001[K,M,N,P,Q,R]

● **S72.413 Displaced unspecified condyle**
fracture of lower end of unspecified
femur A, K, M, N, P, Q, R 🅒, **B, C** 🅜,
🅒, **A, B, C** 🅟
(Ex) **For S72.413[A,B,C]:** See S72.401[B,C]
For S72.413[K,M,N,P,Q,R]:
See S72.001[K,M,N,P,Q,R]

N Newborn Age: 0   P Pediatric Age: 0–17   M Maternity DX: 12–55   A Adult Age: 15–124   ♀ Females Only   ♂ Males Only
🅒 Complication\Comorbidity   🅜 Major C\C   (Ex) CC/MCC Exclusions   🅟 Present on Admission Requirement   🅗 Hospital-Acquired Condition

● **S72.414**   Nondisplaced unspecified condyle fracture of lower end of right femur A, K, M, N, P, Q, R 🔊, B, C 🔊, 🔊, A, B, C 🔊
    (Ex:) **For S72.414[A]:** See S72.401[A]
       For S72.414[B,C]: See S72.401[B,C]
       For S72.414[K,M,N,P,Q,R]:
       See S72.001[K,M,N,P,Q,R]

● **S72.415**   Nondisplaced unspecified condyle fracture of lower end of left femur A, K, M, N, P, Q, R 🔊, B, C 🔊, 🔊, A, B, C 🔊
    (Ex:) **For S72.415[A]:** See S72.402[A]
       For S72.415[B,C]: See S72.401[B,C]
       For S72.415[K,M,N,P,Q,R]:
       See S72.001[K,M,N,P,Q,R]

● **S72.416**   Nondisplaced unspecified condyle fracture of lower end of unspecified femur A, K, M, N, P, Q, R 🔊, B, C 🔊, 🔊, A, B, C 🔊
    (Ex:) **For S72.416[A,B,C]:** See S72.401[B,C]
       For S72.416[K,M,N,P,Q,R]:
       See S72.001[K,M,N,P,Q,R]

● **S72.42**   Fracture of lateral condyle of femur

● **S72.421**   Displaced fracture of lateral condyle of right femur A, K, M, N, P, Q, R 🔊, B, C 🔊, 🔊, A, B, C 🔊
    (Ex:) **For S72.421[A]:** See S72.401[A]
       For S72.421[B,C]: See S72.401[B,C]
       For S72.421[K,M,N,P,Q,R]:
       See S72.001[K,M,N,P,Q,R]

● **S72.422**   Displaced fracture of lateral condyle of left femur A, K, M, N, P, Q, R 🔊, B, C 🔊, 🔊, A, B, C 🔊
    (Ex:) **For S72.422[A]:** See S72.402[A]
       For S72.422[B,C]: See S72.401[B,C]
       For S72.422[K,M,N,P,Q,R]:
       See S72.001[K,M,N,P,Q,R]

● **S72.423**   Displaced fracture of lateral condyle of unspecified femur A, K, M, N, P, Q, R 🔊, B, C 🔊, 🔊, A, B, C 🔊
    (Ex:) **For S72.423[A,B,C]:** See S72.401[B,C]
       For S72.423[K,M,N,P,Q,R]:
       See S72.001[K,M,N,P,Q,R]

● **S72.424**   Nondisplaced fracture of lateral condyle of right femur A, K, M, N, P, Q, R 🔊, B, C 🔊, 🔊, A, B, C 🔊
    (Ex:) **For S72.424[A]:** See S72.401[A]
       For S72.424[B,C]: See S72.401[B,C]
       For S72.424[K,M,N,P,Q,R]:
       See S72.001[K,M,N,P,Q,R]

● **S72.425**   Nondisplaced fracture of lateral condyle of left femur A, K, M, N, P, Q, R 🔊, B, C 🔊, 🔊, A, B, C 🔊
    (Ex:) **For S72.425[A]:** See S72.402[A]
       For S72.425[B,C]: See S72.401[B,C]
       For S72.425[K,M,N,P,Q,R]:
       See S72.001[K,M,N,P,Q,R]

● **S72.426**   Nondisplaced fracture of lateral condyle of unspecified femur A, K, M, N, P, Q, R 🔊, B, C 🔊, 🔊, A, B, C 🔊
    (Ex:) **For S72.426[A,B,C]:** See S72.401[B,C]
       For S72.426[K,M,N,P,Q,R]:
       See S72.001[K,M,N,P,Q,R]

● **S72.43**   Fracture of medial condyle of femur

● **S72.431**   Displaced fracture of medial condyle of right femur A, K, M, N, P, Q, R 🔊, B, C 🔊, 🔊, A, B, C 🔊
    (Ex:) **For S72.431[A]:** See S72.401[A]
       For S72.431[B,C]: See S72.401[B,C]
       For S72.431[K,M,N,P,Q,R]:
       See S72.001[K,M,N,P,Q,R]

● **S72.432**   Displaced fracture of medial condyle of left femur A, K, M, N, P, Q, R 🔊, B, C 🔊, 🔊, A, B, C 🔊
    (Ex:) **For S72.432[A]:** See S72.402[A]
       For S72.432[B,C]: See S72.401[B,C]
       For S72.432[K,M,N,P,Q,R]:
       See S72.001[K,M,N,P,Q,R]

● **S72.433**   Displaced fracture of medial condyle of unspecified femur A, K, M, N, P, Q, R 🔊, B, C 🔊, 🔊, A, B, C 🔊
    (Ex:) **For S72.433[A,B,C]:** See S72.401[B,C]
       For S72.433[K,M,N,P,Q,R]:
       See S72.001[K,M,N,P,Q,R]

● **S72.434**   Nondisplaced fracture of medial condyle of right femur A, K, M, N, P, Q, R 🔊, B, C 🔊, 🔊, A, B, C 🔊
    (Ex:) **For S72.434[A]:** See S72.401[A]
       For S72.434[B,C]: See S72.401[B,C]
       For S72.434[K,M,N,P,Q,R]:
       See S72.001[K,M,N,P,Q,R]

● **S72.435**   Nondisplaced fracture of medial condyle of left femur A, K, M, N, P, Q, R 🔊, B, C 🔊, 🔊, A, B, C 🔊
    (Ex:) **For S72.435[A]:** See S72.402[A]
       For S72.435[B,C]: See S72.401[B,C]
       For S72.435[K,M,N,P,Q,R]:
       See S72.001[K,M,N,P,Q,R]

● **S72.436**   Nondisplaced fracture of medial condyle of unspecified femur A, K, M, N, P, Q, R 🔊, B, C 🔊, 🔊, A, B, C 🔊
    (Ex:) **For S72.436[A,B,C]:** See S72.401[B,C]
       For S72.436[K,M,N,P,Q,R]:
       See S72.001[K,M,N,P,Q,R]

● **S72.44**   Fracture of lower epiphysis (separation) of femur

    Excludes 1   Salter-Harris Type I physeal fracture of lower end of femur (S79.11-)

● **S72.441**   Displaced fracture of lower epiphysis (separation) of right femur A, K, M, N, P, Q, R 🔊, B, C 🔊, 🔊, A, B, C 🔊
    (Ex:) **For S72.441[A]:** See S72.401[A]
       For S72.441[B,C]: See S72.401[B,C]
       For S72.441[K,M,N,P,Q,R]:
       See S72.001[K,M,N,P,Q,R]

● **S72.442**   Displaced fracture of lower epiphysis (separation) of left femur A, K, M, N, P, Q, R 🔊, B, C 🔊, 🔊, A, B, C 🔊
    (Ex:) **For S72.442[A]:** See S72.402[A]
       For S72.442[B,C]: See S72.401[B,C]
       For S72.442[K,M,N,P,Q,R]:
       See S72.001[K,M,N,P,Q,R]

CHAPTER 19 (S00-T88)

◄ New   ◄▥ Revised   ~~deleted~~ Deleted   Excludes 1   Excludes 2   Includes   Use additional   Code first   Code also   Unspecified
OGCR Official Guidelines   ● Unacceptable Principal Diagnosis   X Assign placeholder X   ● Use Additional Character(s)   ▌ Manifestation Code   **Coding Clinic**

● S72.443 Displaced fracture of lower epiphysis
(separation) of unspecified femur
A, K, M, P, Q, R 🞉, B, C 🞉, 🞉,
A, B, C 🞉
(Ex) For S72.443[A,B,C]: See S72.401[B,C]
For S72.443[K,M,N,P,Q,R]:
See S72.001[K,M,N,P,Q,R]

● S72.444 Nondisplaced fracture of lower
epiphysis (separation) of right femur
A, K, M, N, P, Q, R 🞉, B, C 🞉, 🞉,
A, B, C 🞉
(Ex) For S72.444[A]: See S72.401[A]
For S72.444[B,C]: See S72.401[B,C]
For S72.444[K,M,N,P,Q,R]:
See S72.001[K,M,N,P,Q,R]

● S72.445 Nondisplaced fracture of lower
epiphysis (separation) of left femur
A, K, M, N, P, Q, R 🞉, B, C 🞉, 🞉,
A, B, C 🞉
(Ex) For S72.445[A]: See S72.402[A]
For S72.445[B,C]: See S72.401[B,C]
For S72.445[K,M,N,P,Q,R]:
See S72.001[K,M,N,P,Q,R]

● S72.446 Nondisplaced fracture of lower
epiphysis (separation) of unspecified
femur A; K, M, N, P, Q, R 🞉, B, C 🞉,
🞉, A, B, C 🞉
(Ex) For S72.446[A,B,C]: See S72.401[B,C]
For S72.446[K,M,N,P,Q,R]:
See S72.001[K,M,N,P,Q,R]

● S72.45 Supracondylar fracture without intracondylar
extension of lower end of femur
Supracondylar fracture of lower end of femur
NOS
Excludes1 supracondylar fracture with
intracondylar extension of
lower end of femur (S72.46-)

● S72.451 Displaced supracondylar fracture
without intracondylar extension of
lower end of right femur
A, K, M, N, P, Q, R 🞉, B, C 🞉, 🞉,
A, B, C 🞉
(Ex) For S72.451[A]: See S72.401[A]
For S72.451[B,C]: See S72.401[B,C]
For S72.451[K,M,N,P,Q,R]:
See S72.001[K,M,N,P,Q,R]

● S72.452 Displaced supracondylar fracture
without intracondylar extension of
lower end of left femur
A, K, M, N, P, Q, R 🞉, B, C 🞉, 🞉,
A, B, C 🞉
(Ex) For S72.452[A]: See S72.402[A]
For S72.452[B,C]: See S72.401[B,C]
For S72.452[K,M,N,P,Q,R]:
See S72.001[K,M,N,P,Q,R]

● S72.453 Displaced supracondylar fracture
without intracondylar extension of
lower end of unspecified femur
A, K, M, N, P, Q, R 🞉, B, C 🞉, 🞉,
A, B, C 🞉
(Ex) For S72.453[A,B,C]: See S72.401[B,C]
For S72.453[K,M,N,P,Q,R]:
See S72.001[K,M,N,P,Q,R]

● S72.454 Nondisplaced supracondylar fracture
without intracondylar extension of
lower end of right femur
A, K, M, N, P, Q, R 🞉, B, C 🞉, 🞉,
A, B, C 🞉
(Ex) For S72.454[A]: See S72.401[A]
For S72.454[B,C]: See S72.401[B,C]
For S72.454[K,M,N,P,Q,R]:
See S72.001[K,M,N,P,Q,R]

● S72.455 Nondisplaced supracondylar fracture
without intracondylar extension of
lower end of left femur
A, K, M, N, P, Q, R 🞉, B, C 🞉, 🞉,
A, B, C 🞉
(Ex) For S72.455[A]: See S72.402[A]
For S72.455[B,C]: See S72.401[B,C]
For S72.455[K,M,N,P,Q,R]:
See S72.001[K,M,N,P,Q,R]

● S72.456 Nondisplaced supracondylar fracture
without intracondylar extension of
lower end of unspecified femur
A, K, M, N, P, Q, R 🞉, B, C 🞉, 🞉,
A, B, C 🞉
(Ex) For S72.456[A,B,C]: See S72.401[B,C]
For S72.456[K,M,N,P,Q,R]:
See S72.001[K,M,N,P,Q,R]

● S72.46 Supracondylar fracture with intracondylar
extension of lower end of femur
Excludes1 supracondylar fracture without
intracondylar extension of
lower end of femur (S72.45-)

● S72.461 Displaced supracondylar fracture
with intracondylar extension of lower
end of right femur
A, K, M, N, P, Q, R 🞉, B, C 🞉, 🞉,
A, B, C 🞉
(Ex) For S72.461[A]: See S72.401[A]
For S72.461[B,C]: See S72.401[B,C]
For S72.461[K,M,N,P,Q,R]:
See S72.001[K,M,N,P,Q,R]

● S72.462 Displaced supracondylar fracture
with intracondylar extension of lower
end of left femur
A, K, M, N, P, Q, R 🞉, B, C 🞉, 🞉,
A, B, C 🞉
(Ex) For S72.462[A]: See S72.402[A]
For S72.462[B,C]: See S72.401[B,C]
For S72.462[K,M,N,P,Q,R]:
See S72.001[K,M,N,P,Q,R]

● S72.463 Displaced supracondylar fracture
with intracondylar extension of lower
end of unspecified femur
A, K, M, N, P, Q, R 🞉, B, C 🞉, 🞉,
A, B, C 🞉
(Ex) For S72.463[A,B,C]: See S72.401[B,C]
For S72.463[K,M,N,P,Q,R]:
See S72.001[K,M,N,P,Q,R]

● S72.464 Nondisplaced supracondylar fracture
with intracondylar extension of lower
end of right femur
A, K, M, N, P, Q, R 🞉, B, C 🞉, 🞉,
A, B, C 🞉
(Ex) For S72.464[A]: See S72.401[A]
For S72.464[B,C]: See S72.401[B,C]
For S72.464[K,M,N,P,Q,R]:
See S72.001[K,M,N,P,Q,R]

● S72.465 Nondisplaced supracondylar fracture
with intracondylar extension of lower
end of left femur
A, K, M, N, P, Q, R 🞉, B, C 🞉, 🞉,
A, B, C 🞉
(Ex) For S72.465[A]: See S72.402[A]
For S72.465[B,C]: See S72.401[B,C]
For S72.465[K,M,N,P,Q,R]:
See S72.001[K,M,N,P,Q,R]

● S72.466 Nondisplaced supracondylar fracture
with intracondylar extension of lower
end of unspecified femur
A, K, M, N, P, Q, R 🞉, B, C 🞉, 🞉,
A, B, C 🞉
(Ex) For S72.466[A,B,C]: See S72.401[B,C]
For S72.466[K,M,N,P,Q,R]:
See S72.001[K,M,N,P,Q,R]

CHAPTER 19 (S00-T88)

N Newborn Age: 0   **P** Pediatric Age: 0–17   **M** Maternity DX: 12–55   **A** Adult Age: 15–124   ♀ Females Only   ♂ Males Only

🞉 Complication\Comorbidity   🞉 Major C\C   (Ex) CC/MCC Exclusions   🞉 Present on Admission Requirement   🞉 Hospital-Acquired Condition

1441

● **S72.47**   **Torus fracture of lower end of femur**

The appropriate 7th character is to be added to all codes in subcategory S72.47

A	initial encounter for closed fracture
D	subsequent encounter for fracture with routine healing
G	subsequent encounter for fracture with delayed healing
K	subsequent encounter for fracture with nonunion
P	subsequent encounter for fracture with malunion
S	sequela

● **S72.471**   **Torus fracture of lower end of right femur** A, K, P 🔲, 🔲, A 🔲
    Ⓔⓧ **For S72.471[A]:** See S72.401[A]
       For S72.471[K,P]: See S72.001[K,M,N,P,Q,R]

● **S72.472**   **Torus fracture of lower end of left femur** A, K, P 🔲, 🔲, A 🔲
    Ⓔⓧ **For S72.472[A]:** See S72.402[A]
       For S72.472[K,P]: See S72.001[K,M,N,P,Q,R]

● **S72.479**   **Torus fracture of lower end of unspecified femur** A, K, P 🔲, 🔲, A 🔲
    Ⓔⓧ **For S72.479[A]:** See S72.401[B,C]
       For S72.479[K,P]: See S72.001[K,M,N,P,Q,R]

● **S72.49**   **Other fracture of lower end of femur**

● **S72.491**   **Other fracture of lower end of right femur** A, K, M, N, P, Q, R 🔲, B, C 🔲, 🔲, A, B, C 🔲
    Ⓔⓧ **For S72.491[A]:** See S72.401[A]
       For S72.491[B,C]: M80.00X-M80.019[A],
       M80.041-M80.059[A], M80.80X-M80.819[A],
       M80.841-M80.859[A], M84.40X-M84.419[A],
       M84.451-M84.459[A], M84.474-M84.519[A],
       M84.541-M84.559[A], M84.574-M84.619[A],
       M84.641-M84.659[A], M84.674-M84.68X[A],
       S03.8XX-S03.9XX[A], S29.011-S29.019[A],
       S38.3XX[A], S39.011-S39.013[A],
       S72.491-S72.499[B,C], S73.101-S73.199[A],
       S76.001-S76.019[A], S76.091-S76.119[A],
       S76.191-S76.219[A], S76.291-S76.319[A],
       S76.391-S76.819[A], S76.891-S76.919[A],
       S76.991-S76.999[A], S79.811-S79.929[A],
       S82.001-S82.099[A,B,C],
       S82.90X-S82.92X[A,B,C], T14.8-T14.91, T79.
       A9X- T79.9XX[A]
       For S72.491[K,M,N,P,Q,R]:
       See S72.001[K,M,N,P,Q,R]

● **S72.492**   **Other fracture of lower end of left femur** A, K, M, N, P, Q, R 🔲, B, C 🔲, 🔲, A, B, C 🔲
    Ⓔⓧ **For S72.492[A]:** See S72.402[A]
       For S72.492[B,C]: See S72.491[B,C]
       For S72.492[K,M,N,P,Q,R]:
       See S72.001[K,M,N,P,Q,R]

● **S72.499**   **Other fracture of lower end of unspecified femur** A, K, M, N, P, Q, R 🔲, B, C 🔲, 🔲, A, B, C 🔲
    Ⓔⓧ **For S72.499[A]:** See S72.401[B,C]
       For S72.499[B,C]: See S72.491[B,C]
       For S72.499[K,M,N,P,Q,R]:
       See S72.001[K,M,N,P,Q,R]

● **S72.8**   **Other fracture of femur**
    Ⓔⓧ **For category S72.8 CC codes S72.8[A,B,C]:** See S72.001[B,C]
       For S72.8[K,M,N,P,Q,R]: See S72.001[K,M,N,P,Q,R]

● **S72.8X**   **Other fracture of femur**

● **S72.8X1**   **Other fracture of right femur** K, M, N, P, Q, R 🔲, A, B, C 🔲, 🔲, A, B, C 🔲

● **S72.8X2**   **Other fracture of left femur** K, M, N, P, Q, R 🔲, A, B, C 🔲, 🔲, A, B, C 🔲

● **S72.8X9**   **Other fracture of unspecified femur** K, M, N, P, Q, R 🔲, A, B, C 🔲, 🔲, A, B, C 🔲

● **S72.9**   **Unspecified fracture of femur**
Fracture of thigh NOS
Fracture of upper leg NOS

    Excludes1   fracture of hip NOS (S72.00-, S72.01-)
    Ⓔⓧ **For category S72.9 CC codes S72.9[A,B,C]:** See S72.001[B,C]
       For S72.9[K,M,N,P,Q,R]: See S72.001[K,M,N,P,Q,R]

X ● **S72.90**   **Unspecified fracture of unspecified femur** K, M, N, P, Q, R 🔲, A, B, C 🔲, 🔲, A, B, C 🔲
       Coding Clinic: 2012, Q4, P94

X ● **S72.91**   **Unspecified fracture of right femur** K, M, N, P, Q, R 🔲, A, B, C 🔲, 🔲, A, B, C 🔲

X ● **S72.92**   **Unspecified fracture of left femur** K, M, N, P, Q, R 🔲, A, B, C 🔲, 🔲, A, B, C 🔲

● **S73**   **Dislocation and sprain of joint and ligaments of hip**

    Includes   avulsion of joint or ligament of hip
       laceration of cartilage, joint or ligament of hip
       sprain of cartilage, joint or ligament of hip
       traumatic hemarthrosis of joint or ligament of hip
       traumatic rupture of joint or ligament of hip
       traumatic subluxation of joint or ligament of hip
       traumatic tear of joint or ligament of hip

Code also any associated open wound

    Excludes2   strain of muscle, fascia and tendon of hip and thigh (S76.-)

The appropriate 7th character is to be added to each code from category S73

A	initial encounter
D	subsequent encounter
S	sequela

● **S73.0**   **Subluxation and dislocation of hip**
    Out of position

    Excludes2   dislocation and subluxation of hip prosthesis (T84.020, T84.021)

● **S73.00**   **Unspecified subluxation and dislocation of hip**
Dislocation of hip NOS
Subluxation of hip NOS

● **S73.001**   **Unspecified subluxation of right hip** A 🔲, 🔲, A 🔲
    Ⓔⓧ M99.16-M99.17, M99.19, S33.30X-S33.39X[A],
       S73.001[A], S73.003-S73.004[A], S73.006[A],
       S73.041[A], S73.043-S73.044[A], S73.046[A]

● **S73.002**   **Unspecified subluxation of left hip** A 🔲, 🔲, A 🔲
    Ⓔⓧ M99.16-M99.17, M99.19, S33.30X-S33.39X[A],
       S73.002-S73.003[A], S73.005-S73.006[A],
       S73.042-S73.043[A], S73.045-S73.046[A]

● **S73.003**   **Unspecified subluxation of unspecified hip** A 🔲, 🔲, A 🔲
    Ⓔⓧ M99.16-M99.17, M99.19, S33.30X-S33.39X[A],
       S73.001-S73.006[A], S73.041-S73.046[A]

● **S73.004**   **Unspecified dislocation of right hip** A 🔲, 🔲, A 🔲
    Ⓔⓧ See S73.001

● **S73.005**   **Unspecified dislocation of left hip** A 🔲, 🔲, A 🔲
    Ⓔⓧ See S73.002

● **S73.006**   **Unspecified dislocation of unspecified hip** A 🔲, 🔲, A 🔲
    Ⓔⓧ See S73.003

● **S73.01**   Posterior subluxation and dislocation of hip

   ● **S73.011**   Posterior subluxation of right hip A 🔖, 🔖, A 🔖
     (Ex:) M99.16-M99.17, M99.19, S33.30X-S33.39X[A], S73.011[A], S73.013-S73.014[A], S73.016[A]

   ● **S73.012**   Posterior subluxation of left hip A 🔖, 🔖, A 🔖
     (Ex:) M99.16-M99.17, M99.19, S33.30X-S33.39X[A], S73.012-S73.013[A], S73.015-S73.016[A]

   ● **S73.013**   Posterior subluxation of unspecified hip A 🔖, 🔖, A 🔖
     (Ex:) M99.16-M99.17, M99.19, S33.30X-S33.39X[A], S73.011-S73.016[A]

   ● **S73.014**   Posterior dislocation of right hip A 🔖, 🔖, A 🔖
     (Ex:) See S73.011

   ● **S73.015**   Posterior dislocation of left hip A 🔖, 🔖, A 🔖
     (Ex:) See S73.012

   ● **S73.016**   Posterior dislocation of unspecified hip A 🔖, 🔖, A 🔖
     (Ex:) See S73.013

● **S73.02**   Obturator subluxation and dislocation of hip

   ● **S73.021**   Obturator subluxation of right hip A 🔖, 🔖, A 🔖
     (Ex:) M99.16-M99.17, M99.19, S33.30X-S33.39X[A], S73.021[A], S73.023-S73.024[A], S73.026[A]

   ● **S73.022**   Obturator subluxation of left hip A 🔖, 🔖, A 🔖
     (Ex:) M99.16-M99.17, M99.19, S33.30X-S33.39X[A], S73.022-S73.023[A], S73.025-S73.026[A]

   ● **S73.023**   Obturator subluxation of unspecified hip A 🔖, 🔖, A 🔖
     (Ex:) M99.16-M99.17, M99.19, S33.30X-S33.39X[A], S73.021-S73.026[A]

   ● **S73.024**   Obturator dislocation of right hip A 🔖, 🔖, A 🔖
     (Ex:) See S73.021

   ● **S73.025**   Obturator dislocation of left hip A 🔖, 🔖, A 🔖
     (Ex:) See S73.022

   ● **S73.026**   Obturator dislocation of unspecified hip A 🔖, 🔖, A 🔖
     (Ex:) See S73.023

● **S73.03**   Other anterior dislocation of hip

   ● **S73.031**   Other anterior subluxation of right hip A 🔖, 🔖, A 🔖
     (Ex:) M99.16-M99.17, M99.19, S33.30X-S33.39X[A], S73.031[A], S73.033-S73.034[A], S73.036[A]

   ● **S73.032**   Other anterior subluxation of left hip A 🔖, 🔖, A 🔖
     (Ex:) M99.16-M99.17, M99.19, S33.30X-S33.39X[A], S73.032-S73.033[A], S73.035-S73.036[A]

   ● **S73.033**   Other anterior subluxation of unspecified hip A 🔖, 🔖, A 🔖
     (Ex:) M99.16-M99.17, M99.19, S33.30X-S33.39X[A], S73.031-S73.036[A]

   ● **S73.034**   Other anterior dislocation of right hip A 🔖, 🔖, A 🔖
     (Ex:) See S73.031

   ● **S73.035**   Other anterior dislocation of left hip A 🔖, 🔖, A 🔖
     (Ex:) See S73.032

   ● **S73.036**   Other anterior dislocation of unspecified hip A 🔖, 🔖, A 🔖
     (Ex:) See S73.033

● **S73.04**   Central dislocation of hip

   ● **S73.041**   Central subluxation of right hip A 🔖, 🔖, A 🔖
     (Ex:) See S73.001

   ● **S73.042**   Central subluxation of left hip A 🔖, 🔖, A 🔖
     (Ex:) See S73.002

   ● **S73.043**   Central subluxation of unspecified hip A 🔖, 🔖, A 🔖
     (Ex:) See S73.003

   ● **S73.044**   Central dislocation of right hip A 🔖, 🔖, A 🔖
     (Ex:) See S73.001

   ● **S73.045**   Central dislocation of left hip A 🔖, 🔖, A 🔖
     (Ex:) See S73.002

   ● **S73.046**   Central dislocation of unspecified hip A 🔖, 🔖, A 🔖
     (Ex:) See S73.003

● **S73.1**   Sprain of hip

   ● **S73.10**   Unspecified sprain of hip

     ● **S73.101**   Unspecified sprain of right hip 🔖
     ● **S73.102**   Unspecified sprain of left hip 🔖
     ● **S73.109**   Unspecified sprain of unspecified hip 🔖

   ● **S73.11**   Iliofemoral ligament sprain of hip

     ● **S73.111**   Iliofemoral ligament sprain of right hip 🔖
     ● **S73.112**   Iliofemoral ligament sprain of left hip 🔖
     ● **S73.119**   Iliofemoral ligament sprain of unspecified hip 🔖

   ● **S73.12**   Ischiocapsular (ligament) sprain of hip

     ● **S73.121**   Ischiocapsular ligament sprain of right hip 🔖
     ● **S73.122**   Ischiocapsular ligament sprain of left hip 🔖
     ● **S73.129**   Ischiocapsular ligament sprain of unspecified hip 🔖

   ● **S73.19**   Other sprain of hip

     ● **S73.191**   Other sprain of right hip 🔖
     ● **S73.192**   Other sprain of left hip 🔖
     ● **S73.199**   Other sprain of unspecified hip 🔖

● **S74**   **Injury of nerves at hip and thigh level**

   Code also any associated open wound (S71.-)

   Excludes2   injury of nerves at ankle and foot level (S94.-)
              injury of nerves at lower leg level (S84.-)

   The appropriate 7th character is to be added to each code from category S74

     | | |
     A   initial encounter
     D   subsequent encounter
     S   sequela

   ● **S74.0**   Injury of sciatic nerve at hip and thigh level

     X ● **S74.00**   Injury of sciatic nerve at hip and thigh level, unspecified leg 🔖
     X ● **S74.01**   Injury of sciatic nerve at hip and thigh level, right leg 🔖
     X ● **S74.02**   Injury of sciatic nerve at hip and thigh level, left leg 🔖

   ● **S74.1**   Injury of femoral nerve at hip and thigh level

     X ● **S74.10**   Injury of femoral nerve at hip and thigh level, unspecified leg 🔖
     X ● **S74.11**   Injury of femoral nerve at hip and thigh level, right leg 🔖
     X ● **S74.12**   Injury of femoral nerve at hip and thigh level, left leg 🔖

CHAPTER 19 (S00-T88)

● **S74.2**   Injury of cutaneous sensory nerve at hip and thigh level

   X ● **S74.20**   Injury of cutaneous sensory nerve at hip and thigh level, unspecified leg 🐾

   X ● **S74.21**   Injury of cutaneous sensory nerve at hip and high level, right leg 🐾

   X ● **S74.22**   Injury of cutaneous sensory nerve at hip and thigh level, left leg 🐾

● **S74.8**   Injury of other nerves at hip and thigh level

   ● **S74.8X**   Injury of other nerves at hip and thigh level

     ● **S74.8X1**   Injury of other nerves at hip and thigh level, right leg 🐾

     ● **S74.8X2**   Injury of other nerves at hip and thigh level, left leg 🐾

     ● **S74.8X9**   Injury of other nerves at hip and thigh level, unspecified leg 🐾

● **S74.9**   Injury of unspecified nerve at hip and thigh level

   X ● **S74.90**   Injury of unspecified nerve at hip and thigh level, unspecified leg 🐾

   X ● **S74.91**   Injury of unspecified nerve at hip and thigh level, right leg 🐾

   X ● **S74.92**   Injury of unspecified nerve at hip and thigh level, left leg 🐾

● **S75**   **Injury of blood vessels at hip and thigh level**

   Code also any associated open wound (S71.-)

   Excludes2   injury of blood vessels at lower leg level (S85.-)
              injury of popliteal artery (S85.0)

   The appropriate 7th character is to be added to each code from category S75

A	initial encounter
D	subsequent encounter
S	sequela

● **S75.0**   Injury of femoral artery

   ● **S75.00**   Unspecified injury of femoral artery

     ● **S75.001**   Unspecified injury of femoral artery, right leg A 🐾, 🐾

       (Ex:) S75.001[A], S75.009-S75.021[A], S75.029-S75.091[A], S75.099[A], S75.801[A], S75.809-S75.811[A], S75.819-S75.891[A], S75.899-S75.901[A], S75.909-S75.911[A], S75.919-S75.991[A], S75.999[A], S85.201[A], S85.209-S85.211[A], S85.219-S85.291[A], S85.299[A], S85.801[A], S85.809-S85.811[A], S85.819-S85.891[A], S85.899-S85.901[A], S85.909-S85.911[A], S85.919-S85.991[A], S85.999[A], S95.001[A], S95.009-S95.011[A], S95.019-S95.091[A], S95.099[A], S95.201[A], S95.209-S95.211[A], S95.219-S95.291[A], S95.299-S95.801[A], S95.809-S95.811[A], S95.819-S95.891[A], S95.899-S95.901[A], S95.909-S95.911[A], S95.919-S95.991[A], S95.999[A]

     ● **S75.002**   Unspecified injury of femoral artery, left leg A 🐾, 🐾

       (Ex:) S75.002-S75.009[A], S75.012-S75.019[A], S75.022-S75.029[A], S75.092[A], S75.099[A], S75.802-S75.809[A], S75.812-S75.819[A], S75.892-S75.899[A], S75.902-S75.909[A], S75.912-S75.919[A], S75.992-S75.999[A], S85.202-S85.209[A], S85.212-S85.219[A], S85.292-S85.299[A], S85.802-S85.809[A], S85.812-S85.819[A], S85.892-S85.899[A], S85.902-S85.909[A], S85.912-S85.919[A], S85.992-S85.999[A], S95.002-S95.009[A], S95.012-S95.019[A], S95.092-S95.099[A], S95.202-S95.209[A], S95.212-S95.219[A], S95.292-S95.299[A], S95.802-S95.809[A], S95.812-S95.819[A], S95.892-S95.899[A], S95.902-S95.909[A], S95.912-S95.919[A], S95.992-S95.999[A]

● **S75.009**   Unspecified injury of femoral artery, unspecified leg A 🐾, 🐾

   (Ex:) S75.001-S75.099[A], S75.801-S75.999[A], S85.201-S85.299[A], S85.801-S85.999[A], S95.001-S95.099[A], S95.201-S95.999[A]

● **S75.01**   Minor laceration of femoral artery
     Incomplete transection of femoral artery
     Laceration of femoral artery NOS
     Superficial laceration of femoral artery

   ● **S75.011**   Minor laceration of femoral artery, right leg A 🐾, 🐾
     (Ex:) See S75.001

   ● **S75.012**   Minor laceration of femoral artery, left leg A 🐾, 🐾
     (Ex:) See S75.002

   ● **S75.019**   Minor laceration of femoral artery, unspecified leg A 🐾, 🐾
     (Ex:) See S75.009

● **S75.02**   Major laceration of femoral artery
     Complete transection of femoral artery
     Traumatic rupture of femoral artery

   ● **S75.021**   Major laceration of femoral artery, right leg A 🐾, 🐾
     (Ex:) See S75.001

   ● **S75.022**   Major laceration of femoral artery, left leg A 🐾, 🐾
     (Ex:) See S75.002

   ● **S75.029**   Major laceration of femoral artery, unspecified leg A 🐾, 🐾
     (Ex:) See S75.009

● **S75.09**   Other specified injury of femoral artery

   ● **S75.091**   Other specified injury of femoral artery, right leg A 🐾, 🐾
     (Ex:) See S75.001

   ● **S75.092**   Other specified injury of femoral artery, left leg A 🐾, 🐾
     (Ex:) See S75.002

   ● **S75.099**   Other specified injury of femoral artery, unspecified leg A 🐾, 🐾
     (Ex:) See S75.009

● **S75.1**   Injury of femoral vein at hip and thigh level

   ● **S75.10**   Unspecified injury of femoral vein at hip and thigh level

     ● **S75.101**   Unspecified injury of femoral vein at hip and thigh level, right leg A 🐾, 🐾

       (Ex:) S75.101[A], S75.109-S75.111[A], S75.119-S75.121[A], S75.129-S75.191[A], S75.199[A], S75.801[A], S75.809-S75.811[A], S75.819-S75.891[A], S75.899-S75.901[A], S75.909-S75.911[A], S75.919-S75.991[A], S75.999[A], S85.201[A], S85.209-S85.211[A], S85.219-S85.291[A], S85.299[A], S85.801[A], S85.809-S85.811[A], S85.819-S85.891[A], S85.899-S85.901[A], S85.909-S85.911[A], S85.919-S85.991[A], S85.999[A], S95.001[A], S95.009-S95.011[A], S95.019-S95.091[A], S95.099[A], S95.201[A], S95.209-S95.211[A], S95.219-S95.291[A], S95.299-S95.801[A], S95.809-S95.811[A], S95.819-S95.891[A], S95.899-S95.901[A], S95.909-S95.911[A], S95.919-S95.991[A], S95.999[A]

◀ New   ◀⁞⁞ Revised   ~~deleted~~ Deleted   Excludes 1   Excludes 2   Includes   Use additional   Code first   Code also   Unspecified

OGCR Official Guidelines   ● Unacceptable Principal Diagnosis   X Assign placeholder X   🐾 Use Additional Character(s)   ▶ Manifestation Code   **Coding Clinic**

● **S75.102** Unspecified injury of femoral vein at hip and thigh level, left leg A 🗁, 🖿
  (Ex) S75.102-S75.109[A], S75.112-S75.119[A],
    S75.122-S75.129[A], S75.192-S75.199[A],
    S75.802-S75.809[A], S75.812-S75.819[A],
    S75.892-S75.899[A], S75.902-S75.909[A],
    S75.912-S75.919[A], S75.992-S75.999[A],
    S85.202-S85.209[A], S85.212-S85.219[A],
    S85.292-S85.299[A], S85.802-S85.809[A],
    S85.812-S85.819[A], S85.892-S85.899[A],
    S85.902-S85.909[A], S85.912-S85.919[A],
    S85.992-S85.999[A], S95.002-S95.009[A],
    S95.012-S95.019[A], S95.092-S95.099[A],
    S95.202-S95.209[A], S95.212-S95.219[A],
    S95.292-S95.299[A], S95.802-S95.809[A],
    S95.812-S95.819[A], S95.892-S95.899[A],
    S95.902-S95.909[A], S95.912-S95.919[A],
    S95.992-S95.999[A]

● **S75.109** Unspecified injury of femoral vein at hip and thigh level, unspecified leg A 🗁, 🖿
  (Ex) S75.101-S75.199[A], S75.801-S75.999[A],
    S85.201-S85.299[A], S85.801-S85.999[A],
    S95.001-S95.099[A], S95.201-S95.999[A]

● **S75.11** Minor laceration of femoral vein at hip and thigh level
    Incomplete transection of femoral vein at hip and thigh level
    Laceration of femoral vein at hip and thigh level NOS
    Superficial laceration of femoral vein at hip and thigh level

  ● **S75.111** Minor laceration of femoral vein at hip and thigh level, right leg A 🗁, 🖿
    (Ex) See S75.101

  ● **S75.112** Minor laceration of femoral vein at hip and thigh level, left leg A 🗁, 🖿
    (Ex) See S75.102

  ● **S75.119** Minor laceration of femoral vein at hip and thigh level, unspecified leg A 🗁, 🖿
    (Ex) See S75.109

● **S75.12** Major laceration of femoral vein at hip and thigh level
    Complete transection of femoral vein at hip and thigh level
    Traumatic rupture of femoral vein at hip and thigh level

  ● **S75.121** Major laceration of femoral vein at hip and thigh level, right leg A 🗁, 🖿
    (Ex) See S75.101

  ● **S75.122** Major laceration of femoral vein at hip and thigh level, left leg A 🗁, 🖿
    (Ex) See S75.102

  ● **S75.129** Major laceration of femoral vein at hip and thigh level, unspecified leg A 🗁, 🖿
    (Ex) See S75.109

● **S75.19** Other specified injury of femoral vein at hip and thigh level

  ● **S75.191** Other specified injury of femoral vein at hip and thigh level, right leg A 🗁, 🖿
    (Ex) See S75.101

  ● **S75.192** Other specified injury of femoral vein at hip and thigh level, left leg A 🗁, 🖿
    (Ex) See S75.102

  ● **S75.199** Other specified injury of femoral vein at hip and thigh level, unspecified leg A 🗁, 🖿
    (Ex) See S75.109

● **S75.2** Injury of greater saphenous vein at hip and thigh level
    Excludes1   greater saphenous vein NOS (S85.3)

● **S75.20** Unspecified injury of greater saphenous vein at hip and thigh level

  ● **S75.201** Unspecified injury of greater saphenous vein at hip and thigh level, right leg A 🗁, 🖿
    (Ex) S75.201[A], S75.209-S75.211[A],
    S75.219-S75.221[A], S75.229-S75.291[A],
    S75.299-S75.801[A], S75.809-S75.811[A],
    S75.819-S75.891[A], S75.899-S75.901[A],
    S75.909-S75.911[A], S75.919-S75.991[A],
    S75.999[A], S85.201[A], S85.209[A],
    S85.211[A], S85.219-S85.291[A],
    S85.299-S85.301[A], S85.309-S85.311[A],
    S85.319-S85.391[A], S85.399-S85.401[A],
    S85.409-S85.411[A], S85.419-S85.491[A],
    S85.499[A], S85.801-S85.809[A],
    S85.811[A], S85.819-S85.891[A],
    S85.899-S85.901[A], S85.909-S85.911[A],
    S85.919-S85.991[A], S85.999[A], S95.001[A],
    S95.009-S95.011[A], S95.019-S95.091[A],
    S95.099[A], S95.201[A], S95.209-S95.211[A],
    S95.219-S95.291[A], S95.299-S95.801[A],
    S95.809-S95.811[A], S95.819-S95.891[A],
    S95.899-S95.901[A], S95.909-S95.911[A],
    S95.919-S95.991[A], S95.999[A]

  ● **S75.202** Unspecified injury of greater saphenous vein at hip and thigh level, left leg A 🗁, 🖿
    (Ex) S75.202-S75.209[A], S75.212-S75.219[A],
    S75.222-S75.229[A], S75.292-S75.299[A],
    S75.802-S75.809[A], S75.812-S75.819[A],
    S75.892-S75.899[A], S75.902-S75.909[A],
    S75.912-S75.919[A], S75.992-S75.999[A], S85.
    202-S85.209[A],S85.212-S85.219[A],
    S85.292-S85.299[A], S85.302-S85.309[A],
    S85.312-S85.319[A], S85.392-S85.399[A],
    S85.402-S85.409[A], S85.412-S85.419[A],
    S85.492-S85.499[A], S85.802-S85.809[A],
    S85.812-S85.819[A], S85.892-S85.899[A],
    S85.902-S85.909[A], S85.912-S85.919[A],
    S85.992-S85.999[A], S95.002-S95.009[A],
    S95.012-S95.019[A], S95.092-S95.099[A],
    S95.202-S95.209[A], S95.212-S95.219[A],
    S95.292-S95.299[A], S95.802-S95.809[A],
    S95.812-S95.819[A], S95.892-S95.899[A],
    S95.902-S95.909[A], S95.912-S95.919[A],
    S95.992-S95.999[A]

  ● **S75.209** Unspecified injury of greater saphenous vein at hip and thigh level, unspecified leg A 🗁, 🖿
    (Ex) S75.201-S75.999[A], S85.201-S85.499[A],
    S85.801-S85.999[A], S95.001-S95.099[A],
    S95.201-S95.999[A]

● **S75.21** Minor laceration of greater saphenous vein at hip and thigh level
    Incomplete transection of greater saphenous vein at hip and thigh level
    Laceration of greater saphenous vein at hip and thigh level NOS
    Superficial laceration of greater saphenous vein at hip and thigh level

  ● **S75.211** Minor laceration of greater saphenous vein at hip and thigh level, right leg A 🗁, 🖿
    (Ex) See S75.201

  ● **S75.212** Minor laceration of greater saphenous vein at hip and thigh level, left leg A 🗁, 🖿
    (Ex) See S75.202

  ● **S75.219** Minor laceration of greater saphenous vein at hip and thigh level, unspecified leg A 🗁, 🖿
    (Ex) See S75.209

CHAPTER 19 (S00-T88)

N Newborn Age: 0   P Pediatric Age: 0–17   M Maternity DX: 12–55   A Adult Age: 15–124   ♀ Females Only   ♂ Males Only

🗁 Complication\Comorbidity   🖿 Major C\C   (Ex) CC/MCC Exclusions   🖿 Present on Admission Requirement   🖿 Hospital-Acquired Condition

1445

CHAPTER 19 (S00-T88)

● **S75.22** **Major laceration of greater saphenous vein at hip and thigh level**
Complete transection of greater saphenous vein at hip and thigh level
Traumatic rupture of greater saphenous vein at hip and thigh level

● **S75.221** Major laceration of greater saphenous vein at hip and thigh level, right leg
A ⬤, ⬤
Ⓔⓧ See S75.201

● **S75.222** Major laceration of greater saphenous vein at hip and thigh level, left leg
A ⬤, ⬤
Ⓔⓧ See S75.202

● **S75.229** Major laceration of greater saphenous vein at hip and thigh level, unspecified leg A ⬤, ⬤
Ⓔⓧ See S75.209

● **S75.29** **Other specified injury of greater saphenous vein at hip and thigh level**

● **S75.291** Other specified injury of greater saphenous vein at hip and thigh level, right leg A ⬤, ⬤
Ⓔⓧ See S75.201

● **S75.292** Other specified injury of greater saphenous vein at hip and thigh level, left leg A ⬤, ⬤
Ⓔⓧ See S75.202

● **S75.299** Other specified injury of greater saphenous vein at hip and thigh level, unspecified leg A ⬤, ⬤
Ⓔⓧ See S75.209

● **S75.8** **Injury of other blood vessels at hip and thigh level**

● **S75.80** **Unspecified injury of other blood vessels at hip and thigh level**

● **S75.801** Unspecified injury of other blood vessels at hip and thigh level, right leg A ⬤, ⬤
Ⓔⓧ M79.A21-M79.A29, S75.001[A], S75.009-S75.011[A], S75.019-S7.021[A], S75.029-S75.091[A], S75.099-S75.101[A], S75.109-S75.111[A], S75.119-S75.121[A], S75.129-S75.191[A], S75.199-S75.201[A], S75.209-S75.211[A], S75.219-S75.221[A], S75.229-S75.291[A], S75.299-S75.801[A], S75.809-S75.891[A], S75.899-S75.901[A], S75.909-S75.911[A], S75.919-S75.991[A], S75.999[A], S85.001[A], S85.009-S85.011[A], S85.019-S85.091[A], S85.099-S85.101[A], S85.109-S85.111[A], S85.119-S85.121[A], S85.129-S85.131[A], S85.139-S85.141[A], S85.149-S85.151[A], S85.159-S85.161[A], S85.169-S85.171[A], S85.179-S85.181[A], S85.189-S85.201[A], S85.209-S85.211[A], S85.219-S85.291[A], S85.299-S85.301[A], S85.309-S85.311[A], S85.319-S85.391[A], S85.399-S85.401[A], S85.409-S85.411[A], S85.419-S85.491[A], S85.499-S85.501[A], S85.509-S85.511[A], S85.519-S85.591[A], S85.599-S85.801[A], S85.809-S85.811[A], S85.819-S85.891[A], S85.899-S85.901[A] S85.909-S85.911[A], S85.919-S85.991[A], S85.999[A], S95.001[A], S95.009-S95.011[A], S95.019[A], S95.091[A], S95.099-S95.101[A], S95.109-S95.111[A], S95 119-S95.191[A], S95.199-S95.201[A], S95.209-S95.211[A], S95.219-S95.291[A], S95.299-S95.801[A], S95.809-S95.811[A]. S95.819-S95.891[A], S95.899-S95.901[A], S95.909-S95.911[A], S95.919-S95.991[A], S95.999[A]

● **S75.802** Unspecified injury of other blood vessels at hip and thigh level, left leg
A ⬤, ⬤
Ⓔⓧ M79.A21-M79.A29, S75.002-S75.009[A], S75.012-S75.019[A], S75.022-S75.029[A], S75.092-S75.099[A], S75.102-S75.109[A], S75.112-S75.119[A], S75.122-S75.129[A], S75.192-S75.199[A], S75.202-S75.209[A], S75.212-S75.219[A], S75.222-S75.229[A], S75.292-S75.299[A], S75.802-S75.809[A], S75.812-S75.819[A], S75.892-S75.899[A], S75.902-S75.909[A], S75.912-S75.919[A], S75.992-S75.999[A], S85.002-S85.009[A], S85.012-S85.019[A], S85.092-S85.099[A], S85.102-S85.109[A], S85.112-S85.119[A], S85.122-S85.129[A], S85.132-S85.139[A], S85.142-S85.149[A], S85.152-S85.159[A], S85.162-S85.169[A], S85.172-S85.179[A], S85.182-S85.189[A], S85.202-S85.209[A], S85.212-S85.219[A], S85.292-S85.299[A], S85.302-S85.309[A], S85.312-S85.319[A], S85.392-S85.399[A], S85.402-S85.409[A], S85.412-S85.419[A], S85.492-S85.499[A], S85.502-S85.509[A], S85.512-S85.519[A], S85.592-S85.599[A], S85.802-S85.809[A], S85.812-S85.819[A], S85.892-S85.899[A], S85.902-S85.909[A], S85.912-S85.919[A], S85.992-S85.999[A], S95.002-S95.009[A], S95.012-S95.019[A], S95.092-S95.099[A], S95.102-S95.109[A], S95.112-S95.119[A], S95.192-S95.199[A], S95.202-S95.209[A], S95.212-S95.219[A], S95.292-S95.299[A], S95.802-S95.809[A], S95.812-S95.819[A], S95.892-S95.899[A], S95.902-S95.909[A], S95.912-S95.919[A], S95.992-S95.999[A]

● **S75.809** Unspecified injury of other blood vessels at hip and thigh level, unspecified leg A ⬤, ⬤
Ⓔⓧ M79.A21-M79.A29, S75.001-S75.999[A], S85.001-S85.999[A], S95.001-S95.999[A]

● **S75.81** **Laceration of other blood vessels at hip and thigh level**

● **S75.811** Laceration of other blood vessels at hip and thigh level, right leg A ⬤, ⬤
Ⓔⓧ See S75.801

● **S75.812** Laceration of other blood vessels at hip and thigh level, left leg A ⬤, ⬤
Ⓔⓧ See S75.802

● **S75.819** Laceration of other blood vessels at hip and thigh level, unspecified leg A ⬤, ⬤
Ⓔⓧ See S75.809

● **S75.89** **Other specified injury of other blood vessels at hip and thigh level**

● **S75.891** Other specified injury of other blood vessels at hip and thigh level, right leg A ⬤, ⬤
Ⓔⓧ See S75.801

● **S75.892** Other specified injury of other blood vessels at hip and thigh level, left leg A ⬤, ⬤
Ⓔⓧ See S75.802

● **S75.899** Other specified injury of other blood vessels at hip and thigh level, unspecified leg A ⬤, ⬤
Ⓔⓧ See S75.809

◀ New   ◀▥ Revised   ~~deleted~~ Deleted   Excludes 1   Excludes 2   Includes   Use additional   Code first   Code also   Unspecified
OGCR Official Guidelines   ● Unacceptable Principal Diagnosis   X Assign placeholder X   ● Use Additional Character(s)   ▌ Manifestation Code   **Coding Clinic**

● S75.9   Injury of unspecified blood vessel at hip and thigh level
    ● S75.90   Unspecified injury of unspecified blood vessel at hip and thigh level
       ● S75.901   Unspecified injury of unspecified blood vessel at hip and thigh level, right leg A 🦠, 🦠
           (Ex:) See S75.801
       ● S75.902   Unspecified injury of unspecified blood vessel at hip and thigh level, left leg A 🦠, 🦠
           (Ex:) See S75.802
       ● S75.909   Unspecified injury of unspecified blood vessel at hip and thigh level, unspecified leg A 🦠, 🦠
           (Ex:) See S75.809
    ● S75.91   Laceration of unspecified blood vessel at hip and thigh level
       ● S75.911   Laceration of unspecified blood vessel at hip and thigh level, right leg A 🦠, 🦠
           (Ex:) See S75.801
       ● S75.912   Laceration of unspecified blood vessel at hip and thigh level, left leg A 🦠, 🦠
           (Ex:) See S75.802
       ● S75.919   Laceration of unspecified blood vessel at hip and thigh level, unspecified leg A 🦠, 🦠
           (Ex:) See S75.809
    ● S75.99   Other specified injury of unspecified blood vessel at hip and thigh level
       ● S75.991   Other specified injury of unspecified blood vessel at hip and thigh level, right leg A 🦠, 🦠
           (Ex:) See S75.801
       ● S75.992   Other specified injury of unspecified blood vessel at hip and thigh level, left leg A 🦠, 🦠
           (Ex:) See S75.802
       ● S75.999   Other specified injury of unspecified blood vessel at hip and thigh level, unspecified leg A 🦠, 🦠
           (Ex:) See S75.809

● S76   Injury of muscle, fascia and tendon at hip and thigh level
    Code also any associated open wound (S71.-)
    Excludes2   injury of muscle, fascia and tendon at lower leg level (S86)
           sprain of joint and ligament of hip (S73.1)
    The appropriate 7th character is to be added to each code from category S76

> A   initial encounter
> D   subsequent encounter
> S   sequela

    ● S76.0   Injury of muscle, fascia and tendon of hip
       ● S76.00   Unspecified injury of muscle, fascia and tendon of hip
          ● S76.001   Unspecified injury of muscle, fascia and tendon of right hip 🦠
          ● S76.002   Unspecified injury of muscle, fascia and tendon of left hip 🦠
          ● S76.009   Unspecified injury of muscle, fascia and tendon of unspecified hip 🦠

● S76.01   Strain of muscle, fascia and tendon of hip
    ● S76.011   Strain of muscle, fascia and tendon of right hip 🦠
    ● S76.012   Strain of muscle, fascia and tendon of left hip 🦠
    ● S76.019   Strain of muscle, fascia and tendon of unspecified hip 🦠
● S76.02   Laceration of muscle, fascia and tendon of hip
    ● S76.021   Laceration of muscle, fascia and tendon of right hip A 🦠, 🦠
       (Ex:) S71.001[A], S71.009-S71.011[A], S71.019-S71.021[A], S71.029-S71.031[A], S71.039-S71.041[A], S71.049-S71.051[A], S71.059-S71.101[A], S71.109-S71.111[A], S71.119-S71.121[A], S71.129-S71.131[A], S71.139-S71.141[A], S71.149-S71.151[A], S71.159[A], S76.021[A], S76.029[A], S76.121[A], S76.129[A], S76.221[A], S76.229[A], S76.321[A], S76.329[A], S76.821[A], S76.829[A], S76.921[A], S76.929[A]
    ● S76.022   Laceration of muscle, fascia and tendon of left hip A 🦠, 🦠
       (Ex:) S71.002-S71.009[A], S71.012-S71.019[A], S71.022-S71.029[A], S71.032-S71.039[A], S71.042-S71.049[A], S71.052-S71.059[A], S71.102-S71.109[A], S71.112-S71.119[A], S71.122-S71.129[A], S71.132-S71.139[A], S71.142-S71.149[A], S71.152-S71.159[A], S76.022-S76.029[A], S76.122-S76.129[A], S76.222-S76.229[A], S76.322-S76.329[A], S76.822-S76.829[A], S76.922-S76.929[A]
    ● S76.029   Laceration of muscle, fascia and tendon of unspecified hip A 🦠, 🦠
       (Ex:) S71.001-S71.159[A], S76.021-S76.029[A], S76.121-S76.129[A], S76.221-S76.229[A], S76.321-S76.329[A], S76.821-S76.829[A], S76.921-S76.929[A]
● S76.09   Other specified injury of muscle, fascia and tendon of hip
    ● S76.091   Other specified injury of muscle, fascia and tendon of right hip 🦠
    ● S76.092   Other specified injury of muscle, fascia and tendon of left hip 🦠
    ● S76.099   Other specified injury of muscle, fascia and tendon of unspecified hip 🦠
● S76.1   Injury of quadriceps muscle, fascia and tendon
    Injury of patellar ligament (tendon)
    ● S76.10   Unspecified injury of quadriceps muscle, fascia and tendon
       ● S76.101   Unspecified injury of right quadriceps muscle, fascia and tendon 🦠
       ● S76.102   Unspecified injury of left quadriceps muscle, fascia and tendon 🦠
       ● S76.109   Unspecified injury of unspecified quadriceps muscle, fascia and tendon 🦠

N   Newborn Age: 0   P   Pediatric Age: 0–17   M   Maternity DX: 12–55   A   Adult Age: 15–124   ♀   Females Only   ♂   Males Only

🦠 Complication\Comorbidity   🦠 Major C\C   (Ex:) CC/MCC Exclusions   🦠 Present on Admission Requirement   🦠 Hospital-Acquired Condition

1447

● S76.11   Strain of quadriceps muscle, fascia and tendon
    ● S76.111   Strain of right quadriceps muscle, fascia and tendon 🔁
    ● S76.112   Strain of left quadriceps muscle, fascia and tendon 🔁
    ● S76.119   Strain of unspecified quadriceps muscle, fascia and tendon 🔁
● S76.12   Laceration of quadriceps muscle, fascia and tendon
    ● S76.121   Laceration of right quadriceps muscle, fascia and tendon A 🔁, 🔁
        Ex: See S76.021
    ● S76.122   Laceration of left quadriceps muscle, fascia and tendon A 🔁, 🔁
        Ex: See S76.022
    ● S76.129   Laceration of unspecified quadriceps muscle, fascia and tendon A 🔁, 🔁
        Ex: See S76.029
● S76.19   Other specified injury of quadriceps muscle, fascia and tendon
    ● S76.191   Other specified injury of right quadriceps muscle, fascia and tendon 🔁
    ● S76.192   Other specified injury of left quadriceps muscle, fascia and tendon 🔁
    ● S76.199   Other specified injury of unspecified quadriceps muscle, fascia and tendon 🔁

● S76.2   Injury of adductor muscle, fascia and tendon of thigh
● S76.20   Unspecified injury of adductor muscle, fascia and tendon of thigh
    ● S76.201   Unspecified injury of adductor muscle, fascia and tendon of right thigh 🔁
    ● S76.202   Unspecified injury of adductor muscle, fascia and tendon of left thigh 🔁
    ● S76.209   Unspecified injury of adductor muscle, fascia and tendon of unspecified thigh 🔁
● S76.21   Strain of adductor muscle, fascia and tendon of thigh
    ● S76.211   Strain of adductor muscle, fascia and tendon of right thigh 🔁
    ● S76.212   Strain of adductor muscle, fascia and tendon of left thigh 🔁
    ● S76.219   Strain of adductor muscle, fascia and tendon of unspecified thigh 🔁
● S76.22   Laceration of adductor muscle, fascia and tendon of thigh
    ● S76.221   Laceration of adductor muscle, and tendon of right thigh A 🔁, 🔁
        Ex: See S76.021
    ● S76.222   Laceration of adductor muscle, fascia and tendon of left thigh A 🔁, 🔁
        Ex: See S76.022
    ● S76.229   Laceration of adductor muscle, fascia and tendon of unspecified thigh A 🔁, 🔁
        Ex: See S76.029

● S76.29   Other injury of adductor muscle, fascia and tendon of thigh
    ● S76.291   Other injury of adductor muscle, fascia and tendon of right thigh 🔁
    ● S76.292   Other injury of adductor muscle, fascia and tendon of left thigh 🔁
    ● S76.299   Other injury of adductor muscle, fascia and tendon of unspecified thigh 🔁

● S76.3   Injury of muscle, fascia and tendon of the posterior muscle group at thigh level
● S76.30   Unspecified injury of muscle, fascia and tendon of the posterior muscle group at thigh level
    ● S76.301   Unspecified injury of muscle, fascia and tendon of the posterior muscle group at thigh level, right thigh 🔁
    ● S76.302   Unspecified injury of muscle, fascia and tendon of the posterior muscle group at thigh level, left thigh 🔁
    ● S76.309   Unspecified injury of muscle, fascia and tendon of the posterior muscle group at thigh level, unspecified thigh 🔁
● S76.31   Strain of muscle, fascia and tendon of the posterior muscle group at thigh level
    ● S76.311   Strain of muscle, fascia and tendon of the posterior muscle group at thigh level, right thigh 🔁
    ● S76.312   Strain of muscle, fascia and tendon of the posterior muscle group at thigh level, left thigh 🔁
    ● S76.319   Strain of muscle, fascia and tendon of the posterior muscle group at thigh level, unspecified thigh 🔁
● S76.32   Laceration of muscle, fascia and tendon of the posterior muscle group at thigh level
    ● S76.321   Laceration of muscle, fascia and tendon of the posterior muscle group at thigh level, right thigh A 🔁, 🔁
        Ex: See S76.021
    ● S76.322   Laceration of muscle, fascia and tendon of the posterior muscle group at thigh level, left thigh A 🔁, 🔁
        Ex: See S76.022
    ● S76.329   Laceration of muscle, fascia and tendon of the posterior muscle group at thigh level, unspecified thigh A 🔁, 🔁
        Ex: See S76.029
● S76.39   Other specified injury of muscle, fascia and tendon of the posterior muscle group at thigh level
    ● S76.391   Other specified injury of muscle, fascia and tendon of the posterior muscle group at thigh level, right thigh 🔁
    ● S76.392   Other specified injury of muscle, fascia and tendon of the posterior muscle group at thigh level, left thigh 🔁
    ● S76.399   Other specified injury of muscle, fascia and tendon of the posterior muscle group at thigh level, unspecified thigh 🔁

◄ New   ◄ Revised   ~~deleted~~ Deleted   Excludes 1   Excludes 2   Includes   Use additional   Code first   Code also   Unspecified
OGCR Official Guidelines   ● Unacceptable Principal Diagnosis   X Assign placeholder X   ● Use Additional Character(s)   ▌ Manifestation Code   Coding Clinic

● S76.8   Injury of other specified muscles, fascia and tendons at thigh level
- ● S76.80   Unspecified injury of other specified muscles, fascia and tendons at thigh level
  - ● S76.801   Unspecified injury of other specified muscles, fascia and tendons at thigh level, right thigh 🪱
  - ● S76.802   Unspecified injury of other specified muscles, fascia and tendons at thigh level, left thigh 🪱
  - ● S76.809   Unspecified injury of other specified muscles, fascia and tendons at thigh level, unspecified thigh 🪱
- ● S76.81   Strain of other specified specified muscles, fascia and tendons at thigh level
  - ● S76.811   Strain of other specified muscles, fascia and tendons at thigh level, right thigh 🪱
  - ● S76.812   Strain of other specified muscles, fascia and tendons at thigh level, left thigh 🪱
  - ● S76.819   Strain of other specified muscles, fascia and tendons at thigh level, unspecified thigh 🪱
- ● S76.82   Laceration of other specified muscles, fascia and tendons at thigh level
  - ● S76.821   Laceration of other specified muscles, fascia and tendons at thigh level, right thigh A 🪱, 🪱
    (Ex) See S76.021
  - ● S76.822   Laceration of other specified muscles, fascia and tendons at thigh level, left thigh A 🪱, 🪱
    (Ex) See S76.022
  - ● S76.829   Laceration of other specified muscles, fascia and tendons at thigh level, unspecified thigh A 🪱, 🪱
    (Ex) See S76.029
- ● S76.89   Other injury of other specified muscles, fascia and tendons at thigh level
  - ● S76.891   Other injury of other specified muscles, fascia and tendons at thigh level, right thigh 🪱
  - ● S76.892   Other injury of other specified muscles, fascia and tendons at thigh level, left thigh 🪱
  - ● S76.899   Other injury of other specified muscles, fascia and tendons at thigh level, unspecified thigh 🪱
● S76.9   Injury of unspecified muscles, fascia and tendons at thigh level
- ● S76.90   Unspecified injury of unspecified muscles, fascia and tendons at thigh level
  - ● S76.901   Unspecified injury of unspecified muscles, fascia and tendons at thigh level, right thigh 🪱
  - ● S76.902   Unspecified injury of unspecified muscles, fascia and tendons at thigh level, left thigh 🪱
  - ● S76.909   Unspecified injury of unspecified muscles, fascia and tendons at thigh level, unspecified thigh 🪱

● S76.91   Strain of unspecified muscles, fascia and tendons at thigh level
- ● S76.911   Strain of unspecified muscles, fascia and tendons at thigh level, right thigh 🪱
- ● S76.912   Strain of unspecified muscles, fascia and tendons at thigh level, left thigh 🪱
- ● S76.919   Strain of unspecified muscles, fascia and tendons at thigh level, unspecified thigh 🪱
● S76.92   Laceration of unspecified muscles, fascia and tendons at thigh level
- ● S76.921   Laceration of unspecified muscles, fascia and tendons at thigh level, right thigh A 🪱, 🪱
  (Ex) See S76.021
- ● S76.922   Laceration of unspecified muscles, fascia and tendons at thigh level, left thigh A 🪱, 🪱
  (Ex) See S76.022
- ● S76.929   Laceration of unspecified muscles, fascia and tendons at thigh level, unspecified thigh A 🪱, 🪱
  (Ex) See S76.029
● S76.99   Other specified injury of unspecified muscles, fascia and tendons at thigh level
- ● S76.991   Other specified injury of unspecified muscles, fascia and tendons at thigh level, right thigh 🪱
- ● S76.992   Other specified injury of unspecified muscles, fascia and tendons at thigh level, left thigh 🪱
- ● S76.999   Other specified injury of unspecified muscles, fascia and tendons at thigh level, unspecified thigh 🪱

● S77   Crushing injury of hip and thigh
> Use additional code(s) for all associated injuries
> **Excludes2**   crushing injury of ankle and foot (S97.-)
>   crushing injury of lower leg (S87.-)
> The appropriate 7th character is to be added to each code from category S77

A	initial encounter
D	subsequent encounter
S	sequela

- ● S77.0   Crushing injury of hip
  (Ex) **For category S77.0 CC codes:** S77.00X-S77.02X[A], S77.20X-S77.22X[A]
  - X ● S77.00   Crushing injury of unspecified hip A 🪱, 🪱, A 🪱
  - X ● S77.01   Crushing injury of right hip A 🪱, 🪱, A 🪱
  - X ● S77.02   Crushing injury of left hip A 🪱, 🪱, A 🪱
- ● S77.1   Crushing injury of thigh
  (Ex) **For category S77.1 CC codes:** S77.10X-S77.22X[A]
  - X ● S77.10   Crushing injury of unspecified thigh A 🪱, 🪱, A 🪱
  - X ● S77.11   Crushing injury of right thigh A 🪱, 🪱, A 🪱
  - X ● S77.12   Crushing injury of left thigh A 🪱, 🪱, A 🪱
- ● S77.2   Crushing injury of hip with thigh
  - X ● S77.20   Crushing injury of unspecified hip with thigh 🪱
  - X ● S77.21   Crushing injury of right hip with thigh 🪱
  - X ● S77.22   Crushing injury of left hip with thigh 🪱

N   Newborn Age: 0   P   Pediatric Age: 0–17   M   Maternity DX: 12–55   A   Adult Age: 15–124   ♀   Females Only   ♂   Males Only

🪱 Complication\Comorbidity   🪱 Major C\C   (Ex) CC/MCC Exclusions   🪱 Present on Admission Requirement   🪱 Hospital-Acquired Condition

1449

CHAPTER 19 (S00-T88)

● **S78**   **Traumatic amputation of hip and thigh**
> An amputation not identified as partial or complete should be coded to complete
>> **Excludes1**   traumatic amputation of knee (S88.0-)
>
> The appropriate 7th character is to be added to each code from category S78

A	initial encounter
D	subsequent encounter
S	sequela

● **S78.0**   **Traumatic amputation at hip joint**
> ● **S78.01**   **Complete traumatic amputation at hip joint**
>> ● **S78.011**   **Complete traumatic amputation at right hip joint** A 🗪, 🗪
>>
>> Ⓔ S71.001[A], S71.009-S71.011[A],
>> S71.019-S71.021[A], S71.029-S71.031[A],
>> S71.039-S71.041[A], S71.049-S71.051[A],
>> S71.059-S71.101[A], S71.109-S71.111[A],
>> S71.119-S71.121[A], S71.129-S71.131[A],
>> S71.139-S71.141[A], S71.149-S71.151[A],
>> S71.159[A], S76.021[A], S76.029[A],
>> S76.121[A], S76.129[A], S76.221[A],
>> S76.229[A], S76.321[A], S76.329[A],
>> S76.821[A], S76.829[A], S76.921[A],
>> S76.929[A], S78.011[A], S78.019-S78.021[A],
>> S78.029-S78.111[A], S78.119-S78.121[A],
>> S78.129-S78.911[A], S78.919-S78.921[A],
>> S78.929[A], S81.001[A], S81.009-S81.011[A],
>> S81.019-S81.021[A], S81.029-S81.031[A],
>> S81.039-S81.041[A], S81.049-S81.051[A],
>> S81.059-S81.801[A], S81.809-S81.811[A],
>> S81.819-S81.821[A], S81.829-S81.831[A],
>> S81.839-S81.841[A], S81.849-S81.851[A],
>> S81.859[A], S86.021[A], S86.029[A],
>> S86.121[A], S86.129[A], S86.221[A],
>> S86.229[A], S86.321[A], S86.329[A],
>> S86.821[A], S86.829[A], S86.921[A],
>> S86.929[A], S88.011[A], S88.019-S88.021[A],
>> S88.029-S88.111[A], S88.119-S88.121[A],
>> S88.129-S88.911[A], S88.919-S88.921[A],
>> S88.929[A], S91.001[A], S91.009-S91.011[A],
>> S91.019-S91.021[A], S91.029-S91.031[A],
>> S91.039-S91.041[A], S91.049-S91.051[A],
>> S91.059-S91.101[A], S91.103-S91.104[A],
>> S91.106-S91.111[A], S91.113-S91.114[A],
>> S91.116-S91.121[A], S91.123-S91.124[A],
>> S91.126-S91.131[A], S91.133-S91.134[A],
>> S91.136-S91.141[A], S91.143-S91.144[A],
>> S91.146-S91.151[A], S91.153-S91.154[A],
>> S91.156-S91.201[A], S91.203-S91.204[A],
>> S91.206-S91.211[A], S91.213-S91.214[A],
>> S91.216-S91.221[A], S91.223-S91.224[A],
>> S91.226-S91.231[A], S91.233-S91.234[A],
>> S91.236-S91.241[A], S91.243-S91.244[A],
>> S91.246-S91.251[A], S91.253-S91.254[A],
>> S91.256-S91.301[A], S91.309-S91.311[A],
>> S91.319-S91.321[A], S91.329-S91.331[A],
>> S91.339-S91.341[A], S91.349-S91.351[A],
>> S91.359[A], S96.021[A], S96.029[A],
>> S96.121[A], S96.129[A], S96.221[A],
>> S96.229[A], S96.821[A], S96.829[A],
>> S96.921[A], S96.929[A], S98.011[A],
>> S98.019-S98.021[A], S98.029-S98.111[A],
>> S98.119-S98.121[A], S98.129-S98.131[A],
>> S98.139-S98.141[A], S98.149-S98.211[A],
>> S98.219-S98.221[A], S98.229-S98.311[A],
>> S98.319-S98.321[A], S98.329-S98.911[A],
>> S98.919-S98.921[A], S98.929[A],
>> T14.8-T14.91, T79.8XX-T79.9XX[A], T79.
>> A0X-T79.A9X[A]

● **S78.012**   **Complete traumatic amputation at left hip joint** A 🗪, 🗪
> Ⓔ S71.002-S71.009[A], S71.012-S71.019[A],
> S71.022-S71.029[A], S71.032-S71.039[A],
> S71.042-S71.049[A], S71.052-S71.059[A],S71.
> 102-S71.109[A], S71.112-S71.119[A],
> S71.122-S71.129[A], S71.132-S71.139[A],
> S71.142-S71.149[A], S71.152-S71.159[A],
> S76.022-S76.029[A], S76.122-S76.129[A],
> S76.222-S76.229[A], S76.322-S76.329[A],
> S76.822-S76.829[A], S76.922-S76.929[A],
> S78.012-S78.019[A], S78.022-S78.029[A],
> S78.112-S78.119[A], S78.122-S78.129[A],
> S78.912-S78.919[A], S78.922-S78.929[A],
> S81.002-S81.009[A], S81.012-S81.019[A],
> S81.022-S81.029[A], S81.032-S81.039[A],
> S81.042-S81.049[A], S81.052-S81.059[A],
> S81.802-S81.809[A], S81.812-S81.819[A],
> S81.822-S81.829[A], S81.832-S81.839[A],
> S81.842-S81.849[A], S81.852-S81.859[A],
> S86.022-S86.029[A], S86.122-S86.129[A],
> S86.222-S86.229[A], S86.322-S86.329[A],
> S86.822-S86.829[A], S86.922-S86.929[A],
> S88.012-S88.019[A], S88.022-S88.029[A],
> S88.112-S88.119[A], S88.122-S88.129[A],
> S88.912-S88.919[A], S88.922-S88.929[A],
> S91.002-S91.009[A], S91.012-S91.019[A],
> S91.022-S91.029[A], S91.032-S91.039[A],
> S91.042-S91.049[A], S91.052-S91.059[A],
> S91.102-S91.103[A], S91.105-S91.109[A],
> S91.112-S91.113[A], S91.115-S91.119[A],
> S91.122-S91.123[A], S91.125-S91.129[A],
> S91.132-S91.133[A], S91.135-S91.139[A],
> S91.142-S91.143[A], S91.145-S91.149[A],
> S91.152-S91.153[A], S91.155-S91.159[A],
> S91.202-S91.203[A], S91.205-S91.209[A],
> S91.212-S91.213[A], S91.215-S91.219[A],
> S91.222-S91.223[A], S91.225-S91.229[A],
> S91.232-S91.233[A], S91.235-S91.239[A],
> S91.242-S91.243[A], S91.245-S91.249[A],
> S91.252-S91.253[A], S91.255-S91.259[A],
> S91.302-S91.309[A], S91.312-S91.319[A],
> S91.322-S91.329[A], S91.332-S91.339[A],
> S91.342-S91.349[A], S91.352-S91.359[A],
> S96.022-S96.029[A], S96.122-S96.129[A],
> S96.222-S96.229[A], S96.822-S96.829[A],
> S96.922-S96.929[A], S98.012-S98.019[A],
> S98.022-S98.029[A], S98.112-S98.119[A],
> S98.122-S98.129[A], S98.132-S98.139[A],
> S98.142-S98.149[A], S98.212-S98.219[A],
> S98.222-S98.229[A], S98.312-S98.319[A],
> S98.322-S98.329[A], S98.912-S98.919[A],
> S98.922-S98.929[A], T14.8-T14.91,
> T79.8XX-T79.9XX[A], T79.A0X-T79.A9X[A]

● **S78.019**   **Complete traumatic amputation at unspecified hip joint** A 🗪, 🗪
> Ⓔ S71.001-S71.159[A], S76.021-S76.029[A],
> S76.121-S76.129[A], S76.221-S76.229[A],
> S76.321-S76.329[A], S76.821-S76.829[A],
> S76.921-S76.929[A], S78.011-S78.929[A],
> S81.001-S81.859[A], S86.021-S86.029[A],
> S86.121-S86.129[A], S86.221-S86.229[A],
> S86.321-S86.329[A], S86.821-S86.829[A],
> S86.921-S86.929[A], S88.011-S88.929[A],
> S91.001-S91.359[A], S96.021-S96.029[A],
> S96.121-S96.129[A], S96.221-S96.229[A],
> S96.821-S96.829[A], S96.921-S96.929[A],
> S98.011-S98.929[A], T14.8-T14.91,
> T79.8XX-T79.9XX[A], T79.A0X-T79.A9X[A]

- S78.02   Partial traumatic amputation at hip joint
  - S78.021   Partial traumatic amputation at right hip joint A 🦠, 🦠
    - (Ex) See S78.011
  - S78.022   Partial traumatic amputation at left hip joint A 🦠, 🦠
    - (Ex) See S78.012
  - S78.029   Partial traumatic amputation at unspecified hip joint A 🦠, 🦠
    - (Ex) See S78.019
- S78.1   Traumatic amputation at level between hip and knee
  - **Excludes1**   traumatic amputation of knee (S88.0-)
  - S78.11   Complete traumatic amputation at level between hip and knee
    - S78.111   Complete traumatic amputation at level between right hip and knee A 🦠, 🦠
      - (Ex) See S78.011
    - S78.112   Complete traumatic amputation at level between left hip and knee A 🦠, 🦠
      - (Ex) See S78.012
    - S78.119   Complete traumatic amputation at level between unspecified hip and knee A 🦠, 🦠
      - (Ex) See S78.019
  - S78.12   Partial traumatic amputation at level between hip and knee
    - S78.121   Partial traumatic amputation at level between right hip and knee A 🦠, 🦠
      - (Ex) See S78.011
    - S78.122   Partial traumatic amputation at level between left hip and knee A 🦠, 🦠
      - (Ex) See S78.012
    - S78.129   Partial traumatic amputation at level between unspecified hip and knee A 🦠, 🦠
      - (Ex) See S78.019
- S78.9   Traumatic amputation of hip and thigh, level unspecified
  - S78.91   Complete traumatic amputation of hip and thigh, level unspecified
    - S78.911   Complete traumatic amputation of right hip and thigh, level unspecified A 🦠, 🦠
      - (Ex) See S78.011
    - S78.912   Complete traumatic amputation of left hip and thigh, level unspecified A 🦠, 🦠
      - (Ex) See S78.012
    - S78.919   Complete traumatic amputation of unspecified hip and thigh, level unspecified A 🦠, 🦠
      - (Ex) See S78.019
  - S78.92   Partial traumatic amputation of hip and thigh, level unspecified
    - S78.921   Partial traumatic amputation of right hip and thigh, level unspecified A 🦠, 🦠
      - (Ex) See S78.011
    - S78.922   Partial traumatic amputation of left hip and thigh, level unspecified A 🦠, 🦠
      - (Ex) See S78.012
    - S78.929   Partial traumatic amputation of unspecified hip and thigh, level unspecified A 🦠, 🦠
      - (Ex) See S78.019

Item 19–5   SALTER-HARRIS TYPE 1: epiphysis is completely separated from end of bone, or metaphysic growth plate remains attached to epiphysis

SALTER-HARRIS TYPE 2: epiphysis and growth plate are partially separated from metaphysis, which is cracked—most common type

SALTER-HARRIS TYPE 3: fracture occurring through epiphysis and separates part of epiphysis and growth plate from metaphysis fracture, usually at distal end of tibia

SALTER-HARRIS TYPE 4: fracture runs through epiphysis, across growth plate, into metaphysic, surgery is required to restore joint surface to normal and align growth plate

- S79   Other and unspecified injuries of hip and thigh
  - **Note:** A fracture not indicated as open or closed should be coded to closed
  - The appropriate 7th character is to be added to each code from subcategories S79.0 and S79.1

A	initial encounter for closed fracture
D	subsequent encounter for fracture with routine healing
G	subsequent encounter for fracture with delayed healing
K	subsequent encounter for fracture with nonunion
P	subsequent encounter for fracture with malunion
S	sequela

  - S79.0   Physeal fracture of upper end of femur
    - **Excludes1**   apophyseal fracture of upper end of femur (S72.13-)
      - nontraumatic slipped upper femoral epiphysis (M93.0-)
    - S79.00   Unspecified physeal fracture of upper end of femur
      - S79.001   Unspecified physeal fracture of upper end of right femur K, P 🦠, A 🦠, 🦠, A 🦠
        - (Ex) For S79.001[A]: See S72.004[A]
        - For S79.001[K,P]: See S72.001[K,M,N,P,Q,R]
      - S79.002   Unspecified physeal fracture of upper end of left femur K, P 🦠, A 🦠, 🦠, A 🦠
        - (Ex) For S79.002[A]: See S72.002[A]
        - For S79.002[K,P]: See S72.001[K,M,N,P,Q,R]
      - S79.009   Unspecified physeal fracture of upper end of unspecified femur K, P 🦠, A 🦠, 🦠, A 🦠
        - (Ex) For S79.009[A]: See S72.001[B,C]
        - For S79.009[K,P]: See S72.001[K,M,N,P,Q,R]
    - S79.01   Salter-Harris Type I physeal fracture of upper end of femur
      - Acute on chronic slipped capital femoral epiphysis (traumatic)
      - Acute slipped capital femoral epiphysis (traumatic)
      - Capital femoral epiphyseal fracture
      - **Excludes1**   chronic slipped upper femoral epiphysis (nontraumatic) (M93.02-)
      - S79.011   Salter-Harris Type I physeal fracture of upper end of right femur K, P 🦠, A 🦠, 🦠, A 🦠
        - (Ex) For S79.011[A]: See S72.004[A]
        - For S79.011[K,P]: See S72.001[K,M,N,P,Q,R]
      - S79.012   Salter-Harris Type I physeal fracture of upper end of left femur K, P 🦠, A 🦠, 🦠, A 🦠
        - (Ex) For S79.012[A]: See S72.002[A]
        - For S79.012[K,P]: See S72.001[K,M,N,P,Q,R]
      - S79.019   Salter-Harris Type I physeal fracture of upper end of unspecified femur K, P 🦠, A 🦠, A 🦠
        - (Ex) For S79.019[A]: See S72.001[B,C]
        - For S79.019[K,P]: See S72.001[K,M,N,P,Q,R]

● **S79.09**   Other physeal fracture of upper end of femur

   ● **S79.091**   Other physeal fracture of upper end of right femur K, P 🔖, A 🔖, 🔖, A 🔖
       Ⓔⓧ For S79.091[A]: See S72.004[A]
          For S79.091[K,P]: See S72.001[K,M,N,P,Q,R]

   ● **S79.092**   Other physeal fracture of upper end of left femur K, P 🔖, A 🔖, 🔖, A 🔖
       Ⓔⓧ For S79.092[A]: See S72.002[A]
          For S79.092[K,P]: See S72.001[K,M,N,P,Q,R]

   ● **S79.099**   Other physeal fracture of upper end of unspecified femur K, P 🔖, A 🔖, 🔖, A 🔖
       Ⓔⓧ For S79.099[A]: See S72.001[B,C]
          For S79.099[K,P]: See S72.001[K,M,N,P,Q,R]

● **S79.1**   Physeal fracture of lower end of femur

  ● **S79.10**   Unspecified physeal fracture of lower end of femur

   ● **S79.101**   Unspecified physeal fracture of lower end of right femur A, K, P 🔖, 🔖, A 🔖
       Ⓔⓧ For S79.101[A]: See S72.401[A]
          For S79.101[K,P]: See S72.001[K,M,N,P,Q,R]

   ● **S79.102**   Unspecified physeal fracture of lower end of left femur A, K, P 🔖, 🔖, A 🔖
       Ⓔⓧ For S79.102[A]: See S72.402[A]
          For S72.102[K,P]: See S72.001[K,M,N,P,Q,R]

   ● **S79.109**   Unspecified physeal fracture of lower end of unspecified femur A, K, P 🔖, 🔖, A 🔖
       Ⓔⓧ For S79.109[A]: See S72.401[B,C]
          For S79.109[K,P]: See S72.001[K,M,N,P,Q,R]

  ● **S79.11**   Salter-Harris Type I physeal fracture of lower end of femur

   ● **S79.111**   Salter-Harris Type I physeal fracture of lower end of right femur A, K, P 🔖, 🔖, A 🔖
       Ⓔⓧ For S79.111[A]: See S72.401[A]
          For S79.111[K,P]: See S72.001[K,M,N,P,Q,R]

   ● **S79.112**   Salter-Harris Type I physeal fracture of lower end of left femur A, K, P 🔖, 🔖, A 🔖
       Ⓔⓧ For S79.112[A]: See S72.402[A]
          For S72.112[K,P]: See S72.001[K,M,N,P,Q,R]

   ● **S79.119**   Salter-Harris Type I physeal fracture of lower end of unspecified femur A, K, P 🔖, 🔖, A 🔖
       Ⓔⓧ For S79.119[A]: See S72.401[B,C]
          For S79.119[K,P]: See S72.001[K,M,N,P,Q,R]

  ● **S79.12**   Salter-Harris Type II physeal fracture of lower end of femur

   ● **S79.121**   Salter-Harris Type II physeal fracture of lower end of right femur A, K, P 🔖, 🔖, A 🔖
       Ⓔⓧ For S79.121[A]: See S72.401[A]
          For S79.121[K,P]: See S72.001[K,M,N,P,Q,R]

   ● **S79.122**   Salter-Harris Type II physeal fracture of lower end of left femur A, K, P 🔖, 🔖, A 🔖
       Ⓔⓧ For S79.122[A]: See S72.402[A]
          For S72.122[K,P]: See S72.001[K,M,N,P,Q,R]

   ● **S79.129**   Salter-Harris Type II physeal fracture of lower end of unspecified femur A, K, P 🔖, 🔖, A 🔖
       Ⓔⓧ For S79.129[A]: See S72.401[B,C]
          For S79.129[K,P]: See S72.001[K,M,N,P,Q,R]

● **S79.13**   Salter-Harris Type III physeal fracture of lower end of femur

   ● **S79.131**   Salter-Harris Type III physeal fracture of lower end of right femur A, K, P 🔖, 🔖, A 🔖
       Ⓔⓧ For S79.131[A]: See S72.401[A]
          For S79.131[K,P]: See S72.001[K,M,N,P,Q,R]

   ● **S79.132**   Salter-Harris Type III physeal fracture of lower end of left femur A, K, P 🔖, 🔖, A 🔖
       Ⓔⓧ For S79.132[A]: See S72.402[A]
          For S72.132[K,P]: See S72.001[K,M,N,P,Q,R]

   ● **S79.139**   Salter-Harris Type III physeal fracture of lower end of unspecified femur A, K, P 🔖, 🔖, A 🔖
       Ⓔⓧ For S79.139[A]: See S72.401[B,C]
          For S79.139[K,P]: See S72.001[K,M,N,P,Q,R]

● **S79.14**   Salter-Harris Type IV physeal fracture of lower end of femur

   ● **S79.141**   Salter-Harris Type IV physeal fracture of lower end of right femur A, K, P 🔖, 🔖, A 🔖
       Ⓔⓧ For S79.141[A]: See S72.401[A]
          For S79.141[K,P]: See S72.001[K,M,N,P,Q,R]

   ● **S79.142**   Salter-Harris Type IV physeal fracture of lower end of left femur A, K, P 🔖, 🔖, A 🔖
       Ⓔⓧ For S79.142[A]: See S72.402[A]
          For S72.142[K,P]: See S72.001[K,M,N,P,Q,R]

   ● **S79.149**   Salter-Harris Type IV physeal fracture of lower end of unspecified femur A, K, P 🔖, 🔖, A 🔖
       Ⓔⓧ For S79.149[A]: See S72.401[B,C]
          For S79.149[K,P]: See S72.001[K,M,N,P,Q,R]

  ● **S79.19**   Other physeal fracture of lower end of femur

   ● **S79.191**   Other physeal fracture of lower end of right femur A, K, P 🔖, 🔖, A 🔖
       Ⓔⓧ For S79.191[A]: See S72.401[A]
          For S79.191[K,P]: See S72.001[K,M,N,P,Q,R]

   ● **S79.192**   Other physeal fracture of lower end of left femur A, K, P 🔖, 🔖, A 🔖
       Ⓔⓧ For S79.192[A]: See S72.402[A]
          For S72.192[K,P]: See S72.001[K,M,N,P,Q,R]

   ● **S79.199**   Other physeal fracture of lower end of unspecified femur A, K, P 🔖, 🔖, A 🔖
       Ⓔⓧ For S79.199[A]: See S72.401[B,C]
          For S79.199[K,P]: See S72.001[K,M,N,P,Q,R]

● **S79.8**   Other specified injuries of hip and thigh

     The appropriate 7th character is to be added to each code in subcategory S79.8

A	initial encounter
D	subsequent encounter
S	sequela

  ● **S79.81**   Other specified injuries of hip

   ● **S79.811**   Other specified injuries of right hip 🔖

   ● **S79.812**   Other specified injuries of left hip 🔖

   ● **S79.819**   Other specified injuries of unspecified hip 🔖

  ● **S79.82**   Other specified injuries of thigh

   ● **S79.821**   Other specified injuries of right thigh 🔖

   ● **S79.822**   Other specified injuries of left thigh 🔖

   ● **S79.829**   Other specified injuries of unspecified thigh 🔖

◀ New   ◀▥ Revised   ~~deleted~~ Deleted   Excludes 1   Excludes 2   Includes   Use additional   Code first   Code also   Unspecified

OGCR Official Guidelines   ● Unacceptable Principal Diagnosis   X Assign placeholder X   ● Use Additional Character(s)   ▌ Manifestation Code   **Coding Clinic**

● **S79.9   Unspecified injury of hip and thigh**

The appropriate 7th character is to be added to each code in subcategory S79.9

> A   initial encounter
> D   subsequent encounter
> S   sequela

● **S79.91   Unspecified injury of hip**
    ● S79.911   Unspecified injury of right hip 🔖
    ● S79.912   Unspecified injury of left hip 🔖
    ● S79.919   Unspecified injury of unspecified hip 🔖
● **S79.92   Unspecified injury of thigh**
    ● S79.921   Unspecified injury of right thigh 🔖
    ● S79.922   Unspecified injury of left thigh 🔖
    ● S79.929   Unspecified injury of unspecified thigh 🔖

INJURIES TO THE KNEE AND LOWER LEG (S80-S89)

Excludes2   burns and corrosions (T20-T32)
               frostbite (T33-T34)
               injuries of ankle and foot, except fracture of ankle and malleolus (S90-S99)
               insect bite or sting, venomous (T63.4)

● **S80   Superficial injury of knee and lower leg**

Excludes2   superficial injury of ankle and foot (S90.-)

The appropriate 7th character is to be added to each code from category S80

> A   initial encounter
> D   subsequent encounter
> S   sequela

● **S80.0   Contusion of knee**
   X ● S80.00   Contusion of unspecified knee 🔖
   X ● S80.01   Contusion of right knee 🔖
   X ● S80.02   Contusion of left knee 🔖
● **S80.1   Contusion of lower leg**
   X ● S80.10   Contusion of unspecified lower leg 🔖
   X ● S80.11   Contusion of right lower leg 🔖
   X ● S80.12   Contusion of left lower leg 🔖
● **S80.2   Other superficial injuries of knee**
   ● **S80.21   Abrasion of knee**
      ● S80.211   Abrasion, right knee 🔖
      ● S80.212   Abrasion, left knee 🔖
      ● S80.219   Abrasion, unspecified knee 🔖
   ● **S80.22   Blister (nonthermal) of knee**
      ● S80.221   Blister (nonthermal), right knee 🔖
      ● S80.222   Blister (nonthermal), left knee 🔖
      ● S80.229   Blister (nonthermal), unspecified knee 🔖
   ● **S80.24   External constriction of knee**
      ● S80.241   External constriction, right knee 🔖
      ● S80.242   External constriction, left knee 🔖
      ● S80.249   External constriction, unspecified knee 🔖
   ● **S80.25   Superficial foreign body of knee**
        Splinter in the knee
      ● S80.251   Superficial foreign body, right knee 🔖
      ● S80.252   Superficial foreign body, left knee 🔖
      ● S80.259   Superficial foreign body, unspecified knee 🔖

   ● **S80.26   Insect bite (nonvenomous) of knee**
      ● S80.261   Insect bite (nonvenomous), right knee 🔖
      ● S80.262   Insect bite (nonvenomous), left knee 🔖
      ● S80.269   Insect bite (nonvenomous), unspecified knee 🔖
   ● **S80.27   Other superficial bite of knee**
       Excludes1   open bite of knee (S81.05-)
      ● S80.271   Other superficial bite of right knee 🔖
      ● S80.272   Other superficial bite of left knee 🔖
      ● S80.279   Other superficial bite of unspecified knee 🔖
● **S80.8   Other superficial injuries of lower leg**
   ● **S80.81   Abrasion of lower leg**
      ● S80.811   Abrasion, right lower leg 🔖
      ● S80.812   Abrasion, left lower leg 🔖
      ● S80.819   Abrasion, unspecified lower leg 🔖
   ● **S80.82   Blister (nonthermal) of lower leg**
      ● S80.821   Blister (nonthermal), right lower leg 🔖
      ● S80.822   Blister (nonthermal), left lower leg 🔖
      ● S80.829   Blister (nonthermal), unspecified lower leg 🔖
   ● **S80.84   External constriction of lower leg**
      ● S80.841   External constriction, right lower leg 🔖
      ● S80.842   External constriction, left lower leg 🔖
      ● S80.849   External constriction, unspecified lower leg 🔖
   ● **S80.85   Superficial foreign body of lower leg**
        Splinter in the lower leg
      ● S80.851   Superficial foreign body, right lower leg 🔖
      ● S80.852   Superficial foreign body, left lower leg 🔖
      ● S80.859   Superficial foreign body, unspecified lower leg 🔖
   ● **S80.86   Insect bite (nonvenomous) of lower leg**
      ● S80.861   Insect bite (nonvenomous), right lower leg 🔖
      ● S80.862   Insect bite (nonvenomous), left lower leg 🔖
      ● S80.869   Insect bite (nonvenomous), unspecified lower leg 🔖
   ● **S80.87   Other superficial bite of lower leg**
       Excludes1   open bite of lower leg (S81.85-)
      ● S80.871   Other superficial bite, right lower leg 🔖
      ● S80.872   Other superficial bite, left lower leg 🔖
      ● S80.879   Other superficial bite, unspecified lower leg 🔖

N   Newborn Age: 0   P   Pediatric Age: 0–17   M   Maternity DX: 12–55   A   Adult Age: 15–124   ♀   Females Only   ♂   Males Only

🔖   Complication\Comorbidity   🔖   Major C\C   (Ex)   CC/MCC Exclusions   🔖   Present on Admission Requirement   🔖   Hospital-Acquired Condition

1453

● S80.9   Unspecified superficial injury of knee and lower leg
- ● S80.91   Unspecified superficial injury of knee
  - ● S80.911   Unspecified superficial injury of right knee ✎
  - ● S80.912   Unspecified superficial injury of left knee ✎
  - ● S80.919   Unspecified superficial injury of unspecified knee ✎
- ● S80.92   Unspecified superficial injury of lower leg
  - ● S80.921   Unspecified superficial injury of right lower leg ✎
  - ● S80.922   Unspecified superficial injury of left lower leg ✎
  - ● S80.929   Unspecified superficial injury of unspecified lower leg ✎

● S81   Open wound of knee and lower leg

     Code also any associated wound infection

     Excludes1   open fracture of knee and lower leg (S82.-)
                  traumatic amputation of lower leg (S88.-)

     Excludes2   open wound of ankle and foot (S91.-)

     The appropriate 7th character is to be added to each code from category S81

       A   initial encounter
       D   subsequent encounter
       S   sequela

- ● S81.0   Open wound of knee
  - ● S81.00   Unspecified open wound of knee
    - ● S81.001   Unspecified open wound, right knee ✎
    - ● S81.002   Unspecified open wound, left knee ✎
    - ● S81.009   Unspecified open wound, unspecified knee ✎
  - ● S81.01   Laceration without foreign body of knee
    - ● S81.011   Laceration without foreign body, right knee ✎
    - ● S81.012   Laceration without foreign body, left knee ✎
    - ● S81.019   Laceration without foreign body, unspecified knee ✎
  - ● S81.02   Laceration with foreign body of knee
    - ● S81.021   Laceration with foreign body, right knee ✎
    - ● S81.022   Laceration with foreign body, left knee ✎
    - ● S81.029   Laceration with foreign body, unspecified knee ✎
  - ● S81.03   Puncture wound without foreign body of knee
    - ● S81.031   Puncture wound without foreign body, right knee ✎
    - ● S81.032   Puncture wound without foreign body, left knee ✎
    - ● S81.039   Puncture wound without foreign body, unspecified knee ✎

- ● S81.04   Puncture wound with foreign body of knee
  - ● S81.041   Puncture wound with foreign body, right knee ✎
  - ● S81.042   Puncture wound with foreign body, left knee ✎
  - ● S81.049   Puncture wound with foreign body, unspecified knee ✎
- ● S81.05   Open bite of knee
  - Bite of knee NOS
  -      **Excludes1**   superficial bite of knee (S80.27-)
  - ● S81.051   Open bite, right knee ✎
  - ● S81.052   Open bite, left knee ✎
  - ● S81.059   Open bite, unspecified knee ✎
- ● S81.8   Open wound of lower leg
  - ● S81.80   Unspecified open wound of lower leg
    - ● S81.801   Unspecified open wound, right lower leg ✎
    - ● S81.802   Unspecified open wound, left lower leg ✎
    - ● S81.809   Unspecified open wound, unspecified lower leg ✎
  - ● S81.81   Laceration without foreign body of lower leg
    - ● S81.811   Laceration without foreign body, right lower leg ✎
    - ● S81.812   Laceration without foreign body, left lower leg ✎
    - ● S81.819   Laceration without foreign body, unspecified lower leg ✎
  - ● S81.82   Laceration with foreign body of lower leg
    - ● S81.821   Laceration with foreign body, right lower leg ✎
    - ● S81.822   Laceration with foreign body, left lower leg ✎
    - ● S81.829   Laceration with foreign body, unspecified lower leg ✎
  - ● S81.83   Puncture wound without foreign body of lower leg
    - ● S81.831   Puncture wound without foreign body, right lower leg ✎
    - ● S81.832   Puncture wound without foreign body, left lower leg ✎
    - ● S81.839   Puncture wound without foreign body, unspecified lower leg ✎
  - ● S81.84   Puncture wound with foreign body of lower leg
    - ● S81.841   Puncture wound with foreign body, right lower leg ✎
    - ● S81.842   Puncture wound with foreign body, left lower leg ✎
    - ● S81.849   Puncture wound with foreign body, unspecified lower leg ✎
  - ● S81.85   Open bite of lower leg
    - Bite of lower leg NOS
    -      **Excludes1**   superficial bite of lower leg (S80.86-, S80.87-)
    - ● S81.851   Open bite, right lower leg ✎
    - ● S81.852   Open bite, left lower leg ✎
    - ● S81.859   Open bite, unspecified lower leg ✎

CHAPTER 19 (S00-T88)

● **S82**   **Fracture of lower leg, including ankle**

    Note: A fracture not indicated as displaced or nondisplaced should be coded to displaced

        A fracture not indicated as open or closed should be coded to closed

        The open fracture designations are based on the Gustilo open fracture classification

    Includes   fracture of malleolus

    Excludes1   traumatic amputation of lower leg (S88.-)

    Excludes2   fracture of foot, except ankle (S92.-)
             periprosthetic fracture of prosthetic implant of knee (T84.042, T84.043)

    The appropriate 7th character is to be added to all codes from category S82

A	initial encounter for closed fracture
B	initial encounter for open fracture type I or II initial encounter for open fracture NOS
C	initial encounter for open fracture type IIIA, IIIB, or IIIC
D	subsequent encounter for closed fracture with routine healing
E	subsequent encounter for open fracture type I or II with routine healing
F	subsequent encounter for open fracture type IIIA, IIIB, or IIIC with routine healing
G	subsequent encounter for closed fracture with delayed healing
H	subsequent encounter for open fracture type I or II with delayed healing
J	subsequent encounter for open fracture type IIIA, IIIB, or IIIC with delayed healing
K	subsequent encounter for closed fracture with nonunion
M	subsequent encounter for open fracture type I or II with nonunion
N	subsequent encounter for open fracture type IIIA, IIIB, or IIIC with nonunion
P	subsequent encounter for closed fracture with malunion
Q	subsequent encounter for open fracture type I or II with malunion
R	subsequent encounter for open fracture type IIIA, IIIB, or IIIC with malunion
S	sequela

● **S82.0**   **Fracture of patella**
    Knee cap

  ● **S82.00**   **Unspecified fracture of patella**

    ● **S82.001**   `Unspecified` **fracture of right patella**
        A, B, C,K,M, N, P, Q, R 🔵, 🔵,
        A, B, C 🔵
         Ⓔⓧ **For S82.001[A]:** S82.001-S82.099[A,B,C]
          For S82.001[B,C]: M80.00X-M80.019[A],
           M80.041-M80.049[A], M80.80X-M80.819[A],
           M80.841-M80.849[A], M84.40X-M84.419[A],
           M84.441-M84.446[A], M84.454[A],
           M84.474-M84.519[A], M84.541-M84.550[A],
           M84.574-M84.576[A], M84.60X-M84.619[A],
           M84.641-M84.650[A], M84.674-M84.68X[A],
           S03.8XX-S03.9XX[A], S29.011-S29.019[A],
           S38.3XX[A], S39.011-S39.013[A],
           S73.101-S73.199[A], S76.001-S76.019[A],
           S76.091-S76.119[A], S76.191-S76.219[A],
           S76.291-S76.319[A], S76.391-S76.819[A],
           S76.891-S76.919[A], S76.991-S76.999[A],
           S79.811-S79.929[A], S82.001-S82.099[B,C],
           S82.101-S82.156[A,B,C], S82.191-S82.299[A,B,C],
           S82.401-S82.499[A,B,C], S82.831-S82.839[A,B,C],
           S82.861-S82.866[A,B,C], S82.90X-S82.92X[A,B,C],
           S89.001-S89.099[A], S89.201-S89.299[A],
           T14.8-T14.91, T79.8XX-T79.9XX[A], T79.A9X[A]
          For S82.001[K,M,N,P,Q,R]:
          See S72.001[K,M,N,P,Q,R]

    ● **S82.002**   `Unspecified` **fracture of left patella**
        A, B, C,K,M, N, P, Q, R 🔵, 🔵,
        A, B, C 🔵
         Ⓔⓧ **For S82.002[A]:** S82.001[B,C],
          S82.002-S82.009[A,B,C], S82.011[B,C],
          S82.012-S82.013[A,B,C], S82.014-S82.021[A,B,C],
          S82.022-S82.023[A,B,C], S82.024[B,C],
          S82.025-S82.026[A,B,C], S82.031-S82.033[A,B,C],
          S82.034[B,C], S82.035-S82.036[A,B,C],
          S82.041[B,C], S82.042-S82.043[A,B,C],
          S82.044[B,C], S82.045-S82.046[A,B,C],
          S82.091[B,C], S82.092-S82.099[A,B,C]
         For S82.002[B,C]: See S82.001[B,C]
         For S82.002[K,M,N,P,Q,R]:
         See S72.001[K,M,N,P,Q,R]

  ● **S82.009**   `Unspecified` **fracture of unspecified patella** A, B, C,K,M, N, P, Q, R 🔵, 🔵,
     A, B, C 🔵
       Ⓔⓧ **For S82.009[A]:** S82.001-S82.099[A,B,C]
       For S82.009[B,C]: See S82.001[B,C]
       For S82.009[K,M,N,P,Q,R]:
       See S72.001[K,M,N,P,Q,R]

● **S82.01**   **Osteochondral fracture of patella**

  ● **S82.011**   **Displaced osteochondral fracture of right patella**
     A, B, C,K,M, N, P, Q, R 🔵, 🔵,
     A, B, C 🔵
       Ⓔⓧ **For S82.011[A]:** See S82.001[A]
       For S82.011[B,C]: See S82.001[B,C]
       For S82.011[K,M,N,P,Q,R]:
       See S72.001[K,M,N,P,Q,R]

  ● **S82.012**   **Displaced osteochondral fracture of left patella** A, B, C,K,M, N, P, Q, R 🔵,
     🔵, A, B, C 🔵
       Ⓔⓧ **For S82.012[A]:** See S82.002[A]
       For S82.012[B,C]: See S82.001[B,C]
       For S82.012[K,M,N,P,Q,R]:
       See S72.001[K,M,N,P,Q,R]

  ● **S82.013**   **Displaced osteochondral fracture of** `unspecified` **patella**
     A, B, C,K,M, N, P, Q, R 🔵, 🔵,
     A, B, C 🔵
       Ⓔⓧ **For S82.013[A]:** See S82.003
       For S82.013[B,C]: See S82.001[B,C]
       For S82.013[K,M,N,P,Q,R]:
       See S72.001[K,M,N,P,Q,R]

  ● **S82.014**   **Nondisplaced osteochondral fracture of right patella** A, B, C,K,M, N,
     P, Q, R 🔵, 🔵, A, B, C 🔵
       Ⓔⓧ **For S82.014[A]:** See S82.001[A]
       For S82.014[B,C]: See S82.001[B,C]
       For S82.014[K,M,N,P,Q,R]:
       See S72.001[K,M,N,P,Q,R]

  ● **S82.015**   **Nondisplaced osteochondral fracture of left patella** A, B, C,K,M, N,
     P, Q, R 🔵, 🔵, A, B, C 🔵
       Ⓔⓧ **For S82.015[A]:** See S82.002[A]
       For S82.015[B,C]: See S82.001[B,C]
       For S82.015[K,M,N,P,Q,R]:
       See S72.001[K,M,N,P,Q,R]

  ● **S82.016**   **Nondisplaced osteochondral fracture of** `unspecified` **patella** A, B, C,K,M, N,
     P, Q, R 🔵, 🔵, A, B, C 🔵
       Ⓔⓧ **For S82.016[A]:** S82.001-S82.099[A,B,C]
       For S82.016[B,C]: See S82.001[B,C]
       For S82.016[K,M,N,P,Q,R]:
       See S72.001[K,M,N,P,Q,R]

N   Newborn Age: 0   P   Pediatric Age: 0–17   M   Maternity DX: 12–55   A   Adult Age: 15–124   ♀   Females Only   ♂   Males Only

🔵   Complication\Comorbidity   🔵   Major C\C   Ⓔⓧ   CC/MCC Exclusions   🔵   Present on Admission Requirement   🔵   Hospital-Acquired Condition

1455

CHAPTER 19 (S00-T88)

● S82.02   **Longitudinal fracture of patella**

   ● S82.021   **Displaced longitudinal fracture of right patella** A, B, C,K,M, N, P, Q, R 🪙, 🪙, A, B, C 🪙
      Ex: For S82.021[A]: See S82.001[A]
      For S82.021[B,C]: See S82.001[B,C]
      For S82.021[K,M,N,P,Q,R]:
      See S72.001[K,M,N,P,Q,R]

   ● S82.022   **Displaced longitudinal fracture of left patella** A, B, C,K,M, N, P, Q, R 🪙, 🪙, A, B, C 🪙
      Ex: For S82.022[A]: See S82.002[A]
      For S82.022[B,C]: See S82.001[B,C]
      For S82.022[K,M,N,P,Q,R]:
      See S72.001[K,M,N,P,Q,R]

   ● S82.023   **Displaced longitudinal fracture of unspecified patella** A, B, C,K,M, N, P, Q, R 🪙, 🪙, A, B, C 🪙
      Ex: For S82.023[A]: S82.001-S82.099[A,B,C]
      For S82.023[B,C]: See S82.001[B,C]
      For S82.023[K,M,N,P,Q,R]:
      See S72.001[K,M,N,P,Q,R]

   ● S82.024   **Nondisplaced longitudinal fracture of right patella** A, B, C,K,M, N, P, Q, R 🪙, 🪙, A, B, C 🪙
      Ex: For S82.024[A]: See S82.001[A]
      For S82.024[B,C]: See S82.001[B,C]
      For S82.024[K,M,N,P,Q,R]:
      See S72.001[K,M,N,P,Q,R]

   ● S82.025   **Nondisplaced longitudinal fracture of left patella** A, B, C,K,M, N, P, Q, R 🪙, 🪙, A, B, C 🪙
      Ex: For S82.025[A]: See S82.002[A]
      For S82.025[B,C]: See S82.001[B,C]
      For S82.025[K,M,N,P,Q,R]:
      See S72.001[K,M,N,P,Q,R]

   ● S82.026   **Nondisplaced longitudinal fracture of unspecified patella** A, B, C,K,M, N, P, Q, R 🪙, 🪙, A, B, C 🪙
      Ex: For S82.026[A]: S82.001-S82.099[A,B,C]
      For S82.026[B,C]: See S82.001[B,C]
      For S82.026[K,M,N,P,Q,R]:
      See S72.001[K,M,N,P,Q,R]

● S82.03   **Transverse fracture of patella**

   ● S82.031   **Displaced transverse fracture of right patella** A, B, C,K,M, N, P, Q, R 🪙, 🪙, A, B, C 🪙
      Ex: For S82.031[A]: See S82.001[A]
      For S82.031[B,C]: See S82.001[B,C]
      For S82.031[K,M,N,P,Q,R]:
      See S72.001[K,M,N,P,Q,R]

   ● S82.032   **Displaced transverse fracture of left patella** A, B, C,K,M, N, P, Q, R 🪙, 🪙, A, B, C 🪙
      Ex: For S82.032[A]: See S82.002[A]
      For S82.032[B,C]: See S82.001[B,C]
      For S82.032[K,M,N,P,Q,R]:
      See S72.001[K,M,N,P,Q,R]

   ● S82.033   **Displaced transverse fracture of unspecified patella** A, B, C,K,M, N, P, Q, R 🪙, 🪙, A, B, C 🪙
      Ex: For S82.033[A]: S82.001-S82.099[A,B,C]
      For S82.033[B,C]: See S82.001[B,C]
      For S82.033[K,M,N,P,Q,R]:
      See S72.001[K,M,N,P,Q,R]

   ● S82.034   **Nondisplaced transverse fracture of right patella** A, B, C,K,M, N, P, Q, R 🪙, 🪙, A, B, C 🪙
      Ex: For S82.034[A]: See S82.001[A]
      For S82.034[B,C]: See S82.001[B,C]
      For S82.034[K,M,N,P,Q,R]:
      See S72.001[K,M,N,P,Q,R]

   ● S82.035   **Nondisplaced transverse fracture of left patella** A, B, C,K,M, N, P, Q, R 🪙, 🪙, A, B, C 🪙
      Ex: For S82.035[A]: See S82.002[A]
      For S82.035[B,C]: See S82.001[B,C]
      For S82.035[K,M,N,P,Q,R]:
      See S72.001[K,M,N,P,Q,R]

   ● S82.036   **Nondisplaced transverse fracture of unspecified patella** A, B, C,K,M, N, P, Q, R 🪙, 🪙, A, B, C 🪙
      Ex: For S82.036[A]: S82.001-S82.099[A,B,C]
      For S82.036[B,C]: See S82.001[B,C]
      For S82.036[K,M,N,P,Q,R]:
      See S72.001[K,M,N,P,Q,R]

● S82.04   **Comminuted fracture of patella**

   ● S82.041   **Displaced comminuted fracture of right patella** A, B, C,K,M, N, P, Q, R 🪙, 🪙, A, B, C 🪙
      Ex: For S82.041[A]: See S82.001[A]
      For S82.041[B,C]: See S82.001[B,C]
      For S82.041[K,M,N,P,Q,R]:
      See S72.001[K,M,N,P,Q,R]

   ● S82.042   **Displaced comminuted fracture of left patella** A, B, C,K,M, N, P, Q, R 🪙, 🪙, A, B, C 🪙
      Ex: For S82.042[A]: See S82.002[A]
      For S82.042[B,C]: See S82.001[B,C]
      For S82.042[K,M,N,P,Q,R]:
      See S72.001[K,M,N,P,Q,R]

   ● S82.043   **Displaced comminuted fracture of unspecified patella** A, B, C,K,M, N, P, Q, R 🪙, 🪙, A, B, C 🪙
      Ex: For S82.043[A]: S82.001-S82.099[A,B,C]
      For S82.043[B,C]: See S82.001[B,C]
      For S82.043[K,M,N,P,Q,R]:
      See S72.001[K,M,N,P,Q,R]

   ● S82.044   **Nondisplaced comminuted fracture of right patella** A, B, C,K,M, N, P, Q, R 🪙, 🪙, A, B, C 🪙
      Ex: For S82.044[A]: See S82.001[A]
      For S82.044[B,C]: See S82.001[B,C]
      For S82.044[K,M,N,P,Q,R]:
      See S72.001[K,M,N,P,Q,R]

   ● S82.045   **Nondisplaced comminuted fracture of left patella** A, B, C,K,M, N, P, Q, R 🪙, 🪙, A, B, C 🪙
      Ex: For S82.045[A]: See S82.002[A]
      For S82.045[B,C]: See S82.001[B,C]
      For S82.045[K,M,N,P,Q,R]:
      See S72.001[K,M,N,P,Q,R]

   ● S82.046   **Nondisplaced comminuted fracture of unspecified patella** A, B, C,K,M, N, P, Q, R 🪙, 🪙, A, B, C 🪙
      Ex: For S82.046[A]: S82.001-S82.099[A,B,C]
      For S82.046[B,C]: See S82.001[B,C]
      For S82.046[K,M,N,P,Q,R]:
      See S72.001[K,M,N,P,Q,R]

◀ New   ◀ Revised   ~~deleted~~ Deleted   Excludes 1   Excludes 2   Includes   Use additional   Code first   Code also   Unspecified
OGCR Official Guidelines   ● Unacceptable Principal Diagnosis   X Assign placeholder X   ● Use Additional Character(s)   ▶ Manifestation Code   **Coding Clinic**

● S82.09   Other fracture of patella

    ● S82.091   **Other fracture of right patella**
        A, B, C,K,M, N, P, Q, R 🔵, 🔵,
        A, B, C 🔵
         Ⓔ **For S82.091[A]:** See S82.001[A]
           For S82.091[B,C]: See S82.001[B,C]
           For S82.091[K,M,N,P,Q,R]:
           See S72.001[K,M,N,P,Q,R]

    ● S82.092   **Other fracture of left patella**
        A, B, C,K,M, N, P, Q, R 🔵, 🔵,
        A, B, C 🔵
         Ⓔ **For S82.092[A]:** See S82.002[A]
           For S82.092[B,C]: See S82.001[B,C]
           For S82.092[K,M,N,P,Q,R]:
           See S72.001[K,M,N,P,Q,R]

    ● S82.099   **Other fracture of** unspecified **patella**
        A, B, C,K,M, N, P, Q, R 🔵, 🔵,
        A, B, C 🔵
         Ⓔ **For S82.099[A]:** S82.001-S82.099[A,B,C]
           For S82.099[B,C]: See S82.001[B,C]
           For S82.099[K,M,N,P,Q,R]:
           See S72.001[K,M,N,P,Q,R]

● S82.1   **Fracture of upper end of tibia**
    Fracture of proximal end of tibia
    Excludes2   fracture of shaft of tibia (S82.2-)
           physeal fracture of upper end of tibia
           (S89.0-)

    ● S82.10   **Unspecified fracture of upper end of tibia**

       ● S82.101   Unspecified **fracture of upper end of**
          right tibia A, K, M, N, P, Q, R 🔵,
          B, C 🔵, 🔵, A, B, C 🔵
           Ⓔ **For S82.101[A]:** M80.00X-M80.019[A],
           M80.041-M80.049[A], M80.061-M80.819[A],
           M80.841-M80.849[A], M80.861-M80.879[A],
           M84.40X-M84.419[A], M84.441-M84.446[A],
           M84.454[A], M84.461-M84.519[A],
           M84.541-M84.550[A], M84.561-M84.619[A],
           M84.641-M84.650[A], M84.661-M84.68X[A],
           S03.8XX-S03.9XX[A], S29.011-S29.019[A],
           S38.3XX[A], S39.011-S39.013[A], S73.101[A],
           S73.109-S73.111[A], S73.119-S73.121[A],
           S73.129-S73.191[A], S73.199[A], S76.001[A],
           S76.009-S76.011[A], S76.019[A], S76.091[A],
           S76.099-S76.101[A], S76.109-S76.111[A],
           S76.119[A], S76.191[A], S76.199-S76.201[A],
           S76.209-S76.211[A], S76.219[A], S76.291[A],
           S76.299-S76.301[A], S76.309-S76.311[A],
           S76.319[A], S76.391[A], S76.399-S76.801[A],
           S76.809-S76.811[A], S76.819[A], S76.891[A],
           S76.899-S76.901[A], S76.909-S76.911[A],
           S76.919[A], S76.991[A], S76.999[A], S79.811[A],
           S79.819-S79.821[A], S79.829[A], S79.911[A],
           S79.919-S79.921[A], S79.929[A], S82.101[A,B,C],
           S82.102[B,C], S82.109-S82.111[A,B,C],
           S82.112[B,C], S82.113-S82.114[A,B,C],
           S82.115[B,C], S82.116-S82.121[A,B,C],
           S82.122[B,C], S82.123-S82.124[A,B,C],
           S82.125[B,C], S82.126-S82.131[A,B,C],
           S82.132[B,C], S82.133-S82.134[A,B,C],
           S82.135[B,C], S82.136-S82.141[A,B,C],

S82.142[B,C], S82.143-S82.144[A,B,C],
S82.145[B,C], S82.146-S82.151[A,B,C],
S82.152[B,C], S82.153-S82.154[A,B,C],
S82.155[B,C], S82.156[A,B,C], S82.191[A,B,C],
S82.192[B,C], S82.199-S82.201[A,B,C],
S82.202[B,C], S82.209-S82.221[A,B,C],
S82.222[B,C], S82.223-S82.224[A,B,C],
S82.225[B,C], S82.226-S82.231[A,B,C],
S82.232[B,C], S82.233-S82.234[A,B,C],
S82.235[B,C], S82.236-S82.241[A,B,C],
S82.242[B,C], S82.243-S82.244[A,B,C],
S82.245[B,C], S82.246-S82.251[A,B,C],
S82.252[B,C], S82.253-S82.254[A,B,C],
S82.255[B,C], S82.256-S82.261[A,B,C],
S82.262[B,C], S82.263-S82.264[A,B,C],
S82.265[B,C], S82.266-S82.291[A,B,C],
S82.292[B,C], S82.299[A,B,C], S82.401[A,B,C],
S82.402[B,C], S82.409-S82.421[A,B,C],
S82.422[B,C], S82.423-S82.424[A,B,C],
S82.425[B,C], S82.426-S82.431[A,B,C],
S82.432[B,C], S82.433-S82.434[A,B,C],
S82.435[B,C], S82.436-S82.441[A,B,C],
S82.442[B,C], S82.443-S82.444[A,B,C],
S82.445[B,C], S82.446-S82.451[A,B,C],
S82.452[B,C], S82.453-S82.454[A,B,C],
S82.455[B,C], S82.456-S82.461[A,B,C],
S82.462[B,C], S82.463-S82.464[A,B,C],
S82.465[B,C], S82.466-S82.491[A,B,C],
S82.492[B,C], S82.499[A,B,C], S82.831[A,B,C],
S82.831-S82.832[B,C], S82.839[A,B,C],
S82.861[A,B,C], S82.862[B,C],
S82.863-S82.864[A,B,C], S82.865[B,C],
S82.866[A,B,C], S82.90X-S82.92X[A,B,C],
S89.001[A], S89.009-S89.011[A],
S89.019-S89.021[A], S89.029-S89.031[A],
S89.039-S89.041[A], S89.049-S89.091[A],
S89.099[A], S89.201[A], S89.209-S89.211[A],
S89.219-S89.221[A], S89.229-S89.291[A],
S89.299[A], T14.8-T14.91, T79.8XX-T79.9XX[A],
T79.A9X[A] **For S82.101[B,C]:**
M80.00X-M80.019[A], M80.041-M80.049[A],
M80.061-M80.819[A], M80.841-M80.849[A],
M80.861-M80.879[A], M84.40X-M84.419[A],
M84.441-M84.446[A], M84.454[A],
M84.461-M84.519[A], M84.541-M84.550[A],
M84.561-M84.619[A], M84.641-M84.650[A],
M84.661-M84.68X[A], S03.8XX-S03.9XX[A],
S29.011-S29.019[A], S38.3XX[A],
S39.011-S39.013[A], S73.101-S73.199[A],
S76.001-S76.019[A], S76.091-S76.119[A],
S76.191-S76.219[A], S76.291-S76.319[A],
S76.391-S76.819[A], S76.891-S76.919[A],
S76.991-S76.999[A], S79.811-S79.929[A],
S82.101-S82.156[A,B,C], S82.191-S82.299[A,B,C],
S82.401-S82.499[A,B,C], S82.831-S82.839[A,B,C],
S82.861-S82.866[A,B,C],
S82.90X-S82.92X[A,B,C], S89.001-S89.099[A],
S89.201-S89.299[A], T14.8-T14.91,
T79.8XX-T79.9XX[A], T79.A9X[A]
For S82.101[K,M,N,P,Q,R]:
See S72.001[K,M,N,P,Q,R]

● **S82.102**   Unspecified fracture of upper end of left tibia A, K, M, N, P, Q, R 🔗, B, C 🔗, 🔗, A, B, C 🔗

    Ex: For S82.102[A]: M80.00X-M80.019[A], M80.041-M80.049[A], M80.061-M80.819[A], M80.841-M80.849[A], M80.861-M80.879[A], M84.40X-M84.419[A], M84.441-M84.446[A], M84.454[A], M84.461-M84.519[A], M84.541-M84.550[A], M84.561-M84.619[A], M84.641-M84.650[A], M84.661-M84.68X[A], S03.8XX-S03.9XX[A], S29.011-S29.019[A], S38.3XX[A], S39.011-S39.013[A], S73.102-S73.109[A], S73.112-S73.119[A], S73.122-S73.129[A], S73.192-S73.199[A], S76.002-S76.009[A], S76.012-S76.019[A], S76.092-S76.099[A], S76.102-S76.109[A], S76.112-S76.119[A], S76.192-S76.199[A], S76.202-S76.209[A], S76.212-S76.219[A], S76.292-S76.299[A], S76.302-S76.309[A], S76.312-S76.319[A], S76.392-S76.399[A], S76.802-S76.809[A], S76.812-S76.819[A], S76.892-S76.899[A], S76.902-S76.909[A], S76.912-S76.919[A], S76.992-S76.999[A], S79.812-S79.819[A], S79.822-S79.829[A], S79.912-S79.919[A], S79.922-S79.929[A], S82.101[B,C], S82.102-S82.109[A,B,C], S82.111[B,C], S82.112-S82.113[A,B,C], S82.114[B,C], S82.115-S82.116[A,B,C], S82.121[B,C], S82.122-S82.123[A,B,C], S82.124[B,C], S82.125-S82.126[A,B,C], S82.131[B,C], S82.132-S82.133[A,B,C], S82.134[B,C], S82.135-S82.136[A,B,C], S82.141[B,C], S82.142-S82.143[A,B,C], S82.144[B,C], S82.145-S82.146[A,B,C], S82.151[B,C], S82.152-S82.153[A,B,C], S82.154[B,C], S82.155-S82.156[A,B,C], S82.191[B,C], S82.192-S82.199[A,B,C], S82.201[B,C], S82.202-S82.209[A,B,C], S82.221[B,C], S82.222-S82.223[A,B,C], S82.224[B,C], S82.225-S82.226[A,B,C], S82.231[B,C], S82.232-S82.233[A,B,C], S82.234[B,C], S82.235-S82.236[A,B,C], S82.241[B,C], S82.242-S82.243[A,B,C], S82.244[B,C], S82.245-S82.246[A,B,C], S82.251[B,C], S82.252-S82.253[A,B,C], S82.254[B,C], S82.255-S82.256[A,B,C], S82.261[B,C], S82.262-S82.263[A,B,C], S82.264[B,C], S82.265-S82.266[A,B,C], S82.291[B,C], S82.292-S82.299[A,B,C], S82.401[B,C], S82.402-S82.409[A,B,C], S82.421[B,C], S82.422-S82.423[A,B,C], S82.424[B,C], S82.425-S82.426[A,B,C], S82.431[B,C], S82.432-S82.433[A,B,C], S82.434[B,C], S82.435-S82.436[A,B,C], S82.441[B,C], S82.442-S82.443[A,B,C], S82.444[B,C], S82.445-S82.446[A,B,C], S82.451[B,C], S82.452-S82.453[A,B,C], S82.454[B,C], S82.455-S82.456[A,B,C], S82.461[B,C], S82.462-S82.463[A,B,C], S82.464[B,C], S82.465-S82.466[A,B,C], S82.491[B,C], S82.492-S82.499[A,B,C], S82.831[B,C], S82.832-S82.839[A,B,C], S82.861[B,C], S82.862-S82.863[A,B,C], S82.864[B,C], S82.865-S82.866[A,B,C], S82.90X-S82.92X[A,B,C], S89.002-S89.009[A], S89.012-S89.019[A], S89.022-S89.029[A], S89.032-S89.039[A], S89.042-S89.049[A], S89.092-S89.099[A], S89.202-S89.209[A], S89.212-S89.219[A], S89.222-S89.229[A], S89.292-S89.299[A], T14.8-T14.91, T79.8XX-T79.9XX[A], T79.A9X[A]

    For S82.102[B,C]: See S82.101[B,C]
    For S82.102[K,M,N,P,Q,R]: See S72.001[K,M,N,P,Q,R]

● **S82.109**   Unspecified fracture of upper end of unspecified tibia A, K, M, N, P, Q, R 🔗, B, C 🔗, 🔗, A, B, C 🔗

    Ex: For S82.109[A,B,C]: See S82.101[B,C]
    For S82.109[K,M,N,P,Q,R]: See S72.001[K,M,N,P,Q,R]

● **S82.11**   Fracture of tibial spine

   ● **S82.111**   Displaced fracture of right tibial spine A, K, M, N, P, Q, R 🔗, B, C 🔗, 🔗, A, B, C 🔗

     Ex: For S82.111[A]: See S82.101[A]
     For S82.111[B,C]: See S82.101[B,C]
     For S82.111[K,M,N,P,Q,R]: See S72.001[K,M,N,P,Q,R]

   ● **S82.112**   Displaced fracture of left tibial spine A, K, M, N, P, Q, R 🔗, B, C 🔗, 🔗, A, B, C 🔗

     Ex: For S82.112[A]: See S82.102[A]
     For S82.112[B,C]: See S82.101[B,C]
     For S82.112[K,M,N,P,Q,R]: See S72.001[K,M,N,P,Q,R]

   ● **S82.113**   Displaced fracture of unspecified tibial spine A, K, M, N, P, Q, R 🔗, B, C 🔗, 🔗, A, B, C 🔗

     Ex: For S82.113 [A,B,C]: See S82.101[B,C]
     For S82.113[K,M,N,P,Q,R]: See S72.001[K,M,N,P,Q,R]

   ● **S82.114**   Nondisplaced fracture of right tibial spine A, K, M, N, P, Q, R 🔗, B, C 🔗, 🔗, A, B, C 🔗

     Ex: For S82.114[A]: See S82.101[A]
     For S82.114[B,C]: See S82.101[B,C]
     For S82.114[K,M,N,P,Q,R]: See S72.001[K,M,N,P,Q,R]

   ● **S82.115**   Nondisplaced fracture of left tibial spine A, K, M, N, P, Q, R 🔗, B, C 🔗, 🔗, A, B, C 🔗

     Ex: For S82.115[A]: See S82.102[A]
     For S82.115[B,C]: See S82.101[B,C]
     For S82.115[K,M,N,P,Q,R]: See S72.001[K,M,N,P,Q,R]

   ● **S82.116**   Nondisplaced fracture of unspecified tibial spine A, K, M, N, P, Q, R 🔗, B, C 🔗, 🔗, A, B, C 🔗

     Ex: For S82.116[A,B,C]: See S82.101[B,C]
     For S82.116[K,M,N,P,Q,R]: See S72.001[K,M,N,P,Q,R]

● **S82.12**   Fracture of lateral condyle of tibia

   ● **S82.121**   Displaced fracture of lateral condyle of right tibia A, K, M, N, P, Q, R 🔗, B, C 🔗, 🔗, A, B, C 🔗

     Ex: For S82.121[A]: See S82.101[A]
     For S82.121[B,C]: See S82.101[B,C]
     For S82.121[K,M,N,P,Q,R]: See S72.001[K,M,N,P,Q,R]

   ● **S82.122**   Displaced fracture of lateral condyle of left tibia A, K, M, N, P, Q, R 🔗, B, C 🔗, 🔗, A, B, C 🔗

     Ex: For S82.122[A]: See S82.102[A]
     For S82.122[B,C]: See S82.101[B,C]
     For S82.122[K,M,N,P,Q,R]: See S72.001[K,M,N,P,Q,R]

   ● **S82.123**   Displaced fracture of lateral condyle of unspecified tibia A, K, M, N, P, Q, R 🔗, B, C 🔗, 🔗, A, B, C 🔗

     Ex: For S82.123[A,B,C]: See S82.101[B,C]
     For S82.123[K,M,N,P,Q,R]: See S72.001[K,M,N,P,Q,R]

   ● **S82.124**   Nondisplaced fracture of lateral condyle of right tibia A, K, M, N, P, Q, R 🔗, B, C 🔗, 🔗, A, B, C 🔗

     Ex: For S82.124[A]: See S82.101[A]
     For S82.124[B,C]: See S82.101[B,C]
     For S82.124[K,M,N,P,Q,R]: See S72.001[K,M,N,P,Q,R]

◀ New   ◀ᴵᴵᴵᴵ Revised   ~~deleted~~ Deleted   Excludes 1   Excludes 2   Includes   Use additional   Code first   Code also   Unspecified

OGCR Official Guidelines   ● Unacceptable Principal Diagnosis   X Assign placeholder X   ● Use Additional Character(s)   ▶ Manifestation Code   **Coding Clinic**

● **S82.125**   **Nondisplaced fracture of lateral condyle of left tibia** A, K, M, N, P, Q, R ⬤, B, C ⬤, ⬤, A, B, C ⬤
    (Ex:) **For S82.125[A]:** See S82.102[A]
      For S82.125[B,C]: See S82.101[B,C]
      For S82.125[K,M,N,P,Q,R]:
      See S72.001[K,M,N,P,Q,R]

● **S82.126**   **Nondisplaced fracture of lateral condyle of unspecified tibia** A, K, M, N, P, Q, R ⬤, B, C ⬤, ⬤, A, B, C ⬤
    (Ex:) **For S82.126[A,B,C]:** See S82.101[B,C]
      For S82.126[K,M,N,P,Q,R]:
      See S72.001[K,M,N,P,Q,R]

● **S82.13**   **Fracture of medial condyle of tibia**

● **S82.131**   **Displaced fracture of medial condyle of right tibia** A, K, M, N, P, Q, R ⬤, B, C ⬤, ⬤, A, B, C ⬤
    (Ex:) **For S82.131[A]:** See S82.101[A]
      For S82.131[B,C]: See S82.101[B,C]
      For S82.131[K,M,N,P,Q,R]:
      See S72.001[K,M,N,P,Q,R]

● **S82.132**   **Displaced fracture of medial condyle of left tibia** A, K, M, N, P, Q, R ⬤, B, C ⬤, ⬤, A, B, C ⬤
    (Ex:) **For S82.132[A]:** See S82.102[A]
      For S82.132[B,C]: See S82.101[B,C]
      For S82.132[K,M,N,P,Q,R]:
      See S72.001[K,M,N,P,Q,R]

● **S82.133**   **Displaced fracture of medial condyle of unspecified tibia** A, K, M, N, P, Q, R ⬤, B, C ⬤, ⬤, A, B, C ⬤
    (Ex:) **For S82.133[A,B,C]:** See S82.101[B,C]
      For S82.133[K,M,N,P,Q,R]:
      See S72.001[K,M,N,P,Q,R]

● **S82.134**   **Nondisplaced fracture of medial condyle of right tibia** A, K, M, N, P, Q, R ⬤, B, C ⬤, ⬤, A, B, C ⬤
    (Ex:) **For S82.134[A]:** See S82.101[A]
      For S82.134[B,C]: See S82.101[B,C]
      For S82.134[K,M,N,P,Q,R]:
      See S72.001[K,M,N,P,Q,R]

● **S82.135**   **Nondisplaced fracture of medial condyle of left tibia** A, K, M, N, P, Q, R ⬤, B, C ⬤, ⬤, A, B, C ⬤
    (Ex:) **For S82.135[A]:** See S82.102[A]
      For S82.135[B,C]: See S82.101[B,C]
      For S82.135[K,M,N,P,Q,R]:
      See S72.001[K,M,N,P,Q,R]

● **S82.136**   **Nondisplaced fracture of medial condyle of unspecified tibia** A, K, M, N, P, Q, R ⬤, B, C ⬤, ⬤, A, B, C ⬤
    (Ex:) **For S82.136[A,B,C]:** See S82.101[B,C]
      For S82.136[K,M,N,P,Q,R]:
      See S72.001[K,M,N,P,Q,R]

● **S82.14**   **Bicondylar fracture of tibia**
    Fracture of tibial plateau NOS

● **S82.141**   **Displaced bicondylar fracture of right tibia** A, K, M, N, P, Q, R ⬤, B, C ⬤, ⬤, A, B, C ⬤
    (Ex:) **For S82.141[A]:** See S82.101[A]
      For S82.141[B,C]: See S82.101[B,C]
      For S82.141[K,M,N,P,Q,R]:
      See S72.001[K,M,N,P,Q,R]

● **S82.142**   **Displaced bicondylar fracture of left tibia** A, K, M, N, P, Q, R ⬤, B, C ⬤, ⬤, A, B, C ⬤
    (Ex:) **For S82.142[A]:** See S82.102[A]
      For S82.142[B,C]: See S82.101[B,C]
      For S82.142[K,M,N,P,Q,R]:
      See S72.001[K,M,N,P,Q,R]

● **S82.143**   **Displaced bicondylar fracture of unspecified tibia** A, K, M, N, P, Q, R ⬤, B, C ⬤, ⬤, A, B, C ⬤
    (Ex:) **For S82.143[A,B,C]:** See S82.101[B,C]
      For S82.143[K,M,N,P,Q,R]:
      See S72.001[K,M,N,P,Q,R]

● **S82.144**   **Nondisplaced bicondylar fracture of right tibia** A, K, M, N, P, Q, R ⬤, B, C ⬤, ⬤, A, B, C ⬤
    (Ex:) **For S82.144[A]:** See S82.101[A]
      For S82.144[B,C]: See S82.101[B,C]
      For S82.144[K,M,N,P,Q,R]:
      See S72.001[K,M,N,P,Q,R]

● **S82.145**   **Nondisplaced bicondylar fracture of left tibia** A, K, M, N, P, Q, R ⬤, B, C ⬤, ⬤, A, B, C ⬤
    (Ex:) **For S82.145[A]:** See S82.102[A]
      For S82.145[B,C]: See S82.101[B,C]
      For S82.145[K,M,N,P,Q,R]:
      See S72.001[K,M,N,P,Q,R]

● **S82.146**   **Nondisplaced bicondylar fracture of unspecified tibia** A, K, M, N, P, Q, R ⬤, B, C ⬤, ⬤, A, B, C ⬤
    (Ex:) **For S82.146[A,B,C]:** See S82.101[B,C]
      For S82.146[K,M,N,P,Q,R]:
      See S72.001[K,M,N,P,Q,R]

● **S82.15**   **Fracture of tibial tuberosity**

● **S82.151**   **Displaced fracture of right tibial tuberosity** A, K, M, N, P, Q, R ⬤, B, C ⬤, ⬤, A, B, C ⬤
    (Ex:) **For S82.151[A]:** See S82.101[A]
      For S82.151[B,C]: See S82.101[B,C]
      For S82.151[K,M,N,P,Q,R]:
      See S72.001[K,M,N,P,Q,R]

● **S82.152**   **Displaced fracture of left tibial tuberosity** A, K, M, N, P, Q, R ⬤, B, C ⬤, ⬤, A, B, C ⬤
    (Ex:) **For S82.152[A]:** See S82.102[A]
      For S82.152[B,C]: See S82.101[B,C]
      For S82.152[K,M,N,P,Q,R]:
      See S72.001[K,M,N,P,Q,R]

● **S82.153**   **Displaced fracture of unspecified tibial tuberosity** A, K, M, N, P, Q, R ⬤, B, C ⬤, ⬤, A, B, C ⬤
    (Ex:) **For S82.153[A,B,C]:** See S82.101[B,C]
      For S82.153[K,M,N,P,Q,R]:
      See S72.001[K,M,N,P,Q,R]

● **S82.154**   **Nondisplaced fracture of right tibial tuberosity** A, K, M, N, P, Q, R ⬤, B, C ⬤, ⬤, A, B, C ⬤
    (Ex:) **For S82.154[A]:** See S82.101[A]
      For S82.154[B,C]: See S82.101[B,C]
      For S82.154[K,M,N,P,Q,R]:
      See S72.001[K,M,N,P,Q,R]

● **S82.155**   **Nondisplaced fracture of left tibial tuberosity** A, K, M, N, P, Q, R ⬤, B, C ⬤, ⬤, A, B, C ⬤
    (Ex:) **For S82.155[A]:** See S82.102[A]
      For S82.155[B,C]: See S82.101[B,C]
      For S82.155[K,M,N,P,Q,R]:
      See S72.001[K,M,N,P,Q,R]

● **S82.156**   **Nondisplaced fracture of unspecified tibial tuberosity** A, K, M, N, P, Q, R ⬤, B, C ⬤, ⬤, A, B, C ⬤
    (Ex:) **For S82.156[A,B,C]:** See S82.101[B,C]
      For S82.156[K,M,N,P,Q,R]:
      See S72.001[K,M,N,P,Q,R]

N Newborn Age: 0   **P** Pediatric Age: 0–17   **M** Maternity DX: 12–55   **A** Adult Age: 15–124   ♀ Females Only   ♂ Males Only

⬤ Complication\Comorbidity   ⬤ Major C\C   (Ex:) CC/MCC Exclusions   ⬤ Present on Admission Requirement   ⬤ Hospital-Acquired Condition

1459

● **S82.16**   **Torus fracture of upper end of tibia**

The appropriate 7th character is to be added to all codes in subcategory S82.16

A	initial encounter for closed fracture
D	subsequent encounter for fracture with routine healing
G	subsequent encounter for fracture with delayed healing
K	subsequent encounter for fracture with nonunion
P	subsequent encounter for fracture with malunion
S	sequela

● **S82.161**   **Torus fracture of upper end of right tibia** A, K, P 🔖, 🔖, A 🔖

Ⓔ **For S82.161[A]:** S82.101[A,B,C], S82.102[B,C], S82.109-S82.111[A,B,C], S82.112[A,B], S82.113-S82.114[A,B,C], S82.115[B,C], S82.116-S82.121[A,B,C], S82.122[B,C], S82.123-S82.124[A,B,C], S82.125[B,C], S82.126-S82.131[A,B,C], S82.132[B,C], S82.133-S82.134[A,B,C], S82.135[B,C], S82.136-S82.141[A,B,C], S82.142[B,C], S82.143-S82.144[A,B,C], S82.145[B,C], S82.146-S82.151[A,B,C], S82.152[B,C], S82.153-S82.154[A,B,C], S82.155[B,C], S82.156[A,B,C], S82.161[A], S82.169[A], S82.191[A,B,C], S82.192[B,C], S82.199-S82.201[A,B,C], S82.202[B,C], S82.209-S82.221[A,B,C], S82.222[B,C], S82.223-S82.224[A,B,C], S82.225[B,C], S82.226-S82.231[A,B,C], S82.232[B,C], S82.233-S82.234[A,B,C], S82.235[B,C], S82.236-S82.241[A,B,C], S82.242[B,C], S82.243-S82.244[A,B,C], S82.245[B,C], S82.246-S82.251[A,B,C], S82.252[B,C], S82.253-S82.254[A,B,C], S82.255[B,C], S82.256-S82.261[A,B,C], S82.262[B,C], S82.263-S82.264[A,B,C], S82.265[B,C], S82.266-S82.291[A,B,C], S82.292[B,C], S82.299[A,B,C], S82.311[A], S82.319[A], S82.401[A,B,C], S82.402[B,C], S82.409-S82.421[A,B,C], S82.422[B,C], S82.423-S82.424[A,B,C], S82.425[B,C], S82.426-S82.431[A,B,C], S82.432[B,C], S82.433-S82.434[A,B,C], S82.435[B,C], S82.436-S82.441[A,B,C], S82.442[B,C], S82.443-S82.444[A,B,C], S82.445[B,C], S82.446-S82.451[A,B,C], S82.452[B,C], S82.453-S82.454[A,B,C], S82.455[B,C], S82.456-S82.461[A,B,C], S82.462[B,C], S82.463-S82.464[A,B,C], S82.465[B,C], S82.466-S82.491[A,B,C], S82.492[B,C], S82.499[A,B,C], S82.811[A], S82.819-S82.821[A], S82.829[A], S82.831[A,B,C], S82.832[B,C], S82.839[A,B,C], S82.861[A,B,C], S82.862[B,C], S82.863-S82.864[A,B,C], S82.865[B,C], S82.866[A,B,C], S89.001[A], S89.009-S89.011[A], S89.019-S89.021[A], S89.029-S89.031[A], S89.039-S89.041[A], S89.049-S89.091[A], S89.099[A], S89.201[A], S89.209-S89.211[A], S89.219-S89.221[A], S89.229-S89.291[A], S89.299[A] **For S82.161[K,P]:** See S72.001[K,M,N,P,Q,R]

● **S82.162**   **Torus fracture of upper end of left tibia** A, K, P 🔖, 🔖, A 🔖

Ⓔ **For S82.162[A]:** S82.101[B,C], S82.102-S82.109[A,B,C], S82.111[B,C], S82.112-S82.113[A,B,C], S82.114[B,C], S82.115-S82.116[A,B,C], S82.121[B,C], S82.122-S82.123[A,B,C], S82.124[B,C], S82.125-S82.126[A,B,C], S82.131[B,C], S82.132-S82.133[A,B,C], S82.134[B,C], S82.135-S82.136[A,B,C], S82.141[B,C], S82.142-S82.143[A,B,C], S82.144[B,C], S82.145-S82.146[A,B,C], S82.151[B,C], S82.152-S82.153[A,B,C], S82.154[B,C], S82.155-S82.156[A,B,C], S82.162-S82.169[A], S82.191[B,C], S82.192-S82.199[A,B,C], S82.201[B,C], S82.202-S82.209[A,B,C], S82.221[B,C], S82.222-S82.223[A,B,C], S82.224[B,C], S82.225-S82.226[A,B,C], S82.231[B,C], S82.232-S82.233[A,B,C], S82.234[B,C], S82.235-S82.236[A,B,C], S82.241[B,C], S82.242-S82.243[A,B,C], S82.244[B,C], S82.245-S82.246[A,B,C], S82.251[B,C], S82.252-S82.253[A,B,C], S82.254[B,C], S82.255-S82.256[A,B,C], S82.261[B,C], S82.262-S82.263[A,B,C], S82.264[B,C], S82.265-S82.266[A,B,C], S82.291[B,C], S82.292-S82.299[A,B,C], S82.312-S82.319[A], S82.401[B,C], S82.402-S82.409[A,B,C], S82.421[B,C], S82.422-S82.423[A,B,C], S82.424[B,C], S82.425-S82.426[A,B,C], S82.431[B,C], S82.432-S82.433[A,B,C], S82.434[B,C], S82.435-S82.436[A,B,C], S82.441[B,C], S82.442-S82.443[A,B,C], S82.444[B,C], S82.445-S82.446[A,B,C], S82.451[B,C], S82.452-S82.453[A,B,C], S82.454[B,C], S82.455-S82.456[A,B,C], S82.461[B,C], S82.462-S82.463[A,B,C], S82.464[B,C], S82.465-S82.466[A,B,C], S82.491[B,C], S82.492-S82.499[A,B,C], S82.812-S82.819[A], S82.822-S82.829[A], S82.831[B,C], S82.832-S82.839[A,B,C], S82.861[B,C], S82.862-S82.863[A,B,C], S82.864[B,C], S82.865-S82.866[A,B,C], S89.002-S89.009[A], S89.012-S89.019[A], S89.022-S89.029[A], S89.032-S89.039[A], S89.042-S89.049[A], S89.092-S89.099[A], S89.202-S89.209[A], S89.212-S89.219[A], S89.222-S89.229[A], S89.292-S89.299[A] **For S82.162[K,P]:** See S72.001[K,M,N,P,Q,R]

● **S82.169**   **Torus fracture of upper end of unspecified tibia** A, K, P 🔖, 🔖, A 🔖

Ⓔ **For S82.169[A]:** S82.101-S82.156[A,B,C], S82.161-S82.169[A], S82.191-S82.299[A,B,C], S82.311-S82.319[A], S82.401-S82.499[A,B,C], S82.811-S82.829[A], S82.831-S82.839[A,B,C], S82.861-S82.866[A,B,C], S89.001-S89.099[A], S89.201-S89.299[A] **S82.169[K,P]:** See S72.001[K,M,N,P,Q,R]

● **S82.19**   **Other fracture of upper end of tibia**

● **S82.191**   **Other fracture of upper end of right tibia** A, K, M, N, P, Q, R 🔖, B, C 🔖, 🔖, A, B, C 🔖

Ⓔ **For S82.191[A]:** See S82.101[A] **For S82.191[B,C]:** See S82.101[B,C] **For S82.191[K,M,N,P,Q,R]:** See S72.001[K,M,N,P,Q,R]

◀ New   ◀▥ Revised   ~~deleted~~ Deleted   Excludes 1   Excludes 2   Includes   Use additional   Code first   Code also   Unspecified
OGCR Official Guidelines   ● Unacceptable Principal Diagnosis   X Assign placeholder X   ● Use Additional Character(s)   ▶ Manifestation Code   **Coding Clinic**

● S82.192   **Other fracture of upper end of left tibia** A, K, M, N, P, Q, R 🔵, B, C 🔷, 🔶, A, B, C 🔶
    Ⓔⓧ **For S82.192[A]:** See S82.102[A]
    For S82.192[B,C]: See S82.101[B,C]
    For S82.192[K,M,N,P,Q,R]:
    See S72.001[K,M,N,P,Q,R]

● S82.199   **Other fracture of upper end of unspecified tibia** A, K, M, N, P, Q, R 🔵, B, C 🔷, 🔶, A, B, C 🔶
    Ⓔⓧ **For S82.199[A,B,C]:** See S82.101[B,C]
    For S82.199[K,M,N,P,Q,R]:
    See S72.001[K,M,N,P,Q,R]

● **S82.2**   **Fracture of shaft of tibia**

● S82.20   **Unspecified fracture of shaft of tibia**
    Fracture of tibia NOS

● S82.201   **Unspecified fracture of shaft of right tibia** A, K, M, N, P, Q, R 🔵, B, C 🔷, 🔶, A, B, C 🔶
    Ⓔⓧ **For S82.201[A]:** M80.00X-M80.019[A],
    M80.041-M80.049[A], M80.061-M80.819[A],
    M80.841-M80.849[A], M80.861-M80.879[A],
    M84.40X-M84.419[A], M84.441-M84.446[A],
    M84.454[A], M84.461-M84.519[A],
    M84.541-M84.550[A], M84.561-M84.576[A],
    M84.60X-M84.619[A], M84.641-M84.650[A],
    M84.661-M84.68X[A], S03.8XX-S03.9XX[A],
    S29.011-S29.019[A], S38.3XX[A],
    S39.011-S39.013[A], S73.101[A],
    S73.109-S73.111[A], S73.119-S73.121[A],
    S73.129-S73.191[A], S73.199[A], S76.001[A],
    S76.009-S76.011[A], S76.019[A], S76.091[A],
    S76.099-S76.101[A], S76.109-S76.111[A],
    S76.119[A], S76.191[A], S76.199-S76.201[A],
    S76.209-S76.211[A], S76.219[A], S76.291[A],
    S76.299-S76.301[A], S76.309-S76.311[A],
    S76.319[A], S76.391[A], S76.399-S76.801[A],
    S76.809-S76.811[A], S76.819[A], S76.891[A],
    S76.899-S76.901[A], S76.909-S76.911[A],
    S76.919[A], S76.991[A], S76.999[A],
    S79.811[A], S79.819-S79.821[A],
    S79.829-S79.911[A], S79.919-S79.921[A],
    S79.929[A], S82.101[A,B,C], S82.102[B,C],
    S82.109-S82.111[A,B,C], S82.112[B,C],
    S82.113-S82.114[A,B,C], S82.115[B,C],
    S82.116-S82.121[A,B,C], S82.122[B,C],
    S82.123-S82.124[A,B,C], S82.125[B,C],
    S82.126-S82.131[A,B,C], S82.132[B,C],
    S82.133-S82.134[A,B,C], S82.135[B,C],
    S82.136-S82.141[A,B,C], S82.142[B,C],
    S82.143-S82.144[A,B,C], S82.145[B,C],
    S82.146-S82.151[A,B,C], S82.152[B,C],
    S82.153-S82.154[A,B,C], S82.155[B,C],
    S82.156[A,B,C], S82.161[A], S82.169[A],
    S82.191[A,B,C], S82.192[B,C],
    S82.199-S82.201[A,B,C], S82.202[B,C],
    S82.209-S82.221[A,B,C], S82.222[B,C],
    S82.223-S82.224[A,B,C], S82.225[B,C],
    S82.226-S82.231[A,B,C], S82.232[B,C],
    S82.233-S82.234[A,B,C], S82.235[B,C],
    S82.236-S82.241[A,B,C], S82.242[B,C],
    S82.243-S82.244[A,B,C], S82.245[B,C],
    S82.246-S82.251[A,B,C], S82.252[B,C],
    S82.253-S82.254[A,B,C], S82.255[B,C],
    S82.256-S82.261[A,B,C], S82.262[B,C,],
    S82.263-S82.264[A,B,C], S82.265[B,C],
    S82.266-S82.291[A,B,C], S82.292[B,C],
    S82.299[A,B,C], S82.311[A], S82.319[A],
    S82.401[A,B,C], S82.402[B,C],
    S82.409-S82.421[A,B,C], S82.422[B,C],
    S82.423-S82.424[A,B,C], S82.425[B,C],
    S82.426-S82.431[A,B,C], S82.432[B,C],
    S82.433-S82.434[A,B,C], S82.435[B,C],
    S82.436-S82.441[A,B,C], S82.442[B,C],
    S82.443-S82.444[A,B,C], S82.445[B,C],
    S82.446-S82.451[A,B,C], S82.452[B,C,],
    S82.453-S82.454[A,B,C], S82.455[B,C],
    S82.456-S82.461[A,B,C], S82.462[B,C],
    S82.463-S82.464[A,B,C], S82.465[B,C],
    S82.466-S82.491[A,B,C], S82.492[B,C],
    S82.499[A,B,C], S82.811[A],
    S82.819-S82.821[A], S82.829[A],
    S82.831[A,B,C], S82.832[B,C], S82.839[A,B,C],
    S82.861[A,B,C], S82.862[B,C],
    S82.863-S82.864[A,B,C], S82.865[B,C],
    S82.866[A,B,C], S82.90X-S82.92X[A,B,C],
    S89.001[A], S89.009-S89.011[A],
    S89.019-S89.021[A], S89.029-S89.031[A],
    S89.039-S89.041[A], S89.049-S89.091[A],
    S89.099[A], S89.201[A], S89.209[A],
    S89.211-S89.219[A], S89.221-S89.229[A],
    S89.291-S89.299[A], T14.8-T14.1, T79.
    A9X-T79.9XX[A] **For S82.201[B,C]:**
    See S82.101[B,C]
    For S82.201[K,M,N,P,Q,R]:
    See S72.001[K,M,N,P,Q,R]

● S82.202   **Unspecified fracture of shaft of left tibia** A, K, M, N, P, Q, R 🔵, B, C 🔷, 🔶, A, B, C 🔶
    Ⓔⓧ **For S82.202[A]:** See S82.102[A]
    For S82.202[B,C]: See S82.101[B,C]
    For S82.202[K,M,N,P,Q,R]:
    See S72.001[K,M,N,P,Q,R]

● S82.209   **Unspecified fracture of shaft of unspecified tibia** A, K, M, N, P, Q, R 🔵, B, C 🔷, 🔶, A, B, C 🔶
    Ⓔⓧ **For S82.209[A,B,C]:** See S82.101[B,C]
    For S82.209[K,M,N,P,Q,R]:
    See S72.001[K,M,N,P,Q,R]

● S82.22   **Transverse fracture of shaft of tibia**

● S82.221   **Displaced transverse fracture of shaft of right tibia** A, K, M, N, P, Q, R 🔵, B, C 🔷, 🔶, A, B, C 🔶
    Ⓔⓧ **For S82.221[A]:** See S82.101[A]
    For S82.221[B,C]: See S82.101[B,C]
    For S82.221[K,M,N,P,Q,R]:
    See S72.001[K,M,N,P,Q,R]

● S82.222   **Displaced transverse fracture of shaft of left tibia** A, K, M, N, P, Q, R 🔵, B, C 🔷, 🔶, A, B, C 🔶
    Ⓔⓧ **For S82.222[A]:** See S82.102[A]
    For S82.222[B,C]: See S82.101[B,C]
    For S82.222[K,M,N,P,Q,R]:
    See S72.001[K,M,N,P,Q,R]

● S82.223   **Displaced transverse fracture of shaft of unspecified tibia** A, K, M, N, P, Q, R 🔵, B, C 🔷, 🔶, A, B, C 🔶
    Ⓔⓧ **For S82.223[A,B,C]:** See S82.101[B,C]
    For S82.223[K,M,N,P,Q,R]:
    See S72.001[K,M,N,P,Q,R]

● S82.224   **Nondisplaced transverse fracture of shaft of right tibia** A, K, M, N, P, Q, R 🔵, B, C 🔷, 🔶, A, B, C 🔶
    Ⓔⓧ **For S82.224[A]:** See S82.101[A]
    For S82.224[B,C]: See S82.101[B,C]
    For S82.224[K,M,N,P,Q,R]:
    See S72.001[K,M,N,P,Q,R]

● S82.225   **Nondisplaced transverse fracture of shaft of left tibia** A, K, M, N, P, Q, R 🔵, B, C 🔷, 🔶, A, B, C 🔶
    Ⓔⓧ **For S82.225[A]:** See S82.102[A]
    For S82.225[B,C]: See S82.101[B,C]
    For S82.225[K,M,N,P,Q,R]:
    See S72.001[K,M,N,P,Q,R]

● S82.226   **Nondisplaced transverse fracture of shaft of unspecified tibia** A, K, M, N, P, Q, R 🔵, B, C 🔷, 🔶, A, B, C 🔶
    Ⓔⓧ **For S82.226[A,B,C]:** See S82.101[B,C]
    For S82.226[K,M,N,P,Q,R]:
    See S72.001[K,M,N,P,Q,R]

CHAPTER 19 (S00-T88)

N Newborn Age: 0   **P** Pediatric Age: 0–17   **M** Maternity DX: 12–55   **A** Adult Age: 15–124   ♀ Females Only   ♂ Males Only

🔵 Complication\Comorbidity   🔷 Major C\C   Ⓔⓧ CC/MCC Exclusions   🔶 Present on Admission Requirement   🔶 Hospital-Acquired Condition

1461

● S82.23   **Oblique fracture of shaft of tibia**

    ● S82.231   **Displaced oblique fracture of shaft of right tibia** A, K, M, N, P, Q, R, B, C, A, B, C
      Ex: For S82.231[A]: See S82.101[A]
        For S82.231[B,C]: See S82.101[B,C]
        For S82.231[K,M,N,P,Q,R]:
         See S72.001[K,M,N,P,Q,R]

    ● S82.232   **Displaced oblique fracture of shaft of left tibia** A, K, M, N, P, Q, R, B, C, A, B, C
      Ex: For S82.232[A]: See S82.102[A]
        For S82.232[B,C]: See S82.101[B,C]
        For S82.232[K,M,N,P,Q,R]:
         See S72.001[K,M,N,P,Q,R]

    ● S82.233   **Displaced oblique fracture of shaft of unspecified tibia** A, K, M, N, P, Q, R, B, C, A, B, C
      Ex: For S82.233[A,B,C]: See S82.101[B,C]
        For S82.233[K,M,N,P,Q,R]:
         See S72.001[K,M,N,P,Q,R]

    ● S82.234   **Nondisplaced oblique fracture of shaft of right tibia** A, K, M, N, P, Q, R, B, C, A, B, C
      Ex: For S82.234[A]: See S82.101[A]
        For S82.234[B,C]: See S82.101[B,C]
        For S82.234[K,M,N,P,Q,R]:
         See S72.001[K,M,N,P,Q,R]

    ● S82.235   **Nondisplaced oblique fracture of shaft of left tibia** A, K, M, N, P, Q, R, B, C, A, B, C
      Ex: For S82.235[A]: See S82.102[A]
        For S82.235[B,C]: See S82.101[B,C]
        For S82.235[K,M,N,P,Q,R]:
         See S72.001[K,M,N,P,Q,R]

    ● S82.236   **Nondisplaced oblique fracture of shaft of unspecified tibia** A, K, M, N, P, Q, R, B, C, A, B, C
      Ex: For S82.236[A,B,C]: See S82.101[B,C]
        For S82.236[K,M,N,P,Q,R]:
         See S72.001[K,M,N,P,Q,R]

● S82.24   **Spiral fracture of shaft of tibia**
      Toddler fracture

    ● S82.241   **Displaced spiral fracture of shaft of right tibia** A, K, M, N, P, Q, R, B, C, A, B, C
      Ex: For S82.241[A]: See S82.101[A]
        For S82.241[B,C]: See S82.101[B,C]
        For S82.241[K,M,N,P,Q,R]:
         See S72.001[K,M,N,P,Q,R]

    ● S82.242   **Displaced spiral fracture of shaft of left tibia** A, K, M, N, P, Q, R, B, C, A, B, C
      Ex: For S82.242[A]: See S82.102[A]
        For S82.242[B,C]: See S82.101[B,C]
        For S82.242[K,M,N,P,Q,R]:
         See S72.001[K,M,N,P,Q,R]

    ● S82.243   **Displaced spiral fracture of shaft of unspecified tibia** A, K, M, N, P, Q, R, B, C, A, B, C
      Ex: For S82.243[A,B,C]: See S82.101[B,C]
        For S82.243[K,M,N,P,Q,R]:
         See S72.001[K,M,N,P,Q,R]

    ● S82.244   **Nondisplaced spiral fracture of shaft of right tibia** A, K, M, N, P, Q, R, B, C, A, B, C
      Ex: For S82.244[A]: See S82.101[A]
        For S82.244[B,C]: See S82.101[B,C]
        For S82.244[K,M,N,P,Q,R]:
         See S72.001[K,M,N,P,Q,R]

    ● S82.245   **Nondisplaced spiral fracture of shaft of left tibia** A, K, M, N, P, Q, R, B, C, A, B, C
      Ex: For S82.245[A]: See S82.102[A]
        For S82.245[B,C]: See S82.101[B,C]
        For S82.245[K,M,N,P,Q,R]:
         See S72.001[K,M,N,P,Q,R]

    ● S82.246   **Nondisplaced spiral fracture of shaft of unspecified tibia** A, K, M, N, P, Q, R, B, C, A, B, C
      Ex: For S82.246[A,B,C]: See S82.101[B,C]
        For S82.246[K,M,N,P,Q,R]:
         See S72.001[K,M,N,P,Q,R]

● S82.25   **Comminuted fracture of shaft of tibia**

    ● S82.251   **Displaced comminuted fracture of shaft of right tibia** A, K, M, N, P, Q, R, B, C, A, B, C
      Ex: For S82.251[A]: See S82.101[A]
        For S82.251[B,C]: See S82.101[B,C]
        For S82.251[K,M,N,P,Q,R]:
         See S72.001[K,M,N,P,Q,R]

    ● S82.252   **Displaced comminuted fracture of shaft of left tibia** A, K, M, N, P, Q, R, B, C, A, B, C
      Ex: For S82.252[A]: See S82.102[A]
        For S82.252[B,C]: See S82.101[B,C]
        For S82.252[K,M,N,P,Q,R]:
         See S72.001[K,M,N,P,Q,R]

    ● S82.253   **Displaced comminuted fracture of shaft of unspecified tibia** A, K, M, N, P, Q, R, B, C, A, B, C
      Ex: For S82.253[A,B,C]: See S82.101[B,C]
        For S82.253[K,M,N,P,Q,R]:
         See S72.001[K,M,N,P,Q,R]

    ● S82.254   **Nondisplaced comminuted fracture of shaft of right tibia** A, K, M, N, P, Q, R, B, C, A, B, C
      Ex: For S82.254[A]: See S82.101[A]
        For S82.254[B,C]: See S82.101[B,C]
        For S82.254[K,M,N,P,Q,R]:
         See S72.001[K,M,N,P,Q,R]

    ● S82.255   **Nondisplaced comminuted fracture of shaft of left tibia** A, K, M, N, P, Q, R, B, C, A, B, C
      Ex: For S82.255[A]: See S82.102[A]
        For S82.255[B,C]: See S82.101[B,C]
        For S82.255[K,M,N,P,Q,R]:
         See S72.001[K,M,N,P,Q,R]

    ● S82.256   **Nondisplaced comminuted fracture of shaft of unspecified tibia** A, K, M, N, P, Q, R, B, C, A, B, C
      Ex: For S82.256[A,B,C]: See S82.101[B,C]
        For S82.256[K,M,N,P,Q,R]:
         See S72.001[K,M,N,P,Q,R]

CHAPTER 19 (S00-T88)

◀ New   ◀ Revised   deleted Deleted   Excludes 1   Excludes 2   Includes   Use additional   Code first   Code also   Unspecified
OGCR Official Guidelines   ● Unacceptable Principal Diagnosis   X Assign placeholder X   ● Use Additional Character(s)   ▶ Manifestation Code   **Coding Clinic**

- **S82.26**   Segmental fracture of shaft of tibia
  - **S82.261**   Displaced segmental fracture of shaft of right tibia A, K, M, N, P, Q, R 🝔, B, C 🝔, 🝔, A, B, C 🝔
    - (Ex) For S82.261[A]: See S82.101[A]
      For S82.261[B,C]: See S82.101[B,C]
      For S82.261[K,M,N,P,Q,R]:
      See S72.001[K,M,N,P,Q,R]
  - **S82.262**   Displaced segmental fracture of shaft of left tibia A, K, M, N, P, Q, R 🝔, B, C 🝔, 🝔, A, B, C 🝔
    - (Ex) For S82.262[A]: See S82.102[A]
      For S82.262[B,C]: See S82.101[B,C]
      For S82.262[K,M,N,P,Q,R]:
      See S72.001[K,M,N,P,Q,R]
  - **S82.263**   Displaced segmental fracture of shaft of unspecified tibia A, K, M, N, P, Q, R 🝔, B, C 🝔, 🝔, A, B, C 🝔
    - (Ex) For S82.263[A,B,C]: See S82.101[B,C]
      For S82.263[K,M,N,P,Q,R]:
      See S72.001[K,M,N,P,Q,R]
  - **S82.264**   Nondisplaced segmental fracture of shaft of right tibia A, K, M, N, P, Q, R 🝔, B, C 🝔, 🝔, A, B, C 🝔
    - (Ex) For S82.264[A]: See S82.101[A]
      For S82.264[B,C]: See S82.101[B,C]
      For S82.264[K,M,N,P,Q,R]:
      See S72.001[K,M,N,P,Q,R]
  - **S82.265**   Nondisplaced segmental fracture of shaft of left tibia A, K, M, N, P, Q, R 🝔, B, C 🝔, 🝔, A, B, C 🝔
    - (Ex) For S82.265[A]: See S82.102[A]
      For S82.265[B,C]: See S82.101[B,C]
      For S82.265[K,M,N,P,Q,R]:
      See S72.001[K,M,N,P,Q,R]
  - **S82.266**   Nondisplaced segmental fracture of shaft of unspecified tibia A, K, M, N, P, Q, R 🝔, B, C 🝔, 🝔, A, B, C 🝔
    - (Ex) For S82.266[A,B,C]: See S82.101[B,C]
      For S82.266[K,M,N,P,Q,R]:
      See S72.001[K,M,N,P,Q,R]
- **S82.29**   Other fracture of shaft of tibia
  - **S82.291**   Other fracture of shaft of right tibia A, K, M, N, P, Q, R 🝔, B, C 🝔, 🝔, A, B, C 🝔
    - (Ex) For S82.291[A]: See S82.101[A]
      For S82.291[B,C]: See S82.101[B,C]
      For S82.291[K,M,N,P,Q,R]:
      See S72.001[K,M,N,P,Q,R]
  - **S82.292**   Other fracture of shaft of left tibia A, K, M, N, P, Q, R 🝔, B, C 🝔, 🝔, A, B, C 🝔
    - (Ex) For S82.292[A]: See S82.102[A]
      For S82.292[B,C]: See S82.101[B,C]
      For S82.292[K,M,N,P,Q,R]:
      See S72.001[K,M,N,P,Q,R]
  - **S82.299**   Other fracture of shaft of unspecified tibia A, K, M, N, P, Q, R, B, C 🝔, 🝔, A, B, C 🝔
    - (Ex) For S82.299[A,B,C]: See S82.101[B,C]
      For S82.299[K,M,N,P,Q,R]:
      See S72.001[K,M,N,P,Q,R]

- **S82.3**   Fracture of lower end of tibia
  - **Excludes1**   bimalleolar fracture of lower leg (S82.84-)
    fracture of medial malleolus alone (S82.5-)
    Maisonneuve's fracture (S82.86-)
    pilon fracture of distal tibia (S82.87-)
    trimalleolar fractures of lower leg
    (S82.85-)
  - **S82.30**   Unspecified fracture of lower end of tibia
    - (Ex) For category S82.30 CC codes S82.30[B,C]:
      M80.00X-M80.019[A], M80.041-M80.049[A],
      M80.061-M80.819[A], M80.841-M80.849[A],
      M80.861-M80.879[A], M84.40X-M84.419[A],
      M84.441-M84.446[A], M84.454[A], M84.461-M84.519[A],
      M84.541-M84.550[A], M84.561-M84.576[A],
      M84.60X-M84.619[A], M84.641-M84.650[A],
      M84.661-M84.68X[A], S03.8XX-S03.9XX[A],
      S29.011-S29.019[A], S38.3XX[A], S39.011-S39.013[A],
      S73.101-S73.199[A], S76.001-S76.019[A],
      S76.091-S76.119[A], S76.191-S76.219[A],
      S76.291-S76.319[A], S76.391-S76.819[A],
      S76.891-S76.919[A], S76.991-S76.999[A],
      S79.811-S79.929[A], S82.301-S82.309[A,B,C],
      S82.391-S82.399[A,B,C], S82.51X-S82.56X[B,C],
      S82.61X-S82.66X[A,B,C], S82.841-S82.856[A,B,C],
      S82.871-S82.876[B,C], S82.891-S82.92X[A,B,C],
      S89.101-S89.199[A], S89.301-S89.399[A], T14.8-T14.91, T79.
      A9X-T79.9XX[A] For S82.30[K,M,N,P,Q,R]:
      See S72.001[K,M,N,P,Q,R]
  - **S82.301**   Unspecified fracture of lower end of right tibia B, C, K, M, N, P, Q, R 🝔, 🝔, B, C 🝔
  - **S82.302**   Unspecified fracture of lower end of left tibia B, C, K, M, N, P, Q, R 🝔, 🝔, B, C 🝔
  - **S82.309**   Unspecified fracture of lower end of unspecified tibia B, C, K, M, N, P, Q, R 🝔, 🝔, B, C 🝔
  - **S82.31**   Torus fracture of lower end of tibia
    The appropriate 7th character is to be added to all codes in subcategory S82.31

A	initial encounter for closed fracture
D	subsequent encounter for fracture with routine healing
G	subsequent encounter for fracture with delayed healing
K	subsequent encounter for fracture with nonunion
P	subsequent encounter for fracture with malunion
S	sequela

    - **S82.311**   Torus fracture of lower end of right tibia A, K, P 🝔, 🝔, A 🝔
      - (Ex) For S82.311[A]: See S82.161[A]
        For S82.311[K,P]: See S72.001[K,M,N,P,Q,R]
    - **S82.312**   Torus fracture of lower end of left tibia A, K, P 🝔, 🝔, A 🝔
      - (Ex) For S82.312[A]: See S82.162[A]
        For S82.312[K,P]: See S72.001[K,M,N,P,Q,R]
    - **S82.319**   Torus fracture of lower end of unspecified tibia A, K, P 🝔, 🝔, A 🝔
      - (Ex) For S82.319[A]: See S82.169[A]
        S82.319[K,P]: See S72.001[K,M,N,P,Q,R]

N   Newborn Age: 0   P   Pediatric Age: 0–17   M   Maternity DX: 12–55   A   Adult Age: 15–124   ♀   Females Only   ♂   Males Only
🝔   Complication\Comorbidity   🝔   Major C\C   (Ex)   CC/MCC Exclusions   🝔   Present on Admission Requirement   🝔   Hospital-Acquired Condition

● **S82.39** Other fracture of lower end of tibia
Ex: For category S82.39 CC codes S82.39[B,C]:
See S82.30[B,C] For S82.39[K,M,N,P,Q,R]:
See S72.001[K,M,N,P,Q,R]

  ● **S82.391** Other fracture of lower end of right tibia B, C, K, M, N, P, Q, R 🐾, 🐾, B, C 🐾

  ● **S82.392** Other fracture of lower end of left tibia B, C, K, M, N, P, Q, R 🐾, 🐾, B, C 🐾

  ● **S82.399** Other fracture of lower end of unspecified tibia B, C, K, M, N, P, Q, R 🐾, 🐾, B, C 🐾

● **S82.4** Fracture of shaft of fibula
  Excludes2 fracture of lateral malleolus alone (S82.6-)
  Ex: For category S82.4 CC codes S82.4[B,C]: See S82.101[B,C]
  For S82.4[K,M,N,P,Q,R]: See S72.001[K,M,N,P,Q,R]

  ● **S82.40** Unspecified fracture of shaft of fibula

    ● **S82.401** Unspecified fracture of shaft of right fibula K, M, N, P, Q, R 🐾, B, C 🐾, 🐾, B, C 🐾

    ● **S82.402** Unspecified fracture of shaft of left fibula K, M, N, P, Q, R 🐾, B, C 🐾, 🐾, B, C 🐾

    ● **S82.409** Unspecified fracture of shaft of unspecified fibula K, M, N, P, Q, R 🐾, B, C 🐾, 🐾, B, C 🐾

  ● **S82.42** Transverse fracture of shaft of fibula

    ● **S82.421** Displaced transverse fracture of shaft of right fibula K, M, N, P, Q, R 🐾, B, C 🐾, 🐾, B, C 🐾

    ● **S82.422** Displaced transverse fracture of shaft of left fibula K, M, N, P, Q, R 🐾, B, C 🐾, 🐾, B, C 🐾

    ● **S82.423** Displaced transverse fracture of shaft of unspecified fibula K, M, N, P, Q, R 🐾, B, C 🐾, 🐾, B, C 🐾

    ● **S82.424** Nondisplaced transverse fracture of shaft of right fibula K, M, N, P, Q, R 🐾, B, C 🐾, 🐾, B, C 🐾

    ● **S82.425** Nondisplaced transverse fracture of shaft of left fibula K, M, N, P, Q, R 🐾, B, C 🐾, 🐾, B, C 🐾

    ● **S82.426** Nondisplaced transverse fracture of shaft of unspecified fibula K, M, N, P, Q, R 🐾, B, C 🐾, 🐾, B, C 🐾

  ● **S82.43** Oblique fracture of shaft of fibula

    ● **S82.431** Displaced oblique fracture of shaft of right fibula K, M, N, P, Q, R 🐾, B, C 🐾, 🐾, B, C 🐾

    ● **S82.432** Displaced oblique fracture of shaft of left fibula K, M, N, P, Q, R 🐾, B, C 🐾, 🐾, B, C 🐾

    ● **S82.433** Displaced oblique fracture of shaft of unspecified fibula K, M, N, P, Q, R 🐾, B, C 🐾, 🐾, B, C 🐾

    ● **S82.434** Nondisplaced oblique fracture of shaft of right fibula K, M, N, P, Q, R 🐾, B, C 🐾, 🐾, B, C 🐾

    ● **S82.435** Nondisplaced oblique fracture of shaft of left fibula K, M, N, P, Q, R 🐾, B, C 🐾, 🐾, B, C 🐾

    ● **S82.436** Nondisplaced oblique fracture of shaft of unspecified fibula K, M, N, P, Q, R 🐾, B, C 🐾, 🐾, B, C 🐾

● **S82.44** Spiral fracture of shaft of fibula

  ● **S82.441** Displaced spiral fracture of shaft of right fibula K, M, N, P, Q, R 🐾, B, C 🐾, 🐾, B, C 🐾

  ● **S82.442** Displaced spiral fracture of shaft of left fibula K, M, N, P, Q, R 🐾, B, C 🐾, 🐾, B, C 🐾

  ● **S82.443** Displaced spiral fracture of shaft of unspecified fibula K, M, N, P, Q, R 🐾, B, C 🐾, 🐾, B, C 🐾

  ● **S82.444** Nondisplaced spiral fracture of shaft of right fibula K, M, N, P, Q, R 🐾, B, C 🐾, 🐾, B, C 🐾

  ● **S82.445** Nondisplaced spiral fracture of shaft of left fibula K, M, N, P, Q, R 🐾, B, C 🐾, 🐾, B, C 🐾

  ● **S82.446** Nondisplaced spiral fracture of shaft of unspecified fibula K, M, N, P, Q, R 🐾, B, C 🐾, 🐾, B, C 🐾

● **S82.45** Comminuted fracture of shaft of fibula

  ● **S82.451** Displaced comminuted fracture of shaft of right fibula K, M, N, P, Q, R 🐾, B, C 🐾, 🐾, B, C 🐾

  ● **S82.452** Displaced comminuted fracture of shaft of left fibula K, M, N, P, Q, R 🐾, B, C 🐾, 🐾, B, C 🐾

  ● **S82.453** Displaced comminuted fracture of shaft of unspecified fibula K, M, N, P, Q, R 🐾, B, C 🐾, 🐾, B, C 🐾

  ● **S82.454** Nondisplaced comminuted fracture of shaft of right fibula K, M, N, P, Q, R 🐾, B, C 🐾, 🐾, B, C 🐾

  ● **S82.455** Nondisplaced comminuted fracture of shaft of left fibula K, M, N, P, Q, R 🐾, B, C 🐾, 🐾, B, C 🐾

  ● **S82.456** Nondisplaced comminuted fracture of shaft of unspecified fibula K, M, N, P, Q, R 🐾, B, C 🐾, 🐾, B, C 🐾

● **S82.46** Segmental fracture of shaft of fibula

  ● **S82.461** Displaced segmental fracture of shaft of right fibula K, M, N, P, Q, R 🐾, B, C 🐾, 🐾, B, C 🐾

  ● **S82.462** Displaced segmental fracture of shaft of left fibula K, M, N, P, Q, R 🐾, B, C 🐾, 🐾, B, C 🐾

  ● **S82.463** Displaced segmental fracture of shaft of unspecified fibula K, M, N, P, Q, R 🐾, B, C 🐾, 🐾, B, C 🐾

  ● **S82.464** Nondisplaced segmental fracture of shaft of right fibula K, M, N, P, Q, R 🐾, B, C 🐾, 🐾, B, C 🐾

  ● **S82.465** Nondisplaced segmental fracture of shaft of left fibula K, M, N, P, Q, R 🐾, B, C 🐾, 🐾, B, C 🐾

  ● **S82.466** Nondisplaced segmental fracture of shaft of unspecified fibula K, M, N, P, Q, R 🐾, B, C 🐾, 🐾, B, C 🐾

● **S82.49** Other fracture of shaft of fibula

  ● **S82.491** Other fracture of shaft of right fibula K, M, N, P, Q, R 🐾, B, C 🐾, 🐾, B, C 🐾

  ● **S82.492** Other fracture of shaft of left fibula K, M, N, P, Q, R 🐾, B, C 🐾, 🐾, B, C 🐾

  ● **S82.499** Other fracture of shaft of unspecified fibula K, M, N, P, Q, R 🐾, B, C 🐾, 🐾, B, C 🐾

◄ New   ◄█ Revised   ~~deleted~~ Deleted   Excludes 1   Excludes 2   Includes   Use additional   Code first   Code also   Unspecified
OGCR Official Guidelines   ● Unacceptable Principal Diagnosis   X Assign placeholder X   ● Use Additional Character(s)   ▌ Manifestation Code   **Coding Clinic**

● S82.5   Fracture of medial malleolus

     Excludes1   pilon fracture of distal tibia (S82.87-)

           Salter-Harris type III of lower end of tibia (S89.13-)

           Salter-Harris type IV of lower end of tibia (S89.14-)

     (Ex) For category S82.5 CC codes S82.5[B,C]: See S82.30[B,C]
         For S82.5[K,M,N,P,Q,R]: See S72.001[K,M,N,P,Q,R]

X ● S82.51   Displaced fracture of medial malleolus of right tibia B, C, K, M, N, P, Q, R ◑, ◐, B, C ◑

X ● S82.52   Displaced fracture of medial malleolus of left tibia B, C, K, M, N, P, Q, R ◑, ◐, B, C ◑

X ● S82.53   Displaced fracture of medial malleolus of unspecified tibia B, C, K, M, N, P, Q, R ◑, ◐, B, C ◑

X ● S82.54   Nondisplaced fracture of medial malleolus of right tibia B, C, K, M, N, P, Q, R ◑, ◐, B, C ◑

X ● S82.55   Nondisplaced fracture of medial malleolus of left tibia B, C, K, M, N, P, Q, R ◑, ◐, B, C ◑

X ● S82.56   Nondisplaced fracture of medial malleolus of unspecified tibia B, C, K, M, N, P, Q, R ◑, ◐, B, C ◑

● S82.6   Fracture of lateral malleolus

     Excludes1   pilon fracture of distal tibia (S82.87-)

     (Ex) For category S82.6 CC codes S82.6[B,C]: See S82.30[B,C]
         For S82.6[K,M,N,P,Q,R]: See S72.001[K,M,N,P,Q,R]

X ● S82.61   Displaced fracture of lateral malleolus of right fibula B, C, K, M, N, P, Q, R ◑, ◐, B, C ◑

X ● S82.62   Displaced fracture of lateral malleolus of left fibula B, C, K, M, N, P, Q, R ◑, ◐, B, C ◑

X ● S82.63   Displaced fracture of lateral malleolus of unspecified fibula B, C, K, M, N, P, Q, R ◑, ◐, B, C ◑

X ● S82.64   Nondisplaced fracture of lateral malleolus of right fibula B, C, K, M, N, P, Q, R ◑, ◐, B, C ◑

X ● S82.65   Nondisplaced fracture of lateral malleolus of left fibula B, C, K, M, N, P, Q, R ◑, ◐, B, C ◑

X ● S82.66   Nondisplaced fracture of lateral malleolus of unspecified fibula B, C, K, M, N, P, Q, R ◑, ◐, B, C ◑

● S82.8   Other fractures of lower leg

  ● S82.81   Torus fracture of upper end of fibula

       The appropriate 7th character is to be added to all codes in subcategory S82.81

A	initial encounter for closed fracture
D	subsequent encounter for fracture with routine healing
G	subsequent encounter for fracture with delayed healing
K	subsequent encounter for fracture with nonunion
P	subsequent encounter for fracture with malunion
S	sequela

     (Ex) For category S82.81 CC codes: See S72.001[K,M,N,P,Q,R]

  ● S82.811   Torus fracture of upper end of right fibula K, P ◑, ◐

  ● S82.812   Torus fracture of upper end of left fibula K, P ◑, ◐

  ● S82.819   Torus fracture of upper end of unspecified fibula K, P ◑, ◐

● S82.82   Torus fracture of lower end of fibula

       The appropriate 7th character is to be added to all codes in subcategory S82.82

A	initial encounter for closed fracture
D	subsequent encounter for fracture with routine healing
G	subsequent encounter for fracture with delayed healing
K	subsequent encounter for fracture with nonunion
P	subsequent encounter for fracture with malunion
S	sequela

     (Ex) For category S82.82 CC codes: See S72.001[K,M,N,P,Q,R]

  ● S82.821   Torus fracture of lower end of right fibula K, P ◑, ◐

  ● S82.822   Torus fracture of lower end of left fibula K, P ◑, ◐

  ● S82.829   Torus fracture of lower end of unspecified fibula K, P ◑, ◐

● S82.83   Other fracture of upper and lower end of fibula

     (Ex) For category S82.83 CC codes S82.83[B,C]:
       See S82.101[B,C] For S82.83[K,M,N,P,Q,R]:
       See S72.001[K,M,N,P,Q,R]

  ● S82.831   Other fracture of upper and lower end of right fibula K, M, N, P, Q, R ◑, B, C ◑, ◐, B, C ◑

  ● S82.832   Other fracture of upper and lower end of left fibula K, M, N, P, Q, R ◑, B, C ◑, ◐, B, C ◑

  ● S82.839   Other fracture of upper and lower end of unspecified fibula K, M, N, P, Q, R ◑, B, C ◑, ◐, B, C ◑

● S82.84   Bimalleolar fracture of lower leg

     (Ex) For category S82.84 CC codes S82.84[B,C]:
       See S82.30[B,C] For S82.84[K,M,N,P,Q,R]:
       See S72.001[K,M,N,P,Q,R]

  ● S82.841   Displaced bimalleolar fracture of right lower leg B, C, K, M, N, P, Q, R ◑, ◐, B, C ◑

  ● S82.842   Displaced bimalleolar fracture of left lower leg B, C, K, M, N, P, Q, R ◑, ◐, B, C ◑

  ● S82.843   Displaced bimalleolar fracture of unspecified lower leg B, C, K, M, N, P, Q, R ◑, ◐, B, C ◑

  ● S82.844   Nondisplaced bimalleolar fracture of right lower leg B, C, K, M, N, P, Q, R ◑, ◐, B, C ◑

  ● S82.845   Nondisplaced bimalleolar fracture of left lower leg B, C, K, M, N, P, Q, R ◑, ◐, B, C ◑

  ● S82.846   Nondisplaced bimalleolar fracture of unspecified lower leg B, C, K, M, N, P, Q, R ◑, ◐, B, C ◑

● S82.85   Trimalleolar fracture of lower leg

     (Ex) For category S82.85 CC codes S82.85[B,C]:
       See S82.30[B,C] For S82.85[K,M,N,P,Q,R]:
       See S72.001[K,M,N,P,Q,R]

  ● S82.851   Displaced trimalleolar fracture of right lower leg B, C, K, M, N, P, Q, R ◑, ◐, B, C ◑

  ● S82.852   Displaced trimalleolar fracture of left lower leg B, C, K, M, N, P, Q, R ◑, ◐, B, C ◑

N   Newborn Age: 0   P   Pediatric Age: 0–17   M   Maternity DX: 12–55   A   Adult Age: 15–124   ♀   Females Only   ♂   Males Only

◑   Complication\Comorbidity   ◐   Major C\C   (Ex)   CC/MCC Exclusions   ◑   Present on Admission Requirement   ◑   Hospital-Acquired Condition

1465

CHAPTER 19 (S00-T88)

● S82.853   Displaced trimalleolar fracture of unspecified lower leg B, C, K, M, N, P, Q, R 🔲, 🔲, B, C 🔲

● S82.854   Nondisplaced trimalleolar fracture of right lower leg B, C, K, M, N, P, Q, R 🔲, 🔲, B, C 🔲

● S82.855   Nondisplaced trimalleolar fracture of left lower leg B, C, K, M, N, P, Q, R 🔲, 🔲, B, C 🔲

● S82.856   Nondisplaced trimalleolar fracture of unspecified lower leg B, C, K, M, N, P, Q, R 🔲, 🔲, B, C 🔲

● S82.86   Maisonneuve's fracture
    (Ex) For category S82.86 CC codes S82.86[B,C]:
    See S82.101[B,C] For S82.86[K,M,N,P,Q,R]:
    See S72.001[K,M,N,P,Q,R]

● S82.861   Displaced Maisonneuve's fracture of right leg K, M, N, P, Q, R 🔲, B, C 🔲, 🔲, B, C 🔲

● S82.862   Displaced Maisonneuve's fracture of left leg K, M, N, P, Q, R 🔲, B, C 🔲, 🔲, B, C 🔲

● S82.863   Displaced Maisonneuve's fracture of unspecified leg K, M, N, P, Q, R 🔲, B, C 🔲, 🔲, B, C 🔲

● S82.864   Nondisplaced Maisonneuve's fracture of right leg K, M, N, P, Q, R 🔲, B, C 🔲, 🔲, B, C 🔲

● S82.865   Nondisplaced Maisonneuve's fracture of left leg K, M, N, P, Q, R 🔲, B, C 🔲, 🔲, B, C 🔲

● S82.866   Nondisplaced Maisonneuve's fracture of unspecified leg K, M, N, P, Q, R 🔲, B, C 🔲, 🔲, B, C 🔲

● S82.87   Pilon fracture of tibia
    (Ex) For category S82.87 CC codes S82.87[B,C]:
    See S82.30[B,C] For S82.87[K,M,N,P,Q,R]:
    See S72.001[K,M,N,P,Q,R]

● S82.871   Displaced pilon fracture of right tibia B, C, K, M, N, P, Q, R 🔲, 🔲, B, C 🔲

● S82.872   Displaced pilon fracture of left tibia B, C, K, M, N, P, Q, R 🔲, 🔲, B, C 🔲

● S82.873   Displaced pilon fracture of unspecified tibia B, C, K, M, N, P, Q, R 🔲, 🔲, B, C 🔲

● S82.874   Nondisplaced pilon fracture of right tibia B, C, K, M, N, P, Q, R 🔲, 🔲, B, C 🔲

● S82.875   Nondisplaced pilon fracture of left tibia B, C, K, M, N, P, Q, R 🔲, 🔲, B, C 🔲

● S82.876   Nondisplaced pilon fracture of unspecified tibia B, C, K, M, N, P, Q, R 🔲, 🔲, B, C 🔲

● S82.89   Other fractures of lower leg
    Fracture of ankle NOS
    (Ex) For category S82.89 CC codes S82.89[B,C]: See
    S82.30[B,C] For S82.89[K,M,N,P,Q,R]: See
    S72.001[K,M,N,P,Q,R]

● S82.891   Other fracture of right lower leg B, C, K, M, N, P, Q, R 🔲, 🔲, B, C 🔲

● S82.892   Other fracture of left lower leg B, C, K, M, N, P, Q, R 🔲, 🔲, B, C 🔲

● S82.899   Other fracture of unspecified lower leg B, C, K, M, N, P, Q, R 🔲, 🔲, B, C 🔲

● S82.9   Unspecified fracture of lower leg
    (Ex) For category S82.9 CC codes S82.9[B,C]: S72.001-S72.92X[A,B,C],
    S79.001-S79.199[A], S82.001-S82.156[A,B,C], S82.191-S82.309[A,B,C],
    S82.391-S82.66X[A,B,C], S82.831-S82.92X[A,B,C], S89.001-S89.399[A],
    S92.001-S92.919[A,B] For S82.9[K,M,N,P,Q,R]:
    See S72.001[K,M,N,P,Q,R]

X ● S82.90   Unspecified fracture of unspecified lower leg A, K, M, N, P, Q, R 🔲, 🔲, B, C 🔲

X ● S82.91   Unspecified fracture of right lower leg A, K, M, N, P, Q, R 🔲, 🔲, B, C 🔲

X ● S82.92   Unspecified fracture of left lower leg A, K, M, N, P, Q, R 🔲, 🔲, B, C 🔲

● S83   **Dislocation and sprain of joints and ligaments of knee**

    Includes   avulsion of joint or ligament of knee
               laceration of cartilage, joint or ligament of knee
               sprain of cartilage, joint or ligament of knee
               traumatic hemarthrosis of joint or ligament of knee
               traumatic rupture of joint or ligament of knee
               traumatic subluxation of joint or ligament of knee
               traumatic tear of joint or ligament of knee

    Code also any associated open wound

    Excludes1   derangement of patella (M22.0-M22.3)
               injury of patellar ligament (tendon) (S76.1-)
               internal derangement of knee (M23.-)
               old dislocation of knee (M24.36)
               pathological dislocation of knee (M24.36)
               recurrent dislocation of knee (M22.0)

    Excludes2   strain of muscle, fascia and tendon of lower leg (S86.-)

    The appropriate 7th character is to be added to each code from category S83

    | | |
    A   initial encounter
    D   subsequent encounter
    S   sequela

● S83.0   Subluxation and dislocation of patella

● S83.00   Unspecified subluxation and dislocation of patella

● S83.001   Unspecified subluxation of right patella 🔲

● S83.002   Unspecified subluxation of left patella 🔲

● S83.003   Unspecified subluxation of unspecified patella 🔲

● S83.004   Unspecified dislocation of right patella 🔲

● S83.005   Unspecified dislocation of left patella 🔲

● S83.006   Unspecified dislocation of unspecified patella 🔲

● S83.01   Lateral subluxation and dislocation of patella

● S83.011   Lateral subluxation of right patella 🔲

● S83.012   Lateral subluxation of left patella 🔲

● S83.013   Lateral subluxation of unspecified patella 🔲

● S83.014   Lateral dislocation of right patella 🔲

● S83.015   Lateral dislocation of left patella 🔲

● S83.016   Lateral dislocation of unspecified patella 🔲

● S83.09   Other subluxation and dislocation of patella

● S83.091   Other subluxation of right patella 🔲

● S83.092   Other subluxation of left patella 🔲

● S83.093   Other subluxation of unspecified patella 🔲

● S83.094   Other dislocation of right patella 🔲

● S83.095   Other dislocation of left patella 🔲

● S83.096   Other dislocation of unspecified patella 🔲

◀ New   ◀ Revised   ~~deleted~~ Deleted   Excludes 1   Excludes 2   Includes   Use additional   Code first   Code also   Unspecified
OGCR Official Guidelines   ● Unacceptable Principal Diagnosis   X Assign placeholder X   ● Use Additional Character(s)   ▶ Manifestation Code   **Coding Clinic**

● **S83.1**   Subluxation and dislocation of knee
> **Excludes2**   instability of knee prosthesis (T84.022, T84.023)

  ● **S83.10**   Unspecified subluxation and dislocation of knee

    ● **S83.101**   Unspecified subluxation of right knee 🔗

    ● **S83.102**   Unspecified subluxation of left knee 🔗

    ● **S83.103**   Unspecified subluxation of unspecified knee 🔗

    ● **S83.104**   Unspecified dislocation of right knee 🔗

    ● **S83.105**   Unspecified dislocation of left knee 🔗

    ● **S83.106**   Unspecified dislocation of unspecified knee 🔗

  ● **S83.11**   Anterior subluxation and dislocation of proximal end of tibia
> Posterior subluxation and dislocation of distal end of femur

    ● **S83.111**   Anterior subluxation of proximal end of tibia, right knee 🔗

    ● **S83.112**   Anterior subluxation of proximal end of tibia, left knee 🔗

    ● **S83.113**   Anterior subluxation of proximal end of tibia, unspecified knee 🔗

    ● **S83.114**   Anterior dislocation of proximal end of tibia, right knee 🔗

    ● **S83.115**   Anterior dislocation of proximal end of tibia, left knee 🔗

    ● **S83.116**   Anterior dislocation of proximal end of tibia, unspecified knee 🔗

  ● **S83.12**   Posterior subluxation and dislocation of proximal end of tibia
> Anterior dislocation of distal end of femur

    ● **S83.121**   Posterior subluxation of proximal end of tibia, right knee 🔗

    ● **S83.122**   Posterior subluxation of proximal end of tibia, left knee 🔗

    ● **S83.123**   Posterior subluxation of proximal end of tibia, unspecified knee 🔗

    ● **S83.124**   Posterior dislocation of proximal end of tibia, right knee 🔗

    ● **S83.125**   Posterior dislocation of proximal end of tibia, left knee 🔗

    ● **S83.126**   Posterior dislocation of proximal end of tibia, unspecified knee 🔗

  ● **S83.13**   Medial subluxation and dislocation of proximal end of tibia

    ● **S83.131**   Medial subluxation of proximal end of tibia, right knee 🔗

    ● **S83.132**   Medial subluxation of proximal end of tibia, left knee 🔗

    ● **S83.133**   Medial subluxation of proximal end of tibia, unspecified knee 🔗

    ● **S83.134**   Medial dislocation of proximal end of tibia, right knee 🔗

    ● **S83.135**   Medial dislocation of proximal end of tibia, left knee 🔗

    ● **S83.136**   Medial dislocation of proximal end of tibia, unspecified knee 🔗

  ● **S83.14**   Lateral subluxation and dislocation of proximal end of tibia

    ● **S83.141**   Lateral subluxation of proximal end of tibia, right knee 🔗

    ● **S83.142**   Lateral subluxation of proximal end of tibia, left knee 🔗

    ● **S83.143**   Lateral subluxation of proximal end of tibia, unspecified knee 🔗

    ● **S83.144**   Lateral dislocation of proximal end of tibia, right knee 🔗

    ● **S83.145**   Lateral dislocation of proximal end of tibia, left knee 🔗

    ● **S83.146**   Lateral dislocation of proximal end of tibia, unspecified knee 🔗

  ● **S83.19**   Other subluxation and dislocation of knee

    ● **S83.191**   Other subluxation of right knee 🔗

    ● **S83.192**   Other subluxation of left knee 🔗

    ● **S83.193**   Other subluxation of unspecified knee 🔗

    ● **S83.194**   Other dislocation of right knee 🔗

    ● **S83.195**   Other dislocation of left knee 🔗

    ● **S83.196**   Other dislocation of unspecified knee 🔗

● **S83.2**   Tear of meniscus, current injury
> **Excludes1**   old bucket-handle tear (M23.2)

  ● **S83.20**   Tear of unspecified meniscus, current injury
> Tear of meniscus of knee NOS

    ● **S83.200**   Bucket-handle tear of unspecified meniscus, current injury, right knee 🔗

    ● **S83.201**   Bucket-handle tear of unspecified meniscus, current injury, left knee 🔗

    ● **S83.202**   Bucket-handle tear of unspecified meniscus, current injury, unspecified knee 🔗

    ● **S83.203**   Other tear of unspecified meniscus, current injury, right knee 🔗

    ● **S83.204**   Other tear of unspecified meniscus, current injury, left knee 🔗

    ● **S83.205**   Other tear of unspecified meniscus, current injury, unspecified knee 🔗

    ● **S83.206**   Unspecified tear of unspecified meniscus, current injury, right knee 🔗

    ● **S83.207**   Unspecified tear of unspecified meniscus, current injury, left knee 🔗

    ● **S83.209**   Unspecified tear of unspecified meniscus, current injury, unspecified knee 🔗

  ● **S83.21**   Bucket-handle tear of medial meniscus, current injury

    ● **S83.211**   Bucket-handle tear of medial meniscus, current injury, right knee 🔗

    ● **S83.212**   Bucket-handle tear of medial meniscus, current injury, left knee 🔗

    ● **S83.219**   Bucket-handle tear of medial meniscus, current injury, unspecified knee 🔗

  ● **S83.22**   Peripheral tear of medial meniscus, current injury

    ● **S83.221**   Peripheral tear of medial meniscus, current injury, right knee 🔗

    ● **S83.222**   Peripheral tear of medial meniscus, current injury, left knee 🔗

    ● **S83.229**   Peripheral tear of medial meniscus, current injury, unspecified knee 🔗

  ● **S83.23**   Complex tear of medial meniscus, current injury

    ● **S83.231**   Complex tear of medial meniscus, current injury, right knee 🔗

    ● **S83.232**   Complex tear of medial meniscus, current injury, left knee 🔗

    ● **S83.239**   Complex tear of medial meniscus, current injury, unspecified knee 🔗

N   Newborn Age: 0   P   Pediatric Age: 0–17   M   Maternity DX: 12–55   A   Adult Age: 15–124   ♀   Females Only   ♂   Males Only

🔗   Complication\Comorbidity   🔗   Major C\C   (Ex)   CC/MCC Exclusions   🔗   Present on Admission Requirement   🔗   Hospital-Acquired Condition

1467

● S83.24   Other tear of medial meniscus, current injury
  ● S83.241   Other tear of medial meniscus, current injury, right knee 🖎
  ● S83.242   Other tear of medial meniscus, current injury, left knee 🖎
  ● S83.249   Other tear of medial meniscus, current injury, unspecified knee 🖎
● S83.25   Bucket-handle tear of lateral meniscus, current injury
  ● S83.251   Bucket-handle tear of lateral meniscus, current injury, right knee 🖎
  ● S83.252   Bucket-handle tear of lateral meniscus, current injury, left knee 🖎
  ● S83.259   Bucket-handle tear of lateral meniscus, current injury, unspecified knee 🖎
● S83.26   Peripheral tear of lateral meniscus, current injury
  ● S83.261   Peripheral tear of lateral meniscus, current injury, right knee 🖎
  ● S83.262   Peripheral tear of lateral meniscus, current injury, left knee 🖎
  ● S83.269   Peripheral tear of lateral meniscus, current injury, unspecified knee 🖎
● S83.27   Complex tear of lateral meniscus, current injury
  ● S83.271   Complex tear of lateral meniscus, current injury, right knee 🖎
  ● S83.272   Complex tear of lateral meniscus, current injury, left knee 🖎
  ● S83.279   Complex tear of lateral meniscus, current injury, unspecified knee 🖎
● S83.28   Other tear of lateral meniscus, current injury
  ● S83.281   Other tear of lateral meniscus, current injury, right knee 🖎
  ● S83.282   Other tear of lateral meniscus, current injury, left knee 🖎
  ● S83.289   Other tear of lateral meniscus, current injury, unspecified knee 🖎
● S83.3   Tear of articular cartilage of knee, current
  X ● S83.30   Tear of articular cartilage of unspecified knee, current 🖎
  X ● S83.31   Tear of articular cartilage of right knee, current 🖎
  X ● S83.32   Tear of articular cartilage of left knee, current 🖎
● S83.4   Sprain of collateral ligament of knee
  ● S83.40   Sprain of unspecified collateral ligament of knee
    ● S83.401   Sprain of unspecified collateral ligament of right knee 🖎
    ● S83.402   Sprain of unspecified collateral ligament of left knee 🖎
    ● S83.409   Sprain of unspecified collateral ligament of unspecified knee 🖎
  ● S83.41   Sprain of medial collateral ligament of knee
    Sprain of tibial collateral ligament
    ● S83.411   Sprain of medial collateral ligament of right knee 🖎
    ● S83.412   Sprain of medial collateral ligament of left knee 🖎
    ● S83.419   Sprain of medial collateral ligament of unspecified knee 🖎
  ● S83.42   Sprain of lateral collateral ligament of knee
    Sprain of fibular collateral ligament
    ● S83.421   Sprain of lateral collateral ligament of right knee 🖎
    ● S83.422   Sprain of lateral collateral ligament of left knee 🖎
    ● S83.429   Sprain of lateral collateral ligament of unspecified knee 🖎

● S83.5   Sprain of cruciate ligament of knee
  ● S83.50   Sprain of unspecified cruciate ligament of knee
    ● S83.501   Sprain of unspecified cruciate ligament of right knee 🖎
    ● S83.502   Sprain of unspecified cruciate ligament of left knee 🖎
    ● S83.509   Sprain of unspecified cruciate ligament of unspecified knee 🖎
  ● S83.51   Sprain of anterior cruciate ligament of knee
    ● S83.511   Sprain of anterior cruciate ligament of right knee 🖎
    ● S83.512   Sprain of anterior cruciate ligament of left knee 🖎
    ● S83.519   Sprain of anterior cruciate ligament of unspecified knee 🖎
  ● S83.52   Sprain of posterior cruciate ligament of knee
    ● S83.521   Sprain of posterior cruciate ligament of right knee 🖎
    ● S83.522   Sprain of posterior cruciate ligament of left knee 🖎
    ● S83.529   Sprain of posterior cruciate ligament of unspecified knee 🖎
● S83.6   Sprain of the superior tibiofibular joint and ligament
  X ● S83.60   Sprain of the superior tibiofibular joint and ligament, unspecified knee 🖎
  X ● S83.61   Sprain of the superior tibiofibular joint and ligament, right knee 🖎
  X ● S83.62   Sprain of the superior tibiofibular joint and ligament, left knee 🖎
● S83.8   Sprain of other specified parts of knee
  ● S83.8X   Sprain of other specified parts of knee
    ● S83.8X1   Sprain of other specified parts of right knee 🖎
    ● S83.8X2   Sprain of other specified parts of left knee 🖎
    ● S83.8X9   Sprain of other specified parts of unspecified knee 🖎
● S83.9   Sprain of unspecified site of knee
  X ● S83.90   Sprain of unspecified site of unspecified knee 🖎
  X ● S83.91   Sprain of unspecified site of right knee 🖎
  X ● S83.92   Sprain of unspecified site of left knee 🖎

● S84   **Injury of nerves at lower leg level**
  Code also any associated open wound (S81.-)
  Excludes2   injury of nerves at ankle and foot level (S94.-)
  The appropriate 7th character is to be added to each code from category S84

A	initial encounter
D	subsequent encounter
S	sequela

● S84.0   Injury of tibial nerve at lower leg level
  X ● S84.00   Injury of tibial nerve at lower leg level, unspecified leg 🖎
  X ● S84.01   Injury of tibial nerve at lower leg level, right leg 🖎
  X ● S84.02   Injury of tibial nerve at lower leg level, left leg 🖎
● S84.1   Injury of peroneal nerve at lower leg level
  X ● S84.10   Injury of peroneal nerve at lower leg level, unspecified leg 🖎
  X ● S84.11   Injury of peroneal nerve at lower leg level, right leg 🖎
  X ● S84.12   Injury of peroneal nerve at lower leg level, left leg 🖎

◀ New   ◀||| Revised   ~~deleted~~ Deleted   Excludes 1   Excludes 2   Includes   Use additional   Code first   Code also   Unspecified

OGCR Official Guidelines   ● Unacceptable Principal Diagnosis   X Assign placeholder X   ● Use Additional Character(s)   ▌ Manifestation Code   **Coding Clinic**

● S84.2   Injury of cutaneous sensory nerve at lower leg level
   X ● S84.20   Injury of cutaneous sensory nerve at lower leg level, unspecified leg 🔏
   X ● S84.21   Injury of cutaneous sensory nerve at lower leg level, right leg 🔏
   X ● S84.22   Injury of cutaneous sensory nerve at lower leg level, left leg 🔏

● S84.8   Injury of other nerves at lower leg level
   ● S84.80   Injury of other nerves at lower leg level
     ● S84.801   Injury of other nerves at lower leg level, right leg 🔏
     ● S84.802   Injury of other nerves at lower leg level, left leg 🔏
     ● S84.809   Injury of other nerves at lower leg level, unspecified leg 🔏

● S84.9   Injury of unspecified nerve at lower leg level
   X ● S84.90   Injury of unspecified nerve at lower leg level, unspecified leg 🔏
   X ● S84.91   Injury of unspecified nerve at lower leg level, right leg 🔏
   X ● S84.92   Injury of unspecified nerve at lower leg level, left leg 🔏

● S85   Injury of blood vessels at lower leg level
   Code also any associated open wound (S81.-)
   Excludes2   injury of blood vessels at ankle and foot level (S95.-)

   The appropriate 7th character is to be added to each code from category S85

     | | |
     A   initial encounter
     D   subsequent encounter
     S   sequela

● S85.0   Injury of popliteal artery
   ● S85.00   Unspecified injury of popliteal artery
     ● S85.001   Unspecified injury of popliteal artery, right leg A 🔏, 🔏
       (Ex:) S75.801[A], S75.809-S75.811[A], S75.819-S75.891[A], S75.899-S75.901[A], S75.909-S75.911[A], S75.919-S75.991[A], S75.999[A], S85.001[A], S85.009-S85.011[A], S85.019-S85.091[A], S85.099[A], S85.201[A], S85.209-S85.211[A], S85.219-S85.291[A], S85.299[A], S85.801[A], S85.809-S85.811[A], S85.819-S85.891[A], S85.899-S85.901[A], S85.909-S85.911[A], S85.919-S85.991[A], S85.999[A], S95.001[A], S95.009-S95.011[A], S95.019-S95.091[A], S95.099-S95.201[A], S95.209-S95.211[A], S95.219-S95.291[A], S95.299-S95.801[A], S95.809-S95.811[A], S95.819-S95.891[A], S95.899-S95.901[A], S95.909-S95.911[A], S95.919-S95.991[A], S95.999[A]

     ● S85.002   Unspecified injury of popliteal artery, left leg A 🔏, 🔏
       (Ex:) S75.802-S75.809[A], S75.812-S75.819[A], S75.892-S75.899[A], S75.902-S75.909[A], S75.912-S75.919[A], S75.992-S75.999[A], S85.002-S85.009[A], S85.012-S85.019[A], S85.092-S85.099[A], S85.202-S85.209[A], S85.212-S85.219[A], S85.292-S85.299[A], S85.802-S85.809[A], S85.812-S85.819[A], S85.892-S85.899[A], S85.902-S85.909[A], S85.912-S85.919[A], S85.992-S85.999[A], S95.002-S95.009[A], S95.012-S95.019[A], S95.092-S95.099[A], S95.202-S95.209[A], S95.212-S95.219[A], S95.292-S95.299[A], S95.802-S95.809[A], S95.812-S95.819[A], S95.892-S95.899[A], S95.902-S95.909[A], S95.912-S95.919[A], S95.992-S95.999[A]

● S85.009   Unspecified injury of popliteal artery, unspecified leg A 🔏, 🔏
   (Ex:) S75.802-S75.809[A], S75.812-S75.819[A], S75.892-S75.899[A], S75.902-S75.909[A], S75.912-S75.919[A], S75.992-S75.999[A], S85.162-S85.169[A], S85.172-S85.179[A], S85.182-S85.189[A], S85.202-S85.209[A], S85.212-S85.219[A], S85.292-S85.299[A], S85.802-S85.809[A], S85.812-S85.819[A], S85.892-S85.899[A], S85.902-S85.909[A], S85.912-S85.919[A], S85.992-S85.999[A], S95.002-S95.009[A], S95.012-S95.019[A], S95.092-S95.099[A], S95.202-S95.209[A], S95.212-S95.219[A], S95.292-S95.299[A], S95.802-S95.809[A], S95.812-S95.819[A], S95.892-S95.899[A], S95.902-S95.909[A], S95.912-S95.919[A], S95.992-S95.999[A]

● S85.01   Laceration of popliteal artery
   ● S85.011   Laceration of popliteal artery, right leg A 🔏, 🔏
     (Ex:) See S85.001
   ● S85.012   Laceration of popliteal artery, left leg A 🔏, 🔏
     (Ex:) See S85.002
   ● S85.019   Laceration of popliteal artery, unspecified leg A 🔏, 🔏
     (Ex:) See S85.009

● S85.09   Other specified injury of popliteal artery
   ● S85.091   Other specified injury of popliteal artery, right leg A 🔏, 🔏
     (Ex:) See S85.001
   ● S85.092   Other specified injury of popliteal artery, left leg A 🔏, 🔏
     (Ex:) See S85.002
   ● S85.099   Other specified injury of popliteal artery, unspecified leg A 🔏, 🔏
     (Ex:) See S85.009

● S85.1   Injury of tibial artery
   ● S85.10   Unspecified injury of unspecified tibial artery
     Injury of tibial artery NOS
     ● S85.101   Unspecified injury of unspecified tibial artery, right leg A 🔏, 🔏
       (Ex:) S75.801[A], S75.809-S75.811[A], S75.819-S75.891[A], S75.899-S75.901[A], S75.909-S75.911[A], S75.919-S75.991[A], S75.999[A], S85.101[A], S85.109-S85.111[A], S85.119-S85.121[A], S85.129[A], S85.201[A], S85.209-S85.211[A], S85.219-S85.291[A], S85.299[A], S85.801[A], S85.809-S85.811[A], S85.819-S85.891[A], S85.899-S85.901[A], S85.909-S85.911[A], S85.919-S85.991[A], S85.999[A], S95.001[A], S95.009-S95.011[A], S95.019-S95.091[A], S95.099-S95.201[A], S95.209-S95.211[A], S95.219-S95.291[A], S95.299-S95.801[A], S95.809-S95.811[A], S95.819-S95.891[A], S95.899-S95.901[A], S95.909-S95.911[A], S95.919-S95.991[A], S95.999[A]

     ● S85.102   Unspecified injury of unspecified tibial artery, left leg A 🔏, 🔏
       (Ex:) S75.802-S75.809[A], S75.812-S75.819[A], S75.892-S75.899[A], S75.902-S75.909[A], S75.912-S75.919[A], S75.992-S75.999[A], S85.102-S85.109[A], S85.112-S85.119[A], S85.122-S85.129[A], S85.202-S85.209[A], S85.212-S85.219[A], S85.292-S85.299[A], S85.802-S85.809[A], S85.812-S85.819[A], S85.892-S85.899[A], S85.902-S85.909[A], S85.912-S85.919[A], S85.992-S85.999[A], S95.002-S95.009[A], S95.012-S95.019[A], S95.092-S95.099[A], S95.202-S95.209[A], S95.212-S95.219[A], S95.292-S95.299[A], S95.802-S95.809[A], S95.812-S95.819[A], S95.892-S95.899[A], S95.902-S95.909[A], S95.912-S95.919[A], S95.992-S95.999[A]

N   Newborn Age: 0   P   Pediatric Age: 0–17   M   Maternity DX: 12–55   A   Adult Age: 15–124   ♀ Females Only   ♂ Males Only

🔏 Complication\Comorbidity   🔏 Major C\C   (Ex:) CC/MCC Exclusions   🔏 Present on Admission Requirement   🔏 Hospital-Acquired Condition

1469

CHAPTER 19 (S00–T88)

● S85.109   Unspecified injury of unspecified tibial artery, unspecified leg A 🔹, 🔹
    (Ex:) S75.801-S75.999[A], S85.101-S85.129[A], S85.201-S85.299[A], S85.801-S85.999[A], S95.001-S95.099[A], S95.201-S95.999[A]

● S85.11   Laceration of unspecified tibial artery

● S85.111   Laceration of unspecified tibial artery, right leg A 🔹, 🔹
    (Ex:) See S85.101

● S85.112   Laceration of unspecified tibial artery, left leg A 🔹, 🔹
    (Ex:) See S85.102

● S85.119   Laceration of unspecified tibial artery, unspecified leg A 🔹, 🔹
    (Ex:) See S85.109

● S85.12   Other specified injury of unspecified tibial artery

● S85.121   Other specified injury of unspecified tibial artery, right leg A 🔹, 🔹
    (Ex:) See S85.101

● S85.122   Other specified injury of unspecified tibial artery, left leg A 🔹, 🔹
    (Ex:) See S85.102

● S85.129   Other specified injury of unspecified tibial artery, unspecified leg A 🔹, 🔹
    (Ex:) See S85.109

● S85.13   Unspecified injury of anterior tibial artery

● S85.131   Unspecified injury of anterior tibial artery, right leg A 🔹, 🔹
    (Ex:) S75.801[A], S75.809-S75.811[A], S75.819-S75.891[A], S75.899-S75.901[A], S75.909-S75.911[A], S75.919-S75.991[A], S75.999[A], S85.131[A], S85.139-S85.141[A], S85.149-S85.151[A], S85.159[A], S85.201[A], S85.209-S85.211[A], S85.219-S85.291[A], S85.299[A], S85.801[A], S85.809-S85.811[A], S85.819-S85.891[A], S85.899-S85.901[A], S85.909-S85.911[A], S85.919-S85.991[A], S85.999[A], S95.001[A], S95.009-S95.011[A], S95.019-S95.091[A], S95.099-S95.201[A], S95.209-S95.211[A], S95.219-S95.291[A], S95.299-S95.801[A], S95.809-S95.811[A], S95.819-S95.891[A], S95.899-S95.901[A], S95.909-S95.911[A], S95.919-S95.991[A], S95.999[A]

● S85.132   Unspecified injury of anterior tibial artery, left leg A 🔹, 🔹
    (Ex:) S75.802-S75.809[A], S75.812-S75.819[A], S75.892-S75.899[A], S75.902-S75.909[A], S75.912-S75.919[A], S75.992-S75.999[A], S85.132-S85.139[A], S85.142-S85.149[A], S85.152-S85.159[A], S85.202-S85.209[A], S85.212-S85.219[A], S85.292-S85.299[A], S85.802-S85.809[A], S85.812-S85.819[A], S85.892-S85.899[A], S85.902-S85.909[A], S85.912-S85.919[A], S85.992-S85.999[A], S95.002-S95.009[A], S95.012-S95.019[A], S95.092-S95.099[A], S95.202-S95.209[A], S95.212-S95.219[A], S95.292-S95.299[A], S95.802-S95.809[A], S95.812-S95.819[A], S95.892-S95.899[A], S95.902-S95.909[A], S95.912-S95.919[A], S95.992-S95.999[A]

● S85.139   Unspecified injury of anterior tibial artery, unspecified leg A 🔹, 🔹
    (Ex:) S75.801-S75.999[A], S85.131-S85.159[A], S85.201-S85.299[A], S85.801-S85.999[A], S95.001-S95.099[A], S95.201-S95.999[A]

● S85.14   Laceration of anterior tibial artery

● S85.141   Laceration of anterior tibial artery, right leg A 🔹, 🔹
    (Ex:) See S85.131

● S85.142   Laceration of anterior tibial artery, left leg A 🔹, 🔹
    (Ex:) See S85.132

● S85.149   Laceration of anterior tibial artery, unspecified leg A 🔹, 🔹
    (Ex:) See S85.139

● S85.15   Other specified injury of anterior tibial artery

● S85.151   Other specified injury of anterior tibial artery, right leg A 🔹, 🔹
    (Ex:) See S85.131

● S85.152   Other specified injury of anterior tibial artery, left leg A 🔹, 🔹
    (Ex:) See S85.132

● S85.159   Other specified injury of anterior tibial artery, unspecified leg A 🔹, 🔹
    (Ex:) See S85.139

● S85.16   Unspecified injury of posterior tibial artery

● S85.161   Unspecified injury of posterior tibial artery, right leg A 🔹, 🔹
    (Ex:) S75.801[A], S75.809-S75.811[A], S75.819-S75.891[A], S75.899-S75.901[A], S75.909-S75.911[A], S75.919-S75.991[A], S75.999[A], S85.161[A], S85.169-S85.171[A], S85.179-S85.181[A], S85.189[A], S85.201[A], S85.209-S85.211[A], S85.219-S85.291[A], S85.299[A], S85.801[A], S85.809-S85.811[A], S85.819-S85.891[A], S85.899-S85.901[A], S85.909-S85.911[A], S85.919-S85.991[A], S85.999[A], S95.001[A], S95.009-S95.011[A], S95.019-S95.091[A], S95.099-S95.201[A], S95.209-S95.211[A], S95.219-S95.291[A], S95.299-S95.801[A], S95.809-S95.811[A], S95.819-S95.891[A], S95.899-S95.901[A], S95.909-S95.911[A], S95.919-S95.991[A], S95.999[A]

● S85.162   Unspecified injury of posterior tibial artery, left leg A 🔹, 🔹
    (Ex:) S75.802-S75.809[A], S75.812-S75.819[A], S75.892-S75.899[A], S75.902-S75.909[A], S75.912-S75.919[A], S75.992-S75.999[A], S85.162-S85.169[A], S85.172-S85.179[A], S85.182-S85.189[A], S85.202-S85.209[A], S85.212-S85.219[A], S85.292-S85.299[A], S85.802-S85.809[A], S85.812-S85.819[A], S85.892-S85.899[A], S85.902-S85.909[A], S85.912-S85.919[A], S85.992-S85.999[A], S95.002-S95.009[A], S95.012-S95.019[A], S95.092-S95.099[A], S95.202-S95.209[A], S95.212-S95.219[A], S95.292-S95.299[A], S95.802-S95.809[A], S95.812-S95.819[A], S95.892-S95.899[A], S95.902-S95.909[A], S95.912-S95.919[A], S95.992-S95.999[A]

● S85.169   Unspecified injury of posterior tibial artery, unspecified leg A 🔹, 🔹
    (Ex:) S75.801-S75.999[A], S85.161-S85.189[A], S85.201-S85.299[A], S85.801-S85.999[A], S95.001-S95.099[A], S95.201-S95.999[A]

◄ New   ◄ Revised   ~~deleted~~ Deleted   Excludes 1   Excludes 2   Includes   Use additional   Code first   Code also   Unspecified
OGCR Official Guidelines   ● Unacceptable Principal Diagnosis   X Assign placeholder X   ● Use Additional Character(s)   ▶ Manifestation Code   **Coding Clinic**

● **S85.17   Laceration of posterior tibial artery**
   ● S85.171   Laceration of posterior tibial artery, right leg A 🔾, 🔾
               (Ex:) See S85.161
   ● S85.172   Laceration of posterior tibial artery, left leg A 🔾, 🔾
               (Ex:) See S85.162
   ● S85.179   Laceration of posterior tibial artery, unspecified leg A 🔾, 🔾
               (Ex:) See S85.169

● **S85.18   Other specified injury of posterior tibial artery**
   ● S85.181   Other specified injury of posterior tibial artery, right leg A 🔾, 🔾
               (Ex:) See S85.161
   ● S85.182   Other specified injury of posterior tibial artery, left leg A 🔾, 🔾
               (Ex:) See S85.162
   ● S85.189   Other specified injury of posterior tibial artery, unspecified leg A 🔾, 🔾
               (Ex:) See S85.169

● **S85.2   Injury of peroneal artery**
   ● **S85.20   Unspecified injury of peroneal artery**
      ● S85.201   Unspecified injury of peroneal artery, right leg A 🔾, 🔾
                  (Ex:) See S75.801
      ● S85.202   Unspecified injury of peroneal artery, left leg A 🔾, 🔾
                  (Ex:) See S75.802
      ● S85.209   Unspecified injury of peroneal artery, unspecified leg A 🔾, 🔾
                  (Ex:) See S75.809

   ● **S85.21   Laceration of peroneal artery**
      ● S85.211   Laceration of peroneal artery, right leg A 🔾, 🔾
                  (Ex:) See S75.801
      ● S85.212   Laceration of peroneal artery, left leg A 🔾, 🔾
                  (Ex:) See S75.802
      ● S85.219   Laceration of peroneal artery, unspecified leg A 🔾, 🔾
                  (Ex:) See S75.809

   ● **S85.29   Other specified injury of peroneal artery**
      ● S85.291   Other specified injury of peroneal artery, right leg A 🔾, 🔾
                  (Ex:) See S75.801
      ● S85.292   Other specified injury of peroneal artery, left leg A 🔾, 🔾
                  (Ex:) See S75.802
      ● S85.299   Other specified injury of peroneal artery, unspecified leg A 🔾, 🔾
                  (Ex:) See S75.809

● **S85.3   Injury of greater saphenous vein at lower leg level**
   Injury of greater saphenous vein NOS
   Injury of saphenous vein NOS
   ● **S85.30   Unspecified injury of greater saphenous vein at lower leg level**
      ● S85.301   Unspecified injury of greater saphenous vein at lower leg level, right leg A 🔾, 🔾
                  (Ex:) See S75.201
      ● S85.302   Unspecified injury of greater saphenous vein at lower leg level, left leg A 🔾, 🔾
                  (Ex:) See S75.202
      ● S85.309   Unspecified injury of greater saphenous vein at lower leg level, unspecified leg A 🔾, 🔾
                  (Ex:) See S75.209

● **S85.31   Laceration of greater saphenous vein at lower leg level**
   ● S85.311   Laceration of greater saphenous vein at lower leg level, right leg A 🔾, 🔾
               (Ex:) See S75.201
   ● S85.312   Laceration of greater saphenous vein at lower leg level, left leg A 🔾, 🔾
               (Ex:) See S75.202
   ● S85.319   Laceration of greater saphenous vein at lower leg level, unspecified leg A 🔾, 🔾
               (Ex:) See S75.209

● **S85.39   Other specified injury of greater saphenous vein at lower leg level**
   ● S85.391   Other specified injury of greater saphenous vein at lower leg level, right leg A 🔾, 🔾
               (Ex:) See S75.201
   ● S85.392   Other specified injury of greater saphenous vein at lower leg level, left leg A 🔾, 🔾
               (Ex:) See S75.202
   ● S85.399   Other specified injury of greater saphenous vein at lower leg level, unspecified leg A 🔾, 🔾
               (Ex:) See S75.209

● **S85.4   Injury of lesser saphenous vein at lower leg level**
   ● **S85.40   Unspecified injury of lesser saphenous vein at lower leg level**
      ● S85.401   Unspecified injury of lesser saphenous vein at lower leg level, right leg A 🔾, 🔾
                  (Ex:) See S75.201
      ● S85.402   Unspecified injury of lesser saphenous vein at lower leg level, left leg A 🔾, 🔾
                  (Ex:) See S75.202
      ● S85.409   Unspecified injury of lesser saphenous vein at lower leg level, unspecified leg A 🔾, 🔾
                  (Ex:) See S75.209

   ● **S85.41   Laceration of lesser saphenous vein at lower leg level**
      ● S85.411   Laceration of lesser saphenous vein at lower leg level, right leg A 🔾, 🔾
                  (Ex:) See S75.201
      ● S85.412   Laceration of lesser saphenous vein at lower leg level, left leg A 🔾, 🔾
                  (Ex:) See S75.202
      ● S85.419   Laceration of lesser saphenous vein at lower leg level, unspecified leg A 🔾, 🔾
                  (Ex:) See S75.209

   ● **S85.49   Other specified injury of lesser saphenous vein at lower leg level**
      ● S85.491   Other specified injury of lesser saphenous vein at lower leg level, right leg A 🔾, 🔾
                  (Ex:) See S75.201
      ● S85.492   Other specified injury of lesser saphenous vein at lower leg level, left leg A 🔾, 🔾
                  (Ex:) See S75.202
      ● S85.499   Other specified injury of lesser saphenous vein at lower leg level, unspecified leg A 🔾, 🔾
                  (Ex:) See S75.209

N Newborn Age: 0   **P** Pediatric Age: 0–17   **M** Maternity DX: 12–55   **A** Adult Age: 15–124   ♀ Females Only   ♂ Males Only

🔾 Complication\Comorbidity   🔾 Major C\C   (Ex:) CC/MCC Exclusions   🔾 Present on Admission Requirement   🔾 Hospital-Acquired Condition

● S85.5   Injury of popliteal vein
   ● S85.50   Unspecified injury of popliteal vein
      ● S85.501   Unspecified injury of popliteal vein, right leg A 🔖, 🔖
          Ex: S75.801[A], S75.809-S75.811[A], S75.819-S75.891[A], S75.899-S75.901[A], S75.909-S75.911[A], S75.919-S75.991[A], S75.999[A], S85.201[A], S85.209-S85.211[A], S85.219-S85.291[A], S85.299[A], S85.501[A], S85.509-S85.511[A], S85.519-S85.591[A], S85.599[A], S85.801[A], S85.809-S85.811[A], S85.819-S85.891[A], S85.899-S85.901[A], S85.909-S85.911[A], S85.919-S85.991[A], S85.999[A], S95.001[A], S95.009-S95.011[A], S95.019-S95.091[A], S95.099-S95.201[A], S95.209-S95.211[A], S95.219-S95.291[A], S95.299-S95.801[A], S95.809-S95.811[A], S95.819-S95.891[A], S95.899-S95.901[A], S95.909-S95.911[A], S95.919-S95.991[A], S95.999[A]

      ● S85.502   Unspecified injury of popliteal vein, left leg A 🔖, 🔖
          Ex: S75.802-S75.809[A], S75.812-S75.819[A], S75.892-S75.899[A], S75.902-S75.909[A], S75.912-S75.919[A], S75.992-S75.999[A], S85.202-S85.209[A], S85.212-S85.219[A], S85.292-S85.299[A], S85.502-S85.509[A], S85.512-S85.519[A], S85.592-S85.599[A], S85.802-S85.809[A], S85.812-S85.819[A], S85.892-S85.899[A], S85.902-S85.909[A], S85.912-S85.919[A], S85.992-S85.999[A], S95.002-S95.009[A], S95.012-S95.019[A], S95.092-S95.099[A], S95.202-S95.209[A], S95.212-S95.219[A], S95.292-S95.299[A], S95.802-S95.809[A], S95.812-S95.819[A], S95.892-S95.899[A], S95.902-S95.909[A], S95.912-S95.919[A], S95.992-S95.999[A]

      ● S85.509   Unspecified injury of popliteal vein, unspecified leg A 🔖, 🔖
          Ex: S75.801-S75.999[A], S85.201-S85.299[A], S85.501-S85.599[A], S85.801-S85.999[A], S95.001-S95.099[A], S95.201-S95.999[A]

   ● S85.51   Laceration of popliteal vein
      ● S85.511   Laceration of popliteal vein, right leg A 🔖, 🔖
          Ex: See S85.501
      ● S85.512   Laceration of popliteal vein, left leg A 🔖, 🔖
          Ex: See S85.502
      ● S85.519   Laceration of popliteal vein, unspecified leg A 🔖, 🔖
          Ex: See S85.509

   ● S85.59   Other specified injury of popliteal vein
      ● S85.591   Other specified injury of popliteal vein, right leg A 🔖, 🔖
          Ex: See S85.501
      ● S85.592   Other specified injury of popliteal vein, left leg A 🔖, 🔖
          Ex: See S85.502
      ● S85.599   Other specified injury of popliteal vein, unspecified leg A 🔖, 🔖
          Ex: See S85.509

● S85.8   Injury of other blood vessels at lower leg level
   ● S85.80   Unspecified injury of other blood vessels at lower leg level
      ● S85.801   Unspecified injury of other blood vessels at lower leg level, right leg A 🔖, 🔖
          Ex: See S75.801
      ● S85.802   Unspecified injury of other blood vessels at lower leg level, left leg A 🔖, 🔖
          Ex: See S75.802
      ● S85.809   Unspecified injury of other blood vessels at lower leg level, unspecified leg A 🔖, 🔖
          Ex: See S75.809

   ● S85.81   Laceration of other blood vessels at lower leg level
      ● S85.811   Laceration of other blood vessels at lower leg level, right leg A 🔖, 🔖
          Ex: See S75.801
      ● S85.812   Laceration of other blood vessels at lower leg level, left leg A 🔖, 🔖
          Ex: See S75.802
      ● S85.819   Laceration of other blood vessels at lower leg level, unspecified leg A 🔖, 🔖
          Ex: See S75.809

   ● S85.89   Other specified injury of other blood vessels at lower leg level
      ● S85.891   Other specified injury of other blood vessels at lower leg level, right leg A 🔖, 🔖
          Ex: See S75.801
      ● S85.892   Other specified injury of other blood vessels at lower leg level, left leg A 🔖, 🔖
          Ex: See S75.802
      ● S85.899   Other specified injury of other blood vessels at lower leg level, unspecified leg A 🔖, 🔖
          Ex: See S75.809

● S85.9   Injury of unspecified blood vessel at lower leg level
   ● S85.90   Unspecified injury of unspecified blood vessel at lower leg level
      ● S85.901   Unspecified injury of unspecified blood vessel at lower leg level, right leg A 🔖, 🔖
          Ex: See S75.801
      ● S85.902   Unspecified injury of unspecified blood vessel at lower leg level, left leg A 🔖, 🔖
          Ex: See S75.802
      ● S85.909   Unspecified injury of unspecified blood vessel at lower leg level, unspecified leg A 🔖, 🔖
          Ex: See S75.809

   ● S85.91   Laceration of unspecified blood vessel at lower leg level
      ● S85.911   Laceration of unspecified blood vessel at lower leg level, right leg A 🔖, 🔖
          Ex: See S75.801
      ● S85.912   Laceration of unspecified blood vessel at lower leg level, left leg A 🔖, 🔖
          Ex: See S75.802
      ● S85.919   Laceration of unspecified blood vessel at lower leg level, unspecified leg A 🔖, 🔖
          Ex: See S75.809

◀ New   ◀ Revised   ~~deleted~~ Deleted   Excludes 1   Excludes 2   Includes   Use additional   Code first   Code also   Unspecified
OGCR Official Guidelines   ● Unacceptable Principal Diagnosis   X Assign placeholder X   ▶ Use Additional Character(s)   ▶ Manifestation Code   Coding Clinic

- **S85.99** Other specified injury of unspecified blood vessel at lower leg level
  - **S85.991** Other specified injury of unspecified blood vessel at lower leg level, right leg A 🗝, 🗝
    - (Ex:) See S75.801
  - **S85.992** Other specified injury of unspecified blood vessel at lower leg level, left leg A 🗝, 🗝
    - (Ex:) See S75.802
  - **S85.999** Other specified injury of unspecified blood vessel at lower leg level, unspecified leg A 🗝, 🗝
    - (Ex:) See S75.809

- **S86** Injury of muscle, fascia and tendon at lower leg level

  Code also any associated open wound (S81.-)

  Excludes2   injury of muscle, fascia and tendon at ankle (S96.-)

        injury of patellar ligament (tendon) (S76.1-)

        sprain of joints and ligaments of knee (S83.-)

  The appropriate 7th character is to be added to each code from category S86

A	initial encounter
D	subsequent encounter
S	sequela

  - **S86.0** Injury of Achilles tendon
    - **S86.00** Unspecified injury of Achilles tendon
      - **S86.001** Unspecified injury of right Achilles tendon 🗝
      - **S86.002** Unspecified injury of left Achilles tendon 🗝
      - **S86.009** Unspecified injury of unspecified Achilles tendon 🗝
    - **S86.01** Strain of Achilles tendon
      - **S86.011** Strain of right Achilles tendon 🗝
      - **S86.012** Strain of left Achilles tendon 🗝
      - **S86.019** Strain of unspecified Achilles tendon 🗝
    - **S86.02** Laceration of Achilles tendon
      - **S86.021** Laceration of right Achilles tendon A 🗝, 🗝
        - (Ex:) S81.001[A], S81.009-S81.011[A], S81.019-S81.021[A], S81.029-S81.031[A], S81.039-S81.041[A], S81.049-S81.051[A], S81.059-S81.801[A], S81.809-S81.811[A], S81.819-S81.821[A], S81.829-S81.831[A], S81.839-S81.841[A], S81.849-S81.851[A], S81.859[A], S86.021[A], S86.029[A], S86.121[A], S86.129[A], S86.221[A], S86.229[A], S86.321[A], S86.329[A], S86.821[A], S86.829-S86.921[A], S86.929[A], S91.001[A], S91.009[A], S91.011[A], S91.019-S91.021[A], S91.029-S91.031[A], S91.039-S91.041[A], S91.049-S91.051[A], S91.059[A], S96.021[A], S96.029[A], S96.121[A], S96.129[A], S96.221[A], S96.229[A], S96.821[A], S96.829[A], S96.921[A], S96.929[A]

  - **S86.022** Laceration of left Achilles tendon A 🗝, 🗝
    - (Ex:) S81.002-S81.009[A], S81.012-S81.019[A], S81.022-S81.029[A], S81.032-S81.039[A], S81.042-S81.049[A], S81.052-S81.059[A], S81.802-S81.809[A], S81.812-S81.819[A], S81.822-S81.829[A], S81.832-S81.839[A], S81.842-S81.849[A], S81.852-S81.859[A], S86.022-S86.029[A], S86.122-S86.129[A], S86.222-S86.229[A], S86.322-S86.329[A], S86.822-S86.829[A], S86.922-S86.929[A], S91.002-S91.009[A], S91.012-S91.019[A], S91.022-S91.029[A], S91.032-S91.039[A], S91.042-S91.049[A], S91.052-S91.059[A], S96.022-S96.029[A], S96.122-S96.129[A], S96.222-S96.229[A], S96.822-S96.829[A], S96.922-S96.929[A]
  - **S86.029** Laceration of unspecified Achilles tendon A 🗝, 🗝
    - (Ex:) S81.001-S81.859[A], S86.021-S86.029[A], S86.121-S86.129[A], S86.221-S86.229[A], S86.321-S86.329[A], S86.821-S86.829[A], S86.921-S86.929[A], S91.001-S91.059[A], S96.021-S96.029[A], S96.121-S96.129[A], S96.221-S96.229[A], S96.821-S96.829[A], S96.921-S96.929[A]
  - **S86.09** Other specified injury of Achilles tendon
    - **S86.091** Other specified injury of right Achilles tendon 🗝
    - **S86.092** Other specified injury of left Achilles tendon 🗝
    - **S86.099** Other specified injury of unspecified Achilles tendon 🗝

  - **S86.1** Injury of other muscle(s) and tendon(s) of posterior muscle group at lower leg level
    - **S86.10** Unspecified injury of other muscle(s) and tendon(s) of posterior muscle group at lower leg level
      - **S86.101** Unspecified injury of other muscle(s) and tendon(s) of posterior muscle group at lower leg level, right leg 🗝
      - **S86.102** Unspecified injury of other muscle(s) and tendon(s) of posterior muscle group at lower leg level, left leg 🗝
      - **S86.109** Unspecified injury of other muscle(s) and tendon(s) of posterior muscle group at lower leg level, unspecified leg 🗝
    - **S86.11** Strain of other muscle(s) and tendon(s) of posterior muscle group at lower leg level
      - **S86.111** Strain of other muscle(s) and tendon(s) of posterior muscle group at lower leg level, right leg 🗝
      - **S86.112** Strain of other muscle(s) and tendon(s) of posterior muscle group at lower leg level, left leg 🗝
      - **S86.119** Strain of other muscle(s) and tendon(s) of posterior muscle group at lower leg level, unspecified leg 🗝

N   Newborn Age: 0   P   Pediatric Age: 0–17   M   Maternity DX: 12–55   A   Adult Age: 15–124   ♀   Females Only   ♂   Males Only

🗝   Complication\Comorbidity   🗝   Major C\C   (Ex:)   CC/MCC Exclusions   🗝   Present on Admission Requirement   🗝   Hospital-Acquired Condition

1473

● S86.12   Laceration of other muscle(s) and tendon(s) of posterior muscle group at lower leg level

  ● S86.121   Laceration of other muscle(s) and tendon(s) of posterior muscle group at lower leg level, right leg A 🐾, 🐾
             (Ex:) See S86.021

  ● S86.122   Laceration of other muscle(s) and tendon(s) of posterior muscle group at lower leg level, left leg A 🐾, 🐾
             (Ex:) See S86.022

  ● S86.129   Laceration of other muscle(s) and tendon(s) of posterior muscle group at lower leg level, unspecified leg A 🐾, 🐾
             (Ex:) See S86.029

● S86.19   Other injury of other muscle(s) and tendon(s) of posterior muscle group at lower leg level

  ● S86.191   Other injury of other muscle(s) and tendon(s) of posterior muscle group at lower leg level, right leg 🐾

  ● S86.192   Other injury of other muscle(s) and tendon(s) of posterior muscle group at lower leg level, left leg 🐾

  ● S86.199   Other injury of other muscle(s) and tendon(s) of posterior muscle group at lower leg level, unspecified leg 🐾

● S86.2   Injury of muscle(s) and tendon(s) of anterior muscle group at lower leg level

  ● S86.20   Unspecified injury of muscle(s) and tendon(s) of anterior muscle group at lower leg level

    ● S86.201   Unspecified injury of muscle(s) and tendon(s) of anterior muscle group at lower leg level, right leg 🐾

    ● S86.202   Unspecified injury of muscle(s) and tendon(s) of anterior muscle group at lower leg level, left leg 🐾

    ● S86.209   Unspecified injury of muscle(s) and tendon(s) of anterior muscle group at lower leg level, unspecified leg 🐾

  ● S86.21   Strain of muscle(s) and tendon(s) of anterior muscle group at lower leg level

    ● S86.211   Strain of muscle(s) and tendon(s) of anterior muscle group at lower leg level, right leg 🐾

    ● S86.212   Strain of muscle(s) and tendon(s) of anterior muscle group at lower leg level, left leg 🐾

    ● S86.219   Strain of muscle(s) and tendon(s) of anterior muscle group at lower leg level, unspecified leg 🐾

  ● S86.22   Laceration of muscle(s) and tendon(s) of anterior muscle group at lower leg level

    ● S86.221   Laceration of muscle(s) and tendon(s) of anterior muscle group at lower leg level, right leg A 🐾, 🐾
               (Ex:) See S86.021

    ● S86.222   Laceration of muscle(s) and tendon(s) of anterior muscle group at lower leg level, left leg A 🐾, 🐾
               (Ex:) See S86.022

    ● S86.229   Laceration of muscle(s) and tendon(s) of anterior muscle group at lower leg level, unspecified leg A 🐾, 🐾
               (Ex:) See S86.029

● S86.29   Other injury of muscle(s) and tendon(s) of anterior muscle group at lower leg level

  ● S86.291   Other injury of muscle(s) and tendon(s) of anterior muscle group at lower leg level, right leg 🐾

  ● S86.292   Other injury of muscle(s) and tendon(s) of anterior muscle group at lower leg level, left leg 🐾

  ● S86.299   Other injury of muscle(s) and tendon(s) of anterior muscle group at lower leg level, unspecified leg 🐾

● S86.3   Injury of muscle(s) and tendon(s) of peroneal muscle group at lower leg level

  ● S86.30   Unspecified injury of muscle(s) and tendon(s) of peroneal muscle group at lower leg level

    ● S86.301   Unspecified injury of muscle(s) and tendon(s) of peroneal muscle group at lower leg level, right leg 🐾

    ● S86.302   Unspecified injury of muscle(s) and tendon(s) of peroneal muscle group at lower leg level, left leg 🐾

    ● S86.309   Unspecified injury of muscle(s) and tendon(s) of peroneal muscle group at lower leg level, unspecified leg 🐾

  ● S86.31   Strain of muscle(s) and tendon(s) of peroneal muscle group at lower leg level

    ● S86.311   Strain of muscle(s) and tendon(s) of peroneal muscle group at lower leg level, right leg 🐾

    ● S86.312   Strain of muscle(s) and tendon(s) of peroneal muscle group at lower leg level, left leg 🐾

    ● S86.319   Strain of muscle(s) and tendon(s) of peroneal muscle group at lower leg level, unspecified leg 🐾

  ● S86.32   Laceration of muscle(s) and tendon(s) of peroneal muscle group at lower leg level

    ● S86.321   Laceration of muscle(s) and tendon(s) of peroneal muscle group at lower leg level, right leg A 🐾, 🐾
               (Ex:) See S86.021

    ● S86.322   Laceration of muscle(s) and tendon(s) of peroneal muscle group at lower leg level, left leg A 🐾, 🐾
               (Ex:) See S86.022

    ● S86.329   Laceration of muscle(s) and tendon(s) of peroneal muscle group at lower leg level, unspecified leg A 🐾, 🐾
               (Ex:) See S86.029

  ● S86.39   Other injury of muscle(s) and tendon(s) of peroneal muscle group at lower leg level

    ● S86.391   Other injury of muscle(s) and tendon(s) of peroneal muscle group at lower leg level, right leg 🐾

    ● S86.392   Other injury of muscle(s) and tendon(s) of peroneal muscle group at lower leg level, left leg 🐾

    ● S86.399   Other injury of muscle(s) and tendon(s) of peroneal muscle group at lower leg level, unspecified leg 🐾

◀ New   ◀▥ Revised   ~~deleted~~ Deleted   Excludes 1   Excludes 2   Includes   Use additional   Code first   Code also   Unspecified
OGCR Official Guidelines   ● Unacceptable Principal Diagnosis   X Assign placeholder X   ▶ Use Additional Character(s)   ▶ Manifestation Code   Coding Clinic

- S86.8   Injury of other muscles and tendons at lower leg level
  - S86.80   Unspecified injury of other muscles and tendons at lower leg level
    - S86.801   Unspecified injury of other muscle(s) and tendon(s) at lower leg level, right leg 🗝
    - S86.802   Unspecified injury of other muscle(s) and tendon(s) at lower leg level, left leg 🗝
    - S86.809   Unspecified injury of other muscle(s) and tendon(s) at lower leg level, unspecified leg 🗝
  - S86.81   Strain of other muscles and tendons at lower leg level
    - S86.811   Strain of other muscle(s) and tendon(s) at lower leg level, right leg 🗝
    - S86.812   Strain of other muscle(s) and tendon(s) at lower leg level, left leg 🗝
    - S86.819   Strain of other muscle(s) and tendon(s) at lower leg level, unspecified leg 🗝
  - S86.82   Laceration of other muscles and tendons at lower leg level
    - S86.821   Laceration of other muscle(s) and tendon(s) at lower leg level, right leg A 🗝, 🗝
      - (Ex) See S86.021
    - S86.822   Laceration of other muscle(s) and tendon(s) at lower leg level, left leg A 🗝, 🗝
      - (Ex) See S86.022
    - S86.829   Laceration of other muscle(s) and tendon(s) at lower leg level, unspecified leg A 🗝, 🗝
      - (Ex) See S86.029
  - S86.89   Other injury of other muscles and tendons at lower leg level
    - S86.891   Other injury of other muscle(s) and tendon(s) at lower leg level, right leg 🗝
    - S86.892   Other injury of other muscle(s) and tendon(s) at lower leg level, left leg 🗝
    - S86.899   Other injury of other muscle(s) and tendon(s) at lower leg level, unspecified leg 🗝
- S86.9   Injury of unspecified muscle and tendon at lower leg level
  - S86.90   Unspecified injury of unspecified muscle and tendon at lower leg level
    - S86.901   Unspecified injury of unspecified muscle(s) and tendon(s) at lower leg level, right leg 🗝
    - S86.902   Unspecified injury of unspecified muscle(s) and tendon(s) at lower leg level, left leg 🗝
    - S86.909   Unspecified injury of unspecified muscle(s) and tendon(s) at lower leg level, unspecified leg 🗝
  - S86.91   Strain of unspecified muscle and tendon at lower leg level
    - S86.911   Strain of unspecified muscle(s) and tendon(s) at lower leg level, right leg 🗝
    - S86.912   Strain of unspecified muscle(s) and tendon(s) at lower leg level, left leg 🗝
    - S86.919   Strain of unspecified muscle(s) and tendon(s) at lower leg level, unspecified leg 🗝

- S86.92   Laceration of unspecified muscle and tendon at lower leg level
  - S86.921   Laceration of unspecified muscle(s) and tendon(s) at lower leg level, right leg A 🗝, 🗝
    - (Ex) See S86.021
  - S86.922   Laceration of unspecified muscle(s) and tendon(s) at lower leg level, left leg A 🗝, 🗝
    - (Ex) See S86.022
  - S86.929   Laceration of unspecified muscle(s) and tendon(s) at lower leg level, unspecified leg A 🗝, 🗝
    - (Ex) See S86.029
  - S86.99   Other injury of unspecified muscle and tendon at lower leg level
    - S86.991   Other injury of unspecified muscle(s) and tendon(s) at lower leg level, right leg 🗝
    - S86.992   Other injury of unspecified muscle(s) and tendon(s) at lower leg level, left leg 🗝
    - S86.999   Other injury of unspecified muscle(s) and tendon(s) at lower leg level, unspecified leg 🗝

- S87   Crushing injury of lower leg
  - Use additional code(s) for all associated injuries
  - **Excludes2**   crushing injury of ankle and foot (S97.-)
  - The appropriate 7th character is to be added to each code from category S87

A	initial encounter
D	subsequent encounter
S	sequela

  - S87.0   Crushing injury of knee
    - X ● S87.00   Crushing injury of unspecified knee 🗝
    - X ● S87.01   Crushing injury of right knee 🗝
    - X ● S87.02   Crushing injury of left knee 🗝
  - S87.8   Crushing injury of lower leg
    - X ● S87.80   Crushing injury of unspecified lower leg 🗝
    - X ● S87.81   Crushing injury of right lower leg 🗝
    - X ● S87.82   Crushing injury of left lower leg 🗝

- S88   Traumatic amputation of lower leg
  - An amputation not identified as partial or complete should be coded to complete
  - **Excludes1**   traumatic amputation of ankle and foot (S98.-)
  - The appropriate 7th character is to be added to each code from category S88

A	initial encounter
D	subsequent encounter
S	sequela

  - S88.0   Traumatic amputation at knee level
    - S88.01   Complete traumatic amputation at knee level
      - S88.011   Complete traumatic amputation at knee level, right lower leg A 🗝, 🗝
        - (Ex) See S78.011
      - S88.012   Complete traumatic amputation at knee level, left lower leg A 🗝, 🗝
        - (Ex) See S78.012
      - S88.019   Complete traumatic amputation at knee level, unspecified lower leg A 🗝, 🗝
        - (Ex) See S78.019

N Newborn Age: 0   **P** Pediatric Age: 0–17   **M** Maternity DX: 12–55   **A** Adult Age: 15–124   ♀ Females Only   ♂ Males Only

🗝 Complication\Comorbidity   🗝 Major C\C   (Ex) CC/MCC Exclusions   🗝 Present on Admission Requirement   🗝 Hospital-Acquired Condition

1475

S88.02   Partial traumatic amputation at knee level

    S88.021   Partial traumatic amputation at knee level, right lower leg A,
        (Ex:) See S78.011

    S88.022   Partial traumatic amputation at knee level, left lower leg A,
        (Ex:) See S78.012

    S88.029   Partial traumatic amputation at knee level, unspecified lower leg A,
        (Ex:) See S78.019

S88.1   Traumatic amputation at level between knee and ankle

  S88.11   Complete traumatic amputation at level between knee and ankle

    S88.111   Complete traumatic amputation at level between knee and ankle, right lower leg A,
        (Ex:) See S78.011

    S88.112   Complete traumatic amputation at level between knee and ankle, left lower leg A,
        (Ex:) See S78.012

    S88.119   Complete traumatic amputation at level between knee and ankle, unspecified lower leg A,
        (Ex:) See S78.019

  S88.12   Partial traumatic amputation at level between knee and ankle

    S88.121   Partial traumatic amputation at level between knee and ankle, right lower leg A,
        (Ex:) See S78.011

    S88.122   Partial traumatic amputation at level between knee and ankle, left lower leg A,
        (Ex:) See S78.012

    S88.129   Partial traumatic amputation at level between knee and ankle, unspecified lower leg A,
        (Ex:) See S78.019

S88.9   Traumatic amputation of lower leg, level unspecified

  S88.91   Complete traumatic amputation of lower leg, level unspecified

    S88.911   Complete traumatic amputation of right lower leg, level unspecified A,
        (Ex:) See S78.011

    S88.912   Complete traumatic amputation of left lower leg, level unspecified A,
        (Ex:) See S78.012

    S88.919   Complete traumatic amputation of unspecified lower leg, level unspecified A,
        (Ex:) See S78.019

  S88.92   Partial traumatic amputation of lower leg, level unspecified

    S88.921   Partial traumatic amputation of right lower leg, level unspecified A,
        (Ex:) See S78.011

    S88.922   Partial traumatic amputation of left lower leg, level unspecified A,
        (Ex:) See S78.012

    S88.929   Partial traumatic amputation of unspecified lower leg, level unspecified A,
        (Ex:) See S78.019

S89   Other and unspecified injuries of lower leg

  Note: A fracture not indicated as open or closed should be coded to closed

  Excludes2   other and unspecified injuries of ankle and foot (S99.-)

  The appropriate 7th character is to be added to each code from subcategories S89.0, S89.1, S89.2, and S89.3

  A   initial encounter for closed fracture
  D   subsequent encounter for fracture with routine healing
  G   subsequent encounter for fracture with delayed healing
  K   subsequent encounter for fracture with nonunion
  P   subsequent encounter for fracture with malunion
  S   sequela

S89.0   Physeal fracture of upper end of tibia

  S89.00   Unspecified physeal fracture of upper end of tibia

    S89.001   Unspecified physeal fracture of upper end of right tibia A, K, P, , A
        (Ex:) For S89.001[A]: See S82.101[A]
        For S89.001[K,P]: See S72.001[K,M,N,P,Q,R]

    S89.002   Unspecified physeal fracture of upper end of left tibia A, K, P, , A
        (Ex:) For S89.002[A]: See S82.102[A]
        For S89.002[K,P]: See S72.001[K,M,N,P,Q,R]

    S89.009   Unspecified physeal fracture of upper end of unspecified tibia A, K, P, , A
        (Ex:) For S89.009[A]: See S82.101[B,C]
        For S89.009[K,P]: See S72.001[K,M,N,P,Q,R]

  S89.01   Salter-Harris Type I physeal fracture of upper end of tibia

    S89.011   Salter-Harris Type I physeal fracture of upper end of right tibia A, K, P, , A
        (Ex:) For S89.011[A]: See S82.101[A]
        For S89.011[K,P]: See S72.001[K,M,N,P,Q,R]

    S89.012   Salter-Harris Type I physeal fracture of upper end of left tibia A, K, P, , A
        (Ex:) For S89.012[A]: See S82.102[A]
        For S89.012[K,P]: See S72.001[K,M,N,P,Q,R]

    S89.019   Salter-Harris Type I physeal fracture of upper end of unspecified tibia A, K, P, , A
        (Ex:) For S89.019[A]: See S82.101[B,C]
        For S89.019[K,P]: See S72.001[K,M,N,P,Q,R]

  S89.02   Salter-Harris Type II physeal fracture of upper end of tibia

    S89.021   Salter-Harris Type II physeal fracture of upper end of right tibia A, K, P, , A
        (Ex:) For S89.021[A]: See S82.101[A]
        For S89.021[K,P]: See S72.001[K,M,N,P,Q,R]

    S89.022   Salter-Harris Type II physeal fracture of upper end of left tibia A, K, P, , A
        (Ex:) For S89.022[A]: See S82.102[A]
        For S89.022[K,P]: See S72.001[K,M,N,P,Q,R]

    S89.029   Salter-Harris Type II physeal fracture of upper end of unspecified tibia A, K, P, , A
        (Ex:) For S89.029[A]: See S82.101[B,C]
        For S89.029[K,P]: See S72.001[K,M,N,P,Q,R]

● **S89.03**   Salter-Harris Type III physeal fracture of upper end of tibia

     ● **S89.031**   Salter-Harris Type III physeal fracture of upper end of right tibia A, K, P 🝙, 🝙, A 🝙

        (Ex) **For S89.031[A]:** See S82.101[A]
        For S89.031[K,P]: See S72.001[K,M,N,P,Q,R]

     ● **S89.032**   Salter-Harris Type III physeal fracture of upper end of left tibia A, K, P 🝙, 🝙, A 🝙

        (Ex) **For S89.032[A]:** See S82.102[A]
        For S89.032[K,P]: See S72.001[K,M,N,P,Q,R]

     ● **S89.039**   Salter-Harris Type III physeal fracture of upper end of unspecified tibia A, K, P 🝙, 🝙, A 🝙

        (Ex) **For S89.039[A]:** See S82.101[B,C]
        For S89.039[K,P]: See S72.001[K,M,N,P,Q,R]

● **S89.04**   Salter-Harris Type IV physeal fracture of upper end of tibia

     ● **S89.041**   Salter-Harris Type IV physeal fracture of upper end of right tibia A, K, P 🝙, 🝙, A 🝙

        (Ex) **For S89.041[A]:** See S82.101[A]
        For S89.041[K,P]: See S72.001[K,M,N,P,Q,R]

     ● **S89.042**   Salter-Harris Type IV physeal fracture of upper end of left tibia A, K, P 🝙, 🝙, A 🝙

        (Ex) **For S89.042[A]:** See S82.102[A]
        For S89.042[K,P]: See S72.001[K,M,N,P,Q,R]

     ● **S89.049**   Salter-Harris Type IV physeal fracture of upper end of unspecified tibia A, K, P 🝙, 🝙, A 🝙

        (Ex) **For S89.049[A]:** See S82.101[B,C]
        For S89.049[K,P]: See S72.001[K,M,N,P,Q,R]

● **S89.09**   Other physeal fracture of upper end of tibia

     ● **S89.091**   Other physeal fracture of upper end of right tibia A, K, P 🝙, 🝙, A 🝙

        (Ex) **For S89.091[A]:** See S82.101[A]
        For S89.091[K,P]: See S72.001[K,M,N,P,Q,R]

     ● **S89.092**   Other physeal fracture of upper end of left tibia A, K, P 🝙, 🝙, A 🝙

        (Ex) **For S89.092[A]:** See S82.102[A]
        For S89.092[K,P]: See S72.001[K,M,N,P,Q,R]

     ● **S89.099**   Other physeal fracture of upper end of unspecified tibia A, K, P 🝙, 🝙, A 🝙

        (Ex) **For S89.099[A]:** See S82.101[B,C]
        For S89.099[K,P]: See S72.001[K,M,N,P,Q,R]

● **S89.1**   Physeal fracture of lower end of tibia

     (Ex) **For category S89.1 CC codes:** See S72.001[K,M,N,P,Q,R]

● **S89.10**   Unspecified physeal fracture of lower end of tibia

     ● **S89.101**   Unspecified physeal fracture of lower end of right tibia K, P 🝙, 🝙

     ● **S89.102**   Unspecified physeal fracture of lower end of left tibia K, P 🝙, 🝙

     ● **S89.109**   Unspecified physeal fracture of lower end of unspecified tibia K, P 🝙, 🝙

● **S89.11**   Salter-Harris Type I physeal fracture of lower end of tibia

     ● **S89.111**   Salter-Harris Type I physeal fracture of lower end of right tibia K, P 🝙, 🝙

     ● **S89.112**   Salter-Harris Type I physeal fracture of lower end of left tibia K, P 🝙, 🝙

     ● **S89.119**   Salter-Harris Type I physeal fracture of lower end of unspecified tibia K, P 🝙, 🝙

● **S89.12**   Salter-Harris Type II physeal fracture of lower end of tibia

     ● **S89.121**   Salter-Harris Type II physeal fracture of lower end of right tibia K, P 🝙, 🝙

     ● **S89.122**   Salter-Harris Type II physeal fracture of lower end of left tibia K, P 🝙, 🝙

     ● **S89.129**   Salter-Harris Type II physeal fracture of lower end of unspecified tibia K, P 🝙, 🝙

● **S89.13**   Salter-Harris Type III physeal fracture of lower end of tibia

     Excludes1   fracture of medial malleolus (adult) (S82.5-)

     ● **S89.131**   Salter-Harris Type III physeal fracture of lower end of right tibia K, P 🝙, 🝙

     ● **S89.132**   Salter-Harris Type III physeal fracture of lower end of left tibia K, P 🝙, 🝙

     ● **S89.139**   Salter-Harris Type III physeal fracture of lower end of unspecified tibia K, P 🝙, 🝙

● **S89.14**   Salter-Harris Type IV physeal fracture of lower end of tibia

     Excludes1   fracture of medial malleolus (adult) (S82.5-)

     ● **S89.141**   Salter-Harris Type IV physeal fracture of lower end of right tibia K, P 🝙, 🝙

     ● **S89.142**   Salter-Harris Type IV physeal fracture of lower end of left tibia K, P 🝙, 🝙

     ● **S89.149**   Salter-Harris Type IV physeal fracture of lower end of unspecified tibia K, P 🝙, 🝙

● **S89.19**   Other physeal fracture of lower end of tibia

     ● **S89.191**   Other physeal fracture of lower end of right tibia K, P 🝙, 🝙

     ● **S89.192**   Other physeal fracture of lower end of left tibia K, P 🝙, 🝙

     ● **S89.199**   Other physeal fracture of lower end of unspecified tibia K, P 🝙, 🝙

● **S89.2**   Physeal fracture of upper end of fibula

     (Ex) **For category S89.2 CC codes:** See S72.001[K,M,N,P,Q,R]

● **S89.20**   Unspecified physeal fracture of upper end of fibula

     ● **S89.201**   Unspecified physeal fracture of upper end of right fibula K, P 🝙, 🝙

     ● **S89.202**   Unspecified physeal fracture of upper end of left fibula K, P 🝙, 🝙

     ● **S89.209**   Unspecified physeal fracture of upper end of unspecified fibula K, P 🝙, 🝙

● **S89.21**   Salter-Harris Type I physeal fracture of upper end of fibula

     ● **S89.211**   Salter-Harris Type I physeal fracture of upper end of right fibula K, P 🝙, 🝙

     ● **S89.212**   Salter-Harris Type I physeal fracture of upper end of left fibula K, P 🝙, 🝙

     ● **S89.219**   Salter-Harris Type I physeal fracture of upper end of unspecified fibula K, P 🝙, 🝙

● **S89.22**   Salter-Harris Type II physeal fracture of upper end of fibula

     ● **S89.221**   Salter-Harris Type II physeal fracture of upper end of right fibula K, P 🝙, 🝙

     ● **S89.222**   Salter-Harris Type II physeal fracture of upper end of left fibula K, P 🝙, 🝙

     ● **S89.229**   Salter-Harris Type II physeal fracture of upper end of unspecified fibula K, P 🝙, 🝙

N Newborn Age: 0   **P** Pediatric Age: 0–17   **M** Maternity DX: 12–55   **A** Adult Age: 15–124   ♀ Females Only   ♂ Males Only

🝙 Complication\Comorbidity   🝙 Major C\C   (Ex) CC/MCC Exclusions   🝙 Present on Admission Requirement   🝙 Hospital-Acquired Condition

● S89.29   Other physeal fracture of upper end of fibula
   ● S89.291   Other physeal fracture of upper end of right fibula K, P 🐾, 🐾
   ● S89.292   Other physeal fracture of upper end of left fibula K, P 🐾, 🐾
   ● S89.299   Other physeal fracture of upper end of unspecified fibula K, P 🐾, 🐾
● S89.3   Physeal fracture of lower end of fibula
   Ex: For category S89.3 CC codes: See S72.001[K,M,N,P,Q,R]
  ● S89.30   Unspecified physeal fracture of lower end of fibula
   ● S89.301   Unspecified physeal fracture of lower end of right fibula K, P 🐾, 🐾
   ● S89.302   Unspecified physeal fracture of lower end of left fibula K, P 🐾, 🐾
   ● S89.309   Unspecified physeal fracture of lower end of unspecified fibula K, P 🐾, 🐾
  ● S89.31   Salter-Harris Type I physeal fracture of lower end of fibula
   ● S89.311   Salter-Harris Type I physeal fracture of lower end of right fibula K, P 🐾, 🐾
   ● S89.312   Salter-Harris Type I physeal fracture of lower end of left fibula K, P 🐾, 🐾
   ● S89.319   Salter-Harris Type I physeal fracture of lower end of unspecified fibula K, P 🐾, 🐾
  ● S89.32   Salter-Harris Type II physeal fracture of lower end of fibula
   ● S89.321   Salter-Harris Type II physeal fracture of lower end of right fibula K, P 🐾, 🐾
   ● S89.322   Salter-Harris Type II physeal fracture of lower end of left fibula K, P 🐾, 🐾
   ● S89.329   Salter-Harris Type II physeal fracture of lower end of unspecified fibula K, P 🐾, 🐾
  ● S89.39   Other physeal fracture of lower end of fibula
   ● S89.391   Other physeal fracture of lower end of right fibula K, P 🐾, 🐾
   ● S89.392   Other physeal fracture of lower end of left fibula K, P 🐾, 🐾
   ● S89.399   Other physeal fracture of lower end of unspecified fibula K, P 🐾, 🐾
● S89.8   Other specified injuries of lower leg

> The appropriate 7th character is to be added to each code in subcategory S89.8
>
> | A | initial encounter |
> | D | subsequent encounter |
> | S | sequela |

 X● S89.80   Other specified injuries of unspecified lower leg 🐾
 X● S89.81   Other specified injuries of right lower leg 🐾
 X● S89.82   Other specified injuries of left lower leg 🐾
● S89.9   Unspecified injury of lower leg

> The appropriate 7th character is to be added to each code in subcategory S89.9
>
> | A | initial encounter |
> | D | subsequent encounter |
> | S | sequela |

 X● S89.90   Unspecified injury of unspecified lower leg 🐾
 X● S89.91   Unspecified injury of right lower leg 🐾
 X● S89.92   Unspecified injury of left lower leg 🐾

INJURIES TO THE ANKLE AND FOOT (S90-S99)

Excludes2   burns and corrosions (T20-T32)
           fracture of ankle and malleolus (S82.-)
           frostbite (T33-T34)
           insect bite or sting, venomous (T63.4)

● S90   Superficial injury of ankle, foot and toes

> The appropriate 7th character is to be added to each code from category S90
>
> | A | initial encounter |
> | D | subsequent encounter |
> | S | sequela |

 ● S90.0   Contusion of ankle
 X● S90.00   Contusion of unspecified ankle 🐾
 X● S90.01   Contusion of right ankle 🐾
 X● S90.02   Contusion of left ankle 🐾
 ● S90.1   Contusion of toe without damage to nail
  ● S90.11   Contusion of great toe without damage to nail
   ● S90.111   Contusion of right great toe without damage to nail 🐾
   ● S90.112   Contusion of left great toe without damage to nail 🐾
   ● S90.119   Contusion of unspecified great toe without damage to nail 🐾
  ● S90.12   Contusion of lesser toe without damage to nail
   ● S90.121   Contusion of right lesser toe(s) without damage to nail 🐾
   ● S90.122   Contusion of left lesser toe(s) without damage to nail 🐾
   ● S90.129   Contusion of unspecified lesser toe(s) without damage to nail 🐾
         Contusion of toe NOS
 ● S90.2   Contusion of toe with damage to nail
  ● S90.21   Contusion of great toe with damage to nail
   ● S90.211   Contusion of right great toe with damage to nail 🐾
   ● S90.212   Contusion of left great toe with damage to nail 🐾
   ● S90.219   Contusion of unspecified great toe with damage to nail 🐾
  ● S90.22   Contusion of lesser toe with damage to nail
   ● S90.221   Contusion of right lesser toe(s) with damage to nail 🐾
   ● S90.222   Contusion of left lesser toe(s) with damage to nail 🐾
   ● S90.229   Contusion of unspecified lesser toe(s) with damage to nail 🐾
 ● S90.3   Contusion of foot
   Excludes2   contusion of toes (S90.1-, S90.2-)
 ● S90.30   Contusion of unspecified foot 🐾
         Contusion of foot NOS
 ● S90.31   Contusion of right foot 🐾
 ● S90.32   Contusion of left foot 🐾
 ● S90.4   Other superficial injuries of toe
  ● S90.41   Abrasion of toe
   ● S90.411   Abrasion, right great toe 🐾
   ● S90.412   Abrasion, left great toe 🐾
   ● S90.413   Abrasion, unspecified great toe 🐾
   ● S90.414   Abrasion, right lesser toe(s) 🐾
   ● S90.415   Abrasion, left lesser toe(s) 🐾
   ● S90.416   Abrasion, unspecified lesser toe(s) 🐾

● **S90.42**   **Blister (nonthermal) of toe**
    ● S90.421   Blister (nonthermal), right great toe 🔾
    ● S90.422   Blister (nonthermal), left great toe 🔾
    ● S90.423   Blister (nonthermal), unspecified great toe 🔾
    ● S90.424   Blister (nonthermal), right lesser toe(s) 🔾
    ● S90.425   Blister (nonthermal), left lesser toe(s) 🔾
    ● S90.426   Blister (nonthermal), unspecified lesser toe(s) 🔾

● **S90.44**   **External constriction of toe**
    Hair tourniquet syndrome of toe
    ● S90.441   External constriction, right great toe 🔾
    ● S90.442   External constriction, left great toe 🔾
    ● S90.443   External constriction, unspecified great toe 🔾
    ● S90.444   External constriction, right lesser toe(s) 🔾
    ● S90.445   External constriction, left lesser toe(s) 🔾
    ● S90.446   External constriction, unspecified lesser toe(s) 🔾

● **S90.45**   **Superficial foreign body of toe**
    Splinter in the toe
    ● S90.451   Superficial foreign body, right great toe 🔾
    ● S90.452   Superficial foreign body, left great toe 🔾
    ● S90.453   Superficial foreign body, unspecified great toe 🔾
    ● S90.454   Superficial foreign body, right lesser toe(s) 🔾
    ● S90.455   Superficial foreign body, left lesser toe(s) 🔾
    ● S90.456   Superficial foreign body, unspecified lesser toe(s) 🔾

● **S90.46**   **Insect bite (nonvenomous) of toe**
    ● S90.461   Insect bite (nonvenomous), right great toe 🔾
    ● S90.462   Insect bite (nonvenomous), left great toe 🔾
    ● S90.463   Insect bite (nonvenomous), unspecified great toe 🔾
    ● S90.464   Insect bite (nonvenomous), right lesser toe(s) 🔾
    ● S90.465   Insect bite (nonvenomous), left lesser toe(s) 🔾
    ● S90.466   Insect bite (nonvenomous), unspecified lesser toe(s) 🔾

● **S90.47**   **Other superficial bite of toe**
    Excludes1   open bite of toe (S91.15-, S91.25-)
    ● S90.471   Other superficial bite of right great toe 🔾
    ● S90.472   Other superficial bite of left great toe 🔾
    ● S90.473   Other superficial bite of unspecified great toe 🔾
    ● S90.474   Other superficial bite of right lesser toe(s) 🔾
    ● S90.475   Other superficial bite of left lesser toe(s) 🔾
    ● S90.476   Other superficial bite of unspecified lesser toe(s) 🔾

● **S90.5**   **Other superficial injuries of ankle**
   ● **S90.51**   **Abrasion of ankle**
    ● S90.511   Abrasion, right ankle 🔾
    ● S90.512   Abrasion, left ankle 🔾
    ● S90.519   Abrasion, unspecified ankle 🔾
   ● **S90.52**   **Blister (nonthermal) of ankle**
    ● S90.521   Blister (nonthermal), right ankle 🔾
    ● S90.522   Blister (nonthermal), left ankle 🔾
    ● S90.529   Blister (nonthermal), unspecified ankle 🔾
   ● **S90.54**   **External constriction of ankle**
    ● S90.541   External constriction, right ankle 🔾
    ● S90.542   External constriction, left ankle 🔾
    ● S90.549   External constriction, unspecified ankle 🔾
   ● **S90.55**   **Superficial foreign body of ankle**
    Splinter in the ankle
    ● S90.551   Superficial foreign body, right ankle 🔾
    ● S90.552   Superficial foreign body, left ankle 🔾
    ● S90.559   Superficial foreign body, unspecified ankle 🔾
   ● **S90.56**   **Insect bite (nonvenomous) of ankle**
    ● S90.561   Insect bite (nonvenomous), right ankle 🔾
    ● S90.562   Insect bite (nonvenomous), left ankle 🔾
    ● S90.569   Insect bite (nonvenomous), unspecified ankle 🔾
   ● **S90.57**   **Other superficial bite of ankle**
    Excludes1   open bite of ankle (S91.05-)
    ● S90.571   Other superficial bite of ankle, right ankle 🔾
    ● S90.572   Other superficial bite of ankle, left ankle 🔾
    ● S90.579   Other superficial bite of ankle, unspecified ankle 🔾

● **S90.8**   **Other superficial injuries of foot**
   ● **S90.81**   **Abrasion of foot**
    ● S90.811   Abrasion, right foot 🔾
    ● S90.812   Abrasion, left foot 🔾
    ● S90.819   Abrasion, unspecified foot 🔾
   ● **S90.82**   **Blister (nonthermal) of foot**
    ● S90.821   Blister (nonthermal), right foot 🔾
    ● S90.822   Blister (nonthermal), left foot 🔾
    ● S90.829   Blister (nonthermal), unspecified foot 🔾
   ● **S90.84**   **External constriction of foot**
    ● S90.841   External constriction, right foot 🔾
    ● S90.842   External constriction, left foot 🔾
    ● S90.849   External constriction, unspecified foot 🔾
   ● **S90.85**   **Superficial foreign body of foot**
    Splinter in the foot
    ● S90.851   Superficial foreign body, right foot 🔾
    ● S90.852   Superficial foreign body, left foot 🔾
    ● S90.859   Superficial foreign body, unspecified foot 🔾
   ● **S90.86**   **Insect bite (nonvenomous) of foot**
    ● S90.861   Insect bite (nonvenomous), right foot 🔾
    ● S90.862   Insect bite (nonvenomous), left foot 🔾
    ● S90.869   Insect bite (nonvenomous), unspecified foot 🔾

N   Newborn Age: 0   **P**   Pediatric Age: 0–17   **M**   Maternity DX: 12–55   **A**   Adult Age: 15–124   ♀   Females Only   ♂   Males Only

🔾   Complication\Comorbidity   🔾   Major C\C   Ⓔx   CC/MCC Exclusions   🔾   Present on Admission Requirement   🔾   Hospital-Acquired Condition

1479

● **S90.87**   Other superficial bite of foot
       Excludes1   open bite of foot (S91.35-)
     ● **S90.871**   Other superficial bite of right foot 🖢
     ● **S90.872**   Other superficial bite of left foot 🖢
     ● **S90.879**   Other superficial bite of unspecified foot 🖢

● **S90.9**   Unspecified superficial injury of ankle, foot and toe
     ● **S90.91**   Unspecified superficial injury of ankle
         ● **S90.911**   Unspecified superficial injury of right ankle 🖢
         ● **S90.912**   Unspecified superficial injury of left ankle 🖢
         ● **S90.919**   Unspecified superficial injury of unspecified ankle 🖢
     ● **S90.92**   Unspecified superficial injury of foot
         ● **S90.921**   Unspecified superficial injury of right foot 🖢
         ● **S90.922**   Unspecified superficial injury of left foot 🖢
         ● **S90.929**   Unspecified superficial injury of unspecified foot 🖢
     S90.93   Unspecified superficial injury of toes
         ● **S90.931**   Unspecified superficial injury of right great toe 🖢
         ● **S90.932**   Unspecified superficial injury of left great toe 🖢
         ● **S90.933**   Unspecified superficial injury of unspecified great toe 🖢
         ● **S90.934**   Unspecified superficial injury of right lesser toe(s) 🖢
         ● **S90.935**   Unspecified superficial injury of left lesser toe(s) 🖢
         ● **S90.936**   Unspecified superficial injury of unspecified lesser toe(s) 🖢

● **S91**   Open wound of ankle, foot and toes
     Code also any associated wound infection
     Excludes1   open fracture of ankle, foot and toes (S92.-with 7th character B)
                traumatic amputation of ankle and foot (S98.-)
     The appropriate 7th character is to be added to each code from category S91

A	initial encounter
D	subsequent encounter
S	sequela

● **S91.0**   Open wound of ankle
     ● **S91.00**   Unspecified open wound of ankle
         ● **S91.001**   Unspecified open wound, right ankle 🖢
         ● **S91.002**   Unspecified open wound, left ankle 🖢
         ● **S91.009**   Unspecified open wound, unspecified ankle 🖢
     ● **S91.01**   Laceration without foreign body of ankle
         ● **S91.011**   Laceration without foreign body, right ankle 🖢
         ● **S91.012**   Laceration without foreign body, left ankle 🖢
         ● **S91.019**   Laceration without foreign body, unspecified ankle 🖢
     ● **S91.02**   Laceration with foreign body of ankle
         ● **S91.021**   Laceration with foreign body, right ankle 🖢
         ● **S91.022**   Laceration with foreign body, left ankle 🖢
         ● **S91.029**   Laceration with foreign body, unspecified ankle 🖢

● **S91.03**   Puncture wound without foreign body of ankle
     ● **S91.031**   Puncture wound without foreign body, right ankle 🖢
     ● **S91.032**   Puncture wound without foreign body, left ankle 🖢
     ● **S91.039**   Puncture wound without foreign body, unspecified ankle 🖢
● **S91.04**   Puncture wound with foreign body of ankle
     ● **S91.041**   Puncture wound with foreign body, right ankle 🖢
     ● **S91.042**   Puncture wound with foreign body, left ankle 🖢
     ● **S91.049**   Puncture wound with foreign body, unspecified ankle 🖢
● **S91.05**   Open bite of ankle
       Excludes1   superficial bite of ankle (S90.56-, S90.57-)
     ● **S91.051**   Open bite, right ankle 🖢
     ● **S91.052**   Open bite, left ankle 🖢
     ● **S91.059**   Open bite, unspecified ankle 🖢

● **S91.1**   Open wound of toe without damage to nail
     ● **S91.10**   Unspecified open wound of toe without damage to nail
         ● **S91.101**   Unspecified open wound of right great toe without damage to nail 🖢
         ● **S91.102**   Unspecified open wound of left great toe without damage to nail 🖢
         ● **S91.103**   Unspecified open wound of unspecified great toe without damage to nail 🖢
         ● **S91.104**   Unspecified open wound of right lesser toe(s) without damage to nail 🖢
         ● **S91.105**   Unspecified open wound of left lesser toe(s) without damage to nail 🖢
         ● **S91.106**   Unspecified open wound of unspecified lesser toe(s) without damage to nail 🖢
         ● **S91.109**   Unspecified open wound of unspecified toe(s) without damage to nail 🖢
     ● **S91.11**   Laceration without foreign body of toe without damage to nail
         ● **S91.111**   Laceration without foreign body of right great toe without damage to nail 🖢
         ● **S91.112**   Laceration without foreign body of left great toe without damage to nail 🖢
         ● **S91.113**   Laceration without foreign body of unspecified great toe without damage to nail 🖢
         ● **S91.114**   Laceration without foreign body of right lesser toe(s) without damage to nail 🖢
         ● **S91.115**   Laceration without foreign body of left lesser toe(s) without damage to nail 🖢
         ● **S91.116**   Laceration without foreign body of unspecified lesser toe(s) without damage to nail 🖢
         ● **S91.119**   Laceration without foreign body of unspecified toe without damage to nail 🖢

● S91.12   Laceration with foreign body of toe without damage to nail

● S91.121   Laceration with foreign body of right great toe without damage to nail 🖐

● S91.122   Laceration with foreign body of left great toe without damage to nail 🖐

● S91.123   Laceration with foreign body of unspecified great toe without damage to nail 🖐

● S91.124   Laceration with foreign body of right lesser toe(s) without damage to nail 🖐

● S91.125   Laceration with foreign body of left lesser toe(s) without damage to nail 🖐

● S91.126   Laceration with foreign body of unspecified lesser toe(s) without damage to nail 🖐

● S91.129   Laceration with foreign body of unspecified toe(s) without damage to nail 🖐

● S91.13   Puncture wound without foreign body of toe without damage to nail

● S91.131   Puncture wound without foreign body of right great toe without damage to nail 🖐

● S91.132   Puncture wound without foreign body of left great toe without damage to nail 🖐

● S91.133   Puncture wound without foreign body of unspecified great toe without damage to nail 🖐

● S91.134   Puncture wound without foreign body of right lesser toe(s) without damage to nail 🖐

● S91.135   Puncture wound without foreign body of left lesser toe(s) without damage to nail 🖐

● S91.136   Puncture wound without foreign body of unspecified lesser toe(s) without damage to nail 🖐

● S91.139   Puncture wound without foreign body of unspecified toe(s) without damage to nail 🖐

● S91.14   Puncture wound with foreign body of toe without damage to nail

● S91.141   Puncture wound with foreign body of right great toe without damage to nail 🖐

● S91.142   Puncture wound with foreign body of left great toe without damage to nail 🖐

● S91.143   Puncture wound with foreign body of unspecified great toe without damage to nail 🖐

● S91.144   Puncture wound with foreign body of right lesser toe(s) without damage to nail 🖐

● S91.145   Puncture wound with foreign body of left lesser toe(s) without damage to nail 🖐

● S91.146   Puncture wound with foreign body of unspecified lesser toe(s) without damage to nail 🖐

● S91.149   Puncture wound with foreign body of unspecified toe(s) without damage to nail 🖐

● S91.15   Open bite of toe without damage to nail
Bite of toe NOS

Excludes1   superficial bite of toe (S90.46-, S90.47-)

● S91.151   Open bite of right great toe without damage to nail 🖐

● S91.152   Open bite of left great toe without damage to nail 🖐

● S91.153   Open bite of unspecified great toe without damage to nail 🖐

● S91.154   Open bite of right lesser toe(s) without damage to nail 🖐

● S91.155   Open bite of left lesser toe(s) without damage to nail 🖐

● S91.156   Open bite of unspecified lesser toe(s) without damage to nail 🖐

● S91.159   Open bite of unspecified toe(s) without damage to nail 🖐

● S91.2   Open wound of toe with damage to nail

● S91.20   Unspecified open wound of toe with damage to nail

● S91.201   Unspecified open wound of right great toe with damage to nail 🖐

● S91.202   Unspecified open wound of left great toe with damage to nail 🖐

● S91.203   Unspecified open wound of unspecified great toe with damage to nail 🖐

● S91.204   Unspecified open wound of right lesser toe(s) with damage to nail 🖐

● S91.205   Unspecified open wound of left lesser toe(s) with damage to nail 🖐

● S91.206   Unspecified open wound of unspecified lesser toe(s) with damage to nail 🖐

● S91.209   Unspecified open wound of unspecified toe(s) with damage to nail 🖐

● S91.21   Laceration without foreign body of toe with damage to nail

● S91.211   Laceration without foreign body of right great toe with damage to nail 🖐

● S91.212   Laceration without foreign body of left great toe with damage to nail 🖐

● S91.213   Laceration without foreign body of unspecified great toe with damage to nail 🖐

● S91.214   Laceration without foreign body of right lesser toe(s) with damage to nail 🖐

● S91.215   Laceration without foreign body of left lesser toe(s) with damage to nail 🖐

● S91.216   Laceration without foreign body of unspecified lesser toe(s) with damage to nail 🖐

● S91.219   Laceration without foreign body of unspecified toe(s) with damage to nail 🖐

N Newborn Age: 0   **P** Pediatric Age: 0–17   **M** Maternity DX: 12–55   **A** Adult Age: 15–124   ♀ Females Only   ♂ Males Only

🖐 Complication\Comorbidity   🖐 Major C\C   (Ex) CC/MCC Exclusions   🖐 Present on Admission Requirement   🖐 Hospital-Acquired Condition

1481

● S91.22   Laceration with foreign body of toe with damage to nail
   ● S91.221   Laceration with foreign body of right great toe with damage to nail 🖎
   ● S91.222   Laceration with foreign body of left great toe with damage to nail 🖎
   ● S91.223   Laceration with foreign body of unspecified great toe with damage to nail 🖎
   ● S91.224   Laceration with foreign body of right lesser toe(s) with damage to nail 🖎
   ● S91.225   Laceration with foreign body of left lesser toe(s) with damage to nail 🖎
   ● S91.226   Laceration with foreign body of unspecified lesser toe(s) with damage to nail 🖎
   ● S91.229   Laceration with foreign body of unspecified toe(s) with damage to nail 🖎

● S91.23   Puncture wound without foreign body of toe with damage to nail
   ● S91.231   Puncture wound without foreign body of right great toe with damage to nail 🖎
   ● S91.232   Puncture wound without foreign body of left great toe with damage to nail 🖎
   ● S91.233   Puncture wound without foreign body of unspecified great toe with damage to nail 🖎
   ● S91.234   Puncture wound without foreign body of right lesser toe(s) with damage to nail 🖎
   ● S91.235   Puncture wound without foreign body of left lesser toe(s) with damage to nail 🖎
   ● S91.236   Puncture wound without foreign body of unspecified lesser toe(s) with damage to nail 🖎
   ● S91.239   Puncture wound without foreign body of unspecified toe(s) with damage to nail 🖎

● S91.24   Puncture wound with foreign body of toe with damage to nail
   ● S91.241   Puncture wound with foreign body of right great toe with damage to nail 🖎
   ● S91.242   Puncture wound with foreign body of left great toe with damage to nail 🖎
   ● S91.243   Puncture wound with foreign body of unspecified great toe with damage to nail 🖎
   ● S91.244   Puncture wound with foreign body of right lesser toe(s) with damage to nail 🖎
   ● S91.245   Puncture wound with foreign body of left lesser toe(s) with damage to nail 🖎
   ● S91.246   Puncture wound with foreign body of unspecified lesser toe(s) with damage to nail 🖎
   ● S91.249   Puncture wound with foreign body of unspecified toe(s) with damage to nail 🖎

● S91.25   Open bite of toe with damage to nail
   Bite of toe with damage to nail NOS
   Excludes1   superficial bite of toe (S90.46-, S90.47-)
   ● S91.251   Open bite of right great toe with damage to nail 🖎
   ● S91.252   Open bite of left great toe with damage to nail 🖎
   ● S91.253   Open bite of unspecified great toe with damage to nail 🖎
   ● S91.254   Open bite of right lesser toe(s) with damage to nail 🖎
   ● S91.255   Open bite of left lesser toe(s) with damage to nail 🖎
   ● S91.256   Open bite of unspecified lesser toe(s) with damage to nail 🖎
   ● S91.259   Open bite of unspecified toe(s) with damage to nail 🖎

● S91.3   Open wound of foot
  ● S91.30   Unspecified open wound of foot
   ● S91.301   Unspecified open wound, right foot 🖎
   ● S91.302   Unspecified open wound, left foot 🖎
   ● S91.309   Unspecified open wound, unspecified foot 🖎

  ● S91.31   Laceration without foreign body of foot
   ● S91.311   Laceration without foreign body, right foot 🖎
   ● S91.312   Laceration without foreign body, left foot 🖎
   ● S91.319   Laceration without foreign body, unspecified foot 🖎

  ● S91.32   Laceration with foreign body of foot
   ● S91.321   Laceration with foreign body, right foot 🖎
   ● S91.322   Laceration with foreign body, left foot 🖎
   ● S91.329   Laceration with foreign body, unspecified foot 🖎

  ● S91.33   Puncture wound without foreign body of foot
   ● S91.331   Puncture wound without foreign body, right foot 🖎
   ● S91.332   Puncture wound without foreign body, left foot 🖎
   ● S91.339   Puncture wound without foreign body, unspecified foot 🖎

  ● S91.34   Puncture wound with foreign body of foot
   ● S91.341   Puncture wound with foreign body, right foot 🖎
   ● S91.342   Puncture wound with foreign body, left foot 🖎
   ● S91.349   Puncture wound with foreign body, unspecified foot 🖎

  ● S91.35   Open bite of foot
   Excludes1   superficial bite of foot (S90.86-, S90.87-)
   ● S91.351   Open bite, right foot 🖎
   ● S91.352   Open bite, left foot 🖎
   ● S91.359   Open bite, unspecified foot 🖎

CHAPTER 19 (S00-T88)

◄ New   ◄ Revised   ~~deleted~~ Deleted   Excludes 1   Excludes 2   Includes   Use additional   Code first   Code also   Unspecified
OGCR Official Guidelines   ● Unacceptable Principal Diagnosis   X Assign placeholder X   ● Use Additional Character(s)   ▮ Manifestation Code   **Coding Clinic**

● **S92   Fracture of foot and toe, except ankle**

    Note: A fracture not indicated as displaced or nondisplaced should be coded to displaced

    A fracture not indicated as open or closed should be coded to closed

    Excludes1 traumatic amputation of ankle and foot (S98.-)

    Excludes2 fracture of ankle (S82.-)
                     fracture of malleolus (S82.-)

    The appropriate 7th character is to be added to each code from category S92

A	initial encounter for closed fracture
B	initial encounter for open fracture
D	subsequent encounter for fracture with routine healing
G	subsequent encounter for fracture with delayed healing
K	subsequent encounter for fracture with nonunion
P	subsequent encounter for fracture with malunion
S	sequela

● **S92.0   Fracture of calcaneus**

    Heel bone   Os calcis

    (Ex) **For category S92.0 CC codes S92.0[B]:** M80.00X-M80.019[A], M80.041-M80.049[A], M80.061-M80.819[A], M80.841-M80.849[A], M80.861-M80.879[A], M84.40X-M84.419[A], M84.441-M84.446[A], M84.454[A], M84.461-M84.519[A], M84.541-M84.550[A], M84.561-M84.576[A], M84.60X-M84.619[A], M84.641-M84.650[A], M84.661-M84.68X[A], S03.8XX-S03.9XX[A], S29.011-S29.019[A], S38.3XX[A], S39.011-S39.013[A], S73.101-S73.199[A], S76.001-S76.019[A], S76.091-S76.219[A], S76.291-S76.319[A], S76.391-S76.819[A], S76.891-S76.919[A], S76.991-S76.999[A], S79.811-S79.929[A], S82.90X-S82.92X[A,B,C], S92.001-S92.066[B], S92.101-S92.356[A,B], S92.901-S92.909[A,B], T14.8-T14.91, T79. A9X-T79.9XX[A] **For S92.0[K,P]:** See S72.001[K,M,N,P,Q,R]

    ● **S92.00   Unspecified fracture of calcaneus**

        ● **S92.001** Unspecified fracture of right calcaneus B, K, P 🔵, 🔵, B 🔵

        ● **S92.002** Unspecified fracture of left calcaneus B, K, P 🔵, 🔵, B 🔵

        ● **S92.009** Unspecified fracture of unspecified calcaneus B, K, P 🔵, 🔵, B 🔵

    ● **S92.01   Fracture of body of calcaneus**

        ● **S92.011** Displaced fracture of body of right calcaneus B, K, P 🔵, 🔵, B 🔵

        ● **S92.012** Displaced fracture of body of left calcaneus B, K, P 🔵, 🔵, B 🔵

        ● **S92.013** Displaced fracture of body of unspecified calcaneus B, K, P 🔵, 🔵, B 🔵

        ● **S92.014** Nondisplaced fracture of body of right calcaneus B, K, P 🔵, 🔵, B 🔵

        ● **S92.015** Nondisplaced fracture of body of left calcaneus B, K, P 🔵, 🔵, B 🔵

        ● **S92.016** Nondisplaced fracture of body of unspecified calcaneus B, K, P 🔵, 🔵, B 🔵

    ● **S92.02   Fracture of anterior process of calcaneus**

        ● **S92.021** Displaced fracture of anterior process of right calcaneus B, K, P 🔵, 🔵, B 🔵

        ● **S92.022** Displaced fracture of anterior process of left calcaneus B, K, P 🔵, 🔵, B 🔵

        ● **S92.023** Displaced fracture of anterior process of unspecified calcaneus B, K, P 🔵, 🔵, B 🔵

        ● **S92.024** Nondisplaced fracture of anterior process of right calcaneus B, K, P 🔵, 🔵, B 🔵

        ● **S92.025** Nondisplaced fracture of anterior process of left calcaneus B, K, P 🔵, 🔵, B 🔵

        ● **S92.026** Nondisplaced fracture of anterior process of unspecified calcaneus B, K, P 🔵, 🔵, B 🔵

● **S92.03   Avulsion fracture of tuberosity of calcaneus**

    ● **S92.031** Displaced avulsion fracture of tuberosity of right calcaneus B, K, P 🔵, 🔵, B 🔵

    ● **S92.032** Displaced avulsion fracture of tuberosity of left calcaneus B, K, P 🔵, 🔵, B 🔵

    ● **S92.033** Displaced avulsion fracture of tuberosity of unspecified calcaneus B, K, P 🔵, B 🔵

    ● **S92.034** Nondisplaced avulsion fracture of tuberosity of right calcaneus B, K, P 🔵, 🔵, B 🔵

    ● **S92.035** Nondisplaced avulsion fracture of tuberosity of left calcaneus B, K, P 🔵, 🔵, B 🔵

    ● **S92.036** Nondisplaced avulsion fracture of tuberosity of unspecified calcaneus B, K, P 🔵, 🔵, B 🔵

● **S92.04   Other fracture of tuberosity of calcaneus**

    ● **S92.041** Displaced other fracture of tuberosity of right calcaneus B, K, P 🔵, 🔵, B 🔵

    ● **S92.042** Displaced other fracture of tuberosity of left calcaneus B, K, P 🔵, 🔵, B 🔵

    ● **S92.043** Displaced other fracture of tuberosity of unspecified calcaneus B, K, P 🔵, 🔵, B 🔵

    ● **S92.044** Nondisplaced other fracture of tuberosity of right calcaneus B, K, P 🔵, 🔵, B 🔵

    ● **S92.045** Nondisplaced other fracture of tuberosity of left calcaneus B, K, P 🔵, 🔵, B 🔵

    ● **S92.046** Nondisplaced other fracture of tuberosity of unspecified calcaneus B, K, P 🔵, 🔵, B 🔵

● **S92.05   Other extraarticular fracture of calcaneus**

    ● **S92.051** Displaced other extraarticular fracture of right calcaneus B, K, P 🔵, 🔵, B 🔵

    ● **S92.052** Displaced other extraarticular fracture of left calcaneus B, K, P 🔵, 🔵, B 🔵

    ● **S92.053** Displaced other extraarticular fracture of unspecified calcaneus B, K, P 🔵, 🔵, B 🔵

    ● **S92.054** Nondisplaced other extraarticular fracture of right calcaneus B, K, P 🔵, 🔵, B 🔵

    ● **S92.055** Nondisplaced other extraarticular fracture of left calcaneus B, K, P 🔵, 🔵, B 🔵

    ● **S92.056** Nondisplaced other extraarticular fracture of unspecified calcaneus B, K, P 🔵, 🔵, B 🔵

● **S92.06   Intraarticular fracture of calcaneus**

    ● **S92.061** Displaced intraarticular fracture of right calcaneus B, K, P 🔵, 🔵, B 🔵

    ● **S92.062** Displaced intraarticular fracture of left calcaneus B, K, P 🔵, 🔵, B 🔵

    ● **S92.063** Displaced intraarticular fracture of unspecified calcaneus B, K, P 🔵, 🔵, B 🔵

    ● **S92.064** Nondisplaced intraarticular fracture of right calcaneus B, K, P 🔵, 🔵, B 🔵

    ● **S92.065** Nondisplaced intraarticular fracture of left calcaneus B, K, P 🔵, 🔵, B 🔵

    ● **S92.066** Nondisplaced intraarticular fracture of unspecified calcaneus B, K, P 🔵, 🔵, B 🔵

N Newborn Age: 0   **P** Pediatric Age: 0–17   **M** Maternity DX: 12–55   **A** Adult Age: 15–124   ♀ Females Only   ♂ Males Only

🔵 Complication\Comorbidity   🔵 Major C\C   (Ex) CC/MCC Exclusions   🔵 Present on Admission Requirement   🔵 Hospital-Acquired Condition

1483

● **S92.1** Fracture of talus
  Astragalus
  (Ex) For category S92.1 CC codes S92.1[B]: M80.00X-M80.019[A],
  M80.041-M80.049[A], M80.80X-M80.819[A], M80.841-M80.849[A],
  M84.40X-M84.419[A], M84.441-M84.446[A], M84.454[A],
  M84.474-M84.519[A], M84.541-M84.550[A], M84.574-M84.576[A],
  M84.60X-M84.619[A], M84.641-M84.650[A], M84.674-M84.68X[A],
  S03.8XX-S03.9XX[A], S29.011-S29.019[A], S38.3XX[A],
  S39.011-S39.013[A], S73.101-S73.199[A], S76.001-S76.019[A],
  S76.091-S76.219[A], S76.291-S76.319[A], S76.391-S76.819[A],
  S76.891-S76.919[A], S76.991-S76.999[A], S79.821-S79.929[A],
  S82.90X-S82.92X[A,B,C], S92.001-S92.066[B], S92.101-S92.356[A,B],
  S92.901-S92.909[A,B], T14.8-T14.91, T79.A9X-T79.9XX[A]
  For S92.1[K,P]: See S72.001[K,M,N,P,Q,R]

  ● **S92.10** Unspecified fracture of talus
    ● **S92.101** Unspecified fracture of right talus
      B, K, P 🐾, 🐾, B 🐾
    ● **S92.102** Unspecified fracture of left talus
      B, K, P 🐾, 🐾, B 🐾
    ● **S92.109** Unspecified fracture of unspecified
      talus B, K, P 🐾, B 🐾

  ● **S92.11** Fracture of neck of talus
    ● **S92.111** Displaced fracture of neck of right
      talus B, K, P 🐾, 🐾, B 🐾
    ● **S92.112** Displaced fracture of neck of left
      talus B, K, P 🐾, 🐾, B 🐾
    ● **S92.113** Displaced fracture of neck of
      unspecified talus B, K, P 🐾, 🐾, B 🐾
    ● **S92.114** Nondisplaced fracture of neck of
      right talus B, K, P 🐾, 🐾, B 🐾
    ● **S92.115** Nondisplaced fracture of neck of left
      talus B, K, P 🐾, 🐾, B 🐾
    ● **S92.116** Nondisplaced fracture of neck of
      unspecified talus B, K, P 🐾, 🐾, B 🐾

  ● **S92.12** Fracture of body of talus
    ● **S92.121** Displaced fracture of body of right
      talus B, K, P 🐾, 🐾, B 🐾
    ● **S92.122** Displaced fracture of body of left
      talus B, K, P 🐾, 🐾, B 🐾
    ● **S92.123** Displaced fracture of body of
      unspecified talus B, K, P 🐾, 🐾, B 🐾
    ● **S92.124** Nondisplaced fracture of body of
      right talus B, K, P 🐾, 🐾, B 🐾
    ● **S92.125** Nondisplaced fracture of body of left
      talus B, K, P 🐾, 🐾, B 🐾
    ● **S92.126** Nondisplaced fracture of body of
      unspecified talus B, K, P 🐾, 🐾, B 🐾

  ● **S92.13** Fracture of posterior process of talus
    ● **S92.131** Displaced fracture of posterior
      process of right talus B, K, P 🐾, 🐾,
      B 🐾
    ● **S92.132** Displaced fracture of posterior
      process of left talus B, K, P 🐾, 🐾, B 🐾
    ● **S92.133** Displaced fracture of posterior
      process of unspecified talus B, K, P 🐾,
      🐾, B 🐾
    ● **S92.134** Nondisplaced fracture of posterior
      process of right talus B, K, P 🐾, 🐾,
      B 🐾
    ● **S92.135** Nondisplaced fracture of posterior
      process of left talus B, K, P 🐾, 🐾, B 🐾
    ● **S92.136** Nondisplaced fracture of posterior
      process of unspecified talus B, K, P 🐾,
      🐾, B 🐾

● **S92.14** Dome fracture of talus
  Excludes1 osteochondritis dissecans
  (M93.2)
    ● **S92.141** Displaced dome fracture of right talus
      B, K, P 🐾, 🐾, B 🐾
    ● **S92.142** Displaced dome fracture of left talus
      B, K, P 🐾, 🐾, B 🐾
    ● **S92.143** Displaced dome fracture of
      unspecified talus B, K, P 🐾, 🐾, B 🐾
    ● **S92.144** Nondisplaced dome fracture of right
      talus B, K, P 🐾, 🐾, B 🐾
    ● **S92.145** Nondisplaced dome fracture of left
      talus B, K, P 🐾, 🐾, B 🐾
    ● **S92.146** Nondisplaced dome fracture of
      unspecified talus B, K, P 🐾, 🐾, B 🐾

● **S92.15** Avulsion fracture (chip fracture) of talus
    ● **S92.151** Displaced avulsion fracture (chip
      fracture) of right talus B, K, P 🐾, 🐾,
      B 🐾
    ● **S92.152** Displaced avulsion fracture (chip
      fracture) of left talus B, K, P 🐾, 🐾,
      B 🐾
    ● **S92.153** Displaced avulsion fracture (chip
      fracture) of unspecified talus
      B, K, P 🐾, 🐾, B 🐾
    ● **S92.154** Nondisplaced avulsion fracture (chip
      fracture) of right talus B, K, P 🐾, 🐾,
      B 🐾
    ● **S92.155** Nondisplaced avulsion fracture (chip
      fracture) of left talus B, K, P 🐾, 🐾,
      B 🐾
    ● **S92.156** Nondisplaced avulsion fracture (chip
      fracture) of unspecified talus
      B, K, P 🐾, 🐾, B 🐾

● **S92.19** Other fracture of talus
    ● **S92.191** Other fracture of right talus B, K, P 🐾,
      🐾, B 🐾
    ● **S92.192** Other fracture of left talus B, K, P 🐾,
      🐾, B 🐾
    ● **S92.199** Other fracture of unspecified talus
      B, K, P 🐾, 🐾, B 🐾

● **S92.2** Fracture of other and unspecified tarsal bone(s)
  (Ex) For category S92.2 CC codes S92.2[B]: See S92.1[B] For S92.2[K,P]:
  See S72.001[K,M,N,P,Q,R] unless otherwise indicated

  ● **S92.20** Fracture of unspecified tarsal bone(s)
    (Ex) For category S92.20 CC codes S92.20[B]:
    S92.001-S92.919[A,B] For S92.20[K,P]: See
    S72.001[K,M,N,P,Q,R]
    ● **S92.201** Fracture of unspecified tarsal bone(s)
      of right foot B, K, P 🐾, 🐾, B 🐾
    ● **S92.202** Fracture of unspecified tarsal bone(s)
      of left foot B, K, P 🐾, 🐾, B 🐾
    ● **S92.209** Fracture of unspecified tarsal bone(s)
      of unspecified foot B, K, P 🐾, 🐾, B 🐾

  ● **S92.21** Fracture of cuboid bone
    ● **S92.211** Displaced fracture of cuboid bone of
      right foot B, K, P 🐾, 🐾, B 🐾
    ● **S92.212** Displaced fracture of cuboid bone of
      left foot B, K, P 🐾, 🐾, B 🐾
    ● **S92.213** Displaced fracture of cuboid bone of
      unspecified foot B, K, P 🐾, 🐾, B 🐾
    ● **S92.214** Nondisplaced fracture of cuboid bone
      of right foot B, K, P 🐾, 🐾, B 🐾
    ● **S92.215** Nondisplaced fracture of cuboid bone
      of left foot B, K, P 🐾, 🐾, B 🐾
    ● **S92.216** Nondisplaced fracture of cuboid bone
      of unspecified foot B, K, P 🐾, 🐾, B 🐾

◄ New   ◄▦ Revised   d̶e̶l̶e̶t̶e̶d̶ Deleted   Excludes 1   Excludes 2   Includes   Use additional   Code first   Code also   Unspecified
OGCR Official Guidelines   ● Unacceptable Principal Diagnosis   X Assign placeholder X   ● Use Additional Character(s)   ❱ Manifestation Code   Coding Clinic

● S92.22   Fracture of lateral cuneiform
    ● S92.221   Displaced fracture of lateral cuneiform of right foot B, K, P 🪙, 🪙, B 🪙
    ● S92.222   Displaced fracture of lateral cuneiform of left foot B, K, P 🪙, 🪙, B 🪙
    ● S92.223   Displaced fracture of lateral cuneiform of unspecified foot B, K, P 🪙, 🪙, B 🪙
    ● S92.224   Nondisplaced fracture of lateral cuneiform of right foot B, K, P 🪙, 🪙, B 🪙
    ● S92.225   Nondisplaced fracture of lateral cuneiform of left foot B, K, P 🪙, 🪙, B 🪙
    ● S92.226   Nondisplaced fracture of lateral cuneiform of unspecified foot B, K, P 🪙, 🪙, B 🪙

● S92.23   Fracture of intermediate cuneiform
    ● S92.231   Displaced fracture of intermediate cuneiform of right foot B, K, P 🪙, 🪙, B 🪙
    ● S92.232   Displaced fracture of intermediate cuneiform of left foot B, K, P 🪙, 🪙, B 🪙
    ● S92.233   Displaced fracture of intermediate cuneiform of unspecified foot B, K, P 🪙, 🪙, B 🪙
    ● S92.234   Nondisplaced fracture of intermediate cuneiform of right foot B, K, P 🪙, 🪙, B 🪙
    ● S92.235   Nondisplaced fracture of intermediate cuneiform of left foot B, K, P 🪙, 🪙, B 🪙
    ● S92.236   Nondisplaced fracture of intermediate cuneiform of unspecified foot B, K, P 🪙, 🪙, B 🪙

● S92.24   Fracture of medial cuneiform
    ● S92.241   Displaced fracture of medial cuneiform of right foot B, K, P 🪙, 🪙, B 🪙
    ● S92.242   Displaced fracture of medial cuneiform of left foot B, K, P 🪙, 🪙, B 🪙
    ● S92.243   Displaced fracture of medial cuneiform of unspecified foot B, K, P 🪙, 🪙, B 🪙
    ● S92.244   Nondisplaced fracture of medial cuneiform of right foot B, K, P 🪙, 🪙, B 🪙
    ● S92.245   Nondisplaced fracture of medial cuneiform of left foot B, K, P 🪙, 🪙, B 🪙
    ● S92.246   Nondisplaced fracture of medial cuneiform of unspecified foot B, K, P 🪙, 🪙, B 🪙

● S92.25   Fracture of navicular [scaphoid] of foot
    ● S92.251   Displaced fracture of navicular [scaphoid] of right foot B, K, P 🪙, 🪙, B 🪙
    ● S92.252   Displaced fracture of navicular [scaphoid] of left foot B, K, P 🪙, 🪙, B 🪙
    ● S92.253   Displaced fracture of navicular [scaphoid] of unspecified foot B, K, P 🪙, 🪙, B 🪙
    ● S92.254   Nondisplaced fracture of navicular [scaphoid] of right foot B, K, P 🪙, 🪙, B 🪙
    ● S92.255   Nondisplaced fracture of navicular [scaphoid] of left foot B, K, P 🪙, 🪙, B 🪙
    ● S92.256   Nondisplaced fracture of navicular [scaphoid] of unspecified foot B, K, P 🪙, 🪙, B 🪙

● S92.3   Fracture of metatarsal bone(s)
   (Ex) For category S92.3 CC codes S92.3[B]: See S92.1[B] For S92.3[K,P]: See S72.001[K,M,N,P,Q,R]

● S92.30   Fracture of unspecified metatarsal bone(s)
    ● S92.301   Fracture of unspecified metatarsal bone(s), right foot B, K, P 🪙, 🪙, B 🪙
    ● S92.302   Fracture of unspecified metatarsal bone(s), left foot B, K, P 🪙, 🪙, B 🪙
    ● S92.309   Fracture of unspecified metatarsal bone(s), unspecified foot B, K, P 🪙, 🪙, B 🪙

● S92.31   Fracture of first metatarsal bone
    ● S92.311   Displaced fracture of first metatarsal bone, right foot B, K, P 🪙, 🪙, B 🪙
    ● S92.312   Displaced fracture of first metatarsal bone, left foot B, K, P 🪙, 🪙, B 🪙
    ● S92.313   Displaced fracture of first metatarsal bone, unspecified foot B, K, P 🪙, 🪙, B 🪙
    ● S92.314   Nondisplaced fracture of first metatarsal bone, right foot B, K, P 🪙, 🪙, B 🪙
    ● S92.315   Nondisplaced fracture of first metatarsal bone, left foot B, K, P 🪙, 🪙, B 🪙
    ● S92.316   Nondisplaced fracture of first metatarsal bone, unspecified foot B, K, P 🪙, 🪙, B 🪙

● S92.32   Fracture of second metatarsal bone
    ● S92.321   Displaced fracture of second metatarsal bone, right foot B, K, P 🪙, 🪙, B 🪙
    ● S92.322   Displaced fracture of second metatarsal bone, left foot B, K, P 🪙, 🪙, B 🪙
    ● S92.323   Displaced fracture of second metatarsal bone, unspecified foot B, K, P 🪙, 🪙, B 🪙
    ● S92.324   Nondisplaced fracture of second metatarsal bone, right foot B, K, P 🪙, 🪙, B 🪙
    ● S92.325   Nondisplaced fracture of second metatarsal bone, left foot B, K, P 🪙, 🪙, B 🪙
    ● S92.326   Nondisplaced fracture of second metatarsal bone, unspecified foot B, K, P 🪙, 🪙, B 🪙

N Newborn Age: 0   **P** Pediatric Age: 0–17   **M** Maternity DX: 12–55   **A** Adult Age: 15–124   ♀ Females Only   ♂ Males Only

🪙 Complication\Comorbidity   🪙 Major C\C   (Ex) CC/MCC Exclusions   🪙 Present on Admission Requirement   🪙 Hospital-Acquired Condition

● S92.33   Fracture of third metatarsal bone

  ● S92.331   Displaced fracture of third metatarsal bone, right foot B, K, P 🖙, 🖙, B 🖙

  ● S92.332   Displaced fracture of third metatarsal bone, left foot B, K, P 🖙, 🖙, B 🖙

  ● S92.333   Displaced fracture of third metatarsal bone, unspecified foot B, K, P 🖙, 🖙, B 🖙

  ● S92.334   Nondisplaced fracture of third metatarsal bone, right foot B, K, P 🖙, 🖙, B 🖙

  ● S92.335   Nondisplaced fracture of third metatarsal bone, left foot B, K, P 🖙, 🖙, B 🖙

  ● S92.336   Nondisplaced fracture of third metatarsal bone, unspecified foot B, K, P 🖙, 🖙, B 🖙

● S92.34   Fracture of fourth metatarsal bone

  ● S92.341   Displaced fracture of fourth metatarsal bone, right foot B, K, P 🖙, 🖙, B 🖙

  ● S92.342   Displaced fracture of fourth metatarsal bone, left foot B, K, P 🖙, 🖙, B 🖙

  ● S92.343   Displaced fracture of fourth metatarsal bone, unspecified foot B, K, P 🖙, 🖙, B 🖙

  ● S92.344   Nondisplaced fracture of fourth metatarsal bone, right foot B, K, P 🖙, 🖙, B 🖙

  ● S92.345   Nondisplaced fracture of fourth metatarsal bone, left foot B, K, P 🖙, 🖙, B 🖙

  ● S92.346   Nondisplaced fracture of fourth metatarsal bone, unspecified foot B, K, P 🖙, 🖙, B 🖙

● S92.35   Fracture of fifth metatarsal bone

  ● S92.351   Displaced fracture of fifth metatarsal bone, right foot B, K, P 🖙, 🖙, B 🖙

  ● S92.352   Displaced fracture of fifth metatarsal bone, left foot B, K, P 🖙, 🖙, B 🖙

  ● S92.353   Displaced fracture of fifth metatarsal bone, unspecified foot B, K, P 🖙, 🖙, B 🖙

  ● S92.354   Nondisplaced fracture of fifth metatarsal bone, right foot B, K, P 🖙, 🖙, B 🖙

  ● S92.355   Nondisplaced fracture of fifth metatarsal bone, left foot B, K, P 🖙, 🖙, B 🖙

  ● S92.356   Nondisplaced fracture of fifth metatarsal bone, unspecified foot B, K, P 🖙, 🖙, B 🖙

● S92.4   Fracture of great toe

  Ⓔⓧ For category S92.4 CC codes: See S72.001[K,M,N,P,Q,R]

  ● S92.40   Unspecified fracture of great toe

  ● S92.401   Displaced unspecified fracture of right great toe K, P 🖙, 🖙

  ● S92.402   Displaced unspecified fracture of left great toe K, P 🖙, 🖙

  ● S92.403   Displaced unspecified fracture of unspecified great toe K, P 🖙, 🖙

  ● S92.404   Nondisplaced unspecified fracture of right great toe K, P 🖙, 🖙

  ● S92.405   Nondisplaced unspecified fracture of left great toe K, P 🖙, 🖙

  ● S92.406   Nondisplaced unspecified fracture of unspecified great toe K, P 🖙, 🖙

● S92.41   Fracture of proximal phalanx of great toe

  ● S92.411   Displaced fracture of proximal phalanx of right great toe K, P 🖙, 🖙

  ● S92.412   Displaced fracture of proximal phalanx of left great toe K, P 🖙, 🖙

  ● S92.413   Displaced fracture of proximal phalanx of unspecified great toe K, P 🖙, 🖙

  ● S92.414   Nondisplaced fracture of proximal phalanx of right great toe K, P 🖙, 🖙

  ● S92.415   Nondisplaced fracture of proximal phalanx of left great toe K, P 🖙, 🖙

  ● S92.416   Nondisplaced fracture of proximal phalanx of unspecified great toe K, P 🖙, 🖙

● S92.42   Fracture of distal phalanx of great toe

  ● S92.421   Displaced fracture of distal phalanx of right great toe K, P 🖙, 🖙

  ● S92.422   Displaced fracture of distal phalanx of left great toe K, P 🖙, 🖙

  ● S92.423   Displaced fracture of distal phalanx of unspecified great toe K, P 🖙, 🖙

  ● S92.424   Nondisplaced fracture of distal phalanx of right great toe K, P 🖙, 🖙

  ● S92.425   Nondisplaced fracture of distal phalanx of left great toe K, P 🖙, 🖙

  ● S92.426   Nondisplaced fracture of distal phalanx of unspecified great toe K, P 🖙, 🖙

● S92.49   Other fracture of great toe

  ● S92.491   Other fracture of right great toe K, P 🖙, 🖙

  ● S92.492   Other fracture of left great toe K, P 🖙, 🖙

  ● S92.499   Other fracture of unspecified great toe K, P 🖙, 🖙

● S92.5   Fracture of lesser toe(s)

  Ⓔⓧ For category S92.5 CC codes: See S72.001[K,M,N,P,Q,R]

  ● S92.50   Unspecified fracture of lesser toe(s)

  ● S92.501   Displaced unspecified fracture of right lesser toe(s) K, P 🖙, 🖙

  ● S92.502   Displaced unspecified fracture of left lesser toe(s) K, P 🖙, 🖙

  ● S92.503   Displaced unspecified fracture of unspecified lesser toe(s) K, P 🖙, 🖙

  ● S92.504   Nondisplaced unspecified fracture of right lesser toe(s) K, P 🖙, 🖙

  ● S92.505   Nondisplaced unspecified fracture of left lesser toe(s) K, P 🖙, 🖙

  ● S92.506   Nondisplaced unspecified fracture of unspecified lesser toe(s) K, P 🖙, 🖙

● S92.51   Fracture of proximal phalanx of lesser toe(s)

  ● S92.511   Displaced fracture of proximal phalanx of right lesser toe(s) K, P 🖙, 🖙

  ● S92.512   Displaced fracture of proximal phalanx of left lesser toe(s) K, P 🖙, 🖙

  ● S92.513   Displaced fracture of proximal phalanx of unspecified lesser toe(s) K, P 🖙, 🖙

  ● S92.514   Nondisplaced fracture of proximal phalanx of right lesser toe(s) K, P 🖙, 🖙

  ● S92.515   Nondisplaced fracture of proximal phalanx of left lesser toe(s) K, P 🖙, 🖙

  ● S92.516   Nondisplaced fracture of proximal phalanx of unspecified lesser toe(s) K, P 🖙, 🖙

◀ New   ◀ⁱⁱⁱ Revised   ~~deleted~~ Deleted   Excludes 1   Excludes 2   Includes   Use additional   Code first   Code also   Unspecified

OGCR Official Guidelines   ● Unacceptable Principal Diagnosis   X Assign placeholder X   ● Use Additional Character(s)   ▸ Manifestation Code   **Coding Clinic**

● **S92.52**   Fracture of medial phalanx of lesser toe(s)

    ● **S92.521**   Displaced fracture of medial phalanx of right lesser toe(s) K, P 🦵, 🦵

    ● **S92.522**   Displaced fracture of medial phalanx of left lesser toe(s) K, P 🦵, 🦵

    ● **S92.523**   Displaced fracture of medial phalanx of unspecified lesser toe(s) K, P 🦵, 🦵

    ● **S92.524**   Nondisplaced fracture of medial phalanx of right lesser toe(s) K, P 🦵, 🦵

    ● **S92.525**   Nondisplaced fracture of medial phalanx of left lesser toe(s) K, P 🦵, 🦵

    ● **S92.526**   Nondisplaced fracture of medial phalanx of unspecified lesser toe(s) K, P 🦵, 🦵

● **S92.53**   Fracture of distal phalanx of lesser toe(s)

    ● **S92.531**   Displaced fracture of distal phalanx of right lesser toe(s) K, P 🦵, 🦵

    ● **S92.532**   Displaced fracture of distal phalanx of left lesser toe(s) K, P 🦵, 🦵

    ● **S92.533**   Displaced fracture of distal phalanx of unspecified lesser toe(s) K, P 🦵, 🦵

    ● **S92.534**   Nondisplaced fracture of distal phalanx of right lesser toe(s) K, P 🦵, 🦵

    ● **S92.535**   Nondisplaced fracture of distal phalanx of left lesser toe(s) K, P 🦵, 🦵

    ● **S92.536**   Nondisplaced fracture of distal phalanx of unspecified lesser toe(s) K, P 🦵, 🦵

● **S92.59**   Other fracture of lesser toe(s)

    ● **S92.591**   Other fracture of right lesser toe(s) K, P 🦵, 🦵

    ● **S92.592**   Other fracture of left lesser toe(s) K, P 🦵, 🦵

    ● **S92.599**   Other fracture of unspecified lesser toe(s) K, P 🦵, 🦵

● **S92.9**   Unspecified fracture of foot and toe

    ● **S92.90**   Unspecified fracture of foot

      (Ex:) **For category S92.90 CC codes S92.90[B]:** S92.001-S92.919[A,B] **For S92.90[K,P]:** See S72.001[K,M,N,P,Q,R]

    ● **S92.901**   Unspecified fracture of right foot B, K, P 🦵, 🦵, B 🦵

    ● **S92.902**   Unspecified fracture of left foot B, K, P 🦵, 🦵, B 🦵

    ● **S92.909**   Unspecified fracture of unspecified foot B, K, P 🦵, 🦵, B 🦵

    ● **S92.91**   Unspecified fracture of toe

      (Ex:) **For category S92.91 CC codes:** See S72.001[K,M,N,P,Q,R]

    ● **S92.911**   Unspecified fracture of right toe(s) K, P 🦵, 🦵

    ● **S92.912**   Unspecified fracture of left toe(s) K, P 🦵, 🦵

    ● **S92.919**   Unspecified fracture of unspecified toe(s) K, P 🦵, 🦵

● **S93**   Dislocation and sprain of joints and ligaments at ankle, foot and toe level

    Includes   avulsion of joint or ligament of ankle, foot and toe

               laceration of cartilage, joint or ligament of ankle, foot and toe

               sprain of cartilage, joint or ligament of ankle, foot and toe

               traumatic hemarthrosis of joint or ligament of ankle, foot and toe

               traumatic rupture of joint or ligament of ankle, foot and toe

               traumatic subluxation of joint or ligament of ankle, foot and toe

               traumatic tear of joint or ligament of ankle, foot and toe

    Code also any associated open wound

    Excludes2   strain of muscle and tendon of ankle and foot (S96.-)

    The appropriate 7th character is to be added to each code from category S93

      A   initial encounter
      D   subsequent encounter
      S   sequela

● **S93.0**   Subluxation and dislocation of ankle joint

      Subluxation and dislocation of astragalus
      Subluxation and dislocation of fibula, lower end
      Subluxation and dislocation of talus
      Subluxation and dislocation of tibia, lower end

   X ● **S93.01**   Subluxation of right ankle joint 🦵

   X ● **S93.02**   Subluxation of left ankle joint 🦵

   X ● **S93.03**   Subluxation of unspecified ankle joint 🦵

   X ● **S93.04**   Dislocation of right ankle joint 🦵

   X ● **S93.05**   Dislocation of left ankle joint 🦵

   X ● **S93.06**   Dislocation of unspecified ankle joint 🦵

● **S93.1**   Subluxation and dislocation of toe

    ● **S93.10**   Unspecified subluxation and dislocation of toe
       Dislocation of toe NOS
       Subluxation of toe NOS

      ● **S93.101**   Unspecified subluxation of right toe(s) 🦵

      ● **S93.102**   Unspecified subluxation of left toe(s) 🦵

      ● **S93.103**   Unspecified subluxation of unspecified toe(s) 🦵

      ● **S93.104**   Unspecified dislocation of right toe(s) 🦵

      ● **S93.105**   Unspecified dislocation of left toe(s) 🦵

      ● **S93.106**   Unspecified dislocation of unspecified toe(s) 🦵

    ● **S93.11**   Dislocation of interphalangeal joint

      ● **S93.111**   Dislocation of interphalangeal joint of right great toe 🦵

      ● **S93.112**   Dislocation of interphalangeal joint of left great toe 🦵

      ● **S93.113**   Dislocation of interphalangeal joint of unspecified great toe 🦵

      ● **S93.114**   Dislocation of interphalangeal joint of right lesser toe(s) 🦵

      ● **S93.115**   Dislocation of interphalangeal joint of left lesser toe(s) 🦵

      ● **S93.116**   Dislocation of interphalangeal joint of unspecified lesser toe(s) 🦵

      ● **S93.119**   Dislocation of interphalangeal joint of unspecified toe(s) 🦵

CHAPTER 19 (S00-T88)

N   Newborn Age: 0   P   Pediatric Age: 0–17   M   Maternity DX: 12–55   A   Adult Age: 15–124   ♀   Females Only   ♂   Males Only

🦵 Complication\Comorbidity   🦵 Major C\C   (Ex:) CC/MCC Exclusions   🦵 Present on Admission Requirement   🦵 Hospital-Acquired Condition

1487

- ● S93.12   Dislocation of metatarsophalangeal joint
  - ● S93.121   Dislocation of metatarsophalangeal joint of right great toe ✇
  - ● S93.122   Dislocation of metatarsophalangeal joint of left great toe ✇
  - ● S93.123   Dislocation of metatarsophalangeal joint of unspecified great toe ✇
  - ● S93.124   Dislocation of metatarsophalangeal joint of right lesser toe(s) ✇
  - ● S93.125   Dislocation of metatarsophalangeal joint of left lesser toe(s) ✇
  - ● S93.126   Dislocation of metatarsophalangeal joint of unspecified lesser toe(s) ✇
  - ● S93.129   Dislocation of metatarsophalangeal joint of unspecified toe(s) ✇
- ● S93.13   Subluxation of interphalangeal joint
  - ● S93.131   Subluxation of interphalangeal joint of right great toe ✇
  - ● S93.132   Subluxation of interphalangeal joint of left great toe ✇
  - ● S93.133   Subluxation of interphalangeal joint of unspecified great toe ✇
  - ● S93.134   Subluxation of interphalangeal joint of right lesser toe(s) ✇
  - ● S93.135   Subluxation of interphalangeal joint of left lesser toe(s) ✇
  - ● S93.136   Subluxation of interphalangeal joint of unspecified lesser toe(s) ✇
  - ● S93.139   Subluxation of interphalangeal joint of unspecified toe(s) ✇
- ● S93.14   Subluxation of metatarsophalangeal joint
  - ● S93.141   Subluxation of metatarsophalangeal joint of right great toe ✇
  - ● S93.142   Subluxation of metatarsophalangeal joint of left great toe ✇
  - ● S93.143   Subluxation of metatarsophalangeal joint of unspecified great toe ✇
  - ● S93.144   Subluxation of metatarsophalangeal joint of right lesser toe(s) ✇
  - ● S93.145   Subluxation of metatarsophalangeal joint of left lesser toe(s) ✇
  - ● S93.146   Subluxation of metatarsophalangeal joint of unspecified lesser toe(s) ✇
  - ● S93.149   Subluxation of metatarsophalangeal joint of unspecified toe(s) ✇
- ● S93.3   Subluxation and dislocation of foot
  - **Excludes2**   dislocation of toe (S93.1-)
  - ● S93.30   Unspecified subluxation and dislocation of foot
    Dislocation of foot NOS
    Subluxation of foot NOS
    - ● S93.301   Unspecified subluxation of right foot ✇
    - ● S93.302   Unspecified subluxation of left foot ✇
    - ● S93.303   Unspecified subluxation of unspecified foot ✇
    - ● S93.304   Unspecified dislocation of right foot ✇
    - ● S93.305   Unspecified dislocation of left foot ✇
    - ● S93.306   Unspecified dislocation of unspecified foot ✇
  - ● S93.31   Subluxation and dislocation of tarsal joint
    - ● S93.311   Subluxation of tarsal joint of right foot ✇
    - ● S93.312   Subluxation of tarsal joint of left foot ✇

- ● S93.313   Subluxation of tarsal joint of unspecified foot ✇
- ● S93.314   Dislocation of tarsal joint of right foot ✇
- ● S93.315   Dislocation of tarsal joint of left foot ✇
- ● S93.316   Dislocation of tarsal joint of unspecified foot ✇
- ● S93.32   Subluxation and dislocation of tarsometatarsal joint
  - ● S93.321   Subluxation of tarsometatarsal joint of right foot ✇
  - ● S93.322   Subluxation of tarsometatarsal joint of left foot ✇
  - ● S93.323   Subluxation of tarsometatarsal joint of unspecified foot ✇
  - ● S93.324   Dislocation of tarsometatarsal joint of right foot ✇
  - ● S93.325   Dislocation of tarsometatarsal joint of left foot ✇
  - ● S93.326   Dislocation of tarsometatarsal joint of unspecified foot ✇
- ● S93.33   Other subluxation and dislocation of foot
  - ● S93.331   Other subluxation of right foot ✇
  - ● S93.332   Other subluxation of left foot ✇
  - ● S93.333   Other subluxation of unspecified foot ✇
  - ● S93.334   Other dislocation of right foot ✇
  - ● S93.335   Other dislocation of left foot ✇
  - ● S93.336   Other dislocation of unspecified foot ✇
- ● S93.4   Sprain of ankle
  Injury to ligaments when one or more is stretched/torn
  - **Excludes2**   injury of Achilles tendon (S86.0-)
  - ● S93.40   Sprain of unspecified ligament of ankle
    Sprain of ankle NOS
    Sprained ankle NOS
    - ● S93.401   Sprain of unspecified ligament of right ankle ✇
    - ● S93.402   Sprain of unspecified ligament of left ankle ✇
    - ● S93.409   Sprain of unspecified ligament of unspecified ankle ✇
  - ● S93.41   Sprain of calcaneofibular ligament
    - ● S93.411   Sprain of calcaneofibular ligament of right ankle ✇
    - ● S93.412   Sprain of calcaneofibular ligament of left ankle ✇
    - ● S93.419   Sprain of calcaneofibular ligament of unspecified ankle ✇
  - ● S93.42   Sprain of deltoid ligament
    - ● S93.421   Sprain of deltoid ligament of right ankle ✇
    - ● S93.422   Sprain of deltoid ligament of left ankle ✇
    - ● S93.429   Sprain of deltoid ligament of unspecified ankle ✇
  - ● S93.43   Sprain of tibiofibular ligament
    - ● S93.431   Sprain of tibiofibular ligament of right ankle ✇
    - ● S93.432   Sprain of tibiofibular ligament of left ankle ✇
    - ● S93.439   Sprain of tibiofibular ligament of unspecified ankle ✇

◀ New   ◀┅ Revised   ~~deleted~~ Deleted   Excludes 1   Excludes 2   Includes   Use additional   Code first   Code also   Unspecified

OGCR Official Guidelines   ● Unacceptable Principal Diagnosis   X Assign placeholder X   ● Use Additional Character(s)   ❚ Manifestation Code   **Coding Clinic**

● **S93.49**   Sprain of other ligament of ankle
     Sprain of internal collateral ligament
     Sprain of talofibular ligament
   ● **S93.491**   Sprain of other ligament of right ankle 🔖
   ● **S93.492**   Sprain of other ligament of left ankle 🔖
   ● **S93.499**   Sprain of other ligament of unspecified ankle 🔖

● **S93.5**   Sprain of toe
  ● **S93.50**   Unspecified sprain of toe
   ● **S93.501**   Unspecified sprain of right great toe 🔖
   ● **S93.502**   Unspecified sprain of left great toe 🔖
   ● **S93.503**   Unspecified sprain of unspecified great toe 🔖
   ● **S93.504**   Unspecified sprain of right lesser toe(s) 🔖
   ● **S93.505**   Unspecified sprain of left lesser toe(s) 🔖
   ● **S93.506**   Unspecified sprain of unspecified lesser toe(s) 🔖
   ● **S93.509**   Unspecified sprain of unspecified toe(s) 🔖
  ● **S93.51**   Sprain of interphalangeal joint of toe
   ● **S93.511**   Sprain of interphalangeal joint of right great toe 🔖
   ● **S93.512**   Sprain of interphalangeal joint of left great toe 🔖
   ● **S93.513**   Sprain of interphalangeal joint of unspecified great toe 🔖
   ● **S93.514**   Sprain of interphalangeal joint of right lesser toe(s) 🔖
   ● **S93.515**   Sprain of interphalangeal joint of left lesser toe(s) 🔖
   ● **S93.516**   Sprain of interphalangeal joint of unspecified lesser toe(s) 🔖
   ● **S93.519**   Sprain of interphalangeal joint of unspecified toe(s) 🔖
  ● **S93.52**   Sprain of metatarsophalangeal joint of toe
   ● **S93.521**   Sprain of metatarsophalangeal joint of right great toe 🔖
   ● **S93.522**   Sprain of metatarsophalangeal joint of left great toe 🔖
   ● **S93.523**   Sprain of metatarsophalangeal joint of unspecified great toe 🔖
   ● **S93.524**   Sprain of metatarsophalangeal joint of right lesser toe(s) 🔖
   ● **S93.525**   Sprain of metatarsophalangeal joint of left lesser toe(s) 🔖
   ● **S93.526**   Sprain of metatarsophalangeal joint of unspecified lesser toe(s) 🔖
   ● **S93.529**   Sprain of metatarsophalangeal joint of unspecified toe(s) 🔖

● **S93.6**   Sprain of foot
   Excludes2   sprain of metatarsophalangeal joint of toe (S93.52-)
         sprain of toe (S93.5-)
  ● **S93.60**   Unspecified sprain of foot
   ● **S93.601**   Unspecified sprain of right foot 🔖
   ● **S93.602**   Unspecified sprain of left foot 🔖
   ● **S93.609**   Unspecified sprain of unspecified foot 🔖

  ● **S93.61**   Sprain of tarsal ligament of foot
   ● **S93.611**   Sprain of tarsal ligament of right foot 🔖
   ● **S93.612**   Sprain of tarsal ligament of left foot 🔖
   ● **S93.619**   Sprain of tarsal ligament of unspecified foot 🔖
  ● **S93.62**   Sprain of tarsometatarsal ligament of foot
   ● **S93.621**   Sprain of tarsometatarsal ligament of right foot 🔖
   ● **S93.622**   Sprain of tarsometatarsal ligament of left foot 🔖
   ● **S93.629**   Sprain of tarsometatarsal ligament of unspecified foot 🔖
  ● **S93.69**   Other sprain of foot
   ● **S93.691**   Other sprain of right foot 🔖
   ● **S93.692**   Other sprain of left foot 🔖
   ● **S93.699**   Other sprain of unspecified foot 🔖

● **S94**   Injury of nerves at ankle and foot level
   The appropriate 7th character is to be added to each code from category S94

A	initial encounter
D	subsequent encounter
S	sequela

   Code also any associated open wound (S91.-)
  ● **S94.0**   Injury of lateral plantar nerve
  X ● **S94.00**   Injury of lateral plantar nerve, unspecified leg 🔖
  X ● **S94.01**   Injury of lateral plantar nerve, right leg 🔖
  X ● **S94.02**   Injury of lateral plantar nerve, left leg 🔖
  ● **S94.1**   Injury of medial plantar nerve
  X ● **S94.10**   Injury of medial plantar nerve, unspecified leg 🔖
  X ● **S94.11**   Injury of medial plantar nerve, right leg 🔖
  X ● **S94.12**   Injury of medial plantar nerve, left leg 🔖
  ● **S94.2**   Injury of deep peroneal nerve at ankle and foot level
     Injury of terminal, lateral branch of deep peroneal nerve
  X ● **S94.20**   Injury of deep peroneal nerve at ankle and foot level, unspecified leg 🔖
  X ● **S94.21**   Injury of deep peroneal nerve at ankle and foot level, right leg 🔖
  X ● **S94.22**   Injury of deep peroneal nerve at ankle and foot level, left leg 🔖
  ● **S94.3**   Injury of cutaneous sensory nerve at ankle and foot level
  X ● **S94.30**   Injury of cutaneous sensory nerve at ankle and foot level, unspecified leg 🔖
  X ● **S94.31**   Injury of cutaneous sensory nerve at ankle and foot level, right leg 🔖
  X ● **S94.32**   Injury of cutaneous sensory nerve at ankle and foot level, left leg 🔖
  ● **S94.8**   Injury of other nerves at ankle and foot level
   ● **S94.8X**   Injury of other nerves at ankle and foot level
    ● **S94.8X1**   Injury of other nerves at ankle and foot level, right leg 🔖
    ● **S94.8X2**   Injury of other nerves at ankle and foot level, left leg 🔖
    ● **S94.8X9**   Injury of other nerves at ankle and foot level, unspecified leg 🔖
  ● **S94.9**   Injury of unspecified nerve at ankle and foot level
  X ● **S94.90**   Injury of unspecified nerve at ankle and foot level, unspecified leg 🔖
  X ● **S94.91**   Injury of unspecified nerve at ankle and foot level, right leg 🔖
  X ● **S94.92**   Injury of unspecified nerve at ankle and foot level, left leg 🔖

N   Newborn Age: 0   P   Pediatric Age: 0–17   M   Maternity DX: 12–55   A   Adult Age: 15–124   ♀   Females Only   ♂   Males Only

🔖 Complication\Comorbidity   🔖 Major C\C   (Ex)   CC/MCC Exclusions   🔖 Present on Admission Requirement   🔖 Hospital-Acquired Condition

● **S95   Injury of blood vessels at ankle and foot level**

Code also any associated open wound (S91.-)

Excludes2   injury of posterior tibial artery and vein (S85.1-, S85.8-)

The appropriate 7th character is to be added to each code from category S95

> A   initial encounter
> D   subsequent encounter
> S   sequela

● **S95.0   Injury of dorsal artery of foot**

   ● **S95.00   Unspecified injury of dorsal artery of foot**

     ● **S95.001   Unspecified injury of dorsal artery of right foot** A 🖉, 🖉
       Ex: See S75.801

     ● **S95.002   Unspecified injury of dorsal artery of left foot** A 🖉, 🖉
       Ex: See S75.802

     ● **S95.009   Unspecified injury of dorsal artery of unspecified foot** A 🖉, 🖉
       Ex: See S75.809

   ● **S95.01   Laceration of dorsal artery of foot**

     ● **S95.011   Laceration of dorsal artery of right foot** A 🖉, 🖉
       Ex: See S75.801

     ● **S95.012   Laceration of dorsal artery of left foot** A 🖉, 🖉
       Ex: See S75.802

     ● **S95.019   Laceration of dorsal artery of unspecified foot** A 🖉, 🖉
       Ex: See S75.809

   ● **S95.09   Other specified injury of dorsal artery of foot**

     ● **S95.091   Other specified injury of dorsal artery of right foot** A 🖉, 🖉
       Ex: See S75.801

     ● **S95.092   Other specified injury of dorsal artery of left foot** A 🖉, 🖉
       Ex: See S75.802

     ● **S95.099   Other specified injury of dorsal artery of unspecified foot** A 🖉, 🖉
       Ex: See S75.809

● **S95.1   Injury of plantar artery of foot**

   ● **S95.10   Unspecified injury of plantar artery of foot**

     ● **S95.101   Unspecified injury of plantar artery of right foot** A 🖉, 🖉
       Ex: S75.801[A], S75.809-S75.811[A], S75.819-S75.891[A], S75.899-S75.901[A], S75.909-S75.911[A], S75.919-S75.991[A], S75.999[A], S85.201[A], S85.209-S85.211[A], S85.219-S85.291[A], S85.299[A], S85.801[A], S85.809-S85.811[A], S85.819-S85.891[A], S85.899-S85.901[A], S85.909-S85.911[A], S85.919-S85.991[A], S85.999[A], S95.001[A], S95.009-S95.011[A], S95.019-S95.091[A], S95.099-S95.201[A], S95.209-S95.211[A], S95.219-S95.291[A], S95.299-S95.801[A], S95.809-S95.811[A], S95.819-S95.891[A], S95.899-S95.901[A], S95.909-S95.911[A], S95.919-S95.991[A], S95.999[A]

     ● **S95.102   Unspecified injury of plantar artery of left foot** A 🖉, 🖉
       Ex: S75.802-S75.809[A], S75.812-S75.819[A], S75.892-S75.899[A], S75.902-S75.909[A], S75.912-S75.919[A], S75.992-S75.999[A], S85.202-S85.209[A], S85.212-S85.219[A], S85.292-S85.299[A], S85.802-S85.809[A], S85.812-S85.819[A], S85.892-S85.899[A], S85.902-S85.909[A], S85.912-S85.919[A], S85.992-S85.999[A], S95.002-S95.009[A], S95.012-S95.019[A], S95.092-S95.099[A], S95.102-S95.109[A], S95.112-S95.119[A], S95.192-S95.199[A], S95.202-S95.209[A], S95.212-S95.219[A], S95.292-S95.299[A], S95.802-S95.809[A], S95.812-S95.819[A], S95.892-S95.899[A], S95.902-S95.909[A], S95.912-S95.919[A], S95.992-S95.999[A]

     ● **S95.109   Unspecified injury of plantar artery of unspecified foot** A 🖉, 🖉
       Ex: S75.801-S75.999[A], S85.201-S85.299[A], S85.801-S85.999[A], S95.001-S95.099[A], S95.101-S95.999[A]

   ● **S95.11   Laceration of plantar artery of foot**

     ● **S95.111   Laceration of plantar artery of right foot** A 🖉, 🖉
       Ex: See S95.101

     ● **S95.112   Laceration of plantar artery of left foot** A 🖉, 🖉
       Ex: See S95.102

     ● **S95.119   Laceration of plantar artery of unspecified foot** A 🖉, 🖉
       Ex: See S95.109

   ● **S95.19   Other specified injury of plantar artery of foot**

     ● **S95.191   Other specified injury of plantar artery of right foot** A 🖉, 🖉
       Ex: See S95.101

     ● **S95.192   Other specified injury of plantar artery of left foot** A 🖉, 🖉
       Ex: See S95.102

     ● **S95.199   Other specified injury of plantar artery of unspecified foot** A 🖉, 🖉
       Ex: See S95.109

● **S95.2   Injury of dorsal vein of foot**

   ● **S95.20   Unspecified injury of dorsal vein of foot**

     ● **S95.201   Unspecified injury of dorsal vein of right foot** A 🖉, 🖉
       Ex: See S75.801

     ● **S95.202   Unspecified injury of dorsal vein of left foot** A 🖉, 🖉
       Ex: See S75.802

     ● **S95.209   Unspecified injury of dorsal vein of unspecified foot** A 🖉, 🖉
       Ex: See S75.809

   ● **S95.21   Laceration of dorsal vein of foot**

     ● **S95.211   Laceration of dorsal vein of right foot** A 🖉, 🖉
       Ex: See S75.801

     ● **S95.212   Laceration of dorsal vein of left foot** A 🖉, 🖉
       Ex: See S75.802

     ● **S95.219   Laceration of dorsal vein of unspecified foot** A 🖉, 🖉
       Ex: See S75.809

   ● **S95.29   Other specified injury of dorsal vein of foot**

     ● **S95.291   Other specified injury of dorsal vein of right foot** A 🖉, 🖉
       Ex: See S75.801

     ● **S95.292   Other specified injury of dorsal vein of left foot** A 🖉, 🖉
       Ex: See S75.802

     ● **S95.299   Other specified injury of dorsal vein of unspecified foot** A 🖉, 🖉
       Ex: See S75.809

◀ New   ◀▥ Revised   ~~deleted~~ Deleted   Excludes 1   Excludes 2   Includes   Use additional   Code first   Code also   Unspecified

OGCR Official Guidelines   ● Unacceptable Principal Diagnosis   X Assign placeholder X   ● Use Additional Character(s)   ▶ Manifestation Code   **Coding Clinic**

● **S95.8** Injury of other blood vessels at ankle and foot level
  ● **S95.80** Unspecified injury of other blood vessels at ankle and foot level
    ● **S95.801** Unspecified injury of other blood vessels at ankle and foot level, right leg A 🗫, 🗫
      Ⓔⓧ See S75.801
    ● **S95.802** Unspecified injury of other blood vessels at ankle and foot level, left leg A 🗫, 🗫
      Ⓔⓧ See S75.802
    ● **S95.809** Unspecified injury of other blood vessels at ankle and foot level, unspecified leg A 🗫, 🗫
      Ⓔⓧ See S75.809
  ● **S95.81** Laceration of other blood vessels at ankle and foot level
    ● **S95.811** Laceration of other blood vessels at ankle and foot level, right leg A 🗫, 🗫
      Ⓔⓧ See S75.801
    ● **S95.812** Laceration of other blood vessels at ankle and foot level, left leg A 🗫, 🗫
      Ⓔⓧ See S75.802
    ● **S95.819** Laceration of other blood vessels at ankle and foot level, unspecified leg A 🗫, 🗫
      Ⓔⓧ See S75.809
  ● **S95.89** Other specified injury of other blood vessels at ankle and foot level
    ● **S95.891** Other specified injury of other blood vessels at ankle and foot level, right leg A 🗫, 🗫
      Ⓔⓧ See S75.801
    ● **S95.892** Other specified injury of other blood vessels at ankle and foot level, left leg A 🗫, 🗫
      Ⓔⓧ See S75.802
    ● **S95.899** Other specified injury of other blood vessels at ankle and foot level, unspecified leg A 🗫, 🗫
      Ⓔⓧ See S75.809
● **S95.9** Injury of unspecified blood vessel at ankle and foot level
  ● **S95.90** Unspecified injury of unspecified blood vessel at ankle and foot level
    ● **S95.901** Unspecified injury of unspecified blood vessel at ankle and foot level, right leg A 🗫, 🗫
      Ⓔⓧ See S75.801
    ● **S95.902** Unspecified injury of unspecified blood vessel at ankle and foot level, left leg A 🗫, 🗫
      Ⓔⓧ See S75.802
    ● **S95.909** Unspecified injury of unspecified blood vessel at ankle and foot level, unspecified leg A 🗫, 🗫
      Ⓔⓧ See S75.809
  ● **S95.91** Laceration of unspecified blood vessel at ankle and foot level
    ● **S95.911** Laceration of unspecified blood vessel at ankle and foot level, right leg A 🗫, 🗫
      Ⓔⓧ See S75.801
    ● **S95.912** Laceration of unspecified blood vessel at ankle and foot level, left leg A 🗫, 🗫
      Ⓔⓧ See S75.802
    ● **S95.919** Laceration of unspecified blood vessel at ankle and foot level, unspecified leg A 🗫, 🗫
      Ⓔⓧ See S75.809

  ● **S95.99** Other specified injury of unspecified blood vessel at ankle and foot level
    ● **S95.991** Other specified injury of unspecified blood vessel at ankle and foot level, right leg A 🗫, 🗫
      Ⓔⓧ See S75.801
    ● **S95.992** Other specified injury of unspecified blood vessel at ankle and foot level, left leg A 🗫, 🗫
      Ⓔⓧ See S75.802
    ● **S95.999** Other specified injury of unspecified blood vessel at ankle and foot level, unspecified leg A 🗫, 🗫
      Ⓔⓧ See S75.809

● **S96** Injury of muscle and tendon at ankle and foot level
  Code also any associated open wound (S91.-)
  Excludes2 injury of Achilles tendon (S86.0-)
  sprain of joints and ligaments of ankle and foot (S93.-)

  The appropriate 7th character is to be added to each code from category S96

A	initial encounter
D	subsequent encounter
S	sequela

  ● **S96.0** Injury of muscle and tendon of long flexor muscle of toe at ankle and foot level
    ● **S96.00** Unspecified injury of muscle and tendon of long flexor muscle of toe at ankle and foot level
      ● **S96.001** Unspecified injury of muscle and tendon of long flexor muscle of toe at ankle and foot level, right foot 🗫
      ● **S96.002** Unspecified injury of muscle and tendon of long flexor muscle of toe at ankle and foot level, left foot 🗫
      ● **S96.009** Unspecified injury of muscle and tendon of long flexor muscle of toe at ankle and foot level, unspecified foot 🗫
    ● **S96.01** Strain of muscle and tendon of long flexor muscle of toe at ankle and foot level
      ● **S96.011** Strain of muscle and tendon of long flexor muscle of toe at ankle and foot level, right foot 🗫
      ● **S96.012** Strain of muscle and tendon of long flexor muscle of toe at ankle and foot level, left foot 🗫
      ● **S96.019** Strain of muscle and tendon of long flexor muscle of toe at ankle and foot level, unspecified foot 🗫
    ● **S96.02** Laceration of muscle and tendon of long flexor muscle of toe at ankle and foot level
      ● **S96.021** Laceration of muscle and tendon of long flexor muscle of toe at ankle and foot level, right foot A 🗫, 🗫
        Ⓔⓧ See S86.021
      ● **S96.022** Laceration of muscle and tendon of long flexor muscle of toe at ankle and foot level, left foot A 🗫, 🗫
        Ⓔⓧ See S86.022
      ● **S96.029** Laceration of muscle and tendon of long flexor muscle of toe at ankle and foot level, unspecified foot A 🗫, 🗫
        Ⓔⓧ See S86.029

● **S96.09** Other injury of muscle and tendon of long flexor muscle of toe at ankle and foot level
  ● S96.091 Other injury of muscle and tendon of long flexor muscle of toe at ankle and foot level, right foot 🔄
  ● S96.092 Other injury of muscle and tendon of long flexor muscle of toe at ankle and foot level, left foot 🔄
  ● S96.099 Other injury of muscle and tendon of long flexor muscle of toe at ankle and foot level, unspecified foot 🔄

● **S96.1** Injury of muscle and tendon of long extensor muscle of toe at ankle and foot level
  ● **S96.10** Unspecified injury of muscle and tendon of long extensor muscle of toe at ankle and foot level
    ● S96.101 Unspecified injury of muscle and tendon of long extensor muscle of toe at ankle and foot level, right foot 🔄
    ● S96.102 Unspecified injury of muscle and tendon of long extensor muscle of toe at ankle and foot level, left foot 🔄
    ● S96.109 Unspecified injury of muscle and tendon of long extensor muscle of toe at ankle and foot level, unspecified foot 🔄
  ● **S96.11** Strain of muscle and tendon of long extensor muscle of toe at ankle and foot level
    ● S96.111 Strain of muscle and tendon of long extensor muscle of toe at ankle and foot level, right foot 🔄
    ● S96.112 Strain of muscle and tendon of long extensor muscle of toe at ankle and foot level, left foot 🔄
    ● S96.119 Strain of muscle and tendon of long extensor muscle of toe at ankle and foot level, unspecified foot 🔄
  ● **S96.12** Laceration of muscle and tendon of long extensor muscle of toe at ankle and foot level
    ● S96.121 Laceration of muscle and tendon of long extensor muscle of toe at ankle and foot level, right foot A 🔄, 🔄
      (Ex:) See S86.021
    ● S96.122 Laceration of muscle and tendon of long extensor muscle of toe at ankle and foot level, left foot A 🔄, 🔄
      (Ex:) See S86.022
    ● S96.129 Laceration of muscle and tendon of long extensor muscle of toe at ankle and foot level, unspecified foot A 🔄, 🔄
      (Ex:) See S86.029
  ● **S96.19** Other specified injury of muscle and tendon of long extensor muscle of toe at ankle and foot level
    ● S96.191 Other specified injury of muscle and tendon of long extensor muscle of toe at ankle and foot level, right foot 🔄
    ● S96.192 Other specified injury of muscle and tendon of long extensor muscle of toe at ankle and foot level, left foot 🔄
    ● S96.199 Other specified injury of muscle and tendon of long extensor muscle of toe at ankle and foot level, unspecified foot 🔄

● **S96.2** Injury of intrinsic muscle and tendon at ankle and foot level
  ● **S96.20** Unspecified injury of intrinsic muscle and tendon at ankle and foot level
    ● S96.201 Unspecified injury of intrinsic muscle and tendon at ankle and foot level, right foot 🔄
    ● S96.202 Unspecified injury of intrinsic muscle and tendon at ankle and foot level, left foot 🔄
    ● S96.209 Unspecified injury of intrinsic muscle and tendon at ankle and foot level, unspecified foot 🔄
  ● **S96.21** Strain of intrinsic muscle and tendon at ankle and foot level
    ● S96.211 Strain of intrinsic muscle and tendon at ankle and foot level, right foot 🔄
    ● S96.212 Strain of intrinsic muscle and tendon at ankle and foot level, left foot 🔄
    ● S96.219 Strain of intrinsic muscle and tendon at ankle and foot level, unspecified foot 🔄
  ● **S96.22** Laceration of intrinsic muscle and tendon at ankle and foot level
    ● S96.221 Laceration of intrinsic muscle and tendon at ankle and foot level, right foot A 🔄, 🔄
      (Ex:) See S86.021
    ● S96.222 Laceration of intrinsic muscle and tendon at left ankle and foot level, left foot A 🔄, 🔄
      (Ex:) See S86.022
    ● S96.229 Laceration of intrinsic muscle and tendon at ankle and foot level, unspecified foot A 🔄, 🔄
      (Ex:) See S86.029
  ● **S96.29** Other specified injury of intrinsic muscle and tendon at ankle and foot level
    ● S96.291 Other specified injury of intrinsic muscle and tendon at ankle and foot level, right foot 🔄
    ● S96.292 Other specified injury of intrinsic muscle and tendon at ankle and foot level, left foot 🔄
    ● S96.299 Other specified injury of intrinsic muscle and tendon at ankle and foot level, unspecified foot 🔄

● **S96.8** Injury of other specified muscles and tendons at ankle and foot level
  ● **S96.80** Unspecified injury of other specified muscles and tendons at ankle and foot level
    ● S96.801 Unspecified injury of other specified muscles and tendons at ankle and foot level, right foot 🔄
    ● S96.802 Unspecified injury of other specified muscles and tendons at ankle and foot level, left foot 🔄
    ● S96.809 Unspecified injury of other specified muscles and tendons at ankle and foot level, unspecified foot 🔄
  ● **S96.81** Strain of other specified muscles and tendons at ankle and foot level
    ● S96.811 Strain of other specified muscles and tendons at ankle and foot level, right foot 🔄
    ● S96.812 Strain of other specified muscles and tendons at ankle and foot level, left foot 🔄
    ● S96.819 Strain of other specified muscles and tendons at ankle and foot level, unspecified foot 🔄

● **S96.82**   Laceration of other specified muscles and tendons at ankle and foot level

  ● **S96.821**   Laceration of other specified muscles and tendons at ankle and foot level, right foot A 🦠, 🦠
     (Ex:) See S86.021

  ● **S96.822**   Laceration of other specified muscles and tendons at ankle and foot level, left foot A 🦠, 🦠
     (Ex:) See S86.022

  ● **S96.829**   Laceration of other specified muscles and tendons at ankle and foot level, unspecified foot A 🦠, 🦠
     (Ex:) See S86.029

● **S96.89**   Other specified injury of other specified muscles and tendons at ankle and foot level

  ● **S96.891**   Other specified injury of other specified muscles and tendons at ankle and foot level, right foot 🦠

  ● **S96.892**   Other specified injury of other specified muscles and tendons at ankle and foot level, left foot 🦠

  ● **S96.899**   Other specified injury of other specified muscles and tendons at ankle and foot level, unspecified foot 🦠

● **S96.9**   Injury of unspecified muscle and tendon at ankle and foot level

  ● **S96.90**   Unspecified injury of unspecified muscle and tendon at ankle and foot level

    ● **S96.901**   Unspecified injury of unspecified muscle and tendon at ankle and foot level, right foot 🦠

    ● **S96.902**   Unspecified injury of unspecified muscle and tendon at ankle and foot level, left foot 🦠

    ● **S96.909**   Unspecified injury of unspecified muscle and tendon at ankle and foot level, unspecified foot 🦠

  ● **S96.91**   Strain of unspecified muscle and tendon at ankle and foot level

    ● **S96.911**   Strain of unspecified muscle and tendon at ankle and foot level, right foot 🦠

    ● **S96.912**   Strain of unspecified muscle and tendon at ankle and foot level, left foot 🦠

    ● **S96.919**   Strain of unspecified muscle and tendon at ankle and foot level, unspecified foot 🦠

  ● **S96.92**   Laceration of unspecified muscle and tendon at ankle and foot level

    ● **S96.921**   Laceration of unspecified muscle and tendon at ankle and foot level, right foot A 🦠, 🦠
       (Ex:) See S86.021

    ● **S96.922**   Laceration of unspecified muscle and tendon at ankle and foot level, left foot A 🦠, 🦠
       (Ex:) See S86.022

    ● **S96.929**   Laceration of unspecified muscle and tendon at ankle and foot level, unspecified foot A 🦠, 🦠
       (Ex:) See S86.029

● **S96.99**   Other specified injury of unspecified muscle and tendon at ankle and foot level

  ● **S96.991**   Other specified injury of unspecified muscle and tendon at ankle and foot level, right foot 🦠

  ● **S96.992**   Other specified injury of unspecified muscle and tendon at ankle and foot level, left foot 🦠

  ● **S96.999**   Other specified injury of unspecified muscle and tendon at ankle and foot level, unspecified foot 🦠

● **S97**   **Crushing injury of ankle and foot**

  Use additional code(s) for all associated injuries

  The appropriate 7th character is to be added to each code from category S97

A	initial encounter
D	subsequent encounter
S	sequela

  ● **S97.0**   Crushing injury of ankle

   X ● **S97.00**   Crushing injury of unspecified ankle 🦠

   X ● **S97.01**   Crushing injury of right ankle 🦠

   X ● **S97.02**   Crushing injury of left ankle 🦠

  ● **S97.1**   Crushing injury of toe

   ● **S97.10**   Crushing injury of unspecified toe(s)

    ● **S97.101**   Crushing injury of unspecified right toe(s) 🦠

    ● **S97.102**   Crushing injury of unspecified left toe(s) 🦠

    ● **S97.109**   Crushing injury of unspecified toe(s) 🦠
       Crushing injury of toe NOS

   ● **S97.11**   Crushing injury of great toe

    ● **S97.111**   Crushing injury of right great toe 🦠

    ● **S97.112**   Crushing injury of left great toe 🦠

    ● **S97.119**   Crushing injury of unspecified great toe 🦠

   ● **S97.12**   Crushing injury of lesser toe(s)

    ● **S97.121**   Crushing injury of right lesser toe(s) 🦠

    ● **S97.122**   Crushing injury of left lesser toe(s) 🦠

    ● **S97.129**   Crushing injury of lesser toe(s), unspecified toe(s) 🦠

  ● **S97.8**   Crushing injury of foot

   X ● **S97.80**   Crushing injury of foot, unspecified side 🦠
       Crushing injury of foot NOS

   X ● **S97.81**   Crushing injury of right foot 🦠

   X ● **S97.82**   Crushing injury of left foot 🦠

● **S98**   **Traumatic amputation of ankle and foot**

  An amputation not identified as partial or complete should be coded to complete

  The appropriate 7th character is to be added to each code from category S98

A	initial encounter
D	subsequent encounter
S	sequela

  ● **S98.0**   Traumatic amputation of foot at ankle level

   ● **S98.01**   Complete traumatic amputation of foot at ankle level

    ● **S98.011**   Complete traumatic amputation of right foot at ankle level A 🦠, 🦠
       (Ex:) See S78.011

    ● **S98.012**   Complete traumatic amputation of left foot at ankle level A 🦠, 🦠
       (Ex:) See S78.012

    ● **S98.019**   Complete traumatic amputation of unspecified foot at ankle level A 🦠, 🦠
       (Ex:) See S78.019

N Newborn Age: 0   **P** Pediatric Age: 0–17   **M** Maternity DX: 12–55   **A** Adult Age: 15–124   ♀ Females Only   ♂ Males Only

🦠 Complication\Comorbidity   🦠 Major C\C   (Ex:) CC/MCC Exclusions   🦠 Present on Admission Requirement   🦠 Hospital-Acquired Condition

1493

CHAPTER 19 (S00-T88)

CHAPTER 19 (S00-T88)

● S98.02   Partial traumatic amputation of foot at ankle level
   ● S98.021   Partial traumatic amputation of right foot at ankle level A 🐾, 🐾
      (Ex:) See S78.011
   ● S98.022   Partial traumatic amputation of left foot at ankle level A 🐾, 🐾
      (Ex:) See S78.012
   ● S98.029   Partial traumatic amputation of unspecified foot at ankle level A 🐾, 🐾
      (Ex:) See S78.019

● S98.1   Traumatic amputation of one toe
  ● S98.11   Complete traumatic amputation of great toe
   ● S98.111   Complete traumatic amputation of right great toe 🐾
   ● S98.112   Complete traumatic amputation of left great toe 🐾
   ● S98.119   Complete traumatic amputation of unspecified great toe 🐾
  ● S98.12   Partial traumatic amputation of great toe
   ● S98.121   Partial traumatic amputation of right great toe 🐾
   ● S98.122   Partial traumatic amputation of left great toe 🐾
   ● S98.129   Partial traumatic amputation of unspecified great toe 🐾
  ● S98.13   Complete traumatic amputation of one lesser toe
     Traumatic amputation of toe NOS
   ● S98.131   Complete traumatic amputation of one right lesser toe 🐾
   ● S98.132   Complete traumatic amputation of one left lesser toe 🐾
   ● S98.139   Complete traumatic amputation of one unspecified lesser toe 🐾
  ● S98.14   Partial traumatic amputation of one lesser toe
   ● S98.141   Partial traumatic amputation of one right lesser toe 🐾
   ● S98.142   Partial traumatic amputation of one left lesser toe 🐾
   ● S98.149   Partial traumatic amputation of one unspecified lesser toe 🐾

● S98.2   Traumatic amputation of two or more lesser toes
  ● S98.21   Complete traumatic amputation of two or more lesser toes
   ● S98.211   Complete traumatic amputation of two or more right lesser toes 🐾
   ● S98.212   Complete traumatic amputation of two or more left lesser toes 🐾
   ● S98.219   Complete traumatic amputation of two or more unspecified lesser toes 🐾
  ● S98.22   Partial traumatic amputation of two or more lesser toes
   ● S98.221   Partial traumatic amputation of two or more right lesser toes 🐾
   ● S98.222   Partial traumatic amputation of two or more left lesser toes 🐾
   ● S98.229   Partial traumatic amputation of two or more unspecified lesser toes 🐾

● S98.3   Traumatic amputation of midfoot
  ● S98.31   Complete traumatic amputation of midfoot
   ● S98.311   Complete traumatic amputation of right midfoot A 🐾, 🐾
      (Ex:) See S78.011
   ● S98.312   Complete traumatic amputation of left midfoot A 🐾, 🐾
      (Ex:) See S78.012
   ● S98.319   Complete traumatic amputation of unspecified midfoot A 🐾, 🐾
      (Ex:) See S78.019

● S98.32   Partial traumatic amputation of midfoot
   ● S98.321   Partial traumatic amputation of right midfoot A 🐾, 🐾
      (Ex:) See S78.011
   ● S98.322   Partial traumatic amputation of left midfoot A 🐾, 🐾
      (Ex:) See S78.012
   ● S98.329   Partial traumatic amputation of unspecified midfoot A 🐾, 🐾
      (Ex:) See S78.019

● S98.9   Traumatic amputation of foot, level unspecified
  ● S98.91   Complete traumatic amputation of foot, level unspecified
   ● S98.911   Complete traumatic amputation of right foot, level unspecified A 🐾, 🐾
      (Ex:) See S78.011
   ● S98.912   Complete traumatic amputation of left foot, level unspecified A 🐾, 🐾
      (Ex:) See S78.012
   ● S98.919   Complete traumatic amputation of unspecified foot, level unspecified A 🐾, 🐾
      (Ex:) See S78.019
  ● S98.92   Partial traumatic amputation of foot, level unspecified
   ● S98.921   Partial traumatic amputation of right foot, level unspecified A 🐾, 🐾
      (Ex:) See S78.011
   ● S98.922   Partial traumatic amputation of left foot, level unspecified A 🐾, 🐾
      (Ex:) See S78.012
   ● S98.929   Partial traumatic amputation of unspecified foot, level unspecified A 🐾, 🐾
      (Ex:) See S78.019

● S99   Other and unspecified injuries of ankle and foot
    The appropriate 7th character is to be added to each code from category S99

A	initial encounter
D	subsequent encounter
S	sequela

● S99.8   Other specified injuries of ankle and foot
  ● S99.81   Other specified injuries of ankle
   ● S99.811   Other specified injuries of right ankle 🐾
   ● S99.812   Other specified injuries of left ankle 🐾
   ● S99.819   Other specified injuries of unspecified ankle 🐾
  ● S99.82   Other specified injuries of foot
   ● S99.821   Other specified injuries of right foot 🐾
   ● S99.822   Other specified injuries of left foot 🐾
   ● S99.829   Other specified injuries of unspecified foot 🐾
● S99.9   Unspecified injury of ankle and foot
  ● S99.91   Unspecified injury of ankle
   ● S99.911   Unspecified injury of right ankle 🐾
   ● S99.912   Unspecified injury of left ankle 🐾
   ● S99.919   Unspecified injury of unspecified ankle 🐾
  ● S99.92   Unspecified injury of foot
   ● S99.921   Unspecified injury of right foot 🐾
   ● S99.922   Unspecified injury of left foot 🐾
   ● S99.929   Unspecified injury of unspecified foot 🐾

◄ New   ◄▦ Revised   ~~deleted~~ Deleted   Excludes 1   Excludes 2   Includes   Use additional   Code first   Code also   Unspecified
OGCR Official Guidelines   ● Unacceptable Principal Diagnosis   X Assign placeholder X   ● Use Additional Character(s)   ▌ Manifestation Code   Coding Clinic

INJURY, POISONING AND CERTAIN OTHER CONSEQUENCES OF EXTERNAL CAUSES (T07-T88)

INJURIES INVOLVING MULTIPLE BODY REGIONS (T07)

> **Excludes1**   burns and corrosions (T20-T32)
>   frostbite (T33-T34)
>   insect bite or sting, venomous (T63.4)
>   sunburn (L55.-)

● **T07**   Unspecified multiple injuries 🦠
> **Excludes1**   injury NOS (T14)

INJURY OF UNSPECIFIED BODY REGION (T14)

● **T14**   Injury of unspecified body region
> **Excludes1**   multiple unspecified injuries (T07)

     T14.8   **Other injury of unspecified body region** 🦠
> Abrasion NOS   Fracture NOS
> Contusion NOS   Skin injury NOS
> Crush injury NOS   Vascular injury NOS

    ● **T14.9**   **Unspecified injury**
        T14.90   **Injury, unspecified** 🦠
> Injury NOS

        T14.91   **Suicide attempt** 🦠
> Attempted suicide NOS

EFFECTS OF FOREIGN BODY ENTERING THROUGH NATURAL ORIFICE (T15-T19)

> **Excludes2**   foreign body accidentally left in operation wound (T81.5-)
>   foreign body in penetrating wound - see open wound by body region
>   residual foreign body in soft tissue (M79.5)
>   splinter, without open wound - see superficial injury by body region

● **T15**   Foreign body on external eye
> **Excludes2**   foreign body in penetrating wound of orbit and eye ball (S05.4-, S05.5-)
>   open wound of eyelid and periocular area (S01.1-)
>   retained foreign body in eyelid (H02.8-)
>   retained (old) foreign body in penetrating wound of orbit and eye ball (H05.5-, H44.6-, H44.7-)
>   superficial foreign body of eyelid and periocular area (S00.25-)

The appropriate 7th character is to be added to each code from category T15

A	initial encounter
D	subsequent encounter
S	sequela

   ● **T15.0**   **Foreign body in cornea**
     X ● **T15.00**   Foreign body in cornea, unspecified eye 🦠
     X ● **T15.01**   Foreign body in cornea, right eye 🦠
     X ● **T15.02**   Foreign body in cornea, left eye 🦠

   ● **T15.1**   **Foreign body in conjunctival sac**
     X ● **T15.10**   Foreign body in conjunctival sac, unspecified eye 🦠
     X ● **T15.11**   Foreign body in conjunctival sac, right eye 🦠
     X ● **T15.12**   Foreign body in conjunctival sac, left eye 🦠

   ● **T15.8**   **Foreign body in other and multiple parts of external eye**
       Foreign body in lacrimal punctum
     X ● **T15.80**   Foreign body in other and multiple parts of external eye, unspecified eye 🦠
     X ● **T15.81**   Foreign body in other and multiple parts of external eye, right eye 🦠
     X ● **T15.82**   Foreign body in other and multiple parts of external eye, left eye 🦠

   ● **T15.9**   **Foreign body on external eye, part unspecified**
     X ● **T15.90**   Foreign body on external eye, part unspecified, unspecified eye 🦠
     X ● **T15.91**   Foreign body on external eye, part unspecified, right eye 🦠
     X ● **T15.92**   Foreign body on external eye, part unspecified, left eye 🦠

● **T16**   Foreign body in ear
> **Includes**   foreign body in auditory canal

The appropriate 7th character is to be added to each code from category T16

A	initial encounter
D	subsequent encounter
S	sequela

X ● **T16.1**   **Foreign body in right ear** 🦠
X ● **T16.2**   **Foreign body in left ear** 🦠
X ● **T16.9**   **Foreign body in ear, unspecified ear** 🦠

● **T17**   Foreign body in respiratory tract

The appropriate 7th character is to be added to each code from category T17

A	initial encounter
D	subsequent encounter
S	sequela

X ● **T17.0**   **Foreign body in nasal sinus** 🦠
X ● **T17.1**   **Foreign body in nostril** 🦠
       Foreign body in nose NOS

   ● **T17.2**   **Foreign body in pharynx**
       Foreign body in nasopharynx
       Foreign body in throat NOS
    ● **T17.20**   **Unspecified foreign body in pharynx**
      ● **T17.200**   Unspecified foreign body in pharynx causing asphyxiation 🦠
      ● **T17.208**   Unspecified foreign body in pharynx causing other injury 🦠
    ● **T17.21**   **Gastric contents in pharynx**
        Aspiration of gastric contents into pharynx
        Vomitus in pharynx
      ● **T17.210**   Gastric contents in pharynx causing asphyxiation 🦠
      ● **T17.218**   Gastric contents in pharynx causing other injury 🦠
    ● **T17.22**   **Food in pharynx**
        Bones in pharynx
        Seeds in pharynx
      ● **T17.220**   Food in pharynx causing asphyxiation 🦠
      ● **T17.228**   Food in pharynx causing other injury 🦠
    ● **T17.29**   **Other foreign object in pharynx**
      ● **T17.290**   Other foreign object in pharynx causing asphyxiation 🦠
      ● **T17.298**   Other foreign object in pharynx causing other injury 🦠

   ● **T17.3**   **Foreign body in larynx**
    ● **T17.30**   **Unspecified foreign body in larynx**
      ● **T17.300**   Unspecified foreign body in larynx causing asphyxiation 🦠
      ● **T17.308**   Unspecified foreign body in larynx causing other injury 🦠
    ● **T17.31**   **Gastric contents in larynx**
        Aspiration of gastric contents into larynx
        Vomitus in larynx
      ● **T17.310**   Gastric contents in larynx causing asphyxiation 🦠
      ● **T17.318**   Gastric contents in larynx causing other injury 🦠

| N | Newborn Age: 0 | P | Pediatric Age: 0–17 | M | Maternity DX: 12–55 | A | Adult Age: 15–124 | ♀ Females Only | ♂ Males Only |

🦠 Complication\Comorbidity   🦠 Major C\C   (Ex) CC/MCC Exclusions   🦠 Present on Admission Requirement   🦠 Hospital-Acquired Condition

1495

CHAPTER 19 (S00-T88)

- T17.32   **Food in larynx**
  Bones in larynx
  Seeds in larynx
  - T17.320   Food in larynx causing
    asphyxiation 🖉
  - T17.328   Food in larynx causing other injury 🖉
- T17.39   **Other foreign object in larynx**
  - T17.390   Other foreign object in larynx causing
    asphyxiation 🖉
  - T17.398   Other foreign object in larynx causing
    other injury 🖉
- T17.4   **Foreign body in trachea**
  (Ex) For category T17.4 CC codes: T17.400-T17.498[A]
  - T17.40   Unspecified foreign body in trachea
    - T17.400   Unspecified foreign body in trachea
      causing asphyxiation A 🖉, 🖉
    - T17.408   Unspecified foreign body in trachea
      causing injury A 🖉, 🖉
  - T17.41   Gastric contents in trachea
    Aspiration of gastric contents into trachea
    Vomitus in trachea
    - T17.410   Gastric contents in trachea causing
      asphyxiation A 🖉, 🖉
    - T17.418   Gastric contents in trachea causing
      other injury A 🖉, 🖉
  - T17.42   Food in trachea
    Bones in trachea
    Seeds in trachea
    - T17.420   Food in trachea causing asphyxiation
      A 🖉, 🖉
    - T17.428   Food in trachea causing other injury
      A 🖉, 🖉
  - T17.49   Other foreign object in trachea
    - T17.490   Other foreign object in trachea
      causing asphyxiation A 🖉, 🖉
    - T17.498   Other foreign object in trachea
      causing injury A 🖉, 🖉
- T17.5   **Foreign body in bronchus**
  (Ex) For category T17.5 CC codes: T17.400-T17.998[A]
  - T17.50   Unspecified foreign body in bronchus
    - T17.500   Unspecified foreign body in bronchus
      causing asphyxiation A 🖉, 🖉
    - T17.508   Unspecified foreign body in bronchus
      causing other injury A 🖉, 🖉
  - T17.51   Gastric contents in bronchus
    Aspiration of gastric contents into bronchus
    Vomitus in bronchus
    - T17.510   Gastric contents in bronchus causing
      asphyxiation A 🖉, 🖉
    - T17.518   Gastric contents in bronchus causing
      other injury A 🖉, 🖉
  - T17.52   Food in bronchus
    Bones in bronchus
    Seeds in bronchus
    - T17.520   Food in bronchus causing
      asphyxiation A 🖉, 🖉
    - T17.528   Food in bronchus causing other
      injury A 🖉, 🖉
  - T17.59   Other foreign object in bronchus
    - T17.590   Other foreign object in bronchus
      causing asphyxiation A 🖉, 🖉
    - T17.598   Other foreign object in bronchus
      causing other injury A 🖉, 🖉

- T17.8   **Foreign body in other parts of respiratory tract**
  Foreign body in bronchioles
  Foreign body in lung
  (Ex) For category T17.8 CC codes: T17.400-T17.998[A]
  - T17.80   Unspecified foreign body in other parts of
    respiratory tract
    - T17.800   Unspecified foreign body in other
      parts of respiratory tract causing
      asphyxiation A 🖉, 🖉
    - T17.808   Unspecified foreign body in other
      parts of respiratory tract causing other
      injury A 🖉, 🖉
  - T17.81   Gastric contents in other parts of respiratory
    tract
    Aspiration of gastric contents into other parts
    of respiratory tract
    Vomitus in other parts of respiratory tract
    - T17.810   Gastric contents in other parts of
      respiratory tract causing asphyxiation
      A 🖉, 🖉
    - T17.818   Gastric contents in other parts of
      respiratory tract causing other injury
      A 🖉, 🖉
  - T17.82   Food in other parts of respiratory tract
    Bones in other parts of respiratory tract
    Seeds in other parts of respiratory tract
    - T17.820   Food in other parts of respiratory tract
      causing asphyxiation A 🖉, 🖉
    - T17.828   Food in other parts of respiratory tract
      causing other injury A 🖉, 🖉
  - T17.89   Other foreign object in other parts of
    respiratory tract
    - T17.890   Other foreign object in other parts of
      respiratory tract causing asphyxiation
      A 🖉, 🖉
    - T17.898   Other foreign object in other parts of
      respiratory tract causing other injury
      A 🖉, 🖉
- T17.9   **Foreign body in respiratory tract, part unspecified**
  - T17.90   Unspecified foreign body in respiratory tract,
    part unspecified
    - T17.900   Unspecified foreign body in
      respiratory tract, part unspecified
      causing asphyxiation 🖉
    - T17.908   Unspecified foreign body in
      respiratory tract, part unspecified
      causing other injury 🖉
  - T17.91   Gastric contents in respiratory tract, part
    unspecified
    Aspiration of gastric contents into respiratory
    tract, part unspecified
    Vomitus in trachea respiratory tract, part
    unspecified
    - T17.910   Gastric contents in respiratory tract,
      part unspecified causing
      asphyxiation 🖉
    - T17.918   Gastric contents in respiratory tract,
      part unspecified causing other
      injury 🖉
  - T17.92   Food in respiratory tract, part unspecified
    Bones in respiratory tract, part unspecified
    Seeds in respiratory tract, part unspecified
    - T17.920   Food in respiratory tract, part
      unspecified causing asphyxiation 🖉
    - T17.928   Food in respiratory tract, part
      unspecified causing other injury 🖉

◀ New   ◀▥ Revised   ~~deleted~~ Deleted   Excludes 1   Excludes 2   Includes   Use additional   Code first   Code also   Unspecified

1496   OGCR Official Guidelines   ● Unacceptable Principal Diagnosis   X Assign placeholder X   ● Use Additional Character(s)   ▶ Manifestation Code   **Coding Clinic**

● **T17.99**   Other foreign object in respiratory tract, part unspecified

    ● **T17.990**   Other foreign object in respiratory tract, part unspecified in causing asphyxiatio

    ● **T17.998**   Other foreign object in respiratory tract, part unspecified causing other injur 🐾

● **T18**   Foreign body in alimentary tract

   Excludes2   foreign body in pharynx (T17.2-)

   The appropriate 7th character is to be added to each code from category T18

A	initial encounter
D	subsequent encounter
S	sequela

X ● **T18.0**   Foreign body in mouth 🐾

X ● **T18.1**   Foreign body in esophagus

   Excludes2   foreign body in respiratory tract (T17.-)

   ● **T18.10**   Unspecified foreign body in esophagus

    ● **T18.100**   Unspecified foreign body in esophagus causing compression of trachea 🐾

     Unspecified foreign body in esophagus causing obstruction of respiration

    ● **T18.108**   Unspecified foreign body in esophagus causing other injury 🐾

   ● **T18.11**   Gastric contents in esophagus

    Vomitus in esophagus

    ● **T18.110**   Gastric contents in esophagus causing compression of trachea 🐾

     Gastric contents in esophagus causing obstruction of respiration

    ● **T18.118**   Gastric contents in esophagus causing other injury 🐾

   ● **T18.12**   Food in esophagus

    Bones in esophagus

    Seeds in esophagus

    ● **T18.120**   Food in esophagus causing compression of trachea 🐾

     Food in esophagus causing obstruction of respiration

    ● **T18.128**   Food in esophagus causing other injury 🐾

   ● **T18.19**   Other foreign object in esophagus

    ● **T18.190**   Other foreign object in esophagus causing compression of trachea 🐾

     Other foreign body in esophagus causing obstruction of respiration

    ● **T18.198**   Other foreign object in esophagus causing other injury 🐾

X ● **T18.2**   Foreign body in stomach 🐾

X ● **T18.3**   Foreign body in small intestine 🐾

X ● **T18.4**   Foreign body in colon 🐾

X ● **T18.5**   Foreign body in anus and rectum 🐾

   Foreign body in rectosigmoid (junction)

X ● **T18.8**   Foreign body in other parts of alimentary tract 🐾

X ● **T18.9**   Foreign body of alimentary tract, part unspecified 🐾

   Foreign body in digestive system NOS

   Swallowed foreign body NOS

● **T19**   Foreign body in genitourinary tract

   Excludes2   complications due to implanted mesh (T83.7-)

    mechanical complications of contraceptive device (intrauterine) (vaginal) (T83.3-)

    presence of contraceptive device (intrauterine) (vaginal) (Z97.5)

   The appropriate 7th character is to be added to each code from category T19

A	initial encounter
D	subsequent encounter
S	sequela

X ● **T19.0**   Foreign body in urethra 🐾

X ● **T19.1**   Foreign body in bladder 🐾

X ● **T19.2**   Foreign body in vulva and vagina ♀ 🐾

X ● **T19.3**   Foreign body in uterus ♀ 🐾

X ● **T19.4**   Foreign body in penis ♂ 🐾

X ● **T19.8**   Foreign body in other parts of genitourinary tract 🐾

X ● **T19.9**   Foreign body in genitourinary tract, part unspecified 🐾

BURNS AND CORROSIONS (T20-T32)

Includes	burns (thermal) from electrical heating appliances
	burns (thermal) from electricity
	burns (thermal) from flame
	burns (thermal) from friction
	burns (thermal) from hot air and hot gases
	burns (thermal) from hot objects
	burns (thermal) from lightning
	burns (thermal) from radiation chemical
	burn [corrosion] (external) (internal) scalds
Excludes2	erythema [dermatitis] ab igne (L59.0)
	radiation-related disorders of the skin and subcutaneous tissue (L55-L59)
	sunburn (L55.-)

OGCR Section I.C.19.d.

Burns and Corrosions

The ICD-10-CM makes a distinction between burn and corrosions. The burn codes are for thermal burns, except sunburns, that come from a heat source, such as a fire or hot appliance. The burn codes are also for burns resulting from electricity and radiation. Corrosions are burns due to chemicals. The guidelines for burns and corrosions are the same.

Current burns (T20-T25) are classified by depth, extent and by agent (X code). Burns are classified by depth as first degree (erythema), second degree (blistering), and third degree (full-thickness involvement). Burns of the eye and internal organs (T26-T28) are classified by site, but not by degree.

1) Sequencing of burn and related condition codes

Sequence first the code that reflects the highest degree of burn when more than one burn is present.

a. When the reason for the admission or encounter is for treatment of external multiple burns, sequence first the code that reflects the burn of the highest degree.

b. When a patient has both internal and external burns, the circumstances of admission govern the selection of the principal diagnosis or first-listed diagnosis.

c. When a patient is admitted for burn injuries and other related conditions such as smoke inhalation and/or respiratory failure, the circumstances of admission govern the selection of the principal or first-listed diagnosis.

2) Burns of the same local site

Classify burns of the same local site (three-character category level, T20-T28) but of different degrees to the subcategory identifying the highest degree recorded in the diagnosis.

CHAPTER 19 (S00-T88)

N   Newborn Age: 0   P   Pediatric Age: 0–17   M   Maternity DX: 12–55   A   Adult Age: 15–124   ♀   Females Only   ♂   Males Only

🐾 Complication\Comorbidity   🐾 Major C\C   (Ex) CC/MCC Exclusions   🐾 Present on Admission Requirement   🐾 Hospital-Acquired Condition

1497

Figure 19-14 A. Second-degree burn. **B.** Third-degree burn. (From Cummings: Otolaryngology: Head & Neck Surgery, ed 4, Mosby, 2005)

BURNS AND CORROSIONS OF EXTERNAL BODY SURFACE, SPECIFIED BY SITE (T20-T25)

Includes　burns and corrosions of first degree [erythema]
　　　　　　burns and corrosions of second degree [blisters] [epidermal loss]
　　　　　　burns and corrosions of third degree [deep necrosis of underlying tissue] [full-thickness skin loss]

Use additional code from category T31 or T32 to identify extent of body surface involved

● **T20**　**Burn and corrosion of head, face, and neck**

Excludes2　burn and corrosion of ear drum (T28.41, T28.91)
　　　　　　burn and corrosion of eye and adnexa (T26.-)
　　　　　　burn and corrosion of mouth and pharynx (T28.0)

The appropriate 7th character is to be added to each code from category T20

> A　initial encounter
> D　subsequent encounter
> S　sequela

● **T20.0**　Burn of unspecified degree of head, face, and neck

Use additional external cause code to identify the source, place and intent of the burn (X00-X19, X75-X77, X96-X98, Y92)

X● **T20.00**　Burn of **unspecified** degree of head, face, and neck, unspecified site ℞

● **T20.01**　Burn of unspecified degree of ear [any part, except ear drum]

Excludes2　burn of ear drum (T28.41-)

● **T20.011**　Burn of **unspecified** degree of right ear [any part, except ear drum] ℞

● **T20.012**　Burn of **unspecified** degree of left ear [any part, except ear drum] ℞

● **T20.019**　Burn of **unspecified** degree of unspecified ear [any part, except ear drum] ℞

X● **T20.02**　Burn of **unspecified** degree of lip(s) ℞

X● **T20.03**　Burn of **unspecified** degree of chin ℞

X● **T20.04**　Burn of **unspecified** degree of nose (septum) ℞

X● **T20.05**　Burn of **unspecified** degree of scalp [any part] ℞

X● **T20.06**　Burn of **unspecified** degree of forehead and cheek ℞

X● **T20.07**　Burn of **unspecified** degree of neck ℞

X● **T20.09**　Burn of **unspecified** degree of multiple sites of head, face, and neck ℞

● **T20.1**　Burn of first degree of head, face, and neck

Use additional external cause code to identify the source, place and intent of the burn (X00-X19, X75-X77, X96-X98, Y92)

X● **T20.10**　Burn of first degree of head, face, and neck, **unspecified** site ℞

● **T20.11**　Burn of first degree of ear [any part, except ear drum]

Excludes2　burn of ear drum (T28.41-)

● **T20.111**　Burn of first degree of right ear [any part, except ear drum] ℞

● **T20.112**　Burn of first degree of left ear [any part, except ear drum] ℞

● **T20.119**　Burn of first degree of **unspecified** ear [any part, except ear drum] ℞

X● **T20.12**　Burn of first degree of lip(s) ℞

X● **T20.13**　Burn of first degree of chin ℞

X● **T20.14**　Burn of first degree of nose (septum) ℞

X● **T20.15**　Burn of first degree of scalp [any part] ℞

X● **T20.16**　Burn of first degree of forehead and cheek ℞

X● **T20.17**　Burn of first degree of neck ℞

X● **T20.19**　Burn of first degree of multiple sites of head, face, and neck ℞

● **T20.2**　Burn of second degree of head, face, and neck

Use additional external cause code to identify the source, place and intent of the burn (X00-X19, X75-X77, X96-X98, Y92)

X● **T20.20**　Burn of second degree of head, face, and neck, **unspecified** site ℞

● **T20.21**　Burn of second degree of ear [any part, except ear drum]

Excludes2　burn of ear drum (T28.41-)

● **T20.211**　Burn of second degree of right ear [any part, except ear drum] ℞

● **T20.212**　Burn of second degree of left ear [any part, except ear drum] ℞

● **T20.219**　Burn of second degree of **unspecified** ear [any part, except ear drum] ℞

X● **T20.22**　Burn of second degree of lip(s) ℞

X● **T20.23**　Burn of second degree of chin ℞

X● **T20.24**　Burn of second degree of nose (septum) ℞

X● **T20.25**　Burn of second degree of scalp [any part] ℞

X● **T20.26**　Burn of second degree of forehead and cheek ℞

X● **T20.27**　Burn of second degree of neck ℞

X● **T20.29**　Burn of second degree of multiple sites of head, face, and neck ℞

● **T20.3**　Burn of third degree of head, face, and neck

Use additional external cause code to identify the source, place and intent of the burn (X00-X19, X75-X77, X96-X98, Y92)

X● **T20.30**　Burn of third degree of head, face, and neck, **unspecified** site A ℞, ℞, A ℞
Ex: T20.30X[A], T20.39X[A], T20.70X[A], T20.79X[A]

● **T20.31**　Burn of third degree of ear [any part, except ear drum]

Excludes2　burn of ear drum (T28.41-)

Ex: For category T20.31 CC codes: T20.311-T20.319[A], T20.39X[A], T20.711-T20.719[A], T20.79X[A]

● **T20.311**　Burn of third degree of right ear [any part, except ear drum] A ℞, ℞, A ℞

● **T20.312**　Burn of third degree of left ear [any part, except ear drum] A ℞, ℞, A ℞

● **T20.319**　Burn of third degree of **unspecified** ear [any part, except ear drum] A ℞, ℞, A ℞

X● **T20.32**　Burn of third degree of lip(s) A ℞, ℞, A ℞
Ex: T20.32X[A], T20.39X[A], T20.72X[A], T20.79X[A]

X ● **T20.33**   Burn of third degree of chin A 🔾, 🔾, A 🔾
     Ⓔⓧ T20.33X[A], T20.39X[A], T20.73X[A], T20.79X[A]

X ● **T20.34**   Burn of third degree of nose (septum) A 🔾, 🔾, A 🔾
     Ⓔⓧ T20.34X[A], T20.39X[A], T20.74X[A], T20.79X[A]

X ● **T20.35**   Burn of third degree of scalp [any part] A 🔾, 🔾, A 🔾
     Ⓔⓧ T20.35X[A], T20.39X[A], T20.75X[A], T20.79X[A]

X ● **T20.36**   Burn of third degree of forehead and cheek A 🔾, 🔾, A 🔾
     Ⓔⓧ T20.36X[A], T20.39X[A], T20.76X[A], T20.79X[A]

X ● **T20.37**   Burn of third degree of neck A 🔾, 🔾, A 🔾
     Ⓔⓧ T20.37X-T20.39X[A], T20.77X-T20.79X[A]

X ● **T20.39**   Burn of third degree of multiple sites of head, face, and neck A 🔾, 🔾, A 🔾
     Ⓔⓧ T20.30X-T20.39X[A], T20.70X-T20.79X[A]

● **T20.4**   Corrosion of unspecified degree of head, face, and neck
    Code first (T51-T65) to identify chemical and intent
    Use additional external cause code to identify place (Y92)

X ● **T20.40**   Corrosion of unspecified degree of head, face, and neck, unspecified site 🔾

● **T20.41**   Corrosion of unspecified degree of ear [any part, except ear drum]
     Excludes2   corrosion of ear drum (T28.91-)

    ● **T20.411**   Corrosion of unspecified degree of right ear [any part, except ear drum] 🔾

    ● **T20.412**   Corrosion of unspecified degree of left ear [any part, except ear drum] 🔾

    ● **T20.419**   Corrosion of unspecified degree of unspecified ear [any part, except ear drum] 🔾

X ● **T20.42**   Corrosion of unspecified degree of lip(s) 🔾

X ● **T20.43**   Corrosion of unspecified degree of chin 🔾

X ● **T20.44**   Corrosion of unspecified degree of nose (septum) 🔾

X ● **T20.45**   Corrosion of unspecified degree of scalp [any part] 🔾

X ● **T20.46**   Corrosion of unspecified degree of forehead and cheek 🔾

X ● **T20.47**   Corrosion of unspecified degree of neck 🔾

X ● **T20.49**   Corrosion of unspecified degree of multiple sites of head, face, and neck 🔾

● **T20.5**   Corrosion of first degree of head, face, and neck
    Code first (T51-T65) to identify chemical and intent
    Use additional external cause code to identify place (Y92)

X ● **T20.50**   Corrosion of first degree of head, face, and neck, unspecified site 🔾

● **T20.51**   Corrosion of first degree of ear [any part, except ear drum]
     Excludes2   corrosion of ear drum (T28.91-)

    ● **T20.511**   Corrosion of first degree of right ear [any part, except ear drum] 🔾

    ● **T20.512**   Corrosion of first degree of left ear [any part, except ear drum] 🔾

    ● **T20.519**   Corrosion of first degree of unspecified ear [any part, except ear drum] 🔾

X ● **T20.52**   Corrosion of first degree of lip(s) 🔾

X ● **T20.53**   Corrosion of first degree of chin 🔾

X ● **T20.54**   Corrosion of first degree of nose (septum) 🔾

X ● **T20.55**   Corrosion of first degree of scalp [any part] 🔾

X ● **T20.56**   Corrosion of first degree of forehead and cheek 🔾 ◀▥

X ● **T20.57**   Corrosion of first degree of neck 🔾

X ● **T20.59**   Corrosion of first degree of multiple sites of head, face, and neck 🔾

● **T20.6**   Corrosion of second degree of head, face, and neck
    Code first (T51-T65) to identify chemical and intent
    Use additional external cause code to identify place (Y92)

X ● **T20.60**   Corrosion of second degree of head, face, and neck, unspecified site 🔾

● **T20.61**   Corrosion of second degree of ear [any part, except ear drum]
     Excludes2   corrosion of ear drum (T28.91-)

    ● **T20.611**   Corrosion of second degree of right ear [any part, except ear drum] 🔾

    ● **T20.612**   Corrosion of second degree of left ear [any part, except ear drum] 🔾

    ● **T20.619**   Corrosion of second degree of unspecified ear [any part, except ear drum] 🔾

X ● **T20.62**   Corrosion of second degree of lip(s) 🔾

X ● **T20.63**   Corrosion of second degree of chin 🔾

X ● **T20.64**   Corrosion of second degree of nose (septum) 🔾

X ● **T20.65**   Corrosion of second degree of scalp [any part] 🔾

X ● **T20.66**   Corrosion of second degree of forehead and cheek 🔾

X ● **T20.67**   Corrosion of second degree of neck 🔾

X ● **T20.69**   Corrosion of second degree of multiple sites of head, face, and neck 🔾

● **T20.7**   Corrosion of third degree of head, face, and neck
    Code first (T51-T65) to identify chemical and intent
    Use additional external cause code to identify place (Y92)

X ● **T20.70**   Corrosion of third degree of head, face, and neck, unspecified site A 🔾, 🔾, A 🔾
     Ⓔⓧ See T20.30

● **T20.71**   Corrosion of third degree of ear [any part, except ear drum]
     Excludes2   corrosion of ear drum (T28.91-)
     Ⓔⓧ For category T20.71 CC codes: See T20.31

    ● **T20.711**   Corrosion of third degree of right ear [any part, except ear drum] A 🔾, 🔾, A 🔾

    ● **T20.712**   Corrosion of third degree of left ear [any part, except ear drum] A 🔾, 🔾, A 🔾

    ● **T20.719**   Corrosion of third degree of unspecified ear [any part, except ear drum] A 🔾, 🔾, A 🔾

X ● **T20.72**   Corrosion of third degree of lip(s) A 🔾, 🔾, A 🔾
     Ⓔⓧ See T20.32

X ● **T20.73**   Corrosion of third degree of chin A 🔾, 🔾, A 🔾
     Ⓔⓧ See T20.33

X ● **T20.74**   Corrosion of third degree of nose (septum) A 🔾, 🔾, A 🔾
     Ⓔⓧ See T20.34

X ● **T20.75**   Corrosion of third degree of scalp [any part] A 🔾, 🔾, A 🔾
     Ⓔⓧ See T20.35

X ● **T20.76**   Corrosion of third degree of forehead and cheek A 🔾, 🔾, A 🔾
     Ⓔⓧ See T20.36

X ● **T20.77**   Corrosion of third degree of neck A 🔾, 🔾, A 🔾
     Ⓔⓧ See T20.37

X ● **T20.79**   Corrosion of third degree of multiple sites of head, face, and neck A 🔾, 🔾, A 🔾
     Ⓔⓧ See T20.39

CHAPTER 19 (S00-T88)

N   Newborn Age: 0   P   Pediatric Age: 0–17   M   Maternity DX: 12–55   A   Adult Age: 15–124   ♀   Females Only   ♂   Males Only

🔾 Complication\Comorbidity   🔾 Major C\C   Ⓔⓧ CC/MCC Exclusions   🔾 Present on Admission Requirement   🔾 Hospital-Acquired Condition

1499

● **T21**   **Burn and corrosion of trunk**

     Includes   burns and corrosion of hip region

     Excludes2   burns and corrosion of axilla (T22.- with fifth character 4)

                burns and corrosion of scapular region (T22.- with fifth character 6)

                burns and corrosion of shoulder (T22.- with fifth character 5)

     The appropriate 7th character is to be added to each code from category T21

> A   initial encounter
> D   subsequent encounter
> S   sequela

● **T21.0**   **Burn of unspecified degree of trunk**

     Use additional external cause code to identify the source, place and intent of the burn (X00-X19, X75-X77, X96-X98, Y92)

   X ● **T21.00**   Burn of unspecified degree of trunk, unspecified site 🖐

   X ● **T21.01**   Burn of unspecified degree of chest wall 🖐
          Burn of of unspecified degree of breast

   X ● **T21.02**   Burn of unspecified degree of abdominal wall 🖐
          Burn of unspecified degree of flank
          Burn of unspecified degree of groin

   X ● **T21.03**   Burn of unspecified degree of upper back 🖐
          Burn of unspecified degree of interscapular region

   X ● **T21.04**   Burn of unspecified degree of lower back 🖐

   X ● **T21.05**   Burn of unspecified degree of buttock 🖐
          Burn of unspecified degree of anus

   X ● **T21.06**   Burn of unspecified degree of male genital region ♂ 🖐
          Burn of unspecified degree of penis
          Burn of unspecified degree of scrotum
          Burn of unspecified degree of testis

   X ● **T21.07**   Burn of unspecified degree of female genital region ♀ 🖐
          Burn of unspecified degree of labium (majus) (minus)
          Burn of unspecified degree of perineum
          Burn of unspecified degree of vulva
          Excludes2   burn of vagina (T28.3)

   X ● **T21.09**   Burn of unspecified degree of other site of trunk 🖐

● **T21.1**   **Burn of first degree of trunk**

     Use additional external cause code to identify the source, place and intent of the burn (X00-X19, X75-X77, X96-X98, Y92)

   X ● **T21.10**   Burn of first degree of trunk, unspecified site 🖐

   X ● **T21.11**   Burn of first degree of chest wall 🖐
          Burn of first degree of breast

   X ● **T21.12**   Burn of first degree of abdominal wall 🖐
          Burn of first degree of flank
          Burn of first degree of groin

   X ● **T21.13**   Burn of first degree of upper back 🖐
          Burn of first degree of interscapular region

   X ● **T21.14**   Burn of first degree of lower back 🖐

   X ● **T21.15**   Burn of first degree of buttock 🖐
          Burn of first degree of anus

   X ● **T21.16**   Burn of first degree of male genital region ♂ 🖐
          Burn of first degree of penis
          Burn of first degree of scrotum
          Burn of first degree of testis

   X ● **T21.17**   Burn of first degree of female genital region ♀ 🖐
          Burn of first degree of labium (majus) (minus)
          Burn of first degree of perineum
          Burn of first degree of vulva
          Excludes2   burn of vagina (T28.3)

   X ● **T21.19**   Burn of first degree of other site of trunk 🖐

● **T21.2**   **Burn of second degree of trunk**

     Use additional external cause code to identify the source, place and intent of the burn (X00-X19, X75-X77, X96-X98, Y92)

   X ● **T21.20**   Burn of second degree of trunk, unspecified site 🖐

   X ● **T21.21**   Burn of second degree of chest wall 🖐
          Burn of second degree of breast

   X ● **T21.22**   Burn of second degree of abdominal wall 🖐
          Burn of second degree of flank
          Burn of second degree of groin

   X ● **T21.23**   Burn of second degree of upper back 🖐
          Burn of second degree of interscapular region

   X ● **T21.24**   Burn of second degree of lower back 🖐

   X ● **T21.25**   Burn of second degree of buttock 🖐
          Burn of second degree of anus

   X ● **T21.26**   Burn of second degree of male genital region ♂ 🖐
          Burn of second degree of penis
          Burn of second degree of scrotum
          Burn of second degree of testis

   X ● **T21.27**   Burn of second degree of female genital region ♀ 🖐
          Burn of second degree of labium (majus) (minus)
          Burn of second degree of perineum
          Burn of second degree of vulva
          Excludes2   burn of vagina (T28.3)

   X ● **T21.29**   Burn of second degree of other site of trunk 🖐

● **T21.3**   **Burn of third degree of trunk**

     Use additional external cause code to identify the source, place and intent of the burn (X00-X19, X75-X77, X96-X98, Y92)

   X ● **T21.30**   Burn of third degree of trunk, unspecified site A 🖐, 🖐, A 🖐
          (Ex) T21.30X[A], T21.39X[A], T21.70X[A], T21.79X[A],

   X ● **T21.31**   Burn of third degree of chest wall A 🖐, 🖐, A 🖐
          Burn of third degree of breast
          (Ex) T21.30X-T21.31X[A], T21.39X[A], T21.70X-T21.71X[A], T21.79X[A]

   X ● **T21.32**   Burn of third degree of abdominal wall A 🖐, 🖐, A 🖐
          Burn of third degree of flank
          Burn of third degree of groin
          (Ex) T21.30X[A], T21.32X[A], T21.39X[A], T21.70X[A], T21.72X[A], T21.79X[A]

   X ● **T21.33**   Burn of third degree of upper back A 🖐, 🖐, A 🖐
          Burn of third degree of interscapular region
          (Ex) T21.30X[A], T21.33X-T21.35X[A], T21.39X[A], T21.70X[A], T21.73X-T21.75X[A], T21.79X[A]

   X ● **T21.34**   Burn of third degree of lower back A 🖐, 🖐, A 🖐
          (Ex) See T21.33

   X ● **T21.35**   Burn of third degree of buttock A 🖐, 🖐, A 🖐
          Burn of third degree of anus
          (Ex) See T21.33

◀ New   ◀ Revised   ~~deleted~~ Deleted   Excludes 1   Excludes 2   Includes   Use additional   Code first   Code also   Unspecified
OGCR Official Guidelines   ● Unacceptable Principal Diagnosis   X Assign placeholder X   ● Use Additional Character(s)   ▶ Manifestation Code   **Coding Clinic**

CHAPTER 19 (S00-T88)

X● **T21.36** **Burn of third degree of male genital region** ♂
A 🔖, 🔖, A 🔖
Burn of third degree of penis
Burn of third degree of scrotum
Burn of third degree of testis
Ⓔ T21.30X[A], T21.36X-T21.39X[A], T21.70X[A],
T21.76X-T21.79X[A]

X● **T21.37** **Burn of third degree of female genital region** ♀
A 🔖, 🔖, A 🔖
Burn of third degree of labium (majus) (minus)
Burn of third degree of perineum
Burn of third degree of vulva
Excludes2　burn of vagina (T28.3)
Ⓔ See T21.36

X● **T21.39** **Burn of third degree of other site of trunk** A 🔖,
🔖, A 🔖
Ⓔ See T21.30

● **T21.4** **Corrosion of unspecified degree of trunk**
Code first (T51-T65) to identify chemical and intent
Use additional external cause code to identify
place (Y92)

X● **T21.40** **Corrosion of unspecified degree of trunk,
unspecified site** 🔖

X● **T21.41** **Corrosion of unspecified degree of chest wall** 🔖
Corrosion of unspecified degree of breast

X● **T21.42** **Corrosion of unspecified degree of abdominal
wall** 🔖
Corrosion of unspecified degree of flank
Corrosion of unspecified degree of groin

X● **T21.43** **Corrosion of unspecified degree of upper
back** 🔖
Corrosion of unspecified degree of
interscapular region

X● **T21.44** **Corrosion of unspecified degree of lower
back** 🔖

X● **T21.45** **Corrosion of unspecified degree of buttock** 🔖
Corrosion of unspecified degree of anus

X● **T21.46** **Corrosion of unspecified degree of male genital
region** ♂ 🔖
Corrosion of unspecified degree of penis
Corrosion of unspecified degree of scrotum
Corrosion of unspecified degree of testis

X● **T21.47** **Corrosion of unspecified degree of female
genital region** ♀ 🔖
Corrosion of unspecified degree of labium
(majus) (minus)
Corrosion of unspecified degree of perineum
Corrosion of unspecified degree of vulva
Excludes2　corrosion of vagina (T28.8)

X● **T21.49** **Corrosion of unspecified degree of other site of
trunk** 🔖

● **T21.5** **Corrosion of first degree of trunk**
Code first (T51-T65) to identify chemical and intent
Use additional external cause code to identify
place (Y92)

X● **T21.50** **Corrosion of first degree of trunk, unspecified
site** 🔖

X● **T21.51** **Corrosion of first degree of chest wall** 🔖
Corrosion of first degree of breast

X● **T21.52** **Corrosion of first degree of abdominal wall** 🔖
Corrosion of first degree of flank
Corrosion of first degree of groin

X● **T21.53** **Corrosion of first degree of upper back** 🔖
Corrosion of first degree of interscapular
region

X● **T21.54** **Corrosion of first degree of lower back** 🔖

X● **T21.55** **Corrosion of first degree of buttock** 🔖
Corrosion of first degree of anus

X● **T21.56** **Corrosion of first degree of male genital
region** ♂ 🔖
Corrosion of first degree of penis
Corrosion of first degree of scrotum
Corrosion of first degree of testis

X● **T21.57** **Corrosion of first degree of female genital
region** ♀ 🔖
Corrosion of first degree of labium (majus)
(minus)
Corrosion of first degree of perineum
Corrosion of first degree of vulva
Excludes2　corrosion of vagina (T28.8)

X● **T21.59** **Corrosion of first degree of other site of
trunk** 🔖

● **T21.6** **Corrosion of second degree of trunk**
Code first (T51-T65) to identify chemical and intent
Use additional external cause code to identify
place (Y92)

X● **T21.60** **Corrosion of second degree of trunk,
unspecified site** 🔖

X● **T21.61** **Corrosion of second degree of chest wall** 🔖
Corrosion of second degree of breast

X● **T21.62** **Corrosion of second degree of abdominal
wall** 🔖
Corrosion of second degree of flank
Corrosion of second degree of groin

X● **T21.63** **Corrosion of second degree of upper back** 🔖
Corrosion of second degree of interscapular
region

X● **T21.64** **Corrosion of second degree of lower back** 🔖

X● **T21.65** **Corrosion of second degree of buttock** 🔖
Corrosion of second degree of anus

X● **T21.66** **Corrosion of second degree of male genital
region** ♂ 🔖
Corrosion of second degree of penis
Corrosion of second degree of scrotum
Corrosion of second degree of testis

X● **T21.67** **Corrosion of second degree of female genital
region** ♀ 🔖
Corrosion of second degree of labium (majus)
(minus)
Corrosion of second degree of perineum
Corrosion of second degree of vulva
Excludes2　corrosion of vagina (T28.8)

X● **T21.69** **Corrosion of second degree of other site of
trunk** 🔖

● **T21.7** **Corrosion of third degree of trunk**
Code first (T51-T65) to identify chemical and intent
Use additional external cause code to identify
place (Y92)

X● **T21.70** **Corrosion of third degree of trunk, unspecified
site** A 🔖, 🔖, A 🔖
Ⓔ See T21.30

X● **T21.71** **Corrosion of third degree of chest wall** A 🔖, 🔖,
A 🔖
Corrosion of third degree of breast
Ⓔ See T21.31

X● **T21.72** **Corrosion of third degree of abdominal wall**
A 🔖, 🔖, A 🔖
Corrosion of third degree of flank
Corrosion of third degree of groin
Ⓔ See T21.32

X● **T21.73** **Corrosion of third degree of upper back** A 🔖,
🔖, A 🔖
Corrosion of third degree of interscapular
region
Ⓔ See T21.33

X● **T21.74** **Corrosion of third degree of lower back** A 🔖,
🔖, A 🔖
Ⓔ See T21.33

N Newborn Age: 0　　**P** Pediatric Age: 0–17　　**M** Maternity DX: 12–55　　**A** Adult Age: 15–124　　♀ Females Only　　♂ Males Only

🔖 Complication\Comorbidity　　🔖 Major C\C　　Ⓔ CC/MCC Exclusions　　🔖 Present on Admission Requirement　　🔖 Hospital-Acquired Condition

1501

CHAPTER 19 (S00-T88)

X ● **T21.75**   **Corrosion of third degree of buttock** A 🖐, 🖐, A 🖐

Corrosion of third degree of anus

(Ex) See T21.33

X ● **T21.76**   **Corrosion of third degree of male genital region** ♂ A 🖐, 🖐, A 🖐

Corrosion of third degree of penis
Corrosion of third degree of scrotum
Corrosion of third degree of testis

(Ex) See T21.36

X ● **T21.77**   **Corrosion of third degree of female genital region** ♀ A 🖐, 🖐, A 🖐

Corrosion of third degree of labium (majus) (minus)
Corrosion of third degree of perineum
Corrosion of third degree of vulva

Excludes2   corrosion of vagina (T28.8)

(Ex) See T21.36

X ● **T21.79**   **Corrosion of third degree of other site of trunk** A 🖐, 🖐, A 🖐

(Ex) See T21.30

● **T22**   **Burn and corrosion of shoulder and upper limb, except wrist and hand**

Excludes2   burn and corrosion of interscapular region (T21.-)
burn and corrosion of wrist and hand (T23.-)

The appropriate 7th character is to be added to each code from category T22

> A   initial encounter
> D   subsequent encounter
> S   sequela

● **T22.0**   **Burn of unspecified degree of shoulder and upper limb, except wrist and hand**

Use additional external cause code to identify the source, place and intent of the burn (X00-X19, X75-X77, X96-X98, Y92)

X ● **T22.00**   Burn of unspecified degree of shoulder and upper limb, except wrist and hand, unspecified site 🖐

● **T22.01**   Burn of unspecified degree of forearm

  ● **T22.011**   Burn of unspecified degree of right forearm 🖐

  ● **T22.012**   Burn of unspecified degree of left forearm 🖐

  ● **T22.019**   Burn of unspecified degree of unspecified forearm 🖐

● **T22.02**   Burn of unspecified degree of elbow

  ● **T22.021**   Burn of unspecified degree of right elbow 🖐

  ● **T22.022**   Burn of unspecified degree of left elbow 🖐

  ● **T22.029**   Burn of unspecified degree of unspecified elbow 🖐

● **T22.03**   Burn of unspecified degree of upper arm

  ● **T22.031**   Burn of unspecified degree of right upper arm 🖐

  ● **T22.032**   Burn of unspecified degree of left upper arm 🖐

  ● **T22.039**   Burn of unspecified degree of unspecified upper arm 🖐

● **T22.04**   Burn of unspecified degree of axilla

  ● **T22.041**   Burn of unspecified degree of right axilla 🖐

  ● **T22.042**   Burn of unspecified degree of left axilla 🖐

  ● **T22.049**   Burn of unspecified degree of unspecified axilla 🖐

● **T22.05**   Burn of unspecified degree of shoulder

  ● **T22.051**   Burn of unspecified degree of right shoulder

  ● **T22.052**   Burn of unspecified degree of left shoulder 🖐

  ● **T22.059**   Burn of unspecified degree of unspecified shoulder 🖐

● **T22.06**   Burn of unspecified degree of scapular region

  ● **T22.061**   Burn of unspecified degree of right scapular region 🖐

  ● **T22.062**   Burn of unspecified degree of left scapular region 🖐

  ● **T22.069**   Burn of unspecified degree of unspecified scapular region 🖐

● **T22.09**   Burn of unspecified degree of multiple sites of shoulder and upper limb, except wrist and hand

  ● **T22.091**   Burn of unspecified degree of multiple sites of right shoulder and upper limb, except wrist and hand 🖐

  ● **T22.092**   Burn of unspecified degree of multiple sites of left shoulder and upper limb, except wrist and hand 🖐

  ● **T22.099**   Burn of unspecified degree of multiple sites of unspecified shoulder and upper limb, except wrist and hand 🖐

● **T22.1**   **Burn of first degree of shoulder and upper limb, except wrist and hand**

Use additional external cause code to identify the source, place and intent of the burn (X00-X19, X75-X77, X96-X98, Y92)

X ● **T22.10**   Burn of first degree of shoulder and upper limb, except wrist and hand, unspecified site 🖐

● **T22.11**   Burn of first degree of forearm

  ● **T22.111**   Burn of first degree of right forearm 🖐

  ● **T22.112**   Burn of first degree of left forearm 🖐

  ● **T22.119**   Burn of first degree of unspecified forearm 🖐

● **T22.12**   Burn of first degree of elbow

  ● **T22.121**   Burn of first degree of right elbow 🖐

  ● **T22.122**   Burn of first degree of left elbow 🖐

  ● **T22.129**   Burn of first degree of unspecified elbow 🖐

● **T22.13**   Burn of first degree of upper arm

  ● **T22.131**   Burn of first degree of right upper arm 🖐

  ● **T22.132**   Burn of first degree of left upper arm 🖐

  ● **T22.139**   Burn of first degree of unspecified upper arm 🖐

● **T22.14**   Burn of first degree of axilla

  ● **T22.141**   Burn of first degree of right axilla 🖐

  ● **T22.142**   Burn of first degree of left axilla 🖐

  ● **T22.149**   Burn of first degree of unspecified axilla 🖐

● **T22.15**   Burn of first degree of shoulder

  ● **T22.151**   Burn of first degree of right shoulder 🖐

  ● **T22.152**   Burn of first degree of left shoulder 🖐

  ● **T22.159**   Burn of first degree of unspecified shoulder 🖐

◀ New   ◀ⅲ Revised   ~~deleted~~ Deleted   Excludes 1   Excludes 2   Includes   Use additional   Code first   Code also   Unspecified

OGCR Official Guidelines   ● Unacceptable Principal Diagnosis   X Assign placeholder X   ● Use Additional Character(s)   ▶ Manifestation Code   **Coding Clinic**

● T22.16   Burn of first degree of scapular region
    ● T22.161   Burn of first degree of right scapular region 🔖
    ● T22.162   Burn of first degree of left scapular region 🔖
    ● T22.169   Burn of first degree of unspecified scapular region 🔖
● T22.19   Burn of first degree of multiple sites of shoulder and upper limb, except wrist and hand
    ● T22.191   Burn of first degree of multiple sites of right shoulder and upper limb, except wrist and hand 🔖
    ● T22.192   Burn of first degree of multiple sites of left shoulder and upper limb, except wrist and hand 🔖
    ● T22.199   Burn of first degree of multiple sites of unspecified shoulder and upper limb, except wrist and hand 🔖
● T22.2   Burn of second degree of shoulder and upper limb, except wrist and hand
    Use additional external cause code to identify the source, place and intent of the burn (X00-X19, X75-X77, X96-X98, Y92)
    X ● T22.20   Burn of second degree of shoulder and upper limb, except wrist and hand, unspecified site 🔖
    ● T22.21   Burn of second degree of forearm
        ● T22.211   Burn of second degree of right forearm 🔖
        ● T22.212   Burn of second degree of left forearm 🔖
        ● T22.219   Burn of second degree of unspecified forearm 🔖
    ● T22.22   Burn of second degree of elbow
        ● T22.221   Burn of second degree of right elbow 🔖
        ● T22.222   Burn of second degree of left elbow 🔖
        ● T22.229   Burn of second degree of unspecified elbow 🔖
    ● T22.23   Burn of second degree of upper arm
        ● T22.231   Burn of second degree of right upper arm 🔖
        ● T22.232   Burn of second degree of left upper arm 🔖
        ● T22.239   Burn of second degree of unspecified upper arm 🔖
    ● T22.24   Burn of second degree of axilla
        ● T22.241   Burn of second degree of right axilla 🔖
        ● T22.242   Burn of second degree of left axilla 🔖
        ● T22.249   Burn of second degree of unspecified axilla 🔖
    ● T22.25   Burn of second degree of shoulder
        ● T22.251   Burn of second degree of right shoulder 🔖
        ● T22.252   Burn of second degree of left shoulder 🔖
        ● T22.259   Burn of second degree of unspecified shoulder 🔖
    ● T22.26   Burn of second degree of scapular region
        ● T22.261   Burn of second degree of right scapular region 🔖
        ● T22.262   Burn of second degree of left scapular region 🔖
        ● T22.269   Burn of second degree of unspecified scapular region 🔖

● T22.29   Burn of second degree of multiple sites of shoulder and upper limb, except wrist and hand
    ● T22.291   Burn of second degree of multiple sites of right shoulder and upper limb, except wrist and hand 🔖
    ● T22.292   Burn of second degree of multiple sites of left shoulder and upper limb, except wrist and hand 🔖
    ● T22.299   Burn of second degree of multiple sites of unspecified shoulder and upper limb, except wrist and hand 🔖
● T22.3   Burn of third degree of shoulder and upper limb, except wrist and hand
    Use additional external cause code to identify the source, place and intent of the burn (X00-X19, X75-X77, X96-X98, Y92)
    X ● T22.30   Burn of third degree of shoulder and upper limb, except wrist and hand, unspecified site A 🔖, 🔖, A 🔖
        (Ex) T22.30X[A], T22.391-T22.399[A], T22.70X[A], T22.791-T22.799[A]
    ● T22.31   Burn of third degree of forearm
        (Ex) For category T22.31 CC codes: T22.30X-T22.319[A], T22.391-T22.399[A], T22.70X-T22.719[A], T22.791-T22.799[A]
        ● T22.311   Burn of third degree of right forearm A 🔖, 🔖, A 🔖
        ● T22.312   Burn of third degree of left forearm A 🔖, 🔖, A 🔖
        ● T22.319   Burn of third degree of unspecified forearm A 🔖, 🔖, A 🔖
    ● T22.32   Burn of third degree of elbow
        (Ex) For category T22.32 CC codes: T22.30X[A], T22.321-T22.329[A], T22.391-T22.399[A], T22.70X[A], T22.721-T22.729[A], T22.791-T22.799[A]
        ● T22.321   Burn of third degree of right elbow A 🔖, 🔖, A 🔖
        ● T22.322   Burn of third degree of left elbow A 🔖, 🔖, A 🔖
        ● T22.329   Burn of third degree of unspecified elbow A 🔖, 🔖, A 🔖
    ● T22.33   Burn of third degree of upper arm
        (Ex) For category T22.33 CC codes: T22.30X[A], T22.331-T22.339[A], T22.391-T22.399[A], T22.70X[A], T22.731-T22.739[A], T22.791-T22.799[A]
        ● T22.331   Burn of third degree of right upper arm A 🔖, 🔖, A 🔖
        ● T22.332   Burn of third degree of left upper arm A 🔖, 🔖, A 🔖
        ● T22.339   Burn of third degree of unspecified upper arm A 🔖; 🔖, A 🔖
    ● T22.34   Burn of third degree of axilla
        (Ex) For category T22.34 CC codes: T22.30X[A], T22.341-T22.349[A], T22.391-T22.399[A], T22.70X[A], T22.741-T22.749[A], T22.791-T22.799[A]
        ● T22.341   Burn of third degree of right axilla A 🔖, 🔖, A 🔖
        ● T22.342   Burn of third degree of left axilla A 🔖, 🔖, A 🔖
        ● T22.349   Burn of third degree of unspecified axilla A 🔖, 🔖, A 🔖
    ● T22.35   Burn of third degree of shoulder
        (Ex) For category T22.35 CC codes: T22.30X[A], T22.351-T22.359[A], T22.391-T22.399[A], T22.70X[A], T22.751-T22.759[A], T22.791-T22.799[A]
        ● T22.351   Burn of third degree of right shoulder A 🔖, 🔖, A 🔖
        ● T22.352   Burn of third degree of left shoulder A 🔖, 🔖, A 🔖
        ● T22.359   Burn of third degree of unspecified shoulder A 🔖, 🔖, A 🔖

CHAPTER 19 (S00-T88)

N Newborn Age: 0   P Pediatric Age: 0–17   M Maternity DX: 12–55   A Adult Age: 15–124   ♀ Females Only   ♂ Males Only

🔖 Complication\Comorbidity   🔖 Major C\C   (Ex) CC/MCC Exclusions   🔖 Present on Admission Requirement   🔖 Hospital-Acquired Condition

1503

● **T22.36**   Burn of third degree of scapular region
     Ⓔⓧ For category T22.36 CC codes: T22.30X[A], T22.361-T22.369[A], T22.391-T22.399[A], T22.70X[A], T22.761-T22.769[A], T22.791-T22.799[A]

     ● **T22.361**   Burn of third degree of right scapular region A 🖐, 🖐, A 🖐

     ● **T22.362**   Burn of third degree of left scapular region A 🖐, 🖐, A 🖐

     ● **T22.369**   Burn of third degree of unspecified scapular region A 🖐, 🖐, A 🖐

● **T22.39**   Burn of third degree of multiple sites of shoulder and upper limb, except wrist and hand
     Ⓔⓧ For category T22.39 CC codes: See T22.30

     ● **T22.391**   Burn of third degree of multiple sites of right shoulder and upper limb, except wrist and hand A 🖐, 🖐, A 🖐

     ● **T22.392**   Burn of third degree of multiple sites of left shoulder and upper limb, except wrist and hand A 🖐, 🖐, A 🖐

     ● **T22.399**   Burn of third degree of multiple sites of unspecified shoulder and upper limb, except wrist and hand A 🖐, 🖐, A 🖐

● **T22.4**   Corrosion of unspecified degree of shoulder and upper limb, except wrist and hand
     Code first (T51-T65) *to identify chemical and intent*
     Use additional external cause code to identify place (Y92)

  X ● **T22.40**   Corrosion of unspecified degree of shoulder and upper limb, except wrist and hand, unspecified site 🖐

     ● **T22.41**   Corrosion of unspecified degree of forearm

     ● **T22.411**   Corrosion of unspecified degree of right forearm 🖐

     ● **T22.412**   Corrosion of unspecified degree of left forearm 🖐

     ● **T22.419**   Corrosion of unspecified degree of unspecified forearm 🖐

     ● **T22.42**   Corrosion of unspecified degree of elbow

     ● **T22.421**   Corrosion of unspecified degree of right elbow 🖐

     ● **T22.422**   Corrosion of unspecified degree of left elbow 🖐

     ● **T22.429**   Corrosion of unspecified degree of unspecified elbow 🖐

     ● **T22.43**   Corrosion of unspecified degree of upper arm

     ● **T22.431**   Corrosion of unspecified degree of right upper arm 🖐

     ● **T22.432**   Corrosion of unspecified degree of left upper arm 🖐

     ● **T22.439**   Corrosion of unspecified degree of unspecified upper arm 🖐

     ● **T22.44**   Corrosion of unspecified degree of axilla

     ● **T22.441**   Corrosion of unspecified degree of right axilla 🖐

     ● **T22.442**   Corrosion of unspecified degree of left axilla 🖐

     ● **T22.449**   Corrosion of unspecified degree of unspecified axilla 🖐

     ● **T22.45**   Corrosion of unspecified degree of shoulder

     ● **T22.451**   Corrosion of unspecified degree of right shoulder 🖐

     ● **T22.452**   Corrosion of unspecified degree of left shoulder 🖐

     ● **T22.459**   Corrosion of unspecified degree of unspecified shoulder 🖐

● **T22.46**   Corrosion of unspecified degree of scapular region

     ● **T22.461**   Corrosion of unspecified degree of right scapular region 🖐

     ● **T22.462**   Corrosion of unspecified degree of left scapular region 🖐

     ● **T22.469**   Corrosion of unspecified degree of unspecified scapular region 🖐

● **T22.49**   Corrosion of unspecified degree of multiple sites of shoulder and upper limb, except wrist and hand

     ● **T22.491**   Corrosion of unspecified degree of multiple sites of right shoulder and upper limb, except wrist and hand 🖐

     ● **T22.492**   Corrosion of unspecified degree of multiple sites of left shoulder and upper limb, except wrist and hand 🖐

     ● **T22.499**   Corrosion of unspecified degree of multiple sites of unspecified shoulder and upper limb, except wrist and hand 🖐

● **T22.5**   Corrosion of first degree of shoulder and upper limb, except wrist and hand
     Code first (T51-T65) *to identify chemical and intent*
     Use additional external cause code to identify place (Y92)

  X ● **T22.50**   Corrosion of first degree of shoulder and upper limb, except wrist and hand unspecified site 🖐

     ● **T22.51**   Corrosion of first degree of forearm

     ● **T22.511**   Corrosion of first degree of right forearm 🖐

     ● **T22.512**   Corrosion of first degree of left forearm 🖐

     ● **T22.519**   Corrosion of first degree of unspecified forearm 🖐

     ● **T22.52**   Corrosion of first degree of elbow

     ● **T22.521**   Corrosion of first degree of right elbow 🖐

     ● **T22.522**   Corrosion of first degree of left elbow 🖐

     ● **T22.529**   Corrosion of first degree of unspecified elbow 🖐

     ● **T22.53**   Corrosion of first degree of upper arm

     ● **T22.531**   Corrosion of first degree of right upper arm 🖐

     ● **T22.532**   Corrosion of first degree of left upper arm 🖐

     ● **T22.539**   Corrosion of first degree of unspecified upper arm 🖐

     ● **T22.54**   Corrosion of first degree of axilla

     ● **T22.541**   Corrosion of first degree of right axilla 🖐

     ● **T22.542**   Corrosion of first degree of left axilla 🖐

     ● **T22.549**   Corrosion of first degree of unspecified axilla 🖐

     ● **T22.55**   Corrosion of first degree of shoulder

     ● **T22.551**   Corrosion of first degree of right shoulder 🖐

     ● **T22.552**   Corrosion of first degree of left shoulder 🖐

     ● **T22.559**   Corrosion of first degree of unspecified shoulder 🖐

◀ New   ◀▥ Revised   ~~deleted~~ Deleted   Excludes 1   Excludes 2   Includes   Use additional   Code first   Code also   Unspecified

OGCR Official Guidelines   ● Unacceptable Principal Diagnosis   X Assign placeholder X   ● Use Additional Character(s)   ▌ Manifestation Code   **Coding Clinic**

- T22.56 Corrosion of first degree of scapular region
  - T22.561 Corrosion of first degree of right scapular region 🖐
  - T22.562 Corrosion of first degree of left scapular region 🖐
  - T22.569 Corrosion of first degree of unspecified scapular region 🖐
- T22.59 Corrosion of first degree of multiple sites of shoulder and upper limb, except wrist and hand
  - T22.591 Corrosion of first degree of multiple sites of right shoulder and upper limb, except wrist and hand 🖐
  - T22.592 Corrosion of first degree of multiple sites of left shoulder and upper limb, except wrist and hand 🖐
  - T22.599 Corrosion of first degree of multiple sites of unspecified shoulder and upper limb, except wrist and hand 🖐
- T22.6 Corrosion of second degree of shoulder and upper limb, except wrist and hand

  Code first (T51-T65) *to identify chemical and intent*

  Use additional external cause code to identify place (Y92)

  - X T22.60 Corrosion of second degree of shoulder and upper limb, except wrist and hand, unspecified site 🖐
  - T22.61 Corrosion of second degree of forearm
    - T22.611 Corrosion of second degree of right forearm 🖐
    - T22.612 Corrosion of second degree of left forearm 🖐
    - T22.619 Corrosion of second degree of unspecified forearm 🖐
  - T22.62 Corrosion of second degree of elbow
    - T22.621 Corrosion of second degree of right elbow 🖐
    - T22.622 Corrosion of second degree of left elbow 🖐
    - T22.629 Corrosion of second degree of unspecified elbow 🖐
  - T22.63 Corrosion of second degree of upper arm
    - T22.631 Corrosion of second degree of right upper arm 🖐
    - T22.632 Corrosion of second degree of left upper arm 🖐
    - T22.639 Corrosion of second degree of unspecified upper arm 🖐
  - T22.64 Corrosion of second degree of axilla
    - T22.641 Corrosion of second degree of right axilla 🖐
    - T22.642 Corrosion of second degree of left axilla 🖐
    - T22.649 Corrosion of second degree of unspecified axilla 🖐
  - T22.65 Corrosion of second degree of shoulder
    - T22.651 Corrosion of second degree of right shoulder 🖐
    - T22.652 Corrosion of second degree of left shoulder 🖐
    - T22.659 Corrosion of second degree of unspecified shoulder 🖐
  - T22.66 Corrosion of second degree of scapular region
    - T22.661 Corrosion of second degree of right scapular region 🖐
    - T22.662 Corrosion of second degree of left scapular region 🖐
    - T22.669 Corrosion of second degree of unspecified scapular region 🖐

- T22.69 Corrosion of second degree of multiple sites of shoulder and upper limb, except wrist and hand
  - T22.691 Corrosion of second degree of multiple sites of right shoulder and upper limb, except wrist and hand 🖐
  - T22.692 Corrosion of second degree of multiple sites of left shoulder and upper limb, except wrist and hand 🖐
  - T22.699 Corrosion of second degree of multiple sites of unspecified shoulder and upper limb, except wrist and hand 🖐
- T22.7 Corrosion of third degree of shoulder and upper limb, except wrist and hand

  Code first (T51-T65) *to identify chemical and intent*

  Use additional external cause code to identify place (Y92)

  - X T22.70 Corrosion of third degree of shoulder and upper limb, except wrist and hand, unspecified site A 🖐, 🖐, A 🖐
    - (Ex) See T22.30
  - T22.71 Corrosion of third degree of forearm
    - (Ex) For category T22.71 CC codes: See T22.31
    - T22.711 Corrosion of third degree of right forearm A 🖐, 🖐, A 🖐
    - T22.712 Corrosion of third degree of left forearm A 🖐, 🖐, A 🖐
    - T22.719 Corrosion of third degree of unspecified forearm A 🖐, 🖐, A 🖐
  - T22.72 Corrosion of third degree of elbow
    - (Ex) For category T22.72 CC codes: See T22.32
    - T22.721 Corrosion of third degree of right elbow A 🖐, 🖐, A 🖐
    - T22.722 Corrosion of third degree of left elbow A 🖐, 🖐, A 🖐
    - T22.729 Corrosion of third degree of unspecified elbow A 🖐, 🖐, A 🖐
  - T22.73 Corrosion of third degree of upper arm
    - (Ex) For category T22.73 CC codes: T22.33
    - T22.731 Corrosion of third degree of right upper arm A 🖐, 🖐, A 🖐
    - T22.732 Corrosion of third degree of left upper arm A 🖐, 🖐, A 🖐
    - T22.739 Corrosion of third degree of unspecified upper arm A 🖐, 🖐, A 🖐
  - T22.74 Corrosion of third degree of axilla
    - (Ex) For category T22.74 CC codes: T22.34
    - T22.741 Corrosion of third degree of right axilla A 🖐, 🖐, A 🖐
    - T22.742 Corrosion of third degree of left axilla A 🖐, 🖐, A 🖐
    - T22.749 Corrosion of third degree of unspecified axilla A 🖐, 🖐, A 🖐
  - T22.75 Corrosion of third degree of shoulder
    - (Ex) For category T22.75 CC codes: T22.35
    - T22.751 Corrosion of third degree of right shoulder A 🖐, 🖐, A 🖐
    - T22.752 Corrosion of third degree of left shoulder A 🖐, 🖐, A 🖐
    - T22.759 Corrosion of third degree of unspecified shoulder A 🖐, 🖐, A 🖐
  - T22.76 Corrosion of third degree of scapular region
    - (Ex) For category T22.76 CC codes: T22.36
    - T22.761 Corrosion of third degree of right scapular region A 🖐, 🖐, A 🖐
    - T22.762 Corrosion of third degree of left scapular region A 🖐, 🖐, A 🖐
    - T22.769 Corrosion of third degree of unspecified scapular region A 🖐, 🖐, A 🖐

N Newborn Age: 0   **P** Pediatric Age: 0–17   **M** Maternity DX: 12–55   **A** Adult Age: 15–124   ♀ Females Only   ♂ Males Only

🖐 Complication\Comorbidity   🖐 Major C\C   (Ex) CC/MCC Exclusions   🖐 Present on Admission Requirement   🖐 Hospital-Acquired Condition

CHAPTER 19 (S00-T88)

1505

● **T22.79**   Corrosion of third degree of multiple sites of shoulder and upper limb, except wrist and hand
    (Ex) For category T22.79 CC codes: See T22.30

  ● **T22.791**   Corrosion of third degree of multiple sites of right shoulder and upper limb, except wrist and hand A 🔖, 🔖, A 🔖

  ● **T22.792**   Corrosion of third degree of multiple sites of left shoulder and upper limb, except wrist and hand A 🔖, 🔖, A 🔖

  ● **T22.799**   Corrosion of third degree of multiple sites of unspecified shoulder and upper limb, except wrist and hand A 🔖, 🔖, A 🔖

● **T23**   Burn and corrosion of wrist and hand

   The appropriate 7th character is to be added to each code from category T23

     A   initial encounter
     D   subsequent encounter
     S   sequela

● **T23.0**   Burn of unspecified degree of wrist and hand

   Use additional external cause code to identify the source, place and intent of the burn (X00-X19, X75-X77, X96-X98, Y92)

  ● **T23.00**   Burn of unspecified degree of hand, unspecified site

    ● **T23.001**   Burn of unspecified degree of right hand, unspecified site 🔖

    ● **T23.002**   Burn of unspecified degree of left hand, unspecified site 🔖

    ● **T23.009**   Burn of unspecified degree of unspecified hand, unspecified site 🔖

  ● **T23.01**   Burn of unspecified degree of thumb (nail)

    ● **T23.011**   Burn of unspecified degree of right thumb (nail) 🔖

    ● **T23.012**   Burn of unspecified degree of left thumb (nail) 🔖

    ● **T23.019**   Burn of unspecified degree of unspecified thumb (nail) 🔖

  ● **T23.02**   Burn of unspecified degree of single finger (nail) except thumb

    ● **T23.021**   Burn of unspecified degree of single right finger (nail) except thumb 🔖

    ● **T23.022**   Burn of unspecified degree of single left finger (nail) except thumb 🔖

    ● **T23.029**   Burn of unspecified degree of unspecified single finger (nail) except thumb 🔖

  ● **T23.03**   Burn of unspecified degree of multiple fingers (nail), not including thumb

    ● **T23.031**   Burn of unspecified degree of multiple right fingers (nail), not including thumb 🔖

    ● **T23.032**   Burn of unspecified degree of multiple left fingers (nail), not including thumb 🔖

    ● **T23.039**   Burn of unspecified degree of unspecified multiple fingers (nail), not including thumb 🔖

● **T23.04**   Burn of unspecified degree of multiple fingers (nail), including thumb

  ● **T23.041**   Burn of unspecified degree of multiple right fingers (nail), including thumb 🔖

  ● **T23.042**   Burn of unspecified degree of multiple left fingers (nail), including thumb 🔖

  ● **T23.049**   Burn of unspecified degree of unspecified multiple fingers (nail), including thumb 🔖

● **T23.05**   Burn of unspecified degree of palm

  ● **T23.051**   Burn of unspecified degree of right palm 🔖

  ● **T23.052**   Burn of unspecified degree of left palm 🔖

  ● **T23.059**   Burn of unspecified degree of unspecified palm 🔖

● **T23.06**   Burn of unspecified degree of back of hand

  ● **T23.061**   Burn of unspecified degree of back of right hand 🔖

  ● **T23.062**   Burn of unspecified degree of back of left hand 🔖

  ● **T23.069**   Burn of unspecified degree of back of unspecified hand 🔖

● **T23.07**   Burn of unspecified degree of wrist

  ● **T23.071**   Burn of unspecified degree of right wrist 🔖

  ● **T23.072**   Burn of unspecified degree of left wrist 🔖

  ● **T23.079**   Burn of unspecified degree of unspecified wrist 🔖

● **T23.09**   Burn of unspecified degree of multiple sites of wrist and hand

  ● **T23.091**   Burn of unspecified degree of multiple sites of right wrist and hand 🔖

  ● **T23.092**   Burn of unspecified degree of multiple sites of left wrist and hand 🔖

  ● **T23.099**   Burn of unspecified degree of multiple sites of unspecified wrist and hand 🔖

● **T23.1**   Burn of first degree of wrist and hand

   Use additional external cause code to identify the source, place and intent of the burn (X00-X19, X75-X77, X96-X98, Y92)

  ● **T23.10**   Burn of first degree of hand, unspecified site

    ● **T23.101**   Burn of first degree of right hand, unspecified site 🔖

    ● **T23.102**   Burn of first degree of left hand, unspecified site 🔖

    ● **T23.109**   Burn of first degree of unspecified hand, unspecified site 🔖

  ● **T23.11**   Burn of first degree of thumb (nail)

    ● **T23.111**   Burn of first degree of right thumb (nail) 🔖

    ● **T23.112**   Burn of first degree of left thumb (nail) 🔖

    ● **T23.119**   Burn of first degree of unspecified thumb (nail) 🔖

◄ New   ◄▥ Revised   ~~deleted~~ Deleted   Excludes 1   Excludes 2   Includes   Use additional   Code first   Code also   Unspecified
OGCR Official Guidelines   ● Unacceptable Principal Diagnosis   X Assign placeholder X   ● Use Additional Character(s)   ▶ Manifestation Code   **Coding Clinic**

● **T23.12**   Burn of first degree of single finger (nail) except thumb
   ● **T23.121**   Burn of first degree of single right finger (nail) except thumb 🖐
   ● **T23.122**   Burn of first degree of single left finger (nail) except thumb 🖐
   ● **T23.129**   Burn of first degree of unspecified single finger (nail) except thumb 🖐
● **T23.13**   Burn of first degree of multiple fingers (nail), not including thumb
   ● **T23.131**   Burn of first degree of multiple right fingers (nail), not including thumb 🖐
   ● **T23.132**   Burn of first degree of multiple left fingers (nail), not including thumb 🖐
   ● **T23.139**   Burn of first degree of unspecified multiple fingers (nail), not including thumb 🖐
● **T23.14**   Burn of first degree of multiple fingers (nail), including thumb
   ● **T23.141**   Burn of first degree of multiple right fingers (nail), including thumb 🖐
   ● **T23.142**   Burn of first degree of multiple left fingers (nail), including thumb 🖐
   ● **T23.149**   Burn of first degree of unspecified multiple fingers (nail), including thumb 🖐
● **T23.15**   Burn of first degree of palm
   ● **T23.151**   Burn of first degree of right palm 🖐
   ● **T23.152**   Burn of first degree of left palm 🖐
   ● **T23.159**   Burn of first degree of unspecified palm 🖐
● **T23.16**   Burn of first degree of back of hand
   ● **T23.161**   Burn of first degree of back of right hand 🖐
   ● **T23.162**   Burn of first degree of back of left hand 🖐
   ● **T23.169**   Burn of first degree of back of unspecified hand 🖐
● **T23.17**   Burn of first degree of wrist
   ● **T23.171**   Burn of first degree of right wrist 🖐
   ● **T23.172**   Burn of first degree of left wrist 🖐
   ● **T23.179**   Burn of first degree of unspecified wrist 🖐
● **T23.19**   Burn of first degree of multiple sites of wrist and hand
   ● **T23.191**   Burn of first degree of multiple sites of right wrist and hand 🖐
   ● **T23.192**   Burn of first degree of multiple sites of left wrist and hand 🖐
   ● **T23.199**   Burn of first degree of multiple sites of unspecified wrist and hand 🖐
● **T23.2**   Burn of second degree of wrist and hand
   Use additional external cause code to identify the source, place and intent of the burn (X00-X19, X75-X77, X96-X98, Y92)
● **T23.20**   Burn of second degree of hand, unspecified site
   ● **T23.201**   Burn of second degree of right hand, unspecified site 🖐
   ● **T23.202**   Burn of second degree of left hand, unspecified site 🖐
   ● **T23.209**   Burn of second degree of unspecified hand, unspecified site 🖐

● **T23.21**   Burn of second degree of thumb (nail)
   ● **T23.211**   Burn of second degree of right thumb (nail) 🖐
   ● **T23.212**   Burn of second degree of left thumb (nail) 🖐
   ● **T23.219**   Burn of second degree of unspecified thumb (nail) 🖐
● **T23.22**   Burn of second degree of single finger (nail) except thumb
   ● **T23.221**   Burn of second degree of single right finger (nail) except thumb 🖐
   ● **T23.222**   Burn of second degree of single left finger (nail) except thumb 🖐
   ● **T23.229**   Burn of second degree of unspecified single finger (nail) except thumb 🖐
● **T23.23**   Burn of second degree of multiple fingers (nail), not including thumb
   ● **T23.231**   Burn of second degree of multiple right fingers (nail), not including thumb 🖐
   ● **T23.232**   Burn of second degree of multiple left fingers (nail), not including thumb 🖐
   ● **T23.239**   Burn of second degree of unspecified multiple fingers (nail), not including thumb 🖐
● **T23.24**   Burn of second degree of multiple fingers (nail), including thumb
   ● **T23.241**   Burn of second degree of multiple right fingers (nail), including thumb 🖐
   ● **T23.242**   Burn of second degree of multiple left fingers (nail), including thumb 🖐
   ● **T23.249**   Burn of second degree of unspecified multiple fingers (nail), including thumb 🖐
● **T23.25**   Burn of second degree of palm
   ● **T23.251**   Burn of second degree of right palm 🖐
   ● **T23.252**   Burn of second degree of left palm 🖐
   ● **T23.259**   Burn of second degree of unspecified palm 🖐
● **T23.26**   Burn of second degree of back of hand
   ● **T23.261**   Burn of second degree of back of right hand 🖐
   ● **T23.262**   Burn of second degree of back of left hand 🖐
   ● **T23.269**   Burn of second degree of back of unspecified hand 🖐
● **T23.27**   Burn of second degree of wrist
   ● **T23.271**   Burn of second degree of right wrist 🖐
   ● **T23.272**   Burn of second degree of left wrist 🖐
   ● **T23.279**   Burn of second degree of unspecified wrist 🖐
● **T23.29**   Burn of second degree of multiple sites of wrist and hand
   ● **T23.291**   Burn of second degree of multiple sites of right wrist and hand 🖐
   ● **T23.292**   Burn of second degree of multiple sites of left wrist and hand 🖐
   ● **T23.299**   Burn of second degree of multiple sites of unspecified wrist and hand 🖐

CHAPTER 19 (S00-T88)

N   Newborn Age: 0   **P**   Pediatric Age: 0–17   **M**   Maternity DX: 12–55   **A**   Adult Age: 15–124   ♀   Females Only   ♂   Males Only

🖐   Complication\Comorbidity   🖐   Major C\C   (Ex)   CC/MCC Exclusions   🖐   Present on Admission Requirement   🖐   Hospital-Acquired Condition

1507

● **T23.3**   **Burn of third degree of wrist and hand**
Use additional external cause code to identify the source, place and intent of the burn (X00-X19, X75-X77, X96-X98, Y92)

● **T23.30**   Burn of third degree of hand, unspecified site
(Ex) For category T23.30 CC codes: T23.301-T23.309[A], T23.391-T23.399[A], T23.701-T23.709[A], T23.791-T23.799[A]

  ● **T23.301**   Burn of third degree of right hand, unspecified site A 🔖, 🔖, A 🔖

  ● **T23.302**   Burn of third degree of left hand, unspecified site A 🔖, 🔖, A 🔖

  ● **T23.309**   Burn of third degree of unspecified hand, unspecified site A 🔖, 🔖, A 🔖

● **T23.31**   Burn of third degree of thumb (nail)
(Ex) For category T23.31 CC codes: T23.301-T23.319[A], T23.391-T23.399[A], T23.701-T23.719[A], T23.791-T23.799[A]

  ● **T23.311**   Burn of third degree of right thumb (nail) A 🔖, 🔖, A 🔖

  ● **T23.312**   Burn of third degree of left thumb (nail) A 🔖, 🔖, A 🔖

  ● **T23.319**   Burn of third degree of unspecified thumb (nail) A 🔖, 🔖, A 🔖

● **T23.32**   Burn of third degree of single finger (nail) except thumb
(Ex) For category T23.32 CC codes: T23.301-T23.309[A], T23.321-T23.329[A], T23.391-T23.399[A], T23.701-T23.709[A], T23.721-T23.729[A], T23.791-T23.799[A]

  ● **T23.321**   Burn of third degree of single right finger (nail) except thumb A 🔖, 🔖, A 🔖

  ● **T23.322**   Burn of third degree of single left finger (nail) except thumb A 🔖, 🔖, A 🔖

  ● **T23.329**   Burn of third degree of unspecified single finger (nail) except thumb A 🔖, 🔖, A 🔖

● **T23.33**   Burn of third degree of multiple fingers (nail), not including thumb
(Ex) For category T23.33 CC codes: T23.301-T23.309[A], T23.331-T23.339[A], T23.391-T23.399[A], T23.701-709[A], T23.731-T23.739[A], T23.791-T23.799[A]

  ● **T23.331**   Burn of third degree of multiple right fingers (nail), not including thumb A 🔖, 🔖, A 🔖

  ● **T23.332**   Burn of third degree of multiple left fingers (nail), not including thumb A 🔖, 🔖, A 🔖

  ● **T23.339**   Burn of third degree of unspecified multiple fingers (nail), not including thumb A 🔖, 🔖, A 🔖

● **T23.34**   Burn of third degree of multiple fingers (nail), including thumb
(Ex) For category T23.34 CC codes: T23.301-T23.309[A], T23.341-T23.349[A], T23.391-T23.399[A], T23.701-T23.709[A], T23.741-T23.749[A], T23.791-T23.799[A]

  ● **T23.341**   Burn of third degree of multiple right fingers (nail), including thumb A 🔖, 🔖, A 🔖

  ● **T23.342**   Burn of third degree of multiple left fingers (nail), including thumb A 🔖, 🔖, A 🔖

  ● **T23.349**   Burn of third degree of unspecified multiple fingers (nail), including thumb A 🔖, 🔖, A 🔖

● **T23.35**   Burn of third degree of palm
(Ex) For category T23.35 CC codes: T23.301-T23.309[A], T23.351-T23.359[A], T23.391-T23.399[A], T23.701-T23.709[A], T23.751-T23.759[A], T23.791-T23.799[A]

  ● **T23.351**   Burn of third degree of right palm A 🔖, 🔖, A 🔖

  ● **T23.352**   Burn of third degree of left palm A 🔖, 🔖, A 🔖

  ● **T23.359**   Burn of third degree of unspecified palm A 🔖, 🔖, A 🔖

● **T23.36**   Burn of third degree of back of hand
(Ex) For category T23.36 CC codes: T23.301-T23.309[A], T23.361-T23.369[A], T23.391-T23.399[A], T23.701-T23.709[A], T23.761-T23.769[A], T23.791-T23.799[A]

  ● **T23.361**   Burn of third degree of back of right hand A 🔖, 🔖, A 🔖

  ● **T23.362**   Burn of third degree of back of left hand A 🔖, 🔖, A 🔖

  ● **T23.369**   Burn of third degree of back of unspecified hand A 🔖, 🔖, A 🔖

● **T23.37**   Burn of third degree of wrist
(Ex) For category T23.37 CC codes: T23.301-T23.309[A], T23.371-T23.379[A], T23.391-T23.399[A], T23.701-T23.709[A], T23.771-T23.779[A], T23.791-T23.799[A]

  ● **T23.371**   Burn of third degree of right wrist A 🔖, 🔖, A 🔖

  ● **T23.372**   Burn of third degree of left wrist A 🔖, 🔖, A 🔖

  ● **T23.379**   Burn of third degree of unspecified wrist A 🔖, 🔖, A 🔖

● **T23.39**   Burn of third degree of multiple sites of wrist and hand
(Ex) For category T23.39 CC codes: T23.30

  ● **T23.391**   Burn of third degree of multiple sites of right wrist and hand A 🔖, 🔖, A 🔖

  ● **T23.392**   Burn of third degree of multiple sites of left wrist and hand A 🔖, 🔖, A 🔖

  ● **T23.399**   Burn of third degree of multiple sites of unspecified wrist and hand A 🔖, 🔖, A 🔖

● **T23.4**   **Corrosion of unspecified degree of wrist and hand**
Code first (T51-T65) *to identify chemical and intent*
Use additional external cause code to identify place (Y92)

● **T23.40**   Corrosion of unspecified degree of hand, unspecified site

  ● **T23.401**   Corrosion of unspecified degree of right hand, unspecified site 🔖

  ● **T23.402**   Corrosion of unspecified degree of left hand, unspecified site 🔖

  ● **T23.409**   Corrosion of unspecified degree of unspecified hand, unspecified site 🔖

● **T23.41**   Corrosion of unspecified degree of thumb (nail)

  ● **T23.411**   Corrosion of unspecified degree of right thumb (nail) 🔖

  ● **T23.412**   Corrosion of unspecified degree of left thumb (nail) 🔖

  ● **T23.419**   Corrosion of unspecified degree of unspecified thumb (nail) 🔖

● **T23.42**   Corrosion of unspecified degree of single finger (nail) except thumb

  ● **T23.421**   Corrosion of unspecified degree of single right finger (nail) except thumb 🔖

  ● **T23.422**   Corrosion of unspecified degree of single left finger (nail) except thumb 🔖

  ● **T23.429**   Corrosion of unspecified degree of unspecified single finger (nail) except thumb 🔖

◀ New   ◀▥ Revised   ~~deleted~~ Deleted   Excludes 1   Excludes 2   Includes   Use additional   Code first   Code also   Unspecified

OGCR Official Guidelines   ● Unacceptable Principal Diagnosis   X Assign placeholder X   ● Use Additional Character(s)   ▶ Manifestation Code   **Coding Clinic**

- **T23.43** Corrosion of unspecified degree of multiple fingers (nail), not including thumb
  - **T23.431** Corrosion of unspecified degree of multiple right fingers (nail), not including thumb
  - **T23.432** Corrosion of unspecified degree of multiple left fingers (nail), not including thumb
  - **T23.439** Corrosion of unspecified degree of unspecified multiple fingers (nail), not including thumb
- **T23.44** Corrosion of unspecified degree of multiple fingers (nail), including thumb
  - **T23.441** Corrosion of unspecified degree of multiple right fingers (nail), including thumb
  - **T23.442** Corrosion of unspecified degree of multiple left fingers (nail), including thumb
  - **T23.449** Corrosion of unspecified degree of unspecified multiple fingers (nail), including thumb
- **T23.45** Corrosion of unspecified degree of palm
  - **T23.451** Corrosion of unspecified degree of right palm
  - **T23.452** Corrosion of unspecified degree of left palm
  - **T23.459** Corrosion of unspecified degree of unspecified palm
- **T23.46** Corrosion of unspecified degree of back of hand
  - **T23.461** Corrosion of unspecified degree of back of right hand
  - **T23.462** Corrosion of unspecified degree of back of left hand
  - **T23.469** Corrosion of unspecified degree of back of unspecified hand
- **T23.47** Corrosion of unspecified degree of wrist
  - **T23.471** Corrosion of unspecified degree of right wrist
  - **T23.472** Corrosion of unspecified degree of left wrist
  - **T23.479** Corrosion of unspecified degree of unspecified wrist
- **T23.49** Corrosion of unspecified degree of multiple sites of wrist and hand
  - **T23.491** Corrosion of unspecified degree of multiple sites of right wrist and hand
  - **T23.492** Corrosion of unspecified degree of multiple sites of left wrist and hand
  - **T23.499** Corrosion of unspecified degree of multiple sites of unspecified wrist and hand
- **T23.5** Corrosion of first degree of wrist and hand
  Code first (T51-T65) *to identify chemical and intent*
  Use additional external cause code to identify place (Y92)
  - **T23.50** Corrosion of first degree of hand, unspecified site
    - **T23.501** Corrosion of first degree of right hand, unspecified site
    - **T23.502** Corrosion of first degree of left hand, unspecified site
    - **T23.509** Corrosion of first degree of unspecified hand, unspecified site

- **T23.51** Corrosion of first degree of thumb (nail)
  - **T23.511** Corrosion of first degree of right thumb (nail)
  - **T23.512** Corrosion of first degree of left thumb (nail)
  - **T23.519** Corrosion of first degree of unspecified thumb (nail)
- **T23.52** Corrosion of first degree of single finger (nail) except thumb
  - **T23.521** Corrosion of first degree of single right finger (nail) except thumb
  - **T23.522** Corrosion of first degree of single left finger (nail) except thumb
  - **T23.529** Corrosion of first degree of unspecified single finger (nail) except thumb
- **T23.53** Corrosion of first degree of multiple fingers (nail), not including thumb
  - **T23.531** Corrosion of first degree of multiple right fingers (nail), not including thumb
  - **T23.532** Corrosion of first degree of multiple left fingers (nail), not including thumb
  - **T23.539** Corrosion of first degree of unspecified multiple fingers (nail), not including thumb
- **T23.54** Corrosion of first degree of multiple fingers (nail), including thumb
  - **T23.541** Corrosion of first degree of multiple right fingers (nail), including thumb
  - **T23.542** Corrosion of first degree of multiple left fingers (nail), including thumb
  - **T23.549** Corrosion of first degree of unspecified multiple fingers (nail), including thumb
- **T23.55** Corrosion of first degree of palm
  - **T23.551** Corrosion of first degree of right palm
  - **T23.552** Corrosion of first degree of left palm
  - **T23.559** Corrosion of first degree of unspecified palm
- **T23.56** Corrosion of first degree of back of hand
  - **T23.561** Corrosion of first degree of back of right hand
  - **T23.562** Corrosion of first degree of back of left hand
  - **T23.569** Corrosion of first degree of back of unspecified hand
- **T23.57** Corrosion of first degree of wrist
  - **T23.571** Corrosion of first degree of right wrist
  - **T23.572** Corrosion of first degree of left wrist
  - **T23.579** Corrosion of first degree of unspecified wrist
- **T23.59** Corrosion of first degree of multiple sites of wrist and hand
  - **T23.591** Corrosion of first degree of multiple sites of right wrist and hand
  - **T23.592** Corrosion of first degree of multiple sites of left wrist and hand
  - **T23.599** Corrosion of first degree of multiple sites of unspecified wrist and hand

CHAPTER 19 (S00-T88)

● **T23.6** Corrosion of second degree of wrist and hand

　Code first (T51-T65) *to identify chemical and intent*

　Use additional external cause code to identify place (Y92)

　● **T23.60** Corrosion of second degree of hand, unspecified site

　　● **T23.601** Corrosion of second degree of right hand, unspecified site 🔍

　　● **T23.602** Corrosion of second degree of left hand, unspecified site 🔍

　　● **T23.609** Corrosion of second degree of unspecified hand, unspecified site 🔍

　● **T23.61** Corrosion of second degree of thumb (nail)

　　● **T23.611** Corrosion of second degree of right thumb (nail) 🔍

　　● **T23.612** Corrosion of second degree of left thumb (nail) 🔍

　　● **T23.619** Corrosion of second degree of unspecified thumb (nail) 🔍

　● **T23.62** Corrosion of second degree of single finger (nail) except thumb

　　● **T23.621** Corrosion of second degree of single right finger (nail) except thumb 🔍

　　● **T23.622** Corrosion of second degree of single left finger (nail) except thumb 🔍

　　● **T23.629** Corrosion of second degree of unspecified single finger (nail) except thumb 🔍

　● **T23.63** Corrosion of second degree of multiple fingers (nail), not including thumb

　　● **T23.631** Corrosion of second degree of multiple right fingers (nail), not including thumb 🔍

　　● **T23.632** Corrosion of second degree of multiple left fingers (nail), not including thumb 🔍

　　● **T23.639** Corrosion of second degree of unspecified multiple fingers (nail), not including thumb 🔍

　● **T23.64** Corrosion of second degree of multiple fingers (nail), including thumb

　　● **T23.641** Corrosion of second degree of multiple right fingers (nail), including thumb 🔍

　　● **T23.642** Corrosion of second degree of multiple left fingers (nail), including thumb 🔍

　　● **T23.649** Corrosion of second degree of unspecified multiple fingers (nail), including thumb 🔍

　● **T23.65** Corrosion of second degree of palm

　　● **T23.651** Corrosion of second degree of right palm 🔍

　　● **T23.652** Corrosion of second degree of left palm 🔍

　　● **T23.659** Corrosion of second degree of unspecified palm 🔍

　● **T23.66** Corrosion of second degree of back of hand

　　● **T23.661** Corrosion of second degree back of right hand 🔍

　　● **T23.662** Corrosion of second degree back of left hand 🔍

　　● **T23.669** Corrosion of second degree back of unspecified hand 🔍

　● **T23.67** Corrosion of second degree of wrist

　　● **T23.671** Corrosion of second degree of right wrist 🔍

　　● **T23.672** Corrosion of second degree of left wrist 🔍

　　● **T23.679** Corrosion of second degree of unspecified wrist 🔍

　● **T23.69** Corrosion of second degree of multiple sites of wrist and hand

　　● **T23.691** Corrosion of second degree of multiple sites of right wrist and hand 🔍

　　● **T23.692** Corrosion of second degree of multiple sites of left wrist and hand 🔍

　　● **T23.699** Corrosion of second degree of multiple sites of unspecified wrist and hand 🔍

● **T23.7** Corrosion of third degree of wrist and hand

　Code first (T51-T65) *to identify chemical and intent*

　Use additional external cause code to identify place (Y92)

　● **T23.70** Corrosion of third degree of hand, unspecified site

　　Ⓔⓧ For category T23.70 CC codes: T23.30

　　● **T23.701** Corrosion of third degree of right hand, unspecified site A 🔍, 🔍, A 🔍

　　● **T23.702** Corrosion of third degree of left hand, unspecified site A 🔍, 🔍, A 🔍

　　● **T23.709** Corrosion of third degree of unspecified hand, unspecified site A 🔍, 🔍, A 🔍

　● **T23.71** Corrosion of third degree of thumb (nail)

　　Ⓔⓧ For category T23.71 CC codes: See T23.31

　　● **T23.711** Corrosion of third degree of right thumb (nail) A 🔍, 🔍, A 🔍

　　● **T23.712** Corrosion of third degree of left thumb (nail) A 🔍, 🔍, A 🔍

　　● **T23.719** Corrosion of third degree of unspecified thumb (nail) A 🔍, 🔍, A 🔍

　● **T23.72** Corrosion of third degree of single finger (nail) except thumb

　　Ⓔⓧ For category T23.72 CC codes: See T23.32

　　● **T23.721** Corrosion of third degree of single right finger (nail) except thumb A 🔍, 🔍, A 🔍

　　● **T23.722** Corrosion of third degree of single left finger (nail) except thumb A 🔍, 🔍, A 🔍

　　● **T23.729** Corrosion of third degree of unspecified single finger (nail) except thumb A 🔍, 🔍, A 🔍

　● **T23.73** Corrosion of third degree of multiple fingers (nail), not including thumb

　　Ⓔⓧ For category T23.73 CC codes: See T23.33

　　● **T23.731** Corrosion of third degree of multiple right fingers (nail), not including thumb A 🔍, 🔍, A 🔍

　　● **T23.732** Corrosion of third degree of multiple left fingers (nail), not including thumb A 🔍, 🔍, A 🔍

　　● **T23.739** Corrosion of third degree of unspecified multiple fingers (nail), not including thumb A 🔍, 🔍, A 🔍

　● **T23.74** Corrosion of third degree of multiple fingers (nail), including thumb

　　Ⓔⓧ For category T23.74 CC codes: See T23.34

　　● **T23.741** Corrosion of third degree of multiple right fingers (nail), including thumb A 🔍, 🔍, A 🔍

　　● **T23.742** Corrosion of third degree of multiple left fingers (nail), including thumb A 🔍, 🔍, A 🔍

　　● **T23.749** Corrosion of third degree of unspecified multiple fingers (nail), including thumb A 🔍, 🔍, A 🔍

◀ New　◀▥ Revised　~~deleted~~ Deleted　| Excludes 1 |　| Excludes 2 |　| Includes |　| Use additional |　| Code first |　| Code also |　| Unspecified |

OGCR Official Guidelines　● Unacceptable Principal Diagnosis　X Assign placeholder X　● Use Additional Character(s)　▸ Manifestation Code　**Coding Clinic**

● **T23.75** Corrosion of third degree of palm
  (Ex) For category T23.75 CC codes: See T23.35
  ● **T23.751** Corrosion of third degree of right palm A 🔸, 🔸, A 🔸
  ● **T23.752** Corrosion of third degree of left palm A 🔸, 🔸, A 🔸
  ● **T23.759** Corrosion of third degree of unspecified palm A 🔸, 🔸, A 🔸
● **T23.76** Corrosion of third degree of back of hand
  (Ex) For category T23.76 CC codes: See T23.36
  ● **T23.761** Corrosion of third degree of back of right hand A 🔸, 🔸, A 🔸
  ● **T23.762** Corrosion of third degree of back of left hand A 🔸, 🔸, A 🔸
  ● **T23.769** Corrosion of third degree of back of unspecified hand A 🔸, 🔸, A 🔸
● **T23.77** Corrosion of third degree of wrist
  (Ex) For category T23.77 CC codes: See T23.37
  ● **T23.771** Corrosion of third degree of right wrist A 🔸, 🔸, A 🔸
  ● **T23.772** Corrosion of third degree of left wrist A 🔸, 🔸, A 🔸
  ● **T23.779** Corrosion of third degree of unspecified wrist A 🔸, 🔸, A 🔸
● **T23.79** Corrosion of third degree of multiple sites of wrist and hand
  (Ex) For category T23.79 CC codes: T23.30
  ● **T23.791** Corrosion of third degree of multiple sites of right wrist and hand A 🔸, 🔸, A 🔸
  ● **T23.792** Corrosion of third degree of multiple sites of left wrist and hand A 🔸, 🔸, A 🔸
  ● **T23.799** Corrosion of third degree of multiple sites of unspecified wrist and hand A 🔸, 🔸, A 🔸

● **T24** Burn and corrosion of lower limb, except ankle and foot
  Excludes2 burn and corrosion of ankle and foot (T25.-)
  burn and corrosion of hip region (T21.-)

  The appropriate 7th character is to be added to each code from category T24

A	initial encounter
D	subsequent encounter
S	sequela

● **T24.0** Burn of unspecified degree of lower limb, except ankle and foot
  Use additional external cause code to identify the source, place and intent of the burn (X00-X19, X75-X77, X96-X98, Y92)
  ● **T24.00** Burn of unspecified degree of unspecified site of lower limb, except ankle and foot
    ● **T24.001** Burn of unspecified degree of unspecified site of right lower limb, except ankle and foot 🔸
    ● **T24.002** Burn of unspecified degree of unspecified site of left lower limb, except ankle and foot 🔸
    ● **T24.009** Burn of unspecified degree of unspecified site of unspecified lower limb, except ankle and foot 🔸
  ● **T24.01** Burn of unspecified degree of thigh
    ● **T24.011** Burn of unspecified degree of right thigh 🔸
    ● **T24.012** Burn of unspecified degree of left thigh 🔸
    ● **T24.019** Burn of unspecified degree of unspecified thigh 🔸

● **T24.02** Burn of unspecified degree of knee
  ● **T24.021** Burn of unspecified degree of right knee 🔸
  ● **T24.022** Burn of unspecified degree of left knee 🔸
  ● **T24.029** Burn of unspecified degree of unspecified knee 🔸
● **T24.03** Burn of unspecified degree of lower leg
  ● **T24.031** Burn of unspecified degree of right lower leg 🔸
  ● **T24.032** Burn of unspecified degree of left lower leg 🔸
  ● **T24.039** Burn of unspecified degree of unspecified lower leg 🔸
● **T24.09** Burn of unspecified degree of multiple sites of lower limb, except ankle and foot
  ● **T24.091** Burn of unspecified degree of multiple sites of right lower limb, except ankle and foot 🔸
  ● **T24.092** Burn of unspecified degree of multiple sites of left lower limb, except ankle and foot 🔸
  ● **T24.099** Burn of unspecified degree of multiple sites of unspecified lower limb, except ankle and foot 🔸
● **T24.1** Burn of first degree of lower limb, except ankle and foot
  Use additional external cause code to identify the source, place and intent of the burn (X00-X19, X75-X77, X96-X98, Y92)
  ● **T24.10** Burn of first degree of unspecified site of lower limb, except ankle and foot
    ● **T24.101** Burn of first degree of unspecified site of right lower limb, except ankle and foot 🔸
    ● **T24.102** Burn of first degree of unspecified site of left lower limb, except ankle and foot 🔸
    ● **T24.109** Burn of first degree of unspecified site of unspecified lower limb, except ankle and foot 🔸
  ● **T24.11** Burn of first degree of thigh
    ● **T24.111** Burn of first degree of right thigh 🔸
    ● **T24.112** Burn of first degree of left thigh 🔸
    ● **T24.119** Burn of first degree of unspecified thigh 🔸
  ● **T24.12** Burn of first degree of knee
    ● **T24.121** Burn of first degree of right knee 🔸
    ● **T24.122** Burn of first degree of left knee 🔸
    ● **T24.129** Burn of first degree of unspecified knee 🔸
  ● **T24.13** Burn of first degree of lower leg
    ● **T24.131** Burn of first degree of right lower leg 🔸
    ● **T24.132** Burn of first degree of left lower leg 🔸
    ● **T24.139** Burn of first degree of unspecified lower leg 🔸
  ● **T24.19** Burn of first degree of multiple sites of lower limb, except ankle and foot
    ● **T24.191** Burn of first degree of multiple sites of right lower limb, except ankle and foot 🔸
    ● **T24.192** Burn of first degree of multiple sites of left lower limb, except ankle and foot 🔸
    ● **T24.199** Burn of first degree of multiple sites of unspecified lower limb, except ankle and foot 🔸

CHAPTER 19 (S00-T88)

N Newborn Age: 0   **P** Pediatric Age: 0–17   **M** Maternity DX: 12–55   **A** Adult Age: 15–124   ♀ Females Only   ♂ Males Only

🔸 Complication\Comorbidity   🔸 Major C\C   (Ex) CC/MCC Exclusions   🔸 Present on Admission Requirement   🔸 Hospital-Acquired Condition

1511

● **T24.2**   **Burn of second degree of lower limb, except ankle and foot**

> Use additional external cause code to identify the source, place and intent of the burn (X00-X19, X75-X77, X96-X98, Y92)

   ● **T24.20**   Burn of second degree of unspecified site of lower limb, except ankle and foot

      ● **T24.201**   Burn of second degree of unspecified site of right lower limb, except ankle and foot 🐾

      ● **T24.202**   Burn of second degree of unspecified site of left lower limb, except ankle and foot 🐾

      ● **T24.209**   Burn of second degree of unspecified site of unspecified lower limb, except ankle and foot 🐾

   ● **T24.21**   Burn of second degree of thigh

      ● **T24.211**   Burn of second degree of right thigh 🐾

      ● **T24.212**   Burn of second degree of left thigh 🐾

      ● **T24.219**   Burn of second degree of unspecified thigh 🐾

   ● **T24.22**   Burn of second degree of knee

      ● **T24.221**   Burn of second degree of right knee 🐾

      ● **T24.222**   Burn of second degree of left knee 🐾

      ● **T24.229**   Burn of second degree of unspecified knee 🐾

   ● **T24.23**   Burn of second degree of lower leg

      ● **T24.231**   Burn of second degree of right lower leg 🐾

      ● **T24.232**   Burn of second degree of left lower leg 🐾

      ● **T24.239**   Burn of second degree of unspecified lower leg 🐾

   ● **T24.29**   Burn of second degree of multiple sites of lower limb, except ankle and foot

      ● **T24.291**   Burn of second degree of multiple sites of right lower limb, except ankle and foot 🐾

      ● **T24.292**   Burn of second degree of multiple sites of left lower limb, except ankle and foot 🐾

      ● **T24.299**   Burn of second degree of multiple sites of unspecified lower limb, except ankle and foot 🐾

● **T24.3**   **Burn of third degree of lower limb, except ankle and foot**

> Use additional external cause code to identify the source, place and intent of the burn (X00-X19, X75-X77, X96-X98, Y92)

   ● **T24.30**   Burn of third degree of unspecified site of lower limb, except ankle and foot

> Ⓔⓧ **For category T24.30 CC codes:** T24.301-T24.309[A], T24.391-T24.399[A], T24.701-T24.709[A], T24.791-T24.799[A], T25.391-T25.399[A], T25.791-T25.799[A]

      ● **T24.301**   Burn of third degree of unspecified site of right lower limb, except ankle and foot A 🐾, 🐾, A 🐾

      ● **T24.302**   Burn of third degree of unspecified site of left lower limb, except ankle and foot A 🐾, 🐾, A 🐾

      ● **T24.309**   Burn of third degree of unspecified site of unspecified lower limb, except ankle and foot A 🐾, 🐾, A 🐾

   ● **T24.31**   Burn of third degree of thigh

> Ⓔⓧ **For category T24.31 CC codes:** T24.301-T24.309[A], T24.311-T24.319[A], T24.391-T24.399[A], T24.701-T24.709-T24.719[A], T24.791-T24.799[A], T25.391-T25.399[A], T25.791-T25.799[A]

      ● **T24.311**   Burn of third degree of right thigh A 🐾, 🐾, A 🐾

      ● **T24.312**   Burn of third degree of left thigh A 🐾, 🐾, A 🐾

      ● **T24.319**   Burn of third degree of unspecified thigh A 🐾, 🐾, A 🐾

   ● **T24.32**   Burn of third degree of knee

> Ⓔⓧ **For category T24.32 CC codes:** T24.301-T24.309[A], T24.321-T24.329[A], T24.391-T24.399[A], T24.701-T24.709[A], T24.721-T24.729[A], T24.791-T24.799[A], T25.391-T25.399[A], T25.791-T25.799[A]

      ● **T24.321**   Burn of third degree of right knee A 🐾, 🐾, A 🐾

      ● **T24.322**   Burn of third degree of left knee A 🐾, 🐾, A 🐾

      ● **T24.329**   Burn of third degree of unspecified knee A 🐾, 🐾, A 🐾

   ● **T24.33**   Burn of third degree of lower leg

> Ⓔⓧ **For category T24.33 CC codes:** T24.301-T24.309[A], T24.331-T24.339[A], T24.391-T24.399[A], T24.701-T24.709[A], T24.731-T24.739[A], T24.791-T24.799[A], T25.391-T25.399[A], T25.791-T25.799[A]

      ● **T24.331**   Burn of third degree of right lower leg A 🐾, 🐾, A 🐾

      ● **T24.332**   Burn of third degree of left lower leg A 🐾, 🐾, A 🐾

      ● **T24.339**   Burn of third degree of unspecified lower leg A 🐾, 🐾, A 🐾

   ● **T24.39**   Burn of third degree of multiple sites of lower limb, except ankle and foot

> Ⓔⓧ **For category T24.39 CC codes:** See T24.30

      ● **T24.391**   Burn of third degree of multiple sites of right lower limb, except ankle and foot A 🐾, 🐾, A 🐾

      ● **T24.392**   Burn of third degree of multiple sites of left lower limb, except ankle and foot A 🐾, 🐾, A 🐾

      ● **T24.399**   Burn of third degree of multiple sites of unspecified lower limb, except ankle and foot A 🐾, 🐾, A 🐾

● **T24.4**   **Corrosion of unspecified degree of lower limb, except ankle and foot**

> *Code first (T51-T65) to identify chemical and intent*
>
> Use additional external cause code to identify place (Y92)

   ● **T24.40**   Corrosion of unspecified degree of unspecified site of lower limb, except ankle and foot

      ● **T24.401**   Corrosion of unspecified degree of unspecified site of right lower limb, except ankle and foot 🐾

      ● **T24.402**   Corrosion of unspecified degree of unspecified site of left lower limb, except ankle and foot 🐾

      ● **T24.409**   Corrosion of unspecified degree of unspecified site of unspecified lower limb, except ankle and foot 🐾

◄ New   ◄⃫ Revised   ~~deleted~~ Deleted   Excludes 1   Excludes 2   Includes   Use additional   Code first   Code also   Unspecified

OGCR Official Guidelines   ● Unacceptable Principal Diagnosis   X Assign placeholder X   ▶ Use Additional Character(s)   ▶ Manifestation Code   **Coding Clinic**

● **T24.41**   Corrosion of unspecified degree of thigh
> ● **T24.411**   Corrosion of unspecified degree of right thigh
> ● **T24.412**   Corrosion of unspecified degree of left thigh
> ● **T24.419**   Corrosion of unspecified degree of unspecified thigh

● **T24.42**   Corrosion of unspecified degree of knee
> ● **T24.421**   Corrosion of unspecified degree of right knee
> ● **T24.422**   Corrosion of unspecified degree of left knee
> ● **T24.429**   Corrosion of unspecified degree of unspecified knee

● **T24.43**   Corrosion of unspecified degree of lower leg
> ● **T24.431**   Corrosion of unspecified degree of right lower leg
> ● **T24.432**   Corrosion of unspecified degree of left lower leg
> ● **T24.439**   Corrosion of unspecified degree of unspecified lower leg

● **T24.49**   Corrosion of unspecified degree of multiple sites of lower limb, except ankle and foot
> ● **T24.491**   Corrosion of unspecified degree of multiple sites of right lower limb, except ankle and foot
> ● **T24.492**   Corrosion of unspecified degree of multiple sites of left lower limb, except ankle and foot
> ● **T24.499**   Corrosion of unspecified degree of multiple sites of unspecified lower limb, except ankle and foot

● **T24.5**   Corrosion of first degree of lower limb, except ankle and foot
> *Code first (T51-T65) to identify chemical and intent*
> Use additional external cause code to identify place (Y92)

● **T24.50**   Corrosion of first degree of unspecified site of lower limb, except ankle and foot
> ● **T24.501**   Corrosion of first degree of unspecified site of right lower limb, except ankle and foot
> ● **T24.502**   Corrosion of first degree of unspecified site of left lower limb, except ankle and foot
> ● **T24.509**   Corrosion of first degree of unspecified site of unspecified lower limb, except ankle and foot

● **T24.51**   Corrosion of first degree of thigh
> ● **T24.511**   Corrosion of first degree of right thigh
> ● **T24.512**   Corrosion of first degree of left thigh
> ● **T24.519**   Corrosion of first degree of unspecified thigh

● **T24.52**   Corrosion of first degree of knee
> ● **T24.521**   Corrosion of first degree of right knee
> ● **T24.522**   Corrosion of first degree of left knee
> ● **T24.529**   Corrosion of first degree of unspecified knee

● **T24.53**   Corrosion of first degree of lower leg
> ● **T24.531**   Corrosion of first degree of right lower leg
> ● **T24.532**   Corrosion of first degree of left lower leg
> ● **T24.539**   Corrosion of first degree of unspecified lower leg

● **T24.59**   Corrosion of first degree of multiple sites of lower limb, except ankle and foot
> ● **T24.591**   Corrosion of first degree of multiple sites of right lower limb, except ankle and foot
> ● **T24.592**   Corrosion of first degree of multiple sites of left lower limb, except ankle and foot
> ● **T24.599**   Corrosion of first degree of multiple sites of unspecified lower limb, except ankle and foot

● **T24.6**   Corrosion of second degree of lower limb, except ankle and foot
> *Code first (T51-T65) to identify chemical and intent*
> Use additional external cause code to identify place (Y92)

● **T24.60**   Corrosion of second degree of unspecified site of lower limb, except ankle and foot
> ● **T24.601**   Corrosion of second degree of unspecified site of right lower limb, except ankle and foot
> ● **T24.602**   Corrosion of second degree of unspecified site of left lower limb, except ankle and foot
> ● **T24.609**   Corrosion of second degree of unspecified site of unspecified lower limb, except ankle and foot

● **T24.61**   Corrosion of second degree of thigh
> ● **T24.611**   Corrosion of second degree of right thigh
> ● **T24.612**   Corrosion of second degree of left thigh
> ● **T24.619**   Corrosion of second degree of unspecified thigh

● **T24.62**   Corrosion of second degree of knee
> ● **T24.621**   Corrosion of second degree of right knee
> ● **T24.622**   Corrosion of second degree of left knee
> ● **T24.629**   Corrosion of second degree of unspecified knee

● **T24.63**   Corrosion of second degree of lower leg
> ● **T24.631**   Corrosion of second degree of right lower leg
> ● **T24.632**   Corrosion of second degree of left lower leg
> ● **T24.639**   Corrosion of second degree of unspecified lower leg

● **T24.69**   Corrosion of second degree of multiple sites of lower limb, except ankle and foot
> ● **T24.691**   Corrosion of second degree of multiple sites of right lower limb, except ankle and foot
> ● **T24.692**   Corrosion of second degree of multiple sites of left lower limb, except ankle and foot
> ● **T24.699**   Corrosion of second degree of multiple sites of unspecified lower limb, except ankle and foot

N Newborn Age: 0   **P** Pediatric Age: 0–17   **M** Maternity DX: 12–55   **A** Adult Age: 15–124   ♀ Females Only   ♂ Males Only

 Complication\Comorbidity   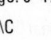 Major C\C   (Ex) CC/MCC Exclusions   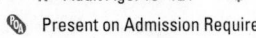 Present on Admission Requirement   Hospital-Acquired Condition

1513

● **T24.7**   **Corrosion of third degree of lower limb, except ankle and foot**

Code first (T51-T65) *to identify chemical and intent*

Use additional external cause code to identify place (Y92)

● **T24.70**   **Corrosion of third degree of unspecified site of lower limb, except ankle and foot**
    (Ex) For category T24.70 CC codes: See T24.30

  ● **T24.701**   Corrosion of third degree of unspecified site of right lower limb, except ankle and foot A 🪙, 🪙, A 🪙

  ● **T24.702**   Corrosion of third degree of unspecified site of left lower limb, except ankle and foot A 🪙, 🪙, A 🪙

  ● **T24.709**   Corrosion of third degree of unspecified site of unspecified lower limb, except ankle and foot A 🪙, 🪙, A 🪙

● **T24.71**   **Corrosion of third degree of thigh**
    (Ex) For category T24.71 CC codes: See T24.31

  ● **T24.711**   Corrosion of third degree of right thigh A 🪙, 🪙, A 🪙

  ● **T24.712**   Corrosion of third degree of left thigh A 🪙, 🪙, A 🪙

  ● **T24.719**   Corrosion of third degree of unspecified thigh A 🪙, 🪙, A 🪙

● **T24.72**   **Corrosion of third degree of knee**
    (Ex) For category T24.72 CC codes: See T24.32

  ● **T24.721**   Corrosion of third degree of right knee A 🪙, 🪙, A 🪙

  ● **T24.722**   Corrosion of third degree of left knee A 🪙, 🪙, A 🪙

  ● **T24.729**   Corrosion of third degree of unspecified knee A 🪙, 🪙, A 🪙

● **T24.73**   **Corrosion of third degree of lower leg**
    (Ex) For category T24.73 CC codes: See T24.33

  ● **T24.731**   Corrosion of third degree of right lower leg A 🪙, 🪙, A 🪙

  ● **T24.732**   Corrosion of third degree of left lower leg A 🪙, 🪙, A 🪙

  ● **T24.739**   Corrosion of third degree of unspecified lower leg A 🪙, 🪙, A 🪙

● **T24.79**   **Corrosion of third degree of multiple sites of lower limb, except ankle and foot**
    (Ex) For category T24.79 CC codes: See T24.30

  ● **T24.791**   Corrosion of third degree of multiple sites of right lower limb, except ankle and foot A 🪙, 🪙, A 🪙

  ● **T24.792**   Corrosion of third degree of multiple sites of left lower limb, except ankle and foot A 🪙, 🪙, A 🪙

  ● **T24.799**   Corrosion of third degree of multiple sites of unspecified lower limb, except ankle and foot A 🪙, 🪙, A 🪙

● **T25**   **Burn and corrosion of ankle and foot**

The appropriate 7th character is to be added to each code from category T25

A	initial encounter
D	subsequent encounter
S	sequela

● **T25.0**   **Burn of unspecified degree of ankle and foot**

Use additional external cause code to identify the source, place and intent of the burn (X00-X19, X75-X77, X96-X98, Y92)

  ● **T25.01**   **Burn of unspecified degree of ankle**

    ● **T25.011**   Burn of unspecified degree of right ankle 🪙

    ● **T25.012**   Burn of unspecified degree of left ankle 🪙

    ● **T25.019**   Burn of unspecified degree of unspecified ankle 🪙

  ● **T25.02**   **Burn of unspecified degree of foot**

    Excludes2   burn of unspecified degree of toe(s) (nail) (T25.03-)

    ● **T25.021**   Burn of unspecified degree of right foot 🪙

    ● **T25.022**   Burn of unspecified degree of left foot 🪙

    ● **T25.029**   Burn of unspecified degree of unspecified foot 🪙

  ● **T25.03**   **Burn of unspecified degree of toe(s) (nail)**

    ● **T25.031**   Burn of unspecified degree of right toe(s) (nail) 🪙

    ● **T25.032**   Burn of unspecified degree of left toe(s) (nail) 🪙

    ● **T25.039**   Burn of unspecified degree of unspecified toe(s) (nail) 🪙

  ● **T25.09**   **Burn of unspecified degree of multiple sites of ankle and foot**

    ● **T25.091**   Burn of unspecified degree of multiple sites of right ankle and foot 🪙

    ● **T25.092**   Burn of unspecified degree of multiple sites of left ankle and foot 🪙

    ● **T25.099**   Burn of unspecified degree of multiple sites of unspecified ankle and foot 🪙

● **T25.1**   **Burn of first degree of ankle and foot**

Use additional external cause code to identify the source, place and intent of the burn (X00-X19, X75-X77, X96-X98, Y92)

  ● **T25.11**   **Burn of first degree of ankle**

    ● **T25.111**   Burn of first degree of right ankle 🪙

    ● **T25.112**   Burn of first degree of left ankle 🪙

    ● **T25.119**   Burn of first degree of unspecified ankle 🪙

  ● **T25.12**   **Burn of first degree of foot**

    Excludes2   burn of first degree of toe(s) (nail) (T25.13-)

    ● **T25.121**   Burn of first degree of right foot 🪙

    ● **T25.122**   Burn of first degree of left foot 🪙

    ● **T25.129**   Burn of first degree of unspecified foot 🪙

◀ New   ◀▥ Revised   ~~deleted~~ Deleted   Excludes 1   Excludes 2   Includes   Use additional   Code first   Code also   Unspecified

OGCR Official Guidelines   ● Unacceptable Principal Diagnosis   X Assign placeholder X   ▶ Use Additional Character(s)   ▶ Manifestation Code   **Coding Clinic**

● T25.13   Burn of first degree of toe(s) (nail)
- ● T25.131   Burn of first degree of right toe(s) (nail) 🐾
- ● T25.132   Burn of first degree of left toe(s) (nail) 🐾
- ● T25.139   Burn of first degree of unspecified toe(s) (nail) 🐾

● T25.19   Burn of first degree of multiple sites of ankle and foot
- ● T25.191   Burn of first degree of multiple sites of right ankle and foot 🐾
- ● T25.192   Burn of first degree of multiple sites of left ankle and foot 🐾
- ● T25.199   Burn of first degree of multiple sites of unspecified ankle and foot 🐾

● T25.2   Burn of second degree of ankle and foot

Use additional external cause code to identify the source, place and intent of the burn (X00-X19, X75-X77, X96-X98, Y92)

● T25.21   Burn of second degree of ankle
- ● T25.211   Burn of second degree of right ankle 🐾
- ● T25.212   Burn of second degree of left ankle 🐾
- ● T25.219   Burn of second degree of unspecified ankle 🐾

● T25.22   Burn of second degree of foot

    Excludes2   burn of second degree of toe(s) (nail) (T25.23-)

- ● T25.221   Burn of second degree of right foot 🐾
- ● T25.222   Burn of second degree of left foot 🐾
- ● T25.229   Burn of second degree of unspecified foot 🐾

● T25.23   Burn of second degree of toe(s) (nail)
- ● T25.231   Burn of second degree of right toe(s) (nail) 🐾
- ● T25.232   Burn of second degree of left toe(s) (nail) 🐾
- ● T25.239   Burn of second degree of unspecified toe(s) (nail) 🐾

● T25.29   Burn of second degree of multiple sites of ankle and foot
- ● T25.291   Burn of second degree of multiple sites of right ankle and foot 🐾
- ● T25.292   Burn of second degree of multiple sites of left ankle and foot 🐾
- ● T25.299   Burn of second degree of multiple sites of unspecified ankle and foot 🐾

● T25.3   Burn of third degree of ankle and foot

Use additional external cause code to identify the source, place and intent of the burn (X00-X19, X75-X77, X96-X98, Y92)

● T25.31   Burn of third degree of ankle

(Ex:) **For category T25.31 CC codes:** T24.301-T24.309[A], T24.391-T24.399[A], T24.701-T24.709[A], T24.791-T24.799[A], T25.311-T25.319[A], T25.391-T25.399[A], T25.711-T25.719[A], T25.791-T25.799[A]

- ● T25.311   Burn of third degree of right ankle A 🐾, 🐾, A 🐾
- ● T25.312   Burn of third degree of left ankle A 🐾, 🐾, A 🐾
- ● T25.319   Burn of third degree of unspecified ankle A 🐾, 🐾, A 🐾

● T25.32   Burn of third degree of foot

    Excludes2   burn of third degree of toe(s) (nail) (T25.33-)

(Ex:) **For category T25.32 CC codes:** T24.301-T24.309[A], T24.391-T24.399[A], T24.701-T24.709[A], T24.791-T24.799[A], T25.321-T25.329[A], T25.391-T25.399[A], T25.721-T25.729[A], T25.791-T25.799[A]

- ● T25.321   Burn of third degree of right foot A 🐾, 🐾, A 🐾
- ● T25.322   Burn of third degree of left foot A 🐾, 🐾, A 🐾
- ● T25.329   Burn of third degree of unspecified foot A 🐾, 🐾, A 🐾

● T25.33   Burn of third degree of toe(s) (nail)

(Ex:) **For category T25.33 CC codes:** T24.301-T24.309[A], T24.391-T24.399[A], T24.701-T24.709[A], T24.791-T24.799[A], T25.331-T25.339[A], T25.391-T25.399[A], T25.731-T25.739[A], T25.791-T25.799[A]

- ● T25.331   Burn of third degree of right toe(s) (nail) A 🐾, 🐾, A 🐾
- ● T25.332   Burn of third degree of left toe(s) (nail) A 🐾, 🐾, A 🐾
- ● T25.339   Burn of third degree of unspecified toe(s) (nail) A 🐾, 🐾, A 🐾

● T25.39   Burn of third degree of multiple sites of ankle and foot

(Ex:) **For category T25.39 CC codes:** See T24.30

- ● T25.391   Burn of third degree of multiple sites of right ankle and foot A 🐾, 🐾, A 🐾
- ● T25.392   Burn of third degree of multiple sites of left ankle and foot A 🐾, 🐾, A 🐾
- ● T25.399   Burn of third degree of multiple sites of unspecified ankle and foot A 🐾, 🐾, A 🐾

● T25.4   Corrosion of unspecified degree of ankle and foot

Code first (T51-T65) to identify chemical and intent

Use additional external cause code to identify place (Y92)

● T25.41   Corrosion of unspecified degree of ankle
- ● T25.411   Corrosion of unspecified degree of right ankle 🐾
- ● T25.412   Corrosion of unspecified degree of left ankle 🐾
- ● T25.419   Corrosion of unspecified degree of unspecified ankle 🐾

● T25.42   Corrosion of unspecified degree of foot

    Excludes2   corrosion of unspecified degree of toe(s) (nail) (T25.43-)

- ● T25.421   Corrosion of unspecified degree of right foot 🐾
- ● T25.422   Corrosion of unspecified degree of left foot 🐾
- ● T25.429   Corrosion of unspecified degree of unspecified foot 🐾

● T25.43   Corrosion of unspecified degree of toe(s) (nail)
- ● T25.431   Corrosion of unspecified degree of right toe(s) (nail) 🐾
- ● T25.432   Corrosion of unspecified degree of left toe(s) (nail) 🐾
- ● T25.439   Corrosion of unspecified degree of unspecified toe(s) (nail) 🐾

N Newborn Age: 0   **P** Pediatric Age: 0–17   **M** Maternity DX: 12–55   **A** Adult Age: 15–124   ♀ Females Only   ♂ Males Only

🐾 Complication\Comorbidity   🐾 Major C\C   (Ex:) CC/MCC Exclusions   🐾 Present on Admission Requirement   🐾 Hospital-Acquired Condition

1515

CHAPTER 19 (S00-T88)

CHAPTER 19 (S00-T88)

- **T25.49**   Corrosion of unspecified degree of multiple sites of ankle and foot
  - **T25.491**   Corrosion of unspecified degree of multiple sites of right ankle and foot 🔗
  - **T25.492**   Corrosion of unspecified degree of multiple sites of left ankle and foot 🔗
  - **T25.499**   Corrosion of unspecified degree of multiple sites of unspecified ankle and foot 🔗
- **T25.5**   Corrosion of first degree of ankle and foot
  - *Code first* (T51-T65) *to identify chemical and intent*
  - Use additional external cause code to identify place (Y92)
  - **T25.51**   Corrosion of first degree of ankle
    - **T25.511**   Corrosion of first degree of right ankle 🔗
    - **T25.512**   Corrosion of first degree of left ankle 🔗
    - **T25.519**   Corrosion of first degree of unspecified ankle 🔗
  - **T25.52**   Corrosion of first degree of foot
    - **Excludes2**   corrosion of first degree of toe(s) (nail) (T25.53-)
    - **T25.521**   Corrosion of first degree of right foot 🔗
    - **T25.522**   Corrosion of first degree of left foot 🔗
    - **T25.529**   Corrosion of first degree of unspecified foot 🔗
  - **T25.53**   Corrosion of first degree of toe(s) (nail)
    - **T25.531**   Corrosion of first degree of right toe(s) (nail) 🔗
    - **T25.532**   Corrosion of first degree of left toe(s) (nail) 🔗
    - **T25.539**   Corrosion of first degree of unspecified toe(s) (nail) 🔗
  - **T25.59**   Corrosion of first degree of multiple sites of ankle and foot
    - **T25.591**   Corrosion of first degree of multiple sites of right ankle and foot 🔗
    - **T25.592**   Corrosion of first degree of multiple sites of left ankle and foot 🔗
    - **T25.599**   Corrosion of first degree of multiple sites of unspecified ankle and foot 🔗
- **T25.6**   Corrosion of second degree of ankle and foot
  - *Code first* (T51-T65) *to identify chemical and intent*
  - Use additional external cause code to identify place (Y92)
  - **T25.61**   Corrosion of second degree of ankle
    - **T25.611**   Corrosion of second degree of right ankle 🔗
    - **T25.612**   Corrosion of second degree of left ankle 🔗
    - **T25.619**   Corrosion of second degree of unspecified ankle 🔗
  - **T25.62**   Corrosion of second degree of foot
    - **Excludes2**   corrosion of second degree of toe(s) (nail) (T25.63-)
    - **T25.621**   Corrosion of second degree of right foot 🔗
    - **T25.622**   Corrosion of second degree of left foot 🔗
    - **T25.629**   Corrosion of second degree of unspecified foot 🔗

- **T25.63**   Corrosion of second degree of toe(s) (nail)
  - **T25.631**   Corrosion of second degree of right toe(s) (nail) 🔗
  - **T25.632**   Corrosion of second degree of left toe(s) (nail) 🔗
  - **T25.639**   Corrosion of second degree of unspecified toe(s) (nail) 🔗
- **T25.69**   Corrosion of second degree of multiple sites of ankle and foot
  - **T25.691**   Corrosion of second degree of right ankle and foot 🔗
  - **T25.692**   Corrosion of second degree of left ankle and foot 🔗
  - **T25.699**   Corrosion of second degree of unspecified ankle and foot 🔗
- **T25.7**   Corrosion of third degree of ankle and foot
  - *Code first* (T51-T65) *to identify chemical and intent*
  - Use additional external cause code to identify place (Y92)
  - **T25.71**   Corrosion of third degree of ankle
    - (Ex) For category T25.71 CC codes: See T25.31
    - **T25.711**   Corrosion of third degree of right ankle A 🔗, 🔗, A 🔗
    - **T25.712**   Corrosion of third degree of left ankle A 🔗, 🔗, A 🔗
    - **T25.719**   Corrosion of third degree of unspecified ankle A 🔗, 🔗, A 🔗
  - **T25.72**   Corrosion of third degree of foot
    - **Excludes2**   corrosion of third degree of toe(s) (nail) (T25.73-)
    - (Ex) For category T25.72 CC codes: See T25.32
    - **T25.721**   Corrosion of third degree of right foot A 🔗, 🔗, A 🔗
    - **T25.722**   Corrosion of third degree of left foot A 🔗, 🔗, A 🔗
    - **T25.729**   Corrosion of third degree of unspecified foot A 🔗, 🔗, A 🔗
  - **T25.73**   Corrosion of third degree of toe(s) (nail)
    - (Ex) For category T25.73 CC codes: See T25.33
    - **T25.731**   Corrosion of third degree of right toe(s) (nail) A 🔗, 🔗, A 🔗
    - **T25.732**   Corrosion of third degree of left toe(s) (nail) A 🔗, 🔗, A 🔗
    - **T25.739**   Corrosion of third degree of unspecified toe(s) (nail) A 🔗, 🔗, A 🔗
  - **T25.79**   Corrosion of third degree of multiple sites of ankle and foot
    - (Ex) For category T25.79 CC codes: See T24.30
    - **T25.791**   Corrosion of third degree of multiple sites of right ankle and foot A 🔗, 🔗, A 🔗
    - **T25.792**   Corrosion of third degree of multiple sites of left ankle and foot A 🔗, 🔗, A 🔗
    - **T25.799**   Corrosion of third degree of multiple sites of unspecified ankle and foot A 🔗, 🔗, A 🔗

◀ New   ◀ Revised   ~~deleted~~ Deleted   Excludes 1   Excludes 2   Includes   Use additional   Code first   Code also   Unspecified

OGCR Official Guidelines   ● Unacceptable Principal Diagnosis   X Assign placeholder X   ● Use Additional Character(s)   ▶ Manifestation Code   **Coding Clinic**

BURNS AND CORROSIONS CONFINED TO EYE AND INTERNAL ORGANS (T26-T28)

● **T26** **Burn and corrosion confined to eye and adnexa**

The appropriate 7th character is to be added to each code from category T26

A	initial encounter
D	subsequent encounter
S	sequela

● **T26.0** **Burn of eyelid and periocular area**

Use additional external cause code to identify the source, place and intent of the burn (X00-X19, X75-X77, X96-X98, Y92)

X ● **T26.00** Burn of unspecified eyelid and periocular area 🔖

X ● **T26.01** Burn of right eyelid and periocular area 🔖

X ● **T26.02** Burn of left eyelid and periocular area 🔖

● **T26.1** **Burn of cornea and conjunctival sac**

Use additional external cause code to identify the source, place and intent of the burn (X00-X19, X75-X77, X96-X98, Y92)

X ● **T26.10** Burn of cornea and conjunctival sac, unspecified eye 🔖

X ● **T26.11** Burn of cornea and conjunctival sac, right eye 🔖

X ● **T26.12** Burn of cornea and conjunctival sac, left eye 🔖

● **T26.2** **Burn with resulting rupture and destruction of eyeball**

Use additional external cause code to identify the source, place and intent of the burn (X00-X19, X75-X77, X96-X98, Y92)

Ⓔ **For category T26.2 CC codes:** No exclusions

X ● **T26.20** Burn with resulting rupture and destruction of unspecified eyeball A 🔖, 🔖, A 🔖

X ● **T26.21** Burn with resulting rupture and destruction of right eyeball A 🔖, 🔖, A 🔖

X ● **T26.22** Burn with resulting rupture and destruction of left eyeball A 🔖, 🔖, A 🔖

● **T26.3** **Burns of other specified parts of eye and adnexa**

Use additional external cause code to identify the source, place and intent of the burn (X00-X19, X75-X77, X96-X98, Y92)

X ● **T26.30** Burns of other specified parts of unspecified eye and adnexa 🔖

X ● **T26.31** Burns of other specified parts of right eye and adnexa 🔖

X ● **T26.32** Burns of other specified parts of left eye and adnexa 🔖

● **T26.4** **Burn of eye and adnexa, part unspecified**

Use additional external cause code to identify the source, place and intent of the burn (X00-X19, X75-X77, X96-X98, Y92)

X ● **T26.40** Burn of unspecified eye and adnexa, part unspecified 🔖

X ● **T26.41** Burn of right eye and adnexa, part unspecified 🔖

X ● **T26.42** Burn of left eye and adnexa, part unspecified 🔖

● **T26.5** **Corrosion of eyelid and periocular area**

Code first (T51-T65) to identify chemical and intent

Use additional external cause code to identify place (Y92)

X ● **T26.50** Corrosion of unspecified eyelid and periocular area 🔖

X ● **T26.51** Corrosion of right eyelid and periocular area 🔖

X ● **T26.52** Corrosion of left eyelid and periocular area 🔖

● **T26.6** **Corrosion of cornea and conjunctival sac**

Code first (T51-T65) to identify chemical and intent

Use additional external cause code to identify place (Y92)

X ● **T26.60** Corrosion of cornea and conjunctival sac, unspecified eye 🔖

X ● **T26.61** Corrosion of cornea and conjunctival sac, right eye 🔖

X ● **T26.62** Corrosion of cornea and conjunctival sac, left eye 🔖

● **T26.7** **Corrosion with resulting rupture and destruction of eyeball**

Code first (T51-T65) to identify chemical and intent

Use additional external cause code to identify place (Y92)

Ⓔ **For category T26.7 CC codes:** No exclusions

X ● **T26.70** Corrosion with resulting rupture and destruction of unspecified eyeball A 🔖, 🔖, A 🔖

X ● **T26.71** Corrosion with resulting rupture and destruction of right eyeball A 🔖, 🔖, A 🔖

X ● **T26.72** Corrosion with resulting rupture and destruction of left eyeball A 🔖, 🔖, A 🔖

● **T26.8** **Corrosions of other specified parts of eye and adnexa**

Code first (T51-T65) to identify chemical and intent

Use additional external cause code to identify place (Y92)

X ● **T26.80** Corrosions of other specified parts of unspecified eye and adnexa 🔖

X ● **T26.81** Corrosions of other specified parts of right eye and adnexa 🔖

X ● **T26.82** Corrosions of other specified parts of left eye and adnexa 🔖

● **T26.9** **Corrosion of eye and adnexa, part unspecified**

Code first (T51-T65) to identify chemical and intent

Use additional external cause code to identify place (Y92)

X ● **T26.90** Corrosion of unspecified eye and adnexa, part unspecified 🔖

X ● **T26.91** Corrosion of right eye and adnexa, part unspecified 🔖

X ● **T26.92** Corrosion of left eye and adnexa, part unspecified 🔖

● **T27** **Burn and corrosion of respiratory tract**

Use additional external cause code to identify the source and intent of the burn (X00-X19, X75-X77, X96-X98) ⬅

Use additional external cause code to identify place (Y92)

The appropriate 7th character is to be added to each code from category T27

A	initial encounter
D	subsequent encounter
S	sequela

Ⓔ **For category T27 CC codes:** T27.0XX-T27.7XX[A], T28.3XX-T28.49X[A], T28.8XX-T28.99X[A]

X ● **T27.0** Burn of larynx and trachea A 🔖, 🔖, A 🔖

X ● **T27.1** Burn involving larynx and trachea with lung A 🔖, 🔖, A 🔖

X ● **T27.2** Burn of other parts of respiratory tract A 🔖, 🔖, A 🔖
Burn of thoracic cavity

X ● **T27.3** Burn of respiratory tract, part unspecified A 🔖, 🔖, A 🔖

Code first (T51-T65) to identify chemical and intent for codes T27.4-T27.7

X ● **T27.4** Corrosion of larynx and trachea A 🔖, 🔖, A 🔖

X ● **T27.5** Corrosion involving larynx and trachea with lung A 🔖, 🔖, A 🔖

X ● **T27.6** Corrosion of other parts of respiratory tract A 🔖, 🔖, A 🔖

X ● **T27.7** Corrosion of respiratory tract, part unspecified A 🔖, 🔖, A 🔖

N Newborn Age: 0   **P** Pediatric Age: 0–17   **M** Maternity DX: 12–55   **A** Adult Age: 15–124   ♀ Females Only   ♂ Males Only

🔖 Complication\Comorbidity   🔖 Major C\C   Ⓔ CC/MCC Exclusions   🔖 Present on Admission Requirement   🔖 Hospital-Acquired Condition

1517

● **T28**   **Burn and corrosion of other internal organs**

     Use additional external cause code to identify the source and intent of the burn (X00-X19, X75-X77, X96-X98) ◄▬▬

     Use additional external cause code to identify place (Y92)

     The appropriate 7th character is to be added to each code from category T28

> A   initial encounter
> D   subsequent encounter
> S   sequela

X ● **T28.0**   Burn of mouth and pharynx 🔍

X ● **T28.1**   Burn of esophagus A 🔍, 🔍, A 🔍
         Ⓔ⒳ T28.1XX[A], T28.3XX-T28.49X[A], T28.6XX[A], T28.8XX-T28.99X[A]

X ● **T28.2**   Burn of other parts of alimentary tract A 🔍, 🔍, A 🔍
         Ⓔ⒳ T28.2XX-T28.49X[A], T28.7XX-T28.99X[A]

X ● **T28.3**   Burn of internal genitourinary organs 🔍

X ● **T28.4**   Burns of other and unspecified internal organs

   X ● **T28.40**   Burn of unspecified internal organ 🔍

   ● **T28.41**   Burn of ear drum

       ● **T28.411**   Burn of right ear drum 🔍

       ● **T28.412**   Burn of left ear drum 🔍

       ● **T28.419**   Burn of unspecified ear drum 🔍

   X ● **T28.49**   Burn of other internal organ 🔍

        Code first (T51-T65) *to identify chemical and intent for T28.5-T28.9-*

X ● **T28.5**   Corrosion of mouth and pharynx 🔍

X ● **T28.6**   Corrosion of esophagus A 🔍, 🔍, A 🔍
         Ⓔ⒳ See T28.1

X ● **T28.7**   Corrosion of other parts of alimentary tract A 🔍, 🔍, A 🔍
         Ⓔ⒳ See T28.2

X ● **T28.8**   Corrosion of internal genitourinary organs 🔍

● **T28.9**   Corrosions of other and unspecified internal organs

   X ● **T28.90**   Corrosions of unspecified internal organs 🔍

   ● **T28.91**   Corrosions of ear drum

       ● **T28.911**   Corrosions of right ear drum 🔍

       ● **T28.912**   Corrosions of left ear drum 🔍

       ● **T28.919**   Corrosions of unspecified ear drum 🔍

   X ● **T28.99**   Corrosions of other internal organs 🔍

BURNS AND CORROSIONS OF MULTIPLE AND UNSPECIFIED BODY REGIONS (T30-T32)

● **T30**   **Burn and corrosion, body region unspecified**

   T30.0   Burn of unspecified body region, unspecified degree 🔍
       This code is not for inpatient use. Code to specified site and degree of burns
       Burn NOS
       Multiple burns NOS

   T30.4   Corrosion of unspecified body region, unspecified degree 🔍
       This code is not for inpatient use. Code to specified site and degree of corrosion
       Corrosion NOS
       Multiple corrosion NOS

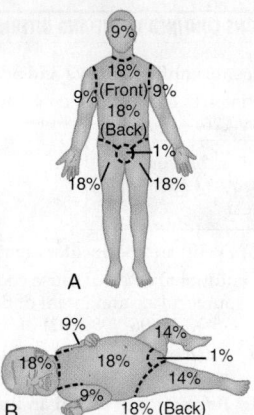

Figure 19-15   Rule of nines: percentages of total body area. (From Marx: Rosen's Emergency Medicine: Concepts and Clinical Practice, ed 6, Mosby, 2006)

OGCR   Section I.C.19.d.5.

> Assign separate code for each burn site
> When coding burns, assign separate codes for each burn site. Category T30, Burn and corrosion, body region unspecified is extremely vague and should rarely be used.

OGCR   See Section III.C.19.d.

● **T31**   **Burns classified according to extent of body surface involved**

     ~~This category is to be used as the primary code only when the site of the burn is unspecified. It should be used as a supplementary code with categories T20-T25 when the site is specified.~~

     Note: This category is to be used as the primary code only when the site of the burn is unspecified. It should be used as a supplementary code with categories T20-T25 when the site is specified. ◄
       Ⓔ⒳ **For category T31 CC codes:** T31.0-T32.99

   T31.0   Burns involving less than 10% of body surface 🔍

● **T31.1**   Burns involving 10-19% of body surface

     T31.10   Burns involving 10-19% of body surface with 0% to 9% third degree burns 🔍 🔍
        Burns involving 10-19% of body surface NOS

     T31.11   Burns involving 10-19% of body surface with 10-19% third degree burns 🔍 🔍

● **T31.2**   Burns involving 20-29% of body surface

     T31.20   Burns involving 20-29% of body surface with 0% to 9% third degree burns 🔍 🔍 🔍
        Burns involving 20-29% of body surface NOS

     T31.21   Burns involving 20-29% of body surface with 10-19% third degree burns 🔍 🔍

     T31.22   Burns involving 20-29% of body surface with 20-29% third degree burns 🔍 🔍

● **T31.3**   Burns involving 30-39% of body surface

     T31.30   Burns involving 30-39% of body surface with 0% to 9% third degree burns 🔍 🔍 🔍
        Burns involving 30-39% of body surface NOS

     T31.31   Burns involving 30-39% of body surface with 10-19% third degree burns 🔍 🔍 🔍

     T31.32   Burns involving 30-39% of body surface with 20-29% third degree burns 🔍 🔍 🔍

     T31.33   Burns involving 30-39% of body surface with 30-39% third degree burns 🔍 🔍 🔍

◄ New   ◄▬ Revised   ~~deleted~~ Deleted   Excludes 1   Excludes 2   Includes   Use additional   Code first   Code also   Unspecified

OGCR Official Guidelines   ● Unacceptable Principal Diagnosis   X Assign placeholder X   ▌ Use Additional Character(s)   ▐ Manifestation Code   **Coding Clinic**

● **T31.4 Burns involving 40-49% of body surface**

T31.40 Burns involving 40-49% of body surface with 0% to 9% third degree burns 🔹🔹🔹
Burns involving 40-49% of body surface NOS

T31.41 Burns involving 40-49% of body surface with 10-19% third degree burns 🔹🔹🔹

T31.42 Burns involving 40-49% of body surface with 20-29% third degree burns 🔹🔹🔹

T31.43 Burns involving 40-49% of body surface with 30-39% third degree burns 🔹🔹🔹

T31.44 Burns involving 40-49% of body surface with 40-49% third degree burns 🔹🔹🔹

● **T31.5 Burns involving 50-59% of body surface**

T31.50 Burns involving 50-59% of body surface with 0% to 9% third degree burns 🔹🔹🔹
Burns involving 50-59% of body surface NOS

T31.51 Burns involving 50-59% of body surface with 10-19% third degree burns 🔹🔹🔹

T31.52 Burns involving 50-59% of body surface with 20-29% third degree burns 🔹🔹🔹

T31.53 Burns involving 50-59% of body surface with 30-39% third degree burns 🔹🔹🔹

T31.54 Burns involving 50-59% of body surface with 40-49% third degree burns 🔹🔹🔹

T31.55 Burns involving 50-59% of body surface with 50-59% third degree burns 🔹🔹🔹

● **T31.6 Burns involving 60-69% of body surface**

T31.60 Burns involving 60-69% of body surface with 0% to 9% third degree burns 🔹🔹🔹
Burns involving 60-69% of body surface NOS

T31.61 Burns involving 60-69% of body surface with 10-19% third degree burns 🔹🔹🔹

T31.62 Burns involving 60-69% of body surface with 20-29% third degree burns 🔹🔹🔹

T31.63 Burns involving 60-69% of body surface with 30-39% third degree burns 🔹🔹🔹

T31.64 Burns involving 60-69% of body surface with 40-49% third degree burns 🔹🔹🔹

T31.65 Burns involving 60-69% of body surface with 50-59% third degree burns 🔹🔹🔹

T31.66 Burns involving 60-69% of body surface with 60-69% third degree burns 🔹🔹🔹

● **T31.7 Burns involving 70-79% of body surface**

T31.70 Burns involving 70-79% of body surface with 0% to 9% third degree burns 🔹🔹🔹
Burns involving 70-79% of body surface NOS

T31.71 Burns involving 70-79% of body surface with 10-19% third degree burns 🔹🔹🔹

T31.72 Burns involving 70-79% of body surface with 20-29% third degree burns 🔹🔹🔹

T31.73 Burns involving 70-79% of body surface with 30-39% third degree burns 🔹🔹🔹

T31.74 Burns involving 70-79% of body surface with 40-49% third degree burns 🔹🔹🔹

T31.75 Burns involving 70-79% of body surface with 50-59% third degree burns 🔹🔹🔹

T31.76 Burns involving 70-79% of body surface with 60-69% third degree burns 🔹🔹🔹

T31.77 Burns involving 70-79% of body surface with 70-79% third degree burns 🔹🔹🔹

● **T31.8 Burns involving 80-89% of body surface**

T31.80 Burns involving 80-89% of body surface with 0% to 9% third degree burns 🔹🔹🔹
Burns involving 80-89% of body surface NOS

T31.81 Burns involving 80-89% of body surface with 10-19% third degree burns 🔹🔹🔹

T31.82 Burns involving 80-89% of body surface with 20-29% third degree burns 🔹🔹🔹

T31.83 Burns involving 80-89% of body surface with 30-39% third degree burns 🔹🔹🔹

T31.84 Burns involving 80-89% of body surface with 40-49% third degree burns 🔹🔹🔹

T31.85 Burns involving 80-89% of body surface with 50-59% third degree burns 🔹🔹🔹

T31.86 Burns involving 80-89% of body surface with 60-69% third degree burns 🔹🔹🔹

T31.87 Burns involving 80-89% of body surface with 70-79% third degree burns 🔹🔹🔹

T31.88 Burns involving 80-89% of body surface with 80-89% third degree burns 🔹🔹🔹

● **T31.9 Burns involving 90% or more of body surface**

T31.90 Burns involving 90% or more of body surface with 0% to 9% third degree burns 🔹🔹🔹
Burns involving 90% or more of body surface NOS

T31.91 Burns involving 90% or more of body surface with 10-19% third degree burns 🔹🔹🔹

T31.92 Burns involving 90% or more of body surface with 20-29% third degree burns 🔹🔹🔹

T31.93 Burns involving 90% or more of body surface with 30-39% third degree burns 🔹🔹🔹

T31.94 Burns involving 90% or more of body surface with 40-49% third degree burns 🔹🔹🔹

T31.95 Burns involving 90% or more of body surface with 50-59% third degree burns 🔹🔹🔹

T31.96 Burns involving 90% or more of body surface with 60-69% third degree burns 🔹🔹🔹

T31.97 Burns involving 90% or more of body surface with 70-79% third degree burns 🔹🔹🔹

T31.98 Burns involving 90% or more of body surface with 80-89% third degree burns 🔹🔹🔹

T31.99 Burns involving 90% or more of body surface with 90% or more third degree burns 🔹🔹🔹

● **T32 Corrosions classified according to extent of body surface involved**

Note: This category is to be used as the primary code only when the site of the corrosion is unspecified. It may be used as a supplementary code with categories T20-T25 when the site is specified.

Ex. For category T32 CC codes: T31.0-T32.99

T32.0 Corrosions involving less than 10% of body surface 🔹

● **T32.1 Corrosions involving 10-19% of body surface**

T32.10 Corrosions involving 10-19% of body surface with 0% to 9% third degree corrosion 🔹🔹🔹
Corrosions involving 10-19% of body surface NOS

T32.11 Corrosions involving 10-19% of body surface with 10-19% third degree corrosion 🔹🔹🔹

● **T32.2 Corrosions involving 20-29% of body surface**

T32.20 Corrosions involving 20-29% of body surface with 0% to 9% third degree corrosion 🔹🔹🔹

T32.21 Corrosions involving 20-29% of body surface with 10-19% third degree corrosion 🔹🔹🔹

T32.22 Corrosions involving 20-29% of body surface with 20-29% third degree corrosion 🔹🔹🔹

● **T32.3 Corrosions involving 30-39% of body surface**

T32.30 Corrosions involving 30-39% of body surface with 0% to 9% third degree corrosion 🔹🔹🔹

T32.31 Corrosions involving 30-39% of body surface with 10-19% third degree corrosion 🔹🔹🔹

T32.32 Corrosions involving 30-39% of body surface with 20-29% third degree corrosion 🔹🔹🔹

T32.33 Corrosions involving 30-39% of body surface with 30-39% third degree corrosion 🔹🔹🔹

CHAPTER 19 (S00-T88)

N Newborn Age: 0   P Pediatric Age: 0–17   M Maternity DX: 12–55   A Adult Age: 15–124   ♀ Females Only   ♂ Males Only

🔹 Complication\Comorbidity   🔹 Major C\C   Ex CC/MCC Exclusions   🔹 Present on Admission Requirement   🔹 Hospital-Acquired Condition

1519

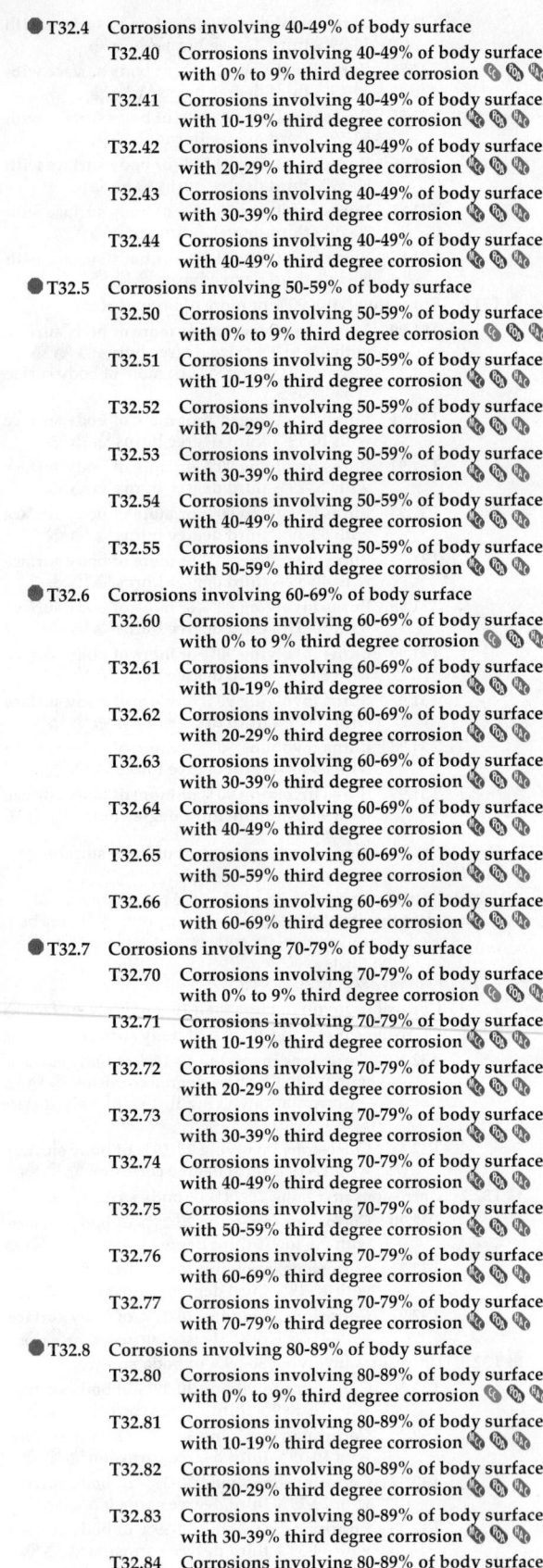

- **T32.4** Corrosions involving 40-49% of body surface
  - T32.40 Corrosions involving 40-49% of body surface with 0% to 9% third degree corrosion
  - T32.41 Corrosions involving 40-49% of body surface with 10-19% third degree corrosion
  - T32.42 Corrosions involving 40-49% of body surface with 20-29% third degree corrosion
  - T32.43 Corrosions involving 40-49% of body surface with 30-39% third degree corrosion
  - T32.44 Corrosions involving 40-49% of body surface with 40-49% third degree corrosion
- **T32.5** Corrosions involving 50-59% of body surface
  - T32.50 Corrosions involving 50-59% of body surface with 0% to 9% third degree corrosion
  - T32.51 Corrosions involving 50-59% of body surface with 10-19% third degree corrosion
  - T32.52 Corrosions involving 50-59% of body surface with 20-29% third degree corrosion
  - T32.53 Corrosions involving 50-59% of body surface with 30-39% third degree corrosion
  - T32.54 Corrosions involving 50-59% of body surface with 40-49% third degree corrosion
  - T32.55 Corrosions involving 50-59% of body surface with 50-59% third degree corrosion
- **T32.6** Corrosions involving 60-69% of body surface
  - T32.60 Corrosions involving 60-69% of body surface with 0% to 9% third degree corrosion
  - T32.61 Corrosions involving 60-69% of body surface with 10-19% third degree corrosion
  - T32.62 Corrosions involving 60-69% of body surface with 20-29% third degree corrosion
  - T32.63 Corrosions involving 60-69% of body surface with 30-39% third degree corrosion
  - T32.64 Corrosions involving 60-69% of body surface with 40-49% third degree corrosion
  - T32.65 Corrosions involving 60-69% of body surface with 50-59% third degree corrosion
  - T32.66 Corrosions involving 60-69% of body surface with 60-69% third degree corrosion
- **T32.7** Corrosions involving 70-79% of body surface
  - T32.70 Corrosions involving 70-79% of body surface with 0% to 9% third degree corrosion
  - T32.71 Corrosions involving 70-79% of body surface with 10-19% third degree corrosion
  - T32.72 Corrosions involving 70-79% of body surface with 20-29% third degree corrosion
  - T32.73 Corrosions involving 70-79% of body surface with 30-39% third degree corrosion
  - T32.74 Corrosions involving 70-79% of body surface with 40-49% third degree corrosion
  - T32.75 Corrosions involving 70-79% of body surface with 50-59% third degree corrosion
  - T32.76 Corrosions involving 70-79% of body surface with 60-69% third degree corrosion
  - T32.77 Corrosions involving 70-79% of body surface with 70-79% third degree corrosion
- **T32.8** Corrosions involving 80-89% of body surface
  - T32.80 Corrosions involving 80-89% of body surface with 0% to 9% third degree corrosion
  - T32.81 Corrosions involving 80-89% of body surface with 10-19% third degree corrosion
  - T32.82 Corrosions involving 80-89% of body surface with 20-29% third degree corrosion
  - T32.83 Corrosions involving 80-89% of body surface with 30-39% third degree corrosion
  - T32.84 Corrosions involving 80-89% of body surface with 40-49% third degree corrosion
  - T32.85 Corrosions involving 80-89% of body surface with 50-59% third degree corrosion
  - T32.86 Corrosions involving 80-89% of body surface with 60-69% third degree corrosion
  - T32.87 Corrosions involving 80-89% of body surface with 70-79% third degree corrosion
  - T32.88 Corrosions involving 80-89% of body surface with 80-89% third degree corrosion
- **T32.9** Corrosions involving 90% or more of body surface
  - T32.90 Corrosions involving 90% or more of body surface with 0% to 9% third degree corrosion
  - T32.91 Corrosions involving 90% or more of body surface with 10-19% third degree corrosion
  - T32.92 Corrosions involving 90% or more of body surface with 20-29% third degree corrosion
  - T32.93 Corrosions involving 90% or more of body surface with 30-39% third degree corrosion
  - T32.94 Corrosions involving 90% or more of body surface with 40-49% third degree corrosion
  - T32.95 Corrosions involving 90% or more of body surface with 50-59% third degree corrosion
  - T32.96 Corrosions involving 90% or more of body surface with 60-69% third degree corrosion
  - T32.97 Corrosions involving 90% or more of body surface with 70-79% third degree corrosion
  - T32.98 Corrosions involving 90% or more of body surface with 80-89% third degree corrosion
  - T32.99 Corrosions involving 90% or more of body surface with 90% or more third degree corrosion

FROSTBITE (T33-T34)

Excludes2   hypothermia and other effects of reduced temperature (T68, T69.-)

- **T33** Superficial frostbite

  Includes   frostbite with partial thickness skin loss

  The appropriate 7th character is to be added to each code from category T33

A	initial encounter
D	subsequent encounter
S	sequela

  - **T33.0** Superficial frostbite of head
    - Ex: For category T33.0 CC codes: T33.011-T33.42X[A], T33.60X-T33.72X[A], T33.90X-T34.42X[A], T34.60X-T34.72X[A], T34.90X-T34.99X[A]
    - **T33.01** Superficial frostbite of ear
      - **T33.011** Superficial frostbite of right ear A, A
      - **T33.012** Superficial frostbite of left ear A, A
      - **T33.019** Superficial frostbite of unspecified ear A, A
    - X **T33.02** Superficial frostbite of nose A, A
    - X **T33.09** Superficial frostbite of other part of head A, A
  - X **T33.1** Superficial frostbite of neck A, A
    - Ex: See T33.0
  - X **T33.2** Superficial frostbite of thorax A, A
    - Ex: T33.011-T34.99X[A], T69.021-T69.029[A]

X ● **T33.3**   **Superficial frostbite of abdominal wall, lower back and pelvis** A 🔖, 🔖, A 🔖
     (Ex) See T33.2

● **T33.4**   **Superficial frostbite of arm**
     Excludes2   superficial frostbite of wrist and hand (T33.5-)
     (Ex) **For category T33.4 CC codes:** See T33.2

     X ● **T33.40**   **Superficial frostbite of** unspecified **arm** A 🔖, 🔖, A 🔖

     X ● **T33.41**   **Superficial frostbite of right arm** A 🔖, 🔖, A 🔖

     X ● **T33.42**   **Superficial frostbite of left arm** A 🔖, 🔖, A 🔖

● **T33.5**   **Superficial frostbite of wrist, hand, and fingers**
     (Ex) **For category T33.5 CC codes:** T33.2XX-T33.72X[A], T33.90X-T33.99X[A], T34.2XX-T34.72X[A], T34.90X-T34.99X[A]

     ● **T33.51**   **Superficial frostbite of wrist**

       ● **T33.511**   **Superficial frostbite of right wrist** A 🔖, 🔖, A 🔖

       ● **T33.512**   **Superficial frostbite of left wrist** A 🔖, 🔖, A 🔖

       ● **T33.519**   **Superficial frostbite of** unspecified **wrist** A 🔖, 🔖, A 🔖

     ● **T33.52**   **Superficial frostbite of hand**
       Excludes2   superficial frostbite of fingers (T33.53-)

       ● **T33.521**   **Superficial frostbite of right hand** A 🔖, 🔖, A 🔖

       ● **T33.522**   **Superficial frostbite of left hand** A 🔖, 🔖, A 🔖

       ● **T33.529**   **Superficial frostbite of** unspecified **hand** A 🔖, 🔖, A 🔖

     ● **T33.53**   **Superficial frostbite of finger(s)**

       ● **T33.531**   **Superficial frostbite of right finger(s)** A 🔖, 🔖, A 🔖

       ● **T33.532**   **Superficial frostbite of left finger(s)** A 🔖, 🔖, A 🔖

       ● **T33.539**   **Superficial frostbite of** unspecified **finger(s)** A 🔖, 🔖, A 🔖

● **T33.6**   **Superficial frostbite of hip and thigh**
     (Ex) **For category T33.6 CC codes:** See T33.2

     X ● **T33.60**   **Superficial frostbite of** unspecified **hip and thigh** A 🔖, 🔖, A 🔖

     X ● **T33.61**   **Superficial frostbite of right hip and thigh** A 🔖, 🔖, A 🔖

     X ● **T33.62**   **Superficial frostbite of left hip and thigh** A 🔖, 🔖, A 🔖

● **T33.7**   **Superficial frostbite of knee and lower leg**
     Excludes2   superficial frostbite of ankle and foot (T33.8-)
     (Ex) **For category T33.7 CC codes:** See T33.2

     X ● **T33.70**   **Superficial frostbite of** unspecified **knee and lower leg** A 🔖, 🔖, A 🔖

     X ● **T33.71**   **Superficial frostbite of right knee and lower leg** A 🔖, 🔖, A 🔖

     X ● **T33.72**   **Superficial frostbite of left knee and lower leg** A 🔖, 🔖, A 🔖

● **T33.8**   **Superficial frostbite of ankle, foot, and toe(s)**
     (Ex) **For category T33.8 CC codes:** T33.2XX-T33.42X[A], T33.60X-T33.99X[A], T34.2XX-T34.42X[A], T34.60X-T34.99X[A]

     ● **T33.81**   **Superficial frostbite of ankle**

       ● **T33.811**   **Superficial frostbite of right ankle** A 🔖, 🔖, A 🔖

       ● **T33.812**   **Superficial frostbite of left ankle** A 🔖, 🔖, A 🔖

       ● **T33.819**   **Superficial frostbite of** unspecified **ankle** A 🔖, 🔖, A 🔖

     ● **T33.82**   **Superficial frostbite of foot**

       ● **T33.821**   **Superficial frostbite of right foot** A 🔖, 🔖, A 🔖

       ● **T33.822**   **Superficial frostbite of left foot** A 🔖, 🔖, A 🔖

       ● **T33.829**   **Superficial frostbite of** unspecified **foot** A 🔖, 🔖, A 🔖

     ● **T33.83**   **Superficial frostbite of toe(s)**

       ● **T33.831**   **Superficial frostbite of right toe(s)** A 🔖, 🔖, A 🔖

       ● **T33.832**   **Superficial frostbite of left toe(s)** A 🔖, 🔖, A 🔖

       ● **T33.839**   **Superficial frostbite of** unspecified **toe(s)** A 🔖, 🔖, A 🔖

● **T33.9**   **Superficial frostbite of other and unspecified sites**
     (Ex) **For category T33.9 CC codes:** See T33.2

     X ● **T33.90**   **Superficial frostbite of** unspecified **sites** A 🔖, 🔖, A 🔖
       Superficial frostbite NOS

     X ● **T33.99**   **Superficial frostbite of other sites** A 🔖, 🔖, A 🔖
       Superficial frostbite of leg NOS
       Superficial frostbite of trunk NOS

● **T34**   **Frostbite with tissue necrosis**
     The appropriate 7th character is to be added to each code from category T34

A	initial encounter
D	subsequent encounter
S	sequela

     ● **T34.0**   **Frostbite with tissue necrosis of head**
       (Ex) **For category T34.0 CC codes:** See T33.0

       ● **T34.01**   **Frostbite with tissue necrosis of ear**

         ● **T34.011**   **Frostbite with tissue necrosis of right ear** A 🔖, 🔖, A 🔖

         ● **T34.012**   **Frostbite with tissue necrosis of left ear** A 🔖, 🔖, A 🔖

         ● **T34.019**   **Frostbite with tissue necrosis of** unspecified **ear** A 🔖, 🔖, A 🔖

       X ● **T34.02**   **Frostbite with tissue necrosis of nose** A 🔖, 🔖, A 🔖

       X ● **T34.09**   **Frostbite with tissue necrosis of other part of head** A 🔖, 🔖, A 🔖

     X ● **T34.1**   **Frostbite with tissue necrosis of neck** A 🔖, 🔖, A 🔖
       (Ex) See T33.0

     X ● **T34.2**   **Frostbite with tissue necrosis of thorax** A 🔖, 🔖, A 🔖
       (Ex) See T33.2

     X ● **T34.3**   **Frostbite with tissue necrosis of abdominal wall, lower back and pelvis** A 🔖, 🔖, A 🔖
       (Ex) See T33.2

     ● **T34.4**   **Frostbite with tissue necrosis of arm**
       Excludes2   frostbite with tissue necrosis of wrist and hand (T34.5-)
       (Ex) **For category T34.4 CC codes:** See T33.2

       X ● **T34.40**   **Frostbite with tissue necrosis of** unspecified **arm** A 🔖, 🔖, A 🔖

       X ● **T34.41**   **Frostbite with tissue necrosis of right arm** A 🔖, 🔖, A 🔖

       X ● **T34.42**   **Frostbite with tissue necrosis of left arm** A 🔖, 🔖, A 🔖

     ● **T34.5**   **Frostbite with tissue necrosis of wrist, hand, and finger(s)**
       (Ex) **For category T34.5 CC codes:** See T33.5

       ● **T34.51**   **Frostbite with tissue necrosis of wrist**

         ● **T34.511**   **Frostbite with tissue necrosis of right wrist** A 🔖, 🔖, A 🔖

         ● **T34.512**   **Frostbite with tissue necrosis of left wrist** A 🔖, 🔖, A 🔖

         ● **T34.519**   **Frostbite with tissue necrosis of** unspecified **wrist** A 🔖, 🔖, A 🔖

N Newborn Age: 0   **P** Pediatric Age: 0–17   **M** Maternity DX: 12–55   **A** Adult Age: 15–124   ♀ Females Only   ♂ Males Only

 Complication\Comorbidity   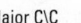 Major C\C   (Ex) CC/MCC Exclusions   Present on Admission Requirement   Hospital-Acquired Condition

1521

CHAPTER 19 (S00-T88)

● **T34.52** **Frostbite with tissue necrosis of hand**

　Excludes2 frostbite with tissue necrosis of finger(s) (T34.53-)

● **T34.521** **Frostbite with tissue necrosis of right hand** A 🖐, 🖐, A 🖐

● **T34.522** **Frostbite with tissue necrosis of left hand** A 🖐, 🖐, A 🖐

● **T34.529** **Frostbite with tissue necrosis of unspecified hand** A 🖐, 🖐, A 🖐

● **T34.53** **Frostbite with tissue necrosis of finger(s)**

● **T34.531** **Frostbite with tissue necrosis of right finger(s)** A 🖐, 🖐, A 🖐

● **T34.532** **Frostbite with tissue necrosis of left finger(s)** A 🖐, 🖐, A 🖐

● **T34.539** **Frostbite with tissue necrosis of unspecified finger(s)** A 🖐, 🖐, A 🖐

● **T34.6** **Frostbite with tissue necrosis of hip and thigh**

　(Ex) For category T34.6 CC codes: See T33.2

X ● **T34.60** **Frostbite with tissue necrosis of unspecified hip and thigh** A 🖐, 🖐, A 🖐

X ● **T34.61** **Frostbite with tissue necrosis of right hip and thigh** A 🖐, 🖐, A 🖐

X ● **T34.62** **Frostbite with tissue necrosis of left hip and thigh** A 🖐, 🖐, A 🖐

● **T34.7** **Frostbite with tissue necrosis of knee and lower leg**

　Excludes2 frostbite with tissue necrosis of ankle and foot (T34.8-)

　(Ex) For category T34.7 CC codes: See T33.2

X ● **T34.70** **Frostbite with tissue necrosis of unspecified knee and lower leg** A 🖐, 🖐, A 🖐

X ● **T34.71** **Frostbite with tissue necrosis of right knee and lower leg** A 🖐, 🖐, A 🖐

X ● **T34.72** **Frostbite with tissue necrosis of left knee and lower leg** A 🖐, 🖐, A 🖐

● **T34.8** **Frostbite with tissue necrosis of ankle, foot, and toe(s)**

　(Ex) For category T34.8 CC codes: See T33.8

● **T34.81** **Frostbite with tissue necrosis of ankle**

● **T34.811** **Frostbite with tissue necrosis of right ankle** A 🖐, 🖐, A 🖐

● **T34.812** **Frostbite with tissue necrosis of left ankle** A 🖐, 🖐, A 🖐

● **T34.819** **Frostbite with tissue necrosis of unspecified ankle** A 🖐, 🖐, A 🖐

● **T34.82** **Frostbite with tissue necrosis of foot**

● **T34.821** **Frostbite with tissue necrosis of right foot** A 🖐, 🖐, A 🖐

● **T34.822** **Frostbite with tissue necrosis of left foot** A 🖐, 🖐, A 🖐

● **T34.829** **Frostbite with tissue necrosis of unspecified foot** A 🖐, 🖐, A 🖐

● **T34.83** **Frostbite with tissue necrosis of toe(s)**

● **T34.831** **Frostbite with tissue necrosis of right toe(s)** A 🖐, 🖐, A 🖐

● **T34.832** **Frostbite with tissue necrosis of left toe(s)** A 🖐, 🖐, A 🖐

● **T34.839** **Frostbite with tissue necrosis of unspecified toe(s)** A 🖐, 🖐, A 🖐

● **T34.9** **Frostbite with tissue necrosis of other and unspecified sites**

　(Ex) For category T34.9 CC codes: See T33.2

X ● **T34.90** **Frostbite with tissue necrosis of unspecified sites** A 🖐, 🖐, A 🖐

　　Frostbite with tissue necrosis NOS

X ● **T34.99** **Frostbite with tissue necrosis of other sites** A 🖐, 🖐, A 🖐

　　Frostbite with tissue necrosis of leg NOS

　　Frostbite with tissue necrosis of trunk NOS

OGCR See Guidelines Section I.C.19.e.

POISONING BY, ADVERSE EFFECTS OF AND UNDERDOSING OF DRUGS, MEDICAMENTS AND BIOLOGICAL SUBSTANCES (T36-T50)

Includes adverse effect of correct substance properly administered

poisoning by overdose of substance

poisoning by wrong substance given or taken in error

underdosing by (inadvertently) (deliberately) taking less substance than prescribed or instructed

Code first, for adverse effects, the nature of the adverse effect, such as:

adverse effect NOS (T88.7)

aspirin gastritis (K29.-)

blood disorders (D56-D76)

contact dermatitis (L23-L25)

dermatitis due to substances taken internally (L27.-)

nephropathy (N14.0-N14.2)

Note: The drug giving rise to the adverse effect should be identified by use of codes from categories T36-T50 with fifth or sixth character 5.

Use additional code(s) to specify:

manifestations of poisoning

underdosing or failure in dosage during medical and surgical care (Y63.6, Y63.8-Y63.9)

underdosing of medication regimen (Z91.12-, Z91.13-)

Excludes1 toxic reaction to local anesthesia in pregnancy (O29.3-)

Excludes2 abuse and dependence of psychoactive substances (F10-F19)

abuse of non-dependence-producing substances (F55.-)

drug reaction and poisoning affecting newborn (P00-P96)

pathological drug intoxication (inebriation) (F10-F19)

● **T36** **Poisoning by, adverse effect of and underdosing of systemic antibiotics**

　Excludes1 antineoplastic antibiotics (T45.1-)

locally applied antibiotic NEC (T49.0)

topically used antibiotic for ear, nose and throat (T49.6)

topically used antibiotic for eye (T49.5)

The appropriate 7th character is to be added to each code from category T36

A	initial encounter
D	subsequent encounter
S	sequela

● **T36.0** **Poisoning by, adverse effect of and underdosing of penicillins**

● **T36.0X** **Poisoning by, adverse effect of and underdosing of penicillins**

● **T36.0X1** **Poisoning by penicillins, accidental (unintentional)** 🖐

　　Poisoning by penicillins NOS

● **T36.0X2** **Poisoning by penicillins, intentional self-harm** 🖐

● **T36.0X3** **Poisoning by penicillins, assault** 🖐

● **T36.0X4** **Poisoning by penicillins, undetermined** 🖐

● **T36.0X5** **Adverse effect of penicillins** 🖐

● **T36.0X6** **Underdosing of penicillins** 🖐

◀ New　◀▥ Revised　~~deleted~~ Deleted　Excludes 1　Excludes 2　Includes　Use additional　Code first　Code also　Unspecified

OGCR Official Guidelines　● Unacceptable Principal Diagnosis　X Assign placeholder X　● Use Additional Character(s)　▌Manifestation Code　**Coding Clinic**

● **T36.1** Poisoning by, adverse effect of and underdosing of cephalosporins and other betalactam antibiotics

　● **T36.1X** Poisoning by, adverse effect of and underdosing of cephalosporins and other beta-lactam antibiotics

　　● **T36.1X1** Poisoning by cephalosporins and other beta-lactam antibiotics, accidental (unintentional) 🗞
　　　　Poisoning by cephalosporins and other beta-lactam antibiotics NOS

　　● **T36.1X2** Poisoning by cephalosporins and other beta-lactam antibiotics, intentional self-harm 🗞

　　● **T36.1X3** Poisoning by cephalosporins and other beta-lactam antibiotics, assault 🗞

　　● **T36.1X4** Poisoning by cephalosporins and other beta-lactam antibiotics, undetermined 🗞

　　● **T36.1X5** Adverse effect of cephalosporins and other beta-lactam antibiotics 🗞

　　● **T36.1X6** Underdosing of cephalosporins and other beta-lactam antibiotics 🗞

● **T36.2** Poisoning by, adverse effect of and underdosing of chloramphenicol group

　● **T36.2X** Poisoning by, adverse effect of and underdosing of chloramphenicol group

　　● **T36.2X1** Poisoning by chloramphenicol group, accidental (unintentional) 🗞
　　　　Poisoning by chloramphenicol group NOS

　　● **T36.2X2** Poisoning by chloramphenicol group, intentional self-harm 🗞

　　● **T36.2X3** Poisoning by chloramphenicol group, assault 🗞

　　● **T36.2X4** Poisoning by chloramphenicol group, undetermined 🗞

　　● **T36.2X5** Adverse effect of chloramphenicol group 🗞

　　● **T36.2X6** Underdosing of chloramphenicol group 🗞

● **T36.3** Poisoning by, adverse effect of and underdosing of macrolides

　● **T36.3X** Poisoning by, adverse effect of and underdosing of macrolides

　　● **T36.3X1** Poisoning by macrolides, accidental (unintentional) 🗞
　　　　Poisoning by macrolides NOS

　　● **T36.3X2** Poisoning by macrolides, intentional self-harm 🗞

　　● **T36.3X3** Poisoning by macrolides, assault 🗞

　　● **T36.3X4** Poisoning by macrolides, undetermined 🗞

　　● **T36.3X5** Adverse effect of macrolides 🗞

　　● **T36.3X6** Underdosing of macrolides 🗞

● **T36.4** Poisoning by, adverse effect of and underdosing of tetracyclines

　● **T36.4X** Poisoning by, adverse effect of and underdosing of tetracyclines

　　● **T36.4X1** Poisoning by tetracyclines, accidental (unintentional) 🗞
　　　　Poisoning by tetracyclines NOS

　　● **T36.4X2** Poisoning by tetracyclines, intentional self-harm 🗞

　　● **T36.4X3** Poisoning by tetracyclines, assault 🗞

　　● **T36.4X4** Poisoning by tetracyclines, undetermined 🗞

　　● **T36.4X5** Adverse effect of tetracyclines 🗞

　　● **T36.4X6** Underdosing of tetracyclines 🗞

● **T36.5** Poisoning by, adverse effect of and underdosing of aminoglycosides
　　Poisoning by, adverse effect of and underdosing of streptomycin

　● **T36.5X** Poisoning by, adverse effect of and underdosing of aminoglycosides

　　● **T36.5X1** Poisoning by aminoglycosides, accidental (unintentional) 🗞
　　　　Poisoning by aminoglycosides NOS

　　● **T36.5X2** Poisoning by aminoglycosides, intentional self-harm 🗞

　　● **T36.5X3** Poisoning by aminoglycosides, assault 🗞

　　● **T36.5X4** Poisoning by aminoglycosides, undetermined 🗞

　　● **T36.5X5** Adverse effect of aminoglycosides 🗞

　　● **T36.5X6** Underdosing of aminoglycosides 🗞

● **T36.6** Poisoning by, adverse effect of and underdosing of rifampicins

　● **T36.6X** Poisoning by, adverse effect of and underdosing of rifampicins

　　● **T36.6X1** Poisoning by rifampicins, accidental (unintentional) 🗞
　　　　Poisoning by rifampicins NOS

　　● **T36.6X2** Poisoning by rifampicins, intentional self-harm 🗞

　　● **T36.6X3** Poisoning by rifampicins, assault 🗞

　　● **T36.6X4** Poisoning by rifampicins, undetermined 🗞

　　● **T36.6X5** Adverse effect of rifampicins 🗞

　　● **T36.6X6** Underdosing of rifampicins 🗞

● **T36.7** Poisoning by, adverse effect of and underdosing of antifungal antibiotics, systemically used

　● **T36.7X** Poisoning by, adverse effect of and underdosing of antifungal antibiotics, systemically used

　　● **T36.7X1** Poisoning by antifungal antibiotics, systemically used, accidental (unintentional) 🗞
　　　　Poisoning by antifungal antibiotics, systemically used NOS

　　● **T36.7X2** Poisoning by antifungal antibiotics, systemically used, intentional self-harm 🗞

　　● **T36.7X3** Poisoning by antifungal antibiotics, systemically used, assault 🗞

　　● **T36.7X4** Poisoning by antifungal antibiotics, systemically used, undetermined 🗞

　　● **T36.7X5** Adverse effect of antifungal antibiotics, systemically used 🗞

　　● **T36.7X6** Underdosing of antifungal antibiotics, systemically used 🗞

● **T36.8** Poisoning by, adverse effect of and underdosing of other systemic antibiotics

　● **T36.8X** Poisoning by, adverse effect of and underdosing of other systemic antibiotics

　　● **T36.8X1** Poisoning by other systemic antibiotics, accidental (unintentional) 🗞
　　　　Poisoning by other systemic antibiotics NOS

　　● **T36.8X2** Poisoning by other systemic antibiotics, intentional self-harm 🗞

　　● **T36.8X3** Poisoning by other systemic antibiotics, assault 🗞

　　● **T36.8X4** Poisoning by other systemic antibiotics, undetermined 🗞

　　● **T36.8X5** Adverse effect of other systemic antibiotics 🗞

　　● **T36.8X6** Underdosing of other systemic antibiotics 🗞

CHAPTER 19 (S00-T88)

N Newborn Age: 0　　**P** Pediatric Age: 0–17　　**M** Maternity DX: 12–55　　**A** Adult Age: 15–124　　♀ Females Only　　♂ Males Only

🗞 Complication\Comorbidity　　🗞 Major C\C　　(Ex) CC/MCC Exclusions　　🗞 Present on Admission Requirement　　🗞 Hospital-Acquired Condition

● **T36.9**   **Poisoning by, adverse effect of and underdosing of unspecified systemic antibiotic**

    X● **T36.91**   **Poisoning by** unspecified **systemic antibiotic, accidental (unintentional)** 🔍
         Poisoning by systemic antibiotic NOS

    X● **T36.92**   **Poisoning by** unspecified **systemic antibiotic, intentional self-harm** 🔍

    X● **T36.93**   **Poisoning by** unspecified **systemic antibiotic, assault** 🔍

    X● **T36.94**   **Poisoning by** unspecified **systemic antibiotic, undetermined** 🔍

    X● **T36.95**   **Adverse effect of** unspecified **systemic antibiotic** 🔍

    X● **T36.96**   **Underdosing of** unspecified **systemic antibiotic** 🔍

● **T37**   **Poisoning by, adverse effect of and underdosing of other systemic anti-infectives and antiparasitics**

    Excludes1   anti-infectives topically used for ear, nose and throat (T49.6-)
               anti-infectives topically used for eye (T49.5-)
               locally applied anti-infectives NEC (T49.0-)

    The appropriate 7th character is to be added to each code from category T37

> | | |
> |---|---|
> | A | initial encounter |
> | D | subsequent encounter |
> | S | sequela |

   ● **T37.0**   **Poisoning by, adverse effect of and underdosing of sulfonamides**

      ● **T37.0X**   **Poisoning by, adverse effect of and underdosing of sulfonamides**

        ● **T37.0X1**   **Poisoning by sulfonamides, accidental (unintentional)** 🔍
                 Poisoning by sulfonamides NOS

        ● **T37.0X2**   **Poisoning by sulfonamides, intentional self-harm** 🔍

        ● **T37.0X3**   **Poisoning by sulfonamides, assault** 🔍

        ● **T37.0X4**   **Poisoning by sulfonamides, undetermined** 🔍

        ● **T37.0X5**   **Adverse effect of sulfonamides** 🔍

        ● **T37.0X6**   **Underdosing of sulfonamides** 🔍

   ● **T37.1**   **Poisoning by, adverse effect of and underdosing of antimycobacterial drugs**

      Excludes1   rifampicins (T36.6-) streptomycin (T36.5-)

      ● **T37.1X**   **Poisoning by, adverse effect of and underdosing of antimycobacterial drugs**

        ● **T37.1X1**   **Poisoning by antimycobacterial drugs, accidental (unintentional)** 🔍
                 Poisoning by antimycobacterial drugs NOS

        ● **T37.1X2**   **Poisoning by antimycobacterial drugs, intentional self-harm** 🔍

        ● **T37.1X3**   **Poisoning by antimycobacterial drugs, assault** 🔍

        ● **T37.1X4**   **Poisoning by antimycobacterial drugs, undetermined** 🔍

        ● **T37.1X5**   **Adverse effect of antimycobacterial drugs** 🔍

        ● **T37.1X6**   **Underdosing of antimycobacterial drugs** 🔍

● **T37.2**   **Poisoning by, adverse effect of and underdosing of antimalarials and drugs acting on other blood protozoa**

    Excludes1   hydroxyquinoline derivatives (T37.8-)

   ● **T37.2X**   **Poisoning by, adverse effect of and underdosing of antimalarials and drugs acting on other blood protozoa**

      ● **T37.2X1**   **Poisoning by antimalarials and drugs acting on other blood protozoa, accidental (unintentional)** 🔍
               Poisoning by antimalarials and drugs acting on other blood protozoa NOS

      ● **T37.2X2**   **Poisoning by antimalarials and drugs acting on other blood protozoa, intentional self-harm** 🔍

      ● **T37.2X3**   **Poisoning by antimalarials and drugs acting on other blood protozoa, assault** 🔍

      ● **T37.2X4**   **Poisoning by antimalarials and drugs acting on other blood protozoa, undetermined** 🔍

      ● **T37.2X5**   **Adverse effect of antimalarials and drugs acting on other blood protozoa** 🔍

      ● **T37.2X6**   **Underdosing of antimalarials and drugs acting on other blood protozoa** 🔍

● **T37.3**   **Poisoning by, adverse effect of and underdosing of other antiprotozoal drugs**

   ● **T37.3X**   **Poisoning by, adverse effect of and underdosing of other antiprotozoal drugs**

      ● **T37.3X1**   **Poisoning by other antiprotozoal drugs, accidental (unintentional)** 🔍
               Poisoning by other antiprotozoal drugs NOS

      ● **T37.3X2**   **Poisoning by other antiprotozoal drugs, intentional self-harm** 🔍

      ● **T37.3X3**   **Poisoning by other antiprotozoal drugs, assault** 🔍

      ● **T37.3X4**   **Poisoning by other antiprotozoal drugs, undetermined** 🔍

      ● **T37.3X5**   **Adverse effect of other antiprotozoal drugs** 🔍

      ● **T37.3X6**   **Underdosing of other antiprotozoal drugs** 🔍

● **T37.4**   **Poisoning by, adverse effect of and underdosing of anthelminthics**

   ● **T37.4X**   **Poisoning by, adverse effect of and underdosing of anthelminthics**

      ● **T37.4X1**   **Poisoning by anthelminthics, accidental (unintentional)** 🔍
               Poisoning by anthelminthics NOS

      ● **T37.4X2**   **Poisoning by anthelminthics, intentional self-harm** 🔍

      ● **T37.4X3**   **Poisoning by anthelminthics, assault** 🔍

      ● **T37.4X4**   **Poisoning by anthelminthics, undetermined** 🔍

      ● **T37.4X5**   **Adverse effect of anthelminthics** 🔍

      ● **T37.4X6**   **Underdosing of anthelminthics** 🔍

● **T37.5**   Poisoning by, adverse effect of and underdosing of antiviral drugs
> **Excludes1**   amantadine (T42.8-)
> cytarabine (T45.1-)

  ● **T37.5X**   Poisoning by, adverse effect of and underdosing of antiviral drugs

    ● **T37.5X1**   Poisoning by antiviral drugs, accidental (unintentional) 🗇
> Poisoning by antiviral drugs NOS

    ● **T37.5X2**   Poisoning by antiviral drugs, intentional self-harm 🗇

    ● **T37.5X3**   Poisoning by antiviral drugs, assault 🗇

    ● **T37.5X4**   Poisoning by antiviral drugs, undetermined 🗇

    ● **T37.5X5**   Adverse effect of antiviral drugs 🗇

    ● **T37.5X6**   Underdosing of antiviral drugs 🗇

● **T37.8**   Poisoning by, adverse effect of and underdosing of other specified systemic anti-infectives and antiparasitics
> Poisoning by, adverse effect of and underdosing of hydroxyquinoline derivatives
> **Excludes1**   antimalarial drugs (T37.2-)

  ● **T37.8X**   Poisoning by, adverse effect of and underdosing of other specified systemic anti-infectives and antiparasitics

    ● **T37.8X1**   Poisoning by other specified systemic anti-infectives and antiparasitics, accidental (unintentional) 🗇
> Poisoning by other specified systemic anti-infectives and antiparasitics NOS

    ● **T37.8X2**   Poisoning by other specified systemic anti-infectives and antiparasitics, intentional self-harm 🗇

    ● **T37.8X3**   Poisoning by other specified systemic anti-infectives and antiparasitics, assault 🗇

    ● **T37.8X4**   Poisoning by other specified systemic anti-infectives and antiparasitics, undetermined 🗇

    ● **T37.8X5**   Adverse effect of other specified systemic anti-infectives and antiparasitics 🗇

    ● **T37.8X6**   Underdosing of other specified systemic anti-infectives and antiparasitics 🗇

● **T37.9**   Poisoning by, adverse effect of and underdosing of unspecified systemic anti-infective and antiparasitics

  X ● **T37.91**   Poisoning by unspecified systemic anti-infective and antiparasitics, accidental (unintentional) 🗇
> Poisoning by, adverse effect of and underdosing of systemic anti-infective and antiparasitics NOS

  X ● **T37.92**   Poisoning by unspecified systemic anti-infective and antiparasitics, intentional self-harm 🗇

  X ● **T37.93**   Poisoning by unspecified systemic anti-infective and antiparasitics, assault 🗇

  X ● **T37.94**   Poisoning by unspecified systemic anti-infective and antiparasitics, undetermined 🗇

  X ● **T37.95**   Adverse effect of unspecified systemic anti-infective and antiparasitic 🗇

  X ● **T37.96**   Underdosing of unspecified systemic anti-infectives and antiparasitics 🗇

● **T38**   Poisoning by, adverse effect of and underdosing of hormones and their synthetic substitutes and antagonists, not elsewhere classified
> **Excludes1**   mineralocorticoids and their antagonists (T50.0-)
> oxytocic hormones (T48.0-)
> parathyroid hormones and derivatives (T50.9-)

The appropriate 7th character is to be added to each code from category T38

> | A | initial encounter |
> |---|---|
> | D | subsequent encounter |
> | S | sequela |

● **T38.0**   Poisoning by, adverse effect of and underdosing of glucocorticoids and synthetic analogues
> **Excludes1**   glucocorticoids, topically used (T49.-)

  ● **T38.0X**   Poisoning by, adverse effect of and underdosing of glucocorticoids and synthetic analogues

    ● **T38.0X1**   Poisoning by glucocorticoids and synthetic analogues, accidental (unintentional) 🗇
> Poisoning by glucocorticoids and synthetic analogues NOS

    ● **T38.0X2**   Poisoning by glucocorticoids and synthetic analogues, intentional self-harm 🗇

    ● **T38.0X3**   Poisoning by glucocorticoids and synthetic analogues, assault 🗇

    ● **T38.0X4**   Poisoning by glucocorticoids and synthetic analogues, undetermined 🗇

    ● **T38.0X5**   Adverse effect of glucocorticoids and synthetic analogues 🗇

    ● **T38.0X6**   Underdosing of glucocorticoids and synthetic analogues 🗇

● **T38.1**   Poisoning by, adverse effect of and underdosing of thyroid hormones and substitutes

  ● **T38.1X**   Poisoning by, adverse effect of and underdosing of thyroid hormones and substitutes

    ● **T38.1X1**   Poisoning by thyroid hormones and substitutes, accidental (unintentional) 🗇
> Poisoning by thyroid hormones and substitutes NOS

    ● **T38.1X2**   Poisoning by thyroid hormones and substitutes, intentional self-harm 🗇

    ● **T38.1X3**   Poisoning by thyroid hormones and substitutes, assault 🗇

    ● **T38.1X4**   Poisoning by thyroid hormones and substitutes, undetermined 🗇

    ● **T38.1X5**   Adverse effect of thyroid hormones and substitutes 🗇

    ● **T38.1X6**   Underdosing of thyroid hormones and substitutes 🗇

● **T38.2**   Poisoning by, adverse effect of and underdosing of antithyroid drugs

  ● **T38.2X**   Poisoning by, adverse effect of and underdosing of antithyroid drugs

    ● **T38.2X1**   Poisoning by antithyroid drugs, accidental (unintentional) 🗇
> Poisoning by antithyroid drugs NOS

    ● **T38.2X2**   Poisoning by antithyroid drugs, intentional self-harm 🗇

    ● **T38.2X3**   Poisoning by antithyroid drugs, assault 🗇

    ● **T38.2X4**   Poisoning by antithyroid drugs, undetermined 🗇

    ● **T38.2X5**   Adverse effect of antithyroid drugs 🗇

    ● **T38.2X6**   Underdosing of antithyroid drugs 🗇

CHAPTER 19 (S00-T88)

N Newborn Age: 0   **P** Pediatric Age: 0–17   **M** Maternity DX: 12–55   **A** Adult Age: 15–124   ♀ Females Only   ♂ Males Only

🗇 Complication\Comorbidity   🗇 Major C\C   (Ex) CC/MCC Exclusions   🗇 Present on Admission Requirement   🗇 Hospital-Acquired Condition

1525

● **T38.3** **Poisoning by, adverse effect of and underdosing of insulin and oral hypoglycemic [antidiabetic] drugs**

　● **T38.3X** Poisoning by, adverse effect of and underdosing of insulin and oral hypoglycemic [antidiabetic] drugs

　　● **T38.3X1** Poisoning by insulin and oral hypoglycemic [antidiabetic] drugs, accidental (unintentional) ✎

　　　Poisoning by insulin and oral hypoglycemic [antidiabetic] drugs NOS

　　● **T38.3X2** Poisoning by insulin and oral hypoglycemic [antidiabetic] drugs, intentional self-harm ✎

　　● **T38.3X3** Poisoning by insulin and oral hypoglycemic [antidiabetic] drugs, assault ✎

　　● **T38.3X4** Poisoning by insulin and oral hypoglycemic [antidiabetic] drugs, undetermined ✎

　　● **T38.3X5** Adverse effect of insulin and oral hypoglycemic [antidiabetic] drugs ✎

　　● **T38.3X6** Underdosing of insulin and oral hypoglycemic [antidiabetic] drugs ✎

● **T38.4** **Poisoning by, adverse effect of and underdosing of oral contraceptives**

　Poisoning by, adverse effect of and underdosing of multiple- and single-ingredient oral contraceptive preparations

　● **T38.4X** Poisoning by, adverse effect of and underdosing of oral contraceptives

　　● **T38.4X1** Poisoning by oral contraceptives, accidental (unintentional) ✎

　　　Poisoning by oral contraceptives NOS

　　● **T38.4X2** Poisoning by oral contraceptives, intentional self-harm ✎

　　● **T38.4X3** Poisoning by oral contraceptives, assault ✎

　　● **T38.4X4** Poisoning by oral contraceptives, undetermined ✎

　　● **T38.4X5** Adverse effect of oral contraceptives ✎

　　● **T38.4X6** Underdosing of oral contraceptives ✎

● **T38.5** **Poisoning by, adverse effect of and underdosing of other estrogens and progestogens**

　Poisoning by, adverse effect of and underdosing of estrogens and progestogens mixtures and substitutes

　● **T38.5X** Poisoning by, adverse effect of and underdosing of other estrogens and progestogens

　　● **T38.5X1** Poisoning by other estrogens and progestogens, accidental (unintentional) ✎

　　　Poisoning by other estrogens and progestogens NOS

　　● **T38.5X2** Poisoning by other estrogens and progestogens, intentional self-harm ✎

　　● **T38.5X3** Poisoning by other estrogens and progestogens, assault ✎

　　● **T38.5X4** Poisoning by other estrogens and progestogens, undetermined ✎

　　● **T38.5X5** Adverse effect of other estrogens and progestogens ✎

　　● **T38.5X6** Underdosing of other estrogens and progestogens ✎

● **T38.6** **Poisoning by, adverse effect of and underdosing of antigonadotrophins, antiestrogens, antiandrogens, not elsewhere classified**

　Poisoning by, adverse effect of and underdosing of tamoxifen

　● **T38.6X** Poisoning by, adverse effect of and underdosing of antigonadotrophins, antiestrogens, antiandrogens, not elsewhere classified

　　● **T38.6X1** Poisoning by antigonadotrophins, antiestrogens, antiandrogens, not elsewhere classified, accidental (unintentional) ✎

　　　Poisoning by antigonadotrophins, antiestrogens, antiandrogens, not elsewhere classified NOS

　　● **T38.6X2** Poisoning by antigonadotrophins, antiestrogens, antiandrogens, not elsewhere classified, intentional self-harm ✎

　　● **T38.6X3** Poisoning by antigonadotrophins, antiestrogens, antiandrogens, not elsewhere classified, assault ✎

　　● **T38.6X4** Poisoning by antigonadotrophins, antiestrogens, antiandrogens, not elsewhere classified, undetermined ✎

　　● **T38.6X5** Adverse effect of antigonadotrophins, antiestrogens, antiandrogens, not elsewhere classified ✎

　　● **T38.6X6** Underdosing of antigonadotrophins, antiestrogens, antiandrogens, not elsewhere classified ✎

● **T38.7** **Poisoning by, adverse effect of and underdosing of androgens and anabolic congeners**

　● **T38.7X** Poisoning by, adverse effect of and underdosing of androgens and anabolic congeners

　　● **T38.7X1** Poisoning by androgens and anabolic congeners, accidental (unintentional) ✎

　　　Poisoning by androgens and anabolic congeners NOS

　　● **T38.7X2** Poisoning by androgens and anabolic congeners, intentional self-harm ✎

　　● **T38.7X3** Poisoning by androgens and anabolic congeners, assault ✎

　　● **T38.7X4** Poisoning by androgens and anabolic congeners, undetermined ✎

　　● **T38.7X5** Adverse effect of androgens and anabolic congeners ✎

　　● **T38.7X6** Underdosing of androgens and anabolic congeners ✎

● **T38.8** **Poisoning by, adverse effect of and underdosing of other and unspecified hormones and synthetic substitutes**

　● **T38.80** Poisoning by, adverse effect of and underdosing of unspecified hormones and synthetic substitutes

　　● **T38.801** Poisoning by unspecified hormones and synthetic substitutes, accidental (unintentional) ✎

　　　Poisoning by unspecified hormones and synthetic substitutes NOS

　　● **T38.802** Poisoning by unspecified hormones and synthetic substitutes, intentional self-harm ✎

　　● **T38.803** Poisoning by unspecified hormones and synthetic substitutes, assault ✎

◀ New　　◀▪ Revised　　~~deleted~~ Deleted　　Excludes 1　　Excludes 2　　Includes　　Use additional　　Code first　　Code also　　Unspecified

OGCR Official Guidelines　　● Unacceptable Principal Diagnosis　　X Assign placeholder X　　● Use Additional Character(s)　　▶ Manifestation Code　　**Coding Clinic**

● T38.804   Poisoning by unspecified hormones and synthetic substitutes, undetermined 🗞

● T38.805   Adverse effect of unspecified hormones and synthetic substitutes 🗞

● T38.806   Underdosing of unspecified hormones and synthetic substitutes 🗞

● T38.81   Poisoning by, adverse effect of and underdosing of anterior pituitary [adenohypophyseal] hormones

   ● T38.811   Poisoning by anterior pituitary [adenohypophyseal] hormones, accidental (unintentional) 🗞
        Poisoning by anterior pituitary [adenohypophyseal] hormones NOS

   ● T38.812   Poisoning by anterior pituitary [adenohypophyseal] hormones, intentional self-harm 🗞

   ● T38.813   Poisoning by anterior pituitary [adenohypophyseal] hormones, assault 🗞

   ● T38.814   Poisoning by anterior pituitary [adenohypophyseal] hormones, undetermined 🗞

   ● T38.815   Adverse effect of anterior pituitary [adenohypophyseal] hormones 🗞

   ● T38.816   Underdosing of anterior pituitary [adenohypophyseal] hormones 🗞

● T38.89   Poisoning by, adverse effect of and underdosing of other hormones and synthetic substitutes

   ● T38.891   Poisoning by other hormones and synthetic substitutes, accidental (unintentional) 🗞
        Poisoning by other hormones and synthetic substitutes NOS

   ● T38.892   Poisoning by other hormones and synthetic substitutes, intentional self-harm 🗞

   ● T38.893   Poisoning by other hormones and synthetic substitutes, assault 🗞

   ● T38.894   Poisoning by other hormones and synthetic substitutes, undetermined 🗞

   ● T38.895   Adverse effect of other hormones and synthetic substitutes 🗞

   ● T38.896   Underdosing of other hormones and synthetic substitutes 🗞

● T38.9   Poisoning by, adverse effect of and underdosing of other and unspecified hormone antagonists

 ● T38.90   Poisoning by, adverse effect of and underdosing of unspecified hormone antagonists

   ● T38.901   Poisoning by unspecified hormone antagonists, accidental (unintentional) 🗞
        Poisoning by unspecified hormone antagonists NOS

   ● T38.902   Poisoning by unspecified hormone antagonists, intentional self-harm 🗞

   ● T38.903   Poisoning by unspecified hormone antagonists, assault 🗞

   ● T38.904   Poisoning by unspecified hormone antagonists, undetermined 🗞

   ● T38.905   Adverse effect of unspecified hormone antagonists 🗞

   ● T38.906   Underdosing of unspecified hormone antagonists 🗞

● T38.99   Poisoning by, adverse effect of and underdosing of other hormone antagonists

   ● T38.991   Poisoning by other hormone antagonists, accidental (unintentional) 🗞
        Poisoning by other hormone antagonists NOS

   ● T38.992   Poisoning by other hormone antagonists, intentional self-harm 🗞

   ● T38.993   Poisoning by other hormone antagonists, assault 🗞

   ● T38.994   Poisoning by other hormone antagonists, undetermined 🗞

   ● T38.995   Adverse effect of other hormone antagonists 🗞

   ● T38.996   Underdosing of other hormone antagonists 🗞

● T39   Poisoning by, adverse effect of and underdosing of nonopioid analgesics, antipyretics and antirheumatics

The appropriate 7th character is to be added to each code from category T39

A	initial encounter
D	subsequent encounter
S	sequela

● T39.0   Poisoning by, adverse effect of and underdosing of salicylates

 ● T39.01   Poisoning by, adverse effect of and underdosing of aspirin
        Poisoning by, adverse effect of and underdosing of acetylsalicylic acid

   ● T39.011   Poisoning by aspirin, accidental (unintentional) 🗞

   ● T39.012   Poisoning by aspirin, intentional self-harm 🗞

   ● T39.013   Poisoning by aspirin, assault 🗞

   ● T39.014   Poisoning by aspirin, undetermined 🗞

   ● T39.015   Adverse effect of aspirin 🗞

   ● T39.016   Underdosing of aspirin 🗞

 ● T39.09   Poisoning by, adverse effect of and underdosing of other salicylates

   ● T39.091   Poisoning by salicylates, accidental (unintentional) 🗞
        Poisoning by salicylates NOS

   ● T39.092   Poisoning by salicylates, intentional self-harm 🗞

   ● T39.093   Poisoning by salicylates, assault 🗞

   ● T39.094   Poisoning by salicylates, undetermined 🗞

   ● T39.095   Adverse effect of salicylates 🗞

   ● T39.096   Underdosing of salicylates 🗞

● T39.1   Poisoning by, adverse effect of and underdosing of 4-Aminophenol derivatives

 ● T39.1X   Poisoning by, adverse effect of and underdosing of 4-Aminophenol derivatives

   ● T39.1X1   Poisoning by 4-Aminophenol derivatives, accidental (unintentional) 🗞
        Poisoning by 4-Aminophenol derivatives NOS

   ● T39.1X2   Poisoning by 4-Aminophenol derivatives, intentional self-harm 🗞

   ● T39.1X3   Poisoning by 4-Aminophenol derivatives, assault 🗞

   ● T39.1X4   Poisoning by 4-Aminophenol derivatives, undetermined 🗞

   ● T39.1X5   Adverse effect of 4-Aminophenol derivatives 🗞

   ● T39.1X6   Underdosing of 4-Aminophenol derivatives 🗞

CHAPTER 19 (S00-T88)

N Newborn Age: 0   P Pediatric Age: 0–17   M Maternity DX: 12–55   A Adult Age: 15–124   ♀ Females Only   ♂ Males Only

🗞 Complication\Comorbidity   🗞 Major C\C   (Ex) CC/MCC Exclusions   🗞 Present on Admission Requirement   🗞 Hospital-Acquired Condition

1527

CHAPTER 19 (S00-T88)

- T39.2   Poisoning by, adverse effect of and underdosing of pyrazolone derivatives
  - T39.2X   Poisoning by, adverse effect of and underdosing of pyrazolone derivatives
    - T39.2X1   Poisoning by pyrazolone derivatives, accidental (unintentional) ✏
      Poisoning by pyrazolone derivatives NOS
    - T39.2X2   Poisoning by pyrazolone derivatives, intentional self-harm ✏
    - T39.2X3   Poisoning by pyrazolone derivatives, assault ✏
    - T39.2X4   Poisoning by pyrazolone derivatives, undetermined ✏
    - T39.2X5   Adverse effect of pyrazolone derivatives ✏
    - T39.2X6   Underdosing of pyrazolone derivatives ✏
- T39.3   Poisoning by, adverse effect of and underdosing of other nonsteroidal anti-inflammatory drugs [NSAID]
  - T39.31   Poisoning by, adverse effect of and underdosing of propionic acid derivatives
    Poisoning by, adverse effect of and underdosing of fenoprofen
    Poisoning by, adverse effect of and underdosing of flurbiprofen
    Poisoning by, adverse effect of and underdosing of ibuprofen
    Poisoning by, adverse effect of and underdosing of ketoprofen
    Poisoning by, adverse effect of and underdosing of naproxen
    Poisoning by, adverse effect of and underdosing of oxaprozin
    - T39.311   Poisoning by propionic acid derivatives, accidental (unintentional) ✏
    - T39.312   Poisoning by propionic acid derivatives, intentional self-harm ✏
    - T39.313   Poisoning by propionic acid derivatives, assault ✏
    - T39.314   Poisoning by propionic acid derivatives, undetermined ✏
    - T39.315   Adverse effect of propionic acid derivatives ✏
    - T39.316   Underdosing of propionic acid derivatives ✏
  - T39.39   Poisoning by, adverse effect of and underdosing of other nonsteroidal anti-inflammatory drugs [NSAID]
    - T39.391   Poisoning by other nonsteroidal anti-inflammatory drugs [NSAID], accidental (unintentional) ✏
      Poisoning by other nonsteroidal anti-inflammatory drugs NOS
    - T39.392   Poisoning by other nonsteroidal anti-inflammatory drugs [NSAID], intentional self-harm ✏
    - T39.393   Poisoning by other nonsteroidal anti-inflammatory drugs [NSAID], assault ✏
    - T39.394   Poisoning by other nonsteroidal anti-inflammatory drugs [NSAID], undetermined ✏
    - T39.395   Adverse effect of other nonsteroidal anti-inflammatory drugs [NSAID] ✏
    - T39.396   Underdosing of other nonsteroidal anti-inflammatory drugs [NSAID] ✏

- T39.4   Poisoning by, adverse effect of and underdosing of antirheumatics, not elsewhere classified
  - **Excludes1**   poisoning by, adverse effect of and underdosing of glucocorticoids (T38.0-)
    poisoning by, adverse effect of and underdosing of salicylates (T39.0-)
  - T39.4X   Poisoning by, adverse effect of and underdosing of antirheumatics, not elsewhere classified
    - T39.4X1   Poisoning by antirheumatics, not elsewhere classified, accidental (unintentional) ✏
      Poisoning by antirheumatics, not elsewhere classified NOS
    - T39.4X2   Poisoning by antirheumatics, not elsewhere classified, intentional self-harm ✏
    - T39.4X3   Poisoning by antirheumatics, not elsewhere classified, assault ✏
    - T39.4X4   Poisoning by antirheumatics, not elsewhere classified, undetermined ✏
    - T39.4X5   Adverse effect of antirheumatics, not elsewhere classified ✏
    - T39.4X6   Underdosing of antirheumatics, not elsewhere classified ✏
- T39.8   Poisoning by, adverse effect of and underdosing of other nonopioid analgesics and antipyretics, not elsewhere classified
  - T39.8X   Poisoning by, adverse effect of and underdosing of other nonopioid analgesics and antipyretics, not elsewhere classified
    - T39.8X1   Poisoning by other nonopioid analgesics and antipyretics, not elsewhere classified, accidental (unintentional) ✏
      Poisoning by other nonopioid analgesics and antipyretics, not elsewhere classified NOS
    - T39.8X2   Poisoning by other nonopioid analgesics and antipyretics, not elsewhere classified, intentional self-harm ✏
    - T39.8X3   Poisoning by other nonopioid analgesics and antipyretics, not elsewhere classified, assault ✏
    - T39.8X4   Poisoning by other nonopioid analgesics and antipyretics, not elsewhere classified, undetermined ✏
    - T39.8X5   Adverse effect of other nonopioid analgesics and antipyretics, not elsewhere classified ✏
    - T39.8X6   Underdosing of other nonopioid analgesics and antipyretics, not elsewhere classified ✏
- T39.9   Poisoning by, adverse effect of and underdosing of unspecified nonopioid analgesic, antipyretic and antirheumatic
  - X T39.91   Poisoning by unspecified nonopioid analgesic, antipyretic and antirheumatic, accidental (unintentional) ✏
    Poisoning by nonopioid analgesic, antipyretic and antirheumatic NOS
  - X T39.92   Poisoning by unspecified nonopioid analgesic, antipyretic and antirheumatic, intentional self-harm ✏
  - X T39.93   Poisoning by unspecified nonopioid analgesic, antipyretic and antirheumatic, assault ✏
  - X T39.94   Poisoning by unspecified nonopioid analgesic, antipyretic and antirheumatic, undetermined ✏

◀ New   ◀▥ Revised   d̶e̶l̶e̶t̶e̶d̶ Deleted   Excludes 1   Excludes 2   Includes   Use additional   Code first   Code also   Unspecified

OGCR Official Guidelines   ● Unacceptable Principal Diagnosis   X Assign placeholder X   ● Use Additional Character(s)   ▶ Manifestation Code   **Coding Clinic**

X ● **T39.95** Adverse effect of unspecified nonopioid analgesic, antipyretic and antirheumatic 🖎

X ● **T39.96** Underdosing of unspecified nonopioid analgesic, antipyretic and antirheumatic 🖎

● **T40** Poisoning by, adverse effect of and underdosing of narcotics and psychodysleptics [hallucinogens]

> **Excludes2** drug dependence and related mental and behavioral disorders due to psychoactive substance use (F10.-F19.-)

> The appropriate 7th character is to be added to each code from category T40

> A　initial encounter
> D　subsequent encounter
> S　sequela

● **T40.0** Poisoning by, adverse effect of and underdosing of opium

　● **T40.0X** Poisoning by, adverse effect of and underdosing of opium

　　T40.0X1 Poisoning by opium, accidental (unintentional) 🖎
　　　　　Poisoning by opium NOS

　　● **T40.0X2** Poisoning by opium, intentional self-harm 🖎

　　● **T40.0X3** Poisoning by opium, assault 🖎

　　● **T40.0X4** Poisoning by opium, undetermined 🖎

　　● **T40.0X5** Adverse effect of opium 🖎

　　● **T40.0X6** Underdosing of opium 🖎

● **T40.1** Poisoning by and adverse effect of heroin

　● **T40.1X** Poisoning by and adverse effect of heroin

　　● **T40.1X1** Poisoning by heroin, accidental (unintentional) 🖎
　　　　　Poisoning by heroin NOS

　　● **T40.1X2** Poisoning by heroin, intentional self-harm 🖎

　　● **T40.1X3** Poisoning by heroin, assault 🖎

　　● **T40.1X4** Poisoning by heroin, undetermined 🖎

　　~~T40.1X5　Adverse effect of heroin~~

● **T40.2** Poisoning by, adverse effect of and underdosing of other opioids

　● **T40.2X** Poisoning by, adverse effect of and underdosing of other opioids

　　● **T40.2X1** Poisoning by other opioids, accidental (unintentional) 🖎
　　　　　Poisoning by other opioids NOS

　　● **T40.2X2** Poisoning by other opioids, intentional self-harm 🖎

　　● **T40.2X3** Poisoning by other opioids, assault 🖎

　　● **T40.2X4** Poisoning by other opioids, undetermined 🖎

　　● **T40.2X5** Adverse effect of other opioids 🖎

　　● **T40.2X6** Underdosing of other opioids 🖎

● **T40.3** Poisoning by, adverse effect of and underdosing of methadone

　● **T40.3X** Poisoning by, adverse effect of and underdosing of methadone

　　● **T40.3X1** Poisoning by methadone, accidental (unintentional) 🖎
　　　　　Poisoning by methadone NOS

　　● **T40.3X2** Poisoning by methadone, intentional self-harm 🖎

　　● **T40.3X3** Poisoning by methadone, assault 🖎

　　● **T40.3X4** Poisoning by methadone, undetermined 🖎

　　● **T40.3X5** Adverse effect of methadone 🖎

　　● **T40.3X6** Underdosing of methadone 🖎

● **T40.4** Poisoning by, adverse effect of and underdosing of other synthetic narcotics

　● **T40.4X** Poisoning by, adverse effect of and underdosing of other synthetic narcotics 🖎

　　● **T40.4X1** Poisoning by other synthetic narcotics, accidental (unintentional) 🖎
　　　　　Poisoning by other synthetic narcotics NOS

　　● **T40.4X2** Poisoning by other synthetic narcotics, intentional self-harm 🖎

　　● **T40.4X3** Poisoning by other synthetic narcotics, assault 🖎

　　● **T40.4X4** Poisoning by other synthetic narcotics, undetermined 🖎

　　● **T40.4X5** Adverse effect of other synthetic narcotics 🖎

　　● **T40.4X6** Underdosing of other synthetic narcotics 🖎

● **T40.5** Poisoning by, adverse effect of and underdosing of cocaine

　● **T40.5X** Poisoning by, adverse effect of and underdosing of cocaine

　　● **T40.5X1** Poisoning by cocaine, accidental (unintentional) 🖎
　　　　　Poisoning by cocaine NOS

　　● **T40.5X2** Poisoning by cocaine, intentional self-harm 🖎

　　● **T40.5X3** Poisoning by cocaine, assault 🖎

　　● **T40.5X4** Poisoning by cocaine, undetermined 🖎

　　● **T40.5X5** Adverse effect of cocaine 🖎

　　● **T40.5X6** Underdosing of cocaine 🖎

● **T40.6** Poisoning by, adverse effect of and underdosing of other and unspecified narcotics

　● **T40.60** Poisoning by, adverse effect of and underdosing of unspecified narcotics

　　● **T40.601** Poisoning by unspecified narcotics, accidental (unintentional) 🖎
　　　　　Poisoning by narcotics NOS

　　● **T40.602** Poisoning by unspecified narcotics, intentional self-harm 🖎

　　● **T40.603** Poisoning by unspecified narcotics, assault 🖎

　　● **T40.604** Poisoning by unspecified narcotics, undetermined 🖎

　　● **T40.605** Adverse effect of unspecified narcotics 🖎

　　● **T40.606** Underdosing of unspecified narcotics 🖎

　● **T40.69** Poisoning by, adverse effect of and underdosing of other narcotics

　　● **T40.691** Poisoning by other narcotics, accidental (unintentional) 🖎
　　　　　Poisoning by other narcotics NOS

　　● **T40.692** Poisoning by other narcotics, intentional self-harm 🖎

　　● **T40.693** Poisoning by other narcotics, assault 🖎

　　● **T40.694** Poisoning by other narcotics, undetermined 🖎

　　● **T40.695** Adverse effect of other narcotics 🖎

　　● **T40.696** Underdosing of other narcotics 🖎

CHAPTER 19 (S00-T88)

N Newborn Age: 0　　P Pediatric Age: 0–17　　M Maternity DX: 12–55　　A Adult Age: 15–124　　♀ Females Only　　♂ Males Only

🖎 Complication\Comorbidity　　🖎 Major C\C　　(Ex) CC/MCC Exclusions　　🖎 Present on Admission Requirement　　🖎 Hospital-Acquired Condition

1529

- **T40.7**   **Poisoning by, adverse effect of and underdosing of cannabis (derivatives)**
  - **T40.7X**   Poisoning by, adverse effect of and underdosing of cannabis (derivatives)
    - **T40.7X1**   Poisoning by cannabis (derivatives), accidental (unintentional) 🔍
      Poisoning by cannabis NOS
    - **T40.7X2**   Poisoning by cannabis (derivatives), intentional self-harm 🔍
    - **T40.7X3**   Poisoning by cannabis (derivatives), assault 🔍
    - **T40.7X4**   Poisoning by cannabis (derivatives), undetermined 🔍
    - **T40.7X5**   Adverse effect of cannabis (derivatives) 🔍
    - **T40.7X6**   Underdosing of cannabis (derivatives) 🔍
- **T40.8**   Poisoning by and adverse effect of lysergide [LSD]
  - **T40.8X**   Poisoning by and adverse effect of lysergide [LSD]
    - **T40.8X1**   Poisoning by lysergide [LSD], accidental (unintentional) 🔍
      Poisoning by lysergide [LSD] NOS
    - **T40.8X2**   Poisoning by lysergide [LSD], intentional self-harm 🔍
    - **T40.8X3**   Poisoning by lysergide [LSD], assault 🔍
    - **T40.8X4**   Poisoning by lysergide [LSD], undetermined 🔍
    - ~~T40.8X5~~   ~~Adverse effect of lysergide [LSD]~~
- **T40.9**   Poisoning by, adverse effect of and underdosing of other and unspecified psychodysleptics [hallucinogens]
  - **T40.90**   Poisoning by, adverse effect of and underdosing of unspecified psychodysleptics [hallucinogens]
    - **T40.901**   Poisoning by unspecified psychodysleptics [hallucinogens], accidental (unintentional) 🔍
    - **T40.902**   Poisoning by unspecified psychodysleptics [hallucinogens], intentional self-harm 🔍
    - **T40.903**   Poisoning by unspecified psychodysleptics [hallucinogens], assault 🔍
    - **T40.904**   Poisoning by unspecified psychodysleptics [hallucinogens], undetermined 🔍
    - **T40.905**   Adverse effect of unspecified psychodysleptics [hallucinogens] 🔍
    - **T40.906**   Underdosing of unspecified psychodysleptics 🔍
  - **T40.99**   Poisoning by, adverse effect of and underdosing of other psychodysleptics [hallucinogens]
    - **T40.991**   Poisoning by other psychodysleptics [hallucinogens], accidental (unintentional) 🔍
      Poisoning by other psychodysleptics [hallucinogens] NOS
    - **T40.992**   Poisoning by other psychodysleptics [hallucinogens], intentional self-harm 🔍
    - **T40.993**   Poisoning by other psychodysleptics [hallucinogens], assault 🔍
    - **T40.994**   Poisoning by other psychodysleptics [hallucinogens], undetermined 🔍
    - **T40.995**   Adverse effect of other psychodysleptics [hallucinogens] 🔍
    - **T40.996**   Underdosing of other psychodysleptics 🔍

- **T41**   Poisoning by, adverse effect of and underdosing of anesthetics and therapeutic gases
  - **Excludes1**   benzodiazepines (T42.4-)
    cocaine (T40.5-)
    complications of anesthesia during pregnancy (O29.-)
    complications of anesthesia during labor and delivery (O74.-)
    complications of anesthesia during the puerperium (O89.-) opioids (T40.0-T40.2-)

  The appropriate 7th character is to be added to each code from category T41

A	initial encounter
D	subsequent encounter
S	sequela

  - **T41.0**   Poisoning by, adverse effect of and underdosing of inhaled anesthetics
    - **Excludes1**   oxygen (T41.5-)
    - **T41.0X**   Poisoning by, adverse effect of and underdosing of inhaled anesthetics
      - **T41.0X1**   Poisoning by inhaled anesthetics, accidental (unintentional) 🔍
        Poisoning by inhaled anesthetics NOS
      - **T41.0X2**   Poisoning by inhaled anesthetics, intentional self-harm 🔍
      - **T41.0X3**   Poisoning by inhaled anesthetics, assault 🔍
      - **T41.0X4**   Poisoning by inhaled anesthetics, undetermined 🔍
      - **T41.0X5**   Adverse effect of inhaled anesthetics 🔍
      - **T41.0X6**   Underdosing of inhaled anesthetics 🔍
  - **T41.1**   Poisoning by, adverse effect of and underdosing of intravenous anesthetics
    Poisoning by, adverse effect of and underdosing of thiobarbiturates
    - **T41.1X**   Poisoning by, adverse effect of and underdosing of intravenous anesthetics
      - **T41.1X1**   Poisoning by intravenous anesthetics, accidental (unintentional) 🔍
        Poisoning by intravenous anesthetics NOS
      - **T41.1X2**   Poisoning by intravenous anesthetics, intentional self-harm 🔍
      - **T41.1X3**   Poisoning by intravenous anesthetics, assault 🔍
      - **T41.1X4**   Poisoning by intravenous anesthetics, undetermined 🔍
      - **T41.1X5**   Adverse effect of intravenous anesthetics 🔍
      - **T41.1X6**   Underdosing of intravenous anesthetics 🔍
  - **T41.2**   Poisoning by, adverse effect of and underdosing of other and unspecified general anesthetics
    - **T41.20**   Poisoning by, adverse effect of and underdosing of unspecified general anesthetics
      - **T41.201**   Poisoning by unspecified general anesthetics, accidental (unintentional) 🔍
        Poisoning by general anesthetics NOS
      - **T41.202**   Poisoning by unspecified general anesthetics, intentional self-harm 🔍
      - **T41.203**   Poisoning by unspecified general anesthetics, assault 🔍
      - **T41.204**   Poisoning by unspecified general anesthetics, undetermined 🔍

◀ New   ◀▦ Revised   ~~deleted~~ Deleted   Excludes 1   Excludes 2   Includes   Use additional   Code first   Code also   Unspecified

OGCR Official Guidelines   ● Unacceptable Principal Diagnosis   X Assign placeholder X   🔍 Use Additional Character(s)   ▌ Manifestation Code   **Coding Clinic**

● T41.205   Adverse effect of unspecified general anesthetics 🔖

● T41.206   Underdosing of unspecified general anesthetics 🔖

● T41.29   Poisoning by, adverse effect of and underdosing of other general anesthetics

     ● T41.291   Poisoning by other general anesthetics, accidental (unintentional) 🔖
         Poisoning by other general anesthetics NOS

     ● T41.292   Poisoning by other general anesthetics, intentional self-harm 🔖

     ● T41.293   Poisoning by other general anesthetics, assault 🔖

     ● T41.294   Poisoning by other general anesthetics, undetermined 🔖

     ● T41.295   Adverse effect of other general anesthetics 🔖

     ● T41.296   Underdosing of other general anesthetics 🔖

● T41.3   Poisoning by, adverse effect of and underdosing of local anesthetics
     Cocaine (topical)

     Excludes2   poisoning by cocaine used as a central nervous system stimulant (T40.5X1-T40.5X4) ◄▥

     ● T41.3X   Poisoning by, adverse effect of and underdosing of local anesthetics

         ● T41.3X1   Poisoning by local anesthetics, accidental (unintentional) 🔖
             Poisoning by local anesthetics NOS

         ● T41.3X2   Poisoning by local anesthetics, intentional self-harm 🔖

         ● T41.3X3   Poisoning by local anesthetics, assault 🔖

         ● T41.3X4   Poisoning by local anesthetics, undetermined 🔖

         ● T41.3X5   Adverse effect of local anesthetics 🔖

         ● T41.3X6   Underdosing of local anesthetics 🔖

● T41.4   Poisoning by, adverse effect of and underdosing of unspecified anesthetic

     X● T41.41   Poisoning by unspecified anesthetic, accidental (unintentional) 🔖
         Poisoning by anesthetic NOS

     X● T41.42   Poisoning by unspecified anesthetic, intentional self-harm 🔖

     X● T41.43   Poisoning by unspecified anesthetic, assault 🔖

     X● T41.44   Poisoning by unspecified anesthetic, undetermined 🔖

     X● T41.45   Adverse effect of unspecified anesthetic 🔖

     X● T41.46   Underdosing of unspecified anesthetics 🔖

● T41.5   Poisoning by, adverse effect of and underdosing of therapeutic gases

     ● T41.5X   Poisoning by, adverse effect of and underdosing of therapeutic gases

         ● T41.5X1   Poisoning by therapeutic gases, accidental (unintentional) 🔖
             Poisoning by therapeutic gases NOS

         ● T41.5X2   Poisoning by therapeutic gases, intentional self-harm 🔖

         ● T41.5X3   Poisoning by therapeutic gases, assault 🔖

         ● T41.5X4   Poisoning by therapeutic gases, undetermined 🔖

         ● T41.5X5   Adverse effect of therapeutic gases 🔖

         ● T41.5X6   Underdosing of therapeutic gases 🔖

● T42   Poisoning by, adverse effect of and underdosing of antiepileptic, sedative-hypnotic and antiparkinsonism drugs

     Excludes2   drug dependence and related mental and behavioral disorders due to psychoactive substance use (F10.--F19.-)

     The appropriate 7th character is to be added to each code from category T42

A	initial encounter
D	subsequent encounter
S	sequela

● T42.0   Poisoning by, adverse effect of and underdosing of hydantoin derivatives

     ● T42.0X   Poisoning by, adverse effect of and underdosing of hydantoin derivatives

         ● T42.0X1   Poisoning by hydantoin derivatives, accidental (unintentional) 🔖
             Poisoning by hydantoin derivatives NOS

         ● T42.0X2   Poisoning by hydantoin derivatives, intentional self-harm 🔖

         ● T42.0X3   Poisoning by hydantoin derivatives, assault 🔖

         ● T42.0X4   Poisoning by hydantoin derivatives, undetermined 🔖

         ● T42.0X5   Adverse effect of hydantoin derivatives 🔖

         ● T42.0X6   Underdosing of hydantoin derivatives 🔖

● T42.1   Poisoning by, adverse effect of and underdosing of iminostilbenes
     Poisoning by, adverse effect of and underdosing of carbamazepine

     ● T42.1X   Poisoning by, adverse effect of and underdosing of iminostilbenes 🔖

         ● T42.1X1   Poisoning by iminostilbenes, accidental (unintentional) 🔖
             Poisoning by iminostilbenes NOS

         ● T42.1X2   Poisoning by iminostilbenes, intentional self-harm 🔖

         ● T42.1X3   Poisoning by iminostilbenes, assault 🔖

         ● T42.1X4   Poisoning by iminostilbenes, undetermined 🔖

         ● T42.1X5   Adverse effect of iminostilbenes 🔖

         ● T42.1X6   Underdosing of iminostilbenes 🔖

● T42.2   Poisoning by, adverse effect of and underdosing of succinimides and oxazolidinediones

     ● T42.2X   Poisoning by, adverse effect of and underdosing of succinimides and oxazolidinediones

         ● T42.2X1   Poisoning by succinimides and oxazolidinediones, accidental (unintentional) 🔖
             Poisoning by succinimides and oxazolidinediones NOS

         ● T42.2X2   Poisoning by succinimides and oxazolidinediones, intentional self-harm 🔖

         ● T42.2X3   Poisoning by succinimides and oxazolidinediones, assault 🔖

         ● T42.2X4   Poisoning by succinimides and oxazolidinediones, undetermined 🔖

         ● T42.2X5   Adverse effect of succinimides and oxazolidinediones 🔖

         ● T42.2X6   Underdosing of succinimides and oxazolidinediones 🔖

N   Newborn Age: 0   P   Pediatric Age: 0–17   M   Maternity DX: 12–55   A   Adult Age: 15–124   ♀   Females Only   ♂   Males Only

🔖 Complication\Comorbidity   🔖 Major C\C   (Ex) CC/MCC Exclusions   🔖 Present on Admission Requirement   🔖 Hospital-Acquired Condition

● **T42.3**   **Poisoning by, adverse effect of and underdosing of barbiturates**

> **Excludes1**   poisoning by, adverse effect of and underdosing of thiobarbiturates (T41.1-)

  ● **T42.3X**   Poisoning by, adverse effect of and underdosing of barbiturates

    ● **T42.3X1**   **Poisoning by barbiturates, accidental (unintentional)** 🔍
> Poisoning by barbiturates NOS

    ● **T42.3X2**   **Poisoning by barbiturates, intentional self-harm** 🔍

    ● **T42.3X3**   **Poisoning by barbiturates, assault** 🔍

    ● **T42.3X4**   **Poisoning by barbiturates, undetermined** 🔍

    ● **T42.3X5**   **Adverse effect of barbiturates** 🔍

    ● **T42.3X6**   **Underdosing of barbiturates** 🔍

● **T42.4**   **Poisoning by, adverse effect of and underdosing of benzodiazepines**

  ● **T42.4X**   Poisoning by, adverse effect of and underdosing of benzodiazepines

    ● **T42.4X1**   **Poisoning by benzodiazepines, accidental (unintentional)** 🔍
> Poisoning by benzodiazepines NOS

    ● **T42.4X2**   **Poisoning by benzodiazepines, intentional self-harm** 🔍

    ● **T42.4X3**   **Poisoning by benzodiazepines, assault** 🔍

    ● **T42.4X4**   **Poisoning by benzodiazepines, undetermined** 🔍

    ● **T42.4X5**   **Adverse effect of benzodiazepines** 🔍

    ● **T42.4X6**   **Underdosing of benzodiazepines** 🔍

● **T42.5**   **Poisoning by, adverse effect of and underdosing of mixed antiepileptics**

  ● **T42.5X**   Poisoning by, adverse effect of and underdosing of antiepileptics

    ● **T42.5X1**   **Poisoning by mixed antiepileptics, accidental (unintentional)** 🔍
> Poisoning by mixed antiepileptics NOS

    ● **T42.5X2**   **Poisoning by mixed antiepileptics, intentional self-harm** 🔍

    ● **T42.5X3**   **Poisoning by mixed antiepileptics, assault** 🔍

    ● **T42.5X4**   **Poisoning by mixed antiepileptics, undetermined** 🔍

    ● **T42.5X5**   **Adverse effect of mixed antiepileptics** 🔍

    ● **T42.5X6**   **Underdosing of mixed antiepileptics** 🔍

● **T42.6**   **Poisoning by, adverse effect of and underdosing of other antiepileptic and sedative-hypnotic drugs**
> Poisoning by, adverse effect of and underdosing of methaqualone
> Poisoning by, adverse effect of and underdosing of valproic acid

> **Excludes1**   poisoning by, adverse effect of and underdosing of carbamazepine (T42.1-)

  ● **T42.6X**   Poisoning by, adverse effect of and underdosing of other antiepileptic and sedative-hypnotic drugs

    ● **T42.6X1**   **Poisoning by other antiepileptic and sedative-hypnotic drugs, accidental (unintentional)** 🔍
> Poisoning by other antiepileptic and sedative-hypnotic drugs NOS

    ● **T42.6X2**   **Poisoning by other antiepileptic and sedative-hypnotic drugs, intentional self-harm** 🔍

    ● **T42.6X3**   **Poisoning by other antiepileptic and sedative-hypnotic drugs, assault** 🔍

    ● **T42.6X4**   **Poisoning by other antiepileptic and sedative-hypnotic drugs, undetermined** 🔍

    ● **T42.6X5**   **Adverse effect of other antiepileptic and sedative-hypnotic drugs** 🔍

    ● **T42.6X6**   **Underdosing of other antiepileptic and sedative-hypnotic drugs** 🔍

● **T42.7**   **Poisoning by, adverse effect of and underdosing of unspecified antiepileptic and sedative-hypnotic drugs**

  X ● **T42.71**   **Poisoning by unspecified antiepileptic and sedative-hypnotic drugs, accidental (unintentional)** 🔍
> Poisoning by antiepileptic and sedative-hypnotic drugs NOS

  X ● **T42.72**   **Poisoning by unspecified antiepileptic and sedative-hypnotic drugs, intentional self-harm** 🔍

  X ● **T42.73**   **Poisoning by unspecified antiepileptic and sedative-hypnotic drugs, assault** 🔍

  X ● **T42.74**   **Poisoning by unspecified antiepileptic and sedative-hypnotic drugs, undetermined** 🔍

  X ● **T42.75**   **Adverse effect of unspecified antiepileptic and sedative-hypnotic drugs** 🔍

  X ● **T42.76**   **Underdosing of unspecified antiepileptic and sedative-hypnotic drugs** 🔍

● **T42.8**   **Poisoning by, adverse effect of and underdosing of antiparkinsonism drugs and other central muscle-tone depressants**
> Poisoning by, adverse effect of and underdosing of amantadine

  ● **T42.8X**   Poisoning by, adverse effect of and underdosing of antiparkinsonism drugs and other central muscle-tone depressants

    ● **T42.8X1**   **Poisoning by antiparkinsonism drugs and other central muscle-tone depressants, accidental (unintentional)** 🔍
> Poisoning by antiparkinsonism drugs and other central muscle-tone depressants NOS

    ● **T42.8X2**   **Poisoning by antiparkinsonism drugs and other central muscle-tone depressants, intentional self-harm** 🔍

    ● **T42.8X3**   **Poisoning by antiparkinsonism drugs and other central muscle-tone depressants, assault** 🔍

    ● **T42.8X4**   **Poisoning by antiparkinsonism drugs and other central muscle-tone depressants, undetermined** 🔍

    ● **T42.8X5**   **Adverse effect of antiparkinsonism drugs and other central muscle-tone depressants** 🔍

    ● **T42.8X6**   **Underdosing of antiparkinsonism drugs and other central muscle-tone depressants** 🔍

● T43 **Poisoning by, adverse effect of and underdosing of psychotropic drugs, not elsewhere classified**

   Excludes1 appetite depressants (T50.5-)
   barbiturates (T42.3-)
   benzodiazepines (T42.4-)
   methaqualone (T42.6-)
   psychodysleptics [hallucinogens] (T40.7-T40.9-)

   Excludes2 drug dependence and related mental and behavioral disorders due to psychoactive substance use (F10.--F19.-)

   The appropriate 7th character is to be added to each code from category T43

A	initial encounter
D	subsequent encounter
S	sequela

● T43.0 **Poisoning by, adverse effect of and underdosing of tricyclic and tetracyclic antidepressants**

   ● T43.01 **Poisoning by, adverse effect of and underdosing of tricyclic antidepressants**

      ● T43.011 Poisoning by tricyclic antidepressants, accidental (unintentional)
      Poisoning by tricyclic antidepressants NOS

      ● T43.012 Poisoning by tricyclic antidepressants, intentional self-harm

      ● T43.013 Poisoning by tricyclic antidepressants, assault

      ● T43.014 Poisoning by tricyclic antidepressants, undetermined

      ● T43.015 Adverse effect of tricyclic antidepressants

      ● T43.016 Underdosing of tricyclic antidepressants

   ● T43.02 **Poisoning by, adverse effect of and underdosing of tetracyclic antidepressants**

      ● T43.021 Poisoning by tetracyclic antidepressants, accidental (unintentional)
      Poisoning by tetracyclic antidepressants NOS

      ● T43.022 Poisoning by tetracyclic antidepressants, intentional self-harm

      ● T43.023 Poisoning by tetracyclic antidepressants, assault

      ● T43.024 Poisoning by tetracyclic antidepressants, undetermined

      ● T43.025 Adverse effect of tetracyclic antidepressants

      ● T43.026 Underdosing of tetracyclic antidepressants

● T43.1 **Poisoning by, adverse effect of and underdosing of monoamine-oxidase-inhibitor antidepressants**

   ● T43.1X **Poisoning by, adverse effect of and underdosing of monoamine-oxidase-inhibitor antidepressants**

      ● T43.1X1 Poisoning by monoamine-oxidase-inhibitor antidepressants, accidental (unintentional)
      Poisoning by monoamine-oxidase-inhibitor antidepressants NOS

      ● T43.1X2 Poisoning by monoamine-oxidase-inhibitor antidepressants, intentional self-harm

      ● T43.1X3 Poisoning by monoamine-oxidase-inhibitor antidepressants, assault

      ● T43.1X4 Poisoning by monoamine-oxidase-inhibitor antidepressants, undetermined

      ● T43.1X5 Adverse effect of monoamine-oxidase-inhibitor antidepressants

      ● T43.1X6 Underdosing of monoamine-oxidase-inhibitor antidepressants

● T43.2 **Poisoning by, adverse effect of and underdosing of other and unspecified antidepressants**

   ● T43.20 **Poisoning by, adverse effect of and underdosing of unspecified antidepressants**

      ● T43.201 Poisoning by unspecified antidepressants, accidental (unintentional)
      Poisoning by antidepressants NOS

      ● T43.202 Poisoning by unspecified antidepressants, intentional self-harm

      ● T43.203 Poisoning by unspecified antidepressants, assault

      ● T43.204 Poisoning by unspecified antidepressants, undetermined

      ● T43.205 Adverse effect of unspecified antidepressants

      ● T43.206 Underdosing of unspecified antidepressants

   ● T43.21 **Poisoning by, adverse effect of and underdosing of selective serotonin and norepinephrine reuptake inhibitors**
   Poisoning by, adverse effect of and underdosing of SSNRI antidepressants

      ● T43.211 Poisoning by selective serotonin and norepinephrine reuptake inhibitors, accidental (unintentional)

      ● T43.212 Poisoning by selective serotonin and norepinephrine reuptake inhibitors, intentional self-harm

      ● T43.213 Poisoning by selective serotonin and norepinephrine reuptake inhibitors, assault

      ● T43.214 Poisoning by selective serotonin and norepinephrine reuptake inhibitors, undetermined

      ● T43.215 Adverse effect of selective serotonin and norepinephrine reuptake inhibitors

      ● T43.216 Underdosing of selective serotonin and norepinephrine reuptake inhibitors

   ● T43.22 **Poisoning by, adverse effect of and underdosing of selective serotonin reuptake inhibitors**
   Poisoning by, adverse effect of and underdosing of SSRI antidepressants

      ● T43.221 Poisoning by selective serotonin reuptake inhibitors, accidental (unintentional)

      ● T43.222 Poisoning by selective serotonin reuptake inhibitors, intentional self-harm

      ● T43.223 Poisoning by selective serotonin reuptake inhibitors, assault

      ● T43.224 Poisoning by selective serotonin reuptake inhibitors, undetermined

      ● T43.225 Adverse effect of selective serotonin reuptake inhibitors

      ● T43.226 Underdosing of selective serotonin reuptake inhibitors

CHAPTER 19 (S00-T88)

- T43.29   **Poisoning by, adverse effect of and underdosing of other antidepressants**
  - T43.291   **Poisoning by other antidepressants, accidental (unintentional)** 🔍
    Poisoning by other antidepressants NOS
  - T43.292   **Poisoning by other antidepressants, intentional self-harm** 🔍
  - T43.293   **Poisoning by other antidepressants, assault** 🔍
  - T43.294   **Poisoning by other antidepressants, undetermined** 🔍
  - T43.295   **Adverse effect of other antidepressants** 🔍
  - T43.296   **Underdosing of other antidepressants** 🔍
- T43.3   **Poisoning by, adverse effect of and underdosing of phenothiazine antipsychotics and neuroleptics**
  - T43.3X   **Poisoning by, adverse effect of and underdosing of phenothiazine antipsychotics and neuroleptics**
    - T43.3X1   **Poisoning by phenothiazine antipsychotics and neuroleptics, accidental (unintentional)** 🔍
      Poisoning by phenothiazine antipsychotics and neuroleptics NOS
    - T43.3X2   **Poisoning by phenothiazine antipsychotics and neuroleptics, intentional self-harm** 🔍
    - T43.3X3   **Poisoning by phenothiazine antipsychotics and neuroleptics, assault** 🔍
    - T43.3X4   **Poisoning by phenothiazine antipsychotics and neuroleptics, undetermined** 🔍
    - T43.3X5   **Adverse effect of phenothiazine antipsychotics and neuroleptics** 🔍
    - T43.3X6   **Underdosing of phenothiazine antipsychotics and neuroleptics** 🔍
- T43.4   **Poisoning by, adverse effect of and underdosing of butyrophenone and thiothixene neuroleptics**
  - T43.4X   **Poisoning by, adverse effect of and underdosing of butyrophenone and thiothixene neuroleptics**
    - T43.4X1   **Poisoning by butyrophenone and thiothixene neuroleptics, accidental (unintentional)** 🔍
      Poisoning by butyrophenone and thiothixene neuroleptics NOS
    - T43.4X2   **Poisoning by butyrophenone and thiothixene neuroleptics, intentional self-harm** 🔍
    - T43.4X3   **Poisoning by butyrophenone and thiothixene neuroleptics, assault** 🔍
    - T43.4X4   **Poisoning by butyrophenone and thiothixene neuroleptics, undetermined** 🔍
    - T43.4X5   **Adverse effect of butyrophenone and thiothixene neuroleptics** 🔍
    - T43.4X6   **Underdosing of butyrophenone and thiothixene neuroleptics** 🔍

- T43.5   **Poisoning by, adverse effect of and underdosing of other and unspecified antipsychotics and neuroleptics**
  > **Excludes1**   poisoning by, adverse effect of and underdosing of rauwolfia (T46.5-)
  - T43.50   **Poisoning by, adverse effect of and underdosing of unspecified antipsychotics and neuroleptics**
    - T43.501   **Poisoning by unspecified antipsychotics and neuroleptics, accidental (unintentional)** 🔍
      Poisoning by antipsychotics and neuroleptics NOS
    - T43.502   **Poisoning by unspecified antipsychotics and neuroleptics, intentional self-harm** 🔍
    - T43.503   **Poisoning by unspecified antipsychotics and neuroleptics, assault** 🔍
    - T43.504   **Poisoning by unspecified antipsychotics and neuroleptics, undetermined** 🔍
    - T43.505   **Adverse effect of unspecified antipsychotics and neuroleptics** 🔍
    - T43.506   **Underdosing of unspecified antipsychotics and neuroleptics** 🔍
  - T43.59   **Poisoning by, adverse effect of and underdosing of other antipsychotics and neuroleptics**
    - T43.591   **Poisoning by other antipsychotics and neuroleptics, accidental (unintentional)** 🔍
      Poisoning by other antipsychotics and neuroleptics NOS
    - T43.592   **Poisoning by other antipsychotics and neuroleptics, intentional self-harm** 🔍
    - T43.593   **Poisoning by other antipsychotics and neuroleptics, assault** 🔍
    - T43.594   **Poisoning by other antipsychotics and neuroleptics, undetermined** 🔍
    - T43.595   **Adverse effect of other antipsychotics and neuroleptics** 🔍
    - T43.596   **Underdosing of other antipsychotics and neuroleptics** 🔍
- T43.6   **Poisoning by, adverse effect of and underdosing of psychostimulants**
  > **Excludes1**   poisoning by, adverse effect of and underdosing of cocaine (T40.5-)
  - T43.60   **Poisoning by, adverse effect of and underdosing of unspecified psychostimulant**
    - T43.601   **Poisoning by unspecified psychostimulants, accidental (unintentional)** 🔍
      Poisoning by psychostimulants NOS
    - T43.602   **Poisoning by unspecified psychostimulants, intentional self-harm** 🔍
    - T43.603   **Poisoning by unspecified psychostimulants, assault** 🔍
    - T43.604   **Poisoning by unspecified psychostimulants, undetermined** 🔍
    - T43.605   **Adverse effect of unspecified psychostimulants** 🔍
    - T43.606   **Underdosing of unspecified psychostimulants** 🔍
  - T43.61   **Poisoning by, adverse effect of and underdosing of caffeine**
    - T43.611   **Poisoning by caffeine, accidental (unintentional)** 🔍
      Poisoning by caffeine NOS
    - T43.612   **Poisoning by caffeine, intentional self-harm** 🔍

◀ New   ◀▥ Revised   ~~deleted~~ Deleted   Excludes 1   Excludes 2   Includes   Use additional   Code first   Code also   Unspecified
OGCR Official Guidelines   ● Unacceptable Principal Diagnosis   X Assign placeholder X   ● Use Additional Character(s)   ▶ Manifestation Code   **Coding Clinic**

● T43.613 Poisoning by caffeine, assault 🔎
● T43.614 Poisoning by caffeine, undetermined 🔎
● T43.615 Adverse effect of caffeine 🔎
● T43.616 Underdosing of caffeine 🔎

● T43.62 Poisoning by, adverse effect of and underdosing of amphetamines
    Poisoning by, adverse effect of and underdosing of methamphetamines

  ● T43.621 Poisoning by amphetamines, accidental (unintentional) 🔎
    Poisoning by amphetamines NOS
  ● T43.622 Poisoning by amphetamines, intentional self-harm 🔎
  ● T43.623 Poisoning by amphetamines, assault 🔎
  ● T43.624 Poisoning by amphetamines, undetermined 🔎
  ● T43.625 Adverse effect of amphetamines 🔎
  ● T43.626 Underdosing of amphetamines 🔎

● T43.63 Poisoning by, adverse effect of and underdosing of methylphenidate

  ● T43.631 Poisoning by methylphenidate, accidental (unintentional) 🔎
    Poisoning by methylphenidate NOS
  ● T43.632 Poisoning by methylphenidate, intentional self-harm 🔎
  ● T43.633 Poisoning by methylphenidate, assault 🔎
  ● T43.634 Poisoning by methylphenidate, undetermined 🔎
  ● T43.635 Adverse effect of methylphenidate 🔎
  ● T43.636 Underdosing of methylphenidate 🔎

● T43.69 Poisoning by, adverse effect of and underdosing of other psychostimulants

  ● T43.691 Poisoning by other psychostimulants, accidental (unintentional) 🔎
    Poisoning by other psychostimulants NOS
  ● T43.692 Poisoning by other psychostimulants, intentional self-harm 🔎
  ● T43.693 Poisoning by other psychostimulants, assault 🔎
  ● T43.694 Poisoning by other psychostimulants, undetermined 🔎
  ● T43.695 Adverse effect of other psychostimulants 🔎
  ● T43.696 Underdosing of other psychostimulants 🔎

● T43.8 Poisoning by, adverse effect of and underdosing of other psychotropic drugs

● T43.8X Poisoning by, adverse effect of and underdosing of other psychotropic drugs

  ● T43.8X1 Poisoning by other psychotropic drugs, accidental (unintentional) 🔎
    Poisoning by other psychotropic drugs NOS
  ● T43.8X2 Poisoning by other psychotropic drugs, intentional self-harm 🔎
  ● T43.8X3 Poisoning by other psychotropic drugs, assault 🔎
  ● T43.8X4 Poisoning by other psychotropic drugs, undetermined 🔎
  ● T43.8X5 Adverse effect of other psychotropic drugs 🔎
  ● T43.8X6 Underdosing of other psychotropic drugs 🔎

● T43.9 Poisoning by, adverse effect of and underdosing of unspecified psychotropic drug

X ● T43.91 Poisoning by unspecified psychotropic drug, accidental (unintentional) 🔎
    Poisoning by psychotropic drug NOS
X ● T43.92 Poisoning by unspecified psychotropic drug, intentional self-harm 🔎
X ● T43.93 Poisoning by unspecified psychotropic drug, assault 🔎
X ● T43.94 Poisoning by unspecified psychotropic drug, undetermined 🔎
X ● T43.95 Adverse effect of unspecified psychotropic drug 🔎
X ● T43.96 Underdosing of unspecified psychotropic drug 🔎

● T44 Poisoning by, adverse effect of and underdosing of drugs primarily affecting the autonomic nervous system

  The appropriate 7th character is to be added to each code from category T44

A	initial encounter
D	subsequent encounter
S	sequela

● T44.0 Poisoning by, adverse effect of and underdosing of anticholinesterase agents

● T44.0X Poisoning by, adverse effect of and underdosing of anticholinesterase agents

  ● T44.0X1 Poisoning by anticholinesterase agents, accidental (unintentional) 🔎
    Poisoning by anticholinesterase agents NOS
  ● T44.0X2 Poisoning by anticholinesterase agents, intentional self-harm 🔎
  ● T44.0X3 Poisoning by anticholinesterase agents, assault 🔎
  ● T44.0X4 Poisoning by anticholinesterase agents, undetermined 🔎
  ● T44.0X5 Adverse effect of anticholinesterase agents 🔎
  ● T44.0X6 Underdosing of anticholinesterase agents 🔎

● T44.1 Poisoning by, adverse effect of and underdosing of other parasympathomimetics [cholinergics]

● T44.1X Poisoning by, adverse effect of and underdosing of other parasympathomimetics [cholinergics]

  ● T44.1X1 Poisoning by other parasympathomimetics [cholinergics], accidental (unintentional) 🔎
    Poisoning by other parasympathomimetics [cholinergics] NOS
  ● T44.1X2 Poisoning by other parasympathomimetics [cholinergics], intentional self-harm 🔎
  ● T44.1X3 Poisoning by other parasympathomimetics [cholinergics], assault 🔎
  ● T44.1X4 Poisoning by other parasympathomimetics [cholinergics], undetermined 🔎
  ● T44.1X5 Adverse effect of other parasympathomimetics [cholinergics] 🔎
  ● T44.1X6 Underdosing of other parasympathomimetics 🔎

N Newborn Age: 0   P Pediatric Age: 0–17   M Maternity DX: 12–55   A Adult Age: 15–124   ♀ Females Only   ♂ Males Only

🔎 Complication\Comorbidity   🔎 Major C\C   (Ex) CC/MCC Exclusions   🔎 Present on Admission Requirement   🔎 Hospital-Acquired Condition

1535

- T44.2 Poisoning by, adverse effect of and underdosing of ganglionic blocking drugs
  - T44.2X Poisoning by, adverse effect of and underdosing of ganglionic blocking drugs
    - T44.2X1 Poisoning by ganglionic blocking drugs, accidental (unintentional)
      Poisoning by ganglionic blocking drugs NOS
    - T44.2X2 Poisoning by ganglionic blocking drugs, intentional self-harm
    - T44.2X3 Poisoning by ganglionic blocking drugs, assault
    - T44.2X4 Poisoning by ganglionic blocking drugs, undetermined
    - T44.2X5 Adverse effect of ganglionic blocking drugs
    - T44.2X6 Underdosing of ganglionic blocking drugs
- T44.3 Poisoning by, adverse effect of and underdosing of other parasympatholytics [anticholinergics and antimuscarinics] and spasmolytics
  Poisoning by, adverse effect of and underdosing of papaverine
  - T44.3X Poisoning by, adverse effect of and underdosing of other parasympatholytics [anticholinergics and antimuscarinics] and spasmolytics
    - T44.3X1 Poisoning by other parasympatholytics [anticholinergics and antimuscarinics] and spasmolytics, accidental (unintentional)
      Poisoning by other parasympatholytics [anticholinergics and antimuscarinics] and spasmolytics NOS
    - T44.3X2 Poisoning by other parasympatholytics [anticholinergics and antimuscarinics] and spasmolytics, intentional self-harm
    - T44.3X3 Poisoning by other parasympatholytics [anticholinergics and antimuscarinics] and spasmolytics, assault
    - T44.3X4 Poisoning by other parasympatholytics [anticholinergics and antimuscarinics] and spasmolytics, undetermined
    - T44.3X5 Adverse effect of other parasympatholytics [anticholinergics and antimuscarinics] and spasmolytics
    - T44.3X6 Underdosing of other parasympatholytics [anticholinergics and antimuscarinics] and spasmolytics
- T44.4 Poisoning by, adverse effect of and underdosing of predominantly alpha-adrenoreceptor agonists
  Poisoning by, adverse effect of and underdosing of metaraminol
  - T44.4X Poisoning by, adverse effect of and underdosing of predominantly alpha-adrenoreceptor agonists
    - T44.4X1 Poisoning by predominantly alpha-adrenoreceptor agonists, accidental (unintentional)
      Poisoning by predominantly alpha-adrenoreceptor agonists NOS
    - T44.4X2 Poisoning by predominantly alpha-adrenoreceptor agonists, intentional self-harm

- T44.4X3 Poisoning by predominantly alpha-adrenoreceptor agonists, assault
- T44.4X4 Poisoning by predominantly alpha-adrenoreceptor agonists, undetermined
- T44.4X5 Adverse effect of predominantly alpha-adrenoreceptor agonists
- T44.4X6 Underdosing of predominantly alpha-adrenoreceptor agonists
- T44.5 Poisoning by, adverse effect of and underdosing of predominantly beta-adrenoreceptor agonists
  > **Excludes1**   poisoning by, adverse effect of and underdosing of beta-adrenoreceptor agonists used in asthma therapy (T48.6-)
  - T44.5X Poisoning by, adverse effect of and underdosing of predominantly beta-adrenoreceptor agonists
    - T44.5X1 Poisoning by predominantly beta-adrenoreceptor agonists, accidental (unintentional)
      Poisoning by predominantly beta-adrenoreceptor agonists NOS
    - T44.5X2 Poisoning by predominantly beta-adrenoreceptor agonists, intentional self-harm
    - T44.5X3 Poisoning by predominantly beta-adrenoreceptor agonists, assault
    - T44.5X4 Poisoning by predominantly beta-adrenoreceptor agonists, undetermined
    - T44.5X5 Adverse effect of predominantly beta-adrenoreceptor agonists
    - T44.5X6 Underdosing of predominantly beta-adrenoreceptor agonists
- T44.6 Poisoning by, adverse effect of and underdosing of alpha-adrenoreceptor antagonists
  > **Excludes1**   poisoning by, adverse effect of and underdosing of ergot alkaloids (T48.0)
  - T44.6X Poisoning by, adverse effect of and underdosing of alpha-adrenoreceptor antagonists
    - T44.6X1 Poisoning by alpha-adrenoreceptor antagonists, accidental (unintentional)
      Poisoning by alpha-adrenoreceptor antagonists NOS
    - T44.6X2 Poisoning by alpha-adrenoreceptor antagonists, intentional self-harm
    - T44.6X3 Poisoning by alpha-adrenoreceptor antagonists, assault
    - T44.6X4 Poisoning by alpha-adrenoreceptor antagonists, undetermined
    - T44.6X5 Adverse effect of alpha-adrenoreceptor antagonists
    - T44.6X6 Underdosing of alpha-adrenoreceptor antagonists
- T44.7 Poisoning by, adverse effect of and underdosing of beta-adrenoreceptor antagonists
  - T44.7X Poisoning by, adverse effect of and underdosing of beta-adrenoreceptor antagonists
    - T44.7X1 Poisoning by beta-adrenoreceptor antagonists, accidental (unintentional)
      Poisoning by beta-adrenoreceptor antagonists NOS
    - T44.7X2 Poisoning by beta-adrenoreceptor antagonists, intentional self-harm

◀ New   ◀⁞ Revised   ~~deleted~~ Deleted   Excludes 1   Excludes 2   Includes   Use additional   Code first   Code also   Unspecified
OGCR Official Guidelines   ● Unacceptable Principal Diagnosis   X Assign placeholder X   ● Use Additional Character(s)   ▶ Manifestation Code   **Coding Clinic**

● T44.7X3   Poisoning by beta-adrenoreceptor antagonists, assault 🅠

● T44.7X4   Poisoning by beta-adrenoreceptor antagonists, undetermined 🅠

● T44.7X5   Adverse effect of beta-adrenoreceptor antagonists 🅠

● T44.7X6   Underdosing of beta-adrenoreceptor antagonists 🅠

● T44.8   Poisoning by, adverse effect of and underdosing of centrally-acting and adrenergic-neuron-blocking agents

   Excludes1   poisoning by, adverse effect of and underdosing of clonidine (T46.5)
   poisoning by, adverse effect of and underdosing of guanethidine (T46.5)

● T44.8X   Poisoning by, adverse effect of and underdosing of centrally-acting and adrenergic-neuron-blocking agents

   ● T44.8X1   Poisoning by centrally-acting and adrenergic-neuron-blocking agents, accidental (unintentional) 🅠
      Poisoning by centrally-acting and adrenergic-neuron-blocking agents NOS

   ● T44.8X2   Poisoning by centrally-acting and adrenergic-neuron-blocking agents, intentional self-harm 🅠

   ● T44.8X3   Poisoning by centrally-acting and adrenergic-neuron-blocking agents, assault 🅠

   ● T44.8X4   Poisoning by centrally-acting and adrenergic-neuron-blocking agents, undetermined 🅠

   ● T44.8X5   Adverse effect of centrally-acting and adrenergic-neuron-blocking agents 🅠

   ● T44.8X6   Underdosing of centrally-acting and adrenergic-neuron-blocking agents 🅠

● T44.9   Poisoning by, adverse effect of and underdosing of other and unspecified drugs primarily affecting the autonomic nervous system
   Poisoning by, adverse effect of and underdosing of drug stimulating both alpha and beta-adrenoreceptors

   ● T44.90   Poisoning by, adverse effect of and underdosing of unspecified drugs primarily affecting the autonomic nervous system

      ● T44.901   Poisoning by unspecified drugs primarily affecting the autonomic nervous system, accidental (unintentional) 🅠
         Poisoning by unspecified drugs primarily affecting the autonomic nervous system NOS

      ● T44.902   Poisoning by unspecified drugs primarily affecting the autonomic nervous system, intentional self-harm 🅠

      ● T44.903   Poisoning by unspecified drugs primarily affecting the autonomic nervous system, assault 🅠

      ● T44.904   Poisoning by unspecified drugs primarily affecting the autonomic nervous system, undetermined 🅠

      ● T44.905   Adverse effect of unspecified drugs primarily affecting the autonomic nervous system 🅠

      ● T44.906   Underdosing of unspecified drugs primarily affecting the autonomic nervous system 🅠

● T44.99   Poisoning by, adverse effect of and underdosing of other drugs primarily affecting the autonomic nervous system

   ● T44.991   Poisoning by other drug primarily affecting the autonomic nervous system, accidental (unintentional) 🅠
      Poisoning by other drugs primarily affecting the autonomic nervous system NOS

   ● T44.992   Poisoning by other drug primarily affecting the autonomic nervous system, intentional self-harm 🅠

   ● T44.993   Poisoning by other drug primarily affecting the autonomic nervous system, assault 🅠

   ● T44.994   Poisoning by other drug primarily affecting the autonomic nervous system, undetermined 🅠

   ● T44.995   Adverse effect of other drug primarily affecting the autonomic nervous system 🅠

   ● T44.996   Underdosing of other drug primarily affecting the autonomic nervous system 🅠

● T45   Poisoning by, adverse effect of and underdosing of primarily systemic and hematological agents, not elsewhere classified

   The appropriate 7th character is to be added to each code from category T45

A	initial encounter
D	subsequent encounter
S	sequela

● T45.0   Poisoning by, adverse effect of and underdosing of antiallergic and antiemetic drugs

   Excludes1   poisoning by, adverse effect of and underdosing of phenothiazine-based neuroleptics (T43.3)

   ● T45.0X   Poisoning by, adverse effect of and underdosing of antiallergic and antiemetic drugs

      ● T45.0X1   Poisoning by antiallergic and antiemetic drugs, accidental (unintentional) 🅠
         Poisoning by antiallergic and antiemetic drugs NOS

      ● T45.0X2   Poisoning by antiallergic and antiemetic drugs, intentional self-harm 🅠

      ● T45.0X3   Poisoning by antiallergic and antiemetic drugs, assault 🅠

      ● T45.0X4   Poisoning by antiallergic and antiemetic drugs, undetermined 🅠

      ● T45.0X5   Adverse effect of antiallergic and antiemetic drugs 🅠

      ● T45.0X6   Underdosing of antiallergic and antiemetic drugs 🅠

● T45.1   Poisoning by, adverse effect of and underdosing of antineoplastic and immunosuppressive drugs

   Excludes1   poisoning by, adverse effect of and underdosing of tamoxifen (T38.6)

   ● T45.1X   Poisoning by, adverse effect of and underdosing of antineoplastic and immunosuppressive drugs

      ● T45.1X1   Poisoning by antineoplastic and immunosuppressive drugs, accidental (unintentional) 🅠
         Poisoning by antineoplastic and immunosuppressive drugs NOS

      ● T45.1X2   Poisoning by antineoplastic and immunosuppressive drugs, intentional self-harm 🅠

N Newborn Age: 0   **P** Pediatric Age: 0–17   **M** Maternity DX: 12–55   **A** Adult Age: 15–124   ♀ Females Only   ♂ Males Only

🅠 Complication\Comorbidity   🅠 Major C\C   (Ex) CC/MCC Exclusions   🅠 Present on Admission Requirement   🅠 Hospital-Acquired Condition

1537

CHAPTER 19 (S00-T88)

● T45.1X3   Poisoning by antineoplastic and immunosuppressive drugs, assault 🔍

● T45.1X4   Poisoning by antineoplastic and immunosuppressive drugs, undetermined 🔍

● T45.1X5   Adverse effect of antineoplastic and immunosuppressive drugs 🔍

● T45.1X6   Underdosing of antineoplastic and immunosuppressive drugs 🔍

● T45.2   Poisoning by, adverse effect of and underdosing of vitamins

> **Excludes2**   poisoning by, adverse effect of and underdosing of nicotinic acid (derivatives) (T46.7)
> poisoning by, adverse effect of and underdosing of iron (T45.4)
> poisoning by, adverse effect of and underdosing of vitamin K (T45.7)

   ● T45.2X   Poisoning by, adverse effect of and underdosing of vitamins

     ● T45.2X1   Poisoning by vitamins, accidental (unintentional) 🔍
> Poisoning by vitamins NOS

     ● T45.2X2   Poisoning by vitamins, intentional self-harm 🔍

     ● T45.2X3   Poisoning by vitamins, assault 🔍

     ● T45.2X4   Poisoning by vitamins, undetermined 🔍

     ● T45.2X5   Adverse effect of vitamins 🔍

     ● T45.2X6   Underdosing of vitamins 🔍
> **Excludes1**   vitamin deficiencies (E50-E56)

● T45.3   Poisoning by, adverse effect of and underdosing of enzymes

   ● T45.3X   Poisoning by, adverse effect of and underdosing of enzymes

     ● T45.3X1   Poisoning by enzymes, accidental (unintentional) 🔍
> Poisoning by enzymes NOS

     ● T45.3X2   Poisoning by enzymes, intentional self-harm 🔍

     ● T45.3X3   Poisoning by enzymes, assault 🔍

     ● T45.3X4   Poisoning by enzymes, undetermined 🔍

     ● T45.3X5   Adverse effect of enzymes 🔍

     ● T45.3X6   Underdosing of enzymes 🔍

● T45.4   Poisoning by, adverse effect of and underdosing of iron and its compounds

   ● T45.4X   Poisoning by, adverse effect of and underdosing of iron and its compounds

     ● T45.4X1   Poisoning by iron and its compounds, accidental (unintentional) 🔍
> Poisoning by iron and its compounds NOS

     ● T45.4X2   Poisoning by iron and its compounds, intentional self-harm 🔍

     ● T45.4X3   Poisoning by iron and its compounds, assault 🔍

     ● T45.4X4   Poisoning by iron and its compounds, undetermined 🔍

     ● T45.4X5   Adverse effect of iron and its compounds 🔍

     ● T45.4X6   Underdosing of iron and its compounds 🔍
> **Excludes1**   iron deficiency (E61.1)

● T45.5   Poisoning by, adverse effect of and underdosing of anticoagulants and antithrombotic drugs

   ● T45.51   Poisoning by, adverse effect of and underdosing of anticoagulants

     T45.511   Poisoning by anticoagulants, accidental (unintentional) 🔍
> Poisoning by anticoagulants NOS

     ● T45.512   Poisoning by anticoagulants, intentional self-harm 🔍

     ● T45.513   Poisoning by anticoagulants, assault 🔍

     ● T45.514   Poisoning by anticoagulants, undetermined 🔍

     ● T45.515   Adverse effect of anticoagulants 🔍

     ● T45.516   Underdosing of anticoagulants 🔍

   ● T45.52   Poisoning by, adverse effect of and underdosing of antithrombotic drugs
> Poisoning by, adverse effect of and underdosing of antiplatelet drugs

> **Excludes2**   poisoning by, adverse effect of and underdosing of aspirin (T39.01-)
> poisoning by, adverse effect of and underdosing of acetylsalicylic acid (T39.01-)

     ● T45.521   Poisoning by antithrombotic drugs, accidental (unintentional) 🔍
> Poisoning by antithrombotic drug NOS

     ● T45.522   Poisoning by antithrombotic drugs, intentional self-harm 🔍

     ● T45.523   Poisoning by antithrombotic drugs, assault 🔍

     ● T45.524   Poisoning by antithrombotic drugs, undetermined 🔍

     ● T45.525   Adverse effect of antithrombotic drugs 🔍

     ● T45.526   Underdosing of antithrombotic drugs 🔍

● T45.6   Poisoning by, adverse effect of and underdosing of fibrinolysis-affecting drugs

   ● T45.60   Poisoning by, adverse effect of and underdosing of unspecified fibrinolysis-affecting drugs

     ● T45.601   Poisoning by unspecified fibrinolysis-affecting drugs, accidental (unintentional) 🔍
> Poisoning by fibrinolysis-affecting drug NOS

     ● T45.602   Poisoning by unspecified fibrinolysis-affecting drugs, intentional self-harm 🔍

     ● T45.603   Poisoning by unspecified fibrinolysis-affecting drugs, assault 🔍

     ● T45.604   Poisoning by unspecified fibrinolysis-affecting drugs, undetermined 🔍

     ● T45.605   Adverse effect of unspecified fibrinolysis-affecting drugs 🔍

     ● T45.606   Underdosing of unspecified fibrinolysis-affecting drugs 🔍

   ● T45.61   Poisoning by, adverse effect of and underdosing of thrombolytic drugs

     ● T45.611   Poisoning by thrombolytic drug, accidental (unintentional) 🔍
> Poisoning by thrombolytic drug NOS

     ● T45.612   Poisoning by thrombolytic drug, intentional self-harm 🔍

◀ New   ◀┅ Revised   ~~deleted~~ Deleted   Excludes 1   Excludes 2   Includes   Use additional   Code first   Code also   Unspecified

OGCR Official Guidelines   ● Unacceptable Principal Diagnosis   X Assign placeholder X   ▶ Use Additional Character(s)   ▶ Manifestation Code   **Coding Clinic**

● T45.613   Poisoning by thrombolytic drug, assault 🦠

● T45.614   Poisoning by thrombolytic drug, undetermined 🦠

● T45.615   Adverse effect of thrombolytic drugs 🦠

● T45.616   Underdosing of thrombolytic drugs 🦠

● T45.62   Poisoning by, adverse effect of and underdosing of hemostatic drugs

    ● T45.621   Poisoning by hemostatic drug, accidental (unintentional) 🦠
        Poisoning by hemostatic drug NOS

    ● T45.622   Poisoning by hemostatic drug, intentional self-harm 🦠

    ● T45.623   Poisoning by hemostatic drug, assault 🦠

    ● T45.624   Poisoning by hemostatic drug, undetermined 🦠

    ● T45.625   Adverse effect of hemostatic drug 🦠

    ● T45.626   Underdosing of hemostatic drugs 🦠

● T45.69   Poisoning by, adverse effect of and underdosing of other fibrinolysis-affecting drugs

    ● T45.691   Poisoning by other fibrinolysis-affecting drugs, accidental (unintentional) 🦠
        Poisoning by other fibrinolysis-affecting drug NOS

    ● T45.692   Poisoning by other fibrinolysis-affecting drugs, intentional self-harm 🦠

    ● T45.693   Poisoning by other fibrinolysis-affecting drugs, assault 🦠

    ● T45.694   Poisoning by other fibrinolysis-affecting drugs, undetermined 🦠

    ● T45.695   Adverse effect of other fibrinolysis-affecting drugs 🦠

    ● T45.696   Underdosing of other fibrinolysis-affecting drugs 🦠

● T45.7   Poisoning by, adverse effect of and underdosing of anticoagulant antagonists, vitamin K and other coagulants

    ● T45.7X   Poisoning by, adverse effect of and underdosing of anticoagulant antagonists, vitamin K and other coagulants

       ● T45.7X1   Poisoning by anticoagulant antagonists, vitamin K and other coagulants, accidental (unintentional) 🦠
          Poisoning by anticoagulant antagonists, vitamin K and other coagulants NOS

       ● T45.7X2   Poisoning by anticoagulant antagonists, vitamin K and other coagulants, intentional self-harm 🦠

       ● T45.7X3   Poisoning by anticoagulant antagonists, vitamin K and other coagulants, assault 🦠

       ● T45.7X4   Poisoning by anticoagulant antagonists, vitamin K and other coagulants, undetermined 🦠

       ● T45.7X5   Adverse effect of anticoagulant antagonists, vitamin K and other coagulants 🦠

       ● T45.7X6   Underdosing of anticoagulant antagonist, vitamin K and other coagulants 🦠
          Excludes1   vitamin K deficiency (E56.1)

● T45.8   Poisoning by, adverse effect of and underdosing of other primarily systemic and hematological agents
    Poisoning by, adverse effect of and underdosing of liver preparations and other antianemic agents
    Poisoning by, adverse effect of and underdosing of natural blood and blood products
    Poisoning by, adverse effect of and underdosing of plasma substitute

    Excludes2   poisoning by, adverse effect of and underdosing of immunoglobulin (T50.Z1)
          poisoning by, adverse effect of and underdosing of iron (T45.4)
          transfusion reactions (T80.-)

    ● T45.8X   Poisoning by, adverse effect of and underdosing of other primarily systemic and hematological agents

       ● T45.8X1   Poisoning by other primarily systemic and hematological agents, accidental (unintentional) 🦠
          Poisoning by other primarily systemic and hematological agents NOS

       ● T45.8X2   Poisoning by other primarily systemic and hematological agents, intentional self-harm 🦠

       ● T45.8X3   Poisoning by other primarily systemic and hematological agents, assault 🦠

       ● T45.8X4   Poisoning by other primarily systemic and hematological agents, undetermined 🦠

       ● T45.8X5   Adverse effect of other primarily systemic and hematological agents 🦠

       ● T45.8X6   Underdosing of other primarily systemic and hematological agents 🦠

● T45.9   Poisoning by, adverse effect of and underdosing of unspecified primarily systemic and hematological agent

    X ● T45.91   Poisoning by unspecified primarily systemic and hematological agent, accidental (unintentional) 🦠
        Poisoning by primarily systemic and hematological agent NOS

    X ● T45.92   Poisoning by unspecified primarily systemic and hematological agent, intentional self-harm 🦠

    X ● T45.93   Poisoning by unspecified primarily systemic and hematological agent, assault 🦠

    X ● T45.94   Poisoning by unspecified primarily systemic and hematological agent, undetermined 🦠

    X ● T45.95   Adverse effect of unspecified primarily systemic and hematological agent 🦠

    X ● T45.96   Underdosing of unspecified primarily systemic and hematological agent 🦠

CHAPTER 19 (S00-T88)

N   Newborn Age: 0   P   Pediatric Age: 0–17   M   Maternity DX: 12–55   A   Adult Age: 15–124   ♀ Females Only   ♂ Males Only

🦠 Complication\Comorbidity   🦠 Major C\C   (Ex) CC/MCC Exclusions   🦠 Present on Admission Requirement   🦠 Hospital-Acquired Condition

1539

● **T46 Poisoning by, adverse effect of and underdosing of agents primarily affecting the cardiovascular system**

> Excludes1   poisoning by, adverse effect of and underdosing of metaraminol (T44.4)

> The appropriate 7th character is to be added to each code from category T46

> A   initial encounter
> D   subsequent encounter
> S   sequela

● **T46.0 Poisoning by, adverse effect of and underdosing of cardiac-stimulant glycosides and drugs of similar action**

  ● **T46.0X Poisoning by, adverse effect of and underdosing of cardiac-stimulant glycosides and drugs of similar action**

    ● **T46.0X1 Poisoning by cardiac-stimulant glycosides and drugs of similar action, accidental (unintentional)** 🔍
      Poisoning by cardiac-stimulant glycosides and drugs of similar action NOS

    ● **T46.0X2 Poisoning by cardiac-stimulant glycosides and drugs of similar action, intentional self-harm** 🔍

    ● **T46.0X3 Poisoning by cardiac-stimulant glycosides and drugs of similar action, assault** 🔍

    ● **T46.0X4 Poisoning by cardiac-stimulant glycosides and drugs of similar action, undetermined** 🔍

    ● **T46.0X5 Adverse effect of cardiac-stimulant glycosides and drugs of similar action** 🔍

    ● **T46.0X6 Underdosing of cardiac-stimulant glycosides and drugs of similar action** 🔍

● **T46.1 Poisoning by, adverse effect of and underdosing of calcium-channel blockers**

  ● **T46.1X Poisoning by, adverse effect of and underdosing of calcium-channel blockers**

    ● **T46.1X1 Poisoning by calcium-channel blockers, accidental (unintentional)** 🔍
      Poisoning by calcium-channel blockers NOS

    ● **T46.1X2 Poisoning by calcium-channel blockers, intentional self-harm** 🔍

    ● **T46.1X3 Poisoning by calcium-channel blockers, assault** 🔍

    ● **T46.1X4 Poisoning by calcium-channel blockers, undetermined** 🔍

    ● **T46.1X5 Adverse effect of calcium-channel blockers** 🔍

    ● **T46.1X6 Underdosing of calcium-channel blockers** 🔍

● **T46.2 Poisoning by, adverse effect of and underdosing of other antidysrhythmic drugs, not elsewhere classified**

> Excludes1   poisoning by, adverse effect of and underdosing of beta-adrenoreceptor antagonists (T44.7-)

  ● **T46.2X Poisoning by, adverse effect of and underdosing of other antidysrhythmic drugs**

    ● **T46.2X1 Poisoning by other antidysrhythmic drugs, accidental (unintentional)** 🔍
      Poisoning by other antidysrhythmic drugs NOS

    ● **T46.2X2 Poisoning by other antidysrhythmic drugs, intentional self-harm** 🔍

    ● **T46.2X3 Poisoning by other antidysrhythmic drugs, assault** 🔍

    ● **T46.2X4 Poisoning by other antidysrhythmic drugs, undetermined** 🔍

    ● **T46.2X5 Adverse effect of other antidysrhythmic drugs** 🔍

    ● **T46.2X6 Underdosing of other antidysrhythmic drugs** 🔍

● **T46.3 Poisoning by, adverse effect of and underdosing of coronary vasodilators**
  Poisoning by, adverse effect of and underdosing of dipyridamole

> Excludes1   poisoning by, adverse effect of and underdosing of calcium-channel blockers (T46.1)

  ● **T46.3X Poisoning by, adverse effect of and underdosing of coronary vasodilators**

    ● **T46.3X1 Poisoning by coronary vasodilators, accidental (unintentional)** 🔍
      Poisoning by coronary vasodilators NOS

    ● **T46.3X2 Poisoning by coronary vasodilators, intentional self-harm** 🔍

    ● **T46.3X3 Poisoning by coronary vasodilators, assault** 🔍

    ● **T46.3X4 Poisoning by coronary vasodilators, undetermined** 🔍

    ● **T46.3X5 Adverse effect of coronary vasodilators** 🔍

    ● **T46.3X6 Underdosing of coronary vasodilators** 🔍

● **T46.4 Poisoning by, adverse effect of and underdosing of angiotensin-converting-enzyme inhibitors**

  ● **T46.4X Poisoning by, adverse effect of and underdosing of angiotensin-converting-enzyme inhibitors**

    ● **T46.4X1 Poisoning by angiotensin-converting-enzyme inhibitors, accidental (unintentional)** 🔍
      Poisoning by angiotensin-converting-enzyme inhibitors NOS

    ● **T46.4X2 Poisoning by angiotensin-converting-enzyme inhibitors, intentional self-harm** 🔍

    ● **T46.4X3 Poisoning by angiotensin-converting-enzyme inhibitors, assault** 🔍

    ● **T46.4X4 Poisoning by angiotensin-converting-enzyme inhibitors, undetermined** 🔍

    ● **T46.4X5 Adverse effect of angiotensin-converting-enzyme inhibitors** 🔍

    ● **T46.4X6 Underdosing of angiotensin-converting-enzyme inhibitors** 🔍

◀ New   ◀▥ Revised   ~~deleted~~ Deleted   Excludes 1   Excludes 2   Includes   Use additional   Code first   Code also   Unspecified

OGCR Official Guidelines   ● Unacceptable Principal Diagnosis   X Assign placeholder X   ● Use Additional Character(s)   ▶ Manifestation Code   **Coding Clinic**

● **T46.5**   Poisoning by, adverse effect of and underdosing of other antihypertensive drugs

> **Excludes2**   poisoning by, adverse effect of and underdosing of beta-adrenoreceptor antagonists (T44.7)
> poisoning by, adverse effect of and underdosing of calcium-channel blockers (T46.1)
> poisoning by, adverse effect of and underdosing of diuretics (T50.0-T50.2)

  ● **T46.5X**   Poisoning by, adverse effect of and underdosing of other antihypertensive drugs

    ● **T46.5X1**   Poisoning by other antihypertensive drugs, accidental (unintentional) 🗪
> Poisoning by other antihypertensive drugs NOS

    ● **T46.5X2**   Poisoning by other antihypertensive drugs, intentional self-harm 🗪

    ● **T46.5X3**   Poisoning by other antihypertensive drugs, assault 🗪

    ● **T46.5X4**   Poisoning by other antihypertensive drugs, undetermined 🗪

    ● **T46.5X5**   Adverse effect of other antihypertensive drugs 🗪

    ● **T46.5X6**   Underdosing of other antihypertensive drugs 🗪

● **T46.6**   Poisoning by, adverse effect of and underdosing of antihyperlipidemic and antiarteriosclerotic drugs

  ● **T46.6X**   Poisoning by, adverse effect of and underdosing of antihyperlipidemic and antiarteriosclerotic drugs

    ● **T46.6X1**   Poisoning by antihyperlipidemic and antiarteriosclerotic drugs, accidental (unintentional) 🗪
> Poisoning by antihyperlipidemic and antiarteriosclerotic drugs NOS

    ● **T46.6X2**   Poisoning by antihyperlipidemic and antiarteriosclerotic drugs, intentional self-harm 🗪

    ● **T46.6X3**   Poisoning by antihyperlipidemic and antiarteriosclerotic drugs, assault 🗪

    ● **T46.6X4**   Poisoning by antihyperlipidemic and antiarteriosclerotic drugs, undetermined 🗪

    ● **T46.6X5**   Adverse effect of antihyperlipidemic and antiarteriosclerotic drugs 🗪

    ● **T46.6X6**   Underdosing of antihyperlipidemic and antiarteriosclerotic drugs 🗪

● **T46.7**   Poisoning by, adverse effect of and underdosing of peripheral vasodilators
> Poisoning by, adverse effect of and underdosing of nicotinic acid (derivatives)

> **Excludes1**   poisoning by, adverse effect of and underdosing of papaverine (T44.3)

  ● **T46.7X**   Poisoning by, adverse effect of and underdosing of peripheral vasodilators

    ● **T46.7X1**   Poisoning by peripheral vasodilators, accidental (unintentional) 🗪
> Poisoning by peripheral vasodilators NOS

    ● **T46.7X2**   Poisoning by peripheral vasodilators, intentional self-harm 🗪

    ● **T46.7X3**   Poisoning by peripheral vasodilators, assault 🗪

    ● **T46.7X4**   Poisoning by peripheral vasodilators, undetermined 🗪

    ● **T46.7X5**   Adverse effect of peripheral vasodilators 🗪

    ● **T46.7X6**   Underdosing of peripheral vasodilators 🗪

● **T46.8**   Poisoning by, adverse effect of and underdosing of antivaricose drugs, including sclerosing agents

  ● **T46.8X**   Poisoning by, adverse effect of and underdosing of antivaricose drugs, including sclerosing agents

    ● **T46.8X1**   Poisoning by antivaricose drugs, including sclerosing agents, accidental (unintentional) 🗪
> Poisoning by antivaricose drugs, including sclerosing agents NOS

    ● **T46.8X2**   Poisoning by antivaricose drugs, including sclerosing agents, intentional self-harm 🗪

    ● **T46.8X3**   Poisoning by antivaricose drugs, including sclerosing agents, assault 🗪

    ● **T46.8X4**   Poisoning by antivaricose drugs, including sclerosing agents, undetermined 🗪

    ● **T46.8X5**   Adverse effect of antivaricose drugs, including sclerosing agents 🗪

    ● **T46.8X6**   Underdosing of antivaricose drugs, including sclerosing agents 🗪

● **T46.9**   Poisoning by, adverse effect of and underdosing of other and unspecified agents primarily affecting the cardiovascular system

  ● **T46.90**   Poisoning by, adverse effect of and underdosing of unspecified agents primarily affecting the cardiovascular system

    ● **T46.901**   Poisoning by unspecified agents primarily affecting the cardiovascular system, accidental (unintentional) 🗪

    ● **T46.902**   Poisoning by unspecified agents primarily affecting the cardiovascular system, intentional self-harm 🗪

    ● **T46.903**   Poisoning by unspecified agents primarily affecting the cardiovascular system, assault 🗪

    ● **T46.904**   Poisoning by unspecified agents primarily affecting the cardiovascular system, undetermined 🗪

    ● **T46.905**   Adverse effect of unspecified agents primarily affecting the cardiovascular system 🗪

    ● **T46.906**   Underdosing of unspecified agents primarily affecting the cardiovascular system 🗪

  ● **T46.99**   Poisoning by, adverse effect of and underdosing of other agents primarily affecting the cardiovascular system

    ● **T46.991**   Poisoning by other agents primarily affecting the cardiovascular system, accidental (unintentional) 🗪

    ● **T46.992**   Poisoning by other agents primarily affecting the cardiovascular system, intentional self-harm 🗪

    ● **T46.993**   Poisoning by other agents primarily affecting the cardiovascular system, assault 🗪

    ● **T46.994**   Poisoning by other agents primarily affecting the cardiovascular system, undetermined 🗪

    ● **T46.995**   Adverse effect of other agents primarily affecting the cardiovascular system 🗪

    ● **T46.996**   Underdosing of other agents primarily affecting the cardiovascular system 🗪

CHAPTER 19 (S00-T88)

N   Newborn Age: 0   P   Pediatric Age: 0–17   M   Maternity DX: 12–55   A   Adult Age: 15–124   ♀ Females Only   ♂ Males Only

🗪 Complication\Comorbidity   🗪 Major C\C   (Ex) CC/MCC Exclusions   🗪 Present on Admission Requirement   🗪 Hospital-Acquired Condition

1541

● T47   Poisoning by, adverse effect of and underdosing of agents primarily affecting the gastrointestinal system

The appropriate 7th character is to be added to each code from category T47

> A   initial encounter
> D   subsequent encounter
> S   sequela

● T47.0   Poisoning by, adverse effect of and underdosing of histamine H2-receptor blockers
  ● T47.0X   Poisoning by, adverse effect of and underdosing of histamine H2-receptor blockers
    ● T47.0X1   Poisoning by histamine H2-receptor blockers, accidental (unintentional) 🔍
        Poisoning by histamine H2-receptor blockers NOS
    ● T47.0X2   Poisoning by histamine H2-receptor blockers, intentional self-harm 🔍
    ● T47.0X3   Poisoning by histamine H2-receptor blockers, assault 🔍
    ● T47.0X4   Poisoning by histamine H2-receptor blockers, undetermined 🔍
    ● T47.0X5   Adverse effect of histamine H2-receptor blockers 🔍
    ● T47.0X6   Underdosing of histamine H2-receptor blockers 🔍

● T47.1   Poisoning by, adverse effect of and underdosing of other antacids and anti-gastric-secretion drugs
  ● T47.1X   Poisoning by, adverse effect of and underdosing of other antacids and anti-gastric-secretion drugs
    ● T47.1X1   Poisoning by other antacids and anti-gastric-secretion drugs, accidental (unintentional) 🔍
        Poisoning by other antacids and anti-gastric-secretion drugs NOS
    ● T47.1X2   Poisoning by other antacids and anti-gastric-secretion drugs, intentional self-harm 🔍
    ● T47.1X3   Poisoning by other antacids and anti-gastric-secretion drugs, assault 🔍
    ● T47.1X4   Poisoning by other antacids and anti-gastric-secretion drugs, undetermined 🔍
    ● T47.1X5   Adverse effect of other antacids and anti-gastric-secretion drugs 🔍
    ● T47.1X6   Underdosing of other antacids and anti-gastric-secretion drugs 🔍

● T47.2   Poisoning by, adverse effect of and underdosing of stimulant laxatives
  ● T47.2X   Poisoning by, adverse effect of and underdosing of stimulant laxatives
    ● T47.2X1   Poisoning by stimulant laxatives, accidental (unintentional) 🔍
        Poisoning by stimulant laxatives NOS
    ● T47.2X2   Poisoning by stimulant laxatives, intentional self-harm 🔍
    ● T47.2X3   Poisoning by stimulant laxatives, assault 🔍
    ● T47.2X4   Poisoning by stimulant laxatives, undetermined 🔍
    ● T47.2X5   Adverse effect of stimulant laxatives 🔍
    ● T47.2X6   Underdosing of stimulant laxatives 🔍

● T47.3   Poisoning by, adverse effect of and underdosing of saline and osmotic laxatives
  ● T47.3X   Poisoning by and adverse effect of saline and osmotic laxatives
    ● T47.3X1   Poisoning by saline and osmotic laxatives, accidental (unintentional) 🔍
        Poisoning by saline and osmotic laxatives NOS
    ● T47.3X2   Poisoning by saline and osmotic laxatives, intentional self-harm 🔍
    ● T47.3X3   Poisoning by saline and osmotic laxatives, assault 🔍
    ● T47.3X4   Poisoning by saline and osmotic laxatives, undetermined 🔍
    ● T47.3X5   Adverse effect of saline and osmotic laxatives 🔍
    ● T47.3X6   Underdosing of saline and osmotic laxatives 🔍

● T47.4   Poisoning by, adverse effect of and underdosing of other laxatives
  ● T47.4X   Poisoning by, adverse effect of and underdosing of other laxatives
    ● T47.4X1   Poisoning by other laxatives, accidental (unintentional) 🔍
        Poisoning by other laxatives NOS
    ● T47.4X2   Poisoning by other laxatives, intentional self-harm 🔍
    ● T47.4X3   Poisoning by other laxatives, assault 🔍
    ● T47.4X4   Poisoning by other laxatives, undetermined 🔍
    ● T47.4X5   Adverse effect of other laxatives 🔍
    ● T47.4X6   Underdosing of other laxatives 🔍

● T47.5   Poisoning by, adverse effect of and underdosing of digestants
  ● T47.5X   Poisoning by, adverse effect of and underdosing of digestants
    ● T47.5X1   Poisoning by digestants, accidental (unintentional) 🔍
        Poisoning by digestants NOS
    ● T47.5X2   Poisoning by digestants, intentional self-harm 🔍
    ● T47.5X3   Poisoning by digestants, assault 🔍
    ● T47.5X4   Poisoning by digestants, undetermined 🔍
    ● T47.5X5   Adverse effect of digestants 🔍
    ● T47.5X6   Underdosing of digestants 🔍

● T47.6   Poisoning by, adverse effect of and underdosing of antidiarrheal drugs

> **Excludes2**   poisoning by, adverse effect of and underdosing of systemic antibiotics and other anti-infectives (T36-T37)

  ● T47.6X   Poisoning by, adverse effect of and underdosing of antidiarrheal drugs
    ● T47.6X1   Poisoning by antidiarrheal drugs, accidental (unintentional) 🔍
        Poisoning by antidiarrheal drugs NOS
    ● T47.6X2   Poisoning by antidiarrheal drugs, intentional self-harm 🔍
    ● T47.6X3   Poisoning by antidiarrheal drugs, assault 🔍
    ● T47.6X4   Poisoning by antidiarrheal drugs, undetermined 🔍
    ● T47.6X5   Adverse effect of antidiarrheal drugs 🔍
    ● T47.6X6   Underdosing of antidiarrheal drugs 🔍

◀ New   ◀━ Revised   deleted Deleted   Excludes 1   Excludes 2   Includes   Use additional   Code first   Code also   Unspecified

OGCR Official Guidelines   ● Unacceptable Principal Diagnosis   X Assign placeholder X   ▸ Use Additional Character(s)   ▸ Manifestation Code   Coding Clinic

● **T47.7**   Poisoning by, adverse effect of and underdosing of emetics

   ● **T47.7X**   Poisoning by, adverse effect of and underdosing of emetics

      ● **T47.7X1**   Poisoning by emetics, accidental (unintentional) 🗈

          Poisoning by emetics NOS

      ● **T47.7X2**   Poisoning by emetics, intentional self-harm 🗈

      ● **T47.7X3**   Poisoning by emetics, assault 🗈

      ● **T47.7X4**   Poisoning by emetics, undetermined 🗈

      ● **T47.7X5**   Adverse effect of emetics 🗈

      ● **T47.7X6**   Underdosing of emetics 🗈

● **T47.8**   Poisoning by, adverse effect of and underdosing of other agents primarily affecting gastrointestinal system

   ● **T47.8X**   Poisoning by, adverse effect of and underdosing of other agents primarily affecting gastrointestinal system

      ● **T47.8X1**   Poisoning by other agents primarily affecting gastrointestinal system, accidental (unintentional) 🗈

          Poisoning by other agents primarily affecting gastrointestinal system NOS

      ● **T47.8X2**   Poisoning by other agents primarily affecting gastrointestinal system, intentional self-harm 🗈

      ● **T47.8X3**   Poisoning by other agents primarily affecting gastrointestinal system, assault 🗈

      ● **T47.8X4**   Poisoning by other agents primarily affecting gastrointestinal system, undetermined 🗈

      ● **T47.8X5**   Adverse effect of other agents primarily affecting gastrointestinal system 🗈

      ● **T47.8X6**   Underdosing of other agents primarily affecting gastrointestinal system 🗈

● **T47.9**   Poisoning by, adverse effect of and underdosing of unspecified agents primarily affecting the gastrointestinal system

   X ● **T47.91**   Poisoning by unspecified agents primarily affecting the gastrointestinal system, accidental (unintentional) 🗈

       Poisoning by agents primarily affecting the gastrointestinal system NOS

   X ● **T47.92**   Poisoning by unspecified agents primarily affecting the gastrointestinal system, intentional self-harm 🗈

   X ● **T47.93**   Poisoning by unspecified agents primarily affecting the gastrointestinal system, assault 🗈

   X ● **T47.94**   Poisoning by unspecified agents primarily affecting the gastrointestinal system, undetermined 🗈

   X ● **T47.95**   Adverse effect of unspecified agents primarily affecting the gastrointestinal system 🗈

   X ● **T47.96**   Underdosing of unspecified agents primarily affecting the gastrointestinal system 🗈

● **T48**   Poisoning by, adverse effect of and underdosing of agents primarily acting on smooth and skeletal muscles and the respiratory system

    The appropriate 7th character is to be added to each code from category T48

A	initial encounter
D	subsequent encounter
S	sequela

● **T48.0**   Poisoning by, adverse effect of and underdosing of oxytocic drugs

    Excludes1   poisoning by, adverse effect of and underdosing of estrogens, progestogens and antagonists (T38.4-T38.6)

   ● **T48.0X**   Poisoning by, adverse effect of and underdosing of oxytocic drugs

      ● **T48.0X1**   Poisoning by oxytocic drugs, accidental (unintentional) 🗈

          Poisoning by oxytocic drugs NOS

      ● **T48.0X2**   Poisoning by oxytocic drugs, intentional self-harm 🗈

      ● **T48.0X3**   Poisoning by oxytocic drugs, assault 🗈

      ● **T48.0X4**   Poisoning by oxytocic drugs, undetermined 🗈

      ● **T48.0X5**   Adverse effect of oxytocic drugs 🗈

      ● **T48.0X6**   Underdosing of oxytocic drugs 🗈

● **T48.1**   Poisoning by, adverse effect of and underdosing of skeletal muscle relaxants [neuromuscular blocking agents]

   ● **T48.1X**   Poisoning by, adverse effect of and underdosing of skeletal muscle relaxants [neuromuscular blocking agents]

      ● **T48.1X1**   Poisoning by skeletal muscle relaxants [neuromuscular blocking agents], accidental (unintentional) 🗈

          Poisoning by skeletal muscle relaxants [neuromuscular blocking agents] NOS

      ● **T48.1X2**   Poisoning by skeletal muscle relaxants [neuromuscular blocking agents], intentional self-harm 🗈

      ● **T48.1X3**   Poisoning by skeletal muscle relaxants [neuromuscular blocking agents], assault 🗈

      ● **T48.1X4**   Poisoning by skeletal muscle relaxants [neuromuscular blocking agents], undetermined 🗈

      ● **T48.1X5**   Adverse effect of skeletal muscle relaxants [neuromuscular blocking agents] 🗈

      ● **T48.1X6**   Underdosing of skeletal muscle relaxants [neuromuscular blocking agents] 🗈

● **T48.2**   Poisoning by, adverse effect of and underdosing of other and unspecified drugs acting on muscles

   ● **T48.20**   Poisoning by, adverse effect of and underdosing of unspecified drugs acting on muscles

      ● **T48.201**   Poisoning by unspecified drugs acting on muscles, accidental (unintentional) 🗈

          Poisoning by unspecified drugs acting on muscles NOS

      ● **T48.202**   Poisoning by unspecified drugs acting on muscles, intentional self-harm 🗈

      ● **T48.203**   Poisoning by unspecified drugs acting on muscles, assault 🗈

      ● **T48.204**   Poisoning by unspecified drugs acting on muscles, undetermined 🗈

CHAPTER 19 (S00-T88)

N Newborn Age: 0   P Pediatric Age: 0–17   M Maternity DX: 12–55   A Adult Age: 15–124   ♀ Females Only   ♂ Males Only

🗈 Complication\Comorbidity   🗈 Major C\C   (Ex) CC/MCC Exclusions   🗈 Present on Admission Requirement   🗈 Hospital-Acquired Condition

1543

● T48.205 Adverse effect of unspecified drugs acting on muscles 🔍

● T48.206 Underdosing of unspecified drugs acting on muscles 🔍

● T48.29 Poisoning by, adverse effect of and underdosing of other drugs acting on muscles

  ● T48.291 Poisoning by other drugs acting on muscles, accidental (unintentional) 🔍
             Poisoning by other drugs acting on muscles NOS

  ● T48.292 Poisoning by other drugs acting on muscles, intentional self-harm 🔍

  ● T48.293 Poisoning by other drugs acting on muscles, assault 🔍

  ● T48.294 Poisoning by other drugs acting on muscles, undetermined 🔍

  ● T48.295 Adverse effect of other drugs acting on muscles 🔍

  ● T48.296 Underdosing of other drugs acting on muscles 🔍

● T48.3 Poisoning by, adverse effect of and underdosing of antitussives

  ● T48.3X Poisoning by, adverse effect of and underdosing of antitussives

    ● T48.3X1 Poisoning by antitussives, accidental (unintentional) 🔍
               Poisoning by antitussives NOS

    ● T48.3X2 Poisoning by antitussives, intentional self-harm 🔍

    ● T48.3X3 Poisoning by antitussives, assault 🔍

    ● T48.3X4 Poisoning by antitussives, undetermined 🔍

    ● T48.3X5 Adverse effect of antitussives 🔍

    ● T48.3X6 Underdosing of antitussives 🔍

● T48.4 Poisoning by, adverse effect of and underdosing of expectorants

  ● T48.4X Poisoning by, adverse effect of and underdosing of expectorants

    ● T48.4X1 Poisoning by expectorants, accidental (unintentional) 🔍
               Poisoning by expectorants NOS

    ● T48.4X2 Poisoning by expectorants, intentional self-harm 🔍

    ● T48.4X3 Poisoning by expectorants, assault 🔍

    ● T48.4X4 Poisoning by expectorants, undetermined 🔍

    ● T48.4X5 Adverse effect of expectorants 🔍

    ● T48.4X6 Underdosing of expectorants 🔍

● T48.5 Poisoning by, adverse effect of and underdosing of other anti-common-cold drugs
         Poisoning by, adverse effect of and underdosing of decongestants

    Excludes2 poisoning by, adverse effect of and underdosing of antipyretics, NEC (T39.9-)
               poisoning by, adverse effect of and underdosing of non-steroidal antiinflammatory drugs (T39.3-)
               poisoning by, adverse effect of and underdosing of salicylates (T39.0-)

  ● T48.5X Poisoning by, adverse effect of and underdosing of other anti-common-cold drugs

    ● T48.5X1 Poisoning by other anti-common-cold drugs, accidental (unintentional) 🔍
               Poisoning by other anti-common-cold drugs NOS

    ● T48.5X2 Poisoning by other anti-common-cold drugs, intentional self-harm 🔍

    ● T48.5X3 Poisoning by other anti-common-cold drugs, assault 🔍

    ● T48.5X4 Poisoning by other anti-common-cold drugs, undetermined 🔍

    ● T48.5X5 Adverse effect of other anti-common-cold drugs 🔍

    ● T48.5X6 Underdosing of other anti-common-cold drugs 🔍

● T48.6 Poisoning by, adverse effect of and underdosing of antiasthmatics, not elsewhere classified
         Poisoning by, adverse effect of and underdosing of beta-adrenoreceptor agonists used in asthma therapy

    Excludes1 poisoning by, adverse effect of and underdosing of beta-adrenoreceptor agonists not used in asthma therapy (T44.5)
               poisoning by, adverse effect of and underdosing of anterior pituitary [adenohypophyseal] hormones (T38.8)

  ● T48.6X Poisoning by, adverse effect of and underdosing of antiasthmatics

    ● T48.6X1 Poisoning by antiasthmatics, accidental (unintentional) 🔍
               Poisoning by antiasthmatics NOS

    ● T48.6X2 Poisoning by antiasthmatics, intentional self-harm 🔍

    ● T48.6X3 Poisoning by antiasthmatics, assault 🔍

    ● T48.6X4 Poisoning by antiasthmatics, undetermined 🔍

    ● T48.6X5 Adverse effect of antiasthmatics 🔍

    ● T48.6X6 Underdosing of antiasthmatics 🔍

● T48.9 Poisoning by, adverse effect of and underdosing of other and unspecified agents primarily acting on the respiratory system

  ● T48.90 Poisoning by, adverse effect of and underdosing of unspecified agents primarily acting on the respiratory system

    ● T48.901 Poisoning by unspecified agents primarily acting on the respiratory system, accidental (unintentional) 🔍

    ● T48.902 Poisoning by unspecified agents primarily acting on the respiratory system, intentional self-harm 🔍

    ● T48.903 Poisoning by unspecified agents primarily acting on the respiratory system, assault 🔍

    ● T48.904 Poisoning by unspecified agents primarily acting on the respiratory system, undetermined 🔍

    ● T48.905 Adverse effect of unspecified agents primarily acting on the respiratory system 🔍

    ● T48.906 Underdosing of unspecified agents primarily acting on the respiratory system 🔍

  ● T48.99 Poisoning by, adverse effect of and underdosing of other agents primarily acting on the respiratory system

    ● T48.991 Poisoning by other agents primarily acting on the respiratory system, accidental (unintentional) 🔍

    ● T48.992 Poisoning by other agents primarily acting on the respiratory system, intentional self-harm 🔍

    ● T48.993 Poisoning by other agents primarily acting on the respiratory system, assault 🔍

    ● T48.994 Poisoning by other agents primarily acting on the respiratory system, undetermined 🔍

- ● T48.995 Adverse effect of other agents primarily acting on the respiratory system ⊛
- ● T48.996 Underdosing of other agents primarily acting on the respiratory system ⊛

● T49 **Poisoning by, adverse effect of and underdosing of topical agents primarily affecting skin and mucous membrane and by ophthalmological, otorhinolaryngological and dental drugs**

Includes poisoning by, adverse effect of and underdosing of glucocorticoids, topically used

The appropriate 7th character is to be added to each code from category T49

> A initial encounter
> D subsequent encounter
> S sequela

- ● T49.0 **Poisoning by, adverse effect of and underdosing of local antifungal, anti-infective and anti-inflammatory drugs**
  - ● T49.0X **Poisoning by, adverse effect of and underdosing of local antifungal, anti-infective and anti-inflammatory drugs**
    - ● T49.0X1 Poisoning by local antifungal, anti-infective and anti-inflammatory drugs, accidental (unintentional) ⊛
      Poisoning by local antifungal, anti-infective and anti-inflammatory drugs NOS
    - ● T49.0X2 Poisoning by local antifungal, anti-infective and anti-inflammatory drugs, intentional self-harm ⊛
    - ● T49.0X3 Poisoning by local antifungal, anti-infective and anti-inflammatory drugs, assault ⊛
    - ● T49.0X4 Poisoning by local antifungal, anti-infective and anti-inflammatory drugs, undetermined ⊛
    - ● T49.0X5 Adverse effect of local antifungal, anti-infective and anti-inflammatory drugs ⊛
    - ● T49.0X6 Underdosing of local antifungal, anti-infective and anti-inflammatory drugs ⊛
- ● T49.1 **Poisoning by, adverse effect of and underdosing of antipruritics**
  - ● T49.1X **Poisoning by, adverse effect of and underdosing of antipruritics**
    - ● T49.1X1 Poisoning by antipruritics, accidental (unintentional) ⊛
      Poisoning by antipruritics NOS
    - ● T49.1X2 Poisoning by antipruritics, intentional self-harm ⊛
    - ● T49.1X3 Poisoning by antipruritics, assault ⊛
    - ● T49.1X4 Poisoning by antipruritics, undetermined ⊛
    - ● T49.1X5 Adverse effect of antipruritics ⊛
    - ● T49.1X6 Underdosing of antipruritics ⊛
- ● T49.2 **Poisoning by, adverse effect of and underdosing of local astringents and local detergents**
  - ● T49.2X **Poisoning by, adverse effect of and underdosing of local astringents and local detergents**
    - ● T49.2X1 Poisoning by local astringents and local detergents, accidental (unintentional) ⊛
      Poisoning by local astringents and local detergents NOS
    - ● T49.2X2 Poisoning by local astringents and local detergents, intentional self-harm ⊛
    - ● T49.2X3 Poisoning by local astringents and local detergents, assault ⊛

- ● T49.2X4 Poisoning by local astringents and local detergents, undetermined ⊛
- ● T49.2X5 Adverse effect of local astringents and local detergents ⊛
- ● T49.2X6 Underdosing of local astringents and local detergents ⊛

- ● T49.3 **Poisoning by, adverse effect of and underdosing of emollients, demulcents and protectants**
  - ● T49.3X **Poisoning by, adverse effect of and underdosing of emollients, demulcents and protectants**
    - ● T49.3X1 Poisoning by emollients, demulcents and protectants, accidental (unintentional) ⊛
      Poisoning by emollients, demulcents and protectants NOS
    - ● T49.3X2 Poisoning by emollients, demulcents and protectants, intentional self-harm ⊛
    - ● T49.3X3 Poisoning by emollients, demulcents and protectants, assault ⊛
    - ● T49.3X4 Poisoning by emollients, demulcents and protectants, undetermined ⊛
    - ● T49.3X5 Adverse effect of emollients, demulcents and protectants ⊛
    - ● T49.3X6 Underdosing of emollients, demulcents and protectants ⊛
- ● T49.4 **Poisoning by, adverse effect of and underdosing of keratolytics, keratoplastics, and other hair treatment drugs and preparations**
  - ● T49.4X **Poisoning by, adverse effect of and underdosing of keratolytics, keratoplastics, and other hair treatment drugs and preparations**
    - ● T49.4X1 Poisoning by keratolytics, keratoplastics, and other hair treatment drugs and preparations, accidental (unintentional) ⊛
      Poisoning by keratolytics, keratoplastics, and other hair treatment drugs and preparations NOS
    - ● T49.4X2 Poisoning by keratolytics, keratoplastics, and other hair treatment drugs and preparations, intentional self-harm ⊛
    - ● T49.4X3 Poisoning by keratolytics, keratoplastics, and other hair treatment drugs and preparations, assault ⊛
    - ● T49.4X4 Poisoning by keratolytics, keratoplastics, and other hair treatment drugs and preparations, undetermined ⊛
    - ● T49.4X5 Adverse effect of keratolytics, keratoplastics, and other hair treatment drugs and preparations ⊛
    - ● T49.4X6 Underdosing of keratolytics, keratoplastics, and other hair treatment drugs and preparations ⊛
- ● T49.5 **Poisoning by, adverse effect of and underdosing of ophthalmological drugs and preparations**
  - ● T49.5X **Poisoning by, adverse effect of and underdosing of ophthalmological drugs and preparations**
    - ● T49.5X1 Poisoning by ophthalmological drugs and preparations, accidental (unintentional) ⊛
      Poisoning by ophthalmological drugs and preparations NOS
    - ● T49.5X2 Poisoning by ophthalmological drugs and preparations, intentional self-harm ⊛

N Newborn Age: 0   P Pediatric Age: 0–17   M Maternity DX: 12–55   A Adult Age: 15–124   ♀ Females Only   ♂ Males Only
⊛ Complication\Comorbidity   ⊛ Major C\C   Ⓔⓧ CC/MCC Exclusions   ⊛ Present on Admission Requirement   ⊛ Hospital-Acquired Condition

1545

● T49.5X3   Poisoning by ophthalmological drugs and preparations, assault 🕮

● T49.5X4   Poisoning by ophthalmological drugs and preparations, undetermined 🕮

● T49.5X5   Adverse effect of ophthalmological drugs and preparations 🕮

● T49.5X6   Underdosing of ophthalmological drugs and preparations 🕮

● T49.6   Poisoning by, adverse effect of and underdosing of otorhinolaryngological drugs and preparations

  ● T49.6X   Poisoning by, adverse effect of and underdosing of otorhinolaryngological drugs and preparations

    ● T49.6X1   Poisoning by otorhinolaryngological drugs and preparations, accidental (unintentional) 🕮
      Poisoning by otorhinolaryngological drugs and preparations NOS

    ● T49.6X2   Poisoning by otorhinolaryngological drugs and preparations, intentional self-harm 🕮

    ● T49.6X3   Poisoning by otorhinolaryngological drugs and preparations, assault 🕮

    ● T49.6X4   Poisoning by otorhinolaryngological drugs and preparations, undetermined 🕮

    ● T49.6X5   Adverse effect of otorhinolaryngological drugs and preparations 🕮

    ● T49.6X6   Underdosing of otorhinolaryngological drugs and preparations 🕮

● T49.7   Poisoning by, adverse effect of and underdosing of dental drugs, topically applied

  ● T49.7X   Poisoning by, adverse effect of and underdosing of dental drugs, topically applied

    ● T49.7X1   Poisoning by dental drugs, topically applied, accidental (unintentional) 🕮
      Poisoning by dental drugs, topically applied NOS

    ● T49.7X2   Poisoning by dental drugs, topically applied, intentional self-harm 🕮

    ● T49.7X3   Poisoning by dental drugs, topically applied, assault 🕮

    ● T49.7X4   Poisoning by dental drugs, topically applied, undetermined 🕮

    ● T49.7X5   Adverse effect of dental drugs, topically applied 🕮

    ● T49.7X6   Underdosing of dental drugs, topically applied 🕮

● T49.8   Poisoning by, adverse effect of and underdosing of other topical agents
  Poisoning by, adverse effect of and underdosing of spermicides

  ● T49.8X   Poisoning by, adverse effect of and underdosing of other topical agents

    ● T49.8X1   Poisoning by other topical agents, accidental (unintentional) 🕮
      Poisoning by other topical agents NOS

    ● T49.8X2   Poisoning by other topical agents, intentional self-harm 🕮

    ● T49.8X3   Poisoning by other topical agents, assault 🕮

    ● T49.8X4   Poisoning by other topical agents, undetermined 🕮

    ● T49.8X5   Adverse effect of other topical agents 🕮

    ● T49.8X6   Underdosing of other topical agents 🕮

● T49.9   Poisoning by, adverse effect of and underdosing of unspecified topical agent

  X ● T49.91   Poisoning by unspecified topical agent, accidental (unintentional) 🕮

  X ● T49.92   Poisoning by unspecified topical agent, intentional self-harm 🕮

  X ● T49.93   Poisoning by unspecified topical agent, assault 🕮

  X ● T49.94   Poisoning by unspecified topical agent, undetermined 🕮

  X ● T49.95   Adverse effect of unspecified topical agent 🕮

  X ● T49.96   Underdosing of unspecified topical agent 🕮

T50   Poisoning by, adverse effect of and underdosing of diuretics and other and unspecified drugs, medicaments and biological substances

  The appropriate 7th character is to be added to each code from category T50

> A   initial encounter
> D   subsequent encounter
> S   sequela

● T50.0   Poisoning by, adverse effect of and underdosing of mineralocorticoids and their antagonists

  ● T50.0X   Poisoning by, adverse effect of and underdosing of mineralocorticoids and their antagonists

    ● T50.0X1   Poisoning by mineralocorticoids and their antagonists, accidental (unintentional) 🕮
      Poisoning by mineralocorticoids and their antagonists NOS

    ● T50.0X2   Poisoning by mineralocorticoids and their antagonists, intentional self-harm 🕮

    ● T50.0X3   Poisoning by mineralocorticoids and their antagonists, assault 🕮

    ● T50.0X4   Poisoning by mineralocorticoids and their antagonists, undetermined 🕮

    ● T50.0X5   Adverse effect of mineralocorticoids and their antagonists 🕮

    ● T50.0X6   Underdosing of mineralocorticoids and their antagonists 🕮

● T50.1   Poisoning by, adverse effect of and underdosing of loop [high-ceiling] diuretics

  ● T50.1X   Poisoning by, adverse effect of and underdosing of loop [high-ceiling] diuretics

    ● T50.1X1   Poisoning by loop [high-ceiling] diuretics, accidental (unintentional) 🕮
      Poisoning by loop [high-ceiling] diuretics NOS

    ● T50.1X2   Poisoning by loop [high-ceiling] diuretics, intentional self-harm 🕮

    ● T50.1X3   Poisoning by loop [high-ceiling] diuretics, assault 🕮

    ● T50.1X4   Poisoning by loop [high-ceiling] diuretics, undetermined 🕮

    ● T50.1X5   Adverse effect of loop [high-ceiling] diuretics 🕮

    ● T50.1X6   Underdosing of loop [high-ceiling] diuretics 🕮

● T50.2   Poisoning by, adverse effect of and underdosing of carbonic-anhydrase inhibitors, benzothiadiazides and other diuretics
      Poisoning by, adverse effect of and underdosing of acetazolamide

   ● T50.2X   Poisoning by, adverse effect of and underdosing of carbonic-anhydrase inhibitors, benzothiadiazides and other diuretics

      ● T50.2X1   Poisoning by carbonic-anhydrase inhibitors, benzothiadiazides and other diuretics, accidental (unintentional) 🗝
            Poisoning by carbonic-anhydrase inhibitors, benzothiadiazides and other diuretics NOS

      ● T50.2X2   Poisoning by carbonic-anhydrase inhibitors, benzothiadiazides and other diuretics, intentional self-harm 🗝

      ● T50.2X3   Poisoning by carbonic-anhydrase inhibitors, benzothiadiazides and other diuretics, assault 🗝

      ● T50.2X4   Poisoning by carbonic-anhydrase inhibitors, benzothiadiazides and other diuretics, undetermined 🗝

      ● T50.2X5   Adverse effect of carbonic-anhydrase inhibitors, benzothiadiazides and other diuretics 🗝

      ● T50.2X6   Underdosing of carbonic-anhydrase inhibitors, benzothiadiazides and other diuretics 🗝

● T50.3   Poisoning by, adverse effect of and underdosing of electrolytic, caloric and water-balance agents
      Poisoning by, adverse effect of and underdosing of oral rehydration salts

   ● T50.3X   Poisoning by, adverse effect of and underdosing of electrolytic, caloric and water-balance agents

      ● T50.3X1   Poisoning by electrolytic, caloric and water-balance agents, accidental (unintentional) 🗝
            Poisoning by electrolytic, caloric and water-balance agents NOS

      ● T50.3X2   Poisoning by electrolytic, caloric and water-balance agents, intentional self-harm 🗝

      ● T50.3X3   Poisoning by electrolytic, caloric and water-balance agents, assault 🗝

      ● T50.3X4   Poisoning by electrolytic, caloric and water-balance agents, undetermined 🗝

      ● T50.3X5   Adverse effect of electrolytic, caloric and water-balance agents 🗝

      ● T50.3X6   Underdosing of electrolytic, caloric and water-balance agents 🗝

● T50.4   Poisoning by, adverse effect of and underdosing of drugs affecting uric acid metabolism

   ● T50.4X   Poisoning by, adverse effect of and underdosing of drugs affecting uric acid metabolism

      ● T50.4X1   Poisoning by drugs affecting uric acid metabolism, accidental (unintentional) 🗝
            Poisoning by drugs affecting uric acid metabolism NOS

      ● T50.4X2   Poisoning by drugs affecting uric acid metabolism, intentional self-harm 🗝

      ● T50.4X3   Poisoning by drugs affecting uric acid metabolism, assault 🗝

      ● T50.4X4   Poisoning by drugs affecting uric acid metabolism, undetermined 🗝

      ● T50.4X5   Adverse effect of drugs affecting uric acid metabolism 🗝

      ● T50.4X6   Underdosing of drugs affecting uric acid metabolism 🗝

● T50.5   Poisoning by, adverse effect of and underdosing of appetite depressants

   ● T50.5X   Poisoning by, adverse effect of and underdosing of appetite depressants

      ● T50.5X1   Poisoning by appetite depressants, accidental (unintentional) 🗝
            Poisoning by appetite depressants NOS

      ● T50.5X2   Poisoning by appetite depressants, intentional self-harm 🗝

      ● T50.5X3   Poisoning by appetite depressants, assault 🗝

      ● T50.5X4   Poisoning by appetite depressants, undetermined 🗝

      ● T50.5X5   Adverse effect of appetite depressants 🗝

      ● T50.5X6   Underdosing of appetite depressants 🗝

● T50.6   Poisoning by, adverse effect of and underdosing of antidotes and chelating agents
      Poisoning by, adverse effect of and underdosing of alcohol deterrents

   ● T50.6X   Poisoning by, adverse effect of and underdosing of antidotes and chelating agents

      ● T50.6X1   Poisoning by antidotes and chelating agents, accidental (unintentional) 🗝
            Poisoning by antidotes and chelating agents NOS

      ● T50.6X2   Poisoning by antidotes and chelating agents, intentional self-harm 🗝

      ● T50.6X3   Poisoning by antidotes and chelating agents, assault 🗝

      ● T50.6X4   Poisoning by antidotes and chelating agents, undetermined 🗝

      ● T50.6X5   Adverse effect of antidotes and chelating agents 🗝

      ● T50.6X6   Underdosing of antidotes and chelating agents 🗝

● T50.7   Poisoning by, adverse effect of and underdosing of analeptics and opioid receptor antagonists

   ● T50.7X   Poisoning by, adverse effect of and underdosing of analeptics and opioid receptor antagonists

      ● T50.7X1   Poisoning by analeptics and opioid receptor antagonists, accidental (unintentional) 🗝
            Poisoning by analeptics and opioid receptor antagonists NOS

      ● T50.7X2   Poisoning by analeptics and opioid receptor antagonists, intentional self-harm 🗝

      ● T50.7X3   Poisoning by analeptics and opioid receptor antagonists, assault 🗝

      ● T50.7X4   Poisoning by analeptics and opioid receptor antagonists, undetermined 🗝

      ● T50.7X5   Adverse effect of analeptics and opioid receptor antagonists 🗝

      ● T50.7X6   Underdosing of analeptics and opioid receptor antagonists 🗝

N Newborn Age: 0   P Pediatric Age: 0–17   M Maternity DX: 12–55   A Adult Age: 15–124   ♀ Females Only   ♂ Males Only

🗝 Complication\Comorbidity   🗝 Major C\C   Ⓔ CC/MCC Exclusions   🗝 Present on Admission Requirement   🗝 Hospital-Acquired Condition

1547

T50.8 Poisoning by, adverse effect of and underdosing of diagnostic agents

T50.8X Poisoning by, adverse effect of and underdosing of diagnostic agents

T50.8X1 Poisoning by diagnostic agents, accidental (unintentional) ✎

Poisoning by diagnostic agents NOS

T50.8X2 Poisoning by diagnostic agents, intentional self-harm ✎

T50.8X3 Poisoning by diagnostic agents, assault ✎

T50.8X4 Poisoning by diagnostic agents, undetermined ✎

T50.8X5 Adverse effect of diagnostic agents ✎

T50.8X6 Underdosing of diagnostic agents ✎

T50.A Poisoning by, adverse effect of and underdosing of bacterial vaccines

T50.A1 Poisoning by, adverse effect of and underdosing of pertussis vaccine, including combinations with a pertussis component

T50.A11 Poisoning by pertussis vaccine, including combinations with a pertussis component, accidental (unintentional) ✎

T50.A12 Poisoning by pertussis vaccine, including combinations with a pertussis component, intentional self-harm ✎

T50.A13 Poisoning by pertussis vaccine, including combinations with a pertussis component, assault ✎

T50.A14 Poisoning by pertussis vaccine, including combinations with a pertussis component, undetermined ✎

T50.A15 Adverse effect of pertussis vaccine, including combinations with a pertussis component ✎

T50.A16 Underdosing of pertussis vaccine, including combinations with a pertussis component ✎

T50.A2 Poisoning by, adverse effect of and underdosing of mixed bacterial vaccines without a pertussis component

T50.A21 Poisoning by mixed bacterial vaccines without a pertussis component, accidental (unintentional) ✎

T50.A22 Poisoning by mixed bacterial vaccines without a pertussis component, intentional self-harm ✎

T50.A23 Poisoning by mixed bacterial vaccines without a pertussis component, assault ✎

T50.A24 Poisoning by mixed bacterial vaccines without a pertussis component, undetermined ✎

T50.A25 Adverse effect of mixed bacterial vaccines without a pertussis component ✎

T50.A26 Underdosing of mixed bacterial vaccines without a pertussis component ✎

T50.A9 Poisoning by, adverse effect of and underdosing of other bacterial vaccines

T50.A91 Poisoning by other bacterial vaccines, accidental (unintentional) ✎

T50.A92 Poisoning by other bacterial vaccines, intentional self-harm ✎

T50.A93 Poisoning by other bacterial vaccines, assault ✎

T50.A94 Poisoning by other bacterial vaccines, undetermined ✎

T50.A95 Adverse effect of other bacterial vaccines ✎

T50.A96 Underdosing of other bacterial vaccines ✎

T50.B Poisoning by, adverse effect of and underdosing of viral vaccines

T50.B1 Poisoning by, adverse effect of and underdosing of smallpox vaccines

T50.B11 Poisoning by smallpox vaccines, accidental (unintentional) ✎

T50.B12 Poisoning by smallpox vaccines, intentional self-harm ✎

T50.B13 Poisoning by smallpox vaccines, assault ✎

T50.B14 Poisoning by smallpox vaccines, undetermined ✎

T50.B15 Adverse effect of smallpox vaccines ✎

T50.B16 Underdosing of smallpox vaccines ✎

T50.B9 Poisoning by, adverse effect of and underdosing of other viral vaccines

T50.B91 Poisoning by other viral vaccines, accidental (unintentional) ✎

T50.B92 Poisoning by other viral vaccines, intentional self-harm ✎

T50.B93 Poisoning by other viral vaccines, assault ✎

T50.B94 Poisoning by other viral vaccines, undetermined ✎

T50.B95 Adverse effect of other viral vaccines ✎

T50.B96 Underdosing of other viral vaccines ✎

T50.Z Poisoning by, adverse effect of and underdosing of other vaccines and biological substances

T50.Z1 Poisoning by, adverse effect of and underdosing of immunoglobulin

T50.Z11 Poisoning by immunoglobulin, accidental (unintentional) ✎

T50.Z12 Poisoning by immunoglobulin, intentional self-harm ✎

T50.Z13 Poisoning by immunoglobulin, assault ✎

T50.Z14 Poisoning by immunoglobulin, undetermined ✎

T50.Z15 Adverse effect of immunoglobulin ✎

T50.Z16 Underdosing of immunoglobulin ✎

◀ New   ◀▥ Revised   ~~deleted~~ Deleted   Excludes 1   Excludes 2   Includes   Use additional   Code first   Code also   Unspecified

OGCR Official Guidelines   ● Unacceptable Principal Diagnosis   X Assign placeholder X   ● Use Additional Character(s)   ▶ Manifestation Code   **Coding Clinic**

- T50.Z9   Poisoning by, adverse effect of and underdosing of other vaccines and biological substances
  - T50.Z91   Poisoning by other vaccines and biological substances, accidental (unintentional) 🖋
  - T50.Z92   Poisoning by other vaccines and biological substances, intentional self-harm 🖋
  - T50.Z93   Poisoning by other vaccines and biological substances, assault 🖋
  - T50.Z94   Poisoning by other vaccines and biological substances, undetermined 🖋
  - T50.Z95   Adverse effect of other vaccines and biological substances 🖋
  - T50.Z96   Underdosing of other vaccines and biological substances 🖋
- T50.9   Poisoning by, adverse effect of and underdosing of other and unspecified drugs, medicaments and biological substances
  - T50.90   Poisoning by, adverse effect of and underdosing of unspecified drugs, medicaments and biological substances
    - T50.901   Poisoning by unspecified drugs, medicaments and biological substances, accidental (unintentional) 🖋
    - T50.902   Poisoning by unspecified drugs, medicaments and biological substances, intentional self-harm 🖋
    - T50.903   Poisoning by unspecified drugs, medicaments and biological substances, assault 🖋
    - T50.904   Poisoning by unspecified drugs, medicaments and biological substances, undetermined 🖋
    - T50.905   Adverse effect of unspecified drugs, medicaments and biological substances 🖋
    - T50.906   Underdosing of unspecified drugs, medicaments and biological substances 🖋
  - T50.99   Poisoning by, adverse effect of and underdosing of other drugs, medicaments and biological substances
    - T50.991   Poisoning by other drugs, medicaments and biological substances, accidental (unintentional) 🖋
    - T50.992   Poisoning by other drugs, medicaments and biological substances, intentional self-harm 🖋
    - T50.993   Poisoning by other drugs, medicaments and biological substances, assault 🖋
    - T50.994   Poisoning by other drugs, medicaments and biological substances, undetermined 🖋
    - T50.995   Adverse effect of other drugs, medicaments and biological substances 🖋
    - T50.996   Underdosing of other drugs, medicaments and biological substances 🖋

TOXIC EFFECTS OF SUBSTANCES CHIEFLY NONMEDICINAL AS TO SOURCE (T51-T65)

Note: When no intent is indicated code to accidental. Undetermined intent is only for use when there is specific documentation in the record that the intent of the toxic effect cannot be determined. ◀▥

Use additional code(s): for all associated manifestations of toxic effect, such as:
respiratory conditions due to external agents (J60-J70)
personal history of foreign body fully removed (Z87.821)
to identify any retained foreign body, if applicable (Z18.-)

Excludes1   contact with and (suspected) exposure to toxic substances (Z77.-)

- T51   Toxic effect of alcohol

  The appropriate 7th character is to be added to each code from category T51

A	initial encounter
D	subsequent encounter
S	sequela

  - T51.0   Toxic effect of ethanol

    Toxic effect of ethyl alcohol

    Excludes2   acute alcohol intoxication or 'hangover' effects (F10.129, F10.229, F10.929)
    drunkenness (F10.129, F10.229, F10.929)
    pathological alcohol intoxication (F10.129, F10.229, F10.929)

    - T51.0X   Toxic effect of ethanol
      - T51.0X1   Toxic effect of ethanol, accidental (unintentional) 🖋
        Toxic effect of ethanol NOS
      - T51.0X2   Toxic effect of ethanol, intentional self-harm 🖋
      - T51.0X3   Toxic effect of ethanol, assault 🖋
      - T51.0X4   Toxic effect of ethanol, undetermined 🖋
  - T51.1   Toxic effect of methanol

    Toxic effect of methyl alcohol

    - T51.1X   Toxic effect of methanol
      - T51.1X1   Toxic effect of methanol, accidental (unintentional) 🖋
        Toxic effect of methanol NOS
      - T51.1X2   Toxic effect of methanol, intentional self-harm 🖋
      - T51.1X3   Toxic effect of methanol, assault 🖋
      - T51.1X4   Toxic effect of methanol, undetermined 🖋
  - T51.2   Toxic effect of 2-Propanol

    Toxic effect of isopropyl alcohol

    - T51.2X   Toxic effect of 2-Propanol
      - T51.2X1   Toxic effect of 2-Propanol, accidental (unintentional) 🖋
        Toxic effect of 2-Propanol NOS
      - T51.2X2   Toxic effect of 2-Propanol, intentional self-harm 🖋
      - T51.2X3   Toxic effect of 2-Propanol, assault 🖋
      - T51.2X4   Toxic effect of 2-Propanol, undetermined 🖋
  - T51.3   Toxic effect of fusel oil

    Toxic effect of amyl alcohol
    Toxic effect of butyl [1-butanol] alcohol
    Toxic effect of propyl [1-propanol] alcohol

    - T51.3X   Toxic effect of fusel oil
      - T51.3X1   Toxic effect of fusel oil, accidental (unintentional) 🖋
        Toxic effect of fusel oil NOS
      - T51.3X2   Toxic effect of fusel oil, intentional self-harm 🖋
      - T51.3X3   Toxic effect of fusel oil, assault 🖋
      - T51.3X4   Toxic effect of fusel oil, undetermined 🖋

CHAPTER 19 (S00-T88)

N   Newborn Age: 0   P   Pediatric Age: 0–17   M   Maternity DX: 12–55   A   Adult Age: 15–124   ♀   Females Only   ♂   Males Only

🖋   Complication\Comorbidity   🖋   Major C\C   (Ex)   CC/MCC Exclusions   🖋   Present on Admission Requirement   🖋   Hospital-Acquired Condition

1549

CHAPTER 19 (S00-T88)

- T51.8 Toxic effect of other alcohols
  - T51.8X Toxic effect of other alcohols
    - T51.8X1 Toxic effect of other alcohols, accidental (unintentional) 🔍
      Toxic effect of other alcohols NOS
    - T51.8X2 Toxic effect of other alcohols, intentional self-harm 🔍
    - T51.8X3 Toxic effect of other alcohols, assault 🔍
    - T51.8X4 Toxic effect of other alcohols, undetermined 🔍
- T51.9 Toxic effect of unspecified alcohol
  - X T51.91 Toxic effect of unspecified alcohol, accidental (unintentional) 🔍
  - X T51.92 Toxic effect of unspecified alcohol, intentional self-harm 🔍
  - X T51.93 Toxic effect of unspecified alcohol, assault 🔍
  - X T51.94 Toxic effect of unspecified alcohol, undetermined 🔍
- T52 Toxic effect of organic solvents

  Excludes1 halogen derivatives of aliphatic and aromatic hydrocarbons (T53.-)

  The appropriate 7th character is to be added to each code from category T52

A	initial encounter
D	subsequent encounter
S	sequela

  - T52.0 Toxic effects of petroleum products
    Toxic effects of gasoline [petrol]
    Toxic effects of kerosene [paraffin oil]
    Toxic effects of paraffin wax
    Toxic effects of ether petroleum
    Toxic effects of naphtha petroleum
    Toxic effects of spirit petroleum
    - T52.0X Toxic effects of petroleum products
      - T52.0X1 Toxic effect of petroleum products, accidental (unintentional) 🔍
        Toxic effects of petroleum products NOS
      - T52.0X2 Toxic effect of petroleum products, intentional self-harm 🔍
      - T52.0X3 Toxic effect of petroleum products, assault 🔍
      - T52.0X4 Toxic effect of petroleum products, undetermined 🔍
  - T52.1 Toxic effects of benzene

    Excludes1 homologues of benzene (T52.2)
    nitroderivatives and aminoderivatives of benzene and its homologues (T65.3)

    - T52.1X Toxic effects of benzene
      - T52.1X1 Toxic effect of benzene, accidental (unintentional) 🔍
        Toxic effects of benzene NOS
      - T52.1X2 Toxic effect of benzene, intentional self-harm 🔍
      - T52.1X3 Toxic effect of benzene, assault 🔍
      - T52.1X4 Toxic effect of benzene, undetermined 🔍
  - T52.2 Toxic effects of homologues of benzene
    Toxic effects of toluene [methylbenzene]
    Toxic effects of xylene [dimethylbenzene]
    - T52.2X Toxic effects of homologues of benzene
      - T52.2X1 Toxic effect of homologues of benzene, accidental (unintentional) 🔍
        Toxic effects of homologues of benzene NOS
      - T52.2X2 Toxic effect of homologues of benzene, intentional self-harm 🔍

- T52.2X3 Toxic effect of homologues of benzene, assault 🔍
- T52.2X4 Toxic effect of homologues of benzene, undetermined 🔍
- T52.3 Toxic effects of glycols
  - T52.3X Toxic effects of glycols
    - T52.3X1 Toxic effect of glycols, accidental (unintentional) 🔍
      Toxic effects of glycols NOS
    - T52.3X2 Toxic effect of glycols, intentional self-harm 🔍
    - T52.3X3 Toxic effect of glycols, assault 🔍
    - T52.3X4 Toxic effect of glycols, undetermined 🔍
- T52.4 Toxic effects of ketones
  - T52.4X Toxic effects of ketones
    - T52.4X1 Toxic effect of ketones, accidental (unintentional) 🔍
      Toxic effects of ketones NOS
    - T52.4X2 Toxic effect of ketones, intentional self-harm 🔍
    - T52.4X3 Toxic effect of ketones, assault 🔍
    - T52.4X4 Toxic effect of ketones, undetermined 🔍
- T52.8 Toxic effects of other organic solvents
  - T52.8X Toxic effects of other organic solvents
    - T52.8X1 Toxic effect of other organic solvents, accidental (unintentional) 🔍
      Toxic effects of other organic solvents NOS
    - T52.8X2 Toxic effect of other organic solvents, intentional self-harm 🔍
    - T52.8X3 Toxic effect of other organic solvents, assault 🔍
    - T52.8X4 Toxic effect of other organic solvents, undetermined 🔍
- T52.9 Toxic effects of unspecified organic solvent
  - X T52.91 Toxic effect of unspecified organic solvent, accidental (unintentional) 🔍
  - X T52.92 Toxic effect of unspecified organic solvent, intentional self-harm 🔍
  - X T52.93 Toxic effect of unspecified organic solvent, assault 🔍
  - X T52.94 Toxic effect of unspecified organic solvent, undetermined 🔍
- T53 Toxic effect of halogen derivatives of aliphatic and aromatic hydrocarbons

  The appropriate 7th character is to be added to each code from category T53

A	initial encounter
D	subsequent encounter
S	sequela

  - T53.0 Toxic effects of carbon tetrachloride
    Toxic effects of tetrachloromethane
    - T53.0X Toxic effects of carbon tetrachloride
      - T53.0X1 Toxic effect of carbon tetrachloride, accidental (unintentional) 🔍
        Toxic effects of carbon tetrachloride NOS
      - T53.0X2 Toxic effect of carbon tetrachloride, intentional self-harm 🔍
      - T53.0X3 Toxic effect of carbon tetrachloride, assault 🔍
      - T53.0X4 Toxic effect of carbon tetrachloride, undetermined 🔍

◀ New ◀ Revised ~~deleted~~ Deleted Excludes 1 Excludes 2 Includes Use additional Code first Code also Unspecified

OGCR Official Guidelines ● Unacceptable Principal Diagnosis X Assign placeholder X ▶ Use Additional Character(s) ▶ Manifestation Code **Coding Clinic**

● **T53.1** **Toxic effects of chloroform**
     Toxic effects of trichloromethane
   ● **T53.1X** **Toxic effects of chloroform**
     ● **T53.1X1** Toxic effect of chloroform, accidental (unintentional) ✎
         Toxic effects of chloroform NOS
     ● **T53.1X2** Toxic effect of chloroform, intentional self-harm ✎
     ● **T53.1X3** Toxic effect of chloroform, assault ✎
     ● **T53.1X4** Toxic effect of chloroform, undetermined ✎

● **T53.2** **Toxic effects of trichloroethylene**
     Toxic effects of trichloroethene
   ● **T53.2X** **Toxic effects of trichloroethylene**
     ● **T53.2X1** Toxic effect of trichloroethylene, accidental (unintentional) ✎
         Toxic effects of trichloroethylene NOS
     ● **T53.2X2** Toxic effect of trichloroethylene, intentional self-harm ✎
     ● **T53.2X3** Toxic effect of trichloroethylene, assault ✎
     ● **T53.2X4** Toxic effect of trichloroethylene, undetermined ✎

● **T53.3** **Toxic effects of tetrachloroethylene**
     Toxic effects of perchloroethylene
     Toxic effect of tetrachloroethene
   ● **T53.3X** **Toxic effects of tetrachloroethylene**
     ● **T53.3X1** Toxic effect of tetrachloroethylene, accidental (unintentional) ✎
         Toxic effects of tetrachloroethylene NOS
     ● **T53.3X2** Toxic effect of tetrachloroethylene, intentional self-harm ✎
     ● **T53.3X3** Toxic effect of tetrachloroethylene, assault ✎
     ● **T53.3X4** Toxic effect of tetrachloroethylene, undetermined ✎

● **T53.4** **Toxic effects of dichloromethane**
     Toxic effects of methylene chloride
   ● **T53.4X** **Toxic effects of dichloromethane**
     ● **T53.4X1** Toxic effect of dichloromethane, accidental (unintentional) ✎
         Toxic effects of dichloromethane NOS
     ● **T53.4X2** Toxic effect of dichloromethane, intentional self-harm ✎
     ● **T53.4X3** Toxic effect of dichloromethane, assault ✎
     ● **T53.4X4** Toxic effect of dichloromethane, undetermined ✎

● **T53.5** **Toxic effects of chlorofluorocarbons**
   ● **T53.5X** **Toxic effects of chlorofluorocarbons**
     ● **T53.5X1** Toxic effect of chlorofluorocarbons, accidental (unintentional) ✎
         Toxic effects of chlorofluorocarbons NOS
     ● **T53.5X2** Toxic effect of chlorofluorocarbons, intentional self-harm ✎
     ● **T53.5X3** Toxic effect of chlorofluorocarbons, assault ✎
     ● **T53.5X4** Toxic effect of chlorofluorocarbons, undetermined ✎

● **T53.6** **Toxic effects of other halogen derivatives of aliphatic hydrocarbons**
   ● **T53.6X** **Toxic effects of other halogen derivatives of aliphatic hydrocarbons**
     ● **T53.6X1** Toxic effect of other halogen derivatives of aliphatic hydrocarbons, accidental (unintentional) ✎
         Toxic effects of other halogen derivatives of aliphatic hydrocarbons NOS
     ● **T53.6X2** Toxic effect of other halogen derivatives of aliphatic hydrocarbons, intentional self-harm ✎
     ● **T53.6X3** Toxic effect of other halogen derivatives of aliphatic hydrocarbons, assault ✎
     ● **T53.6X4** Toxic effect of other halogen derivatives of aliphatic hydrocarbons, undetermined ✎

● **T53.7** **Toxic effects of other halogen derivatives of aromatic hydrocarbons**
   ● **T53.7X** **Toxic effects of other halogen derivatives of aromatic hydrocarbons**
     ● **T53.7X1** Toxic effect of other halogen derivatives of aromatic hydrocarbons, accidental (unintentional) ✎
         Toxic effects of other halogen derivatives of aromatic hydrocarbons NOS
     ● **T53.7X2** Toxic effect of other halogen derivatives of aromatic hydrocarbons, intentional self-harm ✎
     ● **T53.7X3** Toxic effect of other halogen derivatives of aromatic hydrocarbons, assault ✎
     ● **T53.7X4** Toxic effect of other halogen derivatives of aromatic hydrocarbons, undetermined ✎

● **T53.9** **Toxic effects of unspecified halogen derivatives of aliphatic and aromatic hydrocarbons**
   X ● **T53.91** Toxic effect of unspecified halogen derivatives of aliphatic and aromatic hydrocarbons, accidental (unintentional) ✎
   X ● **T53.92** Toxic effect of unspecified halogen derivatives of aliphatic and aromatic hydrocarbons, intentional self-harm ✎
   X ● **T53.93** Toxic effect of unspecified halogen derivatives of aliphatic and aromatic hydrocarbons, assault ✎
   X ● **T53.94** Toxic effect of unspecified halogen derivatives of aliphatic and aromatic hydrocarbons, undetermined ✎

● **T54** **Toxic effect of corrosive substances**
     The appropriate 7th character is to be added to each code from category T54

A	initial encounter
D	subsequent encounter
S	sequela

● **T54.0** **Toxic effects of phenol and phenol homologues**
   ● **T54.0X** **Toxic effects of phenol and phenol homologues**
     ● **T54.0X1** Toxic effect of phenol and phenol homologues, accidental (unintentional) ✎
         Toxic effects of phenol and phenol homologues NOS
     ● **T54.0X2** Toxic effect of phenol and phenol homologues, intentional self-harm ✎
     ● **T54.0X3** Toxic effect of phenol and phenol homologues, assault ✎
     ● **T54.0X4** Toxic effect of phenol and phenol homologues, undetermined ✎

CHAPTER 19 (S00-T88)

N   Newborn Age: 0   P   Pediatric Age: 0–17   M   Maternity DX: 12–55   A   Adult Age: 15–124   ♀   Females Only   ♂   Males Only

✎   Complication\Comorbidity   ✎   Major C\C   (Ex)   CC/MCC Exclusions   ✎   Present on Admission Requirement   ✎   Hospital-Acquired Condition

1551

● **T54.1**   Toxic effects of other corrosive organic compounds

    ● **T54.1X**   Toxic effects of other corrosive organic compounds

        ● **T54.1X1**   Toxic effect of other corrosive organic compounds, accidental (unintentional) 🖎

             Toxic effects of other corrosive organic compounds NOS

        ● **T54.1X2**   Toxic effect of other corrosive organic compounds, intentional self-harm 🖎

        ● **T54.1X3**   Toxic effect of other corrosive organic compounds, assault 🖎

        ● **T54.1X4**   Toxic effect of other corrosive organic compounds, undetermined 🖎

● **T54.2**   Toxic effects of corrosive acids and acid-like substances

     Toxic effects of hydrochloric acid

     Toxic effects of sulfuric acid

    ● **T54.2X**   Toxic effects of corrosive acids and acid-like substances

        ● **T54.2X1**   Toxic effect of corrosive acids and acid-like substances, accidental (unintentional) 🖎

             Toxic effects of corrosive acids and acid-like substances NOS

        ● **T54.2X2**   Toxic effect of corrosive acids and acid-like substances, intentional self-harm 🖎

        ● **T54.2X3**   Toxic effect of corrosive acids and acid-like substances, assault 🖎

        ● **T54.2X4**   Toxic effect of corrosive acids and acid-like substances, undetermined 🖎

● **T54.3**   Toxic effects of corrosive alkalis and alkali-like substances

     Toxic effects of potassium hydroxide

     Toxic effects of sodium hydroxide

    ● **T54.3X**   Toxic effects of corrosive alkalis and alkali-like substances

        ● **T54.3X1**   Toxic effect of corrosive alkalis and alkali-like substances, accidental (unintentional) 🖎

             Toxic effects of corrosive alkalis and alkali-like substances NOS

        ● **T54.3X2**   Toxic effect of corrosive alkalis and alkali-like substances, intentional self-harm 🖎

        ● **T54.3X3**   Toxic effect of corrosive alkalis and alkali-like substances, assault 🖎

        ● **T54.3X4**   Toxic effect of corrosive alkalis and alkali-like substances, undetermined 🖎

● **T54.9**   Toxic effects of unspecified corrosive substance

    X ● **T54.91**   Toxic effect of unspecified corrosive substance, accidental (unintentional) 🖎

    X ● **T54.92**   Toxic effect of unspecified corrosive substance, intentional self-harm 🖎

    X ● **T54.93**   Toxic effect of unspecified corrosive substance, assault 🖎

    X ● **T54.94**   Toxic effect of unspecified corrosive substance, undetermined 🖎

● **T55**   Toxic effect of soaps and detergents

     The appropriate 7th character is to be added to each code from category T55

A	initial encounter
D	subsequent encounter
S	sequela

● **T55.0**   Toxic effect of soaps

    ● **T55.0X**   Toxic effect of soaps

        ● **T55.0X1**   Toxic effect of soaps, accidental (unintentional) 🖎

             Toxic effect of soaps NOS

        ● **T55.0X2**   Toxic effect of soaps, intentional self-harm 🖎

        ● **T55.0X3**   Toxic effect of soaps, assault 🖎

        ● **T55.0X4**   Toxic effect of soaps, undetermined 🖎

● **T55.1**   Toxic effect of detergents

    ● **T55.1X**   Toxic effect of detergents

        ● **T55.1X1**   Toxic effect of detergents, accidental (unintentional) 🖎

             Toxic effect of detergents NOS

        ● **T55.1X2**   Toxic effect of detergents, intentional self-harm 🖎

        ● **T55.1X3**   Toxic effect of detergents, assault 🖎

        ● **T55.1X4**   Toxic effect of detergents, undetermined 🖎

● **T56**   Toxic effect of metals

    Includes   toxic effects of fumes and vapors of metals

             toxic effects of metals from all sources, except medicinal substances

     Use additional code to identify any retained metal foreign body, if applicable (Z18.0-, T18.1-)

    Excludes1   arsenic and its compounds (T57.0)

             manganese and its compounds (T57.2)

     The appropriate 7th character is to be added to each code from category T56

A	initial encounter
D	subsequent encounter
S	sequela

● **T56.0**   Toxic effects of lead and its compounds

    ● **T56.0X**   Toxic effects of lead and its compounds

        ● **T56.0X1**   Toxic effect of lead and its compounds, accidental (unintentional) 🖎

             Toxic effects of lead and its compounds NOS

        ● **T56.0X2**   Toxic effect of lead and its compounds, intentional self-harm 🖎

        ● **T56.0X3**   Toxic effect of lead and its compounds, assault 🖎

        ● **T56.0X4**   Toxic effect of lead and its compounds, undetermined 🖎

● **T56.1**   Toxic effects of mercury and its compounds

    ● **T56.1X**   Toxic effects of mercury and its compounds

        ● **T56.1X1**   Toxic effect of mercury and its compounds, accidental (unintentional) 🖎

             Toxic effects of mercury and its compounds NOS

        ● **T56.1X2**   Toxic effect of mercury and its compounds, intentional self-harm 🖎

        ● **T56.1X3**   Toxic effect of mercury and its compounds, assault 🖎

        ● **T56.1X4**   Toxic effect of mercury and its compounds, undetermined 🖎

◄ New   ◄▬ Revised   ~~deleted~~ Deleted   Excludes 1   Excludes 2   Includes   Use additional   Code first   Code also   Unspecified

OGCR Official Guidelines   ● Unacceptable Principal Diagnosis   X Assign placeholder X   ▌ Use Additional Character(s)   ▌ Manifestation Code   **Coding Clinic**

● **T56.2**   Toxic effects of chromium and its compounds
   ● **T56.2X**   Toxic effects of chromium and its compounds
     ● **T56.2X1**   Toxic effect of chromium and its compounds, accidental (unintentional) 🗫
         Toxic effects of chromium and its compounds NOS
     ● **T56.2X2**   Toxic effect of chromium and its compounds, intentional self-harm 🗫
     ● **T56.2X3**   Toxic effect of chromium and its compounds, assault 🗫
     ● **T56.2X4**   Toxic effect of chromium and its compounds, undetermined 🗫

● **T56.3**   Toxic effects of cadmium and its compounds
   ● **T56.3X**   Toxic effects of cadmium and its compounds
     ● **T56.3X1**   Toxic effect of cadmium and its compounds, accidental (unintentional) 🗫
         Toxic effects of cadmium and its compounds NOS
     ● **T56.3X2**   Toxic effect of cadmium and its compounds, intentional self-harm 🗫
     ● **T56.3X3**   Toxic effect of cadmium and its compounds, assault 🗫
     ● **T56.3X4**   Toxic effect of cadmium and its compounds, undetermined 🗫

● **T56.4**   Toxic effects of copper and its compounds
   ● **T56.4X**   Toxic effects of copper and its compounds
     ● **T56.4X1**   Toxic effect of copper and its compounds, accidental (unintentional) 🗫
         Toxic effects of copper and its compounds NOS
     ● **T56.4X2**   Toxic effect of copper and its compounds, intentional self-harm 🗫
     ● **T56.4X3**   Toxic effect of copper and its compounds, assault 🗫
     ● **T56.4X4**   Toxic effect of copper and its compounds, undetermined 🗫

● **T56.5**   Toxic effects of zinc and its compounds
   ● **T56.5X**   Toxic effects of zinc and its compounds
     ● **T56.5X1**   Toxic effect of zinc and its compounds, accidental (unintentional) 🗫
         Toxic effects of zinc and its compounds NOS
     ● **T56.5X2**   Toxic effect of zinc and its compounds, intentional self-harm 🗫
     ● **T56.5X3**   Toxic effect of zinc and its compounds, assault 🗫
     ● **T56.5X4**   Toxic effect of zinc and its compounds, undetermined 🗫

● **T56.6**   Toxic effects of tin and its compounds
   ● **T56.6X**   Toxic effects of tin and its compounds
     ● **T56.6X1**   Toxic effect of tin and its compounds, accidental (unintentional) 🗫
         Toxic effects of tin and its compounds NOS
     ● **T56.6X2**   Toxic effect of tin and its compounds, intentional self-harm 🗫
     ● **T56.6X3**   Toxic effect of tin and its compounds, assault 🗫
     ● **T56.6X4**   Toxic effect of tin and its compounds, undetermined 🗫

● **T56.7**   Toxic effects of beryllium and its compounds
   ● **T56.7X**   Toxic effects of beryllium and its compounds
     ● **T56.7X1**   Toxic effect of beryllium and its compounds, accidental (unintentional) 🗫
         Toxic effects of beryllium and its compounds NOS
     ● **T56.7X2**   Toxic effect of beryllium and its compounds, intentional self-harm 🗫
     ● **T56.7X3**   Toxic effect of beryllium and its compounds, assault 🗫
     ● **T56.7X4**   Toxic effect of beryllium and its compounds, undetermined 🗫

● **T56.8**   Toxic effects of other metals
   ● **T56.81**   Toxic effect of thallium
     ● **T56.811**   Toxic effect of thallium, accidental (unintentional) 🗫
         Toxic effect of thallium NOS
     ● **T56.812**   Toxic effect of thallium, intentional self-harm 🗫
     ● **T56.813**   Toxic effect of thallium, assault 🗫
     ● **T56.814**   Toxic effect of thallium, undetermined 🗫
   ● **T56.89**   Toxic effects of other metals
     ● **T56.891**   Toxic effect of other metals, accidental (unintentional) 🗫
         Toxic effects of other metals NOS
     ● **T56.892**   Toxic effect of other metals, intentional self-harm 🗫
     ● **T56.893**   Toxic effect of other metals, assault 🗫
     ● **T56.894**   Toxic effect of other metals, undetermined 🗫

● **T56.9**   Toxic effects of unspecified metal
   X ● **T56.91**   Toxic effect of unspecified metal, accidental (unintentional) 🗫
   X ● **T56.92**   Toxic effect of unspecified metal, intentional self-harm 🗫
   X ● **T56.93**   Toxic effect of unspecified metal, assault 🗫
   X ● **T56.94**   Toxic effect of unspecified metal, undetermined 🗫

● **T57**   Toxic effect of other inorganic substances
   The appropriate 7th character is to be added to each code from category T57

> A   initial encounter
> D   subsequent encounter
> S   sequela

● **T57.0**   Toxic effect of arsenic and its compounds
   ● **T57.0X**   Toxic effect of arsenic and its compounds
     ● **T57.0X1**   Toxic effect of arsenic and its compounds, accidental (unintentional) 🗫
         Toxic effect of arsenic and its compounds NOS
     ● **T57.0X2**   Toxic effect of arsenic and its compounds, intentional self-harm 🗫
     ● **T57.0X3**   Toxic effect of arsenic and its compounds, assault 🗫
     ● **T57.0X4**   Toxic effect of arsenic and its compounds, undetermined 🗫

CHAPTER 19 (S00–T88)

N   Newborn Age: 0   P   Pediatric Age: 0–17   M   Maternity DX: 12–55   A   Adult Age: 15–124   ♀   Females Only   ♂   Males Only

🗫 Complication\Comorbidity   🗫 Major C\C   Ⓔⓧ CC/MCC Exclusions   🗫 Present on Admission Requirement   🗫 Hospital-Acquired Condition

1553

● **T57.1** Toxic effect of phosphorus and its compounds
　　Excludes1　organophosphate insecticides (T60.0)
　● **T57.1X** Toxic effect of phosphorus and its compounds
　　● **T57.1X1** Toxic effect of phosphorus and its compounds, accidental (unintentional) %
　　　　Toxic effect of phosphorus and its compounds NOS
　　● **T57.1X2** Toxic effect of phosphorus and its compounds, intentional self-harm %
　　● **T57.1X3** Toxic effect of phosphorus and its compounds, assault %
　　● **T57.1X4** Toxic effect of phosphorus and its compounds, undetermined %
● **T57.2** Toxic effect of manganese and its compounds
　● **T57.2X** Toxic effect of manganese and its compounds
　　● **T57.2X1** Toxic effect of manganese and its compounds, accidental (unintentional) %
　　　　Toxic effect of manganese and its compounds NOS
　　● **T57.2X2** Toxic effect of manganese and its compounds, intentional self-harm %
　　● **T57.2X3** Toxic effect of manganese and its compounds, assault %
　　● **T57.2X4** Toxic effect of manganese and its compounds, undetermined %
● **T57.3** Toxic effect of hydrogen cyanide
　● **T57.3X** Toxic effect of hydrogen cyanide
　　● **T57.3X1** Toxic effect of hydrogen cyanide, accidental (unintentional) %
　　　　Toxic effect of hydrogen cyanide NOS
　　● **T57.3X2** Toxic effect of hydrogen cyanide, intentional self-harm %
　　● **T57.3X3** Toxic effect of hydrogen cyanide, assault %
　　● **T57.3X4** Toxic effect of hydrogen cyanide, undetermined %
● **T57.8** Toxic effect of other specified inorganic substances
　● **T57.8X** Toxic effect of other specified inorganic substances
　　● **T57.8X1** Toxic effect of other specified inorganic substances, accidental (unintentional) %
　　　　Toxic effect of other specified inorganic substances NOS
　　● **T57.8X2** Toxic effect of other specified inorganic substances, intentional self-harm %
　　● **T57.8X3** Toxic effect of other specified inorganic substances, assault %
　　● **T57.8X4** Toxic effect of other specified inorganic substances, undetermined %
● **T57.9** Toxic effect of unspecified inorganic substance
　X● **T57.91** Toxic effect of unspecified inorganic substance, accidental (unintentional) %
　X● **T57.92** Toxic effect of unspecified inorganic substance, intentional self-harm %
　X● **T57.93** Toxic effect of unspecified inorganic substance, assault %
　X● **T57.94** Toxic effect of unspecified inorganic substance, undetermined %

● **T58** Toxic effect of carbon monoxide
　　Includes　asphyxiation from carbon monoxide
　　　　toxic effect of carbon monoxide from all sources
　　The appropriate 7th character is to be added to each code from category T58

A	initial encounter
D	subsequent encounter
S	sequela

● **T58.0** Toxic effect of carbon monoxide from motor vehicle exhaust
　　Toxic effect of exhaust gas from gas engine
　　Toxic effect of exhaust gas from motor pump
　X● **T58.01** Toxic effect of carbon monoxide from motor vehicle exhaust, accidental (unintentional) %
　X● **T58.02** Toxic effect of carbon monoxide from motor vehicle exhaust, intentional self-harm %
　X● **T58.03** Toxic effect of carbon monoxide from motor vehicle exhaust, assault %
　X● **T58.04** Toxic effect of carbon monoxide from motor vehicle exhaust, undetermined %
● **T58.1** Toxic effect of carbon monoxide from utility gas
　　Toxic effect of acetylene
　　Toxic effect of gas NOS used for lighting, heating, cooking
　　Toxic effect of water gas
　X● **T58.11** Toxic effect of carbon monoxide from utility gas, accidental (unintentional) %
　X● **T58.12** Toxic effect of carbon monoxide from utility gas, intentional self-harm %
　X● **T58.13** Toxic effect of carbon monoxide from utility gas, assault %
　X● **T58.14** Toxic effect of carbon monoxide from utility gas, undetermined %
● **T58.2** Toxic effect of carbon monoxide from incomplete combustion of other domestic fuels
　　Toxic effect of carbon monoxide from incomplete combustion of coal, coke, kerosene, wood
　● **T58.2X** Toxic effect of carbon monoxide from incomplete combustion of other domestic fuels
　　● **T58.2X1** Toxic effect of carbon monoxide from incomplete combustion of other domestic fuels, accidental (unintentional) %
　　● **T58.2X2** Toxic effect of carbon monoxide from incomplete combustion of other domestic fuels, intentional self-harm %
　　● **T58.2X3** Toxic effect of carbon monoxide from incomplete combustion of other domestic fuels, assault %
　　● **T58.2X4** Toxic effect of carbon monoxide from incomplete combustion of other domestic fuels, undetermined %
● **T58.8** Toxic effect of carbon monoxide from other source
　　Toxic effect of carbon monoxide from blast furnace gas
　　Toxic effect of carbon monoxide from fuels in industrial use
　　Toxic effect of carbon monoxide from kiln vapor
　● **T58.8X** Toxic effect of carbon monoxide from other source
　　● **T58.8X1** Toxic effect of carbon monoxide from other source, accidental (unintentional) %
　　● **T58.8X2** Toxic effect of carbon monoxide from other source, intentional self-harm %
　　● **T58.8X3** Toxic effect of carbon monoxide from other source, assault %
　　● **T58.8X4** Toxic effect of carbon monoxide from other source, undetermined %

◀ New　◀ Revised　~~deleted~~ Deleted　Excludes 1　Excludes 2　Includes　Use additional　Code first　Code also　Unspecified
OGCR Official Guidelines　● Unacceptable Principal Diagnosis　X Assign placeholder X　● Use Additional Character(s)　❱ Manifestation Code　Coding Clinic

● **T58.9**   Toxic effect of carbon monoxide from unspecified source

    X ● **T58.91**   Toxic effect of carbon monoxide from <mark>unspecified</mark> source, accidental (unintentional) 🔍

    X ● **T58.92**   Toxic effect of carbon monoxide from <mark>unspecified</mark> source, intentional self-harm 🔍

    X ● **T58.93**   Toxic effect of carbon monoxide from <mark>unspecified</mark> source, assault 🔍

    X ● **T58.94**   Toxic effect of carbon monoxide from <mark>unspecified</mark> source, undetermined 🔍

● **T59**   Toxic effect of other gases, fumes and vapors

    Includes   aerosol propellants

    Excludes1   chlorofluorocarbons (T53.5)

    The appropriate 7th character is to be added to each code from category T59

      A   initial encounter
      D   subsequent encounter
      S   sequela

● **T59.0**   Toxic effect of nitrogen oxides

    ● **T59.0X**   Toxic effect of nitrogen oxides

      ● **T59.0X1**   Toxic effect of nitrogen oxides, accidental (unintentional) 🔍
        Toxic effect of nitrogen oxides NOS

      ● **T59.0X2**   Toxic effect of nitrogen oxides, intentional self-harm 🔍

      ● **T59.0X3**   Toxic effect of nitrogen oxides, assault 🔍

      ● **T59.0X4**   Toxic effect of nitrogen oxides, undetermined 🔍

● **T59.1**   Toxic effect of sulfur dioxide

    ● **T59.1X**   Toxic effect of sulfur dioxide

      ● **T59.1X1**   Toxic effect of sulfur dioxide, accidental (unintentional) 🔍
        Toxic effect of sulfur dioxide NOS

      ● **T59.1X2**   Toxic effect of sulfur dioxide, intentional self-harm 🔍

      ● **T59.1X3**   Toxic effect of sulfur dioxide, assault 🔍

      ● **T59.1X4**   Toxic effect of sulfur dioxide, undetermined 🔍

● **T59.2**   Toxic effect of formaldehyde

    ● **T59.2X**   Toxic effect of formaldehyde

      ● **T59.2X1**   Toxic effect of formaldehyde, accidental (unintentional) 🔍
        Toxic effect of formaldehyde NOS

      ● **T59.2X2**   Toxic effect of formaldehyde, intentional self-harm 🔍

      ● **T59.2X3**   Toxic effect of formaldehyde, assault 🔍

      ● **T59.2X4**   Toxic effect of formaldehyde, undetermined 🔍

● **T59.3**   Toxic effect of lacrimogenic gas
    Toxic effect of tear gas

    ● **T59.3X**   Toxic effect of lacrimogenic gas

      ● **T59.3X1**   Toxic effect of lacrimogenic gas, accidental (unintentional) 🔍
        Toxic effect of lacrimogenic gas NOS

      ● **T59.3X2**   Toxic effect of lacrimogenic gas, intentional self-harm 🔍

      ● **T59.3X3**   Toxic effect of lacrimogenic gas, assault 🔍

      ● **T59.3X4**   Toxic effect of lacrimogenic gas, undetermined 🔍

● **T59.4**   Toxic effect of chlorine gas

    ● **T59.4X**   Toxic effect of chlorine gas

      ● **T59.4X1**   Toxic effect of chlorine gas, accidental (unintentional) 🔍
        Toxic effect of chlorine gas NOS

      ● **T59.4X2**   Toxic effect of chlorine gas, intentional self-harm 🔍

      ● **T59.4X3**   Toxic effect of chlorine gas, assault 🔍

      ● **T59.4X4**   Toxic effect of chlorine gas, undetermined 🔍

● **T59.5**   Toxic effect of fluorine gas and hydrogen fluoride

    ● **T59.5X**   Toxic effect of fluorine gas and hydrogen fluoride

      ● **T59.5X1**   Toxic effect of fluorine gas and hydrogen fluoride, accidental (unintentional) 🔍
        Toxic effect of fluorine gas and hydrogen fluoride NOS

      ● **T59.5X2**   Toxic effect of fluorine gas and hydrogen fluoride, intentional self-harm 🔍

      ● **T59.5X3**   Toxic effect of fluorine gas and hydrogen fluoride, assault 🔍

      ● **T59.5X4**   Toxic effect of fluorine gas and hydrogen fluoride, undetermined 🔍

● **T59.6**   Toxic effect of hydrogen sulfide

    ● **T59.6X**   Toxic effect of hydrogen sulfide

      ● **T59.6X1**   Toxic effect of hydrogen sulfide, accidental (unintentional) 🔍
        Toxic effect of hydrogen sulfide NOS

      ● **T59.6X2**   Toxic effect of hydrogen sulfide, intentional self-harm 🔍

      ● **T59.6X3**   Toxic effect of hydrogen sulfide, assault 🔍

      ● **T59.6X4**   Toxic effect of hydrogen sulfide, undetermined 🔍

● **T59.7**   Toxic effect of carbon dioxide

    ● **T59.7X**   Toxic effect of carbon dioxide

      ● **T59.7X1**   Toxic effect of carbon dioxide, accidental (unintentional) 🔍
        Toxic effect of carbon dioxide NOS

      ● **T59.7X2**   Toxic effect of carbon dioxide, intentional self-harm 🔍

      ● **T59.7X3**   Toxic effect of carbon dioxide, assault 🔍

      ● **T59.7X4**   Toxic effect of carbon dioxide, undetermined 🔍

● **T59.8**   Toxic effect of other specified gases, fumes and vapors

    ● **T59.81**   Toxic effect of smoke
      Smoke inhalation

      Excludes2   toxic effect of cigarette (tobacco) smoke (T65.22-)

      ● **T59.811**   Toxic effect of smoke, accidental (unintentional) 🔍
        Toxic effect of smoke NOS

      ● **T59.812**   Toxic effect of smoke, intentional self-harm 🔍

      ● **T59.813**   Toxic effect of smoke, assault 🔍

      ● **T59.814**   Toxic effect of smoke, undetermined 🔍

    ● **T59.89**   Toxic effect of other specified gases, fumes and vapors

      ● **T59.891**   Toxic effect of other specified gases, fumes and vapors, accidental (unintentional) 🔍

      ● **T59.892**   Toxic effect of other specified gases, fumes and vapors, intentional self-harm 🔍

      ● **T59.893**   Toxic effect of other specified gases, fumes and vapors, assault 🔍

      ● **T59.894**   Toxic effect of other specified gases, fumes and vapors, undetermined 🔍

N   Newborn Age: 0   P   Pediatric Age: 0–17   M   Maternity DX: 12–55   A   Adult Age: 15–124   ♀   Females Only   ♂   Males Only

🔍 Complication\Comorbidity   🔍 Major C\C   (Ex) CC/MCC Exclusions   🔍 Present on Admission Requirement   🔍 Hospital-Acquired Condition

CHAPTER 19 (S00-T88)

● T59.9   Toxic effect of unspecified gases, fumes and vapors

   X ● T59.91   Toxic effect of unspecified gases, fumes and vapors, accidental (unintentional) 🔍

   X ● T59.92   Toxic effect of unspecified gases, fumes and vapors, intentional self-harm 🔍

   X ● T59.93   Toxic effect of unspecified gases, fumes and vapors, assault 🔍

   X ● T59.94   Toxic effect of unspecified gases, fumes and vapors, undetermined 🔍

● T60   Toxic effect of pesticides

   Includes   toxic effect of wood preservatives

   The appropriate 7th character is to be added to each code from category T60

     A   initial encounter
     D   subsequent encounter
     S   sequela

● T60.0   Toxic effect of organophosphate and carbamate insecticides

   ● T60.0X   Toxic effect of organophosphate and carbamate insecticides

     ● T60.0X1   Toxic effect of organophosphate and carbamate insecticides, accidental (unintentional) 🔍
         Toxic effect of organophosphate and carbamate insecticides NOS

     ● T60.0X2   Toxic effect of organophosphate and carbamate insecticides, intentional self-harm 🔍

     ● T60.0X3   Toxic effect of organophosphate and carbamate insecticides, assault 🔍

     ● T60.0X4   Toxic effect of organophosphate and carbamate insecticides, undetermined 🔍

● T60.1   Toxic effect of halogenated insecticides

   Excludes1   chlorinated hydrocarbon (T53.-)

   ● T60.1X   Toxic effect of halogenated insecticides

     ● T60.1X1   Toxic effect of halogenated insecticides, accidental (unintentional) 🔍
         Toxic effect of halogenated insecticides NOS

     ● T60.1X2   Toxic effect of halogenated insecticides, intentional self-harm 🔍

     ● T60.1X3   Toxic effect of halogenated insecticides, assault 🔍

     ● T60.1X4   Toxic effect of halogenated insecticides, undetermined 🔍

● T60.2   Toxic effect of other insecticides

   ● T60.2X   Toxic effect of other insecticides

     ● T60.2X1   Toxic effect of other insecticides, accidental (unintentional) 🔍
         Toxic effect of other insecticides NOS

     ● T60.2X2   Toxic effect of other insecticides, intentional self-harm 🔍

     ● T60.2X3   Toxic effect of other insecticides, assault 🔍

     ● T60.2X4   Toxic effect of other insecticides, undetermined 🔍

● T60.3   Toxic effect of herbicides and fungicides

   ● T60.3X   Toxic effect of herbicides and fungicides

     ● T60.3X1   Toxic effect of herbicides and fungicides, accidental (unintentional) 🔍
         Toxic effect of herbicides and fungicides NOS

     ● T60.3X2   Toxic effect of herbicides and fungicides, intentional self-harm 🔍

     ● T60.3X3   Toxic effect of herbicides and fungicides, assault 🔍

     ● T60.3X4   Toxic effect of herbicides and fungicides, undetermined 🔍

● T60.4   Toxic effect of rodenticides

   Excludes1   strychnine and its salts (T65.1)
         thallium (T56.81-)

   ● T60.4X   Toxic effect of rodenticides

     ● T60.4X1   Toxic effect of rodenticides, accidental (unintentional) 🔍
         Toxic effect of rodenticides NOS

     ● T60.4X2   Toxic effect of rodenticides, intentional self-harm 🔍

     ● T60.4X3   Toxic effect of rodenticides, assault 🔍

     ● T60.4X4   Toxic effect of rodenticides, undetermined 🔍

● T60.8   Toxic effect of other pesticides

   ● T60.8X   Toxic effect of other pesticides

     ● T60.8X1   Toxic effect of other pesticides, accidental (unintentional) 🔍
         Toxic effect of other pesticides NOS

     ● T60.8X2   Toxic effect of other pesticides, intentional self-harm 🔍

     ● T60.8X3   Toxic effect of other pesticides, assault 🔍

     ● T60.8X4   Toxic effect of other pesticides, undetermined 🔍

● T60.9   Toxic effect of unspecified pesticide

   ● T60.91   Toxic effect of unspecified pesticide, accidental (unintentional) 🔍

   ● T60.92   Toxic effect of unspecified pesticide, intentional self-harm 🔍

   ● T60.93   Toxic effect of unspecified pesticide, assault 🔍

   ● T60.94   Toxic effect of unspecified pesticide, undetermined 🔍

● T61   Toxic effect of noxious substances eaten as seafood

   Excludes1   allergic reaction to food, such as:
         anaphylactic reaction or shock due to adverse food reaction (T78.0-)
         bacterial foodborne intoxications (A05.-)
         dermatitis (L23.6, L25.4, L27.2)
         gastroenteritis (noninfective) (K52.2)
         ~~anaphylactic shock (T78.02, T78.05)~~
         toxic effect of aflatoxin and other mycotoxins (T64) ◀▥
         ~~aflatoxin and other mycotoxins (T64)~~
         toxic effect of cyanides (T65.0-) ◀▥
         toxic effect of harmful algae bloom (T65.82-) ◀▥
         toxic effect of hydrogen cyanide (T57.3-) ◀▥
         toxic effect of mercury (T56.1-) ◀▥
         toxic effect of red tide (T65.82-) ◀▥

   The appropriate 7th character is to be added to each code from category T61

     A   initial encounter
     D   subsequent encounter
     S   sequela

● T61.0   Ciguatera fish poisoning

   X ● T61.01   Ciguatera fish poisoning, accidental (unintentional) 🔍

   X ● T61.02   Ciguatera fish poisoning, intentional self-harm 🔍

   X ● T61.03   Ciguatera fish poisoning, assault 🔍

   X ● T61.04   Ciguatera fish poisoning, undetermined 🔍

● T61.1   Scombroid fish poisoning
   Histamine-like syndrome

   X ● T61.11   Scombroid fish poisoning, accidental (unintentional) 🔍

   X ● T61.12   Scombroid fish poisoning, intentional self-harm 🔍

   X ● T61.13   Scombroid fish poisoning, assault 🔍

   X ● T61.14   Scombroid fish poisoning, undetermined 🔍

◀ New   ◀▥ Revised   ~~deleted~~ Deleted   Excludes 1   Excludes 2   Includes   Use additional   Code first   Code also   Unspecified

OGCR Official Guidelines   ● Unacceptable Principal Diagnosis   X Assign placeholder X   🔍 Use Additional Character(s)   ▌ Manifestation Code   **Coding Clinic**

● **T61.7**   **Other fish and shellfish poisoning**
   ● **T61.77**   **Other fish poisoning**
      ● **T61.771**   **Other fish poisoning, accidental (unintentional)** 🖐
      ● **T61.772**   **Other fish poisoning, intentional self-harm** 🖐
      ● **T61.773**   **Other fish poisoning, assault** 🖐
      ● **T61.774**   **Other fish poisoning, undetermined** 🖐
   ● **T61.78**   **Other shellfish poisoning**
      ● **T61.781**   **Other shellfish poisoning, accidental (unintentional)** 🖐
      ● **T61.782**   **Other shellfish poisoning, intentional self-harm** 🖐
      ● **T61.783**   **Other shellfish poisoning, assault** 🖐
      ● **T61.784**   **Other shellfish poisoning, undetermined** 🖐
● **T61.8**   **Toxic effect of other seafood**
   ● **T61.8X**   **Toxic effect of other seafood**
      ● **T61.8X1**   **Toxic effect of other seafood, accidental (unintentional)** 🖐
      ● **T61.8X2**   **Toxic effect of other seafood, intentional self-harm** 🖐
      ● **T61.8X3**   **Toxic effect of other seafood, assault** 🖐
      ● **T61.8X4**   **Toxic effect of other seafood, undetermined** 🖐
● **T61.9**   **Toxic effect of unspecified seafood**
   X ● **T61.91**   **Toxic effect of unspecified seafood, accidental (unintentional)** 🖐
   X ● **T61.92**   **Toxic effect of unspecified seafood, intentional self-harm** 🖐
   X ● **T61.93**   **Toxic effect of unspecified seafood, assault** 🖐
   X ● **T61.94**   **Toxic effect of unspecified seafood, undetermined** 🖐

● **T62**   **Toxic effect of other noxious substances eaten as food**

   Excludes1   allergic reaction to food, such as:
          anaphylactic shock (reaction) due to adverse food reaction (T78.0-)
          dermatitis (L23.6, L25.4, L27.2)
          gastroenteritis (noninfective) (K52.2)
          bacterial food borne intoxications (A05.-)
       toxic effect of ~~food contaminants, such as~~ aflatoxin and other mycotoxins (T64) ⬅
          ~~aflatoxin and other mycotoxins (T64)~~
       toxic effect of cyanides (T65.0-) ⬅
       toxic effect of hydrogen cyanide (T57.3-) ⬅
       toxic effect of mercury (T56.1-) ⬅

   The appropriate 7th character is to be added to each code from category T62

A	initial encounter
D	subsequent encounter
S	sequela

● **T62.0**   **Toxic effect of ingested mushrooms**
   ● **T62.0X**   **Toxic effect of ingested mushrooms**
      ● **T62.0X1**   **Toxic effect of ingested mushrooms, accidental (unintentional)** 🖐
          Toxic effect of ingested mushrooms NOS
      ● **T62.0X2**   **Toxic effect of ingested mushrooms, intentional self-harm** 🖐
      ● **T62.0X3**   **Toxic effect of ingested mushrooms, assault** 🖐
      ● **T62.0X4**   **Toxic effect of ingested mushrooms, undetermined** 🖐

● **T62.1**   **Toxic effect of ingested berries**
   ● **T62.1X**   **Toxic effect of ingested berries**
      ● **T62.1X1**   **Toxic effect of ingested berries, accidental (unintentional)** 🖐
          Toxic effect of ingested berries NOS
      ● **T62.1X2**   **Toxic effect of ingested berries, intentional self-harm** 🖐
      ● **T62.1X3**   **Toxic effect of ingested berries, assault** 🖐
      ● **T62.1X4**   **Toxic effect of ingested berries, undetermined** 🖐
● **T62.2**   **Toxic effect of other ingested (parts of) plant(s)**
   ● **T62.2X**   **Toxic effect of other ingested (parts of) plant(s)**
      ● **T62.2X1**   **Toxic effect of other ingested (parts of) plant(s), accidental (unintentional)** 🖐
          Toxic effect of other ingested (parts of) plant(s) NOS
      ● **T62.2X2**   **Toxic effect of other ingested (parts of) plant(s), intentional self-harm** 🖐
      ● **T62.2X3**   **Toxic effect of other ingested (parts of) plant(s), assault** 🖐
      ● **T62.2X4**   **Toxic effect of other ingested (parts of) plant(s), undetermined** 🖐
● **T62.8**   **Toxic effect of other specified noxious substances eaten as food**
   ● **T62.8X**   **Toxic effect of other specified noxious substances eaten as food**
      ● **T62.8X1**   **Toxic effect of other specified noxious substances eaten as food, accidental (unintentional)** 🖐
          Toxic effect of other specified noxious substances eaten as food NOS
      ● **T62.8X2**   **Toxic effect of other specified noxious substances eaten as food, intentional self-harm** 🖐
      ● **T62.8X3**   **Toxic effect of other specified noxious substances eaten as food, assault** 🖐
      ● **T62.8X4**   **Toxic effect of other specified noxious substances eaten as food, undetermined** 🖐
● **T62.9**   **Toxic effect of unspecified noxious substance eaten as food**
   X ● **T62.91**   **Toxic effect of unspecified noxious substance eaten as food, accidental (unintentional)** 🖐
          Toxic effect of unspecified noxious substance eaten as food NOS
   X ● **T62.92**   **Toxic effect of unspecified noxious substance eaten as food, intentional self-harm** 🖐
   X ● **T62.93**   **Toxic effect of unspecified noxious substance eaten as food, assault** 🖐
   X ● **T62.94**   **Toxic effect of unspecified noxious substance eaten as food, undetermined** 🖐

● **T63**   **Toxic effect of contact with venomous animals and plants**

   Includes   bite or touch of venomous animal
          pricked or stuck by thorn or leaf

   Excludes2   ingestion of toxic animal or plant (T61.-, T62.-)

   The appropriate 7th character is to be added to each code from category T63

A	initial encounter
D	subsequent encounter
S	sequela

● **T63.0**   **Toxic effect of snake venom**
   ● **T63.00**   **Toxic effect of unspecified snake venom**
      ● **T63.001**   **Toxic effect of unspecified snake venom, accidental (unintentional)** 🖐
          Toxic effect of unspecified snake venom NOS
      ● **T63.002**   **Toxic effect of unspecified snake venom, intentional self-harm** 🖐

N Newborn Age: 0   **P** Pediatric Age: 0–17   **M** Maternity DX: 12–55   **A** Adult Age: 15–124   ♀ Females Only   ♂ Males Only

🖐 Complication\Comorbidity   🖐 Major C\C   (Ex) CC/MCC Exclusions   🖐 Present on Admission Requirement   🖐 Hospital-Acquired Condition

1557

CHAPTER 19 (S00–T88)

● T63.003   Toxic effect of unspecified snake venom, assault 🖉

● T63.004   Toxic effect of unspecified snake venom, undetermined 🖉

● T63.01   Toxic effect of rattlesnake venom

● T63.011   Toxic effect of rattlesnake venom, accidental (unintentional) 🖉
     Toxic effect of rattlesnake venom NOS

● T63.012   Toxic effect of rattlesnake venom, intentional self-harm 🖉

● T63.013   Toxic effect of rattlesnake venom, assault 🖉

● T63.014   Toxic effect of rattlesnake venom, undetermined 🖉

● T63.02   Toxic effect of coral snake venom

● T63.021   Toxic effect of coral snake venom, accidental (unintentional) 🖉
     Toxic effect of coral snake venom NOS

● T63.022   Toxic effect of coral snake venom, intentional self-harm 🖉

● T63.023   Toxic effect of coral snake venom, assault 🖉

● T63.024   Toxic effect of coral snake venom, undetermined 🖉

● T63.03   Toxic effect of taipan venom

● T63.031   Toxic effect of taipan venom, accidental (unintentional) 🖉
     Toxic effect of taipan venom NOS

● T63.032   Toxic effect of taipan venom, intentional self-harm 🖉

● T63.033   Toxic effect of taipan venom, assault 🖉

● T63.034   Toxic effect of taipan venom, undetermined 🖉

● T63.04   Toxic effect of cobra venom

● T63.041   Toxic effect of cobra venom, accidental (unintentional) 🖉
     Toxic effect of cobra venom NOS

● T63.042   Toxic effect of cobra venom, intentional self-harm 🖉

● T63.043   Toxic effect of cobra venom, assault 🖉

● T63.044   Toxic effect of cobra venom, undetermined 🖉

● T63.06   Toxic effect of venom of other North and South American snake

● T63.061   Toxic effect of venom of other North and South American snake, accidental (unintentional) 🖉
     Toxic effect of venom of other North and South American snake NOS

● T63.062   Toxic effect of venom of other North and South American snake, intentional self-harm 🖉

● T63.063   Toxic effect of venom of other North and South American snake, assault 🖉

● T63.064   Toxic effect of venom of other North and South American snake, undetermined 🖉

● T63.07   Toxic effect of venom of other Australian snake

● T63.071   Toxic effect of venom of other Australian snake, accidental (unintentional) 🖉
     Toxic effect of venom of other Australian snake NOS

● T63.072   Toxic effect of venom of other Australian snake, intentional self-harm 🖉

● T63.073   Toxic effect of venom of other Australian snake, assault 🖉

● T63.074   Toxic effect of venom of other Australian snake, undetermined 🖉

● T63.08   Toxic effect of venom of other African and Asian snake

● T63.081   Toxic effect of venom of other African and Asian snake, accidental (unintentional) 🖉
     Toxic effect of venom of other African and Asian snake NOS

● T63.082   Toxic effect of venom of other African and Asian snake, intentional self-harm 🖉

● T63.083   Toxic effect of venom of other African and Asian snake, assault 🖉

● T63.084   Toxic effect of venom of other African and Asian snake, undetermined 🖉

● T63.09   Toxic effect of venom of other snake

● T63.091   Toxic effect of venom of other snake, accidental (unintentional) 🖉
     Toxic effect of venom of other snake NOS

● T63.092   Toxic effect of venom of other snake, intentional self-harm 🖉

● T63.093   Toxic effect of venom of other snake, assault 🖉

● T63.094   Toxic effect of venom of other snake, undetermined 🖉

● T63.1   Toxic effect of venom of other reptiles

● T63.11   Toxic effect of venom of gila monster

● T63.111   Toxic effect of venom of gila monster, accidental (unintentional) 🖉
     Toxic effect of venom of gila monster NOS

● T63.112   Toxic effect of venom of gila monster, intentional self-harm 🖉

● T63.113   Toxic effect of venom of gila monster, assault 🖉

● T63.114   Toxic effect of venom of gila monster, undetermined 🖉

● T63.12   Toxic effect of venom of other venomous lizard

● T63.121   Toxic effect of venom of other venomous lizard, accidental (unintentional) 🖉
     Toxic effect of venom of other venomous lizard NOS

● T63.122   Toxic effect of venom of other venomous lizard, intentional self-harm 🖉

● T63.123   Toxic effect of venom of other venomous lizard, assault 🖉

● T63.124   Toxic effect of venom of other venomous lizard, undetermined 🖉

● T63.19   Toxic effect of venom of other reptiles

● T63.191   Toxic effect of venom of other reptiles, accidental (unintentional) 🖉
     Toxic effect of venom of other reptiles NOS

● T63.192   Toxic effect of venom of other reptiles, intentional self-harm 🖉

● T63.193   Toxic effect of venom of other reptiles, assault 🖉

● T63.194   Toxic effect of venom of other reptiles, undetermined 🖉

◀ New   ◀▥ Revised   ~~deleted~~ Deleted   Excludes 1   Excludes 2   Includes   Use additional   Code first   Code also   Unspecified

OGCR Official Guidelines   ● Unacceptable Principal Diagnosis   X Assign placeholder X   ● Use Additional Character(s)   ▶ Manifestation Code   **Coding Clinic**

- T63.2   Toxic effect of venom of scorpion
    - T63.2X   Toxic effect of venom of scorpion
        - T63.2X1   Toxic effect of venom of scorpion, accidental (unintentional) 🐾
            Toxic effect of venom of scorpion NOS
        - T63.2X2   Toxic effect of venom of scorpion, intentional self-harm 🐾
        - T63.2X3   Toxic effect of venom of scorpion, assault 🐾
        - T63.2X4   Toxic effect of venom of scorpion, undetermined 🐾
- T63.3   Toxic effect of venom of spider
    - T63.30   Toxic effect of unspecified spider venom
        - T63.301   Toxic effect of unspecified spider venom, accidental (unintentional) 🐾
        - T63.302   Toxic effect of unspecified spider venom, intentional self-harm 🐾
        - T63.303   Toxic effect of unspecified spider venom, assault 🐾
        - T63.304   Toxic effect of unspecified spider venom, undetermined 🐾
    - T63.31   Toxic effect of venom of black widow spider
        - T63.311   Toxic effect of venom of black widow spider, accidental (unintentional) 🐾
        - T63.312   Toxic effect of venom of black widow spider, intentional self-harm 🐾
        - T63.313   Toxic effect of venom of black widow spider, assault 🐾
        - T63.314   Toxic effect of venom of black widow spider, undetermined 🐾
    - T63.32   Toxic effect of venom of tarantula
        - T63.321   Toxic effect of venom of tarantula, accidental (unintentional) 🐾
        - T63.322   Toxic effect of venom of tarantula, intentional self-harm 🐾
        - T63.323   Toxic effect of venom of tarantula, assault 🐾
        - T63.324   Toxic effect of venom of tarantula, undetermined 🐾
    - T63.33   Toxic effect of venom of brown recluse spider
        - T63.331   Toxic effect of venom of brown recluse spider, accidental (unintentional) 🐾
        - T63.332   Toxic effect of venom of brown recluse spider, intentional self-harm 🐾
        - T63.333   Toxic effect of venom of brown recluse spider, assault 🐾
        - T63.334   Toxic effect of venom of brown recluse spider, undetermined 🐾
    - T63.39   Toxic effect of venom of other spider
        - T63.391   Toxic effect of venom of other spider, accidental (unintentional) 🐾
        - T63.392   Toxic effect of venom of other spider, intentional self-harm 🐾
        - T63.393   Toxic effect of venom of other spider, assault 🐾
        - T63.394   Toxic effect of venom of other spider, undetermined 🐾
- T63.4   Toxic effect of venom of other arthropods
    - T63.41   Toxic effect of venom of centipedes and venomous millipedes
        - T63.411   Toxic effect of venom of centipedes and venomous millipedes, accidental (unintentional) 🐾
        - T63.412   Toxic effect of venom of centipedes and venomous millipedes, intentional self-harm 🐾
        - T63.413   Toxic effect of venom of centipedes and venomous millipedes, assault 🐾
        - T63.414   Toxic effect of venom of centipedes and venomous millipedes, undetermined 🐾
    - T63.42   Toxic effect of venom of ants
        - T63.421   Toxic effect of venom of ants, accidental (unintentional) 🐾
        - T63.422   Toxic effect of venom of ants, intentional self-harm 🐾
        - T63.423   Toxic effect of venom of ants, assault 🐾
        - T63.424   Toxic effect of venom of ants, undetermined 🐾
    - T63.43   Toxic effect of venom of caterpillars
        - T63.431   Toxic effect of venom of caterpillars, accidental (unintentional) 🐾
        - T63.432   Toxic effect of venom of caterpillars, intentional self-harm 🐾
        - T63.433   Toxic effect of venom of caterpillars, assault 🐾
        - T63.434   Toxic effect of venom of caterpillars, undetermined 🐾
    - T63.44   Toxic effect of venom of bees
        - T63.441   Toxic effect of venom of bees, accidental (unintentional) 🐾
        - T63.442   Toxic effect of venom of bees, intentional self-harm 🐾
        - T63.443   Toxic effect of venom of bees, assault 🐾
        - T63.444   Toxic effect of venom of bees, undetermined 🐾
    - T63.45   Toxic effect of venom of hornets
        - T63.451   Toxic effect of venom of hornets, accidental (unintentional) 🐾
        - T63.452   Toxic effect of venom of hornets, intentional self-harm 🐾
        - T63.453   Toxic effect of venom of hornets, assault 🐾
        - T63.454   Toxic effect of venom of hornets, undetermined 🐾
    - T63.46   Toxic effect of venom of wasps
        Toxic effect of yellow jacket
        - T63.461   Toxic effect of venom of wasps, accidental (unintentional) 🐾
        - T63.462   Toxic effect of venom of wasps, intentional self-harm 🐾
        - T63.463   Toxic effect of venom of wasps, assault 🐾
        - T63.464   Toxic effect of venom of wasps, undetermined 🐾

CHAPTER 19 (S00-T88)

N Newborn Age: 0   **P** Pediatric Age: 0–17   **M** Maternity DX: 12–55   **A** Adult Age: 15–124   ♀ Females Only   ♂ Males Only

🐾 Complication\Comorbidity   🐾 Major C\C   Ⓔⓧ CC/MCC Exclusions   🐾 Present on Admission Requirement   🐾 Hospital-Acquired Condition

1559

● T63.48 Toxic effect of venom of other arthropod
  ● T63.481 Toxic effect of venom of other arthropod, accidental (unintentional) ⊗
  ● T63.482 Toxic effect of venom of other arthropod, intentional self-harm ⊗
  ● T63.483 Toxic effect of venom of other arthropod, assault ⊗
  ● T63.484 Toxic effect of venom of other arthropod, undetermined ⊗
● T63.5 Toxic effect of contact with venomous fish
    Excludes2 poisoning by ingestion of fish (T61.-) ◀
  ● T63.51 Toxic effect of contact with stingray
    ● T63.511 Toxic effect of contact with stingray, accidental (unintentional) ⊗
    ● T63.512 Toxic effect of contact with stingray, intentional self-harm ⊗
    ● T63.513 Toxic effect of contact with stingray, assault ⊗
    ● T63.514 Toxic effect of contact with stingray, undetermined ⊗
  ● T63.59 Toxic effect of contact with other venomous fish
    ● T63.591 Toxic effect of contact with other venomous fish, accidental (unintentional) ⊗
    ● T63.592 Toxic effect of contact with other venomous fish, intentional self-harm ⊗
    ● T63.593 Toxic effect of contact with other venomous fish, assault ⊗
    ● T63.594 Toxic effect of contact with other venomous fish, undetermined ⊗
● T63.6 Toxic effect of contact with other venomous marine animals
    Excludes1 sea-snake venom (T63.09)
    Excludes2 poisoning by ingestion of shellfish (T61.78-)
  ● T63.61 Toxic effect of contact with Portugese Man-o-war
    Toxic effect of contact with bluebottle
    ● T63.611 Toxic effect of contact with Portugese Man-o-war, accidental (unintentional) ⊗
    ● T63.612 Toxic effect of contact with Portugese Man-o-war, intentional self-harm ⊗
    ● T63.613 Toxic effect of contact with Portugese Man-o-war, assault ⊗
    ● T63.614 Toxic effect of contact with Portugese Man-o-war, undetermined ⊗
  ● T63.62 Toxic effect of contact with other jellyfish
    ● T63.621 Toxic effect of contact with other jellyfish, accidental (unintentional) ⊗
    ● T63.622 Toxic effect of contact with other jellyfish, intentional self-harm ⊗
    ● T63.623 Toxic effect of contact with other jellyfish, assault ⊗
    ● T63.624 Toxic effect of contact with other jellyfish, undetermined ⊗
  ● T63.63 Toxic effect of contact with sea anemone
    ● T63.631 Toxic effect of contact with sea anemone, accidental (unintentional) ⊗
    ● T63.632 Toxic effect of contact with sea anemone, intentional self-harm ⊗
    ● T63.633 Toxic effect of contact with sea anemone, assault ⊗
    ● T63.634 Toxic effect of contact with sea anemone, undetermined ⊗

● T63.69 Toxic effect of contact with other venomous marine animals
  ● T63.691 Toxic effect of contact with other venomous marine animals, accidental (unintentional) ⊗
  ● T63.692 Toxic effect of contact with other venomous marine animals, intentional self-harm ⊗
  ● T63.693 Toxic effect of contact with other venomous marine animals, assault ⊗
  ● T63.694 Toxic effect of contact with other venomous marine animals, undetermined ⊗
● T63.7 Toxic effect of contact with venomous plant
  ● T63.71 Toxic effect of contact with venomous marine plant
    ● T63.711 Toxic effect of contact with venomous marine plant, accidental (unintentional) ⊗
    ● T63.712 Toxic effect of contact with venomous marine plant, intentional self-harm ⊗
    ● T63.713 Toxic effect of contact with venomous marine plant, assault ⊗
    ● T63.714 Toxic effect of contact with venomous marine plant, undetermined ⊗
  ● T63.79 Toxic effect of contact with other venomous plant
    ● T63.791 Toxic effect of contact with other venomous plant, accidental (unintentional) ⊗
    ● T63.792 Toxic effect of contact with other venomous plant, intentional self-harm ⊗
    ● T63.793 Toxic effect of contact with other venomous plant, assault ⊗
    ● T63.794 Toxic effect of contact with other venomous plant, undetermined ⊗
● T63.8 Toxic effect of contact with other venomous animals
  ● T63.81 Toxic effect of contact with venomous frog
    Excludes1 contact with nonvenomous frog (W62.0)
    ● T63.811 Toxic effect of contact with venomous frog, accidental (unintentional) ⊗
    ● T63.812 Toxic effect of contact with venomous frog, intentional self-harm ⊗
    ● T63.813 Toxic effect of contact with venomous frog, assault ⊗
    ● T63.814 Toxic effect of contact with venomous frog, undetermined ⊗
  ● T63.82 Toxic effect of contact with venomous toad
    Excludes1 contact with nonvenomous toad (W62.1)
    ● T63.821 Toxic effect of contact with venomous toad, accidental (unintentional) ⊗
    ● T63.822 Toxic effect of contact with venomous toad, intentional self-harm ⊗
    ● T63.823 Toxic effect of contact with venomous toad, assault ⊗
    ● T63.824 Toxic effect of contact with venomous toad, undetermined ⊗

◀ New ◀ Revised ~~deleted~~ Deleted | Excludes 1 | Excludes 2 | Includes | Use additional | Code first | Code also | Unspecified
OGCR Official Guidelines ● Unacceptable Principal Diagnosis X Assign placeholder X ⊗ Use Additional Character(s) ▌ Manifestation Code **Coding Clinic**

● **T63.83** Toxic effect of contact with other venomous amphibian

> **Excludes1** contact with nonvenomous amphibian (W62.9)

  ● **T63.831** Toxic effect of contact with other venomous amphibian, accidental (unintentional) 🐾

  ● **T63.832** Toxic effect of contact with other venomous amphibian, intentional self-harm 🐾

  ● **T63.833** Toxic effect of contact with other venomous amphibian, assault 🐾

  ● **T63.834** Toxic effect of contact with other venomous amphibian, undetermined 🐾

● **T63.89** Toxic effect of contact with other venomous animals

  ● **T63.891** Toxic effect of contact with other venomous animals, accidental (unintentional) 🐾

  ● **T63.892** Toxic effect of contact with other venomous animals, intentional self-harm 🐾

  ● **T63.893** Toxic effect of contact with other venomous animals, assault 🐾

  ● **T63.894** Toxic effect of contact with other venomous animals, undetermined 🐾

● **T63.9** Toxic effect of contact with unspecified venomous animal

  X ● **T63.91** Toxic effect of contact with unspecified venomous animal, accidental (unintentional) 🐾

  X ● **T63.92** Toxic effect of contact with unspecified venomous animal, intentional self-harm 🐾

  X ● **T63.93** Toxic effect of contact with unspecified venomous animal, assault 🐾

  X ● **T63.94** Toxic effect of contact with unspecified venomous animal, undetermined 🐾

● **T64** Toxic effect of aflatoxin and other mycotoxin food contaminants

The appropriate 7th character is to be added to each code from category T64

A	initial encounter
D	subsequent encounter
S	sequela

● **T64.0** Toxic effect of aflatoxin

  X ● **T64.01** Toxic effect of aflatoxin, accidental (unintentional) 🐾

  X ● **T64.02** Toxic effect of aflatoxin, intentional self-harm 🐾

  X ● **T64.03** Toxic effect of aflatoxin, assault 🐾

  X ● **T64.04** Toxic effect of aflatoxin, undetermined 🐾

● **T64.8** Toxic effect of other mycotoxin food contaminants

  X ● **T64.81** Toxic effect of other mycotoxin food contaminants, accidental (unintentional) 🐾

  X ● **T64.82** Toxic effect of other mycotoxin food contaminants, intentional self-harm 🐾

  X ● **T64.83** Toxic effect of other mycotoxin food contaminants, assault 🐾

  X ● **T64.84** Toxic effect of other mycotoxin food contaminants, undetermined 🐾

● **T65** Toxic effect of other and unspecified substances

The appropriate 7th character is to be added to each code from category T65

A	initial encounter
D	subsequent encounter
S	sequela

● **T65.0** Toxic effect of cyanides

> **Excludes1** hydrogen cyanide (T57.3-)

  ● **T65.0X** Toxic effect of cyanides

    ● **T65.0X1** Toxic effect of cyanides, accidental (unintentional) 🐾
      Toxic effect of cyanides NOS

    ● **T65.0X2** Toxic effect of cyanides, intentional self-harm 🐾

    ● **T65.0X3** Toxic effect of cyanides, assault 🐾

    ● **T65.0X4** Toxic effect of cyanides, undetermined 🐾

● **T65.1** Toxic effect of strychnine and its salts

  ● **T65.1X** Toxic effect of strychnine and its salts

    ● **T65.1X1** Toxic effect of strychnine and its salts, accidental (unintentional) 🐾
      Toxic effect of strychnine and its salts NOS

    ● **T65.1X2** Toxic effect of strychnine and its salts, intentional self-harm 🐾

    ● **T65.1X3** Toxic effect of strychnine and its salts, assault 🐾

    ● **T65.1X4** Toxic effect of strychnine and its salts, undetermined 🐾

● **T65.2** Toxic effect of tobacco and nicotine

> **Excludes2** nicotine dependence (F17.-)

  ● **T65.21** Toxic effect of chewing tobacco

    ● **T65.211** Toxic effect of chewing tobacco, accidental (unintentional) 🐾
      Toxic effect of chewing tobacco NOS

    ● **T65.212** Toxic effect of chewing tobacco, intentional self-harm 🐾

    ● **T65.213** Toxic effect of chewing tobacco, assault 🐾

    ● **T65.214** Toxic effect of chewing tobacco, undetermined 🐾

  ● **T65.22** Toxic effect of tobacco cigarettes
    Toxic effect of tobacco smoke

> Use additional code for exposure to second hand tobacco smoke (Z57.31, Z77.22)

    ● **T65.221** Toxic effect of tobacco cigarettes, accidental (unintentional) 🐾
      Toxic effect of tobacco cigarettes NOS

    ● **T65.222** Toxic effect of tobacco cigarettes, intentional self-harm 🐾

    ● **T65.223** Toxic effect of tobacco cigarettes, assault 🐾

    ● **T65.224** Toxic effect of tobacco cigarettes, undetermined 🐾

  ● **T65.29** Toxic effect of other tobacco and nicotine

    ● **T65.291** Toxic effect of other tobacco and nicotine, accidental (unintentional) 🐾
      Toxic effect of other tobacco and nicotine NOS

    ● **T65.292** Toxic effect of other tobacco and nicotine, intentional self-harm 🐾

    ● **T65.293** Toxic effect of other tobacco and nicotine, assault 🐾

    ● **T65.294** Toxic effect of other tobacco and nicotine, undetermined 🐾

CHAPTER 19 (S00-T88)

N Newborn Age: 0   P Pediatric Age: 0–17   M Maternity DX: 12–55   A Adult Age: 15–124   ♀ Females Only   ♂ Males Only

🐾 Complication\Comorbidity   🐾 Major C\C   (Ex) CC/MCC Exclusions   🐾 Present on Admission Requirement   🐾 Hospital-Acquired Condition

1561

● T65.3   Toxic effect of nitroderivatives and aminoderivatives of benzene and its homologues
    Toxic effect of anilin [benzenamine]
    Toxic effect of nitrobenzene
    Toxic effect of trinitrotoluene

● T65.3X   Toxic effect of nitroderivatives and aminoderivatives of benzene and its homologues

● T65.3X1   Toxic effect of nitroderivatives and aminoderivatives of benzene and its homologues, accidental (unintentional) 🔍
    Toxic effect of nitroderivatives and aminoderivatives of benzene and its homologues NOS

● T65.3X2   Toxic effect of nitroderivatives and aminoderivatives of benzene and its homologues, intentional self-harm 🔍

● T65.3X3   Toxic effect of nitroderivatives and aminoderivatives of benzene and its homologues, assault 🔍

● T65.3X4   Toxic effect of nitroderivatives and aminoderivatives of benzene and its homologues, undetermined 🔍

● T65.4   Toxic effect of carbon disulfide

● T65.4X   Toxic effect of carbon disulfide

● T65.4X1   Toxic effect of carbon disulfide, accidental (unintentional) 🔍
    Toxic effect of carbon disulfide NOS

● T65.4X2   Toxic effect of carbon disulfide, intentional self-harm 🔍

● T65.4X3   Toxic effect of carbon disulfide, assault 🔍

● T65.4X4   Toxic effect of carbon disulfide, undetermined 🔍

● T65.5   Toxic effect of nitroglycerin and other nitric acids and esters
    Toxic effect of 1,2,3-Propanetriol trinitrate

● T65.5X   Toxic effect of nitroglycerin and other nitric acids and esters

● T65.5X1   Toxic effect of nitroglycerin and other nitric acids and esters, accidental (unintentional) 🔍
    Toxic effect of nitroglycerin and other nitric acids and esters NOS

● T65.5X2   Toxic effect of nitroglycerin and other nitric acids and esters, intentional self-harm 🔍

● T65.5X3   Toxic effect of nitroglycerin and other nitric acids and esters, assault 🔍

● T65.5X4   Toxic effect of nitroglycerin and other nitric acids and esters, undetermined 🔍

● T65.6   Toxic effect of paints and dyes, not elsewhere classified

● T65.6X   Toxic effect of paints and dyes, not elsewhere classified

● T65.6X1   Toxic effect of paints and dyes, not elsewhere classified, accidental (unintentional) 🔍
    Toxic effect of paints and dyes NOS

● T65.6X2   Toxic effect of paints and dyes, not elsewhere classified, intentional self-harm 🔍

● T65.6X3   Toxic effect of paints and dyes, not elsewhere classified, assault 🔍

● T65.6X4   Toxic effect of paints and dyes, not elsewhere classified, undetermined 🔍

● T65.8   Toxic effect of other specified substances

● T65.81   Toxic effect of latex

● T65.811   Toxic effect of latex, accidental (unintentional) 🔍
    Toxic effect of latex NOS

● T65.812   Toxic effect of latex, intentional self-harm 🔍

● T65.813   Toxic effect of latex, assault 🔍

● T65.814   Toxic effect of latex, undetermined 🔍

● T65.82   Toxic effect of harmful algae and algae toxins
    Toxic effect of (harmful) algae bloom NOS
    Toxic effect of blue-green algae bloom
    Toxic effect of brown tide
    Toxic effect of cyanobacteria bloom
    Toxic effect of Florida red tide
    Toxic effect of pfiesteria piscicida
    Toxic effect of red tide

● T65.821   Toxic effect of harmful algae and algae toxins, accidental (unintentional) 🔍
    Toxic effect of harmful algae and algae toxins NOS

● T65.822   Toxic effect of harmful algae and algae toxins, intentional self-harm 🔍

● T65.823   Toxic effect of harmful algae and algae toxins, assault 🔍

● T65.824   Toxic effect of harmful algae and algae toxins, undetermined 🔍

● T65.83   Toxic effect of fiberglass

● T65.831   Toxic effect of fiberglass, accidental (unintentional) 🔍
    Toxic effect of fiberglass NOS

● T65.832   Toxic effect of fiberglass, intentional self-harm 🔍

● T65.833   Toxic effect of fiberglass, assault 🔍

● T65.834   Toxic effect of fiberglass, undetermined 🔍

● T65.89   Toxic effect of other specified substances

● T65.891   Toxic effect of other specified substances, accidental (unintentional) 🔍
    Toxic effect of other specified substances NOS

● T65.892   Toxic effect of other specified substances, intentional self-harm 🔍

● T65.893   Toxic effect of other specified substances, assault 🔍

● T65.894   Toxic effect of other specified substances, undetermined 🔍

● T65.9   Toxic effect of unspecified substance

X **● T65.91   Toxic effect of unspecified substance, accidental (unintentional)** 🔍
    Poisoning NOS

X **● T65.92   Toxic effect of unspecified substance, intentional self-harm** 🔍

X **● T65.93   Toxic effect of unspecified substance, assault** 🔍

X **● T65.94   Toxic effect of unspecified substance, undetermined** 🔍

◀ New   ◀ Revised   ~~deleted~~ Deleted   Excludes 1   Excludes 2   Includes   Use additional   Code first   Code also   Unspecified
OGCR Official Guidelines   ● Unacceptable Principal Diagnosis   X Assign placeholder X   ● Use Additional Character(s)   ▌ Manifestation Code   Coding Clinic

OTHER AND UNSPECIFIED EFFECTS OF EXTERNAL CAUSES (T66-T78)

● **T66**　**Radiation sickness, unspecified** 🔶

　　Excludes1　specified adverse effects of radiation, such as:
　　　　　　　　burns (T20-T31)
　　　　　　　　leukemia (C91-C95)
　　　　　　　　radiation gastroenteritis and colitis (K52.0)
　　　　　　　　radiation pneumonitis (J70.0)
　　　　　　　　radiation related disorders of the skin and
　　　　　　　　　subcutaneous tissue (L55-L59)
　　　　　　　　sunburn (L55.-)

　　The appropriate 7th character is to be added to code T66

A	initial encounter
D	subsequent encounter
S	sequela

● **T67**　**Effects of heat and light**

　　Excludes1　erythema [dermatitis] ab igne (L59.0)
　　　　　　　　malignant hyperpyrexia due to anesthesia (T88.3)
　　　　　　　　radiation-related disorders of the skin and
　　　　　　　　　subcutaneous tissue (L55-L59)

　　Excludes2　burns (T20-T31)
　　　　　　　　sunburn (L55.-)
　　　　　　　　sweat disorder due to heat (L74-L75)

　　The appropriate 7th character is to be added to each code from
　　　category T67

A	initial encounter
D	subsequent encounter
S	sequela

X ● **T67.0**　**Heatstroke and sunstroke** A 🔶, 🔶, A 🔶
　　　　Heat apoplexy
　　　　Heat pyrexia
　　　　Siriasis
　　　　Thermoplegia
　　　　Use additional code(s) to identify any associated
　　　　　complications of heatstroke, such as:
　　　　　　coma and stupor (R40.-)
　　　　　　systemic inflammatory response syndrome (R65.1-)
　　　　(Ex:) T67.0XX-T67.9XX[A]

X ● **T67.1**　**Heat syncope** 🔶
　　　　Heat collapse

X ● **T67.2**　**Heat cramp** 🔶

X ● **T67.3**　**Heat exhaustion, anhydrotic** 🔶
　　　　Heat prostration due to water depletion
　　　　　Excludes1　heat exhaustion due to salt depletion
　　　　　　　　　　(T67.4)

X ● **T67.4**　**Heat exhaustion due to salt depletion** 🔶
　　　　Heat prostration due to salt (and water) depletion

X ● **T67.5**　**Heat exhaustion, unspecified** 🔶
　　　　Heat prostration NOS

X ● **T67.6**　**Heat fatigue, transient** 🔶

X ● **T67.7**　**Heat edema** 🔶

X ● **T67.8**　**Other effects of heat and light** 🔶

X ● **T67.9**　**Effect of heat and light, unspecified** 🔶

● **T68**　**Hypothermia** 🔶
　　　　Accidental hypothermia
　　　　Hypothermia NOS
　　　　Use additional code to identify source of exposure:
　　　　　Exposure to excessive cold of man-made origin (W93)
　　　　　Exposure to excessive cold of natural origin (X31)

　　Excludes1　hypothermia following anesthesia (T88.51)
　　　　　　　　hypothermia not associated with low
　　　　　　　　　environmental temperature (R68.0)
　　　　　　　　hypothermia of newborn (P80.-)

　　Excludes2　frostbite (T33-T34)

　　The appropriate 7th character is to be added to code T68

A	initial encounter
D	subsequent encounter
S	sequela

● **T69**　**Other effects of reduced temperature**
　　　　Use additional code to identify source of exposure:
　　　　　Exposure to excessive cold of man-made origin (W93)
　　　　　Exposure to excessive cold of natural origin (X31)

　　Excludes2　frostbite (T33-T34)

　　The appropriate 7th character is to be added to each code from
　　　category T69

A	initial encounter
D	subsequent encounter
S	sequela

● **T69.0**　**Immersion hand and foot**

　● **T69.01**　**Immersion hand**

　　● **T69.011**　**Immersion hand, right hand** 🔶

　　● **T69.012**　**Immersion hand, left hand** 🔶

　　● **T69.019**　**Immersion hand, unspecified hand** 🔶

　● **T69.02**　**Immersion foot**
　　　　Trench foot
　　　　(Ex:) For category T69.02 CC codes: T33.2XX-T33.42X[A],
　　　　　T33.60X-T33.72X[A], T33.90X-T33.99X[A],
　　　　　T34.2XX-T34.42X[A], T34.60X-T34.72X[A],
　　　　　T34.90X-T34.99X[A], T69.021-T69.029[A]

　　● **T69.021**　**Immersion foot, right foot** A 🔶, 🔶,
　　　　　A 🔶

　　● **T69.022**　**Immersion foot, left foot** A 🔶, 🔶,
　　　　　A 🔶

　　● **T69.029**　**Immersion foot, unspecified foot** A 🔶,
　　　　　🔶, A 🔶

X ● **T69.1**　**Chilblains** 🔶

X ● **T69.8**　**Other specified effects of reduced temperature** 🔶

X ● **T69.9**　**Effect of reduced temperature, unspecified** 🔶

● **T70**　**Effects of air pressure and water pressure**
　　The appropriate 7th character is to be added to each code from
　　　category T70

A	initial encounter
D	subsequent encounter
S	sequela

X ● **T70.0**　**Otitic barotrauma** 🔶
　　　　Aero-otitis media
　　　　Effects of change in ambient atmospheric pressure or
　　　　　water pressure on ears

X ● **T70.1**　**Sinus barotrauma** 🔶
　　　　Aerosinusitis
　　　　Effects of change in ambient atmospheric pressure on
　　　　　sinuses

● **T70.2**　**Other and unspecified effects of high altitude**
　　Excludes2　polycythemia due to high altitude (D75.1)

X ● **T70.20**　**Unspecified effects of high altitude** 🔶

X ● **T70.29**　**Other effects of high altitude** 🔶
　　　　Alpine sickness
　　　　Anoxia due to high altitude
　　　　Barotrauma NOS
　　　　Hypobaropathy
　　　　Mountain sickness

X ● **T70.3**　**Caisson disease [decompression sickness]** A 🔶, 🔶, A 🔶
　　　　Compressed-air disease
　　　　Diver's palsy or paralysis
　　　　(Ex:) T70.3XX-T70.9XX[A]

X ● **T70.4**　**Effects of high-pressure fluids** 🔶
　　　　Hydraulic jet injection (industrial)
　　　　Pneumatic jet injection (industrial)
　　　　Traumatic jet injection (industrial)

X ● **T70.8**　**Other effects of air pressure and water pressure** 🔶

X ● **T70.9**　**Effect of air pressure and water pressure, unspecified** 🔶

N Newborn Age: 0　　**P** Pediatric Age: 0–17　　**M** Maternity DX: 12–55　　**A** Adult Age: 15–124　　♀ Females Only　　♂ Males Only

🔶 Complication\Comorbidity　　🔶 Major C\C　　(Ex:) CC/MCC Exclusions　　🔶 Present on Admission Requirement　　🔶 Hospital-Acquired Condition

1563

● **T71 Asphyxiation**
Mechanical suffocation
Traumatic suffocation

Excludes1   acute respiratory distress (syndrome) (J80)
anoxia due to high altitude (T70.2)
asphyxia NOS (R09.01)
asphyxia from carbon monoxide (T58.-)
asphyxia from inhalation of food or foreign body
  (T17.-)
asphyxia from other gases, fumes and vapors
  (T59.-)
respiratory distress (syndrome) in newborn
  (P22.-)

The appropriate 7th character is to be added to each code from
  category T71

> A   initial encounter
> D   subsequent encounter
> S   sequela

(Ex) For category T71 CC codes: T71.111-T71.9XX[A]

● **T71.1 Asphyxiation due to mechanical threat to breathing**
Suffocation due to mechanical threat to breathing

  ● **T71.11 Asphyxiation due to smothering under pillow**

    ● **T71.111 Asphyxiation due to smothering
under pillow, accidental** A 🔾, 🔾, A 🔾
Asphyxiation due to smothering
under pillow NOS

    ● **T71.112 Asphyxiation due to smothering
under pillow, intentional self-harm**
A 🔾, 🔾, A 🔾

    ● **T71.113 Asphyxiation due to smothering
under pillow, assault** A 🔾, 🔾, A 🔾

    ● **T71.114 Asphyxiation due to smothering
under pillow, undetermined** A 🔾, 🔾,
A 🔾

  ● **T71.12 Asphyxiation due to plastic bag**

    ● **T71.121 Asphyxiation due to plastic bag,
accidental** A 🔾, 🔾, A 🔾
Asphyxiation due to plastic bag
NOS

    ● **T71.122 Asphyxiation due to plastic bag,
intentional self-harm** A 🔾, 🔾, A 🔾

    ● **T71.123 Asphyxiation due to plastic bag,
assault** A 🔾, 🔾, A 🔾

    ● **T71.124 Asphyxiation due to plastic bag,
undetermined** A 🔾, 🔾, A 🔾

  ● **T71.13 Asphyxiation due to being trapped in bed
linens**

    ● **T71.131 Asphyxiation due to being trapped in
bed linens, accidental** A 🔾, 🔾, A 🔾
Asphyxiation due to being trapped
in bed linens NOS

    ● **T71.132 Asphyxiation due to being trapped in
bed linens, intentional self-harm**
A 🔾, 🔾, A 🔾

    ● **T71.133 Asphyxiation due to being trapped in
bed linens, assault** A 🔾, 🔾, A 🔾

    ● **T71.134 Asphyxiation due to being trapped in
bed linens, undetermined** A 🔾, 🔾,
A 🔾

● **T71.14 Asphyxiation due to smothering under another
person's body (in bed)**

  ● **T71.141 Asphyxiation due to smothering
under another person's body (in bed),
accidental** A 🔾, 🔾, A 🔾
Asphyxiation due to smothering
under another person's body
(in bed) NOS

  ● **T71.143 Asphyxiation due to smothering
under another person's body (in bed),
assault** A 🔾, 🔾, A 🔾

  ● **T71.144 Asphyxiation due to smothering
under another person's body (in bed),
undetermined** A 🔾, 🔾, A 🔾

● **T71.15 Asphyxiation due to smothering in furniture**

  ● **T71.151 Asphyxiation due to smothering in
furniture, accidental** A 🔾, 🔾, A 🔾
Asphyxiation due to smothering in
furniture NOS

  ● **T71.152 Asphyxiation due to smothering in
furniture, intentional self-harm** A 🔾,
🔾, A 🔾

  ● **T71.153 Asphyxiation due to smothering in
furniture, assault** A 🔾, 🔾, A 🔾

  ● **T71.154 Asphyxiation due to smothering in
furniture, undetermined** A 🔾, 🔾,
A 🔾

● **T71.16 Asphyxiation due to hanging**
Hanging by window shade cord

  Use additional code for any associated injuries,
such as:
crushing injury of neck (S17.-)
fracture of cervical vertebrae (S12.0-S12.2-)
open wound of neck (S11.-)

  ● **T71.161 Asphyxiation due to hanging,
accidental** A 🔾, 🔾, A 🔾
Asphyxiation due to hanging NOS
Hanging NOS

  ● **T71.162 Asphyxiation due to hanging,
intentional self-harm** A 🔾, 🔾, A 🔾

  ● **T71.163 Asphyxiation due to hanging, assault**
A 🔾, 🔾, A 🔾

  ● **T71.164 Asphyxiation due to hanging,
undetermined** A 🔾, 🔾, A 🔾

● **T71.19 Asphyxiation due to mechanical**
Threat to breathing due to other causes

  ● **T71.191 Asphyxiation due to mechanical
threat to breathing due to other
causes, accidental** A 🔾, 🔾, A 🔾
Asphyxiation due to other causes
NOS

  ● **T71.192 Asphyxiation due to mechanical
threat to breathing due to other
causes, intentional self-harm** A 🔾, 🔾,
A 🔾

  ● **T71.193 Asphyxiation due to mechanical
threat to breathing due to other
causes, assault** A 🔾, 🔾, A 🔾

  ● **T71.194 Asphyxiation due to mechanical
threat to breathing due to other
causes, undetermined** A 🔾, 🔾, A 🔾

◀ New   ◀▥ Revised   ~~deleted~~ Deleted   Excludes 1   Excludes 2   Includes   Use additional   Code first   Code also   Unspecified
OGCR Official Guidelines   ● Unacceptable Principal Diagnosis   X Assign placeholder X   ● Use Additional Character(s)   ▷ Manifestation Code   Coding Clinic

● **T71.2**   **Asphyxiation due to systemic oxygen deficiency due to low oxygen content in ambient air**
Suffocation due to systemic oxygen deficiency due to low oxygen content in ambient air

X● **T71.20**   **Asphyxiation due to systemic oxygen deficiency due to low oxygen content in ambient air due to** unspecified **cause** A ◐, ◐, A ◐

X● **T71.21**   **Asphyxiation due to cave-in or falling earth** A ◐, ◐, A ◐
Use additional code for any associated cataclysm (X34-X38)

● **T71.22**   **Asphyxiation due to being trapped in a car trunk**

● **T71.221**   Asphyxiation due to being trapped in a car trunk, accidental A ◐, ◐

● **T71.222**   Asphyxiation due to being trapped in a car trunk, intentional self-harm A ◐, ◐

● **T71.223**   Asphyxiation due to being trapped in a car trunk, assault A ◐, ◐

● **T71.224**   Asphyxiation due to being trapped in a car trunk, undetermined A ◐, ◐

● **T71.23**   **Asphyxiation due to being trapped in a (discarded) refrigerator**

● **T71.231**   Asphyxiation due to being trapped in a (discarded) refrigerator, accidental A ◐, ◐

● **T71.232**   Asphyxiation due to being trapped in a (discarded) refrigerator, intentional self-harm A ◐, ◐

● **T71.233**   Asphyxiation due to being trapped in a (discarded) refrigerator, assault A ◐, ◐

● **T71.234**   Asphyxiation due to being trapped in a (discarded) refrigerator, undetermined A ◐, ◐

X● **T71.29**   **Asphyxiation due to being trapped in other low oxygen environment** A ◐, ◐, A ◐

X● **T71.9**   **Asphyxiation due to** unspecified **cause** A ◐, ◐, A ◐
Suffocation (by strangulation) due to unspecified cause
Suffocation NOS
Systemic oxygen deficiency due to low oxygen content in ambient air due to unspecified cause
Systemic oxygen deficiency due to mechanical threat to breathing due to unspecified cause
Traumatic asphyxia NOS

● **T73**   **Effects of other deprivation**
The appropriate 7th character is to be added to each code from category T73

A	initial encounter
D	subsequent encounter
S	sequela

X● **T73.0**   **Starvation** ◐
Deprivation of food

X● **T73.1**   **Deprivation of water** ◐

X● **T73.2**   **Exhaustion due to exposure** ◐

X● **T73.3**   **Exhaustion due to excessive exertion** ◐
Exhaustion due to overexertion

X● **T73.8**   **Other effects of deprivation** ◐

X● **T73.9**   **Effect of deprivation,** unspecified ◐

● **T74**   **Adult and child abuse, neglect and other maltreatment, confirmed**
Use additional code, if applicable, to identify any associated current injury
external cause code to identify perpetrator, if known (Y07.-)

Excludes1   abuse and maltreatment in pregnancy (O9A.3-, O9A.4-, O9A.5-)
adult and child maltreatment, suspected (T76.-)

The appropriate 7th character is to be added to each code from category T74

A	initial encounter
D	subsequent encounter
S	sequela

(Ex) **For category T74 CC codes unless otherwise indicated:** T74.01X-T74.92X[A], T76.01X-T76.92X[A]

● **T74.0**   **Neglect or abandonment, confirmed**

X● **T74.01**   **Adult neglect or abandonment, confirmed** A ◐, ◐   A

X● **T74.02**   **Child neglect or abandonment, confirmed** A ◐, ◐   P

● **T74.1**   **Physical abuse, confirmed**
Excludes2   sexual abuse (T74.2-)

X● **T74.11**   **Adult physical abuse, confirmed** A ◐, ◐   A

X● **T74.12**   **Child physical abuse, confirmed** A ◐, ◐   P
Excludes2   shaken infant syndrome (T74.4)

● **T74.2**   **Sexual abuse, confirmed**
Rape, confirmed
Sexual assault, confirmed

X● **T74.21**   **Adult sexual abuse, confirmed** A ◐, ◐   A

X● **T74.22**   **Child sexual abuse, confirmed** A ◐, ◐   P

● **T74.3**   **Psychological abuse, confirmed**

X● **T74.31**   **Adult psychological abuse, confirmed** ◐   A

X● **T74.32**   **Child psychological abuse, confirmed** A ◐, ◐   P

X● **T74.4**   **Shaken infant syndrome** A ◐, ◐   P

● **T74.9**   **Unspecified maltreatment, confirmed**

X● **T74.91**   Unspecified **adult maltreatment, confirmed** A ◐, ◐   A
(Ex) T74.91X[A], T76.91X[A]

X● **T74.92**   Unspecified **child maltreatment, confirmed** A ◐, ◐   P

● **T75**   **Other and unspecified effects of other external causes**
Excludes1   adverse effects NEC (T78.-)
Excludes2   burns (electric) (T20-T31)

The appropriate 7th character is to be added to each code from category T75

A	initial encounter
D	subsequent encounter
S	sequela

● **T75.0**   **Effects of lightning**
Struck by lightning

X● **T75.00**   Unspecified **effects of lightning** ◐
Struck by lightning NOS

X● **T75.01**   **Shock due to being struck by lightning** ◐

X● **T75.09**   **Other effects of lightning** ◐
Use additional code for other effects of lightning

X● **T75.1**   Unspecified **effects of drowning and nonfatal submersion** A ◐, ◐, A ◐
Immersion
Excludes1   specified effects of drowning code to effects
(Ex) T75.1XX[A]

N   Newborn Age: 0   P   Pediatric Age: 0–17   M   Maternity DX: 12–55   A   Adult Age: 15–124   ♀ Females Only   ♂ Males Only

◐ Complication\Comorbidity   ◐ Major C\C   (Ex) CC/MCC Exclusions   ◐ Present on Admission Requirement   ◐ Hospital-Acquired Condition

1565

CHAPTER 19 (S00-T88)

CHAPTER 19 (S00–T88)

● **T75.2   Effects of vibration**
   X ● **T75.20   Unspecified effects of vibration** 🔲
   X ● **T75.21   Pneumatic hammer syndrome** 🔲
   X ● **T75.22   Traumatic vasospastic syndrome** 🔲
   X ● **T75.23   Vertigo from infrasound** 🔲
      Excludes1   vertigo NOS (R42)
   X ● **T75.29   Other effects of vibration** 🔲
X ● **T75.3   Motion sickness** 🔲
      Airsickness   Travel sickness
      Seasickness
      Use additional external cause code to identify vehicle or
         type of motion (Y92.81-, Y93.5-)
X ● **T75.4   Electrocution** 🔲
      Shock from electric current
      Shock from electroshock gun (taser)
● **T75.8   Other specified effects of external causes**
   X ● **T75.81   Effects of abnormal gravitation [G] forces** 🔲
   X ● **T75.82   Effects of weightlessness** 🔲
   X ● **T75.89   Other specified effects of external causes** 🔲

● **T76   Adult and child abuse, neglect and other maltreatment,
         suspected**
      Use additional code, if applicable, to identify any associated
         current injury
      Excludes1   adult and child maltreatment, confirmed (T74.-)
                     suspected abuse and maltreatment in pregnancy
                        (O9A.3-, O9A.4-, O9A.5-)
                     suspected adult physical abuse, ruled out
                        (Z04.71)
                     suspected adult sexual abuse, ruled out (Z04.41)
                     suspected child physical abuse, ruled out (Z04.72)
                     suspected child sexual abuse, ruled out (Z04.42)
      The appropriate 7th character is to be added to each code from
         category T76

         | A | initial encounter |
         | D | subsequent encounter |
         | S | sequela |

      (Ex:) **For category T76 CC codes unless otherwise indicated:** T74.01X-T74.92X[A],
         T76.01X-T76.92X[A]

● **T76.0   Neglect or abandonment, suspected**
   X ● **T76.01   Adult neglect or abandonment,
                  suspected** A 🔲, 🔲   A
   X ● **T76.02   Child neglect or abandonment,
                  suspected** A 🔲, 🔲   P
● **T76.1   Physical abuse, suspected**
   X ● **T76.11   Adult physical abuse, suspected** A 🔲, 🔲   A
   X ● **T76.12   Child physical abuse, suspected** A 🔲, 🔲   P
● **T76.2   Sexual abuse, suspected**
      Rape, suspected
      Sexual abuse, suspected
      Excludes1   alleged abuse, ruled out (Z04.7)
   X ● **T76.21   Adult sexual abuse, suspected** A 🔲, 🔲   A
   X ● **T76.22   Child sexual abuse, suspected** A 🔲, 🔲   P
● **T76.3   Psychological abuse, suspected**
   X ● **T76.31   Adult psychological abuse, suspected** 🔲   A
   X ● **T76.32   Child psychological abuse, suspected** A 🔲, 🔲   P
● **T76.9   Unspecified maltreatment, suspected**
   X ● **T76.91   Unspecified adult maltreatment, suspected**
                  A 🔲, 🔲   A
                  (Ex:) T74.91X[A], T76.91X[A]
   X ● **T76.92   Unspecified child maltreatment,
                  suspected** A 🔲, 🔲   P

● **T78   Adverse effects, not elsewhere classified**
      Excludes2   complications of surgical and medical care NEC
                     (T80-T88)
      The appropriate 7th character is to be added to each code from
         category T78

         | A | initial encounter |
         | D | subsequent encounter |
         | S | sequela |

      (Ex:) **For category T78 CC codes:** T78.00X-T78.09X[A]

● **T78.0   Anaphylactic reaction due to food**
      Anaphylactic reaction due to adverse food reaction
      Anaphylactic shock or reaction due to nonpoisonous
         foods
      Anaphylactoid reaction due to food
   X ● **T78.00   Anaphylactic reaction due to unspecified food**
                  A 🔲, 🔲
   X ● **T78.01   Anaphylactic reaction due to peanuts** A 🔲, 🔲
   X ● **T78.02   Anaphylactic reaction due to shellfish
                  (crustaceans)** A 🔲, 🔲
   X ● **T78.03   Anaphylactic reaction due to other fish** A 🔲, 🔲
   X ● **T78.04   Anaphylactic reaction due to fruits and
                  vegetables** A 🔲, 🔲
   X ● **T78.05   Anaphylactic reaction due to tree nuts and
                  seeds** A 🔲, 🔲
         Excludes1   anaphylactic reaction due to
                        peanuts (T78.01)
   X ● **T78.06   Anaphylactic reaction due to food additives**
                  A 🔲, 🔲
   X ● **T78.07   Anaphylactic reaction due to milk and dairy
                  products** A 🔲, 🔲
   X ● **T78.08   Anaphylactic reaction due to eggs** A 🔲, 🔲
   X ● **T78.09   Anaphylactic reaction due to other food
                  products** A 🔲, 🔲
● **T78.1   Other adverse food reactions, not elsewhere classified** 🔲
      Use additional code to identify the type of reaction
      Excludes1   anaphylactic reaction or shock due to
                        adverse food reaction (T78.0-)
                     anaphylactic reaction due to food (T78.0-)
                     bacterial food borne intoxications (A05.-)
      Excludes2   allergic and dietetic gastroenteritis and
                        colitis (K52.2)
                     allergic rhinitis due to food (J30.5)
                     dermatitis due to food in contact with
                        skin (L23.6, L24.6, L25.4)
                     dermatitis due to ingested food (L27.2)
X ● **T78.2   Anaphylactic shock, unspecified** A 🔲, 🔲
      *Occurs when allergic response triggers large quantities of
         histamines, prostaglandins, leukotrienes resulting in
         systemic vasodilation*
      Allergic shock
      Anaphylactic reaction
      Anaphylaxis
      Excludes1   anaphylactic reaction or shock due to
                        adverse effect of correct medicinal
                        substance properly administered
                        (T88.6)
                     anaphylactic reaction or shock due to
                        adverse food reaction (T78.0-)
                     anaphylactic reaction or shock due to
                        serum (T80.5-)
X ● **T78.3   Angioneurotic edema** 🔲
      Allergic angioedema
      Giant urticaria
      *Vascular disorder resulting from abnormalities of autonomic
         nervous system fibers supplying blood vessels*
      Quincke's edema
      Excludes1   serum urticaria (T80.6-)
                     urticaria (L50.-)

◀ New   ◀═ Revised   ~~deleted~~ Deleted   Excludes 1   Excludes 2   Includes   Use additional   Code first   Code also   Unspecified
OGCR Official Guidelines   ● Unacceptable Principal Diagnosis   X Assign placeholder X   ● Use Additional Character(s)   ▶ Manifestation Code   **Coding Clinic**

● **T78.4**   **Other and unspecified allergy**

> **Excludes1**   specified types of allergic reaction such
>   as:
>   allergic diarrhea (K52.2)
>   allergic gastroenteritis and colitis
>   (K52.2)
>   dermatitis (L23-L25, L27.-)
>   hay fever (J30.1)

X ● **T78.40**   **Allergy, unspecified**
>   Allergic reaction NOS
>   Hypersensitivity NOS

X ● **T78.41**   **Arthus phenomenon**
>   Arthus reaction

X ● **T78.49**   **Other allergy**

X ● **T78.8**   **Other adverse effects, not elsewhere classified**

CERTAIN EARLY COMPLICATIONS OF TRAUMA (T79)

● **T79**   **Certain early complications of trauma, not elsewhere classified**

> **Excludes2**   acute respiratory distress syndrome (J80)
>   complications occurring during or following
>   medical procedures (T80-T88)
>   complications of surgical and medical care NEC
>   (T80-T88)
>   newborn respiratory distress syndrome (P22.0)

The appropriate 7th character is to be added to each code from
category T79

> | A | initial encounter |
> |---|---|
> | D | subsequent encounter |
> | S | sequela |

X ● **T79.0**   **Air embolism (traumatic)** A ,

> **Excludes1**   air embolism complicating abortion
>   or ectopic or molar pregnancy
>   (O00-O07, O08.2) ◀
>   ~~abortion or ectopic or molar pregnancy~~
>   ~~(O00-O07, O08.2)~~
>   air embolism complicating pregnancy,
>   childbirth and the puerperium
>   (O88.0) ◀
>   air embolism following infusion,
>   transfusion, and therapeutic injection
>   (T80.0) ◀
>   ~~infusion, transfusion, and therapeutic~~
>   ~~injection (T80.0)~~
>   air embolism following procedure NEC
>   (T81.7-) ◀

(Ex) D78.81-D78.89, E36.8, E89.810-E89.89, H59.011-H59.019,
H59.031-H59.039, H59.091-H59.099, H59.811-H59.89, H95.811-H95.89,
I97.3, L76.81-L76.82, M96.89, N98.1-N98.9, T14.8-T14.91, T79.0XX[A],
T79.A0X- T79.9XX[A], T80.0XX[A], T81.82X[A], T81.89X-T81.9XX[A]

X ● **T79.1**   **Fat embolism (traumatic)** A ,

> **Excludes1**   fat embolism complicating:
>   abortion or ectopic or molar pregnancy
>   (O00-O07, O08.2)
>   pregnancy, childbirth and the
>   puerperium (O88.8)

(Ex) D78.81-D78.89, E36.8, E89.810-E89.89, H59.011-H59.019,
H59.031-H59.039, H59.091-H59.099, H59.811-H59.89, H95.811-H95.89,
I97.3, L76.81-L76.82, M96.89, N98.1-N98.9, T14.8-T14.91, T79.0XX[A],
T79.A0X- T79.9XX[A], T81.82X[A], T81.89X-T81.9XX[A]

X ● **T79.2**   **Traumatic secondary and recurrent hemorrhage and seroma** A ,

(Ex) D78.81-D78.89, E36.8, E89.810-E89.89, H59.011-H59.019,
H59.031-H59.039, H59.091-H59.099, H59.811-H59.89, H95.811-H95.89,
I97.3, L76.81-L76.82, M96.89, N98.1-N98.9, T14.8-T14.91, 79.2XX[A], T79.
A0X-T79.9XX[A], T81.82X-T81.9XX[A]

X ● **T79.4**   **Traumatic shock** A ,
>   Shock (immediate) (delayed) following injury

> **Excludes1**   anaphylactic shock due to adverse food
>   reaction (T78.0-)
>   anaphylactic shock due to correct
>   medicinal substance properly
>   administered (T88.6)
>   anaphylactic shock due to serum (T80.5-)
>   anaphylactic shock NOS (T78.2)
>   anesthetic shock (T88.2)
>   electric shock (T75.4)
>   nontraumatic shock NEC (R57.-)
>   obstetric shock (O75.1)
>   postprocedural shock (T81.1-)
>   septic shock (R65.21)
>   shock complicating abortion or ectopic or
>   molar pregnancy (O00-O07, O08.3)
>   shock due to lightning (T75.01)
>   shock NOS (R57.9)

(Ex) D78.81-D78.89, E36.8, E89.810-E89.89, H59.011-H59.019,
H59.031-H59.039, H59.091-H59.099, H59.811-H59.89, H95.811-H95.89,
I97.3, L76.81-L76.82, M96.89, N98.1-N98.9, T14.8-T14.91, T79.4XX[A],
T79.A0X-T79.9XX[A], T81.82X-T81.9XX[A]

X ● **T79.5**   **Traumatic anuria** A ,
>   Crush syndrome
>   Renal failure following crushing

(Ex) D78.01-D78.02, D78.21-D78.22, D78.81-D78.89, E36.01-E36.02, E36.8,
E89.810-E89.89, G97.51-G97.52, H59.011-H59.019, H59.031-H59.039,
H59.091-H59.099, H59.111-H59.129, H59.311-H59.329, H59.811-H59.819,
H59.88-H59.89, H95.21-H95.22, H95.41-H95.42, H95.811-H95.819,
H95.88-H95.89, I97.3-I97.42, I97.610-I97.62, J95.61-J95.62,
J95.830-J95.831, K91.61-K91.62, K91.840-K91.841, L76.01-L76.02,
L76.21-L76.22, L76.81-L76.82, M96.810-M96.811, M96.830-M96.89,
N98.1-N98.9, N99.61-N99.62, N99.820-N99.821, T14.8-T14.91, T79.5XX[A],
T79.A0X-T79.9XX[A], T81.10X-T81.19X[A], T81.82X-T81.9XX[A], T88.2XX[A]

X ● **T79.6**   **Traumatic ischemia of muscle**
>   Traumatic rhabdomyolysis
>   Volkmann's ischemic contracture

> **Excludes2**   anterior tibial syndrome (M76.8)
>   compartment syndrome (traumatic)
>   (T79.A-)
>   nontraumatic ischemia of muscle (M62.2-)

X ● **T79.7**   **Traumatic subcutaneous emphysema** A ,

> **Excludes1**   emphysema NOS (J43)
>   emphysema (subcutaneous) resulting
>   from a procedure (T81.82)

(Ex) D78.81-D78.89, E36.8, E89.810-E89.89, H59.011-H59.019,
H59.031-H59.039, H59.091-H59.099, H59.811-H59.89, H95.811-H95.89,
I97.3, L76.81-L76.82, M96.89, N98.1-N98.9, S21.101-S21.159[A],
S21.301-S21.459[A], S21.90X-S21.95X[A], S27.0XX-S27.399[A],
S27.50X-S27.809[A], S27.892—S27.9XX[A], S28.1XX[A],
S29.021-S29.029[A], T14.8-T14.91, T79.7XX-T79.9XX[A],
T81.82X-T81.9XX[A]

● **T79.A**   **Traumatic compartment syndrome**

> **Excludes1**   fibromyalgia (M79.7)
>   nontraumatic compartment syndrome
>   (M79.A-)
>   traumatic ischemic infarction of muscle
>   (T79.6)

(Ex) For category T79.A CC codes unless otherwise indicated:
M70.80-M70.99, M79.81-M79.9, R29.898

X ● **T79.A0**   **Compartment syndrome, unspecified** A ,
>   Compartment syndrome NOS

> (Ex) S31.001[A], S31.011[A], S31.021[A], S31.031[A], S31.041[A],
> S31.051[A], S31.600-S31.659[A], S36.81X-S36.899[A]

● **T79.A1**   **Traumatic compartment syndrome of upper extremity**
>   Traumatic compartment syndrome of shoulder,
>   arm, forearm, wrist, hand, and fingers

> ● **T79.A11**   **Traumatic compartment syndrome of right upper extremity** A ,

> ● **T79.A12**   **Traumatic compartment syndrome of left upper extremity** A ,

> ● **T79.A19**   **Traumatic compartment syndrome of unspecified upper extremity** A ,

CHAPTER 19 (S00-T88)

● T79.A2   **Traumatic compartment syndrome of lower extremity**
Traumatic compartment syndrome of hip, buttock, thigh, leg, foot, and toes

    ● T79.A21   **Traumatic compartment syndrome of right lower extremity** A 🔖, 🔖

    ● T79.A22   **Traumatic compartment syndrome of left lower extremity** A 🔖, 🔖

    ● T79.A29   **Traumatic compartment syndrome of unspecified lower extremity** A 🔖, 🔖

X ● T79.A3   **Traumatic compartment syndrome of abdomen** A 🔖, 🔖
    (Ex:) S31.001[A], S31.011[A], S31.021[A], S31.031[A], S31.041[A], S31.051[A], S31.100-S31.159[A], S31.600-S31.659[A], S31.831-S31.839[A], S36.00X-S37.599[A], S37.812-S37.99X[A], S38.3XX[A], S39.021-S39.023[A], T14.8-T14.91, T79.8XX-T79.9XX[A]

X ● T79.A9   **Traumatic compartment syndrome of other sites** A 🔖, 🔖
    (Ex:) See T79.A0

X ● T79.8   **Other early complications of trauma** 🔖

X ● T79.9   **Unspecified early complication of trauma** 🔖

COMPLICATIONS OF SURGICAL AND MEDICAL CARE, NOT ELSEWHERE CLASSIFIED (T80-T88)

Use additional code for adverse effect, if applicable, to identify drug (T36-T50 with fifth or sixth character 5)

Use additional code(s) to identify the specified condition resulting from the complication.

Use additional code to identify devices involved and details of circumstances (Y62-Y82)

Excludes2   any encounters with medical care for postprocedural conditions in which no complications are present, such as:
    artificial opening status (Z93.-)
    closure of external stoma (Z43.-)
    fitting and adjustment of external prosthetic device (Z44.-)
burns and corrosions from local applications and irradiation (T20-T32)
complications of surgical procedures during pregnancy, childbirth and the puerperium (O00-O9A)
mechanical complication of respirator [ventilator] (J95.850)
poisoning and toxic effects of drugs and chemicals (T36-T65 with fifth or sixth character 1-4 or 6)
postprocedural fever (R50.82)
specified complications classified elsewhere, such as:
    cerebrospinal fluid leak from spinal puncture (G97.0)
    colostomy malfunction (K94.0-)
    disorders of fluid and electrolyte imbalance (E86-E87) ◀▥
    functional disturbances following cardiac surgery (I97.0-I97.1)
    intraoperative and postprocedural complications of specified body systems (D78.-, E36.-, E89.-, G97.3-, G97.4, H59.3-, H59.-, H95.2-, H95.3, I97.4-, I97.5, J95.6-, J95.7, K91.6-, L76.-, M96.-, N99.-)
    ostomy complications (J95.0-, K94.-, N99.5-) ◀▥
    postgastric surgery syndromes (K91.1)
    postlaminectomy syndrome NEC (M96.1)
    postmastectomy lymphedema syndrome (I97.2)
    postsurgical blind-loop syndrome (K91.2)
    ventilator associated pneumonia (J95.851)

● T80   **Complications following infusion, transfusion and therapeutic injection**

   Includes   complications following perfusion

   Excludes2   bone marrow transplant rejection (T86.01)
febrile nonhemolytic transfusion reaction (R50.84)
fluid overload due to transfusion (E87.71)
posttransfusion purpura (D69.51)
transfusion associated circulatory overload (TACO) (E87.71)
transfusion (red blood cell) associated hemochromatosis (E83.111)
transfusion related acute lung injury (TRALI) (J95.84)

The appropriate 7th character is to be added to each code from category T80

> A   initial encounter
> D   subsequent encounter
> S   sequela

X ● T80.0   **Air embolism following infusion, transfusion and therapeutic injection** A 🔖, 🔖, A 🔖
    (Ex:) T79.0XX[A], T80.0XX[A]

X ● T80.1   **Vascular complications following infusion, transfusion and therapeutic injection** A 🔖, 🔖
Use additional code to identify the vascular complication

   Excludes2   extravasation of vesicant agent (T80.81-)
infiltration of vesicant agent (T80.81-)
vascular complications specified as due to prosthetic devices, implants and grafts (T82.8- T83.8, T84.8-, T85.8)
postprocedural vascular complications (T81.7-)
    (Ex:) T80.1XX[A], T80.810-T80.818[A], T80.90X[A]

● T80.2   **Infections following infusion, transfusion and therapeutic injection**
Use additional code to identify the specific infection, such as:
    sepsis (A41.9)
Use additional code (R65.2-) to identify severe sepsis, if applicable

   Excludes2   infections specified as due to prosthetic devices, implants and grafts (T82.6-T82.7, T83.5-T83.6, T84.5-T84.7, T85.7)
postprocedural infections (T81.4)
    (Ex:) **For category T80.2 CC codes:** Ex: N98.0, T80.211-T80.29X[A], T82.7XX[A], T88.0XX[A]

    ● T80.21   **Infection due to central venous catheter**

      ● T80.211   **Bloodstream infection due to central venous catheter** A 🔖, 🔖, A 🔖
Catheter-related bloodstream infection (CRBSI) NOS
Central line-associated bloodstream infection (CLABSI)
Bloodstream infection due to Hickman catheter
Bloodstream infection due to peripherally inserted central catheter (PICC)
Bloodstream infection due to portacath (port-a-cath)
Bloodstream infection due to triple lumen catheter
Bloodstream infection due to umbilical venous catheter

◀ New   ◀▥ Revised   ~~deleted~~ Deleted   Excludes 1   Excludes 2   Includes   Use additional   Code first   Code also   Unspecified

OGCR Official Guidelines   ● Unacceptable Principal Diagnosis   X Assign placeholder X   ● Use Additional Character(s)   ▌ Manifestation Code   **Coding Clinic**

● **T80.212** **Local infection due to central venous catheter** A 🔵, 🔵, A 🔵
     Exit or insertion site infection
     Local infection due to Hickman catheter
     Local infection due to peripherally inserted central catheter (PICC)
     Local infection due to portacath (port-a-cath)
     Local infection due to triple lumen catheter
     Local infection due to umbilical venous catheter
     Port or reservoir infection
     Tunnel infection

● **T80.218** **Other infection due to central venous catheter** A 🔵, 🔵, A 🔵
     Other central line-associated infection
     Other infection due to Hickman catheter
     Other infection due to peripherally inserted central catheter (PICC)
     Other infection due to portacath (port-a-cath)
     Other infection due to triple lumen catheter
     Other infection due to umbilical venous catheter

● **T80.219** **Unspecified infection due to central venous catheter** A 🔵, 🔵, A 🔵
     Central line-associated infection NOS
     Unspecified infection due to Hickman catheter
     Unspecified infection due to peripherally inserted central catheter (PICC)
     Unspecified infection due to portacath (port-a-cath)
     Unspecified infection due to triple lumen catheter
     Unspecified infection due to umbilical venous catheter

X● **T80.22** **Acute infection following transfusion, infusion, or injection of blood and blood products** A 🔵, 🔵

X● **T80.29** **Infection following other infusion, transfusion and therapeutic injection** A 🔵, 🔵

● **T80.3** **ABO incompatibility reaction due to transfusion of blood or blood products**
     Excludes1   minor blood group antigens reactions (Duffy) (E) (K(ell)) (Kidd) (Lewis) (M) (N) (P) (S) (T80.A)
     (Ex) **For category T80.3 CC codes:** T80.30X-T80.A9X[A], T80.910-T80.92X[A]

X● **T80.30** **ABO incompatibility reaction due to transfusion of blood or blood products, unspecified** A 🔵, 🔵, A 🔵
     ABO incompatibility blood transfusion NOS
     Reaction to ABO incompatibility from transfusion NOS

● **T80.31** **ABO incompatibility with hemolytic transfusion reaction**

  ● **T80.310** **ABO incompatibility with acute hemolytic transfusion reaction** A 🔵, 🔵, A 🔵
     ABO incompatibility with hemolytic transfusion reaction less than 24 hours after transfusion
     Acute hemolytic transfusion reaction (AHTR) due to ABO incompatibility

  ● **T80.311** **ABO incompatibility with delayed hemolytic transfusion reaction** A 🔵, 🔵, A 🔵
     ABO incompatibility with hemolytic transfusion reaction 24 hours or more after transfusion
     Delayed hemolytic transfusion reaction (DHTR) due to ABO incompatibility

  ● **T80.319** **ABO incompatibility with hemolytic transfusion reaction, unspecified** A 🔵, 🔵, A 🔵
     ABO incompatibility with hemolytic transfusion reaction at unspecified time after transfusion
     Hemolytic transfusion reaction (HTR) due to ABO incompatibility NOS

X● **T80.39** **Other ABO incompatibility reaction due to transfusion of blood or blood products** A 🔵, 🔵, A 🔵
     Delayed serologic transfusion reaction (DSTR) from ABO incompatibility
     Other ABO incompatible blood transfusion
     Other reaction to ABO incompatible blood transfusion

● **T80.4** **Rh incompatibility reaction due to transfusion of blood or blood products**
     Reaction due to incompatibility of Rh antigens (C) (c) (D) (E) (e)
     (Ex) **For category T80.4 CC codes unless otherwise indicated:** See T80.3

X● **T80.40** **Rh incompatibility reaction due to transfusion of blood or blood products, unspecified** A 🔵, 🔵
     Reaction due to Rh factor in transfusion NOS
     Rh incompatible blood transfusion NOS

● **T80.41** **Rh incompatibility with hemolytic transfusion reaction**

  ● **T80.410** **Rh incompatibility with acute hemolytic transfusion reaction** A 🔵, 🔵
     Acute hemolytic transfusion reaction (AHTR) due to Rh incompatibility
     Rh incompatibility with hemolytic transfusion reaction less than 24 hours after transfusion

  ● **T80.411** **Rh incompatibility with delayed hemolytic transfusion reaction** A 🔵, 🔵
     Delayed hemolytic transfusion reaction (DHTR) due to Rh incompatibility
     Rh incompatibility with hemolytic transfusion reaction 24 hours or more after transfusion

  ● **T80.419** **Rh incompatibility with hemolytic transfusion reaction, unspecified** A 🔵, 🔵
     Rh incompatibility with hemolytic transfusion reaction at unspecified time after transfusion
     Hemolytic transfusion reaction (HTR) due to Rh incompatibility NOS

X● **T80.49** **Other Rh incompatibility reaction due to transfusion of blood or blood products** A 🔵, 🔵
     Delayed serologic transfusion reaction (DSTR) from Rh incompatibility
     Other reaction to Rh incompatible blood transfusion
     (Ex) T80.30X-T80.419[A], T80.910-T80.92X[A], T80.A9X[A]

CHAPTER 19 (S00-T88)

N Newborn Age: 0   **P** Pediatric Age: 0–17   **M** Maternity DX: 12–55   **A** Adult Age: 15–124   ♀ Females Only   ♂ Males Only

🔵 Complication\Comorbidity   🔵 Major C\C   (Ex) CC/MCC Exclusions   🔵 Present on Admission Requirement   🔵 Hospital-Acquired Condition

1569

● **T80.A** **Non-ABO incompatibility reaction due to transfusion of blood or blood products**
　Reaction due to incompatibility of minor antigens (Duffy) (Kell) (Kidd) (Lewis) (M) (N) (P) (S)
　Ex: For category T80.A CC codes unless otherwise indicated: See T80.49

X ● **T80.A0** **Non-ABO incompatibility reaction due to transfusion of blood or blood products, unspecified** A 🝙, 🝙
　Non-ABO antigen incompatibility reaction from transfusion NOS

● **T80.A1** **Non-ABO incompatibility with hemolytic transfusion reaction**

● **T80.A10** **Non-ABO incompatibility with acute hemolytic transfusion reaction** A 🝙, 🝙
　Acute hemolytic transfusion reaction (AHTR) due to non-ABO incompatibility
　Non-ABO incompatibility with hemolytic transfusion reaction less than 24 hours after transfusion

● **T80.A11** **Non-ABO incompatibility with delayed hemolytic transfusion reaction** A 🝙, 🝙
　Delayed hemolytic transfusion reaction (DHTR) due to non-ABO incompatibility
　Non-ABO incompatibility with hemolytic transfusion reaction 24 or more hours after transfusion

● **T80.A19** **Non-ABO incompatibility with hemolytic transfusion reaction, unspecified** A 🝙, 🝙
　Hemolytic transfusion reaction (HTR) due to non-ABO incompatibility NOS
　Non-ABO incompatibility with hemolytic transfusion reaction at unspecified time after transfusion

X ● **T80.A9** **Other non-ABO incompatibility reaction due to transfusion of blood or blood products** A 🝙, 🝙
　Delayed serologic transfusion reaction (DSTR) from non-ABO incompatibility
　Other reaction to non-ABO incompatible blood transfusion
　Ex: See T80.3

● **T80.5** **Anaphylactic reaction due to serum**
　Allergic reaction due to serum
　Anaphylactic shock due to serum
　Anaphylactoid reaction due to serum
　Anaphylaxis due to serum
　Excludes1 ABO incompatibility reaction due to transfusion of blood or blood products (T80.3-)
　allergic reaction or shock NOS (T78.2)
　anaphylactic reaction or shock NOS (T78.2)
　anaphylactic reaction or shock due to adverse effect of correct medicinal substance properly administered (T88.6)
　other serum reaction (T80.6-)
　Ex: For category T80.5 CC codes: T80.51X-T80.69X[A]

X ● **T80.51** **Anaphylactic reaction due to administration of blood and blood products** A 🝙, 🝙

X ● **T80.52** **Anaphylactic reaction due to vaccination** A 🝙, 🝙

X ● **T80.59** **Anaphylactic reaction due to other serum** A 🝙, 🝙

● **T80.6** **Other serum reactions**
　Intoxication by serum　　Serum sickness
　Protein sickness　　　　Serum urticaria
　Serum rash
　Excludes2 serum hepatitis (B16.-)
　Ex: For category T80.6 CC codes unless otherwise indicated: T80.51X-T80.69X[A]

X ● **T80.61** **Other serum reaction due to administration of blood and blood products** A 🝙, 🝙

X ● **T80.62** **Other serum reaction due to vaccination** A 🝙, 🝙

X ● **T80.69** **Other serum reaction due to other serum** A 🝙, 🝙
　Ex: T80.61X-T80.69X[A]

● **T80.8** **Other complications following infusion, transfusion and therapeutic injection**

● **T80.81** **Extravasation of vesicant agent**
　Infiltration of vesicant agent
　Ex: For category T80.81 CC codes: T80.1XX[A], T80.810-T80.818[A], T80.90X[A]

● **T80.810** **Extravasation of vesicant antineoplastic chemotherapy** A 🝙, 🝙
　Infiltration of vesicant antineoplastic chemotherapy

● **T80.818** **Extravasation of other vesicant agent** A 🝙, 🝙
　Infiltration of other vesicant agent

X ● **T80.89** **Other complications following infusion, transfusion and therapeutic injection** 🝙
　Delayed serologic transfusion reaction (DSTR), unspecified incompatibility
　Use additional code to identify graft-versus-host reaction, if applicable, (D89.81-)

● **T80.9** **Unspecified complication following infusion, transfusion and therapeutic injection**

X ● **T80.90** **Unspecified complication following infusion and therapeutic injection** 🝙

● **T80.91** **Hemolytic transfusion reaction, unspecified incompatibility**
　Excludes1 ABO incompatibility with hemolytic transfusion reaction (T80.31-)
　Non-ABO incompatibility with hemolytic transfusion reaction (T80.A1-)
　Rh incompatibility with hemolytic transfusion reaction (T80.41-)
　Ex: For category T80.91 CC codes unless otherwise indicated: See T80.3

● **T80.910** **Acute hemolytic transfusion reaction, unspecified incompatibility** A 🝙, 🝙

● **T80.911** **Delayed hemolytic transfusion reaction, unspecified incompatibility** A 🝙, 🝙

● **T80.919** **Hemolytic transfusion reaction, unspecified incompatibility, unspecified as acute or delayed** A 🝙, 🝙
　Hemolytic transfusion reaction NOS

X ● **T80.92** **Unspecified transfusion reaction** 🝙
　Transfusion reaction NOS

◄ New　◄ Revised　̶d̶e̶l̶e̶t̶e̶d̶ Deleted　Excludes 1　Excludes 2　Includes　Use additional　Code first　Code also　Unspecified
OGCR Official Guidelines　● Unacceptable Principal Diagnosis　X Assign placeholder X　● Use Additional Character(s)　▶ Manifestation Code　**Coding Clinic**

● **T81**   **Complications of procedures, not elsewhere classified**

Use additional code for adverse effect, if applicable, to identify drug (T36-T50 with fifth or sixth character 5)

Excludes2   complications following immunization (T88.0-T88.1)

complications following infusion, transfusion and therapeutic injection (T80.-)

complications of transplanted organs and tissue (T86.-)

poisoning and toxic effects of drugs and chemicals (T36-T65 with fifth or sixth character 1-4 or 6)

specified complications classified elsewhere, such as:

complication of prosthetic devices, implants and grafts (T82-T85)

dermatitis due to drugs and medicaments (L23.3, L24.4, L25.1, L27.0-L27.1)

endosseous dental implant failure (M27.6-)

floppy iris syndrome (IFIS) (intraoperative) H21.81

intraoperative and postprocedural complications of specific body system (D78.-, E36.-, E89.-, G97.3-, G97.4, H59.3-, H59.-, H95.2-, H95.3, I97.4-, I97.5, J95, K91.-, L76.-, M96.-, N99.-) ◀▥

ostomy complications (J95.0-, K94.-, N99.5-)

plateau iris syndrome (post-iridectomy) (postprocedural) H21.82

The appropriate 7th character is to be added to each code from category T81

A	initial encounter
D	subsequent encounter
S	sequela

● **T81.1**   **Postprocedural shock**

Shock during or resulting from a procedure, not elsewhere classified

Excludes1   anaphylactic shock NOS (T78.2)

anaphylactic shock due to correct substance properly administered (T88.6)

anaphylactic shock due to serum (T80.5-)

anesthetic shock (T88.2)

electric shock (T75.4)

obstetric shock (O75.1)

septic shock (R65.21)

shock following abortion or ectopic or molar pregnancy (O00-O07, O08.3)

traumatic shock (T79.4)

Ⓔⓧ **For category T81.1 CC codes:** D78.01-D78.02, D78.21-D78.22, D78.81-D78.89, E36.01-E36.02, E36.8, E89.810-E89.89, G97.51-G97.52, H59.011-H59.019, H59.031-H59.039, H59.091-H59.099, H59.111-H59.129, H59.311-H59.329, H59.811-H59.819, H59.88-H59.89, H95.21-H95.22, H95.41-H95.42, H95.811-H95.819, H95.88-H95.89, I97.3-I97.42, I97.610-I97.62, J95.61-J95.62, J95.830-J95.831, K91.61-K91.62, K91.840-K91.841, L76.01-L76.02, L76.21-L76.22, L76.81-L76.82, M96.810-M96.811, M96.830-M96.89, N98.1-N98.9, N99.61-N99.62, N99.820-N99.821, T79.4XX[A], T81.10X-T81.19X[A], T81.82X-T81.9XX[A], T88.2XX[A]

X● **T81.10**   **Postprocedural shock unspecified** A 🅒, 🅜

Collapse NOS during or resulting from a procedure, not elsewhere classified

Postprocedural failure of peripheral circulation

Postprocedural shock NOS

X● **T81.11**   **Postprocedural cardiogenic shock** A 🅒, 🅜

A●X● **T81.12**   **Postprocedural septic shock** A 🅒, 🅜

Postprocedural endotoxic shock during or resulting from a procedure, not elsewhere classified

Postprocedural gram-negative shock during or resulting from a procedure, not elsewhere classified

Code first underlying infection

Use additional code, to identify any associated acute organ dysfunction, if applicable

X● **T81.19**   **Other postprocedural shock** A 🅒, 🅜

Postprocedural hypovolemic shock

● **T81.3**   **Disruption of wound, not elsewhere classified**

Disruption of any suture materials or other closure methods

Excludes1   breakdown (mechanical) of permanent sutures (T85.612)

displacement of permanent sutures (T85.622)

disruption of cesarean delivery wound (O90.0)

disruption of perineal obstetric wound (O90.1)

mechanical complication of permanent sutures NEC (T85.692)

Ⓔⓧ **For category T81.3 CC codes:** D78.81-D78.89, E36.8, E89.810-E89.89, H59.011-H59.019, H59.031-H59.039, H59.091-H59.099, H59.811-H59.89, H95.811-H95.89, I97.3, L76.81-L76.82, M96.89, N98.1-N98.9, T81.30X-T81.33X[A], T81.82X-T81.9XX[A]

X● **T81.30**   **Disruption of wound, unspecified** A 🅒, 🅜

Disruption of wound NOS

X● **T81.31**   **Disruption of external operation (surgical) wound, not elsewhere classified** A 🅒, 🅜

Excludes1   dehiscence of amputation stump (T87.81)

Dehiscence of operation wound NOS

Disruption of operation wound NOS

Disruption or dehiscence of closure of cornea

Disruption or dehiscence of closure of mucosa

Disruption or dehiscence of closure of skin and subcutaneous tissue

Full-thickness skin disruption or dehiscence

Superficial disruption or dehiscence of operation wound

X● **T81.32**   **Disruption of internal operation (surgical) wound, not elsewhere classified** A 🅒, 🅜

Deep disruption or dehiscence of operation wound NOS

Disruption or dehiscence of closure of internal organ or other internal tissue

Disruption or dehiscence of closure of muscle or muscle flap

Disruption or dehiscence of closure of ribs or rib cage

Disruption or dehiscence of closure of skull or craniotomy

Disruption or dehiscence of closure of sternum or sternotomy

Disruption or dehiscence of closure of tendon or ligament

Disruption or dehiscence of closure of superficial or muscular fascia

X● **T81.33**   **Disruption of traumatic injury wound repair** A 🅒, 🅜

Disruption or dehiscence of closure of traumatic laceration (external) (internal)

N Newborn Age: 0   **P** Pediatric Age: 0–17   **M** Maternity DX: 12–55   **A** Adult Age: 15–124   ♀ Females Only   ♂ Males Only

🅒 Complication\Comorbidity   🅜 Major C\C   Ⓔⓧ CC/MCC Exclusions   🄿 Present on Admission Requirement   🄷 Hospital-Acquired Condition   **1571**

X ● **T81.4**   **Infection following a procedure** A 🔵, 🔵, A 🔵
      Intra-abdominal abscess following a procedure
      Postprocedural infection, not elsewhere classified
      Sepsis following a procedure
      Stitch abscess following a procedure
      Subphrenic abscess following a procedure
      Wound abscess following a procedure

      Use additional code to identify infection

      Use additional code (R65.2-) to identify severe sepsis, if
      applicable

      Excludes1   obstetric surgical wound infection (O86.0)
                 postprocedural fever NOS (R50.82)
                 postprocedural retroperitoneal abscess
                     (K68.11)

      Excludes2   bleb associated endophthalmitis (H59.4-)
                 infection due to infusion, transfusion and
                     therapeutic injection (T80.2-)
                 infection due to prosthetic devices,
                     implants and grafts (T82.6-T82.7,
                     T83.5-T83.6, T84.5-T84.7, T85.7)

      (Ex:) D78.81-D78.89, E36.8, E89.810-E89.89, H59.011-H59.019,
          H59.031-H59.099, H59.811-H59.89, H95.811-H95.89, I97.3, K68.11,
          L76.81-L76.82, M96.89, N98.1-N98.9, T81.4XX[A], T81.82X[A],
          T81.89X-T81.9XX[A]

● **T81.5**   **Complications of foreign body accidentally left in body
following procedure**
      (Ex:) **For category T81.5 CC codes:** D78.81-D78.89, E36.8, E89.810-E89.89,
          H59.011-H59.019, H59.031-H59.039, H59.091-H59.099, H59.811-H59.89,
          H95.811-H95.89, I97.3, L76.81-L76.82, M96.89, N98.1-N98.9,
          T81.500-T81.599[A], T81.82X-T81.9XX[A]

  ● **T81.50**   **Unspecified complication of foreign body
accidentally left in body following procedure**

    ● **T81.500**   Unspecified complication of foreign
body accidentally left in body
following surgical operation A 🔵, 🔵,
A 🔵

    ● **T81.501**   Unspecified complication of foreign
body accidentally left in body
following infusion or transfusion
A 🔵, 🔵, A 🔵

    ● **T81.502**   Unspecified complication of foreign
body accidentally left in body
following kidney dialysis A 🔵, 🔵,
A 🔵

    ● **T81.503**   Unspecified complication of foreign
body accidentally left in body
following injection or immunization
A 🔵, 🔵, A 🔵

    ● **T81.504**   Unspecified complication of foreign
body accidentally left in body
following endoscopic examination
A 🔵, 🔵, A 🔵

    ● **T81.505**   Unspecified complication of foreign
body accidentally left in body
following heart catheterization A 🔵,
🔵, A 🔵

    ● **T81.506**   Unspecified complication of foreign
body accidentally left in body
following aspiration, puncture or
other catheterization A 🔵, 🔵, A 🔵

    ● **T81.507**   Unspecified complication of foreign
body accidentally left in body
following removal of catheter or
packing A 🔵, 🔵, A 🔵

    ● **T81.508**   Unspecified complication of foreign
body accidentally left in body
following other procedure A 🔵, 🔵,
A 🔵

    ● **T81.509**   Unspecified complication of foreign
body accidentally left in body
following unspecified procedure A 🔵,
🔵, A 🔵

● **T81.51**   **Adhesions due to foreign body accidentally left
in body following procedure**

  ● **T81.510**   Adhesions due to foreign body
accidentally left in body following
surgical operation A 🔵, 🔵, A 🔵

  ● **T81.511**   Adhesions due to foreign body
accidentally left in body following
infusion or transfusion A 🔵, 🔵, A 🔵

  ● **T81.512**   Adhesions due to foreign body
accidentally left in body following
kidney dialysis A 🔵, 🔵, A 🔵

  ● **T81.513**   Adhesions due to foreign body
accidentally left in body following
injection or immunization A 🔵, 🔵,
A 🔵

  ● **T81.514**   Adhesions due to foreign body
accidentally left in body following
endoscopic examination A 🔵, 🔵, A 🔵

  ● **T81.515**   Adhesions due to foreign body
accidentally left in body following
heart catheterization A 🔵, 🔵, A 🔵

  ● **T81.516**   Adhesions due to foreign body
accidentally left in body following
aspiration, puncture or other
catheterization A 🔵, 🔵, A 🔵

  ● **T81.517**   Adhesions due to foreign body
accidentally left in body following
removal of catheter or packing A 🔵,
🔵, A 🔵

  ● **T81.518**   Adhesions due to foreign body
accidentally left in body following
other procedure A 🔵, 🔵, A 🔵

  ● **T81.519**   Adhesions due to foreign body
accidentally left in body following
unspecified procedure A 🔵, 🔵, A 🔵

● **T81.52**   **Obstruction due to foreign body accidentally
left in body following procedure**

  ● **T81.520**   Obstruction due to foreign body
accidentally left in body following
surgical operation A 🔵, 🔵, A 🔵

  ● **T81.521**   Obstruction due to foreign body
accidentally left in body following
infusion or transfusion A 🔵, 🔵, A 🔵

  ● **T81.522**   Obstruction due to foreign body
accidentally left in body following
kidney dialysis A 🔵, 🔵, A 🔵

  ● **T81.523**   Obstruction due to foreign body
accidentally left in body following
injection or immunization A 🔵, 🔵,
A 🔵

  ● **T81.524**   Obstruction due to foreign body
accidentally left in body following
endoscopic examination A 🔵, 🔵, A 🔵

  ● **T81.525**   Obstruction due to foreign body
accidentally left in body following
heart catheterization A 🔵, 🔵, A 🔵

  ● **T81.526**   Obstruction due to foreign body
accidentally left in body following
aspiration, puncture or other
catheterization A 🔵, 🔵, A 🔵

  ● **T81.527**   Obstruction due to foreign body
accidentally left in body following
removal of catheter or packing A 🔵,
🔵, A 🔵

  ● **T81.528**   Obstruction due to foreign body
accidentally left in body following
other procedure A 🔵, 🔵, A 🔵

  ● **T81.529**   Obstruction due to foreign body
accidentally left in body following
unspecified procedure A 🔵, 🔵, A 🔵

◀ New   ◀▥ Revised   ~~deleted~~ Deleted   Excludes 1   Excludes 2   Includes   Use additional   Code first   Code also   Unspecified

OGCR Official Guidelines   ● Unacceptable Principal Diagnosis   X Assign placeholder X   ▌ Use Additional Character(s)   ▐ Manifestation Code   **Coding Clinic**

CHAPTER 19 (S00-T88)

● **T81.53** Perforation due to foreign body accidentally left in body following procedure

● **T81.530** Perforation due to foreign body accidentally left in body following surgical operation A 🔵, 🔵, A 🔵

● **T81.531** Perforation due to foreign body accidentally left in body following infusion or transfusion A 🔵, 🔵, A 🔵

● **T81.532** Perforation due to foreign body accidentally left in body following kidney dialysis A 🔵, 🔵, A 🔵

● **T81.533** Perforation due to foreign body accidentally left in body following injection or immunization A 🔵, 🔵, A 🔵

● **T81.534** Perforation due to foreign body accidentally left in body following endoscopic examination A 🔵, 🔵, A 🔵

● **T81.535** Perforation due to foreign body accidentally left in body following heart catheterization A 🔵, 🔵, A 🔵

● **T81.536** Perforation due to foreign body accidentally left in body following aspiration, puncture or other catheterization A 🔵, 🔵, A 🔵

● **T81.537** Perforation due to foreign body accidentally left in body following removal of catheter or packing A 🔵, 🔵, A 🔵

● **T81.538** Perforation due to foreign body accidentally left in body following other procedure A 🔵, 🔵, A 🔵

● **T81.539** Perforation due to foreign body accidentally left in body following unspecified procedure A 🔵, 🔵, A 🔵

● **T81.59** Other complications of foreign body accidentally left in body following procedure

Excludes2   obstruction or perforation due to prosthetic devices and implants intentionally left in body (T82.0-T82.5, T83.0-T83.4, T83.7, T84.0-T84.4, T85.0-T85.6)

● **T81.590** Other complications of foreign body accidentally left in body following surgical operation A 🔵, 🔵, A 🔵

● **T81.591** Other complications of foreign body accidentally left in body following infusion or transfusion A 🔵, 🔵, A 🔵

● **T81.592** Other complications of foreign body accidentally left in body following kidney dialysis A 🔵, 🔵, A 🔵

● **T81.593** Other complications of foreign body accidentally left in body following injection or immunization A 🔵, 🔵, A 🔵

● **T81.594** Other complications of foreign body accidentally left in body following endoscopic examination A 🔵, 🔵, A 🔵

● **T81.595** Other complications of foreign body accidentally left in body following heart catheterization A 🔵, 🔵, A 🔵

● **T81.596** Other complications of foreign body accidentally left in body following aspiration, puncture or other catheterization A 🔵, 🔵, A 🔵

● **T81.597** Other complications of foreign body accidentally left in body following removal of catheter or packing A 🔵, 🔵, A 🔵

● **T81.598** Other complications of foreign body accidentally left in body following other procedure A 🔵, 🔵, A 🔵

● **T81.599** Other complications of foreign body accidentally left in body following unspecified procedure A 🔵, 🔵, A 🔵

● **T81.6** Acute reaction to foreign substance accidentally left during a procedure

Excludes2   complications of foreign body accidentally left in body cavity or operation wound following procedure (T81.5-)

(Ex:) **For category T81.6 CC codes:** D78.81-D78.89, E36.8, E89.810-E89.89, H59.011-H59.019, H59.031-H59.039, H59.091-H59.099, H59.811-H59.89, H95.811-H95.89, I97.3, L76.81-L76.82, M96.89, N98.1-N98.9, T81.60X-T81.69X[A], T81.82X-T81.9XX[A]

X ● **T81.60** Unspecified acute reaction to foreign substance accidentally left during a procedure A 🔵, 🔵, A 🔵

X ● **T81.61** Aseptic peritonitis due to foreign substance accidentally left during a procedure A 🔵, 🔵, A 🔵
Chemical peritonitis

X ● **T81.69** Other acute reaction to foreign substance accidentally left during a procedure A 🔵, 🔵, A 🔵

● **T81.7** Vascular complications following a procedure, not elsewhere classified
Air embolism following procedure NEC
Phlebitis or thrombophlebitis resulting from a procedure

Excludes1   embolism complicating abortion or ectopic or molar pregnancy (O00-O07, O08.2)
embolism complicating pregnancy, childbirth and the puerperium (O88.-)
traumatic embolism (T79.0)

Excludes2   embolism due to prosthetic devices, implants and grafts (T82.8, T83.8, T84.8-, T85.8)
embolism following infusion, transfusion and therapeutic injection (T80.0)

● **T81.71** Complication of artery following a procedure, not elsewhere classified
(Ex:) **For category T81.71 CC codes T81.710-T81.711:** D78.81-D78.89, E36.8, E89.810-E89.89, H59.011-H59.019, H59.031-H59.039, H59.091-H59.099, H59.811-H59.89, H95.811-H95.89, I97.3, L76.81-L76.82, M96.89, N98.1-N98.9, T81.710-T81.72X[A], T81.82X-T81.9XX[A] **For T81.718-T81.719:** D78.81-D78.89, E36.8, E89.810-E89.89, H59.011-H59.019, H59.031-H59.039, H59.091-H59.099, H59.811-H59.89, H95.811-H95.89, I97.3, L76.81-L76.82, M96.89, N98.1-N98.9, T81.718-T81.72X[A], T81.82X-T81.9XX[A]

● **T81.710** Complication of mesenteric artery following a procedure, not elsewhere classified A 🔵, 🔵

● **T81.711** Complication of renal artery following a procedure, not elsewhere classified A 🔵, 🔵

● **T81.718** Complication of other artery following a procedure, not elsewhere classified A 🔵, 🔵

● **T81.719** Complication of unspecified artery following a procedure, not elsewhere classified A 🔵, 🔵

X ● **T81.72** Complication of vein following a procedure, not elsewhere classified A 🔵, 🔵
(Ex:) See T81.718-T81.719

N Newborn Age: 0   P Pediatric Age: 0–17   M Maternity DX: 12–55   A Adult Age: 15–124   ♀ Females Only   ♂ Males Only

🔵 Complication\Comorbidity   🔵 Major C\C   (Ex:) CC/MCC Exclusions   🔵 Present on Admission Requirement   🔵 Hospital-Acquired Condition

CHAPTER 19 (S00-T88)

1573

●T81.8   **Other complications of procedures, not elsewhere classified**
     Excludes2   hypothermia following anesthesia (T88.51)
            malignant hyperpyrexia due to anesthesia (T88.3)

X●T81.81   **Complication of inhalation therapy** 🔍
      A MCE: Questionable admission when principal dx

X●T81.82   **Emphysema (subcutaneous) resulting from a procedure** 🔍

X●T81.83   **Persistent postprocedural fistula** A 🔍, 🔍
      (Ex) D78.81-D78.89, E36.8, E89.810-E89.89, H59.011-H59.019, H59.031-H59.039, H59.091-H59.099, H59.811-H59.89, H95.811-H95.89, I97.3, L76.81-L76.82, M96.89, N98.1-N98.9, T81.82X-T81.9XX[A]

X●T81.89   **Other complications of procedures, not elsewhere classified** 🔍
      Use additional code to specify complication, such as:
         postprocedural delirium (F05)

X●T81.9   **Unspecified complication of procedure** 🔍

●T82   **Complications of cardiac and vascular prosthetic devices, implants and grafts**
     Excludes2   failure and rejection of transplanted organs and tissue (T86.-)
     The appropriate 7th character is to be added to each code from category T82

A	initial encounter
D	subsequent encounter
S	sequela

●T82.0   **Mechanical complication of heart valve prosthesis**
     Mechanical complication of artificial heart valve
     Excludes1   mechanical complication of biological heart valve graft (T82.22-)
     (Ex) **For category T82.0 CC codes:** D78.81-D78.89, E36.8, E89.810-E89.89, H59.011-H59.019, H59.031-H59.039, H59.091-H59.099, H59.811-H59.89, H95.811-H95.89, I97.3, L76.81-L76.82, M96.89, N98.1-N98.9, T81.82X-T81.9XX[A], T82.01X-T82.09X[A]

X●T82.01   **Breakdown (mechanical) of heart valve prosthesis** A 🔍, 🔍

X●T82.02   **Displacement of heart valve prosthesis** A 🔍, 🔍
      Malposition of heart valve prosthesis

X●T82.03   **Leakage of heart valve prosthesis** A 🔍, 🔍

X●T82.09   **Other mechanical complication of heart valve prosthesis** A 🔍, 🔍
      Obstruction (mechanical) of heart valve prosthesis
      Perforation of heart valve prosthesis
      Protrusion of heart valve prosthesis

●T82.1   **Mechanical complication of cardiac electronic device**
     (Ex) **For category T82.1 CC codes:** D78.81-D78.89, E36.8, E89.810-E89.89, H59.011-H59.019, H59.031-H59.039, H59.091-H59.099, H59.811-H59.89, H95.811-H95.89, I97.3, L76.81-L76.82, M96.89, N98.1-N98.9, T81.82X-T81.9XX[A], T82.110-T82.199[A]

●T82.11   **Breakdown (mechanical) of cardiac electronic device**

 ●T82.110   **Breakdown (mechanical) of cardiac electrode** A 🔍, 🔍

 ●T82.111   **Breakdown (mechanical) of cardiac pulse generator (battery)** A 🔍, 🔍

 ●T82.118   **Breakdown (mechanical) of other cardiac electronic device** A 🔍, 🔍

 ●T82.119   **Breakdown (mechanical) of unspecified cardiac electronic device** A 🔍, 🔍

●T82.12   **Displacement of cardiac electronic device**
     Malposition of cardiac electronic device

 ●T82.120   **Displacement of cardiac electrode** A 🔍, 🔍

 ●T82.121   **Displacement of cardiac pulse generator (battery)** A 🔍, 🔍

 ●T82.128   **Displacement of other cardiac electronic device** A 🔍, 🔍

 ●T82.129   **Displacement of unspecified cardiac electronic device** A 🔍, 🔍

●T82.19   **Other mechanical complication of cardiac electronic device**
     Leakage of cardiac electronic device
     Obstruction of cardiac electronic device
     Perforation of cardiac electronic device
     Protrusion of cardiac electronic device

 ●T82.190   **Other mechanical complication of cardiac electrode** A 🔍, 🔍

 ●T82.191   **Other mechanical complication of cardiac pulse generator (battery)** A 🔍, 🔍

 ●T82.198   **Other mechanical complication of other cardiac electronic device** A 🔍, 🔍

 ●T82.199   **Other mechanical complication of unspecified cardiac device** A 🔍, 🔍

●T82.2   **Mechanical complication of coronary artery bypass graft and biological heart valve graft**
     Excludes1   mechanical complication of artificial heart valve prosthesis (T82.0-)

●T82.21   **Mechanical complication of coronary artery bypass graft**
     (Ex) **For category T82.21 CC codes:** D78.81-D78.89, E36.8, E89.810-E89.89, H59.011-H59.019, H59.031-H59.039, H59.091-H59.099, H59.811-H59.89, H95.811-H95.89, I97.3, L76.81-L76.82, M96.89, N98.1-N98.9, T81.82X-T81.9XX[A], T82.211-T82.218[A]

 ●T82.211   **Breakdown (mechanical) of coronary artery bypass graft** A 🔍, 🔍

 ●T82.212   **Displacement of coronary artery bypass graft** A 🔍, 🔍
      Malposition of coronary artery bypass graft

 ●T82.213   **Leakage of coronary artery bypass graft** A 🔍, 🔍

 ●T82.218   **Other mechanical complication of coronary artery bypass graft** A 🔍, 🔍
      Obstruction, mechanical of coronary artery bypass graft
      Perforation of coronary artery bypass graft
      Protrusion of coronary artery bypass graft

●T82.22   **Mechanical complication of biological heart valve graft**
     (Ex) **For category T82.22 CC codes:** D78.81-D78.89, E36.8, E89.810-E89.89, H59.011-H59.019, H59.031-H59.039, H59.091-H59.099, H59.811-H59.89, H95.811-H95.89, I97.3, L76.81-L76.82, M96.89, N98.1-N98.9, T81.82X-T81.9XX[A], T82.221-T82.228[A], T82.512-T82.598[A]

 ●T82.221   **Breakdown (mechanical) of biological heart valve graft** A 🔍, 🔍

 ●T82.222   **Displacement of biological heart valve graft** A 🔍, 🔍
      Malposition of biological heart valve graft

● T82.223   Leakage of biological heart valve graft A 🔵, 🔵

● T82.228   Other mechanical complication of biological heart valve graft A 🔵, 🔵
  Obstruction of biological heart valve graft
  Perforation of biological heart valve graft
  Protrusion of biological heart valve graft

● T82.3   Mechanical complication of other vascular grafts
  (Ex) For category T82.3 CC codes: D78.81-D78.89, E36.8, E89.810-E89.89, H59.011-H59.019, H59.031-H59.039, H59.091-H59.099, H59.811-H59.89, H95.811-H95.89, I97.3, L76.81-L76.82, M96.89, N98.1-N98.9, T81.82X-T81.9XX[A], T82.310-T82.538[A], T82.590-T82.595[A]

● T82.31   Breakdown (mechanical) of other vascular grafts

  ● T82.310   Breakdown (mechanical) of aortic (bifurcation) graft (replacement) A 🔵, 🔵

  ● T82.311   Breakdown (mechanical) of carotid arterial graft (bypass) A 🔵, 🔵

  ● T82.312   Breakdown (mechanical) of femoral arterial graft (bypass) A 🔵, 🔵

  ● T82.318   Breakdown (mechanical) of other vascular grafts A 🔵, 🔵

  ● T82.319   Breakdown (mechanical) of unspecified vascular grafts A 🔵, 🔵

● T82.32   Displacement of other vascular grafts
  Malposition of other vascular grafts

  ● T82.320   Displacement of aortic (bifurcation) graft (replacement) A 🔵, 🔵

  ● T82.321   Displacement of carotid arterial graft (bypass) A 🔵, 🔵

  ● T82.322   Displacement of femoral arterial graft (bypass) A 🔵, 🔵

  ● T82.328   Displacement of other vascular grafts A 🔵, 🔵

  ● T82.329   Displacement of unspecified vascular grafts A 🔵, 🔵

● T82.33   Leakage of other vascular grafts

  ● T82.330   Leakage of aortic (bifurcation) graft (replacement) A 🔵, 🔵

  ● T82.331   Leakage of carotid arterial graft (bypass) A 🔵, 🔵

  ● T82.332   Leakage of femoral arterial graft (bypass) A 🔵, 🔵

  ● T82.338   Leakage of other vascular grafts A 🔵, 🔵

  ● T82.339   Leakage of unspecified vascular graft A 🔵, 🔵

● T82.39   Other mechanical complication of other vascular grafts
  Obstruction (mechanical) of other vascular grafts
  Perforation of other vascular grafts
  Protrusion of other vascular grafts

  ● T82.390   Other mechanical complication of aortic (bifurcation) graft (replacement) A 🔵, 🔵

  ● T82.391   Other mechanical complication of carotid arterial graft (bypass) A 🔵, 🔵

  ● T82.392   Other mechanical complication of femoral arterial graft (bypass) A 🔵, 🔵

  ● T82.398   Other mechanical complication of other vascular grafts A 🔵, 🔵

  ● T82.399   Other mechanical complication of unspecified vascular grafts A 🔵, 🔵

● T82.4   Mechanical complication of vascular dialysis catheter
  Mechanical complication of hemodialysis catheter
  Excludes1   mechanical complication of intraperitoneal dialysis catheter (T85.62)
  (Ex) For category T82.4 CC codes: See T82.3

X ● T82.41   Breakdown (mechanical) of vascular dialysis catheter A 🔵, 🔵

X ● T82.42   Displacement of vascular dialysis catheter A 🔵, 🔵
  Malposition of vascular dialysis catheter

X ● T82.43   Leakage of vascular dialysis catheter A 🔵, 🔵

X ● T82.49   Other complication of vascular dialysis catheter A 🔵, 🔵
  Obstruction (mechanical) of vascular dialysis catheter
  Perforation of vascular dialysis catheter
  Protrusion of vascular dialysis catheter

● T82.5   Mechanical complication of other cardiac and vascular devices and implants
  Excludes2   mechanical complication of epidural and subdural infusion catheter (T85.61)
  (Ex) For category T82.5 CC codes unless otherwise indicated: See T82.3

● T82.51   Breakdown (mechanical) of other cardiac and vascular devices and implants

  ● T82.510   Breakdown (mechanical) of surgically created arteriovenous fistula A 🔵, 🔵

  ● T82.511   Breakdown (mechanical) of surgically created arteriovenous shunt A 🔵, 🔵

  ● T82.512   Breakdown (mechanical) of artificial heart A 🔵, 🔵
    (Ex) See T82.22

  ● T82.513   Breakdown (mechanical) of balloon (counterpulsation) device A 🔵, 🔵

  ● T82.514   Breakdown (mechanical) of infusion catheter A 🔵, 🔵

  ● T82.515   Breakdown (mechanical) of umbrella device A 🔵, 🔵

  ● T82.518   Breakdown (mechanical) of other cardiac and vascular devices and implants A 🔵, 🔵

  ● T82.519   Breakdown (mechanical) of unspecified cardiac and vascular devices and implants A 🔵, 🔵
    (Ex) D78.81-D78.89, E36.8, E89.810-E89.89, H59.011-H59.019, H59.031-H59.039, H59.091-H59.099, H59.811-H59.89, H95.811-H95.89, I97.3, L76.81-L76.82, M96.89, N98.1-N98.9, T81.82X-T81.9XX[A], T82.519[A], T82.539[A], T82.599-T82.9XX[A], T85.9XX[A]

● T82.52   Displacement of other cardiac and vascular devices and implants
  Malposition of other cardiac and vascular devices and implants

  ● T82.520   Displacement of surgically created arteriovenous fistula A 🔵, 🔵

  ● T82.521   Displacement of surgically created arteriovenous shunt A 🔵, 🔵

  ● T82.522   Displacement of artificial heart A 🔵, 🔵
    (Ex) See T82.22

  ● T82.523   Displacement of balloon (counterpulsation) device A 🔵, 🔵

  ● T82.524   Displacement of infusion catheter A 🔵, 🔵

  ● T82.525   Displacement of umbrella device A 🔵, 🔵

N Newborn Age: 0   P Pediatric Age: 0–17   M Maternity DX: 12–55   A Adult Age: 15–124   ♀ Females Only   ♂ Males Only

🔵 Complication\Comorbidity   🔵 Major C\C   (Ex) CC/MCC Exclusions   🔵 Present on Admission Requirement   🔵 Hospital-Acquired Condition

1575

● **T82.528** Displacement of other cardiac and vascular devices and implants A 🔾, 🔾

● **T82.529** Displacement of unspecified cardiac and vascular devices and implants A 🔾, 🔾

● **T82.53** Leakage of other cardiac and vascular devices and implants

● **T82.530** Leakage of surgically created arteriovenous fistula A 🔾, 🔾

● **T82.531** Leakage of surgically created arteriovenous shunt A 🔾, 🔾

● **T82.532** Leakage of artificial heart A 🔾, 🔾
Ex: See T82.22

● **T82.533** Leakage of balloon (counterpulsation) device A 🔾, 🔾

● **T82.534** Leakage of infusion catheter A 🔾, 🔾

● **T82.535** Leakage of umbrella device A 🔾, 🔾

● **T82.538** Leakage of other cardiac and vascular devices and implants A 🔾, 🔾

● **T82.539** Leakage of unspecified cardiac and vascular devices and implants A 🔾, 🔾
Ex: See T82.519

● **T82.59** Other mechanical complication of other cardiac and vascular devices and implants
Obstruction (mechanical) of other cardiac and vascular devices and implants
Perforation of other cardiac and vascular devices and implants
Protrusion of other cardiac and vascular devices and implants

● **T82.590** Other mechanical complication of surgically created arteriovenous fistula A 🔾, 🔾

● **T82.591** Other mechanical complication of surgically created arteriovenous shunt A 🔾, 🔾

● **T82.592** Other mechanical complication of artificial heart A 🔾, 🔾
Ex: See T82.22

● **T82.593** Other mechanical complication of balloon (counterpulsation) device A 🔾, 🔾

● **T82.594** Other mechanical complication of infusion catheter A 🔾, 🔾
Ex: See T82.22

● **T82.595** Other mechanical complication of umbrella device A 🔾, 🔾

● **T82.598** Other mechanical complication of other cardiac and vascular devices and implants A 🔾, 🔾
Ex: See T82.22

● **T82.599** Other mechanical complication of unspecified cardiac and vascular devices and implants A 🔾, 🔾
Ex: See T82.519

X ● **T82.6** Infection and inflammatory reaction due to cardiac valve prosthesis A 🔾, 🔾, A 🔾

Use additional code to identify infection
Ex: D78.81-D78.89, E36.8, E89.810-E89.89, H59.011-H59.019,
H59.031-H59.039, H59.091-H59.099, H59.811-H59.89, H95.811-H95.89,
I97.3, L76.81-L76.82, M96.89, N98.1-N98.9, T81.82X-T81.9XX[A],
T82.01X-T82.9XX[A], T85.310-T85.311[A], T85.320-T85.321[A],
T85.390-T85.391[A], T85.510-T85.9XX[A], T86.820-T86.829,
T86.842-T86.849

X ● **T82.7** Infection and inflammatory reaction due to other cardiac and vascular devices, implants and grafts A 🔾, 🔾, A 🔾
Use additional code to identify infection
Ex: See T82.6

● **T82.8** Other specified complications of cardiac and vascular prosthetic devices, implants and grafts

● **T82.81** Embolism of cardiac and vascular prosthetic devices, implants and grafts

● **T82.817** Embolism of cardiac prosthetic devices, implants and grafts A 🔾, 🔾
Ex: D78.81-D78.89, E36.8, E89.810-E89.89,
H59.011-H59.019, H59.031-H59.039,
H59.091-H59.099, H59.811-H59.89,
H95.811-H95.89, I97.3, L76.81-L76.82,
M96.89, N98.1-N98.9, T81.82X-T81.9XX[A],
T82.01X-T82.9XX[A], T85.310-T85.311[A],
T85.320-T85.321[A], T85.390-T85.391[A],
T85.510-T85.9XX[A], T86.820-T86.829,
T86.842-T86.849

● **T82.818** Embolism of vascular prosthetic devices, implants and grafts A 🔾, 🔾
Ex: See T82.6

● **T82.82** Fibrosis of cardiac and vascular prosthetic devices, implants and grafts

● **T82.827** Fibrosis of cardiac prosthetic devices, implants and grafts A 🔾, 🔾
Ex: See T82.817

● **T82.828** Fibrosis of vascular prosthetic devices, implants and grafts A 🔾, 🔾
Ex: See T82.6

● **T82.83** Hemorrhage of cardiac and vascular prosthetic devices, implants and grafts

● **T82.837** Hemorrhage of cardiac prosthetic devices, implants and grafts A 🔾, 🔾
Ex: See T82.817

● **T82.838** Hemorrhage of vascular prosthetic devices, implants and grafts A 🔾, 🔾
Ex: See T82.6

● **T82.84** Pain from cardiac and vascular prosthetic devices, implants and grafts

● **T82.847** Pain from cardiac prosthetic devices, implants and grafts A 🔾, 🔾
Ex: See T82.817

● **T82.848** Pain from vascular prosthetic devices, implants and grafts A 🔾, 🔾
Ex: See T82.6

● **T82.85** Stenosis of cardiac and vascular prosthetic devices, implants and grafts

● **T82.857** Stenosis of cardiac prosthetic devices, implants and grafts A 🔾, 🔾
Ex: See T82.817

● **T82.858** Stenosis of vascular prosthetic devices, implants and grafts A 🔾, 🔾
Ex: See T82.6

● **T82.86** Thrombosis of cardiac and vascular prosthetic devices, implants and grafts

● **T82.867** Thrombosis of cardiac prosthetic devices, implants and grafts A 🔾, 🔾
Ex: See T82.817

● **T82.868** Thrombosis of vascular prosthetic devices, implants and grafts A 🔾, 🔾
Ex: See T82.6

● **T82.89** Other specified complication of cardiac and vascular prosthetic devices, implants and grafts

● **T82.897** Other specified complication of cardiac prosthetic devices, implants and grafts A 🔾, 🔾
Ex: See T82.817

● **T82.898** Other specified complication of vascular prosthetic devices, implants and grafts A 🔾, 🔾
Ex: See T82.6

X ● **T82.9** Unspecified complication of cardiac and vascular prosthetic device, implant and graft A 🔾, 🔾
Ex: See T82.817

◀ New   ◀▥ Revised   deleted Deleted   Excludes 1   Excludes 2   Includes   Use additional   Code first   Code also   Unspecified
OGCR Official Guidelines   ● Unacceptable Principal Diagnosis   X Assign placeholder X   ● Use Additional Character(s)   ▶ Manifestation Code   **Coding Clinic**

CHAPTER 19 (S00-T88)

● **T83** **Complications of genitourinary prosthetic devices, implants and grafts**

Excludes2 failure and rejection of transplanted organs and tissue (T86.-)

The appropriate 7th character is to be added to each code from category T83

> A initial encounter
> D subsequent encounter
> S sequela

(Ex) **For category T83 CC codes unless otherwise indicated:** D78.81-D78.89, E36.8, E89.810-E89.89, H59.011-H59.019, H59.031-H59.039, H59.091-H59.099, H59.811-H59.89, H95.811-H95.89, I97.3, L76.81-L76.82, M96.89, N98.1-N98.9, N99.510-N99.518, T81.82[A], T81.89-T81.9[A], T83.010[A], T83.020[A], T83.030[A], T83.090[A], T83.110-T83.29X[A], T83.410-T83.6XX[A], T83.718[A], T83.728-T83.9XX[A]

● **T83.0** **Mechanical complication of urinary (indwelling) catheter**

Excludes2 complications of stoma of urinary tract (N99.5-)

● **T83.01** **Breakdown (mechanical) of urinary (indwelling) catheter**

● **T83.010** **Breakdown (mechanical) of cystostomy catheter** A 🔹, 🔹

● **T83.018** **Breakdown (mechanical) of other indwelling urethral catheter** 🔹

● **T83.02** **Displacement of urinary (indwelling) catheter**
Malposition of urinary (indwelling) catheter

● **T83.020** **Displacement of cystostomy catheter** A 🔹, 🔹

● **T83.028** **Displacement of other indwelling urethral catheter** 🔹

● **T83.03** **Leakage of urinary (indwelling) catheter**

● **T83.030** **Leakage of cystostomy catheter** A 🔹, 🔹

● **T83.038** **Leakage of other indwelling urethral catheter** 🔹

● **T83.09** **Other mechanical complication of urinary (indwelling) catheter**
Obstruction (mechanical) of urinary (indwelling) catheter
Perforation of urinary (indwelling) catheter
Protrusion of urinary (indwelling) catheter

● **T83.090** **Other mechanical complication of cystostomy catheter** A 🔹, 🔹

● **T83.098** **Other mechanical complication of other indwelling urethral catheter** 🔹

● **T83.1** **Mechanical complication of other urinary devices and implants**

● **T83.11** **Breakdown (mechanical) of other urinary devices and implants**

● **T83.110** **Breakdown (mechanical) of urinary electronic stimulator device** A 🔹, 🔹

● **T83.111** **Breakdown (mechanical) of urinary sphincter implant** A 🔹, 🔹

● **T83.112** **Breakdown (mechanical) of urinary stent** A 🔹, 🔹

● **T83.118** **Breakdown (mechanical) of other urinary devices and implants** A 🔹, 🔹

● **T83.12** **Displacement of other urinary devices and implants**
Malposition of other urinary devices and implants

● **T83.120** **Displacement of urinary electronic stimulator device** A 🔹, 🔹

● **T83.121** **Displacement of urinary sphincter implant** A 🔹, 🔹

● **T83.122** **Displacement of urinary stent** A 🔹, 🔹

● **T83.128** **Displacement of other urinary devices and implants** A 🔹, 🔹

● **T83.19** **Other mechanical complication of other urinary devices and implants**
Leakage of other urinary devices and implants
Obstruction (mechanical) of other urinary devices and implants
Perforation of other urinary devices and implants
Protrusion of other urinary devices and implants

● **T83.190** **Other mechanical complication of urinary electronic stimulator device** A 🔹, 🔹

● **T83.191** **Other mechanical complication of urinary sphincter implant** A 🔹, 🔹

● **T83.192** **Other mechanical complication of urinary stent** A 🔹, 🔹

● **T83.198** **Other mechanical complication of other urinary devices and implants** A 🔹, 🔹

● **T83.2** **Mechanical complication of graft of urinary organ**

X● **T83.21** **Breakdown (mechanical) of graft of urinary organ** A 🔹, 🔹

X● **T83.22** **Displacement of graft of urinary organ** A 🔹, 🔹
Malposition of graft of urinary organ

X● **T83.23** **Leakage of graft of urinary organ** A 🔹, 🔹

X● **T83.29** **Other mechanical complication of graft of urinary organ** A 🔹, 🔹
Obstruction (mechanical) of graft of urinary organ
Perforation of graft of urinary organ
Protrusion of graft of urinary organ

● **T83.3** **Mechanical complication of intrauterine contraceptive device**

X● **T83.31** **Breakdown (mechanical) of intrauterine contraceptive device** ♀ 🔹

X● **T83.32** **Displacement of intrauterine contraceptive device** ♀ 🔹
Malposition of intrauterine contraceptive device

X● **T83.39** **Other mechanical complication of intrauterine contraceptive device** ♀ 🔹
Leakage of intrauterine contraceptive device
Obstruction (mechanical) of intrauterine contraceptive device
Perforation of intrauterine contraceptive device
Protrusion of intrauterine contraceptive device

● **T83.4** **Mechanical complication of other prosthetic devices, implants and grafts of genital tract**

● **T83.41** **Breakdown (mechanical) of other prosthetic devices, implants and grafts of genital tract**

● **T83.410** **Breakdown (mechanical) of penile (implanted) prosthesis** ♂ A 🔹, 🔹

● **T83.418** **Breakdown (mechanical) of other prosthetic devices, implants and grafts of genital tract** A 🔹, 🔹

● **T83.42** **Displacement of other prosthetic devices, implants and grafts of genital tract**
Malposition of other prosthetic devices, implants and grafts of genital tract

● **T83.420** **Displacement of penile (implanted) prosthesis** ♂ A 🔹, 🔹

● **T83.428** **Displacement of other prosthetic devices, implants and grafts of genital tract** A 🔹, 🔹

N Newborn Age: 0   **P** Pediatric Age: 0–17   **M** Maternity DX: 12–55   **A** Adult Age: 15–124   ♀ Females Only   ♂ Males Only

🔹 Complication\Comorbidity   🔹 Major C\C   (Ex) CC/MCC Exclusions   🔹 Present on Admission Requirement   🔹 Hospital-Acquired Condition

1577

● T83.49   **Other mechanical complication of other prosthetic devices, implants and grafts of genital tract**
Leakage of other prosthetic devices, implants and grafts of genital tract
Obstruction, mechanical of other prosthetic devices, implants and grafts of genital tract
Perforation of other prosthetic devices, implants and grafts of genital tract
Protrusion of other prosthetic devices, implants and grafts of genital tract

    ● T83.490   **Other mechanical complication of penile (implanted) prosthesis** ♂
A 🖫, 🖫

    ● T83.498   **Other mechanical complication of other prosthetic devices, implants and grafts of genital tract** A 🖫, 🖫

● T83.5   **Infection and inflammatory reaction due to prosthetic device, implant and graft in urinary system**
Use additional code to identify infection

   X ● T83.51   **Infection and inflammatory reaction due to indwelling urinary catheter** A 🖫, 🖫, A 🖫

      Excludes2   complications of stoma of urinary tract (N99.5-)

      Ⓔ D78.81-D78.89, E36.8, E89.810-E89.89, H59.011-H59.019, H59.031-H59.039, H59.091-H59.099, H59.811-H59.89, H95.811-H95.89, I97.3, L76.81-L76.82, M96.89, N39.0, N98.1-N98.9, N99.510-N99.518, T81.82X-T81.9XX[A], T83.010[A], T83.020[A], T83.030[A], T83.090[A], T83.110-T83.29X[A], T83.410-T83.6XX[A], T83.718[A], T83.728-T83.9XX[A], T85.310-T85.311[A], T85.320-T85.321[A], T85.390-T85.391[A], T85.510-T85.9XX[A], T86.842-T86.849

   X ● T83.59   **Infection and inflammatory reaction due to prosthetic device, implant and graft in urinary system** A 🖫, 🖫

      Ⓔ D78.81-D78.89, E36.8, E89.810-E89.89, H59.011-H59.019, H59.031-H59.039, H59.091-H59.099, H59.811-H59.89, H95.811-H95.89, I97.3, L76.81-L76.82, M96.89, N98.1-N98.9, N99.510-N99.518, T81.82X-T81.9XX[A], T83.010[A], T83.020[A], T83.030[A], T83.090[A], T83.110-T83.29X[A], T83.410-T83.6XX[A], T83.718[A], T83.728-T83.9XX[A], T85.310-T85.311[A], T85.320-T85.321[A], T85.390-T85.391[A], T85.510-T85.9XX[A], T86.820-T86.829, T86.842-T86.849

   X ● T83.6   **Infection and inflammatory reaction due to prosthetic device, implant and graft in genital tract** A 🖫, 🖫
Use additional code to identify infection
Ⓔ See T83.59

● T83.7   **Complications due to implanted mesh and other prosthetic materials**

   ● T83.71   **Erosion of implanted mesh and other prosthetic materials to surrounding organ or tissue**

    ● T83.711   **Erosion of implanted vaginal mesh and other prosthetic materials to surrounding organ or tissue** 🖫
Erosion of implanted vaginal mesh and other prosthetic materials into pelvic floor muscles

    ● T83.718   **Erosion of other implanted mesh and other prosthetic materials to surrounding organ or tissue** A 🖫, 🖫

   ● T83.72   **Exposure of implanted mesh and other prosthetic materials into surrounding organ or tissue**

    ● T83.721   **Exposure of implanted vaginal mesh and other prosthetic materials into vagina** 🖫
Exposure of implanted vaginal mesh and other prosthetic materials through vaginal wall

    ● T83.728   **Exposure of other implanted mesh and other prosthetic materials to surrounding organ or tissue** A 🖫, 🖫

● T83.8   **Other specified complications of genitourinary prosthetic devices, implants and grafts**
Ⓔ **For category T83.8 CC codes: See T83.59**

   X ● T83.81   **Embolism of genitourinary prosthetic devices, implants and grafts** A 🖫, 🖫

   X ● T83.82   **Fibrosis of genitourinary prosthetic devices, implants and grafts** A 🖫, 🖫

   X ● T83.83   **Hemorrhage of genitourinary prosthetic devices, implants and grafts** A 🖫, 🖫

   X ● T83.84   **Pain from genitourinary prosthetic devices, implants and grafts** A 🖫, 🖫

   X ● T83.85   **Stenosis of genitourinary prosthetic devices, implants and grafts** A 🖫, 🖫

   X ● T83.86   **Thrombosis of genitourinary prosthetic devices, implants and grafts** A 🖫, 🖫

   X ● T83.89   **Other specified complication of genitourinary prosthetic devices, implants and grafts** A 🖫, 🖫

  X ● T83.9   Unspecified **complication of genitourinary prosthetic device, implant and graft** A 🖫, 🖫
Ⓔ See T83.59

● T84   **Complications of internal orthopedic prosthetic devices, implants and grafts**

   Excludes2   failure and rejection of transplanted organs and tissues (T86.-)
fracture of bone following insertion of orthopedic implant, joint prosthesis or bone plate (M96.6)

The appropriate 7th character is to be added to each code from category T84

A	initial encounter
D	subsequent encounter
S	sequela

Ⓔ **For category T84 CC codes unless otherwise indicated:** D78.81, D78.89, E36.8, E89.810-E89.89, H59.011-H59.019, H59.031-H59.819, H59.88-H59.89, H95.811-H95.89, I97.3, L76.81-L76.82, M96.621-M96.69, M96.89, N98.1-N98.9, T81.82X[A], T81.89X-T81.9XX[A], T84.010-T84.9XX[A]

● T84.0   **Mechanical complication of internal joint prosthesis**

   ● T84.01   **Broken internal joint prosthesis**
Breakage (fracture) of prosthetic joint
Broken prosthetic joint implant

      Excludes1   periprosthetic joint implant fracture (T84.04)

    ● T84.010   **Broken internal right hip prosthesis** A 🖫, 🖫

    ● T84.011   **Broken internal left hip prosthesis** A 🖫, 🖫

    ● T84.012   **Broken internal right knee prosthesis** A 🖫, 🖫

    ● T84.013   **Broken internal left knee prosthesis** A 🖫, 🖫

    ● T84.018   **Broken internal joint prosthesis, other site** A 🖫, 🖫
Use additional code to identify the joint (Z96.6-)

    ● T84.019   **Broken internal joint prosthesis, unspecified site** A 🖫, 🖫

   ● T84.02   **Dislocation of internal joint prosthesis**
Instability of internal joint prosthesis
Subluxation of internal joint prosthesis

    ● T84.020   **Dislocation of internal right hip prosthesis** A 🖫, 🖫

    ● T84.021   **Dislocation of internal left hip prosthesis** A 🖫, 🖫

    ● T84.022   **Instability of internal right knee prosthesis** A 🖫, 🖫

    ● T84.023   **Instability of internal left knee prosthesis** A 🖫, 🖫

● T84.028   Dislocation of other internal joint prosthesis A 🔾, 🔾
    Use additional code to identify the joint (Z96.6-)

● T84.029   Dislocation of unspecified internal joint prosthesis A 🔾, 🔾

● T84.03   Mechanical loosening of internal prosthetic joint
    Aseptic loosening of prosthetic joint

● T84.030   Mechanical loosening of internal right hip prosthetic joint A 🔾, 🔾

● T84.031   Mechanical loosening of internal left hip prosthetic joint A 🔾, 🔾

● T84.032   Mechanical loosening of internal right knee prosthetic joint A 🔾, 🔾

● T84.033   Mechanical loosening of internal left knee prosthetic joint A 🔾, 🔾

● T84.038   Mechanical loosening of other internal prosthetic joint A 🔾, 🔾
    Use additional code to identify the joint (Z96.6-)

● T84.039   Mechanical loosening of unspecified internal prosthetic joint A 🔾, 🔾

● T84.04   Periprosthetic fracture around internal prosthetic joint
   Excludes2   breakage (fracture) of prosthetic joint (T84.01)

● T84.040   Periprosthetic fracture around internal prosthetic right hip joint A 🔾, 🔾

● T84.041   Periprosthetic fracture around internal prosthetic left hip joint A 🔾, 🔾

● T84.042   Periprosthetic fracture around internal prosthetic right knee joint A 🔾, 🔾

● T84.043   Periprosthetic fracture around internal prosthetic left knee joint A 🔾, 🔾

● T84.048   Periprosthetic fracture around other internal prosthetic joint A 🔾, 🔾
    Use additional code to identify the joint (Z96.6-)

● T84.049   Periprosthetic fracture around unspecified internal prosthetic joint A 🔾, 🔾

● T84.05   Periprosthetic osteolysis of internal prosthetic joint
    Use additional code to identify major osseous defect, if applicable (M89.7-)

● T84.050   Periprosthetic osteolysis of internal prosthetic right hip joint A 🔾, 🔾

● T84.051   Periprosthetic osteolysis of internal prosthetic left hip joint A 🔾, 🔾

● T84.052   Periprosthetic osteolysis of internal prosthetic right knee joint A 🔾, 🔾

● T84.053   Periprosthetic osteolysis of internal prosthetic left knee joint A 🔾, 🔾

● T84.058   Periprosthetic osteolysis of other internal prosthetic joint A 🔾, 🔾
    Use additional code to identify the joint (Z96.6-)

● T84.059   Periprosthetic osteolysis of unspecified internal prosthetic joint A 🔾, 🔾

● T84.06   Wear of articular bearing surface of internal prosthetic joint

● T84.060   Wear of articular bearing surface of internal prosthetic right hip joint A 🔾, 🔾

● T84.061   Wear of articular bearing surface of internal prosthetic left hip joint A 🔾, 🔾

● T84.062   Wear of articular bearing surface of internal prosthetic right knee joint A 🔾, 🔾

● T84.063   Wear of articular bearing surface of internal prosthetic left knee joint A 🔾, 🔾

● T84.068   Wear of articular bearing surface of other internal prosthetic joint A 🔾, 🔾
    Use additional code to identify the joint (Z96.6-)

● T84.069   Wear of articular bearing surface of unspecified internal prosthetic joint A 🔾, 🔾

● T84.09   Other mechanical complication of internal joint prosthesis
    Prosthetic joint implant failure NOS

● T84.090   Other mechanical complication of internal right hip prosthesis A 🔾, 🔾

● T84.091   Other mechanical complication of internal left hip prosthesis A 🔾, 🔾

● T84.092   Other mechanical complication of internal right knee prosthesis A 🔾, 🔾

● T84.093   Other mechanical complication of internal left knee prosthesis A 🔾, 🔾

● T84.098   Other mechanical complication of other internal joint prosthesis A 🔾, 🔾
    Use additional code to identify the joint (Z96.6-)

● T84.099   Other mechanical complication of unspecified internal joint prosthesis A 🔾, 🔾

● T84.1   Mechanical complication of internal fixation device of bones of limb
   Excludes2   mechanical complication of internal fixation device of bones of feet (T84.2-)
      mechanical complication of internal fixation device of bones of fingers (T84.2-)
      mechanical complication of internal fixation device of bones of hands (T84.2-)
      mechanical complication of internal fixation device of bones of toes (T84.2-)

● T84.11   Breakdown (mechanical) of internal fixation device of bones of limb

● T84.110   Breakdown (mechanical) of internal fixation device of right humerus A 🔾, 🔾

● T84.111   Breakdown (mechanical) of internal fixation device of left humerus A 🔾, 🔾

● T84.112   Breakdown (mechanical) of internal fixation device of bone of right forearm A 🔾, 🔾

● T84.113   Breakdown (mechanical) of internal fixation device of bone of left forearm A 🔾, 🔾

● T84.114   Breakdown (mechanical) of internal fixation device of right femur A 🔾, 🔾

● T84.115   Breakdown (mechanical) of internal fixation device of left femur A 🔾, 🔾

● T84.116   Breakdown (mechanical) of internal fixation device of bone of right lower leg A 🔾, 🔾

● T84.117   Breakdown (mechanical) of internal fixation device of bone of left lower leg A 🔾, 🔾

● T84.119   Breakdown (mechanical) of internal fixation device of unspecified bone of limb A 🔾, 🔾

N   Newborn Age: 0   P   Pediatric Age: 0–17   M   Maternity DX: 12–55   A   Adult Age: 15–124   ♀   Females Only   ♂   Males Only

🔾 Complication\Comorbidity   🔾 Major C\C   (Ex) CC/MCC Exclusions   Present on Admission Requirement   🔾 Hospital-Acquired Condition   **1579**

T84.12   Displacement of internal fixation device of bones of limb
　　　　　　Malposition of internal fixation device of bones of limb

- **T84.120**   Displacement of internal fixation device of right humerus A
- **T84.121**   Displacement of internal fixation device of left humerus A
- **T84.122**   Displacement of internal fixation device of bone of right forearm A
- **T84.123**   Displacement of internal fixation device of bone of left forearm A
- **T84.124**   Displacement of internal fixation device of right femur A
- **T84.125**   Displacement of internal fixation device of left femur A
- **T84.126**   Displacement of internal fixation device of bone of right lower leg A
- **T84.127**   Displacement of internal fixation device of bone of left lower leg A
- **T84.129**   Displacement of internal fixation device of unspecified bone of limb A

T84.19   Other mechanical complication of internal fixation device of bones of limb
　　　　　　Obstruction (mechanical) of internal fixation device of bones of limb
　　　　　　Perforation of internal fixation device of bones of limb
　　　　　　Protrusion of internal fixation device of bones of limb

- **T84.190**   Other mechanical complication of internal fixation device of right humerus A
- **T84.191**   Other mechanical complication of internal fixation device of left humerus A
- **T84.192**   Other mechanical complication of internal fixation device of bone of right forearm A
- **T84.193**   Other mechanical complication of internal fixation device of bone of left forearm A
- **T84.194**   Other mechanical complication of internal fixation device of right femur A
- **T84.195**   Other mechanical complication of internal fixation device of left femur A
- **T84.196**   Other mechanical complication of internal fixation device of bone of right lower leg A
- **T84.197**   Other mechanical complication of internal fixation device of bone of left lower leg A
- **T84.199**   Other mechanical complication of internal fixation device of unspecified bone of limb A

T84.2   Mechanical complication of internal fixation device of other bones

T84.21   Breakdown (mechanical) of internal fixation device of other bones

- **T84.210**   Breakdown (mechanical) of internal fixation device of bones of hand and fingers A
- **T84.213**   Breakdown (mechanical) of internal fixation device of bones of foot and toes A
- **T84.216**   Breakdown (mechanical) of internal fixation device of vertebrae A
- **T84.218**   Breakdown (mechanical) of internal fixation device of other bones A

T84.22   Displacement of internal fixation device of other bones
　　　　　　Malposition of internal fixation device of other bones

- **T84.220**   Displacement of internal fixation device of bones of hand and fingers A
- **T84.223**   Displacement of internal fixation device of bones of foot and toes A
- **T84.226**   Displacement of internal fixation device of vertebrae A
- **T84.228**   Displacement of internal fixation device of other bones A

T84.29   Other mechanical complication of internal fixation device of other bones
　　　　　　Obstruction (mechanical) of internal fixation device of other bones
　　　　　　Perforation of internal fixation device of other bones
　　　　　　Protrusion of internal fixation device of other bones

- **T84.290**   Other mechanical complication of internal fixation device of bones of hand and fingers A
- **T84.293**   Other mechanical complication of internal fixation device of bones of foot and toes A
- **T84.296**   Other mechanical complication of internal fixation device of vertebrae A
- **T84.298**   Other mechanical complication of internal fixation device of other bones A

T84.3   Mechanical complication of other bone devices, implants and grafts
　　　　Excludes2   other complications of bone graft (T86.83-)

T84.31   Breakdown (mechanical) of other bone devices, implants and grafts

- **T84.310**   Breakdown (mechanical) of electronic bone stimulator A
- **T84.318**   Breakdown (mechanical) of other bone devices, implants and grafts A

T84.32   Displacement of other bone devices, implants and grafts
　　　　　　Malposition of other bone devices, implants and grafts

- **T84.320**   Displacement of electronic bone stimulator A
- **T84.328**   Displacement of other bone devices, implants and grafts A

◀ New   ◀▥ Revised   ~~deleted~~ Deleted   Excludes 1   Excludes 2   Includes   Use additional   Code first   Code also   Unspecified
OGCR Official Guidelines   ● Unacceptable Principal Diagnosis   X Assign placeholder X   ● Use Additional Character(s)   ▌ Manifestation Code   Coding Clinic

● **T84.39** **Other mechanical complication of other bone devices, implants and grafts**
　　Obstruction (mechanical) of other bone devices, implants and grafts
　　Perforation of other bone devices, implants and grafts
　　Protrusion of other bone devices, implants and grafts

　● **T84.390** **Other mechanical complication of electronic bone stimulator** A 🔘, 🔘

　● **T84.398** **Other mechanical complication of other bone devices, implants and grafts** A 🔘, 🔘

● **T84.4** **Mechanical complication of other internal orthopedic devices, implants and grafts**

　● **T84.41** **Breakdown (mechanical) of other internal orthopedic devices, implants and grafts**

　　● **T84.410** **Breakdown (mechanical) of muscle and tendon graft** A 🔘, 🔘

　　● **T84.418** **Breakdown (mechanical) of other internal orthopedic devices, implants and grafts** A 🔘, 🔘

　● **T84.42** **Displacement of other internal orthopedic devices, implants and grafts**
　　　Malposition of other internal orthopedic devices, implants and grafts

　　● **T84.420** **Displacement of muscle and tendon graft** A 🔘, 🔘

　　● **T84.428** **Displacement of other internal orthopedic devices, implants and grafts** A 🔘, 🔘

　● **T84.49** **Other mechanical complication of other internal orthopedic devices, implants and grafts**
　　　Mechanical complication of other internal orthopedic devices, implants and grafts NOS
　　　Obstruction (mechanical) of other internal orthopedic devices, implants and grafts
　　　Perforation of other internal orthopedic devices, implants and grafts
　　　Protrusion of other internal orthopedic devices, implants and grafts

　　● **T84.490** **Other mechanical complication of muscle and tendon graft** A 🔘, 🔘

　　● **T84.498** **Other mechanical complication of other internal orthopedic devices, implants and grafts** A 🔘, 🔘

● **T84.5** **Infection and inflammatory reaction due to internal joint prosthesis**
　　Use additional code to identify infection
　　(Ex) For category T84.5 CC codes: D78.81-D78.89, E36.8, E89.810-E89.89, H59.011-H59.019, H59.031-H59.039, H59.091-H59.099, H59.811-H59.89, H95.811-H95.89, I97.3, L76.81-L76.82, M96.621-M96.69, M96.89, N98.1-N98.9, T81.82X-T81.9XX[A], T84.010-T84.9XX[A], T85.310-T85.311[A], T85.320-T85.321[A], T85.390-T85.391[A], T85.510-T85.9XX[A], T86.820-T86.829, T86.842-T86.849

　X● **T84.50** **Infection and inflammatory reaction due to unspecified internal joint prosthesis** A 🔘, 🔘

　X● **T84.51** **Infection and inflammatory reaction due to internal right hip prosthesis** A 🔘, 🔘

　X● **T84.52** **Infection and inflammatory reaction due to internal left hip prosthesis** A 🔘, 🔘

　X● **T84.53** **Infection and inflammatory reaction due to internal right knee prosthesis** A 🔘, 🔘

　X● **T84.54** **Infection and inflammatory reaction due to internal left knee prosthesis** A 🔘, 🔘

　X● **T84.59** **Infection and inflammatory reaction due to other internal joint prosthesis** A 🔘, 🔘

● **T84.6** **Infection and inflammatory reaction due to internal fixation device**
　　Use additional code to identify infection
　　(Ex) For category T84.6 CC codes: See T84.5

　X● **T84.60** **Infection and inflammatory reaction due to internal fixation device of unspecified site** A 🔘, 🔘, A 🔘

　● **T84.61** **Infection and inflammatory reaction due to internal fixation device of arm**

　　● **T84.610** **Infection and inflammatory reaction due to internal fixation device of right humerus** A 🔘, 🔘, A 🔘

　　● **T84.611** **Infection and inflammatory reaction due to internal fixation device of left humerus** A 🔘, 🔘, A 🔘

　　● **T84.612** **Infection and inflammatory reaction due to internal fixation device of right radius** A 🔘, 🔘, A 🔘

　　● **T84.613** **Infection and inflammatory reaction due to internal fixation device of left radius** A 🔘, 🔘, A 🔘

　　● **T84.614** **Infection and inflammatory reaction due to internal fixation device of right ulna** A 🔘, 🔘, A 🔘

　　● **T84.615** **Infection and inflammatory reaction due to internal fixation device of left ulna** A 🔘, 🔘, A 🔘

　　● **T84.619** **Infection and inflammatory reaction due to internal fixation device of unspecified bone of arm** A 🔘, 🔘, A 🔘

　● **T84.62** **Infection and inflammatory reaction due to internal fixation device of leg**

　　● **T84.620** **Infection and inflammatory reaction due to internal fixation device of right femur** A 🔘, 🔘

　　● **T84.621** **Infection and inflammatory reaction due to internal fixation device of left femur** A 🔘, 🔘

　　● **T84.622** **Infection and inflammatory reaction due to internal fixation device of right tibia** A 🔘, 🔘

　　● **T84.623** **Infection and inflammatory reaction due to internal fixation device of left tibia** A 🔘, 🔘

　　● **T84.624** **Infection and inflammatory reaction due to internal fixation device of right fibula** A 🔘, 🔘

　　● **T84.625** **Infection and inflammatory reaction due to internal fixation device of left fibula** A 🔘, 🔘

　　● **T84.629** **Infection and inflammatory reaction due to internal fixation device of unspecified bone of leg** A 🔘, 🔘

　X● **T84.63** **Infection and inflammatory reaction due to internal fixation device of spine** A 🔘, 🔘, A 🔘

　X● **T84.69** **Infection and inflammatory reaction due to internal fixation device of other site** A 🔘, 🔘, A 🔘

● **T84.7** **Infection and inflammatory reaction due to other internal orthopedic prosthetic devices, implants and grafts** A 🔘, 🔘, A 🔘
　　Use additional code to identify infection
　　(Ex) See T84.5

N Newborn Age: 0　**P** Pediatric Age: 0–17　**M** Maternity DX: 12–55　**A** Adult Age: 15–124　♀ Females Only　♂ Males Only
🔘 Complication\Comorbidity　🔘 Major C\C　(Ex) CC/MCC Exclusions　🔘 Present on Admission Requirement　🔘 Hospital-Acquired Condition

1581

● **T84.8**   **Other specified complications of internal orthopedic prosthetic devices, implants and grafts**
    Ex: For category T84.8 CC codes: See T84.5

X ● **T84.81**   **Embolism due to internal orthopedic prosthetic devices, implants and grafts** A 🝙, 🝙

X ● **T84.82**   **Fibrosis due to internal orthopedic prosthetic devices, implants and grafts** A 🝙, 🝙

X ● **T84.83**   **Hemorrhage due to internal orthopedic prosthetic devices, implants and grafts** A 🝙, 🝙

X ● **T84.84**   **Pain due to internal orthopedic prosthetic devices, implants and grafts** A 🝙, 🝙

X ● **T84.85**   **Stenosis due to internal orthopedic prosthetic devices, implants and grafts** A 🝙, 🝙

X ● **T84.86**   **Thrombosis due to internal orthopedic prosthetic devices, implants and grafts** A 🝙, 🝙

X ● **T84.89**   **Other specified complication of internal orthopedic prosthetic devices, implants and grafts** A 🝙, 🝙

X ● **T84.9**   Unspecified **complication of internal orthopedic prosthetic device, implant and graft** A 🝙, 🝙
    Ex: See T84.5

● **T85**   **Complications of other internal prosthetic devices, implants and grafts**

    Excludes2   failure and rejection of transplanted organs and tissue (T86.-)

    The appropriate 7th character is to be added to each code from category T85

    | | |
    A   initial encounter
    D   subsequent encounter
    S   sequela

● **T85.0**   **Mechanical complication of ventricular intracranial (communicating) shunt**
    Ex: For category T85.0 CC codes: D78.81-D78.89, E36.8, E89.810-E89.89, H59.011-H59.019, H59.031-H59.039, H59.091-H59.099, H59.811-H59.89, H95.811-H95.89, I97.3, L76.81-L76.82, M96.89, N98.1-N98.9, T81.82X-T81.9XX[A], T85.01X-T85.199[A]

X ● **T85.01**   **Breakdown (mechanical) of ventricular intracranial (communicating) shunt** A 🝙, 🝙

X ● **T85.02**   **Displacement of ventricular intracranial (communicating) shunt** A 🝙, 🝙
    Malposition of ventricular intracranial (communicating) shunt

X ● **T85.03**   **Leakage of ventricular intracranial (communicating) shunt** A 🝙, 🝙

X ● **T85.09**   **Other mechanical complication of ventricular intracranial (communicating) shunt** A 🝙, 🝙
    Obstruction (mechanical) of ventricular intracranial (communicating) shunt
    Perforation of ventricular intracranial (communicating) shunt
    Protrusion of ventricular intracranial (communicating) shunt

● **T85.1**   **Mechanical complication of implanted electronic stimulator of nervous system**
    Ex: For category T85.1 CC codes: See T85.0

● **T85.11**   **Breakdown (mechanical) of implanted electronic stimulator of nervous system**

● **T85.110**   **Breakdown (mechanical) of implanted electronic neurostimulator (electrode) of brain** A 🝙, 🝙

● **T85.111**   **Breakdown (mechanical) of implanted electronic neurostimulator (electrode) of peripheral nerve** A 🝙, 🝙

● **T85.112**   **Breakdown (mechanical) of implanted electronic neurostimulator (electrode) of spinal cord** A 🝙, 🝙

● **T85.118**   **Breakdown (mechanical) of other implanted electronic stimulator of nervous system** A 🝙, 🝙

● **T85.12**   **Displacement of implanted electronic stimulator of nervous system**
    Malposition of implanted electronic stimulator of nervous system

● **T85.120**   **Displacement of implanted electronic neurostimulator (electrode) of brain** A 🝙, 🝙

● **T85.121**   **Displacement of implanted electronic neurostimulator (electrode) of peripheral nerve** A 🝙, 🝙

● **T85.122**   **Displacement of implanted electronic neurostimulator (electrode) of spinal cord** A 🝙, 🝙

● **T85.128**   **Displacement of other implanted electronic stimulator of nervous system** A 🝙, 🝙

● **T85.19**   **Other mechanical complication of implanted electronic stimulator of nervous system**
    Leakage of implanted electronic stimulator of nervous system
    Obstruction (mechanical) of implanted electronic stimulator of nervous system
    Perforation of implanted electronic stimulator of nervous system
    Protrusion of implanted electronic stimulator of nervous system

● **T85.190**   **Other mechanical complication of implanted electronic neurostimulator (electrode) of brain** A 🝙, 🝙

● **T85.191**   **Other mechanical complication of implanted electronic neurostimulator (electrode) of peripheral nerve** A 🝙, 🝙

● **T85.192**   **Other mechanical complication of implanted electronic neurostimulator (electrode) of spinal cord** A 🝙, 🝙

● **T85.199**   **Other mechanical complication of other implanted electronic stimulator of nervous system** A 🝙, 🝙

● **T85.2**   **Mechanical complication of intraocular lens**
    Ex: For category T85.2 CC codes: D78.81-D78.89, E89.810-E89.89, H59.011-H59.019, H59.031-H59.039, H59.091-H59.099, H59.811-H59.89, H95.811-H95.89, I97.3, M96.89, N98.1-N98.9, T85.21X-T85.29X[A]

X ● **T85.21**   **Breakdown (mechanical) of intraocular lens** A 🝙, 🝙

X ● **T85.22**   **Displacement of intraocular lens** A 🝙, 🝙
    Malposition of intraocular lens

X ● **T85.29**   **Other mechanical complication of intraocular lens** A 🝙, 🝙
    Obstruction (mechanical) of intraocular lens
    Perforation of intraocular lens
    Protrusion of intraocular lens

● **T85.3**   **Mechanical complication of other ocular prosthetic devices, implants and grafts**

    Excludes2   other complications of corneal graft (T86.84-)

    Ex: For category T85.3 CC codes: H59.011-H59.019, H59.031-H59.819, H59.88-H59.89, H95.811-H95.89, I97.3, M96.89, N98.1-N98.9, T85.310-T85.311[A], T85.320-T85.321[A], T85.390-T85.391[A], T85.612[A], T85.618[A], T85.622[A], T85.628[A], T85.638[A], T85.692[A], T85.698-T85.9XX[A], T86.842-T86.849

● **T85.31**   **Breakdown (mechanical) of other ocular prosthetic devices, implants and grafts**

● **T85.310**   **Breakdown (mechanical) of prosthetic orbit of right eye** A 🝙, 🝙

● **T85.311**   **Breakdown (mechanical) of prosthetic orbit of left eye** A 🝙, 🝙

● **T85.318**   **Breakdown (mechanical) of other ocular prosthetic devices, implants and grafts** 🝙

● **T85.32**   **Displacement of other ocular prosthetic devices, implants and grafts**
> Malposition of other ocular prosthetic devices, implants and grafts

  ● **T85.320**   **Displacement of prosthetic orbit of right eye** A 🗫, 🗫

  ● **T85.321**   **Displacement of prosthetic orbit of left eye** A 🗫, 🗫

  ● **T85.328**   **Displacement of other ocular prosthetic devices, implants and grafts** 🗫

● **T85.39**   **Other mechanical complication of other ocular prosthetic devices, implants and grafts**
> Obstruction (mechanical) of other ocular prosthetic devices, implants and grafts
> Perforation of other ocular prosthetic devices, implants and grafts
> Protrusion of other ocular prosthetic devices, implants and grafts

  ● **T85.390**   **Other mechanical complication of prosthetic orbit of right eye** A 🗫, 🗫

  ● **T85.391**   **Other mechanical complication of prosthetic orbit of left eye** A 🗫, 🗫

  ● **T85.398**   **Other mechanical complication of other ocular prosthetic devices, implants and grafts** 🗫

● **T85.4**   **Mechanical complication of breast prosthesis and implant**
> Ⓔⓧ **For category T85.4 CC codes:** D78.81-D78.89, E89.810-E89.89, H59.011-H59.019, H59.031-H59.039, H59.091-H59.099, H59.811-H59.89, H95.811-H95.89, I97.3, M96.89, N98.1-N98.9, T85.41X-T85.49X[A]

 X● **T85.41**   **Breakdown (mechanical) of breast prosthesis and implant** A 🗫, 🗫

 X● **T85.42**   **Displacement of breast prosthesis and implant** A 🗫, 🗫
> Malposition of breast prosthesis and implant

 X● **T85.43**   **Leakage of breast prosthesis and implant** A 🗫, 🗫

 X● **T85.44**   **Capsular contracture of breast implant** A 🗫, 🗫

 X● **T85.49**   **Other mechanical complication of breast prosthesis and implant** A 🗫, 🗫
> Obstruction (mechanical) of breast prosthesis and implant
> Perforation of breast prosthesis and implant
> Protrusion of breast prosthesis and implant

● **T85.5**   **Mechanical complication of gastrointestinal prosthetic devices, implants and grafts**
> Ⓔⓧ **For category T85.5 CC codes:** H95.811-H95.89, I97.3, M96.89, N98.1-N98.9, T85.510-T85.598[A], T85.612[A], T85.618[A], T85.622[A], T85.628[A], T85.638[A], T85.692[A], T85.698-T85.9XX[A]

● **T85.51**   **Breakdown (mechanical) of gastrointestinal prosthetic devices, implants and grafts**

  ● **T85.510**   **Breakdown (mechanical) of bile duct prosthesis** A 🗫, 🗫

  ● **T85.511**   **Breakdown (mechanical) of esophageal anti-reflux device** A 🗫, 🗫

  ● **T85.518**   **Breakdown (mechanical) of other gastrointestinal prosthetic devices, implants and grafts** A 🗫, 🗫

● **T85.52**   **Displacement of gastrointestinal prosthetic devices, implants and grafts**
> Malposition of gastrointestinal prosthetic devices, implants and grafts

  ● **T85.520**   **Displacement of bile duct prosthesis** A 🗫, 🗫

  ● **T85.521**   **Displacement of esophageal anti-reflux device** A 🗫, 🗫

  ● **T85.528**   **Displacement of other gastrointestinal prosthetic devices, implants and grafts** A 🗫, 🗫

● **T85.59**   **Other mechanical complication of gastrointestinal prosthetic devices, implants and**
> Obstruction, mechanical of gastrointestinal prosthetic devices, implants and grafts
> Perforation of gastrointestinal prosthetic devices, implants and grafts
> Protrusion of gastrointestinal prosthetic devices, implants and grafts

  ● **T85.590**   **Other mechanical complication of bile duct prosthesis** A 🗫, 🗫

  ● **T85.591**   **Other mechanical complication of esophageal anti-reflux device** A 🗫, 🗫

  ● **T85.598**   **Other mechanical complication of other gastrointestinal prosthetic devices, implants and grafts** A 🗫, 🗫

● **T85.6**   **Mechanical complication of other specified internal and external prosthetic devices, implants and grafts**

● **T85.61**   **Breakdown (mechanical) of other specified internal prosthetic devices, implants and grafts**

  ● **T85.610**   **Breakdown (mechanical) of epidural and subdural infusion catheter** A 🗫, 🗫
> Ⓔⓧ H95.811-H95.89, I97.3, M96.89, N98.1-N98.9, T85.610[A], T85.612[A], T85.618-T85.620[A], T85.622[A], T85.628-T85.630[A], T85.638-T85.690[A], T85.692[A], T85.698-T85.9XX[A]

  ● **T85.611**   **Breakdown (mechanical) of intraperitoneal dialysis catheter** A 🗫, 🗫

> **Excludes1**   mechanical complication of vascular dialysis catheter (T82.4-)

> Ⓔⓧ H95.811-H95.89, I97.3, M96.89, N98.1-N98.9, T85.611-T85.612[A], T85.614-T85.618[A], T85.621-T85.622[A], T85.624-T85.628[A], T85.631-T85.638[A], T85.691-T85.692[A], T85.694-T85.9XX[A]

  ● **T85.612**   **Breakdown (mechanical) of permanent sutures** A 🗫, 🗫

> **Excludes1**   mechanical complication of permanent (wire) suture used in bone repair (T84.1-T84.2)

> Ⓔⓧ D78.81-D78.89, E89.810-E89.89, H59.011-H59.019, H59.031-H59.039, H59.091-H59.099, H59.811-H59.89, H95.811-H95.89, I97.3, M96.89, N98.1-N98.9, T85.310-T85.311[A], T85.320-T85.321[A], T85.390-T85.391[A], T85.510-T85.9XX[A], T86.842-T86.849

  ● **T85.613**   **Breakdown (mechanical) of artificial skin graft and decellularized allodermis** A 🗫, 🗫
> Failure of artificial skin graft and decellularized allodermis
> Non-adherence of artificial skin graft and decellularized allodermis
> Poor incorporation of artificial skin graft and decellularized allodermis
> Shearing of artificial skin graft and decellularized allodermis
> Ⓔⓧ H95.811-H95.89, I97.3, M96.89, N98.1-N98.9, T85.612-T85.613[A], T85.618[A], T85.622-T85.623[A], T85.628[A], T85.638[A], T85.692-T85.693[A], T85.698-T85.9XX[A], T86.820-T86.829

N Newborn Age: 0   **P** Pediatric Age: 0–17   **M** Maternity DX: 12–55   **A** Adult Age: 15–124   ♀ Females Only   ♂ Males Only

🗫 Complication\Comorbidity   🗫 Major C\C   Ⓔⓧ CC/MCC Exclusions   🗫 Present on Admission Requirement   🗫 Hospital-Acquired Condition

1583

CHAPTER 19 (S00-T88)

● **T85.614** **Breakdown (mechanical) of insulin pump** A 🔴, 🔴
Ex: H95.811-H95.89, I97.3, M96.621-M96.89, N98.1-N98.9, N99.510-N99.518, T81.82X-T81.9XX[A], T82.01X-T83.010[A], T83.020[A], T83.030[A], T83.090[A], T83.110-T83.29X[A], T83.410-T83.6XX[A], T83.718[A], T83.728-T83.9XX[A], T84.010-T85.29X[A], T85.41X-T85.49X[A], T85.611-T85.618[A], T85.621-T85.622[A], T85.624-T85.628[A], T85.631-T85.638[A], T85.691-T85.692[A], T85.694-T85.9XX[A], T86.820-T86.829

● **T85.618** **Breakdown (mechanical) of other specified internal prosthetic devices, implants and grafts** A 🔴, 🔴
Ex: See T85.612

● **T85.62** **Displacement of other specified internal prosthetic devices, implants and grafts**
Malposition of other specified internal prosthetic devices, implants and grafts

● **T85.620** **Displacement of epidural and subdural infusion catheter** A 🔴, 🔴
Ex: See T85.610

● **T85.621** **Displacement of intraperitoneal dialysis catheter** A 🔴, 🔴
Excludes1 mechanical complication of vascular dialysis catheter (T82.4-)
Ex: See T85.611

● **T85.622** **Displacement of permanent sutures** A 🔴, 🔴
Excludes1 mechanical complication of permanent (wire) suture used in bone repair (T84.1-T84.2)
Ex: See T85.612

● **T85.623** **Displacement of artificial skin graft and decellularized allodermis** A 🔴, 🔴
Dislodgement of artificial skin graft and decellularized allodermis
Displacement of artificial skin graft and decellularized allodermis
Ex: See T85.613

● **T85.624** **Displacement of insulin pump** A 🔴, 🔴
Ex: See T85.614

● **T85.628** **Displacement of other specified internal prosthetic devices, implants and grafts** A 🔴, 🔴
Ex: See T85.612

● **T85.63** **Leakage of other specified internal prosthetic devices, implants and grafts**

● **T85.630** **Leakage of epidural and subdural infusion catheter** A 🔴, 🔴
Ex: See T85.610

● **T85.631** **Leakage of intraperitoneal dialysis catheter** A 🔴, 🔴
Excludes1 mechanical complication of vascular dialysis catheter (T82.4)
Ex: See T85.611

● **T85.633** **Leakage of insulin pump** A 🔴, 🔴
Ex: See T85.614

● **T85.638** **Leakage of other specified internal prosthetic devices, implants and grafts** A 🔴, 🔴
Ex: See T85.612

● **T85.69** **Other mechanical complication of other specified internal prosthetic devices, implants and grafts**
Obstruction, mechanical of other specified internal prosthetic devices, implants and grafts
Perforation of other specified internal prosthetic devices, implants and grafts
Protrusion of other specified internal prosthetic devices, implants and grafts

● **T85.690** **Other mechanical complication of epidural and subdural infusion catheter** A 🔴, 🔴
Ex: See T85.610

● **T85.691** **Other mechanical complication of intraperitoneal dialysis catheter** A 🔴, 🔴
Excludes1 mechanical complication of vascular dialysis catheter (T82.4)
Ex: See T85.611

● **T85.692** **Other mechanical complication of permanent sutures** A 🔴, 🔴
Excludes1 mechanical complication of permanent (wire) suture used in bone repair (T84.1-T84.2)
Ex: See T85.612

● **T85.693** **Other mechanical complication of artificial skin graft and decellularized allodermis** A 🔴, 🔴
Ex: See T85.613

● **T85.694** **Other mechanical complication of insulin pump** A 🔴, 🔴
Ex: See T85.614

● **T85.698** **Other mechanical complication of other specified internal prosthetic devices, implants and grafts** A 🔴, 🔴
Mechanical complication of nonabsorbable surgical material NOS
Ex: See T85.612

● **T85.7** **Infection and inflammatory reaction due to other internal prosthetic devices, implants and grafts**
Use additional code to identify infection
Ex: For category T85.7 CC codes unless otherwise indicated: D78.81-D78.89, E36.8, E89.810-E89.89, H59.011-H59.019, H59.031-H59.039, H59.091-H59.099, H59.811-H59.89, H95.811-H95.89, I97.3, L76.81-L76.82, M96.621-M96.89, N98.1-N98.9, N99.510-N99.518, T81.82X-T81.9XX[A], T82.01X-T83.29X[A], T83.410-T83.6XX[A], T83.718[A], T83.728-T83.9XX[A], T84.010-T85.9XX[A], T86.820-T86.849

X ● **T85.71** **Infection and inflammatory reaction due to peritoneal dialysis catheter** A 🔴, 🔴
Ex: See T85.612

X ● **T85.72** **Infection and inflammatory reaction due to insulin pump** A 🔴, 🔴

X ● **T85.79** **Infection and inflammatory reaction due to other internal prosthetic devices, implants and grafts** A 🔴, 🔴

● **T85.8** **Other specified complications of internal prosthetic devices, implants and grafts, not elsewhere classified**
Ex: For category T85.8 CC codes: See T85.7

X ● **T85.81** **Embolism due to internal prosthetic devices, implants and grafts, not elsewhere classified** A 🔴

X ● **T85.82** **Fibrosis due to internal prosthetic devices, implants and grafts, not elsewhere classified** A 🔴

◀ New   ◀⁞⁞ Revised   ~~deleted~~ Deleted   Excludes 1   Excludes 2   Includes   Use additional   Code first   Code also   Unspecified
OGCR Official Guidelines   ● Unacceptable Principal Diagnosis   X Assign placeholder X   ● Use Additional Character(s)   ❱ Manifestation Code   **Coding Clinic**

X ● **T85.83**   **Hemorrhage due to internal prosthetic devices, implants and grafts, not elsewhere classified** A 🔾, 🔾

X ● **T85.84**   **Pain due to internal prosthetic devices, implants and grafts, not elsewhere classified** A 🔾, 🔾

X ● **T85.85**   **Stenosis due to internal prosthetic devices, implants and grafts, not elsewhere classified** A 🔾, 🔾

X ● **T85.86**   **Thrombosis due to internal prosthetic devices, implants and grafts, not elsewhere classified** A 🔾, 🔾

X ● **T85.89**   **Other specified complication of internal prosthetic devices, implants and grafts, not elsewhere classified** A 🔾, 🔾

X ● **T85.9**   **Unspecified** complication of internal prosthetic device, implant and graft 🔾
    Complication of internal prosthetic device, implant and graft NOS

● **T86**   **Complications of transplanted organs and tissue**
    Use additional code to identify other transplant complications, such as:
      graft-versus-host disease (D89.81-)
      malignancy associated with organ transplant (C80.2)
      post-transplant lymphoproliferative disorders (PTLD) (D47.Z1)

   ● **T86.0**   **Complications of bone marrow transplant**
     (Ex) **For category T86.0 CC codes:** D78.81-D78.89, D89.810-D89.813, E89.810-E89.89, H59.011-H59.019, H59.031-H59.099, H59.811-H59.89, H95.811-H95.89, I97.3, M96.89, N98.1-N98.9, T86.00-T86.09

     T86.00   **Unspecified** complication of bone marrow transplant 🔾, 🔾

     T86.01   **Bone marrow transplant rejection** 🔾, 🔾

     T86.02   **Bone marrow transplant failure** 🔾, 🔾

     T86.03   **Bone marrow transplant infection** 🔾, 🔾

     T86.09   **Other complications of bone marrow transplant** 🔾, 🔾

   ● **T86.1**   **Complications of kidney transplant**
     (Ex) **For category T86.1 CC codes:** D78.81-D78.89, E89.810-E89.89, H59.011-H59.019, H59.031-H59.039, H59.091-H59.099, H59.811-H59.89, H95.811-H95.89, I97.3, M96.89, N98.1-N98.9, T86.10-T86.19

     T86.10   **Unspecified** complication of kidney transplant 🔾, 🔾

     T86.11   **Kidney transplant rejection** 🔾, 🔾

     T86.12   **Kidney transplant failure** 🔾, 🔾

     T86.13   **Kidney transplant infection** 🔾, 🔾
       Use additional code to specify infection

     T86.19   **Other complication of kidney transplant** 🔾, 🔾

OGCR Section I.C.19.g.3.

Organ Transplant Complications

Transplant Complications

(a) Transplant complications other than kidney

Codes under category T86, Complications of transplanted organs and tissues, are for use for both complications and rejection of transplanted organs. A transplant complication code is only assigned if the complication affects the function of the transplanted organ. Two codes are required to fully describe a transplant complication: the appropriate code from category T86 and a secondary code that identifies the complication.

Pre-existing conditions or conditions that develop after the transplant are not coded as complications unless they affect the function of the transplanted organs.

See I.C.21 for transplant organ removal status

See I.C.2 for malignant neoplasm associated with transplanted organ.

   ● **T86.2**   **Complications of heart transplant**
     Excludes1   complication of:
       artificial heart device (T82.5)
       heart-lung transplant (T86.3)
     (Ex) **For category T86.2 CC codes:** D78.81-D78.89, E89.810-E89.89, H59.011-H59.019, H59.031-H59.039, H59.091-H59.099, H59.811-H59.89, H95.811-H95.89, I97.3, M96.89, N98.1-N98.9, T86.20-T86.39

     T86.20   **Unspecified** complication of heart transplant 🔾, 🔾

     T86.21   **Heart transplant rejection** 🔾, 🔾

     T86.22   **Heart transplant failure** 🔾, 🔾

     T86.23   **Heart transplant infection** 🔾, 🔾
       Use additional code to specify infection

   ● **T86.29**   **Other complications of heart transplant**

     T86.290   **Cardiac allograft vasculopathy** 🔾, 🔾
       Excludes1   atherosclerosis of coronary arteries (I25.75-, I25.76-, I25.81-)

     T86.298   **Other complications of heart transplant** 🔾, 🔾

   ● **T86.3**   **Complications of heart-lung transplant**
     (Ex) **For category T86.3 CC codes:** See T86.2

     T86.30   **Unspecified** complication of heart-lung transplant 🔾, 🔾

     T86.31   **Heart-lung transplant rejection** 🔾, 🔾

     T86.32   **Heart-lung transplant failure** 🔾, 🔾

     T86.33   **Heart-lung transplant infection** 🔾, 🔾
       Use additional code to specify infection

     T86.39   **Other complications of heart-lung transplant** 🔾, 🔾

   ● **T86.4**   **Complications of liver transplant**
     (Ex) **For category T86.4 CC codes:** D78.81-D78.89, E89.810-E89.89, H59.011-H59.019, H59.031-H59.039, H59.091-H59.099, H59.811-H59.89, H95.811-H95.89, I97.3, M96.89, N98.1-N98.9, T86.40-T86.49

     T86.40   **Unspecified** complication of liver transplant 🔾, 🔾

     T86.41   **Liver transplant rejection** 🔾, 🔾

     T86.42   **Liver transplant failure** 🔾, 🔾

     T86.43   **Liver transplant infection** 🔾, 🔾
       Use additional code to identify infection, such as:
        Cytomegalovirus (CMV) infection (B25.-)

     T86.49   **Other complications of liver transplant** 🔾, 🔾

   ● **T86.5**   **Complications of stem cell transplant** 🔾, 🔾
     Complications from stem cells from peripheral blood
     Complications from stem cells from umbilical cord
     (Ex) D78.81-D78.89, E89.810-E89.89, H59.011-H59.019, H59.031-H59.039, H59.091-H59.099, H59.811-H59.89, H95.811-H95.89, I97.3, M96.89, N98.1-N98.9, T86.5, T86.830-T86.839

   ● **T86.8**   **Complications of other transplanted organs and tissues**

     ● **T86.81**   **Complications of lung transplant**
       Excludes1   complication of heart-lung transplant (T86.3-)
       (Ex) **For category T86.81 CC codes:** D78.81-D78.89, E89.810-E89.89, H59.011-H59.019, H59.031-H59.039, H59.091-H59.099, H59.811-H59.89, H95.811-H95.89, I97.3, M96.89, N98.1-N98.9, T86.810-T86.819

       T86.810   **Lung transplant rejection** 🔾, 🔾

       T86.811   **Lung transplant failure** 🔾, 🔾

       T86.812   **Lung transplant infection** 🔾, 🔾
        Use additional code to specify infection

       T86.818   **Other complications of lung transplant** 🔾, 🔾

       T86.819   **Unspecified** complication of lung transplant 🔾, 🔾

N   Newborn Age: 0   P   Pediatric Age: 0–17   M   Maternity DX: 12–55   A   Adult Age: 15–124   ♀ Females Only   ♂ Males Only

🔾 Complication\Comorbidity   🔾 Major C\C   (Ex) CC/MCC Exclusions   🔾 Present on Admission Requirement   Hospital-Acquired Condition

1585

CHAPTER 19 (S00-T88)

CHAPTER 19 (S00–T88)

● T86.82   Complications of skin graft (allograft) (autograft)

    Excludes2   complication of artificial skin graft (T85.693) ◀▨

    Ⓔⓧ **For category T86.82 CC codes:** D78.81–D78.89, E89.810–E89.89, H59.011–H59.019, H59.031–H59.039, H59.091–H59.099, H59.811–H59.89, H95.811–H95.89, I97.3, M96.89, N98.1–N98.9, T85.613[A], T85.623[A], T85.693[A], T86.820–T86.829

   T86.820   Skin graft (allograft) rejection 🖉, 🖉

   T86.821   Skin graft (allograft) (autograft) failure 🖉, 🖉

   T86.822   Skin graft (allograft) (autograft) infection 🖉, 🖉

     Use additional code to specify infection

   T86.828   Other complications of skin graft (allograft) (autograft) 🖉, 🖉

   T86.829   Unspecified complication of skin graft (allograft) (autograft) 🖉, 🖉

● T86.83   Complications of bone graft

    Excludes2   mechanical complications of bone graft (T84.3-)

    Ⓔⓧ **For category T86.83 CC codes:** H95.811–H95.89, I97.3, M96.89, N98.1–N98.9, T86.5, T86.830–T86.839

   T86.830   Bone graft rejection 🖉, 🖉

   T86.831   Bone graft failure 🖉, 🖉

   T86.832   Bone graft infection 🖉, 🖉

     Use additional code to specify infection

   T86.838   Other complications of bone graft 🖉, 🖉

   T86.839   Unspecified complication of bone graft 🖉, 🖉

● T86.84   Complications of corneal transplant

    Excludes2   mechanical complications of corneal graft (T85.3-)

    Ⓔⓧ **For category T86.84 CC codes unless otherwise indicated:** H59.011–H59.019, H59.031–H59.039, H59.091–H59.099, H59.811–H59.89, H95.811–H95.89, I97.3, M96.621–M96.89, N98.1–N98.9, N99.510–N99.518, T81.82X[A], T81.89X–T81.9XX[A], T82.01X–T83.010[A], T83.020[A], T83.030[A], T83.090[A], T83.110–T83.29X[A], T83.410–T83.6XX[A], T83.718[A], T83.728–T85.49X[A], T85.612[A], T85.618[A], T85.622[A], T85.628[A], T85.638[A], T85.692[A], T85.698–T85.9XX[A], T86.820–T86.829, T86.840–T86.849

   T86.840   Corneal transplant rejection 🖉, 🖉

    Ⓔⓧ H59.031–H59.039, H59.091–H59.099, H59.811–H59.89, H95.811–H95.89, I97.3, M96.89, N98.1–N98.9, T85.318[A], T85.328[A], T85.398[A], T86.840–T86.841

   T86.841   Corneal transplant failure 🖉, 🖉

    Ⓔⓧ See T86.840

   T86.842   Corneal transplant infection 🖉, 🖉

     Use additional code to specify infection

   T86.848   Other complications of corneal transplant 🖉, 🖉

   T86.849   Unspecified complication of corneal transplant 🖉, 🖉

● T86.85   Complication of intestine transplant

    Ⓔⓧ **For category T86.85 CC codes:** D47.Z1, D78.81–D78.89, E89.810–E89.89, H59.011–H59.019, H59.031–H59.099, H59.811–H59.89, H95.811–H95.89, I97.3, M96.89, N98.1–N98.9, T86.850–T86.99

   T86.850   Intestine transplant rejection 🖉, 🖉

   T86.851   Intestine transplant failure 🖉, 🖉

   T86.852   Intestine transplant infection 🖉, 🖉

     Use additional code to specify infection

   T86.858   Other complications of intestine transplant 🖉, 🖉

   T86.859   Unspecified complication of intestine transplant 🖉, 🖉

● T86.89   Complications of other transplanted tissue

    Transplant failure or rejection of pancreas

    Ⓔⓧ **For category T86.89 CC codes:** D78.81–D78.89, E89.810–E89.89, H59.011–H59.019, H59.031–H59.039, H59.091–H59.099, H59.811–H59.89, H95.811–H95.89, I97.3, M96.89, N98.1–N98.9, T86.890–T86.899

   T86.890   Other transplanted tissue rejection 🖉, 🖉

   T86.891   Other transplanted tissue failure 🖉, 🖉

   T86.892   Other transplanted tissue infection 🖉, 🖉

     Use additional code to specify infection

   T86.898   Other complications of other transplanted tissue 🖉, 🖉

   T86.899   Unspecified complication of other transplanted tissue 🖉, 🖉

● T86.9   Complication of unspecified transplanted organ and tissue

    Ⓔⓧ **For category T86.9 CC codes:** See T86.85

   T86.90   Unspecified complication of unspecified transplanted organ and tissue 🖉, 🖉

   T86.91   Unspecified transplanted organ and tissue rejection 🖉, 🖉

   T86.92   Unspecified transplanted organ and tissue failure 🖉, 🖉

   T86.93   Unspecified transplanted organ and tissue infection 🖉, 🖉

     Use additional code to specify infection

   T86.99   Other complications of unspecified transplanted organ and tissue 🖉, 🖉

● T87   **Complications peculiar to reattachment and amputation**

 ● T87.0   Complications of reattached (part of) upper extremity

    Ⓔⓧ **For category T87.0 CC codes:** D78.81–D78.89, E36.8, E89.810–E89.89, H59.011–H59.019, H59.031–H59.039, H59.091–H59.099, H59.811–H59.89, H95.811–H95.89, I97.3, L76.81–L76.82, M96.89, N98.1–N98.9, T81.82X–T81.9XX[A], T87.0X1–T87.0X9

 ● T87.0X   Complications of reattached (part of) upper extremity

   T87.0X1   Complications of reattached (part of) right upper extremity 🖉, 🖉

   T87.0X2   Complications of reattached (part of) left upper extremity 🖉, 🖉

   T87.0X9   Complications of reattached (part of) unspecified upper extremity 🖉, 🖉

 ● T87.1   Complications of reattached (part of) lower extremity

    Ⓔⓧ **For category T87.1 CC codes:** D78.81–D78.89, E36.8, E89.810–E89.89, H59.011–H59.019, H59.031–H59.039, H59.091–H59.099, H59.811–H59.89, H95.811–H95.89, I97.3, L76.81–L76.82, M96.89, N98.1–N98.9, T81.82X–T81.9XX[A], T87.1X1–T87.1X9

 ● T87.1X   Complications of reattached (part of) lower extremity

   T87.1X1   Complications of reattached (part of) right lower extremity 🖉, 🖉

   T87.1X2   Complications of reattached (part of) left lower extremity 🖉, 🖉

   T87.1X9   Complications of reattached (part of) unspecified lower extremity 🖉, 🖉

   T87.2   Complications of other reattached body part 🖉, 🖉

    Ⓔⓧ D78.81–D78.89, E36.8, E89.810–E89.89, H59.011–H59.019, H59.031–H59.039, H59.091–H59.099, H59.811–H59.89, H95.811–H95.89, I97.3, L76.81–L76.82, M96.89, N98.1–N98.9, T81.82X–T81.9XX[A], T87.2

 ● T87.3   Neuroma of amputation stump

 ● T87.30   Neuroma of amputation stump, unspecified extremity 🖉

   T87.31   Neuroma of amputation stump, right upper extremity 🖉

◀ New   ◀▨ Revised   ~~deleted~~ Deleted   Excludes 1   Excludes 2   Includes   Use additional   Code first   Code also   Unspecified

OGCR Official Guidelines   ● Unacceptable Principal Diagnosis   X Assign placeholder X   🖉 Use Additional Character(s)   ▌ Manifestation Code   **Coding Clinic**

T87.32   Neuroma of amputation stump, left upper extremity 🕮

T87.33   Neuroma of amputation stump, right lower extremity 🕮

T87.34   Neuroma of amputation stump, left lower extremity 🕮

● T87.4   **Infection of amputation stump**

Ex) For category T87.4 CC codes: D78.81-D78.89, E36.8, E89.810-E89.89, H59.011-H59.019, H59.031-H59.039, H59.091-H59.099, H59.811-H59.89, H95.811-H95.89, I97.3, L76.81-L76.82, M96.89, N98.1-N98.9, T81.82X-T81.9XX[A], T87.40-T87.9

T87.40   Infection of amputation stump, unspecified extremity 🕮, 🕮

T87.41   Infection of amputation stump, right upper extremity 🕮, 🕮

T87.42   Infection of amputation stump, left upper extremity 🕮, 🕮

T87.43   Infection of amputation stump, right lower extremity 🕮, 🕮

T87.44   Infection of amputation stump, left lower extremity 🕮, 🕮

● T87.5   **Necrosis of amputation stump**

T87.50   Necrosis of amputation stump, unspecified extremity 🕮

T87.51   Necrosis of amputation stump, right upper extremity 🕮

T87.52   Necrosis of amputation stump, left upper extremity 🕮

T87.53   Necrosis of amputation stump, right lower extremity 🕮

T87.54   Necrosis of amputation stump, left lower extremity 🕮

● T87.8   **Other complications of amputation stump**

   ● T87.81   **Dehiscence of amputation stump** 🕮

   ● T87.89   **Other complications of amputation stump** 🕮

Amputation stump contracture
Amputation stump contracture of next proximal joint
Amputation stump flexion
Amputation stump edema
Amputation stump hematoma

Excludes2   phantom limb syndrome (G54.6-G54.7)

T87.9   Unspecified complications of amputation stump 🕮

● T88   **Other complications of surgical and medical care, not elsewhere classified**

Excludes2   complication following infusion, transfusion and therapeutic injection (T80.-)
complication following procedure NEC (T81.-)
complications of anesthesia in labor and delivery (O74.-)
complications of anesthesia in pregnancy (O29.-)
complications of anesthesia in puerperium (O89.-)
complications of devices, implants and grafts (T82-T85)
complications of obstetric surgery and procedure (O75.4)
dermatitis due to drugs and medicaments (L23.3, L24.4, L25.1, L27.0-L27.1)
poisoning and toxic effects of drugs and chemicals (T36-T65 with fifth or sixth character 1-4 or 6)
specified complications classified elsewhere

The appropriate 7th character is to be added to each code from category T88

A	initial encounter
D	subsequent encounter
S	sequela

X ● T88.0   **Infection following immunization** A 🕮, 🕮

Sepsis following immunization

Ex) N98.0, T80.211-T80.29X[A], T82.7XX[A], T88.0XX[A]

X ● T88.1   **Other complications following immunization, not elsewhere classified** A 🕮, 🕮

Generalized vaccinia
Rash following immunization

Excludes1   vaccinia not from vaccine (B08.011)

Excludes2   anaphylactic shock due to serum (T80.5-)
other serum reactions (T80.6-)
postimmunization arthropathy (M02.2)
postimmunization encephalitis (G04.02)
postimmunization fever (R50.83)

Ex) T88.1XX[A]

X ● T88.2   **Shock due to anesthesia** A 🕮, 🕮

Use additional code for adverse effect, if applicable, to identify drug (T41.- with fifth or sixth character 5)

Excludes1   complications of anesthesia (in):
labor and delivery (O74.-)
pregnancy (O29.-)
puerperium (O89.-)
postprocedural shock NOS (T81.1-)

Ex) See T81.1

X ● T88.3   **Malignant hyperthermia due to anesthesia** A 🕮, 🕮

Use additional code for adverse effect, if applicable, to identify drug (T41.- with fifth or sixth character 5)

Ex) D78.01-D78.02, D78.21-D78.89, E36.01-E36.02, E36.8, E89.810-E89.89, G97.51-G97.52, H59.011-H59.019, H59.031-H59.039, H59.091-H59.099, H59.111-H59.129, H59.311-H59.329, H59.811-H59.89, H95.21-H95.22, H95.41-H95.42, H95.811-H95.89, I97.3-I97.42, I97.610-I97.62, J95.61-J95.62, J95.830-J95.831, K91.61-K91.62, K91.840-K91.841, L76.01-L76.02, L76.21-L76.22, L76.81-L76.82, M96.810-M96.811, M96.830-M96.89, N98.1-N98.9, N99.61-N99.62, N99.820-N99.821, T79.4XX[A], T81.10X-T81.19X[A], T81.82X[A], T81.89X-T81.9XX[A], T88.2XX-T88.3XX[A]

X ● T88.4   **Failed or difficult intubation** 🕮

A MCE: Questionable admission when principal dx

X ● T88.5   **Other complications of anesthesia**

Use additional code for adverse effect, if applicable, to identify drug (T41.- with fifth or sixth character 5)

X ● T88.51   **Hypothermia following anesthesia** 🕮

X ● T88.52   **Failed moderate sedation during procedure** 🕮

Failed conscious sedation during procedure

Excludes2   personal history of failed moderate sedation (Z92.83)

X ● T88.59   **Other complications of anesthesia** 🕮

X ● T88.6   **Anaphylactic reaction due to adverse effect of correct drug or medicament properly administered** A 🕮, 🕮

Anaphylactic shock due to adverse effect of correct drug or medicament properly administered
Anaphylactoid reaction NOS

Use additional code for adverse effect, if applicable, to identify drug (T36-T50 with fifth or sixth character 5)

Excludes1   anaphylactic reaction due to serum (T80.5-)
anaphylactic shock or reaction due to adverse food reaction (T78.0-)

Ex) T78.00X-T78.09X[A]

X ● T88.7   **Unspecified adverse effect of drug or medicament** 🕮

Drug hypersensitivity NOS
Drug reaction NOS

Use additional code for adverse effect, if applicable, to identify drug (T36-T50 with fifth or sixth character 5)

Excludes1   specified adverse effects of drugs and medicaments (A00-R94 and T80-T88.6, T88.8)

A MCE: Questionable admission when principal dx

X ● T88.8   **Other specified complications of surgical and medical care, not elsewhere classified** 🕮

Use additional code to identify the complication

A MCE: Questionable admission when principal dx

X ● T88.9   **Complication of surgical and medical care, unspecified** 🕮

A MCE: Questionable admission when principal dx

N Newborn Age: 0   **P** Pediatric Age: 0–17   **M** Maternity DX: 12–55   **A** Adult Age: 15–124   ♀ Females Only   ♂ Males Only

🕮 Complication\Comorbidity   🕮 Major C\C   Ex) CC/MCC Exclusions   🕮 Present on Admission Requirement   🕮 Hospital-Acquired Condition

1587

CHAPTER 19 (S00-T88)

CHAPTER 20

EXTERNAL CAUSES OF MORBIDITY (V00-Y99)

Note: This chapter permits the classification of environmental events and circumstances as the cause of injury, and other adverse effects. Where a code from this section is applicable, it is intended that it shall be used secondary to a code from another chapter of the Classification indicating the nature of the condition. Most often, the condition will be classifiable to Chapter 19, Injury, poisoning and certain other consequences of external causes (S00-T88). Other conditions that may be stated to be due to external causes are classified in Chapters I to XVIII. For these conditions, codes from Chapter 20 should be used to provide additional information as to the cause of the condition.

This chapter contains the following blocks:

V00-X58	Accidents
V00-V99	Transport accidents
V00-V09	Pedestrian injured in transport accident
V10-V19	Pedal cycle rider injured in transport accident
V20-V29	Motorcycle rider injured in transport accident
V30-V39	Occupant of three-wheeled motor vehicle injured in transport accident
V40-V49	Car occupant injured in transport accident
V50-V59	Occupant of pick-up truck or van injured in transport accident
V60-V69	Occupant of heavy transport vehicle injured in transport accident
V70-V79	Bus occupant injured in transport accident
V80-V89	Other land transport accidents
V90-V94	Water transport accidents
V95-V97	Air and space transport accidents
V98-V99	Other and unspecified transport accidents
W00-X58	Other external causes of accidental injury
W00-W19	Slipping, tripping, stumbling and falls
W20-W49	Exposure to inanimate mechanical forces
W50-W64	Exposure to animate mechanical forces
W65-W74	Accidental non-transport drowning and submersion
W85-W99	Exposure to electric current, radiation and extreme ambient air temperature and pressure
X00-X08	Exposure to smoke, fire and flames
X10-X19	Contact with heat and hot substances
X30-X39	Exposure to forces of nature
X52, X58	Accidental exposure to other specified factors
X71-X83	Intentional self-harm
X92-Y08	Assault
Y21-Y33	Event of undetermined intent
Y35-Y38	Legal intervention, operations of war, military operations, and terrorism
Y62-Y84	Complications of medical and surgical care
Y62-Y69	Misadventures to patients during surgical and medical care
Y70-Y82	Medical devices associated with adverse incidents in diagnostic and therapeutic use
Y83-Y84	Surgical and other medical procedures as the cause of abnormal reaction of the patient, or of later complication, without mention of misadventure at the time of the procedure
Y90-Y99	Supplementary factors related to causes of morbidity classified elsewhere

ACCIDENTS (V00-X58)

TRANSPORT ACCIDENTS (V00-V99)

Note: This section is structured in 12 groups. Those relating to land transport accidents (V01-V89) reflect the victim's mode of transport and are subdivided to identify the victim's 'counterpart' or the type of event. The vehicle of which the injured person is an occupant is identified in the first two characters since it is seen as the most important factor to identify for prevention purposes. A transport accident is one in which the vehicle involved must be moving or running or in use for transport purposes at the time of the accident. ◀▥▥

Use additional code to identify:
Airbag injury (W22.1)
Type of street or road (Y92.4-)
Use of cellular telephone and other electronic equipment at the time of the transport accident (Y93.C-)

Excludes1 agricultural vehicles in stationary use or maintenance (W31.-)
assault by crashing of motor vehicle (Y03.-)
automobile or motor cycle in stationary use or maintenance - code to type of accident
crashing of motor vehicle, undetermined intent (Y32)
intentional self-harm by crashing of motor vehicle (X82)

Excludes2 transport accidents due to cataclysm (X34-X38)

Note: Definitions of transport vehicles:

(a) A transport accident is any accident involving a device designed primarily for, or used at the time primarily for, conveying persons or good from one place to another.

(b) A public highway [trafficway] or street is the entire width between property lines (or other boundary lines) of land open to the public as a matter of right or custom for purposes of moving persons or property from one place to another. A roadway is that part of the public highway designed, improved and customarily used for vehicular traffic.

(c) A traffic accident is any vehicle accident occurring on the public highway [i.e., originating on, terminating on, or involving a vehicle partially on the highway]. A vehicle accident is assumed to have occurred on the public highway unless another place is specified, except in the case of accidents involving only off-road motor vehicles, which are classified as nontraffic accidents unless the contrary is stated.

(d) A nontraffic accident is any vehicle accident that occurs entirely in any place other than a public highway.

(e) A pedestrian is any person involved in an accident who was not at the time of the accident riding in or on a motor vehicle, railway train, streetcar or animal-drawn or other vehicle, or on a pedal cycle or animal. This includes, a person changing a tire or working on a parked car. It also includes the use of a pedestrian conveyance such as a baby carriage, ice-skates, roller skates, a skateboard, nonmotorized or motorized wheelchair, motorized mobility scooter, or nonmotorized scooter.

(f) A driver is an occupant of a transport vehicle who is operating or intending to operate it.

(g) A passenger is any occupant of a transport vehicle other than the driver, except a person traveling on the outside of the vehicle.

(h) A person on the outside of a vehicle is any person being transported by a vehicle but not occupying the space normally reserved for the driver or passengers, or the space intended for the transport of property. This includes the body, bumper, fender, roof, running board or step of a vehicle.

(i) A pedal cycle is any land transport vehicle operated solely by nonmotorized pedals including a bicycle or tricycle.

(j)   A pedal cyclist is any person riding a pedal cycle or in a sidecar or trailer attached to a pedal cycle.

(k)   A motorcycle is a two-wheeled motor vehicle with one or two riding saddles and sometimes with a third wheel for the support of a sidecar. The sidecar is considered part of the motorcycle.

(l)   A motorcycle rider is any person riding a motorcycle or in a sidecar or trailer attached to the motorcycle.

(m)   A three-wheeled motor vehicle is a motorized tricycle designed primarily for on-road use. This includes a motor-driven tricycle, a motorized rickshaw, or a three-wheeled motor car.

(n)   A car [automobile] is a four-wheeled motor vehicle designed primarily for carrying up to 7 persons. A trailer being towed by the car is considered part of the car.

(o)   A pick-up truck or van is a four or six-wheeled motor vehicle designed for carrying passengers as well as property or cargo weighing less than the local limit for classification as a heavy goods vehicle, and not requiring a special driver's license. This includes a minivan and a sport-utility vehicle (SUV).

(p)   A heavy transport vehicle is a motor vehicle designed primarily for carrying property, meeting local criteria for classification as a heavy goods vehicle in terms of weight and requiring a special driver's license.

(q)   A bus (coach) is a motor vehicle designed or adapted primarily for carrying more than 10 passengers, and requiring a special driver's license.

(r)   A railway train or railway vehicle is any device, with or without freight or passenger cars coupled to it, designed for traffic on a railway track. This includes subterranean (subways) or elevated trains.

(s)   A streetcar is a device designed and used primarily for transporting passengers within a municipality, running on rails, usually subject to normal traffic control signals, and operated principally on a right-of-way that forms part of the roadway. This includes a tram or trolley that runs on rails. A trailer being towed by a streetcar is considered part of the streetcar.

(t)   A special vehicle mainly used on industrial premises is a motor vehicle designed primarily for use within the buildings and premises of industrial or commercial establishments. This includes battery-powered trucks, forklifts, coal-cars in a coal mine, logging cars and trucks used in mines or quarries.

(u)   A special vehicle mainly used in agriculture is a motor vehicle designed specifically for use in farming and agriculture (horticulture), to work the land, tend and harvest crops and transport materials on the farm. This includes harvesters, farm machinery and tractor and trailers.

(v)   A special construction vehicle is a motor vehicle designed specifically for use on construction and demolition sites. This includes bulldozers, diggers, earth levellers, dump trucks, backhoes, front-end loaders, pavers, and mechanical shovels.

(w)   A special all-terrain vehicle is a motor vehicle of special design to enable it to negotiate over rough or soft terrain, snow or sand. This includes snow mobiles, all-terrain vehicles (ATV), and dune buggies. It does not include passenger vehicle designated as sport utility vehicles (SUV).

(x)   A watercraft is any device designed for transporting passengers or goods on water. This includes motor or sail boats, ships, and hovercraft.

(y)   An aircraft is any device for transporting passengers or goods in the air. This includes hot-air balloons, gliders, helicopters and airplanes.

(z)   A military vehicle is any motorized vehicle operating on a public roadway owned by the military and being operated by a member of the military.

PEDESTRIAN INJURED IN TRANSPORT ACCIDENT (V00-V09)

Includes   person changing tire on transport vehicle
person examining engine of vehicle broken down in (on side of) road

Excludes1   fall due to non-transport collision with other person (W03)
pedestrian on foot falling (slipping) on ice and snow (W00.-)
struck or bumped by another person (W51)

● **V00**   **Pedestrian conveyance accident**

Use additional place of occurrence and activity external cause codes, if known (Y92.-, Y93.-)

Excludes1   collision with another person without fall (W51)
fall due to person on foot colliding with another person on foot (W03)
fall from non-moving wheelchair, nonmotorized scooter and motorized mobility scooter without collision (W05.-)
pedestrian (conveyance) collision with other land transport vehicle (V01-V09)
pedestrian on foot falling (slipping) on ice and snow (W00.-)

The appropriate 7th character is to be added to each code from category V00

> A   initial encounter
> D   subsequent encounter
> S   sequela

● **V00.0**   **Pedestrian on foot injured in collision with pedestrian conveyance**

   X ● **V00.01**   **Pedestrian on foot injured in collision with roller-skater** 🔍

   X ● **V00.02**   **Pedestrian on foot injured in collision with skateboarder** 🔍

   X ● **V00.09**   **Pedestrian on foot injured in collision with other pedestrian conveyance** 🔍

● **V00.1**   **Rolling-type pedestrian conveyance accident**

   Excludes1   accident with babystroller (V00.82-)
accident with wheelchair (powered) (V00.81-)
accident with motorized mobility scooter (V00.83-)

   ● **V00.11**   **In-line roller-skate accident**

     ● **V00.111**   **Fall from in-line roller-skates** 🔍

     ● **V00.112**   **In-line roller-skater colliding with stationary object** 🔍

     ● **V00.118**   **Other in-line roller-skate accident** 🔍

       Excludes1   roller-skater collision with other land transport vehicle (V01-V09 with 5th character 1)

   ● **V00.12**   **Non-in-line roller-skate accident**

     ● **V00.121**   **Fall from non-in-line roller-skates** 🔍

     ● **V00.122**   **Non-in-line roller-skater colliding with stationary object** 🔍

     ● **V00.128**   **Other non-in-line roller-skating accident** 🔍

       Excludes1   roller-skater collision with other land transport vehicle (V01-V09 with 5th character 1)

N   Newborn Age: 0   P   Pediatric Age: 0–17   M   Maternity DX: 12–55   A   Adult Age: 15–124   ♀   Females Only   ♂   Males Only

🔍 Complication\Comorbidity   🔍 Major C\C   (Ex) CC/MCC Exclusions   🔍 Present on Admission Requirement   🔍 Hospital-Acquired Condition

1589

- ● V00.13   **Skateboard accident**
  - ● V00.131   **Fall from skateboard** 🗸
  - ● V00.132   **Skateboarder colliding with stationary object** 🗸
  - ● V00.138   **Other skateboard accident** 🗸
    - **Excludes1**   skateboarder collision with other land transport vehicle (V01-V09 with 5th character 2)
- ● V00.14   **Scooter (nonmotorized) accident**
  - **Excludes1**   motorscooter accident (V20-V29)
  - ● V00.141   **Fall from scooter (nonmotorized)** 🗸
  - ● V00.142   **Scooter (nonmotorized) colliding with stationary object** 🗸
  - ● V00.148   **Other scooter (nonmotorized) accident** 🗸
    - **Excludes1**   scooter (non-motorized) collision with other land transport vehicle (V01-V09 with fifth character 9)
- ● V00.15   **Heelies accident**
  - Rolling shoe
  - Wheeled shoe
  - Wheelies accident
  - ● V00.151   **Fall from heelies** 🗸
  - ● V00.152   **Heelies colliding with stationary object** 🗸
  - ● V00.158   **Other heelies accident** 🗸
- ● V00.18   **Accident on other rolling-type pedestrian conveyance**
  - ● V00.181   **Fall from other rolling-type pedestrian conveyance** 🗸
  - ● V00.182   **Pedestrian on other rolling-type pedestrian conveyance colliding with stationary object** 🗸
  - ● V00.188   **Other accident on other rolling-type pedestrian conveyance** 🗸
- ● V00.2   **Gliding-type pedestrian conveyance accident**
  - ● V00.21   **Ice-skates accident**
    - ● V00.211   **Fall from ice-skates** 🗸
    - ● V00.212   **Ice-skater colliding with stationary object** 🗸
    - ● V00.218   **Other ice-skates accident** 🗸
      - **Excludes1**   ice-skater collision with other land transport vehicle (V01-V09 with 5th digit 9)
  - ● V00.22   **Sled accident**
    - ● V00.221   **Fall from sled** 🗸
    - ● V00.222   **Sledder colliding with stationary object** 🗸
    - ● V00.228   **Other sled accident** 🗸
      - **Excludes1**   sled collision with other land transport vehicle (V01-V09 with 5th digit 9)

- ● V00.28   **Other gliding-type pedestrian conveyance accident**
  - ● V00.281   **Fall from other gliding-type pedestrian conveyance** 🗸
  - ● V00.282   **Pedestrian on other gliding-type pedestrian conveyance colliding with stationary object** 🗸
  - ● V00.288   **Other accident on other gliding-type pedestrian conveyance** 🗸
    - **Excludes1**   gliding-type pedestrian conveyance collision with other land transport vehicle (V01-V09 with 5th digit 9)
- ● V00.3   **Flat-bottomed pedestrian conveyance accident**
  - ● V00.31   **Snowboard accident**
    - ● V00.311   **Fall from snowboard** 🗸
    - ● V00.312   **Snowboarder colliding with stationary object** 🗸
    - ● V00.318   **Other snowboard accident** 🗸
      - **Excludes1**   snowboarder collision with other land transport vehicle (V01-V09 with 5th digit 9)
  - ● V00.32   **Snow-ski accident**
    - ● V00.321   **Fall from snow-skis** 🗸
    - ● V00.322   **Snow-skier colliding with stationary object** 🗸
    - ● V00.328   **Other snow-ski accident** 🗸
      - **Excludes1**   snow-skier collision with other land transport vehicle (V01-V09 with 5th digit 9)
  - ● V00.38   **Other flat-bottomed pedestrian conveyance accident**
    - ● V00.381   **Fall from other flat-bottomed pedestrian conveyance** 🗸
    - ● V00.382   **Pedestrian on other flat-bottomed pedestrian conveyance colliding with stationary object** 🗸
    - ● V00.388   **Other accident on other flat-bottomed pedestrian conveyance** 🗸
- ● V00.8   **Accident on other pedestrian conveyance**
  - ● V00.81   **Accident with wheelchair (powered)**
    - ● V00.811   **Fall from moving wheelchair (powered)** 🗸
      - **Excludes1**   fall from non-moving wheelchair (W05.0)
    - ● V00.812   **Wheelchair (powered) colliding with stationary object** 🗸
    - ● V00.818   **Other accident with wheelchair (powered)** 🗸
  - ● V00.82   **Accident with babystroller**
    - ● V00.821   **Fall from babystroller** 🗸
    - ● V00.822   **Babystroller colliding with stationary object** 🗸
    - ● V00.828   **Other accident with babystroller** 🗸

◀ New   ◀░ Revised   ~~deleted~~ Deleted   Excludes 1   Excludes 2   Includes   Use additional   Code first   Code also   Unspecified

OGCR Official Guidelines   ● Unacceptable Principal Diagnosis   X Assign placeholder X   ▶ Use Additional Character(s)   ▶ Manifestation Code   **Coding Clinic**

● **V00.83**   **Accident with motorized mobility scooter**
    ● **V00.831**   **Fall from motorized mobility scooter** 🏥
        Excludes1   fall from non-moving motorized mobility scooter (W05.2)
    ● **V00.832**   **Motorized mobility scooter colliding with stationary object** 🏥
    ● **V00.838**   **Other accident with motorized mobility scooter** 🏥
● **V00.89**   **Accident on other pedestrian conveyance**
    ● **V00.891**   **Fall from other pedestrian conveyance** 🏥
    ● **V00.892**   **Pedestrian on other pedestrian conveyance colliding with stationary object** 🏥
    ● **V00.898**   **Other accident on other pedestrian conveyance** 🏥
        Excludes1   other pedestrian (conveyance) collision with other land transport vehicle (V01-V09 with 5th digit 9)

● **V01**   **Pedestrian injured in collision with pedal cycle**
    The appropriate 7th character is to be added to each code from category V01

> A   initial encounter
> D   subsequent encounter
> S   sequela

● **V01.0**   **Pedestrian injured in collision with pedal cycle in nontraffic accident**
    X ● **V01.00**   **Pedestrian on foot injured in collision with pedal cycle in nontraffic accident** 🏥
        Pedestrian NOS injured in collision with pedal cycle in nontraffic accident
    X ● **V01.01**   **Pedestrian on roller-skates injured in collision with pedal cycle in nontraffic accident** 🏥
    X ● **V01.02**   **Pedestrian on skateboard injured in collision with pedal cycle in nontraffic accident** 🏥
    X ● **V01.09**   **Pedestrian with other conveyance injured in collision with pedal cycle in nontraffic accident** 🏥
        Pedestrian with babystroller injured in collision with pedal cycle in nontraffic accident
        Pedestrian in wheelchair (powered) injured in collision with pedal cycle in nontraffic accident
        Pedestrian in motorized mobility scooter injured in collision with pedal cycle in nontraffic accident
        Pedestrian on ice-skates injured in collision with pedal cycle in nontraffic accident
        Pedestrian on nonmotorized scooter injured in collision with pedal cycle in nontraffic accident
        Pedestrian on sled injured in collision with pedal cycle in nontraffic accident
        Pedestrian on snowboard injured in collision with pedal cycle in nontraffic accident
        Pedestrian on snow-skis injured in collision with pedal cycle in nontraffic accident

● **V01.1**   **Pedestrian injured in collision with pedal cycle in traffic accident**
    X ● **V01.10**   **Pedestrian on foot injured in collision with pedal cycle in traffic accident** 🏥
        Pedestrian NOS injured in collision with pedal cycle in traffic accident
    X ● **V01.11**   **Pedestrian on roller-skates injured in collision with pedal cycle in traffic accident** 🏥
    X ● **V01.12**   **Pedestrian on skateboard injured in collision with pedal cycle in traffic accident** 🏥
    X ● **V01.19**   **Pedestrian with other conveyance injured in collision with pedal cycle in traffic accident** 🏥
        Pedestrian with babystroller injured in collision with pedal cycle in traffic accident
        Pedestrian in wheelchair (powered) injured in collision with pedal cycle in traffic accident
        Pedestrian in motorized mobility scooter injured in collision with pedal cycle in traffic accident
        Pedestrian on ice-skates injured in collision with pedal cycle in traffic accident
        Pedestrian on nonmotorized scooter injured in collision with pedal cycle in traffic accident
        Pedestrian on sled injured in collision with pedal cycle in traffic accident
        Pedestrian on snowboard injured in collision with pedal cycle in traffic accident
        Pedestrian on snow-skis injured in collision with pedal cycle in traffic accident

● **V01.9**   **Pedestrian injured in collision with pedal cycle, unspecified whether traffic or nontraffic accident**
    X ● **V01.90**   **Pedestrian on foot injured in collision with pedal cycle, unspecified whether traffic or nontraffic accident** 🏥
        Pedestrian NOS injured in collision with pedal cycle, unspecified whether traffic or nontraffic accident
    X ● **V01.91**   **Pedestrian on roller-skates injured in collision with pedal cycle, unspecified whether traffic or nontraffic accident** 🏥
    X ● **V01.92**   **Pedestrian on skateboard injured in collision with pedal cycle, unspecified whether traffic or nontraffic accident** 🏥
    X ● **V01.99**   **Pedestrian with other conveyance injured in collision with pedal cycle, unspecified whether traffic or nontraffic accident** 🏥
        Pedestrian with babystroller injured in collision with pedal cycle, unspecified whether traffic or nontraffic accident
        Pedestrian in wheelchair (powered) injured in collision with pedal cycle, unspecified whether traffic or nontraffic accident
        Pedestrian in motorized mobility scooter injured in collision with pedal cycle, unspecified whether traffic or nontraffic accident
        Pedestrian on ice-skates injured in collision with pedal cycle unspecified, whether traffic or nontraffic accident
        Pedestrian on nonmotorized scooter injured in collision with pedal cycle, unspecified whether traffic or nontraffic accident
        Pedestrian on sled injured in collision with pedal cycle unspecified, whether traffic or nontraffic accident
        Pedestrian on snowboard injured in collision with pedal cycle, unspecified whether traffic or nontraffic accident
        Pedestrian on snow-skis injured in collision with pedal cycle, unspecified whether traffic or nontraffic accident

CHAPTER 20 (V01-Y99)

N Newborn Age: 0   P Pediatric Age: 0–17   M Maternity DX: 12–55   A Adult Age: 15–124   ♀ Females Only   ♂ Males Only
🏥 Complication\Comorbidity   🏥 Major C\C   (Ex) CC/MCC Exclusions   🏥 Present on Admission Requirement   🏥 Hospital-Acquired Condition

1591

CHAPTER 20 (V01-Y99)

● V02   Pedestrian injured in collision with two- or three-wheeled motor vehicle

> The appropriate 7th character is to be added to each code from category V02

> | A | initial encounter |
> |---|---|
> | D | subsequent encounter |
> | S | sequela |

● V02.0   Pedestrian injured in collision with two- or three-wheeled motor vehicle in nontraffic accident

X ● V02.00   Pedestrian on foot injured in collision with two- or three-wheeled motor vehicle in nontraffic accident ✎

> Pedestrian NOS injured in collision with two- or three-wheeled motor vehicle in nontraffic accident

X ● V02.01   Pedestrian on roller-skates injured in collision with two- or three-wheeled motor vehicle in nontraffic accident ✎

X ● V02.02   Pedestrian on skateboard injured in collision with two- or three-wheeled motor vehicle in nontraffic accident ✎

X ● V02.09   Pedestrian with other conveyance injured in collision with two- or three-wheeled motor vehicle in nontraffic accident ✎

> Pedestrian with babystroller injured in collision with two- or three-wheeled motor vehicle in nontraffic accident
>
> Pedestrian on ice-skates injured in collision with two- or three-wheeled motor vehicle in nontraffic accident
>
> Pedestrian in wheelchair (powered) injured in collision with two- or three-wheeled motor vehicle in nontraffic accident
>
> Pedestrian in motorized mobility scooter injured in collision with two- or three-wheeled motor vehicle in nontraffic accident
>
> Pedestrian on nonmotorized scooter injured in collision with two- or three-wheeled motor vehicle in nontraffic accident
>
> Pedestrian on sled injured in collision with two- or three-wheeled motor vehicle in nontraffic accident
>
> Pedestrian on snowboard injured in collision with two- or three-wheeled motor vehicle in nontraffic accident
>
> Pedestrian on snow-skis injured in collision with two- or three-wheeled motor vehicle in nontraffic accident

● V02.1   Pedestrian injured in collision with two- or three-wheeled motor vehicle in traffic accident

X ● V02.10   Pedestrian on foot injured in collision with two- or three-wheeled motor vehicle in traffic accident ✎

> Pedestrian NOS injured in collision with two- or three-wheeled motor vehicle in traffic accident

X ● V02.11   Pedestrian on roller-skates injured in collision with two- or three-wheeled motor vehicle in traffic accident ✎

X ● V02.12   Pedestrian on skateboard injured in collision with two- or three-wheeled motor vehicle in traffic accident ✎

X ● V02.19   Pedestrian with other conveyance injured in collision with two- or three-wheeled motor vehicle in traffic accident ✎

> Pedestrian with babystroller injured in collision with two- or three-wheeled motor vehicle in traffic accident
>
> Pedestrian in wheelchair (powered) injured in collision with two- or three-wheeled motor vehicle in traffic accident
>
> Pedestrian in motorized mobility scooter injured in collision with two- or three-wheeled motor vehicle in traffic accident
>
> Pedestrian on ice-skates injured in collision with two- or three-wheeled motor vehicle in traffic accident
>
> Pedestrian on nonmotorized scooter injured in collision with two- or three-wheeled motor vehicle in traffic accident
>
> Pedestrian on sled injured in collision with two- or three-wheeled motor vehicle in traffic accident
>
> Pedestrian on snowboard injured in collision with two- or three-wheeled motor vehicle in traffic accident
>
> Pedestrian on snow-skis injured in collision with two- or three-wheeled motor vehicle in traffic accident

● V02.9   Pedestrian injured in collision with two- or three-wheeled motor vehicle, unspecified whether traffic or nontraffic accident

X ● V02.90   Pedestrian on foot injured in collision with two- or three-wheeled motor vehicle, unspecified whether traffic or nontraffic accident ✎

> Pedestrian NOS injured in collision with two- or three-wheeled motor vehicle, unspecified whether traffic or nontraffic accident

X ● V02.91   Pedestrian on roller-skates injured in collision with two- or three-wheeled motor vehicle, unspecified whether traffic or nontraffic accident ✎

X ● V02.92   Pedestrian on skateboard injured in collision with two- or three-wheeled motor vehicle, unspecified whether traffic or nontraffic accident ✎

◀ New   ◀◀ Revised   ~~deleted~~ Deleted   Excludes 1   Excludes 2   Includes   Use additional   Code first   Code also   Unspecified

OGCR Official Guidelines   ● Unacceptable Principal Diagnosis   X Assign placeholder X   ● Use Additional Character(s)   ▷ Manifestation Code   **Coding Clinic**

X ● **V02.99** **Pedestrian with other conveyance injured in collision with two- or three-wheeled motor vehicle, unspecified whether traffic or nontraffic accident** 🔖

Pedestrian with babystroller injured in collision with two- or three-wheeled motor vehicle, unspecified whether traffic or nontraffic accident

Pedestrian in wheelchair (powered) injured in collision with two- or three-wheeled motor vehicle, unspecified whether traffic or nontraffic accident

Pedestrian in motorized mobility scooter injured in collision with two- or three-wheeled motor vehicle, unspecified whether traffic or nontraffic accident

Pedestrian on ice-skates injured in collision with two- or three-wheeled motor vehicle, unspecified whether traffic or nontraffic accident

Pedestrian on nonmotorized scooter injured in collision with two- or three-wheeled motor vehicle, unspecified whether traffic or nontraffic accident

Pedestrian on sled injured in collision with two- or three-wheeled motor vehicle, unspecified whether traffic or nontraffic accident

Pedestrian on snowboard injured in collision with two- or three-wheeled motor vehicle, unspecified whether traffic or nontraffic accident

Pedestrian on snow-skis injured in collision with two- or three-wheeled motor vehicle, unspecified whether traffic or nontraffic accident

● **V03** **Pedestrian injured in collision with car, pick-up truck or van**

The appropriate 7th character is to be added to each code from category V03

A	initial encounter
D	subsequent encounter
S	sequela

● **V03.0** **Pedestrian injured in collision with car, pick-up truck or van in nontraffic accident**

X ● **V03.00** **Pedestrian on foot injured in collision with car, pick-up truck or van in nontraffic accident** 🔖

Pedestrian NOS injured in collision with car, pick-up truck or van in nontraffic accident

X ● **V03.01** **Pedestrian on roller-skates injured in collision with car, pick-up truck or van in nontraffic accident** 🔖

X ● **V03.02** **Pedestrian on skateboard injured in collision with car, pick-up truck or van in nontraffic accident** 🔖

X ● **V03.09** **Pedestrian with other conveyance injured in collision with car, pick-up truck or van in nontraffic accident** 🔖

Pedestrian with babystroller injured in collision with car, pick-up truck or van in nontraffic accident

Pedestrian in wheelchair (powered) injured in collision with car, pick-up truck or van in nontraffic accident

Pedestrian in motorized mobility scooter injured in collision with car, pick-up truck or van in nontraffic accident

Pedestrian on ice-skates injured in collision with car, pick-up truck or van in nontraffic accident

Pedestrian on nonmotorized scooter injured in collision with car, pick-up truck or van in nontraffic accident

Pedestrian on sled injured in collision with car, pick-up truck or van in nontraffic accident

Pedestrian on snowboard injured in collision with car, pick-up truck or van in nontraffic accident

Pedestrian on snow-skis injured in collision with car, pick-up truck or van in nontraffic accident

● **V03.1** **Pedestrian injured in collision with car, pick-up truck or van in traffic accident**

X ● **V03.10** **Pedestrian on foot injured in collision with car, pick-up truck or van in traffic accident** 🔖

Pedestrian NOS injured in collision with car, pick-up truck or van in traffic accident

X ● **V03.11** **Pedestrian on roller-skates injured in collision with car, pick-up truck or van in traffic accident** 🔖

X ● **V03.12** **Pedestrian on skateboard injured in collision with car, pick-up truck or van in traffic accident** 🔖

X ● **V03.19** **Pedestrian with other conveyance injured in collision with car, pick-up truck or van in traffic accident** 🔖

Pedestrian with babystroller injured in collision with car, pick-up truck or van in traffic accident

Pedestrian in wheelchair (powered) injured in collision with car, pick-up truck or van in traffic accident

Pedestrian in motorized mobility scooter injured in collision with car, pick-up truck or van in traffic accident

Pedestrian on ice-skates injured in collision with car, pick-up truck or van in traffic accident

Pedestrian on nonmotorized scooter injured in collision with car, pick-up truck or van in traffic accident

Pedestrian on sled injured in collision with car, pick-up truck or van in traffic accident

Pedestrian on snowboard injured in collision with car, pick-up truck or van in traffic accident

Pedestrian on snow-skis injured in collision with car, pick-up truck or van in traffic accident

CHAPTER 20 (V01-Y99)

N Newborn Age: 0   **P** Pediatric Age: 0–17   **M** Maternity DX: 12–55   **A** Adult Age: 15–124   ♀ Females Only   ♂ Males Only

🔖 Complication\Comorbidity   🔖 Major C\C   (Ex) CC/MCC Exclusions   🔖 Present on Admission Requirement   🔖 Hospital-Acquired Condition

1593

● **V03.9**   **Pedestrian injured in collision with car, pick-up truck or van, unspecified whether traffic or nontraffic accident**

X● **V03.90**   **Pedestrian on foot injured in collision with car, pick-up truck or van, unspecified whether traffic or nontraffic accident**

Pedestrian NOS injured in collision with car, pick-up truck or van, unspecified whether traffic or nontraffic accident

X● **V03.91**   **Pedestrian on roller-skates injured in collision with car, pick-up truck or van, unspecified whether traffic or nontraffic accident** 🕮

X● **V03.92**   **Pedestrian on skateboard injured in collision with car, pick-up truck or van, unspecified whether traffic or nontraffic accident** 🕮

X● **V03.99**   **Pedestrian with other conveyance injured in collision with car, pick-up truck or van, unspecified whether traffic or nontraffic accident** 🕮

Pedestrian with babystroller injured in collision with car, pick-up truck or van, unspecified whether traffic or nontraffic accident

Pedestrian in wheelchair (powered) injured in collision with car, pick-up truck or van, unspecified whether traffic or nontraffic accident

Pedestrian in motorized mobility scooter injured in collision with car, pick-up truck or van, unspecified whether traffic or nontraffic accident

Pedestrian on ice-skates injured in collision with car, pick-up truck or van, unspecified whether traffic or nontraffic accident

Pedestrian on nonmotorized scooter injured in collision with car, pick-up truck or van, unspecified whether traffic or nontraffic accident

Pedestrian on sled injured in collision with car, pick-up truck or van in nontraffic accident

Pedestrian on snowboard injured in collision with car, pick-up truck or van, unspecified whether traffic or nontraffic accident

Pedestrian on snow-skis injured in collision with car, pick-up truck or van, unspecified whether traffic or nontraffic accident

● **V04**   **Pedestrian injured in collision with heavy transport vehicle or bus**

Excludes1   pedestrian injured in collision with military vehicle (V09.01, V09.21)

The appropriate 7th character is to be added to each code from category V04

> A   initial encounter
> D   subsequent encounter
> S   sequela

● **V04.0**   **Pedestrian injured in collision with heavy transport vehicle or bus in nontraffic accident**

X● **V04.00**   **Pedestrian on foot injured in collision with heavy transport vehicle or bus in nontraffic accident** 🕮

Pedestrian NOS injured in collision with heavy transport vehicle or bus in nontraffic accident

X● **V04.01**   **Pedestrian on roller-skates injured in collision with heavy transport vehicle or bus in nontraffic accident** 🕮

X● **V04.02**   **Pedestrian on skateboard injured in collision with heavy transport vehicle or bus in nontraffic accident** 🕮

X● **V04.09**   **Pedestrian with other conveyance injured in collision with heavy transport vehicle or bus in nontraffic accident** 🕮

Pedestrian with babystroller injured in collision with heavy transport vehicle or bus in nontraffic accident

Pedestrian in wheelchair (powered) injured in collision with heavy transport vehicle or bus in nontraffic accident

Pedestrian in motorized mobility scooter injured in collision with heavy transport vehicle or bus in nontraffic accident

Pedestrian on ice-skates injured in collision with heavy transport vehicle or bus in nontraffic accident

Pedestrian on nonmotorized scooter injured in collision with heavy transport vehicle or bus in nontraffic accident

Pedestrian on sled injured in collision with heavy transport vehicle or bus in nontraffic accident

Pedestrian on snowboard injured in collision with heavy transport vehicle or bus in nontraffic accident

Pedestrian on snow-skis injured in collision with heavy transport vehicle or bus in nontraffic accident

● **V04.1**   **Pedestrian injured in collision with heavy transport vehicle or bus in traffic accident**

X● **V04.10**   **Pedestrian on foot injured in collision with heavy transport vehicle or bus in traffic accident** 🕮

Pedestrian NOS injured in collision with heavy transport vehicle or bus in traffic accident

X● **V04.11**   **Pedestrian on roller-skates injured in collision with heavy transport vehicle or bus in traffic accident** 🕮

X● **V04.12**   **Pedestrian on skateboard injured in collision with heavy transport vehicle or bus in traffic accident** 🕮

X● **V04.19**   **Pedestrian with other conveyance injured in collision with heavy transport vehicle or bus in traffic accident** 🕮

Pedestrian with babystroller injured in collision with heavy transport vehicle or bus in traffic accident

Pedestrian in wheelchair (powered) injured in collision with heavy transport vehicle or bus in traffic accident

Pedestrian in motorized mobility scooter injured in collision with heavy transport vehicle or bus in traffic accident

Pedestrian on ice-skates injured in collision with heavy transport vehicle or bus in traffic accident

Pedestrian on nonmotorized scooter injured in collision with heavy transport vehicle or bus in traffic accident

Pedestrian on sled injured in collision with heavy transport vehicle or bus in traffic accident

Pedestrian on snowboard injured in collision with heavy transport vehicle or bus in traffic accident

Pedestrian on snow-skis injured in collision with heavy transport vehicle or bus in traffic accident

◄ New   ◄═ Revised   ~~deleted~~ Deleted   Excludes 1   Excludes 2   Includes   Use additional   Code first   Code also   Unspecified

OGCR Official Guidelines   ● Unacceptable Principal Diagnosis   X Assign placeholder X   ● Use Additional Character(s)   🕮 Manifestation Code   **Coding Clinic**

● V04.9 **Pedestrian injured in collision with heavy transport vehicle or bus, unspecified whether traffic or nontraffic accident**

X● V04.90 **Pedestrian on foot injured in collision with heavy transport vehicle or bus, unspecified whether traffic or nontraffic accident** 🔍

Pedestrian NOS injured in collision with heavy transport vehicle or bus, unspecified whether traffic or nontraffic accident

X● V04.91 **Pedestrian on roller-skates injured in collision with heavy transport vehicle or bus, unspecified whether traffic or nontraffic accident** 🔍

X● V04.92 **Pedestrian on skateboard injured in collision with heavy transport vehicle or bus, unspecified whether traffic or nontraffic accident** 🔍

X● V04.99 **Pedestrian with other conveyance injured in collision with heavy transport vehicle or bus, unspecified whether traffic or nontraffic accident** 🔍

Pedestrian with babystroller injured in collision with heavy transport vehicle or bus, unspecified whether traffic or nontraffic accident

Pedestrian in wheelchair (powered) injured in collision with heavy transport vehicle or bus, unspecified whether traffic or nontraffic accident

Pedestrian in motorized mobility scooter injured in collision with heavy transport vehicle or bus, unspecified whether traffic or nontraffic accident

Pedestrian on ice-skates injured in collision with heavy transport vehicle or bus, unspecified whether traffic or nontraffic accident

Pedestrian on nonmotorized scooter injured in collision with heavy transport vehicle or bus, unspecified whether traffic or nontraffic accident

Pedestrian on sled injured in collision with heavy transport vehicle or bus, unspecified whether traffic or nontraffic accident

Pedestrian on snowboard injured in collision with heavy transport vehicle or bus, unspecified whether traffic or nontraffic accident

Pedestrian on snow-skis injured in collision with heavy transport vehicle or bus, unspecified whether traffic or nontraffic accident

● V05 **Pedestrian injured in collision with railway train or railway vehicle**

The appropriate 7th character is to be added to each code from category V05

A	initial encounter
D	subsequent encounter
S	sequela

● V05.0 **Pedestrian injured in collision with railway train or railway vehicle in nontraffic accident**

X● V05.00 **Pedestrian on foot injured in collision with railway train or railway vehicle in nontraffic accident** 🔍

Pedestrian NOS injured in collision with railway train or railway vehicle in nontraffic accident

X● V05.01 **Pedestrian on roller-skates injured in collision with railway train or railway vehicle in nontraffic accident** 🔍

X● V05.02 **Pedestrian on skateboard injured in collision with railway train or railway vehicle in nontraffic accident** 🔍

X● V05.09 **Pedestrian with other conveyance injured in collision with railway train or railway vehicle in nontraffic accident** 🔍

Pedestrian with babystroller injured in collision with railway train or railway vehicle in nontraffic accident

Pedestrian in wheelchair (powered) injured in collision with railway train or railway vehicle in nontraffic accident

Pedestrian in motorized mobility scooter injured in collision with railway train or railway vehicle in nontraffic accident

Pedestrian on ice-skates injured in collision with railway train or railway vehicle in nontraffic accident

Pedestrian on nonmotorized scooter injured in collision with railway train or railway vehicle in nontraffic accident

Pedestrian on sled injured in collision with railway train or railway vehicle in nontraffic accident

Pedestrian on snowboard injured in collision with railway train or railway vehicle in nontraffic accident

Pedestrian on snow-skis injured in collision with railway train or railway vehicle in nontraffic accident

● V05.1 **Pedestrian injured in collision with railway train or railway vehicle in traffic accident**

X● V05.10 **Pedestrian on foot injured in collision with railway train or railway vehicle in traffic accident** 🔍

Pedestrian NOS injured in collision with railway train or railway vehicle in traffic accident

X● V05.11 **Pedestrian on roller-skates injured in collision with railway train or railway vehicle in traffic accident** 🔍

X● V05.12 **Pedestrian on skateboard injured in collision with railway train or railway vehicle in traffic accident** 🔍

X● V05.19 **Pedestrian with other conveyance injured in collision with railway train or railway vehicle in traffic accident** 🔍

Pedestrian with babystroller injured in collision with railway train or railway vehicle in traffic accident

Pedestrian in wheelchair (powered) injured in collision with railway train or railway vehicle in traffic accident

Pedestrian in motorized mobility scooter injured in collision with railway train or railway vehicle in traffic accident

Pedestrian on ice-skates injured in collision with railway train or railway vehicle in traffic accident

Pedestrian on nonmotorized scooter injured in collision with railway train or railway vehicle in traffic accident

Pedestrian on sled injured in collision with railway train or railway vehicle in traffic accident

Pedestrian on snowboard injured in collision with railway train or railway vehicle in traffic accident

Pedestrian on snow-skis injured in collision with railway train or railway vehicle in traffic accident

N Newborn Age: 0   P Pediatric Age: 0–17   M Maternity DX: 12–55   A Adult Age: 15–124   ♀ Females Only   ♂ Males Only

🔍 Complication\Comorbidity   🔍 Major C\C   (Ex) CC/MCC Exclusions   🔍 Present on Admission Requirement   🔍 Hospital-Acquired Condition

1595

● **V05.9**   Pedestrian injured in collision with railway train or railway vehicle, unspecified whether traffic or nontraffic accident

   X ● **V05.90**   Pedestrian on foot injured in collision with railway train or railway vehicle, unspecified whether traffic or nontraffic accident 🔍

      Pedestrian NOS injured in collision with railway train or railway vehicle, unspecified whether traffic or nontraffic accident

   X ● **V05.91**   Pedestrian on roller-skates injured in collision with railway train or railway vehicle, unspecified whether traffic or nontraffic accident 🔍

   X ● **V05.92**   Pedestrian on skateboard injured in collision with railway train or railway vehicle, unspecified whether traffic or nontraffic accident 🔍

   X ● **V05.99**   Pedestrian with other conveyance injured in collision with railway train or railway vehicle, unspecified whether traffic or nontraffic accident 🔍

      Pedestrian with babystroller injured in collision with railway train or railway vehicle, unspecified whether traffic or nontraffic

      Pedestrian in wheelchair (powered) injured in collision with railway train or railway vehicle, unspecified whether traffic or nontraffic

      Pedestrian in motorized mobility scooter injured in collision with railway train or railway vehicle, unspecified whether traffic or nontraffic

      Pedestrian on ice-skates injured in collision with railway train or railway vehicle, unspecified whether traffic or nontraffic

      Pedestrian on nonmotorized scooter injured in collision with railway train or railway vehicle, unspecified whether traffic or nontraffic

      Pedestrian on sled injured in collision with railway train or railway vehicle, unspecified whether traffic or nontraffic

      Pedestrian on snowboard injured in collision with railway train or railway vehicle, unspecified whether traffic or nontraffic

      Pedestrian on snow-skis injured in collision with railway train or railway vehicle, unspecified whether traffic or nontraffic

● **V06**   Pedestrian injured in collision with other nonmotor vehicle

   Includes   collision with animal-drawn vehicle, animal being ridden, nonpowered streetcar

   Excludes1   pedestrian injured in collision with pedestrian conveyance (V00.0-)

The appropriate 7th character is to be added to each code from category V06

   A   initial encounter
   D   subsequent encounter
   S   sequela

● **V06.0**   Pedestrian injured in collision with other nonmotor vehicle in nontraffic accident

   X ● **V06.00**   Pedestrian on foot injured in collision with other nonmotor vehicle in nontraffic accident 🔍

      Pedestrian NOS injured in collision with other nonmotor vehicle in nontraffic accident

   X ● **V06.01**   Pedestrian on roller-skates injured in collision with other nonmotor vehicle in nontraffic accident 🔍

   X ● **V06.02**   Pedestrian on skateboard injured in collision with other nonmotor vehicle in nontraffic accident 🔍

   X ● **V06.09**   Pedestrian with other conveyance injured in collision with other nonmotor vehicle in nontraffic accident 🔍

      Pedestrian with babystroller injured in collision with other nonmotor vehicle in nontraffic accident

      Pedestrian in wheelchair (powered) injured in collision with other nonmotor vehicle in nontraffic accident

      Pedestrian in motorized mobility scooter injured in collision with other nonmotor vehicle in nontraffic accident

      Pedestrian on ice-skates injured in collision with other nonmotor vehicle in nontraffic accident

      Pedestrian on nonmotorized scooter injured in collision with other nonmotor vehicle in nontraffic accident

      Pedestrian on sled injured in collision with other nonmotor vehicle in nontraffic accident

      Pedestrian on snowboard injured in collision with other nonmotor vehicle in nontraffic accident

      Pedestrian on snow-skis injured in collision with other nonmotor vehicle in nontraffic accident

● **V06.1**   Pedestrian injured in collision with other nonmotor vehicle in traffic accident

   X ● **V06.10**   Pedestrian on foot injured in collision with other nonmotor vehicle in traffic accident 🔍

      Pedestrian NOS injured in collision with other nonmotor vehicle in traffic accident

   X ● **V06.11**   Pedestrian on roller-skates injured in collision with other nonmotor vehicle in traffic accident 🔍

   X ● **V06.12**   Pedestrian on skateboard injured in collision with other nonmotor vehicle in traffic accident 🔍

   X ● **V06.19**   Pedestrian with other conveyance injured in collision with other nonmotor vehicle in traffic accident 🔍

      Pedestrian with babystroller injured in collision with other nonmotor vehicle in nontraffic accident

      Pedestrian in wheelchair (powered) injured in collision with other nonmotor vehicle in traffic accident

      Pedestrian in motorized mobility scooter injured in collision with other nonmotor vehicle in traffic accident

      Pedestrian on ice-skates injured in collision with other nonmotor vehicle in traffic accident

      Pedestrian on nonmotorized scooter injured in collision with other nonmotor vehicle in traffic accident

      Pedestrian on sled injured in collision with other nonmotor vehicle in traffic accident

      Pedestrian on snowboard injured in collision with other nonmotor vehicle in traffic accident

      Pedestrian on snow-skis injured in collision with other nonmotor vehicle in traffic accident

● **V06.9**   Pedestrian injured in collision with other nonmotor vehicle, unspecified whether traffic or nontraffic accident

   X ● **V06.90**   Pedestrian on foot injured in collision with other nonmotor vehicle, unspecified whether traffic or nontraffic accident 🔍

      Pedestrian NOS injured in collision with other nonmotor vehicle, unspecified whether traffic or nontraffic accident

   X ● **V06.91**   Pedestrian on roller-skates injured in collision with other nonmotor vehicle, unspecified whether traffic or nontraffic accident 🔍

◄ New   ◄▬ Revised   ~~deleted~~ Deleted   Excludes 1   Excludes 2   Includes   Use additional   Code first   Code also   Unspecified

OGCR Official Guidelines   ● Unacceptable Principal Diagnosis   X Assign placeholder X   ▌ Use Additional Character(s)   ▌ Manifestation Code   **Coding Clinic**

X ● **V06.92**   **Pedestrian on skateboard injured in collision with other nonmotor vehicle, unspecified whether traffic or nontraffic accident** 🔖

X ● **V06.99**   **Pedestrian with other conveyance injured in collision with other nonmotor vehicle, unspecified whether traffic or nontraffic accident** 🔖

> Pedestrian with babystroller injured in collision with other nonmotor vehicle, unspecified whether traffic or nontraffic accident
>
> Pedestrian in wheelchair (powered) injured in collision with other nonmotor vehicle, unspecified whether traffic or nontraffic accident
>
> Pedestrian in motorized mobility scooter injured in collision with other nonmotor vehicle, unspecified whether traffic or nontraffic accident
>
> Pedestrian on ice-skates injured in collision with other nonmotor vehicle, unspecified whether traffic or nontraffic accident
>
> Pedestrian on nonmotorized scooter injured in collision with other nonmotor vehicle, unspecified whether traffic or nontraffic accident
>
> Pedestrian on sled injured in collision with other nonmotor vehicle, unspecified whether traffic or nontraffic accident
>
> Pedestrian on snowboard injured in collision with other nonmotor vehicle, unspecified whether traffic or nontraffic accident
>
> Pedestrian on snow-skis injured in collision with other nonmotor vehicle, unspecified whether traffic or nontraffic accident

● **V09**   **Pedestrian injured in other and unspecified transport accidents**

The appropriate 7th character is to be added to each code from category V09

A	initial encounter
D	subsequent encounter
S	sequela

● **V09.0**   **Pedestrian injured in nontraffic accident involving other and unspecified motor vehicles**

X ● **V09.00**   **Pedestrian injured in nontraffic accident involving unspecified motor vehicles** 🔖

X ● **V09.01**   **Pedestrian injured in nontraffic accident involving military vehicle** 🔖

X ● **V09.09**   **Pedestrian injured in nontraffic accident involving other motor vehicles** 🔖

> Pedestrian injured in nontraffic accident by special vehicle

X ● **V09.1**   **Pedestrian injured in unspecified nontraffic accident** 🔖

● **V09.2**   **Pedestrian injured in traffic accident involving other and unspecified motor vehicles**

X ● **V09.20**   **Pedestrian injured in traffic accident involving unspecified motor vehicles** 🔖

X ● **V09.21**   **Pedestrian injured in traffic accident involving military vehicle** 🔖

X ● **V09.29**   **Pedestrian injured in traffic accident involving other motor vehicles** 🔖

X ● **V09.3**   **Pedestrian injured in unspecified traffic accident** 🔖

X ● **V09.9**   **Pedestrian injured in unspecified transport accident** 🔖

PEDAL CYCLE RIDER INJURED IN TRANSPORT ACCIDENT (V10-V19)

Includes   any non-motorized vehicle, excluding an animal-drawn vehicle, or a sidecar or trailer attached to the pedal cycle

Excludes2   rupture of pedal cycle tire (W37.0)

● **V10**   **Pedal cycle rider injured in collision with pedestrian or animal**

Excludes1   pedal cycle rider collision with animal-drawn vehicle or animal being ridden (V16.-) ◀▦

The appropriate 7th character is to be added to each code from category V10

A	initial encounter
D	subsequent encounter
S	sequela

X ● **V10.0**   **Pedal cycle driver injured in collision with pedestrian or animal in nontraffic accident** 🔖

X ● **V10.1**   **Pedal cycle passenger injured in collision with pedestrian or animal in nontraffic accident** 🔖

X ● **V10.2**   **Unspecified pedal cyclist injured in collision with pedestrian or animal in nontraffic accident** 🔖

X ● **V10.3**   **Person boarding or alighting a pedal cycle injured in collision with pedestrian or animal** 🔖

X ● **V10.4**   **Pedal cycle driver injured in collision with pedestrian or animal in traffic accident** 🔖

X ● **V10.5**   **Pedal cycle passenger injured in collision with pedestrian or animal in traffic accident** 🔖

X ● **V10.9**   **Unspecified pedal cyclist injured in collision with pedestrian or animal in traffic accident** 🔖

● **V11**   **Pedal cycle rider injured in collision with other pedal cycle**

The appropriate 7th character is to be added to each code from category V11

A	initial encounter
D	subsequent encounter
S	sequela

X ● **V11.0**   **Pedal cycle driver injured in collision with other pedal cycle in nontraffic accident** 🔖

X ● **V11.1**   **Pedal cycle passenger injured in collision with other pedal cycle in nontraffic accident** 🔖

X ● **V11.2**   **Unspecified pedal cyclist injured in collision with other pedal cycle in nontraffic accident** 🔖

X ● **V11.3**   **Person boarding or alighting a pedal cycle injured in collision with other pedal cycle** 🔖

X ● **V11.4**   **Pedal cycle driver injured in collision with other pedal cycle in traffic accident** 🔖

X ● **V11.5**   **Pedal cycle passenger injured in collision with other pedal cycle in traffic accident** 🔖

X ● **V11.9**   **Unspecified pedal cyclist injured in collision with other pedal cycle in traffic accident** 🔖

● **V12**   **Pedal cycle rider injured in collision with two- or three-wheeled motor vehicle**

The appropriate 7th character is to be added to each code from category V12

A	initial encounter
D	subsequent encounter
S	sequela

X ● **V12.0**   **Pedal cycle driver injured in collision with two- or three-wheeled motor vehicle in nontraffic accident** 🔖

X ● **V12.1**   **Pedal cycle passenger injured in collision with two- or three-wheeled motor vehicle in nontraffic accident** 🔖

CHAPTER 20 (V01-Y99)

N   Newborn Age: 0   P   Pediatric Age: 0–17   M   Maternity DX: 12–55   A   Adult Age: 15–124   ♀   Females Only   ♂   Males Only

🔖 Complication\Comorbidity   🔖 Major C\C   (Ex) CC/MCC Exclusions   🔖 Present on Admission Requirement   🔖 Hospital-Acquired Condition

1597

X ● **V12.2** Unspecified pedal cyclist injured in collision with two- or three-wheeled motor vehicle in nontraffic accident 🔍

X ● **V12.3** Person boarding or alighting a pedal cycle injured in collision with two- or three-wheeled motor vehicle 🔍

X ● **V12.4** Pedal cycle driver injured in collision with two- or three-wheeled motor vehicle in traffic accident 🔍

X ● **V12.5** Pedal cycle passenger injured in collision with two- or three-wheeled motor vehicle in traffic accident 🔍

X ● **V12.9** Unspecified pedal cyclist injured in collision with two- or three-wheeled motor vehicle in traffic accident 🔍

● **V13** Pedal cycle rider injured in collision with car, pick-up truck or van

The appropriate 7th character is to be added to each code from category V13

> A   initial encounter
> D   subsequent encounter
> S   sequela

X ● **V13.0** Pedal cycle driver injured in collision with car, pick-up truck or van in nontraffic accident 🔍

X ● **V13.1** Pedal cycle passenger injured in collision with car, pick-up truck or van in nontraffic accident 🔍

X ● **V13.2** Unspecified pedal cyclist injured in collision with car, pick-up truck or van in nontraffic accident 🔍

X ● **V13.3** Person boarding or alighting a pedal cycle injured in collision with car, pick-up truck or van 🔍

X ● **V13.4** Pedal cycle driver injured in collision with car, pick-up truck or van in traffic accident 🔍

X ● **V13.5** Pedal cycle passenger injured in collision with car, pick-up truck or van in traffic accident 🔍

X ● **V13.9** Unspecified pedal cyclist injured in collision with car, pick-up truck or van in traffic accident 🔍

● **V14** Pedal cycle rider injured in collision with heavy transport vehicle or bus

> Excludes1   pedal cycle rider injured in collision with military vehicle (V19.81)

The appropriate 7th character is to be added to each code from category V14

> A   initial encounter
> D   subsequent encounter
> S   sequela

X ● **V14.0** Pedal cycle driver injured in collision with heavy transport vehicle or bus in nontraffic accident 🔍

X ● **V14.1** Pedal cycle passenger injured in collision with heavy transport vehicle or bus in nontraffic accident 🔍

X ● **V14.2** Unspecified pedal cyclist injured in collision with heavy transport vehicle or bus in nontraffic accident 🔍

X ● **V14.3** Person boarding or alighting a pedal cycle injured in collision with heavy transport vehicle or bus 🔍

X ● **V14.4** Pedal cycle driver injured in collision with heavy transport vehicle or bus in traffic accident 🔍

X ● **V14.5** Pedal cycle passenger injured in collision with heavy transport vehicle or bus in traffic accident 🔍

X ● **V14.9** Unspecified pedal cyclist injured in collision with heavy transport vehicle or bus in traffic accident 🔍

● **V15** Pedal cycle rider injured in collision with railway train or railway vehicle

The appropriate 7th character is to be added to each code from category V15

> A   initial encounter
> D   subsequent encounter
> S   sequela

X ● **V15.0** Pedal cycle driver injured in collision with railway train or railway vehicle in nontraffic accident 🔍

X ● **V15.1** Pedal cycle passenger injured in collision with railway train or railway vehicle in nontraffic accident 🔍

X ● **V15.2** Unspecified pedal cyclist injured in collision with railway train or railway vehicle in nontraffic accident 🔍

X ● **V15.3** Person boarding or alighting a pedal cycle injured in collision with railway train or railway vehicle 🔍

X ● **V15.4** Pedal cycle driver injured in collision with railway train or railway vehicle in traffic accident 🔍

X ● **V15.5** Pedal cycle passenger injured in collision with railway train or railway vehicle in traffic accident 🔍

X ● **V15.9** Unspecified pedal cyclist injured in collision with railway train or railway vehicle in traffic accident 🔍

● **V16** Pedal cycle rider injured in collision with other nonmotor vehicle

> Includes   collision with animal-drawn vehicle, animal being ridden, streetcar

The appropriate 7th character is to be added to each code from category V16

> A   initial encounter
> D   subsequent encounter
> S   sequela

X ● **V16.0** Pedal cycle driver injured in collision with other nonmotor vehicle in nontraffic accident 🔍

X ● **V16.1** Pedal cycle passenger injured in collision with other nonmotor vehicle in nontraffic accident 🔍

X ● **V16.2** Unspecified pedal cyclist injured in collision with other nonmotor vehicle in nontraffic accident 🔍

X ● **V16.3** Person boarding or alighting a pedal cycle injured in collision with other nonmotor vehicle in nontraffic accident 🔍

X ● **V16.4** Pedal cycle driver injured in collision with other nonmotor vehicle in traffic accident 🔍

X ● **V16.5** Pedal cycle passenger injured in collision with other nonmotor vehicle in traffic accident 🔍

X ● **V16.9** Unspecified pedal cyclist injured in collision with other nonmotor vehicle in traffic accident 🔍

● **V17** Pedal cycle rider injured in collision with fixed or stationary object

The appropriate 7th character is to be added to each code from category V17

> A   initial encounter
> D   subsequent encounter
> S   sequela

X ● **V17.0** Pedal cycle driver injured in collision with fixed or stationary object in nontraffic accident 🔍

X ● **V17.1** Pedal cycle passenger injured in collision with fixed or stationary object in nontraffic accident 🔍

X ● **V17.2** Unspecified pedal cyclist injured in collision with fixed or stationary object in nontraffic accident 🔍

X ● **V17.3** Person boarding or alighting a pedal cycle injured in collision with fixed or stationary object 🔍

X ● **V17.4** Pedal cycle driver injured in collision with fixed or stationary object in traffic accident 🔍

X ● **V17.5** Pedal cycle passenger injured in collision with fixed or stationary object in traffic accident 🔍

X ● **V17.9** Unspecified pedal cyclist injured in collision with fixed or stationary object in traffic accident 🔍

● **V18**   **Pedal cycle rider injured in noncollision transport accident**

Includes	fall or thrown from pedal cycle (without antecedent collision)
	overturning pedal cycle NOS
	overturning pedal cycle without collision

The appropriate 7th character is to be added to each code from category V18

A	initial encounter
D	subsequent encounter
S	sequela

X● **V18.0**   Pedal cycle driver injured in noncollision transport accident in nontraffic accident 🔖

X● **V18.1**   Pedal cycle passenger injured in noncollision transport accident in nontraffic accident 🔖

X● **V18.2**   Unspecified pedal cyclist injured in noncollision transport accident in nontraffic accident 🔖

X● **V18.3**   Person boarding or alighting a pedal cycle injured in noncollision transport accident 🔖

X● **V18.4**   Pedal cycle driver injured in noncollision transport accident in traffic accident 🔖

X● **V18.5**   Pedal cycle passenger injured in noncollision transport accident in traffic accident 🔖

X● **V18.9**   Unspecified pedal cyclist injured in noncollision transport accident in traffic accident 🔖

● **V19**   **Pedal cycle rider injured in other and unspecified transport accidents**

The appropriate 7th character is to be added to each code from category V19

A	initial encounter
D	subsequent encounter
S	sequela

● **V19.0**   Pedal cycle driver injured in collision with other and unspecified motor vehicles in nontraffic accident

     X● **V19.00**   Pedal cycle driver injured in collision with unspecified motor vehicles in nontraffic accident 🔖

     X● **V19.09**   Pedal cycle driver injured in collision with other motor vehicles in nontraffic accident 🔖

● **V19.1**   Pedal cycle passenger injured in collision with other and unspecified motor vehicles in nontraffic accident

     X● **V19.10**   Pedal cycle passenger injured in collision with unspecified motor vehicles in nontraffic accident 🔖

     X● **V19.19**   Pedal cycle passenger injured in collision with other motor vehicles in nontraffic accident 🔖

● **V19.2**   Unspecified pedal cyclist injured in collision with other and unspecified motor vehicles in nontraffic accident

     X● **V19.20**   Unspecified pedal cyclist injured in collision with unspecified motor vehicles in nontraffic accident 🔖

         Pedal cycle collision NOS, nontraffic

     X● **V19.29**   Unspecified pedal cyclist injured in collision with other motor vehicles in nontraffic accident 🔖

X● **V19.3**   Pedal cyclist (driver) (passenger) injured in unspecified nontraffic accident 🔖

     Pedal cycle accident NOS, nontraffic

     Pedal cyclist injured in nontraffic accident NOS

● **V19.4**   Pedal cycle driver injured in collision with other and unspecified motor vehicles in traffic accident

     X● **V19.40**   Pedal cycle driver injured in collision with unspecified motor vehicles in traffic accident 🔖

     X● **V19.49**   Pedal cycle driver injured in collision with other motor vehicles in traffic accident 🔖

● **V19.5**   Pedal cycle passenger injured in collision with other and unspecified motor vehicles in traffic accident

     X● **V19.50**   Pedal cycle passenger injured in collision with unspecified motor vehicles in traffic accident 🔖

     X● **V19.59**   Pedal cycle passenger injured in collision with other motor vehicles in traffic accident 🔖

● **V19.6**   Unspecified pedal cyclist injured in collision with other and unspecified motor vehicles in traffic accident

     X● **V19.60**   Unspecified pedal cyclist injured in collision with unspecified motor vehicles in traffic accident 🔖

         Pedal cycle collision NOS (traffic)

     X● **V19.69**   Unspecified pedal cyclist injured in collision with other motor vehicles in traffic accident 🔖

● **V19.8**   Pedal cyclist (driver) (passenger) injured in other specified transport accidents

     X● **V19.81**   Pedal cyclist (driver) (passenger) injured in transport accident with military vehicle 🔖

     X● **V19.88**   Pedal cyclist (driver) (passenger) injured in other specified transport accidents 🔖

X● **V19.9**   Pedal cyclist (driver) (passenger) injured in unspecified traffic accident 🔖

     Pedal cycle accident NOS

MOTORCYCLE RIDER INJURED IN TRANSPORT ACCIDENT (V20-V29)

| **Includes** | moped motorcycle with sidecar motorized bicycle |
| | motor scooter |

| **Excludes 1** | three-wheeled motor vehicle (V30-V39) |

● **V20**   **Motorcycle rider injured in collision with pedestrian or animal**

| **Excludes 1** | motorcycle rider collision with animal-drawn vehicle or animal being ridden (V26.-) |

The appropriate 7th character is to be added to each code from category V20

A	initial encounter
D	subsequent encounter
S	sequela

X● **V20.0**   Motorcycle driver injured in collision with pedestrian or animal in nontraffic accident 🔖

X● **V20.1**   Motorcycle passenger injured in collision with pedestrian or animal in nontraffic accident 🔖

X● **V20.2**   Unspecified motorcycle rider injured in collision with pedestrian or animal in nontraffic accident 🔖

X● **V20.3**   Person boarding or alighting a motorcycle injured in collision with pedestrian or animal 🔖

X● **V20.4**   Motorcycle driver injured in collision with pedestrian or animal in traffic accident 🔖

X● **V20.5**   Motorcycle passenger injured in collision with pedestrian or animal in traffic accident 🔖

X● **V20.9**   Unspecified motorcycle rider injured in collision with pedestrian or animal in traffic accident 🔖

● **V21**   **Motorcycle rider injured in collision with pedal cycle**

The appropriate 7th character is to be added to each code from category V21

A	initial encounter
D	subsequent encounter
S	sequela

X● **V21.0**   Motorcycle driver injured in collision with pedal cycle in nontraffic accident 🔖

X● **V21.1**   Motorcycle passenger injured in collision with pedal cycle in nontraffic accident 🔖

X● **V21.2**   Unspecified motorcycle rider injured in collision with pedal cycle in nontraffic accident 🔖

X● **V21.3**   Person boarding or alighting a motorcycle injured in collision with pedal cycle 🔖

N Newborn Age: 0   **P** Pediatric Age: 0–17   **M** Maternity DX: 12–55   **A** Adult Age: 15–124   ♀ Females Only   ♂ Males Only

🔖 Complication\Comorbidity   🔖 Major C\C   (Ex) CC/MCC Exclusions   🔖 Present on Admission Requirement   🔖 Hospital-Acquired Condition

1599

CHAPTER 20 (V01-Y99)

X● **V21.4** Motorcycle driver injured in collision with pedal cycle in traffic accident ✎

X● **V21.5** Motorcycle passenger injured in collision with pedal cycle in traffic accident ✎

X● **V21.9** Unspecified motorcycle rider injured in collision with pedal cycle in traffic accident ✎

● **V22** Motorcycle rider injured in collision with two- or three-wheeled motor vehicle

The appropriate 7th character is to be added to each code from category V22

A	initial encounter
D	subsequent encounter
S	sequela

X● **V22.0** Motorcycle driver injured in collision with two- or three-wheeled motor vehicle in nontraffic accident ✎

X● **V22.1** Motorcycle passenger injured in collision with two- or three-wheeled motor vehicle in nontraffic accident ✎

X● **V22.2** Unspecified motorcycle rider injured in collision with two- or three-wheeled motor vehicle in nontraffic accident ✎

X● **V22.3** Person boarding or alighting a motorcycle injured in collision with two- or three-wheeled motor vehicle ✎

X● **V22.4** Motorcycle driver injured in collision with two- or three-wheeled motor vehicle in traffic accident ✎

X● **V22.5** Motorcycle passenger injured in collision with two- or three-wheeled motor vehicle in traffic accident ✎

X● **V22.9** Unspecified motorcycle rider injured in collision with two- or three-wheeled motor vehicle in traffic accident ✎

● **V23** Motorcycle rider injured in collision with car, pick-up truck or van

The appropriate 7th character is to be added to each code from category V23

A	initial encounter
D	subsequent encounter
S	sequela

X● **V23.0** Motorcycle driver injured in collision with car, pick-up truck or van in nontraffic accident ✎

X● **V23.1** Motorcycle passenger injured in collision with car, pick-up truck or van in nontraffic accident ✎

X● **V23.2** Unspecified motorcycle rider injured in collision with car, pick-up truck or van in nontraffic accident ✎

X● **V23.3** Person boarding or alighting a motorcycle injured in collision with car, pick-up truck or van ✎

X● **V23.4** Motorcycle driver injured in collision with car, pick-up truck or van in traffic accident ✎

X● **V23.5** Motorcycle passenger injured in collision with car, pick-up truck or van in traffic accident ✎

X● **V23.9** Unspecified motorcycle rider injured in collision with car, pick-up truck or van in traffic accident ✎

● **V24** Motorcycle rider injured in collision with heavy transport vehicle or bus

     Excludes1   motorcycle rider injured in collision with military vehicle (V29.81)

The appropriate 7th character is to be added to each code from category V24

A	initial encounter
D	subsequent encounter
S	sequela

X● **V24.0** Motorcycle driver injured in collision with heavy transport vehicle or bus in nontraffic accident ✎

X● **V24.1** Motorcycle passenger injured in collision with heavy transport vehicle or bus in nontraffic accident ✎

X● **V24.2** Unspecified motorcycle rider injured in collision with heavy transport vehicle or bus in nontraffic accident ✎

X● **V24.3** Person boarding or alighting a motorcycle injured in collision with heavy transport vehicle or bus ✎

X● **V24.4** Motorcycle driver injured in collision with heavy transport vehicle or bus in traffic accident ✎

X● **V24.5** Motorcycle passenger injured in collision with heavy transport vehicle or bus in traffic accident ✎

X● **V24.9** Unspecified motorcycle rider injured in collision with heavy transport vehicle or bus in traffic accident ✎

● **V25** Motorcycle rider injured in collision with railway train or railway vehicle

The appropriate 7th character is to be added to each code from category V25

A	initial encounter
D	subsequent encounter
S	sequela

X● **V25.0** Motorcycle driver injured in collision with railway train or railway vehicle in nontraffic accident ✎

X● **V25.1** Motorcycle passenger injured in collision with railway train or railway vehicle in nontraffic accident ✎

X● **V25.2** Unspecified motorcycle rider injured in collision with railway train or railway vehicle in nontraffic accident ✎

X● **V25.3** Person boarding or alighting a motorcycle injured in collision with railway train or railway vehicle ✎

X● **V25.4** Motorcycle driver injured in collision with railway train or railway vehicle in traffic accident ✎

X● **V25.5** Motorcycle passenger injured in collision with railway train or railway vehicle in traffic accident ✎

X● **V25.9** Unspecified motorcycle rider injured in collision with railway train or railway vehicle in traffic accident ✎

● **V26** Motorcycle rider injured in collision with other nonmotor vehicle

     Includes   collision with animal-drawn vehicle, animal being ridden, streetcar

The appropriate 7th character is to be added to each code from category V26

A	initial encounter
D	subsequent encounter
S	sequela

X● **V26.0** Motorcycle driver injured in collision with other nonmotor vehicle in nontraffic accident ✎

X● **V26.1** Motorcycle passenger injured in collision with other nonmotor vehicle in nontraffic accident ✎

X● **V26.2** Unspecified motorcycle rider injured in collision with other nonmotor vehicle in nontraffic accident ✎

X● **V26.3** Person boarding or alighting a motorcycle injured in collision with other nonmotor vehicle ✎

X● **V26.4** Motorcycle driver injured in collision with other nonmotor vehicle in traffic accident ✎

X● **V26.5** Motorcycle passenger injured in collision with other nonmotor vehicle in traffic accident ✎

X● **V26.9** Unspecified motorcycle rider injured in collision with other nonmotor vehicle in traffic accident ✎

● **V27** Motorcycle rider injured in collision with fixed or stationary object

The appropriate 7th character is to be added to each code from category V27

A	initial encounter
D	subsequent encounter
S	sequela

X● **V27.0** Motorcycle driver injured in collision with fixed or stationary object in nontraffic accident ✎

X● **V27.1** Motorcycle passenger injured in collision with fixed or stationary object in nontraffic accident ✎

X● **V27.2** Unspecified motorcycle rider injured in collision with fixed or stationary object in nontraffic accident ✎

◀ New   ◀ Revised   ~~deleted~~ Deleted   Excludes 1   Excludes 2   Includes   Use additional   Code first   Code also   Unspecified

OGCR Official Guidelines   ● Unacceptable Principal Diagnosis   X Assign placeholder X   ● Use Additional Character(s)   ▶ Manifestation Code   **Coding Clinic**

X ● **V27.3** Person boarding or alighting a motorcycle injured in collision with fixed or stationary object %

X ● **V27.4** Motorcycle driver injured in collision with fixed or stationary object in traffic accident %

X ● **V27.5** Motorcycle passenger injured in collision with fixed or stationary object in traffic accident %

X ● **V27.9** Unspecified motorcycle rider injured in collision with fixed or stationary object in traffic accident %

● **V28** Motorcycle rider injured in noncollision transport accident

> **Includes**   fall or thrown from motorcycle (without antecedent collision)
> overturning motorcycle NOS
> overturning motorcycle without collision

The appropriate 7th character is to be added to each code from category V28

> A   initial encounter
> D   subsequent encounter
> S   sequela

X ● **V28.0** Motorcycle driver injured in noncollision transport accident in nontraffic accident %

X ● **V28.1** Motorcycle passenger injured in noncollision transport accident in nontraffic accident %

X ● **V28.2** Unspecified motorcycle rider injured in noncollision transport accident in nontraffic accident %

X ● **V28.3** Person boarding or alighting a motorcycle injured in noncollision transport accident %

X ● **V28.4** Motorcycle driver injured in noncollision transport accident in traffic accident %

X ● **V28.5** Motorcycle passenger injured in noncollision transport accident in traffic accident %

X ● **V28.9** Unspecified motorcycle rider injured in noncollision transport accident in traffic accident %

● **V29** Motorcycle rider injured in other and unspecified transport accidents

The appropriate 7th character is to be added to each code from category V29

> A   initial encounter
> D   subsequent encounter
> S   sequela

● **V29.0** Motorcycle driver injured in collision with other and unspecified motor vehicles in nontraffic accident

X ● **V29.00** Motorcycle driver injured in collision with unspecified motor vehicles in nontraffic accident %

X ● **V29.09** Motorcycle driver injured in collision with other motor vehicles in nontraffic accident %

● **V29.1** Motorcycle passenger injured in collision with other and unspecified motor vehicles in nontraffic accident

X ● **V29.10** Motorcycle passenger injured in collision with unspecified motor vehicles in nontraffic accident %

X ● **V29.19** Motorcycle passenger injured in collision with other motor vehicles in nontraffic accident %

● **V29.2** Unspecified motorcycle rider injured in collision with other and unspecified motor vehicles in nontraffic accident

X ● **V29.20** Unspecified motorcycle rider injured in collision with unspecified motor vehicles in nontraffic accident %
> Motorcycle collision NOS, nontraffic

X ● **V29.29** Unspecified motorcycle rider injured in collision with other motor vehicles in nontraffic accident %

X ● **V29.3** Motorcycle rider (driver) (passenger) injured in unspecified nontraffic accident %
> Motorcycle accident NOS, nontraffic
> Motorcycle rider injured in nontraffic accident NOS

● **V29.4** Motorcycle driver injured in collision with other and unspecified motor vehicles in traffic accident

X ● **V29.40** Motorcycle driver injured in collision with unspecified motor vehicles in traffic accident %

X ● **V29.49** Motorcycle driver injured in collision with other motor vehicles in traffic accident %

● **V29.5** Motorcycle passenger injured in collision with other and unspecified motor vehicles in traffic accident

X ● **V29.50** Motorcycle passenger injured in collision with unspecified motor vehicles in traffic accident %

X ● **V29.59** Motorcycle passenger injured in collision with other motor vehicles in traffic accident %

● **V29.6** Unspecified motorcycle rider injured in collision with other and unspecified motor vehicles in traffic accident

X ● **V29.60** Unspecified motorcycle rider injured in collision with unspecified motor vehicles in traffic accident %
> Motorcycle collision NOS (traffic)

X ● **V29.69** Unspecified motorcycle rider injured in collision with other motor vehicles in traffic accident %

● **V29.8** Motorcycle rider (driver) (passenger) injured in other specified transport accidents

X ● **V29.81** Motorcycle rider (driver) (passenger) injured in transport accident with military vehicle %

X ● **V29.88** Motorcycle rider (driver) (passenger) injured in other specified transport accidents %

X ● **V29.9** Motorcycle rider (driver) (passenger) injured in unspecified traffic accident %
> Motorcycle accident NOS

OCCUPANT OF THREE-WHEELED MOTOR VEHICLE INJURED IN TRANSPORT ACCIDENT (V30-V39)

> **Includes**   motorized tricycle
> motorized rickshaw
> three-wheeled motor car

> **Excludes1**   all-terrain vehicles (V86.-)
> motorcycle with sidecar (V20-V29)
> vehicle designed primarily for off-road use (V86.-)

● **V30** Occupant of three-wheeled motor vehicle injured in collision with pedestrian or animal

> **Excludes1**   three-wheeled motor vehicle collision with animal-drawn vehicle or animal being ridden (V36.-)

The appropriate 7th character is to be added to each code from category V30

> A   initial encounter
> D   subsequent encounter
> S   sequela

X ● **V30.0** Driver of three-wheeled motor vehicle injured in collision with pedestrian or animal in nontraffic accident %

X ● **V30.1** Passenger in three-wheeled motor vehicle injured in collision with pedestrian or animal in nontraffic accident %

X ● **V30.2** Person on outside of three-wheeled motor vehicle injured in collision with pedestrian or animal in nontraffic accident %

X ● **V30.3** Unspecified occupant of three-wheeled motor vehicle injured in collision with pedestrian or animal in nontraffic accident %

X ● **V30.4** Person boarding or alighting a three-wheeled motor vehicle injured in collision with pedestrian or animal %

X ● **V30.5** Driver of three-wheeled motor vehicle injured in collision with pedestrian or animal in traffic accident %

X ● **V30.6** Passenger in three-wheeled motor vehicle injured in collision with pedestrian or animal in traffic accident %

N Newborn Age: 0   **P** Pediatric Age: 0–17   **M** Maternity DX: 12–55   **A** Adult Age: 15–124   ♀ Females Only   ♂ Males Only

% Complication\Comorbidity   % Major C\C   (Ex) CC/MCC Exclusions   % Present on Admission Requirement   % Hospital-Acquired Condition   1601

CHAPTER 20 (V01-Y99)

X ● **V30.7** Person on outside of three-wheeled motor vehicle injured in collision with pedestrian or animal in traffic accident 🔍

X ● **V30.9** Unspecified occupant of three-wheeled motor vehicle injured in collision with pedestrian or animal in traffic accident 🔍

● **V31** Occupant of three-wheeled motor vehicle injured in collision with pedal cycle

The appropriate 7th character is to be added to each code from category V31

A	initial encounter
D	subsequent encounter
S	sequela

X ● **V31.0** Driver of three-wheeled motor vehicle injured in collision with pedal cycle in nontraffic accident 🔍

X ● **V31.1** Passenger in three-wheeled motor vehicle injured in collision with pedal cycle in nontraffic accident 🔍

X ● **V31.2** Person on outside of three-wheeled motor vehicle injured in collision with pedal cycle in nontraffic accident 🔍

X ● **V31.3** Unspecified occupant of three-wheeled motor vehicle injured in collision with pedal cycle in nontraffic accident 🔍

X ● **V31.4** Person boarding or alighting a three-wheeled motor vehicle injured in collision with pedal cycle 🔍

X ● **V31.5** Driver of three-wheeled motor vehicle injured in collision with pedal cycle in traffic accident 🔍

X ● **V31.6** Passenger in three-wheeled motor vehicle injured in collision with pedal cycle in traffic accident 🔍

X ● **V31.7** Person on outside of three-wheeled motor vehicle injured in collision with pedal cycle in traffic accident 🔍

X ● **V31.9** Unspecified occupant of three-wheeled motor vehicle injured in collision with pedal cycle in traffic accident 🔍

● **V32** Occupant of three-wheeled motor vehicle injured in collision with two- or three-wheeled motor vehicle

The appropriate 7th character is to be added to each code from category V32

A	initial encounter
D	subsequent encounter
S	sequela

X ● **V32.0** Driver of three-wheeled motor vehicle injured in collision with two- or three-wheeled motor vehicle in nontraffic accident 🔍

X ● **V32.1** Passenger in three-wheeled motor vehicle injured in collision with two- or three-wheeled motor vehicle in nontraffic accident 🔍

X ● **V32.2** Person on outside of three-wheeled motor vehicle injured in collision with two- or three-wheeled motor vehicle in nontraffic accident 🔍

X ● **V32.3** Unspecified occupant of three-wheeled motor vehicle injured in collision with two- or three-wheeled motor vehicle in nontraffic accident 🔍

X ● **V32.4** Person boarding or alighting a three-wheeled motor vehicle injured in collision with two- or three-wheeled motor vehicle 🔍

X ● **V32.5** Driver of three-wheeled motor vehicle injured in collision with two- or three-wheeled motor vehicle in traffic accident 🔍

X ● **V32.6** Passenger in three-wheeled motor vehicle injured in collision with two- or three-wheeled motor vehicle in traffic accident 🔍

X ● **V32.7** Person on outside of three-wheeled motor vehicle injured in collision with two- or three-wheeled motor vehicle in traffic accident 🔍

X ● **V32.9** Unspecified occupant of three-wheeled motor vehicle injured in collision with two- or three-wheeled motor vehicle in traffic accident 🔍

● **V33** Occupant of three-wheeled motor vehicle injured in collision with car, pick-up truck or van

The appropriate 7th character is to be added to each code from category V33

A	initial encounter
D	subsequent encounter
S	sequela

X ● **V33.0** Driver of three-wheeled motor vehicle injured in collision with car, pick-up truck or van in nontraffic accident 🔍

X ● **V33.1** Passenger in three-wheeled motor vehicle injured in collision with car, pick-up truck or van in nontraffic accident 🔍

X ● **V33.2** Person on outside of three-wheeled motor vehicle injured in collision with car, pick-up truck or van in nontraffic accident 🔍

X ● **V33.3** Unspecified occupant of three-wheeled motor vehicle injured in collision with car, pick-up truck or van in nontraffic accident 🔍

X ● **V33.4** Person boarding or alighting a three-wheeled motor vehicle injured in collision with car, pick-up truck or van 🔍

X ● **V33.5** Driver of three-wheeled motor vehicle injured in collision with car, pick-up truck or van in traffic accident 🔍

X ● **V33.6** Passenger in three-wheeled motor vehicle injured in collision with car, pick-up truck or van in traffic accident 🔍

X ● **V33.7** Person on outside of three-wheeled motor vehicle injured in collision with car, pick-up truck or van in traffic accident 🔍

X ● **V33.9** Unspecified occupant of three-wheeled motor vehicle injured in collision with car, pick-up truck or van in traffic accident 🔍

● **V34** Occupant of three-wheeled motor vehicle injured in collision with heavy transport vehicle or bus

Excludes1 occupant of three-wheeled motor vehicle injured in collision with military vehicle (V39.81)

The appropriate 7th character is to be added to each code from category V34

A	initial encounter
D	subsequent encounter
S	sequela

X ● **V34.0** Driver of three-wheeled motor vehicle injured in collision with heavy transport vehicle or bus in nontraffic accident 🔍

X ● **V34.1** Passenger in three-wheeled motor vehicle injured in collision with heavy transport vehicle or bus in nontraffic accident 🔍

X ● **V34.2** Person on outside of three-wheeled motor vehicle injured in collision with heavy transport vehicle or bus in nontraffic accident 🔍

X ● **V34.3** Unspecified occupant of three-wheeled motor vehicle injured in collision with heavy transport vehicle or bus in nontraffic accident 🔍

X ● **V34.4** Person boarding or alighting a three-wheeled motor vehicle injured in collision with heavy transport vehicle or bus 🔍

X ● **V34.5** Driver of three-wheeled motor vehicle injured in collision with heavy transport vehicle or bus in traffic accident 🔍

X ● **V34.6** Passenger in three-wheeled motor vehicle injured in collision with heavy transport vehicle or bus in traffic accident 🔍

X ● **V34.7** Person on outside of three-wheeled motor vehicle injured in collision with heavy transport vehicle or bus in traffic accident 🔍

X ● **V34.9** Unspecified occupant of three-wheeled motor vehicle injured in collision with heavy transport vehicle or bus in traffic accident 🔍

◀ New   ◀▥ Revised   ~~deleted~~ Deleted   Excludes 1   Excludes 2   Includes   Use additional   Code first   Code also   Unspecified

OGCR Official Guidelines   ● Unacceptable Principal Diagnosis   X Assign placeholder X   ● Use Additional Character(s)   ▌ Manifestation Code   **Coding Clinic**

● **V35**   **Occupant of three-wheeled motor vehicle injured in collision with railway train or railway vehicle**

The appropriate 7th character is to be added to each code from category V35

A	initial encounter
D	subsequent encounter
S	sequela

X● **V35.0**   Driver of three-wheeled motor vehicle injured in collision with railway train or railway vehicle in nontraffic accident 🔖

X● **V35.1**   Passenger in three-wheeled motor vehicle injured in collision with railway train or railway vehicle in nontraffic accident 🔖

X● **V35.2**   Person on outside of three-wheeled motor vehicle injured in collision with railway train or railway vehicle in nontraffic accident 🔖

X● **V35.3**   Unspecified occupant of three-wheeled motor vehicle injured in collision with railway train or railway vehicle in nontraffic accident 🔖

X● **V35.4**   Person boarding or alighting a three-wheeled motor vehicle injured in collision with railway train or railway vehicle 🔖

X● **V35.5**   Driver of three-wheeled motor vehicle injured in collision with railway train or railway vehicle in traffic accident 🔖

X● **V35.6**   Passenger in three-wheeled motor vehicle injured in collision with railway train or railway vehicle in traffic accident 🔖

X● **V35.7**   Person on outside of three-wheeled motor vehicle injured in collision with railway train or railway vehicle in traffic accident 🔖

X● **V35.9**   Unspecified occupant of three-wheeled motor vehicle injured in collision with railway train or railway vehicle in traffic accident 🔖

● **V36**   **Occupant of three-wheeled motor vehicle injured in collision with other nonmotor vehicle**

> **Includes**   collision with animal-drawn vehicle, animal being ridden, streetcar

The appropriate 7th character is to be added to each code from category V36

A	initial encounter
D	subsequent encounter
S	sequela

X● **V36.0**   Driver of three-wheeled motor vehicle injured in collision with other nonmotor vehicle in nontraffic accident 🔖

X● **V36.1**   Passenger in three-wheeled motor vehicle injured in collision with other nonmotor vehicle in nontraffic accident 🔖

X● **V36.2**   Person on outside of three-wheeled motor vehicle injured in collision with other nonmotor vehicle in nontraffic accident 🔖

X● **V36.3**   Unspecified occupant of three-wheeled motor vehicle injured in collision with other nonmotor vehicle in nontraffic accident 🔖

X● **V36.4**   Person boarding or alighting a three-wheeled motor vehicle injured in collision with other nonmotor vehicle 🔖

X● **V36.5**   Driver of three-wheeled motor vehicle injured in collision with other nonmotor vehicle in traffic accident 🔖

X● **V36.6**   Passenger in three-wheeled motor vehicle injured in collision with other nonmotor vehicle in traffic accident 🔖

X● **V36.7**   Person on outside of three-wheeled motor vehicle injured in collision with other nonmotor vehicle in traffic accident 🔖

X● **V36.9**   Unspecified occupant of three-wheeled motor vehicle injured in collision with other nonmotor vehicle in traffic accident 🔖

● **V37**   **Occupant of three-wheeled motor vehicle injured in collision with fixed or stationary object**

The appropriate 7th character is to be added to each code from category V37

A	initial encounter
D	subsequent encounter
S	sequela

X● **V37.0**   Driver of three-wheeled motor vehicle injured in collision with fixed or stationary object in nontraffic accident 🔖

X● **V37.1**   Passenger in three-wheeled motor vehicle injured in collision with fixed or stationary object in nontraffic accident 🔖

X● **V37.2**   Person on outside of three-wheeled motor vehicle injured in collision with fixed or stationary object in nontraffic accident 🔖

X● **V37.3**   Unspecified occupant of three-wheeled motor vehicle injured in collision with fixed or stationary object in nontraffic accident 🔖

X● **V37.4**   Person boarding or alighting a three-wheeled motor vehicle injured in collision with fixed or stationary object 🔖

X● **V37.5**   Driver of three-wheeled motor vehicle injured in collision with fixed or stationary object in traffic accident 🔖

X● **V37.6**   Passenger in three-wheeled motor vehicle injured in collision with fixed or stationary object in traffic accident 🔖

X● **V37.7**   Person on outside of three-wheeled motor vehicle injured in collision with fixed or stationary object in traffic accident 🔖

X● **V37.9**   Unspecified occupant of three-wheeled motor vehicle injured in collision with fixed or stationary object in traffic accident 🔖

● **V38**   **Occupant of three-wheeled motor vehicle injured in noncollision transport accident**

> **Includes**   fall or thrown from three-wheeled motor vehicle
> overturning of three-wheeled motor vehicle NOS
> overturning of three-wheeled motor vehicle without collision

The appropriate 7th character is to be added to each code from category V38

A	initial encounter
D	subsequent encounter
S	sequela

X● **V38.0**   Driver of three-wheeled motor vehicle injured in noncollision transport accident in nontraffic accident 🔖

X● **V38.1**   Passenger in three-wheeled motor vehicle injured in noncollision transport accident in nontraffic accident 🔖

X● **V38.2**   Person on outside of three-wheeled motor vehicle injured in noncollision transport accident in nontraffic accident 🔖

X● **V38.3**   Unspecified occupant of three-wheeled motor vehicle injured in noncollision transport accident in nontraffic accident 🔖

X● **V38.4**   Person boarding or alighting a three-wheeled motor vehicle injured in noncollision transport accident 🔖

X● **V38.5**   Driver of three-wheeled motor vehicle injured in noncollision transport accident in traffic accident 🔖

X● **V38.6**   Passenger in three-wheeled motor vehicle injured in noncollision transport accident in traffic accident 🔖

X● **V38.7**   Person on outside of three-wheeled motor vehicle injured in noncollision transport accident in traffic accident 🔖

X● **V38.9**   Unspecified occupant of three-wheeled motor vehicle injured in noncollision transport accident in traffic accident 🔖

CHAPTER 20 (V01-Y99)

N Newborn Age: 0   P Pediatric Age: 0–17   M Maternity DX: 12–55   A Adult Age: 15–124   ♀ Females Only   ♂ Males Only

🔖 Complication\Comorbidity   🔖 Major C\C   (Ex) CC/MCC Exclusions   🔖 Present on Admission Requirement   🔖 Hospital-Acquired Condition

1603

- ● **V39** **Occupant of three-wheeled motor vehicle injured in other and unspecified transport accidents**

  The appropriate 7th character is to be added to each code from category V39

A	initial encounter
D	subsequent encounter
S	sequela

  - ● **V39.0** Driver of three-wheeled motor vehicle injured in collision with other and unspecified motor vehicles in nontraffic accident
    - X ● **V39.00** Driver of three-wheeled motor vehicle injured in collision with unspecified motor vehicles in nontraffic accident 🔎
    - X ● **V39.09** Driver of three-wheeled motor vehicle injured in collision with other motor vehicles in nontraffic accident 🔎
  - ● **V39.1** Passenger in three-wheeled motor vehicle injured in collision with other and unspecified motor vehicles in nontraffic accident
    - X ● **V39.10** Passenger in three-wheeled motor vehicle injured in collision with unspecified motor vehicles in nontraffic accident 🔎
    - X ● **V39.19** Passenger in three-wheeled motor vehicle injured in collision with other motor vehicles in nontraffic accident 🔎
  - ● **V39.2** Unspecified occupant of three-wheeled motor vehicle injured in collision with other and unspecified motor vehicles in nontraffic accident
    - X ● **V39.20** Unspecified occupant of three-wheeled motor vehicle injured in collision with unspecified motor vehicles in nontraffic accident 🔎
      Collision NOS involving three-wheeled motor vehicle, nontraffic
    - X ● **V39.29** Unspecified occupant of three-wheeled motor vehicle injured in collision with other motor vehicles in nontraffic accident 🔎
  - X ● **V39.3** Occupant (driver) (passenger) of three-wheeled motor vehicle injured in unspecified nontraffic accident 🔎
    Accident NOS involving three-wheeled motor vehicle, nontraffic
    Occupant of three-wheeled motor vehicle injured in nontraffic accident NOS
  - ● **V39.4** Driver of three-wheeled motor vehicle injured in collision with other and unspecified motor vehicles in traffic accident
    - X ● **V39.40** Driver of three-wheeled motor vehicle injured in collision with unspecified motor vehicles in traffic accident 🔎
    - X ● **V39.49** Driver of three-wheeled motor vehicle injured in collision with other motor vehicles in traffic accident 🔎
  - ● **V39.5** Passenger in three-wheeled motor vehicle injured in collision with other and unspecified motor vehicles in traffic accident
    - X ● **V39.50** Passenger in three-wheeled motor vehicle injured in collision with unspecified motor vehicles in traffic accident 🔎
    - X ● **V39.59** Passenger in three-wheeled motor vehicle injured in collision with other motor vehicles in traffic accident 🔎
  - ● **V39.6** Unspecified occupant of three-wheeled motor vehicle injured in collision with other and unspecified motor vehicles in traffic accident
    - X ● **V39.60** Unspecified occupant of three-wheeled motor vehicle injured in collision with unspecified motor vehicles in traffic accident 🔎
      Collision NOS involving three-wheeled motor vehicle (traffic)
    - X ● **V39.69** Unspecified occupant of three-wheeled motor vehicle injured in collision with other motor vehicles in traffic accident 🔎

- ● **V39.8** Occupant (driver) (passenger) of three-wheeled motor vehicle injured in other specified transport accidents
  - X ● **V39.81** Occupant (driver) (passenger) of three-wheeled motor vehicle injured in transport accident with military vehicle 🔎
  - X ● **V39.89** Occupant (driver) (passenger) of three-wheeled motor vehicle injured in other specified transport accidents 🔎
- X ● **V39.9** Occupant (driver) (passenger) of three-wheeled motor vehicle injured in unspecified traffic accident 🔎
  Accident NOS involving three-wheeled motor vehicle

CAR OCCUPANT INJURED IN TRANSPORT ACCIDENT (V40-V49)

Includes	a four-wheeled motor vehicle designed primarily for carrying passengers
	automobile (pulling a trailer or camper)
Excludes 1	bus (V50-V59)
	minibus (V50-V59)
	minivan (V50-V59)
	motorcoach (V70-V79)
	pick-up truck (V50-V59)
	sport utility vehicle (SUV) (V50-V59)

- ● **V40** **Car occupant injured in collision with pedestrian or animal**

Excludes 1	car collision with animal-drawn vehicle or animal being ridden (V46.-)

  The appropriate 7th character is to be added to each code from category V40

A	initial encounter
D	subsequent encounter
S	sequela

  - X ● **V40.0** Car driver injured in collision with pedestrian or animal in nontraffic accident 🔎
  - X ● **V40.1** Car passenger injured in collision with pedestrian or animal in nontraffic accident 🔎
  - X ● **V40.2** Person on outside of car injured in collision with pedestrian or animal in nontraffic accident 🔎
  - X ● **V40.3** Unspecified car occupant injured in collision with pedestrian or animal in nontraffic accident 🔎
  - X ● **V40.4** Person boarding or alighting a car injured in collision with pedestrian or animal 🔎
  - X ● **V40.5** Car driver injured in collision with pedestrian or animal in traffic accident 🔎
  - X ● **V40.6** Car passenger injured in collision with pedestrian or animal in traffic accident 🔎
  - X ● **V40.7** Person on outside of car injured in collision with pedestrian or animal in traffic accident 🔎
  - X ● **V40.9** Unspecified car occupant injured in collision with pedestrian or animal in traffic accident 🔎

- ● **V41** **Car occupant injured in collision with pedal cycle**

  The appropriate 7th character is to be added to each code from category V41

A	initial encounter
D	subsequent encounter
S	sequela

  - X ● **V41.0** Car driver injured in collision with pedal cycle in nontraffic accident 🔎
  - X ● **V41.1** Car passenger injured in collision with pedal cycle in nontraffic accident 🔎
  - X ● **V41.2** Person on outside of car injured in collision with pedal cycle in nontraffic accident 🔎
  - X ● **V41.3** Unspecified car occupant injured in collision with pedal cycle in nontraffic accident 🔎
  - X ● **V41.4** Person boarding or alighting a car injured in collision with pedal cycle 🔎
  - X ● **V41.5** Car driver injured in collision with pedal cycle in traffic accident 🔎
  - X ● **V41.6** Car passenger injured in collision with pedal cycle in traffic accident 🔎

◀ New   ◀▥ Revised   ~~deleted~~ Deleted   Excludes 1   Excludes 2   Includes   Use additional   Code first   Code also   Unspecified

1604   **OGCR** Official Guidelines   ● Unacceptable Principal Diagnosis   X Assign placeholder X   ● Use Additional Character(s)   ▶ Manifestation Code   **Coding Clinic**

CHAPTER 20 (V01-Y99)

X ● **V41.7**   Person on outside of car injured in collision with pedal cycle in traffic accident 🔍

X ● **V41.9**   Unspecified car occupant injured in collision with pedal cycle in traffic accident 🔍

● **V42**   Car occupant injured in collision with two- or three-wheeled motor vehicle

> The appropriate 7th character is to be added to each code from category V42
>
> | | |
> |---|---|
> | A | initial encounter |
> | D | subsequent encounter |
> | S | sequela |

X ● **V42.0**   Car driver injured in collision with two- or three-wheeled motor vehicle in nontraffic accident 🔍

X ● **V42.1**   Car passenger injured in collision with two- or three-wheeled motor vehicle in nontraffic accident 🔍

X ● **V42.2**   Person on outside of car injured in collision with two- or three-wheeled motor vehicle in nontraffic accident 🔍

X ● **V42.3**   Unspecified car occupant injured in collision with two- or three-wheeled motor vehicle in nontraffic accident 🔍

X ● **V42.4**   Person boarding or alighting a car injured in collision with two- or three-wheeled motor vehicle 🔍

X ● **V42.5**   Car driver injured in collision with two- or three-wheeled motor vehicle in traffic accident 🔍

X ● **V42.6**   Car passenger injured in collision with two- or three-wheeled motor vehicle in traffic accident 🔍

X ● **V42.7**   Person on outside of car injured in collision with two- or three-wheeled motor vehicle in traffic accident 🔍

X ● **V42.9**   Unspecified car occupant injured in collision with two- or three-wheeled motor vehicle in traffic accident 🔍

● **V43**   Car occupant injured in collision with car, pick-up truck or van

> The appropriate 7th character is to be added to each code from category V43
>
> | | |
> |---|---|
> | A | initial encounter |
> | D | subsequent encounter |
> | S | sequela |

● **V43.0**   Car driver injured in collision with car, pick-up truck or van in nontraffic accident

X ● **V43.01**   Car driver injured in collision with sport utility vehicle in nontraffic accident 🔍

X ● **V43.02**   Car driver injured in collision with other type car in nontraffic accident 🔍

X ● **V43.03**   Car driver injured in collision with pick-up truck in nontraffic accident 🔍

X ● **V43.04**   Car driver injured in collision with van in nontraffic accident 🔍

● **V43.1**   Car passenger injured in collision with car, pick-up truck or van in nontraffic accident

X ● **V43.11**   Car passenger injured in collision with sport utility vehicle in nontraffic accident 🔍

X ● **V43.12**   Car passenger injured in collision with other type car in nontraffic accident 🔍

X ● **V43.13**   Car passenger injured in collision with pick-up in nontraffic accident 🔍

X ● **V43.14**   Car passenger injured in collision with van in nontraffic accident 🔍

● **V43.2**   Person on outside of car injured in collision with car, pick-up truck or van in nontraffic accident

X ● **V43.21**   Person on outside of car injured in collision with sport utility vehicle in nontraffic accident 🔍

X ● **V43.22**   Person on outside of car injured in collision with other type car in nontraffic accident 🔍

X ● **V43.23**   Person on outside of car injured in collision with pick-up truck in nontraffic accident 🔍

X ● **V43.24**   Person on outside of car injured in collision with van in nontraffic accident 🔍

● **V43.3**   Unspecified car occupant injured in collision with car, pick-up truck or van in nontraffic accident

X ● **V43.31**   Unspecified car occupant injured in collision with sport utility vehicle in nontraffic accident 🔍

X ● **V43.32**   Unspecified car occupant injured in collision with other type car in nontraffic accident 🔍

X ● **V43.33**   Unspecified car occupant injured in collision with pick-up truck in nontraffic accident 🔍

X ● **V43.34**   Unspecified car occupant injured in collision with van in nontraffic accident 🔍

● **V43.4**   Person boarding or alighting a car injured in collision with car, pick-up truck or van

X ● **V43.41**   Person boarding or alighting a car injured in collision with sport utility vehicle 🔍

X ● **V43.42**   Person boarding or alighting a car injured in collision with other type car 🔍

X ● **V43.43**   Person boarding or alighting a car injured in collision with pick-up truck 🔍

X ● **V43.44**   Person boarding or alighting a car injured in collision with van 🔍

● **V43.5**   Car driver injured in collision with car, pick-up truck or van in traffic accident

X ● **V43.51**   Car driver injured in collision with sport utility vehicle in traffic accident 🔍

X ● **V43.52**   Car driver injured in collision with other type car in traffic accident 🔍

X ● **V43.53**   Car driver injured in collision with pick-up truck in traffic accident 🔍

X ● **V43.54**   Car driver injured in collision with van in traffic accident 🔍

● **V43.6**   Car passenger injured in collision with car, pick-up truck or van in traffic accident

X ● **V43.61**   Car passenger injured in collision with sport utility vehicle in traffic accident 🔍

X ● **V43.62**   Car passenger injured in collision with other type car in traffic accident 🔍

X ● **V43.63**   Car passenger injured in collision with pick-up truck in traffic accident 🔍

X ● **V43.64**   Car passenger injured in collision with van in traffic accident 🔍

● **V43.7**   Person on outside of car injured in collision with car, pick-up truck or van in traffic accident

X ● **V43.71**   Person on outside of car injured in collision with sport utility vehicle in traffic accident 🔍

X ● **V43.72**   Person on outside of car injured in collision with other type car in traffic accident 🔍

X ● **V43.73**   Person on outside of car injured in collision with pick-up truck in traffic accident 🔍

X ● **V43.74**   Person on outside of car injured in collision with van in traffic accident 🔍

● **V43.9**   Unspecified car occupant injured in collision with car, pick-up truck or van in traffic accident

X ● **V43.91**   Unspecified car occupant injured in collision with sport utility vehicle in traffic accident 🔍

X ● **V43.92**   Unspecified car occupant injured in collision with other type car in traffic accident 🔍

X ● **V43.93**   Unspecified car occupant injured in collision with pick-up truck in traffic accident 🔍

X ● **V43.94**   Unspecified car occupant injured in collision with van in traffic accident 🔍

CHAPTER 20 (V01-Y99)

N Newborn Age: 0   **P** Pediatric Age: 0–17   **M** Maternity DX: 12–55   **A** Adult Age: 15–124   ♀ Females Only   ♂ Males Only

🔍 Complication\Comorbidity   🔍 Major C\C   (Ex) CC/MCC Exclusions   🔍 Present on Admission Requirement   🔍 Hospital-Acquired Condition

1605

CHAPTER 20 (V01–Y99)

● V44   Car occupant injured in collision with heavy transport vehicle or bus

> Excludes1   car occupant injured in collision with military vehicle (V49.81)

> The appropriate 7th character is to be added to each code from category V44

> | A | initial encounter |
> |---|---|
> | D | subsequent encounter |
> | S | sequela |

X ● V44.0   Car driver injured in collision with heavy transport vehicle or bus in nontraffic accident 🔍

X ● V44.1   Car passenger injured in collision with heavy transport vehicle or bus in nontraffic accident 🔍

X ● V44.2   Person on outside of car injured in collision with heavy transport vehicle or bus in nontraffic accident 🔍

X ● V44.3   Unspecified car occupant injured in collision with heavy transport vehicle or bus in nontraffic accident 🔍

X ● V44.4   Person boarding or alighting a car injured in collision with heavy transport vehicle or bus 🔍

X ● V44.5   Car driver injured in collision with heavy transport vehicle or bus in traffic accident 🔍

X ● V44.6   Car passenger injured in collision with heavy transport vehicle or bus in traffic accident 🔍

X ● V44.7   Person on outside of car injured in collision with heavy transport vehicle or bus in traffic accident 🔍

X ● V44.9   Unspecified car occupant injured in collision with heavy transport vehicle or bus in traffic accident 🔍

● V45   Car occupant injured in collision with railway train or railway vehicle

> The appropriate 7th character is to be added to each code from category V45

> | A | initial encounter |
> |---|---|
> | D | subsequent encounter |
> | S | sequela |

X ● V45.0   Car driver injured in collision with railway train or railway vehicle in nontraffic accident 🔍

X ● V45.1   Car passenger injured in collision with railway train or railway vehicle in nontraffic accident 🔍

X ● V45.2   Person on outside of car injured in collision with railway train or railway vehicle in nontraffic accident 🔍

X ● V45.3   Unspecified car occupant injured in collision with railway train or railway vehicle in nontraffic accident 🔍

X ● V45.4   Person boarding or alighting a car injured in collision with railway train or railway vehicle 🔍

X ● V45.5   Car driver injured in collision with railway train or railway vehicle in traffic accident 🔍

X ● V45.6   Car passenger injured in collision with railway train or railway vehicle in traffic accident 🔍

X ● V45.7   Person on outside of car injured in collision with railway train or railway vehicle in traffic accident 🔍

X ● V45.9   Unspecified car occupant injured in collision with railway train or railway vehicle in traffic accident 🔍

● V46   Car occupant injured in collision with other nonmotor vehicle

> Includes   collision with animal-drawn vehicle, animal being ridden, streetcar

> The appropriate 7th character is to be added to each code from category V46

> | A | initial encounter |
> |---|---|
> | D | subsequent encounter |
> | S | sequela |

X ● V46.0   Car driver injured in collision with other nonmotor vehicle in nontraffic accident 🔍

X ● V46.1   Car passenger injured in collision with other nonmotor vehicle in nontraffic accident 🔍

X ● V46.2   Person on outside of car injured in collision with other nonmotor vehicle in nontraffic accident 🔍

X ● V46.3   Unspecified car occupant injured in collision with other nonmotor vehicle in nontraffic accident 🔍

X ● V46.4   Person boarding or alighting a car injured in collision with other nonmotor vehicle 🔍

X ● V46.5   Car driver injured in collision with other nonmotor vehicle in traffic accident 🔍

X ● V46.6   Car passenger injured in collision with other nonmotor vehicle in traffic accident 🔍

X ● V46.7   Person on outside of car injured in collision with other nonmotor vehicle in traffic accident 🔍

X ● V46.9   Unspecified car occupant injured in collision with other nonmotor vehicle in traffic accident 🔍

● V47   Car occupant injured in collision with fixed or stationary object

> The appropriate 7th character is to be added to each code from category V47

> | A | initial encounter |
> |---|---|
> | D | subsequent encounter |
> | S | sequela |

● V47.0   Car driver injured in collision with fixed or stationary object in nontraffic accident

X ● V47.01   Driver of sport utility vehicle injured in collision with fixed or stationary object in nontraffic accident 🔍

X ● V47.02   Driver of other type car injured in collision with fixed or stationary object in nontraffic accident 🔍

● V47.1   Car passenger injured in collision with fixed or stationary object in nontraffic accident

X ● V47.11   Passenger of sport utility vehicle injured in collision with fixed or stationary object in nontraffic accident 🔍

X ● V47.12   Passenger of other type car injured in collision with fixed or stationary object in nontraffic accident 🔍

X ● V47.2   Person on outside of car injured in collision with fixed or stationary object in nontraffic accident 🔍

● V47.3   Unspecified car occupant injured in collision with fixed or stationary object in nontraffic accident

X ● V47.31   Unspecified occupant of sport utility vehicle injured in collision with fixed or stationary object in nontraffic accident 🔍

X ● V47.32   Unspecified occupant of other type car injured in collision with fixed or stationary object in nontraffic accident 🔍

X ● V47.4   Person boarding or alighting a car injured in collision with fixed or stationary object 🔍

● V47.5   Car driver injured in collision with fixed or stationary object in traffic accident

X ● V47.51   Driver of sport utility vehicle injured in collision with fixed or stationary object in traffic accident 🔍

X ● V47.52   Driver of other type car injured in collision with fixed or stationary object in traffic accident 🔍

● V47.6   Car passenger injured in collision with fixed or stationary object in traffic accident

X ● V47.61   Passenger of sport utility vehicle injured in collision with fixed or stationary object in traffic accident 🔍

X ● V47.62   Passenger of other type car injured in collision with fixed or stationary object in traffic accident 🔍

X ● V47.7   Person on outside of car injured in collision with fixed or stationary object in traffic accident 🔍

● **V47.9** Unspecified car occupant injured in collision with fixed or stationary object in traffic accident

   X ● **V47.91** Unspecified occupant of sport utility vehicle injured in collision with fixed or stationary object in traffic accident 🔖

   X ● **V47.92** Unspecified occupant of other type car injured in collision with fixed or stationary object in traffic accident 🔖

● **V48** Car occupant injured in noncollision transport accident

   Includes   overturning car NOS
                 overturning car without collision

   The appropriate 7th character is to be added to each code from category V48

> A   initial encounter
> D   subsequent encounter
> S   sequela

X ● **V48.0** Car driver injured in noncollision transport accident in nontraffic accident 🔖

X ● **V48.1** Car passenger injured in noncollision transport accident in nontraffic accident 🔖

X ● **V48.2** Person on outside of car injured in noncollision transport accident in nontraffic accident 🔖

X ● **V48.3** Unspecified car occupant injured in noncollision transport accident in nontraffic accident 🔖

X ● **V48.4** Person boarding or alighting a car injured in noncollision transport accident 🔖

X ● **V48.5** Car driver injured in noncollision transport accident in traffic accident 🔖

X ● **V48.6** Car passenger injured in noncollision transport accident in traffic accident 🔖

X ● **V48.7** Person on outside of car injured in noncollision transport accident in traffic accident 🔖

X ● **V48.9** Unspecified car occupant injured in noncollision transport accident in traffic accident 🔖

● **V49** Car occupant injured in other and unspecified transport accidents

   The appropriate 7th character is to be added to each code from category V49

> A   initial encounter
> D   subsequent encounter
> S   sequela

● **V49.0** Driver injured in collision with other and unspecified motor vehicles in nontraffic accident

   X ● **V49.00** Driver injured in collision with unspecified motor vehicles in nontraffic accident 🔖

   X ● **V49.09** Driver injured in collision with other motor vehicles in nontraffic accident 🔖

● **V49.1** Passenger injured in collision with other and unspecified motor vehicles in nontraffic accident

   X ● **V49.10** Passenger injured in collision with unspecified motor vehicles in nontraffic accident 🔖

   X ● **V49.19** Passenger injured in collision with other motor vehicles in nontraffic accident 🔖

● **V49.2** Unspecified car occupant injured in collision with other and unspecified motor vehicles in nontraffic accident

   X ● **V49.20** Unspecified car occupant injured in collision with unspecified motor vehicles in nontraffic accident 🔖
        Car collision NOS, nontraffic

   X ● **V49.29** Unspecified car occupant injured in collision with other motor vehicles in nontraffic accident 🔖

X ● **V49.3** Car occupant (driver) (passenger) injured in unspecified nontraffic accident 🔖
      Car accident NOS, nontraffic
      Car occupant injured in nontraffic accident NOS

● **V49.4** Driver injured in collision with other and unspecified motor vehicles in traffic accident

   X ● **V49.40** Driver injured in collision with unspecified motor vehicles in traffic accident 🔖

   X ● **V49.49** Driver injured in collision with other motor vehicles in traffic accident 🔖

● **V49.5** Passenger injured in collision with other and unspecified motor vehicles in traffic accident

   X ● **V49.50** Passenger injured in collision with unspecified motor vehicles in traffic accident 🔖

   X ● **V49.59** Passenger injured in collision with other motor vehicles in traffic accident 🔖

● **V49.6** Unspecified car occupant injured in collision with other and unspecified motor vehicles in traffic accident

   X ● **V49.60** Unspecified car occupant injured in collision with unspecified motor vehicles in traffic accident 🔖
        Car collision NOS (traffic)

   X ● **V49.69** Unspecified car occupant injured in collision with other motor vehicles in traffic accident 🔖

● **V49.8** Car occupant (driver) (passenger) injured in other specified transport accidents

   X ● **V49.81** Car occupant (driver) (passenger) injured in transport accident with military vehicle 🔖

   X ● **V49.88** Car occupant (driver) (passenger) injured in other specified transport accidents 🔖

X ● **V49.9** Car occupant (driver) (passenger) injured in unspecified traffic accident 🔖
      Car accident NOS

OCCUPANT OF PICK-UP TRUCK OR VAN INJURED IN TRANSPORT ACCIDENT (V50-V59)

   Includes   a four- or six-wheel motor vehicle designed primarily for carrying passengers and property but weighing less than the local limit for classification as a heavy goods vehicle
               minibus
               minivan
               sport utility vehicle (SUV)
               truck
               van

   Excludes1   heavy transport vehicle (V60-V69)

● **V50** Occupant of pick-up truck or van injured in collision with pedestrian or animal

   Excludes1   pick-up truck or van collision with animal-drawn vehicle or animal being ridden (V56.-)

   The appropriate 7th character is to be added to each code from category V50

> A   initial encounter
> D   subsequent encounter
> S   sequela

X ● **V50.0** Driver of pick-up truck or van injured in collision with pedestrian or animal in nontraffic accident 🔖

X ● **V50.1** Passenger in pick-up truck or van injured in collision with pedestrian or animal in nontraffic accident 🔖

X ● **V50.2** Person on outside of pick-up truck or van injured in collision with pedestrian or animal in nontraffic accident 🔖

X ● **V50.3** Unspecified occupant of pick-up truck or van injured in collision with pedestrian or animal in nontraffic accident 🔖

X ● **V50.4** Person boarding or alighting a pick-up truck or van injured in collision with pedestrian or animal 🔖

X ● **V50.5** Driver of pick-up truck or van injured in collision with pedestrian or animal in traffic accident 🔖

X ● **V50.6** Passenger in pick-up truck or van injured in collision with pedestrian or animal in traffic accident 🔖

N Newborn Age: 0   **P** Pediatric Age: 0–17   **M** Maternity DX: 12–55   **A** Adult Age: 15–124   ♀ Females Only   ♂ Males Only

🔖 Complication\Comorbidity   🔖 Major C\C   (Ex) CC/MCC Exclusions   🔖 Present on Admission Requirement   🔖 Hospital-Acquired Condition

1607

X ● V50.7   Person on outside of pick-up truck or van injured in collision with pedestrian or animal in traffic accident 🔍

X ● V50.9   Unspecified occupant of pick-up truck or van injured in collision with pedestrian or animal in traffic accident 🔍

● V51   Occupant of pick-up truck or van injured in collision with pedal cycle

The appropriate 7th character is to be added to each code from category V51

A	initial encounter
D	subsequent encounter
S	sequela

X ● V51.0   Driver of pick-up truck or van injured in collision with pedal cycle in nontraffic accident 🔍

X ● V51.1   Passenger in pick-up truck or van injured in collision with pedal cycle in nontraffic accident 🔍

X ● V51.2   Person on outside of pick-up truck or van injured in collision with pedal cycle in nontraffic accident 🔍

X ● V51.3   Unspecified occupant of pick-up truck or van injured in collision with pedal cycle in nontraffic accident 🔍

X ● V51.4   Person boarding or alighting a pick-up truck or van injured in collision with pedal cycle 🔍

X ● V51.5   Driver of pick-up truck or van injured in collision with pedal cycle in traffic accident 🔍

X ● V51.6   Passenger in pick-up truck or van injured in collision with pedal cycle in traffic accident 🔍

X ● V51.7   Person on outside of pick-up truck or van injured in collision with pedal cycle in traffic accident 🔍

X ● V51.9   Unspecified occupant of pick-up truck or van injured in collision with pedal cycle in traffic accident 🔍

● V52   Occupant of pick-up truck or van injured in collision with two- or three-wheeled motor vehicle

The appropriate 7th character is to be added to each code from category V52

A	initial encounter
D	subsequent encounter
S	sequela

X ● V52.0   Driver of pick-up truck or van injured in collision with two- or three-wheeled motor vehicle in nontraffic accident 🔍

X ● V52.1   Passenger in pick-up truck or van injured in collision with two- or three-wheeled motor vehicle in nontraffic accident 🔍

X ● V52.2   Person on outside of pick-up truck or van injured in collision with two- or three-wheeled motor vehicle in nontraffic accident 🔍

X ● V52.3   Unspecified occupant of pick-up truck or van injured in collision with two- or three-wheeled motor vehicle in nontraffic accident 🔍

X ● V52.4   Person boarding or alighting a pick-up truck or van injured in collision with two- or three-wheeled motor vehicle 🔍

X ● V52.5   Driver of pick-up truck or van injured in collision with two- or three-wheeled motor vehicle in traffic accident 🔍

X ● V52.6   Passenger in pick-up truck or van injured in collision with two- or three-wheeled motor vehicle in traffic accident 🔍

X ● V52.7   Person on outside of pick-up truck or van injured in collision with two- or three-wheeled motor vehicle in traffic accident 🔍

X ● V52.9   Unspecified occupant of pick-up truck or van injured in collision with two- or three-wheeled motor vehicle in traffic accident 🔍

● V53   Occupant of pick-up truck or van injured in collision with car, pick-up truck or van

The appropriate 7th character is to be added to each code from category V53

A	initial encounter
D	subsequent encounter
S	sequela

X ● V53.0   Driver of pick-up truck or van injured in collision with car, pick-up truck or van in nontraffic accident 🔍

X ● V53.1   Passenger in pick-up truck or van injured in collision with car, pick-up truck or van in nontraffic accident 🔍

X ● V53.2   Person on outside of pick-up truck or van injured in collision with car, pick-up truck or van in nontraffic accident 🔍

X ● V53.3   Unspecified occupant of pick-up truck or van injured in collision with car, pick-up truck or van in nontraffic accident 🔍

X ● V53.4   Person boarding or alighting a pick-up truck or van injured in collision with car, pick-up truck or van 🔍

X ● V53.5   Driver of pick-up truck or van injured in collision with car, pick-up truck or van in traffic accident 🔍

X ● V53.6   Passenger in pick-up truck or van injured in collision with car, pick-up truck or van in traffic accident 🔍

X ● V53.7   Person on outside of pick-up truck or van injured in collision with car, pick-up truck or van in traffic accident 🔍

X ● V53.9   Unspecified occupant of pick-up truck or van injured in collision with car, pick-up truck or van in traffic accident 🔍

● V54   Occupant of pick-up truck or van injured in collision with heavy transport vehicle or bus

Excludes1   occupant of pick-up truck or van injured in collision with military vehicle (V59.81)

The appropriate 7th character is to be added to each code from category V54

A	initial encounter
D	subsequent encounter
S	sequela

X ● V54.0   Driver of pick-up truck or van injured in collision with heavy transport vehicle or bus in nontraffic accident 🔍

X ● V54.1   Passenger in pick-up truck or van injured in collision with heavy transport vehicle or bus in nontraffic accident 🔍

X ● V54.2   Person on outside of pick-up truck or van injured in collision with heavy transport vehicle or bus in nontraffic accident 🔍

X ● V54.3   Unspecified occupant of pick-up truck or van injured in collision with heavy transport vehicle or bus in nontraffic accident 🔍

X ● V54.4   Person boarding or alighting a pick-up truck or van injured in collision with heavy transport vehicle or bus 🔍

X ● V54.5   Driver of pick-up truck or van injured in collision with heavy transport vehicle or bus in traffic accident 🔍

X ● V54.6   Passenger in pick-up truck or van injured in collision with heavy transport vehicle or bus in traffic accident 🔍

X ● V54.7   Person on outside of pick-up truck or van injured in collision with heavy transport vehicle or bus in traffic accident 🔍

X ● V54.9   Unspecified occupant of pick-up truck or van injured in collision with heavy transport vehicle or bus in traffic accident 🔍

● V55 Occupant of pick-up truck or van injured in collision with railway train or railway vehicle

The appropriate 7th character is to be added to each code from category V55

A	initial encounter
D	subsequent encounter
S	sequela

X ● **V55.0** Driver of pick-up truck or van injured in collision with railway train or railway vehicle in nontraffic accident 🕭

X ● **V55.1** Passenger in pick-up truck or van injured in collision with railway train or railway vehicle in nontraffic accident 🕭

X ● **V55.2** Person on outside of pick-up truck or van injured in collision with railway train or railway vehicle in nontraffic accident 🕭

X ● **V55.3** Unspecified occupant of pick-up truck or van injured in collision with railway train or railway vehicle in nontraffic accident 🕭

X ● **V55.4** Person boarding or alighting a pick-up truck or van injured in collision with railway train or railway vehicle 🕭

X ● **V55.5** Driver of pick-up truck or van injured in collision with railway train or railway vehicle in traffic accident 🕭

X ● **V55.6** Passenger in pick-up truck or van injured in collision with railway train or railway vehicle in traffic accident 🕭

X ● **V55.7** Person on outside of pick-up truck or van injured in collision with railway train or railway vehicle in traffic accident 🕭

X ● **V55.9** Unspecified occupant of pick-up truck or van injured in collision with railway train or railway vehicle in traffic accident 🕭

● V56 Occupant of pick-up truck or van injured in collision with other nonmotor vehicle

Includes   collision with animal-drawn vehicle, animal being ridden, streetcar

The appropriate 7th character is to be added to each code from category V56

A	initial encounter
D	subsequent encounter
S	sequela

X ● **V56.0** Driver of pick-up truck or van injured in collision with other nonmotor vehicle in nontraffic accident 🕭

X ● **V56.1** Passenger in pick-up truck or van injured in collision with other nonmotor vehicle in nontraffic accident 🕭

X ● **V56.2** Person on outside of pick-up truck or van injured in collision with other nonmotor vehicle in nontraffic accident 🕭

X ● **V56.3** Unspecified occupant of pick-up truck or van injured in collision with other nonmotor vehicle in nontraffic accident 🕭

X ● **V56.4** Person boarding or alighting a pick-up truck or van injured in collision with other nonmotor vehicle 🕭

X ● **V56.5** Driver of pick-up truck or van injured in collision with other nonmotor vehicle in traffic accident 🕭

X ● **V56.6** Passenger in pick-up truck or van injured in collision with other nonmotor vehicle in traffic accident 🕭

X ● **V56.7** Person on outside of pick-up truck or van injured in collision with other nonmotor vehicle in traffic accident 🕭

X ● **V56.9** Unspecified occupant of pick-up truck or van injured in collision with other nonmotor vehicle in traffic accident 🕭

● V57 Occupant of pick-up truck or van injured in collision with fixed or stationary object

The appropriate 7th character is to be added to each code from category V57

A	initial encounter
D	subsequent encounter
S	sequela

X ● **V57.0** Driver of pick-up truck or van injured in collision with fixed or stationary object in nontraffic accident 🕭

X ● **V57.1** Passenger in pick-up truck or van injured in collision with fixed or stationary object in nontraffic accident 🕭

X ● **V57.2** Person on outside of pick-up truck or van injured in collision with fixed or stationary object in nontraffic accident 🕭

X ● **V57.3** Unspecified occupant of pick-up truck or van injured in collision with fixed or stationary object in nontraffic accident 🕭

X ● **V57.4** Person boarding or alighting a pick-up truck or van injured in collision with fixed or stationary object 🕭

X ● **V57.5** Driver of pick-up truck or van injured in collision with fixed or stationary object in traffic accident 🕭

X ● **V57.6** Passenger in pick-up truck or van injured in collision with fixed or stationary object in traffic accident 🕭

X ● **V57.7** Person on outside of pick-up truck or van injured in collision with fixed or stationary object in traffic accident 🕭

X ● **V57.9** Unspecified occupant of pick-up truck or van injured in collision with fixed or stationary object in traffic accident 🕭

● V58 Occupant of pick-up truck or van injured in noncollision transport accident

Includes   overturning pick-up truck or van NOS
overturning pick-up truck or van without collision

The appropriate 7th character is to be added to each code from category V58

A	initial encounter
D	subsequent encounter
S	sequela

X ● **V58.0** Driver of pick-up truck or van injured in noncollision transport accident in nontraffic accident 🕭

X ● **V58.1** Passenger in pick-up truck or van injured in noncollision transport accident in nontraffic accident 🕭

X ● **V58.2** Person on outside of pick-up truck or van injured in noncollision transport accident in nontraffic accident 🕭

X ● **V58.3** Unspecified occupant of pick-up truck or van injured in noncollision transport accident in nontraffic accident 🕭

X ● **V58.4** Person boarding or alighting a pick-up truck or van injured in noncollision transport accident 🕭

X ● **V58.5** Driver of pick-up truck or van injured in noncollision transport accident in traffic accident 🕭

X ● **V58.6** Passenger in pick-up truck or van injured in noncollision transport accident in traffic accident 🕭

X ● **V58.7** Person on outside of pick-up truck or van injured in noncollision transport accident in traffic accident 🕭

X ● **V58.9** Unspecified occupant of pick-up truck or van injured in noncollision transport accident in traffic accident 🕭

CHAPTER 20 (V01-Y99)

N Newborn Age: 0   **P** Pediatric Age: 0–17   **M** Maternity DX: 12–55   **A** Adult Age: 15–124   ♀ Females Only   ♂ Males Only

🕭 Complication\Comorbidity   🕭 Major C\C   Ⓔⱼ CC/MCC Exclusions   🕭 Present on Admission Requirement   🕭 Hospital-Acquired Condition

1609

● **V59**   **Occupant of pick-up truck or van injured in other and unspecified transport accidents**

The appropriate 7th character is to be added to each code from category V59

> A   initial encounter
> D   subsequent encounter
> S   sequela

● **V59.0**   Driver of pick-up truck or van injured in collision with other and unspecified motor vehicles in nontraffic accident

   X● **V59.00**   Driver of pick-up truck or van injured in collision with unspecified motor vehicles in nontraffic accident

   X● **V59.09**   Driver of pick-up truck or van injured in collision with other motor vehicles in nontraffic accident 🖐

● **V59.1**   Passenger in pick-up truck or van injured in collision with other and unspecified motor vehicles in nontraffic accident

   X● **V59.10**   Passenger in pick-up truck or van injured in collision with unspecified motor vehicles in nontraffic accident 🖐

   X● **V59.19**   Passenger in pick-up truck or van injured in collision with other motor vehicles in nontraffic accident 🖐

● **V59.2**   Unspecified occupant of pick-up truck or van injured in collision with other and unspecified motor vehicles in nontraffic accident

   X● **V59.20**   Unspecified occupant of pick-up truck or van injured in collision with unspecified motor vehicles in nontraffic accident 🖐

> Collision NOS involving pick-up truck or van, nontraffic

   X● **V59.29**   Unspecified occupant of pick-up truck or van injured in collision with other motor vehicles in nontraffic accident 🖐

X● **V59.3**   Occupant (driver) (passenger) of pick-up truck or van injured in unspecified nontraffic accident 🖐

> Accident NOS involving pick-up truck or van, nontraffic
> Occupant of pick-up truck or van injured in nontraffic accident NOS

● **V59.4**   Driver of pick-up truck or van injured in collision with other and unspecified motor vehicles in traffic accident

   X● **V59.40**   Driver of pick-up truck or van injured in collision with unspecified motor vehicles in traffic accident 🖐

   X● **V59.49**   Driver of pick-up truck or van injured in collision with other motor vehicles in traffic accident 🖐

● **V59.5**   Passenger in pick-up truck or van injured in collision with other and unspecified motor vehicles in traffic accident

   X● **V59.50**   Passenger in pick-up truck or van injured in collision with unspecified motor vehicles in traffic accident 🖐

   X● **V59.59**   Passenger in pick-up truck or van injured in collision with other motor vehicles in traffic accident 🖐

● **V59.6**   Unspecified occupant of pick-up truck or van injured in collision with other and unspecified motor vehicles in traffic accident

   X● **V59.60**   Unspecified occupant of pick-up truck or van injured in collision with unspecified motor vehicles in traffic accident 🖐

> Collision NOS involving pick-up truck or van (traffic)

   X● **V59.69**   Unspecified occupant of pick-up truck or van injured in collision with other motor vehicles in traffic accident 🖐

● **V59.8**   Occupant (driver) (passenger) of pick-up truck or van injured in other specified transport accidents

   X● **V59.81**   Occupant (driver) (passenger) of pick-up truck or van injured in transport accident with military vehicle 🖐

   X● **V59.88**   Occupant (driver) (passenger) of pick-up truck or van injured in other specified transport accidents 🖐

X● **V59.9**   Occupant (driver) (passenger) of pick-up truck or van injured in unspecified traffic accident 🖐

> Accident NOS involving pick-up truck or van

OCCUPANT OF HEAVY TRANSPORT VEHICLE INJURED IN TRANSPORT ACCIDENT (V60-V69)

Includes   18 wheeler
              armored car
              panel truck

Excludes1   bus
              motorcoach

● **V60**   Occupant of heavy transport vehicle injured in collision with pedestrian or animal

> **Excludes1**   heavy transport vehicle collision with animal-drawn vehicle or animal being ridden (V66.-)

The appropriate 7th character is to be added to each code from category V60

> A   initial encounter
> D   subsequent encounter
> S   sequela

X● **V60.0**   Driver of heavy transport vehicle injured in collision with pedestrian or animal in nontraffic accident 🖐

X● **V60.1**   Passenger in heavy transport vehicle injured in collision with pedestrian or animal in nontraffic accident 🖐

X● **V60.2**   Person on outside of heavy transport vehicle injured in collision with pedestrian or animal in nontraffic accident 🖐

X● **V60.3**   Unspecified occupant of heavy transport vehicle injured in collision with pedestrian or animal in nontraffic accident 🖐

X● **V60.4**   Person boarding or alighting a heavy transport vehicle injured in collision with pedestrian or animal 🖐

X● **V60.5**   Driver of heavy transport vehicle injured in collision with pedestrian or animal in traffic accident 🖐

X● **V60.6**   Passenger in heavy transport vehicle injured in collision with pedestrian or animal in traffic accident 🖐

X● **V60.7**   Person on outside of heavy transport vehicle injured in collision with pedestrian or animal in traffic accident 🖐

X● **V60.9**   Unspecified occupant of heavy transport vehicle injured in collision with pedestrian or animal in traffic accident 🖐

● **V61**   Occupant of heavy transport vehicle injured in collision with pedal cycle

The appropriate 7th character is to be added to each code from category V61

> A   initial encounter
> D   subsequent encounter
> S   sequela

X● **V61.0**   Driver of heavy transport vehicle injured in collision with pedal cycle in nontraffic accident 🖐

X● **V61.1**   Passenger in heavy transport vehicle injured in collision with pedal cycle in nontraffic accident 🖐

X● **V61.2**   Person on outside of heavy transport vehicle injured in collision with pedal cycle in nontraffic accident 🖐

X● **V61.3**   Unspecified occupant of heavy transport vehicle injured in collision with pedal cycle in nontraffic accident 🖐

◄ New   ◄ Revised   ~~deleted~~ Deleted   Excludes 1   Excludes 2   Includes   Use additional   Code first   Code also   Unspecified

OGCR Official Guidelines   ● Unacceptable Principal Diagnosis   X Assign placeholder X   ● Use Additional Character(s)   ▶ Manifestation Code   **Coding Clinic**

X● **V61.4** Person boarding or alighting a heavy transport vehicle injured in collision with pedal cycle while boarding or alighting ●

X● **V61.5** Driver of heavy transport vehicle injured in collision with pedal cycle in traffic accident ●

X● **V61.6** Passenger in heavy transport vehicle injured in collision with pedal cycle in traffic accident ●

X● **V61.7** Person on outside of heavy transport vehicle injured in collision with pedal cycle in traffic accident ●

X● **V61.9** Unspecified occupant of heavy transport vehicle injured in collision with pedal cycle in traffic accident ●

● **V62** Occupant of heavy transport vehicle injured in collision with two- or three-wheeled motor vehicle

The appropriate 7th character is to be added to each code from category V62

> A   initial encounter
> D   subsequent encounter
> S   sequela

X● **V62.0** Driver of heavy transport vehicle injured in collision with two- or three-wheeled motor vehicle in nontraffic accident ●

X● **V62.1** Passenger in heavy transport vehicle injured in collision with two- or three-wheeled motor vehicle in nontraffic accident ●

X● **V62.2** Person on outside of heavy transport vehicle injured in collision with two- or three-wheeled motor vehicle in nontraffic accident ●

X● **V62.3** Unspecified occupant of heavy transport vehicle injured in collision with two- or three-wheeled motor vehicle in nontraffic accident ●

X● **V62.4** Person boarding or alighting a heavy transport vehicle injured in collision with two- or three-wheeled motor vehicle ●

X● **V62.5** Driver of heavy transport vehicle injured in collision with two- or three-wheeled motor vehicle in traffic accident ●

X● **V62.6** Passenger in heavy transport vehicle injured in collision with two- or three-wheeled motor vehicle in traffic accident ●

X● **V62.7** Person on outside of heavy transport vehicle injured in collision with two- or three-wheeled motor vehicle in traffic accident ●

X● **V62.9** Unspecified occupant of heavy transport vehicle injured in collision with two- or three-wheeled motor vehicle in traffic accident ●

● **V63** Occupant of heavy transport vehicle injured in collision with car, pick-up truck or van

The appropriate 7th character is to be added to each code from category V63

> A   initial encounter
> D   subsequent encounter
> S   sequela

X● **V63.0** Driver of heavy transport vehicle injured in collision with car, pick-up truck or van in nontraffic accident ●

X● **V63.1** Passenger in heavy transport vehicle injured in collision with car, pick-up truck or van in nontraffic accident ●

X● **V63.2** Person on outside of heavy transport vehicle injured in collision with car, pick-up truck or van in nontraffic accident ●

X● **V63.3** Unspecified occupant of heavy transport vehicle injured in collision with car, pick-up truck or van in nontraffic accident ●

X● **V63.4** Person boarding or alighting a heavy transport vehicle injured in collision with car, pick-up truck or van ●

X● **V63.5** Driver of heavy transport vehicle injured in collision with car, pick-up truck or van in traffic accident ●

X● **V63.6** Passenger in heavy transport vehicle injured in collision with car, pick-up truck or van in traffic accident ●

X● **V63.7** Person on outside of heavy transport vehicle injured in collision with car, pick-up truck or van in traffic accident ●

X● **V63.9** Unspecified occupant of heavy transport vehicle injured in collision with car, pick-up truck or van in traffic accident ●

● **V64** Occupant of heavy transport vehicle injured in collision with heavy transport vehicle or bus

> **Excludes1** occupant of heavy transport vehicle injured in collision with military vehicle (V69.81)

The appropriate 7th character is to be added to each code from category V64

> A   initial encounter
> D   subsequent encounter
> S   sequela

X● **V64.0** Driver of heavy transport vehicle injured in collision with heavy transport vehicle or bus in nontraffic accident ●

X● **V64.1** Passenger in heavy transport vehicle injured in collision with heavy transport vehicle or bus in nontraffic accident ●

X● **V64.2** Person on outside of heavy transport vehicle injured in collision with heavy transport vehicle or bus in nontraffic accident ●

X● **V64.3** Unspecified occupant of heavy transport vehicle injured in collision with heavy transport vehicle or bus in nontraffic accident ●

X● **V64.4** Person boarding or alighting a heavy transport vehicle injured in collision with heavy transport vehicle or bus while boarding or alighting ●

X● **V64.5** Driver of heavy transport vehicle injured in collision with heavy transport vehicle or bus in traffic accident ●

X● **V64.6** Passenger in heavy transport vehicle injured in collision with heavy transport vehicle or bus in traffic accident ●

X● **V64.7** Person on outside of heavy transport vehicle injured in collision with heavy transport vehicle or bus in traffic accident ●

X● **V64.9** Unspecified occupant of heavy transport vehicle injured in collision with heavy transport vehicle or bus in traffic accident ●

● **V65** Occupant of heavy transport vehicle injured in collision with railway train or railway vehicle

The appropriate 7th character is to be added to each code from category V65

> A   initial encounter
> D   subsequent encounter
> S   sequela

X● **V65.0** Driver of heavy transport vehicle injured in collision with railway train or railway vehicle in nontraffic accident ●

X● **V65.1** Passenger in heavy transport vehicle injured in collision with railway train or railway vehicle in nontraffic accident ●

X● **V65.2** Person on outside of heavy transport vehicle injured in collision with railway train or railway vehicle in nontraffic accident ●

X● **V65.3** Unspecified occupant of heavy transport vehicle injured in collision with railway train or railway vehicle in nontraffic accident ●

X● **V65.4** Person boarding or alighting a heavy transport vehicle injured in collision with railway train or railway vehicle ●

X● **V65.5** Driver of heavy transport vehicle injured in collision with railway train or railway vehicle in traffic accident ●

CHAPTER 20 (V01-Y99)

X ● **V65.6** Passenger in heavy transport vehicle injured in collision with railway train or railway vehicle in traffic accident 🖉

X ● **V65.7** Person on outside of heavy transport vehicle injured in collision with railway train or railway vehicle in traffic accident 🖉

X ● **V65.9** Unspecified occupant of heavy transport vehicle injured in collision with railway train or railway vehicle in traffic accident 🖉

● **V66** Occupant of heavy transport vehicle injured in collision with other nonmotor vehicle

     Includes   collision with animal-drawn vehicle, animal being ridden, streetcar

     The appropriate 7th character is to be added to each code from category V66

A	initial encounter
D	subsequent encounter
S	sequela

X ● **V66.0** Driver of heavy transport vehicle injured in collision with other nonmotor vehicle in nontraffic accident 🖉

X ● **V66.1** Passenger in heavy transport vehicle injured in collision with other nonmotor vehicle in nontraffic accident 🖉

X ● **V66.2** Person on outside of heavy transport vehicle injured in collision with other nonmotor vehicle in nontraffic accident 🖉

X ● **V66.3** Unspecified occupant of heavy transport vehicle injured in collision with other nonmotor vehicle in nontraffic accident 🖉

X ● **V66.4** Person boarding or alighting a heavy transport vehicle injured in collision with other nonmotor vehicle 🖉

X ● **V66.5** Driver of heavy transport vehicle injured in collision with other nonmotor vehicle in traffic accident 🖉

X ● **V66.6** Passenger in heavy transport vehicle injured in collision with other nonmotor vehicle in traffic accident 🖉

X ● **V66.7** Person on outside of heavy transport vehicle injured in collision with other nonmotor vehicle in traffic accident 🖉

X ● **V66.9** Unspecified occupant of heavy transport vehicle injured in collision with other nonmotor vehicle in traffic accident 🖉

● **V67** Occupant of heavy transport vehicle injured in collision with fixed or stationary object

     The appropriate 7th character is to be added to each code from category V67

A	initial encounter
D	subsequent encounter
S	sequela

X ● **V67.0** Driver of heavy transport vehicle injured in collision with fixed or stationary object in nontraffic accident 🖉

X ● **V67.1** Passenger in heavy transport vehicle injured in collision with fixed or stationary object in nontraffic accident 🖉

X ● **V67.2** Person on outside of heavy transport vehicle injured in collision with fixed or stationary object in nontraffic accident 🖉

X ● **V67.3** Unspecified occupant of heavy transport vehicle injured in collision with fixed or stationary object in nontraffic accident 🖉

X ● **V67.4** Person boarding or alighting a heavy transport vehicle injured in collision with fixed or stationary object 🖉

X ● **V67.5** Driver of heavy transport vehicle injured in collision with fixed or stationary object in traffic accident 🖉

X ● **V67.6** Passenger in heavy transport vehicle injured in collision with fixed or stationary object in traffic accident 🖉

X ● **V67.7** Person on outside of heavy transport vehicle injured in collision with fixed or stationary object in traffic accident 🖉

X ● **V67.9** Unspecified occupant of heavy transport vehicle injured in collision with fixed or stationary object in traffic accident 🖉

● **V68** Occupant of heavy transport vehicle injured in noncollision transport accident

     Includes   overturning heavy transport vehicle NOS
                    overturning heavy transport vehicle without collision

     The appropriate 7th character is to be added to each code from category V68

A	initial encounter
D	subsequent encounter
S	sequela

X ● **V68.0** Driver of heavy transport vehicle injured in noncollision transport accident in nontraffic accident 🖉

X ● **V68.1** Passenger in heavy transport vehicle injured in noncollision transport accident in nontraffic accident 🖉

X ● **V68.2** Person on outside of heavy transport vehicle injured in noncollision transport accident in nontraffic accident 🖉

X ● **V68.3** Unspecified occupant of heavy transport vehicle injured in noncollision transport accident in nontraffic accident 🖉

X ● **V68.4** Person boarding or alighting a heavy transport vehicle injured in noncollision transport accident 🖉

X ● **V68.5** Driver of heavy transport vehicle injured in noncollision transport accident in traffic accident 🖉

X ● **V68.6** Passenger in heavy transport vehicle injured in noncollision transport accident in traffic accident 🖉

X ● **V68.7** Person on outside of heavy transport vehicle injured in noncollision transport accident in traffic accident 🖉

X ● **V68.9** Unspecified occupant of heavy transport vehicle injured in noncollision transport accident in traffic accident 🖉

● **V69** Occupant of heavy transport vehicle injured in other and unspecified transport accidents

     The appropriate 7th character is to be added to each code from category V69

A	initial encounter
D	subsequent encounter
S	sequela

● **V69.0** Driver of heavy transport vehicle injured in collision with other and unspecified motor vehicles in nontraffic accident

   X ● **V69.00** Driver of heavy transport vehicle injured in collision with unspecified motor vehicles in nontraffic accident 🖉

   X ● **V69.09** Driver of heavy transport vehicle injured in collision with other motor vehicles in nontraffic accident 🖉

● **V69.1** Passenger in heavy transport vehicle injured in collision with other and unspecified motor vehicles in nontraffic accident

   X ● **V69.10** Passenger in heavy transport vehicle injured in collision with unspecified motor vehicles in nontraffic accident 🖉

   X ● **V69.19** Passenger in heavy transport vehicle injured in collision with other motor vehicles in nontraffic accident 🖉

● **V69.2** Unspecified occupant of heavy transport vehicle injured in collision with other and unspecified motor vehicles in nontraffic accident

   X ● **V69.20** Unspecified occupant of heavy transport vehicle injured in collision with unspecified motor vehicles in nontraffic accident 🖉

       Collision NOS involving heavy transport vehicle, nontraffic

   X ● **V69.29** Unspecified occupant of heavy transport vehicle injured in collision with other motor vehicles in nontraffic accident 🖉

◄ New   ◀ Revised   ~~deleted~~ Deleted   Excludes 1   Excludes 2   Includes   Use additional   Code first   Code also   Unspecified

OGCR Official Guidelines   ● Unacceptable Principal Diagnosis   X Assign placeholder X   ● Use Additional Character(s)   ▶ Manifestation Code   **Coding Clinic**

X● **V69.3** Occupant (driver) (passenger) of heavy transport vehicle injured in unspecified nontraffic accident 🅗
     Accident NOS involving heavy transport vehicle, nontraffic
     Occupant of heavy transport vehicle injured in nontraffic accident NOS ◄▥

● **V69.4** Driver of heavy transport vehicle injured in collision with other and unspecified motor vehicles in traffic accident

     X● **V69.40** Driver of heavy transport vehicle injured in collision with unspecified motor vehicles in traffic accident 🅗

     X● **V69.49** Driver of heavy transport vehicle injured in collision with other motor vehicles in traffic accident 🅗

● **V69.5** Passenger in heavy transport vehicle injured in collision with other and unspecified motor vehicles in traffic accident

     X● **V69.50** Passenger in heavy transport vehicle injured in collision with unspecified motor vehicles in traffic accident 🅗

     X● **V69.59** Passenger in heavy transport vehicle injured in collision with other motor vehicles in traffic accident 🅗

● **V69.6** Unspecified occupant of heavy transport vehicle injured in collision with other and unspecified motor vehicles in traffic accident

     X● **V69.60** Unspecified occupant of heavy transport vehicle injured in collision with unspecified motor vehicles in traffic accident 🅗
         Collision NOS involving heavy transport vehicle (traffic)

     X● **V69.69** Unspecified occupant of heavy transport vehicle injured in collision with other motor vehicles in traffic accident 🅗

● **V69.8** Occupant (driver) (passenger) of heavy transport vehicle injured in other specified transport accidents

     X● **V69.81** Occupant (driver) (passenger) of heavy transport vehicle injured in transport accidents with military vehicle 🅗

     X● **V69.88** Occupant (driver) (passenger) of heavy transport vehicle injured in other specified transport accidents 🅗

X● **V69.9** Occupant (driver) (passenger) of heavy transport vehicle injured in unspecified traffic accident 🅗
     Accident NOS involving heavy transport vehicle

BUS OCCUPANT INJURED IN TRANSPORT ACCIDENT (V70-V79)

Includes   motorcoach
Excludes1   minibus (V50-V59)

● **V70** Bus occupant injured in collision with pedestrian or animal

     Excludes1   bus collision with animal-drawn vehicle or animal being ridden (V76.-)

The appropriate 7th character is to be added to each code from category V70

A	initial encounter
D	subsequent encounter
S	sequela

X● **V70.0** Driver of bus injured in collision with pedestrian or animal in nontraffic accident 🅗

X● **V70.1** Passenger on bus injured in collision with pedestrian or animal in nontraffic accident 🅗

X● **V70.2** Person on outside of bus injured in collision with pedestrian or animal in nontraffic accident 🅗

X● **V70.3** Unspecified occupant of bus injured in collision with pedestrian or animal in nontraffic accident 🅗

X● **V70.4** Person boarding or alighting from bus injured in collision with pedestrian or animal 🅗

X● **V70.5** Driver of bus injured in collision with pedestrian or animal in traffic accident 🅗

X● **V70.6** Passenger on bus injured in collision with pedestrian or animal in traffic accident 🅗

X● **V70.7** Person on outside of bus injured in collision with pedestrian or animal in traffic accident 🅗

X● **V70.9** Unspecified occupant of bus injured in collision with pedestrian or animal in traffic accident 🅗

● **V71** Bus occupant injured in collision with pedal cycle

The appropriate 7th character is to be added to each code from category V71

A	initial encounter
D	subsequent encounter
S	sequela

X● **V71.0** Driver of bus injured in collision with pedal cycle in nontraffic accident 🅗

X● **V71.1** Passenger on bus injured in collision with pedal cycle in nontraffic accident 🅗

X● **V71.2** Person on outside of bus injured in collision with pedal cycle in nontraffic accident 🅗

X● **V71.3** Unspecified occupant of bus injured in collision with pedal cycle in nontraffic accident 🅗

X● **V71.4** Person boarding or alighting from bus injured in collision with pedal cycle 🅗

X● **V71.5** Driver of bus injured in collision with pedal cycle in traffic accident 🅗

X● **V71.6** Passenger on bus injured in collision with pedal cycle in traffic accident 🅗

X● **V71.7** Person on outside of bus injured in collision with pedal cycle in traffic accident 🅗

X● **V71.9** Unspecified occupant of bus injured in collision with pedal cycle in traffic accident 🅗

● **V72** Bus occupant injured in collision with two- or three-wheeled motor vehicle

The appropriate 7th character is to be added to each code from category V72

A	initial encounter
D	subsequent encounter
S	sequela

X● **V72.0** Driver of bus injured in collision with two- or three-wheeled motor vehicle in nontraffic accident 🅗

X● **V72.1** Passenger on bus injured in collision with two- or three-wheeled motor vehicle in nontraffic accident 🅗

X● **V72.2** Person on outside of bus injured in collision with two- or three-wheeled motor vehicle in nontraffic accident 🅗

X● **V72.3** Unspecified occupant of bus injured in collision with two- or three-wheeled motor vehicle in nontraffic accident 🅗

X● **V72.4** Person boarding or alighting from bus injured in collision with two- or three-wheeled motor vehicle 🅗

X● **V72.5** Driver of bus injured in collision with two- or three-wheeled motor vehicle in traffic accident 🅗

X● **V72.6** Passenger on bus injured in collision with two- or three-wheeled motor vehicle in traffic accident 🅗

X● **V72.7** Person on outside of bus injured in collision with two- or three-wheeled motor vehicle in traffic accident 🅗

X● **V72.9** Unspecified occupant of bus injured in collision with two- or three-wheeled motor vehicle in traffic accident 🅗

N Newborn Age: 0   **P** Pediatric Age: 0–17   **M** Maternity DX: 12–55   **A** Adult Age: 15–124   ♀ Females Only   ♂ Males Only

🅗 Complication\Comorbidity   🅗 Major C\C   (Ex) CC/MCC Exclusions   🅗 Present on Admission Requirement   🅗 Hospital-Acquired Condition

1613

● V73   Bus occupant injured in collision with car, pick-up truck or van

The appropriate 7th character is to be added to each code from category V73

> A   initial encounter
> D   subsequent encounter
> S   sequela

X ● V73.0   Driver of bus injured in collision with car, pick-up truck or van in nontraffic accident 🖐

X ● V73.1   Passenger on bus injured in collision with car, pick-up truck or van in nontraffic accident 🖐

X ● V73.2   Person on outside of bus injured in collision with car, pick-up truck or van in nontraffic accident 🖐

X ● V73.3   Unspecified occupant of bus injured in collision with car, pick-up truck or van in nontraffic accident 🖐

X ● V73.4   Person boarding or alighting from bus injured in collision with car, pick-up truck or van 🖐

X ● V73.5   Driver of bus injured in collision with car, pick-up truck or van in traffic accident 🖐

X ● V73.6   Passenger on bus injured in collision with car, pick-up truck or van in traffic accident 🖐

X ● V73.7   Person on outside of bus injured in collision with car, pick-up truck or van in traffic accident 🖐

X ● V73.9   Unspecified occupant of bus injured in collision with car, pick-up truck or van in traffic accident 🖐

● V74   Bus occupant injured in collision with heavy transport vehicle or bus

> Excludes1   bus occupant injured in collision with military vehicle (V79.81)

The appropriate 7th character is to be added to each code from category V74

> A   initial encounter
> D   subsequent encounter
> S   sequela

X ● V74.0   Driver of bus injured in collision with heavy transport vehicle or bus in nontraffic accident 🖐

X ● V74.1   Passenger on bus injured in collision with heavy transport vehicle or bus in nontraffic accident 🖐

X ● V74.2   Person on outside of bus injured in collision with heavy transport vehicle or bus in nontraffic accident 🖐

X ● V74.3   Unspecified occupant of bus injured in collision with heavy transport vehicle or bus in nontraffic accident 🖐

X ● V74.4   Person boarding or alighting from bus injured in collision with heavy transport vehicle or bus 🖐

X ● V74.5   Driver of bus injured in collision with heavy transport vehicle or bus in traffic accident 🖐

X ● V74.6   Passenger on bus injured in collision with heavy transport vehicle or bus in traffic accident 🖐

X ● V74.7   Person on outside of bus injured in collision with heavy transport vehicle or bus in traffic accident 🖐

X ● V74.9   Unspecified occupant of bus injured in collision with heavy transport vehicle or bus in traffic accident 🖐

● V75   Bus occupant injured in collision with railway train or railway vehicle

The appropriate 7th character is to be added to each code from category V75

> A   initial encounter
> D   subsequent encounter
> S   sequela

X ● V75.0   Driver of bus injured in collision with railway train or railway vehicle in nontraffic accident 🖐

X ● V75.1   Passenger on bus injured in collision with railway train or railway vehicle in nontraffic accident 🖐

X ● V75.2   Person on outside of bus injured in collision with railway train or railway vehicle in nontraffic accident 🖐

X ● V75.3   Unspecified occupant of bus injured in collision with railway train or railway vehicle in nontraffic accident 🖐

X ● V75.4   Person boarding or alighting from bus injured in collision with railway train or railway vehicle 🖐

X ● V75.5   Driver of bus injured in collision with railway train or railway vehicle in traffic accident 🖐

X ● V75.6   Passenger on bus injured in collision with railway train or railway vehicle in traffic accident 🖐

X ● V75.7   Person on outside of bus injured in collision with railway train or railway vehicle in traffic accident 🖐

X ● V75.9   Unspecified occupant of bus injured in collision with railway train or railway vehicle in traffic accident 🖐

● V76   Bus occupant injured in collision with other nonmotor vehicle

> Includes   collision with animal-drawn vehicle, animal being ridden, streetcar

The appropriate 7th character is to be added to each code from category V76

> A   initial encounter
> D   subsequent encounter
> S   sequela

X ● V76.0   Driver of bus injured in collision with other nonmotor vehicle in nontraffic accident 🖐

X ● V76.1   Passenger on bus injured in collision with other nonmotor vehicle in nontraffic accident 🖐

X ● V76.2   Person on outside of bus injured in collision with other nonmotor vehicle in nontraffic accident 🖐

X ● V76.3   Unspecified occupant of bus injured in collision with other nonmotor vehicle in nontraffic accident 🖐

X ● V76.4   Person boarding or alighting from bus injured in collision with other nonmotor vehicle 🖐

X ● V76.5   Driver of bus injured in collision with other nonmotor vehicle in traffic accident 🖐

X ● V76.6   Passenger on bus injured in collision with other nonmotor vehicle in traffic accident 🖐

X ● V76.7   Person on outside of bus injured in collision with other nonmotor vehicle in traffic accident 🖐

X ● V76.9   Unspecified occupant of bus injured in collision with other nonmotor vehicle in traffic accident 🖐

● V77   Bus occupant injured in collision with fixed or stationary object

The appropriate 7th character is to be added to each code from category V77

> A   initial encounter
> D   subsequent encounter
> S   sequela

X ● V77.0   Driver of bus injured in collision with fixed or stationary object in nontraffic accident 🖐

X ● V77.1   Passenger on bus injured in collision with fixed or stationary object in nontraffic accident 🖐

X ● V77.2   Person on outside of bus injured in collision with fixed or stationary object in nontraffic accident 🖐

X ● V77.3   Unspecified occupant of bus injured in collision with fixed or stationary object in nontraffic accident 🖐

X ● V77.4   Person boarding or alighting from bus injured in collision with fixed or stationary object 🖐

X ● V77.5   Driver of bus injured in collision with fixed or stationary object in traffic accident 🖐

X ● V77.6   Passenger on bus injured in collision with fixed or stationary object in traffic accident 🖐

X ● V77.7   Person on outside of bus injured in collision with fixed or stationary object in traffic accident 🖐

X ● V77.9   Unspecified occupant of bus injured in collision with fixed or stationary object in traffic accident 🖐

◄ New   ◄▪▪ Revised   ~~deleted~~ Deleted   Excludes 1   Excludes 2   Includes   Use additional   Code first   Code also   Unspecified

OGCR Official Guidelines   ● Unacceptable Principal Diagnosis   X Assign placeholder X   ● Use Additional Character(s)   ▌ Manifestation Code   **Coding Clinic**

CHAPTER 20 (V01-Y99)

● **V78   Bus occupant injured in noncollision transport accident**

     Includes   overturning bus NOS
                    overturning bus without collision

     The appropriate 7th character is to be added to each code from category V78

A	initial encounter
D	subsequent encounter
S	sequela

X● **V78.0**   Driver of bus injured in noncollision transport accident in nontraffic accident 🔖

X● **V78.1**   Passenger on bus injured in noncollision transport accident in nontraffic accident 🔖

X● **V78.2**   Person on outside of bus injured in noncollision transport accident in nontraffic accident 🔖

X● **V78.3**   Unspecified occupant of bus injured in noncollision transport accident in nontraffic accident 🔖

X● **V78.4**   Person boarding or alighting from bus injured in noncollision transport accident 🔖

X● **V78.5**   Driver of bus injured in noncollision transport accident in traffic accident 🔖

X● **V78.6**   Passenger on bus injured in noncollision transport accident in traffic accident 🔖

X● **V78.7**   Person on outside of bus injured in noncollision transport accident in traffic accident 🔖

X● **V78.9**   Unspecified occupant of bus injured in noncollision transport accident in traffic accident 🔖

● **V79   Bus occupant injured in other and unspecified transport accidents**

     The appropriate 7th character is to be added to each code from category V79

A	initial encounter
D	subsequent encounter
S	sequela

● **V79.0**   Driver of bus injured in collision with other and unspecified motor vehicles in nontraffic accident

     X● **V79.00**   Driver of bus injured in collision with unspecified motor vehicles in nontraffic accident 🔖

     X● **V79.09**   Driver of bus injured in collision with other motor vehicles in nontraffic accident 🔖

● **V79.1**   Passenger on bus injured in collision with other and unspecified motor vehicles in nontraffic accident

     X● **V79.10**   Passenger on bus injured in collision with unspecified motor vehicles in nontraffic accident 🔖

     X● **V79.19**   Passenger on bus injured in collision with other motor vehicles in nontraffic accident 🔖

● **V79.2**   Unspecified bus occupant injured in collision with other and unspecified motor vehicles in nontraffic accident

     X● **V79.20**   Unspecified bus occupant injured in collision with unspecified motor vehicles in nontraffic accident 🔖
           Bus collision NOS, nontraffic

     X● **V79.29**   Unspecified bus occupant injured in collision with other motor vehicles in nontraffic accident 🔖

X● **V79.3**   Bus occupant (driver) (passenger) injured in unspecified nontraffic accident 🔖
       Bus accident NOS, nontraffic
       Bus occupant injured in nontraffic accident NOS

● **V79.4**   Driver of bus injured in collision with other and unspecified motor vehicles in traffic accident

     X● **V79.40**   Driver of bus injured in collision with unspecified motor vehicles in traffic accident 🔖

     X● **V79.49**   Driver of bus injured in collision with other motor vehicles in traffic accident 🔖

● **V79.5**   Passenger on bus injured in collision with other and unspecified motor vehicles in traffic accident

     X● **V79.50**   Passenger on bus injured in collision with unspecified motor vehicles in traffic accident 🔖

     X● **V79.59**   Passenger on bus injured in collision with other motor vehicles in traffic accident 🔖

● **V79.6**   Unspecified bus occupant injured in collision with other and unspecified motor vehicles in traffic accident

     X● **V79.60**   Unspecified bus occupant injured in collision with unspecified motor vehicles in traffic accident 🔖
           Bus collision NOS (traffic)

     X● **V79.69**   Unspecified bus occupant injured in collision with other motor vehicles in traffic accident 🔖

● **V79.8**   Bus occupant (driver) (passenger) injured in other specified transport accidents

     X● **V79.81**   Bus occupant (driver) (passenger) injured in transport accidents with military vehicle 🔖

     X● **V79.88**   Bus occupant (driver) (passenger) injured in other specified transport accidents 🔖

X● **V79.9**   Bus occupant (driver) (passenger) injured in unspecified traffic accident 🔖
       Bus accident NOS

OTHER LAND TRANSPORT ACCIDENTS (V80-V89)

● **V80   Animal-rider or occupant of animal-drawn vehicle injured in transport accident**

     The appropriate 7th character is to be added to each code from category V80

A	initial encounter
D	subsequent encounter
S	sequela

● **V80.0**   Animal-rider or occupant of animal drawn vehicle injured by fall from or being thrown from animal or animal-drawn vehicle in noncollision accident

     ● **V80.01**   Animal-rider injured by fall from or being thrown from animal in noncollision accident

         ● **V80.010**   Animal-rider injured by fall from or being thrown from horse in noncollision accident 🔖

         ● **V80.018**   Animal-rider injured by fall from or being thrown from other animal in noncollision accident 🔖

     X● **V80.02**   Occupant of animal-drawn vehicle injured by fall from or being thrown from animal-drawn vehicle in noncollision accident 🔖
           Overturning animal-drawn vehicle NOS
           Overturning animal-drawn vehicle without collision

● **V80.1**   Animal-rider or occupant of animal-drawn vehicle injured in collision with pedestrian or animal

     Excludes1   animal-rider or animal-drawn vehicle collision with animal-drawn vehicle or animal being ridden (V80.7)

     X● **V80.11**   Animal-rider injured in collision with pedestrian or animal 🔖

     X● **V80.12**   Occupant of animal-drawn vehicle injured in collision with pedestrian or animal 🔖

● **V80.2**   Animal-rider or occupant of animal-drawn vehicle injured in collision with pedal cycle

     X● **V80.21**   Animal-rider injured in collision with pedal cycle 🔖

     X● **V80.22**   Occupant of animal-drawn vehicle injured in collision with pedal cycle 🔖

N Newborn Age: 0   P Pediatric Age: 0–17   M Maternity DX: 12–55   A Adult Age: 15–124   ♀ Females Only   ♂ Males Only

🔖 Complication\Comorbidity   🔖 Major C\C   (Ex) CC/MCC Exclusions   🔖 Present on Admission Requirement   🔖 Hospital-Acquired Condition

1615

CHAPTER 20 (V01-Y99)

● **V80.3** Animal-rider or occupant of animal-drawn vehicle injured in collision with two- or three-wheeled motor vehicle

  X● **V80.31** Animal-rider injured in collision with two- or three-wheeled motor vehicle ✎

  X● **V80.32** Occupant of animal-drawn vehicle injured in collision with two- or three-wheeled motor vehicle ✎

● **V80.4** Animal-rider or occupant of animal-drawn vehicle injured in collision with car, pick-up truck, van, heavy transport vehicle or bus

    Excludes1   animal-rider injured in collision with military vehicle (V80.910)

               occupant of animal-drawn vehicle injured in collision with military vehicle (V80.920)

  X● **V80.41** Animal-rider injured in collision with car, pick-up truck, van, heavy transport vehicle or bus ✎

  X● **V80.42** Occupant of animal-drawn vehicle injured in collision with car, pick-up truck, van, heavy transport vehicle or bus ✎

● **V80.5** Animal-rider or occupant of animal-drawn vehicle injured in collision with other specified motor vehicle

  X● **V80.51** Animal-rider injured in collision with other specified motor vehicle ✎

  X● **V80.52** Occupant of animal-drawn vehicle injured in collision with other specified motor vehicle ✎

● **V80.6** Animal-rider or occupant of animal-drawn vehicle injured in collision with railway train or railway vehicle

  X● **V80.61** Animal-rider injured in collision with railway train or railway vehicle ✎

  X● **V80.62** Occupant of animal-drawn vehicle injured in collision with railway train or railway vehicle ✎

● **V80.7** Animal-rider or occupant of animal-drawn vehicle injured in collision with other nonmotor vehicles

  ● **V80.71** Animal-rider or occupant of animal-drawn vehicle injured in collision with animal being ridden

    ● **V80.710** Animal-rider injured in collision with other animal being ridden ✎

    ● **V80.711** Occupant of animal-drawn vehicle injured in collision with animal being ridden ✎

  ● **V80.72** Animal-rider or occupant of animal-drawn vehicle injured in collision with other animal-drawn vehicle

    ● **V80.720** Animal-rider injured in collision with animal-drawn vehicle ✎

    ● **V80.721** Occupant of animal-drawn vehicle injured in collision with other animal-drawn vehicle ✎

  ● **V80.73** Animal-rider or occupant of animal-drawn vehicle injured in collision with streetcar

    ● **V80.730** Animal-rider injured in collision with streetcar ✎

    ● **V80.731** Occupant of animal-drawn vehicle injured in collision with streetcar ✎

  ● **V80.79** Animal-rider or occupant of animal-drawn vehicle injured in collision with other nonmotor vehicles

    ● **V80.790** Animal-rider injured in collision with other nonmotor vehicles ✎

    ● **V80.791** Occupant of animal-drawn vehicle injured in collision with other nonmotor vehicles ✎

● **V80.8** Animal-rider or occupant of animal-drawn vehicle injured in collision with fixed or stationary object

  X● **V80.81** Animal-rider injured in collision with fixed or stationary object ✎

  X● **V80.82** Occupant of animal-drawn vehicle injured in collision with fixed or stationary object ✎

● **V80.9** Animal-rider or occupant of animal-drawn vehicle injured in other and unspecified transport accidents

  ● **V80.91** Animal-rider injured in other and unspecified transport accidents

    ● **V80.910** Animal-rider injured in transport accident with military vehicle ✎

    ● **V80.918** Animal-rider injured in other transport accident ✎

    ● **V80.919** Animal-rider injured in unspecified transport accident ✎

         Animal rider accident NOS

  ● **V80.92** Occupant of animal-drawn vehicle injured in other and unspecified transport accidents

    ● **V80.920** Occupant of animal-drawn vehicle injured in transport accident with military vehicle ✎

    ● **V80.928** Occupant of animal-drawn vehicle injured in other transport accident ✎

    ● **V80.929** Occupant of animal-drawn vehicle injured in unspecified transport accident ✎

         Animal-drawn vehicle accident NOS

● **V81** Occupant of railway train or railway vehicle injured in transport accident

    Includes   derailment of railway train or railway vehicle

               person on outside of train

    Excludes1   streetcar (V82.-)

     The appropriate 7th character is to be added to each code from category V81

       A   initial encounter

       D   subsequent encounter

       S   sequela

  X● **V81.0** Occupant of railway train or railway vehicle injured in collision with motor vehicle in nontraffic accident ✎

    Excludes1   occupant of railway train or railway vehicle injured due to collision with military vehicle (V81.83)

  X● **V81.1** Occupant of railway train or railway vehicle injured in collision with motor vehicle in traffic accident ✎

    Excludes1   occupant of railway train or railway vehicle injured due to collision with military vehicle (V81.83)

  X● **V81.2** Occupant of railway train or railway vehicle injured in collision with or hit by rolling stock ✎

  X● **V81.3** Occupant of railway train or railway vehicle injured in collision with other object ✎

       Railway collision NOS

  X● **V81.4** Person injured while boarding or alighting from railway train or railway vehicle ✎

  X● **V81.5** Occupant of railway train or railway vehicle injured by fall in railway train or railway vehicle ✎

  X● **V81.6** Occupant of railway train or railway vehicle injured by fall from railway train or railway vehicle ✎

  X● **V81.7** Occupant of railway train or railway vehicle injured in derailment without antecedent collision ✎

◀ New   ⬅ Revised   ~~deleted~~ Deleted   Excludes 1   Excludes 2   Includes   Use additional   Code first   Code also   Unspecified

OGCR Official Guidelines   ● Unacceptable Principal Diagnosis   X Assign placeholder X   ● Use Additional Character(s)   ▶ Manifestation Code   **Coding Clinic**

● **V81.8** **Occupant of railway train or railway vehicle injured in other specified railway accidents**
- X● **V81.81** **Occupant of railway train or railway vehicle injured due to explosion or fire on train** 🔊
- X● **V81.82** **Occupant of railway train or railway vehicle injured due to object falling onto train** 🔊
  - Occupant of railway train or railway vehicle injured due to falling earth onto train
  - Occupant of railway train or railway vehicle injured due to falling rocks onto train
  - Occupant of railway train or railway vehicle injured due to falling snow onto train
  - Occupant of railway train or railway vehicle injured due to falling trees onto train
- X● **V81.83** **Occupant of railway train or railway vehicle injured due to collision with military vehicle** 🔊
- X● **V81.89** **Occupant of railway train or railway vehicle injured due to other specified railway accident** 🔊

X● **V81.9** **Occupant of railway train or railway vehicle injured in** unspecified **railway accident** 🔊
- Railway accident NOS

● **V82** **Occupant of powered streetcar injured in transport accident**

Includes	interurban electric car
	person on outside of streetcar
	tram (car)
	trolley (car)

Excludes1	bus (V70-V79)
	motorcoach (V70-V79)
	nonpowered streetcar (V76.-)
	train (V81.-)

The appropriate 7th character is to be added to each code from category V82

A	initial encounter
D	subsequent encounter
S	sequela

X● **V82.0** **Occupant of streetcar injured in collision with motor vehicle in nontraffic accident** 🔊
X● **V82.1** **Occupant of streetcar injured in collision with motor vehicle in traffic accident** 🔊
X● **V82.2** **Occupant of streetcar injured in collision with or hit by rolling stock** 🔊
X● **V82.3** **Occupant of streetcar injured in collision with other object** 🔊

Excludes1	collision with animal-drawn vehicle or animal being ridden (V82.8)

X● **V82.4** **Person injured while boarding or alighting from streetcar** 🔊
X● **V82.5** **Occupant of streetcar injured by fall in streetcar** 🔊

Excludes1	fall in streetcar:
	while boarding or alighting (V82.4)
	with antecedent collision (V82.0-V82.3)

X● **V82.6** **Occupant of streetcar injured by fall from streetcar** 🔊

Excludes1	fall from streetcar:
	while boarding or alighting (V82.4)
	with antecedent collision (V82.0-V82.3)

X● **V82.7** **Occupant of streetcar injured in derailment without antecedent collision** 🔊

Excludes1	occupant of streetcar injured in derailment with antecedent collision (V82.0-V82.3)

X● **V82.8** **Occupant of streetcar injured in other specified transport accidents** 🔊
- Streetcar collision with military vehicle
- Streetcar collision with train or nonmotor vehicles

X● **V82.9** **Occupant of streetcar injured in** unspecified **traffic accident** 🔊
- Streetcar accident NOS

● **V83** **Occupant of special vehicle mainly used on industrial premises injured in transport accident**

Includes	battery-powered airport passenger vehicle
	battery-powered truck (baggage) (mail)
	coal-car in mine
	forklift (truck)
	logging car
	self-propelled industrial truck
	station baggage truck (powered)
	tram, truck, or tub (powered) in mine or quarry

Excludes1	special construction vehicles (V85.-)
	special industrial vehicle in stationary use or maintenance (W31.-)

The appropriate 7th character is to be added to each code from category V83

A	initial encounter
D	subsequent encounter
S	sequela

X● **V83.0** **Driver of special industrial vehicle injured in traffic accident** 🔊
X● **V83.1** **Passenger of special industrial vehicle injured in traffic accident** 🔊
X● **V83.2** **Person on outside of special industrial vehicle injured in traffic accident** 🔊
X● **V83.3** Unspecified **occupant of special industrial vehicle injured in traffic accident** 🔊
X● **V83.4** **Person injured while boarding or alighting from special industrial vehicle** 🔊
X● **V83.5** **Driver of special industrial vehicle injured in nontraffic accident** 🔊
X● **V83.6** **Passenger of special industrial vehicle injured in nontraffic accident** 🔊
X● **V83.7** **Person on outside of special industrial vehicle injured in nontraffic accident** 🔊
X● **V83.9** Unspecified **occupant of special industrial vehicle injured in nontraffic accident** 🔊
- Special-industrial-vehicle accident NOS

● **V84** **Occupant of special vehicle mainly used in agriculture injured in transport accident**

Includes	self-propelled farm machinery
	tractor (and trailer)

Excludes1	animal-powered farm machinery accident (W30.8-)
	contact with combine harvester (W30.0)
	special agricultural vehicle in stationary use or maintenance (W30.-)

The appropriate 7th character is to be added to each code from category V84

A	initial encounter
D	subsequent encounter
S	sequela

X● **V84.0** **Driver of special agricultural vehicle injured in traffic accident** 🔊
X● **V84.1** **Passenger of special agricultural vehicle injured in traffic accident** 🔊
X● **V84.2** **Person on outside of special agricultural vehicle injured in traffic accident** 🔊
X● **V84.3** Unspecified **occupant of special agricultural vehicle injured in traffic accident** 🔊
X● **V84.4** **Person injured while boarding or alighting from special agricultural vehicle** 🔊
X● **V84.5** **Driver of special agricultural vehicle injured in nontraffic accident** 🔊
X● **V84.6** **Passenger of special agricultural vehicle injured in nontraffic accident** 🔊
X● **V84.7** **Person on outside of special agricultural vehicle injured in nontraffic accident** 🔊
X● **V84.9** Unspecified **occupant of special agricultural vehicle injured in nontraffic accident** 🔊
- Special-agricultural vehicle accident NOS

CHAPTER 20 (V01-Y99)

N Newborn Age: 0   P Pediatric Age: 0–17   M Maternity DX: 12–55   A Adult Age: 15–124   ♀ Females Only   ♂ Males Only

🔊 Complication\Comorbidity   🔊 Major C\C   Ⓔⓧ CC/MCC Exclusions   🔊 Present on Admission Requirement   🔊 Hospital-Acquired Condition

1617

● **V85**   Occupant of special construction vehicle injured in transport accident

> **Includes**   bulldozer
> digger
> dump truck
> earth-leveller
> mechanical shovel
> road-roller

> **Excludes1**   special industrial vehicle (V83.-)
> special construction vehicle in stationary use or maintenance (W31.-)

The appropriate 7th character is to be added to each code from category V85

> A   initial encounter
> D   subsequent encounter
> S   sequela

X● **V85.0**   Driver of special construction vehicle injured in traffic accident 🔖

X● **V85.1**   Passenger of special construction vehicle injured in traffic accident 🔖

X● **V85.2**   Person on outside of special construction vehicle injured in traffic accident 🔖

X● **V85.3**   Unspecified occupant of special construction vehicle injured in traffic accident 🔖

X● **V85.4**   Person injured while boarding or alighting from special construction vehicle 🔖

X● **V85.5**   Driver of special construction vehicle injured in nontraffic accident 🔖

X● **V85.6**   Passenger of special construction vehicle injured in nontraffic accident 🔖

X● **V85.7**   Person on outside of special construction vehicle injured in nontraffic accident 🔖

X● **V85.9**   Unspecified occupant of special construction vehicle injured in nontraffic accident 🔖
> Special-construction-vehicle accident NOS

● **V86**   Occupant of special all-terrain or other off-road motor vehicle, injured in transport accident

> **Excludes1**   special all-terrain vehicle in stationary use or maintenance (W31.-)
> sport-utility vehicle (V50-V59)
> three-wheeled motor vehicle designed for on-road use (V30-V39)

The appropriate 7th character is to be added to each code from category V86

> A   initial encounter
> D   subsequent encounter
> S   sequela

● **V86.0**   Driver of special all-terrain or other off-road motor vehicle injured in traffic accident

X● **V86.01**   Driver of ambulance or fire engine injured in traffic accident 🔖

X● **V86.02**   Driver of snowmobile injured in traffic accident 🔖

X● **V86.03**   Driver of dune buggy injured in traffic accident 🔖

X● **V86.04**   Driver of military vehicle injured in traffic accident 🔖

X● **V86.09**   Driver of other off-road special all-terrain or other off-road vehicle injured in traffic accident 🔖
> Driver of dirt bike injured in traffic accident
> Driver of go cart injured in traffic accident
> Driver of golf cart injured in traffic accident

● **V86.1**   Passenger of special all-terrain or other off-road motor vehicle injured in traffic accident

X● **V86.11**   Passenger of ambulance or fire engine injured in traffic accident 🔖

X● **V86.12**   Passenger of snowmobile injured in traffic accident 🔖

X● **V86.13**   Passenger of dune buggy injured in traffic accident 🔖

X● **V86.14**   Passenger of military vehicle injured in traffic accident 🔖

X● **V86.19**   Passenger of other off-road special all-terrain or other off-road off-road motor vehicle injured in traffic accident 🔖
> Passenger of dirt bike injured in traffic accident
> Passenger of go cart injured in traffic accident
> Passenger of golf cart injured in traffic accident

● **V86.2**   Person on outside of special all-terrain or other off-road motor vehicle injured in traffic accident

X● **V86.21**   Person on outside of ambulance or fire engine injured in traffic accident 🔖

X● **V86.22**   Person on outside of snowmobile injured in traffic accident 🔖

X● **V86.23**   Person on outside of dune buggy injured in traffic accident 🔖

X● **V86.24**   Person on outside of military vehicle injured in traffic accident 🔖

X● **V86.29**   Person on outside of other special all-terrain or other off-road motor vehicle injured in traffic accident 🔖
> Person on outside of dirt bike injured in traffic accident
> Person on outside of go cart in traffic accident
> Person on outside of golf cart injured in traffic accident

● **V86.3**   Unspecified occupant of special all-terrain or other off-road motor vehicle injured in traffic accident

X● **V86.31**   Unspecified occupant of ambulance or fire engine injured in traffic accident 🔖

X● **V86.32**   Unspecified occupant of snowmobile injured in traffic accident 🔖

X● **V86.33**   Unspecified occupant of dune buggy injured in traffic accident 🔖

X● **V86.34**   Unspecified occupant of military vehicle injured in traffic accident 🔖

X● **V86.39**   Unspecified occupant of other special all-terrain or other off-road motor vehicle injured in traffic accident 🔖
> Unspecified occupant of dirt bike injured in traffic accident
> Unspecified occupant of go cart injured in traffic accident
> Unspecified occupant of golf cart injured in traffic accident

● **V86.4**   Person injured while boarding or alighting from special all-terrain or other off-road motor vehicle

X● **V86.41**   Person injured while boarding or alighting from ambulance or fire engine 🔖

X● **V86.42**   Person injured while boarding or alighting from snowmobile 🔖

X● **V86.43**   Person injured while boarding or alighting from dune buggy 🔖

X● **V86.44**   Person injured while boarding or alighting from military vehicle 🔖

X● **V86.49**   Person injured while boarding or alighting from other special all-terrain or other off-road motor vehicle 🔖
> Person injured while boarding or alighting from dirt bike
> Person injured while boarding or alighting from go cart
> Person injured while boarding or alighting from golf cart

◀ New   ◀⎯ Revised   ~~deleted~~ Deleted   Excludes 1   Excludes 2   Includes   Use additional   Code first   Code also   Unspecified

OGCR Official Guidelines   ● Unacceptable Principal Diagnosis   X Assign placeholder X   ● Use Additional Character(s)   🔖 Manifestation Code   **Coding Clinic**

● **V86.5**   **Driver of special all-terrain or other off-road motor vehicle injured in nontraffic accident**

   X● **V86.51**   Driver of ambulance or fire engine injured in nontraffic accident 🖐

   X● **V86.52**   Driver of snowmobile injured in nontraffic accident 🖐

   X● **V86.53**   Driver of dune buggy injured in nontraffic accident 🖐

   X● **V86.54**   Driver of military vehicle injured in nontraffic accident 🖐

   X● **V86.59**   Driver of other off-road special all-terrain or other off-road motor vehicle injured in nontraffic accident 🖐
      Driver of dirt bike injured in nontraffic accident
      Driver of go cart injured in nontraffic accident
      Driver of golf cart injured in nontraffic accident

● **V86.6**   **Passenger of special all-terrain or other off-road motor vehicle injured in nontraffic accident**

   X● **V86.61**   Passenger of ambulance or fire engine injured in nontraffic accident 🖐

   X● **V86.62**   Passenger of snowmobile injured in nontraffic accident 🖐

   X● **V86.63**   Passenger of dune buggy injured in nontraffic accident 🖐

   X● **V86.64**   Passenger of military vehicle injured in nontraffic accident 🖐

   X● **V86.69**   Passenger of other special all-terrain or other off-road vehicle injured in nontraffic accident 🖐
      Passenger of dirt bike injured in nontraffic accident
      Passenger of go cart injured in nontraffic accident
      Passenger of golf cart injured in nontraffic accident

● **V86.7**   **Person on outside of special all-terrain or other off-road motor vehicle injured in nontraffic accident**

   X● **V86.71**   Person on outside of ambulance or fire engine injured in nontraffic accident 🖐

   X● **V86.72**   Person on outside of snowmobile injured in nontraffic accident 🖐

   X● **V86.73**   Person on outside of dune buggy injured in nontraffic accident 🖐

   X● **V86.74**   Person on outside of military vehicle injured in nontraffic accident 🖐

   X● **V86.79**   Person on outside of other special all-terrain or other off-road motor vehicles injured in nontraffic accident 🖐
      Person on outside of dirt bike injured in nontraffic accident
      Person on outside of go cart injured in nontraffic accident
      Person on outside of golf cart injured in nontraffic accident

● **V86.9**   **Unspecified occupant of special all-terrain or other off-road motor vehicle injured in nontraffic accident**

   X● **V86.91**   Unspecified occupant of ambulance or fire engine injured in nontraffic accident 🖐

   X● **V86.92**   Unspecified occupant of snowmobile injured in nontraffic accident 🖐

   X● **V86.93**   Unspecified occupant of dune buggy injured in nontraffic accident 🖐

   X● **V86.94**   Unspecified occupant of military vehicle injured in nontraffic accident 🖐

   X● **V86.99**   Unspecified occupant of other off-road special all-terrain or other off-road motor vehicle injured in nontraffic accident 🖐
      All-terrain motor-vehicle accident NOS
      Off-road motor-vehicle accident NOS
      Other motor-vehicle accident NOS
      Unspecified occupant of dirt bike injured in nontraffic accident
      Unspecified occupant of go cart injured in nontraffic accident
      Unspecified occupant of golf cart injured in nontraffic accident
      Unspecified occupant of race car injured in nontraffic accident

● **V87**   **Traffic accident of specified type but victim's mode of transport unknown**

   Excludes1   collision involving:
        pedal cycle (V10-V19)
        pedestrian (V01-V09)

   The appropriate 7th character is to be added to each code from category V87

A	initial encounter
D	subsequent encounter
S	sequela

   X● **V87.0**   Person injured in collision between car and two- or three-wheeled powered vehicle (traffic) 🖐

   X● **V87.1**   Person injured in collision between other motor vehicle and two- or three-wheeled motor vehicle (traffic) 🖐

   X● **V87.2**   Person injured in collision between car and pick-up truck or van (traffic) 🖐

   X● **V87.3**   Person injured in collision between car and bus (traffic) 🖐

   X● **V87.4**   Person injured in collision between car and heavy transport vehicle (traffic) 🖐

   X● **V87.5**   Person injured in collision between heavy transport vehicle and bus (traffic) 🖐

   X● **V87.6**   Person injured in collision between railway train or railway vehicle and car (traffic) 🖐

   X● **V87.7**   Person injured in collision between other specified motor vehicles (traffic) 🖐

   X● **V87.8**   Person injured in other specified noncollision transport accidents involving motor vehicle (traffic) 🖐

   X● **V87.9**   Person injured in other specified (collision) (noncollision) transport accidents involving nonmotor vehicle (traffic) 🖐

● **V88**   **Nontraffic accident of specified type but victim's mode of transport unknown**

   Excludes1   collision involving:
        pedal cycle (V10-V19)
        pedestrian (V01-V09)

   The appropriate 7th character is to be added to each code from category V88

A	initial encounter
D	subsequent encounter
S	sequela

   X● **V88.0**   Person injured in collision between car and two- or three-wheeled motor vehicle, nontraffic 🖐

   X● **V88.1**   Person injured in collision between other motor vehicle and two- or three-wheeled motor vehicle, nontraffic 🖐

   X● **V88.2**   Person injured in collision between car and pick-up truck or van, nontraffic 🖐

N   Newborn Age: 0   **P**   Pediatric Age: 0–17   **M**   Maternity DX: 12–55   **A**   Adult Age: 15–124   ♀   Females Only   ♂   Males Only

🖐   Complication\Comorbidity   🖐   Major C\C   ⓔⓧ   CC/MCC Exclusions   🖐   Present on Admission Requirement   🖐   Hospital-Acquired Condition

1619

CHAPTER 20 (V01-Y99)

X ● **V88.3**   **Person injured in collision between car and bus, nontraffic** 🔍

X ● **V88.4**   **Person injured in collision between car and heavy transport vehicle, nontraffic** 🔍

X ● **V88.5**   **Person injured in collision between heavy transport vehicle and bus, nontraffic** 🔍

X ● **V88.6**   **Person injured in collision between railway train or railway vehicle and car, nontraffic** 🔍

X ● **V88.7**   **Person injured in collision between other specified motor vehicle, nontraffic** 🔍

X ● **V88.8**   **Person injured in other specified noncollision transport accidents involving motor vehicle, nontraffic** 🔍

X ● **V88.9**   **Person injured in other specified (collision) (noncollision) transport accidents involving nonmotor vehicle, nontraffic** 🔍

● **V89**   **Motor- or nonmotor-vehicle accident, type of vehicle unspecified**

> The appropriate 7th character is to be added to each code from category V89

> | | |
> |---|---|
> | A | initial encounter |
> | D | subsequent encounter |
> | S | sequela |

X ● **V89.0**   **Person injured in** unspecified **motor-vehicle accident, nontraffic** 🔍
> Motor-vehicle accident NOS, nontraffic

X ● **V89.1**   **Person injured in** unspecified **nonmotor-vehicle accident, nontraffic** 🔍
> Nonmotor-vehicle accident NOS (nontraffic)

X ● **V89.2**   **Person injured in** unspecified **motor-vehicle accident, traffic** 🔍
> Motor-vehicle accident [MVA] NOS
> Road (traffic) accident [RTA] NOS

X ● **V89.3**   **Person injured in** unspecified **nonmotor-vehicle accident, traffic** 🔍
> Nonmotor-vehicle traffic accident NOS

X ● **V89.9**   **Person injured in** unspecified **vehicle accident** 🔍
> Collision NOS

WATER TRANSPORT ACCIDENTS (V90-V94)

● **V90**   **Drowning and submersion due to accident to watercraft**
> **Excludes1**   civilian water transport accident involving military watercraft (V94.81-)
>   fall into water not from watercraft (W16.-)
>   military watercraft accident in military or war operations (Y36.0-, Y37.0-)
>   water-transport–related drowning or submersion without accident to watercraft (V92.-)

> The appropriate 7th character is to be added to each code from category V90

> | | |
> |---|---|
> | A | initial encounter |
> | D | subsequent encounter |
> | S | sequela |

● **V90.0**   **Drowning and submersion due to watercraft overturning**

X ● **V90.00**   **Drowning and submersion due to merchant ship overturning**

X ● **V90.01**   **Drowning and submersion due to passenger ship overturning** 🔍
> Drowning and submersion due to ferry-boat overturning
> Drowning and submersion due to liner overturning

X ● **V90.02**   **Drowning and submersion due to fishing boat overturning** 🔍

X ● **V90.03**   **Drowning and submersion due to other powered watercraft overturning** 🔍
> Drowning and submersion due to hovercraft (on open water) overturning
> Drowning and submersion due to jet ski overturning

X ● **V90.04**   **Drowning and submersion due to sailboat overturning** 🔍

X ● **V90.05**   **Drowning and submersion due to canoe or kayak overturning** 🔍

X ● **V90.06**   **Drowning and submersion due to (nonpowered) inflatable craft overturning** 🔍

X ● **V90.08**   **Drowning and submersion due to other unpowered watercraft overturning**
> Drowning and submersion due to windsurfer overturning

X ● **V90.09**   **Drowning and submersion due to** unspecified **watercraft overturning** 🔍
> Drowning and submersion due to boat NOS overturning
> Drowning and submersion due to ship NOS overturning
> Drowning and submersion due to watercraft NOS overturning

● **V90.1**   **Drowning and submersion due to watercraft sinking**

X ● **V90.10**   **Drowning and submersion due to merchant ship sinking** 🔍

X ● **V90.11**   **Drowning and submersion due to passenger ship sinking** 🔍
> Drowning and submersion due to ferry-boat sinking
> Drowning and submersion due to liner sinking

X ● **V90.12**   **Drowning and submersion due to fishing boat sinking** 🔍

X ● **V90.13**   **Drowning and submersion due to other powered watercraft sinking** 🔍
> Drowning and submersion due to hovercraft (on open water) sinking
> Drowning and submersion due to jet ski sinking

X ● **V90.14**   **Drowning and submersion due to sailboat sinking** 🔍

X ● **V90.15**   **Drowning and submersion due to canoe or kayak sinking** 🔍

X ● **V90.16**   **Drowning and submersion due to (nonpowered) inflatable craft sinking** 🔍

X ● **V90.18**   **Drowning and submersion due to other unpowered watercraft sinking** 🔍

X ● **V90.19**   **Drowning and submersion due to** unspecified **watercraft sinking** 🔍
> Drowning and submersion due to boat NOS sinking
> Drowning and submersion due to ship NOS sinking
> Drowning and submersion due to watercraft NOS sinking

● **V90.2**   **Drowning and submersion due to falling or jumping from burning watercraft**

X ● **V90.20**   **Drowning and submersion due to falling or jumping from burning merchant ship** 🔍

X ● **V90.21**   **Drowning and submersion due to falling or jumping from burning passenger ship** 🔍
> Drowning and submersion due to falling or jumping from burning ferry-boat
> Drowning and submersion due to falling or jumping from burning liner

X ● **V90.22**   **Drowning and submersion due to falling or jumping from burning fishing boat** 🔍

X ● **V90.23**   **Drowning and submersion due to falling or jumping from other burning powered watercraft** 🔍
> Drowning and submersion due to falling and jumping from burning hovercraft (on open water)
> Drowning and submersion due to falling and jumping from burning jet ski

X ● **V90.24**   **Drowning and submersion due to falling or jumping from burning sailboat** 🔍

X ● **V90.25**   **Drowning and submersion due to falling or jumping from burning canoe or kayak** 🔍

◄ New   ◄▩ Revised   ~~deleted~~ Deleted   Excludes 1   Excludes 2   Includes   Use additional   Code first   Code also   Unspecified

OGCR Official Guidelines   ● Unacceptable Principal Diagnosis   X Assign placeholder X   🔍 Use Additional Character(s)   ▌ Manifestation Code   **Coding Clinic**

X⬤ **V90.26** **Drowning and submersion due to falling or jumping from burning (nonpowered) inflatable craft** 🦠

X⬤ **V90.27** **Drowning and submersion due to falling or jumping from burning water-skis** 🦠

X⬤ **V90.28** **Drowning and submersion due to falling or jumping from other burning unpowered watercraft** 🦠
　　　Drowning and submersion due to falling and jumping from burning surf-board
　　　Drowning and submersion due to falling and jumping from burning windsurfer

X⬤ **V90.29** **Drowning and submersion due to falling or jumping from unspecified burning watercraft** 🦠
　　　Drowning and submersion due to falling or jumping from burning boat NOS
　　　Drowning and submersion due to falling or jumping from burning ship NOS
　　　Drowning and submersion due to falling or jumping from burning watercraft NOS

⬤ **V90.3** **Drowning and submersion due to falling or jumping from crushed watercraft**

X⬤ **V90.30** **Drowning and submersion due to falling or jumping from crushed merchant ship** 🦠

X⬤ **V90.31** **Drowning and submersion due to falling or jumping from crushed passenger ship** 🦠
　　　Drowning and submersion due to falling and jumping from crushed ferry-boat
　　　Drowning and submersion due to falling and jumping from crushed liner

X⬤ **V90.32** **Drowning and submersion due to falling or jumping from crushed fishing boat** 🦠

X⬤ **V90.33** **Drowning and submersion due to falling or jumping from other crushed powered watercraft** 🦠
　　　Drowning and submersion due to falling and jumping from crushed hovercraft
　　　Drowning and submersion due to falling and jumping from crushed jet ski

X⬤ **V90.34** **Drowning and submersion due to falling or jumping from crushed sailboat** 🦠

X⬤ **V90.35** **Drowning and submersion due to falling or jumping from crushed canoe or kayak** 🦠

X⬤ **V90.36** **Drowning and submersion due to falling or jumping from crushed (nonpowered) inflatable craft** 🦠

X⬤ **V90.37** **Drowning and submersion due to falling or jumping from crushed water-skis** 🦠

X⬤ **V90.38** **Drowning and submersion due to falling or jumping from other crushed unpowered watercraft** 🦠
　　　Drowning and submersion due to falling and jumping from crushed surf-board
　　　Drowning and submersion due to falling and jumping from crushed windsurfer

X⬤ **V90.39** **Drowning and submersion due to falling or jumping from crushed unspecified watercraft** 🦠
　　　Drowning and submersion due to falling and jumping from crushed boat NOS
　　　Drowning and submersion due to falling and jumping from crushed ship NOS
　　　Drowning and submersion due to falling and jumping from crushed watercraft NOS

⬤ **V90.8** **Drowning and submersion due to other accident to watercraft**

X⬤ **V90.80** **Drowning and submersion due to other accident to merchant ship** 🦠

X⬤ **V90.81** **Drowning and submersion due to other accident to passenger ship** 🦠
　　　Drowning and submersion due to other accident to ferry-boat
　　　Drowning and submersion due to other accident to liner

X⬤ **V90.82** **Drowning and submersion due to other accident to fishing boat** 🦠

X⬤ **V90.83** **Drowning and submersion due to other accident to other powered watercraft** 🦠
　　　Drowning and submersion due to other accident to hovercraft (on open water)
　　　Drowning and submersion due to other accident to jet ski

X⬤ **V90.84** **Drowning and submersion due to other accident to sailboat** 🦠

X⬤ **V90.85** **Drowning and submersion due to other accident to canoe or kayak** 🦠

X⬤ **V90.86** **Drowning and submersion due to other accident to (nonpowered) inflatable craft** 🦠

X⬤ **V90.87** **Drowning and submersion due to other accident to water-skis** 🦠

X⬤ **V90.88** **Drowning and submersion due to other accident to other unpowered watercraft** 🦠
　　　Drowning and submersion due to other accident to surf-board
　　　Drowning and submersion due to other accident to windsurfer

X⬤ **V90.89** **Drowning and submersion due to other accident to unspecified watercraft** 🦠
　　　Drowning and submersion due to other accident to boat NOS
　　　Drowning and submersion due to other accident to ship NOS
　　　Drowning and submersion due to other accident to watercraft NOS

⬤ **V91** **Other injury due to accident to watercraft**

　Includes　any injury except drowning and submersion as a result of an accident to watercraft

　Excludes1　civilian water transport accident involving military watercraft (V94.81-)
　　　military watercraft accident in military or war operations (Y36, Y37.-) ◀▥

　Excludes2　drowning and submersion due to accident to watercraft (V90.-)

The appropriate 7th character is to be added to each code from category V91

A	initial encounter
D	subsequent encounter
S	sequela

⬤ **V91.0** **Burn due to watercraft on fire**

　Excludes1　burn from localized fire or explosion on board ship without accident to watercraft (V93.-)

X⬤ **V91.00** **Burn due to merchant ship on fire** 🦠

X⬤ **V91.01** **Burn due to passenger ship on fire** 🦠
　　　Burn due to ferry-boat on fire
　　　Burn due to liner on fire

X⬤ **V91.02** **Burn due to fishing boat on fire** 🦠

X⬤ **V91.03** **Burn due to other powered watercraft on fire** 🦠
　　　Burn due to hovercraft (on open water) on fire
　　　Burn due to jet ski on fire

X⬤ **V91.04** **Burn due to sailboat on fire** 🦠

X⬤ **V91.05** **Burn due to canoe or kayak on fire** 🦠

X⬤ **V91.06** **Burn due to (nonpowered) inflatable craft on fire** 🦠

X⬤ **V91.07** **Burn due to water-skis on fire** 🦠

X⬤ **V91.08** **Burn due to other unpowered watercraft on fire** 🦠

X⬤ **V91.09** **Burn due to unspecified watercraft on fire** 🦠
　　　Burn due to boat NOS on fire
　　　Burn due to ship NOS on fire
　　　Burn due to watercraft NOS on fire

N Newborn Age: 0　　**P** Pediatric Age: 0–17　　**M** Maternity DX: 12–55　　**A** Adult Age: 15–124　　♀ Females Only　　♂ Males Only

🦠 Complication\Comorbidity　　🦠 Major C\C　　(Ex) CC/MCC Exclusions　　🦠 Present on Admission Requirement　　🦠 Hospital-Acquired Condition

1621

CHAPTER 20 (V01-Y99)

● **V91.1 Crushed between watercraft and other watercraft or other object due to collision**
Crushed by lifeboat after abandoning ship in a collision
Note: Select the specified type of watercraft that the victim was on at the time of the collision.
X ● **V91.10 Crushed between merchant ship and other watercraft or other object due to collision** 🅠
X ● **V91.11 Crushed between passenger ship and other watercraft or other object due to collision** 🅠
Crushed between ferry-boat and other watercraft or other object due to collision
Crushed between liner and other watercraft or other object due to collision
X ● **V91.12 Crushed between fishing boat and other watercraft or other object due to collision** 🅠
X ● **V91.13 Crushed between other powered watercraft and other watercraft or other object due to collision** 🅠
Crushed between hovercraft (on open water) and other watercraft or other object due to collision
Crushed between jet ski and other watercraft or other object due to collision
X ● **V91.14 Crushed between sailboat and other watercraft or other object due to collision** 🅠
X ● **V91.15 Crushed between canoe or kayak and other watercraft or other object due to collision** 🅠
X ● **V91.16 Crushed between (nonpowered) inflatable craft and other watercraft or other object due to collision** 🅠
X ● **V91.18 Crushed between other unpowered watercraft and other watercraft or other object due to collision** 🅠
Crushed between surfboard and other watercraft or other object due to collision
Crushed between windsurfer and other watercraft or other object due to collision
X ● **V91.19 Crushed between unspecified watercraft and other watercraft or other object due to collision** 🅠
Crushed between boat NOS and other watercraft or other object due to collision
Crushed between ship NOS and other watercraft or other object due to collision
Crushed between watercraft NOS and other watercraft or other object due to collision

● **V91.2 Fall due to collision between watercraft and other watercraft or other object**
Fall while remaining on watercraft after collision
Note: Select the specified type of watercraft that the victim was on at the time of the collision.
Excludes1 crushed between watercraft and other watercraft and other object due to collision (V91.1-)
drowning and submersion due to falling from crushed watercraft (V90.3-)
X ● **V91.20 Fall due to collision between merchant ship and other watercraft or other object** 🅠
X ● **V91.21 Fall due to collision between passenger ship and other watercraft or other object** 🅠
Fall due to collision between ferry-boat and other watercraft or other object
Fall due to collision between liner and other watercraft or other object
X ● **V91.22 Fall due to collision between fishing boat and other watercraft or other object** 🅠

X ● **V91.23 Fall due to collision between other powered watercraft and other watercraft or other object** 🅠
Fall due to collision between hovercraft (on open water) and other watercraft or other object
Fall due to collision between jet ski and other watercraft or other object
X ● **V91.24 Fall due to collision between sailboat and other watercraft or other object** 🅠
X ● **V91.25 Fall due to collision between canoe or kayak and other watercraft or other object** 🅠
X ● **V91.26 Fall due to collision between (nonpowered) inflatable craft and other watercraft or other object** 🅠
X ● **V91.29 Fall due to collision between unspecified watercraft and other watercraft or other object** 🅠
Fall due to collision between boat NOS and other watercraft or other object
Fall due to collision between ship NOS and other watercraft or other object
Fall due to collision between watercraft NOS and other watercraft or other object

● **V91.3 Hit or struck by falling object due to accident to watercraft**
Hit or struck by falling object (part of damaged watercraft or other object) after falling or jumping from damaged watercraft
Excludes2 drowning or submersion due to fall or jumping from damaged watercraft (V90.2-, V90.3-)
X ● **V91.30 Hit or struck by falling object due to accident to merchant ship** 🅠
X ● **V91.31 Hit or struck by falling object due to accident to passenger ship** 🅠
Hit or struck by falling object due to accident to ferry-boat
Hit or struck by falling object due to accident to liner
X ● **V91.32 Hit or struck by falling object due to accident to fishing boat** 🅠
X ● **V91.33 Hit or struck by falling object due to accident to other powered watercraft** 🅠
Hit or struck by falling object due to accident to hovercraft (on open water)
Hit or struck by falling object due to accident to jet ski
X ● **V91.34 Hit or struck by falling object due to accident to sailboat** 🅠
X ● **V91.35 Hit or struck by falling object due to accident to canoe or kayak** 🅠
X ● **V91.36 Hit or struck by falling object due to accident to (nonpowered) inflatable craft** 🅠
X ● **V91.37 Hit or struck by falling object due to accident to water-skis** 🅠
Hit by water-skis after jumping off of waterskis
X ● **V91.38 Hit or struck by falling object due to accident to other unpowered watercraft** 🅠
Hit or struck by surf-board after falling off damaged surf-board
Hit or struck by object after falling off damaged windsurfer
X ● **V91.39 Hit or struck by falling object due to accident to unspecified watercraft** 🅠
Hit or struck by falling object due to accident to boat NOS
Hit or struck by falling object due to accident to ship NOS
Hit or struck by falling object due to accident to watercraft NOS

◄ New ◄▦ Revised ~~deleted~~ Deleted Excludes 1 Excludes 2 Includes Use additional Code first Code also Unspecified
OGCR Official Guidelines ● Unacceptable Principal Diagnosis X Assign placeholder X ● Use Additional Character(s) ▌ Manifestation Code **Coding Clinic**

● V91.8   Other injury due to other accident to watercraft

   X ● V91.80   **Other injury due to other accident to merchant ship** 🔍

   X ● V91.81   **Other injury due to other accident to passenger ship** 🔍
      Other injury due to other accident to ferry-boat
      Other injury due to other accident to liner

   X ● V91.82   **Other injury due to other accident to fishing boat** 🔍

   X ● V91.83   **Other injury due to other accident to other powered watercraft** 🔍
      Other injury due to other accident to hovercraft (on open water)
      Other injury due to other accident to jet ski

   X ● V91.84   **Other injury due to other accident to sailboat** 🔍

   X ● V91.85   **Other injury due to other accident to canoe or kayak** 🔍

   X ● V91.86   **Other injury due to other accident to (nonpowered) inflatable craft** 🔍

   X ● V91.87   **Other injury due to other accident to water-skis** 🔍

   X ● V91.88   **Other injury due to other accident to other unpowered watercraft** 🔍
      Other injury due to other accident to surf-board
      Other injury due to other accident to windsurfer

   X ● V91.89   **Other injury due to other accident to unspecified watercraft** 🔍
      Other injury due to other accident to boat NOS
      Other injury due to other accident to ship NOS
      Other injury due to other accident to watercraft NOS

● V92   **Drowning and submersion due to accident on board watercraft, without accident to watercraft**

   Excludes1   civilian water transport accident involving military watercraft (V94.81-)
      drowning or submersion due to accident to watercraft (V90-V91)
      drowning or submersion of diver who voluntarily jumps from boat not involved in an accident (W16.711, W16.721)
      fall into water without watercraft (W16.-)
      military watercraft accident in military or war operations (Y36, Y37)

   The appropriate 7th character is to be added to each code from category V92

     | | |
     A   initial encounter
     D   subsequent encounter
     S   sequela

● V92.0   **Drowning and submersion due to fall off watercraft**
      Drowning and submersion due to fall from gangplank of watercraft
      Drowning and submersion due to fall overboard watercraft

   Excludes2   hitting head on object or bottom of body of water due to fall from watercraft (V94.0-)

   X ● V92.00   **Drowning and submersion due to fall off merchant ship** 🔍

   X ● V92.01   **Drowning and submersion due to fall off passenger ship** 🔍
      Drowning and submersion due to fall off ferry-boat
      Drowning and submersion due to fall off liner

   X ● V92.02   **Drowning and submersion due to fall off fishing boat** 🔍

   X ● V92.03   **Drowning and submersion due to fall off other powered watercraft** 🔍
      Drowning and submersion due to fall off hovercraft (on open water)
      Drowning and submersion due to fall off jet ski

   X ● V92.04   **Drowning and submersion due to fall off sailboat** 🔍

   X ● V92.05   **Drowning and submersion due to fall off canoe or kayak** 🔍

   X ● V92.06   **Drowning and submersion due to fall off (nonpowered) inflatable craft** 🔍

   X ● V92.07   **Drowning and submersion due to fall off water-skis** 🔍

     Excludes1   drowning and submersion due to falling off burning water-skis (V90.27)
      drowning and submersion due to falling off crushed water-skis (V90.37)
      hit by boat while water-skiing NOS (V94.X) ◀▥

   X ● V92.08   **Drowning and submersion due to fall off other unpowered watercraft** 🔍
      Drowning and submersion due to fall off surf-board
      Drowning and submersion due to fall off windsurfer

     Excludes1   drowning and submersion due to fall off burning unpowered watercraft (V90.28)
      drowning and submersion due to fall off crushed unpowered watercraft (V90.38)
      drowning and submersion due to fall off damaged unpowered watercraft (V90.88)
      drowning and submersion due to rider of nonpowered watercraft being hit by other watercraft (V94.-) ◀▥
      other injury due to rider of nonpowered watercraft being hit by other watercraft (V94.-) ◀▥

   X ● V92.09   **Drowning and submersion due to fall off unspecified watercraft** 🔍
      Drowning and submersion due to fall off boat NOS
      Drowning and submersion due to fall off ship
      Drowning and submersion due to fall off watercraft NOS

● V92.1   **Drowning and submersion due to being thrown overboard by motion of watercraft**

   Excludes1   drowning and submersion due to fall off surf-board (V92.08)
      drowning and submersion due to fall off water-skis (V92.07)
      drowning and submersion due to fall off windsurfer (V92.08)

   X ● V92.10   **Drowning and submersion due to being thrown overboard by motion of merchant ship** 🔍

   X ● V92.11   **Drowning and submersion due to being thrown overboard by motion of passenger ship** 🔍
      Drowning and submersion due to being thrown overboard by motion of ferry-boat
      Drowning and submersion due to being thrown overboard by motion of liner

N   Newborn Age: 0   P   Pediatric Age: 0–17   M   Maternity DX: 12–55   A   Adult Age: 15–124   ♀   Females Only   ♂   Males Only

🔍 Complication\Comorbidity   🔍 Major C\C   (Ex) CC/MCC Exclusions   🔍 Present on Admission Requirement   🔍 Hospital-Acquired Condition

1623

X ● **V92.12** **Drowning and submersion due to being thrown overboard by motion of fishing boat** 🖐

X ● **V92.13** **Drowning and submersion due to being thrown overboard by motion of other powered watercraft** 🖐

    Drowning and submersion due to being thrown overboard by motion of hovercraft

X ● **V92.14** **Drowning and submersion due to being thrown overboard by motion of sailboat** 🖐

X ● **V92.15** **Drowning and submersion due to being thrown overboard by motion of canoe or kayak** 🖐

X ● **V92.16** **Drowning and submersion due to being thrown overboard by motion of (nonpowered) inflatable craft** 🖐

X ● **V92.19** **Drowning and submersion due to being thrown overboard by motion of** `unspecified` **watercraft** 🖐

    Drowning and submersion due to being thrown overboard by motion of boat NOS

    Drowning and submersion due to being thrown overboard by motion of ship NOS

    Drowning and submersion due to being thrown overboard by motion of watercraft NOS

● **V92.2** **Drowning and submersion due to being washed overboard from watercraft**

    Code first any associated cataclysm (X37.0-)

X ● **V92.20** **Drowning and submersion due to being washed overboard from merchant ship** 🖐

X ● **V92.21** **Drowning and submersion due to being washed overboard from passenger ship** 🖐

    Drowning and submersion due to being washed overboard from ferry-boat

    Drowning and submersion due to being washed overboard from liner

X ● **V92.22** **Drowning and submersion due to being washed overboard from fishing boat** 🖐

X ● **V92.23** **Drowning and submersion due to being washed overboard from other powered watercraft** 🖐

    Drowning and submersion due to being washed overboard from hovercraft (on open water)

    Drowning and submersion due to being washed overboard from jet ski

X ● **V92.24** **Drowning and submersion due to being washed overboard from sailboat** 🖐

X ● **V92.25** **Drowning and submersion due to being washed overboard from canoe or kayak** 🖐

X ● **V92.26** **Drowning and submersion due to being washed overboard from (nonpowered) inflatable craft** 🖐

X ● **V92.27** **Drowning and submersion due to being washed overboard from water-skis** 🖐

    `Excludes1`   drowning and submersion due to fall off water-skis (V92.07)

X ● **V92.28** **Drowning and submersion due to being washed overboard from other unpowered watercraft** 🖐

    Drowning and submersion due to being washed overboard from surf-board

    Drowning and submersion due to being washed overboard from windsurfer

X ● **V92.29** **Drowning and submersion due to being washed overboard from** `unspecified` **watercraft** 🖐

    Drowning and submersion due to being washed overboard from boat NOS

    Drowning and submersion due to being washed overboard from ship NOS

    Drowning and submersion due to being washed overboard from watercraft NOS

● **V93** **Other injury due to accident on board watercraft, without accident to watercraft**

    `Excludes1`   civilian water transport accident involving military watercraft (V94.81-)

        other injury due to accident to watercraft (V91.-)

        military watercraft accident in military or war operations (Y36, Y37.-) ◀━

    `Excludes2`   drowning and submersion due to accident on board watercraft, without accident to watercraft (V92.-)

    The appropriate 7th character is to be added to each code from category V93

A	initial encounter
D	subsequent encounter
S	sequela

● **V93.0** **Burn due to localized fire on board watercraft**

    `Excludes1`   burn due to watercraft on fire (V91.0-)

X ● **V93.00** **Burn due to localized fire on board merchant vessel** 🖐

X ● **V93.01** **Burn due to localized fire on board passenger vessel** 🖐

    Burn due to localized fire on board ferry-boat

    Burn due to localized fire on board liner

X ● **V93.02** **Burn due to localized fire on board fishing boat** 🖐

X ● **V93.03** **Burn due to localized fire on board other powered watercraft** 🖐

    Burn due to localized fire on board hovercraft

    Burn due to localized fire on board jet ski

X ● **V93.04** **Burn due to localized fire on board sailboat** 🖐

X ● **V93.09** **Burn due to localized fire on board** `unspecified` **watercraft** 🖐

    Burn due to localized fire on board boat NOS

    Burn due to localized fire on board ship NOS

    Burn due to localized fire on board watercraft NOS

● **V93.1** **Other burn on board watercraft**

    Burn due to source other than fire on board watercraft

    `Excludes1`   burn due to watercraft on fire (V91.0-)

X ● **V93.10** **Other burn on board merchant vessel** 🖐

X ● **V93.11** **Other burn on board passenger vessel** 🖐

    Other burn on board ferry-boat

    Other burn on board liner

X ● **V93.12** **Other burn on board fishing boat** 🖐

X ● **V93.13** **Other burn on board other powered watercraft** 🖐

    Other burn on board hovercraft

    Other burn on board jet ski

X ● **V93.14** **Other burn on board sailboat** 🖐

X ● **V93.19** **Other burn on board** `unspecified` **watercraft** 🖐

    Other burn on board boat NOS

    Other burn on board ship NOS

    Other burn on board watercraft NOS

● **V93.2** **Heat exposure on board watercraft**

    `Excludes1`   exposure to man-made heat not aboard watercraft (W92)

        exposure to natural heat while on board watercraft (X30)

        exposure to sunlight while on board watercraft (X32)

    `Excludes2`   burn due to fire on board watercraft (V93.0-)

X ● **V93.20** **Heat exposure on board merchant ship** 🖐

X ● **V93.21** **Heat exposure on board passenger ship** 🖐

    Heat exposure on board ferry-boat

    Heat exposure on board liner

X ● **V93.22** **Heat exposure on board fishing boat** 🖐

X ● **V93.23** **Heat exposure on board other powered watercraft** 🖐

    Heat exposure on board hovercraft

◀ New   ◀━ Revised   ~~deleted~~ Deleted   `Excludes 1`   `Excludes 2`   `Includes`   `Use additional`   `Code first`   `Code also`   `Unspecified`

OGCR Official Guidelines   ● Unacceptable Principal Diagnosis   X Assign placeholder X   🖐 Use Additional Character(s)   ▌ Manifestation Code   **Coding Clinic**

X ● **V93.24** **Heat exposure on board sailboat** 🔲

X ● **V93.29** **Heat exposure on board** unspecified **watercraft** 🔲
  Heat exposure on board boat NOS
  Heat exposure on board ship NOS
  Heat exposure on board watercraft NOS

● **V93.3** **Fall on board watercraft**
  Excludes1   fall due to collision of watercraft (V91.2-)

X ● **V93.30** **Fall on board merchant ship** 🔲

X ● **V93.31** **Fall on board passenger ship** 🔲
  Fall on board ferry-boat
  Fall on board liner

X ● **V93.32** **Fall on board fishing boat** 🔲

X ● **V93.33** **Fall on board other powered watercraft** 🔲
  Fall on board hovercraft (on open water)
  Fall on board jet ski

X ● **V93.34** **Fall on board sailboat** 🔲

X ● **V93.35** **Fall on board canoe or kayak** 🔲

X ● **V93.36** **Fall on board (nonpowered) inflatable craft** 🔲

X ● **V93.38** **Fall on board other unpowered watercraft** 🔲

X ● **V93.39** **Fall on board** unspecified **watercraft** 🔲
  Fall on board boat NOS
  Fall on board ship NOS
  Fall on board watercraft NOS

● **V93.4** **Struck by falling object on board watercraft**
  Hit by falling object on board watercraft
  Excludes1   struck by falling object due to accident to watercraft (V91.3)

X ● **V93.40** **Struck by falling object on merchant ship** 🔲

X ● **V93.41** **Struck by falling object on passenger ship** 🔲
  Struck by falling object on ferry-boat
  Struck by falling object on liner

X ● **V93.42** **Struck by falling object on fishing boat** 🔲

X ● **V93.43** **Struck by falling object on other powered watercraft** 🔲
  Struck by falling object on hovercraft

X ● **V93.44** **Struck by falling object on sailboat** 🔲

X ● **V93.48** **Struck by falling object on other unpowered watercraft** 🔲

X ● **V93.49** **Struck by falling object on** unspecified **watercraft** 🔲

● **V93.5** **Explosion on board watercraft**
  Boiler explosion on steamship
  Excludes2   fire on board watercraft (V93.0-)

X ● **V93.50** **Explosion on board merchant ship** 🔲

X ● **V93.51** **Explosion on board passenger ship** 🔲
  Explosion on board ferry-boat
  Explosion on board liner

X ● **V93.52** **Explosion on board fishing boat** 🔲

X ● **V93.53** **Explosion on board other powered watercraft** 🔲
  Explosion on board hovercraft
  Explosion on board jet ski

X ● **V93.54** **Explosion on board sailboat** 🔲

X ● **V93.59** **Explosion on board** unspecified **watercraft** 🔲
  Explosion on board boat NOS
  Explosion on board ship NOS
  Explosion on board watercraft NOS

● **V93.6** **Machinery accident on board watercraft**
  Excludes1   machinery explosion on board watercraft (V93.4-)
       machinery fire on board watercraft (V93.0-)

X ● **V93.60** **Machinery accident on board merchant ship** 🔲

X ● **V93.61** **Machinery accident on board passenger ship** 🔲
  Machinery accident on board ferry-boat
  Machinery accident on board liner

X ● **V93.62** **Machinery accident on board fishing boat** 🔲

X ● **V93.63** **Machinery accident on board other powered watercraft** 🔲
  Machinery accident on board hovercraft

X ● **V93.64** **Machinery accident on board sailboat** 🔲

X ● **V93.69** **Machinery accident on board** unspecified **watercraft** 🔲
  Machinery accident on board boat NOS
  Machinery accident on board ship NOS
  Machinery accident on board watercraft NOS

● **V93.8** **Other injury due to other accident on board watercraft**
  Accidental poisoning by gases or fumes on watercraft

X ● **V93.80** **Other injury due to other accident on board merchant ship** 🔲

X ● **V93.81** **Other injury due to other accident on board passenger ship** 🔲
  Other injury due to other accident on board ferry-boat
  Other injury due to other accident on board liner

X ● **V93.82** **Other injury due to other accident on board fishing boat** 🔲

X ● **V93.83** **Other injury due to other accident on board other powered watercraft** 🔲
  Other injury due to other accident on board hovercraft
  Other injury due to other accident on board jet ski

X ● **V93.84** **Other injury due to other accident on board sailboat** 🔲

X ● **V93.85** **Other injury due to other accident on board canoe or kayak** 🔲

X ● **V93.86** **Other injury due to other accident on board (nonpowered) inflatable craft** 🔲

X ● **V93.87** **Other injury due to other accident on board water-skis** 🔲
  Hit or struck by object while waterskiing

X ● **V93.88** **Other injury due to other accident on board other unpowered watercraft** 🔲
  Hit or struck by object while surfing
  Hit or struck by object while on board windsurfer

X ● **V93.89** **Other injury due to other accident on board** unspecified **watercraft** 🔲
  Other injury due to other accident on board boat NOS
  Other injury due to other accident on board ship NOS
  Other injury due to other accident on board watercraft NOS

● **V94** **Other and unspecified water transport accidents**
  Excludes1   military watercraft accidents in military or war operations (Y36, Y37)

  The appropriate 7th character is to be added to each code from category V94

A	initial encounter
D	subsequent encounter
S	sequela

X ● **V94.0** **Hitting object or bottom of body of water due to fall from watercraft** 🔲
  Excludes2   drowning and submersion due to fall from watercraft (V92.0-)

● **V94.1** **Bather struck by watercraft**
  Swimmer hit by watercraft

X ● **V94.11** **Bather struck by powered watercraft** 🔲

X ● **V94.12** **Bather struck by nonpowered watercraft** 🔲

N Newborn Age: 0   **P** Pediatric Age: 0–17   **M** Maternity DX: 12–55   **A** Adult Age: 15–124   ♀ Females Only   ♂ Males Only

 Complication\Comorbidity   Major C\C   (Ex) CC/MCC Exclusions   🔲 Present on Admission Requirement   🔲 Hospital-Acquired Condition

1625

● V94.2   **Rider of nonpowered watercraft struck by other watercraft**

    X● V94.21   **Rider of nonpowered watercraft struck by other nonpowered watercraft** 🔍
       Canoer hit by other nonpowered watercraft
       Surfer hit by other nonpowered watercraft
       Windsurfer hit by other nonpowered watercraft

    X● V94.22   **Rider of nonpowered watercraft struck by powered watercraft** 🔍
       Canoer hit by motorboat
       Surfer hit by motorboat
       Windsurfer hit by motorboat

● V94.3   **Injury to rider of (inflatable) watercraft being pulled behind other watercraft**

    X● V94.31   **Injury to rider of (inflatable) recreational watercraft being pulled behind other watercraft** 🔍
       Injury to rider of inner-tube pulled behind motor boat

    X● V94.32   **Injury to rider of non-recreational watercraft being pulled behind other watercraft** 🔍
       Injury to occupant of dingy being pulled behind boat or ship
       Injury to occupant of life-raft being pulled behind boat or ship

    X● V94.4   **Injury to barefoot water-skier** 🔍
       Injury to person being pulled behind boat or ship

● V94.8   **Other water transport accident**

    ● V94.81   **Water transport accident involving military watercraft**

       ● V94.810   **Civilian watercraft involved in water transport accident with military watercraft** 🔍
         Passenger on civilian watercraft injured due to accident with military watercraft

       ● V94.811   **Civilian in water injured by military watercraft** 🔍

       ● V94.818   **Other water transport accident involving military watercraft** 🔍

    X● V94.89   **Other water transport accident** 🔍

● X● V94.9   Unspecified **water transport accident** 🔍
       Water transport accident NOS

AIR AND SPACE TRANSPORT ACCIDENTS (V95-V97)

   Excludes1   military aircraft accidents in military or war operations (Y36, Y37) ◀▥

● V95   **Accident to powered aircraft causing injury to occupant**
      The appropriate 7th character is to be added to each code from category V95

A	initial encounter
D	subsequent encounter
S	sequela

   ● V95.0   **Helicopter accident injuring occupant**

    X● V95.00   Unspecified **helicopter accident injuring occupant** 🔍

    X● V95.01   **Helicopter crash injuring occupant** 🔍

    X● V95.02   **Forced landing of helicopter injuring occupant** 🔍

    X● V95.03   **Helicopter collision injuring occupant** 🔍
       Helicopter collision with any object, fixed, movable or moving

    X● V95.04   **Helicopter fire injuring occupant** 🔍

    X● V95.05   **Helicopter explosion injuring occupant** 🔍

    X● V95.09   **Other helicopter accident injuring occupant** 🔍

● V95.1   **Ultralight, microlight or powered-glider accident injuring occupant**

    X● V95.10   Unspecified **ultralight, microlight or powered-glider accident injuring occupant** 🔍

    X● V95.11   **Ultralight, microlight or powered-glider crash injuring occupant** 🔍

    X● V95.12   **Forced landing of ultralight, microlight or powered-glider injuring occupant** 🔍

    X● V95.13   **Ultralight, microlight or powered-glider collision injuring occupant** 🔍
       Ultralight, microlight or powered-glider collision with any object, fixed, movable or moving

    X● V95.14   **Ultralight, microlight or powered-glider fire injuring occupant** 🔍

    X● V95.15   **Ultralight, microlight or powered-glider explosion injuring occupant** 🔍

    X● V95.19   **Other ultralight, microlight or powered-glider accident injuring occupant** 🔍

● V95.2   **Other private fixed-wing aircraft accident injuring occupant**

    X● V95.20   Unspecified **accident to other private fixed-wing aircraft, injuring occupant** 🔍

    X● V95.21   **Other private fixed-wing aircraft crash injuring occupant** 🔍

    X● V95.22   **Forced landing of other private fixed-wing aircraft injuring occupant** 🔍

    X● V95.23   **Other private fixed-wing aircraft collision injuring occupant** 🔍
       Other private fixed-wing aircraft collision with any object, fixed, movable or moving

    X● V95.24   **Other private fixed-wing aircraft fire injuring occupant** 🔍

    X● V95.25   **Other private fixed-wing aircraft explosion injuring occupant** 🔍

    X● V95.29   **Other accident to other private fixed-wing aircraft injuring occupant** 🔍

● V95.3   **Commercial fixed-wing aircraft accident injuring occupant**

    X● V95.30   Unspecified **accident to commercial fixed-wing aircraft injuring occupant** 🔍

    X● V95.31   **Commercial fixed-wing aircraft crash injuring occupant** 🔍

    X● V95.32   **Forced landing of commercial fixed-wing aircraft injuring occupant** 🔍

    X● V95.33   **Commercial fixed-wing aircraft collision injuring occupant** 🔍
       Commercial fixed-wing aircraft collision with any object, fixed, movable or moving

    X● V95.34   **Commercial fixed-wing aircraft fire injuring occupant** 🔍

    X● V95.35   **Commercial fixed-wing aircraft explosion injuring occupant** 🔍

    X● V95.39   **Other accident to commercial fixed-wing aircraft injuring occupant** 🔍

● V95.4   **Spacecraft accident injuring occupant**

    X● V95.40   Unspecified **spacecraft accident injuring occupant** 🔍

    X● V95.41   **Spacecraft crash injuring occupant** 🔍

    X● V95.42   **Forced landing of spacecraft injuring occupant** 🔍

    X● V95.43   **Spacecraft collision injuring occupant** 🔍
       Spacecraft collision with any object, fixed, moveable or moving

    X● V95.44   **Spacecraft fire injuring occupant** 🔍

    X● V95.45   **Spacecraft explosion injuring occupant** 🔍

    X● V95.49   **Other spacecraft accident injuring occupant** 🔍

◀ New   ◀▥ Revised   ~~deleted~~ Deleted   Excludes 1   Excludes 2   Includes   Use additional   Code first   Code also   Unspecified

OGCR Official Guidelines   ● Unacceptable Principal Diagnosis   X Assign placeholder X   ● Use Additional Character(s)   ▌ Manifestation Code   **Coding Clinic**

X ● **V95.8**   Other powered aircraft accidents injuring occupant 🏥
X ● **V95.9**   Unspecified aircraft accident injuring occupant 🏥
     Aircraft accident NOS
     Air transport accident NOS

● **V96**   Accident to nonpowered aircraft causing injury to occupant
     The appropriate 7th character is to be added to each code from category V96

A	initial encounter
D	subsequent encounter
S	sequela

   ● **V96.0**   Balloon accident injuring occupant
     X ● **V96.00**   Unspecified balloon accident injuring occupant 🏥
     X ● **V96.01**   Balloon crash injuring occupant 🏥
     X ● **V96.02**   Forced landing of balloon injuring occupant 🏥
     X ● **V96.03**   Balloon collision injuring occupant 🏥
         Balloon collision with any object, fixed, moveable or moving
     X ● **V96.04**   Balloon fire injuring occupant 🏥
     X ● **V96.05**   Balloon explosion injuring occupant 🏥
     X ● **V96.09**   Other balloon accident injuring occupant 🏥
   ● **V96.1**   Hang-glider accident injuring occupant
     X ● **V96.10**   Unspecified hang-glider accident injuring occupant 🏥
     X ● **V96.11**   Hang-glider crash injuring occupant 🏥
     X ● **V96.12**   Forced landing of hang-glider injuring occupant 🏥
     X ● **V96.13**   Hang-glider collision injuring occupant 🏥
         Hang-glider collision with any object, fixed, moveable or moving
     X ● **V96.14**   Hang-glider fire injuring occupant 🏥
     X ● **V96.15**   Hang-glider explosion injuring occupant 🏥
     X ● **V96.19**   Other hang-glider accident injuring occupant 🏥
   ● **V96.2**   Glider (nonpowered) accident injuring occupant
     X ● **V96.20**   Unspecified glider (nonpowered) accident injuring occupant 🏥
     X ● **V96.21**   Glider (nonpowered) crash injuring occupant 🏥
     X ● **V96.22**   Forced landing of glider (nonpowered) injuring occupant 🏥
     X ● **V96.23**   Glider (nonpowered) collision injuring occupant 🏥
         Glider (nonpowered) collision with any object, fixed, moveable or moving
     X ● **V96.24**   Glider (nonpowered) fire injuring occupant 🏥
     X ● **V96.25**   Glider (nonpowered) explosion injuring occupant 🏥
     X ● **V96.29**   Other glider (nonpowered) accident injuring occupant 🏥
X ● **V96.8**   Other nonpowered-aircraft accidents injuring occupant 🏥
     Kite carrying a person accident injuring occupant
X ● **V96.9**   Unspecified nonpowered-aircraft accident injuring occupant 🏥
     Nonpowered-aircraft accident NOS

● **V97**   Other specified air transport accidents
     The appropriate 7th character is to be added to each code from category V97

A	initial encounter
D	subsequent encounter
S	sequela

X ● **V97.0**   Occupant of aircraft injured in other specified air transport accidents 🏥
     Fall in, on or from aircraft in air transport accident
     Excludes1   accident while boarding or alighting aircraft (V97.1)
X ● **V97.1**   Person injured while boarding or alighting from aircraft 🏥
   ● **V97.2**   Parachutist accident
     X ● **V97.21**   Parachutist entangled in object 🏥
         Parachutist landing in tree
     X ● **V97.22**   Parachutist injured on landing 🏥
     X ● **V97.29**   Other parachutist accident 🏥
   ● **V97.3**   Person on ground injured in air transport accident
     X ● **V97.31**   Hit by object falling from aircraft 🏥
         Hit by crashing aircraft
         Injured by aircraft hitting house
         Injured by aircraft hitting car
     X ● **V97.32**   Injured by rotating propeller 🏥
     X ● **V97.33**   Sucked into jet engine 🏥
     X ● **V97.39**   Other injury to person on ground due to air transport accident 🏥
   ● **V97.8**   Other air transport accidents, not elsewhere classified
     Excludes1   aircraft accident NOS (V95.9)
         exposure to changes in air pressure during ascent or descent (W94.-)
     ● **V97.81**   Air transport accident involving military aircraft
       ● **V97.810**   Civilian aircraft involved in air transport accident with military aircraft 🏥
         Passenger in civilian aircraft injured due to accident with military aircraft
       ● **V97.811**   Civilian injured by military aircraft 🏥
       ● **V97.818**   Other air transport accident involving military aircraft 🏥
     X ● **V97.89**   Other air transport accidents, not elsewhere classified 🏥
         Injury from machinery on aircraft

OTHER AND UNSPECIFIED TRANSPORT ACCIDENTS (V98-V99)

Excludes1   vehicle accident, type of vehicle unspecified (V89.-)

● **V98**   Other specified transport accidents
     The appropriate 7th character is to be added to each code from category V98

A	initial encounter
D	subsequent encounter
S	sequela

X ● **V98.0**   Accident to, on or involving cable-car, not on rails 🏥
     Caught or dragged by cable-car, not on rails
     Fall or jump from cable-car, not on rails
     Object thrown from or in cable-car, not on rails
X ● **V98.1**   Accident to, on or involving land-yacht 🏥
X ● **V98.2**   Accident to, on or involving ice yacht 🏥
X ● **V98.3**   Accident to, on or involving ski lift 🏥
     Accident to, on or involving ski chair-lift
     Accident to, on or involving ski-lift with gondola
X ● **V98.8**   Other specified transport accidents 🏥

N Newborn Age: 0   **P** Pediatric Age: 0–17   **M** Maternity DX: 12–55   **A** Adult Age: 15–124   ♀ Females Only   ♂ Males Only
🏥 Complication\Comorbidity   🏥 Major C\C   (Ex) CC/MCC Exclusions   🏥 Present on Admission Requirement   🏥 Hospital-Acquired Condition

1627

X ● **V99**   Unspecified **transport accident** 🔊

     The appropriate 7th character is to be added to code V99

        A   initial encounter
        D   subsequent encounter
        S   sequela

OTHER EXTERNAL CAUSES OF ACCIDENTAL INJURY (W00-X58)

SLIPPING, TRIPPING, STUMBLING AND FALLS (W00-W19)

     Excludes1   assault involving a fall (Y01-Y02)
                 fall from animal (V80.-) ◀▥
                 ~~animal (V80.-)~~
                 fall (in) (from) machinery (in operation)
                       (W28-W31) ◀▥
                 fall (in) (from) transport vehicle (V01-V99) ◀▥
                 intentional self-harm involving a fall (X80-X81)
     Excludes2   at risk for fall (history of fall) Z91.81
                 fall (in) (from) burning building (X00.-) ◀▥
                 ~~burning building (X00.-)~~
                 fall into fire (X00-X04, X08-X09) ◀▥

● **W00**   **Fall due to ice and snow**
      Includes   pedestrian on foot falling (slipping) on ice and
                       snow
      Excludes1   fall on (from) ice and snow involving pedestrian
                       conveyance (V00.-)
                     fall from stairs and steps not due to ice and snow
                       (W10.-)

     The appropriate 7th character is to be added to each code from
        category W00

        A   initial encounter
        D   subsequent encounter
        S   sequela

X ● **W00.0**   **Fall on same level due to ice and snow**

X ● **W00.1**   **Fall from stairs and steps due to ice and snow**

X ● **W00.2**   **Other fall from one level to another due to ice and snow**

X ● **W00.9**   Unspecified **fall due to ice and snow**

● **W01**   **Fall on same level from slipping, tripping and stumbling**
      Includes   fall on moving sidewalk
      Excludes1   fall due to bumping (striking) against object
                       (W18.0-)
                     fall in shower or bathtub (W18.2-)
                     fall on same level NOS (W18.30)
                     fall on same level from slipping, tripping and
                       stumbling due to ice or snow (W00.0)
                     fall off or from toilet (W18.1-)
                     slipping, tripping and stumbling NOS (W18.40)
                     slipping, tripping and stumbling without falling
                       (W18.4-)

     The appropriate 7th character is to be added to each code from
        category W01

        A   initial encounter
        D   subsequent encounter
        S   sequela

X ● **W01.0**   **Fall on same level from slipping, tripping and
             stumbling without subsequent striking against object**
             Falling over animal

● **W01.1**   **Fall on same level from slipping, tripping and
             stumbling with subsequent striking against object**

X ● **W01.10**   **Fall on same level from slipping, tripping and
                 stumbling with subsequent striking against
                ** unspecified **object**

● **W01.11**   **Fall on same level from slipping, tripping and
                 stumbling with subsequent striking against
                 sharp object**

     ● **W01.110**   **Fall on same level from slipping,
                      tripping and stumbling with
                      subsequent striking against sharp
                      glass**

     ● **W01.111**   **Fall on same level from slipping,
                      tripping and stumbling with
                      subsequent striking against power
                      tool or machine**

     ● **W01.118**   **Fall on same level from slipping,
                      tripping and stumbling with
                      subsequent striking against other
                      sharp object**

     ● **W01.119**   **Fall on same level from slipping,
                      tripping and stumbling with
                      subsequent striking against
                     ** unspecified **sharp object**

● **W01.19**   **Fall on same level from slipping, tripping and
                 stumbling with subsequent striking against
                 other object**

     ● **W01.190**   **Fall on same level from slipping,
                      tripping and stumbling with
                      subsequent striking against furniture**

     ● **W01.198**   **Fall on same level from slipping,
                      tripping and stumbling with
                      subsequent striking against other
                      object**

X ● **W03**   **Other fall on same level due to collision with another person**
        Fall due to non-transport collision with other person
      Excludes1   collision with another person without fall (W51)
                     crushed or pushed by a crowd or human
                       stampede (W52)
                   fall involving pedestrian conveyance (V00-V09)
                   fall due to ice or snow (W00)
                   fall on same level NOS (W18.30)

     The appropriate 7th character is to be added to code W03

        A   initial encounter
        D   subsequent encounter
        S   sequela

Coding Clinic: 2012, Q4, P108

X ● **W04**   **Fall while being carried or supported by other persons**
        Accidentally dropped while being carried

     The appropriate 7th character is to be added to code W04

        A   initial encounter
        D   subsequent encounter
        S   sequel

● **W05**   **Fall from non-moving wheelchair, nonmotorized scooter and
        motorized mobility scooter**
      Excludes1   fall from moving wheelchair (powered) (V00.811)
                     fall from moving motorized mobility scooter
                       (V00.831)
                   fall from nonmotorized scooter (V00.141)

     The appropriate 7th character is to be added to each code from
        category W05

        A   initial encounter
        D   subsequent encounter
        S   sequela

X ● **W05.0**   **Fall from non-moving wheelchair**

X ● **W05.1**   **Fall from non-moving nonmotorized scooter**

X ● **W05.2**   **Fall from non-moving motorized mobility scooter**

◀ New   ◀▥ Revised   ~~deleted~~ Deleted   Excludes 1   Excludes 2   Includes   Use additional   Code first   Code also   Unspecified

OGCR Official Guidelines   ● Unacceptable Principal Diagnosis   X Assign placeholder X   ▐ Use Additional Character(s)   ▷ Manifestation Code   **Coding Clinic**

X ● **W06 Fall from bed**
  The appropriate 7th character is to be added to code W06

A	initial encounter
D	subsequent encounter
S	sequela

X ● **W07 Fall from chair**
  The appropriate 7th character is to be added to code W07

A	initial encounter
D	subsequent encounter
S	sequela

X ● **W08 Fall from other furniture**
  The appropriate 7th character is to be added to code W08

A	initial encounter
D	subsequent encounter
S	sequela

● **W09 Fall on and from playground equipment**
  Excludes1 fall involving recreational machinery (W31)
  The appropriate 7th character is to be added to each code from category W09

A	initial encounter
D	subsequent encounter
S	sequela

  X ● **W09.0 Fall on or from playground slide** 🔖
  X ● **W09.1 Fall from playground swing** 🔖
  X ● **W09.2 Fall on or from jungle gym** 🔖
  X ● **W09.8 Fall on or from other playground equipment** 🔖

● **W10 Fall on and from stairs and steps**
  Excludes1 fall from stairs and steps due to ice and snow (W00.1)
  The appropriate 7th character is to be added to each code from category W10

A	initial encounter
D	subsequent encounter
S	sequela

  X ● **W10.0 Fall (on) (from) escalator**
  X ● **W10.1 Fall (on) (from) sidewalk curb**
  X ● **W10.2 Fall (on) (from) incline**
       Fall (on) (from) ramp
  X ● **W10.8 Fall (on) (from) other stairs and steps**
  X ● **W10.9 Fall (on) (from) unspecified stairs and steps**

X ● **W11 Fall on and from ladder**
  The appropriate 7th character is to be added to code W11

A	initial encounter
D	subsequent encounter
S	sequela

X ● **W12 Fall on and from scaffolding**
  The appropriate 7th character is to be added to code W12

A	initial encounter
D	subsequent encounter
S	sequela

● **W13 Fall from, out of or through building or structure**
  The appropriate 7th character is to be added to each code from category W13

A	initial encounter
D	subsequent encounter
S	sequela

  X ● **W13.0 Fall from, out of or through balcony**
       Fall from, out of or through railing
  X ● **W13.1 Fall from, out of or through bridge**
  X ● **W13.2 Fall from, out of or through roof**
  X ● **W13.3 Fall through floor**
  X ● **W13.4 Fall from, out of or through window**
       Excludes2 fall with subsequent striking against sharp glass (W01.110)
  X ● **W13.8 Fall from, out of or through other building or structure**
       Fall from, out of or through viaduct
       Fall from, out of or through wall
       Fall from, out of or through flag-pole
  X ● **W13.9 Fall from, out of or through building, not otherwise specified**
       Excludes1 collapse of a building or structure (W20.-)
                    fall or jump from burning building or structure (X00.-)

X ● **W14 Fall from tree** 🔖
  The appropriate 7th character is to be added to code W14

A	initial encounter
D	subsequent encounter
S	sequela

X ● **W15 Fall from cliff** 🔖
  The appropriate 7th character is to be added to code W15

A	initial encounter
D	subsequent encounter
S	sequela

● **W16 Fall, jump or diving into water**
  Excludes1 accidental non-watercraft drowning and submersion not involving fall (W65-W74)
               effects of air pressure from diving (W94.-)
               fall into water from watercraft (V90-V94)
               hitting an object or against bottom when falling from watercraft (V94.0)
  Excludes2 striking or hitting diving board (W21.4) ◀▥
  The appropriate 7th character is to be added to each code from category W16

A	initial encounter
D	subsequent encounter
S	sequela

  ● **W16.0 Fall into swimming pool**
       Fall into swimming pool NOS
       Excludes1 fall into empty swimming pool (W17.3)
  ● **W16.01 Fall into swimming pool striking water surface**
       ● **W16.011 Fall into swimming pool striking water surface causing drowning and submersion**
            Excludes1 drowning and submersion while in swimming pool without fall (W67)
       ● **W16.012 Fall into swimming pool striking water surface causing other injury**

N Newborn Age: 0   **P** Pediatric Age: 0–17   **M** Maternity DX: 12–55   **A** Adult Age: 15–124   ♀ Females Only   ♂ Males Only

🔖 Complication\Comorbidity   🔖 Major C\C   Ⓔⓧ CC/MCC Exclusions   🔖 Present on Admission Requirement   🔖 Hospital-Acquired Condition

1629

● W16.02   Fall into swimming pool striking bottom
    ● W16.021   Fall into swimming pool striking bottom causing drowning and submersion
        Excludes1   drowning and submersion while in swimming pool without fall (W67)
    ● W16.022   Fall into swimming pool striking bottom causing other injury
● W16.03   Fall into swimming pool striking wall
    ● W16.031   Fall into swimming pool striking wall causing drowning and submersion
        Excludes1   drowning and submersion while in swimming pool without fall (W67)
    ● W16.032   Fall into swimming pool striking wall causing other injury
● W16.1   Fall into natural body of water
    Fall into lake
    Fall into open sea
    Fall into river
    Fall into stream
    ● W16.11   Fall into natural body of water striking water surface
        ● W16.111   Fall into natural body of water striking water surface causing drowning and submersion
            Excludes1   drowning and submersion while in natural body of water without fall (W69)
        ● W16.112   Fall into natural body of water striking water surface causing other injury
    ● W16.12   Fall into natural body of water striking bottom
        ● W16.121   Fall into natural body of water striking bottom causing drowning and submersion
            Excludes1   drowning and submersion while in natural body of water without fall (W69)
        ● W16.122   Fall into natural body of water striking bottom causing other injury
    ● W16.13   Fall into natural body of water striking side
        ● W16.131   Fall into natural body of water striking side causing drowning and submersion
            Excludes1   drowning and submersion while in natural body of water without fall (W69)
        ● W16.132   Fall into natural body of water striking side causing other injury
● W16.2   Fall in (into) filled bathtub or bucket of water
    ● W16.21   Fall in (into) filled bathtub
        Excludes1   fall into empty bathtub (W18.2)
        ● W16.211   Fall in (into) filled bathtub causing drowning and submersion
            Excludes1   drowning and submersion while in filled bathtub without fall (W65)
        ● W16.212   Fall in (into) filled bathtub causing other injury

● W16.22   Fall in (into) bucket of water
    ● W16.221   Fall in (into) bucket of water causing drowning and submersion
    ● W16.222   Fall in (into) bucket of water causing other injury
● W16.3   Fall into other water
    Fall into fountain
    Fall into reservoir
    ● W16.31   Fall into other water striking water surface
        ● W16.311   Fall into other water striking water surface causing drowning and submersion
            Excludes1   drowning and submersion while in other water without fall (W73)
        ● W16.312   Fall into other water striking water surface causing other injury
    ● W16.32   Fall into other water striking bottom
        ● W16.321   Fall into other water striking bottom causing drowning and submersion
            Excludes1   drowning and submersion while in other water without fall (W73)
        ● W16.322   Fall into other water striking bottom causing other injury
    ● W16.33   Fall into other water striking wall
        ● W16.331   Fall into other water striking wall causing drowning and submersion
            Excludes1   drowning and submersion while in other water without fall (W73)
        ● W16.332   Fall into other water striking wall causing other injury
● W16.4   Fall into unspecified water
  X ● W16.41   Fall into unspecified water causing drowning and submersion
  X ● W16.42   Fall into unspecified water causing other injury
● W16.5   Jumping or diving into swimming pool
    ● W16.51   Jumping or diving into swimming pool striking water surface
        ● W16.511   Jumping or diving into swimming pool striking water surface causing drowning and submersion
            Excludes1   drowning and submersion while in swimming pool without jumping or diving (W67)
        ● W16.512   Jumping or diving into swimming pool striking water surface causing other injury
    ● W16.52   Jumping or diving into swimming pool striking bottom
        ● W16.521   Jumping or diving into swimming pool striking bottom causing drowning and submersion
            Excludes1   drowning and submersion while in swimming pool without jumping or diving (W67)
        ● W16.522   Jumping or diving into swimming pool striking bottom causing other injury

◄ New   ◄═ Revised   ~~deleted~~ Deleted   Excludes 1   Excludes 2   Includes   Use additional   Code first   Code also   Unspecified
OGCR Official Guidelines   ● Unacceptable Principal Diagnosis   X Assign placeholder X   ▌ Use Additional Character(s)   ▌ Manifestation Code   Coding Clinic

● **W16.53** **Jumping or diving into swimming pool striking wall**

  ● **W16.531** **Jumping or diving into swimming pool striking wall causing drowning and submersion**

     Excludes1   drowning and submersion while in swimming pool without jumping or diving (W67)

  ● **W16.532** **Jumping or diving into swimming pool striking wall causing other injury**

● **W16.6** **Jumping or diving into natural body of water**

   Jumping or diving into lake
   Jumping or diving into open sea
   Jumping or diving into river
   Jumping or diving into stream

  ● **W16.61** **Jumping or diving into natural body of water striking water surface**

    ● **W16.611** **Jumping or diving into natural body of water striking water surface causing drowning and submersion**

       Excludes1   drowning and submersion while in natural body of water without jumping or diving (W69)

    ● **W16.612** **Jumping or diving into natural body of water striking water surface causing other injury**

  ● **W16.62** **Jumping or diving into natural body of water striking bottom**

    ● **W16.621** **Jumping or diving into natural body of water striking bottom causing drowning and submersion**

       Excludes1   drowning and submersion while in natural body of water without jumping or diving (W69)

    ● **W16.622** **Jumping or diving into natural body of water striking bottom causing other injury**

● **W16.7** **Jumping or diving from boat**

   Excludes1   fall from boat into water - see watercraft accident (V90-V94)

  ● **W16.71** **Jumping or diving from boat striking water surface**

    ● **W16.711** **Jumping or diving from boat striking water surface causing drowning and submersion**

    ● **W16.712** **Jumping or diving from boat striking water surface causing other injury**

  ● **W16.72** **Jumping or diving from boat striking bottom**

    ● **W16.721** **Jumping or diving from boat striking bottom causing drowning and submersion**

    ● **W16.722** **Jumping or diving from boat striking bottom causing other injury**

● **W16.8** **Jumping or diving into other water**

   Jumping or diving into fountain
   Jumping or diving into reservoir

  ● **W16.81** **Jumping or diving into other water striking water surface**

    ● **W16.811** **Jumping or diving into other water striking water surface causing drowning and submersion**

       Excludes1   drowning and submersion while in other water without jumping or diving (W73)

    ● **W16.812** **Jumping or diving into other water striking water surface causing other injury**

  ● **W16.82** **Jumping or diving into other water striking bottom**

    ● **W16.821** **Jumping or diving into other water striking bottom causing drowning and submersion**

       Excludes1   drowning and submersion while in other water without jumping or diving (W73)

    ● **W16.822** **Jumping or diving into other water striking bottom causing other injury**

  ● **W16.83** **Jumping or diving into other water striking wall**

    ● **W16.831** **Jumping or diving into other water striking wall causing drowning and submersion**

       Excludes1   drowning and submersion while in other water without jumping or diving (W73)

    ● **W16.832** **Jumping or diving into other water striking wall causing other injury**

● **W16.9** **Jumping or diving into unspecified water**

  X ● **W16.91** **Jumping or diving into unspecified water causing drowning and submersion**

  X ● **W16.92** **Jumping or diving into unspecified water causing other injury**

● **W17** **Other fall from one level to another**

   The appropriate 7th character is to be added to each code from category W17

     | | |
     A   initial encounter
     D   subsequent encounter
     S   sequela

X ● **W17.0** **Fall into well**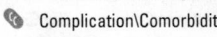

X ● **W17.1** **Fall into storm drain or manhole**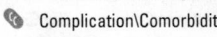

X ● **W17.2** **Fall into hole**

   Fall into pit

X ● **W17.3** **Fall into empty swimming pool**

   Excludes1   fall into filled swimming pool (W16.0-)

X ● **W17.4** **Fall from dock**

● **W17.8** **Other fall from one level to another**

  X ● **W17.81** **Fall down embankment (hill)**

  X ● **W17.82** **Fall from (out of) grocery cart**

     Fall due to grocery cart tipping over

  X ● **W17.89** **Other fall from one level to another**

     Fall from cherry picker
     Fall from lifting device
     Fall from mobile elevated work platform [MEWP]
     Fall from sky lift

CHAPTER 20 (V01-Y99)

N Newborn Age: 0   **P** Pediatric Age: 0–17   **M** Maternity DX: 12–55   **A** Adult Age: 15–124   ♀ Females Only   ♂ Males Only

 Complication\Comorbidity   Major C\C   CC/MCC Exclusions   Present on Admission Requirement   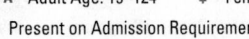 Hospital-Acquired Condition   **1631**

● **W18   Other slipping, tripping and stumbling and falls**

The appropriate 7th character is to be added to each code from category W18

> A   initial encounter
> D   subsequent encounter
> S   sequela

● **W18.0   Fall due to bumping against object**

Striking against object with subsequent fall

> **Excludes1**   fall on same level due to slipping, tripping, or stumbling with subsequent striking against object (W01.1-)

X ● **W18.00   Striking against unspecified object with subsequent fall**

X ● **W18.01   Striking against sports equipment with subsequent fall** 🔍

X ● **W18.02   Striking against glass with subsequent fall**

X ● **W18.09   Striking against other object with subsequent fall**

● **W18.1   Fall from or off toilet**

X ● **W18.11   Fall from or off toilet without subsequent striking against object**

Fall from (off) toilet NOS

X ● **W18.12   Fall from or off toilet with subsequent striking against object**

X ● **W18.2   Fall in (into) shower or empty bathtub**

> **Excludes1**   fall in full bathtub causing drowning or submersion (W16.21-)

● **W18.3   Other and unspecified fall on same level**

X ● **W18.30   Fall on same level, unspecified**

X ● **W18.31   Fall on same level due to stepping on an object**

Fall on same level due to stepping on an animal

> **Excludes1**   slipping, tripping and stumbling without fall due to stepping on animal (W18.41)

X ● **W18.39   Other fall on same level**

● **W18.4   Slipping, tripping and stumbling without falling**

> **Excludes1**   collision with another person without fall (W51)

X ● **W18.40   Slipping, tripping and stumbling without falling, unspecified**

X ● **W18.41   Slipping, tripping and stumbling without falling due to stepping on object**

Slipping, tripping and stumbling without falling due to stepping on animal

> **Excludes1**   slipping, tripping and stumbling with fall due to stepping on animal (W18.31)

X ● **W18.42   Slipping, tripping and stumbling without falling due to stepping into hole or opening**

X ● **W18.43   Slipping, tripping and stumbling without falling due to stepping from one level to another**

X ● **W18.49   Other slipping, tripping and stumbling without falling**

X ● **W19   Unspecified fall**

Accidental fall NOS

The appropriate 7th character is to be added to code W19

> A   initial encounter
> D   subsequent encounter
> S   sequela

Coding Clinic: 2012, Q4, P95

EXPOSURE TO INANIMATE MECHANICAL FORCES (W20-W49)

> **Excludes1**   assault (X92-Y08)
> contact or collision with animals or persons (W50-W64)
> exposure to inanimate mechanical forces involving military or war operations (Y36.-, Y37.-)
> intentional self-harm (X71-X83)

● **W20   Struck by thrown, projected or falling object**

Code first any associated:
cataclysm (X34-X39)
lightning strike (T75.00)

> **Excludes1**   falling object in machinery accident (W24, W28-W31) ◀
> ~~machinery accident (W24, W28-W31)~~
> falling object in transport accident (V01-V99) ◀
> object set in motion by explosion (W35-W40) ◀
> ~~explosion (W35-W40)~~
> object set in motion by firearm (W32-W34) ◀
> struck by thrown sports equipment (W21.-)

The appropriate 7th character is to be added to each code from category W20

> A   initial encounter
> D   subsequent encounter
> S   sequela

X ● **W20.0   Struck by falling object in cave-in**

> **Excludes2**   asphyxiation due to cave-in (T71.21)

X ● **W20.1   Struck by object due to collapse of building**

> **Excludes1**   struck by object due to collapse of burning building (X00.2, X02.2)

X ● **W20.8   Other cause of strike by thrown, projected or falling object**

> **Excludes1**   struck by thrown sports equipment (W21.-)

● **W21   Striking against or struck by sports equipment**

> **Excludes1**   assault with sports equipment (Y08.0-)
> striking against or struck by sports equipment with subsequent fall (W18.01)

The appropriate 7th character is to be added to each code from category W21

> A   initial encounter
> D   subsequent encounter
> S   sequela

● **W21.0   Struck by hit or thrown ball**

X ● **W21.00   Struck by hit or thrown ball, unspecified type** 🔍

X ● **W21.01   Struck by football** 🔍

X ● **W21.02   Struck by soccer ball** 🔍

X ● **W21.03   Struck by baseball** 🔍

X ● **W21.04   Struck by golf ball** 🔍

X ● **W21.05   Struck by basketball** 🔍

X ● **W21.06   Struck by volleyball** 🔍

X ● **W21.07   Struck by softball** 🔍

X ● **W21.09   Struck by other hit or thrown ball** 🔍

● **W21.1   Struck by bat, racquet or club**

X ● **W21.11   Struck by baseball bat** 🔍

X ● **W21.12   Struck by tennis racquet** 🔍

X ● **W21.13   Struck by golf club** 🔍

X ● **W21.19   Struck by other bat, racquet or club** 🔍

◀ New   ◀▦ Revised   ~~deleted~~ Deleted   Excludes 1   Excludes 2   Includes   Use additional   Code first   Code also   Unspecified

OGCR Official Guidelines   ● Unacceptable Principal Diagnosis   X Assign placeholder X   ● Use Additional Character(s)   ▸ Manifestation Code   **Coding Clinic**

● W21.2 Struck by hockey stick or puck
  ● W21.21 Struck by hockey stick
    ● W21.210 Struck by ice hockey stick 🗅
    ● W21.211 Struck by field hockey stick 🗅
  ● W21.22 Struck by hockey puck
    ● W21.220 Struck by ice hockey puck 🗅
    ● W21.221 Struck by field hockey puck 🗅
● W21.3 Struck by sports foot wear
 X ● W21.31 Struck by shoe cleats 🗅
    Stepped on by shoe cleats
 X ● W21.32 Struck by skate blades 🗅
    Skated over by skate blades
 X ● W21.39 Struck by other sports foot wear 🗅
X ● W21.4 Striking against diving board 🗅
    Use additional code for subsequent falling into water, if applicable (W16.-)
● W21.8 Striking against or struck by other sports equipment
 X ● W21.81 Striking against or struck by football helmet 🗅
 X ● W21.89 Striking against or struck by other sports equipment 🗅
X ● W21.9 Striking against or struck by `unspecified` sports equipment 🗅

● W22 Striking against or struck by other objects
  `Excludes1` striking against or struck by object with subsequent fall (W18.09)
  The appropriate 7th character is to be added to each code from category W22

A	initial encounter
D	subsequent encounter
S	sequela

● W22.0 Striking against stationary object
  `Excludes1` striking against stationary sports equipment (W21.8)
 X ● W22.01 Walked into wall
 X ● W22.02 Walked into lamppost
 X ● W22.03 Walked into furniture
  ● W22.04 Striking against wall of swimming pool
    ● W22.041 Striking against wall of swimming pool causing drowning and submersion
      `Excludes1` drowning and submersion while swimming without striking against wall (W67)
    ● W22.042 Striking against wall of swimming pool causing other injury
 X ● W22.09 Striking against other stationary object
● W22.1 Striking against or struck by automobile airbag
 X ● W22.10 Striking against or struck by `unspecified` automobile airbag
 X ● W22.11 Striking against or struck by driver side automobile airbag
 X ● W22.12 Striking against or struck by front passenger side automobile airbag
 X ● W22.19 Striking against or struck by other automobile airbag
X ● W22.8 Striking against or struck by other objects
  Striking against or struck by object NOS
  `Excludes1` struck by thrown, projected or falling object (W20.-)

● W23 Caught, crushed, jammed or pinched in or between objects
  `Excludes1` injury caused by cutting or piercing instruments (W25-W27)
    injury caused by firearms malfunction (W32.1, W33.1-, W34.1-)
    injury caused by lifting and transmission devices (W24.-)
    injury caused by machinery (W28-W31)
    injury caused by nonpowered hand tools (W27.-)
    injury caused by transport vehicle being used as a means of transportation (V01-V99)
    injury caused by struck by thrown, projected or falling object (W20.-)
  The appropriate 7th character is to be added to each code from category W23

A	initial encounter
D	subsequent encounter
S	sequela

X ● W23.0 Caught, crushed, jammed, or pinched between moving objects
X ● W23.1 Caught, crushed, jammed, or pinched between stationary objects

● W24 Contact with lifting and transmission devices, not elsewhere classified
  `Excludes1` transport accidents (V01-V99)
  The appropriate 7th character is to be added to each code from category W24

A	initial encounter
D	subsequent encounter
S	sequela

X ● W24.0 Contact with lifting devices, not elsewhere classified
  Contact with chain hoist
  Contact with drive belt
  Contact with pulley (block)
X ● W24.1 Contact with transmission devices, not elsewhere classified
  Contact with transmission belt or cable

X ● W25 Contact with sharp glass
  Code first any associated:
    injury due to flying glass from explosion or firearm discharge (W32-W40)
    transport accident (V00-V99)
  `Excludes1` fall on same level due to slipping, tripping and stumbling with subsequent striking against sharp glass (W01.10)
    striking against sharp glass with subsequent fall (W18.02)
  The appropriate 7th character is to be added to code W25

A	initial encounter
D	subsequent encounter
S	sequela

● W26 Contact with knife, sword or dagger
  The appropriate 7th character is to be added to each code from category W26

A	initial encounter
D	subsequent encounter
S	sequela

X ● W26.0 Contact with knife
  `Excludes1` contact with electric knife (W29.1)
X ● W26.1 Contact with sword or dagger

N Newborn Age: 0   P Pediatric Age: 0–17   M Maternity DX: 12–55   A Adult Age: 15–124   ♀ Females Only   ♂ Males Only

🗅 Complication\Comorbidity   🗅 Major C\C   (Ex) CC/MCC Exclusions   🗅 Present on Admission Requirement   🗅 Hospital-Acquired Condition   **1633**

● **W27 Contact with nonpowered hand tool**

The appropriate 7th character is to be added to each code from category W27

A	initial encounter
D	subsequent encounter
S	sequela

X● **W27.0 Contact with workbench tool**
Contact with auger
Contact with axe
Contact with chisel
Contact with handsaw
Contact with screwdriver

X● **W27.1 Contact with garden tool**
Contact with hoe
Contact with nonpowered lawn mower
Contact with pitchfork
Contact with rake

X● **W27.2 Contact with scissors**

X● **W27.3 Contact with needle (sewing)**
Excludes1 contact with hypodermic needle (W46.-)

X● **W27.4 Contact with kitchen utensil**
Contact with fork
Contact with ice-pick
Contact with can-opener NOS

X● **W27.5 Contact with paper-cutter**

X● **W27.8 Contact with other nonpowered hand tool**
Contact with nonpowered sewing machine
Contact with shovel

X● **W28 Contact with powered lawn mower**
Powered lawn mower (commercial) (residential)
Excludes1 contact with nonpowered lawn mower (W27.1)
Excludes2 exposure to electric current (W86.-)
The appropriate 7th character is to be added to code W28

A	initial encounter
D	subsequent encounter
S	sequela

● **W29 Contact with other powered hand tools and household machinery**
Excludes1 contact with commercial machinery (W31.82)
contact with hot household appliance (X15)
contact with nonpowered hand tool (W27.-)
exposure to electric current (W86)

The appropriate 7th character is to be added to each code from category W29

A	initial encounter
D	subsequent encounter
S	sequela

X● **W29.0 Contact with powered kitchen appliance**
Contact with blender
Contact with can-opener
Contact with garbage disposal
Contact with mixer

X● **W29.1 Contact with electric knife**

X● **W29.2 Contact with other powered household machinery**
Contact with electric fan
Contact with powered dryer (clothes) (powered) (spin)
Contact with washing-machine
Contact with sewing machine

X● **W29.3 Contact with powered garden and outdoor hand tools and machinery**
Contact with chainsaw
Contact with edger
Contact with garden cultivator (tiller)
Contact with hedge trimmer
Contact with other powered garden tool
Excludes1 contact with powered lawn mower (W28)

X● **W29.4 Contact with nail gun**

X● **W29.8 Contact with other powered powered hand tools and household machinery**
Contact with do-it-yourself tool NOS

● **W30 Contact with agricultural machinery**
Includes animal-powered farm machine
Excludes1 agricultural transport vehicle accident (V01-V99)
explosion of grain store (W40.8)
exposure to electric current (W86.-)

The appropriate 7th character is to be added to each code from category W30

A	initial encounter
D	subsequent encounter
S	sequela

X● **W30.0 Contact with combine harvester** 🔖
Contact with reaper
Contact with thresher

X● **W30.1 Contact with power take-off devices (PTO)** 🔖

X● **W30.2 Contact with hay derrick** 🔖

X● **W30.3 Contact with grain storage elevator** 🔖
Excludes1 explosion of grain store (W40.8)

● **W30.8 Contact with other specified agricultural machinery**

X● **W30.81 Contact with agricultural transport vehicle in stationary use** 🔖
Contact with agricultural transport vehicle under repair, not on public roadway
Excludes1 agricultural transport vehicle accident (V01-V99)

X● **W30.89 Contact with other specified agricultural machinery** 🔖

X● **W30.9 Contact with unspecified agricultural machinery** 🔖
Contact with farm machinery NOS

● **W31 Contact with other and unspecified machinery**
Excludes1 contact with agricultural machinery (W30.-)
contact with machinery in transport under own power or being towed by a vehicle (V01-V99)
exposure to electric current (W86)

The appropriate 7th character is to be added to each code from category W31

A	initial encounter
D	subsequent encounter
S	sequela

X● **W31.0 Contact with mining and earth-drilling machinery** 🔖
Contact with bore or drill (land) (seabed)
Contact with shaft hoist
Contact with shaft lift
Contact with undercutter

X● **W31.1 Contact with metalworking machines** 🔖
Contact with abrasive wheel
Contact with forging machine
Contact with lathe
Contact with mechanical shears
Contact with metal drilling machine
Contact with milling machine
Contact with power press
Contact with rolling-mill
Contact with metal sawing machine

X● **W31.2 Contact with powered woodworking and forming machines** 🔖
Contact with band saw
Contact with bench saw
Contact with circular saw
Contact with molding machine
Contact with overhead plane
Contact with powered saw
Contact with radial saw
Contact with sander
Excludes1 nonpowered woodworking tools (W27.0)

◀ New ◄═ Revised ~~deleted~~ Deleted Excludes 1 Excludes 2 Includes Use additional Code first Code also Unspecified
OGCR Official Guidelines ● Unacceptable Principal Diagnosis X Assign placeholder X ● Use Additional Character(s) ▶ Manifestation Code **Coding Clinic**

X● **W31.3**   **Contact with prime movers** 🖐
     Contact with gas turbine
     Contact with internal combustion engine
     Contact with steam engine
     Contact with water driven turbine

● **W31.8**   **Contact with other specified machinery**

   X● **W31.81**   **Contact with recreational machinery** 🖐
       Contact with roller-coaster

   X● **W31.82**   **Contact with other commercial machinery** 🖐
       Contact with commercial electric fan
       Contact with commercial kitchen appliances
       Contact with commercial powered dryer
         (clothes) (powered) (spin)
       Contact with commercial washing-machine
       Contact with commercial sewing machine

       Excludes1   contact with household
                 machinery (W29.-)
              contact with powered lawn
                 mower (W28)

   X● **W31.83**   **Contact with special construction vehicle in stationary use** 🖐
       Contact with special construction vehicle
         under repair, not on public roadway

       Excludes1   special construction vehicle
                 accident (V01-V99)

   X● **W31.89**   **Contact with other specified machinery** 🖐

X● **W31.9**   **Contact with unspecified machinery** 🖐
     Contact with machinery NOS

● **W32**   **Accidental handgun discharge and malfunction**

     Includes   accidental discharge and malfunction of gun for
          single hand use
         accidental discharge and malfunction of pistol
         accidental discharge and malfunction of revolver
         handgun discharge and malfunction NOS

     Excludes1   accidental airgun discharge and malfunction
          (W34.010, W34.110)
         accidental BB gun discharge and malfunction
          (W34.010, W34.110)
         accidental pellet gun discharge and malfunction
          (W34.010, W34.110)
         accidental shotgun discharge and malfunction
          (W33.01, W33.11)
         assault by handgun discharge (X93)
         handgun discharge involving legal intervention
          (Y35.0-)
         handgun discharge involving military or war
          operations (Y36.4-)
         intentional self-harm by handgun discharge (X72)
         Very pistol discharge and malfunction (W34.09,
          W34.19)

The appropriate 7th character is to be added to each code from
   category W32

A	initial encounter
D	subsequent encounter
S	sequela

X● **W32.0**   **Accidental handgun discharge** 🖐
X● **W32.1**   **Accidental handgun malfunction** 🖐
     Injury due to explosion of handgun (parts)
     Injury due to malfunction of mechanism or component
       of handgun
     Injury due to recoil of handgun
     Powder burn from handgun

● **W33**   **Accidental rifle, shotgun and larger firearm discharge and malfunction**

     Includes   rifle, shotgun and larger firearm discharge and
          malfunction NOS

     Excludes1   accidental airgun discharge and malfunction
          (W34.010, W34.110)
         accidental BB gun discharge and malfunction
          (W34.010, W34.110)
         accidental handgun discharge and malfunction
          (W32.-) ◀▥
         accidental pellet gun discharge and malfunction
          (W34.010, W34.110)
         assault by rifle, shotgun and larger firearm
          discharge (X94)
         firearm discharge involving legal intervention
          (Y35.0-)
         firearm discharge involving military or war
          operations (Y36.4-)
         intentional self-harm by rifle, shotgun and larger
          firearm discharge (X73)

The appropriate 7th character is to be added to each code from
   category W33

A	initial encounter
D	subsequent encounter
S	sequela

● **W33.0**   **Accidental rifle, shotgun and larger firearm discharge**

   X● **W33.00**   **Accidental discharge of unspecified larger firearm** 🖐
       Discharge of unspecified larger firearm NOS

   X● **W33.01**   **Accidental discharge of shotgun** 🖐
       Discharge of shotgun NOS

   X● **W33.02**   **Accidental discharge of hunting rifle** 🖐
       Discharge of hunting rifle NOS

   X● **W33.03**   **Accidental discharge of machine gun** 🖐
       Discharge of machine gun NOS

   X● **W33.09**   **Accidental discharge of other larger firearm** 🖐
       Discharge of other larger firearm NOS

● **W33.1**   **Accidental rifle, shotgun and larger firearm malfunction**
     Injury due to explosion of rifle, shotgun and larger
       firearm (parts)
     Injury due to malfunction of mechanism or component
       of rifle, shotgun and larger firearm
     Injury due to piercing, cutting, crushing or pinching
       due to (by) slide trigger mechanism, scope or other
       gun part
     Injury due to recoil of rifle, shotgun and larger firearm
     Powder burn from rifle, shotgun and larger firearm

   X● **W33.10**   **Accidental malfunction of unspecified larger firearm** 🖐
       Malfunction of unspecified larger firearm NOS

   X● **W33.11**   **Accidental malfunction of shotgun** 🖐
       Malfunction of shotgun NOS

   X● **W33.12**   **Accidental malfunction of hunting rifle** 🖐
       Malfunction of hunting rifle NOS

   X● **W33.13**   **Accidental malfunction of machine gun** 🖐
       Malfunction of machine gun NOS

   X● **W33.19**   **Accidental malfunction of other larger firearm** 🖐
       Malfunction of other larger firearm NOS

N Newborn Age: 0   **P** Pediatric Age: 0–17   **M** Maternity DX: 12–55   **A** Adult Age: 15–124   ♀ Females Only   ♂ Males Only

🖐 Complication\Comorbidity   🖐 Major C\C   (Ex) CC/MCC Exclusions   🖐 Present on Admission Requirement   🖐 Hospital-Acquired Condition

1635

● **W34** **Accidental discharge and malfunction from other and unspecified firearms and guns**

> The appropriate 7th character is to be added to each code from category W34

> | A | initial encounter |
> |---|---|
> | D | subsequent encounter |
> | S | sequela |

   ● **W34.0** **Accidental discharge from other and unspecified firearms and guns**

     X ● **W34.00** **Accidental discharge from unspecified firearms or gun** 🔍

>> Discharge from firearm NOS
>> Gunshot wound NOS
>> Shot NOS

     ● **W34.01** **Accidental discharge of gas, air or spring-operated guns**

       ● **W34.010** **Accidental discharge of airgun** 🔍
>>> Accidental discharge of BB gun
>>> Accidental discharge of pellet gun

       ● **W34.011** **Accidental discharge of paintball gun** 🔍
>>> Accidental injury due to paintball discharge

       ● **W34.018** **Accidental discharge of other gas, air or spring-operated gun** 🔍

     X ● **W34.09** **Accidental discharge from other specified firearms** 🔍
>> Accidental discharge from Very pistol [flare]

   ● **W34.1** **Accidental malfunction from other and unspecified firearms and guns**

     X ● **W34.10** **Accidental malfunction from unspecified firearms or gun** 🔍
>> Firearm malfunction NOS

     ● **W34.11** **Accidental malfunction of gas, air or spring-operated guns**

       ● **W34.110** **Accidental malfunction of airgun** 🔍
>>> Accidental malfunction of BB gun
>>> Accidental malfunction of pellet gun

       ● **W34.111** **Accidental malfunction of paintball gun** 🔍
>>> Accidental injury due to paintball gun malfunction

       ● **W34.118** **Accidental malfunction of other gas, air or spring-operated gun** 🔍

     X ● **W34.19** **Accidental malfunction from other specified firearms** 🔍
>> Accidental malfunction from Very pistol [flare]

● **W35** **Explosion and rupture of boiler** 🔍

> **Excludes1**   explosion and rupture of boiler on watercraft (V93.4)

> The appropriate 7th character is to be added to code W35

> | A | initial encounter |
> |---|---|
> | D | subsequent encounter |
> | S | sequela |

● **W36** **Explosion and rupture of gas cylinder**

> The appropriate 7th character is to be added to each code from category W36

> | A | initial encounter |
> |---|---|
> | D | subsequent encounter |
> | S | sequela |

   X ● **W36.1** **Explosion and rupture of aerosol can** 🔍
   X ● **W36.2** **Explosion and rupture of air tank** 🔍
   X ● **W36.3** **Explosion and rupture of pressurized-gas tank** 🔍
   X ● **W36.8** **Explosion and rupture of other gas cylinder** 🔍
   X ● **W36.9** **Explosion and rupture of unspecified gas cylinder** 🔍

● **W37** **Explosion and rupture of pressurized tire, pipe or hose**

> The appropriate 7th character is to be added to each code from category W37

> | A | initial encounter |
> |---|---|
> | D | subsequent encounter |
> | S | sequela |

   X ● **W37.0** **Explosion of bicycle tire** 🔍
   X ● **W37.8** **Explosion and rupture of other pressurized tire, pipe or hose** 🔍

X ● **W38** **Explosion and rupture of other specified pressurized devices** 🔍

> The appropriate 7th character is to be added to code W38

> | A | initial encounter |
> |---|---|
> | D | subsequent encounter |
> | S | sequela |

X ● **W39** **Discharge of firework** 🔍

> The appropriate 7th character is to be added to code W39

> | A | initial encounter |
> |---|---|
> | D | subsequent encounter |
> | S | sequela |

● **W40** **Explosion of other materials**

> **Excludes1**   assault by explosive material (X96)
> explosion involving legal intervention (Y35.1-)
> explosion involving military or war operations (Y36.0-, Y36.2-)
> intentional self-harm by explosive material (X75)

> The appropriate 7th character is to be added to each code from category W40

> | A | initial encounter |
> |---|---|
> | D | subsequent encounter |
> | S | sequela |

   X ● **W40.0** **Explosion of blasting material** 🔍
>> Explosion of blasting cap
>> Explosion of detonator
>> Explosion of dynamite
>> Explosion of explosive (any) used in blasting operations

   X ● **W40.1** **Explosion of explosive gases** 🔍
>> Explosion of acetylene
>> Explosion of butane
>> Explosion of coal gas
>> Explosion in mine NOS
>> Explosion of explosive gas
>> Explosion of fire damp
>> Explosion of gasoline fumes
>> Explosion of methane
>> Explosion of propane

   X ● **W40.8** **Explosion of other specified explosive materials** 🔍
>> Explosion in dump NOS
>> Explosion in factory NOS
>> Explosion in grain store
>> Explosion in munitions

>> **Excludes1**   explosion involving legal intervention (Y35.1-)
>> explosion involving military or war operations (Y36.0-, Y36.2-)

   X ● **W40.9** **Explosion of unspecified explosive materials** 🔍
>> Explosion NOS

● **W42** **Exposure to noise**

> The appropriate 7th character is to be added to each code from category W42

> | A | initial encounter |
> |---|---|
> | D | subsequent encounter |
> | S | sequela |

   X ● **W42.0** **Exposure to supersonic waves**
   X ● **W42.9** **Exposure to other noise**
>> Exposure to sound waves NOS

◄ New   ◄▬ Revised   ~~deleted~~ Deleted   Excludes 1   Excludes 2   Includes   Use additional   Code first   Code also   Unspecified

OGCR Official Guidelines   ● Unacceptable Principal Diagnosis   X Assign placeholder X   ● Use Additional Character(s)   ▌Manifestation Code   **Coding Clinic**

● **W45　Foreign body or object entering through skin**

> **Excludes2**　contact with hand tools (nonpowered) (powered)
> (W27-W29)
> contact with knife, sword or dagger (W26.-)
> contact with sharp glass (W25.-)
> struck by objects (W20-W22)

The appropriate 7th character is to be added to each code from category W45

A	initial encounter
D	subsequent encounter
S	sequela

X ● **W45.0　Nail entering through skin**

X ● **W45.1　Paper entering through skin**
Paper cut

X ● **W45.2　Lid of can entering through skin**

X ● **W45.8　Other foreign body or object entering through skin**
Splinter in skin NOS

● **W46　Contact with hypodermic needle**

The appropriate 7th character is to be added to each code from category W46

A	initial encounter
D	subsequent encounter
S	sequela

X ● **W46.0　Contact with hypodermic needle**
Hypodermic needle stick NOS

X ● **W46.1　Contact with contaminated hypodermic needle**

● **W49　Exposure to other inanimate mechanical forces**

> **Includes**　exposure to abnormal gravitational [G] forces
> exposure to inanimate mechanical forces NEC

> **Excludes1**　exposure to inanimate mechanical forces involving military or war operations (Y36.-, Y37.-)

The appropriate 7th character is to be added to each code from category W49

A	initial encounter
D	subsequent encounter
S	sequela

● **W49.0　Item causing external constriction**

X ● **W49.01　Hair causing external constriction**

X ● **W49.02　String or thread causing external constriction**

X ● **W49.03　Rubber band causing external constriction**

X ● **W49.04　Ring or other jewelry causing external constriction**

X ● **W49.09　Other item causing external constriction**

X ● **W49.9　Exposure to other inanimate mechanical forces**

EXPOSURE TO ANIMATE MECHANICAL FORCES (W50-W64)

> **Excludes1**　toxic effect of contact with venomous animals and plants (T63.-)

● **W50　Accidental hit, strike, kick, twist, bite or scratch by another person**

> **Includes**　hit, strike, kick, twist, bite, or scratch by another person NOS

> **Excludes1**　assault by bodily force (Y04)
> struck by objects (W20-W22)

The appropriate 7th character is to be added to each code from category W50

A	initial encounter
D	subsequent encounter
S	sequela

X ● **W50.0　Accidental hit or strike by another person**
Hit or strike by another person NOS

X ● **W50.1　Accidental kick by another person**
Kick by another person NOS

X ● **W50.2　Accidental twist by another person**
Twist by another person NOS

X ● **W50.3　Accidental bite by another person**
Human bite
Bite by another person NOS

X ● **W50.4　Accidental scratch by another person**
Scratch by another person NOS

X ● **W51　Accidental striking against or bumped into by another person**

> **Excludes1**　assault by striking against or bumping into by another person (Y04.2)
> fall due to collision with another person (W03)

The appropriate 7th character is to be added to code W51

A	initial encounter
D	subsequent encounter
S	sequela

X ● **W52　Crushed, pushed or stepped on by crowd or human stampede** 🔖
Crushed, pushed or stepped on by crowd or human stampede with or without fall

The appropriate 7th character is to be added to code W52

A	initial encounter
D	subsequent encounter
S	sequela

● **W53　Contact with rodent**

> **Includes**　contact with saliva, feces or urine of rodent

The appropriate 7th character is to be added to each code from category W53

A	initial encounter
D	subsequent encounter
S	sequela

● **W53.0　Contact with mouse**

X ● **W53.01　Bitten by mouse**

X ● **W53.09　Other contact with mouse**

● **W53.1　Contact with rat**

X ● **W53.11　Bitten by rat**

X ● **W53.19　Other contact with rat**

● **W53.2　Contact with squirrel**

X ● **W53.21　Bitten by squirrel**

X ● **W53.29　Other contact with squirrel**

● **W53.8　Contact with other rodent**

X ● **W53.81　Bitten by other rodent**

X ● **W53.89　Other contact with other rodent**

● **W54　Contact with dog**

> **Includes**　contact with saliva, feces or urine of dog

The appropriate 7th character is to be added to each code from category W54

A	initial encounter
D	subsequent encounter
S	sequela

X ● **W54.0　Bitten by dog**

X ● **W54.1　Struck by dog**
Knocked over by dog

X ● **W54.8　Other contact with dog**

N　Newborn Age: 0　　P　Pediatric Age: 0–17　　M　Maternity DX: 12–55　　A　Adult Age: 15–124　　♀ Females Only　　♂　Males Only

🔖 Complication\Comorbidity　　🔖 Major C\C　　(Ex) CC/MCC Exclusions　　🔖 Present on Admission Requirement　　🔖 Hospital-Acquired Condition

● **W55 Contact with other mammals**

    Includes   contact with saliva, feces or urine of mammal

    Excludes1   animal being ridden - see transport accidents

              bitten or struck by dog (W54)

              bitten or struck by rodent (W53.-)

              contact with marine mammals (W56.X-) ◄▦

    The appropriate 7th character is to be added to each code from category W55

      A   initial encounter
      D   subsequent encounter
      S   sequela

  ● **W55.0 Contact with cat**

    X● **W55.01 Bitten by cat**

    X● **W55.03 Scratched by cat**

    X● **W55.09 Other contact with cat**

  ● **W55.1 Contact with horse**

    X● **W55.11 Bitten by horse**

    X● **W55.12 Struck by horse**

    X● **W55.19 Other contact with horse**

  ● **W55.2 Contact with cow**

    Contact with bull

    X● **W55.21 Bitten by cow**

    X● **W55.22 Struck by cow**

           Gored by bull

    X● **W55.29 Other contact with cow**

  ● **W55.3 Contact with other hoof stock**

    Contact with goats

    Contact with sheep

    X● **W55.31 Bitten by other hoof stock**

    X● **W55.32 Struck by other hoof stock**

           Gored by goat

           Gored by ram

    X● **W55.39 Other contact with other hoof stock**

  ● **W55.4 Contact with pig**

    X● **W55.41 Bitten by pig**

    X● **W55.42 Struck by pig**

    X● **W55.49 Other contact with pig**

  ● **W55.5 Contact with raccoon**

    X● **W55.51 Bitten by raccoon**

    X● **W55.52 Struck by raccoon**

    X● **W55.59 Other contact with raccoon**

  ● **W55.8 Contact with other mammals**

    X● **W55.81 Bitten by other mammals**

    X● **W55.82 Struck by other mammals**

    X● **W55.89 Other contact with other mammals**

● **W56 Contact with nonvenomous marine animal**

    Excludes1   contact with venomous marine animal (T63.-)

    The appropriate 7th character is to be added to each code from category W56

      A   initial encounter
      D   subsequent encounter
      S   sequela

  ● **W56.0 Contact with dolphin**

    X● **W56.01 Bitten by dolphin** 🔍

    X● **W56.02 Struck by dolphin** 🔍

    X● **W56.09 Other contact with dolphin** 🔍

  ● **W56.1 Contact with sea lion**

    X● **W56.11 Bitten by sea lion** 🔍

    X● **W56.12 Struck by sea lion** 🔍

    X● **W56.19 Other contact with sea lion** 🔍

  ● **W56.2 Contact with orca**

    Contact with killer whale

    X● **W56.21 Bitten by orca** 🔍

    X● **W56.22 Struck by orca** 🔍

    X● **W56.29 Other contact with orca** 🔍

  ● **W56.3 Contact with other marine mammals**

    X● **W56.31 Bitten by other marine mammals** 🔍

    X● **W56.32 Struck by other marine mammals** 🔍

    X● **W56.39 Other contact with other marine mammals** 🔍

  ● **W56.4 Contact with shark**

    X● **W56.41 Bitten by shark** 🔍

    X● **W56.42 Struck by shark** 🔍

    X● **W56.49 Other contact with shark** 🔍

  ● **W56.5 Contact with other fish**

    X● **W56.51 Bitten by other fish** 🔍

    X● **W56.52 Struck by other fish** 🔍

    X● **W56.59 Other contact with other fish** 🔍

  ● **W56.8 Contact with other nonvenomous marine animals**

    X● **W56.81 Bitten by other nonvenomous marine animals** 🔍

    X● **W56.82 Struck by other nonvenomous marine animals** 🔍

    X● **W56.89 Other contact with other nonvenomous marine animals** 🔍

X● **W57 Bitten or stung by nonvenomous insect and other nonvenomous arthropods**

    Excludes1   contact with venomous insects and arthropods (T63.2-, T63.3-, T63.4-)

    The appropriate 7th character is to be added to code W57

      A   initial encounter
      D   subsequent encounter
      S   sequela

● **W58 Contact with crocodile or alligator**

    The appropriate 7th character is to be added to each code from category W58

      A   initial encounter
      D   subsequent encounter
      S   sequela

  ● **W58.0 Contact with alligator**

    X● **W58.01 Bitten by alligator** 🔍

    X● **W58.02 Struck by alligator** 🔍

    X● **W58.03 Crushed by alligator** 🔍

    X● **W58.09 Other contact with alligator** 🔍

  ● **W58.1 Contact with crocodile**

    X● **W58.11 Bitten by crocodile** 🔍

    X● **W58.12 Struck by crocodile** 🔍

    X● **W58.13 Crushed by crocodile** 🔍

    X● **W58.19 Other contact with crocodile** 🔍

● **W59 Contact with other nonvenomous reptiles**

    Excludes1   contact with venomous reptile (T63.0-, T63.1-)

    The appropriate 7th character is to be added to each code from category W59

      A   initial encounter
      D   subsequent encounter
      S   sequela

  ● **W59.0 Contact with nonvenomous lizards**

    X● **W59.01 Bitten by nonvenomous lizards**

    X● **W59.02 Struck by nonvenomous lizards**

    X● **W59.09 Other contact with nonvenomous lizards**

           Exposure to nonvenomous lizards

◄ New   ▦ Revised   ~~deleted~~ Deleted   Excludes 1   Excludes 2   Includes   Use additional   Code first   Code also   Unspecified

OGCR Official Guidelines   ● Unacceptable Principal Diagnosis   X Assign placeholder X   ▶ Use Additional Character(s)   ▶ Manifestation Code   **Coding Clinic**

● **W59.1 Contact with nonvenomous snakes**
  X● **W59.11 Bitten by nonvenomous snake**
  X● **W59.12 Struck by nonvenomous snake**
  X● **W59.13 Crushed by nonvenomous snake**
  X● **W59.19 Other contact with nonvenomous snake**
● **W59.2 Contact with turtles**
  > **Excludes1**   contact with tortoises (W59.8-)
  X● **W59.21 Bitten by turtle**
  X● **W59.22 Struck by turtle**
  X● **W59.29 Other contact with turtle**
  > Exposure to turtles
● **W59.8 Contact with other nonvenomous reptiles**
  X● **W59.81 Bitten by other nonvenomous reptiles**
  X● **W59.82 Struck by other nonvenomous reptiles**
  X● **W59.83 Crushed by other nonvenomous reptiles**
  X● **W59.89 Other contact with other nonvenomous reptiles**

X● **W60 Contact with nonvenomous plant thorns and spines and sharp leaves**
  > **Excludes1**   contact with venomous plants (T63.X7-) ◄▥
  > The appropriate 7th character is to be added to code W60

A	initial encounter
D	subsequent encounter
S	sequela

● **W61 Contact with birds (domestic) (wild)**
  > **Includes**   contact with excreta of birds
  > The appropriate 7th character is to be added to each code from category W61

A	initial encounter
D	subsequent encounter
S	sequela

● **W61.0 Contact with parrot**
  X● **W61.01 Bitten by parrot** 🦠
  X● **W61.02 Struck by parrot** 🦠
  X● **W61.09 Other contact with parrot** 🦠
  > Exposure to parrots
● **W61.1 Contact with macaw**
  X● **W61.11 Bitten by macaw** 🦠
  X● **W61.12 Struck by macaw** 🦠
  X● **W61.19 Other contact with macaw** 🦠
  > Exposure to macaws
● **W61.2 Contact with other psittacines**
  X● **W61.21 Bitten by other psittacines** 🦠
  X● **W61.22 Struck by other psittacines** 🦠
  X● **W61.29 Other contact with other psittacines** 🦠
  > Exposure to other psittacines
● **W61.3 Contact with chicken**
  X● **W61.32 Struck by chicken** 🦠
  X● **W61.33 Pecked by chicken** 🦠
  X● **W61.39 Other contact with chicken** 🦠
  > Exposure to chickens
● **W61.4 Contact with turkey**
  X● **W61.42 Struck by turkey** 🦠
  X● **W61.43 Pecked by turkey** 🦠
  X● **W61.49 Other contact with turkey** 🦠
● **W61.5 Contact with goose**
  X● **W61.51 Bitten by goose** 🦠
  X● **W61.52 Struck by goose** 🦠
  X● **W61.59 Other contact with goose** 🦠
● **W61.6 Contact with duck**
  X● **W61.61 Bitten by duck** 🦠
  X● **W61.62 Struck by duck** 🦠
  X● **W61.69 Other contact with duck** 🦠

● **W61.9 Contact with other birds**
  X● **W61.91 Bitten by other birds** 🦠
  X● **W61.92 Struck by other birds** 🦠
  X● **W61.99 Other contact with other birds** 🦠
  > Contact with bird NOS

● **W62 Contact with nonvenomous amphibians**
  > **Excludes1**   contact with venomous amphibians (T63.81-R63.83)
  > The appropriate 7th character is to be added to each code from category W62

A	initial encounter
D	subsequent encounter
S	sequela

  X● **W62.0 Contact with nonvenomous frogs** 🦠
  X● **W62.1 Contact with nonvenomous toads** 🦠
  X● **W62.9 Contact with other nonvenomous amphibians** 🦠

X● **W64 Exposure to other animate mechanical forces**
  > **Includes**   exposure to nonvenomous animal NOS
  > **Excludes1**   contact with venomous animal (T63.-)
  > The appropriate 7th character is to be added to code W64

A	initial encounter
D	subsequent encounter
S	sequela

ACCIDENTAL NON-TRANSPORT DROWNING AND SUBMERSION (W65-W74)

> **Excludes1**   accidental drowning and submersion due to fall into water (W16.-)
> accidental drowning and submersion due to water transport accident (V90.-, V92.-)
> **Excludes2**   accidental drowning and submersion due to cataclysm (X34-X39)

X● **W65 Accidental drowning and submersion while in bathtub**
  > **Excludes1**   accidental drowning and submersion due to fall in (into) bathtub (W16.211)
  > The appropriate 7th character is to be added to code W65

A	initial encounter
D	subsequent encounter
S	sequela

X● **W67 Accidental drowning and submersion while in swimming pool**
  > **Excludes1**   accidental drowning and submersion due to fall into swimming pool (W16.011, W16.021, W16.031)
  > accidental drowning and submersion due to striking into wall of swimming pool (W22.041)
  > The appropriate 7th character is to be added to code W67

A	initial encounter
D	subsequent encounter
S	sequela

X● **W69 Accidental drowning and submersion while in natural water**
  > Accidental drowning and submersion while in lake
  > Accidental drowning and submersion while in open sea
  > Accidental drowning and submersion while in river
  > Accidental drowning and submersion while in stream
  > **Excludes1**   accidental drowning and submersion due to fall into natural body of water (W16.111, W16.121, W16.131)
  > The appropriate 7th character is to be added to code W69

A	initial encounter
D	subsequent encounter
S	sequela

N Newborn Age: 0   **P** Pediatric Age: 0–17   **M** Maternity DX: 12–55   **A** Adult Age: 15–124   ♀ Females Only   ♂ Males Only

🦠 Complication\Comorbidity   🦠 Major C\C   (Ex) CC/MCC Exclusions   🦠 Present on Admission Requirement   🦠 Hospital-Acquired Condition

1639

CHAPTER 20 (V01-Y99)

X⬤**W73** **Other specified cause of accidental non-transport drowning and submersion**
    Accidental drowning and submersion while in quenching tank
    Accidental drowning and submersion while in reservoir

    Excludes1   accidental drowning and submersion due to
                   fall into other water (W16.311, W16.321,
                   W16.331)

    The appropriate 7th character is to be added to code W73

A	initial encounter
D	subsequent encounter
S	sequela

X⬤**W74** **Unspecified** **cause of accidental drowning and submersion**
    Drowning NOS

    The appropriate 7th character is to be added to code W74

A	initial encounter
D	subsequent encounter
S	sequela

EXPOSURE TO ELECTRIC CURRENT, RADIATION AND EXTREME AMBIENT AIR TEMPERATURE AND PRESSURE (W85-W99)

    Excludes1   exposure to:
            failure in dosage of radiation or temperature
               during surgical and medical care
               (Y63.2-Y63.5)
            lightning (T75.0-)
            natural cold (X31)
            natural heat (X30)
            natural radiation NOS (X39)
            radiological procedure and radiotherapy
               (Y84.2)
            sunlight (X32)

X⬤**W85** **Exposure to electric transmission lines**
    Broken power line

    The appropriate 7th character is to be added to code W85

A	initial encounter
D	subsequent encounter
S	sequela

⬤**W86** **Exposure to other specified electric current**
    The appropriate 7th character is to be added to each code from category W86

A	initial encounter
D	subsequent encounter
S	sequela

X⬤**W86.0** **Exposure to domestic wiring and appliances**
X⬤**W86.1** **Exposure to industrial wiring, appliances and electrical machinery**
    Exposure to conductors
    Exposure to control apparatus
    Exposure to electrical equipment and machinery
    Exposure to transformers
X⬤**W86.8** **Exposure to other electric current**
    Exposure to wiring and appliances in or on farm (not farmhouse)
    Exposure to wiring and appliances outdoors
    Exposure to wiring and appliances in or on public building
    Exposure to wiring and appliances in or on residential institutions
    Exposure to wiring and appliances in or on schools

⬤**W88** **Exposure to ionizing radiation**
    Excludes1   exposure to sunlight (X32)

    The appropriate 7th character is to be added to each code from category W88

A	initial encounter
D	subsequent encounter
S	sequela

X⬤**W88.0** **Exposure to X-rays**
X⬤**W88.1** **Exposure to radioactive isotopes**
X⬤**W88.8** **Exposure to other ionizing radiation**

⬤**W89** **Exposure to man-made visible and ultraviolet light**
    Includes   exposure to welding light (arc)
    Excludes2   exposure to sunlight (X32)

    The appropriate 7th character is to be added to each code from category W89

A	initial encounter
D	subsequent encounter
S	sequela

X⬤**W89.0** **Exposure to welding light (arc)** 🔖
X⬤**W89.1** **Exposure to tanning bed** 🔖
X⬤**W89.8** **Exposure to other man-made visible and ultraviolet light** 🔖
X⬤**W89.9** **Exposure to** **unspecified** **man-made visible and ultraviolet light** 🔖

⬤**W90** **Exposure to other nonionizing radiation**
    Excludes1   exposure to sunlight (X32)

    The appropriate 7th character is to be added to each code from category W90

A	initial encounter
D	subsequent encounter
S	sequela

X⬤**W90.0** **Exposure to radiofrequency**
X⬤**W90.1** **Exposure to infrared radiation**
X⬤**W90.2** **Exposure to laser radiation**
X⬤**W90.8** **Exposure to other nonionizing radiation**

X⬤**W92** **Exposure to excessive heat of man-made origin**
    The appropriate 7th character is to be added to code W92

A	initial encounter
D	subsequent encounter
S	sequela

⬤**W93** **Exposure to excessive cold of man-made origin**
    The appropriate 7th character is to be added to each code from category W93

A	initial encounter
D	subsequent encounter
S	sequela

⬤**W93.0** **Contact with or inhalation of dry ice**
    X⬤**W93.01** **Contact with dry ice**
    X⬤**W93.02** **Inhalation of dry ice**
⬤**W93.1** **Contact with or inhalation of liquid air**
    X⬤**W93.11** **Contact with liquid air**
        Contact with liquid hydrogen
        Contact with liquid nitrogen
    X⬤**W93.12** **Inhalation of liquid air**
        Inhalation of liquid hydrogen
        Inhalation of liquid nitrogen
X⬤**W93.2** **Prolonged exposure in deep freeze unit or refrigerator**
X⬤**W93.8** **Exposure to other excessive cold of man-made origin**

◀ New   ◀ Revised   ~~deleted~~ Deleted   Excludes 1   Excludes 2   Includes   Use additional   Code first   Code also   Unspecified

OGCR Official Guidelines   ⬤ Unacceptable Principal Diagnosis   X Assign placeholder X   🔖 Use Additional Character(s)   ▶ Manifestation Code   **Coding Clinic**

● **W94　Exposure to high and low air pressure and changes in air pressure**

The appropriate 7th character is to be added to each code from category W94

> A　initial encounter
> D　subsequent encounter
> S　sequela

X● **W94.0　Exposure to prolonged high air pressure**

● **W94.1　Exposure to prolonged low air pressure**

X● **W94.11　Exposure to residence or prolonged visit at high altitude**

X● **W94.12　Exposure to other prolonged low air pressure**

● **W94.2　Exposure to rapid changes in air pressure during ascent**

X● **W94.21　Exposure to reduction in atmospheric pressure while surfacing from deep-water diving**

X● **W94.22　Exposure to reduction in atmospheric pressure while surfacing from underground**

X● **W94.23　Exposure to sudden change in air pressure in aircraft during ascent**

X● **W94.29　Exposure to other rapid changes in air pressure during ascent**

● **W94.3　Exposure to rapid changes in air pressure during descent**

X● **W94.31　Exposure to sudden change in air pressure in aircraft during descent** ◀▥

X● **W94.32　Exposure to high air pressure from rapid descent in water**

X● **W94.39　Exposure to other rapid changes in air pressure during descent**

X● **W99　Exposure to other man-made environmental factors**

The appropriate 7th character is to be added to code W99

> A　initial encounter
> D　subsequent encounter
> S　sequela

EXPOSURE TO SMOKE, FIRE AND FLAMES (X00-X08)

Excludes1　arson (X97)

Excludes2　explosions (W35-W40)
　　　　　　lightning (T75.0-)
　　　　　　transport accident (V01-V99)

● **X00　Exposure to uncontrolled fire in building or structure**

Includes　conflagration in building or structure

Code first any associated cataclysm

Excludes2　exposure to ignition or melting of nightwear (X05)
　　　　　　exposure to ignition or melting of other clothing and apparel (X06.-) ◀▥
　　　　　　exposure to other specified smoke, fire and flames (X08.-)

The appropriate 7th character is to be added to each code from category X00

> A　initial encounter
> D　subsequent encounter
> S　sequela

X● **X00.0　Exposure to flames in uncontrolled fire in building or structure**

X● **X00.1　Exposure to smoke in uncontrolled fire in building or structure**

X● **X00.2　Injury due to collapse of burning building or structure in uncontrolled fire**

Excludes1　injury due to collapse of building not on fire (W20.1)

X● **X00.3　Fall from burning building or structure in uncontrolled fire**

X● **X00.4　Hit by object from burning building or structure in uncontrolled fire**

X● **X00.5　Jump from burning building or structure in uncontrolled fire**

X● **X00.8　Other exposure to uncontrolled fire in building or structure**

● **X01　Exposure to uncontrolled fire, not in building or structure**

Includes　exposure to forest fire

The appropriate 7th character is to be added to each code from category X01

> A　initial encounter
> D　subsequent encounter
> S　sequela

X● **X01.0　Exposure to flames in uncontrolled fire, not in building or structure**

X● **X01.1　Exposure to smoke in uncontrolled fire, not in building or structure**

X● **X01.3　Fall due to uncontrolled fire, not in building or structure**

X● **X01.4　Hit by object due to uncontrolled fire, not in building or structure**

X● **X01.8　Other exposure to uncontrolled fire, not in building or structure**

● **X02　Exposure to controlled fire in building or structure**

Includes　exposure to fire in fireplace exposure to fire in stove

The appropriate 7th character is to be added to each code from category X02

> A　initial encounter
> D　subsequent encounter
> S　sequela

X● **X02.0　Exposure to flames in controlled fire in building or structure** 🗓

X● **X02.1　Exposure to smoke in controlled fire in building or structure** 🗓

X● **X02.2　Injury due to collapse of burning building or structure in controlled fire** 🗓

Excludes1　injury due to collapse of building not on fire (W20.1)

X● **X02.3　Fall from burning building or structure in controlled fire** 🗓

X● **X02.4　Hit by object from burning building or structure in controlled fire** 🗓

X● **X02.5　Jump from burning building or structure in controlled fire** 🗓

X● **X02.8　Other exposure to controlled fire in building or structure** 🗓

● **X03　Exposure to controlled fire, not in building or structure**

Includes　exposure to bon fire exposure to camp fire exposure to trash fire

The appropriate 7th character is to be added to each code from category X03

> A　initial encounter
> D　subsequent encounter
> S　sequela

X● **X03.0　Exposure to flames in controlled fire, not in building or structure** 🗓

X● **X03.1　Exposure to smoke in controlled fire, not in building or structure** 🗓

X● **X03.3　Fall due to controlled fire, not in building or structure** 🗓

X● **X03.4　Hit by object due to controlled fire, not in building or structure** 🗓

X● **X03.8　Other exposure to controlled fire, not in building or structure** 🗓

N Newborn Age: 0　　**P** Pediatric Age: 0–17　　**M** Maternity DX: 12–55　　**A** Adult Age: 15–124　　♀ Females Only　　♂ Males Only

🗓 Complication\Comorbidity　　🗓 Major C\C　　(Ex) CC/MCC Exclusions　　🗓 Present on Admission Requirement　　🗓 Hospital-Acquired Condition

1641

X ● **X04**   **Exposure to ignition of highly flammable material** 🔗
     Exposure to ignition of gasoline
     Exposure to ignition of kerosene
     Exposure to ignition of petrol

     Excludes2   exposure to ignition or melting of nightwear (X05)
           exposure to ignition or melting of other clothing and apparel (X06)

     The appropriate 7th character is to be added to code X04

A	initial encounter
D	subsequent encounter
S	sequela

X ● **X05**   **Exposure to ignition or melting of nightwear**

     Excludes2   exposure to uncontrolled fire in building or structure (X00.-)
           exposure to uncontrolled fire, not in building or structure (X01.-)
           exposure to controlled fire in building or structure (X02.-)
           exposure to controlled fire, not in building or structure (X03.-)
           exposure to ignition of highly flammable materials (X04.-)

     The appropriate 7th character is to be added to code X05

A	initial encounter
D	subsequent encounter
S	sequela

● **X06**   **Exposure to ignition or melting of other clothing and apparel**

     Excludes2   exposure to uncontrolled fire in building or structure (X00.-)
           exposure to uncontrolled fire, not in building or structure (X01.-)
           exposure to controlled fire in building or structure (X02.-)
           exposure to controlled fire, not in building or structure (X03.-)
           exposure to ignition of highly flammable materials (X04.-)

     The appropriate 7th character is to be added to each code from category X06

A	initial encounter
D	subsequent encounter
S	sequela

X ● **X06.0**   **Exposure to ignition of plastic jewelry**
X ● **X06.1**   **Exposure to melting of plastic jewelry**
X ● **X06.2**   **Exposure to ignition of other clothing and apparel**
X ● **X06.3**   **Exposure to melting of other clothing and apparel**

● **X08**   **Exposure to other specified smoke, fire and flames**

     The appropriate 7th character is to be added to each code from category X08

A	initial encounter
D	subsequent encounter
S	sequela

● **X08.0**   **Exposure to bed fire**
     Exposure to mattress fire

X ● **X08.00**   **Exposure to bed fire due to unspecified burning material**
X ● **X08.01**   **Exposure to bed fire due to burning cigarette**
X ● **X08.09**   **Exposure to bed fire due to other burning material**

● **X08.1**   **Exposure to sofa fire**

X ● **X08.10**   **Exposure to sofa fire due to unspecified burning material**
X ● **X08.11**   **Exposure to sofa fire due to burning cigarette**
X ● **X08.19**   **Exposure to sofa fire due to other burning material**

● **X08.2**   **Exposure to other furniture fire**

X ● **X08.20**   **Exposure to other furniture fire due to unspecified burning material**
X ● **X08.21**   **Exposure to other furniture fire due to burning cigarette**
X ● **X08.29**   **Exposure to other furniture fire due to other burning material**

X ● **X08.8**   **Exposure to other specified smoke, fire and flames**

CONTACT WITH HEAT AND HOT SUBSTANCES (X10-X19)

     Excludes1   exposure to excessive natural heat (X30)
           exposure to fire and flames (X00-X09)

● **X10**   **Contact with hot drinks, food, fats and cooking oils**

     The appropriate 7th character is to be added to each code from category X10

A	initial encounter
D	subsequent encounter
S	sequela

X ● **X10.0**   **Contact with hot drinks**
X ● **X10.1**   **Contact with hot food**
X ● **X10.2**   **Contact with fats and cooking oils**

● **X11**   **Contact with hot tap-water**

     Includes   contact with boiling tap-water
           contact with boiling water NOS

     Excludes1   contact with water heated on stove (X12)

     The appropriate 7th character is to be added to each code from category X11

A	initial encounter
D	subsequent encounter
S	sequela

X ● **X11.0**   **Contact with hot water in bath or tub**

     Excludes1   contact with running hot water in bath or tub (X11.1)

X ● **X11.1**   **Contact with running hot water**
     Contact with hot water running out of hose
     Contact with hot water running out of tap

X ● **X11.8**   **Contact with other hot tap-water**
     Contact with hot water in bucket
     Contact with hot tap-water NOS

X ● **X12**   **Contact with other hot fluids**
     Contact with water heated on stove

     Excludes1   hot (liquid) metals (X18)

     The appropriate 7th character is to be added to code X12

A	initial encounter
D	subsequent encounter
S	sequela

● **X13**   **Contact with steam and other hot vapors**

     The appropriate 7th character is to be added to each code from category X13

A	initial encounter
D	subsequent encounter
S	sequela

X ● **X13.0**   **Inhalation of steam and other hot vapors**
X ● **X13.1**   **Other contact with steam and other hot vapors**

◄ New   ◄ Revised   ~~deleted~~ Deleted   Excludes 1   Excludes 2   Includes   Use additional   Code first   Code also   Unspecified

OGCR Official Guidelines   ● Unacceptable Principal Diagnosis   X Assign placeholder X   ● Use Additional Character(s)   ▶ Manifestation Code   **Coding Clinic**

● X14 Contact with hot air and other hot gases

The appropriate 7th character is to be added to each code from category X14

A	initial encounter
D	subsequent encounter
S	sequela

X ● **X14.0 Inhalation of hot air and gases**

X ● **X14.1 Other contact with hot air and other hot gases**

● X15 Contact with hot household appliances

> **Excludes1** contact with heating appliances (X16)
> contact with powered household appliances (W29.-)
> exposure to controlled fire in building or structure due to household appliance (X02.8)
> exposure to household appliances electrical current (W86.0)

The appropriate 7th character is to be added to each code from category X15

A	initial encounter
D	subsequent encounter
S	sequela

X ● **X15.0 Contact with hot stove (kitchen)**

X ● **X15.1 Contact with hot toaster**

X ● **X15.2 Contact with hotplate**

X ● **X15.3 Contact with hot saucepan or skillet**

X ● **X15.8 Contact with other hot household appliances**
Contact with cooker
Contact with kettle
Contact with light bulbs

X ● **X16 Contact with hot heating appliances, radiators and pipes**

> **Excludes1** contact with powered appliances (W29.-)
> exposure to controlled fire in building or structure due to appliance (X02.8)
> exposure to industrial appliances electrical current (W86.1)

The appropriate 7th character is to be added to code X16

A	initial encounter
D	subsequent encounter
S	sequela

X ● **X17 Contact with hot engines, machinery and tools**

> **Excludes1** contact with hot heating appliances, radiators and pipes (X16)
> contact with hot household appliances (X15)

The appropriate 7th character is to be added to code X17

A	initial encounter
D	subsequent encounter
S	sequela

X ● **X18 Contact with other hot metals**
Contact with liquid metal

The appropriate 7th character is to be added to code X18

A	initial encounter
D	subsequent encounter
S	sequela

X ● **X19 Contact with other heat and hot substances**

> **Excludes1** objects that are not normally hot, e.g., an object made hot by a house fire (X00-X09)

The appropriate 7th character is to be added to code X19

A	initial encounter
D	subsequent encounter
S	sequela

EXPOSURE TO FORCES OF NATURE (X30-X39)

X ● **X30 Exposure to excessive natural heat**
Exposure to excessive heat as the cause of sunstroke
Exposure to heat NOS

> **Excludes1** excessive heat of man-made origin (W92)
> exposure to man-made radiation (W89)
> exposure to sunlight (X32)
> exposure to tanning bed (W89)

The appropriate 7th character is to be added to code X30

A	initial encounter
D	subsequent encounter
S	sequela

X ● **X31 Exposure to excessive natural cold**
Excessive cold as the cause of chilblains NOS
Excessive cold as the cause of immersion foot or hand
Exposure to cold NOS
Exposure to weather conditions

> **Excludes1** cold of man-made origin (W93.-)
> contact with or inhalation of dry ice (W93.-) ◄▥
> contact with or inhalation of liquefied gas (W93.-) ◄▥
> ~~liquefied gas (W93.-)~~

The appropriate 7th character is to be added to code X31

A	initial encounter
D	subsequent encounter
S	sequela

X ● **X32 Exposure to sunlight**

> **Excludes1** radiation-related disorders of the skin and subcutaneous tissue (L55-L59)
> man-made radiation (tanning bed) (W89)

The appropriate 7th character is to be added to code X32

A	initial encounter
D	subsequent encounter
S	sequela

X ● **X34 Earthquake**

> **Excludes2** tidal wave (tsunami) due to earthquake (X37.41)

The appropriate 7th character is to be added to code X34

A	initial encounter
D	subsequent encounter
S	sequela

X ● **X35 Volcanic eruption**

> **Excludes2** tidal wave (tsunami) due to volcanic eruption (X37.41)

The appropriate 7th character is to be added to code X35

A	initial encounter
D	subsequent encounter
S	sequela

● **X36 Avalanche, landslide and other earth movements**

> **Includes** victim of mudslide of cataclysmic nature
> **Excludes1** earthquake (X34)
> **Excludes2** transport accident involving collision with avalanche or landslide not in motion (V01-V99)

The appropriate 7th character is to be added to each code from category X36

A	initial encounter
D	subsequent encounter
S	sequela

X ● **X36.0 Collapse of dam or man-made structure causing earth movement**

X ● **X36.1 Avalanche, landslide, or mudslide**

N Newborn Age: 0   P Pediatric Age: 0–17   M Maternity DX: 12–55   A Adult Age: 15–124   ♀ Females Only   ♂ Males Only

🔖 Complication\Comorbidity   🔖 Major C\C   (Ex) CC/MCC Exclusions   🔖 Present on Admission Requirement   🔖 Hospital-Acquired Condition

CHAPTER 20 (V01-Y99)

● **X37   Cataclysmic storm**
The appropriate 7th character is to be added to each code from
category X37

> A   initial encounter
> D   subsequent encounter
> S   sequela

X ● **X37.0   Hurricane**
Storm surge   Typhoon

X ● **X37.1   Tornado**
Cyclone   Twister

X ● **X37.2   Blizzard (snow) (ice)**

X ● **X37.3   Dust storm**

● **X37.4   Tidalwave**

X ● **X37.41   Tidal wave due to earthquake or volcanic
eruption**
Tidal wave NOS
Tsunami

X ● **X37.42   Tidal wave due to storm**

X ● **X37.43   Tidal wave due to landslide**

X ● **X37.8   Other cataclysmic storms**
Cloudburst
Torrential rain

> **Excludes2**   flood (X38)

X ● **X37.9   Unspecified cataclysmic storm**
Storm NOS

> **Excludes1**   collapse of dam or man-made structure
> causing earth movement (X39.0)

X ● **X38   Flood**
Flood arising from remote storm
Flood of cataclysmic nature arising from melting snow
Flood resulting directly from storm

> **Excludes1**   collapse of dam or man-made structure causing
> earth movement (X39.0)
> tidal wave NOS (X37.41)
> tidal wave caused by storm (X37.2)

The appropriate 7th character is to be added to code X38

> A   initial encounter
> D   subsequent encounter
> S   sequela

● **X39   Exposure to other forces of nature**
The appropriate 7th character is to be added to each code from
category X39

> A   initial encounter
> D   subsequent encounter
> S   sequela

● **X39.0   Exposure to natural radiation**

> **Excludes1**   contact with and (suspected) exposure to
> radon and other naturally occuring
> radiation (Z77.122)
> exposure to man-made radiation
> (W88-W90)
> exposure to sunlight (X32)

X ● **X39.01   Exposure to radon**

X ● **X39.08   Exposure to other natural radiation**

X ● **X39.8   Other exposure to forces of nature**

X ● **X52   Prolonged stay in weightless environment** 🖐
Weightlessness in spacecraft (simulator)

The appropriate 7th character is to be added to code X52

> A   initial encounter
> D   subsequent encounter
> S   sequela

X ● **X58   Exposure to other specified factors**
Accident NOS
Exposure NOS

The appropriate 7th character is to be added to code X58

> A   initial encounter
> D   subsequent encounter
> S   sequela

INTENTIONAL SELF-HARM (X71-X83)
Purposely self-inflicted injury
Suicide (attempted)

● **X71   Intentional self-harm by drowning and submersion**
The appropriate 7th character is to be added to each code from
category X71

> A   initial encounter
> D   subsequent encounter
> S   sequela

X ● **X71.0   Intentional self-harm by drowning and submersion
while in bathtub**

X ● **X71.1   Intentional self-harm by drowning and submersion
while in swimming pool** 🖐

X ● **X71.2   Intentional self-harm by drowning and submersion after
jump into swimming pool** 🖐

X ● **X71.3   Intentional self-harm by drowning and submersion in
natural water** 🖐

X ● **X71.8   Other intentional self-harm by drowning and
submersion** 🖐

X ● **X71.9   Intentional self-harm by drowning and submersion,
unspecified** 🖐

X ● **X72   Intentional self-harm by handgun discharge** 🖐
Intentional self-harm by gun for single hand use
Intentional self-harm by pistol
Intentional self-harm by revolver

> **Excludes1**   Very pistol (X74.8)

The appropriate 7th character is to be added to code X72

> A   initial encounter
> D   subsequent encounter
> S   sequela

● **X73   Intentional self-harm by rifle, shotgun and larger firearm
discharge**

> **Excludes1**   airgun (X74.01)

The appropriate 7th character is to be added to each code from
category X73

> A   initial encounter
> D   subsequent encounter
> S   sequela

X ● **X73.0   Intentional self-harm by shotgun discharge** 🖐

X ● **X73.1   Intentional self-harm by hunting rifle discharge** 🖐

X ● **X73.2   Intentional self-harm by machine gun discharge** 🖐

X ● **X73.8   Intentional self-harm by other larger firearm
discharge** 🖐

X ● **X73.9   Intentional self-harm by unspecified larger firearm
discharge** 🖐

◄ New   ◄▬ Revised   ~~deleted~~ Deleted   Excludes 1   Excludes 2   Includes   Use additional   Code first   Code also   Unspecified
OGCR Official Guidelines   ● Unacceptable Principal Diagnosis   X Assign placeholder X   ▶ Use Additional Character(s)   ▷ Manifestation Code   Coding Clinic

● **X74**   **Intentional self-harm by other and unspecified firearm and gun discharge**

> The appropriate 7th character is to be added to each code from category X74

> | | |
> |---|---|
> | A | initial encounter |
> | D | subsequent encounter |
> | S | sequela |

  ● **X74.0**   **Intentional self-harm by gas, air or spring-operated guns**

    X● **X74.01**   **Intentional self-harm by airgun** 🔖
         Intentional self-harm by BB gun discharge
         Intentional self-harm by pellet gun discharge

    X● **X74.02**   **Intentional self-harm by paintball gun** 🔖

    X● **X74.09**   **Intentional self-harm by other gas, air or spring-operated gun** 🔖

  X● **X74.8**   **Intentional self-harm by other firearm discharge** 🔖
       Intentional self-harm by Very pistol [flare] discharge

  X● **X74.9**   **Intentional self-harm by unspecified firearm discharge** 🔖

X●**X75**   **Intentional self-harm by explosive material** 🔖

> The appropriate 7th character is to be added to code X75

> | | |
> |---|---|
> | A | initial encounter |
> | D | subsequent encounter |
> | S | sequela |

X●**X76**   **Intentional self-harm by smoke, fire and flames** 🔖

> The appropriate 7th character is to be added to code X76

> | | |
> |---|---|
> | A | initial encounter |
> | D | subsequent encounter |
> | S | sequela |

● **X77**   **Intentional self-harm by steam, hot vapors and hot objects**

> The appropriate 7th character is to be added to each code from category X77

> | | |
> |---|---|
> | A | initial encounter |
> | D | subsequent encounter |
> | S | sequela |

  X● **X77.0**   **Intentional self-harm by steam or hot vapors** 🔖
  X● **X77.1**   **Intentional self-harm by hot tap water** 🔖
  X● **X77.2**   **Intentional self-harm by other hot fluids** 🔖
  X● **X77.3**   **Intentional self-harm by hot household appliances** 🔖
  X● **X77.8**   **Intentional self-harm by other hot objects** 🔖
  X● **X77.9**   **Intentional self-harm by unspecified hot objects** 🔖

● **X78**   **Intentional self-harm by sharp object**

> The appropriate 7th character is to be added to each code from category X78

> | | |
> |---|---|
> | A | initial encounter |
> | D | subsequent encounter |
> | S | sequela |

  X● **X78.0**   **Intentional self-harm by sharp glass**
  X● **X78.1**   **Intentional self-harm by knife**
  X● **X78.2**   **Intentional self-harm by sword or dagger**
  X● **X78.8**   **Intentional self-harm by other sharp object**
  X● **X78.9**   **Intentional self-harm by unspecified sharp object**

X●**X79**   **Intentional self-harm by blunt object**

> The appropriate 7th character is to be added to code X79

> | | |
> |---|---|
> | A | initial encounter |
> | D | subsequent encounter |
> | S | sequela |

X●**X80**   **Intentional self-harm by jumping from a high place**
> Intentional fall from one level to another

> The appropriate 7th character is to be added to code X80

> | | |
> |---|---|
> | A | initial encounter |
> | D | subsequent encounter |
> | S | sequela |

● **X81**   **Intentional self-harm by jumping or lying in front of moving object**

> The appropriate 7th character is to be added to each code from category X81

> | | |
> |---|---|
> | A | initial encounter |
> | D | subsequent encounter |
> | S | sequela |

  X● **X81.0**   **Intentional self-harm by jumping or lying in front of motor vehicle** 🔖
  X● **X81.1**   **Intentional self-harm by jumping or lying in front of (subway) train** 🔖
  X● **X81.8**   **Intentional self-harm by jumping or lying in front of other moving object** 🔖

● **X82**   **Intentional self-harm by crashing of motor vehicle**

> The appropriate 7th character is to be added to each code from category X82

> | | |
> |---|---|
> | A | initial encounter |
> | D | subsequent encounter |
> | S | sequela |

  X● **X82.0**   **Intentional collision of motor vehicle with other motor vehicle** 🔖
  X● **X82.1**   **Intentional collision of motor vehicle with train** 🔖
  X● **X82.2**   **Intentional collision of motor vehicle with tree** 🔖
  X● **X82.8**   **Other intentional self-harm by crashing of motor vehicle** 🔖

● **X83**   **Intentional self-harm by other specified means**

> **Excludes1**   intentional self-harm by poisoning or contact with toxic substance - see Table of Drugs and Chemicals

> The appropriate 7th character is to be added to each code from category X83

> | | |
> |---|---|
> | A | initial encounter |
> | D | subsequent encounter |
> | S | sequela |

  X● **X83.0**   **Intentional self-harm by crashing of aircraft** 🔖
  X● **X83.1**   **Intentional self-harm by electrocution** 🔖
  X● **X83.2**   **Intentional self-harm by exposure to extremes of cold** 🔖
  X● **X83.8**   **Intentional self-harm by other specified means** 🔖

ASSAULT (X92-Y08)

> **Includes**   homicide injuries inflicted by another person with intent to injure or kill, by any means

> **Excludes1**   injuries due to legal intervention (Y35.-)
> injuries due to operations of war (Y36.-)
> injuries due to terrorism (Y38.-)

● **X92**   **Assault by drowning and submersion**

> The appropriate 7th character is to be added to each code from category X92

> | | |
> |---|---|
> | A | initial encounter |
> | D | subsequent encounter |
> | S | sequela |

  X● **X92.0**   **Assault by drowning and submersion while in bathtub**
  X● **X92.1**   **Assault by drowning and submersion while in swimming pool**

N   Newborn Age: 0   P   Pediatric Age: 0–17   M   Maternity DX: 12–55   A   Adult Age: 15–124   ♀   Females Only   ♂   Males Only

🔖 Complication\Comorbidity   🔖 Major C\C   (Ex) CC/MCC Exclusions   🔖 Present on Admission Requirement   🔖 Hospital-Acquired Condition

1645

CHAPTER 20 (V01-Y99)

X● **X92.2** **Assault by drowning and submersion after push into swimming pool**

X● **X92.3** **Assault by drowning and submersion in natural water**

X● **X92.8** **Other assault by drowning and submersion**

X● **X92.9** **Assault by drowning and submersion, unspecified**

X● **X93** **Assault by handgun discharge**
Assault by discharge of gun for single hand use
Assault by discharge of pistol
Assault by discharge of revolver

> **Excludes1**   Very pistol (X95.8)

The appropriate 7th character is to be added to code X93

A	initial encounter
D	subsequent encounter
S	sequela

● **X94** **Assault by rifle, shotgun and larger firearm discharge**

> **Excludes1**   airgun (X95.01)

The appropriate 7th character is to be added to each code from category X94

A	initial encounter
D	subsequent encounter
S	sequela

X● **X94.0** **Assault by shotgun**

X● **X94.1** **Assault by hunting rifle**

X● **X94.2** **Assault by machine gun**

X● **X94.8** **Assault by other larger firearm discharge**

X● **X94.9** **Assault by unspecified larger firearm discharge**

● **X95** **Assault by other and unspecified firearm and gun discharge**

The appropriate 7th character is to be added to each code from category X95

A	initial encounter
D	subsequent encounter
S	sequela

● **X95.0** **Assault by gas, air or spring-operated guns**

    X● **X95.01** **Assault by airgun discharge**
Assault by BB gun discharge
Assault by pellet gun discharge

    X● **X95.02** **Assault by paintball gun discharge**

    X● **X95.09** **Assault by other gas, air or spring-operated gun**

X● **X95.8** **Assault by other firearm discharge**
Assault by very pistol [flare] discharge

X● **X95.9** **Assault by unspecified firearm discharge**

● **X96** **Assault by explosive material**

> **Excludes1**   incendiary device (X97)
> terrorism involving explosive material (Y38.2-)

The appropriate 7th character is to be added to each code from category X96

A	initial encounter
D	subsequent encounter
S	sequela

X● **X96.0** **Assault by antipersonnel bomb**

> **Excludes1**   antipersonnel bomb use in military or war (Y36.2-)

X● **X96.1** **Assault by gasoline bomb**

X● **X96.2** **Assault by letter bomb**

X● **X96.3** **Assault by fertilizer bomb**

X● **X96.4** **Assault by pipe bomb**

X● **X96.8** **Assault by other specified explosive**

X● **X96.9** **Assault by unspecified explosive**

X● **X97** **Assault by smoke, fire and flames**
Assault by arson
Assault by cigarettes
Assault by incendiary device

The appropriate 7th character is to be added to code X97

A	initial encounter
D	subsequent encounter
S	sequela

● **X98** **Assault by steam, hot vapors and hot objects**

The appropriate 7th character is to be added to each code from category X98

A	initial encounter
D	subsequent encounter
S	sequela

X● **X98.0** **Assault by steam or hot vapors**

X● **X98.1** **Assault by hot tap water**

X● **X98.2** **Assault by hot fluids**

X● **X98.3** **Assault by hot household appliances**

X● **X98.8** **Assault by other hot objects**

X● **X98.9** **Assault by unspecified hot objects**

● **X99** **Assault by sharp object**

> **Excludes1**   assault by strike by sports equipment (Y08.0-)

The appropriate 7th character is to be added to each code from category X99

A	initial encounter
D	subsequent encounter
S	sequela

X● **X99.0** **Assault by sharp glass**

X● **X99.1** **Assault by knife**

X● **X99.2** **Assault by sword or dagger**

X● **X99.8** **Assault by other sharp object**

X● **X99.9** **Assault by unspecified sharp object**
Assault by stabbing NOS

X● **Y00** **Assault by blunt object**

> **Excludes1**   assault by strike by sports equipment (Y08.0)

The appropriate 7th character is to be added to code Y00

A	initial encounter
D	subsequent encounter
S	sequela

X● **Y01** **Assault by pushing from high place**

The appropriate 7th character is to be added to code Y01

A	initial encounter
D	subsequent encounter
S	sequela

● **Y02** **Assault by pushing or placing victim in front of moving object**

The appropriate 7th character is to be added to each code from category Y02

A	initial encounter
D	subsequent encounter
S	sequela

X● **Y02.0** **Assault by pushing or placing victim in front of motor vehicle**

X● **Y02.1** **Assault by pushing or placing victim in front of (subway) train**

X● **Y02.8** **Assault by pushing or placing victim in front of other moving object**

◀ New   ⬛◀ Revised   ~~deleted~~ Deleted   Excludes 1   Excludes 2   Includes   Use additional   Code first   Code also   Unspecified

OGCR Official Guidelines   ● Unacceptable Principal Diagnosis   X Assign placeholder X   ▶ Use Additional Character(s)   ▶ Manifestation Code   **Coding Clinic**

● **Y03**   **Assault by crashing of motor vehicle**

The appropriate 7th character is to be added to each code from category Y03

A	initial encounter	
D	subsequent encounter	
S	sequela	

X ● **Y03.0**   **Assault by being hit or run over by motor vehicle**

X ● **Y03.8**   **Other assault by crashing of motor vehicle**

● **Y04**   **Assault by bodily force**

> **Excludes1**   assault by:
> submersion (X92.-)
> use of weapon (X93-X95, X99, Y00)

The appropriate 7th character is to be added to each code from category Y04

A	initial encounter	
D	subsequent encounter	
S	sequela	

X ● **Y04.0**   **Assault by unarmed brawl or fight**

X ● **Y04.1**   **Assault by human bite**

X ● **Y04.2**   **Assault by strike against or bumped into by another person**

X ● **Y04.8**   **Assault by other bodily force**
       Assault by bodily force NOS

OGCR   Section I.C.19.f.

> Adult and child abuse, neglect and other maltreatment
>
> Sequence first the appropriate code from categories T74.- or T76.- for abuse, neglect and other maltreatment, followed by any accompanying mental health or injury code(s).
>
> If the documentation in the medical record states abuse or neglect it is coded as confirmed. It is coded as suspected if it is documented as suspected.
>
> For cases of confirmed abuse or neglect an external cause code from the assault section (X92-Y08) should be added to identify the cause of any physical injuries. A perpetrator code (Y07) should be added when the perpetrator of the abuse is known. For suspected cases of abuse or neglect, do not report external cause or perpetrator code.
>
> If a suspected case of abuse, neglect or mistreatment is ruled out during an encounter code Z04.71, Encounter for examination and observation following alleged physical adult abuse, ruled out, or code Z04.72, Encounter for examination and observation following alleged child physical abuse, ruled out, should be used, not a code from T76.
>
> If a suspected case of alleged rape or sexual abuse is ruled out during an encounter code Z04.41, Encounter for examination and observation following alleged physical adult abuse, ruled out, or code Z04.42, Encounter for examination and observation following alleged rape or sexual abuse, ruled out, should be used, not a code from T76.

● **Y07**   **Perpetrator of assault, maltreatment and neglect**

Note: Codes from this category are for use only in cases of confirmed abuse (T74.-)

Selection of the correct perpetrator code is based on the relationship between the perpetrator and the victim

> **Includes**   perpetrator of abandonment
> perpetrator of emotional neglect
> perpetrator of mental cruelty
> perpetrator of physical abuse
> perpetrator of physical neglect
> perpetrator of sexual abuse
> perpetrator of torture

● **Y07.0**   **Spouse or partner, perpetrator of maltreatment and neglect**
       Spouse or partner, perpetrator of maltreatment and neglect against spouse or partner

     Y07.01   **Husband, perpetrator of maltreatment and neglect**

     Y07.02   **Wife, perpetrator of maltreatment and neglect**

     Y07.03   **Male partner, perpetrator of maltreatment and neglect**

     Y07.04   **Female partner, perpetrator of maltreatment and neglect**

● **Y07.1**   **Parent (adoptive) (biological), perpetrator of maltreatment and neglect**

     Y07.11   **Biological father, perpetrator of maltreatment and neglect**

     Y07.12   **Biological mother, perpetrator of maltreatment and neglect**

     Y07.13   **Adoptive father, perpetrator of maltreatment and neglect**

     Y07.14   **Adoptive mother, perpetrator of maltreatment and neglect**

● **Y07.4**   **Other family member, perpetrator of maltreatment and neglect**

● **Y07.41**   **Sibling, perpetrator of maltreatment and neglect**

> **Excludes1**   stepsibling, perpetrator of maltreatment and neglect (Y07.435, Y07.436)

     Y07.410   **Brother, perpetrator of maltreatment and neglect**

     Y07.411   **Sister, perpetrator of maltreatment and neglect**

● **Y07.42**   **Foster parent, perpetrator of maltreatment and neglect**

     Y07.420   **Foster father, perpetrator of maltreatment and neglect**

     Y07.421   **Foster mother, perpetrator of maltreatment and neglect**

● **Y07.43**   **Stepparent or stepsibling, perpetrator of maltreatment and neglect**

     Y07.430   **Stepfather, perpetrator of maltreatment and neglect**

     Y07.432   **Male friend of parent (co-residing in household), perpetrator of maltreatment and neglect**

     Y07.433   **Stepmother, perpetrator of maltreatment and neglect**

     Y07.434   **Female friend of parent (co-residing in household), perpetrator of maltreatment and neglect**

     Y07.435   **Stepbrother, perpetrator or maltreatment and neglect**

     Y07.436   **Stepsister, perpetrator of maltreatment and neglect**

● **Y07.49**   **Other family member, perpetrator of maltreatment and neglect**

     Y07.490   **Male cousin, perpetrator of maltreatment and neglect**

     Y07.491   **Female cousin, perpetrator of maltreatment and neglect**

     Y07.499   **Other family member, perpetrator of maltreatment and neglect**

● **Y07.5**   **Non-family member, perpetrator of maltreatment and neglect**

     Y07.50   **Unspecified non-family member, perpetrator of maltreatment and neglect**

● **Y07.51**   **Daycare provider, perpetrator of maltreatment and neglect**

     Y07.510   **At-home childcare provider, perpetrator of maltreatment and neglect**

     Y07.511   **Daycare center childcare provider, perpetrator of maltreatment and neglect**

     Y07.512   **At-home adultcare provider, perpetrator of maltreatment and neglect**

N   Newborn Age: 0   P   Pediatric Age: 0–17   M   Maternity DX: 12–55   A   Adult Age: 15–124   ♀   Females Only   ♂   Males Only

⚲   Complication\Comorbidity   ⚲   Major C\C   (Ex)   CC/MCC Exclusions   ⚲   Present on Admission Requirement   ⚲   Hospital-Acquired Condition

1647

CHAPTER 20 (V01-Y99)

Y07.513　Adultcare center provider, perpetrator of maltreatment and neglect

Y07.519　Unspecified daycare provider, perpetrator of maltreatment and neglect

● Y07.52　Healthcare provider, perpetrator of maltreatment and neglect

Y07.521　Mental health provider, perpetrator of maltreatment and neglect

Y07.528　Other therapist or healthcare provider, perpetrator of maltreatment and neglect

　　　Nurse perpetrator of maltreatment and neglect

　　　Occupational therapist perpetrator of maltreatment and neglect

　　　Physical therapist perpetrator of maltreatment and neglect

　　　Speech therapist perpetrator of maltreatment and neglect

Y07.529　Unspecified healthcare provider, perpetrator of maltreatment and neglect

Y07.53　Teacher or instructor, perpetrator of maltreatment and neglect

　　　Coach, perpetrator of maltreatment and neglect

Y07.59　Other non-family member, perpetrator of maltreatment and neglect

● Y07.9　Unspecified perpetrator of maltreatment and neglect

● Y08　Assault by other specified means

The appropriate 7th character is to be added to each code from category Y08

A	initial encounter
D	subsequent encounter
S	sequela

● Y08.0　Assault by strike by sport equipment

X ● Y08.01　Assault by strike by hockey stick

X ● Y08.02　Assault by strike by baseball bat

X ● Y08.09　Assault by strike by other specified type of sport equipment

● Y08.8　Assault by other specified means

X ● Y08.81　Assault by crashing of aircraft

X ● Y08.89　Assault by other specified means

● Y09　Assault by unspecified means

Assassination (attempted) NOS
Homicide (attempted) NOS
Manslaughter (attempted) NOS
Murder (attempted) NOS

EVENT OF UNDETERMINED INTENT (Y21-Y33)

Undetermined intent is only for use when there is specific documentation in the record that the intent of the injury cannot be determined. If no such documentation is present, code to accidental (unintentional)

● Y21　Drowning and submersion, undetermined intent

The appropriate 7th character is to be added to each code from category Y21

A	initial encounter
D	subsequent encounter
S	sequela

X ● Y21.0　Drowning and submersion while in bathtub, undetermined intent 🖲

X ● Y21.1　Drowning and submersion after fall into bathtub, undetermined intent 🖲

X ● Y21.2　Drowning and submersion while in swimming pool, undetermined intent 🖲

X ● Y21.3　Drowning and submersion after fall into swimming pool, undetermined intent 🖲

X ● Y21.4　Drowning and submersion in natural water, undetermined intent 🖲

X ● Y21.8　Other drowning and submersion, undetermined intent 🖲

X ● Y21.9　Unspecified drowning and submersion, undetermined intent 🖲

X ● Y22　Handgun discharge, undetermined intent 🖲

Discharge of gun for single hand use, undetermined intent
Discharge of pistol, undetermined intent
Discharge of revolver, undetermined intent

Excludes2　very pistol (Y24.8)

The appropriate 7th character is to be added to code Y22

A	initial encounter
D	subsequent encounter
S	sequela

● Y23　Rifle, shotgun and larger firearm discharge, undetermined intent

Excludes2　airgun (Y24.0)

The appropriate 7th character is to be added to each code from category Y23

A	initial encounter
D	subsequent encounter
S	sequela

X ● Y23.0　Shotgun discharge, undetermined intent 🖲

X ● Y23.1　Hunting rifle discharge, undetermined intent 🖲

X ● Y23.2　Military firearm discharge, undetermined intent 🖲

X ● Y23.3　Machine gun discharge, undetermined intent 🖲

X ● Y23.8　Other larger firearm discharge, undetermined intent 🖲

X ● Y23.9　Unspecified larger firearm discharge, undetermined intent 🖲

● Y24　Other and unspecified firearm discharge, undetermined intent

The appropriate 7th character is to be added to each code from category Y24

A	initial encounter
D	subsequent encounter
S	sequela

X ● Y24.0　Airgun discharge, undetermined intent 🖲

BB gun discharge, undetermined intent
Pellet gun discharge, undetermined intent

X ● Y24.8　Other firearm discharge, undetermined intent 🖲

Paintball gun discharge, undetermined intent
Very pistol [flare] discharge, undetermined intent

X ● Y24.9　Unspecified firearm discharge, undetermined intent 🖲

X ● Y25　Contact with explosive material, undetermined intent

The appropriate 7th character is to be added to code Y25

A	initial encounter
D	subsequent encounter
S	sequela

X ● Y26　Exposure to smoke, fire and flames, undetermined intent

The appropriate 7th character is to be added to code Y26

A	initial encounter
D	subsequent encounter
S	sequela

● **Y27**   **Contact with steam, hot vapors and hot objects, undetermined intent**

> The appropriate 7th character is to be added to each code from category Y27

> | | |
> |---|---|
> | A | initial encounter |
> | D | subsequent encounter |
> | S | sequela |

X ● **Y27.0**   Contact with steam and hot vapors, undetermined intent

X ● **Y27.1**   Contact with hot tap water, undetermined intent

X ● **Y27.2**   Contact with hot fluids, undetermined intent

X ● **Y27.3**   Contact with hot household appliance, undetermined intent

X ● **Y27.8**   Contact with other hot objects, undetermined intent

X ● **Y27.9**   Contact with unspecified hot objects, undetermined intent

● **Y28**   **Contact with sharp object, undetermined intent**

> The appropriate 7th character is to be added to each code from category Y28

> | | |
> |---|---|
> | A | initial encounter |
> | D | subsequent encounter |
> | S | sequela |

X ● **Y28.0**   Contact with sharp glass, undetermined intent

X ● **Y28.1**   Contact with knife, undetermined intent

X ● **Y28.2**   Contact with sword or dagger, undetermined intent

X ● **Y28.8**   Contact with other sharp object, undetermined intent

X ● **Y28.9**   Contact with unspecified sharp object, undetermined intent

X ● **Y29**   **Contact with blunt object, undetermined intent**

> The appropriate 7th character is to be added to code Y29

> | | |
> |---|---|
> | A | initial encounter |
> | D | subsequent encounter |
> | S | sequela |

X ● **Y30**   **Falling, jumping or pushed from a high place, undetermined intent** 🖐

> Victim falling from one level to another, undetermined intent

> The appropriate 7th character is to be added to code Y30

> | | |
> |---|---|
> | A | initial encounter |
> | D | subsequent encounter |
> | S | sequela |

X ● **Y31**   **Falling, lying or running before or into moving object, undetermined intent**

> The appropriate 7th character is to be added to code Y31

> | | |
> |---|---|
> | A | initial encounter |
> | D | subsequent encounter |
> | S | sequela |

X ● **Y32**   **Crashing of motor vehicle, undetermined intent**

> The appropriate 7th character is to be added to code Y32

> | | |
> |---|---|
> | A | initial encounter |
> | D | subsequent encounter |
> | S | sequela |

X ● **Y33**   **Other specified events, undetermined intent**

> The appropriate 7th character is to be added to code Y33

> | | |
> |---|---|
> | A | initial encounter |
> | D | subsequent encounter |
> | S | sequela |

LEGAL INTERVENTION, OPERATIONS OF WAR, MILITARY OPERATIONS, AND TERRORISM (Y35-Y38)

● **Y35**   **Legal intervention**

> **Includes**   any injury sustained as a result of an encounter with any law enforcement official, serving in any capacity at the time of the encounter, whether on-duty or off-duty. Includes: injury to law enforcement official, suspect and bystander ◀▥

> The appropriate 7th character is to be added to each code from category Y35

> | | |
> |---|---|
> | A | initial encounter |
> | D | subsequent encounter |
> | S | sequela |

● **Y35.0**   Legal intervention involving firearm discharge

   ● **Y35.00**   Legal intervention involving unspecified firearm discharge

> Legal intervention involving gunshot wound
> Legal intervention involving shot NOS

     ● **Y35.001**   Legal intervention involving unspecified firearm discharge, law enforcement official injured 🖐

     ● **Y35.002**   Legal intervention involving unspecified firearm discharge, bystander injured 🖐

     ● **Y35.003**   Legal intervention involving unspecified firearm discharge, suspect injured 🖐

   ● **Y35.01**   Legal intervention involving injury by machine gun

     ● **Y35.011**   Legal intervention involving injury by machine gun, law enforcement official injured 🖐

     ● **Y35.012**   Legal intervention involving injury by machine gun, bystander injured 🖐

     ● **Y35.013**   Legal intervention involving injury by machine gun, suspect injured 🖐

   ● **Y35.02**   Legal intervention involving injury by handgun

     ● **Y35.021**   Legal intervention involving injury by handgun, law enforcement official injured 🖐

     ● **Y35.022**   Legal intervention involving injury by handgun, bystander injured 🖐

     ● **Y35.023**   Legal intervention involving injury by handgun, suspect injured 🖐

   ● **Y35.03**   Legal intervention involving injury by rifle pellet

     ● **Y35.031**   Legal intervention involving injury by rifle pellet, law enforcement official injured 🖐

     ● **Y35.032**   Legal intervention involving injury by rifle pellet, bystander injured 🖐

     ● **Y35.033**   Legal intervention involving injury by rifle pellet, suspect injured 🖐

   ● **Y35.04**   Legal intervention involving injury by rubber bullet

     ● **Y35.041**   Legal intervention involving injury by rubber bullet, law enforcement official injured 🖐

     ● **Y35.042**   Legal intervention involving injury by rubber bullet, bystander injured 🖐

     ● **Y35.043**   Legal intervention involving injury by rubber bullet, suspect injured 🖐

CHAPTER 20 (V01-Y99)

N Newborn Age: 0	**P** Pediatric Age: 0–17	**M** Maternity DX: 12–55	**A** Adult Age: 15–124	♀ Females Only	♂ Males Only
🖐 Complication\Comorbidity	🖐 Major C\C	(Ex) CC/MCC Exclusions	🖐 Present on Admission Requirement		🖐 Hospital-Acquired Condition

1649

● Y35.09   Legal intervention involving other firearm discharge
     ● Y35.091   Legal intervention involving other firearm discharge, law enforcement official injured 🖎
     ● Y35.092   Legal intervention involving other firearm discharge, bystander injured 🖎
     ● Y35.093   Legal intervention involving other firearm discharge, suspect injured 🖎

● Y35.1   Legal intervention involving explosives
   ● Y35.10   Legal intervention involving unspecified explosives
     ● Y35.101   Legal intervention involving unspecified explosives, law enforcement official injured 🖎
     ● Y35.102   Legal intervention involving unspecified explosives, bystander injured 🖎
     ● Y35.103   Legal intervention involving unspecified explosives, suspect injured 🖎

   ● Y35.11   Legal intervention involving injury by dynamite
     ● Y35.111   Legal intervention involving injury by dynamite, law enforcement official injured 🖎
     ● Y35.112   Legal intervention involving injury by dynamite, bystander injured 🖎
     ● Y35.113   Legal intervention involving injury by dynamite, suspect injured 🖎

   ● Y35.12   Legal intervention involving injury by explosive shell
     ● Y35.121   Legal intervention involving injury by explosive shell, law enforcement official injured 🖎
     ● Y35.122   Legal intervention involving injury by explosive shell, bystander injured 🖎
     ● Y35.123   Legal intervention involving injury by explosive shell, suspect injured 🖎

   ● Y35.19   Legal intervention involving other explosives
       Legal intervention involving injury by grenade
       Legal intervention involving injury by mortar bomb
     ● Y35.191   Legal intervention involving other explosives, law enforcement official injured 🖎
     ● Y35.192   Legal intervention involving other explosives, bystander injured 🖎
     ● Y35.193   Legal intervention involving other explosives, suspect injured 🖎

● Y35.2   Legal intervention involving gas
       Legal intervention involving asphyxiation by gas
       Legal intervention involving poisoning by gas
   ● Y35.20   Legal intervention involving unspecified gas
     ● Y35.201   Legal intervention involving unspecified gas, law enforcement official injured 🖎
     ● Y35.202   Legal intervention involving unspecified gas, bystander injured 🖎
     ● Y35.203   Legal intervention involving unspecified gas, suspect injured 🖎

● Y35.21   Legal intervention involving injury by tear gas
     ● Y35.211   Legal intervention involving injury by tear gas, law enforcement official injured 🖎
     ● Y35.212   Legal intervention involving injury by tear gas, bystander injured 🖎
     ● Y35.213   Legal intervention involving injury by tear gas, suspect injured 🖎

   ● Y35.29   Legal intervention involving other gas
     ● Y35.291   Legal intervention involving other gas, law enforcement official injured 🖎
     ● Y35.292   Legal intervention involving other gas, bystander injured 🖎
     ● Y35.293   Legal intervention involving other gas, suspect injured 🖎

● Y35.3   Legal intervention involving blunt objects
       Legal intervention involving being hit or struck by blunt object
   ● Y35.30   Legal intervention involving unspecified blunt objects
     ● Y35.301   Legal intervention involving unspecified blunt objects, law enforcement official injured 🖎
     ● Y35.302   Legal intervention involving unspecified blunt objects, bystander injured 🖎
     ● Y35.303   Legal intervention involving unspecified blunt objects, suspect injured 🖎

   ● Y35.31   Legal intervention involving baton
     ● Y35.311   Legal intervention involving baton, law enforcement official injured 🖎
     ● Y35.312   Legal intervention involving baton, bystander injured 🖎
     ● Y35.313   Legal intervention involving baton, suspect injured 🖎

   ● Y35.39   Legal intervention involving other blunt objects
     ● Y35.391   Legal intervention involving other blunt objects, law enforcement official injured 🖎
     ● Y35.392   Legal intervention involving other blunt objects, bystander injured 🖎
     ● Y35.393   Legal intervention involving other blunt objects, suspect injured 🖎

● Y35.4   Legal intervention involving sharp objects
       Legal intervention involving being cut by sharp objects
       Legal intervention involving being stabbed by sharp objects
   ● Y35.40   Legal intervention involving unspecified sharp objects
     ● Y35.401   Legal intervention involving unspecified sharp objects, law enforcement official injured 🖎
     ● Y35.402   Legal intervention involving unspecified sharp objects, bystander injured 🖎
     ● Y35.403   Legal intervention involving unspecified sharp objects, suspect injured 🖎

● Y35.41   Legal intervention involving bayonet
   ● Y35.411   Legal intervention involving bayonet, law enforcement official injured 🔘
   ● Y35.412   Legal intervention involving bayonet, bystander injured 🔘
   ● Y35.413   Legal intervention involving bayonet, suspect injured 🔘
● Y35.49   Legal intervention involving other sharp objects
   ● Y35.491   Legal intervention involving other sharp objects, law enforcement official injured 🔘
   ● Y35.492   Legal intervention involving other sharp objects, bystander injured 🔘
   ● Y35.493   Legal intervention involving other sharp objects, suspect injured 🔘
● Y35.8   Legal intervention involving other specified means
   ● Y35.81   Legal intervention involving manhandling
     ● Y35.811   Legal intervention involving manhandling, law enforcement official injured 🔘
     ● Y35.812   Legal intervention involving manhandling, bystander injured 🔘
     ● Y35.813   Legal intervention involving manhandling, suspect injured 🔘
   ● Y35.89   Legal intervention involving other specified means
     ● Y35.891   Legal intervention involving other specified means, law enforcement official injured 🔘
     ● Y35.892   Legal intervention involving other specified means, bystander injured 🔘
     ● Y35.893   Legal intervention involving other specified means, suspect injured 🔘
● Y35.9   Legal intervention, means unspecified
   X ● Y35.91   Legal intervention, means unspecified, law enforcement official injured 🔘
   X ● Y35.92   Legal intervention, means unspecified, bystander injured 🔘
   X ● Y35.93   Legal intervention, means unspecified, suspect injured 🔘

● Y36   Operations of war

Includes	injuries to military personnel and civilians caused by war, civil insurrection, and peacekeeping missions
Excludes1	injury to military personnel occurring during peacetime military operations (Y37.-)
	military vehicles involved in transport accidents with non-military vehicle during peacetime (V09.01, V09.21, V19.81, V29.81, V39.81, V49.81, V59.81, V69.81, V79.81)

The appropriate 7th character is to be added to each code from category Y36

> A   initial encounter
> D   subsequent encounter
> S   sequela

● Y36.0   War operations involving explosion of marine weapons
   Weapons and military watercraft
   ● Y36.00   War operations involving explosion of unspecified marine weapon
     War operations involving underwater blast NOS
     ● Y36.000   War operations involving explosion of unspecified marine weapon, military personnel 🔘
     ● Y36.001   War operations involving explosion of unspecified marine weapon, civilian 🔘

● Y36.01   War operations involving explosion of depth-charge
   ● Y36.010   War operations involving explosion of depth-charge, military personnel 🔘
   ● Y36.011   War operations involving explosion of depth-charge, civilian 🔘
● Y36.02   War operations involving explosion of marine mine
   War operations involving explosion of marine mine, at sea or in harbor
   ● Y36.020   War operations involving explosion of marine mine, military personnel 🔘
   ● Y36.021   War operations involving explosion of marine mine, civilian 🔘
● Y36.03   War operations involving explosion of sea-based artillery shell
   ● Y36.030   War operations involving explosion of sea-based artillery shell, military personnel 🔘
   ● Y36.031   War operations involving explosion of sea-based artillery shell, civilian 🔘
● Y36.04   War operations involving explosion of torpedo
   ● Y36.040   War operations involving explosion of torpedo, military personnel 🔘
   ● Y36.041   War operations involving explosion of torpedo, civilian 🔘
● Y36.05   War operations involving accidental detonation of onboard marine weapons
   ● Y36.050   War operations involving accidental detonation of onboard marine weapons, military personnel 🔘
   ● Y36.051   War operations involving accidental detonation of onboard marine weapons, civilian 🔘
● Y36.09   War operations involving explosion of other marine weapons
   ● Y36.090   War operations involving explosion of other marine weapons, military personnel 🔘
   ● Y36.091   War operations involving explosion of other marine weapons, civilian 🔘
● Y36.1   War operations involving destruction of aircraft
   ● Y36.10   War operations involving unspecified destruction of aircraft
     ● Y36.100   War operations involving unspecified destruction of aircraft, military personnel 🔘
     ● Y36.101   War operations involving unspecified destruction of aircraft, civilian 🔘
   ● Y36.11   War operations involving destruction of aircraft due to enemy fire or explosives
     War operations involving destruction of aircraft due to air to air missile
     War operations involving destruction of aircraft due to explosive placed on aircraft
     War operations involving destruction of aircraft due to rocket propelled grenade [RPG]
     War operations involving destruction of aircraft due to small arms fire
     War operations involving destruction of aircraft due to surface to air missile
     ● Y36.110   War operations involving destruction of aircraft due to enemy fire or explosives, military personnel 🔘
     ● Y36.111   War operations involving destruction of aircraft due to enemy fire or explosives, civilian 🔘

N Newborn Age: 0   **P** Pediatric Age: 0–17   **M** Maternity DX: 12–55   **A** Adult Age: 15–124   ♀ Females Only   ♂ Males Only

🔘 Complication\Comorbidity   🔘 Major C\C   (Ex) CC/MCC Exclusions   🔘 Present on Admission Requirement   🔘 Hospital-Acquired Condition

1651

● Y36.12   War operations involving destruction of aircraft due to collision with other aircraft
     ● Y36.120   War operations involving destruction of aircraft due to collision with other aircraft, military personnel 🖎
     ● Y36.121   War operations involving destruction of aircraft due to collision with other aircraft, civilian 🖎

● Y36.13   War operations involving destruction of aircraft due to onboard fire
     ● Y36.130   War operations involving destruction of aircraft due to onboard fire, military personnel 🖎
     ● Y36.131   War operations involving destruction of aircraft due to onboard fire, civilian 🖎

● Y36.14   War operations involving destruction of aircraft due to accidental detonation of onboard munitions and explosives
     ● Y36.140   War operations involving destruction of aircraft due to accidental detonation of onboard munitions and explosives, military personnel 🖎
     ● Y36.141   War operations involving destruction of aircraft due to accidental detonation of onboard munitions and explosives, civilian 🖎

● Y36.19   War operations involving other destruction of aircraft
     ● Y36.190   War operations involving other destruction of aircraft, military personnel 🖎
     ● Y36.191   War operations involving other destruction of aircraft, civilian 🖎

● Y36.2   War operations involving other explosions and fragments
     Excludes1   war operations involving explosion of aircraft (Y36.1-)
         war operations involving explosion of marine weapons (Y36.0-)
         war operations involving explosion of nuclear weapons (Y36.5-)
         war operations involving explosion occurring after cessation of hostilities (Y36.8-)

     ● Y36.20   War operations involving unspecified explosion and fragments
         War operations involving air blast NOS
         War operations involving blast NOS
         War operations involving blast fragments NOS
         War operations involving blast wave NOS
         War operations involving blast wind NOS
         War operations involving explosion NOS
         War operations involving explosion of bomb NOS
        ● Y36.200   War operations involving unspecified explosion and fragments, military personnel 🖎
        ● Y36.201   War operations involving unspecified explosion and fragments, civilian 🖎

     ● Y36.21   War operations involving explosion of aerial bomb
        ● Y36.210   War operations involving explosion of aerial bomb, military personnel 🖎
        ● Y36.211   War operations involving explosion of aerial bomb, civilian 🖎

     ● Y36.22   War operations involving explosion of guided missile
        ● Y36.220   War operations involving explosion of guided missile, military personnel 🖎
        ● Y36.221   War operations involving explosion of guided missile, civilian 🖎

● Y36.23   War operations involving explosion of improvised explosive device [IED]
     War operations involving explosion of person-borne improvised explosive device [IED]
     War operations involving explosion of vehicle-borne improvised explosive device [IED]
     War operations involving explosion of roadside improvised explosive device [IED]
     ● Y36.230   War operations involving explosion of improvised explosive device [IED], military personnel 🖎
     ● Y36.231   War operations involving explosion of improvised explosive device [IED], civilian 🖎

● Y36.24   War operations involving explosion due to accidental detonation and discharge of own munitions or munitions launch device
     ● Y36.240   War operations involving explosion due to accidental detonation and discharge of own munitions or munitions launch device, military personnel 🖎
     ● Y36.241   War operations involving explosion due to accidental detonation and discharge of own munitions or munitions launch device, civilian 🖎

● Y36.25   War operations involving fragments from munitions
     ● Y36.250   War operations involving fragments from munitions, military personnel 🖎
     ● Y36.251   War operations involving fragments from munitions, civilian 🖎

● Y36.26   War operations involving fragments of improvised explosive device [IED]
     War operations involving fragments of person-borne improvised explosive device [IED]
     War operations involving fragments of vehicle-borne improvised explosive device [IED]
     War operations involving fragments of roadside improvised explosive device [IED]
     ● Y36.260   War operations involving fragments of improvised explosive device [IED], military personnel 🖎
     ● Y36.261   War operations involving fragments of improvised explosive device [IED], civilian 🖎

● Y36.27   War operations involving fragments from weapons
     ● Y36.270   War operations involving fragments from weapons, military personnel 🖎
     ● Y36.271   War operations involving fragments from weapons, civilian 🖎

● Y36.29   War operations involving other explosions and fragments
     War operations involving explosion of grenade
     War operations involving explosions of land mine
     War operations involving shrapnel NOS
     ● Y36.290   War operations involving other explosions and fragments, military personnel 🖎
     ● Y36.291   War operations involving other explosions and fragments, civilian 🖎

◀ New   ⬅ Revised   ~~deleted~~ Deleted   Excludes 1   Excludes 2   Includes   Use additional   Code first   Code also   Unspecified
OGCR Official Guidelines   ● Unacceptable Principal Diagnosis   X Assign placeholder X   ● Use Additional Character(s)   🖎 Manifestation Code   **Coding Clinic**

- **Y36.3** **War operations involving fires, conflagrations and hot substances**

  War operations involving smoke, fumes, and heat from fires, conflagrations and hot substances

  Excludes1   war operations involving fires and conflagrations aboard military aircraft (Y36.1-)

  war operations involving fires and conflagrations aboard military watercraft (Y36.0-)

  war operations involving fires and conflagrations caused indirectly by conventional weapons (Y36.2-)

  war operations involving fires and thermal effects of nuclear weapons (Y36.53-)

  - **Y36.30** **War operations involving unspecified fire, conflagration and hot substance**

    - **Y36.300** War operations involving unspecified fire, conflagration and hot substance, military personnel 🔖

    - **Y36.301** War operations involving unspecified fire, conflagration and hot substance, civilian 🔖

  - **Y36.31** **War operations involving gasoline bomb**

    War operations involving incendiary bomb
    War operations involving petrol bomb

    - **Y36.310** War operations involving gasoline bomb, military personnel 🔖

    - **Y36.311** War operations involving gasoline bomb, civilian 🔖

  - **Y36.32** **War operations involving incendiary bullet**

    - **Y36.320** War operations involving incendiary bullet, military personnel 🔖

    - **Y36.321** War operations involving incendiary bullet, civilian 🔖

  - **Y36.33** **War operations involving flamethrower**

    - **Y36.330** War operations involving flamethrower, military personnel 🔖

    - **Y36.331** War operations involving flamethrower, civilian 🔖

  - **Y36.39** **War operations involving other fires, conflagrations and hot substances**

    - **Y36.390** War operations involving other fires, conflagrations and hot substances, military personnel 🔖

    - **Y36.391** War operations involving other fires, conflagrations and hot substances, civilian 🔖

- **Y36.4** **War operations involving firearm discharge and other forms of conventional warfare**

  - **Y36.41** **War operations involving rubber bullets**

    - **Y36.410** War operations involving rubber bullets, military personnel 🔖

    - **Y36.411** War operations involving rubber bullets, civilian 🔖

  - **Y36.42** **War operations involving firearms pellets**

    - **Y36.420** War operations involving firearms pellets, military personnel 🔖

    - **Y36.421** War operations involving firearms pellets, civilian 🔖

- **Y36.43** **War operations involving other firearms discharge**

  War operations involving bullets NOS

  Excludes1   war operations involving munitions fragments (Y36.25-)

  war operations involving incendiary bullets (Y36.32-)

  - **Y36.430** War operations involving other firearms discharge, military personnel 🔖

  - **Y36.431** War operations involving other firearms discharge, civilian 🔖

- **Y36.44** **War operations involving unarmed hand to hand combat**

  Excludes1   war operations involving combat using blunt or piercing object (Y36.45-)

  war operations involving intentional restriction of air and airway (Y36.46-)

  war operations involving unintentional restriction of air and airway (Y36.47-)

  - **Y36.440** War operations involving unarmed hand to hand combat, military personnel 🔖

  - **Y36.441** War operations involving unarmed hand to hand combat, civilian 🔖

- **Y36.45** **War operations involving combat using blunt or piercing object**

  - **Y36.450** War operations involving combat using blunt or piercing object, military personnel 🔖

  - **Y36.451** War operations involving combat using blunt or piercing object, civilian 🔖

- **Y36.46** **War operations involving intentional restriction of air and airway**

  - **Y36.460** War operations involving intentional restriction of air and airway, military personnel 🔖

  - **Y36.461** War operations involving intentional restriction of air and airway, civilian 🔖

- **Y36.47** **War operations involving unintentional restriction of air and airway**

  - **Y36.470** War operations involving unintentional restriction of air and airway, military personnel 🔖

  - **Y36.471** War operations involving unintentional restriction of air and airway, civilian 🔖

- **Y36.49** **War operations involving other forms of conventional warfare**

  - **Y36.490** War operations involving other forms of conventional warfare, military personnel 🔖

  - **Y36.491** War operations involving other forms of conventional warfare, civilian 🔖

- **Y36.5** **War operations involving nuclear weapons**

  War operations involving dirty bomb NOS

  - **Y36.50** **War operations involving unspecified effect of nuclear weapon**

    - **Y36.500** War operations involving unspecified effect of nuclear weapon, military personnel 🔖

    - **Y36.501** War operations involving unspecified effect of nuclear weapon, civilian 🔖

● Y36.51   War operations involving direct blast effect of nuclear weapon
    War operations involving blast pressure of nuclear weapon
   ● Y36.510   War operations involving direct blast effect of nuclear weapon, military personnel 🔍
   ● Y36.511   War operations involving direct blast effect of nuclear weapon, civilian 🔍

● Y36.52   War operations involving indirect blast effect of nuclear weapon
    War operations involving being thrown by blast of nuclear weapon
    War operations involving being struck or crushed by blast debris of nuclear weapon
   ● Y36.520   War operations involving indirect blast effect of nuclear weapon, military personnel 🔍
   ● Y36.521   War operations involving indirect blast effect of nuclear weapon, civilian 🔍

● Y36.53   War operations involving thermal radiation effect of nuclear weapon
    War operations involving direct heat from nuclear weapon
    War operation involving fireball effects from nuclear weapon
   ● Y36.530   War operations involving thermal radiation effect of nuclear weapon, military personnel 🔍
   ● Y36.531   War operations involving thermal radiation effect of nuclear weapon, civilian 🔍

● Y36.54   War operation involving nuclear radiation effects of nuclear weapon
    War operation involving acute radiation exposure from nuclear weapon
    War operation involving exposure to immediate ionizing radiation from nuclear weapon
    War operation involving fallout exposure from nuclear weapon
    War operation involving secondary effects of nuclear weapons
   ● Y36.540   War operation involving nuclear radiation effects of nuclear weapon, military personnel 🔍
   ● Y36.541   War operation involving nuclear radiation effects of nuclear weapon, civilian 🔍

● Y36.59   War operation involving other effects of nuclear weapons
   ● Y36.590   War operation involving other effects of nuclear weapons, military personnel 🔍
   ● Y36.591   War operation involving other effects of nuclear weapons, civilian 🔍

● Y36.6   War operations involving biological weapons
   ● Y36.6X   War operations involving biological weapons
     ● Y36.6X0   War operations involving biological weapons, military personnel 🔍
     ● Y36.6X1   War operations involving biological weapons, civilian 🔍

● Y36.7   War operations involving chemical weapons and other forms of unconventional warfare
   Excludes 1   war operations involving incendiary devices (Y36.3-, Y36.5-)
   ● Y36.7X   War operations involving chemical weapons and other forms of unconventional warfare
     ● Y36.7X0   War operations involving chemical weapons and other forms of unconventional warfare, military personnel 🔍
     ● Y36.7X1   War operations involving chemical weapons and other forms of unconventional warfare, civilian 🔍

● Y36.8   War operations occurring after cessation of hostilities
    War operations classifiable to categories Y36.0-Y36.8 but occurring after cessation of hostilities
   ● Y36.81   Explosion of mine placed during war operations but exploding after cessation of hostilities
     ● Y36.810   Explosion of mine placed during war operations but exploding after cessation of hostilities, military personnel 🔍
     ● Y36.811   Explosion of mine placed during war operations but exploding after cessation of hostilities, civilian 🔍
   ● Y36.82   Explosion of bomb placed during war operations but exploding after cessation of hostilities
     ● Y36.820   Explosion of bomb placed during war operations but exploding after cessation of hostilities, military personnel 🔍
     ● Y36.821   Explosion of bomb placed during war operations but exploding after cessation of hostilities, civilian 🔍
   ● Y36.88   Other war operations occurring after cessation of hostilities
     ● Y36.880   Other war operations occurring after cessation of hostilities, military personnel 🔍
     ● Y36.881   Other war operations occurring after cessation of hostilities, civilian 🔍
   ● Y36.89   Unspecified war operations occurring after cessation of hostilities
     ● Y36.890   Unspecified war operations occurring after cessation of hostilities, military personnel 🔍
     ● Y36.891   Unspecified war operations occurring after cessation of hostilities, civilian 🔍

● Y36.9   Other and unspecified war operations
   X ● Y36.90   War operations, unspecified 🔍
   X ● Y36.91   War operations involving unspecified weapon of mass destruction [WMD] 🔍
   X ● Y36.92   War operations involving friendly fire 🔍

◀ New   ◀▥ Revised   ~~deleted~~ Deleted   Excludes 1   Excludes 2   Includes   Use additional   Code first   Code also   Unspecified
OGCR Official Guidelines   ● Unacceptable Principal Diagnosis   X Assign placeholder X   ▶ Use Additional Character(s)   ▶ Manifestation Code   **Coding Clinic**

● **Y37   Military operations**

   Includes   Injuries to military personnel and civilians occurring during peacetime on military property and during routine military exercises and operations

   Excludes1   military aircraft involved in aircraft accident with civilian aircraft (V97.81-)

         military vehicles involved in transport accident with civilian vehicle (V09.01, V09.21, V19.81, V29.81, V39.81, V49.81, V59.81, V69.81, V79.81)

         military watercraft involved in water transport accident with civilian watercraft (V94.81-)

         war operations (Y36.-)

   The appropriate 7th character is to be added to each code from category Y37

> A   initial encounter
> D   subsequent encounter
> S   sequela

● **Y37.0   Military operations involving explosion of marine weapons**

   ● **Y37.00   Military operations involving explosion of unspecified marine weapon**

       Military operations involving underwater blast NOS

     ● **Y37.000   Military operations involving explosion of unspecified marine weapon, military personnel** 🏥

     ● **Y37.001   Military operations involving explosion of unspecified marine weapon, civilian** 🏥

   ● **Y37.01   Military operations involving explosion of depth-charge**

     ● **Y37.010   Military operations involving explosion of depth-charge, military personnel** 🏥

     ● **Y37.011   Military operations involving explosion of depth-charge, civilian** 🏥

   ● **Y37.02   Military operations involving explosion of marine mine**

       Military operations involving explosion of marine mine, at sea or in harbor

     ● **Y37.020   Military operations involving explosion of marine mine, military personnel** 🏥

     ● **Y37.021   Military operations involving explosion of marine mine, civilian** 🏥

   ● **Y37.03   Military operations involving explosion of sea-based artillery shell**

     ● **Y37.030   Military operations involving explosion of sea-based artillery shell, military personnel** 🏥

     ● **Y37.031   Military operations involving explosion of sea-based artillery shell, civilian** 🏥

   ● **Y37.04   Military operations involving explosion of torpedo**

     ● **Y37.040   Military operations involving explosion of torpedo, military personnel** 🏥

     ● **Y37.041   Military operations involving explosion of torpedo, civilian** 🏥

● **Y37.05   Military operations involving accidental detonation of onboard marine weapons**

   ● **Y37.050   Military operations involving accidental detonation of onboard marine weapons, military personnel** 🏥

   ● **Y37.051   Military operations involving accidental detonation of onboard marine weapons, civilian** 🏥

● **Y37.09   Military operations involving explosion of other marine weapons**

   ● **Y37.090   Military operations involving explosion of other marine weapons, military personnel** 🏥

   ● **Y37.091   Military operations involving explosion of other marine weapons, civilian** 🏥

● **Y37.1   Military operations involving destruction of aircraft**

   ● **Y37.10   Military operations involving unspecified destruction of aircraft**

     ● **Y37.100   Military operations involving unspecified destruction of aircraft, military personnel** 🏥

     ● **Y37.101   Military operations involving unspecified destruction of aircraft, civilian** 🏥

   ● **Y37.11   Military operations involving destruction of aircraft due to enemy fire or explosives**

       Military operations involving destruction of aircraft due to air to air missile

       Military operations involving destruction of aircraft due to explosive placed on aircraft

       Military operations involving destruction of aircraft due to rocket propelled grenade [RPG]

       Military operations involving destruction of aircraft due to small arms fire

       Military operations involving destruction of aircraft due to surface to air missile

     ● **Y37.110   Military operations involving destruction of aircraft due to enemy fire or explosives, military personnel** 🏥

     ● **Y37.111   Military operations involving destruction of aircraft due to enemy fire or explosives, civilian** 🏥

   ● **Y37.12   Military operations involving destruction of aircraft due to collision with other aircraft**

     ● **Y37.120   Military operations involving destruction of aircraft due to collision with other aircraft, military personnel** 🏥

     ● **Y37.121   Military operations involving destruction of aircraft due to collision with other aircraft, civilian** 🏥

   ● **Y37.13   Military operations involving destruction of aircraft due to onboard fire**

     ● **Y37.130   Military operations involving destruction of aircraft due to onboard fire, military personnel** 🏥

     ● **Y37.131   Military operations involving destruction of aircraft due to onboard fire, civilian** 🏥

N Newborn Age: 0   **P** Pediatric Age: 0–17   **M** Maternity DX: 12–55   **A** Adult Age: 15–124   ♀ Females Only   ♂ Males Only

🏥 Complication\Comorbidity   🏥 Major C\C   (Ex) CC/MCC Exclusions   🏥 Present on Admission Requirement   🏥 Hospital-Acquired Condition   **1655**

● **Y37.14**   **Military operations involving destruction of aircraft due to accidental detonation of onboard munitions and explosives**

    ● **Y37.140**   **Military operations involving destruction of aircraft due to accidental detonation of onboard munitions and explosives, military personnel** 🔍

    ● **Y37.141**   **Military operations involving destruction of aircraft due to accidental detonation of onboard munitions and explosives, civilian** 🔍

● **Y37.19**   **Military operations involving other destruction of aircraft**

    ● **Y37.190**   **Military operations involving other destruction of aircraft, military personnel** 🔍

    ● **Y37.191**   **Military operations involving other destruction of aircraft, civilian** 🔍

● **Y37.2**   **Military operations involving other explosions and fragments**

    Excludes1   military operations involving explosion of aircraft (Y37.1-)
                military operations involving explosion of marine weapons (Y37.0-)
                military operations involving explosion of nuclear weapons (Y37.5-)

    ● **Y37.20**   **Military operations involving unspecified explosion and fragments**
         Military operations involving air blast NOS
         Military operations involving blast NOS
         Military operations involving blast fragments NOS
         Military operations involving blast wave NOS
         Military operations involving blast wind NOS
         Military operations involving explosion NOS
         Military operations involving explosion of bomb NOS

        ● **Y37.200**   **Military operations involving unspecified explosion and fragments, military personnel** 🔍

        ● **Y37.201**   **Military operations involving unspecified explosion and fragments, civilian** 🔍

    ● **Y37.21**   **Military operations involving explosion of aerial bomb**

        ● **Y37.210**   **Military operations involving explosion of aerial bomb, military personnel** 🔍

        ● **Y37.211**   **Military operations involving explosion of aerial bomb, civilian** 🔍

    ● **Y37.22**   **Military operations involving explosion of guided missile**

        ● **Y37.220**   **Military operations involving explosion of guided missile, military personnel** 🔍

        ● **Y37.221**   **Military operations involving explosion of guided missile, civilian** 🔍

● **Y37.23**   **Military operations involving explosion of improvised explosive device [IED]**
     Military operations involving explosion of person-borne improvised explosive device [IED]
     Military operations involving explosion of vehicle-borne improvised explosive device [IED]
     Military operations involving explosion of roadside improvised explosive device [IED]

    ● **Y37.230**   **Military operations involving explosion of improvised explosive device [IED], military personnel** 🔍

    ● **Y37.231**   **Military operations involving explosion of improvised explosive device [IED], civilian** 🔍

● **Y37.24**   **Military operations involving explosion due to accidental detonation and discharge of own munitions or munitions launch device**

    ● **Y37.240**   **Military operations involving explosion due to accidental detonation and discharge of own munitions or munitions launch device, military personnel** 🔍

    ● **Y37.241**   **Military operations involving explosion due to accidental detonation and discharge of own munitions or munitions launch device, civilian** 🔍

● **Y37.25**   **Military operations involving fragments from munitions**

    ● **Y37.250**   **Military operations involving fragments from munitions, military personnel** 🔍

    ● **Y37.251**   **Military operations involving fragments from munitions, civilian** 🔍

● **Y37.26**   **Military operations involving fragments of improvised explosive device [IED]**
     Military operations involving fragments of person-borne improvised explosive device [IED]
     Military operations involving fragments of vehicle-borne improvised explosive device [IED]
     Military operations involving fragments of roadside improvised explosive device [IED]

    ● **Y37.260**   **Military operations involving fragments of improvised explosive device [IED], military personnel** 🔍

    ● **Y37.261**   **Military operations involving fragments of improvised explosive device [IED], civilian** 🔍

● **Y37.27**   **Military operations involving fragments from weapons**

    ● **Y37.270**   **Military operations involving fragments from weapons, military personnel** 🔍

    ● **Y37.271**   **Military operations involving fragments from weapons, civilian** 🔍

● **Y37.29**   **Military operations involving other explosions and fragments**
     Military operations involving explosion of grenade
     Military operations involving explosions of land mine
     Military operations involving shrapnel NOS

    ● **Y37.290**   **Military operations involving other explosions and fragments, military personnel** 🔍

    ● **Y37.291**   **Military operations involving other explosions and fragments, civilian** 🔍

◀ New   ◀▦ Revised   ~~deleted~~ Deleted   Excludes 1   Excludes 2   Includes   Use additional   Code first   Code also   Unspecified
OGCR Official Guidelines   ● Unacceptable Principal Diagnosis   X Assign placeholder X   ● Use Additional Character(s)   ▶ Manifestation Code   **Coding Clinic**

● **Y37.3** **Military operations involving fires, conflagrations and hot substances**
  Military operations involving smoke, fumes, and heat from fires, conflagrations and hot substances
  Excludes1 military operations involving fires and conflagrations aboard military aircraft (Y37.1-)
  military operations involving fires and conflagrations aboard military watercraft (Y37.0-)
  military operations involving fires and conflagrations caused indirectly by conventional weapons (Y37.2-)
  military operations involving fires and thermal effects of nuclear weapons (Y36.53-)

● **Y37.30** **Military operations involving unspecified fire, conflagration and hot substance**
  ● **Y37.300** **Military operations involving unspecified fire, conflagration and hot substance, military personnel** 🔖
  ● **Y37.301** **Military operations involving unspecified fire, conflagration and hot substance, civilian** 🔖

● **Y37.31** **Military operations involving gasoline bomb**
  Military operations involving incendiary bomb
  Military operations involving petrol bomb
  ● **Y37.310** **Military operations involving gasoline bomb, military personnel** 🔖
  ● **Y37.311** **Military operations involving gasoline bomb, civilian** 🔖

● **Y37.32** **Military operations involving incendiary bullet**
  ● **Y37.320** **Military operations involving incendiary bullet, military personnel** 🔖
  ● **Y37.321** **Military operations involving incendiary bullet, civilian** 🔖

● **Y37.33** **Military operations involving flamethrower**
  ● **Y37.330** **Military operations involving flamethrower, military personnel** 🔖
  ● **Y37.331** **Military operations involving flamethrower, civilian** 🔖

● **Y37.39** **Military operations involving other fires, conflagrations and hot substances**
  ● **Y37.390** **Military operations involving other fires, conflagrations and hot substances, military personnel** 🔖
  ● **Y37.391** **Military operations involving other fires, conflagrations and hot substances, civilian** 🔖

● **Y37.4** **Military operations involving firearm discharge and other forms of conventional warfare**
  ● **Y37.41** **Military operations involving rubber bullets**
    ● **Y37.410** **Military operations involving rubber bullets, military personnel** 🔖
    ● **Y37.411** **Military operations involving rubber bullets, civilian** 🔖
  ● **Y37.42** **Military operations involving firearms pellets**
    ● **Y37.420** **Military operations involving firearms pellets, military personnel** 🔖
    ● **Y37.421** **Military operations involving firearms pellets, civilian** 🔖

● **Y37.43** **Military operations involving other firearms discharge**
  Military operations involving bullets NOS
  Excludes1 military operations involving munitions fragments (Y37.25-)
  military operations involving incendiary bullets (Y37.32-)
  ● **Y37.430** **Military operations involving other firearms discharge, military personnel** 🔖
  ● **Y37.431** **Military operations involving other firearms discharge, civilian** 🔖

● **Y37.44** **Military operations involving unarmed hand to hand combat**
  Excludes1 military operations involving combat using blunt or piercing object (Y37.45-)
  military operations involving intentional restriction of air and airway (Y37.46-)
  military operations involving unintentional restriction of air and airway (Y37.47-)
  ● **Y37.440** **Military operations involving unarmed hand to hand combat, military personnel** 🔖
  ● **Y37.441** **Military operations involving unarmed hand to hand combat, civilian** 🔖

● **Y37.45** **Military operations involving combat using blunt or piercing object**
  ● **Y37.450** **Military operations involving combat using blunt or piercing object, military personnel** 🔖
  ● **Y37.451** **Military operations involving combat using blunt or piercing object, civilian** 🔖

● **Y37.46** **Military operations involving intentional restriction of air and airway**
  ● **Y37.460** **Military operations involving intentional restriction of air and airway, military personnel** 🔖
  ● **Y37.461** **Military operations involving intentional restriction of air and airway, civilian** 🔖

● **Y37.47** **Military operations involving unintentional restriction of air and airway**
  ● **Y37.470** **Military operations involving unintentional restriction of air and airway, military personnel** 🔖
  ● **Y37.471** **Military operations involving unintentional restriction of air and airway, civilian** 🔖

● **Y37.49** **Military operations involving other forms of conventional warfare**
  ● **Y37.490** **Military operations involving other forms of conventional warfare, military personnel** 🔖
  ● **Y37.491** **Military operations involving other forms of conventional warfare, civilian** 🔖

- Y37.5 **Military operations involving nuclear weapons**
  Military operation involving dirty bomb NOS
  - Y37.50 **Military operations involving unspecified effect of nuclear weapon**
    - Y37.500 **Military operations involving unspecified effect of nuclear weapon, military personnel** �填
    - Y37.501 **Military operations involving unspecified effect of nuclear weapon, civilian** �填
  - Y37.51 **Military operations involving direct blast effect of nuclear weapon**
    Military operations involving blast pressure of nuclear weapon
    - Y37.510 **Military operations involving direct blast effect of nuclear weapon, military personnel** �填
    - Y37.511 **Military operations involving direct blast effect of nuclear weapon, civilian** �填
  - Y37.52 **Military operations involving indirect blast effect of nuclear weapon**
    Military operations involving being thrown by blast of nuclear weapon
    Military operations involving being struck or crushed by blast debris of nuclear weapon
    - Y37.520 **Military operations involving indirect blast effect of nuclear weapon, military personnel** �填
    - Y37.521 **Military operations involving indirect blast effect of nuclear weapon, civilian** �填
  - Y37.53 **Military operations involving thermal radiation effect of nuclear weapon**
    Military operations involving direct heat from nuclear weapon
    Military operation involving fireball effects from nuclear weapon
    - Y37.530 **Military operations involving thermal radiation effect of nuclear weapon, military personnel** �填
    - Y37.531 **Military operations involving thermal radiation effect of nuclear weapon, civilian** �填
  - Y37.54 **Military operation involving nuclear radiation effects of nuclear weapon**
    Military operation involving acute radiation exposure from nuclear weapon
    Military operation involving exposure to immediate ionizing radiation from nuclear weapon
    Military operation involving fallout exposure from nuclear weapon
    Military operation involving secondary effects of nuclear weapons
    - Y37.540 **Military operation involving nuclear radiation effects of nuclear weapon, military personnel** �填
    - Y37.541 **Military operation involving nuclear radiation effects of nuclear weapon, civilian** �填
  - Y37.59 **Military operation involving other effects of nuclear weapons**
    - Y37.590 **Military operation involving other effects of nuclear weapons, military personnel** �填
    - Y37.591 **Military operation involving other effects of nuclear weapons, civilian** �填

- Y37.6 **Military operations involving biological weapons**
  - Y37.6X **Military operations involving biological weapons**
    - Y37.6X0 **Military operations involving biological weapons, military personnel** �填
    - Y37.6X1 **Military operations involving biological weapons, civilian** �填
- Y37.7 **Military operations involving chemical weapons and other forms of unconventional warfare**
  Excludes1 military operations involving incendiary devices (Y36.3-, Y36.5-)
  - Y37.7X **Military operations involving chemical weapons and other forms of unconventional warfare**
    - Y37.7X0 **Military operations involving chemical weapons and other forms of unconventional warfare, military personnel** �填
    - Y37.7X1 **Military operations involving chemical weapons and other forms of unconventional warfare, civilian** �填
- Y37.9 **Other and unspecified military operations**
  - X Y37.90 **Military operations, unspecified** �填
  - X Y37.91 **Military operations involving unspecified weapon of mass destruction [WMD]** �填
  - X Y37.92 **Military operations involving friendly fire** �填

- Y38 **Terrorism**
  These codes are for use to identify injuries resulting from the unlawful use of force or violence against persons or property to intimidate or coerce a government, the civilian population, or any segment thereof, in furtherance of political or social objective

  Use additional code for place of occurrence (Y92.-)

  The appropriate 7th character is to be added to each code from category Y38

A	initial encounter
D	subsequent encounter
S	sequela

- Y38.0 **Terrorism involving explosion of marine weapons**
  Terrorism involving depth-charge
  Terrorism involving marine mine
  Terrorism involving mine NOS, at sea or in harbor
  Terrorism involving sea-based artillery shell
  Terrorism involving torpedo
  Terrorism involving underwater blast
  - Y38.0X **Terrorism involving explosion of marine weapons**
    - Y38.0X1 **Terrorism involving explosion of marine weapons, public safety official injured** �填
    - Y38.0X2 **Terrorism involving explosion of marine weapons, civilian injured** �填
    - Y38.0X3 **Terrorism involving explosion of marine weapons, terrorist injured** 🔲
- Y38.1 **Terrorism involving destruction of aircraft**
  Terrorism involving aircraft burned
  Terrorism involving aircraft exploded
  Terrorism involving aircraft being shot down
  Terrorism involving aircraft used as a weapon
  - Y38.1X **Terrorism involving destruction of aircraft**
    - Y38.1X1 **Terrorism involving destruction of aircraft, public safety official injured** 🔲
    - Y38.1X2 **Terrorism involving destruction of aircraft, civilian injured** 🔲
    - Y38.1X3 **Terrorism involving destruction of aircraft, terrorist injured** 🔲

◀ New ◀ Revised ~~deleted~~ Deleted | Excludes 1 | Excludes 2 | Includes | Use additional | Code first | Code also | Unspecified

OGCR Official Guidelines ● Unacceptable Principal Diagnosis X Assign placeholder X ● Use Additional Character(s) ▶ Manifestation Code **Coding Clinic**

● **Y38.2** **Terrorism involving other explosions and fragments**
Terrorism involving antipersonnel (fragments) bomb
Terrorism involving blast NOS
Terrorism involving explosion NOS
Terrorism involving explosion of breech block
Terrorism involving explosion of cannon block
Terrorism involving explosion (fragments) of artillery shell
Terrorism involving explosion (fragments) of bomb
Terrorism involving explosion (fragments) of grenade
Terrorism involving explosion (fragments) of guided missile
Terrorism involving explosion (fragments) of land mine
Terrorism involving explosion of mortar bomb
Terrorism involving explosion of munitions
Terrorism involving explosion (fragments) of rocket
Terrorism involving explosion (fragments) of shell
Terrorism involving shrapnel
Terrorism involving mine NOS, on land

> **Excludes1**   terrorism involving explosion of nuclear weapon (Y38.5)
> terrorism involving suicide bomber (Y38.81)

● **Y38.2X** **Terrorism involving other explosions and fragments**

● **Y38.2X1** **Terrorism involving other explosions and fragments, public safety official injured** 🗞

● **Y38.2X2** **Terrorism involving other explosions and fragments, civilian injured** 🗞

● **Y38.2X3** **Terrorism involving other explosions and fragments, terrorist injured** 🗞

● **Y38.3** **Terrorism involving fires, conflagration and hot substances**
Terrorism involving conflagration NOS
Terrorism involving fire NOS
Terrorism involving petrol bomb

> **Excludes1**   terrorism involving fire or heat of nuclear weapon (Y38.5)

● **Y38.3X** **Terrorism involving fires, conflagration and hot substances**

● **Y38.3X1** **Terrorism involving fires, conflagration and hot substances, public safety official injured** 🗞

● **Y38.3X2** **Terrorism involving fires, conflagration and hot substances, civilian injured** 🗞

● **Y38.3X3** **Terrorism involving fires, conflagration and hot substances, terrorist injured** 🗞

● **Y38.4** **Terrorism involving firearms**
Terrorism involving carbine bullet
Terrorism involving machine gun bullet
Terrorism involving pellets (shotgun)
Terrorism involving pistol bullet
Terrorism involving rifle bullet
Terrorism involving rubber (rifle) bullet

● **Y38.4X** **Terrorism involving firearms**

● **Y38.4X1** **Terrorism involving firearms, public safety official injured** 🗞

● **Y38.4X2** **Terrorism involving firearms, civilian injured** 🗞

● **Y38.4X3** **Terrorism involving firearms, terrorist injured** 🗞

● **Y38.5** **Terrorism involving nuclear weapons**
Terrorism involving blast effects of nuclear weapon
Terrorism involving exposure to ionizing radiation from nuclear weapon
Terrorism involving fireball effect of nuclear weapon
Terrorism involving heat from nuclear weapon

● **Y38.5X** **Terrorism involving nuclear weapons**

● **Y38.5X1** **Terrorism involving nuclear weapons, public safety official injured** 🗞

● **Y38.5X2** **Terrorism involving nuclear weapons, civilian injured** 🗞

● **Y38.5X3** **Terrorism involving nuclear weapons, terrorist injured** 🗞

● **Y38.6** **Terrorism involving biological weapons**
Terrorism involving anthrax
Terrorism involving cholera
A serious, often deadly, infectious disease of small intestine
Terrorism involving smallpox

● **Y38.6X** **Terrorism involving biological weapons**

● **Y38.6X1** **Terrorism involving biological weapons, public safety official injured** 🗞

● **Y38.6X2** **Terrorism involving biological weapons, civilian injured** 🗞

● **Y38.6X3** **Terrorism involving biological weapons, terrorist injured** 🗞

● **Y38.7** **Terrorism involving chemical weapons**
Terrorism involving gases, fumes, chemicals
Terrorism involving hydrogen cyanide
Terrorism involving phosgene
Terrorism involving sarin

● **Y38.7X** **Terrorism involving chemical weapons**

● **Y38.7X1** **Terrorism involving chemical weapons, public safety official injured** 🗞

● **Y38.7X2** **Terrorism involving chemical weapons, civilian injured** 🗞

● **Y38.7X3** **Terrorism involving chemical weapons, terrorist injured** 🗞

● **Y38.8** **Terrorism involving other and unspecified means**

● **Y38.80** **Terrorism involving unspecified means** 🗞
Terrorism NOS

● **Y38.81** **Terrorism involving suicide bomber**

● **Y38.811** **Terrorism involving suicide bomber, public safety official injured** 🗞

● **Y38.812** **Terrorism involving suicide bomber, civilian injured** 🗞

● **Y38.89** **Terrorism involving other means**
Terrorism involving drowning and submersion
Terrorism involving lasers
Terrorism involving piercing or stabbing instruments

● **Y38.891** **Terrorism involving other means, public safety official injured** 🗞

● **Y38.892** **Terrorism involving other means, civilian injured** 🗞

● **Y38.893** **Terrorism involving other means, terrorist injured** 🗞

● **Y38.9** **Terrorism, secondary effects**

> **Note:** This code is for use to identify conditions occurring subsequent to a terrorist attack not those that are due to the initial terrorist attack.

● **Y38.9X** **Terrorism, secondary effects**

● **Y38.9X1** **Terrorism, secondary effects, public safety official injured** 🗞

● **Y38.9X2** **Terrorism, secondary effects, civilian injured categories** 🗞

N Newborn Age: 0   **P** Pediatric Age: 0–17   **M** Maternity DX: 12–55   **A** Adult Age: 15–124   ♀ Females Only   ♂ Males Only

🗞 Complication\Comorbidity   🗞 Major C\C   (Ex) CC/MCC Exclusions   🗞 Present on Admission Requirement   🗞 Hospital-Acquired Condition

1659

COMPLICATIONS OF MEDICAL AND SURGICAL CARE (Y62-Y84)

Includes   complications of medical devices surgical and medical procedures as the cause of abnormal reaction of the patient, or of later complication, without mention of misadventure at the time of the procedure

MISADVENTURES TO PATIENTS DURING SURGICAL AND MEDICAL CARE (Y62-Y69)

Excludes2   breakdown or malfunctioning of medical device (during procedure) (after implantation) (ongoing use) (Y70-Y82)
surgical and medical procedures as the cause of abnormal reaction of the patient, without mention of misadventure at the time of the procedure (Y83-Y84)

● **Y62   Failure of sterile precautions during surgical and medical care**

Y62.0   Failure of sterile precautions during surgical operation

Y62.1   Failure of sterile precautions during infusion or transfusion

Y62.2   Failure of sterile precautions during kidney dialysis and other perfusion

Y62.3   Failure of sterile precautions during injection or immunization

Y62.4   Failure of sterile precautions during endoscopic examination

Y62.5   Failure of sterile precautions during heart catheterization

Y62.6   Failure of sterile precautions during aspiration, puncture and other catheterization

Y62.8   Failure of sterile precautions during other surgical and medical care

Y62.9   Failure of sterile precautions during unspecified surgical and medical care

● **Y63   Failure in dosage during surgical and medical care**

Excludes2   accidental overdose of drug or wrong drug given in error (T36-T50)

Y63.0   Excessive amount of blood or other fluid given during transfusion or infusion

Y63.1   Incorrect dilution of fluid used during infusion

Y63.2   Overdose of radiation given during therapy

Y63.3   Inadvertent exposure of patient to radiation during medical care

Y63.4   Failure in dosage in electroshock or insulin-shock therapy

Y63.5   Inappropriate temperature in local application and packing

Y63.6   Underdosing and nonadministration of necessary drug, medicament or biological substance

Y63.8   Failure in dosage during other surgical and medical care

Y63.9   Failure in dosage during unspecified surgical and medical care

● **Y64   Contaminated medical or biological substances**

Y64.0   Contaminated medical or biological substance, transfused or infused

Y64.1   Contaminated medical or biological substance, injected or used for immunization

Y64.8   Contaminated medical or biological substance administered by other means

Y64.9   Contaminated medical or biological substance administered by unspecified means
Administered contaminated medical or biological substance NOS

● Y65   **Other misadventures during surgical and medical care**

Y65.0   Mismatched blood in transfusion

Y65.1   Wrong fluid used in infusion

Y65.2   Failure in suture or ligature during surgical operation

Y65.3   Endotracheal tube wrongly placed during anesthetic procedure

Y65.4   Failure to introduce or to remove other tube or instrument

● Y65.5   Performance of wrong procedure (operation)

● Y65.51   **Performance of wrong procedure (operation) on correct patient**
Wrong device implanted into correct surgical site

Excludes1   performance of correct procedure (operation) on wrong side or body part (Y65.53)

MCE: Wrong procedure performed

● Y65.52   **Performance of procedure (operation) on patient not scheduled for surgery**
Performance of procedure (operation) intended for another patient
Performance of procedure (operation) on wrong patient

MCE: Wrong procedure performed

● Y65.53   **Performance of correct procedure (operation) on wrong side or body part**
Performance of correct procedure (operation) on wrong side
Performance of correct procedure (operation) on wrong site

MCE: Wrong procedure performed

Y65.8   Other specified misadventures during surgical and medical care

Y66   **Nonadministration of surgical and medical care**
Premature cessation of surgical and medical care

Excludes1   DNR status (Z66)
palliative care (Z51.5)

Y69   Unspecified misadventure during surgical and medical care

MEDICAL DEVICES ASSOCIATED WITH ADVERSE INCIDENTS IN DIAGNOSTIC AND THERAPEUTIC USE (Y70-Y82)

Includes   breakdown or malfunction of medical devices (during use) (after implantation) (ongoing use)

Excludes1   misadventure to patients during surgical and medical care, classifiable to (Y62-Y69)
later complications following use of medical devices without breakdown or malfunctioning of device (Y83-Y84)

● Y70   **Anesthesiology devices associated with adverse incidents**

Y70.0   Diagnostic and monitoring anesthesiology devices associated with adverse incidents

Y70.1   Therapeutic (nonsurgical) and rehabilitative anesthesiology devices associated with adverse incidents

Y70.2   Prosthetic and other implants, materials and accessory anesthesiology devices associated with adverse incidents

Y70.3   Surgical instruments, materials and anesthesiology devices (including sutures) associated with adverse incidents

Y70.8   Miscellaneous anesthesiology devices associated with adverse incidents, not elsewhere classified

◀ New   ◀▥ Revised   ~~deleted~~ Deleted   Excludes 1   Excludes 2   Includes   Use additional   Code first   Code also   Unspecified
OGCR Official Guidelines   ● Unacceptable Principal Diagnosis   X Assign placeholder X   ◗ Use Additional Character(s)   ▸ Manifestation Code   **Coding Clinic**

● **Y71 Cardiovascular devices associated with adverse incidents**

Y71.0 Diagnostic and monitoring cardiovascular devices associated with adverse incidents

Y71.1 Therapeutic (nonsurgical) and rehabilitative cardiovascular devices associated with adverse incidents

Y71.2 Prosthetic and other implants, materials and accessory cardiovascular devices associated with adverse incidents

Y71.3 Surgical instruments, materials and cardiovascular devices (including sutures) associated with adverse incidents

Y71.8 Miscellaneous cardiovascular devices associated with adverse incidents, not elsewhere classified

● **Y72 Otorhinolaryngological devices associated with adverse incidents**

Y72.0 Diagnostic and monitoring otorhinolaryngological devices associated with adverse incidents

Y72.1 Therapeutic (nonsurgical) and rehabilitative otorhinolaryngological devices associated with adverse incidents

Y72.2 Prosthetic and other implants, materials and accessory otorhinolaryngological devices associated with adverse incidents

Y72.3 Surgical instruments, materials and otorhinolaryngological devices (including sutures) associated with adverse incidents

Y72.8 Miscellaneous otorhinolaryngological devices associated with adverse incidents, not elsewhere classified

● **Y73 Gastroenterology and urology devices associated with adverse incidents**

Y73.0 Diagnostic and monitoring gastroenterology and urology devices associated with adverse incidents

Y73.1 Therapeutic (nonsurgical) and rehabilitative gastroenterology and urology devices associated with adverse incidents

Y73.2 Prosthetic and other implants, materials and accessory gastroenterology and urology devices associated with adverse incidents

Y73.3 Surgical instruments, materials and gastroenterology and urology devices (including sutures) associated with adverse incidents

Y73.8 Miscellaneous gastroenterology and urology devices associated with adverse incidents, not elsewhere classified

● **Y74 General hospital and personal-use devices associated with adverse incidents**

Y74.0 Diagnostic and monitoring general hospital and personal-use devices associated with adverse incidents

Y74.1 Therapeutic (nonsurgical) and rehabilitative general hospital and personal-use devices associated with adverse incidents

Y74.2 Prosthetic and other implants, materials and accessory general hospital and personal-use devices associated with adverse incidents

Y74.3 Surgical instruments, materials and general hospital and personal-use devices (including sutures) associated with adverse incidents

Y74.8 Miscellaneous general hospital and personal-use devices associated with adverse incidents, not elsewhere classified

● **Y75 Neurological devices associated with adverse incidents**

Y75.0 Diagnostic and monitoring neurological devices associated with adverse incidents

Y75.1 Therapeutic (nonsurgical) and rehabilitative neurological devices associated with adverse incidents

Y75.2 Prosthetic and other implants, materials and neurological devices associated with adverse incidents

Y75.3 Surgical instruments, materials and neurological devices (including sutures) associated with adverse incidents

Y75.8 Miscellaneous neurological devices associated with adverse incidents, not elsewhere classified

● **Y76 Obstetric and gynecological devices associated with adverse incidents**

Y76.0 Diagnostic and monitoring obstetric and gynecological devices associated with adverse incidents ♀

Y76.1 Therapeutic (nonsurgical) and rehabilitative obstetric and gynecological devices associated with adverse incidents ♀

Y76.2 Prosthetic and other implants, materials and accessory obstetric and gynecological devices associated with adverse incidents ♀

Y76.3 Surgical instruments, materials and obstetric and gynecological devices (including sutures) associated with adverse incidents ♀

Y76.8 Miscellaneous obstetric and gynecological devices associated with adverse incidents, not elsewhere classified ♀

● **Y77 Ophthalmic devices associated with adverse incidents**

Y77.0 Diagnostic and monitoring ophthalmic devices associated with adverse incidents

Y77.1 Therapeutic (nonsurgical) and rehabilitative ophthalmic devices associated with adverse incidents

Y77.2 Prosthetic and other implants, materials and accessory ophthalmic devices associated with adverse incidents

Y77.3 Surgical instruments, materials and ophthalmic devices (including sutures) associated with adverse incidents

Y77.8 Miscellaneous ophthalmic devices associated with adverse incidents, not elsewhere classified

● **Y78 Radiological devices associated with adverse incidents**

Y78.0 Diagnostic and monitoring radiological devices associated with adverse incidents

Y78.1 Therapeutic (nonsurgical) and rehabilitative radiological devices associated with adverse incidents

Y78.2 Prosthetic and other implants, materials and accessory radiological devices associated with adverse incidents

Y78.3 Surgical instruments, materials and radiological devices (including sutures) associated with adverse incidents

Y78.8 Miscellaneous radiological devices associated with adverse incidents, not elsewhere classified

● **Y79 Orthopedic devices associated with adverse incidents**

Y79.0 Diagnostic and monitoring orthopedic devices associated with adverse incidents

Y79.1 Therapeutic (nonsurgical) and rehabilitative orthopedic devices associated with adverse incidents

Y79.2 Prosthetic and other implants, materials and accessory orthopedic devices associated with adverse incidents

Y79.3 Surgical instruments, materials and orthopedic devices (including sutures) associated with adverse incidents

Y79.8 Miscellaneous orthopedic devices associated with adverse incidents, not elsewhere classified

CHAPTER 20 (V01–Y99)

CHAPTER 20 (V01–Y99)

● Y80 Physical medicine devices associated with adverse incidents

Y80.0 Diagnostic and monitoring physical medicine devices associated with adverse incidents

Y80.1 Therapeutic (nonsurgical) and rehabilitative physical medicine devices associated with adverse incidents

Y80.2 Prosthetic and other implants, materials and accessory physical medicine devices associated with adverse incidents

Y80.3 Surgical instruments, materials and physical medicine devices (including sutures) associated with adverse incidents

Y80.8 Miscellaneous physical medicine devices associated with adverse incidents, not elsewhere classified

● Y81 General- and plastic-surgery devices associated with adverse incidents

Y81.0 Diagnostic and monitoring general- and plastic-surgery devices associated with adverse incidents

Y81.1 Therapeutic (nonsurgical) and rehabilitative general- and plastic-surgery devices associated with adverse incidents

Y81.2 Prosthetic and other implants, materials and accessory general- and plastic-surgery devices associated with adverse incidents

Y81.3 Surgical instruments, materials and general- and plastic-surgery devices (including sutures) associated with adverse incidents

Y81.8 Miscellaneous general- and plastic-surgery devices associated with adverse incidents, not elsewhere classified

● Y82 Other and unspecified medical devices associated with adverse incidents

Y82.8 Other medical devices associated with adverse incidents

Y82.9 Unspecified medical devices associated with adverse incidents

---

SURGICAL AND OTHER MEDICAL PROCEDURES AS THE CAUSE OF ABNORMAL REACTION OF THE PATIENT, OR OF LATER COMPLICATION, WITHOUT MENTION OF MISADVENTURE AT THE TIME OF THE PROCEDURE (Y83–Y84)

Excludes1 misadventures to patients during surgical and medical care, classifiable to (Y62–Y69)

● Y83 Surgical operation and other surgical procedures as the cause of abnormal reaction of the patient, or of later complication, without mention of misadventure at the time of the procedure

Y83.0 Surgical operation with transplant of whole organ as the cause of abnormal reaction of the patient, or of later complication, without mention of misadventure at the time of the procedure

Y83.1 Surgical operation with implant of artificial internal device as the cause of abnormal reaction of the patient, or of later complication, without mention of misadventure at the time of the procedure

Y83.2 Surgical operation with anastomosis, bypass or graft as the cause of abnormal reaction of the patient, or of later complication, without mention of misadventure at the time of the procedure

Y83.3 Surgical operation with formation of external stoma as the cause of abnormal reaction of the patient, or of later complication, without mention of misadventure at the time of the procedure

Y83.4 Other reconstructive surgery as the cause of abnormal reaction of the patient, or of later complication, without mention of misadventure at the time of the procedure

Y83.5 Amputation of limb(s) as the cause of abnormal reaction of the patient, or of later complication, without mention of misadventure at the time of the procedure

Y83.6 Removal of other organ (partial) (total) as the cause of abnormal reaction of the patient, or of later complication, without mention of misadventure at the time of the procedure

Y83.8 Other surgical procedures as the cause of abnormal reaction of the patient, or of later complication, without mention of misadventure at the time of the procedure

Y83.9 Surgical procedure, unspecified as the cause of abnormal reaction of the patient, or of later complication, without mention of misadventure at the time of the procedure

● Y84 Other medical procedures as the cause of abnormal reaction of the patient, or of later complication, without mention of misadventure at the time of the procedure

Y84.0 Cardiac catheterization as the cause of abnormal reaction of the patient, or of later complication, without mention of misadventure at the time of the procedure

Y84.1 Kidney dialysis as the cause of abnormal reaction of the patient, or of later complication, without mention of misadventure at the time of the procedure

Y84.2 Radiological procedure and radiotherapy as the cause of abnormal reaction of the patient, or of later complication, without mention of misadventure at the time of the procedure

Y84.3 Shock therapy as the cause of abnormal reaction of the patient, or of later complication, without mention of misadventure at the time of the procedure

Y84.4 Aspiration of fluid as the cause of abnormal reaction of the patient, or of later complication, without mention of misadventure at the time of the procedure

Y84.5 Insertion of gastric or duodenal sound as the cause of abnormal reaction of the patient, or of later complication, without mention of misadventure at the time of the procedure

Y84.6 Urinary catheterization as the cause of abnormal reaction of the patient, or of later complication, without mention of misadventure at the time of the procedure

Y84.7 Blood-sampling as the cause of abnormal reaction of the patient, or of later complication, without mention of misadventure at the time of the procedure

Y84.8 Other medical procedures as the cause of abnormal reaction of the patient, or of later complication, without mention of misadventure at the time of the procedure

Y84.9 Medical procedure, unspecified as the cause of abnormal reaction of the patient, or of later complication, without mention of misadventure at the time of the procedure

---

SUPPLEMENTARY FACTORS RELATED TO CAUSES OF MORBIDITY CLASSIFIED ELSEWHERE (Y90–Y99)

Note: These categories may be used to provide supplementary information concerning causes of morbidity. They are not to be used for single-condition coding.

● Y90 Evidence of alcohol involvement determined by blood alcohol level

Code first any associated alcohol related disorders (F10)

Y90.0 Blood alcohol level of less than 20 mg/100 ml

Y90.1 Blood alcohol level of 20-39 mg/100 ml

Y90.2 Blood alcohol level of 40-59 mg/100 ml

Y90.3 Blood alcohol level of 60-79 mg/100 ml

Y90.4 Blood alcohol level of 80-99 mg/100 ml

Y90.5 Blood alcohol level of 100-119 mg/100 ml

Y90.6 Blood alcohol level of 120-199 mg/100 ml

Y90.7 Blood alcohol level of 200-239 mg/100 ml

Y90.8 Blood alcohol level of 240 mg/100 ml or more

Y90.9 Presence of alcohol in blood, level not specified

◄ New   ◄▥ Revised   ~~deleted~~ Deleted   Excludes 1   Excludes 2   Includes   Use additional   Code first   Code also   Unspecified

OGCR Official Guidelines   ● Unacceptable Principal Diagnosis   X Assign placeholder X   ● Use Additional Character(s)   ▌ Manifestation Code   **Coding Clinic**

OGCR Section I.C.20.b.

20.9 Place of Occurrence

Place of Occurrence Guideline

Codes from category Y92, Place of occurrence of the external cause, are secondary codes for use after other external cause codes to identify the location of the patient at the time of injury or other condition.

A place of occurrence code is used only once, at the initial encounter for treatment. No 7th characters are used for Y92. Only one code from Y92 should be recorded on a medical record. A place of occurrence code should be used in conjunction with an activity code, Y93.

Do not use place of occurrence code Y92.9 if the place is not stated or is not applicable.

● **Y92**   **Place of occurrence of the external cause**

The following category is for use, when relevant, to identify the place of occurrence of the external cause. Use in conjunction with an activity code.

Place of occurrence should be recorded only at the initial encounter for treatment

● **Y92.0**   **Non-institutional (private) residence as the place of occurrence of the external cause**

Excludes1   abandoned or derelict house (Y92.89)
home under construction but not yet occupied (Y92.6-)
institutional place of residence (Y92.1-)

● **Y92.00**   **Unspecified non-institutional (private) residence as the place of occurrence of the external cause**

Y92.000   Kitchen of unspecified non-institutional (private) residence as the place of occurrence of the external cause 🔖

Y92.001   Dining room of unspecified non-institutional (private) residence as the place of occurrence of the external cause 🔖

Y92.002   Bathroom of unspecified non-institutional (private) residence single-family (private) house as the place of occurrence of the external cause 🔖 ◀▥

Y92.003   Bedroom of unspecified non-institutional (private) residence as the place of occurrence of the external cause 🔖

Y92.007   Garden or yard of unspecified non-institutional (private) residence as the place of occurrence of the external cause 🔖

Y92.008   Other place in unspecified non-institutional (private) residence as the place of occurrence of the external cause 🔖

Y92.009   Unspecified place in unspecified non-institutional (private) residence as the place of occurrence of the external cause 🔖
Home (NOS) as the place of occurrence of the external cause

● **Y92.01**   **Single-family non-institutional (private) house as the place of occurrence of the external cause**
Farmhouse as the place of occurrence of the external cause

Excludes1   barn (Y92.71)
chicken coop or hen house (Y92.72)
farm field (Y92.73)
orchard (Y92.74)
single family mobile home or trailer (Y92.02-)
slaughter house (Y92.86)

Y92.010   Kitchen of single-family (private) house as the place of occurrence of the external cause 🔖

Y92.011   Dining room of single-family (private) house as the place of occurrence of the external cause 🔖

Y92.012   Bathroom of single-family (private) house as the place of occurrence of the external cause 🔖

Y92.013   Bedroom of single-family (private) house as the place of occurrence of the external cause 🔖

Y92.014   Private driveway to single-family (private) house as the place of occurrence of the external cause 🔖

Y92.015   Private garage of single-family (private) house as the place of occurrence of the external cause 🔖

Y92.016   Swimming pool in single-family (private) house or garden as the place of occurrence of the external cause 🔖

Y92.017   Garden or yard in single-family (private) house as the place of occurrence of the external cause 🔖

Y92.018   Other place in single-family (private) house as the place of occurrence of the external cause 🔖

Y92.019   Unspecified place in single-family (private) house as the place of occurrence of the external cause 🔖

● **Y92.02**   **Mobile home as the place of occurrence of the external cause**

Y92.020   Kitchen in mobile home as the place of occurrence of the external cause 🔖

Y92.021   Dining room in mobile home as the place of occurrence of the external cause 🔖

Y92.022   Bathroom in mobile home as the place of occurrence of the external cause 🔖

Y92.023   Bedroom in mobile home as the place of occurrence of the external cause 🔖

Y92.024   Driveway of mobile home as the place of occurrence of the external cause 🔖

Y92.025   Garage of mobile home as the place of occurrence of the external cause 🔖

Y92.026   Swimming pool of mobile home as the place of occurrence of the external cause 🔖

Y92.027   Garden or yard of mobile home as the place of occurrence of the external cause 🔖

Y92.028   Other place in mobile home as the place of occurrence of the external cause 🔖

Y92.029   Unspecified place in mobile home as the place of occurrence of the external cause 🔖

N Newborn Age: 0   P Pediatric Age: 0–17   M Maternity DX: 12–55   A Adult Age: 15–124   ♀ Females Only   ♂ Males Only

🔖 Complication\Comorbidity   🔖 Major C\C   (Ex) CC/MCC Exclusions   🔖 Present on Admission Requirement   🔖 Hospital-Acquired Condition   **1663**

● **Y92.03** **Apartment as the place of occurrence of the external cause**
　　Condominium as the place of occurrence of the external cause
　　Co-op apartment as the place of occurrence of the external cause

　Y92.030　Kitchen in apartment as the place of occurrence of the external cause 🔖

　Y92.031　Bathroom in apartment as the place of occurrence of the external cause 🔖

　Y92.032　Bedroom in apartment as the place of occurrence of the external cause 🔖

　Y92.038　Other place in apartment as the place of occurrence of the external cause 🔖

　Y92.039　Unspecified place in apartment as the place of occurrence of the external cause 🔖

● **Y92.04** **Boarding-house as the place of occurrence of the external cause**

　Y92.040　Kitchen in boarding-house as the place of occurrence of the external cause 🔖

　Y92.041　Bathroom in boarding-house as the place of occurrence of the external cause 🔖

　Y92.042　Bedroom in boarding-house as the place of occurrence of the external cause 🔖

　Y92.043　Driveway of boarding-house as the place of occurrence of the external cause 🔖

　Y92.044　Garage of boarding-house as the place of occurrence of the external cause 🔖

　Y92.045　Swimming pool of boarding-house as the place of occurrence of the external cause 🔖

　Y92.046　Garden or yard of boarding-house as the place of occurrence of the external cause 🔖

　Y92.048　Other place in boarding-house as the place of occurrence of the external cause 🔖

　Y92.049　Unspecified place in boarding-house as the place of occurrence of the external cause 🔖

● **Y92.09** **Other non-institutional residence as the place of occurrence of the external cause**

　Y92.090　Kitchen in other non-institutional residence as the place of occurrence of the external cause 🔖

　Y92.091　Bathroom in other non-institutional residence as the place of occurrence of the external cause 🔖

　Y92.092　Bedroom in other non-institutional residence as the place of occurrence of the external cause 🔖

　Y92.093　Driveway of other non-institutional residence as the place of occurrence of the external cause 🔖

　Y92.094　Garage of other non-institutional residence as the place of occurrence of the external cause 🔖

　Y92.095　Swimming pool of other non-institutional residence as the place of occurrence of the external cause 🔖

　Y92.096　Garden or yard of other non-institutional residence as the place of occurrence of the external cause 🔖

　Y92.098　Other place in other non-institional residence as the place of occurrence of the external cause 🔖

　Y92.099　Unspecified place in other non-institutional residence as the place of occurrence of the external cause 🔖

● **Y92.1** **Institutional (nonprivate) residence as the place of occurrence of the external cause**

　Y92.10　Unspecified residential institution as the place of occurrence of the external cause 🔖

● **Y92.11** **Children's home and orphanage as the place of occurrence of the external cause**

　Y92.110　Kitchen in children's home and orphanage as the place of occurrence of the external cause 🔖

　Y92.111　Bathroom in children's home and orphanage as the place of occurrence of the external cause 🔖

　Y92.112　Bedroom in children's home and orphanage as the place of occurrence of the external cause 🔖

　Y92.113　Driveway of children's home and orphanage as the place of occurrence of the external cause 🔖

　Y92.114　Garage of children's home and orphanage as the place of occurrence of the external cause 🔖

　Y92.115　Swimming pool of children's home and orphanage as the place of occurrence of the external cause 🔖

　Y92.116　Garden or yard of children's home and orphanage as the place of occurrence of the external cause 🔖

　Y92.118　Other place in children's home and orphanage as the place of occurrence of the external cause 🔖

　Y92.119　Unspecified place in children's home and orphanage as the place of occurrence of the external cause 🔖

● **Y92.12** **Nursing home as the place of occurrence of the external cause**
　　Home for the sick as the place of occurrence of the external cause
　　Hospice as the place of occurrence of the external cause

　Y92.120　Kitchen in nursing home as the place of occurrence of the external cause 🔖

　Y92.121　Bathroom in nursing home as the place of occurrence of the external cause 🔖

　Y92.122　Bedroom in nursing home as the place of occurrence of the external cause 🔖

　Y92.123　Driveway of nursing home as the place of occurrence of the external cause 🔖

　Y92.124　Garage of nursing home as the place of occurrence of the external cause 🔖

　Y92.125　Swimming pool of nursing home as the place of occurrence of the external cause 🔖

　Y92.126　Garden or yard of nursing home as the place of occurrence of the external cause 🔖

　Y92.128　Other place in nursing home as the place of occurrence of the external cause 🔖

　Y92.129　Unspecified place in nursing home as the place of occurrence of the external cause 🔖

◀ New　◀▥ Revised　̶d̶e̶l̶e̶t̶e̶d̶ Deleted　Excludes 1　Excludes 2　Includes　Use additional　Code first　Code also　Unspecified

OGCR Official Guidelines　● Unacceptable Principal Diagnosis　X Assign placeholder X　● Use Additional Character(s)　▌Manifestation Code　**Coding Clinic**

● Y92.13   Military base as the place of occurrence of the external cause

      Excludes1   military training grounds (Y92.83)

    Y92.130   Kitchen on military base as the place of occurrence of the external cause

    Y92.131   Mess hall on military base as the place of occurrence of the external cause

    Y92.133   Barracks on military base as the place of occurrence of the external cause

    Y92.135   Garage on military base as the place of occurrence of the external cause

    Y92.136   Swimming pool on military base as the place of occurrence of the external cause

    Y92.137   Garden or yard on military base as the place of occurrence of the external cause

    Y92.138   Other place on military base as the place of occurrence of the external cause

    Y92.139   Unspecified place military base as the place of occurrence of the external cause

● Y92.14   Prison as the place of occurrence of the external cause

    Y92.140   Kitchen in prison as the place of occurrence of the external cause

    Y92.141   Dining room in prison as the place of occurrence of the external cause

    Y92.142   Bathroom in prison as the place of occurrence of the external cause

    Y92.143   Cell of prison as the place of occurrence of the external cause

    Y92.146   Swimming pool of prison as the place of occurrence of the external cause

    Y92.147   Courtyard of prison as the place of occurrence of the external cause

    Y92.148   Other place in prison as the place of occurrence of the external cause

    Y92.149   Unspecified place in prison as the place of occurrence of the external cause

● Y92.15   Reform school as the place of occurrence of the external cause

    Y92.150   Kitchen in reform school as the place of occurrence of the external cause

    Y92.151   Dining room in reform school as the place of occurrence of the external cause

    Y92.152   Bathroom in reform school as the place of occurrence of the external cause

    Y92.153   Bedroom in reform school as the place of occurrence of the external cause

    Y92.154   Driveway of reform school as the place of occurrence of the external cause

    Y92.155   Garage of reform school as the place of occurrence of the external cause

    Y92.156   Swimming pool of reform school as the place of occurrence of the external cause

    Y92.157   Garden or yard of reform school as the place of occurrence of the external cause

    Y92.158   Other place in reform school as the place of occurrence of the external cause

    Y92.159   Unspecified place in reform school as the place of occurrence of the external cause

● Y92.16   School dormitory as the place of occurrence of the external cause

      Excludes1   reform school as the place of occurrence of the external cause (Y92.15-)
              school buildings and grounds as the place of occurrence of the external cause (Y92.2-)
              school sports and athletic areas as the place of occurrence of the external cause (Y92.3-)

    Y92.160   Kitchen in school dormitory as the place of occurrence of the external cause

    Y92.161   Dining room in school dormitory as the place of occurrence of the external cause

    Y92.162   Bathroom in school dormitory as the place of occurrence of the external cause

    Y92.163   Bedroom in school dormitory as the place of occurrence of the external cause

    Y92.168   Other place in school dormitory as the place of occurrence of the external cause

    Y92.169   Unspecified place in school dormitory as the place of occurrence of the external cause

● Y92.19   Other specified residential institution as the place of occurrence of the external cause

    Y92.190   Kitchen in other specified residential institution as the place of occurrence of the external cause

    Y92.191   Dining room in other specified residential institution as the place of occurrence of the external cause

    Y92.192   Bathroom in other specified residential institution as the place of occurrence of the external cause

    Y92.193   Bedroom in other specified residential institution as the place of occurrence of the external cause

    Y92.194   Driveway of other specified residential institution as the place of occurrence of the external cause

    Y92.195   Garage of other specified residential institution as the place of occurrence of the external cause

    Y92.196   Pool of other specified residential institution as the place of occurrence of the external cause

    Y92.197   Garden or yard of other specified residential institution as the place of occurrence of the external cause

    Y92.198   Other place in other specified residential institution as the place of occurrence of the external cause

    Y92.199   Unspecified place in other specified residential institution as the place of occurrence of the external cause

CHAPTER 20 (V01-Y99)

N Newborn Age: 0   P Pediatric Age: 0–17   M Maternity DX: 12–55   A Adult Age: 15–124   ♀ Females Only   ♂ Males Only

Complication\Comorbidity   Major C\C   (Ex) CC/MCC Exclusions   Present on Admission Requirement   Hospital-Acquired Condition   **1665**

● Y92.2 **School, other institution and public administrative area as the place of occurrence of the external cause**
Building and adjacent grounds used by the general public or by a particular group of the public

> **Excludes1** building under construction as the place of occurrence of the external cause (Y92.6)
> residential institution as the place of occurrence of the external cause (Y92.1)
> school dormitory as the place of occurrence of the external cause (Y92.16-)
> sports and athletics area of schools as the place of occurrence of the external cause (Y92.3-)

● Y92.21 **School (private) (public) (state) as the place of occurrence of the external cause**

Y92.210 Daycare center as the place of occurrence of the external cause ✎

Y92.211 Elementary school as the place of occurrence of the external cause ✎
Kindergarten as the place of occurrence of the external cause

Y92.212 Middle school as the place of occurrence of the external cause ✎

Y92.213 High school as the place of occurrence of the external cause ✎
Coding Clinic: 2012, Q4, P108

Y92.214 College as the place of occurrence of the external cause ✎
University as the place of occurrence of the external cause

Y92.215 Trade school as the place of occurrence of the external cause ✎

Y92.218 Other school as the place of occurrence of the external cause ✎

Y92.219 Unspecified school as the place of occurrence of the external cause ✎

Y92.22 **Religious institution as the place of occurrence of the external cause** ✎
Church as the place of occurrence of the external cause
Mosque as the place of occurrence of the external cause
Synagogue as the place of occurrence of the external cause

● Y92.23 **Hospital as the place of occurrence of the external cause**

> **Excludes1** ambulatory (outpatient) health services establishments (Y92.53-)
> home for the sick as the place of occurrence of the external cause (Y92.12-)
> hospice as the place of occurrence of the external cause (Y92.12-)
> nursing home as the place of occurrence of the external cause (Y92.12-)

Y92.230 Patient room in hospital as the place of occurrence of the external cause ✎

Y92.231 Patient bathroom in hospital as the place of occurrence of the external cause ✎

Y92.232 Corridor of hospital as the place of occurrence of the external cause ✎

Y92.233 Cafeteria of hospital as the place of occurrence of the external cause ✎

Y92.234 Operating room of hospital as the place of occurrence of the external cause ✎

Y92.238 Other place in hospital as the place of occurrence of the external cause ✎

Y92.239 Unspecified place in hospital as the place of occurrence of the external cause ✎

● Y92.24 **Public administrative building as the place of occurrence of the external cause**

Y92.240 Courthouse as the place of occurrence of the external cause ✎

Y92.241 Library as the place of occurrence of the external cause ✎

Y92.242 Post office as the place of occurrence of the external cause ✎

Y92.243 City hall as the place of occurrence of the external cause ✎

Y92.248 Other public administrative building as the place of occurrence of the external cause ✎

● Y92.25 **Cultural building as the place of occurrence of the external cause**

Y92.250 Art gallery as the place of occurrence of the external cause ✎

Y92.251 Museum as the place of occurrence of the external cause ✎

Y92.252 Music hall as the place of occurrence of the external cause ✎

Y92.253 Opera house as the place of occurrence of the external cause ✎

Y92.254 Theater (live) as the place of occurrence of the external cause ✎

Y92.258 Other cultural public building as the place of occurrence of the external cause ✎

Y92.26 **Movie house or cinema as the place of occurrence of the external cause** ✎

Y92.29 **Other specified public building as the place of occurrence of the external cause** ✎
Assembly hall as the place of occurrence of the external cause
Clubhouse as the place of occurrence of the external cause

● Y92.3 **Sports and athletics area as the place of occurrence of the external cause**

● Y92.31 **Athletic court as the place of occurrence of the external cause**

> **Excludes1** tennis court in private home or garden (Y92.09)

Y92.310 Basketball court as the place of occurrence of the external cause ✎

Y92.311 Squash court as the place of occurrence of the external cause ✎

Y92.312 Tennis court as the place of occurrence of the external cause ✎

Y92.318 Other athletic court as the place of occurrence of the external cause ✎

● Y92.32 **Athletic field as the place of occurrence of the external cause**

Y92.320 Baseball field as the place of occurrence of the external cause ✎

Y92.321 Football field as the place of occurrence of the external cause ✎

Y92.322 Soccer field as the place of occurrence of the external cause ✎

Y92.328 Other athletic field as the place of occurrence of the external cause ✎
Cricket field as the place of occurrence of the external cause
Hockey field as the place of occurrence of the external cause

◄ New ◄▮ Revised ~~deleted~~ Deleted | Excludes 1 | Excludes 2 | Includes | Use additional | Code first | Code also | Unspecified
OGCR Official Guidelines ● Unacceptable Principal Diagnosis X Assign placeholder X ● Use Additional Character(s) ▮ Manifestation Code **Coding Clinic**

● **Y92.33**   **Skating rink as the place of occurrence of the external cause**

    Y92.330   **Ice skating rink (indoor) (outdoor) as the place of occurrence of the external cause** 🔍

    Y92.331   **Roller skating rink as the place of occurrence of the external cause** 🔍

Y92.34   **Swimming pool (public) as the place of occurrence of the external cause** 🔍

    Excludes1   swimming pool in private home or garden (Y92.016)

Y92.39   **Other specified sports and athletic area as the place of occurrence of the external cause** 🔍

    Golf-course as the place of occurrence of the external cause

    Gymnasium as the place of occurrence of the external cause

    Riding-school as the place of occurrence of the external cause

    Stadium as the place of occurrence of the external cause

● **Y92.4**   **Street, highway and other paved roadways as the place of occurrence of the external cause**

    Excludes1   private driveway of residence (Y92.014, Y92.024, Y92.043, Y92.093, Y92.113, Y92.123, Y92.154, Y92.194) ◄▥

● **Y92.41**   **Street and highway as the place of occurrence of the external cause**

    Y92.410   **Unspecified street and highway as the place of occurrence of the external cause** 🔍

       Road NOS as the place of occurrence of the external cause

    Y92.411   **Interstate highway as the place of occurrence of the external cause** 🔍

       Freeway as the place of occurrence of the external cause

       Motorway as the place of occurrence of the external cause

    Y92.412   **Parkway as the place of occurrence of the external cause** 🔍

    Y92.413   **State road as the place of occurrence of the external cause** 🔍

    Y92.414   **Local residential or business street as the place of occurrence of the external cause** 🔍

    Y92.415   **Exit ramp or entrance ramp of street or highway as the place of occurrence of the external cause** 🔍

● **Y92.48**   **Other paved roadways as the place of occurrence of the external cause**

    Y92.480   **Sidewalk as the place of occurrence of the external cause** 🔍

    Y92.481   **Parking lot as the place of occurrence of the external cause** 🔍

    Y92.482   **Bike path as the place of occurrence of the external cause** 🔍

    Y92.488   **Other paved roadways as the place of occurrence of the external cause** 🔍

● **Y92.5**   **Trade and service area as the place of occurrence of the external cause**

    Excludes1   garage in private home (Y92.015) schools and other public administration buildings (Y92.2-)

● **Y92.51**   **Private commercial establishments as the place of occurrence of the external cause**

    Y92.510   **Bank as the place of occurrence of the external cause** 🔍

    Y92.511   **Restaurant or café as the place of occurrence of the external cause** 🔍

    Y92.512   **Supermarket, store or market as the place of occurrence of the external cause** 🔍

    Y92.513   **Shop (commercial) as the place of occurrence of the external cause** 🔍

● **Y92.52**   **Service areas as the place of occurrence of the external cause**

    Y92.520   **Airport as the place of occurrence of the external cause** 🔍

    Y92.521   **Bus station as the place of occurrence of the external cause** 🔍

    Y92.522   **Railway station as the place of occurrence of the external cause** 🔍

    Y92.523   **Highway rest stop as the place of occurrence of the external cause** 🔍

    Y92.524   **Gas station as the place of occurrence of the external cause** 🔍

       Petroleum station as the place of occurrence of the external cause

       Service station as the place of occurrence of the external cause

● **Y92.53**   **Ambulatory health services establishments as the place of occurrence of the external cause**

    Y92.530   **Ambulatory surgery center as the place of occurrence of the external cause** 🔍

       Outpatient surgery center, including that connected with a hospital as the place of occurrence of the external cause

       Same day surgery center, including that connected with a hospital as the place of occurrence of the external cause

    Y92.531   **Health care provider office as the place of occurrence of the external cause** 🔍

       Physician office as the place of occurrence of the external cause

    Y92.532   **Urgent care center as the place of occurrence of the external cause** 🔍

    Y92.538   **Other ambulatory health services establishments as the place of occurrence of the external cause** 🔍

Y92.59   **Other trade areas as the place of occurrence of the external cause** 🔍

    Office building as the place of occurrence of the external cause

    Casino as the place of occurrence of the external cause

    Garage (commercial) as the place of occurrence of the external cause

    Hotel as the place of occurrence of the external cause

    Radio or television station as the place of occurrence of the external cause

    Shopping mall as the place of occurrence of the external cause

    Warehouse as the place of occurrence of the external cause

CHAPTER 20 (V01-Y99)

N   Newborn Age: 0   P   Pediatric Age: 0–17   M   Maternity DX: 12–55   A   Adult Age: 15–124   ♀   Females Only   ♂   Males Only

🔍 Complication\Comorbidity   🔍 Major C\C   (Ex) CC/MCC Exclusions   🔍 Present on Admission Requirement   🔍 Hospital-Acquired Condition

1667

● Y92.6   **Industrial and construction area as the place of occurrence of the external cause**

   Y92.61   **Building [any] under construction as the place of occurrence of the external cause** 🖐

   Y92.62   **Dock or shipyard as the place of occurrence of the external cause** 🖐
             Dockyard as the place of occurrence of the external cause
             Dry dock as the place of occurrence of the external cause
             Shipyard as the place of occurrence of the external cause

   Y92.63   **Factory as the place of occurrence of the external cause** 🖐
             Factory building as the place of occurrence of the external cause
             Factory premises as the place of occurrence of the external cause
             Industrial yard as the place of occurrence of the external cause

   Y92.64   **Mine or pit as the place of occurrence of the external cause** 🖐
             Mine as the place of occurrence of the external cause

   Y92.65   **Oil rig as the place of occurrence of the external cause** 🖐
             Pit (coal) (gravel) (sand) as the place of occurrence of the external cause

   Y92.69   **Other specified industrial and construction area as the place of occurrence of the external cause** 🖐
             Gasworks as the place of occurrence of the external cause
             Power-station (coal) (nuclear) (oil) as the place of occurrence of the external cause
             Tunnel under construction as the place of occurrence of the external cause
             Workshop as the place of occurrence of the external cause

● Y92.7   **Farm as the place of occurrence of the external cause**
           Ranch as the place of occurrence of the external cause
           Excludes1   farmhouse and home premises of farm (Y92.01-)

   Y92.71   **Barn as the place of occurrence of the external cause** 🖐

   Y92.72   **Chicken coop as the place of occurrence of the external cause** 🖐
             Hen house as the place of occurrence of the external cause

   Y92.73   **Farm field as the place of occurrence of the external cause** 🖐

   Y92.74   **Orchard as the place of occurrence of the external cause** 🖐

   Y92.79   **Other farm location as the place of occurrence of the external cause** 🖐

● Y92.8   **Other places as the place of occurrence of the external cause**

● Y92.81   **Transport vehicle as the place of occurrence of the external cause**
           Excludes1   transport accidents (V00-V99)

   Y92.810   **Car as the place of occurrence of the external cause** 🖐

   Y92.811   **Bus as the place of occurrence of the external cause** 🖐

   Y92.812   **Truck as the place of occurrence of the external cause** 🖐

   Y92.813   **Airplane as the place of occurrence of the external cause** 🖐

   Y92.814   **Boat as the place of occurrence of the external cause** 🖐

   Y92.815   **Train as the place of occurrence of the external cause** 🖐

   Y92.816   **Subway car as the place of occurrence of the external cause** 🖐

   Y92.818   **Other transport vehicle as the place of occurrence of the external cause** 🖐

● Y92.82   **Wilderness area**

   Y92.820   **Desert as the place of occurrence of the external cause** 🖐

   Y92.821   **Forest as the place of occurrence of the external cause** 🖐

   Y92.828   **Other wilderness area as the place of occurrence of the external cause** 🖐
             Swamp as the place of occurrence of the external cause
             Mountain as the place of occurrence of the external cause
             Marsh as the place of occurrence of the external cause
             Prairie as the place of occurrence of the external cause

● Y92.83   **Recreation area as the place of occurrence of the external cause**

   Y92.830   **Public park as the place of occurrence of the external cause** 🖐

   Y92.831   **Amusement park as the place of occurrence of the external cause** 🖐

   Y92.832   **Beach as the place of occurrence of the external cause** 🖐
             Seashore as the place of occurrence of the external cause

   Y92.833   **Campsite as the place of occurrence of the external cause** 🖐

   Y92.834   **Zoological garden (zoo) as the place of occurrence of the external cause** 🖐

   Y92.838   **Other recreation area as the place of occurrence of the external cause** 🖐

   Y92.84   **Military training ground as the place of occurrence of the external cause** 🖐

   Y92.85   **Railroad track as the place of occurrence of the external cause** 🖐

   Y92.86   **Slaughter house as the place of occurrence of the external cause** 🖐

   Y92.89   **Other specified places as the place of occurrence of the external cause** 🖐
             Derelict house as the place of occurrence of the external cause

● Y92.9   **Unspecified place or not applicable** 🖐

◀ New   ◀📖 Revised   ~~deleted~~ Deleted | Excludes 1 | | Excludes 2 | | Includes | | Use additional | | Code first | | Code also | | Unspecified |

OGCR Official Guidelines   ● Unacceptable Principal Diagnosis   ✗ Assign placeholder X   ● Use Additional Character(s)   ▶ Manifestation Code   **Coding Clinic**

OGCR See Section I.C.20.c.

Activity code

● **Y93   Activity codes**

     Note: Category Y93 is provided for use to indicate the activity of the person seeking healthcare for an injury or health condition, such as a heart attack while shoveling snow, which resulted from, or was contributed to, by the activity. These codes are appropriate for use for both acute injuries, such as those from chapter 19, and conditions that are due to the long-term, cumulative effects of an activity, such as those from chapter 13. They are also appropriate for use with external cause codes for cause and intent if identifying the activity provides additional information on the event. These codes should be used in conjunction with codes for external cause status (Y99) and place of occurrence (Y92).

     This section contains the following broad activity categories:

        Y93.0   Activities involving walking and running

        Y93.1   Activities involving water and water craft

        Y93.2   Activities involving ice and snow

        Y93.3   Activities involving climbing, rappelling, and jumping off

        Y93.4   Activities involving dancing and other rhythmic movement

        Y93.5   Activities involving other sports and athletics played individually

        Y93.6   Activities involving other sports and athletics played as a team or group

        Y93.7   Activities involving other specified sports and athletics

        Y93.A   Activities involving other cardiorespiratory exercise

        Y93.B   Activities involving other muscle strengthening exercises

        Y93.C   Activities involving computer technology and electronic devices

        Y93.D   Activities involving arts and handcrafts

        Y93.E   Activities involving personal hygiene and interior property and clothing maintenance

        Y93.F   Activities involving caregiving

        Y93.G   Activities involving food preparation, cooking and grilling

        Y93.H   Activities involving exterior property and land maintenance, building and construction

        Y93.I   Activities involving roller coasters and other types of external motion

        Y93.J   Activities involving playing musical instrument

        Y93.K   Activities involving animal care

        Y93.8   Activities, other specified

        Y93.9   Activity, unspecified

● **Y93.0   Activities involving walking and running**

     Excludes1   Activity, walking an animal (Y93.K1)
                 Activity, walking or running on a treadmill (Y93.A1)

     Y93.01   Activity, walking, marching and hiking 🗐
         Activity, walking, marching and hiking on level or elevated terrain

         Excludes1   activity, mountain climbing (Y93.31)

     Y93.02   Activity, running 🗐

● **Y93.1   Activities involving water and water craft**

     Excludes1   activities involving ice (Y93.2-)

     Y93.11   Activity, swimming 🗐

     Y93.12   Activity, springboard and platform diving 🗐

     Y93.13   Activity, water polo 🗐

     Y93.14   Activity, water aerobics and water exercise 🗐

     Y93.15   Activity, underwater diving and snorkeling 🗐
         Activity, SCUBA diving

     Y93.16   Activity, rowing, canoeing, kayaking, rafting and tubing 🗐
         Activity, canoeing, kayaking, rafting and tubing in calm and turbulent water

     Y93.17   Activity, water skiing and wake boarding 🗐

     Y93.18   Activity, surfing, windsurfing and boogie boarding 🗐
         Activity, water sliding

     Y93.19   Activity, other involving water and watercraft 🗐
         Activity involving water NOS
         Activity, parasailing
         Activity, water survival training and testing

● **Y93.2   Activities involving ice and snow**

     Excludes1   activity, shoveling ice and snow (Y93.H1)

     Y93.21   Activity, ice skating 🗐
         Activity, figure skating (singles) (pairs)
         Activity, ice dancing

         Excludes1   activity, ice hockey (Y93.22)

     Y93.22   Activity, ice hockey 🗐

     Y93.23   Activity, snow (alpine) (downhill) skiing, snow boarding, sledding, tobogganing and snow tubing 🗐

         Excludes1   activity, cross country skiing (Y93.24)

     Y93.24   Activity, cross country skiing 🗐
         Activity, nordic skiing

     Y93.29   Activity, other activity involving ice and snow 🗐
         Activity, activity involving ice and snow NOS

● **Y93.3   Activities involving climbing, rappelling and jumping off**

     Excludes1   activity, hiking on level or elevated terrain (Y93.01)
                 activity, jumping rope (Y93.56)
                 activity, trampoline jumping (Y93.44)

     Y93.31   Activity, mountain climbing, rock climbing and wall climbing 🗐

     Y93.32   Activity, rappelling 🗐

     Y93.33   Activity, BASE jumping 🗐
         Activity, building, Antenna, Span, Earth jumping

     Y93.34   Activity, bungee jumping 🗐

     Y93.35   Activity, hang gliding 🗐

     Y93.39   Activity, other activity involving climbing, rappelling and jumping off 🗐

● **Y93.4   Activities involving dancing and other rhythmic movement**

     Excludes1   activity, martial arts (Y93.75)

     Y93.41   Activity, dancing 🗐
         Coding Clinic: 2012, Q4, P108

     Y93.42   Activity, yoga 🗐

     Y93.43   Activity, gymnastics 🗐
         Activity, rhythmic gymnastics

         Excludes1   activity, trampolining (Y93.44)

     Y93.44   Activity, trampolining 🗐

     Y93.45   Activity, cheerleading 🗐

     Y93.49   Activity, other involving dancing and other rhythmic movements 🗐

N Newborn Age: 0   **P** Pediatric Age: 0–17   **M** Maternity DX: 12–55   **A** Adult Age: 15–124   ♀ Females Only   ♂ Males Only

🗐 Complication\Comorbidity   🗐 Major C\C   (Ex) CC/MCC Exclusions   🗐 Present on Admission Requirement   🗐 Hospital-Acquired Condition

1669

● **Y93.5**   **Activities involving other sports and athletics played individually**
> **Excludes1**   activity, dancing (Y93.41)
> activity, gymnastic (Y93.43)
> activity, trampolining (Y93.44)
> activity, yoga (Y93.42)

Y93.51   **Activity, roller skating (inline) and skateboarding** ✎

Y93.52   **Activity, horseback riding** ✎

Y93.53   **Activity, golf** ✎

Y93.54   **Activity, bowling** ✎

Y93.55   **Activity, bike riding** ✎

Y93.56   **Activity, jumping rope** ✎

Y93.57   **Activity, non-running track and field events** ✎
> **Excludes1**   activity, running (any form) (Y93.02)

Y93.59   **Activity, other involving other sports and athletics played individually** ✎
> **Excludes1**   activities involving climbing, rappelling, and jumping (Y93.3-)
> activities involving ice and snow (Y93.2-)
> activities involving walking and running (Y93.0-)
> activities involving water and watercraft (Y93.1-)

● **Y93.6**   **Activities involving other sports and athletics played as a team or group**
> **Excludes1**   activity, ice hockey (Y93.22)
> activity, water polo (Y93.13)

Y93.61   **Activity, American tackle football** ✎
> Activity, football NOS

Y93.62   **Activity, American flag or touch football** ✎

Y93.63   **Activity, rugby** ✎

Y93.64   **Activity, baseball** ✎
> Activity, softball

Y93.65   **Activity, lacrosse and field hockey** ✎

Y93.66   **Activity, soccer** ✎

Y93.67   **Activity, basketball** ✎

Y93.68   **Activity, volleyball (beach) (court)** ✎

Y93.6A   **Activity, physical games generally associated with school recess, summer camp and children** ✎   P
> Activity, capture the flag
> Activity, dodge ball
> Activity, four square
> Activity, kickball

Y93.69   **Activity, other involving other sports and athletics played as a team or group** ✎
> Cricket

● **Y93.7**   **Activities involving other specified sports and athletics**

Y93.71   **Activity, boxing** ✎

Y93.72   **Activity, wrestling** ✎

Y93.73   **Activity, racquet and hand sports** ✎
> Activity, handball
> Activity, racquetball
> Activity, squash
> Activity, tennis

Y93.74   **Activity, frisbee** ✎
> Activity, ultimate frisbee

Y93.75   **Activity, martial arts** ✎
> Activity, combatives

Y93.79   **Activity, other specified sports and athletics** ✎
> **Excludes1**   sports and athletics activities specified in categories Y93.0-Y93.6

● **Y93.A**   **Activities involving other cardiorespiratory exercise**
> Activities involving physical training

Y93.A1   **Activity, exercise machines primarily for cardiorespiratory conditioning** ✎
> Activity, elliptical and stepper machines
> Activity, stationary bike
> Activity, treadmill

Y93.A2   **Activity, calisthenics** ✎
> Activity, jumping jacks
> Activity, warm up and cool down

Y93.A3   **Activity, aerobic and step exercise** ✎

Y93.A4   **Activity, circuit training** ✎

Y93.A5   **Activity, obstacle course** ✎
> Activity, challenge course
> Activity, confidence course

Y93.A6   **Activity, grass drills** ✎
> Activity, guerilla drills

Y93.A9   **Activity, other involving other cardiorespiratory exercise** ✎
> **Excludes1**   activities involving cardiorespiratory exercise specified in categories Y93.0-Y93.7

● **Y93.B**   **Activity involving other muscle strengthening exercises**

Y93.B1   **Activity, exercise machines primarily for muscle strengthening** ✎

Y93.B2   **Activity, push-ups, pull-ups, sit-ups** ✎

Y93.B3   **Activity, free weights** ✎
> Activity, barbells
> Activity, dumbbells

Y93.B4   **Activity, pilates** ✎

Y93.B9   **Activity, other involving other muscle strengthening exercises** ✎
> **Excludes1**   activities involving muscle strengthening specified in categories Y93.0-Y93.A

● **Y93.C**   **Activities involving computer technology and electronic devices**
> **Excludes1**   activity, electronic musical keyboard or instruments (Y93.J-)

Y93.C1   **Activity, computer keyboarding** ✎
> Activity, electronic game playing using keyboard or other stationary device

Y93.C2   **Activity, hand held interactive electronic device** ✎
> Activity, cellular telephone and communication device
> Activity, electronic game playing using interactive device
> **Excludes1**   activity, electronic game playing using keyboard or other stationary device (Y93.C1)

Y93.C9   **Activity, other involving computer technology and electronic devices** ✎

● **Y93.D**   **Activities involving arts and handcrafts**
> **Excludes1**   activities involving playing musical instrument (Y93.J-)

Y93.D1   **Knitting and crocheting** ✎

Y93.D2   **Sewing** ✎

Y93.D3   **Furniture building and finishing** ✎
> Furniture repair

Y93.D9   **Activity, other involving arts and handcrafts** ✎

● **Y93.E**   Activities involving personal hygiene and interior property and clothing maintenance

> **Excludes1**   activities involving cooking and grilling (Y93.G-)
> activities involving exterior property and land maintenance, building and construction (Y93.H-)
> activity involving caregiving (Y93.F-)
> activity, dishwashing (Y93.G1)
> activity, food preparation (Y93.G1)
> activity, gardening (Y93.H2)

   Y93.E1   Activity, personal bathing and showering ⬠

   Y93.E2   Activity, laundry ⬠

   Y93.E3   Activity, vacuuming ⬠

   Y93.E4   Activity, ironing ⬠

   Y93.E5   Activity, floor mopping and cleaning ⬠

   Y93.E6   Activity, residential relocation ⬠
> Activity, packing up and unpacking involved in moving to a new residence

   Y93.E8   Activity, other personal hygiene activity ⬠

   Y93.E9   Activity, other household maintenance ⬠

● **Y93.F**   Activities involving person providing caregiving
> Activity involving the provider of caregiving

   Y93.F1   Activity, caregiving involving bathing ⬠

   Y93.F2   Activity, caregiving involving lifting ⬠

   Y93.F9   Activity, other caregiving ⬠

● **Y93.G**   Activities involving food preparation, cooking and grilling

   Y93.G1   Activity, food preparation and clean up ⬠
> Activity, dishwashing

   Y93.G2   Activity, grilling and smoking food ⬠

   Y93.G3   Activity, cooking and baking ⬠
> Activity, use of stove, oven and microwave oven

   Y93.G9   Activity, other activity involving cooking and grilling ⬠

● **Y93.H**   Activities involving property and land maintenance, building and construction

   Y93.H1   Activity, digging, shoveling and raking ⬠
> Activity, dirt digging
> Activity, raking leaves
> Activity, snow shoveling

   Y93.H2   Activity, gardening and landscaping ⬠
> Activity, pruning, trimming shrubs, weeding

   Y93.H3   Activity, building and construction ⬠

   Y93.H9   Activity, other activity involving property and land maintenance, building and construction ⬠

● **Y93.I**   Activities involving roller coasters and other types of external motion

   Y93.I1   Activity, rollercoaster riding ⬠

   Y93.I9   Activity, other involving external motion ⬠

● **Y93.J**   Activities involving playing musical instrument
> Activity involving playing electric musical instrument

   Y93.J1   Activity, piano playing ⬠
> Activity, musical keyboard (electronic) playing

   Y93.J2   Activity, drum and other percussion instrument playing ⬠

   Y93.J3   Activity, string instrument playing ⬠

   Y93.J4   Activity, winds and brass instrument playing ⬠

● **Y93.K**   Activities involving animal care

> **Excludes1**   activity, horseback riding (Y93.52)

   Y93.K1   Activity, walking an animal ⬠

   Y93.K2   Activity, milking an animal ⬠

   Y93.K3   Activity, grooming and shearing an animal ⬠

   Y93.K9   Activity, other activity involving animal care ⬠

● **Y93.8**   Other activity

   Y93.81   Activity, refereeing a sports activity ⬠

   Y93.82   Activity, spectator at an event ⬠

   Y93.83   Activity, rough housing and horseplay ⬠

   Y93.84   Activity, sleeping ⬠

   Y93.89   Activity, other specified ⬠

● **Y93.9**   Activity, unspecified ⬠

Y95   Nosocomial condition

● **Y99**   External cause status

> **Note:** A single code from category Y99 should be used in conjunction with the external cause code(s) assigned to a record to indicate the status of the person at the time the event occurred.

   Y99.0   Civilian activity done for income or pay ⬠
> Civilian activity done for financial or other compensation

> **Excludes1**   military activity (Y99.1)
> volunteer activity (Y99.2)

   Y99.1   Military activity ⬠

> **Excludes1**   activity of off duty military personnel (Y99.8) ◄

> ~~Excludes~~   ~~activity of off duty military personnel (Y99.8)~~

   Y99.2   Volunteer activity ⬠

> **Excludes1**   activity of child or other family member assisting in compensated work of other family member (Y99.8)

   Y99.8   Other external cause status ⬠
> Activity NEC
> Activity of child or other family member assisting in compensated work of other family member
> Hobby not done for income
> Leisure activity
> Off-duty activity of military personnel
> Recreation or sport not for income or while a student
> Student activity

> **Excludes1**   civilian activity done for income or compensation (Y99.0)
> military activity (Y99.1)

> **Coding Clinic:** 2012, Q4, P108

   Y99.9   Unspecified external cause status ⬠

N Newborn Age: 0   **P** Pediatric Age: 0–17   **M** Maternity DX: 12–55   **A** Adult Age: 15–124   ♀ Females Only   ♂ Males Only

⬠ Complication\Comorbidity   ⬠ Major C\C   Ⓔⓧ CC/MCC Exclusions   ⬠ Present on Admission Requirement   ⬠ Hospital-Acquired Condition   **1671**

CHAPTER 21

FACTORS INFLUENCING HEALTH STATUS AND CONTACT WITH HEALTH SERVICES (Z00-Z99)

Note: Z codes represent reasons for encounters. A corresponding procedure code must accompany a Z code if a procedure is performed. Categories Z00-Z99 are provided for occasions when circumstances other than a disease, injury or external cause classifiable to categories A00-Y89 are recorded as 'diagnoses' or 'problems.' This can arise in two main ways:

(a) When a person who may or may not be sick encounters the health services for some specific purpose, such as to receive limited care or service for a current condition, to donate an organ or tissue, to receive prophylactic vaccination (immunization), or to discuss a problem which is in itself not a disease or injury.

(b) When some circumstance or problem is present which influences the person's health status but is not in itself a current illness or injury.

This chapter contains the following blocks:

Z00-Z13	Persons encountering health services for examination
Z14-Z15	Genetic carrier and genetic susceptibility to disease
Z16	Resistance to antimicrobial drugs
Z17	Estrogen receptor status
Z18	Retained foreign body fragments
Z20-Z28	Persons with potential health hazards related to communicable diseases
Z30-Z39	Persons encountering health services in circumstances related to reproduction
Z40-Z53	Encounters for other specific health care
Z55-Z65	Persons with potential health hazards related to socioeconomic and psychosocial circumstances
Z66	Do not resuscitate status
Z67	Blood type
Z68	Body mass index (BMI)
Z69-Z76	Persons encountering health services in other circumstances
Z77-Z99	Persons with potential health hazards related to family and personal history and certain conditions influencing health status

PERSONS ENCOUNTERING HEALTH SERVICES FOR EXAMINATIONS (Z00-Z13)

Note: Nonspecific abnormal findings disclosed at the time of these examinations are classified to categories R70-R94.

Excludes1 examinations related to pregnancy and reproduction (Z30-Z36, Z39.-)

● **Z00 Encounter for general examination without complaint, suspected or reported diagnosis**

Excludes1 encounter for examination for administrative purposes (Z02.-)

Excludes2 encounter for pre-procedural examinations (Z01.81-)
special screening examinations (Z11-Z13)

● **Z00.0 Encounter for general adult medical examination**
Encounter for adult periodic examination (annual) (physical) and any associated laboratory and radiologic examinations

Excludes1 encounter for examination of sign or symptom - code to sign or symptom general health check-up of infant or child (Z00.12.-)

● **Z00.00 Encounter for general adult medical examination without abnormal findings** 🐾   A
Encounter for adult health check-up NOS

● **Z00.01 Encounter for general adult medical examination with abnormal findings** 🐾   A

Use additional code to identify abnormal findings

● **Z00.1 Encounter for newborn, infant and child health examinations**

● **Z00.11 Newborn health examination**
Health check for child under 29 days old

Use additional code to identify any abnormal findings

Excludes1 health check for child over 28 days old (Z00.12-)

● **Z00.110 Health examination for newborn under 8 days old** 🐾   N
Health check for newborn under 8 days old

● **Z00.111 Health examination for newborn 8 to 28 days old** 🐾   N
Health check for newborn 8 to 28 days old
Newborn weight check

● **Z00.12 Encounter for routine child health examination**
Encounter for development testing of infant or child
Health check (routine) for child over 28 days old

Excludes1 health check for child under 29 days old (Z00.11-) ◀
health supervision of foundling or other healthy infant or child (Z76.1-Z76.2)
newborn health examination (Z00.11-)

● **Z00.121 Encounter for routine child health examination with abnormal findings** 🐾   P
Use additional code to identify abnormal findings

● **Z00.129 Encounter for routine child health examination without abnormal findings** 🐾   P
Encounter for routine child health examination NOS

● **Z00.2 Encounter for examination for period of rapid growth in childhood** 🐾   P

● **Z00.3 Encounter for examination for adolescent development state** 🐾   P
Encounter for puberty development state

● **Z00.5 Encounter for examination of potential donor of organ and tissue** 🐾

Z00.6 Encounter for examination for normal comparison and control in clinical research program 🐾
Examination of participant or control in clinical research program

● **Z00.7 Encounter for examination for period of delayed growth in childhood**

● **Z00.70 Encounter for examination for period of delayed growth in childhood without abnormal findings** 🐾   P

● **Z00.71 Encounter for examination for period of delayed growth in childhood with abnormal findings** 🐾   P
Use additional code to identify abnormal findings

● **Z00.8 Encounter for other general examination** 🐾
Encounter for health examination in population surveys

● **Z01   Encounter for other special examination without complaint, suspected or reported diagnosis**

     Includes   routine examination of specific system

     Note: Codes from category Z01 represent the reason for the encounter. A separate procedure code is required to identify any examinations or procedures performed.

     Excludes1   encounter for examination for administrative purposes (Z02.-)

                encounter for examination for suspected conditions, proven not to exist (Z03.-)

                encounter for laboratory and radiologic examinations as a component of general medical examinations (Z00.0-)

                encounter for laboratory, radiologic and imaging examinations for sign(s) and symptom(s) - code to the sign(s) or symptom(s)

     Excludes2   screening examinations (Z11-Z13)

● **Z01.0   Encounter for examination of eyes and vision**

     Excludes1   examination for driving license (Z02.4)

     Z01.00   Encounter for examination of eyes and vision without abnormal findings 🔖

           Encounter for examination of eyes and vision NOS

     Z01.01   Encounter for examination of eyes and vision with abnormal findings 🔖

           Use additional code to identify abnormal findings

● **Z01.1   Encounter for examination of ears and hearing**

   ● **Z01.10   Encounter for examination of ears and hearing without abnormal findings** 🔖

           Encounter for examination of ears and hearing NOS

   ● **Z01.11   Encounter for examination of ears and hearing with abnormal findings**

     ● **Z01.110   Encounter for hearing examination following failed hearing screening** 🔖

     ● **Z01.118   Encounter for examination of ears and hearing with other abnormal findings** 🔖

           Use additional code to identify abnormal findings

   ● **Z01.12   Encounter for hearing conservation and treatment** 🔖

● **Z01.2   Encounter for dental examination and cleaning**

   ● **Z01.20   Encounter for dental examination and cleaning without abnormal findings** 🔖

           Encounter for dental examination and cleaning NOS

   ● **Z01.21   Encounter for dental examination and cleaning with abnormal findings** 🔖

           Use additional code to identify abnormal findings

● **Z01.3   Encounter for examination of blood pressure**

   ● **Z01.30   Encounter for examination of blood pressure without abnormal findings** 🔖

           Encounter for examination of blood pressure NOS

   ● **Z01.31   Encounter for examination of blood pressure with abnormal findings** 🔖

           Use additional code to identify abnormal findings

● **Z01.4   Encounter for gynecological examination**

     Excludes2   pregnancy examination or test (Z32.0-) routine examination for contraceptive maintenance (Z30.4-)

   ● **Z01.41   Encounter for routine gynecological examination**

           Encounter for general gynecological examination with or without cervical smear

           Encounter for gynecological examination (general) (routine) NOS

           Encounter for pelvic examination (annual) (periodic)

           Use additional code:

              for screening for human papillomavirus, if applicable (Z11.51)

              for screening vaginal pap smear, if applicable (Z12.72)

              to identify acquired absence of uterus, if applicable (Z90.71-)

           Excludes1   gynecologic examination status-post hysterectomy for malignant condition (Z08)

                screening cervical pap smear not a part of a routine gynecological examination (Z12.4)

     Z01.411   Encounter for gynecological examination (general) (routine) with abnormal findings ♀ 🔖

     Z01.419   Encounter for gynecological examination (general) (routine) without abnormal findings ♀ 🔖

           Use additional code to identify abnormal findings

   Z01.42   Encounter for cervical smear to confirm findings of recent normal smear following initial abnormal smear ♀ 🔖

● **Z01.8   Encounter for other specified special examinations**

   ● **Z01.81   Encounter for preprocedural examinations**

           Encounter for preoperative examinations

           Encounter for radiological and imaging examinations as part of preprocedural examination

     Z01.810   Encounter for preprocedural cardiovascular examination 🔖

     Z01.811   Encounter for preprocedural respiratory examination 🔖

     ● **Z01.812   Encounter for preprocedural laboratory examination** 🔖

           Blood and urine tests prior to treatment or procedure

     ● **Z01.818   Encounter for other preprocedural examination** 🔖

           Encounter for preprocedural examination NOS

           Encounter for examinations prior to antineoplastic chemotherapy

   ● **Z01.82   Encounter for allergy testing** 🔖

     Excludes1   encounter for antibody response examination (Z01.84)

   ● **Z01.83   Encounter for blood typing** 🔖

     Encounter for Rh typing

   ● **Z01.84   Encounter for antibody response examination** 🔖

     Encounter for immunity status testing

     Excludes1   encounter for allergy testing (Z01.82)

   ● **Z01.89   Encounter for other specified special examinations** 🔖

N Newborn Age: 0   **P** Pediatric Age: 0–17   **M** Maternity DX: 12–55   **A** Adult Age: 15–124   ♀ Females Only   ♂ Males Only

🔖 Complication\Comorbidity   🔖 Major C\C   (Ex) CC/MCC Exclusions   🔖 Present on Admission Requirement   🔖 Hospital-Acquired Condition   **1673**

CHAPTER 21 (Z00–Z99)

● **Z02** **Encounter for administrative examination**

  ● **Z02.0** **Encounter for examination for admission to educational institution** 🔒

    Encounter for examination for admission to preschool (education)

    Encounter for examination for re-admission to school following illness or medical treatment

  ● **Z02.1** **Encounter for pre-employment examination** 🔒

  ● **Z02.2** **Encounter for examination for admission to residential institution** 🔒

    Excludes1 examination for admission to prison (Z02.89)

  Z02.3 **Encounter for examination for recruitment to armed forces** 🔒

  ● **Z02.4** **Encounter for examination for driving license** 🔒

  ● **Z02.5** **Encounter for examination for participation in sport** 🔒

    Excludes1 blood-alcohol and blood-drug test (Z02.83)

  ● **Z02.6** **Encounter for examination for insurance purposes** 🔒

  ● **Z02.7** **Encounter for issue of medical certificate**

    Excludes1 encounter for general medical examination (Z00-Z01, Z02.0-Z02.6, Z02.8-Z02.9)

    ● **Z02.71** **Encounter for disability determination** 🔒

      Encounter for issue of medical certificate of incapacity

      Encounter for issue of medical certificate of invalidity

    ● **Z02.79** **Encounter for issue of other medical certificate** 🔒

  ● **Z02.8** **Encounter for other administrative examinations**

    Z02.81 **Encounter for paternity testing** 🔒

    ● **Z02.82** **Encounter for adoption services** 🔒

    Z02.83 **Encounter for blood-alcohol and blood-drug test** 🔒

      Use additional code for findings of alcohol or drugs in blood (R78.-)

    ● **Z02.89** **Encounter for other administrative examinations** 🔒

      Encounter for examination for admission to prison

      Encounter for examination for admission to summer camp

      Encounter for immigration examination

      Encounter for naturalization examination

      Encounter for premarital examination

      Excludes1 health supervision of foundling or other healthy infant or child (Z76.1-Z76.2)

  ● **Z02.9** **Encounter for administrative examinations, unspecified** 🔒

● **Z03** **Encounter for medical observation for suspected diseases and conditions ruled out**

  This category is to be used when a person without a diagnosis is suspected of having an abnormal condition, without signs or symptoms, which requires study, but after examination and observation, is ruled out. This category is also for use for administrative and legal observation status.

  Excludes1 contact with and (suspected) exposures hazardous to health (Z77.-)

    newborn observation for suspected condition, ruled out (P00-P04)

    person with feared complaint in whom no diagnosis is made (Z71.1)

    signs or symptoms under study - code to signs or symptoms

  Z03.6 **Encounter for observation for suspected toxic effect from ingested substance ruled out** 🔒

    Encounter for observation for suspected adverse effect from drug

    Encounter for observation for suspected poisoning

◀ New ◀ Revised ~~deleted~~ Deleted Excludes 1 Excludes 2 Includes Use additional Code first Code also Unspecified

OGCR Official Guidelines ● Unacceptable Principal Diagnosis X Assign placeholder X ● Use Additional Character(s) ▌ Manifestation Code **Coding Clinic**

● **Z03.7**   **Encounter for suspected maternal and fetal conditions ruled out**
     Encounter for suspected maternal and fetal conditions not found
     Excludes1   known or suspected fetal anomalies affecting management of mother, not ruled out (O26.-, O35.-, O36.-, O40.-, O41.-)

  ● **Z03.71**   **Encounter for suspected problem with amniotic cavity and membrane ruled out** ♀ 🐾   M
     Encounter for suspected oligohydramnios ruled out
     Encounter for suspected polyhydramnios ruled out

  ● **Z03.72**   **Encounter for suspected placental problem ruled out** ♀ 🐾   M

  ● **Z03.73**   **Encounter for suspected fetal anomaly ruled out** ♀ 🐾   M

  ● **Z03.74**   **Encounter for suspected problem with fetal growth ruled out** ♀ 🐾   M

  ● **Z03.75**   **Encounter for suspected cervical shortening ruled out** ♀ 🐾   M

  ● **Z03.79**   **Encounter for other suspected maternal and fetal conditions ruled out** ♀ 🐾   M

● **Z03.8**   **Encounter for observation for other suspected diseases and conditions ruled out**

  ● **Z03.81**   **Encounter for observation for suspected exposure to biological agents ruled out**

     Z03.810   **Encounter for observation for suspected exposure to anthrax ruled out** 🐾

     Z03.818   **Encounter for observation for suspected exposure to other biological agents ruled out** 🐾

  ● **Z03.89**   **Encounter for observation for other suspected diseases and conditions ruled out** 🐾

● **Z04**   **Encounter for examination and observation for other reasons**
     Includes   encounter for examination for medicolegal reasons
     This category is to be used when a person without a diagnosis is suspected of having an abnormal condition, without signs or symptoms, which requires study, but after examination and observation, is ruled-out. This category is also for use for administrative and legal observation status.

   Z04.1   **Encounter for examination and observation following transport accident**
     Excludes1   encounter for examination and observation following work accident (Z04.2)

   Z04.2   **Encounter for examination and observation following work accident**

   Z04.3   **Encounter for examination and observation following other accident**

● **Z04.4**   **Encounter for examination and observation following alleged rape**
     Encounter for examination and observation of victim following alleged rape
     Encounter for examination and observation of victim following alleged sexual abuse

     Z04.41   **Encounter for examination and observation following alleged adult rape**   A
     Suspected adult rape, ruled out
     Suspected adult sexual abuse, ruled out

     Z04.42   **Encounter for examination and observation following alleged child rape**   P
     Suspected child rape, ruled out
     Suspected child sexual abuse, ruled out

   Z04.6   **Encounter for general psychiatric examination, requested by authority**

● **Z04.7**   **Encounter for examination and observation following alleged physical abuse**

     Z04.71   **Encounter for examination and observation following alleged adult physical abuse**   A
     Suspected adult physical abuse, ruled out
     Excludes1   confirmed case of adult physical abuse (T74.-)
     encounter for examination and observation following alleged adult sexual abuse (Z04.41)
     suspected case of adult physical abuse, not ruled out (T76.-)

     Z04.72   **Encounter for examination and observation following alleged child physical abuse**   P
     Suspected child physical abuse, ruled out
     Excludes1   confirmed case of child physical abuse (T74.-)
     encounter for examination and observation following alleged child sexual abuse (Z04.42)
     suspected case of child physical abuse, not ruled out (T76.-)

● **Z04.8**   **Encounter for examination and observation for other specified reasons**
     Encounter for examination and observation for request for expert evidence

● **Z04.9**   **Encounter for examination and observation for unspecified reason**
     Encounter for observation NOS

OGCR   See Section II.C.21.c.7.

> The follow-up codes are used to explain continuing surveillance following completed treatment of a disease, condition, or injury. They imply that the condition has been fully treated and no longer exists. They should not be confused with aftercare codes, or injury codes with 7th character "D," that explain ongoing care of a healing condition or its sequelae. Follow-up codes may be used in conjunction with history codes to provide the full picture of the healed condition and its treatment. The follow-up code is sequenced first, followed by the history code.
>
> A follow-up code may be used to explain multiple visits. Should a condition be found to have recurred on the follow-up visit, then the diagnosis code for the condition should be assigned in place of the follow-up code.
>
> The follow-up Z code categories:
>
> Z08   Encounter for follow-up examination after completed treatment for malignant neoplasm
>
> Z09   Encounter for follow-up examination after completed treatment for conditions other than malignant neoplasm
>
> Z39   Encounter for maternal postpartum care and examination

● **Z08**   **Encounter for follow-up examination after completed treatment for malignant neoplasm** 🐾
     Medical surveillance following completed treatment
     Use additional code to identify any acquired absence of organs (Z90.-)
     Use additional code to identify the personal history of malignant neoplasm (Z85.-)
     Excludes1   aftercare following medical care (Z43-Z49, Z51)

● **Z09**   **Encounter for follow-up examination after completed treatment for conditions other than malignant neoplasm** 🐾
     Medical surveillance following completed treatment
     Use additional code to identify any applicable history of disease code (Z86.-. Z87.-)
     Excludes1   aftercare following medical care (Z43-Z49, Z51)
     surveillance of contraception (Z30.4-)
     surveillance of prosthetic and other medical devices (Z44-Z46)

CHAPTER 21 (Z00-Z99)

N   Newborn Age: 0   **P**   Pediatric Age: 0–17   **M**   Maternity DX: 12–55   **A**   Adult Age: 15–124   ♀   Females Only   ♂   Males Only

🐾   Complication\Comorbidity   🐾   Major C\C   (Ex)   CC/MCC Exclusions   🐾   Present on Admission Requirement   🐾   Hospital-Acquired Condition   **1675**

● **Z11**   **Encounter for screening for infectious and parasitic diseases**
Screening is the testing for disease or disease precursors in asymptomatic individuals so that early detection and treatment can be provided for those who test positive for the disease.

> **Excludes1**   encounter for diagnostic examination - code to sign or symptom

  ● **Z11.0**   **Encounter for screening for intestinal infectious diseases** 🔍

OGCR Section II.C.21.c.5.

> Screening
>
> Screening is the testing for disease or disease precursors in seemingly well individuals so that early detection and treatment can be provided for those who test positive for the disease (e.g., screening mammogram).
>
> The testing of a person to rule out or confirm a suspected diagnosis because the patient has some sign or symptom is a diagnostic examination, not a screening. In these cases, the sign or symptom is used to explain the reason for the test.
>
> A screening code may be a first listed code if the reason for the visit is specifically the screening exam. It may also be used as an additional code if the screening is done during an office visit for other health problems. A screening code is not necessary if the screening is inherent to a routine examination, such as a pap smear done during a routine pelvic examination.
>
> Should a condition be discovered during the screening then the code for the condition may be assigned as an additional diagnosis.
>
> The Z code indicates that a screening exam is planned. A procedure code is required to confirm that the screening was performed.
>
> The screening Z codes /categories:
>
> Z11   Encounter for screening for infectious and parasitic diseases
> Z12   Encounter for screening for malignant neoplasms
> Z13   Encounter for screening for other diseases and disorders
>   Except: Z13.9, Encounter for screening, unspecified
> Z36   Encounter for antenatal screening for mother

  ● **Z11.1**   **Encounter for screening for respiratory tuberculosis** 🔍
  ● **Z11.2**   **Encounter for screening for other bacterial diseases** 🔍
  ● **Z11.3**   **Encounter for screening for infections with a predominantly sexual mode of transmission** 🔍

> **Excludes2**   encounter for screening for human immunodeficiency virus [HIV] (Z11.4)
> encounter for screening for human papillomavirus (Z11.51)

  ● **Z11.4**   **Encounter for screening for human immunodeficiency virus [HIV]** 🔍
  ● **Z11.5**   **Encounter for screening for other viral diseases**

> **Excludes2**   encounter for screening for viral intestinal disease (Z11.0)

    ● **Z11.51**   **Encounter for screening for human papillomavirus (HPV)** 🔍
    ● **Z11.59**   **Encounter for screening for other viral diseases** 🔍

  ● **Z11.6**   **Encounter for screening for other protozoal diseases and helminthiases** 🔍
> *Diseases or infestations caused by parasitic worms*

> **Excludes2**   encounter for screening for protozoal intestinal disease (Z11.0)

  ● **Z11.8**   **Encounter for screening for other infectious and parasitic diseases** 🔍
> Encounter for screening for chlamydia
> Encounter for screening for rickettsial
> Encounter for screening for spirochetal
> Encounter for screening for mycoses

  ● **Z11.9**   **Encounter for screening for infectious and parasitic diseases, unspecified** 🔍

● **Z12**   **Encounter for screening for malignant neoplasms**
Screening is the testing for disease or disease precursors in asymptomatic individuals so that early detection and treatment can be provided for those who test positive for the disease.

> Use additional code to identify any family history of malignant neoplasm (Z80.-)

> **Excludes1**   encounter for diagnostic examination - code to sign or symptom

  ● **Z12.0**   **Encounter for screening for malignant neoplasm of stomach** 🔍
  ● **Z12.1**   **Encounter for screening for malignant neoplasm of intestinal tract**

    ● **Z12.10**   **Encounter for screening for malignant neoplasm of intestinal tract, unspecified** 🔍
    ● **Z12.11**   **Encounter for screening for malignant neoplasm of colon** 🔍
> Encounter for screening colonoscopy NOS
    ● **Z12.12**   **Encounter for screening for malignant neoplasm of rectum** 🔍
    ● **Z12.13**   **Encounter for screening for malignant neoplasm of small intestine** 🔍

  ● **Z12.2**   **Encounter for screening for malignant neoplasm of respiratory organs** 🔍
  ● **Z12.3**   **Encounter for screening for malignant neoplasm of breast**

    ● **Z12.31**   **Encounter for screening mammogram for malignant neoplasm of breast** 🔍
> **Excludes1**   inconclusive mammogram (R92.2)
    ● **Z12.39**   **Encounter for other screening for malignant neoplasm of breast** 🔍

  ● **Z12.4**   **Encounter for screening for malignant neoplasm of cervix** ♀ 🔍
> Encounter for screening pap smear for malignant neoplasm of cervix
> **Excludes1**   encounter for screening for human papillomavirus (Z11.51)
> when screening is part of general gynecological examination (Z01.4-)

  ● **Z12.5**   **Encounter for screening for malignant neoplasm of prostate** ♂ 🔍
  ● **Z12.6**   **Encounter for screening for malignant neoplasm of bladder** 🔍
  ● **Z12.7**   **Encounter for screening for malignant neoplasm of other genitourinary organs**

    ● **Z12.71**   **Encounter for screening for malignant neoplasm of testis** ♂ 🔍
    ● **Z12.72**   **Encounter for screening for malignant neoplasm of vagina** ♀ 🔍
> Vaginal pap smear status - post hysterectomy for non-malignant condition
> Use additional code to identify acquired absence of uterus (Z90.71-)
> **Excludes1**   vaginal pap smear status - post hysterectomy for malignant conditions (Z08)
    ● **Z12.73**   **Encounter for screening for malignant neoplasm of ovary** ♀ 🔍
    ● **Z12.79**   **Encounter for screening for malignant neoplasm of other genitourinary organs** 🔍

  ● **Z12.8**   **Encounter for screening for malignant neoplasm of other sites**

    ● **Z12.81**   **Encounter for screening for malignant neoplasm of oral cavity** 🔍
    ● **Z12.82**   **Encounter for screening for malignant neoplasm of nervous system** 🔍
    ● **Z12.83**   **Encounter for screening for malignant neoplasm of skin** 🔍

◄ New   ◄▦ Revised   ~~deleted~~ Deleted   Excludes 1   Excludes 2   Includes   Use additional   Code first   Code also   Unspecified
OGCR Official Guidelines   ● Unacceptable Principal Diagnosis   X Assign placeholder X   ● Use Additional Character(s)   ▸ Manifestation Code   **Coding Clinic**

● **Z12.89** Encounter for screening for malignant neoplasm of other sites 🔍

● **Z12.9** Encounter for screening for malignant neoplasm, site **unspecified** 🔍

● **Z13** **Encounter for screening for other diseases and disorders**
Screening is the testing for disease or disease precursors in asymptomatic individuals so that early detection and treatment can be provided for those who test positive for the disease.

> **Excludes1** encounter for diagnostic examination - code to sign or symptom

● **Z13.0** Encounter for screening for diseases of the blood and blood-forming organs and certain disorders involving the immune mechanism 🔍

● **Z13.1** Encounter for screening for diabetes mellitus 🔍

● **Z13.2** Encounter for screening for nutritional, metabolic and other endocrine disorders

  ● **Z13.21** Encounter for screening for nutritional disorder 🔍

  ● **Z13.22** Encounter for screening for metabolic disorder

   ● **Z13.220** Encounter for screening for lipoid disorders 🔍
Encounter for screening for cholesterol level
Encounter for screening for hypercholesterolemia
Encounter for screening for hyperlipidemia

   ● **Z13.228** Encounter for screening for other metabolic disorders 🔍

  ● **Z13.29** Encounter for screening for other suspected endocrine disorder 🔍

   > **Excludes1** encounter for screening for diabetes mellitus (Z13.1)

● **Z13.4** Encounter for screening for certain developmental disorders in childhood 🔍   P
Encounter for screening for developmental handicaps in early childhood

  > **Excludes1** routine development testing of infant or child (Z00.1-)

● **Z13.5** Encounter for screening for eye and ear disorders 🔍

  > **Excludes2** encounter for general hearing examination (Z01.1-)
encounter for general vision examination (Z01.0-)

● **Z13.6** Encounter for screening for cardiovascular disorders 🔍

● **Z13.7** Encounter for screening for genetic and chromosomal anomalies

  > **Excludes1** genetic testing for procreative management (Z31.4-)

  ● **Z13.71** Encounter for nonprocreative screening for genetic disease carrier status 🔍

  ● **Z13.79** Encounter for other screening for genetic and chromosomal anomalies 🔍

● **Z13.8** Encounter for screening for other specified diseases and disorders

  > **Excludes2** screening for malignant neoplasms (Z12.-)

  ● **Z13.81** Encounter for screening for digestive system disorders

   ● **Z13.810** Encounter for screening for upper gastrointestinal disorder 🔍

   ● **Z13.811** Encounter for screening for lower gastrointestinal disorder 🔍

    > **Excludes1** encounter for screening for intestinal infectious disease (Z11.0)

   ● **Z13.818** Encounter for screening for other digestive system disorders 🔍

  ● **Z13.82** Encounter for screening for musculoskeletal disorder

   ● **Z13.820** Encounter for screening for osteoporosis 🔍

   ● **Z13.828** Encounter for screening for other musculoskeletal disorder 🔍

  ● **Z13.83** Encounter for screening for respiratory disorder NEC 🔍

   > **Excludes1** encounter for screening for respiratory tuberculosis (Z11.1)

  ● **Z13.84** Encounter for screening for dental disorders 🔍

  ● **Z13.85** Encounter for screening for nervous system disorders

   ● **Z13.850** Encounter for screening for traumatic brain injury 🔍

   ● **Z13.858** Encounter for screening for other nervous system disorders 🔍

  ● **Z13.88** Encounter for screening for disorder due to exposure to contaminants 🔍

   > **Excludes1** those exposed to contaminants without suspected disorders (Z57-Z77.-)

  ● **Z13.89** Encounter for screening for other disorder 🔍
Encounter for screening for genitourinary disorders

● **Z13.9** Encounter for screening, **unspecified** 🔍

GENETIC CARRIER AND GENETIC SUSCEPTIBILITY TO DISEASE (Z14-Z15)

● **Z14** **Genetic carrier**

  ● **Z14.0** Hemophilia A carrier

   ● **Z14.01** Asymptomatic hemophilia A carrier 🔍

   ● **Z14.02** Symptomatic hemophilia A carrier 🔍

  ● **Z14.1** Cystic fibrosis carrier 🔍

  ● **Z14.8** Genetic carrier of other disease 🔍

● **Z15** **Genetic susceptibility to disease**

  > **Excludes1** chromosomal anomalies (Q90-Q99)
  > **Includes** confirmed abnormal gene

Use additional code, if applicable, for any associated family history of the disease (Z80-Z84)

  ● **Z15.0** Genetic susceptibility to malignant neoplasm
Code first if applicable, any current malignant neoplasm (C00-C75, C81-C96)
Use additional code, if applicable, for any personal history of malignant neoplasm (Z85.-)

   ● **Z15.01** Genetic susceptibility to malignant neoplasm of breast 🔍

   ● **Z15.02** Genetic susceptibility to malignant neoplasm of ovary ♀ 🔍

   ● **Z15.03** Genetic susceptibility to malignant neoplasm of prostate ♂ 🔍

   ● **Z15.04** Genetic susceptibility to malignant neoplasm of endometrium ♀ 🔍

   ● **Z15.09** Genetic susceptibility to other malignant neoplasm 🔍

  ● **Z15.8** Genetic susceptibility to other disease

   ● **Z15.81** Genetic susceptibility to multiple endocrine neoplasia [MEN] 🔍

    > **Excludes1** multiple endocrine neoplasia [MEN] syndromes (E31.2-)

   ● **Z15.89** Genetic susceptibility to other disease 🔍

N Newborn Age: 0   **P** Pediatric Age: 0–17   **M** Maternity DX: 12–55   **A** Adult Age: 15–124   ♀ Females Only   ♂ Males Only

🔍 Complication\Comorbidity   🔍 Major C\C   (Ex) CC/MCC Exclusions   🔍 Present on Admission Requirement   🔍 Hospital-Acquired Condition

1677

RESISTANCE TO ANTIMICROBIAL DRUGS (Z16)

● Z16   Resistance to antimicrobial drugs
        Note: The codes in this category are provided for use
              as additional codes to identify the resistance and
              non-responsiveness of a condition to antimicrobial drugs.
        Code first the infection
        Excludes1 Methicillin resistant Staphylococcus aureus
                        infection (A49.02)
                      Methicillin resistant Staphylococcus aureus
                        infection in diseases classified elsewhere
                        (B95.62)
                      Methicillin resistant Staphylococcus aureus
                        pneumonia (J15.212)
                      Sepsis due to Methicillin resistant Staphylococcus
                        aureus (A41.02)

● Z16.1   Resistance to beta lactam antibiotics
   ● Z16.10   Resistance to unspecified beta lactam
              antibiotics
   ● Z16.11   Resistance to penicillins
              Resistance to amoxicillin
              Resistance to ampicillin
   ● Z16.12   Extended spectrum beta lactamase (ESBL)
              resistance
   ● Z16.19   Resistance to other specified beta lactam
              antibiotics
              Resistance to cephalosporins

● Z16.2   Resistance to other antibiotics
   ● Z16.20   Resistance to unspecified antibiotic
              Resistance to antibiotics NOS
   ● Z16.21   Resistance to vancomycin
   ● Z16.22   Resistance to vancomycin related antibiotics
   ● Z16.23   Resistance to quinolones and fluoroquinolones
   ● Z16.24   Resistance to multiple antibiotics
   ● Z16.29   Resistance to other single specified antibiotic
              Resistance to aminoglycosides
              Resistance to macrolides
              Resistance to sulfonamides
              Resistance to tetracyclines

● Z16.3   Resistance to other antimicrobial drugs
        Excludes1 resistance to antibiotics (Z16.1-, Z16.2-)
   ● Z16.30   Resistance to unspecified antimicrobial drugs
              Drug resistance NOS
   ● Z16.31   Resistance to antiparasitic drug(s)
              Resistance to quinine and related compounds
   ● Z16.32   Resistance to antifungal drug(s)
   ● Z16.33   Resistance to antiviral drug(s)
   ● Z16.34   Resistance to antimycobacterial drug(s)
              Resistance to tuberculostatics
      ● Z16.341   Resistance to single antimycobacterial
                  drug
                  Resistance to antimycobacterial drug
                    NOS
      ● Z16.342   Resistance to multiple
                  antimycobacterial drugs
   ● Z16.35   Resistance to multiple antimicrobial drugs
        Excludes1 Resistance to multiple antibiotics
                        only (Z16.24)
   ● Z16.39   Resistance to other specified antimicrobial drug

ESTROGEN RECEPTOR STATUS (Z17)

● Z17   Estrogen receptor status
        Code first malignant neoplasm of breast (C50.-)
   ● Z17.0   Estrogen receptor positive status [ER+] 🖐
   ● Z17.1   Estrogen receptor negative status [ER-] 🖐

RETAINED FOREIGN BODY FRAGMENTS (Z18)

● Z18   Retained foreign body fragments
        Includes   embedded fragment (status)
                      embedded splinter (status)
                      retained foreign body status
        Excludes1 artificial joint prosthesis status (Z96.6-)
                      foreign body accidentally left during a procedure
                        (T81.5-)
                      foreign body entering through orifice (T15-T19)
                      in situ cardiac device (Z95.-)
                      organ or tissue replaced by means other than
                        transplant (Z96.-, Z97.-)
                      organ or tissue replaced by transplant (Z94.-)
                      personal history of retained foreign body fully
                        removed Z87.821
                      superficial foreign body (non-embedded splinter)
                        - code to superficial foreign body, by site

● Z18.0   Retained radioactive fragments
   ● Z18.01   Retained depleted uranium fragments 🖐
   ● Z18.09   Other retained radioactive fragments 🖐
              Other retained depleted isotope fragments
              Retained nontherapeutic radioactive fragments

● Z18.1   Retained metal fragments
        Excludes1 retained radioactive metal fragments
                        (Z18.01-Z18.09)
   ● Z18.10   Retained metal fragments, unspecified 🖐
              Retained metal fragment NOS
   ● Z18.11   Retained magnetic metal fragments 🖐
   ● Z18.12   Retained nonmagnetic metal fragments 🖐

● Z18.2   Retained plastic fragments 🖐
              Acrylics fragments
              Diethylhexylphthalates fragments
              Isocyanate fragments

● Z18.3   Retained organic fragments
   ● Z18.31   Retained animal quills or spines 🖐
   ● Z18.32   Retained tooth 🖐
   ● Z18.33   Retained wood fragments 🖐
   ● Z18.39   Other retained organic fragments 🖐

● Z18.8   Other specified retained foreign body
   ● Z18.81   Retained glass fragments 🖐
   ● Z18.83   Retained stone or crystalline fragments 🖐
              Retained concrete or cement fragments
   ● Z18.89   Other specified retained foreign body
              fragments 🖐

● Z18.9   Retained foreign body fragments, unspecified
          material 🖐

PERSONS WITH POTENTIAL HEALTH HAZARDS RELATED TO COMMUNICABLE DISEASES (Z20-Z28)

● Z20   Contact with and (suspected) exposure to communicable
        diseases
        Excludes1 carrier of infectious disease (Z22.-)
                      diagnosed current infectious or parasitic disease -
                        see Alphabetic Index
        Excludes2 personal history of infectious and parasitic
                        diseases (Z86.1-)

● Z20.0   Contact with and (suspected) exposure to intestinal
          infectious diseases
        Z20.01   Contact with and (suspected) exposure to
                 intestinal infectious diseases due to Escherichia
                 coli (E. coli)
   ● Z20.09   Contact with and (suspected) exposure to other
              intestinal infectious diseases

● Z20.1   Contact with and (suspected) exposure to tuberculosis
● Z20.2   Contact with and (suspected) exposure to infections with
          a predominantly sexual mode of transmission
● Z20.3   Contact with and (suspected) exposure to rabies

- Z20.4   Contact with and (suspected) exposure to rubella
- Z20.5   Contact with and (suspected) exposure to viral hepatitis
- Z20.6   Contact with and (suspected) exposure to human immunodeficiency virus [HIV]

  > **Excludes1**   asymptomatic human immunodeficiency virus [HIV]
  > HIV infection status (Z21)

- Z20.7   Contact with and (suspected) exposure to pediculosis, acariasis and other infestations
- Z20.8   Contact with and (suspected) exposure to other communicable diseases
  - Z20.81   Contact with and (suspected) exposure to other bacterial communicable diseases
    - Z20.810   Contact with and (suspected) exposure to anthrax
    - Z20.811   Contact with and (suspected) exposure to meningococcus
    - Z20.818   Contact with and (suspected) exposure to other bacterial communicable diseases
  - Z20.82   Contact with and (suspected) exposure to other viral communicable diseases
    - Z20.820   Contact with and (suspected) exposure to varicella
    - Z20.828   Contact with and (suspected) exposure to other viral communicable diseases
  - Z20.89   Contact with and (suspected) exposure to other communicable diseases
- Z20.9   Contact with and (suspected) exposure to unspecified communicable disease

- Z21   **Asymptomatic human immunodeficiency virus [HIV] infection status**

  HIV positive NOS

  Code first Human immunodeficiency virus [HIV] disease complicating pregnancy, childbirth and the puerperium, if applicable (O98.7-)

  > **Excludes1**   acquired immunodeficiency syndrome (B20)
  > contact with human immunodeficiency virus [HIV] (Z20.6)
  > exposure to human immunodeficiency virus [HIV] (Z20.6)
  > human immunodeficiency virus [HIV] disease (B20)
  > inconclusive laboratory evidence of human immunodeficiency virus [HIV] (R75)

  MCE: Questionable admission when principal dx

- Z22   **Carrier of infectious disease**

  > **Includes**   colonization status
  > suspected carrier

  - Z22.0   Carrier of typhoid
  - Z22.1   Carrier of other intestinal infectious diseases
  - Z22.2   Carrier of diphtheria
  - Z22.3   Carrier of other specified bacterial diseases
    - Z22.31   Carrier of bacterial disease due to meningococci
    - Z22.32   Carrier of bacterial disease due to staphylococci
      - Z22.321   Carrier or suspected carrier of Methicillin susceptible Staphylococcus aureus
        MSSA colonization
      - Z22.322   Carrier or suspected carrier of Methicillin resistant Staphylococcus aureus
        MRSA colonization
    - Z22.33   Carrier of bacterial disease due to streptococci
      - Z22.330   Carrier of Group B streptococcus
      - Z22.338   Carrier of other streptococcus
    - Z22.39   Carrier of other specified bacterial diseases

- Z22.4   Carrier of infections with a predominantly sexual mode of transmission
- Z22.5   Carrier of viral hepatitis
  - Z22.50   Carrier of unspecified viral hepatitis
  - Z22.51   Carrier of viral hepatitis B
    Hepatitis B surface antigen [HBsAg] carrier
  - Z22.52   Carrier of viral hepatitis C
  - Z22.59   Carrier of other viral hepatitis
- Z22.6   Carrier of human T-lymphotropic virus type-1 [HTLV-1] infection
- Z22.8   Carrier of other infectious diseases
- Z22.9   Carrier of infectious disease, unspecified

- Z23   Encounter for immunization

  Code first any routine childhood examination

  Note: Procedure codes are required to identify the types of immunizations given.

- Z28   Immunization not carried out and underimmunization status

  > **Includes**   vaccination not carried out

  - Z28.0   Immunization not carried out because of contraindication
    - Z28.01   Immunization not carried out because of acute illness of patient
    - Z28.02   Immunization not carried out because of chronic illness or condition of patient
    - Z28.03   Immunization not carried out because of immune compromised state of patient
    - Z28.04   Immunization not carried out because of patient allergy to vaccine or component
    - Z28.09   Immunization not carried out because of other contraindication
  - Z28.1   Immunization not carried out because of patient decision for reasons of belief or group pressure
    Immunization not carried out because of religious belief
  - Z28.2   Immunization not carried out because of patient decision for other and unspecified reason
    - Z28.20   Immunization not carried out because of patient decision for unspecified reason
    - Z28.21   Immunization not carried out because of patient refusal
    - Z28.29   Immunization not carried out because of patient decision for other reason
  - Z28.3   Underimmunization status
    Delinquent immunization status
    Lapsed immunization schedule status
  - Z28.8   Immunization not carried out for other reason
    - Z28.81   Immunization not carried out due to patient having had the disease
    - Z28.82   Immunization not carried out because of caregiver refusal
      Immunization not carried out because of guardian refusal
      Immunization not carried out because of parent refusal

      > **Excludes1**   immunization not carried out because of caregiver refusal because of religious belief (Z28.1)

    - Z28.89   Immunization not carried out for other reason
  - Z28.9   Immunization not carried out for unspecified reason

N   Newborn Age: 0   P   Pediatric Age: 0–17   M   Maternity DX: 12–55   A   Adult Age: 15–124   ♀ Females Only   ♂ Males Only

Complication\Comorbidity   Major C\C   (Ex) CC/MCC Exclusions   Present on Admission Requirement   Hospital-Acquired Condition   1679

CHAPTER 21 (Z00-Z99)

PERSONS ENCOUNTERING HEALTH SERVICES IN CIRCUMSTANCES RELATED TO REPRODUCTION (Z30-Z39)

● **Z30   Encounter for contraceptive management**
● **Z30.0   Encounter for general counseling and advice on contraception**
● **Z30.01   Encounter for initial prescription of contraceptives**
    Excludes1   encounter for surveillance of contraceptives (Z30.4-)
● **Z30.011   Encounter for initial prescription of contraceptive pills** ♀
● **Z30.012   Encounter for prescription of emergency contraception** ♀ 🔳
    Encounter for postcoital contraception
● **Z30.013   Encounter for initial prescription of injectable contraceptive** ♀ 🔳
● **Z30.014   Encounter for initial prescription of intrauterine contraceptive device** ♀ 🔳
    Excludes1   encounter for insertion of intrauterine contraceptive device (Z30.430, Z30.432)
● **Z30.018   Encounter for initial prescription of other contraceptives** ♀ 🔳
● **Z30.019   Encounter for initial prescription of contraceptives, unspecified** ♀ 🔳
● **Z30.02   Counseling and instruction in natural family planning to avoid pregnancy** 🔳
● **Z30.09   Encounter for other general counseling and advice on contraception** 🔳
    Encounter for family planning advice NOS
Z30.2   Encounter for sterilization 🔳
Z30.4   Encounter for surveillance of contraceptives
● **Z30.40   Encounter for surveillance of contraceptives, unspecified** 🔳
● **Z30.41   Encounter for surveillance of contraceptive pills** ♀ 🔳
    Encounter for repeat prescription for contraceptive pill
● **Z30.42   Encounter for surveillance of injectable contraceptive** ♀ 🔳
● **Z30.43   Encounter for surveillance of intrauterine contraceptive device**
● **Z30.430   Encounter for insertion of intrauterine contraceptive device** ♀ 🔳
● **Z30.431   Encounter for routine checking of intrauterine contraceptive device** ♀ 🔳
● **Z30.432   Encounter for removal of intrauterine contraceptive device** ♀ 🔳
● **Z30.433   Encounter for removal and reinsertion of intrauterine contraceptive device** ♀ 🔳
    Encounter for replacement of intrauterine contraceptive device
● **Z30.49   Encounter for surveillance of other contraceptives** ♀ 🔳
● **Z30.8   Encounter for other contraceptive management** ♀ 🔳
    Encounter for postvasectomy sperm count
    Encounter for routine examination for contraceptive maintenance
    Excludes1   sperm count following sterilization reversal (Z31.42)
    sperm count for fertility testing (Z31.41)
● **Z30.9   Encounter for contraceptive management, unspecified** 🔳

● **Z31   Encounter for procreative management**
    Excludes1   complications associated with artificial fertilization (N98.-)
    female infertility (N97.-)
    male infertility (N46.-)
● **Z31.0   Encounter for reversal of previous sterilization** 🔳
● **Z31.4   Encounter for procreative investigation and testing**
    Excludes1   postvasectomy sperm count (Z30.8)
● **Z31.41   Encounter for fertility testing** 🔳
    Encounter for fallopian tube patency testing
    Encounter for sperm count for fertility testing
● **Z31.42   Aftercare following sterilization reversal** 🔳
    Sperm count following sterilization reversal
● **Z31.43   Encounter for genetic testing of female for procreative management**
    Use additional code for recurrent pregnancy loss, if applicable (N96, O26.2-)
    Excludes1   nonprocreative genetic testing (Z13.7-)
● **Z31.430   Encounter of female for testing for genetic disease carrier status for procreative management** ♀ 🔳
● **Z31.438   Encounter for other genetic testing of female for procreative management** ♀ 🔳
● **Z31.44   Encounter for genetic testing of male for procreative management**
    Excludes1   nonprocreative genetic testing (Z13.7-)
● **Z31.440   Encounter of male for testing for genetic disease carrier status for procreative management** ♂ 🔳
● **Z31.441   Encounter for testing of male partner of patient with recurrent pregnancy loss** ♂ 🔳   A
● **Z31.448   Encounter for other genetic testing of male for procreative management** ♂ 🔳   A
● **Z31.49   Encounter for other procreative investigation and testing** 🔳
● **Z31.5   Encounter for genetic counseling** 🔳
● **Z31.6   Encounter for general counseling and advice on procreation**
● **Z31.61   Procreative counseling and advice using natural family planning** 🔳
● **Z31.62   Encounter for fertility preservation counseling** 🔳
    Encounter for fertility preservation counseling prior to cancer therapy
    Encounter for fertility preservation counseling prior to surgical removal of gonads
● **Z31.69   Encounter for other general counseling and advice on procreation** 🔳
● **Z31.8   Encounter for other procreative management**
● **Z31.81   Encounter for male factor infertility in female patient** ♀ 🔳
● **Z31.82   Encounter for Rh incompatibility status** ♀ 🔳
● **Z31.83   Encounter for assisted reproductive fertility procedure cycle** ♀ 🔳
    Patient undergoing in vitro fertilization cycle
    Use additional code to identify the type of infertility
    Excludes1   pre-cycle diagnosis and testing - code to reason for encounter
● **Z31.84   Encounter for fertility preservation procedure** 🔳
    Encounter for fertility preservation procedure prior to cancer therapy
    Encounter for fertility preservation procedure prior to surgical removal of gonads
● **Z31.89   Encounter for other procreative management** 🔳
● **Z31.9   Encounter for procreative management, unspecified** 🔳

◄ New   ◄■ Revised   d̶e̶l̶e̶t̶e̶d̶ Deleted   Excludes 1   Excludes 2   Includes   Use additional   Code first   Code also   Unspecified
OGCR Official Guidelines   ● Unacceptable Principal Diagnosis   X Assign placeholder X   ▶ Use Additional Character(s)   ▶ Manifestation Code   Coding Clinic

● **Z32   Encounter for pregnancy test and childbirth and childcare instruction**

    ● **Z32.0   Encounter for pregnancy test**

        Z32.00   Encounter for pregnancy test, result unknown ♀ 🖐

            Encounter for pregnancy test NOS

        Z32.01   Encounter for pregnancy test, result positive ♀ 🖐   M

        Z32.02   Encounter for pregnancy test, result negative ♀ 🖐

    ● **Z32.2   Encounter for childbirth instruction 🖐**

    ● **Z32.3   Encounter for childcare instruction 🖐**

        Encounter for prenatal or postpartum childcare instruction

● **Z33   Pregnant state**

    ● **Z33.1   Pregnant state, incidental ♀ 🖐**   M

        Pregnant state NOS

        Excludes1   complications of pregnancy (O00-O9A)

    Z33.2   Encounter for elective termination of pregnancy ♀   M

        Excludes1   early fetal death with retention of dead fetus (O02.1)

            late fetal death (O36.4)

            spontaneous abortion (O03)

● **Z34   Encounter for supervision of normal pregnancy**

    Excludes1   any complication of pregnancy (O00-O9A)

        encounter for pregnancy test (Z32.0-)

        encounter for supervision of high risk pregnancy (O09.-)

    ● **Z34.0   Encounter for supervision of normal first pregnancy**

        ● **Z34.00   Encounter for supervision of normal first pregnancy, unspecified trimester ♀ 🖐**   M

        ● **Z34.01   Encounter for supervision of normal first pregnancy, first trimester ♀ 🖐**   M

        ● **Z34.02   Encounter for supervision of normal first pregnancy, second trimester ♀ 🖐**   M

        ● **Z34.03   Encounter for supervision of normal first pregnancy, third trimester ♀ 🖐**   M

    ● **Z34.8   Encounter for supervision of other normal pregnancy**

        ● **Z34.80   Encounter for supervision of other normal pregnancy, unspecified trimester ♀ 🖐**   M

        ● **Z34.81   Encounter for supervision of other normal pregnancy, first trimester ♀ 🖐**   M

        ● **Z34.82   Encounter for supervision of other normal pregnancy, second trimester ♀ 🖐**   M

        ● **Z34.83   Encounter for supervision of other normal pregnancy, third trimester ♀ 🖐**   M

    ● **Z34.9   Encounter for supervision of normal pregnancy, unspecified**

        ● **Z34.90   Encounter for supervision of normal pregnancy, unspecified, unspecified trimester ♀ 🖐**   M

        ● **Z34.91   Encounter for supervision of normal pregnancy, unspecified, first trimester ♀ 🖐**   M

        ● **Z34.92   Encounter for supervision of normal pregnancy, unspecified, second trimester ♀ 🖐**   M

        ● **Z34.93   Encounter for supervision of normal pregnancy, unspecified, third trimester ♀ 🖐**   M

● **Z36   Encounter for antenatal screening of mother ♀ 🖐**   M

    Excludes1   abnormal findings on antenatal screening of mother (O28.-)

        diagnostic examination - code to sign or symptom

        encounter for suspected maternal and fetal conditions ruled out (Z03.7-)

        suspected fetal condition affecting management of pregnancy - code to condition in Chapter 15

    Excludes2   genetic counseling and testing (Z31.43-, Z31.5)

        routine prenatal care (Z34)

● **Z3A   Weeks of gestation**

    Note: Codes from category Z3A are for use, only on the maternal record, to indicate the weeks of gestation of the pregnancy.

    Code first complications of pregnancy, childbirth and the puerperium (O00-O9A)

    ● **Z3A.0   Weeks of gestation of pregnancy, unspecified or less than 10 weeks**

        Z3A.00   Weeks of gestation of pregnancy not specified ♀ 🖐   M

        Z3A.01   Less than 8 weeks gestation of pregnancy ♀ 🖐   M

        Z3A.08   8 weeks gestation of pregnancy ♀ 🖐   M

        Z3A.09   9 weeks gestation of pregnancy ♀ 🖐   M

    ● **Z3A.1   Weeks of gestation of pregnancy, weeks 10-19**

        ● **Z3A.10   10 weeks gestation of pregnancy ♀**   M

        ● **Z3A.11   11 weeks gestation of pregnancy ♀**   M

        ● **Z3A.12   12 weeks gestation of pregnancy ♀**   M

        ● **Z3A.13   13 weeks gestation of pregnancy ♀**   M

        ● **Z3A.14   14 weeks gestation of pregnancy ♀**   M

        ● **Z3A.15   15 weeks gestation of pregnancy ♀**   M

        ● **Z3A.16   16 weeks gestation of pregnancy ♀**   M

        ● **Z3A.17   17 weeks gestation of pregnancy ♀**   M

        ● **Z3A.18   18 weeks gestation of pregnancy ♀**   M

        ● **Z3A.19   19 weeks gestation of pregnancy ♀**   M

    ● **Z3A.2   Weeks of gestation of pregnancy, weeks 20-29**

        ● **Z3A.20   20 weeks gestation of pregnancy ♀**   M

        ● **Z3A.21   21 weeks gestation of pregnancy ♀**   M

        ● **Z3A.22   22 weeks gestation of pregnancy ♀**   M

        ● **Z3A.23   23 weeks gestation of pregnancy ♀**   M

        ● **Z3A.24   24 weeks gestation of pregnancy ♀**   M

        ● **Z3A.25   25 weeks gestation of pregnancy ♀**   M

        ● **Z3A.26   26 weeks gestation of pregnancy ♀**   M

        ● **Z3A.27   27 weeks gestation of pregnancy ♀**   M

        ● **Z3A.28   28 weeks gestation of pregnancy ♀**   M

        ● **Z3A.29   29 weeks gestation of pregnancy ♀**   M

    ● **Z3A.3   Weeks of gestation of pregnancy, weeks 30-39**

        ● **Z3A.30   30 weeks gestation of pregnancy ♀**   M

        ● **Z3A.31   31 weeks gestation of pregnancy ♀**   M

        ● **Z3A.32   32 weeks gestation of pregnancy ♀**   M

        ● **Z3A.33   33 weeks gestation of pregnancy ♀**   M

        ● **Z3A.34   34 weeks gestation of pregnancy ♀**   M

        ● **Z3A.35   35 weeks gestation of pregnancy ♀**   M

        ● **Z3A.36   36 weeks gestation of pregnancy ♀**   M

        ● **Z3A.37   37 weeks gestation of pregnancy ♀**   M

        ● **Z3A.38   38 weeks gestation of pregnancy ♀**   M

        ● **Z3A.39   39 weeks gestation of pregnancy ♀**   M

    ● **Z3A.4   Weeks of gestation of pregnancy, weeks 40 or greater**

        ● **Z3A.40   40 weeks gestation of pregnancy ♀**   M

        ● **Z3A.41   41 weeks gestation of pregnancy ♀**   M

        ● **Z3A.42   42 weeks gestation of pregnancy ♀**   M

        ● **Z3A.49   Greater than 42 weeks gestation of pregnancy ♀**   M

CHAPTER 21 (Z00-Z99)

N Newborn Age: 0   **P** Pediatric Age: 0–17   **M** Maternity DX: 12–55   **A** Adult Age: 15–124   ♀ Females Only   ♂ Males Only

🖐 Complication\Comorbidity   ◆ Major C\C   (Ex) CC/MCC Exclusions   🖐 Present on Admission Requirement   ◆ Hospital-Acquired Condition

1681

● **Z37   Outcome of delivery**
This category is intended for use as an additional code to identify the outcome of delivery on the mother's record. It is not for use on the newborn record.

Excludes1   stillbirth (P95)

● **Z37.0   Single live birth** ♀ ✎   M
● **Z37.1   Single stillbirth** ♀ ✎   M
● **Z37.2   Twins, both liveborn** ♀ ✎   M
● **Z37.3   Twins, one liveborn and one stillborn** ♀ ✎   M
● **Z37.4   Twins, both stillborn** ♀ ✎   M
● **Z37.5   Other multiple births, all liveborn**
   ● **Z37.50   Multiple births, unspecified, all liveborn** ♀ ✎ M
   ● **Z37.51   Triplets, all liveborn** ♀ ✎   M
   ● **Z37.52   Quadruplets, all liveborn** ♀ ✎   M
   ● **Z37.53   Quintuplets, all liveborn** ♀ ✎   M
   ● **Z37.54   Sextuplets, all liveborn** ♀ ✎   M
   ● **Z37.59   Other multiple births, all liveborn** ♀ ✎   M
● **Z37.6   Other multiple births, some liveborn**
   ● **Z37.60   Multiple births, unspecified, some liveborn** ♀ ✎   M
   ● **Z37.61   Triplets, some liveborn** ♀ ✎   M
   ● **Z37.62   Quadruplets, some liveborn** ♀ ✎   M
   ● **Z37.63   Quintuplets, some liveborn** ♀ ✎   M
   ● **Z37.64   Sextuplets, some liveborn** ♀ ✎   M
   ● **Z37.69   Other multiple births, some liveborn** ♀ ✎   M
● **Z37.7   Other multiple births, all stillborn** ♀ ✎   M
● **Z37.9   Outcome of delivery, unspecified** ♀ ✎   M
   Multiple birth NOS
   Single birth NOS

● **Z38   Liveborn infants according to place of birth and type of delivery**
This category is for use as the principal code on the initial record of a newborn baby. It is to be used for the initial birth record only. It is not to be used on the mother's record.

● **Z38.0   Single liveborn infant, born in hospital**
   Single liveborn infant, born in birthing center or other health care facility
   Z38.00   Single liveborn infant, delivered vaginally ✎ N
   Z38.01   Single liveborn infant, delivered by cesarean ✎   N
● **Z38.1   Single liveborn infant, born outside hospital** ✎   N
   Z38.2   Single liveborn infant, unspecified as to place of birth ✎   N
   Single liveborn infant NOS
● **Z38.3   Twin liveborn infant, born in hospital**
   Z38.30   Twin liveborn infant, delivered vaginally ✎   N
   Z38.31   Twin liveborn infant, delivered by cesarean ✎ N
● **Z38.4   Twin liveborn infant, born outside hospital** ✎   N
   Z38.5   Twin liveborn infant, unspecified as to place of birth ✎ N
● **Z38.6   Other multiple liveborn infant, born in hospital**
   Z38.61   Triplet liveborn infant, delivered vaginally ✎   N
   Z38.62   Triplet liveborn infant, delivered by cesarean ✎   N
   Z38.63   Quadruplet liveborn infant, delivered vaginally ✎   N
   Z38.64   Quadruplet liveborn infant, delivered by cesarean ✎   N
   Z38.65   Quintuplet liveborn infant, delivered vaginally ✎   N
   Z38.66   Quintuplet liveborn infant, delivered by cesarean ✎   N
   Z38.68   Other multiple liveborn infant, delivered vaginally ✎   N
   Z38.69   Other multiple liveborn infant, delivered by cesarean ✎   N

   Z38.7   Other multiple liveborn infant, born outside hospital ✎   N
   Z38.8   Other multiple liveborn infant, unspecified as to place of birth ✎   N

● **Z39   Encounter for maternal postpartum care and examination**
   Z39.0   Encounter for care and examination of mother immediately after delivery ♀ ✎   M
      Care and observation in uncomplicated cases when the delivery occurs outside a healthcare facility
      Excludes1   care for postpartum complication - see Alphabetic index
   ● **Z39.1   Encounter for care and examination of lactating mother** ♀ ✎   M
      Encounter for supervision of lactation
      Excludes1   disorders of lactation (O92.-)
   ● **Z39.2   Encounter for routine postpartum follow-up** ♀ ✎   M

ENCOUNTERS FOR OTHER SPECIFIC HEALTH CARE (Z40-Z53)

Categories Z40-Z53 are intended for use to indicate a reason for care. They may be used for patients who have already been treated for a disease or injury, but who are receiving aftercare or prophylactic care, or care to consolidate the treatment, or to deal with a residual state

Excludes2   follow-up examination for medical surveillance after treatment (Z08-Z09)

● **Z40   Encounter for prophylactic surgery**
   Excludes1   organ donations (Z52.-)
      therapeutic organ removal - code to condition
   ● **Z40.0   Encounter for prophylactic surgery for risk factors related to malignant neoplasms**
      Admission for prophylactic organ removal
      Use additional code to identify risk factor
      Z40.00   Encounter for prophylactic removal of unspecified organ
      Z40.01   Encounter for prophylactic removal of breast
      Z40.02   Encounter for prophylactic removal of ovary ♀
      Z40.09   Encounter for prophylactic removal of other organ
   ● **Z40.8   Encounter for other prophylactic surgery**
   ● **Z40.9   Encounter for prophylactic surgery, unspecified**

● **Z41   Encounter for procedures for purposes other than remedying health state**
   Z41.1   Encounter for cosmetic surgery ✎
      Encounter for cosmetic breast implant
      Encounter for cosmetic procedure
      Excludes1   encounter for plastic and reconstructive surgery following medical procedure or healed injury (Z42.-)
         encounter for post-mastectomy breast implantation (Z42.1)
   Z41.2   Encounter for routine and ritual male circumcision ♂ ✎
   ● **Z41.3   Encounter for ear piercing** ✎
   ● **Z41.8   Encounter for other procedures for purposes other than remedying health state** ✎
   ● **Z41.9   Encounter for procedure for purposes other than remedying health state, unspecified** ✎

● **Z42   Encounter for plastic and reconstructive surgery following medical procedure or healed injury**
   Excludes1   encounter for cosmetic plastic surgery (Z41.1)
      encounter for plastic surgery for treatment of current injury - code to relevent injury
   Z42.1   Encounter for breast reconstruction following mastectomy ✎   A
      Excludes1   deformity and disproportion of reconstructed breast (N65.1-)
   Z42.8   Encounter for other plastic and reconstructive surgery following medical procedure or healed injury ✎

● **Z43** Encounter for attention to artificial openings

| Includes | closure of artificial openings |

passage of sounds or bougies through artificial openings

reforming artificial openings

removal of catheter from artificial openings

toilet or cleansing of artificial openings

| Excludes1 | artificial opening status only, without need for care (Z93.-) |

complications of external stoma (J95.0-, K94.-, N99.5-)

| Excludes2 | fitting and adjustment of prosthetic and other devices (Z44-Z46) |

Z43.0 Encounter for attention to tracheostomy 🗐

Z43.1 Encounter for attention to gastrostomy 🗐 🗐

(Ex) Z43.1

Z43.2 Encounter for attention to ileostomy 🗐

Z43.3 Encounter for attention to colostomy 🗐

Z43.4 Encounter for attention to other artificial openings of digestive tract 🗐

Z43.5 Encounter for attention to cystostomy 🗐

Z43.6 Encounter for attention to other artificial openings of urinary tract 🗐

Encounter for attention to nephrostomy

Encounter for attention to ureterostomy

Encounter for attention to urethrostomy

Z43.7 Encounter for attention to artificial vagina 🗐

Z43.8 Encounter for attention to other artificial openings 🗐

● Z43.9 Encounter for attention to unspecified artificial opening 🗐

● **Z44** Encounter for fitting and adjustment of external prosthetic device

| Includes | removal or replacement of external prosthetic device |

| Excludes1 | malfunction or other complications of device - see Alphabetical Index presence of prosthetic device (Z97.-) |

● Z44.0 Encounter for fitting and adjustment of artificial arm

● Z44.00 Encounter for fitting and adjustment of unspecified artificial arm

Z44.001 Encounter for fitting and adjustment of unspecified right artificial arm 🗐

Z44.002 Encounter for fitting and adjustment of unspecified left artificial arm 🗐

Z44.009 Encounter for fitting and adjustment of unspecified artificial arm, unspecified arm 🗐

● Z44.01 Encounter for fitting and adjustment of complete artificial arm

Z44.011 Encounter for fitting and adjustment of complete right artificial arm 🗐

Z44.012 Encounter for fitting and adjustment of complete left artificial arm 🗐

Z44.019 Encounter for fitting and adjustment of complete artificial arm, unspecified arm 🗐

● Z44.02 Encounter for fitting and adjustment of partial artificial arm

Z44.021 Encounter for fitting and adjustment of partial artificial right arm 🗐

Z44.022 Encounter for fitting and adjustment of partial artificial left arm 🗐

Z44.029 Encounter for fitting and adjustment of partial artificial arm, unspecified arm 🗐

● Z44.1 Encounter for fitting and adjustment of artificial leg

● Z44.10 Encounter for fitting and adjustment of unspecified artificial leg

Z44.101 Encounter for fitting and adjustment of unspecified right artificial leg 🗐

Z44.102 Encounter for fitting and adjustment of unspecified left artificial leg 🗐

Z44.109 Encounter for fitting and adjustment of unspecified artificial leg, unspecified leg 🗐

● Z44.11 Encounter for fitting and adjustment of complete artificial leg

Z44.111 Encounter for fitting and adjustment of complete right artificial leg 🗐

Z44.112 Encounter for fitting and adjustment of complete left artificial leg 🗐

Z44.119 Encounter for fitting and adjustment of complete artificial leg, unspecified leg 🗐

● Z44.12 Encounter for fitting and adjustment of partial artificial leg

Z44.121 Encounter for fitting and adjustment of partial artificial right leg 🗐

Z44.122 Encounter for fitting and adjustment of partial artificial left leg 🗐

Z44.129 Encounter for fitting and adjustment of partial artificial leg, unspecified leg 🗐

● Z44.2 Encounter for fitting and adjustment of artificial eye

| Excludes1 | mechanical complication of ocular prosthesis (T85.3) |

Z44.20 Encounter for fitting and adjustment of artificial eye, unspecified 🗐

Z44.21 Encounter for fitting and adjustment of artificial right eye 🗐

Z44.22 Encounter for fitting and adjustment of artificial left eye 🗐

● Z44.3 Encounter for fitting and adjustment of external breast prosthesis

| Excludes1 | complications of breast implant (T85.4-) |

encounter for adjustment or removal of breast implant (Z45.81-)

encounter for initial breast implant insertion for cosmetic breast augmentation (Z41.1)

encounter for breast reconstruction following mastectomy (Z42.1)

Z44.30 Encounter for fitting and adjustment of external breast prosthesis, unspecified breast ♀ 🗐

Z44.31 Encounter for fitting and adjustment of external right breast prosthesis ♀ 🗐

Z44.32 Encounter for fitting and adjustment of external left breast prosthesis ♀ 🗐

Z44.8 Encounter for fitting and adjustment of other external prosthetic devices 🗐

● Z44.9 Encounter for fitting and adjustment of unspecified external prosthetic device 🗐

N Newborn Age: 0   P Pediatric Age: 0–17   M Maternity DX: 12–55   A Adult Age: 15–124   ♀ Females Only   ♂ Males Only

🗐 Complication\Comorbidity   🗐 Major C\C   (Ex) CC/MCC Exclusions   🗐 Present on Admission Requirement   🗐 Hospital-Acquired Condition

ICD-10-CM DRAFT

● **Z45** **Encounter for adjustment and management of implanted device**

Includes removal or replacement of implanted device

Excludes1 malfunction or other complications of device - see Alphabetical Index

presence of prosthetic and other devices (Z95-Z97)

Excludes2 encounter for fitting and adjustment of non-implanted device (Z46.-)

● **Z45.0** **Encounter for adjustment and management of cardiac device**

● **Z45.01** **Encounter for adjustment and management of cardiac pacemaker**

Excludes1 encounter for adjustment and management of automatic implantable cardiac defibrillator with synchronous cardiac pacemaker (Z45.02)

Z45.010 **Encounter for checking and testing of cardiac pacemaker pulse generator [battery]** 🖉

Encounter for replacing cardiac pacemaker pulse generator [battery]

MCE: Questionable admission when principal dx

Z45.018 **Encounter for adjustment and management of other part of cardiac pacemaker** 🖉

MCE: Questionable admission when principal dx

Z45.02 **Encounter for adjustment and management of automatic implantable cardiac defibrillator** 🖉

Encounter for adjustment and management of automatic implantable cardiac defibrillator with synchronous cardiac pacemaker

MCE: Questionable admission when principal dx

Z45.09 **Encounter for adjustment and management of other cardiac device** 🖉

MCE: Questionable admission when principal dx

Z45.1 **Encounter for adjustment and management of infusion pump** 🖉

Z45.2 **Encounter for adjustment and management of vascular access device** 🖉

Encounter for adjustment and management of vascular catheters

Excludes1 encounter for adjustment and management of renal dialysis catheter (Z49.01)

● **Z45.3** **Encounter for adjustment and management of implanted devices of the special senses**

Z45.31 **Encounter for adjustment and management of implanted visual substitution device** 🖉

● **Z45.32** **Encounter for adjustment and management of implanted hearing device** 🖉

Excludes1 encounter for fitting and adjustment of hearing aide (Z46.1)

Z45.320 **Encounter for adjustment and management of bone conduction device** 🖉

Z45.321 **Encounter for adjustment and management of cochlear device** 🖉

Z45.328 **Encounter for adjustment and management of other implanted hearing device** 🖉

● **Z45.4** **Encounter for adjustment and management of implanted nervous system device**

Z45.41 **Encounter for adjustment and management of cerebrospinal fluid drainage device** 🖉

Encounter for adjustment and management of cerebral ventricular (communicating) shunt

Z45.42 **Encounter for adjustment and management of neuropacemaker (brain) (peripheral nerve) (spinal cord)** 🖉

Z45.49 **Encounter for adjustment and management of other implanted nervous system device** 🖉

● **Z45.8** **Encounter for adjustment and management of other implanted devices**

● **Z45.81** **Encounter for adjustment or removal of breast implant**

Encounter for elective implant exchange (different material) (different size)

Encounter removal of tissue expander without synchronous insertion of permanent implant

Excludes1 complications of breast implant (T85.4-)

encounter for initial breast implant insertion for cosmetic breast augmentation (Z41.1)

encounter for breast reconstruction following mastectomy (Z42.1)

Z45.811 **Encounter for adjustment or removal of right breast implant** ♀ 🖉

Z45.812 **Encounter for adjustment or removal of left breast implant** ♀ 🖉

Z45.819 **Encounter for adjustment or removal of unspecified breast implant** ♀ 🖉

● **Z45.82** **Encounter for adjustment or removal of myringotomy device (stent) (tube)** 🖉

● **Z45.89** **Encounter for adjustment and management of other implanted devices** 🖉

● **Z45.9** **Encounter for adjustment and management of unspecified implanted device** 🖉

● **Z46** **Encounter for fitting and adjustment of other devices**

Includes removal or replacement of other device

Excludes1 malfunction or other complications of device - see Alphabetical Index

Excludes2 encounter for fitting and management of implanted devices (Z45.-)

issue of repeat prescription only (Z76.0)

presence of prosthetic and other devices (Z95-Z97)

● **Z46.0** **Encounter for fitting and adjustment of spectacles and contact lenses** 🖉

● **Z46.1** **Encounter for fitting and adjustment of hearing aid** 🖉

Excludes1 encounter for adjustment and management of implanted hearing device (Z45.32-)

Z46.2 **Encounter for fitting and adjustment of other devices related to nervous system and special senses** 🖉

Excludes2 encounter for adjustment and management of implanted nervous system device (Z45.4-)

encounter for adjustment and management of implanted visual substitution device (Z45.31)

Z46.3 **Encounter for fitting and adjustment of dental prosthetic device** 🖉

Encounter for fitting and adjustment of dentures

● **Z46.4** **Encounter for fitting and adjustment of orthodontic device** 🖉

◄ New ◄ Revised ~~deleted~~ Deleted Excludes 1 Excludes 2 Includes Use additional Code first Code also Unspecified

OGCR Official Guidelines ● Unacceptable Principal Diagnosis X Assign placeholder X ● Use Additional Character(s) ▶ Manifestation Code **Coding Clinic**

● **Z46.5**   **Encounter for fitting and adjustment of other gastrointestinal appliance and device**

> **Excludes1**   encounter for attention to artificial openings of digestive tract (Z43.1-Z43.4)

   ● **Z46.51**   Encounter for fitting and adjustment of gastric lap band 🔲

   ● **Z46.59**   Encounter for fitting and adjustment of other gastrointestinal appliance and device 🔲

● **Z46.6**   **Encounter for fitting and adjustment of urinary device** 🔲

> **Excludes2**   attention to artificial openings of urinary tract (Z43.5, Z43.6)

● **Z46.8**   **Encounter for fitting and adjustment of other specified devices**

   ● **Z46.81**   Encounter for fitting and adjustment of insulin pump 🔲
> Encounter for insulin pump instruction and training ◀
> Encounter for insulin pump titration ◀

   Z46.82   Encounter for fitting and adjustment of non-vascular catheter 🔲

   ● **Z46.89**   Encounter for fitting and adjustment of other specified devices 🔲
> Encounter for fitting and adjustment of wheelchair

● **Z46.9**   **Encounter for fitting and adjustment of unspecified device** 🔲

● **Z47**   **Orthopedic aftercare**

> **Excludes1**   aftercare for healing fracture - code to fracture with 7th character D

   Z47.1   **Aftercare following joint replacement surgery**
> Use additional code to identify the joint (Z96.6-)

   Z47.2   **Encounter for removal of internal fixation device**

> **Excludes1**   encounter for adjustment of internal fixation device for fracture treatment - code to fracture with appropriate 7th character
> encounter for removal of external fixation device - code to fracture with 7th character D
> infection or inflammatory reaction to internal fixation device (T84.6-)
> mechanical complication of internal fixation device (T84.1-)

● **Z47.3**   **Aftercare following explantation of joint prosthesis**
> Aftercare following explantation of joint prosthesis, staged procedure
> Encounter for joint prosthesis insertion following prior explantation of joint prosthesis

   Z47.31   **Aftercare following explantation of shoulder joint prosthesis**

> **Excludes1**   acquired absence of shoulder joint following prior explantation of shoulder joint prosthesis (Z89.23-)
> shoulder joint prosthesis explantation status (Z89.23-)

   Z47.32   **Aftercare following explantation of hip joint prosthesis**

> **Excludes1**   acquired absence of hip joint following prior explantation of hip joint prosthesis (Z89.62-)
> hip joint prosthesis explantation status (Z89.62-)

   Z47.33   **Aftercare following explantation of knee joint prosthesis**

> **Excludes1**   acquired absence of knee joint following prior explantation of knee prosthesis (Z89.52-)
> knee joint prosthesis explantation status (Z89.52-)

● **Z47.8**   **Encounter for other orthopedic aftercare**

   Z47.81   **Encounter for orthopedic aftercare following surgical amputation**
> Use additional code to identify the limb amputated (Z89.-)

   Z47.82   **Encounter for orthopedic aftercare following scoliosis surgery** 🔲

   Z47.89   **Encounter for other orthopedic aftercare** 🔲

● **Z48**   **Encounter for other postprocedural aftercare**

> **Excludes1**   encounter for follow-up examination after completed treatment (Z08-Z09)

> **Excludes2**   encounter for attention to artificial openings (Z43.-)
> encounter for fitting and adjustment of prosthetic and other devices (Z44-Z46)

● **Z48.0**   **Encounter for attention to dressings, sutures and drains**

> **Excludes1**   encounter for planned postprocedural wound closure (Z48.1)

   ● **Z48.00**   Encounter for change or removal of nonsurgical wound dressing
> Encounter for change or removal of wound dressing NOS

   ● **Z48.01**   Encounter for change or removal of surgical wound dressing

   ● **Z48.02**   Encounter for removal of sutures
> Encounter for removal of staples

   Z48.03   Encounter for change or removal of drains

   Z48.1   **Encounter for planned postprocedural wound closure** 🔲

> **Excludes1**   encounter for attention to dressings and sutures (Z48.0-)

● **Z48.2**   **Encounter for aftercare following organ transplant**

   ● **Z48.21**   Encounter for aftercare following heart transplant 🔲
> CC when PDx is its own CC
> (Ex:) D47.Z1, T86.20-T86.39, T86.850-T86.859, T86.90-T86.99, Z94.1, Z94.3, Z94.89-Z94.9

   ● **Z48.22**   Encounter for aftercare following kidney transplant 🔲
> CC when PDx is its own CC
> (Ex:) D47.Z1, T86.10-T86.19, T86.850-T86.859, T86.90-T86.99, Z94.0, Z94.89-Z94.9

   ● **Z48.23**   Encounter for aftercare following liver transplant 🔲
> CC when PDx is its own CC
> (Ex:) D47.Z1, T86.40-T86.49, T86.850-T86.859, T86.90-T86.99, Z94.4, Z94.89, Z94.9

   ● **Z48.24**   Encounter for aftercare following lung transplant 🔲
> CC when PDx is its own CC
> (Ex:) D47.Z1, T86.810-T86.819, T86.850-T86.859, T86.90-T86.99, Z94.2, Z94.89-Z94.9

   ● **Z48.28**   Encounter for aftercare following multiple organ transplant

     ● **Z48.280**   Encounter for aftercare following heart-lung transplant 🔲
> CC when PDx is its own CC
> (Ex:) See Z48.21

     ● **Z48.288**   Encounter for aftercare following multiple organ transplant

   ● **Z48.29**   Encounter for aftercare following other organ transplant

     ● **Z48.290**   Encounter for aftercare following bone marrow transplant 🔲
> CC when PDx is its own CC
> (Ex:) D47.Z1, D89.810-D89.813, T86.00-T86.09, T86.850-T86.859, T86.90-T86.99, Z94.9

     ● **Z48.298**   Encounter for aftercare following other organ transplant

CHAPTER 21 (Z00-Z99)

N   Newborn Age: 0   P   Pediatric Age: 0–17   M   Maternity DX: 12–55   A   Adult Age: 15–124   ♀   Females Only   ♂   Males Only

🔲 Complication\Comorbidity   🔲 Major C\C   (Ex:) CC/MCC Exclusions   🔲 Present on Admission Requirement   🔲 Hospital-Acquired Condition

1685

Z48.3   Aftercare following surgery for neoplasm
Use additional code to identify the neoplasm

● **Z48.8   Encounter for other specified postprocedural aftercare**

    ● **Z48.81   Encounter for surgical aftercare following surgery on specified body systems**
These codes identify the body system requiring aftercare. They are for use in conjunction with other aftercare codes to fully explain the aftercare encounter. The condition treated should also be coded if still present.

       Excludes1   aftercare for injury - code the injury with 7th character D
aftercare following surgery for neoplasm (Z48.3)

       Excludes2   aftercare following organ transplant (Z48.2-)
orthopedic aftercare (Z47.-)

      Z48.810   Encounter for surgical aftercare following surgery on the sense organs

      Z48.811   Encounter for surgical aftercare following surgery on the nervous system

         Excludes2   encounter for surgical aftercare following surgery on the sense organs (Z48.810)

      Z48.812   Encounter for surgical aftercare following surgery on the circulatory system
Coding Clinic: 2012, Q4, P96

      Z48.813   Encounter for surgical aftercare following surgery on the respiratory system

      Z48.814   Encounter for surgical aftercare following surgery on the teeth or oral cavity

      Z48.815   Encounter for surgical aftercare following surgery on the digestive system

      Z48.816   Encounter for surgical aftercare following surgery on the genitourinary system

         Excludes1   encounter for aftercare following sterilization reversal (Z31.42)

      Z48.817   Encounter for surgical aftercare following surgery on the skin and subcutaneous tissue

    Z48.89   Encounter for other specified surgical aftercare

● **Z49   Encounter for care involving renal dialysis**
Code also associated end stage renal disease (N18.6)

   ● **Z49.0   Preparatory care for renal dialysis**
Encounter for dialysis instruction and training

     Z49.01   Encounter for fitting and adjustment of extracorporeal dialysis catheter 🔍
Removal or replacement of renal dialysis catheter
Toilet or cleansing of renal dialysis catheter

    ● **Z49.02   Encounter for fitting and adjustment of peritoneal dialysis catheter** 🔍

   ● **Z49.3   Encounter for adequacy testing for dialysis**

    ● **Z49.31   Encounter for adequacy testing for hemodialysis** 🔍

    ● **Z49.32   Encounter for adequacy testing for peritoneal dialysis** 🔍
Encounter for peritoneal equilibration test

● **Z51   Encounter for other aftercare**
Code also condition requiring care

      Excludes1   follow-up examination after treatment (Z08-Z09)

   Z51.0   Encounter for antineoplastic radiation therapy 🔍

   ● **Z51.1   Encounter for antineoplastic chemotherapy and immunotherapy**

      Excludes2   encounter for chemotherapy and immunotherapy for nonneoplastic condition-code to condition

     Z51.11   Encounter for antineoplastic chemotherapy 🔍

     Z51.12   Encounter for antineoplastic immunotherapy 🔍

   ● **Z51.5   Encounter for palliative care** 🔍

   ● **Z51.8   Encounter for other specified aftercare**

      Excludes1   holiday relief care (Z75.5)

     Z51.81   Encounter for therapeutic drug level monitoring 🔍
Code also any long-term (current) drug therapy (Z79.-)

         Excludes1   encounter for blood-drug test for administrative or medicolegal reasons (Z02.83)

    ● **Z51.89   Encounter for other specified aftercare** 🔍
Coding Clinic: 2012, Q4, P96-97

● **Z52   Donors of organs and tissues**

    Includes   autologous and other living donors

    Excludes1   cadaveric donor - omit code
examination of potential donor (Z00.5)
Coding Clinic: 2012, Q4, P100

   ● **Z52.0   Blood donor**

    ● **Z52.00   Unspecified blood donor**

     ● **Z52.000   Unspecified donor, whole blood** 🔍

     ● **Z52.001   Unspecified donor, stem cells** 🔍

     ● **Z52.008   Unspecified donor, other blood** 🔍

    ● **Z52.01   Autologous blood donor**

     ● **Z52.010   Autologous donor, whole blood** 🔍

     ● **Z52.011   Autologous donor, stem cells** 🔍

     ● **Z52.018   Autologous donor, other blood** 🔍

    ● **Z52.09   Other blood donor**
Volunteer donor

     ● **Z52.090   Other blood donor, whole blood** 🔍

     ● **Z52.091   Other blood donor, stem cells** 🔍

     ● **Z52.098   Other blood donor, other blood** 🔍

   ● **Z52.1   Skin donor**

     Z52.10   Skin donor, unspecified 🔍

     Z52.11   Skin donor, autologous 🔍

     Z52.19   Skin donor, other 🔍

   ● **Z52.2   Bone donor**

     Z52.20   Bone donor, unspecified 🔍

     Z52.21   Bone donor, autologous 🔍

     Z52.29   Bone donor, other 🔍

   Z52.3   Bone marrow donor 🔍

   Z52.4   Kidney donor 🔍

   Z52.5   Cornea donor 🔍

   Z52.6   Liver donor 🔍
Coding Clinic: 2012, Q4, P100

● **Z52.8**   Donor of other specified organs or tissues
   ● **Z52.81**   Egg (Oocyte) donor
     ● **Z52.810**   Egg (Oocyte) donor under age 35, anonymous recipient ♀ 🩺
       Egg donor under age 35 NOS
     ● **Z52.811**   Egg (Oocyte) donor under age 35, designated recipient ♀ 🩺
     ● **Z52.812**   Egg (Oocyte) donor age 35 and over, anonymous recipient ♀ 🩺
       Egg donor age 35 and over NOS
     ● **Z52.813**   Egg (Oocyte) donor age 35 and over, designated recipient ♀ 🩺
     ● **Z52.819**   Egg (Oocyte) donor, unspecified ♀ 🩺
   Z52.89   Donor of other specified organs or tissues 🩺
  Z52.9   Donor of unspecified organ or tissue 🩺
     Donor NOS

● **Z53**   Persons encountering health services for specific procedures and treatment, not carried out
  ● **Z53.0**   Procedure and treatment not carried out because of contraindication
   ● **Z53.01**   Procedure and treatment not carried out due to patient smoking
   ● **Z53.09**   Procedure and treatment not carried out because of other contraindication
  ● **Z53.1**   Procedure and treatment not carried out because of patient's decision for reasons of belief and group pressure
  ● **Z53.2**   Procedure and treatment not carried out because of patient's decision for other and unspecified reasons
   ● **Z53.20**   Procedure and treatment not carried out because of patient's decision for unspecified reasons
   ● **Z53.21**   Procedure and treatment not carried out due to patient leaving prior to being seen by health care provider
   ● **Z53.29**   Procedure and treatment not carried out because of patient's decision for other reasons
  ● **Z53.8**   Procedure and treatment not carried out for other reasons
  ● **Z53.9**   Procedure and treatment not carried out, unspecified reason

---

PERSONS WITH POTENTIAL HEALTH HAZARDS RELATED TO SOCIOECONOMIC AND PSYCHOSOCIAL CIRCUMSTANCES (Z55-Z65)

● **Z55**   Problems related to education and literacy
   Excludes1   disorders of psychological development (F80-F89)
  ● **Z55.0**   Illiteracy and low-level literacy
  ● **Z55.1**   Schooling unavailable and unattainable
  ● **Z55.2**   Failed school examinations
  ● **Z55.3**   Underachievement in school
  ● **Z55.4**   Educational maladjustment and discord with teachers and classmates
  ● **Z55.8**   Other problems related to education and literacy
     Problems related to inadequate teaching
  ● **Z55.9**   Problems related to education and literacy, unspecified
     Academic problems NOS

● **Z56**   Problems related to employment and unemployment
   Excludes2   occupational exposure to risk factors (Z57.-)
     problems related to housing and economic circumstances (Z59.-)
  ● **Z56.0**   Unemployment, unspecified
  ● **Z56.1**   Change of job
  ● **Z56.2**   Threat of job loss
  ● **Z56.3**   Stressful work schedule

● **Z56.4**   Discord with boss and workmates
● **Z56.5**   Uncongenial work environment
     Difficult conditions at work
● **Z56.6**   Other physical and mental strain related to work
● **Z56.8**   Other problems related to employment
   ● **Z56.81**   Sexual harassment on the job
   ● **Z56.82**   Military deployment status
     Individual (civilian or military) currently deployed in theater or in support of military war, peacekeeping and humanitarian operations
   ● **Z56.89**   Other problems related to employment
● **Z56.9**   Unspecified problems related to employment
     Occupational problems NOS

● **Z57**   Occupational exposure to risk factors
  ● **Z57.0**   Occupational exposure to noise
  ● **Z57.1**   Occupational exposure to radiation
  ● **Z57.2**   Occupational exposure to dust
  ● **Z57.3**   Occupational exposure to other air contaminants
   ● **Z57.31**   Occupational exposure to environmental tobacco smoke
     Excludes2   exposure to environmental tobacco smoke (Z77.22)
   ● **Z57.39**   Occupational exposure to other air contaminants
  ● **Z57.4**   Occupational exposure to toxic agents in agriculture
     Occupational exposure to solids, liquids, gases or vapors in agriculture
  ● **Z57.5**   Occupational exposure to toxic agents in other industries
     Occupational exposure to solids, liquids, gases or vapors in other industries
  ● **Z57.6**   Occupational exposure to extreme temperature
  ● **Z57.7**   Occupational exposure to vibration
  ● **Z57.8**   Occupational exposure to other risk factors
  ● **Z57.9**   Occupational exposure to unspecified risk factor

● **Z59**   Problems related to housing and economic circumstances
   Excludes2   problems related to upbringing (Z62.-)
  ● **Z59.0**   Homelessness 🩺
  ● **Z59.1**   Inadequate housing 🩺
     Lack of heating
     Restriction of space
     Technical defects in home preventing adequate care
     Unsatisfactory surroundings
     Excludes1   problems related to the natural and physical environment (Z77.1-)
  ● **Z59.2**   Discord with neighbors, lodgers and landlord 🩺
  ● **Z59.3**   Problems related to living in residential institution 🩺
     Boarding-school resident
     Excludes1   institutional upbringing (Z62.2)
  ● **Z59.4**   Lack of adequate food and safe drinking water 🩺
     Inadequate drinking water supply
     Excludes1   effects of hunger (T73.0)
       inappropriate diet or eating habits (Z72.4)
       malnutrition (E40-E46)
  ● **Z59.5**   Extreme poverty 🩺
  ● **Z59.6**   Low income 🩺
  ● **Z59.7**   Insufficient social insurance and welfare support 🩺
  ● **Z59.8**   Other problems related to housing and economic circumstances 🩺
     Foreclosure on loan
     Isolated dwelling
     Problems with creditors
  ● **Z59.9**   Problem related to housing and economic circumstances, unspecified 🩺

A

N Newborn Age: 0   **P** Pediatric Age: 0–17   **M** Maternity DX: 12–55   **A** Adult Age: 15–124   ♀ Females Only   ♂ Males Only

🩺 Complication\Comorbidity   🩺 Major C\C   (Ex) CC/MCC Exclusions   🩺 Present on Admission Requirement   🩺 Hospital-Acquired Condition   **1687**

CHAPTER 21 (Z00-Z99)

● **Z60   Problems related to social environment**
  ● **Z60.0   Problems of adjustment to life-cycle transitions**
    Empty nest syndrome
    Phase of life problem
    Problem with adjustment to retirement [pension]
  ● **Z60.2   Problems related to living alone**
  ● **Z60.3   Acculturation difficulty**
    Problem with migration
    Problem with social transplantation
  ● **Z60.4   Social exclusion and rejection**
    Exclusion and rejection on the basis of personal characteristics, such as unusual physical appearance, illness or behavior.
    Excludes1   target of adverse discrimination such as for racial or religious reasons (Z60.5)
  ● **Z60.5   Target of (perceived) adverse discrimination and persecution**
    Excludes1   social exclusion and rejection (Z60.4)
  ● **Z60.8   Other problems related to social environment**
  ● **Z60.9   Problem related to social environment, unspecified**

● **Z62   Problems related to upbringing**
  Includes   current and past negative life events in childhood
    current and past problems of a child related to upbringing
  Excludes2   maltreatment syndrome (T74.-)
    problems related to housing and economic circumstances (Z59.-)
  ● **Z62.0   Inadequate parental supervision and control**
  ● **Z62.1   Parental overprotection**
  ● **Z62.2   Upbringing away from parents**
    Excludes1   problems with boarding school (Z59.3)
    ● **Z62.21   Child in welfare custody**   P
      Child in care of non-parental family member
      Child in foster care
      Excludes2   problem for parent due to child in welfare custody (Z63.5)
    ● **Z62.22   Institutional upbringing**
      Child living in orphanage or group home
    ● **Z62.29   Other upbringing away from parents**
  ● **Z62.3   Hostility towards and scapegoating of child**   P
  ● **Z62.6   Inappropriate (excessive) parental pressure**
  ● **Z62.8   Other specified problems related to upbringing**
    ● **Z62.81   Personal history of abuse in childhood**
      ● **Z62.810   Personal history of physical and sexual abuse in childhood**
        Excludes1   current child physical abuse (T74.12, T76.12)
          current child sexual abuse (T74.22, T76.22)
      ● **Z62.811   Personal history of psychological abuse in childhood**
        Excludes1   current child psychological abuse (T74.32, T76.32)
      ● **Z62.812   Personal history of neglect in childhood**
        Excludes1   current child neglect (T74.02, T76.02)
      ● **Z62.819   Personal history of unspecified abuse in childhood**
        Excludes1   current child abuse NOS (T74.92, T76.92)

    ● **Z62.82   Parent-child conflict**
      ● **Z62.820   Parent-biological child conflict**
        Parent-child problem NOS
      ● **Z62.821   Parent-adopted child conflict**
      ● **Z62.822   Parent-foster child conflict**
    ● **Z62.89   Other specified problems related to upbringing**
      ● **Z62.890   Parent-child estrangement NEC**
      ● **Z62.891   Sibling rivalry**
      ● **Z62.898   Other specified problems related to upbringing**
  ● **Z62.9   Problem related to upbringing, unspecified**

● **Z63   Other problems related to primary support group, including family circumstances**
  Excludes2   maltreatment syndrome (T74.-, T76)
    parent-child problems (Z62.-)
    problems related to negative life events in childhood (Z62.-)
    problems related to upbringing (Z62.-)
  ● **Z63.0   Problems in relationship with spouse or partner** 🔍
    Excludes1   counseling for spousal or partner abuse problems (Z69.1)
      counseling related to sexual attitude, behavior, and orientation (Z70.-)
  ● **Z63.1   Problems in relationship with in-laws** 🔍
  ● **Z63.3   Absence of family member**
    Excludes1   absence of family member due to disappearance and death (Z63.4)
      absence of family member due to separation and divorce (Z63.5)
    ● **Z63.31   Absence of family member due to military deployment** 🔍
      Individual or family affected by other family member being on military deployment
      Excludes1   family disruption due to return of family member from military deployment (Z63.71)
    ● **Z63.32   Other absence of family member** 🔍
  ● **Z63.4   Disappearance and death of family member** 🔍
    Assumed death of family member
    Bereavement
  ● **Z63.5   Disruption of family by separation and divorce** 🔍
    Marital estrangement
  ● **Z63.6   Dependent relative needing care at home** 🔍
  ● **Z63.7   Other stressful life events affecting family and household**
    ● **Z63.71   Stress on family due to return of family member from military deployment** 🔍
      Individual or family affected by family member having returned from military deployment (current or past conflict)
    ● **Z63.72   Alcoholism and drug addiction in family** 🔍
    ● **Z63.79   Other stressful life events affecting family and household** 🔍
      Anxiety (normal) about sick person in family
      Health problems within family
      Ill or disturbed family member
      Isolated family
  ● **Z63.8   Other specified problems related to primary support group** 🔍
    Family discord NOS
    Family estrangement NOS
    High expressed emotional level within family
    Inadequate family support NOS
    Inadequate or distorted communication within family
  ● **Z63.9   Problem related to primary support group, unspecified** 🔍
    Relationship disorder NOS

◀ New   ◀ Revised   ~~deleted~~ Deleted   Excludes 1   Excludes 2   Includes   Use additional   Code first   Code also   Unspecified
OGCR Official Guidelines   ● Unacceptable Principal Diagnosis   X Assign placeholder X   ▶ Use Additional Character(s)   ▶ Manifestation Code   **Coding Clinic**

● **Z64   Problems related to certain psychosocial circumstances**
   ● **Z64.0   Problems related to unwanted pregnancy** ♀   M
   ● **Z64.1   Problems related to multiparity** ♀
   ● **Z64.4   Discord with counselors**
       Discord with probation officer
       Discord with social worker

● **Z65   Problems related to other psychosocial circumstances**
   ● **Z65.0   Conviction in civil and criminal proceedings without imprisonment** 🖐
   ● **Z65.1   Imprisonment and other incarceration** 🖐
   ● **Z65.2   Problems related to release from prison** 🖐
   ● **Z65.3   Problems related to other legal circumstances** 🖐
       Arrest
       Child custody or support proceedings
       Litigation
       Prosecution
   ● **Z65.4   Victim of crime and terrorism** 🖐
       Victim of torture
   ● **Z65.5   Exposure to disaster, war and other hostilities** 🖐   A
      Excludes1   target of perceived discrimination or persecution (Z60.5)
   ● **Z65.8   Other specified problems related to psychosocial circumstances** 🖐
   ● **Z65.9   Problem related to unspecified psychosocial circumstances** 🖐

DO NOT RESUSCITATE STATUS (Z66)

● **Z66   Do not resuscitate**
     DNR status

BLOOD TYPE (Z67)

● **Z67   Blood type**
   ● **Z67.1   Type A blood**
     ● **Z67.10   Type A blood, Rh positive** 🖐
     ● **Z67.11   Type A blood, Rh negative** 🖐
   ● **Z67.2   Type B blood**
     ● **Z67.20   Type B blood, Rh positive** 🖐
     ● **Z67.21   Type B blood, Rh negative** 🖐
   ● **Z67.3   Type AB blood**
     ● **Z67.30   Type AB blood, Rh positive** 🖐
     ● **Z67.31   Type AB blood, Rh negative** 🖐
   ● **Z67.4   Type O blood**
     ● **Z67.40   Type O blood, Rh positive** 🖐
     ● **Z67.41   Type O blood, Rh negative** 🖐
   ● **Z67.9   Unspecified blood type**
     ● **Z67.90   Unspecified blood type, Rh positive** 🖐
     ● **Z67.91   Unspecified blood type, Rh negative** 🖐

BODY MASS INDEX [BMI] (Z68)

● **Z68   Body mass index [BMI]**
     Kilograms per meters squared
     Note: BMI adult codes are for use for persons 21 years of age or older.
       BMI pediatric codes are for use for persons 2-20 years of age. These percentiles are based on the growth charts published by the Centers for Disease Control and Prevention (CDC)
   ● **Z68.1   Body mass index (BMI) 19 or less, adult** 🖐 🖐   A
      (Ex) E66.01-E66.1, E66.8-E66.9, Z68.1-Z68.54
   ● **Z68.2   Body mass index (BMI) 20-29, adult**
     ● **Z68.20   Body mass index (BMI) 20.0-20.9, adult** 🖐   A
     ● **Z68.21   Body mass index (BMI) 21.0-21.9, adult** 🖐   A
     ● **Z68.22   Body mass index (BMI) 22.0-22.9, adult** 🖐   A
     ● **Z68.23   Body mass index (BMI) 23.0-23.9, adult** 🖐   A

     ● **Z68.24   Body mass index (BMI) 24.0-24.9, adult** 🖐   A
     ● **Z68.25   Body mass index (BMI) 25.0-25.9, adult** 🖐   A
     ● **Z68.26   Body mass index (BMI) 26.0-26.9, adult** 🖐   A
     ● **Z68.27   Body mass index (BMI) 27.0-27.9, adult** 🖐   A
     ● **Z68.28   Body mass index (BMI) 28.0-28.9, adult** 🖐   A
     ● **Z68.29   Body mass index (BMI) 29.0-29.9, adult** 🖐   A
   ● **Z68.3   Body mass index (BMI) 30-39, adult**
     ● **Z68.30   Body mass index (BMI) 30.0-30.9, adult** 🖐   A
     ● **Z68.31   Body mass index (BMI) 31.0-31.9, adult** 🖐   A
     ● **Z68.32   Body mass index (BMI) 32.0-32.9, adult** 🖐   A
     ● **Z68.33   Body mass index (BMI) 33.0-33.9, adult** 🖐   A
     ● **Z68.34   Body mass index (BMI) 34.0-34.9, adult** 🖐   A
     ● **Z68.35   Body mass index (BMI) 35.0-35.9, adult** 🖐   A
     ● **Z68.36   Body mass index (BMI) 36.0-36.9, adult** 🖐   A
     ● **Z68.37   Body mass index (BMI) 37.0-37.9, adult** 🖐   A
     ● **Z68.38   Body mass index (BMI) 38.0-38.9, adult** 🖐   A
     ● **Z68.39   Body mass index (BMI) 39.0-39.9, adult** 🖐   A
   ● **Z68.4   Body mass index (BMI) 40 or greater, adult**
     (Ex) For category **Z68.4** CC codes: E65-E66.1, E66.8-E66.9, Z68.1-Z68.54
     ● **Z68.41   Body mass index (BMI) 40.0-44.9, adult** 🖐 🖐   A
     ● **Z68.42   Body mass index (BMI) 45.0-49.9, adult** 🖐 🖐   A
     ● **Z68.43   Body mass index (BMI) 50-59.9, adult** 🖐 🖐   A
     ● **Z68.44   Body mass index (BMI) 60.0-69.9, adult** 🖐 🖐   A
     ● **Z68.45   Body mass index (BMI) 70 or greater, adult** 🖐 🖐   A
   ● **Z68.5   Body mass index (BMI) pediatric**
     ● **Z68.51   Body mass index (BMI) pediatric, less than 5th percentile for age** 🖐   P
     ● **Z68.52   Body mass index (BMI) pediatric, 5th percentile to less than 85th percentile for age** 🖐   P
     ● **Z68.53   Body mass index (BMI) pediatric, 85th percentile to less than 95th percentile for age** 🖐   P
     ● **Z68.54   Body mass index (BMI) pediatric, greater than or equal to 95th percentile for age** 🖐   P

PERSONS ENCOUNTERING HEALTH SERVICES IN OTHER CIRCUMSTANCES (Z69-Z76)

● **Z69   Encounter for mental health services for victim and perpetrator of abuse**
     Includes   counseling for victims and perpetrators of abuse
   ● **Z69.0   Encounter for mental health services for child abuse problems**
     ● **Z69.01   Encounter for mental health services for parental child abuse**
       Z69.010   Encounter for mental health services for victim of parental child abuse   P
       ● **Z69.011   Encounter for mental health services for perpetrator of parental child abuse**
         Excludes1   encounter for mental health services for non-parental child abuse (Z69.02-)
     ● **Z69.02   Encounter for mental health services for non-parental child abuse**
       Z69.020   Encounter for mental health services for victim of non-parental child abuse   P
       ● **Z69.021   Encounter for mental health services for perpetrator of non- parental child abuse**
   ● **Z69.1   Encounter for mental health services for spousal or partner abuse problems**
     ● **Z69.11   Encounter for mental health services for victim of spousal or partner abuse**
     ● **Z69.12   Encounter for mental health services for perpetrator of spousal or partner abuse**

N Newborn Age: 0   **P** Pediatric Age: 0–17   **M** Maternity DX: 12–55   **A** Adult Age: 15–124   ♀ Females Only   ♂ Males Only

🖐 Complication\Comorbidity   🖐 Major C\C   (Ex) CC/MCC Exclusions   Present on Admission Requirement   Hospital-Acquired Condition   1689

CHAPTER 21 (Z00-Z99)

- **Z69.8** **Encounter for mental health services for victim or perpetrator of other abuse**
  - **Z69.81** **Encounter for mental health services for victim of other abuse**
    Encounter for rape victim counseling
  - **Z69.82** **Encounter for mental health services for perpetrator of other abuse**
- **Z70** **Counseling related to sexual attitude, behavior and orientation**
  - **Includes** encounter for mental health services for sexual attitude, behavior and orientation
  - **Excludes2** contraceptive or procreative counseling (Z30-Z31)
  - **Z70.0** **Counseling related to sexual attitude**
  - **Z70.1** **Counseling related to patient's sexual behavior and orientation**
    Patient concerned regarding impotence
    Patient concerned regarding non-responsiveness
    Patient concerned regarding promiscuity
    Patient concerned regarding sexual orientation
  - **Z70.2** **Counseling related to sexual behavior and orientation of third party**
    Advice sought regarding sexual behavior and orientation of child
    Advice sought regarding sexual behavior and orientation of partner
    Advice sought regarding sexual behavior and orientation of spouse
  - **Z70.3** **Counseling related to combined concerns regarding sexual attitude, behavior and orientation**
  - **Z70.8** **Other sex counseling**
    Encounter for sex education
  - **Z70.9** **Sex counseling, unspecified**
- **Z71** **Persons encountering health services for other counseling and medical advice, not elsewhere classified**
  - **Excludes2** contraceptive or procreation counseling (Z30-Z31)
    sex counseling (Z70.-)
  - **Z71.0** **Person encountering health services to consult on behalf of another person**
    Person encountering health services to seek advice or treatment for non-attending third party
    - **Excludes2** anxiety (normal) about sick person in family (Z63.7)
      expectant (adoptive) parent(s) pre-birth pediatrician visit (Z76.81)
  - **Z71.1** **Person with feared health complaint in whom no diagnosis is made**
    Person encountering health services with feared condition which was not demonstrated
    Person encountering health services in which problem was normal state
    'Worried well'
    - **Excludes1** medical observation for suspected diseases and conditions proven not to exist (Z03.-)
  - **Z71.2** **Person consulting for explanation of examination or test findings**
  - **Z71.3** **Dietary counseling and surveillance**
    Use additional code for any associated underlying medical condition
    Use additional code to identify body mass index (BMI), if known (Z68.-)
  - **Z71.4** **Alcohol abuse counseling and surveillance**
    Use additional code for alcohol abuse or dependence (F10.-)
    - **Z71.41** **Alcohol abuse counseling and surveillance of alcoholic**
    - **Z71.42** **Counseling for family member of alcoholic**
      Counseling for significant other, partner, or friend of alcoholic

- **Z71.5** **Drug abuse counseling and surveillance**
  Use additional code for drug abuse or dependence (F11-F16, F18-F19)
  - **Z71.51** **Drug abuse counseling and surveillance of drug abuser**
  - **Z71.52** **Counseling for family member of drug abuser**
    Counseling for significant other, partner, or friend of drug abuser
- **Z71.6** **Tobacco abuse counseling**
  Use additional code for nicotine dependence (F17.-)
- **Z71.7** **Human immunodeficiency virus [HIV] counseling**
- **Z71.8** **Other specified counseling**
  - **Excludes2** counseling for contraception (Z30.0-)
    counseling for genetics (Z31.5)
    counseling for procreative management (Z31.6-)
  - **Z71.81** **Spiritual or religious counseling**
  - **Z71.89** **Other specified counseling**
- **Z71.9** **Counseling, unspecified**
  Encounter for medical advice NOS
- **Z72** **Problems related to lifestyle**
  - **Excludes2** problems related to life-management difficulty (Z73.-)
    problems related to socioeconomic and psychosocial circumstances (Z55-Z65)
  - **Z72.0** **Tobacco use** 🖐
    Tobacco use NOS
    - **Excludes1** history of tobacco dependence (Z87.891)
      nicotine dependence (F17.2-)
      tobacco dependence (F17.2-)
      tobacco use during pregnancy (O99.33-)
  - **Z72.3** **Lack of physical exercise** 🖐
  - **Z72.4** **Inappropriate diet and eating habits** 🖐
    - **Excludes1** behavioral eating disorders of infancy or childhood (F98.2.-F98.3) ◀
      eating disorders (F50.-)
      lack of adequate food (Z59.4)
      malnutrition and other nutritional deficiencies (E40-E64)
  - **Z72.5** **High risk sexual behavior**
    Promiscuity
    - **Excludes1** paraphilias (F65)
    - **Z72.51** **High risk heterosexual behavior** 🖐
    - **Z72.52** **High risk homosexual behavior** 🖐
    - **Z72.53** **High risk bisexual behavior** 🖐
  - **Z72.6** **Gambling and betting** 🖐
    - **Excludes1** compulsive or pathological gambling (F63.0)
  - **Z72.8** **Other problems related to lifestyle**
    - **Z72.81** **Antisocial behavior**
      - **Excludes1** conduct disorders (F91.-)
      - **Z72.810** **Child and adolescent antisocial behavior** 🖐   P
        Antisocial behavior (child) (adolescent) without manifest psychiatric disorder
        Delinquency NOS
        Group delinquency
        Offenses in the context of gang membership
        Stealing in company with others
        Truancy from school
      - **Z72.811** **Adult antisocial behavior** 🖐   A
        Adult antisocial behavior without manifest psychiatric disorder

◀ New   ◀▪▪ Revised   ~~deleted~~ Deleted   Excludes 1   Excludes 2   Includes   Use additional   Code first   Code also   Unspecified
OGCR Official Guidelines   ● Unacceptable Principal Diagnosis   X Assign placeholder X   🖐 Use Additional Character(s)   ▸ Manifestation Code   **Coding Clinic**

● **Z72.82** **Problems related to sleep**

    Z72.820 **Sleep deprivation** 🔖

        Lack of adequate sleep

        Excludes1 insomnia (G47.0-)

    ● **Z72.821** **Inadequate sleep hygiene** 🔖

        Bad sleep habits

        Irregular sleep habits

        Unhealthy sleep wake schedule

        Excludes1 insomnia (F51.0-, G47.0-)

  ● **Z72.89** **Other problems related to lifestyle** 🔖

    Self-damaging behavior

● **Z72.9** **Problem related to lifestyle, unspecified** 🔖

● **Z73** **Problems related to life management difficulty**

  Excludes2 problems related to socioeconomic and psychosocial circumstances (Z55-Z65)

  ● **Z73.0** **Burn-out**

  ● **Z73.1** **Type A behavior pattern**

  ● **Z73.2** **Lack of relaxation and leisure**

  ● **Z73.3** **Stress, not elsewhere classified**

    Physical and mental strain NOS

    Excludes1 stress related to employment or unemployment (Z56.-)

  ● **Z73.4** **Inadequate social skills, not elsewhere classified**

  ● **Z73.5** **Social role conflict, not elsewhere classified**

  ● **Z73.6** **Limitation of activities due to disability**

    Excludes1 care-provider dependency (Z74.-)

  ● **Z73.8** **Other problems related to life management difficulty**

    ● **Z73.81** **Behavioral insomnia of childhood**

      ● **Z73.810** **Behavioral insomnia of childhood, sleep-onset association type**   P

      ● **Z73.811** **Behavioral insomnia of childhood, limit setting type**   P

      ● **Z73.812** **Behavioral insomnia of childhood, combined type**   P

      ● **Z73.819** **Behavioral insomnia of childhood, unspecified type**   P

    ● **Z73.82** **Dual sensory impairment**

    ● **Z73.89** **Other problems related to life management difficulty**

  ● **Z73.9** **Problem related to life management difficulty, unspecified** 🔖

● **Z74** **Problems related to care provider dependency**

  Excludes2 dependence on enabling machines or devices NEC (Z99.-)

  ● **Z74.0** **Reduced mobility**

    ● **Z74.01** **Bed confinement status** 🔖

      Bedridden

    ● **Z74.09** **Other reduced mobility**

      Chairridden

      Reduced mobility NOS

      Excludes2 wheelchair dependence (Z99.3)

  ● **Z74.1** **Need for assistance with personal care**

  ● **Z74.2** **Need for assistance at home and no other household member able to render care**

  ● **Z74.3** **Need for continuous supervision**

  ● **Z74.8** **Other problems related to care provider dependency**

  ● **Z74.9** **Problem related to care provider dependency, unspecified**

● **Z75** **Problems related to medical facilities and other health care**

  ● **Z75.0** **Medical services not available in home**

    Excludes1 no other household member able to render care (Z74.2)

  ● **Z75.1** **Person awaiting admission to adequate facility elsewhere**

  ● **Z75.2** **Other waiting period for investigation and treatment**

  ● **Z75.3** **Unavailability and inaccessibility of health care facilities**

    Excludes1 bed unavailable (Z75.1)

  ● **Z75.4** **Unavailability and inaccessibility of other helping agencies**

  ● **Z75.5** **Holiday relief care**

  ● **Z75.8** **Other problems related to medical facilities and other health care**

  ● **Z75.9** **Unspecified problem related to medical facilities and other health care**

● **Z76** **Persons encountering health services in other circumstances**

  ● **Z76.0** **Encounter for issue of repeat prescription** 🔖

    Encounter for issue of repeat prescription for appliance

    Encounter for issue of repeat prescription for medicaments

    Encounter for issue of repeat prescription for spectacles

    Excludes2 issue of medical certificate (Z02.7)

      repeat prescription for contraceptive (Z30.4-)

  Z76.1 **Encounter for health supervision and care of foundling** 🔖

  ● **Z76.2** **Encounter for health supervision and care of other healthy infant and child** 🔖   P

    Encounter for medical or nursing care or supervision of healthy infant under circumstances such as adverse socioeconomic conditions at home

    Encounter for medical or nursing care or supervision of healthy infant under circumstances such as awaiting foster or adoptive placement

    Encounter for medical or nursing care or supervision of healthy infant under circumstances such as maternal illness

    Encounter for medical or nursing care or supervision of healthy infant under circumstances such as number of children at home preventing or interfering with normal care

  Z76.3 **Healthy person accompanying sick person** 🔖

  Z76.4 **Other boarder to healthcare facility** 🔖

    Excludes1 homelessness (Z59.0)

  Z76.5 **Malingerer [conscious simulation]** 🔖

    Person feigning illness (with obvious motivation)

    Excludes1 factitious disorder (F68.1-)

      peregrinating patient (F68.1-)

  ● **Z76.8** **Persons encountering health services in other specified circumstances**

    ● **Z76.81** **Expectant parent(s) prebirth pediatrician visit** 🔖

      Pre-adoption pediatrician visit for adoptive parent(s)

    ● **Z76.82** **Awaiting organ transplant status** 🔖

      Patient waiting for organ availability

    ● **Z76.89** **Persons encountering health services in other specified circumstances** 🔖

      Persons encountering health services NOS

N Newborn Age: 0   P Pediatric Age: 0–17   M Maternity DX: 12–55   A Adult Age: 15–124   ♀ Females Only   ♂ Males Only

Complication\Comorbidity   🔖 Major C\C   (Ex) CC/MCC Exclusions   🔖 Present on Admission Requirement   🔖 Hospital-Acquired Condition

1691

PERSONS WITH POTENTIAL HEALTH HAZARDS RELATED TO FAMILY AND PERSONAL HISTORY AND CERTAIN CONDITIONS INFLUENCING HEALTH STATUS (Z77-Z99)

Code also any follow-up examination (Z08-Z09)

● **Z77   Other contact with and (suspected) exposures hazardous to health**

Includes   contact with and (suspected) exposures to potential hazards to health

Excludes2   contact with and (suspected) exposure to communicable diseases (Z20.-)
exposure to (parental) (environmental) tobacco smoke in the perinatal period (P96.81)
newborn (suspected to be) affected by noxious substances transmitted via placenta or breast milk (P04.-)
occupational exposure to risk factors (Z57.-)
retained foreign body (Z18.-)
retained foreign body fully removed (Z87.821)
toxic effects of substances chiefly nonmedicinal as to source (T51-T65)

● **Z77.0   Contact with and (suspected) exposure to hazardous, chiefly nonmedicinal, chemicals**

● **Z77.01   Contact with and (suspected) exposure to hazardous metals**

● **Z77.010   Contact with and (suspected) exposure to arsenic**

● **Z77.011   Contact with and (suspected) exposure to lead**

● **Z77.012   Contact with and (suspected) exposure to uranium**

Excludes1   retained depleted uranium fragments (Z18.01)

● **Z77.018   Contact with and (suspected) exposure to other hazardous metals**
Contact with and (suspected) exposure to chromium compounds
Contact with and (suspected) exposure to nickel dust

● **Z77.02   Contact with and (suspected) exposure to hazardous aromatic compounds**

● **Z77.020   Contact with and (suspected) exposure to aromatic amines**

● **Z77.021   Contact with and (suspected) exposure to benzene**

● **Z77.028   Contact with and (suspected) exposure to other hazardous aromatic compounds**
Aromatic dyes NOS
Polycyclic aromatic hydrocarbons

● **Z77.09   Contact with and (suspected) exposure to other hazardous, chiefly nonmedicinal, chemicals**

● **Z77.090   Contact with and (suspected) exposure to asbestos**

● **Z77.098   Contact with and (suspected) exposure to other hazardous, chiefly nonmedicinal, chemicals**
Dyes NOS

● **Z77.1   Contact with and (suspected) exposure to environmental pollution and hazards in the physical environment**

● **Z77.11   Contact with and (suspected) exposure to environmental pollution**

● **Z77.110   Contact with and (suspected) exposure to air pollution**

● **Z77.111   Contact with and (suspected) exposure to water pollution**

● **Z77.112   Contact with and (suspected) exposure to soil pollution**

● **Z77.118   Contact with and (suspected) exposure to other environmental pollution**

● **Z77.12   Contact with and (suspected) exposure to hazards in the physical environment**

● **Z77.120   Contact with and (suspected) exposure to mold (toxic)**

● **Z77.121   Contact with and (suspected) exposure to harmful algae and algae toxins**
Contact with and (suspected) exposure to (harmful) algae bloom NOS
Contact with and (suspected) exposure to blue-green algae bloom
Contact with and (suspected) exposure to brown tide
Contact with and (suspected) exposure to cyanobacteria bloom
Contact with and (suspected) exposure to Florida red tide
Contact with and (suspected) exposure to pfiesteria piscicida
Contact with and (suspected) exposure to red tide

● **Z77.122   Contact with and (suspected) exposure to noise**

● **Z77.123   Contact with and (suspected) exposure to radon and other naturally occuring radiation**

Excludes2   radiation exposure as the cause of a confirmed condition (W88-W90, X39.0-)
radiation sickness NOS (T66)

● **Z77.128   Contact with and (suspected) exposure to other hazards in the physical environment**

● **Z77.2   Contact with and (suspected) exposure to other hazardous substances**

● **Z77.21   Contact with and (suspected) exposure to potentially hazardous body fluids**

● **Z77.22   Contact with and (suspected) exposure to environmental tobacco smoke (acute) (chronic)**
Exposure to second hand tobacco smoke (acute) (chronic)
Passive smoking (acute) (chronic)

Excludes1   nicotine dependence (F17.-)
tobacco use (Z72.0)

Excludes2   occupational exposure to environmental tobacco smoke (Z57.31)

● **Z77.29   Contact with and (suspected) exposure to other hazardous substances**

● **Z77.9   Other contact with and (suspected) exposures hazardous to health**

◀ New   ◀▥ Revised   ~~deleted~~ Deleted   Excludes 1   Excludes 2   Includes   Use additional   Code first   Code also   Unspecified
OGCR Official Guidelines   ● Unacceptable Principal Diagnosis   X Assign placeholder X   ● Use Additional Character(s)   ▶ Manifestation Code   **Coding Clinic**

● **Z78   Other specified health status**

    Excludes2   asymptomatic human immunodeficiency virus
        [HIV] infection status (Z21)
        postprocedural status (Z93-Z99) ◀▥
        sex reassignment status (Z87.890)

● **Z78.0   Asymptomatic menopausal state ♀ 🦠**   A
    Menopausal state NOS
    Postmenopausal status NOS

    Excludes2   symptomatic menopausal state (N95.1)

● **Z78.1   Physical restraint status 🦠**

    Excludes1   physical restraint due to a procedure -
        omit code

● **Z78.9   Other specified health status 🦠**

● **Z79   Long term (current) drug therapy**

    Includes   long term (current) drug use for prophylactic
        purposes

    Code also any therapeutic drug level monitoring (Z51.81)

    Excludes2   drug abuse and dependence (F11-F19)
        drug use complicating pregnancy, childbirth, and
        the puerperium (O99.32-)

● **Z79.0   Long term (current) use of anticoagulants and
    antithrombotics/antiplatelets**

    Excludes2   long term (current) use of aspirin (Z79.82)

    Z79.01   Long term (current) use of anticoagulants 🦠

●   **Z79.02   Long term (current) use of antithrombotics/
       antiplatelets 🦠**

● **Z79.1   Long term (current) use of non-steroidal
    anti-inflammatories (NSAID) 🦠**

    Excludes2   long term (current) use of aspirin (Z79.82)

● **Z79.2   Long term (current) use of antibiotics 🦠**

   Z79.3   Long term (current) use of hormonal contraceptives 🦠
    Long term (current) use of birth control pill or patch

   Z79.4   Long term (current) use of insulin 🦠

● **Z79.5   Long term (current) use of steroids**

●   **Z79.51   Long term (current) use of inhaled steroids 🦠**

●   **Z79.52   Long term (current) use of systemic steroids 🦠**

● **Z79.8   Other long term (current) drug therapy**

●   **Z79.81   Long term (current) use of agents affecting
       estrogen receptors and estrogen levels**

      Code first, *if applicable:*
      malignant neoplasm of breast (C50.-)
      malignant neoplasm of prostate (C61)

      Use additional code, if applicable, to identify:
      estrogen receptor positive status (Z17.0)
      family history of breast cancer (Z80.3)
      genetic susceptibility to malignant neoplasm
        (cancer) (Z15.0-)
      personal history of breast cancer (Z85.3)
      personal history of prostate cancer (Z85.46)
      postmenopausal status (Z78.0)

      Excludes1   hormone replacement therapy
        (postmenopausal) (Z79.890)

●   **Z79.810   Long term (current) use of selective
       estrogen receptor modulators
       (SERMs) 🦠**
        Long term (current) use of raloxifene
         (Evista)
        Long term (current) use of tamoxifen
         (Nolvadex)
        Long term (current) use of
         toremifene (Fareston)

●   **Z79.811   Long term (current) use of aromatase
       inhibitors 🦠**
        Long term (current) use of
         anastrozole (Arimidex)
        Long term (current) use of
         exemestane (Aromasin)
        Long term (current) use of letrozole
         (Femara)

●   **Z79.818   Long term (current) use of other
       agents affecting estrogen receptors
       and estrogen levels 🦠**
        Long term (current) use of estrogen
         receptor downregulators
        Long term (current) use of
         fulvestrant (Faslodex)
        Long term (current) use of
         gonadotropin-releasing
         hormone (GnRH) agonist
        Long term (current) use of goserelin
         acetate (Zoladex)
        Long term (current) use of
         leuprolide acetate (leuprorelin)
         (Lupron)
        Long term (current) use of megestrol
         acetate (Megace)

    Z79.82   Long term (current) use of aspirin 🦠

●   **Z79.83   Long term (current) use of bisphosphonates**

●   **Z79.89   Other long term (current) drug therapy**

●   **Z79.890   Hormone replacement therapy
       (postmenopausal) ♀ 🦠**

    **Z79.891   Long term (current) use of opiate
       analgesic 🦠**
        Long term (current) use of
         methadone for pain
         management

      Excludes1   methadone use NOS
        (F11.2-)
        use of methodone
        for treatment of
        heroin addiction
        (F11.2-)

    **Z79.899   Other long term (current) drug
       therapy 🦠**

● **Z80   Family history of primary malignant neoplasm**

● **Z80.0   Family history of malignant neoplasm of digestive
    organs 🦠**
    Conditions classifiable to C15-C26

● **Z80.1   Family history of malignant neoplasm of trachea,
    bronchus and lung 🦠**
    Conditions classifiable to C33-C34

● **Z80.2   Family history of malignant neoplasm of other
    respiratory and intrathoracic organs 🦠**
    Conditions classifiable to C30-C32, C37-C39

● **Z80.3   Family history of malignant neoplasm of breast 🦠**
    Conditions classifiable to C50.-

● **Z80.4   Family history of malignant neoplasm of genital organs**
    Conditions classifiable to C51-C63

●   **Z80.41   Family history of malignant neoplasm of
      ovary ♀ 🦠**

●   **Z80.42   Family history of malignant neoplasm of
      prostate ♂ 🦠**

●   **Z80.43   Family history of malignant neoplasm of
      testis ♂ 🦠**

●   **Z80.49   Family history of malignant neoplasm of other
      genital organs 🦠**

● **Z80.5   Family history of malignant neoplasm of urinary tract**
    Conditions classifiable to C64-C68

  **Z80.51   Family history of malignant neoplasm of
      kidney 🦠**

●   **Z80.52   Family history of malignant neoplasm of
      bladder 🦠**

●   **Z80.59   Family history of malignant neoplasm of other
      urinary tract organ 🦠**

● **Z80.6   Family history of leukemia 🦠**
    Conditions classifiable to C91-C95

N Newborn Age: 0   P Pediatric Age: 0–17   M Maternity DX: 12–55   A Adult Age: 15–124   ♀ Females Only   ♂ Males Only

🦠 Complication\Comorbidity   🦠 Major C\C   (Ex) CC/MCC Exclusions   🦠 Present on Admission Requirement   🦠 Hospital-Acquired Condition

CHAPTER 21 (Z00-Z99)

● **Z80.7** **Family history of other malignant neoplasms of lymphoid, hematopoietic and related tissues** 🖋
Conditions classifiable to C81-C90, C96.-

● **Z80.8** **Family history of malignant neoplasm of other organs or systems** 🖋
Conditions classifiable to C00-C14, C40-C49, C69-C79

● **Z80.9** **Family history of malignant neoplasm, unspecified** 🖋
Conditions classifiable to C80.1

● **Z81** **Family history of mental and behavioral disorders**

● **Z81.0** **Family history of intellectual disabilities** 🖋
Conditions classifiable to F70-F79

● **Z81.1** **Family history of alcohol abuse and dependence** 🖋
Conditions classifiable to F10.-

● **Z81.2** **Family history of tobacco abuse and dependence** 🖋
Conditions classifiable to F17.-

● **Z81.3** **Family history of other psychoactive substance abuse and dependence** 🖋
Conditions classifiable to F11-F16, F18-F19

● **Z81.4** **Family history of other substance abuse and dependence** 🖋
Conditions classifiable to F55

● **Z81.8** **Family history of other mental and behavioral disorders** 🖋
Conditions classifiable elsewhere in F01-F99

● **Z82** **Family history of certain disabilities and chronic diseases (leading to disablement)**

● **Z82.0** **Family history of epilepsy and other diseases of the nervous system** 🖋
Conditions classifiable to G00-G99

● **Z82.1** **Family history of blindness and visual loss** 🖋
Conditions classifiable to H54.-

● **Z82.2** **Family history of deafness and hearing loss** 🖋
Conditions classifiable to H90-H91

● **Z82.3** **Family history of stroke** 🖋
Conditions classifiable to I60-I64

● **Z82.4** **Family history of ischemic heart disease and other diseases of the circulatory system** 🖋
Conditions classifiable to I00-I52, I65-I99

● **Z82.41** **Family history of sudden cardiac death** 🖋

● **Z82.49** **Family history of ischemic heart disease and other diseases of the circulatory system** 🖋

● **Z82.5** **Family history of asthma and other chronic lower respiratory diseases** 🖋
Conditions classifiable to J40-J47

     Excludes2   family history of other diseases of the respiratory system (Z83.6)

● **Z82.6** **Family history of arthritis and other diseases of the musculoskeletal system and connective tissue**
Conditions classifiable to M00-M99

● **Z82.61** **Family history of arthritis** 🖋

● **Z82.62** **Family history of osteoporosis** 🖋

● **Z82.69** **Family history of other diseases of the musculoskeletal system and connective tissue** 🖋

● **Z82.7** **Family history of congenital malformations, deformations and chromosomal abnormalities**
Conditions classifiable to Q00-Q99

● **Z82.71** **Family history of polycystic kidney** 🖋

● **Z82.79** **Family history of other congenital malformations, deformations and chromosomal abnormalities** 🖋

● **Z82.8** **Family history of other disabilities and chronic diseases leading to disablement, not elsewhere classified** 🖋

● **Z83** **Family history of other specific disorders**

     Excludes2   contact with and (suspected) exposure to communicable disease in the family (Z20.-)

● **Z83.0** **Family history of human immunodeficiency virus [HIV] disease** 🖋
Conditions classifiable to B20

● **Z83.1** **Family history of other infectious and parasitic diseases** 🖋
Conditions classifiable to A00-B19, B25-B94, B99

● **Z83.2** **Family history of diseases of the blood and blood-forming organs and certain disorders involving the immune mechanism** 🖋
Conditions classifiable to D50-D89

● **Z83.3** **Family history of diabetes mellitus** 🖋
Conditions classifiable to E08-E13

● **Z83.4** **Family history of other endocrine, nutritional and metabolic diseases**
Conditions classifiable to E00-E07, E15-E88

● **Z83.41** **Family history of multiple endocrine neoplasia [MEN] syndrome** 🖋

● **Z83.49** **Family history of other endocrine, nutritional and metabolic diseases** 🖋

● **Z83.5** **Family history of eye and ear disorders**

● **Z83.51** **Family history of eye disorders**
Conditions classifiable to H00-H53, H55-H59

     Excludes2   family history of blindness and visual loss (Z82.1)

● **Z83.511** **Family history of glaucoma** 🖋

● **Z83.518** **Family history of other specified eye disorder** 🖋

● **Z83.52** **Family history of ear disorders** 🖋
Conditions classifiable to H60-H83, H92-H95

     Excludes2   family history of deafness and hearing loss (Z82.2)

● **Z83.6** **Family history of other diseases of the respiratory system**
Conditions classifiable to J00-J39, J60-J99

     Excludes2   family history of asthma and other chronic lower respiratory diseases (Z82.5)

● **Z83.7** **Family history of diseases of the digestive system**
Conditions classifiable to K00-K93

● **Z83.71** **Family history of colonic polyps** 🖋

     Excludes1   family history of malignant neoplasm of digestive organs (Z80.0)

● **Z83.79** **Family history of other diseases of the digestive system** 🖋

● **Z84** **Family history of other conditions**

● **Z84.0** **Family history of diseases of the skin and subcutaneous tissue** 🖋
Conditions classifiable to L00-L99

● **Z84.1** **Family history of disorders of kidney and ureter** 🖋
Conditions classifiable to N00-N29

● **Z84.2** **Family history of other diseases of the genitourinary system** 🖋
Conditions classifiable to N30-N99

● **Z84.3** **Family history of consanguinity** 🖋

● **Z84.8** **Family history of other specified conditions**

● **Z84.81** **Family history of carrier of genetic disease** 🖋

● **Z84.89** **Family history of other specified conditions** 🖋

◀ New   ◀▬ Revised   ~~deleted~~ Deleted   Excludes 1   Excludes 2   Includes   Use additional   Code first   Code also   Unspecified

OGCR Official Guidelines   ● Unacceptable Principal Diagnosis   X Assign placeholder X   🖋 Use Additional Character(s)   ▶ Manifestation Code   **Coding Clinic**

● **Z85**   **Personal history of malignant neoplasm**

     Code first any follow-up examination after treatment of malignant neoplasm (Z08)

     Use additional code to identify:
       alcohol use and dependence (F10.-)
       exposure to environmental tobacco smoke (Z77.22)
       history of tobacco use (Z87.891)
       occupational exposure to environmental tobacco smoke (Z57.31)
       tobacco dependence (F17.-)
       tobacco use (Z72.0)

     Excludes2   personal history of benign neoplasm (Z86.01-)
                  personal history of carcinoma-in-situ (Z86.00-)

● **Z85.0**   **Personal history of malignant neoplasm of digestive organs**

    ● **Z85.00**   Personal history of malignant neoplasm of unspecified digestive organ

    ● **Z85.01**   Personal history of malignant neoplasm of esophagus
           Conditions classifiable to C15

    ● **Z85.02**   Personal history of malignant neoplasm of stomach

       ● **Z85.020**   Personal history of malignant carcinoid tumor of stomach
              Conditions classifiable to C7A.092

       ● **Z85.028**   Personal history of other malignant neoplasm of stomach
              Conditions classifiable to C16

    ● **Z85.03**   Personal history of malignant neoplasm of large intestine

       ● **Z85.030**   Personal history of malignant carcinoid tumor of large intestine
              Conditions classifiable to C7A.022-C7A.025, C7A.029

       ● **Z85.038**   Personal history of other malignant neoplasm of large intestine
              Conditions classifiable to C18

    ● **Z85.04**   Personal history of malignant neoplasm of rectum, rectosigmoid junction, and anus

       ● **Z85.040**   Personal history of malignant carcinoid tumor of rectum
              Conditions classifiable to C7A.026

       ● **Z85.048**   Personal history of other malignant neoplasm of rectum, rectosigmoid junction, and anus
              Conditions classifiable to C19-C21

    ● **Z85.05**   Personal history of malignant neoplasm of liver
           Conditions classifiable to C22

    ● **Z85.06**   Personal history of malignant neoplasm of small intestine

       ● **Z85.060**   Personal history of malignant carcinoid tumor of small intestine
              Conditions classifiable to C7A.01-

       ● **Z85.068**   Personal history of other malignant neoplasm of small intestine
              Conditions classifiable to C17

    ● **Z85.07**   Personal history of malignant neoplasm of pancreas
           Conditions classifiable to C25

    ● **Z85.09**   Personal history of malignant neoplasm of other digestive organs

● **Z85.1**   **Personal history of malignant neoplasm of trachea, bronchus and lung**

    ● **Z85.11**   Personal history of malignant neoplasm of bronchus and lung

       ● **Z85.110**   Personal history of malignant carcinoid tumor of bronchus and lung
              Conditions classifiable to C7A.090

       ● **Z85.118**   Personal history of other malignant neoplasm of bronchus and lung
              Conditions classifiable to C34

    ● **Z85.12**   Personal history of malignant neoplasm of trachea
           Conditions classifiable to C33

● **Z85.2**   **Personal history of malignant neoplasm of other respiratory and intrathoracic organs**

    ● **Z85.20**   Personal history of malignant neoplasm of unspecified respiratory organ

    ● **Z85.21**   Personal history of malignant neoplasm of larynx
           Conditions classifiable to C32

    ● **Z85.22**   Personal history of malignant neoplasm of nasal cavities, middle ear, and accessory sinuses
           Conditions classifiable to C30-C31

    ● **Z85.23**   Personal history of malignant neoplasm of thymus

       ● **Z85.230**   Personal history of malignant carcinoid tumor of thymus
              Conditions classifiable to C7A.091

       ● **Z85.238**   Personal history of other malignant neoplasm of thymus
              Conditions classifiable to C37

    ● **Z85.29**   Personal history of malignant neoplasm of other respiratory and intrathoracic organs

● **Z85.3**   **Personal history of malignant neoplasm of breast**
       Conditions classifiable to C50.-

● **Z85.4**   **Personal history of malignant neoplasm of genital organs**
       Conditions classifiable to C51-C63

    ● **Z85.40**   Personal history of malignant neoplasm of unspecified female genital organ ♀

    ● **Z85.41**   Personal history of malignant neoplasm of cervix uteri ♀

    ● **Z85.42**   Personal history of malignant neoplasm of other parts of uterus ♀

    ● **Z85.43**   Personal history of malignant neoplasm of ovary ♀

    ● **Z85.44**   Personal history of malignant neoplasm of other female genital organs ♀

    ● **Z85.45**   Personal history of malignant neoplasm of unspecified male genital organ ♂

    ● **Z85.46**   Personal history of malignant neoplasm of prostate ♂

    ● **Z85.47**   Personal history of malignant neoplasm of testis ♂

    ● **Z85.48**   Personal history of malignant neoplasm of epididymis ♂

    ● **Z85.49**   Personal history of malignant neoplasm of other male genital organs ♂

CHAPTER 21 (Z00-Z99)

N Newborn Age: 0   P Pediatric Age: 0–17   M Maternity DX: 12–55   A Adult Age: 15–124   ♀ Females Only   ♂ Males Only

Complication\Comorbidity   Major C\C   (Ex) CC/MCC Exclusions   Present on Admission Requirement   Hospital-Acquired Condition   **1695**

● **Z85.5   Personal history of malignant neoplasm of urinary tract**
Conditions classifiable to C64-C68

● **Z85.50   Personal history of malignant neoplasm of unspecified urinary tract organ** 🖉

● **Z85.51   Personal history of malignant neoplasm of bladder** 🖉

● **Z85.52   Personal history of malignant neoplasm of kidney**

　　Excludes1   personal history of malignant neoplasm of renal pelvis (Z85.53)

● **Z85.520   Personal history of malignant carcinoid tumor of kidney** 🖉
　Conditions classifiable to C7A.093

● **Z85.528   Personal history of other malignant neoplasm of kidney** 🖉
　Conditions classifiable to C64

● **Z85.53   Personal history of malignant neoplasm of renal pelvis** 🖉

● **Z85.54   Personal history of malignant neoplasm of ureter** 🖉

● **Z85.59   Personal history of malignant neoplasm of other urinary tract organ** 🖉

● **Z85.6   Personal history of leukemia** 🖉
Conditions classifiable to C91-C95

　　Excludes1   leukemia in remission C91.0-C95.9 with 5th character 1

● **Z85.7   Personal history of other malignant neoplasms of lymphoid, hematopoietic and related tissues**

● **Z85.71   Personal history of Hodgkin lymphoma** 🖉
　Conditions classifiable to C81

● **Z85.72   Personal history of non-Hodgkin lymphomas** 🖉
　Conditions classifiable to C82-C85

● **Z85.79   Personal history of other malignant neoplasms of lymphoid, hematopoietic and related tissues** 🖉
　Conditions classifiable to C88-C90, C96

　　Excludes1   multiple myeloma in remission (C90.01)
　　　　plasma cell leukemia in remission (C90.11)
　　　　plasmacytoma in remission (C90.21)

● **Z85.8   Personal history of malignant neoplasms of other organs and systems**
Conditions classifiable to C00-C14, C40-C49, C69-C79, C7A.098

● **Z85.81   Personal history of malignant neoplasm of lip, oral cavity, and pharynx**

● **Z85.810   Personal history of malignant neoplasm of tongue** 🖉

● **Z85.818   Personal history of malignant neoplasm of other sites of lip, oral cavity, and pharynx** 🖉

● **Z85.819   Personal history of malignant neoplasm of unspecified site of lip, oral cavity, and pharynx** 🖉

● **Z85.82   Personal history of malignant neoplasm of skin**

● **Z85.820   Personal history of malignant melanoma of skin** 🖉
　Conditions classifiable to C43

● **Z85.821   Personal history of Merkel cell carcinoma** 🖉
　Conditions classifiable to C4A

● **Z85.828   Personal history of other malignant neoplasm of skin** 🖉
　Conditions classifiable to C44

● **Z85.83   Personal history of malignant neoplasm of bone and soft tissue**

● **Z85.830   Personal history of malignant neoplasm of bone** 🖉

● **Z85.831   Personal history of malignant neoplasm of soft tissue** 🖉

　　Excludes2   personal history of malignant neoplasm of skin (Z85.82-)

● **Z85.84   Personal history of malignant neoplasm of eye and nervous tissue**

● **Z85.840   Personal history of malignant neoplasm of eye** 🖉

● **Z85.841   Personal history of malignant neoplasm of brain** 🖉

● **Z85.848   Personal history of malignant neoplasm of other parts of nervous tissue** 🖉

● **Z85.85   Personal history of malignant neoplasm of endocrine glands**

● **Z85.850   Personal history of malignant neoplasm of thyroid** 🖉

● **Z85.858   Personal history of malignant neoplasm of other endocrine glands** 🖉

● **Z85.89   Personal history of malignant neoplasm of other organs and systems** 🖉

● **Z85.9   Personal history of malignant neoplasm, unspecified** 🖉
Conditions classifiable to C7A.00, C80.1

● **Z86   Personal history of certain other diseases**
Code first any follow-up examination after treatment (Z09)

● **Z86.0   Personal history of in-situ and benign neoplasms and neoplasms of uncertain behavior**

　　Excludes2   personal history of malignant neoplasms (Z85.-)

● **Z86.00   Personal history of in-situ neoplasm**

● **Z86.000   Personal history of in-situ neoplasm of breast** 🖉

● **Z86.001   Personal history of in-situ neoplasm of cervix uteri ♀** 🖉

● **Z86.008   Personal history of in-situ neoplasm of other site** 🖉

● **Z86.01   Personal history of benign neoplasm**

● **Z86.010   Personal history of colonic polyps** 🖉

● **Z86.011   Personal history of benign neoplasm of the brain** 🖉

● **Z86.012   Personal history of benign carcinoid tumor** 🖉

● **Z86.018   Personal history of other benign neoplasm** 🖉

● **Z86.03   Personal history of neoplasm of uncertain behavior** 🖉

● **Z86.1   Personal history of infectious and parasitic diseases**
Conditions classifiable to A00-B89, B99

　　Excludes1   personal history of infectious diseases specific to a body system sequelae of infectious and parasitic diseases (B90-B94)

● **Z86.11   Personal history of tuberculosis** 🖉

● **Z86.12   Personal history of poliomyelitis** 🖉

● **Z86.13   Personal history of malaria** 🖉

● **Z86.14   Personal history of Methicillin resistant Staphylococcus aureus infection** 🖉
Personal history of MRSA infection

● **Z86.19   Personal history of other infectious and parasitic diseases** 🖉

● **Z86.2   Personal history of diseases of the blood and blood-forming organs and certain disorders involving the immune mechanism** 🖐
Conditions classifiable to D50-D89

● **Z86.3   Personal history of endocrine, nutritional and metabolic diseases**
Conditions classifiable to E00-E88

● **Z86.31   Personal history of diabetic foot ulcer** 🖐
Excludes2   current diabetic foot ulcer (E08.621, E09.621, E10.621, E11.621, E13.621)

● **Z86.32   Personal history of gestational diabetes** ♀ 🖐
Personal history of conditions classifiable to O24.4-
Excludes1   gestational diabetes mellitus in current pregnancy (O24.4-)

● **Z86.39   Personal history of other endocrine, nutritional and metabolic disease** 🖐

● **Z86.5   Personal history of mental and behavioral disorders**
Conditions classifiable to F40-F59

● **Z86.51   Personal history of combat and operational stress reaction** 🖐   A

● **Z86.59   Personal history of other mental and behavioral disorders** 🖐

● **Z86.6   Personal history of diseases of the nervous system and sense organs**
Conditions classifiable to G00-G99, H00-H95

● **Z86.61   Personal history of infections of the central nervous system** 🖐
Personal history of encephalitis
Personal history of meningitis

● **Z86.69   Personal history of other diseases of the nervous system and sense organs** 🖐

● **Z86.7   Personal history of diseases of the circulatory system**
Conditions classifiable to I00-I99
Excludes2   old myocardial infarction (I25.2)
personal history of anaphylactic shock (Z87.892)
postmyocardial infarction syndrome (I24.1)

● **Z86.71   Personal history of venous thrombosis and embolism**

● **Z86.711   Personal history of pulmonary embolism** 🖐

● **Z86.718   Personal history of other venous thrombosis and embolism** 🖐

● **Z86.72   Personal history of thrombophlebitis** 🖐

● **Z86.73   Personal history of transient ischemic attack (TIA), and cerebral infarction without residual deficits** 🖐
Personal history of prolonged reversible ischemic neurological deficit (PRIND)
Personal history of stroke NOS without residual deficits
Excludes1   personal history of traumatic brain injury (Z87.820)
sequelae of cerebrovascular disease (I69.-)
Coding Clinic: 2012, Q4, P3

● **Z86.74   Personal history of sudden cardiac arrest** 🖐
Personal history of sudden cardiac death successfully resuscitated

● **Z86.79   Personal history of other diseases of the circulatory system** 🖐

● **Z87   Personal history of other diseases and conditions**
Code first any follow-up examination after treatment (Z09)

● **Z87.0   Personal history of diseases of the respiratory system**
Conditions classifiable to J00-J99

● **Z87.01   Personal history of pneumonia (recurrent)** 🖐

● **Z87.09   Personal history of other diseases of the respiratory system** 🖐

● **Z87.1   Personal history of diseases of the digestive system**
Conditions classifiable to K00-K93

● **Z87.11   Personal history of peptic ulcer disease** 🖐

● **Z87.19   Personal history of other diseases of the digestive system** 🖐

● **Z87.2   Personal history of diseases of the skin and subcutaneous tissue** 🖐
Conditions classifiable to L00-L99
Excludes2   personal history of diabetic foot ulcer (Z86.31)

● **Z87.3   Personal history of diseases of the musculoskeletal system and connective tissue**
Conditions classifiable to M00-M99
Excludes2   personal history of (healed) traumatic fracture (Z87.81)

● **Z87.31   Personal history of (healed) nontraumatic fracture**

● **Z87.310   Personal history of (healed) osteoporosis fracture** 🖐
Personal history of (healed) fragility fracture
Personal history of (healed) collapsed vertebra due to osteoporosis

● **Z87.311   Personal history of (healed) other pathological fracture** 🖐
Personal history of (healed) collapsed vertebra NOS
Excludes2   personal history of osteoporosis fracture (Z87.310)

● **Z87.312   Personal history of (healed) stress fracture** 🖐
Personal history of (healed) fatigue fracture

● **Z87.39   Personal history of other diseases of the musculoskeletal system and connective tissue** 🖐

● **Z87.4   Personal history of diseases of genitourinary system**
Conditions classifiable to N00-N99

● **Z87.41   Personal history of dysplasia of the female genital tract**
Excludes1   personal history of malignant neoplasm of female genital tract (Z85.40-Z85.44)

● **Z87.410   Personal history of cervical dysplasia** ♀ 🖐

● **Z87.411   Personal history of vaginal dysplasia** ♀ 🖐

● **Z87.412   Personal history of vulvar dysplasia** ♀ 🖐

● **Z87.42   Personal history of other diseases of the female genital tract** ♀ 🖐

N Newborn Age: 0   **P** Pediatric Age: 0–17   **M** Maternity DX: 12–55   **A** Adult Age: 15–124   ♀ Females Only   ♂ Males Only

🖐 Complication\Comorbidity   🖐 Major C\C   (Ex) CC/MCC Exclusions   🖐 Present on Admission Requirement   🖐 Hospital-Acquired Condition   **1697**

● **Z87.43**   **Personal history of diseases of male genital organs**

    ● **Z87.430**   **Personal history of prostatic dysplasia** 🖉

       Excludes1   personal history of malignant neoplasm of prostate (Z85.46)

    ● **Z87.438**   **Personal history of other diseases of male genital organs** 🖉

● **Z87.44**   **Personal history of diseases of urinary system**

    Excludes1   personal history of malignant neoplasm of cervix uteri (Z85.41)

    ● **Z87.440**   **Personal history of urinary (tract) infections** 🖉

    ● **Z87.441**   **Personal history of nephrotic syndrome** 🖉

    ● **Z87.442**   **Personal history of urinary calculi** 🖉
       Personal history of kidney stones

    ● **Z87.448**   **Personal history of other diseases of urinary system** 🖉

● **Z87.5**   **Personal history of complications of pregnancy, childbirth and the puerperium**
    Conditions classifiable to O00-O9A

    Excludes2   recurrent pregnancy loss (N96)

    ● **Z87.51**   **Personal history of pre-term labor** ♀ 🖉

       Excludes1   current pregnancy with history of pre-term labor (O09.21-)

    ● **Z87.59**   **Personal history of other complications of pregnancy, childbirth and the puerperium** ♀ 🖉
       Personal history of trophoblastic disease

● **Z87.7**   **Personal history of (corrected) congenital malformations**
    Conditions classifiable to Q00-Q89 that have been repaired or corrected

    Excludes1   congenital malformations that have been partially corrected or repair but which still require medical treatment - code to condition

    Excludes2   other postprocedural states (Z98.-)
       personal history of medical treatment (Z92.-)
       presence of cardiac and vascular implants and grafts (Z95.-)
       presence of other devices (Z97.-)
       presence of other functional implants (Z96.-)
       transplanted organ and tissue status (Z94.-)

    ● **Z87.71**   **Personal history of (corrected) congenital malformations of genitourinary system**

      ● **Z87.710**   **Personal history of (corrected) hypospadias** ♂ 🖉

      ● **Z87.718**   **Personal history of other specified (corrected) congenital malformations of genitourinary system** 🖉

    ● **Z87.72**   **Personal history of (corrected) congenital malformations of nervous system and sense organs**

      ● **Z87.720**   **Personal history of (corrected) congenital malformations of eye** 🖉

      ● **Z87.721**   **Personal history of (corrected) congenital malformations of ear** 🖉

      ● **Z87.728**   **Personal history of other specified (corrected) congenital malformations of nervous system and sense organs** 🖉

● **Z87.73**   **Personal history of (corrected) congenital malformations of digestive system**

    ● **Z87.730**   **Personal history of (corrected) cleft lip and palate** 🖉

    ● **Z87.738**   **Personal history of other specified (corrected) congenital malformations of digestive system** 🖉

● **Z87.74**   **Personal history of (corrected) congenital malformations of heart and circulatory system** 🖉

● **Z87.75**   **Personal history of (corrected) congenital malformations of respiratory system** 🖉

● **Z87.76**   **Personal history of (corrected) congenital malformations of integument, limbs and musculoskeletal system** 🖉

● **Z87.79**   **Personal history of other (corrected) congenital malformations**

    ● **Z87.790**   **Personal history of (corrected) congenital malformations of face and neck** 🖉

    ● **Z87.798**   **Personal history of other (corrected) congenital malformations** 🖉

● **Z87.8**   **Personal history of other specified conditions**

    Excludes2   personal history of self harm (Z91.5)

    ● **Z87.81**   **Personal history of (healed) traumatic fracture** 🖉

       Excludes2   personal history of (healed) nontraumatic fracture (Z87.31-)

    ● **Z87.82**   **Personal history of other (healed) physical injury and trauma**
       Conditions classifiable to S00-T88, except traumatic fractures

      ● **Z87.820**   **Personal history of traumatic brain injury** 🖉

         Excludes1   personal history of transient ischemic attack (TIA), and cerebral infarction without residual deficits (Z86.73)

      ● **Z87.821**   **Personal history of retained foreign body fully removed** 🖉

      ● **Z87.828**   **Personal history of other (healed) physical injury and trauma** 🖉

    ● **Z87.89**   **Personal history of other specified conditions**

      Z87.890   **Personal history of sex reassignment** 🖉

      ● **Z87.891**   **Personal history of nicotine dependence** 🖉

        Excludes1   current nicotine dependence (F17.2-)

      ● **Z87.892**   **Personal history of anaphylaxis** 🖉
       Code also allergy status such as:
         allergy status to drugs, medicaments and biological substances (Z88.-)
         allergy status, other than to drugs and biological substances (Z91.0-)

      ● **Z87.898**   **Personal history of other specified conditions** 🖉

◀ New   ◀▥ Revised   ~~deleted~~ Deleted   Excludes 1   Excludes 2   Includes   Use additional   Code first   Code also   Unspecified

OGCR Official Guidelines   ● Unacceptable Principal Diagnosis   X Assign placeholder X   ● Use Additional Character(s)   ▶ Manifestation Code   **Coding Clinic**

- **Z88 Allergy status to drugs, medicaments and biological substances**
  - **Excludes2** allergy status, other than to drugs and biological substances (Z91.0-)
  - Z88.0 Allergy status to penicillin 🖐
  - Z88.1 Allergy status to other antibiotic agents status 🖐
  - Z88.2 Allergy status to sulfonamides status 🖐
  - Z88.3 Allergy status to other anti-infective agents status 🖐
  - Z88.4 Allergy status to anesthetic agent status 🖐
  - Z88.5 Allergy status to narcotic agent status 🖐
  - Z88.6 Allergy status to analgesic agent status 🖐
  - Z88.7 Allergy status to serum and vaccine status 🖐
  - Z88.8 Allergy status to other drugs, medicaments and biological substances status 🖐
  - Z88.9 Allergy status to unspecified drugs, medicaments and biological substances status 🖐

- **Z89 Acquired absence of limb**
  - **Includes** amputation status
    postprocedural loss of limb
    post-traumatic loss of limb
  - **Excludes1** acquired deformities of limbs (M20-M21)
    congenital absence of limbs (Q71-Q73)
  - Z89.0 Acquired absence of thumb and other finger(s)
    - Z89.01 Acquired absence of thumb
      - Z89.011 Acquired absence of right thumb 🖐
      - Z89.012 Acquired absence of left thumb 🖐
      - Z89.019 Acquired absence of unspecified thumb 🖐
    - Z89.02 Acquired absence of other finger(s)
      - **Excludes2** acquired absence of thumb (Z89.01-)
      - Z89.021 Acquired absence of right finger(s) 🖐
      - Z89.022 Acquired absence of left finger(s) 🖐
      - Z89.029 Acquired absence of unspecified finger(s) 🖐
  - Z89.1 Acquired absence of hand and wrist
    - Z89.11 Acquired absence of hand
      - Z89.111 Acquired absence of right hand 🖐
      - Z89.112 Acquired absence of left hand 🖐
      - Z89.119 Acquired absence of unspecified hand 🖐
    - Z89.12 Acquired absence of wrist
      Disarticulation at wrist
      - Z89.121 Acquired absence of right wrist 🖐
      - Z89.122 Acquired absence of left wrist 🖐
      - Z89.129 Acquired absence of unspecified wrist 🖐
  - Z89.2 Acquired absence of upper limb above wrist
    - Z89.20 Acquired absence of upper limb, unspecified level
      - Z89.201 Acquired absence of right upper limb, unspecified level 🖐
      - Z89.202 Acquired absence of left upper limb, unspecified level 🖐
      - Z89.209 Acquired absence of unspecified upper limb, unspecified level 🖐
        Acquired absence of arm NOS
    - Z89.21 Acquired absence of upper limb below elbow
      - Z89.211 Acquired absence of right upper limb below elbow 🖐
      - Z89.212 Acquired absence of left upper limb below elbow 🖐
      - Z89.219 Acquired absence of unspecified upper limb below elbow 🖐

- Z89.22 Acquired absence of upper limb above elbow
  Disarticulation at elbow
  - Z89.221 Acquired absence of right upper limb above elbow 🖐
  - Z89.222 Acquired absence of left upper limb above elbow 🖐
  - Z89.229 Acquired absence of unspecified upper limb above elbow 🖐
- Z89.23 Acquired absence of shoulder
  Acquired absence of shoulder joint following explantation of shoulder joint prosthesis, with or without presence of antibiotic-impregnated cement spacer
  - Z89.231 Acquired absence of right shoulder 🖐
  - Z89.232 Acquired absence of left shoulder 🖐
  - Z89.239 Acquired absence of unspecified shoulder 🖐
- **Z89.4 Acquired absence of toe(s), foot, and ankle**
  - Z89.41 Acquired absence of great toe
    - Z89.411 Acquired absence of right great toe 🖐
    - Z89.412 Acquired absence of left great toe 🖐
    - Z89.419 Acquired absence of unspecified great toe 🖐
  - Z89.42 Acquired absence of other toe(s)
    - **Excludes2** acquired absence of great toe (Z89.41-)
    - Z89.421 Acquired absence of other right toe(s) 🖐
    - Z89.422 Acquired absence of other left toe(s) 🖐
    - Z89.429 Acquired absence of other toe(s), unspecified side 🖐
  - Z89.43 Acquired absence of foot
    - Z89.431 Acquired absence of right foot 🖐
    - Z89.432 Acquired absence of left foot 🖐
    - Z89.439 Acquired absence of unspecified foot 🖐
  - Z89.44 Acquired absence of ankle
    Disarticulation of ankle
    - Z89.441 Acquired absence of right ankle 🖐
    - Z89.442 Acquired absence of left ankle 🖐
    - Z89.449 Acquired absence of unspecified ankle 🖐
- **Z89.5 Acquired absence of leg below knee**
  - Z89.51 Acquired absence of leg below knee
    - Z89.511 Acquired absence of right leg below knee 🖐
    - Z89.512 Acquired absence of left leg below knee 🖐
    - Z89.519 Acquired absence of unspecified leg below knee 🖐
  - Z89.52 Acquired absence of knee
    Acquired absence of knee joint following explantation of knee joint prosthesis, with or without presence of antibiotic-impregnated cement spacer
    - Z89.521 Acquired absence of right knee 🖐
    - Z89.522 Acquired absence of left knee 🖐
    - Z89.529 Acquired absence of unspecified knee 🖐

CHAPTER 21 (Z00-Z99)

● **Z89.6 Acquired absence of leg above knee**
    ● **Z89.61 Acquired absence of leg above knee**
        Acquired absence of leg NOS
        Disarticulation at knee
        ● **Z89.611 Acquired absence of right leg above knee** 🔍
        ● **Z89.612 Acquired absence of left leg above knee** 🔍
        ● **Z89.619 Acquired absence of unspecified leg above knee** 🔍
    ● **Z89.62 Acquired absence of hip**
        Acquired absence of hip joint following explantation of hip joint prosthesis, with or without presence of antibiotic-impregnated cement spacer
        Disarticulation at hip
        ● **Z89.621 Acquired absence of right hip joint** 🔍
        ● **Z89.622 Acquired absence of left hip joint** 🔍
        ● **Z89.629 Acquired absence of unspecified hip joint** 🔍
● **Z89.9 Acquired absence of limb, unspecified** 🔍

● **Z90 Acquired absence of organs, not elsewhere classified**
    Includes   postprocedural or post-traumatic loss of body part NEC
    Excludes1   congenital absence - see Alphabetical Index
    Excludes2   postprocedural absence of endocrine glands (E89.-)
    ● **Z90.0 Acquired absence of part of head and neck**
        ● **Z90.01 Acquired absence of eye**
        ● **Z90.02 Acquired absence of larynx**
        ● **Z90.09 Acquired absence of other part of head and neck**
            Acquired absence of nose
            Excludes2   teeth (K08.1)
    ● **Z90.1 Acquired absence of breast and nipple**
        Z90.10 Acquired absence of unspecified breast and nipple
        Z90.11 Acquired absence of right breast and nipple
        Z90.12 Acquired absence of left breast and nipple
        Z90.13 Acquired absence of bilateral breasts and nipples
    ● **Z90.2 Acquired absence of lung [part of]**
    ● **Z90.3 Acquired absence of stomach [part of]**
    ● **Z90.4 Acquired absence of other specified parts of digestive tract**
        ● **Z90.41 Acquired absence of pancreas**
            Use additional code to identify any associated:
                insulin use (Z79.4)
                diabetes mellitus, postpancreatectomy (E13.-)
            ● **Z90.410 Acquired total absence of pancreas**
                Acquired absence of pancreas NOS
            ● **Z90.411 Acquired partial absence of pancreas**
        ● **Z90.49 Acquired absence of other specified parts of digestive tract**
    ● **Z90.5 Acquired absence of kidney**
    ● **Z90.6 Acquired absence of other parts of urinary tract**
        Acquired absence of bladder

● **Z90.7 Acquired absence of genital organ(s)**
    Excludes1   personal history of sex reassignment (Z87.890)
    Excludes2   female genital mutilation status (N90.81-)
    ● **Z90.71 Acquired absence of cervix and uterus**
        ● **Z90.710 Acquired absence of both cervix and uterus** ♀ 🔍
            Acquired absence of uterus NOS
            Status post total hysterectomy
        ● **Z90.711 Acquired absence of uterus with remaining cervical stump** ♀
            Status post partial hysterectomy with remaining cervical stump
        ● **Z90.712 Acquired absence of cervix with remaining uterus** ♀
    ● **Z90.72 Acquired absence of ovaries**
        ● **Z90.721 Acquired absence of ovaries, unilateral** ♀
        ● **Z90.722 Acquired absence of ovaries, bilateral** ♀
    ● **Z90.79 Acquired absence of other genital organ(s)**
● **Z90.8 Acquired absence of other organs**
    ● **Z90.81 Acquired absence of spleen**
    ● **Z90.89 Acquired absence of other organs**

● **Z91 Personal risk factors, not elsewhere classified**
    Excludes2   contact with and (suspected) exposures hazardous to health (Z77.-)
            exposure to pollution and other problems related to physical environment (Z77.1-)
            occupational exposure to risk factors (Z57.-)
            personal history of physical injury and trauma (Z87.81, Z87.82-)
    ● **Z91.0 Allergy status, other than to drugs and biological substances**
        Excludes2   allergy status to drugs, medicaments, and biological substances (Z88.-)
        ● **Z91.01 Food allergy status**
            Excludes2   food additives allergy status (Z91.02)
            ● **Z91.010 Allergy to peanuts** 🔍
            ● **Z91.011 Allergy to milk products** 🔍
                Excludes1   lactose intolerance (E73.-)
            ● **Z91.012 Allergy to eggs** 🔍
            ● **Z91.013 Allergy to seafood** 🔍
                Allergy to shellfish
                Allergy to octopus or squid ink
            ● **Z91.018 Allergy to other foods** 🔍
                Allergy to nuts other than peanuts
        ● **Z91.02 Food additives allergy status** 🔍
        ● **Z91.03 Insect allergy status**
            ● **Z91.030 Bee allergy status** 🔍
            ● **Z91.038 Other insect allergy status** 🔍
        ● **Z91.04 Nonmedicinal substance allergy status**
            ● **Z91.040 Latex allergy status** 🔍
                Latex sensitivity status
            ● **Z91.041 Radiographic dye allergy status** 🔍
                Allergy status to contrast media used for diagnostic X-ray procedure
            ● **Z91.048 Other nonmedicinal substance allergy status**
        ● **Z91.09 Other allergy status, other than to drugs and biological substances** 🔍

◀ New   ⬅ Revised   ~~deleted~~ Deleted   Excludes 1   Excludes 2   Includes   Use additional   Code first   Code also   Unspecified
OGCR Official Guidelines   ● Unacceptable Principal Diagnosis   X Assign placeholder X   ● Use Additional Character(s)   ▶ Manifestation Code   **Coding Clinic**

● **Z91.1**   **Patient's noncompliance with medical treatment and regimen**
   ● **Z91.11**   Patient's noncompliance with dietary regimen
   ● **Z91.12**   Patient's intentional underdosing of medication regimen

> *Code first underdosing of medication (T36-T50) with fifth or sixth character 6*

Excludes1   adverse effect of prescribed drug taken as directed - code to adverse effect
     poisoning (overdose) - code to poisoning

     ● **Z91.120**   Patient's intentional underdosing of medication regimen due to financial hardship
     ● **Z91.128**   Patient's intentional underdosing of medication regimen for other reason
   ● **Z91.13**   Patient's unintentional underdosing of medication regimen

> *Code first underdosing of medication (T36-T50) with fifth or sixth character 6*

Excludes1   adverse effect of prescribed drug taken as directed - code to adverse effect
     poisoning (overdose) - code to poisoning

     ● **Z91.130**   Patient's unintentional underdosing of medication regimen due to age-related debility
     ● **Z91.138**   Patient's unintentional underdosing of medication regimen for other reason
   ● **Z91.14**   Patient's other noncompliance with medication regimen
      Patient's underdosing of medication NOS
   ● **Z91.15**   Patient's noncompliance with renal dialysis
   ● **Z91.19**   Patient's noncompliance with other medical treatment and regimen
● **Z91.4**   **Personal history of psychological trauma, not elsewhere classified**
   ● **Z91.41**   Personal history of adult abuse

Excludes2   personal history of abuse in childhood (Z62.81-)

     ● **Z91.410**   Personal history of adult physical and sexual abuse 🔲   A

Excludes1   current adult physical abuse (T74.11, T76.11)
     current adult sexual abuse (T74.21, T76.11) ◀▥

     ● **Z91.411**   Personal history of adult psychological abuse 🔲   A
     ● **Z91.412**   Personal history of adult neglect 🔲   A

Excludes1   current adult neglect (T74.01, T76.01)

     ● **Z91.419**   Personal history of unspecified adult abuse 🔲   A
   ● **Z91.49**   Other personal history of psychological trauma, not elsewhere classified 🔲
● **Z91.5**   **Personal history of self-harm** 🔲
     Personal history of parasuicide
     Personal history of self-poisoning
     Personal history of suicide attempt

● **Z91.8**   **Other specified personal risk factors, not elsewhere classified**
   ● **Z91.81**   History of falling 🔲
     At risk for falling
   ● **Z91.82**   Personal history of military deployment 🔲
     Individual (civilian or military) with past history of military war, peacekeeping and humanitarian deployment (current or past conflict)
     Returned from military deployment
   ▶ **Z91.83**   *Wandering in diseases classified elsewhere* 🔲

> *Code first underlying disorder such as:*
>   Alzheimer's disease (G30.-) ◀▥
>   autism or pervasive developmental disorder (F84.-) ◀▥
>   intellectual disabilities (F70-F79)
>   unspecified dementia with behavioral disturbance (F03.9-)

   ● **Z91.89**   Other specified personal risk factors, not elsewhere classified 🔲
● **Z92**   **Personal history of medical treatment**

Excludes2   postprocedural states (Z98.-)

   ● **Z92.0**   Personal history of contraception 🔲

Excludes1   counseling or management of current contraceptive practices (Z30.-)
     long term (current) use of contraception (Z79.3)
     presence of (intrauterine) contraceptive device (Z97.5)

   ● **Z92.2**   Personal history of drug therapy

Excludes2   long term (current) drug therapy (Z79.-)

     ● **Z92.21**   Personal history of antineoplastic chemotherapy 🔲
     ● **Z92.22**   Personal history of monoclonal drug therapy 🔲
     ● **Z92.23**   Personal history of estrogen therapy 🔲
     ● **Z92.24**   Personal history of steroid therapy 🔲
       ● **Z92.240**   Personal history of inhaled steroid therapy 🔲
       ● **Z92.241**   Personal history of systemic steroid therapy 🔲
        Personal history of steroid therapy NOS
     ● **Z92.25**   Personal history of immunosupression therapy 🔲

Excludes2   personal history of steroid therapy (Z92.24)

     ● **Z92.29**   Personal history of other drug therapy 🔲
   ● **Z92.3**   Personal history of irradiation 🔲
     Personal history of exposure to therapeutic radiation

Excludes1   exposure to radiation in the physical environment (Z77.12)
     occupational exposure to radiation (Z57.1)

   ● **Z92.8**   Personal history of other medical treatment
     ● **Z92.81**   Personal history of extracorporeal membrane oxygenation (ECMO) 🔲
     ● **Z92.82**   Status post administration of tPA (rtPA) in a different facility within the last 24 hours prior to admission to current facility 🔲

> *Code first condition requiring tPA administration, such as:*
>   acute cerebral infarction (I63.-)
>   acute myocardial infarction (I21.-, I22.-)

     ● **Z92.83**   Personal history of failed moderate sedation 🔲
      Personal history of failed conscious sedation

Excludes2   failed moderate sedation during procedure (T88.52)

     ● **Z92.89**   Personal history of other medical treatment 🔲

N Newborn Age: 0   **P** Pediatric Age: 0–17   **M** Maternity DX: 12–55   **A** Adult Age: 15–124   ♀ Females Only   ♂ Males Only

🔲 Complication\Comorbidity   🔲 Major C\C   (Ex) CC/MCC Exclusions   🔲 Present on Admission Requirement   Hospital-Acquired Condition   **1701**

CHAPTER 21 (Z00-Z99)

● **Z93** **Artificial opening status**

> **Excludes1** artificial openings requiring attention or management (Z43.-)
>
> complications of external stoma (J95.0-, K94.-, N99.5-)

- ● **Z93.0** **Tracheostomy status** 🔎
- ● **Z93.1** **Gastrostomy status** 🔎
- ● **Z93.2** **Ileostomy status** 🔎
- ● **Z93.3** **Colostomy status** 🔎
- ● **Z93.4** **Other artificial openings of gastrointestinal tract status** 🔎
- ● **Z93.5** **Cystostomy status**
  - ● **Z93.50** **Unspecified cystostomy status** 🔎
  - ● **Z93.51** **Cutaneous-vesicostomy status** 🔎
  - ● **Z93.52** **Appendico-vesicostomy status** 🔎
  - ● **Z93.59** **Other cystostomy status** 🔎
- ● **Z93.6** **Other artificial openings of urinary tract status** 🔎

  Nephrostomy status
  Ureterostomy status
  Urethrostomy status
- ● **Z93.8** **Other artificial opening status** 🔎
- ● **Z93.9** **Artificial opening status, unspecified** 🔎

● **Z94** **Transplanted organ and tissue status**

> **Includes** organ or tissue replaced by heterogenous or homogenous transplant
>
> **Excludes1** complications of transplanted organ or tissue - see Alphabetical Index
>
> **Excludes2** presence of vascular grafts (Z95.-)

- ● **Z94.0** **Kidney transplant status** 🔎 🔎

  (Ex:) D47.Z1, T86.10-T86.19, T86.850-T86.859, T86.90-T86.99, Z94.0, Z94.89-Z94.9
- ● **Z94.1** **Heart transplant status** 🔎 🔎

  > **Excludes1** artificial heart status (Z95.812) ◀━
  > heart-valve replacement status (Z95.2-Z95.4)

  (Ex:) D47.Z1, T86.20-T86.39, T86.850-T86.859, T86.90-T86.99, Z94.1, Z94.3, Z94.89-Z94.9
- ● **Z94.2** **Lung transplant status** 🔎 🔎

  (Ex:) D47.Z1, T86.810-T86.819, T86.850-T86.859, T86.90-T86.99, Z94.2, Z94.89-Z94.9
- ● **Z94.3** **Heart and lungs transplant status** 🔎 🔎

  CC when PDx is its own CC
  (Ex:) See Z94.1
- ● **Z94.4** **Liver transplant status** 🔎 🔎

  (Ex:) D47.Z1, T86.40-T86.49, T86.850-T86.859, T86.90-T86.99, Z94.4, Z94.89, Z94.9
- ● **Z94.5** **Skin transplant status** 🔎

  Autogenous skin transplant status
- ● **Z94.6** **Bone transplant status** 🔎
- ● **Z94.7** **Corneal transplant status** 🔎
- ● **Z94.8** **Other transplanted organ and tissue status**
  - ● **Z94.81** **Bone marrow transplant status** 🔎 🔎

    (Ex:) D47.Z1, D89.810-D89.813, T86.00-T86.09, T86.850-T86.859, T86.90-T86.99, Z94.9
  - ● **Z94.82** **Intestine transplant status** 🔎 🔎

    (Ex:) D47.Z1, T86.830-T86.839, T86.90-T86.99, Z94.82, Z94.89-Z94.9
  - ● **Z94.83** **Pancreas transplant status** 🔎 🔎

    (Ex:) D47.Z1, T86.850-T86.859, T86.890-T86.99, Z94.83, Z94.9
  - ● **Z94.84** **Stem cells transplant status** 🔎 🔎

    (Ex:) D47.Z1, T86.850-T86.859, T86.90-T86.99, Z94.9
  - ● **Z94.89** **Other transplanted organ and tissue status** 🔎
- ● **Z94.9** **Transplanted organ and tissue status, unspecified** 🔎

● **Z95** **Presence of cardiac and vascular implants and grafts**

> **Excludes1** complications of cardiac and vascular devices, implants and grafts (T82.-)

- ● **Z95.0** **Presence of cardiac pacemaker** 🔎

  > **Excludes1** adjustment or management of cardiac pacemaker (Z45.0)
  > presence of automatic (implantable) cardiac defibrillator with synchronous cardiac pacemaker (Z95.810) ◀━
- ● **Z95.1** **Presence of aortocoronary bypass graft** 🔎
- ● **Z95.2** **Presence of prosthetic heart valve** 🔎

  Presence of heart valve NOS
- ● **Z95.3** **Presence of xenogenic heart valve** 🔎
- ● **Z95.4** **Presence of other heart-valve replacement** 🔎
- ● **Z95.5** **Presence of coronary angioplasty implant and graft** 🔎

  > **Excludes1** coronary angioplasty status without implant and graft (Z98.61)
- ● **Z95.8** **Presence of other cardiac and vascular implants and grafts**
  - ● **Z95.81** **Presence of other cardiac implants and grafts**

    (Ex:) **For category Z95.81 CC codes:** D47.Z1, T86.20-T86.39, T86.850-T86.99, Z94.1, Z94.3, Z95.811-Z95.812
    - ● **Z95.810** **Presence of automatic (implantable) cardiac defibrillator** 🔎

      Presence of automatic (implantable) cardiac defibrillator with synchronous cardiac pacemaker
    - ● **Z95.811** **Presence of heart assist device** 🔎 🔎
    - ● **Z95.812** **Presence of fully implantable artificial heart** 🔎
    - ● **Z95.818** **Presence of other cardiac implants and grafts** 🔎
  - ● **Z95.82** **Presence of other vascular implants and grafts**
    - ● **Z95.820** **Peripheral vascular angioplasty status with implants and grafts** 🔎

      > **Excludes1** peripheral vascular angioplasty without implant and graft (Z98.62)
    - ● **Z95.828** **Presence of other vascular implants and grafts** 🔎

      Presence of intravascular prosthesis NEC
- ● **Z95.9** **Presence of cardiac and vascular implant and graft, unspecified** 🔎

● **Z96** **Presence of other functional implants**

> **Excludes2** complications of internal prosthetic devices, implants and grafts (T82-T85)
>
> fitting and adjustment of prosthetic and other devices (Z44-Z46)

- ● **Z96.0** **Presence of urogenital implants**
- ● **Z96.1** **Presence of intraocular lens**

  Presence of pseudophakia
- ● **Z96.2** **Presence of otological and audiological implants**
  - ● **Z96.20** **Presence of otological and audiological implant, unspecified**
  - ● **Z96.21** **Cochlear implant status**
  - ● **Z96.22** **Myringotomy tube(s) status**
  - ● **Z96.29** **Presence of other otological and audiological implants**

    Presence of bone-conduction hearing device
    Presence of eustachian tube stent
    Stapes replacement

- **Z96.3**   Presence of artificial larynx
- **Z96.4**   Presence of endocrine implants
  - **Z96.41**   Presence of insulin pump (external) (internal)
  - **Z96.49**   Presence of other endocrine implants
- **Z96.5**   Presence of tooth-root and mandibular implants
- **Z96.6**   Presence of orthopedic joint implants
  - **Z96.60**   Presence of unspecified orthopedic joint implant
  - **Z96.61**   Presence of artificial shoulder joint
    - **Z96.611**   Presence of right artificial shoulder joint
    - **Z96.612**   Presence of left artificial shoulder joint
    - **Z96.619**   Presence of unspecified artificial shoulder joint
  - **Z96.62**   Presence of artificial elbow joint
    - **Z96.621**   Presence of right artificial elbow joint
    - **Z96.622**   Presence of left artificial elbow joint
    - **Z96.629**   Presence of unspecified artificial elbow joint
  - **Z96.63**   Presence of artificial wrist joint
    - **Z96.631**   Presence of right artificial wrist joint
    - **Z96.632**   Presence of left artificial wrist joint
    - **Z96.639**   Presence of unspecified artificial wrist joint
  - **Z96.64**   Presence of artificial hip joint
    Hip-joint replacement (partial) (total)
    - **Z96.641**   Presence of right artificial hip joint
    - **Z96.642**   Presence of left artificial hip joint
    - **Z96.643**   Presence of artificial hip joint, bilateral
    - **Z96.649**   Presence of unspecified artificial hip joint
  - **Z96.65**   Presence of artificial knee joint
    - **Z96.651**   Presence of right artificial knee joint
    - **Z96.652**   Presence of left artificial knee joint
    - **Z96.653**   Presence of artificial knee joint, bilateral
    - **Z96.659**   Presence of unspecified artificial knee joint
  - **Z96.66**   Presence of artificial ankle joint
    - **Z96.661**   Presence of right artificial ankle joint
    - **Z96.662**   Presence of left artificial ankle joint
    - **Z96.669**   Presence of unspecified artificial ankle joint
  - **Z96.69**   Presence of other orthopedic joint implants
    - **Z96.691**   Finger-joint replacement of right hand
    - **Z96.692**   Finger-joint replacement of left hand
    - **Z96.693**   Finger-joint replacement, bilateral
    - **Z96.698**   Presence of other orthopedic joint implants
- **Z96.7**   Presence of other bone and tendon implants
  Presence of skull plate
- **Z96.8**   Presence of other specified functional implants
  - **Z96.81**   Presence of artificial skin
  - **Z96.89**   Presence of other specified functional implants
- **Z96.9**   Presence of functional implant, unspecified

- **Z97**   **Presence of other devices**
  - **Excludes1**   complications of internal prosthetic devices, implants and grafts (T82-T85)
    fitting and adjustment of prosthetic and other devices (Z44-Z46)
  - **Excludes2**   presence of cerebrospinal fluid drainage device (Z98.2)
  - **Z97.0**   Presence of artificial eye 🔷
  - **Z97.1**   Presence of artificial limb (complete) (partial)
    - **Z97.10**   Presence of artificial limb (complete) (partial), unspecified 🔷
    - **Z97.11**   Presence of artificial right arm (complete) (partial) 🔷
    - **Z97.12**   Presence of artificial left arm (complete) (partial) 🔷
    - **Z97.13**   Presence of artificial right leg (complete) (partial) 🔷
    - **Z97.14**   Presence of artificial left leg (complete) (partial) 🔷
    - **Z97.15**   Presence of artificial arms, bilateral (complete) (partial) 🔷
    - **Z97.16**   Presence of artificial legs, bilateral (complete) (partial) 🔷
  - **Z97.2**   Presence of dental prosthetic device (complete) (partial) 🔷
    Presence of dentures (complete) (partial)
  - **Z97.3**   Presence of spectacles and contact lenses 🔷
  - **Z97.4**   Presence of external hearing-aid 🔷
  - **Z97.5**   Presence of (intrauterine) contraceptive device ♀ 🔷
    - **Excludes1**   checking, reinsertion or removal of contraceptive device (Z30.43)
  - **Z97.8**   Presence of other specified devices 🔷

- **Z98**   **Other postprocedural states**
  - **Excludes2**   aftercare (Z43-Z49, Z51)
    follow-up medical care (Z08-Z09)
    postprocedural complication - see Alphabetical Index
  - **Z98.0**   Intestinal bypass and anastomosis status 🔷
    - **Excludes2**   bariatric surgery status (Z98.84)
      gastric bypass status (Z98.84)
      obesity surgery status (Z98.84)
  - **Z98.1**   Arthrodesis status 🔷
  - **Z98.2**   Presence of cerebrospinal fluid drainage device 🔷
    Presence of CSF shunt
  - **Z98.3**   Post therapeutic collapse of lung status 🔷
    Code first underlying disease
  - **Z98.4**   Cataract extraction status
    Use additional code to identify intraocular lens implant status (Z96.1)
    - **Excludes1**   aphakia (H27.0)
    - **Z98.41**   Cataract extraction status, right eye 🔷
    - **Z98.42**   Cataract extraction status, left eye 🔷
    - **Z98.49**   Cataract extraction status, unspecified eye 🔷
  - **Z98.5**   Sterilization status
    - **Excludes1**   female infertility (N97.-)
      male infertility (N46.-)
    - **Z98.51**   Tubal ligation status ♀ 🔷
    - **Z98.52**   Vasectomy status ♂ 🔷   A

CHAPTER 21 (Z00-Z99)

N   Newborn Age: 0   P   Pediatric Age: 0–17   M   Maternity DX: 12–55   A   Adult Age: 15–124   ♀   Females Only   ♂   Males Only

🔷 Complication\Comorbidity   🔷 Major C\C   Ⓔⓧ CC/MCC Exclusions   🔷 Present on Admission Requirement   🔷 Hospital-Acquired Condition

1703

● **Z98.6 Angioplasty status**
  ● **Z98.61 Coronary angioplasty status** 🔲
    Excludes1 coronary angioplasty status with implant and graft (Z95.5)
  ● **Z98.62 Peripheral vascular angioplasty status** 🔲
    Excludes1 peripheral vascular angioplasty status with implant and graft (Z95.820)
● **Z98.8 Other specified postprocedural states**
  ● **Z98.81 Dental procedure status**
    ● **Z98.810 Dental sealant status** 🔲
    ● **Z98.811 Dental restoration status** 🔲
      Dental crown status
      Dental fillings status
    ● **Z98.818 Other dental procedure status** 🔲
  ● **Z98.82 Breast implant status** 🔲
    Excludes1 breast implant removal status (Z98.86)
  ● **Z98.83 Filtering (vitreous) bleb after glaucoma surgery status** 🔲
    Excludes1 inflammation (infection) of postprocedural bleb (H59.4-)
  ● **Z98.84 Bariatric surgery status**
    Gastric banding status
    Gastric bypass status for obesity
    Obesity surgery status
    Excludes1 bariatric surgery status complicating pregnancy, childbirth, or the puerperium (O99.84)
    Excludes2 intestinal bypass and anastomosis status (Z98.0)
  ● **Z98.85 Transplanted organ removal status** 🔲
    Transplanted organ previously removed due to complication, failure, rejection or infection
    Excludes1 encounter for removal of transplanted organ
      -code to complication of transplanted organ (T86.-)
  ● **Z98.86 Personal history of breast implant removal** 🔲
  ● **Z98.87 Personal history of in utero procedure**
    ● **Z98.870 Personal history of in utero procedure during pregnancy** ♀ 🔲
      Excludes2 complications from in utero procedure for current pregnancy (O35.7)
      supervision of current pregnancy with history of in utero procedure during previous pregnancy (O09.82-)
    ● **Z98.871 Personal history of in utero procedure while a fetus** 🔲
  ● **Z98.89 Other specified postprocedural states** 🔲
    Personal history of surgery, not elsewhere classified

● **Z99 Dependence on enabling machines and devices, not elsewhere classified**
    Excludes1 cardiac pacemaker status (Z95.0)
  ● **Z99.0 Dependence on aspirator** 🔲
  ● **Z99.1 Dependence on respirator** 🔲
    Dependence on ventilator
    (Ex) For category Z99.1 CC codes: J95.850, Z99.0-Z99.12, Z99.81-Z99.89
    Z99.11 Dependence on respirator [ventilator] status 🔲 🔲
    Z99.12 Encounter for respirator [ventilator] dependence during power failure 🔲 🔲
      Excludes1 mechanical complication of respirator [ventilator] (J95.850)
  ● **Z99.2 Dependence on renal dialysis** 🔲
    Hemodialysis status
    Peritoneal dialysis status
    Presence of arteriovenous shunt for dialysis
    Renal dialysis status NOS
    Excludes1 encounter for fitting and adjustment of dialysis catheter (Z49.0-)
    noncompliance with renal dialysis (Z91.15)
  ● **Z99.3 Dependence on wheelchair** 🔲
    Wheelchair confinement status
    Code first cause of dependence, such as:
      muscular dystrophy (G71.0)
      obesity (E66.-)
  ● **Z99.8 Dependence on other enabling machines and devices**
    ● **Z99.81 Dependence on supplemental oxygen** 🔲
      Dependence on long-term oxygen
    ● **Z99.89 Dependence on other enabling machines and devices** 🔲
      Dependence on machine or device NOS

Trust Carol J. Buck and Elsevier
to take you through the levels
of coding success

Step 4:
Professional Resources

Step 3:
Certify

With the resources you need for every
level of coding success, Carol J. Buck
and Elsevier are with you every step
of your coding career. From beginning
to advanced, from the classroom to
the workplace, from application to
certification, the Step Series products
are your guides to greater opportunities
and successful career advancement.

Step 2:
Practice

Step 1:
Learn

Keep climbing with the most trusted name in medical coding.

Author and Educator
Carol J. Buck, MS, CPC, CPC-H, CCS-P

Trust Carol J. Buck and Elsevier for the resources you need at each step of your coding career!

Track your progress toward complete coding success!

2014

Step 1: Learn

☐ Step-by-Step Medical Coding, 2014 Edition • ISBN: 978-1-4557-4635-4
☐ Workbook for Step-by-Step Medical Coding, 2014 Edition • ISBN: 978-1-4557-4630-9
☐ Medical Coding Online for Step-by-Step Medical Coding, 2014 Edition • ISBN: 978-1-4557-4631-6

Step 2: Practice

☐ The Next Step: Advanced Medical Coding and Auditing, 2014 Edition • ISBN: 978-1-4557-5897-5
☐ E/M Auditing Step, Third Edition • ISBN: 978-1-4557-5199-0
☐ *Capstone* Online Internship for Medical Coding, 2014 Edition • ISBN: 978-0-323-23937-0

Step 3: Certify

☐ Physician Coding Exam Review 2014: The Certification Step with ICD-9-CM • ISBN: 978-1-4557-2287-7
☐ Facility Coding Exam Review 2014: The Certification Step with ICD-10-CM/PCS • ISBN: 978-1-4557-4574-6

Author and Educator
Carol J. Buck, MS, CPC, CPC-H, CCS-P

Step 4: Professional Resources

☐ 2014 ICD-9-CM for Physicians, Volumes 1 & 2, Professional Edition • ISBN: 978-0-323-18676-6
☐ 2014 ICD-9-CM for Hospitals, Volumes 1, 2, & 3, Professional Edition • ISBN: 978-0-323-18674-2
☐ 2014 ICD-9-CM for Physicians, Volumes 1 & 2, Standard Edition • ISBN: 978-0-323-18677-3
☐ 2014 ICD-9-CM for Hospitals, Volumes 1, 2, & 3, Standard Edition • ISBN: 978-0-323-18675-9
☐ 2014 HCPCS Level II Professional Edition • ISBN: 978-1-4557-7504-0
☐ 2014 HCPCS Level II Standard Edition • ISBN: 978-1-4557-7505-7
☐ 2014 ICD-10-CM Draft Manual • ISBN: 978-1-4557-2290-7
☐ 2014 ICD-10-PCS Draft Manual • ISBN: 978-1-4557-2289-1
☐ ICD-10-CM Online Training Modules (by Buck) • ISBN: 978-0-323-22145-0
☐ ICD-10-PCS Online Training Modules (by Lovaasen) • ISBN: 978-0-323-22811-4

Order today!

- Order securely at **www.us.elsevierhealth.com.**
- Call toll-free **1-800-545-2522.**
- Visit your **local bookstore.**

CL-0